COLOR ATLASES

HARRISON'S 15TH EDITION

PRINCIPLES OF
INTERNAL MEDICINE

EDITORS OF PREVIOUS EDITIONS

T. R. HARRISON
Editor-in-Chief, Editions 1, 2, 3, 4, 5

W. R. RESNICK
Editor, Editions 1, 2, 3, 4, 5

M. M. WINTROBE
Editor, Editions 1, 2, 3, 4, 5
Editor-in-Chief, Editions 6, 7

G. W. THORN
Editor, Editions 1, 2, 3, 4, 5, 6, 7
Editor-in-Chief, Edition 8

R. D. ADAMS
Editor, Editions 2, 3, 4, 5, 6, 7, 8, 9, 10

P. B. BEESON
Editor, Editions 1, 2

I. L. BENNETT, JR.
Editor, Editions 3, 4, 5, 6

E. BRAUNWALD
Editor, Editions 6, 7, 8, 9, 10, 12, 13, 14
Editor-in-Chief, Edition 11

K. J. ISSELBACHER
Editor, Editions 6, 7, 8, 10, 11, 12, 14
Editor-in-Chief, Editions 9, 13

R. G. PETERSDORF
Editor, Editions 6, 7, 8, 9, 11, 12, 13
Editor-in-Chief, Edition 10

J. D. WILSON
Editor, Editions 9, 10, 11, 13, 14
Editor-in-Chief, Edition 12

J. B. MARTIN
Editor, Editions 10, 11, 12, 13, 14

A. S. FAUCI
Editor, Editions 11, 12, 13
Editor-in-Chief, Edition 14

R. ROOT
Editor, Edition 12

D. L. KASPER
Editor, Editions 13, 14

S. L. HAUSER
Editor, Edition 14

D. L. LONGO
Editor, Edition 14

HARRISON'S 15TH EDITION

PRINCIPLES OF INTERNAL MEDICINE

EDITORS

EUGENE BRAUNWALD, MD,
MD(Hon), ScD(Hon)

Distinguished Hersey Professor of Medicine,
Faculty Dean for Academic Programs at Brigham and
Women's Hospital and Massachusetts General Hospital,
Harvard Medical School; Vice-President for Academic
Programs, Partners HealthCare Systems, Boston

ANTHONY S. FAUCI, MD,
ScD(Hon)

Chief, Laboratory of Immunoregulation; Director,
National Institute of Allergy and Infectious Diseases,
National Institutes of Health, Bethesda

DENNIS L. KASPER, MD,
MA(Hon)

William Ellery Channing Professor of Medicine,
Professor of Microbiology and Molecular Genetics,
Executive Dean for Academic Programs, Harvard
Medical School; Director, Channing Laboratory,
Department of Medicine, Brigham and Women's
Hospital, Boston

STEPHEN L. HAUSER, MD

Betty Anker Fife Professor and Chairman,
Department of Neurology,
University of California San Francisco,
San Francisco

DAN L. LONGO, MD

Scientific Director, National Institute on Aging,
National Institutes of Health,
Bethesda and Baltimore

J. LARRY JAMESON, MD, PhD

Irving S. Cutter Professor and Chairman,
Department of Medicine,
Northwestern University Medical School;
Physician-in-Chief, Northwestern
Memorial Hospital, Chicago

VOLUME 1

McGraw-Hill
MEDICAL PUBLISHING DIVISION

New York   San Francisco   Washington, DC   Auckland   Bogotá   Caracas   Lisbon   London
Madrid   Mexico City   Milan   Montreal   New Delhi   San Juan   Singapore   Sydney   Tokyo   Toronto

McGraw-Hill

A Division of The McGraw·Hill Companies

Harrison's
PRINCIPLES OF INTERNAL MEDICINE
Fifteenth Edition

1234567890 DOWDOW 0987654321
ISBN 0-07-007272-8 (Combo)
0-07-007273-6 (Vol. 1)
0-07-007274-4 (Vol. 2)
0-07-913686-9 (Set)

FOREIGN LANGUAGE EDITIONS
Arabic (13e)—McGraw-Hill Libri Italia srl (est. 1996)
Chinese (12e)—McGraw-Hill Book Company—Singapore © 1994
Croatian (13e)—Placebo, Split, Croatia
French (14e)—McGraw-Hill Publishing Co., Maidenhead, UK © 1999
German (14e)—McGraw-Hill Publishing Co., Maidenhead, UK © 1999
Greek (14e)—Parissianos, Athens, Greece © 2000
Italian (14e)—McGraw-Hill Libri Italia srl, Milan © 1999

Japanese (11e)—Hirokawa © 1991
Polish (14e)—Czelej Publishing Company, Lubin, Poland (est. 2000)
Portuguese (14e)—McGraw-Hill Interamericana do Brasil Ltda © 1998
Romania (14e)—Teora Publishers, Bucharest, Romania (est. 2000)
Spanish (14e)—McGraw-Hill Interamericana de Espana, Madrid © 1998
Turkish (13e)—McGraw-Hill Libri Italia srl (est. 1996)

This book was set in Times Roman by Progressive Information Technologies. The editors were Martin Wonsiewicz and Mariapaz Ramos Englis. The production director was Robert Laffler. The index was prepared by Irving C. Tullar. The text and cover designer was Marsha Cohen/Parallelogram Graphics.

R. R. Donnelley and Sons, Inc. was the printer and binder.

Library of Congress Cataloging-in-Publication Data

Harrison's principles of internal medicine—15th ed./editors, Eugene Braunwald . . . [et al.].   p. cm.
   Includes bibliographical references and index.
   ISBN 0-07-913686-9 (set)—ISBN 0-07-007273-6 (v. 1)—ISBN 0-07-0072744-4 (v. 2)
      1. Internal medicine. I. Braunwald, Eugene, date
RC46.H333 2001
616—dc21

00-063809

INTERNATIONAL EDITION ISBN 0-07-118319-1 (Set); 0-07-118320-5 (Vol 1); 0-07-118321-3 (Vol 2)
Copyright © 2001. Exclusive rights by *The McGraw-Hill Companies, Inc.*, for manufacture and export. This book cannot be re-exported from the country to which it is consigned by McGraw-Hill. The International Edition is not available in North America.

DEDICATION

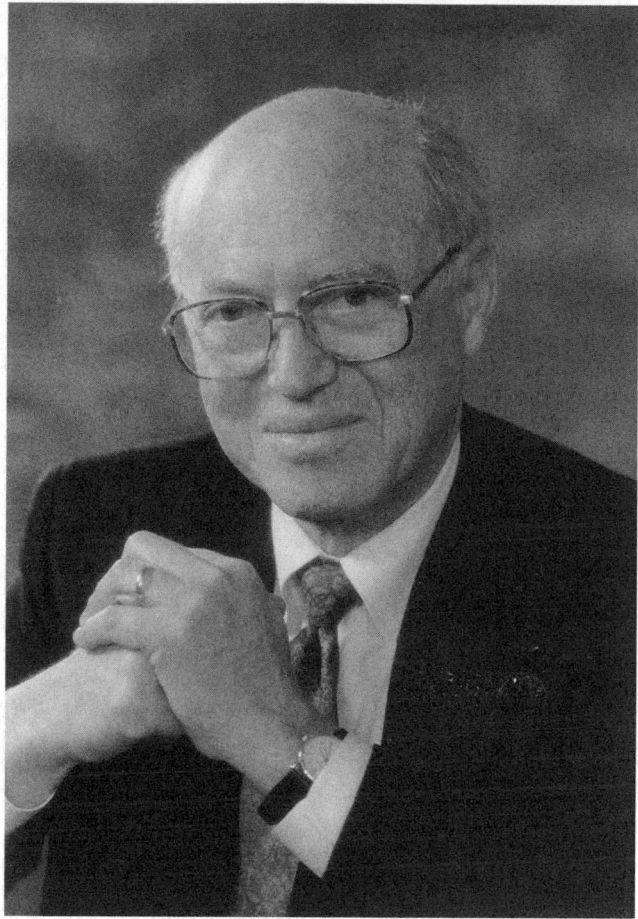

KURT J. ISSELBACHER

With this edition, the editors acknowledge the many contributions of our colleague Kurt J. Isselbacher, who served as an editor of *Harrison's* for nine editions, the sixth through the fourteenth, including Editor-in-Chief of the ninth and thirteenth editions. For more than three decades Dr. Isselbacher played a decisive role in ensuring that *Harrison's* epitomized the state of the art and science of internal medicine and the essence of accuracy and clarity. His indelible contributions to *Harrison's* are felt in the fifteenth edition and will endure into the future.

Dr. Isselbacher is a graduate of Harvard College and of the Harvard Medical School. His further training included a residency in medicine at the Massachusetts General Hospital and a research fellowship at the National Institutes of Health. Chosen to lead the Gastrointestinal Unit of the MGH at the remarkable age of 31, over the ensuing 30 years as Chief of that Unit, he was a leader in advancing both the clinical specialty of gastroenterology and the basic understanding of gastrointestinal disease. Under his leadership, the MGH Gastrointestinal Unit became renowned for its training program in academic gastroenterology as well as for being one of the world's leading centers for clinical and research activities in gastroenterology. In 1987, Dr. Isselbacher undertook new challenges as the first Director of the Cancer Center at the MGH, bringing his characteristic insight and leadership to this new task. In a relatively short time, the MGH Cancer Center has emerged as a premier cancer research institute. Dr. Isselbacher holds the Mallinckrodt Distinguished Professorship of Medicine at Harvard Medical School, and he has been a powerful force for excellence in scholarship at this institution since his graduation. For almost 30 years he served as Chairman of the

Executive Committee of Harvard's Departments of Medicine and played a pivotal role in the departments' growth and quest for excellence.

Dr. Isselbacher combines the attributes of an excellent scientist with those of a superb clinician and teacher. He has trained generations of physicians and investigators, including many who are now leaders in academic medicine. As the author of more than 400 scientific articles in leading journals, his research contributions include definition of enzymatic defects in absorptive disorders, and delineation of biochemical mechanisms of absorption, malabsorption, protein synthesis, derangements of metabolism, and immunologic aspects of hepatic gastrointestinal disease. Kurt Isselbacher has been a recipient of many well-earned honors, including the Distinguished Achievement Award and the Friedenwald Medal of the American Gastroenterological Association, the John Phillips Memorial Award for distinguished contributions to clinical medicine from the American College of Physicians, as well as the Kober Medal of the Association of American Physicians. He is a member of the National Academy of Sciences and of its Institute of Medicine and has served as President of the American Gastroenterological Association, the American Association for the Study of Liver Disease, and the Association of American Physicians.

Kurt Isselbacher exemplifies the highest values of medicine. A caring, empathic physician, he consistently combines compassion with incisive analysis in the care of patients. With contributions as a clinician, teacher, scientist, and editor, he has advanced the care of patients with gastrointestinal disorders and cancer while educating generations of physicians.

DEDICATION

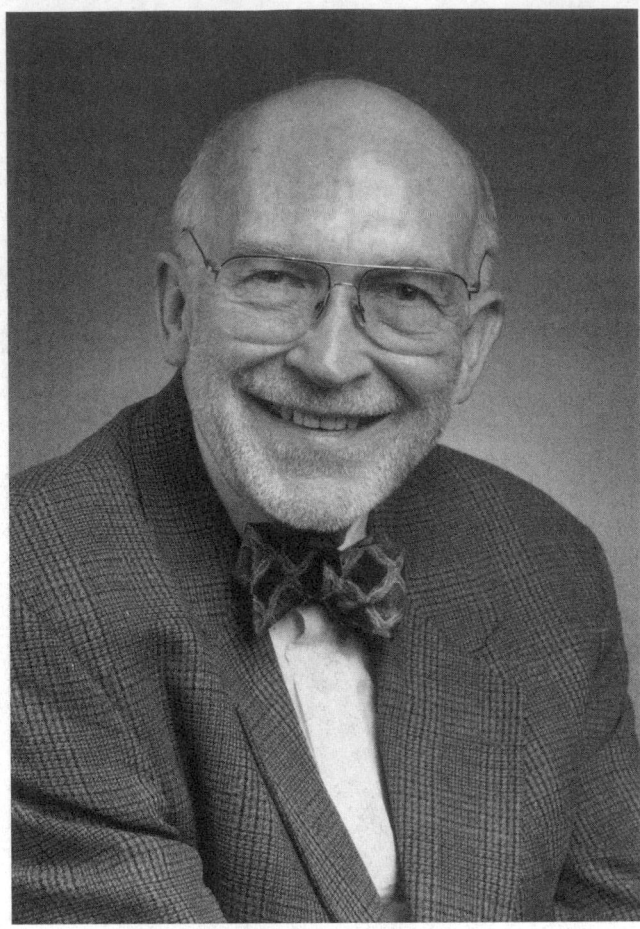

JEAN DONALD WILSON

Jean Wilson served as editor of the ninth through the fourteenth editions of *Harrison's Principles of Internal Medicine* from 1978 to 1998; he was Editor-in-Chief of the twelfth edition. A native of Texas, Jean Wilson attended the University of Texas at Austin and the University of Texas Southwestern Medical School in Dallas. He trained as a resident in internal medicine and as a fellow in endocrinology and metabolism at Parkland Hospital. With the exception of 2 years of research in biochemistry in the intramural program of the National Institutes of Health, Dr. Wilson spent his entire career at the University of Texas Southwestern Medical School, where he now holds the Charles Cameron Sprague Distinguished Chair in Biomedical Science.

Dr. Wilson is one of America's most distinguished biomedical scientists and is largely responsible for working out the mechanism of action and physiology of the male sex hormones from the embryo to the normal and diseased adult. Among his many important discoveries has been the 5α-reductase reaction, whereby male target tissues convert testosterone to the more active androgen, dihydrotestosterone. He has been honored many times for his research, having received the Ernst Oppenheimer Memorial Award of the Endocrine Society, the Amory Prize of the American Academy of Arts and Sciences, the Lita Annenberg Hazen Award for Excellence in Clinical Research, the Henry Dale Medal of the Society for Endocrinology, the Gregory Pincus Award of the Worcester Foundation for Experimental Biology, the Fred Conrad Koch Award of the Endocrine Society, and the Kober Medal of the Association of American Physicians.

Amongst his memberships are the National Academy of Sciences, the Institute of Medicine of the National Academy of Sciences, and the American Academy of Arts and Sciences. He is a Fellow of the Royal College of Physicians. He has served as President of the American Society for Clinical Investigation, the Association of American Physicians, and the Endocrine Society. For two decades, Dr. Wilson directed the enormously successful MD/PhD program and for 8 years, the highly esteemed Endocrine-Metabolism Division at Southwestern.

Perhaps the finest thing that can be said of Jean Wilson is that he is a professor of internal medicine in the complete sense. He is, and always has been, a superb teacher and exemplary clinician while constantly maintaining a sterling career in research. Perhaps nothing describes him better than the enduring image of this renowned academic physician trimming callouses and ulcers in the Diabetic Foot Care Clinic at Parkland Memorial Hospital, his teaching hospital, where the patients are the medically indigent of Dallas.

Dr. Wilson is a man of diverse interests, a true intellectual. One of his great gifts and loves is scientific and medical editing. He served as Editor-in-Chief of the *Journal of Clinical Investigation* and of *Williams Textbook of Endocrinology*. As an editor of *Harrison's* for two decades, Dr. Wilson made ample use of his conspicuous strengths as clinician, teacher, and scientist. His meticulous scholarship and high standards have had an enormous impact, not only on the Endocrinology, Metabolism, and Genetics sections, for which he had primary responsibility, but on the entire book.

DEDICATION

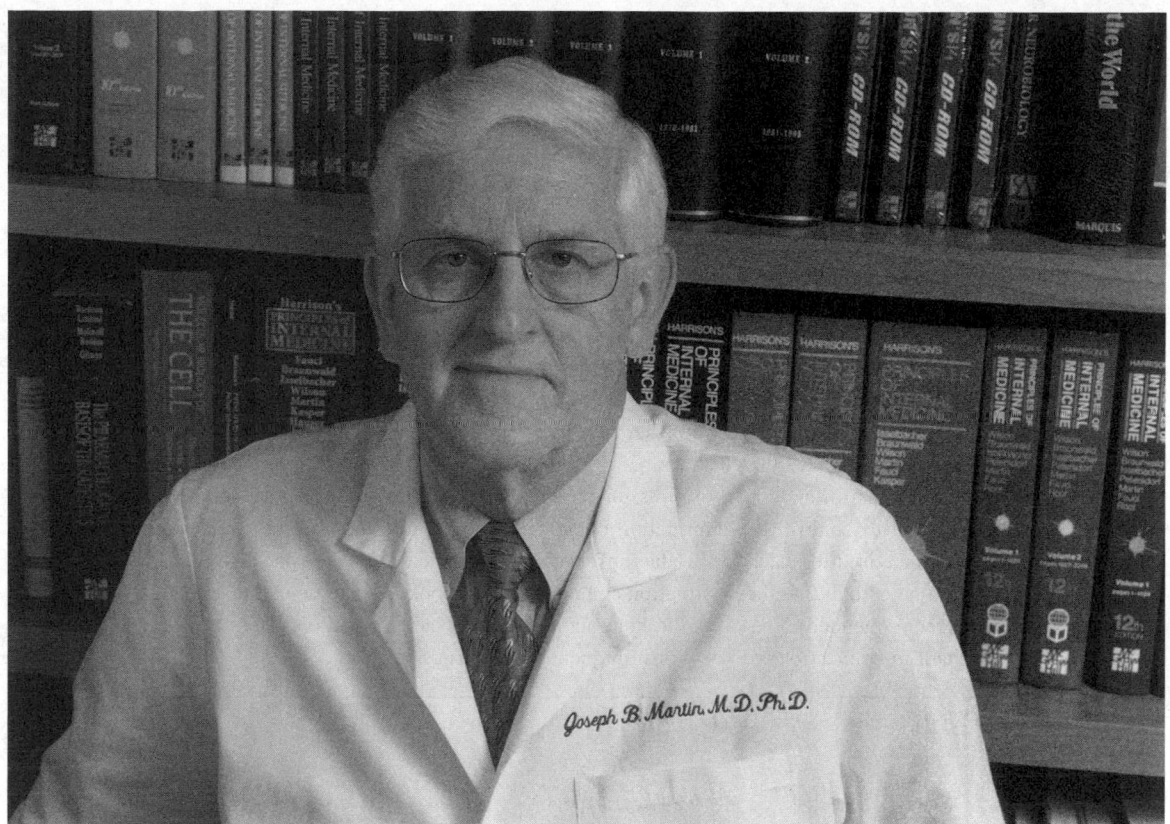

JOSEPH B. MARTIN

The editors wish to acknowledge the enormous contributions made by Joseph B. Martin, who edited the Neurology section of *Harrison's* from the tenth to the fourteenth editions. Dr. Martin followed Dr. Raymond D. Adams as editor of the Neurology section. In retrospect, the choice of Joseph Martin to replace Adams was prescient. It foresaw the transformation of neurology in the 1980s and 1990s from a largely descriptive discipline to one of the most dynamic and rapidly evolving areas of internal medicine. With his appointment as editor, the textbook had secured the foremost leader in the new field of molecular neurology to its ranks. Beginning with the tenth edition, Martin built upon the powerful didactic structure of the "syndromic approach" to neurology created by Adams and emphasized advances in molecular genetics and cell biology that reclassify neurologic diseases, clarify disease mechanisms, and offer new insights into clinical diagnosis and therapy. During his tenure, the neurology section of *Harrison's* became the best resource of its kind for the exposition of new discoveries in neurology and contributed substantially to the growing overall success of the textbook.

Born in Bassano, Alberta, Canada, Dr. Martin received his premedical and medical education at the University of Alberta, Edmonton, trained in neurology at Case Western University, and received the PhD from the University of Rochester. His career in academic medicine began in 1971 at McGill University in Montreal, where he established an independent laboratory focused on hypothalamic regulation of pituitary hormone secretion, and where he quickly rose to become Chair of the Department of Neurology and Neurosurgery. In 1978, he joined the faculty at Harvard Medical School as Bullard (later Julianne Dorn) Professor of Neurology and Chief of the Neurology Service at Massachusetts General Hospital. While at Harvard,

he established the Huntington's Disease Center Without Walls, which in 1983 reported the spectacular finding of a genetic marker linked to Huntington's disease, thereby inaugurating the modern era of molecular neurogenetics. In 1989 Dr. Martin joined the University of California, San Francisco, initially serving as Dean of the School of Medicine and subsequently as Chancellor. Among his many achievements at UCSF was the conception of a major new research campus in San Francisco, which is fast becoming a reality. In July 1997, he returned to Harvard as the Caroline Shields Walker Professor of Neurobiology and Clinical Neuroscience and Dean of the Faculty of Medicine. A wonderful teacher and physician, Joe Martin has inspired a generation of housestaff, students, and colleagues at Harvard and UCSF.

Dr. Martin has received many honors, including honorary degrees from five distinguished universities and the Abraham Flexner Award of the Association of American Medical Colleges. He serves or has served on the editorial boards of nineteen medical and neurology journals. He is a member of the Institute of Medicine of the National Academy of Sciences and has served as President of the American Neurological Association.

Dr. Martin's many contributions to this textbook were enhanced by his extraordinary organizational skills and by a clear and direct style of writing and editing that permitted him to distill complex concepts into easily readable prose accessible to a general medical readership. As an example, his chapter on neurogenetics has become an instant classic and a highlight of each new edition of the book. The editors greatly value their friendship with this remarkable man whose integrity and intellectual strengths have served *Harrison's* so well during the past two decades.

CONTENTS

Part Ten
DISORDERS OF THE KIDNEY AND URINARY TRACT

Part Eleven
DISORDERS OF THE GASTROINTESTINAL SYSTEM

SECTION 1
DISORDERS OF THE ALIMENTARY TRACT

SECTION 2
LIVER AND BILIARY TRACT DISEASE

Part Fourteen

NEUROLOGIC DISORDERS

SECTION 1
DIAGNOSIS OF NEUROLOGIC DISORDERS

SECTION 2
DISEASES OF THE CENTRAL NERVOUS SYSTEM

SECTION 3
DISORDERS OF NERVE AND MUSCLES

SECTION 4
CHRONIC FATIGUE SYNDROME

SECTION 5
PSYCHIATRIC DISORDERS

SECTION 6
ALCOHOLISM AND DRUG DEPENDENCY

Part Fifteen

ENVIRONMENTAL AND OCCUPATIONAL HAZARDS

SECTION 1
SPECIFIC ENVIRONMENTAL AND OCCUPATIONAL HAZARDS

SECTION 2
ILLNESSES DUE TO POISONS, DRUG OVERDOSAGE, AND ENVENOMATION

APPENDICES

INDEX

CONTRIBUTORS

Numbers in brackets refer to chapters written or co-written by the contributor.

ELIAS ABRUTYN, MD
Professor of Medicine and Public Health; Associate Provost and Associate Dean for Faculty Affairs, Department of Medicine, Division of Infectious Diseases, MCP Hahnemann University School of Medicine, Philadelphia [143, 144]

JOHN W. ADAMSON, MD
Director, Blood Research Institute, Blood Center of Southeastern Wisconsin, Milwaukee [61, 105]

DAVID A. AHLQUIST, MD
Professor of Medicine, Mayo Medical School; Consultant in Gastroenterology, Mayo Clinic and Foundation, Rochester [42]

LEENA ALA-KOKKO, MD
Collagen Research Unit, Biocenter Oulu and Department of Medical Biochemistry, University of Oulu, Finland [351]

MUHAMMAD T. AL-LOZI, MBBS
Assistant Professor of Neurology, Washington University, St. Louis [101]

MICHAEL J. AMINOFF, MD
Professor of Neurology, University of California San Francisco, San Francisco [22, 357, 363]

KENNETH C. ANDERSON, MD
Associate Professor of Medicine, Harvard Medical School; Medical Director, Blood Component Laboratory, Dana-Farber Cancer Institute, Boston [114]

ELLIOTT M. ANTMAN, MD
Associate Professor of Medicine, Harvard Medical School; Director, Samuel A. Levine Cardiac Unit, Brigham and Women's Hospital, Boston [243]

FREDERICK R. APPELBAUM, MD
Member and Director, Clinical Research Division Fred Hutchinson Cancer Research Center; Professor and Head, Division of Medical Oncology, University of Washington School of Medicine, Seattle [115]

GORDON L. ARCHER, MD
Chairman, Division of Infectious Diseases, Department of Internal Medicine; Professor of Medicine and Microbiology/Immunology, Medical College of Virginia, Campus of Virginia Commonwealth University, Richmond [137]

JAMES O. ARMITAGE, MD
Dean, College of Medicine, and Professor of Internal Medicine, Section of Oncology/Hematology, University of Nebraska, Omaha [112]

ARTHUR K. ASBURY, MD
Van Meter Professor of Neurology Emeritus, University of Pennsylvania School of Medicine, Philadelphia [23, 377, 378]

JOHN R. ASPLIN, MD
Assistant Professor of Medicine, Section of Nephrology, University of Chicago, Pritzker School of Medicine, Chicago [276, 279]

JOHN C. ATHERTON, MRCP
Lecturer, Department of Medicine, Division of Gastroenterology and Institute of Infections and Immunity, University of Nottingham, Nottingham, England [154]

PAUL S. AUERBACH, MD
Clinical Professor of Surgery, Division of Emergency Medicine, Stanford University School of Medicine, Los Altos [397]

K. FRANK AUSTEN, MD
Theodore Bevier Bayles Professor of Medicine, Harvard Medical School; Director, Inflammation and Allergic Diseases Research Section, Division of Rheumatology, Immunology and Allergy, Brigham and Women's Hospital, Boston [310]

BERNARD M. BABIOR, MD, PhD
Head, Division of Biochemistry, Department of Molecular and Experimental Medicine, The Scripps Research Institute; Professor and Staff Physician, Division of Hematology and Oncology, Department of Medicine, Scripps Clinic and Research Foundation, La Jolla [107]

KAMAL F. BADR, MD
Professor and Chair, Department of Internal Medicine, American University of Beirut (Lebanon); Attending Physician, American University of Beirut Medical Center, Beirut, Lebanon [278]

DONALD S. BAIM, MD
Professor of Medicine, Harvard Medical School; Director, Center for Minimally Invasive Therapy, Brigham and Women's Hospital, Boston [228, 245]

ROBERT L. BARBIERI, MD
Kate Macy Ladd Professor Obstetrics, Gynecology and Reproductive Biology, Harvard Medical School; Chairman, Department of Obstetrics and Gynecology, Brigham and Women's Hospital, Boston [7]

TAMAR F. BARLAM, MD
Assistant Professor of Medicine, Harvard Medical School; Senior Associate Physician, Beth Israel Deaconess Medical Center, Boston; Director, Project on Antibiotic Resistance, Center for Science in the Public Interest, Washington, D.C. [19, 150]

KENNETH J. BART, MD, MPH, MSHPM
Director, Graduate School of Public Health, San Diego State University, San Diego [122]

M. FLINT BEAL, MD
Anne Parrish Titzel Professor and Chairman of Neurology, Weill Medical College; Neurologist-in-Chief, New York Presbyterian Hospital, New York [367, 376]

ROBERT S. BENJAMIN, MD
Internist and Professor of Medicine, Chairman, Department of Melanoma/Sarcoma Medical Oncology; Medical Director, Multidisciplinary Sarcoma Center, The University of Texas M.D. Anderson Cancer Center, Houston [98]

JOHN E. BENNETT, MD
Head, Clinical Mycology Section, Laboratory of Clinical Investigation, National Institute of Allergy and Infectious Diseases, National Institutes of Health, Potomac [200, 201, 202, 203, 204, 205, 206, 207, 208]

EDWARD J. BENZ, JR., MD
Richard and Susan Smith Professor of Medicine, Professor of Pediatrics and Pathology, Harvard Medical School; President, Dana-Farber Cancer Institute, Boston [106]

PAUL D. BERK, MD
Department of Medicine, Division of Liver Disease, Mount Sinai School of Medicine, New York [294]

DAVID R. BICKERS, MD
Carl Truman Nelson Professor and Chairman, Department of Dermatology, Columbia University, New York [60]

HENRY J. BINDER, MD
Professor of Medicine, Section of Digestive Diseases, Yale University, New Haven [286]

THOMAS D. BIRD, MD
Professor of Neurology, University of Washington; Chief of Neurology, Veterans Affairs Medical Center, Seattle [26, 362, 379]

NEIL R. BLACKLOW, MD
Richard M. Haidack Distinguished Professor of Medicine, Molecular Genetics and Microbiology, University of Massachusetts Medical School, Worcester [187]

MARTIN J. BLASER, MD
Frederick J. King Professor of Internal Medicine, Chairman, Department of Medicine, and Professor of Microbiology, New York University School of Medicine, New York [154, 158]

CLARA D. BLOOMFIELD, MD
Director, The Ohio State University Comprehensive Cancer Center; Deputy Director, The Arthur G. James Cancer Hospital and Richard J. Solove Research Institute; William G. Pace III Endowed Chair in Cancer Research; Director and Professor, Division of Hematology and Oncology, Department of Internal Medicine, College of Medicine and Public Health, The Ohio State University, Columbus [111]

RICHARD S. BLUMBERG, MD
Associate Professor of Medicine, Harvard Medical School; Chief, Division of Gastroenterology, Department of Medicine, Brigham and Women's Hospital, Boston [287]

JEAN L. BOLOGNIA, MD
Professor of Dermatology, Yale University School of Medicine, New Haven [57]

GEORGE J. BOSL, MD
Chairman, Department of Medicine, Memorial Sloan-Kettering Cancer Center; Professor of Medicine, Cornell University Medical College, New York [96]

PATRICK BOSQUE, MD
Assistant Professor of Neurology, Institute for Neurodegenerative Diseases, University of California San Francisco, San Francisco [375]

RICHARD C. BOUCHER, MD
William Rand Kenan Professor of Medicine, University of North Carolina at Chapel Hill; Director, Cystic Fibrosis/Pulmonary Research & Treatment Center, Chapel Hill [257]

KAREN D. BRADSHAW, MD
Associate Professor of Obstetrics and Gynecology, The University of Texas Southwestern Medical Center, Dallas [52, 336]

HUGH R. BRADY, MD, PhD
Professor of Medicine and Therapeutics, University College Dublin; Mater Misericordiae Hospital, Dublin, Ireland [269, 273, 274, 275]

KENNETH D. BRANDT, MD
Professor of Medicine and Head, Rheumatology Division, Indiana University School of Medicine; Director, Indiana University Multipurpose Arthritis and Musculoskeletal Disease Center, Indianapolis [321]

EUGENE BRAUNWALD, MD, MD(Hon), ScD(Hon)
Distinguished Hersey Professor of Medicine; Faculty Dean for Academic Programs at Brigham and Women's Hospital and Massachusetts General Hospital, Harvard Medical School; Vice-President for Academic Programs, Partners HealthCare System, Boston [32, 33, 34, 36, 37, 224, 225, 231, 232, 236, 237, 238, 239, 243, 244]

IRWIN M. BRAVERMAN, MD
Professor of Dermatology, Yale University School of Medicine, New Haven [57]

OTIS W. BRAWLEY, MD
Assistant Director, Office of Special Populations Research, Office of the Director, National Cancer Institute, National Institutes of Health, Bethesda [80]

JOEL G. BREMAN, MD, DTPH
Deputy Director, Division of International Training and Research, Fogarty International Center, National Institutes of Health, Bethesda [214]

BARRY M. BRENNER, MD, DSc(Hon), DMSc(Hon)
Samuel A. Levine Professor of Medicine, Harvard Medical School; Director, Renal Division, Brigham and Women's Hospital, Boston [47, 49, 268, 269, 270, 271, 273, 274, 275, 277, 278, 281]

ROBERT M. BRENNER, MD
Associate Medical Director, Clinical Research, Amgen Inc., Thousand Oaks, California [268]

CHARLES G. D. BROOK, MA, MD
Emeritus Professor of Pediatric Endocrinology, University College London, London, UK [8]

CLAIRE V. BROOME, MD
Senior Advisor to the Director, Integrated Health Information Systems, Centers for Disease Control and Prevention, Atlanta [142]

ROBERT H. BROWN, JR., DPhil, MD
Associate Neurologist, Massachusetts General Hospital; Professor of Neurology, Harvard Medical School, Boston [365, 383]

ROBERT C. BRUNHAM, MD
Professor of Medicine; Director and Medical Director, University of British Columbia Centre for Disease Control, Vancouver, BC, Canada [133]

H. FRANKLIN BUNN, MD
Professor of Medicine, Harvard Medical School; Physician, Brigham and Women's Hospital, Boston [107, 108]

DAVID M. BURNS, MD
Professor of Medicine, University of California San Diego, San Diego [390]

MICHAEL J. BURNS, MD
Instructor of Medicine, Harvard Medical School; Department of Emergency Medicine, Division of Toxicology, Beth Israel Deaconess Medical Center, Boston [396]

JOAN R. BUTTERTON, MD
Assistant Professor of Medicine, Harvard Medical School; Assistant in Medicine, Infectious Disease Division, Massachusetts General Hospital, Boston [131]

JOHN C. BYRD, MD
Director of Clinical Research, Hematology-Oncology Service, Department of Medicine, Walter Reed Army Medical Center, Washington, D.C. [111]

STEPHEN B. CALDERWOOD, MD
Chief, Division of Infectious Diseases, Massachusetts General Hospital; Associate Professor of Medicine (Microbiology and Molecular Genetics), Harvard Medical School, Boston [131]

MICHAEL CAMILLERI, MD
Professor of Medicine and Physiology, Mayo Medical School; Consultant in Gastroenterology, Physiology and Biophysics, Mayo Clinic and Mayo Foundation, Rochester [42]

GRANT L. CAMPBELL, MD, PhD
Division of Vector-Borne Infectious Diseases, National Center for Infectious Diseases, Centers for Disease Control and Prevention, Fort Collins [162, 175]

MARK D. CARLSON, MD
Vice Chair, Department of Medicine, University Hospitals of Cleveland; Associate Professor of Medicine, Case Western Reserve University School of Medicine, Cleveland [21]

CHARLES B. CARPENTER, MD
Professor of Medicine, Harvard Medical School; Senior Physician, Brigham and Women's Hospital, Boston [272]

BRUCE R. CARR, MD
Professor and Director, Division of Reproductive Endocrinology, and Holder, Paul C. MacDonald Distinguished Chair in Obstetrics and Gynecology, The University of Texas Southwestern Medical Center, Dallas [52, 336]

AGUSTIN CASTELLANOS, MD
Professor of Medicine and Director, Clinical Electrophysiology, University of Miami School of Medicine, Miami [39]

PHILLIP F. CHANCE, MD
Professor of Pediatrics and Neurology, University of Washington School of Medicine; Chief, Division of Genetics and Development, Children's Hospital and Regional Medical Center, Seattle [379]

FENG-YEE CHANG, MD, DSc
Associate Professor of Medicine, National Defense Medical Center; Chief, Division of Infectious Diseases, Tri-Service General Hospital, Taipei, Taiwan [151]

YUAN-TSONG CHEN, MD, PhD
Professor of Pediatrics and Genetics, and Chief, Division of Medical Genetics, Duke University Medical Center, Durham [350]

JOHN S. CHILD, MD
Professor of Medicine, University of California, Los Angeles; Co-Chief, Cardiology and Co-Director, Ahmanson/UCLA Adult Congenital Heart Disease Center, UCLA Medical Center, Los Angeles [234]

OLIVIER M. CHOSIDOW, MD
Department of Internal Medicine, Pitie-Salpêtrière Hospital, Paris, France [59]

RAYMOND T. CHUNG, MD
Medical Director, Liver Transplant Program; Director, Liver Service, Gastrointestinal Unit, Massachusetts General Hospital; Assistant Professor of Medicine, Harvard Medical School, Boston [299]

FREDRIC L. COE, MD
Professor of Medicine and Physiology and Director, Clinical Research Training Program, University of Chicago Pritzker School of Medicine, Chicago [276, 279]

ALAN S. COHEN, MD
Distinguished Professor of Medicine in Rheumatology, Emeritus, and Conrad Wesselhoeft Professor of Medicine, Emeritus, Boston University School of Medicine; Chief of Medicine and Director, Emeritus, Thorndike Memorial Laboratory, Boston City Hospital, Boston [319]

JEFFREY I. COHEN, MD
Head, Medical Virology Section, Laboratory of Clinical Investigation, National Institute of Allergy and Infectious Diseases, National Institutes of Health, Bethesda [184, 193]

FRANCIS S. COLLINS, MD, PhD
Director, National Human Genome Research Institute, National Institutes of Health, Bethesda [81]

WILSON S. COLUCCI, MD
Professor of Medicine, and Chief, Cardiovascular Medicine, Boston University School of Medicine, Boston [240]

GERALD A. COLVIN, DO
Assistant Professor of Medicine and Medical Research Scientist, University of Massachusetts Memorial Medical Center, Worcester [104]

MAUREEN T. CONNELLY, MD, MPH
Instructor in Medicine, Harvard Medical School; Harvard Pilgrim Health Care, Boston [10]

MAX D. COOPER, MD
Professor of Medicine, Pediatrics and Howard Hughes Medical Institute Investigator, University of Alabama at Birmingham, Birmingham [308]

LAWRENCE COREY, MD
Professor, Medicine and Laboratory Medicine, and Head, Virology Division, University of Washington; Head, Program in Infectious Diseases, Fred Hutchinson Cancer Research Center, Seattle [182, 197]

FELICIA COSMAN, MD
Associate Professor of Clinical Medicine, Columbia University; Medical Director, Clinical Research Center, Helen Hayes Hospital, West Haverstraw [342]

MARK A. CREAGER, MD
Associate Professor of Medicine, Harvard Medical School; Director, Vascular Center, Brigham and Women's Hospital, Boston [247, 248]

PHILIP E. CRYER, MD
Irene E. and Michael M. Karl Professor of Endocrinology and Metabolism, and Director, Division of Endocrinology, Diabetes and Metabolism, Washington University School of Medicine, St. Louis [334]

RONALD G. CRYSTAL, MD
Bruce Webster Professor of Medicine, Director, Institute of Geriatric Medicine, and Director, The Arthur and Rochelle Belfer Gene Therapy Care Facility, Weill Medical College of Cornell University, New York [318]

JOHN J. CUSH, MD
Medical Director, Arthritis Center, Presbyterian Hospital of Dallas, Dallas [320]

CHARLES A. CZEISLER, MD, PhD
Professor of Medicine, Harvard Medical School; Director, Sleep Disorders and Circadian Medicine, Brigham and Women's Hospital, Boston [27]

MARINOS C. DALAKAS, JR., MD
Chief, Neuromuscular Diseases Section, National Institute of Neurological Disorders and Stroke, National Institutes of Health, Bethesda [382]

DANIEL F. DANZL, MD
Professor and Chair, Department of Emergency Medicine, University of Louisville School of Medicine, Floyd Knobs, IN [20]

ROBERT B. DAROFF, MD
Chief of Staff and Senior Vice President for Academic Affairs, University Hospitals of Cleveland; Professor of Neurology and Associate Dean, Case Western Reserve University School of Medicine, Cleveland [21]

MEHUL T. DATTANI, MD
Senior Lecturer/Honorary Consultant in Pediatric Endocrinology, Institute of Child Health and Great Ormond Street Children's Hospital, London, UK [8]

CHARLES E. DAVIS, MD
Professor of Pathology and Medicine, University of California - San Diego School of Medicine; Director Emeritus, Microbiology Laboratory, UCSD Medical Center, San Diego [211]

JOHN DEL VALLE, MD
Professor of Medicine, Division of Gastroenterology, Department of Medicine, University of Michigan School of Medicine, Ann Arbor [285]

BRADLEY M. DENKER, MD
Assistant Professor of Medicine, Harvard Medical School; Associate Physician, Brigham and Women's Hospital, Boston [47]

DAVID T. DENNIS, MD, MPH
Chief, Bacterial Zoonoses Branch, Centers for Disease Control and Prevention, Fort Collins [162, 175]

ROBERT L. DERESIEWICZ, MD
Assistant Professor of Medicine, Harvard Medical School, Boston [139]

ROBERT J. DESNICK, PhD, MD
Professor and Chairman, Department of Human Genetics, Mount Sinai School of Medicine, New York [346]

BETTY DIAMOND, MD
Chief, Division of Rheumatology, Department of Microbiology and Immunology, Albert Einstein College of Medicine, New York [307]

JULES L. DIENSTAG, MD
Associate Professor of Medicine, Harvard Medical School; Physician, Massachusetts General Hospital, Boston [91, 295, 296, 297, 301]

WILLIAM P. DILLON, MD
Professor of Radiology, Neurology and Neurosurgery; Chief, Diagnostic Neuroradiology, University of California San Francisco, San Francisco [358]

CHARLES A. DINARELLO, MD
Professor of Medicine, University of Colorado Health Sciences Center, Denver [17]

ROBERT G. DLUHY, MD
Professor of Medicine, Harvard Medical School, Brigham and Women's Hospital, Boston [331]

RAPHAEL DOLIN, MD
Maxwell Finland Professor of Medicine, and Dean for Clinical Programs, Harvard Medical School, Boston [181, 189, 190]

DANIEL B. DRACHMAN, MD
Professor of Neurology and Neurosciences; Director, Neuromuscular Unit, The Johns Hopkins University School of Medicine, Baltimore [380]

JEFFREY M. DRAZEN, MD
Professor of Medicine, Harvard Medical School; Senior Physician, Brigham and Women's Hospital, Boston [249, 250, 251, 266]

THOMAS D. DuBOSE, JR., MD
Peter T. Bohan Professor and Chairman, Department of Internal Medicine; Professor of Molecular and Integrative Physiology, University of Kansas School of Medicine, Kansas City [50]

J. STEPHEN DUMLER, MD
Associate Professor and Associate Director, Division of Medical Microbiology, Department of Pathology, The Johns Hopkins Medical Institutions, Baltimore [177]

ANDREA E. DUNAIF, MD
Associate Professor of Medicine, Director, Center of Excellence in Women's Health, Harvard Medical School; Chief, Division of Women's Health and Senior Physician, Brigham and Women's Hospital, Boston [6]

MARLENE DURAND, MD
Assistant Professor of Medicine, Harvard Medical School, Boston [30]

JANICE DUTCHER, MD
Professor of Medicine, New York Medical College; Associate Director for Clinical Affairs, Our Lady of Mercy Comprehensive Cancer Center, New York [102]

JOHANNA DWYER, MD
Professor of Medicine and Community Health, Tufts University School of Medicine; Professor, Tufts University School of Nutrition Science and Policy; Senior Scientist, Jean Mayer USDA Human Nutrition Research Center at Tufts University, Boston [73]

VICTOR J. DZAU, MD
Hersey Professor of the Theory and Practice of Physic (Medicine), Harvard Medical School; Chairman, Department of Medicine, and Director of Research, Brigham and Women's Hospital, Boston [247, 248]

JEFFERY S. DZIECZKOWSKI, MD
Assistant Professor, Departments of Pathology and Internal Medicine, Wayne State University School of Medicine, Detroit [114]

J. DONALD EASTON, MD
Professor and Chair, Department of Clinical Neurosciences, Brown University School of Medicine; Neurologist-in-Chief, Rhode Island Hospital, Providence [361]

DAVID A. EHRMANN, MD
Associate Professor, Section of Endocrinology, Department of Medicine, University of Chicago, Chicago [53]

JOHN W. ENGSTROM, MD
Associate Professor of Neurology, and Vice Chairman, Department of Neurology, University of California San Francisco, San Francisco [16, 366]

ALAN EPSTEIN, MD
Assistant Professor of Medicine, Brown University School of Medicine, Providence [289]

ANTHONY S. FAUCI, MD
Chief, Laboratory of Immunoregulation; Director, National Institute of Allergy and Infectious Diseases, National Institutes of Health, Bethesda [191, 305, 309, 317]

MURRAY J. FAVUS, MD
Professor of Medicine, University of Chicago Pritzker School of Medicine; Director, General Clinical Research Center; Director, Bone Program, Chicago [279]

ROBERT G. FENTON, MD, PhD
Associate Professor of Medicine, University of Maryland Greenebaum Cancer Center, Baltimore [82]

HOWARD L. FIELDS, MD, PhD
Professor of Neurology and Physiology, University of California San Francisco, San Francisco [12]

GREGORY A. FILICE, MD
Associate Professor of Medicine, University of Minnesota; Chief, Infectious Disease Section, Veterans Affairs Medical Center, Minneapolis [165]

ROBERT FINBERG, MD
Professor of Medicine, and Chair Department of Medicine, University of Massachusetts Medical School, Worcester [85, 136]

JOYCE D. FINGEROTH, MD
Assistant Professor of Medicine, Harvard Medical School; Physician, Beth Israel Deaconess Medical Center, Boston [136]

JEFFREY S. FLIER, MD
George C. Reisman Professor of Medicine, Harvard Medical School; Vice-Chair for Research, and Chief, Division of Endocrinology, Department of Medicine, Beth Israel Deaconess Medical Center, Boston [77]

JUDAH FOLKMAN, MD
Surgeon-in-Chief, Emeritus, Director, Surgical Research Laboratory, Children's Hospital; Andrus Professor of Pediatric Surgery, Professor of Cell Biology, Department of Surgery, Harvard Medical School, Boston [83]

SONIA FRIEDMAN, MD
Instructor in Medicine, Harvard Medical School; Associate Physician in Medicine, Brigham and Women's Hospital, Boston [287]

WILLIAM F. FRIEDMAN, MD
J.H. Nicholson Professor of Pediatrics (Cardiology); Associate Dean for Academic Affairs, University of California, Los Angeles School of Medicine and UCLA Medical Center, Los Angeles [234]

ADRIANE FUGH-BERMAN, MD
Assistant Clinical Professor, Department of Health Care Sciences, George Washington University School of Medicine, Washington, D.C. [11]

ROBERT F. GAGEL, MD
Chairman, Department of Internal Medicine Specialties, and Chief, Section of Endocrine Neoplasia and Hormonal Disorders, University of Texas M.D. Anderson Cancer Center, Houston [339]

JOHN I. GALLIN, MD
Director, NIH Warren Grant G. Magnuson Clinical Center; NIH Associate Director for Clinical Research; Chief Laboratory of Host Defenses, National Institute of Allergy and Infectious Diseases, National Institutes of Health, Bethesda [64]

ABHIMANYU GARG, MD
Professor, Department of Internal Medicine, Center for Human Nutrition, University of Texas Southwestern Medical Center at Dallas; Director, Diabetes Clinic, Department of Veterans Affairs Medical Center, Dallas [354]

ROBERT H. GELBER, MD
Clinical Professor of Medicine and Dermatology, University of California San Francisco, San Anselmo [170]

JEFFREY A. GELFAND, MD
Visiting Professor of Medicine, Harvard Medical School; Distinguished Professor of Medicine, Tufts University School of Medicine; Attending Physician in Infectious Diseases, Massachusetts General Hospital, Boston [17, 125]

ANNE A. GERSHON, MD
Professor of Pediatrics, and Director of Division of Pediatric Infectious Diseases, Columbia University College of Physicians and Surgeons, New York [194, 195, 196]

MARC GHANY, MD
Medical Staff Fellow, Liver Diseases Section, Digestive Diseases Branch, National Institute of Diabetes and Digestive and Kidney Diseases, National Institutes of Health, Bethesda [292]

RAYMOND J. GIBBONS, MD
Arthur M. and Glady D. Gray Professor of Medicine, Mayo Medical School, Rochester [227]

BRUCE C. GILLILAND, MD
Professor of Medicine and Laboratory Medicine, University of Washington School of Medicine, Seattle [313, 325, 326]

HENRY N. GINSBERG, MD
Irving Professor of Medicine, Columbia University College of Physicians and Surgeons, New York [344]

ELI GLATSTEIN, MD
Vice-Chairman and Clinical Director, Radiation Oncology, University of Pennsylvania Medical Center, Philadelphia [394]

ROBERT M. GLICKMAN, MD
Professor of Medicine and Dean, New York University School of Medicine, New York [46]

IRA J. GOLDBERG, MD
Professor of Medicine, Division of Preventive Medicine and Nutrition, Columbia University College of Physicians and Surgeons, New York [344]

ARY L. GOLDBERGER, MD
Associate Professor of Medicine, Harvard Medical School; Director, Margret and H.A. Rey Laboratory for Nonlinear Dynamics in Medicine, Beth Israel Deaconess Medical Center, Boston [226]

SAMUEL Z. GOLDHABER, MD
Associate Professor of Medicine, Harvard Medical School; Director, Venous Thromboembolism Research Group; Director, Cardiac Center's Anticoagulation Service, Brigham and Women's Hospital, Boston [261]

DONALD E. GOODKIN, MD
San Rafael, California [371]

RAJ K. GOYAL, MD
Associate Chief of Staff for Research and Development, VA Medical Center; Mallinckrodt Professor of Medicine, Harvard Medical School, West Roxbury [40, 284]

GREGORY A. GRABOWSKI, MD
Professor of Pediatrics; Director, Division and Program in Human Genetics, Children's Hospital Research Foundation, Cincinnati [349]

JACOB GREEN, MD
Associate Professor of Medicine, Department of Nephrology, Technion Faculty of Medicine, Haifa, Israel [270]

HARRY B. GREENBERG, MD
Senior Associate Dean for Research, Professor of Medicine, Microbiology and Immunology, and ACOS for Research VAPAHCS, Stanford University, Stanford [192]

NORTON J. GREENBERGER, MD
Professor of Medicine, and Senior Associate Dean for Medical Education, University of Kansas School of Medicine, Kansas City [302, 303, 304]

JOHN S. GREENSPAN, BDS, PhD
Professor and Chair, Department of Stomatology and Director, Oral AIDS Center, School of Dentistry; Professor, Department of Pathology, and Director, AIDS Clinical Research Center, School of Medicine, University of California San Francisco, San Francisco [31]

DARYL R. GRESS, MD
Associate Professor of Neurology and Neurosurgery; Director, Neurovascular Service, University of California San Francisco, San Francisco [376]

JAMES E. GRIFFIN, MD
Diana and Richard C. Strauss Professor in Biomedical Research, and Professor of Internal Medicine, University of Texas Southwestern Medical Center, Dallas [335, 338]

WILLIAM GROSSMAN, MD
Myer Friedman Distinguished Professor of Medicine, University of California San Francisco; Chief of Cardiology, University of California San Francisco Medical Center, San Francisco [228]

RASIM GUCALP, MD
Associate Professor of Medicine, Department of Oncology, Montefiore Medical Center, Albert Einstein College of Medicine, New York [102]

BEVRA HANNAHS HAHN, MD
Professor of Medicine, Chief of Rheumatology, and Vice-Chair, Department of Medicine, University of California, Los Angeles, Los Angeles [311]

STEPHEN M. HAHN, MD
Assistant Professor of Medicine, Department of Radiation Oncology, University of Pennsylvania Medical Center, Philadelphia [394]

JANET E. HALL, MD
Associate Professor of Medicine, Harvard Medical School; Assistant Chief, Reproductive Endocrine Unit, Massachusetts General Hospital, Boston [54]

SCOTT A. HALPERIN, MD
Professor of Pediatrics, and Associate Professor of Microbiology and Immunology, Dalhousie University; Head, Pediatric Infectious Diseases, IWK-Grace Health Center, Halifax, Nova Scotia, Canada [152]

CHARLES H. HALSTED, MD
Professor of Internal Medicine, Division of Clinical Nutrition and Metabolism, University of California-Davis School of Medicine, Davis [74]

ROBERT I. HANDIN, MD
Professor of Medicine, Harvard Medical School; Co-Director, Hematology Division, and Executive Vice Chairman, Department of Medicine, Brigham and Women's Hospital, Boston [62, 116, 117, 118]

GAVIN HART, MD, MPH
Director, STD Services, Royal Adelaide Hospital; Clinical Associate Professor, School of Medicine, Flinders University, Adelaide South Australia, Australia [164]

WILLIAM L. HASLER, MD
Associate Professor of Internal Medicine, Division of Gastroenterology, University of Michigan Medical Center, Ann Arbor [41]

TERRY HASSOLD, PhD
Professor, Department of Genetics, Case Western Reserve University and the Center for Human Genetics, University Hospitals of Cleveland, Cleveland [66]

STEPHEN L. HAUSER, MD
Betty Anker Fife Professor and Chairman, Department of Neurology, University of California San Francisco, San Francisco [355, 356, 361, 367, 368, 371, 378]

BARTON F. HAYNES, MD
Frederic M. Hanes Professor of Medicine, and Chair, Department of Medicine, Duke University Medical Center, Durham [305]

J. CLAUDE HEMPHILL III, MD
Assistant Professor of Neurology, University of California San Francisco; Director, Neurovascular and Neurocritical Care Program, San Francisco General Hospital, San Francisco [376]

PATRICK H. HENRY, MD
Chairman, Department of Medicine, St. John's Mercy Medical Center, St. Louis [63]

BARBARA L. HERWALDT, MD, MPH
Medical Epidemiologist, Division of Parasitic Diseases, Centers for Disease Control Prevention, Atlanta [215]

MARTIN S. HIRSCH, MD
Professor of Medicine, Harvard Medical School; Director, AIDS Clinical Research, Massachusetts General Hospital, Boston [185]

BERNARD HIRSCHEL, MD
Associate Professor of Medicine; Head, HIV/AIDS Section, Division of Infectious Diseases, University Hospital, Geneva [171]

MICHAEL F. HOLICK, MD, PhD
Professor of Medicine, Department of Endocrinology, Diabetes and Metabolism, Boston University School of Medicine, Boston [340]

STEVEN M. HOLLAND, MD
Senior Investigator and Head, Immunopathogenesis Unit, Clinical Pathophysiology Section, Laboratory of Host Defenses, National Institute of Allergy and Infectious Diseases, National Institute of Health, Bethesda [64]

KING K. HOLMES, MD, PhD
Professor of Medicine, and Director, Center for AIDS and Sexually Transmitted Diseases, University of Washington; Head, Infectious Diseases, Harborview Medical Center, Seattle [132, 133]

RANDALL K. HOLMES, MD, PhD
Professor and Chair, Department of Microbiology, University of Colorado School of Medicine, Denver [141]

ERIC G. HONIG, MD
Professor of Medicine, Emory University School of Medicine, Atlanta [258]

JAY H. HOOFNAGLE, MD
Director, Division of Digestive Diseases and Nutrition, National Institute of Diabetes and Digestive and Kidney Diseases, National Institutes of Health, Bethesda [292]

JONATHAN C. HORTON, MD, PhD
Associate Professor of Ophthalmology, Neurology, and Physiology, University of California San Francisco, San Francisco [28]

LYN HOWARD, MB
Professor of Medicine, Associate Professor of Pediatrics, and Head-Division of Clinical Nutrition in Department of Medicine, Albany Medical College, Albany [76]

HOWARD HU, MD, DPH
Associate Professor of Occupational Medicine, Harvard School of Public Health; Assistant Professor of Medicine, Harvard Medical School; Associate Physician, Channing Laboratory, Brigham and Women's Hospital, Boston [5, 391, 395]

GARY W. HUNNINGHAKE, MD
Professor, Department of Internal Medicine, and Director, Division of Pulmonary, Critical Care, and Occupational Medicine, University of Iowa College of Medicine, Iowa City [253]

EDWARD P. INGENITO, MD
Assistant Professor of Medicine, Harvard Medical School; Director, Pulmonary Function Laboratory, Brigham and Women's Hospital, Boston [266]

ROLAND H. INGRAM, JR., MD
Martha West Looney Professor Emeritus, Emory University School of Medicine, Atlanta [32, 258, 265]

THOMAS S. INUI, ScM, MD
President and CEO, The Fetzer Institute, Kalamazoo, Michigan [10]

MARK A. ISRAEL, MD
Professor, Departments of Neurological Surgery and Pediatrics; Director, Preuss Laboratory of Molecular Neuro-Oncology, University of California San Francisco, San Francisco [370]

KURT J. ISSELBACHER, MD
Distinguished Mallinckrodt Professor of Medicine, Harvard Medical School; Physician and Director, Massachusetts General Hospital Cancer Center, Boston [91, 282, 289, 295, 296, 297, 345]

RICHARD F. JACOBS, MD, FAAP
Horace C. Cabe Professor of Pediatrics, University of Arkansas for Medical Sciences; Chief, Pediatric Infectious Diseases, Arkansas Children's Hospital, Little Rock [161]

J. LARRY JAMESON, MD, PhD
Irving S. Cutter Professor and Chairman, Department of Medicine, Northwestern University Medical School; Physician-in-Chief, Northwestern Memorial Hospital, Chicago [65, 68, 327, 330]

ROBERT T. JENSEN, MD
Digestive Diseases Branch, National Institute of Diabetes and Digestive and Kidney Diseases, National Institutes of Health, Bethesda [93]

DONALD R. JOHNS, MD
Associate Professor of Neurology and Ophthalmology; Harvard Medical School; Director, Division of Neuromuscular Disease, Beth Israel Deaconess Medical Center, Boston [67]

BRUCE E. JOHNSON, MD
Associate Professor of Medicine, Brigham and Women's Hospital and Harvard Medical School; Program Director, Lowe Center for Thoracic Oncology, Dana-Farber Cancer Institute, Boston [100]

MICHAEL JOSEPH, MD
Physician, Weber Medical Clinic, Ltd., Olney, Illinois [30]

MARK E. JOSEPHSON, MD
Professor of Medicine, Harvard Medical School; Director of the Harvard Thorndike Electrophysiology Institute and Arrhythmia Services, Beth Israel Deaconess Medical Center, Boston [229, 230]

EDWARD L. KAPLAN, MD
Professor of Pediatrics, Department of Pediatrics, University of Minnesota Medical School, Minneapolis [235]

MARSHALL M. KAPLAN, MD
Professor of Medicine, Tufts University School of Medicine; Chief, Gastroenterology Department, New England Medical Center, Boston [45, 293]

ADOLF W. KARCHMER, MD
Chief, Division of Infectious Diseases, Beth Israel Deaconess Medical Center; Professor of Medicine, Harvard Medical School, Boston [126]

DENNIS L. KASPER, MD, MA (Hon)
William Ellery Channing Professor of Medicine, Professor of Microbiology and Molecular Genetics, Executive Dean for Academic Programs, Harvard Medical School; Director, Channing Laboratory, Department of Medicine, Brigham and Women's Hospital, Boston [19, 119, 130, 145, 150, 160, 167]

LLOYD H. KASPER, MD
Professor of Medicine (Neurology) and Microbiology, Dartmouth Medical School, Hanover [217]

MARK A. KAY, MD, PhD
Director, Program in Human Gene Therapy, and Associate Professor, Departments of Pediatrics and Genetics, Stanford University School of Medicine, Stanford [69]

ELAINE T. KAYE, MD
Clinical Instructor in Dermatology, Harvard Medical School; Assistant in Medicine, Department of Medicine, Children's Hospital Medical Center, Weston [18]

KENNETH M. KAYE, MD
Assistant Professor of Medicine, Harvard Medical School; Associate Physician, Division of Infectious Diseases, Brigham and Women's Hospital, Boston [18]

GERALD T. KEUSCH, MD
Associate Director for International Research; Director, Fogarty International Center, National Institutes of Health; Professor of Medicine, Tufts University School of Medicine; New England Medical Center, Bethesda [122, 157, 159]

J. S. KEYSTONE, MD
Professor of Medicine, University of Toronto; Centre for Travel and Tropical Medicine, Division of Infectious Disease, Toronto General Hospital, Toronto, Ontario, Canada [123]

ELLIOTT KIEFF, MD, PhD
Albee Professor of Medicine and Microbiology and Molecular Genetics, Harvard Medical School, Boston [180]

TALMADGE E. KING, JR., MD
Constance B. Wofsy Distinguished Professor and Vice Chairman, Department of Medicine, University of California San Francisco; Chief, Medical Services, San Francisco General Hospital, San Francisco [259]

LOUIS V. KIRCHHOFF, MD, MPH
Professor, Department of Internal Medicine, University of Iowa; Staff Physician, Department of Veterans Affairs Medical Center, Iowa City [216]

JOEL N. KLINE, MD
Assistant Professor, University of Iowa College of Medicine, Iowa City [253]

HOWARD K. KOH, MD, PhD
Professor of Dermatology, Medicine and Public Health, Boston University Schools of Medicine and Public Health; Co-Director, Skin Oncology Program, Director, Cancer Prevention and Control Center, Boston [86]

ANTHONY L. KOMAROFF, MD
Professor of Medicine, Harvard Medical School; Senior Physician, Brigham and Women's Hospital, Boston [6]

PETER KOPP, MD
Assistant Professor of Medicine, Division of Endocrinology, Metabolism and Molecular Medicine, Northwestern University, Chicago [65]

WALTER J. KOROSHETZ, MD
Associate Professor of Neurology and Medicine; Associate Director, Stroke and Clinical Neurology Services, Massachusetts General Hospital, Harvard Medical School, Boston [374]

P. E. KOZARSKY, MD
Associate Professor of Medicine, Emory University School of Medicine; Adjunct Assistant Professor of Medicine, Emory University School of Public Health, Atlanta [123]

BARNETT S. KRAMER, MD, MPH
Director, Office of Medical Applications of Research, National Institutes of Health, Bethesda [80]

STEPHEN M. KRANE, MD
Persis, Cyrus and Marlow B. Harrison Professor of Medicine, Harvard Medical School; Physician and Chief, Arthritis Unit, Massachusetts General Hospital, Boston [340, 343]

HELENA KUIVANIEMI, MD, PhD
Associate Professor, Wayne State University School of Medicine, Detroit [351]

LOREN LAINE, MD
Professor of Medicine, University of Southern California School of Medicine, Los Angeles [44]

ANIL K. LALWANI, MD
Associate Professor, Department of Otolaryngology- Head and Neck Surgery, University of California San Francisco, San Francisco [29]

LEWIS LANDSBERG, MD
Professor of Medicine, Vice-President for Medical Affairs, and Dean, Northwestern University Medical School, Chicago [72, 332]

H. CLIFFORD LANE, MD
Head, Clinical and Molecular Retrovirology Section, Laboratory of Immunoregulation; Clinical Director, National Institute of Allergy and Infectious Diseases, National Institutes of Health, Bethesda [309]

THOMAS J. LAWLEY, MD
Professor, Department of Dermatology, and Dean, Emory University School of Medicine, Atlanta [55, 56, 58]

RAPHAEL C. LEE, MBME, MD, ScD, PhD(Hon)
Professor of Surgery (Plastic), Professor of Organismal Biology and Anatomy (Biomechanics) and, Director, Electrical Injury Research Program, University of Chicago; Attending Surgeon, Ancilla / St. Mary's Burn Center, Chicago [393]

THOMAS H. LEE, MD, MSc
Associate Professor, Harvard Medical School; Medical Director, Partners Community Health Care, Inc., Boston [13]

CAMMIE F. LESSER, MD, PhD
Infectious Disease Fellow, University of Washington, Seattle [156]

MATTHEW E. LEVISON, MD
Professor of Medicine and Public Health, and Chief, Division of Infectious Diseases, Allegheny University of the Health Sciences, Philadelphia [255]

PETER LIBBY, MD
Mallinckrodt Professor of Medicine, Harvard Medical School; Chief, Cardiovascular Medicine, Brigham and Women's Hospital, Boston [241, 242]

RICHARD W. LIGHT, MD
Professor of Medicine, Vanderbilt University; Director, Pulmonary Diseases, Saint Thomas Hospital, Nashville [262]

CHRISTOPHER H. LINDEN, MD
Associate Professor, Department of Emergency Medicine, University of Massachusetts Medical School, Worcester [396]

ROBERT LINDSAY, MBChB, PhD
Professor of Clinical Medicine, Columbia University College of Physicians and Surgeons; Chief, Internal Medicine, Helen Hayes Hospital, West Haverstraw, New York [342]

MARC E. LIPPMAN, MD
John G. Searle Professor and Chairman, Department of Internal Medicine, University of Michigan Health Science System, Ann Arbor [89]

PETER E. LIPSKY, MD
Scientific Director, National Institute of Arthritis and Musculoskeletal and Skin Diseases, National Institutes of Health, Bethesda [307, 312, 315, 320]

LEO X. LIU, MD, DTMH
Assistant Professor of Medicine, Harvard Medical School; Division of Infectious Diseases, Department of Medicine, Beth Israel Deaconess Medical Center, Boston [219]

BERNARD LO, MD
Professor of Medicine and Director, Program in Medical Ethics, University of California San Francisco, San Francisco [2]

DAN L. LONGO, MD
Scientific Director, National Institute on Aging, National Institutes of Health, Bethesda and Baltimore [61, 63, 79, 82, 84, 103, 112, 113, 191]

FRANK M. LONGO, MD, PhD
Professor of Neurology, University of California San Francisco; Chief of Neurology, Veterans Affairs Medical Center, Department of Neurology, San Francisco [359]

NICOLA LONGO, MD, PhD
Associate Professor, Division of Medical Genetics, Department of Pediatrics, Emory University School of Medicine Atlanta [352, 353]

DANIEL H. LOWENSTEIN, MD
Carl W. Walter Professor of Neurology and Dean for Medical Education, Harvard Medical School, Boston [360]

SHEILA A. LUKEHART, PhD
Research Professor of Medicine, Division of Allergy and Infectious Diseases, University of Washington School of Medicine, Seattle [172, 173]

M. MONIR MADKOUR, DM
Military Hospital, Riyadh, Saudi Arabia; Faculty of Medicine, Ain Shams University, Cairo, Egypt, Riyadh, Saudi Arabia [160]

LAWRENCE C. MADOFF, MD
Assistant Professor of Medicine, Harvard Medical School; Associate Physician, Channing Laboratory and Division of Infectious Diseases, Brigham and Women's Hospital, Boston [119, 127]

JAMES H. MAGUIRE, MD
Associate Professor of Medicine, Harvard Medical School; Department of Immunology and Infectious Diseases, Harvard School of Public Health, Boston [129, 323, 398]

ADEL A.F. MAHMOUD, MD, PhD
President, Merck Vaccines, Merck & Co., Inc., Whitehouse Station, New Jersey [222]

RONALD V. MAIER, MD
Professor and Vice Chairman of Surgery, University of Washington; Surgeon in Chief, Harborview Medical Center, Seattle [38]

MARK E. MAILLIARD, MD
Associate Professor of Medicine, Division of Gastroenterology and Hepatology, University of Nebraska Medical Center, Omaha [298]

DANIEL B. MARK, MD, MPH
Professor of Medicine, Duke University Medical Center; Director, Outcomes Research and Assessment Group, Durham [3, 4]

THOMAS MARRIE, MD
Professor and Chair, Department of Medicine, University of Alberta, Edmonton, Alberta, Canada [177]

JOSEPH B. MARTIN, MD, PhD, MA (Hon)
Dean of the Faculty of Medicine; Caroline Shields Walker Professor of Neurobiology and Clinical Neuroscience, Harvard Medical School, Boston [12, 356, 359, 366]

JANET R. MAURER, MD
Head, Section of Advanced Lung Disease and Lung Transplantation, Division of Pulmonary and Critical Care Medicine, and Medical Director, Transplant Center, The Cleveland Clinic Foundation, Cleveland [267]

ROBERT J. MAYER, MD
Professor of Medicine, Harvard Medical School; Vice-Chair for Academic Affairs, Department of Adult Oncology, Dana-Farber Cancer Institute, Boston [90, 92]

JOHN D. MCCONNELL, MD
Professor and Chairman, Department of Urology, The University of Texas Southwestern Medical Center, Dallas [48]

WILLIAM M. MCCORMACK, MD
Professor of Medicine and of Obstetrics and Gynecology, and Chief, Division of Infectious Diseases, State University of New York, New York [178]

E. REGIS MCFADDEN, JR., MD
Argyl J. Beams Professor of Medicine, Director, Division of Pulmonary and Critical Care Medicine, University Hospitals of Cleveland, Cleveland [252]

KEVIN T. MCVARY, MD
Associate Professor, Department of Urology, Northwestern University Medical School, Chicago [51]

NANCY K. MELLO, PhD
Professor of Psychology (Neuroscience), Harvard Medical School; Alcohol and Drug Abuse Research Center, McLean Hospital, Belmont [389]

SHLOMO MELMED, MD
Professor and Director, Cedars Sinai Research Institute, University of California Los Angeles School of Medicine, Los Angeles [328]

JERRY R. MENDELL, MD
Chairman and Professor of Neurology; Director, Neuromuscular Disease Center, The Ohio State University, Columbus [381, 383]

JACK H. MENDELSON, MD
Professor of Psychiatry (Neuroscience), Harvard Medical School; Alcohol and Drug Abuse Research Center, McLean Hospital, Belmont [389]

ROBERT O. MESSING, MD
Associate Professor of Neurology, and Associate Director, Ernest Gallo Clinic and Research Center, University of California San Francisco, San Francisco [386]

M. -MARSEL MESULAM, MD
Ruth and Evelyn Dunbar Professor of Neurology and Psychiatry; Director, Center for Behavioral and Cognitive Neurology; Director, Alzheimer's Program, Northwestern University Medical School, Chicago [25]

SUSAN MIESFELDT, MD
Assistant Professor of Medicine, Division of Hematology and Oncology, University of Virginia Health System, Charlottesville [68]

EDGAR L. MILFORD, MD
Associate Professor of Medicine, Harvard Medical School; Director of Renal Transplantation, Brigham and Women's Hospital, Boston [272]

SAMUEL I. MILLER, MD
Professor of Medicine and Microbiology, University of Washington, Seattle [156]

JOHN D. MINNA, MD
Professor, Internal Medicine and Pharmacology; Director, Hamon Center for Therapeutic Oncology Research, University of Texas Southwestern Medical Center, Dallas [88]

JEROME H. MODELL, MD
Associate Vice President for Health Affairs, and Professor of Anesthesiology, College of Medicine, University of Florida, Gainesville [392]

THOMAS A. MOORE, MD
Clinical Assistant Professor, Department of Internal Medicine, University of Kansas School of Medicine, Wichita [212]

MARC MOSS, MD
Assistant Professor of Medicine, Emory University School of Medicine; Director, Medical Intensive Care Unit, Grady Memorial Hospital, Atlanta [265]

ROBERT J. MOTZER, MD
Associate Attending Physician, Division of Solid Tumor Oncology, Department of Medicine, Memorial Sloan-Kettering Cancer Center; Associate Professor of Medicine, Cornell University Medical College, New York [94, 96]

HARALAMPOS M. MOUTSOPOULOS, MD
Professor and Director, Department of Pathophysiology, National University School of Medicine; President of the National Organization for Medicines, Athens, Greece [314, 316]

ROBERT S. MUNFORD, MD
Jan and Henri Bromberg Professor of Internal Medicine, and Professor of Microbiology, University of Texas Southwestern Medical Center, Dallas [124, 146]

TIMOTHY F. MURPHY, MD
Professor of Medicine and Microbiology, and Chief, Division of Infectious Diseases, State University of New York at Buffalo, Buffalo [149]

DANIEL M. MUSHER, MD
Professor of Medicine, and Professor of Molecular Virology, Baylor College of Medicine; Chief, Infectious Diseases, Veterans Affairs Medical Center, Houston [138, 148]

ROBERT J. MYERBURG, MD
Professor of Medicine and Physiology; Director, Division of Cardiology, University of Miami School of Medicine, Miami [39]

GERALD T. NEPOM, MD, PhD
Professor, Department of Immunology, University of Washington School of Medicine; Director, Virginia Mason Research Center, Seattle [306]

RICHARD A. NISHIMURA, MD
Professor of Medicine, Mayo Medical School, Rochester [227]

ROBERT L. NORRIS, MD
Associate Professor of Surgery, Department of Surgery; Chief, Division of Emergency Medicine, Stanford University, Stanford [397]

THOMAS B. NUTMAN, MD
Head, Helminth Immunology Section, Laboratory of Parasitic Diseases, National Institute of Allergy and Infectious Diseases, National Institutes of Health, Bethesda [220, 221]

JOHN A. OATES, MD
The Thomas F. Frist, Sr. Professor of Medicine, and Professor of Pharmacology, Vanderbilt University School of Medicine, Nashville [70]

RICHARD J. O'BRIEN, MD
Chief, Research and Evaluation Branch Division of Tuberculosis Elimination, Centers for Diseases Control and Prevention, Atlanta [169]

PATRICK T. O'GARA, MD
Associate Professor of Medicine, Harvard Medical School; Director, Clinical Cardiology, Brigham & Women's Hospital, Boston [34]

CHRISTOPHER A. OHL, MD
Assistant Professor of Medicine, Section on Infectious Diseases, Wake Forest University School of Medicine; Director, Center for Antimicrobial Utilization, Stewardship and Epidemiology, Baptist Medical Center, Winston-Salem [155]

RICHARD K. OLNEY, MD
Professor of Neurology, University of California San Francisco, San Francisco [22]

YVONNE M. O'MEARA, MD, FRCPI
Senior Lecturer in Medicine, University College Dublin; Consultant Nephrologist, Mater Misericordiae Hospital, Dublin, Ireland [274, 275]

ANDREW B. ONDERDONK, PhD
Professor of Pathology, Harvard Medical School; Director of Clinical Microbiology, Brigham and Women's Hospital, Boston [121]

ROBERT A. O'ROURKE, MD
Charles Conrad Brown Distinguished Professor of Cardiovascular Science, University of Texas Health Science Center at San Antonio, San Antonio [225]

CHUNG OWYANG, MD
Professor of Internal Medicine, H. Marvin Pollard Collegiate Professor and Chief, Division of Gastroenterology, Department of Internal Medicine, University of Michigan Medical Center, Ann Arbor [288]

JEFFREY PARSONNET, MD
Associate Professor of Medicine and of Microbiology, Dartmouth Medical School; Staff Physician, Infectious Diseases Section, Dartmouth-Hitchcock Medical Center, Lebanon [139]

SHREYASKUMAR R. PATEL, MD
Associate Professor of Medicine, Department of Melanoma/Sarcoma, Medical Oncology, University of Texas, MD Anderson Cancer Center, Houston [98]

GUSTAV PAUMGARTNER, MD
Professor of Medicine, Ludwig Maximiliam University of Munich, Durchwal, Germany [302]

STEPHEN J. PEROUTKA, MD
Burlingame, California [15]

MICHAEL C. PERRY, MD, MS
Professor of Internal Medicine; Director, Division of Hematology/Oncology, Nellie B. Smith Professor of Oncology, University of Missouri/Ellis Fischel Cancer Center; Consultant, Harry S. Truman VA Hospital, Columbia [103]

ALAN PESTRONK, MD
Professor of Neurology, Washington University, St. Louis [101]

CLARENCE J. PETERS, MD
Chief, Special Pathogens Branch, Centers for Disease Control and Prevention; Adjunct Professor of Microbiology and Immunology, Emory University, Atlanta [198, 199]

ELIOT A. PHILLIPSON, MD
Sir John and Lady Eaton Professor and Chair, Department of Medicine, University of Toronto, Toronto, Ontario, Canada [263, 264]

GERALD B. PIER, PhD
Professor of Medicine (Microbiology and Molecular Genetics), Harvard Medical School; Microbiologist, Brigham and Women's Hospital, Boston [120]

DANIEL K. PODOLSKY, MD
Mallinckrodt Professor of Medicine, Harvard Medical School; Chief of Gastrointestinal Unit; Director, Center for the Study of Inflammatory Bowel Disease, Massachusetts General Hospital, Boston [282, 299, 300]

RONALD E. POLK, Pharm. D.
Professor, Pharmacy and Medicine, School of Pharmacy Medical College of Virginia Campus, Virginia Commonwealth University, Richmond [137]

MATTHEW POLLACK, MD
Professor of Medicine, Uniformed Services University; F. Edward He'bert School of Medicine; Attending Staff Physician, Internal Medicine and Infectious Diseases, National Naval Medical Center, Bethesda [155]

JOHN T. POTTS, JR., MD
Distinguished Jackson Professor of Clinical Medicine, Harvard Medical School; Director of Research, Massachusetts General Hospital, Boston [341]

LAWRIE W. POWELL, MD, PhD
Professor of Medicine, The University of Queensland and Royal Brisbane Hospital, Brisbane, Queensland, Australia [345]

ALVIN C. POWERS, MD
Associate Professor of Medicine, Molecular Physiology and Biophysics, Vanderbilt University School of Medicine; Chief, Section of Endocrinology and Diabetes, VA Medical Center, Nashville [333]

DANIEL S. PRATT, MD
Assistant Professor of Medicine, Tufts University School of Medicine; Medical Director of Liver Transplantation, New England Medical Center, Boston [45, 293]

DARWIN J. PROCKOP, MD, PhD
Professor and Director, Center for Gene Therapy, Philadelphia [351]

DANIEL T. PRICE, MD
Assistant Professor of Medicine, Boston University School of Medicine; Staff Physician, Boston Veterans Affairs Medical Center, West Roxbury [240]

STANLEY B. PRUSINER, MD
Director, Institute for Neurodegenerative Diseases; Professor, Departments of Neurology, Biochemistry and Biophysics, University of California San Francisco, San Francisco [375]

PETER J. QUESENBERRY, MD
Professor of Medicine, University of Massachusetts School of Medicine, Worcester [104]

SANJAY RAM, MD
Assistant Professor of Medicine, Section of Infectious Diseases, Boston University School of Medicine and Boston Medical Center, Boston [147]

DIDIER RAOULT, MD
Professor of Medicine, Unité des Rickettsies, School of Medicine, University of Aux-Marseille, Marseille, France [177]

NEIL H. RASKIN, MD
Professor of Neurology, University of California San Francisco, San Francisco [15]

MARIO RAVIGLIONE, MD
TB Coordinator, Communicable Disease Programme, World Health Organization, Geneva, Switzerland [169]

SHARON L. REED, MD
Professor of Pathology and Medicine, and Director, Microbiology and Virology Laboratories, University of California, San Diego Medical Center, San Diego [213]

ANTONIO J. REGINATO, MD
Professor of Medicine, and Head, Division of Rheumatology, Cooper University Medical Center, Robert Wood Johnson Medical School at Camden, Camden [322]

RICHARD C. REICHMAN, MD
Professor of Medicine, Microbiology and Immunology, Head Infectious Diseases Unit, Senior Associate Dean for Clinical Research, University of Rochester School of Medicine and Dentistry, Rochester [188]

CAROL M. REIFE, MD
Clinical Assistant Professor of Medicine, Jefferson Medical College, Thomas Jefferson University, Philadelphia [43]

JOHN T. REPKE, MD
Chris J. and Marie A. Olson Professor of Obstetrics and Gynecology, and Chairman, Department of Obstetrics and Gynecology, University of Nebraska Medical Center, Omaha [7]

NEIL M. RESNICK, MD
Professor of Medicine, University of Pittsburgh School of Medicine; Chief, Division of Gerontology and Geriatric Medicine, University of Pittsburgh Healthcare System, Pittsburgh [9]

VICTOR I. REUS, MD
Professor of Psychiatry, University of California San Francisco; Medical Director, Langley Porter Hospital, San Francisco [385]

PETER A. RICE, MD
Professor of Medicine and Chief, Section of Infectious Diseases, Boston University School of Medicine and Boston Medical Center, Boston [147]

STUART RICH, MD
Professor of Medicine, Rush Medical College; Director, Rush Heart Institute Center for Pulmonary Heart Disease, Chicago [260]

GARY S. RICHARDSON, MD
Assistant Professor of Psychiatry, Case Western Reserve University; Senior Research Scientist, Sleep Disorders and Research Center, Henry Ford Hospital, Cleveland [27]

CELESTE ROBB-NICHOLSON, MD
Assistant Professor of Medicine, Harvard Medical School; Assistant Physician, Massachusetts General Hospital, Boston [6]

GARY L. ROBERTSON, MD
Professor of Medicine and Neurology, Northwestern University Medical School, Chicago [329]

DAN M. RODEN, MD
Professor of Medicine and Pharmacology; Director, Division of Clinical Pharmacology, Vanderbilt University School of Medicine, Nashville [70]

KAREN L. ROOS, MD
Professor of Neurology, Indiana University School of Medicine, Indianapolis [372]

ALLAN H. ROPPER, MD
Professor and Chairman of Neurology, Tufts University School of Medicine; Chief, Division of Neurology, St. Elizabeth's Medical Center, Boston [24, 369]

ROGER N. ROSENBERG, MD
Zale Distinguished Chair in Neurology; Professor of Neurology and Physiology, University of Texas Southwestern Medical Center; Attending Neurologist, Parkland Hospital and Zale-Lipsky University Hospital, Dallas [364]

WENDELL ROSSE, MD
Florence Reynaud McAlister Professor of Medicine and Medical Research, Department of Medicine, Duke University Medical School, Durham [108]

DAVID W. RUSSELL, MD, PhD
Associate Professor of Medicine, Division of Hematology University of Washington School of Medicine, Seattle [69]

ROBERT M. RUSSELL, MD
Professor of Medicine and Nutrition, Tufts University; Associate Director, USDA Human Nutrition Research Center, Tufts University, Boston [75]

THOMAS A. RUSSO, MD, CM
Assistant Professor of Medicine, Division of Infectious Diseases, Department of Medicine, State University of New York at Buffalo, Buffalo [153, 166]

STEPHEN M. SAGAR, MD
Professor of Neurology, Case Western Reserve School of Medicine, Cleveland [370]

EDWARD A. SAUSVILLE, MD, PhD
Associate Director, Developmental Therapeutics Program, Division of Cancer Treatment and Diagnosis, National Cancer Institute, Bethesda [84]

MOHAMED H. SAYEGH, MD
Associate Professor of Medicine, Harvard Medical School; Research Director, Laboratory of Immunogenetics and Transplantation, Brigham and Women's Hospital, Boston [272]

I. HERBERT SCHEINBERG, MD
Senior Lecturer in Medicine, College of Physicians and Surgeons, Columbia University, New York [348]

HOWARD I. SCHER, MD
Attending Physician, Chief, Genitourinary Oncology Service, Division of Solid Tumor Oncology, Department of Medicine, Memorial Sloan-Kettering Cancer Center; Professor of Medicine, Department of Medicine, Weill Medical College, New York [94, 95]

ALAN L. SCHILLER, MD
Irene Heinz Given and John LaPorte Given Professor and Chairman of Pathology, Mount Sinai School of Medicine; Chairman of Pathology, The Mount Sinai Hospital, New York [343]

HARRY W. SCHROEDER, JR., MD, PhD
Professor of Medicine and Microbiology, University of Alabama at Birmingham, Birmingham [308]

JOHN S. SCHROEDER, MD
Professor of Medicine, Cardiovascular Medicine, Stanford University School of Medicine, Stanford [233]

ANNE SCHUCHAT, MD
Chief, Respiratory Diseases Branch, Division of Bacterial and Mycotic Diseases, National Center for Infectious Diseases, Centers for Disease Control and Prevention, Atlanta [142]

MARC A. SCHUCKIT, MD
Professor of Psychiatry, University of California San Diego, and Veterans Affairs Medical Center, San Diego [387, 388]

PETER H. SCHUR, MD
Professor of Medicine, Harvard Medical School; Physician, Brigham and Women's Hospital, Boston [324]

STUART SCHWARTZ, PhD
Professor, Department of Genetics, Case Western Reserve University and the Center for Human Genetics, University Hospitals of Cleveland, Cleveland [66]

DAVID S. SEGAL, PhD
Professor of Psychiatry, University of California San Diego, La Jolla [388]

JULIAN L. SEIFTER, MD
Associate Professor of Medicine, Harvard Medical School; Physician, Brigham and Women's Hospital, Boston [281]

ANDREW P. SELWYN, MA, MD
Professor of Medicine, Harvard Medical School, Boston [244]

STEVEN I. SHERMAN, MD
Associate Professor, Section of Endocrine Neoplasia and Hormonal Disorders, University of Texas M.D. Anderson Cancer Center, Houston [339]

KARL SKORECKI, MD
Annie Chutick Professor of Medicine, Bruce Rappaport Faculty of Medicine, Technion-Israel Institute of Technology; Director, Department of Nephrology and Molecular Medicine, Rambam Medical Center, Haifa, Israel [270]

WILLIAM SILEN, MD
Johnson and Johnson Distinguished Professor of Surgery, and Dean for Faculty Development and Diversity, Harvard Medical School; Physician, Brigham and Women's Hospital, Boston [14, 290, 291]

GARY G. SINGER, MD
Assistant Professor of Medicine, Washington University School of Medicine; Associate Director, Transplant Nephrology, Barnes Jewish Hospital, St. Louis [49]

AJAY K. SINGH, MD
Associate Professor of Medicine, Harvard Medical School; Directory of Clinical Nephrology, Brigham and Women's Hospital, Boston [271]

JEAN D. SIPE, PhD
Scientific Review Administrator, Center for Scientific Review, National Institutes of Health; Adjunct Professor, Department of Biochemistry, Boston University School of Medicine, Bethesda [319]

WADE S. SMITH, MD, PhD
Assistant Professor of Neurology; Director, Stroke Service, University of California San Francisco, San Francisco [361]

JAMES B. SNOW, JR., MD
Professor Emeritus, Department of Otorhinolaryngology, University of Pennsylvania; former Director, National Institute on Deafness and Other Communication Disorders, National Institutes of Health, Bethesda [29]

ARTHUR J. SOBER, MD
Associate Professor of Dermatology, Harvard Medical School; Associate Chief of Dermatology, Massachusetts General Hospital, Boston [86]

MICHAEL F. SORRELL, MD
Robert L. Grissom Professor of Medicine; Medical Director, Liver Transplant Program, University of Nebraska Medical Center, Omaha [298]

PETER SPEELMAN, MD
Division of Infectious Diseases, Tropical Medicine and AIDS, Department of Internal Medicine, Academic Medical Center, University of Amsterdam, Amsterdam, The Netherlands [174]

FRANK E. SPEIZER, MD
Edward H. Kass Professor of Medicine, Harvard Medical School; Co-Director, Channing Laboratory, Brigham and Women's Hospital, Boston [5, 254, 391]

ANDREW SPIELMAN, ScD
Professor of Tropical Public Health, Harvard School of Public Health, Boston [398]

JERRY L. SPIVAK, MD
Professor of Medicine and Oncology, The Johns Hopkins University School of Medicine, Baltimore [110]

WALTER E. STAMM, MD
Professor of Medicine and Head, Division of Allergy and Infectious Diseases, University of Washington School of Medicine, Seattle [179, 280]

ALLEN C. STEERE, MD
Zucker Professor of Medicine, Tufts University School of Medicine; Chief, Rheumatology/Immunology, New England Medical Center, Boston [176]

ROBERT S. STERN, MD
Carl J. Herzog Professor of Dermatology, Harvard Medical School; Dermatologist-in-Chief, Beth Israel Deaconess Medical Center, Boston [59]

DENNIS L. STEVENS, MD, PhD
Professor of Medicine, University of Washington School of Medicine, Seattle; Chief, Infectious Diseases, VA Medical Center, Boise [128]

RICHARD M. STONE, MD
Associate Professor of Medicine, Harvard Medical School; Clinical Director, Adult Leukemia Program, Dana-Farber Cancer Institute, Brigham and Women's Hospital, Boston [99]

STEPHEN E. STRAUS, MD
Chief, Laboratory of Clinical Investigation, National Institute of Allergy and Infectious Diseases, National Institutes of Health, Bethesda [384]

MORTON N. SWARTZ, MD
Professor, Department of Medicine, Harvard Medical School; Chief, James Jackson Firm Medical Services, Massachusetts General Hospital, Boston [374]

ROBERT A. SWERLICK, MD
Associate Professor, Department of Dermatology, Emory University School of Medicine, Atlanta [56]

A. JAMIL TAJIK, MD
Thomas J. Walker Jr. Professor of Medicine and Pediatrics, Mayo Medical School; Chair, Division of Cardiovascular Diseases, Mayo Clinic, Rochester [227]

JOEL D. TAUROG, MD
Professor of Internal Medicine, and William M. and Gay Burnett Professor for Arthritis Research, University of Texas Southwestern Medical Center; Interim Chief, Division of Rheumatic Diseases and Interim Director, Harold C. Simmons Arthritis Research Center, Dallas [306, 315]

SCOTT J. THALER, MD
Director, Clinical Monitor, Clinical Research, Vaccines, Merck Research Laboratories, Merck & Co., Inc., Blue Bell [323]

LUCY STUART TOMPKINS, MD, PhD
Professor of Medicine (Infectious Diseases and Geographic Medicine), Professor of Microbiology, Immunology and Pathology, Stanford University School of Medicine, Stanford [163]

MARK TOPAZIAN, MD
Associate Professor of Medicine, Yale University School of Medicine; Assistant Director, Gastrointestinal Procedure Center, Yale New Haven Hospital, New Haven [283]

PHILLIP P. TOSKES, MD
Professor of Medicine and Director, Division of Gastroenterology, Hepatology and Nutrition; Associate Chairman for Clinical Affairs, Department of Medicine, University of Florida, Gainesville [303, 304]

JEFFREY M. TRENT, PhD
Chief, Laboratory of Cancer Genetics; Director, Division of Intramural Research, National Human Genome Research Institute, National Institutes of Health, Bethesda [81]

GERARD TROMP, PhD
Assistant Professor, Wayne State University School of Medicine, Detroit [351]

KENNETH L. TYLER, MD
Vice Chairman and Professor of Neurology, Professor of Medicine, Microbiology and Immunology, University of Colorado Health Sciences Center; Chief, Neurology Service, Denver VA Medical Center, Denver [372, 373]

EVERETT E. VOKES, MD
Duchossois Professor, Departments of Medicine and Radiation Oncology; Director, Section of Hematology/Oncology, University of Chicago Medical Center, Chicago [87]

MATTHEW K. WALDOR, MD
Assistant Professor of Medicine, New England Medical Center, Tufts University School of Medicine, Boston [159]

DAVID WALKER, MD
Professor and Chairman, Department of Pathology, University of Texas Medical Branch, Galveston [177]

RICHARD J. WALLACE, JR., MD
Professor and Chairman, Department of Microbiology and Research, University of Texas Health Center at Tyler, Tyler [168]

B. TIMOTHY WALSH, MD
William and Joy Ruane Professor of Pediatric Psychopharmacology, Department of Psychiatry, College of Physicians and Surgeons, Columbia University; Director, Eating Disorders Research Unit, New York State Psychiatric Institute, New York [78]

PETER D. WALZER, MD
Professor of Medicine, University of Cincinnati College of Medicine; Chief, Infectious Diseases, VA Medical Center, Cincinnati [209]

FREDERICK C.S. WANG, MD
Associate Professor of Medicine, Harvard Medical School; Physician, Brigham and Women's Hospital, Boston [180, 186]

CARL V. WASHINGTON, JR., MD
Assistant Professor of Dermatology, Emory University School of Medicine; Director, Mohs Surgery Unit, The Emory Clinic, Atlanta [86]

ANTHONY P. WEETMAN, MD, DSC
Professor of Medicine and Dean, University of Sheffield Medical School; Consultant Physician, Northern General Hospital, Sheffield, UK [330]

STEVEN E. WEINBERGER, MD
Professor of Medicine, Harvard Medical School; Vice-Chairman, Department of Medicine, Beth Israel Deaconess Medical Center, Boston [33, 249, 250, 251, 256]

ROBERT A. WEINSTEIN, MD
Professor of Medicine, Rush Medical College; Chairman of Infectious Diseases, Cook County Hospital, Chicago [134]

PETER F. WELLER, MD
Professor of Medicine, Harvard Medical School; Co-Chief, Division of Infectious Diseases, Chief, Division of Allergy and Inflammation, Department of Medicine, Beth Israel Deaconess Medical Center, Boston [210, 218, 219, 220, 221, 223]

MICHAEL R. WESSELS, MD
Associate Professor of Pediatrics and Medicine, Harvard Medical School; Chief, Division of Infectious Diseases, Children's Hospital; Channing Laboratory, Brigham and Women's Hospital, Boston [140]

MEIR WETZLER, MD
Assistant Professor of Medicine, State University of New York at Buffalo, Buffalo [111]

A. CLINTON WHITE, JR., MD
Associate Professor of Medicine, Department of Medicine, Microbiology and Immunology, Baylor College of Medicine, Houston [223]

NICHOLAS J. WHITE, DSC, MD
Professor of Tropical Medicine, Mahidol University, Thailand and Oxford University, UK, Bangkok, Thailand [214]

RICHARD J. WHITLEY, MD
Loeb Eminent Scholar Chair in Pediatrics, Professor of Pediatrics, Microbiology and Medicine, University of Alabama at Birmingham, Birmingham [183]

GRANT R. WILKINSON, PhD
Professor of Pharmacology, Vanderbilt University School of Medicine, Nashville [70]

GORDON H. WILLIAMS, MD
Professor of Medicine, Harvard Medical School; Chief, Endocrine-Hypertension Division, Brigham & Women's Hospital, Boston [35, 246, 331]

JEAN D. WILSON, MD
Charles Cameron Sprague Distinguished Chair and Clinical Professor of Internal Medicine, The University of Texas Southwestern Medical Center, Dallas [335, 337, 338]

JOHN W. WINKELMAN, MD, PhD
Assistant Professor of Psychiatry, Harvard Medical School; Medical Director, Sleep Health Center, Brigham and Women's Hospital, Boston [27]

BRUCE U. WINTROUB, MD
Associate Dean, Professor and Chair of Dermatology, University of California at San Francisco, San Francisco [59]

GREGORY P. WITTENBERG, MD
Rapid City Medical Center, LLP, Rapid City [86]

ALLAN W. WOLKOFF, MD
Department of Medicine and Marion Bessin Liver Center, Albert Einstein College of Medicine, New York [294]

ALASTAIR J.J. WOOD, MB, ChB
Assistant Vice Chancellor, Professor of Medicine, Professor of Pharmacology, Vanderbilt University, School of Medicine, Nashville [71]

ROBERT L. WORTMANN, MD
Professor and Chairman, Department of Internal Medicine, University of Oklahoma College of Medicine, Tulsa [347]

PAUL W. WRIGHT, MD
Director of Predoctoral Education and Professor of Family Practice, University of Texas Health Center, Tyler [168]

JOSHUA WYNNE, MD, MBA
Professor of Internal Medicine, Wayne State University, Detroit [238]

KIM B. YANCEY, MD
Senior Investigator, Dermatology Branch, Division of Clinical Sciences, National Cancer Institute, National Institutes of Health; Adjunct Professor, Department of Dermatology, Uniformed Services University of the Health Sciences, Bethesda [55, 58]

JAMES B. YOUNG, MD
Professor of Medicine, Northwestern University Medical School; Attending Physician, Northwestern Memorial Hospital, Chicago [72, 332]

NEAL S. YOUNG, MD
Chief, Hematology Branch, National Heart, Lung and Blood Institute, National Institutes of Health, Bethesda [109]

ROBERT C. YOUNG, MD
President, Fox Chase Cancer Center, Philadelphia [97]

ALAN S.L. YU, MB, BChir
Assistant Professor of Medicine, Harvard Medical School; Associate Physician, Renal Division, Brigham and Women's Hospital, Boston [277]

VICTOR L. YU, MD
Professor of Medicine, University of Pittsburgh; Chief, Infectious Disease Section, VA Medical Center, Pittsburgh [151]

DORI F. ZALEZNIK, MD
Assistant Professor of Medicine, Harvard Medical School; Senior Physician, Beth Israel Deaconess Medical Center, Wellesley, Boston [130, 135, 145]

PETER ZIMETBAUM, MD
Instructor in Medicine, Harvard Medical School; Cardiovascular Division, Beth Israel Deaconess Medical Center, Boston [229, 230]

PHILIPPE E. ZIMMERN, MD
Associate Professor of Urology, The University of Texas Southwestern Medical School, Dallas [48]

PREFACE

The first edition of *Harrison's Principles of Internal Medicine* was published in the middle of the twentieth century, more than 50 years ago. In this fifteenth edition, the first of the new century, the text has undergone major revision to reflect further understanding of the biology and pathophysiology of disease and at the same time to retain those facts that, while not new, remain clinically useful and important. Virtually every chapter in this new edition has been completely or substantially rewritten, and a record 86 are new or have new authors. In this preface, we cannot describe all of these changes; however, we would like to call to the reader's attention those that are particularly noteworthy.

Part One, "Introduction to Clinical Medicine," contains new chapters dealing with decision making and cost awareness in clinical medicine. A growing number of patients are turning to alternative therapies, and these are discussed in a new chapter. New authors describe contemporary approaches to medical problems associated with pregnancy and the peripartum period. The chapters on medical ethics and on segments of the population that often present special problems—adolescents, women, and the elderly—have been revised and updated.

Part Two, "Cardinal Manifestations and Presentation of Disease," serves as a comprehensive introduction to clinical medicine, examining current concepts of the pathophysiology and differential diagnosis to be considered in patients with these manifestations. Major symptoms are reviewed and correlated with specific disease states, and clinical approaches to patients presenting with these symptoms are summarized. New chapters have been prepared on chest discomfort, headache, hypothermia, shock, and disorders of smell, taste, and hearing. A new chapter succinctly outlines a rational approach to the febrile patient presenting to the emergency department. The sections on alterations in gastrointestinal and sexual function are almost entirely new.

Given the explosive advances in human genetics, including the completion of a working draft of the sequence of the entire human genome and its growing relevance to clinical practice, Part Three, "Genetics and Disease," has been expanded and completely rewritten with new chapters on human genetics, chromosomal genetics, genetic defects, mitochondrial dysfunction, genetic screening and counseling, as well as gene therapy.

Part Four, "Clinical Pharmacology," provides a sound theoretical basis for pharmacotherapy, so critical to every aspect of medical practice.

Part Five, "Nutrition," has been extensively revised, with five new authors contributing chapters. This section covers nutritional considerations related to clinical medicine, including nutritional requirements, assessment of nutritional status, protein-energy malnutrition, and enteral and parenteral nutrition. It contains a new chapter on obesity, which incorporates the results of rapidly developing basic research in this important field.

The core of *Harrison's* encompasses the disorders of the organ systems and is contained in Parts Six through Fifteen. These sections include succinct accounts of the pathophysiology of the diseases involving the major organ systems and emphasize clinical manifestations, diagnostic procedures, differential diagnosis, and treatment strategies. The treatment sections of virtually every chapter have been amplified and updated. They are supplemented by the liberal use of algorithms, and are clearly highlighted. Guidelines for disease management prepared by specialty societies are included for the first time.

Part Six, "Oncology and Hematology," includes twelve chapters with new authors, including a new chapter by Judah Folkman on angiogenesis. In addition, a new chapter has been added on the medical problems that can arise in patients cured of cancer, including disease-related and treatment-related sequelae. The chapters on myeloid and lymphoid neoplasms include the new World Health Organization classification schemes. A conscientious effort has been made to provide specific, up-to-date treatment recommendations. Where appropriate, diagnostic and management algorithms have been incorporated.

Changes in Part Seven, "Infectious Diseases," include the latest information on the pathology, genetics, and epidemiology of infectious diseases while focusing sharply on the needs of clinicians who must accurately diagnose and treat infections in their patients. Specific recommendations are offered for therapeutic regimens, including the drug of choice, dose, duration, and alternatives. Current figures and trends in antimicrobial resistance are presented and considered in light of their impact on therapeutic choices. New authors cover the latest advances in the management of diseases such as infective endocarditis, meningococcal and gonococcal infections, and schistosomiasis. The overview of pathogenesis from earlier editions has been expanded to encompass viruses, fungi, and parasites as well as bacteria. The Atlas of Hematology includes a complete diagnostic set of spectacular color plates showing malaria-infected red blood cells.

In Part Eight, "Disorders of the Cardiovascular System," a new chapter on the prevention of atherosclerosis focuses not only on the importance of the traditional risk factors but also on the novel risk factors that influence plaque stability. Global risk assessment and management are described. Both primary and secondary prevention of atherosclerosis are discussed. Myocardial imaging by means of ultrasound or radionuclide techniques, at rest and during stress, plays an ever more critical role in assessment of patients with ischemic heart disease, and a new chapter focuses on the clinical use of these important technologies.

Despite major advances in its diagnosis and therapy, acute myocardial infarction remains the most common cause of death in industrialized nations. The chapter on acute myocardial infarction provides important new information on myocardial reperfusion therapy, thrombolysis, and primary coronary angioplasty and summarizes guidelines for acute coronary care and for risk stratification in the postinfarct patient. Unstable angina and congestive heart failure have emerged as two of the most common conditions leading to hospital admission in Western nations. Important advances in pathophysiology and therapy of these two very important conditions are included.

Enormous strides have been made in the use of lung transplantation for selected patients with end-stage, irreversible, pulmonary parenchymal and vascular disease, and Part Nine, "Disorders of the Respiratory System," provides a chapter that focuses on patient selection for this therapy. New chapters on interstitial and granulomatous lung diseases as well as on sleep apnea provide contemporary views of these conditions at the interface between basic science and clinical pulmonology.

In Part Ten, "Disorders of the Kidney and Urinary Tract," there has been considerable revision, with a new chapter on dialysis, incorporating the most recent advances.

In Part Eleven, "Disorders of the Gastrointestinal System," several new authors have contributed to the section on liver and biliary tract disease, and all chapters have been extensively revised. The section is pivoted by a new chapter on "Approach to the Patient with Liver Disease." Recent advances in the therapy of hepatitis B and C have been highlighted. New authors have contributed chapters on endoscopy, peptic ulcer disease, disorders of absorption, inflammatory bowel disease, and irritable bowel syndrome. Our new contributors include the leaders in gastroenterology and hepatology.

In Part Twelve, "Disorders of the Immune System, Connective Tissue, and Joints," the updating focuses on therapy. The chapter on

"Introduction to the Immune System" has been completely rewritten and provides a comprehensive review of the human immune system, using the modern designations of innate versus adaptive immunity. The chapter on HIV disease and AIDS is comprehensive and up-to-date and includes coverage of the natural history, epidemiology, and immunopathogenic mechanisms of HIV disease. In addition, the chapter contains both an organ system by organ system approach and a delineation of the major complications of HIV disease. The sections on therapy include a state-of-the-art discussion of the striking treatment advances of HIV infection with combinations of antiretroviral agents as well as the complications of such therapy.

Profound changes can be found in Part Thirteen, "Endocrinology and Metabolism." Many new authors have been recruited, and all chapters have been extensively revised under the direction of our new editor, Dr. J. Larry Jameson. Nine of these chapters are completely new, including those on the pituitary, thyroid, diabetes mellitus, and osteoporosis. These clinically demanding topics retain a traditional pathophysiologic approach that characterizes the field of endocrinology. In addition, new insights from genetics permeate this section, and the results of evidence-based medicine provide a firm foundation for medical decision making and treatment.

Part Fourteen, "Neurologic Disorders," has been thoroughly updated and expanded. The theme of genetics is emphasized throughout the section, and new chapters highlight the remarkable progress made during the "decade of the brain" in the 1990s that has elucidated the molecular basis of many neurologic and psychiatric diseases. One of the new chapters, written by 1997 Nobel Laureate Stanley B. Prusiner, summarizes the unique biology of prions and the clinical features of human prion disorders, including "mad cow disease."

The very latest information can be found on treatment of epilepsy, Parkinson's disease, and Alzheimer's disease. Coverage of immune-mediated disorders of the nervous system has been greatly expanded to include the many new insights into pathogenesis and treatment that have appeared since the fourteenth edition. The chapter on cerebrovascular diseases offers state-of-the-art information on prevention and treatment of stroke, the third leading killer in the developed world; this chapter is a mini-textbook of stroke and stroke therapy. Another feature of the fifteenth edition is a discussion of the acute neurologic disorders encountered in the setting of critical illness; this chapter should be of value to all physicians who care for hospitalized patients.

Throughout the book, there is an emphasis on the use of neuroimaging figures to illustrate the various disorders discussed. Harrison's exceptional collection of high-quality neuroimaging photographs sets a new standard for textbooks of medicine.

Finally, Part Fifteen, "Environmental and Occupational Hazards," has been expanded and reorganized.

In view of the requirements for continuing education for licensure and relicensure, as well as the emphasis on certification and recertification, a revision of the Pre-Test Self-Assessment and Review will again be published with this edition. It consists of several hundred questions based on Harrison's, along with answers and explanations for the answers. The Companion Handbook that was pioneered as a supplement to the eleventh edition of Harrison's has been updated and will appear shortly after the publication of this edition. A CD-ROM version of Harrison's has been available since the thirteenth edition. An expanded CD-ROM version of the fifteenth edition will be available and will be regularly updated. In 1998, Harrison's went online to provide a "living" textbook of internal medicine. In addition to providing full search capabilities of the text, Harrison's Online offers daily updating, reports of clinical trials, practice guidelines, and concise reviews of timely topics, as well as new references with links to MEDLINE abstracts.

The fifteenth edition of Harrison's welcomes a new editor, Dr. J. Larry Jameson, who has taken on principal responsibility for the sections on Nutrition, Genetics, Endocrinology, and Metabolism and whose impact on this edition is already clear. Dr. Kurt J. Isselbacher, Dr. Jean D. Wilson, and Dr. Joseph B. Martin have left the editorial group. Their enormous contributions to Harrison's are cited elsewhere. Special thanks go to Dr. Robert F. Schrier who has prepared biographies of Nobel Prize Laureates in Physiology or Medicine. These brief essays remind us how deeply our current knowledge and practice of medicine depends on seminal contributions to biomedical science and informs about the lives of some of the most outstanding contributors.

We wish to express our appreciation to our many associates and colleagues, who, as experts in their fields, have helped us with constructive criticism and helpful suggestions. We acknowledge especially the contributions of:

Donna Ambrosino, Peter Banks, Richard Blumberg, Douglas Brust, Myron Cohen, Jonathan Edlow, Christopher Fanta, Mary Gillam, Douglas Golenbach, Fred Gorelick, Charles Halsted, Lee Kaplan, Peter Kopp, Bruce Levy, Leo Liu, William Lowe, Lawrence Madoff, Josh Meeks, Mark Molitch, Chung Owyang, Eugene Pergament, Alice Pau, Gerald Pier, Peter Rice, Paul Sax, Tom Schnitzer, Julian Seifter, Anushua Sinha, Steven Weinberger, Michael Wessels, and Lee Wetzler.

This book could not have been edited without the dedicated help of our co-workers in the editorial offices of the individual editors. We are especially indebted to Scott Cromer, Pat Duffey, Sarah Anne Matero, Julie McCoy, Elizabeth Robbins, Kathryn Saxon, Marie Scurti, and Julieta Tayco.

Finally, we continue to be indebted to two outstanding members of the McGraw-Hill organization: Mariapaz Ramos Englis, Senior Managing Editor, and Martin J. Wonsiewicz, Publisher. They are an effective team who have given the editors constant encouragement and sage advice and have been of enormous help in bringing this edition to fruition in a timely manner.

The Editors

<table>
1 | *The Editors*
</table>

THE PRACTICE OF MEDICINE

WHAT IS EXPECTED OF THE PHYSICIAN The practice of medicine combines both science and art. The role of *science in medicine* is clear. Science-based technology and deductive reasoning form the foundation for the solution to many clinical problems; the spectacular advances in genetics, biochemistry, and imaging techniques allow access to the innermost parts of the cell and the most remote recesses of the body. Highly advanced therapeutic maneuvers are increasingly a major part of medical practice. Yet skill in the most sophisticated application of laboratory technology and in the use of the latest therapeutic modality alone does not make a good physician. One must be able to identify the crucial elements in a complex history and physical examination and extract the key laboratory results from the crowded computer printouts of laboratory data in order to determine in a difficult case whether to "treat" or to "watch." Deciding when a clinical clue is worth pursuing, or when it should be dismissed as a "red herring," and estimating in any given patient whether a proposed treatment entails a greater risk than the disease are essential to the decision-making process that the skilled clinician must exercise many times each day. This combination of medical knowledge, intuition, and judgment defines the *art of medicine*, which is as necessary to the practice of medicine as is a sound scientific base.

The editors of the first edition of this book articulated what is expected of the physician in words that, although they reflect the gender bias of that era, still ring true as a universal principle:

No greater opportunity, responsibility, or obligation can fall to the lot of a human being than to become a physician. In the care of the suffering he needs technical skill, scientific knowledge, and human understanding. He who uses these with courage, with humility, and with wisdom will provide a unique service for his fellow man, and will build an enduring edifice of character within himself. The physician should ask of his destiny no more than this; he should be content with no less.

Tact, sympathy and understanding are expected of the physician, for the patient is no mere collection of symptoms, signs, disordered functions, damaged organs, and disturbed emotions. He is human, fearful, and hopeful, seeking relief, help and reassurance.

THE PATIENT-PHYSICIAN RELATIONSHIP It may seem trite to emphasize that physicians need to approach patients not as "cases" or "diseases" but as individuals whose problems all too often transcend their physical complaints. Most patients are anxious and frightened. Physicians should instill confidence and reassurance, overtly and in their demeanor, but without an air of arrogance. A professional attitude, coupled with warmth and openness, can do much to alleviate the patients' anxiety and to encourage them to share parts of their history that may be embarrassing. Some patients "use" illness to gain attention or to serve as a crutch to extricate themselves from a stressful situation; some even feign physical illness; others may be openly hostile. Whatever the patient's attitude, the physician needs to consider the setting in which an illness occurs—in terms not only of the patients themselves but also of their families and social and cultural backgrounds. The ideal patient-physician relationship is based on thorough knowledge of the patient, on mutual trust, and on the ability to communicate with one another.

The direct, one-to-one patient-physician relationship, which has traditionally characterized the practice of medicine, is increasingly in jeopardy because of the increasing complexity of medicine and change in health care delivery systems. Often the management of the individual patient is a team effort involving a number of several different physicians and professional personnel. The patient can benefit greatly from such collaboration, but *it is the duty of the patient's principal physician to guide them through an illness*. To carry out this difficult task, this physician must be familiar with the techniques, skills, and objectives of specialist physicians and of colleagues in the fields allied to medicine. In giving the patient an opportunity to benefit from scientific advances, the primary physician must, in the last analysis, retain responsibility for the major decisions concerning diagnosis and treatment.

Patients are increasingly cared for by groups of physicians in clinics, hospitals, integrated health care delivery systems, and health maintenance organizations (HMOs). Whatever the potential advantages of such organized medical groups, there are also drawbacks, chiefly the loss of the clear identification of the physician who is primarily and continuously responsible for the patient. Even under these circumstances, it is essential for each patient to have a physician who has an overview of the problems and who is familiar with the patient's reaction to the illness, to the drugs given, and to the challenges that the patient faces.

The practice of medicine in a "managed care" setting puts additional stress on the classic paradigm of the patient-physician relationship. Many physicians must deal with a patient within a restricted time frame, with limited access to specialists, and under organizational guidelines that may compromise their ability to exercise their individual clinical judgment. As difficult as these restrictions may be, it is the ultimate responsibility of the physician to determine what is best for the patient. This responsibility cannot be relinquished in the name of compliance with organizational guidelines.

The physician must also bear in mind that the modern hospital constitutes an intimidating environment for most patients. Lying in a bed surrounded by air jets, buttons, and lights; invaded by tubes and wires; beset by the numerous members of the health care team—nurses, nurses' aides, physicians' assistants, social workers, technologists, physical therapists, medical students, house officers, attending and consulting physicians, and many others; sharing rooms with other patients who have their own problems, visitors, and physicians; transported to special laboratories and imaging facilities replete with blinking lights, strange sounds, and unfamiliar personnel—it is little wonder that patients may lose their sense of reality. In fact, the physician is often the only tenuous link between the patient and the real world, and a strong personal relationship with the physician helps to sustain the patient in such a stressful situation.

Many trends in contemporary society tend to make medical care impersonal. Some of these have been mentioned already and include (1) vigorous efforts to reduce the escalating costs of health care; (2) the growing number of managed care programs, which are intended to reduce costs but in which the patient may have little choice in selecting a physician; (3) increasing reliance on technologic advances and computerization for many aspects of diagnosis and treatment; (4) increased geographic mobility of both patients and physicians; (5) the need for numerous physicians to be involved in the care of most patients who are seriously ill; and (6) an increasing tendency on the part of patients to express their frustrations with the health care system by legal means (i.e., by malpractice litigation). Given these changes in the medical care system, it is a major challenge for physicians to maintain the *humane* aspects of medical care. The American Board of Internal Medicine has defined humanistic qualities as encompassing integrity, respect, and compassion. Availability, the expression of sincere concern, the willingness to take the time to explain all aspects of the illness, and a nonjudgmental attitude when dealing with patients whose cultures, lifestyles, attitudes, and values differ from those of the physician are just a few of the characteristics of the humane physician. Every physician will, at times, be challenged by patients who evoke strongly negative (or strongly positive) emotional responses. Physicians should be alert to their own reactions to such patients and situations and should consciously monitor and control their behavior so that the patients' best interests remain the principal motivation for their actions at all times.

An important aspect of patient care involves an appreciation of the "quality of life," a subjective assessment of what each patient values most. Such an assessment requires detailed, sometimes intimate knowledge of the patient, which can usually be obtained only through deliberate, unhurried, and often repeated conversations. It is in these situations that the time constraints of a managed care setting may prove problematic.

The famous statement of Dr. Francis Peabody is even more relevant today than when delivered more than three-quarters of a century ago:

The significance of the intimate personal relationship between physician and patient cannot be too strongly emphasized, for in an extraordinarily large number of cases both the diagnosis and treatment are directly dependent on it. One of the essential qualities of the clinician is interest in humanity, **for the secret of the care of the patient is in caring for the patient.**

CLINICAL SKILLS   History Taking   The written history of an illness should embody all the facts of medical significance in the life of the patient. Recent events should be given the most attention. The patient should, at some point, have the opportunity to tell his or her own story of the illness without frequent interruption and, when appropriate, receive expressions of interest, encouragement, and empathy from the physician. The physician must be alert to the possibility that any event related by the patient, however trivial or apparently remote, may be the key to the solution of the medical problem.

An informative history is more than an orderly listing of symptoms; something is always gained by listening to patients and noting the way in which they describe their symptoms. Inflections of voice, facial expression, gestures, and attitude may reveal important clues to the meaning of the symptoms to the patient. Taking history often involves much data gathering. Patients vary in their medical sophistication and ability to recall facts. Medical history should therefore be corroborated whenever possible. The family and social history can also provide important insights into the types of diseases that should be considered. In listening to the history, the physician discovers not only something about the disease but also something about the patient. The process of history taking provides an opportunity to observe the patient's behavior and to watch for features to be pursued more thoroughly during the physical examination.

The very act of eliciting the history provides the physician with the opportunity to establish or enhance the unique bond that is the basis for the ideal patient-physician relationship. It is helpful to develop an appreciation of the patient's perception of the illness, the patient's expectations of the physician and the medical care system, and the financial and social implications of the illness to the patient. The confidentiality of the patient-physician relationship should be emphasized, and the patient should be given the opportunity to identify any aspects of the history that should not be disclosed.

Physical Examination   Physical signs are objective indications of disease whose significance is enhanced when they confirm a functional or structural change already suggested by the patient's history. At times, however, the physical signs may be the only evidence of disease.

The physical examination should be performed methodically and thoroughly, with consideration for the patient's comfort and modesty. Although attention is often directed by the history to the diseased organ or part of the body, the examination of a new patient must extend from head to toe in an objective search for abnormalities. Unless the physical examination is systematic, important segments may be omitted. The results of the examination, like the details of the history, should be recorded at the time they are elicited, not hours later when they are subject to the distortions of memory. Skill in physical diagnosis is acquired with experience, but it is not merely technique that determines success in eliciting signs. The detection of a few scattered petechiae, a faint diastolic murmur, or a small mass in the abdomen is not a question of keener eyes and ears or more sensitive fingers but of a mind alert to these findings. Since physical findings are subject to changes, the physical examination should be repeated as frequently as the clinical situation warrants.

Laboratory Tests   The availability of a wide array of laboratory tests has increased our reliance on these studies for the solution of clinical problems. The accumulation of laboratory data does not relieve the physician from the responsibility of careful observation, examination, and study of the patient. It is also essential to bear in mind the limitations of such tests. By virtue of their impersonal quality, complexity, and apparent precision, they often gain an aura of authority regardless of the fallibility of the tests themselves, the instruments used in the tests, and the individuals performing or interpreting them. Physicians must weigh the expense involved in the laboratory procedures they order relative to the value of the information they are likely to provide.

Single laboratory tests are rarely ordered. Rather, they are generally obtained as "batteries" of multiple tests, which are often useful. For example, abnormalities of hepatic function may provide the clue to such nonspecific symptoms as generalized weakness and increased fatigability, suggesting the diagnosis of chronic liver disease. Sometimes a single abnormality, such as an elevated serum calcium level, points to particular diseases, such as hyperparathyroidism or underlying malignancy.

The thoughtful use of screening tests should not be confused with indiscriminate laboratory testing. The use of screening tests is based on the fact that a group of laboratory determinations can be carried out conveniently on a single specimen of blood at relatively low cost. Screening tests are most useful when they are directed towards common diseases or disorders in which the result directs other useful tests or interventions that would otherwise be costly to perform. Biochemical measurements, together with simple laboratory examinations such as blood count, urinalysis, and sedimentation rate, often provide the major clue to the presence of a pathologic process. At the same time, the physician must learn to evaluate occasional abnormalities among the screening tests that may not necessarily connote significant disease. An in-depth workup following a report of an isolated laboratory abnormality in a person who is otherwise well is almost invariably wasteful and unproductive. Among the more than 40 tests that are routinely performed on patients, one or two are often slightly abnormal. If there is no suspicion of an underlying illness, these tests are ordinarily repeated to ensure that the abnormality does not represent a laboratory error. If an abnormality is confirmed, it is important to consider its potential significance in the context of the patient's condition and other test results.

Imaging Techniques   The availability of ultrasonography, a variety of scans that employ isotopes to visualize organs heretofore inaccessible, computed tomography, and magnetic resonance imaging has opened new diagnostic vistas and has benefited patients because these new techniques have largely supplanted more invasive ones. While the enthusiasm for noninvasive technology is understandable, the expense entailed in performing these tests is often substantial and should be considered when assessing the potential benefits of the information provided.

PRINCIPLES OF PATIENT CARE   Medical Decision-Making   Both during and in particular after the physician has taken the history, performed the physical examination, and reviewed the laboratory and imaging data, the challenging process of the differential diagnosis and medical decision-making begins. Formulating a differential diagnosis requires not only a broad knowledge base but also the ability to assess the relative probabilities of various diseases and to understand the significance of missing diagnoses that may be less likely. Arriving at a diagnosis requires the application of the scientific method. Hypotheses are formed, data are collected, and objective conclusions are reached concerning whether to accept or reject a particular diagnosis. Analysis of the differential diagnosis is an iterative process. As new information or test results are acquired, the group of disease processes being considered can be contracted or expanded appropriately. Medical decision-making occurs throughout the diagnostic and treatment process. It involves the ordering of additional tests, requests for consults, and decisions regarding prognosis and treatment. This process requires an in-depth understanding of the natural history and pathophysiology of disease, explaining why these features are strongly emphasized in this textbook. As described below, medical decision-making should be evidence-based, thereby ensuring that patients derive the full benefit of the scientific knowledge available to physicians.

Evidence-Based Medicine Sackett has defined evidence-based medicine as "the conscientious, explicit and judicious use of current best evidence in making decisions about the care of individual patients." Rigorously obtained evidence is contrasted with anecdotal experience, which is often biased. Even the most experienced physicians can be influenced by recent experiences with selected patients, unless they are attuned to the importance of using larger, more objective studies for making decisions. The prospectively designed, double-blind, randomized clinical trial represents the "gold standard" for providing evidence regarding therapeutic decisions, but it is not the only source. Valuable evidence about the natural history of disease and prognosis can come from prospective cohort studies and analytic surveys. Persuasive evidence on the accuracy of diagnostic tests can be derived from cross-sectional studies of patients in whom a specific disorder is suspected. Evidence is strengthened immensely when it has been confirmed by multiple investigations, which can be compared with one another and presented in a meta-analysis or systemic overview.

In failing to apply the best and most current evidence, the physician places the patient at unnecessary risk. However, a knowledge of or rapid access to the best available evidence is not sufficient for optimal care. The physician must know whether the evidence is relevant to the patient in question and, when it is, the consequences of applying it in any particular situation. The skills and judgment required to apply sound evidence represent an increasing challenge. Indeed, one might redefine a "good doctor" as one who uses the ever-growing body of rigorously obtained evidence (the science of medicine) in a sensible, compassionate manner (the art of medicine).

While an understanding of biologic and physiologic mechanisms forms the basis of contemporary medicine, when a therapeutic modality is selected, the highest priority must often be placed on improving *clinical outcome* rather than interrupting what is believed to be the underlying process. For example, for decades patients who had suffered myocardial infarction were treated intuitively with drugs that suppress frequent ventricular extrasystoles, since these were believed to be harbingers of ventricular fibrillation and sudden death. Clinical trials, however, have provided firm evidence that the antiarrhythmic agents actually increase the risk of death in such patients. This finding suggests that the extrasystoles are *markers* of high risk rather than the *cause* of fatal events.

Practice Guidelines Physicians are faced with a large, increasing, and often bewildering body of evidence pointing to potentially useful diagnostic techniques and therapeutic choices. The intelligent and cost-effective practice of medicine consists of making selections most appropriate to a particular patient and clinical situation. Professional organizations and government agencies are developing formal clinical practice guidelines in an effort to aid physicians and other caregivers in this endeavor. When guidelines are current and properly applied, they can provide a useful framework for managing patients with particular diagnoses or symptoms. They can protect patients—

particularly those with inadequate health care benefits—from receiving substandard care. Guidelines can also protect conscientious caregivers from inappropriate charges of malpractice and society from the excessive costs associated with the overuse of medical resources. On the other hand, clinical guidelines tend to oversimplify the complexities of medicine. Different groups with differing perspectives may develop divergent recommendations regarding issues as basic as the need for periodic sigmoidoscopy in middle-aged persons. Furthermore, guidelines do not—and cannot be expected to—take into account the uniqueness of each individual and of his or her illness. The challenge for the physician is to integrate into clinical practice the useful recommendations offered by the experts who prepare clinical practice guidelines without accepting them blindly or being inappropriately constrained by them.

Assessing the Outcome of Treatment Clinicians generally use *objective* and readily measurable parameters to judge the outcome of a therapeutic intervention. For example, findings on physical or laboratory examination—such as the level of blood pressure, the patency of a coronary artery on an angiogram, or the size of a mass on a radiologic examination—can provide information of critical importance. However, patients usually seek medical attention for *subjective* reasons; they wish to obtain relief from pain, to preserve or regain function, and to enjoy life. The components of a patient's health status or quality of life can include bodily comfort, capacity for physical activity, personal and professional function, sexual function, cognitive function, and overall perception of health. Each of these important areas can be assessed by means of structured interviews or specially designed questionnaires. Such assessments also provide useful parameters by which the physician can judge the patient's subjective view of his or her disability and the response to treatment, particularly in chronic illness. The practice of medicine requires consideration and integration of both objective and subjective outcomes.

Care of the Elderly Over the next several decades, the practice of medicine will be greatly influenced by the health care needs of the growing elderly population. In the United States the population over age 65 will almost triple over the next 30 years. It is essential that we understand and appreciate the physiologic processes associated with aging; the different responses of the elderly to common diseases; and disorders that occur commonly with aging, such as depression, dementia, frailty, urinary incontinence, and fractures. The elderly have more adverse reactions to drugs, in large part due to altered pharmacokinetics and pharmacodynamics. Commonly used medications such as digoxin and aminoglycosides have prolonged half-lives in the elderly, and tissues such as the central nervous system are more sensitive to certain drugs, such as the benzodiazepines and narcotics. The large number of drugs used by the elderly increases the risk of unwanted interactions, especially when care is provided by several physicians in an uncoordinated manner.

Diseases in Women versus Men In the past, many epidemiologic studies and clinical trials focused on men. It is now appreciated that there are significant gender differences in diseases that afflict both men and women. Mortality rates are substantially higher in women than in men under the age of 50 suffering acute myocardial infarction. Hypertension is more prevalent in African-American women than in their male counterparts (and in African-American than in white males); osteoporosis is more common in women, reflecting the menopausal loss of estrogen; diseases involving the immune system, such as lupus erythematosus, multiple sclerosis, and primary biliary cirrhosis, occur more frequently in women; and the average life expectancy of women is greater than that of men. Recently, considerable attention has been paid to women's health issues, a subject that regrettably did not receive sufficient attention in the past. Ongoing study should enhance our understanding of the mechanisms of gender differences in the course and outcome of certain diseases.

Iatrogenic Disorders In an *iatrogenic disorder*, the deleterious effects of a therapeutic or diagnostic maneuver cause pathology independent of the condition for which the intervention was performed. Adverse drug reactions occur in at least 5% of hospitalized patients, and the incidence increases with use of a large number of drugs. No matter what the clinical situation, it is the responsibility of the physician to use powerful therapeutic measures wisely, with due regard for their beneficial action, potential dangers, and cost. Every medical procedure, whether diagnostic or therapeutic, has the potential for harm, but it would be impossible to provide the benefits of modern scientific medicine if reasonable steps in diagnosis and therapy were withheld because of possible risks. *Reasonable* implies that the physician has weighed the pros and cons of a procedure and has concluded, on the basis of objective evidence whenever possible, that it is necessary for establishing a diagnosis, for the relief of discomfort, or for the cure of disease. However, the harm that a physician can do is not limited to the imprudent use of medication or procedures. Equally important are ill-considered or unjustified remarks. Many a patient has developed a cardiac neurosis because the physician ventured a grave prognosis on the basis of a misinterpreted finding of a heart murmur. Not only the diagnostic procedure or the treatment but the physician's words and behavior are capable of causing injury.

Informed Consent   Patients often require diagnostic and therapeutic procedures that are painful and that pose some risk. For many such procedures, patients are required to sign a consent form. The patient must understand clearly the risks entailed in these procedures; this is the definition of *informed consent*. It is incumbent on the physician to explain the procedures in a clear and understandable manner and to ascertain that the patient comprehends both the nature of the procedure and the attendant risks. The dread of the unknown that is inherent in hospitalization can be mitigated by such explanations.

Incurability and Death   No problem is more distressing than that presented by the patient with an incurable disease, particularly when premature death is inevitable. What should the patient and family be told, what measures should be taken to maintain life, what can be done to maintain the quality of life, and how is death to be defined?

The concept of incurable illness and terminal care often evokes examples of cancer. However, patients with many other end-stage diseases including chronic obstructive pulmonary disease, congestive heart failure, renal or hepatic failure, and overwhelming infection face similar issues. The same principles of terminal care should be applied in each of these cases. Doing seemingly small things, focused on the needs of the patient, can do much to restore comfort or dignity during a person's final weeks or days. In the same way that pain should be attentively managed with analgesia, every effort should be made to alleviate shortness of breath and to provide good skin care.

Although some would argue otherwise, there is no ironclad rule that the patient must immediately be told "everything," even if the patient is an adult with substantial family responsibilities. How much is told should depend on the individual's ability to deal with the possibility of imminent death; often this capacity grows with time, and whenever possible, gradual rather than abrupt disclosure is the best strategy. A wise and insightful physician is often guided by an understanding of what a patient wants to know and when he or she wants to know it. The patient's religious beliefs may also be taken into consideration. The patient must be given an opportunity to talk with the physician and ask questions. Patients may find it easier to share their feelings about death with their physician, who is likely to be more objective and less emotional, than with family members. As William Osler wrote:

> One thing is certain; it is not for you to don the black cap and, assuming the judicial function, take hope away from any patient . . . hope that comes to us all.

Even when the patient directly inquires, "Am I dying?" the physician must attempt to determine whether this is a request for information or a demand for reassurance. Only open communication between the patient and the physician can resolve this question and guide the physician in what to say and how to say it.

The physician should provide or arrange for emotional, physical, and spiritual support and must be compassionate, unhurried, and open. There is much to be gained by the laying on of hands. Pain should be adequately controlled, human dignity maintained, and isolation from the family avoided. These aspects of care tend to be overlooked in hospitals, where the intrusion of life-sustaining apparatus can so easily detract from attention to the whole person and encourage concentration instead on the life-threatening disease, against which the battle will ultimately be lost in any case. In the face of terminal illness, the goal of medicine must shift from *cure* to *care*, in the broadest sense of the term. In offering care to the dying patient, the physician must be prepared to provide information to family members and to deal with their guilt and grief. It is important for the doctor to assure the family that everything possible has been done.

"Do Not Resuscitate" Orders and Cessation of Therapy When carried out in a timely and expert manner, cardiopulmonary resuscitation is often useful in the prevention of sudden, unexpected death. However, unless there are reasons to the contrary, this procedure should not be used merely to prolong the life of a patient with terminal, incurable disease. The decision whether or not to resuscitate or even to treat an incurably and terminally ill patient must be reviewed frequently and must take into consideration any unexpected changes in the patient's condition. In this context, the administration of fluids or food is considered therapy that may be withdrawn or withheld. These decisions must also take into account both the underlying medical condition, especially its reversibility, and the wishes of the patient, especially if these have been expressed in a living will or advance directive. If the patient's wishes cannot be ascertained directly, a close relative or another surrogate who can be relied on to transmit the patient's wishes and to be guided by the patient's best interests should be consulted. The patient's autonomy—whether the choice is to continue or discontinue treatment or to be resuscitated or not in the event of a cardiopulmonary arrest—must be paramount. The courts have ruled that competent patients may refuse therapy and that an incompetent patient's previously stated wishes regarding life support should therefore be respected. The issues involving death and dying are among the most difficult in medicine. In approaching them rationally and consistently, the physician must combine both the science and the art of medicine.

THE EXPANDING ROLE OF THE PHYSICIAN   Genetics and Medicine   The genomic era is likely to lead to a revolution in the practice of medicine. Obtaining the DNA sequence of the entire human genome may help to elucidate the genetic components of common chronic diseases—hypertension, diabetes, atherosclerosis, many cancers, dementias, and behavioral and autoimmune disorders. This information should make it possible to determine individual susceptibility to these conditions early in life and to implement individualized prevention programs. Subclassification of many diseases on a genetic basis may allow the selection of appropriate therapy for each patient. As the response to drugs becomes more predictable, pharmacotherapy should become more rational. In short, the completion of the Human Genome Project is likely to lead to a substantial increase in physicians' ability to influence their patient's health and well-being.

Patients will be best served if physicians play an active role in applying this powerful, sensitive new information rather than being passive bystanders who are intimidated by the new technology. This is a rapidly evolving field, and physicians and other health care professionals must remain updated to apply this new knowledge. Genetic testing requires wise counsel based on an understanding of the value and limitations of the tests as well as the implications of their results for specific individuals.

Medicine on the Internet   The explosion in use of the Internet through personal computers is having an important impact on many practicing physicians. The Internet makes a wide range of information available to physicians almost instantaneously at any time of the day or night and from anywhere in the world. This medium holds enormous potential for delivering up-to-date information, practice guidelines, state-of-the-art conferences, journal contents, textbooks (including this text), and direct communications with other physicians and specialists, thereby expanding the depth and breadth of information available to the physician about the diagnosis and care of patients. Most medical journals are now accessible on-line, providing rapid and comprehensive sources of information. Patients, too, are turning to the Internet in increasing numbers to derive information about their illnesses and therapies and to join Internet-based support groups. Physicians are increasingly challenged by dealing with patients who are becoming more sophisticated in their understanding of illness. At this time, there is one critically important caveat. Virtually anything can be published on the Internet, thus circumventing the peer-review process that is an essential feature of quality publications. Physicians or patients who search the Internet for medical information must be aware of this danger. Notwithstanding this limitation, appropriate use of the Internet is revolutionizing information access for physicians and is a positive force in the practice of medicine.

Delivering Cost-Effective Medical Care As the cost of medical care has risen, it has become necessary to establish priorities in the expenditure of resources. In some instances, preventive measures offer the greatest return for the expenditure; outstanding examples include vaccination, improved sanitation, reduction in accidents and occupational hazards, and biochemical- and DNA-based screening of newborns. For example, the detection of phenylketonuria by newborn screening may result in a net saving of many thousands of dollars.

As resources become increasingly constrained, the physician must weigh the possible benefits of performing costly procedures that provide only a limited life expectancy against the pressing need for more primary care for those persons who do not have adequate access to medical services. For the individual patient, it is important to reduce costly hospital admissions as much as possible if total health care is to be provided at a cost that most can afford. This policy, of course, implies and depends on close cooperation among patients, their physicians, employers, payers, and government. It is equally important for physicians to know the cost of the diagnostic procedures they order and the drugs and other therapies they prescribe and to monitor both costs and effectiveness. The medical profession should provide leadership and guidance to the public in matters of cost control, and physicians must take this responsibility seriously without being or seeming to be self-serving. However, the economic aspects of health care delivery must not interfere with the welfare of patients. The patient must be able to rely on the individual physician as his or her principal advocate in matters of health care.

Accountability Medicine is a satisfying but demanding profession. Physicians must understand the characteristics of the populations they serve, and they must appreciate their patients' social and cultural attitudes to health, disease, and death. As the public has become more educated and more sophisticated regarding health matters, their expectations of the health system in general and of their physicians in particular have risen. Physicians are expected to maintain mastery of their rapidly advancing fields (the *science* of medicine) while considering their patient's unique needs (the *art* of medicine). Thus, physicians are held accountable not only for the technical aspects of the care that they provide but also for their patient's satisfaction with the delivery and costs of care.

In the United States, there are increasing demands for physicians to account for the way in which they practice medicine by meeting certain standards prescribed by federal and state governments. The hospitalization of patients whose health care costs are reimbursed by the government and other third parties is subjected to utilization review. Thus the physician must defend the cause for and duration of a patient's hospitalization if it falls outside certain "average" standards. Authorization for reimbursement is increasingly based on documentation of the nature and complexity of an illness, as reflected by recorded elements of the history and physical examination. The purpose of these regulations is both to improve standards of health care and to contain spiraling health care costs. This type of review is being extended to all phases of medical practice and is profoundly altering the practice of medicine. Physicians are also expected to give evidence of

their continuing competence through mandatory continuing education, patient-record audits, recertification by examination, or relicensing.

Continued Learning The conscientious physician must be a perpetual student because the body of medical knowledge is constantly expanding and being refined. The profession of medicine should be inherently linked to a career-long thirst for new knowledge that can be used for the good of the patient. It is the responsibility of a physician to pursue continually the acquisition of new knowledge by reading, attending conferences and courses, and consulting colleagues and the Internet. This is often a difficult task for a busy practitioner; however, such a commitment to continued learning is an integral part of being a physician and must be given the highest priority.

Research and Teaching The title *doctor* is derived from the Latin *docere*, "to teach," and physicians should share information and medical knowledge with colleagues, with students of medicine and related professions, and with their patients. The practice of medicine is dependent on the sum total of medical knowledge, which in turn is based on an unending chain of scientific discovery, clinical observation, analysis, and interpretation. Advances in medicine depend on the acquisition of new information, i.e., on research, which often involves patients; improved medical care requires the transmission of this information. As part of broader societal responsibilities, the physician should encourage patients to participate in ethical and properly approved clinical investigations if they do not impose undue hazard, discomfort, or inconvenience. To quote Osler once more:

To wrest from nature the secrets which have perplexed philosophers in all ages, to track to their sources the causes of disease, to correlate the vast stores of knowledge, that they may be quickly available for the prevention and cure of disease—these are our ambitions.

BIBLIOGRAPHY

COLLINS FS: Shattuck Lecture: Medical and Societal Consequences of the Human Genome Project. N Engl J Med 341:28, 1999

COUNCIL ON GRADUATE MEDICAL EDUCATION: *Thirteenth Report: Physician Education for a Changing Health Care Environment*. US Department of Health and Human Services, March 1999

SACKETT DL et al: *Evidence Based Medicine: How to Practise and Teach EBM*. London. Churchill Livingstone, 1997

TAUBES G: Looking for the evidence in medicine. Science 272:22, 1996

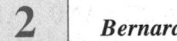

| **2** | *Bernard Lo* |

ETHICAL ISSUES IN CLINICAL MEDICINE

Physicians frequently confront ethical issues in clinical practice that are perplexing, time-consuming, and emotionally draining. Experience, common sense, and simply being a good person do not guarantee that physicians can identify or resolve ethical dilemmas. Knowledge about common ethical dilemmas is also essential.

FUNDAMENTAL ETHICAL GUIDELINES

Physicians should follow two fundamental but frequently conflicting ethical guidelines: respecting patient autonomy and acting in the patient's best interests.

RESPECTING PATIENT AUTONOMY Competent, informed patients may refuse recommended interventions and choose among reasonable alternatives.

Informed Consent Informed consent requires physicians to discuss with patients the nature of the proposed care, the alternatives, the risks and benefits of each, the likely consequences, and to obtain the patient's agreement to care. Informed consent involves more than obtaining signatures on consent forms. Physicians need to educate patients, answer questions, make recommendations, and help them deliberate. Patients can be overwhelmed with medical jargon, needlessly complicated explanations, or too much information at once.

Nondisclosure of Information Physicians may consider withholding a serious diagnosis, misrepresenting it, or limiting discussions of prognosis or risks because they fear that a patient will develop severe anxiety or depression or refuse needed care. Patients should not be forced to receive information against their will. Most people, however, want to know their diagnosis and prognosis, even if they are terminally ill. Generally, physicians should provide relevant information, offer empathy and hope, and help patients cope with bad news.

Emergency Care Informed consent is not required when patients cannot give consent and when delay of treatment would place their life or health in peril. People are presumed to want such emergency care, unless they have previously indicated otherwise.

Futile Interventions Autonomy does not entitle patients to insist on whatever care they want. Physicians are not obligated to provide futile interventions that have no physiologic rationale or have already failed. For example, cardiopulmonary resuscitation would be futile in a patient with progressive hypotension despite maximal therapy. But physicians should be wary of using the term "futile" in looser senses to justify unilateral decisions to forego interventions when they believe that the probability of success is too low, no worthwhile goals can be achieved, the patient's quality of life is unacceptable, or the costs are too high. Such looser usages of the term are problematic because they may be inconsistent and mask value judgments.

ACTING IN THE BEST INTERESTS OF PATIENTS The guideline of *beneficence* requires physicians to act for the patient's benefit. Laypeople do not possess medical expertise and may be vulnerable because of their illness. They justifiably rely on physicians to provide sound advice and to promote their well-being. Physicians encourage such trust. Hence, physicians have a fiduciary duty to act in the best interests of their patients. The interests of the patient should prevail over physicians' self-interest or the interests of third parties, such as hospitals or insurers. These fiduciary obligations of physicians contrast sharply with business relationships, which are characterized by "let the buyer beware," not by trust and reliance. The guideline of "*do no harm*" forbids physicians from providing ineffective interventions or acting without due care. This precept, while often cited, provides only limited guidance, because many beneficial interventions also have serious risks.

CONFLICTS BETWEEN BENEFICENCE AND AUTONOMY Patients' refusals of care may thwart their own goals or cause them serious harm. For example, a young man with asthma may refuse mechanical ventilation for reversible respiratory failure. Simply to accept such refusals, in the name of respecting autonomy, seems morally constricted. Physicians can elicit patients' expectations and concerns, correct misunderstandings, and try to persuade them to accept beneficial therapies. If disagreements persist after discussions, the patient's informed choices and view of his or her best interests should prevail. While refusing recommended care does not render a patient incompetent, it may lead the physician to probe further to ensure that the patient is able to make informed decisions.

PATIENTS WHO LACK DECISION-MAKING CAPACITY

Patients may not be able to make informed decisions because of unconsciousness, dementia, delirium, or other conditions. Physicians should ask two questions regarding such patients: Who is the appropriate surrogate? What would the patient want done?

ASSESSING CAPACITY TO MAKE MEDICAL DECISIONS All adults are considered legally competent unless declared incompetent by a court. In practice, physicians usually determine that patients lack the capacity to make health care decisions and arrange for surrogates to make them, without involving the courts. By definition, competent patients can express a choice and appreciate the medical situation, the nature of the proposed care, the alternatives, and the risks, benefits, and consequences of each. Their choices should be consistent with their values and should not result from delusions or hallucinations. Psychiatrists may help in difficult cases because they are skilled at interviewing mentally impaired patients and can identify treatable depression or psychosis. When impairments are fluctuating or reversible, decisions should be postponed if possible until the patient recovers decision-making capacity.

CHOICE OF SURROGATE If a patient lacks decision-making capacity, physicians routinely ask family members to serve as surrogates. Most patients want their family members to be surrogates, and family members generally know the patient's preferences and have the patient's best interests at heart. Patients may designate a particular individual to serve as proxy; such choices should be respected. Some states have established a prioritized list of which relative may serve as surrogate if the patient has not designated a proxy.

STANDARDS FOR SURROGATE DECISION MAKING **Advance Directives** These are statements by competent patients to direct care if they lose decision-making capacity. They may indicate (1) what interventions they would refuse or accept or (2) who should serve as surrogate. Following the patient's advance directives, surrogate respects patients' autonomy.

Oral conversations are the most frequent form of advance directives. While such conversations are customarily followed in clinical practice, casual or vague comments may not be trustworthy.

Living wills direct physicians to forego or provide life-sustaining interventions if the patient develops a terminal condition or persistent vegetative state. Generally patients may refuse only interventions that "merely prolong the process of dying."

A health care proxy is someone appointed by the patient to make health care decisions if he or she loses decision-making capacity. It is more flexible and comprehensive than the living will, applying whenever the patient is unable to make decisions.

Physicians can encourage patients to provide advance directives, to indicate both what they would want and who should be surrogate, and to discuss their preferences with surrogates. In discussions with patients, physicians can ensure that advance directives are informed, up-to-date, and address likely clinical scenarios. Such discussions are best carried out in the ambulatory setting. The federal Patient Self-Determination Act requires hospitals and health maintenance organizations to inform patients of their right to make health care decisions and to provide advance directives.

Substituted Judgment In the absence of clear advance directives, surrogates and physicians should try to decide as the patient would under the circumstances, using all information that they know about the patient. While such substituted judgments try to respect the patient's values, they may be speculative or inaccurate. A surrogate may be mistaken about the patient's preferences, particularly when they have not been discussed explicitly.

Best Interests When the patient's preferences are unclear or unknown, decisions should be based on the patient's best interests. Patients generally take into account the quality of life as well as the duration of life when making decisions for themselves. It is understandable that surrogates would also consider quality of life of patients who lack decision-making capacity. Judgments about quality of life are appropriate if they reflect the patient's own values. Bias or discrimination may occur, however, if others project their values onto the patient or weigh the perceived social worth of the patient. Most patients with chronic illness rate their quality of life higher than their family members and physicians do.

Legal Issues Physicians need to know pertinent state laws regarding patients who lack decision-making capacity. A few state courts allow doctors to forego life-sustaining interventions only if patients have provided written advance directives or very specific oral ones.

Disagreements Disagreements may occur among potential surrogates or between the physician and surrogate. Physicians can remind everyone to base decisions on what the patient would want, not what they would want for themselves. Consultation with the hospital ethics committee or with another physician often helps resolve disputes. Such consultation is also helpful when patients have no surrogate and no advance directives. The courts should be used only as a last resort when disagreements cannot be resolved in the clinical setting.

DECISIONS ABOUT LIFE-SUSTAINING INTERVENTIONS

Although medical technology can save lives, it can also prolong the process of dying. Competent, informed patients may refuse life-sustaining interventions. Such interventions may also be withheld from patients who lack decision-making capacity on the basis of advance directives or decisions by appropriate surrogates. Courts have ruled that foregoing life-sustaining interventions is neither suicide nor murder.

MISLEADING DISTINCTIONS People commonly draw distinctions that are intuitively plausible but prove untenable on closer analysis.

Extraordinary and Ordinary Care Some physicians are willing to forego "extraordinary" or "heroic" interventions, such as surgery, mechanical ventilation, or renal dialysis, but insist on providing "ordinary" ones, such as antibiotics, intravenous fluids, or feeding tubes. However, this distinction is not logical because all medical interventions have both risks and benefits. Any intervention may be withheld, if the burdens for the individual patient outweigh the benefits.

Withdrawing and Withholding Interventions Many health care providers find it more difficult to discontinue interventions than to withhold them in the first place. Although such emotions need to be acknowledged, there is no logical distinction between the two acts. Justifications for withholding interventions, such as refusal by patients or surrogates, are also justifications for withdrawing them. In addition, an intervention may prove unsuccessful or new information about the patient's preferences or condition may become available after the intervention is started. If interventions could not be discontinued, patients and surrogates might not even attempt treatments that might prove beneficial.

DO NOT RESUSCITATE (DNR) ORDERS When a patient suffers a cardiopulmonary arrest, cardiopulmonary resuscitation (CPR) is initiated unless a DNR order has been made. Although CPR can restore people to vigorous health, it can also disrupt a peaceful death. After CPR is attempted on a general hospital service, only 14% of patients survive to discharge, and even fewer in certain subgroups. DNR orders are appropriate if the patient or surrogate requests them or if CPR would be futile. To prevent misunderstandings, physicians should write DNR orders and the reasons for them in the medical record. "Slow" or "show" codes that merely appear to provide CPR are deceptive and therefore unacceptable. Although a DNR order signifies only that CPR will be withheld, the reasons that justify DNR orders may lead to a reconsideration of other plans for care.

ASSISTED SUICIDE AND ACTIVE EUTHANASIA Proponents of these controversial acts believe that competent, terminally ill patients should have control over the end of life and that physicians should relieve refractory suffering. Opponents assert that such actions violate the sanctity of life, that suffering can generally be relieved, that abuses are inevitable, and that such actions are outside the physician's proper role. These actions are illegal throughout the United States, except that physician-assisted suicide is legal in Oregon under certain circumstances. Whatever their personal views, physicians should respond to patients' inquiries with compassion and concern. Physicians should elicit and address any underlying problems, such as physical symptoms, loss of control, or depression. Often, additional efforts to relieve distress are successful, and after this is done patients generally withdraw their requests for these acts.

CARE OF DYING PATIENTS Patients often suffer unrelieved pain and other symptoms during their final days of life. Physicians may hesitate to order high doses of narcotics and sedatives, fearing they will hasten death. Relieving pain in terminal illness and alleviating dyspnea when patients forego mechanical ventilation enhances patient comfort and dignity. If lower doses of narcotics and sedatives have failed to relieve suffering, increasing the dose to levels that may suppress respiratory drive is ethically appropriate because the physician's intention is to relieve suffering, not hasten death. Physicians can also relieve suffering by spending time with dying patients, listening to them, and attending to their psychological distress.

CONFLICTS OF INTEREST

Acting in the patient's best interests may conflict with the physician's self-interest or the interests of third parties such as insurers or hospitals. The ethical ideal is to keep the patient's interests paramount. Even the appearance of a conflict of interest may undermine trust in the profession.

FINANCIAL INCENTIVES In managed care systems, physicians may serve as gatekeepers or bear financial risk for expenditures. Although such incentives are intended to reduce inefficiency and waste, there is concern that physicians may withhold beneficial care in order to control costs. In contrast, physicians have incentives to provide more care than indicated when they receive fee-for-service reimbursement or when they refer patients to medical facilities in which they have invested. Regardless of financial incentives, physicians should recommend available care that is in the patient's best interests—no more and no less.

DENIALS OF COVERAGE Utilization review programs designed to reduce unnecessary services may also deny coverage for care that the physician believes will benefit the patient. Physicians should inform patients when a plan is not covering standard care and act as patient advocates by appealing such denials of coverage. Patients may ask physicians to misrepresent their condition to help them obtain insurance coverage or disability. While physicians understandably want to help patients, such misrepresentation undermines physicians' credibility and violates their integrity.

GIFTS FROM PHARMACEUTICAL COMPANIES Physicians may be offered gifts ranging from pens and notepads to lavish entertainment. Critics worry that any gift from drug companies may impair objectivity, increase the cost of health care, and give the appearance of conflict of interest. A helpful rule of thumb is to consider whether patients would approve if they knew physicians had accepted such gifts.

OCCUPATIONAL RISKS Some health care workers, fearing fatal occupational infections, refuse to care for persons with HIV infection or multidrug-resistant tuberculosis. Such fears about personal safety need to be acknowledged, and institutions should reduce occupational risk by providing proper training, equipment, and supervision. Physicians should provide appropriate care within their clinical expertise, despite personal risk.

MISTAKES Mistakes are inevitable in clinical medicine. They may cause serious harm to patients or result in substantial changes in management. Physicians and students may fear that disclosing such mistakes could damage their careers. Without disclosure, however, patients cannot understand their clinical situation or make informed choices about subsequent care. Similarly, unless attending physicians are informed of trainees' mistakes, they cannot provide optimal care and help trainees learn from mistakes.

LEARNING CLINICAL SKILLS Learning clinical medicine, particularly learning to perform invasive procedures, may present inconvenience or risk to patients. To ensure patient cooperation, students may be introduced as physicians, or patients may not be told that trainees will be performing procedures. Such misrepresentation undermines trust, may lead to more elaborate deception, and makes it difficult for patients to make informed choices about their care. Patients should be told who is providing care, what benefits and burdens can be attributed to trainees, and how trainees are supervised. Most patients, when informed, allow trainees to play an active role in their care.

IMPAIRED PHYSICIANS   Physicians may hesitate to intervene when colleagues impaired by alcohol abuse, drug abuse, or psychiatric or medical illness place patients at risk. However, society relies on physicians to regulate themselves. If colleagues of an impaired physician do not take steps to protect patients, no one else may be in a position to do so.

CONFLICTS FOR TRAINEES   Medical students and residents may fear that they will receive poor grades or evaluations if they act on the patient's behalf by disclosing mistakes, avoiding misrepresentation of their role, and reporting impaired colleagues. Discussing such dilemmas with more senior physicians can help trainees check their interpretation of the situation and obtain advice and assistance.

ADDITIONAL ETHICAL ISSUES

MAINTAINING CONFIDENTIALITY   Maintaining the confidentiality of medical information respects patients' autonomy and privacy, encourages them to seek treatment and to discuss their problems candidly, and prevents discrimination. Physicians need to guard against inadvertent breaches of confidentiality, as when talking about patients in elevators. Maintaining confidentiality is not an absolute rule. The law may require physicians to override confidentiality in order to protect third parties, for example, reporting to government officials persons with specified infectious conditions, such as tuberculosis and syphilis; persons with gunshot wounds; and victims of elder abuse and domestic violence. Computerized medical records raise additional concerns because breaches of confidentiality may affect many patients.

ALLOCATING RESOURCES JUSTLY   Allocation of limited health care resources is problematic. Ideally, allocation decisions should be made as public policy, with physician input. At the bedside, physicians generally should act as patient advocates within constraints set by society, reasonable insurance coverage, and sound practice. *Ad hoc* rationing by the individual physician at the bedside may be inconsistent, discriminatory, and ineffective. In some cases, however, two patients may compete for the same limited resources, such as physician time or a bed in intensive care. When this occurs, physicians should ration their time and resources according to patients' medical needs and the probability of benefit.

ASSISTANCE WITH ETHICAL ISSUES   Discussing perplexing ethical issues with other members of the health care team, colleagues, or the hospital ethics committee often clarifies issues and suggests ways to improve communication and to deal with strong emotions. When struggling with difficult ethical issues, physicians may need to reevaluate their basic convictions, tolerate uncertainty, and maintain their integrity while respecting the opinions of others.

BIBLIOGRAPHY

ALPERS A, LO B: When is CPR futile? JAMA 273:156, 1995

AMERICAN COLLEGE OF PHYSICIANS: *American College of Physicians Ethics Manual.* Ann Intern Med, 128:576, 1998

BEAUCHAMP TL, CHILDRESS JF: *Principles of Biomedical Ethics*, 5th ed. New York, Oxford University Press, 2000

EMANUEL EJ et al: The practice of euthanasia and physician-assisted suicide in the United States: Adherence to proposed safeguards and effects on physicians. JAMA 280:507, 1998

GRISSO T, APPELBAUM P: *Assessing Competence to Consent to Treatment: A Guide for Physicians and Other Health Professionals.* New York, Oxford University Press, 1998

KASSIRER JP: Managed care and the morality of the marketplace. N Engl J Med 333:50, 1995

LO B: *Resolving Ethical Dilemmas: A Guide for Clinicians*, 2d ed. Philadelphia, Lippincott Williams & Wilkins, 2000

MEISEL A: *The Right to Die*, 2d ed. New York, Wiley, 1995

QUILL TE et al: Palliative options of last resort: A comparison of voluntarily stopping eating and drinking, terminal sedation, physician-assisted suicide, and voluntary active euthanasia. JAMA 278:2099, 1997

TULSKY JA et al: Opening the black box: How do physicians communicate about advance directives. Ann Intern Med 129:441, 1998

3   *Daniel B. Mark*

DECISION-MAKING IN CLINICAL MEDICINE

To the medical student who requires 2 h to collect a patient's history and perform a physical examination, and several additional hours to organize them into a coherent presentation, the experienced clinician's ability to reach a diagnosis and decide on a management plan in a fraction of the time seems extraordinary. While medical knowledge and experience play a significant role in the senior clinician's ability to arrive at a differential diagnosis and plan quickly, much of the process involves skill in clinical decision-making. The first goal of this chapter is to provide an introduction to the study of clinical reasoning.

Equally bewildering to the student are the proper use of diagnostic tests and the integration of the results into the clinical assessment. The novice medical practitioner typically uses a "shotgun" approach to testing, hoping to a hit a target without knowing exactly what that target is. The expert, on the other hand, usually has a specific target in mind and efficiently adjusts the testing strategy to it. The second goal of this chapter is to review briefly some of the crucial basic statistical concepts that govern the proper interpretation and use of diagnostic tests; quantitative tools available to assist in clinical decision-making will also be discussed.

CLINICAL DECISION-MAKING

CLINICAL REASONING   The most important clinical actions are not procedures or prescriptions but the judgments from which all other aspects of clinical medicine flow. In the modern era of large randomized trials, it is easy to overlook the importance of this elusive mental activity and focus instead on the algorithmic practice guidelines constructed to improve care. One reason for this apparent neglect is that much more research has been done on how doctors *should* make decisions (e.g., using a Bayesian model discussed below) than on how they actually *do*. Thus, much of what we know about clinical reasoning comes from empirical studies of nonmedical problem-solving behavior.

Despite the great technological advances of the twentieth century, uncertainty still plays a pivotal role in all aspects of medical decision-making. We may know that a patient does not have long to live, but we cannot be certain how long. We may prescribe a potent new receptor blocker to reverse the course of a patient's illness, but we cannot be certain that the therapy will do so without side effects. Uncertainty in medical outcomes creates the need for probabilities and other mathematical/statistical tools to help guide decision-making. (These tools are reviewed later in the chapter.)

Uncertainty is compounded by the information overload that characterizes modern medicine. Today's experienced clinician needs close to 2 million pieces of information to practice medicine. Doctors subscribe to an average of 7 journals, representing over 2500 new articles each year. Computers offer the obvious solution both for management of information and for better quantitation and management of the daily uncertainties of medical care. While the technology to computerize medical practice is available, many practical problems remain to be solved before patient information can be standardized and integrated with medical evidence on a single electronic platform.

The following three examples introduce the subject of clinical reasoning:

- A 46-year-old man presents to his internist with a chief complaint of hemoptysis. The physician knows that the differential diagnosis of hemoptysis includes over 100 different conditions, including cancer and tuberculosis (Chap. 33). The examination begins with some general background questions, and the patient is asked to describe his symptoms and their chronology. By the time the examination is completed, and even before any tests are run, the physician has formulated a working diagnostic hypothesis and planned a series of steps to test it. In an otherwise healthy and nonsmoking patient recovering from a viral bronchitis, the doctor's hypothesis would be that the acute bronchitis is responsible for the small amount of blood-streaked sputum the patient observed. In this case, a chest x-ray and purified protein derivative (PPD) skin test may be sufficient.
- A second 46-year-old patient with the same chief complaint who has a 100-pack-year smoking history, a productive morning cough, and episodes of blood-streaked sputum may generate the principal diagnostic hypothesis of carcinoma of the lung. Consequently, along with the chest x-ray and PPD skin test, the physician refers this patient for bronchoscopy.
- A third 46-year-old patient with hemoptysis who is from a developing country is evaluated with an echocardiogram as well, because the physician thinks she hears a soft diastolic rumble at the apex on cardiac auscultation, suggesting rheumatic mitral stenosis.

These three vignettes illustrate two aspects of expert clinical reasoning: (1) the use of cognitive shortcuts, or *heuristics*, as a way to organize the complex unstructured material that is collected in the clinical evaluation; and (2) the use of diagnostic hypotheses to consolidate the information and indicate appropriate management steps.

THE USE OF COGNITIVE SHORTCUTS Heuristics reduce the complexity of a problem to a manageable level. Psychologists have found that people rely on three basic types of heuristics. For example, when assessing a patient, clinicians often weigh the probability that this patient's clinical features match those of the class of patients with the leading diagnostic hypotheses being considered. In other words, the clinician is searching for the diagnosis for which the patient appears to be a representative example; this cognitive shortcut is called the *representativeness heuristic*. It may take only a few characteristics from the history for an expert clinician using the representativeness heuristic to arrive at a sound diagnostic hypothesis. For example, an elderly patient with new-onset fever, cough productive of copious sputum, unilateral pleuritic chest pain, and dyspnea is readily identified as fitting the pattern for acute pneumonia, probably of bacterial origin. Evidence of focal pulmonary consolidation on the physical examination will increase the clinician's confidence in the diagnosis because it fits the expected pattern of acute bacterial pneumonia. Knowing this allows the experienced clinician to conduct an efficient, directed, and therapeutically productive patient evaluation although there may be little else in the history or physical examination of direct relevance. The inexperienced medical student or resident, who has not yet learned the patterns most prevalent in clinical medicine, must work much harder to achieve the same result and is often at risk of missing the important clinical problem in a sea of compulsively collected but unhelpful data.

However, physicians using the representativeness heuristic can reach erroneous conclusions if they fail to consider the underlying prevalence of two competing diagnoses. Consider a patient with pleuritic chest pain, dyspnea, and a low-grade fever. A clinician might consider acute pneumonia and acute pulmonary embolism to be the two leading diagnostic alternatives. Clinicians using the representativeness heuristic might judge both diagnostic candidates to be equally likely, although to do so would be wrong if pneumonia was much more prevalent in the underlying population. Mistakes may also result from a failure to consider that a pattern based on a small number of prior observations will likely be less reliable than one based on larger samples.

A second commonly used cognitive shortcut, the *availability heuristic*, involves judgments made on the basis of how easily prior similar cases or outcomes can be brought to mind. For example, the experienced clinician may recall 20 elderly patients seen over the past few years who presented with painless dyspnea of acute onset and were found to have acute myocardial infarction. The novice clinician may spend valuable time seeking a pulmonary cause for the symptoms before considering and discovering the cardiac diagnosis. In this situation, the patient's clinical pattern does not fit the expected pattern of acute myocardial infarction, but experience with this atypical presentation, and the ability to recall it, can help direct the physician to the diagnosis.

Errors with the availability heuristic can come from several sources of recall bias. For example, rare catastrophes are likely to be remembered with a clarity and force out of proportion to their value, and recent experience is, of course, easier to recall and therefore more influential on clinical judgments.

The third commonly used cognitive shortcut, the *anchoring heuristic*, involves estimating a probability by starting from a familiar point (the anchor) and adjusting to the new case from there. For example, a clinician may judge the probability of colorectal cancer to be extremely high after an elevated screening carcinoembryonic antigen (CEA) result because the prediction of colorectal cancer is anchored to the test result. Yet, as discussed below, this prediction would be inaccurate if the clinical picture of the patient being tested indicates a low probability of disease (for example, a 30-year-old woman with no risk factors). Anchoring can be a powerful tool for diagnosis but is often used incorrectly (see "Measures of Disease Probability and Bayes' Theorem," below).

DIAGNOSTIC HYPOTHESIS GENERATION Cognitive scientists studying the thought processes of expert clinicians have observed that clinicians group data into packets or "chunks," which are stored in their memories and manipulated to generate diagnostic hypotheses. Because short-term memory can typically hold only 7 to 10 items at a time, the number of packets that can be actively integrated into hypothesis-generating activities is similarly limited. The cognitive shortcuts discussed above play a key role in the generation of diagnostic hypotheses, many of which are discarded as rapidly as they are formed.

A diagnostic hypothesis sets a context for diagnostic steps to follow and provides testable predictions. For example, if the enlarged and quite tender liver felt on physical examination is due to acute hepatitis (the hypothesis), certain specific liver function tests should be markedly elevated (the prediction). If the tests come back normal, the hypothesis may need to be discarded or substantially modified.

One of the factors that makes teaching diagnostic reasoning so difficult is that expert clinicians do not follow a fixed pattern in patient examinations. From the outset, they are generating, refining, and discarding diagnostic hypotheses. The questions they ask in the history are driven by the hypotheses they are working with at the moment. Even the physical examination is driven by specific questions rather than a preordained checklist. While the student is palpating the abdomen of the alcoholic patient, waiting for a finding to strike him, the expert clinician is on a focused search mission. Is the spleen enlarged? How big is the liver? Is it tender? Are there any palpable masses or nodules? Each question focuses the attention of the examiner to the exclusion of all other inputs until answered, allowing the examiner to move on to the next specific question.

Negative findings are often as important as positive ones in establishing and refining diagnostic hypotheses. Chest discomfort that is not provoked or worsened by exertion in an active patient reduces the likelihood that chronic ischemic heart disease is the underlying cause. The absence of a resting tachycardia and thyroid gland enlargement reduces the likelihood of hyperthyroidism in a patient with paroxysmal atrial fibrillation.

While the representativeness and availability heuristics may play the major roles in shaping early diagnostic hypotheses, the acuity of a patient's illness can also be very influential. For example, clinicians are taught to consider aortic dissection routinely as a possible cause of acute severe chest discomfort along with myocardial infarction, even though the typical history of dissection is different from myocardial infarction and dissection is far less prevalent (Chap. 247). This recommendation is based on the recognition that a relatively rare but catastrophic diagnosis like aortic dissection is very difficult to make unless it is explicitly considered. If the clinician fails to elicit any of the characteristic features of dissection by history and finds equivalent blood pressures in both arms and no pulse deficits, he or she may feel comfortable in discarding the aortic dissection hypothesis. If, however, the chest x-ray shows a widened mediastinum, the hypothesis may be reinstated and a diagnostic test ordered [e.g., thoracic computed tomography (CT) scan, transesophageal echocardiogram] to evaluate it more fully. In noncritical situations, the prevalence of potential alternative diagnoses should play a much more prominent role in diagnostic hypothesis generation. The value of conducting a rapid systematic clinical survey of symptoms and organ systems to avoid missing important but inapparent clues cannot be overstated.

Because the generation and evaluation of appropriate diagnostic hypotheses is a skill that not all clinicians possess to an equal degree, errors in this process can occur, and in the patient with serious acute illness these may lead to tragic consequences. Consider the following hypothetical example. A 45-year-old male patient with a 3-week history of a "flulike" upper respiratory infection (URI) presented to his physician with symptoms of dyspnea and a productive cough. Based on the presenting complaint, the clinician pulled out a "URI Assessment Form" to improve quality and efficiency of care. The physician quickly completed the examination components outlined on this structured form, noting in particular the absence of fever and a clear chest examination. He then prescribed an antibiotic for presumed bronchitis, showed the patient how to breathe into a paper bag to relieve his "hyperventilation," and sent him home with the reassurance that his illness was not serious. After a sleepless night with significant dyspnea unrelieved by rebreathing into a bag, the patient developed nausea and vomiting and collapsed. He was brought into the Emergency Department in cardiac arrest and could not be resuscitated. Autopsy showed a posterior wall myocardial infarction and a fresh thrombus in an atherosclerotic right coronary artery. What went wrong? The clinician decided, even before starting the history, that the patient's complaints were not serious. He therefore felt confident that he could perform an abbreviated and focused examination using the URI assessment protocol rather than considering the full range of possibilities and performing appropriate tests to confirm or refute his initial hypotheses. In particular, by concentrating on the "URI," the clinician failed to elicit the full dyspnea history, which would have suggested a far more serious disorder, and did not even search for other symptoms that could have directed him to the correct diagnosis.

This example illustrates how patients can diverge from textbook symptoms and the potential consequences of being unable to adapt the diagnostic process to real-world challenges. The expert, while recognizing that common things occur commonly, approaches each evaluation on high alert for clues that the initial diagnosis may be wrong. Patients often provide information that "does not fit" with any of the leading diagnostic hypotheses being considered. Distinguishing real clues from false trails can only be achieved by practice and experience. A less experienced clinician who tries to be too efficient (as in the above example) can make serious judgment errors.

MAJOR INFLUENCES ON CLINICAL DECISION-MAKING More than a decade of research on variations in clinician practice patterns has shed much light on forces that shape clinical decisions. The use of heuristic "shortcuts," as detailed above, provides a partial explanation, but several other key factors play an important role in shaping diagnostic hypotheses and management decisions. These factors can be grouped conceptually into three overlapping categories: (1) factors related to physician personal characteristics and practice style, (2) factors related to the practice setting, and (3) economic incentive factors.

Practice Style Factors One of the key roles of the physician in medical care is to serve as the patient's agent to ensure that necessary care is provided at a high level of quality. Factors that influence this role include the physician's knowledge, training, and experience. It is obvious that physicians cannot practice evidence-based medicine if they are unfamiliar with the evidence. As would be expected, specialists generally know the evidence in their field better than do generalists. Surgeons may be more enthusiastic about recommending surgery than medical doctors because their belief in the beneficial effects of surgery is stronger. For the same reason, invasive cardiologists are much more likely to refer chest pain patients for diagnostic catheterization than are noninvasive cardiologists or generalists. The physician beliefs that drive these different practice styles are based on personal experience, recollection, and interpretation of the available medical evidence. For example, heart failure specialists are much more likely than generalists to achieve target angiotensin-converting enzyme (ACE) inhibitor therapy in their heart failure patients because they are more familiar with what the targets are (as defined by large clinical trials), have more familiarity with the specific drugs (including dosages and side effects), and are less likely to overreact to foreseeable problems in therapy such as a rise in creatinine levels or symptomatic hypotension. Other intriguing research has shown a wide distribution of acceptance times of antibiotic therapy for peptic ulcer disease following widespread dissemination of the "evidence" in the medical literature. Some gastroenterologists accepted this new therapy before the evidence was clear (reflecting, perhaps, an aggressive practice style), and some gastroenterologists lagged behind (a conservative practice style, associated in this case with older physicians). As a group, internists lagged several years behind gastroenterologists.

The opinion of influential leaders can also have an important effect on practice patterns. Such influence can occur at both the national level (e.g., expert physicians teaching at national meetings) and the local level (e.g., local educational programs, "curbside consultants"). Opinion leaders do not have to be physicians. When conducting rounds with clinical pharmacists, physicians are less likely to make medication errors and more likely to use target levels of evidence-based therapies.

The patient's welfare is not the only concern that drives clinical decisions. The physician's perception about the risk of a malpractice suit resulting from either an erroneous decision or a bad outcome creates a style of practice referred to as *defensive medicine*. This practice involves using tests and therapies with very small marginal returns to preclude future criticism in the event of an adverse outcome. For example, a 40-year-old woman who presents with a long-standing history of intermittent headache and a new severe headache along with a normal neurologic examination has a very low likelihood of structural intracranial pathology. Performance of a head CT or magnetic resonance imaging (MRI) scan in this situation would constitute defensive medicine. On the other hand, the results of the test could provide reassurance to an anxious patient.

Practice Setting Factors Factors in this category relate to the physical resources available to the physician's practice and the practice environment. *Physician-induced demand* is a term that refers to the repeated observation that physicians have a remarkable ability to accommodate to and employ the medical facilities available to them. A classic early study in this area showed that physicians in Boston had an almost 50% higher hospital admission rate than did physicians in New Haven, despite there being no obvious differences in the health of the cities' inhabitants. The physicians in New Haven were not aware of using fewer hospital beds for their patients, nor were the Boston physicians aware of using less stringent criteria to admit patients.

Other environmental factors that can influence decision-making include the local availability of specialists for consultations and procedures, "high tech" facilities such as angiography suites, a heart surgery program, and MRI machines.

Economic Incentives Economic incentives are closely related to the other two categories of practice-modifying factors. Financial issues can exert both stimulatory and inhibitory influences on clinical practice. In general, physicians are paid on a fee-for-service, capitation, or salary basis (Chap. 4). In fee-for-service, the more the physician does, the more the physician gets paid. The incentive in this case is to do more. When fees are reduced (discounted fee-for-service), doctors tend to increase the number of services billed for. Capitation, in contrast, provides a fixed payment per patient per year, encouraging physicians to take on more patients but to provide each patient with fewer services. Expensive services are more likely to be affected by this type of incentive than inexpensive preventive services. Salary compensation plans pay physicians the same regardless of the amount of clinical work performed. The incentive here is to see fewer patients. Recognizing these powerful shapers of physician behavior, managed care plans have begun to explore combinations of the three reimbursement types with the goal of improving individual physician productivity while restraining their use of expensive tests and therapies.

In summary, expert clinical decision-making can be appreciated as a complex interplay between cognitive devices used to simplify large amounts of complex information interacting with physician biases reflecting education, training, and experience, all of which are shaped by powerful, sometimes perverse, external forces. In the next section, we will review a set of statistical tools and concepts that can assist in making clinical decisions under uncertainty.

QUANTITATIVE METHODS TO AID CLINICAL DECISION-MAKING

The process of medical decision-making can be divided into two parts: (1) defining the available courses of action and estimating the likely outcomes with each, and (2) assessing the desirability of the outcomes. The former task involves integrating key information about the patient along with relevant evidence from the medical literature to create the structure of a decision problem. The remainder of this chapter will present some quantitative tools to assist the clinician in these activities. These tools can be divided into those that assist the clinician in making better outcome predictions, which are then used to make decisions, and those that support the decision process directly. While these tools are not yet used routinely in daily clinical practice, the computerization of medicine is creating the required substrate for their future widespread dissemination.

QUANTITATIVE MEDICAL PREDICTIONS **Diagnostic Testing** The purpose of performing a test on a patient is to reduce uncertainty about the patient's diagnosis or prognosis and to aid the clinician in making management decisions. Although diagnostic tests are commonly thought of as laboratory tests (e.g., measurement of serum amylase level) or procedures (e.g., colonoscopy or bronchoscopy), any technology that changes our understanding of the patient's problem qualifies as a diagnostic test. Thus, even the history and physical examination can be considered a form of diagnostic test. In clinical medicine, it is common to reduce the results of a test to a dichotomous outcome, such as positive or negative, normal or abnormal. In many cases, this simplification results in the waste of useful information. However, such simplification makes it easier to demonstrate some of the quantitative ways in which test data can be used.

To characterize the accuracy of diagnostic tests, four terms are routinely used (Table 3-1). The *true-positive rate*, i.e., the sensitivity, provides a measure of how well the test correctly identifies patients with disease. The *false-negative rate* is calculated as (1 − sensitivity). The *true-negative rate*, i.e., the specificity, reflects how well the test correctly identifies patients without disease. The *false-positive rate* is

Table 3-1 Measures of Diagnostic Test Accuracy

	Disease Status	
Test Result	**Present**	**Absent**
Positive	True-positive (*TP*)	False-positive (*FP*)
Negative	False-negative (*FN*)	True-negative (*TN*)

IDENTIFICATION OF PATIENTS WITH DISEASE

True-positive rate (sensitivity) = $TP/(TP + FN)$
False-negative rate = $FN/(TP + FN)$
True-positive rate = $1 -$ false-negative rate

IDENTIFICATION OF PATIENTS WITHOUT DISEASE

True-negative rate (specificity) = $TN/(TN + FP)$
False-positive rate = $FP/(TN + FP)$
True-negative rate = $1 -$ false-positive rate

(1 − specificity). A perfect test would have a sensitivity of 100% and a specificity of 100% and would completely separate patients with disease from those without it.

Calculating sensitivity and specificity require selection of a cutpoint value for the test to separate "normal" from "diseased" subjects. As the cutpoint is moved to improve sensitivity, specificity typically falls and vice versa. This dynamic tradeoff between more accurate identification of subjects with versus those without disease is often displayed graphically as a receiver operating characteristic (ROC) curve. An ROC curve plots sensitivity (*y*-axis) versus 1 − specificity (*x*-axis). Each point on the curve represents a potential cutpoint with an associated sensitivity and specificity value. The area under the ROC curve is often used as a quantitative measure of the information content of a test. Values range from 0.5 (no diagnostic information at all, test is equivalent to flipping a coin) to 1.0 (perfect test).

In the diagnostic testing literature, ROC areas are often used to compare alternative tests. The test with the highest area (i.e., closest to 1.0) is presumed to be the most accurate. However, ROC curves are not a panacea for evaluation of diagnostic test utility. Like Bayes' theorem, they are typically focused on only one possible test parameter (e.g., ST segment response in a treadmill exercise test) to the exclusion of other potentially relevant data. In addition, ROC area comparisons do not simulate the way test information is actually used in clinical practice. Finally, biases in the underlying population used to generate the ROC curves (e.g., related to an unrepresentative test sample) can bias the ROC area and the validity of a comparison among tests.

Measures of Disease Probability and Bayes' Theorem Unfortunately, there are no perfect tests; after every test is completed the true disease state of the patient remains uncertain. Quantitating this residual uncertainty can be done with Bayes' theorem. This theorem provides a simple mathematical way to calculate the posttest probability of disease from three parameters: the pretest probability of disease, the test sensitivity, and the test specificity (Table 3-2). The pretest probability is a quantitative expression of the confidence in a diagnosis before the test is performed. In the absence of more relevant information it is usually estimated from the prevalence of the disease in the underlying population. For some common conditions, such as coronary artery disease (CAD), nomograms and statistical models have been created to generate better estimates of pretest probability from elements of the history and physical examination. The posttest probability, then, is a revised statement of the confidence in the diagnosis, taking into account both what was known before and after the test.

To understand how Bayes' theorem creates this revised confidence statement, it is useful to examine a nomogram version of Bayes' theorem that uses the same three parameters to predict the posttest probability of disease (Fig. 3-1). In this nomogram, the accuracy of the diagnostic test in question is summarized by the likelihood ratio for a

Table 3-2   Measures of Disease Probability

Pretest probability of disease = probability of disease before test is done; may use population prevalence of disease or more patient-specific data to generate this probability estimate.

Posttest probability of disease = probability of disease accounting for both pretest probability and test results; also called predictive value of the test.

Bayes' theorem
Computational version:

$$\text{Posttest probability} = \frac{\text{Pretest probability} \times \text{test sensitivity}}{\begin{array}{c}\text{Pretest probability} \times \text{test sensitivity} + \\ (1 - \text{disease prevalence}) \times \text{test false-positive rate}\end{array}}$$

Example [with a pretest probability of 0.50 and a "positive" diagnostic test result (test sensitivity = 0.90, test specificity = 0.90)]:

$$\text{Posttest probability} = \frac{(0.50)(0.90)}{(0.50)(0.90) + (0.50)(0.10)}$$
$$= 0.90$$

positive test, which is the ratio of the true-positive rate to the false-positive rate [or sensitivity/(1 − specificity)]. For example, a test with a sensitivity of 0.90 and a specificity of 0.90 has a likelihood ratio of 0.90/(1 − 0.90), or 9. Thus, for this hypothetical test, a "positive"

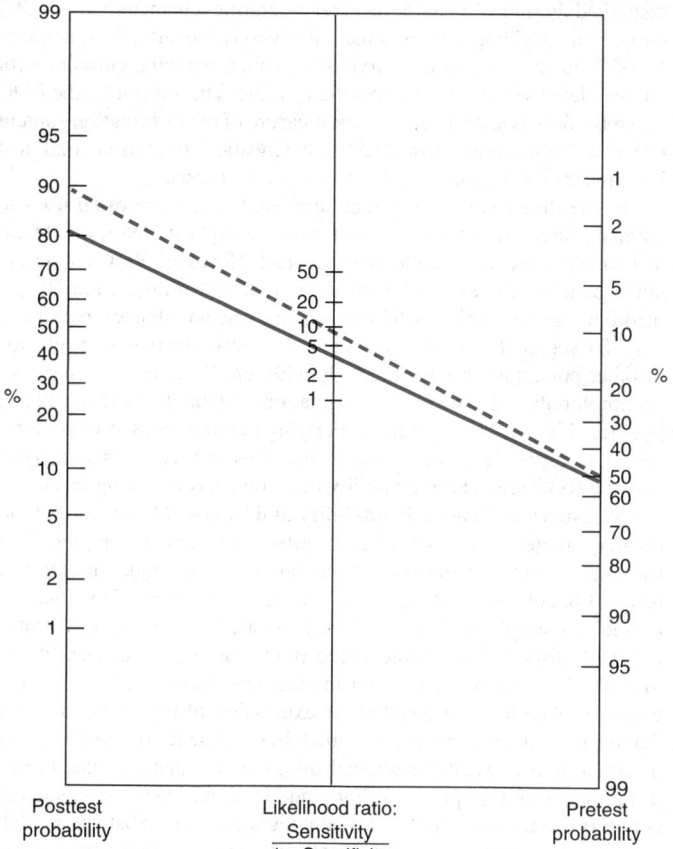

FIGURE 3-1 Nomogram version of Bayes' theorem used to predict the posttest probability of disease (left-hand scale) using the pretest probability of disease (right-hand scale) and the likelihood ratio for a positive test (middle scale). The likelihood ratio is calculated as the sensitivity/(1 − specificity). To use, place a straight edge connecting the pretest probability and the likelihood ratio, and read off the posttest probability. This figure illustrates the value of a positive exercise treadmill test (likelihood ratio 4) and a positive exercise thallium SPECT study (likelihood ratio 9) in the patient with a pretest probability of coronary artery disease of 50%. Treadmill results shown in solid line; thallium results in dashed line. *(Adapted from Fagan TJ: N Engl J Med 293:257, 1975.)*

result is 9 times more likely in a patient with the disease than in a patient without it. The more accurate the test, the higher the likelihood ratio. However, if sensitivity is excellent but specificity is less so, the likelihood ratio will be substantially reduced (e.g., with a 90% sensitivity but a 60% specificity, the likelihood ratio is 2.25). Most tests in medicine have likelihood ratios for a positive result between 1.5 and 20.

Consider two tests commonly used in the diagnosis of CAD, an exercise treadmill and an exercise thallium-201 single photon emission CT (SPECT) test (Chap. 244). Meta-analysis has shown the treadmill to have an average sensitivity of 66% and an average specificity of 84%, yielding a likelihood ratio of 4.1 [0.66/(1 − 0.84)]. If we use this test on a patient with a pretest probability of CAD of 10%, the posttest probability of disease following a positive result rises only to about 30%. If a patient with a pretest probability of CAD of 80% has a positive test result, the posttest probability of disease is about 95%.

The exercise thallium SPECT test is a more accurate test for the diagnosis of CAD. For our purposes, assume that it has both a sensitivity and specificity of 90%, yielding a likelihood ratio of 9.0 [0.90/(1 − 0.90)]. If we again test our low pretest probability patient and he has a positive test, using Fig. 3-1 we can demonstrate that the posttest probability of CAD rises from 10 to 50%. However, from a decision-making point of view, the more accurate test has not been able to improve diagnostic confidence enough to change management. In fact, the test has moved us from being fairly certain that the patient did not have CAD to being completely undecided (a 50:50 chance of disease). In a patient with a pretest probability of 80%, using the more accurate thallium SPECT test raises the posttest probability to 97% (compared with 95% for the exercise treadmill). Again, the more accurate test does not provide enough improvement in posttest confidence to alter management, and neither test has improved much upon what was known from clinical data alone.

If the pretest probability is low (e.g., ≤20%), even a positive result on a very accurate test will not move the posttest probability to a range high enough to rule in disease (e.g., ≥80%). Conversely, with a high pretest probability, a negative test will not adequately rule out disease. Thus, the largest gain in diagnostic confidence from a test occurs when the clinician is most uncertain before performing it (e.g., pretest probability between 30 and 70%). For example, if a patient has a pretest probability for CAD of 50%, a positive exercise treadmill test will move the posttest probability to 80% and a positive exercise thallium SPECT test will move it to 90% (Fig. 3-1).

Bayes' theorem, as presented above, employs a number of important simplifications that should be considered. First, few tests have only two useful outcomes, positive or negative, and many tests provide numerous pieces of data about the patient. Even if these can be integrated into a summary result, multiple levels of useful information may be present (e.g., strongly positive, positive, indeterminate, negative, strongly negative). While Bayes' theorem can be adapted to this more detailed test result format, it is computationally complex to do so. Second, Bayes' theorem assumes that the information from the test is completely unique and nonoverlapping with information used to estimate the pretest probability. This independence assumption, however, is often wrong. In many cases, test results are correlated with patient characteristics. For example, the findings of cardiomegaly and pulmonary edema on chest x-ray are correlated with the historic features of heart failure and with the physical findings of a displaced left ventricular apical impulse, an S_3 gallop, and rales. The unique predictive information contributed by the test in this case (the chest x-ray) is only a fraction of its total information because much had already been learned about the probability of heart failure before the test was done.

Finally, it has long been thought that sensitivity and specificity are prevalence-independent parameters of test accuracy, and many texts still make this assertion. This statistically useful assumption, however, is clinically wrong. For example, a treadmill exercise test has a sensitivity in a population of patients with one-vessel CAD of around 30%, whereas the sensitivity in severe three-vessel CAD approaches

80%. Thus, the best estimate of sensitivity to use in a particular decision will often vary depending on the distribution of disease stages present in the tested population. A hospitalized population typically has a higher prevalence of disease and in particular a higher prevalence of more advanced disease stages than an outpatient population. As a consequence, test sensitivity will tend to be higher in hospitalized patients, whereas test specificity will be higher in outpatients.

Statistical Prediction Models Bayes' theorem, as presented above, deals with a clinical prediction problem that is unrealistically simple relative to most problems a clinician faces. Prediction models, based on multivariable statistical models, can handle much more complex problems and substantially enhance predictive accuracy for specific situations. Their particular advantage is the ability to take into account many overlapping pieces of information and assign a relative weight to each based on its unique contribution to the prediction in question. For example, a logistic regression model to predict the probability of CAD takes into account all of the relevant independent factors from the clinical examination and diagnostic testing instead of the small handful of data that clinicians can manage in their heads or with Bayes' theorem. However, despite this strength, the models are too complex computationally to use without a calculator or computer (although this limit may be overcome when medicine is practiced from a fully computerized platform.) To date, only a handful of prediction models have been developed and properly validated. The importance of independent validation in a population separate from the one used to develop the model cannot be overstated. Unfortunately, most published models have not been properly validated, making their utility in clinical practice uncertain at best.

When statistical models have been compared directly with expert clinicians, they have been found to be more consistent, as would be expected, but not significantly more accurate. Their biggest promise, then, would seem to be to make less-experienced clinicians more accurate predictors of outcome.

DECISION SUPPORT TOOLS

DECISION SUPPORT SYSTEMS Over the past 30 years, many attempts have been made to develop computer systems to help clinicians make decisions and manage patients. Conceptually, computers offer a very attractive way to handle the vast information load that today's physicians face. The computer can help by making accurate predictions of outcome, simulating the whole decision process, or providing algorithmic guidance. Computer-based predictions using Bayesian or statistical regression models inform a clinical decision but do not actually reach a "conclusion" or "recommendation." Artificial intelligence systems attempt to simulate or replace human reasoning with a computer-based analogue. To date, such approaches have achieved only limited success. Reminder or protocol-directed systems do not make predictions but use existing algorithms, such as practice guidelines, to guide clinical practice. In general, however, decision

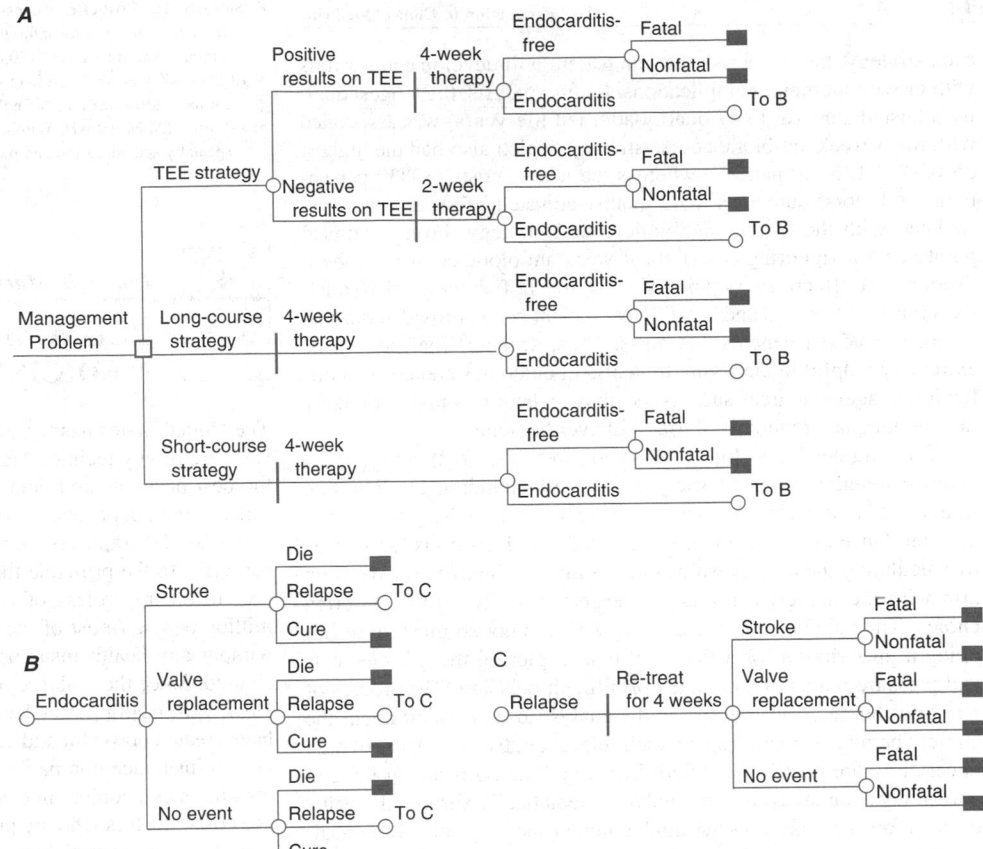

FIGURE 3-2 Decision model used to evaluate strategies for management of the risk of infective endocarditis after catheter-associated *Staphylococcus aureus* bacteremia. The square node indicates a decision between possible management strategies, round nodes represent chance events, and rectangular (or terminal) nodes indicate the outcomes of interest. All nonterminal chance nodes in the main tree (structure *A*) enter substructure *B*. All nonterminal chance nodes in substructure *B* enter substructure *C*. TEE, transesophageal echocardiography. (*From Rosen et al.*)

support systems have shown little impact on practice. Reminder systems, although not yet in widespread use, have shown the most promise, particularly in correcting drug dosing and in promoting guideline adherence. The full potential of these approaches will only be achieved when computers are fully integrated into medical practice.

DECISION ANALYSIS Compared with the methods discussed above, decision analysis represents a completely different approach to decision support. Its principal application is in decision problems that are complex and involve a substantial risk, a high degree of uncertainty in some key area, or an idiosyncratic feature that does not "fit" the available evidence. Three general steps are involved. First, the decision problem must be clearly defined. Second, the elements of the decision must be made explicit. This involves specifying the alternatives being considered, their relevant outcomes, the probabilities attached to each outcome, and the relative desirability (called "utility") of each outcome. Cost can also be assigned to each branch of the decision tree, allowing calculation of cost-effectiveness (Chap. 4).

An example of a decision tree used to evaluate strategies for management of the risk of infective endocarditis after catheter-associated *Staphylococcus aureus* bacteremia is shown in Fig. 3-2. Approximately 35,000 cases of *S. aureus* bacteremia occur each year in the United States. The development of complicating endocarditis, which occurs in about 6% of cases, is associated with high morbidity (31% mortality, 21% stroke rate) and medical costs. The three choices for management of the bacteremia are (1) transesophageal echocardiography (TEE), (2) a 4-week course of intravenous antibiotics (long-course), or (3) a 2-week course of intravenous antibiotics (short-course). In the TEE strategy, a 4-week course of antibiotics is given if endocarditis is evident and a 2-week course is given if it is not. With each strategy, there is a risk that the patient will develop endocarditis with or without major complications. In this analysis, the longest quality-adjusted survival (5.47 quality-adjusted life-years) was associated with the 4-week antibiotic course strategy, which also had the highest costs ($14,136 per patient), whereas the lowest costs ($9830 per patient) and worst outcomes (5.42 quality-adjusted life-years) were associated with the 2-week antibiotic course strategy. From a clinical point of view (ignoring costs), the 4-week antibiotic course was best. From a cost-effectiveness point of view, the TEE strategy (5.46 quality-adjusted life-years and $10,051 per patient costs) provided the best balance of added benefits and costs. Thus, decision analysis can be extremely helpful in clarifying tradeoffs in outcomes and costs in difficult management areas such as the above where it is highly unlikely that an adequate randomized trial will ever be done.

The data needed to fill in a decision tree (Fig. 3-2) are typically cobbled together from a variety of sources, including the literature (randomized trials, meta-analyses, observational studies) and expert opinion. Once the decision tree is finished, the decision is "analyzed" by calculating the average value of each limb of the tree. The decision arm with the highest net value (or expected utility) is the preferred choice. The value of this exercise, however, is not so much in developing a prescription for action as it is in exploring the key elements and pressure points of a complex or difficult decision. The process of building the decision tree forces the analyst to be explicit about the choices being considered and all their relevant outcomes. Areas of high uncertainty are readily identified. Sensitivity analyses are an integral part of decision analysis and involve systematically varying the value of each key parameter in the model alone (one-way sensitivity analysis,) in pairs (two-way), or in higher combinations (multivariable) to assess the impact on choice of preferred management strategy. In the above example, varying the incidence of endocarditis resulting from *S. aureus* bacteremia from 3% to over 50% had no impact on the choice of TEE as the preferred strategy.

User friendly personal computer–based software packages now make the creation and analysis of decision trees much more straightforward than in the past. However, the process is still too cumbersome and time-consuming to be used on a routine basis. When medicine is practiced from a fully computerized platform, a library of prestructured decision trees with user modifiable values can be made available to support practitioners working with individual patients.

CONCLUSIONS

In this era of evidence-based medicine, it is tempting to think that all the difficult decisions practitioners face have been or soon will be solved and digested into practice guidelines and computerized reminders. For the foreseeable future, however, such is not the case. Meta-analyses cannot generate evidence where there are no adequate randomized trials, and most of what clinicians face will never be thoroughly tested in a randomized trial. Excellent clinical reasoning skills and experience supplemented by well-designed quantitative tools and a keen appreciation for individual patient preferences will continue to be of paramount importance in the professional life of medical practitioners for years to come.

BIBLIOGRAPHY

AYANIAN JZ et al: Knowledge and practices of generalist and specialist physicians regarding drug therapy for acute myocardial infarction. N Engl J Med 331:1136, 1994

EDDY DM: Anatomy of a decision. JAMA 263:441, 1990

HIRTH RA et al: Specialist and generalist physicians' adoption of antibiotic therapy to eradicate *Helicobacter pylori* infection. Med Care 34:1199, 1996

KASSIRER JP, KOPELMAN RI: *Learning Clinical Reasoning*. Baltimore, Williams & Wilkins, 1991

NAYLOR CD: Gray zones of clinical practice: Some limits to evidence-based medicine. Lancet 345:840, 1995

ROSEN AB et al: Cost-effectiveness of transesophageal echocardiography to determine the duration of therapy for intravascular catheter-associated *Staphylococcus aureus* bacteremia. Ann Intern Med 130:810, 1999

SCHULMAN KA et al: The effect of race and sex on physicians' recommendations for cardiac catheterization. N Engl J Med 340:618, 1999

SEKKARIE MA, MOSS AH: Withholding and withdrawing dialysis: The role of physician specialty and education and patient functional status. Am J Kidney Dis 31:464, 1998

---

4   *Daniel B. Mark*

ECONOMIC ISSUES IN CLINICAL MEDICINE

The United States has the distinction of having some of the best medical care of any technologically advanced country. We have many of the best hospitals and doctors in the world. The research pipeline is full of significant new therapeutic advances, with revolutionary genetic-based therapies perhaps only a decade away. Our citizens largely subscribe to the principle that excellent medical care should be available to all, regardless of ability to pay. Yet we also have over 43 million people (most of them employed and earning minimal wages) without any health insurance and many more who are inadequately insured. Since the collapse of the Clinton health care reform efforts in 1994, U.S. health policy has been directed by marketplace forces that have created powerful and sometimes perverse incentives in medicine: Health insurance companies that use every available means to avoid insuring sick people; "managed care" programs that really only manage costs; doctors who are provided incentives to provide less medical care; and pharmaceutical companies that develop powerful and expensive new drugs priced beyond the reach of many of the elderly and chronically ill who need them most.

Facing such powerful and chaotic forces, physicians tend to focus narrowly on what they are most comfortable with, taking care of individual patients and conducting academic investigations. Many doctors consider economics too arcane for them to grasp and therefore do not even try. Consequently, when presented with economic arguments and evidence they are often unable to discriminate the legitimate from the fallacious. More importantly, they are ill equipped to defend their patients' interests in the crucible of cost containment that characterizes the modern managed care era.

This chapter has two goals: first, to provide a brief introduction to some of the larger economic forces that shape modern medical practices, and second, to introduce the economic tools that are used for assessing the value of medical practices, including cost effectiveness analysis.

HEALTH CARE SPENDING AND FINANCING

HOW MUCH IS SPENT ON HEALTH CARE? In 1997, the United States spent $1.1 trillion on its health care system, representing 13.5% of the gross domestic product (GDP) (a crude measure of national income). Most of this ($969 billion) was spent on personal health care: 34% went to hospitals, 20% to physicians, 7% to nursing homes, and 8% to outpatient pharmaceuticals. In comparison, Canada and Western European countries spend a substantially smaller portion (6 to 10%) of their national income on health care but their citizens appear to be equally healthy, at least by crude metrics such as life expectancy and infant mortality rates. Economists and politicians have for years used such data to argue that the United States spends too much on health care. The issue of how much to spend is an inherently political one, however, and the discipline of economics has little to say about it.

WHO PAYS FOR HEALTH CARE? Two major factors are continually driving up the costs of medical care: introduction into medical practice of new medical technologies (drugs, devices, procedures) that have a high price tag, and the aging of the U.S. population (since older people require more medical care than younger ones). These costs are distributed unevenly across society. In 1997, the government paid about 47% of the total national health care bill (75% federal, 25% states), private insurance paid about 32%, and individuals paid 17%. The government, of course, gets its money from taxpayers and uses the health care segment of its budget to pay for the Medicare and Medicaid programs (discussed below). To respond to rising medical costs, the government can increase taxes or redistribute funds from other programs such as defense and education. Neither of these options are politically attractive. Alternatively, because of its size in the medical marketplace, the government can impose lower prices on providers to make the available funds go farther (see "Cost-Containment Strategies," below). Much of the private insurance bill is subsidized by employers through their employee benefits packages. As medical costs go up, health insurance costs also rise and businesses must either pass on higher premium and copayment costs to their employees, raise their prices (potentially impairing their competitive position in the marketplace), or reduce their profit margin (a very unpopular move with stockholders). Like the government, businesses may also negotiate lower prices with health care providers and/or health insurance plans.

PUBLIC FINANCING OF HEALTH CARE The public sector (i.e., government as an agent for society) finances the Medicare and Medicaid programs as well as the Veteran's Administration Hospital system, the Department of Defense military care system, the Public Health Service, and the Indian Health Service. Of these, Medicare is by far the largest and most influential, with 39 million people receiving health insurance at a total cost in 1997 of $214.6 billion (20% of total national health expenditures). The Medicare program was enacted in 1965 by Congress as an amendment to the Social Security Act of 1935 and was envisioned by President Lyndon B. Johnson as a first step toward universal health insurance in the United States, a key part of his "great society" plan. Its impact on the evolution of the U.S. health care system has been profound. The original congressional act provided health care insurance for the elderly (defined as those 65 and older) who were eligible for social security (i.e., retired workers who had paid into the system during their working years and their dependents). Amendments in 1972 extended coverage to the disabled of all ages (currently numbering around 5 million) and to patients with chronic renal failure (who currently number about 284,000).

Medicare consists of two related insurance programs. The Medicare Hospital Insurance Trust Fund (also known as Part A) covers hospital care and skilled nursing home care and is funded by compulsory federal payroll taxes on employers and employees. Medicare Part B, the Medical Supplementary Insurance Program, covers physician fees as well as laboratory and other diagnostic tests and is funded by general federal tax revenues and patient premiums. Both programs have substantial gaps in coverage, necessitating supplemental insurance (so-called Medigap policies) for those who can afford them. Because of its compulsory income redistribution feature, taking tax money from current workers to pay for health care for elderly citizens (many of whom are on fixed income close to the poverty level), Medicare is both a health insurance program and a social welfare program designed to combat poverty in the disabled and elderly. In exchange for their tax money, the 150 million workers funding the program are promised the same type of social security when they become elderly (paid for by future generations of workers).

Medicaid is a social insurance program for the poor that is jointly run by the federal and state governments. The federal government gives each state a grant of money for the program based on that state's per capita income (in 1997, this amount totaled $95 billion), and the states pay for the rest ($65 billion in 1997). The program, like Medicare, was enacted by Congress in 1965 as a part of President Johnson's "great society" program. It is larger than Medicare in terms of eligible beneficiaries (41 million people) but smaller in terms of budget ($160 billion, or 12% of the total national health expenditures). Because the requirements to qualify for Medicaid are stringent, many low-income individuals under age 65 (especially the working poor) do not qualify. Eligibility criteria are set by each state within general federal guidelines, and the income and asset tests individuals must meet to qualify vary widely among states. Many of the dollars in the Medicaid program actually pay for care for elderly and disabled Medicare beneficiaries who also qualify for Medicaid on the basis of poverty.

PRIVATE FINANCING OF HEALTH CARE Approximately 70% of the non-elderly U.S. population is covered by some form of private medical insurance. The feasibility of group insurance for medical care was initially demonstrated in the 1930s by Blue Cross, a franchise of nonprofit groups providing hospitalization insurance in order to help prop up the financially strapped U.S. hospital industry. Blue Shield, a separate organization modeled after Blue Cross, started providing insurance for in-hospital physician services in 1939. During World War II, employee wages were frozen by the government and to entice workers, who were in short supply, some employers started offering health insurance as a fringe benefit. With the feasibility of employer-sponsored group health insurance demonstrated by the experience of the "Blues," commercial insurers began to enter the market. To win the support of doctors and hospitals, insurers agreed to pay "reasonable and customary charges" and to defer all medical management decisions to doctors. This "fee-for-service" reimbursement system, created in the post–World War II era, sowed the seeds of the tremendous inflation observed in the U.S. medical system during the 1970s and 1980s.

The original focus of indemnity insurance plans was to cover individuals against catastrophic financial losses from high medical care bills. Insurance is a contract for protection against specific hazards that are unpredictable for individuals but can be defined with confidence for large groups. "Major medical" health insurance was designed to provide coverage for catastrophic illness, a relatively rare event in most populations. Group coverage is less expensive than individual coverage because it allows the insurance company to diffuse the risk of a large payout among a big pool of individuals who will pay premiums but make no claims. When coverage is shifted from a focus on rare catastrophes to routine maintenance medical care (comprehensive insurance policies), health insurance becomes a means for payment of expected rather than unexpected care. The consequence is higher health insurance premiums. The early appeal of health maintenance organizations (HMOs) was that they appeared to offer an economically efficient way to provide routine preventive care and to manage the occasional catastrophic illness.

MANAGED CARE Managed care is a generic term that embraces a wide spectrum of systems for integrating the financing and delivery of health care. Managed care organizations (MCOs) contract with doctors and hospitals to provide comprehensive care to enrolled members for a fixed, prospectively set, premium. HMOs are a form of managed care originally organized between the 1940s and 1960s as an alternative to the prevailing fee-for-service–based private insurance. With the advent of serious medical inflation in the 1970s, the HMO model was promoted by the federal government as a way to control the growth in medical spending. Early enthusiasm for this initiative was limited; in 1984, only 5% of individuals with employer-based health insurance were in an HMO. However, by 1998 that figure had risen to 85%. The exponential growth of managed care started in the 1990s in part as an employer-driven response to the uncontrolled medical inflation of the previous two decades.

The massive increase in demand for managed care by employers and by the Medicare program produced a rapid, and sometimes bewildering, evolution in the managed care industry. One important trend has been the growth of for-profit (i.e., investor owned) managed care companies. Over half of HMO members now belong to a for-profit plan. Investment dollars from Wall Street have made it easier for these plans to respond quickly to increased employer demand for managed care options. However, compared with their not-for-profit counterparts, for-profit HMOs spend a smaller proportion of each premium dollar paying for health care for members (the paradoxically named "medical loss ratio"), since stockholders also have to be paid. As a result, for-profit HMOs are less successful than not-for-profit plans in providing preventive care (a presumed strength of managed care).

Another prevalent trend of the 1990s was the move from traditional HMO models to virtual HMOs, built from contractual relationships with community physicians and hospitals. The three HMO models are the staff model, the group model, and the Independent Practice Association (IPA). The staff model HMO is a vertically integrated organization. That is, it owns its own hospitals, employs all its physicians full time for a set salary, and is focused in a particular geographic area. The group model HMO, exemplified by Group Health Cooperative of Puget Sound, contracts with one or more large multispecialty group practices to care for its patients for a preset capitated reimbursement. These physicians do not care for non-HMO patients. In the IPA model, the HMO contracts with an association of self-employed physicians who maintain their own offices and see both HMO and non-HMO patients. The network model refers to a hybrid of the other three forms of HMO. IPA and network model HMOs now have the majority of HMO membership in the United States.

The other portion of the managed care industry is represented by point of service (POS) plans and preferred provider organizations (PPOs). POS plans incorporate key features of both HMOs and traditional fee-for-service plans. A patient may choose care from a provider network or go outside the network. Care within network requires only a minimal copayment, while care outside the network requires a deductible and a large (e.g., 30%) copayment. The goal of the plan is to offer patients a choice but to provide major financial incentives to stay within the HMO portion of the plan. PPOs use a defined provider network (physicians, hospitals) that has agreed to accept discounted fee-for-service to care for enrolled members. PPOs may incorporate various managed care features, such as physician gatekeepers and utilization review.

THE UNINSURED AND UNDERINSURED Data from the U.S. Census Bureau indicate that 43.4 million people had no health insurance for all of 1997 and 71.5 million people were without insurance for at least part of the year. The great majority of uninsured individuals either work for small employers who do not offer a health insurance benefit or, more commonly, cannot afford the premiums of the plan(s) that are offered. Underinsurance also has a significant impact on the working poor by requiring them to pay an excessive proportion of their family's income for health insurance premiums and out-of-pocket medical costs (deductibles, copayments, and uninsured care). Outpatient prescription medications are a major source of underinsurance. Prescription drug costs are now the fastest growing segment of the national medical budget and the least likely segment to be covered by insurance. The elderly are particularly affected, since Medicare does not currently cover outpatient prescriptions and even Medigap policies have limited coverage.

Some states have experimented with expanded coverage through their Medicaid programs to help the uninsured poor (such as the Oregon Medicaid program). For the forseeable future, however, it does not appear that the federal government will address this problem comprehensively.

COST-CONTAINMENT STRATEGIES Current projections from the federal government's Health Care Finance Administration (HCFA) are that health care expenditures will double (to $2.2 trillion, or 16.2% of the GDP) by 2008. Over the past 30 years, the U.S. health care system has experimented with a vast array of cost-containment approaches. Conceptually, there are four major ways to control medical spending: (1) control prices, (2) control volume of care provided, (3) control the total budget available to pay for care, and (4) shift costs to another payer.

Two of the most important price control initiatives in medicine have been the Medicare Hospital Prospective Payment System and the Medicare Fee Schedule for physicians. In 1983, Medicare replaced its retrospective cost-based hospital reimbursement system with a pro-

spective payment system. In this system, all hospitalizations are classified into one of approximately 500 Diagnosis Related Groups (DRGs) based on the principal discharge diagnosis for the hospitalization and a few selected additional factors such as age, the performance of surgery, and the presence of complications. Each DRG is assigned an average reimbursement (adjusted annually). If the hospital can provide care for less than this amount, they make a profit. If they spend more than this amount, they lose money. The DRG system was designed to promote efficiency and cost containment in hospital-based care. While it has helped to control Medicare costs, it has not reduced overall U.S. health care costs, probably because of substantial cost-shifting by hospitals to the private insurance sector.

Between 1975 and 1987, Medicare payments to physicians increased at an annual rate of 18%, well above the rate of inflation. While total spending for physician services accounts for less than 25% of the Medicare budget, physicians have control over aspects of care (use of procedures, length of stay, hospital admission) that extend their direct influence to over 75% of the Medicare budget. Recognizing the importance of physicians in cost containment, Congress directed the development of a new physician payment system based on the use of a resource-based relative value scale (RBRVS). The Medicare Fee Schedule, which was first used in 1992, has three components: (1) a measure of the total work (time and complexity) involved in each physician service and standardized across all specialties, (2) a practice expense to cover the cost of running an office, and (3) an amount to cover malpractice insurance costs. The Medicare Fee Schedule classifies all physician services using the American Medical Association's Current Procedural Terminology (CPT) codes. Each CPT code has an associated relative value units (RVUs) weight. The RVU weights are multiplied by a national conversion factor to generate the actual physician fee associated with the service in question.

Price controls are attractive for cost containment because they are less expensive administratively than volume controls and don't involve micromanagement of clinical care. Price controls alone, however, don't generally achieve control of costs because of compensatory responses of providers. For example, under Medicare prospective payment, hospitals have shifted much care to the outpatient setting, where DRGs are not used. Physicians have responded to lower fees by an increased volume and intensity of service.

Volume controls include various programs to limit the diffusion of expensive technologies (such as heart surgery) or extra hospital beds. Limits can be operationalized using either a regulatory approach [such as certificate of need (CON) programs] or a budgetary approach. Utilization review approaches attempt to discern which expensive care items are medically necessary and which are not.

Budgetary controls are simpler than either price or volume control approaches. In Canada, for example, hospitals have global annual budgets. How the money is spent is decided by each hospital. If the budget is exceeded, there are no guarantees that the shortfall will be covered.

Finally, payers can control their costs by cost-shifting to other willing payers. For example, as health insurance premiums rise, employers can choose to pass these costs on to employees. Hospitals and doctors who lose money caring for Medicare patients can try to make up their losses by charging more to private insurance patients. Insurance companies can choose to offer limited or no coverage for outpatient pharmaceuticals, shifting the full cost of expensive new medicines directly to patients.

MEDICAL ECONOMIC CONCEPTS AND TOOLS

MEDICAL COST CONCEPTS Medical cost analysis is a field that borrows heavily from both economics and accounting. Economics provides the theoretical structure that defines the key questions to be addressed, and accounting provides many of the measurement tools. Traditional economics has as one of its major axioms that societal resources are finite. For this reason, society must choose from among the many ways that resources can be used and not all of society's goals can be fulfilled. Economics has devised a theoretical framework and a set of tools (including cost-effectiveness analysis) to help define the major competing goals for societal resources and to assist in selecting from among the ones that most efficiently fulfill societal needs. "Cost" in economics refers not so much to money but rather to the lost opportunities that occur when the limited societal resources are expended in a particular way. For example, if our medical armamentarium is enhanced over the next decade by discovery of powerful but expensive therapies and these are incorporated into standard clinical practice, the ability of the country to invest in education, defense, or transportation may be compromised. This notion of cost as a lost opportunity to use resources in alternative ways is referred to as *opportunity cost*. While representing the purest economic notion of cost, there is no practical way to measure it.

Accountants, who are much more concerned with issues of measurement, have proposed a "gold standard" of cost measurement, *true accounting cost*, that involves enumerating all the individual resources consumed in the production of a particular medical good or service and assigning market prices for each of them. The total cost is then the sum of the dollar costs for all the component resources. Even this calculation, however, may be prohibitively difficult in "real world" applications, for several reasons. First, all medical care requires not only the easily identifiable components of personnel time and disposable supplies but also the infrastructure components such as the rent on the office building where the care is provided, the cost of utilities, and the expense of an office staff. Second, even if all the components can be identified, enumeration of exactly what is used may be prohibitively expensive. Finally, medicine does not have publicly available "market prices" that can be readily obtained for a medical cost analysis, the way one can obtain prices for automobiles or refrigerators. The reasons for this relate to the lack of a true competitive free market in medicine along with the severe price distortion created in medical charges by cost-shifting practices.

KEY COST TERMS Several key sets of cost terms are used in medicine. As the volume of health care produced is increased or decreased, costs may exhibit either variable or fixed "behavior." *Variable costs* change with each unit shift in production volume (up or down). For example, each vaccination administered to a group of children increases costs (related to the dose of vaccine and the disposable syringe) in a predictable linear fashion. *Fixed costs* do not shift with short-term changes in the volume of care provided. For example, the rent on the clinical building and the cost of heating, lighting, and so forth do not change according to the number of individuals vaccinated per day. Some types of costs display hybrid features of both variable and fixed components. For example, clinic personnel costs (e.g., nurses, secretaries) may be fixed if these personnel are paid a salary regardless of clinic volume. If the clinic volume goes up so much that evening hours must be added, either new personnel must be hired or existing personnel must work overtime. Either of these changes would graft a variable component onto the fixed personnel costs.

Marginal cost is a concept often used by economists to refer to the cost of producing one more unit of a given health care good or service. For example, the costs of doing one more or one less diagnostic cardiac catheterization would be its marginal cost. For all practical purposes, this is the same as its variable costs (since fixed costs do not change with small changes in volume). While the concept of unit changes in volume is theoretically interesting, a more pragmatic issue is the cost effect of changing a group of patients from one strategy to another. Many experts use the term *incremental costs* to refer to this type of shift (although some use marginal and incremental synonymously). Incremental analysis is a key component of cost-effectiveness analysis (see below).

Another set of cost terms relates to the traceability of costs to the production of health care goods and services. *Direct costs*, such as nursing and physician personnel and disposable supplies, can be clearly linked to the health care provided and are under the control of the health care providers. *Indirect costs*, sometimes known as *overhead*, cannot. For example, the utility, laundry, maintenance, and administration costs of a hospital cannot be linked with the care of an individual patient and are generally not under the control of the physicians and nurses providing the medical care. The distinction of direct versus indirect is useful in cost-containment efforts, where the first step is to identify all major cost components and decide how they are to be controlled.

One common error in the evaluation of medical costs is to focus on the cost of a test or therapy in isolation. Virtually every major medical management decision creates downstream consequences. For example, if physicians order a screening diagnostic test and the result is abnormal, they will need to do a confirmatory or more definitive test. If they order a potent new antibiotic and a fraction of patients develop liver failure as an unexpected toxicity, the total cost of that course of antibiotic includes not only the cost of the drug itself but also the costs of treating the liver failure in the fraction of patients who develop it. Extra costs added as a consequence of some diagnostic or therapeutic decision are referred to as *induced costs*. Similarly, if a management decision produces downstream savings, these would be referred to as *induced savings*. For example, administration of HMG CoA reductase inhibitors to patients with hypercholesterolemia can prevent future myocardial infarctions and revascularization procedures, both of which entail expensive hospitalizations.

One final important cost concept relates to the societal costs of lost productivity (primarily lost time from work) due to illness. While economists often refer to these as indirect costs, confusion with the accounting concept of indirect costs (overhead) has led many to prefer the alternative term, *productivity costs*.

COST MEASUREMENT Using varying degrees of simplification, medical costs can be measured using either bottom-up or top-down approaches. Bottom-up approaches build from component resources to calculate total cost for an episode or type of care. Microcosting is the gold standard approach. It involves careful enumeration of all resources consumed and detailed cost-accounting estimation of the costs for each component resource. A number of medical centers have now installed computer-based cost-accounting systems that perform a modified type of microcosting analysis. For difficult-to-obtain resource use data (such as time required for a particular type of care by a given type of personnel), these systems use expert opinion in place of empirical data. The other extreme of the bottom-up category of approaches involves enumeration and costing for only the "big ticket" or expensive items, such as hospitalization episodes and costly tests and procedures.

The top-down methods of medical cost estimation calculate a cost estimate from aggregated data. One such approach uses hospital billing charge data and charge-to-cost conversion ratios (which each hospital produces annually in its Medicare Cost Report) to estimate hospital costs. Despite the approximations involved, this approach, which can be used for most nonfederal U.S. hospitals, has provided good agreement with bottom-up estimates in the few instances where formal comparisons have been made. The other top-down approach is the use of DRG assignments and reimbursement rates to provide standard cost weights for hospitalization episodes.

COST-EFFECTIVENESS ANALYSIS Given a finite budget (for health care overall or for a particular health system), how can we use the available money to provide the most health benefits for our patients? For the clinician, who is less concerned with such policy issues, a prevalent question is whether a new treatment is economically attractive. The analysis method used to address this question is dependent on how the effectiveness and costs of the new therapy compare with those of "standard care" (Fig. 4-1). *Cost-effectiveness analysis* is used when effectiveness of the new treatment is greater and its costs are higher. This analysis calculates the ratio of added (or incremental)

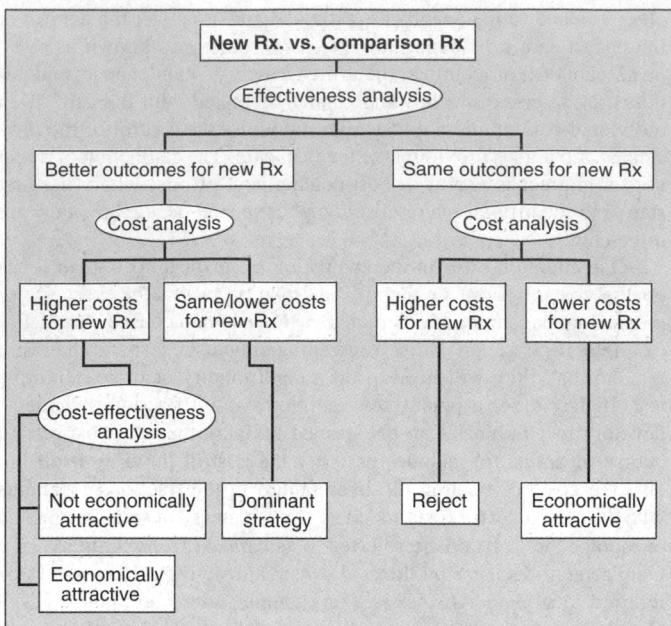

FIGURE 4-1   Schematic representation of patterns of outcome and cost differences that may result when a new therapy or strategy is compared with an existing standard. Effectiveness is always considered first because if the new therapy is less effective, its cost is rarely of concern. If effectiveness is better, or at least equivalent, then costs are prepared. If the outcomes are better but the net costs are higher, cost effectiveness analysis is then performed. If the costs are equivalent or lower, the therapy is said to be *dominant* (i.e., it becomes the preferred option). If outcomes are equivalent, cost analysis is used to select the more efficient, less costly option. This form of cost analysis is sometimes referred to as *cost minimization* or *cost-efficiency analysis*.

health benefits to added costs produced by a new therapy or strategy relative to some reference standard. The general formula is:

$$\text{Cost-effectiveness ratio} = \frac{C_{\text{new}} - C_{\text{usual care}}}{E_{\text{new}} - E_{\text{usual care}}}$$

where C = costs and E = effectiveness.

The cost-effectiveness ratio provides a quantitative statement of the amount of money required to produce a single extra unit of benefit with the new therapy relative to usual care or some other relevant reference standard. The benefit can be calculated in any meaningful clinical unit, such as added survivors or extra patients with a correct diagnosis. However, the vast majority of cost-effectiveness analyses use the epidemiologic concept of life-years to express incremental benefit. Virtually all benchmarks for cost effectiveness relate to this endpoint. Because some therapies affect quality of life but not quantity, a more generally relevant effectiveness measure combines qualify of life and life expectancy into a single composite metric, the quality-adjusted life year (QALY). Calculation of incremental dollars required to add an extra QALY is called *cost-utility analysis*. The QALY is a useful concept, but many details regarding measurement and interpretation remain controversial. The third form of economic efficiency analysis, *cost-benefit analysis*, requires conversion of health benefits into monetary equivalents. Because such conversions are controversial, this form of analysis is rarely used in medicine. In theory, the time horizon of a cost-effectiveness analysis should be long enough to capture all important cost and health consequences of the therapy or strategy being evaluated. Most often, analysts use a lifetime time frame. Because very few empirical studies are long enough to observe lifetime outcomes (especially when chronic diseases are being studied), models are required to extrapolate from available data.

A cost-effectiveness analysis can be done from a variety of perspectives, but the most widely applicable perspective is societal. Other perspectives are often much narrower and may include unattractive qualities. For example, a managed care organization may be interested only in short-term costs and outcomes, knowing that patients tend to change their health insurance every few years.

The benchmarks for cost-effectiveness ratios are determined by comparison with other well-accepted therapies in widespread medical use. A useful benchmark is hemodialysis for chronic renal failure, since the federal government has paid for all renal failure patients to get dialysis since 1973 through the End Stage Renal Disease Program. Recent estimates are that it costs this Medicare program about $50,000 to add 1 life-year to a chronic renal failure patient. Partly for this reason, many analysts use a cost-effectiveness ratio of <$50,000 per added life-year to identify therapies that are economically attractive (i.e., have a favorable balance of extra costs to extra benefits), while therapies with ratios >$100,000 per added life-year are deemed economically unattractive and therapies between $50,000 and $100,000 per added life-year are in the economic "gray zone."

Several caveats about cost-effectiveness analysis should be noted. First, cost-effectiveness analysis is descriptive, not prescriptive. It measures value that could be produced with available health care dollars but does not mandate how these dollars are to be used. If an expensive new therapy is introduced and is found to be very economically attractive by the above benchmarks, it will still not get used if there is no money in the budget to pay for it. Second, a cost-effectiveness ratio is only as good as the data that were used to calculate it. High-quality results can be obtained if economic analysis is prospectively incorporated into the design of large-scale multicenter randomized trials. Third, although cost-effectiveness ratios are often presented as deterministic (i.e., no variability), they often incorporate large amounts of uncertainty. This should be examined either with sensitivity analyses (varying each key parameter through a plausible range to see if the results are materially changed) or calculation of confidence limits.

MEDICAL ECONOMICS AND CLINICAL PRACTICE

In evaluating new therapies, three issues must be addressed: (1) is the new therapy significantly better than what is currently available? (2) how much does it cost and is it economically attractive? and (3) how many patients will need this therapy and is it affordable? The clinician should be primarily concerned with the answer to the first question. Although cost issues are now a reality of daily clinical life and cost-containment pressures are often substantial, decisions by clinicians that are based primarily on economic rather than clinical considerations put the physician in the role of the double agent (i.e., acting on behalf of both the patient and the payer) and compromise our fiduciary obligation to patients. The second question addresses cost effectiveness and, if favorable, can be used to support an argument by clinicians for adoption of the therapy. In the ideal world, at least, therapies that have a large database of evidence demonstrating effectiveness and economic attractiveness should be given preference over therapies that do not have such supporting data. The final question is of primary concern to payers and health policy analysts. An effective therapy that is too expensive to use is of little more value than a therapy that has yet to be discovered.

BIBLIOGRAPHY

AZIMA NA, WELCH HG: The effectiveness of cost effectiveness analysis in containing costs. J Gen Intern Med 13:664, 1998

BODENHEIMER T: The American health care system: Physicians and the changing medical marketplace. N Engl J Med 340:584, 1999

CANTOR SB, GANIATS TG: Incremental cost effectiveness analysis: The optimal strategy depends on the strategy set. J Clin Epidemiol 52:517, 1999

GRANATA AV, HILLMAN AL: Competing practice guidelines: Using cost effectiveness analysis to make optimal decisions. Ann Intern Med 128:56, 1998

HLATKY MA et al: for the BARI Investigators: Medical care costs and quality of life after randomization to coronary angioplasty or coronary bypass surgery. N Engl J Med 336:92, 1997

KUTTNER R: The American health care system: Health insurance coverage. N Engl J Med 340:163, 1999

MARK DB et al: Cost effectiveness of thrombolytic therapy with tissue plasminogen activator as compared with streptokinase for acute myocardial infarction. N Engl J Med 332:1418, 1995

5   Howard Hu, Frank E. Speizer

INFLUENCE OF ENVIRONMENTAL AND OCCUPATIONAL HAZARDS ON DISEASE

Exposures to hazardous materials and processes in the home, the workplace, and the community can cause or exacerbate a multitude of diseases. Physicians commonly treat the sequelae of such diseases in the practice of medicine; however, unless the underlying connection with hazardous exposures is identified and mitigated, treatment of manifestations rather than the cause at best only ameliorates the condition. At worst, the neglect of hazardous exposures may lead to both failure of treatment and failure to recognize a public health problem with wide significance.

No existing surveillance or reporting system can estimate the total contribution of hazardous exposures to morbidity and mortality. However, careful histories have identified occupational factors as etiologic in more than 10% of all admissions to general internal medicine wards in hospitals, with even higher percentages when the primary illness is either respiratory or musculoskeletal. Estimates of the number of new cases of disease due to work in the United States range from 125,000 to 350,000 per year; these cases do not include 5.3 million work-related injuries.

Environmental exposures are increasingly associated with decrements in measures of health whose outcomes range from subclinical to clinically catastrophic. For example, exposure to lead at levels that are common in the general population has been associated with increased blood pressure and decreased creatinine clearance. Ambient air pollution with respect to levels of ozone and fine-particulate matter has been related to increased rates of hospital admission for respiratory and cardiovascular diseases and to increased mortality rates, respectively. Indoor exposure to radon and passive indoor exposure to environmental tobacco smoke have been linked with an increased risk of lung cancer. There is pressure on clinicians to be aware of and act on this type of information, which is suggestive but not necessarily conclusive with respect to causation.

Patients are becoming increasingly concerned about hazardous exposures. More than 15% of patients seen in one study conducted in a primary care clinic expressed the opinion that their health problems were work-related, and 75% of this subgroup of patients reported exposure to one or more recognized toxic agents. Patients often want answers to very specific questions, such as: Is the water in our town safe to drink? Could my breathing problem be related to the new roofing sealant used in my building at work? Physicians are consulted because they are the most trusted sources of information on health risks, including chemical risks. Unfortunately, few physicians have more than rudimentary training in environmental and occupational medicine. Therefore, it becomes important for primary care physicians to be able to recognize symptoms precipitated by exposure to environmental or occupational hazards and either to manage these cases or to make appropriate referrals.

Many manifestations of exposure-related illnesses are nonspecific (e.g., dizziness, headache) or are commonly encountered in general internal medicine (e.g., myocardial infarction, cancer). The establishment of a connection with an environmental or occupational hazard requires a high index of suspicion and the application of fundamental concepts of environmental/occupational medicine. Furthermore, early recognition by physicians of unusual patterns of illness or of evidence of asymptomatic exposure to toxins with low-level effects (e.g., an elevated blood lead level) can alert health officials to the need for control measures. Case reports either sent to local authorities or published in the literature often prompt follow-up studies that can lead to the identification of new hazards. In many states and countries, the reporting by physicians of occupational/environmental diseases is mandatory. For instance, beginning in 1992, physicians in Massachusetts were required to report cases of pneumoconiosis, occupational asthma, carpal tunnel syndrome, and carbon monoxide poisoning, among other conditions. Identification of an environmental/occupational etiology of an illness may have important economic ramifications for the patient (e.g., the awarding of worker's compensation, which covers medical bills as well as lost wages). Finally, physicians are frequently asked to provide expert medical testimony during litigation on the causal relationship between toxic exposures and diseases. In this setting, the more knowledgeable the physician is about potential hazardous exposures, the better prepared he or she is to serve the patient.

THE ENVIRONMENTAL/OCCUPATIONAL HISTORY

For a physician, the most critical steps toward recognizing these disorders are remembering to consider them in the differential diagnosis and taking an appropriate environmental/occupational history as part of the medical workup. The level of detail that is called for depends on the clinical situation. *Information should always be obtained on current and major past occupations, and patients should be asked whether they think their health problem is related to their work or to any particular environment or exposure.* In the review of systems, patients should be asked if they have been exposed to dusts, fumes, chemicals, radiation, or loud noise. When patient and physician are confronted with an illness of uncertain etiology, these factors should be explored in more detail, with the environmental/occupational history as the point of departure. (A brief outline of a sample history is shown in Table 5-1.)

The identification of specific chemical exposures can be difficult. Household products must list chemical ingredients on their labels, and this information may prove useful. For workplace exposures, the U.S. Occupational Safety and Health Administration (OSHA) requires chemical suppliers to provide material safety data sheets with their products and requires employers to retain these sheets and make them available to employees. The data sheets can be obtained by the physician or employee by a telephoned or written request; failure of an

Table 5-1   Initial Clinical Approach to the Recognition of Illness Caused by Environmental or Occupational Hazards

1. Screening questions
    a. Chief symptom and history of present illness
        • What kind of work do you do?
        • Do you think your health problems are related to your work, home, or any other particular environment or exposure?
        • Does the timing of your symptoms have any relation to being at work or at home or to any other particular exposures or activities?
    b. Review of systems
        • Are you now or have you previously been exposed to dusts, fumes, chemicals, radiation, or loud noise?
2. Detailed questioning based on initial suspicion
    • Chronology of jobs: Job title, type of industry, dates of work, description of job, a typical day, potentially hazardous exposures, protective equipment used
    • Chronology of residences: Description of potentially hazardous exposures (e.g., furnaces, pesticide application, home hobbies involving chemicals)
    • Identification of other employees or household members who have similar health problems
    • Exploration in detail of the temporal link between potential exposures and chief symptoms
    • Clinical clues (suspicious scenarios; see text)

SOURCE: Adapted from Newman, 1995.

employer to provide them within 30 days of such a request is a violation of OSHA regulations and is punishable by fines. In addition to providing information on chemical ingredients and percent composition, the material safety data sheets provide basic information on toxicity. This information is seldom adequate from a clinical perspective but may indicate the general type of toxicity to be anticipated.

EVALUATION OF POSSIBLE CHEMICAL OR ENVIRONMENTAL HAZARDS Given the wide variety of toxic exposures that may be uncovered during a workup, a clinician should routinely consult additional reference material to evaluate whether particular hazards may be associated with the illness at hand. Many sources of information exist. OSHA and some regional poison-control centers have extensive information on hazards and brief summary documents that can be transmitted over the Internet or by telephone or facsimile. Depending on the area, other resources may include county and state health departments; regional offices of the National Institute for Occupational Safety and Health and the Environmental Protection Agency; the Consumer Products Safety Commission in Washington, DC; academic institutions; websites of these institutions; and individual toxicologists, occupational/environmental medicine specialists, or industrial hygienists. Sophisticated computerized databases are also available, including detailed listings on CD-ROM information systems. MEDLARS, the electronic database maintained by the National Library of Medicine, is accessible by modem or the Internet and is familiar to many physicians. Files other than MEDLINE, such as the Hazardous Substances Databank, provide specific toxicity information on chemicals and include toxicologic references not covered by MEDLINE. Many of these databases can also be accessed through the Internet.

As with any other illness, laboratory investigation may be crucial. For example, tests of carboxyhemoglobin level to document carbon monoxide exposure or of serum anticholinesterase level to document organophosphate pesticide absorption should be performed within hours of exposure. As in cases of acute drug overdose, it is useful to freeze samples of urine and serum from any patient suspected of having had an acute chemical exposure; such specimens can be analyzed at a later date by sensitive methods of detection. Use of other tests must rely on knowledge of the specific hazard or illness in question.

SUSPICIOUS SCENARIOS Some medical problems or clinical scenarios demand a particularly high degree of suspicion of occupational or environmental factors as causative or contributing agents.

Respiratory Disease The contribution of occupational/environmental factors to respiratory disease is generally underrecognized, particularly among patients who smoke and among the elderly (Chap. 254). For instance, asthma related to chemical exposure may be treated without regard to cause or may be erroneously diagnosed as acute tracheobronchitis. A study of new-onset asthma among HMO members in Massachusetts found that 21% of these individuals met criteria for clinically significant asthma attributable to occupational exposures. The types of exposures and jobs in these cases varied widely; examples include exposure to smoke in a firefighter, to welding fumes in a technical school student, to cleaning compounds in a bartender, and to epoxy in an archery repairman. No single type of job or exposure predominated. Other examples of etiologic errors include shortness of breath from asbestosis that is attributed to chronic obstructive pulmonary disease and chemical pneumonitis that is misdiagnosed as a bacterial infection.

Cancer Many cancers are thought to be causally related to occupational and environmental factors in addition to tobacco. Some are particularly likely to have a chemical etiology or another environmental cause, including cancers of the skin (solar radiation, arsenic, coal tar, soot); lung (asbestos, arsenic, nickel, radon); pleura (almost exclusively asbestos); nasal cavity and sinuses (chromium, nickel, wood

and leather dusts); liver (arsenic, vinyl chloride); bone marrow (benzene, ionizing radiation); and bladder (aromatic amines).

Coronary Disease and Hypertension Carbon monoxide exposure is common, particularly in homes with malfunctioning furnaces or in workplaces close to motor vehicle exhaust. By reducing oxygen transport by hemoglobin and inhibiting mitochondrial metabolism, carbon monoxide can aggravate coronary disease. Methylene chloride, a solvent used in paint stripping, is converted to carbon monoxide and thus poses the same risk. Exposure to carbon disulfide, a chemical used in the production of rayon, accelerates the rate of atherosclerotic plaque formation. Chronic lead exposure, even at modest levels, is a risk factor for the development of hypertension as well as abnormalities of cardiac conduction.

Hepatitis/Chronic Liver Disease In the absence of evidence that a viral infection, alcohol ingestion, or drug use is the main cause of hepatitis (Chaps. 295, 296, and 297), the involvement of a toxin must be considered. Toxin-induced hepatic injury may be cytotoxic, cholestatic, or both. The list of hepatotoxic agents is long, including organic synthetic compounds such as carbon tetrachloride (used in solvents and cleaning fluids) and methylene diamine (a resin hardener); pesticides such as chlordecone (Kepone); metals, particularly arsenic (used in pesticides and paints and found in well water); and natural toxins such as the pyrrolidizine alkaloids.

Kidney Disease Many chemical and environmental factors can cause renal injury (Chap. 269). The etiology of much chronic kidney disease, however, remains unknown. An increasing body of evidence now links chronic renal failure with hypertension to lead exposure. One study demonstrated that chelation therapy with EDTA slowed the progression of renal insufficiency in patients with a mildly elevated body lead burden. Some studies suggest that chronic exposure to hydrocarbons (e.g., gasoline, paints, solvents) may lead to various types of glomerulonephritis, including Goodpasture's syndrome. Environmental cadmium exposure has been found to promote calcium loss via urinary excretion, which results in skeletal demineralization and thus in an increased risk of fractures.

Peripheral Neuropathy Organic solvents such as *n*-hexane, heavy metals such as lead and arsenic, and some organophosphate compounds can damage the axons of peripheral nerves. Dimethylaminopropionitrile, an industrial catalyst, causes bladder neuropathy. Nerve entrapment syndromes of the upper extremity, such as carpal tunnel syndrome, may be caused by jobs that involve repetitive motion, especially those requiring the maintenance of awkward positions.

Central Nervous System Disorders Fatigue, memory loss, difficulty in concentration, and emotional lability have been linked to chronic exposure to solvents such as toluene and perchloroethylene. Painters, metal degreasers, plastics workers, and cleaners are commonly exposed to solvents and develop these symptoms at a high rate. Among the features that distinguish these patients are characteristic patterns on formal neurobehavioral testing and stabilization of symptoms with gradual improvement after discontinuation of the exposure. Other substances associated with neurobehavioral dysfunction include metals, particularly lead, mercury, arsenic, and manganese; pesticides, such as organophosphates and organochlorines; polychlorinated biphenyls (PCBs); and gases such as carbon monoxide.

Environmental factors are also suspected of contributing to other neurologic diseases, such as degenerative disorders, motor neuron diseases, and extrapyramidal disorders. For example, a study in monozygotic and dizygotic twin pairs found a similarity in concordance indicating that environmental (as opposed to genetic) factors play a major etiologic role in cases of typical Parkinson's disease beginning after the age of 50 years.

Teratogenesis and Reproductive Problems Toxins can impair successful reproduction at a variety of levels. Examples include insecticides and herbicides, PCBs and polybrominated biphenyls (PBBs), ethylene oxide (a sterilizing gas used in hospitals), metals (lead, arsenic, cadmium, mercury), and solvents. Dibromochloropropane, a nematocide, suppresses spermatogenesis. Some toxins, such as PCBs,

PBBs, and chlorinated pesticides, are concentrated in milk. Concern has arisen over the ability of specific organic pollutants, particularly pesticides, to persist in the environment and accumulate in human tissues. Some of these chemicals may disrupt endocrine function, and these effects may be related to phenomena such as the observed increases in the incidences of testicular cancer, breast cancer, and hypospadias.

Immunosuppression, Autoimmunity, and Hypersensitivity Evidence is increasing that exposures to some chemical agents can compromise the immune system, thereby leading to a generalized increase in the incidence of tumors (e.g., exposure to PBBs) or infections (e.g., respiratory infections after exposure to common air pollutants). Mercury, dieldrin, and methylcholanthrene are known to elicit autoimmune responses. Some chemicals are potent allergic sensitizers that cause dermal and respiratory problems (Chaps. 60 and 254).

BIOLOGICAL MARKERS An increasing number of methods are available for measuring and interpreting toxic exposure, including (1) the internal dose of specific toxins and (2) markers of the biologic effects of toxins. Internal-dose markers are relevant for toxins that are sequestered in the human body, such as lead (in blood), arsenic (in hair), and other metals (Chap. 395), and for halogenated compounds (such as PCBs). Examples of markers of the biologic effects of toxins include depressed levels of acetylcholinesterase in serum after exposure to organophosphate pesticides, sister chromatid exchanges in peripheral lymphocytes after exposure to the carcinogen ethylene oxide, and DNA adducts after exposure to tobacco smoke carcinogens.

MANAGING A HAZARD-RELATED ILLNESS Once a chemical or another environmental hazard has been identified as an important contributor to an illness, the next step is to prevent further exposure. Although for chronic diseases such as cancer this step may be irrelevant for the patient in question, prevention of further exposure may still be critical for other persons who have been similarly exposed. When prevention of further exposure is important, *the physician must be willing to become an active advocate for the patient*. This advocacy may involve writing a letter stating that the patient should no longer be exposed to a hazard or should remain out of work. Alternatively, it may involve contacting appropriate officials in government, industry, or labor or other advocates who can deal with a hazardous exposure. Treatment is dependent on the specific hazard.

In few areas of medicine does a physician deal with more scientific uncertainty. Comprehensive information on toxicants is available for only a small percentage of chemicals. In general, the physician should take a conservative approach (i.e., advise the patient to avoid a hazard likely to have contributed to illness) and should use common sense and up-to-date information to evaluate causal relationships.

LOW-LEVEL EXPOSURES AND THEIR EFFECTS The subclinical effects of toxins that are widespread in our environment and our workplaces are of increasing concern. Given the absence of any demonstrable effect threshold, low-level exposure to carcinogens should be avoided; not only carcinogenic but also noncarcinogenic effects of chronic low-level exposure to these substances are important.

Perhaps lead provides the most important example of low-level noncarcinogenic effects that constitute a major public health problem. Multiple pathways of exposure, including the combustion of leaded gasoline, the use of lead-based paints and solder, and the presence of lead in cans containing food, have contributed to exposure of the entire population. Such low-level exposures can impair neurobehavioral development in infants and children and can raise blood pressure in adults. Furthermore, absorbed lead is stored in the skeleton and may reenter the circulation at times of heightened bone turnover (e.g., pregnancy, lactation, osteoporosis, hyperthyroidism). Subclinical toxic effects can be prevented if chronic low-level exposure is detected early and curtailed. In the case of lead, such exposure is detected by tests of blood lead level, which should be performed regularly in young children living in old housing and as a precautionary measure in adults with a history of lead exposure.

BIBLIOGRAPHY

DeRosa C et al: Environmental exposures that affect the endocrine system: Public health implications. J Toxicol Environ Health B Crit Rev 1:3, 1998

Dockery DW et al: An association between air pollution and mortality in six U.S. cities. N Engl J Med 329:1753, 1993

Gennart J-P et al: Importance of accurate employment histories of patients admitted to units of internal medicine. Scand J Work Environ Health 17:386, 1991

Institutes of Medicine: *Role of the Primary Care Physician in Occupational and Environmental Medicine*. Washington, DC, National Academy Press, 1988

Lin JL et al: Chelation therapy for patients with elevated body lead burden and progressive renal insufficiency. A randomized, controlled trial. Ann Intern Med 5:7, 1999

Milton DK et al: Risk and incidence of asthma attributable to occupational exposure among HMO members. Am J Ind Med 33:1, 1998

Newman LS: Current concepts: Occupational illness. N Engl J Med 333:1128, 1995

Paul M (ed): *Occupational/Environmental Hazards and Reproductive Health: A Guide for Clinicians*. Baltimore, Williams & Wilkins, 1992

Rom WN: *Environmental and Occupational Medicine*. Philadelphia, Lippincott-Raven, 1998

Staessen JA et al: Environmental exposure to cadmium, forearm bone density, and risk of fractures: Prospective population study. Lancet 353:1140, 1999

Tanner CM et al: Parkinson disease in twins. An etiologic study. JAMA 281:341, 1999

6 **Anthony L. Komaroff, Celeste Robb-Nicholson, Andrea E. Dunaif**

WOMEN'S HEALTH

In recent years, the medical problems and health care of women have received increasing attention. There are poorly understood differences between men and women, both in morbidity and mortality and in the expression of diseases. Many research studies of disease prevention and pathophysiology have included only male subjects; most illnesses that can affect both sexes have not been as well studied in women. It also appears that women receive different care than men for certain common health problems. Finally, an increasing number of women are seeking health care in multidisciplinary women's health units that combine the expertise of gynecology, psychiatry, and internal medicine or family medicine.

MORBIDITY AND MORTALITY IN WOMEN **Morbidity** Past studies have found that women experience more days of restricted activity than men at all ages, over and above the restricted activity caused by obstetric and gynecologic conditions. However, a study in 1998 concluded differently. Women make more visits to physicians, particularly for acute self-limited illnesses.

Mortality In the developed nations, women live longer than men. In the United States, as of 1996, the projected average life expectancy from birth is 79.1 years for females, and 73.1 years for males. Although there are more male fetuses conceived than female fetuses, females have a survival advantage when compared to males, in all age groups. The longer life expectancy of women versus men in developed countries is due in large part to the difference in mortality caused by ischemic heart disease (IHD).

As shown in Table 6-1, the leading causes of death among young women in the United States are accidents, homicide, and suicide. During the middle years, breast cancer is a slightly more common cause of death than IHD and lung cancer. In women between ages 65 and 74, IHD, lung cancer, and cerebrovascular disease supercede breast cancer as the leading causes of death. Among women of all ages, IHD is the leading cause of death by a substantial margin, with a mortality rate five to sixfold higher than the rate for either lung or breast cancer. Nevertheless, polls find that U.S. women believe breast cancer poses the greatest threat to their lives.

Table 6-1   Death Rates (per 100,000) for the Leading Causes of Death in U.S. Women, 1996

Ages 25–34 Total: 74.7	Ages 45–54 Total: 323.3	Ages 65–74 Total: 1,979.0	All Ages Total: 806.5
1. Motor vehicle accidents (10.7)	1. Breast cancer (38.8)	1. Ischemic heart disease (452.6)	1. Ischemic heart disease (172.8)
2. HIV infection (8.5)	2. Ischemic heart disease (30.2)	2. Lung cancer[a] (209.0)	2. Cerebrovascular disease (71.9)
3. Homicide (5.5)	3. Lung cancer[a] (29.0)	3. GI cancer[b] (147.1)	3. Lung cancer[a] (45.6)
4. Non-motor vehicle accidents (5.0)	4. GI cancer[b] (20.2)	4. COPD[c] (136.7)	4. GI cancer[b] (20.2)
5. Suicide (5.0)	5. Cancer of the genital organs (16.4)	5. Cerebrovascular disease (120.1)	5. COPD[c] (38.0)

[a] Cancer of respiratory and intrathoracic organs, predominantly lung cancer.
[b] Cancer of digestive organs and peritoneum.
[c] Chronic obstructive pulmonary disease, including asthma, and allied conditions.
SOURCE: Adapted from National Center for Health Statistics Web site, Vital Statistics of the United States, 1996, general mortality table GMWK290. URL: www.cdc.gov/nchswww/data/gm290.pdf

Social Factors Influencing Morbidity and Mortality Gender differences in morbidity and mortality may be explained in part by psychosocial factors such as socially-defined gender roles, poverty, participation in the work force, health insurance, and lifestyle.

In the past 30 years in the United States, there has been a "feminization of poverty." One-third of families headed by women currently live in poverty, and the fraction is greater than one-half for African-American and Latino women. Almost a fifth of women over age 65 live below the poverty level. People of lower socioeconomic status experience poorer health and a higher mortality rate than those in higher income groups. The poor are more likely to smoke and less likely to have recommended preventive measures, including cancer screening. Lack of adequate health insurance is a major problem for many women; in general, they are more likely than men to have low-paying, part-time, non-union jobs that do not provide health insurance. Women who are divorced or widowed may also lose health insurance that they had through their husbands.

PREVENTION (See also Chap. 10) Primary prevention and screening are crucial elements in improving the health of women. Based upon available literature and the consensus of experts, various authoritative organizations have published guidelines on preventive practices in women.

Most physicians believe that a baseline history and physical examination is useful to set the stage for preventive measures appropriate to each patient. In general, authorities recommend that blood pressure be measured every other year throughout life. Counseling on diet, smoking cessation, exercise, and use of seatbelts are of demonstrated value in the primary prevention of diseases and accidents. Counseling about safe sexual practices, alcohol abuse, and violence are also recommended.

Screening for glaucoma is recommended for African-American women over age 40 and for Caucasian women over age 50. Yearly examinations to test visual acuity are recommended for women over age 70.

Regular screening for breast, cervical, and colorectal cancer is recommended, but how often tests should be performed and which tools to use are still being debated. Most authorities recommend annual clinical breast examination in all women beginning at age 35 to 40. There is strong evidence to support the efficacy of annual mammography in women age 50 to 59. For women age 60 or older, the evidence for screening is less strong. The benefits of screening for women between the ages of 40 and 49 are still being debated.

Most authorities recommend Pap smear screening beginning at age 18 or when a woman becomes sexually active. After two or three consecutive normal Pap smears, most groups recommend Pap smear testing every three years. If Pap smears have been normal for 10 years, they can be discontinued in women after age 65.

Recommendations for colorectal cancer screening vary. For patients over 50, the American Cancer Society recommends yearly fecal occult blood testing and rectal examination combined with flexible sigmoidoscopy every 5 years, colonoscopy every 10 years, or double-contrast barium enema every 5 to 10 years.

Bone mineral testing has gained rapid acceptance as a screening tool for detecting osteoporosis, as well as for predicting the likelihood of the condition in the future. With the advent of multiple preventive and therapeutic strategies for osteoporosis, many authorities now recommend bone mineral testing to screen for the condition. A bone mineral density test is recomended for all women over age 65 as well as for all postmenopausal women who are at increased risk for developing osteoporosis (Chap. 342).

Cigarette smoking, a major risk factor for cardiovascular diseases and cancers in women, has been well studied (Chap. 390). Over the past 60 years there has been a sharp decline in smoking among men, but not among women; teenage women smoke at higher rates than their male counterparts. "Low-yield" cigarettes are marketed heavily to women. The Nurses' Health Study showed that one-third of the excess risk of ischemic heart disease was eliminated two years after smoking cessation, and that all of the excess risk was eliminated by 10 to 14 years after smoking cessation.

The National Cholesterol Education Program recommends that total cholesterol and high-density lipoprotein (HDL) levels be measured once. If both are normal, a repeat test after 5 years is recommended. A meta-analysis of several small studies of women showed an increased risk of IHD in women with serum cholesterol greater than 265, a ratio of total cholesterol to HDL cholesterol greater than 4, or an elevated fasting triglyceride.

In various case-control and observational studies, postmenopausal estrogen therapy is associated with a 40 to 50% reduction in deaths due to IHD, but its value in a prospective, randomized trial has not yet been documented.

Calcium and estrogen, as well as alendronate and the selective estrogen receptor modulators, tamoxifen and raloxifene, slow the development of osteoporosis and reduce the frequency of hip and vertebral fracture in postmenopausal women. In randomized clinical trials, both tamoxifen and raloxifene have been shown to reduce the risk of breast cancer in postmenopausal women.

Considerable research indicates that a relatively high dietary intake of various antioxidants (including vitamins E and C) is associated with lower rates of vascular disease and malignancies. Randomized trials of supplemental antioxidants are under way. Preliminary research indicates that regular aspirin use is associated with reduced rates of IHD and colorectal carcinoma.

GENDER DIFFERENCES IN DISEASE Obviously, some diseases and conditions occur exclusively (or nearly exclusively) in women—e.g., menopause and various breast and gynecological disorders. These are discussed elsewhere in this book (Chaps. 52, 89, 336, 337). In this chapter, we seek to highlight some gender differences in diseases that occur in both women and men.

Ischemic Heart Disease (See also Chap. 244) Many persons think of IHD as a primary problem for men rather than women, perhaps because men have more than twice the total incidence of cardiovascular morbidity and mortality between the ages of 35 and 84. However, as stated earlier, in the United States IHD is among the leading causes of death among women as well as men (Table 6-1). The curve for the IHD mortality rate in women lags behind that for men by about a decade. Nevertheless, nearly 250,000 women die annually from IHD; after age 40, one in three women will die from heart disease. Although IHD mortality has been falling in men in the United States over the past 30 years, it has been increasing in women.

Why are IHD rates lower in women? They have a more favorable risk profile in some respects: higher HDL cholesterol levels, lower triglyceride levels, and less upper-body obesity than men. But women also have a less favorable risk profile in other respects: more obesity, higher blood pressure, higher plasma cholesterol levels, higher fibrinogen levels, and more diabetes. The simplest explanation for the sex differential in IHD is the "cardioprotective" effect of estrogen, which can be due to improvement of the lipid profile, a direct vasodilatory effect, and perhaps other factors. HDL cholesterol levels appear to be a particularly important risk factor for IHD in women. HDL levels are higher in all age groups in women compared to men, and are higher in premenopausal and estrogen-treated postmenopausal women. Smoking is the most important risk factor for IHD in women.

IHD presents differently in men and women. In the Framingham study, angina was the most frequent initial symptom of IHD in females, occurring in 47% of women, whereas myocardial infarction was the most frequent initial symptom in males, occurring in 46% of men. The exercise electrocardiogram has a substantial false positive as well as false negative rate for women, compared to men.

Women, particularly African-American women, have a higher risk of morbidity and mortality than men following a myocardial infarction. Compared to men, women who obtain coronary artery bypass graft surgery have more advanced disease, a higher perioperative mortality rate, less relief of angina, and less graft patency; however, 5- and 10-year survival rates are similar. Women undergoing percutaneous transluminal coronary angioplasty have lower rates of clinical and angiographic success than men, but also a lower rate of restenosis and a better long-term outcome. Women may benefit less and have more frequent serious bleeding complications from thrombolytic therapy than do men. Factors such as older age, more comorbid conditions, and more severe IHD in women at the time of events or procedures appear to account for at least part of the gender differences observed. Women with IHD benefit at least as much as men, and perhaps more, from reductions in cholesterol level.

The incidence of IHD increases markedly at menopause, consistent with the hypothesis that estrogens are cardioprotective. A number of observational studies have supported this hypothesis by demonstrating significant decreases in IHD in women on hormone replacement therapy (HRT), both estrogen alone and estrogen-progestin combination therapy. However, the HERS, a recent clinical trial of HRT for the *secondary* prevention of IHD, showed no significant difference in cardiovascular events between therapy with combined continuous conjugated equine estrogen (0.625 mg qd) and that with medroxyprogesterone acetate (2.5 mg qd), compared to placebo over four years. Indeed, in the HRT group, there was about a 50% increase in cardiovascular events in the first year of the trial. The Women's Health Initiative is investigating directly the impact of various HRT modalities as a *primary* prevention of IHD risk. Until further data are available, caution should be exercised in prescribing HRT to women with a history of IHD, or for cardioprotection alone.

Hypertension (See also Chap. 246)   Hypertension is more common in U.S. women than men, largely owing to the high prevalence of hypertension in older age groups and the longer survival rate for women. Both the effectiveness and the adverse effects of various antihypertensive drugs appear to be comparable in women and men. Benefits of treatment for severe hypertension have been dramatic in both women and men. However, in clinical trials of the treatment of mild to moderate hypertension, women have had a smaller decrease in morbidity and mortality than men, perhaps because women have a lower risk of myocardial infarction and stroke than men to begin with. Older women benefit at least as much as men from treatment, as demonstrated by the Systolic Hypertension in Elderly study. The incidence of hypertension (above 140/90) appears to be low (less than 5%) with the current low-dose oral contraceptives. Postmenopausal estrogen therapy is not associated with increases in blood pressure.

Immunologically Mediated Diseases   Several immunologically mediated diseases—e.g., rheumatoid arthritis, systemic lupus erythematosus, multiple sclerosis, Graves' disease, and thyroiditis—oc-cur much more frequently in women than in men. In animal models of rheumatoid arthritis—lupus and multiple sclerosis, for example—it is the females of the species that are predominantly affected. On the other hand, animal studies indicate that females are less susceptible to infection.

In short, female animals appear to have more vigorous immune responses, with both beneficial and adverse consequences. Increasing evidence indicates that estrogens upregulate both cellular and humoral immunity. Also, some immunocytes contain estrogen, progestin and androgen receptors, and the uterus produces a variety of cytokines, suggesting a complex interaction between the reproductive and immune systems.

Osteoporosis (See also Chap. 342)   This condition is much more prevalent in postmenopausal women than in men of similar age. Osteoporotic hip fractures are a major cause of morbidity in elderly women. Men accumulate more bone mass and lose bone more slowly than women. Gender differences in bone mass are found as early as infancy. Calcium intake, vitamin D and estrogen all play important roles in osteoporosis; calcium intake is an important determinant of peak bone mass, particularly during adolescence. Vitamin D deficiency is surprisingly common in elderly women. Receptors for estrogens and androgens have been identified in bone. The aromatase enzyme system, which converts androgens to estrogens, is also present in bone.

Therapy with HRT, or with calcium and vitamin D, has been shown to reduce the risk of osteoporotic fractures. Newer modalities, such as bisphosphonates (alendronate), calcitonin, and raloxifene, a selective estrogen receptor modulator, prevent bone loss and reduce the risk of osteoporotic fractures.

Alzheimer's Disease (See also Chap. 362)   Alzheimer's disease (AD) affects approximately twice as many women as men, in part because women live longer. Several observational studies suggest that HRT may decrease the risk of AD and improve cognitive function in older women. These benefits are seen in both current as well as past HRT users. In a few experimental studies, estrogen replacement has been shown to be associated with improved memory compared to placebo treatment. Estrogens enhance neuronal growth and activity, providing a biologic basis for these putative cognitive effects of HRT. Prospective clinical trials, including the Women's Health Initiative, are underway to pursue these intriguing observations.

Diabetes Mellitus (See also Chap. 333)   Estrogens enhance insulin sensitivity in women but not in men. Despite this, the prevalence of type 2 diabetes mellitus (DM) is higher in women, which is related in part to the higher prevalence of female obesity. Premenopausal women with DM lose the cardioprotective effect of female gender and have identical rates of IHD to those in males. This is partially explained by the presence of several IHD risk factors in women with DM: obesity, hypertension and dysplipidemia. Recent evidence suggests that vascular responses differ in women with DM, as compared to normal women. Polycystic ovary syndrome and gestational diabetes mellitus—common conditions in premenopausal women—are associated with a significantly increased risk for type 2 DM.

Psychological Disorders (See also Chap. 385)   Depression, anxiety panic disorder and eating disorders (bulimia and anorexia nervosa) occur more often in women than in men. Epidemiologic studies from both developed and developing nations consistently find major depression to be twice as common in women as in men, with the gender disparity becoming evident in early adolescence. Depression occurs in 10% of women during pregnancy and in 10 to 15% of women during the first several months of the postpartum period. The incidence of major depression diminishes after age 45, and does not increase with the onset of menopause. Depression in women also appears to have a worse prognosis than in men; episodes of depression last longer and there is a lower rate of spontaneous remission.

Social factors may account for the greater prevalence of some disorders in women; the traditionally subordinate role of women in society may generate feelings of helplessness and frustration which contribute to psychiatric illness. In addition, it is likely that biological factors, including hormonally influenced neurochemical changes, also play a role. The limbic system and hypothalamus—areas of the brain thought to subserve appetite, satiety and emotion—contain estradiol and testosterone receptors.

Alcohol and Drug Abuse (See also Chap. 387)   One-third of Americans who suffer from alcoholism are women. Women alcoholics are less likely to be diagnosed than men; a greater proportion of men than women seek help for alcohol and drug abuse. Men are more likely to go to an alcohol or drug treatment facility, while women tend to approach a primary care physician or mental health professional for help under the guise of a psychosocial problem. Late-life alcoholism is more common in women than men. In 1997, an epidemiologic survey reported that, among women over age 59, an estimated 1.8 million were addicted to or abused alcohol, and over 2.8 million were addicted to or abused psychoactive or mood-altering prescription drugs.

On average, alcoholic women drink less than alcoholic men, but exhibit the same degree of impairment. Blood alcohol levels are higher in women than in men after drinking equivalent amounts of alcohol, adjusted for body weight. This greater bioavailability of alcohol in women is probably due to the higher proportion of body fat and lower total body water. Women also have a lower gastric "first-pass metabolism" of alcohol, associated with lower activity of gastric alcohol dehydrogenase. In addition, alcoholic women are more likely than alcoholic men to abuse tranquilizers, sedatives, and amphetamines. Women alcoholics have a higher mortality rate than do nonalcoholic women and alcoholic men. Compared to men, women also appear to develop alcoholic liver disease and other alcohol-related diseases with shorter drinking histories and lower levels of alcohol consumption. Alcohol abuse also poses special risks to women who are or wish to become pregnant, adversely affecting fertility and the health of the baby (fetal alcohol syndrome).

Finally, there is growing evidence that for several illicit drugs, women proceed more rapidly to drug dependence than do men.

Human Immunodeficiency Virus Infection (See also Chap. 309) As of September 1998, the Centers for Disease Control and Prevention estimate that between 120,000 and 160,000 adolescent and adult women in the United States were living with HIV infection, including those with AIDS (Table 6-1). Between 1985 and 1998, the proportion of all U.S. AIDS cases reported among women more than tripled, from 7 to 23%. HIV infection was the fourth leading cause of death among U.S. women age 25 to 44 in 1997, and the second leading cause of death among African-American women in this age group. The CDC estimates that 30% of the approximately 40,000 new HIV infections in the United States each year are among women.

Between 1996 and 1997 the incidence of new AIDS cases in the United States decreased by 18% and that of AIDS-related deaths by 42%, largely because of advances in HIV therapies. The decline continued between 1997 and 1998, albeit at a slower rate. AIDS incidence and AIDS-related mortality fell by 11 and 20%, respectively. However, AIDS incidence and deaths are not decreasing as rapidly among women as among men. HIV and AIDS continue to affect women in racial/ethnic minorities and lower socioeconomic classes disproportionately. CDC estimates that 64% of new HIV infections in 1998 occured among African-American women, 18% among Hispanic women, and 18% among white women. Of the new HIV infections among women in the United States in 1998, CDC estimates that 75% of women were infected through heterosexual sex and 25% of women through injection drug use.

Violence Against Women   Violence against women in the United States is an enormous problem. Incidents of both rape and domestic violence are vastly underreported. Sexual assault is one of the most common crimes against women. One in five adult women in the United States reports having experienced sexual assault during her lifetime. Adult women are much more likely to be raped by a spouse, ex-spouse, or acquaintance than by a stranger.

Domestic violence is defined in the American Medical Association guidelines as "an ongoing, debilitating experience of physical, psychologic, and/or sexual abuse in the home, associated with increasing isolation from the outside world and limited personal freedom and accessibility to resources." It affects women of all ages, ethnic orientations, and socioeconomic groups. Based upon national crime statistics, every year an estimated 2 million women in the United States are severely injured and more than 1000 are killed by their current or former male partner. Domestic violence is the most common cause of physical injury in women, exceeding the combined incidence of all other types of injury (such as from rape, mugging, and auto accidents). Women who are young, single, pregnant, recently separated or divorced, or who have a history of substance abuse or mental illness, or a partner with substance abuse or mental illness, are at increased risk of domestic violence.

Domestic violence and sexual assault are associated with increased rates of physical and psychologic symptoms, medical office visits, and hospitalizations. Given this indirect presentation of the consequences of violence, and the high prevalence of unreported violence, clinicians should have a low threshold for pursuing the possibility of violence in female patients, particularly those with vague symptoms and psychological disorders.

The immediate treatment of rape and domestic violence focuses on assessing and treating physical injuries; providing emotional support; assessing and dealing with the risks of sexually transmitted infection and pregnancy; evaluating the safety of the patient and other family members; and documenting the patient's history and physical examination findings. In addition to dealing with the medical and psychological issues, appropriate care includes providing information about legal services, shelters and safe houses, hotlines, support groups, and counseling services.

RESEARCH IN WOMEN'S HEALTH   The growing recognition of the importance of women's health has spawned a number of research efforts, including large observational studies and clinical trials. The U.S. National Institutes of Health has introduced guidelines to mandate the inclusion of women in clinical studies, and the reporting of gender-specific data.

Studies of Prevention   Large observational studies of men and women, such as the Rancho Bernardo Study and the Framingham Study, designed to analyze data specific to women have been on the increase. The Nurses' Health Study has been following more than 200,000 women, many for more than 20 years, prospectively collecting data to study the impact of smoking, diet, physical activity, medications, prevention and screening behaviors, and some psychosocial factors on the risk of various medical disorders, including breast cancer, IHD, stroke, diabetes, and fracture, as well as causes of mortality.

These studies have set the stage for clinical trials such as the Postmenopausal Estrogens/Progestins Intervention (PEPI) Trial, the first multicenter, randomized, double-blind, placebo-control trial of the effects of three estrogen/progestin regimens on risk factors for cardiovascular disease, bone mineral density, and endometrial hyperplasia. The study found that estrogen, alone or in combination with progestin, increased serum levels of HDL and decreased low-density lipoprotein (LDL) and fibrinogen levels. While unopposed estrogen (without progestins) resulted in the most beneficial effects on lipids, it was also associated with an increased risk of endometrial hyperplasia.

In 1992, the NIH funded the Women's Health Initiative (WHI), a study of the health of postmenopausal women. The WHI, the largest research study ever funded by the NIH, involves over 160,000 postmenopausal women participating at 45 clinical centers across the United States through the year 2002. The WHI study includes both a prospective observational study and an interventional randomized trial involving over 63,000 women, which is designed to test the effects of a low-fat diet, hormone replacement therapy, and calcium and vitamin

D supplementation on the risks for cardiovascular disease, breast cancer, and osteoporotic fractures.

Many other studies currently in progress promise new insights into the health of women within the next decade.

Pharmacologic Studies Historically, women have been underrepresented in drug trials, even though the majority of pharmaceuticals sold in the United States each year are used by women. However, this has been rapidly changing. The FDA requires information on the safety and effectiveness of experimental drugs in women, on the effects of the menstrual cycle and menopause on a drug's pharmacokinetics, and on a drug's influence on the effectiveness of oral contraceptives. The increased emphasis on entering women into drug trials is likely to yield important information. Studies that have included women indicate that there are clinically significant differences in the way women respond to a number of frequently prescribed pharmaceuticals, including sedative-hypnotics, antidepressants, antipsychotics, anticonvulsants, and β-adrenergic blocking agents. The 1992 FDA Adverse Experience Report found that women have a higher frequency of adverse drug reactions than men. Other studies suggest that the efficacy of many drugs may be different in women compared to men. For example, women require lower doses of neuroleptics to control schizophrenia than men do. Women awaken from anesthesia faster than do men who are given the same doses of anesthetics, and they have a more powerful response to certain classes of analgesics than men. The reasons for these differences are not clear. However, these observations have spurred researchers to consider separating out the effects of gender in future clinical research in an effort to define "gender-based" biologic processes.

CONCLUSION At the same time that the health of women is undergoing more rigorous study and women's clinics are becoming increasingly common and popular, a growing fraction of health professionals are women. The number of women physicians has increased by 300% between 1970 and 1990, and more than 40% of all U.S. medical students now are women. This infusion of women into the physician work force is likely to lead to a still greater recognition of the unique aspects of health and disease in women.

BIBLIOGRAPHY

CDC FACT SHEET, September 99. HIV/AIDS among U.S. women: Minority and young women at continuing risk. www.cdc.gov/nchstp/hiv_aids/pubs/facts/women.htm

COLDITZ GA: The Nurses' Health Study: A cohort of U.S. women followed since 1976. J Am Med Women's Assoc 50:40, 1995

COUNCIL ON SCIENTIFIC AFFAIRS, AMERICAN MEDICAL ASSOCIATION: Violence against women. Relevance for medical practitioners. JAMA 267:3184, 1992

GIJSBERS VAN WIJK CMT et al: Symptom sensitivity and sex differences in physical morbidity: A review of health surveys in the United States and the Netherlands. Women Health 17:91, 1991

HULLY S et al: Randomized trial of estrogen plus progestin for secondary prevention of coronary heart disease in postmenopausal women. Heart and Estrogen/Progestin Replacement Study (HERS) Research Group. JAMA 280: 605, 1998

KAPLAN NM: The treatment of hypertension in women. Arch Intern Med 185:563, 1995

MINKOFF HL, DEHOVITZ JA: Care of women infected with the human immunodeficiency virus. JAMA 266:2253, 1991

MURABITO JM: Women and cardiovascular disease: Contributions from the Framingham Heart Study. J Am Med Women's Assoc 50:35, 1995

MUSTARD CA et al: Sex differences in the use of health care services. N Engl J Med 338: 1678, 1998

RICH-EDWARDS JW et al: The primary prevention of coronary heart disease in women. N Engl J Med 332:1758, 1995

RODIN J, ICKOVICS JR: Women's health. Review and research agenda as we approach the 21st century. Am Psychol 45:1018, 1990

SHAYWITZ SE et al: Effects of estrogen on brain activation patterns in postmenopausal women during working memory tasks. JAMA 281:1197, 1999

VERBRUGGE LM, WINGARD DL: Sex differentials in health and mortality. Women Health 12:103, 1987

WEISSMAN MM, OLFSON M: Depression in women: Implications for health care research. Science 269:799, 1995

WINKLEBY MA et al: Ethnic and socioeconomic differences in cardiovascular disease risk factors: findings for women from the Third National Health and Nutrition Examination Survey, 1988–1994. JAMA 280:356, 1998

WRITING GROUP FOR THE PEPI TRIAL: Effects of estrogen or estrogen/progestin regimens on heart disease risk factors in postmenopausal women: The Postmenopausal Estrogen/Progestin Interventions Trial. JAMA 273:199, 1995

| 7 | *Robert L. Barbieri, John T. Repke* |

MEDICAL DISORDERS DURING PREGNANCY

Approximately 4 million births occur in the United States each year. A significant proportion of these are complicated by one or more medical disorders. Two decades ago, many medical disorders were contraindications to pregnancy. Advances in obstetrics, neonatology, obstetric anesthesiology, and medicine have increased the expectation that pregnancy will result in an excellent outcome for both mother and fetus despite most of these conditions. Successful pregnancy requires important physiologic adaptations, such as a marked increase in cardiac output. Medical problems that interfere with the physiologic adaptations of pregnancy increase the risk for poor pregnancy outcome; conversely, in some instances pregnancy may adversely impact an underlying medical disorder.

HYPERTENSION (See also Chap. 246)

In pregnancy, cardiac output increases by 40%, most of which is due to an increase in stroke volume. Heart rate increases by approximately 10 beats per minute during the third trimester. In the second trimester of pregnancy, systemic vascular resistance decreases and this is associated with a fall in blood pressure. During pregnancy, a blood pressure of 140/90 mmHg is considered to be abnormally elevated and is associated with a marked increase in perinatal morbidity and mortality. In all pregnant women, the measurement of blood pressure should be performed in the sitting position, because for many the lateral recumbent position is associated with a blood pressure lower than that recorded in the sitting position. The diagnosis of hypertension requires the measurement of two elevated blood pressures, at least 6 h apart. Hypertension during pregnancy is usually caused by preeclampsia, chronic hypertension, gestational hypertension, or renal disease.

PREECLAMPSIA Approximately 5 to 7% of all pregnant women develop *preeclampsia*, the new onset of hypertension (blood pressure > 140/90 mmHg), proteinuria (>300 mg per 24 h), and pathologic edema. Although the precise placental factors that cause preeclampsia are unknown, the end result is vasospasm and endothelial injury in multiple organs. Preeclampsia is associated with abnormalities of cerebral circulatory autoregulation, which increase the risk of stroke at near-normal blood pressures. Risk factors for the development of preeclampsia include nulliparity, diabetes mellitus, a history of renal disease or chronic hypertension, a prior history of preeclampsia, extremes of maternal age (>35 years or <15 years), obesity, factor V Leiden mutation, angiotensinogen gene T235, antiphospholipid antibody syndrome, and multiple gestation.

There are no well-established strategies for the prevention of preeclampsia. Clinical trials have demonstrated that low-dose aspirin treatment does *not* prevent preeclampsia in either low- or high-risk women. Two meta-analyses reported that dietary calcium supplementation appeared to be effective in reducing the risk of developing preeclampsia. Subsequently, however, a large randomized clinical trial in low-risk women did not demonstrate a protective effect of calcium supplementation. Therefore, calcium supplementation may be considered in women at high risk for preeclampsia (see above). The observation that dietary intervention may reduce the risk of hypertension in men and nonpregnant women raises the possibility that dietary manipulations will be discovered that reduce the risk of preeclampsia.

Severe preeclampsia is the presence of new-onset hypertension and proteinuria accompanied by central nervous system dysfunction (headaches, blurred vision, seizures, coma), marked elevations of blood pressure (>160/110 mmHg), severe proteinuria (>5 g per 24 h), oliguria or renal failure, pulmonary edema, hepatocellular injury (ALT > 2× the upper limits of normal), thrombocytopenia (platelet count < 100,000/μL), or disseminated intravascular coagulation. Women with *mild preeclampsia* are those with the diagnosis of new-onset hypertension, proteinuria, and edema without evidence of severe preeclampsia. The *HELLP* (*h*emolysis, *e*levated *l*iver enzymes, *l*ow *p*latelets) syndrome is a special subgroup of severe preeclampsia and is a major cause of morbidity and mortality in this disease. The presence of platelet dysfunction and coagulation disorders further increases the risk of stroke.

℞ **TREATMENT**   Preeclampsia resolves within a few weeks after delivery. For pregnant women with preeclampsia prior to 37 weeks' gestation, delivery reduces the mother's morbidity but exposes the fetus to the risk of premature delivery. The management of preeclampsia is challenging because it requires the clinician to balance the health of both mother and fetus simultaneously and to make management decisions that afford both the best opportunities for infant survival. In general, prior to term, women with *mild* preeclampsia can be managed conservatively with bed rest, close monitoring of blood pressure and renal function, and careful fetal surveillance. For women with *severe* preeclampsia, delivery is recommended after 32 weeks' gestation. This reduces maternal morbidity and slightly increases the risks associated with prematurity for the newborn. Prior to 32 weeks' gestation, the risks of prematurity for the fetus are great, and some authorities recommend conservative management to allow for continued fetal maturation. Expectant management of severe preeclampsia remote from term affords some benefits for the fetus with significant risks for the mother. Such management should be restricted to tertiary care centers where maternal-fetal medicine, neonatal medicine, and critical care medicine expertise are available.

The definitive treatment of preeclampsia is delivery of the fetus and placenta. For women with severe preeclampsia, aggressive management of blood pressures > 160/110 mmHg reduces the risk of cerebrovascular accidents.

Intravenous labetalol or hydralazine are the drugs most commonly used to manage preeclampsia. Alternative agents such as calcium channel blockers may be used. Elevated arterial pressure should be reduced slowly to avoid hypotension and a decrease in blood flow to the fetus. *Angiotensin-converting enzyme (ACE) inhibitors as well as angiotensin-receptor blockers should be avoided in the second and third trimesters of pregnancy because of their adverse effects on fetal development.* Pregnant women treated with ACE inhibitors often develop oligohydramnios, which may be caused by decreased fetal renal function.

Magnesium sulfate is the treatment of choice for the prevention and treatment of eclamptic seizures. Two large randomized clinical trials have demonstrated the superiority of magnesium sulfate over phenytoin and diazepam. Magnesium may prevent seizures by interacting with *N*-methyl-D-asparate (NMDA) receptors in the central nervous system. Given the difficulty of predicting eclamptic seizures on the basis of disease severity, it is recommended that once the decision to proceed with delivery is made, all patients carrying a diagnosis of preeclampsia be treated with magnesium sulfate (see Guideline).

CHRONIC ESSENTIAL HYPERTENSION   Pregnancy complicated by chronic essential hypertension is associated with intrauterine growth restriction and increased perinatal mortality. Pregnant women with chronic hypertension are at increased risk for superimposed preeclampsia and abruptio placenta. Women with chronic hypertension should have a thorough prepregnancy evaluation, both to identify remediable causes of hypertension and to ensure that the

Regimens for the Administration of Magnesium Sulfate for Seizure Prophylaxis in Women in Labor with Preeclampsia	
Intramuscular	**Intravenous**
10 g (5 g IM deep in each buttock)[a]	6-g bolus over 15 min
5 g IM deep q4h, alternating sides	1–3 g/h by continuous infusion pump
	May be mixed in 100 mL crystalloid; if given by intravenous push, make up as 20% solution; push at maximum rate of 1g/min
	40-g $MgSO_4 \cdot 7H_2O$ in 1000 mL Ringers lactate; run at 25–75 mL/h (1–3 g/h)[a]

[a] Made up as 50% solution

prescribed antihypertensive agents are not associated with adverse pregnancy outcome (e.g., ACE inhibitors, angiotensin-receptor blockers). α-Methyldopa and labetalol are the most commonly used medications for the treatment of chronic hypertension in pregnancy. Baseline evaluation of renal function is necessary to help differentiate the effects of chronic hypertension versus superimposed preeclampsia should the hypertension worsen during pregnancy. There are no convincing data that demonstrate that treatment of mild chronic hypertension improves perinatal outcome.

GESTATIONAL HYPERTENSION   This is the development of elevated blood pressure during pregnancy or in the first 24 h post partum in the absence of preexisting chronic hypertension and other signs of preeclampsia. Uncomplicated gestational hypertension that does not progress to preeclampsia has not been associated with adverse pregnancy outcome or adverse long-term prognosis.

RENAL DISEASE (See also Chap. 268)

Normal pregnancy is characterized by an increase in glomerular filtration rate and creatinine clearance. This occurs secondary to a rise in renal plasma flow and increase glomerular filtration pressures. Patients with underlying renal disease and hypertension may expect a worsening of hypertension during pregnancy. If superimposed preeclampsia develops, the additional endothelial injury results in a capillary leak syndrome that may make the management of these patients challenging. In general, patients with underlying renal disease and hypertension benefit from more aggressive management of blood pressure than do those with gestational hypertension. Preconception counseling is also essential for these patients so that accurate risk assessment can occur prior to the establishment of pregnancy and important medication changes and adjustments be made. In general, a prepregnancy serum creatinine level <133 μmol/L (<1.5 mg/dL) is associated with a favorable prognosis. When renal disease worsens during pregnancy, close collaboration between the nephrologist and the maternal-fetal medicine specialist is essential so that decisions regarding delivery can be weighed in the context of sequelae of prematurity for the neonate versus long-term sequelae for the mother with respect to future renal function.

Successful pregnancy after renal transplantation has been reported increasingly. Predictors for success include a normal-functioning transplanted kidney, absence of rejection for at least 2 years prior to the pregnancy, absence of hypertension, and preferably minimal doses of immunosuppressant medications. Pregnancies in women using cyclosporine are more likely to be complicated by renal insufficiency and/or the development of hypertension. Such patients require very careful maternal and fetal surveillance. Nearly half of these pregnancies deliver preterm, and 20% of neonates are small for their gestational age. Rejection occurs in approximately 10% of pregnancies, and approximately 15% of patients will have deterioration in their renal function that persists after delivery. While pregnancy is generally well tolerated in renal transplant recipients, controversy remains as to whether or not deterioration of graft function is accelerated by pregnancy. More aggressive management of blood pressure has been suggested in this group of patients in an effort to protect the grafted kidney.

Another subset of patients with chronic renal disease and hypertension are those patients whose pregnancies are complicated by systemic lupus erythematosus (SLE) (Chap. 311). In the past, SLE was considered to be a contraindication to pregnancy. With improved understanding of the effects of SLE on pregnancy, and vice versa, and with improved pharmacologic methods for managing SLE, successful pregnancy outcome is likely. Good prognostic factors for establishment of pregnancy in the presence of SLE are as follows:

1. Disease quiescence > 6 months
2. Normal blood pressure (with or without medication)
3. Normal renal function [creatinine < 133 μmol/L (< 1.5 mg/dL)]
4. Absence of antiphospholipid antibodies
5. Minimal or no need for immunosuppressive drugs
6. Absence of prior adverse reproductive outcome

Previously a point of controversy, there is now increasing consensus that pregnancy and the postpartum period are times of increased lupus activity. In severe flares early in gestation, pregnancy termination is often recommended. If pregnancy termination is not an option, then medical therapy to manage the lupus flare should not be influenced by the pregnancy, provided informed consent for treatment is obtained from the patient. Pulsed glucocorticoid therapy, azathioprine, hydroxychloroquine, and cyclophosphamide have all been used successfully in pregnancy.

CARDIAC DISEASE

VALVULAR HEART DISEASE (See also Chap. 236) This is the most common cardiac problem complicating pregnancy.

Mitral Stenosis This is the valvular disease most likely to cause death during pregnancy. The pregnancy-induced increase in blood volume and cardiac output can cause pulmonary edema in women with mitral stenosis. Pregnancy associated with long-standing mitral stenosis may result in pulmonary hypertension. Sudden death has been reported when hypovolemia has been allowed to occur in this condition. Careful control of heart rate, especially during labor and delivery, minimizes the impact of tachycardia and reduced ventricular filling times on cardiac function. Pregnant women with mitral stenosis are at increased risk for the development of atrial fibrillation and other tachyarrythmias. Medical management of severe mitral stenosis and atrial fibrillation with digoxin and beta blockers is recommended. Balloon valvulotomy can be carried out during pregnancy.

Mitral Regurgitation and Aortic Regurgitation These are both generally well tolerated during pregnancy. The pregnancy-induced decrease in systemic vascular resistance reduces the risk of cardiac failure with these conditions. As a rule, mitral valve prolapse does not present problems for the pregnant patient and aortic stenosis, unless very severe, is also well tolerated. In the most severe cases of aortic stenosis, limitation of activity or balloon valvuloplasty may be indicated.

For women with artificial valves contemplating pregnancy, it is important that warfarin be stopped and heparin initiated prior to conception. Warfarin therapy during the first trimester of pregnancy has been associated with fetal chondrodysplasia punctata. In the second and third trimester of pregnancy, warfarin may cause fetal optic atrophy and mental retardation.

CONGENITAL HEART DISEASE (See also Chap. 234) The presence of a congenital cardiac lesion in the mother increases the risk of congenital cardiac disease in the newborn. Prenatal screening of the fetus for congenital cardiac disease with ultrasound is recommended. Atrial or ventricular septal defect is usually well tolerated during pregnancy in the absence of pulmonary hypertension, provided that the woman's prepregnancy cardiac status is favorable. Use of air filters on intravenous sets during labor and delivery in patients with intracardiac shunts is generally recommended.

OTHER CARDIAC DISORDERS Supraventricular tachycardia (Chap. 230) is a common cardiac complication of pregnancy. Treatment is the same as in the nonpregnant patient, and fetal tolerance of medications such as adenosine and calcium channel blockers is acceptable. When necessary, electrocardioversion may be performed and is generally well tolerated by mother and fetus.

Peripartum cardiomyopathy (Chap. 238) is a rare disorder of pregnancy associated with myocarditis, and its etiology remains unknown. Treatment is directed toward symptomatic relief and improvement of cardiac function. Many patients recover completely; others are left with a progressive dilated cardiomyopathy. Recurrence in a subsequent pregnancy has been reported, and women should be counseled to avoid pregnancy after a diagnosis of peripartum cardiomyopathy.

SPECIFIC HIGH RISK CARDIAC LESIONS **Marfan Syndrome** (See also Chap. 351) This is an autosomal dominant disease, associated with a high risk of maternal morbidity. Approximately 15% of pregnant women with Marfan syndrome develop a major cardiovascular manifestation during pregnancy, with almost all women surviving. An aortic root diameter <40 mm is considered to be associated with a favorable outcome of pregnancy. Prophylactic therapy with beta blockers has been advocated, although large-scale clinical trials in pregnancy have not been performed.

Pulmonary Hypertension (See also Chap. 260) Maternal mortality in the setting of severe pulmonary hypertension is high, and primary pulmonary hypertension is a contraindication to pregnancy. Termination of pregnancy may be advisable in these circumstances to preserve the life of the mother. In the Eisenmenger syndrome, i.e., the combination of pulmonary hypertension with right-to-left shunting due to congenital abnormalities (Chap. 234), maternal and fetal death occur frequently. Systemic hypotension may occur after blood loss, prolonged Valsalva maneuver, or regional anesthesia; sudden death secondary to hypotension is a dreaded complication. Management of these patients is challenging, and invasive hemodynamic monitoring during labor and delivery is generally recommended.

In patients with pulmonary hypertension, vaginal delivery is less stressful hemodynamically than Cesarean section, which should be reserved for accepted obstetric indications.

DEEP VENOUS THROMBOSIS AND PULMONARY EMBOLISM
(See also Chaps. 248 and 261)

A hypercoagulable state is characteristic of pregnancy, and deep venous thrombosis (DVT) is a common complication. Indeed, pulmonary embolism is the most common cause of maternal death in the United States. Activated protein C resistance caused by the factor V Leiden mutation increases the risk for DVT and pulmonary embolism during pregnancy. Approximately 25% of women with DVT during pregnancy carry the factor V Leiden allele. The presence of the factor V Leiden mutation also increases the risk for severe preeclampsia. If the fetus carries a factor V Leiden mutation, the risk of extensive placental infarction is very high. Additional genetic mutations associated with DVT during pregnancy include the prothrombin G20210A mutation (heterozygotes and homozygotes) and the methylenetetrahydrofolate reductase C677T mutation (homozygotes).

TREATMENT Aggressive diagnosis and management of DVT and suspected pulmonary embolism optimize the outcome for mother and fetus. In general, all diagnostic and therapeutic modalities afforded the nonpregnant patient should be utilized in pregnancy. Anticoagulant therapy with heparin is indicated in pregnant women with DVT. Warfarin therapy is contraindicated in the first trimester due to its association with fetal chondrodysplasia punctata. In the second and third trimesters, warfarin may cause fetal optic atrophy and mental retardation. In the initial treatment of DVT, heparin, which does not cross the placenta, may be administered as an intravenous bolus of approximately 100 IU per kilogram of body weight. Continuous heparin infusion is generally initiated at 1000 IU/h and then titrated to achieve a target activated partial thromboplastin time of 50 to 80 s. After initial intravenous anticoagulation, intermittent subcutaneous heparin therapy with 10,000 IU two or three times daily may be employed. When deep venous thromboembolism occurs in the postpartum period, heparin therapy for 7 to 10 days may be followed by warfarin therapy for 3 to 6 months. Warfarin is not contraindicated in breast-feeding women.

Low-molecular-weight heparins are of sufficient size and charge that they do not cross the placenta and may be substituted for unfractionated heparin in the pregnant patient. Recent concerns about low-molecular-weight heparin use and epidural hematoma suggest that caution be used in the anesthetic management of patients who had been receiving low-molecular-weight heparin near the onset of labor.

ENDOCRINE DISORDERS

DIABETES MELLITUS (See also Chap. 333)   In pregnancy, the fetoplacental unit induces major metabolic changes, the purpose of which is to shunt glucose and amino acids to the fetus while the mother uses ketones and triglycerides to fuel her metabolic needs. These metabolic changes are accompanied by maternal insulin resistance, caused in part by placental production of steroids, a growth hormone variant, and placental lactogen. Although pregnancy has been referred to as a state of accelerated starvation, it is better characterized as accelerated ketosis. In pregnancy, after an overnight fast, plasma glucose is lower by 0.8 to 1.1 mmol/L (15 to 20 mg/dL) than in the nonpregnant state. This is due to the use of glucose by the fetus. In early pregnancy, fasting may result in circulating glucose concentrations in the range of 2.2 mmol/L (40 mg/dL) and may be associated with symptoms of hypoglycemia. In contrast to the decrease in maternal glucose concentration, plasma hydroxybutyrate and acetoacetate levels rise to two to four times normal after a fast.

℞ TREATMENT   Pregnancy complicated by diabetes mellitus is associated with higher maternal and perinatal morbidity and mortality rates. Preconception counseling and treatment are important for the diabetic patient contemplating pregnancy. Optimizing preconception glucose control and attention to other dietary needs such as appropriate levels of folate can significantly reduce the risk of congenital fetal malformations. Folate supplementation reduces the incidence of fetal neural tube defects, which occur with greater frequency in fetuses of diabetic mothers. In addition, optimizing glucose control during key periods of organogenesis reduces other congenital anomalies including sacral agenesis, caudal dysplasia, renal agenesis, and ventricular septal defect.

Once pregnancy is established, glucose control should be managed more aggressively than in the nonpregnant state. In addition to dietary changes, this requires more frequent blood glucose monitoring and often involves additional injections of insulin or conversion to an insulin pump. Fasting blood glucose levels should be maintained at <5.8 mmol/L (<105 mg/dL) with no values exceeding 7.8 mmol/L (140 mg/dL). Commencing in the third trimester, regular surveillance of maternal glucose control as well as assessment of fetal growth (obstetric sonography) and fetoplacental oxygenation (fetal heart rate monitoring or biophysical profile) optimize pregnancy outcome. Pregnant diabetic patients without vascular disease are at greater risk for delivering a macrosomic fetus, and attention to fetal growth via clinical and ultrasound examinations is important. Fetal macrosomia is associated with an increased risk of maternal and fetal birth trauma. Pregnant women with diabetes have an increased risk of developing preeclampsia, and those with vascular disease are at greater risk for developing intrauterine growth restriction, which is associated with an increased risk of fetal and neonatal death. Excellent pregnancy outcomes in patients with diabetic nephropathy and proliferative retinopathy have been reported with aggressive glucose control and intensive maternal and fetal surveillance.

Glycemic control may become more difficult to achieve as pregnancy progresses. Because of delayed pulmonary maturation of the fetuses of diabetic mothers, early delivery should be avoided unless there is biochemical evidence of fetal lung maturity. In general, efforts to control glucose and maintain the pregnancy until the estimated date of delivery result in the best overall outcome for both mother and newborn.

GESTATIONAL DIABETES   All pregnant women should be screened for gestational diabetes unless they are in a low-risk group. Women at low risk for gestational diabetes are those <25 years of age; those with a body mass index < 25 kg/m², no maternal history of macrosomia or gestational diabetes, and no diabetes in a first-degree relative; and those not members of a high-risk ethnic group (African American, Hispanic, Native American). A typical two-step strategy for establishing the diagnosis of gestational diabetes involves administration of a 50-g oral glucose challenge with a single serum glucose measurement at 60 min. If the serum glucose is < 7.8 mmol/L (<140 mg/dL), the test is considered normal. Serum glucose > 7.8 mmol/L (>140 mg/dL) warrants administration of a 100-g oral glucose challenge with serum glucose measurements obtained in the fasting state, and at 1, 2, and 3 h. Normal values are serum glucose concentrations <5.8 mmol/L (<105 mg/dL), 10.5 mmol/L (190 mg/dL), 9.1 mmol/L (165 mg/dL), and 8.0 mmol/L (145 mg/dL), respectively.

Pregnant women with gestational diabetes are at increased risk of preeclampsia, delivering infants who are large for their gestational age, and birth lacerations. Their fetuses are at risk of hypoglycemia and birth trauma (brachial plexus) injury.

℞ TREATMENT   Gestational diabetes is first treated with dietary measures. Inability to maintain fasting glucose concentrations <5.8 mmol/L (<105 mg/dL) or 2-h postprandial glucose concentrations <6.7 mmol/L (<120 mg/dL) should prompt initiation of insulin therapy. Oral agents should not be used to treat diabetes in pregnancy. Patients with a diagnosis of gestational diabetes will benefit from postpartum follow-up as they are at increased risk for developing type 2 diabetes.

THYROID DISEASE (See also Chap. 330)   In pregnancy, the estrogen-induced increase in thyroxine-binding globulin causes an increase in circulating levels of total T_3 and total T_4. The normal range of circulating levels of free T_4, free T_3, and thyroid stimulating hormone (TSH) remain unaltered by pregnancy.

The thyroid gland normally enlarges during pregnancy. Maternal hyperthyroidism occurs at a rate of approximately 2 per 1000 pregnancies and is generally well tolerated by pregnant women. Clinical signs and symptoms should alert the physician to the occurrence of this disease. Many of the physiologic adaptations to pregnancy may mimic subtle signs of hyperthyroidism. Although pregnant women are able to tolerate mild hyperthyroidism without adverse sequelae, more severe hyperthyroidism can cause spontaneous abortion or premature labor, and thyroid storm is associated with a significant risk of maternal mortality.

℞ TREATMENT   *Hyperthyroidism* in pregnancy should be aggressively evaluated and treated. The treatment of choice is propylthiouracil. Because it crosses the placenta, the minimum effective dose should be used to maintain free T_4 in the upper normal range. Methimazole crosses the placenta to a greater degree than propylthiouracil and has been associated with fetal aplasia cutis. Radioiodine should not be used during pregnancy, either for scanning or treatment, because of effects on the fetal thyroid. In emergent circumstances, additional treatment with beta blockers and a saturated solution of potassium iodide may be necessary. Hyperthyroidism is most difficult to control in the first trimester of pregnancy and easiest to control in the third trimester.

The goal of therapy for *hypothyroidism* is to maintain the serum TSH in the normal range, and thyroxine is the drug of choice. Children born to women with an elevated serum TSH (and a normal total thyroxine) during pregnancy have impaired performance on neuropsychologic tests. During pregnancy, the dose of thyroxine required to keep the TSH in the normal range rises. In one study, the mean replacement dose of thyroxine required to maintain the TSH in the normal range was 0.1 mg daily before pregnancy, and it increased to 0.15 mg daily during pregnancy.

DISORDERS OF CALCIUM METABOLISM (See also Chap. 340)   Serum *total* calcium concentration decreases throughout gestation due to a reduction in serum albumin concentration, while serum *ionized* calcium remains unchanged during pregnancy. Circulating parathyroid hormone concentration is slightly reduced throughout the course of pregnancy. Pregnancy has been described as a state of physiologic absorptive hypercalciuria. Estrogen and increased production of 1,25-dihydroxyvitamin D by both the kidney and the placenta mediate the increased absorption of calcium during pregnancy. Due to the fetal requirements for calcium, the National Institutes of Health has recommended that pregnant women receive 1500 mg/d of elemental calcium, slightly higher than the recommended daily intake of 1200 mg/d for nonpregnant adults.

HEMATOLOGIC DISORDERS

Pregnancy has been described as a state of physiologic anemia. Part of the reduction in hemoglobin concentration is dilutional, but iron and folate deficiencies are the major causes of correctable anemia during pregnancy. Folic acid food supplementation implemented in 1998 has reduced the risk of fetal neural tube defects.

In populations at high risk for hemoglobinopathies (Chap. 106), hemoglobin electrophoresis should be performed as part of the prenatal screen. Hemoglobinopathies can be associated with increased maternal and fetal morbidity and mortality. Management is tailored to the specific hemoglobinopathy and is generally the same for both pregnant and nonpregnant women. Prenatal diagnosis of hemoglobinopathies in the fetus is readily available and should be discussed with prospective parents either prior to or early in pregnancy.

Thrombocytopenia occurs commonly during pregnancy. The majority of cases are benign gestational thrombocytopenias, but the differential diagnosis should include immune thrombocytopenia (Chap. 116) and preeclampsia. Maternal thrombocytopenia may also be caused by catastrophic obstetric events such as retention of a dead fetus, sepsis, abruptio placenta, and amniotic fluid embolism.

NEOPLASTIC DISEASES

Maternal neoplasms are rarely, if ever, transmitted to the fetus. The three most common cancers in pregnant women are cervical cancer (~1 case per 1000 pregnancies, depending on the country), breast cancer (~2 cases per 10,000 pregnancies), and lymphomas (Hodgkin's disease or non-Hodgkin's lymphomas). Cervical cancer may be missed when its early sign, vaginal bleeding, is attributed to the pregnancy. Pregnant women with vaginal bleeding should be examined, and suspicious cervical lesions biopsied. Conization is generally performed only after the first trimester because of the abortion risk.

Breast lumps may also be attributed to change associated with pregnancy. However, women with a dominant mass should undergo diagnostic evaluation (mammogram, ultrasound, biopsy). Resection of the primary lesion is safe, but radiation therapy is unsafe at any time during pregnancy. The fetus cannot be shielded from internal scattering of radiation; therapeutic doses are associated with spontaneous abortion, increased perinatal death, and defects in central nervous system and/or cognitive function. Tamoxifen is not safe for pregnant women.

Lymphoma is usually diagnosed on the basis of adenopathy or constitutional symptoms (fever, sweats, or weight loss). Staging eval-

uation is not undertaken during the first trimester; women in the first trimester should be counseled about termination of the pregnancy. Single-agent chemotherapy can be used in the second or third trimester as a temporizing measure. Vinblastine or doxorubicin have been used most commonly. Early induction of labor may permit the physician to maximize the survival chances of both the fetus and the mother. Survival rates for 28-week-old fetuses are about 75% and about 90% for 32-week-old fetuses.

Cancer survivors of reproductive age may desire children. Pregnancy may increase the risk of melanoma recurrence but does not influence breast cancer recurrence. Cancer treatment may deplete oocytes. Oocyte retrieval and storage of fertilized or nonfertilized eggs before cancer treatment may permit conception after the cancer has been treated successfully.

GASTROINTESTINAL AND LIVER DISEASE

Up to 90% of pregnant women experience nausea and vomiting during the first trimester of pregnancy. Occasionally, hyperemesis gravidarum requires hospitalization to prevent dehydration, and sometimes parenteral nutrition is required.

Crohn's disease may be associated with exacerbations in the second and third trimesters. Ulcerative colitis is associated with disease exacerbations in the first trimester and during the early postpartum period. Medical management of these diseases during pregnancy is identical to the management in the nonpregnant state (Chap. 287).

Exacerbation of gall bladder disease is commonly observed during pregnancy. In part this may be due to pregnancy-induced alteration in the metabolism of bile and fatty acids. Intrahepatic cholestasis of pregnancy is generally a third-trimester event. Profound pruritus may accompany this condition and may be associated with increased fetal mortality. It has been suggested that placental bile salt deposition may contribute to progressive uteroplacental insufficiency. Therefore, regular fetal surveillance should be undertaken once the diagnosis of intrahepatic cholestasis is made. Favorable results with ursodiol have been reported.

Acute fatty liver is a rare complication of pregnancy. Frequently confused with the HELLP syndrome (see "Preeclampsia," above) and severe preeclampsia, the diagnosis of acute fatty liver of pregnancy may be facilitated by imaging studies and laboratory evaluation. Acute fatty liver of pregnancy is generally characterized by markedly increased levels of bilirubin and ammonia and by hypoglycemia. Management of acute fatty liver of pregnancy is supportive; recurrence in subsequent pregnancies has been reported.

All pregnant women should be screened for hepatitis B. This information is important for pediatricians after delivery of the infant. All infants receive hepatitis B vaccine. Infants born to mothers who are carriers of hepatitis B surface antigen should also receive hepatitis B immune globulin as soon after birth as possible and preferably within the first 72 h.

INFECTIONS

BACTERIAL INFECTIONS   Other than bacterial vaginosis, the most common bacterial infections during pregnancy involve the urinary tract (Chap. 280). Many pregnant women have asymptomatic bacteriuria, most likely due to stasis caused by progestational effects on ureteral and bladder smooth muscle and to compression effects of the enlarging uterus. In itself, this condition is not associated with an adverse outcome of pregnancy. However, if asymptomatic bacteriuria is left untreated, symptomatic pyelonephritis may occur. Indeed, approximately 75% of cases of pregnancy-associated pyelonephritis are the result of untreated asymptomatic bacteriuria. All pregnant women should be screened with a urine culture for asymptomatic bacteriuria at the first prenatal visit. Subsequent screening with nitrite/leukocyte esterase strips is indicated for high-risk women, such as those with sickle cell trait or a history of urinary tract infections. All women with positive screens should be treated.

Because of the association between bacterial vaginosis and preterm delivery, screening for bacterial vaginosis has been used in an effort to reduce risk. However, standard treatment for bacterial vaginosis does not reduce the risk of preterm delivery.

Abdominal pain and fever during pregnancy create a clinical dilemma. The diagnosis of greatest concern is intrauterine amniotic infection. While amniotic infection most commonly follows rupture of the membranes, this is not always the case. In general, antibiotic therapy is not recommended as a temporizing measure in these circumstances. If intrauterine infection is suspected, induced delivery with concomitant antibiotic therapy is generally indicated. Intrauterine amniotic infection is most often caused by pathogens such as *Escherichia coli* and group B streptococcus. In high-risk patients at term or in preterm patients, routine intrapartum prophylaxis of group B streptococcal disease is recommended. Penicillin G and ampicillin are the drugs of choice. In penicillin-allergic patients, clindamycin is recommended.

Postpartum infection is a significant cause of maternal morbidity and mortality. While rare after vaginal delivery, postpartum endomyometritis develops in 5% of patients having elective repeat cesarean section and in 25% of patients after emergency cesarean section following prolonged labor. Prophylactic antibiotics should be given to all patients undergoing cesarean section. As most cases of postpartum endomyometritis are polymicrobial, broad-spectrum antibiotic coverage with a penicillin, aminoglycoside, and metronidazole is recommended (Chap. 167). Most cases resolve within 72 h. Women who do not respond to antibiotic treatment for postpartum endomyometritis should be evaluated for septic pelvic thrombophlebitis. Imaging studies may be helpful in establishing the diagnosis, which is primarily a clinical diagnosis of exclusion. Patients with septic pelvic thrombophlebitis generally have tachycardia out of proportion to their fever and respond rapidly to intravenous administration of heparin.

All patients are screened prenatally for gonorrhea and chlamydial infections, and the detection of either should result in prompt treatment. Ceftriaxone and azithromycin are the agents of choice (Chaps. 147 and 179).

VIRAL INFECTIONS Cytomegalovirus Infection   Viral infection in pregnancy presents a significant challenge. The most common cause of congenital viral infection in the United States is cytomegalovirus (CMV) (Chap. 185). As many as 50 to 90% of women of childbearing age have antibodies to CMV, but only rarely does CMV reactivation result in neonatal infection. More commonly, primary CMV infection during pregnancy creates a risk of congenital CMV. No currently accepted treatment of CMV during pregnancy has been demonstrated to protect the fetus effectively. Moreover, it is impossible to predict which fetus will sustain life-threatening CMV infection. Severe CMV disease in the newborn is characterized most often by petechiae, hepatosplenomegaly, and jaundice. Chorioretinitis, microcephaly, intracranial calcifications, hepatitis, hemolytic anemia, and purpura may also develop. Central nervous system involvement resulting in the development of psychomotor, ocular, auditory, and dental abnormalities over time have been described.

Rubella (See also Chap. 195)   Rubella virus is a known teratogen; first-trimester rubella carries a high risk of fetal anomalies, though the risk decreases significantly later in pregnancy. Congenital rubella may be diagnosed by percutaneous umbilical blood sampling with the detection of IgM antibodies in fetal blood. All pregnant women should be screened for their immune status to rubella. Indeed, all women of childbearing age, regardless of pregnancy status, should have their immune status for rubella verified and be immunized if necessary. The incidence of congenital rubella in the United States is extremely low.

Herpesvirus (See also Chap. 182)   The acquisition of genital herpes during pregnancy is associated with spontaneous abortion, pre-

maturity, and congenital and neonatal herpes. A recent cohort study of pregnant women without evidence of previous herpes infection demonstrated that approximately 2% of the women acquired a new herpes infection during the pregnancy. Approximately 60% of the newly infected women had no clinical symptoms. Infection occurred equally in all three trimesters. If herpes seroconversion occurred early in pregnancy, the risk of transmission to the newborn was very low. In women who acquired genital herpes shortly before delivery, the risk of transmission was high. The risk of active genital herpes lesions at term can be reduced by prescribing acyclovir for the last 4 weeks of pregnancy to women who have had their first episode of genital herpes during the pregnancy. However, whether or not this strategy results in less viral shedding or enhanced fetal protection at delivery remains to be determined.

Herpesvirus infection in the newborn can be devastating. Disseminated neonatal herpes carries with it high mortality and morbidity rates from central nervous system involvement. It is recommended that pregnant women with active genital herpes lesions at the time of presentation in labor be delivered by cesarean section.

Parvovirus (See also Chap. 187)   Parvovirus infection (human parvovirus B19) may occur during pregnancy. It rarely causes sequelae, but susceptible women infected during pregnancy may be at risk for fetal hydrops secondary to erythroid aplasia and profound anemia.

Toxoplasmosis (See also Chap. 217)   In the United States, approximately 70% of women of childbearing age are susceptible to *Toxoplasma*. Most primary infections of toxoplasmosis in the United States come from eating undercooked meat. The diagnosis of congenital toxoplasmosis is possible through sampling of fetal umbilical blood. If there is no evidence of placental/fetal infection, single-drug treatment with spiramycin is recommended. Triple-drug therapy with spiramycin, pyrimethamine, and sulfa is recommended if there is evidence of fetal infection and the woman does not wish to terminate the pregnancy or cannot terminate it because of advanced gestational age. Prenatal treatment has been shown to reduce the number of infants with severe infection.

Human Immunodeficiency Virus (See also Chap. 309)   The predominant cause of HIV infection in children is transmission of the virus from the mother to the newborn during the perinatal period. Exposures, which increase the risk of mother-to-child transmission, include vaginal delivery, preterm delivery, trauma to the fetal skin, and maternal bleeding. Additionally, recent infection with high maternal viral load, low maternal CD4+T cell count, prolonged labor, prolonged length of membrane rupture, and the presence of other genital tract infections, such as syphilis or herpes, increase the risk of transmission. Breast feeding may also transmit HIV to the newborn and is therefore contraindicated in most developed countries for HIV-infected mothers. There is no clear evidence to suggest that the course of HIV disease is altered by pregnancy. There is also no clear evidence to suggest that uncomplicated HIV disease adversely impacts pregnancy other than by its inherent infection risk.

℞ **TREATMENT**   The majority of cases of mother-to-child (vertical) transmission of HIV-1 occur during the intrapartum period. Mechanisms of vertical transmission include infection after rupture of the membranes and direct contact of the fetus with infected secretions or blood from the maternal genital tract. In women with HIV infection who are not receiving antiretroviral therapy, the rate of vertical transmission is approximately 25%. Cesarean section and treatment with zidovudine, administered both before and during delivery, decrease the rate of vertical transmission. In a meta-analysis, zidovudine treatment of both the mother during the prenatal and intrapartum periods and of the neonate at birth reduced the risk of vertical transmission to 7.3%. The combination of elective cesarean section plus zidovudine treatment reduced the risk of vertical transmission to 2%. The role of multiple drug therapy during pregnancy has not yet been established, pending safety data for the neonate.

SUMMARY

Maternal mortality has decreased steadily during the past 60 years. The maternal death rate has decreased from nearly 600/100,000 live births in 1935 to 8.5/100,000 live births in 1996. The most common causes of maternal death in the United States today are, in decreasing order of frequency, thromboembolic disease, hypertension, ectopic pregnancy, and hemorrhage. With improved diagnostic and therapeutic modalities as well as with advances in the treatment of infertility, more patients with medical complications will be seeking, and be in need of, complex obstetric care. Improving outcome of pregnancy in these women will be best obtained by assembling a team of internists and specialists in maternal-fetal medicine (high-risk obstetrics) to counsel these patients about the risks of pregnancy and to plan their treatment prior to conception. The importance of preconception counseling cannot be overstated. It is the responsibility of all physicians caring for women in the reproductive age group to assess their patient's reproductive plans as part of their overall health evaluation.

BIBLIOGRAPHY

Brown ZA et al: The acquisition of herpes simplex virus during pregnancy. N Engl J Med 337:509, 1997

Caritis S et al: Low dose aspirin to prevent preeclampsia in women at high risk. N Engl J Med 338:701, 1998

Gleicher N (ed): *Principles and Practice of Medical Therapy in Pregnancy*, 3d ed. Stamford, CT, Appleton/Lange, 1998

Haddow JE et al: Maternal thyroid deficiency during pregnancy and subsequent neuropsychological development of the child. N Engl J Med 41:549, 1999

Hirsch DR et al: Pulmonary embolism and deep venous thrombosis during pregnancy or oral contraceptive use: Prevalence of factor V Leiden. Am Heart J 131:1145, 1996

International Perinatal HIV Group: The mode of delivery and the risk of vertical transmission of human immunodeficiency virus type 1—a meta-analysis of 15 prospective cohort studies. N Engl J Med 325:1371, 1999

Jones DC, Hayslett JP: Outcome of pregnancy in women with moderate or severe renal insufficiency. N Engl J Med 335:226, 1996

Lipscomb KJ et al: Outcome of pregnancy in women with Marfan's syndrome. Br J Obstet Gynecol 104:201, 1997

Mandel SJ et al: Increased need for thyroxine during pregnancy in women with primary hypothyroidism. N Engl J Med 323:91, 1990

Ridker PM et al: Factor V Leiden mutation as a risk factor for recurrent pregnancy loss. Ann Intern Med 128:1000, 1998

Scott LL et al: Acyclovir suppression to prevent cesarean delivery after first episode genital herpes. Obstet Gynecol 87:69, 1996

8

Mehul T. Dattani, Charles G. D. Brook

ADOLESCENT HEALTH PROBLEMS

Adolescence marks the transition from childhood to adulthood. It is a time of dramatic physical and psychological change. Adolescents are particularly prone to risk-taking behaviors. In the United States, 73% of deaths among adolescents and young adults result from motor vehicle and other accidents, homicide, and suicide. As a result of sexual maturation, adolescents begin to experiment sexually and, consequently, are susceptible to sexually transmitted diseases (STDs) and unwanted pregnancies. For adolescents with underlying disease, the psychological consequences can be as important as the physical disabilities; denial or resentment of disease is common and can hamper treatment. Adolescence is also a time when many lifelong health-relevant behaviors are established, including dietary habits, exercise patterns, tobacco and alcohol use, and interactions with the health care system. The physician, working together with parents, can help to guide adolescents through this dynamic period of life.

PUBERTY

Puberty encompasses (1) the adolescent growth spurt, (2) development of secondary sexual characteristics, (3) attainment of fertility, and (4) establishment of individual sexual identity.

There is wide variation in the timing of puberty. Signs of puberty are first evident between 9 and 14 years of age (mean 11.5) in 95% of American boys (Fig. 8-1A). In girls, puberty begins earlier, with 95% of American girls entering puberty between 8 and 12 years of age (mean 10.5) (Fig. 8-1B). The age of menarche in girls from developed countries has decreased by approximately 2 to 3 months per decade over the past 100 to 150 years. This trend is likely the result of improvements in socioeconomic conditions, nutritional status, and general health and well-being. Currently in the United States, the average age of menarche is 12.8 years. Genetic factors also influence the course of puberty. Data from twin studies indicate that the average age of

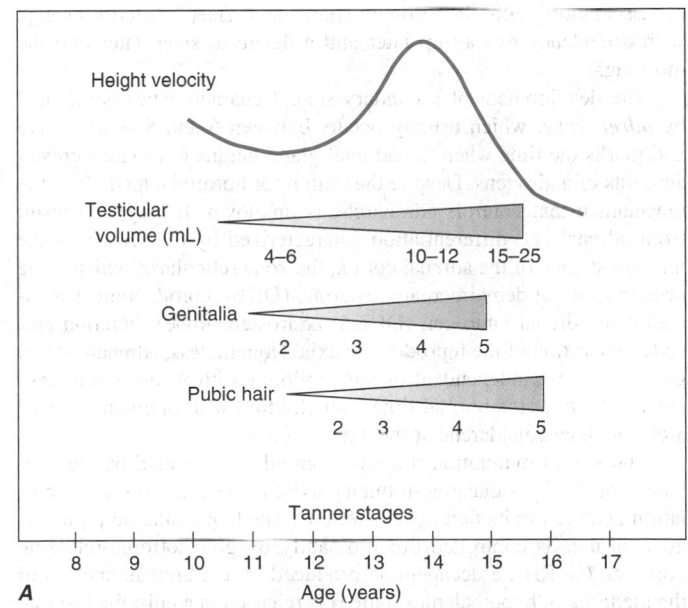

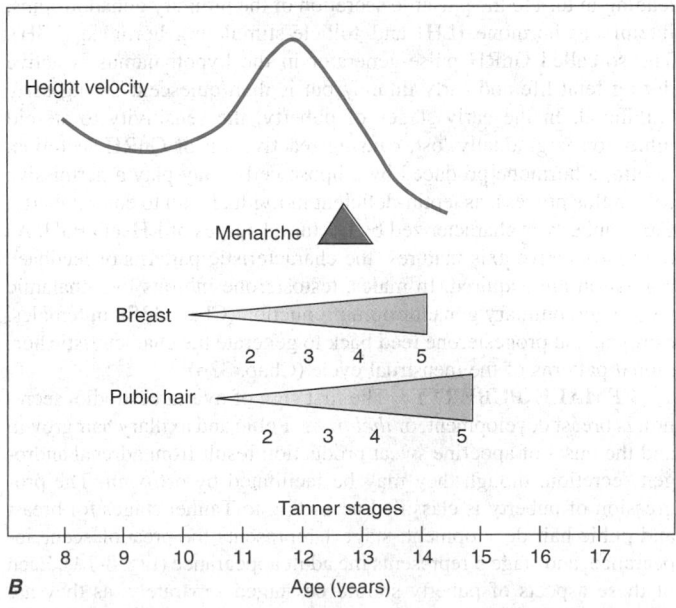

FIGURE 8-1 *A.* Pubertal events in males. Sexual maturity ratings for genitalia and pubic hair and divided into five stages *(From Marshall and Tanner, 1970).* *B.* Pubertal events in females. Sexual maturity ratings for breast development and pubic hair are divided into five stages *(From Marshall and Tanner, 1969).*

menarche is more similar in identical twin sisters than in nonidentical twins. Secondary sexual development occurs earlier in girls of Asian and African-Caribbean heritage than in girls of European heritage. Recognition of the progressively earlier onset of puberty, the ethnic variations, and wide age distribution in the timing of puberty is important for identifying precocious or delayed puberty and for counseling adolescents and parents about the natural course of physiologic changes.

HORMONAL CHANGES Puberty is accompanied by dramatic changes in multiple hormonal systems including alterations in adrenal steroid production, maturation of the reproductive axis, and increased production and action of growth hormone (GH). Serum GH levels increase early in puberty as a consequence of the rise in gonadal steroids. GH in turn increases the level of insulin-like growth factor 1 (IGF-1), which enhances linear bone growth (Chap. 328). The prolonged pubertal exposure to gonadal steroids ultimately causes epiphyseal closure and limits further bone growth. Appetite increases in association with the growth spurt, and sleep patterns change with a tendency to stay up later and a desire to sleep later into the morning.

The development of secondary sexual characteristics is initiated by *adrenarche*, which usually occurs between 6 and 8 years of age and marks the time when the adrenal gland begins to produce greater amounts of androgens. Despite the search for hormonal mediators, the mechanism that controls adrenarche is unknown. It may well result from adrenal cell differentiation, characterized by the growth of the innermost zone of the adrenal cortex, the zona reticularis, which is the principal site of dehydroepiandrosterone (DHEA) production. The increase in adrenal androgen (DHEA, androstenedione) secretion precedes activation of the reproductive axis. Nonetheless, adrenarche and gonadarche are independent events: children with Addison's disease enter puberty at the normal time, and children with premature adrenarche achieve gonadarche at the expected age.

The sexual maturation process is greatly accelerated by the activation of the hypothalamic-pituitary axis, leading to gonadal stimulation and the production of sex steroids. The hypothalamic-pituitary-gonadal axis is controlled predominantly by gonadotropin-releasing hormone (GnRH), a decapeptide produced by the arcuate nucleus of the mediobasal hypothalamus. GnRH is released in a pulsatile fashion, leading in turn to the pulsatile secretion of the pituitary gonadotropins, luteinizing hormone (LH) and follicle-stimulating hormone (FSH). The so-called GnRH pulse-generator in the hypothalamus is active during fetal life and early infancy but is then quiescent during early childhood. In the early stages of puberty, the sensitivity to steroid inhibition is gradually lost, causing reactivation of GnRH secretion. Leptin, a hormone produced by adipose cells, may play a permissive role in this process, as leptin-deficient individuals fail to enter puberty. Early puberty is characterized by nocturnal surges of LH and FSH. As the reproductive axis matures, the characteristic patterns of feedback regulation are acquired. In males, testosterone inhibits hypothalamic GnRH and pituitary gonadotropin production (Chap. 335); in females, estrogen and progesterone feed back to generate the characteristic hormonal patterns of the menstrual cycle (Chap. 336).

FEMALE PUBERTY The first sign of ovarian estradiol secretion is breast development, or *thelarche*. Pubic and axillary hair growth and the onset of apocrine sweat production result from adrenal androgen secretion, though they may be facilitated by estrogen. The progression of puberty is classified according to Tanner stages for breast and pubic hair development: stage 1 represents the preadolescent appearance, and stage 5 represents the adult appearance (Fig. 8-1*A*). Each of these aspects of puberty should be staged separately, as they are controlled by different underlying endocrine mechanisms. Concurrent with these outward signs of puberty are the changes in the size and shape of the uterus. The pubertal growth spurt is dependent on estradiol secretion, which leads to increased GH secretion. This in turn results in a doubling of the growth rate, and peak height velocity is usually coincident with breast stage 3. After menarche, a girl usually grows only an additional 5 cm.

MALE PUBERTY In boys, growth of the testes is usually the first sign of puberty, reflecting the effects of pulsatile gonadotropin secretion on seminiferous tubule volume and, to some degree, Leydig cell mass. Testosterone is converted to dihydrotestosterone by 5-α reductase. Both hormones act via the androgen receptor to induce growth of the external genitalia and pubic hair (Fig. 8-1; Chap. 338). The growth spurt in boys occurs at a testicular volume of about 10 to 12 mL (as measured by a Prader orchidometer). Testosterone also deepens the voice and increases muscle growth. Dihydrotestosterone stimulates prostate growth and beard growth and initiates recession of the temporal hairline. Although boys enter puberty approximately 6 to 12 months later than girls, they are potentially fertile at an earlier stage of puberty. Aromatization of testosterone to estradiol increases GH secretion, which acts synergistically with testosterone to induce a greater peak height velocity in boys than in girls.

DISORDERS OF PUBERTY *Precocious puberty* is usually defined as an early onset of puberty in boys younger than 9 years or in girls younger than 8 years of age. Some authorities suggest that the lower limits of normal in girls be revised downward to age 7 for Caucasians and age 6 for African-American girls. *Premature thelarche* refers to breast development in the absence of other signs of puberty. It occurs most commonly in girls between infancy and 3 years of age and usually resolves spontaneously. Causes of precocious puberty are divided into central *gonadotropin-dependent* forms and peripheral *gonadotropin-independent* forms (Table 8-1). Central precocious puberty is much more common in girls than in boys, and the majority of these cases involve idiopathic activation of spontaneous GnRH pulses. It

Table 8-1 Causes of Precocious and Delayed Puberty

I. Causes of precocious puberty
  A. Central (gonadotropin-dependent)
    1. Idiopathic
    2. CNS tumor or inflammatory states
    3. Hypothalamic hamartoma
  B. Peripheral (gonadotropin-independent)
    1. Females
      a. McCune-Albright syndrome
      b. Congenital adrenal hyperplasia
      c. Aromatase excess syndrome
      d. Exogenous estrogen
      e. Hypothyroidism
    2. Males
      a. Congenital adrenal hyperplasia
      b. Activating LH receptor mutations
      c. hCG-secreting tumor
      d. Exogenous androgens
      e. Hypothyroidism
II. Causes of pubertal delay
  A. Constitutional delay
  B. Chronic diseases (asthma, gastrointestinal problems, renal failure)
  C. Malnutrition
  D. Excessive exercise
  E. Anorexia nervosa
  F. Hypothalamic-pituitary causes of pubertal failure (low gonadotropins)
    1. Congenital defects (Kallmann syndrome, congenital adrenal hypoplasia, pituitary hypoplasia)
    2. CNS tumors and their treatment (radiotherapy and surgery)
    3. Hemochromatosis
  G. Gonadal causes of pubertal failure (elevated gonadotropins)
    1. Females
      a. Chemotherapy or radiotherapy
      b. Turner syndrome
      c. Premature menopause
    2. Males
      a. Chemotherapy or radiotherapy
      b. Anorchia
      c. Bilateral undescended testes
      d. Orchitis

NOTE: CNS, central nervous system; hCG, human chorionic gonadotropin; LH, luteinizing hormone.

can also be caused by a variety of central nervous system tumors, structural lesions, and inflammatory conditions.

Delayed puberty is defined as the 3% of girls and boys who have not developed the first signs of puberty by 13.2 and 14.2 years, respectively. It is most commonly due to delayed activation of the hypothalamic-pituitary-gonadal axis (Table 8-1). Most individuals who meet this definition will progress through puberty normally, but at a later age. Short stature and delayed skeletal maturation are commonly seen in association with delayed puberty. Growth delay may have been evident earlier in childhood; the diagnosis of *constitutional delay of growth and puberty* can be suspected from a delayed bone age in a short child who is otherwise well. Individuals who experience delays in puberty may be emotionally as well as physically immature relative to their peers.

The main diagnostic challenge in delayed puberty is to distinguish those with constitutional delay, who will progress through puberty at a later age, from those with an underlying pathologic process. LH and FSH responses to GnRH do not differentiate constitutional delay from pathologic causes of *hypogonadotropic hypogonadism* (Chap. 335). Thus, constitutional delay is a diagnosis of exclusion and requires ongoing evaluation during development to assure that normal growth and development occur at a later time. Reassurance without hormonal treatment is appropriate for most individuals with presumed constitutional delay of puberty. Alternatively, an anabolic steroid (e.g., 50 to 100 mg per month testosterone enanthate, intramuscularly) in boys or estrogen (5 to 10 mg/d ethinyl estradiol, orally) in girls may be useful to induce growth and secondary sexual characteristics appropriate for age. Low-dose oral oxandrolone (2.5 mg/d), an anabolic steroid that is not aromatized to estrogen, is also used for boys because it does not accelerate skeletal maturation when used for short periods. After treatment for a year or more, hormonal treatments can be stopped and the function of the reproductive axis can be reassessed.

PSYCHOLOGICAL CHANGES AND SOCIAL FACTORS

The adolescent years are characterized by a multitude of psychological changes, including (1) the development of abstract thinking, (2) greater independence from family, (3) the formation of a personal and sexual identity, (4) the establishment of a system of values, and (5) an increase in socialization. For most adolescents, these transitions occur relatively smoothly. For others, however, these years can be frustrating and tumultuous; parents and clinicians must be attuned to the needs of those who show signs of struggling with emotional, sexual, and social issues.

Young people tend to share their feelings openly, one of which is ambivalence. These contradictory feelings most often involve both a desire for greater autonomy and, at the same time, a need to cling to the emotional and physical security provided by the family. Adolescents are granted increasing responsibilities but still lack some of the social and legal privileges of adults. This feature of adolescence can lead to conflict and challenges to parental authority.

Adolescents have a strong desire to establish an identity that is increasingly independent of the family. This new identity is strongly influenced by peer groups, some of which are institutionalized (e.g., team sports). Role confusion is quite common in adolescence, and some young people move from one intense allegiance to another with alarming speed. These transitional arrangements are eventually replaced by more permanent attachments to individuals.

In an attempt to alleviate some of the transitions associated with adolescence, many cultures have traditionally used "rites of passage" to acknowledge and accelerate an adolescent's evolution to adulthood. Among Native American Great Plains cultures, for example, a boy was sent away from the village at the time of puberty to fast and receive a vision from a spirit; upon returning to the community, he took his place among the adult men. Similarly, it was traditional in many societies for girls to be secluded at the time of the first menstruation before returning a "full-grown woman." These rites provide a public recognition of the end of childhood, and the ritual leaves the young

person with the conviction that he or she has undergone a personal transformation. A relative lack of these coming-of-age rituals in western cultures may contribute to the sense of alienation experienced by some adolescents in this part of the world.

During adolescence, gender identity must be renegotiated. Though prepubertal children have a relatively secure view of themselves as either a boy or a girl, experimentation with gender roles is a common feature of adolescence. For example, adolescents may explore, at least in fantasy, alternative gender roles (e.g., cross-dressing), homosexuality, or relationships with older men or women.

The hormonal changes of puberty influence behavior as well as causing physical changes. Rising levels of testosterone in boys and the increase in adrenal and ovarian androgens in girls increase libido. The mean age of sexual intercourse varies widely within and among cultures, but ranges between ages 15 and 18 for most groups. Boys generally report sexual intercourse about 1 year earlier than girls.

ADOLESCENT VIOLENCE

Adolescents and young adults are subject to much greater rates of violence, both as victims and perpetrators. Males are involved in violence much more commonly than females and account for >90% of homicides involving those 10 to 17 years of age. Ethnic and racial differences in rates of adolescent violence have been noted consistently. African Americans, Hispanics, and Native Americans are much more likely to be victims and perpetrators of lethal violence than are people of Asian or European ancestry. The origins of different rates of violence are complex. Higher rates of lethal aggression are associated with low socioeconomic status, high housing density, increased population turnover in neighborhoods, single-parent households, and socially disorganized communities. In many cases, these factors interact; increased violence leads to high population turnover and social disorganization.

Gangs represent a potentially volatile environment that is characterized by power struggles, initiation and detachment rituals, battles over territory, and escalating violence associated with retaliation. The increase in lethal violence has been attributed in part to easier access to firearms and a greater willingness to use firearms. A Centers for Disease Control and Prevention study in 1995 found that about one-fourth of students had carried a weapon to school during the preceding month and 8 to 10% had carried a gun. Many adolescents lack the abstract reasoning skills required to understand social mores and the consequence of gun use. Though firearms do not cause violence, handguns in particular provide a facile means to a lethal outcome; widespread reduction in access to handguns is essential to curb the current trend in adolescent homicide and serious injury.

Aggressive behavior can often be recognized in early childhood; bullying is a precursor to later antisocial behavior. Child abuse, antisocial parents, inadequate child-rearing practices, and dysfunctional interpersonal interactions between parents or among siblings are associated with aggressive behavior. The physician, along with teachers, clergy, and others in positions of authority, should be alert to a pattern of aggressive behavior or problems in the home. Though these issues are not easily remedied, appropriate interventions to improve family functioning and parenting may interrupt a pattern of violence, which is all too often perpetuated by the adolescent.

HEALTH PROBLEMS

Adolescence is generally a healthy period and is often accompanied by a feeling of immortality, which leads to risk-taking. When diseases of childhood or the consequences of their treatment extend into adolescence, or when disease strikes during adolescence, the sense of unfairness may be overwhelming. Anger and denial can lead to poor compliance with therapeutic regimens.

Table 8-2 Medical Disorders for Which Adolescents Are at Increased Risk

Cancer and hematologic disorders	Orthopedic disorders
Hodgkin's disease, lymphomas	Osteosarcoma, Ewing's sarcoma
Acute myelogenous leukemia, acute	Fractures
lymphoblastic leukemia	Legg-Calvé-Perthes disease (slipped capital
Ovarian cysts/cancer, testicular cancer	femoral epiphysis)
Survivors of childhood cancers, secondary	Osgood-Schlatter disease (osteochondrosis of
cancers	tibial tuberosity)
Sickle cell anemia	Scoliosis
Hemophilias	Rheumatologic disorders
Infectious diseases	Juvenile rheumatoid arthritis
Sexually transmitted diseases (see text)	Connective tissue diseases (e.g., systemic
HIV	lupus erythematosus)
Chlamydia, gonorrhea, syphilis	Vasculitis (e.g., Takayasu's arteritis,
Human papilloma virus	Kawasaki's disease)
Pelvic inflammatory disease	Endocrine disorders
Toxic shock syndrome	Type 1 diabetes mellitus
Meningococcal infection	Polycystic ovarian syndrome
Tuberculosis	Delayed puberty
Infectious mononucleosis	Turner syndrome
Pertussis	Klinefelter syndrome
Rubella	Graves' disease
Parvovirus	Neurologic disorders
Cardiac disorders	Becker muscular dystrophy
Survivors of congenital heart disease	Migraine headaches
Atrial septal defect, bicuspid aortic valve,	Temporal lobe epilepsy
pulmonary stenosis	Multiple sclerosis
Hypertrophic cardiomyopathy	Friedreich's ataxia
Marfan syndrome	Germinomas
Hypertension	Meningitis
Respiratory disorders	Psychiatric and behavioral disorders
Asthma	Depression
Cystic fibrosis	Substance abuse
Tobacco abuse	Antisocial behavior
Renal disorders	Excessive risk-taking
Survivors of childhood renal failure	Eating disorders
Glomerulonephritis, interstitial nephritis	
Gastrointestinal disorders	
Celiac disease	
Crohn's disease	

Relatively few diseases are unique to adolescents. Rather, diseases of childhood, including many inherited disorders and infectious diseases, extend into the adolescent period. Similarly, many of the disorders that affect teenagers are also seen in the adult population. The presentation and management of asthma, for example, is similar in adolescents and adults. Some of the diseases with relatively increased prevalence during adolescence are summarized in Table 8-2. These diseases should be borne in mind when considering the differential diagnosis. For example, when an adolescent presents with exertional chest pain, dyspnea, and syncope, hypertrophic cardiomyopathy or congenital heart disease should be considered as likely diagnoses, whereas coronary artery disease would be more likely in an adult.

SEXUALLY TRANSMITTED DISEASES Sexually active adolescents are at greater risk of acquiring STDs than their adult counterparts (Chap. 132). Prevention of STDs in adolescence depends on adequate sexual education coupled with access to appropriate clinical services. Early age of first sexual intercourse is associated with (1) an increased number of lifetime sexual partners; (2) an increased risk of acquiring chronic STDs, such as herpes simplex, HIV, and hepatitis B; and (3) cervical cancer in women. In addition, pelvic inflammatory disease in adolescent females increases the likelihood of future ectopic pregnancy, tubal infertility, and chronic pelvic inflammation. A low rate of barrier contraceptive use, combined with ignorance about the acquisition and prevention of infectious diseases, also contributes to the increased risk of STDs among adolescents. Screening for STDs is recommended in sexually active teens (Table 8-3). Adolescents with sexually transmitted infections, particularly those who deny sexual activity, may be victims of sexual abuse.

CHILD SEXUAL ABUSE Child sexual abuse is defined as the involvement of developmentally immature children and adoles-

cents in sexual activities they do not comprehend, to which they are unable to give consent, or that violate social taboos or family roles. In a U.S. study in 1985, sexual abuse during childhood was reported by 27% of adult females and 16% of adult males. Females are more likely than males to have been sexually abused by a family member. Although there is a paucity of literature on male sexual abuse, it is probably more common than generally recognized. The psychological trauma appears to be similar for boys and girls. Sexual abuse during adolescence may merge with peer sexual assault, or "date rape." Sexual abuse in adolescent girls can be associated with a constant fear of pregnancy. Teenage pregnancy or STD may, in fact, be the first indication of ongoing abuse.

Psychological consequences of child sexual abuse often involve behavioral problems, psychiatric disturbances, or adjustment difficulties at the onset of adolescence, even though the actual abuse may have taken place at a younger age. Child sexual abuse may lead to low self-esteem and/or a degree of sexual disinhibition. The cognitive maturation that occurs with adolescence may bring about the realization and expression of these feelings. Young women who have been sexually abused have significantly higher rates of early-onset consensual sexual activity, teenage pregnancy, multiple sexual partners, unprotected intercourse, STDs, and later sexual assault. Poor psychological outcome is related to the duration of abuse, the extent to which the abuse involves violence or coercion, and the perception that the child has cooperated with the abuser, with ensuing feelings of guilt. The impact of these sequelae can be reduced by supportive peer and family relationships. Disclosure of the abuse may help to ameliorate some of the psychological traumas associated with abuse.

SUBSTANCE ABUSE Substance abuse and drug misuse among adolescents is a significant cause of morbidity and mortality (Chaps. 386 to 389). The prevalence rates vary widely by region, ethnic group, age, and gender. The age of initiation into substance abuse has gradually declined. In 1997, rates among American teenagers for substance use or abuse, at some stage during their lifetimes, were: cigarettes smoking (70%), alcohol use (79%), marijuana use (47%), cocaine use (8%), anabolic steroids (4%), injected illegal drugs (2%), and other illegal drugs (17%), e.g., lysergic acid (LSD), phencyclidine (PCP), methylenedioxymethamphetamine (ecstasy), methamphetamine (ice), or heroin.

The forms of substance abuse change continuously. Anabolic steroids, for example, are now used by 3 to 5% of male high school seniors, with a 10% prevalence rate among male adolescent athletes. In addition to their use by athletes in an effort to increase muscle strength, nonathletes use anabolic steroids with a goal of achieving a more virile appearance. In contrast to popular views, anabolic steroids do not appear to enhance performance except at very high doses, which are associated with significant side effects (Chap. 335). Other performance-enhancing agents include human growth hormone and erythropoietin (EPO), but the high cost of these hormones limits their use.

In addition to the direct effect on health, substance abuse is associated with other risk-taking behaviors. The relationship of alcohol use and motor vehicle accidents, for example, is well documented. However, drug and alcohol use are also correlated with many other problems during adolescence including violence, suicide, depression, STD,

Table 8-3   Health Maintenance during Adolescence

History/counseling
  Review physical and psychological changes associated with puberty and adolescence
  Assess habits including tobacco, alcohol, anabolic steroids, illegal drugs
  Inquire about sexual activity and preference
  Review strategies to prevent unwanted pregnancies and STDs
  Provide guidance regarding injury prevention, particularly related to motor vehicles, sports and recreation, weapons
  Encourage development of health maintenance including diet and exercise
  Inquire regarding history of emotional, sexual, or physical abuse
  Review school attendance; assess decline in performance or evidence of learning disabilities
Examination
  Comprehensive physical examination at least every 3 years
  Evaluate progression of growth and puberty
  Yearly screening for hypertension[a]
  Yearly body mass index (BMI),[b] consider features of eating disorders
  Review symptoms and signs of depression or risk of suicide
Laboratory testing
  Screen for hyperlipidemia in those at increased risk[c]
  Screen sexually active adolescents for STDs,[d] including chlamydia, gonorrhea using urinary tests or pelvic examination; consider syphilis in those with other STDs
  HIV in those at increased risk (Chap. 309)
Immunizations[e] (Chaps. 122, 132)
  Review previous immunizations and tuberculin testing
  Measles/mumps/rubella (MMR), tetanus toxoid at age 11 to 12, if indicated
  Varicella vaccine, in the absence of childhood chickenpox
  Hepatitis B
  Influenza vaccine in those with underlying respiratory or cardiac disease

---

[a] See Update on the Task Force Report (1987) on High Blood Pressure in Children and Adolescents: A Working Group Report from the High Blood Pressure Education Program. NIH Publication No. 96-3790, 1996 (www.nhibi.nih.gov/health/prof/heart/hbp/hbp_ped.pdf).
[b] See Clinical guidelines on the identification, evaluation, and treatment of overweight and obesity in adults (www.nhibi.nih.gov/guidelines/obesity/ob_gdlns.pdf).
[c] See protocol developed by the Expert Panel on Blood Cholesterol Levels in Children and Adolescents (amhrt.org/Heart_and_Stroke_A_Z_Guide/cholk.html).
[d] See Centers for Disease Control and Prevention 1998 Guidelines for Treatment of Sexually Transmitted Diseases (aepo-xdv-www.epo.cdc.gov/wonder/prevguid/p0000480/body002.htm).
[e] See Centers for Disease Control and Prevention Recommendations of the Advisory Committee on Immunization Practices (ACIP) www.cdc.gov/nip/publications/ACIP-list.htm.
NOTE: STDs, sexually tansmitted diseases.
SOURCE: Adapted from Guidelines for Adolescent Preventive Services (GAPS) (www.ama-assn.org/adolhlth/recomend/monogrf1.htm)

and unwanted pregnancies. Therefore, the presence of one form of risky behavior should prompt consideration of others.

SUICIDAL BEHAVIOR AND DEPRESSION   After motor vehicle accidents and homicide, suicide is the third leading cause of death in adolescents, and the rate has risen almost fourfold over the past 50 years. In 1988, the suicide rate among 15- to 19-year olds was 11.3 in 100,000. The causes for increased rates of suicide are not well understood, but one theory holds that modern society fosters increased social isolation and alienation. Nearly one-fourth of adolescents acknowledge seriously considering suicide, and 8% have actually attempted it. Attempted suicide is three times more common in females than males, with drug overdose or wrist-cutting being the most common means of suicide attempt. Completed suicide is three to five times more common in teenage boys than girls and usually involves firearms, hanging, or jumping from heights. Suicide is rare before puberty. Risk factors for suicide among adolescents include prior attempt of suicide, a history of depression or other major psychiatric disorder, history of substance abuse, medical illness, family history of suicidal behavior, and knowing someone who has committed suicide. Unfortunately, these and other risk factors are relatively common among nonsuicidal youth as well, making suicide difficult to predict in individual cases. Stressful events can precipitate depression and increase risk of suicide; these can include the death of a relative or friend, disciplinary crisis,

rejection or humiliation, school difficulty, and anxiety about homosexuality. Apparently impulsive actions may be harbingers of more serious underlying mood disturbances, personality disorders, or substance abuse.

Major depression occurs in 4 to 6% of adolescents, and the *DSM-IV* criteria for diagnosis are the same as in adults (Chap. 385). Every depressed or suicidal adolescent should undergo psychiatric examination, whether hospitalized or not. Comprehensive evaluation requires exploration of the adolescent's history of mental health problems, symptoms of depression, level of functioning in school, interactions with friends and family, and evaluation for comorbid disorders. Indications for hospitalization include imminent risk of suicide as evidenced by an identified plan and access to lethal means, recurrent suicide attempts, the presence of severe depression or psychosis, substance abuse, and the need to remove the individual from an overwhelmingly stressful environment.

ADOLESCENT EATING DISORDERS   Many adolescents have voracious appetites in response to the increased energy and caloric requirements generated by the growth spurt. The unique physical, psychological, and social transitions of adolescence provide a context for the development and perpetuation of eating patterns. Adolescents with a body mass index (BMI), measured as weight (kg)/height (m²), greater than the 95th percentile for age and gender are overweight, and those between the 85th and 94th percentiles are at risk for becoming overweight. Based on the NHANES III survey for 1988 to 1994, there was evidence for a 6% increase in the prevalence of overweight adolescents compared to the previous decade. The increasing prevalence of obesity is multifactorial and involves patterns of eating behavior as well as alterations in activity level (Chap. 77). Physical activity among both girls and boys tends to decline steadily during adolescence. Regular involvement in enjoyable forms of exercise should be encouraged to help promote lifelong habits that involve physical activity.

Eating disorders such as anorexia nervosa or bulimia nervosa often have their onset during adolescence (Chap. 78). Control over dietary intake is perhaps one of the first mechanisms that adolescents use to establish autonomy and achieve independence from family. The majority of female adolescents and young adults in western cultures report feeling discontented with their body shape. Surveys of normal adolescent populations disclose a surprisingly high frequency of dieting and abnormal eating patterns. For instance, up to 79% binge, 70% consider themselves fat, 11% induce vomiting, 5% abuse laxatives, and about 3% meet diagnostic criteria for anorexia or bulimia nervosa. Eating disorders also occur in males, but much less frequently than in females.

PHYSICIAN–ADOLESCENT RELATIONSHIP

The transition from the pediatrician to an adult medical practice can be difficult for adolescents, their parents, and their physicians. The emergence of adolescent medicine as a specialty practice has helped to facilitate this transition and to focus on the special needs of this group. When adolescents transfer to an adult-based practice, the physician should first establish a relationship with the patient and his or her parents. Previous medical history should be reviewed and medical records obtained. The need for the teenager to be seen alone, and office policies concerning confidentiality, should be discussed and agreed to with the parent(s) and adolescent together.

Legal issues related to the medical care of minors arise frequently, and laws vary in different countries and from state to state (Chap. 2). As a general rule, anyone who has reached the age of majority (usually 18 years) may consent to treatment. Under this age, a parent or legal guardian must consent for medical intervention. However, there are several exceptions to this requirement. The delivery of medical care is generally accepted in an emergency, but it is important to document the nature of the emergency and any efforts to notify parents. Emancipated minors may also provide consent. This group includes those fulfilling adult roles (e.g., military service), married teens, and those who are financially independent and living separately from their parents. In addition, when the health of a minor is potentially endangered by disorders for which they may be reluctant to seek parental consent, such as substance abuse, pregnancy, or STD, mature minors may generally provide consent. In these circumstances, the caregiver must assess the minor's maturity, ability to understand the risks and benefits of treatment, and capacity to provide informed consent. Mature or emancipated minors do not need to reveal consent or treatment to their parents.

Obtaining a medical history from an adolescent includes many elements that are distinct from an adult history. It should include, for example, schoolwork, home environment, and relationships with parents, siblings, and peers. Adolescents often lack knowledge about medical issues and may be reluctant to discuss sensitive topics with authority figures. Most will be nervous, even when these issues do not pertain. It can be useful, therefore, to provide printed forms or questionnaires. These not only serve to gather information in a relatively nonthreatening manner but also provide an indication of the kinds of issues that might be discussed with the physician. It is difficult to predict the topics that are paramount to the adolescent. Some may be preoccupied with concerns about the onset of acne, whereas others fear HIV or pregnancy. Adolescents may harbor guilt about sexual abuse or feel overwhelmed by peer pressure to engage in certain activities. The physician is well positioned to assist with many of these issues, if there is trust and an indication of interest and understanding. Because of these types of questions, it is important to interview the adolescent in private. Some parents will resist this approach, but it is necessary if the adolescent is to volunteer information that he or she is unwilling to discuss in the presence of parents. It is useful to reinforce the fact that conversations will be kept confidential. Adolescents are sometimes willing to bring concerns to the attention of nurses or other caregivers before raising these issues with a physician. It is helpful, therefore, to have another health care provider interact with the patient, if only briefly. In addition to direct questioning, general conversation about topical issues or inquiries about school or peers may provide insight into an adolescent's interests, activities, and potential risk factors. Because of the prevalence of substance abuse, risk-taking behavior, suicide, sexual orientation crises, STDs, unwanted pregnancies, sexual abuse, depression, and eating disorders in the teenage years, these topics warrant specific inquiry as part of routine health assessment. The interview should also include adequate time for education, health care guidance, and counseling. It is also useful to provide written information about topics that are pertinent to the care of the adolescent.

The physical examination of the adolescent, while incorporating many elements of the adult examination, has several unique features. Foremost among these is the assessment of growth and sexual development. In addition to questionnaires that allow the adolescent an opportunity to self-assess stages of pubertal development, the examination can be made less stressful by using it as opportunity to explain normal physiology. The issue of when to perform a pelvic examination as part of the routine health maintenance is controversial. Some advocate pelvic examinations in all sexually active young women as a means to detect STDs and for Pap smears. With the advent of urinary screening tests for chlamydia and gonorrhea, others suggest that pelvic examinations are not routinely necessary in the absence of specific indications. When a pelvic examination is performed, the patient should be asked whether she prefers her mother or a member of the health care team as an observer. The physical examination should also focus on diseases that tend to present during adolescence (Table 8-2).

Disorders such as hypertension, hyperlipidemia, and obesity are often first detected during adolescence. Strategies for disease prevention also include immunization, avoidance of cigarette smoking or excessive alcohol use, establishing good dietary habits, and engaging in regular exercise. General guidelines for adolescent preventive services (GAPS) are summarized in Table 8-3.

SUMMARY

The term *adolescent* is derived from a Latin phrase meaning "to grow up." Adolescence is, in many ways, the culmination of development, with the achievement of identity and reproductive competence. Though these processes are triggered by internal physiologic events, they are intimately intertwined with the family and social environment. Physicians have an important role to facilitate these transitions by providing information and managing the diseases of adolescents. Moreover, it should be remembered that many adolescents view physicians as role models and will seek objective and informed advice about issues that reach beyond medicine.

BIBLIOGRAPHY

ELLIOTT DS et al: *Violence in American Schools: A New Perspective*. New York, Cambridge University Press, 1998

EMANS SJ et al: *Pediatric and Adolescent Gynecology*, 4th ed. Philadelphia, Lippincott-Raven, 1998

FINKELHOR D et al: Sexual abuse in a national survey of adult men and women: Prevalence, characteristics, and risk factors. Child Abuse Negl 14:19, 1990

GRUMBACH MM, STYNE DM: Puberty: Ontogeny, neuroendocrinology, physiology, and disorders, in *Williams Textbook of Endocrinology*, 9th ed, JD Wilson, DW Foster, HM Kronenberg, PR Larsen (eds). Philadelphia, Saunders, 1998, pp 1509–1625

Guidelines for adolescent preventive services (GAPS). Arch Pediatr Adolesc Med 51:123, 1997

JELLINEK MS, SNYDER JB: Depression and suicide in children and adolescents. Pediatr Rev 19:255, 1998

KANN L et al: Youth risk behavior surveillance—United States, 1997. MMWR CDC Surveill Summ 47:1, 1998

KAPLOWITZ PB et al: Reexamination of the age limit for defining when puberty is precocious in girls in the United States: Implications from evaluation and treatment. Pediatrics 104:936, 1999

MARSHALL WA, TANNER JM: Variations in pattern of pubertal changes in girls. Arch Dis Child 44:291, 1969

———, ———: Variations in the pattern of pubertal changes in boys. Arch Dis Child 45:13, 1970

SHAFER MB: Annual pelvic examination in the sexually active adolescent female: What are we doing and why are we doing it? J Adolesc Health 23:68, 1998

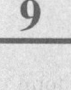

9   *Neil M. Resnick*

GERIATRIC MEDICINE

Of all the people who have ever lived to age 65, more than half are now alive. This statistic has important demographic and economic implications, and its impact on medical care is also substantial.

BIOLOGY OF AGING

Numerous molecular concomitants of aging have been described. For instance, there is an increase in chromosome structural abnormalities, DNA cross-linking, and frequency of single-strand breaks; a decline in DNA methylation; and loss of DNA telomeric sequences. The primary structure of proteins is unaltered, but posttranslational changes, such as deamidation, oxidation, cross-linking, and nonenzymatic glycation, increase. Mitochondrial structure also deteriorates, albeit not universally.

However, the biologic changes are clearer than the mechanisms that mediate them. In fact, although the senescent phenotype appears to be ubiquitous, biologists disagree about whether senescence even exists beyond zoos and civilized societies and whether it occurs at all in many species. There is little evolutionary rationale for a process that happens after reproduction is complete, particularly one associated with such a long and complex course. In nature, senescence is most notable for its absence; nearly all animals die of predation, disease, or environmental hazards rather than aging. The argument that different species have different maximum life spans can be explained without invoking a specific aging process: while growth and development are based on a genetic template, aging may reflect merely the accumulation of random damage rather than a specific mechanism.

If aging exists as a distinct process, there is consensus that the mechanisms are likely multifactorial, environmentally influenced, and species-specific, if not organ- and cell-specific, making the paucity of available human data particularly problematic. As a result, there are nearly as many theories of aging as investigators. Most theories overlap or are not mutually exclusive, and none is completely compatible with the dearth of data. As a group, the theories can be divided into two broad categories, based on whether they attribute aging to a genetic program or to progressive and random damage to homeostatic systems.

Enthusiasm for genetic theories of aging is fueled by several observations, including the dramatic species-specific differences in maximal life span, the strong correlation with survival among monozygotic compared to dizygotic twins, and the fact that single mutations can prolong life span by more than 50% in some nematodes and mice. However, all genetic theories must account for the fact that evolutionary selection pressure is minimal following completion of reproduction. Three genetic theories have recently been advanced, but few relevant data have yet been accrued. The first theory suggests that, since animals usually succumb to natural forces long before reaching their maximal life span, aging might reflect mutations that impair long-term survival. These mutations would accumulate in the genome because there is no selection pressure to delete them. A second theory, "pleiotropic antagonism," proposes that aging may be caused by the late and deleterious effects of genes that are conserved because of the survival advantages they confer prior to reproduction. The third theory applies to ecological niches where extrinsic hazards are relatively low. In such an environment, evolution might select for mutations that retard the aging process since these might allow an animal to produce and protect many more litters. In support of this theory, the rate of aging in an isolated clan of Virginia opossums was calculated to be roughly half of that seen in their less fortunate cousins.

The "random damage" theories are based on the possibility that the balance between ongoing damage and repair is disrupted. The theories differ in the emphasis placed on increased damage (e.g., by free radicals, oxidation, or glycation) versus deficient repair, as well as in the mechanisms that might mediate each. However, all share the observation that cell and organ repair capacity declines with age. Some 40 years ago, Hayflick and Moorehead observed that the number of replications among cultured cells is finite. Subsequent research revealed that this replicative senescence was due to arrest of the cell cycle at the G_1/S phase, the point at which DNA synthesis begins. Recently, cell replication has also been linked to the length of telomeric DNA. Present at the termini of chromosomes, telomeric DNA prevents chromosomal instability, fragmentation, and rearrangement; anchors chromosomes to nuclear matrix; and provides a buffer between coding regions of DNA and the ends of the chromosomes. In addition, telomeric DNA is necessary for cell division. With each cell division, however, roughly 50 of the total 2000 base pairs of the telomere are lost. Telomeric shortening might thus result in loss of gene accessibility, which is necessary to repair ongoing cell damage caused by metabolism. Together with cytoplasmic factors mediating arrest of DNA synthesis, telomeric shortening could also limit the cell's ability to divide and thereby replace cells lost to apoptosis.

Many mechanisms previously postulated to mediate aging have not been borne out, including the somatic mutation theory (in which aging would result from cumulative spontaneous mutations), the error catastrophe theory (in which aging would result from errors in the synthesis of proteins critical to the synthesis of genetic material or protein-synthesizing machinery), and the intrinsic mutagenesis theory (in which aging is the result of ongoing intrinsic DNA rearrangements).

To date, the only intervention known to delay aging is caloric restriction. The salutary effect of restricting caloric intake by 30 to 40% has been documented in multiple species, from single-cell organisms to rodents. In rodents, it not only increases average life expectancy and maximum life span but also delays the onset of some typical age-associated diseases as well as deterioration of physiologic systems (e.g., immune responsiveness, glucose metabolism, muscle atrophy). Moreover, its impact is evident in both mitotic and postmitotic cells, in gene expression, and in protein turnover and cross-linking. Although the mechanism is still not determined, it is specific to caloric restriction rather than to reduction of any dietary component (e.g., fat intake) or supplements with vitamins or antioxidants. Unfortunately, adequate data from primates are not yet available, and the effect of caloric restriction in humans is still unknown.

PRINCIPLES OF GERIATRIC MEDICINE

Despite the biologic controversy, from a physiologic standpoint human aging is characterized by progressive constriction of the homeostatic reserve of every organ system. This decline, often referred to as *homeostenosis*, is evident by the third decade and is gradual and progressive, although the rate and extent of decline vary. The decline of each organ system (Table 9-1) appears to occur independently of changes in other organ systems and is influenced by diet, environment, and personal habits as well as by genetic factors.

Several important principles follow from these facts: (1) Individuals become more dissimilar as they age, belying any stereotype of aging; (2) an *abrupt* decline in any system or function is always due to disease and not to "normal aging"; (3) "normal aging" can be attenuated by modification of risk factors (e.g., increased blood pressure, smoking, sedentary lifestyle); and (4) "healthy old age" is not an oxymoron. In fact, *in the absence of disease, the decline in homeostatic reserve causes no symptoms and imposes few restrictions on activities of daily living regardless of age.*

Appreciation of these facts may make it easier to understand the striking increases that have occurred in life expectancy. Average life expectancy is now 17 years at age 65, 11 years at age 75, 6 years at age 85, 4 years at age 90, and 2 years at age 100. Moreover, the bulk of these years is characterized by a lack of significant impairment (Table 9-2). Even beyond age 85, only 30% of people are impaired in any activity required for daily living and only 20% reside in a nursing home. Yet, as individuals age they are more likely to suffer from disease, disability, and the side effects of drugs, all of which, when combined with the decrease in physiologic reserve, make the older person more vulnerable to environmental, pathologic, and pharmacologic challenges.

The following concepts underlie the remainder of the chapter:

1. Disease presentation is often atypical in the elderly, especially in those more than 75 to 80 years old. Homeostatic strain caused by onset of a new disease often leads to symptoms associated with a different organ system, particularly one compromised by preexisting disease. For example, fewer than one-fourth of older patients with hyperthyroidism present with goiter, tremor, and exophthalmos; more likely are atrial fibrillation, confusion, depression, syncope, and weakness. Significantly, because the "weakest link" is so often the brain, the lower urinary tract, or the cardiovascular or musculoskeletal system, a limited number of presenting symptoms predominate—acute confusion, depression, incontinence, falling, and syncope—no matter what the underlying disease. Thus for the most common geriatric syndromes, regardless of the presenting symptom, the differential diagnosis is often largely similar. The corollary is equally important: The organ system usually associated with a particular symptom is less likely to be the source of that symptom in older individuals than in younger ones. Compared with middle-aged individuals, for example, acute confusion in older patients is less often due to a new brain lesion,

Table 9-1 Selected Age-Related Changes and Their Consequences

Organ/System	Age-Related Physiologic Change[a]	Consequences of Age-Related Physiologic Change	Consequences of Disease, not Age
General	↑ Body fat	↑ Volume of distribution for fat-soluble drugs	Obesity
	↓ Total body water	↓ Volume of distribution for water-soluble drugs	Anorexia
Eyes/ears	Presbyopia	↓ Accommodation	
	Lens opacification	↑ Susceptibility to glare	Blindness
		Need for increased illumination	
	↓ High-frequency acuity	Difficulty discriminating words if background noise is present	Deafness
Endocrine	Impaired glucose homeostasis	↑ Glucose level in response to acute illness	Diabetes mellitus
	↓ Thyroxine clearance (and production)	↓ T_4 dose required in hypothyroidism	Thyroid dysfunction
	↑ ADH, ↓ renin, and ↓ aldosterone		↓ Na⁺, ↑ K⁺
	↓ Testosterone		Impotence
	↓ Vitamin D absorption and activation	Osteopenia	Osteomalacia, fracture
Respiratory	↓ Lung elasticity and ↑ chest wall stiffness	Ventilation/perfusion mismatch and ↓ P_{O_2}	Dyspnea, hypoxia
Cardiovascular	↓ Arterial compliance and ↑ systolic BP →LVH	Hypotensive response to ↑ HR, volume depletion, or loss of atrial contraction	Syncope
	↓ β-adrenergic responsiveness	↓ Cardiac output and HR response to stress	Heart failure
	↓ Baroreceptor sensitivity and ↓ SA node automaticity	Impaired blood pressure response to standing, volume depletion	Heart block
Gastrointestinal	↓ Hepatic function	Delayed metabolism of some drugs	Cirrhosis
	↓ Gastric acidity	↓ Ca^{2+} absorption on empty stomach	Osteoporosis, B_{12} deficiency
	↓ Colonic motility	Constipation	Fecal impaction
	↓ Anorectal function		Fecal incontinence
Hematologic/immune system	↓ Bone marrow reserve(?)		Anemia
	↓ T cell function	False-negative PPD response	
	↑ Autoantibodies	False-positive rheumatoid factor, antinuclear antibody	Autoimmune disease
Renal	↓ GFR	Impaired excretion of some drugs	↑ Serum creatinine
	↓ Urine concentration/dilution (see also "Endocrine")	Delayed response to salt or fluid restriction/overload; nocturia	↓ ↑ Na⁺
Genitourinary	Vaginal/urethral mucosal atrophy	Dyspareunia, bacteriuria	Symptomatic UTI
	Prostate enlargement	↑ Residual urine volume	Urinary incontinence; urinary retention
Musculoskeletal	↓ Lean body mass, muscle		Functional impairment
	↓ Bone density	Osteopenia	Hip fracture
Nervous system	Brain atrophy	Benign senescent forgetfulness	Dementia, delirium
	↓ Brain catechol synthesis		Depression
	↓ Brain dopaminergic synthesis	Stiffer gait	Parkinson's disease
	↓ Righting reflexes	↑ Body sway	Falls
	↓ Stage 4 sleep	Early wakening, insomnia	Sleep apnea

[a] Changes generally observed in healthy elderly subjects free of symptoms and detectable disease in the organ system studied. The changes are usually important only when the system is stressed or other factors are added (e.g., drugs, disease, or environmental challenge); they rarely result in symptoms otherwise. Abbreviations: T_4, thyroxine; BP, blood pressure; HR, heart rate; ADH, antidiuretic hormone; GFR, glomerular filtration rate.

depression to a psychiatric disorder, incontinence to bladder dysfunction, falling to a neuropathy, or syncope to heart disease.

2. Because of decreased physiologic reserve, older patients often develop symptoms at an earlier stage of their disease (Fig. 9-1). For example, heart failure may be precipitated by mild hyperthyroidism, cognitive dysfunction by mild hyperparathyroidism, urinary retention by mild prostatic enlargement, and nonketotic hyperosmolar coma by mild glucose intolerance. Paradoxically, therefore, treatment of the underlying disease may be easier because it is frequently less advanced at the time of presentation. A corollary is that drug side effects can occur with drugs and drug doses unlikely to produce side effects in younger people (Chap. 71). For instance, an antihistamine (e.g., diphenhydramine) may cause confusion, loop diuretics may precipitate urinary incontinence, digoxin may induce depression even with normal serum levels, and over-the-counter sympathomimetics may precipitate urinary retention in men with mild prostatic obstruction.

Table 9-2 Life Expectancy and Number of Remaining Years Free of Dependency in Activities of Daily Living

Age	Life Expectancy[a], av		Disability-Free Years Remaining	
	Men	Women	Men	Women
65–69	13	20	9	11
70–74	12	16	8	8
75–79	10	13	7	7
80–84	7	10	5	5
≥85	7	8	3	3

[a] For independent noninstitutionalized elderly men and women in Massachusetts. Longevity and disability-free longevity are surprisingly long and must be incorporated into treatment decisions. All figures rounded to nearest year. See text for more recent data on longevity alone.

SOURCE: S Katz et al: N Engl J Med 309:1218, 1983.

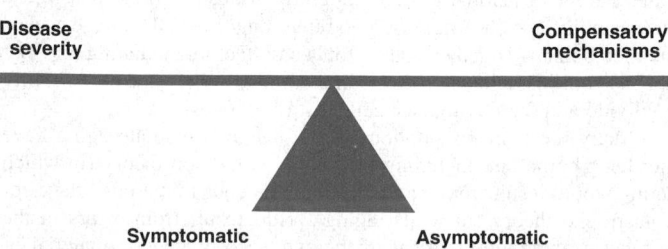

FIGURE 9-1 Even mild organ system dysfunction may cause symptoms if compensatory mechanisms are impaired. (*From NM Resnick: JAMA 276:1832, 1996.*)

Unfortunately, the predisposition to develop symptoms at an earlier stage of disease is often offset by the change in illness behavior that occurs with age. Raised at a time when symptoms and debility were accepted as normal consequences of aging, the elderly are less likely to seek attention until symptoms become disabling. Thus, any symptom, particularly those associated with a change in functional status, must be taken seriously and evaluated promptly.

3. Since many homeostatic mechanisms may be compromised concurrently, there are usually multiple abnormalities amenable to treatment, and small improvements in each may yield dramatic benefits overall. For instance, cognitive impairment in patients with Alzheimer's disease may respond much better to interventions that alleviate comorbidity than to prescription of donepezil (Fig. 9-2). Similar approaches apply to most other geriatric syndromes, including falls, incontinence, depression, delirium, syncope, and fracture. In each case, substantial functional improvement can result from treating the contributing factors even if—as in Alzheimer's disease—the disease itself is largely untreatable.

4. Many findings that are abnormal in younger patients are relatively common in older people—e.g., bacteriuria, premature ventricular contractions, low bone mineral density, impaired glucose tolerance, and uninhibited bladder contractions. However, they may not be responsible for a particular symptom but only be incidental findings that result in missed diagnoses and misdirected therapy. For instance, the finding of bacteriuria should not end the search for a source of fever in an acutely ill older patient, nor should an elevated random blood sugar—especially in an acutely ill patient—be incriminated as the cause of neuropathy. On the other hand, certain other abnormalities must not be dismissed as due to old age—e.g., there is no anemia, impotence, depression, or confusion of old age.

5. Because symptoms in older people are often due to multiple causes, the diagnostic "law of parsimony" often does not apply. For instance, fever, anemia, retinal embolus, and a heart murmur prompt almost a reflex diagnosis of infective endocarditis in a younger patient but may reflect aspirin-induced blood loss, a cholesterol embolus, insignificant aortic sclerosis, and a viral illness in an older patient. Moreover, even when the diagnosis is correct, treatment of a single disease in an older patient is unlikely to result in cure. For instance, in a younger patient, incontinence due to involuntary bladder contractions is treated effectively with a bladder relaxant medication. However, in an older patient with the same condition but who also has fecal impaction, takes medications that cloud the sensorium, and suffers from arthritis-associated impairments of mobility and manual dexterity, treatment of the bladder spasms alone is unlikely to restore continence. On the other hand, disimpaction, discontinuation of the offending medications, and treatment of the arthritis are likely to restore continence without the need for a bladder relaxant. Failure to recognize these principles often leads to prescribing "ineffective" therapy and to unjustified therapeutic nihilism towards older patients.

6. Because the older patient is more likely to suffer the adverse consequences of disease, treatment—and even prevention—may be equally or even more effective. For instance, the survival benefits of exercise, as well as thrombolysis and beta-blocker therapy after a myocardial infarction, are as impressive in older patients as in younger ones; and treatment of hypertension and transient ischemic attacks, as well as immunization against influenza and pneumococcal pneumonia, are more effective in older patients. In addition, prevention in older patients must often be seen in a broader context. For instance, although interventions to increase bone density may be limited in older patients, fracture may still be prevented by efforts to improve balance, strengthen legs, reduce peripheral edema, treat other contributing medical conditions, replete nutritional deficits, eliminate environmental hazards, and remove adverse medications—not so much those that affect bone metabolism, but rather those that induce orthostasis, confusion, and extrapyramidal stiffness.

In summary, optimal treatment of the older patient generally requires treating much more than the organ system usually associated

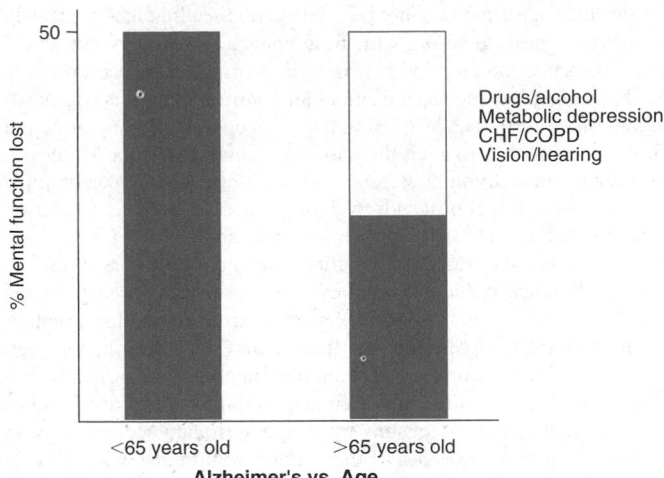

FIGURE 9-2 Although young and old patients may appear to suffer equally from Alzheimer's disease, its extent in older patients is often magnified by comorbidity and drug use. Identification and treatment of these contributing factors will improve the older patient's function even though the Alzheimer's disease is inadequately treatable. CHF, congestive heart failure; COPD, chronic obstructive pulmonary disease. *(From Resnick and Marcantonio.)*

with the disease or symptom, and often permits ignoring that system entirely.

EVALUATION   Evaluation of the older patient can be time-consuming, even when it is tailored to the problem. Yet, such initial investment can reduce subsequent morbidity and resource utilization and enhance patient and physician satisfaction. Additionally, the assessment can often be accomplished over several visits. Moreover, much can be gleaned from questionnaires filled out by the patient or caregiver in advance as well as from observation. For instance, greeting the patient in the waiting room allows the physician to note affective and cognitive response, the strength of the handshake, the ease of rising from a chair without using the arms, the length and steadiness of the stride, and the ability to follow directions to the examining room and to sit down safely in the examining room chair. Observing the patient dress or undress can also enhance detection of impaired cognition, fine motor skills, balance, and judgment. Such observations often provide more information than standard examinations and can shorten the clinical evaluation.

HISTORY TAKING IN ELDERLY PATIENTS   Most older patients are able to provide a reliable medical history; however, a multitude of complaints may make obtaining a history more difficult. If the patient is unable to comprehend or communicate, data should be sought from family, friends, and caregivers. The history should also include drug ingestion; dietary patterns; falling, incontinence, sexual dysfunction, depression and anxiety.

Advance Directives   All older patients should be asked whether they have drafted advance health care directives, and, if they have, a copy should be placed in the record. Such directives may consist of a health care proxy or durable power of attorney for health care, in which patients designate a surrogate decision-maker who makes health care decisions if the patient cannot, and/or a living will or medical directive, in which patients specify their desires for treatment in specific situations if they cannot communicate at the critical time.

Whether or not the patient has formally drafted these directives, it is useful to indicate in the record who should make health care decisions if the patient is no longer able to do so. Patients should then be encouraged to discuss their thoughts with the physician as well as the designated proxy. It is not feasible to cover all possible future complications in such discussions. Ascertaining patients' perspectives on specific interventions, such as resuscitation or intubation, is also difficult because preferences will likely differ depending on prognosis.

For instance, a patient may not be interested in feeding tube placement following a massive stroke with little chance of recovery but would prefer the same intervention if it is short-term and helps ensure more rapid and complete recovery from an intercurrent illness such as pneumonia. More useful is a discussion that uses open-ended questions and empathic comments to elicit the patient's values and goals. Moreover, for any given condition, preferences may differ depending on baseline clinical status. For robust elderly individuals, recovery is a realistic goal, albeit the odds of complications are higher than for younger individuals. For the frail elderly patient with comorbidity that impairs functional status, reduction or alleviation of symptoms may be the goal. For patients with advanced dementia or terminal illness, palliation may be the most appropriate strategy. In each situation, however, early elicitation of a patient's preferences and values—when the patient can still state them—can often help both physicians and families in subsequent difficult decisions by giving surrogate decision-makers the sense that they are doing as the patient would have wanted.

PHYSICAL EXAMINATION   Certain features of the examination should receive special attention, depending in part on clues from the history. Weight and postural blood pressure should be measured at most visits. Vision and hearing should be checked; if hearing is impaired, excess cerumen should be removed from the external auditory canals prior to audiologic referral. Denture fit should be assessed, and the oral cavity should be inspected with the dentures removed. Although thyroid disease becomes more common with age, the sensitivity and specificity of related findings are substantially lower than in younger individuals; consequently, the physical examination can rarely corroborate or exclude thyroid dysfunction in older patients. The breasts should not be overlooked, since older women are more likely to have breast cancer and less likely to do breast self-examination. The systolic murmur of aortic sclerosis is common and may be difficult to differentiate from aortic stenosis, especially since the presence of a fourth heart sound in an elderly person does not imply significant cardiac disease, and the carotid upstroke normally increases owing to age-related arterial stiffening.

In inactive patients and those with fecal or urinary incontinence, one should check for fecal impaction. In patients with urinary incontinence—especially men—a distended bladder must be looked for, since it may be the only finding in urinary retention; perineal sensation and the bulbocavernosus reflex should also be tested. Patients who fall should be observed standing up from a chair, bending down, reaching up, walking 10 feet, turning, returning, and sitting again; abnormalities of gait and balance should be evaluated with the patient's eyes open and closed and in response to a sternal push. It should be appreciated that "frontal release signs" (e.g., "snout," "glabellar," or palmomental reflexes) and absent ankle jerks and vibratory sense in the feet may be normal in the elderly.

MENTAL STATUS EXAMINATION   In addition to evaluating mood and affect, some form of cognitive testing is essential in all elderly patients, even if it involves only checking different components of the history for consistency. People with mild degrees of dementia usually retain their social graces and may mask intellectual impairment by a cheerful and cooperative manner. Thus, the examiner should always probe for content. For patients who follow the news, one can ask what stories they are particularly interested in and why; the same applies to reading, social events—even the soap operas on television.

If there is any suspicion of a cognitive deficit after this kind of conversational probing, further questioning is indicated. An examination that tests only orientation as to person, place, and time is insufficient to detect mild or moderate intellectual impairment. As a quick screen, simply assessing orientation and asking the patient to draw a clock with the hands at a set time (e.g., 10 min before 2:00) can be very informative regarding cognitive status, visuospatial deficits, ability to comprehend and execute instructions in logical sequence, and presence or absence of perseveration. For slightly more

detailed examinations, many practical mental status tests are available. The most widely used is the Mini-Mental Status Examination of Folstein (Chap. 24), which provides a numerical score that can be obtained in 5 to 10 min. Regardless of the test employed, the total score is less useful diagnostically than is knowledge of the specific domain of the deficit. As a general rule, disproportionate difficulty with immediate recall (e.g., of a list of three items) suggests depression, while predominant difficulty with recalling the items 5 min later suggests dementia. For patients with deficits of attention—recognized by inability to spell simple words backwards, repeat five digits, or recite the months of the year backwards—delirium is probably present, and the accuracy of the remainder of the test is dubious. However, the test can be interpreted accurately only in the context of a comprehensive evaluation.

EVALUATION OF FUNCTIONAL CAPACITY   Medical problem lists, a standard tool for assessing and following younger patients, often prove inadequate for older patients. Heart failure, stroke, and prostate cancer can describe a bedbound institutionalized person as well as a Supreme Court justice. Thus, it is essential to ascertain the patient's degree of functional incapacity owing to both medical and psychosocial problems. The functional assessment includes determination of the patient's ability to perform basic activities of daily life (ADL), which are those needed for personal self-care, as well as the ability to perform more complex tasks required for independent living, the instrumental activities of daily living (IADL). ADLs include bathing, dressing, toileting, feeding, getting in and out of chairs and bed, and walking. IADLs include shopping, cooking, money management, housework, using a telephone, and traveling outside the home. For frail patients, an assessment in the home by a trained observer may be required, but for most patients a questionnaire dealing with these activities can be completed by the family or patient. In either case, the physician must determine the cause of any impairment and whether it can be treated. Assessment should conclude with determination of the socioeconomic circumstances and social support systems.

MANAGEMENT OF COMMON GERIATRIC CONDITIONS

Diseases more common in the elderly are covered elsewhere in the text. The medical problems discussed below do not usually present as clear-cut organ-specific diagnoses and are most common in the frail elderly, especially those over 80 years of age.

INTELLECTUAL IMPAIRMENT   The predominant causes of impaired mentation in older patients are delirium, dementia, and depression. Each condition is covered elsewhere in the text in detail (Chaps. 24 and 362), but their management in the elderly is discussed here.

Differentiating the causes of impaired mentation is important, but in older patients they frequently coexist. Thus, the most important first step is to search for and correct all factors that may contribute to cognitive impairment, even in patients with dementia (Fig. 9-2). Evidence of dangerous behavior should also be sought (e.g., leaving the stove on, wandering, and getting lost), and plans should be devised to deal with it. Although there is no specific pharmacologic treatment for Alzheimer's disease and agents such as donepezil are of limited efficacy, this does not mean that the physician has no further role in treating the patient and family. In addition to discontinuing all nonessential medications and treating new intercurrent illness, the physician should help the family and patient predict and deal with the disease; indeed, the family often needs the physician's support more than the patient does.

℞ **TREATMENT**   Community services should be suggested as needed, including a visiting nurse, a home health aide to assist with personal hygiene, a homemaker to assist with housework, meal delivery, transportation services, day health centers, and respite care to ease the burden on family members. Support groups such as the

Alzheimer's Association are often of value to the family and help them to anticipate problems. Signs of patient abuse by an overstressed caregiver should be watched for. Legal counsel should be recommended to help the patient and family devise plans for ongoing management and ultimate disposition of assets not already obtained; advance directives should be sought as soon as possible while the patient can still participate.

Finally, abrupt worsening of mentation or the onset of disruptive behavior should always prompt a search for new illness or medication. Exacerbation of cognitive dysfunction may occur with mild infections (e.g., subungual toe abscess, vaginitis, or pressure ulcer); with "therapeutic" levels of many drugs; with use of nonprescribed drugs or alcohol; with modest abnormalities of serum sodium, calcium, glucose, or thyroxine; with mild hypoxia; with borderline nutritional deficiencies; with subdural hematoma or "minor" stroke; and with the development of fecal impaction, urinary retention, pain, or change in environment, particularly in frail older patients. However, if a cause is not found and behavior does not respond to environmental manipulation (e.g., ignoring the behavior, distracting the patient, addressing situational "triggers," and providing a calm environment), low doses of an antipsychotic medication may be helpful (e.g., haloperidol 0.25 to 2 mg/d orally; see below).

DEPRESSION   Depression of significant degree occurs in 5 to 10% of community-dwelling elderly but is often overlooked. At highest risk are individuals with recent medical illness (e.g., stroke or fracture), bereavement, lack of social supports, recent nursing home admission, or psychiatric history (including alcohol abuse). The diagnosis requires the presence of a depressed mood for at least two consecutive weeks plus at least four of the following eight symptoms: sleep disturbance, lack of interest, feelings of guilt, decreased energy, decreased concentration, decreased appetite, psychomotor agitation/retardation, and suicidal ideation. Also helpful diagnostically are a personal or family history of depression, anhedonia (loss of pleasure), and past response to an antidepressant. It is essential to bear in mind that depression in older patients is often caused or contributed to by drugs or a systemic illness. Although "subsyndromal" depression (fewer than four of the above symptoms) also causes substantial morbidity and health resource utilization, it appears to be less responsive than major depression to therapy.

℞ **TREATMENT**   For the hospitalized patient in whom acute depression delays recovery or rehabilitation—when correction of medical and pharmacologic contributing factors is ineffective and there is no prior history of mania or major depression—methylphenidate, 5 to 10 mg at 8 A.M. and noon (to avoid insomnia) is often very effective, with benefits discernible within a few days. For patients with major depression, there is no ideal antidepressant drug. All are about equally effective, but the side effects differ (see below and Chap. 385). Consequently, one should become familiar with one or two agents for patients with psychomotor retardation (e.g., sertaline, desipramine) and for those with agitation (e.g., nortriptyline or nefazodone). Because of its potent anticholinergic and orthostatic side effects, amitriptyline should be avoided whenever possible in older patients. Initial low dosages should be increased slowly to avoid serious side effects; low doses of each medication (e.g., nortriptyline, 10 to 50 mg daily; desipramine, 25 to 75 mg daily; or sertraline 50 to 150 mg daily) are often effective in the elderly. Careful follow-up is required to anticipate and minimize anticholinergic side effects, orthostatic hypotension, sedating effects, confusion, bizarre mental symptoms, cardiovascular complications, and drug overdose with suicidal intent. Adverse drug reactions should not be assumed to be due to the aging process.

Cautious use of the monoamine oxidase inhibitors is sometimes of benefit when other antidepressants are ineffective. Neither monoamine oxidase inhibitors nor selective serotonin reuptake inhibitors should be used in combination with the cyclic compounds. Electroconvulsive therapy has been successful and is usually well tolerated by elderly patients who remain severely depressed despite drug treatment, particularly if they also have delusions.

URINARY INCONTINENCE   Transient Incontinence (Table 9-3)   Because urinary continence requires adequate mobility, mentation, motivation, and manual dexterity—in addition to integrated control of the lower urinary tract—problems outside the bladder can result in incontinence.

1. *Delirium.* A clouded sensorium impedes recognition of both the need to void and the location of the nearest toilet; once delirium clears, incontinence resolves.
2. *Infection.* Symptomatic urinary tract infection commonly causes or contributes to incontinence; asymptomatic infection does not.
3. *Atrophic urethritis/vaginitis.* Atrophic urethritis/vaginitis, characterized by the presence of vaginal telangiectasia, petechiae, erythema, or friability, commonly contributes to incontinence in women and responds to a several-month course of low-dose estrogen or vaginal estrogen creams.
4. *Pharmaceutical.* The drugs most commonly causing transient incontinence are listed in Table 9-4.
5. *Psychologic.* Depression and psychosis are uncommon but treatable causes.
6. *Excess urine output.* Excess urine output may overwhelm the ability to reach a toilet in time. Causes include diuretics, alcohol, excess fluid intake, and metabolic abnormalities (e.g., hyperglycemia, hypercalcemia, diabetes insipidus); nocturnal incontinence may also result from mobilization of peripheral edema.
7. *Restricted mobility.* If mobility cannot be improved, access to a urinal or commode may restore continence. (See "Immobility," below.)
8. *Stool impaction.* This is a common cause of urinary incontinence, especially in hospitalized or immobile patients. Although the mechanism is unknown, a clue to its presence is the coexistence of both urinary and fecal incontinence. Disimpaction restores continence.

Established Incontinence (Table 9-3)   The causes of established incontinence include irreversible functional deficits, such as *end-stage* Alzheimer's disease, and intrinsic lower urinary tract dysfunction. Lower urinary tract dysfunction should be sought after transient causes have been excluded.

Detrusor Overactivity   This disorder (involuntary bladder contraction) accounts for two-thirds of geriatric incontinence in both sexes, regardless of whether patients are demented. Detrusor overactivity can be diagnosed presumptively in a woman when leakage occurs in the absence of stress maneuvers or urinary retention and is preceded by the abrupt onset of an intense urge to urinate that cannot

Table 9-3   Classification of Incontinence

TRANSIENT

Delirium/confusional state
Infection—urinary (symptomatic)
Atrophic urethritis/vaginitis
Pharmaceuticals
Psychological, especially depression
Excessive urine output (e.g., CHF, hyperglycemia)
Restricted mobility
Stool impaction

ESTABLISHED

Detrusor overactivity
Detrusor underactivity
Urethral obstruction
Urethral incompetence

NOTE: CHF, congestive heart failure.
SOURCE: Adapted from NM Resnick: Medical Grand Rounds 3:281, 1984.

Table 9-4 Commonly Used Medications that May Affect Continence

Type of Medication	Examples	Potential Effects on Continence
Sedatives/hypnotics	Long-acting benzodi-azepines (e.g., diaz-epam, flurazepam)	Sedation, delirium, immobility
Alcohol		Polyuria, frequency, urgency, sedation, delirium, immobility
Anticholinergics	Dicyclomine, diso-pyramide, sedating antihistamines	Urinary retention, overflow inconti-nence, delirium, im-paction
Antipsychotics	Thioridazine, haloper-idol	Anticholinergic ac-tions, sedation, ri-gidity, immobility
Tricyclic antidepres-sants	Amitriptyline, desi-pramine	Anticholinergic ac-tions, sedation
Antiparkinsonians	Trihexyphenidyl, benztropine mesyl-ate (not L-dopa/sele-giline)	Anticholinergic ac-tions, sedation
Narcotic analgesics	Opiates	Urinary retention, fe-cal impaction, seda-tion, delirium
α-Adrenergic antago-nists	Prazosin, terazosin, doxazosin	Urethral relaxation may precipitate stress incontinence in women
α-Adrenergic agonists	Nasal decongestants	Urinary retention in men
Calcium channel blockers	All dihydropyridines[a]	Urinary retention; nocturnal diuresis due to fluid retention
Potent diuretics	Furosemide, bumet-anide	Polyuria, frequency, urgency
Angiotensin-convert-ing enzyme inhibi-tors	Captopril, enalapril, lisinopril	Drug-induced cough can precipitate stress incontinence in women and in some men with prior pros-tatectomy
Vincristine		Urinary retention

[a] Examples include nifedipine, nicardipine, israpidine, felodipine, nimodipine.
SOURCE: Adapted from NM Resnick, in *Current Medical Diagnosis and Treatment*, LT Tierney et al (eds), Norwalk, Appleton & Lange, 1993.

be forestalled. In men, the symptoms are similar, but since detrusor overactivity often coexists with urethral obstruction, urodynamic test-ing should be done if prescription of a bladder relaxant is planned. Because detrusor overactivity may also be due to bladder stones or tumor, the abrupt onset of otherwise unexplained urge incontinence—especially if accompanied by perineal/suprapubic discomfort or sterile hematuria—should prompt cystoscopy and cytologic examination.

℞ TREATMENT The cornerstone of treatment is behavioral therapy with or without biofeedback. Patients without dementia are instructed to void every 1 to 2 h (while awake only) and to suppress urgency in between; once daytime continence is restored, the interval between voiding can be progressively increased. Demented patients are "prompted" to void at similar intervals. When drugs are necessary, they should be added to these regimens and monitored to avoid in-ducing urinary retention. Effective drugs include oxybutynin (2.5 to 5 mg three or four times daily, or sustained release, 5 to 20 mg once daily), dicyclomine (10 to 30 mg three times daily), tolterodine (1 to 2 mg twice daily), and imipramine or doxepin (25 to 100 mg at bed-time). If prescribed for older patients, DDAVP should be used cau-tiously—especially in the setting of renal insufficiency or heart fail-ure—and it probably should not be given to patients with

hyponatremia or urine output >2500 mL/d. Alternative treatments, such as neuromodulation, are under investigation.

Indwelling catheterization is rarely indicated for detrusor overac-tivity. If all measures fail, an external collection device or protective pad or undergarment may be required.

Stress Incontinence This disorder, the second most common cause of established incontinence in older women (it is rare in men), is characterized by symptoms and evidence of *instantaneous* leakage of urine in response to stress. Leakage is worse or occurs only during the day unless another abnormality (e.g., detrusor overactivity) is also present. On examination, with the bladder full and the perineum re-laxed, instantaneous leakage upon coughing strongly suggests stress incontinence, especially if it reproduces symptoms and if urinary re-tention has been excluded by a postvoiding residual determination; a several-second delay suggests that leakage is instead caused by an involuntary bladder contraction induced by coughing.

℞ TREATMENT Surgery is the most effective treatment. For women who can comply indefinitely, pelvic muscle exercises are an option for mild to moderate stress incontinence, but they often require specialized training using vaginal cones or biofeedback. If not contraindicated, an α-adrenergic agonist (e.g., phenylpropanolamine) is also helpful in such cases, especially if combined with estrogen. Occasionally, a pessary or even a tampon (for women with vaginal stenosis) provides some relief.

Urethral Obstruction Rarely present in women, urethral ob-struction (due to prostatic enlargement, urethral stricture, bladder neck contracture, or prostate cancer) is the second most common cause of established incontinence in older men. It can present as dribbling in-continence after voiding, urge incontinence due to detrusor overactiv-ity (which coexists in two-thirds of cases), or overflow incontinence due to urinary retention. Renal ultrasound is recommended to exclude hydronephrosis in men whose postvoiding residual volume exceeds 100 to 200 mL; in older men for whom surgery is planned, urodynamic confirmation of obstruction is strongly advised.

℞ TREATMENT Surgical decompression is the most effective treatment for obstruction, especially if there is urinary retention. For a nonoperative candidate, intermittent or indwelling catheteriza-tion is used; a condom catheter is contraindicated when urinary reten-tion is present. For a man with prostatic obstruction who is not in retention, treatment with an α-adrenergic antagonist (e.g., terazosin 5 to 10 mg daily) may lessen symptoms in a few weeks. The 5α-reduc-tase inhibitor finasteride may also ameliorate symptoms in a third or more of patients, but its impact is modest and not apparent for many months. Combined treatment with both agents has proved no better than treatment with an alpha blocker alone in most men.

Detrusor Underactivity Whether idiopathic or due to sacral lower motor nerve dysfunction, this is the least common cause of in-continence (<10% of cases). When it causes incontinence, detrusor underactivity is associated with urinary frequency, nocturia, and fre-quent leakage of small amounts. The elevated postvoiding residual volume (generally >450 mL) distinguishes it from detrusor overactiv-ity and stress incontinence, but only urodynamic testing (rather than cystoscopy or intravenous urography) differentiates it from urethral obstruction in men; such testing is not usually required in women, in whom obstruction is rare.

℞ TREATMENT For the patient with a poorly contractile blad-der, augmented voiding techniques (e.g., double voiding or ap-plying suprapubic pressure) are often effective; pharmacologic agents (e.g., bethanechol) are rarely effective. If further emptying is needed or for the patient with an acontractile bladder, intermittent or indwell-ing catheterization is the only option. Antibiotics should be used for symptomatic upper tract infection, or as prophylaxis for recurrent symptomatic infections only in a patient using intermittent catheterization; they should not be used as prophylaxis with an indwelling catheter.

FALLS Falls are a major problem for elderly people, especially women. Some 30% of community-dwelling elderly individuals fall each year, and the proportion increases with age. Nonetheless, falling must *not* be viewed as accidental, inevitable, or untreatable.

Causes of Falls Balance and ambulation require a complex interplay of cognitive, neuromuscular, and cardiovascular function and the ability to adapt rapidly to an environmental challenge. With age, balance becomes impaired and sway increases. The resulting vulnerability predisposes the older person to fall when challenged by an additional insult to *any* of these systems. Thus, a seemingly minor fall may be due to a serious problem, such as pneumonia or a myocardial infarction.

Much more commonly, however, falls are due to the complex interaction between a variably impaired patient and an environmental challenge. While a warped floorboard may pose little problem for a vigorous, unmedicated, alert person, it may be sufficient to precipitate a fall and hip fracture in the patient with impaired vision, strength, balance, or cognition. Thus, falls in older people are rarely due to a single cause, and effective prevention entails a comprehensive assessment of the patient's intrinsic deficits (usually diseases and medications), the routine activities, and the environmental obstacles.

Intrinsic deficits are those that impair sensory input, judgment, blood pressure regulation, reaction time, and balance and gait (Table 9-5). Medications and alcohol use are among the most common, significant, and reversible causes of falling. Other treatable contributors include postprandial hypotension (which peaks 30 to 60 min after a meal), insomnia, urinary urgency, foot problems, and peripheral edema [which can burden impaired leg strength and gait with an additional 2 to 5 kg (5 to 10 lb)].

Environmental obstacles are listed in Table 9-6. Since most falls occur in or around the home, a visit by a visiting nurse, physical therapist, or physician often reaps substantial dividends.

Complications of Falls and Treatment One out of four people who fall suffers serious injury. About 5% of falls result in fractures, and an equal proportion cause serious soft tissue damage. Falls are the sixth leading cause of death for older people and a contributing factor in 40% of admissions to nursing homes. Resultant hip problems and fear of falls are major causes of loss of independence.

Subdural hematoma is a treatable but easily overlooked complication of falls that must be considered in any elderly patient presenting with new neurologic signs, including confusion alone, even in the absence of a headache. Dehydration, electrolyte imbalance, pressure sores, rhabdomyolysis, and hypothermia may also occur and endanger the patient's life following a fall.

The risk of falling is related to the number of contributory conditions. Because the relationship is multiplicative rather than additive, however, even minor improvement in a number of these factors will reduce the risk substantially. In addition, gait training by a physical therapist often alleviates fear of falling. Ensuring the availability of phones at floor level, a portable phone, or a lightweight radio call system is also important, as is detection and treatment of osteoporosis.

IMMOBILITY The main causes of immobility are weakness, stiffness, pain, imbalance, and psychological problems. Weakness may result from disuse of muscles, malnutrition, electrolyte disturbances, anemia, neurologic disorders, or myopathies. The most common cause of stiffness in the elderly is osteoarthritis; however, Parkinson's disease, rheumatoid arthritis, gout, pseudogout, and antipsychotic drugs such as haloperidol may also contribute. Pain, whether from bone (e.g., osteoporosis, osteomalacia, Paget's disease, metastatic bone cancer, trauma), joints (e.g., osteoarthritis, rheumatoid arthritis, gout), bursa, muscle (e.g., polymyalgia rheumatica, intermittent claudication, or "pseudoclaudication"), or foot problems may immobilize the patient.

Imbalance and fear of falling are major causes of immobilization. Imbalance may result from general debility, neurologic causes (e.g., stroke; loss of postural reflexes; peripheral neuropathy due to diabetes mellitus, alcohol, or malnutrition; and vestibulocerebellar abnormalities), orthostatic or postprandial hypotension, or drugs (e.g., diuretics, antihypertensives, neuroleptics, and antidepressants) or may occur following prolonged bed rest. Psychological conditions such as severe anxiety or depression may also contribute to immobilization.

Consequences In addition to thrombophlebitis and pulmonary embolus, there are multiple hazards of bed rest in the elderly. Decon-

Table 9-5 Intrinsic Risk Factors for Falling, and Possible Interventions

Risk Factor	Interventions	
	Medical	Rehabilitative or Environmental
Reduced visual acuity, dark adaptation, and perception	Refraction; cataract extraction	Home safety assessment
Reduced hearing	Removal of cerumen; audiologic evaluation	Hearing aid if appropriate (with training); reduction in background noise
Vestibular dysfunction	Avoidance of drugs affecting the vestibular system; neurologic or ear, nose, and throat evaluation, if indicated	Habituation exercises
Proprioceptive dysfunction, cervical degenerative disorders, and peripheral neuropathy	Screening for vitamin B_{12} deficiency and cervical spondylosis	Balance exercises; appropriate walking aid; correctly sized footwear with firm soles; home safety assessment
Dementia	Detection of reversible causes; avoidance of sedative or centrally acting drugs	Supervised exercise and ambulation; home safety assessment
Musculoskeletal disorders	Appropriate diagnostic evaluation	Balance-and-gait training; muscle-strengthening exercises; appropriate walking aid; home safety assessment
Foot disorders (calluses, bunions, deformities, edema)	Shaving of calluses; bunionectomy; treatment of edema	Trimming of nails; appropriate footwear
Postural hypotension	Assessment of medications; rehydration; possible alteration in situational factors (e.g., meals, change of position)	Dorsiflexion exercises; pressure-graded stockings; elevation of head of bed; use of tilt table if condition is severe
Use of medications (sedatives: benzodiazepines, phenothiazines, antidepressants; antihypertensives; others: antiarrhythmics, anticonvulsants, diuretics, alcohol)	Steps to be taken: 1. Attempted reduction in the total number of medications taken 2. Assessment of risks and benefits of each medication 3. Selection of medication, if needed, that is least centrally acting, least associated with postural hypotension, and has shortest action 4. Prescription of lowest effective dose 5. Frequent reassessment of risks and benefits	

SOURCE: After ME Tinetti and M Speechley, N Engl J Med 320:1055, 1989.

Table 9-6 Environmental Factors Affecting the Risk of Falling

Environmental Area or Factor	Objective and Recommendations
All areas	
Lighting	Adequacy of illumination (older people need twice as much as younger people); absence of glare and shadows; accessible switches at room entrances; night light in bedroom, hall, bathroom
Floors	Nonskid backing for throw rugs; carpet edges tacked down; carpets with shallow pile; nonskid wax on floors; cords out of walking path; small objects (e.g., clothes, shoes) off floor
Stairs	Lighting sufficient, with switches at top and bottom of stairs; securely fastened bilateral handrails that stand out from wall; top and bottom steps marked with bright, contrasting tape; stair rises of no more than 6 in; steps in good repair; no objects stored on steps
Kitchen	Items stored so that reaching up and bending over are not necessary; secure step stool available if climbing is necessary; firm, nonmovable table
Bathroom	Grab bars for tub, shower, and toilet; nonskid decals or rubber mat in tub or shower; shower chair with handheld shower; nonskid rugs; raised toilet seat; door locks removed to ensure access in an emergency
Yard and entrances	Repair of cracks in pavement, holes in lawn; removal of rocks, tools, and other tripping hazards; well-lit walkways, free of ice and wet leaves; stairs and steps as above
Institutions	All the above; bed at proper height (not too high or low); spills on floor cleaned up promptly; appropriate use of walking aids and wheelchairs
Footwear	Shoes with firm, nonskid, nonfriction soles; low heels (unless person is accustomed to high heels); avoidance of walking in stocking feet or loose slippers

SOURCE: After ME Tinetti and M Speechley, N Engl J Med 320:1055, 1989.

ditioning of the cardiovascular system occurs within days and involves fluid shifts, fluid loss, decreased cardiac output, decreased peak oxygen uptake, and increased resting heart rate. Striking changes also occur in skeletal muscle. At the cellular level, intracellular ATP and glycogen concentrations decrease, rates of protein degradation increase, and contractile velocity and strength decline, while at the whole-muscle level, atrophy, weakness, and shortening are seen. Pressure sores are another serious complication; mechanical pressure, moisture, friction, and shearing forces all predispose to their development. As a result, within days of being confined to bed, the risk of postural hypotension, falls, and skin breakdown rises. Moreover, these changes usually take weeks to months to reverse.

℞ **TREATMENT** The most important step is preventive—to avoid bedrest whenever possible. When it cannot be avoided, several measures can be employed to minimize its consequences. Patients should be positioned as close to the upright position as possible several times daily. Range-of-motion exercises should begin immediately, and the skin over pressure points should be inspected frequently. Isometric and isotonic exercises should be performed while the patient is in bed, and whenever possible patients should assist their own positioning, transferring, and self-care. As mobility becomes feasible, graduated ambulation should begin. For individuals confined to a wheelchair, ring-shaped devices ("donuts") should not be used to prevent pressure ulcers since they cause venous congestion and edema and actually increase the risk.

If a pressure ulcer develops, therapy depends on its stage. Stage 1 ulcers are characterized by nonblanchable erythema of intact skin; stage 2 lesions involve an ulcer of the epidermis, dermis, or both; stage 3 ulcers extend to the subcutaneous tissue; and stage 4 lesions involve muscle, bone, and/or the supporting tissues. For stage 1 lesions, eliminating excess pressure and ensuring adequate nutrition and hygiene

are sufficient. For the remaining types, the caregiver must also ensure that the wound stays clean and moist; thus, if saline dressings are used they should be changed when they are damp rather than dry. Synthetic dressings are more expensive than saline but are more effective because they require fewer changes (with less disruption of reepithelialization) and protect against contamination. Because bacterial colonization of pressure ulcers is universal, swab cultures should not be performed and topical treatment should be considered only for patients whose ulcers have not healed after 2 weeks of therapy. By contrast, associated cellulitis, osteomyelitis, or sepsis requires systemic therapy after cultures of blood and the wound border (by needle aspiration or biopsy) have been obtained. Surgical or enzymatic debridement is required for stage 3 and 4 lesions. In addition to a daily multivitamin, prescribing vitamin C (500 mg twice daily) is also useful. For debilitated patients, special mattresses are beneficial, including those that reduce pressure (e.g., static air mattress or foam) and those that relieve it (e.g., dynamic units that sequentially inflate and deflate).

In addition to treating all identified factors that contribute to immobility, consultation with a physical therapist should be sought. Installing handrails, lowering the bed, and providing chairs of proper height with arms and rubber skid guards may allow the patient to be safely mobile in the home. A properly fitted cane or walker may be helpful.

IATROGENIC DRUG REACTIONS For several reasons, older patients are two or three times more likely to have adverse drug reactions (Chap. 71). Drug clearance is often markedly reduced. This is due to a decrease in renal plasma flow and glomerular filtration rate and a reduced hepatic clearance. The last is due to a decrease in activity of the drug-metabolizing microsomal enzymes and an overall decline in blood flow to the liver with aging. The volume of distribution of drugs is also affected, since the elderly have a decrease in total-body water and a relative increase in body fat. Thus, water-soluble drugs become more concentrated, and fat-soluble drugs have longer half-lives. In addition, serum albumin levels decline, particularly in sick patients, so that there is a decrease in protein binding of some drugs (e.g., warfarin, phenytoin), leaving more free (active) drug available.

In addition to impaired drug clearance, which alters pharmacokinetics, older patients have altered responses to similar serum drug levels, a phenomenon known as *altered pharmacodynamics*. They are more sensitive to some drugs (e.g., opiates, anticoagulants) and less sensitive to others (e.g., β-adrenergic agents). Finally, the older patient with multiple chronic conditions is likely to be taking several drugs, including nonprescribed agents. Thus, adverse drug reactions and dosage errors are more likely to occur, especially if the patient has visual, hearing, or memory deficits.

Precautions to Avoid Drug Toxicity • *Drug selection and administration* Before initiating treatment, the physician should first ensure that the symptom requiring treatment is not itself due to another drug. For example, antipsychotic agents can cause symptoms that mimic depression (flat affect, restlessness, and pacing); such symptoms should prompt lowering of the dose rather than initiation of an antidepressant. In addition, drug therapy should be employed only after nonpharmacologic means have been considered or tried and only when the benefit clearly outweighs the risk.

Once pharmacotherapy has been decided upon, it should begin at less than the usual adult dosage and the dose should be increased slowly. However, given the marked variability in pharmacokinetics and pharmacodynamics in the elderly, dose escalation should continue until either a successful endpoint is reached or an intolerable side effect is encountered. The final dosage schedule should be kept as simple as possible, and the number of pills should be kept as low as possible. Serum drug levels are often useful in older patients, especially for monitoring drugs with narrow therapeutic indices such as phenytoin, theophylline, quinidine, aminoglycosides, lithium, and psychotropic agents such as nortriptyline. However, toxicity can occur even with "normal" therapeutic levels of some drugs (e.g., digoxin, phenytoin).

Over-the-counter agents Nearly three-quarters of the elderly regularly use nonprescribed drugs, many of which cause significant symptoms and/or interact with other medications. Frequent offenders include nonprescribed agents for insomnia (all of which are anticholinergics), and nonsteroidal anti-inflammatory drugs (NSAIDs), which can hamper control of hypertension in addition to causing renal dysfunction and gastrointestinal bleeding. Gingko biloba, increasingly used as a "memory booster," may interfere with previously stable anticoagulation regimens. Because older patients often consider such agents "nostrums" rather than drugs, the physician must ask about them directly.

Sedative-hypnotics If nonpharmacologic treatment of insomnia is unsuccessful, low-dose and short-term or intermittent use of an intermediate-acting agent whose metabolism is not affected by age (e.g., oxazepam, 10 to 30 mg/d) may be useful. Because of the increased risk of confusion and other adverse effects, benzodiazepines with either short (e.g., triazolam) or long duration of action (e.g., flurazepam and diazepam) should be avoided. Barbiturates should be avoided for the same reasons. An antidepressant should not be prescribed for insomnia unless the patient is depressed.

Antibiotics Serum creatinine is not a good index of renal function in old people; however, when it is elevated, special care must be taken with the administration of drugs normally excreted by the kidneys. Concentrations of relevant antibiotics should be measured directly.

Cardiac drugs In older patients, digitalis, procainamide, and quinidine have prolonged half-lives and narrow therapeutic windows; toxicity is common at the usual dosages. For example, digoxin toxicity—especially anorexia, confusion, or depression—can occur even with therapeutic digoxin levels.

H_2 receptor antagonists Most of these agents interfere with hepatic metabolism of other drugs, and all can produce confusion in the elderly. Because they are renally excreted, lower doses should be used to minimize the risk of toxicity in older individuals.

Antipsychotics and tricyclic antidepressants These drugs can produce anticholinergic side effects in old people (e.g., confusion, urinary retention, constipation, dry mouth). These can be minimized by switching to a nonanticholinergic agent (e.g., sertraline or nefazodone) or one with less anticholinergic effect (e.g., olanzapine, desipramine). In general, the least potent agents for psychosis (e.g., chlorpromazine) have the most sedating and anticholinergic effects and are the most likely to induce postural hypotension. By contrast, the most potent antipsychotic agents (e.g., haloperidol) have the least sedating, anticholinergic, and hypotensive side effects but cause extrapyramidal side effects, including dystonia, akathisia, rigidity, and tardive dyskinesia. The newer potent antipsychotics (e.g., risperidone, olanzapine, quetiapine, and clozapine) are relative exceptions to this rule. More specific for serotonin than dopamine D_2 receptors, these medications may be safer for older demented patients, especially those with hallucinations associated with Lewy body dementia or in those receiving therapy for Parkinson's disease. Unfortunately, even these newer drugs lose their specificity at the higher doses that are commonly required in clinical practice. Thus all of these agents are potentially toxic. Moreover, since both depression and agitation often remit spontaneously, cautious discontinuation of these drugs should be considered periodically.

Glaucoma medications Both topical beta blockers and carbonic anhydrase inhibitors can cause systemic side effects. The latter can cause malaise and anorexia independent of the induced metabolic acidosis.

Anticoagulants Elderly patients benefit from anticoagulation as much as do younger individuals but are more vulnerable to serious bleeding and drug interactions. Hence, more careful monitoring and less aggressive anticoagulation are advisable.

Analgesics Both propoxyphene and meperidine are associated with a disproportionate risk of delirium, and propoxyphene also increases the risk of hip fracture. Of the NSAIDs, indomethacin is most likely to induce confusion, fluid retention, and gastrointestinal bleeding. Each of these agents should be avoided in the elderly.

Avoidance of overtreatment Drugs are frequently not indicated in some common clinical situations. For instance, antibiotics need not be given for asymptomatic bacteriuria unless obstructive uropathy, other anatomic abnormalities, or stones are also present. Ankle edema is often due to venous insufficiency, drugs such as NSAIDs or some calcium antagonists, or even inactivity or malnutrition in chairbound patients. Diuretics are usually not indicated unless edema is associated with heart failure. Fitted, pressure gradient stockings are often helpful. Regular exercise is much more useful for claudication than is pentoxifylline. Finally, since older patients generally tolerate aspirin and other NSAIDs less well than do younger patients, localized pain should be treated when possible with local measures such as injection, physical therapy, heat, ultrasound, or transcutaneous electrical stimulation (Chap. 12).

PREVENTION

Much can be done to prevent the progression and even the onset of disease in older people. Dietary inadequacies should be corrected. Daily calcium intake should approximate 1500 mg, and most elderly people should take 400 to 800 IU of vitamin D daily (contained in one to two multivitamin tablets). Tobacco and alcohol use should be minimized, since the benefits of discontinuing these accrue even to individuals over age 65. The importance of reviewing all of a patient's medications and discontinuing them whenever feasible cannot be overemphasized.

Hypertension, whether isolated systolic hypertension or combined systolic and diastolic hypertension, should be treated. Treatment reduces the risk of stroke and the risk of death due to cardiovascular causes substantially in this age group and may also reduce the risk of cognitive impairment. These benefits have been achieved using *low doses* of a thiazide-like diuretic (e.g., chlorthalidone, 12.5 to 25 mg/d) as the first step (alone effective in almost half of patients) and adding low-dose reserpine (0.05 to 0.1 mg/d) or atenolol (25 to 50 mg/d) only as needed. Benefits are dramatic, side effects are minimal, cost is trivial, and concerns about potential toxicity have not been borne out.

Because of the prevalence, functional impact, and ease of treatment, glaucoma should be screened for, and visual and auditory impairment should be corrected. Dentures should be assessed for their fit, and oral lesions beneath them should be detected.

Because thyroid dysfunction is more prevalent in the elderly, difficult to detect clinically, and treatable, serum levels of thyroid-stimulating hormone should be measured at least once in asymptomatic older people and probably every 3 to 5 years thereafter. Serum cholesterol is worth measuring in patients with established coronary heart disease, but in those without apparent disease, screening for hypercholesterolemia is controversial. It seems reasonable to screen those who would be willing to comply with therapy, whose quality of life is good (from the patient's viewpoint), whose life expectancy exceeds several years (long enough to potentially benefit from therapy), and whose other risk factors—for which benefit of treatment has been definitely established—have already been addressed. A Papanicolaou test should be done in women who have not had one before, since the incidence of both preventable cervical carcinoma and associated death increases with age, especially in this group; it should be repeated triennially in all older women unless two previous tests have been normal. Screening for colon cancer is warranted until a minimum age of 80 to 85, at least in the community-dwelling elderly, although the optimal method is unclear. Immunizations for influenza, pneumococcal pneumonia, and tetanus should be current. Purified protein derivative (PPD) testing should be done on residents of chronic care facilities and on others at high risk of tuberculosis; those who have recently converted probably should be treated. Since responsiveness wanes with age, the test, if negative, should be repeated in a week to increase the chances of detecting all exposed patients. Because older women with breast cancer are more likely to die *of* it than *with* it, screening mammography is indicated every 1 to 2 years at least until age 75 and thereafter if a positive finding would result in therapeutic intervention. The relative risks and benefits of low-dose aspirin and (for women) estrogen replacement therapy have not yet been elucidated sufficiently in the elderly to warrant routine use, but they should be considered on an individual basis.

Exercise should be encouraged not only because of its beneficial effects on blood pressure, cardiovascular conditioning, glucose homeostasis, bone density, insomnia, functional status, and even longevity, but also because it may improve mood and social interaction, reduce constipation, and prevent falls. Resistance training should be encouraged as much as a walking program. Spinal flexion exercises should be avoided in patients with osteopenia; consultation with a physical therapist may be helpful.

Measures should be taken to prevent falling, as outlined in Tables 9-5 and 9-6. Now that alendronate has proved effective in preventing vertebral and hip fractures in older women, bone density should be measured in women who are willing to take the drug and who do not already take estrogen. Counseling about driving is important, especially for patients with cognitive impairment.

Perhaps the most valuable preventive measure in old people is to take a careful history, focusing not only on the "chief complaint" but also on common and often hidden conditions such as falls, confusion, depression, alcohol abuse, sexual dysfunction, and incontinence. In addition, one should always identify the complications for which the specific patient is at risk and take steps to avert them. For instance, a patient with cognitive impairment who smokes is at risk not only for lung cancer but also for starting a fire, and a patient who requires narcotics is at risk for fecal impaction, delirium, urinary retention, and confusion. Community-dwelling patients who are at highest risk of rapid deterioration and institutionalization and who should be monitored more closely include those over age 80, those who live alone, those who are bereaved or depressed, and those who are intellectually impaired.

BIBLIOGRAPHY

BURGIO KL et al: Behavioral vs. drug treatment for urge urinary incontinence in older women: A randomized controlled trial. JAMA 280:1995, 1998

Clinical Practice Guideline: *Recognition and Initial Assessment of Alzheimer's Disease and Related Dementias.* AHCPR Publication No. 97-0702. U.S. Dept. Health and Human Services, Public Health Service. Rockville, MD, Agency for Health Care Policy and Research, 1997

CLOSE J et al: Prevention of Falls in the Elderly Trial (PROFET). A randomized controlled trial. Lancet 353:93, 1999

COUNCIL ON ETHICAL AND JUDICIAL AFFAIRS, AMA: Medical futility in end-of-life care. JAMA 281:937, 1999

ERSHLER WB, LONGO DL: The biology of aging. Cancer 80:1284, 1997

GILLICK M et al: A patient-centered approach to advance medical planning in the nursing home. J Am Geriatr Soc 47:227, 1999

GUI Z et al: Cognitive impairment, drug use, and the risk of hip fracture in persons over 75 years old: A community-based prospective study. Am J Epidemiol 148:887, 1998

GUEYFFIER F et al: Antihypertensive drugs in very old people: A subgroup meta-analysis of randomised controlled trials. Lancet 353:793, 1999

IKEGAMI N: Functional assessment and its place in health care. N Engl J Med 332:598, 1995

INOUYE S et al: A multicomponent intervention to prevent delirium in hospitalized older patients. N Engl J Med 340:669, 1999

LEBOWITZ BD et al: Diagnosis and treatment of depression in late life. Consensus statement update. JAMA 278:1186, 1997

MILLER KE et al: The geriatric patient: A systematic approach to maintaining health. Am Family Phys 61:1089, 2000

OUSLANDER JG, SCHNELLE JF: Incontinence in the nursing home. Ann Intern Med 122:438, 1995

REYNOLDS CF et al: Treating insomnia in older adults. JAMA 281:1034, 1999

RESNICK NM, MARCANTONIO ER: How should clinical care of the aged differ? Lancet 350:1157, 1997

SALZMAN C: *Clinical Geriatric Psychopharmacology,* 3d ed. Baltimore, Williams & Wilkins, 1998

SINGER PA et al: Quality end-of-life care. Patients' perspectives. JAMA 281:163, 1999

VESTAL R: Aging and pharmacology. Cancer 80:1302, 1997

YANCIK R, RIES LA: Aging and cancer in America: Demographic and epidemiologic perspectives. Hem Onc Clin N Am 14:17, 2000

10   *Maureen T. Connelly, Thomas S. Inui*

PRINCIPLES OF DISEASE PREVENTION

PERSPECTIVES ON PREVENTION

The primary goals of prevention in medicine are to prolong life, to decrease morbidity, and to improve quality of life—all with the available resources. Working in partnership with patients, physicians play critical roles as educators, managers of access to screening and intervention services, and interpreters of divergent recommendations for promoting health. Despite evidence of the effectiveness of many preventive services in prolonging healthy life and decreasing medical costs, physicians frequently do not integrate appropriate preventive practices into their care. Obstacles to providing optimal preventive care include lack of appropriate training, doubt about the effectiveness of preventive interventions, skepticism about patients' commitment to change, limited reimbursement and time, and conflicting professional recommendations. Success achieved for populations may not be visible to individuals, and physicians may not appreciate the cumulative benefit of their efforts. Despite considerable success in some areas, such as the reduction of smoking by U.S. adults from 40 to 25% in the last 35 years, effective behavior change in other domains is often elusive, challenging and frustrating physicians and patients alike.

DEFINITIONS This chapter will be devoted to a discussion of *primary* and *secondary* prevention. *Primary prevention,* including various forms of health promotion and vaccination, is care intended to minimize risk factors and the subsequent incidence of disease. *Secondary prevention* is screening for detection of early disease, for example the use of mammography to detect preclinical breast cancer. While the term secondary prevention is also sometimes used for the prevention of recurrent episodes of an existing illness, most would consider this activity to be *tertiary prevention,* care intended to ameliorate the course of established disease.

Deciding what types of primary and secondary preventive care clinicians should offer to their patients is not a trivial matter. The United States Preventive Services Task Force (USPSTF), The Canadian Task Force on the Periodic Health Examination, and the American College of Physicians, among other organizations, have critically reviewed the strength of available evidence for preventive practices and have made recommendations. Adopting an evidence-based approach to the development of preventive practices policy is an essential step to assuaging provider concerns about the validity of particular recommendations, to identifying the specific basis of controversies in prevention, and to reassuring patients that certain interventions will do more good than harm.

PRIMARY PREVENTION

RISK MODIFICATION Of the more than 2 million deaths that occur in the United States each year, as many as half may be due to preventable causes (Table 10-1). Life-style and behavior play a central role in the primary causes of morbidity and mortality for adults—coronary heart disease, cancer, and injuries.

Tobacco The largest potentially modifiable risk to health is the abuse of tobacco products. Responsible for more than 400,000 deaths each year and an estimated annual cost to society as high as $50 billion, tobacco abuse accounts for a substantial fraction of cardiovascular, cancer, and pulmonary morbidity and mortality. Recent evidence also suggests that passive exposure to tobacco smoke results in chronic pulmonary disease, cardiovascular disease, and lung cancer for some adults. Because of the addictive properties of nicotine, preventing the initiation of tobacco abuse is the tobacco control intervention of choice. Most adult smokers acquire their habit as teenagers, and primary efforts to discourage initial tobacco use must engage younger

Cause	Deaths	
	Estimated No.*	Percentage of Total Deaths
Tobacco	400,000	19
Diet/activity patterns	300,000	14
Alcohol	100,000	5
Microbial agents	90,000	4
Toxic agents	60,000	3
Firearms	35,000	2
Sexual behavior	30,000	1
Motor vehicles	25,000	1
Illicit use of drugs	20,000	<1
TOTAL	1,060,000	50

* Composite approximation drawn from studies that use different approaches to derive estimates, ranging from actual counts (e.g., firearms) to population attributable risk calculations (e.g., tobacco). Numbers over 100,000 are rounded to the nearest 100,000; those over 50,000 are rounded to the nearest 10,000; those below 50,000 are rounded to the nearest 5000.
SOURCE: McGinnis JM, Foege WH: Actual cases of death in the United States. JAMA 270:2207, 1993.

audiences. However, smoking cessation extends life, even in individuals who quit after age 65 or those with established disease.

Counseling regarding the health risks of tobacco and methods for quitting is advised by all prevention advisory panels. Because 70% of smokers come into contact with health professionals each year, the medical encounter provides an opportunity to address the health implications of tobacco abuse. Although 70% of smokers say that they want to stop smoking, many are not ready to make an immediate change. The role of the provider is to motivate smokers to attempt cessation, reduce barriers to smoking cessation, and advise effective methods for cessation, including an expanding array of pharmacotherapeutic agents. Ninety percent of successful quitters will stop smoking without the aid of programmatic interventions. Setting a date to quit, arranging follow-up visits or phone calls during the initial quitting period, providing literature, and considering the use of nicotine replacement systems and other effective medications, such as bupropion, are all interventions that may improve the quitting success rate. Compared to placebo, nicotine replacement systems and bupropion have approximately twice the success rate at 6 months.

Diet   Mounting evidence suggests that modification of caloric intake, particularly the quality of calories, can result in decreased morbidity and mortality from cardiovascular disease, cancer, and diabetes. Excess weight is an independent risk factor for coronary disease, in addition to its contribution to the incidence of diabetes, hyperlipidemia, and hypertension. Between 20 and 30% of Americans are overweight, defined as 20% above the acceptable body-mass index (kg/m^2), and more than 40% of certain subpopulations, such as black, Native American, and Mexican-American women, are overweight. Despite concern about the risk of weight cycling, the health hazards of obesity appear to outweigh the potential harm of repeated weight loss and gain.

Americans derive excess calories from fats, particularly saturated fats, rather than from more beneficial sources such as complex carbohydrates, monounsaturated fats, and fiber. Since intake of saturated fat correlates with cholesterol level, and coronary heart disease is reduced by 2 to 3% for every 1% reduction in plasma cholesterol level, dietary modification will play a central role in decreasing the primary cause of mortality in America. Excess dietary fat intake has also been associated with breast, colon, prostate, and lung cancer in epidemiologic studies. The once widely accepted goals of reducing calories from all fats to 30% and from saturated fat to 10% have been challenged as the impact of types of fat (not simply fat itself) on morbidity and mortality is further elucidated. Increasing the intake of dietary fiber, such as from plant, legume, and grain sources, may contribute specifically to a decrease in colon cancer incidence.

Dietary sodium restriction may benefit those who have salt-sensitive hypertension, although the need for such restriction in the general population is unclear. Calcium and vitamin D are protective against osteoporosis, particularly in young women prior to reaching menopause, and evidence suggests that females at all ages have an inadequate intake. Menstruating women are at risk for iron-deficiency anemia. To achieve the recommended daily intake of vitamins and minerals, a varied diet including fish, lean meats, dairy products, whole grains, and five to six servings of fruits and vegetables daily is recommended, rather than the use of vitamin supplements. However, certain nutrients, such as adequate folate to prevent neural tube defects in developing fetuses, are not readily obtained from the typical American diet and may be best found in supplements. While evidence supporting the use of antioxidants such as vitamins E and C is still incomplete, the recommended quantities of these micronutrients can be obtained from a balanced diet.

Alcohol and Drugs   The use of alcohol and drugs accounts for more than 100,000 deaths annually. While the ability of health care providers to prevent the initiation of such behaviors has not been proven, screening for exposure and addiction could potentially direct medical effort to the prevention of alcohol and drug-associated problems such as injury, violence, and medical complications of drug abuse. Although instruments such as the CAGE questionnaire have proven to be valuable for detection of alcohol abuse, no comparable brief screening strategy is available for the routine identification of illicit drug abuse. Health care providers screen inadequately for both disorders, despite evidence for effective early treatment of addictions and their complications. Reviewing recent data that moderate alcohol consumption may lower the risk of heart disease may open a discussion with patients about appropriate use. Legal implications of identifying illicit drug use may hinder detection of this problem. When screening for these disorders is feasible, interventions that have proven effective include brief counseling, referral to ambulatory and in-patient treatment programs, use of 12-step and other community organizations, and appropriate use of medications such as methadone for heroin abuse.

Physical Activity   Not only can increased physical activity decrease obesity, but avoiding a sedentary life-style can also decrease the incidence of cardiac disease, hypertension, diabetes, and osteoporotic fracture. It is estimated that only 22% of U.S. adults engage in at least light to moderate physical activity, such as walking for 30 min three to five times per week. A full quarter of the population pursues no vigorous physical activity at all. The magnitude of benefit derived from physical activity may be as great as a 35% reduction in coronary heart disease, and even light exercise is preferable to no exercise. At present, the intensity, frequency, duration, and type of physical activity required to achieve optimal cardiac benefit remain unclear. While earlier studies suggested that vigorous exercise was needed to achieve maximal risk reduction, recent studies suggest that regular moderate-intensity activity, such as walking for exercise on most days, is associated with a reduced risk of cardiac events. A sudden onset of vigorous activity in the unfit may increase the risk for myocardial infarction and sudden death. Patients should be informed that, despite previous physical inactivity, the incremental adoption of a regular fitness program can decrease their risk of cardiovascular and other diseases to the level of those who have remained fit throughout their lives. Successful exercise programs are integrated into daily routines, self-directed, and injury-free.

Sexual Behavior   Because of the substantial risks of infectious diseases and unwanted pregnancy from unprotected sexual activity, patients should be strongly advised to use barrier methods for all high-risk practices such as oral, anal, and vaginal intercourse as well as additional contraceptive methods when pregnancy would not be welcome.

Environment   Physicians should adopt a broad construction of environmental risks to health, considering the physical, social, and occupational environments of their patients. Taking a complete exposure history, focusing on home, work, neighborhood, hobbies, and

Table 10-2 Recommendations for Preventive Medical Care for the General Population, Age 25 and Older

Screening
  Blood pressure
  Height and weight
  Pap smear if history of sexual activity and cervix present
  FOBT and/or sigmoidoscopy[a]
  Mammography ± breast exam[b]
  Assess for problem drinking
  Total blood cholesterol (men age 35 to 64, women age 45 to 64)
  Vision screening[c]
  Assess for hearing impairment[c]
Counseling
  Tobacco cessation
  Avoidance of alcohol and drugs when driving, swimming, boating
  Limitation of fat, cholesterol
  Maintenance of caloric balance
  Emphasis on grains, fruits, vegetables in diet
  Adequate calcium
  Physical activity
  Lap/shoulder belts
  Motorcycle and bicycle helmets
  Smoke detectors
  Storage or removal of firearms
  STD prevention
  Dental visits, fluoride, flossing
  Contraception
  Fall prevention[c]
  CPR training for household[c]
  Hot water heater at <120°[c]
Immunization
  Tetanus-diphtheria (Td)
  Pneumococcal vaccine[c]
  Influenza vaccine[c]
  Rubella serology or vaccination[d]
Chemoprophylaxis
  Discussion of hormone replacement therapy with perimenopausal women
  Multivitamin with folic acid[d]

[a] After age 49
[b] After age 49; evidence conflicting after age 69[d]
[c] Ages 65+
[d] Women of childbearing years
SOURCE: Adapted from the U.S. Preventive Services Task Force *Guide to Clinical Preventive Services.* Consult full report for details and recommendations for high-risk individuals.

dietary habits, can help direct interventions and recommendations. While local circumstances will dictate specific risks to which patients should be alerted, such as regional infectious diseases or particular toxic exposures produced by local industry, certain general recommendations should be adopted universally for health promotion.

Since skin cancers, the vast majority of them secondary to sun exposure, constitute the most common form of malignancy, all patients should be counseled to avoid sun overexposure and to use sunscreens. Patients should be encouraged to consider potential toxin exposures, such as those due to air pollution, household smoking, or carbon monoxide and radon gases, and be informed of the medical symptoms and consequences of such exposures. Proper food preparation and storage decrease the incidence of food-borne infectious disease.

Unintended injury constitutes a significant preventable burden of morbidity and mortality and is the leading cause of death for the general population under 40. Automobile accidents are the leading cause of unintentional injuries. The risk of being involved in a disabling traffic accident may be as high as 30% in the course of an individual's lifetime, and 50% of deaths from automobile accidents could be prevented with regular seatbelt use. Physicians should recommend seatbelt use, as well as helmet use for motorcycle and bicycle riders, since evidence supports a higher likelihood of use among patients who receive such advice. Clinicians should also recommend against operating

a motor vehicle after drinking, since alcohol (and illicit drugs) is a clear-cut risk cofactor.

Smoke detectors are underused, being found in only 80% of homes. Since most deaths due to fire occur in the residential setting, patients should be encouraged to install at least one on each floor of their home.

Attention to health hazards in the workplace can identify those at risk and prevent long-term consequences of exposure. Evaluation of the work environment should include questions about exposure to metals, dusts, fibers, chemicals, fumes, radiation, loud noises, extreme temperatures, and biologic agents.

Community and family violence, particularly through the misuse of firearms, is the second leading cause of death from unintentional injury. Firearms, especially handguns, are far more likely to injure a family member than an intruder and are associated with increased rates of suicide and harm to children. Patients should be encouraged to remove their weapons from the home and should be informed of the risks associated with improper security and storage of firearms. At a minimum, trigger locks may prevent accidental injury from firearms. While community and family violence are epidemic in the United States, interventions to curtail violent behavior are not well established. Screening for exposure to relationship violence, developing plans for safe havens, and referrals to appropriate community and government agencies can prevent continued abuse.

IMMUNIZATION As many as 70,000 deaths due to influenza, pneumococcal infections, and hepatitis B occur in the United States annually. Despite good availability and evidence for the cost-effectiveness of recommended vaccinations for adults, only 40% or fewer members of target populations are immunized. Factors explaining poor adherence to adult immunization guidelines include lack of confidence in vaccine efficacy among providers and patients, underestimation of the severity of the target diseases, incomplete reimbursement, lack of systems to identify and vaccinate high-risk populations, and the absence of an adult requirement for vaccination equivalent to our vaccination policies for school-age children. Table 10-2 lists recommended adult immunizations.

CHEMOPROPHYLAXIS There is significant supportive evidence for the use of certain medications in primary prevention. Therapy of this nature in the otherwise healthy person, however, is not risk-free. The use of aspirin for the prevention of cardiovascular disease or colorectal cancer, for example, is supported by evidence from cohort and, in the case of cardiovascular disease, randomized controlled trials. The potential for cerebral bleeds and gastrointestinal intolerance, however, must be balanced against a patient's individual risk for the target diseases. Although no randomized trials have measured the impact on mortality, postmenopausal hormone replacement therapy is another therapy given to healthy women for the prevention of future disease (coronary heart disease and osteoporosis), as well as to control menopausal symptoms. These benefits must be weighed against the risks of possible breast and endometrial cacinoma. Patient involvement in the decision-making process, perhaps even informed consent, is recommended to ensure compliance, proper use of medication, and sustained monitoring for side effects.

SECONDARY PREVENTION

SCREENING Widespread screening for the presence of existing diseases should meet the following criteria:

1. The targeted disease must be sufficiently burdensome to the population that a screening program is warranted. Minor changes in relative risk should have a substantial impact on the absolute risk within the population.
2. The target disease must have a well-understood natural history with a long preclinical latent period.
3. The screening method must have acceptable technical performance parameters, detecting the disease at an earlier stage than would be possible without screening and minimizing false-positive and false-negative results.
4. Efficacious treatment for the target illness must be available.

5. Early detection must improve disease outcome.

6. Cost, feasibility, and acceptability of screening and early treatment should be established.

While physicians under-provide certain screening services that have met these criteria (for example, regular mammograms for women over age 50 years), it is also the case that some prevalent screening practices today are not solidly rooted in evidence. Screening tests such as mammography in women under 50 and measurement of prostate-specific antigen have been adopted for use by many clinicians despite lack of complete current evidence that these services will decrease the risk of morbidity or mortality or improve the quality of life. See Table 10-2 recommendations of the USPSTF for screening of adults who are at average risk for target conditions. Recommendations for special-risk and vulnerable populations are available in the USPSTF *Guide*.

COMMUNITY HEALTH ADVOCACY

In addition to the direct clinical provision of preventive and health-promoting services, physicians can bring their knowledge, expertise, clinical experience, and influence to bear at the community level to promote health. Whether arguing for the denormalization of tobacco use or providing data about the health risks of local incinerators, physicians are important sources of information and support for improving health beyond the clinical office. Such activities are consistent with the overall objective of caring for patients and may have a substantial impact on decreasing the prevalence of the root causes of disease.

BIBLIOGRAPHY

BROWN AI, GARBER AM: A concise review of the cost effectiveness of coronary heart disease prevention. Med Clin N Am 84:279, 2000

FEDSON DS: Adult immunization: Summary of the National Vaccine Advisory Committee Report. JAMA 272:1133, 1994

GOLDSTEIN MG, NIAURA R: Methods to enhance smoking cessation after myocardial infarction. Med Clin N Am 84:63, 2000

HENSRUD DD: Clinical preventive medicine in primary care: Background and practice. Mayo Clin Proc 75:165, 2000

LEMAITRE RN et al: Leisure-time physical activity and the risk of primary cardiac arrest. Arch Intern Med 159:686, 1999

POPE AM, RALL DP (eds): *Environmental Medicine: Integrating a Missing Element into Medical Education*. Washington, DC, National Academy Press, 1995

SMOKING CESSATION CLINICAL PRACTICE GUIDELINE PANEL AND STAFF. The Agency for Health Care Policy and Research Smoking Cessation Clinical Practice Guideline. JAMA 275:1270, 1996

SOX HC: Preventive health services in adults. N Engl J Med 330:1589, 1994

U.S. PREVENTIVE SERVICES TASK FORCE: *Guide to Clinical Preventive Services*, 2d ed. Baltimore, Williams & Wilkins, 1995

WILLETT WC: Diet and health: What should we eat? Science 264:532, 1994

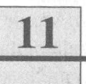

11

Adriane Fugh-Berman

ALTERNATIVE MEDICINE

Alternatives to conventional medicine will always exist. Defined by its outsider status, alternative therapies of one era may be conventional therapies in another. Radiation treatment and the use of transcutaneous electrical nerve stimulation (TENS), now widely used in medicine, were once unconventional therapies. Even leeches have made a minor comeback; hirudin, a potent anticoagulant secreted by leeches, has been approved by the U.S. Food and Drug Administration (FDA) as an antithrombotic agent. Alternative medicine is any approach to a health problem that is different from those used by conventional medical practitioners; many alternative therapies complement rather than supplant conventional medicine.

Alternative medicine ranges from systems with distinct disease theories, diagnostic methods, and multiple treatment options (including traditional Chinese medicine and Ayurvedic medicine) to single-

component panaceas, such as bee pollen (Table 11-1). While conventional western medicine is primarily based upon physiology and pathophysiology, alternative therapies may be based on alternative paradigms (e.g., eastern concepts of energy, called "qi" in Chinese medicine or "prana" in Ayurvedic medicine) or may be based on unproven biochemical hypotheses (e.g., high doses of vitamin C). Although many unconventional therapies are not supported by rigorous prospective clinical trials, "alternative" is not synonymous with "unproven." Data from well-designed and well-executed clinical studies support the use of certain alternative medicines in some settings (see below).

The use of unconventional therapies is widespread. In 1997, a telephone survey found that 42% of English-speaking adults in the United States used some sort of alternative therapy. Usage is especially high among people of color, reflecting the fact that, for many, alternative therapies *are* traditional medicine. Patients who use alternative medicine do so most often at opposite ends of the disease spectrum: either for symptom relief in mild or chronic illnesses or for life-threatening conditions (typically as adjuncts to conventional medicine).

PLACEBO OR NONSPECIFIC EFFECTS To what extent does the *placebo effect* explain the popularity of alternative medicine? Now more commonly called *nonspecific effects*, this phenomenon encompasses numerous factors including the environment, the relationship between the patient and the practitioner, beliefs and expectations (of both the patient and practitioner), natural history of the disease, and individual variability. The nature of the placebo effect is itself under investigation.

It may be assumed that nonspecific effects enhance positive outcomes of both unconventional and conventional therapies. However, scientific evaluation must be the primary determinant of the physician's attitude toward alternative therapies.

HERBAL MEDICINE Herbalism (also called *phytomedicine*, *phytotherapy*, or *botanical medicine*) is the medicinal use of plants or plant constituents. The use of plants as medicine predates even human evolution; great apes have been noted to consume specific medicinal plants when they are ill. Many of the drugs in clinical practice are derived from plants, as are the majority of analgesics: lidocaine and novocaine from the coca plant (*Erythroxylum coca*); opioids from the poppy (*Papaver somniferum*); aspirin from meadowsweet (*Spirea ulmaria*), whence the "spir" part of its name derives. The progestin component of oral contraceptives comes from the Mexican yam (*Diascorea villosa*); digoxin comes from foxglove (*Digitalis lanata*); cromolyn sodium is a khellin derivative from the Ayurvedic herb *Ammi visnaga*; and warfarin is a derivative of dicoumarin, from sweet clover (*Melilotus officinalis*). The ipecac that is kept in the medicine cabinet for poisonings comes from the root of a South American shrub (*Cephaelis ipecacuanha*); the benzoin that attaches bandages to skin is a gum resin from *Styrax benzoin*; and the witch hazel used to soothe hemorrhoids is an extract of *Hamamelis virginiana*. Fungi also have contributed to pharmaceuticals: penicillin was isolated from the fungus *Penicillium notatum*, cephalosporins were derived from a marine fungus (*Cephalosporium acremonium*), and lovastatin was derived from the fungus *Aspergillus terreus*.

Essentially every culture has a tradition of herbal medicine. In western herbalism, herbs are often used singly but may sometimes be combined. Chinese herbal medicine utilizes complex mixtures of many herbs, sometimes combined with animal materials. Herbs may be used to treat or prevent disease. As preventives, "tonics" support the function of specific organs, and "adaptogens" are nonspecific treatments that facilitate a return to homeostasis.

Some clinical trial data support the use of Saint John's wort (SJW) for depression, kava for anxiety, saw palmetto for benign prostatic hyperplasia (BPH), and ginkgo for increasing cerebral blood flow. Evidence also supports the use of garlic for lowering cholesterol, hawthorn to improve cardiac function, and echinacea for treating (but not preventing) upper respiratory infections.

Saint John's Wort (*Hypericum perforatum*) A meta-analysis of the use of SJW for mild to moderate depression examined 23 ran-

Table 11-1 Some Alternative Medicines

Type	Description
Ayurvedic medicine	The major East Indian traditional medicine system, utilizing pulse and tongue diagnosis; treatments include diet, exercise, herbs, oil massages, and elimination regimens (utilizing emetics, diarrheals, etc.)
Aromatherapy	The use of essential plant oils (distilled concentrates) in massage, baths, or inhalation
Alexander technique	A movement therapy that emphasizes efficient use of muscles to relieve pain, decrease skeletal strain, and improve posture
Acupuncture	A Chinese medical practice that involves the insertion of hair-thin needles into non-anatomic energy channels called meridians
Anthroposophic medicine	A spiritually based system of medicine that incorporates herbs, homeopathy, diet, and a movement therapy called eurythmy
Bach flower remedies	Dilute flower infusions used to treat emotional conditions
Biofeedback	The use of machinery that translates physiologic processes into audio or visual signals
Chiropractic	Adjustment of spinal vertebrae in an effort to affect neuromuscular function
Cranial sacral therapy	Gentle manipulation of the cranium and spine
Curanderismo	A spiritual healing tradition common in Mexican-American communities that utilizes ritual cleansing, herbs, and incantations
Espiritismo/Mesa Blanca/spiritism	A religious system, common in Puerto Rico and Cuba, that utilizes mediums; therapies include herbs and oils
Dance therapy	Therapeutic method that uses movement to facilitate emotional expression and release
Feldenkrais bodywork	Highly structured movement sequences that emphasize proper head positioning
Guided imagery	The use of imagination to invoke specific images that affect physiologic function
Hydropathy	Treatment utilizing water at various temperatures, sometimes aerated or under pressure, sometimes with added salts or other substances
Hypnosis	The induction of an altered state of mind within which a subject becomes receptive to specific suggestions
Massage	The use of specific gliding and kneading strokes and friction to achieve muscle relaxation
Meditation	A process by which one tries to achieve awareness without thought
Music therapy	Singing, playing instruments, or listening to music
Naturopathy	A mixture of modalities that may include herbs, homeopathy, acupuncture, hydropathy, diet, and exercise
Native American medicine	Diverse systems, many of which incorporate prayer, chant, music, healing ceremonies, counseling, herbs, laying on of hands, and smudging (ritual cleansing with smoke from sacred plants)
Reflexology/zone therapy	Manual stimulation of points on the hands or feet, believed to affect distant organs
Rolfing/structural integration	A manual therapy that attempts to realign the body by deep tissue manipulation of fasciae
Santeria	A Latin American spiritist system derived from the Yoruba tribe (of southern Nigeria); santeros are believed to communicate with saints
Shiatsu/acupressure	Finger pressure at points along nonanatomic meridians
Siddha medicine	An East Indian medical system (prevalent among Tamil-speaking people) utilizing breathing techniques, incantations, herbs, and muppu (a tri-salt preparation)
T'ai chi ch'uan	Chinese dance-like exercises described as a "moving meditation"
Therapeutic touch	Secular version of the laying on of hands, described as a "healing meditation"
Tibetan medicine	A medical system that utilizes diagnosis by pulse and urine examination; therapies include herbs, diet, and massage
Traditional Chinese medicine	A medical system that utilizes examination of the tongue and pulses for diagnosis and acunpuncture, herbal mixtures, massage, exercise, and diet as therapeutics
Trager bodywork	Light massage combined with gentle passive movements to help patients maximize freedom of movement
Unani medicine	An East Indian medical system, derived from Persian medicine, practiced primarily in the Muslim community
Yoga	An Indian practice that includes postures (asanas), breathing exercises (pranayama), and cleansing practices (kriyas)

tops standardized to 0.3% hypericin (long thought to be the most active compound in SJW). However, hyperforin is most likely the prime active agent, and extracts standardized to 3% hyperforin have been tested in clinical trials and are available. The usual dose of both of these preparations is 300 mg tid.

In vitro, a high concentration of SJW inhibits the uptake of serotonin, norepinephrine, and dopamine. Among neurotransmitters, its strongest binding affinity is to γ-aminobutyric acid (GABA) A and B receptors. Although SJW demonstrates monoamine oxidase (MAO) inhibition in vitro, this effect has not been demonstrated in vivo, nor have there been any reported cases of MAO inhibitor–associated hypertensive crises in humans using SJW (the herb may, however, potentiate serotonin reuptake inhibitors). Side effects of SJW include gastrointestinal symptoms, fatigue, and photosensitization.

Ginkgo (*Ginkgo biloba*) Ginkgo leaf extracts have been proposed for treating Alzheimer's or multi-infarct dementia. In several randomized controlled trials, a small but statistically significant effect after 3 to 6 months of treatment with 40 to 80 mg tid of standardized *G. biloba* extract (containing 22 to 27% flavonoid glycosides and 5 to 7% terpene lactones) was noted on objective measures of cognitive function in patients with Alzheimer's disease. Ginkgo appears to have vasoregulatory and antioxidant effects as well as inhibiting platelet-activating factor (PAF). Serious intracerebral bleeding associated with ginkgo use has been reported, including two subdural hematomas, one intracerebral hemorrhage, one subarachnoid hemorrhage, and one case of spontaneous hyphema. In most cases, these patients were receiving concurrent anticoagulant drugs.

Kava (*Piper methysticum*) Used in Polynesia as a ceremonial beverage, the roots and rhizomes of kava are used medicinally for anxiety and insomnia in Europe and in North America. Several placebo-controlled trials have shown significant anxiolytic activity of kava products (standardized to 70% kavalactones), usually in a dose of 70 mg tid. *Kavalactones* (also called *kavapyrones*) are muscle relaxants; they include kawain, dihydrokawain, methysticin, and dihydromethysticin (the latter two are potent inhibitors of norepinephrine uptake).

Therapeutic doses may result in mild gastrointestinal complaints or allergic skin reactions (incidence ~1.5%). Chronic use of high-dose kava may result in *kava dermopathy*, a reversible ichthyosiform eruption that is often accompanied by eye irritation.

Ginseng (*Panax ginseng* and other *Panax* species) Ginseng is a popular herb in both western and eastern medicine. The place of ginseng root in the treatment of specific conditions remains to be shown in clinical trials. Ginseng contains ginsenosides, polyacetylenes, and sesquiterpenes. It appears to have some glucocorticoid-like actions and hypoglycemic activity and also affects neurotransmitter activity. Glucocorticoid administration blocks the effect of ginsenosides both in vitro and in vivo; ginsenosides increase adrenal cyclic AMP in intact but not hypophysectomized rats,

domized trials (20 were double-blind) with a total of 1757 outpatients. In 15 placebo-controlled trials, SJW was found to be significantly more effective than placebo. In eight treatment-controlled trials, clinical improvement in those receiving SJW did not differ significantly from those receiving tricyclic antidepressants. The trials in this meta-analysis were heterogeneous and used varying diagnostic criteria and dosages of SJW.

Most clinical trials have been done with extracts of the flowering-

so effects on adrenal secretion appear to be through the pituitary gland. Several cases of postmenopausal uterine bleeding have been reported from ginseng use, although ginseng does not contain known phytoestrogens.

Saw Palmetto (*Serenoa repens*) Saw palmetto fruits were used as food by Native Americans; their most common use today is to treat BPH. A systemic review of randomized controlled trials of extracts of the fruit *S. repens* (alone or in combination with other herbs) identified 18 randomized trials (16 double-blind) that included 2939 men and lasted 4 to 48 weeks. Compared with placebo, *S. repens* improved urinary symptom scores, nocturia, and peak urine flow. In two studies that compared finasteride with *S. repens*, improvements in urinary symptoms scores were similar. Adverse effects due to *S. repens* were mild and infrequent.

Saw palmetto is usually administered in liposterolic extracts standardized to 70 to 95% free fatty acids; the usual dose is 160 mg bid. Saw palmetto appears to have multiple mechanisms of action including inhibition of 5α-reductase and inhibition of dihydrotestosterone binding to cytosolic androgen receptors.

Pollen/Bee Pollen Pollen may be collected directly from plants or their pollinators; bee pollen is flower pollen collected from bees. A double-blind placebo-controlled trial of a mixed-pollen extract in 60 patients with BPH found that subjective improvement was significantly better in the treated group; there was a significant decrease in residual urine and in diameter of the prostate on ultrasound. However, flow rate and volume were unchanged. Allergic reactions, hypereosinophilia, and eosinophilic gastroenteritis have been associated with bee pollen intake.

Echinacea Species Echinacea roots are used to treat or prevent infections. The three species used commercially are *Echinacea purpurea*, *E. angustifolia*, and *E. pallida*. A systemic review of 16 trials (8 prevention and 8 treatment trials on upper respiratory tract infections) with a total of 3396 participants found a wide variation in preparations and methodologic quality of trials. Although many available studies reported positive results of echinacea compared to placebo, reviewers concluded that the evidence is not strong enough to recommend a specific dose, product, or preparation.

Immunomodulatory effects are attributed to five classes of compounds in echinacea preparations: caffeic acid derivatives, alkylamides, polyacetylenes, glycoproteins, and polysaccharides. The alkylamides are regarded as the most active chemical constituent. Echinacea stimulates both humoral and cellular immunity; theoretically, it could worsen symptoms in atopic individuals or those with autoimmune disease.

Adverse Effects of Herbs Herbs have pharmacologic effects and can be associated with adverse effects or interactions. Many medicinal herbs (and pharmaceutical drugs) are therapeutic at one dose and toxic at another. The relative dearth of reports of adverse events and interactions attributed to herbal products reflects a combination of underreporting and the relatively nontoxic nature of most herbal usage.

The most dangerous plants used medicinally are aconite and any herbs containing unsaturated pyrrolizidine alkaloids (saturated pyrrolizidine alkaloids lack toxicity). Several herbs that do not contain pyrrolizidine alkaloids have also shown hepatotoxicity.

Aconite (*Aconitum* spp.), sometimes used in Chinese herb mixtures to treat pain or heart failure, contains aconitine and other C_{19} diterpenoid alkaloids. Proper curing of aconite reduces alkaloids by 90%, but even appropriately cured aconite can result in serious, sometimes fatal, cardiac arrhythmias. The first symptoms of aconite poisoning occur within 90 min of ingestion; the majority of patients present with neurologic symptoms (most commonly oral numbness or burning), progressing to peripheral paresthesia and generalized muscle weakness. Nausea and vomiting are also common.

Cardiovascular effects include bradycardia, hypotension, and arrhythmias (including ventricular or supraventricular tachycardia, bidirectional tachycardia, sinus bradycardia with first-degree heart block, bundle branch block with junctional escape rhythm, or torsade de pointes). Other symptoms may include chest pain, abdominal pain,

diarrhea, hyperventilation, respiratory distress, dizziness, sweating, confusion, headache, and excessive lacrimation. No specific antidote for aconite is known, and treatment is mainly supportive. Atropine may be given if symptoms of cholinergic excess are apparent. Antiarrhythmics are often helpful, but characteristically, electrical cardioversion is markedly unsuccessful in aconite poisoning.

Unsaturated pyrrolizidine alkaloids are hepatotoxic; children may be especially sensitive. Unsaturated pyrrolizidine alkaloids occur in comfrey (*Symphytum*), borage (*Borago officinalis*) leaf (seed oils are safe), coltsfoot (*Tussilago farfara*), and species of *Crotalaria* and *Senecio*. Liver toxicity has also been associated with chaparral (*Larrea divaricata*), germander (*Teucrium chamaedrys*), and a Chinese medicine called *jin bu huan* (which contains 36% levo-tetrahydropalmitine, a chemical present in *Stephania* and *Corydalis* genera).

Drug Interactions One of the most serious herb-drug interactions is increased risk of bleeding when warfarin is combined with anticoagulant herbs: cases of bleeding have been reported with ginkgo (*G. biloba*), garlic (*Allium sativum*), and the Chinese herbs danshen (*Salvia miltiorrhiza*) and dong quai (*Angelica sinensis*). The soluble fibers guar gum and psyllium can slow or reduce the absorption of many drugs, and anthranoid-containing laxatives, including senna (*Cassia senna* and *C. angustifolia*) and cascara sagrada (*Rhamnus purshiana*), can also reduce the absorption of many drugs. An Ayurvedic syrup, shankhapushpi, has been associated with reduced levels of phenytoin. Licorice (*Glycyrrhiza glabra*) can potentiate both oral and topical glucocorticoids.

Several herbs can interact with psychotropic drugs; the herb yohimbe (*Pausinystalia yohimbe*) (also available as the drug yohimbine; both forms are used to treat impotence) increases the risk of hypertension when combined with tricyclic antidepressants. Extrapyramidal effects have occurred in patients ingesting neuroleptics and betel nut (*Areca catechu*); mania has been induced in depressed patients who mix antidepressants and *P. ginseng*; and SJW (*H. perforatum*) combined with a serotonin reuptake inhibitor may produce a mild "serotonin syndrome" (with symptoms of nausea, vomiting, and confusion); the full-blown syndrome may include myoclonus, agitation, fever, abdominal cramping, and hypertension (Chap. 385).

Adulterants and Contaminants Herbal products may be contaminated, mislabeled, or contain misidentified plants. Medicinal plants from India and Sri Lanka can be contaminated with toxigenic fungi, including *Aspergillus* and *Fusarium*. Heavy metals have been detected in some Asian herbal products (metals are sometimes deliberately used in the preparation of Ayurvedic herbal medicines). Without any mention on the label, pharmaceutical drugs may also be incorporated into herbal products, a particular problem in Chinese herbal preparations imported from Hong Kong and Taiwan. Nonsteroidal anti-inflammatory drugs and benzodiazepines have been found in Chinese herbal products, including Miracle Herb, Tung Shueh, and Chuifong Toukuwan (since 1974 this notorious brand has incorporated at least 10 different drugs into the preparation). The absence of standard manufacturing practices creates risks that are difficult to quantify.

ACUPUNCTURE Acupuncture was recognized in western medical texts a century ago; Sir William Osler's *Principles and Practice of Medicine*, first published in 1892, recommended acupuncture for both sciatica and lumbago; and the 1901 edition of *Gray's Anatomy* noted the use of acupuncture for sciatica.

Stimulation of acupuncture points may be done by needles, finger pressure, electrical stimulation, or heat (usually applied by a smoldering cone or rod of "moxa," made of the herb mugwort, *Artemisia vulgaris*). Acupuncture is effective in the treatment of nausea and vomiting. In 27 of 33 controlled trials, superiority of acupuncture point stimulation over placebo for nausea and vomiting of various etiologies was demonstrated. In substance abusers, the therapy may reduce withdrawal symptoms, but evidence is lacking about whether acupuncture has any long-term effect in preventing recidivism. An analysis of 16 randomized controlled trials of acupuncture for smoking cessation showed no beneficial effect of acupuncture over sham or no treatment. Limited preliminary data suggest a possible beneficial effect for acupuncture in stroke rehabilitation. Although acupuncture is known to stimulate endorphin release, and its use for pain is better accepted than for other conditions, controlled clinical trials of pain treatment have had mixed results.

Risks Inadequately sterilized acupuncture needles have been linked to infections, including HIV infection and an epidemic of hepatitis B. Two cases of fatal *Staphylococcus* sepsis have been reported. More than 100 cases of pneumothorax have been reported. Rare cases both of spinal trauma and cardiac tamponade (caused by penetration of a congenital sternal foramen) have been reported.

HOMEOPATHY Originated in the early nineteenth century by Samuel Hahnemann, a German physician, homeopathy is based on the "doctrine of similars"; animal, vegetable, or mineral substances that cause symptoms in a well person are used to treat those same symptoms in a sick person. For example, poison ivy (*Rhus toxicodendron*) is used to treat varicella (chickenpox). Because conventional treatments aim to counter rather than reproduce symptoms, practitioners of homeopathy refer to conventional medicine as "allopathy."

Usually, remedies are used in highly dilute concentrations, and homeopaths believe that the most dilute remedies are the most potent. If analyzed chemically, many homeopathic remedies contain no detectable levels of the original substance. It is difficult to conceive of a scientifically testable hypothesis that could explain the putative effects of homeopathic medicine where a preparation containing few or no molecules of an active agent are said to have pharmacologic effects. A meta-analysis of 89 placebo-controlled trials of homeopathy found that the odds ratio was 2.45 (CI, 2.05 to 2.93) in favor of homeopathy over placebo. The quality of these studies was not uniform, and the studies with the best methodologic quality yielded significantly less positive results.

Risks A case of pancreatitis associated with intake of homeopathic medication has been reported. Potentially toxic levels of arsenic and cadmium have been found in "low potency" (less dilute) homeopathic preparations.

SPINAL MANIPULATION Therapeutic manipulation of the body has ancient roots; Hippocrates, Aesculapius, and Galen all used some form of it. A physician, Andrew Taylor Still, originated osteopathy in 1892. Daniel David Palmer invented chiropractic in 1895. A meta-analysis of nine methodologically acceptable studies of spinal manipulation for low-back pain found a definite improvement at 3 weeks for patients with uncomplicated, acute back pain. For patients with chronic pain or sciatic nerve irritation, chiropractic was not helpful.

A meta-analysis of cervical manipulation for neck pain concluded that manipulation, in combination with other treatment, may produce short-term pain relief.

Risks Complications of spinal manipulation include vertebrobasilar accidents, disc herniations, vertebral fracture, spinal cord compression, and cauda equina syndrome. More than 80% of serious complications from chiropractic occur after cervical manipulation. It is impossible to determine the true rate of complications from chiropractic manipulations, but estimates vary from 1 in 400,000 to between 3 and 6 per 10 million. The incidence of cauda equina syndrome is thought to be less than 1 per 10 million manipulations.

MASSAGE Several studies support the use of massage for reducing lymphedema; the technique matches the effectiveness of uniform-pressure pneumatic devices.

Numerous studies in hospital settings describe the use of infant massage to decrease hospital stays of premature babies. A meta-analysis of randomized trials found that massage interventions improved daily weight gain by 5 g, while gentle, still touch did not show a benefit. Methodologic concerns about the blinding undermine the conclusions.

Risks Massage has been used in an effort to prevent pressure sores, but it is not clearly effective and may increase tissue trauma when done over bony prominences.

MIND/BODY THERAPIES Biofeedback Biofeedback uses instruments to translate information on physiologic function into audio or visual signals that patients use as cues to help them learn to affect functions not normally thought to be under voluntary control. Commonly used modalities include electromyographic (EMG) feedback of skeletal muscle contraction, thermal feedback of skin temperature (an indirect measure of peripheral blood flow), electroencephalographic (EEG) feedback, electrodermal response (EDR) (feedback of sweat gland activity on the fingers), and perineometry (feedback of contraction of pelvic floor muscles and anal sphincter).

Biofeedback treatment modalities may be combined. For example, for urinary incontinence, biofeedback may be used to measure pelvic muscle activity through urethral sphincter pressure and electromyography, circumvaginal muscle manometry and electromyography, and anorectal manometry and electromyography. Detrusor pressure feedback may be measured by cystometry, and feedback on intraabdominal pressure may be used to help patients learn to simultaneously contract pelvic muscles while relaxing abdominal muscles (to avoid putting excess pressure on the bladder). Clinical trials support the use of biofeedback in the treatment of urinary incontinence (stress, urge, or mixed), fecal incontinence, migraine, tension headaches, and in stroke rehabilitation.

Hypnosis Traditional hypnosis utilizes the induction of a deep trance state to enhance suggestibility. Several clinical trials indicate that hypnosis is effective in chemotherapy-associated nausea and may be helpful in the treatment of irritable bowel syndrome and pain syndromes. Numerous uncontrolled trials suggest a beneficial effect of hypnosis on smoking cessation, but controlled trials are less impressive. A meta-analysis of hypnosis in nine randomized controlled trials of hypnotherapy found significant heterogeneity among the results of the individual studies, with conflicting results for the effectiveness of hypnotherapy compared to no treatment or to advice. Hypnotherapy was not more effective than rapid smoking (an aversive therapy in which cigarettes are smoked in quick succession) or psychological treatment.

DIETARY SUPPLEMENTS The fundamental principles of good nutrition are to eat a balanced variety of foods and to maintain a balance of calories taken in with calories burned through activity. Dietary supplements have become a large and lucrative business that promotes the idea that our food is somehow lacking in specific nutrients and that additional intake of any number of food components will treat or prevent specific diseases, improve athletic and sexual performance, and make us live longer. These claims are largely either untested or unproven (Table 11-2). Unfortunately, the *Dietary Supplement Health and Education Act* (DSHEA) of 1994 prevents the FDA from monitoring the quality or safety of dietary supplements before marketing. Supplements do not even have to be dietary components to be sold as dietary supplements (the availability of over-the-counter hormones, including DHEA, progesterone topical creams, and organ extracts is particularly worrisome).

Even vitamin and mineral supplementation may have unexpected results. For example, high dietary consumption of carrots, sweet potatoes, greens, and other foods rich in β-carotene is associated with decreased risk of cardiovascular disease and cancer. However, two large prospective randomized controlled trials of β-carotene [the Alpha Tocopherol Beta Carotene (ATBC) Cancer Prevention Study and the Beta-Carotene and Retinal Efficacy Trial (CARET)] found that β-carotene increased rates of lung cancer in supplemented groups. The ATBC trial also failed to show a benefit in terms of cardiovascular disease, and β-carotene supplementation has been disappointing in other trials. β-carotene may well be a dietary marker for more beneficial carotenoids (including lycopene, lutein, α-carotene, and β-cryptoxanthin) that typically occur in mixtures in foods.

Similarly, while dietary intake of vitamin E is associated with a reduced risk of coronary heart disease and several observational studies (including the Health Professionals Follow-Up Study and the Nurses Health Study) found a protective effect of supplemental vitamin E, prospective placebo-controlled trials have had mixed results.

Table 11-2 Some Commonly Used Dietary Supplements

Supplement	Clinical Trial Evidence	Toxicities	Comments
Arginine	Preliminary evidence of improvement in intermittent claudication and improved endothelial function in arteries.	Very safe.	
Vitamin A	Derivatives used to treat certain epithelial cell cancers, acne, and psoriasis. Decreases childhood mortality and measles mortality (in developing countries).	Headaches, nausea, bone pain; liver toxicity at high doses (>50,000 IU qd). Teratogenic; pregnant women should avoid supplements containing >5000 IU qd.	Vitamin A deficiency is unusual in North America. Megadoses have significant toxicity.
Riboflavin (vitamin B_2)	High doses of riboflavin may help in migraine prophylaxis.	Very safe	
Pantothenic acid	Preliminary evidence of benefit in hyperlipidemia.	Very safe. High doses can cause diarrhea.	
Vitamin B_6 (pyridoxine)	Improves symptoms in carpal tunnel syndrome, premenstrual syndrome, and nausea and vomiting of pregnancy.	Although more common at doses >200 mg qd, doses as low as 50 mg qd can cause sensory neuropathy.	
Vitamin B_{12} (cobalamin)	With folic acid, preliminary evidence that B_{12} may decrease bronchial squamous metaplasia in smokers.	Very safe.	B_{12} deficiency is common in North America, especially in the elderly and those on proton pump inhibitors. In the absence of macrocytosis or anemia, deficiency may cause psychiatric symptoms.
Thiamine (B_1)	Possible benefit in CHF but no large prospective trials.	Very safe.	Marginal deficiency is common (symptoms include weakness, parasthesia, and depression). Administer thiamine IV first when treating alcohol toxicity (IV glucose may cause life-threatening lactic acidosis in a thiamine-deficient patient).
Niacin (vitamin B_3)	Nicotinic acid lowers serum triglycerides, lowers LDL, and increases HDL.	Flushing, itching, rashes, gastrointestinal effects, and fatigue. Should not be used by those with impaired hepatic function or in those on beta blockers. Sustained-release preparations are hepatotoxic and should never be used.	Niacinamide is ineffective for hypercholesterolemia
Vitamin C	Preliminary evidence of improved endothelial function in arteries of patients with CHF. No evidence of benefit in advanced cancer or colds.	Diarrhea at high doses; increases iron absorption.	Epidemiologically, vitamin C intake or serum levels are associated with lower risk of nephrolithiasis, gall bladder disease, and some cancers. High serum levels are associated with lower serum lead levels.
Calcium	Reduces bone loss; lowers risk of recurrence of colorectal adenomas; may help premenstrual syndrome. Mixed results on treatment of hypertension; reduces risk of pregnancy-induced hypertension.	Relatively safe. Extremely high doses can cause milk alkali syndrome or hypercalcemia (symptoms may include lax muscle tone, nausea, constipation, large urine volume, later confusion, coma, death).	Although dietary intake of calcium reduces renal stone formation, supplemental calcium (especially taken between meals) may increase risk.
β-Carotene	Increases risk of lung cancer in smokers; may increase risk of cardiovascular disease; no effect on risk of type 2 diabetes; mixed results on prevention of cervical intraepithelial neoplasia; may decrease oral leukoplakia.	Hypercarotenosis (benign yellowing of the skin). In general, supplementation appears harmful; there is no risk to consuming foods high in β-carotene.	Dietary intake of foods high in carotenoids associated with decreased risk of cardiovascular disease and cancer (see text).
Vitamin D (calciferol)	Analogues are used to treat osteoporosis, renal osteodystrophy, hypocalcemia, and psoriasis and are being studied as cancer treatments.	In high doses may cause weakness, fatigue, headache, vomiting, hypercalcemia, hypercalciuria, and impaired renal function.	Marginal deficiency is common. Sunscreen use prevents vitamin D conversion in the skin. Fortification is required in milk but not other dairy products.
Vitamin E (α-tocopherol)	Ineffective in preventing lung cancer, reducing cardiovascular deaths, or reducing angina; may increase risk of pancreatic cancer; may reduce risk of myocardial infarction and risk of prostate cancer	Increases risk of hemorrhagic stroke.	Large doses of α-tocopherol displace γ-tocopherol in tissues.
Dehydroepiandrosterone (DHEA)	May be helpful in lupus and menopausal symptoms.	Acne and hirsutism (in women).	High serum levels are associated with decreased cardiovascular disease in men; increased cardiovascular disease in women; and increased risk of postmenopausal breast cancer.
Coenzyme Q10	Trials are mixed on whether it benefits CHF.	Very safe. Occasionally causes gastrointestinal upset.	
Iron	In iron-deficient individuals, supplementation reduces symptoms in restless legs syndrome; increases verbal learning and memory in adolescents, and increases growth in children.	High body stores of iron are associated with increased risk of cardiovascular disease. In iron-replete young children, supplementation may impair growth.	Supplementation should be discouraged unless deficiency exists.
Melatonin	Mixed results in jet lag or sleep disorders, not well examined in other indications	May cause depression. Safety of long-term use not established.	High-dose melatonin is under study as an adjunctive cancer treatment.
Magnesium	Mixed results in trials on hypertension and cardiovascular disease; may decrease arrhythmias; may help in migraine prophylaxis.	Toxic in high doses (causing hyporeflexia), later cardiac arrest; can cause diarrhea at relatively low doses; renal patients should avoid supplementation	

(continued)

Table 11-2 Some Commonly Used Dietary Supplements—*(continued)*

Supplement	Clinical Trial Evidence	Toxicities	Comments
Glucosamine	Effective in osteoarthritis	Very safe; may cause gastrointestinal discomfort.	
Chondroitin	Preliminary evidence of benefit in osteoarthritis	Very safe	
Fish oil	Lowers blood pressure in hypertensives; mixed results on reduction of coronary restenosis, may help psoriasis and rheumatoid arthritis, retards renal failure in IgA nephropathy, improved lung function in cystic fibrosis; improves symptoms in inflammatory bowel disease. Lowers VLDL, increases LDL, no effect on HDL or total cholesterol.	Relatively safe. May cause gastrointestinal discomfort, fishy breath, anticoagulant effects.	Dietary sources of fish oil include salmon, mackerel, sardines, and bluefish.
Selenium	Reduces prostate, lung, and colon cancer incidence; no effect on skin cancer.	Dizziness, nausea, metallic taste, garlicky breath. Very high doses (>4 mg qd) can cause loss of hair and nails, skin lesions, tooth decay, and peripheral neuropathy.	
Carnitine	Improves exercise tolerance and time to ST-segment depression in patients with angina; preliminary evidence of improvement in left ventricular dysfunction.	Relatively safe; L-carnitine occasionally causes diarrhea or agitation. D-carnitine can cause muscle pain and weakness	
Zinc	No evidence of benefit in leg ulcers. Mixed results on zinc lozenges for cold symptoms. Reduces respiratory infections and diarrhea in developing countries. Preliminary evidence of increased cell-mediated immunity in elderly.	In high doses, nausea, vomiting, diarrhea, abdominal pain; can cause copper depletion.	
Chromium	Preliminary evidence of benefit in diabetes; appears to increase HDL. No effect on body composition or strength in nondeficient individuals.	Oral chromium is safe. Occupational exposure to high doses of airborne chromium may cause dermatitis, skin and nasal septum lesions, and increased incidence of lung cancer.	

NOTE: CHF, congestive heart failure; HDL, high-density lipoprotein; LDL, low-density lipoprotein; VLDL, very low density lipoprotein.

In the Cambridge Heart Antioxidant Study (CHAOS), a placebo-controlled trial of vitamin E supplementation in patients with coronary artery disease, vitamin E supplementation reduced nonfatal myocardial infarction but did not appear to decrease cardiovascular deaths or all-cause mortality. In the ATBC study, vitamin E failed to protect male smokers with a previous myocardial infarction from major coronary events and significantly increased risk of death from hemorrhagic stroke. Although vitamin E improves endothelium-dependent vasodilation significantly and attenuates the development of nitrate tolerance, prospective trials have found no benefit of vitamin E for angina.

Vitamin E is not a single compound; the term applies to eight related compounds in two groups, the tocopherols and the tocotrienols. Most North American dietary sources of vitamin E are composed of two-thirds γ-tocopherol and one-third α-tocopherol. γ-Tocopherol neutralizes both oxygen and nitrogen free radicals, while α-tocopherol is selective for oxygen free radicals. Most vitamin E supplements, however, contain only D- or D,L-α-tocopherol, and large doses of α-tocopherol displace γ-tocopherol in plasma and tissues.

While it is possible that tomorrow's trendy carotenoid or tocopherol will be more successful than yesterday's, it is more likely that carotenoids and tocopherols are most beneficial when consumed in the naturally occurring mixtures of nutrients found in foods.

Dietary supplements that are safe under one set of conditions may be harmful under other conditions. For example, nearly all physiologic reactions that generate free radicals are oxidation-reduction reactions, capable of either generating free radicals or reducing free radicals. While low doses of vitamin C and other substances have antioxidant effects, high levels may actually have a prooxidant effect.

There is clinical trial evidence supporting the supplemental use of some vitamins, minerals, and amino acids (Table 11-2); but at high doses these supplements should be treated with the same respect given pharmaceuticals.

SUMMARY The incorporation of science into medicine began only in the middle of the nineteenth century; *evidence-based medicine* is a recent term and still not necessarily standard practice. There is no such thing as objective care of a patient. There are many ways in which we physicians communicate goals and our own beliefs in our therapies; it is likely that a substantial proportion of benefit from even rational interventions is due to nonspecific effects.

Many of our patients take alternative medicines; physicians need to adopt an open-minded, nonjudgmental attitude toward the practice. Inquire about all the medications and supplements a patient is taking. Increasingly, data are available to help guide decision-making about alternative medicines. A thorough knowledge of all therapies a patient is utilizing may help explain unexpected findings and is an important component of a holistic approach to patient care.

Conventional medicine often casts a wary eye on therapies outside its boundaries, but it is incumbent upon physicians to evaluate evidence regarding alternative therapies with the same rigor with which we evaluate conventional therapies. Scientific evidence from controlled clinical trials supports specific applications of alternative medicine, and some therapies considered alternative today may well be incorporated into conventional medicine in the future.

BIBLIOGRAPHY

DeSMet AGM et al: *Adverse Effects of Herbal Drugs*, vol. 3. Berlin, Springer-Verlag, 1997

ERNST E (ed): *Complementary Medicine: An Objective Appraisal*. Oxford, Butterworth-Heinemann, 1996

FUGH-BERMAN A: *5 Minute Clinical Consult to Herbs and Dietary Supplements*. Philadelphia, Lippincott, Williams & Wilkins, in press

———: *Alternative Medicine: What Works*. Baltimore, Williams & Wilkins, 1997

JONAS WB, LEVIN JS (eds): *Essentials of Complementary and Alternative Medicine*. Philadelphia, Lippincott Williams & Wilkins, 1999

KAPTCHUK TJ, EISENBERG DM: Chiropractic: Origins, controversies, and contributions. Arch Intern Med 158:2215, 1998

LINDE K et al: Are the clinical effects of homeopathy placebo effects? A meta-analysis of placebo-controlled trials. Lancet 350:834, 1997

SCHULZ V et al: *Rational Phytotherapy*, 3d ed. Berlin, Springer, 1998

SHILS ME et al: *Modern Nutrition in Health and Disease*, 9th ed. Baltimore, Williams & Wilkins, 1999

VANDENBROUCKE JP: Medical journals and the shaping of medical knowledge. Lancet 352:2001, 1998

Section 1
PAIN

12

Howard L. Fields, Joseph B. Martin

PAIN: PATHOPHYSIOLOGY AND MANAGEMENT

The task of medicine is to preserve and restore health and to relieve suffering. Understanding pain is essential to both these goals. Because pain is universally understood as a signal of disease, it is the most common symptom that brings a patient to a physician's attention. The function of the pain sensory system is to detect, localize, and identify tissue-damaging processes. Since different diseases produce characteristic patterns of tissue damage, the quality, time course, and location of a patient's pain complaint and the location of tenderness provide important diagnostic clues and are used to evaluate the response to treatment.

THE PAIN SENSORY SYSTEM

Pain is an unpleasant sensation localized to a part of the body. It is often described in terms of a penetrating or tissue-destructive process (e.g., stabbing, burning, twisting, tearing, squeezing) and/or of a bodily or emotional reaction (e.g., terrifying, nauseating, sickening). Furthermore, any pain of moderate or higher intensity is accompanied by anxiety and the urge to escape or terminate the feeling. These properties illustrate the duality of pain: it is both sensation and emotion. When acute, pain is characteristically associated with behavioral arousal and a stress response consisting of increased blood pressure, heart rate, pupil diameter, and plasma cortisol levels. In addition, local muscle contraction (e.g., limb flexion, abdominal wall rigidity) is often present.

THE PRIMARY AFFERENT NOCICEPTOR A peripheral nerve consists of the axons of three different types of neurons: primary sensory afferents, motor neurons, and sympathetic postganglionic neurons (Fig. 12-1). The cell bodies of primary afferents are located in the dorsal root ganglia in the vertebral foramina. The primary afferent axon bifurcates to send one process into the spinal cord and the other to innervate tissues. Primary afferents are classified by their diameter, degree of myelination, and conduction velocity. The largest-diameter fibers, A-beta (Aβ), respond maximally to light touch and/or moving stimuli; they are present primarily in nerves that innervate the skin. In normal individuals, the activity of these fibers does not produce pain. There are two other classes of primary afferents: the small-diameter myelinated A-delta (Aδ) and the unmyelinated (C fiber) axons (Fig. 12-1). These fibers are present in nerves to the skin and to deep somatic and visceral structures. Some tissues, such as the cornea, are innervated only by Aδ and C afferents. Most Aδ and C

afferents respond maximally only to intense (painful) stimuli and produce the subjective experience of pain when they are electrically stimulated; this defines them as *primary afferent nociceptors (pain receptors)*. The ability to detect painful stimuli is completely abolished when Aδ and C axons are blocked.

Individual primary afferent nociceptors can respond to several different types of noxious stimuli. For example, most nociceptors respond to heating, intense mechanical stimuli such as a pinch, and application of irritating chemicals.

Sensitization When intense, repeated, or prolonged stimuli are applied in the presence of damaged tissue or inflammation, the threshold for activating primary afferent nociceptors is lowered and the frequency of firing is higher for all stimulus intensities. Inflammatory mediators such as bradykinin, some prostaglandins, and leukotrienes contribute to this process, which is called *sensitization*. In sensitized tissues normally innocuous stimuli can produce pain. Sensitization is a clinically important process that contributes to tenderness, soreness, and hyperalgesia. A striking example of sensitization is sunburned skin, in which severe pain can be produced by a gentle slap on the back or a warm shower.

Under normal conditions, viscera are relatively insensitive to noxious mechanical and thermal stimuli. Hollow viscera do generate significant discomfort when distended. Furthermore, when affected by a disease process with an inflammatory component, deep structures such as joints or hollow viscera characteristically become exquisitely sensitive to mechanical stimulation.

A large proportion of Aδ and C afferents innervating viscera are completely insensitive in normal noninjured, noninflamed tissue. That is, they cannot be activated by known mechanical or thermal stimuli and are not spontaneously active. However, in the presence of inflammatory mediators, these afferents become sensitive to mechanical stimuli. Such afferents have been termed *silent nociceptors*, and their characteristic properties may explain how under pathologic conditions the relatively insensitive deep structures can become the source of severe and debilitating pain and tenderness.

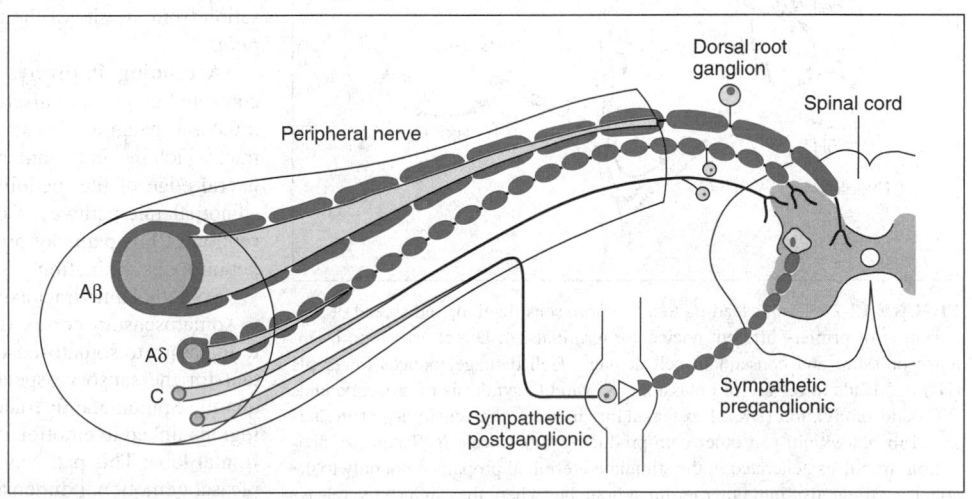

FIGURE 12-1 Components of a typical cutaneous nerve. There are two distinct functional categories of axons: primary afferents with cell bodies in the dorsal root ganglion, and sympathetic postganglionic fibers with cell bodies in the sympathetic ganglion. Primary afferents include those with large-diameter myelinated (Aβ), small-diameter myelinated (Aδ), and unmyelinated (C) axons. All sympathetic postganglionic fibers are unmyelinated.

Nociceptor-Induced Inflammation   One important concept to emerge in recent years is that afferent nociceptors also have a neuroeffector function. Most nociceptors contain polypeptide mediators that are released from their peripheral terminals when they are activated (Fig. 12-2). An example is substance P, an 11-amino-acid peptide. Substance P is released from primary afferent nociceptors and has multiple biologic activities. It is a potent vasodilator, degranulates mast cells, is a chemoattractant for leukocytes, and increases the production and release of inflammatory mediators. Interestingly, depletion of substance P from joints reduces the severity of experimental arthritis. Primary afferent nociceptors are not simply passive messengers of threats to tissue injury but also play an active role in tissue protection through these neuroeffector functions.

CENTRAL PATHWAYS FOR PAIN   The Spinal Cord and Referred Pain   The axons of primary afferent nociceptors enter the spinal cord via the dorsal root. They terminate in the dorsal horn of the spinal gray matter (Fig. 12-3). The terminals of primary afferent

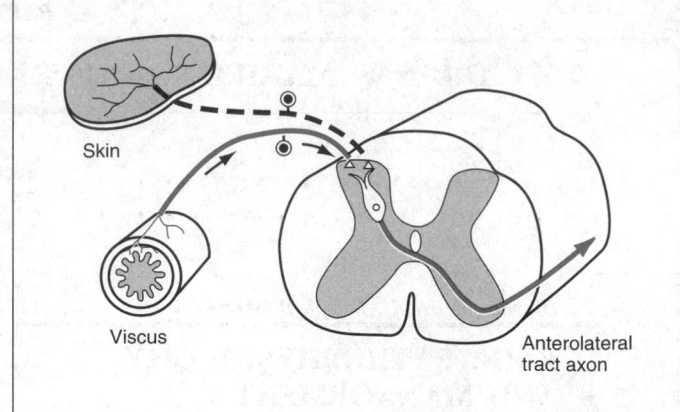

FIGURE 12-3   The convergence-projection hypothesis of referred pain. According to this hypothesis, visceral afferent nociceptors converge on the same pain-projection neurons as the afferents from the somatic structures in which the pain is perceived. The brain has no way of knowing the actual source of input and mistakenly "projects" the sensation to the somatic structure.

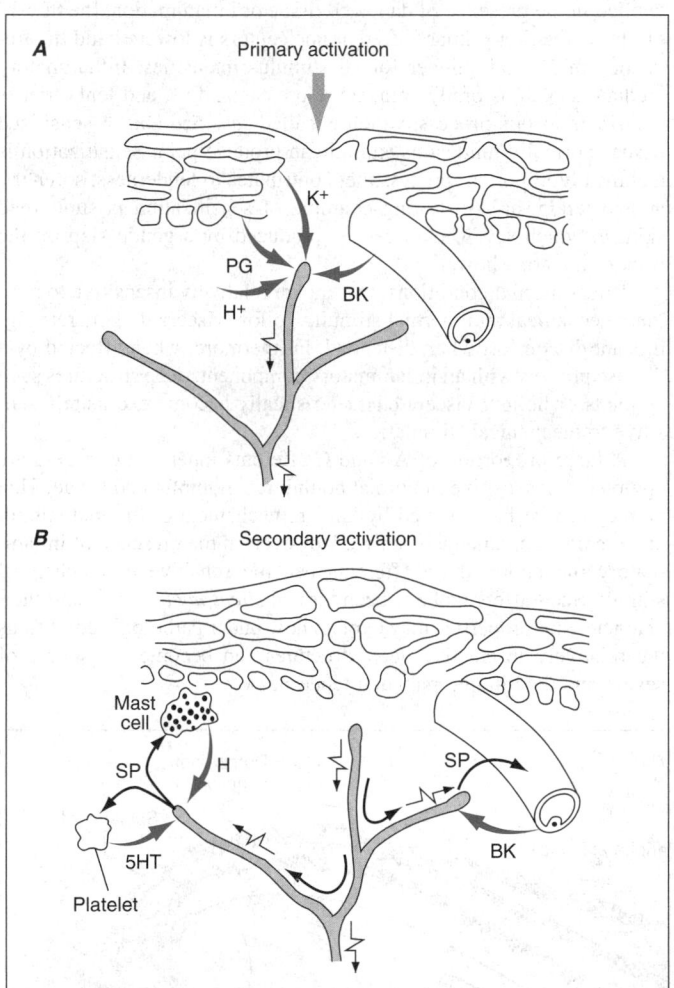

FIGURE 12-2   Events leading to activation, sensitization, and spread of sensitization of primary afferent nociceptor terminals. *A.* Direct activation by intense pressure and consequent cell damage. Cell damage induces lower pH (H$^+$) and leads to release of potassium (K$^+$) and to synthesis of prostaglandins (PG) and bradykinin (BK). Prostaglandins increase the sensitivity of the terminal to bradykinin and other pain-producing substances. *B.* Secondary activation. Impulses generated in the stimulated terminal propagate not only to the spinal cord but also into other terminal branches where they induce the release of peptides, including substance P (SP). Substance P causes vasodilation and neurogenic edema with further accumulation of bradykinin. Substance P also causes the release of histamine (H) from mast cells and serotonin (5HT) from platelets.

axons contact spinal neurons that transmit the pain signal to brain sites involved in pain perception. The axon of each primary afferent contacts many spinal neurons, and each spinal neuron receives convergent inputs from many primary afferents.

From a clinical standpoint, the convergence of many sensory inputs to a single spinal pain-transmission neuron is of great importance because it underlies the phenomenon of referred pain. All spinal neurons that receive input from the viscera and deep musculoskeletal structures also receive input from the skin. The convergence patterns are determined by the spinal segment of the dorsal root ganglion that supplies the afferent innervation of a structure. For example, the afferents that supply the central diaphragm are derived from the third and fourth cervical dorsal root ganglia. Primary afferents with cell bodies in these same ganglia supply the skin of the shoulder and lower neck. Thus sensory inputs from both the shoulder skin and the central diaphragm converge on pain-transmission neurons in the third and fourth cervical spinal segments. *Because of this convergence and the fact that the spinal neurons are most often activated by inputs from the skin, activity evoked in spinal neurons by input from deep structures is mislocalized by the patient to a place that is roughly coextensive with the region of skin innervated by the same spinal segment.* Thus inflammation near the central diaphragm is usually reported as discomfort near the shoulder. This spatial displacement of pain sensation from the site of the injury that produces it is known as *referred pain.*

Ascending Pathways for Pain   A majority of spinal neurons contacted by primary afferent nociceptors send their axons to the contralateral thalamus. These axons form the contralateral spinothalamic tract which lies in the anterolateral white matter of the spinal cord, the lateral edge of the medulla, and the lateral pons and midbrain. The spinothalamic pathway is crucial for pain sensation in humans. Interruption of this pathway produces permanent deficits in pain and temperature discrimination.

Spinothalamic tract axons connect to thalamic neurons that project to somatosensory cortex (Fig. 12-4). This pathway from spinal cord to thalamus to somatosensory cortex appears to be particularly important for the sensory aspects of pain, i.e., its location, intensity, and quality. Spinothalamic tract axons also connect to thalamic and cortical regions linked to emotional responses, such as the cingulate gyrus and frontal lobe. This pathway is thought to subserve the affective or unpleasant emotional dimension of pain.

PAIN MODULATION   The pain produced by similar injuries is remarkably variable in different situations and in different people. For example, athletes have been known to sustain serious fractures with only minor pain, and Beecher's classic World War II survey

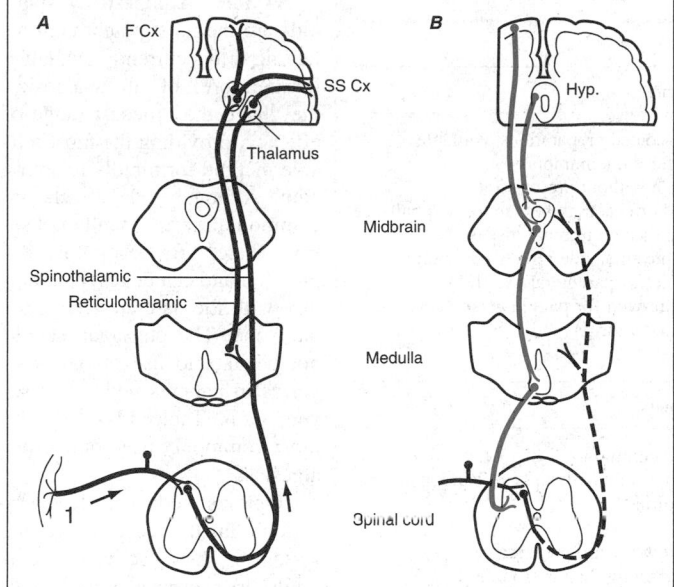

FIGURE 12-4 *A.* Transmission system for nociceptive messages. Noxious stimuli activate the sensitive peripheral ending of the primary afferent nociceptor by the process of transduction (1). The message is then transmitted over the peripheral nerve to the spinal cord, where it synapses with cells of origin of the two major ascending pain pathways, the spinothalamic and spinoreticulothalamic. The message is relayed in the thalamus to both the frontal (F Cx) and the somatosensory cortex (SS Cx). *B.* Pain-modulation network. Inputs from frontal cortex and hypothalamus (Hyp.) activate cells in the midbrain that control spinal pain-transmission cells via cells in the medulla.

revealed that many men were unbothered by battle injuries that would have produced agonizing pain in civilian patients. Furthermore, even the suggestion of relief can have a significant analgesic effect (placebo). On the other hand, many patients find even minor injuries (such as venipuncture) unbearable, and the expectation of pain has been demonstrated to induce pain *without a noxious stimulus.*

The powerful effect of expectation and other psychological variables on the perceived intensity of pain implies the existence of brain circuits that can modulate the activity of the pain-transmission pathways. Although there are probably several circuits that can modulate pain, only one has been studied extensively. This circuit has links in the hypothalamus, midbrain, and medulla, and it selectively controls spinal pain-transmission neurons through a descending pathway (Fig. 12-4).

There is good evidence that this pain-modulating circuit contributes to the pain-relieving effect of opioid analgesic medications. Each of the component structures of the pathway contains opioid receptors and is sensitive to the direct application of opioid drugs. Furthermore, lesions of the system reduce the analgesic effect of systemically administered opioids such as morphine. Along with the opioid receptor, the component nuclei of this pain-modulating circuit contain endogenous opioid peptides such as the enkephalins and β-endorphin.

The most reliable way to activate this endogenous opioid-mediated modulating system is by prolonged pain and/or fear. There is evidence that pain-relieving endogenous opioids are released following operative procedures and in patients given a placebo for pain relief.

Pain modulation is bidirectional. Pain-modulating circuits not only produce analgesia but are also capable of increasing pain. Both pain-inhibiting and pain-facilitating neurons in the medulla project to and control spinal pain-transmission neurons. Since pain-transmission neurons can be activated by modulatory neurons, it is theoretically possible to generate a pain signal with no peripheral noxious stimulus. Some such mechanism could account for the finding that pain can be induced by suggestion alone and may provide a framework for understanding how psychological factors can contribute to chronic pain.

NEUROPATHIC PAIN   The normal nervous system transmits coded signals that result in pain. Thus lesions of the peripheral or central nervous system may result in a loss or impairment of pain sensation. Paradoxically, damage or dysfunction of the nervous system can produce pain. For example, damage to peripheral nerves, as occurs in diabetic neuropathy, or to primary afferents, as in herpes zoster, can result in pain that is referred to the body region innervated by the damaged nerves. Though rare, pain may also be produced by damage to the central nervous system, particularly the spinothalamic pathway or thalamus. Such neuropathic pains are often severe and are notoriously intractable to standard treatments for pain.

Neuropathic pains typically have an unusual burning, tingling, or electric shock-like quality and may be triggered by very light touch. These features are rare in other types of pain. On examination, a sensory deficit is characteristically present in the area of the patient's pain.

A variety of mechanisms contribute to neuropathic pain. As with sensitized primary afferent nociceptors, damaged primary afferents, including nociceptors, become highly sensitive to mechanical stimulation and begin to generate impulses in the absence of stimulation. There is evidence that this increased sensitivity and spontaneous activity is due to an increased concentration of sodium channels. Damaged primary afferents may also develop sensitivity to norepinephrine. Interestingly, spinal pain-transmission neurons cut off from their normal input may also become spontaneously active. Thus both central and peripheral nervous system changes may contribute to neuropathic pain.

Sympathetically Maintained Pain   A certain percentage of patients with peripheral nerve injury develop a severe burning pain (causalgia) in the region innervated by the nerve. The pain typically begins after a delay of hours to days or even weeks. The pain is accompanied by swelling of the extremity, periarticular osteoporosis, and arthritic changes in the distal joints. A similar syndrome called *reflex sympathetic dystrophy* can be produced without obvious nerve damage by a variety of injuries, including fractures of bone, soft tissue trauma, myocardial infarction, and stroke (Chap. 366). Although the pathophysiology of this condition is poorly understood, the pain can be relieved within minutes by blocking the sympathetic nervous system. This implies that sympathetic activity activates nociceptors even if they are not obviously damaged. These results also suggest that the sympathetic nervous system can, under some circumstances, play an active role in inflammation.

℞ **TREATMENT**   The ideal treatment for any pain is to remove the cause. Sometimes this is possible, but more often after diagnosis and initiation of appropriate treatments for the cause, there is a lag period before the pain subsides. Furthermore, some conditions are so painful that rapid and effective analgesia is essential (e.g., the postoperative state, burns, trauma, cancer, sickle cell crisis). Analgesic medications are a first line of treatment in these cases, and their use should be familiar to all practitioners.

Aspirin, Acetaminophen, and Nonsteroidal Anti-Inflammatory Agents (NSAIDS)   These drugs are considered together because they are used for similar problems and may have a similar mechanism of action (Table 12-1). All these compounds inhibit cyclooxygenase (COX), and, except for acetaminophen, all have anti-inflammatory actions, especially at higher dosages. They are particularly effective for mild to moderate headache and for pain of musculoskeletal origin.

Since they are effective for these common types of pains and are available without prescription, COX inhibitors are by far the most commonly used analgesics. They are absorbed well from the gastrointestinal tract and, with occasional use, side effects are minimal. With chronic use, gastric irritation is a common side effect of aspirin and NSAIDs and is the problem that most frequently limits the dose that can be given. Gastric irritation is most severe with aspirin, which may cause erosion of the gastric mucosa, and because aspirin irreversibly acetylates platelets and interferes with coagulation of the blood, gas-

Table 12-1 Drugs for Relief of Pain

NONNARCOTIC ANALGESICS: USUAL DOSES AND INTERVALS

Generic Name	Dose, mg	Interval	Comments
Acetylsalicylic acid	650 PO	q 4 h	Enteric-coated preparations available
Acetaminophen	650 PO	q 4 h	Side effects uncommon
Ibuprofen	400 PO	q 4–6 h	Available without prescription
Naproxen	250–500 PO	q 12 h	Delayed effects may be due to long half-life
Fenoprofen	200 PO	q 4–6 h	Contraindicated in renal disease
Indomethacin	25–50 PO	q 8 h	Gastrointestinal side effects common
Ketorolac	15–60 IM	q 4–6 h	Available for parenteral use (IM)
Rofecoxib	12.5–25 PO	q 24 h	FDA approved for pain management
Celecoxib	100–200 PO	q 12–24 h	Useful for arthritis

NARCOTIC ANALGESICS: USUAL DOSES AND INTERVALS

Generic Name	Parenteral Dose, mg	PO Dose, mg	Comments
Codeine	30–60 q 4 h	30–60 q 4 h	Nausea common
Oxycodone	—	5–10 q 4–6 h	Usually available with acetaminophen or aspirin
Morphine	10 q 4 h	60 q 4 h	
Morphine sustained release	—	30–200 bid to tid	Oral slow-release preparation
Hydromorphone	1–2 q 4 h	2–4 q 4 h	Shorter acting than morphine sulfate
Levorphanol	2 q 6–8 h	4 q 6–8 h	Longer acting than morphine sulfate; absorbed well PO
Methadone	10 q 6–8 h	20 q 6–8 h	Delayed sedation due to long half-life
Meperidine	75–100 q 3–4 h	300 q 4 h	Poorly absorbed PO; normeperidine a toxic metabolite
Butorphanol	—	1–2 q 4 h	Intranasal spray
Fentanyl	2.5–10 q 72 h	—	Transdermal patch
Tramadol	—	50–100 q4–6 h	Mixed opioid/adrenergic action

ANTICONVULSANTS AND ANTIARRHYTHMICS

Generic Name	PO Dose, mg	Interval
Phenytoin	300	daily/qhs
Carbamazepine	200–300	q 6 h
Clonazepam	1	q 6 h
Mexiletine	150–300	q 6–12 h
Gabapentin	600–1200	q 8 h

ANTIDEPRESSANTS

Generic Name	Uptake Blockade 5-HT	NE	Sedative Potency	Anticholinergic Potency	Orthostatic Hypotension	Cardiac Arrhythmia	Average Dose, mg/day	Range, mg/day
Doxepin	++	+	High	Moderate	Moderate	Less	200	75–400
Amitriptyline	++++	++	High	Highest	Moderate	Yes	150	25–300
Imipramine	++++	++	Moderate	Moderate	High	Yes	200	75–400
Nortriptyline	+++	++	Moderate	Moderate	Low	Yes	100	40–150
Desipramine	+++	++++	Low	Low	Low	Yes	150	50–300
Venlafaxine	+++	++	Low	None	None	No	150	75–400

NOTE: 5-HT, serotonin; NE, norepinephrine.

trointestinal bleeding is a risk. The NSAIDs are less problematic in this regard. Although toxic to the liver when taken in a high dose, acetaminophen rarely produces gastric irritation and does not interfere with platelet function. Table 12-1 lists the dosages and durations of action of the commonly used drugs of this class.

The introduction of a parenteral form of NSAID, ketorolac, extends the usefulness of this class of compounds in the management of acute severe pain. Ketorolac is sufficiently potent and rapid in onset to supplant opioids for many patients with acute severe headache and musculoskeletal pain.

There are two major classes of COX: COX 1 is constitutively expressed, and COX 2 is induced in the inflammatory state. COX 2–selective drugs have recently been introduced for the treatment of arthritis and are associated with a significant reduction of gastric irritation. Whether COX 2-selective drugs have analgesic actions equivalent to other NSAIDs remains to be demonstrated.

Opioid Analgesics Opioids are the most potent pain-relieving drugs currently available. Furthermore, of all analgesics, they have the broadest range of efficacy, providing the most reliable method for rapidly relieving pain. Although side effects are common, they are usually not serious except for respiratory depression and can be reversed rapidly with the narcotic antagonist naloxone. The physician should not hesitate to use opioid analgesics in patients with acute severe pain. Table 12-1 lists the most commonly used opioid analgesics.

Opioids produce analgesia by actions in the central nervous system. They activate pain-inhibitory neurons and directly inhibit pain-transmission neurons. Most of the commercially available opioid analgesics act at the same opioid receptor (mu receptor), differing mainly in potency, speed of onset, duration of action, and optimal route of administration. Although the dose-related side effects (sedation, respiratory depression, pruritus, constipation) are similar among the different opioids, some side effects are due to accumulation of nonopioid metabolites that are unique to individual drugs. One striking example of this is normeperidine, a metabolite of meperidine. Normeperidine produces hyperexcitability and seizures that are not reversible with naloxone. Normeperidine accumulation is much greater in patients with renal failure.

The most rapid relief with opioids is obtained by intravenous administration; relief with oral administration is significantly slower. Common acute side effects include nausea, vomiting, and sedation. The most serious side effect is respiratory depression. Patients with any form of respiratory compromise must be kept under close observation following opioid administration; an oxygen saturation monitor may be useful. The opioid antagonist, naloxone, should be readily available. These effects are dose-related, and there is great variability among patients in the doses that relieve pain and produce side effects. Because of this, initiation of therapy requires titration to optimal dose and interval. The most important principle is to provide adequate pain relief. This requires asking the patient whether the drug has relieved the pain and, if so, when the relief wears off. *The most common error made by physicians in managing severe pain with opioids is to prescribe an inadequate dose. Since many patients are reluctant to complain, this practice leads to needless suffering.* In the absence of sedation at the expected time of peak effect, a physician should not hesitate to repeat the initial dose to achieve satisfactory pain relief.

An innovative approach to the problem of achieving adequate pain relief is the use of patient-controlled analgesia (PCA). PCA requires a device that delivers a baseline continuous dose of an opioid drug, and preprogrammed additional doses whenever the patient pushes a button. The device can be programmed to limit the total hourly dose so that overdosing is impossible. The patient can then titrate the dose to the optimal level. This approach is used most extensively for the management of postoperative pain, but there is no reason why it should not be used for any hospitalized patient with persistent severe pain. PCA is also used for short-term home care of patients with intractable pain, such as is caused by metastatic cancer.

Many physicians, nurses, and patients have a certain trepidation about using opioids that is based on an exaggerated fear of patients becoming addicted. In fact, there is a vanishingly small chance of patients becoming addicted to narcotics as a result of their appropriate medical use.

The availability of new routes of administration has extended the usefulness of opioid analgesics. Most important is the availability of spinal administration. Opioids can be infused through a spinal catheter placed either intrathecally or epidurally. By applying opioids directly to the spinal cord, regional analgesia can be obtained using a relatively low total dose. In this way, such side effects as sedation, nausea, and respiratory depression can be minimized. This approach has been used extensively in obstetric procedures and for lower-body postoperative pain. Opioids can also be given intranasally (butorphanol), rectally, and transdermally (fentanyl), thus avoiding the discomfort of frequent injections in patients who cannot be given oral medication.

Opioid and cyclooxygenase inhibitor combinations When used in combination, opioids and COX inhibitors have additive effects. Because a lower dose of each can be used to achieve the same degree of pain relief and their side effects are nonadditive, such combinations can be used to lower the severity of dose-related side effects. Fixed-ratio combinations of an opioid with acetaminophen carry a special risk. Dose escalation as a result of increased severity of pain or decreased opioid effect as a result of tolerance may lead to levels of acetaminophen that are toxic to the liver.

CHRONIC PAIN

PATIENT EVALUATION Managing patients with chronic pain is intellectually and emotionally challenging. The patient's problem is often difficult to diagnose: such patients are demanding of the physician's time and often appear emotionally distraught. The traditional medical approach of seeking an obscure organic pathology is usually unhelpful. On the other hand, psychological evaluation and behaviorally based treatment paradigms are frequently helpful, particularly in the setting of a multidisciplinary pain-management center.

There are several factors that can cause, perpetuate, or exacerbate chronic pain. First, of course, the patient may simply have a disease that is characteristically painful for which there is presently no cure. Arthritis, cancer, migraine headaches, fibromyalgia, and diabetic neuropathy are examples of this. Second, there may be secondary perpetuating factors that are initiated by disease and persist after that disease has resolved. Examples include damaged sensory nerves, sympathetic efferent activity, and painful reflex muscle contraction. Finally, a variety of psychological conditions can exacerbate or even cause pain.

There are certain areas to which special attention should be paid in the medical history. Because depression is the most common emotional disturbance in patients with chronic pain, patients should be questioned about their mood, appetite, sleep patterns, and daily activity. A simple standardized questionnaire, such as the Beck Depression Inventory, can be a useful screening device. It is important to remember that major depression is a common, treatable, and potentially fatal illness.

Other clues that a significant emotional disturbance is contributing to a patient's chronic pain complaint include: pain that occurs in multiple unrelated sites; a pattern of recurrent, but separate, pain problems beginning in childhood or adolescence; pain beginning at a time of

emotional trauma, such as the loss of a parent or spouse; a history of physical or sexual abuse; and past or present substance abuse.

On examination, special attention should be paid to whether the patient guards the painful area and whether certain movements or postures are avoided because of pain. Discovering a mechanical component to the pain can be useful both diagnostically and therapeutically. Painful areas should be examined for deep tenderness, noting whether this is localized to muscle, ligamentous structures, or joints. Chronic myofascial pain is very common, and in these patients deep palpation may reveal highly localized trigger points that are firm bands or knots in muscle. If injection of local anesthetic into these trigger points relieves the pain, it supports the diagnosis. A neuropathic component to the pain is indicated by evidence of nerve damage, such as sensory impairment, exquisitely sensitive skin, weakness and muscle atrophy, or loss of deep tendon reflexes. Evidence suggesting sympathetic nervous system involvement includes the presence of diffuse swelling, changes in skin color and temperature, and hypersensitive skin and joint tenderness compared with the normal side. Relief of the pain with a sympathetic block is diagnostic.

A guiding principle in evaluating patients with chronic pain is to assess both emotional and organic factors before initiating therapy. Addressing these issues together, rather than waiting to "rule out" organic causes of the pain, improves compliance in part because it assures patients that a psychological evaluation does not mean that the physician is questioning the validity of their complaint. Even when an organic cause for a patient's pain can be found, it is still wise to look for other factors. For example, cancer patients with painful bony metastases may also have pain due to nerve damage and significant depression. Optimal therapy requires that each of these factors be looked for and treated.

℞ TREATMENT Once the evaluation process has been completed and the likely causative and exacerbating factors identified, an explicit treatment plan should be developed. An important part of this process is to identify specific and realistic functional goals for therapy, such as getting a good night's sleep, being able to go shopping, or returning to work. A multidisciplinary approach that utilizes medications, counseling, physical therapy, nerve blocks, and even surgery may be required to improve the patient's quality of life. This may require referral to a pain clinic; however, this is not necessary for all chronic pain patients. For some, pharmacologic management alone can provide significant help.

Antidepressant Medications The tricyclic antidepressants (Table 12-1) are extremely useful for the management of patients with chronic pain. Although developed for the treatment of depression, the tricyclics have a spectrum of dose-related biologic activities that include the production of analgesia in a variety of clinical conditions. Although the mechanism is unknown, the analgesic effect of tricyclics has a more rapid onset and occurs at a lower dose than is typically required for the treatment of depression. Furthermore, patients with chronic pain who are not depressed obtain pain relief with antidepressants. There is evidence that tricyclic drugs potentiate opioid analgesia, so they are useful adjuncts for the treatment of severe persistent pain such as occurs with malignant tumors. Table 12-2 lists some of the painful conditions that respond to tricyclics. Tricyclics are of particular

Table 12-2   Painful Conditions That Respond to Tricyclic Antidepressants

Postherpetic neuralgia[a]	Rheumatoid arthritis[a,b]
Diabetic neuropathy[a]	Chronic low back pain[b]
Tension headache[a]	Cancer
Migraine headache[a]	

[a] Controlled trials demonstrate analgesia.
[b] Controlled studies indicate benefit but not analgesia.
SOURCE: From HL Fields: *Pain.* New York, McGraw-Hill, 1987.

value in the management of neuropathic pain such as occurs in diabetic neuropathy and postherpetic neuralgia, for which there are few other therapeutic options.

The tricyclics that have been shown to relieve pain have significant side effects (Table 12-1; Chap 385). Unfortunately, some of the serotonin-selective reuptake inhibitors such as fluoxetine (Prozac) that have fewer and less serious side effects have not been shown to provide pain relief. On the other hand, venlafaxine (Effexor), a nontricyclic antidepressant that blocks both serotonin and norepinephrine reuptake, appears to be useful in patients who cannot tolerate tricyclics.

Anticonvulsants and Antiarrhythmics (Table 12-1) These drugs are useful primarily for patients with neuropathic pain. Phenytoin (Dilantin) and carbamazepine (Tegretol) were first shown to relieve the pain of trigeminal neuralgia. This pain has a characteristic brief, shooting, electric shock-like quality. In fact, anticonvulsants seem to be helpful largely for pains that have such a lancinating quality. A new-generation anticonvulsant, gabapentin (Neurontin), which increases brain γ-aminobutyric acid levels, is effective for a broad range of neuropathic pains.

Antiarrhythmic drugs such as low-dose lidocaine and mexiletine (Mexitil) are also effective for neuropathic pains. These drugs block the spontaneous activity of primary afferent nociceptors that appears when they are damaged.

Chronic Opioid Medication The long-term use of opioids is accepted for patients with pain due to malignant disease. Although its use for chronic pain of nonmalignant origin is controversial, it is clear that for many such patients opioid analgesics are the only option available for obtaining effective relief. This is understandable since opioids are the most potent and have the broadest range of efficacy of any analgesic medications. Although addiction is rare in patients who first use opioids for pain relief, some degree of tolerance and physical dependence are likely to occur with long-term use. Therefore, before embarking on opioid therapy, other options should be explored, and the limitations and risks of opioids should be explained to the patient. It is also important to point out that some opioid analgesic medications have mixed agonist-antagonist properties (e.g., pentazocine and butorphanol). From a practical standpoint, this means that they may worsen pain by inducing an abstinence syndrome in patients who are physically dependent on other opioid analgesics.

With long-term outpatient use of orally administered opioids it is desirable to use long-acting compounds such as levorphanol, methadone, or sustained-release morphine (Table 12-1). The pharmacokinetic profile of these drugs enables prolonged pain relief, minimizes side effects such as sedation that are associated with high peak plasma levels, and, perhaps, reduces the likelihood of rebound pain associated with a rapid fall in plasma opioid concentration. Constipation is a virtually universal side effect of opioid use and should be treated expectantly.

It is worth emphasizing, in conclusion, that many patients, especially those with chronic pain, seek medical attention primarily because they are suffering and because only physicians can provide the medications required for their relief. A primary responsibility of all physicians is to minimize the physical and emotional discomfort of their patients. Familiarity with pain mechanisms and analgesic medications is an important step toward accomplishing this aim.

BIBLIOGRAPHY

BARON R et al: Causalgia and reflex sympathetic dystrophy: Does the sympathetic nervous system contribute to the generation of pain? Muscle Nerve 22:678, 1999

DEVOR M et al (eds): Proceedings of the Ninth World Congress on Pain. Seattle IASP Press, 1160 pp, 2000

FIELDS HL et al: Postherpetic neuralgia: Irritable nociceptors and deafferentation. Neurobiol Dis 5:209, 1998

——— et al: Peripheral neuropathic pain: An approach to management, in *Textbook of Pain*, 4th ed, PD Wall, R Melzack (eds). London, Churchill Livingston, 1999

FORT J: Celecoxib, a COX-2–specific inhibitor: The clinical data. Am J Orthop 28(3 Suppl):13, 1999

GEBHART GF (ed): *Visceral Pain*. Seattle, IASP Press, 1995

MARKOWITZ JS, PATRICK KS: Venlafaxine-tramadol similarities. Med Hypotheses 51: 167, 1998

ROWBOTHAM MC et al: Gabapentin for the treatment of postherpetic neuralgia: A randomized controlled trial. JAMA 280:1837, 1998

STEIN C: The control of pain in peripheral tissue by opioids. N Engl J Med 332:1685, 1995

WALL PD, MELZACK R (eds): *Textbook of Pain*, 4th ed. London, Churchill Livingstone, 1999

WILLIS WD (ed): *Hyperalgesia and Allodynia*. New York, Raven, 1992

———, COGGESHALL RE: *Sensory Mechanism of the Spinal Cord*. New York, Plenum, 1991

---

13 *Thomas H. Lee*

CHEST DISCOMFORT AND PALPITATIONS

CHEST DISCOMFORT

Chest discomfort is one of the most common challenges for clinicians in the office or emergency department. The differential diagnosis includes conditions affecting organs throughout the thorax and abdomen, with prognostic implications that vary from benign to life-threatening (Table 13-1). Failure to recognize potentially serious conditions such as acute ischemic heart disease, aortic dissection, or pulmonary embolism can lead to serious complications, including death. Conversely, overly conservative management of low-risk patients leads to unnecessary hospital admissions, tests, and procedures.

CAUSES OF CHEST DISCOMFORT Myocardial Ischemia and Injury (See also Chap. 244) Myocardial ischemia occurs when the oxygen supply to the heart is not sufficient to meet metabolic needs. This mismatch can result from a decrease in oxygen supply, a rise in demand, or both. The most common underlying cause of myocardial ischemia is obstruction of coronary arteries by atherosclerosis; in the presence of such obstruction, transient ischemic episodes are usually precipitated by an increase in oxygen demand as a result of physical exertion. However, ischemia can also result from psychological stress, fever, or large meals or from compromised oxygen delivery due to anemia, hypoxia, or hypotension. Ventricular hypertrophy due to valvular heart disease, hypertrophic cardiomyopathy, or hypertension can predispose the myocardium to ischemia because of impaired penetration of blood flow from epicardial coronary arteries to the endocardium.

Angina pectoris The chest discomfort of myocardial ischemia is a visceral discomfort that is usually described as a heaviness, pressure,

Table 13-1 Differential Diagnoses of Patients Admitted to Hospital with Acute Chest Pain Ruled Not Myocardial Infarction

Diagnosis	Percent
Gastroesophageal disease	42
Gastroesophageal reflux	(30)
Esophageal motility disorders	(13)
Peptic ulcer	(10)
Gallstones	(5)
Ischemic heart disease	31
Chest wall syndromes	28
Pericarditis	4
Pleuritis/pneumonia	2
Pulmonary embolism	2
Lung cancer	1.5
Aortic aneurysm	1
Aortic stenosis	1
Herpes zoster	1

SOURCE: Fruergaard P et al: Eur Heart J 17:1028, 1996.

or squeezing (Table 13-2). Other common adjectives for anginal pain are burning and aching. Some patients deny any "pain" but may admit to dyspnea or a vague sense of anxiety. The word "sharp" is sometimes used by patients to describe intensity rather than quality.

The location of angina pectoris is usually retrosternal; most patients do not localize the pain to any small area. The discomfort may radiate to the neck, jaw, teeth, arms, or shoulders, reflecting the common origin in the posterior horn of the spinal cord of sensory neurons supplying the heart and these areas. Some patients present with aching in sites of radiated pain as their only symptoms of ischemia. Occa-

Table 13-2   Typical Clinical Features of Major Causes of Acute Chest Discomfort

Condition	Duration	Quality	Location	Associated Features
Angina	More than 2 and less than 10 min	Pressure, tightness, squeezing, heaviness, burning	Retrosternal, often with radiation to or isolated discomfort in neck, jaw, shoulders, or arms—frequently on left	Precipitated by exertion, exposure to cold, psychologic stress S4 gallop or mitral regurgitation murmur during pain
Unstable angina	10–20 min	Similar to angina but often more severe	Similar to angina	Similar to angina, but occurs with low levels of exertion or even at rest
Acute myocardial infarction	Variable; often more than 30 min	Similar to angina but often more severe	Similar to angina	Unrelieved by nitroglycerin May be associated with evidence of heart failure or arrhythmia
Aortic stenosis	Recurrent episodes as described for angina	As described for angina	As described for angina	Late-peaking systolic murmur radiating to carotid arteries
Pericarditis	Hours to days; may be episodic	Sharp	Retrosternal or toward cardiac apex; may radiate to left shoulder	May be relieved by sitting up and leaning forward Pericardial friction rub
Aortic dissection	Abrupt onset of unrelenting pain	Tearing or ripping sensation; knifelike	Anterior chest, often radiating to back, between shoulder blades	Associated with hypertension and/or underlying connective tissue disorder, e.g., Marfan syndrome Murmur of aortic insufficiency, pericardial rub, pericardial tamponade, or loss of peripheral pulses
Pulmonary embolism	Abrupt onset; several minutes to a few hours	Pleuritic	Often lateral, on the side of the embolism	Dyspnea, tachypnea, tachycardia, and hypotension
Pulmonary hypertension	Variable	Pressure	Substernal	Dyspnea, signs of increased venous pressure including edema and jugular venous distention
Pneumonia or pleuritis	Variable	Pleuritic	Unilateral, often localized	Dyspnea, cough, fever, rales, occasional rub
Spontaneous pneumothorax	Sudden onset; several hours	Pleuritic	Lateral to side of pneumothorax	Dyspnea, decreased breath sounds on side of pneumothorax
Esophageal reflux	10–60 min	Burning	Substernal, epigastric	Worsened by postprandial recumbency Relieved by antacids
Esophageal spasm	2–30 min	Pressure, tightness, burning	Retrosternal	Can closely mimic angina
Peptic ulcer	Prolonged	Burning	Epigastric, substernal	Relieved with food or antacids
Gallbladder disease	Prolonged	Burning, pressure	Epigastric, right upper quadrant, substernal	May follow meal
Musculoskeletal disease	Variable	Aching	Variable	Aggravated by movement May be reproduced by localized pressure on examination
Herpes zoster	Variable	Sharp or burning	Dermatomal distribution	Vesicular rash in area of discomfort
Emotional and psychiatric conditions	Variable; may be fleeting	Variable	Variable; may be retrosternal	Situational factors may precipitate symptoms Anxiety or depression often detectable with careful history

sional patients report epigastric distress with ischemic episodes. Less common is radiation to below the umbilicus or to the back.

Stable angina pectoris usually develops gradually with exertion, emotional excitement, or after heavy meals. Rest or treatment with sublingual nitroglycerin typically leads to relief within several minutes. In contrast, pain that is fleeting (lasting only a few seconds) is rarely ischemic in origin. Similarly, pain that lasts for several hours is unlikely to represent angina, particularly if the patient's electrocardiogram does not show evidence of ischemia.

Anginal episodes can be precipitated by any physiologic or psychological stress that induces tachycardia. Most myocardial perfusion occurs during diastole, when there is minimal pressure opposing coronary artery flow from within the left ventricle. Since tachycardia decreases the percentage of the time in which the heart is in diastole, it decreases myocardial perfusion.

Unstable angina and myocardial infarction (See also Chaps. 243 and 244)   Patients with these acute ischemic syndromes usually complain of symptoms similar in quality to angina pectoris, but more prolonged and severe. The onset of these syndromes may occur with the patient at rest, and sublingual nitroglycerin may lead to transient or no relief. Accompanying symptoms may include diaphoresis, dyspnea, nausea, and light-headedness.

The physical examination may be completely normal in patients with chest discomfort due to ischemic heart disease. Careful auscultation during ischemic episodes may reveal a third or fourth heart sound, reflecting myocardial systolic or diastolic dysfunction. A transient murmur of mitral regurgitation suggests ischemic papillary muscle dysfunction. Severe episodes of ischemia can lead to pulmonary congestion and even pulmonary edema.

Other cardiac causes   Myocardial ischemia caused by hypertrophic cardiomyopathy, aortic stenosis, or other conditions leads to angina pectoris similar to that caused by coronary atherosclerosis. In such cases, a systolic murmur or other findings usually suggest abnormalities other than coronary atherosclerosis that may be contributing to the patient's symptoms.

Pericarditis (See also Chap. 239)   The pain in pericarditis is believed to be due to inflammation of the adjacent parietal pleura, since most of the pericardium is believed to be insensitive to pain. Thus, infectious pericarditis, which usually involves adjoining pleura surfaces, tends to be associated with pain, while conditions that cause only local inflammation (e.g., myocardial infarction or uremia) and cardiac tamponade tend to result in mild or no chest pain.

The adjacent parietal pleura receives its sensory supply from several sources, so the pain of pericarditis can be experienced in areas ranging from the shoulder and neck to the abdomen and back. Most typically, the pain is retrosternal and is aggravated by coughing, deep breaths, or changes in position—all of which lead to movements of pleural surfaces. The pain is often worse in the supine position and relieved by sitting upright and leaning forward. Less common is a steady aching discomfort that mimics acute myocardial infarction.

Diseases of the Aorta (See also Chap. 247)   *Aortic dissection* is a potentially catastrophic condition that is due to spread within the wall of the aorta of a subintimal hematoma. The hematoma may begin with a tear in the intima of the aorta or with rupture of the vasa vasorum within the aortic media. This syndrome can occur with trauma to the aorta, including motor vehicle accidents or medical procedures in which catheters or intraaortic balloon pumps damage the intima of the aorta. Nontraumatic aortic dissections are rare in the absence of hypertension and/or conditions associated with deterioration of the elastic or muscular components of the media within the aorta's wall. Cystic medial degeneration is a feature of several inherited connective tissue diseases, including Marfan and Ehlers-Danlos syndromes. About half of all aortic dissections in women under 40 years of age occur during pregnancy.

Almost all patients with acute dissections present with severe chest pain, although some patients with chronic dissections are identified without associated symptoms. Unlike the pain of ischemic heart disease, symptoms of aortic dissection tend to reach peak severity immediately, often causing the patient to collapse from its intensity. The adjectives used to describe the pain reflect the process occurring within the wall of the aorta—"ripping" and "tearing"—and the location usually correlates with the site and extent of the dissection. Thus, dissections that begin in the ascending aorta and extend to the descending aorta tend to cause pain in the front of the chest that extends into the back, between the shoulder blades.

Physical findings may also reflect extension of the aortic dissection that compromises flow into arteries branching off the aorta. Thus, loss of a pulse in one or both arms, cerebrovascular accident, or paraplegia can all be catastrophic consequences of aortic dissection. Hematomas that extend proximally and undermine the coronary arteries or aortic valve apparatus may lead to acute myocardial infarction or acute aortic insufficiency. Rupture of the hematoma into the pericardial space leads to pericardial tamponade.

Another abnormality of the aorta that can cause chest pain is a *thoracic aortic aneurysm*. Aortic aneurysms are frequently asymptomatic but can cause chest pain and other symptoms by compressing adjacent structures. This pain tends to be steady, deep, and sometimes severe.

Pulmonary Embolism (See also Chap. 261)   Chest pain due to pulmonary embolism is believed to be due to distention of the pulmonary artery or infarction of a segment of the lung adjacent to the pleura. Massive pulmonary emboli may lead to substernal pain that is suggestive of acute myocardial infarction. More commonly, smaller emboli lead to focal pulmonary infarctions that cause pain that is lateral and pleuritic. Associated symptoms include dyspnea and, occasionally, hemoptysis. Tachycardia is usually present.

Pneumonia or Pleuritis   Lung diseases that damage and cause inflammation of the pleura of the lung usually cause a sharp, knifelike pain that is aggravated by inspiration or coughing.

Gastrointestinal Conditions   Esophageal pain from acid reflux from the stomach, spasm, obstruction, or injury can be difficult to discern from myocardial syndromes. Acid reflux typically causes a deep burning discomfort that may be exacerbated by alcohol, aspirin, or some foods; this discomfort is often relieved by antacid or other acid-reducing therapies. Acid reflux tends to be exacerbated by lying down and may be worse in early morning when the stomach is empty of food that might otherwise absorb gastric acid.

Esophageal spasm may occur in the presence or absence of acid reflux, and leads to a squeezing pain indistinguishable from angina. Prompt relief of esophageal spasm is often provided by antianginal therapies such as sublingual nifedipine, further promoting confusion between these syndromes. Chest pain can also result from injury to the esophagus, such as a Mallory-Weiss tear caused by severe vomiting.

Chest pain can result from diseases of the gastrointestinal tract below the diaphragm, including *peptic ulcer disease*, *biliary disease*, and *pancreatitis*. These conditions usually cause abdominal pain as well as chest discomfort; symptoms are not likely to be associated with exertion. The pain of ulcer disease typically occurs 60 to 90 min after meals, when postprandial acid production is no longer neutralized by food in the stomach. Cholecystitis usually causes a pain that is described as aching, occurring an hour or more after meals.

Neuromusculoskeletal Conditions   *Cervical disk disease* can cause chest pain by compression of nerve roots. Pain in a dermatomal distribution can also be caused by *intercostal muscle cramps* or by *herpes zoster*. Chest pain symptoms due to herpes zoster may occur before skin lesions are apparent.

Costochondral and chondrosternal syndromes are the most common causes of anterior chest musculoskeletal pain. Only occasionally are physical signs of costochondritis such as swelling, redness, and warmth (Tietze's syndrome) present. The pain of such syndromes is usually fleeting and sharp, but some patients experience a dull ache that lasts for hours. Direct pressure on the chondrosternal and costochondral junctions may reproduce the pain from these and other musculoskeletal syndromes. Arthritis of the shoulder and spine and bursitis may also cause chest pain. Some patients who have these conditions and myocardial ischemia blur and confuse symptoms of these syndromes.

Emotional and Psychiatric Conditions As many as 10% of patients who present to emergency departments with acute chest pain have panic disorder or other emotional conditions. The symptoms in these populations are highly variable, but frequently the discomfort is described as visceral tightness or aching that lasts more than 30 min. Some patients offer other atypical descriptions, such as pain that is fleeting, sharp, and/or localized to a small region. The electrocardiogram in patients with emotional conditions may be difficult to interpret if hyperventilation causes ST-T-wave abnormalities. A careful history may elicit clues of depression, prior panic attacks, somatization, agoraphobia, or other phobias.

Approach to the Patient

The evaluation of the patient with chest discomfort must accommodate two goals—determining the diagnosis and assessing the safety of the immediate management plan. The latter issue is often dominant when the patient has acute chest discomfort, such as patients seen in the emergency department. In such settings, the clinician must focus on questions such as the safety of discharge to home, admission to a non-coronary care unit facility, or immediate exercise testing. Table 13-3 displays a sequence of questions that can be used in the evaluation of the patient with chest discomfort, with the diagnostic entities that are most important for consideration at each stage of the evaluation.

Acute Chest Discomfort In patients with acute chest discomfort, the clinician must first assess the patient's respiratory and hemodynamic status. If either is compromised, initial management should focus on stabilizing the patient before the diagnostic evaluation is pursued. If, however, the patient does not require emergent interventions, then a focused history, physical examination, and laboratory evaluation should be performed to assess the patient's risk of life-threatening conditions, including acute ischemic heart disease, aortic dissection, and pulmonary embolism.

The *history* should include questions about the quality and location of the chest discomfort (Table 13-2). The patient should also be asked about the nature of onset of the pain and its duration. Myocardial ischemia is usually associated with a gradual intensification of symptoms over a period of minutes. Pain that is fleeting or that lasts hours without being associated with electrocardiographic changes is not likely to be ischemic in origin.

The *physical examination* should include evaluation of blood pressure in both arms and of pulses in both legs. Poor perfusion of a limb

may be due to an aortic dissection that has compromised flow to an artery branching from the aorta. Chest auscultation may reveal diminished breath sounds; a pleural rub; or evidence of pneumothorax, pulmonary embolism, pneumonia, or pleurisy. The cardiac examination should seek pericardial rubs, systolic and diastolic murmurs, and third or fourth heart sounds.

An *electrocardiogram* is an essential test for adults with chest discomfort that is not due to an obvious traumatic cause. The presence of electrocardiographic changes consistent with ischemia or infarction (Chap. 226) is associated with high risks of acute myocardial infarction or unstable angina (Table 13-4); such patients should be admitted to a unit with electrocardiographic monitoring and the capacity to respond to a cardiac arrest. The absence of such changes does not exclude acute ischemic heart disease, but the risk of life-threatening complications is low for patients with normal electrocardiograms or only nonspecific ST-T-wave changes. If these patients are not considered appropriate for immediate discharge, they are often candidates for early or immediate exercise testing.

Markers of myocardial injury are often obtained in the emergency department evaluation of acute chest discomfort. The most commonly used markers are creatine kinase (CK), CK-MB, and the cardiac troponins (I and T). Single values of these markers do not have high sensitivity for acute myocardial infarction or for prediction of complications. Hence, decisions to discharge patients home should not be made on the basis of single negative values of these tests.

Provocative tests for coronary artery disease are not appropriate for patients with ongoing chest pain. In such patients, rest myocardial perfusion scans can be considered; a normal scan reduces the likelihood of coronary artery disease. Clinicians frequently employ therapeutic trials with sublingual nitroglycerin or antacids, and a common error is to assume that a response to either of these interventions clarifies the diagnosis. While such information is often helpful, the patient's response may be due to the placebo effect. Hence, myocardial ischemia should never be considered excluded solely because of a response to antacid therapy. Similarly, failure of nitroglycerin to relieve pain does not exclude the diagnosis of coronary disease.

If the patient's history or examination is consistent with aortic dissection, imaging studies to evaluate the aorta must be pursued promptly because of the high risk of catastrophic complications with this condition. A chest x-ray is not sufficient to exclude this diagnosis. Appropriate tests include a chest computed tomography scan with contrast or a magnetic resonance imaging scan in patients who are hemodynamically stable, or a transesophageal echocardiogram in pa-

---

Table 13-3 Considerations in the Assessment of the Patient with Chest Pain

1. Could the chest discomfort be due to an acute, potentially life-threatening condition that warrants immediate hospitalization and aggressive evaluation?

   Acute ischemic heart disease Pulmonary embolism
   Aortic dissection Spontaneous pneumothorax

2. If not, could the discomfort be due to a chronic condition likely to lead to serious complications?

   Stable angina
   Aortic stenosis
   Pulmonary hypertension

3. If not, could the discomfort be due to an acute condition that warrants specific treatment?

   Pericarditis
   Pneumonia/pleuritis
   Herpes zoster

4. If not, could the discomfort be due to another treatable chronic condition?

   Esophageal reflux Cervical disk disease
   Esophageal spasm Arthritis of the shoulder or spine
   Peptic ulcer disease Costochondritis
   Gallbladder disease Other musculoskeletal disorders
   Other gastrointestinal conditions Anxiety state

Table 13-4 Prevalence of Myocardial Infarction and Unstable Angina Among Subsets of Patients with Acute Chest Pain in the Emergency Department

Finding	Prevalence of Myocardial Infarction, %	Prevalence of Unstable Angina, %
ST elevation (≥ 1 mm) or Q waves on ECG not known to be old	79	12
Ischemia or strain on ECG not known to be old (ST depression ≥ 1 mm or ischemic T waves)	20	41
None of the preceding ECG changes but a prior history of angina or myocardial infarction (history of heart attack or nitroglycerin use)	4	51
None of the preceding ECG changes and no prior history of angina or myocardial infarction (history of heart attack or nitroglycerin use)	2	14

NOTE: ECG, electrocardiogram.
SOURCE: Unpublished data from Brigham and Women's Hospital Chest Pain Study, 1997–1999.

tients who are less stable. Aortic angiography is no longer a first test at most institutions.

Acute pulmonary embolism should be considered in patients with respiratory symptoms, pleuritic chest pain, hemoptysis, or a history of venous thromboembolism or coagulation abnormalities. Initial tests usually include a lung scan and/or pulmonary arteriography.

If patients with acute chest discomfort show no evidence of life-threatening conditions, the clinician should then focus on serious chronic conditions with the potential to cause major complications, the most common of which is stable angina. Early use of treadmill exercise testing for such patients, whether in the office or the emergency department, is now an accepted management strategy for low-risk patients. Exercise testing is not appropriate, however, for patients who (1) report pain that is believed to be ischemic occurring at rest or (2) have electrocardiographic changes consistent with ischemia not known to be old.

Patients with sustained chest discomfort who do not have evidence for life-threatening conditions should be evaluated for evidence of conditions likely to benefit from acute treatment (Table 13-3). Pericarditis may be suggested by the history, physical examination, and electrocardiogram (Table 13-2). Clinicians should carefully assess blood pressure patterns and consider echocardiography in such patients to detect evidence of impending pericardial tamponade. Chest x-rays can be used to evaluate the possibility of pulmonary disease.

GUIDELINES AND CRITICAL PATHWAYS FOR ACUTE CHEST PAIN

Guidelines for the initial evaluation for patients with acute chest pain have been developed by the American College of Emergency Physicians (ACEP) and other organizations. The ACEP statement describes *rules* and *guidelines* about the data that should be recorded as part of the evaluation, and the actions that should follow from certain findings (Table 13-5). In the ACEP framework, *rules* are actions that are general principles of good practice, while *guidelines* are actions that should be considered but are not always followed. Hence, failure to follow a guideline is not necessarily improper care.

Other organizations, including the Agency for Health Care Policy and Research (AHCPR) and the National Heart Attack Alert Program, have also issued guidelines for management of patients with a high probability of acute ischemic heart disease. In these and other guidelines, patients with possible or probable acute myocardial infarction as suggested by the description of their pain or electrocardiographic findings are expected to be admitted to the hospital. The AHCPR guidelines for unstable angina note that not all patients with that syndrome require admission but recommend that patients with unstable angina be monitored electrocardiographically during their evaluation; that those with ongoing rest pain should be placed at bed rest during the initial phase of stabilization. The ACEP policy statement indicates that patients who are discharged should be given a referral for follow-up care and instructions regarding treatment and circumstances that require a return to the emergency department.

Many medical centers have adopted critical pathways and other forms of guidelines to increase efficiency. These guidelines emphasize two strategies:

- Triage to non-coronary care unit monitored facilities such as intermediate care units or chest pain units of patients with a low risk for complications, such as patients without new ischemic changes on their electrocardiograms and without ongoing chest pain. Such patients can usually be safely observed in non-coronary care unit settings, undergo early exercise testing, or be discharged home. Risk stratification can be assisted through use of prospectively validated multivariate algorithms that have been published for acute ischemic heart disease and its complications.
- Shortening lengths of stay in the coronary care unit and hospital. Recommendations regarding the minimum length of stay in a monitored bed for a patient who has no further symptoms have decreased in recent years to 12 h or less if exercise testing or other risk stratification technologies are available.

NONACUTE CHEST DISCOMFORT   The management of patients who do not require admission to the hospital or who no longer require inpatient observation should seek to identify the cause of the symptoms and the likelihood of major complications. Cost-effectiveness analyses support use of noninvasive testing for coronary disease, such as exercise electrocardiography and stress echocardiography. These tests serve both to diagnose coronary disease and to identify patients with high-risk forms of coronary disease who may benefit from revascularization. Gastrointestinal causes of chest pain can be evaluated via endoscopy or radiology studies. Emotional and psychiatric conditions warrant appropriate evaluation and treatment; randomized trial data indicate that cognitive therapy and group interventions lead to decreases in symptoms for such patients.

PALPITATIONS

Palpitations are characterized by an awareness of the beating of the heart. Patients commonly describe "pounding" or "fluttering" heart beats or report a sensation that the heart is stopping or skipping beats. These symptoms may be caused by a change in the heart's rhythm or rate or by an increase in the force of its contractions. In many cases, this awareness reflects lack of competing sensory stimuli, such as when a person is lying in bed, unable to sleep.

Palpitations are often manifestations of psychiatric conditions, the most common of which are depression and panic disorder. For example, in one study of outpatients referred for ambulatory electrocardiographic monitoring to evaluate palpitations, 19% were found to have a psychiatric disorder. Patients with psychiatric disorders were more likely than other patients to report that their palpitations lasted longer than 15 min or were accompanied by ancillary symptoms. In this study, physicians usually recognized the emotional basis of the patients' symptoms but frequently did not refer the patient for specific therapy.

Palpitations can also be caused by virtually any cardiac arrhythmia as well as by other cardiac and noncardiac conditions. A markedly enlarged left ventricle can cause awareness of the heart beat by contact with the chest wall. Any condition associated with increased catecholamine levels can lead to palpitations both by increasing the forcefulness of cardiac contractions and by increasing the rate of premature beats.

Palpitations can be intermittent or sustained and regular or irregular. Patients with this complaint should be asked to describe their palpitations' onset, duration, associated symptoms and the circumstances in which they occur. Abrupt onset and termination after several minutes may reflect a sustained ventricular or supraventricular tachyarrhythmia. Gradual onset and termination of a pounding heart beat is more consistent with sinus tachycardia. Patients should try to replicate the rhythm of their palpitations by tapping on a table. This maneuver can help the physician determine the nature of any cardiac arrhythmia. Patients should also be taught to take their pulse so that they can more accurately report their approximate heart rate and whether the rhythm was regular.

DIFFERENTIAL DIAGNOSIS   Patients who report "skipped" beats or a "flopping" sensation often have atrial or ventricular extrasystoles (Chap. 230). These premature beats are followed by a compensatory pause, and the first heart beat after the pause may be unusually strong due to increased left ventricular volume and enhanced contractility (a phenomenon called *postextrasystolic potentiation*). Sustained bursts of rapid heart beats may be due to ventricular or supraventricular tachyarrhythmias. A sustained irregular rhythm suggests atrial fibrillation.

Conditions that cause marked left ventricular enlargement such as aortic regurgitation can cause an awareness of the heart beat that is sometimes positional. Presumably because of associated arrhythmias, hypertrophic cardiomyopathy, mitral valve prolapse, and other cardiac structural abnormalities are also associated with palpitations.

Palpitations can also be a prominent symptom in noncardiac conditions, including thyrotoxicosis, hypoglycemia, pheochromocytoma,

Table 13-5   Evaluation of Acute Chest Pain: Excerpts from the Clinical Policy of the American College of Emergency Physicians (1995)

		Action	
Variable	Finding	Rule[a]	Guideline[b]
HISTORY			
Pain	Ongoing *and* severe *and* crushing *and* substernal *or* same as previous pain diagnosed as MI	IV access Supplemental oxygen ECG Aspirin Nitrates Management of ongoing pain Admit	Serum cardiac markers CXR Anticoagulation
	Severe *or* pressure *or* substernal *or* exertional *or* radiating to jaw, neck, shoulder, or arm	ECG	IV access Supplemental oxygen Cardiac monitor Serum cardiac markers CXR Nitrates Management of ongoing pain Admit
	Tearing, severe, and radiating to back	Large-bore IV access Supplemental oxygen Cardiac monitor CXR ECG	Differential upper extremity blood pressures Aortic imaging Management of ongoing pain Admit
	Similar to that of previous pulmonary embolus	IV access Supplemental oxygen Cardiac monitor ABG and oximetry Anticoagulation/pulmonary vascular imaging ECG	CXR Admit
	Indigestion or burning epigastric	None	ECG
	Pleuritic	None	CXR ECG
ASSESSMENT			
Associated symptoms	Syncope or near-syncope	ECG	Cardiac monitor Hct
	Shortness of breath, dyspnea on exertion, paroxysmal nocturnal dyspnea, or orthopnea	ECG	ABG/oximetry CXR
Past medical history	Previous MI, coronary artery bypass surgery, angioplasty, cocaine use within last 96 h, previous positive cardiac diagnostic studies	ECG	
	Major risk factors for coronary artery disease		ECG
	Pericarditis/myocarditis	ECG	Serum cardiac markers CXR Echocardiography Consult/admit
	Unstable angina—new-onset, exertional	ECG Aspirin	IV access Supplemental oxygen Cardiac monitor Nitrates Consult/admit
	Unstable angina—ongoing or recurrent ischemia	IV access Supplemental oxygen Cardiac monitor	Serial serum cardiac markers CXR Cardiac imaging
	ECG showing new ST segment depressions or T wave inversions consistent with ischemia	Anticoagulation Aspirin Nitrates Management of ongoing pain Admit	Serial ECGs Beta blockers

(continued)

Table 13-5—*(continued)*

Variable	Finding	Action Rule[a]	Action Guideline[b]
	High clinical suspicion of MI with nondiagnostic ECG	IV access Supplemental oxygen Cardiac monitor Anticoagulation Aspirin Nitrates Management of ongoing pain Admit	Serial serum cardiac markers CXR Cardiac imaging Serial ECGs Magnesium therapy Beta blockers
	High clinical suspicion of MI with diagnostic ECG of bundle branch block	IV access Supplemental oxygen Cardiac monitor Assessment for thrombolytic therapy or other reperfusion techniques Anticoagulation Aspirin Nitrates Management of ongoing pain Admit	Serial serum cardiac markers CXR Cardiac imaging Serial ECGs Magnesium therapy if not given thrombolytics Beta blockers
	Aortic dissection	Large-bore IV access Supplemental oxygen Cardiac monitor Blood type and cross-match ECG Management of blood pressure/cardiac contractility Management of ongoing pain Immediate surgical consultation Admit	Aortic imaging

[a] Rule: An action reflecting principles of good practice in most situations. There may be circumstances when a rule need not or cannot be followed; in these situations, it is advisable that deviation from the rule be justified in writing. Inability to comply with rules should be incorporated in institutional policies.

[b] Guideline: An action that may be considered, depending on the patient, the circumstances, or other factors. Thus, guidelines are not always followed, and there is no implication that failure to follow a guideline is improper.

NOTE: MI, myocardial infarction; ECG, electrocardiogram; CXR, chest x-ray; ABG, arterial blood gases; Hct, hematocrit.

SOURCE: American College of Emergency Physicians.

and fever. The physiologic basis of palpitations with these conditions is either arrhythmia or increased catecholamine levels leading to greater myocardial contractility. Drugs that can precipitate arrhythmias and palpitations include tobacco, coffee, tea, alcohol, epinephrine, ephedrine, aminophylline, and atropine.

Approach to the Patient

The first goal in the evaluation of patients with palpitations is to exclude the possibility of life-threatening arrhythmias. The risk for such arrhythmias is highest in patients with coronary artery disease, congestive heart failure, or other structural cardiac abnormalities. The history, physical examination, and electrocardiogram should therefore be focused on stratifying patients according to the risk of such conditions. Palpitations are also more likely to reflect serious arrhythmias if they are associated with symptoms that suggest hemodynamic compromise, such as syncope, light-headedness, dizziness, or shortness of breath.

The most common first test after the initial evaluation of palpitations is continuous electrocardiographic (Holter) monitoring. This test is especially useful if patients have palpitations on a daily basis. For patients with more sporadic palpitations, a variety of new technologies have become available to allow capture of electrocardiographic tracings at the time of their symptoms. These technologies include loop recorders, that can freeze the last several minutes of data when the patient presses a button, and telephonic monitors, which can be used to "call in" tracings when symptoms occur. If episodes are associated with physical stress, exercise electrocardiography can be used in an attempt to elicit an arrhythmia.

Most patients with palpitations do not have evidence of major arrhythmias or abnormal physiologic conditions associated with increased catecholamine levels. Patients with emotional or psychological causes of palpitations should be evaluated for possible cognitive and pharmaceutical therapy. Drugs and medications that may precipitate palpitations should be eliminated or reduced. A trial of beta blockers is often successful in reducing premature beats and symptoms. Regardless of the cause and treatment, the clinician should remain aware that palpitations are extremely bothersome symptoms for patients. Reassurance that a comprehensive evaluation has been performed and that the palpitations do not adversely affect the patient's prognosis is a critical part of the patient's care.

BIBLIOGRAPHY

AMERICAN COLLEGE OF EMERGENCY PHYSICIANS: Clinical policy for the initial approach to adults presenting with a chief complaint of chest pain, with no history of trauma. Ann Emerg Med 25:274, 1995

BARSKY AJ et al: Somatized psychiatric disorder presenting as palpitations. Arch Intern Med 156:1102, 1996

BRAUNWALD E et al: *Unstable Angina: Diagnosis and Management. Clinical Practice Guideline Number 10* (amended). AHCPR Publication No. 94-0602. Rockville, MD, Agency for Health Care Policy and Research and National Heart, Lung, and Blood Institute, Public Health Service, U.S. Department of Health and Human Services, May 1994

FARKOUH ME et al: A clinical trial of a chest-pain observation unit for patients with unstable angina. N Engl J Med 339:1882, 1998

KUNTZ KM et al: Cost-effectiveness of diagnostic strategies for patients with chest pain. Ann Intern Med 130:709, 1999

NICHOL G et al: A critical pathway for management of patients with acute chest pain at low risk for myocardial ischemia. Recommendations and potential impact. Ann Intern Med 127:996, 1997

VAN PESKI-OOSTERBAAN AS et al: Cognitive-behavioral therapy for noncardiac chest pain: A randomized trial. Am J Med 106:424, 1999

WEBER BE, KAPOOR WN: Evaluation and outcomes of patients with palpitations. Am J Med 100:138, 1996

14   *William Silen*

ABDOMINAL PAIN

The correct interpretation of acute abdominal pain is challenging. Since proper therapy may require urgent action, the unhurried approach suitable for the study of other conditions is sometimes denied. Few other clinical situations demand greater judgment, because the most catastrophic of events may be forecast by the subtlest of symptoms and signs. A meticulously executed, detailed history and physical examination is of great importance. The etiologic classification in Table 14-1, although not complete, forms a useful basis for the evaluation of patients with abdominal pain.

The diagnosis of "acute or surgical abdomen" is not an acceptable one because of its often misleading and erroneous connotation. The most obvious of "acute abdomens" may not require operative intervention, and the mildest of abdominal pains may herald an urgently correctable lesion. Any patient with abdominal pain of recent onset requires early and thorough evaluation and accurate diagnosis.

SOME MECHANISMS OF PAIN ORIGINATING IN THE ABDOMEN Inflammation of the Parietal Peritoneum The pain of parietal peritoneal inflammation is steady and aching in character and is located directly over the inflamed area, its exact reference being possible because it is transmitted by somatic nerves supplying the parietal peritoneum. The intensity of the pain is dependent

Table 14-1   Some Important Causes of Abdominal Pain

PAIN ORIGINATING IN THE ABDOMEN

1. Parietal peritoneal inflammation
   a. Bacterial contamination, e.g., perforated appendix, pelvic inflammatory disease
   b. Chemical irritation, e.g., perforated ulcer, pancreatitis, mittelschmerz
2. Mechanical obstruction of hollow viscera
   a. Obstruction of the small or large intestine
   b. Obstruction of the biliary tree
   c. Obstruction of the ureter
3. Vascular disturbances
   a. Embolism or thrombosis
   b. Vascular rupture
   c. Pressure or torsional occlusion
   d. Sickle cell anemia
4. Abdominal wall
   a. Distortion or traction of mesentery
   b. Trauma or infection of muscles
5. Distention of visceral surfaces, e.g., hepatic or renal capsules

PAIN REFERRED FROM EXTRAABDOMINAL SOURCE

1. Thorax, e.g., pneumonia, referred pain from coronary occlusion
2. Spine, e.g., radiculitis from arthritis
3. Genitalia, e.g., torsion of the testicle

METABOLIC CAUSES

1. Exogenous
   a. Black widow spider bite
   b. Lead poisoning and others
2. Endogenous
   a. Uremia
   b. Diabetic ketoacidosis
   c. Porphyria
   d. Allergic factors (C′1 esterase inhibitor deficiency)

NEUROGENIC CAUSES

1. Organic
   a. Tabes dorsalis
   b. Herpes zoster
   c. Causalgia and others
2. Functional

on the type and amount of material to which the peritoneal surfaces are exposed in a given time period. For example, the sudden release into the peritoneal cavity of a small quantity of *sterile* acid gastric juice causes much more pain than the same amount of grossly contaminated neutral feces. Enzymatically active pancreatic juice incites more pain and inflammation than does the same amount of sterile bile containing no potent enzymes. Blood and urine are often so bland as to go undetected if exposure of the peritoneum has not been sudden and massive. In the case of bacterial contamination, such as in pelvic inflammatory disease, the pain is frequently of low intensity early in the illness until bacterial multiplication has caused the elaboration of irritating substances.

The rate at which the irritating material is applied to the peritoneum is important. Perforated peptic ulcer may be associated with entirely different clinical pictures dependent only on the rapidity with which the gastric juice enters the peritoneal cavity.

The pain of peritoneal inflammation is invariably accentuated by pressure or changes in tension of the peritoneum, whether produced by palpation or by movement, as in coughing or sneezing. The patient with peritonitis lies quietly in bed, preferring to avoid motion, in contrast to the patient with colic, who may writhe incessantly.

Another characteristic feature of peritoneal irritation is tonic reflex spasm of the abdominal musculature, localized to the involved body segment. The intensity of the tonic muscle spasm accompanying peritoneal inflammation is dependent on the location of the inflammatory process, the rate at which it develops, and the integrity of the nervous system. Spasm over a perforated retrocecal appendix or perforated ulcer into the lesser peritoneal sac may be minimal or absent because of the protective effect of overlying viscera. A slowly developing process often greatly attenuates the degree of muscle spasm. Catastrophic abdominal emergencies such as a perforated ulcer may be associated with minimal or no detectable pain or muscle spasm in obtunded, seriously ill, debilitated elderly patients or in psychotic patients.

Obstruction of Hollow Viscera The pain of obstruction of hollow abdominal viscera is classically described as intermittent, or colicky. Yet the lack of a truly cramping character should not be misleading, because distention of a hollow viscus may produce steady pain with only very occasional exacerbations. It is not nearly as well localized as the pain of parietal peritoneal inflammation.

The colicky pain of obstruction of the small intestine is usually periumbilical or supraumbilical and is poorly localized. As the intestine becomes progressively dilated with loss of muscular tone, the colicky nature of the pain may diminish. With superimposed strangulating obstruction, pain may spread to the lower lumbar region if there is traction on the root of the mesentery. The colicky pain of colonic obstruction is of lesser intensity than that of the small intestine and is often located in the infraumbilical area. Lumbar radiation of pain is common in colonic obstruction.

Sudden distention of the biliary tree produces a steady rather than colicky type of pain; hence the term *biliary colic* is misleading. Acute distention of the gallbladder usually causes pain in the right upper quadrant with radiation to the right posterior region of the thorax or to the tip of the right scapula, and distention of the common bile duct is often associated with pain in the epigastrium radiating to the upper part of the lumbar region. Considerable variation is common, however, so that differentiation between these may be impossible. The typical subscapular pain or lumbar radiation is frequently absent. Gradual dilatation of the biliary tree, as in carcinoma of the head of the pancreas, may cause no pain or only a mild aching sensation in the epigastrium or right upper quadrant. The pain of distention of the pancreatic ducts is similar to that described for distention of the common bile duct but, in addition, is very frequently accentuated by recumbency and relieved by the upright position.

Obstruction of the urinary bladder results in dull suprapubic pain, usually low in intensity. Restlessness without specific complaint of pain may be the only sign of a distended bladder in an obtunded patient. In contrast, acute obstruction of the intravesicular portion of the ureter is characterized by severe suprapubic and flank pain that radiates to the penis, scrotum, or inner aspect of the upper thigh. Obstruction of the ureteropelvic junction is felt as pain in the costovertebral angle, whereas obstruction of the remainder of the ureter is associated with flank pain that often extends into the same side of the abdomen.

Vascular Disturbances   A frequent misconception, despite abundant experience to the contrary, is that pain associated with intraabdominal vascular disturbances is sudden and catastrophic in nature. The pain of embolism or thrombosis of the superior mesenteric artery or that of impending rupture of an abdominal aortic aneurysm certainly may be severe and diffuse. Yet, just as frequently, the patient with occlusion of the superior mesenteric artery has only mild continuous diffuse pain for 2 or 3 days before vascular collapse or findings of peritoneal inflammation appear. The early, seemingly insignificant discomfort is caused by hyperperistalsis rather than peritoneal inflammation. Indeed, absence of tenderness and rigidity in the presence of continuous, diffuse pain in a patient likely to have vascular disease is quite characteristic of occlusion of the superior mesenteric artery. Abdominal pain with radiation to the sacral region, flank, or genitalia should always signal the possible presence of a rupturing abdominal aortic aneurysm. This pain may persist over a period of several days before rupture and collapse occur.

Abdominal Wall   Pain arising from the abdominal wall is usually constant and aching. Movement, prolonged standing, and pressure accentuate the discomfort and muscle spasm. In the case of hematoma of the rectus sheath, now most frequently encountered in association with anticoagulant therapy, a mass may be present in the lower quadrants of the abdomen. Simultaneous involvement of muscles in other parts of the body usually serves to differentiate myositis of the abdominal wall from an intraabdominal process that might cause pain in the same region.

REFERRED PAIN IN ABDOMINAL DISEASES   Pain referred to the abdomen from the thorax, spine, or genitalia may prove a vexing diagnostic problem, because diseases of the upper part of the abdominal cavity such as acute cholecystitis or perforated ulcer are frequently associated with intrathoracic complications. A most important, yet often forgotten, dictum is that the possibility of intrathoracic disease must be considered in every patient with abdominal pain, especially if the pain is in the upper part of the abdomen. Systematic questioning and examination directed toward detecting myocardial or pulmonary infarction, pneumonia, pericarditis, or esophageal disease (the intrathoracic diseases that most often masquerade as abdominal emergencies) will often provide sufficient clues to establish the proper diagnosis. Diaphragmatic pleuritis resulting from pneumonia or pulmonary infarction may cause pain in the right upper quadrant and pain in the supraclavicular area, the latter radiation to be distinguished from the referred subscapular pain caused by acute distention of the extrahepatic biliary tree. The ultimate decision as to the origin of abdominal pain may require deliberate and planned observation over a period of several hours, during which repeated questioning and examination will provide the diagnosis.

Referred pain of thoracic origin is often accompanied by splinting of the involved hemithorax with respiratory lag and decrease in excursion more marked than that seen in the presence of intraabdominal disease. In addition, apparent abdominal muscle spasm caused by referred pain will diminish during the inspiratory phase of respiration, whereas it is persistent throughout both respiratory phases if it is of abdominal origin. Palpation over the area of referred pain in the abdomen also does not usually accentuate the pain and in many instances actually seems to relieve it. Thoracic and abdominal disease frequently coexist and may be difficult or impossible to differentiate.

For example, the patient with known biliary tract disease often has epigastric pain during myocardial infarction, or biliary colic may be referred to the precordium or left shoulder in a patient who has suffered previously from angina pectoris. →*For an explanation of the radiation of pain to a previously diseased area, see Chap. 12.*

Referred pain from the spine, which usually involves compression or irritation of nerve roots, is characteristically intensified by certain motions such as cough, sneeze, or strain and is associated with hyperesthesia over the involved dermatomes. Pain referred to the abdomen from the testicles or seminal vesicles is generally accentuated by the slightest pressure on either of these organs. The abdominal discomfort is of dull aching character and is poorly localized.

METABOLIC ABDOMINAL CRISES   Pain of metabolic origin may simulate almost any other type of intraabdominal disease. Several mechanisms may be at work. In certain instances, such as hyperlipidemia, the metabolic disease itself may be accompanied by an intraabdominal process such as pancreatitis, which can lead to unnecessary laparotomy unless recognized. C'1 esterase deficiency associated with angioneurotic edema is often associated with episodes of severe abdominal pain. Whenever the cause of abdominal pain is obscure, a metabolic origin always must be considered. Abdominal pain is also the hallmark of familial Mediterranean fever (Chap. 289).

The problem of differential diagnosis is often not readily resolved. The pain of porphyria and of lead colic is usually difficult to distinguish from that of intestinal obstruction, because severe hyperperistalsis is a prominent feature of both. The pain of uremia or diabetes is nonspecific, and the pain and tenderness frequently shift in location and intensity. Diabetic acidosis may be precipitated by acute appendicitis or intestinal obstruction, so if prompt resolution of the abdominal pain does not result from correction of the metabolic abnormalities, an underlying organic problem should be suspected. Black widow spider bites produce intense pain and rigidity of the abdominal muscles and back, an area infrequently involved in intraabdominal disease.

NEUROGENIC CAUSES   Causalgic pain may occur in diseases that injure sensory nerves. It has a burning character and is usually limited to the distribution of a given peripheral nerve. Normal stimuli such as touch or change in temperature may be transformed into this type of pain, which is frequently present in a patient at rest. The demonstration of irregularly spaced cutaneous pain spots may be the only indication of an old nerve lesion underlying causalgic pain. Even though the pain may be precipitated by gentle palpation, rigidity of the abdominal muscles is absent, and the respirations are not disturbed. Distention of the abdomen is uncommon, and the pain has no relationship to the intake of food.

Pain arising from spinal nerves or roots comes and goes suddenly and is of a lancinating type (Chap. 16). It may be caused by herpes zoster, impingement by arthritis, tumors, herniated nucleus pulposus, diabetes, or syphilis. It is not associated with food intake, abdominal distention, or changes in respiration. Severe muscle spasm, as in the gastric crises of tabes dorsalis, is common but is either relieved or is not accentuated by abdominal palpation. The pain is made worse by movement of the spine and is usually confined to a few dermatomes. Hyperesthesia is very common.

Psychogenic pain conforms to none of the aforementioned patterns. Mechanism is hard to define. The most common problem is the hysterical adolescent or young person who develops abdominal pain and who frequently loses an appendix or other organs because of it. Ovulation or some other natural event that causes brief mild abdominal discomfort may be experienced as an abdominal catastrophe.

Psychogenic pain varies enormously in type and location but usually has no relation to meals. It is often markedly accentuated during the night. Nausea and vomiting are rarely observed. Spasm is seldom induced in the abdominal musculature and, if present, does not persist, especially if the attention of the patient can be distracted. Persistent localized tenderness is rare, and if found, the muscle spasm in the area is inconsistent or absent. Shallow respiration is the most common breathing abnormality; anxiety may produce a smothering or choking sensation. It occurs in the absence of thoracic splinting or change in the respiratory rate.

Approach to the Patient

Few abdominal conditions require such urgent operative intervention that an orderly approach need be abandoned, no matter how ill the patient. Only those patients with exsanguinating hemorrhage must be rushed to the operating room immediately, but in such instances, only a few minutes are required to assess the critical nature of the problem. Under these circumstances, all obstacles must be swept aside, adequate venous access for fluid replacement obtained, and the operation begun. Many patients of this type have died in the radiology department or the emergency room while awaiting such unnecessary examinations as electrocardiograms or abdominal films. *There are no contraindications to operation when massive hemorrhage is present.* This situation fortunately is relatively rare.

Nothing will supplant an orderly, painstakingly *detailed history*, which is far more valuable than any laboratory or radiographic examination. This kind of history is laborious and time-consuming, making it not especially popular, even though a reasonably accurate diagnosis can be made on the basis of the history alone in the majority of cases. Computer-aided diagnosis of abdominal pain provides no advantage over clinical assessment alone. In cases of *acute* abdominal pain, a diagnosis is readily established in most instances, whereas success is not so frequent in patients with *chronic* pain. Irritable bowel syndrome is one of the most common causes of abdominal pain and must always be kept in mind (Chap. 288). The *chronological sequence of events* in the patient's history is often more important than emphasis on the location of pain. If the examiner is sufficiently open-minded and unhurried, asks the proper questions, and listens, the patient will usually provide the diagnosis. Careful attention should be paid to the extraabdominal regions that may be responsible for abdominal pain. An accurate menstrual history in a female patient is essential. Narcotics or analgesics should *not* be withheld until a definitive diagnosis or a definitive plan has been formulated; obfuscation of the diagnosis by adequate analgesia is unlikely.

In the examination, simple critical inspection of the patient, e.g., of facies, position in bed, and respiratory activity, may provide valuable clues. The amount of information to be gleaned is directly proportional to the *gentleness* and thoroughness of the examiner. Once a patient with peritoneal inflammation has been examined brusquely, accurate assessment by the next examiner becomes almost impossible. Eliciting rebound tenderness by sudden release of a deeply palpating hand in a patient with suspected peritonitis is cruel and unnecessary. The same information can be obtained by gentle percussion of the abdomen (rebound tenderness on a miniature scale), a maneuver that can be far more precise and localizing. Asking the patient to cough will elicit true rebound tenderness without the need for placing a hand on the abdomen. Furthermore, the forceful demonstration of rebound tenderness will startle and induce protective spasm in a nervous or worried patient in whom true rebound tenderness is not present. A palpable gallbladder will be missed if palpation is so brusque that voluntary muscle spasm becomes superimposed on involuntary muscular rigidity.

As in history taking, there is no substitute for sufficient time spent in the examination. Abdominal signs may be minimal but nevertheless, if accompanied by consistent symptoms, may be exceptionally meaningful. Abdominal signs may be virtually or totally absent in cases of pelvic peritonitis, so careful *pelvic and rectal examinations are mandatory in every patient with abdominal pain.* Tenderness on pelvic or rectal examination in the absence of other abdominal signs can be caused by operative indications such as perforated appendicitis, diverticulitis, twisted ovarian cyst, and many others.

Much attention has been paid to the presence or absence of peristaltic sounds, their quality, and their frequency. Auscultation of the abdomen is one of the least revealing aspects of the physical examination of a patient with abdominal pain. Catastrophes such as strangulating small intestinal obstruction or perforated appendicitis may occur in the presence of normal peristalsis. Conversely, when the proximal part of the intestine above an obstruction becomes markedly distended and edematous, peristaltic sounds may lose the characteristics of borborygmi and become weak or absent, even when peritonitis is not present. It is usually the severe chemical peritonitis of sudden onset that is associated with the truly silent abdomen. Assessment of the patient's state of hydration is important.

Laboratory examinations may be of great value in assessment of the patient with abdominal pain, yet with few exceptions they rarely establish a diagnosis. Leukocytosis should never be the single deciding factor as to whether or not operation is indicated. A white blood cell count greater than $20,000/\mu L$ may be observed with perforation of a viscus, but pancreatitis, acute cholecystitis, pelvic inflammatory disease, and intestinal infarction may be associated with marked leukocytosis. A normal white blood cell count is not rare in cases of perforation of abdominal viscera. The diagnosis of anemia may be more helpful than the white blood cell count, especially when combined with the history.

The urinalysis may reveal the state of hydration or rule out severe renal disease, diabetes, or urinary infection. Blood urea nitrogen, glucose, and serum bilirubin levels may be helpful. Serum amylase levels may be increased by many diseases other than pancreatitis, e.g., perforated ulcer, strangulating intestinal obstruction, and acute cholecystitis; thus, elevations of serum amylase do not rule out the need for an operation. The determination of the serum lipase may have greater accuracy than that of the serum amylase.

Plain and upright or lateral decubitus radiographs of the abdomen may be of value in cases of intestinal obstruction, perforated ulcer, and a variety of other conditions. They are usually unnecessary in patients with acute appendicitis or strangulated external hernias. In rare instances, barium or water-soluble contrast study of the upper part of the gastrointestinal tract may demonstrate partial intestinal obstruction that may elude diagnosis by other means. If there is any question of obstruction of the colon, oral administration of barium sulfate should be avoided. On the other hand, in cases of suspected colonic obstruction (with perforation), contrast enema may be diagnostic.

In the absence of trauma, peritoneal lavage has been replaced as a diagnostic tool by ultrasound, computed tomography (CT), and laparoscopy. Ultrasonography has proved to be useful in detecting an enlarged gallbladder or pancreas, the presence of gallstones, an enlarged ovary, or a tubal pregnancy. Laparoscopy is especially helpful in diagnosing pelvic conditions, such as ovarian cysts, tubal pregnancies, salpingitis, and acute appendicitis. Radioisotopic scans (HIDA) may help differentiate acute cholecystitis from acute pancreatitis. A CT scan may demonstrate an enlarged pancreas, ruptured spleen, or thickened colonic or appendiceal wall and streaking of the mesocolon or mesoappendix characteristic of diverticulitis or appendicitis.

Sometimes, even under the best circumstances with all available aids and with the greatest of clinical skill, a definitive diagnosis cannot be established at the time of the initial examination. Nevertheless, despite lack of a clear anatomic diagnosis, it may be abundantly clear to an experienced and thoughtful physician and surgeon that on clinical grounds alone operation is indicated. Should that decision be questionable, watchful waiting with repeated questioning and examination will often elucidate the true nature of the illness and indicate the proper course of action.

BIBLIOGRAPHY

BOHNER H et al: Simple data from history and physical examination help to exclude bowel obstruction and to avoid radiographic studies in patients with acute abdominal pain. Eur J Surg 164:777, 1998

CERVERO F, LAIRD JM: Visceral pain. Lancet 353:2145, 1999

DAVIES AH et al: Ultrasonography in the acute abdomen. Br J Surg 78:1178, 1991

MARCO CA et al: Abdominal pain in geriatric emergency patients: Variables associated with adverse outcome. Acad Emerg Med 5:1163, 1998

SCOTT HJ, ROSIN RD: The influence of diagnostic and therapeutic laparoscopy on patients presenting with an acute abdomen. J R Soc Med 86:699, 1993

TAIT IS et al: Do patients with abdominal pain wait unduly long for analgesia? J R Coll Surg Edinb 44:181, 1999

TAOUREL P et al: Acute abdomen of unknown origin: Impact of CT on diagnosis and management. Gastrointest Radiol 17:287, 1992

---

15   *Neil H. Raskin, Stephen J. Peroutka*

HEADACHE, INCLUDING MIGRAINE AND CLUSTER HEADACHE

CSF cerebrospinal fluid	MELAS *m*itochondrial
CT computed tomography	*e*ncephalomyopathy, *l*actic *a*cidosis, and
ESR erythrocyte sedimentation rate	*s*troke-like episodes
FDA Food and Drug Administration	MRI magnetic resonance imaging
FHM Familial hemiplegic migraine	NSAIDs nonsteroidal anti-
5-HT 5-hydroxytryptamine	inflammatory drugs
MAOIs monoamine oxidase	PET positron emission tomography
inhibitors	SNS sympathetic nervous system

Few of us are spared the experience of head pain. As many as 90% of individuals have at least one headache per year. Severe, disabling headache is reported to occur at least annually by 40% of individuals worldwide. A useful classification of the many causes of headache is shown in Table 15-1. Headache is usually a benign symptom, but occasionally it is the manifestation of a serious illness such as brain tumor, subarachnoid hemorrhage, meningitis, or giant cell arteritis. In emergency settings, approximately 5% of patients with headache are found to have a serious underlying neurologic disorder. Therefore, it is imperative that the serious causes of headache be diagnosed rapidly and accurately.

PAIN-SENSITIVE STRUCTURES OF THE HEAD

Pain is most commonly due to tissue injury resulting in stimulation of peripheral nociceptors in an intact nervous system. Pain can also result from damage to or anomalous activation of pain-sensitive pathways of the peripheral or central nervous system. Headache may originate from either or both mechanisms. Relatively few cranial structures are pain-sensitive: the scalp, middle meningeal artery, dural sinuses, falx cerebri, and the proximal segments of the large pial arteries. The ventricular ependyma, choroid plexus, pial veins, and much of the brain parenchyma are pain-insensitive. Electrical stimulation of the midbrain in the region of the dorsal raphe has resulted in migraine-like headaches. Thus, whereas most of the brain is insensitive to electrode probing, a site in the midbrain represents a possible source of headache generation. Sensory stimuli from the head are conveyed to the central nervous system via the trigeminal nerves for structures above the tentorium in the anterior and middle fossae of the skull and via the first three cervical nerves for those in the posterior fossa and the inferior surface of the tentorium.

Headache can occur as the result of (1) distention, traction, or dilation of intracranial or extracranial arteries; (2) traction or displacement of large intracranial veins or their dural envelope; (3) compression, traction, or inflammation of cranial and spinal nerves; (4) spasm, inflammation, or trauma to cranial and cervical muscles; (5) meningeal irritation and raised intracranial pressure; or (6) other possible mechanisms such as activation of brainstem structures.

GENERAL CLINICAL CONSIDERATIONS

The quality, location, duration, and time course of the headache and the conditions that produce, exacerbate, or relieve it should be carefully reviewed. Ascertaining the *quality* of cephalic pain is occasionally helpful for diagnosis. Most tension-type headaches are described as tight "bandlike" pain or as dull, deeply located, and aching pain. Jabbing, brief, sharp cephalic pain, often occurring multifocally (ice pick–like pain), is the signature of a benign, nondescript disorder. A throbbing quality and tight muscles about the head, neck, and shoulder girdle are common nonspecific accompaniments of vascular headaches.

Pain *intensity* rarely has diagnostic value, although from the patient's perspective, it is the single aspect of pain that is most important. Although meningitis, subarachnoid hemorrhage, and cluster headache produce intense cranial pain, most patients entering emergency departments with the most severe headache of their lives usually have migraine. Contrary to common belief, the headache produced by a brain tumor is not usually distinctive or severe.

Data regarding *location* of headache may be informative. If the source is an extracranial structure, as in giant cell arteritis, the correspondence with the site of pain is fairly precise. Inflammation of an extracranial artery causes pain and exquisite tenderness localized to the site of the vessel. Lesions of paranasal sinuses, teeth, eyes, and upper cervical vertebrae induce less sharply localized pain, but pain that is still referred in a regional distribution. Intracranial lesions in the posterior fossa cause pain that is usually occipitonuchal, and supratentorial lesions most often induce frontotemporal pain.

Duration and *time-intensity* curves of headaches are diagnostically useful. A ruptured aneurysm results in head pain that peaks in an instant, thunderclap-like; much less often, unruptured aneurysms may signal their presence in the same way. Cluster headache attacks reach their peak over 3 to 5 min, remain at maximal levels for about 45 min, and then taper off. Migraine attacks build up over hours, are maintained for several hours to days, and are characteristically relieved by sleep. Sleep disruption and early morning headaches that improve during the day are characteristics of headaches produced by brain tumors.

The analysis of facial pain requires a different approach. Trigeminal and, less commonly, glossopharyngeal neuralgia are frequent causes of facial pain (Chap. 367). "Neuralgias" are painful disorders characterized by paroxysmal, fleeting, often electric shock–like episodes that are frequently caused by demyelinating lesions of nerves (the trigeminal or glossopharyngeal nerves in cranial neuralgias). Certain maneuvers characteristically trigger paroxysms of pain. However, the most common cause of facial pain by far is dental; provocation by hot, cold, or sweet foods is typical. The application of a cold stimulus will repeatedly induce dental pain, whereas in neuralgic disorders, a refractory period usually occurs after the initial response so that pain cannot be repeatedly induced.

The effect of eating on facial pain may provide insight into its cause. Is it the chewing, swallowing, or taste of the food that elicits pain? Chewing points toward trigeminal neuralgia, temporomandibular joint dysfunction, or giant cell arteritis ("jaw claudication"), whereas swallowing *and* taste provocation point toward glossopharyngeal neuralgia. Pain upon swallowing is common among patients with carotidynia (see below) because the inflamed, tender carotid artery abuts the esophagus during deglutition.

Many patients with facial pain do not experience stereotypic neuralgias; the term *atypical facial pain* has been used in this setting.

Table 15-1 International Headache Society Classification of Headache

1. **Migraine**
   Migraine without aura
   Migraine with aura
   Ophthalmoplegic migraine
   Retinal migraine
   Childhood periodic syndromes that may be precursors to or associated
     with migraine
   Migrainous disorder not fulfilling above criteria
2. **Tension-type headache**
   Episodic tension-type headache
   Chronic tension-type headache
3. **Cluster headache and chronic paroxysmal hemicrania**
   Cluster headache
   Chronic paroxysmal hemicrania
4. **Miscellaneous headaches not associated with structural lesion**
   Idiopathic stabbing headache
   External compression headache
   Cold stimulus headache
   Benign cough headache
   Benign exertional headache
   Headache associated with sexual activity
5. **Headache associated with head trauma**
   Acute posttraumatic headache
   Chronic posttraumatic headache
6. **Headache associated with vascular disorders**
   Acute ischemic cerebrovascular disorder
   Intracranial hematoma
   Subarachnoid hemorrhage
   Unruptured vascular malformation
   Arteritis
   Carotid or vertebral artery pain
   Venous thrombosis
   Arterial hypertension
   Other vascular disorder
7. **Headache associated with nonvascular intracranial disorder**
   High CSF pressure
   Low CSF pressure
   Intracranial infection

7. **Headache associated with nonvascular intracranial disorder (cont.)**
   Sarcoidosis and other noninfectious inflammatory diseases
   Related to intrathecal injections
   Intracranial neoplasm
   Associated with other intracranial disorder
8. **Headache associated with substances or their withdrawal**
   Headache induced by acute substance use or exposure
   Headache induced by chronic substance use or exposure
   Headache from substance withdrawal (acute use)
   Headache from substance withdrawal (chronic use)
9. **Headache associated with noncephalic infection**
   Viral infection
   Bacterial infection
   Other infection
10. **Headache associated with metabolic disorder**
   Hypoxia
   Hypercapnia
   Mixed hypoxia and hypercapnia
   Hypoglycemia
   Dialysis
   Other metabolic abnormality
11. **Headache or facial pain associated with disorder of facial or cranial
    structures**
   Cranial bone
   Eyes
   Ears
   Nose and sinuses
   Teeth, jaws, and related structures
   Temporomandibular joint disease
12. **Cranial neuralgias, nerve trunk pain, and deafferentation pain**
   Persistent (in contrast to ticlike) pain of cranial nerve origin
   Trigeminal neuralgia
   Glossopharyngeal neuralgia
   Nervus intermedius neuralgia
   Superior laryngeal neuralgia
   Occipital neuralgia
   Central causes of head and facial pain other than tic douloureux
13. **Headache not classifiable**

NOTE: CSF, cerebrospinal fluid.
SOURCE: After Olesen, 1988.

Vague, poorly localized, continuous facial pain is characteristic of nasopharyngeal carcinoma; a burning pain often develops as deafferentation occurs and evidence of cranial neuropathy appears. Burning facial pain may also occur with tumors of the fifth cranial nerve (meningioma or schwannoma) or with lesions of the pons that interrupt the dorsal root entry zone of the nerve (multiple sclerosis). In patients with facial pain, the finding of objective sensory loss is an important clue to a serious underlying disorder. Occasionally, the cause of a pain problem cannot be resolved promptly, necessitating periodic follow-up until further signs appear.

CLINICAL EVALUATION OF ACUTE, NEW-ONSET HEADACHE

Patients who present with their first severe headache raise entirely different diagnostic possibilities than those with recurrent headaches over many years. In new-onset and severe headaches, the probability of finding a potentially serious cause is considerably greater than in recurrent headache. When a patient complains of an acute, new-onset headache, a number of causes should be considered including meningitis, subarachnoid hemorrhage, epidural or subdural hematoma, glaucoma, and purulent sinusitis. Clinical features of acute, new-onset headache caused by serious underlying conditions are summarized in Table 15-2.

A complete neurologic examination is an essential first step in the evaluation. In most cases, an abnormal examination should be followed by a computed tomography (CT) or a magnetic resonance imaging (MRI) study. As a screening procedure for intracranial pathology in this setting, CT and MRI methods appear to be equally sensitive.

A general evaluation of acute headache might include the investigation of cardiovascular and renal status by blood pressure monitoring and urine examination; eyes by fundoscopy, intraocular pressure measurement, and refraction; cranial arteries by palpation; and cervical spine by the effect of passive movement of the head and imaging.

The psychological state of the patient should also be evaluated since a relationship exists between head pain and depression. Many patients in chronic daily pain cycles become depressed; moreover, there is a greater-than-chance coincidence of migraine with both bipolar (manic depressive) and unipolar major depressive disorders. Drugs with antidepressant actions are also effective in the prophylactic treatment of both tension-type headache and migraine.

Underlying recurrent headache disorders may be activated by pain that follows otologic or endodontic surgical procedures. Treatment of the headache problem is largely ineffective until the cause of the primary problem is addressed. Thus, pain about the head as the result of

Table 15-2 Headache Symptoms That Suggest a Serious Underlying Disorder

"Worst" headache ever
First severe headache
Subacute worsening over days or weeks
Abnormal neurologic examination
Fever or unexplained systemic signs
Vomiting precedes headache
Induced by bending, lifting, cough
Disturbs sleep or present immediately upon awakening
Known systemic illness
Onset after age 55

diseased tissue or trauma may reawaken an otherwise quiescent migrainous syndrome.

Serious underlying conditions that are associated with headache are described below and in Table 15-3.

MENINGITIS   In general, acute, severe headache with stiff neck and fever suggests meningitis. Lumbar puncture is mandatory. Often there is striking accentuation of pain with eye movement. Meningitis is particularly easy to mistake for migraine in that the cardinal symptoms of pounding headache, photophobia, nausea, and vomiting are present. →*A detailed discussion of meningitis can be found in Chaps. 372 to 374.*

INTRACRANIAL HEMORRHAGE   In general, acute, severe headache with stiff neck but without fever suggests subarachnoid hemorrhage. A ruptured aneurysm, arteriovenous malformation, or intraparenchymal hemorrhage may also present with only headache. Rarely, if the hemorrhage is small or below the foramen magnum, the head CT scan can be normal. Therefore, a lumbar puncture may be required to make the definitive diagnosis of a subarachnoid hemorrhage. →*A detailed discussion of intracranial hemorrhage can be found in Chap. 361.*

BRAIN TUMOR   Approximately 30% of patients with brain tumors consider headache to be their chief complaint. The head pain is usually nondescript—an intermittent deep, dull aching of moderate intensity, which may worsen with exertion or change in position and may be associated with nausea and vomiting. This pattern of symptoms results from migraine far more often than from brain tumor. Headache of brain tumor disturbs sleep in about 10% of patients. Vomiting that precedes the appearance of headache by weeks is highly characteristic of posterior fossa brain tumors. A history of amenorrhea or galactorrhea should lead one to question whether a prolactin-secreting pituitary adenoma (or the polycystic ovary syndrome) is the source of headache. Headache arising de novo in a patient with known malignancy suggests either cerebral metastases and/or carcinomatous meningitis. Head pain appearing abruptly after bending, lifting, or coughing can be the clue to a posterior fossa mass (or a Chiari malformation). →*A detailed discussion of brain tumors can be found in Chap. 370.*

TEMPORAL ARTERITIS   (See also Chaps. 28 and 317) Temporal (giant cell) arteritis is an inflammatory disorder of arteries that frequently involves the extracranial carotid circulation. This is a common disorder of the elderly; its annual incidence is 77:100,000 in individuals aged 50 and older. The average age of onset is 70 years,

and women account for 65% of cases. About half of patients with untreated temporal arteritis develop blindness due to involvement of the ophthalmic artery and its branches; indeed, the ischemic optic neuropathy induced by giant cell arteritis is the major cause of rapidly developing bilateral blindness in patients over 60 years of age. Because treatment with glucocorticoids is effective in preventing this complication, prompt recognition of this disorder is important.

Typical presenting symptoms include headache, polymyalgia rheumatica (Chap. 317), jaw claudication, fever, and weight loss. Headache is the dominant symptom and often appears in association with malaise and muscle aches. Head pain may be unilateral or bilateral and is located temporally in 50% of patients but may involve any and all aspects of the cranium. Pain usually appears gradually over a few hours before peak intensity is reached; occasionally, it is explosive in onset. The quality of pain is only seldom throbbing; it is almost invariably described as dull and boring with superimposed episodic ice pick–like lancinating pains similar to the sharp pains that appear in migraine. Most patients can recognize that the origin of their head pain is superficial, external to the skull, rather than originating deep within the cranium (the pain site for migraineurs). Scalp tenderness is present, often to a marked degree; brushing the hair or resting the head on a pillow may be impossible because of pain. Headache is usually worse at night and is often aggravated by exposure to cold. Reddened, tender nodules or red streaking of the skin overlying the temporal arteries may be found in patients with headache, as is tenderness of the temporal or, less commonly, the occipital arteries.

The erythrocyte sedimentation rate (ESR) is often, though not always, elevated; a normal ESR does not exclude giant cell arteritis. A temporal artery biopsy and the initiation of prednisone at 80 mg daily for the first 4 to 6 weeks should be instituted when clinical suspicion is high. The prevalence of migraine among the elderly is substantial, considerably higher than that of giant cell arteritis. Migraineurs often report amelioration of their headaches with prednisone, so that one must be cautious about interpreting the therapeutic response.

GLAUCOMA   Glaucoma may present with a prostrating headache associated with nausea and vomiting. The history will usually reveal that the headache started with severe eye pain. On physical examination, the eye is often red with a fixed, moderately dilated pupil. →*A detailed discussion of glaucoma can be found in Chap. 28.*

OTHER CAUSES OF HEADACHE   **Systemic Illness** There is hardly any illness that is never manifested by headache; however, some illnesses are frequently associated with headache. These include infectious mononucleosis, systemic lupus erythematosus, chronic pulmonary failure with hypercapnia (early morning headaches), Hashimoto's thyroiditis, inflammatory bowel disease, many of the illnesses associated with HIV, and the acute blood pressure elevations that occur in pheochromocytoma and in malignant hypertension. The last two examples are the exceptions to the generalization that hypertension per se is a very uncommon cause of headache; diastolic pressures of at least 120 mmHg are requisite for hypertension to cause headache. Persistent headache and fever are often the manifestations of an acute systemic viral infection; if the neck is supple in such a patient, lumbar puncture may be deferred. Some drugs and drug-withdrawal states, e.g., oral contraceptives, ovulation-promoting medications, and glucocorticoid withdrawal, are also associated with headache in some individuals.

Idiopathic Intracranial Hypertension (Pseudotumor Cerebri)
Headache, clinically resembling that of brain tumor, is a common presenting symptom of pseudotumor cerebri, a disorder of raised intracranial pressure probably resulting from impaired cerebrospinal fluid CSF absorption by the arachnoid villi. Transient visual obscurations and papilledema with enlarged blind spots and loss of peripheral visual fields are additional manifestations. Most patients are young, female, and obese. They often have a history of exposure to provoking agents such as vitamin A and glucocorticoids. →*Treatment of idiopathic intracranial hypertension is discussed in Chap. 28.*

Table 15-3   Symptoms of Serious Underlying Causes of Headache

Cause	Symptoms
Meningitis	Nuchal rigidity, headache, photophobia, and prostration; may not be febrile. Lumbar puncture is diagnostic.
Intracranial hemorrhage	Nuchal rigidity and headache; may not have clouded consciousness or seizures. Hemorrhage may not be seen on CT scan. Lumbar puncture shows "bloody tap" that does not clear by the last tube. A fresh hemorrhage may not be xanthochromic.
Brain tumor	May present with prostrating pounding headaches that are associated with nausea and vomiting. Should be suspected in progressively severe new "migraine" that is invariably unilateral.
Temporal arteritis	May present with a unilateral pounding headache. Onset generally in older patients (>50 years) and frequently associated with visual changes. The erythrocyte sedimentation rate is the best screening test and is usually markedly elevated (i.e., >50). Definitive diagnosis can be made by arterial biopsy.
Glaucoma	Usually consists of severe eye pain. May have nausea and vomiting. The eye is usually painful and red. The pupil may be partially dilated.

Cough A male-dominated (4:1) syndrome, cough headache is characterized by transient, severe head pain upon coughing, bending, lifting, sneezing, or stooping. Head pain persists for seconds to a few minutes. Many patients date the origins of the syndrome to a lower respiratory infection accompanied by severe coughing or to strenuous weight-lifting programs. Headache is usually diffuse but is lateralized in about one-third of patients. The incidence of serious intracranial structural anomalies causing this condition is about 25%; the Chiari malformation (Chap. 368) is a common cause. Thus, MRI is indicated for most patients with cough headache. The benign disorder may persist for a few years; it responds dramatically to indomethacin at doses ranging from 50 to 200 mg daily. Approximately half of patients will also show a response to therapeutic lumbar puncture with removal of 40 mL of CSF.

Many patients with migraine note that attacks of headache may be provoked by *sustained* physical exertion, such as during the third mile of a 5-mile run. Such headaches build up over hours, in contrast to cough headache. The term *effort migraine* has been used for this syndrome to avoid the ambiguous term *exertional headache*.

Lumbar Puncture Headache following lumbar puncture (Chap. 356) usually begins within 48 h but may be delayed for up to 12 days. Its incidence is between 10 and 30%. Head pain is dramatically positional; it begins when the patient sits or stands upright; there is relief upon reclining or with abdominal compression. The longer the patient is upright, the longer the latency before head pain subsides. It is worsened by head shaking and jugular vein compression. The pain is usually a dull ache but may be throbbing; its location is occipitofrontal. Nausea and stiff neck often accompany headache, and occasional patients report blurred vision, photophobia, tinnitus, and vertigo. The symptoms resolve over a few days but may on occasion persist for weeks to months.

Loss of CSF volume decreases the brain's supportive cushion, so that when a patient is upright there is probably dilation and tension placed on the brain's anchoring structures, the pain-sensitive dural sinuses, resulting in pain. Intracranial hypotension often occurs, but severe lumbar puncture headache may be present even in patients who have normal CSF pressure.

Treatment with intravenous caffeine sodium benzoate given over a few minutes as a 500-mg dose will promptly terminate headache in 75% of patients; a second dose given in 1 h brings the total success rate to 85%. An epidural blood patch accomplished by injection of 15 mL of autologous whole blood rarely fails for those who do not respond to caffeine. The mechanism for these treatment effects is not straightforward. The blood patch has an *immediate* effect, making it unlikely that sealing off a dural hole with blood clot is its mechanism of action.

Postconcussion Following seemingly trivial head injuries and particularly after rear-end motor vehicle collisions, many patients report varying combinations of headache, dizziness, vertigo, and impaired memory. Anxiety, irritability and difficulty with concentration are other hallmarks of this syndrome. Symptoms may remit after several weeks or persist for months and even years after the injury. Postconcussion headaches may occur whether or not a person was rendered unconscious by head trauma. Typically, the neurologic examination is normal with the exception of the behavioral abnormalities, and CT or MRI studies are unrevealing. Chronic subdural hematoma may on occasion mimic this disorder. Although the cause of postconcussive headache disorder is not known, it should not in general be viewed as a primary psychological disturbance. It often persists long after the settlement of pending lawsuits. The treatment is symptomatic support. Repeated encouragement that the syndrome eventually remits is important.

Coital Headache This is another male-dominated (4:1) syndrome. Attacks occur periorgasmically, are very abrupt in onset, and subside in a few minutes if coitus is interrupted. These are nearly always benign events and usually occur sporadically; if they persist for hours or are accompanied by vomiting, subarachnoid hemorrhage must be excluded (Chap. 361).

PRINCIPAL CLINICAL VARIETIES OF RECURRENT HEADACHE

There is usually little difficulty in diagnosing the serious types of headaches listed above because of the clues provided by the associated symptoms and signs. It is when headache is chronic, recurrent, and unattended by other important signs of disease that the physician faces a challenging and unique medical problem. The following sections describe a variety of headache types, ranging from the most common (e.g., tension-type headache) to rare causes of recurrent headache.

TENSION-TYPE HEADACHE The term *tension-type headache* is still commonly used to describe a chronic head pain syndrome characterized by bilateral tight, bandlike discomfort. Patients may report that the head feels as if it is in a vise or that the posterior neck muscles are tight. The pain typically builds slowly, fluctuates in severity, and may persist more or less continuously for many days. Exertion does not usually worsen the headache. The headache may be episodic or chronic (i.e., present more than 15 days per month). Tension-type headache is common in all age groups, and females tend to predominate. In some patients, anxiety or depression coexist with tension headache.

The pathophysiologic basis of tension-type headache remains unknown. Some investigators believe that periodic tension headache is biologically indistinguishable from migraine, whereas others believe that tension-type headache and migraine are two distinct clinical entities. Abnormalities of cervical and temporal muscle contraction are likely to exist, but the exact nature of the dysfunction has not yet been elucidated.

Relaxation almost always relieves tension-type headaches. Patients should be encouraged to find a means of relaxation, which, for a given individual, could include bed rest, massage, and/or formal biofeedback training. Pharmacologic treatment consists of either simple analgesics and/or muscle relaxants. Ibuprofen and naproxen sodium are useful treatments for most individuals. When simple over-the-counter analgesics such as acetaminophen, aspirin, ibuprofen, and/or other nonsteroidal anti-inflammatory drugs (NSAIDs) alone fail, the addition of butalbital and caffeine (in a combination compound such as Fiorinal, Fioricet) to these analgesics may be effective. A list of commonly used analgesics for tension-type headaches is presented in Table 15-4. For chronic tension-type headache, prophylactic therapy is recommended. Low doses of amitriptyline (10 to 50 mg at bedtime) can provide effective prophylaxis.

MIGRAINE Migraine, the most common cause of vascular headache, afflicts approximately 15% of women and 6% of men. A useful definition of migraine is a benign and recurring syndrome of headache, nausea, vomiting, and/or other symptoms of neurologic dysfunction in varying admixtures (Table 15-5). Migraine can often be recognized by its activators (red wine, menses, hunger, lack of sleep, glare, estrogen, worry, perfumes, let-down periods) and its deactivators (sleep, pregnancy, exhiliration, sumatriptan). A classification of the many subtypes of migraine, as defined by the International Headache Society, is shown in Table 15-1.

Severe headache attacks, regardless of cause, are more likely to be described as throbbing and associated with vomiting and scalp tenderness. Milder headaches tend to be nondescript—tight, bandlike discomfort often involving the entire head—the profile of tension-type headache.

Pathogenesis • *Genetic basis of migraine* Migraine has a definite genetic predisposition. Specific mutations leading to *rare* causes of vascular headache have been identified (Table 15-6). For example, the MELAS syndrome consists of a *m*itochondrial *e*ncephalomyopathy, *l*actic *a*cidosis, and *s*troke-like episodes and is caused by an A → G point mutation in the mitochondrial gene encoding for tRNA$^{\text{Leu(UUR)}}$ at nucleotide position 3243. Episodic migraine-like headaches are another common clinical feature of this syndrome, especially early in the

Table 15-4 Drugs Effective in the Treatment of Tension-Type Headache

Drug	Trade Name	Dosage
NONSTEROIDAL ANTI-INFLAMMATORY AGENTS		
Acetaminophen	Tylenol, generic	650 mg PO q4–6h
Aspirin	Generic	650 mg PO q4–6h
Diclofenac	Cataflam, generic	50–100 mg q4–6h (max 200 mg/d)
Ibuprofen	Advil, Motrin, Nuprin, Generic	400 mg PO q3–4h
Naprosyn sodium	Aleve, Anaprox, generic	220–550 mg bid
COMBINATION ANALGESICS		
Acetaminophen, 325 mg, *plus* butalbital, 50 mg	Phrenelin, generic	1–2 tablets; max 6 per day
Acetaminophen, 650 mg, *plus* butalbital, 50 mg	Phrenelin Forte	1 tablet; max 6 per day
Acetaminophen, 325 mg, *plus* butalbital, 50 mg, *plus* caffeine, 40 mg	Fioricet; Esgic, generic	1–2 tablets; max 6 per day
Acetaminophen, 500 mg, *plus* butalbital, 50 mg, *plus* caffeine, 40 mg	Esgicplus	1–2 tablets; max 6 per day
Aspirin, 325 mg, *plus* butalbital, 50 mg, *plus* caffeine, 40 mg	Fiorinal	1–2 tablets; max 6 per day
Aspirin, 650 mg, *plus* butalbital, 50 mg	Axotal	1 tablet q4h; max 6 per day
PROPHYLACTIC MEDICATIONS		
Amitriptyline	Elavil, generic	10–50 mg at bedtime
Doxepin	Sinequan, generic	10–75 mg at bedtime
Nortriptyline	Pamelor, generic	25–75 mg at bedtime

course of the disease. The genetic pattern of mitochondrial disorders is unique, since only mothers transmit mitochondrial DNA. Thus, all children of mothers with MELAS syndrome are affected with the disorder.

Familial hemiplegic migraine (FHM) is characterized by episodes of recurrent hemiparesis or hemiplegia during the aura phase of a migraine headache. Other associated symptoms may include hemianesthesia or paresthesia; hemianopic visual field disturbances; dysphasia; and variable degrees of drowsiness, confusion, and/or coma. In severe attacks, these symptoms can be quite prolonged and persist for days or weeks, but characteristically they last for only 30 to 60 min and are followed by a unilateral throbbing headache.

Approximately 50% of cases of FHM appear to be caused by mutations within the CACNL1A4 gene on chromosome 19, which encodes a P/Q type calcium channel subunit expressed only in the central nervous system. The gene is very large (>300 kb in length) and consists of 47 exons. Four distinct point mutations have been identified within the gene (in five different families) that cosegregate with the clinical diagnosis of FHM. Analysis of haplotypes in the two families with the same mutation suggest that each mutation arose independently

Table 15-5 Symptoms Accompanying Severe Migraine Attacks in a Group of 500 Patients

Symptom	Patients Affected, %
Nausea	87
Photophobia	82
Lightheadedness	72
Scalp tenderness	65
Vomiting	56
Visual disturbances	36
Photopsia	26
Fortification spectra	10
Paresthesias	33
Vertigo	33
Alteration of consciousness	18
Syncope	10
Seizure	4
Confusional state	4
Diarrhea	16

SOURCE: From Raskin, 1988.

rather than representing a founder effect. Thus, certain subtypes of FHM are caused by mutations in the CACNL1A4 gene. The function of the CACNL1A4 gene remains unknown, but it is likely to play a role in calcium-induced neurotransmitter release and/or contraction of smooth muscle. Different mutations within this gene are the cause of another neurogenetic disorder, episodic ataxia type 2 (Chap. 364).

In a genetic association study, a *Nco*I polymorphism in the gene encoding the D_2 dopamine receptor (DRD2) was overrepresented in a population of patients with migraine with aura compared to a control group of nonmigraineurs, suggesting that susceptibility to migraine with aura is modified by certain DRD2 alleles. In a Sardinian population, an association between different DRD2 alleles and migraine has also been demonstrated. Therefore, these initial studies suggest that variations in dopamine receptor regulation and/or function may alter susceptibility to migraine since molecular variations within the DRD2 gene have been associated with variations in dopaminergic function. However, since not all individuals with certain DRD2 genotypes suffer from migraine with aura, additional genes or factors must also be involved. Migraine is likely to be a complex disorder with polygenic inheritance and a strong environmental component.

The vascular theory of migraine   It was widely held for many years that the headache phase of migrainous attacks was caused by extracranial vasodilatation and that the neurologic symptoms were produced by intracranial vasoconstriction (i.e., the "vascular" hypothesis of migraine). Regional cerebral blood flow studies have shown that in patients with classic migraine there is, during attacks, a modest cortical hypoperfusion that begins in the visual cortex and spreads forward at a rate of 2 to 3 mm/min. The decrease in blood flow averages 25 to 30% (insufficient to explain symptoms on the basis of ischemia) and progresses anteriorly in a wavelike fashion independent of the topography of cerebral arteries. The wave of hypoperfusion persists for 4 to 6 h, appears to follow the convolutions of the cortex, and does not cross the central or lateral sulcus, progressing to the frontal lobe via the insula. Perfusion of subcortical structures is normal. Contralateral neurologic symptoms appear during temporoparietal hypoperfusion; at times, hypoperfusion persists in these regions after symptoms cease. More often, frontal spread continues as the headache phase begins. A few patients with classic migraine show no flow abnormalities; an occasional patient has developed focal ischemia sufficient to cause symptoms. However, focal ischemia does not appear to be *necessary* for focal symptoms to occur.

The ability of these changes to induce the symptoms of migraine has been questioned. Specifically, the decrease in blood flow that is observed does not appear to be significant enough to cause focal neurologic symptoms. Second, the increase in blood flow per se is not painful, and vasodilatation alone cannot account for the local edema and focal tenderness often observed in migraineurs. Moreover, in migraine without aura, no flow abnormalities are usually seen. Thus, it is unlikely that simple vasoconstriction and vasodilatation are the fundamental pathophysiologic abnormalities in migraine. However, it is clear that cerebral blood flow is altered during certain migraine attacks, and these changes may explain some, but clearly not all, of the clinical syndrome of migraine.

The neuronal theory of migraine   In 1941, the psychologist KS Lashley charted his own *fortification spectrum*, which is a migraine aura characterized by a slowly enlarging visual scotoma with luminous edges (see below). He was able to estimate that the evolution of his own scotoma proceeded across the occipital cortex at a rate of 3 mm/

min. He speculated that a wavefront of intense excitation followed by a wave of complete inhibition of activity were propagated across the visual cortex. In 1944, the phenomenon that has come to be known as *spreading depression* was described by the Brazilian physiologist Leão in the cerebral cortex of laboratory animals. It is a slowly moving (2 to 3 mm/min), potassium-liberating depression of cortical activity, preceded by a wavefront of increased metabolic activity that can be produced by a variety of experimental stimuli, including hypoxia, mechanical trauma, and the topical application of potassium. These observations suggest that neuronal abnormalities, most likely initiated in the brainstem, could be the cause of a migraine attack. More recently, both cortical and brainstem changes have been observed in positron emission tomography (PET) scan studies of migraine. Thus, the existence of a specific "brainstem generator" for migraine remains an intriguing possibility that might represent the pathophysiologic basis of migraine.

The trigeminovascular system in migraine Activation of cells in the trigeminal nucleus caudalis in the medulla (a pain-processing center for the head and face region) results in the release of vasoactive neuropeptides, including substance P and calcitonin gene–related peptide (CGRP), at vascular terminations of the trigeminal nerve. These peptide neurotransmitters have been proposed to induce a sterile inflammation that activates trigeminal nociceptive afferents originating on the vessel wall, further contributing to the production of pain. This mechanism also provides a potential mechanism for the soft tissue swelling and tenderness of blood vessels that attend migraine attacks. However, numerous pharmacologic agents that are effective in preventing or reducing inflammation in this animal model (e.g., selective 5-HT$_{1D}$ agonists, NK-1 antagonists, endothelin antagonists) have failed to demonstrate any clinical efficacy in recent migraine trials.

5-Hydroxytryptamine in migraine Pharmacologic and other data point to the involvement of the neurotransmitter 5-hydroxytryptamine (5-HT; also know as serotonin) in migraine. Approximately 40 years ago, methysergide was found to antagonize certain peripheral actions of 5-HT and was introduced as the first drug capable of preventing migraine attacks. Subsequently, it was found that platelet levels of 5-HT fall consistently at the onset of headache and that drugs that cause 5-HT to be released may trigger migrainous episodes. Such changes in circulating 5-HT levels proved to be pharmacologically trivial, however, and interest in the humoral role of 5-HT in migraine declined.

More recently, interest in the role of 5-HT in migraine has been renewed due to the introduction of the triptan class of antimigraine drugs. The triptans are designed to stimulate selectively a particular subpopulation of 5-HT receptors. Molecular cloning studies have demonstrated that at least 14 specific 5-HT receptors exist in humans. The triptans (e.g., naratriptan, rizatriptan, sumatriptan, and zolmitriptan) are potent agonists of 5-HT$_{1B}$, 5-HT$_{1D}$, and 5-HT$_{1F}$ receptors and are less potent at 5-HT$_{1A}$ and 5-HT$_{1E}$ receptors. A growing body of data indicates that the antimigraine efficacy of the triptans relates to their ability to stimulate 5-HT$_{1B}$ receptors, which are located both on blood vessels and nerve terminals. Selective 5-HT$_{1D}$ receptor agonists have, thus far, failed to demonstrate clinical efficacy in migraine. Triptans that are weak 5-HT$_{1F}$ agonists are also effective in migraine; however, only 5-HT$_{1B}$ efficacy is currently thought to be essential for antimigraine efficacy.

Physiologically, electrical stimulation near dorsal raphe neurons can result in migraine-like headaches. Blood flow in the pons and midbrain increases focally during migraine headache episodes; this alteration probably results from increased activity of cells in the dorsal raphe and locus caeruleus. There are projections from the dorsal raphe that terminate on cerebral arteries and alter cerebral blood flow. There are also major projections from the dorsal raphe to important visual centers, including the lateral geniculate body, superior colliculus, ret-

Table 15-6   Status of Migraine Genetics

Gene (Locus)	Function of Gene	Clinical Syndrome	Comment
tRNA$^{Leu(UUR)}$ (mitochondrial)	Unknown	MELAS syndrome	Extremely rare syndrome
CACNL1A4 (19p13)	P/Q calcium channel regulating neurotransmitter release	Familial hemiplegic migraine (FHM)	Mutations account for approximately 50% of FHM cases
DRD2 (11q23)	G protein–coupled D$_2$ receptor for dopamine	Migraine	Positive association reported in two independent laboratories

ina, and visual cortex. These various serotonergic projections may represent the neural substrate for the circulatory and visual characteristics of migraine. The dorsal raphe cells stop firing during deep sleep, and sleep is known to ameliorate migraine; the antimigraine prophylactic drugs also inhibit activity of the dorsal raphe cells through a direct or indirect agonist effect.

Recent PET scan studies have demonstrated that midbrain structures near the dorsal raphe are differentially activated during a migraine attack. In one study of acute migraine, an injection of sumatriptan relieved the headache, but did not alter the brainstem changes noted on the PET scan. These data suggest that a "brainstem generator" may be the cause of migraine and that certain antimigraine medications may not interfere with the underlying pathologic process in migraine.

Dopamine in migraine A growing body of biologic, pharmacologic, and genetic data support a role for dopamine in the pathophysiology of certain subtypes of migraine. Most migraine symptoms can be induced by dopaminergic stimulation. Moreover, there is dopamine receptor hypersensitivity in migraineurs, as demonstrated by the induction of yawning, nausea, vomiting, hypotension, and other symptoms of a migraine attack by dopaminergic agonists at doses that do not affect nonmigraineurs. Conversely, dopamine receptor antagonists are effective therapeutic agents in migraine, especially when given parenterally or concurrently with other antimigraine agents. As noted above, recent genetic data also suggest that molecular variations within dopamine receptor genes play a modifying role in the pathophysiology of migraine with aura. Therefore, modulation of dopaminergic neurotransmission should be considered in the therapeutic management of migraine.

The sympathetic nervous system in migraine Biochemical changes occur within the sympathetic nervous system (SNS) of migraineurs before, during, and between migraine attacks. Factors that activate the SNS are all trigger factors for migraine. Specific examples include environmental changes (e.g., stress, sleep patterns, hormonal shifts, hypoglycemia) and agents that cause release and a secondary depletion of peripheral catecholamines [e.g., tyramine, phenylethylamine, fenfluramine, m-chlorophenylpiperazine (mCPP) and reserpine]. By contrast, effective therapeutic approaches to migraine share an ability to mimic and/or enhance the effects of norepinephrine in the peripheral SNS. For example, norepinephrine itself, sympathomimetics (e.g., isometheptene), monoamine oxidase inhibitors (MAOIs) and reuptake blockers alleviate migraine. Dopamine antagonists, prostaglandin synthesis inhibitors, and adenosine antagonists are pharmacologic agents effective in the acute treatment of migraine. These drugs block the negative feedback inhibition or norepinephrine release induced by endogenous dopamine, prostaglandins, and adenosine. Therefore, migraine susceptibility may relate to genetically based variations in the ability to maintain adequate concentrations of certain neurotransmitters within postganglionic sympathetic nerve terminals. This hypothesis has been called the *empty neuron theory* of migraine.

Clinical Features • *Migraine without aura (common migraine)* In this syndrome no focal neurologic disturbance precedes the recurrent headaches. Migraine without aura is by far the more frequent type of vascular headache. The International Headache Society criteria for migraine include moderate to severe head pain, pulsating quality, unilateral location, aggravation by walking stairs or similar routine activity, attendant nausea and/or vomiting, photophobia and phonophobia, and multiple attacks, each lasting 4 to 72 h.

Migraine with aura (classic migraine)   In this syndrome headache is associated with characteristic premonitory sensory, motor, or visual symptoms. Focal neurologic disturbances are more common during headache attacks than as prodromal symptoms. Focal neurologic disturbances without headache or vomiting have come to be known as *migraine equivalents* or *migraine accompaniments* and appear to occur more commonly in patients between the ages of 40 and 70 years. The term *complicated migraine* has generally been used to describe migraine with dramatic transient focal neurologic features or a migraine attack that leaves a persisting residual neurologic deficit.

The most common premonitory symptoms reported by migraineurs are visual, arising from dysfunction of occipital lobe neurons. Scotomas and/or hallucinations occur in about one-third of migraineurs and usually appear in the central portions of the visual fields. A highly characteristic syndrome occurs in about 10% of patients; it usually begins as a small paracentral scotoma, which slowly expands into a "C" shape. Luminous angles appear at the enlarging outer edge, becoming colored as the scintillating scotoma expands and moves toward the periphery of the involved half of the visual field, eventually disappearing over the horizon of peripheral vision. The entire process lasts 20 to 25 min. This phenomenon is pathognomonic for migraine, and has never been described in association with a cerebral structural anomaly. It is commonly referred to as a *fortification spectrum* because the serrated edges of the hallucinated "C" seemed to resemble a "fortified town with bastions all round it"; "spectrum" is used in the sense of an apparition or specter.

Basilar migraine   Symptoms referable to a disturbance in brainstem function, such as vertigo, dysarthria, or diplopia, occur as the only neurologic symptoms of the attack in about 25% of patients. A dramatic form of basilar migraine (Bickerstaff's migraine) occurs primarily in adolescent females. Episodes begin with total blindness accompanied or followed by admixtures of vertigo, ataxia, dysarthria, tinnitus, and distal and perioral paresthesia. In about one-quarter of patients, a confusional state supervenes. The neurologic symptoms usually persist for 20 to 30 min and are generally followed by a throbbing occipital headache. This basilar migraine syndrome is now known also to occur in children and in adults over age 50. An altered sensorium may persist for as long as 5 days and may take the form of confusional states superficially resembling psychotic reactions. Full recovery after the episode is the rule.

Carotidynia   The carotidynia syndrome, sometimes called *lower-half headache* or *facial migraine*, is most common among older patients, with the incidence peaking in the fourth through sixth decades. Pain is usually located at the jaw or neck, although sometimes periorbital or maxillary pain occurs; it may be continuous, deep, dull, and aching, and it becomes pounding or throbbing episodically. There are often superimposed sharp, ice pick–like jabs. Attacks occur one to several times per week, each lasting several minutes to hours. Tenderness and prominent pulsations of the cervical carotid artery and soft tissue swelling overlying the carotid are usually present ipsilateral to the pain; many patients also report throbbing ipsilateral headache concurrent with carotidynia attacks as well as between attacks. Dental trauma is a common precipitant of this syndrome. Carotid artery involvement also appears to be common in the more traditional forms of migraine; over 50% of patients with frequent migraine attacks are found to have carotid tenderness at several points on the side most often involved during hemicranial migraine attacks.

℞ TREATMENT

Nonpharmacologic Approaches for All Migraineurs   Migraine can often be managed to some degree by a variety of nonpharmacologic approaches (Table 15-7). The measures that apply to a given individual should be used routinely since they provide a simple, cost-effective approach to migraine management. Patients with mi-

Table 15-7   Nonpharmacologic Approaches to Migraine

Identify and then avoid trigger factors such as:
  Alcohol (e.g., red wine)
  Foods (e.g., chocolate, certain cheeses, monosodium glutamate, nitrate-containing foods)
  Hunger (avoid missing meals)
  Irregular sleep patterns (both lack of sleep and excessive sleep)
  Organic odors
  Sustained exertion
  Acute changes in stress levels
  Miscellaneous (glare, flashing lights)
Attempt to manage environmental shifts
  Time zone shifts
  High altitude
  Barometric pressure changes
  Weather changes
Assess menstrual cycle relationship

graine do not encounter more stress than headache-free individuals; overresponsiveness to stress appears to be the issue. Since the stresses of everyday living cannot be eliminated, lessening one's response to stress by various techniques is helpful for many patients. These include yoga, transcendental meditation, hypnosis, and conditioning techniques such as biofeedback. For most patients, this approach is, at best, an adjunct to pharmacotherapy. Avoidance of migraine trigger factors may also provide significant prophylactic benefits (Table 15-7). Unfortunately, these measures are unlikely to prevent all migraine attacks. When these measures fail to prevent an attack, then pharmacologic approaches are needed to abort an attack.

Pharmacologic Treatment of Acute Migraine   The mainstay of pharmacologic therapy is the judicious use of one or more of the many drugs that are effective in migraine. The selection of the optimal regimen for a given patient depends on a number of factors, the most important of which is the severity of the attack (Table 15-8). Mild migraine attacks can usually be managed by oral agents; the average efficacy rate is 50–70%. Severe migraine attacks may require parenteral therapy. Most drugs effective in the treatment of migraine are members of one of three major pharmacologic classes: anti-inflammatory agents, 5-HT1 agonists, and dopamine antagonists.

Table 15-9 lists specific drugs effective in migraine. In general, an adequate dose of whichever agent is chosen should be used as soon as possible after the onset of an attack. If additional medication is required within 60 min because symptoms return or have not abated, the initial dose should be increased for subsequent attacks. Migraine therapy must be individualized for each patient; a standard approach for all patients is not possible. A therapeutic regimen may need to be constantly refined and personalized until one is identified that provides

Table 15-8   A Staged Approach to Migraine Pharmacotherapy

Stage	Diagnosis	Therapies
Mild migraine	Occasional throbbing headaches	NSAIDs
	No major impairment of functioning	Combination analgesics
		Oral 5-HT$_1$ agonists
Moderate migraine	Moderate or severe headaches	Oral, nasal, or SC 5-HT$_1$ agonists
	Nausea common	Oral dopamine antagonists
	Some impairment of functioning	
Severe migraine	Severe headaches >3 times per month	SC, IM, or IV 5-HT$_1$ agonists
	Significant functional impairment	IM or IV dopamine antagonists
	Marked nausea and/or vomiting	Prophylactic medications

NOTE: NSAIDs, nonsteroidal anti-inflammatory drugs; 5-HT, 5-hydroxytryptamine.

Table 15-9 Drugs Effective in Acute Treatment of Migraine

Drug	Trade Name	Dosage
NSAIDs		
Acetaminophen, aspirin, caffeine	Excedrin Migraine	Two tablets or caplets q6h (max 8 per day)
5-HT₁ AGONISTS		
Oral		
Ergotamine	Ergomar	One 2-mg sublingual tablet at onset and q1/2h (max 3 per day, 5 per week)
Ergotamine 1 mg, caffeine 100 mg	Ercaf, Wigraine	One or two tablets at onset, then one tablet q1/2h (max 6 per day, 10 per week)
Naratriptan	Amerge	2.5-mg tablet at onset; may repeat once after 4 h
Rizatriptan	Maxalt Maxalt-MLT	5- to 10-mg tablet at onset; may repeat after 2 h (max 30 mg/d)
Sumatriptan	Imitrex	50- to 100-mg tablet at onset; may repeat after 2 h (max 200 mg/d)
Zolmitriptan	Zomig Zomig Rapimelt	2.5-mg tablet at onset; may repeat after 2 h (max 10 mg/d)
Nasal		
Dihydroergotamine	Migranal Nasal Spray	Prior to nasal spray, the pump must be primed 4 times; one spray (0.5 mg) per nostril is administered followed by, in 15 min, by a second spray per nostril
Sumatriptan	Imitrex Nasal Spray	5- to 20-mg spray as 4 sprays of 5 mg per nostril or a single 20-mg spray (may repeat once after 2 h, not to exceed a dose of 40 mg/d)
Parenteral		
Dihydroergotamine	DHE-45	1 mg IV, IM, or SC at onset and q1h (max 3 mg/d, 6 mg per week)
Sumatriptan	Imitrex Injection	6 mg SC at onset (may repeat once after 1 h for max of two doses in 24 h)
DOPAMINE ANTAGONISTS		
Oral		
Metoclopramide	Reglan,ᵃ genericᵃ	5–10 mg/d
Prochlorperazine	Compazine,ᵃ genericᵃ	1–25 mg/d
Parenteral		
Chlorpromazine	Genericᵃ	0.1 mg/kg IV at 2 mg/min; max 35 mg/d
Metoclopramide	Reglan,ᵃ generic	10 mg IV
Prochlorperazine	Compazine,ᵃ genericᵃ	10 mg IV
OTHER		
Oral		
Acetaminophen, 325 mg, *plus* dichloralphenazone, 100 mg, *plus* isometheptene, 65 mg	Midrin, Duradrin, generic	Two capsules at onset followed by 1 capsule q1h (max 5 capsules)
Nasal		
Butorphanol	Stadolᵃ	1 mg (1 spray in 1 nostril), may repeat if necessary in 1–2 h
Parenteral		
Narcotics	Genericᵃ	Multiple preparations and dosages; see Table 12-1.

ᵃ Not specifically indicated by the U.S. Food and Drug Administration for migraine.
NOTE: NSAIDs, nonsteroidal anti-inflammatory drugs; 5-HT, 5-hydroxytryptamine.

the patient with rapid, complete, and consistent relief with minimal side effects.

Nonsteroidal anti-inflammatory agents Both the severity and duration of a migraine attack can be reduced significantly by anti-inflammatory agents. Indeed, many undiagnosed migraineurs are self-treated with nonprescription anti-inflammatory agents (Table 15-4). A general consensus is that NSAIDs are most effective when taken early in the migraine attack. However, the effectiveness of anti-inflammatory agents in migraine is usually less than optimal in moderate or severe migraine attacks. The combination of acetaminophen, aspirin, and caffeine (Excedrin Migraine) has been approved for use by the U.S. Food and Drug Administration (FDA) for the treatment of mild to moderate migraine. The combination of aspirin and metoclopramide has been show to be equivalent to a single dose of sumatriptan. Major side effects of NSAIDs include dyspepsia and gastrointestinal irritation.

5-HT₁ agonists • *ORAL* Stimulation of 5-HT₁ receptors can stop an acute migraine attack. Ergotamine and dihydroergotamine are nonselective receptor agonists, while the series of drugs known as triptans are selective 5-HT₁ receptor agonists. A variety of triptans (e.g., naratriptan, rizatriptan, sumatriptan, zolmitriptan) are now available for the treatment of migraine (Table 15-9).

Each of the triptan class of drugs has similar pharmacologic properties, but varies slightly in terms of clinical efficacy. Rizatriptan appears to be the fastest acting and most efficacious of the triptans currently available in the United States. Sumatriptan and zolmitriptan have similar rates of efficacy as well as time to onset, whereas naratriptan is the slowest acting and the least efficacious. Clinical efficacy appears to be related more to the t_{max} (time to peak plasma level) than to the potency, half-life, or bioavailability (Table 15-10). This observation is in keeping with a significant body of data indicating that faster-acting analgesics are more efficacious than slower-acting agents.

Unfortunately, monotherapy with a selective oral 5-HT₁ agonist does not result in rapid, consistent, and complete relief of migraine in all patients. Triptans are not effective in migraine with aura unless given after the aura is completed and the headache initiated. Side effects, although often mild and transient, occur in up to 89% of patients. Moreover, 5-HT₁ agonists are contraindicated in individuals with a history of cardiovascular disease. Recurrence of headache is a major limitation of triptan use, and occurs at least occasionally in 40 to 78% of patients.

Ergotamine preparations offer a nonselective means of stimulating 5-HT₁ receptors. A nonnauseating dose of ergotamine should be sought since a dose that provokes nausea is too high and may intensify head pain. Except for a sublingual formulation of ergotamine (Ergomar), oral formulations of ergotamine also contain 100 mg caffeine (theoretically to enhance ergotamine absorption and possibly to add additional vasoconstrictor activity). The average oral ergotamine dose for a migraine attack is 2 mg. Since the clinical studies demonstrating the efficacy of ergotamine in migraine predated the clinical trial methodologies used with the triptans, it is difficult to assess the clinical efficacy of ergotamine versus the triptans. In general, ergotamine appears to have a much higher incidence of nausea than triptans, but less headache recurrence.

NASAL The fastest acting nonparenteral antimigraine therapies that can be self-administered include nasal formulations of dihydroer-

Table 15-10 Comparative Pharmacology of Oral Triptansᵃ

Drug and Dose	t_{max}, h	$t_{1/2}$, h	Oral Bioavailability, %	Clinical Efficacy at 2 h, %
Rizatriptan, 10 mg	1–2	2–3	45	71
Zolmitriptan, 2.5 mg	2	2.5–3	44	65
Sumatriptan, 50 mg	2–3	2	14	61
Naratriptan, 2.5 mg	2–4	5–6	68	45

ᵃ Data adapted from package inserts approved by the U.S. Food and Drug Administration.

gotamine (Migranal) or sumatriptan (Imitrex Nasal). The nasal sprays result in substantial blood levels within 30 to 60 min. However, the nasal formulations suffer from inconsistent dosing, poor taste, and variable efficacy. Although in theory the nasal sprays might provide faster and more effective relief of a migraine attack than oral formulations, their reported efficacy is only approximately 50 to 60%.

PARENTERAL   Parenteral administration of drugs such as dihydroergotamine (DHE-45 Injectable) and sumatriptan (Imitrex SC) is approved by the FDA for the rapid relief of a migraine attack. Peak plasma levels of dihydroergotamine are achieved 3 min after intravenous dosing, 30 min after intramuscular dosing, and 45 min after subcutaneous dosing. If an attack has not already peaked, subcutaneous or intramuscular administration of 1 mg dihydroergotamine suffices for about 80 to 90% of patients. Sumatriptan, 6 mg subcutaneously is effective in approximately 70 to 80% of patients.

Dopamine antagonists • ORAL   Oral dopamine antagonists should be considered as adjunctive therapy in migraine. Drug absorption is impaired during migrainous attacks because of reduced gastrointestinal motility. Delayed absorption occurs in the absence of nausea and is related to the severity of the attack and not its duration. Therefore, when oral NSAIDs and/or triptan agents fail, the addition of a dopamine antagonist such as metoclopramide, 10 mg, should be considered to enhance gastric absorption. In addition, dopamine antagonists decrease nausea/vomiting and restore normal gastric motility.

PARENTERAL   Parenteral dopamine antagonists (e.g., chlorpromazine, prochlorperazine, metoclopramide) can also provide significant acute relief of migraine; they can be used in combination with parenteral 5-HT$_1$ agonists. A common intravenous protocol used for the treatment of severe migraine is the administration over 2 min of a mixture of 5 mg of prochlorperazine and 0.5 mg of dihydroergotamine.

Other medications for acute migraine • ORAL   The combination of acetaminophen, dichloralphenazone, and isometheptene (i.e., Midrin, Duradrin, generic), one to two capsules, has been classified by the FDA as "possibly" effective in the treatment of migraine. Since the clinical studies demonstrating the efficacy of this combination analgesic in migraine predated the clinical trial methodologies used with the triptans, it is difficult to assess the clinical efficacy of this sympathomimetic compound in comparison to other agents.

NASAL   A nasal preparation of butorphanol is available for the treatment of acute pain. As with all narcotics, the use of nasal butorphanol should be limited to a select group of migraineurs, as described below.

PARENTERAL   Narcotics are effective in the acute treatment of migraine. For example, intravenous meperidene (Demerol), 50 to 100 mg, is given frequently in the emergency room. This regimen "works" in the sense that the pain of migraine is eliminated. However, this regimen is clearly suboptimal in patients with recurrent headache for two major reasons. First, narcotics do not treat the underlying headache mechanism; rather, they act at the thalamic level to alter pain sensation. Second, the recurrent use of narcotics can lead to significant problems. In patients taking oral narcotics such as oxycodone (Percodan) or hydrocodone (Vicoden), narcotic addiction can greatly confuse the treatment of migraine. The headache that results from narcotic craving and/or withdrawal can be difficult to distinguish from chronic migraine. Therefore, it is recommended that narcotic use in migraine be limited to patients with severe, but infrequent, headaches that are unresponsive to other pharmacologic approaches.

Prophylactic Treatment of Migraine   A substantial number of drugs are now available that have the capacity to stabilize migraine (Table 15-11). The decision of whether to use this approach depends on the frequency of attacks and on how well acute treatment is working. The occurrence of at least three attacks per month could be an indication for this approach. Drugs must be taken daily and there is usually a lag of at least 2 to 6 weeks before an effect is seen. The

Table 15-11   Drugs Effective in the Prophylactic Treatment of Migraine

Drug	Trade Name	Dosage
β-Adrenergic agents		
Propranolol	Inderal	80–320 mg qd
	Inderal LA	
Timolol	Blocadren	20–60 mg qd
Anticonvulsants		
Sodium valproate	Depakote	250 mg bid (max 1000 mg/d)
Tricyclic antidepressants		
Amitriptyline	Elavil,[a] generic	10–50 mg qhs
Nortriptyline	Pamelor,[a] generic	25–75 mg qhs
Monoamine oxidase inhibitors		
Phenelzine	Nardil[a]	15 mg tid
Isocarboxazid	Marplan[a]	10 mg qid
Serotonoergic drugs		
Methysergide	Sansert	4–8 mg qd
Cyproheptadine	Periactin[a]	4–16 mg qd
Other		
Verapamil	Calan[a]	40–240 mg qd
	Isoptin[a]	

[a] Not specifically indicated for migraine by the U.S. Food and Drug Administration.

drugs that have been approved by the FDA for the prophylactic treatment of migraine include propranolol, timolol, sodium valproate, and methysergide. In addition, a number of other drugs appear to display prophylactic efficacy. This group of drugs includes amitriptyline, nortriptyline, verapamil, phenelzine, isocarbazid, and cyproheptadine. Phenelzine and methysergide are usually reserved for recalcitrant cases because of their serious potential side effects. Phenelzine is an MAOI; therefore, tyramine-containing foods, decongestants, and meperidine are contraindicated. Methysergide may cause retroperitoneal or cardiac valvular fibrosis when it is used for more than 8 months, thus monitoring is required for patients using this drug; the risk of the fibrotic complication is about 1:1500 and is likely to reverse after the drug is stopped.

The probability of success with any one of the antimigraine drugs is 50 to 75%; thus, if one drug is assessed each month, there is a good chance that effective stabilization will be achieved within a few months. Many patients are managed adequately with low-dose amitriptyline, propranolol, or valproate. If these agents fail or lead to unacceptable side effects, then methysergide or phenelzine can be used. Once effective stabilization is achieved, the drug is continued for 5 to 6 months and then slowly tapered to assess the continued need. Many patients are able to discontinue medication and experience fewer and milder attacks for long periods, suggesting that these drugs may alter the natural history of migraine.

CLUSTER HEADACHE   A variety of names have been used for this condition, including *Raeder's syndrome*, *histamine cephalalgia*, and *sphenopalatine neuralgia*. *Cluster headache* is a distinctive and treatable vascular headache syndrome. The episodic type is most common and is characterized by one to three short-lived attacks of periorbital pain per day over a 4- to 8-week period, followed by a pain-free interval that averages 1 year. The chronic form, which may begin de novo or several years after an episodic pattern has become established, is characterized by the absence of sustained periods of remission. Each type may transform into the other. Men are affected seven to eight times more often than women; hereditary factors are usually absent. Although the onset is generally between ages 20 and 50, it may occur as early as the first decade of life. Propranolol and amitriptyline are largely ineffective. Lithium is beneficial for cluster headache and ineffective in migraine. The cluster syndrome is thus clinically, genetically, and therapeutically different from migraine. Nevertheless, mixed features of the two disorders are occasionally present, suggesting some common elements to their pathogenesis.

Clinical Features   Periorbital or, less commonly, temporal pain begins without warning and reaches a crescendo within 5 min. It is often excruciating in intensity and is deep, nonfluctuating, and explosive in quality; only rarely is it pulsatile. Pain is strictly unilateral and usually affects the same side in subsequent months. Attacks last from 30 min to 2 h; there are often associated symptoms of homolateral lacrimation, reddening of the eye, nasal stuffiness, lid ptosis, and nausea. Alcohol provokes attacks in about 70% of patients but ceases to be provocative when the bout remits; this on-off vulnerability to alcohol is pathognomonic of cluster headache. Only rarely do foods or emotional factors precipitate pain, in contrast to migraine.

There is a striking periodicity of attacks in at least 85% of patients. At least one of the daily attacks of pain recurs at about the same hour each day for the duration of a cluster bout. Onset is nocturnal in about 50% of the cases, and then the pain usually awakens the patient within 2 h of falling asleep.

Pathogenesis   No consistent cerebral blood flow changes accompany attacks of pain. Perhaps the strongest evidence for a central mechanism is the periodicity of attacks; the existence of a central mechanism is also suggested by the observation that autonomic symptoms that accompany the pain are bilateral and are more severe on the painful side. The hypothalamus may be the site of activation in this disorder. The posterior hypothalamus contains cells that regulate autonomic functions, and the anterior hypothalamus contains cells (in the suprachiasmatic nuclei) that constitute the principal circadian pacemaker in mammals. Activation of both is necessary to explain the symptoms of cluster headache. The pacemaker is modulated via serotonergic dorsal raphe projections. It can be concluded tentatively that both migraine and cluster headache result from abnormal serotonergic neurotransmission, albeit at different loci.

℞   **TREATMENT**   The most satisfactory treatment is the administration of drugs to prevent cluster attacks until the bout is over. Effective prophylactic drugs are prednisone, lithium, methysergide, ergotamine, sodium valproate, and verapamil. Lithium (600 to 900 mg daily) appears to be particularly useful for the chronic form of the disorder. A 10-day course of prednisone, beginning at 60 mg daily for 7 days followed by a rapid taper, may interrupt the pain bout for many patients. When ergotamine is used, it is most effective when given 1 to 2 h before an expected attack. Patients must be educated regarding the early symptoms of ergotism when ergotamine is used daily; a weekly limit of 14 mg should be adhered to.

For the attacks themselves, oxygen inhalation (9 L/min via a loose mask) is the most effective modality; 15 min of inhalation of 100% oxygen is often necessary. Sumatriptan, 6 mg subcutaneously, will usually shorten an attack to 10 to 15 min.

BIBLIOGRAPHY

BRESLAU N: Psychiatric comorbidity in migraine. Cephalalgia 18(Suppl 22): 56, 1998

CAO Y et al: Functional MRI-BOLD of visually triggered headache in patients with migraine. Arch Neurol 56:548, 1999

COUCH JR: Headache to worry about. Med Clin North Am 77:141, 1993

EDLOW JA, CAPLAN LR: Avoiding pitfalls in the diagnosis of subarachnoid hemorrhage. N Engl J Med 342:29, 2000

FRISHBERG BM: The utility of neuroimaging in the evaluation of headache in patients with normal examination. Neurology 44:1191, 1994

GERVIL et al: The relative role of genetic and environmental factors in migraine without aura. Neurology 53:995, 1999

GOADSBY PJ: Serotonin 5-HT 1B/1D receptor agonists in migraine. CNS Drugs 10:271, 1998

LANCE JW, GOADSBY PJ: *Mechanism and Management of Headache*, 6th ed. London, Butterworth Scientific, 1998

LIPTON RB: Pharmacologic profile and clinical efficacy of rizatriptan. Headache 39 (Suppl 1):S9, 1999

———— et al: Efficacy and safety of acetaminophen, aspirin and caffeine in alleviating migraine pain. Three double-blind, randomized, placebo-controlled trials. Arch Neurol 55:210, 1998

MAY A et al: Hypothalamic activation in cluster headache attacks. Lancet 352:275, 1998

———— et al: Correlation between structural and functional changes in brain in an idiopathic headache syndrome. Nature Med 5:836, 1999

MOSKOWITZ MA, COUTRER FM: Attacking migraine headache from beginning to end. Neurology 49:1193, 1997

OLESEN C et al: Pregnancy outcome following prescription for sumatriptan. Headache 40: 20, 2000

OLESEN J: Headache Classification Committee of the International Headache Society. Classification and diagnostic criteria for headache disorders, cranial neuralgia, and facial pain. Cephalalgia 8(Suppl 7): 1, 1988

OPHOFF RA et al: Familial hemiplegic migraine and episodic ataxia type-2 are caused by mutations in the Ca²⁺ channel gene CACNL1A4. Cell 87:543, 1996

PASCUAL J et al: Cough, exertional, and sexual headaches: An analysis of 72 benign and symptomatic cases. Neurology 46:1520, 1996

PEROUTKA SJ: Dopamine and migraine. Neurology 49:650, 1997

———— et al: Clinical susceptibility to migraine with aura is modified by dopamine D2 receptor (DRD2) NcoI alleles. Neurology 49:201, 1997

RASKIN NH: *Headache*, 2d ed. New York, Churchill Livingstone, 1988

SCHWARTZ BS et al: Epidemiology of tension-type headache. JAMA 279:381, 1998

SILBERSTEIN SD et al: Classification of daily and near-daily headaches: Field trial of revised IHS criteria. Neurology 47:871, 1996

TOUNIER-LASSERVE E: CACNA1A mutations: Hemiplegic migraine, episodic ataxia type 2, and the others. Neurology 53:3, 1999

---

16   *John W. Engstrom*

BACK AND NECK PAIN

AAA	abdominal aortic aneurysm	MRI	magnetic resonance imaging
ALBP	acute low back pain	NSAIDs	nonsteroidal anti-inflammatory
CLBP	chronic low back pain		drugs
CPGs	clinical practice guidelines	PT	physical therapy
CSF	cerebrospinal fluid	RA	rheumatoid arthritis
CT	computed tomography	SLR	straight leg–raising
EMG	electromyography	TOS	thoracic outlet syndrome

The importance of back and neck pain in our society is underscored by the following: (1) the annual societal cost of back pain in the United States is estimated to be between $20 and $50 billion; (2) back symptoms are the most common cause of disability in patients under 45 years of age; (3) 50% of working adults, in one survey, admitted to having a back injury each year; and (4) approximately 1% of the U.S. population is chronically disabled because of back pain.

The enormous economic pressure to provide rational and efficient care of patients with back pain has resulted in clinical practice guidelines (CPGs) for these patients. CPGs are algorithms which guide evaluation or treatment at specific steps in patient care. CPGs for *acute low back pain* (ALBP) are based upon incomplete evidence (see algorithms, Fig. 16-6) but represent an attempt to standardize common medical practice. Major revisions in CPGs for back pain can be anticipated in the future. Management of patients with *chronic low back pain* (CLBP) is complex and not amenable to a simple algorithmic approach at this time.

ANATOMY OF THE SPINE

The anterior portion of the spine consists of cylindrical vertebral bodies separated by intervertebral disks and held together by the anterior and posterior longitudinal ligaments. The intervertebral disks are composed of a central gelatinous nucleus pulposus surrounded by a tough cartilagenous ring, the annulus fibrosis; disks are responsible for 25% of spinal column length (Figs. 16-1 and 16-2). The disks are largest in the cervical and lumbar regions where movements of the spine are greatest. The disks are elastic in youth and allow the bony vertebrae to move easily upon each other. Elasticity is lost with age. The function of the anterior spine is to absorb the shock of typical body movements such as walking and running.

The posterior portion of the spine consists of the vertebral arches and seven processes. Each arch consists of paired cylindrical pedicles anteriorly and paired laminae posteriorly (Fig. 16-1). The vertebral arch gives rise to two transverse processes laterally, one spinous pro-

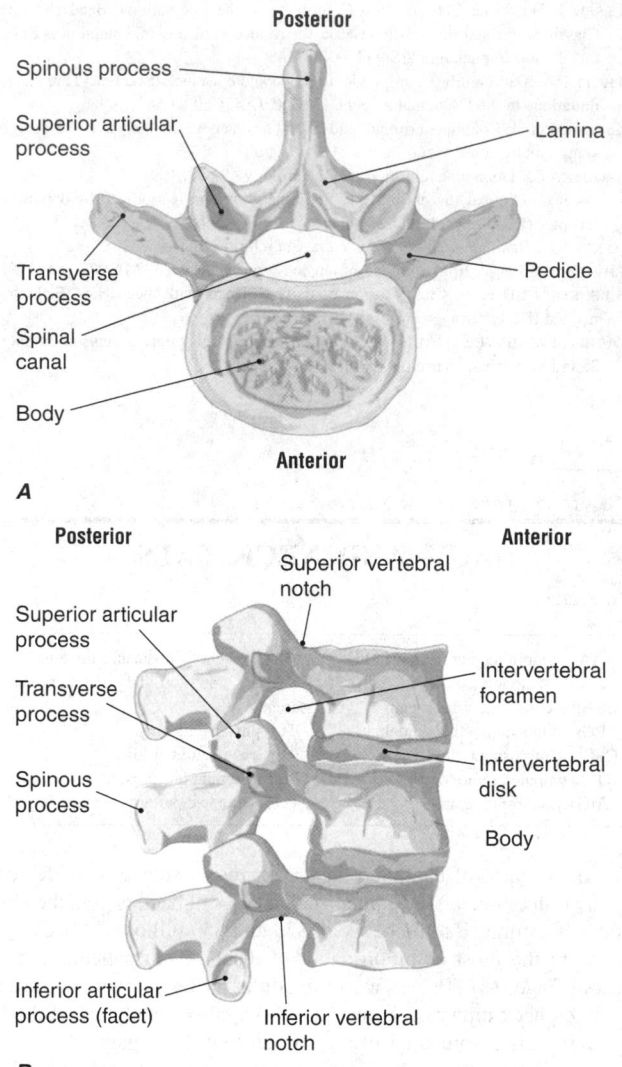

Posterior

Spinous process

Superior articular
process

Lamina

Transverse
process

Pedicle

Spinal
canal

Body

Anterior

A

Posterior   Anterior

Superior vertebral
notch

Superior articular
process

Transverse
process

Intervertebral
foramen

Intervertebral
disk

Spinous
process

Body

Inferior articular
process (facet)

Inferior vertebral
notch

B

FIGURE 16-1 Vertebral anatomy. (*From Andrea Gauthier Cornuelle and Diane H. Gronefeld, Radiographic Anatomy Positioning. New York, McGraw-Hill, 1998, with permission.*)

cess posteriorly, plus two superior and two inferior articular facets. The functions of the posterior spine are to protect the spinal cord and nerves within the spinal canal and to stabilize the spine by providing sites for the attachment of muscles and ligaments. The contraction of muscles attached to the spinous and transverse processes produces a system of pulleys and levers that results in flexion, extension, and lateral bending movements of the spine. Normal upright posture in humans places the center of gravity anterior to the spine. The graded contraction of well-developed paraspinal muscles attached to the laminae, transverse processes, and spinous processes is necessary to maintain normal upright posture.

The nerve roots exit at a level above their respective vertebral bodies in the cervical region (the C7 nerve root exits at the C6-C7 level) and below their respective vertebral bodies in the thoracic and lumbar regions (the T1 nerve root exits at the T1-T2 level). The spinal cord ends at the L1 or L2 level of the bony spine. Consequently, the lumbar nerve roots follow a long intraspinal course and can be injured anywhere from the upper lumbar spine to their exit at the intervertebral foramen. For example, it is common for disk herniation at the L4-L5 level to produce compression of the S1 nerve root (Fig. 16-3). In contrast, cervical nerve roots follow a short intraspinal course and exit at the level of their respective spinal cord segments (upper cervical) or one segment below the corresponding levels (lower cervical cord).

Cervical spine pathology can result in spinal cord compression, but lumbar spine pathology cannot.

Pain-sensitive structures in the spine include the vertebral body periosteum, dura, facet joints, annulus fibrosus of the intervertebral disk, epidural veins, and the posterior longitudinal ligament. Damage to these nonneural structures may cause pain. The nucleus pulposus of the intervertebral disk is not pain-sensitive under normal circumstances. Pain sensation is conveyed by the sinuvertebral nerve that arises from the spinal nerve at each spine segment and reenters the spinal canal through the intervertebral foramen at the same level. Disease of these diverse pain-sensitive spine structures may explain many cases of back pain without nerve root compression. The lumbar and cervical spine possess the greatest potential for movement and injury.

Approach to the Patient

Types of Back Pain   An understanding of the nature of the pain as described by the patient is the essential first step in evaluation. Attention is also focused on identification of risk factors for serious underlying diseases that require specific evaluation.

Local pain is caused by stretching of pain-sensitive structures that compress or irritate sensory nerve endings. The site of the pain is near the affected part of the back.

Pain referred to the back may arise from abdominal or pelvic viscera. The pain is usually described as primarily abdominal or pelvic but is accompanied by back pain and usually unaffected by posture. The patient may occasionally complain of back pain only.

Pain of spine origin may be located in the back or referred to the buttocks or legs. Diseases affecting the upper lumbar spine tend to refer pain to the lumbar region, groin, or anterior thighs. Diseases affecting the lower lumbar spine tend to produce pain referred to the buttocks, posterior thighs, or rarely the calves or feet. Provocative injections into pain-sensitive structures of the spine (diskography) may produce leg pain that does not follow a dermatomal distribution. The exact pathogenesis of this "sclerotomal" pain is unclear, but it may explain many instances in which combined back and leg pain is unaccompanied by evidence of nerve root compression.

Radicular back pain is typically sharp and radiates from the spine to the leg within the territory of a nerve root (see "Lumbar Disk Disease," below). Coughing, sneezing, or voluntary contraction of abdominal muscles (lifting heavy objects or straining at stool) may elicit the radiating pain. The pain may increase in postures that stretch the nerves and nerve roots. Sitting stretches the sciatic nerve (L5 and S1 roots) because the nerve passes posterior to the hip. The femoral nerve (L2, L3, and L4 roots) passes anterior to the hip and is not stretched by sitting. The description of the pain alone often fails to distinguish clearly between sclerotomal pain and radiculopathy.

Pain associated with muscle spasm, although of obscure origin, is commonly associated with many spine disorders. The spasms are accompanied by abnormal posture, taut paraspinal muscles, and dull pain.

Back pain at rest or unassociated with specific postures should raise the index of suspicion for an underlying serious cause (e.g., spine tumor, fracture, infection, or referred pain from visceral structures). Knowledge of the circumstances associated with the onset of back pain is important when weighing possible serious underlying causes for the pain. Some patients involved in accidents or work-related injuries may exaggerate their pain for the purpose of compensation or for psychological reasons.

Examination of the Back   A physical examination that includes the abdomen and rectum is advisable. Back pain referred from visceral organs may be reproduced during palpation of the abdomen (pancreatitis, abdominal aortic aneurysm) or percussion over the costovertebral angles (pyelonephritis, adrenal disease, L1-L2 transverse process fracture).

The normal spine (Fig. 16-2) displays a thoracic kyphosis, lumbar lordosis, and cervical lordosis. Exaggeration of these normal alignments may result in hyperkyphosis (lameback) of the thoracic spine or hyperlordosis (swayback) of the lumbar spine. Spasm of lumbar paraspinal muscles results in flattening of the usual lumbar lordosis. Inspection may reveal lateral curvature of the spine (scoliosis) or an asymmetry in the appearance of the paraspinal muscles, suggesting muscle spasm. Taut paraspinal muscles limit the motion of the lumbar spine. Back pain of bony spine origin is often reproduced by palpation or percussion over the spinous process of the affected vertebrae.

Forward bending is frequently limited by paraspinal muscle spasm. Flexion of the hips is normal in patients with lumbar spine disease, but flexion of the lumbar spine is limited and sometimes painful. Lateral bending to the side opposite the injured spinal element may stretch the damaged tissues, worsen pain, and limit motion. Hyperextension of the spine (with the patient prone or standing) is limited when nerve root compression or bony spine disease is present.

Pain from hip disease may mimic the pain of lumbar spine disease. The first movement is typically internal rotation of the hip. Manual internal and external rotation at the hip with the knee and hip in flexion (Patrick sign) may reproduce the pain, as may percussion of the heel (of an outstretched leg) with the palm of the examiner's hand.

In the supine position passive flexion of the thigh on the abdomen while the knee is extended produces stretching of the L5 and S1 nerve roots and the sciatic nerve because the nerve passes posterior to the hip. Passive dorsiflexion of the foot during the maneuver adds to the stretch. While flexion to at least 80° is normally possible without causing pain, tight hamstrings commonly limit motion, may result in pain, and are readily identified by the patient. This *straight leg–raising* (SLR) *sign* is positive if the maneuver reproduces the patient's usual back or limb pain. Eliciting the SLR sign in the sitting position may help determine if the finding is reproducible. The patient may describe pain in the low back, buttocks, posterior thigh, or lower leg, but the key feature is reproduction of the patient's usual pain. The *crossed* SLR sign is positive when performance of the maneuver on one leg reproduces the patient's pain symptoms in the opposite leg or buttocks. The nerve or nerve root lesion is always on the side of the pain. The *reverse* SLR sign is elicited by standing the patient next to the examination table and passively extending each leg while the patient continues to stand. This maneuver stretches the L2-L4 nerve roots and the femoral nerve because the nerves pass anterior to the hip. The reverse SLR test is positive if the maneuver reproduces the patient's usual back or limb pain.

The neurologic examination includes a search for weakness, muscle atrophy, focal reflex changes, diminished sensation in the legs, and signs of spinal cord injury. Findings with specific nerve root lesions are shown in Table 16-1 and are discussed below.

Laboratory Studies   Routine laboratory studies such as a complete blood count, erythrocyte sedimentation rate, chemistry panel, and urinalysis are rarely needed for the initial evaluation of acute (<3 months), nonspecific, low back pain. If risk factors for a serious underlying disease are present, then laboratory studies (guided by the history and examination) are indicated (Fig. 16-6B).

Plain films of the lumbar or cervical spine are helpful when risk factors for vertebral fracture (trauma, chronic steroid use) are present. *In the absence of risk factors, routine x-rays of the lumbar spine in the setting of acute, nonspecific, low back pain are expensive and rarely helpful.* Magnetic resonance imaging (MRI) and computed tomography (CT)-myelography have emerged as the radiologic tests of choice for evaluation of most serious diseases involving the spine. In general, the definition of soft tissue structures by MRI is superior, whereas CT-myelography provides optimal imaging of bony lesions in the region of the lateral recess and intervertebral foramen and is tolerated by claustrophobic patients. With rare exceptions, conventional myelography and bone scan are inferior to MRI and CT-myelography.

Electromyography (EMG) can be used to assess the functional

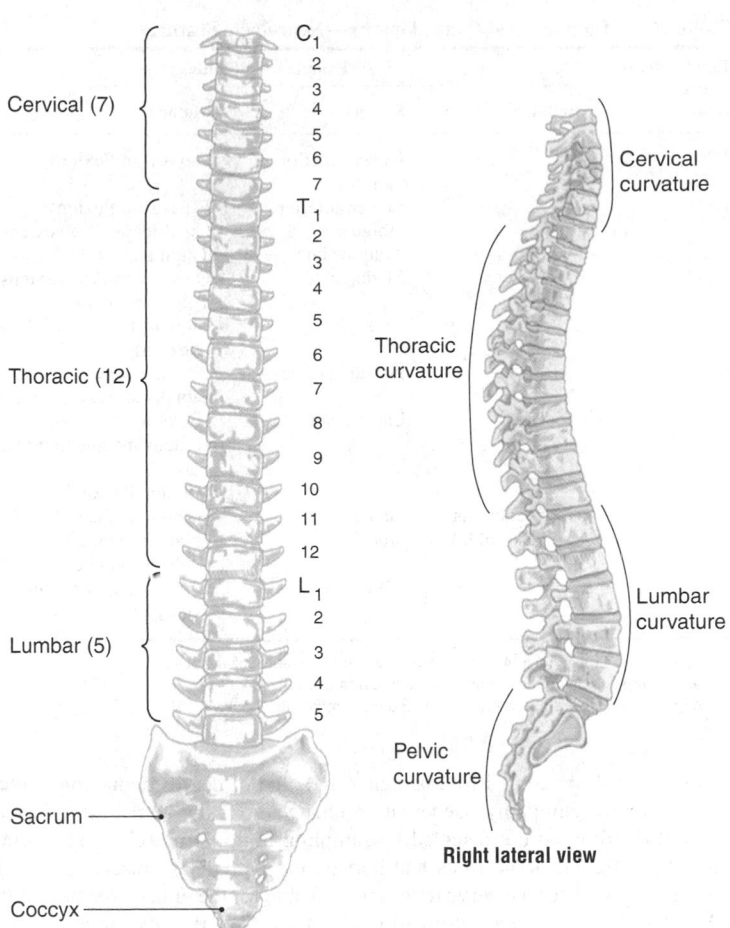

FIGURE 16-2   Spinal column. (*From Andrea Gauthier Cornuelle and Diane H. Gronefeld, Radiographic Anatomy Positioning. New York, McGraw-Hill, 1998, with permission.*)

integrity of the peripheral nervous system (Chap. 357) in the setting of back pain. Sensory nerve conduction studies are normal when focal sensory loss is due to nerve root damage because the nerve roots are proximal to the nerve cell bodies in the dorsal root ganglia. The di-

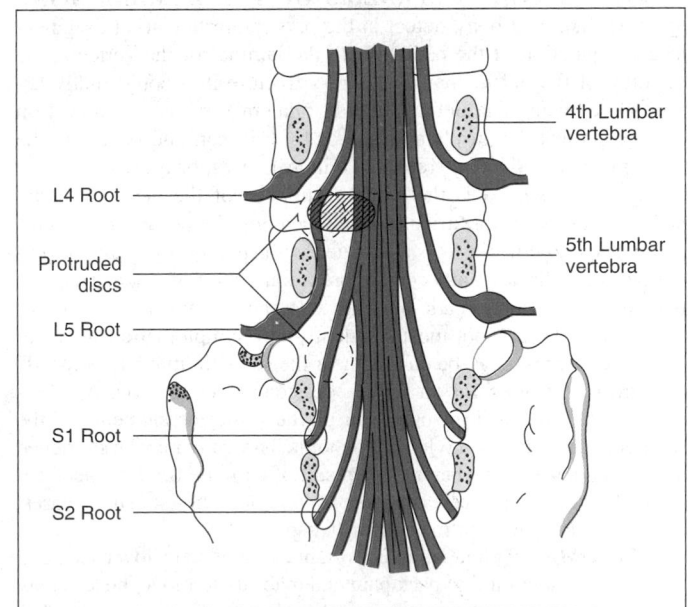

FIGURE 16-3   Locations of compression of lumbar and sacral roots by herniated disks. (*From RD Adams, M Victor, A Ropper, Principles of Neurology, 7th ed. New York, McGraw-Hill, 1997, with permission.*)

Table 16-1 Lumbosacral Radiculopathy—Neurologic Features

Lumbosacral Nerve Roots	Examination Findings			Pain Distribution
	Reflex	Sensory	Motor	
L2[a]	—	Upper anterior thigh	Psoas (hip flexion)	Anterior thigh
L3[a]	—	Lower anterior thigh	Psoas (hip flexion)	Anterior thigh, knee
		Anterior knee	Quadriceps (knee extension)	
			Thigh adduction	
L4[a]	Quadriceps (knee)	Medial calf	Quadriceps (knee extension)[b]	Knee, medial calf
			Thigh adduction	
			Tibialis anterior (foot dorsiflexion)	
L5[c]	—	Dorsal surface—foot	Peroneii (foot eversion)[b]	Lateral calf, dorsal foot, posterolateral thigh, buttocks
		Lateral calf	Tibialis anterior (foot dorsiflexion)	
			Gluteus medius (hip abduction)	
			Toe dorsiflexors	
S1[c]	Gastrocnemius/soleus (ankle)	Plantar surface—foot	Gastrocnemius/soleus (foot plantar flexion)[b]	Bottom foot, posterior calf, posterior thigh, buttocks
		Lateral aspect—foot	Abductor hallucis (toe flexors)[b]	
			Gluteus maximus (hip extension)	

[a] Reverse straight leg–raising sign present—see "Examination of the Back."
[b] These muscles receive the majority of innervation from this root.
[c] Straight leg–raising sign present—see "Examination of the Back."

agnostic yield of needle EMG is higher than that of nerve conduction studies for radiculopathy. Denervation changes in a myotomal (segmental) distribution are detected by sampling multiple muscles supplied by different nerve roots and nerves; the pattern of muscle involvement indicates the nerve root(s) responsible for the injury. Needle EMG provides objective information about motor nerve fiber injury when the clinical evaluation of weakness is limited by pain or poor effort. EMG and nerve conduction studies will be normal when only limb pain or sensory nerve root injury or irritation is present. Mixed nerve somatosensory evoked potentials and F-wave studies are of uncertain value in the evaluation of radiculopathy.

CAUSES OF BACK PAIN

CONGENITAL ANOMALIES OF THE LUMBAR SPINE
Spondylolysis is a bony defect in the pars interarticularis (a segment near the junction of the pedicle with the lamina) of the vertebra; the etiology of the defect may be a stress fracture in a congenitally abnormal segment. The defect (usually bilateral) is best visualized on oblique projections in plain x-rays or by CT scan and occurs in the setting of a single injury, repeated minor injuries, or growth.

Spondylolisthesis is the anterior slippage of the vertebral body, pedicles, and superior articular facets, leaving the posterior elements behind. Spondylolisthesis is associated with spondylolysis and degenerative spine disease and occurs more frequently in women. The slippage may be asymptomatic but may also cause low back pain, nerve root injury (the L5 root most frequently), or symptomatic spinal stenosis. Tenderness may be elicited near the segment that has "slipped" forward (most often L4 on L5 or occasionally L5 on S1). A "step" may be present on deep palpation of the posterior elements of the segment above the spondylolisthetic joint. The trunk may be shortened and the abdomen protuberant as a result of extreme forward displacement of L4 on L5 in severe degrees of spondylolisthesis. In these cases, cauda equina syndrome may occur (Chap. 368).

TRAUMA
Trauma is an important cause of acute low back pain. A patient complaining of back pain and inability to move the legs may have a spinal fracture or dislocation, and, with fractures above L1, spinal cord compression. In such cases care must be taken to avoid further damage to the spinal cord or nerve roots. The back should be immobilized pending results of plain x-rays.

Sprains and Strains The terms *low back sprain, strain,* or *mechanically induced muscle spasm* are used for minor, self-limited injuries associated with lifting a heavy object, a fall, or a sudden deceleration such as occurs in an automobile accident. These terms are used loosely and do not clearly describe a specific anatomic lesion. The pain is usually confined to the lower back, and there is no radiation to the buttocks or legs. Patients with low back pain and paraspinal muscle spasm often assume unusual postures.

Vertebral Fractures Most traumatic fractures of the lumbar vertebral bodies result from compression or flexion injuries producing anterior wedging or compression. With more severe trauma, the patient may sustain a fracture-dislocation or a "burst" fracture involving not only the vertebral body but posterior elements as well. Traumatic vertebral fractures are caused by falls from a height (a pars interarticularis fracture of the L5 vertebra is common), sudden deceleration in an automobile accident, or direct injury. Neurologic impairment is commonly associated with these injuries, and early surgical treatment is indicated (Chap. 369).

When fractures are atraumatic, the bone is presumed to be weakened by a pathologic process. The cause is usually postmenopausal (type 1) or senile (type 2) osteoporosis (Chap. 342). Underlying systemic disorders such as osteomalacia, hyperparathyroidism, hyperthyroidism, multiple myeloma, metastatic carcinoma, or glucocorticoid use may also weaken the vertebral body. The clinical context, neurologic signs, and x-ray appearance of the spine establish the diagnosis. Antiresorptive drugs including biphosphatonates, alendronate, transdermal estrogen, and tamoxifen have been shown to reduce the risk of osteoporotic fractures.

LUMBAR DISK DISEASE
This disorder is a common cause of chronic or recurrent low back and leg pain. Disk disease is most likely to occur at the L4-L5 and L5-S1 levels, but upper lumbar levels are involved occasionally. The cause of the disk injury is often unknown; the risk is increased in overweight individuals. Degeneration of the nucleus pulposus and the annulus fibrosus increases with age and may be asymptomatic or painful. A sneeze, cough, or trivial movement may cause the nucleus pulposus to prolapse, pushing the frayed and weakened annulus posteriorly. In severe disk disease, the nucleus may protrude through the annulus (herniation) or become extruded to lie as a free fragment in the spinal canal.

The mechanism by which intervertebral disk injury causes back pain is controversial. The inner annulus fibrosus and nucleus pulposis are normally devoid of innervation. Inflammation and production of proinflammatory cytokines within the protruding or ruptured disk may trigger or perpetuate back pain. Ingrowth of nociceptive (pain) nerve fibers into inner portions of diseased intervertebral disk may be responsible for chronic "diskogenic" pain. Nerve root injury (*radiculopathy*) from disk herniation may be due to compression, inflammation, or both; pathologically, varying degrees of demyelination and axonal loss are usually present.

The symptoms of a ruptured intervertebral disk include back pain, abnormal posture, limitation of spine motion (particularly flexion), or radicular pain. A dermatomal pattern of sensory loss or a reduction in or loss of a deep tendon reflex is more suggestive of a specific root lesion than the pattern of pain. Motor findings (focal weakness, muscle atrophy, or fasciculations) occur less frequently than sensory or reflex changes, but a myotomal pattern of involvement can suggest specific nerve root injury. Lumbar disk disease is usually unilateral (Fig. 16-4), but bilateral involvement does occur with large central disk herniations that compress several nerve roots at the same level. Clinical manifestations of specific lumbosacral nerve root lesions are summarized in Table 16-1. There is evidence to suggest that lumbar disk herniation with a nonprogressive nerve root deficit can be managed conservatively (i.e., nonsurgically) with a successful outcome. The size of the disk protrusion may naturally decrease over time.

Degeneration of the intervertebral disk without frank extrusion of disk tissue may give rise to low back pain only. There may be referred pain in the leg, buttock, or hip with little or no discomfort in the back and no signs of nerve root involvement. Lumbar disk syndromes are usually unilateral, but large central disk herniations can cause bilateral symptoms and signs and may produce a cauda equina syndrome.

Breakaway weakness describes a variable power of muscle contraction by a patient who is asked to provide maximal effort. The weakness may be due to pain or a combination of pain and underlying true weakness. Breakaway weakness without pain is due to lack of effort; patients who exhibit breakaway weakness should be asked if testing a specific muscle is painful. In uncertain cases, EMG can determine whether or not true weakness is present.

The differential diagnosis of lumbar disk disease includes a variety of serious and treatable conditions, including epidural abscess, hematoma, or tumor. Fever, constant pain uninfluenced by position, sphincter abnormalities, or signs of spinal cord disease suggest an etiology other than lumbar disk disease. Bilateral absence of ankle reflexes can be a normal finding in old age or a sign of bilateral S1 radiculopathy. An absent deep tendon reflex or focal sensory loss may reflect injury to a nerve root, but other sites of injury along the nerve must also be considered. For example, an absent knee reflex may be due to a femoral neuropathy rather than an L4 nerve root injury. A focal decrease in sensation over the foot and distal lateral calf may result from a peroneal or lateral sciatic neuropathy rather than an L5 nerve root injury. Focal muscle atrophy may reflect loss of motor axons from a nerve root or peripheral nerve injury, an anterior horn cell disease, or disuse.

An MRI scan or CT-myelogram is necessary to establish the location and type of pathology. Simple MRI yields exquisite views of intraspinal and adjacent soft tissue anatomy and is more likely to establish a specific anatomic diagnosis than plain films or myelography. Bony lesions of the lateral recess or intervertebral foramen may be seen with optimal clarity on CT-myelographic studies.

The correlation of neuroradiologic findings to symptoms, particularly pain, is often problematic. As examples, contrast-enhancing tears in the annulus fibrosus or disk protrusions are widely accepted as common sources of back pain. However, one recent study found that over half of asymptomatic adults have annular tears on lumbar spine MR imaging, nearly all of which demonstrate contrast enhancement. Furthermore, asymptomatic disk protrusions are common in adults, and many of these abnormalities enhance with contrast. These observations strongly suggest that MRI findings of disk protrusion, tears in the annulus fibrosus, or contrast enhancement are common incidental findings that by themselves should not dictate management decisions for patients with back pain. The presence or absence of persistent disk herniation 10 years after surgical or conservative treatment has no bearing on a successful clinical outcome.

There are four indications for intervertebral disk surgery: (1) progressive motor weakness from nerve root injury demonstrated on clinical examination or EMG, (2) bowel or bladder disturbance or other signs of spinal cord disease, (3) incapacitating nerve root pain despite conservative treatment for at least 4 weeks, and (4) recurrent incapacitating pain despite conservative treatment. The latter two criteria are more subjective and less well established than the others. Surgical treatment should also be considered if the pain and/or neurologic findings do not substantially improve over 4 to 12 weeks.

Surgery is preceded by MRI scan or CT-myelogram to define the

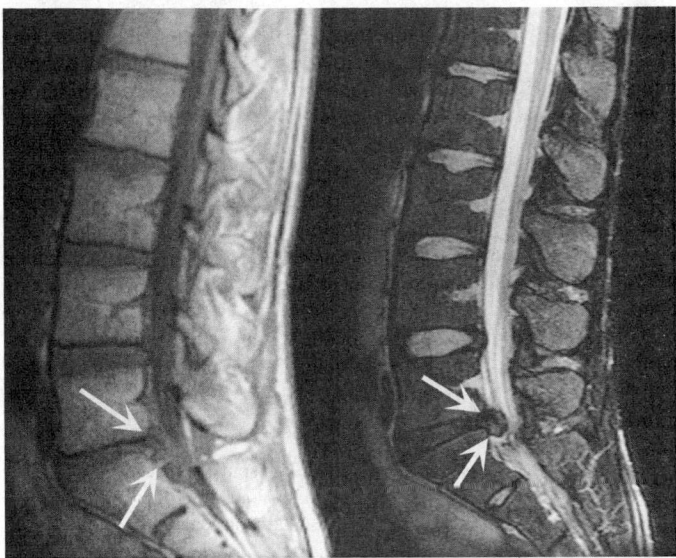

FIGURE 16-4   Lumbar herniated disk; left S1 radiculopathy. Sagittal T1-weighted image on the left with arrows outlining disk margins. Sagittal T2 image on the right reveals a protruding disk at the L5-S1 level (*arrows*), which displaces the central thecal sac.

location and type of pathology. The usual surgical procedure is a partial hemilaminectomy with excision of the involved and prolapsed intervertebral disk. Arthrodesis of the involved lumbar segments is considered only in the presence of significant spinal instability (i.e., degenerative spondylolisthesis or isthmic spondylolysis).

OTHER CAUSES OF LOW BACK PAIN   *Spinal stenosis* is an anatomic diagnosis reflecting a narrowed lumbar or cervical spinal canal. Classic *neurogenic claudication* occurs in the setting of moderate to severe spinal stenosis and typically consists of back and buttock or leg pain induced by walking or standing. The pain is relieved by sitting. Symptoms in the legs are usually bilateral. Focal weakness, sensory loss, or reflex changes may occur when associated with radiculopathy. Unlike vascular claudication, the symptoms are often provoked by standing without walking. Unlike lumbar disk disease, the symptoms are usually relieved by sitting. Severe neurologic deficits, including paralysis and urinary incontinence, occur rarely. Spinal stenosis usually results from acquired (75%), congenital, or mixed acquired/congenital factors. Congenital forms (achondroplasia, idiopathic) are characterized by short, thick pedicles that produce both spinal canal and lateral recess stenosis. Acquired factors that may contribute to spinal stenosis include degenerative diseases (spondylosis, spondylolisthesis, scoliosis), trauma, spine surgery (postlaminectomy, fusion), metabolic or endocrine disorders (epidural lipomatosis, osteoporosis, acromegaly, renal osteodystrophy, hypoparathyroidism), and Paget's disease. MRI or CT-myelography provide the best definition of the abnormal anatomy (Fig. 16-5).

Conservative treatment includes nonsteroidal anti-inflammatory drugs (NSAIDs), exercise programs, and symptomatic treatment of acute pain exacerbations. Surgical therapy is considered when medical therapy does not relieve pain sufficiently to allow for activities of daily living or when significant focal neurologic signs are present. Between 65 and 80% of properly selected patients treated surgically experience >75% relief of back and leg pain. Up to 25% develop recurrent stenosis at the same spinal level or an adjacent level 5 years after the initial surgery; recurrent symptoms usually respond to a second surgical decompression.

Facet joint hypertrophy can produce unilateral radicular symptoms, due to bony compression, that are indistinguishable from disk-related radiculopathy. Patients may exhibit stretch signs, focal motor weakness, hyporeflexia, or sensory loss. Hypertrophic superior or in-

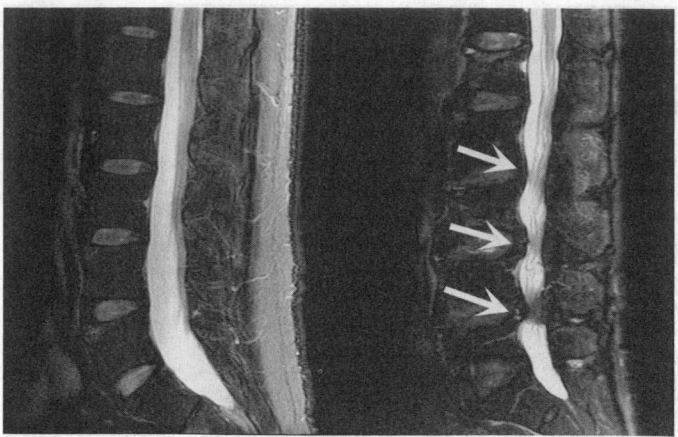

FIGURE 16-5 Spinal stenosis. Sagittal T2 fast spin echo magnetic resonance imaging of a normal (left) and stenotic (right) lumbar spine, revealing multifocal narrowing (arrows) of the cerebrospinal fluid spaces surrounding the nerve roots within the thecal sac.

ferior facets can often be visualized radiologically. Foraminotomy results in long-term relief of leg and back pain in 80 to 90% of patients.

Lumbar adhesive arachnoiditis with radiculopathy is the result of a fibrotic process following an inflammatory response to local tissue injury within the subarachnoid space. The fibrosis results in nerve root adhesions, producing back and leg pain associated with motor, sensory, and reflex changes. Myelography-induced arachnoiditis has become rare with the abandonment of oil-based contrast. Other causes of arachnoiditis include multiple lumbar operations, chronic spinal infections, spinal cord injury, intrathecal hemorrhage, intrathecal injection of steroids and anesthetics, and foreign bodies. The spine MRI appearance of arachnoiditis includes nerve roots clumping together centrally and adherent to the dura peripherally, or loculations of cerebrospinal fluid (CSF) within the thecal sac that obscure nerve root visualization. Treatment is often unsatisfactory. Microsurgical lysis of adhesions, dorsal rhizotomy, and dorsal root ganglionectomy have resulted in poor outcomes. Dorsal column stimulation for pain relief has produced varying results. Epidural steroid injections have been of limited value.

ARTHRITIS   Arthritis is a major cause of spine pain.

Spondylosis   Osteoarthritic spine disease typically occurs in later life and primarily involves the cervical and lumbosacral spine. Patients often complain of back pain that is increased by motion and associated with stiffness or limitation of motion. The relationship between clinical symptoms and radiologic findings is usually not straightforward. Pain may be prominent when x-ray findings are minimal; alternatively, large osteophytes can be seen in asymptomatic patients in middle and later life. Hypertrophied facets and osteophytes may compress nerve roots in the lateral recess or intervertebral foramen. Osteophytes arising from the vertebral body may cause or contribute to central spinal canal stenosis. Loss of intervertebral disk height reduces the vertical dimensions of the intervertebral foramen; the descending pedicle may compress the nerve root exiting at that level. Osteoarthritic changes in the lumbar spine may rarely compress the cauda equina.

Ankylosing Spondylitis (See also Chap. 315)   This distinctive arthritic spine disease typically presents with the insidious onset of low back and buttock pain. Patients are often males below age 40. Associated features include morning back stiffness, nocturnal pain, pain unrelieved by rest, an elevated sedimentation rate, and the histocompatibility antigen HLA-B27. The differential diagnosis includes tumor and infection. Onset at a young age and back pain characteristically improving with exercise suggest ankylosing spondylitis. Loss of the normal lumbar lordosis and exaggeration of thoracic kyphosis are seen as the disease progresses. Inflammation and erosion of the outer fibers of the annulus fibrosus at the point of contact with the vertebral body are followed by ossification and bone growth. Bony growth (syndesmophyte) bridges adjacent vertebral bodies and results in reduced spine mobility in all planes. The radiologic hallmarks of the disease are periarticular destructive changes, sclerosis of the sacroiliac joints, and bridging of vertebral bodies by bone to produce the fused "bamboo spine." Similar restricted movement may accompany Reiter's syndrome, psoriatic arthritis, and chronic inflammatory bowel disease. Stress fractures through the spontaneously ankylosed posterior bony elements of the rigid, osteoporotic spine may result in focal spine pain, spinal cord compression or cauda equina syndrome. Occasional atlantoaxial subluxation with spinal cord compression occurs. Bilateral ankylosis of the ribs to the spine and a decrease in the height of axial thoracic structures may cause marked impairment of respiratory function.

OTHER DESTRUCTIVE DISEASES **Neoplasm** (See also Chap. 370)   Back pain is the most common neurologic symptom among patients with systemic cancer. One-third of patients with undiagnosed back or neck pain and known systemic cancer have epidural extension or metastasis of tumor, and one-third have pain associated with vertebral metastases alone. About 11% have back pain unrelated to metastatic disease. Metastatic carcinoma (breast, lung, prostate, thyroid, kidney, gastrointestinal tract), multiple myeloma, and non-Hodgkin's and Hodgkin's lymphomas frequently involve the spine. Back pain may be the presenting symptom because the primary tumor site may be overlooked or asymptomatic. The pain tends to be constant, dull, unrelieved by rest, and worse at night. In contrast, mechanical low back pain is usually improved with rest. Plain x-rays usually, though not always, show destructive lesions in one or several vertebral bodies without disk space involvement. MRI or CT-myelography are the studies of choice in the setting of suspected spinal metastasis, but the trend of evidence favors the use of MRI. The procedure of choice is the study most rapidly available because the patient may worsen during a diagnostic delay.

Infection   *Vertebral osteomyelitis* is usually caused by staphylococci, but other bacteria or the tubercle bacillus (Pott's disease) may be the responsible organism. A primary source of infection, most often from the urinary tract, skin, or lungs, can be identified in 40% of patients. Intravenous drug use is a well-recognized risk factor. Back pain exacerbated by motion and unrelieved by rest, spine tenderness over the involved spine segment, and an elevated erythrocyte sedimentation rate are the most common findings. Fever or elevated white blood cell count are found in a minority of patients. Plain radiographs may show a narrowed disk space with erosion of adjacent vertebrae; these diagnostic changes may take weeks or months to appear. MRI and CT are sensitive and specific for osteomyelitis; MRI definition of soft tissue detail is exquisite. CT scan may be more readily available and better tolerated by some patients with severe back pain.

Spinal epidural abscess (Chap. 368) presents with back pain (aggravated by palpation or movement) and fever. The patient may exhibit nerve root injury or spinal cord compression accompanied by a sensory level, incontinence, or paraplegia. The abscess may track over multiple spinal levels and is best delineated by spine MRI.

Osteoporosis and Osteosclerosis   Considerable loss of bone may occur with or without symptoms in association with medical disorders, including hyperparathyroidism, chronic glucocorticoid use, or immobilization. Compression fractures occur in up to half of patients with severe osteoporosis. The risk of osteoporotic vertebral fracture is 4.5 times greater over 3 years among patients with a baseline fracture compared with osteoporotic controls. The sole manifestation of a compression fracture may be focal lumbar or thoracic aching (often after a trivial injury) that is exacerbated by movement. Other patients experience thoracic or upper lumbar radicular pain. Focal spine tenderness is common. When compression fractures are found, treatable risk factors should be sought. Compression fractures above the midthoracic region suggest malignancy.

Osteosclerosis is readily identifiable on routine x-ray studies (e.g., Paget's disease) and may or may not produce back pain. Spinal cord or nerve root compression may result from bony encroachment on the spinal canal or intervertebral foramina. Single dual-beam photon absorptiometry or quantitative CT can be used to detect small changes in bone mineral density. →*For further discussion of these bone disorders, see Chaps. 341 to 343.*

REFERRED PAIN FROM VISCERAL DISEASE Diseases of the pelvis, abdomen, or thorax may produce referred pain to the posterior portion of the spinal segment that innervates the diseased organ. Occasionally, back pain may be the first and only sign. In general, pelvic diseases refer pain to the sacral region, lower abdominal diseases to the lumbar region (around the second to fourth lumbar vertebrae), and upper abdominal diseases to the lower thoracic or upper lumbar region (eighth thoracic to the first and second lumbar vertebrae). Local signs (pain with spine palpation, paraspinal muscle spasm) are absent, and minimal or no pain accompanies normal spine movements.

Low Thoracic and Upper Lumbar Pain in Abdominal Disease Peptic ulcer or tumor of the posterior stomach or duodenum typically produces epigastric pain (Chaps. 285 and 90), but midline back or paraspinal pain may occur if retroperitoneal extension is present. Back pain due to peptic ulcer may be precipitated by ingestion of an orange, alcohol, or coffee and relieved by food or antacids. Fatty foods are more likely to induce back pain associated with biliary disease. Diseases of the pancreas may produce back pain to the right of the spine (head of the pancreas involved) or to the left (body or tail involved). Pathology in retroperitoneal structures (hemorrhage, tumors, pyelonephritis) may produce paraspinal pain with radiation to the lower abdomen, groin, or anterior thighs. A mass in the iliopsoas region often produces unilateral lumbar pain with radiation toward the groin, labia, or testicle. The sudden appearance of lumbar pain in a patient receiving anticoagulants suggests retroperitoneal hemorrhage.

Isolated low back pain occurs in 15 to 20% of patients with a contained rupture of an abdominal aortic aneurysm (AAA). The classic clinical triad of abdominal pain, shock, and back pain in an elderly man occurs in fewer than 20% of patients. Two of these three features are present in two-thirds of patients, and hypotension is present in half. Ruptured AAA has a high mortality rate; the typical patient is an elderly male smoker with back pain. The diagnosis is initially missed in at least one-third of patients because the symptoms and signs can be nonspecific. Common misdiagnoses include nonspecific back pain, diverticulitis, renal colic, sepsis, and myocardial infarction. A careful abdominal examination revealing a pulsatile mass (present in 50 to 75% of patients) is an important physical finding.

Lumbar Pain with Lower Abdominal Diseases Inflammatory bowel disorders (colitis, diverticulitis) or colonic neoplasms may produce lower abdominal pain, midlumbar back pain, or both. The pain may have a beltlike distribution around the body. A lesion in the transverse or initial descending colon may refer pain to the middle or left back at the L2-L3 level. Sigmoid colon disease may refer pain to the upper sacral or midline suprapubic regions or left lower quadrant of the abdomen.

Sacral Pain in Gynecologic and Urologic Disease Pelvic organs rarely cause low back pain, except for gynecologic disorders involving the uterosacral ligaments. The pain is referred to the sacral region. Endometriosis or uterine carcinoma may invade the uterosacral ligaments; malposition of the uterus may cause uterosacral ligament traction. The pain associated with endometriosis begins during the premenstrual phase and often continues until it merges with menstrual pain. Malposition of the uterus (retroversion, descensus, and prolapse) may lead to sacral pain after standing for several hours.

Menstrual pain may be felt in the sacral region. The poorly localized, cramping pain can radiate down the legs. Other pelvic sources of low back pain include neoplastic invasion of pelvic nerves, radiation necrosis, and pregnancy. Pain due to neoplastic infiltration of nerves is typically continuous, progressive in severity, and unrelieved by rest at night. Radiation therapy of pelvic tumors may produce sacral pain from late radiation necrosis of tissue or nerves. Low back pain with radiation into one or both thighs is common in the last weeks of pregnancy.

Urologic sources of lumbosacral back pain include chronic prostatitis, prostate carcinoma with spinal metastasis, and diseases of the kidney and ureter. Lesions of the bladder and testes do not usually produce back pain. The diagnosis of metastatic prostate carcinoma is established by rectal examination, spine imaging studies (MRI or CT), and measurement of prostate-specific antigen (PSA) (Chap. 95). Infectious, inflammatory, or neoplastic renal diseases may result in ipsilateral lumbosacral pain, as can renal artery or vein thrombosis. Ureteral obstruction due to renal stones may produce paraspinal lumbar pain.

Postural Back Pain There is a group of patients with chronic, nonspecific low back pain in whom no anatomic or pathologic lesion can be found despite exhaustive investigation. These individuals complain of vague, diffuse back pain with prolonged sitting or standing that is relieved by rest. The physical examination is unrevealing except for "poor posture." Imaging studies and laboratory evaluations are normal. Exercises to strengthen the paraspinal and abdominal muscles are sometimes therapeutic.

Psychiatric Disease Chronic low back pain (CLBP) may be encountered in patients with compensation hysteria, malingering, substance abuse, chronic anxiety states, or depression. Many patients with CLBP have a history of psychiatric illness (depression, anxiety, substance abuse) or childhood trauma (physical or sexual abuse) that antedates the onset of back pain. Preoperative psychological assessment has been used to exclude patients with marked psychological impairment who are at high risk for a poor surgical outcome. It is important to be certain that the back pain in these patients does not represent serious spine or visceral pathology in addition to the impaired psychological state.

Unidentified The cause of low back pain occasionally remains unclear. Some patients have had multiple operations for disk disease but have persistent pain and disability. The original indications for surgery may have been questionable with back pain only, no definite neurologic signs, or a minor disk bulge noted on CT or MRI. Scoring systems based upon neurologic signs, psychological factors, physiologic studies, and imaging studies have been devised to minimize the likelihood of unsuccessful surgical explorations and to avoid selection of patients with psychological profiles that predict poor functional outcomes.

TREATMENT Acute Low Back Pain A practical approach to the management of low back pain is to consider acute and chronic presentations separately. ALBP is defined as pain of less than 3 months' duration. Full recovery can be expected in 85% of adults with ALBP unaccompanied by leg pain. Most of these patients exhibit "mechanical" symptoms—pain that is aggravated by motion and relieved by rest.

Observational, population-based studies have been used to justify a minimalist approach to individual patient care. These studies share a number of limitations: (1) a true placebo control group is often lacking; (2) patients who consult different provider groups (generalists, orthopedists, neurologists) are assumed to have similar etiologies for their back pain; (3) no information is provided about the details of treatment within each provider group or between provider groups; and (4) no attempt to tabulate serious causes of ALBP is made. The appropriateness of specific diagnostic procedures or therapeutic interventions for low back pain cannot be assessed from these studies.

The proposed algorithms (Fig. 16-6) for management of ALBP in adults draw considerably from published guidelines. However, it must be emphasized that current CPGs for the treatment of low back pain are based on incomplete evidence—for example, there is a paucity of well-designed studies documenting the natural history of disk lesions associated with a focal neurologic deficit. Guidelines should not substitute for sound clinical judgment.

The initial assessment excludes serious causes of spine pathology that require urgent intervention, including infection, cancer, and

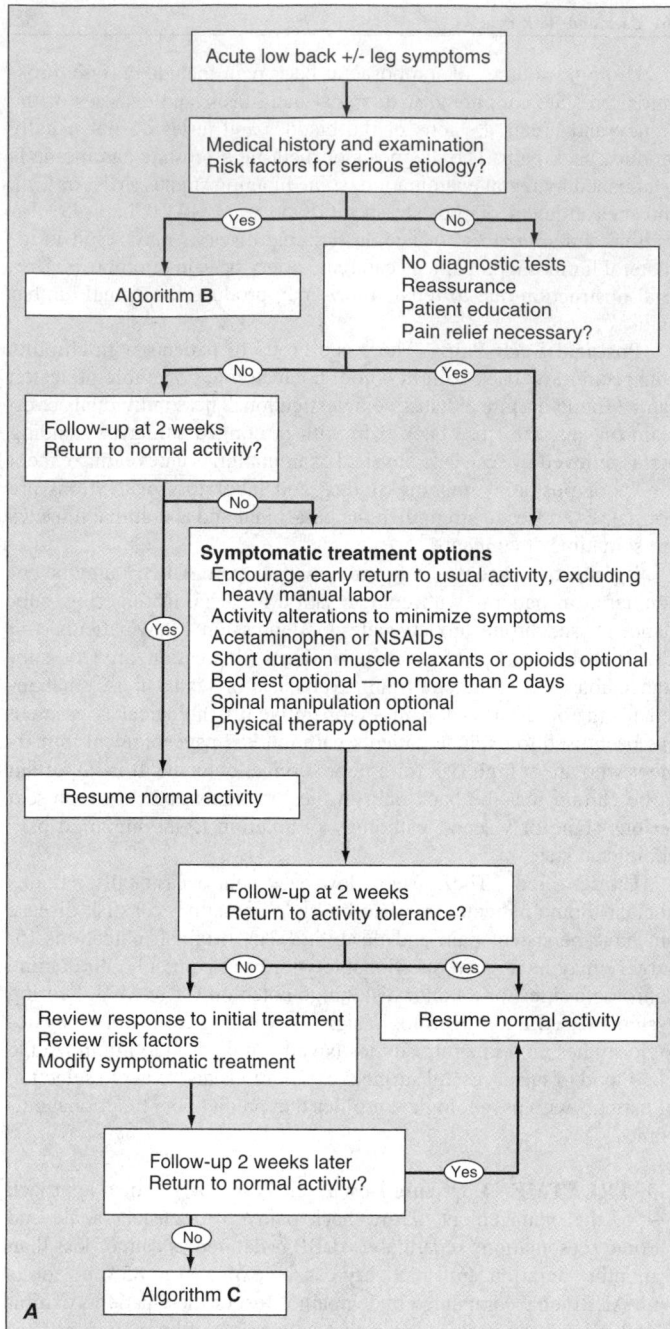

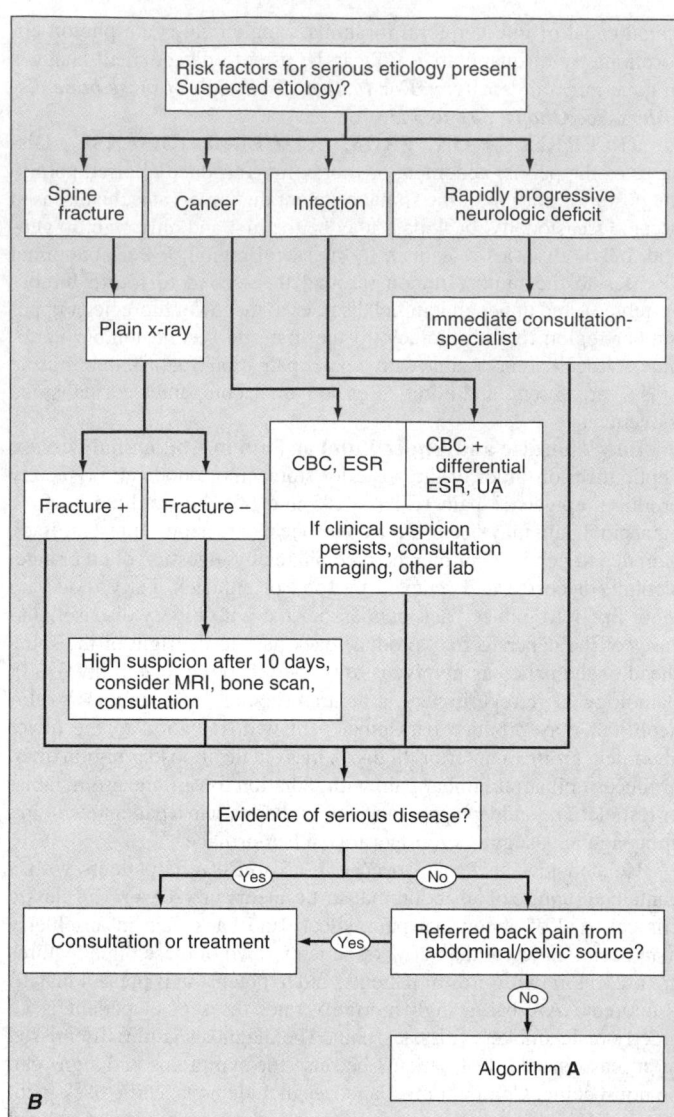

FIGURE 16-6 Algorithms for management of acute low back pain, age ≥18 years. *A.* Symptoms <3 months, first 4 weeks. *B.* Possible serious etiology.

trauma. Risks factors for a possible serious underlying cause of back pain include: age > 50 years, prior diagnosis of cancer or other serious medical illness, bed rest without relief, duration of pain >1 month, urinary incontinence or recent nocturia, focal leg weakness or numbness, pain radiating into the leg(s) from the back, intravenous drug use, chronic infection (pulmonary or urinary), pain increasing with standing and relieved by sitting, history of spine trauma, and glucocorticoid use. Clinical signs associated with a possible serious etiology include unexplained fever, well-documented and unexplained weight loss, positive SLR sign or reverse SLR sign, crossed SLR sign, percussion tenderness over the spine or costovertebral angle, an abdominal mass (pulsatile or nonpulsatile), a rectal mass, focal sensory loss (saddle anesthesia or focal limb sensory loss), true leg weakness, spasticity, and asymmetric leg reflexes. Laboratory studies are unnecessary unless a serious underlying cause (Fig. 16-6, Algorithms *A* and *B*) is suspected. Plain spine films are rarely indicated in the first month of symptoms unless a spine fracture is suspected.

The roles of bed rest, early exercise, and traction in the treatment of acute uncomplicated low back pain have been the subject of recent prospective studies. Clinical trials fail to demonstrate any benefit of prolonged (>2 days) bed rest for ALBP. There is evidence that bed rest is also ineffective for patients with sciatica or for acute back pain with findings of nerve root injury. Theoretical advantages of early ambulation for ALBP include maintenance of cardiovascular conditioning, improved disk and cartilage nutrition, improved bone and muscle strength, and increased endorphin levels. A recent trial did not show benefit from an early vigorous exercise program, but the benefits of less vigorous exercise or other exercise programs remain unknown. The early resumption of normal physical activity (without heavy manual labor) is likely to be beneficial. Well-designed clinical studies of traction that include a sham traction group have failed to show a benefit of traction for ALBP. Despite this knowledge, one survey of physicians' perceptions of effective treatment identified strict bed rest for >3 days, trigger point injections (see below), and physical therapy (PT) as beneficial for more than 50% of patients with ALBP. In many instances, the behavior of treating physicians does not reflect the current medical literature.

Proof is lacking to support the treatment of acute back and neck pain with acupuncture, transcutaneous electrical nerve stimulation, massage, ultrasound, diathermy, or electrical stimulation. Cervical collars can be modestly helpful by limiting spontaneous and reflex neck movements that exacerbate pain. Evidence regarding the efficacy of ice or heat is lacking, but these interventions are optional given the

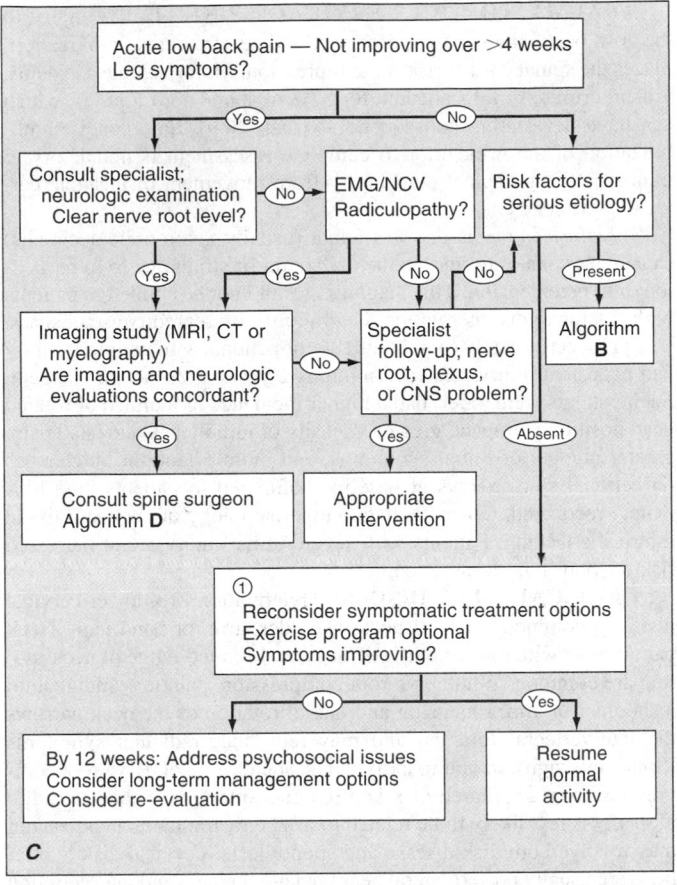

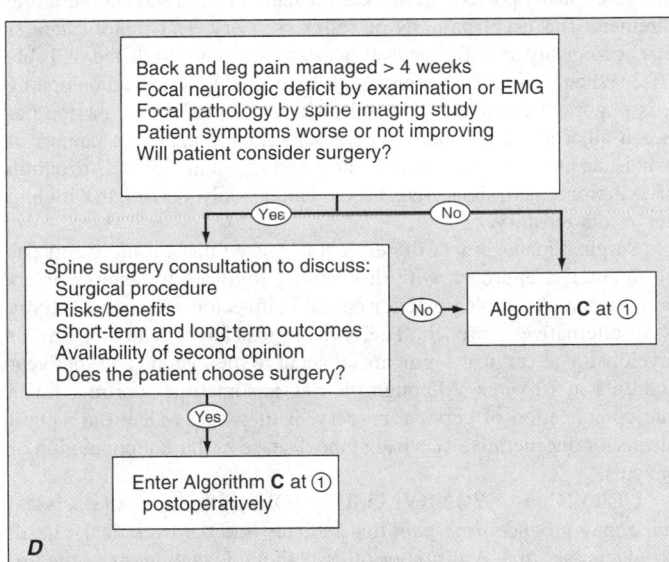

FIGURE 16-6—*(continued)* *C*. Management weeks 4–12. ①, entry point from Algorithm D postoperatively or if patient declines surgery. *D*. Surgical options. (NSAIDs, nonsteroidal anti-inflammatory drugs; CBC, complete blood count; ESR, erythrocyte sedimentation rate; UA, urinalysis; EMG, electromyography; NCV, nerve conduction velocity studies; MRI, magnetic resonance imaging; CT, computed tomography; CNS, central nervous system.)

lack of negative evidence, low cost, and low risk. Biofeedback has not been studied rigorously. Facet joint, trigger point, and ligament injections are not recommended in the treatment of ALBP.

A beneficial role for specific exercises or modification of posture has not been validated by rigorous clinical studies. As a practical matter, temporary suspension of activity known to increase mechanical stress on the spine (heavy lifting, prolonged sitting, bending or twisting, straining at stool) may be helpful.

Patient education is an important part of treatment. Studies reveal that patient satisfaction and the likelihood of follow-up increase when patients are educated about prognosis, treatment methods, activity modifications, and strategies to prevent future exacerbations. In one study, patients who felt they did not receive an adequate explanation for their symptoms wanted more diagnostic tests. Evidence for the efficacy of structured education programs ("back school") is inconclusive; in one controlled study, patients attending back school had a shorter duration of sick leave during the initial episode but not during subsequent episodes. Recent large, controlled, randomized studies of back school for primary prevention of low back injury and pain have failed to demonstrate a benefit.

Medications used in the treatment of ALBP include NSAIDs, acetaminophen, muscle relaxants, and opioids. NSAIDs are superior to placebo for back pain relief. Acetaminophen is superior to placebo in the treatment of other types of pain but has not been compared against placebo for low back pain. Muscle relaxants provide short-term (4 to 7 days) benefit compared with placebo, but drowsiness often limits their daytime use. The efficacy of muscle relaxants compared to NSAIDs or in combination with NSAIDs is unclear. Opioid analgesics have not been shown to be more effective than NSAIDs or acetaminophen for relief of ALBP or likelihood of return to work. Short-term use of opioids in selected patients unresponsive to or intolerant of acetaminophen or NSAIDs may be helpful. There is no evidence to support the use of oral glucocorticoids or tricyclic antidepressants in treatment of ALBP.

The role of diagnostic and therapeutic nerve root blocks for patients with acute back or neck pain remains controversial. Equivocal data suggests that epidural steroids may occasionally produce short-term pain relief in patients with ALBP and radiculopathy, but proof is lacking for pain relief beyond 1 month. Epidural anesthetics, steroids, or opioids are not indicated as initial treatment for ALBP without radiculopathy. Diagnostic selective nerve root blocks have been advocated to determine if pain originates from a nerve root. However, these studies may be falsely positive due to a placebo effect, in patients with a painful lesion located distally along the peripheral nerve, or from anesthesia of the sinuvertebral nerve. Therapeutic selective nerve root blocks are an option after brief conservative measures fail, particularly when temporary relief of pain may be important for patient function. Needle position is confirmed under fluoroscopic guidance with nonionic contrast before injection of glucocorticoid and local anesthetic.

A short course of spinal manipulation or PT for symptomatic relief of uncomplicated ALBP is an option. A prospective, randomized study comparing PT, chiropractic manipulation, and education interventions for patients with ALBP found modest trends toward benefit with both PT and chiropractic manipulation at 1 year. Costs per year were equivalent in the PT/chiropractic group and ~$280 less for the group treated with the education booklet alone. The extent to which this modest improvement in symptoms and outcome is worth the cost must be determined for each patient. Extended duration of treatment or treatment of patients with radiculopathy is of unknown value and carries potential risk. The appropriate frequency or duration of spinal manipulation has not been addressed adequately.

Chronic Low Back Pain CLBP is defined as pain lasting longer than 12 weeks. Patients with CLBP account for 50% of back pain costs. Overweight individuals appear to be at particular risk. Other risk factors include: female gender, older age, prior history of back pain, restricted spinal mobility, pain radiating into a leg, high levels of psychological distress, poor self-rated health, minimal physical activity, smoking, job dissatisfaction, and widespread pain. Combinations of these premorbid factors have been used to predict which individuals with ALBP are likely to develop CLBP. The initial approach to these patients is similar to that for ALBP, and the differential diagnosis of CLBP includes most of the conditions described in this chapter. Treatment of this heterogeneous group of patients is directed toward the underlying cause when possible; the ultimate goal is to restore function to the greatest extent possible.

Many conditions that produce CLBP can be identified by the combination of neuroimaging and electrophysiologic studies. Spine MRI or CT-myelography are the techniques of choice but are generally not indicated within the first month after initial evaluation in the absence of risk factors for a serious underlying cause. Imaging studies should be performed only in circumstances where the results are likely to influence surgical or medical treatment.

Diskography is of questionable value in the evaluation of back pain. No additional anatomic information is provided beyond what is available by MRI. Reproduction of the patient's typical pain with the injection is often used as evidence that a specific disk is the pain generator, but it is not known whether this information has any value in selecting candidates for surgery. There is no proven role for thermography in the assessment of radiculopathy.

The diagnosis of nerve root injury is most secure when the history, examination, results of imaging studies, and the EMG are concordant. The correlation between CT and EMG for localization of nerve root injury is between 65 and 73%. Up to one-third of asymptomatic adults have a disk protrusion detected by CT or MRI scans. Thus, surgical intervention based solely upon radiologic findings and pain increases the likelihood of an unsuccessful outcome.

CLBP can be treated with a variety of conservative measures. Acute and subacute exacerbations are managed with NSAIDs and comfort measures. There is no good evidence to suggest that one NSAID is more effective than another. Bed rest should not exceed 2 days. Activity tolerance is the primary goal, while pain relief is secondary. Exercise programs can reverse type II muscle fiber atrophy in paraspinal muscles and strengthen trunk extension. Supervised, intensive physical exercise or "work hardening" regimens (under the guidance of a physical therapist) have been effective in returning some patients to work, improving walking distances, and diminishing pain. The benefit can be sustained with home exercise regimens; compliance with the exercise regimen strongly influences outcome. The role of manipulation, back school, or epidural steroid injections in the treatment of CLBP is unclear. Up to 30% of "blind" epidural steroid injections miss the epidural space even when performed by an experienced anesthesiologist. There is no strong evidence to support the use of acupuncture or traction in this setting. A reduction in sick leave days, long-term health care utilization, and pension expenditures may offset the initial expense of multidisciplinary treatment programs. In one study comparing 3 weeks of hydrotherapy versus routine ambulatory care, hydrotherapy resulted in diminished duration and intensity of back pain, reduced analgesic drug consumption, improved spine mobility, and improved functional score. Functional score returned to baseline at the 9-month follow-up, but all other beneficial effects were sustained. Percutaneous electrical nerve stimulation (PENS) has been shown to provide significant short-term relief of CLBP, but additional studies regarding long-term efficacy and cost are necessary.

PAIN IN THE NECK AND SHOULDER

Approach to the Patient

In one recent epidemiologic survey, the 6-month prevalence of disabling neck pain was 4.6% among adults. Neck pain commonly arises from diseases of the cervical spine and soft tissues of the neck. Neck pain arising from the cervical spine is typically precipitated by neck movements and may be accompanied by focal spine tenderness and limitation of motion. Pain arising from the brachial plexus, shoulder, or peripheral nerves can be confused with cervical spine disease, but the history and examination usually identify a more distal origin for the pain. Cervical spine trauma, disk disease, or spondylosis may be asymptomatic or painful and can produce a myelopathy, radiculopathy, or both. The nerve roots most commonly affected are C7 and C6.

TRAUMA TO THE CERVICAL SPINE   Unlike injury to the low back, trauma to the cervical spine (fractures, subluxation) places the spinal cord at risk for compression. Motor vehicle accidents, violent crimes, or falls account for 87% of spinal cord injuries, which can have devastating consequences (Chap. 369). Emergency immobilization of the neck prior to complete assessment is mandatory to minimize further spinal cord injury from movement of unstable cervical spine segments.

Whiplash injury is due to trauma (usually automobile accidents) causing cervical musculoligamental sprain or strain due to hyperflexion or hyperextension. This diagnosis should not be applied to patients with fractures, disk herniation, head injury, or altered consciousness. One prospective study found that 18% of patients with whiplash injury had persistent injury-related symptoms 2 years after the car accident. Such patients were older, had a higher incidence of inclined or rotated head position at impact, greater intensity of initial neck and head pain, greater number of initial symptoms, and more osteoarthritic changes on cervical spine x-rays at baseline compared to patients who ultimately recovered. Objective data on the pathology of neck soft tissue injuries is lacking. Patients with severe initial injury are at increased risk for poor long-term outcome.

CERVICAL DISK DISEASE   Herniation of a lower cervical disk is a common cause of neck, shoulder, arm, or hand pain. Neck pain (worse with movement), stiffness, and limited range of neck motion are common. With nerve root compression, pain may radiate into a shoulder or arm. Extension and lateral rotation of the neck narrows the intervertebral foramen and may reproduce radicular symptoms (Spurling's sign). In young individuals, acute cervical nerve root compression from a ruptured disk is often due to trauma. Subacute radiculopathy is less likely to be related to a specific traumatic incident and may involve both disk disease and spondylosis. Cervical disk herniations are usually posterolateral near the lateral recess and intervertebral foramen. The usual patterns of reflex, sensory, and motor changes that accompany specific cervical nerve root lesions are listed in Table 16-2. When evaluating patients with suspected cervical radiculopathy it is important to consider the following: (1) overlap in function between adjacent nerve roots is common, (2) the anatomic pattern of pain is the most variable of the clinical features, and (3) the distribution of symptoms and signs may be evident in only part of the injured nerve root territory.

Surgical management of cervical herniated disks usually consists of an anterior approach with diskectomy followed by anterior interbody fusion. A simple posterior partial laminectomy with diskectomy is an alternative approach. The risk of subsequent radiculopathy or myelopathy at cervical segments adjacent to the fusion is 3% per year and 26% at 10 years. Although the risk is sometimes portrayed as a late complication of cervical surgery, it may also reflect the natural history of degenerative cervical spine disease in this subpopulation of patients.

CERVICAL SPONDYLOSIS   Osteoarthritis of the cervical spine may produce neck pain that radiates into the back of the head, shoulders, or arms. Arthritic or other pathologic conditions of the upper cervical spine may be the source of headaches in the posterior occipital region (supplied by the C2-C4 nerve roots). Cervical spondylosis with osteophyte formation in the lateral recess or hypertrophic facet joints may produce a monoradiculopathy (Fig. 16-7). Narrowing of the spinal canal by osteophytes, ossification of the posterior longitudinal ligament, or a large central disk may compress the cervical spinal cord. In some patients, a combination of radiculopathy and myelopathy occur. An electrical sensation elicited by neck flexion and radiating down the spine from the neck (Lhermitte's symptom) usually indicates cervical or upper thoracic (T1-T2) spinal cord involvement. When little or no neck pain accompanies the cord compression, the diagnosis may be confused with amyotrophic lateral sclerosis (Chap. 365), multiple sclerosis (Chap. 371), spinal cord tumors (Chap. 368), or syringomyelia (Chap. 368). The possibility of this treatable cervical spinal cord disease must be considered even when the patient presents with leg complaints only. Furthermore, lumbar radiculopathy or polyneuropathy may mask an associated cervical myelopathy. MRI or CT-myelography can define the anatomic abnormalities, and EMG and nerve conduction studies can quantify the severity and localize the levels of motor nerve root injury.

OTHER CAUSES OF NECK PAIN Rheumatoid arthritis (RA) (Chap. 312) of the cervical apophyseal joints results in neck pain, stiffness, and limitation of motion. In typical cases with symmetric inflammatory polyarthritis, the diagnosis of RA is straightforward. In advanced RA, synovitis of the atlantoaxial joint (C1 C2; Fig. 16-2) may damage the transverse ligament of the atlas, producing forward displacement of the atlas on the axis (atlantoaxial subluxation). Radiologic evidence of atlantoaxial subluxation occurs in 30% of patients with RA. Not surprisingly, the degree of subluxation correlates with the severity of erosive disease. When subluxation is present, careful neurologic assessment is important to identify early signs of myelopathy. Occasional patients develop high spinal cord compression leading to quadriparesis, respiratory insufficiency, and death. Although low back pain is common among RA patients, the frequency of facet disease, fracture, and spondylolisthesis is no greater than among age- and sex-matched controls with mechanical low back pain.

Ankylosing spondylitis can cause neck pain and on occasion atlantoaxial subluxation; when spinal cord compression is present or threatened, surgical intervention is indicated. Herpes zoster produces neck and posterior occipital pain in a C2-C3 distribution prior to the outbreak of vesicles. Neoplasms metastatic to the cervical spine, infections (osteomyelitis and epidural abscess), and metabolic bone diseases may also be the cause of neck pain. Neck pain may also be referred from the heart in the setting of coronary artery ischemia (cervical angina syndrome).

THORACIC OUTLET The thoracic outlet is an anatomic region containing the first rib, the subclavian artery and vein, the brachial plexus, the clavicle, and the lung apex. Injury to these structures may result in posture or task-related pain around the shoulder and supraclavicular region. There are at least three subtypes of thoracic outlet syndrome (TOS). *True neurogenic TOS* results from compression of the lower trunk of the brachial plexus by an anomalous band of tissue connecting an elongate transverse process at C7 with the first rib. Neurologic deficits include weakness of intrinsic muscles of the hand and diminished sensation on the palmar aspect of the fourth and fifth digits. EMG and nerve conduction studies confirm the diagnosis. Definitive treatment consists of surgical division of the anomalous band compressing either the lower trunk of the brachial plexus or ventral rami of the C8 or T1 nerve roots. The weakness and wasting of intrinsic hand muscles typically does not improve, but surgery halts the insidious progression of weakness. The *arterial TOS* results from compression of the subclavian artery by a cervical rib; the compression results in poststenotic dilatation of the artery and thrombus formation. Blood pressure is reduced in the affected limb, and signs of emboli may be present in the hand; neurologic signs are absent. Noninvasive ultrasound techniques confirm the diagnosis. Treatment is with thrombolysis or anticoagulation (with or without embolectomy) and surgical excision of the cervical rib compressing the subclavian artery or vein. The *disputed TOS* includes a large number of patients with chronic arm and shoulder pain of unclear cause. The lack of sensitive and specific findings on physical examination or laboratory markers for this condition frequently results in diagnostic uncertainty. The role of surgery in disputed TOS is controversial; conservative approaches often include multidisciplinary pain management. Treatment is often unsuccessful.

BRACHIAL PLEXUS AND NERVES Pain from injury to the brachial plexus or arm peripheral nerves can occasionally be confused with pain of cervical spine origin. Neoplastic infiltration of the lower trunk of the brachial plexus may produce shoulder pain radiating down the arm, numbness of the fourth and fifth fingers, and weakness of intrinsic hand muscles innervated by the ulnar and median nerves.

Table 16-2 Cervical Radiculopathy—Neurologic Features

Cervical Nerve Roots	Examination Findings			
	Reflex	Sensory	Motor	Pain Distribution
C5	Biceps	Over lateral deltoid	Supraspinatus[a] (initial arm abduction) Infraspinatus[a] (arm external rotation) Deltoid[a] (arm abduction) Biceps (arm flexion)	Lateral arm, medial scapula
C6	Biceps	Thumb, index fingers Radial hand/ forearm	Biceps (arm flexion) Pronator teres (internal forearm rotation)	Lateral forearm, thumb, index finger
C7	Triceps	Middle fingers Dorsum forearm	Triceps[a] (arm extension) Wrist extensors[a] Extensor digitorum[a] (finger extension)	Posterior arm, dorsal forearm, lateral hand
C8	Finger flexors	Little finger Medial hand and forearm	Abductor pollicis brevis (abduction D1) First dorsal interosseous (abduction D2) Abductor digiti minimi (abduction D5)	4th and 5th fingers, medial forearm
T1	Finger flexors	Axilla and medial arm	Abductor pollicis brevis (abduction D1) First dorsal interosseous (abduction D2) Abductor digiti minimi (abduction D5)	Medial arm, axilla

[a] These muscles receive the majority of innervation from this root.

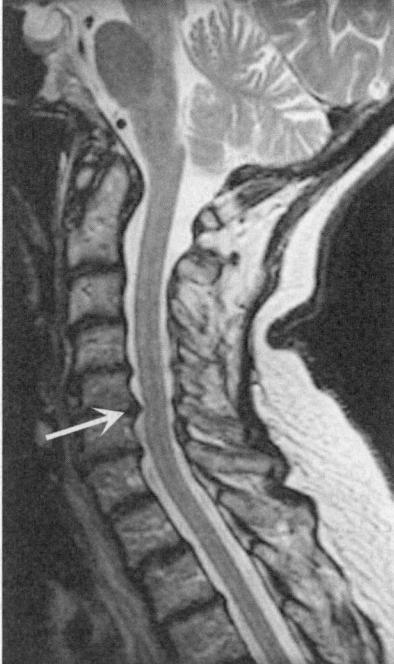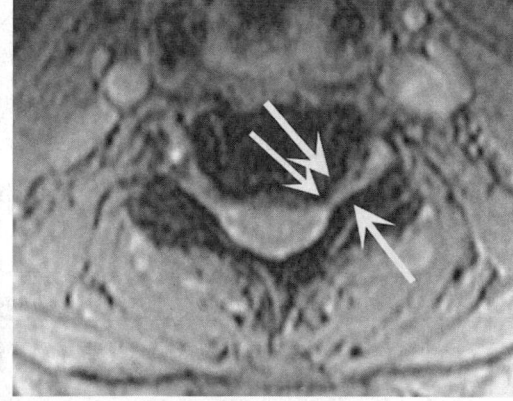

FIGURE 16-7 Cervical spondylosis; left C6 radiculopathy. *A.* Sagittal T2 fast spin echo magnetic resonance imaging reveals a hypointense osteophyte that protrudes from the C5-C6 level into the thecal sac, displacing the spinal cord posteriorly (*white arrow*). *B.* Axial 2-mm section from a 3-D volume gradient echo sequence of the cervical spine. The high signal of the right C5-C6 intervertebral foramen contrasts with the narrow high signal of the left C5-C6 intervertebral foramen produced by osteophytic spurring (*arrows*).

Postradiation fibrosis (breast carcinoma is the most common setting) or a Pancoast tumor of the lung (Chap. 88) may produce similar findings. A Horner's syndrome is present in two-thirds of patients with a Pancoast tumor. Suprascapular neuropathy may produce severe shoulder pain, weakness, and wasting of the supraspinatous and infraspinatous muscles. *Acute brachial neuritis* is often confused with radiculopathy. It consists of the acute onset of severe shoulder or scapular pain followed over days to weeks by weakness of the proximal arm and shoulder girdle muscles innervated by the upper or middle trunks or cords of the brachial plexus. The onset is often preceeded by an infection or immunization. Separation of this syndrome from cervical radiculopathy is important because slow, complete recovery of brachial neuritis occurs in 75% of patients after 2 years and in 89% after 3 years. Occasional cases of carpal tunnel syndrome produce pain and paresthesia extending into the forearm, arm, and shoulder resembling a C5 or C6 root lesion. Lesions of the radial or ulnar nerve can mimic a radiculopathy at C7 or C8, respectively. EMG and nerve conduction studies can accurately localize lesions to the nerve roots, brachial plexus, or nerves. →*For further discussion of peripheral nerve disorders, see Chap. 377.*

SHOULDER   Pain in the shoulder region can be difficult to separate clearly from neck pain. If the symptoms and signs of radiculopathy are absent, then the differential diagnosis includes mechanical shoulder pain (tendonitis, bursitis, rotator cuff tear, dislocation, adhesive capsulitis, and cuff impingement under the acromion) and referred pain (subdiaphragmatic irritation, angina, Pancoast tumor). Mechanical pain is often worse at night, associated with local shoulder tenderness, and aggravated by abduction, internal rotation, or extension of the arm. The pain of shoulder disease may at times radiate into the arm or hand, but the sensory, motor, and reflex changes that indicate disease of the nerve roots, plexus, or peripheral nerves are absent.

℞ **TREATMENT**   A paucity of well-designed clinical trials exists for the treatment of neck pain. Symptomatic treatment of neck pain can include the use of analgesic medications and/or a soft cervical collar. Current indications for cervical disk surgery are similar to those for lumbar disk surgery; because of the risk of spinal cord injury with cervical spine disease, an aggressive approach is generally indicated whenever spinal cord injury is threatened. Surgical management of cervical herniated disks usually consists of an anterior approach with diskectomy followed by anterior interbody fusion. A simple posterior partial laminectomy with diskectomy is an acceptable alternative approach. The cumulative risk of subsequent radiculopathy or myelopathy at cervical segments adjacent to the fusion is approximately 3% per year and 26% per decade. Although this risk is sometimes portrayed as a late complication of surgery, it may also reflect the natural history of degenerative cervical spine disease. Nonprogressive cervical radiculopathy (associated with a focal neurologic deficit) due to a herniated cervical disk may be treated conservatively with a high rate of success. Cervical spondylosis with bony, compressive cervical radiculopathy is generally treated with surgical decompression to interrupt the progression of neurologic signs. Cervical spondylotic myelopathy is typically managed with either anterior decompression and fusion or laminectomy. Outcomes in both surgical groups vary, but late functional deterioration occurs in 20 to 30% of patients; a prospective, controlled study comparing different surgical interventions is sorely needed.

BIBLIOGRAPHY

ANDERSSON GBJ et al: A comparison of osteopathic spinal manipulation with standard care for patients with low back pain. N Engl J Med 341(19):1426, 1999

BEURSKENS AJ et al: Efficacy of traction for non-specific low back pain: A randomised clinical trial. Lancet 346:1596, 1995

BIGOS SJ: Perils, pitfalls, and accomplishments of guidelines for treatment of back problems. Neurol Clin North Am 17(1):179, 1999

CAREY TS et al: The outcomes and costs of care for acute low back pain among patients seen by primary care practitioners, chiropractors, and orthopedic surgeons. N Engl J Med 333:913, 1995

CASSIDY JD et al: Effect of eliminating compensation for pain and suffering on the outcome of insurance claims for whiplash injury. N Engl J Med 342:1179, 2000

CHERKIN DC et al: A comparison of physical therapy, chiropractic manipulation, and provision of an educational booklet for the treatment of patients with low back pain. JAMA 339(15):1021, 1998

DALTROY LH et al: A controlled trial of an educational program to prevent low back injuries. N Engl J Med 337:322, 1998

FRANKLIN GM et al: Outcome of surgery for thoracic outlet syndrome in Washington state workers' compensation. Neurology 54:1252, 2000

LAUDER TD et al: Effect of history and exam in predicting electrodiagnostic outcome among patients with suspected lumbosacral radiculopathy. Am J Phys Med Rehabil 79(1):60, 75, 2000

MALMIVAARA A et al: The treatment of acute low back pain—bed rest, exercises, or ordinary activity? N Engl J Med 332:351, 1995

STADNIK TW et al: Annular tears and disk herniation: Prevalence and contrast enhancement on MR images in the absence of low back pain or sciatica. Radiology 206(1):49, 1998

VROOMEN PCAJ et al: Lack of effectiveness of bed rest for sciatica. N Engl J Med 40(6):418, 1999

Section 2
ALTERATIONS IN BODY TEMPERATURE

17   *Charles A. Dinarello, Jeffrey A. Gelfand*

FEVER AND HYPERTHERMIA

Body temperature is controlled by the hypothalamus. Neurons in both the preoptic anterior hypothalamus and the posterior hypothalamus receive two kinds of signals: one from peripheral nerves that reflect warmth/cold receptors and the other from the temperature of the blood bathing the region. These two types of signals are integrated by the thermoregulatory center of the hypothalamus to maintain normal temperature. In a neutral environment, the metabolic rate of humans consistently produces more heat than is necessary to maintain the core body temperature at 37°C. Therefore, the hypothalamus controls temperature by mechanisms of heat loss.

A normal body temperature is ordinarily maintained, despite environmental variations, because the hypothalamic thermoregulatory center balances the excess heat production derived from metabolic activity in muscle and the liver with heat dissipation from the skin and lungs. According to recent studies of healthy individuals 18 to 40 years of age, the mean oral temperature is 36.8° ± 0.4°C (98.2° ± 0.7°F), with low levels at 6 A.M. and higher levels at 4 to 6 P.M. The maximum normal oral temperature is 37.2°C (98.9°F) at 6 A.M. and 37.7°C (99.9°F) at 4 P.M.; these values define the 99th percentile for healthy individuals. In light of these studies, *an A.M. temperature of >37.2°C (98.9°F) or a P.M. temperature of >37.7°C (99.9°F) would define a fever.* The normal daily temperature variation is typically 0.5°C (0.9°F). However, in some individuals recovering from a febrile illness, this daily variation can be as great as 1.0°C. During a febrile illness, diurnal variations are usually maintained but at higher levels. Daily temperature swings do not occur in patients with hyperthermia (see below). Rectal temperatures are generally 0.4°C (0.7°F) higher than oral readings. The lower oral readings are probably attributable to mouth breathing, which is a particularly important factor in patients with respiratory infections and rapid breathing. Lower esophageal temperatures closely reflect core temperature. Tympanic membrane (TM) thermometers measure radiant heat energy from the tympanic membrane and nearby ear canal and display that absolute value (unadjusted mode) or a value automatically calculated from the absolute reading on the basis of nomograms relating the radiant temperature measured to actual core temperatures obtained in clinical studies (adjusted mode). These measurements, although convenient, may be more variable than directly determined oral or rectal values. Studies in adults show that readings are lower with unadjusted-mode than with adjusted-mode TM thermometers and that unadjusted-mode TM values are 0.8°C (1.6°F) lower than rectal temperatures.

In women who menstruate, the A.M. temperature is generally lower in the 2 weeks before ovulation; it then rises by about 0.6°C (1°F) with ovulation and remains at that level until menses occur. Seasonal variation in body temperature has been described but may reflect a metabolic change and is not common. Body temperature is elevated in the postprandial state, but this elevation does not represent fever. Pregnancy and endocrinologic dysfunction also affect body temperature. The daily temperature variation appears to be fixed in early childhood; in contrast, elderly individuals can exhibit a reduced ability to develop fever, with only a modest fever even in severe infections.

FEVER VERSUS HYPERTHERMIA

FEVER Fever is an elevation of body temperature that exceeds the normal daily variation and occurs *in conjunction with an increase in the hypothalamic set point*—for example, from 37°C to 39°C. This shift of the set point from "normothermic" to febrile levels very much resembles the resetting of the home thermostat to a higher level in order to raise the ambient temperature in a room. Once the hypothalamic set point is raised, neurons in the vasomotor center are activated and vasoconstriction commences. The individual first notices vasoconstriction in the hands and feet. Shunting of blood away from the periphery to the internal organs essentially decreases heat loss from the skin, and the person feels cold. For most fevers, body temperature increases by 1 to 2°C. Shivering, which increases heat production from the muscles, may begin at this time; however, shivering is not required if heat conservation mechanisms raise blood temperature sufficiently. Heat production from the liver also increases. In humans, behavioral instincts (e.g., putting on more clothing or bedding) lead to a reduction of exposed surfaces, which helps raise body temperature.

The processes of heat conservation (vasoconstriction) and heat production (shivering and increased metabolic activity) continue until the temperature of the blood bathing the hypothalamic neurons matches the new thermostat setting. Once that point is reached, the hypothalamus maintains the temperature at the febrile level by the same mechanisms of heat balance that are operative in the afebrile state. When the hypothalamic set point is again reset downward (due to either a reduction in the concentration of pyrogens or the use of antipyretics), the processes of heat loss through vasodilation and sweating are initiated. Behavioral changes triggered at this time include the removal of insulating clothing or bedding. Loss of heat by sweating and vasodilation continues until the blood temperature at the hypothalamic level matches the lower setting.

A fever of >41.5°C (106.7°F) is called *hyperpyrexia*. This extraordinarily high fever can develop in patients with severe infections but most commonly occurs in patients with central nervous system hemorrhages. In the preantibiotic era, fever due to a variety of infectious diseases rarely exceeded 106°F, and there has been speculation that this natural "thermal ceiling" is mediated by neuropeptides functioning as central antipyretics.

In some rare cases, the hypothalamic set point is elevated as a result of local trauma, hemorrhage, tumor, or intrinsic hypothalamic malfunction. The term *hypothalamic fever* is sometimes used to describe elevated temperature caused by abnormal hypothalamic function. However, most patients with hypothalamic damage have *sub*normal, not *supra*normal, body temperatures. These patients do not respond properly to mild environmental temperature changes. For example, when exposed to only mildly cold conditions, their core temperature falls quickly rather than over the normal period of a few hours. In the very few patients in whom elevated core temperature is suspected to be due to hypothalamic damage, diagnosis depends on the demonstration of other abnormalities in hypothalamic function, such as the production of hypothalamic releasing factors, abnormal response to cold, and absence of circadian temperature and hormonal rhythms.

HYPERTHERMIA Hyperthermia is characterized by *an unchanged (normothermic) setting of the thermoregulatory center* in conjunction with an uncontrolled increase in body temperature that exceeds the body's ability to lose heat. Exogenous heat exposure and endogenous heat production are two mechanisms by which hyperthermia can result in dangerously high internal temperatures. Excessive heat production can easily cause hyperthermia despite physiologic and behavioral control of body temperature. For example, over-insulating clothing can result in an elevated core temperature, and work or exercise in hot environments can produce heat faster than peripheral mechanisms can lose it.

Although most patients with elevated body temperature have fever, there are a few circumstances in which elevated temperature represents not fever but hyperthermia (Table 17-1). *Heat stroke*, caused by thermoregulatory failure in association with a warm environment, may be categorized as exertional or nonexertional. *Exertional heat stroke* typically occurs in younger individuals exercising at ambient temperatures and/or humidities that are higher than normal. Even in normal individuals, dehydration or the use of common medications (e.g., over-the-counter antihistamines with anticholinergic side effects) may help to precipitate exertional heat stroke. *Nonexertional* or *classic heat stroke* typically occurs in elderly individuals, particularly during heat waves. For example, in Chicago in July 1995, 465 deaths were certified as heat related. The elderly, the bedridden, persons taking anticholinergic or antiparkinsonian drugs or diuretics, and individuals confined to poorly ventilated and non-air-conditioned environments are most susceptible.

Drug-induced hyperthermia has become increasingly common as a result of the increased use of prescription psychotropic drugs and illicit drugs. Drug-induced hyperthermia may be caused by monoamine oxidase inhibitors, tricyclic antidepressants, and amphetamines and by the illicit use of phencyclidine, lysergic acid diethylamide (LSD), or cocaine.

Table 17-1 Causes of Hyperthermia Syndromes

Heat stroke
    Exertional: Exercise in higher-than-normal heat and/or humidity
    Nonexertional: Anticholinergics, including antihistamines; antiparkinsonian drugs; diuretics; phenothiazines
Drug-induced hyperthermia
    Amphetamines; monoamine oxidase inhibitors; cocaine; phencyclidine; tricyclic antidepressants; LSD
Neuroleptic malignant syndrome
    Phenothiazines; butyrophenones, including haloperidol and bromperidol; fluoxetine; loxapine; tricyclic dibenzodiazepines; metoclopramide; domperidone; thiothixene; molindone
Malignant hyperthermia
    Inhalational anesthetics; succinylcholine
Endocrinopathy
    Thyrotoxicosis
    Pheochromocytoma

SOURCE: After FJ Curley, RS Irwin, JM Rippe et al (eds): *Intensive Care Medicine*, 3d ed. Boston, Little, Brown, 1996.

Malignant hyperthermia occurs in individuals with an inherited abnormality of skeletal-muscle sarcoplasmic reticulum that causes a rapid increase in intracellular calcium levels in response to halothane and other inhalational anesthetics or to succinylcholine. Elevated temperature, increased muscle metabolism, rigidity, rhabdomyolysis, acidosis, and cardiovascular instability develop rapidly. This condition is often fatal. The *neuroleptic malignant syndrome* can occur with phenothiazines and other drugs such as haloperidol and is characterized by muscle rigidity, autonomic dysregulation, and hyperthermia. This disorder appears to be caused by the inhibition of central dopamine receptors in the hypothalamus, which results in increased heat generation and decreased heat dissipation. Thyrotoxicosis and pheochromocytoma can also cause increased thermogenesis.

It is important to distinguish between fever and hyperthermia since hyperthermia can be rapidly fatal and characteristically does not respond to antipyretics. However, there is no rapid way to make this distinction. Hyperthermia is often diagnosed on the basis of the events immediately preceding the elevation of core temperature—e.g., heat exposure or treatment with drugs that interfere with thermoregulation. However, in addition to the clinical history of the patient, the physical aspects of some forms of hyperthermia may alert the clinician. For example, in patients with heat stroke syndromes and in those taking drugs that block sweating, the skin is hot but dry. Moreover, antipyretics do not reduce the elevated temperature in hyperthermia, whereas in fever—and even in hyperpyrexia—adequate doses of either aspirin or acetaminophen usually result in some decrease in body temperature.

PYROGENS   The term *pyrogen* is used to describe any substance that causes fever. *Exogenous* pyrogens are derived from outside the patient; most are microbial products, microbial toxins, or whole microorganisms. The classic example of an exogenous pyrogen is the lipopolysaccharide endotoxin produced by all gram-negative bacteria. Endotoxins are potent not only as pyrogens but also as inducers of various pathologic changes in gram-negative infections. Another group of potent bacterial pyrogens is produced by gram-positive organisms and includes the enterotoxins of *Staphylococcus aureus* and the group A and B streptococcal toxins, also called *superantigens*. One staphylococcal toxin of clinical importance is the toxic shock syndrome toxin associated with isolates of *S. aureus* from patients with toxic shock syndrome. Like the endotoxins of gram-negative bacteria, the toxins produced by staphylococci and streptococci cause fever in experimental animals when injected intravenously at concentrations of <1 μg/kg of body weight. Endotoxin is a highly pyrogenic molecule in humans: a dose of 2 to 3 ng/kg produces fever and generalized symptoms of malaise in volunteers.

PYROGENIC CYTOKINES   Cytokines are small proteins (molecular mass, 10,000 to 20,000 Da) that regulate immune, inflammatory, and hematopoietic processes. For example, stimulation of lymphocyte proliferation during an immune response to vaccination is the result of the cytokines interleukin (IL) 2, IL-4, and IL-6. Another cytokine, granulocyte colony-stimulating factor, stimulates granulocytopoiesis in the bone marrow. Some cytokines cause fever and hence are called *pyrogenic cytokines*. From a historic point of view, the field of cytokine biology began in the 1940s with laboratory investigations into fever induction by products of activated leukocytes. These fever-producing molecules were called *endogenous pyrogens*. When endogenous pyrogens were purified from activated leukocytes, they were shown to possess various biologic activities, which are now recognized as the properties of the various cytokines.

The known pyrogenic cytokines include IL-1, IL-6, tumor necrosis factor (TNF), ciliary neurotropic factor (CNTF), and interferon (IFN) α. Others probably exist. Each cytokine is encoded by a separate gene, and each pyrogenic cytokine has been shown to cause fever in laboratory animals and in humans. When injected into humans, IL-1, IL-6, and TNF produce fever at low doses (10 to 100 ng/kg).

The synthesis and release of endogenous pyrogenic cytokines are induced by a wide spectrum of exogenous pyrogens, most of which have recognizable bacterial or fungal sources. Viruses also induce pyrogenic cytokines by infecting cells. However, in the absence of microbial infection, inflammation, trauma, tissue necrosis, or antigen-antibody complexes can induce the production of IL-1, TNF, and/or IL-6, which—individually or in combination—trigger the hypothalamus to raise the set point to febrile levels. The cellular sources of pyrogenic cytokines are primarily monocytes, neutrophils, and lymphocytes, although many other types of cells can synthesize these molecules when stimulated.

ELEVATION OF THE HYPOTHALAMIC SET POINT BY CYTOKINES   During fever, levels of prostaglandin E$_2$ (PGE$_2$) are elevated in hypothalamic tissue and the third cerebral ventricle. The concentrations of PGE$_2$ are highest near the circumventricular vascular organs (organum vasculosum of lamina terminalis)—networks of enlarged capillaries surrounding the hypothalamic regulatory centers. Destruction of these organs reduces the ability of pyrogens to produce fever. Most studies in animals have failed to show, however, that pyrogenic cytokines pass from the circulation into the brain itself. Thus, it appears that both exogenous and endogenous pyrogens interact with the endothelium of these capillaries and that this interaction is the first step in initiating fever—i.e., in raising the set point to febrile levels.

The key events in the production of fever are illustrated in Fig. 17-1. As has been mentioned, several cell types can produce pyrogenic cytokines. Pyrogenic cytokines such as IL-1, IL-6, and TNF are released from the cells and enter the systemic circulation. Although the systemic effects of these circulating cytokines lead to fever by inducing the synthesis of PGE$_2$, they also induce PGE$_2$ in peripheral tissues. The increase in PGE$_2$ in the periphery accounts for the nonspecific myalgias and arthralgias that often accompany fever. However, it is the induction of PGE$_2$ in the brain that starts the process of raising the hypothalamic set point for core temperature.

There are four receptors for PGE$_2$, and each signals the cell in different ways. Of the four receptors, the third (EP-3) is essential for fever: when the gene for this receptor is deleted in mice, no fever follows the injection of IL-1 or endotoxin. Deletion of the other PGE$_2$ receptor genes leaves the fever mechanism intact. Although PGE$_2$ is essential for fever, it is not a neurotransmitter. Rather, the release of PGE$_2$ from the brain side of the hypothalamic endothelium triggers the PGE$_2$ receptor on glial cells, and this stimulation results in the rapid release of cyclic adenosine 5′-monophosphate (cyclic AMP), which is a neurotransmitter. As shown in Fig. 17-1, the release of cyclic AMP from the glial cells activates neuronal endings from the thermoregulatory center that extend into the area. The elevation of cyclic AMP is thought to account for changes in the hypothalamic set point either directly or indirectly by inducing the release of monoamine

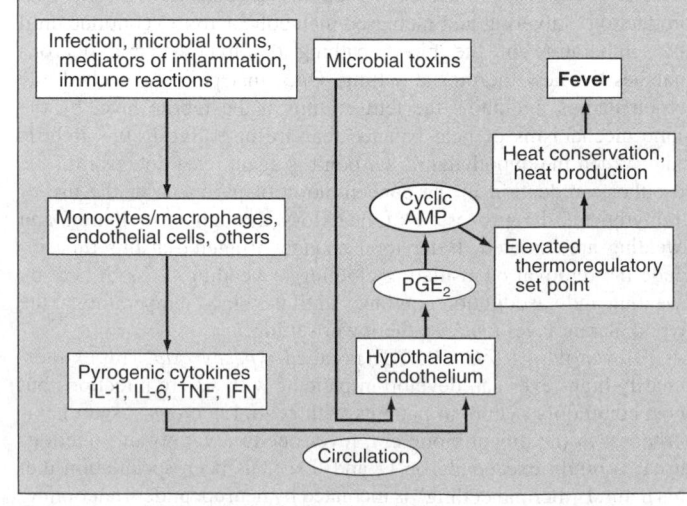

FIGURE 17-1 Chronology of events required for the induction of fever.

neurotransmitters. Since receptors for endotoxin are in many ways similar to IL-1 receptors, the activation of endotoxin receptors on the hypothalamic endothelium also results in PGE_2 production and fever.

PRODUCTION OF CYTOKINES IN THE CENTRAL NERVOUS SYSTEM Several viral diseases produce active infection in the brain. Glial and possibly neuronal cells synthesize IL-1, TNF, and IL-6. CNTF is also synthesized by neural as well as neuronal cells. What role in the production of fever is played by these cytokines produced in the brain itself? In experimental animals, the concentrations of cytokine required to cause fever are several orders of magnitude lower with direct injection into the brain than with intravenous injection. Therefore, central nervous system production of these cytokines apparently can raise the hypothalamic set point, bypassing the circumventricular organs involved in fever caused by circulating cytokines. Central nervous system cytokines may account for the hyperpyrexia of central nervous system hemorrhage, trauma, or infection.

Approach to the Patient

History It is in the diagnosis of a febrile illness that the science and art of medicine come together. In no other clinical situation is a meticulous history more important. Painstaking attention must be paid to the chronology of symptoms in relation to the use of prescription drugs (including drugs or herbs taken without a physician's supervision) or treatments such as surgical or dental procedures. The exact nature of any prosthetic materials and/or implanted devices should be ascertained. A careful occupational history should include exposures to animals; toxic fumes; potential infectious agents; possible antigens; or other febrile or infected individuals in the home, workplace, or school. A history of the geographic areas in which the patient has lived and a travel history should include locations during military service. Information on unusual hobbies, dietary proclivities (such as raw or poorly cooked meat, raw fish, and unpasteurized milk or cheeses), and household pets should be elicited, as should that on sexual orientation and practices, including precautions taken or omitted. Attention should be directed to the use of tobacco, marijuana, intravenous drugs, or alcohol; trauma; animal bites; tick or other insect bites; and prior transfusions, immunizations, drug allergies, or hypersensitivities. A careful family history should include information on family members with tuberculosis, other febrile or infectious diseases, arthritis or collagen vascular disease, or unusual familial symptomatology such as deafness, urticaria, fevers and polyserositis, bone pain, or anemia. Ethnic origin may be critical. For example, blacks are more likely than persons in other groups to have hemoglobinopathies. Turks, Arabs, Armenians, and Sephardic Jews are especially likely to have familial Mediterranean fever.

Physical Examination A meticulous physical examination should be repeated on a regular basis. All the vital signs are relevant. The temperature may be taken orally or rectally, but the site used should be consistent. Axillary temperatures are notoriously unreliable. Particular attention should be paid to daily (or sometimes more frequent) physical examination, which should continue until the diagnosis is certain and the anticipated response has been achieved. Special attention should be paid to the skin, lymph nodes, eyes, nail beds, cardiovascular system, chest, abdomen, musculoskeletal system, and nervous system. Rectal examination is imperative. The penis, prostate, scrotum, and testes should be examined carefully and the foreskin, if present, retracted. Pelvic examination must be part of every complete physical examination of a woman, with a search for such causes of fever as pelvic inflammatory disease and tubo-ovarian abscess.

Laboratory Tests Few signs and symptoms in medicine have as many diagnostic possibilities as fever. If the history, epidemiologic situation, or physical examination suggests more than a simple viral illness or streptococcal pharyngitis, then laboratory testing is indicated. The tempo and complexity of the workup will depend on the pace of the illness, diagnostic considerations, and the immune status of the host. If findings are focal or if the history, epidemiologic setting, or physical examination suggests certain diagnoses, the laboratory examination can be focused. If fever is undifferentiated, the diagnostic nets must be cast farther, and certain guidelines are indicated, as follows.

Clinical pathology The workup should include a complete blood count; a differential count should be performed manually or with an instrument sensitive to the identification of eosinophils, juvenile or band forms, toxic granulations, and Döhle bodies, the last three of which are suggestive of bacterial infection. Neutropenia may be present with some viral infections, particularly parvovirus B19 infection; drug reactions; systemic lupus erythematosus; typhoid; brucellosis; and infiltrative diseases of the bone marrow, including lymphoma, leukemia, tuberculosis, and histoplasmosis. Lymphocytosis may occur with typhoid, brucellosis, tuberculosis, and viral disease. Atypical lymphocytes are documented in many viral diseases, including infection with Epstein-Barr virus, cytomegalovirus, or HIV; dengue; rubella; varicella; measles; and viral hepatitis. This abnormality also occurs in serum sickness and toxoplasmosis. Monocytosis is a feature of typhoid, tuberculosis, brucellosis, and lymphoma. Eosinophilia may be associated with hypersensitivity drug reactions, Hodgkin's disease, adrenal insufficiency, and certain metazoan infections. If the febrile illness appears to be severe or is prolonged, the smear should be examined carefully for malarial or babesial pathogens (where appropriate) as well as for classic morphologic features, and the erythrocyte sedimentation rate should be determined. Urinalysis, with examination of urinary sediment, is indicated. It is axiomatic that any abnormal fluid accumulation (pleural, peritoneal, joint), even if previously sampled, merits reexamination in the presence of undiagnosed fever. Joint fluids should be examined for bacteria as well as crystals. Bone marrow biopsy (not simple aspiration) for histopathologic studies (as well as culture) is indicated when marrow infiltration by pathogens or tumor cells is possible. Stool should be inspected for occult blood; an inspection for fecal leukocytes, ova, or parasites also may be indicated.

Chemistry Electrolyte, glucose, blood urea nitrogen, and creatinine levels should be measured. Liver function tests are usually indicated if efforts to identify the cause of fever do not point to the involvement of another organ. Additional assessments (e.g., measurement of creatinine phosphokinase or amylase) can be added as the workup progresses.

Microbiology Smears and cultures of specimens from the throat, urethra, anus, cervix, and vagina should be assessed when there are no localizing findings or when findings suggest the involvement of the pelvis or the gastrointestinal tract. If respiratory tract infection is suspected, sputum evaluation (Gram's staining, staining for acid-fast bacilli, culture) is indicated. Cultures of blood, abnormal fluid collections, and urine are indicated when fever is thought to reflect more than uncomplicated viral illness. Cerebrospinal fluid should be examined and cultured if meningismus, severe headache, or a change in mental status is noted.

Radiology A chest x-ray is usually part of the evaluation for any significant febrile illness.

Outcome of Diagnostic Efforts In most cases of fever, either the patient recovers spontaneously or the history, physical examination, and initial screening laboratory studies lead to a diagnosis. When fever continues for 2 to 3 weeks, during which time repeat physical examinations and laboratory tests are unrevealing, the patient is provisionally diagnosed as having fever of unknown origin (Chap. 125).

℞ **TREATMENT The Decision to Treat Fever** Most fevers are associated with self-limited infections, most commonly of viral origin. In these cases, the general cause of the fever is easily identified. The routine use of antipyretics given automatically as "standing," "routine," or "prn" orders to treat low-grade fevers in adult patients on hospital wards is entirely unacceptable. This practice masks not only fever but also other important clinical indicators of a patient's course. The assumption underlying any decision to reduce fever with antipyretics is that there is no diagnostic benefit to be gained by allowing the fever to persist. However, there may be such a diagnostic benefit. For example, the daily highs and lows of normal temperature are exaggerated in most fevers, but the usual times of peak and trough temperatures may be reversed in typhoid fever and disseminated tuberculosis. Temperature-pulse dissociation (relative bradycardia) occurs in typhoid fever, brucellosis, leptospirosis, some drug-induced fevers, and factitious fever. In newborns, the elderly, patients with chronic renal failure, and patients taking glucocorticoids, fever may not be present despite infection, or core temperature may be hypothermic. Hypothermia is observed in patients with septic shock.

Some febrile diseases have characteristic patterns. With *relapsing* fevers, febrile episodes are separated by intervals of normal temperature; when paroxysms occur on the first and third days, the fever is called *tertian. Plasmodium vivax* causes tertian fevers. *Quartan* fevers are associated with paroxysms on the first and fourth days and are seen with *P. malariae*. Other relapsing fevers are related to *Borrelia* infections and rat-bite fever, which are both associated with days of fever followed by a several-day afebrile period and then a relapse of days of fever. Pel-Ebstein fever, with fevers lasting 3 to 10 days followed by afebrile periods of 3 to 10 days, is classic for Hodgkin's disease and other lymphomas. Another characteristic fever is that of cyclic neutropenia, in which fevers occur every 21 days and accompany the neutropenia. There is no periodicity of fever in patients with familial Mediterranean fever.

Mechanisms of Antipyretic Agents   The synthesis of PGE_2 depends on the constitutively expressed enzyme cyclooxygenase. The substrate for cyclooxygenase is arachidonic acid released from the cell membrane, and this release is the rate-limiting step in the synthesis of PGE_2. Inhibitors of cyclooxygenase are potent antipyretics. The antipyretic potency of various drugs is directly correlated with the inhibition of brain cyclooxygenase. Acetaminophen is a poor cyclooxygenase inhibitor in peripheral tissue and is without noteworthy anti-inflammatory activity; in the brain, however, acetaminophen is oxidized by the p450 cytochrome system, and the oxidized form inhibits cyclooxygenase activity.

Oral aspirin and acetaminophen are equally effective in reducing fever in humans. Nonsteroidal anti-inflammatory agents (NSAIDs) such as indomethacin and ibuprofen are also excellent antipyretics. Chronic high-dose therapy with antipyretics such as aspirin or the NSAIDs used in arthritis does not reduce normal core body temperature. Thus, PGE_2 appears to play no role in normal thermoregulation.

As effective antipyretics, glucocorticoids act at two levels. First, similar to the cyclooxygenase inhibitors, glucocorticoids reduce PGE_2 synthesis by inhibiting the activity of phospholipase A_2, which is needed to release arachidonic acid from the cell membrane. Second, glucocorticoids block the transcription of the mRNA for the pyrogenic cytokines.

Drugs that interfere with vasoconstriction (phenothiazines, for example) can act as antipyretics, as can drugs that block muscle contractions. However, these agents are not true antipyretics since they can also reduce core temperature independently of hypothalamic control.

Indications and Regimens for the Treatment of Fever   The objectives in treating fever are first to reduce the elevated hypothalamic set point and second to facilitate heat loss. There is no evidence that fever itself facilitates the recovery from infection or acts as an adjuvant to the immune system. In fact, peripheral PGE_2 production is a potent immunosuppressant. Hence, treating fever and its symptoms does no harm and does not slow the resolution of common viral and bacterial infections. Reducing fever with antipyretics also reduces systemic symptoms of headache, myalgias, and arthralgias.

Oral aspirin and NSAIDs effectively reduce fever but can adversely affect platelets and the gastrointestinal tract. Therefore, acetaminophen is preferred to all of these agents as an antipyretic. In children, acetaminophen must be used because aspirin increases the risk of Reye's syndrome. If the patient cannot take oral antipyretics, parenteral preparations of NSAIDs and rectal suppository preparations of various antipyretics can be used.

Treatment of fever in some patient groups is recommended. Fever increases the demand for oxygen (i.e., for every increase of 1°C over 37°C, there is a 13% increase in oxygen consumption) and can aggravate preexisting cardiac, cerebrovascular, or pulmonary insufficiency. Elevated temperature can induce mental changes in patients with organic brain disease. Children with a history of febrile or nonfebrile seizure should be aggressively treated to reduce fever, although it is unclear what triggers the febrile seizure and there is no correlation between absolute temperature elevation and onset of a febrile seizure in susceptible children.

In hyperpyrexia, the use of cooling blankets facilitates the reduction of temperature; however, cooling blankets should not be used without oral antipyretics. In hyperpyretic patients with central nervous system disease or trauma, reducing core temperature mitigates the ill effects of high temperature on the brain.

Treating Hyperthermia   A high core temperature in a patient with an appropriate history (e.g., environmental heat exposure or treatment with anticholinergic or neuroleptic drugs, tricyclic antidepressants, succinylcholine, or halothane) along with appropriate clinical findings (dry skin, hallucinations, delirium, pupil dilation, muscle rigidity, and/or elevated levels of creatine phosphokinase) suggests hyperthermia. The attempt to lower the already normal hypothalamic set point is of little use. Physical cooling with sponging, fans, cooling blankets, and even ice baths should be initiated immediately in conjunction with the administration of intravenous fluids and appropriate pharmacologic agents (see below). If insufficient cooling is achieved by external means, internal cooling can be achieved by gastric or peritoneal lavage with iced saline. In extreme circumstances, hemodialysis or even cardiopulmonary bypass with cooling of blood may be performed.

Malignant hyperthermia should be treated immediately with cessation of anesthesia and intravenous administration of dantrolene sodium. The recommended dose of dantrolene is 1 to 2.5 mg/kg of body weight given intravenously every 6 h for at least 24 to 48 h—until oral dantrolene can be administered, if needed. Procainamide should also be administered to patients with malignant hyperthermia because of the likelihood of ventricular fibrillation in this syndrome. Dantrolene at similar doses is indicated in the neuroleptic malignant syndrome and in drug-induced hyperthermia and may even be useful in the hyperthermia of thyrotoxicosis. The neuroleptic malignant syndrome may also be treated with bromocriptine, levodopa, amantadine, or nifedipine or by induction of muscle paralysis with curare and pancuronium. Tricyclic antidepressant overdose may be treated with physostigmine.

BIBLIOGRAPHY

ATKINS E: Pathogenesis of fever. Physiol Rev 40:580, 1960

BREDER CD et al: Interleukin-1 immunoreactive innervation of the human hypothalamus. Science 240:321, 1988

COCEANI F et al: Prostaglandin E_2 fever: A continuing debate. Yale J Biol Med 59:169, 1986

FLOWER RJ et al: Inhibition of prostaglandin synthetase in brain explains the anti-pyretic activity of paracetamol (4-acetamidophenol). Nature 240:410, 1972

MACKOWIAK PA: Carl Reinhold August Wunderlich and the evolution of clinical thermometry. Clin Infect Dis 18:458, 1994

———: Concepts of fever. Arch Intern Med 158:1870, 1998

——— et al: A critical appraisal of 98.6°F, the upper limit of the normal body temperature, and other legacies of Carl Reinhold August Wunderlich. JAMA 268:1578, 1992

USHIKUBI F et al: Impaired febrile response in mice lacking the prostaglandin E receptor subtype EP3. Nature 395:281, 1998

WOLFF SM: Biological effects of bacterial endotoxins in man. J Infect Dis 128:733, 1973

YANG RB et al: Toll-like receptor-2 mediates lipopolysaccharide-induced cellular signalling. Nature 395:284, 1998

18

Elaine T. Kaye, Kenneth M. Kaye

FEVER AND RASH

The acutely ill patient with fever and rash often presents a diagnostic challenge for physicians. The distinctive appearance of an eruption in concert with a clinical syndrome may facilitate a prompt diagnosis and the institution of life-saving therapy or critical infection-control interventions.

Approach to the Patient

A thorough history of patients with fever and rash includes the following relevant information: immune status, medications taken within the previous month, specific travel history, immunization status, exposure to domestic pets and other animals, history of animal or arthropod bites, existence of cardiac abnormalities, presence of prosthetic material, recent exposure to ill individuals, and exposure to sexually transmitted diseases. The history should also include the site of onset of the rash and its direction and rate of spread.

A thorough physical examination entails close attention to the rash, with an assessment and precise definition of its salient features. First, it is critical to determine the *type* of lesions that make up the eruption. *Macules* are flat lesions defined by an area of changed color (i.e., a blanchable erythema). *Papules* are raised, solid lesions <5 mm in diameter; *plaques* are lesions >5 mm in diameter with a flat, plateau-like surface; and *nodules* are lesions >5 mm in diameter with a more rounded configuration. *Wheals* (urticaria, hives) are papules or plaques that are pale pink and may appear annular (ringlike) as they enlarge; classic (nonvasculitic) wheals are transient, lasting only 24 to 48 h in any defined area. *Vesicles* (<5 mm) and *bullae* (>5 mm) are circumscribed, elevated lesions containing fluid. *Pustules* are raised lesions containing purulent exudate; vesicular processes such as varicella or herpes simplex may evolve to pustules. *Nonpalpable purpura* is a flat lesion that is due to bleeding into the skin; if <3 mm in diameter, the purpuric lesions are termed *petechiae*; if >3 mm, they are termed *ecchymoses*. *Palpable purpura* is a raised lesion that is due to inflammation of the vessel wall (vasculitis) with subsequent hemorrhage. An *ulcer* is a defect in the skin extending at least into the upper layer of the dermis, and an *eschar* (tâche noire) is a necrotic lesion covered with a black crust.

Other pertinent features of rashes include their *configuration* (i.e., annular or target), the *arrangement* of their lesions, and their *distribution* (i.e., central or peripheral). →*For further discussion, see Chaps. 55 and 57.*

CLASSIFICATION OF RASH This chapter reviews rashes that reflect systemic disease but does not include localized skin eruptions (i.e., cellulitis, impetigo) that may also be associated with fever (Chap. 128). Rashes are classified herein on the basis of the morphology and distribution of lesions. For practical purposes, this classification system is based on the most typical disease presentations. However, morphology may vary as rashes evolve, and the presentation of diseases with rashes is subject to many variations (Chap. 57). For instance, the classic petechial rash of Rocky Mountain spotted fever (RMSF) may initially consist of blanchable erythematous macules distributed peripherally; at times, the rash associated with RMSF may not be predominantly acral, or a rash may not develop at all.

Diseases with fever and rash may be classified by type of eruption: centrally distributed maculopapular, peripheral, confluent desquamative erythematous, vesiculobullous, urticarial, nodular, purpuric, ulcerated, or eschars (Table 18-1). For a more detailed discussion of each disease associated with a rash, the reader is referred to the chapter dealing with that specific disease. (Reference chapters and color plates are cited in the text and listed in Table 18-1.)

Centrally Distributed Maculopapular Eruptions Centrally distributed rashes, in which lesions are primarily truncal, are the most common type of eruption. The rash of *measles* (rubeola) starts at the hairline 2 to 3 days into the illness and moves down the body, sparing the palms and soles (Chap. 194). It begins as discrete erythematous lesions, which become confluent as the rash spreads. Koplik's spots (1- to 2-mm white or bluish lesions with an erythematous halo on the buccal mucosa) are pathognomonic for measles and are generally seen during the first 2 days of symptoms. They should not be confused with Fordyce's spots (ectopic sebaceous glands), which have no erythematous halos and are found in the mouth of healthy individuals. Koplik's spots may briefly overlap with the measles exanthem.

German measles (rubella) also spreads from the hairline downward; unlike that of measles, however, the rash of rubella tends to clear from originally affected areas as it migrates and may be pruritic (Chap. 195). Forchheimer spots (palatal petechiae) may develop but are nonspecific since they also develop in mononucleosis (Chap. 184) and scarlet fever (Chap. 140). Postauricular and suboccipital adenopathy and arthritis are common among adults with German measles. Exposure of pregnant women to ill individuals should be avoided, as rubella causes severe congenital abnormalities. Numerous strains of enteroviruses (Chap. 193), primarily echoviruses and coxsackieviruses, cause nonspecific syndromes of fever and eruptions that may mimic rubella or measles. Patients with infectious mononucleosis caused by Epstein-Barr virus or with primary infection caused by HIV (Chap. 309) may exhibit pharyngitis, lymphadenopathy, and a nonspecific maculopapular exanthem.

The rash of *erythema infectiosum* (fifth disease), which is caused by human parvovirus B19, primarily affects children 3 to 12 years old; it develops after fever has resolved as a bright blanchable erythema on the cheeks ("slapped cheeks") with perioral pallor (Chap. 187). A more diffuse rash (often pruritic) appears the next day on the trunk and extremities and then rapidly develops into a lacy reticular eruption that may wax and wane (especially with temperature change) over 3 weeks. Adults with fifth disease often have arthritis, and fetal hydrops can develop in association with this condition in pregnant women.

Exanthem subitum (roseola) is most common among children under 3 years of age (Chap. 185). As in erythema infectiosum, the rash usually appears after fever has subsided. It consists of 2- to 3-mm rose-pink macules and papules that rarely coalesce, occur initially on the trunk and sometimes on the extremities (sparing the face), and fade within 2 days.

Though drug reactions have many manifestations, including urticaria, exanthematous *drug-induced eruptions* (Chap. 59) are most common and are often difficult to distinguish from viral exanthems. Eruptions elicited by drugs are usually more intensely erythematous and pruritic than viral exanthems, but this distinction is not reliable. A history of new medications and an absence of prostration may help to distinguish a drug-related rash from an eruption of another etiology. Rashes may persist for up to 2 weeks after administration of the offending agent is discontinued. Certain populations are more prone than others to drug rashes. Of HIV-infected patients, 50 to 60% develop a rash in response to sulfa drugs; 50 to 100% of patients with mononucleosis due to Epstein-Barr virus develop a rash when given ampicillin.

Rickettsial illnesses (Chap. 177) should be considered in the evaluation of individuals with centrally distributed maculopapular eruptions. The usual setting for *epidemic typhus* is a site of war or natural disaster in which people are exposed to body lice. A diagnosis of recrudescent typhus should be considered in European immigrants to the United States. However, an indigenous form of typhus, presumably transmitted by flying squirrels, has been reported in the southeastern United States. *Endemic typhus* or *leptospirosis* (the latter caused by a spirochete; Chap. 174) may be seen in urban environments where rodents proliferate. Outside the United States, other rickettsial diseases cause a spotted-fever syndrome and should be considered in residents

Table 18-1   Diseases Associated with Fever and Rash

Disease	Etiology	Description	Group Affected/ Epidemiologic Factors	Clinical Syndrome	Chapter/Color Atlas Reference
CENTRALLY DISTRIBUTED MACULOPAPULAR ERUPTIONS					
Measles (rubeola, first disease)	Paramyxovirus	Discrete lesions that become confluent as rash spreads from hairline downward, sparing palms and soles; lasts ≥3 days; Koplik's spots	Nonimmune individuals	Cough, conjunctivitis, coryza, severe prostration	194
German measles (rubella, third disease)	Togavirus	Spreads from hairline downward, clearing as it spreads; Forchheimer spots	Nonimmune individuals	Adenopathy, arthritis	195
Erythema infectiosum (fifth disease)	Human parvovirus B19	Bright-red "slapped-cheek" appearance followed by diffuse lacy reticular rash that waxes and wanes over 3 weeks	Most common in children aged 3–12 years; occurs in winter and spring	Mild fever; arthritis in adults	187/IID-40
Exanthem subitum (roseola, sixth disease)	Human herpesvirus 6	Diffuse maculopapular eruption (sparing face); resolves within 2 days	Usually affects children <3 years old	Rash following resolution of fever; similar to Boston exanthem (echovirus 16)	185
Primary HIV infection	HIV	Nonspecific diffuse macules and papules; may be urticarial; oral or genital ulcers in some cases	Individuals recently infected with HIV	Pharyngitis, adenopathy, arthralgias	309
Infectious mononucleosis	Epstein-Barr virus	Diffuse maculopapular eruption (10–15% of cases; 90% if ampicillin is given); urticaria in some cases; periorbital edema (50%); palatal petechiae (25%)	Adolescents, young adults	Hepatosplenomegaly, pharyngitis, cervical lymphadenopathy, atypical lymphocytosis, heterophile antibody	184
Other viral exanthems	Echoviruses 2, 4, 9, 11, 16, 19, and 25; coxsackieviruses A9, B1, and B5	Skin findings mimicking rubella or measles	Affect children more commonly than adults	Nonspecific viral syndromes	193
Exanthematous drug-induced eruption	Drugs (antibiotics, anticonvulsants, diuretics, etc.)	Intensely pruritic, bright-red macules and papules, symmetric on trunk and extremities; may become confluent	Occurs 2–3 d after exposure in those previously sensitized; otherwise, after 2–3 weeks (but can occur anytime, even after drug is discontinued)	Variable findings: fever and eosinophilia	59
Epidemic typhus	*Rickettsia prowazekii*	Maculopapular eruption appears in axillae, spreads to trunk and later to extremities; usually spares face, palms, soles; evolves from blanchable macules to confluent eruption with petechiae; rash evanescent in recrudescent typhus (Brill-Zinsser disease)	Exposure to body lice; occurrence of recrudescent typhus as relapse after 30–50 years	Headache, myalgias; 10–40% mortality if untreated; milder clinical presentation in recrudescent form	177
Endemic (murine) typhus	*Rickettsia typhi*	Maculopapular eruption, usually sparing palms, soles	Exposure to rat or cat fleas	Headache, myalgias	177
Scrub typhus	*Rickettsia tsutsugamushi*	Diffuse macular rash starting on trunk; eschar at site of mite bite	Endemic in South Pacific, Australia, Asia; transmitted by mites	Headache, myalgias, regional adenopathy; mortality up to 30% if untreated	177
Rickettsial spotted fevers	*Rickettsia conorii* (boutonneuse fever), *Rickettsia australis* (North Queensland tick typhus), *Rickettsia sibirica* (Siberian tick typhus)	Eschar at site of bite; maculopapular (rarely, vesicular and petechial) eruption on proximal extremities, spreading to trunk and face	Exposure to ticks; *R. conorii* in Mediterranean region, India, Africa; *R. australis* in Australia; *R. sibirica* in Siberia, Mongolia	Headache, myalgias, regional adenopathy	177
Ehrlichiosis	*Ehrlichia* spp.	Maculopapular eruption (40% of cases), involves trunk and extremities; may be petechial	Tick-borne; most common in U.S. Southeast and southern Midwest	Headache, myalgias, leukopenia	177
Leptospirosis	*Leptospira interrogans*	Maculopapular eruption; conjunctivitis; scleral hemorrhage in some cases	Exposure to water contaminated with animal urine	Myalgias; aseptic meningitis; *fulminant form*: icterohemorrhagic fever (Weil's disease)	174

(continued)

Table 18-1—*(continued)*

Disease	Etiology	Description	Group Affected/ Epidemiologic Factors	Clinical Syndrome	Chapter/Color Atlas Reference
Lyme disease	*Borrelia burgdorferi*	Papule expanding to erythematous annular lesion with central clearing (ECM; average diameter, 15 cm), sometimes with concentric rings, sometimes with indurated or vesicular center; multiple secondary ECM lesions in some cases	Bite of tick vector	Headache, myalgias, chills, photophobia occurring acutely; CNS disease, myocardial disease, arthritis weeks to months later in some cases	176/IID-46
Typhoid fever	*Salmonella typhi*	Blanchable erythematous macules and papules, 2–4 mm, usually on trunk (rose spots)	Ingestion of contaminated food or water (rare in U.S.)	Variable abdominal pain and diarrhea; headache, myalgias, hepatosplenomegaly	156
Rat-bite fever (sodoku)	*Spirillum minus*	Eschar at site of bite; then blotchy violaceous or red-brown rash involving trunk and extremities	Rate bite; primarily found in Asia; rare in U.S.	Regional adenopathy, recurrent fevers if untreated	127
Relapsing fever	*Borrelia* spp.	Central rash at end of febrile episode; petechiae in some cases	Exposure to ticks or body lice	Recurrent fever, headache, myalgias, hepatosplenomegaly	175
Erythema marginatum (rheumatic fever)	Group A *Streptococcus*	Erythematous annular papules and plaques occurring as polycyclic lesions in waves over trunk, proximal extremities; evolving and resolving within hours	Patients with rheumatic fever	Pharyngitis preceding polyarthritis, carditis, subcutaneous nodules, chorea	235
Systemic lupus erythematosus	Autoimmune disease	Macular and papular erythema, often in sun-exposed areas; discoid lupus lesions (local atrophy, scale, pigmentary changes); periungual telangiectasis; malar rash; vasculitis sometimes causing urticaria, palpable purpura; oral erosions in some cases	Most common in young to middle-aged women; flares precipitated by sun exposure	Arthritis; cardiac, pulmonary, renal, hematologic, and vasculitic disease	311/IIE-61, IIE-62
Still's disease	Autoimmune disease	Transient 2- to 5-mm erythematous papules appearing at height of fever on trunk, proximal extremities; lesions evanescent	Children and young adults	High spiking fever, polyarthritis, splenomegaly; erythrocyte sedimentation rate, >100 mm/h	326
Arcanobacterial pharyngitis	*Arcanobacterium (Corynebacterium) haemolyticum*	Diffuse, erythematous, maculopapular eruption involving trunk and proximal extremities; may desquamate	Children and young adults	Exudative pharyngitis, lymphadenopathy	141

PERIPHERAL ERUPTIONS

Disease	Etiology	Description	Group Affected/ Epidemiologic Factors	Clinical Syndrome	Chapter/Color Atlas Reference
Chronic meningococcemia, disseminated gonococcal infection[a]	—	—	—	—	146, 147
RMSF	*Rickettsia rickettsii*	Rash beginning on wrists and ankles and spreading centripetally; appears on palms and soles later in disease; lesion evolution from blanchable macules to petechiae	Tick vector; widespread but more common in southeastern and southwest-central U.S.	Headache, myalgias, abdominal pain; mortality up to 40% if untreated	177/IID-45
Secondary syphilis	*Treponema pallidum*	Coincident primary chancre in 10% of cases; copper-colored, scaly papular eruption, diffuse but prominent on palms and soles; rash never vesicular in adults; condyloma latum, mucous patches, and alopecia in some cases	Sexually transmitted	Fever, constitutional symptoms	172/IID-48, IID-50
Atypical measles	Paramyxovirus	Maculopapular eruption beginning on distal extremities and spreading centripetally; may evolve into vesicles or petechiae; edema of extremities; Koplik's spots absent	Individuals contracting measles who received killed measles vaccine between 1963 and 1967 in U.S.	Headache, nodular pneumonia	194
Hand-foot-and-mouth disease	Coxsackievirus A16	Tender vesicles, erosions in mouth; 0.25-cm papules on hands and feet with rim of erythema evolving into tender vesicles	Summer and fall; primarily children under 10 years; multiple family members	Transient fever	193/IID-39

(continued)

Table 18-1 Diseases Associated with Fever and Rash—*(continued)*

Disease	Etiology	Description	Group Affected/ Epidemiologic Factors	Clinical Syndrome	Chapter/Color Atlas Reference
Erythema multiforme	Drugs, infection, idiopathic causes	Target lesions (central erythema surrounded by area of clearing and another rim of erythema) up to 2 cm; symmetric on knees, elbows, palms, soles; may become diffuse; may involve mucosal surfaces	Drug intake (i.e., sulfa, phenytoin, penicillin); herpes simplex or *Mycoplasma pneumoniae* infection	Varies with predisposing factor	—,[b] IIE-67
Rat-bite fever (Haverhill fever)	*Streptobacillus moniliformis*	Maculopapular eruption over palms, soles, and extremities, tends to be more severe at joints; eruption may become generalized; may be purpuric; may desquamate	Rat bite, ingestion of contaminated food	Myalgias; arthritis (50%); fever recurrence in some cases	127
Bacterial endocarditis	*Streptococcus, Staphylococcus,* etc.	*Subacute course:* Osler's nodes (tender pink nodules on finger or toe pads); petechiae on skin and mucosa; splinter hemorrhages. *Acute course (S. aureus):* Janeway lesions (painless erythematous or hemorrhagic macules, usually on palms and soles)	Abnormal heart valve, intravenous drug use	New heart murmur	126/IID-58

CONFLUENT DESQUAMATIVE ERYTHEMAS

Disease	Etiology	Description	Group Affected/ Epidemiologic Factors	Clinical Syndrome	Chapter/Color Atlas Reference
Scarlet fever (second disease)	Group A *Streptococcus* (pyrogenic exotoxins A, B, C)	Diffuse blanchable erythema beginning on face and spreading to trunk and extremities; circumoral pallor; "sandpaper" texture to skin; accentuation of linear erythema in skin folds (Pastia's lines); enanthem of white evolving into red "strawberry" tongue; desquamation in second week	Most common in children aged 2–10 years; usually follows group A streptococcal pharyngitis	Fever, pharyngitis, headache	140
Kawasaki disease	Idiopathic causes	Rash similar to scarlet fever (scarlatiniform) or erythema multiforme; fissuring of lips, strawberry tongue; conjunctivitis; edema of hands, feet; desquamation later in disease	Children under 8 years	Cervical adenopathy, pharyngitis, coronary artery vasculitis	57, 317
Streptococcal toxic shock syndrome	Group A *Streptococcus* (associated with pyrogenic exotoxin A or certain M types)	When present, rash often scarlatiniform	May occur in setting of severe group A streptococcal infections, such as necrotizing fasciitis, bacteremia, pneumonia	Multiorgan failure, hypotension; 30% mortality rate	140
Staphylococcal toxic shock syndrome	*S. aureus* (toxic shock syndrome toxin 1, enterotoxin B or C)	Diffuse erythema involving palms; pronounced erythema of mucosal surfaces, conjunctivitis; desquamation 7–10 days into illness	Colonization with toxin-producing *S. aureus*	Fever >39°C (102°F), hypotension, multiorgan dysfunction	139
Staphylococcal scalded-skin syndrome	*S. aureus,* phage group II	Diffuse tender erythema, often with bullae and desquamation; Nikolsky's sign	Colonization with toxin-producing *S. aureus*; occurs in children under 10 (termed "Ritter's disease" in neonates) or adults with renal dysfunction	Irritability; nasal or conjunctival secretions	139
Exfoliative erythroderma syndrome	Underlying psoriasis, eczema, drug eruption, mycosis fungoides	Diffuse erythema (often scaling) interspersed with lesions of underlying condition	Usually occurs in adults over age 50; more common in men	Fever, chills (i.e., difficulty with thermoregulation); lymphadenopathy	56, 59
Toxic epidermal necrolysis	Drugs, other causes (infection, neoplasm, graft-vs.-host disease)	Diffuse erythema or target-like lesions progressing to bullae, with sloughing and necrosis of entire epidermis; Nikolsky's sign	Uncommon in children; more common in patients with HIV infection or graft-vs.-host disease	Dehydration, sepsis sometimes resulting from lack of normal skin integrity; 25% mortality	59

(continued)

Table 18-1—*(continued)*

Disease	Etiology	Description	Group Affected/ Epidemiologic Factors	Clinical Syndrome	Chapter/Color Atlas Reference
VESICULOBULLOUS ERUPTIONS					
Hand-foot-and-mouth syndrome[c]; staphylococcal scalded-skin syndrome, toxic epidermal necrolysis[d]	—	—	—	—	—[b]
Varicella (chickenpox)	Varicella-zoster virus	Macules (2–3 mm) evolving into papules, then vesicles (sometimes umbilicated), on an erythematous base ("dewdrops on a rose petal"); pustules then forming and crusting; lesions appearing in crops; may involve scalp, mouth; intensely pruritic	Usually affects children; 10% of adults susceptible; most common in late winter and spring	Malaise; mild disease in healthy children; more severe disease with complications in adults and immuno-compromised children	183/IID-36
Disseminated herpesvirus infection	Varicella-zoster virus or herpes simplex virus (HSV)	Individual lesions similar for varicella-zoster and HSV; *zoster cutaneous dissemination*: >25 lesions extending outside involved dermatome; *HSV*: extensive, progressive mucocutaneous lesions in some cases; HSV lesions sometimes disseminate in eczematous skin (eczema herpeticum); HSV visceral dissemination may occur with only limited skin lesions	Immunosuppressed individuals, eczema	Visceral organ involvement (especially of liver) may occur	183, 373/IID-37
Rickettsialpox	*Rickettsia akari*	Eschar found at site of mite bite; generalized rash involving face, trunk, extremities; may involve palms and soles; <100 papules and plaques (2–10 mm); top of lesions develop vesicles that may evolve into pustules	Seen in urban settings; transmitted by mouse mites	Headache, myalgias, regional adenopathy; mild disease	177
Disseminated *Vibrio vulnificus* infection	*V. vulnificus*	Erythematous lesions evolving into hemorrhagic bullae and then into necrotic ulcers	Patients with cirrhosis, diabetes, renal failure; exposure by ingestion of contaminated saltwater seafood	Hypotension; 50% mortality	159
Ecthyma gangrenosum	*Pseudomonas aeruginosa*, other gram-negative rods, fungi	Indurated plaque evolving into hemorrhagic bulla or pustule that sloughs, resulting in eschar formation; erythematous halo; most common in axillary, groin, perianal regions	Usually affects neutropenic patients; occurs in up to 28% of individuals with *Pseudomonas* bacteremia	Clinical signs of sepsis	155/IID-57C
URTICARIAL ERUPTIONS					
Urticarial vasculitis	Serum sickness, often due to infection (including hepatitis B, enterovirus, parasitic), drugs (including penicillins, sulfonamides, salicylates, barbiturates); connective-tissue disease; idiopathic causes	Erythematous, circumscribed areas of edema; occasionally indurated; pruritic or burning; lesions sometimes purpuric; individual lesions lasting up to 5 days	In serum sickness, occurs 8–14 days after antigen exposure in nonsensitized individuals; may occur within 36 h in sensitized individuals	Malaise, lymphadenopathy, myalgias, arthralgias	317[b]/IIA-14A
NODULAR ERUPTIONS					
Disseminated infection	Fungi (e.g., candidiasis, histoplasmosis, cryptococcosis, sporotrichosis, coccidioidomycosis); mycobacteria	Subcutaneous nodules (up to 3 cm); fluctuance, draining common with mycobacteria; necrotic nodules (extremities, periorbital or nasal regions) common with *Aspergillus*, *Mucor*	Immunocompromised hosts (i.e., bone marrow transplant recipients, patients undergoing chemotherapy, HIV-infected patients, alcoholics)	Features vary with organism	—[b]

(continued)

Table 18-1 Diseases Associated with Fever and Rash—*(continued)*

Disease	Etiology	Description	Group Affected/ Epidemiologic Factors	Clinical Syndrome	Chapter/Color Atlas Reference
Erythema nodosum (septal panniculitis)	Infections (e.g., streptococcal, fungal, mycobacterial, yersinial); drugs (e.g., sulfas, penicillins, oral contraceptives); sarcoidosis; idiopathic causes	Large, violaceous, nonulcerative, subcutaneous nodules; exquisitely tender; usually on lower legs but also on upper extremities	More common in females aged 15–30	Arthralgias (50%); features vary with associated condition	—[b], IIE-70
Sweet's syndrome (acute febrile neutrophilic dermatosis)	Yersinial infection; lymphoproliferative disorders; idiopathic causes	Tender red or blue edematous nodules giving impression of vesiculation; usually on face, neck, upper extremities; when on lower extremities, may mimic erythema nodosum	More common in women and in persons aged 30–60; 20% of cases associated with malignancy (men and women equally affected in this group)	Headache, arthralgias, leukocytosis	57
Bacillary angiomatosis	*Bartonella henselae* or *Bartonella quintana*	Many forms, including erythematous, smooth vascular nodules; friable, exophytic lesions; erythematous plaques (may be dry, scaly); subcutaneous nodules (may be erythematous)	Usually in HIV infection	Peliosis of liver and spleen in some cases; lesions may involve multiple organs; bacteremia	163

PURPURIC ERUPTIONS

Disease	Etiology	Description	Group Affected/ Epidemiologic Factors	Clinical Syndrome	Chapter/Color Atlas Reference
RMSF, rat-bite fever, endocarditis[c]; epidemic typhus[e]	—	—	—	—	—[b]
Acute meningococcemia	*Neisseria meningitidis*	Petechiae rapidly becoming numerous, sometimes enlarging and becoming vesicular; trunk, extremities most commonly involved; may appear on face, hands, feet; may include purpura fulminans reflecting DIC (see below)	Most common in children, individuals with asplenia or terminal complement component deficiency (C5-C8)	Hypotension, meningitis (sometimes preceded by upper respiratory infection)	146/IID-44
Purpura fulminans	Severe DIC	Large ecchymoses with sharply irregular shapes evolving into hemorrhagic bullae and then into black necrotic lesions	Individuals with sepsis (e.g., involving *N. meningitidis*), malignancy, or massive trauma; asplenic patients at high risk for sepsis	Hypotension	124, 146
Chronic meningococcemia	*N. meningitidis*	Variety of recurrent eruptions, including pink maculopapular; nodular (usually on lower extremities); petechial (sometimes developing vesicular centers); purpuric areas with pale blue-gray centers	Individuals with complement deficiencies	Fevers, sometimes intermittent; arthritis, myalgias, headache	146
Disseminated gonococcal infection	*Neisseria gonorrhoeae*	Papules (1–5 mm) evolving over 1–2 days into hemorrhagic pustules with gray necrotic centers; hemorrhagic bullae occurring rarely; lesions (usually fewer than 40) distributed peripherally near joints (more commonly on upper extremities)	Sexually active individuals (more often females), some with complement deficiency	Low-grade fever, tenosynovitis, arthritis	147/IID-60
Enteroviral petechial rash	Usually echovirus 9 or coxsackievirus A9	Disseminated petechial lesions (may also be maculopapular, vesicular, or urticarial)	Often occurs in outbreaks	Pharyngitis, headache; aseptic meningitis with echovirus 9	193
Viral hemorrhagic fever	Arboviruses and arenaviruses	Petechial rash	Residence in or travel to endemic areas	Triad of fever, shock, hemorrhage from mucosa or gastrointestinal tract	198, 199
Thrombotic thrombocytopenic purpura	Idiopathic causes	Petechiae	Usually affects young adults; more common in women; hemolytic-uremic syndrome seen in children after gastroenteritis caused by *Escherichia coli* O157:H7	Fever, hemolytic anemia, thrombocytopenia, neurologic and renal dysfunction; coagulation studies normal	57, 108, 116

(continued)

Table 18-1—*(continued)*

Disease	Etiology	Description	Group Affected/ Epidemiologic Factors	Clinical Syndrome	Chapter/Color Atlas Reference
Cutaneous small-vessel vasculitis (leukocytoclastic vasculitis)	Infections (including group A *Streptococcus*, viral hepatitis), drugs, chemicals, food allergens, idiopathic causes	Palpable purpuric lesions appearing in crops on legs or other dependent areas; may become vesicular or ulcerative; usually resolve over 3–4 weeks	Occurs in a wide spectrum of diseases, including connective tissue disease, cryoglobulinemia, malignancy, Henoch-Schönlein purpura (HSP; more common in children)	Fever, malaise, arthralgias, myalgias; systemic vasculitis in some cases; renal, joint, and gastrointestinal involvement commonly seen in HSP	57/IIE-71
ERUPTIONS WITH ULCERS AND/OR ESCHARS					
Scrub typhus, rickettsial spotted fevers, rat-bite fever[e]; rickettsialpox, ecthyma gangrenosum[f]	—	—	—	—	—[b]
Tularemia	*Francisella tularensis*	Ulceroglandular form. erythematous, tender papule evolves into necrotic, tender ulcer with raised borders; in 35% of cases, eruptions (maculopapular, vesiculopapular, acneiform, urticarial, erythema nodosum, or erythema multiforme) may occur	Exposure to ticks, biting flies, infected animals	Fever, headache, lymphadenopathy	161
Anthrax	*Bacillus anthracis*	Pruritic papule enlarging and evolving into a 1- to 3-cm painless ulcer surrounded by vesicles and then developing a central eschar with edema; residual scar	Exposure to infected animals or animal products	Lymphadenopathy, headache	141

[a] See "Purpuric eruptions."
[b] See etiology-specific chapters.
[c] See "Peripheral eruptions."
[d] See "Confluent desquamative erythemas."

[e] See "Centrally distributed maculopapular eruptions."
[f] See "Vesiculobullous eruptions."
NOTE: DIC, disseminated intravascular coagulation; ECM, erythema chronicum migrans; RMSF, Rocky Mountain spotted fever.

of or travelers to endemic areas. Similarly, *typhoid fever*, a nonrickettsial disease caused by *Salmonella typhi* (Chap. 156), is usually acquired during travel outside the United States.

Some centrally distributed maculopapular eruptions have distinctive features. Erythema chronicum migrans (ECM), the rash of Lyme disease (Chap. 176), typically manifests as singular or multiple annular plaques. Untreated ECM lesions usually fade within a month but may persist for more than a year. *Erythema marginatum*, the rash of acute rheumatic fever (Chap. 235), has a distinctive pattern of enlarging and shifting transient annular lesions.

Collagen vascular diseases may cause fever and rash. Patients with *systemic lupus erythematosus* (Chap. 311) typically develop a sharply defined, erythematous eruption in a butterfly distribution on the cheeks (malar rash) as well as many other skin manifestations. *Still's disease* (Chap. 326) manifests as an evanescent salmon-colored rash on the trunk and proximal extremities that coincides with fever spikes.

Peripheral Eruptions These rashes are alike in that they are most prominent peripherally or begin in peripheral (acral) areas before spreading centripetally. Early diagnosis and therapy are critical in RMSF (Chap. 177) because of its grave prognosis if untreated. Lesions evolve from macular to petechial, start on the wrists and ankles, spread centripetally, and appear on the palms and soles only later in the disease. The rash of *secondary syphilis* (Chap. 172), which may be diffuse but is prominent on the palms and soles, should be considered in the differential diagnosis of pityriasis rosea, especially in sexually active patients. *Atypical measles* (Chap. 194) is seen in individuals contracting measles who received the killed measles vaccine between 1963 and 1967 in the United States and who were not subsequently protected with the live vaccine. *Hand-foot-and-mouth disease* (Chap. 193) is distinguished by tender vesicles distributed peripherally and in the mouth; outbreaks commonly occur within families. The classic target lesions of *erythema multiforme* appear symmetrically on the elbows, knees, palms, and soles. In relatively severe cases, these lesions may spread diffusely and involve mucosal surfaces. Lesions may develop on the hands and feet in *endocarditis* (Chap. 126).

Confluent Desquamative Erythemas These eruptions consist of diffuse erythema frequently followed by desquamation. The eruptions caused by group A *Streptococcus* or *Staphylococcus aureus* are toxin mediated. Certain disease features may provide diagnostic clues. *Scarlet fever* (Chap. 140) usually follows pharyngitis; patients have a facial flush, a "strawberry" tongue, and accentuated petechiae in body folds (Pastia's lines). *Kawasaki disease* (Chaps. 57 and 317) presents in the pediatric population as fissuring of the lips, a strawberry tongue, conjunctivitis, adenopathy, and sometimes cardiac abnormalities. *Streptococcal toxic shock syndrome* (Chap. 140) manifests with hypotension, multiorgan failure, and often a severe group A streptococcal infection (e.g., necrotizing fasciitis). *Staphylococcal toxic shock syndrome* (Chap. 139) also presents with hypotension and multiorgan failure, but usually only *S. aureus* colonization—not a severe *S. aureus* infection—is documented. *Staphylococcal scalded-skin syndrome* (Chap. 139) is seen primarily in children and in immunocompromised adults. Generalized erythema is often evident during the prodrome of fever and malaise; profound tenderness of the skin is distinctive. In the exfoliative stage, the skin can be induced to form bullae with light lateral pressure (Nikolsky's sign). In a mild form, a scarlatiniform eruption mimics scarlet fever, but the patient does not exhibit a strawberry tongue or circumoral pallor. In contrast to the staphylococcal scalded-skin syndrome, in which the cleavage plane is superficial in the epidermis, *toxic epidermal necrolysis* (Chap. 59) involves sloughing of the entire epidermis, resulting in severe disease. *Exfoliative erythroderma syndrome* (Chaps. 56 and 59) is a serious reaction associated with systemic toxicity that is often due to eczema, psoriasis, mycosis fungoides, or a severe drug reaction.

Vesiculobullous Eruptions *Varicella* (Chap. 183) is highly contagious, often occurring in winter or spring. At a given time within a given region of the body, varicella lesions are in different stages of development. In immunocompromised hosts, varicella vesicles may lack the characteristic erythematous base or may appear hemorrhagic. *Rickettsialpox* (Chap. 177) is often documented in urban settings and is characterized by vesicles. It can be distinguished from varicella by an eschar at the site of the mouse-mite bite and the papule/plaque base of each vesicle. Disseminated *Vibrio vulnificus* infection (Chap. 159) or *ecthyma gangrenosum* due to *Pseudomonas aeruginosa* (Chap. 155) should be considered in immunosuppressed individuals with sepsis and hemorrhagic bullae.

Urticarial Eruptions Individuals with classic urticaria ("hives") usually have a hypersensitivity reaction without associated fever. In the presence of fever, urticarial eruptions are usually due to *urticarial vasculitis* (Chap. 317). Unlike individual lesions of classic urticaria, which last up to 48 h, these lesions may last up to 5 days. Etiologies include serum sickness (often induced by drugs such as penicillins, sulfas, salicylates, or barbiturates), connective-tissue disease (e.g., systemic lupus erythematosus or Sjögren's syndrome), and infection (e.g., with hepatitis B virus, coxsackievirus A9, or parasites). Malignancy may be associated with fever and chronic urticaria (Chap. 57).

Nodular Eruptions In immunocompromised hosts, nodular lesions often represent disseminated infection. Patients with disseminated *candidiasis* (often due to *Candida tropicalis*) may have a triad of fever, myalgias, and eruptive nodules (Chap. 205). Disseminated *cryptococcosis* lesions (Chap. 204) may resemble molluscum contagiosum. Necrosis of nodules should raise the suspicion of *aspergillosis* (Chap. 206) or *mucormycosis* (Chap. 207). *Erythema nodosum* presents with exquisitely tender nodules on the lower extremities. *Sweet's syndrome* (Chap. 57) should be considered in individuals with multiple nodules and plaques, often so edematous that they give the appearance of vesicles or bullae. Sweet's syndrome may affect either healthy individuals or persons with lymphoproliferative disease.

Purpuric Eruptions *Acute meningococcemia* (Chap. 146) classically presents in children as a petechial eruption, but initial lesions may appear as blanchable macules or urticaria. RMSF should be considered in the differential diagnosis of acute meningococcemia. *Echovirus 9 infection* (Chap. 193) may mimic acute meningococcemia; patients should be treated as if they have bacterial sepsis since prompt differentiation of these conditions may be impossible. Large ecchymotic areas of *purpura fulminans* (Chaps. 124 and 146) reflect severe underlying disseminated intravascular coagulation, which may be due to infectious or noninfectious causes. The lesions of *chronic meningococcemia* (Chap. 146) may have a variety of morphologies, including petechial. Purpuric nodules may develop on the legs and resemble erythema nodosum but lack its exquisite tenderness. Lesions of *disseminated gonococcemia* (Chap. 147) are distinctive, sparse, countable hemorrhagic pustules, usually located near joints. The lesions of chronic meningococcemia and those of gonococcemia may be indistinguishable in terms of appearance and distribution. *Viral hemorrhagic fever* (Chaps. 198 and 199) should be considered in patients with an appropriate travel history and a petechial rash. *Thrombotic thrombocytopenic purpura* (Chaps. 57, 108, and 116) is a noninfectious cause of fever and petechiae. *Cutaneous small-vessel vasculitis* (*leukocytoclastic vasculitis*) typically manifests as palpable purpura and has a wide variety of causes (Chap. 57).

Eruptions with Ulcers or Eschars The presence of an ulcer or eschar in the setting of a more widespread eruption can provide an important diagnostic clue. For example, the presence of an eschar may suggest the diagnosis of scrub typhus or rickettsialpox in the appropriate setting. In other illnesses (e.g., anthrax), an ulcer or eschar may be the only skin manifestation.

BIBLIOGRAPHY

CHERRY JD: Contemporary infectious exanthems. Clin Infect Dis 16:199, 1993

———: Cutaneous manifestations of systemic infections, in *Textbook of Pediatric Infectious Diseases*, vol. 1, 3d ed, RD Feigin and JD Cherry (eds). Philadelphia, Saunders, 1992, pp 755–782

FREEDBERG IM et al (eds): *Fitzpatrick's Dermatology in General Medicine*, 5th ed. New York, McGraw-Hill, 1999

HURWITZ S (ed): *Clinical Pediatric Dermatology*. Philadelphia, Saunders, 1981

LEVIN S, GOODMAN LJ: An approach to acute fever and rash (AFR) in the adult. Curr Clin Top Infect Dis 15:19, 1995

LOTTI T et al: Cutaneous small-vessel vasculitis. J Am Acad Dermatol 39:667, 1998

SCHLOSSBERG D: Fever and rash. Infect Dis Clin North Am 10:101, 1996

WEBER DJ, COHEN MS: The acutely ill patient with fever and rash, in *Principles and Practice of Infectious Diseases*, vol 1, 4th ed, GL Mandell et al (eds). New York, Churchill Livingstone, 1995, pp 549–561

WENNER HA: Virus diseases associated with cutaneous eruptions. Prog Med Virol 16: 269, 1973

---

19   *Tamar F. Barlam, Dennis L. Kasper*

APPROACH TO THE ACUTELY ILL INFECTED FEBRILE PATIENT

The physician treating the acutely ill febrile patient must be able to recognize infections that require emergent attention. If such infections are not adequately evaluated and treated at initial presentation, the opportunity to alter an adverse outcome may be lost. In this chapter, the clinical presentations of and approach to patients with relatively common infectious disease emergencies are discussed. These infectious processes are discussed in detail in other chapters. →*Noninfectious causes of fever are not covered in this chapter; information on the approach to fever of unknown origin, including that eventually shown to be of noninfectious etiology, is presented in Chap. 125.*

GENERAL CONSIDERATIONS

APPEARANCE A physician must have a consistent approach to acutely ill patients. Even before the history is elicited and a physical examination performed, an immediate assessment of the patient's general appearance yields valuable information. The perceptive physician's subjective sense that a patient is septic or toxic often proves accurate. Visible agitation or anxiety in a febrile patient can be a harbinger of critical illness.

HISTORY Presenting symptoms are frequently nonspecific. In addition to a general description of symptoms, it is important to obtain a sense of disease progression. Detailed questions should be asked about the onset and duration of symptoms and about changes in severity or rate of progression over time. Host factors and comorbid conditions may enhance the risk of infection with certain organisms or of a more fulminant course than is usually seen. Lack of splenic function, alcoholism with significant liver disease, intravenous drug use, HIV infection, diabetes, malignancy, and chemotherapy all predispose to specific infections and frequently to increased severity. The patient should be questioned about factors that might help identify a nidus for invasive infection, such as recent upper respiratory tract infections, influenza, or varicella; prior trauma; disruption of cutaneous barriers due to lacerations, burns, surgery, or decubiti; and the presence of foreign bodies, such as nasal packing after rhinoplasty, barrier contraceptives, tampons, arteriovenous fistulas, or prosthetic joints. Travel, contact with pets or other animals, or activities that might result in tick exposure can lead to diagnoses that would not otherwise be considered. Recent dietary intake, medication use, social contact with ill individuals, vaccination history, and menstrual history may be relevant. A review of systems should focus on any neurologic signs or sensorium alterations, rashes or skin lesions, and focal pain or tenderness and should also include a general review of respiratory, gastrointestinal, or genitourinary symptoms. It is especially important to determine the duration and progression of these symptoms in order to gain an appreciation of the pace and urgency of the process.

PHYSICAL EXAMINATION A complete physical examination should be performed, with special attention to some areas that are sometimes given short shrift in routine examinations. Assessment of the patient's general appearance and vital signs, skin and soft tissue examination, and the neurologic evaluation are of particular importance.

The patient may appear either anxious and agitated or lethargic and apathetic. Fever is usually present, although the elderly and compromised hosts, such as those who are uremic or cirrhotic and patients who are taking glucocorticoids or nonsteroidal anti-inflammatory agents, may be afebrile despite serious underlying infection. Measurement of blood pressure, heart rate, and respiratory rate helps determine the degree of hemodynamic and metabolic compromise. The patient's airway must be evaluated to rule out the risk of obstruction from an invasive oropharyngeal infection.

The etiologic diagnosis may become evident in the context of a thorough skin examination. Petechial rashes are typically seen with meningococcemia or Rocky Mountain spotted fever (RMSF); erythroderma is usual with toxic shock syndrome (TSS) and drug fever. The soft tissue and muscle examination is critical. Areas of erythema or duskiness, edema, and tenderness may indicate underlying necrotizing fasciitis, myositis, or myonecrosis. The neurologic examination must include a careful assessment of mental status for signs of early encephalopathy. Evidence of nuchal rigidity or focal neurologic findings should be sought. Focal findings, depressed mental status, or papilledema should be evaluated by brain imaging prior to lumbar puncture, which, in this setting, could initiate herniation.

SPECIFIC PRESENTATIONS

For most infections, there is time for careful evaluation, diagnostic testing, and consultation with other physicians. However, the infections considered below according to common clinical presentation can have rapidly catastrophic outcomes, and their immediate recognition can be life-saving. Recommended therapeutic regimens are presented in Table 19-1.

SEPSIS WITHOUT AN OBVIOUS FOCUS OF PRIMARY INFECTION These patients initially have a brief prodrome of nonspecific symptoms and signs that progresses quickly to hemodynamic instability with hypotension, tachycardia, tachypnea, or respiratory distress. A patient may display altered mental status. Disseminated intravascular coagulation (DIC) with clinical evidence of a hemorrhagic diathesis is a poor prognostic sign.

Septic Shock (See also Chap. 124) Patients with bacteremia leading to septic shock may have a primary site of infection (e.g., pneumonia, pyelonephritis, or cholangitis) that is not evident initially. Elderly patients with comorbid conditions, hosts compromised by malignancy and neutropenia, or patients who have recently undergone a surgical procedure or hospitalization are at increased risk for an adverse outcome. Gram-negative bacteremia with organisms such as *Pseudomonas aeruginosa, Aeromonas hydrophila,* or *Escherichia coli* and gram-positive infection with organisms such as *Staphylococcus aureus* or group A streptococci can present as intractable hypotension and multiorgan failure. Treatment can usually be initiated empirically on the basis of the presentation (Table 124-3).

Overwhelming Infection in Asplenic Patients (See also Chap. 124) Patients without splenic function are at risk for overwhelming bacterial sepsis. Asplenic patients succumb to sepsis at 600 times the rate of the general population; 50 to 70% of cases occur within the first 2 years after splenectomy, with a mortality rate of up to 80%. However, in the asplenic individual, an increased risk of overwhelming sepsis continues throughout life. In asplenia, encapsulated bacteria cause the majority of infections, and adults are at lower risk than children because they are more likely to have antibody to these organisms. *Streptococcus pneumoniae* infection is most common, but the risk of infection with *Haemophilus influenzae* or *Neisseria meningitidis* is also high. Severe clinical manifestations of infections due to *E. coli, S. aureus,* group B streptococci, *P. aeruginosa, Capnocytophaga, Babesia,* and *Plasmodium* have been described.

Babesiosis (See also Chap. 214) A history of recent travel to endemic areas should raise the possibility of infection with *Babesia.* Between 1 and 4 weeks after a tick bite, the patient experiences chills, fatigue, anorexia, myalgia, arthralgia, nausea, and headache; ecchymosis and/or petechiae are occasionally seen. The tick that most commonly transmits *Babesia, Ixodes scapularis,* also transmits *Borrelia burgdorferi* (the agent of Lyme disease) and *Ehrlichia,* and co-infection can occur, resulting in more severe disease. Infection with the European species *Babesia divergens* is more frequently fulminant than that due to the U.S. species *B. microti,* causing a febrile syndrome with hemolysis, jaundice, hemoglobinemia, and renal failure and a mortality rate of >50%. Severe babesiosis is especially common in asplenic hosts but does occur in hosts with normal splenic function.

Other Sepsis Syndromes Tularemia (Chap. 161) is seen throughout the United States, but primarily in Arkansas, Oklahoma, and Missouri, in association with wild rabbit, tick, and tabanid fly contact. The uncommon typhoidal form can be associated with gram-negative septic shock and a mortality rate of >30%. In the United States, plague (Chap. 162) is found primarily in New Mexico, Arizona, and Colorado after contact with ground squirrels, prairie dogs, or chipmunks. The septic form is particularly rare and is associated with shock, multiorgan failure, and a 30% mortality rate. These rare infections should be considered in the appropriate epidemiologic setting.

SEPSIS WITH SKIN MANIFESTATIONS (See also Chap. 18) Maculopapular rashes may reflect early meningococcal or rickettsial disease but are usually associated with nonemergent infections. Exanthems are usually viral.

Petechiae Petechial rashes caused by viruses are seldom associated with hypotension or a toxic appearance, although severe measles can be an exception. In other settings, petechial rashes require more urgent attention.

Meningococcemia (See also Chap. 146) Almost three-quarters of patients with bacteremic *N. meningitidis* infection have a rash. Meningococcemia most often affects young children (i.e., those 6 months to 5 years old, often in daycare). However, sporadic cases and outbreaks occur in schools (grade school through college) and army barracks. Between 10 and 20% of all cases have a fulminant course, with shock, DIC, and multiorgan failure. Of these patients, 50 to 60% die, and survivors often require extensive debridement or amputation of gangrenous extremities. Patients may exhibit fever, headache, nausea, vomiting, myalgias, change in mental status, and meningismus. However, the rapidly progressive form of disease is not usually associated with meningitis. The rash is initially pink, blanching, and maculopapular, appearing on the trunk and extremities, but then becomes hemorrhagic, forming petechiae. Petechiae are first seen at the ankles, wrists, axillae, mucosal surfaces, and palpebral and bulbar conjunctiva, with subsequent spread to the lower extremities and trunk. A cluster of petechiae may be seen at pressure points, e.g., where a blood pressure cuff has been inflated. In rapidly progressive meningococcemia, the petechial rash quickly becomes purpuric **(Plate IID-44)** and patients develop DIC. Hypotension with petechiae for <12 h is associated with significant mortality. The mortality rate can exceed 90% in patients without meningitis who have rash, hypotension, and a normal or low white blood cell count and erythrocyte sedimentation rate. A better prognosis has been reported in cases where antibiotics are given before admission by the primary care provider. This observation suggests that early initiation of treatment may be life-saving.

Rocky Mountain spotted fever (See also Chap. 177) RMSF occurs throughout the United States. A history of tick bite is common; however, if such a history is lacking, a history of travel or outdoor activity (e.g., camping in tick-infested areas) can be ascertained. RMSF is caused by *Rickettsia rickettsii.* For the first 3 days, headache, fever, malaise, myalgias, nausea, vomiting, and anorexia are present. By day 3, half of patients have skin findings. Blanching macules develop initially on the wrists and ankles and then spread over the legs and trunk. The lesions become hemorrhagic and are frequently pete-

Table 19-1 Common Infectious Disease Emergencies

Clinical Syndrome	Possible Etiologies	Treatment	Comments	Reference Chapter(s)
Sepsis without a clear focus				
Gram-negative sepsis	*Pseudomonas* spp., gram-negative enteric bacilli	Piperacillin/tazobactam (3.75 g q4h) *or* Ceftazidime (2 g q8h) *plus* Tobramycin (5 mg/kg per day)	See Table 124-3.	124, 155
Gram-positive sepsis	*Staphylococcus* spp., *Streptococcus* spp.	Vancomycin (1 g q12h) *plus* Gentamicin (5 mg/kg per day)	If a β-lactam-sensitive strain is identified, antibiotics should be altered.	124, 139, 140
Overwhelming post-splenectomy sepsis	*Streptococcus pneumoniae, Haemophilus influenzae, Neisseria meningitidis*	Ceftriaxone (2 g q12h)[a]	If the isolate is penicillin-sensitive, penicillin is the drug of choice.	124
Babesiosis	*Babesia microti* (U.S.), *B. divergens* (Europe)	Clindamycin (600 mg tid) *plus* Quinine (650 mg tid)	Treatment with doxycycline (100 mg bid) for potential coinfection with *Borrelia burgdorferi* or *Ehrlichia* spp. may be prudent.	212, 214
Sepsis with skin findings				
Petechiae				
Meningococcemia	*N. meningitidis*	Penicillin (4 million units q4h) *or* Ceftriaxone (2 g q12h)	If both meningococcemia and Rocky Mountain spotted fever are being considered, use chloramphenicol (50–75 mg/kg per day in four divided doses). *Do not add doxycycline to a regimen including a β-lactam agent.*	146, 177
Rocky Mountain spotted fever	*Rickettsia rickettsii*	Doxycycline (100 mg bid)		
Purpura fulminans	*S. pneumoniae, H. influenzae, N. meningitidis*	Ceftriaxone (2 g q12h)[a]	If the isolate is penicillin-sensitive, penicillin is the drug of choice.	124, 146
Erythroderma: toxic shock syndrome	Group A *Streptococcus, Staphylococcus aureus*	Penicillin (2 million units q4h) *or* Oxacillin (2 g q4h) *plus* Clindamycin (600 mg q8h)	Site of toxigenic bacteria should be debrided; if necessary, intravenous immunoglobulin can be used in severe cases.	139, 140
Sepsis with soft tissue findings				
Necrotizing fasciitis	Group A *Streptococcus*, mixed aerobic/anaerobic flora	Penicillin (2 million units q4h) *plus* Clindamycin (600 mg q8h) *plus* Gentamicin (5 mg/kg per day)	Urgent surgical evaluation is critical.	128, 140
Clostridial myonecrosis	*Clostridium perfringens*	Penicillin (2 million units q4h) *plus* Clindamycin (600 mg q8h)	Urgent surgical evaluation is critical.	145
Neurologic infections				
Bacterial meningitis	*S. pneumoniae, N. meningitidis*	Ceftriaxone (2 g q12h)[a]	If the isolate is penicillin-sensitive, penicillin is the drug of choice. If the patient is >50 years old, add ampicillin for *Listeria* coverage.	372
Suppurative intracranial infections	*Staphylococcus* spp., *Streptococcus* spp., anaerobes, gram-negative bacilli	Oxacillin (2 g q4h)[b] *plus* Metronidazole (500 mg tid) *plus* Ceftriaxone (2 g q12h)	Urgent surgical evaluation is critical.	372
Brain abscess	*Streptococcus* spp., anaerobes, *Staphylococcus* spp.	Penicillin (4 million units q4h) *or* Oxacillin (2 g q4h)[b] *plus* Metronidazole (500 mg tid)	Surgical evaluation is essential.	372
Cerebral malaria	*Plasmodium falciparum*	Quinine (650 mg tid for 3 days) *plus* Tetracycline (250 mg tid for 7 days)	Do not use glucocorticoids.	212, 214
Spinal epidural abscess	*Staphylococcus* spp.	Oxacillin (2 g q4h)[c]	Surgical evaluation is essential.	368
Focal infections				
Acute bacterial endocarditis	*S. aureus*, β-hemolytic streptococci, HACEK group,[d] *Neisseria* spp., *S. pneumoniae*	Ceftriaxone (2 g q12h) *plus* Vancomycin (1 g q12h)	Adjust treatment when culture data become available. Surgical evaluation is essential.	126

[a] If resistant pneumococci are prevalent, add vancomycin (1 g q12h).
[b] Vancomycin (1 g q12h) should replace oxacillin if methicillin-resistant strains are highly prevalent.
[c] In HIV-infected intravenous drug users with suspected spinal epidural abscess, empirical therapy must cover gram-negative rods and methicillin-resistant *S. aureus*.

[d] *Haemophilus aphrophilus, H. paraphrophilus, H. parainfluenzae, Actinobacillus actinomycetemcomitans, Cardiobacterium hominis, Eikenella corrodens,* and *Kingella kingae.*

chial. The rash spreads to palms and soles later in the course (**Plate IID-45**). The centripetal spread is a classic feature of RMSF. However, 10 to 15% of patients with RMSF never develop a rash. The patient can be hypotensive and develop noncardiogenic pulmonary edema, confusion, lethargy, and encephalitis progressing to coma. The cerebrospinal fluid (CSF) contains 10 to 100 cells/μL, usually with a predominance of mononuclear cells. The CSF glucose level is often normal; the protein concentration may be slightly elevated. Renal and hepatic injury and bleeding secondary to vascular damage are noted. Untreated infection has a mortality rate of 30%.

Purpura Fulminans (See also Chaps. 124 and 146) This is the cutaneous manifestation of DIC and presents as large ecchymotic areas and hemorrhagic bullae. Progression of petechiae to purpura and ecchymoses is associated with congestive heart failure, septic shock, acute renal failure, acidosis, hypoxia, hypotension, and death. Purpura fulminans has primarily been associated with *N. meningitidis* but, in the splenectomized patient, has been described in association with *S. pneumoniae* and *H. influenzae*.

Ecthyma Gangrenosum Septic shock caused by *P. aeruginosa* and *A. hydrophila* can be associated with ecthyma gangrenosum (**Plate IID-57C**): hemorrhagic vesicles surrounded by a rim of erythema with central necrosis and ulceration. These gram-negative bacteremias are most common among patients with neutropenia, extensive burns, and hypogammaglobulinemia.

Other Emergent Infections Associated with Rash *Vibrio vulnificus* and other noncholera *Vibrio* bacteremic infections (Chap. 159) can cause focal skin lesions and overwhelming sepsis in the host with liver disease. After ingestion of contaminated shellfish, there is a sudden onset of malaise, chills, fever, and hypotension. The patient develops bullous or hemorrhagic skin lesions, usually on the lower extremities, and 75% of patients have leg pain. The mortality rate can be as high as 50%. *Capnocytophaga canimorsus* (Chap. 127) can cause septic shock in asplenic patients. Infection with this fastidious gram-negative rod typically presents after a dog bite as fever, chills, myalgia, vomiting, diarrhea, dyspnea, confusion, and headache. Findings can include an exanthem or erythema multiforme (**Plate IIE-67**), cyanotic mottling or peripheral cyanosis, petechiae, and ecchymosis. About 30% of patients with this fulminant form die of overwhelming sepsis and DIC, and survivors may require amputation to treat gangrene.

Erythroderma TSS (Chaps. 139 and 140) is usually associated with erythroderma. The patient presents with fever, malaise, myalgias, nausea, vomiting, diarrhea, and confusion. There is a sunburn-type rash that may be subtle and patchy but is usually diffuse and is found on the face, trunk, and extremities. Erythroderma, which desquamates after 1 to 2 weeks, is more common in *Staphylococcus*-associated than in *Streptococcus*-associated TSS. Hypotension develops rapidly after onset of symptoms, often within hours. Multiorgan failure is seen. Often there is no indication of a primary focal infection. Colonization rather than overt infection of the vagina or a postoperative wound, for example, is typical with staphylococcal TSS, and the mucosal areas appear hyperemic but not infected. Early renal failure may distinguish this syndrome from other septic shock syndromes. Clinical evaluation constitutes the diagnosis because TSS is defined by the clinical criteria of fever, rash, hypotension, and multiorgan involvement. The mortality rate is 5% for menstruation-associated TSS, 10 to 15% for nonmenstrual TSS, and 30 to 70% for streptococcal TSS.

SEPSIS WITH A SOFT TISSUE/MUSCLE PRIMARY FOCUS (See also Chap. 128) **Necrotizing Fasciitis** This infection may arise at a site of minimal trauma or postoperative incision and may also be associated with recent varicella, childbirth, or muscle strain. The most common causes of necrotizing fasciitis are group A streptococci alone (Chap. 140) and a mixed facultative and anaerobic flora (Chap. 128). Diabetes mellitus, peripheral vascular disease, and intravenous drug use are associated risk factors. Use of nonsteroidal anti-inflammatory agents adversely affects granulocyte chemotaxis, phagocytosis, and bacterial killing, allowing progression of skin or soft tissue infections. The patient may have bacteremia and hypotension without other organ-system failure. Physical findings are minimal

compared to the severity of pain and the degree of fever. The examination is often unremarkable except for soft tissue edema and erythema. The infected area is red, hot, shiny, swollen, and exquisitely tender. In untreated infection, the overlying skin develops blue-gray patches after 36 h, and cutaneous bullae and necrosis develop after 3 to 5 days. Necrotizing fasciitis due to a mixed flora, but not that due to group A streptococci, can be associated with gas production. Without treatment, pain decreases because of thrombosis of the small blood vessels and destruction of the peripheral nerves—an ominous sign. The mortality rate is >30% overall, >70% in association with TSS, and nearly 100% without surgical intervention. Life-threatening necrotizing fasciitis may also be due to *Clostridium perfringens* (Chap. 145); in this condition, the patient is extremely toxic and the mortality rate is high. Within 48 h, rapid tissue invasion and systemic toxicity associated with hemolysis and death ensue. The distinction between this entity and clostridial myonecrosis is made by muscle biopsy.

Clostridial Myonecrosis (See also Chap. 145) Myonecrosis is often associated with trauma or surgery but can be spontaneous. The incubation period is usually 12 to 24 h long, and massive necrotizing gangrene develops within hours of onset. Systemic toxicity, shock, and death can occur within 12 h. The patient's pain and toxic appearance are out of proportion to physical findings. On examination, the patient is febrile, apathetic, tachycardic, and tachypneic and may express a feeling of impending doom. Hypotension and renal failure develop later, and hyperalertness is evident preterminally. The skin over the affected area is bronze-brown, mottled, and edematous. Bullous lesions with serosanguineous drainage and a mousy or sweet odor can be present. Crepitus can occur secondary to gas production in muscle tissue. The mortality rate is >65% with spontaneous myonecrosis, which is often associated with *C. septicum* and underlying malignancy. The mortality rates associated with trunk and limb infection are 63% and 12%, respectively, and any delay in surgical treatment increases the risk of death.

NEUROLOGIC INFECTIONS WITH OR WITHOUT SEPTIC SHOCK **Bacterial Meningitis** (See also Chap. 372) Bacterial meningitis is one of the most common infectious emergencies involving the central nervous system. Although hosts with cell-mediated immune deficiency, including transplant recipients, diabetic patients, the elderly, and cancer patients treated with certain chemotherapeutic agents, are at particular risk for *Listeria monocytogenes* meningitis, most cases in adults are due to *S. pneumoniae* (30 to 50%) and *N. meningitidis* (10 to 35%). An early presentation of headache, meningismus, and fever is classic but is seen in only half of patients. The elderly can present without fever or meningeal signs despite lethargy and confusion. Cerebral dysfunction is evidenced by confusion, delirium, and lethargy that can progress to coma. The presentation is fulminant, with sepsis and brain edema, in some cases; papilledema at presentation is unusual and suggests another diagnosis (e.g., an intracranial lesion). Focal signs, including cranial nerve palsies (IV, VI, VII), can be seen in 10 to 20% of cases; 50 to 60% of patients have bacteremia. A poor neurologic outcome is associated with coma at any time during the course or with a CSF glucose level of <0.6 mmol/L (<10 mg/dL). Mortality is associated with coma, respiratory distress, shock, a CSF protein level of >2.5 g/L, a peripheral white blood cell count of <5000/μL, and a serum sodium level of <135 mmol/L.

Suppurative Intracranial Infections (See also Chap. 372) Other rare intracranial lesions that present with sepsis and hemodynamic instability are subdural empyema, septic cavernous sinus thrombosis, and septic superior sagittal sinus thrombosis. Rapid recognition of the toxic patient with central neurologic signs is crucial to improvement of the dismal prognosis of these entities.

Subdural empyema This infection arises from the paranasal sinus in 60 to 70% of cases. Microaerophilic streptococci and staphylococci are the predominant etiologic organisms. The patient is toxic, with fever, headache, and nuchal rigidity. Of all patients, 75% have focal signs and 6 to 20% die.

Septic cavernous sinus thrombosis   This condition follows a facial or sphenoid sinus infection; 70% of cases are due to staphylococci and the remainder to aerobic or anaerobic streptococci. A unilateral or retroorbital headache progresses to a toxic appearance and fever within days. Three-quarters of patients have unilateral periorbital edema that becomes bilateral and then progresses to ptosis, proptosis, ophthalmoplegia, and papilledema. The mortality rate is as high as 30%.

Septic thrombosis of the superior sagittal sinus   This infection spreads from the ethmoid or maxillary sinuses. Its bacterial causes include *S. pneumoniae*, other streptococci, and staphylococci. The fulminant course is characterized by headache, nausea, vomiting, rapid progression to confusion and coma, nuchal rigidity, and brainstem signs. If the sinus is totally thrombosed, the mortality rate exceeds 80%.

Brain Abscess (See also Chap. 372)   Brain abscess often occurs without systemic signs. Almost half of patients are afebrile, and presentations are more consistent with a space-occupying lesion in the brain; 70% have headache, 50% have focal neurologic signs, and 25% have papilledema. Abscesses can present as single or multiple lesions resulting from contiguous foci or hematogenous infection, such as unrecognized endocarditis. The infection progresses over several days from cerebritis to an abscess with a mature capsule. Abscesses arising hematogenously are especially apt to rupture into the ventricular space, causing a sudden and severe deterioration in clinical status and high mortality. Otherwise, mortality is low but morbidity is high (30 to 55%). Patients presenting with stroke and a parameningeal infectious focus, such as sinusitis or otitis, may have a brain abscess, and physicians must maintain a high level of suspicion. Prognosis worsens in patients with a fulminant course, delayed diagnosis, abscess rupture into the ventricles, multiple abscesses, or abnormal neurologic status at presentation.

Cerebral Malaria (See also Chap. 214)   This entity should be urgently considered if patients who have recently traveled to areas endemic for malaria present with a febrile illness and lethargy or other neurologic signs. Fulminant malaria is caused by *Plasmodium falciparum* and is associated with temperatures of $>40°C$ ($>104°F$), hypotension, jaundice, adult respiratory distress syndrome, and bleeding. By definition, any patient with a change in mental status or repeated seizure in the setting of fulminant malaria has cerebral malaria. In adults this nonspecific febrile illness progresses to coma over several days; occasionally, coma occurs within hours and death within 24 h. Nuchal rigidity and photophobia are rare. On physical examination, symmetric encephalopathy is typical, and upper motor neuron dysfunction with decorticate and decerebrate posturing can be seen with advanced disease. Unrecognized infection results in a 30% mortality rate.

Spinal Epidural Abscesses (See also Chap. 368)   Patients with spinal epidural abscesses often present with back pain and develop neurologic deficits late in their course. At-risk patients include those with diabetes mellitus; intravenous drug use; recent spinal trauma, surgery, or epidural anesthesia; and other comorbid conditions, such as HIV infection. The thoracic or lumbar spine is the most common location, and staphylococci are the most common etiologic agents; in HIV-infected intravenous drug users, therapy must cover gram-negative rods and methicillin-resistant *S. aureus*. If a patient gives a history of antecedent back pain and has new neurologic symptoms, this diagnosis must immediately be considered. Almost 60% of patients have fever and almost 90% have back pain. Paresthesia, bowel and bladder dysfunction, radicular pain, and weakness are frequent neurologic complaints, and examination of the patient may reveal abnormal reflexes and motor and sensory deficits. Rapid recognition and treatment, including immediate drainage, can prevent or minimize permanent neurologic sequelae.

FOCAL SYNDROMES WITH A FULMINANT COURSE
Infection at virtually any primary focus (e.g., osteomyelitis, pneumonia, pyelonephritis, or cholangitis) can result in bacteremia and sepsis.

TSS has been associated with focal infections such as septic arthritis, peritonitis, sinusitis, and wound infection. Death occurs secondary to septic shock or toxin production with hemodynamic instability and multiorgan failure. Rapid clinical deterioration and death can be associated with destruction of the primary site of infection, as is seen in endocarditis and in necrotizing infections of the oropharynx (in which edema suddenly compromises the airway).

Rhinocerebral Mucormycosis (See also Chap. 207)   Patients with diabetes or malignancy are at risk for invasive rhinocerebral mucormycosis. Patients present with low-grade fever, dull sinus pain, diplopia, decreased mental status, decreased ocular motion, chemosis, proptosis, dusky or necrotic nasal turbinates, and necrotic hard-palate lesions that respect the midline. Without rapid recognition and intervention, the process continues an inexorable invasive course with high mortality.

Acute Bacterial Endocarditis (See also Chap. 126)   This entity presents with a much more aggressive course than subacute endocarditis. Bacteria such as *S. aureus, S. pneumoniae, L. monocytogenes, Haemophilus* spp., and streptococci of groups A, B, and G attack native valves. Mortality rates range from 10 to 40%. The host may have comorbid conditions such as underlying malignancy, diabetes mellitus, intravenous drug use, or alcoholism. The patient presents with fever, fatigue, and malaise <2 weeks after onset of infection. On physical examination, a changing murmur and congestive heart failure may be noted. Hemorrhagic macules on palms or soles (*Janeway lesions*) sometimes develop. Petechiae, Roth's spots, splinter hemorrhages, and splenomegaly are unusual. Rapid valvular destruction, particularly of the aortic valve, results in pulmonary edema and hypotension. Myocardial abscesses can form, eroding through the septum or into the conduction system and causing life-threatening arrhythmias or high-degree conduction block. Large friable vegetations can result in major arterial emboli, metastatic infection, or tissue infarction. Emboli can lead to stroke, change in mental status, visual disturbances, aphasia, ataxia, headache, meningismus, brain abscess, cerebritis, spinal cord infarct with paraplegia, arthralgia, osteomyelitis, splenic abscess, septic arthritis, and hematuria. Rapid intervention is crucial for a successful outcome.

DIAGNOSTIC WORKUP OF THE ACUTELY ILL PATIENT

After a quick clinical assessment, diagnostic material should be obtained rapidly and antibiotic and supportive treatment begun. In the sepsis syndromes, blood (for cultures; baseline complete blood count with differential; measurement of serum electrolytes, blood urea nitrogen, serum creatinine, and serum glucose; and liver function tests) can be obtained at the time an intravenous line is placed and before antibiotics are administered. For patients with possible acute endocarditis, three sets of blood cultures should be performed. Asplenic patients should have a blood smear examined to confirm the presence of Howell-Jolly bodies (indicating the absence of splenic function) and a buffy coat examined for bacteria; these patients can have $>10^6$ organisms per milliliter of blood (compared to 10^4/mL in patients with an intact spleen). Blood smears from patients with possible cerebral malaria or babesiosis must be examined for the diagnosis and quantitation of parasitemia. Blood smears may also be diagnostic in ehrlichiosis.

Patients with meningitis should have CSF obtained before the initiation of antibiotic therapy. *If focal neurologic signs, abnormal mental status, or papilledema mandates brain imaging before a lumbar puncture, antibiotics should be administered prior to imaging but after blood for cultures has been drawn.* If CSF cultures are negative, laboratory examination of CSF by latex agglutination or immunoprecipitation can be attempted to make an etiologic diagnosis. However, blood cultures will provide the diagnosis in 50 to 70% of cases.

Focal abscesses necessitate immediate computed tomography or magnetic resonance imaging as part of an evaluation for surgical intervention. Other diagnostic procedures, such as cultures of wounds or scraping of skin lesions, should not delay the initiation of treatment for more than minutes. Once emergent evaluation, diagnostic procedures, and (if appropriate) surgical consultation (see below) have been completed, other laboratory tests can be conducted. Appropriate radiography, computed axial tomography, magnetic resonance imaging, urinalysis, erythrocyte sedimentation rate determination, and transthoracic or transesophageal echocardiography may all prove important.

℞ **TREATMENT** Table 19-1 lists first-line treatments for the infections considered in this chapter. (For a more detailed discussion of treatment, see specific chapters.) In addition to the initiation of parenteral antibiotic therapy, several of these infections require urgent surgical attention. General surgery for possible necrotizing fasciitis or myonecrosis, neurosurgical evaluation for subdural empyema or spinal epidural abscess, otolaryngologic surgery for possible mucormycosis, and cardiothoracic surgery for critically ill patients with acute endocarditis are as important as the rapid commencement of antibiotic therapy. For infections such as necrotizing fasciitis and clostridial myonecrosis, rapid surgical intervention supercedes other diagnostic or therapeutic maneuvers.

Acutely ill febrile patients require close observation, aggressive supportive measures, and—in most cases—admission to intensive care units. Adjunctive treatments, such as intravenous immunoglobulin administration for TSS, can be considered after initial stabilization. The most important task of the physician is to recognize the acute infectious emergency and proceed with appropriate urgency.

BIBLIOGRAPHY

ASTIZ ME et al: Septic shock. Lancet 351:1501, 1998

BARQUET N et al: Prognostic factors in meningococcal disease—development of a bedside predictive model and scoring system. JAMA 278:491, 1997

DAVIES HD et al: Invasive group A streptococcal infections in Ontario, Canada. N Engl J Med 335:547, 1996

DRAGE LA: Life-threatening rashes: Dermatologic signs of four infectious diseases. Mayo Clin Proc 74:68, 1999

MATHISEN GE et al: Brain abscess. Clin Infect Dis 25:763, 1997

NEWTON CRJC et al: Neurological manifestations of falciparum malaria. Ann Neurol 43:695, 1998

QUAGLIARELLO VJ et al: Treatment of bacterial meningitis. N Engl J Med 336:709, 1997

20   *Daniel F. Danzl*

HYPOTHERMIA AND FROSTBITE

HYPOTHERMIA

Accidental hypothermia occurs when there is an unintentional drop in the body's core temperature below 35°C (95°F). At this temperature, many of the compensatory physiologic mechanisms to conserve heat begin to fail. *Primary accidental hypothermia* is a result of the direct exposure of a previously healthy individual to the cold. The mortality rate is much higher for those patients who develop *secondary hypothermia* as a complication of a serious systemic disorder.

CAUSES   Primary accidental hypothermia is geographically and seasonally pervasive. Although most cases occur in the winter months and in colder climates, it is surprisingly common in warmer regions as well. In the United States, hypothermia accounts for more than 700 deaths each year, half of which occur in people age 65 or older.

Multiple variables make individuals at the extremes of age, the elderly and neonates, particularly vulnerable to hypothermia (Table 20-1). The elderly have diminished thermal proprioception and are more susceptible to immobility, malnutrition, and systemic illnesses that interfere with heat generation or conservation. Dementia, psychiatric illness, and socioeconomic factors often compound these problems by impeding adequate measures to prevent hypothermia. Neonates have high rates of heat loss because of their increased

Table 20-1   Risk Factors for Hypothermia

Age extremes	Endocrine-related
Elderly	Hypoglycemia
Neonates	Hypothyroidism
Outdoor exposure	Adrenal insufficiency
Occupational	Hypopituitarism
Sports-related	Neurologic-related
Inadequate clothing	Stroke
Drugs and intoxicants	Hypothalamic disorders
Ethanol	Parkinson's disease
Phenothiazines	Spinal cord injury
Barbiturates	Multisystem
Anesthetics	Malnutrition
Neuromuscular blockers	Sepsis
Others	Shock
	Hepatic or renal failure
	Burns and exfoliative dermatologic disorders
	Immobility or debilitation

surface-to-mass ratio and their lack of effective shivering and adaptive behavioral responses. In addition, malnutrition can contribute to heat loss because of diminished subcutaneous fat and because of its association with depleted energy stores used for thermogenesis.

Individuals whose occupations or hobbies entail extensive exposure to cold weather are clearly at increased risk for hypothermia. Military history is replete with hypothermic tragedies. Hunters, sailors, skiers, and climbers also are at great risk of exposure, whether it involves injury, changes in weather, or lack of preparedness.

Ethanol causes vasodilatation (which increases heat loss), reduces thermogenesis and gluconeogenesis, and may impair judgment or lead to obtundation. Hypothermia is not an uncommon feature in Wernicke's encephalopathy and may mask its other manifestations. A number of medications are associated with altered thermal regulation. Phenothiazines, barbiturates, benzodiazepines, cyclic antidepressants, and many other medications reduce centrally-mediated vasoconstriction. Up to one-quarter of patients admitted to an intensive care unit because of drug overdose are hypothermic. Anesthetics can block the shivering responses; their effects may be compounded when patients are not covered adequately in the operating or recovery rooms.

Several types of endocrine dysfunction can lead to hypothermia. Hypothyroidism—particularly when extreme, as in myxedema coma—reduces the metabolic rate and impairs thermogenesis and behavioral responses. Myxedema is more common in women than in men and may be occult. Adrenal insufficiency and hypopituitarism can also increase susceptibility to hypothermia. Hypoglycemia, most commonly caused by insulin or oral hypoglycemic drugs, is associated with hypothermia, in part the result of neuroglycopenic effects on hypothalamic function. Increased osmolality and metabolic derangements associated with uremia, diabetic ketoacidosis, and lactic acidosis can lead to altered hypothalamic thermoregulation.

Neurologic injury from trauma, cerebrovascular accident, subarachnoid hemorrhage, or hypothalamic lesions increases susceptibility to hypothermia. Agenesis of the corpus callosum, or Shapiro syndrome, is one cause of episodic hypothermia, characterized by profuse perspiration followed by a rapid fall in temperature. Acute spinal cord injury disrupts the autonomic pathways that lead to shivering and prevents cold-induced reflex vasoconstrictive responses.

Hypothermia associated with sepsis is a poor prognostic sign. Hepatic failure causes decreased glycogen stores and gluconeogenesis, as well as a diminished shivering response. In acute myocardial infarction associated with low cardiac output, hypothermia may be reversed after adequate resuscitation. With extensive burns, psoriasis, erythrodermas, and other skin diseases, increased peripheral blood flow leads to excessive heat loss.

THERMOREGULATION   Heat loss occurs through five mechanisms: radiation (55 to 65% of heat loss), conduction (10 to 15% of heat loss, but much greater in cold water), convection (increase in the wind), respiration, and evaporation (which are affected by the ambient temperature and the relative humidity).

The preoptic anterior hypothalamus normally orchestrates thermoregulation (Chap. 17). The immediate defense of thermoneutrality is via the autonomic nervous system (Chap. 72), whereas delayed control is mediated by the endocrine system. Autonomic nervous system responses include the release of norepinephrine, increased muscle tone, and shivering, leading to thermogenesis and an increase in the basal metabolic rate. Cutaneous cold thermoreception causes direct reflex vasoconstriction to converse heat. Prolonged exposure to cold also stimulates hypothalamic release of thyrotropin releasing hormone; this leads to increased levels of thyroid stimulating hormone (TSH), which stimulates the thyroid gland to produce thyroxine, a hormone that increases metabolic rate.

CLINICAL PRESENTATION   In most cases of hypothermia, the history of exposure to environmental factors, such as prolonged exposure to the outdoors without adequate clothing, makes the diagnosis straightforward. In urban settings, however, the presentation is often more subtle and the clinician may focus on other disease processes, toxin exposures, or psychiatric diagnoses.

After initial stimulation by hypothermia, there is progressive depression of all organ systems. The timing of the appearance of these clinical manifestations varies widely (Table 20-2). Without knowing the core temperature, it can be difficult to interpret other vital signs. For example, a tachycardia disproportionate to the core temperature suggests secondary hypothermia resulting from hypoglycemia, hypovolemia, or a toxin overdose. Because carbon dioxide production declines progressively, the respiratory rate should be low; persistent hyperventilation suggests a central nervous system (CNS) lesion or one of the organic acidoses. A markedly depressed level of consciousness in a patient with mild hypothermia should raise suspicion of an overdose or CNS dysfunction due to infection or trauma.

Physical examination findings can also be altered by hypothermia. For instance, the assumption that areflexia is solely attributable to hypothermia can obscure and delay the diagnosis of a spinal cord injury. Patients with hypothermia may be confused or combative; these symptoms abate more rapidly with rewarming than with the use of restraints. A classic example of maladaptive behavior in patients with hypothermia is paradoxical undressing, which involves the inappropriate removal of clothing in response to a cold stress. The cold-induced ileus and abdominal rectus spasm can mimic, or mask, the presentation of an acute abdomen (Chap. 14).

When a patient in hypothermic cardiac arrest is first discovered, cardiopulmonary resuscitation is indicated, unless (1) a do-not-resuscitate status is verified, (2) obviously lethal injuries are identified, or (3) the depression of a frozen chest wall is not possible. As the resuscitation proceeds, the prognosis is grave if there is evidence of widespread cell lysis, as reflected by potassium levels exceeding 10 mEq/L. Other findings that may preclude continuing resuscitation include a core temperature <12°C, a pH <6.5, or evidence of intravascular thrombosis with a fibrinogen value <50 mg/dL. The decision to terminate resuscitation before rewarming the patient to 35°C is extremely difficult. There are no validated prognostic indicators for recovery from hypothermia. A history of asphyxia with secondary cooling is the most important negative predictor of survival.

DIAGNOSIS AND STABILIZATION   Hypothermia is confirmed by measuring the core temperature, preferably at two sites. Rectal probes should be placed to a depth of 15 cm and not adjacent to cold feces. A simultaneous esophageal measurement will be falsely high during heated inhalation therapy. The probe should be placed 24 cm below the larynx. The greatest discordance between the readings is usually during the transition phase before effective rewarming. Relying solely on infrared tympanic thermography is not advisable.

After a diagnosis of hypothermia is established, cardiac monitoring should be instituted, along with attempts to limit further heat loss. If the patient is in ventricular fibrillation, one sequence of 3 defibrillation attempts (2 J/kg) should be administered. If unsuccessful, active re-

Table 20-2 Physiologic Changes Associated with Hypothermia

Severity of Hypothermia	Body Temperature	Central Nervous System	Cardiovascular	Respiratory	Renal and Endocrine	Neuromuscular
Mild	35°C (95°F)–32.2°C (90°F)	Linear depression of cerebral metabolism; amnesia; apathy; dysarthria; impaired judgment; maladaptive behavior	Tachycardia, then progressive bradycardia; cardiac-cycle prolongation; vasoconstriction; increase in cardiac output and blood pressure	Tachypnea, then progressive decrease in respiratory minute volume; declining oxygen consumption; bronchorrhea; bronchospasm	Diuresis; increase in catecholamines, adrenal steroids, triiodothyronine and thyroxine; increase in metabolism with shivering	Increased preshivering muscle tone, then fatiguing, shivering-induced thermogenesis; ataxia
Moderate	<32.2°C (90°F)–28°C (82.4°F)	EEG abnormalities; progressive depression of level of consciousness; pupillary dilatation; paradoxical undressing; hallucinations	Progressive decrease in pulse and cardiac output; increased atrial and ventricular arrhythmias; nonspecific and suggestive (J-wave) electrocardiographic changes; prolonged systole	Hypoventilation; 50% decrease in carbon dioxide production per 8°C drop in temperature; absence of protective airway reflexes; 50% decrease in oxygen consumption	50% increase in renal blood flow; renal autoregulation intact; impaired insulin action	Hyporeflexia; diminishing shivering-induced thermogenesis; rigidity
Severe	<28°C (82.4°F)	Loss of cerebrovascular autoregulation; decline in cerebral blood flow; coma; loss of ocular reflexes; progressive decrease in EEG	Progressive decreases in blood pressure, heart rate, and cardiac output; reentrant dysrhythmias; decreased ventricular arrhythmia threshold; asystole	Pulmonic congestion and edema; 75% decrease in oxygen consumption; apnea	Decrease in renal blood flow parallels decrease in cardiac output; extreme oliguria; poikilothermia; 80% decrease in basal metabolism	No motion; decreased nerve-conduction velocity; peripheral areflexia

warming should be continued past 30° to 32°C. Supplemental oxygenation is always warranted, since tissue oxygenation is adversely affected by the leftward shift of the oxyhemoglobin dissociation curve. Pulse oximetry may be unreliable in patients with vasoconstriction. If protective airway reflexes are absent, gentle endotracheal intubation should be performed. Adequate pre-oxygenation will prevent ventricular arrhythmias.

Insertion of a gastric tube prevents dilatation secondary to decreased bowel motility. Indwelling bladder catheters facilitate monitoring of cold-induced diuresis. Dehydration is commonly encountered with chronic hypothermia, and most patients benefit from a bolus of crystalloid. Normal saline containing 5% dextrose is preferable to lactated Ringer's solution, as the liver in hypothermic patients inefficiently metabolizes lactate. The placement of a pulmonary artery catheter, although of potential value, risks perforation of the less compliant pulmonary artery. The use of a central venous catheter should be avoided because of right atrial irritability.

Arterial blood gases should not be corrected for temperature (Chap. 30). This is termed the ectothermic or alpha-stat approach, which maximizes enzymatic function and maintains the normal distribution of charged metabolic intermediates. An uncorrected pH of 7.42 and a P_{CO_2} of 40 mmHg reflects appropriate alveolar ventilation and acid-base balance at any core temperature. Acid-base imbalances should be corrected gradually, since the bicarbonate buffering system is inefficient. When the P_{CO_2} increases 10 mmHg at 28°C, it doubles the pH decline of 0.08 that is normally induced at 37°C.

The severity of anemia may be underestimated because the hematocrit increases 2% for each 1°C drop in temperature. White blood cell sequestration and bone marrow suppression are common, potentially masking an infection. Although hypokalemia is more common in chronic hypothermia, hyperkalemia also occurs; the expected electrocardiographic changes can be obscured by hypothermia. Patients with renal insufficiency, metabolic acidoses, or rhabdomyolysis are most at risk for electrolyte disturbances.

Coagulopathies are common because cold inhibits the enzymatic reactions required for activation of the intrinsic cascade. In addition, the production of thromboxane B_2 by platelets is temperature-dependent, and platelet function is impaired. The administration of platelets and fresh frozen plasma is, therefore, not effective. The prothrombin or partial thromboplastin times reported by the laboratory appear deceptively normal and contrast with the observed coagulopathy. This contradiction appears because all coagulation tests are routinely performed at 37°C, and the enzymes are thus rewarmed.

REWARMING STRATEGIES The key initial decision is whether to rewarm the patient passively or actively. *Passive external rewarming* simply involves covering and insulating the patient in a warm environment. With the head covered, the rate of rewarming is usually 0.5° to 2.0°C per hour. This technique is ideal for previously healthy patients who develop acute, mild primary accidental hypothermia. The patient must have sufficient fuel and glycogen to support endogenous thermogenesis.

There are reservations about the application of heat directly to the extremities of patients with chronic severe hypothermia. Extinguishing peripheral vasoconstriction in the dehydrated patient may precipitate core temperature "afterdrop"—the continual decline in the core temperature after removal of the patient from the cold. This phenomenon results from conductive temperature equilibration and a circulatory convective mechanism. Rewarming frostbitten extremities before stabilization of the core temperature causes a significant core temperature afterdrop. In contrast, truncal heat application may minimize the risk of afterdrop.

Active rewarming is necessary under the following circumstances: core temperature <32°C (poikilothermia), cardiovascular instability, age extremes, CNS dysfunction, endocrine insufficiency, or any suspicion of secondary hypothermia. *Active external rewarming* is best accomplished with forced-air heating blankets. Other options include radiant heat sources and hot packs. Monitoring a patient with hypothermia in a heated tub is extremely difficult. Electric blankets should be avoided because vasoconstricted skin is easily burned. Widely available *active core rewarming* options include heated inhalation, heated infusion, and lavage (gastric, colonic, mediastinal, thoracic, pleural). The therapeutic options also include hemodialysis, venovenous, and continuous arteriovenous rewarming, in addition to formal cardiopulmonary bypass.

Arteriovenous anastomoses (AVA) rewarming provides exogenous heat by immersion of the hands, forearms, feet, and calves in 44° to 45°C water. Airway rewarming with heated humidified oxygen (40° to 45°C) is a convenient option via mask or endotracheal tube. Although airway rewarming provides less heat than some other forms of active core rewarming, it eliminates respiratory heat loss and adds 1° to 2°C to the overall rewarming rate. Crystalloids should be heated to 40° to 42°C. The quantity of heat provided is significant only during massive volume resuscitations. The most efficient method for heating and delivering fluid or blood is with a countercurrent in-line heat exchanger. Heated irrigation of the gastrointestinal tract or bladder transfers minimal heat because of the limited available surface area. These methods should be reserved for patients in cardiac arrest and then used in combination with all available active rewarming techniques. Closed thoracic lavage is far more efficient in severely hypothermic patients with cardiac arrest. The hemithoraces are irrigated through two large-bore thoracostomy tubes that are inserted into the left or both of the hemithoraces. Thoracostomy tubes should not be placed in the left chest of a spontaneously perfusing patient for purposes of rewarming. Peritoneal lavage with the dialysate at 40° to 45°C efficiently transfers heat when delivered through two catheters with outflow suction. Like peritoneal dialysis, standard hemodialysis is especially useful for patients with electrolyte abnormalities, rhabdomyolysis, or toxin ingestions.

With extracorporeal venovenous rewarming, the blood is removed from a central venous catheter, heated to 40°C, and returned through a second central or peripheral venous catheter. Continuous arteriovenous rewarming involves the use of percutaneously inserted femoral arterial and contralateral femoral venous 8.5 Fr catheters. The blood pressure must be at least 60 mmHg. Heparin-bonded tubing obviates the need for systemic anticoagulation. Full circulatory support with an oxygenator can only be provided through formal cardiopulmonary bypass (CPB). Femoral flow rates of 2 to 3 L/min elevate the core temperature 1° to 2°C every 3 to 5 min. CPB should be considered in nonperfusing patients without documented contraindications to resuscitation. Circulatory support may also be the only effective option in patients with completely frozen extremities, or those with significant tissue destruction coupled with rhabdomyolysis.

There is no evidence that extremely rapid rewarming improves survival in perfusing patients. The best strategy is usually a combination of passive, truncal active, and active core rewarming techniques.

DRUG THERAPY When a patient is hypothermic, target organs and the cardiovascular system respond minimally to most medications. Moreover, cumulative doses can cause toxicity during rewarming because of increased binding of drugs to proteins, and impaired metabolism and excretion. As an example, the administration of repeated doses of digoxin or insulin would be ineffective while the patient is hypothermic, and the residual drugs are potentially toxic during rewarming.

Any pharmacologic manipulation of the depressed and vasoconstricted cardiovascular system should generally be avoided. If the hypotension does not respond to crystalloid infusion and rewarming, low-dose dopamine (2 to 5 μg/kg per min) support should be considered. Atrial arrhythmias should initially be monitored without intervention, as the ventricular response will be slow, and most will convert spontaneously during rewarming. When indicated, bretylium tosylate is the class III ventricular antiarrhythmic of choice. During ventricular fibrillation, it should initially be administered at a dose of 10 mg/kg. Bretylium uniquely increases the ventricular arrhythmia threshold at low temperatures, although the wisdom of prophylaxis is unresolved.

Initiating empirical therapy for adrenal insufficiency is usually not warranted unless there is a history suggesting steroid dependence, hypoadrenalism, or a failure to rewarm with standard therapy. However, the administration of parenteral levothyroxine to euthyroid patients with hypothermia is potentially hazardous. Because laboratory results can be delayed and confounded by the presence of the sick euthyroid syndrome (Chap. 330), historical clues or physical findings suggestive of hypothyroidism should be sought. When myxedema is the cause of hypothermia, the relaxation phase of the Achilles reflex is prolonged more than the contraction phase.

Hypothermia obscures most of the symptoms and signs of infection, notably fever and leukocytosis. Shaking rigors from infection may be mistaken for shivering. Except in mild cases, extensive cultures and repeated physical examinations are essential. Unless an infectious source is identified, empirical antibiotic prophylaxis is most warranted in the elderly, neonates, and immunocompromised patients.

Preventive measures should be discussed with high-risk individuals, such as the elderly or people whose work frequently exposes them to extreme cold. The importance of layered clothing and headgear, adequate shelter, increased caloric intake, and the avoidance of ethanol should be emphasized, along with access to rescue services.

FROSTBITE

Peripheral cold injuries include both freezing and nonfreezing injuries to tissue. Frostbite occurs when the tissue temperature drops below 0°C. Ice crystal formation subsequently distorts and destroys the cellular architecture. Once the vascular endothelium is damaged, stasis progresses rapidly to microvascular thrombosis. Tissue freezes quickly when in contact with thermal conductors such as metal or volatile solutions. Other predisposing factors include constrictive clothing or boots, immobility, or vasoconstrictive medications.

Clinically, it is most practical to classify frostbite as superficial or deep. Superficial does not entail tissue loss. Classically, frostbite is retrospectively graded like a burn once the resultant pathology is demarcated over time. First-degree frostbite causes only anesthesia and erythema. The appearance of superficial vesiculation surrounded by edema and erythema is considered second degree (**Plates IIA-18, IIA-19**). Hemorrhagic vesicles reflect a serious injury to the microvasculature, and indicate third-degree frostbite. Fourth-degree injuries damage subcuticular, muscular, and osseous tissues.

PATHOPHYSIOLOGY   Peripheral cold injury involves a cascade of events. Endothelial cells are very susceptible to cold injury. In the prefreeze phase, plasma leaks and there is the development of microvascular vasoconstriction. The radiation of heat from underlying tissues initially prevents crystallization. The freeze phase usually begins with extracellular fluid crystallization. Water exits the cell and causes intracellular dehydration, hyperosmolality, and ultimately cellular shrinkage and demise. Damaged tissue releases thromboxane A_2 and prostaglandin $F_{2\alpha}$, which produce platelet aggregation, leukocyte immobilization, and vasoconstriction.

After the tissue thaws, the second phase of the cascade causes progressive dermal ischemia. The microvasculature begins to collapse, arteriovenous shunting increases tissue pressures, and there is progressive formation of edema. Finally, thrombosis, ischemia, and superficial necrosis appear. The development of mummification and demarcation may take weeks to months.

CLINICAL PRESENTATION   The initial presentation of frostbite can be deceptively benign. The symptoms always include a sensory deficiency affecting light touch, pain, and temperature perception. The acral areas and distal extremities are the most common insensate areas. Some patients complain of a clumsy or "chunk of wood" sensation in the extremity.

Deep frostbitten tissue can appear waxy, mottled, yellow, or violaceous-white. Favorable presenting signs include some warmth or sensation with normal color. The injury is often superficial if the subcutaneous tissue is pliable or if the dermis can be rolled over boney prominences.

The two most common nonfreezing peripheral cold injuries are *chilblain (pernio)* and *immersion (trench) foot*. Chilblain results from neuronal and endothelial damage induced by repetitive exposure to dry cold. Young females, particularly those with a history of Raynaud's phenomenon, are most at risk. Persistent vasospasticity and vasculitis can cause erythema, mild edema, and pruritus. Eventually plaques, blue nodules, and ulcerations develop. These lesions typically involve the dorsa of the hands and feet. In contrast, immersion (trench) foot results from repetitive exposure to wet cold above the freezing point. The feet initially appear cyanotic, cold, and edematous. The subsequent development of bullae is often indistinguishable from frostbite. This vesiculation rapidly progresses to ulceration and liquefaction gangrene. Patients with milder cases complain of hyperhidrosis, cold sensitivity, and painful ambulation for many years.

Various ancillary tests have been used in an attempt to diagnose the severity of peripheral cold injuries. None consistently predicts the extent of injury at presentation. For example, angiography and magnetic resonance imaging can demonstrate the patency of large vessels but not the microvasculature. Ultrasonography and digital plethysmography are also insensitive. Thermography and technetium scintigraphy help evaluate perfusion several days after rewarming.

℞ TREATMENT   Frozen tissue should be rapidly and completely thawed by immersion in circulating water at 37° to 40°C. Rapid rewarming often produces an initial hyperemia. The early formation of clear distal large blebs is more favorable than smaller proximal dark hemorrhagic blebs. A common error is the premature termination of thawing, since the reestablishment of perfusion is intensely painful. Parenteral narcotics will be necessary with deep frostbite. If cyanosis persists after rewarming, the tissue compartment pressures should be monitored carefully.

Numerous experimental antithrombotic and vasodilatory treatment regimens have been evaluated. There is no conclusive evidence that dextran, heparin, steroids, calcium channel blockers, or hyperbaric oxygen salvage tissue. A treatment protocol for frostbite is summarized in Table 20-3.

Unless infection develops,

Table 20-3   Treatment for Frostbite

Before Thawing	During Thawing	After Thawing
Remove from environment	Consider parenteral analgesia and ketorolac	Gently dry and protect part; elevate; pledgets between toes, if macerated
Prevent partial thawing and refreezing	Administer ibuprofen, 400 mg PO	If clear vesicles are intact, the fluid will reabsorb in days; if broken, debride and dress with antibiotic or sterile aloe vera ointment
Stabilize core temperature and treat hypothermia	Immerse part in 37°–40°C (thermometer-monitored) circulating water containing an antiseptic soap until distal flush (10–45 min)	Leave hemorrhagic vesicles intact to prevent infection
Protect frozen part—no friction or massage	Encourage patient to gently move part	Continue ibuprofen 400 mg PO (12 mg/kg per day) q8–12h
Address medical or surgical conditions	If pain is refractory, reduce water temperature to 33°–37°C	Consider tetanus and streptococcal prophylaxis; elevate part Hydrotherapy at 37°C

any decision regarding debridement or amputation should be deferred until there is clear evidence of demarcation, mummification, and sloughing. The most common symptomatic sequelae reflect neuronal injury and the persistently abnormal sympathetic tone, including paresthesias, thermal misperception, and hyperhidrosis. Delayed findings include nail deformities, cutaneous carcinomas, and epiphyseal damage in children.

BIBLIOGRAPHY

DANZL DF: Accidental hypothermia, in *Emergency Medicine: Concepts and Clinical Practice*, 4th ed, P Rosen et al (eds). St. Louis, Mosby, 1998, p 963

DANZL DF, POZOS RS: Current concepts: Accidental hypothermia. N Engl J Med 331:1756, 1994

GIESBRECHT GG, BRISTOW GK: Recent advances in hypothermia research. Ann NY Acad Sci 813:676, 1997

MCADAMS TR et al: Frostbite: An orthopedic perspective. Am J Orthop 28:21, 1999

WEINBERG AD: The role of inhalation rewarming in the early management of hypothermia. Resuscitation 36:101, 1998

Section 3
NERVOUS SYSTEM DYSFUNCTION

21 *Robert B. Daroff, Mark D. Carlson*

FAINTNESS, SYNCOPE, DIZZINESS, AND VERTIGO

Syncope is defined as transient loss of consciousness due to reduced cerebral blood flow. Syncope is associated with postural collapse and spontaneous recovery. It may occur suddenly, without warning, or may be preceded by symptoms of varying duration. These include faintness or lightheadedness, "dizziness" without true vertigo, a feeling of warmth, diaphoresis, nausea, and visual blurring occasionally proceeding to blindness. These presyncopal symptoms may increase in severity until loss of consciousness occurs or may resolve prior to loss of consciousness if the cerebral ischemia is corrected. The differentiation of syncope from seizure is an important, sometimes difficult, diagnostic problem.

Syncope may be benign when it occurs as a result of normal cardiovascular reflex effects on heart rate and vascular tone or malignant when due to a life-threatening arrhythmia. Syncope may occur as a single event or may be recurrent. Recurrent, unexplained syncope, particularly in an individual with structural heart disease, is associated with a high risk for death (40% mortality within 2 years).

SYNCOPE

At the beginning of a syncopal attack, the patient is nearly always in the upright position, either sitting or standing. A cardiac etiology, such as an arrhythmia, is exceptional in this respect. The patient is warned of the impending faint by a sense of "feeling bad," of giddiness, and of movement or swaying of the floor or surrounding objects. The patient becomes confused and may yawn, visual spots and dimming may occur, and the ears may ring. Nausea and vomiting sometimes accompany these symptoms. There is a striking pallor or ashen gray color of the face, and generalized perspiration ensues. In some patients, a gradual onset with presyncopal symptoms may allow time for protection against injury; in others the syncope is sudden and without warning. The onset varies from instantaneous to 10 to 30 s, rarely longer.

The depth and duration of unconsciousness vary. Sometimes the patient remains partly aware of the surroundings, or there may be profound coma. The patient may remain in this state for seconds or minutes. Usually the patient lies motionless with skeletal muscles relaxed, but a few clonic jerks of the limbs and face may occur shortly after consciousness is lost. Sphincter control is usually maintained, in contrast to a seizure. The pulse is feeble or apparently absent, the blood pressure may be low or undetectable, and breathing may be almost imperceptible. Once the patient is in a horizontal position, gravity no longer hinders the flow of blood to the brain. The strength of the pulse may then improve, color begins to return to the face, breathing becomes quicker and deeper, and consciousness is regained. There is usually an immediate recovery of consciousness. Some patients, however, may be keenly aware of physical weakness, and rising too soon may precipitate another faint. In other patients, particularly those with tachyarrhythmias, there may be no residual symptoms following the initial syncope. Headache and drowsiness, which with mental confusion are the usual sequelae of a seizure, do not follow a syncopal attack.

PATHOPHYSIOLOGY The more common types of faint are reducible to a few simple mechanisms. Syncope results from a sudden impairment of brain metabolism, usually brought about by hypotension with reduction of cerebral blood flow. Several mechanisms subserve circulatory adjustments to the upright posture. Approximately three-fourths of the systemic blood volume is contained in the venous bed, and any interference in venous return may lead to a reduction in cardiac output. Cerebral blood flow may still be maintained, as long as systemic arterial vasoconstriction occurs, but when this adjustment fails, serious hypotension with resultant cerebral underperfusion to less than half of normal results in syncope. Normally, the pooling of blood in the lower parts of the body is prevented by: (1) pressor reflexes that induce constriction of peripheral arterioles and venules, (2) reflex acceleration of the heart by means of aortic and carotid reflexes, and (3) improvement of venous return to the heart by activity of the muscles of the limbs. Placing a normal person on a tilt table to relax the muscles and tilting upright slightly diminishes cardiac output and allows the blood to accumulate in the legs to a slight degree; this may then be followed by a slight transitory fall in systolic arterial pressure and, in patients with defective vasomotor reflexes, may produce faints.

CAUSES OF SYNCOPE Transiently decreased cerebral blood flow is usually due to one of three general mechanisms: disorders of vascular tone or blood volume, cardiovascular disorders including cardiac arrhythmias, or cerebrovascular disease (Table 21-1). Not infrequently, however, the cause of syncope is multifactorial.

Disorders of Vascular Tone or Blood Volume Disorders of autonomic control of the heart and circulation account for at least half of syncopal episodes. These disorders share common pathophysiologic mechanisms: a cardioinhibitory component (e.g., bradycardia due to increased efferent vagal activity), a vasodepressor component (e.g., inappropriate vasodilatation due to sympathetic withdrawal), or both.

Vasovagal (vasodepressor, neurocardiogenic) syncope This form of syncope is the common faint that may be experienced by normal persons and accounts for approximately half of all episodes of syncope. It is frequently recurrent and commonly precipitated by a hot or crowded environment, alcohol, extreme fatigue, severe pain, hunger, prolonged standing, and emotional or stressful situations. Episodes are often preceded by a presyncopal prodrome lasting seconds

Table 21-1   Causes of Syncope

I. Disorders of vascular tone or blood volume
  A. Vasovagal (vasodepressor, neurocardiogenic)
  B. Postural (orthostatic) hypotension
    1. Drug induced (especially antihypertensive or vasodilator drugs)
    2. Peripheral neuropathy (diabetic, alcoholic, nutritional, amyloid)
    3. Idiopathic postural hypotension
    4. Multisystem atrophies
    5. Physical deconditioning
    6. Sympathectomy
    7. Acute dysautonomia (Guillain-Barré syndrome variant)
    8. Decreased blood volume (adrenal insufficiency, acute blood loss, etc.)
  C. Carotid sinus hypersensitivity
  D. Situational
    1. Cough
    2. Micturition
    3. Defecation
    4. Valsalva
    5. Deglutition
  E. Glossopharyngeal Neuralgia
II. Cardiovascular disorders
  A. Cardiac arrhythmias (Chaps. 229 and 230)
    1. Bradyarrhythmias
      a. Sinus bradycardia, sinoatrial block, sinus arrest, sick-sinus syndrome
      b. Atrioventricular block
    2. Tachyarrhythmias
      a. Supraventricular tachycardia with structural cardiac disease
      b. Atrial fibrillation associated with the Wolff-Parkinson-White syndrome
      c. Atrial flutter with 1:1 atrioventricular conduction
      d. Ventricular tachycardia
  B. Other cardiopulmonary etiologies
    1. Pulmonary embolism
    2. Pulmonary hypertension
    3. Atrial myxoma
    4. Myocardial disease (massive myocardial infarction)
    5. Left ventricular myocardial restriction or constriction
    6. Pericardial constriction or tamponade
    7. Aortic outflow tract obstruction
    8. Aortic valvular stenosis
    9. Hypertrophic obstructive cardiomyopathy
III. Cerebrovascular disease (Chap. 361)
  A. Vertebrobasilar insufficiency
  B. Basilar artery migraine
IV. Other disorders that may resemble syncope
  A. Metabolic
    1. Hypoxia
    2. Anemia
    3. Diminished carbon dioxide due to hyperventilation
    4. Hypoglycemia
  B. Psychogenic
    1. Anxiety attacks
    2. Hysterical fainting
  C. Seizures

to minutes. Vasovagal syncope rarely occurs in the supine position. The individual is usually sitting or standing and experiences weakness, nausea, diaphoresis, lightheadedness, blurred vision, and often a forceful heart beat with tachycardia followed by cardiac slowing prior to loss of consciousness. The individual appears pallid and has decreasing blood pressure prior to syncope. The duration of unconsciousness is rarely longer than a few minutes if the conditions that provoke the episode are reversed. Consciousness is usually regained shortly after assuming a recumbent posture, but unconsciousness may be prolonged if an individual remains upright. Although commonly benign, vasovagal syncope can be associated with prolonged asystole and hypotension, resulting in injury.

Vasovagal syncope occurs in the setting of increased sympathetic activity and venous pooling. Under these conditions, vigorous myocardial contraction of a relatively empty left ventricle activates ven-

tricular mechanoreceptors and vagal afferent nerve fibers, inhibiting sympathetic efferent activity and increasing parasympathetic efferent activity. The resultant vasodilatation and bradycardia induce hypotension and syncope.

The central nervous system (CNS) mechanisms responsible for vasovagal syncope are not clear. Animal studies, not confirmed in humans, suggest that endogenous opiates (endorphins) may play a role. Serotonin (5-hydroxytryptamine) participates in blood pressure regulation and may also be involved in inhibition of sympathetic efferent activity (and arterial vasodilatation) associated with vasovagal syncope.

Although the reflex involving myocardial mechanoreceptors is the mechanism usually accepted as responsible for vasovagal syncope, other reflexes may also be operative. Patients with transplanted (denervated) hearts have experienced cardiovascular responses identical to those present during vasovagal syncope. This should not be possible if the response depends solely on the reflex mechanisms described above unless the transplanted heart has become reinnervated. Moreover, vasovagal syncope often occurs in response to stimuli (fear, emotional stress, or pain) that may not be associated with venous pooling in the lower extremities, which suggests a cognitive or cortical component to the reflex. Thus, a variety of afferent and efferent responses may cause vasovagal syncope.

Postural (orthostatic) hypotension   This occurs in patients who have a chronic defect in, or variable instability of, vasomotor reflexes. Systemic arterial blood pressure falls on assumption of upright posture due to loss of vasoconstriction reflexes in resistance and capacitance vessels of the lower extremities. Although the syncopal attack differs little from vasodepressor syncope, the effect of posture is critical. Sudden rising from a recumbent position or standing quietly are precipitating circumstances. *Orthostatic hypotension may be the cause of syncope in up to 30% of the elderly; polypharmacy with antihypertensive or antidepressant drugs is often a contributor in these patients.*

Postural syncope may occur in otherwise normal persons with defective postural reflexes. Patients with *idiopathic postural hypotension* may be identified by a characteristic response to upright tilt on a table. Initially, the blood pressure diminishes slightly before stabilizing at a lower level. Shortly thereafter, the compensatory reflexes fail and the systemic arterial pressure falls precipitously. The condition is often familial.

Orthostatic hypotension, often accompanied by disturbances in sweating, impotence, and sphincter difficulties, is also a primary feature of the autonomic nervous system disorders discussed in Chap. 366 and listed in Table 366-1. The most common causes of neurogenic orthostatic hypotension are chronic diseases of the peripheral nervous system that involve postganglionic unmyelinated fibers (e.g., diabetic, nutritional, and amyloid polyneuropathy). Much less common are the multisystem atrophies, which are CNS disorders in which orthostatic hypotension is associated with (1) parkinsonism (Shy-Drager syndrome), (2) progressive cerebellar degeneration, or (3) a more variable parkinsonian and cerebellar syndrome (striatonigral degeneration). Very rarely, an acute postganglionic dysautonomia has been reported that appears to represent a variant of Guillain-Barré syndrome (Chap. 378).

There are several additional causes of postural syncope: (1) After physical deconditioning (such as after prolonged illness with recumbency, especially in elderly individuals with reduced muscle tone) or after prolonged weightlessness, as in space flight; (2) after sympathectomy that has abolished vasopressor reflexes; and (3) in patients receiving antihypertensive or vasodilator drugs and those who are hypovolemic because of diuretics, excessive sweating, diarrhea, vomiting, hemorrhage, or adrenal insufficiency.

Carotid sinus hypersensitivity   Syncope due to carotid sinus hypersensitivity is precipitated by pressure on the carotid sinus baroreceptors, which are located just cephalad to the bifurcation of the common carotid artery. This typically occurs in the setting of shaving, a tight collar, or turning the head to one side. Carotid sinus hypersensitivity occurs predominantly in men, most of whom are 50 years of age or older. Activation of carotid sinus baroreceptors gives rise to impulses carried via the nerve of Hering, a branch of the glossopharyngeal nerve, to the medulla oblongata. These afferent impulses activate efferent sympathetic nerve fibers to the heart and blood vessels, cardiac vagal efferent nerve fibers, or both. In patients with carotid sinus hypersensitivity, these responses may cause sinus arrest or atrioventricular (AV) block (a cardioinhibitory response), vasodilatation (a vasodepressor response), or both (a mixed response). Although originally described in 1933, the mechanisms responsible for the syndrome are not clear, and validated diagnostic criteria do not exist; some authorities have questioned its very existence.

Situational syncope A variety of activities, including cough, deglutition, micturition, and defecation, are associated with syncope in susceptible individuals. These syndromes are caused, at least in part, by abnormal autonomic control and may involve a cardioinhibitory response, a vasodepressor response, or both. Cough, micturition, and defecation are associated with maneuvers (such as Valsalva, straining, and coughing) that may contribute to hypotension and syncope by decreasing venous return. Increased intracranial pressure secondary to the increased intrathoracic pressure may also contribute by decreasing cerebral blood flow.

Cough syncope typically occurs in men with chronic bronchitis or chronic obstructive lung disease during or immediately after prolonged coughing fits. Micturition syncope occurs predominantly in middle-aged and older men, particularly those with prostatic hypertrophy and obstruction of the bladder neck; loss of consciousness usually occurs at night during or immediately after voiding. Deglutition and defecation syncope occur in men and women. Deglutition syncope may be associated with esophageal disorders, particularly esophageal spasm. In some individuals, particular foods and carbonated or cold beverages initiate episodes by activating esophageal sensory receptors that trigger reflex sinus bradycardia or AV block. Defecation syncope is probably secondary to a Valsalva maneuver in older individuals with constipation.

Glossopharyngeal neuralgia Syncope due to glossopharyngeal neuralgia is preceded by pain in the oropharynx, tonsillar fossa, or tongue. Loss of consciousness is usually associated with asystole rather than vasodilatation. The mechanism is thought to involve activation of afferent impulses in the glossopharyngeal nerve which terminate in the nucleus solitarius of the medulla and, via collaterals, activate the dorsal motor nucleus of the vagus nerve.

Cardiovascular Disorders Cardiac syncope results from a sudden reduction in cardiac output, caused most commonly by a cardiac arrhythmia. In normal individuals, heart rates between 30 and 180 beats per minutes (bpm) do not reduce cerebral blood flow, especially if the person is in the supine position. As the heart rate decreases, ventricular filling time and stroke volume increase to maintain normal cardiac output. At rates below 30 bpm, stroke volume can no longer increase to compensate adequately for the decreased heart rate. At rates greater than approximately 180 bpm, ventricular filling time is inadequate to maintain adequate stroke volume. In either case, cerebral hypoperfusion and syncope may occur. Upright posture, cerebrovascular disease, anemia, and coronary, myocardial, or valvular disease all reduce the tolerance to alterations in rate.

Bradyarrhythmias (Chap. 229) may occur as a result of an abnormality of impulse generation (e.g., sinoatrial arrest) or impulse conduction (e.g., AV block). Either may cause syncope if the escape pacemaker rate is insufficient to maintain cardiac output. Syncope due to bradyarrhythmias may occur abruptly, without presyncopal symptoms, and recur several times daily. Patients with *sick sinus syndrome* may have sinus pauses (>3 s), and those with syncope due to high-degree AV block (*Stokes-Adams-Morgagni syndrome*) may have evidence of conduction system disease (e.g., prolonged PR interval, bundle branch block). However, the arrhythmia is often transitory, and the surface electrocardiogram or continuous electrocardiographic monitor (Holter monitor) taken later may not reveal the abnormality. The *bradycardia-tachycardia syndrome* is a common form of sinus node dysfunction in which syncope generally occurs as a result of marked sinus pauses

following termination of paroxysmal supraventricular tachycardia. Drugs are a common cause for bradyarrhythmias, particularly in patients with underlying structural heart disease. Digoxin, β-adrenergic receptor antagonists, calcium channel blockers, and many antiarrhythmic drugs may suppress sinoatrial node impulse generation or slow AV nodal conduction.

Syncope due to a *tachyarrhythmia* (Chap. 230) is usually preceded by palpitation or lightheadedness but may occur abruptly with no warning symptoms. *Supraventricular tachyarrhythmias* are unlikely to cause syncope in individuals with structurally normal hearts but may do so if they occur in patients with: (1) heart disease that also compromises cardiac output, (2) cerebrovascular disease, (3) a disorder of vascular tone or blood volume, or (4) a rapid ventricular rate. These tachycardias result most commonly from paroxysmal atrial flutter, atrial fibrillation, or reentry involving the AV node or accessory pathways that bypass part or all of the AV conduction system. Patients with the *Wolff-Parkinson-White syndrome* may experience syncope when a very rapid ventricular rate occurs due to reentry across an accessory AV connection.

In patients with structural heart disease, ventricular tachycardia, sometimes associated with ventricular fibrillation, is a common cause of syncope, particularly in patients with a prior myocardial infarction. Patients with aortic valvular stenosis and hypertrophic obstructive cardiomyopathy are also at risk for ventricular tachycardia. Individuals with abnormalities of ventricular repolarization (prolongation of the QT interval) are at risk to develop polymorphic ventricular tachycardia (*torsade de pointes*). Those with the inherited form of this syndrome often have a family history of sudden death in young individuals. Genetic markers can identify some patients with familial long-QT syndrome but the clinical utility of these markers remains unproven. Drugs (i.e., certain antiarrhythmics and erythromycin) and electrolyte disorders (i.e., hypokalemia, hypocalcemia, hypomagnesemia) can prolong the QT interval and predispose to torsade de pointes. Antiarrhythmic medications may precipitate ventricular tachycardia, particularly in patients with structural heart disease.

In addition to arrythmias, syncope may also occur with a variety of structural cardiovascular disorders. Episodes are usually precipitated when the cardiac output cannot increase to compensate adequately for peripheral vasodilatation. Peripheral vasodilatation may be appropriate, such as following exercise, or may occur due to inappropriate activation of left ventricular mechanoreceptor reflexes, as occurs in aortic outflow tract obstruction (aortic valvular stenosis or hypertrophic obstructive cardiomyopathy). Obstruction to forward flow is the most common reason that cardiac output cannot increase. Pericardial tamponade is a rare cause of syncope. Syncope occurs in up to 10% of patients with massive pulmonary embolism and may occur with exertion in patients with severe primary pulmonary hypertension. The cause is an inability of the right ventricle to provide appropriate cardiac output in the presence of obstruction or increased pulmonary vascular resistance. Loss of consciousness is usually accompanied by other symptoms such as chest pain and dyspnea. Atrial myxoma, a prosthetic valve thrombus, and, rarely, mitral stenosis may impair left ventricular filling, decrease cardiac output, and cause syncope.

Cerebrovascular Disease Cerebrovascular disease alone rarely causes syncope but may lower the threshold for syncope in patients with other causes. The vertebrobasilar arteries, which supply brainstem centers responsible for maintaining consciousness, are usually involved when cerebrovascular disease causes or contributes to syncope. An exception is the rare patient with tight bilateral carotid stenosis and recurrent syncope, often precipitated by standing or walking. Most patients who experience lightheadedness or syncope due to cerebrovascular disease also have symptoms of focal neurologic ischemia, such as arm or leg weakness, diplopia, ataxia, dysarthria, or sensory disturbances. Basilar artery migraine is a rare disorder that causes syncope in adolescents.

DIFFERENTIAL DIAGNOSIS Anxiety Attacks and the Hyperventilation Syndrome Anxiety, such as occurs in panic attacks, is frequently interpreted as a feeling of faintness or dizziness resembling presyncope. The symptoms are not accompanied by facial pallor and are not relieved by recumbency. The diagnosis is made on the basis of the associated symptoms such as a feeling of impending doom, air hunger, palpitations, and tingling of the fingers and perioral region. Attacks can often be reproduced by hyperventilation, resulting in hypocapnia, alkalosis, increased cerebrovascular resistance, and decreased cerebral blood flow. The release of epinephrine in anxiety states also contributes to the symptoms.

Seizures A seizure may be heralded by an aura, which is caused by a focal seizure discharge and hence has localizing significance. The aura is usually followed by a rapid return to normal or by a loss of consciousness. Injury from falling is frequent in a seizure and rare in syncope, because only in seizures are protective reflexes abolished instantaneously. Tonic-convulsive movements are characteristic of seizures and usually do not occur with syncope, although, as stated above, brief tonic-clonic seizure-like activity can accompany fainting episodes. The period of unconsciousness tends to be longer in seizures than in syncope. Urinary incontinence is frequent in seizures and rare in syncope. The return of consciousness is prompt in syncope, slow after a seizure. Mental confusion, headache, and drowsiness are common sequelae of seizures; physical weakness with a clear sensorium characterizes the postsyncopal state. Repeated spells of unconsciousness in a young person at a rate of several per day or month are more suggestive of epilepsy than syncope.

Hypoglycemia Severe hypoglycemia is usually due to a serious disease such as a tumor of the islets of Langerhans; advanced adrenal, pituitary, or hepatic disease; or to excessive administration of insulin.

Acute Hemorrhage Hemorrhage, usually within the gastrointestinal tract, is an occasional cause of syncope. In the absence of pain and hematemesis, the cause of the weakness, faintness, or even unconsciousness may remain obscure until the passage of a black stool.

Hysterical Fainting The attack is usually unattended by an outward display of anxiety. Lack of change in pulse and blood pressure or color of the skin and mucous membranes distinguish it from the vasodepressor faint.

_____ *Approach to the Patient* _____

The diagnosis of syncope is often challenging. The cause may only be apparent at the time of the event, leaving few, if any, clues when the patient is seen later by the physician. In dealing with patients who have fainted, the physician should think first of those causes of fainting that constitute a therapeutic emergency. Among them are massive internal hemorrhage or myocardial infarction, which may be painless, and cardiac arrythmias. In elderly persons, a sudden faint, without obvious cause, should arouse the suspicion of complete heart block or a tachyarrhythmia, even though all findings are negative when the patient is seen.

An algorithmic approach to syncope is presented in Fig. 21-1. A careful history is the most important diagnostic tool, both to suggest the correct cause and to exclude other important potential causes (Table 21-1). Although no single element of the history is specific for a particular etiology of syncope, the nature of the events and their time course immediately prior to, during, and after an episode often provide valuable etiologic clues. Loss of consciousness in particular situations, such as during venipuncture, micturition, or in association with volume depletion, suggests an abnormality of vascular tone. The position of the patient at the time of the syncopal episode is very important; syncope in the supine position is unlikely to be vasovagal and suggests an arrhythmia or a seizure. Syncope due to carotid sinus syndrome may occur when the individual is wearing a shirt with a tight collar, turning the head (turning to look while driving in reverse), or manipulating the neck (as in shaving). The patient's medications must be

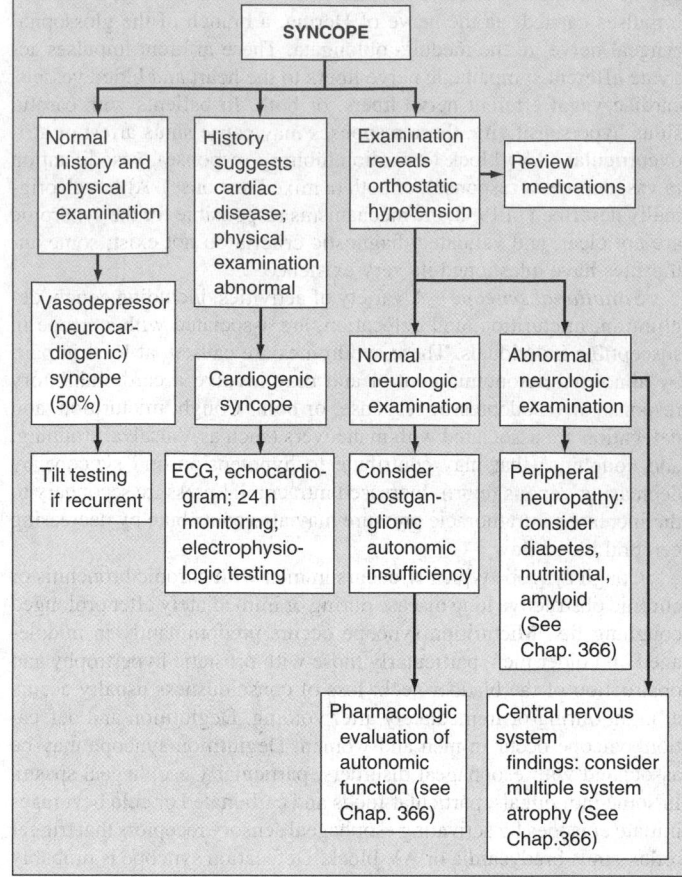

FIGURE 21-1 Approach to the patient with syncope.

noted, including nonprescription drugs or health store supplements, with particular attention to recent changes.

The physical examination should include evaluation of heart rate and blood pressure in the supine, sitting, and standing positions. In patients with unexplained recurrent syncope, an attempt to reproduce an attack may assist in diagnosis. Anxiety attacks induced by hyperventilation can be reproduced readily by having the patient breathe rapidly and deeply for 2 to 3 min. Cough syncope may be reproduced by inducing the Valsalva maneuver. Carotid sinus massage should generally be avoided, even in patients with suspected carotid sinus hypersensitivity; it is a risky procedure that can cause a transient ischemic attack (TIA) or stroke in susceptible individuals.

Diagnostic Tests The choice of diagnostic tests should be guided by the history and the physical examination. Measurements of serum electrolytes, glucose, and the hematocrit may help to establish the cause of syncope. Cardiac enzymes should be evaluated if myocardial ischemia is suspected. Blood and urine toxicology screens may reveal the presence of alcohol or other drugs. In patients with possible adrenocortical insufficiency, plasma aldosterone and mineralocorticoid levels should be obtained.

Although the surface electrocardiogram is unlikely to provide a definitive diagnosis, it may provide clues to the cause of syncope *and should be performed in almost all patients*. The presence of conduction abnormalities (PR prolongation and bundle branch block) suggests a bradyarrhythmia, whereas pathologic Q waves or prolongation of the QT interval suggests a ventricular tachyarrhythmia. Inpatients should undergo continuous electrocardiographic monitoring; outpatients should wear a Holter monitor for 24 to 48 h. Whenever possible, symptoms should be correlated with the occurrence of arrhythmias. Continuous electrocardiographic monitoring may establish the cause of syncope in as many as 15% of patients. Cardiac event monitors may be useful in patients with infrequent symptoms, particularly in patients with presyncope. The presence of a late potential on a signal-averaged electrocardiogram is associated with increased risk for ventricular tacharrhythmias in patients with a prior myocardial infarction. Low-voltage (visually inapparent) T wave alternans is also associated with development of sustained ventricular arrhythmias.

Invasive cardiac electrophysiologic testing provides diagnostic and prognostic information regarding sinus node function, AV conduction, and supraventricular and ventricular arrhythmias. Abnormal findings include prolongation of the sinus node recovery time, prolongation of the histoventricle (HV) interval, induction of a supraventricular arrhythmia associated with hypotension, or induction of a supraventricular arrhythmia. Prolongation of the sinus node recovery time (>1500 ms) is a specific finding (85 to 100%) for diagnosis of sinus node dysfunction but has a low sensitivity; continuous electrocardiographic monitoring is usually more effective for diagnosing this abnormality. Prolongation of the HV interval and conduction block below the His bundle indicate that His-Purkinje disease may be responsible for syncope. Although an HV interval >100 ms is abnormal, this finding is not common in patients with syncope, and some patients with shorter intervals are also at risk for AV block. Programmed stimulation for ventricular arrhythmias is most useful in patients who have experienced a myocardial infarction; the sensitivity and specificity of this technique is lower in patients with normal hearts or those with heart disease other than coronary artery disease.

Upright tilt table testing is indicated for recurrent syncope, a single syncopal episode that caused injury, or a single syncopal event in a "high-risk" setting (pilot, commercial vehicle driver, etc.), whether or not there is a history of preexisting heart disease or prior vasovagal episodes. In susceptible patients, upright tilt at an angle between 60 and 80° for 30 to 60 min induces a vasovagal episode. The protocol can be shortened if upright tilt is combined with intravenous administration of drugs that cause venous pooling or increase adrenergic stimulation (isoproterenol, nitroglycerin, edrophonium, or adenosine). The sensitivity and specificity of tilt table testing is difficult to ascertain because of the lack of validated criteria. Moreover, the reflexes responsible for vasovagal syncope can be elicited in most, if not all, individuals given the appropriate stimulus. The reported accuracy of the test ranges from 30 to 80%, depending on the population studied and the techniques used. Whereas the reproducibility of a negative test is 85 to 100%, the reproducibility of a positive tilt table test is only between 62 and 88%.

A variety of other tests may be useful to determine the presence of structural heart disease that may cause syncope. The echocardiogram with Doppler examination detects valvular, myocardial, and pericardial abnormalities. The echocardiogram is the "gold standard" for the diagnosis of hypertrophic cardiomyopathy and atrial myxoma. Cardiac cine magnetic resonance (MR) imaging provides an alternative noninvasive modality that may be useful for patients in whom diagnostic-quality echocardiographic images cannot be obtained. This test is also indicated for patients suspected of having arrhythmogenic right ventricular dysplasia or right ventricular outflow tract ventricular tachycardia. Both are associated with right ventricular structural abnormalities that are better visualized on MR imaging than by echocardiogram. Exercise testing may detect ischemia or exercise-induced arrhythmias. In some patients, cardiac catheterization may be necessary to diagnose the presence or severity of coronary artery disease or valvular abnormalities. Ultrafast computed tomographic scan, ventilation-perfusion scan, or pulmonary angiography are indicated in patients in whom syncope may be due to pulmonary embolus.

In possible cases of cerebrovascular syncope, a variety of neuroimaging tests may be indicated, including Doppler ultrasound studies of the carotid and vertebrobasilar systems, MR imaging, MR angiography, and x-ray angiography of the cerebral vasculature (Chaps. 358 and 361). Electroencephalography is indicated if seizures are suspected.

℞ **TREATMENT** The treatment of syncope is directed toward the underlying cause. This discussion will focus on the treatment

of disorders of autonomic control. →*Arrythmias are discussed in Chaps. 229 and 230, valvular heart diseases in Chap. 236, and cerebrovascular disorders in Chap. 361.*

Certain precautions should be taken regardless of the cause of syncope. At the first sign of symptoms, patients should make every effort to avoid injury should they lose consciousness. Patients with frequent episodes, or those who have experienced syncope without warning symptoms should avoid situations in which sudden loss of consciousness might result in injury (e.g., climbing ladders, swimming alone, operating heavy machinery, driving). Patients should lower their head to the extent possible, and preferably should lie down. Lowering the head by bending at the waist should be avoided because it may further compromise venous return to the heart. When appropriate, family members or other close contacts should be educated as to the problem. This will ensure appropriate therapy and may prevent delivery of inappropriate therapy (chest compressions associated with cardiopulmonary resuscitation) that may inflict trauma.

Patients who have lost consciousness should be placed in a position that maximizes cerebral blood flow, offers protection from trauma, and secures the airway. Whenever possible, the patient should be placed supine with the head turned to the side to prevent aspiration and the tongue from blocking the airway. Assessment of the pulse and direct cardiac auscultation may assist in determining if the episode is associated with a bradyarrhythmia or tachyarrhythmia. Clothing that fits tightly around the neck or waist should be loosened. Peripheral stimulation, such as by sprinkling cold water on the face, may be helpful. Patients should not be given anything by mouth or be permitted to rise until the sense of physical weakness has passed.

Patients with vasovagal syncope should be instructed to avoid situations or stimuli that have caused them to lose consciousness. Episodes associated with intravascular volume depletion may be prevented by salt and fluid loading prior to provocative events. β-Adrenoceptor antagonists, the most widely used agents, mitigate the increase in myocardial contractility that stimulates left ventricular mechanoreceptors and also block central serotonin receptors. Disopyramide, a vagolytic with negative inotropic properties, and another vagolytic, transdermal scopolamine, are used to treat vasovagal syncope. Paroxetine, a serotonin reuptake inhibitor used for depression, appears to be an effective treatment, as are theophylline and ephedrine. Midodrine, an α agonist, has been a first-line agent for some patients. Permanent cardiac pacing is effective for patients with frequent episodes of vasovagal syncope and is indicated for those with prolonged asystole associated with vasovagal episodes.

Patients with orthostatic hypotension should be instructed to rise slowly and systematically (supine to seated, seated to standing) from the bed or a chair. Movement of the legs prior to rising facilitates venous return from the lower extremities. Whenever possible, medications that aggravate the problem (vasodilators, diuretics, etc.) should be discontinued. Elevation of the head of the bed [20 to 30 cm (8 to 12 in.)] and use of elastic stockings may help.

Therapeutic modalities include devices that prevent lower limb blood pooling, such as an antigravity or g suit or elastic stockings; salt loading; and a variety of pharmacologic agents including sympathomimetic amines, monamine oxidase inhibitors, beta blockers, and levodopa. →*The treatment of orthostatic hypotension secondary to central or peripheral disorders of the autonomic nervous system is discussed in Chap. 366.*

Glossopharyngeal neuralgia is treated with carbamazepine, which is effective for the syncope as well as for the pain. Patients with carotid sinus syndrome should be instructed to avoid clothing and situations that stimulate carotid sinus baroreceptors. Patients should turn their entire body, rather than just their head, to look to one side. Those with intractable syncope due to the cardioinhibitory response to carotid sinus stimulation should undergo permanent pacemaker implantation.

Patients with syncope should be hospitalized when the episode may have resulted from a life-threatening abnormality or if recurrence with significant injury seems likely. These individuals should be admitted to a bed with continuous electrocardiographic monitoring. Patients who are known to have a normal heart and for whom the history strongly suggests vasovagal or situational syncope may be treated as outpatients if the episodes are neither frequent nor severe.

DIZZINESS AND VERTIGO

Dizziness is a common and often vexing symptom. Patients use the term to encompass a variety of sensations, including those that seem semantically appropriate (e.g., lightheadedness, faintness, spinning, giddiness, etc.) and those that are misleadingly inappropriate, such as mental confusion, blurred vision, headache, or tingling. Moreover, some individuals with gait disorders complain of dizziness despite the absence of vertigo or other abnormal cephalic sensations. The causes include peripheral neuropathy, myelopathy, spasticity, parkinsonian rigidity, and cerebellar ataxia. In this context, the term *dizziness* is being used to describe disturbed mobility. There may be mild associated lightheadedness, particularly with impaired sensation from the feet or poor vision; this is known as *multiple-sensory-defect dizziness* and occurs in elderly individuals who complain of dizziness only during ambulation. Decreased position sense (secondary to neuropathy or myelopathy) and poor vision (from cataracts or retinal degeneration) create an overreliance on the aging vestibular apparatus. A less precise but sometimes comforting designation to patients is *benign dysequilibrium of aging*. Thus, a careful history is necessary to determine exactly what a patient who states, "Doctor, I'm dizzy," is experiencing. After eliminating the misleading symptoms or gait disturbance, "dizziness" usually means either *faintness* (presyncope) or *vertigo* (an illusory or hallucinatory sense of movement of the body or environment, most often a feeling of spinning). Operationally, dizziness is classified into three categories: (1) faintness, (2) vertigo, and (3) miscellaneous head sensations.

FAINTNESS   Prior to an actual faint (syncope), there are often prodromal presyncopal symptoms (faintness) reflecting ischemia to a degree insufficient to impair consciousness (see above).

VERTIGO   Vertigo is usually due to a disturbance in the vestibular system. The end organs of this system, situated in the bony labyrinths of the inner ears, consist of the three semicircular canals and the otolithic apparatus (utricle and saccule) on each side. The canals transduce angular acceleration, while the otoliths transduce linear acceleration and static gravitational forces, the latter providing a sense of head position in space. The neural output of the end organs is conveyed to the vestibular nuclei in the brainstem via the eighth cranial nerve. The principal projections from the vestibular nuclei are to the nuclei of cranial nerves III, IV, and VI, the spinal cord, the cerebral cortex, and the cerebellum. The vestibuloocular reflex (VOR) serves to maintain visual stability during head movement and depends on direct projections from the vestibular nuclei to the sixth cranial nerve (abducens) nuclei in the pons and, via the medial longitudinal fasciculus, to the third (oculomotor) and fourth (trochlear) cranial nerve nuclei in the midbrain. These connections account for the nystagmus (to-and-fro oscillation of the eyes) that is an almost invariable accompaniment of vestibular dysfunction. The vestibular nerves and nuclei project to areas of the cerebellum (primarily the flocculus and nodulus) that modulate the VOR. The vestibulospinal pathways assist in the maintenance of postural stability. Projections to the cerebral cortex, via the thalamus, provide conscious awareness of head position and movement.

The vestibular system is one of three sensory systems subserving spatial orientation and posture; the other two are the visual system (retina to occipital cortex) and the somatosensory system that conveys peripheral information from skin, joint, and muscle receptors. The three stabilizing systems overlap sufficiently to compensate (partially or completely) for each other's deficiencies. Vertigo may represent either physiologic stimulation or pathologic dysfunction in any of the three systems.

Physiologic Vertigo   This occurs when (1) the brain is confronted with a mismatch among the three stabilizing sensory systems; (2) the vestibular system is subjected to unfamiliar head movements to which it has never adapted, such as in seasickness; or (3) unusual head/neck positions, such as the extreme extension when painting a ceiling. Intersensory mismatch explains carsickness, height vertigo, and the visual vertigo most commonly experienced during motion picture chase scenes; in the latter, the visual sensation of environmental movement is unaccompanied by concomitant vestibular and somatosensory movement cues. *Space sickness*, a frequent transient effect of active head movement in the weightless zero-gravity environment, is another example of physiologic vertigo.

Pathologic Vertigo   This results from lesions of the visual, somatosensory, or vestibular systems. Visual vertigo is caused by new or incorrect spectacles or by the sudden onset of an extraocular muscle paresis with diplopia; in either instance, CNS compensation rapidly counteracts the vertigo. Somatosensory vertigo, rare in isolation, is usually due to a peripheral neuropathy that reduces the sensory input necessary for central compensation when there is dysfunction of the vestibular or visual systems.

The most common cause of pathologic vertigo is vestibular dysfunction. The vertigo is frequently accompanied by nausea, jerk nystagmus, postural unsteadiness, and gait ataxia. Since vertigo increases with rapid head movements, patients tend to hold their heads still.

Labyrinthine dysfunction   This causes severe rotational or linear vertigo. When rotational, the hallucination of movement, whether of environment or self, is directed away from the side of the lesion. The fast phases of nystagmus beat away from the lesion side, and the tendency to fall is toward the side of the lesion.

When the head is straight and immobile, the vestibular end organs generate a tonic resting firing frequency that is equal from the two sides. With any rotational acceleration, the anatomic positions of the semicircular canals on each side necessitate an increased firing rate from one and a commensurate decrease from the other. This change in neural activity is ultimately projected to the cerebral cortex, where it is summed with inputs from the visual and somatosensory systems to produce the appropriate conscious sense of rotational movement. After cessation of movement, the firing frequencies of the two end organs reverse; the side with the initially increased rate decreases, and the other side increases. A sense of rotation in the opposite direction is experienced; since there is no actual head movement, this hallucinatory sensation is *physiologic postrotational vertigo*.

Any disease state that changes the firing frequency of an end organ, producing unequal neural input to the brainstem and ultimately the cerebral cortex, causes vertigo. The symptom can be conceptualized as the cortex inappropriately interpreting the abnormal neural input from the brainstem as indicating actual head rotation. Transient abnormalities produce short-lived symptoms. With a fixed unilateral deficit, central compensatory mechanisms ultimately diminish the vertigo. Since compensation depends on the plasticity of connections between the vestibular nuclei and the cerebellum, patients with brainstem or cerebellar disease have diminished adaptive capacity, and symptoms may persist indefinitely. Compensation is always inadequate for severe fixed bilateral lesions despite normal cerebellar connections: these patients are permanently symptomatic.

Acute unilateral labyrinthine dysfunction is caused by infection, trauma, and ischemia. Often, no specific etiology is uncovered, and the nonspecific terms *acute labyrinthitis*, *acute peripheral vestibulopathy*, or *vestibular neuritis* are used to describe the event. The attacks are brief and leave the patient for some days with a mild positional vertigo. Infection with herpes simplex virus type 1 has been implicated. It is impossible to predict whether a patient recovering from the first bout of vertigo will have recurrent episodes.

Acute bilateral labyrinthine dysfunction is usually the result of toxins such as drugs or alcohol. The most common offending drugs are the aminoglycoside antibiotics which damage the fine hair cells of the vestibular end organs and may cause a permanent disorder of equilibrium.

Recurrent unilateral labyrinthine dysfunction, in association with signs and symptoms of cochlear disease (progressive hearing loss and tinnitus), is usually due to Ménière's disease (Chap. 29). When auditory manifestations are absent, the term *vestibular neuronitis* denotes recurrent monosymptomatic vertigo. TIAs of the posterior cerebral circulation (vertebrobasilar insufficiency) very infrequently cause recurrent vertigo without concomitant motor, sensory, visual, cranial nerve, or cerebellar signs.

Positional vertigo is precipitated by a recumbent head position, either to the right or to the left. Benign paroxysmal positional (or positioning) vertigo (BPPV) of the posterior semicircular canal is particularly common. Although the condition may be due to head trauma, usually no precipitating factors are identified. It generally abates spontaneously after weeks or months. The vertigo and accompanying nystagmus have a distinct pattern of latency, fatigability, and habituation that differs from the less common central positional vertigo (Table 21-2) due to lesions in and around the fourth ventricle. Moreover, the pattern of nystagmus in posterior canal BPPV is distinctive. The lower eye displays a large-amplitude torsional nystagmus, and the upper eye has a lesser degree of torsion combined with upbeating nystagmus. If the eyes are directed to the upper ear, the vertical nystagmus in the upper eye increases in amplitude.

Vertigo of vestibular nerve origin may occur with diseases that involve the nerve in the petrous bone or the cerebellopontine angle. Except that it is less severe and less frequently paroxysmal, it has many of the characteristics of labyrinthine vertigo. The adjacent auditory division of the eighth cranial nerve also may be affected, which explains the frequent association of vertigo with tinnitus and deafness. The function of the eighth cranial nerve may be disturbed by tumors of the lateral recess (especially schwannomas), less frequently by meningeal inflammation in this region and, rarely, by an abnormal vessel that compresses the nerve.

Schwannomas involving the eighth cranial nerve (*acoustic neuroma*) grow slowly and produce such a gradual reduction of labyrinthine output that central compensatory mechanisms can prevent or minimize the vertigo; auditory symptoms of hearing loss and tinnitus are the most common manifestations. While lesions of the brainstem or cerebellum can cause acute vertigo, associated signs and symptoms usually permit distinction from a labyrinthine etiology (Table 21-3). However, labyrinthine ischemia, presumably due to occlusion of the labyrinthine branch of the internal auditory artery, may be the sole manifestation of vertebrobasilar insufficiency; patients with this syndrome present with the abrupt onset of severe vertigo, nausea and vomiting without tinnitus or hearing loss. Occasionally, an acute lesion of the vestibulocerebellum may present with monosymptomatic vertigo indistinguishable from a labyrinthopathy.

Vestibular epilepsy, vertigo secondary to temporal lobe epileptic activity, is rare and almost always intermixed with other epileptic manifestations.

Psychogenic vertigo, usually a concomitant of panic attacks or

Table 21-2 Benign Paroxysmal Positional Vertigo (BPPV) and Central Positional Vertigo

Features	BPPV	Central
Latency[a]	3–40 s	None: immediate vertigo and nystagmus
Fatigability[b]	Yes	No
Habituation[c]	Yes	No
Intensity of vertigo	Severe	Mild
Reproducibility[d]	Variable	Good

[a] Time between attaining head position and onset of symptoms.
[b] Disappearance of symptoms with maintenance of offending position.
[c] Lessening of symptoms with repeated trials.
[d] Likelihood of symptom production during any examination session.

Table 21-3 Differentiation of Peripheral and Central Vertigo

Sign or Symptom	Peripheral (Labyrinth)	Central (Brainstem or Cerebellum)
Direction of associated nystagmus	Unidirectional; fast phase opposite lesion[a]	Bidirectional or unidirectional
Purely horizontal nystagmus without torsional component	Uncommon	Common
Vertical or purely torsional nystagmus	Never present	May be present
Visual fixation	Inhibits nystagmus and vertigo	No inhibition
Severity of vertigo	Marked	Often mild
Direction of spin	Toward fast phase	Variable
Direction of fall	Toward slow phase	Variable
Duration of symptoms	Finite (minutes, days, weeks) but recurrent	May be chronic
Tinnitus and/or deafness	Often present	Usually absent
Associated central abnormalities	None	Extremely common
Common causes	Infection (labyrinthitis), Ménière's, neuronitis, ischemia, trauma, toxin	Vascular, demyelinating, neoplasm

[a] In Ménière's disease, the direction of the fast phase is variable.

agoraphobia (fear of large open spaces, crowds, or leaving the safety of home), should be suspected in patients so "incapacitated" by their symptoms that they adopt a prolonged housebound status. Most patients with organic vertigo attempt to function despite their discomfort. Organic vertigo is accompanied by nystagmus; a psychogenic etiology is almost certain when nystagmus is absent during a vertiginous episode.

Miscellaneous Head Sensations This designation is used, primarily for purposes of initial classification, to describe dizziness that is neither faintness nor vertigo. Cephalic ischemia or vestibular dysfunction may be of such low intensity that the usual symptomatology is not clearly identified. For example, a small decrease in blood pressure or a slight vestibular imbalance may cause sensations different from distinct faintness or vertigo but that may be identified properly during provocative testing techniques. Other causes of dizziness in this category are hyperventilation syndrome, hypoglycemia, and the somatic symptoms of a clinical depression; these patients should have normal neurologic examinations and vestibular function tests.

Approach to the Patient

The most important diagnostic tool is a careful history focused on the meaning of "dizziness" to the patient. Is it faintness? Is there a sensation of spinning? If either of these is affirmed and the neurologic examination is normal, appropriate investigations for the multiple etiologies of cephalic ischemia or vestibular dysfunction are undertaken.

When the meaning of "dizziness" is uncertain, provocative tests may be helpful. These office procedures simulate either cephalic ischemia or vestibular dysfunction. Cephalic ischemia is obvious if the dizziness is duplicated during maneuvers that produce orthostatic hypotension. Further provocation involves the Valsalva maneuver, which decreases cerebral blood flow and should reproduce ischemic symptoms.

The simplest provocative test for vestibular dysfunction is rapid rotation and abrupt cessation of movement in a swivel chair. This always induces vertigo that the patients can compare with their symptomatic dizziness. The intense induced vertigo may be unlike the spontaneous symptoms, but shortly thereafter, when the vertigo has all but subsided, a lightheadedness supervenes that may be identified as "my dizziness." When this occurs, the dizzy patient, originally classified as suffering from "miscellaneous head sensations," is now properly diagnosed as having mild vertigo secondary to a vestibulopathy.

Patients with symptoms of positional vertigo should be appropriately tested (Table 21-2); positional testing is more sensitive with special spectacles that preclude visual fixation (Frenzel lenses).

A final provocative test, requiring the use of Frenzel lenses, is vigorous head shaking in the horizontal plane for about 10 s. If nystagmus develops after the shaking stops, even in the absence of vertigo, vestibular dysfunction is demonstrated. The maneuver can then be repeated in the vertical plane. If the provocative tests establish the dizziness as a vestibular symptom, an evaluation of vestibular vertigo is undertaken.

Evaluation of Patients with Pathologic Vestibular Vertigo
The evaluation depends on whether a central etiology is suspected (Table 21-3). If so, MR imaging of the head is mandatory. Such an examination is rarely helpful in cases of recurrent monosymptomatic vertigo with a normal neurologic examination. Typical BPPV requires no investigation after the diagnosis is made (Table 21-2).

Vestibular function tests serve to (1) demonstrate an abnormality when the distinction between organic and psychogenic is uncertain, (2) establish the side of the abnormality, and (3) distinguish between peripheral and central etiologies. The standard test is electronystagmography (calorics), where warm and cold water (or air) are applied, in a prescribed fashion, to the tympanic membranes, and the slow-phase velocities of the resultant nystagmus from the right and left ears are compared. A velocity decrease from one side indicates hypofunction ("canal paresis"). An inability to induce nystagmus with ice water denotes a "dead labyrinth." Some institutions have the capability of quantitatively determining various aspects of the vestibuloocular reflex using computer-driven rotational chairs and precise oculographic recording of the eye movements.

Hyperventilation is the cause of dizziness in many anxious individuals; tingling of the hands and face may be absent. Forced hyperventilation for 1 min is indicated for patients with enigmatic dizziness and normal neurologic examinations. Similarly, depressive symptoms (which patients usually insist are "secondary" to the dizziness) must alert the examiner to a clinical depression as the *cause*, rather than the effect, of the dizziness.

CNS disease can produce dizzy sensations of all types. Consequently, a neurologic examination is always required even if the history or provocative tests suggest a cardiac, peripheral vestibular, or psychogenic etiology. Any abnormality on the neurologic examination should prompt appropriate neurodiagnostic studies.

℞ **TREATMENT**   Treatment of acute vertigo consists of bed rest and vestibular suppressant drugs such as antihistaminics (meclizine, dimenhydrinate, promethazine), or a tranquilizer with GABA-ergic effects (diazepam). If the vertigo persists beyond a few days, most authorities advise ambulation in an attempt to induce central compensatory mechanisms, despite the short-term discomfort to the patient. Chronic vertigo of labyrinthine origin may be treated with a systematized vestibular rehabilitation program to facilitate central compensation (see also Table 21-4).

BPPV is often self-limited but, when persistent, responds dramatically to specific repositioning exercise programs designed to empty particulate debris from the posterior semicircular canal. One of these exercises, the Epley procedure, is graphically demonstrated, in four languages, on a website for use in both physician's offices and self-treatment (www.charite.de/ch/neuro/vertigo.html).

Prophylactic measures to prevent recurrent vertigo are variably effective. Antihistamines are commonly utilized. Ménière's disease may respond to a diuretic or, more effectively, to a very low salt diet (1 g/day).

There are a variety of inner ear surgical procedures for refractory Ménière's disease, but these are only rarely necessary.

Table 21-4   Treatment of Vertigo

Agent	Dose[a]
Antihistamines	
Meclizine	25–50 mg 3 times/day
Dimenhydrinate	50 mg 1–2 times/day
Promethazine[b]	25–50 mg/d
Anticholinergic[c]	
Scopolamine transdermal patch	1.5 mg over 3 days
Sympathomimetic	
Ephedrine	25 mg/d
Benzodiazepine	
Diazepam	2.5 mg 1–3 times/day
Combination preparation	
Ephedrine and promethazine	25 mg/d of each
Exercise therapy	
Repositioning maneuvers[d]	
Vestibular rehabilitation[e]	
Other	
Diuretics or low-salt (1 g/d) diet[f]	
Inner ear surgery[g]	

[a] Usual starting dose in adults; maintenance dose can be increased by a factor of 2–3.
[b] Also has strong antiemetic effect.
[c] For motion sickness only.
[d] For benign paroxysmal positional vertigo.
[e] For vertigo other than Ménière's and positional.
[f] For Ménière's disease.
[g] For refractory cases of Ménière's disease.

BIBLIOGRAPHY

Arbusow V et al: Distribution of herpes simplex virus Type I in human geniculate and vestibular ganglia: Implications for vestibular neuritis. Ann Neurol 46:416, 1999

Baloh RW: Vertigo. Lancet 352:1841, 1998

Baloh RW: The dizzy patient: Presence of vertigo points to vestibular cause. Post Grad Med 105:161, 1999

Büttner U et al: The direction of nystagmus is important for the diagnosis of central paroxysmal positional nystagmus (cPPV). Neuro-ophthalmology 21:97, 1999

Connolly SJ et al: The North American Vasovagal Pacemaker Study (VPS). A randomized trial of permanent cardiac pacing for the prevention of vasovagal syncope. J Am Coll Cardiol 33:16, 1999

DiGirolamo E et al: Effects of paroxetine hydrochloride, a selective serotonin reuptake inhibitor, on refractory vasovagal syncope: A randomized double-blind, placebo controlled study. J Am Coll Cardiol 33:1227, 1999

Furman JM, Cass SP: Benign paroxysmal positional vertigo. N Engl J Med 3418:590, 1999

Herdman SJ et al: Vestibular rehabilitation of patients with vestibular hypofunction or with benign positional vertigo. Curr Opin Neurol 13:39, 2000

Hoffman RM et al: Evaluating dizziness. Am J Med 107:468, 1999

Linzer M et al: Diagnosing syncope—Part 1: Value of history, physical examination, and electrocardiography. Ann Intern Med 126:989, 1997

———— et al: Diagnosing syncope—Part 2: Unexplained syncope. Ann Intern Med 127: 76, 1997

Radtke A et al: A modified Epley's procedure for self-treatment of benign paroxysmal positional vertigo. Neurology 53:1358, 1999

Troost BT: Dizziness and vertigo, in *Neurology in Clinical Practice*, 3d ed, WG Bradley et al (eds). Boston, Butterworth-Heinemann, 2000, chap 18

Tusa RJ: The dizzy patient: Disturbances of the vestibular system. In *Neuro-ophthalmology*, 3d ed, JS Glaser (ed). New York, Lippincott Williams & Wilkins, 2000, chap 18

22   *Richard K. Olney, Michael J. Aminoff*

WEAKNESS, MYALGIAS, DISORDERS OF MOVEMENT, AND IMBALANCE

Normal motor function requires integrated muscle activity with appropriate modulation by neuronal activity in the cerebral cortex, basal ganglia, cerebellum, and spinal cord. Symptoms and signs of motor system dysfunction may include weakness, fatigue, myalgias, spasms, cramps, dyskinetic movement, ataxia, imbalance, or disorders in the initiation or planning of movement.

WEAKNESS

Weakness is a reduction in normal power of one or more muscles. Patients may use the term differently; thus one or more specific examples of weakness should be elicited during the history. Increased fatigability or limitation in function due to pain is often confused with weakness by patients. *Increased fatigability* is the inability to sustain the performance of an activity that should be normal for a person of the same age, gender, and size.

Weakness is described commonly by severity and distribution. Paralysis and the suffix "-plegia" indicate weakness that is so severe that it is complete or nearly complete. "Paresis" refers to weakness that is mild or moderate. The prefix "hemi-" refers to one half of the body, "para-" to both legs, and "quadri-" to all four limbs.

Tone is the resistance of a muscle to passive stretch. Central nervous system (CNS) abnormalities that cause weakness generally produce *spasticity*, an increase in tone due to upper motor neuron disease. Spasticity is velocity-dependent, has a sudden release after reaching a maximum (the "clasp-knife" phenomenon), and predominantly affects antigravity muscles (i.e., upper limb flexors and lower limb extensors). Spasticity is distinct from rigidity and paratonia, two other types of increased tone. *Rigidity* is increased tone that is present throughout the range of motion (a "lead pipe" or "plastic" stiffness) and affects flexors and extensors equally. In some patients, rigidity has a cogwheel quality that is enhanced by voluntary movement of the contralateral limb (reinforcement). Rigidity occurs with certain extrapyramidal disorders. *Paratonia*, also referred to as *gegenhalten*, is increased tone that varies irregularly in a manner that may seem related to the degree of relaxation, is present throughout the range of motion, and affects flexors and extensors equally. Paratonia usually results from disease of the frontal lobes. Weakness with decreased tone (flaccidity) or normal tone occurs with disorders of the *motor unit*, that is, a single lower motor neuron and all of the muscle fibers it innervates.

Three basic patterns of weakness can usually be recognized based on the signs summarized in Table 22-1. One results from upper motor neuron pathology, and the other two from disorders of the motor unit (lower motor neuron and myopathic weakness). Fasciculations and early atrophy help to distinguish lower motor neuron (neurogenic) weakness from myopathic weakness. A *fasciculation* is a visible or palpable twitch within a single muscle due to the spontaneous discharge of one motor unit. Neurogenic weakness also produces more prominent hypotonia and greater depression of tendon reflexes than myopathic weakness.

PATHOGENESIS Upper Motor Neuron Weakness This pattern of weakness results from disorders that affect the upper motor neurons or their axons in the cerebral cortex, subcortical white matter, internal capsule, brainstem, or spinal cord (Fig. 22-1). Both the pyramidal and bulbospinal pathways contribute to normal strength, tone, coordination, and gait. Upper motor neuron lesions produce weakness through decreased activation of the lower motor neurons. In general, distal muscle groups are affected more severely than proximal ones, and axial movements are spared unless the lesion is severe and bilateral. With corticobulbar involvement, weakness is usually observed

Table 22-1 Signs That Distinguish Patterns of Weakness

Sign	Upper Motor Neuron	Lower Motor Neuron	Myopathic
Atrophy	None	Severe	Mild
Fasciculations	None	Common	None
Tone	Spastic	Decreased	Normal/decreased
Distribution of weakness	Pyramidal/regional	Distal/segmental	Proximal
Tendon reflexes	Hyperactive	Hypoactive/absent	Normal/hypoactive
Babinski's sign	Present	Absent	Absent

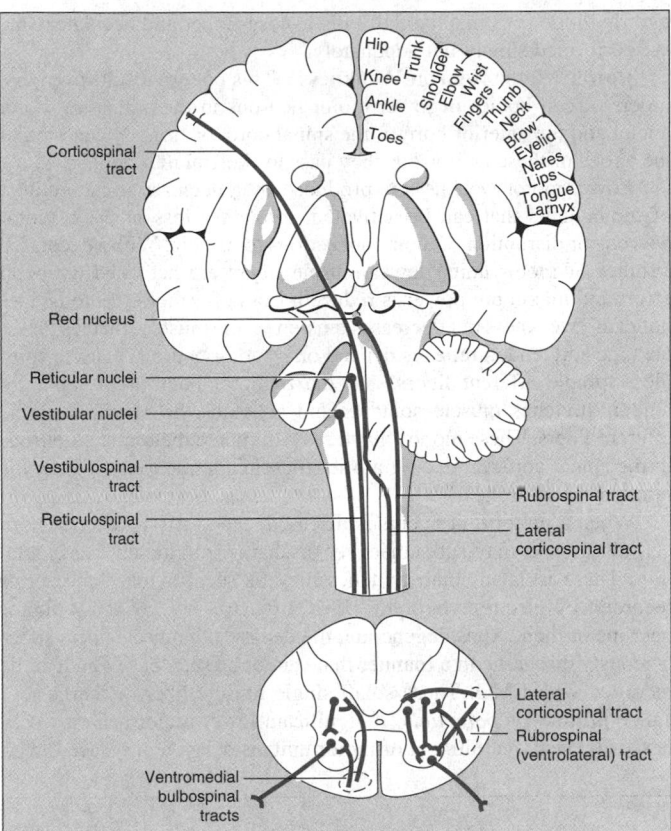

FIGURE 22-1 The corticospinal and bulbospinal upper motor neuron pathways. Upper motor neurons have their cell bodies in layer V of the primary motor cortex (the precentral gyrus, or Brodmann's area 4) and in the premotor and supplemental motor cortex (area 6). The upper motor neurons in the primary motor cortex are somatotopically organized as illustrated on the right side of the figure.

Axons of the upper motor neurons descend through the subcortical white matter and the posterior limb of the internal capsule. Axons of the *pyramidal* or *corticospinal system* descend through the brainstem in the cerebral peduncle of the midbrain, the basis pontis, and the medullary pyramids. At the cervicomedullary junction, most pyramidal axons decussate into the contralateral corticospinal tract of the lateral spinal cord, but 10 to 30% remain ipsilateral in the anterior spinal cord. Pyramidal neurons make direct monosynaptic connections with lower motor neurons. They innervate most densely the lower motor neurons of hand muscles and are involved in the execution of learned, fine movements. Corticobulbar neurons are similar to corticospinal neurons but innervate brainstem motor nuclei.

Bulbospinal upper motor neurons influence strength and tone but are not part of the pyramidal system. The descending *ventromedial bulbospinal pathways* originate in the tectum of the midbrain (tectospinal pathway), the vestibular nuclei (vestibulospinal pathway), and the reticular formation (reticulospinal pathway). These pathways influence axial and proximal muscles and are involved in the maintenance of posture and integrated movements of the limbs and trunk. The descending *ventrolateral bulbospinal pathways*, which originate predominantly in the red nucleus (rubrospinal pathway), facilitate distal limb muscles. The bulbospinal system is sometimes referred to as the *extrapyramidal upper motor neuron system*. In all figures, nerve cell bodies and axon terminals are shown, respectively, as closed circles and forks.

only in the lower face and tongue; extraocular, upper facial, pharyngeal, and jaw muscles are almost always spared. With bilateral corticobulbar lesions, *pseudobulbar palsy* often develops, in which dysarthria, dysphagia, dysphonia, and emotional lability accompany bilateral facial weakness. Spasticity accompanies upper motor neuron weakness but may not be present in the acute phase.

Upper motor neuron lesions also affect the ability to perform rapid repetitive movements. Such movements are slow and coarse, but normal rhythmicity is maintained. Finger-nose-finger and heel-knee-shin are performed slowly but adequately.

Lower Motor Neuron Weakness This pattern results from disorders of cell bodies of lower motor neurons in the brainstem motor nuclei and the anterior horn of the spinal cord, or from dysfunction of the axons of these neurons as they pass to skeletal muscle (Fig. 22-2).

Lower motor weakness is produced by a decrease in the number of motor units that can be activated, through a loss of the α motor neurons or disruption of their connections to muscle. With a decreased number of motor units, fewer muscle fibers are activated with full effort and maximum power is reduced. Loss of γ motor neurons does not cause weakness but decreases tension on the muscle spindles. Muscle tone and tendon reflexes depend on γ motor neurons, muscle spindles, spindle afferent fibers, and the α motor neurons. A tap on a tendon stretches muscle spindles and activates the primary spindle afferent fibers. These monosynaptically stimulate the α motor neurons in the spinal cord, producing a brief muscle contraction, which is the familiar tendon reflex.

When a motor unit becomes diseased, especially in anterior horn cell diseases, it may spontaneously discharge, producing a fasciculation. These isolated small twitches may be seen or felt clinically or recorded by electromyography (EMG) (Chap. 357). When α motor neurons or their axons degenerate, the denervated muscle fibers spontaneously discharge in a manner that cannot be seen or felt but can be recorded with EMG. These small single muscle fiber discharges are called *fibrillation potentials*. If significant lower motor neuron weakness is present, recruitment of motor units is delayed or reduced, with

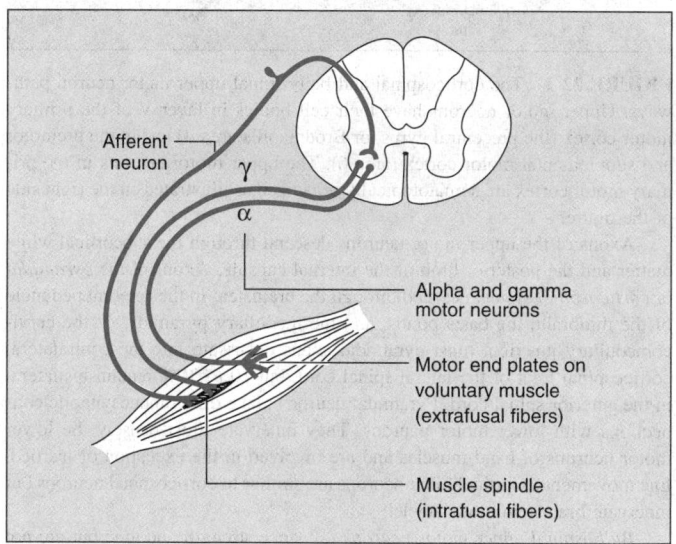

Afferent neuron
γ
α
Alpha and gamma motor neurons
Motor end plates on voluntary muscle (extrafusal fibers)
Muscle spindle (intrafusal fibers)

FIGURE 22-2 Lower motor neurons are divided into α and γ types. γ motor neurons are smaller than α motor neurons and innervate the intrafusal muscle fibers of the muscle spindle. Activation of the γ motor neuron increases the tension on muscle spindles and facilitates stretch reflexes and other local reflex mechanisms that activate a muscle through the α motor neurons. Each muscle is innervated by many (usually several hundred) α motor neurons.

Lower motor axons exit the brainstem in certain cranial nerves and the spinal cord in the ventral roots. The ventral roots fuse with the dorsal roots at the intervertebral foramen to form spinal nerves. For innervation of limb muscles, several adjacent spinal nerves fuse to form plexuses before dividing into peripheral nerves. Most peripheral nerves branch one or more times as they innervate different muscles. Each α motor axon extensively arborizes just before reaching the many muscle fibers that it innervates.

The α motor neuron receives direct excitatory input from corticomotoneurons and primary muscle spindle afferents. The α and γ motor neurons also receive excitatory input from other descending upper motor neuron pathways, segmental sensory inputs, and interneurons. The α motor neurons receive direct inhibition from Renshaw cell interneurons, and other interneurons indirectly inhibit the α and γ motor neurons.

fewer than normal activated at a given discharge frequency. This contrasts with upper motor neuron weakness, in which a normal number of motor units are activated at a given frequency but in which the maximum discharge frequency is decreased.

Myopathic Weakness This pattern of weakness is produced by disorders within the motor unit that affect the muscle fibers or the neuromuscular junctions.

Two types of muscle fibers exist. Type I muscle fibers are rich in mitochondria and oxidative enzymes, produce relatively low force, but have low energy demands that can be supplied by ongoing aerobic metabolism. They produce sustained postural and nonforceful movements. Type II muscle fibers are rich in glycolytic enzymes, can produce relatively high force, but have high energy demands that cannot be supplied for long by ongoing aerobic metabolism. Thus, these units can be activated maximally for only brief periods of time to produce high-force movements.

For graded voluntary movements, type I muscle fibers are activated earlier in recruitment. For each muscle fiber, if the nerve terminal releases a normal number of acetylcholine molecules presynaptically and a sufficient number of postsynaptic acetylcholine receptors are opened, the end plate reaches threshold and thereby generates an action potential that spreads across the muscle fiber membrane and into the transverse tubular system. This electrical excitation activates intracellular events that produce an energy-dependent contraction of the muscle fiber (excitation-contraction coupling).

Myopathic weakness is produced by a decrease in the number or contractile force of muscle fibers activated within the motor unit. With muscular dystrophies, inflammatory myopathies, or myopathies with muscle fiber necrosis, decreased numbers of muscle fibers survive within many motor units. As demonstrated with EMG, the size of each motor unit action potential is decreased so that motor units must be recruited more rapidly than normal to produce the power necessary for a certain movement. Neuromuscular junction diseases, such as myasthenia gravis, produce weakness in a similar manner, although the loss of muscle fibers within the motor unit is functional rather than actual. Furthermore, the number of muscle fibers activated can vary over time, depending on the state of rest of the neuromuscular junctions. Thus, fatigable weakness is suggestive of myasthenia gravis or another neuromuscular junction disease. Some myopathies produce weakness through loss of contractile force of muscle fibers or through relatively selective involvement of the type II muscle fibers. These may not affect the size of individual motor unit action potentials observed with EMG and are detected by a discrepancy between the electrical activity and force of a muscle.

Integrated Movements Most purposeful movements require the integrated coordination of many muscle groups. Consider a simple movement, such as grasping a ball. The primary movement is a flexion of the thumb and fingers of one hand, with opposition of the thumb and little finger. This requires the contraction of several muscles, including flexor digitorum superficialis, flexor digitorum profundus, flexor pollicis longus, flexor pollicis brevis, opponens pollicis, and opponens digiti minimi. These prime movers for this action are called *agonists*. In order for the grasping to be smooth and forceful, the thumb and finger extensors need to relax at the same rate as the flexors contract. The muscles that act in a directly opposing manner to the agonists are *antagonists*. A secondary action of the thumb and finger flexors is to flex the wrist; because wrist flexion tends to weaken finger flexion if both occur, activation of wrist extensors assists the grasping movement. Muscles that produce such complementary movements are *synergists*. Finally, the arm needs to be held in a stable position as the grasp occurs, so that the ball is not knocked away before it is secured. Muscles that stabilize the arm position are *fixators*.

The coordination of activity by agonists, antagonists, synergists, and fixators is regulated by a three-level hierarchy of motor control. The lowest level of control is mediated through segmental reflexes in the spinal cord. These reflexes facilitate agonists and reciprocally inhibit the antagonists. Spinal segments also control rhythmic patterns of movement that involve more than a single pair of agonists and antagonists. For example, the lumbosacral spinal cord contains the basic programming for cyclical stepping movements that involve the synergistic activation of different muscle groups over time. The intermediate level of control is mediated through the descending bulbo-spinal pathways, which integrate visual, proprioceptive, and vestibular feedback into the execution of an action. For example, the locomotor center in the midbrain is required to modify the cyclical stepping movements in order that balance be maintained and forward movement occur. The highest level of control is mediated by the cerebral cortex. Superimposition of this highest level of control is necessary for activities such as walking to be goal-directed. Precise movements that are learned and improved through practice are also initiated and controlled by the motor cortex. Although only the agonists are directly activated, during the course of a complex sequence of actions such as playing the piano, the sequential activation of different groups of agonists for each note or chord is a part of the learned motor program. Further, the execution of these actions also involves input from the basal ganglia and cerebellar hemispheres to facilitate agonists, synergists, and fixators and to inhibit undesired antagonists.

Apraxia is a disorder of planning and initiating a skilled or learned movement (Chap. 25). Unilateral apraxia of the right hand may be due to a lesion of the left frontal lobe (especially anterior or inferior), the left temporoparietal region (especially the supramarginal gyrus), or their connections. Left body apraxia is produced by lesions of these regions in the right hemisphere or by lesions in the corpus callosum that disconnect the right temporoparietal or frontal regions from those on the left. Bilateral apraxia is often due to bilateral frontal lobe lesions or diffuse bilateral hemispheric disease.

Approach to the Patient

The mode of onset, distribution, and associated features of weakness should be carefully defined. When there is a discrepancy between the history and physical findings, it is usually because the patient complains of weakness, whereas symptoms are actually due to other causes, such as incoordination or pain limiting effort. Power may be examined in a variety of ways. The patient is asked to push or pull in a specified direction against resistance, and the strength in each muscle group is graded from 0 to 5 by the scale developed by the Medical Research Council (Table 22-2). A second method is indirect testing through observation of task performance such as holding the arms outstretched. This is especially useful in detecting mild, asymmetric upper motor neuron weakness through the observation of a downward drift with pronation of the forearm on one side. A third method is functional testing, which involves quantitation of activities. Common tests include counting the number of times a person can perform a deep-knee bend or step on a stool or chair, or timing the length of time the arms can be held abducted to 90 degrees. When performed serially, functional tests provide useful estimates of changes in the patient's status over time.

Other elements of the motor examination include appraisal of muscular bulk, inspection for fasciculations, and assessment of tone. Fasciculations are most easily determined by observing relaxed limbs that are illuminated from behind, but they can also be palpated as irregular low-amplitude twitches within the muscle. Tone is assessed by passive movement of each limb at its various joints and at several different speeds. In the clinical context of weakness, tone may be spastic or

Table 22-2 Medical Research Council Grading of Strength

Grade	Definition
5	Normal strength
4	Active movement against gravity and resistance
3	Active movement against gravity (no resistance from physician)
2	Active movement with gravity eliminated (no resistance from physician)
1	Flicker or trace contraction
0	No visible or palpable contraction

flaccid. The presence of cogwheel rigidity, lead-pipe rigidity, or paratonia suggests a disorder of integrated movements, rather than true weakness.

Hemiparesis Hemiparesis results from an upper motor neuron lesion above the midcervical spinal cord; most lesions that produce hemiparesis are located above the foramen magnum. The presence of language disorders, cortical sensory disturbances, cognitive abnormalities, disorders of visual-spatial integration, apraxia, or seizures indicates a cortical lesion. Homonymous visual field defects reflect either a cortical or a subcortical hemispheric lesion. A "pure motor" hemiparesis of the face, arm, and/or leg is due to a small, discrete lesion in the posterior limb of the internal capsule, cerebral peduncle, or upper pons. Some brainstem lesions produce the classic findings of ipsilateral cranial nerve signs and contralateral hemiparesis. These "crossed paralyses" are discussed further in Chap. 361. The absence of cranial nerve signs or facial weakness suggests that a hemiparesis is due to a lesion in the high cervical spinal cord, especially if associated with ipsilateral loss of proprioception and contralateral loss of pain and temperature sense (the Brown-Séquard syndrome). However, most spinal cord lesions produce quadriparesis or paraparesis.

Acute or episodic hemiparesis usually has a vascular pathogenesis, either ischemia or a primary hemorrhage (Chap. 361). Less commonly, hemorrhage may occur into brain tumors (Chap. 370) or from rupture of normal vessels due to trauma (Chap. 369); the trauma may be trivial in patients who are anticoagulated or elderly. Less likely possibilities include a focal inflammatory lesion from multiple sclerosis (Chap. 371), abscess, or sarcoidosis (Chap. 318). Evaluation begins immediately with a computed tomography (CT) scan of the brain (Fig. 22-3). If CT is normal and an ischemic stroke is unlikely, magnetic resonance imaging (MRI) of the brain or cervical spine may be indicated.

Subacute hemiparesis that evolves over days or weeks has a long differential diagnosis. A common cause is subdural hematoma; this readily treatable condition must always be considered, especially in elderly or anticoagulated patients, even in the absence of a history of trauma (Chap. 369). Infectious possibilities include cerebral bacterial abscess (Chap. 372), fungal granuloma or meningitis (Chap. 374), and parasitic infection. Weakness from malignant primary and metastatic neoplasms may evolve over days to weeks (Chap. 370). AIDS (Chap. 309) may present with subacute hemiparesis due to toxoplasmosis or primary CNS lymphoma. Noninfectious inflammatory processes, such as multiple sclerosis (Chap. 371) or, less commonly, sarcoidosis, are further considerations. If the brain MRI is normal and if cortical and hemispheric signs are not present, MRI of the cervical spine may be required.

Chronic hemiparesis that evolves over months is usually due to a neoplasm (Chap. 370), an unruptured arteriovenous malformation (Chap. 361), a chronic subdural hematoma (Chap. 369), or a degenerative disease (Chaps. 363 to 366). The initial diagnostic test is often an MRI of the brain, especially if the clinical findings suggest brainstem pathology. If MRI of the brain is normal, the possibility of a foramen magnum or high cervical spinal cord lesion should be considered.

Paraparesis An intraspinal lesion at or below the upper thoracic spinal cord level is most commonly responsible. A sensory level over the trunk identifies the approximate level of the cord lesion. Paraparesis can also result from lesions at other locations that disturb upper motor neurons (especially parasagittal lesions and hydrocephalus) and lower motor neurons (anterior horn cell disorders, cauda equina syndromes, and occasionally peripheral neuropathies).

Acute or episodic paraparesis due to spinal cord disease may be difficult to distinguish from disorders affecting lower motor neurons or cerebral hemispheres. Recurrent episodes of paraparesis are often due to multiple sclerosis or to vascular malformations of the spinal cord. With acute spinal cord disease, the upper motor neuron deficit

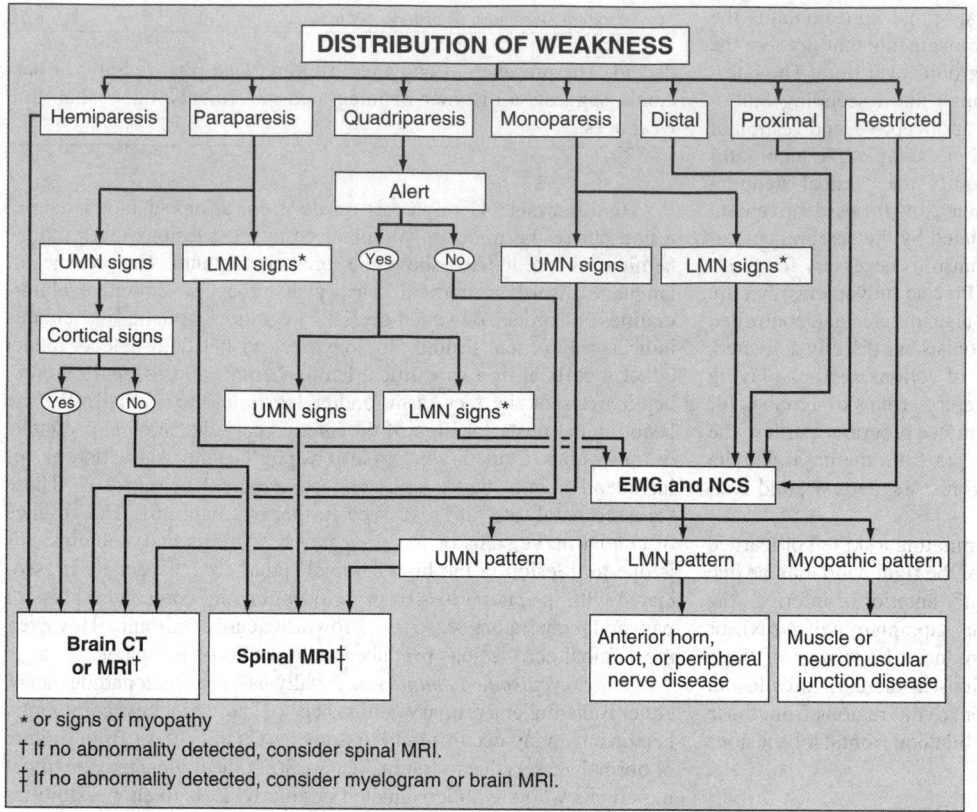

FIGURE 22-3 An algorithm for the initial work-up of a patient with weakness. CT, computed tomography; EMG, electromyography; LMN, lower motor neuron; MRI, magnetic resonance imaging; NCS, nerve conduction studies; UMN, upper motor neuron.

The algorithm (DISTRIBUTION OF WEAKNESS) includes the following notes:

* or signs of myopathy
† If no abnormality detected, consider spinal MRI.
‡ If no abnormality detected, consider myelogram or brain MRI.

is usually associated with incontinence and a sensory disturbance of the lower limbs that extends rostrally to a level on the trunk; tone is typically flaccid, and tendon reflexes absent. In such cases, the diagnostic approach starts with an imaging study of the spinal cord (Fig. 22-3). Compressive lesions (particularly epidural tumor, abscess, or hematoma), spinal cord infarction (proprioception is usually spared), an arteriovenous fistula or other vascular anomaly, and transverse myelitis, among other causes may be responsible (Chap. 368). Diseases of the cerebral hemispheres that produce acute paraparesis include anterior cerebral artery ischemia (shoulder shrug also affected), superior sagittal sinus or cortical venous thrombosis, and acute hydrocephalus. If upper motor neuron signs are associated with drowsiness, confusion, seizures, or other hemispheric signs but not a sensory level over the trunk, the diagnostic approach starts with an MRI of the brain. Paraparesis is part of the cauda equina syndrome, which may result from trauma to the low back, a midline disk herniation, or intraspinal tumor; although sphincters are affected, hip flexion is often spared, as is sensation over the anterolateral thighs. Rarely, paraparesis is caused by a rapidly evolving peripheral neuropathy such as Guillain-Barré syndrome or by a myopathy. In such cases, electrophysiologic studies are diagnostically helpful and refocus the subsequent evaluation (Chaps. 378 and 381).

Subacute or chronic paraparesis with spasticity is caused by upper motor neuron disease. When paraparesis evolves over weeks or months with lower limb sensory loss and sphincter involvement, possible spinal cord disorders include multiple sclerosis, intraparenchymal tumor, chronic spinal cord compression from degenerative disease of the spine, subacute combined degeneration due to vitamin B_{12} deficiency, viral infections (especially human T cell leukemia/lymphoma virus I), and hereditary or other degenerative diseases. Primary progressive multiple sclerosis usually presents in the fourth or fifth decade as progressive paraparesis (Chap. 371). Gliomas of the spinal cord typically produce a progressive myelopathy that is painful (Chap. 370). The clinical approach begins with an MRI of the spinal cord. If the imaging study is normal and spasticity is present, MRI of the brain may be indicated. If hemispheric signs are present, parasagittal meningioma or chronic hydrocephalus is likely and MRI of the brain is the initial test. Progression over months to years is typical of degenerative disorders such as primary lateral sclerosis (Chap. 365) and hereditary disorders such as familial spastic paraparesis and adrenomyeloneuropathy (Chap. 368). In the rare situations when a chronic paraparesis is due to a lower motor neuron or myopathic etiology, the localization is usually suspected on clinical grounds by the absence of spasticity and confirmed by EMG and nerve conduction tests.

Quadriparesis or Generalized Weakness Generalized weakness may be due to disorders of the central nervous system or of the motor unit. Although the terms *quadriparesis* and *generalized weakness* are often used interchangeably, quadriparesis is more often chosen when an upper motor neuron cause is suspected and generalized weakness when a disease of the motor unit is likely. Weakness from CNS disorders is usually associated with changes in consciousness or cognition, with increased muscle tone and muscle stretch reflexes, and with alterations of sensation. Most neuromuscular causes of intermittent weakness are associated with normal mental function, diminished muscle tone, and hypoactive muscle stretch reflexes. Exceptions are some causes of acute quadriparesis due to upper motor neuron disorders in which transient hypotonia is present. The major causes of intermittent weakness are listed in Table 22-3. A patient with generalized fatigability without objective weakness may have the *chronic fatigue syndrome* (Chap. 384).

Acute quadriparesis Acute quadriparesis with onset over minutes may result from disorders of upper motor neurons (e.g., anoxia, hypotension, brainstem or cervical cord ischemia, trauma, and systemic metabolic abnormalities) or muscle (electrolyte disturbances, certain inborn errors of muscle energy metabolism, toxins, or periodic paralyses). Onset over hours to weeks may, in addition to the above, be due to lower motor neuron disorders. Guillain-Barré syndrome (Chap. 378) is the most common lower motor neuron weakness that progresses over days to several weeks; the finding of an elevated protein level in the cerebrospinal fluid is helpful but may be absent early in the course. If stupor or coma is present, the evaluation begins with

Table 22-3   Causes of Episodic Generalized Weakness

1. Electrolyte disturbances, e.g., a. hypokalemia, b. hyperkalemia, c. hypercalcemia, d. hypernatremia, e. hyponatremia, f. hypophosphatemia, g. hypermagnesemia
2. Muscle disorders
   a. Channelopathies (periodic paralyses)
   b. Metabolic defects of muscle (impaired carbohydrate or fatty acid utilization; abnormal mitochondrial function
3. Neuromuscular junction disorders
   a. Myasthenia gravis
   b. Lambert-Eaton myasthenic syndrome
4. Central nervous system disorders
   a. Transient ischemic attacks of the brainstem
   b. Transient global cerebral ischemia
   c. Multiple sclerosis

a CT scan of the brain. If upper motor neuron signs are present but the patient is alert, the initial test is usually an MRI of the cervical cord. If weakness is lower motor neuron, myopathic, or uncertain in origin, the clinical approach starts with blood studies for muscle enzymes and electrolytes and an EMG and nerve conduction study.

Subacute or chronic quadriparesis When quadriparesis due to upper motor neuron disease develops over weeks, months, or years, the distinction between disorders of the cerebral hemispheres, brainstem, and cervical spinal cord is usually possible by clinical criteria alone. The diagnostic approach begins with an MRI of the clinically suspected site of pathology. Lower motor neuron disease usually presents with weakness that is most profound distally, whereas myopathic weakness is typically proximal; the evaluation then begins with EMG and nerve conduction studies.

Monoparesis This is usually due to lower motor neuron disease, with or without associated sensory involvement. Upper motor neuron weakness occasionally presents with a monoparesis of distal and nonantigravity muscles. Myopathic weakness is rarely limited to one limb.

Acute monoparesis Distinguishing between upper and lower motor neuron disorders may be difficult clinically because tone and reflexes are frequently decreased in both at presentation. If the weakness is predominantly in distal and nonantigravity muscles and not associated with sensory impairment or pain, focal cortical ischemia is likely (Chap. 361); in this setting, diagnostic possibilities are similar to those for acute hemiparesis. Sensory loss and pain usually accompany acute lower motor neuron weakness. The distribution of weakness is commonly localized to a single nerve root or peripheral nerve within one limb but occasionally reflects involvement of the brachial or lumbosacral plexus. If lower motor neuron weakness is suspected, or if the pattern of weakness is uncertain, the clinical approach begins with an EMG and nerve conduction study.

Subacute or chronic monoparesis Weakness with atrophy of one limb that develops over weeks or months is almost always lower motor neuron in origin. If the weakness is associated with numbness, a peripheral nerve or spinal root origin is likely; uncommonly, the brachial or lumbosacral plexus is affected. If numbness is absent, anterior horn cell disease is likely. In either case, an electrodiagnostic study is indicated. If upper rather than lower motor neuron signs are present, a tumor, vascular malformation, or other cortical lesion affecting the precentral gyrus may be responsible. Alternatively, if the leg is affected, a small thoracic cord lesion, often a tumor or multiple sclerosis, may be present. In these situations, the approach begins with an imaging study of the suspicious area.

Distal Weakness Involvement of two or four limbs distally suggests lower motor neuron or peripheral nerve disease. Acute distal lower limb weakness occurs occasionally from an acute toxic polyneuropathy or cauda equina syndrome. Distal symmetric weakness usually develops over weeks, months, or years and is due to metabolic, toxic, hereditary, degenerative, or inflammatory diseases of peripheral nerves (Chap. 377). With peripheral nerve disease, weakness is usually less severe than numbness. Anterior horn cell disease may begin distally but is typically asymmetric and is not associated with numbness (Chap. 365). Rarely, myopathies also present with distal weakness (Chap. 381). The first step in evaluation is an electrodiagnostic study (Fig. 22-3).

Proximal Weakness Proximal weakness of two or four limbs suggests a disorder of muscle or, less commonly, neuromuscular junction or anterior horn cell. Myopathy often produces symmetric weakness of the pelvic or shoulder girdle muscles (Chap. 381). Diseases of the neuromuscular junction (such as myasthenia gravis) may present with symmetric proximal weakness (Chap. 380), often associated with ptosis, diplopia, or bulbar weakness and fluctuating in severity during the day. Extreme fatigability present in some cases of myasthenia gravis may even suggest episodic weakness, but strength rarely returns fully to normal. The proximal weakness of anterior horn cell disease is most often asymmetric, but may be symmetric if familial (Chap. 365). Numbness does not occur with any of these diseases. The eval-

uation usually begins with determination of the serum creatine kinase level and electrophysiologic studies.

Weakness in a Restricted Distribution In some patients, weakness does not fit any of the above patterns. Examples include weakness limited to the extraocular, hemifacial, bulbar, or respiratory muscles. If unilateral, restricted weakness is usually due to lower motor neuron or peripheral nerve disease, such as in a facial palsy (Chap. 367) or an isolated superior oblique muscle paresis (Chap. 28). Relatively symmetric weakness of extraocular or bulbar muscles is usually due to a myopathy (Chap. 381) or neuromuscular junction disorder (Chap. 380). Bilateral facial palsy with areflexia suggests Guillain-Barré syndrome (Chap. 378). Worsening of relatively symmetric weakness with fatigue is characteristic of neuromuscular junction disorders (Chap. 380). Asymmetric bulbar weakness is usually due to motor neuron disease. Weakness limited to respiratory muscles is uncommon and is usually due to motor neuron disease, myasthenia gravis, or polymyositis/dermatomyositis (Chap. 382).

MYALGIAS, SPASMS, AND CRAMPS

Spontaneous or exercise-related discomfort from muscles is usually benign and is rarely caused by a definable neuromuscular disease. However, a number of disorders of the motor system are characteristically painful. Some terms for muscular discomfort or involuntary contractions, such as myalgias, spasms, and cramps, are often used interchangeably by patients but have a more specific meaning to physicians. Other terms, such as aching, heaviness, and stiffness, are less specific. *Myalgias* are pains that are felt in muscle; the term does not imply an involuntary contraction. *Spasms* and *cramps* refer to episodes of involuntary contraction of one or more muscles. Cramps are usually painful, whereas spasms are not necessarily uncomfortable.

MYALGIAS Proximal or generalized weakness associated with myalgias is usually due to an inflammatory, metabolic, endocrine, or toxic myopathy (Chap. 381). Spontaneous myalgias not accompanied by objective weakness are often without a clear cause unless associated with a well-defined systemic illness. Myalgias are a common manifestation of fever or infection, especially influenza. Muscle pains and stiffness with elevated serum creatine kinase concentration is common in hypothyroidism, even in patients without objective weakness. *Polymyalgia rheumatica* (Chap. 317) is characterized by diffuse myalgias and joint stiffness that predominantly affect the pelvic and shoulder girdles in a patient over 50 years of age who has anorexia, mild weight loss, and low-grade fever. Limitation of activity from the myalgias and joint stiffness also leads to disuse atrophy and may give the impression of weakness. However, EMG, serum creatine kinase levels, and muscle biopsy are normal. The erythrocyte sedimentation rate is elevated in most patients, and features of giant-cell arteritis are present in 25%. Diffuse myalgias are common in many rheumatologic diseases, in which the diagnosis and treatment are based on other symptoms and signs. Myalgias are occasionally present in dermatomyositis/polymyositis, but most patients have weakness without significant pain. *Fibromyalgia* (fibrositis, fibromyositis) is associated with pain and tenderness of muscle and adjacent connective tissue (Chap. 325). Fatigue, insomnia, and depression are often present, but objective weakness, elevation of serum creatine kinase level, or elevation of the erythrocyte sedimentation rate does not occur. The diagnosis is dependent upon identifying characteristic focal "trigger points."

Focal Myalgias Focal muscle pain is often traumatic. Rupture of muscle tendons such as the biceps or gastrocnemius muscle may produce visible muscle shortening. Many such tears resolve without surgery but leave an abnormal appearance to the muscle belly. Nontraumatic focal muscle pain is often related to adjacent nonmuscular disorders (e.g., unilateral gastrocnemius pain due to deep venous thrombosis). Rarely, focal muscle pain may be caused by ischemic infarction or bacterial myositis, if acute, or by neoplasm, parasitic infection, sarcoidosis, or other inflammation or infection, if subacute or chronic.

Exertional Myalgias Myalgias following unaccustomed, strenuous physical activity occur in normal individuals are often associated with laboratory evidence for muscle damage, such as an elevation of serum creatine kinase, edema of muscles on MRI, necrosis of muscle fibers on biopsy, and rarely myoglobinuria. Similar symptoms and laboratory abnormalities characterize certain metabolic disorders of muscle, such as carnitine palmitoyl transferase and glycolytic pathway enzyme deficiencies. The association of objective weakness during an episode of myalgias suggests a metabolic muscle disease. The development of an acute contracture (the inability to relax a muscle due to energy depletion) with the myalgias suggests a metabolic muscle disease with a glycolytic enzyme deficiency (Chap. 383). Exertional myalgias with muscle fiber necrosis also occur in muscular dystrophy with partial deficiency of dystrophin, and certain mitochondrial cytopathies (Chap. 383). Exertional myalgias with elevated creatine kinase concentration but without weakness also occur in hypothyroidism, and when confined to the legs may be due to vascular or neurogenic intermittent claudication. Most patients with exertional myalgias and no weakness do not have a definable abnormality.

SPASMS AND CRAMPS Involuntary contraction of muscle may occur with disorders of the CNS, lower motor neuron, or muscle. Contractions that originate within the CNS and are associated with upper motor neuron signs are usually referred to as spasms and generally affect the flexors or extensors of one or more limbs. Those that originate within the CNS and are not associated with upper motor neuron signs include movement disorders discussed below, as well as the rare stiff-person syndrome and tetanus. Muscle rigidity from active muscle contraction can occur in the malignant hyperthermia syndrome, usually associated with general anesthesia. In the neuroleptic malignant syndrome, muscle rigidity arises from CNS overactivity and is present in muscle. Involuntary contractions that originate in the lower motor neurons are usually cramps, occasionally tetany, or rarely neuromyotonia. Spasms that originate in muscle or muscle membrane are usually a delayed relaxation after voluntary contraction, either myotonia or rarely a contracture. These conditions may be difficult to distinguish clinically but are often well characterized by EMG studies.

Stiff-Person Syndrome This rare syndrome is characterized by slowly progressive muscle stiffness and superimposed spasms. The stiffness commonly begins in the low back and spreads over months up the spine and into the limbs but not into the jaw. The gait becomes stiff, and there is hyperlordosis of the lumbar spine. Spasms are often produced by startle. Emotional stress tends to worsen the stiffness as well as the frequency and severity of spasms. The spontaneous motor activity disappears during sleep. The syndrome is often associated with diabetes mellitus and can be paraneoplastic, accompanying Hodgkin's lymphoma, small cell cancer of the lung, and breast cancer. Most patients have a serum antibody against glutamic acid decarboxylase, an enzyme responsible for synthesis of the inhibitory neurotransmitter γ-aminobutyric acid (GABA). Stiffness results from loss of descending brainstem or segmental spinal inhibitory influences on the lower motor neurons. EMG studies reveal continuous motor unit activity that is similar to voluntary effort with preservation of the silent period to muscle stretch. Stiffness and spasms typically respond partially to treatment with baclofen or benzodiazepines.

Tetanus This rare hyperexcitable state results from exposure to tetanus toxin in patients infected with *Clostridium tetani* (Chap. 143). Painful spasms typically begin with jaw closure (trismus) and soon become generalized. EMG studies reveal continuous motor unit activity that is similar to voluntary effort except for loss of the silent period to muscle stretch.

Cramps These are the most common type of involuntary muscle contraction. Cramps are a painful contraction of a single muscle that produces a palpable knot within the muscle for seconds to minutes and is relieved by passive stretch of the muscle or spontaneously. EMG

studies reveal motor unit activity that has too high a discharge frequency to be voluntary. If cramps are associated with weakness, the weakness is almost always lower motor neuron in origin. When strength is normal, no definable condition is usually found, although dehydration, hypothyroidism, or uremia is occasionally present. If prominent, membrane stabilizing drugs, such as carbamazepine, may provide symptomatic benefit.

Tetany Tetany is characterized by contraction of distal muscles of the hands (carpal spasm with extension of interphalangeal joints and adduction and flexion of the metacarpophalangeal joints) and feet (pedal spasm) and is associated with tingling around the mouth and distally in the limbs. Tetany with carpopedal spasms is a common manifestation of hypocalcemia or respiratory alkalosis (even from hyperventilation). EMG studies reveal single or more often grouped motor unit discharges at low discharge frequency.

Neuromyotonia (Isaac's Syndrome) Neuromyotonia is characterized by muscle stiffness at rest that persists during sleep and by delayed relaxation after voluntary effort. Distal limb muscles are usually affected most severely, but all skeletal muscle may be involved. Gait may be stiff, and close inspection of the muscle reveals undulation of the overlying skin due to continuous muscle fiber contractions (myokymia). The continuous muscle fiber activity generates heat, and excessive sweating is common. EMG studies commonly reveal myokymic discharges, especially in familial cases. Rarely, EMGs record high-frequency neuromyotonic discharges. Autoantibodies against voltage-gated potassium channels have been demonstrated in some cases, and plasma exchange may be effective.

Myotonia This is a nonpainful delay in the relaxation of muscle after voluntary activity. Delay in opening the hand after a forceful grip (grip myotonia) is common. These disorders are usually familial and worsen in cold weather. EMG demonstrates a waxing and waning discharge of individual muscle fibers.

Contracture A painful inability to relax a muscle after voluntary activity due to energy depletion characterizes certain metabolic disorders with failure of energy production, such as myophosphorylase deficiency (McArdle's disease). EMG studies reveal electrical silence.

MOVEMENT DISORDERS

Movement disorders are neurologic syndromes in which abnormal movements (or *dyskinesias*) occur due to a disturbance of fluency and speed of voluntary movement or the presence of unintended extra movements. Because they are so distinct from the pyramidal disorders that cause upper motor neuron weakness, movement disorders are often referred to as *extrapyramidal diseases. Hyperkinetic movement disorders* are those in which an excessive amount of spontaneous motor activity is seen or in which abnormal involuntary movements occur. *Hypokinetic movement disorders* are characterized by *akinesia* or *bradykinesia*, in which purposeful motor activity is absent or reduced. This is often described as "poverty of movement."

PATHOGENESIS Movement disorders result from disease of the basal ganglia, paired subcortical gray matter structures consisting of the caudate and the putamen (which together are called the striatum), the internal and external segments of the globus pallidus, the subthalamic nucleus, and the substantia nigra. The major interconnections and neurotransmitters involved in basal ganglia circuits are illustrated in Fig. 22-4A. An understanding of this circuitry can explain, in part, the perturbation that occurs in both the hypo- and hyperkinetic disorders.

Parkinson's disease (Chap. 363), the prototypic hypokinetic movement disorder, results from a loss of dopaminergic neurons in the substantia nigra pars compacta. This leads to less excitation of striatal neurons that express the D_1 type of dopamine receptors and less inhibition of D_2 striatal neurons, both contributing to reduced facilitation of cortically initiated movement (Fig. 22-4B). The resting tremor of Parkinson's disease is less readily explained by this model but may result from effects on cholinergic interneurons in the striatum. *Huntington's disease* (Chap. 362), a hyperkinetic movement disorder, may be explained by selective loss of D_2 striatal neurons, resulting in

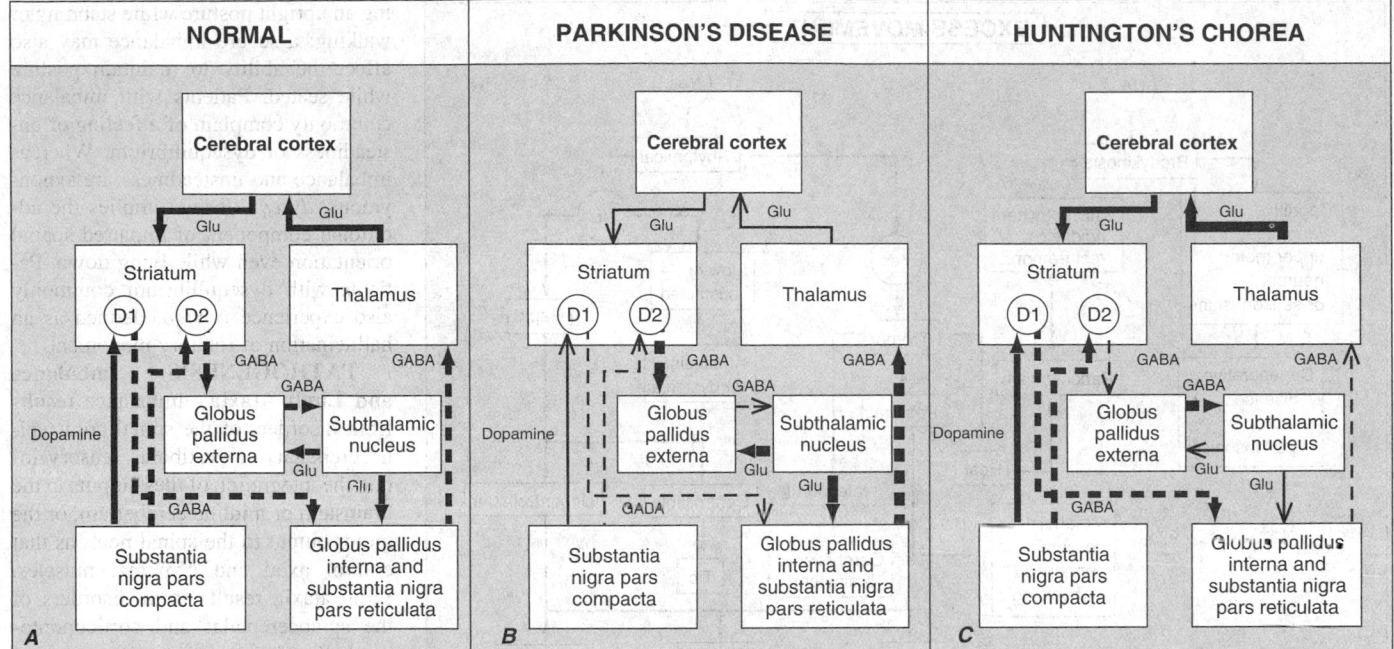

FIGURE 22-4 Basal ganglia circuits. *A.* Normal interaction. The striatum (caudate and putamen) receives glutamatergic afferents from the sensorimotor cortex and dopaminergic afferents from the substantia nigra pars compacta. The striatum has direct and indirect projections to the major outflow nuclei of the basal ganglia, the globus pallidus interna and the substantia nigra pars reticulata. The direct pathway from the striatum is GABA-ergic and inhibits the output nuclei. By contrast, the indirect pathway, which is more complex, facilitates the output nuclei. The output nuclei project to the ventral anterior and ventral lateral nuclei of the thalamus via inhibitory GABA neurotransmission. The thalamic nuclei in turn have glutamatergic, excitatory projections to cortical neurons. Thus, the direct pathway disinhibits (facilitates) thalamocortical projections that reinforce cortically initiated movement, whereas the indirect pathway is more complex and has the opposite effect. The direct and indirect pathways are influenced also by input from the substantia nigra pars compacta. This dopaminergic input on the striatum excites the direct pathway

neurons that predominantly express D_1 dopamine receptors and inhibits the indirect pathway neurons that predominantly express D_2 dopamine receptors. Striatal activity is further modulated by cholinergic interneurons within the striatum, which are functionally antagonistic to the dopaminergic projections.

B. Parkinson's disease results from a loss of dopaminergic projections from the substantia nigra pars compacta to the striatum. Loss of D_1 receptor stimulation results in disinhibition of the output nuclei by the direct pathway. Loss of D_2 receptor inhibition results in excitation of the output nuclei by the indirect pathway. Thus, inhibition of the thalamus is abnormally increased, and cortically initiated movements are not facilitated.

C. Huntington's chorea results from loss of striatal neurons that express D_2 receptors and normally project GABA-ergic inhibition to the globus pallidus externa. This causes disinhibition of the thalamus and excess thalamocortical excitation of movements. GABA, γ-aminobutyric acid; Glu, glutamate; ⟶ excitatory; dashed arrow, ┄┄➤, inhibitory.

disinhibition of cortically initiated movements without normal feedback control. The pathogenesis of hemiballismus is similar—a direct lesion of the glutamatergic neurons in the subthalamic nucleus (usually from a stroke) leads to disinhibition of thalamocortical projections.

Approach to the Patient

An algorithm for the interpretation of abnormal movements is illustrated in Fig. 22-5. The initial step is to determine if the movement disorder is due to an excess or a poverty of movement (i.e., a hyperkinetic or a hypokinetic movement disorder).

Hyperkinetic Movement Disorders Abnormal involuntary movements are divided into those that are rhythmical and those that are irregular. Those that are rhythmical are termed *tremors*, with the uncommon exception of *palatal and segmental myoclonus*. Tremors are divided into three types: rest, postural, and intention tremor. A *rest tremor* is maximal at rest and becomes less prominent with activity. It is characteristic of parkinsonism, a hypokinetic movement disorder, and is therefore commonly associated with bradykinesia and cogwheel rigidity. A rest tremor that develops acutely is usually due to toxins [such as exposure to 1-methyl-4-phenyl-1,2,3,6-tetrahydropyridine (MPTP)] or dopamine blocking drugs (such as phenothiazines). If insidious in onset, the diagnostic approach is the same as for Parkinson's disease (Chap. 363). A *postural tremor* is maximal while limb posture is actively maintained against gravity; it is lessened by rest and is not markedly enhanced during voluntary movement toward a target. A postural tremor that develops acutely is usually due to toxic or metabolic factors (for example, hyperthyroidism) or stress. The insidious onset of a postural tremor suggests a benign or familial essential tremor

(Chap. 363). An *intention tremor* is most prominent during voluntary movement toward a target and is not present during postural maintenance or at rest. It is a sign of cerebellar disease (Chap. 364). *Asterixis*, which may superficially resemble a tremor, is an intermittent inhibition of muscle contraction that occurs with metabolic encephalopathy (Chap. 376). This leads, for example, to a momentary and repetitive partial flexion of the wrists during attempted sustained wrist extension.

Involuntary movements that are irregular are characterized further by their speed and site of occurrence and by whether they can be suppressed voluntarily. The slowest are athetosis and dystonia. *Athetosis* is a slow, writhing, sinuous movement that occurs nearly continuously in distal muscles. *Dystonia* is a slowly varying but nearly continuous deviation of posture about one or more joints; it may occur in a proximal or distal limb or in axial structures. Dystonia is a more sustained deviation of posture than athetosis, although these two phenomena overlap considerably. The further evaluation of athetosis and dystonia are discussed in Chap. 363.

Among the rapid irregular movements, *tics* are controlled with voluntary effort, while the others are not. Tics often occur repetitively in a single location but are sometimes multifocal (Chap. 363).

Chorea, hemiballismus, and myoclonus are rapid, irregular jerks that cannot be consciously suppressed. *Hemiballismus* is the most distinctive among them. It is manifest as a sudden and often violent flinging movement of a proximal limb, usually an arm (Chap. 363). Hemiballismus usually develops acutely due to infarction of the contralateral subthalamic nucleus but occasionally develops subacutely or chronically due to other lesions of this nucleus.

Chorea is a rapid, jerky, irregular movement that tends to occur

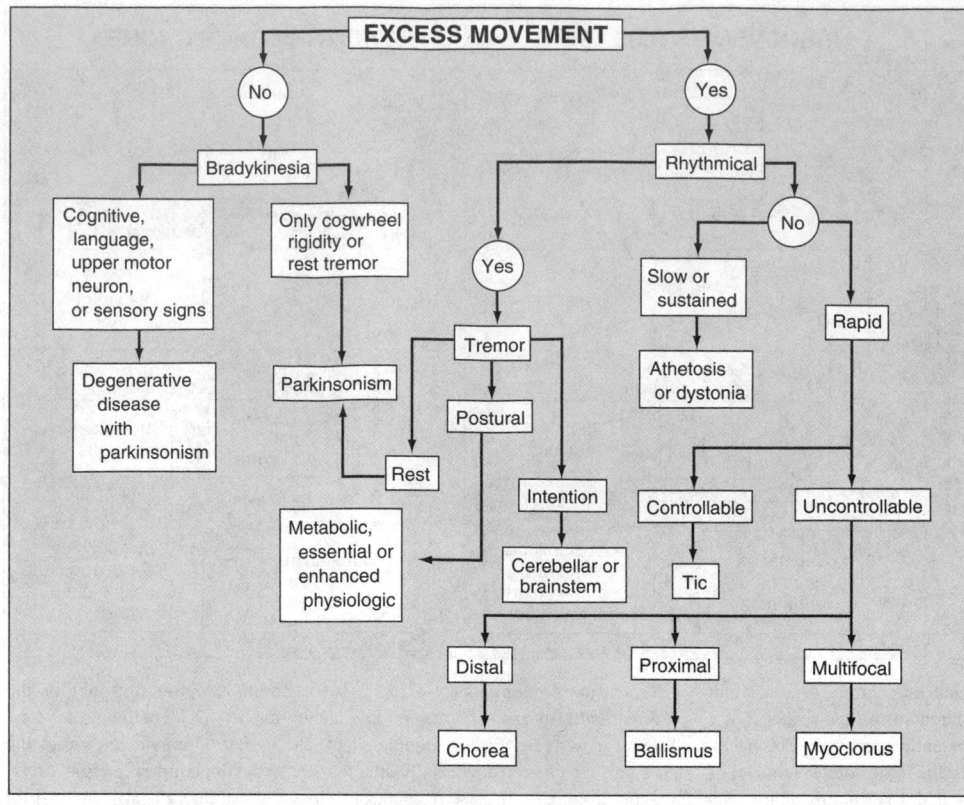

FIGURE 22-5 An algorithm for interpretation of abnormal movements.

in the distal limbs or face but may also occur in proximal limb and axial structures. Acute or subacute onset is usually toxic due to excess levodopa or dopamine-agonist therapy or, less often, neuroleptics, birth control pills, pregnancy (chorea gravidarum), hyperthyroidism, or the antiphospholipid syndrome. In children, it may be associated with rheumatic fever and, in such cases, is referred to as *Sydenham's chorea*. The gradual onset of chorea is typical of degenerative neurologic diseases, such as Huntington's chorea (Chap. 362).

Myoclonus is a rapid, brief, irregular movement that is usually multifocal. Myoclonus can occur spontaneously at rest, in response to sensory stimuli, or with voluntary movements. It is a symptom that occurs in a wide variety of metabolic and neurologic disorders. Posthypoxic intention myoclonus is a special myoclonic syndrome that occurs as a sequel to transient cerebral anoxia. Myoclonus may result from lipid storage disease, encephalitis, Creutzfeldt-Jakob disease, or metabolic encephalopathies due to respiratory failure, chronic renal failure, hepatic failure, or electrolyte imbalance. Myoclonus is also a feature of certain types of epilepsy, as discussed in Chap. 360. *Palatal and segmental myoclonus* are uncommon rhythmic forms of myoclonus that may resemble tremor; they are caused by structural disease of the brainstem or spinal cord at the level of the abnormal movement.

Hypokinetic Movement Disorders These syndromes are manifest as bradykinesia, with a masked, expressionless facial appearance, loss of associated limb movements during walking, and rigid en bloc turning. If bradykinesia is associated only with a rest tremor, cogwheel rigidity, or impairment of postural reflexes (especially with a tendency to fall backwards), Parkinson's disease is likely (Chap. 363). If cognitive, language, upper motor neuron, sensory, or autonomic signs are also present, a *multisystem degenerative neurologic disease* is present. →*These disorders are discussed in Chaps. 363, 364, and 366.*

IMBALANCE AND DISORDERS OF GAIT

Imbalance is the impaired ability to maintain the intended orientation of the body in space. It is generally manifest as difficulty in maintain-

ing an upright posture while standing or walking; a severe imbalance may also affect the ability to maintain posture while seated. Patients with imbalance commonly complain of a feeling of unsteadiness or dysequilibrium. Whereas imbalance and unsteadiness are synonymous, *dysequilibrium* implies the additional component of impaired spatial orientation even while lying down. Patients with dysequilibrium commonly also experience *vertigo*, defined as an hallucination of rotatory movement.

PATHOGENESIS   Imbalance and Limb Ataxia Imbalance results from disorders of the spinal cord (spinocerebellar) or vestibular sensory input, the integration of these inputs in the brainstem or midline cerebellum, or the motor output to the spinal neurons that control axial and proximal muscles. Limb ataxia results from disorders of the spinocerebellar and corticopontocerebellar inputs, the integration of these inputs in the intermediate and lateral cerebellum, or the output to the spinal neurons (via the red nucleus and rubrospinal tract) or to the cortex. These pathways ensure adequate speed, fluency, and integration of limb movements. The lateral cerebellar hemispheres coordinate a complex feedback circuit that modulates cortically initiated limb movement.

Sensory ataxia is caused by lesions that affect the peripheral sensory fibers, dorsal root ganglia cells, posterior columns of the spinal cord, lemniscal system in the brainstem, thalamus, or parietal cortex; relevant anatomy is discussed in Chap. 23. Impairment of the proprioceptive sensory feedback to the cerebellum, basal ganglia, and cortex produces sensory ataxia. Sensory ataxia results in imbalance and disturbs the fluency and integration of movements that can be partially alleviated by visual feedback.

Disorders of Gait Walking is one of the most complicated motor activities. Essentially all structures discussed in this chapter participate in normal walking. Cyclical stepping movements produced by the lumbosacral spinal cord centers are modified by cortical, basal ganglionic, brainstem, and cerebellar influences based on proprioceptive, vestibular, and visual feedback.

―――――― Approach to the Patient ――――――

Examination of coordination, balance, and gait is typically performed at the same time. The finger-nose-finger and the heel-knee-shin maneuvers are observed for signs of incoordination in general and dysmetria in particular. *Dysmetria* consists of irregular errors in the amplitude and force of limb movements. This is accentuated near the target or point of intention and hence termed *intention tremor*. The patient is also asked to maintain the arms outstretched against a resistance that is suddenly removed; excessive *rebound* indicates cerebellar dysfunction. The ability of the patient to rapidly and repetitively tap the hands and feet is assessed for speed and rhythmicity. Errors in rhythm (irregular rate, velocity, or force) indicate *dysdiadochokinesia*. Slow, coarse, but rhythmical movements indicate upper motor neuron disorders. The patient is asked to demonstrate how to comb the hair or brush the teeth to assess the ability to initiate and execute a simple sequence of activity. Balance is examined by having the patient stand stationary with the feet together. If this position can be maintained, the eyes are closed for 5 to 10 s. Accentuation of sway or actual loss of balance is assessed. If balance is momentarily lost, several trials may be necessary to determine if the loss is consistently in the same direction. Walking along an uncrowded space, such as a hallway, is observed. Symmetry of arm swing and various phases of the gait cycle are observed. Walking is then performed for several steps on the heels, on the toes, and in tandem.

Imbalance An algorithm for interpretation of imbalance is presented in Fig. 22-6.

Cerebellar ataxia results from disorders of the cerebellum or of its afferent inputs or efferent projections. Abnormalities of the midline cerebellar vermis or the flocculonodular lobe produce truncal ataxia which is usually revealed during the process of rising from a chair, assuming the upright stance with the feet together, or performing some other activity while standing. Once a desired position is reached, imbalance may be surprisingly mild. As walking begins, the imbalance recurs. Patients usually learn to lessen the imbalance by walking with the legs widely separated. The imbalance is usually not lateralized and may be accompanied by symmetric nystagmus.

Abnormalities of the intermediate and lateral portions of the cerebellum typically produce impaired limb movements rather than truncal ataxia. If involvement is asymmetric, lateralized imbalance is common and usually associated with asymmetric nystagmus. Clinical signs of cerebellar limb ataxia include dysmetria, intention tremor, dysdiadochokinesia, and abnormal rebound. Muscle tone is often modestly reduced; this contributes to the abnormal rebound due to decreased activation of segmental spinal cord reflexes and also to pendular reflexes, i.e., a tendency for a tendon reflex to produce multiple swings to and fro after a single tap. →*For further discussion of cerebellar diseases, see Chap. 364.*

Imbalance with vestibular dysfunction is characterized by a consistent tendency to fall to one side. The patient commonly complains of vertigo rather than imbalance, especially if the onset is acute. Acute vertigo associated with lateralized imbalance but no other neurologic signs is often due to disorders of the semicircular canal (Chap. 21); the presence of other neurologic signs suggests brainstem ischemia (Chap. 361) or multiple sclerosis (Chap. 371). When the vestibular dysfunction is peripheral, positional nystagmus and vertigo tend to resolve if a provocative position is maintained (extinction) or repeated (habituation). Lateralized imbalance of gradual onset or persisting for more than 2 weeks, accompanied by nystagmus, may result from lesions of the semicircular canal or vestibular nerve, brainstem, or cerebellum.

Imbalance with sensory ataxia is characterized by marked worsening when visual feedback is removed. The patient can often assume the upright stance with feet together cautiously with eyes open. With eye closure, balance is rapidly lost (positive Romberg sign) in various directions at random. Sensory examination reveals impairment of proprioception at the toes and ankles, usually associated with an even more prominent abnormality of vibratory perception. Prompt evaluation for vitamin B_{12} deficiency is important, as this disorder is reversible if recognized early (Chap. 368). Depression or absence of reflexes

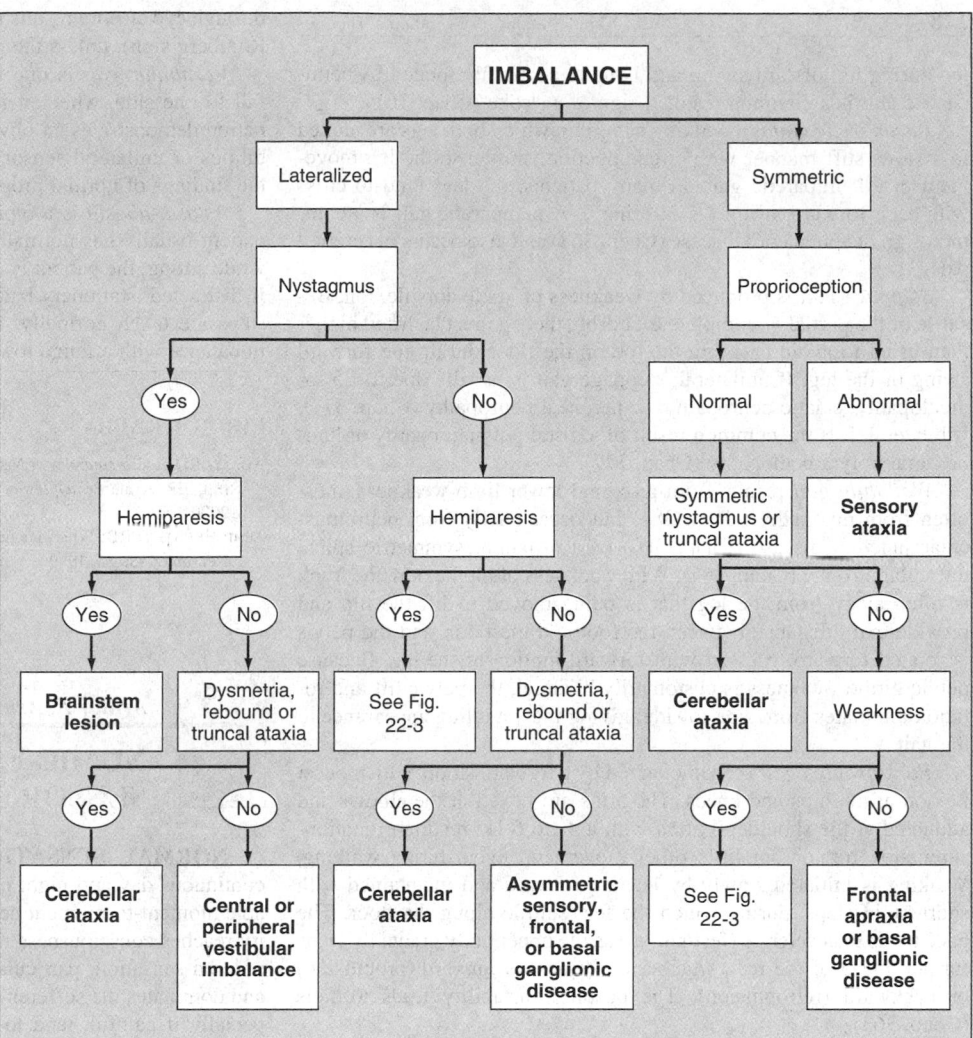

FIGURE 22-6 An algorithm for evaluation of imbalance.

points to peripheral nerve disorders (Chap. 377). Spasticity with extensor plantar responses suggests posterior column and spinal cord disorders (Chap. 368). Rarely, sensory ataxia produces lateralized imbalance. In these cases, the disorder is usually in the parietal lobe or thalamus (Chap. 23), but may also be due to an asymmetric sensory neuropathy (Chap. 377) or posterior column disease (Chap. 368).

Sensory limb ataxia is similar to cerebellar limb ataxia but is markedly worse when the eyes are closed. Examination also reveals abnormal proprioception and vibratory perception. The approach focuses on localizing the proprioceptive impairment to the peripheral nerves (Chap. 377), the posterior columns of the spinal cord (Chap. 368), or rarely the parietal lobe.

Other forms of imbalance occur, but the fundamental problem is usually a primary disorder of strength, extrapyramidal function, or cortical initiation of movement.

Abnormal Gait Each of the disorders discussed in this chapter produces a characteristic gait disturbance. If the neurologic examination is normal except for an abnormal gait, diagnosis may be difficult even for the experienced clinician.

Hemiparetic gait characterizes spastic hemiparesis. In its most severe form, an abnormal posture of the limbs is produced by spasticity. The arm is adducted and internally rotated, with flexion of the elbow, wrist, and fingers and with extension of the hip, knee, and ankle. Forward swing of the spastic leg during walking requires abduction and circumduction at the hip, often with contralateral tilt of the trunk to prevent the toes catching on the floor as the leg is advanced. In its mildest form, the affected arm is held in a normal position, but swings less than the normal arm. The affected leg is flexed less than the normal leg during its forward swing and is more externally rotated. A hemiparetic gait is a common residual sign of a stroke (Chap. 361).

Paraparetic gait is a walking pattern in which both legs are moved in a slow, stiff manner with circumduction, similar to the leg movement in a hemiparetic gait. In many patients, the legs tend to cross with each forward swing ("scissoring"). A paraparetic gait is a common sign of spinal cord disease (Chap. 368) and also occurs in cerebral palsy.

Steppage gait is produced by weakness of ankle dorsiflexion. Because of the partial or complete foot drop, the leg must be lifted higher than usual to avoid catching the toe on the floor during the forward swing of the leg. If unilateral, steppage gait is usually due to L5 radiculopathy, sciatic neuropathy, or peroneal neuropathy (Chap. 377). If bilateral, it is the common result of a distal polyneuropathy or lumbosacral polyradiculopathy (Chap. 377).

Waddling gait results from proximal lower limb weakness, most often from myopathy (Chap. 381) but occasionally from neuromuscular junction disease (Chap. 380) or a proximal symmetric spinal muscular atrophy (Chap. 365). With weakness of hip flexion, the trunk is tilted away from the leg that is being moved to lift the hip and provide extra distance between the foot and the floor, and the pelvis is rotated forward to assist with forward motion of the leg. Because pelvic girdle weakness is customarily bilateral, the pelvic lift and rotation alternates from side to side, giving the waddling appearance to the gait.

Parkinsonian gait is characterized by a forward stoop, with modest flexion at the hips and knees. The arms are flexed at the elbows and adducted at the shoulders, often with a 4- to 6-Hz resting pronation-supination tremor but little other movement, even during walking. Walking is initiated slowly by leaning forward and maintained with short rapid steps, during which the feet shuffle along the floor. The pace tends to accelerate (festination) as the upper body gradually leans further ahead of the feet, whether movement is forward (propulsion) or backward (retropulsion). The postural instability leads to falls (Chap. 363).

Apraxic gait results from bilateral frontal lobe disease with impaired ability to plan and execute sequential movements. This gait superficially resembles that of parkinsonism, in that the posture is stooped and any steps taken are short and shuffling. However, initiation and maintenance of walking are impaired in a different manner. Each movement that is required for walking can usually be performed, if tested in isolation while sitting or lying. However, when asked to step forward while standing, a long pause often occurs before any attempt is made to flex at the hip and advance, as if the patient is "glued to the ground." Once walking is initiated, it is not maintained, even in an abnormal festinating manner. Rather, after one or several steps are taken, walking is stopped for several seconds or longer. The process is then repeated. Dementia and incontinence may coexist.

Choreoathetotic gait is characterized by an intermittent, irregular movement that disrupts the smooth flow of a normal gait. Flexion or extension movements at the hip are common and unpredictable but readily observed as a pelvic lurch (Chap. 363).

Cerebellar ataxic gait is a broad-based gait disorder in which the speed and length of stride varies irregularly from step to step. With midline cerebellar disease, as in alcoholics, posture is erect but the feet are separated; lower limb ataxia is commonly present as well. Assumption of a particular stance or a change in position may cause instability, yet balance can usually be maintained well with the eyes open or closed. Walking may be rapid, but cadence is irregular. Although patients commonly lack confidence in the stability of their walking, only minimal support is often required for reassurance. With disease of the cerebellar hemispheres, limb ataxia and nystagmus are commonly present as well (Chap. 364).

Sensory ataxic gait may resemble a cerebellar gait, with its broad-based stance and difficulty with change in position. However, although balance may be maintained with the eyes open, loss of visual input

through eye closure results in rapid loss of balance with a fall (positive Romberg sign), unless the physician assists the patient.

Vestibular gait is one in which the patient consistently tends to fall to one side, whether walking or standing. Cranial nerve examination demonstrates an obviously asymmetric nystagmus. The possibilities of unilateral sensory ataxia and hemiparesis are excluded by the findings of normal proprioception and strength (Chap. 21).

Astasia-abasia is a typical hysterical gait disorder. Although the patient usually has normal coordination of leg movements in bed or while sitting, the patient is unable to stand or walk without assistance. If distracted, stationary balance is sometimes maintained and several steps are taken normally, followed by a dramatic demonstration of imbalance with a lunge toward the examiner's arms or a nearby bed.

BIBLIOGRAPHY

ADAMS RD et al: *Principles of Neurology*, 6th ed. McGraw-Hill, New York, 1997

KANDEL ER et al: *Principles of Neural Science*, 4th ed, McGraw-Hill, New York, 2000

ZEHR EP, STEIN RB: What functions do reflexes serve during human locomotion? Prog Neurobiol 58:185, 1999

23   *Arthur K. Asbury*

NUMBNESS, TINGLING, AND SENSORY LOSS

NORMAL SENSATION   Normal somatic sensation reflects a continuous day and night monitoring process that occupies considerable moment-to-moment nervous system capacity. Little of this activity reaches consciousness under ordinary conditions. In contrast, disordered sensation, particularly if experienced as painful, is alarming and dominates the sufferer's attention. Abnormalities of sensation, especially if painful, tend to make those suffering seek medical help. The physician must be able to recognize abnormal sensations by how they are described, know their type and likely site of origin, and understand their implications. →*For a consideration of pain, see Chap. 12.*

Positive and Negative Phenomena   Abnormal sensory phenomena may be divided into two categories, positive and negative. The prototypical positive phenomenon is tingling (pins-and-needles), and the principal negative phenomenon is numbness. In addition to tingling, positive sensory phenomena include other altered sensations that are often described as pricking, bandlike, lightning-like shooting feelings (lancinations), aching, knifelike, twisting, drawing, pulling, tightening, burning, searing, electrical, or raw feelings. These descriptors are frequently the actual words used by patients. Such sensations may or may not be experienced as painful.

Positive phenomena usually result from trains of impulses generated at a site or sites of lowered threshold or heightened excitability along a sensory pathway, either peripheral or central. The nature and severity of an abnormal sensation depend on the number, rate, timing, and distribution of ectopic impulses and the type and function of nervous tissue in which they arise. Because positive phenomena represent excessive activity in sensory pathways, they are not necessarily associated with any sensory deficit (loss) upon examination.

Negative phenomena represent loss of sensory function and are characterized by diminished or absent feeling, often experienced as numbness. In contrast to positive phenomena, negative phenomena are accompanied by abnormal findings on sensory examination. In disorders affecting peripheral sensation, it is estimated that at least half the afferent axons innervating a given site are lost or functionless before sensory deficit can be demonstrated by clinical examination. This estimate probably varies according to how rapidly sensory nerve fibers have lost function. If the rate of loss is slow and chronic, lack of cutaneous feeling may be unnoticed by the patient and difficult to demonstrate on examination, even though few sensory fibers are functioning. Rapidly evolving sensory abnormality usually evokes both positive and negative phenomena and is readily recognized by patients. Subclinical degrees of sensory dysfunction not demonstrable on clinical sensory examination may be revealed by sensory nerve conduction studies or somatosensory cerebral evoked potentials (Chap. 357). Sensory symptoms may be either positive or negative, but sensory signs on examination are always a measure of negative phenomena.

Terminology Words used to characterize sensory disturbance are descriptive and have been arrived at mainly by convention. Paresthesia and dysesthesia are general terms used to denote sensory symptoms (positive phenomena) and are usually stated in the plural form. *Paresthesias* usually refer to tingling or pins-and-needles sensations but may also include a wide variety of other abnormal sensations, excepting pain. Sometimes "paresthesias" carry the implication that the abnormal sensations are perceived without an apparent stimulus. *Dysesthesia* is a more general term used to subsume all types of abnormal sensations, even painful ones, whether a stimulus is evident or not.

While dysesthesias and paresthesias refer to sensations described by patients, another set of terms refers to sensory abnormalities found on examination. These include *hypesthesia* or *hypoesthesia* (reduction of cutaneous sensation to a specific type of testing such as pressure, light touch, and warm or cold stimuli); *anesthesia* (complete absence of skin sensation to the same stimuli plus pinprick); and *hypalgesia* (referring to reduced pain perception, i.e., nociception, such as the pricking quality elicited by a pin). *Hyperesthesia* means pain in response to touch. Similarly, *allodynia* describes the situation in which a nonpainful stimulus, once perceived, is experienced as painful, even excruciating. An example is elicitation of a painful sensation by application of a vibrating tuning fork. *Hyperalgesia* denotes severe pain in response to a mildly noxious stimulus, and *hyperpathia*, a broad term, encompasses all the phenomena described by hyperesthesia, allodynia, and hyperalgesia. With hyperpathia, the threshold for a sensory stimulus is increased and the perception is delayed but once felt, is unduly painful.

Disorders of deep sensation, arising from muscle spindles, tendons, and joints, affect proprioception (position sense). Manifestations include imbalance (particularly with eyes closed or in the dark), clumsiness of precision movements, and unsteadiness of gait, which are referred to collectively as *sensory ataxia* (Chap. 22). Other findings on examination usually, but not invariably, include reduced or absent joint position and vibratory sensibility and absent deep tendon reflexes in the affected limbs. Romberg's sign is positive, which means that the patient sways or topples when asked to stand with feet close together and eyes closed. In severe states of deafferentation involving deep sensation, the patient cannot walk or stand unaided or even sit unsupported. Continuous, sometimes wormlike involuntary movements, called *pseudoathetosis*, of the outstretched hands and fingers occur, particularly with eyes closed. Such patients are severely disabled.

Anatomy of Sensation Cutaneous afferent innervation is conveyed by a rich variety of receptors, both naked nerve endings (nociceptors and thermoreceptors) and encapsulated terminals (mechanoreceptors). Each type of receptor has its own set of sensitivities to specific stimuli, size and distinctness of receptive fields, and adaptational qualities. Much of the knowledge about these receptors has come from the development of techniques to study single intact nerve fibers intraneurally in awake unanesthetized human subjects. It is possible not only to record from single nerve fibers, large or small, but also to stimulate single fibers in isolation. A single impulse, whether elicited by a natural stimulus or evoked by electrical microstimulation, in a large myelinated afferent fiber may be both perceived and localized.

Afferent fibers of all sizes in peripheral nerve trunks traverse the dorsal roots and enter the dorsal horn of the spinal cord (Fig. 23-1). From there the smaller fibers take a different route to the parietal cortex than the larger fibers. The polysynaptic projections of the smaller fibers

(unmyelinated and small myelinated), which subserve mainly nociception, temperature sensibility, and touch, cross and ascend in the opposite anterior and lateral columns of the spinal cord, through the brainstem, to the ventral posterolateral (VPL) nucleus of the thalamus, and ultimately project to the postcentral gyrus of the parietal cortex (Chap. 12). This is referred to as the *spinothalamic pathway*, or *anterolateral system*. The larger fibers, which subserve tactile and position sense and kinesthesia, project rostrally in the posterior column on the same side of the spinal cord and make their first synapse in the gracile or cuneate nuclei of the lower medulla. The second-order neuron decussates and ascends in the medial lemniscus located medially in the medulla and in the tegmentum of the pons and midbrain and synapses in the VPL. The third-order neuron projects to parietal cortex; this large fiber system is referred to as the *posterior column–medial lemniscal pathway* (lemniscal, for short). Note that although the lemniscal and the anterolateral pathways both project up the spinal cord to the thalamus, it is the (crossed) anterolateral pathway that is referred to as the *spinothalamic tract*, by convention.

Although the fiber types and functions that make up the spinothalamic and lemniscal systems are relatively well known, it has been found that many other fibers, particularly those associated with touch, pressure, and position sense, ascend in a diffusely distributed pattern both ipsilaterally and contralaterally in the anterolateral quadrants of the spinal cord. This explains why an individual with a complete lesion of the posterior columns of the spinal cord may have little sensory deficit on examination.

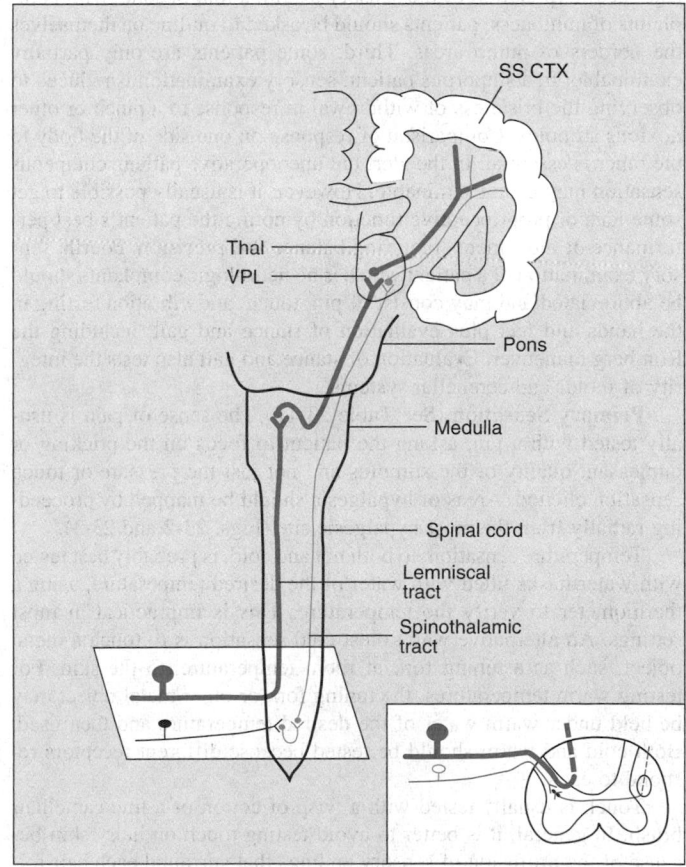

FIGURE 23-1 Schematic diagram of lemniscal and spinothalamic pathways. Note that the large fibers that subserve proprioception and discriminative touch ascend ipsilaterally as the lemniscal pathway in the posterior column of the spinal cord, and that the small fibers that subserve pain, thermal sensation, and crude touch ascend contralaterally as the spinothalamic pathway in the anterior and lateral columns of the spinal cord (insert). SS CTX, somatosensory cortex; Thal, thalamus; VPL, ventral posterolateral nucleus.

Table 23-1 Testing Primary Sensation

Sense	Test Device	Endings Activated	Fiber Size Mediating	Central Pathway
Pain	Pinprick	Cutaneous nociceptors	Small	SpTh, also D
Temperature, heat	Warmed metal object	Cutaneous thermoreceptors for hot	Small	SpTh
Temperature, cold	Cold metal object	Cutaneous thermoreceptors for cold	Small	SpTh
Touch	Cotton wisp, fine brush	Cutaneous mechanoreceptors, also naked endings	Large and small	Lem, also D and SpTh
Vibration	Tuning fork, 128 Hz	Mechanoreceptors, especially pacinian corpuscles	Large	Lem, also D
Joint position	Passive movement of specific joints	Joint capsule and tendon endings, muscle spindles	Large	Lem, also D

NOTE: D, diffuse ascending projections in ipsilateral and contralateral anterolateral columns; SpTh, spinothalamic projection, contralateral; Lem, posterior column and lemniscal projection, ipsilateral.

EXAMINATION OF SENSATION The main tasks of the sensory examination are tests of primary sensation. By convention these include the sense of pain, touch, vibration, joint position, and thermal sensation, both hot and cold (Table 23-1). Detailed descriptions of how to perform the various tests of the sensory examination can be found in standard texts (see "Bibliography").

Some general principles pertain. First, the examiner must depend on subjective patient response, particularly when using cutaneous stimuli (pin, touch, vibration, warm or cold). This factor may complicate the interpretation of the sensory examination. Second, with complaints of numbness, patients should be asked to outline on themselves the borders of numb areas. Third, some patients are only partially examinable. In a stuporous patient, sensory examination is reduced to observing the briskness of withdrawal in response to a pinch or other noxious stimulus. Comparison of response on one side of the body to the other is essential. In the alert but uncooperative patient, cutaneous sensation may be unexaminable. However, it is usually possible to get some idea of proprioceptive function by noting the patient's best performance of movements requiring balance and precision. Fourth, sensory examination of a patient who has no neurologic complaints should be abbreviated and may consist of pin, touch, and vibration testing in the hands and feet plus evaluation of stance and gait, including the Romberg maneuver. Evaluation of stance and gait also tests the integrity of motor and cerebellar systems.

Primary Sensation (See Table 23-1) The sense of pain is usually tested with a pin, asking the patient to focus on the pricking or unpleasant quality of the stimulus and not just the pressure or touch sensation elicited. Areas of hypalgesia should be mapped by proceeding radially from the most hypalgesic site (Figs. 23-2 and 23-3).

Temperature sensation, to both hot and cold, is probably best tested with water flasks filled with water of the desired temperature, using a thermometer to verify the temperature. This is impractical in most settings. An alternative way to test cold sensation is to touch a metal object, such as a tuning fork at room temperature, to the skin. For testing warm temperatures, the tuning fork or other metal object may be held under warm water of the desired temperature and then used. Both cold and warm should be tested because different receptors respond to each.

Touch is usually tested with a wisp of cotton or a fine camelhair brush. In general, it is better to avoid testing touch on hairy skin because of the profusion of sensory endings that surround each hair follicle.

Joint position testing is a measure of proprioception, one of the most important functions of the sensory system. With the patient keeping eyes closed, joint position is tested in the great toe and in the fingers. If errors are made in recognizing the direction of passive movements of the toe or the finger, more proximal joints should be

tested. A test of proximal joint position sense, primarily at the shoulder, is performed by asking the patient to bring the two index fingers together with the arms extended and the eyes closed. Normal individuals should be able to do this quite accurately, with errors of a centimeter or less.

The sense of vibration is tested with a tuning fork, preferably a large one that vibrates at 128 Hz. Vibration is usually tested at bony prominences, beginning distally at the malleoli of the ankles, and at the knuckles. If abnormalities are found, more proximal sites can be examined. Vibratory theshelds at the same site in the patient and the examiner can be compared for control purposes.

Quantitative Sensory Testing Effective sensory testing devices have been developed over the past two decades. Quantitative sensory testing is particularly useful for serial evaluation of cutaneous sensation in clinical trials. Threshold testing for touch and vibratory and thermal sensation is the most widely used application.

Cortical Sensation Cortical sensory testing includes two-point discrimination, touch localization, and bilateral simultaneous stimu-

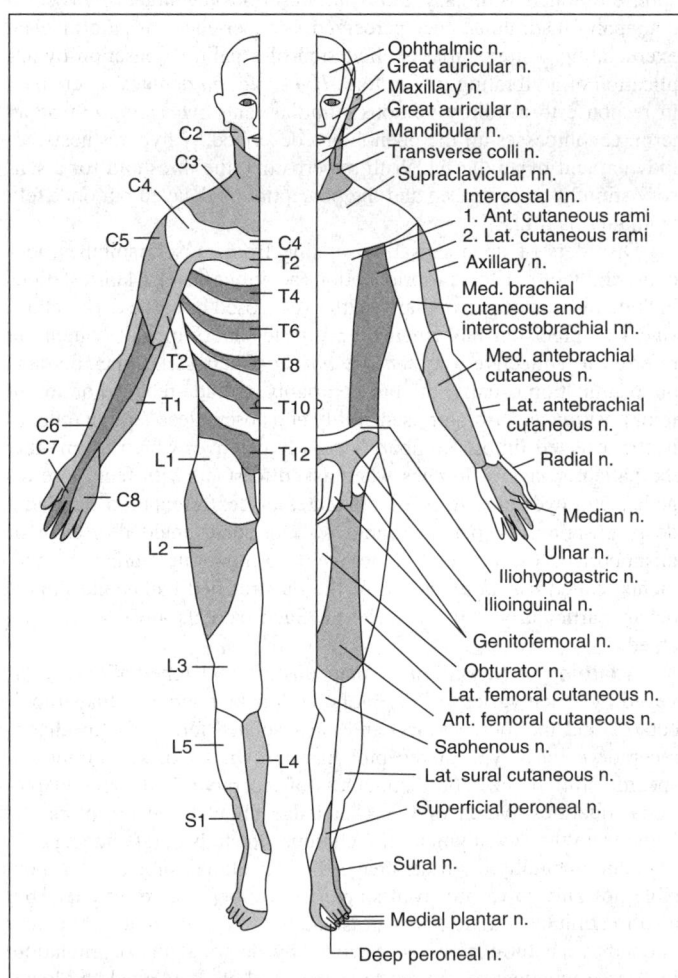

FIGURE 23-2 Anterior view of dermatomes *(left)* and cutaneous areas supplied by individual peripheral nerves *(right)*. *(Modified from MB Carpenter and J Sutin, in Human Neuroanatomy, 8th ed, Baltimore, Williams & Wilkins, 1983.)*

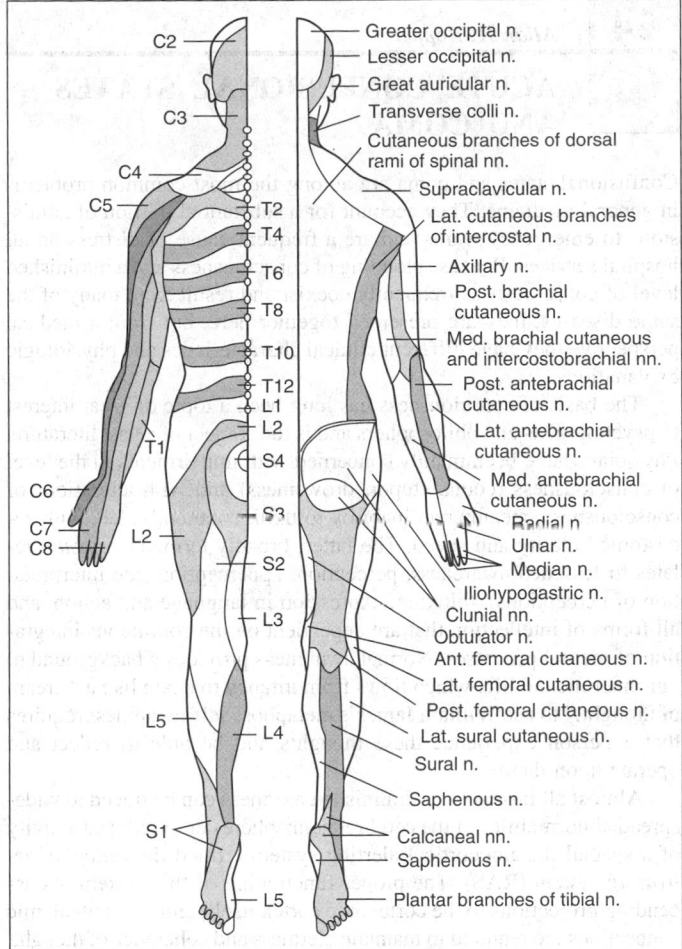

FIGURE 23-3 Posterior view of dermatomes *(left)* and cutaneous areas supplied by individual peripheral nerves *(right)*. *(Modified from MB Carpenter and J Sutin, in Human Neuroanatomy, 8th ed, Baltimore, Williams & Wilkins, 1983.)*

lation and tests for graphesthesia and stereognosis, to name the most commonly used methods. Abnormalities of these sensory tests, in the presence of normal primary sensation in an alert cooperative patient, signify a lesion of the parietal cortex or thalamocortical projections to the parietal lobe. If primary sensation is altered, these cortical discriminative functions will usually be abnormal, too. Comparisons should always be made between analogous sites on the two sides of the body because the deficit with a specific parietal lesion is likely to be hemilateral. Side-to-side comparisons hold true for all cortical sensory testing.

Two-point discrimination is tested by special calipers, the points of which may be set from 2 mm to several centimeters apart and then applied simultaneously to the site to be tested. The pulp of the fingertips is a common site to test; a normal individual can distinguish about 3-mm separation of points there.

Touch localization is usually carried out by light pressure with the examiner's fingertip, asking the patient, whose eyes are closed, to identify the site of touch. It is usual to ask the patient to touch the same site with a fingertip.

Bilateral simultaneous stimulation at analogous sites (e.g., the dorsa of both hands) can be carried out to determine whether the perception of touch is extinguished consistently on one side or the other. The phenomenon is referred to as *extinction* on bilateral simultaneous stimulation.

Graphesthesia means the capacity to recognize with eyes closed letters or numbers drawn by the examiner's fingertip on the palm of the hand. Once again, the comparison of one side with the other is of prime importance. Inability to recognize numbers or letters is termed *agraphesthesia.*

Stereognosis refers to the ability to identify common objects by palpation, recognizing their shape, texture, and size. Common standard objects are the best test objects, such as a marble, a paper clip, or coins. Patients with normal stereognosis should be able to distinguish a dime from a penny and a nickel from a quarter without looking. Patients should only be allowed to feel the object with one hand at a time. If they are unable to identify it in one hand, it should be placed in the other for comparison. Individuals unable to identify common objects and coins in one hand who can do so in the other are said to have *astereognosis* of the abnormal hand.

LOCALIZATION OF SENSORY ABNORMALITIES

Sensory symptoms and signs can result from lesions at almost any level of the nervous system, including parietal cortex, deep white matter, thalamus, brainstem, spinal cord, spinal root, peripheral nerve, and sensory receptor. Noting the distribution and nature of sensory symptoms and signs is the most important way to localize their source. The extent, configuration, symmetry, quality, and severity are the key observations.

Dysesthesias without sensory findings by examination can be difficult to interpret. To illustrate, tingling dysesthesias in an acral distribution (hands and feet) can have more than one interpretation. Distal dysesthesias can be systemic in origin, e.g., secondary to hyperventilation, or can be induced by a medication, such as the diuretic acetazolamide. Distal dysesthesias can also be an early event in an evolving polyneuropathy or can herald a myelopathy, such as with vitamin B_{12} deficiency. Sometimes distal dysesthesias have no definable basis. In contrast, dysesthesias that correspond to a particular peripheral nerve territory denote a lesion of that nerve trunk. For instance, dysesthesias restricted to the fifth digit and the adjacent one-half of the fourth finger on one hand reliably point to disorder of the ulnar nerve, most commonly at the elbow.

Nerve and Root In focal nerve trunk lesions severe enough to cause a deficit, sensory abnormalities are readily mapped and generally have discrete boundaries (Figs. 23-2 and 23-3). Root lesions, referred to as radicular, are frequently accompanied by deep, aching pain along the course of the related nerve trunk. With compression of a fifth lumbar (L5) or first sacral (S1) root, as may occur with a ruptured intervertebral disc, sciatica is a frequent manifestation. With a lesion affecting a single root, sensory deficit in the distribution of that root is often minimal or not demonstrable at all. This is because adjacent root territories overlap extensively.

Polyneuropathies are generally graded, distal, and symmetric in distribution of deficit (Chap. 377). Dysesthesias begin in the toes and ascend symmetrically, followed by numbness. When dysesthesias reach the knees, they have usually also appeared in the fingertips. The process appears to be nerve length–dependent, and the deficit is often described as "stocking-glove" in type. Although most polyneuropathies are pansensory and affect all modalities of sensation, selective sensory dysfunction according to nerve fiber size may occur. In polyneuropathies that affect small nerve fibers selectively, the hallmark is burning, painful dysesthesias with reduced pinprick and thermal sensation but with sparing of proprioception, motor function, and even deep tendon jerks. Touch is variably involved, but when spared, the sensory pattern is referred to as *sensory dissociation*. Sensory dissociation patterns can be seen with spinal cord lesions (see below) as well as with small fiber neuropathies. In contrast to small fiber polyneuropathies, large fiber polyneuropathies are characterized by position sense deficit, imbalance, absent tendon jerks, and variable motor dysfunction but preservation of most cutaneous sensation. Dysesthesias, if present at all, tend to be tingling or bandlike.

Spinal Cord (See Chap. 368) If the spinal cord is transected, all sensation is lost below the level of transection. Bladder and bowel function are also lost, as is motor function. Hemisection of the spinal cord produces the Brown-Séquard syndrome, which involves absent pain and temperature sensation on the opposite side below the lesion, and loss of proprioceptive sensation and loss of motor power on the same side below the lesion (see Figs. 23-1 and 368-1). Dissociated sensory deficit patterns (see above) are also a sign of spinothalamic tract involvement in the spinal cord, especially if the deficit is unilateral and has an upper level on the torso. Bilateral spinothalamic tract involvement occurs with lesions affecting the center of the spinal cord, such as happens with expansion of the central canal in syringomyelia. Sensory dissociation is characteristic of syringomyelia.

Brainstem   Harlequin patterns of sensory disturbance, in which one side of the face and the opposite side of the body are affected, localize to the lateral medulla. Here a small lesion may damage both the ipsilateral descending trigeminal tract and ascending spinothalamic fibers subserving the opposite arm, leg, and hemitorso (see "Lateral medullary syndrome" in Fig. 361-7). In the tegmentum of the pons and midbrain, where the lemniscal and spinothalamic tracts merge, a lesion here causes pansensory loss on the contralateral body.

Thalamus   Hemisensory disturbance with tingling numbness from head to foot is often thalamic in origin but can also be anterior parietal. If abrupt in onset, the lesion is likely to be due to a small stroke (lacunar infarction), particularly if localized to the thalamus. Occasionally, with lesions affecting the VPL or adjacent white matter, a syndrome of thalamic pain, also called *Déjerine-Roussy syndrome*, may ensue. This persistent unrelenting hemipainful state is often described in dramatic terms such as "like the flesh is being torn from my limbs" or "as though that side is bathed in acid" (Chap. 12).

Cortex   With lesions of the parietal lobe, either of the cortex or of subjacent white matter, the most prominent symptoms are contralateral hemineglect, hemi-inattention, and a tendency not to use the affected hand and arm. Tests of primary sensation may be normal or altered. Anterior parietal infarction may present as a pseudothalamic syndrome with crossed hemilateral loss of primary sensation. Dysesthesias or a sense of numbness may also occur, and rarely a painful state.

Focal Sensory Seizures   These are generally due to lesions in or near the postcentral gyrus. Symptoms of focal sensory seizures are usually combinations of numbness and tingling, but frequently additional more complex sensations are present, such as a rushing feeling, a sense of warmth, a sense of movement without visible motion, or other unpleasant dysesthesias. Duration of seizures is variable; they may be transient, lasting only seconds, or they may persist for hours. Focal motor features (clonic jerking) may supervene, and seizures can become generalized with loss of consciousness. Likely sites of symptoms are unilaterally in the lips, face, digits, or foot, and symptoms may spread as in a Jacksonian march. On occasion, symptoms may occur in a symmetric bilateral fashion, for instance, in both hands; this results from involvement of the second sensory area (unilaterally) located in the rolandic area at and just above the Sylvian fissure.

BIBLIOGRAPHY

ADAMS RD et al: *Principles of Neurology*, 6th ed. New York, McGraw-Hill, 1997

BASSETTI C et al: Sensory syndromes in parietal stroke. Neurology 43:1942, 1993

MOGYDROS I et al: Mechanisms of paresthesias arising from healthy axons. Muscle Nerve 23:310, 2000

OCHOA JL: Positive sensory symptoms in neuropathy: Mechanisms and aspects of treatment, in *Peripheral Nerve Disorders*, AK Asbury, PK Thomas (eds). Oxford, Butterworth-Heinemann, 1995, pp 44–58

REMY P et al: Somatosensory cortical activations are suppressed in patients with tactile extinction. Neurology 52:571, 1999

ROSS RT: *How to Examine the Nervous System*, 3d ed. Stamford, Appleton & Lange, 1999

ROWBOTHAM MC, FIELDS HL: The relationship of pain, allodynia and thermal sensation in post-herpetic neuralgia. Brain 119:347, 1996

SIMON RP et al: *Clinical Neurology*, 4th ed. Stamford, Appleton & Lange, 1999

YARNITSKY D: Quantitative sensory testing. Muscle Nerve 20:198, 1997

24   *Allan H. Ropper*

ACUTE CONFUSIONAL STATES AND COMA

Confusional states and coma are among the most common problems in general medicine. They account for a substantial portion of admissions to emergency wards and are a frequent cause of distress on all hospital services. Because clouding of consciousness and a diminished level of consciousness frequently coexist and result from many of the same diseases, they are presented together here, but from a medical perspective they have different clinical characteristics and physiologic explanations.

The basis of consciousness has long been a topic of great interest to psychologists and philosophers and is the subject of a vast literature. Physicians have been mainly concerned with impairments in the level of consciousness (coma, stupor, drowsiness) and with alterations of consciousness, meaning an inability to think coherently, i.e., with accustomed clarity and speed. The latter, broadly termed *confusion* relates to lessened awareness, perception, apperception (the interpretation of perceptions), thinking, expression in language and action, and all forms of intellection that are dependent on the continuous integration of mental processes. Normal awareness provides a background to our inner mental life, which flows from infancy to death like a "stream of thought," to use William James's metaphor. Self-awareness requires that a person experience these thoughts and be able to reflect and operate upon them.

Almost all instances of diminished alertness can be traced to widespread abnormalities of the cerebral hemispheres or to reduced activity of a special thalamocortical alerting system termed the *reticular activating system* (RAS). The proper functioning of this system, its ascending projections to the cortex, the cortex itself, and corticothalamic connections are required to maintain alertness and coherence of thought.

THE CONFUSIONAL STATE   Confusion is a mental and behavioral state of reduced comprehension, coherence, and capacity to reason. Inattention, as defined by the inability to sustain uninterrupted thought and actions, and disorientation are its earliest outward signs. As the state of confusion worsens, there are more global mental failings, including impairments of memory, perception, comprehension, problem solving, language, praxis, visuospatial function, and various aspects of emotional behavior that are each attributable to particular regions of the brain. In other instances an apparent confusional state may arise from an isolated deficit in mental function such as an impairment of language (*aphasia*), loss of memory (*amnesia*), or lack of appreciation of spatial relations of self and the external environment (*agnosia*), but the attributes of the problem are then quite different (Chap. 25). Confusion is also a feature of dementia, in which case the chronicity of the process, as in the instance of Alzheimer's disease, distinguishes it from an acute encephalopathy (Chap. 26).

The confused patient is usually subdued, not inclined to speak, and is physically inactive. A state of confusion that is accompanied by agitation, hallucinations, tremor, and illusions (misperceptions of environmental sight, sound, or touch) is termed *delirium*, as typified by delirium tremens from alcohol or drug withdrawal. In psychiatric circles, delirium often refers, albeit imprecisely, to all acute states of confusion with clouding of consciousness and incoherence of thought.

—————— *Approach to the Patient* ——————

Confusion and delirium always signify a disorder of the nervous system. They may be the major manifestation of a head injury; a seizure; drug toxicity (or drug withdrawal); a metabolic disorder resulting from hepatic, renal, pulmonary or cardiac failure; a systemic infection; meningitis or encephalitis; or a chronic dementing disease.

The search for these manifold causes begins with a careful history emphasizing the patient's condition before the onset of confusion. The clinical examination should focus on signs of diminished attentiveness, disorientation, and drowsiness and on the presence of localizing neurologic signs. From the clinical data the clinician is directed to the appropriate laboratory tests discussed further on. Often, even after all diagnostic tests are completed, one may still not know the cause of a confusional state. The proper approach is to observe the patient in the hospital for a number of days under stable conditions. New clues may appear or an obscure confusion perhaps related to a medication, may clear up, while other causes such as renal or hepatic failure may worsen and lead to coma.

Orientation and memory are tested by asking the patient in a forthright manner the date, inclusive of month, day, year, and day of week; the precise place; and some items of generally acknowledged and universally known information (the names of the President and Vice President, a recent national catastrophe, the state capital). Further probing may be necessary to reveal a defect—why is the patient in the hospital; what is his or her address, zip code, telephone number, social security number? Problems of increasing complexity may be pursued, but they usually provide little additional information. Attention and coherence of thought can be gauged by the clarity of and speed of responses while the history is being given but are examined more explicitly by having the patient repeat strings of numbers (most adults easily retain seven digits forward and four backward), spell a word such as "world" backwards, and perform serial calculations—tests of serial subtraction of 3 from 30 or 7 from 100 are useful. It is the inability to sustain coherent mental activity in performing tasks such as these that exposes the most subtle confusional states.

Other salient neurologic findings are the level of alertness, which fluctuates if there is drowsiness; indications of focal damage of the cerebrum such as hemiparesis, hemianopia, and aphasia; or adventitious movements of myoclonus or partial convulsions. The language of the confused patient may be disorganized and rambling, even to the extent of incorporating paraphasic words. These features, along with impaired comprehension that is due mainly to inattention, may be mistaken for aphasia.

One of the most specific signs of a metabolic encephalopathy is asterixis, which is an arrhythmic flapping tremor that is typically elicited by asking the patient to hold the arms outstretched with the wrists and hands fully extended. After a few seconds, there is a large jerking lapse in the posture of the hand and then a rapid return to the original position. The same movements can be appreciated in any tonically held posture, even of the tongue, and in extreme form the movements may intrude on voluntary limb motion. Bilateral asterixis always signifies a metabolic encephalopathy, e.g., from hepatic failure, hypercapnia, or from drug ingestion, especially with anticonvulsant medications. Myoclonic jerking and tremor in an awake patient are typical of uremic encephalopathy or the use of antipsychotic drugs such as lithium, phenothiazines, or butyrophenones; myoclonus with coma may also signify anoxic cerebral damage.

Confusion in the postoperative period is common but at times so subtle as to escape attention. Cardiac and orthopedic procedures are particularly likely to produce disorientation or delirium in susceptible patients. Often a careful history will reveal that a mild but compensated dementia existed prior to the operation. Medications, particularly those with anticholinergic activity (including meperidine), inadvertent withdrawal from sleeping pills or alcohol, fever, and any of the endogenous metabolic derangements listed above may be responsible, or a stroke may have occurred.

Frequently confusion cannot be attributed to any single factor and it clears in several days. In many cases, particularly in the elderly, transient confusion and drowsiness arise with a febrile infection of the urinary tract, lungs, blood, or peritoneum. The term *septic encephalopathy* is currently used to describe this association, but the mechanism by which infection or inflammation leads to cerebral dysfunction is unknown. Fever can also alter brain function in a way that makes preexisting focal signs worse.

Distinguishing dementia from an acute confusional state is a great problem, especially in the elderly, since the two may coexist if a fever, other acute medical problem, or a poorly tolerated medication supervenes in a mildly demented patient, producing a so-called beclouded dementia. The memory loss of dementia brings about a confusional state that varies little in severity from hour to hour and day to day. Poor mental performance is derived mainly from incomplete recollection, inadequate access to names and ideas, and the inability to retain new information, thus affecting orientation and factual knowledge. In contrast to the acute confusional states, attention, alertness, and coherence are preserved until the most advanced stages. Eventually dementia produces a chronic confusion with breakdown of all types of mental performance, and the distinction from an acute encephalopathy depends mainly on the longstanding nature of the condition.

Treatment of the confusional state requires that all unnecessary medication be stopped, metabolic alterations be rectified, and infection be treated. Skilled nursing and a quiet room with a window are important. Careful explanations should be given at regular intervals to the family. In the elderly, regular reorientation and active measures to avoid risk factors (sleep deprivation, immobility, and vision and hearing impairments) reduce the number and severity of episodes of delirium in hospitalized patients.

COMA AND RELATED DISORDERS OF CONSCIOUSNESS The unnatural situation of reduced alertness and responsiveness represents a continuum that in severest form is called *coma*, a deep sleeplike state from which the patient cannot be aroused. *Stupor* defines lesser degrees of unarousability in which the patient can be awakened only by vigorous stimuli, accompanied by motor behavior that leads to avoidance of uncomfortable or aggravating stimuli. *Drowsiness*, which is familiar to all persons, simulates light sleep and is characterized by easy arousal and the persistence of alertness for brief periods. Drowsiness and stupor are usually attended by some degree of confusion. In clinical practice these terms should be supplemented by a narrative description of the level of arousal and of the type of responses evoked by various stimuli precisely as observed at the bedside. Such an account is preferable to ambiguous terms such as semicoma or obtundation, the definitions of which differ between physicians.

Several other neurologic conditions render patients apparently unresponsive and simulate coma, and certain other subsyndromes of coma must be considered separately because of their special significance. Among the latter, the *vegetative state* signifies an awake but unresponsive state. Most of these patients were earlier comatose and after a period of days or weeks emerge to an unresponsive state in which their eyelids are open, giving the appearance of wakefulness. Yawning, grunting, swallowing, as well as limb and head movements persist, but there are few, if any, meaningful responses to the external and internal environment—in essence, an "awake coma." Although respiratory and autonomic functions are retained, the term "vegetative" is nonetheless unfortunate as it is subject to misinterpretation by lay persons. Always there are accompanying signs that indicate extensive damage in both cerebral hemispheres, e.g., decerebrate or decorticate limb posturing and absent responses to visual stimuli (see below). Cardiac arrest and head injuries are the most common causes of the vegetative state (Chaps. 369 and 376). The prognosis for regaining mental faculties once the vegetative state has supervened for several months is almost nil hence the term *persistent vegetative state*. Most instances of dramatic recovery, when investigated carefully, are found to yield to the usual rules for prognosis, but it must be acknowledged that rare instances of awakening to a condition of dementia and paralysis have been documented.

Certain other clinical states are prone to be misinterpreted as stupor or coma. *Akinetic mutism* refers to a partially or fully awake patient who is able to form impressions and think but remains immobile and mute, particularly when unstimulated. The condition may result from damage in the regions of the medial thalamic nuclei, the frontal lobes (particularly situated deeply or on the orbitofrontal surfaces), or from hydrocephalus. The term *abulia* is used to describe a mental and physical slowness and lack of impulse to activity that is in essence a mild form of akinetic mutism, with the same anatomic origins. *Catatonia* is a curious hypomobile and mute syndrome associated with a major psychosis. In the typical form patients appear awake with eyes open but make no voluntary or responsive movements, although they blink spontaneously, swallow, and may not appear distressed. As often, the eyes are half-open as if the patient is in a fog or light sleep. There are signs that indicate voluntary attempts to appear less than fully responsive, though it may take some ingenuity on the part of the examiner to demonstrate these. Eyelid elevation is actively resisted, blinking occurs in response to a visual threat, and the eyes move concomitantly with head rotation, all signs belying a brain lesion. It is characteristic but not invariable for the limbs to retain the posture, no matter how bizarre, in which they have been placed by the examiner ("waxy flexibility," or catalepsy.) Upon recovery, such patients have some memory of events that occurred during their catatonic stupor. The appearance is superficially similar to akinetic mutism, but clinical evidence of brain damage is lacking.

The *locked-in state* describes a pseudocoma in which an awake patient has no means of producing speech or volitional limb, face, and pharyngeal movements in order to indicate that he or she is awake, but vertical eye movements and lid elevation remain unimpaired, thus allowing the patient to signal. Such individuals have written entire treatises using Morse code. Infarction or hemorrhage of the ventral pons, which transects all descending corticospinal and corticobulbar pathways, is the usual cause. A similar awake but deefferented state occurs as a result of total paralysis of the musculature in severe cases of Guillain-Barré syndrome (Chap. 378), critical illness neuropathy (Chap. 376), and pharmacologic neuromuscular blockade.

THE ANATOMY AND PHYSIOLOGY OF UNCONSCIOUSNESS   To the extent that all complex waking behaviors require the widespread participation of the cerebral cortex, consciousness cannot exist without the activity of these structures. A loosely grouped aggregation of neurons located in the upper brainstem and medial thalamus, the RAS, maintains the cerebral cortex in a state of wakeful consciousness. It follows that the principal causes of coma are (1) lesions that damage a substantial portion of the RAS; (2) destruction of large portions of both cerebral hemispheres; and (3) suppression of thalamocerebral function by drugs, toxins, or by internal metabolic derangements such as hypoglycemia, anoxia, azotemia, or hepatic failure.

The classic animal experiments of Moruzzi and Magoun, published in 1949, and subsequent human clinicopathologic observations have established that the regions of the reticular formation that are critical to the maintenance of wakefulness extend from the caudal midbrain to the lower thalamus. A most important practical consideration derives from the anatomic proximity of the RAS to structures that are concerned with pupillary function and eye movements. Pupillary enlargement and loss of vertical and adduction movements of the globes suggest that upper brainstem damage may be the source of coma. Although circumscribed lesions confined to one or both cerebral hemispheres do not affect the brainstem RAS, a large mass on one side of the brain may cause coma by secondarily compressing the upper brainstem and consequently producing abnormalities of the pupils and eye movements (see discussion of transtentorial herniation below). This type of indirect effect is most typical of cerebral hemorrhages and of rapidly expanding tumors within a cerebral hemisphere. In all cases the degree of diminished alertness also relates to the rapidity of evolution and the extent of compression of the RAS.

The neurons of the RAS are thought to project rostrally to the cortex primarily via thalamic relay nuclei that in turn exert a tonic influence on the activity of the entire cerebral cortex. The behavioral arousal effected by somesthetic, auditory, and visual stimuli depends upon the rich reciprocal innervation that the RAS receives from these sensory systems. The relays between the RAS and the thalamic and

cortical areas utilize a variety of neurotransmittors. Of these, the effect of arousal on acetylcholine and on the biogenic amines has been studied more extensively. Cholinergic fibers connect the midbrain to other areas of the upper brainstem, thalamus, and cortex. Serotonin and norepinephrine also subserve important functions in regulation of the sleep-wake cycle (Chap. 27). Their roles in arousal and coma have not been clearly established, although the alerting effects of amphetamines are likely to be mediated by catecholamine release.

Coma Due to Cerebral Mass Lesions and Herniations   The cranial cavity is separated into compartments by infoldings of the dura—the two cerebral hemispheres are separated by the falx, and the anterior and posterior fossae by the tentorium. *Herniation* refers to displacement of brain tissue away from a mass and into a compartment that it normally does not occupy. Many of the signs associated with coma, and indeed coma itself, can be attributed to these tissue shifts. Herniation can be *transfalcial* (displacement of the cingulate gyrus under the falx and across the midline), *transtentorial* (displacement of the medial temporal lobe into the tentorial opening), and *foraminal* (downward forcing of the cerebellar tonsils into the foramen magnum; Fig. 24-1).

Uncal transtentorial herniation refers to impaction of the anterior medial temporal gyrus (the uncus) into the anterior portion of the tentorial opening. The displaced tissue compresses the third nerve as it traverses the subarachnoid space and results in enlargement of the ipsilateral pupil (putatively because the fibers subserving parasympathetic pupillary function are located peripherally in the nerve). The coma that follows may be due to lateral compression of the midbrain against the opposite tentorial edge by the displaced parahippocampal gyrus (Fig. 24-2). In some cases the lateral displacement causes compression of the opposite cerebral peduncle, producing a Babinski response and hemiparesis contralateral to the original hemiparesis (the Kernohan-Woltman sign). In addition to compressing the upper brainstem, tissue shifts, including herniations, may compress major blood vessels, particularly the anterior and posterior cerebral arteries as they pass over the tentorial reflections, thus producing brain infarctions. The distortions may also entrap portions of the ventricular system, resulting in regional hydrocephalus.

Central transtentorial herniation denotes a symmetric downward movement of the upper thalamic region through the tentorial opening. Miotic pupils and drowsiness are the heralding signs. Both temporal and central herniations are thought to cause progressive compression of the brainstem from above: first the midbrain, then the pons, and finally the medulla. The result is a sequential appearance of neurologic signs that corresponds to the affected level.

A direct relationship between the various configurations of transtentorial herniations and coma is, at best, tenuous. The orderly pro-

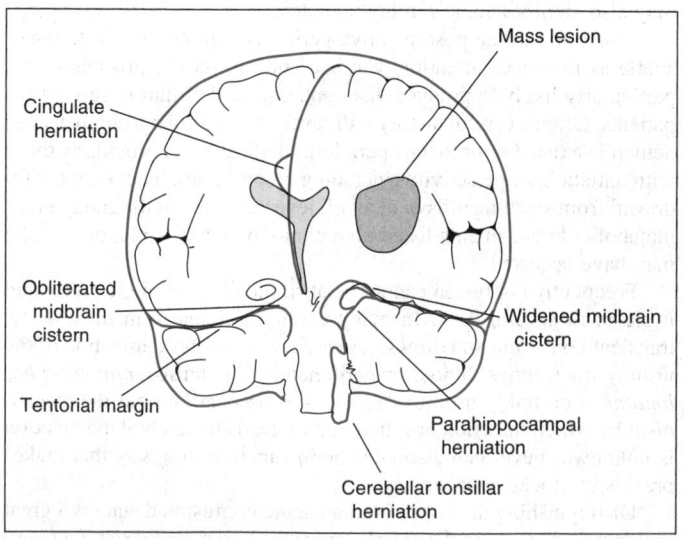

FIGURE 24-1   Herniation.

gression of signs from midbrain to medulla is often bypassed in catastrophic lesions where all brainstem functions are lost almost simultaneously. It is also clear that displacement of deep brain structures by a mass in any direction, with or without herniation, compresses the region of the RAS and results in coma. Furthermore, drowsiness and stupor typically occur with moderate lateral shifts at the level of the diencephalon (thalami) well before transtentorial or other herniations are evident. Lateral shift is easily quantified on axial images of computed tomography (CT) and magnetic resonance imaging (MRI) scans (Fig. 24-2). In cases of *acutely appearing masses*, a fairly consistent and simple relationship exists between the degree of horizontal displacement of midline structures and the level consciousness. Specifically, horizontal displacement of the pineal calcification of 3 to 5 mm is generally associated with drowsiness, 6 to 8 mm with stupor, and >9 mm with coma. At the same time, intrusion of the medial temporal lobe into the tentorial opening may be apparent as an obliteration of the cisterns that surround the upper brainstem.

Coma and Confusional States Due to Metabolic Disorders A large variety of systemic metabolic abnormalities cause coma by interrupting the delivery of energy substrates (hypoxia, ischemia, hypoglycemia) or by altering neuronal excitability (drug and alcohol intoxication, anesthesia, and epilepsy). The same metabolic abnormalities that produce coma may in milder form induce widespread cortical dysfunction and an acute confusional state. Thus, in metabolic encephalopathies, clouded consciousness and coma are a continuum. Neuropathologic changes in the various metabolic failures are variable—very evident in hypoxia-ischemia, manifest as astrocytic changes in hepatic coma, and negligible in renal and other metabolic encephalopathies.

Cerebral neurons are fully dependent on cerebral blood flow (CBF) and the related delivery of oxygen and glucose. CBF approximates 75 mL per 100 g/min in gray matter and 30 mL per 100 g/min in white matter (mean = 55 mL per 100 g/min); oxygen consumption is 3.5 mL per 100 g/min, and glucose utilization is 5 mg per 100 g/min. Brain stores of glucose provide energy for approximately 2 min after blood flow is interrupted, and oxygen stores last 8 to 10 s after the cessation of blood flow. Simultaneous hypoxia and ischemia exhaust glucose more rapidly. The electroencephalogram (EEG) rhythm in these circumstances becomes diffusely slowed, typical of metabolic encephalopathies, and as conditions of substrate delivery worsen, eventually all recordable brain electrical activity ceases. In almost all instances of metabolic encephalopathy, the global metabolic activity of the brain is reduced in proportion to the degree of unconsciousness.

Conditions such as hyponatremia, hyperosmolarity, hypercapnia, hypercalcemia, and hepatic and renal failure are associated with a variety of alterations in neurons and astrocytes. It should be stated at the outset that the reversible effects of these conditions on the brain are not understood, but they may in different circumstances impair energy supplies, change ion fluxes across neuronal membranes, and cause neurotransmitter abnormalities. For example, the high brain ammonia concentration that is associated with hepatic coma interferes with cerebral energy metabolism and with the Na⁺, K⁺-ATPase pump, increases the number and size of astrocytes, alters nerve cell function, and causes increased concentrations of potentially toxic products of ammonia metabolism; it may also result in abnormalities of neurotransmitters, including possible "false" neurotransmitters that may be active at receptor sites. Apart from hyperammonemia, which of these mechanisms is of critical importance is not clear. The mechanism of the encephalopathy of renal failure is also not known. Unlike ammonia, urea itself does not produce central nervous system (CNS) toxicity. A multifactorial causation has been proposed, including increased per-

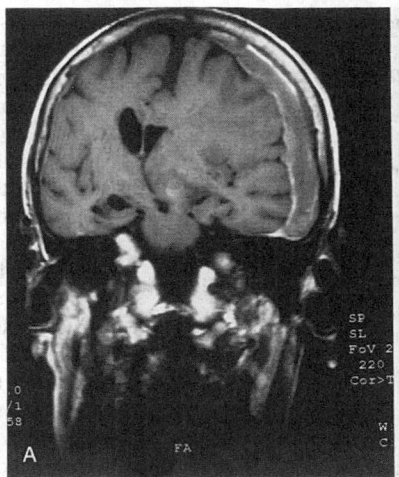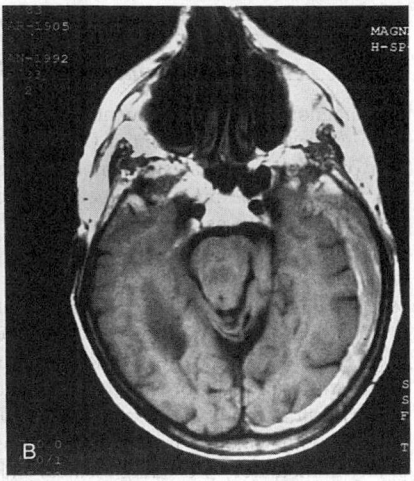

FIGURE 24-2 Coronal *(A)* and axial *(B)* magnetic resonance images from a stuporous patient with a left third nerve palsy as a result of large left-sided subdural hematoma (seen as a gray-white rim). The upper midbrain and lower thalamic regions are compressed and displaced laterally to the right, and there is transtentorial herniation of the medial temporal lobe structures, including the uncus anteriorly. The lateral ventricle opposite to the hematoma has become enlarged as a result of compression of the third ventricle.

meability of the blood-brain barrier to toxic substances such as organic acids and an increase in brain calcium or cerebrospinal fluid (CSF) phosphate content. Likewise, the basis of confusion and drowsiness that commonly accompanies the septic state has not been clarified.

Coma and seizures are a common accompaniment of any large shifts in sodium and water balance. These changes in osmolarity may be the result of a number of systemic medical disorders including diabetic ketoacidosis, the nonketotic hyperosmolar state, and hyponatremia from any cause (e.g., water intoxication, excessive secretion of antidiuretic hormone or atrial natriuretic peptides). The volume of brain water correlates with the level of consciousness in these states, but other factors also play a role. Sodium levels below 125 mmol/L induce confusion, and below 115 mmol/L are associated with coma and convulsions. In hyperosmolar coma the serum osmolarity generally exceeds 350 mosmol/L. *As in most other metabolic encephalopathies, the severity of neurologic change depends to a large degree on the rapidity with which the serum changes occur.* Hypercapnia depresses the level of consciousness in proportion to the rise in CO_2 tension in the blood and depends very much on the rapidity of change. The pathophysiology of other metabolic encephalopathies such as hypercalcemia, hypothyroidism, vitamin B_{12} deficiency, and hypothermia are incompletely understood but must also reflect derangements of CNS biochemistry and membrane function.

Epileptic Coma Although all metabolic derangements in some way alter neuronal electrophysiologic function, epilepsy is the only primary excitatory disturbance of brain electrical activity that is encountered in clinical practice. Continuous, generalized electrical discharges of the cortex (*seizures*) are associated with coma even in the absence of epileptic motor activity (*convulsions*). The self-limited coma that follows seizures, termed the *postictal state*, may be due to exhaustion of energy reserves or effects of locally toxic molecules that are the byproduct of seizures. The postictal state produces a pattern of continuous, generalized slowing of the background EEG activity similar to that of other metabolic encephalopathies.

Pharmacologic Coma This class of encephalopathy is in large measure reversible and leaves no residual damage providing hypoxia does not supervene. Many drugs and toxins are capable of depressing nervous system function. Some produce coma by affecting both the brainstem nuclei, including the RAS, and the cerebral cortex. The combination of cortical and brainstem signs, which occurs in certain drug overdoses, may lead to an incorrect diagnosis of structural brainstem disease.

_____ *Approach to the Patient* _____

The diagnosis and management of coma depend on knowledge of its main causes (see "Differential Diagnosis," below) and on interpretation of salient clinical signs, notably brainstem reflexes and motor function. Acute respiratory and cardiovascular problems should be attended to prior to neurologic assessment. A complete medical evaluation, except for the vital signs, funduscopy, and examination for nuchal rigidity, may be deferred until the neurologic evaluation has established the severity and nature of coma.

History   In many cases, the cause of coma is immediately evident (e.g., trauma, cardiac arrest, or known drug ingestion). In the remainder, historic information about the onset of coma is often sparse, but certain historic points are especially useful: (1) the circumstances and rapidity with which neurologic symptoms developed; (2) the details of any immediately preceding medical and neurologic symptoms (confusion, weakness, headache, fever, seizures, dizziness, double vision, or vomiting); (3) the use of medications, illicit drugs, or alcohol; and (4) chronic liver, kidney, lung, heart, or other medical disease. Direct interrogation or telephone calls to family and observers on the scene are an important part of the initial evaluation. Ambulance technicians often provide the most useful information in an enigmatic case.

General Physical Examination   The temperature, pulse, respiratory rate and pattern, and blood pressure should be measured quickly as the evaluation is getting under way. Fever suggests a systemic infection, bacterial meningitis, or encephalitis; only rarely is it attributable to a brain lesion that has disturbed temperature-regulating centers. A slight elevation in temperature may follow vigorous convulsions. High body temperature, 42 to 44°C, associated with dry skin should arouse the suspicion of heat stroke or anticholinergic drug intoxication. Hypothermia is observed with bodily exposure to lowered environmental temperature; alcoholic, barbiturate, sedative, or phenothiazine intoxication; hypoglycemia; peripheral circulatory failure; or hypothyroidism. Hypothermia itself causes coma only when the temperature is <31°C. Tachypnea may indicate acidosis or pneumonia. Aberrant respiratory patterns that may reflect brainstem disorders are discussed below. Marked hypertension, a sign of hypertensive encephalopathy or a rapid rise in intracranial pressure, may occur acutely after head injury. Hypotension is characteristic of coma from alcohol or barbiturate intoxication, internal hemorrhage, myocardial infarction, sepsis, profound hypothyroidism, or Addisonian crisis. The funduscopic examination is invaluable in detecting subarachnoid hemorrhage (subhyaloid hemorrhages), hypertensive encephalopathy (exudates, hemorrhages, vessel-crossing changes, papilledema), and increased intracranial pressure (papilledema). Generalized cutaneous petechiae suggest thrombotic thrombocytopenic purpura, meningococcemia, or a bleeding diathesis from which an intracerebral hemorrhage arises.

Neurologic Assessment   The patient should be observed first without examiner intervention. Patients who toss about, reach up toward the face, cross their legs, yawn, swallow, cough, or moan are close to being awake. Lack of restless movements on one side or an outturned leg at rest suggests a hemiplegia. Intermittent twitching movements of a foot, finger, or facial muscle may be the only sign of seizures. Multifocal myoclonus almost always indicates a metabolic disorder, particularly azotemia, anoxia, or drug ingestion (lithium and haloperidol are particularly prone to cause this sign), or the rarer conditions of spongiform encephalopathy and Hashitmoto disease. In a drowsy and confused patient bilateral asterixis is a certain sign of metabolic encephalopathy or drug ingestion.

The terms *decorticate rigidity* and *decerebrate rigidity*, or "posturing," describe stereotyped arm and leg movements occurring spontaneously or elicited by sensory stimulation. Flexion of the elbows and wrists and supination of the arm (decortication) suggests severe bilateral damage rostral to the midbrain, whereas extension of the elbows and wrists with pronation (decerebration) indicates damage to motor tracts in the midbrain or caudal diencephalon. The less frequent combination of arm extension with leg flexion or flaccid legs is associated

with lesions in the pons. These concepts have been adapted from animal work and cannot be applied with the same precision to coma in humans. In fact, acute and widespread cerebral disorders of any type, regardless of location, frequently cause limb extension, and almost all such extensor posturing becomes predominantly flexor as time passes. Thus, posturing alone cannot be utilized for precise anatomic localization. Posturing may also be unilateral and may coexist with purposeful limb movements, usually reflecting incomplete damage to the motor system.

Level of Arousal and Elicited Movements   If the patient is not aroused by a conversational volume of voice, a sequence of increasingly intense stimuli is used to determine the patient's threshold of arousal and the optimal motor response of each limb. It should be recognized that the results of this testing may vary from minute to minute and that serial examinations are most useful. Tickling the nostrils with a cotton wisp is a moderate stimulus to arousal—all but deeply stuporous and comatose patients will move the head away and rouse to some degree. Using the hand to remove an offending stimulus such as this one represents an even lesser degree of unresponsiveness.

Responses to noxious stimuli should be appraised critically. Stereotyped posturing indicates severe dysfunction of the corticospinal system. Abduction-avoidance movement of a limb is usually purposeful and denotes an intact corticospinal system extending from the contralateral cortex to the ipsilateral spinal cord. Pressure on the knuckles or bony prominences and pinprick are humane forms of noxious stimulus; pinching the skin causes unsightly ecchymoses and is generally not necessary but may be useful in eliciting abduction withdrawal movements of the limbs. Conversely, consistent (obligatory) adduction and flexion of stimulated limbs may be reflexive in origin and implies damage to the corticospinal system. Brief clonus or twitching may occur at the end of extensor posturing movements and should not be mistaken for convulsions.

Brainstem Reflexes   Assessment of brainstem damage is essential to the localization of the lesion in coma (Fig. 24-3). The brainstem reflexes that are conveniently assessed are pupillary responses to light, spontaneous and elicited eye movements, corneal responses, and the respiratory pattern. As a rule, when these brainstem activities are preserved, particularly the pupil reactions and eye movements, coma must necessarily be ascribed to bilateral hemispheral disease. The converse, however, is not always true as a mass in the hemispheres may be the proximate cause of coma but nonetheless produce brainstem signs.

Pupils   Pupillary reactions are examined with a bright, diffuse light (not an ophthalmoscope); if the response is absent, this should be confirmed by observation through a magnifying lens. Reaction to light is often difficult to appreciate in pupils <2 mm in diameter, and bright room lighting mutes pupillary reactivity. Normally reactive and round pupils of midsize (2.5 to 5 mm) essentially exclude midbrain damage, either primary or secondary to compression. One unreactive and enlarged pupil (>6 mm) or one that is poorly reactive signifies a compression or stretching of the third nerve from the effects of a mass above. Enlargement of the pupil contralateral to a mass may occur but is infrequent. It may be found in cases of subdural hematoma or brain hemorrhage, possibly as a result of compression of the midbrain or third nerve against the opposite tentorial margin. An oval and slightly eccentric pupil is a transitional sign that accompanies early midbrain–third nerve compression. The most extreme pupillary sign, bilaterally dilated and unreactive pupils, indicates severe midbrain damage, usually from compression by a mass or from ingestion of drugs with anticholinergic activity. The use of mydriatic eye drops, by a previous examiner or self-administered by the patient, and direct ocular trauma are among the causes of misleading pupillary enlargement.

Unilateral miosis in coma has been attributed to dysfunction of sympathetic efferents originating in the posterior hypothalamus and descending in the tegmentum of the brainstem to the cervical cord. Reactive and bilaterally small (1 to 2.5 mm) but not pinpoint pupils are seen in metabolic encephalopathies or in deep bilateral hemispheral lesions such as hydrocephalus or thalamic hemorrhage. Very small but reactive pupils (<1 mm) characterize narcotic or barbiturate overdoses

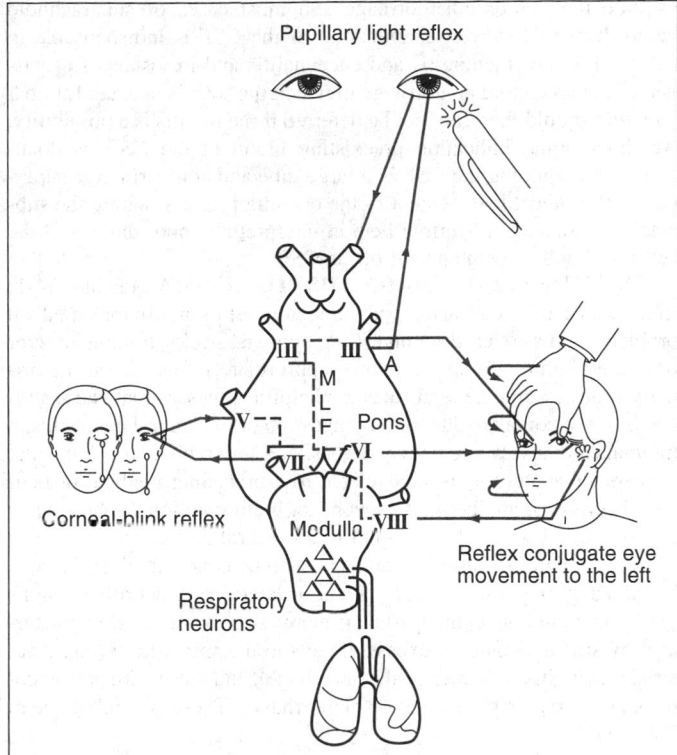

Pupillary light reflex

Corneal-blink reflex

Pons

M
L
F

III III
M   A

V

VII VI

Medulla VIII

Respiratory
neurons

Reflex conjugate eye
movement to the left

FIGURE 24-3 Brainstem reflexes in the coma examination. Midbrain and third nerve function are tested by pupillary reaction to light, pontine function by spontaneous and reflex eye movements and corneal responses, and medullary function by respiratory and pharyngeal responses.

Reflex conjugate, horizontal eye movements are dependent on the medial longitudinal fasciculus (MLF) interconnecting the sixth and contralateral third nerve nuclei. Head rotation (oculocephalic reflex) or caloric stimulation of the labyrinths (oculovestibular reflex) elicits contraversive eye movements (for details see text).

but also occur with extensive pontine hemorrhage. The response to naloxone and the presence of reflex eye movements (see below) distinguish these. The unilaterally small pupil of the Horner syndrome is detected by failure of the pupil to enlarge in the dark. It is an occasional finding with a large cerebral hemorrhage that affects the thalamus.

Ocular movements Eye movements are the second sign of importance in determining if the brainstem has been damaged. Abnormalities, implicate both midbrain and pontine functions, thus permitting the analysis of a large portion of the brainstem. The eyes are first observed by elevating the lids and noting the resting position and spontaneous movements of the globes. Lid tone, tested by lifting the eyelids and noting their resistance to opening and the speed of closure, is reduced progressively as coma deepens. Horizontal divergence of the eyes at rest is normal in drowsiness. As coma deepens, the ocular axes may become parallel again. An abducted eye indicates a medial rectus paresis due to third nerve dysfunction and has the same significance as pupillary enlargement. An adducted eye indicates lateral rectus paresis due to a sixth nerve lesion and, when bilateral, is often a sign of increased intracranial pressure. With few exceptions, vertical separation of the ocular axes (one eye lower than the other, i.e. skew deviation) results from pontine or cerebellar lesions but may also be a manifestation of a partial third nerve palsy.

Spontaneous eye movements in coma often take the form of conjugate horizontal roving. This finding alone exonerates the midbrain and pons and has the same meaning as normal reflex eye movements (see below). Cyclic vertical downward movements are seen in some circumstances. "Ocular bobbing" describes a brisk downward and slow upward movement of the eyes associated with loss of horizontal eye movements and is diagnostic of bilateral pontine damage, characteristically from thrombosis of the basilar artery. "Ocular dipping" is a

slower, arrhythmic downward movement followed by a faster upward movement in patients with normal reflex horizontal gaze; it usually indicates diffuse cortical anoxic damage. The eyes may turn down and inward as a result of thalamic and upper midbrain lesions, typically with thalamic hemorrhage or dilatation of the third ventricle from hydrocephalus. Conjugate horizontal ocular deviation to one extreme at rest indicates damage to the pons on the side of the gaze paresis or a lesion in the frontal lobe on the opposite side. This phenomenon may be summarized by the following maxim: *The eyes look toward a hemispheral lesion and away from a brainstem lesion.* On rare occasions, the eyes may turn paradoxically away from the side of a deep hemispheral lesion ("wrong-way eyes"). Many other complex and interesting eye movements are known but do not have the same salience in coma as the ones already mentioned.

Oculocephalic reflexes are automatic movements of the eyes elicited by moving the head from side to side or vertically. As the activity of the hemispheres is subdued from whatever cause, eye movements are evoked in the direction opposite to the head movement (Fig. 24-3). These movements, called somewhat inappropriately "doll's eyes" (which more accurately refers to the reflex elevation of the eyelids with flexion of the neck) are suppressed by visual fixation, which requires the patient to be awake. Induced adduction of the globes tends to be less complete than abduction, hence subtle abnormalities in the doll's-eye maneuver should be interpreted with caution. Oculocephalic reflexes are generated by brainstem mechanisms originating in the labyrinths and in cervical proprioceptors and require the undiminished activity of the third nerve nucleus in the midbrain, the contralateral sixth nerve nucleus in the pons, and the medial longitudinal fasciculus (MLF) that runs virtually the length of the brainstem and links the two. Preservation of reflex eye movements (particularly adduction) therefore informs the examiner that coma is probably not due to an upper brainstem lesion and by implication that the origin of unconsciousness lies in the cerebral diencephalic structures. However, the opposite—the absence of eye movements—may signify either damage within the brainstem or profound metabolic depression of all neuronal function including the brainstem nuclei. Metabolic causes of depressed neuronal function include overdoses of phenytoin, tricyclic antidepressants, barbiturates, alcohol, phenothiazines, diazepam, and neuromuscular blocking agents. The presence of normal pupillary size and light reaction will distinguish most drug-induced comas from structural brainstem damage.

Thermal, or "caloric," stimulation of the vestibular apparatus (oculovestibular response) provides a more intense stimulus that may be used to confirm the absence of the oculocephalic reflex but gives fundamentally the same information. The test is performed by irrigating the external auditory canal with cool water in order to induce convection currents in the labyrinths. After a brief latency, the result is tonic deviation of both eyes (lasting 30 to 120 s) to the side of cool-water irrigation. The integrity of the third and sixth nerve complexes and brainstem pathways from the labyrinths to the midbrain are thereby confirmed, thus excluding a brainstem lesion as the cause of coma. If the cerebral hemispheres are functioning, as in catatonic or hysterical pseudocoma, an obligate rapid corrective nystagmus is generated away from the side of tonic deviation. (The acronym "COWS" has been used to remind generations of medical students of the direction of compensatory nystagmus—"cold water opposite, warm water same"). The absence of this nystagmus despite conjugate deviation of the globes signifies that the cerebral hemispheres are damaged or profoundly suppressed.

By touching the cornea with a wisp of cotton, a response consisting of brief bilateral lid closure is normally observed. Although the corneal reflexes are rarely useful alone, they may corroborate eye-movement abnormalities because they also depend on the integrity of pontine pathways. The response is lost if the reflex connections between the fifth (afferent) and both seventh (efferent) cranial nerves within the pons are damaged. CNS depressant drugs diminish or eliminate the corneal responses soon after reflex eye movements are paralyzed but before the pupils become unreactive to light. The corneal (and pharyngeal) response may be lost for a time on the side of an acute hemiplegia.

Respiration   Respiratory patterns have received much attention in coma diagnosis but are of less localizing value in comparison to other brainstem signs. Shallow, slow, but regular breathing suggests metabolic or drug depression. Cheyne-Stokes respiration in its classic cyclic form, ending with a brief apneic period, signifies bihemispheral damage or metabolic suppression and commonly accompanies light coma. Rapid, deep (Kussmaul) breathing usually implies metabolic acidosis but may also occur with pontomesencephalic lesions and, of course, severe pneumonia. Agonal gasps reflect bilateral lower brainstem damage and are well known as the terminal respiratory pattern of severe brain damage. A number of other cyclic breathing variations are of lesser significance for localization.

LABORATORY STUDIES AND IMAGING   The following studies are most useful in the diagnosis of confusional states and coma: chemical-toxicologic analysis of blood and urine, cranial CT or MRI, EEG, and CSF examination. Arterial blood-gas analysis is helpful in patients with lung disease and acid-base disorders. Chemical blood determinations are obtained routinely to disclose metabolic, toxic, or drug-induced encephalopathies. The metabolic aberrations commonly encountered in clinical practice require measurements of electrolytes, glucose, calcium, osmolarity, and renal (blood urea nitrogen) and hepatic (NH_3) function. Toxicologic analysis is necessary in any case of coma where the diagnosis is not immediately clear. However, the presence of exogenous drugs or toxins, especially alcohol, does not exclude the possibility that other factors, particularly head trauma, are also contributing to the clinical state. An ethanol level of 43 mmol/L (200 mg/dL) in nonhabituated patients generally causes confusion and impaired mental activity and of >65 mmol/L (300 mg/dL) is associated with stupor. The development of tolerance may allow the chronic alcoholic to remain awake at levels >87 mmol/L (400 mg/dL).

The increased availability of CT and MRI has focused attention on causes of coma that are radiologically detectable (e.g., hemorrhages, tumors, or hydrocephalus). Resorting primarily to this approach, although at times expedient, is imprudent because most cases of coma (and confusion) are metabolic or toxic in origin. The notion that a normal CT scan excludes anatomic lesions as the cause of coma is also erroneous. Bilateral hemisphere infarction, small brainstem lesions, encephalitis, meningitis, mechanical shearing of axons as a result of closed head trauma, absent cerebral perfusion associated with brain death, sagittal sinus thrombosis, and subdural hematomas that are isodense to adjacent brain are some of the lesions that may not be visible. Nevertheless, if the source of coma remains unknown, a scan should be obtained.

The EEG is useful in metabolic or drug-induced confusional states but is rarely diagnostic, with the important exceptions of coma due to clinically unrecognized seizures, to herpesvirus encephalitis and Creutzfeldt-Jakob disease. The amount of background slowing of the EEG is a useful reflection of the severity of any diffuse encephalopathy. Predominant high-voltage slowing (δ or triphasic waves) in the frontal regions is typical of metabolic coma, as from hepatic failure, and widespread fast (β) activity implicates sedative drugs (diazepines, barbiturates). A pattern of "α coma," defined by widespread, variable 8- to 12-Hz activity, superficially resembles the normal α rhythm of waking but is unresponsive to environmental stimuli. It results from pontine or diffuse cortical damage and has a poor prognosis. Most importantly, EEG recordings reveal coma that is due to persistent epileptic discharges that are not clinically manifested as convulsions. Normal α activity on the EEG may also alert the clinician to the locked-in syndrome or to hysteria or catatonia.

Lumbar puncture is used more judiciously than in prior decades in cases of coma or confusion because neuroimaging scans effectively exclude intracerebral hemorrhage and most cases of subarachnoid hemorrhages. However, examination of the CSF is indispensable in the diagnosis of meningitis and encephalitis and in instances of suspected subarachnoid hemorrhage in which the scan is normal. Lumbar puncture should therefore not be deferred if meningitis is a possibility. Xanthochromia, indicating preexisting blood in the CSF, is documented by spinning the CSF in a large tube and comparing the supernatant to water. Measurement of the opening pressure within the subarachnoid space is of further help in interpreting abnormalities of the cell count and protein content of the CSF.

DIFFERENTIAL DIAGNOSIS OF COMA   (Table 24-1) In most instances confusion and coma are part of an obvious medical problem such as overt drug ingestion, hypoxia, stroke, trauma, or liver or kidney failure. Attention is then appropriately focused on the primary illness. Some general rules are helpful. Illnesses that cause sudden onset of coma are due to drug ingestion or to cerebral hemorrhage, trauma, cardiac arrest, epilepsy, or basilar artery embolism. Coma that appears subacutely is usually related to a preceding medical or neurologic problem, including the secondary brain swelling that surrounds a preexisting lesion such as a tumor or cerebral infarction.

The structural causes of coma can also be conceptualized in three broad categories: those without focal or lateralizing neurologic signs (e.g., metabolic encephalopathies); meningitis syndromes, characterized by stiff neck and an excess of cells in the spinal fluid (e.g., bacterial meningitis, subarachnoid hemorrhage); and those with prominent focal signs (e.g., stroke, cerebral hemorrhage). These are elaborated in Table 24-1.

Table 24-1   Approach to the Differential Diagnosis of Coma

1. Diseases that cause no focal or lateralizing neurologic signs, usually with normal brainstem functions; CT scan and cellular content of the CSF are normal
   a. Intoxications: alcohol, sedative drugs, opiates, etc.
   b. Metabolic disturbances: anoxia, hyponatremia, hypernatremia, hypercalcemia, diabetic acidosis, nonketotic hyperosmolar hyperglycemia, hypoglycemia, uremia, hepatic coma, hypercarbia, addisonian crisis, hypo- and hyperthyroid states, profound nutritional deficiency
   c. Severe systemic infections: pneumonia, septicemia, typhoid fever, malaria, Waterhouse-Friderichsen syndrome
   d. Shock from any cause
   e. Postseizure states, status epilepticus, subclinical epilepsy
   f. Hypertensive encephalopathy, eclampsia
   g. Severe hyperthermia, hypothermia
   h. Concussion
   i. Acute hydrocephalus
2. Diseases that cause meningeal irritation with or without fever, and with an excess of WBCs or RBCs in the CSF, usually without focal or lateralizing cerebral or brainstem signs; CT or MRI shows no mass lesion
   a. Subarachnoid hemorrhage from ruptured aneurysm, arteriovenous malformation, occasionally trauma
   b. Acute bacterial meningitis
   c. Some forms of viral encephalitis
   d. Miscellaneous: Fat embolism, cholesterol embolism, carcinomatous and lymphamatous meningitis, etc.
3. Diseases that cause focal brainstem or lateralizing cerebral signs, with or without changes in the CSF; CT and MRI are abnormal
   a. Hemispheral hemorrhage (basal ganglionic, thalamic) or infarction (large middle cerebral artery territory) with secondary brainstem compression
   b. Brainstem infarction due to basilar artery thrombosis or embolism
   c. Brain abscess, subdural empyema
   d. Epidural and subdural hemorrhage, brain contusion
   e. Brain tumor with surrounding edema
   f. Cerebellar and pontine hemorrhage and infarction
   g. Widespread traumatic brain injury
   h. Metabolic coma (see above) with preexisting focal damage
   i. Miscellaneous: cortical vein thrombosis, herpes simplex encephalitis, multiple cerebral emboli due to bacterial endocarditis, acute hemorrhagic leukoencephalitis, acute disseminated (postinfectious) encephalomyelitis, thrombotic thrombocytopenic purpura, cerebral vasculitis, gliomatous cerebri, pituitary apoplexy, intravascular lymphoma, etc.

NOTE: CT, computed tomography; CSF, cerebrospinal fluid; WBCs, white blood cells; RBCs, red blood cells; MRI, magnetic resonance imaging.

Cerebrovascular diseases cause the greatest difficulty in coma diagnosis. These are described in more detail in Chap. 361 but may be summarized as follows: (1) basal ganglia and thalamic hemorrhage (acute but not instantaneous onset, vomiting, headache, hemiplegia, and characteristic eye signs); (2) pontine hemorrhage (sudden onset, pinpoint pupils, loss of reflex eye movements and corneal responses, ocular bobbing, posturing, hyperventilation, and excessive sweating); (3) cerebellar hemorrhage (occipital headache, vomiting, gaze paresis, and inability to stand); (4) basilar artery thrombosis (neurologic prodrome or warning spells, diplopia, dysarthria, vomiting, eye movement and corneal response abnormalities, and asymmetric limb paresis); and (5) subarachnoid hemorrhage (precipitous coma after headache and vomiting). The most common stroke, infarction in the territory of the middle cerebral artery, does not cause coma acutely but the surrounding edema may expand and act as a mass in a limited number of patients with large infarcts. The syndrome of acute hydrocephalus may accompany many intracranial diseases, particularly subarachnoid hemorrhage. Acute symmetric enlargement of both lateral ventricles causes headache and sometimes vomiting that may progress quickly to coma, with extensor posturing of the limbs, bilateral Babinski signs, small nonreactive pupils, and impaired vertical oculocephalic movements in the vertical direction.

If the history and examination do not suggest a large cerebral lesion or meningitic syndrome or a metabolic or drug cause, then information obtained from CT or MRI may be needed as outlined in Table 24-1. As mentioned earlier, the majority of medical causes of coma can be established without a neuroimaging study.

BRAIN DEATH This is a state in which there has been cessation of cerebral blood flow; as a result, global ischemia of the brain occurs while respiration is maintained by artificial means and the heart continues to function. It is the only type of brain damage that is unequivocally recognized as death. Many roughly equivalent criteria have been advanced for the diagnosis of brain death, and it is essential to adhere to those endorsed as standards by the local medical community. Ideal criteria are simple, can be conducted at the bedside, and allow no chance of diagnostic error. They contain three essential elements: (1) widespread cortical destruction shown by deep coma—unresponsiveness to all forms of stimulation; (2) global brainstem damage demonstrated by absent pupillary light reaction and the loss of oculovestibular and corneal reflexes; and (3) lower brainstem destruction indicated by complete apnea. The pulse rate is also invariant and unresponsive to atropine. Most patients have diabetes insipidus, but in some it develops only hours or days after the clinical signs of brain death. The pupils are often enlarged and may be mid-sized but should not be constricted. The absence of deep tendon reflexes is not required because the spinal cord may remain functional.

The proof that apnea is due to irreversible medullary damage requires that the P_{CO_2} be high enough to stimulate respiration during a test of spontaneous breathing (apnea test). This can be done safely in most patients by the use, prior to removing the ventilator, of diffusion oxygenation. This is accomplished by preoxygenation with 100% oxygen and then sustained during the test by a tracheal cannula connected to an oxygen supply. CO_2 tension increases approximately 0.3 to 0.4 kPa/min (2 to 3 mmHg/min) during apnea. At the end of the period of observation, typically several minutes in duration, arterial P_{CO_2} should be at least >6.6 to 8.0 kPa (50 to 60 mmHg) for the test to be valid.

The possibility of profound drug-induced or hypothermic depression of the nervous system should be excluded, and some period of observation, usually 6 to 24 h, is desirable during which this state is shown to be sustained. It is particularly advisable to delay clinical testing for up to 24 h if a cardiac arrest has caused brain death or if the inciting disease is not known. An isoelectric EEG may be used as a confirmatory test for total cerebral damage but is not absolutely necessary. Radionuclide brain scanning, cerebral angiography, or transcranial Doppler measurements may also be used to demonstrate the absence of cerebral blood flow, but with the exception of the latter, they are cumbersome and have not been correlated extensively with pathology.

There is no compelling reason to demonstrate brain death except when organ transplantation is involved. Although it is largely accepted in western society that the respirator can be disconnected from a brain-dead patient, problems frequently arise because of inadequate explanation and preparation of the family by the physician. Moreover, there is no proscription in reasonable medical practice to removing such support from patients who are not brain dead but whose condition is nonetheless hopeless and are likely to live for only a brief time.

℞ **TREATMENT** The immediate goal in acute coma is the prevention of further nervous system damage. Hypotension, hypoglycemia, hypercalcemia, hypoxia, hypercapnia, and hyperthermia should be corrected rapidly and assiduously. An oropharyngeal airway is adequate to keep the pharynx open in drowsy patients who are breathing normally. Tracheal intubation is indicated if there is apnea, upper airway obstruction, hypoventilation, or emesis, or if the patient is liable to aspirate because of coma. Mechanical ventilation is required if there is hypoventilation or if there is an intracranial mass and a need to induce hypocapnia in order to lower intracranial pressure (ICP) as described below. Intravenous access is established and naloxone and dextrose are administered if narcotic overdose or hypoglycemia are even remote possibilities, and thiamine is given with glucose in order to avoid eliciting Wernicke disease in malnourished patients. In cases of suspected basilar thrombosis with brainstem ischemia, intravenous heparin or a thrombolytic agent is often utilized, keeping in mind that cerebellar and pontine hemorrhages resemble basilar artery occlusion. Physostigmine, when used by experienced physicians and with careful monitoring, may awaken patients with anticholinergic-type drug overdose, but many physicians believe that this is justified only to treat cardiac arrhythmias resulting from these overdoses. The use of benzodiazepine antagonists offers some prospect of improvement after overdoses of soporific drugs and has transient benefit in hepatic encephalopathy. Intravenous administration of hypotonic solutions should be monitored carefully in any serious acute brain illness because of the potential for exacerbating brain swelling. Cervical spine injuries must not be overlooked, particularly prior to attempting intubation or the evaluation of oculocephalic responses. Headache accompanied by fever and meningismus indicates an urgent need for examination of the CSF to diagnose meningitis, and it is worth reemphasizing that lumbar puncture should not be delayed while awaiting a CT scan. If the lumbar puncture in a case of suspected meningitis is delayed for any reason, an antibiotic such as a third-generation cephalosporin should be administered as soon as possible, preferably after obtaining blood cultures.

Enlargement of one pupil usually indicates secondary midbrain or third nerve compression by a hemispherical mass and requires that ICP be reduced (Chap. 376). Surgical evacuation of the mass may be appropriate in some cases (e.g., subdural and epidural hematoma.). Medical management to reduce ICP begins with the infusion of normal saline (safe because it is slightly hyperosmolar to serum). Therapeutic hyperventilation may be used to reduce ICP by inducing an arterial P_{CO_2} of 3.7 to 4.2 kPa (28 to 32 mmHg), but its effects are brief. Hyperosmolar therapy with mannitol or an equivalent agent is the mainstay of ICP reduction. It is used simultaneously with hyperventilation in critical cases. A ventricular puncture is necessary to decompress hydrocephalus if medical measures fail to improve alertness. The routine use of high-dose barbiturates and other neuronal-sparing agents soon after cardiac arrest or head trauma has not been shown in clinical studies to be beneficial, and glucocorticoids, although often still used, have no proven value except in cases of brain tumor with edema.

PROGNOSIS The prediction of the outcome of coma must be considered in reference to long-term care and medical resources. One hopes to avoid the emotionally painful, hopeless outcomes associated with patients who are left severely disabled or vegetative. Several general rules pertain. The uniformly pessimistic outcome of the persistent vegetative state has already been mentioned. Children and young adults may have ominous early clinical findings such as abnormal brainstem reflexes and yet recover, so that temporization in offering a prognosis in this group of patients is wise. Metabolic comas have a far better prognosis than traumatic comas. All schemes for prognosis in adults should be taken as approximate indicators, and medical judgments must be tempered by factors such as age, underlying systemic disease, and general medical condition. In an attempt to collect prognostic information from large numbers of patients with head injury, the Glasgow Coma Scale was devised; empirically it has predictive value in cases of brain trauma (Chap. 369). For anoxic and metabolic coma, clinical signs such as the pupillary and motor responses after 1 day, 3 days, and 1 week have been shown to have predictive value (Chap. 376). The absence of the cortical waves of the somatosensory evoked potentials has also proved a strong indicator of poor outcome in coma from any cause.

BIBLIOGRAPHY

CELESIA GG et al: Persistent vegetative state—report of the American Neurological Association Committee on Ethical Affairs. Ann Neurol 33:386, 1993

FISHER CM: The neurological examination of the comatose patient. Acta Neurol Scand 45(Suppl 36):4, 1969

INOUYE SK et al: A multicomponent intervention to prevent delirium in hospitalized older patients. N Engl J Med 340:669, 1999

IVAN L, BRUCE D: *Coma*. Springfield, IL, Charles C Thomas, 1982

JENNETT B, PLUM F: Persistent vegetative state after brain damage. Lancet 1:734, 1972

PLUM F, POSNER J: *The Diagnosis of Stupor and Coma*, 3d ed. Philadelphia, Davis, 1980

ROPPER AH: Lateral displacement of the brain and level of consciousness in patients with an acute hemispheral mass. N Engl J Med 314:953, 1986

———: *Neurological and Neurosurgical Intensive Care*, 3d ed. New York, Raven, 1992

SAPOSNIK G et al: Spontaneous and reflex movements in brain death. Neurol 54:221, 2000

YOUNG BY, PIGOTT SE: Neurobiological basis of consciousness. Arch Neurol 56:153, 1999

——— et al: *Coma and Impaired Consciousness*. New York, McGraw-Hill, 1998

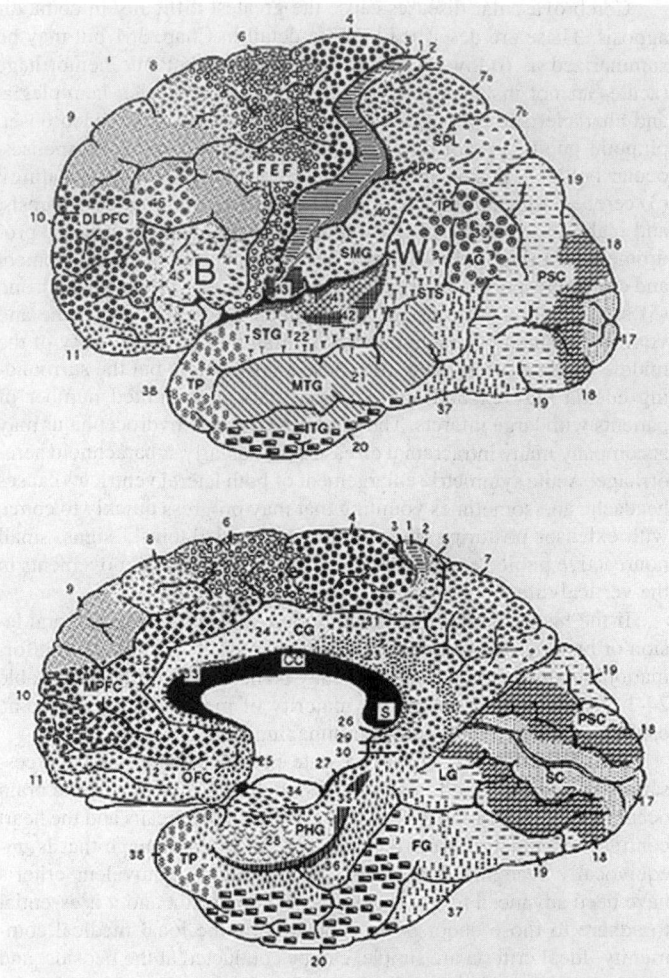

FIGURE 25-1 Lateral (*top*) and medial (*bottom*) views of the cerebral hemispheres. The numbers refer to the Brodmann cytoarchitectonic designations. Area 17 corresponds to primary visual cortex, 41–42 to primary auditory cortex, 1–3 to primary somatosensory cortex, and 4 to primary motor cortex. The rest of the cerebral cortex contains association areas. AG, angular gyrus; B, Broca's area; CC, corpus callosum; CG, cingulate cortex; DLPFC, dorsolateral prefrontal cortex; FEF, frontal eye fields (premotor cortex); FG, fusiform gyrus; IPL, inferior parietal lobule; ITG, inferior temporal gyrus; LG, lingual gyrus; MPFC, medial prefrontal cortex; MTG, middle temporal gyrus; OFC, orbitofrontal cortex; PHG, parahippocampal gyrus; PPC, posterior parietal cortex; PSC, peristriate cortex; SC, striate cortex; SMG, supramarginal gyrus; SPL, superior parietal lobule; STG, superior temporal gyrus; STS, superior temporal sulcus; TP, temporopolar cortex; W, Wernicke's area.

| **25** | *M.-Marsel Mesulam* |

APHASIAS AND OTHER FOCAL CEREBRAL DISORDERS

The cerebral cortex of the human brain contains approximately 20 billion neurons spread over an area of 2 m². The *primary sensory* areas provide an obligatory portal for the entry of sensory information into cortical circuitry, whereas the *primary motor* areas provide a final common pathway for coordinating complex motor acts. The primary sensory and motor areas constitute <10% of the cerebral cortex. The rest is subsumed by unimodal, heteromodal, paralimbic, and limbic areas, collectively known as the *association cortex* (Fig. 25-1). The association cortex mediates the integrative processes that subserve cognition, emotion, and comportment. A systematic testing of these mental functions is necessary for the effective clinical assessment of the association cortex and its diseases.

According to current thinking, there are no centers for "hearing words," "perceiving space," or "storing memories." Cognitive and behavioral functions (domains) are coordinated by intersecting *large-scale neural networks* that contain interconnected cortical and subcortical components. The network approach to higher cerebral function has at least four implications of clinical relevance: (1) a single domain such as language or memory can be disrupted by damage to any one of several areas, as long as these areas belong to the same network; (2) damage confined to a single area can give rise to multiple deficits, involving the functions of all networks that intersect in that region; (3) damage to a network component may give rise to minimal or tran-

sient deficits if other parts of the network undergo compensatory reorganization; and (4) individual anatomic sites within a network display a relative (but not absolute) specialization for different behavioral aspects of the relevant function. Five anatomically defined large-scale networks are most relevant to clinical practice: a perisylvian network for language; a parietofrontal network for spatial cognition; an occipitotemporal network for face and object recognition; a limbic network for retentive memory; and a prefrontal network for attention and comportment.

THE LEFT PERISYLVIAN NETWORK FOR LANGUAGE: APHASIAS AND RELATED CONDITIONS Language allows the communication and reshaping of thoughts and experiences by linking them to arbitrary symbols known as words. The neural substrate of language is composed of a distributed network centered in the perisylvian region of the *left* hemisphere. The posterior pole of this network is known as *Wernicke's area* and includes the posterior third of the superior temporal gyrus and a surrounding rim of the inferior parietal lobule. An essential function of Wernicke's area is to transform sensory inputs into their neural word representations so that these can establish the distributed associations that give the word its meaning. The anterior pole of the language network, known as *Broca's area*, includes the posterior part of the inferior frontal gyrus and a surrounding rim of prefrontal heteromodal cortex. An essential function of this area is to transform neural word representations into their articulatory sequences so that the words can be uttered in the form of spoken language. The sequencing function of Broca's area also appears to involve the ordering of words into sentences that contain a meaning-appropriate *syntax* (grammar). Wernicke's and Broca's areas are

Table 25-1 Clinical Features of Aphasias and Related Conditions

	Comprehension	Repetition of Spoken Language	Naming	Fluency
Wernicke's	Impaired	Impaired	Impaired	Preserved or increased
Broca's	Preserved (except grammar)	Impaired	Impaired	Decreased
Global	Impaired	Impaired	Impaired	Decreased
Conduction	Preserved	Impaired	Impaired	Preserved
Nonfluent (motor) transcortical	Preserved	Preserved	Impaired	Impaired
Fluent (sensory) transcortical	Impaired	Preserved	Impaired	Preserved
Isolation	Impaired	Echolalia	Impaired	No purposeful speech
Anomic	Preserved	Preserved	Impaired	Preserved except for word-finding pauses
Pure word deafness	Impaired only for spoken language	Impaired	Preserved	Preserved
Pure alexia	Impaired only for reading	Preserved	Preserved	Preserved

interconnected with each other and with additional perisylvian, temporal, prefrontal, and posterior parietal regions, making up a neural network subserving the various aspects of language function. Damage to any one of these components or to their interconnections can give rise to language disturbances (*aphasia*). Aphasia should be diagnosed only when there are deficits in the formal aspects of language such as naming, word choice, comprehension, spelling, and syntax. Dysarthria and mutism do not, by themselves, lead to a diagnosis of aphasia. The language network shows a left hemisphere dominance pattern in the vast majority of the population. In approximately 90% of right handers and 60% of left handers, aphasia occurs only after lesions of the left hemisphere. In some individuals no hemispheric dominance for language can be discerned, and in some others (including a small minority of right handers) there is a right hemisphere dominance for language. A language disturbance occurring after a right hemisphere lesion in a right hander is called *crossed aphasia*.

Clinical Examination The clinical examination of language should include the assessment of naming, spontaneous speech, comprehension, repetition, reading, and writing. A deficit of naming (*anomia*) is the single most common finding in aphasic patients. When asked to name common objects (pencil or wristwatch) or their parts (eraser, lead, stem, band), the patient may fail to come up with the appropriate word, may provide a circumlocutious description of the object ("the thing for writing"), or may come up with the wrong word (*paraphasia*). If the patient offers an incorrect but legitimate word ("pen" for "pencil"), the naming error is known as a *semantic paraphasia*; if the word approximates the correct answer but is phonetically inaccurate ("plentil" for "pencil"), it is known as a *phonemic paraphasia*. Asking the patient to name body parts, geometric shapes, and component parts of objects (lapel of coat, cap of pen) can elicit mild forms of anomia in patients who can otherwise name common objects. In most anomias, the patient cannot retrieve the appropriate name when shown an object but can point to the appropriate object when the name is provided by the examiner. This is known as a one-way (or retrieval-based) naming deficit. A two-way naming deficit exists if the patient can neither provide nor recognize the correct name, indicating the presence of a language comprehension impairment. *Spontaneous speech* is described as "fluent" if it maintains appropriate output volume, phrase length, and melody or as "nonfluent" if it is sparse, halting, and average phrase length is below four words. The examiner should also note if the speech is paraphasic or circumlocutious; if it shows a relative paucity of substantive nouns and action verbs versus function words (prepositions, conjunctions); and if word order, tenses, suffixes, prefixes, plurals, and possessives are appropriate. *Comprehension* can be tested by assessing the patient's ability to follow conversation, by asking yes-no questions ("Can a dog fly?", "Does it snow

in summer?") or asking the patient to point to appropriate objects ("Where is the source of illumination in this room?"). Statements with embedded clauses or passive voice construction ("If a tiger is eaten by a lion, which animal stays alive?") help to assess the ability to comprehend complex syntactic structure. Commands to close or open the eyes, stand up, sit down, or roll over should not be used to assess overall comprehension since appropriate responses aimed at such axial movements can be preserved in patients who otherwise have profound comprehension deficits.

Repetition is assessed by asking the patient to repeat single words, short sentences, or strings of words such as "No ifs, ands, or buts." The testing of repetition with tongue-twisters such as "hippopotamus" or "Irish constabulary" provides a better assessment of dysarthria and pallilalia than aphasia. Aphasic patients may have little difficulty with tongue-twisters but have a particularly hard time repeating a string of function words. It is important to make sure that the number of words does not exceed the patient's attention span. Otherwise, the failure of repetition becomes a reflection of the narrowed attention span rather than an indication of an aphasic deficit. *Reading* should be assessed for deficits in reading aloud as well as comprehension. *Writing* is assessed for spelling errors, word order, and grammar. *Alexia* describes an inability to either read aloud or comprehend single words and simple sentences; *agraphia* (or dysgraphia) is used to describe an acquired deficit in the spelling or grammar of written language.

The correspondence between individual deficits of language function and lesion location does not display a rigid one-to-one relationship and should be conceptualized within the context of the distributed network model. Nonetheless, the classification of aphasic patients into specific clinical syndromes helps to determine the most likely anatomic distribution of the underlying neurologic disease and has implications for etiology and prognosis (Table 25-1). Aphasic syndromes can be divided into "central" syndromes, which result from damage to the two epicenters of the language network (Broca's and Wernicke's areas), and "disconnection" syndromes, which arise from lesions that interrupt the functional connectivity of these centers with each other and with the other components of the language network. The syndromes outlined below are idealizations; pure syndromes occur rarely.

Wernicke's aphasia Comprehension is impaired for spoken and written language. Language output is fluent but is highly paraphasic and circumlocutious. The tendency for paraphasic errors may be so pronounced that it leads to strings of neologisms, which form the basis of what is known as "jargon aphasia." Speech contains large numbers of function words (e.g., prepositions, conjunctions) but few substantive nouns or verbs that refer to specific actions. The output is therefore voluminous but uninformative. For example, a patient attempts to describe how his wife accidentally threw away something important, perhaps his dentures: "We don't need it anymore, she says. And with it when that was downstairs was my teethtick . . . a . . . den . . . dentith . . . my dentist. And they happened to be in that bag . . . see? How could this have happened? How could a thing like this happen . . . So she says we won't need it anymore . . . I didn't think we'd use it. And now if I have any problems anybody coming a month from now, four months from now, or six months from now, I have a new dentist. Where my two . . . two little pieces of dentist that I use . . . that I . . . all gone. If she throws the whole thing away . . . visit some friends of hers and she can't throw them away."

Gestures and pantomime do not improve communication. The patient does not seem to realize that his or her language is incomprehensible and may appear angry and impatient when the examiner fails to decipher the meaning of a severely paraphasic statement. In some patients this type of aphasia can be associated with severe agitation and paranoid behaviors. One area of comprehension that may be preserved is the ability to follow commands aimed at axial musculature. The dissociation between the failure to understand simple questions ("What is your name") in a patient who rapidly closes his or her eyes, sits up, or rolls over when asked to do so is characteristic of Wernicke's aphasia and helps to differentiate it from deafness, psychiatric disease, or malingering. Patients with Wernicke's aphasia cannot express their thoughts in meaning-appropriate words and cannot decode the meaning of words in any modality of input. This aphasia therefore has expressive as well as receptive components. Repetition, naming, reading, and writing are also impaired.

The lesion site most commonly associated with Wernicke's aphasia is the posterior portion of the language network and tends to involve at least parts of Wernicke's area. An embolus to the inferior division of the middle cerebral artery, and to the posterior temporal or angular branches in particular, is the most common etiology (Chap. 361). Intracerebral hemorrhage, severe head trauma, or neoplasm are other causes. A coexisting right hemi- or superior quadrantanopia is common, and mild right nasolabial flattening may be found, but otherwise the examination is often unrevealing. The paraphasic, neologistic speech in an agitated patient with an otherwise unremarkable neurologic examination may lead to the suspicion of a primary psychiatric disorder such as schizophrenia or mania, but the other components characteristic of acquired aphasia and the absence of prior psychiatric disease usually settle the issue. Some patients with Wernicke's aphasia due to intracerebral hemorrhage or head trauma may improve as the hemorrhage or the injury heals. In most other patients, prognosis for recovery is guarded.

Broca's aphasia   Speech is nonfluent, labored, interrupted by many word-finding pauses, and usually dysarthric. It is impoverished in function words but enriched in meaning-appropriate nouns and verbs. Abnormal word order and the inappropriate deployment of *bound morphemes* (word endings used to denote tenses, possessives, or plurals) lead to a characteristic agrammatism. Speech is telegraphic and pithy but quite informative. In the following passage, a patient with Broca's aphasia describes his medical history: "I see . . . the dotor, dotor sent me . . . Bosson. Go to hospital. Dotor . . . kept me beside. Two, tee days, doctor send me home."

Output may be reduced to a grunt or single word ("yes" or "no"), which is emitted with different intonations in an attempt to express approval or disapproval. In addition to fluency, naming and repetition are also impaired. Comprehension of spoken language is intact, except for syntactically difficult sentences with passive voice structure or embedded clauses. Reading comprehension is also preserved, with the occasional exception of a specific inability to read small grammatical words such as conjunctions and pronouns. The last two features indicate that Broca's aphasia is not just an "expressive" or "motor" disorder and that it may also involve a comprehension deficit for function words and syntax. Patients with Broca's aphasia can be tearful, easily frustrated, and profoundly depressed. Insight into their condition is

preserved, in contrast to Wernicke's aphasia. Even when spontaneous speech is severely dysarthric, the patient may be able to display a relatively normal articulation of words when singing. This dissociation has been used to develop specific therapeutic approaches (melodic intonation therapy) for Broca's aphasia. Additional neurologic deficits usually include right facial weakness, hemiparesis or hemiplegia, and a buccofacial apraxia characterized by an inability to carry out motor commands involving oropharyngeal and facial musculature (e.g., patients are unable to demonstrate how to blow out a match or suck through a straw). Visual fields are intact. The cause is most often infarction of Broca's area (the inferior frontal convolution; Fig. 25-1) and surrounding anterior perisylvian and insular cortex, due to occlusion of the superior division of the middle cerebral artery (Chap. 361). Mass lesions including tumor, intracerebral hemorrhage, or abscess may also be responsible. Small lesions confined to the posterior part of Broca's area may lead to a nonaphasic and often reversible deficit of speech articulation, usually accompanied by mild right facial weakness. When the cause of Broca's aphasia is stroke, recovery of language function generally peaks within 2 to 6 months, after which time further progress is limited.

Global aphasia   Speech output is nonfluent, and comprehension of spoken language is severely impaired. Naming, repetition, reading, and writing are also impaired. This syndrome represents the combined dysfunction of Broca's and Wernicke's areas and usually results from strokes that involve the entire middle cerebral artery distribution in the left hemisphere. Most patients are initially mute or say a few words, such as "hi" or "yes." Related signs include right hemiplegia, hemisensory loss, and homonymous hemianopia. Occasionally, a patient with a lesion in Wernicke's area will present with a global aphasia that soon resolves into Wernicke's aphasia.

Conduction aphasia   Speech output is fluent but paraphasic, comprehension of spoken language is intact, and repetition is severely impaired. Naming and writing are also impaired. Reading aloud is impaired, but reading comprehension is preserved. The lesion sites spare Broca's and Wernicke's areas but may induce a functional disconnection between the two so that neural word representations formed in Wernicke's area and adjacent regions cannot be conveyed to Broca's area for assembly into corresponding articulatory patterns. Occasionally, a Wernicke's area lesion gives rise to a transient Wernicke's aphasia that rapidly resolves into a conduction aphasia. The paraphasic output in conduction aphasia interferes with the ability to express meaning, but this deficit is not nearly as severe as the one displayed by patients with Wernicke's aphasia. Associated neurologic signs in conduction aphasia vary according to the primary lesion site.

Nonfluent transcortical aphasia (transcortical motor aphasia)   The features are similar to Broca's aphasia, but repetition is intact and agrammatism may be less pronounced. The neurologic examination may be otherwise intact, but a right hemiparesis can also exist. The lesion site disconnects the intact language network from prefrontal areas of the brain and usually involves the anterior watershed zone between anterior and middle cerebral artery territories or the supplementary motor cortex in the territory of the anterior cerebral artery.

Fluent transcortical aphasia (transcortical sensory aphasia)   Clinical features are similar to those of Wernicke's aphasia, but repetition is intact. The lesion site disconnects the intact core of the language network from other temporoparietal association areas. Associated neurologic findings may include hemianopia. Cerebrovascular lesions (e.g., infarctions in the posterior watershed zone) or neoplasms that involve the temporoparietal cortex posterior to Wernicke's area are the most common causes.

Isolation aphasia   This rare syndrome represents a combination of the two transcortical aphasias. Comprehension is severely impaired, and there is no purposeful speech output. The patient may parrot fragments of heard conversations (*echolalia*), indicating that the neural mechanisms for repetition are at least partially intact. This condition represents the pathologic function of the language network when it is isolated from other regions of the brain. Broca's and Wernicke's areas tend to be spared, but there is damage in surrounding frontal, parietal, and temporal cortex. Lesions are patchy and can be associated with anoxia, carbon monoxide poisoning, or complete watershed zone infarctions.

Anomic aphasia This form of aphasia may be considered the "minimal dysfunction" syndrome of the language network. Articulation, comprehension, and repetition are intact, but confrontation naming, word finding, and spelling are impaired. Speech is enriched in function words but impoverished in substantive nouns and verbs denoting specific actions. Language output is fluent but paraphasic, circumlocutious, and uninformative. The lesion sites can be anywhere within the left hemisphere language network, including the middle and inferior temporal gyri. *Anomic aphasia is the single most common language disturbance seen in head trauma, metabolic encephalopathy, and Alzheimer's disease.* The language impairment of Alzheimer's disease almost always leads to fluent aphasias (e.g., anomic, Wernicke's, conduction, or fluent transcortical aphasia). The insidious onset and relentless progression of nonfluent language disturbances (Broca's or nonfluent transcortical aphasia) can be seen in *primary progressive aphasia*, a degenerative syndrome most commonly associated with focal nonspecific neuronal loss or Pick's disease.

Pure word deafness This is not a true aphasic syndrome because the language deficit is modality-specific. The most common lesions are either bilateral or left-sided in the superior temporal gyrus. The net effect of the underlying lesion is to interrupt the flow of information from the unimodal auditory association cortex to Wernicke's area. Patients have no difficulty understanding written language and can express themselves well in spoken or written language. They have no difficulty interpreting and reacting to environmental sounds since primary auditory cortex and subcortical auditory relays are intact. Since auditory information cannot be conveyed to the language network, however, it cannot be decoded into neural word representations and the patient reacts to speech as if it were in an alien tongue that cannot be deciphered. Patients cannot repeat spoken language but have no difficulty naming objects. In time, patients with pure word deafness teach themselves lip reading and may appear to have improved. There may be no additional neurologic findings, but agitated paranoid reactions are frequent in the acute stages. Cerebrovascular lesions are the most frequent cause.

Pure alexia without agraphia This is the visual equivalent of pure word deafness. The lesions (usually a combination of damage to the left occipital cortex and to a posterior sector of the corpus callosum—the splenium) interrupt the flow of visual input into the language network. There is usually a right hemianopia, but the core language network remains unaffected. The patient can understand and produce spoken language, name objects in the left visual hemifield, repeat, and write. However, the patient acts as if illiterate when asked to read even the simplest sentence because the visual information from the written words (presented to the intact left visual hemifield) cannot reach the language network. Objects in the left hemifield may be named accurately because they activate nonvisual associations in the right hemisphere, which, in turn, can access the language network through transcallosal pathways anterior to the splenium. Patients with this syndrome may also lose the ability to name colors, although they can match colors. This is known as a *color anomia*. The most common etiology of pure alexia is a vascular lesion in the territory of the posterior cerebral artery or an infiltrating neoplasm in the left occipital cortex that involves the optic radiations as well as the crossing fibers of the splenium. Since the posterior cerebral artery also supplies medial temporal components of the limbic system, the patient with pure alexia may also experience an amnesia, but this is usually transient because the limbic lesion is unilateral.

Aphemia There is an acute onset of severely impaired fluency (often mutism), which cannot be accounted by corticobulbar, cerebellar, or extrapyramidal dysfunction. Recovery is the rule and involves an intermediate stage of hoarse whispering. Writing, reading, and comprehension are intact, so this is not a true aphasic syndrome. Partial lesions of Broca's area or subcortical lesions that undercut its connections with other parts of the brain may be present. Occasionally, the

lesion site is on the medial aspects of the frontal lobes and may involve the supplementary motor cortex of the left hemisphere.

Apraxia This generic term designates a complex motor deficit that cannot be attributed to pyramidal, extrapyramidal, cerebellar, or sensory dysfunction and that does not arise from the patient's failure to understand the nature of the task. The form that is most frequently encountered in clinical practice is known as *ideomotor apraxia*. Commands to perform a specific motor act ("cough," "blow out a match") or to pantomime the use of a common tool (a comb, hammer, straw, or toothbrush) in the absence of the real object cannot be followed. The patient's ability to comprehend the command is ascertained by demonstrating multiple movements and establishing that the correct one can be recognized. Some patients with this type of apraxia can imitate the appropriate movement (when it is demonstrated by the examiner) and show no impairment when handed the real object, indicating that the sensorimotor mechanisms necessary for the movement are intact. Some forms of ideomotor apraxia represent a disconnection of the language network from pyramidal motor systems: commands to execute complex movements are understood but cannot be conveyed to the appropriate motor areas, even though the relevant motor mechanisms are intact. *Buccofacial apraxia* involves apraxic deficits in movements of the face and mouth. *Limb apraxia* encompasses apraxic deficits in movements of the arms and legs. Ideomotor apraxia is almost always caused by lesions in the left hemisphere and is commonly associated with aphasic syndromes, especially Broca's aphasia and conduction aphasia. Its presence cannot be ascertained in patients with language comprehension deficits. The ability to follow commands aimed at axial musculature ("close the eyes," "stand up") is subserved by different pathways and may be intact in otherwise severely aphasic and apraxic patients. Patients with lesions of the anterior corpus callosum can display a special type of ideomotor apraxia confined to the left side of the body. Since the handling of real objects is not impaired, ideomotor apraxia, by itself, causes no limitation of daily living activities.

Ideational apraxia refers to a deficit in the execution of a goal-directed sequence of movements in patients who have no difficulty executing the individual components of the sequence. For example, when asked to pick up a pen and write, the sequence of uncapping the pen, placing the cap at the opposite end, turning the point towards the writing surface, and writing may be disrupted, and the patient may be seen trying to write with the wrong end of the pen or even with the removed cap. These motor sequencing problems are usually seen in the context of confusional states and dementias rather than focal lesions associated with aphasic conditions. *Limb-kinetic apraxia* involves a clumsiness in the actual use of tools that cannot be attributed to sensory, pyramidal, extrapyramidal, or cerebellar dysfunction. This condition can emerge in the context of focal premotor cortex lesions or *corticobasal ganglionic degeneration*.

Gerstmann's syndrome The combination of *acalculia* (impairment of simple arithmetic), *dysgraphia* (impaired writing), *finger anomia* (an inability to name individual fingers such as the index or thumb), and *right-left confusion* (an inability to tell whether a hand, foot, or arm of the patient or examiner is on the right or left side of the body) is known as Gerstmann's syndrome. In making this diagnosis it is important to establish that the finger and left-right naming deficits are not part of a more generalized anomia and that the patient is not otherwise aphasic. When Gerstmann's syndrome is seen in isolation, it is commonly associated with damage to the inferior parietal lobule (especially the angular gyrus) in the left hemisphere.

Aprosodia Variations of melodic stress and intonation influence the meaning and impact of spoken language. For example, the two statements "He *is* clever." and "He is clever?" contain an identical word choice and syntax but convey vastly different messages because of differences in the intonation and stress with which the statements are uttered. This aspect of language is known as *prosody*. Damage to perisylvian areas in the right hemisphere can interfere with speech prosody and can lead to syndromes of aprosodia. Ross has pointed out that damage to right hemisphere regions corresponding to Wernicke's area yields a greater impairment in the decoding of speech prosody, whereas damage to right hemisphere regions corresponding to Broca's area yields a greater impairment in the ability to introduce meaning-appropriate prosody into spoken language. The latter deficit is the most common type of aprosodia identified in clinical practice—the patient produces grammatically correct language with accurate word choice but the statements are uttered in a monotone that interferes with the ability to convey the intended stress and affect. Patients with this type of aprosodia give the mistaken impression of being depressed or indifferent.

Subcortical aphasias   Damage to subcortical components of the language network (e.g., the striatum and thalamus of the left hemisphere) can also lead to aphasia. The resulting syndromes contain combinations of deficits in the various aspects of language but rarely fit the specific patterns described in Table 25-1. An anomic aphasia accompanied by dysarthria or a fluent aphasia with hemiparesis should raise the suspicion of a subcortical lesion site.

THE PARIETOFRONTAL NETWORK FOR SPATIAL ORIENTATION: NEGLECT AND RELATED CONDITIONS

Hemispatial Neglect   Adaptive orientation to significant events within the extrapersonal space is subserved by a large-scale network containing three major cortical components. The *cingulate cortex* provides access to a limbic-motivational mapping of the extrapersonal space, the *posterior parietal cortex* to a sensorimotor representation of salient extrapersonal events, and the *frontal eye fields* to motor strategies for attentional behaviors (Fig. 25-2). Subcortical components of this network include the striatum and the thalamus. Contralesional hemispatial neglect represents one outcome of damage to any of the cortical or subcortical components of this network. *The traditional view that hemispatial neglect always denotes a parietal lobe lesion is inaccurate.* In keeping with this anatomic organization, the clinical manifestations of neglect display three behavioral components: sensory events (or their mental representations) within the neglected hemispace have a lesser impact on overall awareness; there is a paucity of exploratory and orienting acts directed toward the neglected hemispace; and the patient behaves as if the neglected hemispace was motivationally devalued.

According to one model of spatial cognition, the right hemisphere directs attention within the *entire* extrapersonal space, whereas the left hemisphere directs attention mostly within the contralateral right hemispace. Consequently, unilateral left hemisphere lesions do not give rise to much contralesional neglect since the ipsilateral attentional mechanisms of the right hemisphere can compensate for the loss of the *contralaterally* directed attentional functions of the left hemisphere. Unilateral right hemisphere lesions, however, give rise to severe contralesional left hemispatial neglect because the unaffected left hemisphere does not contain ipsilateral attentional mechanisms. This model is consistent with clinical experience, which shows that contralesional neglect is more common, severe, and lasting after damage to the right hemisphere than after damage to the left hemisphere. Severe neglect for the right hemispace is rare, even in left handers with left hemisphere lesions.

Patients with severe neglect may fail to dress, shave, or groom the left side of the body; may fail to eat food placed on the left side of the tray; and may fail to read the left half of sentences. When the examiner draws a large circle [12 to 16 cm (5 to 6 in.) in diameter] and asks the patient to place the numbers 1 to 12 as if the circle represented the face of a clock, there is a tendency to crowd the numbers on the right side and leave the left side empty. When asked to copy a simple line drawing, the patient fails to copy detail on the left; and when asked to write, there is a tendency to leave an unusually wide margin on the left.

Two bedside tests that are useful in assessing neglect are *simultaneous bilateral stimulation* and *visual target cancellation*. In the former, the examiner provides either unilateral or simultaneous bilat-

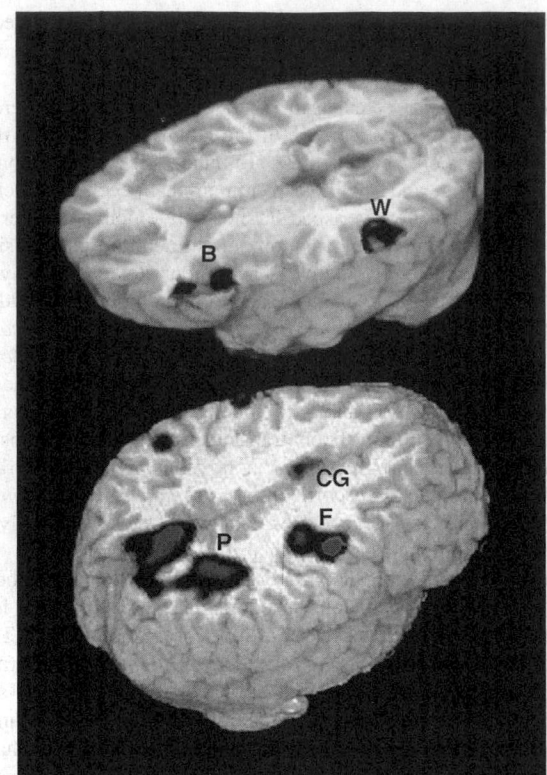

FIGURE 25-2   Functional magnetic resonance imaging of language and spatial attention in neurologically intact subjects. The dark areas show regions of task-related significant activation. (*Top*) The subjects were asked to determine if two words were synonymous. This language task led to the simultaneous activation of the two epicenters of the language network, Broca's area (B) and Wernicke's area (W). The activations are exclusively in the left hemisphere. (*Bottom*) The subjects were asked to shift spatial attention to a peripheral target. This task led to the simultaneous activation of the three epicenters of the attentional network, the posterior parietal cortex (P), the frontal eye fields (F), and the cingulate gyrus (CG). The activations are predominantly in the right hemisphere. (*Figure courtesy of Darren Gitelman, MD.*)

eral stimulation in the visual, auditory, and tactile modalities. Following right hemisphere injury, patients who have no difficulty detecting unilateral stimuli on either side experience the bilaterally presented stimulus as coming only from the right. This phenomenon is known as *extinction* and is a manifestation of the sensory-representational aspect of hemispatial neglect. In the target detection task, targets (e.g., A's) are interspersed with foils (e.g., other letters of the alphabet) on a 21.5 × 28.0 cm (8.5 × 11 in.) sheet of paper and the patient is asked to circle all the targets. A failure to detect targets on the left is a manifestation of the exploratory deficit in hemispatial neglect. Hemianopia, by itself, does not interfere with performance in this task since the patient is free to turn the head and eyes to the left. The normal tendency in target detection tasks is to start from the left upper quadrant and move systematically in horizontal or vertical sweeps. Some patients show a tendency to start the process from the right and proceed in a haphazard fashion. This represents a subtle manifestation of left neglect, even if the patient eventually manages to detect all the appropriate targets. Some patients with neglect may also deny the existence of hemiparesis and may even deny ownership of the paralyzed limb, a condition known as *anosognosia.*

Cerebrovascular lesions and neoplasms in the right hemisphere are the most common causes of hemispatial neglect. Depending on the site of the lesion, the patient with neglect may also have hemiparesis, hemihypesthesia, and hemianopia on the left, but these are not invariant findings. The majority of patients display considerable improvement of hemispatial neglect, usually within the first several weeks.

Bálint's Syndrome, Simultanagnosia, Dressing Apraxia, and Construction Apraxia   Bilateral involvement of the network for spatial attention, especially its parietal components, leads to a state of severe spatial disorientation known as *Bálint's syndrome*. Bálint's syndrome involves deficits in the orderly visuomotor scanning of the environment (*oculomotor apraxia*) and in accurate manual reaching toward visual targets (*optic ataxia*). The third and most dramatic component of Bálint's syndrome is known as *simultanagnosia* and reflects an inability to integrate visual information in the center of gaze with more peripheral information. The patient gets stuck on the detail that falls in the center of gaze without attempting to scan the visual environment for additional information. The patient with simultanagnosia "misses the forest for the trees." Complex visual scenes cannot be grasped in their entirety, leading to severe limitations in the visual identification of objects and scenes. For example, a patient who is shown a table lamp and asked to name the object may look at its circular base and call it an ash tray. Some patients with simultanagnosia report that objects they look at may suddenly vanish, probably indicating an inability to look back at the original point of gaze after brief saccadic displacements. Movement and distracting stimuli greatly exacerbate the difficulties of visual perception. Simultanagnosia can sometimes occur without the other two components of Bálint's syndrome.

A modification of the letter cancellation task described above can be used for the bedside diagnosis of simultanagnosia. In this modification, some of the targets (e.g., A's) are made to be much larger than the others [7.5 to 10 cm vs. 2.5 cm (3 to 4 in. vs. 1 in.) in height], and all targets are embedded among foils. Patients with simultanagnosia display a counterintuitive but characteristic tendency to miss the larger targets (Fig. 25-3). This occurs because the information needed for the identification of the larger targets cannot be confined to the immediate line of gaze and requires the integration of visual information across a more extensive field of view. The greater difficulty in the detection of the larger targets also indicates that poor acuity is not responsible for the impairment of visual function and that the problem is central rather than peripheral. Bálint's syndrome results from bilateral dorsal parietal lesions; common settings include watershed infarction between the middle and posterior cerebral artery territories, hypoglycemia, sagittal sinus thrombosis, or atypical forms of Alzheimer's disease. In patients with Bálint's syndrome due to stroke, bilateral visual field defects (usually inferior quadrantanopias) are common.

Another manifestation of bilateral (or right sided) dorsal parietal lobe lesions is *dressing apraxia*. The patient with this condition is unable to align the body axis with the axis of the garment and can be seen struggling as he or she holds a coat from its bottom or extends his or her arm into a fold of the garment rather than into its sleeve. Lesions that involve the posterior parietal cortex also lead to severe

difficulties in copying simple line drawings. This is known as a *construction apraxia* and is much more severe if the lesion is in the right hemisphere. In some patients with right hemisphere lesions, the drawing difficulties are confined to the left side of the figure and represent a manifestation of hemispatial neglect; in others, there is a more universal deficit in reproducing contours and three-dimensional perspective. Dressing apraxia and construction apraxia represent special instances of a more general disturbance in spatial orientation.

THE OCCIPITOTEMPORAL NETWORK FOR FACE AND OBJECT RECOGNITION: PROSOPAGNOSIA AND OBJECT AGNOSIA Perceptual information about faces and objects is initially encoded in primary (striate) visual cortex and adjacent (upstream) peristriate visual association areas. This information is subsequently relayed first to the downstream visual association areas of occipitotemporal cortex and then to other heteromodal and paralimbic areas of the cerebral cortex. Bilateral lesions in the fusiform and lingual gyri of occipitotemporal cortex disrupt this process and interfere with the ability of otherwise-intact perceptual information to activate the distributed multimodal associations that lead to the recognition of faces and objects. The resultant face and object recognition deficits are known as *prosopagnosia* and *visual object agnosia*.

The patient with prosopagnosia cannot recognize familiar faces, including, sometimes, the reflection of his or her own face in the mirror. This is not a perceptual deficit since prosopagnosic patients can easily tell if two faces are identical or not. Furthermore, a prosopagnosic patient who cannot recognize a familiar face by visual inspection alone can use auditory cues to reach appropriate recognition if allowed to listen to the person's voice. The deficit in prosopagnosia is therefore modality-specific and reflects the existence of a lesion that prevents the activation of otherwise intact multimodal templates by relevant visual input. Damasio has pointed out that the deficit in prosopagnosia is not limited to the recognition of faces but that it can also extend to the recognition of individual members of larger generic object groups. For example, prosopagnosic patients characteristically have no difficulty with the generic identification of a face as a face or of a car as a car, but they cannot recognize the identity of an individual face or the make of an individual car. This reflects a visual recognition deficit for proprietary features that characterize individual members of an object class. When recognition problems become more generalized and extend to the generic identification of common objects, the condition is known as visual object agnosia. In contrast to prosopagnosic patients, those with object agnosia cannot recognize a face as a face or a car as a car. It is important to distinguish visual object agnosia from anomia. The patient with anomia cannot name the object but can describe its use. In contrast, the patient with visual agnosia is unable either to name a visually presented object or to describe its use. The characteristic lesions in prosopagnosia and visual object agnosia consist of bilateral infarctions in the territory of the posterior cerebral arteries. Associated deficits can include visual field defects (especially superior quadrantanopias) or a centrally based color blindness known as achromatopsia. Rarely, the responsible lesion is unilateral. In such cases, prosopagnosia is associated with lesions in the right hemisphere and object agnosia with lesions in the left.

THE LIMBIC NETWORK FOR MEMORY: AMNESIAS Limbic and paralimbic areas (such as the hippocampus, amygdala, and entorhinal cortex), the anterior and medial nuclei of the thalamus, the medial and basal parts of the striatum, and the hypothalamus collectively constitute a distributed network known as the *limbic system*. The behavioral affiliations of this network include the coordination of emotion, motivation, autonomic tone, and endocrine function. An additional area of specialization for the limbic network, and the one which is of most relevance to clinical practice, is that of declarative (conscious) memory for recent episodes and experiences. A disturbance in this function is known as *amnestic state*. In the absence of deficits in motivation, attention, language, or visuospatial function, the clinical diagnosis of a persistent global amnestic state is always as-

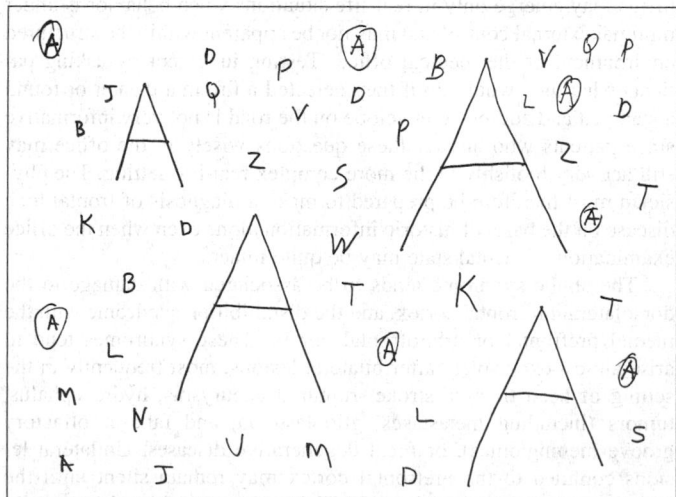

FIGURE 25-3 A 70-year-old woman with a 2-year history of degenerative dementia was asked to circle all the A's. She detects most of the small targets but ignores the larger ones. This is a manifestation of simultanagnosia.

sociated with bilateral damage to the limbic network, usually within the hippocampo-entorhinal complex or the thalamus.

The memory disturbance in the amnestic state is multimodal and includes retrograde and anterograde components. The *retrograde amnesia* involves an inability to recall experiences that occurred before the onset of the amnestic state. Relatively recent events are more vulnerable to retrograde amnesia than more remote events. A patient who comes to the emergency room complaining that he cannot remember his identity but who can remember the events of the previous day is almost certainly not suffering from a neurologic cause of memory disturbance. The second and most important component of the amnestic state is the *anterograde amnesia*, which indicates an inability to store, retain, and recall new knowledge. Patients with amnestic states cannot remember what they ate a few minutes ago or the details of an important event they may have experienced a few hours ago. In the acute stages, there may also be a tendency to fill in memory gaps with inaccurate, fabricated, and often implausible information. This is known as *confabulation*. Patients with the amnestic syndrome forget that they forget and tend to deny the existence of a memory problem when questioned.

The patient with an amnestic state is almost always disoriented, especially to time. Accurate temporal orientation and accurate knowledge of current news rule out a major amnestic state. Memory can be tested with a list of four to five words read aloud by the examiner up to five times or until the patient can immediately repeat the entire list without intervening delay. In the next phase of testing, the patient is allowed to concentrate on the words and to rehearse them internally for 1 min before being asked to recall them. Accurate performance in this phase indicates that the patient is motivated and sufficiently attentive to hold the words on-line for at least 1 min. The final phase of the testing involves a retention period of 5 to 10 min, during which the patient is engaged in other tasks. Adequate recall at the end of this interval requires off-line storage, retention, and retrieval. Amnestic patients fail this phase of the task and may even forget that they were given a list of words to remember. Accurate recognition of the words by multiple choice in a patient who cannot recall them indicates a less severe memory disturbance that affects mostly the retrieval stage of memory.

Many neurologic diseases can give rise to an amnestic state. These include tumors (of the sphenoid wing, posterior corpus callosum, thalamus, or medial temporal lobe), infarctions (in the territories of the anterior or posterior cerebral arteries), head trauma, herpes simplex encephalitis, Wernicke-Korsakoff encephalopathy, paraneoplastic limbic encephalitis, and degenerative dementias such as Alzheimer's or Pick's disease. The one common denominator of all these diseases is that they lead to the bilateral lesions within one or more components in the limbic network, most commonly the hippocampus, entorhinal cortex, the mammillary bodies of the hypothalamus, and the limbic thalamus. Occasionally, unilateral left-sided lesions can give rise to an amnestic state, but the memory disorder tends to be transient. Depending on the nature and distribution of the underlying neurologic disease, the patient may also have visual field deficits, eye movement limitations, or cerebellar findings. In many patients, such as those with *transient global amnesia* (Chap. 26), there are no associated neurologic findings; this sometimes leads incorrectly to the diagnosis of a psychiatric disorder.

Although the limbic network is the site of damage for amnestic states, it is almost certainly not the storage site for memories. Memories are stored in widely distributed form throughout the association cortex. The role attributed to the limbic network is to bind these distributed fragments into coherent events and experiences that can sustain conscious recall. Damage to the limbic network does not necessarily destroy memories but interferes with their conscious (declarative) recall in coherent form. The individual fragments of information remain preserved despite the limbic lesions and can sustain what is known as *implicit memory*. For example, patients with amnestic states can acquire new motor or perceptual skills, even though they may have no conscious knowledge of the experiences that led to the acquisition of these skills.

THE PREFRONTAL NETWORK FOR ATTENTION AND COMPORTMENT Approximately one-third of all the cerebral cortex in the human brain is located in the frontal lobes. The frontal lobes can be subdivided into motor-premotor, dorsolateral prefrontal, medial prefrontal, and orbitofrontal components. The terms *frontal lobe syndrome* and *prefrontal cortex* refer only to the last three of these four components. These are the parts of the cerebral cortex that show the greatest phylogenetic expansion in primates and especially in humans. The dorsolateral prefrontal, medial prefrontal, and orbitofrontal areas, and the subcortical structures with which they are interconnected (i.e., the head of the caudate and the dorsomedial nucleus of the thalamus), collectively make up a large-scale network that coordinates exceedingly complex aspects of human cognition and comportment.

The prefrontal network plays an important role in behaviors that require an integration of thought with emotion and motivation. There is no simple formula for summarizing the diverse functional affiliations of the prefrontal network. Its integrity appears important for the simultaneous awareness of context, options, consequences, relevance, and emotional impact so as to allow the formulation of adaptive inferences, decisions, and actions. Damage to this part of the brain impairs mental flexibility, reasoning, hypothesis formation, abstract thinking, foresight, judgment, the on-line (attentive) holding of information, and the ability to inhibit inappropriate responses. Behaviors impaired by prefrontal cortex lesions, especially those related to the manipulation of mental content, are often referred to as "executive functions."

Even very large bilateral prefrontal lesions may leave all sensory, motor, and basic cognitive functions intact while leading to isolated but dramatic alterations of personality and comportment. The most common clinical manifestations of damage to the prefrontal network take the form of two relatively distinct syndromes. In the *frontal abulic syndrome*, the patient shows a loss of initiative, creativity, and curiosity and displays a pervasive emotional blandness and apathy. In the *frontal disinhibition syndrome*, the patient becomes socially disinhibited and shows severe impairments of judgment, insight, and foresight. The dissociation between intact intellectual function and a total lack of even rudimentary common sense is striking. Despite the preservation of all essential memory functions, the patient cannot learn from experience and continues to display inappropriate behaviors without appearing to feel emotional pain, guilt, or regret when such behaviors repeatedly lead to disastrous consequences. The impairments may emerge only in real-life situations when behavior is under minimal external control and may not be apparent within the structured environment of the medical office. Testing judgment by asking patients what they would do if they detected a fire in a theater or found a stamped and addressed envelope on the road is not very informative since patients who answer these questions wisely in the office may still act very foolishly in the more complex real-life setting. The physician must therefore be prepared to make a diagnosis of frontal lobe disease on the basis of historic information alone even when the office examination of mental state may be quite intact.

The abulic syndrome tends to be associated with damage to the dorsolateral prefrontal cortex, and the disinhibition syndrome with the medial prefrontal or orbitofrontal cortex. These syndromes tend to arise almost exclusively after bilateral lesions, most frequently in the setting of head trauma, stroke, ruptured aneurysms, hydrocephalus, tumors (including metastases, glioblastoma, and falx or olfactory groove meningiomas), or focal degenerative diseases. Unilateral lesions confined to the prefrontal cortex may remain silent until the pathology spreads to the other side. The emergence of developmentally primitive reflexes such as grasping, rooting, and sucking are seen primarily in patients with large structural lesions that extend into the premotor components of the frontal lobes or in the context of metabolic encephalopathies. The vast majority of patients with prefrontal lesions and frontal lobe behavioral syndromes do not display these reflexes.

Damage to the frontal lobe disrupts a variety of attention-related functions including working memory (the transient on-line holding of information), concentration span, verbal fluency, the scanning and retrieval of stored information, the inhibition of immediate but inappropriate responses, and mental flexibility. The capacity for focusing on a trend of thought and the ability to voluntarily shift the focus of attention from one thought or stimulus to another can become impaired. Digit span (which should be seven forward and five reverse) is decreased; the recitation of the months of the year in reverse order (which should take less than 15 s) is slowed; and the number of words starting with a, f, or s that can be generated in 1 min (normally 12 or more per letter) is diminished even in nonaphasic patients. Characteristically, there is a progressive slowing of performance as the task proceeds; e.g., the patient asked to count backwards by 3s may say "100, 97, 94 . . . 91, . . . 88," etc., and may not complete the task. In go–no go tasks (where the instruction is to raise the finger upon hearing one tap but to keep it still upon hearing two taps), the patient shows a characteristic inability to keep still in response to the "no go" stimulus; mental flexibility (tested by the ability to shift from one criterion to another in sorting or matching tasks) is impoverished; distractibility by irrelevant stimuli is increased; and there is a pronounced tendency for impersistence and perseveration.

These attentional deficits disrupt the orderly registration and retrieval of new information and lead to *secondary* memory deficits. Such memory deficits can be differentiated from the *primary* memory impairments of the amnestic state by showing that they improve when the attentional load of the task is decreased. Working memory (also known as immediate memory) is an attentional function based on the temporary on-line holding of information. It is closely associated with the integrity of the prefrontal network and the ascending reticular activating system. Retentive memory, on the other hand, depends on the stable (off-line) storage of information and is associated with the integrity of the limbic network. The distinction of the underlying neural mechanisms is illustrated by the observation that severely amnestic patients who cannot remember events that occurred a few minutes ago may have intact if not superior working memory capacity as shown in tests of digit span.

Lesions in the caudate nucleus or in the dorsomedial nucleus of the thalamus (subcortical components of the prefrontal network) can also produce a frontal lobe syndrome. This is one reason why the mental state changes associated with degenerative basal ganglia diseases, such as Parkinson's or Huntington's disease, may take the form of a frontal lobe syndrome. Because of its widespread connections with other regions of association cortex, one essential computational role of the prefrontal network is to function as an integrator, or "orchestrator," for other networks. Bilateral multifocal lesions of the cerebral hemispheres, none of which are individually large enough to cause specific cognitive deficits such as aphasia or neglect, can collectively interfere with the connectivity and integrating function of prefrontal cortex. A frontal lobe syndrome is the single most common behavioral profile associated with a variety of bilateral multifocal brain diseases including metabolic encephalopathy, multiple sclerosis, vitamin B_{12} deficiency, and others. In fact, the vast majority of patients with the clinical diagnosis of a frontal lobe syndrome tend to have lesions that do not involve prefrontal cortex but involve either the subcortical components of the prefrontal network or its connections with other parts of the brain. In order to avoid making a diagnosis of "frontal lobe syndrome" in a patient with no evidence of frontal cortex disease, it is advisable to use the diagnostic term *frontal network syndrome*, with the understanding that the responsible lesions can lie anywhere within this distributed network.

The patient with frontal lobe disease raises potential dilemmas in differential diagnosis: the abulia and blandness may be misinterpreted as depression, and the disinhibition as mania or acting-out. Appropri-

ate intervention may be delayed while a treatable tumor keeps expanding. An informed approach to frontal lobe disease and its comportmental manifestations may help to avoid such errors.

CARING FOR THE PATIENT WITH DEFICITS OF HIGHER CEREBRAL FUNCTION Some of the deficits described in this chapter are so complex that they may bewilder not only the patient and family but also the physician. It is imperative to carry out a systematic clinical evaluation in order to characterize the nature of the deficits and explain them in lay terms to the patient and family. Such an explanation can allay at least some of the anxieties, address the mistaken impression that the deficit (e.g., social disinhibition or inability to recognize family members) is psychologically motivated, and lead to practical suggestions for daily living activities. The consultation of a skilled neuropsychologist may aid in the formulation of diagnosis and management. Patients with simultanagnosia, for example, may benefit from the counterintuitive instruction to stand back when they cannot find an item so that a greater search area falls within the immediate field of gaze. In some patients, the history may be more important than the bedside examination. For example, patients with frontal lobe disease can be extremely irritable and abusive to spouses and yet display all the appropriate social graces during the visit to the medical office.

Reactive depression is common in patients with higher cerebral dysfunction and should be treated. These patients may be sensitive to the usual doses of antidepressants or anxiolytics and deserve a careful titration of dosage. Brain damage may cause a dissociation between feeling states and their expression, so that a patient who may superficially appear jocular could still be suffering from an underlying depression that deserves to be treated. In many cases, agitation may be controlled with reassurance. In other cases, treatment with benzodiazepines or sedating antidepressants may become necessary. The use of neuroleptics for the control of agitation should be reserved for refractory cases since extrapyramidal side effects are frequent in patients with coexisting brain damage.

Spontaneous improvement of cognitive deficits due to acute neurologic lesions is common. It is most rapid in the first few weeks but may continue for up to 2 years, especially in young individuals with single brain lesions. The mechanisms for this recovery are incompletely understood. Some of the initial deficits appear to arise from remote dysfunction (diaschisis) in parts of the brain that are interconnected with the site of initial injury. Improvement in these patients may reflect, at least in part, a normalization of the remote dysfunction. Other mechanisms may involve functional reorganization in surviving neurons adjacent to the injury or the compensatory use of homologous structures, e.g., the right superior temporal gyrus with recovery from Wernicke's aphasia. In some patients with large lesions involving Broca's and Wernicke's areas, only Wernicke's area may show contralateral compensatory reorganization (or bilateral functionality), giving rise to a situation where a lesion that should have caused a global aphasia becomes associated with a residual Broca aphasia. Prognosis for recovery from aphasia is best when Wernicke's area is spared. Cognitive rehabilitation procedures have been used in the treatment of higher cortical deficits. There are few controlled studies, but some do show a benefit of rehabilitation in the recovery from hemispatial neglect and aphasia. Some types of deficits may be more prone to recovery than others. For example, patients with nonfluent aphasias are more likely to benefit from speech therapy than patients with fluent aphasias and comprehension deficits. In general, lesions that lead to a denial of illness (e.g., anosognosia) are associated with cognitive deficits that are more resistant to rehabilitation. The recovery of higher cortical dysfunction is rarely complete. Periodic neuropsychological assessment is necessary for quantifying the pace of the improvement and for generating specific recommendations for cognitive rehabilitation, modifications in the home environment, and the timetable for returning to school or work.

BIBLIOGRAPHY

DAMASIO AR, DAMASIO H: Aphasia and the neural basis of language, in *Principles of Behavioral and Cognitive Neurology*, 2d ed. M-M Mesulam (ed). New York, Oxford University Press, 2000, pp 294–315

GITELMAN DR et al: A large-scale distributed network for covert spatial attention. Further anatomical delineation based on stringent behavioral and cognitive controls. Brain 122:1093, 1999

HEISS W-D et al: Differential capacity of left and right hemispheric areas for compensation of poststroke aphasia. Ann Neurol 45:430, 1999

LEIGUARDA RC, MARSDEN CD: Limb apraxias. Higher-order disorders of sensorimotor integration. Brain 123:860, 2000

MESULAM M-M: Behavioral neuroanatomy: Large-scale networks, association cortex, frontal syndromes, the limbic system and hemispheric specializations, in *Principles of Behavioral and Cognitive Neurology*, 2d ed, M-M Mesulam (ed). New York, Oxford University Press, 2000, pp 1–120

———: From sensation to cognition. Brain 121:1031, 1998

26	*Thomas D. Bird*

MEMORY LOSS AND DEMENTIA

AD Alzheimer's disease	EEG electroencephalogram
CADASIL cerebral autosomal dominant arteriopathy with subcortical infarcts and leukoencephalopathy	FTD Frontotemporal dementia
	HD Huntington's disease
CJD Creutzfeldt-Jakob disease	LTP Long-term potentiation
CNS central nervous system	MMSE mini-mental status exam
CREB cyclic AMP-responsive element binding protein	MRI magnetic resonance imaging
	PD Parkinson's disease
CSF cerebrospinal fluid	SPECT single photon emission computed tomography
CT Computed tomography	TGA Transient global amnesia
EDTA ethylene diaminetetraacetic acid	VDRL Venereal Disease Research Laboratory

DEFINITION Dementia is a serious and common problem that affects more than 4 million Americans and costs society more than $50 billion annually. Ten percent of persons over age 70 and 20 to 40% of individuals over age 85 have clinically identifiable memory loss. Dementia is a syndrome with many causes. A simple definition of dementia is a deterioration in cognitive abilities that impairs the previously successful performance of activities of daily living. Memory is the most common and most important cognitive ability that is lost. Other mental faculties may also be affected such as attention, judgment, comprehension, orientation, learning, calculation, problem solving, mood, and behavior. Agitation or withdrawal, hallucinations, delusions, insomnia, and loss of inhibitions are also common. Individuals with mental retardation and psychosis may become demented if a decline in intellectual function occurs. Many common forms of dementia are progressive, but some dementing illnesses are static and unchanging. Dementia is a chronic condition, whereas delirium is an acute confusional state associated with a change in level of consciousness (ranging from lethargy to agitation).

Memory is a complex function of the brain that has fascinated philosophers and scientists for centuries. Memory is currently viewed as a mental process that uses several storage buffers of differing capacity and duration (Table 26-1). Sensory memory lasts for about 250 ms in the visual mode (iconic memory) and 1 to 2 s in the auditory mode (echoic memory). Immediate (short-term or primary) memory has a duration of about half a minute and a limited capacity of approximately 5 to 10 items. Immediate memory is highly vulnerable to distraction, requiring attention and vigilance to maintain the content. It is often tested at the bedside by asking the patient to recall several digits forward and backward. Recent, or secondary, memory has been called both "short-term" and "long-term." It has a duration of minutes to weeks and exhibits a larger storage capacity than immediate memory. On entering this buffer, information undergoes a process of consolidation of variable duration. Recent memory is commonly tested in the clinical setting by asking a patient to recall three words after 3 to 5 min. Remote, or long-term, memory stores information lasting weeks to a lifetime and contains most of our personal experiences and knowledge. Some information appears to be stored accurately for an indefinite time, whereas other items fade or become distorted. Memory function includes registration (encoding or acquisition), retention (storage or consolidation), stabilization, and retrieval (decoding or recall). Registration and retrieval are conscious processes. Animal experiments have shown that long-term memory requires new protein synthesis, and the stabilization process probably involves physical changes at neuronal synapses.

Several additional classifications of memory are sometimes used by psychologists, particularly in reference to the content or use of the memory stores. Reference memory refers to a filing system that contains recent and remote information gained from previous experience. Working memory refers to an active process that is being updated continually by current experience. Episodic memory contains information about events occurring in a specific place and time. Semantic memory contains unchanging facts, principles, associations, and rules (for example, state capitals and the number of days in a week). Declarative (explicit) memory refers to facts about the world and past personal events that must be consciously retrieved to be remembered. Procedural (implicit) memory, in contrast, is involved in learning and retaining a skill or procedure such as how to ride a bicycle, get dressed, or drive a car. Abilities stored in procedural memory become automatic and do not require conscious implementation.

Finally, the term *executive function* refers to mental activity involved in planning, initiating, and regulating behavior. It is considered the central organizing function of the brain that results in systematic, goal-directed activity. Executive functions are active in nonroutine situations where reflex or automatic behavior is not adequate. The anatomic and physiologic substrates of executive function are presumed to involve the frontal lobes (Chap. 25). Deficits in executive function occur frequently in patients with dementia.

FUNCTIONAL ANATOMY AND PATHOGENESIS Dementia results from disorders of cerebral neuronal circuits and is a result of the total quantity of neuronal loss combined with the specific location of such loss (Chap. 25). The anatomic basis of memory was initially clarified from study of the alcohol/thiamine deficiency syndrome of Korsakoff and the consequences of temporal lobe surgery performed for the treatment of epilepsy. In Korsakoff's syndrome lesions in the hypothalamus, mammillary bodies, and dorsomedial nuclei of the thalamus showed that these areas were important for learning, recall, and recognition. Unilateral temporal lobe surgery for epilepsy produced mild to moderate amnesia for either verbal or nonverbal material. Bilateral medial temporal lobe excision involving the hippocampal formation, the parahippocampal gyrus, and part of the amygdala produced a severe anterograde learning disorder, i.e., an inability to store new memories, often with retained ability to recall old ones. The components of the medial temporal lobe memory system include the hippocampus and adjacent cortex, including the entorhinal, perirhinal, and parahippocampal regions (Fig. 26-1). This includes a circular pathway of neurons from the entorhinal cortex to the dentate gyrus, CA3 and CA1 neurons of the hippocampus to the subiculum, and back to the entorhinal cortex; this pathway is heavily damaged in Alzheimer's disease (AD). This system is fast, has limited capacity, and performs a crucial function at the time of learning and establishing declarative memory. Its role continues after learning during a lengthy period of reorganization and consolidation whereby memory stored in neocortex eventually becomes independent of the medial temporal lobe memory system. This process, by which the burden of long-term (permanent) memory storage is gradually assumed by neocortex, assures that the medial temporal lobe system is always available for the acquisition of new information. Recent functional brain imaging studies indicate that learning and memory involve many of the same regions of the cortex that process sensory information and control motor output. The forms of perceptual and motor learning that can occur without conscious recollections are mediated in part by contractions and expansions of representations in the sensory and motor cortex. One study, for example, has shown that the cortical representation of the fingers of the left hand of musical string players is larger than that in control individuals, suggesting that the representation of different parts of the body in the primary somatosensory cortex of humans depends on use and changes to conform to the current needs and experiences of the individual. Discrete cortical regions exist in which object knowledge (such as words related to color, animals, tools, or action) is organized as a distributed system in which the attributes of an object are stored close to the regions of the cortex that mediate perception of those attributes (Chap. 25). That is, brain regions active during object identification are partly dependent on the intrinsic properties of the object. Procedural (implicit) memory appears to involve centers outside the hippocampus such as amygdala, cerebellum, and sensory cortex. Different frontal regions are activated for different kinds of memory storage. Functional magnetic resonance imaging (MRI) studies show that the magnitude of focal activation in left prefrontal-temporal regions or right prefrontal-bilateral parahippocampal regions predicts how well verbal or visual stimuli, respectively, will be remembered.

Biochemically, the cholinergic system plays an important role in memory. Anticholinergic agents such as atropine and scopolamine interfere with memory. Choline acetyl transferase (the enzyme catalyzing the formation of acetylcholine) and nicotinic cholinergic receptors are known to be deficient in the cortex of patients with AD. The brains of patients with AD show severe neuronal loss in the nucleus basalis of Meynert, a major source of cholinergic input to the cerebral cortex. These findings form the basis for the use of cholinesterase inhibitors in the treatment of AD, with benefit presumably arising from increased available levels of acetylcholine. Behavior and mood are modulated by noradrenergic, serotonergic, and dopaminergic pathways; and norepinephrine has been shown to be reduced in the brainstem locus coeruleus in patients with AD. Neurotrophins are also postulated to play a role in memory in part by preserving cholinergic neurons.

Long-term potentiation (LTP), which refers to a long-lasting enhancement of synaptic transmission resulting from repetitive stimulation of excitatory synapses, is presumed to be involved in memory acquisition and storage. LTP occurs in hippocampus and is mediated by N-methyl-D-aspartate (NMDA) receptors as well as cyclic AMP-responsive element

binding protein (CREB). Gene knockout mouse models have been useful in the definition of secondary messenger systems that play a role in hippocampal LTP. For example, disruption of either calcium/calmodulin-dependent protein kinase or cytoplasmic tyrosine kinase (fyn) results in deficient hippocampal LTP and impaired spatial learning. In contrast, mice in which a neuronal glycoprotein thy-1 has been inactivated show regionally selective impairment of LTP but intact spatial learning, suggesting that LTP in the entorhinal projection to the dentate gyrus of the hippocampus (Fig. 26-1) may not be necessary for some forms of spatial learning. Disruption of hippocampal levels of CREB impairs long-term memory in rats.

Most diseases causing dementia do not have highly restricted regions of pathology. Disorders such as AD appear to eventually rep-

Table 26-1   Classification of Memory

Type	Time Interval	Test/Example	Probable Cerebral Location
Sensory			
Iconic (visual)	<1 s	After image	Visual cortex
Echoic (auditory)	1–2 s	Cough/dog bark	Auditory cortex
Immediate (primary/working)	30 s	Digit span	Perisylvian cortex, frontal lobe
Recent (secondary/reference)	Minutes–weeks/months	Recall 3 words after 3–5 min	Hippocampus, mamillothalamic tract, dorsomedial thalamus
Declarative (explicit)			
Episodic		Recall trip last week	Limbic system and association cortex
Semantic		Recall names of months	
Procedural (implicit)		Ride a bike Get dressed	Amygdala, cerebellum, association cortex, frontal lobe, ? other
Remote (reference)	Months–years	Recall high school graduation	Association cortex, ? other

SOURCE: Modified from K. Erickson: West J Med 152:159, 1990.

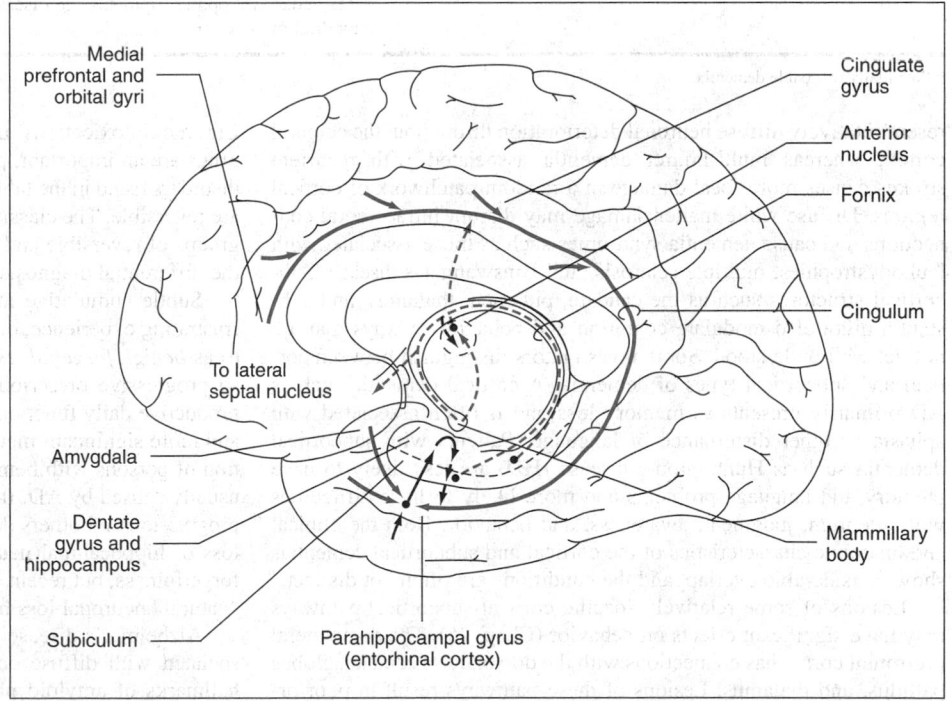

FIGURE 26-1   The principal connections of the hippocampus. Afferent connections (*blue arrows*) from the cingulate gyrus (cortical association fibers) and amygdala converge on the entorhinal cortex (part of the parahippocampal gyrus) and connect with the hippocampus via a polysynaptic circuit (*black arrows*) from dentate to CA3, CA1, and subiculum neurons with output back to the entorhinal cortex. Efferent connections (*broken arrows*) are principally via the fornix to the anterior nucleus of the thalamus, septal nuclei, and mamillary body.

Table 26-2 Differential Diagnosis of Dementia

MOST COMMON CAUSES OF DEMENTIA

Alzheimer's disease	Alcoholism[a]
Vascular dementia	Parkinson's disease
Multi-infarct	Drug/medication intoxication[a]
Diffuse white matter disease (Binswanger's)	

LESS COMMON CAUSES OF DEMENTIA

Vitamin deficiencies	Toxic disorders
Thiamine (B$_1$): Wernicke's encephalopathy[a]	Drug, medication, and narcotic poisoning[a]
B$_{12}$ (pernicious anemia)[a]	Heavy metal intoxication[a]
Nicotinic acid (pellagra)[a]	Dialysis dementia (aluminum)
Endocrine and other organ failure	Organic toxins
Hypothyroidism[a]	Psychiatric
Adrenal insufficiency and Cushing's syndrome[a]	Depression (pseudodementia)[a]
Hypo- and hyperparathyroidism[a]	Schizophrenia[a]
Renal failure[a]	Conversion reaction[a]
Liver failure[a]	Degenerative disorders
Pulmonary failure[a]	Huntington's disease
Chronic infections	Pick's disease
HIV	Diffuse Lewy body disease
Neurosyphilis[a]	Progressive supranuclear palsy (Steel-Richardson
Papovavirus (progressive multifocal leukoencepha-	syndrome)
lopathy)	Multisystem degeneration (Shy-Drager syndrome)
Prion (Creutzfeldt-Jakob and Gerstmann-Sträussler-	Hereditary ataxias (some forms)
Scheinker diseases)	Motor neuron disease [amyotrophic lateral sclerosis
Tuberculosis, fungal, and protozoal[a]	(ALS); some forms]
Sarcoidosis[a]	Frontotemporal dementia
Whipple's disease[a]	Cortical basal degeneration
Head trauma and diffuse brain damage	Multiple sclerosis
Dementia pugilistica	Adult Down's syndrome with Alzheimer's
Chronic subdural hematoma[a]	ALS–Parkinson's–Dementia complex of Guam
Postanoxia	Miscellaneous
Postencephalitis	Vasculitis[a]
Normal-pressure hydrocephalus[a]	CADASIL
Neoplastic	Acute intermittent porphyria[a]
Primary brain tumor[a]	Recurrent nonconvulsive seizures[a]
Metastatic brain tumor[a]	Additional conditions in children or adolescents
Paraneoplastic limbic encephalitis	Hallervorden-Spatz disease
	Subacute sclerosing panencephalitis
	Metabolic disorders (e.g., Wilson's and Leigh's dis-
	eases, leukodystrophies, lipid storage diseases, mito-
	chondrial mutations)

[a] Potentially reversible dementia.

resent relatively diffuse neuronal deterioration throughout the cerebral cortex, whereas multi-infarct dementia associated with recurrent strokes causes more focal damage in a random patchwork of cortical regions. Diffuse white matter damage may disrupt intracerebral connections and cause dementia syndromes such as those associated with leukodystrophies, multiple sclerosis, and Binswanger's disease. Subcortical structures such as the caudate, putamen, thalamus, and substantia nigra also modulate cognition and behavior in ways that are not yet well understood. Some investigators distinguish between cortical and subcortical types of dementia. A cortical dementia such as AD primarily presents as memory loss and is often associated with aphasia or other disturbance of language. Patients with subcortical dementia such as Huntington's disease (HD) are less likely to have memory and language problems and more likely to have difficulties with attention, judgment, awareness, and behavior. Both the clinical and anatomic characteristics of the cortical and subcortical dementias show considerable overlap, and the conditions are often not distinct.

Lesions of some relatively specific cortical-subcortical pathways may have significant effects on behavior (Chap. 25). The dorsolateral prefrontal cortex has connections with the dorsolateral caudate, globus pallidus, and thalamus. Lesions of these pathways result in poor organization and planning, perseveration, and decreased cognitive flexibility with impaired judgment. The lateral orbital frontal cortex connects with the ventromedial caudate, globus pallidus, and thalamus. Lesions of these connections cause irritability, impulsiveness, and distractibility. The anterior cingulate cortex connects with the nucleus accumbens, globus pallidus, and thalamus. Interruption of these con-

nections produces apathy and poverty of speech or even akinetic mutism.

The single strongest risk factor for dementia is increasing age. The prevalence of disabling memory loss increases with each decade over age 50 and is associated most often with the microscopic changes of AD at autopsy. Slow accumulation of mutations in neuronal mitochondria is also hypothesized to contribute to the increasing prevalence of dementia with age. Yet many centenarians have intact memory function and no evidence of clinically significant dementia. Whether dementia is an inevitable consequence of normal human aging remains controversial.

DIFFERENTIAL DIAGNOSIS The many causes of dementia are listed in Table 26-2. The frequency of each condition depends on the age group under study, the country of origin, and perhaps racial or ethnic variations. AD is the most common cause of dementia in western countries, affecting more than half of demented patients. Vascular disease is the second most common cause of dementia in the United States, affecting 10 to 20%; but it is more common than AD in some Asian countries. Dementia associated with chronic alcoholism and Parkinson's disease (PD) represent the next two most common categories. Chronic intoxications including those resulting from prescription drugs are an important, potentially treatable cause of dementia. Other disorders listed in the table are uncommon but important because many are reversible. The classification of dementing illnesses into two broad groups of reversible and irreversible disorders is a useful approach to the differential diagnosis of dementia.

Subtle cumulative memory loss is a natural part of aging. This frustrating experience, often the source of jokes and humor, is referred to as *benign forgetfulness of the elderly*. Benign means that it is not so progressive or serious that it impairs reasonably successful and productive daily functioning, although the distinction between benign and more significant memory loss can be difficult to make. A proportion of persons with benign memory loss progress to frank dementia, usually caused by AD. It remains unclear why some individuals show progression and others do not. It was once assumed that a cumulative loss of hippocampal neurons with normal aging might underlie this forgetfulness, but recent quantitative neuronal counts indicate that this "natural" neuronal loss may not occur.

Alzheimer's disease is a slowly progressive dementing illness associated with diffuse cortical atrophy and specific neuropathologic hallmarks of amyloid plaques and neurofibrillary tangles. Although quite common in the elderly, it remains a diagnosis of exclusion to be confirmed definitively only at autopsy. The clinical diagnosis of AD established by experienced neurologists proves to be correct at autopsy approximately 85 to 90% of the time. →*This condition is described in greater detail in Chap. 362.*

Two major types of vascular dementia can be identified (Chap.

362). The first, often called multi-infarct dementia, results from an accumulation of discrete cerebral strokes that produce disabling deficits of memory, behavior, and other cognitive abilities. Such patients usually give a history of sudden, separate stroke episodes with stepwise deterioration. On examination, focal neurologic deficits such as hemiparesis, unilateral Babinski reflex, aphasia, or visual field defect are common. Brain imaging shows multiple areas of stroke, which may have been ischemic or hemorrhagic. A second, more subtle and insidious type of vascular dementia, Binswanger's disease, is a dementing illness associated with diffuse, subcortical white matter damage often occurring in patients with chronic hypertension and/or severe atherosclerosis. The white matter changes are dramatically visualized by MRI and have also been called leukoareosis. The pathogenesis of Binswanger's disease is unknown. Because AD and vascular dementia are common, occasional patients may have both conditions.

An inherited form of vascular dementia is CADASIL (cerebral autosomal dominant arteriopathy with subcortical infarcts and leuko-encephalopathy). It is caused by a mutation in the notch 3 gene and produces characteristic dense bodies in the media of arterioles in brain and skin. Affected persons have diffuse white matter deficits on brain MRI associated with migraine and recurrent stroke without hypertension.

Frontotemporal dementia (FTD) may represent 10 to 20% of persons with presenile dementia (onset before age 65). Initial symptoms are behavioral, such as disinhibition, apathy, or agitation with relatively intact memory. Brain imaging studies show focal lobar atrophy of the frontal and/or temporal lobes. Pick's disease is a form of FTD. Some cases are familial and associated with neuronal neurofibrillary tangle formation and mutations in the tau gene.

Dementia commonly accompanies chronic alcoholism (Chap. 387). This situation may be a result of associated malnutrition, especially of B vitamins and particularly thiamine. However, other as yet poorly defined aspects of chronic alcohol ingestion may also produce cerebral damage and atrophy. A rare idiopathic syndrome of dementia and seizures with degeneration of the corpus callosum has been reported primarily in male Italian drinkers of red wine (Marchiafava-Bignami disease).

Thiamine (vitamin B_1) deficiency causes Wernicke's encephalopathy. The clinical presentation is a malnourished individual (frequently but not necessarily alcoholic) with confusion, ataxia, and diplopia from ophthalmoplegia (Charcot's triad). Thiamine deficiency damages the thalamus, mammillary bodies, midline cerebellum, periaquaductal gray matter of the midbrain, and peripheral nerves. Damage to medial thalamic regions correlates most closely with memory loss. Prompt administration of parenteral thiamine (100 mg intravenously for 3 days followed by daily oral dosage) may reverse the disease if given in the first few days of symptom onset. However, prolonged untreated thiamine deficiency can result in an irreversible dementia/amnestic syndrome (Korsakoff's psychosis) or even death.

In Korsakoff's syndrome, the patient is unable to recall new information despite normal immediate memory, attention span, and level of consciousness. Memory for new events is seriously impaired, whereas memory of knowledge prior to the illness is relatively intact. Patients are easily confused, disoriented, and incapable of recalling new information for more than a brief interval. Superficially, they may be conversant, entertaining, able to perform simple tasks, and follow immediate commands. Confabulation is common, although not always present, and may result in obviously erroneous statements and elaborations. There is no specific treatment because the previous thiamine deficiency has produced irreversible damage to the medial thalamic nuclei and mammillary bodies. Mammillary body atrophy may be visible on high-resolution MRI.

Vitamin B_{12} deficiency, as can occur in pernicious anemia, causes a macrocytic anemia and may also damage the nervous system (Chaps. 107 and 368). Neurologically it most commonly produces a spinal cord syndrome (myelopathy) affecting the posterior columns (loss of position and vibratory sense) and the lateral corticospinal tracts (hyperactive tendon reflexes and Babinski responses); it also damages pe-

ripheral nerves, resulting in sensory loss with depressed tendon reflexes. Damage to cerebral myelinated fibers may also cause dementia. The mechanism of neurologic damage is unclear but may be related to a deficiency of S-adenosylmethionine (required for methylation of myelin phospholipids) due to reduced methionine synthase activity or accumulation of methylmalonate and propionate, providing abnormal substrates for fatty acid synthesis in myelin. The neurologic signs of vitamin B_{12} deficiency are usually associated with macrocytic anemia, but on occasion may occur in its absence. Treatment with parenteral vitamin B_{12} (1000 μg intramuscularly daily for a week, weekly for a month, and monthly for life for pernicious anemia) stops progression of the disease if instituted promptly, but reversal of advanced nervous system damage will not occur.

Deficiency of nicotinic acid (pellagra) is associated with sun-exposed skin rash, glossitis, and angular stomatitis (Chap. 75). Severe dietary deficiency of nicotinic acid along with other B vitamins such as pyridoxine may result in spastic paraparesis, peripheral neuropathy, fatigue, irritability, and dementia. This syndrome has been seen in prisoner-of-war and concentration camps. Low serum folate levels appear to be a rough index of malnutrition, but isolated folate deficiency has not been proven to be a specific cause of dementia.

Approximately 20% of patients with PD (Chap. 363) eventually develop dementia. Treatment with L-dopa neither accelerates nor prevents this process. Some PD patients with dementia have cytoplasmic neuronal inclusions (Lewy bodies) or AD changes in the cerebral cortex, but others have no specific identifiable cortical pathology. Progressive supranuclear palsy is a dementing illness associated with parkinsonian features of rigidity, bradykinesia, and postural instability. Resting tremor is often absent, there is a vertical gaze palsy, and patients are resistant to treatment with L-dopa.

Infections of the central nervous system (CNS) usually cause delirium and other acute neurologic syndromes (Chap. 24). However, some chronic CNS infections such as tuberculosis or cryptococcosis may produce a dementing illness (Chap. 374). Between 20 and 30% of patients in the advanced stages of infection with HIV become demented (Chap. 309). Cardinal features include psychomotor retardation, apathy, and impaired memory. This condition may result from secondary opportunistic infections but can also be caused by direct involvement of CNS neurons with HIV, where there is a multinucleated giant cell encephalitis and diffuse pallor of white matter. The neuronal toxicity may be mediated by cytokines or the direct neurotoxic effect of the gp 120 envelope glycoprotein. In the absence of CNS opportunistic infection, elevated β_2-microglobulin in cerebrospinal fluid (CSF) is a useful marker for HIV dementia. Herpes simplex encephalitis (Chap. 373) has a predilection for the inferior temporal lobes and may present as subacute confusion and disorientation but more often as an acute syndrome rather than a chronic dementia. Computed tomography (CT), MRI, and electroencephalogram (EEG) may all demonstrate the temporal lobe location of the lesions. CSF usually shows increased protein and a lymphocytic pleocytosis. CNS syphilis (Chap. 172) was a common cause of dementia in the preantibiotic era; it is uncommon now but can still be encountered in individuals with multiple sex partners. Characteristic CSF changes consist of pleocytosis, increased protein, and a positive Venereal Disease Research Laboratory (VDRL) test.

Prion disorders such as Creutzfeldt-Jakob disease (CJD) (Chap. 375) are rare conditions (approximately 1 per million population) that commonly produce dementia. CJD is typically a rapidly progressive disease associated with dementia, rigidity, and myoclonus, causing death in less than 1 to 2 years. These clinical characteristics may also rarely be seen in AD, and the differential diagnosis usually depends on the slower progression of AD and the markedly abnormal periodic EEG discharges seen in CJD. Ataxia or cortical blindness may also accompany CJD. The transmissible agent, or prion, consists principally of an abnormal isoform of a host-encoded protein, the prion protein, which has undergone a physical conformational change and accumulates in affected brains. Bovine spongiform encephalopathy in the United Kingdom is thought to have resulted from cattle feed containing sheep tissues contaminated with infectious prions. Immunoassay for a 14-3-3 brain protein in CSF may be a useful marker for transmissible spongiform encephalopathies in patients with dementia.

Primary and metastatic neoplasms of the CNS (Chap. 370) usually produce focal neurologic findings and seizures rather than dementia. However, if tumor growth begins in the frontal or temporal lobes, the initial manifestations may be memory loss or behavioral changes. A rare paraneoplastic syndrome of dementia associated with occult carcinoma (usually small cell lung cancer) has been termed *limbic encephalitis* (Chap. 101). In this syndrome, confusion, agitation, seizures, poor memory, and frank dementia may occur in association with sensory neuropathy. The CSF often shows an increase in cells and protein. There is neuronal loss and perivascular lymphocytic infiltration in the hippocampus, amygdala, and cingulate and frontal cortex. Circulating antineuronal nuclear antibodies may be present. There is no specific treatment.

The syndrome of normal-pressure hydrocephalus (Chap. 362) is frequently discussed but difficult to diagnose. Clinically, a triad of memory loss, gait disturbance, and bladder incontinence is typical. The gait abnormality is often the initial symptom, and the dementia is usually mild. On imaging studies, the lateral ventricles are enlarged but there is minimal or no cortical atrophy. Lumbar puncture shows a normal or slightly elevated opening pressure with normal CSF. The condition may be idiopathic or the result of previous meningitis or subarachnoid blood from a ruptured aneurysm or head trauma. The pathogenetic mechanism is presumably a block of normal CSF flow over the convexity and delayed absorption into the venous system, with resulting stretch and distortion of white matter tracts within the corona radiata. Some individuals improve with ventricular shunting but many do not. The condition is difficult to distinguish from AD (Chap. 362).

A nonconvulsive seizure disorder may underlie a syndrome of confusion, clouding of consciousness, and garbled speech. Psychiatric disease is often suspected, but an EEG demonstrates the seizure discharges. If recurrent or persistent, the condition may be termed *complex partial status epilepticus.* The cognitive disturbance often responds to anticonvulsant therapy. The etiology may be previous small strokes or head trauma; some cases are idiopathic.

It is important to recognize systemic diseases that indirectly affect the brain and produce chronic confusion or dementia. Such conditions include dysthyroid states (especially hypothyroidism), vasculitis, and hepatic, renal, or pulmonary disease. Hepatic encephalopathy may begin with irritability and confusion and slowly progress to agitation, lethargy, and coma (Chap. 376).

Isolated angiitis of the CNS (CNS granulomatous angiitis) (Chaps. 317 and 361) occasionally causes a chronic encephalopathy associated with confusion, disorientation, and clouding of consciousness. Headache is common, and strokes and cranial neuropathies may occur. Brain imaging studies may be normal or nonspecifically abnormal. Studies of CSF reveal a mild pleocytosis or elevation in the protein level in half of the cases. Cerebral angiography often shows multifocal stenosis and narrowing of vessels. A few patients have only small-vessel disease that is not revealed on angiography. The angiographic appearance is not specific and may be mimicked by atherosclerosis, infection, or other causes of vascular disease. Brain or meningeal biopsy demonstrates abnormal arteries with endothelial cell proliferation and infiltrates of mononuclear cells. Autoantibodies and immune complexes are not present, and a cell-mediated process appears most likely. The prognosis is poor, but some patients respond to glucocorticoids or chemotherapy.

Chronic metal intoxications may also produce a dementing syndrome. The key to diagnosis is the elicitation of a history of exposure at work, home, or even as a consequence of a medical procedure such as dialysis. Lead poisoning has highly variable neurologic manifesta-

tions. Fatigue, depression, and confusion may be associated with episodic abdominal pain and peripheral neuropathy. Gray lead lines may appear in the gums. There is usually an associated anemia with basophilic stippling of red cells. The clinical presentation can resemble that of acute intermittent porphyria, including elevated levels of urine porphyrins as a result of the inhibition of δ-aminolevulinic acid dehydratase. Chronic lead poisoning from inadequately fired glazed pottery has been reported. The treatment is chelation therapy with agents such as ethylene diaminetetraacetic acid (EDTA). Chronic mercury poisoning may produce dementia, peripheral neuropathy, ataxia, and a fine tremulousness that may progress to a cerebellar intention tremor or choreoathetosis. The confusion and memory loss of chronic arsenic intoxication is also associated with nausea, weight loss, peripheral neuropathy, pigmentation and scaling of the skin, and transverse white lines of the fingernails (Mee's lines). Treatment is chelation therapy with dimercaprol (BAL). Aluminum poisoning has been best documented with the dialysis dementia syndrome in which water used during renal dialysis was contaminated with excessive amounts of aluminum. This resulted in a progressive encephalopathy associated with confusion, memory loss, agitation, and, later, lethargy and stupor. Speech arrest and myoclonic jerking was common and associated with severe and generalized EEG changes. The condition was often fatal. There were no specific pathologic findings, but elevated brain aluminum content was documented. The condition has been eliminated by use of deionized water for dialysis. Although aluminum injected into experimental animals may produce neurofibrillary tangles, patients with dialysis dementia had neither tangles nor amyloid plaques, and there has been no direct association of aluminum poisoning with AD.

Recurrent head trauma in professional boxers may lead to dementia, sometimes called the "punch drunk" syndrome or *dementia pugilistica.* The symptoms can be progressive and may begin late in a boxer's career or even long after retirement. The severity of the syndrome correlates with the length of the boxing career and the total number of bouts. Early in the condition there occurs a personality change associated with social instability and sometimes paranoia and delusions. Later, memory loss progresses to full dementia, often associated with parkinsonian signs and ataxia or intention tremor. At autopsy, the cerebral cortex may show changes similar to AD, although neurofibrillary tangles are usually more predominant than amyloid plaques (which are usually diffuse rather than neuritic). There may also be loss of neurons in the substantia nigra. Chronic subdural hematoma is also occasionally associated with dementia, often in the context of underlying cortical atrophy from conditions such as AD or HD. In these latter cases, evacuation of the subdural hematoma does not alter the underlying degenerative process.

Head injury (Chap. 369) may also be associated with temporary amnesia. The memory disturbance may include events that occurred both before the injury (retrograde amnesia) and during the postinjury period (posttraumatic or anterograde amnesia). Retrograde amnesia after severe head injury may extend back for hours or weeks before the injury; remote memory is usually intact. As patients recover, the extent of retrograde amnesia shrinks and may disappear. Often, retrograde amnesia causes permanent inability to recall the few minutes before the head injury, implying disruption of the immediate memory system and failure to register long-term memory. The length of posttraumatic amnesia generally corresponds to the length of the postconcussive confusional state, but posttraumatic amnesia may persist even in the presence of normal immediate memory and digit span. The duration of posttraumatic amnesia indicates the severity of head injury; the ability to learn new material is often the last cognitive deficit to recover. There are reports of recovery from retrograde amnesia occurring months or years after the initial brain insult; the recovery is sometimes stimulated by hypnosis, amobarbital interview, or electrical stimulation. One theory of such recovery envisions a resetting of distorted patterns of neuronal matrices subserving memory.

Transient global amnesia (TGA) is characterized by sudden onset of complete anterograde loss of memory and learning abilities, usually occurring in persons over age 50. Onset of memory loss may occur in the context of an emotional stimulus or physical exertion. During the attack the individual is alert and communicative, general cognition seems intact, and there are no other neurologic signs or symptoms. The patient may seem confused and repeatedly ask about present events. The ability to form new memories returns after a period of hours, and the individual returns to normal but has no recall for the period of the attack. Frequently no cause can be determined, but cerebrovascular disease, epilepsy (7% in one study), migraine, or cardiac arrhythmia sometimes may be implicated. A Mayo Clinic review of 277 patients with TGA found a past history of migraine in 14% and cerebrovascular disease in 11%, but these conditions were not temporally related to the TGA episodes. About one-fourth of the patients had recurrent attacks, but they were not at increased risk for subsequent stroke. Rare instances of permanent memory loss after sudden onset have been reported.

Psychogenic amnesia for personally important memories is common, although whether this amnesia results from deliberate avoidance of unpleasant memories or from unconscious repression may be impossible to establish. The event-specific amnesia is particularly common after violent crimes such as homicide of a close relative or friend or sexual abuse. It also may occur with severe drug or alcohol intoxication and sometimes with schizophrenia. More prolonged psychogenic amnesia occurs in fugue states that also commonly follow severe emotional stress. The patient with a fugue state suffers from a sudden loss of personal identity and may be found wandering far from home. In contrast to organic amnesia, fugue states are associated with amnesia for personal identity and events closely associated with the personal past. At the same time, memory for other recent events and the ability to learn and use new information are preserved. The episodes usually last hours or days and occasionally weeks or months while the patient takes on a new identity. On recovery, there is a residual amnesic gap for the period of the fugue.

Psychiatric diseases may mimic dementia. Severely depressed individuals may appear demented, a phenomenon called *pseudodementia*. Unlike cortical dementias, memory and language are usually intact when carefully tested in depressed persons. The patients may feel confused and are unable to accomplish routine tasks. Vegetative symptoms are common, such as insomnia, lack of energy, poor appetite, and concern with bowel function. The psychosocial milieu may suggest prominent reasons for depression. The patients respond to antidepressant treatment. Schizophrenia is usually not difficult to distinguish from dementia, but occasionally the distinction can be problematic. (Kraepelin's original term for schizophrenia was *dementia praecox*.) Schizophrenia usually has a much earlier age of onset (second and third decades) than most dementing illnesses. It is associated with intact memory, and the delusions and hallucinations of schizophrenia are usually more complex and bizarre than those of dementia. Some individuals with chronic schizophrenia develop an unexplained progressive dementia late in life that is not related to AD. Memory loss may also be part of a conversion reaction. In this situation, patients commonly complain bitterly of memory loss, but careful cognitive testing either does not confirm the deficits or demonstrates inconsistent or unusual patterns of cognitive problems. The patients' behavior and "wrong" answers to questions often indicate that they both understand the question and know the answer.

Clouding of cognition by chronic drug or medication use, often prescribed by physicians, is an important cause of dementia. Sedatives, tranquilizers, and analgesics used to treat insomnia, pain, anxiety, or agitation may cause confusion, memory loss, and lethargy, especially in the elderly. Discontinuation of such medication often improves mentation.

Approach to the Patient

The approach to the patient with dementia should always keep two major questions in the forefront: What is the most accurate diagnosis, and is there a treatable or reversible condition? A broad overview of this approach is shown in Table 26-3.

History The history should concentrate on the onset, duration, and tempo of the memory loss. Acute or subacute confusion may represent delirium and suggests intoxication, infection, or metabolic derangement. An elderly person with slowly progressive memory loss over several years is likely to have AD. Initial symptoms often are difficulty with managing money, driving, shopping, following instructions, or finding one's way around town. A change in personality with disinhibition and intact memory may suggest FTD. A history of sudden stroke with an irregular stepwise progression suggests multi-infarct dementia. Stroke is also commonly associated with a history of hypertension, atrial fibrillation, peripheral vascular disease, and diabetes. Rapid progression with rigidity and myoclonus suggests CJD. Seizures may indicate stroke or neoplasm. Trouble in walking may suggest PD or normal-pressure hydrocephalus, especially the latter when associated with bladder incontinence. A history of multiple sex partners or intravenous drug use may indicate CNS infection, especially with HIV. A history of recurrent head trauma could indicate chronic subdural hematoma, dementia pugilistica, or normal-pressure hydrocephalus. Alcoholism may suggest malnutrition and thiamine deficiency. A remote history of gastric surgery resulting in loss of intrinsic factor might indicate vitamin B_{12} deficiency. Certain occupations such as working in a battery or chemical factory might indicate heavy metal intoxication. Careful review of medication intake, especially of sedatives and tranquilizers, may raise the issue of chronic drug intoxication. A positive family history of dementia would be

Table 26-3 Evaluation of the Patient with Dementia

Routine Evaluation	Optional Focused Tests	Occasionally Helpful Tests
History	HIV	EEG
Physical examination	Chest x-ray	Parathyroid function
Laboratory tests	Lumbar puncture	Adrenal function
Thyroid function (TSH)	Liver function	Urine heavy metals
Vitamin B_{12}	Renal function	RBC sedimentation rate
Complete blood count	Urine toxin screen	Angiogram
Electrolytes	Psychometric testing	Brain biopsy
VDRL	Apolipoprotein E	SPECT
CT/MRI		

DIAGNOSTIC CATEGORIES

Reversible Causes	Irreversible/Degenerative Dementias	Psychiatric Disorders
Examples	Examples	Depression
Hypothyroidism	Alzheimer's	Schizophrenia
Thiamine deficiency	Pick's	Conversion reaction
Vitamin B_{12} deficiency	Huntington's	
Normal-pressure	Diffuse Lewy body disease	
hydrocephalus	Multi-infarct	
Chronic infection	Leukoencephalopathies	
Brain tumor	Parkinson's	
Drug intoxication		

Associated Treatable Conditions
Depression
Seizures
Insomnia
Agitation
Caregiver "burnout"
Drug side effects

elicited in HD, familial AD, and inherited FTD. The recent death of a loved one, insomnia, or poor appetite suggest depression.

Physical Examination A careful examination is essential to document the dementia, look for other signs of nervous system involvement, and search for clues suggesting other systemic disease. Cognitive function should be assessed in terms of orientation, recent and remote memory, and calculation. Many of the simple, commonly used bedside tests of cognitive function (such as serial 7s, digits forward and backward) are most useful when they are performed normally; this makes the diagnosis of dementia unlikely. Mistakes on these simple tests are more difficult to interpret and are of less diagnostic importance. Drawing a clock and the trail-making test are frequently used tests of immediate memory and visual-spatial abilities. The mini-mental status exam (MMSE) is an easily administered 30-points test of cognitive function (Table 26-4). It is used to quickly indicate a dementing process, provide a rough assessment of its severity, and follow progression of the illness. The MMSE is influenced by culture and education and is less useful in the early and late stages of dementia. Language function should be tested by the ability to read, write, comprehend, and name objects. Resting tremor, cogwheel rigidity, bradykinesia, and festinating gait indicate a parkinsonian syndrome. Gait ataxia or apraxia (inability to initiate and coordinate steps in a sequential fashion) suggests normal-pressure hydrocephalus. Confusion, sixth cranial nerve paresis, and ataxia suggests thiamine deficiency. Myoclonic jerks are present in CJD but also occur in AD. Hemiparesis or other focal neurologic deficits may occur in multiinfarct dementia or brain tumor. Bilateral hyperactive tendon reflexes, Babinski responses, and loss of vibration and position sensation suggest a myelopathy, such as occurs in vitamin B_{12} deficiency. Stocking-glove sensory loss and diminished tendon reflexes suggest a peripheral neuropathy, which could indicate underlying diabetes, vitamin deficiency, or heavy metal intoxication. Dry cool skin, hair loss, and bradycardia suggest hypothyroidism. Confusion associated with repetitive stereotyped movements may indicate ongoing seizure activity. Hearing impairment or visual loss may produce confusion and disorientation misinterpreted as dementia. Such sensory deficits are common in the elderly.

Laboratory Tests The use of multiple laboratory tests in the evaluation of dementia is controversial. The physician does not want to miss a treatable cause, yet no single treatable cause stands out as common; thus a screen must employ multiple different tests, each of

which has a low yield. Therefore, cost/benefit ratios are difficult to assess, and many laboratory screening algorithms for dementia discourage multiple tests. Nevertheless, even a test with only a 1 to 2% positive rate is probably worth undertaking if the alternative is missing a reversible or treatable cause of dementia. Table 26-3 lists most screening tests for dementia. Neuroimaging studies (CT and MRI) are especially controversial because of their cost. However, they are clearly of value to identify primary and secondary neoplasms, locate areas of infarction, or suggest normal-pressure hydrocephalus or diffuse white matter disease. They also lend support to the diagnosis of AD, especially if there is hippocampal atrophy in addition to diffuse cortical atrophy, and focal lobar atrophy may suggest FTD. However, attempts to relate cognition to neuroimaging measures of atrophy and white matter changes have shown only modest correlations. A diagnosis of AD is reached primarily by exclusion of other causes of dementia. (The indications for apolipoprotein E testing for AD are discussed in Chap. 362.) Serum levels of vitamin B_{12} and TSH, complete blood count, electrolyte measurements, and a VDRL test are reasonable routine screening measures because they detect treatable conditions. Lumbar puncture need not be done routinely in the evaluation of dementia but is indicated if CNS infection is a serious consideration, for example, in patients with delirium, fever, or nuchal rigidity. CSF levels of tau protein are increased and those of $A\beta$ amyloid are decreased in some patients with AD; however, the clinical usefulness of these changes is not yet clear. Formal psychometric testing is not necessary in every patient with dementia but can be used to document the severity of dementia, suggest psychogenic causes, and provide a semiquantitative method for following the disease course. EEG is rarely helpful except to suggest CJD (repetitive bursts of diffuse high voltage sharp waves) or an underlying nonconvulsive seizure disorder (epileptiform discharges). Brain biopsy (including meninges) is not commonly advised except to diagnose vasculitis, potentially treatable neoplasms, unusual infections (such as sarcoid), or in young persons where the diagnosis is in doubt. Angiography is not likely to be of use except when multiple strokes or cerebral vasculitis is a possible cause of the dementia.

℞ **TREATMENT** The two major goals of management are, first, to treat any correctable cause of the dementia and, second, to provide comfort and support to the patient and caregivers. Treatment of underlying causes might include thyroid replacement for hypothyroidism; vitamin therapy for thiamine and B_{12} deficiency; antibiotics for opportunistic infections; ventricular shunting for normal-pressure hydrocephalus; and appropriate surgical, radiation, and/or chemotherapy for CNS neoplasms. Removal of sedating or cognition-impairing drugs and medications is often beneficial. If the patient is depressed rather than demented (pseudodementia), the depression should be vigorously treated. Patients with degenerative diseases such as AD and HD may also be depressed, and that portion of their condition may respond to antidepressant therapy. Antidepressants should be used with caution in demented patients because they may produce delirium. Antidepressants that have a low incidence of cognitive side effects, such as selective serotonin reuptake inhibitors, and tricyclic antidepressants with low anticholinergic activity such as desipramine and nortriptyline, are advisable. Anticonvulsants are used to control seizures. Agitation, hallucinations, delusions, and confusion are difficult to treat. These behavioral problems represent major causes for nursing home placement and institutionalization. Drugs such as phenothiazines, resperidone, haloperidol, and benzodiazepines may ameliorate the behavior problems but have untoward side effects such as sedation, rigidity, and dyskinesias. Medications that may calm agitation and insomnia without worsening dementia include low-dose haloperidol (0.5 to 2 mg), trazodone, buspirone, and propranolol. Olanzapine is increasingly used for patients with hallucinations. When patients do not respond, it is usually a mistake to advance to higher doses or to use anticholinergics or sedatives (such as barbiturates or benzodiazepines).

Table 26-4 The Mini-Mental Status Examination

	Points
Orientation	
Name: season/date/day/month/year	5 (1 for each name)
Name: hospital/floor/town/state/country	5 (1 for each name)
Registration	
Identify three objects by name and ask patient to repeat	3 (1 for each object)
Attention and calculation	
Serial 7s; subtract from 100 (e.g., 93–86–79–72–65)	5 (1 for each subtraction)
Recall	
Recall the three objects presented earlier	3 (1 for each object)
Language	
Name pencil and watch	2 (1 for each object)
Repeat ''No ifs, ands, or buts''	1
Follow a 3-step command (e.g., ''Take this paper, fold it in half, and place it on the table'')	3 (1 for each command)
Write ''close your eyes'' and ask patient to obey written command	1
Ask patient to write a sentence	1
Ask patient to copy a design (e.g., intersecting pentagons)	1
Total	30

Cholinesterase inhibitors are being used to treat AD, and other drugs, such as estrogen, anti-inflammatory agents, and vitamin E are being investigated for the treatment or prevention of AD. These approaches are reviewed in Chap. 362.

A proactive approach has been shown to reduce the occurrence of delirium in hospitalized patients. This scheme includes frequent orientation, cognitive activities, sleep enhancement measures, vision and hearing aids, and correction of dehydration.

Nondrug behavior therapy has an important place in the management of dementia. The primary goal is to make the life of the patient with dementia comfortable, uncomplicated, and safe. Preparing lists, schedules, calendars, and labels can be helpful. It is also useful to stress familiar routines, short-term tasks, brief walks, and simple physical exercises. For many patients with dementia, the memory for facts is worse than that for routine activities, and they still may be able to take part in remembered physical activities such as walking, bowling, dancing, and golf. Patients with dementia usually object to losing control over familiar tasks such as driving, cooking, and handling finances. Attempts to help or take over may be greeted with complaints, depression, or anger. Hostile responses on the part of the caretaker are useless and sometimes harmful. Explanation, reassurance, distraction, and calm statements are more productive responses in this setting. Eventually, tasks such as finances and driving must be assumed by others, and the patient will conform and adjust. Safety is an important issue that includes not only driving but the environment of the kitchen, bathroom, and sleeping area. These areas need to be monitored, supervised, and made as safe as possible. A move to a retirement home, assisted-living center, or nursing home can initially increase confusion and agitation. Repeated reassurance, reorientation, and careful introduction to the new personnel will help to smooth the process. Provision of activities that are known to be enjoyable to the patient can be of considerable benefit. Attention should also be paid to frustration and depression in family members and caregivers. Caregiver guilt and burn-out are common. Family members often feel overwhelmed and helpless and may vent their frustrations on the patient, each other, and healthcare providers. Caregivers should be encouraged to take advantage of day-care facilities and respite breaks. Education and counseling about dementia are important. Local and national support groups can be of considerable help, such as the Alzheimer's Disease and Related Disorders Association.

BIBLIOGRAPHY

BOWEN J et al: Progression to dementia in patients with isolated memory loss. Lancet 349:763, 1998

CHUI H, ZHANG Q: Evaluation of dementia: A systematic study of the usefulness of the American Academy of Neurology's Practice Parameters. Neurology 49:925, 1997

COREY-BLOOD J et al: Diagnosis and evaluation of dementia. Neurology 45:211, 1995

DESMOND DW et al: Frequency and clinical determinants of Dementia after ischemic stroke. Neurology 54:1124, 2000

FLEMING KC, EVANS JM: Pharmacologic therapies in dementia. Mayo Clin Proc 70:1116, 1995

GALTON CJ et al: Atypical and typical presentations of Alzheimer's disease: A clinical, neuropsychological, neuroimaging and pathological study of 13 cases. Brain 123:484, 2000

INOUYE S et al: A multicomponent intervention to prevent delirium in hospitalized older patients. N Engl J Med 340:669, 1999

JIANG Y et al: Complementary neural mechanisms for tracking items in human working memory. Science 287:643, 2000

KAYE J: Diagnostic challenges in dementia. Neurology 51(Suppl 1):S45, 1998

MARTIN LM, FLEMING KC et al: Recognition and management of anxiety and depression in elderly patients. Mayo Clin Proc 70:999, 1995

MILNER B et al: Cognitive neuroscience and the study of memory. Neuron 20:445, 1998

PICCINI C et al: Treatable and reversible dementias: An update. J Neurol Sci 153:172, 1998

27   *Charles A. Czeisler, John W. Winkelman, Gary S. Richardson*

SLEEP DISORDERS

EEG electroencephalogram	NREM non-rapid-eye-movement
EMG electromyogram	RBD REM sleep behavior disorder
EOG electrooculogram	REM rapid-eye-movement
FDA Food and Drug	RLS restless legs syndrome
Administration	SCN suprachiasmatic nuclei
GABA γ-aminobutyric acid	SSRIs selective serotonin reuptake
LH luteinizing hormone	inhibitors
MSLT multiple sleep latency test	VLPO ventrolateral preoptic

Disturbed sleep is among the most frequent health complaints physicians encounter. More than one-half of adults in the United States experience at least intermittent sleep disturbances. For most, it is an occasional night of poor sleep and/or daytime sleepiness. However, at least 15 to 20% of adults report chronic sleep disturbance or misalignment of circadian timing, which can lead to serious impairment of daytime functioning. In addition, such problems may contribute to or exacerbate medical or psychiatric conditions. Thirty years ago, many such complaints were treated with hypnotic medications without further diagnostic evaluation. Since then, a distinct class of sleep and arousal disorders has been identified, and the field of sleep disorders medicine is now an established clinical discipline. However, most physicians still only receive, on average, 1 h of education in sleep disorders in their medical school curriculum.

PHYSIOLOGY OF SLEEP AND WAKEFULNESS

Most adults sleep 7 to 8 h per night, although the timing, duration, and internal structure of sleep vary among healthy individuals and as a function of age. At the extremes, infants and the elderly have frequent interruptions of sleep. In the United States, adults of intermediate age tend to have one consolidated sleep episode per day, although in some cultures sleep may be divided into a midafternoon nap and a shortened night sleep. Two principal neurobiologic systems govern the sleep-wake cycle: one that actively generates sleep and sleep-related processes and another that times sleep within the 24-h day. Either intrinsic abnormalities in these systems or extrinsic disturbances (environmental, drug- or illness-related) can lead to sleep or circadian rhythm disorders.

STATES AND STAGES OF SLEEP States and stages of human sleep are defined on the basis of characteristic patterns in the electroencephalogram (EEG), the electrooculogram (EOG—a measure of eye-movement activity), and the surface electromyogram (EMG) measured on the chin and neck. The continuous recording of this array of electrophysiologic parameters to define sleep and wakefulness is termed *polysomnography*.

Polysomnographic profiles define two states of sleep: (1) rapid-eye-movement (REM) sleep, and (2) non-rapid-eye-movement (NREM) sleep. NREM sleep is in turn subdivided into four stages, characterized by increasing arousal threshold and slowing of the cortical EEG. REM sleep is characterized by a low-amplitude, mixed-frequency EEG similar to that of NREM stage 1 sleep. The EOG shows bursts of REM similar to those seen during eyes-open wakefulness. Chin EMG activity is absent, reflecting the brainstem-mediated muscle atonia that is characteristic of that state.

ORGANIZATION OF HUMAN SLEEP Normal nocturnal sleep in adults displays a consistent organization from night to night (Fig. 27-1). After sleep onset, sleep usually progresses through NREM stages 1 to 4 within 45 to 60 min. Slow-wave sleep predominates in the first third of the night and comprises 15 to 25% of total nocturnal

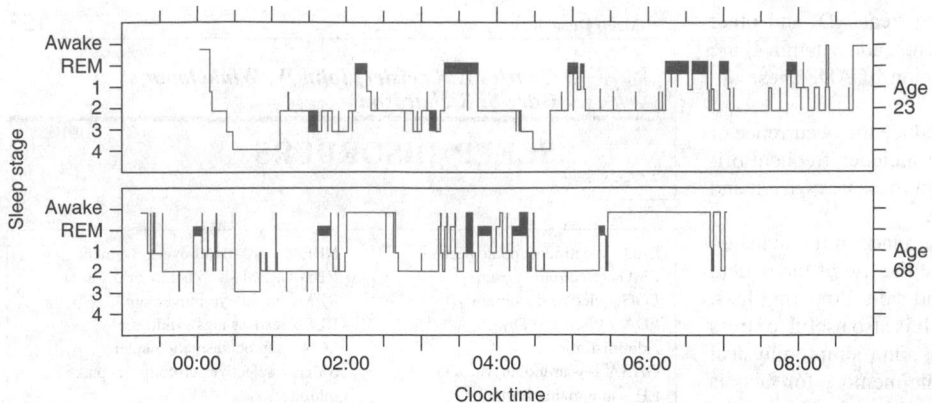

FIGURE 27-1 Plots of the stages of REM sleep (solid bars), the four stages of NREM sleep, and wakefulness over the course of the entire night for representative young (*upper panel*, age 23) and older (*lower panel*, age 68) adult men. The recording in the older subject illustrates the reduction of slow-wave sleep, frequent spontaneous awakenings, early sleep onset, and early morning awakening that are characteristic features of sleep in older people, even in the absence of specific medical or psychiatric pathology. (*From the Circadian, Neuroendocrine, and Sleep Disorders Section, Endocrine Division, Brigham and Womens' Hospital.*)

sleep time in young adults. The percentage of slow-wave sleep is influenced by several factors, most notably age (see below). Prior sleep deprivation increases the rapidity of sleep onset and both the intensity and amount of slow-wave sleep.

The first REM sleep episode usually occurs in the second hour of sleep. More rapid onset of REM sleep in a young adult (particularly if less than 30 min) may suggest pathology such as endogenous depression, narcolepsy, circadian rhythm disorders, or drug withdrawal. NREM and REM alternate through the night with an average period of 90 to 110 min (the "ultradian" sleep cycle). Overall, REM sleep constitutes 20 to 25% of total sleep, and NREM stages 1 and 2 are 50 to 60% (increasing in elderly subjects).

Age has a profound impact on sleep state organization (Fig. 27-1). Slow-wave sleep is most intense and prominent during childhood, decreasing sharply at puberty and across the second and third decades of life. After age 30, there is a progressive, almost linear decline in the amount of slow-wave sleep, and the amplitude of delta EEG activity comprising slow-wave sleep is reduced. In the otherwise healthy older person, slow-wave sleep may be completely absent, particularly in males.

A different age profile exists for REM sleep. In infancy, REM sleep may comprise 50% of total sleep time, and the percentage is inversely proportional to developmental age. The amount of REM sleep falls off sharply over the first postnatal year as a mature REM-NREM cycle develops. During the rest of life into extreme old age, REM sleep occupies a relatively constant percentage of total sleep time.

NEUROANATOMY OF SLEEP Lesion studies in animals and neurologic diseases in humans have suggested distinct neuroanatomic sites in the generation of normal sleep and wakefulness. Experimental studies in animals have variously implicated the medullary reticular formation, the thalamus, and the basal forebrain in the generation of sleep, while the brainstem reticular formation, the midbrain, the subthalamus, the thalamus, and the basal forebrain have all been suggested to play a role in the generation of wakefulness or EEG arousal (Chap. 24).

Current hypotheses suggest that the capacity for sleep and wakefulness generation is distributed along an axial "core" of neurons extending from the brainstem rostrally to the basal forebrain. Complex commingling of neuronal groups occurs at many points along this brainstem-forebrain axis. It was recently discovered that a cluster of γ-aminobutyric acid (GABA) and galaninergic ventrolateral preoptic (VLPO) neurons, which innervate monoaminergic cell groups in the tuberomammilary nucleus that contribute to the ascending arousal system, are activated during sleep. This has led to the hypothesis that

these hypothalamic VLPO neurons may play a key role in sleep regulation.

Moreover, the neuroanatomic correlates of REM sleep appear to be discretely localized. Specific regions in the pons are associated with the neurophysiologic correlates of REM sleep. Small lesions in the dorsal pons result in the loss of the descending muscle inhibition normally associated with REM sleep; microinjections of the cholinergic agonist carbachol into the pontine reticular formation appear to produce a state with all of the features of REM sleep. These experimental manipulations are mimicked by pathologic conditions in humans and animals. In narcolepsy, for example, abrupt, complete, or partial paralysis (cataplexy) occurs in response to a variety of stimuli. In dogs with this condition, physostigmine, a central cholinesterase inhibitor, increases the frequency of cataplectic attacks, while atropine decreases their frequency. Conversely, in REM sleep behavior disorder (see below), patients suffer from incomplete motor inhibition during REM sleep, resulting in involuntary, occasionally violent movement during REM sleep.

NEUROCHEMISTRY OF SLEEP Early experimental studies that focused on the raphe nuclei of the brainstem appeared to implicate serotonin as the primary sleep-promoting neurotransmitter, while catecholamines were considered to be responsible for wakefulness. Subsequent work has demonstrated that the raphe-serotonin system may facilitate sleep but is not necessary for its expression. Extensive pharmacologic studies of sleep and wakefulness suggest roles for other neurotransmitters as well. Cholinergic neurotransmission is known to play a role in REM sleep generation. The alerting influence of caffeine implicates adenosine, whereas the hypnotic effect of benzodiazepines and barbiturates suggests a role for endogenous ligands of the GABA$_A$ receptor complex.

A variety of sleep-promoting substances have been identified, although it is not known whether or not they are involved in the endogenous sleep-wake regulatory process. These include prostaglandin D$_2$, delta sleep–inducing peptide, muramyl dipeptide, interleukin 1, fatty acid primary amides, and melatonin. The hypnotic effect of these substances is commonly limited to NREM or slow-wave sleep, although peptides that increase REM sleep have also been reported. Many putative "sleep factors," including interleukin 1 and prostaglandin D$_2$, are immunologically active as well, suggesting a link between immune function and sleep-wake states.

PHYSIOLOGY OF CIRCADIAN RHYTHMICITY The sleep-wake cycle is the most evident of the many 24-h rhythms in humans. Prominent daily variations also occur in endocrine, thermoregulatory, cardiac, pulmonary, renal, gastrointestinal, and neurobehavioral functions. However, in evaluating a daily variation, it is important to distinguish between those rhythmic components passively evoked by periodic environmental or behavioral changes (e.g., the increase in blood pressure and heart rate upon assumption of the upright posture) and those actively driven by an endogenous oscillatory process (e.g., the circadian variation in plasma cortisol that persists under a variety of environmental and behavioral conditions).

The suprachiasmatic nuclei (SCN) of the hypothalamus act as the central neural pacemaker driving endogenous circadian rhythms in mammals. Bilateral destruction of these nuclei results in a loss of endogenous circadian rhythmicity that can only be restored by transplantation of the same structure from a donor animal. The genetically determined period of this endogenous neural oscillator, which averages ~24.2 h in humans, is normally synchronized to the 24-h period of the environmental light-dark cycle. Entrainment of mammalian circadian rhythms by the light-dark cycle is mediated via the retinohypothalamic tract, a monosynaptic pathway that links the retina to the SCN. Humans are exquisitely sensitive to the resetting effects of light, even at low intensity.

The timing and internal architecture of sleep are directly coupled to the output of the endogenous pacemaker. Paradoxically, the endogenous circadian rhythms of sleep tendency, sleepiness, and REM sleep propensity all peak near the habitual wake time, just after the nadir of the endogenous circadian temperature cycle, whereas the circadian wake propensity rhythm peaks 1 to 3 h before the habitual bedtime. These rhythms are thus timed to oppose the homeostatic decline of sleep tendency during the habitual sleep episode and the rise of sleep tendency throughout the usual waking day, respectively. Misalignment of the output of the endogenous circadian pacemaker with the desired sleep-wake cycle can, therefore, induce insomnia, as well as decrements of alertness and neurobehavioral performance in night-shift workers and after jet lag.

BEHAVIORAL CORRELATES OF SLEEP STATES AND STAGES Polysomnographic staging of sleep correlates with behavioral changes during specific states and stages. During the transitional state between wakefulness and sleep (stage 1 sleep), subjects may respond to faint auditory or visual signals without "awakening." Furthermore, memory incorporation is inhibited at the onset of NREM stage 1 sleep, and individuals aroused from that transitional sleep stage frequently deny having been asleep. Such transitions occur spontaneously after chronic partial sleep deprivation (e.g., 4 to 6 h of sleep per night) and acute total sleep deprivation (e.g., 24 h of wakefulness), notwithstanding attempts to remain continuously awake (see "Shift-Work Sleep Disorder," below).

Awakenings from REM sleep are associated with recall of vivid dream imagery more than 80% of the time. The reliability of dream recall increases with REM sleep episodes occurring later in the night. Imagery may also be reported after NREM sleep interruptions, though these typically lack the detail and vividness of REM sleep dreams. The incidence of NREM sleep dream recall can be increased by selective REM sleep deprivation, suggesting that REM sleep and dreaming per se are not inexorably linked.

PHYSIOLOGIC CORRELATES OF SLEEP STATES AND STAGES All major physiologic systems are influenced by sleep. Changes in cardiovascular function include a decrease in blood pressure and heart rate during NREM, and particularly during slow-wave sleep. During REM sleep, phasic activity (bursts of eye movements) is associated with variability in both blood pressure and heart rate mediated principally by the vagus. Cardiac dysrhythmias may occur selectively during REM sleep. Respiratory function also changes (Chap. 263). In comparison to relaxed wakefulness, respiratory rate becomes more regular during NREM sleep (especially slow-wave sleep) and tonic REM sleep and becomes very irregular during phasic REM sleep. Minute ventilation decreases in NREM sleep out of proportion to the decrease in metabolic rate at sleep onset, resulting in a higher P_{CO_2}.

Endocrine function also varies with sleep. The most prominent changes are apparent in neuroendocrine parameters. Slow-wave sleep is associated with secretion of growth hormone, while sleep in general is associated with augmented secretion of prolactin. Sleep has a complex effect on the secretion of luteinizing hormone (LH): during puberty, sleep is associated with increased LH secretion, whereas sleep in the mature woman inhibits LH secretion in the early follicular phase of the menstrual cycle. Sleep onset (and probably slow-wave sleep) is associated with inhibition of thyroid-stimulating hormone and of the adrenocorticotropic hormone–cortisol axis, an effect that is superimposed on the circadian rhythms in the two systems.

The pineal hormone melatonin is secreted predominantly at night in both day- and night-active species, reflecting the direct modulation of pineal activity by the circadian pacemaker through a circuitous neural pathway from the SCN to the pineal gland. Melatonin secretion is not dependent upon the occurrence of sleep, persisting in individuals kept awake at night. In addition, exogenous melatonin increases sleepiness and may potentiate sleep when administered to good sleepers

attempting to sleep during daylight hours at a time when endogenous melatonin levels are low. However, there is little evidence to support the use of melatonin as a hypnotic in such individuals during nighttime hours, when endogenous melatonin levels are high and sleep is already consolidated. A large-scale, double-blind clinical trial is needed to evaluate the efficacy of melatonin as a sleep-promoting therapeutic for patients with insomnia.

Sleep is also associated with alterations of thermoregulatory function. NREM sleep is associated with an attenuation of thermoregulatory responses to either heat or cold stress, and animal studies of thermosensitive neurons in the hypothalamus document an NREM-sleep-dependent reduction of the thermoregulatory set-point. REM sleep is associated with complete absence of thermoregulatory responsiveness, effectively resulting in functional poikilothermy. However, the potential adverse impact of this failure of thermoregulation is blunted by inhibition of REM sleep by extreme ambient temperatures.

DISORDERS OF SLEEP AND WAKEFULNESS

Approach to the Patient

Patients may seek help from a physician because of one of several symptoms: (1) an acute or chronic inability to sleep adequately at night (insomnia); (2) chronic fatigue, sleepiness, or tiredness during the day; or (3) a behavioral manifestation associated with sleep itself. Complaints of insomnia or excessive daytime sleepiness should be viewed as symptoms (much like fever or pain) of underlying disorders. Knowledge of the differential diagnosis of these presenting complaints is essential to identify the underlying medical disorder. Only then can appropriate treatment, rather than nonspecific approaches (e.g., over-the-counter sleeping aids) be applied. Diagnoses of exclusion, such as primary insomnia, should be made only after other diagnoses have been ruled out. Table 27-1 outlines the diagnostic and therapeutic approach to the patient with a complaint of excessive daytime sleepiness.

A careful history is essential in the evaluation of the patient with a sleep complaint. In particular, the duration, severity, and consistency of the complaint are important, along with the patient's estimate—in the case of an insomnia complaint—of the consequences of reported sleep loss on subsequent waking function. Information from a friend or family member can be an invaluable aid in assessing the symptoms and the severity of the complaint for daytime functioning, as some patients may be unaware of, or will underreport, such potentially embarrassing symptoms as heavy snoring or falling asleep while driving.

Completion by the patient of a day-by-day sleep-work-drug log for at least 2 weeks can help the physician better understand the nature of the complaint. Work times and sleep times (including daytime naps and nocturnal awakenings) as well as drug and alcohol use, including caffeine and hypnotics, should be noted each day. The sleep times should be plotted to facilitate recognition of circadian rhythm sleep disorders such as delayed sleep phase syndrome (see below).

Polysomnography is necessary for the diagnosis of specific disorders such as narcolepsy and sleep apnea and may be of utility in other settings as well. In addition to the three electrophysiologic variables used to define sleep states and stages, the standard clinical polysomnogram includes measures of respiration (respiratory effort, air flow, and oxygen saturation), anterior tibialis EMG, and electrocardiogram. Evaluation of penile tumescence during nocturnal sleep can also help determine whether the cause of erectile dysfunction in a patient is psychogenic or organic (Chap. 51).

INSOMNIA Insomnia is the complaint of inadequate sleep; it can be classified according to the nature of sleep disruption and the duration of the complaint. The nature of the sleep disruption provides important information about the possible etiology of the insomnia and is also central to the selection of specific and appropriate treatment.

Table 27-1 Evaluation of the Patient with the Complaint of Excessive Daytime Somnolence

Findings on History and Physical Examination	Diagnostic Evaluation	Diagnosis	Therapy
Obesity, snoring, hypertension	Polysomnography with respiratory monitoring	Obstructive sleep apnea	Continuous positive airway pressure; ENT surgery (e.g., uvulopalatopharyngoplasty); dental appliance; pharmacologic therapy (e.g., protriptyline); weight loss; (see Chap. 264)
Cataplexy, hypnogogic hallucinations, sleep paralysis, family history	Polysomnography with multiple sleep latency test	Narcolepsy-cataplexy syndrome	Stimulants (e.g., methylphenidate, pemoline); REM-suppressant antidepressants (e.g., protriptyline); genetic counseling
Restless legs syndrome, disturbed sleep, predisposing medical condition (e.g., anemia or renal failure)	Polysomnography with bilateral anterior tibialis EMG	Periodic limb movements of sleep	Treatment of predisposing condition, if possible; dopamine agonists (e.g., levodopa-carbidopa); benzodiazepines (e.g., clonazepam)
Disturbed sleep, predisposing medical conditions (e.g., asthma) and/or predisposing medical therapies (e.g., theophylline)	Sleep-wake diary	Insomnias (see text)	Treatment of predisposing condition and/or change in therapy, if possible; behavioral therapy; short-acting benzodiazepine receptor agonist (e.g., zolpidem)

NOTE: ENT, ears, nose, throat; REM, rapid eye movement; EMG, electromyogram.

Insomnia is subdivided into difficulty falling asleep (*sleep onset insomnia*), frequent or sustained awakenings (*sleep maintenance insomnia*), early morning awakenings (*sleep offset insomnia*), or persistent sleepiness despite sleep of adequate duration (*nonrestorative sleep*). Similarly, the duration of the symptom is an important determinant of the nature of appropriate treatment. An insomnia complaint lasting one to several nights (within a single episode) is termed *transient insomnia*. Transient insomnia is typically the result of situational stress or a change in sleep schedule or environment (e.g., jet lag). *Short-term insomnia* lasts from a few days to 3 weeks. Disruption of this duration is usually associated with more protracted stress, such as recovery from surgery or short-term illness. *Long-term insomnia*, or *chronic insomnia*, lasts for months or years and, in contrast with short-term insomnia, requires a thorough evaluation of underlying causes (see below). Chronic insomnia is often a waxing and waning disorder, with spontaneous or stressor-induced exacerbations.

While an occasional night of poor sleep, typically in the setting of stress or excitement about external events, is both common and without lasting consequences, persistent insomnia can have important adverse consequences in the form of impaired daytime function and increased risk of injury due to accidents. There is also clear evidence of increased risk of the development of major depression with insomnia of at least 1 year's duration. In addition, there is emerging evidence that individuals with chronic insomnia have increased utilization of health care resources, even after controlling for comorbid medical and psychiatric disorders.

Extrinsic Insomnia A number of sleep disorders are the result of extrinsic factors that interfere with sleep. *Transient situational insomnia* can occur after a change in the sleeping environment (e.g., in an unfamiliar hotel or hospital bed) or before or after a significant life event, such as a change of occupation, loss of a loved one, illness, or anxiety over a deadline or examination. Increased sleep latency, frequent awakenings from sleep, and early morning awakening can all occur. Recovery generally occurs rapidly, usually within a few weeks. Treatment is usually symptomatic, with intermittent use of hypnotics and resolution of the underlying stress. *Inadequate sleep hygiene* is characterized by a behavior pattern prior to sleep and/or a bedroom environment that is not conducive to sleep. Noise and/or light in the bedroom can interfere with sleep, as can a bed partner with periodic limb movements during sleep or one who snores loudly. Clocks can heighten the anxiety about the time it has taken to fall asleep. Drugs that act on the central nervous system, large meals, vigorous exercise, or hot showers just before sleep may interfere with sleep onset. Many individuals participate in stressful work-related activities in the evening, producing a state incompatible with sleep onset. In preference to hypnotic medications, patients should be counseled to avoid stressful activities before bed, develop a soporific bedtime ritual, and to prepare and reserve the bedroom environment for sleeping. Consistent, regular rising times should be maintained daily, including weekends.

Psychophysiologic Insomnia Persistent *psychophysiologic insomnia* is a behavioral disorder in which patients are preoccupied with a perceived inability to sleep adequately at night. The sleep disturbance is often triggered by an emotionally stressful event; however, the poor sleep habits and beliefs about sleep acquired during the stressful period persist long after the initial incident. Such patients become hyperaroused by their own persistent efforts to sleep and/or the sleep environment, and the insomnia is a conditioned or learned response. They may be able to fall asleep more easily at unscheduled times (when not trying) or outside the home environment. Polysomnographic recording in patients with psychophysiologic insomnia reveals an objective sleep disturbance, often with an abnormally long sleep latency; frequent nocturnal awakenings; and an increased amount of stage 1 transitional sleep. Rigorous attention should be paid to sleep hygiene and correction of counterproductive, arousing behaviors before bedtime. Behavioral therapies are the treatment modality of choice for psychophysiologic insomnia, with only intermittent use of medications. When patients are awake longer than 20 min, they should read or perform other relaxing activities to distract themselves from insomnia-related anxiety. In addition, bedtime and waketime should be scheduled to restrict time in bed to be equal to their perceived total sleep time. This will generally produce sleep deprivation, greater sleep drive, and, eventually, better sleep. Time in bed can then be gradually expanded.

Medication-, Drug-, or Alcohol-Dependent Insomnia Disturbed sleep can result from ingestion of a wide variety of agents. Caffeine is perhaps the most common pharmacologic cause of insomnia. It produces increased latency to sleep onset, more frequent arousals during sleep, and a reduction in total sleep time for up to 8 to 14 h after ingestion. As few as three to five cups of coffee can significantly disturb sleep in some patients; therefore, a 1- to 2-month trial without caffeine should be attempted in patients with these symptoms. Similarly, alcohol and nicotine can interfere with sleep, despite the fact that many patients use them to relax and promote sleep. Although alcohol can increase drowsiness and shorten sleep latency, even moderate amounts of alcohol increase awakenings in the second half of the night. In addition, alcohol ingestion prior to sleep is contraindicated in patients with sleep apnea because of the inhibitory effects of alcohol on upper airway muscle tone. Acutely, amphetamines and cocaine suppress both REM sleep and total sleep time, which return to normal with chronic use. Withdrawal leads to a REM sleep rebound.

A number of prescribed medications can produce insomnia. Antidepressants, sympathomimetics, and glucocorticoids are common causes. In addition, severe rebound insomnia can result from the acute withdrawal of hypnotics, especially following the use of high doses of benzodiazepines with a short half-life. For this reason, hypnotic doses should be low to moderate, the total duration of hypnotic therapy should usually be limited to 2 to 3 weeks, and prolonged drug tapering is encouraged.

Altitude Insomnia Sleep disturbance is a common consequence of exposure to high altitude. Periodic breathing of the Cheyne-Stokes type occurs during NREM sleep about half the time at high altitude, with restoration of a regular breathing pattern during REM sleep. Both hypoxia and hypocapnia are thought to be involved in the development of periodic breathing. Frequent awakenings and poor quality sleep characterize altitude insomnia, which is generally worst on the first few nights at high altitude but may persist. Treatment with acetazolamide can decrease time spent in periodic breathing and substantially reduce hypoxia during sleep.

Restless Legs Syndrome (RLS) Patients with this sensory-motor disorder report a creeping or crawling dysesthesia deep within the calves or feet, or sometimes even in the upper extemities, that is associated with an irresistible urge to move the affected limbs. For most patients with RLS, the dysesthesias and restlessness are much worse in the evening or night compared to the daytime and frequently interfere with the ability to fall asleep. The disorder is exacerbated by inactivity and temporarily relieved by movement. In contrast, paresthesia secondary to peripheral neuropathy persists with activity. The severity of this chronic disorder may wax and wane with time and can be exacerbated by sleep deprivation, caffeine, and pregnancy. The prevalence is thought to be 5% of adults. Roughly one-third of patients will have multiple affected family members, possibly with an autosomal dominant pattern. Iron deficiency and renal failure may actually cause RLS, which is then considered secondary RLS. The symptoms of RLS are exquisitely sensitive to dopaminergic drugs (e.g., L-dopa or dopamine agonists). Narcotics, benzodiazepines, and certain anticonvulsants may also be of therapeutic value. Most patients with restless legs also experience periodic limb movement disorder during sleep, although the reverse is not the case.

Periodic Limb Movement Disorder *Periodic limb movement disorder*, previously known as *nocturnal myoclonus*, is the principal objective polysomnographic finding in 17% of patients with insomnia and 11% of those with excessive daytime somnolence (Fig. 27-2). It is often unclear whether it is an incidental finding or the cause of disturbed sleep. Stereotyped, 0.5- to 5.0-s extensions of the great toe and dorsiflexion of the foot recur every 20 to 40 s during NREM sleep, in episodes lasting from minutes to hours. Most such episodes occur during the first half of the night. The disorder occurs in a wide variety of sleep disorders (including narcolepsy, sleep apnea, REM sleep behavior disorder, and various forms of insomnia) and may be associated with frequent arousals and an increased number of sleep-stage transitions. The incidence increases with age: 44% of people over age 65 without a sleep complaint have >five periodic leg movements per hour of sleep. The pathophysiology is not well understood, though individuals with high spinal transections can exhibit periodic leg movements during sleep, suggesting the existence of a spinal generator. Polysomnography with bilateral surface EMG recording of the anterior tibialis is used to establish the diagnosis. Treatment options include dopaminergic medications or benzodiazepines.

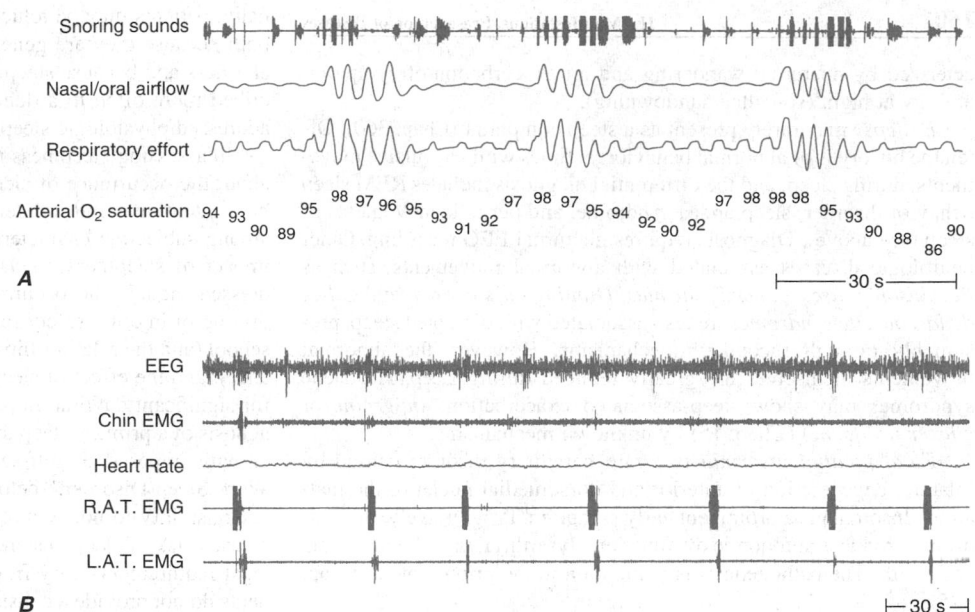

FIGURE 27-2 Polysomnographic recordings of a patient with (*A*) obstructive sleep apnea and one with (*B*) periodic limb movement of sleep. Note the snoring and reduction in air flow in the presence of continued respiratory effort, associated with the subsequent oxygen desaturation (upper panel). Periodic limb movements occur with a relatively constant intermovement interval and are associated with changes in the EEG and heart rates acceleration (lower panel). Abbreviations: R.A.T., right anterior tibialis; L.A.T., left anterior tibialis. (*From the Circadian, Neuroendocrine, and Sleep Disorders Section, Endocrine Division, Brigham and Womens' Hospital.*)

Insomnia Associated with Mental Disorders Approximately 80% of patients with psychiatric disorders describe sleep complaints. There is considerable heterogeneity, however, in the nature of the sleep disturbance both between conditions and among patients with the same condition.

Depression can be associated with sleep onset insomnia, sleep maintenance insomnia, and/or early morning wakefulness. However, hypersomnia occurs in some depressed patients, especially adolescents and those with either bipolar or seasonal (fall/winter) depression (Chap. 385). Indeed, sleep disturbance is an important vegetative sign of depression and may commence before any mood changes are perceived by the patient. Consistent polysomnographic findings in depression include decreased REM sleep latency, lengthened first REM sleep episode, and shortened first NREM sleep episode; however, these findings are not specific for depression, and the extent of these changes varies with age and symptomatology. Depressed patients also show decreased slow-wave sleep and reduced sleep continuity.

In *mania* and *hypomania*, sleep latency is increased and total sleep time can be reduced. Patients with *anxiety disorders* tend not to show the changes in REM sleep and slow-wave sleep seen in endogenously depressed patients. Finally, *chronic alcoholics* lack slow-wave sleep, have decreased amounts of REM sleep (as an acute response to alcohol), and have frequent arousals throughout the night. This is associated with impaired daytime alertness. The sleep of chronic alcoholics may remain disturbed for years after discontinuance of alcohol usage. Sleep architecture and physiology are disturbed in *schizophrenia* (with a decreased amount of stage 4 sleep and a lack of augmentation of REM sleep following REM sleep deprivation); chronic schizophrenics often show day-night reversal, sleep fragmentation, and insomnia.

Insomnia Associated with Neurologic Disorders A variety of neurologic diseases result in sleep disruption through both indirect, nonspecific mechanisms (e.g., pain in cervical spondylosis or low back pain) or by impairment of central neural structures involved in the generation and control of sleep itself.

For example, *dementia* from any cause has long been associated with disturbances in the timing of the sleep-wake cycle, often characterized by nocturnal wandering and an exacerbation of symptomatology at night (so-called sundowning).

Epilepsy may rarely present as a sleep complaint (Chap. 360). Often the history is of abnormal behavior, at times with convulsive movements, during sleep, and the differential diagnosis includes REM sleep behavior disorder, sleep apnea syndrome, and periodic movements of sleep (see above). Diagnosis requires nocturnal EEG recording. Other neurologic diseases associated with abnormal movements, such as *Parkinson's disease, hemiballismus, Huntington's chorea,* and *Gilles de la Tourette syndrome,* are also associated with disrupted sleep, presumably through secondary mechanisms. However, the abnormal movements themselves are greatly reduced during sleep. Headache syndromes may show sleep-associated exacerbations (*migraine* or *cluster headache*) (Chap. 15) by unknown mechanisms.

Fatal familial insomnia is a rare hereditary disorder caused by bilateral degeneration of anterior and dorsomedial nuclei of the thalamus. Insomnia is a prominent early symptom. Progressively, the syndrome produces autonomic dysfunction, dysarthria, myoclonus, coma, and death. The pathogenesis is a mutation in the prion protein (Chap. 375).

Insomnia Associated with Other Medical Disorders   A number of medical conditions are associated with disruptions of sleep. The association is frequently nonspecific, e.g., that between sleep disruption and chronic pain from rheumatologic disorders. Attention to this association is important in that sleep-associated symptoms are the presenting complaint of many such patients. Treatment of the underlying medical disorder or symptom is the most useful approach to such patients. As noted above, sleep disruption can also result from the appropriate use of drugs such as glucocorticoids.

Among the most prominent associations is that between sleep disruption and *asthma.* In many asthmatics there is a prominent daily variation in airway resistance that results in marked increases in asthmatic symptoms at night, especially during sleep. In addition, treatment of asthma with theophylline-based compounds, adrenergic agonists, or glucocorticoids can independently disrupt sleep. When sleep disruption is a prominent side effect of asthma treatment, inhaled steroids (e.g., beclomethasone) that do not disrupt sleep may provide a useful alternative.

Cardiac ischemia may also be associated with sleep disruption. The ischemia itself may result from increases in sympathetic tone as a result of sleep apnea. Patients may present with complaints of nightmares or vivid, disturbing dreams, with or without awareness of the more classic symptoms of angina or of the sleep disordered breathing. Treatment of the sleep apnea may substantially improve the angina and the nocturnal sleep quality. *Paroxysmal nocturnal dyspnea* can also occur as a consequence of sleep-associated cardiac ischemia that causes pulmonary congestion exacerbated by the recumbent posture.

Chronic obstructive pulmonary disease is also associated with sleep disruption, as is *cystic fibrosis, menopause, hyperthyroidism, gastroesophageal reflux, chronic renal failure,* and *liver failure.*

EVALUATION OF DAYTIME SLEEPINESS   Daytime impairment due to sleep loss may be difficult to quantify in the clinical setting for several reasons. First, sleepiness is not necessarily proportional to subjectively assessed sleep deprivation. In obstructive sleep apnea, for example, the repeated brief interruptions of sleep associated with resumption of respiration at the end of apneic episodes result in significant waking impairment, despite the fact that the patient may be unaware of the sleep fragmentation. Second, subjective descriptions of waking impairment vary from patient to patient. Patients may describe themselves as "sleepy," "fatigued," or "tired" and may have a clear sense of the meaning of those terms, while others may use the same terms to describe a completely different condition. Third, sleepiness, particularly when profound, may affect judgment in a manner analogous to ethanol, such that subjective awareness of the condition and the consequent cognitive and motor impairment is reduced. Fi-

nally, patients may be reluctant to admit that sleepiness is a problem, both because they are generally unaware of what constitutes normal alertness and because sleepiness is generally viewed pejoratively, ascribed more often to a deficit in motivation than to an inadequately addressed physiologic sleep need.

In assessing sleepiness in the clinical setting, specific questioning about the occurrence of sleep episodes during normal waking hours, both intentional and unintentional, can overcome the inconsistencies among subjective characterizations and help to interpret the adverse impact of sleepiness on daytime function. Specific areas to be addressed include the occurrence of inadvertent sleep episodes while driving or in other safety-related settings, sleepiness while at work or school (and the relationship of sleepiness to work and school performance), and the effect of sleepiness on social and family life. Evidence for significant daytime impairment [in association either with the diagnosis of a primary sleep disorder, such as narcolepsy or sleep apnea, or with imposed or self-selected sleep-wake schedules (see "Shift-Work Sleep Disorder," below)] raises the question of the physician's responsibility to notify motor vehicle licensing authorities of the increased risk of sleepiness-related vehicle accidents. As with epilepsy, legal requirements vary from state to state, and existing legal precedents do not provide a consistent interpretation of the balance between the physician's responsibility and the patient's right to privacy. At a minimum, physicians should document discussions with the patient regarding the increased risk of operating a vehicle, as well as a recommendation that driving be suspended until successful treatment or schedule modification can be instituted.

The distinction between fatigue and sleepiness can be useful in the differentiation of patients with complaints of fatigue or tiredness in the setting of disorders such as fibromyalgia, chronic fatigue syndrome (Chap. 384), or endocrine deficiencies such as hypothyroidism or Addison's disease. While patients with these disorders can typically distinguish their daytime symptoms from the sleepiness that occurs with sleep deprivation, substantial overlap can occur. This is particularly true when the primary disorder also results in chronic sleep disruption (e.g., sleep apnea in hypothyroidism) or in abnormal sleep (e.g., fibromyalgia).

While clinical evaluation of the complaint of excessive sleepiness is usually adequate, objective quantification is sometimes necessary for diagnostic purposes or for the evaluation of treatment response. Assessment of daytime functioning as an index of the adequacy of sleep can be made with the multiple sleep latency test (MSLT), which involves repeated measurement of sleep latency (time to onset of sleep) under standardized conditions during a day following quantified nocturnal sleep. The average latency across four to six tests (administered every 2 h across the waking day) is taken as an objective measure of daytime sleep tendency. Disorders of sleep that result in pathologic daytime somnolence can be reliably distinguished with the MSLT. In addition, the multiple measurements of sleep onset may identify direct transitions from wakefulness to REM sleep that are suggestive of specific pathologic conditions (e.g., narcolepsy).

NARCOLEPSY   Narcolepsy is both a disorder of the ability to sustain wakefulness voluntarily and a disorder of REM sleep regulation (Table 27-2). The classic "narcolepsy tetrad" consists of excessive daytime somnolence plus three specific symptoms related to an intrusion of REM sleep characteristics (e.g., muscle atonia, vivid dream imagery) into the transition between wakefulness and sleep: (1) sudden weakness or loss of muscle tone without loss of consciousness, often elicited by emotion (cataplexy); (2) hallucinations at sleep onset (hypnogogic hallucinations) or upon awakening (hypnopompic hallucinations); and (3) muscular paralysis upon awakening (sleep paralysis). The severity of cataplexy varies, as patients may have two to three attacks per day or per decade. The extent and duration of an attack may also vary, from a transient sagging of the jaw lasting a few seconds to rare cases of flaccid paralysis of the entire voluntary musculature for up to 20 to 30 min. Symptoms of narcolepsy typically begin in the second decade, although the onset ranges from ages 5 to 50.

Table 27-2   Prevalence of Symptoms in Narcolepsy

Symptom	Prevalence, %
Excessive daytime somnolence	100
Disturbed sleep	87
Cataplexy	76
Hypnagogic hallucinations	68
Sleep paralysis	64
Memory problems	50

SOURCE: Modified from TA Roth, L Merlotti in SA Burton et al (eds), *Narcolepsy 3rd International Symposium: Selected Symposium Proceedings,* Chicago, Matrix Communications, 1989.

Once established, the disease is chronic without remissions. Secondary forms of narcolepsy have been described (e.g., after head trauma).

Narcolepsy affects about 1 in 4000 people in the United States and appears to have a genetic basis. Recently, two independent discoveries have revealed that hypothalamic neurons containing the neuropeptide orexin (hypocretin) may play an important role in the regulation of sleep/wakefulness: (1) a mutation in the orexin (hypocretin) receptor 2 gene has been associated with canine narcolepsy; and (2) orexin "knockout" mice that are genetically unable to produce this neuropeptide exhibit a phenotype, as assessed by behavioral and electrophysiologic criteria, that is similar to human narcolepsy. In addition, modafinil, a drug recently approved by the U.S. Food and Drug Administration (FDA) for the treatment of narcolepsy, activates orexin-containing neurons. However, the inheritance pattern of narcolepsy in humans is more complex than that of the canine model. A high rate of discordance in identical twins indicates that one or more nonheritable factors contributes to its development. First-degree relatives of narcoleptic patients nonetheless have about a 1% incidence of narcolepsy, much higher than the general population but much lower than is seen in the animal models. Of note, nearly all narcoleptics with cataplexy are positive for the human leukocyte antigen DQB*0106 (ordinarily found in 20 to 30% of the general population) (Chap. 306).

Diagnosis   Definition of the essential and distinctive features of narcolepsy has continued to evolve, and the diagnostic criteria continue to be a matter of debate. Certainly, objective verification of excessive daytime somnolence, typically with MSLT mean sleep latencies <8 min, is an essential if nonspecific diagnostic feature. Other conditions that cause excessive sleepiness, such as sleep apnea or chronic sleep restriction, must be rigorously excluded. The other objective diagnostic feature of narcolepsy is the presence of REM sleep in at least two of the naps during the MSLT. This excessive REM "pressure" is also manifested by the appearance of REM sleep immediately or within minutes after sleep onset in 50% of narcoleptic patients, a rarity in unaffected individuals maintaining a conventional sleep-wake schedule. The REM-related symptoms of the classic narcolepsy tetrad are variably present. There is increasing evidence that narcoleptics with cataplexy (one-half to two-thirds of patients) may represent a more homogeneous group than those without this symptom. However, a history of cataplexy can be difficult to establish reliably. Hypnogogic and hypnopompic hallucinations and sleep paralysis are often found in nonnarcoleptic individuals and may be present in only one-half of narcoleptics. Nocturnal sleep disruption is commonly observed in narcolepsy but is also a nonspecific symptom. Similarly, history of "automatic behavior" during wakefulness (a trance-like state during which simple motor behaviors persist) is not specific for narcolepsy and serves principally to corroborate the presence of daytime somnolence.

℞   **TREATMENT**   The treatment of narcolepsy is symptomatic. Somnolence is treated with stimulants. Methylphenidate has long been considered the drug of choice by most; the usual initial dose is 10 mg bid, increasing as needed to a maximum of 20 mg qid. Pemoline, frequently used as an alternative due to its longer half-life, may be less effective and has recently been associated with fatal hepatic failure in several children. Dextroamphetamine, 10 mg bid, and methamphetamine are also frequently used alternatives. Recently, modafinil, a novel wake-promoting agent, has been approved by the FDA for treatment of the excessive daytime somnolence in narcolepsy; the dose is 200–400 mg/d given as a single dose. It is a long-acting agent that may cause fewer side effects than other medications.

Treatment of the REM-related phenomena cataplexy, hypnogogic hallucinations, and sleep paralysis requires the potent REM sleep suppression produced by antidepressant medications. The tricyclic antidepressants [e.g., protriptyline (10–40 mg/d) and clomipramine (25–50 mg/d)] and the selective serotonin reuptake inhibitors (SSRIs) [e.g., fluoxetine (10–20 mg/d)] are commonly used for this purpose in the United States. Efficacy of the antidepressants is limited largely by anticholinergic side effects (tricyclics) and by sleep disturbance and sexual dysfunction (SSRIs). Adequate nocturnal sleep time and planned daytime naps (when possible) are important preventative measures in narcolepsy.

SLEEP APNEA SYNDROMES   Respiratory dysfunction during sleep is a common, serious cause of excessive daytime somnolence as well as of disturbed nocturnal sleep. An estimated 2 to 5 million people in the United States have a reduction or cessation of breathing for 10 to 150 s, from thirty to several hundred times every night during sleep. These episodes may be due to either an occlusion of the airway (*obstructive sleep apnea*), absence of respiratory effort (*central sleep apnea*), or a combination of these factors (*mixed sleep apnea*) (Fig. 27-2). Failure to recognize and treat these conditions appropriately may lead to: significant, and often disabling, impairment of daytime alertness; increased risk of sleep-related motor vehicle accidents; hypertension and other serious cardiovascular complications; and increased mortality. Sleep apnea is particularly prevalent in overweight men and in the elderly, yet it is estimated to remain undiagnosed in 80 to 90% of affected individuals. This is unfortunate since effective treatments are available. →*Readers are referred to Chap. 263 for a comprehensive review of the diagnosis and treatment of patients with these conditions.*

PARASOMNIAS   The term *parasomnia* refers to abnormal behaviors that arise from, or occur during, sleep. A continuum of parasomnias arise from NREM sleep, from brief confusional arousals to sleepwalking and night terrors. The presenting complaint is usually related to the behavior itself, but the parasomnias can disturb sleep continuity or lead to mild impairments in daytime alertness. Only one parasomnia is known to occur in REM sleep, i.e., REM sleep behavior disorder (RBD; see below).

Sleepwalking (Somnambulism)   Patients affected by this disorder carry out automatic motor activities that range from simple to complex. Individuals may leave the bed, walk, urinate inappropriately, eat, or exit from the house while remaining only partially aware. Full arousal may be difficult, and some patients may respond to attempted awakening with agitation or even violence. Sleepwalking arises from stage 3 or 4 NREM sleep and is most common in children and adolescents, when these sleep stages are most robust. Episodes are usually isolated but may be recurrent in 1 to 6% of patients. The cause is unknown, though it has a familial basis in roughly one-third of cases.

Sleep Terrors   This disorder, also called *pavor nocturnus,* occurs primarily in young children during the first several hours after sleep onset, in stages 3 and 4 of NREM sleep. The child suddenly screams, exhibiting autonomic arousal with sweating, tachycardia, and hyperventilation. The individual may be difficult to arouse and rarely recalls the episode on awakening in the morning. Recurrent attacks are rare, and treatment is usually by way of reassurance of parents. Both sleep terrors and sleepwalking represent abnormalities of arousal. In contrast, *nightmares* (dream anxiety attacks) occur during REM sleep and cause full arousal, with intact memory for the unpleasant episode.

REM Sleep Behavior Disorder   RBD is a rare condition that is distinct from other parasomnias in that it occurs during REM sleep. It primarily afflicts men of middle age or older, many of whom have a history of prior neurologic disease. In fact, over one-third of patients will go on to develop Parkinson's disease within 10 to 20 years. Presenting symptoms are of agitated or violent behavior during sleep, reported by a bed partner. In contrast to typical somnambulism, injury to patient or bed partner is not uncommon, and, upon awakening, the patient reports vivid, often unpleasant, dream imagery. The principal differential diagnosis is that of nocturnal seizures, which can be excluded with polysomnography. In RBD, seizure activity is absent on the EEG, and disinhibition of the usual motor atonia is observed in the EMG during REM sleep, at times associated with complex motor behaviors. The pathogenesis is unclear, but damage to brainstem areas mediating descending motor inhibition during REM sleep may be responsible. In support of this hypothesis are the remarkable similarities between RBD and the sleep of animals with bilateral lesions of the pontine tegmentum in areas controlling REM sleep motor inhibition. Treatment with clonazepam provides sustained improvement in almost all reported cases.

Sleep Bruxism   Bruxism is an involuntary, forceful grinding of teeth during sleep that affects 10 to 20% of the population. The patient is usually unaware of the problem. The typical age of onset is 17 to 20 years, and spontaneous remission usually occurs by age 40. Sex distribution appears to be equal. Treatment is dictated by the risk of dental injury. In many cases, the diagnosis is made during dental examination, damage is minor, and no treatment is indicated. In more severe cases, treatment with a rubber tooth guard is necessary to prevent disfiguring tooth injury. Stress management or, in some cases, biofeedback can be useful when bruxism is a manifestation of psychological stress. There are anecdotal reports of benefit using benzodiazepines.

Sleep Enuresis   Bedwetting, like sleepwalking and night terrors, is another parasomnia that occurs during slow-wave sleep in the young. Before age 5 or 6, nocturnal enuresis should probably be considered a normal feature of development. The condition usually improves spontaneously at puberty, has a prevalence in late adolescence of 1 to 3%, and is rare in adulthood. The age threshold for initiation of treatment depends on parental and patient concern about the problem. Persistence of enuresis into adolescence or adulthood may reflect a variety of underlying conditions. In older patients with enuresis a distinction must be made between primary and secondary enuresis, the latter being defined as bedwetting in patients who have been fully continent for 6 to 12 months. Treatment of primary enuresis is reserved for patients of appropriate age (older than 5 or 6 years) and consists of bladder training exercises and behavioral therapy. Urologic abnormalities are more common in primary enuresis and must be assessed by urologic examination. Important causes of secondary enuresis include emotional disturbances, urinary tract infections or malformations, cauda equina lesions, epilepsy, sleep apnea, and certain medications. Symptomatic pharmacotherapy is usually accomplished with intranasal desmopressin, or oral oxybutynin chloride or imipramine.

Miscellaneous Parasomnias   Other clinical entities fulfill the definition of a parasomnia in that they occur selectively during sleep and are associated with some degree of sleep disruption. Examples include *jactatio capitis nocturna* (nocturnal headbanging), sleep talking, nocturnal paroxysmal dystonia, and nocturnal leg cramps.

CIRCADIAN RHYTHM SLEEP DISORDERS

A subset of patients presenting with either insomnia or hypersomnia may have a disorder of sleep *timing* rather than sleep *generation*. Disorders of sleep timing can either be organic (i.e., due to an intrinsic defect in the circadian pacemaker or its input from entraining stimuli) or environmental (i.e., due to a disruption of exposure to entraining

stimuli from the environment). Regardless of etiology, the symptoms reflect the influence of the underlying circadian pacemaker on sleep-wake function. Thus, effective therapeutic approaches should aim to entrain the oscillator at an appropriate phase.

RAPID TIME-ZONE CHANGE (JET LAG) SYNDROME More than 60 million people experience transmeridian air travel annually, which is often associated with excessive daytime sleepiness, sleep onset insomnia, and frequent arousals from sleep, particularly in the latter half of the night. Gastrointestinal discomfort is common. The syndrome is transient, typically lasting 2 to 14 d depending on the number of time zones crossed, the direction of travel, and the traveler's age and phase-shifting capacity. Travelers who spend more time outdoors reportedly adapt more quickly than those who remain in hotel rooms, presumably due to bright (outdoor) light exposure.

SHIFT-WORK SLEEP DISORDER   More than 7 million workers in the United States regularly work at night, either on a permanent or rotating schedule. In addition, each week millions of Americans elect to remain awake at night to meet deadlines, drive long distances, or participate in recreational activities, leading to both sleep loss and misalignment of their circadian rhythms with respect to their sleep-wake cycle. Chronic shift workers have higher rates of cardiac, gastrointestinal, and reproductive disorders. Studies of regular night-shift workers indicate that the circadian timing system usually fails to adapt successfully to such inverted schedules. This leads to a misalignment between the desired work-rest schedule and the output of the pacemaker and in disturbed daytime sleep. Consequent sleep deprivation, increased length of time awake prior to work, and misalignment of circadian phase produce decreased alertness and performance, increased reaction time, and increased risk of performance lapses, thereby resulting in greater safety hazards among night workers and other sleep-deprived individuals.

Sleep onset is associated with marked attenuation in perception of both auditory and visual stimuli and lapses of consciousness. The sleepy individual may thus attempt to perform routine and familiar motor tasks during the transition state between wakefulness and sleep (stage 1 sleep) in the absence of adequate sensory input from the environment. Motor vehicle operators are especially vulnerable to sleep-related accidents since the sleep-deprived driver or operator often fails to heed the warning signs of fatigue. Such attempts to override the powerful biologic drive for sleep by the sheer force of will can yield a catastrophic outcome when sleep processes intrude involuntarily upon the waking brain. Such intrusions typically last only seconds but are known on occasion to persist for longer durations. These frequent brief intrusions of stage 1 sleep into behavioral wakefulness are a major component of the impaired psychomotor performance seen with sleepiness. Such intrusions and their associated performance lapses, which are preceded by a markedly increased subjective sense of sleepiness, will inevitably occur if the need for sleep is not satiated. There is a marked increase in the risk of sleep-related, fatal-to-the-driver highway crashes in the early morning and late afternoon hours, coincident with peaks in the daily rhythm of sleep tendency.

Safety programs should promote education about sleep and increase awareness of the hazards associated with night work and should be aimed at minimizing both circadian disruption and sleep deprivation. The work schedule should minimize: (1) exposure to night work, (2) the frequency of shift rotation so that shifts do not rotate more than once every 2 to 3 weeks, (3) the number of consecutive night shifts, and (4) the duration of night shifts. In fact, shift durations of greater than 18 h should be universally recognized as increasing the risk of sleep-related errors and performance lapses. Caffeine is undoubtedly the most widely used wake-promoting drug, but it cannot forestall sleep indefinitely and does not protect users from sleep-related performance lapses. Postural changes, exercise, and strategic placement of nap opportunities can sometimes temporarily reduce the risk of fatigue-related performance lapses. Properly timed exposure to bright light can facilitate rapid adaptation to night-shift work, where feasible. An adequate number of safe highway rest areas, shoulder rumble strips, and strict enforcement and compliance monitoring of hours-of-service policies are needed to reduce the risk of sleep-related transportation crashes. Such steps can lead to improvements in performance and to reduced accident rates both at work and on the roadways.

DELAYED SLEEP PHASE SYNDROME Delayed sleep phase syndrome is characterized by: (1) reported sleep onset and wake times intractably later than desired, (2) actual sleep times at nearly the same clock hours daily, and (3) essentially normal all-night polysomnography except for delayed sleep onset. Patients exhibit an abnormally delayed endogenous circadian phase, with the temperature minimum during the constant routine occurring later than normal. This delayed phase could be due to: (1) an abnormally long intrinsic period of the endogenous circadian pacemaker; (2) an abnormally reduced phase-advancing capacity of the pacemaker; or (3) an irregular prior sleep-wake schedule, characterized by frequent nights when the patient chooses to remain awake well past midnight (for social, school, or work reasons). In most cases, it is difficult to distinguish among these factors, since patients with an abnormally long intrinsic period are more likely to "choose" such late-night activities because they are unable to sleep at that time. Patients tend to be young adults. This self-perpetuating condition can persist for years and does not usually respond to attempts to reestablish normal bedtime hours.

Treatment methods involving bright-light phototherapy during the morning hours or melatonin administration in the evening hours show promise in these patients, although the relapse rate among such patients is very high.

ADVANCED SLEEP PHASE SYNDROME Advanced sleep phase syndrome is the converse of the delayed sleep phase syndrome and tends to occur in the elderly. Patients with this condition report excessive daytime sleepiness during the evening hours, when they have great difficulty remaining awake, even in social settings. The patients awaken from 3 to 5 A.M. each day, often several hours before their desired wake times. Although such patients have not been studied extensively, familial inheritance of this condition has been reported. Some of these patients may benefit from bright-light phototherapy during the evening hours, designed to reset the circadian pacemaker to a later hour.

NON-24-H SLEEP-WAKE DISORDER This condition can occur when the maximal phase-advancing capacity of the circadian pacemaker is not adequate to accommodate the difference between the 24-h geophysical day and the intrinsic period of the pacemaker in the patient. Alternatively, patients' self-selected exposure to artificial light may drive the circadian pacemaker to a longer than 24-h schedule. Affected patients are not able to maintain a stable phase relationship between the output of the pacemaker and the 24-h day. Such patients typically present with an incremental pattern of successive delays in sleep onsets and wake times, progressing in and out of phase with local time. When the patient's endogenous rhythms are out of phase with the local environment, insomnia coexists with excessive daytime sleepiness. Conversely, when the endogenous rhythms are in phase with the local environment, symptoms remit. The intervals between symptomatic periods may last several weeks to several months. Blind individuals unable to perceive light are particularly susceptible to this disorder. Melatonin administration has been reported to improve sleep, and in some cases even to induce synchronization of the circadian pacemaker.

MEDICAL IMPLICATIONS OF CIRCADIAN RHYTHMICITY Understanding the role of circadian rhythmicity in the pathophysiology of illness may lead to improvements in diagnosis and treatment. For example, prominent circadian variations have been reported in the incidence of *acute myocardial infarction*, *sudden cardiac death*, and *stroke*, the leading causes of death in the United States. Platelet aggregability is increased after arising in the early morning hours, coincident with the peak incidence of these cardiovascular events. A better understanding of the possible role of circadian rhythmicity in the acute destabilization of a chronic condition such as atherosclerotic disease could improve the understanding of the pathophysiology.

Diagnostic and therapeutic procedures may also be affected by the time of day at which data are collected. Examples include blood pressure, body temperature, the dexamethasone suppression test, and plasma cortisol levels. The timing of chemotherapy administration has been reported to have an effect on the outcome of treatment. Few physicians realize the extent to which routine measures are affected by the time (or sleep/wake state) when the measurement is made.

In addition, both the toxicity and effectiveness of drugs can vary during the day. For example, more than a fivefold difference has been observed in mortality rates following administration of toxic agents to experimental animals at different times of day. Anesthetic agents are particularly sensitive to time-of-day effects. Finally, the physician must be increasingly aware of the public health risks associated with the ever-increasing demands made by the duty-rest-recreation schedules in our round-the-clock society.

BIBLIOGRAPHY

ALDRICH MS: Diagnostic aspects of narcolepsy. Neurology 50:S2, 1998

CAJOCHEN C et al: EEG and ocular correlates of circadian melatonin phase and human performance decrements during sleep loss. Am J Physiol 277:R640, 1999

CHEMELLI RM et al: Narcolepsy in orexin knockout mice: Molecular genetics of sleep regulation. Cell 98:437, 1999

CHESSON A JR et al: Practice parameters for the evaluation of chronic insomnia. An American Academy of Sleep Medicine report. Standards of Practice Committee of the American Academy of Sleep Medicine. Sleep 23:237, 2000

CZEISLER CA et al: Exposure to bright light and darkness to treat physiologic maladaptation to night work. N Engl J Med 322:1253, 1990

—— et al: Stability, precision, and near-24-hour period of the human circadian pacemaker. Science 284:2177, 1999

DIJK D-J et al: Ageing and the circadian and homeostatic regulation of human sleep during forced desynchrony of rest, melatonin and temperature rhythms. J Physiol (Lond) 516:611, 1999

DUNLAP JC: Molecular bases for circadian clocks. Cell 96:271, 1999

FARNEY RJ, WALKER JM: Office management of common sleep-wake disorders. Med Clin North Am 79:391, 1995

FOGEL RB, WHITE DP: Obstructive sleep apnea. Adv Int Med 45:351, 2000

FRANKLIN KA et al: Sleep apnea and nocturnal angina. Lancet 345:1085, 1995

KRYGER MH et al (eds): *Principles and Practice of Sleep Medicine*, 3d ed. Philadelphia, Saunders, 2000

LIN L et al: The sleep disorder canine narcolepsy is caused by a mutation in the hypocretin (orexin) receptor 2 gene. Cell 98:365, 1999

MORIN CM et al: Behavioral and pharmacological therapies for late-life insomnia: A randomized controlled trial. JAMA 28:991, 1999

MONTPLAISIR J et al: Restless legs syndrome improved by pramipexole: A double-blind randomized trial. Neurology 52:938, 1999

OLSON EJ et al: Rapid eye movement sleep behavior disorder: Demographic, clinical and laboratory findings in 93 cases. Brain 123:331, 2000

REDLINE S, STROHL KP: Recognition and consequences of obstructive sleep apnea hypopnea syndrome. Clin Chest Med 19:1, 1998

SCHENCK CH, MAHOWALD MW: Long-term, nightly benzodiazepine treatment of injurious parasomnias and other disorders of disrupted nocturnal sleep in 170 adults. Am J Med 100:333, 1996

28 *Jonathan C. Horton*

DISORDERS OF THE EYE

THE HUMAN VISUAL SYSTEM

The visual system provides a supremely efficient means for the rapid assimilation of information from the environment to aid in the guidance of behavior. The act of seeing begins with the capture of images focused by the cornea and lens upon a light-sensitive membrane in the back of the eye, called the *retina*. The retina is actually part of the brain, banished to the periphery to serve as a transducer for the conversion of patterns of light energy into neuronal signals. Light is absorbed by photopigment in two types of receptors: rods and cones. In the human retina there are 100 million rods and 5 million cones. The rods operate in dim (scotopic) illumination. The cones function under daylight (photopic) conditions. The cone system is specialized for color perception and high spatial resolution. The majority of cones are located within the macula, the portion of the retina serving the central 10° of vision. In the middle of the macula a small pit termed the *fovea*, packed exclusively with cones, provides best visual acuity.

Photoreceptors hyperpolarize in response to light, activating bipolar, amacrine, and horizontal cells in the inner nuclear layer. After processing of photoreceptor responses by this complex retinal circuit, the flow of sensory information ultimately converges upon a final common pathway: the ganglion cells. These cells translate the visual image impinging upon the retina into a continuously varying barrage of action potentials that propagates along the primary optic pathway to visual centers within the brain. There are a million ganglion cells in each retina, and hence a million fibers in each optic nerve.

Ganglion cell axons sweep along the inner surface of the retina in the nerve fiber layer, exit the eye at the optic disc, and travel through the optic nerve, optic chiasm, and optic tract to reach targets in the brain. The majority of fibers synapse upon cells in the lateral geniculate body, a thalamic relay station. Cells in the lateral geniculate body project in turn to the primary visual cortex. This massive afferent retinogeniculocortical sensory pathway provides the neural substrate for visual perception. Although the lateral geniculate body is the main target of the retina, separate classes of ganglion cells project to other subcortical visual nuclei involved in different functions. The pupillary reflex is mediated by input to the pretectal olivary nuclei in the midbrain. These pretectal nuclei send their output to the ipsilateral and contralateral Edinger-Westphal nuclei of the oculomotor nuclear complex. Cells in the Edinger-Westphal nuclei provide parasympathetic innervation to the iris sphincter via an interneuron in the ciliary ganglion. Circadian rhythms are timed by a retinal projection to the suprachiasmatic nucleus. Visual orientation and eye movements are served by retinal input to the superior colliculus. Gaze stabilization and optokinetic reflexes are governed by a group of small retinal targets known collectively as the *brainstem accessory optic system*. Finally, there is a sizeable retinal projection to the pulvinar, a large thalamic visual nucleus of obscure function.

The eyes must be rotated constantly within their orbits to place and maintain targets of visual interest upon the fovea. This activity, called *foveation*, or looking, is governed by an elaborate efferent motor system. Each eye is moved by six extraocular muscles, supplied by cranial nerves from the oculomotor (III), trochlear (IV), and abducens (VI) nuclei. Activity in these ocular motor nuclei is coordinated by pontine and midbrain mechanisms for smooth pursuit, saccades, and gaze stabilization during head and body movements. Large regions of the frontal and parietooccipital cortex control these brainstem eye movement centers by providing descending supranuclear input.

Visual function can be disturbed in myriad ways. The eyes are mounted in a prominent position on the head, where they are vulnerable to trauma, exposure, and infection. Vision can be damaged by diseases intrinsic to the eye, such as glaucoma, cataract, or retinal detachment. Many neurologic diseases produce ocular symptoms, because extensive areas of the cortex, thalamus, cerebellum, and brainstem are devoted to visual perception or to the execution of eye movements. In genetic disorders, eye manifestations are common and often help the clinician to recognize a rare syndrome. Finally, the eyes are affected frequently by acquired systemic diseases.

The eye is a specialized organ, requiring unique optical instruments for proper examination. The slit lamp and ophthalmoscope proffer a beautiful, magnified view of the transparent anatomy of the eye and afford the only opportunity for direct inspection of blood vessels in a living subject. Some physicians do not acquire sufficient facility with these instruments to care for patients with eye problems. This is regrettable, for although it may be determined that a patient requires referral to an ophthalmologist, the initial evaluation of ocular symptoms lies within the purview of all physicians, and the assessment of visual acuity, pupils, eye movements, visual fields, and the fundi remain part of any general physical examination.

CLINICAL ASSESSMENT OF VISUAL FUNCTION

REFRACTIVE STATE In approaching the patient with reduced vision, the first step is to decide whether refractive error is responsible. In *emmetropia*, parallel rays from infinity are focused perfectly upon the retina. Sadly, this condition is enjoyed by only a minority of the population. In *myopia*, the globe is too long, and light rays come to a focal point in front of the retina. Near objects can be seen clearly, but distant objects require a diverging lens in front of the eye. In *hyperopia*, the globe is too short, and hence a converging lens is used to supplement the refractive power of the eye. In *astigmatism*, the corneal surface is not perfectly spherical, necessitating a cylindrical corrective lens. In recent years it has become possible to correct refractive error with the excimer laser by performing either LASIK (laser in situ keratomileusis) or PRK (photorefractive keratectomy) to alter the curvature of the cornea.

With the onset of middle age, *presbyopia* develops as the lens within the eye becomes unable to increase its refractive power to accommodate upon near objects. To compensate for presbyopia, the emmetropic patient must use reading glasses. The patient already wearing glasses for distance correction usually switches to bifocals. The only exception is the myopic patient, who may achieve clear vision at near simply by removing glasses containing the distance prescription.

Refractive errors usually develop slowly and remain stable after adolescence, except in unusual circumstances. For example, the acute onset of diabetes mellitus can produce sudden myopia because of fluid imbibition and swelling of the lens induced by hyperglycemia. Testing vision through a pinhole aperture is a useful way to screen quickly for refractive error. If the visual acuity is better through a pinhole than with the unaided eye, the patient needs a refraction to obtain best corrected visual acuity.

VISUAL ACUITY The Snellen chart is used to test acuity at a distance of 6 m (20 ft). For convenience, a scale version of the Snellen chart, called the Rosenbaum card, is held at 36 cm (14 in) from the patient (Fig. 28-1). All subjects should be able to read the 6/6 m (20/20 ft) line with each eye using their refractive correction, if any. Patients who need reading glasses because of presbyopia must wear them for accurate testing with the Rosenbaum card. If 6/6 (20/20) acuity is

ROSENBAUM POCKET VISION SCREENER

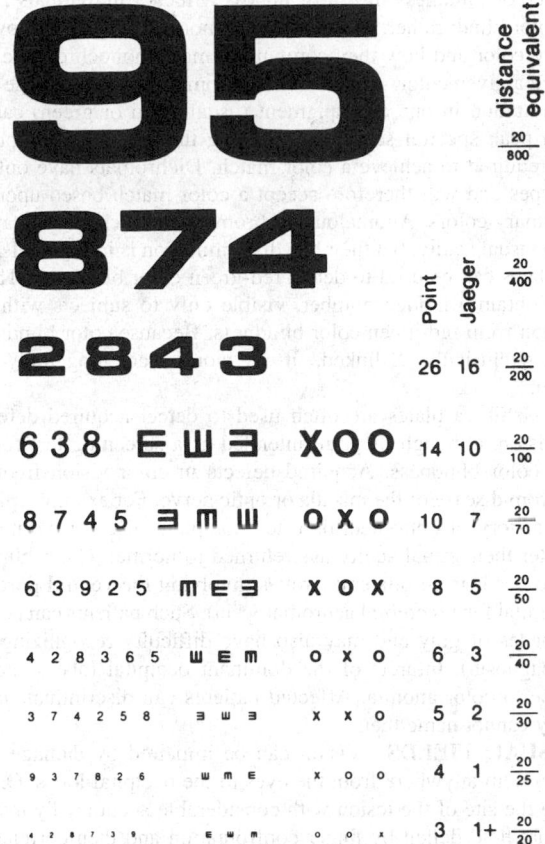

distance equivalent

		Point	Jaeger	
95				$\frac{20}{800}$
874				$\frac{20}{400}$
2843		26	16	$\frac{20}{200}$
638 EШƎ XOO		14	10	$\frac{20}{100}$
8745 ƎШШ OXO		10	7	$\frac{20}{70}$
63925 ШEƎ XOX		8	5	$\frac{20}{50}$
428365 ШEШ OXO		6	3	$\frac{20}{40}$
374258 ƎШШ XXO		5	2	$\frac{20}{30}$
937826 ШШE XOO		4	1	$\frac{20}{25}$
		3	1+	$\frac{20}{20}$

Card is held in good light 14 inches from eye. Record vision for each eye separately with and without glasses. Presbyopic patients should read thru bifocal segment. Check myopes with glasses only.

DESIGN COURTESY J. G. ROSENBAUM. M.D.

PUPIL GAUGE (mm.)

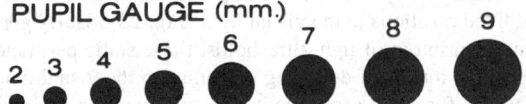

2 3 4 5 6 7 8 9

FIGURE 28-1 The Rosenbaum card is a miniature, scale version of the Snellen chart for testing visual acuity at near. When the visual acuity is recorded, the Snellen distance equivalent should bear a notation indicating that vision was tested at near, not at 6 m (20 ft), or else the Jaeger number system should be used to report the acuity.

not present in each eye, the deficiency in vision must be explained. For acuity worse than 6/240 (20/800), the ability to count fingers, see hand motions, or perceive a bright light should be recorded. Legal blindness is defined by the Internal Revenue Service as a best corrected acuity of 6/60 (20/200) or less in the better eye, or a binocular visual field subtending 20° or less. For driving the laws vary by state, but most require a corrected acuity of 6/12 (20/40) in at least one eye. Patients with a homonymous hemianopia should not drive.

PUPILS The pupils should be tested individually in dim light with the patient fixating upon a distant target. If they respond briskly to light, there is no need to check the near response, because isolated loss of constriction (miosis) to accommodation does not occur. For this reason, the ubiquitous abbreviation PERRLA (pupils equal, round, and reactive to light and accommodation) implies a wasted effort with the last step. However, it is important to test the near response if the light response is poor or absent. Light-near dissociation occurs with neurosyphilis (Argyll Robertson pupil), lesions of the dorsal midbrain (obstructive hydrocephalus, pineal region tumors), and after aberrant regeneration (oculomotor nerve palsy, Adie's tonic pupil).

An eye with no light perception has no pupillary response to direct light stimulation. If the retina or optic nerve is only partially injured, the direct pupillary response will be weaker than the consensual pupillary response evoked by shining a light into the other eye. This *relative afferent pupillary defect* (Marcus Gunn pupil) can be elicited with the swinging flashlight test (Fig. 28-2). It is an extremely useful sign in retrobulbar optic neuritis and other optic nerve diseases, where it may be the sole objective evidence for disease.

Subtle inequality in pupil size, up to 0.5 mm, is a fairly common finding in normal persons. The diagnosis of essential or physiologic anisocoria is secure as long as the relative pupil asymmetry remains constant as ambient lighting varies. Anisocoria that increases in dim light indicates a sympathetic paresis of the iris dilator muscle. The triad of miosis with ipsilateral ptosis and anhidrosis constitutes Horner's syndrome, although anhidrosis is an inconstant feature. Brainstem stroke, carotid dissection, or neoplasm impinging upon the sympathetic chain are occasionally identified as the cause of Horner's syndrome, but most of cases are idiopathic.

Anisocoria that increases in bright light suggests a parasympathetic palsy. The first concern is an oculomotor nerve paresis. This possibility is excluded if the eye movements are full and the patient has no ptosis or diplopia. Acute pupillary dilation (mydriasis) can occur from damage to the ciliary ganglion in the orbit. Common mechanisms are in-

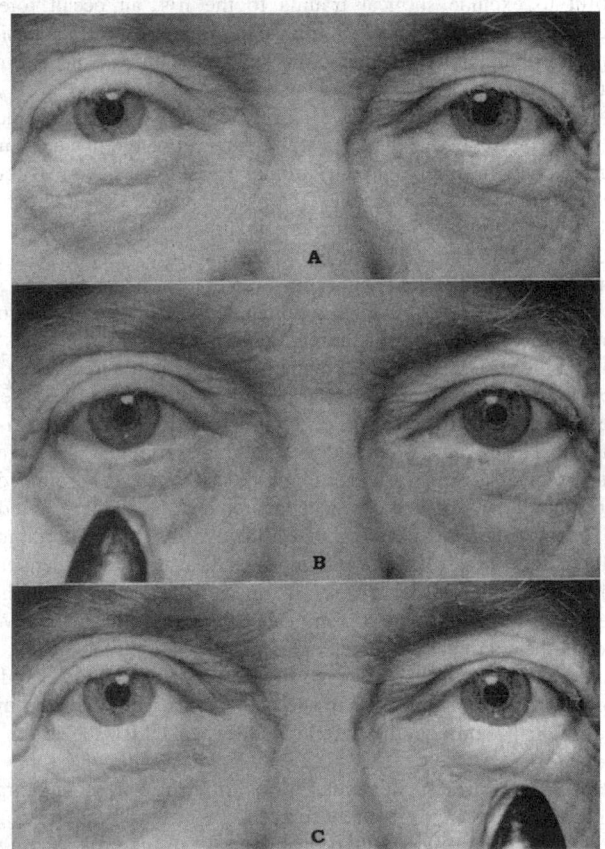

FIGURE 28-2 The swinging flashlight test shows a relative afferent pupil defect (Marcus Gunn pupil) in the left eye. *A.* With the patient fixating on a distant target and background lighting dim, the pupils are equal and relatively large. *B.* Shining a flashlight into the right eye evokes equal, strong constriction of both pupils. *C.* Swinging the flashlight over to the damaged left eye causes dilation of both pupils, although they remain smaller than in *A.* Swinging the flashlight back over to the healthy right eye would result in symmetric constriction back to the appearance shown in *B.* Note that the pupils always remain equal; the damage to the left retina/optic nerve is revealed by weaker bilateral pupil constriction to a flashlight in the left eye compared with the right eye. *(From P Levatin, Arch Ophthalmol 62:768, 1959.)*

fection (herpes zoster, influenza), trauma (blunt, penetrating, surgical), or ischemia (diabetes, temporal arteritis). After denervation of the iris sphincter the pupil does not respond well to light, but the response to near is often relatively intact. When the near stimulus is removed, the pupil redilates very slowly compared with the normal pupil, hence the term *tonic pupil*. In Adie's syndrome, a tonic pupil occurs in conjunction with weak or absent tendon reflexes in the lower extremities. This benign disorder, which occurs predominantly in healthy young women, is assumed to represent a mild dysautonomia. Tonic pupils are also associated with Shy-Drager syndrome, segmental hypohidrosis, diabetes, and amyloidosis. Occasionally, a tonic pupil is discovered incidentally in an otherwise completely normal, asymptomatic individual. The diagnosis is confirmed by placing a drop of dilute (0.125%) pilocarpine into each eye. Denervation hypersensitivity produces pupillary constriction in a tonic pupil, whereas the normal pupil shows no response. Pharmacologic dilation from accidental or deliberate instillation of anticholinergic agents (atropine, scopolamine drops) into the eye can also produce pupillary mydriasis. In this situation, normal strength (1%) pilocarpine causes no constriction.

Both pupils are affected equally by systemic medications. They are small with narcotic use (morphine, heroin) and large with anticholinergics (scopolamine). Parasympathetic agents (pilocarpine, demecarium bromide) used to treat glaucoma produce miosis. In any patient with an unexplained pupillary abnormality, a slit-lamp examination is helpful to exclude surgical trauma to the iris, an occult foreign body, perforating injury, intraocular inflammation, adhesions (synechia), angle-closure glaucoma, and iris sphincter rupture from blunt trauma.

EYE MOVEMENTS AND ALIGNMENT   Eye movements are tested by asking the patient with both eyes open to pursue a small target such as a penlight into the cardinal fields of gaze. Normal ocular versions are smooth, symmetric, full, and maintained in all directions without nystagmus. Saccades, or quick refixation eye movements, are assessed by having the patient look back and forth between two stationary targets. The eyes should move rapidly and accurately in a single jump to their target. Ocular alignment can be judged by holding a penlight directly in front of the patient at about 1 m. If the eyes are straight, the corneal light reflex will be centered in the middle of each pupil. To test eye alignment more precisely, the cover test is useful. The patient is instructed to gaze upon a small fixation target in the distance. One eye is covered suddenly while observing the second eye. If the second eye shifts to fixate upon the target, it was misaligned. If it does not move, the first eye is uncovered and the test is repeated on the second eye. If neither eye moves, the eyes are aligned orthotropically. If the eyes are orthotropic in primary gaze but the patient complains of diplopia, the cover test should be performed with the head tilted or turned in whatever direction elicits the patient's diplopia. With practice the examiner can detect an ocular deviation (heterotropia) as small as 1 to 2° with the cover test. Deviations can be measured by placing prisms in front of the misaligned eye to determine the power required to neutralize the fixation shift evoked by covering the other eye.

STEREOPSIS   Stereoacuity is determined by presenting targets with retinal disparity separately to each eye using polarized images. The most popular office tests measure a range of thresholds from 800 to 40 seconds of arc. Normal stereoacuity is 40 seconds of arc. If a patient achieves this level of stereoacuity, one is assured that the eyes are aligned orthotropically and that vision is intact in each eye. Random dot stereograms have no monocular depth cues and provide an excellent screening test for strabismus and amblyopia in children.

COLOR VISION   The retina contains three classes of cones, with visual pigments of differing peak spectral sensitivity: red (560 nm), green (530 nm), and blue (430 nm). The red and green cone pigments are encoded on the X chromosome; the blue cone pigment on chromosome 7. Mutations of the blue cone pigment are exceedingly

rare. Mutations of the red and green pigments cause congenital X-linked color blindness in 8% of males. Affected individuals are not truly color blind; rather, they differ from normal subjects in how they perceive color and how they combine primary monochromatic lights to match a given color. Anomalous trichromats have three cone types, but a mutation in one cone pigment (usually red or green) causes a shift in peak spectral sensitivity, altering the proportion of primary colors required to achieve a color match. Dichromats have only two cone types and will therefore accept a color match based upon only two primary colors. Anomalous trichromats and dichromats have 6/6 (20/20) visual acuity, but their hue discrimination is impaired. Ishihara color plates can be used to detect red-green color blindness. The test plates contain a hidden number, visible only to subjects with color confusion from red-green color blindness. Because color blindness is almost exclusively X-linked, it is worth screening only male children.

The Ishihara plates are often used to detect acquired defects in color vision, although they are intended as a screening test for congenital color blindness. Acquired defects in color vision frequently result from disease of the macula or optic nerve. For example, patients with a history of optic neuritis often complain of color desaturation long after their visual acuity has returned to normal. Color blindness can also occur from bilateral strokes involving the ventral portion of the occipital lobe (cerebral achromatopsia). Such patients can perceive only shades of gray and may also have difficulty recognizing faces (prosopagnosia). Infarcts of the dominant occipital lobe sometimes give rise to color anomia. Affected patients can discriminate colors, but they cannot name them.

VISUAL FIELDS   Vision can be impaired by damage to the visual system anywhere from the eyes to the occipital lobes. One can localize the site of the lesion with considerable accuracy by mapping the visual field deficit by finger confrontation and then correlating it with the topographic anatomy of the visual pathway (Fig. 28-3). More quantitative data can be obtained by formal perimetric examination of the visual fields. In kinetic perimetry, the patient faces a tangent screen or a hemispheric bowl (Goldmann perimeter) while the examiner moves a small light target from the periphery towards the center. Such manual techniques have largely been supplanted by computer-driven perimeters (Humphrey, Octopus) that present a target of variable intensity at fixed positions in the visual field (Fig. 28-3A). By generating an automated printout of light thresholds, these static perimeters provide a sensitive means of detecting scotomas in the visual field. They are also useful for serial assessment of visual function in chronic diseases such as glaucoma or pseudotumor cerebri.

The crux of visual field analysis is to decide whether a lesion is before, at, or behind the optic chiasm. If a scotoma is confined to one eye, it must be due to a lesion anterior to the chiasm, involving either the optic nerve or retina. Retinal lesions produce scotomas that correspond optically to their location in the fundus. For example, a superior-nasal retinal detachment results in an inferior-temporal field cut. Damage to the macula causes a central scotoma (Fig. 28-3B).

Optic nerve disease produces characteristic patterns of visual field loss. Glaucoma selectively destroys axons that enter the superotemporal or inferotemporal poles of the optic disc, resulting in arcuate scotomas shaped like a Turkish scimitar, which emanate from the blind spot and curve around fixation to end flat against the horizontal meridian (Fig. 28-3C). This type of field defect mirrors the arrangement of the nerve fiber layer in the temporal retina. The superb acuity of humans is achieved by thrusting aside all retinal elements at the fovea except photoreceptors, to minimize absorption and scattering of light. To avoid passing over the fovea, axons from cells in the temporal retina must follow an indirect course arching around the fovea to reach the optic disc. Arcuate or nerve fiber layer scotomas also occur from optic neuritis, ischemic optic neuropathy, optic disc drusen, and branch retinal artery or vein occlusion.

Damage to the entire upper or lower pole of the optic disc causes an altitudinal field cut that follows the horizontal meridian (Fig. 28-3D). This pattern of visual field loss is typical of ischemic optic

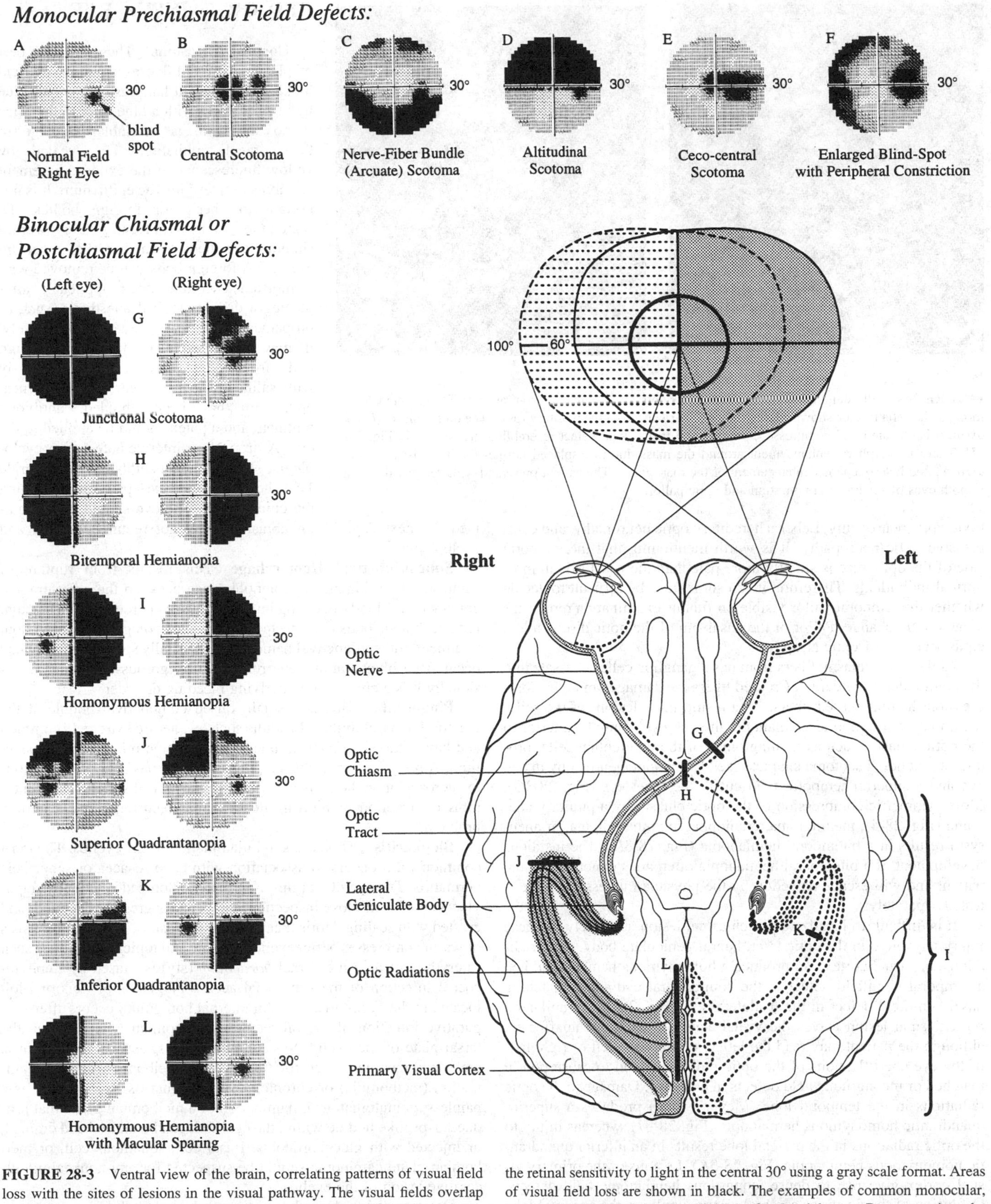

Monocular Prechiasmal Field Defects:

A — Normal Field Right Eye (blind spot) — 30°
B — Central Scotoma — 30°
C — Nerve-Fiber Bundle (Arcuate) Scotoma — 30°
D — Altitudinal Scotoma — 30°
E — Ceco-central Scotoma — 30°
F — Enlarged Blind-Spot with Peripheral Constriction — 30°

Binocular Chiasmal or Postchiasmal Field Defects:

(Left eye) (Right eye)

G — Junctional Scotoma — 30°
H — Bitemporal Hemianopia — 30°
I — Homonymous Hemianopia — 30°
J — Superior Quadrantanopia — 30°
K — Inferior Quadrantanopia — 30°
L — Homonymous Hemianopia with Macular Sparing — 30°

100° — 60°

Right   Left

Optic Nerve
Optic Chiasm
Optic Tract
Lateral Geniculate Body
Optic Radiations
Primary Visual Cortex

FIGURE 28-3 Ventral view of the brain, correlating patterns of visual field loss with the sites of lesions in the visual pathway. The visual fields overlap partially, creating 120° of central binocular field flanked by a 40° monocular crescent on either side. The visual field maps in this figure were done with a computer-driven perimeter (Humphrey Instruments, Carl Zeiss, Inc.). It plots the retinal sensitivity to light in the central 30° using a gray scale format. Areas of visual field loss are shown in black. The examples of common monocular, prechiasmal field defects are all shown for the right eye. By convention, the visual fields are always recorded with the left eye's field on the left, and the right eye's field on the right, just as the patient sees the world.

neuropathy but also occurs from retinal vascular occlusion, advanced glaucoma, and optic neuritis.

About half the fibers in the optic nerve originate from ganglion cells serving the macula. Damage to papillomacular fibers causes a cecocentral scotoma encompassing the blind spot and macula (Fig. 28-3E). If the damage is irreversible, pallor eventually appears in the temporal portion of the optic disc. Temporal pallor from a cecocentral scotoma may develop in optic neuritis, nutritional optic neuropathy,

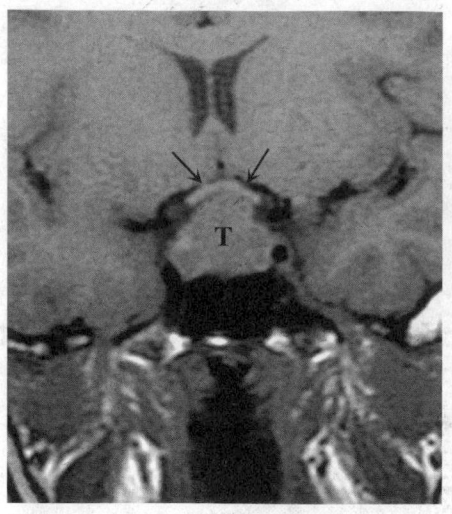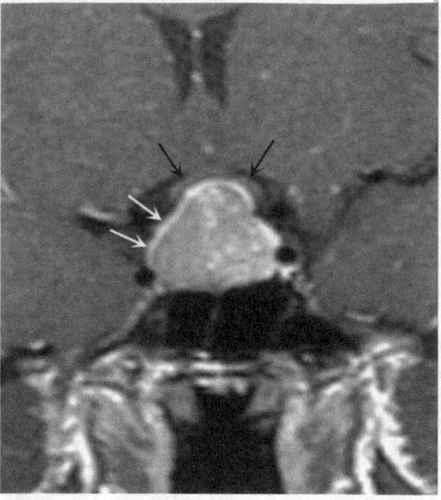

A   **B**

FIGURE 28-4 Pituitary adenoma: Coronal precontrast (*A*) and postcontrast (*B*) T1-weighted MRI through the sella turcica shows a large tumor (T) arising from the pituitary fossa. The optic chiasm (*black arrows*) is elevated and compressed, producing a visual field defect resembling that shown in Fig. 28-3*H*. There is peripheral enhancement around the mass due to displaced normal pituitary tissue (*white arrows*) and heterogeneous enhancement of the mass itself. The patient presented with decreased vision in both eyes of several years duration and optic pallor.

toxic optic neuropathy, Leber's hereditary optic neuropathy, and compressive optic neuropathy. It is worth mentioning that the temporal side of the optic disc is slightly more pale than the nasal side in most normal individuals. Therefore, it can sometimes be difficult to decide whether the temporal pallor visible on fundus examination represents a pathologic change. Pallor of the nasal rim of the optic disc is a less equivocal sign of optic atrophy.

At the optic chiasm, fibers from nasal ganglion cells decussate into the contralateral optic tract. Crossed fibers are damaged more by compression than uncrossed fibers. As a result, mass lesions of the sellar region cause a temporal hemianopia in each eye. Tumors anterior to the optic chiasm, such as meningiomas of the tuberculum sella, produce a junctional scotoma characterized by an optic neuropathy in one eye and a superior temporal field cut in the other eye (Fig. 28-3*G*). More symmetric compression of the optic chiasm by a pituitary adenoma (Fig. 28-4), meningioma, craniopharyngioma, glioma, or aneurysm results in a bitemporal hemianopia (Fig. 28-3*H*). The insidious development of a bitemporal hemianopia often goes unnoticed by the patient and will escape detection by the physician unless each eye is tested separately.

It is difficult to localize a postchiasmal lesion accurately, because injury anywhere in the optic tract, lateral geniculate body, optic radiations, or visual cortex can produce a homonymous hemianopia, i.e., a temporal hemifield defect in the contralateral eye and a matching nasal hemifield defect in the ipsilateral eye (Fig. 28-3*I*). A unilateral postchiasmal lesion leaves the visual acuity in each eye unaffected, although the patient may read the letters on only the left or right half of the eye chart. Lesions of the optic radiations tend to cause poorly matched or incongruous field defects in each eye. Damage to the optic radiations in the temporal lobe (Meyer's loop) produces a superior quandrantic homonymous hemianopia (Fig. 28-3*J*), whereas injury to the optic radiations in the parietal lobe results in an inferior quandrantic homonymous hemianopia (Fig. 28-3*K*). Lesions of the primary visual cortex give rise to dense, congruous hemianopic field defects. Occlusion of the posterior cerebral artery supplying the occipital lobe is a frequent cause of total homonymous hemianopia. Some patients with hemianopia after occipital stroke have macular sparing, because the macular representation at the tip of the occipital lobe is supplied by collaterals from the middle cerebral artery (Fig. 28-3*L*). Destruction of both occipital lobes produces cortical blindness. This condition can be distinguished from bilateral prechiasmal visual loss by noting that the pupil responses and optic fundi remain normal.

RED OR PAINFUL EYE

Corneal Abrasions These are seen best by placing a drop of fluorescein in the eye and looking with the slit lamp using a cobalt-blue light. A penlight with a blue filter will suffice if no slit lamp is available. Damage to the corneal epithelium is revealed by yellow fluorescence of the exposed basement membrane underlying the epithelium. It is important to check for foreign bodies. To search the conjunctival fornices, the lower lid should be pulled down and the upper lid everted. A foreign body can be removed with a moistened cotton-tipped applicator after placing a drop of topical anesthetic, such as proparacaine, in the eye. Alternatively, it may be possible to flush the foreign body from the eye by irrigating copiously with saline or artificial tears. If the corneal epithelium has been abraded, antibiotic ointment and a patch should be applied to the eye. A drop of an intermediate-acting cycloplegic, such as cyclopentolate hydrochloride 1%, helps to reduce pain by relaxing the ciliary body. The eye should be reexamined the next day. Minor abrasions may not require patching and cycloplegia.

Subconjunctival Hemorrhage This results from rupture of small vessels bridging the potential space between the episclera and conjunctiva. Blood dissecting into this space can produce a spectacular red eye, but vision is not affected and the hemorrhage resolves without treatment. Subconjunctival hemorrhage is usually spontaneous but can occur from blunt trauma, eye rubbing, or vigorous coughing. Occasionally it is a clue to an underlying bleeding disorder.

Pinguecula This is a small, raised conjunctival nodule at the temporal or nasal limbus. In adults such lesions are extremely common and have little significance, unless they become inflamed (pingueculitis). A *pterygium* resembles a pinguecula but has crossed the limbus to encroach upon the corneal surface. Removal is justified when symptoms of irritation or blurring develop, but recurrence is a common problem.

Blepharitis This refers to inflammation of the eyelids. The most common form occurs in association with acne rosacea or seborrheic dermatitis. The eyelid margins are usually colonized heavily by staphylococcus. Upon close inspection, they appear greasy, ulcerated, and crusted with scaling debris that clings to the lashes. Treatment consists of warm compresses, strict eyelid hygiene, and topical antibiotics such as erythromycin. An external *hordeolum* (sty) is caused by staphylococcal infection of the superficial accessory glands of Zeis or Moll located in the eyelid margins. An internal hordeolum occurs after suppurative infection of the oil-secreting meibomian glands within the tarsal plate of the eyelid. Systemic antibiotics, usually tetracyclines, are sometimes necessary for treatment of meibomian gland inflammation (meibomitis) or chronic, severe blepharitis. A *chalazion* is a painless, granulomatous inflammation of a meibomian gland that produces a pealike nodule within the eyelid. It can be incised and drained, or injected with glucocorticoids. Basal cell, squamous cell, or meibomian gland carcinoma should be suspected for any nonhealing, ulcerative lesion of the eyelids.

Dacrocystitis An inflammation of the lacrimal drainage system, this can produce epiphora (tearing) and ocular injection. Gentle pressure over the lacrimal sac evokes pain and reflux of mucus or pus from the tear puncta. Dacrocystitis usually occurs after obstruction of the lacrimal system. It is treated with topical and systemic antibiotics, followed by probing or surgery to reestablish patency. *Entropion* (inversion of the eyelid) or *ectropion* (sagging or eversion of the eyelid) can also lead to epiphora and ocular irritation.

Conjunctivitis This is the most common cause of a red, irritated eye. Pain is minimal, and the visual acuity is reduced only slightly. The most common viral etiology is adenovirus infection. It causes a watery discharge, mild foreign-body sensation, and photophobia. Bacterial infection tends to produce a more mucopurulent exudate. Mild cases of infectious conjunctivitis are usually treated empirically with broad-spectrum topical ocular antibiotics, such as sulfacetamide 10%, polymixin-bacitracin-neomycin, or trimethoprim-polymixin combination. Smears and cultures are usually reserved for severe, resistant, or recurrent cases of conjunctivitis. To prevent contagion, patients should be admonished to wash their hands frequently, not to touch their eyes, and to avoid direct contact with others.

Allergic Conjunctivitis This condition is extremely common and often mistaken for infectious conjunctivitis. Three forms of allergic conjunctivitis are recognized, with closely overlapping manifestations. *Hay fever conjunctivitis* has a seasonal incidence, related to the release of airborne antigens into the air by plants. IgE-mediated activation of mast cells in the conjunctiva causes itching, redness, and edema. *Vernal conjunctivitis* is also seasonal, becoming worse during warm months. It affects exclusively children or adolescents and is more common in boys. The cause is unknown, but airborne antigens are thought to trigger symptoms. Itching, photophobia, epiphora, and mucous discharge are typical. The palpebral conjunctiva may become hypertropic with giant excrescences called cobblestone papillae. Irritation from contact lenses or any chronic foreign body can also induce formation of cobblestone papillae. *Atopic conjunctivitis* occurs in subjects with atopic dermatitis or asthma. Symptoms caused by allergic conjunctivitis can be alleviated with cold compresses, topical vasoconstrictors, antihistamines, and mast-cell stabilizers such as cromolyn sodium. Topical glucocorticoid solutions provide dramatic relief of immune-mediated forms of conjunctivitis, but their long-term use is ill-advised because of the complications of glaucoma, cataract, and secondary infection. Topical nonsteroidal anti-inflammatory agents (NSAIDs) such as ketorolac tromethamine are a better alternative.

Keratoconjunctivitis Sicca Also known as dry eye, it produces a burning, foreign-body sensation, injection, and photophobia. In mild cases the eye appears surprisingly normal, but tear production measured by wetting of a filter paper (Schirmer strip) is deficient. A variety of systemic drugs, including antihistaminic, anticholinergic, and psychotropic medications, result in dry eye by reducing lacrimal secretion. Disorders that involve the lacrimal gland directly, such as sarcoidosis or Sjögren's syndrome, also cause dry eye. Patients may develop dry eye after radiation therapy if the treatment field includes the orbits. Problems with ocular drying are also common after lesions affecting cranial nerves V or VII. Corneal anesthesia is particularly dangerous, because the absence of a normal blink reflex exposes the cornea to injury without pain to warn the patient. Dry eye is managed by frequent and liberal application of artificial tears and ocular lubricants. In severe cases the tear puncta can be plugged or cauterized to reduce lacrimal outflow.

Keratitis This is a threat to vision because of the risk of corneal clouding, scarring, and perforation. Worldwide, the two leading causes of blindness from keratitis are trachoma from chlamydial infection and vitamin A deficiency related to malnutrition. In the United States, contact lenses play a major role in corneal infection and ulceration. They should not be worn by anyone with an active eye infection. In evaluating the cornea, it is important to differentiate between a superficial infection (*keratoconjunctivitis*) and a deeper, more serious ulcerative process. The latter is accompanied by greater visual loss, pain, photophobia, redness, and discharge. Slit-lamp examination shows disruption of the corneal epithelium, a cloudy infiltrate or abscess in the stroma, and an inflammatory cellular reaction in the anterior chamber. In severe cases, pus settles at the bottom of the anterior chamber, giving rise to a hypopyon. Immediate empirical antibiotic therapy should be initiated after corneal scrapings are obtained for Gram's stain, Giemsa stain, and cultures. Fortified topical antibiotics are most effective, supplemented with subconjunctival antibiotics as required. The most frequent bacterial pathogens are *Staphylococcus, Strepto-*

coccus (particularly *S. pneumoniae*), *Pseudomonas*, Enterobacteriaceae, *Haemophilus*, and *Neisseria*. For *Neisseria*, systemic antibiotics should be given in addition to topical antibiotics to eliminate systemic infection. A fungal etiology should always be considered in the patient with keratitis. Fungal infection is common in warm humid climates, especially after penetration of the cornea by plant or vegetable material.

Herpes Simplex The *herpes viruses* are a major cause of blindness from keratitis. Most adults in the United States have serum antibodies to herpes simplex, indicating prior viral infection (Chap. 182). Primary ocular infection is generally caused by herpes simplex type 1, rather than type 2. It manifests as a unilateral follicular blepharoconjunctivitis, easily confused with adenoviral conjunctivitis unless telltale vesicles appear on the periocular skin or conjunctiva. A dendritic pattern of corneal epithelial ulceration revealed by fluorescein staining is pathognomonic for herpes infection but is seen in only a minority of primary infections. Recurrent ocular infection arises from reactivation of the latent herpes virus. Viral eruption in the corneal epithelium may result in the characteristic herpes dendrite. Involvement of the corneal stroma produces edema, vascularization, and iridocyclitis. Herpes keratitis is treated with topical antiviral agents, cycloplegics, and oral acyclovir. Topical glucocorticoids are effective in mitigating corneal scarring but must be used with extreme caution because of the danger of corneal melting and perforation. Topical glucocorticoids also carry the risk of prolonging infection and inducing glaucoma.

Herpes Zoster Herpes zoster from reactivation of latent varicella (chickenpox) virus causes a dermatomal pattern of painful vesicular dermatitis. Ocular symptoms can occur after zoster eruption in any branch of the trigeminal nerve but are particularly common when vesicles form on the nose, reflecting nasociliary (V1) nerve involvement (Hutchinson's sign). Herpes zoster ophthalmicus produces corneal dendrites, which can be difficult to distinguish from those seen in herpes simplex. Stromal keratitis, anterior uveitis, raised intraocular pressure, ocular motor nerve palsies, acute retinal necrosis, and postherpetic scarring and neuralgia are other common sequelae. Herpes zoster ophthalmicus is treated with antiviral agents and cycloplegics. In severe cases, glucocorticoids may be added to prevent permanent visual loss from corneal scarring.

Episcleritis This is an inflammation of the episclera, a thin layer of connective tissue between the conjunctiva and sclera. Episcleritis resembles conjunctivitis but is a more localized process and discharge is absent. Most cases of episcleritis are idiopathic, but some occur in the setting of an autoimmune disease. *Scleritis* refers to a deeper, more severe inflammatory process, frequently associated with a connective tissue disease such as rheumatoid arthritis, lupus erythematosus, polyarteritis nodosa, Wegener's granulomatosis, or relapsing polychondritis. The inflammation and thickening of the sclera can be diffuse or nodular. In anterior forms of scleritis, the globe assumes a violet hue and the patient complains of severe ocular tenderness and pain. With posterior scleritis the pain and redness may be less marked, but there is often proptosis, choroidal effusion, reduced motility, and visual loss. Episcleritis and scleritis should be treated with NSAIDs. If these agents fail, topical or even systemic glucocorticoid therapy may be necessary, especially if an underlying autoimmune process is active.

Uveitis Involving the anterior structures of the eye, this is called *iritis* or *iridocyclitis*. The diagnosis requires slit-lamp examination to identify inflammatory cells floating in the aqueous humor or deposited upon the corneal endothelium (keratic precipitates). Anterior uveitis develops in sarcoidosis, ankylosing spondylitis, juvenile rheumatoid arthritis, inflammatory bowel disease, psoriasis, Reiter's syndrome, and Behçet's disease. It is also associated with herpes infections, syphilis, Lyme disease, onchocerciasis, tuberculosis, and leprosy. Although anterior uveitis can occur in conjunction with many diseases, no cause is found to explain the majority of cases. For this reason, laboratory evaluation is usually reserved for patients with recurrent or severe anterior uveitis. Treatment is aimed at reducing inflammation and scarring by judicious use of topical glucocorticoids. Dilation of the pupil reduces pain and prevents the formation of synechiae.

Posterior Uveitis   This is diagnosed by observing inflammation of the vitreous, retina, or choroid on fundus examination. It is more likely than anterior uveitis to be associated with an identifiable systemic disease. Some patients have panuveitis, or inflammation of both the anterior and posterior segments of the eye. Posterior uveitis is a manifestation of autoimmune diseases such as sarcoidosis, Behçet's disease, Vogt-Koyanagi-Harada syndrome, and inflammatory bowel disease (**see Plate IV-1**). It also accompanies diseases such as toxoplasmosis, onchocerciasis, cysticercosis, coccidioidomycosis, toxocariasis, and histoplasmosis; infections caused by organisms such as *Candida*, *Pneumocystis carinii*, *Cryptococcus*, *Aspergillus*, herpes, and cytomegalovirus (**see Plate IV-2**); and other diseases such as syphilis, Lyme disease, tuberculosis, cat-scratch disease, Whipple's disease, and brucellosis. In multiple sclerosis, chronic inflammatory changes can develop in the extreme periphery of the retina (pars planitis or intermediate uveitis).

Acute Angle-Closure Glaucoma   This is a rare and frequently misdiagnosed cause of a red, painful eye. Susceptible eyes have a shallow anterior chamber, either because the eye has a short axial length (hyperopia) or a lens enlarged by the gradual development of cataract. When the pupil becomes mid-dilated, the peripheral iris blocks aqueous outflow via the anterior chamber angle and the intraocular pressure rises abruptly, producing pain, injection, corneal edema, obscurations, and blurred vision. In some patients, ocular symptoms are overshadowed by nausea, vomiting, or headache, prompting a fruitless workup for abdominal or neurologic disease. The diagnosis is made by measuring the intraocular pressure during an acute attack or by performing gonioscopy to reveal the narrowed chamber angle by means of a specially mirrored contact lens. Acute angle closure is treated with oral or intravenous acetazolamide, topical beta blockers, apraclonidine, and pilocarpine to induce miosis. If these measures fail, a laser can be used to create a hole in the peripheral iris to relieve pupillary block. Many physicians are reluctant to dilate patients routinely for fundus examination because they fear precipitating an angle-closure glaucoma. The risk is actually remote and more than outweighed by the potential benefit to patients of discovering a hidden fundus lesion visible only through a fully dilated pupil. Moreover, a single attack of angle closure after pharmacologic dilation rarely causes any permanent damage to the eye and serves as an inadvertent provocative test to identify patients with narrow angles who would benefit from prophylactic laser iridectomy.

Endophthalmitis   This occurs from bacterial, viral, fungal, or parasitic infection of the internal structures of the eye. It is usually acquired by hematogenous seeding from a remote site. Chronically ill, diabetic, or immunosuppressed patients, especially those with a history of indwelling intravenous catheters or positive blood cultures, are at greatest risk for endogenous endophthalmitis. Although most patients have ocular pain and injection, visual loss is sometimes the only symptom. Septic emboli, from a diseased heart valve or a dental abscess, that lodge in the retinal circulation can give rise to endophthalmitis. White-centered retinal hemorrhages (Roth's spots) are considered pathognomonic for subacute bacterial endocardititis, but they also appear in leukemia, diabetes, and many other conditions. Endophthalmitis also occurs as a complication of ocular surgery, occasionally months or even years after the operation. An occult penetrating foreign body or unrecognized trauma to the globe should be considered in any patient with unexplained intraocular infection or inflammation.

TRANSIENT OR SUDDEN VISUAL LOSS

Amaurosis Fugax   This term refers to a transient ischemic attack of the retina. Because neural tissue has a high rate of metabolism,

interruption of blood flow to the retina for more than a few seconds results in *transient monocular blindness*, a term used interchangeably with amaurosis fugax. Patients describe a rapid fading of vision like a curtain descending, sometimes affecting only a portion of the visual field. Amaurosis fugax usually occurs from an embolus that becomes stuck within a retinal arteriole (**see Plate IV-3**). If the embolus breaks up or passes, flow is restored and vision returns quickly to normal without permanent damage. With prolonged interruption of blood flow, the inner retina suffers infarction. Ophthalmoscopy reveals zones of whitened, edematous retina following the distribution of branch retinal arterioles. Complete occlusion of the central retinal artery produces arrest of blood flow and a milky retina with a cherry-red fovea (**see Plate IV-4**). Emboli are composed of either cholesterol (Hollenhorst plaque), calcium, or platelet-fibrin debris. The most common source is an atherosclerotic plaque in the carotid artery or aorta, although emboli can also arise from the heart, especially in patients with diseased valves, atrial fibrillation, or wall motion abnormalities.

In rare instances, amaurosis fugax occurs from low central retinal artery perfusion pressure in a patient with a critical stenosis of the ipsilateral carotid artery and poor collateral flow via the circle of Willis. In this situation, amaurosis fugax develops when there is a dip in systemic blood pressure or a slight worsening of the carotid stenosis. Sometimes there is contralateral motor or sensory loss, indicating concomitant hemispheric cerebral ischemia.

Retinal arterial occlusion also occurs rarely in association with retinal migraine, lupus erythematosus, anticardiolipin antibodies (**see Plate IV-4**), anticoagulant deficiency states (protein S, protein C, and antithrombin III deficiency), pregnancy, intravenous drug abuse, blood dyscrasias, dysproteinemias, and temporal arteritis.

Amaurosis fugax warns of a patient at high risk for stroke. The carotid arteries should be studied by ultrasound. Endarterectomy for a stenosis of $\geq 60\%$, even in asymptomatic patients, has been shown to reduce the subsequent rate of ipsilateral stroke (Chap. 361). Therapy with aspirin, warfarin, or other anticoagulants is appropriate in selected patients. If no carotid lesion is found, cardiac ultrasound should be performed. Ambulatory electrocardiographic monitoring may reveal that intermittent atrial fibrillation is giving rise to emboli.

Marked *systemic hypertension* causes sclerosis of retinal arterioles, splinter hemorrhages, focal infarcts of the nerve fiber layer (cottonwool spots), and leakage of lipid and fluid (hard exudate) into the macula (**see Plate IV-5**). In hypertensive crisis, sudden visual loss can result from vasospasm of retinal arterioles and consequent retinal ischemia. In addition, acute hypertension may produce visual loss from ischemic swelling of the optic disc. Patients with acute hypertensive retinopathy should be treated by lowering the blood pressure. However, the blood pressure should not be reduced precipitously, because there is a danger of optic disc infarction from sudden hypoperfusion.

Impending *branch* or *central retinal vein occlusion* can produce prolonged visual obscurations that resemble those described by patients with amaurosis fugax. The veins appear engorged and phlebitic, with numerous retinal hemorrhages (**see Plate IV-6**). In some patients, venous blood flow recovers spontaneously, while others evolve a frank obstruction with extensive retinal bleeding ("blood and thunder" appearance), infarction, and visual loss. Venous occlusion of the retina is often idiopathic, but hypertension, diabetes, and glaucoma are prominent risk factors. The benefit of treatment with anticoagulants is unproven and carries the risk of hemorrhage into the vitreous. Polycythemia, thrombocythemia, or other factors leading to an underlying hypercoagulable state should be corrected.

Anterior Ischemic Optic Neuropathy (AION)   This is caused by insufficient blood flow through the posterior ciliary arteries supplying the optic disc. It produces sudden, painless, monocular visual loss, although patients occasionally report premonitory obscurations. The optic disc appears swollen and surrounded by nerve fiber layer splinter hemorrhages (**see Plate IV-7**). AION is divided into two forms: arteritic and nonarteritic. The nonarteritic form of AION is most common. No specific cause can be identified, although diabetes and hypertension are frequent risk factors. No treatment is available. About

5% of patients, especially those over age 60, develop the arteritic form of AION in conjunction with giant cell (temporal) arteritis (Chap. 317). It is urgent to recognize arteritic AION so that high doses of glucocorticoids can be instituted immediately to prevent blindness in the second eye. Symptoms of polymyalgia rheumatica may be present, and the sedimentation rate is usually elevated. In a patient with visual loss from suspected arteritic AION, temporal artery biopsy is helpful to confirm the diagnosis, but glucocorticoids should be started without waiting for the biopsy to be completed. The diagnosis of arteritic AION is difficult to sustain in the face of a normal sedimentation rate and a negative temporal artery biopsy, but such cases do occur rarely.

Posterior Ischemic Optic Neuropathy This is an infrequent cause of acute visual loss. It is induced by the combination of severe anemia and hypotension, causing infarction of the retrobulbar optic nerve. Cases have been reported after major blood loss during surgery, exsanguinating trauma, gastrointestinal bleeding, and renal dialysis. The fundus usually appears normal, although optic disc swelling develops if the process extends far enough anteriorly. Vision can be salvaged in some patients by prompt blood transfusion and reversal of hypotension.

Optic Neuritis This is a common inflammatory disease of the optic nerve. In the Optic Neuritis Treatment Trial (ONTT), the mean age of patients was 32 years, 77% were female, 92% had ocular pain (especially with eye movements), and 35% had optic disc swelling. In most patients, the demyelinating event was retrobulbar and the ocular fundus appeared normal on initial examination (see Plate IV-8), although optic disc pallor slowly developed over subsequent months.

Virtually all patients experience a gradual recovery of vision after a single episode of optic neuritis, even without treatment. This rule is so reliable that failure of vision to improve considerably after a first attack of optic neuritis casts doubt upon the original diagnosis. Treatment of optic neuritis is controversial because the favorable prognosis for visual recovery has made it difficult to demonstrate any benefit from glucocorticoids. The ONTT showed that patients treated with a conventional dose of oral glucocorticoids (prednisone, 1 mg/kg per day for 14 days) did no better than patients treated with a placebo. A recent Danish trial of oral high-dose methylprednisolone (500 mg daily for 5 days, followed by a 10-day taper) reported a slight response at 1 and 3 weeks but none at 8 weeks. From these studies, it is apparent that oral glucocorticoids have little to offer in the treatment of optic neuritis. According to the ONTT, even high-dose intravenous methylprednisolone (250 mg every 6 h for 3 days) followed by oral prednisone (1 mg/kg per day for 11 days) makes no difference in final acuity (measured 6 months after the attack), although the recovery of visual function occurs more rapidly.

For some patients, optic neuritis remains an isolated event. However, the ONTT showed that the 5-year cumulative probability of developing clinically definite multiple sclerosis following optic neuritis is 30%. Remarkably, intravenous glucocorticoids were associated with a reduced rate of development of multiple sclerosis over a 2-year follow-up period, especially in the subgroup of patients with multiple foci of demyelination on their magnetic resonance (MR) scan. However, by the end of a 3-year follow-up period, patients treated with intravenous glucocorticoids versus placebo showed no difference in the rate of multiple sclerosis. Moreover, intravenous glucocorticoids did not reduce the likelihood of subsequent attacks of optic neuritis. To summarize, the organizers of the ONTT recommend an MR scan in patients with optic neuritis. If two or more foci of demyelination are found or visual loss is severe, they suggest treatment with intravenous glucocorticoids. The potential benefits of intravenous glucocorticoids are: (1) a slightly faster recovery of visual function, and (2) a potential reduction in the risk of subsequent neurologic events that would signify multiple sclerosis. Critics of the ONTT have questioned these recommendations, pointing out that: (1) visual outcome is the same in the long run, (2) evidence indicating a reduced risk of eventual multiple sclerosis with intravenous glucocorticoid treatment is based upon follow-up data in a rather small number of patients, and (3) the protection against multiple sclerosis is transient, and no longer apparent beyond 2 years of follow-up. In cases of unilateral optic neuritis, the decision whether to obtain an MR scan or to treat with intravenous glucocorticoids should be based upon clinical judgment and careful discussion with the patient. In cases of bilateral, simultaneous optic neuritis, the rationale for intravenous glucocorticoids is stronger.

Leber's Hereditary Optic Neuropathy This is a disease of young men, characterized by onset over a few weeks of painless, severe, central visual loss in one eye, followed weeks or months later by the same process in the other eye. Acutely, the optic disc appears mildly plethoric with surface capillary telangiectases, but no vascular leakage on fluorescein angiography. Eventually optic atrophy ensues. There is no treatment. Leber's optic neuropathy is caused by a point mutation at codon 11778 in the mitochondrial gene encoding nicotinamide adenine dinucleotide dehydrogenase (NADH) subunit 4. Subsequently, additional mutations responsible for the disease have been identified, most in mitochondrial genes encoding proteins involved in electron transport. Mitochrondrial mutations causing Leber's neuropathy are inherited from the mother by all her children, but usually only sons develop symptoms. This curious male predilection is a mystery.

Toxic Optic Neuropathy This can result in acute visual loss with bilateral optic disc swelling and central or cecocentral scotomas. Such cases have been reported to result from exposure to ethambutol, methyl alcohol (moonshine), ethylene glycol (antifreeze), or carbon monoxide. In toxic optic neuropathy, visual loss can also develop gradually and produce optic atrophy without a phase of acute optic disc edema (see Plate IV-9). Many agents have been implicated as a cause of toxic optic neuropathy, but the evidence supporting the association for many is weak. The following is a partial list of potential offending drugs or toxins: disulfiram, ethchlorvynol, chloramphenicol, amiodarone, monoclonal anti-CD3 antibody, ciprofloxacin, digitalis, streptomycin, lead, arsenic, thallium, D-penicillamine, isoniazid, emetine, and sulfonamides. Deficiency states, induced either by starvation, malabsorption, or alcoholism, can lead to insidious visual loss. Thiamine, vitamin B_{12}, and folate levels should be checked in any patient with unexplained, bilateral central scotomas and optic pallor.

Papilledema This connotes bilateral optic disc swelling from raised intracranial pressure (see Plate IV-10). Headache is a frequent, but not invariable, accompaniment. All other forms of optic disc swelling, e.g., from optic neuritis or ischemic optic neuropathy, should be called "optic disc edema." This convention is arbitrary but serves to avoid confusion. Often it is difficult to differentiate papilledema from other forms of optic disc edema by fundus examination alone. Transient visual obscurations are a classic symptom of papilledema. They can occur in only one eye or simultaneously in both eyes. They usually last seconds but can persist for minutes if the papilledema is fulminant. Obscurations follow abrupt shifts in posture or happen spontaneously. When obscurations are prolonged or spontaneous, the papilledema is more threatening. Visual acuity is not affected by papilledema unless the papilledema is severe, long-standing, or accompanied by macular edema and hemorrhage. Visual field testing shows enlarged blind spots and peripheral constriction (Fig. 28-3F). With unremitting papilledema, peripheral visual field loss progresses in an insidious fashion while the optic nerve develops atrophy. In this setting, reduction of optic disc swelling is an ominous sign of a dying nerve rather than an encouraging indication of resolving papilledema.

Evaluation of papilledema requires computed tomography (CT) or MR imaging to exclude an intracranial lesion. MR angiography is appropriate in selected cases to search for a dural venous sinus occlusion or an arteriovenous shunt. If neuroradiologic studies are negative, the subarachnoid opening pressure should be measured by lumbar puncture. An elevated pressure, with normal cerebrospinal fluid, points by exclusion to the diagnosis of *pseudotumor cerebri* (idiopathic intracranial hypertension). The majority of patients are young, female, and obese. Treatment with a carbonic anhydrase inhibitor such as acetazolamide lowers intracranial pressure by reducing the production of cerebrospinal fluid. Weight reduction is vital but often unsuccessful.

If acetazolamide and weight loss fail, and visual field loss is progressive, lumboperitoneal shunting or optic nerve sheath fenestration should be undertaken without delay to prevent blindness. Occasionally, emergency surgery is required for sudden blindness caused by fulminant papilledema.

Optic Disc Drusen   These are refractile deposits within the substance of the optic nerve head (**see Plate IV-11**). They are unrelated to drusen of the retina, which occur in age-related macular degeneration. Optic disc drusen are most common in people of northern European descent, with an incidence of 0.3 to 0.4%. Their diagnosis is obvious when they are visible as glittering particles upon the surface of the optic disc. However, in many patients they are hidden beneath the surface, producing an elevated optic disc with blurred margins that is easily mistaken for papilledema. It is important to recognize pseudopapilledema due to optic disc drusen to avoid an unneccessary evaluation for papilledema. Ultrasound or CT scanning are sensitive for detection of buried optic disc drusen because they contain calcium. In most patients, optic disc drusen are an incidental, innocuous finding, but they can produce visual obscurations. On perimetry they give rise to enlarged blind spots and arcuate scotomas from damage to the optic disc. With increasing age, drusen tend to become more exposed on the disc surface as optic atrophy develops. Hemorrhage, choroidal neovascular membrane, and AION are more likely to occur in patients with optic disc drusen. No treatment for drusen is available.

Vitreous Degeneration   This occurs in all individuals with advancing age, leading to chronic and acute visual symptoms. Opacities develop in the vitreous, casting annoying shadows upon the retina. As the eye moves, these distracting "floaters" move synchronously, with a slight lag caused by inertia of the vitreous gel. Vitreous traction upon the retina causes mechanical stimulation, resulting in perception of flashing lights. This photopsia is brief and confined to one eye, in contrast to the bilateral, prolonged scintillations of cortical migraine. Contraction of the vitreous can result in sudden separation from the retina, heralded by an alarming shower of floaters and photopsia. This process, known as *vitreous detachment*, is a frequent involutional event in the elderly. It is not harmful unless it damages the retina. A careful examination of the dilated fundus is mandatory in any patient complaining of floaters or photopsia to search for peripheral tears or holes. If such a lesion is found, laser application or cryotherapy can forestall a retinal detachment. Occasionally a tear ruptures a retinal blood vessel, causing vitreous hemorrhage and sudden loss of vision. On attempted ophthalmoscopy the fundus is hidden by a dark red haze of blood. Ultrasound is required to examine the interior of the eye for a retinal tear or detachment. If the hemorrhage does not resolve spontaneously, the vitreous can be removed surgically. Vitreous hemorrhage also occurs from the fragile neovascular vessels that proliferate on the surface of the retina in diabetes, sickle cell anemia, and other ischemic ocular diseases.

Retinal Detachment   This produces symptoms of floaters, flashing lights, and a scotoma in the peripheral visual field corresponding to the detachment (**see Plate IV-12**). If the detachment includes the fovea, there is an afferent pupil defect and the visual acuity is reduced. In most eyes, retinal detachment starts with a hole, flap, or tear in the peripheral retina (rhegmatogenous retinal detachment). Patients with peripheral retinal thinning (lattice degeneration) are particularly vulnerable to this process. Once a break has developed in the retina, liquified vitreous is free to enter the subretinal space, separating the retina from the pigment epithelium. The combination of vitreous traction upon the retinal surface and passage of fluid behind the retina leads inexorably to detachment. Patients with a history of myopia, trauma, or prior cataract extraction are at greatest risk for retinal detachment. The diagnosis is confirmed by ophthalmoscopic examination of the dilated eye.

Classic Migraine (See also Chap. 15)   This usually occurs with a visual aura lasting about 20 min. In a typical attack, a small central disturbance in the field of vision marches toward the periphery, leaving a transient scotoma in its wake. The expanding border of migraine scotoma has a scintillating, dancing, or zig-zag edge, resembling the bastions of a fortified city, hence the term "fortification spectra." Patients' descriptions of fortification spectra vary widely and can be confused with amaurosis fugax. Migraine patterns usually last longer and are perceived in both eyes, whereas amaurosis fugax is briefer and occurs in only one eye. Migraine phenomena also remain visible in the dark or with the eyes closed. Generally they are confined to either the right or left visual hemifield, but sometimes both fields are involved simultaneously. Patients often have a long history of stereotypic attacks. After the visual symptoms recede, headache develops in most patients.

Transient ischemic attacks from *vertebrobasilar insufficiency* result in acute homonymous visual symptoms. Many patients mistakenly describe symptoms in their left or right eye, when in fact they are occurring in the left or right hemifield of both eyes. Interruption of blood supply to the visual cortex causes a sudden fogging or graying of vision, occasionally with flashing lights or other positive phenomena that mimic migraine. Cortical ischemic attacks are briefer in duration than migraine, occur in older patients, and are not followed by headache. There may be associated signs of brainstem ischemia, such as diplopia, vertigo, numbness, weakness, or dysarthria.

Stroke   This occurs when interruption of blood supply from the posterior cerebral artery to the visual cortex is prolonged. The only finding on examination is a homonymous visual field defect that stops abruptly at the vertical meridian. Occipital lobe stroke is usually due to thrombotic occlusion of the vertebrobasilar system, embolus, or dissection. Lobar hemorrhage, tumor, abscess, and arteriovenous malformation are other common causes of hemianopic cortical visual loss.

Factitious (Functional, Nonorganic) Visual Loss   This is claimed by hysterics or malingerers. The latter comprise the vast majority, seeking sympathy, special treatment, or financial gain by feigning loss of sight. The diagnosis is suspected when the history is atypical, physical findings are lacking or contradictory, inconsistencies emerge on testing, and a secondary motive can be identified. In our litigious society, the fraudulent pursuit of recompense has spawned an epidemic of factitious visual loss.

CHRONIC VISUAL LOSS

Cataract   This is a clouding of the lens sufficient to reduce vision. Most cataracts develop slowly as a result of aging, leading to gradual impairment of vision. The formation of cataract occurs more rapidly in patients with a history of ocular trauma, uveitis, or diabetes mellitus. Cataracts are acquired in a variety of genetic diseases, such as myotonic dystrophy, neurofibromatosis type 2, and galactosemia. Radiation therapy and glucocorticoid treatment can induce cataract as a side effect. The cataracts associated with radiation or glucocorticoids have a typical posterior subcapsular location. Cataract can be detected by noting an impaired red reflex when viewing light reflected from the fundus with an ophthalmoscope or by examining the dilated eye using the slit lamp.

The only treatment for cataract is surgical extraction of the opacified lens. Over a million cataract operations are performed each year in the United States. The operation is generally done under local anesthesia on an outpatient basis. Remarkable technical innovations have made it possible to aspirate the cataract while leaving the lens capsule intact (extracapsular cataract extraction), rather than removing the entire lens with its capsule (intracapsular cataract extraction). A plastic or silicone intraocular lens is then placed within the empty lens capsule in the posterior chamber, substituting for the natural lens, and leading to rapid recovery of sight. More than 95% of patients who undergo cataract extraction can expect an improvement in vision. In many patients, the lens capsule remaining in the eye after cataract extraction eventually turns cloudy, causing a secondary loss of vision. A small opening is made in the lens capsule with a laser to restore clarity.

Glaucoma   This is a slowly progressive, insidious optic neuropathy, usually associated with chronic elevation of intraocular pressure.

In Americans of African descent it is the leading cause of blindness. The mechanism whereby raised intraocular pressure injures the optic nerve is not understood. Axons entering the inferotemporal and superotemporal aspects of the optic disc are damaged first, producing typical nerve fiber bundle or arcuate scotomas on perimetric testing. As fibers are destroyed, the neural rim of the optic disc shrinks and the physiologic cup within the optic disc enlarges (see Plate IV-13). This process is referred to colloquially as pathologic "cupping." The cup-to-disc diameter is expressed as a ratio, e.g., 0.2/1. The cup-to-disc ratio ranges widely in normal individuals, making it difficult to diagnose glaucoma reliably simply by observing an unusually large or deep optic cup. Careful documentation of serial prospective examinations is helpful. In the patient with physiologic cupping, the large cup remains stable, whereas in the patient with glaucoma it expands relentlessly over the years. Detection of visual field loss on formal perimetry also contributes to the diagnosis of glaucoma. Finally, most patients with glaucoma have raised intraocular pressure. However, a surprising number of patients with typical glaucomatous cupping and visual field loss have intraocular pressures that apparently never exceed the normal limit of 20 mmHg (so-called low-tension glaucoma).

In acute angle-closure glaucoma, the eye is red and painful due to abrupt, severe elevation of intraocular pressure. Such cases account for only a handful of patients with glaucoma. Most patients with glaucoma have open, nonoccludable anterior chamber angles. The cause of raised intraocular pressure in these patients is uncertain. Recent studies have implicated mutations in a gene encoding a glycoprotein expressed in the trabecular meshwork. This structure serves as a filter to drain aqueous from the eye. Because the elevation of intraocular pressure develops gradually and is less marked than in angle-closure glaucoma, there is no pain or ocular injection. The central visual field and foveal acuity are spared until end-stage disease is reached. For these reasons, severe and irreversible damage can occur before either the patient or physician recognizes the diagnosis. Screening of patients for glaucoma by noting the cup-to-disc ratio on ophthalmoscopy and by measuring intraocular pressure (using a Schiotz, Tonopen, air-puff, or Goldmann tonometer) is vital. Glaucoma is treated with topical adrenergic agonists (epinephrine, dipivefrin, apraclonidine, brimonidine), cholinergic agonists (pilocarpine), beta blockers (betaxolol, carteolol, levobunolol, metipranolol, and timolol), and prostaglandin analogues (latanaprost). Occasionally, systemic absorption of beta blocker from eye drops can be sufficient to cause side effects of bradycardia, hypotension, heart block, bronchospasm, impotence, or depression. Topical or oral carbonic anhydrase inhibitors are used to lower intraocular pressure by reducing aqueous production. Laser treatment of the trabecular meshwork in the anterior chamber angle improves aqueous outflow from the eye. If medical or laser treatments fail to halt optic nerve damage from glaucoma, a filter must be constructed surgically (trabeculectomy) to release aqueous from the eye in a controlled fashion.

Macular Degeneration This is a major cause of gradual, painless, bilateral central visual loss in the elderly. The old term, "senile macular degeneration," misinterpreted by many patients as an unflattering reference, has been replaced with "age-related macular degeneration." It occurs in a nonexudative (dry) form and an exudative (wet) form. The nonexudative process begins with the accumulation of extracellular deposits, called drusen, underneath the retinal pigment epithelium. On ophthalmoscopy, they are pleomorphic but generally appear as small discrete yellow lesions clustered in the macula (see Plate IV-14). With time they become larger, more numerous, and confluent. The retinal pigment epithelium becomes focally detached and atrophic, causing visual loss by interfering with photoreceptor function. There is currently no way to prevent the development of age-related macular degeneration. Concoctions of various vitamins (A, C, and E) and minerals (zinc, copper, and selenium) have been marketed, without good evidence that they retard the process of macular degeneration.

Exudative macular degeneration, which develops in only a minority of patients, occurs when neovascular vessels from the choroid grow through defects in Bruch's membrane into the potential space beneath

the retinal pigment epithelium. Leakage from these vessels produces elevation of the retina and pigment epithelium, with distortion (metamorphopsia) and blurring of vision. Although onset of these symptoms is usually gradual, bleeding from subretinal choroidal neovascular membranes sometimes causes acute visual loss. The neovascular membranes can be difficult to see on fundus examination because they are beneath the retina. Fluorescein or indocyanine green angiography is extremely useful for their detection. In some patients, prompt laser ablation of choroidal neovascular membranes seen on fluorescein angiography can halt the exudative process. However, the neovascular membranes frequently recur, requiring constant vigilance and repeated photocoagulation.

Major or repeated hemorrhage under the retina from neovascular membranes results in fibrosis, development of a round (disciform) macular scar, and permanent loss of central vision. Surgical attempts to remove subretinal membranes in age-related macular degeneration have not improved vision in most patients. However, outcomes have been more encouraging for patients with choroidal neovascular membranes from ocular histoplasmosis syndrome.

Central Serous Chorioretinopathy This primarily affects males between the ages of 20 and 50. Leakage of serous fluid from the choroid causes small, localized detachment of the retinal pigment epithelium and the neurosensory retina. These detachments produce acute or chronic symptoms of metamorphopsia and blurred vision when the macula is involved. They are difficult to visualize with a direct ophthalmoscope because the detached retina is transparent and only slightly elevated. Diagnosis of central serous chorioretinopathy is made easily by fluorescein angiography, which shows dye streaming into the subretinal space. The cause of central serous chorioretinopathy is unknown. Symptoms may resolve spontaneously if the retina reattaches, but recurrent detachment is common. Laser photocoagulation has benefited some patients with this condition.

Diabetic Retinopathy A rare disease until 1921, when the discovery of insulin resulted in a dramatic improvement in life expectancy for patients with diabetes mellitus, it is now a leading cause of blindness in the United States. The retinopathy of diabetes takes years to develop but eventually appears in nearly all cases. Regular surveillance of the dilated fundus is crucial for any patient with diabetes. In advanced diabetic retinopathy, the proliferation of neovascular vessels leads to blindness from vitreous hemorrhage, retinal detachment, and glaucoma (see Plate IV-15). These complications can be avoided in most patients by administration of panretinal laser photocoagulation at the appropriate point in the evolution of the disease. →*For further discussion of the manifestations and management of diabetic retinopathy, see Chap. 333.*

Retinitis Pigmentosa This is a general term for a disparate group of rod and cone dystrophies characterized by progressive night blindness (nyctalopia), visual field constriction with a ring scotoma, loss of acuity, and an abnormal electroretinogram (ERG). It occurs sporadically or in an autosomal recessive, dominant, or X-linked pattern. Irregular black deposits of clumped pigment in the peripheral retina, called bone spicules because of their vague resemblance to the spicules of cancellous bone, give the disease its name (see Plate IV-16). The name is actually a misnomer because retinitis pigmentosa is not an inflammatory process. Most cases are due to a mutation in the gene for rhodopsin, the rod photopigment, or in the gene for peripherin, a glycoprotein located in photoreceptor outer segments. There is no effective treatment for retinitis pigmentosa. Vitamin A (15,000 IU/day) slightly retards the deterioration of the ERG but has no beneficial effect upon visual acuity or visual fields. Some forms of retinitis pigmentosa occur in association with rare, hereditary systemic diseases (olivopontocerebellar degeneration, Bassen-Kornzweig disease, Kearns-Sayre syndrome, Refsum's disease). Chronic treatment with chloroquine, hydroxychloroquine, and phenothiazines (especially thioridazine) can produce visual loss from a toxic retinopathy that resembles retinitis pigmentosa.

Epiretinal Membrane   This is a fibrocellular tissue that grows across the inner surface of the retina, causing metamorphopsia and reduced visual acuity from distortion of the macula. With the ophthalmoscope one can see a crinkled, cellophane-like membrane on the retina. Epiretinal membrane is most common in patients over 50 years of age and is usually unilateral. Most cases are idiopathic, but some occur as a result of hypertensive retinopathy, diabetes, retinal detachment, or trauma. When visual acuity is reduced to the level of about 6/24 (20/80), vitrectomy and surgical peeling of the membrane to relieve macular puckering are recommended. Contraction of an epiretinal membrane sometimes gives rise to a *macular hole*. Most macular holes, however, are caused by local vitreous traction within the fovea. Vision is usually depressed to the level of 6/30 (20/100) or worse. Vitrectomy may improve visual acuity in some patients with macular hole. Fortunately, fewer than 10% of patients with a macular hole develop a hole in their other eye.

Melanoma and Other Tumors   Melanoma is the most common primary tumor of the eye (see Plate IV-17). It causes photopsia, an enlarging scotoma, and loss of vision. A small melanoma is often difficult to differentiate from a benign choroidal nevus. Careful serial examinations are required to document a malignant pattern of growth. Treatment of melanoma is controversial. Options include enucleation, local resection, and irradiation. *Metastatic tumors* to the eye outnumber primary tumors of uveal origin. Breast and lung carcinoma have a special propensity to spread to the choroid or iris. Leukemia and lymphoma also commonly invade ocular tissues. Sometimes their only sign on eye examination is cellular debris in the vitreous, which can masquerade as a chronic posterior uveitis. *Retrobulbar tumor* of the optic nerve (meningioma, glioma) or *chiasmal tumor* (pituitary adenoma, meningioma) produces gradual visual loss with few objective findings, except for optic disc pallor. Rarely, sudden expansion of a pituitary adenoma from infarction and bleeding (*pituitary apoplexy*) causes acute retrobulbar visual loss, with headache, nausea, and ocular motor nerve palsies. In any patient with visual field loss or optic atrophy, CT or MR scanning should be considered if the cause remains unknown after careful review of the history and thorough examination of the eye (Fig. 28-4).

PROPTOSIS

When the globes appear asymmetric, the clinician must first decide which eye is abnormal. Is one eye recessed within the orbit (*enophthalmos*) or is the other eye protuberant (*exophthalmos*, or *proptosis*)? A small globe or a Horner's syndrome can give the appearance of enophthalmos. True enophthalmos occurs commonly after trauma, from atrophy of retrobulbar fat, or fracture of the orbital floor. The position of the eyes within the orbits is measured using a Hertel exophthalmometer, a hand-held instrument that records the position of the anterior corneal surface relative to the lateral orbital rim. If this instrument is not available, relative eye position can be judged by bending the patient's head forward and looking down upon the orbits. A proptosis of only 2 mm in one eye is detectable from this perspective. The development of proptosis implies a space-occupying lesion in the orbit. A CT or MR scan should be obtained in any patient with proptosis, unless the diagnosis of Graves' ophthalmopathy is certain.

Graves' Ophthalmopathy   This is the leading cause of proptosis in adults (Chap. 330). The proptosis is often asymmetric and can even appear to be unilateral. Orbital inflammation and engorgement of the extraocular muscles, particularly the medial rectus and the inferior rectus, account for the protrusion of the globe. Corneal exposure, lid retraction, conjunctival injection, restriction of gaze, diplopia, and visual loss from optic nerve compression are cardinal symptoms. Acute Graves' ophthalmopathy should be treated with oral prednisone (60 mg/day) for 1 month, followed by a taper over several months. Chronic manifestations can be managed by topical lubricants, eyelid surgery,

eye muscle surgery, or radiation treatment. Optic nerve compression should be relieved promptly with glucocorticoids and orbital decompression to prevent permanent visual loss.

Orbital Pseudotumor   This is an idiopathic, inflammatory orbital syndrome, frequently confused with Graves' ophthalmopathy. Symptoms are pain, limited eye movements, proptosis, and congestion. Evaluation for sarcoidosis, Wegener's granulomatosis, and other types of orbital vasculitis or collagen-vascular disease is negative. Imaging often shows swollen eye muscles (orbital myositis) with enlarged tendons. By contrast, in Graves' ophthalmopathy the tendons of the eye muscles are usually spared. The Tolosa-Hunt syndrome may be regarded as an extension of orbital pseudotumor through the superior orbital fissure into the cavernous sinus. The diagnosis of orbital pseudotumor is difficult. Biopsy of the orbit frequently yields nonspecific evidence of fat infiltration by lymphocytes, plasma cells, and eosinophils. A dramatic response to a therapeutic trial of systemic glucocorticoids indirectly provides the best confirmation of the diagnosis.

Orbital Cellulitis   This causes pain, lid erythema, proptosis, conjunctival chemosis, restricted motility, decreased acuity, afferent pupillary defect, fever, and leukocytosis. It often arises from a paranasal sinus, especially by contiguous spread of infection from the ethmoid sinus through the thin lamina papyracea of the medial orbit. A history of recent upper respiratory tract infection, chronic sinusitis, thick mucous secretions, or dental disease is significant in any patient with suspected orbital cellulitis. Blood cultures should be obtained, but they are usually negative. Most patients respond to empiric therapy with broad-spectrum intravenous antibiotics. Occasionally, orbital cellulitis follows an overwhelming course, with massive proptosis, blindness, septic cavernous sinus thrombosis, and meningitis. To avert this disaster, orbital cellulitis should be managed aggressively in the early stages, with immediate antibiotic therapy and imaging of the orbits. Prompt surgical drainage of an orbital abscess or paranasal sinusitis is indicated if optic nerve function deteriorates despite antibiotics.

Tumors   Tumors of the orbit cause painless, progressive proptosis. The most common primary tumors are hemangioma, lymphangioma, neurofibroma, dermoid cyst, adenoid cystic carcinoma, optic nerve glioma, optic nerve meningioma, and benign mixed tumor of the lacrimal gland. Metastatic tumor to the orbit occurs frequently in breast carcinoma, lung carcinoma, and lymphoma. Diagnosis by fine-needle aspiration followed by urgent radiation therapy can sometimes preserve vision.

Carotid Cavernous Fistulas   With anterior drainage through the orbit these produce proptosis, diplopia, glaucoma, and tortuous, red conjunctival vessels. Direct fistulas usually result from trauma. They are easily diagnosed because of the dramatic signs produced by high-flow, high-pressure shunting. Indirect fistulas, or dural arteriovenous malformations, are more likely to occur spontaneously, especially in older women. The signs are more subtle and the diagnosis is frequently missed. The combination of slight proptosis, diplopia, enlarged muscles, and an injected eye is often mistaken for thyroid ophthalmopathy. A bruit heard upon auscultation of the head, or reported by the patient, is a valuable diagnostic clue. Imaging shows an enlarged superior ophthalmic vein in the orbits. Carotid cavernous shunts can be eliminated by intravascular embolization.

PTOSIS

Blepharoptosis   This is an abnormal drooping of the eyelid. Unilateral or bilateral ptosis can be congenital, from dysgenesis of the levator palpebrae superioris, or from abnormal insertion of its aponeurosis into the eyelid. Acquired ptosis can develop so gradually that the patient is unaware of the problem. Inspection of old photographs is helpful in dating the onset. A history of prior trauma, eye surgery, contact lens use, diplopia, systemic symptoms (e.g., dysphagia or peripheral muscle weakness), or a family history of ptosis should be sought. Fluctuating ptosis that worsens late in the day is typical of myasthenia gravis. Examination should focus upon evidence for proptosis, eyelid masses or deformities, inflammation, pupil inequality, or limitation of motility. The width of the palpebral fissures is measured in primary gaze to quantitate the degree of ptosis. The ptosis will be underestimated if the patient is compensating by lifting the brow with the frontalis muscle.

Mechanical Ptosis This occurs in many elderly patients from stretching and redundancy of eyelid skin and subcutaneous fat (dermatochalasis). The extra weight of these sagging tissues causes the lid to droop. Enlargement or deformation of the eyelid from infection, tumor, trauma, or inflammation also results in ptosis on a purely mechanical basis.

Aponeurotic Ptosis This is an acquired dehiscence or stretching of the aponeurotic tendon, which connects the levator muscle to the tarsal plate of the eyelid. It occurs commonly in older patients, presumably from loss of connective tissue elasticity. Aponeurotic ptosis is also a frequent sequela of eyelid swelling from infection or blunt trauma to the orbit, cataract surgery, or hard contact lens usage.

Myogenic Ptosis The causes of *myogenic ptosis* include myasthenia gravis (Chap. 380) and a number of rare myopathies that manifest with ptosis. The term *chronic progressive external ophthalmoplegia* refers to a spectrum of systemic diseases caused by mutations of mitochrondrial DNA. As the name implies, the most prominent findings are symmetric, slowly progressive ptosis and limitation of eye movements. In general, diplopia is a late symptom because all eye movements are reduced equally. In the *Kearns-Sayre* variant, retinal pigmentary changes and abnormalities of cardiac conduction develop. Peripheral muscle biopsy shows characteristic "ragged-red fibers." *Oculopharyngeal dystrophy* is a distinct autosomal dominant disease with onset in middle age, characterized by ptosis, limited eye movements, and trouble swallowing. *Myotonic dystrophy*, another autosomal dominant disorder, causes ptosis, ophthalmoparesis, cataract, and pigmentary retinopathy. Patients have muscle wasting, myotonia, frontal balding, and cardiac abnormalities.

Neurogenic Ptosis This results from a lesion affecting the innervation to either of the two muscles that open the eyelid: Müller's muscle or the levator palpebrae superioris. Examination of the pupil helps to distinguish between these two possibilities. In Horner's syndrome, the eye with ptosis has a smaller pupil and the eye movements are full. In an oculomotor nerve palsy, the eye with the ptosis has a larger, or a normal, pupil. If the pupil is normal but there is limitation of adduction, elevation, and depression, a pupil-sparing oculomotor nerve palsy is likely (see next section). Rarely, a lesion affecting the small, central subnucleus of the oculomotor complex will cause bilateral ptosis with normal eye movements and pupils.

DOUBLE VISION

The first point to clarify is whether diplopia persists in either eye after covering the fellow eye. If it does, the diagnosis is monocular diplopia. The cause is usually intrinsic to the eye and therefore has no dire implications for the patient. Corneal aberrations (e.g., keratoconus, pterygium), uncorrected refractive error, cataract, or foveal traction may give rise to monocular diplopia. Occasionally it is a symptom of malingering or psychiatric disease. Diplopia alleviated by covering one eye is binocular diplopia and is caused by disruption of ocular alignment. Inquiry should be made into the nature of the double vision (purely side-by-side versus partial vertical displacement of images), mode of onset, duration, intermittency, diurnal variation, and associated neurologic or systemic symptoms. If the patient has diplopia while being examined, motility testing should reveal a deficiency corresponding to the patient's symptoms. However, subtle limitation of ocular excursions is often difficult to detect. For example, a patient with a slight left abducens nerve paresis may appear to have full eye movements, despite a complaint of horizontal diplopia upon looking to the left. In this situation, the cover test provides a more sensitive method for demonstrating the ocular malalignment. It should be conducted in primary gaze, and then with the head turned and tilted in each direction. In the above example, a cover test with the head

turned to the right will maximize the fixation shift evoked by the cover test.

Occasionally, a cover test performed in an asymptomatic patient during a routine examination will reveal an ocular deviation. If the eye movements are full and the ocular misalignment is equal in all directions of gaze (concomitant deviation), the diagnosis is strabismus. In this condition, which affects about 1% of the population, fusion is disrupted in infancy or early childhood. To avoid diplopia, vision is suppressed from the nonfixating eye. In some children, this leads to impaired vision (amblyopia, or "lazy" eye) in the deviated eye.

Binocular diplopia occurs from a wide range of processes: infectious, neoplastic, metabolic, degenerative, inflammatory, and vascular. One must decide if the diplopia is neurogenic in origin or due to restriction of globe rotation by local disease in the orbit. Orbital pseudotumor, myositis, infection, tumor, thyroid disease, and muscle entrapment (e.g., from a blowout fracture) cause restrictive diplopia. The diagnosis is confirmed by performing a forced duction test in the office. After applying topical anesthesia, the physician grasps the eye with forceps and pulls it toward the direction of deficient motion. If rotation of the globe is prevented by tethering, a restrictive process is at work. The utility of this test is limited by its unpopularity with patients; in practice, the diagnosis of restriction is made by recognizing other associated signs and symptoms of local orbital disease.

Myasthenia Gravis (See also Chap. 380) This is a major cause of diplopia. The diplopia is often intermittent, variable, and not confined to any single ocular motor nerve distribution. The pupils are always normal. Fluctuating ptosis may be present. Many patients have a purely ocular form of the disease, with no evidence of systemic muscular weakness. The diagnosis can be confirmed by an intravenous edrophonium injection or by an assay for antiacetylcholine receptor antibodies. Negative results from these tests do not exclude the diagnosis. *Botulism* from food or wound poisoning can mimic ocular myasthenia.

After restrictive orbital disease and myasthenia gravis are excluded, a lesion of a cranial nerve supplying innervation to the extraocular muscles is the most likely cause of binocular diplopia.

Oculomotor Nerve The third cranial nerve innervates the medial, inferior, and superior recti; inferior oblique; levator palpebrae superioris; and the iris sphincter. Total palsy of the oculomotor nerve causes ptosis, a dilated pupil, and leaves the eye "down and out" because of the unopposed action of the lateral rectus and superior oblique. This combination of findings is obvious. More challenging is the diagnosis of an early or partial oculomotor nerve palsy. In this setting, any combination of ptosis, pupil dilation, and weakness of the eye muscles supplied by the oculomotor nerve may be encountered. Frequent serial examinations during the evolving phase of the palsy and a high index of suspicion help ensure that the diagnosis is not missed. The advent of an oculomotor nerve palsy with any degree of pupil involvement in an otherwise healthy patient, especially when accompanied by pain, raises the specter of a circle of Willis aneurysm. If an MR scan shows no compressive lesion, an arteriogram must be performed to rule out an aneurysm of either the posterior communicating artery or the basilar artery. If the pupil is entirely normal, with all other components of an oculomotor palsy present, aneurysm is so rare that an angiogram is seldom indicated.

A lesion of the oculomotor nucleus in the rostral midbrain produces signs that differ from those caused by a lesion of the nerve itself. There is bilateral ptosis because the levator muscle is innervated by a single central subnucleus. There is also weakness of the contralateral superior rectus, because it is supplied by the oculomotor nucleus on the other side. Occasionally both superior recti are weak. Isolated nuclear oculomotor palsy is quite rare. Usually neurologic examination reveals additional signs to suggest brainstem damage from infarction, hemorrhage, tumor, or infection.

Injury to structures surrounding fascicles of the oculomotor nerve descending through the midbrain has given rise to a number of classic eponymic designations. In *Nothnagel's syndrome*, injury to the superior cerebellar peduncle causes ipsilateral oculomotor palsy and contralateral cerebellar ataxia. In *Benedikt's syndrome*, injury to the red nucleus results in ipsilateral oculomotor palsy and contralateral tremor, chorea, and athetosis. *Claude's syndrome* incorporates features of both the aforementioned syndromes, by injury to both the red nucleus and the superior cerebellar peduncle. Finally, in *Weber's syndrome*, injury to the cerebral peduncle causes ipsilateral oculomotor palsy with contralateral hemiparesis.

In the subarachnoid space the oculomotor nerve is vulnerable to aneurysm, meningitis, tumor, infarction, and compression. In cerebral herniation the nerve becomes trapped between the edge of the tentorium and the uncus of the temporal lobe. Oculomotor palsy can also occur from midbrain torsion and hemorrhages during herniation. In the cavernous sinus, oculomotor palsy arises from carotid aneurysm, carotid cavernous fistula, cavernous sinus thrombosis, tumor (pituitary adenoma, meningioma, metastasis), herpes zoster infection, and the Tolosa-Hunt syndrome.

The etiology of an isolated, pupil-sparing oculomotor palsy often remains obscure, even after neuroimaging and extensive laboratory testing. Most cases are thought to result from microvascular infarction of the nerve, somewhere along its course from the brainstem to the orbit. Usually the patient complains of pain. Diabetes, hypertension, and vascular disease are major risk factors. Spontaneous recovery over a period of months is the rule. If this fails to occur, or if new findings develop, the diagnosis of microvascular oculomotor nerve palsy should be reconsidered. Aberrant regeneration is common when the oculomotor nerve is injured by trauma or compression (tumor, aneurysm). Miswiring of sprouting fibers to the levator muscle and the rectus muscles results in elevation of the eyelid upon downgaze or adduction. The pupil also constricts upon attempted adduction, elevation, or depression of the globe. Aberrant regeneration is not seen after oculomotor palsy from microvascular infarct and hence vitiates that diagnosis.

Trochlear Nerve   The fourth cranial nerve originates in the midbrain, just caudal to the oculomotor nerve complex. Fibers exit the brainstem dorsally and cross to innervate the contralateral superior oblique. The principal actions of this muscle are to depress and to intort the globe. A palsy therefore results in hypertropia and excyclotorsion. The cyclotorsion is seldom noticed by patients. Instead, they complain of vertical diplopia, especially upon reading or looking down. The vertical diplopia is also exacerbated by tilting the head toward the side with the muscle palsy, and alleviated by tilting it away. This "head tilt test" is a cardinal diagnostic feature.

Isolated trochlear nerve palsy occurs from all the causes listed above for the oculomotor nerve, except aneurysm. The trochlear nerve is particularly apt to suffer injury after closed head trauma. The mechanism is unknown, but the free edge of the tentorium may impinge upon the nerve during a concussive blow. Most isolated trochlear nerve palsies are idiopathic and hence diagnosed by exclusion as "microvascular." Spontaneous improvement occurs over a period of months in most patients. A base-down prism (conveniently applied to the patient's glasses as a stick-on Fresnel lens) may serve as a temporary measure to alleviate diplopia. If the palsy does not resolve, the eyes can be realigned by surgically adjusting other eye muscles.

Abducens Nerve   The sixth cranial nerve innervates the lateral rectus muscle. A palsy produces horizontal diplopia, worse on gaze to the side of the lesion. A nuclear lesion has different consequences, because the abducens nucleus contains interneurons that project via the medial longitudinal fasciculus to the medial rectus subnucleus of the contralateral oculomotor complex. Therefore, an abducens nuclear lesion produces a complete lateral gaze palsy, from weakness of both the ipsilateral lateral rectus and the contralateral medial rectus. *Foville's syndrome* following dorsal pontine injury includes lateral gaze palsy, ipsilateral facial palsy, and contralateral hemiparesis in-

curred by damage to descending corticospinal fibers. *Millard-Gubler syndrome* from ventral pontine injury is similar, except for the eye findings. There is lateral rectus weakness only, instead of gaze palsy, because the abducens fascicle is injured rather than the nucleus. Infarct, tumor, hemorrhage, vascular malformation, and multiple sclerosis are the most common etiologies of brainstem abducens palsy.

After leaving the ventral pons, the abducens nerve runs forward along the clivus to pierce the dura at the petrous apex, where it enters the cavernous sinus. Along its subarachnoid course it is susceptible to meningitis, tumor (meningioma, chordoma, carcinomatous meningitis), subarachnoid hemorrhage, trauma, and compression by aneurysm or dolichoectatic vessels. At the petrous apex, mastoiditis can produce deafness, pain, and ipsilateral abducens palsy (*Gradenigo's syndrome*). In the cavernous sinus, the nerve can be affected by carotid aneurysm, carotid cavernous fistula, tumor (pituitary adenoma, meningioma, nasopharyngeal carcinoma), herpes infection, and Tolosa-Hunt syndrome.

Unilateral or bilateral abducens palsy is a classic sign of raised intracranial pressure. The diagnosis can be confirmed if papilledema is observed on fundus examination. The mechanism is still debated but is probably related to rostral-caudal displacement of the brainstem. The same phenomenon accounts for abducens palsy from low intracranial pressure (e.g., after lumbar puncture, spinal anesthesia, or spontaneous dural cerebrospinal fluid leak).

Treatment of abducens palsy is aimed at prompt correction of the underlying cause. However, the cause remains obscure in many instances, despite diligent evaluation. As mentioned above for isolated trochlear or oculomotor palsy, most cases are assumed to represent microvascular infarcts because they often occur in the setting of diabetes or other vascular risk factors. Some cases may develop as a postinfectious mononeuritis (e.g., following a viral flu). Patching one eye or applying a temporary prism will provide relief of diplopia until the palsy resolves. If recovery is incomplete, eye muscle surgery can nearly always realign the eyes, at least in primary position. A patient with an abducens palsy that fails to improve should be reevaluated for an occult etiology (e.g., chordoma, carcinomatous meningitis, carotid cavernous fistula, myasthenia gravis).

Multiple Ocular Motor Nerve Palsies   These should not be attributed to spontaneous microvascular events affecting more than one cranial nerve at a time. This remarkable coincidence does occur, especially in diabetic patients, but the diagnosis is made only in retrospect after exhausting all other diagnostic alternatives. Neuroimaging should focus on the cavernous sinus, superior orbital fissure, and orbital apex, where all three ocular motor nerves are in close proximity. In the diabetic or compromised host, fungal infection (*Aspergillus*, Mucorales, *Cryptococcus*) is a frequent cause of multiple nerve palsies. In the patient with systemic malignancy, carcinomatous meningitis is a likely diagnosis. Cytologic examination may be negative despite repeated sampling of the cerebrospinal fluid. The cancer-associated Lambert-Eaton myasthenic syndrome can also produce ophthalmoplegia. Giant cell (temporal) arteritis occasionally manifests as diplopia from ischemic palsies of extraocular muscles. Fisher syndrome, an ocular variant of Guillain-Barré, can produce ophthalmoplegia with areflexia and ataxia. Often the ataxia is mild, and the areflexia is overlooked because the physician's attention is focused upon the eyes.

Supranuclear Disorders of Gaze   These are often mistaken for multiple ocular motor nerve palsies. For example, Wernicke's encephalopathy can produce nystagmus and a partial deficit of horizontal and vertical gaze that mimics a combined abducens and oculomotor nerve palsy. The disorder occurs in malnourished or alcoholic patients and can be reversed by giving thiamine. Infarct, hemorrhage, tumor, multiple sclerosis, encephalitis, vasculitis, and Whipple's disease are other important causes of supranuclear gaze palsy.

The *frontal eye field* of the cerebral cortex is involved in generation of saccades to the contralateral side. After hemispheric stroke, the eyes usually deviate towards the lesioned side because of the unopposed action of the frontal eye field in the normal hemisphere. With time, this deficit resolves. Seizures generally have the opposite effect: the eyes deviate conjugately away from the irritative focus. *Parietal lesions* disrupt smooth pursuit of targets moving toward the side of the lesion. Bilateral parietal lesions produce *Balint's syndrome*, characterized by impaired eye-hand coordination (optic ataxia), difficulty initiating voluntary eye movements (ocular apraxia), and visuospatial disorientation (simultanagnosia).

Horizontal Gaze Descending cortical inputs mediating horizontal gaze ultimately converge at the level of the pons. Neurons in the paramedian pontine reticular formation are responsible for controlling conjugate gaze toward the same side. They project directly to the ipsilateral abducens nucleus. A lesion of either the paramedian pontine reticular formation or the abducens nucleus causes an ipsilateral conjugate gaze palsy. Lesions at either locus produce nearly identical clinical syndromes, with the following exception: vestibular stimulation (oculocephalic maneuver or caloric) will succeed in driving the eyes conjugately to the side in a patient with a lesion of the paramedian pontine reticular formation, but not in a patient with a lesion of the abducens nucleus.

Internuclear ophthalmoplegia This results from damage to the medial longitudinal fasciculus ascending from the abducens nucleus in the pons to the oculomotor nucleus in the midbrain (hence, "internuclear"). Damage to fibers carrying the conjugate signal from abducens interneurons to the contralateral medial rectus motoneurons results in a failure of adduction on attempted lateral gaze. For example, a patient with a left internuclear ophthalmoplegia will have slowed or absent adducting movements of the left eye. A patient with bilateral injury to the medial longitudinal fasciculus will have bilateral internuclear ophthalmoplegia. Multiple sclerosis is the most common cause, although tumor, stroke, trauma, or any brainstem process may be responsible. *One-and-a half syndrome* is due to a combined lesion of the medial longitudinal fasciculus and the abducens nucleus on the same side. The patient's only horizontal eye movement is abduction of the eye on the other side.

Vertical Gaze This is controlled at the level of the midbrain. The neuronal circuits affected in disorders of vertical gaze are not well elucidated, but lesions of the rostral interstitial nucleus of the medial longitudinal fasciculus and the interstitial nucleus of Cajal cause supranuclear paresis of upgaze, downgaze, or all vertical eye movements. Distal basilar artery ischemia is the most common etiology. *Skew deviation* refers to a vertical misalignment of the eyes, usually constant in all positions of gaze. The finding has poor localizing value because skew deviation has been reported after lesions in widespread regions of the brainstem and cerebellum.

Parinaud's syndrome Also known as dorsal midbrain syndrome, this is a distinct supranuclear vertical gaze disorder from damage to the posterior commissure. It is a classic sign of hydrocephalus from aqueductal stenosis. Pineal region tumors (germinoma, pineoblastoma), cysticercosis, and stroke also cause Parinaud's syndrome. Features include loss of upgaze (and sometimes downgaze), convergence-retraction nystagmus on attempted upgaze, downwards ocular deviation ("setting sun" sign), lid retraction (Collier's sign), skew deviation, pseudoabducens palsy, and light-near dissociation of the pupils. Disorders of vertical gaze, especially downwards saccades, are an early feature of progressive supranuclear palsy. Smooth pursuit is affected later in the course of the disease. Parkinson's disease, Huntington's chorea, and olivopontocerebellar degeneration can also affect vertical gaze.

Nystagmus This is a rhythmical oscillation of the eyes, occurring physiologically from vestibular and optokinetic stimulation or pathologically in a wide variety of diseases. Abnormalities of the eyes or optic nerves, present at birth or acquired in childhood, can produce a complex, searching nystagmus with irregular pendular (sinusoidal) and jerk features. This nystagmus is commonly referred to as *congenital sensory nystagmus*. It is a poor term, because even in children with congenital lesions, the nystagmus does not appear until several months

of age. *Congenital motor nystagmus*, which looks similar to congenital sensory nystagmus, develops in the absence of any abnormality of the sensory visual system. Visual acuity is also reduced in congenital motor nystagmus, probably by the nystagmus itself, but seldom below a level of 20/200.

Jerk nystagmus This is characterized by a slow drift off the target, followed by a fast corrective saccade. By convention, the nystagmus is named after the quick phase. Jerk nystagmus can be downbeat, upbeat, horizontal (left or right), and torsional. The pattern of nystagmus may vary with gaze position. Some patients will be oblivious to their nystagmus. Others will complain of blurred vision, or a subjective, to-and-fro movement of the environment (oscillopsia) corresponding to their nystagmus. Fine nystagmus may be difficult to see upon gross examination of the eyes. Observation of nystagmoid movements of the optic disc on ophthalmoscopy is a sensitive way to detect subtle nystagmus. The slit lamp is also useful.

Gaze-evoked nystagmus This is the most common form of jerk nystagmus. When the eyes are held eccentrically in the orbits, they have a natural tendency to drift back to primary position. The subject compensates by making a corrective saccade to maintain the deviated eye position. Many normal patients have mild gaze-evoked nystagmus. Exaggerated gaze-evoked nystagmus can be induced by drugs (sedatives, anticonvulsants, alcohol); muscle paresis; myasthenia gravis; demyelinating disease; and cerebellopontine angle, brainstem, and cerebellar lesions.

Vestibular nystagmus Vestibular nystagmus results from dysfunction of the labyrinth (Méniére's disease), vestibular nerve, or vestibular nucleus in the brainstem. Peripheral vestibular nystagmus often occurs in discrete attacks, with symptoms of nausea and vertigo. There may be associated tinnitus and hearing loss. Sudden shifts in head position may provoke or exacerbate symptoms.

Downbeat nystagmus Downbeat nystagmus occurs from lesions near the craniocervical junction (Chiari malformation, basilar invagination). It has also been reported in brainstem or cerebellar stroke, lithium or anticonvulsant intoxication, alcoholism, and multiple sclerosis. *Upbeat nystagmus* is associated with damage to the pontine tegmentum, from stroke, demyelination, or tumor.

Opsoclonus This rare, dramatic disorder of eye movements consists of bursts of consecutive saccades (saccadomania). When the saccades are confined to the horizontal plane, the term *ocular flutter* is preferred. It can occur from viral encephalitis, trauma, or a paraneoplastic effect of neurobastoma, breast carcinoma, and other malignancies. It has also been reported as a benign, transient phenomenon in otherwise healthy patients.

BIBLIOGRAPHY

ALBERT DM, JAKOBIEC FA (eds): *Principles and Practice of Ophthalmology*, 2d ed. Philadelphia, Saunders, 1999

AVERBUCH-HELLER L et al: A double-blind controlled study of gabapentin and baclofen as treatment of acquired nystagmus. Ann Neurol 41:818, 1997

BARTALENA L et al: Relation between therapy for hyperthyroidism and the course of Graves' ophthalmopathy. N Engl J Med 338:73, 1998

BECK RW et al: A randomized controlled trial of corticosteroids in the treatment of acute optic neuritis. N Engl J Med 326:581, 1992

BURDE RM et al: *Clinical Decisions in Neuro-ophthalmology*, 2d ed. St. Louis, Mosby, 1992

GASS JD: *Stereoscopic Atlas of Macular Diseases*, 4th ed. St. Louis, Mosby, 1996

GOLD DH, WEINGEIST TA (eds): *The Eye in Systemic Disease*. Philadelphia, Lippincott, 1990

INZITARI D et al for the North American Symptomatic Carotid Endarterectomy Trial Collaborators: The causes and risks of stroke in patients with asymptomatic internal carotid artery stenosis. N Engl J Med 342:1693, 2000

KRACHMER JH et al: *Cornea*. St. Louis, Mosby, 1997

LEIBOWITZ HM, WARING GO (eds): *Corneal Disorders. Clinical Diagnosis and Management*. Philadelphia, Saunders, 1998

LEIBOWITZ HM: The red eye. N Engl J Med 343:345, 2000

LEIGH RJ, ZEE DS: *The Neurology of Eye Movements*, 3d ed. Oxford, Oxford Univ Press, 1999

MILLER NR, NEWMAN NJ: *Walsh and Hoyt's Clinical Neuroophthalmology*, 5th ed. Baltimore, Williams & Wilkins, 1998

NATHAN J et al: Molecular genetics of inherited variation in human color vision. Science 232:203, 1986

NEITZ M, NEITZ J: Molecular genetics of color vision and color vision defects. Arch Ophthal 118:691, 2000

OPTIC NEURITIS STUDY GROUP: The 5-year risk of MS after optic neuritis. Experience of the optic neuritis treatment trial. Neurology 49:1404, 1997

————: Visual function 5 years after optic neuritis. Experience of the optic neuritis treatment trial. Arch Ophthalmol 115:1545, 1997

POLANSKY JR, NGUYEN TD: The TIGR gene, pathogenic mechanisms, and other recent advances in glaucoma genetics. Curr Opin Ophthalmol 9:15, 1998

SELLEBJERG F et al: A randomized, controlled trial of oral high-dose methylprednisolone in acute optic neuritis. Neurology 52:1479, 1999

SINGH G et al: A mitochondrial DNA mutation as a cause of Leber's hereditary optic neuropathy. N Engl J Med 320:1300, 1989

SPENCER WH (ed): Ophthalmic Pathology. An Atlas and Textbook, 4th ed. Philadelphia, Saunders, 1996

THOMKE F, HOPF HC: Isolated superior oblique palsies with electrophysiologically documented brainstem lesions. Muscle Nerve 23:267, 2000

VAUGHN D et al: *General Ophthalmology*, 15th ed. Norwalk, Appleton & Lange, 1999

WEBER J et al: Selective intra-arterial fibrinolysis of acute central retinal artery occlusion. Stroke 29:2076, 1998

---

29   *Anil K. Lalwani, James B. Snow, Jr.*

DISORDERS OF SMELL, TASTE, AND HEARING

SMELL

The sense of smell determines the flavor and palatability of food and drink. It serves, along with the trigeminal system, as a monitor of inhaled chemicals, including dangerous substances such as natural gas, smoke, and air pollutants. Loss of or decreased ability to smell affects approximately 1% of people under age 60 and more than half of the population beyond this age.

DEFINITIONS   *Smell* is the perception of odor by the nose. *Taste* is the perception of salty, sweet, sour, or bitter by the tongue. Related sensations during eating such as somatic sensations of coolness, warmth, and irritation are mediated through the trigeminal, glossopharyngeal, and vagal afferents in the nose, oral cavity, tongue, pharynx, and larynx. *Flavor* is the complex interaction of taste, smell, and somatic sensation.

Terms relating to disorders of smell include *anosmia*, an absence of the ability to smell; *hyposmia*, a decreased ability to smell; *hyperosmia* (an increased sensitivity to an odorant); *dysosmia* (distortion in the perception of an odor); *phantosmia*, perception of an odorant where none is present; and *agnosia*, inability to classify, contrast, or identify odor sensations verbally, even though the ability to distinguish between odorants or to recognize them may be normal. An odor stimulus is referred to as an *odorant*. Each category of smell dysfunction can be further subclassified as total (applying to all odorants) or partial (dysfunction of only select odorants).

PHYSIOLOGY OF SMELL   The *olfactory neuroepithelium* is located in the superior part of the nasal cavities. It contains an orderly arrangement of bipolar olfactory receptor cells, microvillar cells, sustentacular cells, and basal cells. The dendritic process of the bipolar cell has a bulb-shaped knob, or vesicle, that projects into the mucous layer and bears six to eight cilia. It is the cilia that contain the odorant receptors. The arrangement of cilia increases overall exposure to the environment and translates into each bipolar cell containing 56 cm² (9 in.²) of surface area to receive stimulus.

The microvillar cells are located adjacent to the receptor cells on the surface of the neuroepithelium. The sustentacular cells, unlike their counterparts in the respiratory epithelium, are not specialized to secrete mucus. Although they form a tight barrier separating the neurons from the outside environment, their complete function is unknown. The basal cells are progenitors of other cell types in the olfactory neuroepithelium, including the bipolar receptor cells. There is a regular turnover of the bipolar receptor cells, which function as the primary sensory neurons. In addition, with injury to the cell body or its axon, the receptor cell is replaced by a differentiated basal cell which reestablishes a central neural connection. Hence these primary sensory neurons are unique among sensory systems in that they are regularly replaced and regenerate after injury.

The unmyelinated axons of the receptor cells form the fila of the olfactory nerve, pass through the cribriform plate, and terminate within spherical masses of neuropil, termed *glomeruli*, in the olfactory bulb. The glomeruli are the focus of a high degree of convergence of information, since many more fibers enter than leave them. The main second-order neurons are the mitral cells. The primary dendrite of each mitral cell extends into a single glomerulus. Axons of the mitral cells project along with the axons of adjacent tufted cells to the limbic system, including the anterior olfactory nucleus, the prepiriform cortex, the periamygdaloid cortex, the olfactory tubercle, the nucleus of the lateral olfactory tract, and the corticomedial nucleus of the amygdala. Cognitive awareness of smell requires stimulation of the prepiriform cortex or the amygdaloid nuclei.

A secondary potential site of olfactory chemosensation is located in the epithelium of the vomeronasal organ, a tubular structure that opens on the ventral aspect of the nasal septum. Sensory neurons located in the vomeronasal organ detect pheromones, nonvolatile chemical signals that in lower mammals trigger innate and stereotyped reproductive and social behaviors, as well as neuroendocrine changes. The neurons from the organ project to the accessory olfactory bulbs and not the main olfactory bulb, as in the olfactory neuroepithelium. Whether humans use the vomeronasal organ to detect and respond to chemical signals from others remains controversial. Recent work in delineating the molecular pathology of Kallman syndrome suggests that development of the olfactory and vomeronasal system is required for normal sexual maturation (Chap. 335).

The sensation of smell begins with introduction of an odorant to the cilia of the bipolar neuron. Most odorants are hydrophobic; as they move from the air phase of the nasal cavity to the aqueous phase of the olfactory mucous, they are transported toward the cilia by small water-soluble proteins called *odorant-binding proteins* and reversibly bind to receptors on the cilia surface. Binding causes conformational changes in the receptor protein, which induces a chain of biochemical events and results in generation of action potentials in the primary neurons. Transduction depends on the activation of G protein–coupled second messengers. Intensity appears to be coded by the amount of firing in the afferent neurons.

Basic elements of the genetic coding involved in smell are now becoming understood. Olfactory receptor proteins belong to the large family of G protein–coupled receptors that also includes rhodopsins; α- and β-adrenergic receptors; muscarinic acetylcholine receptors; and neurotransmitter receptors for dopamine, serotonin, and substance P. Members of the G protein–coupled receptors are characterized by the presence of 7 putative α-helical transmembrane domains composed of 20 to 28 hydrophobic amino acid residues. In mammals, there are probably 300 to 1000 olfactory receptor genes belonging to 20 different families located on various chromosomes in clusters. The receptor genes are present at more than 25 different human chromosomal locations. The gene clusters have likely risen as a result of repeated duplication of individual genes or clusters of genes. Each olfactory neuron seems to express only one or, at most, a few receptor genes thus providing the molecular basis of odor discrimination. While the receptors are expressed in several tissues, including the olfactory neuroepithelium and mammalian germ cells, their primary role appears to be odorant recognition and discrimination. Bipolar cells that express similar receptors appear to be scattered across discrete spatial zones.

These similar cells converge on a select few number of glomeruli in the olfactory bulb. The result is a potential spatial map of how we receive odor stimulus, much like the tonotopic organization of how we perceive sound.

DISORDERS OF THE SENSE OF SMELL Disorders of the sense of smell are caused by conditions that interfere with the access of the odorant to the olfactory neuroepithelium (transport loss), injure the receptor region (sensory loss), or damage central olfactory pathways (neural loss). At the present time, there are no clinical tests to differentiate these different types of olfactory losses. Fortunately, the history of the disease provides important clues to the cause. The leading causes of olfactory disorders are summarized in Table 29-1; the most common etiologies are head trauma and viral infections. Head trauma is a frequent cause of anosmia in children and young adults, whereas viral etiologies predominate in older adults.

Cranial trauma is followed by unilateral or bilateral impairment of smell in up to 15% of cases; anosmia is more common than hyposmia. Olfactory dysfunction is more common when trauma is associated with loss of consciousness, moderately severe head injury (grades II to V), and skull fracture. Frontal injuries and fractures disrupt the cribriform plate and olfactory axons that perforate it. Sometimes there is an associated cerebrospinal fluid (CSF) rhinorrhea resulting from a tearing of the dura overlying the cribriform plate and paranasal sinuses. Anosmia may also follow blows to the occiput. Once traumatic anosmia develops, it is usually permanent; only 10% of patients ever improve or recover. Perversion of the sense of smell may occur as a transient phase in the recovery process.

Viral infections destroy the olfactory neuroepithelium, which is replaced by respiratory epithelium. Parainfluenza virus type 3 appears to be especially detrimental to human olfaction. HIV infection is associated with subjective distortion of taste and smell, which may become more severe as the disease progresses. The loss of taste and smell may play an important role in the development and progression of HIV-associated wasting. Congenital anosmias are rare but important. Kallmann syndrome is an X-linked disorder characterized by congenital anosmia and hypogonadotropic hypogonadism resulting from a failure of migration from the olfactory placode of olfactory receptor neurons and neurons synthesizing gonadotropin-releasing hormone (Chap. 328). The responsible gene (*KAL*) has been cloned. Anosmia can also occur in albinos. The receptor cells are present but are hypoplastic, lack cilia, and do not project above the surrounding supporting cells.

Meningioma of the inferior frontal region is the most frequent neoplastic cause of anosmia; loss of smell may be the only neurologic abnormality at presentation. Rarely, anosmia can occur with glioma of the frontal lobe. Occasionally, pituitary adenomas, craniopharyngiomas, suprasellar meningiomas, and aneurysms of the anterior part of the circle of Willis extend forward and damage olfactory structures. These tumors and hamartomas may also induce seizures with olfactory hallucinations, indicating involvement of the uncus of the temporal lobe.

Dysosmia, subjective distortions of olfactory perception, may occur with intranasal disease that partially impairs smell or may represent a phase in the recovery from a neurogenic anosmia. Most dysosmic disorders consist of disagreeable or foul odors, and they may be accompanied by distortions of taste. Dysosmia is associated with depression.

Approach to the Patient

The history of the onset and course of the disorder is often paramount in establishing an etiology. Unilateral anosmia is rarely a complaint and is only recognized by separate testing of smell in each nasal cavity. Bilateral anosmia, on the other hand, brings patients to medical attention. Anosmic patients usually complain of a loss of the sense of taste even though their taste thresholds may be within normal limits. In actuality, they are complaining of a loss of flavor detection, which is mainly an olfactory function. The physical examination should include a complete examination of the ears, upper respiratory tract, and head and neck. A neurologic examination emphasizing the cranial nerves and cerebellar and sensorimotor function is essential. The patient's general mood should be assessed, and any signs of depression should be noted.

The sensory evaluation of olfactory function is necessary to corroborate the patient's complaint, evaluate the efficacy of treatment, and assess the degree of permanent impairment. The degree to which qualitative sensations are present can be assessed by any of several methods. The Odor Stix test uses a commercially available odor-producing magic marker–like pen held approximately 8 to 15 cm (3 to 6 in.) from the patient's nose to check for gross perception of the odorant. Another gross perception of odorant test, the 30-cm alcohol test, uses a freshly opened isopropyl alcohol packet held approximately 30 cm (12 in.) from the patient's nose. There is a commercially available scratch-and-sniff card containing three odors available for testing olfaction grossly. A superior test is the University of Pennsylvania Smell Identification Test (UPSIT). This consists of a 40-item, forced choice, microencapsulated odor, scratch-and-sniff paradigm. For example, one of the items reads, "This odor smells most like (a) chocolate, (b) banana, (c) onion, or (d) fruit punch," and the patient is instructed to answer one of the alternatives. The test is highly reliable, is sensitive to age and sex differences, and provides an accurate quantitative determination of the olfactory deficit. Persons with a total loss of smell function score in the range of 7 to 19 out of 40. The average score for total anosmics is slightly higher than that expected on the basis of chance because of the inclusion of some odorants that act by trigeminal stimulation.

The second step is to establish a detection threshold for the odorant phenyl ethyl alcohol, using a graduated stimulus. Sensitivity for each side of the nose is determined with a detection threshold for phenyl ethyl methyl ethyl carbinol. Nasal resistance can also be measured with anterior rhinomanometry for each side of the nose.

Computed tomography (CT) or magnetic resonance imaging (MRI) of the head is required to rule out paranasal sinusitis, neoplasms of the anterior cranial fossa, nasal cavity, or paranasal sinuses and unsuspected fractures of the anterior cranial fossa. Bone abnormalities are best seen with CT. MRI is useful in evaluating olfactory bulbs, ventricles, and other soft tissue of the brain. Coronal CT is optimal for assessing cribriform plate, anterior cranial fossa, and sinus anatomy.

Techniques have been developed to biopsy the olfactory neuroepithelium, but in view of the widespread degeneration of the olfactory neuroepithelium and intercalation of respiratory epithelium in the ol-

---

Table 29-1 Causes of Olfactory Dysfunction

Transport Olfactory Losses	Neural Olfactory Losses
Allergic rhinitis	AIDS
Bacterial rhinitis and sinusitis	Alcoholism
Congenital Abnormality (encephalocele)	Alzheimer's disease
Nasal neoplasms	Chemical toxins
Nasal polyps	Cigarette smoke
Nasal septal deviation	Depression
Nasal surgery	Diabetes mellitus
Viral infections	Drugs
Sensory Olfactory Losses	Huntington's chorea
Drugs	Hypothyroidism
Neoplasms	Kallmann syndrome
Radiation therapy	Korsakoff's psychosis
Toxic chemical exposure	Malnutrition
Viral infections	Neoplasm
	Neurosurgery
	Parkinson's disease
	Trauma
	Vitamin B_{12} deficiency
	Zinc deficiency

factory area of adults with no apparent olfactory dysfunction, biopsy material must be interpreted cautiously.

R̲x̲ **TREATMENT**   Therapy for patients with transport olfactory losses due to allergic rhinitis, bacterial rhinitis and sinusitis, polyps, neoplasms, and structural abnormalities of the nasal cavities can be undertaken rationally and with a high likelihood for improvement. Allergy management, antibiotic therapy, topical and systemic glucocorticoid therapy, and surgery for nasal polyps, deviation of the nasal septum, and chronic hyperplastic sinusitis are frequently effective in restoring the sense of smell.

There is no treatment with demonstrated efficacy for sensorineural olfactory losses. Fortunately, spontaneous recovery often occurs. Zinc and vitamin therapy (especially with vitamin A) are advocated by some. Profound zinc deficiency can produce loss and distortion of the sense of smell but is not a clinically important problem except in very limited geographic areas (Chap. 75). The epithelial degeneration associated with vitamin A deficiency can cause anosmia, but in western societies the prevalence of vitamin A deficiency is low. Exposure to cigarette smoke and other airborne toxic chemicals can cause metaplasia of the olfactory epithelium. Spontaneous recovery can occur if the insult is discontinued. Patient counseling is therefore helpful in these cases.

As mentioned above, more than half of people over age 60 suffer from olfactory dysfunction. No effective treatment exists for presbyosmia, but patients are often reassured to learn that this problem is common in their age group. In addition, early recognition and counseling can help patients to compensate for the loss of smell. The incidence of natural gas–related accidents is disproportionately high in the elderly, perhaps due in part to the gradual loss of smell. Mercaptan, the pungent odor in natural gas, is an olfactory stimulant and does not activate taste receptors. Many elderly with olfactory dysfunction experience a decrease in flavor sensation and find it necessary to hyperflavor food, usually by increasing the amount of salt in their diet. The physician can assist patients in developing healthy strategies to deal with the decreased sense of smell.

TASTE

Compared with disorders of smell, gustatory disorders are uncommon and their pathogenesis poorly understood. Many patients with a loss of olfactory sensitivity also complain of a loss of the sense of taste. On testing, most of these patients have normal detection thresholds for taste.

DEFINITIONS   Disturbances of the sense of taste may be categorized as *total ageusia*—total absence of gustatory function or inability to detect the qualities of sweet, salt, bitter, or sour; *partial ageusia*—ability to detect some of but not all the qualitative gustatory sensations; *specific ageusia*—inability to detect the taste quality of certain substances; *total hypogeusia*—decreased sensitivity to all tastants; *partial hypogeusia*—decreased sensitivity to some tastants; and *dysgeusia* or *phantogeusia*—distortion in the perception of a tastant, i.e., the perception of the wrong quality when a tastant is presented or the perception of a taste when there has been no tastant ingested. Confusions of sour and bitter are common and, at times, may be semantic misunderstandings. Frequently, however, they have physiologic or pathophysiologic bases. Other taste quality confusions occur between sour and salty and bitter. It may be possible to differentiate between the loss of flavor recognition in patients with olfactory losses who complain of a loss of taste as well as smell by asking if they are able to taste sweetness in sodas, saltiness in potato chips, etc.

PHYSIOLOGY OF TASTE   The taste receptor cells are located in the taste buds, spherical groups of cells arranged in a pattern resembling the segments of a citrus fruit. At the surface, the taste bud has a pore into which microvilli of the receptor cells project. Unlike the olfactory system, the receptor cell is not the primary neuron. Instead, gustatory afferent nerve fibers contact individual taste receptor cells. Transduction depends on activation of G protein–coupled second messengers but differs in details for each taste quality.

The sense of taste is mediated through the facial, glossopharyngeal, and vagal nerves. The gustatory system consists of at least five receptor populations. Taste buds are located in the papillae along the lateral margin and dorsum of the tongue at the junction of the dorsum and the base of the tongue, and in the palate, epiglottis, larynx, and esophagus. The chorda tympani branch of the facial nerve subserves taste from the anterior two-thirds of the tongue. The posterior third of the tongue is supplied by the lingual branch of the glossopharyngeal nerve. Afferents from the palate travel with the greater superficial petrosal nerve to the geniculate ganglion and then via the facial nerve to the brainstem. The internal branch of the superior laryngeal nerve of the vagus nerve contains the taste afferents from the larynx, including the epiglottis and esophagus.

The central connections of the nerves terminate in the brainstem in the nucleus of the tractus solitarius. The central pathway from the nucleus of the tractus solitarius projects to the ipsilateral parabrachial nuclei of the pons. Two divergent pathways project from the parabrachial nuclei. One ascends to the gustatory relay in the dorsal thalamus, synapses, and continues to the cortex of the insula. There is also evidence for a direct pathway from the parabrachial nuclei to the cortex. (Olfaction and gustation appear to be unique among sensory systems in that at least some fibers bypass the thalamus.) The other pathway from the parabrachial nuclei goes to the ventral forebrain, including the lateral hypothalamus, substantia innominata, central nucleus of the amygdala, and the stria terminalis.

Tastants gain access to the receptor cells through the taste pore. Four classes of taste are recognized: sweet, salt, sour, and bitter. Individual gustatory afferent fibers almost always respond to a number of different chemicals. Response patterns of gustatory afferent axons can be grouped into classes based on the stimulus chemical that produces the largest response. For example, for sucrose–best response neurons, the second-best stimulus is almost always sodium chloride. The fact that individual gustatory afferent fibers respond to a large number of different chemicals led to the *across-fiber-pattern* theory of gustatory coding, while the best-stimulus analysis led to the concept of *labeled* afferents. It appears that labeled fibers are important for establishing gross quality, but the across-fiber pattern within a best-stimulus category, and perhaps among categories, is needed for discriminating chemicals within qualities. For example, sweetness may be carried by sucrose-best neurons, but the differentiation of sucrose and fructose may require a comparison of the relative activity among sucrose-best, salt-best, and quinine-best neurons. As with olfaction and other sensory systems, intensity appears to be encoded by the quantity of neural activity.

DISORDERS OF THE SENSE OF TASTE   Disorders of the sense of taste are caused by conditions that interfere with the access of the tastant to the receptor cells in the taste bud (transport loss), injure receptor cells (sensory loss), or damage gustatory afferent nerves and central gustatory pathways (neural loss) (Table 29-2). *Transport gustatory losses* result from xerostomia due to many causes, including Sjögren's syndrome, radiation therapy, heavy-metal intoxication, and bacterial colonization of the taste pore. *Sensory gustatory losses* are caused by inflammatory and degenerative diseases in the oral cavity; a vast number of drugs, particularly those that interfere with cell turnover such as antithyroid and antineoplastic agents; radiation therapy to the oral cavity and pharynx; viral infections; endocrine disorders; neoplasms; and aging. *Neural gustatory losses* occur with neoplasms, trauma, and surgical procedures in which the gustatory afferents are injured. Taste buds degenerate when their gustatory afferents are transected but remain when their somatosensory afferents are severed. Patients with renal disease have increased thresholds for sweet and sour tastes, which resolves with dialysis.

A side effect of medication is the single most common cause of taste dysfunction in clinical practice. The mechanism may be a change

Table 29-2 Causes of Gustatory Dysfunction

Transport Gustatory Losses	Neural Gustatory Losses
Drugs	Diabetes mellitus
Heavy-metal intoxication	Hypothyroidism
Radiation therapy	Oral neoplasms
Sjögren's syndrome	Oral surgery
Xerostomia	Radiation therapy
Sensory Gustatory Losses	Renal disease
Aging	Trauma
Candidiasis	Upper respiratory tract infections
Drugs (antithyroid and antineoplastic)	
Endocrine disorders	
Herpes infection	
Oral neoplasm	
Pemphigus	
Radiation therapy	
Viral infections	

in the composition of saliva, an effect on receptor function or signal transduction, or disruption of the central processing of gustatory input. Unfortunately, the responsible mechanism is not well understood for most medications. Xerostomia, regardless of the etiology, can be associated with taste dysfunction. It is associated with poor oral clearance, poor dental hygeine, and can adversely affect the oral mucosa, all leading to dysgeusia. However, severe salivary gland failure does not necessarily lead to taste complaints. Xerostomia, along with the use of antibiotics or glucocorticoids, and compromised immune function can lead to overgrowth of *Candida*; overgrowth alone, without thrush or overt signs of infection can be associated with bad taste or hypogeusia. When taste dysfunction occurs in a patient at risk for fungal overgrowth, a trial of nystatin or other anti-fungal medication is warranted.

Upper respiratory infections and head trauma can lead to both smell and taste dysfunction; taste is more likely to improve than smell. The mechanism of taste disturbance in these situations is not well understood. Trauma to the chorda tympani branch of the facial nerve during middle ear surgery or third molar extractions is relatively common and can cause dysgeusia. Bilateral chorda tympani injuries are usually associated with hypogeusia, whereas unilateral lesions produce only limited symptoms, perhaps because responses from taste receptors are disinhibited by the glossopharyngeal nerve.

Finally, aging itself may be associated with reduced taste sensitivity. The taste dysfunction may be limited to a single compound and may be mild. While many older patients may acknowledge loss of taste when asked, they are unlikely to seek medical attention for taste disturbance alone.

Approach to the Patient

Patients who complain of loss of taste should be evaluated for both gustatory and olfactory function. Clinical assessment of taste is not as well developed or standardized as that of smell. The first step is to perform suprathreshold whole-mouth taste testing for quality, intensity, and pleasantness perception of four taste qualities: sweet, salty, sour, and bitter. Most commonly used reagents for taste testing are sucrose, citric acid or hydrochloric acid, caffeine or quinine (sulfate or hydrochloride), and sodium chloride. The taste stimuli should be freshly prepared. For quantification, detection thresholds are obtained by applying graduated dilutions to the tongue quandrants or by whole-mouth sips. Electric taste testing (*electrogustometry*) is used clinically to identify taste deficits in specific quadrants of the tongue, following precise applications of stimuli. Regional gustatory testing may also be performed to assess for the possibility of loss localized to one or more receptor fields as a result of a peripheral or central lesion.

Once there is objective evidence of a disorder of taste, it is important to establish an anatomic diagnosis before proceeding to an etiologic diagnosis. The history of the disease often provides important clues to the cause. For example, absence of taste on the anterior two-thirds of the tongue associated with a facial paralysis indicates that the

lesion is proximal to the juncture of the chorda tympani branch with the facial nerve in the mastoid.

℞ TREATMENT Therapy for gustatory loss is limited. Nonetheless, some etiologies of taste dysfunction are amenable to intervention. Taste disturbance related to drugs can often be resolved by changing the prescribed medication. Xerostomia can be treated with artificial saliva, providing some benefits to patients with a disturbed salivary milieu. Oral pilocarpine may be beneficial for a variety of forms of xerostomia. Appropriate treatment of bacterial and fungal infections of the oral cavity can be of great help in improving taste function. Taste dysfunction following trauma may resolve spontaneously without intervention and is more likely to do so than posttraumatic smell dysfunction. Altered taste due to surgical stretch injury of chorda tympani nerve usually improves within 3 to 4 months, while dysfunction is usually permanent with transection of the nerve. In most patients with idiopathic cases of altered taste sensitivity, the problem either remains stable or worsens. Zinc and vitamin therapy for gustatory losses is advocated by some but lacks demonstrated efficacy. No effective therapeutic strategies exist for the sensorineural disorders of taste.

HEARING

Hearing loss is one of the most common sensory disorders in humans. Nearly 10% of the adult population has some hearing loss. For many, this impairment presents early in life. However, hearing loss can present at any age. Between 30 and 35% of individuals over the age of 65 have a hearing loss of sufficient magnitude to require a hearing aid.

PHYSIOLOGY OF HEARING (Fig. 29-1) Hearing occurs by air conduction and bone conduction. In air conduction, sound waves reach the ear by propagation in air, enter the external auditory canal, and set the tympanic membrane in motion, which in turn moves the malleus, incus, and stapes of the middle ear. Movement of the footplate of the stapes causes pressure changes in the fluid-filled inner ear eliciting a traveling wave in the basilar membrane of the cochlea. The tympanic membrane and the ossicular chain in the middle ear serve as an impedence-matching mechanism, improving the efficiency of energy transfer from air to the fluid-filled inner ear. Hearing by bone conduction occurs when the sounding source, in contact with the head, results in vibration of the bones of the skull, including the temporal bone, producing a traveling wave in the basilar membrane.

Stereocilia of the hair cells of the organ of Corti, which rests on the basilar membrane, are in contact with the tectorial membrane and are deformed by the traveling wave. A point of maximal displacement of the basilar membrane is determined by the frequency of the stimulating tone. High-frequency tones cause maximal displacement of the basilar membrane near the base of the cochlea. As the frequency of the stimulating tone decreases, the point of maximal displacement moves toward the apex of the cochlea.

The inner and outer hair cells of the organ of Corti have different innervation patterns, but both are mechanoreceptors. The afferent innervation relates principally to the inner hair cells, and the efferent innervation relates principally to outer hair cells. The motility of the outer hair cells alters the micromechanics of the inner hair cells creating a cochlear amplifier, which explains the exquisite sensitivity and frequency selectivity of the cochlea.

The current concept of cochlear transduction is that displacement of the tips of the stereocilia allows potassium to flow into the cell, resulting in its depolarization. The potassium influx opens calcium channels near the base of the cell, stimulating transmitter release. The neurotransmitter at the hair cell and cochlear nerve dendrite interface is thought to be glutamate. The action potential in the eighth nerve occurs 0.5 ms after the onset of the cochlear microphonic potential.

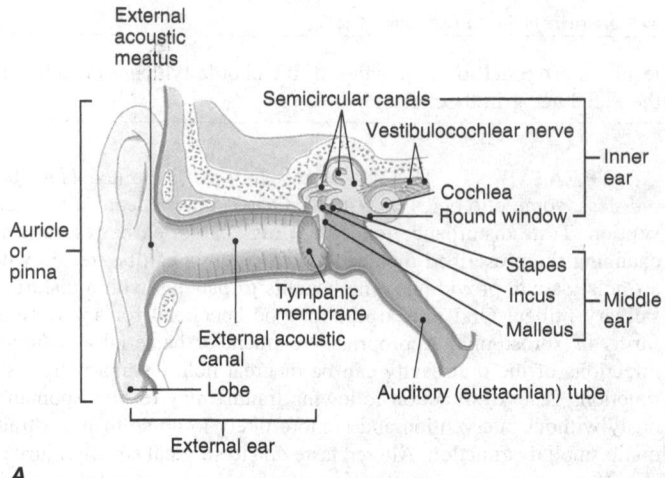

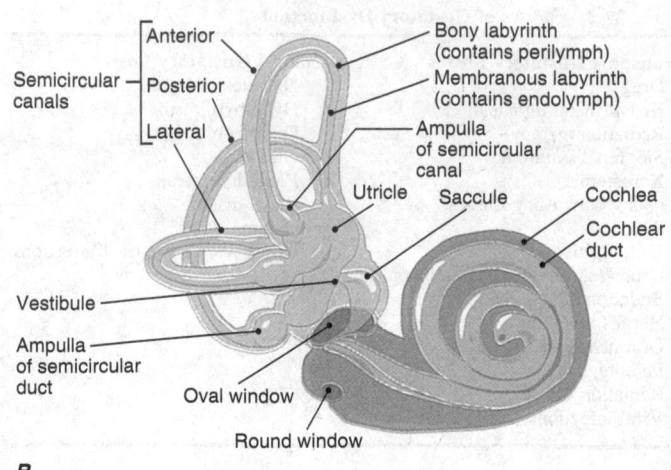

FIGURE 29-1 *A*. Drawing of modified coronal section through external ear and temporal bone, with structures of the middle and inner ear demonstrated.

B. High-resolution view of inner ear.

Each of the cochlear nerve neurons can be activated at a frequency and intensity specific for that cell. This specificity is maintained at each point of the central auditory pathway: dorsal and ventral cochlear nuclei, trapezoid body, superior olivary complex, lateral lemniscus, inferior colliculus, medial geniculate body, and auditory cortex. At low frequencies, individual auditory nerve fibers can respond more or less synchronously with the stimulating tone. At higher frequencies, phase-locking occurs so that neurons alternate in response to particular phases of the cycle of the sound wave. Intensity is encoded by the amount of neural activity in individual neurons, the number of neurons that are active, and the specific neurons that are activated.

GENETIC CAUSES OF HEARING LOSS More than half of childhood hearing impairment is thought to be hereditary; hereditary hearing impairment (HHI) can also manifest later in life. HHI may be classified as either nonsyndromic, when hearing loss is the only clinical abnormality, or syndromic, when hearing loss is associated with anomalies in other organ systems. Nearly two-thirds of HHIs are nonsyndromic and the remaining one-third are syndromic. Between 70 and 80% of nonsyndromic HHI is inherited in an autosomal recessive manner; another 15 to 20% is autosomal dominant. Less than 5% is X-linked or maternally inherited via the mitochondria.

Over 60 loci harboring genes for nonsyndromic HHI have been mapped, with equal numbers of dominant and recessive modes of inheritance; 14 different genes have been cloned (Table 29-3). The hearing genes fall into the categories of structural proteins (MYO7A, MYO15, TECTA, DIAPH1), transcription factors (POU3F4, POU4F3), ion channels (KCNQ4, PDS), and gap junction proteins (Cx26, Cx30, Cx31). Several of these genes, including connexin 26 (Cx26), TECTA, and MYO7A, cause both autosomal dominant and recessive forms of nonsyndromic HHI. In general, the hearing loss associated with dominant genes has its onset in adolescence or adulthood and varies in severity, whereas the hearing loss associated with recessive inheritance is congenital and profound. Connexin 26 is particularly important because it is associated with nearly 20% of cases of childhood deafness; in heterozygotes the onset of hearing loss may be in adolescence or adulthood. Two frame-shift mutations, 30delG and 167delT, account for >50% of the cases, making population screening feasible. The 167delT mutation is highly prevalent in Ashkenazi Jews; it is predicted that 1 in 1765 individuals in this population will be homozygous and affected. The hearing loss can also vary among the members of the same family, suggesting that other genes or factors likely influence the auditory phenotype.

The contribution of genetics to presbycusis (see below) is also becoming better understood. In addition to connexin 26, several other nonsyndromic genes are associated with hearing loss that progresses with age. It is likely that presbycusis has both environmental and genetic components.

Over 200 syndromes are associated with hearing loss. Common syndromic forms of hearing loss include Usher syndrome (retinitis pigmentosa and hearing loss), Waardenburg syndrome (pigmentary abnormality and hearing loss), Pendred syndrome (thyroid organification defect and hearing loss), Alport syndrome (renal disease and hearing loss), Jervell and Lange-Nielsen syndrome (prolonged QT interval and hearing loss), neurofibromatosis type 2 (bilateral acoustic schwannoma), and mitochondrial disorders [mitochondrial encephalopathy, lactic acidosis, and stroke-like episodes (MELAS); myoclonic epilepsy and ragged red fibers (MERRF); progressive external ophthalmoplegia (PEO)].

Rapid progress in understanding the basis of these and related disorders has revealed a fascinating complexity, including evidence for genetic heterogeneity (different genes resulting in a similar clinical phenotype), allelic disorders (distinct phenotypes associated with different mutations in the same gene), and polygenic modifiers (Chap. 65).

DISORDERS OF THE SENSE OF HEARING Hearing loss can result from disorders of the auricle, external auditory canal, middle ear, inner ear, or central auditory pathways (Fig. 29-2). *In general, lesions in the auricle, external auditory canal, or middle ear cause conductive hearing losses, whereas lesions in the inner ear or eighth nerve cause sensorineural hearing losses.*

Conductive Hearing Loss This results from obstruction of the external auditory canal by cerumen, debris, and foreign bodies; swelling of the lining of the canal; atresia of the ear canal; neoplasms of the canal; perforations of the tympanic membrane; disruption of the ossicular chain, as occurs with necrosis of the long process of the incus in trauma or infection; otosclerosis; or fluid, scarring, or neoplasms in the middle ear.

Cholesteatoma, i.e., the presence of stratified squamous epithelium in the middle ear or mastoid, occurs frequently in adults. A cholesteatoma is a benign, slowly growing lesion that destroys bone and normal ear tissue. Major theories of pathogenesis of acquired cholesteatoma include traumatic implantation and invasion, immigration and invasion through a perforation, and metaplasia following chronic infection and irritation. On examination, there is often a perforation filled with cheesy white squamous debris. A chronically draining ear that fails to respond to appropriate antibiotic therapy should raise the suspicion of a cholesteatoma. Conductive hearing loss secondary to ossicular erosion is common. Surgery is required to remove this insidiously growing and destructive disease process.

Conductive hearing loss in the presence of a normal ear canal and intact tympanic membrane is suggestive of ossicular pathology. Fixation of the stapes from *otosclerosis* is a common cause of low-frequency conductive hearing loss. It occurs with equal frequency in men and women and has a simple autosomal dominant inheritance with incomplete penetrance. Hearing impairment usually presents between the late teens to the forties. In women, the hearing loss is often first noticeable during pregnancy, as the otosclerotic process is accelerated during pregnancy. A hearing aid or a short outpatient surgical procedure (stapedectomy) can provide adequate auditory rehabilitation. Extension of otosclerosis beyond the stapes footplate to involve the cochlea (cochlear otosclerosis) can lead to mixed or sensorineural hearing loss. Fluoride therapy to prevent hearing loss associated with cochlear otosclerosis remains controversial.

Eustachian tube dysfunction is extremely common in adults and may predispose to acute otitis media (AOM) or serous otitis media (SOM). Trauma, AOM, or chronic otitis media are the usual factors responsible for tympanic membrane perforation. While small perforations often heal spontaneously, larger defects usually require surgical intervention. Tympanoplasty is highly effective (>90%) in the repair of tympanic membrane perforations. Otoscopy is usually sufficient to diagnose AOM, SOM, chronic otitis media, cerumen impaction, tympanic membrane perforation, and eustachian tube dysfunction.

Table 29-3 Nonsyndromic Genes and Loci

Locus	Gene	Function	Inheritance
DFNB1	GBJ2 (Cx26)	Forms gap junctions, or plasma membrane channels, with connexins	AR
DFNB2	MYO7A	Moves different macromolecular structures relative to actin filaments	AR
DFNB3	MYO15	Organizes actin in hair cells	AR
DFNB4	PDS	Encodes highly hydrophobic proteins containing the sulphate transporter signature	AR
DFNB9	OTOF	Involved in trafficking of membrane vesicles	AR
DFNB21	TECTA	Includes an amino-terminal hydrophobic signal sequence for translocation across the membrane and a carboxy-terminal hydrophobic region characteristic of precursors of glycosylphosphatidyl-inositol-linked membrane-bound proteins	AR
DFNA1	DIAPH1	Involved in cytokinesis and establishment of cell polarity	AD
DFNA2	GJB3 (Cx31)	Forms gap junction protein	AD
	KCNQ4	Forms potassium channel	
DFNA3	GJB2 (Cx26)	Forms gap junctions, or plasma membrane channels, with connexins	AD
	GBJ6 (Cx30)		
DFNA5	DFNA5	Unknown; related to a gene that is upregulated in estrogen receptor–negative breast carcinomas	AD
DFNA8/12	TECTA	Includes an amino-terminal hydrophobic signal sequence for translocation across the membrane and a carboxy-terminal hydrophobic region characteristic of precursors of glycosylphosphatidyl-inositol-linked membrane-bound proteins	AD
DFNA9	COCH	Involved in hemostasis, complement system, immune system, and extracellular matrix assembly	AD
DFNA11	MYO7A	Moves different macromolecular structures relative to actin filaments	AD
DFNA15	POU4F3	Serves as a critical developmental regulator for the determination of cellular phenotypes	AD
DFN3	POU3F4	Serves as a critical developmental regulator for the determination of cellular phenotypes	X-linked

NOTE: AD, autosomal dominant; AR, autosomal recessive.

Sensorineural Hearing Loss Damage to the hair cells of the organ of Corti may be caused by intense noise, viral infections, ototoxic drugs (e.g., salicylates, quinine and its synthetic analogues, aminoglycoside antibiotics, loop diuretics such as furosemide and ethacrynic acid, and cancer chemotherapeutic agents such as cisplatin), fractures of the temporal bone, meningitis, cochlear otosclerosis (see above), Ménière's disease, and aging. Congenital malformations of the inner ear may be the cause of hearing loss in some adults. Genetic predisposition alone or in concert with environmental influences may also be responsible.

Presbycusis (age-associated hearing loss) is the most common cause of sensorineural hearing loss in adults. In the early stages, it is characterized by symmetric, gentle to sharply sloping high-frequency hearing loss. With progression, the hearing loss involves all frequencies. More importantly, the hearing impairment is associated with significant loss in clarity. There is a loss of discrimination for phonemes, recruitment (abnormal growth of loudness), and particular difficulty in understanding speech in noisy environments. Hearing aids may provide limited rehabilitation once the word recognition score deteriorates below 50%. Significant advancements and improvements in cochlear implants have made them the treatment of choice when hearing aids prove inadequate (<30% word recognition score with optimal amplification).

Ménière's disease is characterized by episodic vertigo, fluctuating sensorineural hearing loss, tinnitus, and aural fullness. Tinnitus and/or deafness may be absent during the initial attacks of vertigo, but they invariably appear as the disease progresses and are increased in severity during an acute attack. The annual incidence of Ménière's disease is 0.5 to 7.5 per 1000; onset is most frequently in the fifth decade of life but may also occur in young adults or the elderly. Histologically, there is distention of the endolymphatic system (endolymphatic hydrops) leading to degeneration of vestibular and cochlear hair cells. This may result from endolymphatic sac dysfunction secondary to infection, trauma, autoimmune disease, inflammatory causes, or tumor; an idiopathic etiology constitutes the largest category and is most accurately referred to as Ménière's disease. Although any pattern of hearing loss can be observed, typically, low-frequency, unilateral sensorineural hearing impairment is present. MRI should be obtained to exclude retrocochlear pathology such as cerebellopontine angle tumors or demyelinating disorders. Therapy is directed towards the control of vertigo. A low-salt diet is the mainstay of treatment of the control of rotatory vertigo. Diuretics, a short course of glucocorticoids, and intratympanic gentamicin may also be useful adjuncts in recalcitrant cases. Surgical therapy of vertigo is reserved for unresponsive cases and includes endolymphatic sac decompression, labyrinthectomy, and vestibular nerve section. Both labyrinthectomy and vestibular nerve section abolish rotatory vertigo in >90% of the cases. Unfortunately, there is no effective therapy for hearing loss, tinnitus, or aural fullness associated with Ménière's disease.

Sensorineural hearing loss may also result from any neoplastic, vascular, demyelinating, infectious, or degenerative disease or trauma affecting the central auditory pathways. Human immunodeficiency virus leads to both peripheral and central auditory system pathology and is associated with sensorineural hearing impairment.

An individual can have both conductive and sensory hearing loss termed *mixed hearing loss*. Mixed hearing losses are due to pathology that can affect the middle and inner ear simultaneously such as otosclerosis involving the ossicles and the cochlea, head trauma, chronic otitis media, cholesteatoma, middle ear tumors, and some inner ear malformations.

Trauma resulting in temporal bone fractures may be associated

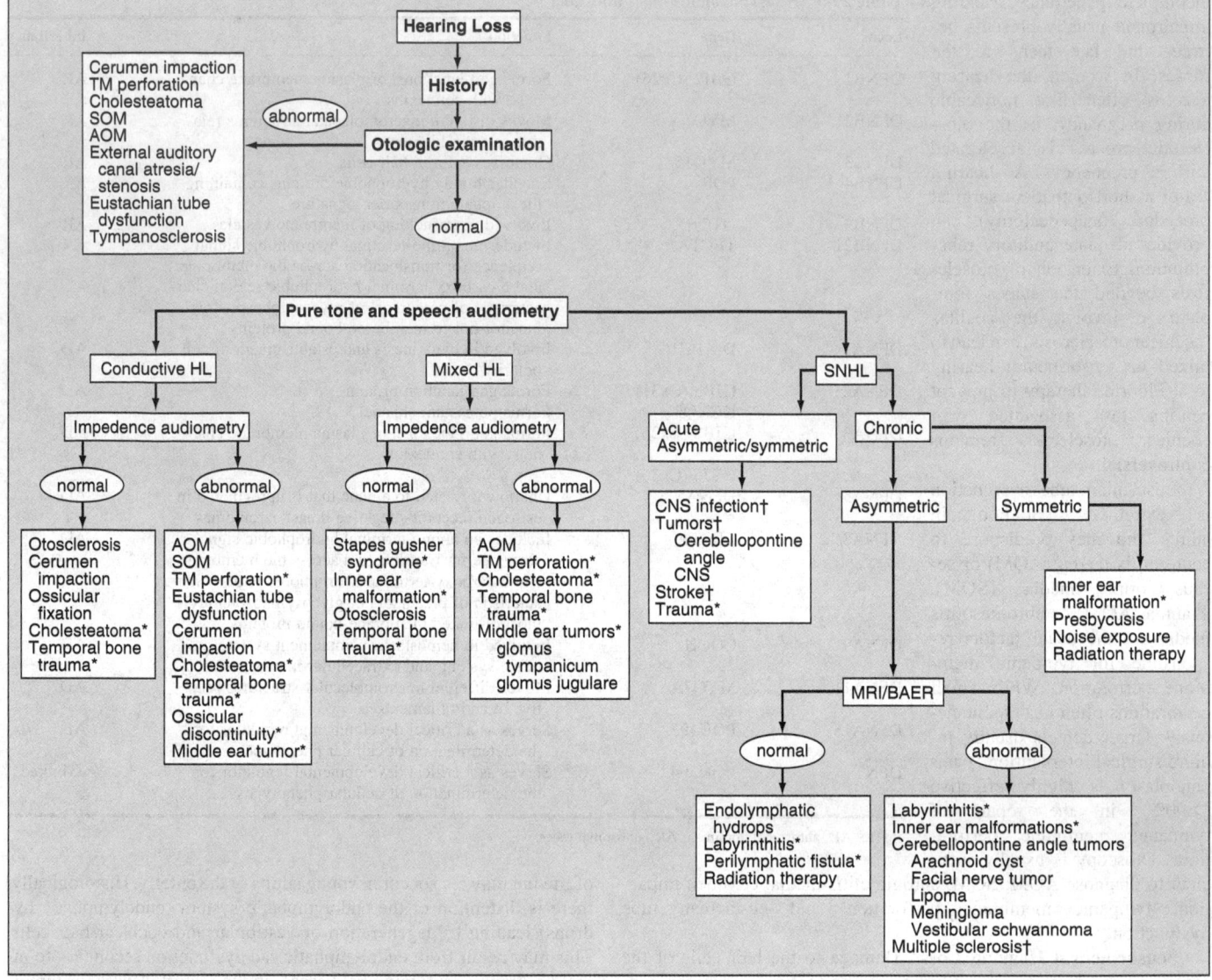

FIGURE 29-2 An algorithm for the approach to hearing loss. HL, hearing loss; SNHL, sensorineural hearing loss; TM, tympanic membrane; SOM, serous otitis media; AOM, acute otitis media; *, CT scan of temporal bone; †, MRI scan.

with conductive, sensorineural, and mixed hearing loss. If the fracture spares the inner ear, there may simply be conductive hearing loss due to rupture of the tympanic membrane or disruption of the ossicular chain. These abnormalities are amenable to surgical correction. Profound hearing loss and severe vertigo are associated with temporal bone fractures involving the inner ear. A perilymphatic fistula associated with leakage of inner-ear fluid into the middle ear can occur and may require surgical repair. An associated facial nerve injury is not uncommon. CT is best suited to assess fracture of the traumatized temporal bone, evaluate the ear canal, and determine the integrity of the ossicular chain and the involvement of the inner ear. CSF leaks that accompany temporal bone fractures are usually self-limited; the use of prophylactic antibiotics is controversial.

Tinnitus is defined as the perception of a sound when there is no sound in the environment. It may have a buzzing, roaring, or ringing quality and may be pulsatile (synchronous with the heartbeat). Tinnitus is often associated with either a conductive or sensorineural hearing loss. The pathophysiology of tinnitus is not well understood. The cause of the tinnitus can usually be determined by finding the cause of the associated hearing loss. Tinnitus may be the first symptom of a serious condition such as a vestibular schwannoma. Pulsatile tinnitus requires evaluation of the vascular system of the head to exclude vascular tumors such as glomus jugulare tumors, aneurysms, and stenotic arterial lesions; it may also occur with SOM.

Approach to the Patient

The goals in the evaluation of a patient with auditory complaints are to determine: (1) the nature of the hearing impairment (conductive vs. sensorineural), (2) the severity of the impairment (mild, moderate, severe, profound), (3) the anatomy of the impairment (external ear, middle ear, inner ear, or central auditory pathway pathology, and (4) the etiology. Initially, the history and the physical examination are critical in the identification of the underlying pathology leading to the auditory deficit. The history should elicit characteristics of the hearing loss, including the duration of deafness, nature of onset (sudden vs. insidious), rate of progression (rapid vs. slow), and involvement of the ear (unilateral vs. bilateral). The presence or absence of tinnitus, vertigo, imbalance, aural fullness, otorrhea, headache, facial nerve dysfunction, and head and neck paresthesias should be ascertained. Information regarding head trauma, exposure to ototoxins, occupational or recreational noise exposure, and family history of hearing impairment may also be important. A sudden onset of unilateral hearing loss, with or without tinnitus, may represent a viral infection of the inner ear or a vascular accident. Patients with unilateral hearing loss (sensory or conductive) usually complain of reduced hearing, poor sound localization, and difficulty hearing clearly with background noise. Gradual progression of a hearing deficit is common with otosclerosis, noise-induced hearing loss, vestibular schwannoma, or Ménière's disease.

Small vestibular schwannomas typically present with asymmetric hearing impairment, tinnitus, and imbalance (rarely vertigo); cranial neuropathy, in particular of the trigeminal or facial nerve, may accompany larger tumors. In addition to hearing loss, Ménière's disease may be associated with episodic vertigo, tinnitus, and aural fullness. Hearing loss with otorrhea is most likely due to chronic otitis media or cholesteatoma.

Family history may be crucial in delineating a genetic basis of hearing impairment. The history may also help identify environmental risk factors that lead to hearing impairment in a family. Sensitivity to aminoglycoside ototoxicity, maternally transmitted through a mitochondrial mutation, can be ascertained through a careful family history (Chap. 67). Susceptibility to noise-induced hearing loss or age-related hearing loss (presbycusis) may also be genetically determined.

The physical examination should evaluate the auricle, external ear canal, and tympanic membrane. The external ear canal of the elderly is often dry and fragile; it is preferable to clean cerumen with wall-mounted suction and cerumen loops and to avoid irrigation. In examining the eardrum, the topography of the tympanic membrane is more critical than the presence or absence of the highly touted light reflex. In addition to the pars tensa (the lower two-thirds of the eardrum), the pars flaccida above the short process of the malleus should also be examined for retraction pockets that may be evidence of chronic eustachian tube dysfunction or cholesteatoma. Insufflation of the ear canal is necessary to assess tympanic membrane mobility and compliance. Careful inspection of the nose, nasopharynx, and upper respiratory tract is indicated. Unilateral serous effusion in the adult should prompt a fiberoptic examination of the nasopharynx to exclude neoplasms. Cranial nerves should be carefully evaluated with special attention to facial and trigeminal nerves, which are commonly disturbed with tumors involving the cerebellopontine angle.

The Weber and Rinne tuning fork tests are used to differentiate conductive from sensorineural hearing losses and to confirm the findings of audiologic evaluation. Rinne's test compares the ability to hear by air conduction with the ability to hear by bone conduction. The tines of a vibrating tuning fork are held near the opening of the external auditory canal, and then the stem is placed on the mastoid process; for direct contact, it may be placed on teeth or dentures. The patient is asked to indicate whether the tone is louder by air conduction or bone conduction. Normally, and in the presence of sensorineural hearing loss, a tone is heard louder by air conduction than by bone conduction; however, with conductive hearing loss of ≥30 dB (see "Audiologic Assessment," below), the bone-conduction stimulus is perceived as louder than the air-conduction stimulus. The Rinne test is most sensitive in detecting mild conductive hearing losses if a 256-Hz tuning fork is used. The Weber test may be performed with a 256- or 512-Hz fork. The stem of a vibrating tuning fork is placed on the head in the midline and the patient asked whether the tone is heard in both ears or better in one ear than in the other. With a unilateral conductive hearing loss, the tone is perceived in the affected ear. With a unilateral sensorineural hearing loss, the tone is perceived in the unaffected ear. As a general rule, a 5-dB difference in hearing between the two ears is required for lateralization. The combined information from the Weber and Rinne tests permits a tentative conclusion as to whether a conductive or sensorineural hearing loss is present; however, these tests are associated with significant false-positive and -negative responses and therefore should be utilized only as screening tools.

LABORATORY ASSESSMENT OF HEARING **Audiologic Assessment** The minimum audiologic assessment for hearing loss should include the measurement of pure tone air-conduction and bone-conduction thresholds, speech reception threshold, discrimination score, tympanometry, acoustic reflexes, and acoustic-reflex decay. This test battery provides a comprehensive screening evaluation of the whole auditory system and allows one to determine whether further differentiation of a sensory (cochlear) from a neural (retrocochlear) hearing loss is indicated.

Pure tone audiometry assesses hearing acuity for pure tones. The test is administered by an audiologist and is performed in a sound-attenuated chamber. The pure tone stimulus is delivered with an audiometer, an electronic device that allows the presentation of specific frequencies (generally between 250 and 8000 Hz) at specific intensities. Air and bone conduction thresholds are established for each ear. Air conduction thresholds are established by presenting the stimulus in air with the use of headphones. Bone conduction thresholds are accomplished by placing the stem of a vibrating tuning fork or an oscillator of an audiometer in contact with the head. In the presence of a hearing loss, broad-spectrum noise is presented to the nontest ear for *masking* purposes so that responses are based on perception from the ear under test.

The responses are measured in decibels. An *audiogram* is a plot of intensity in decibels required to achieve threshold versus frequency. A decibel (dB) is equal to 20 times the logarithm of the ratio of the sound pressure required to achieve threshold in the patient to the sound pressure required to achieve threshold in a normal hearing person. Therefore, a change of 6 dB represents doubling of sound pressure, and a change of 20 dB represents a ten-fold change in sound pressure. Loudness, which depends on the frequency, intensity, and duration of a sound, doubles with approximately each 10-dB increase in sound pressure level. Pitch, on the other hand, does not directly correlate with frequency. The perception of pitch changes slowly in the low and high frequencies. In the middle tones, which are important for human speech, pitch varies more rapidly with changes in frequency.

Pure tone audiometry establishes the presence and severity of hearing impairment, unilateral vs. bilateral involvement, and the type of hearing loss. Conductive hearing losses with a large mass component, as is often seen in middle-ear effusions, produce elevation of thresholds that predominate in the higher frequencies. Conductive hearing losses with a large stiffness component, as in fixation of the footplate of the stapes in early otosclerosis, produce threshold elevations in the lower frequencies. Often, the conductive hearing loss involves all frequencies, suggesting involvement of both stiffness and mass. In general, sensorineural hearing losses such as presbycusis affect higher frequencies more than lower frequencies. An exception is Ménière's disease, which is characteristically associated with low-frequency sensorineural hearing loss. Noise-induced hearing loss has an unusual pattern of hearing impairment in which the loss at 4000 Hz is greater than at higher frequencies. Vestibular schwannomas characteristically affect the higher frequencies, but any pattern of hearing loss can be observed.

Speech recognition requires greater synchronous neural firing than is necessary for appreciation of pure tones. *Speech audiometry* tests the clarity with which one hears. The *speech reception threshold* (SRT) is defined as the intensity at which speech is recognized as a meaningful symbol and is obtained by presenting two-syllable words with an equal accent on each syllable. The intensity at which the patient can repeat 50% of the words correctly is the SRT. Once the SRT is determined, discrimination or word recognition ability is tested by presenting one-syllable words at 25 to 40 dB above the speech reception threshold. The words are phonetically balanced in that the phonemes (speech sounds) occur in the list of words at the same frequency that they occur in ordinary conversational English. An individual with normal hearing or conductive hearing loss can repeat 88 to 100% of the phonetically balanced words correctly. Patients with a sensorineural hearing loss have variable loss of discrimination depending on the severity of hearing loss and the site of lesion. Further, as a general rule, neural lesions are associated with more deterioration in discrimination ability than are lesions in the inner ear. For example, in a patient with mild asymmetric sensorineural hearing loss, a clue to the diagnosis of vestibular schwannoma is the presence of greater than expected deterioration in discrimination ability. Deterioration in discrimination ability at higher intensities above the SRT also suggests a lesion in the eighth nerve or central auditory pathways.

Tympanometry measures the impedance of the middle ear to sound and is particularly useful in the identification and diagnosis of middle-ear effusions. A sounding source and microphone are introduced into the ear canal with an airtight seal. The amount of sound that is absorbed through the middle ear or reflected from the middle ear is measured at the microphone. In conductive hearing losses, more sound is reflected than in the normal middle ear. The pressure in the ear canal can be increased or decreased from atmospheric pressure. A *tympanogram* is the graphic representation of change in impedance or compliance as the pressure in the ear canal is changed. It provides information about the status of the tympanic membrane and the ossicular chain. Normally, the middle ear is most compliant at atmospheric pressure, and the compliance decreases as the pressure is increased or decreased; this pattern is seen with normal hearing or in the presence of sensorineural hearing loss. Compliance that does not change with change in pressure suggests middle-ear effusion. With a negative pressure in the middle ear, as with eustachian tube obstruction, the point of maximal compliance occurs with negative pressure in the ear canal. A tympanogram in which no point of maximal compliance can be obtained is most commonly seen with discontinuity of the ossicular chain. A reduction in the maximal compliance peak can be seen in otosclerosis.

During tympanometry, an intense tone (80 dB above the hearing threshold) elicits contraction of the stapedius muscle. The change in compliance of the middle ear with contraction of the stapedius muscle can be detected. The presence or absence of this *acoustic reflex* is important in the anatomic localization of facial nerve paralysis as well as hearing loss. Normal or elevated acoustic reflex thresholds in an individual with significant sensorineural hearing impairment suggests a cochlear hearing loss. Assessment of *acoustic reflex decay* helps differentiate sensory from neural hearing losses. In neural hearing loss, the reflex adapts or decays with time.

Otoacoustic emissions (OAE) can be measured with sensitive microphones inserted into the external auditory canal. The emissions may be spontaneous or evoked with sound stimulation. The presence of OAEs indicates that the outer hair cells of the organ of Corti are intact and can be used to assess auditory thresholds and to distinguish sensory from neural hearing losses.

Evoked Responses *Electrocochleography* measures the earliest evoked potentials generated in the cochlea and the auditory nerve. Receptor potentials recorded include the cochlear microphonic, generated by the outer hair cells of the organ of Corti, and the summating potential, generated by the inner hair cells in response to sound. The whole nerve action potential representing the composite firing of the first-order neurons can also be recorded during electrocochleography. Clinically, the test is useful in the diagnosis of Ménière's disease where an elevation of the ratio of summating potential to action potential is seen.

Brainstem auditory evoked responses (BAERs) are useful in differentiating the site of sensorineural hearing loss (Chap. 356). In response to sound, five distinct electrical potentials arising from different stations along the peripheral and central auditory pathway can be recorded with computer averaging from scalp surface electrodes. BAERs are valuable in situations in which patients cannot or will not give reliable voluntary thresholds. They are also used to assess the integrity of the auditory nerve and brainstem in various clinical situations, including intraoperative monitoring and in determination of brain death.

Imaging Studies The choice of radiologic tests is largely determined by whether the goal is to evaluate the bony anatomy of the external, middle, and inner ear or to image the auditory nerve and brain. Axial and coronal CT of the temporal bone with fine 1-mm cuts is ideal for determining the caliber of the external auditory canal, integrity of the ossicular chain, and presence of middle-ear or mastoid disease; it can also detect inner-ear malformations. CT is also ideal for the detection of bone erosion often seen in the presence of chronic otitis media and cholesteatoma. MRI is superior to CT for imaging of retrocochlear pathology such as vestibular schwannoma, meningioma, other lesions of the cerebellopontine angle, demyelinating lesions of the brainstem, and brain tumors. Recent experience suggests that both CT and MRI are equally capable of identifying inner-ear malformations and assessing cochlear patency for preoperative evaluation of patients for cochlear implantation.

℞ TREATMENT In general, conductive hearing losses are amenable to surgical intervention and correction, while sensorineural hearing losses are permanent. The diagnosis of conductive hearing loss is usually straightforward, and the etiology of the conductive deficit is often apparent on physical examination. Atresia of the ear canal can be surgically repaired, often with significant improvement in hearing. Tympanic membrane perforations due to chronic otitis media or trauma can be repaired with an outpatient tympanoplasty. Likewise, conductive hearing loss associated with otosclerosis can be treated by stapedectomy, which is successful in 90 to 95% of cases. Tympanostomy tubes allow the prompt return of normal hearing in individuals with middle-ear effusions. Hearing aids are effective and well-tolerated in patients with conductive hearing losses.

Patients with mild, moderate, and severe sensorineural hearing losses are regularly rehabilitated with hearing aids of varying configuration and strength. Hearing aids have been improved to provide greater fidelity and have been miniaturized. The current generation of hearing aids can be placed entirely within the ear canal, thus reducing the stigma associated with their use. In general, the more severe the hearing impairment, the larger the hearing aid required for auditory rehabilitation. Digital hearing aids lend themselves to individual programming, and multiple and directional microphones at the ear level may be helpful in noisy surroundings. Since all hearing aids amplify noise as well as speech, the only absolute solution to the problem found thus far is to place the microphone closer to the speaker than the noise source. This arrangement is not possible with a self-contained, cosmetically acceptable device. It is cumbersome and requires a user-friendly environment.

In many situations, including lectures and the theater, hearing-impaired persons benefit from assistive devices that are based on the principle of having the speaker closer to the microphone than any source of noise. Assistive devices include infrared and FM transmission as well as an electromagnetic loop around the room for transmission to the individual's hearing aid. Hearing aids with telecoils can also be used with properly equipped telephones in the same way.

In the event that the hearing aid provides inadequate rehabilitation, cochlear implants are appropriate. Criteria for implantation include severe to profound hearing loss with word recognition score ≤30% under best aided conditions. Children with congenital and acquired profound hearing impairment are also appropriate candidates for cochlear implantation. Worldwide, more than 20,000 deaf individuals (including 4000 children) have received cochlear implants. Cochlear implants are neural prostheses that convert sound energy to electrical energy and can be used to stimulate the auditory division of the eighth nerve directly. In most cases of profound hearing impairment, the auditory hair cells are lost but the ganglionic cells of the auditory division of the eighth nerve are preserved. Cochlear implants consist of electrodes that are inserted into the cochlea through the round window, speech processors that extract acoustical elements of speech for conversion to electrical currents, and a means of transmitting the electrical energy through the skin. Patients with implants experience sound that helps with speech reading, allows open-set word recognition, and helps in modulating the person's own voice. Usually, within 3 months after implantation, adult patients can understand speech without visual cues. With the current generation of multichannel cochlear implants, nearly 75% of patients are able to converse on the telephone. It is anticipated that improvements in the electrode design and speech processors will permit further enhancement in understanding speech, especially in the presence of background noise.

For individuals who have had both eighth nerves destroyed by trauma or bilateral vestibular schwannomas (e.g., neurofibromatosis type 2), brainstem auditory implants placed near the cochlear nucleus may provide auditory rehabilitation. It is hoped that additional advances may provide benefits similar to those with the cochlear implant.

Tinnitus can often accompany hearing loss. The treatment of tinnitus is particularly problematic. Therapy is usually directed towards minimizing the appreciation of tinnitus. Relief of the tinnitus may be obtained by masking it with background music. Hearing aids are also helpful in tinnitus suppression, as are tinnitus maskers, devices that present a sound to the affected ear that is more pleasant to listen to than the tinnitus. The use of a tinnitus masker is often followed by several hours of inhibition of the tinnitus. Antidepressants have also shown beneficial effect in helping patients deal with tinnitus.

Tinnitus and background noise can significantly affect understanding of speech in individuals with hearing impairment. Hard-of-hearing individuals often benefit from a reduction in unnecessary noise (e.g., radio or television) to enhance the signal-to-noise ratio. Speech comprehension is aided by lip reading; therefore, the impaired listener should be seated so that the face of the speaker is well illuminated and can be seen at all times. Speaking directly into the ear is occasionally helpful, but usually more is lost in communication than gained when the speaker's face cannot be seen. Speech should be slow enough to make each word distinct, but overly slow speech is distracting and loses contextual and speech-reading benefits. Although speech should be in a loud, clear voice, one should be aware that in sensorineural hearing losses in general and in elderly hard-of-hearing persons in particular, recruitment (the ability to hear loud sounds normally loud) may be troublesome. Above all, optimal communication cannot take place without both parties giving it their full and undivided attention.

PREVENTION Conductive hearing losses may be prevented by prompt and appropriate antibiotic therapy of adequate duration for AOM and by ventilation of the middle ear with tympanostomy tubes in middle-ear effusions lasting 12 weeks or longer. Loss of vestibular function and deafness due to aminoglycoside antibiotics can largely be prevented by careful monitoring of serum peak and trough levels.

Some 10 million Americans have noise-induced hearing loss, and 20 million are exposed to hazardous noise in their employment. Noise-induced hearing loss can be prevented by avoidance of exposure to loud noise or by regular use of ear plugs or fluid-filled car muffs to attenuate intense sound. Noise-induced hearing loss results from recreational as well as occupational activities and begins in adolescence. High-risk activities for noise-induced hearing loss include wood and metal working with electrical equipment and target practice and hunting with small firearms. All internal-combustion and electric engines, including snow and leaf blowers, snowmobiles, outboard motors, and chain saws, require protection of the user with hearing protectors. Virtually all noise-induced hearing loss is preventable through education, which should begin before the teenage years. Programs of industrial conservation of hearing are required when the exposure over an 8-h period averages 85 dB on the A scale. Workers in such noisy environments can be protected with preemployment audiologic assessment, the mandatory use of hearing protectors, and annual audiologic assessments.

ACKNOWLEDGMENT
The authors wish to acknowledge Dr. Joseph B. Martin, who was the co-author of this chapter in the 14th edition.

BIBLIOGRAPHY

AIBA T et al: Effect of zinc sulfate on sensorineural olfactory disorder. Acta Otolaryngol Suppl (Stockh) 538:202, 1998

BALLENGER JJ, SNOW JB (eds): *Otorhinolaryngology Head and Neck Surgery*, 15th ed. Baltimore, Williams & Wilkins, 1995

DOTY RL et al: Smell identification ability: Changes with age. Science 226:1441, 1984

FIRESTEIN S, SHEPHERD GM: Interaction of anionic and cationic currents leads to a voltage dependence in the odor response of olfactory receptor neurons. J Neurophysiol 73:562, 1995

GETCHELL TV et al: *Smell and Taste in Health and Disease.* New York, Raven, 1991

KALINEC F et al: A membrane-based force generation mechanism in auditory sensory cells. Proc Natl Acad Sci USA 89:8671, 1992

LALWANI AK, CASTELEIN CM: Cracking the auditory genetic code: Nonsyndromic hereditary hearing impairment. Am J Otol 20(1):115, 1999

MORELL RJ et al: Mutations in the connexin 26 gene (GJB2) among Ashkenazi Jews with nonsyndromic recessive deafness. N Engl J Med 339:1500, 1998

OGAWA T, RUTKA J: Olfactory dysfunction in head injured workers. Acta Otolaryngol Suppl (Stockh) 540:50, 1999

RUGARLI EI et al: Kallmann syndrome and the link between olfactory and reproductive development. Am J Hum Genet 65:943, 1999

RUSSLER KJ et al: A zonal organization of odorant receptor gene expression in the olfactory epithelium. Cell 73:597, 1993

SHARON D et al: Primate evolution of an olfactory receptor cluster: Diversification by gene conversion and recent emergence of pseudogenes. Genomics 61:24, 1999

WARCHOL ME et al: Regenerative proliferation in inner ear sensory epithelia from adult guinea pigs and humans. Science 259:1619, 1993

WILLEMS PJ: Genetic causes of hearing loss. N Engl J Med 342:1101, 2000

30 *Marlene Durand, Michael Joseph*

INFECTIONS OF THE UPPER RESPIRATORY TRACT

Infections of the upper respiratory tract include some of the most common infectious diseases encountered by internists and other primary-care physicians. Pharyngitis, laryngitis, rhinitis, sinusitis, otitis externa, and otitis media account for millions of visits to physicians annually. Although these infections are usually mild enough to be treated on an outpatient basis, the primary-care physician must be able to recognize their serious complications, such as peritonsillar abscess from pharyngitis, subperiosteal abscess from frontal sinusitis, and temporal-bone osteomyelitis from invasive otitis externa. The physician must also identify potentially life-threatening infections of the head and neck, such as epiglottitis, Ludwig's angina, and rhinocerebral mucormycosis.

INFECTIONS OF THE NOSE AND FACE

Skin infections that commonly affect the nose and face include folliculitis, furunculosis, impetigo, and erysipelas. These are discussed in detail elsewhere (Chap. 128, in particular Table 128-1).

Infection of the mucosal surface of the nose is most commonly due to respiratory viruses (e.g., rhinovirus) and presents as acute rhinitis. There are several rare, chronic intranasal infections. *Ozena*, or atrophic rhinitis, is characterized by atrophied mucosa overlaid by foul-smelling dry crusts (Greek *ozein*, "stench"). *Klebsiella ozaenae* is often isolated from nasal cultures, but whether it is a cause of illness or merely a colonizer is unclear. Intranasal irrigation with aminoglycosides (e.g., tobramycin ophthalmic solution) or oral administration of ciprofloxacin has resulted in clinical improvement in some cases. *Klebsiella rhinoscleromatis* causes *rhinoscleroma*, a chronic granulomatous disease of the upper respiratory tract mucosa that is seen in inhabitants of parts of Africa, Asia, and Latin America; it has been described in two patients positive for HIV. Mikulicz cells (foamy histiocytes) are seen in the submucosa of biopsy specimens. Rhinoscleroma can be treated with streptomycin, trimethoprim-sulfamethoxazole, a quinolone, or tetracycline for 2 months. *Pseudomonas mallei* causes *glanders*, a respiratory disease of horses. Infection is rare in humans; nasal inoculation may produce a purulent nasal discharge followed by granulomatous intranasal lesions that ulcerate. Treatment is with sulfadiazine.

Neonatal congenital syphilis may present as rhinitis (snuffles), and the generalized osteochondritis that follows may result in a "saddle-nose" deformity. In *leprosy*, *Mycobacterium leprae* infiltrates the nasal mucosa and may cause chronic nasal congestion and nosebleeds. Involvement of the nasal cartilage may also result in a saddle nose.

Rhinosporidium seeberi is a fungus-like organism, not yet cultured, that causes *rhinosporidiosis*. Pedunculated nasal masses that grow over months or years cause obstruction and a foul odor and must be surgically excised. *Blastomyces dermatitidis*, a fungus prevalent in the Mississippi and Ohio River valleys, usually causes pulmonary disease but may cause chronic ulcerative lesions of the skin and nasal mucosa. *Mucormycosis*, a life-threatening fungal illness that occurs primarily in diabetic patients, may present as black eschars in the nasal cavity (see "Fungal Sinusitis").

THE COMMON COLD

The common cold is a mild, self-limited viral infection of the upper respiratory tract. Adults average two to four colds per year and children six to eight. The most common causes are rhinovirus (40% of cases) and coronavirus (at least 10%), but parainfluenza virus, respiratory syncytial virus, influenza virus, and adenoviruses also account for some cases. Rhinovirus alone has more than 100 different immunotypes, and this diversity has hampered efforts to identify an effective therapy or vaccine. There is no specific treatment for the common cold, although antihistamines, decongestants, and ipratropium bromide nasal spray provide some relief of symptoms. One study found that zinc gluconate lozenges, taken every 2 h, may reduce the duration of symptoms but are associated with nausea in 20% of patients. The value of vitamin C in preventing colds has not been proved.

SINUSITIS

The paranasal sinuses are aerated cavities in the bones of the face that develop as outpouches of the nasal cavity and communicate with this cavity throughout life. The maxillary and ethmoid sinuses are present at birth; the frontal and sphenoid sinuses develop after ages 2 and 7, respectively. Like the nose, the sinuses are lined with respiratory epithelium that includes mucus-producing goblet cells and ciliated cells. The mucous blanket is carried toward the sinus openings (ostia) at a speed of up to 1 cm/min by the beating of the cilia. The ostia are small; the ethmoid sinus ostia, for example, are only 1 to 2 mm in diameter. Delay in the mucociliary transport time or—more important—obstruction of the ostia may lead to retained secretions and sinusitis.

Sinusitis is a common problem. In the United States, this infection accounts for millions of office visits annually. The most common type, maxillary sinusitis, is followed in frequency by ethmoid, frontal, and sphenoid sinusitis. A viral infection of the upper respiratory tract is the most common precursor of sinusitis, although only about 0.5% of such infections are complicated by clinically evident acute bacterial sinusitis. Sinusitis develops primarily through ostial obstruction due to mucosal edema. Viral upper respiratory infections also increase the amount of mucus produced and may damage ciliated cells, thereby delaying mucus transport time. Allergic rhinitis is another common cause of ostial obstruction, either by mucosal edema or by polyps. Nasotracheal or nasogastric intubation can result in obstruction of the ostia and is a major risk factor for nosocomial sinusitis in intensive care units. Dental infections may cause 5 to 10% of all cases of maxillary sinusitis; the roots of the upper back teeth (second bicuspid, first and second molars) abut the floor of the maxillary sinus. Other causes of sinusitis include barotrauma from deep-sea diving or airplane travel, mucus abnormalities (e.g., cystic fibrosis), and chemical irritants. Foreign bodies, tumors (e.g., midline granuloma, intranasal lymphoma, or squamous cell carcinoma), and granulomatous diseases (e.g., Wegener's granulomatosis or rhinoscleroma) may all cause sinusitis secondary to obstruction.

ACUTE BACTERIAL SINUSITIS **Manifestations** Symptoms of acute sinusitis include purulent nasal or postnasal drainage, nasal congestion, and sinus pain or pressure whose location depends on the sinus involved. Maxillary sinus pain is often perceived as being located in the cheek or upper teeth; ethmoid sinus pain, between the eyes or retroorbital; frontal sinus pain, above the eyebrow; and sphenoid sinus pain, in the upper half of the face or retroorbital with radiation to the occiput. Sinus pain is frequently worse when the patient bends over or is supine. Fever develops in about half of patients with acute maxillary sinusitis.

Diagnosis The diagnosis of bacterial sinusitis may be difficult, as symptoms may resemble those of the inciting viral upper respiratory infection. The persistence of cold symptoms for 7 to 10 days (or longer than usual for a particular patient) is the most consistent clinical feature of bacterial sinusitis, according to some authors. Four-view sinus x-rays are helpful in the diagnosis of acute sinusitis: radiologic opacity, an air-fluid level, or ≥4 mm of sinus mucosal thickening correlates well with active bacterial infection. Computed tomography (CT) of the sinus is much more sensitive than routine radiography, particularly for ethmoid and sphenoid disease. Its use should be reserved for complicated cases and for cases in hospitalized patients, however. In light of the finding that sinus CT often shows reversible acute changes in patients with common colds, it is apparent that routine early use of CT would lead to overdiagnosis of bacterial sinusitis.

Etiology The bacteriology of acute community-acquired maxillary sinusitis has been well defined by studies using direct sinus puncture and aspiration. In children and adults, *Streptococcus pneumoniae* and *Haemophilus influenzae* (not type b), the most common pathogens, cause about one-third and one-fourth of cases, respectively. In children, *Moraxella catarrhalis* is also important, accounting for 20% of cases. Rhinoviruses, influenza viruses, and parainfluenza viruses are found alone or with bacteria in one-fifth of adult cases.

℞ TREATMENT Empirical therapy for acute bacterial sinusitis should be directed against the common bacterial pathogens; sinus puncture is not indicated in routine cases, and cultures of nasal drainage are not very reliable. Amoxicillin (500 mg orally, three times daily for 10 to 14 days) or trimethoprim-sulfamethoxazole may be effective in the treatment of first-time cases.[1] Other effective but more expensive antibiotics include amoxicillin/clavulanate, cefuroxime axetil, and clarithromycin. Treatment should be given for 1 to 2 weeks. Intravenous administration of antibiotics may be necessary for the treatment of patients with severe disease who appear toxic. In nosocomial sinusitis, *Staphylococcus aureus* and gram-negative bacilli are most common, and sinus cultures are indicated as an aid in tailoring therapy. Initial broad-spectrum intravenous therapy (e.g., with nafcillin and ceftriaxone) should be adjusted on the basis of culture results. Surgery to widen the ostia and drain thick secretions may be essential in severe acute sinusitis, particularly when ethmoid, frontal, or sphenoid disease fails to respond to initial intravenous therapy.

CHRONIC BACTERIAL SINUSITIS **Manifestations** Chronic sinusitis is characterized by symptoms of sinus inflammation lasting ≥3 months. Most experts believe that this condition is caused by dysfunction of the mucociliary blanket, usually as a result of repeated past infections, rather than by the persistence of bacterial infection. Patients report constant sinus pressure, nasal congestion, and postnasal drainage, especially in the morning. A temperature of ≥38°C (≥100.5°F) is rare and may signify a superimposed acute bacterial infection. Many patients also note a change in nasal discharge (to thick and green) with acute exacerbations.

---

[1]The dosages and durations of antimicrobial therapy given in this chapter are appropriate for adults with normal renal function and should be adjusted for children, for patients with impaired renal function, and in light of the response to treatment.

Diagnosis Sinus CT should be used in all cases of chronic sinusitis to define the extent of disease and to help exclude other diagnoses, such as an obstructing tumor. Patients should be evaluated for allergies and immunodeficiencies (e.g., hypogammaglobulinemia). Evaluation by an otolaryngologist is essential, as this specialist will be able to obtain additional information by an office nasal endoscopic examination. Surgery, now usually done endoscopically, may be necessary to correct blockage of the sinus ostia. This blockage occurs most often in the osteomeatal complex that drains the maxillary, frontal, and anterior ethmoid sinuses. Samples of sinus secretions obtained intraoperatively should be cultured for anaerobes, aerobes, and fungi. Fungal sinusitis may mimic chronic bacterial infection (see "Fungal Sinusitis").

Etiology The bacteriology of chronic sinusitis is not well defined. Nearly all patients with chronic disease, especially those who have had prior sinus surgery, have sinus cultures positive for bacteria. Such cultures may represent colonization rather than infection, however. Patients who have received multiple courses of antibiotics may be colonized by *S. aureus* or by *Pseudomonas* and other gram-negative bacilli. Anaerobes have been isolated from 100% of sinus specimens in some studies but from as few as 2% in others.

℞ **TREATMENT** The need for antibiotic therapy must be assessed on an individual basis, with antibiotics chosen in light of recent culture results.

COMPLICATIONS OF BACTERIAL SINUSITIS Orbital complications of sinusitis, such as orbital cellulitis and orbital abscess, usually arise from ethmoid sinusitis, since the ethmoid is separated from the orbit by only a very thin bone (the lamina papyracea). Patients present with fever, unilateral periorbital edema and erythema, conjunctival injection and chemosis, and proptosis. Eye movement may be decreased; with orbital abscess, the eye is often fixed in the "down and out" position. CT or magnetic resonance imaging (MRI) should be used to rule out an orbital abscess. Treatment of orbital infections should include immediate drainage of any abscess, intravenous administration of broad-spectrum antibiotics—e.g., nafcillin (1.5 to 2.0 g every 4 h) plus ceftriaxone (2 g/d)—for at least 7 days, and a consideration of sinus drainage surgery.

Another extracranial complication of sinusitis is frontal subperiosteal abscess (Pott's puffy tumor) from frontal sinusitis. Patients present with a tender doughy swelling over the forehead. Treatment consists of surgical drainage of the abscess and the frontal sinus and 6 weeks of intravenous antibiotic therapy directed at the isolated organisms.

Intracranial complications such as epidural abscess, subdural empyema, meningitis, cerebral abscess, and dural-vein thrombophlebitis may result from sinusitis, particularly from frontal or sphenoid infections. Because the sphenoid sinus sits between the two cavernous sinuses, sphenoid sinusitis is a major cause of cavernous sinus thrombophlebitis.

FUNGAL SINUSITIS Fungal sinusitis is categorized as noninvasive or invasive. *Noninvasive* disease is chronic and occurs in immunocompetent hosts. It has two forms that are analogous to the noninvasive pulmonary diseases of aspergilloma and allergic bronchopulmonary aspergillosis. A fungus ball (aspergilloma) inside a sinus may cause symptoms of obstruction without invading the mucosa. Typically, only one sinus (often maxillary) is affected, and patients have unilateral symptoms and opacification of only that sinus on CT. Treatment is surgical only, unless special fungal stains show tissue invasion on histopathology. Allergic fungal sinusitis was first described in 1983 and is seen mainly in patients with a history of nasal polyposis and asthma. It is characterized by extremely thick sinus mucus ("allergic mucin") that, on histopathologic examination, is found to contain numerous Charcot-Leyden crystals, eosinophils, and rare fungal hyphae. There is no evidence of tissue invasion. Surgical removal of the inspissated mucus is often curative. Antifungal therapy is not indicated.

Invasive fungal sinusitis presents differently in immunocompetent and immunocompromised hosts. In immunocompromised individuals, fungal disease has an acute presentation. Rhinocerebral mucormycosis is a life-threatening infection due to fungi of the order Mucorales (*Rhizopus, Rhizomucor, Mucor, Absidia, Cunninghamella*). Mucormycosis usually involves diabetic patients (70% of cases), half of whom are in ketoacidosis at presentation. Other patients at risk include those with hematologic malignancies, transplant recipients, and patients receiving chronic glucocorticoid or iron chelation (deferoxamine) therapy. Mucormycosis in patients taking deferoxamine is generally due to *Cunninghamella* and is almost always fatal. Symptoms and signs of mucormycosis may be explained by the fungal predilection for blood vessels and nerves and for invasion into the orbital apex and cavernous sinus, with consequent compromise of cranial nerves II through VI. Patients most frequently present with unilateral ocular findings of 1 to 5 days' duration that may mimic bacterial orbital cellulitis: lid swelling and erythema (sometimes bluish in appearance), ptosis, proptosis, decreased extraocular movement, and impaired vision. Retroorbital or periorbital pain is a prominent complaint. There may be either increased or decreased sensation in the first division of the fifth cranial nerve on the involved side; facial palsy with involvement of cranial nerve VII has also been described. Patients may be afebrile and appear nontoxic. Individuals in whom mucormycosis is a consideration should undergo an immediate examination by an otolaryngologist, who will look for intranasal black eschars or necrotic turbinates. If found, these sites should be biopsied and frozen tissue sections examined by a pathologist. In rare cases, the nasal passage appears normal, but biopsy of the middle turbinate reveals invasive fungi. The finding of tissue invasion by broad-based, nonseptate hyphae necessitates extensive surgical debridement and intravenous therapy with amphotericin B or liposomal amphotericin (Chaps. 200 and 207). *Aspergillus* and other filamentous fungi may also cause invasive sinus disease.

Immunocompetent hosts with invasive fungal sinusitis, in contrast, have slowly progressive disease. Fungi in ethmoid and sphenoid sinuses may invade the orbital apex, causing proptosis, ptosis, limitation of eye movement, and decreased vision. Patients may mistakenly be treated with glucocorticoids for presumed optic neuritis or orbital pseudotumor until sinus disease is recognized and biopsies are undertaken. Treatment consists of surgical debridement of the involved sinuses and prolonged intravenous therapy with amphotericin B. In all cases of invasive fungal sinusitis, follow-up CT and MRI should be conducted frequently to evaluate the progression of disease.

Mortality from invasive fungal sinusitis is high, even among immunocompetent hosts.

EAR AND MASTOID INFECTIONS

AURICULAR CELLULITIS AND PERICHONDRITIS *Auricular cellulitis* usually presents as a swollen, erythematous, hot, tender ear. The lobule is especially swollen and red. There may be a history of minor trauma to the ear (e.g., involving earrings, cotton swabs, or scratching). Treatment consists of warm compresses and intravenous administration of antibiotics active against *S. aureus* and streptococci—e.g., cefazolin (1 g every 8 h) or nafcillin.

Perichondritis, an infection of the perichondrium of the ear, is often accompanied by infection of the underlying cartilage of the pinna (chondritis). Associated interruption of the blood supply to the cartilage may lead to ear deformity. Patients present with a swollen, hot, red, and exquisitely tender pinna, usually with sparing of the lobule. The most common antecedents of the infection are burns, significant trauma to the ear (e.g., as a result of boxing), or ear piercing through the pinna. *Pseudomonas aeruginosa* and *S. aureus* are the most common pathogens. Perichondritis should be treated with antibiotics, such as intravenous ticarcillin/clavulanic acid (3.1 g every 4 h) or intravenous nafcillin plus oral ciprofloxacin, for several weeks. Incision and drainage may be helpful for culture and for resolution of infection, which is often slow. This infection must be distinguished from relapsing polychondritis, a rheumatologic condition (Chap. 325).

OTITIS EXTERNA The external auditory canal is about 2.5 cm long and is lined by skin. Beneath this skin is cartilage in the lateral half of the canal, temporal bone in the medial half. The skin in the bony portion lacks a subcutaneous layer and is attached directly to the periosteum, an important feature in the pathogenesis of invasive otitis externa (see below). Cerumen, secreted by glands, acidifies the canal and suppresses bacterial growth. However, desquamated skin and retained moisture make the canal especially susceptible to the hydrophilic organism *P. aeruginosa.*

Acute otitis externa, or swimmer's ear, occurs mostly in the summer and may be due to a decrease in canal acidity and resulting bacterial overgrowth. The ear is pruritic and painful, and the canal appears swollen and red. The most common pathogens are *P. aeruginosa, S. aureus*, and streptococci. Treatment consists of cleansing of the ear with alcohol–acetic acid mixtures and the administration of topical antibiotic ear drops, such as polymyxin-neomycin (4 drops four times daily for 5 days). Herpes zoster in the external canal causes severe otalgia and is often accompanied by ipsilateral facial paralysis due to the involvement of the geniculate ganglion of cranial nerve VII (Ramsay Hunt syndrome). Reports suggest that treatment with intravenous acyclovir decreases the incidence of permanent facial-nerve palsy, but the results of relevant controlled trials have not yet been published.

Chronic otitis externa causes pruritus rather than ear pain and is often due to irritation from either repeated minor trauma to the canal (e.g., scratching or use of cotton swabs) or drainage of a chronic middle-ear infection. In the latter situation, treatment of chronic otitis media with oral antibiotics will also cover this condition.

Invasive ("malignant") otitis externa is a potentially life-threatening infection, almost always due to *P. aeruginosa*, that slowly invades from the external canal into adjacent soft tissues, mastoid, and temporal bone and eventually spreads across the base of the skull. It occurs primarily in diabetic patients whose diabetes, unlike that of patients with mucormycosis, is usually under control. There is a history of weeks to months of ear pain and drainage, often misdiagnosed as chronic otitis media (an entity that is rarely painful). Examination reveals an edematous canal, with granulation tissue in the posterior wall about halfway down the canal (the region of the cartilage-bone junction). Trismus or partial facial paralysis (cranial nerve VII) is evident in some instances. Cranial nerves IX, X, and XI are occasionally affected as well. Fever is rare in invasive otitis externa and, when it does develop, is usually low-grade.

Laboratory studies generally reveal a normal white blood cell count but a high erythrocyte sedimentation rate. CT and MRI studies are essential for defining the extent of bone and soft-tissue involvement. CT shows bony destruction of the skull base in advanced cases. For culture, biopsies of granulation tissue in the canal or of deeper tissues are preferable to swab specimens of ear drainage, which may be unreliable. In nearly all cases, antibiotics should be withheld until a deep-tissue specimen is obtained for culture and pathologic examination. Once this specimen has been collected, empirical therapy with intravenous antibiotics active against *Pseudomonas*—e.g., ticarcillin (3 g every 4 h), piperacillin, or ceftazidime, plus an aminoglycoside)—may be started intraoperatively. To avoid ototoxicity, ciprofloxacin should be substituted for the aminoglycoside if cultures grow a *Pseudomonas* strain that is sensitive to this drug. In more than 95% of cases, *P. aeruginosa* is the pathogen involved; in the remaining cases, the pathogens include *Staphylococcus epidermidis, Aspergillus, Fusobacterium*, and *Actinomyces*. Systemic antibiotic treatment should be continued for 6 to 8 weeks. In early cases due to sensitive *Pseudomonas* strains, oral ciprofloxacin alone (750 mg twice daily for 6 weeks) may follow the initial 2 weeks of combination intravenous therapy.

ACUTE OTITIS MEDIA The middle ear is connected to the nasopharynx via the eustachian tube. When this tube is blocked, fluid collects in the middle-ear and mastoid cavities, providing a culture medium for any bacteria present. Acute otitis media (AOM), or middle-ear infection, may result. Viral upper respiratory infections, which can cause edema of the eustachian tube mucosa, often precede or accompany episodes of AOM. Otitis media, like upper respiratory tract infections, is most common in fall, winter, and spring. The incidence of AOM declines with age. More than two-thirds of children under age 3 have had at least one episode of AOM; the prevalence among adults is only 0.25%.

Symptoms include ear pain, fever, and decreased hearing acuity. On examination, the tympanic membrane moves poorly with insufflation and is usually red, opaque, bulging, or retracted. Spontaneous perforations of the tympanic membrane and otorrhea are occasionally documented.

The bacteriology of AOM has been delineated for pediatric disease: *S. pneumoniae* (35%), *H. influenzae* (25%), and *M. catarrhalis* (15%) are the most common organisms. Viruses, either alone or with bacteria, are found in one-quarter of pediatric cases. Small studies of AOM in adults have also found *S. pneumoniae* (21%) and *H. influenzae* (26%) to be the most common pathogens. More than 90% of *H. influenzae* infections are due to nontypable strains: those due to type b may be accompanied by bacteremia or meningitis.

TREATMENT Treatment of otitis media is empirical, as diagnostic tympanocentesis is indicated only for patients who appear toxic, who are immunocompromised, or whose infection is refractory to initial therapy. Although about one-third of *H. influenzae* strains and at least three-quarters of *M. catarrhalis* strains are β-lactamase producers, most authorities still find amoxicillin therapy to be successful in routine cases. Other drugs effective against most β-lactamase-positive strains include amoxicillin/clavulanate (875 mg by mouth twice daily for 7 to 10 days), trimethoprim-sulfamethoxazole, erythromycin/sulfisoxazole, clarithromycin, and second-generation oral cephalosporins (e.g., loracarbef, cefpodoxime proxetil, and cefuroxime axetil). Penicillin resistance in pneumococci, now a major problem, is not mediated by β-lactamase (Chap. 138). Strains exhibiting intermediate resistance may respond to therapy with high-dose amoxicillin or to clindamycin, erythromycin, or trimethoprim-sulfamethoxazole. Quinolones such as levofloxacin, although not approved for use in children, may be effective in adults. Serious infections or those due to highly resistant strains require treatment with parenteral ceftriaxone or vancomycin. Adjunctive treatment of AOM with antihistamines is of no proven benefit.

Recurrent episodes of AOM in children are due to the same pathogens that cause primary AOM (*S. pneumoniae, H. influenzae*, and *M. catarrhalis*). Most early recurrences (75%), however, are not relapses but are due to different organisms or to different strains of the organism that caused the initial episode. The pattern of recurrent AOM in adults is presumably similar but has not been well studied. Treatment for recurrent AOM should include drugs with activity against resistant strains. Patients with frequent recurrences (e.g., three episodes within 6 months) may benefit from antibiotic prophylaxis with once-daily amoxicillin or sulfisoxazole during the winter months, although this benefit must be weighed against the risk of selecting more antibiotic-resistant strains of bacteria.

SEROUS OTITIS MEDIA Otitis media with effusion, or serous otitis media, is characterized by the persistence of middle-ear fluid for several months without other signs of infection. This condition is associated with a 25-dB hearing loss in the affected ear. Cultures of middle-ear fluid are usually negative. Although some clinical trials have found that effusions resolve sooner in antibiotic-treated children than in controls, antibiotics are generally not recommended because the risk of increasing antibiotic resistance in the population is thought to outweigh the small benefit observed. Adenoidectomy, myringotomy, or tympanostomy tubes have been shown to decrease the duration of effusion in children.

CHRONIC SUPPURATIVE OTITIS MEDIA In chronic suppurative otitis media, patients have painless hearing loss and intermittent purulent ear drainage. On examination, there is a central perforation in the tympanic membrane and purulent drainage from the middle ear. If a cholesteatoma is present, the perforation is peripheral. Culture of draining fluid reveals *P. aeruginosa* (40%), *S. aureus* (20%), *Klebsiella* (20%), and other enteric gram-negative bacilli. Anaerobes are found in 50% of cases, usually in mixed culture with aerobes. CT should be used to help evaluate a surgically treatable nidus of infection, such as a cholesteatoma or mastoid sequestrum. For therapeutic purposes, patients are divided into two groups: those with and without cholesteatoma. Those in the former group are cured with surgical excision of the cholesteatoma. Those without cholesteatoma require repeated courses of topical antibiotic drops for relapse of "active" (draining) disease, and true cures are rare. The role of systemic antibiotics is unclear. In one study, a course of intravenous antibiotics produced long-term success in 78% of children without cholesteatoma who had persistent otorrhea despite topical and oral antibiotic therapy.

Tuberculous otitis media is rare and is frequently misdiagnosed. It mimics nontuberculous chronic suppurative otitis media, but ear drainage fails to respond to routine antibiotics. On examination, the tympanic membrane often has multiple perforations, and "pearly" or "flabby" tissue is seen in the middle ear. Only 30% of patients have evidence of active tuberculosis on chest x-ray. Treatment is the same as for other types of extrapulmonary tuberculosis.

MASTOIDITIS The mastoid is the portion of the temporal bone posterior to the ear that contains a honeycomb of air cells lined with respiratory epithelium. These air cells connect with the middle ear. Fluid in the middle ear, a prelude to otitis media, is almost always accompanied by fluid in the mastoid. True mastoiditis, however, has become rare in the antibiotic era, probably because of prompt treatment of otitis media.

Mastoiditis is characterized by erosion of the bony partitions between the mastoid air cells. Patients with acute mastoiditis present with pain, tenderness, and swelling over the mastoid. When there is an overlying subperiosteal abscess or cellulitis, the pinna is pushed out and forward. CT may show bony destruction or a drainable mastoid abscess.

The reported bacteriology of mastoiditis has varied. Some cases involve organisms similar to those implicated in AOM (*S. pneumoniae, H. influenzae*); others are attributable to *S. aureus* and gram-negative bacilli, including *Pseudomonas*. Ideally, therapy should be guided by the results of cultures of middle-ear fluid obtained by tympanocentesis. Initial broad-spectrum therapy, such as that with intravenous ticarcillin/clavulanate plus gentamicin or ciprofloxacin, can later be narrowed.

COMPLICATIONS OF OTITIS MEDIA AND MASTOIDITIS Extracranial complications include hearing loss, labyrinthitis and resulting vertigo, and facial-nerve palsy. Additional complications from mastoiditis develop when infection tracks under the periosteum of the temporal bone to cause a subperiosteal abscess or breaks through the mastoid tip to cause a neck abscess deep to the sternocleidomastoid muscle (Bezold's abscess). Intracranial complications include epidural abscess, dural venous thrombophlebitis (usually sigmoid sinus), meningitis, and brain abscess.

INFECTIONS OF THE ORAL CAVITY AND PHARYNX

ORAL CAVITY INFECTIONS The oral cavity extends from the lips to the circumvallate papillae of the tongue and is heavily colonized with viridans streptococci and anaerobes. These organisms can cause several infections in this area. *Gingivitis* is an infection of the gums, the earliest form of periodontal disease. Anaerobes residing in the mouth, especially anaerobic gram-negative rods such as *Prevotella*

intermedia, are the most common pathogens. Patients with *Vincent's angina,* also called *acute necrotizing ulcerative gingivitis* or *trench mouth,* have halitosis and ulcerations of the interdental papillae. Oral anaerobes are the cause, and therapy with oral penicillin plus metronidazole or with clindamycin alone is effective in both this condition and gingivitis.

Ludwig's angina is a rapidly spreading, life-threatening cellulitis of the sublingual and submandibular spaces that usually starts in an infected lower molar. Patients are febrile and may drool the secretions they cannot swallow. A brawny, boardlike edema in the sublingual area pushes the tongue up and back. Airway obstruction may result as the infection spreads to the supraglottic tissues. Treatment with intravenous antibiotics active against streptococci and oral anaerobes—e.g., ampicillin/sulbactam (3 g every 6 h) or high-dose penicillin plus metronidazole—should be followed by oral antibiotic therapy, with a total treatment duration of 14 days. Airway monitoring is also essential. Intubation or tracheostomy may be necessary.

Noma, or *cancrum oris,* is a fulminant gangrenous infection of the oral and facial tissues that occurs in severely malnourished and debilitated patients and is especially common among children. Beginning as a necrotic ulcer in the gingiva of the mandible, noma is caused by oral anaerobes, especially fusospirochetal organisms (e.g., *Fusobacterium nucleatum*). It is treated with high-dose penicillin, debridement, and correction of the underlying malnutrition.

Herpes simplex commonly causes cold sores of the lips but may also cause painful vesicles on the tongue and buccal mucosa. Primary infection may require intravenous hydration and should be treated with acyclovir. *Thrush,* or oropharyngeal candidiasis, is an infection caused by *Candida* spp. such as *C. albicans.* It occurs in neonates, patients who have received prolonged antibiotic therapy, and immunocompromised patients. More than 90% of patients with AIDS develop thrush. Patients with thrush report a "burning" tongue or "raw" throat and, on examination, have white plaques on the tongue and oral mucosa. Treatment consists of topical antifungal agents (clotrimazole, nystatin) or oral fluconazole. Therapy for fluconazole-resistant thrush in patients with AIDS may be difficult; itraconazole oral solution or amphotericin B oral suspension may be effective.

PHARYNGITIS Most cases of pharyngitis are thought to be viral. Many occur as part of common colds caused by rhinovirus, coronavirus, or parainfluenza virus. Patients have a scratchy or sore throat as well as coryza and cough. The pharynx is inflamed and edematous, but no exudate is evident. Influenza virus and adenovirus may cause a particularly severe sore throat, along with fever and myalgias. In infection with either of the latter viruses, there is pharyngeal erythema and edema; however, adenovirus infection also commonly causes an exudate, thus mimicking streptococcal pharyngitis. *Infectious mononucleosis* due to Epstein-Barr virus often causes a severe sore throat. Exudative pharyngitis or tonsillitis is documented in half of mononucleosis cases and may also mimic streptococcal infection. *Herpangina,* caused by coxsackievirus, is characterized by fever, sore throat, myalgias, and a vesicular enanthem on the soft palate between the uvula and the tonsils. There are usually only two to six lesions, which begin as small papules that vesicate and then ulcerate. Fever and nonexudative pharyngitis are common symptoms of the acute retroviral syndrome that develops several weeks after infection with HIV.

The most important bacterial cause of pharyngitis is group A *Streptococcus (S. pyogenes).* This organism is responsible for about 15% of all cases of pharyngitis and can cause important complications, both suppurative (peritonsillar and retropharyngeal abscess) and nonsuppurative (scarlet fever, streptococcal toxic shock syndrome, rheumatic fever, acute poststreptococcal glomerulonephritis). Fever, severe sore throat, cervical adenopathy, and inflammation of the tonsils and pharynx (which are covered with exudate) are classic findings. However, many cases of streptococcal pharyngitis are mild, with minimal erythema and no exudate, and mimic the pharyngitis of the common cold. Although some patients may in fact have viral pharyngitis and may simply be colonized with group A streptococci, these individuals must nevertheless be treated for presumed streptococcal pharyngitis. Diagnosis is made by culture. Rapid antigen tests are now available. These tests are less sensitive than they are specific: a positive test may be considered equivalent to a positive culture, but a negative test requires culture confirmation. Either a single dose of intramuscular benzathine penicillin (1.2 million units) or a 10-day course of oral penicillin (250 mg four times daily) or erythromycin is necessary to eradicate the organism. Sensitivity to erythromycin should be verified if this agent is used, as an increase in erythromycin resistance has been noted, especially in Europe. Other antibiotics active against streptococci may be used (e.g., amoxicillin, cefuroxime), and one trial showed that 4 days of cefuroxime therapy was as effective as 10 days of penicillin treatment in eradicating the organism. However, studies of the prevention of rheumatic fever are available only for penicillin (Chap. 235).

Other bacterial causes of pharyngitis include groups C and G *Streptococcus*, *Neisseria gonorrhoeae* (Chap. 147), *Arcanobacterium haemolyticum*, *Yersinia enterocolitica*, and—very rarely—*Corynebacterium diphtheriae* (Chap. 141). In addition, *Mycoplasma pneumoniae* (Chap. 178) and *Chlamydia pneumoniae* (Chap. 179) can cause pharyngitis.

A peritonsillar abscess (*quinsy*) may follow untreated streptococcal pharyngitis. Oral anaerobes also play a role in quinsy. Patients have a severe sore throat and speak with a "hot-potato" voice. Examination reveals pronounced unilateral peritonsillar swelling and erythema causing deviation of the uvula. Immediate aspiration by an otolaryngologist is required in conjunction with antibiotic therapy—e.g., ampicillin/sulbactam (3 g intravenously every 6 h), penicillin plus metronidazole, or clindamycin.

LARYNGITIS, CROUP, AND EPIGLOTTITIS

LARYNGITIS   Laryngitis is characterized by hoarseness. Most cases of acute laryngitis are caused by viruses (rhinovirus, influenza virus, parainfluenza virus, coxsackievirus, adenovirus, or respiratory syncytial virus). Acute laryngitis may also be associated with group A *Streptococcus* and *M. catarrhalis*. Laryngitis must be differentiated from epiglottitis (see below). The goal of treatment is merely the relief of symptoms except when throat cultures are positive for group A *Streptococcus* (in which case penicillin should be used).

Chronic laryngitis due to infection is rare and must be distinguished from hoarseness of neoplastic etiology. *Tuberculous laryngitis* may be mistaken for laryngeal cancer when assessed by direct laryngoscopy. Laryngeal and supraglottic lesions include mucosal hyperemia and thickening, nodules, and ulcerations. In one study, a history of fever and night sweats was rare, and the most common chest radiographic finding was apical thickening and fibrosis. Biopsy reveals granulomas with acid-fast bacilli. Cultures should be performed to confirm the diagnosis and evaluate the sensitivities of the pathogen. Laryngeal tuberculosis is highly contagious and should be managed with the same precautions and therapy used for active pulmonary disease (Chap. 169). Fungal infections causing laryngitis include histoplasmosis (Chap. 201), blastomycosis (Chap. 203), and candidiasis (Chap. 205). *Histoplasma* and *Blastomyces* may cause nodules on the larynx, with or without ulcerations. *Candida* may cause laryngitis, along with thrush, in immunosuppressed patients or in patients with chronic mucocutaneous candidiasis.

CROUP   Croup, or acute laryngotracheobronchitis, is an infection of the upper and lower respiratory tract that causes marked subglottic edema. It mainly affects 2- and 3-year-old children and usually follows the onset of upper respiratory tract infection by 1 to 2 days. Symptoms include fever, hoarseness, a "seal's bark" cough, and in-

spiratory stridor. The most common etiology is parainfluenza virus, although croup may also be caused by other respiratory viruses (e.g., influenza or respiratory syncytial virus).

Croup must be differentiated from epiglottitis (see below). Epiglottitis usually progresses more rapidly and produces a more toxic appearance. Neck x-rays may be helpful but do not reliably exclude epiglottitis. In croup, the anterior-posterior neck x-ray shows subglottic edema (the "hourglass sign"); in epiglottitis, the lateral neck view shows a thick epiglottis.

Patients with severe croup should be hospitalized, monitored for hypoxemia through pulse oximetry, and watched for airway obstruction requiring intubation. Humidification is commonly prescribed, but few controlled trials have assessed its benefit. Nebulized racemic epinephrine provides temporary (2-h) improvement in patients with marked stridor, but such patients must be observed for rebound edema. Glucocorticoid therapy, either nebulized or parenteral, is clearly beneficial, and its effects are often evident within 1 h. One trial found that treatment with a single dose of either intramuscular dexamethasone or nebulized budesonide reduced the need for hospitalization of children with moderately severe croup by more than 50%.

EPIGLOTTITIS   Acute epiglottitis (supraglottitis) is a life-threatening, rapidly progressive cellulitis of the epiglottis that may cause complete airway obstruction. It begins as a cellulitis between the tongue base and the epiglottis that pushes the epiglottis posteriorly. The epiglottis itself then becomes swollen, threatening the airway. Before the introduction of *H. influenzae* type b (Hib) vaccine, epiglottitis was most common among children 2 to 4 years old. The disease is now rare in children, since the vaccine has reduced the incidence of invasive disease due to Hib by more than 95%. The incidence in adults has not changed.

The typical young child with epiglottitis has a several-hour history of fever, irritability, dysphonia, and dysphagia and presents sitting forward and drooling. Adolescents and adults usually have a less fulminant presentation, with symptoms (especially sore throat) of 1 or 2 days' duration. Adults may present with dyspnea (25%), drooling (15%), and stridor (10%). Epiglottitis constitutes a medical emergency, as airway occlusion may occur suddenly. Lateral neck films showing an enlarged epiglottis (the "thumb sign") are helpful if positive but may be falsely negative. The value of obtaining these films has also been questioned because doing so may cause a critical delay in securing the airway. Direct viewing of the pharynx by use of a tongue blade should not be attempted, as immediate laryngospasm and airway obstruction may result. Instead, a child with suspected epiglottitis should be transported—while sitting up—to the operating room for visualization of the epiglottis with a fiberoptic laryngoscope, with preparations made for immediate airway control. If the epiglottis is cherry-red, an uncuffed endotracheal tube should be placed. Diagnosis in adults is also made by direct viewing of the epiglottis with a flexible fiberoptic laryngoscope, again only after preparations are made to secure the airway.

All patients must be closely monitored in an intensive care unit and should be given antibiotics active against *H. influenzae*. Before Hib vaccine became available, this organism was responsible for nearly all pediatric cases and was isolated from the blood of almost 100% of the affected children. In adults, blood cultures are positive in about 25% of cases, all of which are due to *H. influenzae*. Other pathogens isolated from the pharynx of adults with epiglottitis include *H. parainfluenzae*, *S. pneumoniae*, group A *Streptococcus*, and (rarely) *S. aureus*; the correlation between throat and epiglottis cultures is unclear, however. Children may be treated with intravenous cefuroxime, ceftriaxone, ampicillin/sulbactam, or trimethoprim-sulfamethoxazole. Adults may be treated for at least 7 days with cefuroxime, ampicillin/sulbactam (3 g intravenously every 6 h), or nafcillin plus ceftriaxone; those highly allergic to penicillin may be given clindamycin plus either trimethoprim-sulfamethoxazole or ciprofloxacin. If the patient with *H. influenzae* epiglottitis has household contacts that include an unvaccinated child under age 4, all members of the household and the patient should receive prophylactic rifampin to eradicate the carriage of *H. influenzae.*

DEEP NECK INFECTIONS

Deep neck infections may be life-threatening because of airway compromise, involvement of the carotid sheath, or spread into the mediastinum.

SUBMANDIBULAR SPACE INFECTIONS See *Ludwig's angina* above (under "Oral Cavity Infections").

LATERAL PHARYNGEAL SPACE INFECTIONS The lateral pharyngeal space, also called the parapharyngeal or pharyngomaxillary space, is in the superior lateral portion of the neck and extends from the hyoid bone to the base of the skull. It lies deep to the lateral wall of the pharynx and is lateral to the tonsil and carotid sheath and medial to the parotid gland. Infection in this space may follow tonsillitis, pharyngitis with adenoid involvement, parotitis, mastoiditis, or periodontal infection.

On presentation, most patients appear toxic and have fever, sore throat, pain on swallowing, and leukocytosis. Infection confined to the posterior (retrostyloid) portion of the lateral pharyngeal space causes swelling of the lateral pharyngeal wall, which may be missed because it is behind the palatopharyngeal arch. Involvement of the anterior portion of this space causes medial displacement of the tonsil, swelling over the parotid gland, and trismus. Rigidity of the neck or torticollis toward the opposite side may develop. Diagnosis is confirmed by CT with contrast.

Treatment includes securing of the airway, surgical drainage in the operating room, and administration for at least 10 days of intravenous antibiotics active against streptococci and oral anaerobes (e.g., ampicillin/sulbactam, 3 g every 6 h). Major complications result from involvement of the carotid sheath and the vessels it contains. These complications are frequently fatal and include jugular vein thrombophlebitis, erosion into the carotid artery, and mediastinitis. Jugular vein thrombophlebitis is characterized by high fevers, chills, and neck tenderness at the angle of the mandible. When it is caused by *Fusobacterium necrophorum,* it may be accompanied by sepsis and septic pulmonary emboli (*Lemierre's syndrome*). Erosion into the carotid artery is usually heralded by repeated small bleeds into the mouth. The involvement of adjacent cranial nerves may result in ipsilateral Horner's syndrome, hoarseness, or unilateral tongue paresis. Extension of infection along the carotid sheath into the posterior mediastinum results in mediastinitis and a mortality of 50%. MRI is useful in delineating carotid and jugular involvement.

RETROPHARYNGEAL SPACE INFECTIONS The retropharyngeal space lies between the pharynx and the prevertebral fascia and extends from the base of the skull into the mediastinum. Infection in this space may result from the spread of lateral pharyngeal space infection or from the lymphatic spread of infection in more cephalad sites (posterior sinuses, adenoids, nasopharynx) to the retropharyngeal lymph nodes. Retropharyngeal abscess is most common among infants and young children, probably because the retropharyngeal nodes later involute. Retropharyngeal abscess may also follow trauma to the posterior pharynx (e.g., endoscopy in adults, lollipop-stick perforation in children) or may result from anterior extension of infection from cervical osteomyelitis.

Symptoms include fever, marked difficulty and pain with swallowing, and a "hot-potato" voice. Physical examination may document drooling, nuchal rigidity, and bulging of the posterior pharyngeal wall. Advanced cases include dyspnea and stridor. Diagnosis may be confirmed by a lateral neck soft-tissue x-ray or CT scan. Treatment requires securing of the airway and emergency surgical drainage. Intravenous antibiotics should be given; the agents chosen should be active against streptococci, oral anaerobes, *S. aureus,* and *H. influenzae* (e.g., ampicillin/sulbactam alone or clindamycin plus ceftriaxone). Potential complications include airway obstruction, intraoral rupture of the abscess causing aspiration pneumonia, and mediastinitis.

BIBLIOGRAPHY

CHOW AW: Life-threatening infections of the head and neck. Clin Infect Dis 14:991, 1992

DEL BECCARO MA et al: Bacteriology of acute otitis media: A new perspective. J Pediatr 120:81, 1992

DESHAZO RD et al: Fungal sinusitis. N Engl J Med 337:254, 1997

HARRIS JP, DARROW DH: Complications of chronic otitis media, in *Surgery of the Ear and Temporal Bone,* JB Nadol Jr, HF Schuknecht (eds). New York, Raven Press, 1993, p 171

JOHNSON DW et al: A comparison of nebulized budesonide, intramuscular dexamethasone, and placebo for moderately severe croup. N Engl J Med 339:498, 1998

KLEIN JO: Otitis externa, otitis media, mastoiditis, in *Principles and Practice of Infectious Diseases,* 4th ed, GL Mandell et al (eds). New York, Churchill Livingstone, 1995, p 579

LIM DJ (ed): Recent advances in otitis media: Report of the Sixth Research Conference. Ann Otol Rhinol Laryngol 107(Suppl 174):1, 1998

MAYO-SMITH MF et al: Acute epiglottitis. An 18-year experience in Rhode Island. Chest 108:1640, 1995

TALMOR M et al: Acute paranasal sinusitis in critically ill patients: Guidelines for prevention, diagnosis, and treatment. Clin Infect Dis 25:1441, 1997

TIERNEY MR, BAKER AS: Infections of the head and neck in diabetes mellitus. Infect Dis Clin North Am 9:195, 1995

John S. Greenspan

ORAL MANIFESTATIONS OF DISEASE

A thorough oral examination, to include the oral and pharyngeal soft tissues as well as the teeth, is an important part of the physical examination. The common oral diseases are due to infection by bacteria, fungi, or viruses. The complex development of the orofacial structures leads to close interposition of diverse tissues, which are prone to developmental anomalies, growth disturbances, and neoplasia.

DISEASES OF THE TEETH

DENTAL CARIES, PULPAL AND PERIAPICAL DISEASE, AND COMPLICATIONS Dental caries is a destructive disease of the hard tissues of the teeth due to infection with *Streptococcus mutans* and other bacteria. In the United States, fewer than half of those 17 years and younger now have carious lesions, although in many segments of the population and in developing countries the disease is more common. Artificial fluoridation of water to a level of 1 part per million, fluoride-containing toothpastes, and topical fluoride administration have reduced the incidence. Conversely, retention of teeth and the aging of the population have led to an increase in root caries. Increasing numbers of individuals surviving cancer therapy and other special populations (diabetic patients and those with xerostomia due to Sjögren's syndrome or to medications) may experience severe caries unless appropriate topical fluoride prophylaxis is used. Treatment of caries involves removal of the softened and infected hard tissues, sealing of the exposed dentine, and restoration of the lost tooth structure with silver amalgam, composite plastic, gold, or porcelain.

If the carious lesion progresses, infection of the dental pulp may occur, causing *acute pulpitis.* The tooth may become sensitive to hot or cold. When severe continuous throbbing pain ensues, pulp damage is irreversible, and root canal therapy becomes necessary. The contents of the pulp chamber and root canals are removed, followed by thorough cleaning, antisepsis, and filling with an inert material. Alternatively, extraction of the tooth may be indicated.

If the pulpitis is not treated successfully, infection may spread beyond the tooth apex into the periodontal ligament. Acute inflammation causes pain on chewing or on percussion, and a *periapical abscess* may form. Chronic inflammation may be painless or produce only slight pain, and a *periapical granuloma* may form within the alveolar bone. Proliferation of epithelial cell rests may convert the granuloma into a *periapical cyst.* Periapical radiolucencies may occur with the granuloma or the cyst but not with the abscess, unless it forms as a complication of one or two lesions. The pus in the periapical abscess may track through the alveolar bone into soft tissues, causing cellulitis and bacteremia, or may discharge into the oral cavity (*parulis* or *gumboil*), into the maxillary sinus, or through the skin of the face or submandibular area. A severe form of cellulitis, *Ludwig's angina,* originates from an infected mandibular molar, involves the submandibular space, and extends throughout the floor of the mouth, with elevation of the tongue, dysphagia, and difficulty breathing. Glottal edema may occur, necessitating tracheotomy.

EFFECT OF SYSTEMIC FACTORS ON TEETH
Enamel hypoplasia of the primary and/or permanent teeth, manifested by alterations ranging from white spots to gross defects in the surface structure of the crowns, may be caused by disturbances of calcium and phosphate metabolism such as are found in vitamin D–resistant rickets, hypoparathyroidism, gastroenteritis, and celiac disease. Premature birth or high fevers may also give rise to enamel hypoplasia. Tetracycline, when given during the second half of pregnancy, in infancy, and in childhood up to 8 years of age, causes both a permanent discoloration of the teeth and enamel hypoplasia. Daily ingestion of more than 1.5 mg fluoride can result in enamel discoloration (*mottling*). Larger teeth are associated with maternal diabetes, maternal hypothyroidism, and large birth size. Tooth size is reduced in Down's syndrome. Systemic disease may give rise to pain that simulates pulpal disease. Maxillary sinusitis is frequently manifested as pain in the maxillary teeth, including sensitivity to thermal changes and percussion. Angina pectoris may result in pain referred to the lower jaw, probably through the vagus nerve.

PERIODONTAL DISEASES

In adults, chronic destructive periodontal disease (*pyorrhea*) is responsible for more loss of teeth than caries, particularly in the aged. However, the prevalence and incidence of periodontal disease also appears to be declining in the United States. The most common form of periodontal disease starts as inflammation of the marginal gingiva (*gingivitis*), which is painless, although the gingiva may bleed on brushing. The disease spreads to involve the periodontal ligament, alveolar bone is slowly resorbed, and periodontal ligament attachment between tooth and bone is lost. The soft tissue separates from the tooth surface, causing "pocket" formation with bleeding on probing and during chewing. Acute inflammation may become superimposed on this chronic process, with the production of pus and the formation of a *periodontal abscess.* Ultimately, extreme bone loss, tooth mobility, and recurrent abscess formation lead to tooth exfoliation or may mandate tooth extraction.

Gingivitis and periodontitis are infections associated with the accumulation of *bacterial plaque,* which may become mineralized (*calculus*) and can be prevented by appropriate *oral hygiene* measures, including tooth brushing, flossing, antibacterial mouth rinses, and the removal of impacted food debris. Poorly fabricated or deteriorated restorations may contribute through overextended or inadequate margins. Therapy consists of removal of plaque and calculus, debridement of the pocket lining and superficial infected cementum, and elimination of other contributing factors.

Periodontal disease appears to be a group of conditions, including *adult periodontitis,* associated with *Porphyromonas gingivalis, Prevotella intermedia,* and other gram-negative organisms. *Localized juvenile periodontitis* (LJP) causes rapid, severe pocketing and bone loss and is associated with *Actinobacillus actinomycetemcomitans, Capnocytophaga, Eikenella corrodens,* and other anaerobes. *Acute necrotizing ulcerative gingivitis* (ANUG) involves sudden inflammation

of the gingivae with necrosis, tissue loss, pain, bleeding, and halitosis and is associated with *P. intermedia* and spirochetes. ANUG and an aggressive and rapid form of periodontitis (*necrotizing ulcerative periodontitis*) are seen in association with HIV infection. Some of these cases progress to a destructive gangrene-like lesion of oral soft tissues and bone (*necrotizing stomatitis*) resembling the *noma* seen in severely malnourished populations. Therapy involves local antibacterial measures, debridement, and, in severe cases, systemic antibiotics effective against anaerobes.

Host factors may be involved in the pathogenesis of periodontal disease in other populations as well. Severe periodontal disease may occur in persons with *Down's syndrome* and *diabetes mellitus.* During pregnancy there may be severe gingivitis and the formation of localized *pyogenic granulomas.* Certain drugs, notably the anticonvulsant *phenytoin* and the calcium channel blocker *nifedipine,* cause *fibrous hyperplasia* of the gingiva, which may cover the teeth, interfere with eating, and be unsightly. *Idiopathic familial gingival fibromatosis* may appear similar. Surgery may correct both conditions; change in medication may reverse the drug-induced form. The oral cavity is a significant reservoir for *Helicobacter pylori.* Uncontrolled diabetes mellitus leads to an exacerbation of oral infection, notably periodontal disease. In individuals genetically predisposed to diabetes, periodontal disease may also precipitate or exacerbate the diabetes. Oral infection has been proposed to contribute to coronary atherosclerosis as well as pregnancy outcomes such as premature labor and low birthweight.

Periapical and periodontal bacterial infections can cause transient bacteremia after tooth extraction and even routine dental prophylaxis. Antibiotic coverage is appropriate in patients with heart valves susceptible to infection or those with prosthetic joints.

DISEASES OF THE ORAL MUCOSA

INFECTIONS   Most oral mucosal diseases involve microorganisms (Table 31-1).

PIGMENTED LESIONS See Table 31-2.

DERMATOLOGIC DISEASES See Tables 31-1, -2, and -3 and Chaps. 55 to 60

DISEASES OF THE TONGUE See Table 31-4

HALITOSIS See Table 31-5

HIV DISEASE AND AIDS (See Table 31-6 and also Chaps. 191 and 309)   Immunosuppression induced by HIV infection predisposes to numerous oral infections, neoplasms, and autoimmune and idiopathic lesions. *Oral candidiasis* (**Plate IID-43**) and *hairy leukoplakia* (**Plate IID-42**) [a benign epithelial hyperplasia associated with Epstein-Barr virus (EBV)] are common features of HIV disease and often precede or accompany full-blown AIDS. Oral Kaposi's sarcoma and lymphoma are diagnostic of AIDS. Oral candidiasis is easily treated with topical or systemic antifungals: nystatin oral pastilles, clotrimazole oral troches, nystatin vaginal tablets used orally, fluconazole, and ketoconazole. While most oral lesions of HIV disease are also found in the general population. Necrotizing ulcerative periodontal disease and hairy leukoplakia are strongly associated with HIV infection and are otherwise very rare.

HEMATOLOGIC AND NUTRITIONAL DISEASE   Gingival bleeding, necrotic ulcers, and enlargement due to malignant infiltrates are seen in all forms of leukemia, particularly *monocytic leukemia.* In *agranulocytosis* severe oral mucosal ulcers are seen, while in *thrombocytopenia* oral petechiae, ecchymoses, and gingival bleeding occur. In *Plummer-Vinson syndrome* (Chap. 105), atrophy of oral mucosa, particularly the tongue papillae, causes redness and soreness as well as dysphagia and is associated with increased susceptibility to oral cancer. A smooth tongue can also be seen in *pernicious anemia* (Chap. 107). Severe oral mucositis with ulcers, candidiasis, bacterial infections, and xerostomia complicate radiation therapy for head and neck cancers. Chemotherapy may also cause mucositis. Although now rarely seen in the United States, oral features of vitamin deficiency include oral mucositis and ulcers, glossitis, and burning sensations in the tongue (*B group vitamin deficiency*) and petechiae, gingival swell-

Table 31-1 Vesicular, Bullous, or Ulcerative Lesions of the Oral Mucosa

Condition	Usual Location	Clinical Features	Course
VIRAL DISEASES			
Primary acute herpetic gingivo-stomatitis (herpes simplex virus type 1, rarely type 2)	Lip and oral mucosa	Labial vesicles that rupture and crust, and intraoral vesicles that quickly ulcerate; extremely painful; acute gingivitis, fever, malaise, foul odor, and cervical lymphadenopathy; occurs primarily in infants, children, and young adults	Heals spontaneously in 10–14 days unless secondarily infected
Recurrent herpes labialis	Mucocutaneous junction of lip, perioral skin	Eruption of groups of vesicles that may coalesce then rupture and crust; painful to pressure or spicy foods	Lasts about 1 week, but condition may be prolonged if secondary infection occurs
Recurrent intraoral herpes simplex	Palate and gingiva	Small vesicles that rupture and coalesce; painful	Heal spontaneously in about 1 week
Chickenpox (varicella-zoster virus)	Gingiva and oral mucosa	Skin lesions may be accompanied by small vesicles on oral mucosa that rupture to form shallow ulcers; may coalesce to form large bullous lesions that ulcerate; mucosa may have generalized erythema	Lesions heal spontaneously within 2 weeks
Herpes zoster (reactivation of varicella-zoster virus)	Cheek, tongue, gingiva, or palate	Unilateral vesicular eruption and ulceration in linear pattern following sensory distribution of trigeminal nerve or one of its branches	Gradual healing without scarring; postherpetic neuralgia is common
Infectious mononucleosis (Epstein-Barr virus)	Oral mucosa	Fatigue, sore throat, malaise, low-grade fever, and enlarged cervical lymph nodes; numerous small ulcers usually appear several days before lymphadenopathy; gingival bleeding and multiple petechiae at junction of hard and soft palates	Oral lesions disappear during convalescence
Warts (papillomavirus)	Anywhere on skin and oral mucosa	Single or multiple papillary lesions, with thick, white keratinized surfaces containing many pointed projections; cauliflower lesions covered with normal-colored mucosa or multiple pink or pale bumps (focal epithelial hyperplasia)	Lesions grow rapidly and spread
Herpangina (coxsackievirus A; also possibly coxsackievirus B and echovirus)	Oral mucosa, pharynx, tongue	Sudden onset of fever, sore throat, and oropharyngeal vesicles, usually in children under 4 years, during summer months; diffuse pharyngeal congestion and vesicles (1–2 mm), grayish-white surrounded by red areola; vesicles enlarge and ulcerate	Incubation period 2–9 days; fever for 1–4 days; recovery uneventful
Hand, foot, and mouth disease (type A coxsackicviruses)	Oral mucosa, pharynx, palms, and soles	Fever, malaise, headache with oropharyngeal vesicles that become painful, shallow ulcers	Incubation period 2–18 days; lesions heal spontaneously in 2–4 weeks
Primary HIV infection	Gingiva, palate, and pharynx	Acute gingivitis and oropharyngeal ulceration, associated with febrile illness resembling mononucleosis and including lymphadenopathy	Followed by HIV seroconversion, asymptomatic HIV infection, and usually ultimately by HIV disease
BACTERIAL OR FUNGAL DISEASES			
Acute necrotizing ulcerative gingivitis ("trench mouth," Vincent's infection)	Gingiva	Painful, bleeding gingiva characterized by necrosis and ulceration of gingival papillae and margins plus lymphadenopathy and foul odor	Continued destruction of tissue followed by remission, but may recur
Prenatal (congenital) syphilis	Palate, jaws, tongue, and teeth	Gummatous involvement of palate, jaws, and facial bones; Hutchinson's incisors, mulberry molars, glossitis, mucous patches, and fissures of corners of mouth	Tooth deformities in permanent dentition irreversible
Primary syphilis (chancre)	Lesion appears where organism enters body; may occur on lips, tongue, or tonsillar area	Small papule developing rapidly into a large, painless ulcer with indurated border; unilateral lymphadenopathy; chancre and lymph nodes containing spirochetes; serologic tests positive by third to fourth weeks	Healing of chancre in 1–2 months, followed by secondary syphilis in 6–8 weeks
Secondary syphilis	Oral mucosa frequently involved with mucous patches, primarily on palate, also at commissures of mouth	Maculopapular lesions of oral mucosa, 5–10 mm in diameter with central ulceration covered by grayish membrane; eruptions occurring on various mucosal surfaces and skin accompanied by fever, malaise, and sore throat	Lesions may persist from several weeks to a year
Tertiary syphilis	Palate and tongue	Gummatous infiltration of palate or tongue followed by ulceration and fibrosis; atrophy of tongue papillae produces characteristic bald tongue and glossitis	Gumma may destroy palate, causing complete perforation

(continued)

Condition	Usual Location	Clinical Features	Course
Gonorrhea	Lesions may occur in mouth at site of inoculation or secondarily by hematogenous spread from a primary focus elsewhere	Earliest symptoms are burning or itching sensation, dryness, or heat in mouth followed by acute pain on eating or speaking; tonsils and oropharynx most frequently involved; oral tissues may be diffusely inflamed or ulcerated; saliva develops increased viscosity and fetid odor; submaxillary lymphadenopathy with fever in severe cases	Lesions may resolve with appropriate antibiotic therapy
Tuberculosis	Tongue, tonsillar area, soft palate	A solitary, irregular ulcer covered by a persistent exudate; ulcer has an undermined, firm border	Lesions may persist
Cervicofacial actinomycosis	Swellings in region of face, neck, and floor of mouth	Infection may be associated with an extraction, jaw fracture, or eruption of molar tooth; in acute form resembles an acute pyogenic abscess, but contains yellow "sulfur granules" (gram-positive mycelia and their hyphae)	Acute form may last a few weeks; chronic form lasts months or years; prognosis excellent; actinomycetes respond to antibiotics (tetracyclines or penicillin) but not to antifungal drugs
Histoplasmosis	Any area in mouth, particularly tongue, gingiva, or palate	Numerous small nodules that may ulcerate; hoarseness and dysphagia may occur because of lesions in larynx, usually associated with fever and malaise	May be fatal
Candidiasis	Any area of oral mucosa	Pseudomembranous form has white patches that are easily wiped off leaving red, bleeding, sore surface; erythematous form is flat and red; rarely, candidal leukoplakia appears as white patch in tongue that does not rub off; angular cheilitis due to *Candida* involves sore cracks and redness at angle of mouth; *Candida* seen on KOH preparation in all forms	Responds to antifungals
DERMATOLOGIC DISEASES			
Mucous membrane pemphigoid	Primarily mucous membranes of the oral cavity, but may also involve the eyes, urethra, vagina, and rectum	Painful, grayish-white collapsed vesicles or bullae with peripheral erythematous zone; gingival lesions desquamate, leaving ulcerated area	Protracted course with remissions and exacerbations; involvement of different sites occurs slowly; glucocorticoids may temporarily reduce symptoms but do not control the disease
Erythema multiforme (Stevens-Johnson syndrome)	Primarily the oral mucosa and skin of hands and feet	Intraoral ruptured bullae surrounded by an inflammatory area; lips may show hemorrhagic crusts; the "iris," or "target," lesion on the skin is pathognomonic; patient may have severe signs of toxicity	Onset very rapid; condition may last 1–2 weeks; may be fatal; acute episodes respond to steroids
Pemphigus vulgaris	Oral mucosa and skin	Ruptured bullae and ulcerated oral areas; mostly in older adults	With repeated recurrence of bullae, toxicity may lead to cachexia, infection, and death within 2 years; often controllable with steroids
Lichen planus	Oral mucosa and skin	White striae in mouth; purplish nodules on skin at sites of friction; occasionally causes oral mucosal ulcers and erosive gingivitis	Protracted course, may respond to topical steroids
OTHER CONDITIONS			
Recurrent aphthous ulcers	Anywhere on nonkeratinized oral mucosa (lips, tongue, buccal mucosa, floor of mouth, soft palate, oropharynx)	Single or clusters of painful ulcers with surrounding erythematous border; lesions may be 1–2 mm in diameter in crops (herpetiform), 1–5 mm (minor), or 5–15 mm (major)	Lesions heal in 1–2 weeks but may recur monthly or several times a year; topical steroids give symptomatic relief; systemic glucocorticoids may be needed in severe cases; a tetracycline oral suspension may decrease severity of herpetiform ulcers
Behçet's syndrome	Oral mucosa, eyes, genitalia, gut, and CNS	Multiple aphthous ulcers in mouth; inflammatory ocular changes, ulcerative lesions on genitalia; inflammatory bowel disease and CNS disease	Ulcers may persist for several weeks and heal without scarring
Traumatic ulcers	Anywhere on oral mucosa; dentures frequently responsible for ulcers in vestibule	Localized, discrete ulcerated lesion with red border; produced by accidental biting of mucosa, penetration by a foreign object, or chronic irritation by a denture	Lesions usually heal in 7–10 days when irritant is removed, unless secondarily infected

Table 31-2 Pigmented Lesions of the Oral Mucosa

Condition	Usual Location	Clinical Features	Course
Oral melanotic macule	Any area of the mouth	Discrete or diffuse localized, brown to black macule	Remains indefinitely
Diffuse melanin pigmentation	Any area of the mouth	Diffuse pale to dark-brown pigmentation; may be physiologic ("racial") or due to smoking	Remains indefinitely
Nevi	Any area of the mouth	Discrete, localized, brown to black pigmentation	Remains indefinitely
Malignant melanoma	Any area of the mouth	Can be flat and diffuse, painless, brown to black, or can be raised and nodular	Expands and invades early; metastasis leads to death
Addison's disease	Any area in mouth but mostly on buccal mucosa	Blotches or spots of bluish-black to dark-brown pigmentation occurring early in the disease, accompanied by diffuse pigmentation of skin; other symptoms of adrenal insufficiency	Condition controlled by steroid therapy
Peutz-Jeghers syndrome	Any area in mouth	Dark-brown spots on lips, buccal mucosa, with characteristic distribution of pigment around lips, nose, eyes, and on hands; concomitant intestinal polyposis	Pigmented lesions remain indefinitely; polyps may become malignant
Drug ingestion (tranquilizers, oral contraceptives, antimalarials)	Any area in mouth	Brown, black, or gray areas of pigmentation	Disappears following cessation of drug
Amalgam tattoo	Gingiva and mucobuccal fold	Small blue-black pigmented areas associated with embedded amalgam particles in soft tissues; these may show up on radiographs as radiopaque particles in some cases	Remains indefinitely
Heavy metal pigmentation (bismuth, mercury, lead)	Gingival margin	Thin blue-black pigmented line along gingival margin; due to prior treatment for syphilis with bismuth or mercury or to accidental absorption of lead	Long-lasting
Black hairy tongue	Dorsum of tongue	Elongation of filiform papillae of tongue, which take on a brown to black coloration	Long-lasting but may disappear spontaneously
Fordyce's "disease"	Buccal and labial mucosa	Aggregation of numerous small yellowish spots just beneath mucosal surface; no symptoms; due to hyperplasia of sebaceous glands	Remains without apparent change indefinitely

Table 31-3 White Lesions of Oral Mucosa

Condition	Usual Location	Clinical Features	Course
Lichen planus	Buccal mucosa, tongue, gingiva, and lips; skin	Striae, white plaques, red areas, ulcers in mouth; purplish papules on skin; may be asymptomatic, sore, or painful; lichenoid drug reactions may look similar	Protracted; responds to topical steroids
White sponge nevus	Oral mucosa, vagina, anal mucosa	Painless white thickening of epithelium; adolescent/early adult onset; familial	Benign and permanent
Smoker's leukoplakia and smokeless tobacco lesions	Any area of oral mucosa, sometimes related to location of habit	White patch that may become firm, rough, or red-fissured and ulcerated; may become sore and painful but usually painless	Occasionally premalignant; may or may not resolve on cessation of habit
Nicotinic stomatitis	Palate in pipe smokers	White nodular elevations on hard palate with central red areas	Benign; usually resolves on cessation of pipe smoking
Frictional keratosis	Any area in mouth	Elevated white lesion due to hyperkeratosis and thickening of the oral epithelium secondary to chronic irritation	Removal of irritant leads to healing in 2–3 weeks
Candidiasis ("candidosis," "moniliasis")	Any area in mouth	*Pseudomembranous type* ("thrush"): creamy white curdlike patches that reveal a raw, bleeding surface when scraped; found in sick infants, debilitated elderly patients receiving high doses of glucocorticoids or broad-spectrum antibiotics, or in patients with AIDS	Responds favorably to antifungal therapy and correction of predisposing causes where possible
		Erythematous type: flat, red, sometimes sore areas, same groups of patients	Course same as for pseudomembranous type
		Candidal leukoplakia: nonremovable white thickening of epithelium due to *Candida*	Responds to prolonged antifungals
		Angular cheilitis: sore fissures at corner of mouth	Responds to topical antifungals
Hairy leukoplakia	Usually lateral tongue, rarely elsewhere on oral mucosa	White areas ranging from small and flat to extensive and "hairy"; found in HIV carriers in all risk groups for AIDS; rarely causes discomfort	Due to EBV; many patients develop AIDS; responds to high dose acyclovir but recurs
Chemical burns	Any area in mouth	White slough due to necrosis of epithelium and underlying connective tissue caused by contact with agents (e.g., aspirin) applied locally or the use of undiluted sodium perborate or hydrogen peroxide as a mouthwash; removal of slough leaves a raw, painful surface	Lesion heals in several weeks if not secondarily infected

Table 31-4 Alterations of the Tongue

Type of Change	Clinical Features
SIZE OR MORPHOLOGY CHANGES	
Macroglossia	Enlarged tongue that may be part of a syndrome found in developmental conditions such as Down's syndrome; may be due to tumor (hemangioma or lymphangioma), metabolic disease (such as primary amyloidosis), or endocrine disturbance (such as acromegaly or cretinism)
Fissured ("scrotal") tongue	Dorsal surface and sides of tongue covered by painless shallow or deep fissures that may collect debris and become irritated
Median rhomboid glossitis	Congenital abnormality of tongue with ovoid, denuded area in median posterior portion of the tongue; may be associated with candidiasis and may respond to antifungals
COLOR CHANGES	
"Geographic" tongue (benign migratory glossitis)	Asymptomatic inflammatory condition of the tongue, with rapid loss and regrowth of filiform papillae, leading to appearance of denuded red patches "wandering" across the surface of the tongue
Hairy tongue	Elongation of filiform papillae of the medial dorsal surface area due to failure of keratin layer of the papillae to desquamate normally; brownish-black coloration may be due to staining by tobacco, food, or chromogenic organisms
"Strawberry" and "raspberry" tongue	Appearance of tongue during scarlet fever due to the hypertrophy of fungiform papillae plus changes in the filiform papillae
"Bald" tongue	Atrophy may be associated with xerostomia, pernicious anemia, iron-deficiency anemia, pellagra, or syphilis; may be accompanied by painful burning sensation; may be an expression of erythmematous candidiasis and respond to antifungals

ing, bleeding, and ulceration as well as loosening of teeth (*scurvy* of vitamin C deficiency).

DISEASES OF THE SALIVARY GLANDS

The major and minor salivary glands can be involved in mumps, sarcoidosis, tuberculosis, lymphoma, and Sjögren's syndrome (Chap. 314). The latter may cause dry eyes and dry mouth (*xerostomia*) and be associated with features of connective tissue diseases, including rheumatoid arthritis or systemic lupus erythematosus. Xerostomia may also be due to medications such as diuretics, antihistamines, or tricylic antidepressants as well as radiation therapy for head and neck cancer. Without lysozyme-rich saliva, *cervical or incisal caries* and oral candidiasis may develop. Management includes fluoride mouth rinses and topical applications, saliva substitutes, salivary stimulation with sugarless candies, and the avoidance of sugar-containing drinks or food. Candidiasis is treated with nystatin or other antifungals. Salivary stones (*sialolithiasis*), usually in the duct of a major salivary gland, cause *sialoadenitis* with pain and swelling, often on eating, especially tart foods such as lemons.

The most common neoplasm of the salivary glands is the *pleomorphic adenoma*, which is benign but will recur unless fully resected; malignant tumors include *mucoepidermoid carcinoma*, *adenoid cystic carcinoma*, and *adenocarcinoma*. The pleomorphic adenoma causes a firm, slowly growing mass in the parotid, palate, or cheek, whereas malignant tumors grow faster and can cause ulceration and invade

Table 31-5 Causes of Halitosis

1. Lower respiratory tract infection
   a. Bronchiectasis
   b. Lung abscess
2. Oral infection
   a. Acute primary herpetic gingivostomatitis
   b. Acute necrotizing ulcerative gingivitis
   c. Periodontal disease
   d. Caries
3. Smoking
4. Hepatic failure (fishy odor)
5. Azotemia (ammoniacal or urinary odor)
6. Diabetic ketoacidosis (sweet, fruity odor)
7. *H. pylori* gastric infection
8. Esophageal cancer
9. Metal poisoning (garlicky)

nerves, producing numbness or facial paralysis.

NEUROLOGIC DISTURBANCES AND OROFACIAL PAIN

The mouth and face may be the site of pain from a number of vascular, neurologic, muscle/connective tissue, or joint conditions. Interdisciplinary diagnosis and management programs involving neurologists, restorative dentists, oral surgeons, otorhinolaryngologists, and other specialists, together with new imaging techniques to diagnose or exclude organic lesions, have begun to clarify this complex field. *Temporal arteritis* causes pain in the face, jaws, and tongue and may mimic temporomandibular joint disease. Glucocorticoids may provide relief. *Myofascial pain* is a dull, constant ache with local tenderness in the muscles of the jaws and difficulty in opening the mouth. Teeth clenching and grinding (*bruxism*) may play a role. *Arthralgia* of the temporomandibular joint causes local pain, which may extend to the face and head. Both myofascial pain and arthralgia can be relieved with heat, rest, and anti-inflammatory agents. Displacement of the meniscus or condyle may cause pain, clenching, or locking of the mandible in the open position. The joint may become involved in *osteoarthritis* with minimal symptoms, whereas *rheumatoid arthritis* causes pain and swelling in the joint and limitation of movement. *Ankylosis* may occur, necessitating condylectomy (Chap. 312).

Trigeminal neuralgia (tic douloureux) causes sudden, severe, unilateral lancinating pain initiated by touching a "trigger zone" or occurring spontaneously. Confusion with pulpal or periapical pain is common, leading to inappropriate endodontic or surgical therapy. Many cases respond to carbamazepine and phenytoin, but for a few,

Table 31-6 Oral Lesions of HIV Disease and AIDS

I. Fungal
   A. Candidiasis
      1. Pseudomembranous
      2. Erythematous
      3. Angular cheilitis
   B. Histoplasmosis
   C. Cryptococcosis
II. Bacterial
   A. Acute necrotizing ulcerative gingivitis
   B. Necrotizing ulcerative periodontitis
   C. Necrotizing stomatitis
   D. *Mycoabacterium avium* complex and tuberculosis
   E. Stomatitis due to enteric organisms
III. Viral
   A. Herpes simplex
   B. Herpes zoster
   C. Hairy leukoplakia
   D. Warts
IV. Neoplastic
   A. Kaposi's sarcoma
   B. Lymphoma
V. Other
   A. Recurrent aphthous ulcers
   B. Immune thrombocytopenic purpura
   C. Xerostomia
   D. Salivary gland enlargement

surgical intervention to decompress the trigeminal nerve is indicated. Similar symptoms in the distribution of the ninth cranial nerve (tongue, pharynx, soft palate) are due to *glossopharyngeal neuralgia*, which may be triggered by swallowing and may produce referred pain in the temporomandibular joint. *Postherpetic neuralgia* may follow trigeminal herpes zoster (Chap. 367) and cause burning, aching, and long-lasting pain. *Facial palsy* is usually unilateral and may be due to trauma, surgical intervention, tumor, or infection of the seventh cranial nerve. *Bell's palsy* is a form with acute onset and unknown cause, possibly viral infection such as herpes zoster. The corner of the mouth droops, and there may be difficulty in speech, eating, and in closing the eye. The symptoms usually disappear spontaneously, but residual facial immobility and lip drooping may persist. Abnormal or reduced *taste sensation* may be due to xerostomia, disturbances of the facial and glossopharyngeal nerves or their central connections, aging, or the wearing of dentures. Disease involving the hypoglossal nerve may

cause atrophy of the tongue muscles with protrusion, if bilateral, or deviation toward the affected side, if unilateral. Numb chin (mental neuropathy) may be a sign of primary neural disease, but in the cancer patient it is often a harbinger of tumor relapse or progression.

BIBLIOGRAPHY

BARKER FG et al: The long-term outcome of microvascular decompression for trigeminal neuralgia. N Engl J Med 334:1077, 1996

GREENSPAN D, GREENSPAN JS: HIV-related oral disease. Lancet 348:729, 1996

REGEZI JA, SCIUBBA JJ (eds): *Oral Pathology: Clinical Pathologic Correlations*. 3d ed. Philadelphia, Saunders, 1999

STAMM JW (ed): Periodontal diseases and human health: New directions in periodontal medicine. Ann Periodontal 3:1, 1998

THYLSTRUP A, FEJERSKOV O (eds): *Textbook of Clinical Cariology*, 2d ed. Copenhagen, Munksgaard, 1994

Section 5
ALTERATIONS IN CIRCULATORY AND RESPIRATORY FUNCTIONS

32

Roland H. Ingram, Jr., Eugene Braunwald

DYSPNEA AND PULMONARY EDEMA

DYSPNEA

Breathing is controlled by central and peripheral mechanisms that adjust ventilation appropriate to increased metabolic demands during physical activity and increase ventilation in excess of metabolic demands in conditions such as anxiety and fear. A normal resting person is unaware of the act of breathing, and while he or she may become conscious of breathing during mild to moderate exertion, no discomfort is experienced. However, during and following exhausting exertion, an individual may become unpleasantly aware of breathing yet feel reasonably assured that the sensation will be transitory and is appropriate to the level of exercise. Therefore, as a cardinal symptom of diseases affecting the cardiorespiratory system, *dyspnea* is defined as an *abnormally uncomfortable awareness of breathing*.

Although dyspnea is not painful in the usual sense of the word, it is, like pain, involved with both the perception of a sensation and the reaction to that perception. Patients experience a number of uncomfortable sensations related to breathing and use an even larger number of verbal expressions to describe these sensations, such as "cannot get enough air," "air does not go all the way down," "smothering feeling or tightness or tiredness in the chest," and a "choking sensation." It may be necessary, therefore, to review the patient's history meticulously in order to ascertain whether the more abstruse descriptions do, in fact, represent dyspnea. Once it is established that a patient does have dyspnea, it is of paramount importance to define the circumstances in which it occurs and to assess associated symptoms. There are situations in which breathing appears labored but in which dyspnea does not occur. For example, the hyperventilation associated with metabolic acidemia is rarely accompanied by dyspnea. On the other hand, patients with apparently normal breathing patterns may complain of shortness of breath.

QUANTITATION OF DYSPNEA The gradation of dyspnea is based on the amount of physical exertion required to produce the sensation. In assessing the severity of dyspnea, it is important to obtain a clear understanding of the patient's general physical condition, work history, and recreational habits. For example, the development of dyspnea in a trained runner upon running 2 mi may signify a much more

serious disturbance than a similar degree of breathlessness in a sedentary person upon running a fraction of this distance. Interindividual variation in perception must also be considered. Some patients with severe disease may complain of only mild dyspnea; others with mild disease may experience more severe shortness of breath. Some patients with lung or heart disease may have such reduced capabilities due to other disease (e.g., peripheral vascular insufficiency or severe osteoarthritis of the hips or knees) that exertional dyspnea is precluded despite serious impairment of pulmonary or cardiac function.

Some patterns of dyspnea are not directly related to physical exertion. Sudden and unexpected dyspneic episodes at rest can be associated with pulmonary emboli, spontaneous pneumothorax, hypercapnea secondary to breath holding, or anxiety. Nocturnal episodes of severe paroxysmal dyspnea are characteristic of left ventricular failure. Dyspnea upon assuming the supine posture, *orthopnea* (see below and Chap. 232), thought to be mainly characteristic of congestive heart failure, may also occur in some patients with asthma and chronic obstruction of the airways and is a regular finding in the rare occurrence of bilateral diaphragmatic paralysis. *Trepopnea* is used to describe the unusual circumstance in which dyspnea occurs only in a lateral decubitus position, most often in patients with heart disease, while *platypnea* is dyspnea that occurs only in the upright position. Positional alterations in ventilation-perfusion relationships (Chap. 250) have been invoked to explain these patterns.

MECHANISMS OF DYSPNEA (See Fig. 32-1) Dyspnea occurs whenever the work of breathing is excessive. Increased force generation is required of the respiratory muscles to produce a given volume change if the chest wall or lungs are less compliant or if resistance to airflow is increased. Increased work of breathing also occurs when the ventilation is excessive for the level of activity. Although an individual is more apt to become dyspneic when the work of breathing is increased, the work theory does not account for the perceptual difference between a deep breath with a normal mechanical load and a normal-sized breath with an increased mechanical load. The work might be the same with both breaths, but the normal one with the increased load will be associated with discomfort. In fact, with respiratory loading, such as adding a resistance at the mouth, there is an increase in respiratory center output that is disproportionate to the increase in the work of breathing. It has been postulated that whenever the force that muscles actually generate during breathing approaches some fraction of their maximal force-generating ability, which may vary among individuals, dyspnea ensues due to transduction of mechanical to neural stimuli.

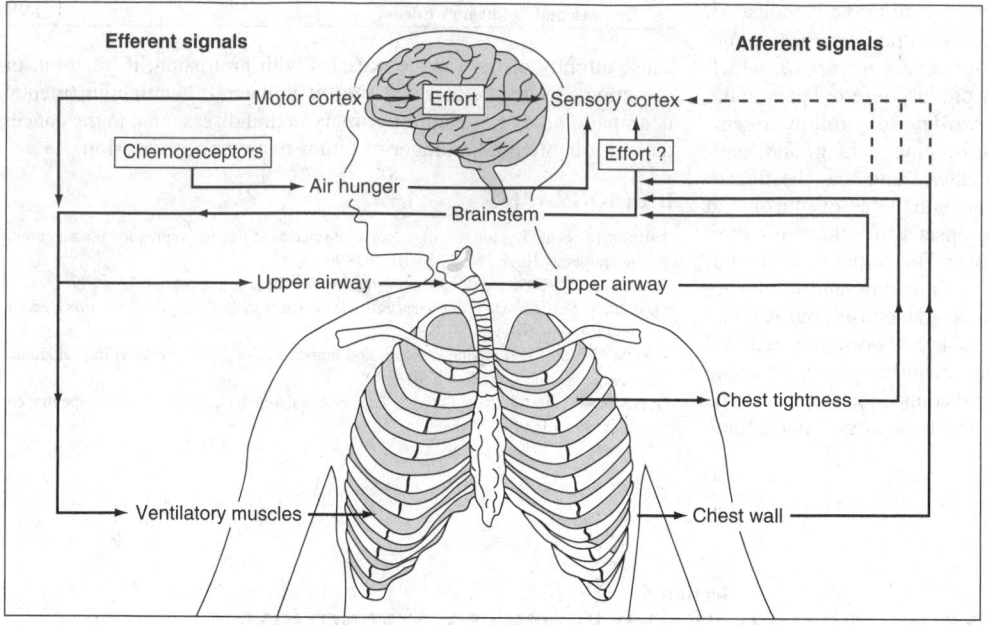

Efferent signals   **Afferent signals**

Motor cortex — Effort — Sensory cortex

Chemoreceptors

Effort ?

Air hunger

Brainstem

Upper airway → Upper airway

Chest tightness

Ventilatory muscles → Chest wall

FIGURE 32-1 Efferent and afferent signals that contribute to the sensation of dyspnea. There is evidence that the sense of respiratory effort arises from a signal transmitted from the motor cortex to the sensory cortex simultaneously with the outgoing motor command to the ventilatory muscles. The motor output of the brainstem may also contribute to the sense of effort, as shown in the arrow from the brainstem to the sensory cortex. The sense of air hunger arises, in part, from increased respiratory activity within the brainstem, and the sensation of chest tightness probably results from stimulation of vagal-irritant receptors. While afferent information from airway, lung, and chest-wall receptors probably passes through the brainstem before reaching the sensory cortex, the dashed lines indicate uncertainty about whether some afferents bypass the brainstem and project directly to the sensory cortex. *(From HL Manning, RM Schwartzstein, Pathophysiology of dyspnea. N Engl J Med 333:1547, 1995, with permission.)*

In all likelihood, several different mechanisms operate to different degrees in the various clinical situations in which dyspnea occurs. In some circumstances, dyspnea is evoked by stimulation of receptors in the upper respiratory tract; in others it may originate from receptors in the lungs, airways, respiratory muscles, chest wall, or some combination of these structures. In any event, dyspnea is characterized by an excessive or abnormal activation of the respiratory centers in the brainstem. This activation comes about from stimuli transmitted from or through a variety of structures and pathways, including (1) intrathoracic receptors via the vagi; (2) afferent somatic nerves, particularly from the respiratory muscles and chest wall, but also from other skeletal muscles and joints; (3) chemoreceptors in the brain, aortic and carotid bodies, and elsewhere in the circulation; (4) higher (cortical) centers; and perhaps (5) afferent fibers in the phrenic nerves. In general, despite the interindividual variations described above, there is a reasonable correlation between the severity of dyspnea and the magnitude of disturbances of pulmonary or cardiac function that are responsible.

The mechanisms responsible for dyspnea may vary in different conditions (Table 32-1).

DIFFERENTIAL DIAGNOSIS   **Obstructive Disease of Airways** (See also Chaps. 252 and 258) Obstruction to airflow can be present anywhere from the extrathoracic airways out to the small airways in the periphery of the lung. Large extrathoracic airway obstruction can occur acutely, as with aspiration of food or a foreign body or with angioedema of the glottis. An allergic history together with a few scattered hives should raise the possibility of glottic edema. Acute upper airway obstruction is a medical emergency. More chronic forms can occur with tumors or with fibrotic stenosis following tracheostomy or prolonged endotracheal intubation. Whether acute or chronic, the cardinal symptom is dyspnea, and the characteristic signs are stridor and retraction of the supraclavicular fossae with *inspiration*.

Obstruction of intrathoracic airways can occur acutely and intermittently or can be present chronically with worsening during respi-

ratory infections. Acute intermittent obstruction with wheezing is typical of *asthma* (Chap. 252). Chronic cough with expectoration is typical of *chronic bronchitis* (Chap. 258) and *bronchiectasis* (Chap. 256). Most often there are prolongation of expiration and coarse rhonchi that are generalized in chronic bronchitis and may be localized in the case of bronchiectasis. Intercurrent infection results in worsening of the cough, increased expectoration of purulent sputum, and more severe dyspnea. During such episodes, the patient may complain of nocturnal paroxysms of dyspnea with wheezing relieved by cough and expectoration of sputum. Despite the fact that severe limitation of expiratory flow and hyperinflation of the lung are characteristic of these diseases, the sensory experience is often that of an inability to take in a sufficiently deep breath rather than difficulty in exhaling.

The patient with predominant *emphysema* is characterized by many years of exertional dyspnea progressing to dyspnea at rest (Chap. 258). Although a parenchymal disease by definition, emphysema is invariably accompanied by obstruction of airways.

Diffuse Parenchymal Lung Diseases (See also Chap. 259) This category includes a large number of diseases ranging from acute pneumonia to chronic disorders such as sarcoidosis and the various forms of *pneumoconiosis* (Chap. 254). History, physical findings, and radiographic abnormalities often provide clues to the diagnosis. The patients are often tachypneic with arterial P_{CO_2} and P_{O_2} values below normal. Exertion often further reduces the arterial P_{O_2}. Lung volumes are decreased, and the lungs are stiffer, i.e., less compliant than normal.

Pulmonary Vascular Occlusive Diseases (See also Chap. 261) Repeated episodes of dyspnea at rest often occur with recurrent pulmonary emboli. Evidence of a source for emboli, such as phlebitis of a lower extremity or the pelvis, is quite helpful in leading the physician to suspect the diagnosis. Arterial blood gases are most often abnormal, but lung volumes are frequently normal or only minimally abnormal.

Diseases of the Chest Wall or Respiratory Muscles (See also Chap. 263) The physical examination establishes the presence of a

Table 32-1 Possible Mechanisms of Dyspnea in Selected Conditions

Condition	Mechanism
Asthma	Increased sense of effort
	Stimulation of irritant receptors in airways
Neuromuscular disease	Increased sense of effort
COPD	Increased sense of effort
	Hypoxia
	Hypercapnia
	Dynamic airway compression
Mechanical ventilation	Afferent mismatch
	Factors associated with the underlying condition
Pulmonary embolism	Stimulation of pressure receptors in pulmonary vasculature or right atrium (possible)

NOTE: COPD, chronic obstructive pulmonary disease.
SOURCE: From HL Manning, RM Schwartzstein, Pathophysiology of dyspnea. N Engl J Med 333:1547, 1995, with permission.

chest wall disease such as severe kyphoscoliosis, pectus excavatum, or ankylosing spondylitis. Although all three of these deformities may be associated with dyspnea, only severe kyphoscoliosis regularly interferes with ventilation sufficiently to produce chronic cor pulmonale and respiratory failure.

Both weakness and paralysis of respiratory muscles can lead to respiratory failure and dyspnea (Chap. 263), but most often the signs and symptoms of the neurologic or muscular disorder are more prominently manifested in other systems.

Heart Disease In patients with cardiac disease, exertional dyspnea occurs most commonly as a consequence of an elevated pulmonary capillary pressure, which in turn may be due to left ventricular dysfunction (Chaps. 231 and 232), reduced left ventricular compliance, and mitral stenosis. The elevation of hydrostatic pressure in the pulmonary vascular bed tends to upset the Starling equilibrium (see "Pulmonary Edema," below) with resulting transudation of liquid into the interstitial space, reducing the compliance of the lungs and stimulating J (juxtacapillary) receptors in the alveolar interstitial space. When it is prolonged, pulmonary venous hypertension results in thickening of the walls of small pulmonary vessels and an increase in perivascular cells and fibrous tissue, causing a further reduction in compliance. The competition for space among vessels, airways, and increased liquid within the interstitial space compromises the lumina of small airways, increasing the airways' resistance. Diminution in compliance and an increase in the airways' resistance increase the work of breathing. In advanced congestive heart failure, usually involving elevation of both pulmonary and systemic venous pressures, hydrothorax may develop, interfering further with pulmonary function and intensifying dyspnea.

Orthopnea, i.e., dyspnea in the supine position, is the result of the alteration of gravitational forces when this position is assumed, which elevates pulmonary venous and capillary pressures. These, in turn, increase the pulmonary closing volume (Chap. 250) and reduce the vital capacity.

Paroxysmal (nocturnal) dyspnea Also known as *cardiac asthma*, this condition is characterized by attacks of severe shortness of breath that generally occur at night and usually awaken the patient from sleep. The attack is precipitated by stimuli that aggravate previously existing pulmonary congestion; frequently, the total blood volume is augmented at night because of the reabsorption of edema from dependent portions of the body during recumbency. A sleeping patient can tolerate relatively severe pulmonary engorgement and may awaken only when actual pulmonary edema and bronchospasm have developed, with the feeling of suffocation and with wheezing respirations.

Two other forms of nocturnal dyspnea must be distinguished from that due to heart failure. Chronic bronchitis is characterized by mucus hypersecretion and, after a few hours sleep, secretions can accumulate and produce dyspnea and wheezing, both of which are relieved by cough and expectoration of sputum. Asthma patients have circadian variations in their degree of airway obstruction. The obstruction becomes most severe between 2 A.M. and 4 A.M. and can be sufficiently severe that the patient awakens with a sense of suffocation, extreme dyspnea, and wheezing. Although there is a prominent inflammatory component to nocturnal asthma, inhaled bronchodilators usually improve symptoms quickly.

Cheyne-Stokes respiration → *See Chap. 232*

Diagnosis The diagnosis of cardiac dyspnea depends on the recognition of heart disease on the basis of the clinical examination supplemented by noninvasive testing. There may be a history of antecedent myocardial infarction; third and fourth heart sounds may be audible; and/or there may be evidence of left ventricular enlargement, jugular neck vein distention, and/or peripheral edema. Often there are radiographic signs of heart failure, with evidence of interstitial edema, pulmonary vascular redistribution, and accumulation of liquid in the septal planes and pleural cavity. Transthoracic echocardiography is particularly useful in establishing the diagnosis of structural heart disease, which can be responsible for dyspnea. Specifically, left atrial and/or left ventricular dilatation, left ventricular hypertrophy, a reduced left ventricular ejection fraction, and disorders of left ventricular

wall motion may be clues to the presence of a cardiac etiology of otherwise unexplained dyspnea.

DIFFERENTIATION BETWEEN CARDIAC AND PULMONARY DYSPNEA In most patients with dyspnea there is obvious clinical evidence of disease of the heart and/or lungs. Like patients with cardiac dyspnea, patients with chronic obstructive lung disease may also waken at night with dyspnea, but, as pointed out above, this is usually associated with sputum production; the dyspnea is relieved after these patients rid themselves of secretions. The difficulty in the distinction between cardiac and pulmonary dyspnea may be compounded by the coexistence of diseases involving both organ systems.

In patients in whom the etiology of dyspnea is not clear, it is desirable to carry out pulmonary function testing, for these tests may be helpful in determining whether dyspnea is produced by heart disease, lung disease, abnormalities of the chest wall, or anxiety (Chap. 250). In addition to the usual means of assessing patients for heart disease, determination of the ejection fraction at rest and during exercise by echocardiography or radionuclide ventriculography is helpful in the differential diagnosis of dyspnea. The left ventricular ejection fraction is depressed in left ventricular failure, while the right ventricular ejection fraction may be low at rest or may decline during exercise in patients with severe lung disease. Both left and right ventricular ejection fractions are normal at rest and during exercise in dyspnea due to anxiety or malingering. Careful observation during the performance of an exercise treadmill test will often help in the identification of the patient who is malingering or whose dyspnea is secondary to anxiety. Under these circumstances, the patient usually complains of severe shortness of breath but appears to be breathing either effortlessly or totally irregularly. Cardiopulmonary testing, in which the patient's maximal functional exercise capacity is assessed while measurements of the electrocardiogram, blood pressure, oxygen consumption, arterial saturation (oximetry), and ventilation are carried out, is useful in the differentiation between cardiac and pulmonary dyspnea (Table 32-2).

ANXIETY NEUROSIS Dyspnea experienced by a patient with an anxiety neurosis is difficult to evaluate. The signs and symptoms of acute and chronic hyperventilation do not serve to distinguish between anxiety neurosis and other processes, such as recurrent pulmonary emboli. Another potentially confusing situation is seen when chest pain and electrocardiographic changes accompany the hyperventilation syndrome. When present and attributable to this condition, often referred to as *neurocirculatory asthenia* (Chap. 13), the chest pain is often sharp, fleeting, and in various loci, and the electrocardio-

Table 32-2 Patterns of Abnormality in Cardiopulmonary Exercise Testing[a]

Cardiovascular limitation
    Heart rate ≥85% of predicted maximum
    Low anaerobic threshold
    Reduced maximal oxygen consumption
    Drop in blood pressure with exercise
    Arrhythmias or ischemic changes on ECG
    Does not achieve maximal predicted ventilation
    Does not have significant desaturation
Respiratory limitation
    Achieves or exceeds maximal predicted ventilation
    Significant desaturation (<90%)
    Stable or increase dead space–to–tidal volume ratio
    Development or bronchospasm with falling FEV_1
    Does not achieve 85% of predicted maximal heart rate
    No ischemic ECG changes

[a] All features will not be present in a particular case, and there may be elements of both cardiovascular and respiratory causes of shortness of breath. One looks for the predominant pattern in assessing the etiology of the patient's exercise limitation.
NOTE: ECG, electrocardiogram; FEV_1, forced expiratory volume in 1 s.
SOURCE: From RM Schwartzstein, GE Thibault, in L Goldman, E Braunwald (eds): *Primary Cardiology.* Philadelphia, Saunders, 1998

graphic changes are most often seen during repolarization. Frequent sighing respirations and an irregular breathing pattern point to a psychogenic origin of the dyspnea. Anxiety and depression in association with heart or lung disease can serve to intensify dyspnea symptoms beyond what would be expected for a given degree of dysfunction.

PULMONARY EDEMA (See Table 32-3)

CARDIOGENIC PULMONARY EDEMA (See Table 32-3, IA) An increase in pulmonary venous pressure, which results initially in engorgement of the pulmonary vasculature, is common in most instances of dyspnea in association with congestive heart failure. The lungs become less compliant, the resistance of small airways increases, and there is an increase in lymphatic flow that apparently serves to maintain a constant pulmonary extravascular liquid volume. Mild tachypnea is present. If the increase in intravascular pressure is sufficient both in magnitude and duration, there is a net gain of liquid in the extravascular space, i.e., *interstitial* edema. At this point symptoms worsen, tachypnea increases, gas exchange deteriorates further, and radiographic changes, such as Kerley B lines and loss of distinct vascular margins, are seen. At this stage, the capillary endothelial intercellular junctions widen and allow passage of macromolecules into the interstices.

Table 32-3 Classification of Pulmonary Edema Based on Initiating Mechanism

I. Imbalance of Starling forces
  A. Increased pulmonary capillary pressure
    1. Increased pulmonary venous pressure without left ventricular failure (e.g., mitral stenosis)
    2. Increased pulmonary venous pressure secondary to left ventricular failure
    3. Increased pulmonary capillary pressure secondary to increased pulmonary arterial pressure (so-called overperfusion pulmonary edema)
  B. Decreased plasma oncotic pressure
    1. Hypoalbuminemia
  C. Increased negativity of interstitial pressure
    1. Rapid removal of pneumothorax with large applied negative pressures (unilateral)
    2. Large negative pleural pressures due to acute airway obstruction alone with increased end-expiratory volumes (asthma)
II. Altered alveolar-capillary membrane permeability (acute respiratory distress syndrome)
  A. Infectious pneumonia—bacterial, viral, parasitic
  B. Inhaled toxins (e.g., phosgene, ozone, chlorine, Teflon fumes, nitrogen dioxide, smoke)
  C. Circulating foreign substances (e.g., snake venom, bacterial endotoxins)
  D. Aspiration of acidic gastric contents
  E. Acute radiation pneumonitis
  F. Endogenous vasoactive substances (e.g., histamine, kinins)
  G. Disseminated intravascular coagulation
  H. Immunologic—hypersensitivity pneumonitis, drugs (nitrofurantoin), leukoagglutinins
  I. Shock lung in association with nonthoracic trauma
  J. Acute hemorrhagic pancreatitis
III. Lymphatic insufficiency
  A. After lung transplant
  B. Lymphangitic carcinomatosis
  C. Fibrosing lymphangitis (e.g., silicosis)
IV. Unknown or incompletely understood
  A. High-altitude pulmonary edema
  B. Neurogenic pulmonary edema
  C. Narcotic overdose
  D. Pulmonary embolism
  E. Eclampsia
  F. After cardioversion
  G. After anesthesia
  H. After cardiopulmonary bypass

SOURCE: From Braunwald et al., with permission.

Further elevations in intravascular pressure disrupt the tight junctions between alveolar lining cells, and *alveolar* edema ensues, with outpouring of liquid that contains both red blood cells and macromolecules. With yet more severe disruption of the alveolar-capillary membrane, edematous liquid floods the alveoli and airways. At this point, full-blown clinical pulmonary edema with bilateral wet rales and rhonchi occurs, and the chest radiograph may show diffuse haziness of the lung fields with greater density in the more proximal hilar regions. Typically, the patient is anxious and perspires freely, and the sputum is frothy and blood-tinged. Gas exchange is more severely compromised with worsening hypoxia. Without effective treatment (described in Chap. 232), progressive acidemia, hypercapnia, and respiratory arrest ensue.

The earlier sequence of liquid accumulation described above follows the Starling law of capillary–interstitial liquid exchange:

$$\text{Liquid accumulation} = K[(P_c - P_{IF}) - \sigma(\pi_{pl} - \pi_{IF})] - Q_{lymph}$$

where K = hydraulic conductance (directly proportional to membrane surface area and inversely proportional to membrane thickness)
P_c = mean intracapillary pressure
π_{IF} = oncotic pressure of interstitial liquid
σ = reflection coefficient of macromolecules
P_{IF} = mean interstitial liquid pressure
π_{pl} = oncotic pressure of the plasma
Q_{lymph} = lymphatic flow

The pressures tending to move liquid out of the vessel are P_c and π_{IF}, which are normally more than offset by pressures tending to move liquid back into the vasculature, i.e., the algebraic sum of P_{IF} and π_{pl}. Implicit in the preceding equation is that lymphatic flow can increase in the case of imbalance of forces and result in no net accumulation of interstitial liquid. Further elevations in P_c not only increase the outward movement of liquid in each capillary region but also recruit more of the capillary bed, which increases K. These two effects lead to liquid filtration that exceeds clearance capability by the lymphatics, and liquid accumulates in the loose interstitial spaces of the lung. Even greater increases in P_c open first the loose endothelial intercellular junctions and later the tight alveolar intercellular junctions with an increase in permeability to macromolecules. This secondary disruption of both the function and structure of the alveolar-capillary membrane leads to alveolar flooding.

NONCARDIOGENIC PULMONARY EDEMA (See Table 32-3, IB IC, II, III, and IV) Several clinical conditions are associated with pulmonary edema based on an imbalance of Starling forces other than through primary elevations of pulmonary capillary pressure. Although diminished plasma oncotic pressure in hypoalbuminemic states (e.g., severe liver disease, nephrotic syndrome, protein-losing enteropathy) might be expected to lead to pulmonary edema, the balance of forces normally so strongly favors resorption that even in these conditions some elevation of capillary pressure is usually necessary before interstitial edema develops. Increased negativity of interstitial pressure has been implicated in the genesis of unilateral pulmonary edema following rapid evacuation of a large pneumothorax. In this situation, the findings may be apparent only by radiography, but occasionally the patient experiences dyspnea with physical findings localized to the edematous lung. It has been proposed that large negative intrapleural pressures during acute severe asthma may be associated with the development of interstitial edema. Lymphatic blockade secondary to fibrotic and inflammatory diseases or lymphangitic carcinomatosis may lead to interstitial edema. In such instances, both clinical and radiographic manifestations are dominated by the underlying disease process.

Other conditions characterized by increases in the interstitial liquid content of the lungs appear to be associated primarily with disruption of the alveolar-capillary membranes. Any number of spontaneously occurring or environmental toxic insults, including diffuse pulmonary infections, aspiration, and shock (particularly due to sepsis and hemorrhagic pancreatitis and following cardiopulmonary bypass), are associated with diffuse pulmonary edema that clearly does not have a hemodynamic origin. →*These conditions, which may lead to the acute respiratory distress syndrome, are discussed in Chap. 265.*

Other Forms of Pulmonary Edema There are three forms of pulmonary edema whose precise mechanism remains unexplained. *Narcotic overdose* is a well-recognized antecedent to pulmonary edema. Although illicit use of parenteral heroin is the most frequent cause, parenteral and oral overdoses of legitimate preparations of morphine, methadone, and dextropropoxyphene have also been associated with pulmonary edema. The earlier idea that injected impurities lead to the disorder is untenable. Available evidence suggests that there are alterations in the permeability of alveolar and capillary membranes rather than an elevation of pulmonary capillary pressure.

Exposure to high altitude in association with severe physical exertion is a well-recognized setting for pulmonary edema in unacclimatized yet otherwise healthy persons. Acclimatized high-altitude natives also develop this syndrome upon return to high altitude after a relatively brief sojourn at low altitudes. The syndrome is far more common in persons under the age of 25 years. The mechanism for high-altitude pulmonary edema (HAPE) remains obscure, and studies have been conflicting, some suggesting pulmonary venous constriction and others indicating pulmonary arteriolar constriction as the prime mechanisms. A role for hypoxia at high altitude is suggested by the fact that patients respond to the administration of oxygen and/or return to lower altitudes. Hypoxia per se does not alter permeability of the alveolar-capillary membrane. Hence increased cardiac output and pulmonary arterial pressures with exercise combined with hypoxic pulmonary arteriolar constriction, which is more prominent in young persons, may combine to make this an example of prearteriolar, high-pressure pulmonary edema.

Neurogenic pulmonary edema has been described in patients with central nervous system disorders and without apparent preexisting left ventricular dysfunction. Although most experimental equivalents have implicated sympathetic nervous system activity, the mechanism whereby sympathetic efferent activity leads to pulmonary edema is a matter of speculation. It is known that a massive adrenergic nervous discharge leads to peripheral vasoconstriction with elevation of blood pressure and shifts of blood to the central circulation. In addition, it is probable that a reduction in left ventricular compliance also occurs, and both factors serve to increase left atrial pressures sufficiently to induce pulmonary edema on a hemodynamic basis. Some experimental evidence suggests that stimulation of adrenergic receptors increases capillary permeability directly, but this effect is relatively minor as compared with the imbalance of Starling forces.

TREATMENT OF PULMONARY EDEMA See Chap. 232

BIBLIOGRAPHY

BARTSCH P. High altitude pulmonary edema. Respiration 64:435, 1997

BRAUNWALD E et al: Clinical aspects of heart failure; High-output heart failure; Pulmonary edema, in *Heart Disease*, 6th ed, E Braunwald, D Zipes, P Libby (eds). Philadelphia, Saunders, 2001

KOSOWSKY JM et al: Continuous and bilevel positive airway pressure in the treatment of acute cardiogenic pulmonary edema. Am J Emerg Med 18:91, 2000

MANNING HL, SCHWARTZSTEIN RM: Mechanisms of dyspnea, in *Dyspnea*, DA Mahler (ed), *Lung Biology in Health and Disease*, vol III. New York, Marcel Dekker, 1998, pp 63–95

RIETVELD S: Symptom perception in asthma: A multidisciplinary review. J Asthma 35: 13, 1998

SACCHETTI AD, HARRIS RH. Acute cardiogenic pulmonary edema. What's the latest in emergency treatment? Postgrad Med 103:145–7, 153–4, 160–2, 1998

SCHWARTZSTEIN RM: Language of dyspnea, in *Dyspnea*, DA Mahler (ed), *Lung Biology in Health and Disease*, vol III. New York, Marcel Dekker, 1998, pp 35–62

STULBARG MS, ADAMS L: Dyspnea, in *Textbook of Respiratory Medicine*, 3d ed. Murray JF, Nadel JA (eds). Philadelphia, Saunders, 2000, pp 541–552

33 *Steven E. Weinberger, Eugene Braunwald*

COUGH AND HEMOPTYSIS

COUGH

Cough is an explosive expiration that provides a normal protective mechanism for clearing the tracheobronchial tree of secretions and foreign material. When excessive or bothersome, it is also one of the most common symptoms for which medical attention is sought. Reasons for the latter include discomfort from the cough itself, interference with normal lifestyle, and concern for the cause of the cough, especially fear of cancer or AIDS.

MECHANISM Coughing may be initiated either voluntarily or reflexively. As a defensive reflex it has both afferent and efferent pathways. The *afferent limb* includes receptors within the sensory distribution of the trigeminal, glossopharyngeal, superior laryngeal, and vagus nerves. The *efferent limb* includes the recurrent laryngeal nerve and the spinal nerves. The cough starts with a deep inspiration followed by glottic closure, relaxation of the diaphragm, and muscle contraction against a closed glottis. The resulting markedly positive intrathoracic pressure causes narrowing of the trachea. Once the glottis opens, the large pressure differential between the airways and the atmosphere coupled with tracheal narrowing produces rapid flow rates through the trachea. The shearing forces that develop aid in the elimination of mucus and foreign materials.

ETIOLOGY Cough can be initiated by a variety of airway irritants, which enter the tracheobronchial tree by inhalation (smoke, dust, fumes) or by aspiration (upper airway secretions, gastric contents, foreign bodies). When cough is due to irritation by upper airway secretions (as with postnasal drip) or gastric contents (as with gastroesophageal reflux), the initiating factor may go unrecognized and the cough can be persistent. Additionally, prolonged exposure to such irritants may initiate airway inflammation, which can itself trigger cough and sensitize the airway to other irritants. Cough associated with gastroesophageal reflux is due only in part to aspiration of gastric contents, whereas vagally mediated reflex mechanisms appear to be responsible in many patients.

Any disorder resulting in inflammation, constriction, infiltration, or compression of airways can be associated with cough. Inflammation commonly results from airway infections, ranging from viral or bacterial bronchitis to bronchiectasis. In viral bronchitis, airway inflammation sometimes persists long after resolution of the typical acute symptoms, thereby producing a prolonged cough, lasting for weeks. Pertussis infection is also a possible cause of persistent cough in adults; however, diagnosis is generally made on clinical grounds (Chap. 152). Asthma is a common cause of cough. Although the clinical setting commonly suggests when a cough is secondary to asthma, some patients present with cough in the absence of wheezing or dyspnea, thus making the diagnosis more subtle ("cough variant asthma"). A neoplasm infiltrating the airway wall, such as bronchogenic carcinoma or a carcinoid tumor, is commonly associated with cough. Airway infiltration with granulomas may also trigger a cough, as seen with endobronchial sarcoidosis or tuberculosis. Compression of airways results from extrinsic masses, including lymph nodes, mediastinal tumors, and aortic aneurysms.

Examples of parenchymal lung disease potentially producing cough include interstitial lung disease, pneumonia, and lung abscess. Congestive heart failure may be associated with cough, probably as a consequence of interstitial as well as peribronchial edema. A nonproductive cough complicates the use of angiotensin-converting enzyme (ACE) inhibitors in 5 to 20% of patients taking these agents. Onset is usually within 1 week of starting the drug but can be delayed up to 6 months. Although the mechanism is not known with certainty, it may

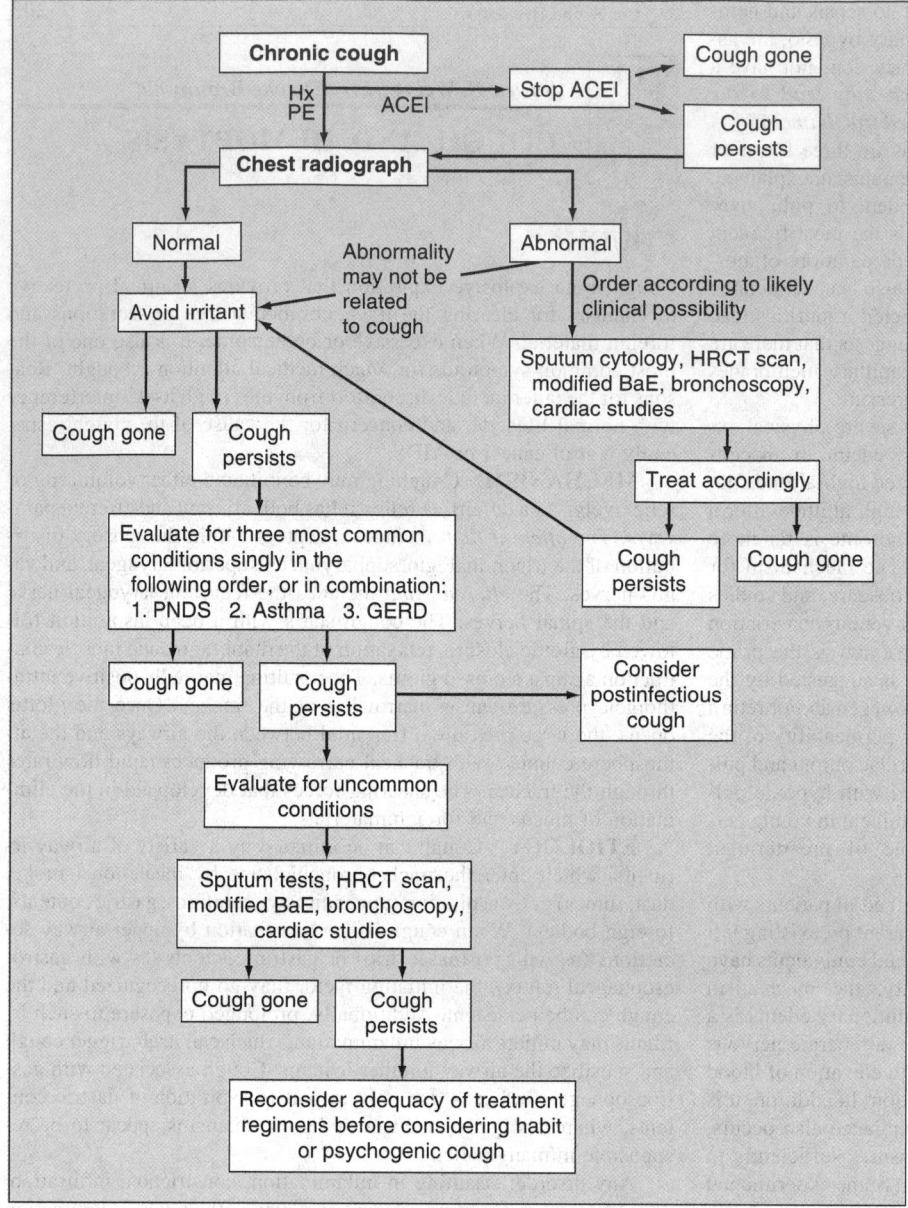

FIGURE 33-1 An algorithm for the evaluation of chronic cough. ACEI, angiotensin-converting enzyme inhibitor; BaE, barium esophagography; GERD, gastroesophageal reflux disease; HRCT, high-resolution computed tomography; Hx, history; PE, physical examination; PNDS, postnasal drip syndrome. *(Reproduced from Irwin, with permission.)*

relate to accumulation of bradykinin or substance P, both of which are degraded by ACE.

The most common causes of cough can be categorized according to the duration of the cough. Acute cough (<3 weeks) is most often due to upper respiratory infection (especially the common cold, acute bacterial sinusitis, and pertussis), but more serious disorders, such as pneumonia, pulmonary embolus, and congestive heart failure, can also present in this fashion. Chronic cough (>3 weeks) in a smoker raises the possibilities of chronic obstructive lung disease or bronchogenic carcinoma. In a nonsmoker who has a normal chest radiograph and is not taking an ACE inhibitor, the most common causes of chronic cough are postnasal drip, asthma, and gastroesophageal reflux.

Approach to the Patient

A detailed *history* frequently provides the most valuable clues for etiology of the cough. Particularly important questions include:

1. Is the cough acute or chronic?
2. At its onset, were there associated symptoms suggestive of a respiratory infection?
3. Is it seasonal or associated with wheezing?
4. Is it associated with symptoms suggestive of postnasal drip (nasal discharge, frequent throat clearing, a "tickle in the throat") or gastroesophageal reflux (heartburn or sensation of regurgitation)? (The absence of such suggestive symptoms does not exclude either of these diagnoses, particularly in the case of gastroesophageal reflux.)
5. Is it associated with fever or sputum? If sputum is present, what is its character?
6. Does the patient have any associated diseases or risk factors for disease (e.g., cigarette smoking, risk factors for infection with HIV, environmental exposures)?
7. Is the patient taking an ACE inhibitor?

The general *physical examination* may point to a nonpulmonary cause of cough, such as heart failure, primary nonpulmonary neoplasm, or AIDS. Examination of the oropharynx may provide suggestive evidence for postnasal drip, including oropharyngeal mucus or erythema, or a "cobblestone" appearance to the mucosa. Auscultation of the chest may demonstrate inspiratory stridor (indicative of upper airway disease), rhonchi or expiratory wheezing (indicative of lower airway disease), or inspiratory crackles (suggestive of a process involving the pulmonary parenchyma, such as interstitial lung disease, pneumonia, or pulmonary edema).

Chest radiography may be particularly helpful in suggesting or confirming the cause of the cough. Important potential findings include the presence of an intrathoracic mass lesion, a localized pulmonary parenchymal infiltrate, or diffuse interstitial or alveolar disease. An area of honeycombing or cyst formation may suggest bronchiectasis, while symmetric bilateral hilar adenopathy may suggest sarcoidosis.

Pulmonary function testing (Chap. 250) is useful for assessing the functional abnormalities that accompany certain disorders producing cough. Measurement of forced expiratory flow rates can demonstrate reversible airflow obstruction characteristic of asthma. When asthma is considered but flow rates are normal, bronchoprovocation testing with methacholine or cold-air inhalation can demonstrate hyperreactivity of the airways to a bronchoconstrictive stimulus. Measurement of lung volumes and diffusing capacity is useful primarily for demonstration of a restrictive pattern, often seen with any of the diffuse interstitial lung diseases.

If *sputum* is produced, gross and microscopic examination may provide useful information. Purulent sputum suggests chronic bronchitis, bronchiectasis, pneumonia, or lung abscess. Blood in the sputum may be seen in the same disorders, but its presence also raises the question of an endobronchial tumor. Gram and acid-fast stains and cultures may demonstrate a particular infectious pathogen, while sputum cytology may provide a diagnosis of a pulmonary malignancy.

More specialized studies are helpful in specific circumstances. *Fiberoptic bronchoscopy* is the procedure of choice for visualizing an endobronchial tumor and collecting cytologic and histologic specimens. Inspection of the tracheobronchial mucosa can demonstrate endobronchial granulomas often seen in sarcoidosis, and endobronchial biopsy of such lesions or transbronchial biopsy of the lung interstitium can confirm the diagnosis. Inspection of the airway mucosa by bronchoscopy can also demonstrate the characteristic appearance of endobronchial Kaposi's sarcoma in patients with AIDS. *High-resolution computed tomography* (HRCT) can confirm the presence of interstitial disease and frequently suggests a diagnosis based on the pattern of disease. It is the procedure of choice for demonstrating dilated airways and confirming the diagnosis of bronchiectasis.

A diagnostic algorithm for evaluation of chronic cough is presented in Fig. 33-1.

COMPLICATIONS Common complications of coughing include chest and abdominal wall soreness, urinary incontinence, and exhaustion. On occasion, paroxysms of coughing may precipitate syncope (cough syncope; Chap. 21), consequent to markedly positive intrathoracic and alveolar pressures, diminished venous return, and decreased cardiac output. Although cough fractures of the ribs may occur in otherwise normal patients, their occurrence should at least raise the possibility of pathologic fractures, which are seen with multiple myeloma, osteoporosis, and osteolytic metastases.

℞ **TREATMENT** Definitive treatment of cough depends on determining the underlying cause and then initiating specific therapy. Elimination of an exogenous inciting agent (cigarette smoke, ACE inhibitors) or an endogenous trigger (postnasal drip, gastroesophageal reflux) is usually effective when such a precipitant can be identified. Other important management considerations are treatment of specific respiratory tract infections, bronchodilators for potentially reversible airflow obstruction, chest physiotherapy to enhance clearance of secretions in patients with bronchiectasis, and treatment of endobronchial tumors or interstitial lung disease when such therapy is available and appropriate.

Symptomatic or nonspecific therapy of cough should be considered when: (1) the cause of the cough is not known or specific treatment is not possible, and (2) the cough performs no useful function or causes marked discomfort. An irritative, nonproductive cough may be suppressed by an antitussive agent, which increases the latency or threshold of the cough center. Such agents include codeine (15 mg qid) or nonnarcotics such as dextromethorphan (15 mg qid). These drugs provide symptomatic relief by interrupting prolonged, self-perpetuating paroxysms. However, a cough productive of significant quantities of sputum should usually not be suppressed, since retention of sputum in the tracheobronchial tree may interfere with the distribution of ventilation, alveolar aeration, and the ability of the lung to resist infection.

Other agents working by a variety of mechanisms have also been used to control cough, but objective information assessing their benefit is meager. The inhaled anticholinergic agent, ipratropium bromide (2 to 4 puffs qid), has been used with the rationale of inhibiting the efferent limb of the cough reflex. Inhaled glucocorticoids, ideally administered with a spacer and dosed according to the particular agent, have been used for patients in whom airway inflammation is thought to be playing a role in the cough.

HEMOPTYSIS

Hemoptysis is defined as the expectoration of blood from the respiratory tract, a spectrum that varies from blood-streaking of sputum to coughing up large amounts of pure blood. *Massive hemoptysis* is variably defined as the expectoration of >100 to >600 mL over a 24-h period, although the patient's estimation of the amount of blood is notoriously unreliable. Expectoration of even relatively small amounts of blood is a frightening symptom and can be a marker for potentially serious disease, such as bronchogenic carcinoma. Massive hemoptysis, on the other hand, can represent an acutely life-threatening problem. Large amounts of blood can fill the airways and the alveolar spaces, not only seriously disturbing gas exchange but potentially causing the patient to suffocate.

ETIOLOGY Because blood originating from the nasopharynx or the gastrointestinal tract can mimic blood coming from the lower respiratory tract, it is important to determine initially that the blood is not coming from one of these alternative sites. Clues that the blood is originating from the gastrointestinal tract include a dark red appearance and an acidic pH, in contrast to the typical bright red appearance and alkaline pH of true hemoptysis.

The bronchial arteries, which are part of the high-pressure systemic circulation, originate either from the aorta or from intercostal arteries and are the source of bleeding in bronchitis or bronchiectasis or with endobronchial tumors.

An etiologic classification of hemoptysis can be based on the site of origin within the lungs (Table 33-1). The most common site of bleeding is the airways, i.e., the tracheobronchial tree, which can be affected by inflammation (acute or chronic bronchitis, bronchiectasis) or by neoplasm (bronchogenic carcinoma, endobronchial metastatic carcinoma, or bronchial carcinoid tumor). Blood originating from the pulmonary parenchyma can be either from a localized source, such as an infection (pneumonia, lung abscess, tuberculosis), or from a process diffusely affecting the parenchyma (as with a coagulopathy or with an autoimmune process such as Goodpasture's syndrome). Disorders primarily affecting the pulmonary vasculature include pulmonary embolic disease and those conditions associated with elevated pulmonary venous and capillary pressures, such as mitral stenosis or left ventricular failure.

Although the relative frequency of the different etiologies of hemoptysis varies from series to series, most recent studies indicate that bronchitis and bronchogenic carcinoma are the two most common causes. Despite the lower frequency of tuberculosis and bronchiectasis seen in recent compared to older series, these two disorders still represent the most common causes of massive hemoptysis in several series. Even after extensive evaluation, a sizable proportion of patients (up to 30% in some series) have no identifiable etiology for their hemoptysis. These patients are classified as having idiopathic or cryp-

Table 33-1 Differential Diagnosis of Hemoptysis

Source other than the lower respiratory tract
    Upper airway (nasopharyngeal) bleeding
    Gastrointestinal bleeding
Tracheobronchial source
    Neoplasm (bronchogenic carcinoma, endobronchial metastatic tumor, Kaposi's sarcoma, bronchial carcinoid)
    Bronchitis (acute or chronic)
    Bronchiectasis
    Broncholithiasis
    Airway trauma
    Foreign body
Pulmonary parenchymal source
    Lung abscess
    Pneumonia
    Tuberculosis
    Mycetoma ("fungus ball")
    Goodpasture's syndrome
    Idiopathic pulmonary hemosiderosis
    Wegener's granulomatosis
    Lupus pneumonitis
    Lung contusion
Primary vascular source
    Arteriovenous malformation
    Pulmonary embolism
    Elevated pulmonary venous pressure (esp. mitral stenosis)
    Pulmonary artery rupture secondary to balloon-tip pulmonary artery catheter manipulation
Miscellaneous/rare causes
    Pulmonary endometriosis
    Systemic coagulopathy or use of anticoagulants or thrombolytic agents

SOURCE: Adapted from SE Weinberger, *Principles of Pulmonary Medicine*, 3d ed, Philadelphia, Saunders, 1998.

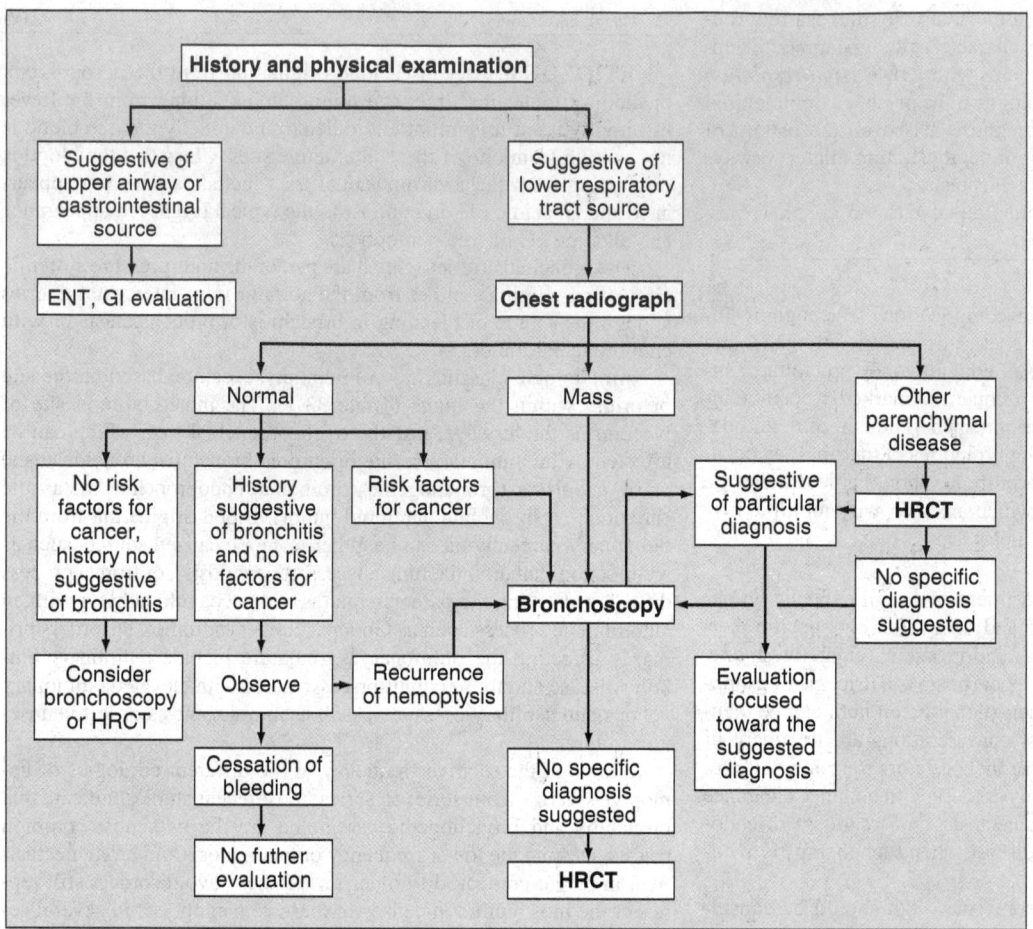

FIGURE 33-2 An algorithm for the evaluation of non-massive hemoptysis. HRCT, high-resolution computed tomography.

chitis), or prominent rhonchi, with or without wheezing or crackles (bronchiectasis). Cardiac examination may demonstrate findings of pulmonary arterial hypertension, mitral stenosis, or heart failure. Skin examination may reveal Kaposi's sarcoma, arteriovenous malformations of Osler-Rendu-Weber disease, or lesions suggestive of systemic lupus erythematosus.

Diagnostic evaluation of hemoptysis starts with a chest radiograph to look for a mass lesion, findings suggestive of bronchiectasis (Chap. 256), or focal or diffuse parenchymal disease (representing either focal or diffuse bleeding or a focal area of pneumonitis). Additional initial screening evaluation often includes a complete blood count, a coagulation profile, and assessment for renal disease with a urinalysis and measurement of blood urea nitrogen and creatinine levels. When sputum is present, examination by Gram and acid-fast stains (along with the corresponding cultures) is indicated.

Fiberoptic bronchoscopy is particularly useful for localizing the site of bleeding and for visualization of endobronchial lesions. When bleeding is massive, rigid bronchoscopy is often preferable to fiberoptic bronchoscopy because of better airway control and greater suction capability. In patients with suspected bronchiectasis, HRCT is now the diagnostic procedure of choice, having replaced bronchography.

A diagnostic algorithm for evaluation of nonmassive hemoptysis is presented in Fig. 33-2.

togenic hemoptysis, and subtle airway or parenchymal disease is presumably responsible for the bleeding.

Approach to the Patient

The *history* is extremely valuable. Hemoptysis that is described as blood-streaking of mucopurulent or purulent sputum often suggests bronchitis. Chronic production of sputum with a recent change in quantity or appearance favors an acute exacerbation of chronic bronchitis. Fever or chills accompanying blood-streaked purulent sputum suggests pneumonia, whereas a putrid smell to the sputum raises the possibility of lung abscess. When sputum production has been chronic and copious, the diagnosis of bronchiectasis should be considered. Hemoptysis following the acute onset of pleuritic chest pain and dyspnea is suggestive of pulmonary embolism.

A history of previous or coexisting disorders should be sought, such as renal disease (seen with Goodpasture's syndrome or Wegener's granulomatosis), lupus erythematosus (with associated pulmonary hemorrhage from lupus pneumonitis), or a previous malignancy (either recurrent lung cancer or endobronchial metastasis from a nonpulmonary primary tumor). In a patient with AIDS, endobronchial or pulmonary parenchymal Kaposi's sarcoma should be considered. Risk factors for bronchogenic carcinoma, particularly smoking and asbestos exposure, should be sought. Patients should be questioned about previous bleeding disorders, treatment with anticoagulants, or use of drugs that can be associated with thrombocytopenia.

The *physical examination* may also provide helpful clues to the diagnosis. For example, examination of the lungs may demonstrate a pleural friction rub (pulmonary embolism), localized or diffuse crackles (parenchymal bleeding or an underlying parenchymal process associated with bleeding), evidence of airflow obstruction (chronic bron-

℞ TREATMENT The rapidity of bleeding and its effect on gas exchange determine the urgency of management. When the bleeding is confined to either blood-streaking of sputum or production of small amounts of pure blood, gas exchange is usually preserved; establishing a diagnosis is the first priority. When hemoptysis is massive, maintaining adequate gas exchange, preventing blood from spilling into unaffected areas of lung, and avoiding asphyxiation are the highest priorities. Keeping the patient at rest and partially suppressing cough may help the bleeding to subside. If the origin of the blood is known and is limited to one lung, the bleeding lung should be placed in the dependent position, so that blood is not aspirated into the unaffected lung.

With massive bleeding, the need to control the airway and maintain adequate gas exchange may necessitate endotracheal intubation and mechanical ventilation. In patients in danger of flooding the lung contralateral to the side of hemorrhage despite proper positioning, isolation of the right and left mainstem bronchi from each other can be achieved by selectively intubating the nonbleeding lung (often with bronchoscopic guidance) or by using specially designed double-lumen endotracheal tubes. Another option involves inserting a balloon catheter through a bronchoscope by direct visualization and inflating the balloon to occlude the bronchus leading to the bleeding site. This technique not only prevents aspiration of blood into unaffected areas but also may promote tamponade of the bleeding site and cessation of bleeding.

Other available techniques for control of significant bleeding include laser phototherapy, electrocautery, embolotherapy, and surgical resection of the involved area of lung. With bleeding from an endobronchial tumor, the neodymium:yttrium-aluminum-garnet (Nd:YAG) laser can often achieve at least temporary hemostasis by coagulating the bleeding site. Electrocautery, which uses an electric current for thermal destruction of tissue, can be used similarly for management of bleeding from an endobronchial tumor. Embolotherapy involves an arteriographic procedure in which a vessel proximal to the bleeding site is cannulated, and a material such as Gelfoam is injected to occlude the bleeding vessel. Surgical resection is a therapeutic option either for the emergent therapy of life-threatening hemoptysis that fails to respond to other measures or for the elective but definitive management of localized disease subject to recurrent bleeding.

BIBLIOGRAPHY

Cough

FAHEY T et al: Quantitative systematic review of randomized control trials comparing antibiotic with placebo for acute cough in adults. BMJ 316:906, 1998

IRWIN RS (ed): Managing cough as a defense mechanism and as a symptom: A consensus panel report of the American College of Chest Physicians. Chest 114 (Suppl): 133S, 1998

——— et al: Appropriate use of antitussives and protussives. A practical review. Drugs 46:80, 1993

IRWIN RS et al: The cough reflex and its relation to gastroesophageal reflux. Am J Med 108:735, 2000

IRWIN RS, WIDDICOMBE J: Cough, in *Textbook of Respiratory Medicine*, 3d ed., Murray JF, Nadel JA (eds). Philadelphia, Saunders, 2000, pp 553–566

ISRAILI ZH, HALL WD: Cough and angioneurotic edema associated with angiotensin-converting enzyme inhibitor therapy. Ann Intern Med 117:234, 1992

WRIGHT SW et al: Pertussis infection in adults with persistent cough. JAMA 273:1044, 1995

Hemoptysis

CAHILL BC, INGBAR DH: Massive hemoptysis: Assessment and management. Clin Chest Med 15:147, 1994

FERNANDO HC et al: Role of bronchial artery embolization in the management of hemoptysis. Arch Surg 133:862, 1998

HIRSHBERG B et al: Hemoptysis: Etiology, evaluation, and outcome in a tertiary referral hospital. Chest 112:440, 1997

PRIMACH SL et al: Diffuse pulmonary hemorrhage: Clinical, pathologic and imaging features. AJR 164:295, 1995

---

34   *Patrick T. O'Gara, Eugene Braunwald*

APPROACH TO THE PATIENT WITH A HEART MURMUR

Auscultation of the heart constitutes the final step in the cardiovascular examination and, for many patients with established or suspected cardiac disease, represents a defining moment in the doctor-patient relationship. The examiner must bring to this exercise an integrated approach that incorporates pertinent information from several sources. The auscultatory findings must be interpreted in the context of the history and general physical examination and with the observations made regarding the venous wave forms and major arterial pulses. In this way, abnormalities of heart sounds, adventitious sounds, and murmurs can be placed in their proper perspective.

In many patients, a heart murmur is the only or the most conspicuous finding on physical examination. The recognition of a heart murmur usually leads to additional testing, such as electrocardiography, chest radiography, and echocardiography, and may result in referral to a cardiologist. The differential diagnosis of a heart murmur should

begin with an unbiased and systematic evaluation of its major attributes: timing, duration, intensity, quality, frequency, configuration, location, radiation, and response to maneuvers (see Table 225-1). Laboratory testing can be pursued thereafter to clarify any remaining ambiguity and to provide additional anatomic and physiologic information that will impact on patient management.

Heart murmurs are defined in terms of their timing within the cardiac cycle. *Systolic murmurs* begin with or after the first heart sound (S_1) and terminate at or before the component (A_2 or P_2) of the second heart sound (S_2) that corresponds to their side of origin (left or right). *Diastolic murmurs* begin with or after the associated component of S_2 and end at or before the subsequent S_1. *Continuous murmurs* are not confined to either phase of the cardiac cycle but rather begin in systole and proceed through S_2 into all or part of diastole.

The appropriate timing of heart murmurs is the first critical step in their identification. The distinction between S_1 and S_2, and, therefore, systole and diastole, is usually a straightforward process but can be difficult in the setting of a tachyarrhythmia, in which case the heart sounds can be distinguished by simultaneous palpation of the carotid arterial pulse. The upstroke should closely follow S_1. The principal causes of heart murmurs are shown in Table 34-1, and the critical importance of the timing of heart murmurs in the differential diagnosis is shown in Fig. 34-1.

SYSTOLIC HEART MURMURS

Systolic heart murmurs derive from the increased turbulence associated with (1) enhanced or accelerated flow across a normal semilunar valve, through a normal ventricular outflow tract, or into a dilated great vessel, (2) normal flow across a structurally abnormal semilunar valve or through a narrowed ventricular outflow tract, (3) flow across an incompetent atrioventricular valve, and (4) flow across the interventricular septum. One approach to their differential diagnosis further subdivides these murmurs according to their time of onset and duration within the systolic phase of the cardiac cycle.

EARLY SYSTOLIC MURMURS Early systolic murmurs begin with S_1 and extend for a variable period of time, ending well before S_2. Their causes are relatively few in number. *Acute severe mitral regurgitation* into a normal-sized, relatively noncompliant left atrium results in an early and attenuated systolic murmur that is decrescendo in configuration and usually best heard at or just medial to the apical impulse (Chap. 236). These characteristics reflect the rapid rise in left atrial pressure caused by the sudden volume load into a nondilated chamber and contrast sharply with the auscultatory features of chronic mitral regurgitation. Clinical settings in which this occurs include: (1) papillary muscle rupture complicating acute myocardial infarction, (2) infective endocarditis, (3) rupture of chordae tendineae, and (4) blunt chest wall trauma.

Acute mitral regurgitation from papillary muscle rupture usually accompanies an inferior, posterior, or lateral infarction. The murmur is associated with a precordial thrill in approximately one-half of cases and is to be distinguished from that associated with postinfarction ventricular septal rupture. The latter is more commonly (90%) accompanied by a thrill at the left sternal edge, is holosystolic, and complicates anterior infarctions as often as inferior-posterior damage. The recognition of either of these mechanical defects mandates aggressive medical stabilization and emergent surgical intervention (Chap. 243).

The other potential causes of acute severe mitral regurgitation may be distinguished on the basis of associated findings. Spontaneous chordal rupture usually occurs on a substrate of myxomatous replacement, such as that underlying most forms of mitral valve prolapse (Chap. 236). This lesion may be part of a more generalized process, as can occur with the Marfan or Ehlers-Danlos syndromes, or it may be an isolated phenomenon. Infective endocarditis is associated with fever, peripheral embolic lesions, and positive blood cultures and most

Table 34-1   Principal Causes of Heart Murmurs

ORGANIC SYSTOLIC MURMURS

Midsystolic
  Aortic
    Obstructive
      Supravalvular—supraaortic stenosis, coarctation of the aorta
      Valvular—AS and sclerosis
      Subvalvular—discrete or HOCM
    Increased flow, hyperkinetic states, AR, complete heart block
    Dilatation of ascending aorta, atheroma, aortitis, aneurysm of aorta
  Pulmonary
    Obstructive
      Supravalvular—pulmonary arterial stenosis
      Valvular—pulmonic valve stenosis
      Subvalvular—infundibular stenosis
    Increased flow, hyperkinetic states, left-to-right shunt (e.g., ASD, VSD)
    Dilatation of pulmonary artery
Holosystolic (regurgitant)
  Atrioventricular valve regurgitation (MR, TR)
  Left-to-right shunt at ventricular level (VSD)

EARLY DIASTOLIC MURMURS

Aortic regurgitation
  Valvular; rheumatic deformity; perforation, postendocarditis, posttrau-
    matic, postvalvulotomy
  Dilatation of valve ring: aorta dissection, annuloectasia, cystic medial ne-
    crosis, hypertension
  Widening of commissures: syphilis
  Congenital: bicuspid valve, with VSD
Pulmonic regurgitation
  Valvular: postvalvulotomy, endocarditis, rheumatic fever, carcinoid
  Dilatation of valve ring: pulmonary hypertension; Marfan syndrome
  Congenital: isolated or associated with tetralogy of Fallot, VSD, pulmonic
    stenosis

MIDDIASTOLIC MURMURS

Mitral stenosis
Carey-Coombs murmur (middiastolic apical murmur in acute rheumatic fe-
  ver)
Increased flow across nonstenotic mitral valve (e.g., MR, VSD, PDA, high-
  output states, and complete heart block)
Tricuspid stenosis
Increased flow across nonstenotic tricuspid valve (e.g., TR, ASD, and anom-
  alous pulmonary venous return)
Left and right atrial tumors

CONTINUOUS MURMURS

Patent ductus arteriosus	Proximal coronary artery stenosis
Coronary AV fistula	Mammary souffle
Ruptured aneurysm of sinus of Valsalva	Pulmonary artery branch stenosis
Aortic septal defect	Bronchial collateral circulation
Cervical venous hum	Small (restrictive) ASD with MS
Anomalous left coronary artery	Intercostal AV fistula

NOTE: AR, aortic regurgitation; AS, aortic stenosis; ASD, atrial septal defect; AV, arteriovenous; HOCM, hypertrophic obstructive cardiomyopathy; MR, mitral regurgitation;
MS, mitral stenosis; PDA, patent ductus arteriosus; TR, tricuspid regurgitation; VSD, ventricular septal defect.
SOURCE: E Braunwald, in *Heart Disease*, 4th ed, E. Braunwald (ed), Philadelphia, Saunders, 1992.

commonly occurs on a previously abnormal valvular apparatus (Chap.
126). Trauma is usually self-evident but may be disarmingly trivial
(Chap. 240). It can result in papillary muscle contusion and rupture,
chordal interruption, or leaflet avulsion or perforation.

Echocardiography should be performed in all cases of suspected
acute severe mitral regurgitation to define the responsible mechanism,
estimate the severity, and provide a preliminary assessment as to the
feasibility of surgical repair (versus replacement).

Other causes of early systolic murmurs include congenital, small
muscular ventricular septal defects. The duration of the murmur is
attenuated by the closure of the defect during systolic contraction. The
murmur is localized to the left sternal edge and is commonly of grade

IV/VI or V/VI intensity. Signs of pulmonary hypertension or left ventricular volume overload are absent. Patients with anatomically large,
uncorrected ventricular septal defects accompanied by pulmonary hypertension may also have murmurs confined to early systole. The elevated pulmonary vascular resistance attenuates the degree of shunting
as pressures within the right and left ventricles equalize during the
latter half of systole.

Tricuspid regurgitation with normal pulmonary artery pressures,
such as that caused by infective endocarditis in injection drug users,
may produce an early systolic murmur. The murmur is soft, best heard
at the lower left sternal edge, and may accentuate with inspiration
(Carvallo's sign). Regurgitant $c-v$ waves may be visible in the jugular
venous pulse.

MIDSYSTOLIC MURMURS   Midsystolic murmurs begin at a
short interval following S_1, end before S_2, and are usually crescendo-
decrescendo in configuration (Fig. 34-1C). Semilunar valve stenosis
is the classic prototype. With aortic valve stenosis, the murmur is
usually loudest in the second right intercostal space (aortic area) and
radiates along the carotid arteries (Chap. 236). The intensity of the
murmur varies directly with the cardiac output; aortic valve stenosis
with severe heart failure may produce a misleadingly soft systolic murmur. With a normal cardiac output, a systolic thrill is usually indicative
of severe stenosis with a peak gradient in excess of 50 to 60 mmHg.
An accompanying early systolic ejection click may be audible in
younger patients with a bicuspid valve; its presence localizes the ob-

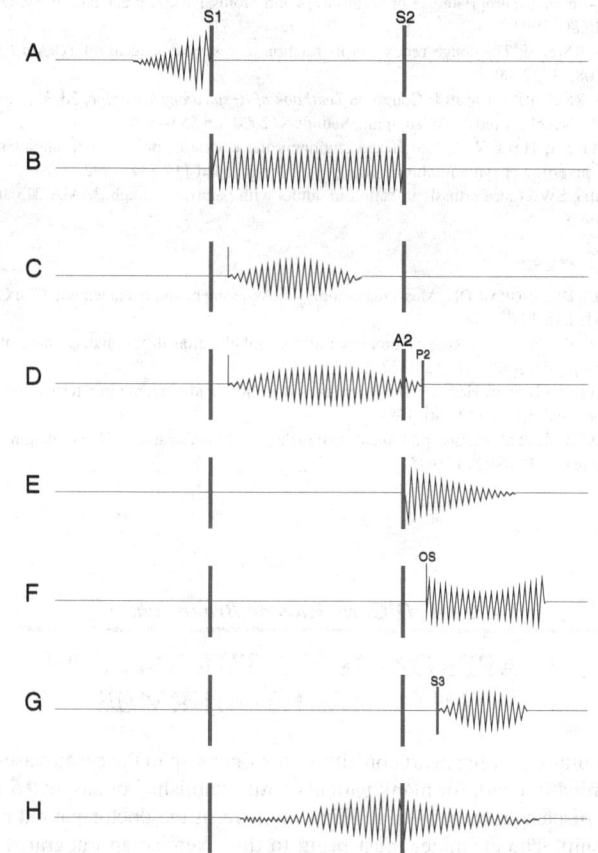

FIGURE 34-1   Diagram depicting principal heart murmurs. *A*. Presystolic
murmur of mitral or tricuspid stenosis. *B*. Holosystolic (pansystolic) murmur
of mitral or tricuspid regurgitation or of ventricular septal defect. *C*. Aortic
ejection murmur beginning with an ejection click and fading before the second
heart sound. *D*. Systolic murmur in pulmonic stenosis spilling through the aortic
second sound, pulmonic valve closure being delayed. *E*. Aortic or pulmonary
diastolic murmur. *F*. Long diastolic murmur of mitral stenosis following the
opening snap. *G*. Short middiastolic inflow murmur following a third heart
sound. *H*. Continuous murmur of patent ductus arteriosus. *(Adapted from P
Wood, Diseases of the Heart and Circulation, Philadelphia, Lippincott, 1968,
with permission.)*

struction to the valvular (as opposed to the sub- or supravalvular) level. The midsystolic murmur of aortic stenosis may be well transmitted to the apex, especially in older patients, where it becomes less harsh and slightly higher pitched (Gallavardin effect). The murmur of aortic stenosis should increase following a postpremature beat, whereas a mitral regurgitant murmur would not be expected to change in intensity.

Sclerosis of the aortic valve produces a murmur of similar location, radiation, and configuration, albeit without the usual signs of hemodynamic significance. The carotid upstroke is well preserved, the murmur peaks in midsystole and is not accompanied by a thrill, and only a modest gradient is estimated by Doppler echocardiography. Noncritical sclerodegenerative thickening of the aortic valve leaflets is perhaps the most common cause of a midsystolic murmur in older adults. The similar midsystolic murmur of pulmonic valve stenosis, usually introduced by an ejection click, is best appreciated in the second and third left intercostal spaces (pulmonic area). The murmur lengthens and the intensity of P_2 diminishes with increasing degrees of stenosis. A midsystolic murmur in the aortic position can also be detected in hyperdynamic states (fever, thyrotoxicosis, pregnancy, anemia) and in the presence of isolated aortic regurgitation with the augmented flow into a dilated proximal aorta.

Crescendo-decrescendo midsystolic murmurs usually of grade II/VI intensity heard in the pulmonic area may be innocent if unaccompanied by any other signs of cardiac disease in children or young adults. They may also reflect enhanced flow into a normal pulmonary artery in hyperkinetic states or augmented flow into a dilated pulmonary artery. The latter may occur with an atrial septal defect, in which case splitting of S_2 is usually abnormal (fixed). Still's murmur is a vibratory, medium frequency, mid-systolic murmur heard best between the lower left sternal edge and the apex in normal children and young adults. It is generated by vibrations of the pulmonic valve leaflets at their attachments or by vibrations of a left ventricular false tendon.

The midsystolic murmur of hypertrophic cardiomyopathy (Chap. 238) is usually loudest between the left sternal edge and apex, of grade II/VI to III/VI intensity, and crescendo-decrescendo in configuration. In contrast to aortic valve stenosis, the murmur does *not* radiate into the neck and the carotid upstrokes are brisk and full and may even be bifid. The intensity of the murmur associated with hypertrophic cardiomyopathy increases following maneuvers that decrease left ventricular volume (strain phase of the Valsalva maneuver, standing, amyl nitrite) or increase myocardial contractility (inotropic therapy). Conversely, the intensity of the systolic murmur decreases with maneuvers that increase ventricular volume (squatting, passive leg raising), impair contractility (beta-adrenoreceptor blockade), or raise preload and systemic afterload (squatting). Among these several maneuvers, auscultation in the standing and squatting positions, if possible, is perhaps the most sensitive technique to elicit a dynamic change in the intensity of the murmur associated with hypertrophic obstructive cardiomyopathy.

LATE SYSTOLIC MURMURS A late systolic murmur begins well after the onset of ejection and is usually best heard at the left ventricular apex or between the apex and the left sternal edge. When introduced by a nonejection click, it is usually indicative of systolic prolapse of the mitral valve leaflet(s) into the left atrium. The click and murmur move closer to S_1 following maneuvers that decrease left ventricular volume (standing, Valsalva) and move oppositely upon increases in volume (leg raising, squatting). The intensity of the murmur augments with increases in systemic afterload (squatting, pressor agents) and decrease with vasodilation (amyl nitrite). Isometric exercise, which also delays the onset of the murmur, accentuates the intensity.

HOLOSYSTOLIC MURMURS These murmurs, also termed *pansystolic murmurs*, begin with S_1 and continue through systole to S_2 (Fig. 34-1*B*). They are, with rare exception, indicative of atrioventricular valve regurgitation or of a ventricular septal defect; the differential diagnosis is shown in Fig. 34-2. The murmur of mitral regurgitation is loudest at the left ventricular apex. Its radiation reflects the direction of the regurgitant jet. With a flail posterior mitral leaflet

due to ruptured chordae tendineae, for example, the jet is directed anterosuperiorly, and the murmur radiates prominently to the base of the heart, where it might be confused with aortic valve stenosis unless the carotid upstrokes are carefully examined. Conversely, a flail anterior leaflet is associated with a posteriorly directed jet, which radiates into the axilla and the back. It may even strike the spine and be transmitted to the base of the neck. Severe mitral regurgitation is usually associated with a systolic thrill, a soft S_3, and a short diastolic rumbling murmur best appreciated in the left lateral decubitus position.

The holosystolic murmur of tricuspid regurgitation is generally softer (grades I to III/VI) than that of mitral regurgitation, is loudest at the left lower sternal edge, and increases in intensity upon inspiration. Associated signs include prominent "$c-v$" waves in the jugular venous pulse, systolic hepatic pulsations, and peripheral edema. Among the several causes of tricuspid regurgitation, annular dilatation from right ventricular enlargement in the setting of pulmonary artery hypertension is the most common.

Ventricular septal defect (Chap. 234) also produces a holosystolic murmur, the intensity of which varies inversely with the anatomic size of the defect. It is usually accompanied by a palpable thrill along the mid-left sternal border. The murmur of a ventricular septal defect is louder than that due to tricuspid regurgitation and does not share the latter's inspiratory increase in intensity or associated peripheral signs.

DIASTOLIC HEART MURMURS

Like systolic murmurs, diastolic murmurs also can be subcategorized according to their time of onset.

EARLY DIASTOLIC MURMURS (Fig. 34-1*E*) Early diastolic murmurs result from semilunar valve incompetence and begin at the valve closure sound (A_2 or P_2), which reflects their site of origin. They are generally high pitched and decrescendo in configuration, especially in states of chronic regurgitation, in which their duration is a crude index of the severity of the lesion. The murmur of aortic regurgitation is generally, but not always, best heard in the second intercostal space at the left sternal edge. There is a tendency for the murmur associated with primary valvular pathology (e.g., rheumatic deformity, congenital bicuspid valve, endocarditis) to radiate more prominently along the *left* sternal border and to be well transmitted to the apex, while the murmur associated with primary aortic root pathology (e.g., annuloaortic ectasia, aortic dissection) radiates more often along the right sternal edge. It is occasionally necessary to examine the patient sitting forward in full expiration to appreciate the murmur, a maneuver that brings the aortic root closer to the anterior chest wall. Severe aortic regurgitation may be accompanied by a lower-pitched mid- to late-diastolic murmur at the apex (Austin Flint murmur), which is generally thought to reflect turbulence at the mitral inflow area from the mixing of the regurgitant (aortic) and forward (mitral) streams, and should be distinguished from mitral stenosis (see above). In the absence of significant heart failure, chronic severe aortic regurgitation is accompanied by several peripheral signs of significant diastolic runoff, including a wide systemic pulse pressure and water-hammer carotid upstrokes (Corrigan's pulse).

The murmur associated with *acute* aortic regurgitation is notably shorter in duration, lower pitched, and can be difficult to appreciate in the presence of tachycardia. Peripheral signs of significant diastolic runoff may be absent. These attributes reflect the abrupt rise in diastolic pressure within the noncompliant left ventricle, with a correspondingly rapid decline in the aortic diastolic–left ventricular pressure gradient.

The murmur of pulmonic valve regurgitation (Graham Steell murmur) begins with a loud (palpable) pulmonic closure sound (P_2) and is best heard in the pulmonic area with radiation along the left sternal border. Typically, it is high pitched, with a decrescendo quality, and is indicative of significant pulmonary artery hypertension with a diastolic pulmonary artery–right ventricular pressure gradient. Its in-

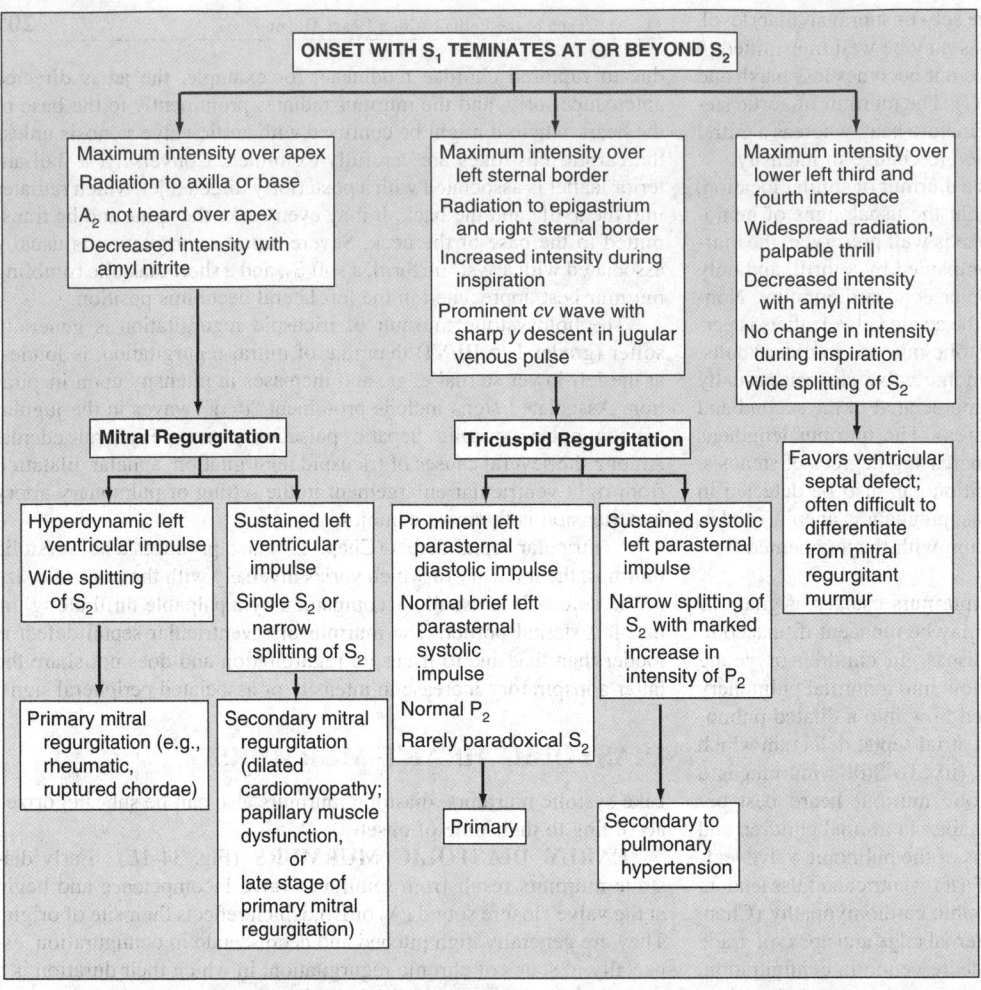

FIGURE 34-2 Differential diagnosis of holosystolic murmur (regurgitant). S_1, first heart sound; S_2, second heart sound; A_2, aortic component of the second heart sound; P_2, pulmonary component of the second heart sound (echo-Doppler evaluation should be considered for differential diagnosis). [*From C Chatterjee, in K Chatterjee et al (eds), Cardiology: An Illustrated Text/Reference, Philadelphia, Lippincott, 1991, with permission.*]

crease in intensity upon inspiration is one means by which to distinguish it from aortic regurgitation. Signs of right ventricular pressure and volume overload are also usually present. With significant mitral stenosis, an early decrescendo diastolic murmur along the left sternal border is not uncommon and is almost always due to aortic rather than

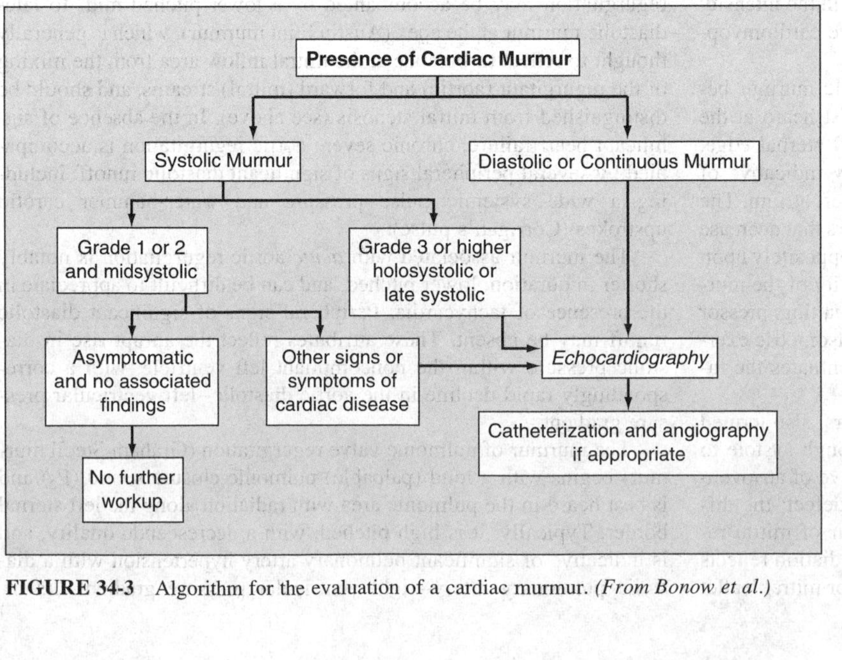

FIGURE 34-3 Algorithm for the evaluation of a cardiac murmur. (*From Bonow et al.*)

pulmonic regurgitation, despite the co-existence of pulmonary artery hypertension.

Pulmonic valve regurgitation in the absence of pulmonary artery hypertension can occur on a congenital basis and rarely with infective endocarditis. In these instances, the early diastolic murmur is softer and lower pitched than the classic Graham Steell murmur. It begins at or even after P_2, which should be easily separable from A_2 and thus produce appreciation of an early diastolic pause.

MIDDIASTOLIC MURMURS Middiastolic murmurs usually result from obstruction and/or augmented flow across the antrioventricular valves. The classic example is that of mitral stenosis due to rheumatic deformity (Fig. 34-1*F*). In the absence of extensive calcification, the first heart sound (S_1) is loud and the murmur begins after the opening snap; the time interval between S_2 and the opening snap is inversely related to the left atrial–left ventricular pressure gradient. The murmur is low pitched and best heard with the bell of the stethoscope over the apex, particularly in the left lateral decubitus position. While its intensity does not reflect the severity of the obstruction accurately, the duration of the murmur does provide some indication as to the magnitude of the obstruction. A longer murmur denotes persistence of a left atrioventricular pressure gradient over a greater proportion of the diastolic time interval. Presystolic accentuation of the murmur (Fig. 34-1*A*) is frequently appreciated in the presence of sinus rhythm and reflects a further increase in transmitral flow consequent to mechanical atrial systole.

The murmur associated with tricuspid stenosis shares many of these features, but it is best heard at the lower left sternal border and, like most right-sided events, increases in intensity upon inspiration. The observant examiner may discern a prolonged *y* descent in the jugular venous pulse. Signs of right heart failure may predominate.

There are several other causes of mid-diastolic murmurs that are important to distinguish from mitral stenosis. *Left atrial myxomas* (Chap. 240) may masquerade as mitral stenosis, but the diastolic murmur is not accompanied by an opening snap or pre-systolic accentuation. Augmented flow across the mitral valve in diastole, such as occurs with severe mitral regurgitation or with large left to right intra-cardiac (ventricular septal defect) or great vessel (patent ductus arteriosus) shunts may produce a short, low pitched mid-diastolic apical murmur. The murmur usually follows a soft S_3 that is lower pitched and later in timing than the opening snap (Fig. 34-1*G*). Severe tricuspid regurgitation can also result in enhanced diastolic tricuspid flow and produce a right-sided filling complex similar to that which accompanies severe mitral regurgitation. The Austin Flint murmur of severe aortic regurgitation has been previously described and occurs in the presence of chronic severe aortic regurgitation.

CONTINUOUS MURMURS

Continuous murmurs begin in systole, peak near S_2, and continue into all or part of diastole (Fig. 34-1*H*). Accordingly, they reflect the persistence of flow between two chambers during both phases of the cardiac cycle. The differential diagnosis of continuous murmurs is shown in Table 34-1. Two innocent variants are the cervical venous hum and the mammary souffle. The former is audible in healthy children and young adults in the right supraclavicular fossa and can be abolished by compression over the internal jugular vein. Its diastolic component may be louder than its systolic counterpart. A mammary souffle represents augmented arterial flow through engorged breasts and becomes audible during the late third trimester of pregnancy or in the early postpartum period. Firm pressure with the diaphragm of the stethoscope can eliminate the diastolic portion of the murmur. The murmur dissipates with time after delivery.

The classic continuous murmur is that due to a patent ductus arteriosus. It is best heard at or just above and to the left of the pulmonic area and may be audible in the back. Over time, a large uncorrected shunt may lead to elevation of the pulmonary vascular resistance, with resultant pulmonary artery hypertension and diminution or elimination of the diastolic component. A continuous murmur can also signify a ruptured congenital sinus of Valsalva aneurysm, which occurs either spontaneously or as a complication of infective endocarditis. Here, a high-pressure fistula is created between the aorta and a cardiac chamber, usually the right atrium or ventricle. The murmur is loudest along the right or left sternal border and is frequently accompanied by a thrill. Notably, the diastolic component is louder than the systolic component. It can be difficult to distinguish continuous murmurs from the temporally separate systolic and diastolic murmurs of mixed aortic valve disease or isolated severe aortic regurgitation. The emphasis is on the envelopment of S_2 by continuous murmurs and a gap between the to-and-fro murmurs of aortic valve disease.

A variety of other lesions can result in continuous murmurs. A coronary arteriovenous fistula sometimes produces a faint, continuous murmur with a louder diastolic component at the left sternal border or left ventricular apex. Severe atherosclerotic disease of a major systemic artery may produce a continuous bruit, the presence of which signifies very high-grade obstruction. Patients with peripheral pulmonary (branch) stenosis or with pulmonary atresia with extensive bronchial collaterals may also have continuous murmurs best heard in the back or along the lateral thoracic cage. Similar findings are present in patients with severe aortic coarctation, a lesion that should be identifiable on the basis of weak and delayed lower extremity pulses and upper extremity hypertension. The continuous murmurs emanate from the enlarged collateral (intercostal) arteries.

Approach to the Patient

It is widely recognized that, despite the importance placed on them by medical schools and training program directors, the auscultatory skills of medical students and residents have declined considerably since the advent of Doppler echocardiography. Recent surveys indicate that trainees fail to correctly identify up to 80% of adventitious sounds and murmurs. Diagnostic errors are as frequent among third-year medical residents as they are for first-year residents. Few training programs provide a dedicated educational curriculum for cardiac auscultation. In the aggregate, these deficiencies lead to an over-reliance on the use of echocardiography and increase the costs of evaluating patients with heart murmurs.

In many patients the cause of a heart murmur can be readily elucidated from careful assessment of the murmur itself, as described in this chapter, when considered in the light of the history, general physical examination, and other features of the cardiac examination, as described in Chap. 225. When the diagnosis is in doubt, or when additional pathoanatomic and physiologic data are necessary in assessing the patient and planning treatment, transthoracic Doppler echocardiography is of great value in identifying not only the etiology of the murmur but also the severity of the responsible lesion (Fig. 34-3).

The majority of heart murmurs are midsystolic and soft (Grades I to II/VI). When such a murmur occurs in an asymptomatic child or young adult *without* other evidence of heart disease on clinical examination, it is usually benign and echocardiography is not generally required. On the other hand, echocardiographic examination is indicated in patients with loud systolic murmurs ($\geq$III/VI), especially those that are holosystolic or late systolic, in most patients with diastolic or continuous murmurs, and in patients with additional unexplained abnormal physical findings on cardiac examination.

BIBLIOGRAPHY

BRAUNWALD E, PERLOFF JK: Physical examination of the heart, in *Heart Disease*, 6th ed, E Braunwald, D Zipes, P Libby (eds). Philadelphia, Saunders, 2001

BONOW RO et al: ACC/AHA guidelines for the management of patients with valvular heart disease: a report of the American College of Cardiology/American Heart Association Task Force on Practice Guidelines (committee on Management of Patients with Valvular Heart Disease). J Am Coll Cardiol 32(5):1486, 1998

ETCHELLS E et al: Does this patient have an abnormal systolic heart murmur? JAMA 277(7):564, 1997

GREWE K et al: Differentiation of cardiac murmurs by auscultation. Curr Probl Cardiol 13:699, 1988

LEMBO NJ et al: Bedside diagnosis of systolic murmurs. N Engl J Med 318(24):1572, 1988

MANGIONE S, NIEMAN LZ: Cardiac auscultatory skills of internal medicine and family practice trainees. A comparison of diagnostic proficiency. JAMA 278(9):717, 1997

MURGO JP: Systolic ejection murmurs in the era of modern cardiology. What do we really know? J Am Coll Cardiol 32:1596, 1998

O'ROURKE RA: Approach to the patient with a heart murmur, in *Primary Cardiology*, L Goldman, E Braunwald (eds). Philadelphia, Saunders, 1998

SHAVER JA: Cardiac auscultation: A cost-effective diagnostic skill. Curr Probl Cardiol 20:441, 1995

| 35 | *Gordon H. Williams* |

APPROACH TO THE PATIENT WITH HYPERTENSION

DEFINITION   Since there is no dividing line between normal and high blood pressure, arbitrary levels have been established to define persons who have an increased risk of developing a morbid cardiovascular event and/or will benefit from medical therapy. These definitions should take into account not only the level of diastolic pressure but also systolic pressure, age, sex, race, and concomitant diseases. For example, patients with a diastolic pressure >90 mmHg have a significant reduction in morbidity and mortality rate if they receive adequate therapy. These, then, are patients who have hypertension and who should be considered for treatment.

The level of *systolic* pressure is also important in assessing the influence of arterial pressure on cardiovascular morbidity. Some data suggest that it may be more important than diastolic pressure. For example, males with normal diastolic pressures (<82 mmHg) but elevated systolic pressures (>158 mmHg) have a cardiovascular mortality rate 2.5 times higher than individuals who have similar diastolic pressures but whose systolic pressures clearly are normal (<130 mmHg). A reduction in mortality and morbidity with treatment, specifically in the elderly, has been documented in these patients. This beneficial effect results mainly from a reduction in strokes and occurs in women as well. Other significant demographic factors that modify the influence of blood pressure on the frequency of morbid cardiovascular events are age, race, and sex, with young black males being most adversely affected by hypertension.

When hypertension is suspected, blood pressure should be measured at least twice during two separate examinations after the initial screening. In adults, a *diastolic* pressure below 85 mmHg is considered to be normal; one between 85 and 89 mmHg is high normal; one of 90 to 99 mmHg represents stage 1 or mild hypertension; one of 100 to 109 mmHg represents stage 2 or moderate hypertension; and one of $\geq$110 mmHg represents stage 3 or severe hypertension. A *systolic* pressure below 130 mmHg indicates normal blood pressure; one between 130 and 139 mmHg indicates high normal; one between 140 and 159 mmHg indicates stage 1 or mild hypertension; one between 160 and 179 mmHg indicates stage 2 or moderate hypertension; and one $\geq$180 mmHg indicates stage 3 or severe hypertension. Increasing use of 12- or 24-h blood pressure monitoring may provide additional useful information in patients who are difficult to classify. However, normal values for this procedure and its usefulness in relation to therapeutic outcomes are not currently known. A useful classification of hypertension derived from the Joint Committee on Detection, Evaluation, and Treatment of High Blood Pressure is shown in Table 35-1.

Arterial pressure fluctuates in most persons, whether they are normotensive or hypertensive. Patients who are classified as having *labile hypertension* are those who sometimes, but not always, have arterial pressures in the hypertensive range. These patients are often considered to have borderline hypertension.

Sustained hypertension can become accelerated or enter a malignant phase, although that is unusual in treated patients. Though a patient with *malignant hypertension* often has a blood pressure above 200/140, the condition is defined by the presence of papilledema, usually accompanied by retinal hemorrhages and exudates, rather than by the absolute pressure level. *Accelerated hypertension* is defined as a significant recent increase over previous hypertensive levels associated with evidence of vascular damage on funduscopic examination but without papilledema.

PATIENT EVALUATION   In evaluating patients with hypertension, the initial history, physical examination, and laboratory tests should be directed at (1) uncovering correctable secondary forms of hypertension (Chap. 246), (2) establishing a pretreatment baseline, (3) assessing factors that may influence the type of therapy or be changed adversely by therapy, (4) determining if target organ damage is present, and (5) determining whether other risk factors for the development of arteriosclerotic cardiovascular disease are present (Chap. 241). Ideally, this evaluation would also determine the underlying mechanism(s) in essential hypertension, particularly if such information leads to a more specific therapeutic program. Unfortunately, at present this aspect of the evaluation is limited by lack of knowledge of some of the underlying mechanisms, by uncertainty as to the correct treatment for a distinct subset even if the underlying mechanisms are known, or by the prohibitive cost of defining a subset of hypertensive patients even if specific therapy were available. However, with the accumulation of additional information, this sixth component of the

evaluation of patients with hypertension may become increasingly important.

Symptoms and Signs   Most patients with hypertension have no specific symptoms referable to their blood pressure elevation and are identified only in the course of a physical examination. When symptoms do bring the patient to the physician, they fall into three categories. They are related to (1) the elevated pressure itself, (2) the hypertensive vascular disease, and (3) the underlying disease, in the case of secondary hypertension. Though popularly considered a symptom of elevated arterial pressure, headache is characteristic only of severe hypertension; most commonly such headaches are localized to the occipital region and are present when the patient awakens in the morning but subside spontaneously after several hours. Other complaints that may be related to elevated blood pressure include dizziness, palpitations, easy fatigability, and impotence. Complaints referable to vascular disease include epistaxis, hematuria, blurring of vision owing to retinal changes, episodes of weakness or dizziness due to transient cerebral ischemia, angina pectoris, and dyspnea due to cardiac failure. Pain due to dissection of the aorta or to a leaking aneurysm is an occasional presenting symptom.

Examples of symptoms related to the underlying disease in secondary hypertension are polyuria, polydipsia, and muscle weakness secondary to hypokalemia in patients with primary aldosteronism or weight gain, and emotional lability in patients with Cushing's syndrome. The patient with a pheochromocytoma may present with episodic headaches, palpitations, diaphoresis, and postural dizziness.

History   A strong family history of hypertension, along with the reported finding of intermittent pressure elevation in the past, favors the diagnosis of essential hypertension. Secondary hypertension often develops before the age of 35 or after 55. A history of use of adrenal steroids or estrogens is of obvious significance. A history of repeated urinary tract infections suggests chronic pyelonephritis, although this condition may occur in the absence of symptoms; nocturia and polydipsia suggest renal or endocrine disease, while trauma to either flank or an episode of acute flank pain may be a clue to the presence of renal injury. A history of weight gain is compatible with Cushing's syndrome, and one of weight loss is compatible with pheochromocytoma. A number of aspects of the history aid in determining whether vascular disease has progressed to a dangerous stage. These include angina pectoris and symptoms of cerebrovascular insufficiency, congestive heart failure, and/or peripheral vascular insufficiency. Other risk factors that should be asked about include cigarette smoking, diabetes mellitus, lipid disorders, and a family history of early deaths due to cardiovascular disease. Finally, aspects of the patient's lifestyle that could contribute to the hypertension or affect its treatment should be assessed, including diet, physical activity, family status, work, and educational level.

Physical Examination   The physical examination starts with the patient's general appearance. For instance, are the round face and truncal obesity of Cushing's syndrome present? Is muscular development in the upper extremities out of proportion to that in the lower extremities, suggesting coarctation of the aorta? The next step is to compare the blood pressures and pulses in the two upper extremities and in the supine and standing positions (for at least 2 min). A rise in diastolic pressure when the patient goes from the supine to the standing position is most compatible with essential hypertension; a fall, in the absence of antihypertensive medications, suggests secondary forms of hypertension. The patient's height and weight should be recorded. Detailed examination of the ocular fundi is mandatory, as funduscopic findings provide one of the best indications of the duration of hypertension and of prognosis. A useful guide is the Keith-Wagener-Barker classification of funduscopic changes (Table 35-2); the specific changes in each fundus should be recorded and a grade assigned. Palpation and auscultation of the carotid arteries for evidence of stenosis or occlusion are important; narrowing of a carotid artery may be a manifestation of hypertensive vascular disease, and it may also be a clue to the presence of a renal arterial lesion, since these two lesions may occur together. In examination of the heart and lungs, evidence of left ventricular

Table 35-1 Classification of Blood Pressure for Adults Aged 18 Years and Older

Category	Systolic Pressure, mmHg	Diastolic Pressure, mmHg
Optimal	<120	<80
Normal	<130	<85
High normal	130–139	85–89
Hypertension[a]		
Stage 1 (mild)	140–159	90–99
Stage 2 (moderate)	160–179	100–109
Stage 3 (severe)	180–209	110–119

[a] Based on the average of $\geq$2 readings taken at each of two or more visits after an initial screening.

NOTE: Classification of blood pressure for adults aged 18 years and older not taking antihypertensive drugs and not acutely ill. When systolic and diastolic pressures fall into different categories, the higher category should be selected to classify the individual's blood pressure status.

SOURCE: The Sixth Report of the Joint National Committee on Prevention, Detection, Evaluation, and Treatment of High Blood Pressure.

Table 35-2 Classification of Hypertensive and Arteriolosclerotic Retinopathy

| | Hypertension | | | | | Arteriolosclerosis | |
| | Arterioles | | | | | | |
Degree	General Narrowing, AV ratio[a]	Focal Spasm[b]	Hemorrhages	Exudates	Papilledema	Arteriolar Light Reflex	AV Crossing Defects[c]
Normal	3:4	1:1	0	0	0	Fine yellow line, red blood column	None
Grade I	1:2	1:1	0	0	0	Broadened yellow line, red blood column	Mild depression of vein
Grade II	1:3	2:3	0	0	0	Broad yellow line, "copper wire," blood column not visible	Depression or humping of vein
Grade III	1:4	1:3	+	+	0	Broad white line, "silver wire," blood column not visible	Right-angle deviation, tapering, and disappearance of vein under arteriole; distal dilation of vein
Grade IV	Fine, fibrous cords	Obliteration of distal flow	+	+	+	Fibrous cords, blood column not visible	Same as grade III

[a] Ratio of arteriolar to venous diameters.
[b] Ratio of diameters of region of spasm to proximal arteriole.
[c] Arteriolar length and tortuosity increase with severity.

hypertrophy and cardiac decompensation should be sought. Is there a left ventricular lift? Are third and fourth heart sounds present? Are there pulmonary rales? A third heart sound and pulmonary rales are unusual in uncomplicated hypertension. Their presence suggests ventricular dysfunction. Chest examination also includes a search for extracardiac murmurs and palpable collateral vessels that may result from coarctation of the aorta.

The most important part of the abdominal examination is auscultation for bruits originating in stenotic renal arteries. Bruits due to renal arterial narrowing nearly always have a diastolic component or may be continuous and are best heard just to the right or left of the midline above the umbilicus or in the flanks; they are present in many patients with renal artery stenosis due to fibrous dysplasia and in 40 to 50% of those with functionally significant stenosis due to arteriosclerosis. The abdomen should also be palpated for an abdominal aneurysm and for the enlarged kidneys of polycystic renal disease. The femoral pulses must be carefully felt, and, if they are decreased and/or delayed in comparison with the radial pulse, the blood pressure in the lower extremities must be measured. Even if the femoral pulse is normal to palpation, arterial pressure in the lower extremities should be recorded at least once in patients in whom hypertension is discovered before the age of 30 years. Finally, examination of the extremities for edema and a search for evidence of a previous cerebrovascular accident and/or other intracranial pathology should be performed.

Laboratory Investigation There is controversy as to what laboratory studies should be performed in patients presenting with hypertension. In general, the disagreement centers on how extensively the patient should be evaluated for secondary forms of hypertension or subsets of essential hypertension. The *basic* laboratory studies that should be performed in all patients with sustained hypertension are described in (Table 35-3). →*The secondary studies that should be added if (1) the initial evaluation indicates a form of secondary hypertension and/or (2) arterial pressure is not controlled after initial therapy are discussed in Chap. 246.*

Renal status is evaluated by assessing the presence of protein, blood, and glucose in the urine and measuring serum creatinine and/or blood urea nitrogen. Microscopic examination of the urine is also helpful. The serum potassium level should be measured both as a screen for mineralocorticoid-induced hypertension and to provide a baseline before diuretic therapy is begun. A blood glucose determination is helpful both because diabetes mellitus may be associated with accelerated arteriosclerosis, renal vascular disease, and diabetic nephropathy in patients with hypertension and because primary aldosteronism, Cushing's syndrome, and pheochromocytoma all may be associated with hyperglycemia. Furthermore, since antihypertensive therapy with diuretics, for example, can raise the blood glucose level,

it is important to establish a baseline. The possibility of hypercalcemia may also be investigated. Serum cholesterol, high-density lipoprotein cholesterol, and triglyceride levels identify other factors that predispose to the development of arteriosclerosis.

An electrocardiogram should be obtained in all cases to permit assessment of cardiac status, particularly if left ventricular hypertrophy is present, and to provide a baseline. The echocardiogram is more sensitive than either the electrocardiogram or physical examination in determining whether cardiac hypertrophy is present. However, a complete, detailed echocardiographic study is expensive. Thus, in some circumstances, a cheaper, limited echocardiogram may be a useful addition to the *baseline* evaluation of a hypertensive patient, particularly as left ventricular hypertrophy is an independent cardiovascular risk factor and its presence suggests the need for vigorous antihypertensive therapy. Furthermore, while a substantial increase in arterial pressure usually correlates with the presence of left ventricular hypertrophy, a mild increase may not. Thus, one cannot use the blood pressure as a surrogate marker for the presence or absence of left ventricular hypertrophy. On the other hand, because of the cost of an echo-

Table 35-3 Laboratory Tests for Evaluation of Hypertension

BASIC TESTS FOR INITIAL EVALUATION

1. Always included
   a. Urine for protein, blood, and glucose
   b. Microscopic urinalysis
   c. Hematocrit
   d. Serum potassium
   e. Serum creatinine and/or blood urea nitrogen
   f. Fasting glucose
   g. Total cholesterol
   h. Electrocardiogram
2. Usually included, depending on cost and other factors
   a. Thyroid-stimulating hormone
   b. White blood cell count
   c. HDL and LDL cholesterol and triglycerides
   d. Serum calcium and phosphate
   e. Chest x-ray; limited echocardiogram

SPECIAL STUDIES TO SCREEN FOR SECONDARY HYPERTENSION

1. Renovascular disease: angiotensin-converting enzyme inhibitor radionuclide renal scan, renal duplex Doppler flow studies, and MRI angiography
2. Pheochromocytoma: 24-h urine assay for creatinine, metanephrines, and catecholamines
3. Cushing's syndrome: overnight dexamethasone suppression test or 24-h urine cortisol and creatinine
4. Primary aldosteronism: plasma aldosterone: renin activity ratio

NOTE: HDL, high-density lipoprotein; LDL, low-density lipoprotein; MRI, magnetic resonance imaging.

cardiogram and the uncertainty as to whether the resultant information would modify therapy, it is unclear that routine *follow-up* echocardiograms during therapy are justified. Furthermore, there are no data to suggest that reversal of left ventricular hypertrophy produces benefits beyond that conferred by blood pressure reduction. The chest roentgenogram may also be helpful by providing the opportunity to identify aortic dilation or elongation and the rib notching that occurs in coarctation of the aorta.

Certain clues from the history, physical examination, and basic laboratory studies may suggest an unusual cause for the hypertension and dictate the need for special studies as outlined in Chap 246.

℞ **TREATMENT**   See Chap. 246.

BIBLIOGRAPHY

BERLOWITZ DR et al: Inadequate management of blood pressure in a hypertensive population. N Engl J Med 339:1967, 1998

KAPLAN N: Systemic hypertension: Mechanisms and diagnosis, in *Heart Disease*, 6th ed, E Braunwald, D Zipes, P Libby (eds). Philadelphia, Saunders 2001

MOSTERD A et al: Trends in the prevalence of hypertension, antihypertensive therapy, and left ventricular hypertrophy from 1950 to 1989. N Engl J Med 340:1221, 1999

REEVES RA: Does this patient have hypertension? How to measure blood pressure. JAMA 273:1211, 1995

THE SIXTH REPORT OF THE JOINT NATIONAL COMMITTEE ON PREVENTION, DETECTION, EVALUATION, AND TREATMENT OF HIGH BLOOD PRESSURE. Arch Intern Med. 157:2413, 1997

WEBER MA et al: Diagnosis of mild hypertension by ambulatory blood pressure monitoring. Circulation 90:2291, 1994

1999 WORLD HEALTH ORGANIZATION—INTERNATIONAL SOCIETY OF HYPERTENSION GUIDELINES FOR THE MANAGEMENT OF HYPERTENSION. J Hypertens 17:151, 1999

36   *Eugene Braunwald*

HYPOXIA AND CYANOSIS

HYPOXIA

The fundamental purpose of the cardiorespiratory system is to deliver O_2 (and substrates) to the cells and to remove CO_2 (and other metabolic products) from them. Proper maintenance of this function depends on intact cardiovascular and respiratory systems and a supply of inspired gas containing adequate O_2. When hypoxia occurs consequent to respiratory failure, Pa_{CO_2} usually rises (Chap. 250), and the hemoglobin-oxygen ($Hb-O_2$) dissociation curve (see Fig. 106-2) is displaced to the right. Under these conditions, the Pa_{O_2} declines. Arterial hypoxemia, i.e., a reduction of O_2 saturation of arterial blood (Sa_{O_2}), and consequent cyanosis are likely to be more marked when such depression of Pa_{O_2} results from pulmonary disease than when the depression occurs as the result of a decline in the fraction of oxygen in inspired air (FI_{O_2}). In this situation Pa_{CO_2} falls secondary to anoxia-induced hyperventilation and the $Hb-O_2$ dissociation curve is displaced to the left, limiting the decline in Sa_{O_2}.

CAUSES OF HYPOXIA   **Anemic Hypoxia**   Any reduction in the hemoglobin concentration of the blood is attended by a corresponding decline in the O_2-carrying capacity of the blood. In anemic hypoxia, the Pa_{O_2} is normal; but as a consequence of the reduction of the hemoglobin concentration, the absolute quantity of O_2 transported per unit volume of blood is diminished. As the anemic blood passes through the capillaries and the usual quantity of O_2 is removed from it, the P_{O_2} in the venous blood declines to a greater degree than would normally be the case.

Carbon Monoxide Intoxication   (See also Chap. 396)   Hemoglobin that is combined with carbon monoxide (carboxyhemoglobin, COHb) is unavailable for O_2 transport. In addition, the presence of COHb shifts the $Hb-O_2$ dissociation curve to the left (see Fig. 106-2) so that O_2 is unloaded only at lower tensions. By such formation of COHb, a given degree of reduction in O_2-carrying power produces a far greater degree of tissue hypoxia than the equivalent reduction in hemoglobin due to simple anemia.

Respiratory Hypoxia   Arterial unsaturation is a common finding in advanced pulmonary disease. The most common cause of respiratory hypoxia is ventilation-perfusion mismatch, which results from perfusion of poorly ventilated alveoli. As discussed in Chap. 250, it may also be caused by hypoventilation, and it is then associated with an elevation of Pa_{CO_2}. These two forms of respiratory hypoxia may be recognized because they are usually correctable by inspiring 100% O_2 for several minutes. A third cause is shunting of blood across the lung from right to left by perfusion of nonventilated portions of the lung, as in pulmonary atelectasis or through arteriovenous connections in the lung. The low Pa_{O_2} in this situation is correctable only in part by an FI_{O_2} of 100%.

Hypoxia Secondary to High Altitude   As one ascends rapidly to 3000 m (approximately 10,000 ft), the alveolar P_{O_2} declines to about 60 mmHg, and impaired memory and other cerebral symptoms of hypoxia may develop. At higher altitudes, arterial saturation declines rapidly and symptoms become more serious; and at 5000 m (approximately 15,000 ft) unacclimatized individuals usually cease to be able to function normally.

Hypoxia Secondary to Right-to-Left Extrapulmonary Shunting   From a physiologic viewpoint, this cause of hypoxia resembles intrapulmonary right-to-left shunting but is caused by congenital cardiac malformations such as tetralogy of Fallot, transposition of the great arteries, and Eisenmenger's syndrome (Chap. 234). As in pulmonary right-to-left shunting, the Pa_{O_2} cannot be restored to normal with inspiration of 100% O_2.

Circulatory Hypoxia   As in anemic hypoxia, the Pa_{O_2} is usually normal, but venous and tissue P_{O_2} values are reduced as a consequence of reduced tissue perfusion. Generalized circulatory hypoxia occurs in heart failure (Chap. 232) and in most forms of shock (Chap. 38).

Specific Organ Hypoxia   Decreased perfusion of any organ resulting in localized circulatory hypoxia may occur secondary to organic arterial obstruction or as a consequence of vasoconstriction (Chap. 248). The latter is seen in the upper extremities in Raynaud's phenomenon. Ischemic hypoxia with accompanying pallor occurs in organic arterial obliterative disease. Localized hypoxia also may result from venous obstruction and the resultant congestion and reduced arterial inflow. Edema, which increases the distance through which O_2 diffuses before it reaches cells, also can cause localized hypoxia. In an attempt to maintain adequate perfusion to more vital organs, constriction may reduce perfusion in all limbs in patients with heart failure or hypovolemic shock.

Increased O_2 Requirements   If the O_2 consumption of the tissues is elevated without a corresponding increase in perfusion, tissue hypoxia ensues and the P_{O_2} in venous blood becomes reduced. Ordinarily, the clinical picture of patients with hypoxia due to an elevated metabolic rate is quite different from that in other types of hypoxia; the skin is warm and flushed, owing to increased cutaneous blood flow that dissipates the excessive heat produced, and cyanosis is usually absent.

Exercise is a classic example of increased tissue O_2 requirements. These increased demands are normally met by several mechanisms operating simultaneously: (1) increasing the cardiac output and ventilation and thus O_2 delivery to the tissues; (2) preferentially directing the blood to the exercising muscles by changing vascular resistances in various circulatory beds, directly and/or reflexly; (3) increasing O_2 extraction from the delivered blood and widening the arteriovenous O_2 difference; and (4) reducing the pH of the tissues and capillary blood, thereby unloading more O_2 from hemoglobin. If the capacity of these mechanisms is exceeded, then hypoxia, especially of the exercising muscles, will result.

Improper Oxygen Utilization   Cyanide (Chap. 396) and several other similarly acting poisons cause cellular hypoxia. The tissues are unable to utilize O_2, and as a consequence, the venous blood tends to have a high O_2 tension. This condition has been termed *histotoxic hypoxia*.

EFFECTS OF HYPOXIA Changes in the central nervous system, particularly the higher centers, are especially important consequences of hypoxia. Acute hypoxia causes impaired judgment, motor incoordination, and a clinical picture closely resembling that of acute alcoholism. When hypoxia is long-standing, fatigue, drowsiness, apathy, inattentiveness, delayed reaction time, and reduced work capacity occur. As hypoxia becomes more severe, the centers of the brainstem are affected, and death usually results from respiratory failure. With the reduction of Pa_{O_2}, cerebrovascular resistance decreases and cerebral blood flow increases, increasing O_2 delivery to the brain as a compensatory mechanism. However, when the reduction of Pa_{O_2} is accompanied by hyperventilation and a reduction of Pa_{CO_2}, cerebrovascular resistance rises, cerebral blood flow falls, and hypoxia is intensified. Hypoxia also causes pulmonary arterial constriction, which shunts blood away from poorly ventilated areas toward better-ventilated portions of the lung. However, it also increases pulmonary vascular resistance and right ventricular afterload.

Glucose is normally broken down to pyruvic acid. However, the further breakdown of pyruvate and the generation of adenosine triphosphate (ATP) consequent to it require O_2; and in the presence of hypoxia increasing proportions of pyruvate are reduced to lactic acid, which cannot be broken down further, causing metabolic acidosis. Under these circumstances, the total energy obtained from the breakdown of carbohydrate is greatly reduced, and the quantity of energy available for the production of ATP becomes inadequate.

An important component of the respiratory response to hypoxia originates in special chemosensitive cells in the carotid and aortic bodies, and in the respiratory center in the brainstem. The stimulation of these cells by hypoxia increases ventilation, with a loss of CO_2, and leads to respiratory alkalosis. When combined with the metabolic acidosis resulting from the production of lactic acid, the serum bicarbonate level declines (Chap. 50).

Diminished P_{O_2} in any tissue results in local vasodilatation, and the diffuse vasodilatation that occurs in generalized hypoxia raises the cardiac output. In patients with underlying heart disease, the requirements of the peripheral tissues for an increase of cardiac output with hypoxia may precipitate congestive heart failure. In patients with ischemic heart disease, a reduced Pa_{O_2} may intensify myocardial ischemia and further impair left ventricular function.

One of the important mechanisms of compensation for chronic hypoxia is an increase in the hemoglobin concentration and in the number of red blood cells in the circulating blood, i.e., the development of polycythemia secondary to erythropoietin production (Chap. 110).

CYANOSIS

Cyanosis refers to a bluish color of the skin and mucous membranes resulting from an increased quantity of reduced hemoglobin, or of hemoglobin derivatives, in the small blood vessels of those areas. It is usually most marked in the lips, nail beds, ears, and malar eminences. Cyanosis, especially if developed recently, is more commonly detected by a family member than the patient. The florid skin characteristic of polycythemia vera (Chap. 110) must be distinguished from the true cyanosis discussed here. A cherry-colored flush, rather than cyanosis, is caused by COHb (Chap. 396). The degree of cyanosis is modified by the color of the cutaneous pigment and the thickness of the skin, as well as by the state of the cutaneous capillaries. The accurate clinical detection of the presence and degree of cyanosis is difficult, as proved by oximetric studies. In some instances, central cyanosis can be detected reliably when the Sa_{O_2} has fallen to 85%; in others, particularly in dark-skinned persons, it may not be detected until it has declined to 75%. In the latter case, examination of the mucous membranes in the oral cavity and the conjunctivae rather than examination of the skin is more helpful in the detection of cyanosis.

The increase in the quantity of reduced hemoglobin in the mucocutaneous vessels that produces cyanosis may be brought about either by an increase in the quantity of venous blood as the result of dilatation of the venules and venous ends of the capillaries or by a reduction in the Sa_{O_2} in the capillary blood. In general, cyanosis becomes apparent when the mean capillary concentration of reduced hemoglobin exceeds 40 g/L (4 g/dL). It is the *absolute* rather than the *relative* quantity of reduced hemoglobin that is important in producing cyanosis. Thus, in a patient with severe anemia, the relative amount of reduced hemoglobin in the venous blood may be very large when considered in relation to the total amount of hemoglobin in the blood. However, since the concentration of the latter is markedly reduced, the *absolute* quantity of reduced hemoglobin may still be small, and therefore patients with severe anemia and even *marked* arterial desaturation do not display cyanosis. Conversely, the higher the total hemoglobin content, the greater is the tendency toward cyanosis; thus, patients with marked polycythemia tend to be cyanotic at higher levels of Sa_{O_2} than patients with normal hematocrit values. Likewise, local passive congestion, which causes an increase in the total amount of reduced hemoglobin in the vessels in a given area, may cause cyanosis. Cyanosis also is observed when nonfunctional hemoglobin such as methemoglobin or sulfhemoglobin (Chap. 106) is present in blood.

Cyanosis may be subdivided into central and peripheral types. In the *central* type, the Sa_{O_2} is reduced or an abnormal hemoglobin derivative is present, and the mucous membranes and skin are both affected. *Peripheral* cyanosis is due to a slowing of blood flow and abnormally great extraction of O_2 from normally saturated arterial blood. It results from vasoconstriction and diminished peripheral blood flow, such as occurs in cold exposure, shock, congestive failure, and peripheral vascular disease. Often in these conditions the mucous membranes of the oral cavity or those beneath the tongue may be spared. Clinical differentiation between central and peripheral cyanosis may not always be simple, and in conditions such as cardiogenic shock with pulmonary edema there may be a mixture of both types.

DIFFERENTIAL DIAGNOSIS Central Cyanosis (Table 36-1) Decreased Sa_{O_2} results from a marked reduction in the Pa_{O_2}. This reduction may be brought about by a decline in the FI_{O_2} without sufficient compensatory alveolar hyperventilation to maintain alveolar P_{O_2}. Cyanosis does not occur to a significant degree in an ascent to an altitude of 2500 m (8000 ft) but is marked in a further ascent to 5000 m (16,000 ft). The reason for this difference becomes clear on studying

Table 36-1 Causes Of Cyanosis

CENTRAL CYANOSIS

Decreased arterial oxygen saturation
  Decreased atmospheric pressure—high altitude
  Impaired pulmonary function
    Alveolar hypoventilation
    Uneven relationships between pulmonary ventilation and perfusion
     (perfusion of hypoventilated alveoli)
    Impaired oxygen diffusion
  Anatomic shunts
    Certain types of congenital heart disease
    Pulmonary arteriovenous fistulas
    Multiple small intrapulmonary shunts
  Hemoglobin with low affinity for oxygen
Hemoglobin abnormalities
  Methemoglobinemia—hereditary, acquired
  Sulfhemoglobinema—acquired
  Carboxyhemoglobinemia (not true cyanosis)

PERIPHERAL CYANOSIS

Reduced cardiac output
Cold exposure
Redistribution of blood flow from extremities
Arterial obstruction
Venous obstruction

the *S* shape of the Hb-O$_2$ dissociation curve (see Fig. 106-1). At 2500 m (8000 ft) the F$_{IO_2}$ is about 120 mmHg, the alveolar P$_{O_2}$ is approximately 80 mmHg, and the Sa$_{O_2}$ is nearly normal. However, at 5000 m (16,000 ft) the F$_{IO_2}$ and alveolar P$_{O_2}$ are about 85 and 50 mmHg, respectively, and the Sa$_{O_2}$ is only about 75%. This leaves 25% of the hemoglobin in the arterial blood in the reduced form, an amount likely to be associated with cyanosis in the absence of anemia. Similarly, a mutant hemoglobin with a low affinity for O$_2$ (e.g., Hb Kansas) causes lowered Sa$_{O_2}$ saturation and resultant central cyanosis (Chap. 106).

Seriously *impaired pulmonary function*, through perfusion of unventilated or poorly ventilated areas of the lung or alveolar hypoventilation, is a common cause of central cyanosis (Chap. 250). This condition may occur acutely, as in extensive pneumonia or pulmonary edema, or chronically with chronic pulmonary diseases (e.g., emphysema). In the last situation, secondary polycythemia is generally present, and clubbing of the fingers may occur. However, in many types of chronic pulmonary disease with fibrosis and obliteration of the capillary vascular bed, cyanosis does not occur because there is relatively little perfusion of underventilated areas.

Another cause of reduced Sa$_{O_2}$ is *shunting of systemic venous blood into the arterial circuit*. Certain forms of congenital heart disease are associated with cyanosis (Chap. 234). Since blood flows from a higher-pressure to a lower-pressure region, for a cardiac defect to result in a right-to-left shunt, it must ordinarily be combined with an obstructive lesion distal to the defect or with elevated pulmonary vascular resistance. The most common congenital cardiac lesion associated with cyanosis in the adult is the combination of ventricular septal defect and pulmonary outflow tract obstruction (*tetralogy of Fallot*). The more severe the obstruction, the greater the degree of right-to-left shunting and resultant cyanosis. In patients with patent ductus arteriosus, pulmonary hypertension, and right-to-left shunt, *differential cyanosis* results; that is, cyanosis occurs in the lower but not in the upper extremities. →*The mechanisms for the elevated pulmonary vascular resistance that may produce cyanosis in the presence of intra- and extracardiac communications without pulmonic stenosis (Eisenmenger syndrome) are discussed in Chap. 234.*

Pulmonary arteriovenous fistulae (Chap. 57) may be congenital or acquired, solitary or multiple, microscopic or massive. The severity of cyanosis produced by these fistulae depends on their size and number. They occur with some frequency in hereditary hemorrhagic telangiectasia. Sa$_{O_2}$ reduction and cyanosis may also occur in some patients with cirrhosis, presumably as a consequence of pulmonary arteriovenous fistulas or portal vein–pulmonary vein anastomoses.

In patients with cardiac or pulmonary right-to-left shunts, the presence and severity of cyanosis depend on the size of the shunt relative to the systemic flow as well as on the Hb-O$_2$ saturation of the venous blood. With increased extraction of O$_2$ from the blood by the exercising muscles, the venous blood returning to the right side of the heart is more unsaturated than at rest, and shunting of this blood or its passage through lungs incapable of normal oxygenation intensifies the cyanosis. Also, since the systemic vascular resistance falls with exercise, the right-to-left shunt is augmented by exercise in patients with congenital heart disease and communications between the two sides of the heart. Secondary polycythemia occurs frequently in patients with arterial O$_2$ unsaturation and contributes to the cyanosis.

Cyanosis can be caused by small amounts of circulating methemoglobin and by even smaller amounts of sulfhemoglobin (Chap. 106). Although they are uncommon causes of cyanosis, these abnormal hemoglobin pigments should be sought by spectroscopy when cyanosis is not readily explained by malfunction of the circulatory or respiratory systems. Generally, digital clubbing does not occur with them. The diagnosis of methemoglobinemia can be suspected if the patient's blood remains brown after being mixed in a test tube and exposed to air.

Peripheral Cyanosis   Probably the most common cause of peripheral cyanosis is the normal vasoconstriction resulting from exposure to cold air or water. When cardiac output is low, as in severe congestive heart failure or shock, cutaneous vasoconstriction occurs as a compensatory mechanism so that blood is diverted from the skin to more vital areas such as the central nervous system and heart (Chap. 232), and intense cyanosis associated with cool extremities may result. Even though the arterial blood is normally saturated, the reduced volume flow through the skin and the reduced P$_{O_2}$ at the venous end of the capillary result in cyanosis.

Arterial obstruction to an extremity, as with an embolus, or arteriolar constriction, as in cold-induced vasospasm (Raynaud's phenomenon, Chap. 248), generally results in pallor and coldness, but there may be associated cyanosis. Venous obstruction, as in thrombophlebitis, dilates the subpapillary venous plexuses and thereby intensifies cyanosis.

Approach to the Patient

Certain features are important in arriving at the cause of cyanosis:

1.   The history, particularly the onset (cyanosis present since birth is usually due to congenital heart disease), and possible exposure to drugs or chemicals that may produce abnormal types of hemoglobin.

2.   Clinical differentiation of central as opposed to peripheral cyanosis. Objective evidence by physical or radiographic examination of disorders of the respiratory or cardiovascular systems. Massage or gentle warming of a cyanotic extremity will increase peripheral blood flow and abolish peripheral but not central cyanosis.

3.   The presence or absence of clubbing of the digits (see below). Clubbing without cyanosis is frequent in patients with infective endocarditis and ulcerative colitis; it may occasionally occur in healthy persons, and in some instances it may be occupational, e.g., in jackhammer operators. The combination of cyanosis and clubbing is frequent in patients with congenital heart disease and right-to-left shunting and is seen occasionally in persons with pulmonary disease such as lung abscess or pulmonary arteriovenous fistulae. In contrast, peripheral cyanosis or acutely developing central cyanosis is *not* associated with clubbed digits.

4.   Determination of Pa$_{O_2}$ tension and Sa$_{O_2}$ and spectroscopic and other examinations of the blood for abnormal types of hemoglobin (critical in the differential diagnosis of cyanosis).

CLUBBING

The selective bullous enlargement of the distal segments of the fingers and toes due to proliferation of connective tissue, particularly on the dorsal surface, is termed *clubbing*; there is increased sponginess of the soft tissue at the base of the nail. Clubbing may be hereditary, idiopathic, or acquired and associated with a variety of disorders, including cyanotic congenital heart disease, infective endocarditis, and a variety of pulmonary conditions (among them primary and metastatic lung cancer, bronchiectasis, lung abscess, cystic fibrosis, and mesothelioma), as well as with some gastrointestinal diseases (including regional enteritis, chronic ulcerative colitis, and hepatic cirrhosis).

Clubbing in patients with primary and metastatic lung cancer, mesothelioma, bronchiectasis, and hepatic cirrhosis may be associated with *hypertrophic osteoarthropathy*. In this condition, the subperiosteal formation of new bone in the distal diaphyses of the long bones of the extremities causes pain and symmetric arthritis-like changes in the shoulders, knees, ankles, wrists, and elbows. The diagnosis of hypertrophic osteoarthropathy may be confirmed by bone radiographs. Although the mechanism of clubbing is unclear, it appears to be secondary to a humoral substance that causes dilation of the vessels of the fingertip.

BIBLIOGRAPHY

BEALL CM: Tibetan and Andean patterns of adaptation to high-altitude hypoxia. Hum Biol 72:201, 2000

BEITNER-JOHNSON D et al: Regulation of gene expression by hypoxia: A molecular approach. Respir Physiol 110:87, 1997

FISHMAN AP: Approach to the patient with respiratory symptoms: Cyanosis and clubbing, in *Fishman's Pulmonary Diseases and Disorders*, 3d ed, Fishman AP et al (eds). Philadelphia, Saunders, 1998, pp 382–3

GALLEY HF, WEBSTER NR: Acidosis and tissue hypoxia in the critically ill: How to measure it and what does it mean? Crit Rev Clin Lab Sci 36:35, 1999

GRIFFEY RT et al: Cyanosis. J Emerg Med 18:369, 2000

GRIFKA RG: Cyanotic congenital heart disease with increased pulmonary blood flow. Pediatr Clin North Am 46:405, 1999

SEVERINHAUS JW: Uses of high altitude for studies of effects of hypoxia. Adv Exp Med Biol 454:17, 1998

TISSUE HYPOXIA: How to detect, how to correct, how to prevent? Third European Consensus Conference in Intensive Care Medicine. J Crit Care 12:39, 1997

WALDMAN JD, WERNLY JA. Cyanotic congenital heart disease with decreased pulmonary blood flow in children. Pediatr Clin North Am 46:385, 1999

| 37 | *Eugene Braunwald* |

EDEMA

Edema is defined as a clinically apparent increase in the interstitial fluid volume, which may expand by several liters before the abnormality is evident. Therefore, a weight gain of several kilograms usually precedes overt manifestations of edema, and a similar weight loss from diuresis can be induced in a slightly edematous patient before "dry weight" is achieved. *Ascites* (Chap. 46) and *hydrothorax* refer to accumulation of excess fluid in the peritoneal and pleural cavities, respectively, and are considered to be special forms of edema. *Anasarca* refers to gross, generalized edema.

Depending on its cause and mechanism, edema may be localized or have a generalized distribution; it is recognized in its generalized form by puffiness of the face, which is most readily apparent in the periorbital areas, and by the persistence of an indentation of the skin following pressure; this is known as "pitting" edema. In its more subtle form, it may be detected by noting that after the stethoscope is removed from the chest wall, the rim of the bell leaves an indentation on the skin of the chest for a few minutes. When the ring on a finger fits more snugly than in the past or when a patient complains of difficulty in putting on shoes, particularly in the evening, edema may be present.

PATHOGENESIS About one-third of the total-body water is confined to the extracellular space. Approximately 25% of the latter, in turn, is composed of the plasma volume, and the remainder is interstitial fluid.

Starling Forces The forces that regulate the disposition of fluid between these two components of the extracellular compartment are frequently referred to as the *Starling forces* (see p. 202). The hydrostatic pressure within the vascular system and the colloid oncotic pressure in the interstitial fluid tend to promote movement of fluid from the vascular to the extravascular space. In contrast, the colloid oncotic pressure contributed by the plasma proteins and the hydrostatic pressure within the interstitial fluid, referred to as the *tissue tension*, promote the movement of fluid into the vascular compartment. Consequently there is a movement of water and diffusible solutes from the vascular space at the arteriolar end of the capillaries.

Fluid is returned from the interstitial space into the vascular system at the venous end of the capillary and by way of the lymphatics, and unless these channels are obstructed, lymph flow tends to increase with increases in net movement of fluid from the vascular compartment to the interstitium. These flows are usually balanced so that a steady state exists in the sizes of the intravascular and interstitial compartments, and yet a large exchange between them occurs. However, should any one of the hydrostatic or oncotic pressure gradients be altered significantly, a further net movement of fluid between the two components of the extracellular space will take place. The development of edema then depends on one or more alterations in the Starling forces so that there is increased flow of fluid from the vascular system into the interstitium or into a body cavity.

Edema due to increase in capillary pressure may result from an elevation of venous pressure due to obstruction in venous drainage. This increase in capillary pressure may be generalized, as occurs in congestive heart failure. The Starling forces may be imbalanced when the colloid oncotic pressure of the plasma is reduced, owing to any factor that may induce hypoalbuminemia, such as saline expansion, malnutrition, liver disease, loss of protein into the urine or into the gastrointestinal tract, or a severe catabolic state.

Capillary Damage Edema may also result from damage to the capillary endothelium, which increases its permeability and permits the transfer of protein into the interstitial compartment. Injury to the capillary wall can result from drugs, viral or bacterial agents, and thermal or mechanical trauma. Increased capillary permeability may also be a consequence of a hypersensitivity reaction and is characteristic of immune injury. Damage to the capillary endothelium is presumably responsible for inflammatory edema, which is usually nonpitting, localized, and accompanied by other signs of inflammation—redness, heat, and tenderness.

To formulate a hypothesis about the pathophysiology of an edematous state, it is important to discriminate between the *primary* events, such as localized or generalized venous or lymphatic obstruction, reduction of cardiac output, hypoalbuminemia, trapping of fluid in spaces such as the pleural or peritoneal cavities, or an increase in capillary permeability, and the predictable *secondary* consequences, which include the renal retention of salt and water in an attempt to restore the plasma volume when the latter has been reduced, as in venous obstruction (see below). Both the primary event and the secondary consequences contribute to the formation of edema. In some cases the primary event is the renal retention of salt and water. Examples are renal failure, nephrotic syndrome, glomerulonephritis, and early hepatic failure.

Reduction of Effective Arterial Volume In many forms of edema the *effective arterial blood volume*, an as yet poorly defined parameter of the filling of the arterial tree, is reduced, and as a consequence a series of physiologic responses designed to restore it to normal are set into motion. A key element of these responses is the retention of salt and therefore of water, principally by the renal proximal tubule (Fig. 37-1), and in many instances this repairs the deficit of the effective arterial blood volume; often this deficit is repaired without the development of overt edema. If, however, the retention of salt and water is insufficient to restore and maintain the effective arterial blood volume, the stimuli are not dissipated, the retention of salt and water continues, and edema may ultimately develop. This sequence of events is operative in dehydration and hemorrhage. Although in these conditions there is a reduction of effective arterial blood volume and activation of the entire sequence shown in the center of Fig. 37-2, including the diminished excretion of salt and water, because the net sodium and water balance is negative rather than positive, edema does *not* occur. In most conditions that lead to edema, the mechanisms responsible for maintaining a normal effective osmolality in the body fluids operate efficiently so that sodium retention promotes thirst and secretion of the antidiuretic hormone. In edematous states, isotonic expansion of the extracellular fluid space may be massive, while the intracellular fluid volume is unchanged.

Reduced Cardiac Output A reduction of cardiac output, whatever the cause, is associated with a lowering of the effective arterial blood volume as well as of renal blood flow, constriction of the efferent renal arterioles, and an elevation of the filtration fraction, i.e., the ratio of glomerular filtration rate to renal plasma flow. In severe heart failure

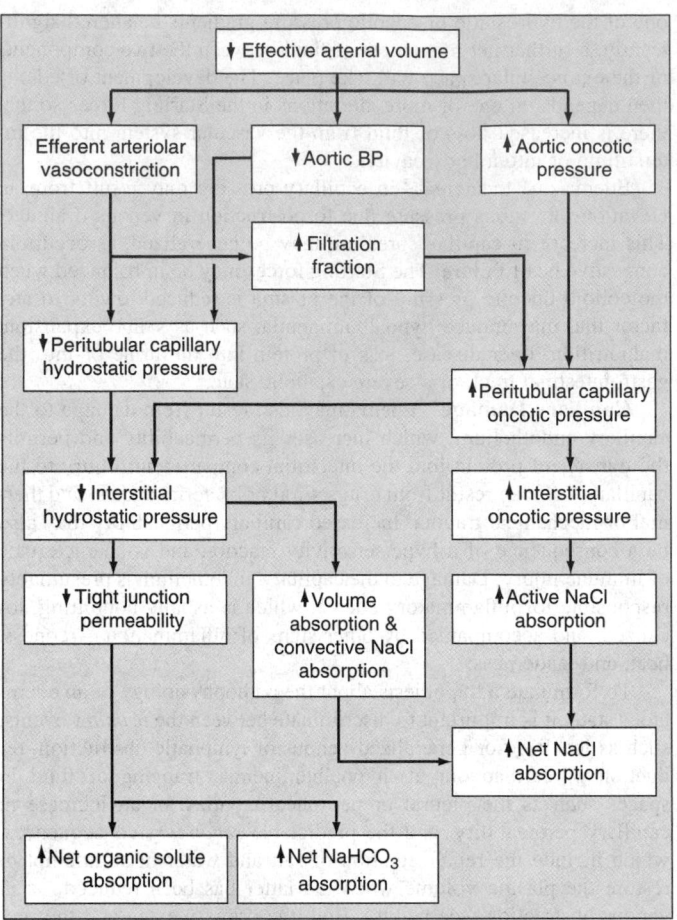

FIGURE 37-1 Effect of hemodynamic changes on proximal tubule solute transport: a summary. Hemodynamic mechanisms by which a reduction of effective arterial volume causes salt and water retention and thereby contributes to the formation of edema. *(From Seldin DW et al, Semin Nephrol 11:212, 1991, with permission.)*

there is a reduction in the glomerular filtration rate. Activation of the sympathetic nervous system and of the renin-angiotensin systems are responsible for renal vasoconstriction. The finding that α-adrenergic blocking agents and/or angiotensin-converting enzyme (ACE) inhibitors augment renal blood flow and induce diuresis supports the role of these two systems in elevating renal vascular resistance and salt and water retention.

Renal Factors Reduced cardiac output lowers effective arterial blood volume. There is increased tubular reabsorption of glomerular filtrate in both the proximal and distal tubules (Fig. 37-1). Alterations in intrarenal hemodynamics appear to play a significant role. Heart failure and other conditions, such as nephrotic syndrome and cirrhosis that reduce effective arterial blood volume, cause renal efferent arteriolar constriction. This, in turn, reduces the hydrostatic pressure while the increased filtration fraction raises the colloid osmotic pressure in the peritubular capillaries, thus enhancing salt and water reabsorption in the proximal tubule as well as in the ascending limb of the loop of Henle.

In addition, the diminished renal blood flow characteristic of states in which the effective arterial blood volume is reduced is translated by the renal juxtaglomerular cells into a signal for increased renin release (Chap. 331). The mechanisms responsible for this release include a baroreceptor response: reduced renal perfusion results in incomplete filling of the renal arterioles and diminished stretch of the juxtaglomerular cells, a signal that provides for the elaboration or release, or both, of renin. A second mechanism for renin release involves the macula densa; as a result of reduced glomerular filtration, the so-

dium chloride load reaching the distal renal tubules is reduced. This is sensed by the macula densa, which signals the neighboring juxtaglomerular cells to secrete renin. A third mechanism involves the sympathetic nervous system and circulating catecholamines. Activation of the β-adrenergic receptors in the juxtaglomerular cells stimulates renin release. These three mechanisms generally act in concert.

The Renin-Angiotensin-Aldosterone (RAA) System (See Chap. 331) Renin, an enzyme with a molecular weight of about 40,000, acts on its substrate, angiotensinogen, an α_2 globulin synthesized by the liver, to release angiotensin I, a decapeptide, which is broken down to angiotensin II (AII), an octapeptide. This has generalized vasoconstrictor properties; it is especially active on the efferent arterioles and independently increases Na^+ reabsorption in the proximal tubule. The RAA system has long been recognized as a hormone system. However, it also operates locally. Both circulating and intrarenally produced AII contribute to renal vasoconstriction and to salt and water retention. These renal effects of AII are mediated by activation of AII type 1 receptors, which can be blocked by specific antagonists such as losartan. AII also enters the circulation and stimulates the production of aldosterone by the zona glomerulosa of the adrenal cortex. In patients with heart failure, not only is aldosterone secretion elevated but the biologic half-life of aldosterone is prolonged, which further increases the plasma level of the hormone. A depression of hepatic blood flow, particularly during exercise, secondary to a reduction in cardiac output, is responsible for the reduced hepatic catabolism of aldosterone. Aldosterone, in turn, enhances Na^+ reabsorption (and K^+ excretion) by the collecting tubule. The activation of the RAA system is most striking in the early phase of acute, severe heart failure and is less intense in patients with chronic, stable, compensated heart failure.

Although increased quantities of aldosterone are secreted in heart failure and in other edematous states and although blockade of the action of aldosterone by spironolactone (an aldosterone antagonist) or amiloride (a blocker of epithelial Na^+ channels) often induces a moderate diuresis in edematous states, persistent augmented levels of aldosterone (or other mineralocorticoids) alone do not always promote accumulation of edema, as witnessed by the lack of striking fluid retention in most instances of primary aldosteronism (Chap. 331). Furthermore, although normal individuals retain some salt and water with the administration of potent mineralocorticoids, such as deoxycorticosterone acetate or fludrocortisone, this accumulation is self-limiting, despite continued exposure to the steroid, a phenomenon known as *mineralocorticoid escape*. The failure of normal individuals who receive large doses of mineralocorticoids to accumulate large quantities of extracellular fluid and to develop edema is probably a consequence of an increase in glomerular filtration rate (pressure natriuresis) and through the action of natriuretic substance(s) (see below). The continued secretion of aldosterone may be more important in the accumulation of fluid in edematous states because patients with edema secondary to heart failure, nephrotic syndrome, and cirrhosis are generally unable to repair the deficit in effective arterial blood volume. As a consequence they do not develop pressure natriuresis.

Blockade of the RAA system, by blocking AII receptors or inhibiting ACE, reduces efferent arteriolar resistance and increases renal blood flow. This action (combined in patients with heart failure with a rise in cardiac output secondary to afterload reduction) as well as reduction in the secretion of aldosterone cause diuresis. However, in patients with moderate or severe impairment of renal function or with renal artery stenosis, interference with the RAA system can cause paradoxical sodium retention due to intensification of renal failure.

Arginine Vasopressin (AVP) and Endothelin (See also Chap. 329) The secretion of AVP occurs in response to increased intracellular osmolar concentration and by stimulating V_2 receptors increases the reabsorption of free water in the renal distal tubule and collecting duct, thereby increasing total-body water. Circulating AVP is elevated in many patients with heart failure secondary to a nonosmotic stimulus associated with decreased effective arterial volume. Such patients fail to show the normal reduction of AVP with a reduction of osmolality, contributing to hyponatremia and edema formation.

Endothelin This is a potent peptide vasoconstrictor released by endothelial cells; its concentration is elevated in heart failure and contributes to renal vasoconstriction, Na$^+$ retention, and edema in heart failure.

Natriuretic Peptides Atrial distention and/or a sodium load cause release into the circulation of atrial natriuretic peptide (ANP), a polypeptide; a high-molecular-weight precursor of ANP is stored in secretory granules within atrial myocytes. Release of ANP causes (1) excretion of sodium and water by augmenting glomerular filtration rate, inhibiting sodium reabsorption in the proximal tubule, and inhibiting release of renin and aldosterone; and (2) arteriolar and venous dilatation by antagonizing the vasoconstrictor actions of AII, AVP, and sympathetic stimulation. Thus, ANP has the capacity to oppose sodium retention and arterial pressure elevation in hypervolemic states.

The closely related brain natriuretic peptide (BNP) is stored primarily in cardiac ventricular myocardium and is released when ventricular diastolic pressure rises. Its actions are similar to those of ANP. Circulating levels of ANP and BNP are elevated in congestive heart failure but obviously not sufficient to prevent edema formation. In addition, in edematous states (particularly heart failure), there is abnormal resistance to the actions of natriuretic peptides.

CLINICAL CAUSES OF EDEMA Obstruction of Venous (and Lymphatic) Drainage of a Limb In this condition the hydrostatic pressure in the capillary bed upstream to the obstruction increases so that an abnormal quantity of fluid is transferred from the vascular to the interstitial space. Since the alternative route (i.e., the lymphatic channels) may also be obstructed, an increased volume of interstitial fluid in the limb develops, i.e., there is a trapping of fluid in the extremity, causing local edema at the expense of the blood volume in the remainder of the body, thereby reducing effective arterial blood volume and leading to the consequences shown in Fig. 37-2.

When venous and lymphatic drainage are obstructed in a limb, fluid accumulates in the interstitium at the expense of plasma volume. The latter stimulates the retention of salt and water until the deficit in plasma volume has been corrected. Tissue tension rises in the affected limb until it counterbalances the primary alterations in the Starling forces, at which time no further fluid accumulates. The net effect is a local increase in the volume of interstitial fluid. This same sequence occurs in ascites and hydrothorax, in which fluid is trapped or accumulates in the cavitary space, depleting the intravascular volume and leading to secondary salt and fluid retention, as already described.

Congestive Heart Failure (See also Chap. 232) In this disorder the defective systolic emptying of the chambers of the heart and/or the impairment of ventricular relaxation promotes an accumulation of blood in the heart and venous circulation at the expense of the effective arterial volume, and the aforementioned sequence of events (Fig. 37-2) is initiated. In mild heart failure, a small increment of total blood volume may repair the deficit of arterial volume and establish a new steady state. Through the operation of Starling's law of the heart, an increase in the volume of blood within the chambers of the heart promotes a more forceful contraction and may thereby increase the cardiac output (See Fig. 232-1). However, if the cardiac disorder is more severe, retention of fluid cannot repair the deficit in effective arterial blood volume. The increment in blood volume accumulates in the venous circulation, and the increase in capillary and lymphatic hydrostatic pressures promotes the formation of edema. In heart failure, a reduction occurs in baroreflex-mediated inhibition of the vasomotor center, which causes activation of renal vasoconstrictor nerves and the RAA system, causing sodium and water retention.

Incomplete ventricular emptying (systolic heart failure) and/or inadequate ventricular relaxation (diastolic heart failure) both lead to an elevation of ventricular diastolic pressure. If the impairment of cardiac function involves the right ventricle, pressures in the systemic veins and capillaries may rise, thereby augmenting the transudation of fluid into the interstitial space and enhancing the likelihood of peripheral edema in the presence of the accumulation of sodium and water, as described above. The elevated systemic venous pressure is transmitted to the thoracic duct with consequent reduction of lymph drainage, further increasing the accumulation of edema.

If the impairment of cardiac function (incomplete ventricular emptying and/or inadequate relaxation) involves the left ventricle primarily, then pulmonary venous and capillary pressures rise [leading in

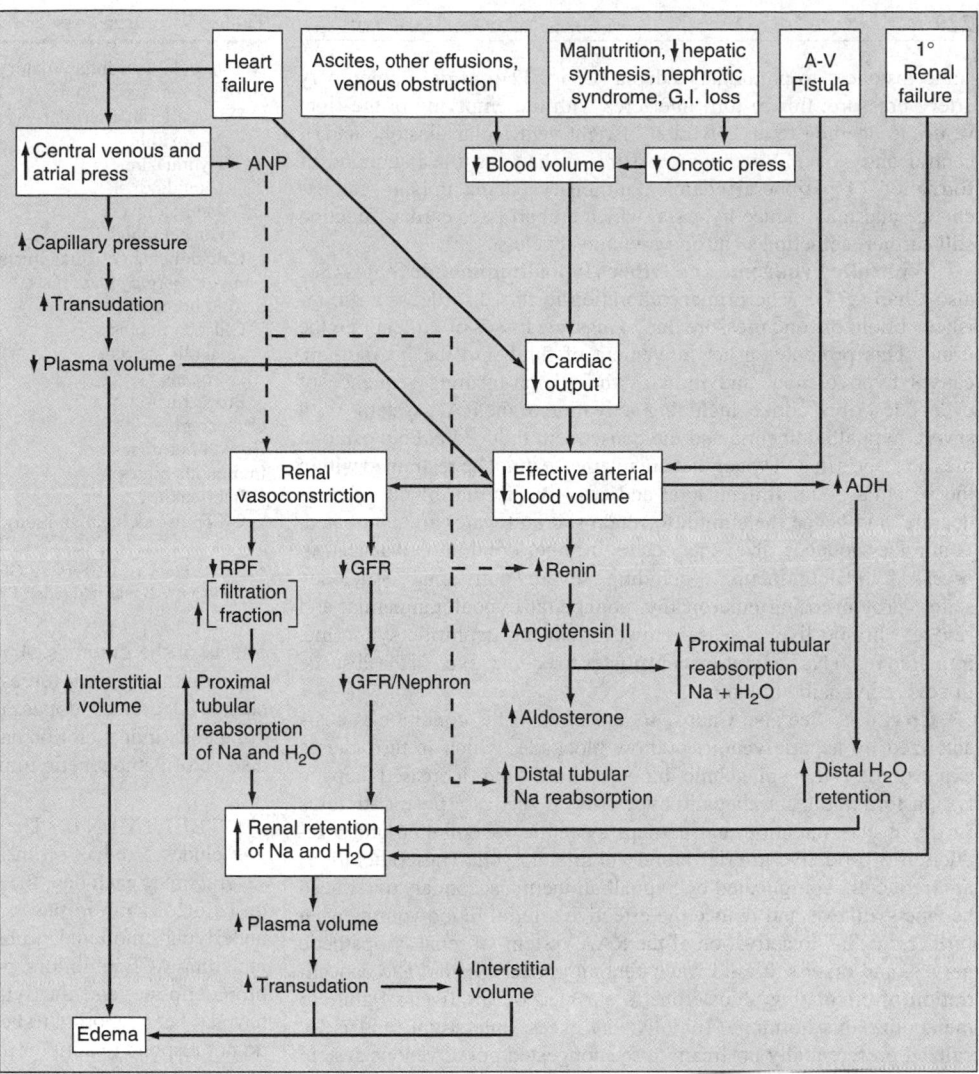

FIGURE 37-2 Sequence of events leading to the formation and retention of salt and water and the development of edema. ANP, atrial natriuretic peptide; RPF, renal plasma flow; GFR, glomerular filtration rate. Inhibitory influences are shown by broken lines. ADH, antidiuretic hormone.

some instances to pulmonary edema (Chap. 32)], as does pulmonary artery pressure; this in turn interferes with the emptying of the right ventricle, leading to an elevation of right ventricular diastolic and of central and systemic venous pressures, enhancing the likelihood of formation of peripheral edema. Pulmonary edema impairs gas exchange and may induce hypoxia, which embarrasses cardiac function still further, sometimes causing a vicious cycle.

Nephrotic Syndrome and Other Hypoalbuminemic States (See also Chap. 274)   The primary alteration in this disorder is a diminished colloid oncotic pressure due to massive losses of protein into the urine. This promotes a net movement of fluid into the interstitium, causes hypovolemia, and initiates the edema-forming sequence of events described above, including activation of the RAA system. With severe hypoalbuminemia and the consequent reduced colloid osmotic pressure, the salt and water that are retained cannot be restrained within the vascular compartment, total and effective arterial blood volumes decline, and hence the stimuli to retain salt and water are not abated. A similar sequence of events occurs in other conditions that lead to *severe* hypoalbuminemia, including severe nutritional deficiency states, protein-losing enteropathy, congenital hypoalbuminemia, and severe, chronic liver disease. However, in the nephrotic syndrome, impaired renal Na^+ excretion contributes to edema, even in the absence of severe hypoalbuminemia.

Cirrhosis (See also Chaps. 46 and 299)   This condition is characterized by hepatic venous outflow blockade, which in turn causes expansion of the splanchnic blood volume and increased hepatic lymph formation. Intrahepatic hypertension acts as a potent stimulus for renal Na^+ retention and perhaps systemic vasodilation and a reduction of effective arterial blood volume as well. These alterations are frequently complicated by hypoalbuminemia secondary to reduced hepatic synthesis and reduce the effective arterial blood volume even further, leading to activation of the RAA system, of renal sympathetic nerves, and other salt- and water-retaining mechanisms. The concentration of circulating aldosterone is elevated by the liver's failure to metabolize this hormone. Initially, the excess interstitial fluid is localized preferentially upstream to the congested portal venous system and obstructed hepatic lymphatics, i.e., in the peritoneal cavity. In later stages, particularly when there is severe hypoalbuminemia, peripheral edema may develop. The excess production of prostaglandins (PGE_2 and PGI_2) in cirrhosis attenuates renal Na^+ retention. When the synthesis of these substances is inhibited by nonsteroidal anti-inflammatory agents, renal function deteriorates and Na^+ retention increases.

Drug-Induced Edema   A large number of widely used drugs can cause edema (Table 37-1). Mechanisms include renal vasoconstriction (nonsteroidal anti-inflammatory agents and cyclosporine), arteriolar dilatation (vasodilators), augmented renal sodium reabsorption (steroid hormones) and capillary damage (interleukin 2).

Idiopathic Edema   This syndrome, which occurs almost exclusively in women, is characterized by periodic episodes of edema (unrelated to the menstrual cycle), frequently accompanied by abdominal distention. Diurnal alterations in weight occur with orthostatic retention of sodium and water, so that the patient may weigh several pounds more after having been in the upright posture for several hours. Such large diurnal weight changes suggest an increase in capillary permeability that appears to fluctuate in severity and to be aggravated by hot weather. There is some evidence that a reduction in plasma volume occurs in this condition with secondary activation of the RAA system and impaired suppression of AVP release. Idiopathic edema should be distinguished from cyclical or premenstrual edema, in which the sodium and water retention may be secondary to excessive estrogen stimulation. There are also some cases in which the edema appears to be "diuretic-induced." It has been postulated that in these patients, chronic diuretic administration leads to mild blood volume depletion, which causes chronic hyperreninemia and juxtaglomerular hyperplasia. Salt-retaining mechanisms appear to overcompensate for the direct

Table 37-1 Drugs Associated with Edema Formation

Nonsteroidal anti-inflammatory drugs
Antihypertensive agents
  Direct arterial/arteriolar vasodilators
    Minoxidil
    Hydralazine
    Clonidine
    Methyldopa
    Guanethidine
  Calcium channel antagonists
  α-Adrenergic antagonists
Steroid hormones
  Glucocorticoids
  Anabolic steroids
  Estrogens
  Progestins
Cyclosporine
Growth hormone
Immunotherapies
  Interleukin 2
  OKT3 monoclonal antibody

SOURCE: From GM Chertow, GE Thibault, Approach to the patient with edema, in L Goldman, E Braunwald (eds): *Primary Cardiology.* Philadelphia, Saunders, 1998.

effects of the diuretics. *Acute* withdrawal of diuretics can then leave the sodium-retaining forces unopposed, leading to fluid retention and edema. Decreased dopaminergic activity and reduced urinary kallikrein and kinin excretion have been reported in this condition and may also be of pathogenetic importance.

TREATMENT   The treatment of idiopathic cyclic edema includes a reduction in salt intake, rest in the supine position for several hours each day, the wearing of elastic stockings (which are put on before arising in the morning), and an attempt to understand any underlying emotional problems. A variety of pharmacologic agents including ACE inhibitors, progesterone, the dopamine receptor agonist bromocriptine, and the sympathomimetic amine dextroamphetamine have all been reported to be useful when administered to patients who do not respond to simpler measures. Diuretics may be helpful initially but may lose their effectiveness with continuous administration; accordingly, they should be employed sparingly, if at all. Discontinuation of diuretics paradoxically leads to diuresis in "diuretic-induced" edema, described above.

DIFFERENTIAL DIAGNOSIS

The differences between the three major causes of generalized edema are shown in Table 37-2.

Localized edema can usually be readily differentiated from generalized edema. The great majority of patients with generalized edema suffer from advanced cardiac, renal, hepatic, or nutritional disorders. Consequently, the differential diagnosis of generalized edema should be directed toward identifying or excluding these several conditions.

LOCALIZED EDEMA (See also Chap. 248)   Edema originating from inflammation or hypersensitivity is usually readily identified. Localized edema due to venous or lymphatic obstruction may be caused by thrombophlebitis, chronic lymphangitis, resection of regional lymph nodes, filariasis, etc. Lymphedema is particularly intractable because restriction of lymphatic flow results in increased protein concentration in the interstitial fluid, a circumstance that aggravates retention of fluid.

EDEMA OF HEART FAILURE (See also Chap. 232)   The presence of heart disease, as manifested by cardiac enlargement and gallop rhythm, together with evidence of cardiac failure, such as dyspnea, basilar rales, venous distention, and hepatomegaly, usually provides an indication on clinical examination that edema results from heart failure. Noninvasive tests such as echocardiography and radionuclide angiography may be helpful in establishing the diagnosis of heart failure.

Table 37-2 Principal Causes of Generalized Edema: History, Physical Examination, and Laboratory Findings

Organ System	History	Physical Examination	Laboratory Findings
Cardiac	Dyspnea with exertion prominent—often associated with orthopnea—or paroxysmal nocturnal dyspnea	Elevated jugular venous pressure, ventricular (S_3) gallop; occasionally with displaced or dyskinetic apical pulse; peripheral cyanosis, cool extremities, small pulse pressure when severe	Elevated urea nitrogen–to–creatinine ratio common; elevated uric acid; serum sodium often diminished; liver enzymes occasionally elevated with hepatic congestion
Hepatic	Dyspnea infrequent, except if associated with significant degree of ascites; most often a history of ethanol abuse	Frequently associated with ascites; jugular venous pressure normal or low; blood pressure lower than in renal or cardiac disease; one or more additional signs of chronic liver disease (jaundice, palmar erythema, Dupuytren's contracture, spider angiomata, male gynecomastia; asterixis and other signs of encephalopathy) may be present	If severe, reductions in serum albumin, cholesterol, other hepatic proteins (transferrin, fibrinogen); liver enzymes elevated, depending on the cause and acuity of liver injury; tendency toward hypokalemia, respiratory alkalosis; macrocytosis from folate deficiency
Renal	Usually chronic: may be associated with uremic signs and symptoms, including decreased appetite, altered (metallic or fishy) taste, altered sleep pattern, difficulty concentrating, restless legs or myoclonus: dyspnea can be present, but generally less prominent than in heart failure	Blood pressure may be elevated; hypertensive or diabetic retinopathy in selected cases; nitrogenous fetor; periorbital edema may predominate; pericardial friction rub in advanced cases with uremia	Albuminuria, hypoalbuminemia; sometimes, elevation of serum creatinine and urea nitrogen; hyperkalemia, metabolic acidosis, hyperphosphatemia, hypocalcemia, anemia (usually normocytic)

NOTE: S_3, third heart sound.

SOURCE: From GM Chertow, GE Thibault, Approach to the patient with edema, in L Goldman, E Braunwald (eds): *Primary Cardiology.* Philadelphia, Saunders, 1998.

EDEMA OF THE NEPHROTIC SYNDROME (See also Chap. 274) Marked proteinuria (>3.5 g/d), hypoalbuminemia (<35 g/L), and in some instances hypercholesterolemia are present. This syndrome may occur during the course of a variety of kidney diseases, which include glomerulonephritis, diabetic glomerulosclerosis, and hypersensitivity reactions. A history of previous renal disease may or may not be elicited.

EDEMA OF ACUTE GLOMERULONEPHRITIS AND OTHER FORMS OF RENAL FAILURE The edema occurring during the acute phases of glomerulonephritis is characteristically associated with hematuria, proteinuria, and hypertension. Although some evidence supports the view that the fluid retention is due to increased capillary permeability, in most instances the edema in this disease results from primary retention of sodium and water by the kidneys owing to renal insufficiency. This state differs from congestive heart failure in that it is characterized by a normal (or sometimes even increased) cardiac output and a normal arterial–mixed venous oxygen difference. Patients with edema due to renal failure commonly have evidence of pulmonary congestion on chest roentgenograms before cardiac enlargement is significant, but they usually do not develop orthopnea. Patients with chronic impairment of renal function may also develop edema due to primary renal retention of sodium and water.

EDEMA OF CIRRHOSIS (See also Chap. 299) Ascites and biochemical and clinical evidence of hepatic disease (collateral venous channels, jaundice, and spider angiomas) characterize edema of hepatic origin. The ascites is frequently refractory to treatment because it collects as a result of a combination of obstruction of hepatic lymphatic drainage, portal hypertension, and hypoalbuminemia. Edema may also occur in other parts of the body in these patients as a result of hypoalbuminemia. Furthermore, the sizable accumulation of ascitic fluid may increase intraabdominal pressure and impede venous return from the lower extremities; hence, it tends to promote accumulation of edema in this region as well.

EDEMA OF NUTRITIONAL ORIGIN A diet grossly deficient in protein over a prolonged period may produce hypoproteinemia and edema. The latter may be intensified by the development of beriberi heart disease, also of nutritional origin, in which multiple peripheral arteriovenous fistulas result in reduced effective systemic perfusion and effective arterial blood volume, thereby enhancing edema formation (Chap. 75). Edema may actually become intensified when these famished subjects are first provided with an adequate diet. The ingestion of more food may increase the quantity of salt ingested, which is then retained along with water. So-called "refeeding edema" may also be linked to increased release of insulin, which directly increases tubular sodium reabsorption. In addition to hypoalbuminemia, hypokalemia and caloric deficits may be involved in the edema of starvation.

OTHER CAUSES OF EDEMA These include hypothyroidism, in which the edema (myxedema) may be located typically in the pretibial region and which may also be associated with periorbital puffiness. Exogenous hyperadrenocortism, pregnancy, and administration of estrogens and vasodilators, particularly the calcium antagonist nifedipine, may also all cause edema.

DISTRIBUTION OF EDEMA The distribution of edema is an important guide to the cause. Thus, edema limited to one leg or to one or both arms is usually the result of venous and/or lymphatic obstruction. Edema resulting from hypoproteinemia characteristically is generalized, but it is especially evident in the very soft tissues of the eyelids and face and tends to be most pronounced in the morning because of the recumbent posture assumed during the night. Less common causes of facial edema include trichinosis, allergic reactions, and myxedema. Edema associated with heart failure, on the other hand, tends to be more extensive in the legs and to be accentuated in the evening, a feature also determined largely by posture. When patients with heart failure have been confined to bed, edema may be most prominent in the presacral region. Unilateral edema occasionally results from lesions in the central nervous system affecting the vasomotor fibers on one side of the body; paralysis also reduces lymphatic and venous drainage on the affected side.

ADDITIONAL FACTORS IN DIAGNOSIS The color, thickness, and sensitivity of the skin are significant. Local tenderness and increase in temperature suggest inflammation. Local cyanosis may signify a venous obstruction. In individuals who have had repeated episodes of prolonged edema, the skin over the involved areas may be thickened, indurated, and often red.

Measurement or estimation of the venous pressure is of importance in evaluating edema. Elevation in an isolated part of the body usually reflects localized venous obstruction. Generalized elevation of systemic venous pressure usually indicates the presence of congestive heart failure. Ordinarily, a significant generalized increase in venous pressure can be recognized by the level at which cervical veins collapse (Chap. 225). In patients with obstruction of the superior vena cava, edema is confined to the face, neck, and upper extremities, where the venous pressure is elevated compared with that in the lower extremities. Measurement of venous pressure in the upper extremities is also useful in patients with massive edema of the lower extremities and ascites; it is elevated in the upper extremities when the edema is on a cardiac basis (e.g., constrictive pericarditis or tricuspid stenosis) but is normal when it is secondary to cirrhosis. Severe heart failure may cause ascites that may be distinguished from the ascites caused by hepatic cirrhosis by the jugular venous pressure, which usually is elevated in heart failure and normal in cirrhosis.

Determination of the concentration of serum albumin aids importantly in identifying those patients in whom edema is due, at least in part, to diminished intravascular colloid oncotic pressure. The presence of proteinuria also affords useful clues. The absence of proteinuria excludes nephrotic syndrome but cannot exclude nonproteinuric causes of renal failure. Slight to moderate proteinuria is the rule in patients with heart failure.

Approach to the Patient

An important first question is whether the edema is localized or generalized. If it is localized, those phenomena that may be responsible should be concentrated upon. Hydrothorax and ascites are forms of localized edema. Either may be a consequence of local venous or lymphatic obstruction, as in inflammatory or neoplastic disease.

If the edema is generalized, it should be determined, first, if there is serious hypoalbuminemia, e.g., serum albumin <25 g/L. If so, the history, physical examination, urinalysis, and other laboratory data will help evaluate the question of cirrhosis, severe malnutrition, protein-losing gastroenteropathy, or the nephrotic syndrome as the underlying disorder. If hypoalbuminemia is not present, it should be determined if there is evidence of congestive heart failure of a severity to promote generalized edema. Finally, it should be determined whether the patient has an adequate urine output, or if there is significant oliguria or even anuria.→*These abnormalities are discussed in Chaps. 47, 269, and 270.*

BIBLIOGRAPHY

ANAND IS et al: Studies of body water and sodium, renal function, hemodynamic indexes, and plasma hormones in untreated congestive heart failure. Circulation 80:299, 1989
BRATER DC: Diuretic therapy. N Engl J Med 339:387, 1998
DISKIN CJ et al: Edema, oncotic pressure, and free entropy: Novel considerations for treatment of edema through attention to thermodynamics. Nephron 78:131, 1998
GOLDEN MHN: Protein deficiency, energy deficiency, and the oedema of malnutrition. Lancet 1:1261, 1982
LEIER C, BOUDOULAS H: Renal disorders and heart disease, in *Heart Disease*, 6th ed, E Braunwald, D Zipes, P Libby (eds). Philadelphia, Saunders, 2001
MILLER JA et al: Control of extracellular fluid volume and the pathophysiology of edema formation, in *The Kidney*, 6th ed, BM Brenner (ed). Philadelphia, Saunders, 2000, pp 795–865
SCHRIER RW, FASSETT RG: A critique of the overfill hypothesis of sodium and water retention in the nephrotic syndrome. Kidney Int 53:1111, 1998
STREETEN DH: Idiopathic edema. Pathogenesis, clinical features, and treatment. Endocrinol Metab Clin North Am 24:531, 1995

38   *Ronald V. Maier*

SHOCK

Shock is the clinical syndrome that results from inadequate tissue perfusion. Irrespective of cause, the hypoperfusion-induced imbalance between the delivery of and requirements for oxygen and substrate leads to cellular dysfunction. The cellular injury created by the inadequate delivery of oxygen and substrates also induces the production and release of inflammatory mediators that further compromise perfusion through functional and structural changes within the microvasculature. This leads to a vicious cycle in which impaired perfusion is responsible for cellular injury which causes maldistribution of blood flow, further

Table 38-1   Classification of Shock

Hypovolemic	Septic
Traumatic	Hyperdynamic
Cardiogenic	Hypodynamic
Intrinsic	Neurogenic
Compressive	Hypoadrenal

compromising cellular perfusion; the latter causes multiple organ failure and, if the process is not interrupted, leads to the death of the patient. The clinical manifestations of shock are the result, in part, of sympathetic neuroendocrine responses to hypoperfusion as well as the breakdown in organ function induced by severe cellular dysfunction.

When very severe and/or persistent, inadequate oxygen delivery leads to irreversible cell injury, and only rapid restoration of oxygen delivery can reverse the progression of the shock state. The fundamental approach to management, therefore, is to recognize overt and impending shock in a timely fashion and to intervene emergently to restore perfusion. Except in cases of cardiogenic shock, this requires the expansion or reexpansion of blood volume. Control of any inciting pathologic process, e.g., continued hemorrhage, impairment of cardiac function, or infection, must occur simultaneously.

Clinical shock is usually accompanied by hypotension, i.e., a mean arterial pressure <60 mmHg in previously normotensive persons. Multiple classification schemes have been developed in an attempt to synthesize the seemingly dissimilar processes leading to shock. Strict adherence to a classification scheme may be difficult from a clinical standpoint because of the frequent combination of two or more causes of shock in any individual patient, but the classification shown in Table 38-1 provides a useful reference point from which to discuss and further delineate the underlying processes. The individual classes are discussed below.

PATHOGENESIS AND ORGAN RESPONSE

MICROCIRCULATION   Normally when cardiac output falls, systemic vascular resistance rises to maintain a level of systemic pressure that is adequate to allow perfusion of the heart and brain at the expense of other tissues, especially muscle, skin, and the gastrointestinal tract. Systemic vascular resistance is determined primarily by the luminal diameter of arterioles. The metabolic rates of the heart and brain are high, and their stores of energy substrate are low. These organs are critically dependent on a continuous supply of oxygen and nutrients, and neither tolerates severe ischemia for more than brief periods. Autoregulation, i.e., the maintenance of blood flow over a wide range of perfusion pressures, is critical in sustaining cerebral and coronary perfusion despite significant hypotension. However, when mean arterial pressure drops to ≤60 mmHg, flow to these organs falls and their function deteriorates.

Arteriolar vascular smooth muscle has both α- and β-adrenergic receptors (Chap. 72). The α_1 receptors mediate vasoconstriction, while the β_2 receptors mediate vasodilation. Efferent sympathetic fibers release norepinephrine, which acts primarily on α_1 receptors in one of the most fundamental compensatory responses to reduced perfusion pressure. Other constrictor substances that are increased in most forms of shock include angiotensin II, vasopressin, endothelin-1, and thromboxane A_2. Both norepinephrine and epinephrine are released by the adrenal medulla, and the concentrations of these catecholamines in the blood stream rise. Circulating vasodilators in shock include prostacyclin (PGI_2), nitric oxide (NO), and, importantly, products of local metabolism such as adenosine that match flow to the metabolic needs of the tissue. The balance between these various vasoconstrictor and vasodilator influences acting upon the microcirculation determines local perfusion.

Transport to cells depends on microcirculatory flow; capillary permeability; the diffusion of oxygen, carbon dioxide, nutrients, and products of metabolism through the interstitium; and the exchange of these products across cell membranes. Impairment of the microcirculation, which is central to the pathophysiologic responses in the late stages of all forms of shock, results in the derangement of cellular metabolism, which is ultimately responsible for organ failure.

The normal response to mild or moderate hypovolemia is an attempt at restitution of intravascular volume through alterations in hydrostatic pressure and osmolarity. Constriction of arterioles leads to reductions in both the capillary hydrostatic pressure and the number of capillary beds perfused, thereby limiting the capillary surface area across which filtration occurs. When filtration is reduced while intravascular oncotic pressure remains constant or rises, there is net reabsorption of fluid into the vascular bed, in accord with Starling's law of capillary-interstitial liquid exchange (Chap. 32). Metabolic changes (including hyperglycemia and elevations in the products of glycolysis, lipolysis, and proteolysis) raise extracellular osmolarity, leading to an osmotic gradient between cells and interstitium that increases interstitial and intravascular volume at the expense of intracellular volume.

CELLULAR RESPONSES Interstitial transport of nutrients is impaired, leading to a decline of intracellular high-energy phosphate stores. Mitochondrial dysfunction and uncoupling of oxidative phosphorylation are the most likely causes for decreased amounts of ATP. As a consequence, there is an accumulation of anaerobic metabolites including hydrogen ions, lactate, and other products of anaerobic metabolism. As shock progresses, these vasodilator metabolites override vasomotor tone, causing further hypotension and hypoperfusion. Dysfunction of cell membranes is thought to represent a common end-stage pathophysiologic pathway in the various forms of shock. Normal cellular transmembrane potential falls, and there is an associated increase in intracellular sodium and water, leading to cell swelling, which interferes further with microvascular perfusion.

NEUROENDOCRINE RESPONSE Hypovolemia, hypotension, and hypoxia are sensed by baroreceptors and chemoreceptors, which contribute further to an autonomic response that attempts to restore blood volume, maintain central perfusion, and mobilize metabolic substrates. Hypotension disinhibits the vasomotor center, resulting in increased adrenergic output and reduced vagal activity. Release of norepinephrine induces peripheral and splanchnic vasoconstriction, a major contributor to the maintenance of central organ perfusion, while reduced vagal activity increases the heart rate and cardiac output. The effects of circulating epinephrine released by the adrenal medulla in shock are largely metabolic, causing increased glycogenolysis and gluconeogenesis and reduced pancreatic insulin release.

Severe pain and other severe stress cause the hypothalamic release of adrenocorticotropic hormone (ACTH). This stimulates cortisol secretion, which contributes to decreased peripheral uptake of glucose and amino acids, enhances lipolysis, and increases gluconeogenesis. Increased pancreatic secretion of glucagon during stress accelerates hepatic gluconeogenesis and further elevates blood glucose concentration. These hormonal actions act synergistically in the maintenance of blood volume. The importance of the cortisol response to stress is illustrated by the profound circulatory collapse that occurs in hypoadrenal patients (see below).

Renin release is increased in response to adrenergic discharge and reduced perfusion of the juxtaglomerular apparatus in the kidney. Renin induces the formation of angiotensin I, which is then converted to angiotensin II, an extremely potent vasoconstrictor and stimulator of aldosterone release by the adrenal cortex and of vasopressin by the posterior pituitary. Aldosterone contributes to the maintainance of intravascular volume by enhancing renal tubular reabsorption of sodium, resulting in the excretion of a low-volume, concentrated, sodium-free urine. Vasopressin has a direct action on vascular smooth muscle, contributing to vasoconstriction, and acts on the distal renal tubules to enhance water reabsorption.

CARDIOVASCULAR RESPONSE Three variables—ventricular filling (preload), the resistance to ventricular ejection (afterload), and myocardial contractility—are paramount in controlling stroke volume (Chap. 231). Cardiac output, the major determinant of tissue perfusion, is the product of stroke volume and heart rate. Hy-

povolemia leads to decreased ventricular preload, which in turn reduces the stroke volume. An increase in heart rate is a useful but limited compensatory mechanism to maintain cardiac output. A shock-induced reduction in myocardial compliance is frequent, reducing ventricular end-diastolic volume and hence stroke volume at any given ventricular filling pressure. Restoration of intravascular volume then returns stroke volume to normal but only at elevated filling pressures. In addition, sepsis, ischemia, myocardial infarction, severe tissue trauma, hypothermia, general anesthesia, prolonged hypotension, and acidemia may all impair myocardial contractility and also reduce the stroke volume at any given ventricular end-diastolic volume. The resistance to ventricular ejection is influenced importantly by the systemic vascular resistance, which is elevated in most forms of shock. However, resistance is depressed in the early hyperdynamic stage of septic shock (see below), thereby allowing the cardiac output to be maintained.

The venous system contains nearly two-thirds of the total circulating blood volume, most in the small veins, and serves as a dynamic reservoir for autoinfusion of blood. Active venoconstriction as a consequence of α-adrenergic activity is an important compensatory mechanism for the maintenance of venous return and therefore of ventricular filling during shock. On the other hand, venous dilatation, as occurs in neurogenic shock, reduces ventricular filling and hence stroke volume and cardiac output (see below).

PULMONARY RESPONSE The response of the pulmonary vascular bed to shock parallels that of the systemic vascular bed, and the relative increase in pulmonary vascular resistance, particularly in septic shock, may exceed that of the systemic vascular resistance. Shock-induced tachypnea reduces tidal volume and increases both dead space and minute ventilation. Relative hypoxia and the subsequent tachypnea induce a respiratory alkalosis. Recumbency and involuntary restriction of ventilation secondary to pain reduce functional residual capacity and may lead to atelectasis. Shock is recognized as a major cause of acute lung injury and subsequent acute respiratory distress syndrome (ARDS; Chap. 265). These disorders are characterized by noncardiogenic pulmonary edema secondary to diffuse pulmonary capillary endothelial and alveolar epithelial injury, hypoxemia, and bilateral diffuse pulmonary infiltrates. Hypoxemia results from perfusion of underventilated and nonventilated alveoli. Loss of surfactant and lung volume in combination with increased interstitial and alveolar edema reduce lung compliance. The work of breathing and the oxygen requirements of respiratory muscles increase.

RENAL RESPONSE Acute renal failure (Chap. 269), a serious complication of shock and hypoperfusion, occurs less frequently than heretofore because of early aggressive volume repletion. Acute tubular necrosis is now more frequently seen as a result of the interactions of shock, sepsis, the administration of nephrotoxic agents (such as aminoglycosides and angiographic contrast media), and rhabdomyolysis; the latter may be particularly severe in skeletal muscle trauma. The physiologic response of the kidney to hypoperfusion is to conserve salt and water. In addition to decreased renal blood flow, increased afferent arteriolar resistance accounts for diminished glomerular filtration rate, which together with increased ADH and aldosterone is responsible for reduced urine formation. Toxic injury causes necrosis of tubular epithelium and tubular obstruction by cellular debris with back-leak of filtrate. The depletion of renal ATP stores that occurs with prolonged renal hypoperfusion is related to subsequent impairment of renal function.

METABOLIC DERANGEMENTS During shock, there is disruption of the normal cycles of carbohydrate, lipid, and protein metabolism. Through the citric acid cycle, alanine in conjunction with lactate (which is converted from pyruvate in the periphery in the presence of oxygen deprivation) enhances the hepatic production of glucose. With reduced availability of oxygen, the breakdown of glucose to pyruvate and ultimately lactate represents an inefficient cycling of substrate with minimal net energy production. An elevated plasma

Table 38-2 Normal Hemodynamic Parameters

Parameter	Calculation	Normal Values
Cardiac output (CO)	SV × HR	4–8 L/min
Cardiac index (CI)	CO/BSA	2.6–4.2 (L/min)/m^2
Stroke volume (SV)	CO/HR	50–100 mL/beat
Systemic vascular resistance (SVR)	[(MAP − RAP)/CO] × 80	700–1600 dynes · s/cm^5
Pulmonary vascular resistance (PVR)	[(PAP$_m$ − PCWP)/CO] × 80	20–130 dynes · s/cm^5
Left ventricular stroke work (LVSW)	SV(MAP − PCWP) × 0.0136	60–80 g-m/beat
Right ventricular stroke work (RVSW)	SV(PAP$_m$ − RAP)	10–15 g-m/beat

NOTE: HR, heart rate; BSA, body surface area; MAP, mean arterial pressure; RAP, right atrial pressure; PAP$_m$, pulmonary artery pressure—mean; PCWP, pulmonary capillary wedge pressure.

lactate/pyruvate ratio is consistent with anaerobic metabolism and reflects inadequate tissue perfusion. Decreased clearance of exogenous triglycerides coupled with increased hepatic lipogenesis causes a significant rise in serum triglyceride concentrations. There is increased protein catabolism, a negative nitrogen balance, and, if the process is prolonged, severe muscle wasting.

INFLAMMATORY RESPONSES Activation of an extensive network of proinflammatory mediator systems plays a significant role in the progression of shock and contributes importantly to the development of organ injury and failure.

Multiple humoral mediators are activated during shock and tissue injury. The complement cascade, activated through both the classic and alternate pathways, generates the anaphylatoxins C3a and C5a. Direct complement fixation to injured tissues can progress to the C5-C9 attack complex, causing further cell damage. Activation of the coagulation cascade causes microvascular thrombosis, with subsequent lysis leading to repeated episodes of ischemia and reperfusion. Components of the coagulation system, such as thrombin, are potent proinflammatory mediators that cause expression of adhesion molecules on endothelial cells and activation of neutrophils, leading to microvascular injury. Coagulation also activates the kallekrein-kininogen cascade, contributing to hypotension.

Eicosanoids are vasoactive and immunomodulatory products of arachidonic acid metabolism that include cyclooxygenase-derived prostaglandins and thromboxane A$_2$ as well as lipoxygenase-derived leukotrienes and lipoxins. Thromboxane A$_2$ is a potent vasoconstrictor that contributes to the pulmonary hypertension and acute tubular necrosis of shock. PGI$_2$ and prostaglandin E$_2$ are potent vasodilators that enhance capillary permeability and edema formation. The cysteinyl leukotrienes LTC$_4$ and LTD$_4$ are pivotal mediators of the vascular sequelae of anaphylaxis, as well as of shock states resulting from sepsis or tissue injury. LTB$_4$ is a potent neutrophil chemoattractant and secretagogue that stimulates the formation of reactive oxygen species. Lipoxins are endogenous autocoids that inhibit leukotriene-mediated responses. Platelet-activating factor, an ether-linked, arachidonyl-containing phospholipid mediator, also carries potent bioactivities that include pulmonary vasoconstriction, bronchoconstriction, systemic vasodilation, increased capillary permeability, and the priming of macrophages and neutrophils to produce enhanced levels of inflammatory mediators.

Tumor necrosis factor (TNF) α, produced by activated macrophages, reproduces many components of the shock state including hypotension, lactic acidosis, and respiratory failure. Interleukin (IL) 1 is also produced by tissue-fixed macrophages and is critical to the inflammatory response occurring in hypoperfusion and septic states. Chemokines also participate in the systemic inflammatory response. For example, IL-8 is a potent neutrophil chemoattractant and activator that upregulates adhesion molecules on the neutrophil to enhance aggregation and adherence to the vascular endothelium. The endothelium normally produces nitric oxide (NO), a potent vasodilator. The inflammatory response stimulates the inducible isoform of NO synthase (iNOS), which is thought to overexpress toxic NO and oxygen-derived free radicals and contributes to the hyperdynamic cardiovascular response that occurs in sepsis.

Multiple inflammatory cells, including neutrophils, macrophages, and platelets, are a major contributor to inflammation-induced injury. Margination of activated neutrophils in the microcirculation is a common pathologic finding in shock, causing secondary injury due to the release of potentially toxic oxygen radicals and proteases. Adhesion molecules are expressed on the surface of the endothelium and on cytokine-stimulated neutrophils. Tissue-fixed macrophages produce virtually all major components of the inflammatory response and orchestrate the progression and duration of the response.

Approach to the Patient

The underlying problem in all forms of shock is inadequate tissue perfusion and an imbalance between delivery and cellular needs of oxygen and metabolic substrate. It is important to recognize the onset of hypoperfusion at the earliest possible time in order to institute aggressive resuscitation and correction of the underlying etiology.

Monitoring Patients in shock require care in an intensive care unit. Careful and continuous assessment of the physiologic status is necessary. Arterial pressure through an indwelling line, pulse, and respiratory rate should be monitored continuously; a Foley catheter should be inserted to follow urine flow; and mental status assessed frequently.

Although there is ongoing debate as to the indications for using the flow-directed pulmonary artery catheter (PAC, Swan-Ganz catheter) in the management of patients in shock, most intensivists believe that the ability to predict the hemodynamic profiles of patients in shock accurately without a PAC is poor. The PAC is placed percutaneously via the subclavian or jugular vein through the central venous circulation and right heart into the pulmonary artery. There are ports both proximal in the right atrium and distal in the pulmonary artery to provide access for infusions and for cardiac output measurements. Right atrial and pulmonary artery pressures are measured, and the pulmonary capillary wedge pressure (PCWP) serves as an approximation of the left atrial pressure. Normal hemodynamic parameters are shown in Table 228-3 and Table 38-2.

Cardiac output is determined by the thermodilution technique, and high-resolution thermistors can also be used to determine right ventricular end-diastolic volume to monitor further the response of the right heart to fluid resuscitation. A PAC with an oximeter port offers the additional advantage of on-line monitoring of the mixed venous oxygen saturation, an important index of tissue perfusion. Systemic and pulmonary vascular resistances are calculated as the ratio of the pressure drop across these vascular beds to the cardiac output (Chap. 228). Determinations of oxygen content in arterial and venous blood, together with cardiac output and hemoglobin concentration allow calculation of oxygen delivery, oxygen consumption, and oxygen-extraction ratio (Table 38-3). The hemodynamic patterns associated with the various form of shock are shown in Table 38-4.

In resuscitation from shock, it is critical to restore tissue perfusion and optimize oxygen delivery, hemodynamics, and cardiac function rapidly. A goal of therapy is to achieve normal mixed venous oxygen saturation and arteriovenous oxygen-extraction ratio. To enhance oxygen delivery, red cell mass, arterial oxygen saturation, and cardiac output may be augmented singly or simultaneously. An increase in oxygen delivery not accompanied by an increase in oxygen consumption implies that oxygen availability is adequate and that oxygen consumption is not flow-dependent. Conversely, an elevation of oxygen consumption with increased cardiac output implies that the oxygen supply is inadequate. A reduction in systemic vascular resistance accompanying an increase in cardiac output indicates that compensatory vasoconstriction is reversing due to improved tissue perfusion. The determination of stepwise expansion of blood volume on cardiac performance allows identification of the optimum preload.

SPECIFIC FORMS OF SHOCK

HYPOVOLEMIC SHOCK This most common form of shock results either from the loss of red blood cell mass and plasma from hemorrhage or from the loss of plasma volume alone arising from extravascular fluid sequestration or gastrointestinal, urinary, and insensible losses. The signs and symptoms of nonhemorrhagic hypovolemic shock are the same as those of hemorrhagic shock, although they may have a more insidious onset. The normal physiologic response to hypovolemia is to maintain perfusion of the brain and heart while restoring an effective circulating blood volume. There is an increase in sympathetic activity, hyperventilation, collapse of venous capacitance vessels, release of stress hormones, and expansion of intravascular volume through the recruitment of interstitial and intracellular fluid and reduction of urine output.

Mild hypovolemia ($\leq 20\%$ of the blood volume) generates mild tachycardia but relatively few external signs, especially in a supine resting young patient (Table 38-5). With moderate hypovolemia (~ 20 to 40% of the blood volume) the patient becomes increasingly anxious and tachycardic; although normal blood pressure may be maintained in the supine position, there may be significant postural hypotension and tachycardia. If hypovolemia is severe ($\geq \sim 40\%$ of the blood volume), the classic signs of shock appear; the blood pressure declines and becomes unstable even in the supine position, and the patient develops marked tachycardia, oliguria, and agitation or confusion. Perfusion of the central nervous system is well maintained until shock becomes severe. Hence, mental obtundation is an ominous clinical sign. The transition from mild to severe hypovolemic shock can be insidious or extremely rapid. If severe shock is not reversed rapidly, especially in elderly patients and those with comorbid illnesses, death is imminent. A very narrow time frame separates the derangements found in severe shock that can be reversed with aggressive resuscitation from those of progressive decompensation and irreversible cell injury.

Diagnosis Hypovolemic shock is readily diagnosed when there are signs of hemodynamic instability and the source of volume loss is obvious. The diagnosis is more difficult when the source of blood loss is occult, as into the gastrointestinal tract, or when plasma volume alone is depleted. After acute hemorrhage, hemoglobin and hematocrit values do not change until compensatory fluid shifts have occurred or exogenous fluid is administered. Thus, an initial normal hematocrit does not disprove the presence of significant blood loss. Plasma losses cause hemoconcentration, and free water loss leads to hypernatremia. These findings should suggest the presence of hypovolemia.

It is essential to distinguish between hypovolemic and cardiogenic shock (see below) because definitive therapy differs significantly. Both forms are associated with a reduced cardiac output and a compensatory sympathetic mediated response characterized by tachycardia and elevated systemic vascular resistance. However, the findings in cardiogenic shock of jugular venous distention, rales, and an S_3 gallop distinguish it from hypovolemic shock and signify that volume expansion is undesirable.

℞ **TREATMENT** Initial resuscitation requires rapid reexpansion of the circulating blood volume along with interventions to control ongoing losses. In accordance with Starling's law (Chap. 231), stroke volume and cardiac output rise with the increase in preload. After resuscitation, the compliance of the ventricles may remain re-

Table 38-3 Oxygen Transport Calculations

Parameter	Calculation	Normal Values
Oxygen-carrying capacity of hemoglobin		1.39 mL/g
Plasma O_2 concentration		$P_{O_2} \times 0.0031$
Arterial O_2 concentration (Ca_{O_2})	$1.39\ SaO_2 + 0.0031\ Pa_{O_2}$	20 vol%
Venous O_2 concentration (Cv_{O_2})	$1.39\ Sv_{O_2} + 0.0031\ Pv_{O_2}$	15.5 vol%
Arteriovenous O_2 difference ($Ca_{O_2} - Cv_{O_2}$)	$1.39\ (Sa_{O_2} - Sv_{O_2}) + 0.0031\ (Pa_{O_2} - Pv_{O_2})$	3.5 vol%
Oxygen delivery (D_{O_2})	$Ca_{O_2} \times CO\ (L/min) \times 10\ (dL/L)$ $1.39\ Sa_{O_2} \times CO \times 10$	800–1600 mL/min
Oxygen uptake (V_{O_2})	$(Ca_{O_2} - Cv_{O_2}) \times CO \times 10$ $1.39\ (Sa_{O_2} - Sv_{O_2}) \times CO \times 10$	150–400 mL/min
Oxygen delivery index ($D_{O_2}I$)	D_{O_2}/BSA	520–720 (mL/min)/m²
Oxygen uptake index ($V_{O_2}I$)	V_{O_2}/BSA	115–165 (mL/min)/m²
Oxygen extraction ratio (O_2ER)	$[1 - (\dot{V}_{O_2}/\dot{D}_{O_2})] \times 100$	22–32%

NOTE: P_{O_2}, partial pressure of oxygen; Sa_{O_2}, saturation of hemoglobin with O_2 in arterial blood; Pa_{O_2}, partial pressure of O_2 in arterial blood; Sv_{O_2}, saturation of hemoglobin with O_2 in venous blood; Pv_{O_2}, partial pressure of O_2 in venous blood; CO, Cardiac output; BSA, body surface area.

Table 38-4 Physiologic Characteristics of the Various Forms of Shock

Type of Shock	CVP and PCWP	Cardiac Output	Systemic Vascular Resistance	Venous O_2 Saturation
Hypovolemic	↓	↓	↑	↓
Cardiogenic	↑	↓	↑	↓
Septic				
Hyperdynamic	↓ ↑	↑	↓	↑
Hypodynamic	↓ ↑	↓	↑	↑ ↓
Traumatic	↓	↓ ↑	↑ ↓	↓
Neurogenic	↓	↓	↓	↓
Hypoadrenal	↓ ↑	↓	= ↓	↓

NOTE: CVP, central venous pressure; PCWP, pulmonary capillary wedge pressure.

Table 38-5 Hypovolemic Shock

Mild (<20% Blood Volume)	Moderate (20–40% Blood Volume)	Severe (>40% Blood Volume)
Cool extremities	Same, plus:	Same, plus:
Increased capillary refill time	Tachycardia	Hemodynamic instability
Diaphoresis	Tachypnea	Marked tachycardia
Collapsed veins	Oliguria	Hypotension
Anxiety	Postural changes	Mental status deterioration (coma)

duced due to increased interstitial fluid in the myocardium. Therefore, elevated filling pressures are required to maintain adequate ventricular performance.

Volume resuscitation is initiated with the rapid infusion of isotonic saline or a balanced salt solution such as Ringer's lactate through large-bore intravenous lines. No distinct benefit from the use of colloid has been demonstrated. The infusion of 2 to 3 L over 10 to 30 min should restore normal hemodynamic parameters. Continued hemodynamic instability implies that shock has not been reversed and/or that there are significant ongoing blood or volume losses. Continuing blood loss, with hemoglobin concentrations declining to ≤ 100 g/L (10 g/dL), should initiate blood transfusion, preferably as fully cross-matched blood. In extreme emergencies, type-specific or O-negative packed red cells may be transfused. In the presence of severe and/or prolonged hypovolemia, inotropic support with dopamine or dobutamine (Chap. 72) may be required to maintain adequate ventricular performance, after blood volume has been restored. Infusion of norepinephrine to increase arterial pressure by raising peripheral resistance is inappropriate, other than as a temporizing measure in severe shock while blood volume is reexpanded.

Successful resuscitation also requires support of respiratory function. Supplemental oxygen should be provided, and endotracheal intubation may be necessary to maintain arterial oxygenation. Following resuscitation from isolated hemorrhagic shock, end-organ damage is frequently less than following septic or traumatic shock. This may be due to the absence of the massive activation of inflammatory mediator response systems and the consequent nonspecific organ injury seen in the latter conditions.

TRAUMATIC SHOCK   Shock following trauma is, in large measure, due to hypovolemia. However, even when hemorrhage has been controlled, patients can continue to suffer loss of plasma volume into the interstitium of injured tissues. These fluid losses are compounded by injury-induced inflammatory responses, which contribute to the secondary microcirculatory injury. This causes secondary tissue injury and maldistribution of blood flow, intensifying tissue ischemia and leading to multiple organ system failure. Trauma to the heart, chest, or head can also contribute to the shock. For example, pericardial tamponade or tension pneumothorax impairs ventricular filling, while myocardial contusion depresses myocardial contractility.

℞ **TREATMENT**   Inability to maintain a systolic blood pressure ≥90 mmHg after trauma-inudced hypovolemia is associated with a mortality rate of ~50%. To prevent decompensation of homeostatic mechanisms, therapy must be promptly administered.

The initial management of the seriously injured patient requires attention to the "ABCs" of resuscitation: assurance of an airway (A), adequate ventilation (breathing, B), and establishment of an adequate blood volume to support the circulation (C). Control of hemorrhage requires immediate attention. Early stabilization of fractures, debridement of devitalized or contaminated tissues, and evacuation of hematomata all reduce the subsequent inflammatory response to the initial insult and minimize subsequent organ injury.

INTRINSIC CARDIOGENIC SHOCK   This form of shock is caused by failure, often sudden, of the heart as an effective pump. It occurs most commonly as a complication of acute myocardial infarction (AMI; Chap. 243), but it may also be seen in patients with severe brady- or tachyarrhythmias, valvular heart disease, or in the terminal stage of chronic heart failure of any cause, including ischemic heart disease and dilated cardiomyopathy. Cardiogenic shock is characterized by a low cardiac output, diminished peripheral perfusion, pulmonary congestion, and elevation of systemic vascular resistance and pulmonary vascular pressures. Acute right heart failure can arise as the result of right ventricular infarction or may complicate the acute respiratory distress syndrome and severe pulmonary hypertension of any etiology. As a consequence of right ventricular failure, left ventricular preload falls, and this, in turn, reduces systemic perfusion. In contrast to other forms of shock, absolute or relative hypovolemia is usually not present in cardiogenic shock.

The ineffective contractile activity of either the right or left side of the heart leads to the accumulation of blood in the venous circulation upstream to the failing ventricle. Cardiogenic shock with left-sided heart failure increases fluid in the lungs that can overwhelm the capacity of the pulmonary lymphatics and causes interstitial and sometimes alveolar edema. Interstitial lung edema usually occurs at pulmonary capillary pressures >18 mmHg, and overt pulmonary alveolar edema develops at pressures >24 mmHg (Chap. 32). Pulmonary edema impacts cardiac function further by impairing diffusion of oxygen, setting up a vicious cycle. The increase in interstitial and intraalveolar fluid causes a progressive reduction in lung compliance, thereby increasing the work of ventilation while increasing perfusion of poorly ventilated alveoli.

In establishing the diagnosis of cardiogenic shock, a history of cardiac disease or of AMI is of value. Associated physical findings include those of hemodynamic instability, peripheral vasoconstriction, and pulmonary and/or systemic venous congestion, as well as findings specific to the underlying cardiac abnormalities. An electrocardiogram may provide evidence of AMI or preexisting cardiac disease. The chest

x-ray may show pulmonary edema and cardiomegaly. Transthoracic or transesophageal echocardiograms assist in the diagnosis of structural abnormalities and/or functional impairment of contractility. Serum cardiac markers will support the diagnosis of acute cardiac injury. Hemodynamic monitoring is usually necessary. Placement of a PAC is helpful and will show a reduced cardiac output and an elevated PCWP, and direct measurement of right atrial pressure allows calculation of systemic vascular resistance which is elevated.

℞ **TREATMENT**   For all forms of cardiogenic shock, preload, afterload, and contractility should be modified using the information provided by the PAC. A PCWP of 15 to 20 mmHg should be the initial goal. If the PCWP is excessively elevated, inotropic agents may provide significant reduction. The goal is to increase contractility without significant increases in heart rate. Dopamine and norepinephrine exert both inotropic and vasoconstrictor actions (Chap. 72) that are useful in the presence of persistent hypotension. Dobutamine, a positive inotropic agent with vasodilator properties, may be substituted when arterial pressure has been restored. Pulmonary congestion may be responsive to intravenous furosemide. Patients with an inadequate response to these measures can be supported by using intraaortic balloon counterpulsation to permit recovery of myocardial function. Additional measures to consider in cases of refractory cardiogenic shock include urgent myocardial revascularization in patients with AMI (Chap. 243), correction of anatomic cardiac defects such as rupture of the papillary muscles of the interventricular septum, the placement of ventricular assist devices, and even urgent cardiac transplantation.

COMPRESSIVE CARDIOGENIC SHOCK   With compression, the heart and surrounding structures are less compliant and, thus, normal filling pressures generate inadequate diastolic filling. Blood or fluid within the poorly distensible pericardial sac may cause tamponade (Chap. 239). Any cause of increased intrathoracic pressure, such as tension pneumothorax, herniation of abdominal viscera through a diaphragmatic hernia, or excessive positive pressure ventilation to support pulmonary function, can also cause compressive cardiogenic shock. Acute right heart failure with a sudden decline in cardiac output can be caused by pulmonary embolism obstructing right ventricular outflow and impairing left ventricular filling. Although initially responsive to increased filling pressures produced by volume expansion, as compression increases, cardiogenic shock occurs.

The diagnosis of compressive cardiogenic shock is most frequently based on clinical findings, the chest radiograph, and an echocardiogram. The diagnosis of compressive cardiac shock may be more difficult to establish in the setting of trauma when hypovolemia and cardiac compression are present simultaneously. The classic findings of pericardial tamponade include the triad of hypotension, neck vein distention, and muffled heart sounds (Chap. 239). Pulsus paradoxus, i.e., an inspiratory reduction in systolic pressure >10 mmHg, may also be noted. The diagnosis is confirmed by echocardiography, and treatment consists of immediate pericardiocentesis. A tension pneumothorax produces ipsilateral decreased breath sounds, tracheal deviation away from the affected thorax, and jugular venous distention. Radiographic findings include increased intrathoracic volume, depression of the diaphragm of the affected hemithorax, and shifting of the mediastinum to the contralateral side. Chest decompression must be carried out immediately. Release of air and restoration of normal cardiovascular dynamics is both diagnostic and therapeutic.

SEPTIC SHOCK   (See also Chap. 124)   This form of shock is caused by the systemic response to a severe infection. It occurs most frequently in elderly or immunocompromised patients and in those who have undergone an invasive procedure in which bacterial contamination has occurred. Infections of the lung, abdomen, or urinary tract are most common, and approximately half of the patients have bacteremia. Gram-positive and -negative bacteria, viruses, fungi, rickettsiae, and protozoa have all been reported to produce the clinical picture of septic shock, and the overall response is generally independent of the specific type of invading organism. The clinical findings in septic shock are a consequence of the combination of metabolic and circulatory derangements driven by the systemic infection and the release of toxic components of the infectious organisms, e.g., the endotoxin of gram-negative bacteria or the exotoxins and enterotoxins of gram-positive bacteria. Organism toxins lead to the release of cytokines, including IL-1 and TNF-α, from tissue macrophages. Tissue factor expression and fibrin deposition are increased, and disseminated intravascular coagulation may develop. The inducible form of NO synthase is stimulated, and NO, a powerful vasodilator, is released. Hemodynamic changes in septic shock occur in two characteristic patterns: early, or hyperdynamic, and late, or hypodynamic, septic shock.

Hyperdynamic Response In hyperdynamic septic shock, tachycardia is present, the cardiac output is normal, and the systemic vascular resistance is reduced while the pulmonary vascular resistance is elevated. The extremities are usually warm. However, splanchnic vasoconstriction with decreased visceral flow is present. The venous capacitance is increased, which decreases venous return. With volume expansion cardiac output becomes supranormal. Myocardial contractility is depressed in septic shock by mediators including NO, IL-1, and/or TNF-α. Inflammatory mediator–induced processes include increased capillary permeability and continued loss of intravascular volume.

In septic shock, in contrast to other types of shock, total oxygen delivery may be increased while oxygen extraction is reduced due to maldistribution of microcirculatory perfusion and impaired utilization. In this setting the presence of a normal mixed venous oxygen saturation is not indicative of adequate peripheral perfusion, and even though the cardiac output may be elevated, it is still inadequate to meet the total metabolic needs. The toxicity of the infectious agents and their byproducts and the subsequent metabolic dysfunction drive the progressive deterioration of cellular and organ function. Acute respiratory distress syndrome, thrombocytopenia, and neutropenia are common complications.

Hypodynamic Response As sepsis progresses, vasoconstriction occurs and the cardiac output declines. The patient usually becomes markedly tachypneic, febrile, diaphoretic, and obtunded, with cool, mottled, and often cyanotic extremities. Oliguria, renal failure, and hypothermia develop; there may be striking increases in serum lactate.

℞ TREATMENT Aggressive volume expansion with a crystalloid solution to a PCWP of approximately 15 mmHg and the restoration of arterial oxygenation with inspired oxygen and frequently with mechanical ventilation are the highest priorities. In the presence of hypodynamic septic shock, augmentation of cardiac output may require inotropic support with dopamine or norepinephrine in the presence of hypotension or with dobutamine if arterial pressure is normal. Antibiotics should be administered, either appropriate for the results of cultures or empirical therapy based on the likely source of infection. Surgical debridement or drainage may also be necessary to control the infection.

NEUROGENIC SHOCK Interruption of sympathetic vasomotor input after a high cervical spinal cord injury, inadvertent cephalad migration of spinal anesthesia, or severe head injury may result in neurogenic shock. In addition to arteriolar dilatation, venodilation causes pooling in the venous system, which decreases venous return and cardiac output. The extremities are often warm, in contrast to the usual vasoconstriction-induced coolness in hypovolemic or cardiogenic shock. Treatment involves a simultaneous approach to the relative hypovolemia and to the loss of vasomotor tone. Large volumes of fluid may be required to restore normal hemodynamics. Once hemorrhage has been ruled out, norepinephrine may be necessary to augment vascular resistance.

HYPOADRENAL SHOCK (See also Chap. 331) The normal host response to the stress of illness, operation, or trauma requires that the adrenal glands hypersecrete cortisol in excess of that normally required. Hypoadrenal shock occurs in settings in which unrecognized adrenal insufficiency complicates the host response to the stress induced by acute illness or major surgery. Adrenocortical insufficiency

may occur as a consequence of the chronic administration of high doses of exogenous glucocorticoids. Recent studies have shown that prolonged stays in a critical state in an intensive care setting may also induce a relative hypoadrenal state. Other, less common causes include adrenal insufficiency secondary to idiopathic atrophy, tuberculosis, metastatic disease, bilateral hemorrhage, and amyloidosis. The shock produced by adrenal insufficiency is characterized by reductions in systemic vascular resistance, hypovolemia, and reduced cardiac output. The diagnosis of adrenal insufficiency may be established by means of an ACTH stimulation test (Chap. 331).

℞ TREATMENT In the hemodynamically unstable patient, dexamethasone sodium phosphate, 4 mg, should be given intravenously. This agent is preferred because unlike hydrocortisone it does not interfere with the ACTH stimulation test. If the diagnosis of adrenal insufficiency has been established, hydrocortisone, 100 mg every 6 to 8 h, can be given and tapered to a maintenance level as the patient achieves hemodynamic stability. Simultaneous volume resuscitation and pressor support is required.

ADJUNCTIVE THERAPIES

As described above, the sympathomimetic amines dobutamine, dopamine, and norepinephrine are widely used in the treatment of all forms of shock. The clinical pharmacology of these agents is described in Chap. 72.

POSITIONING Positioning of the patient may be a valuable adjunct in the initial treatment of hypovolemic shock. Elevating the foot of the bed (i.e., placing it on "shock blocks") and assumption of the Trendelenburg position without flexion at the knees are effective but may increase work of breathing and risk for aspiration. Simply elevating both legs may be the optimal approach.

PNEUMATIC ANTISHOCK GARMENT (PASG) The PASG and the military antishock trousers (MAST) are inflatable external compression devices that can be wrapped around the legs and abdomen and have been widely used in the prehospital setting as a means of providing temporary support of central hemodynamics in shock. They cause an increase in systemic vascular resistance and blood pressure by arterial compression, without causing a significant change in cardiac output. While the use of PASG has been recommended in noncardiogenic forms of shock, the most appropriate use appears to be as a means to tamponade bleeding and augment hemostasis. Inflation of the suit provides splinting of fractures of the pelvis and lower extremities and arrests hemorrhage from fractures.

REWARMING Hypothermia is a potential adverse consequence of massive volume resuscitation. The infusion of large volumes of refrigerated blood products and room-temperature crystalloid solutions can rapidly drop core temperatures if fluid is not run through warming devices. Hypothermia may depress cardiac contractility and thereby further impair cardiac output and oxygen delivery. Hypothermia, particularly temperatures <35° C, directly impairs the coagulation pathway, sometimes causing a significant coagulopathy. Rapid rewarming significantly decreases the requirement for blood products and an improvement in cardiac function. The most effective method for rewarming is extracorporeal countercurrent warmers through femoral artery and vein cannulation. This process does not require a pump and can rewarm from 30° to 36°C in <30 min.

BIBLIOGRAPHY

ASTIZ ME, RACKOW EC: Septic shock. Lancet 351:1501, 1998

CHOI PT et al: Crystalloids vs. colloids in fluid resuscitation: A systematic review. Crit Care Med 27:200, 1999

CONNORS AF JR et al: The effectiveness of right heart catheterization in the initial care of critically ill patients. JAMA 276:889, 1996

DRIES DJ: Hypotensive resuscitation [editorial]. Shock 6:311, 1996

HEBERT PC et al: A multicenter, randomized, controlled clinical trial of transfusion requirements in critical care. Transfusion Requirements in Critical Care Investigators, Canadian Critical Care Trials Group. N Engl J Med 340:409, 1999

HECKBERT SR et al: Outcome after hemorrhagic shock in trauma patients. J Trauma 45: 545, 1998

LEVY B et al: Comparison of norepinephrine and dobutamine to epinephrine for hemodynamics, lactate metabolism, and gastric tonometric variables in septic shock: A prospective, randomized study. Intensive Care Med 23:282, 1997

MIRA JP et al: Association of TNF2, a TNF-alpha promoter polymorphism, with septic shock susceptibility and mortality: A multicenter study. JAMA 282:561, 1999

Practice parameters for hemodynamic support of sepsis in adult patients in sepsis. Task Force of the American College of Critical Care Medicine, Society of Critical Care Medicine. Crit Care Med. 27:639, 1999

WHEELER AP, BERNARD GR: Treating patients with severe sepsis. N Engl J Med 340: 207, 1999

39 Robert J. Myerburg, Agustin Castellanos

CARDIOVASCULAR COLLAPSE, CARDIAC ARREST, AND SUDDEN CARDIAC DEATH

CPR	cardiopulmonary resuscitation	PEA	pulseless electrical activity
EF	ejection fraction	PVCs	premature ventricular
ICD	implantable cardioverter-		contractions
	defibrillator	SCD	sudden *cardiac* death
LV	left ventricular	VF	ventricular fibrillation
MIs	myocardial infarctions	VT	ventricular tachycardia

OVERVIEW AND DEFINITIONS

The vast majority of naturally occurring sudden deaths are caused by cardiac disorders. The magnitude of sudden *cardiac* death (SCD) as a public health problem is highlighted by estimates that more than 300,000 deaths occur each year in the United States by this mechanism, accounting for 50% of all cardiac deaths. SCD is a direct consequence of cardiac arrest, which is often reversible if responded to promptly. Since resuscitation techniques and emergency rescue systems are available to save patients who have out-of-hospital cardiac arrest, which was uniformly fatal in the past, understanding the SCD problem has practical importance.

SCD must be defined carefully. In the context of time, "sudden" is defined, for most clinical and epidemiologic purposes, as 1 h or less between the onset of the terminal clinical event, or an abrupt change in clinical status, and death. An exception is unwitnessed deaths in which pathologists may expand the definition of time to 24 h after the victim was last seen to be alive and stable.

Because of community-based interventions, victims may remain biologically alive for days or even weeks after a cardiac arrest that has resulted in irreversible central nervous system damage. Confusion in terms can be avoided by adhering strictly to definitions of death, cardiac arrest, and cardiovascular collapse (Table 39-1). Death is biologically, legally, and literally an absolute and irreversible event. Death may be delayed in a survivor of cardiac arrest, but "survival after sudden death" is an irrational term. Currently, the accepted definition of SCD is *natural death due to cardiac causes*, heralded by abrupt loss of consciousness within *1 h* of the onset of acute symptoms, in an individual who may have known *preexisting* heart disease but in whom the *time* and *mode* of death are *unexpected*. When biologic death of the cardiac arrest victim is delayed because of interventions, the relevant pathophysiologic event remains the sudden and unexpected cardiac arrest that leads ultimately to death, even though delayed by artificial methods. The language used should reflect the fact that the index event was a cardiac arrest and that death was due to its delayed consequences.

Table 39-1 Distinction Between Death, Cardiac Arrest, and Cardiovascular Collapse

Term	Definition	Qualifiers or Exceptions
Death	Irreversible cessation of all biologic functions	None
Cardiac arrest	Abrupt cessation of cardiac pump function which may be reversible by a prompt intervention but will lead to death in its absence	Rare spontaneous reversions; likelihood of successful interventions relates to mechanism of arrest, clinical setting, and prompt return of circulation
Cardiovascular collapse	A sudden loss of effective blood flow due to cardiac and/or peripheral vascular factors which may reverse spontaneously (e.g., neurocardiogenic syncope; vasovagal syncope) or only with interventions (e.g., cardiac arrest)	Nonspecific term which includes cardiac arrest and its consequences and also events which characteristically revert spontaneously

ETIOLOGY, INITIATING EVENTS, AND CLINICAL EPIDEMIOLOGY

Clinical and epidemiologic studies have identified populations at high risk for SCD. In addition, a large body of pathologic data provides information on the underlying *structural abnormalities* in victims of SCD, and studies of clinical physiology have begun to identify a group of *transient functional factors* that may convert a long-standing underlying structural abnormality from a stable to an unstable state (Table 39-2). This information is developing into an understanding of the causes and mechanisms of SCD.

Cardiac disorders constitute the most common causes of sudden *natural* death. After an initial peak incidence of sudden death between birth and 6 months of age (the sudden infant death syndrome), the incidence of sudden death declines sharply and remains low through childhood and adolescence. Among adolescents and young adults, the incidence of SCD is approximately 1 per 100,000 population per year. The incidence begins to increase in adults over the age of 30 years, reaching a second peak in the age range of 45 to 75 years, when the incidence approximates 1 to 2 per 1000 per year among the unselected adult population. Increasing age within this range is a powerful risk factor for sudden *cardiac* death, and the proportion of cardiac causes among all sudden natural deaths increases dramatically with advancing years. From 1 to 13 years of age, only one of five sudden *natural* deaths is due to cardiac causes. Between 14 and 21 years of age, the proportion increases to 30%, and then to 88% in the middle-aged and elderly.

Young and middle-aged men and women have very different susceptibilities to SCD, but the gender differences decrease with advancing age. In the 45- to 64-year-old age group, the male SCD excess is nearly 7:1. It falls to 2:1 or less in the 65- to 74-year-old age group. The difference in risk for SCD parallels the risks for other manifestations of coronary heart disease in men and women. As the gender gap for manifestations of coronary heart disease closes in the seventh and eighth decades of life, the excess risk of SCD in males also narrows. Despite the lower incidence among younger women, coronary risk factors such as cigarette smoking, diabetes, hyperlipidemia, and hypertension are highly influential, and SCD remains an important clinical and epidemiologic problem.

Hereditary factors contribute to the risk of SCD, but largely in a nonspecific manner; they represent expressions of the hereditary predisposition to coronary heart disease. A few specific syndromes, such as congenital long QT interval syndromes (Chap. 230), right ventricular dysplasia, and the syndrome of right bundle branch block and non-ischemic ST-segment elevations (Brugada syndrome), are char-

STRUCTURAL CAUSES

I. Coronary heart disease
   A. Coronary artery abnormalities
      1. Chronic atherosclerotic lesions
      2. Acute (active) lesions (plaque fissuring, platelet aggregation, acute thrombosis)
      3. Anomalous coronary artery anatomy
   B. Myocardial infarction
      1. Healed
      2. Acute
II. Myocardial hypertrophy
   A. Secondary
   B. Hypertrophic cardiomyopathy
      1. Obstructive
      2. Nonobstructive
III. Dilated cardiomyopathy—primary muscle disease
IV. Inflammatory and infiltrative disorders
   A. Myocarditis
   B. Noninfectious inflammatory diseases
   C. Infiltrative diseases
V. Valvular heart disease
VI. Electrophysiologic abnormalities, structural
   A. Anomalous pathways in Wolff-Parkinson-White syndrome
   B. Conducting system disease
   C. Membrane channel structure (e.g., congenital long QT syndrome)

FUNCTIONAL CONTRIBUTING FACTORS

I. Alterations of coronary blood flow
   A. Transient ischemia
   B. Reperfusion after ischemia
II. Low cardiac output states
   A. Heart failure
      1. Chronic
      2. Acute decompensation
   B. Shock
III. Systemic metabolic abnormalities
   A. Electrolyte imbalance (e.g., hypokalemia)
   B. Hypoxemia, acidosis
IV. Neurophysiologic disturbances
   A. Autonomic fluctuations: central, neural, humoral
   B. Receptor function
V. Toxic responses
   A. Proarrhythmic drug effects
   B. Cardiac toxins (e.g., cocaine, digitalis intoxication)
   C. Drug interactions

acterized by specific hereditary risk of SCD. There are also recent data suggesting a familial predispositon to SCD as a specific pattern of coronary heart disease expression.

The major categories of structural causes of, and functional factors contributing to, the SCD syndrome are listed in Table 39-2. Worldwide, and especially in western cultures, coronary atherosclerotic heart disease is the most common structural abnormality associated with SCD. Up to 80% of all SCDs in the United States are due to the consequences of coronary atherosclerosis. The cardiomyopathies (dilated and hypertrophic, collectively; Chap. 239) account for another 10 to 15% of SCDs, and all the remaining diverse etiologies cause only 5 to 10% of these events. Transient ischemia in the previously scarred or hypertrophied heart, hemodynamic and fluid and electrolyte disturbances, fluctuations in autonomic nervous system activity, and transient electrophysiologic changes caused by drugs or other chemicals (e.g., proarrhythmia) have all been implicated as mechanisms responsible for transition from electrophysiologic stability to instability. In addition, reperfusion of ischemic myocardium may cause transient electrophysiologic instability and arrhythmias.

PATHOLOGY Data from postmortem examinations of SCD victims parallel the clinical observations on the prevalence of coronary heart disease as the major structural etiologic factor. More than 80% of SCD victims have pathologic findings of coronary heart disease. The pathologic description often includes a combination of long-standing, extensive atherosclerosis of the epicardial coronary arteries and

acute active coronary lesions, which include a combination of fissured or ruptured plaques, platelet aggregates, hemorrhage, and thombosis. In one study, chronic coronary atherosclerosis involving two or more major vessels with ≥75% stenosis was observed in 75% of the victims. In another study, atherosclerotic plaque fissuring, platelet aggregates, and/or acute thrombosis were observed in 95 of 100 individuals who had pathologic studies after SCD.

As many as 70 to 75% of males who die suddenly have prior myocardial infarctions (MIs), but only 20 to 30% have recent acute MIs. A high incidence of left ventricular (LV) hypertrophy coexists with prior MIs.

CLINICAL DEFINITION OF FORMS OF CARDIOVASCULAR COLLAPSE (Table 39-1) *Cardiovascular collapse* is a general term connoting loss of effective blood flow due to acute dysfunction of the heart and/or peripheral vasculature. Cardiovascular collapse may be caused by vasodepressor syncope (vasovagal syncope, postural hypotension with syncope, neurocardiogenic syncope—Chap. 21), a transient severe bradycardia, or cardiac arrest. The latter is distinguished from the transient forms of cardiovascular collapse in that it usually requires an intervention to achieve resuscitation. In contrast, vasodepressor syncope and many primary bradyarrhythmic syncopal events are transient and non-life-threatening, with spontaneous return of consciousness.

The most common electrical mechanism for true cardiac arrest is ventricular fibrillation (VF), which is responsible for 65 to 80% of cardiac arrests. Severe persistent bradyarrhythmias, asystole, and pulseless electrical activity (an organized electrical activity without mechanical response, formerly called electomechanical dissociation) cause another 20 to 30%. Sustained ventricular tachycardia (VT) with hypotension is a less common cause. Acute low cardiac output states, having precipitous onset, also may present clinically as a cardiac arrest. The causes include massive acute pulmonary emboli, internal blood loss from ruptured aortic aneurysm, intense anaphylaxis, cardiac rupture after myocardial infarction, and unexpected fatal arrhythmia due to electrolyte disturbances.

CLINICAL CHARACTERISTICS OF CARDIAC ARREST

PRODROME, ONSET, ARREST, DEATH SCD may be presaged by days, weeks, or months of increasing angina, dyspnea, palpitations, easy fatigability, and other nonspecific complaints. However, these *prodromal complaints* are generally predictive of any major cardiac event; they are not specific for predicting SCD.

The *onset of the terminal event*, leading to cardiac arrest, is defined as an acute change in cardiovascular status preceding cardiac arrest by up to 1 h. When the onset is instantaneous or abrupt, the probability that the arrest is cardiac in origin is >95%. Continuous ECG recordings, fortuitously obtained at the onset of a cardiac arrest, commonly demonstrate changes in cardiac electrical activity in the minutes or hours before the event. There is a tendency for the heart rate to increase and for advanced grades of premature ventricular contractions (PVCs) to evolve. Most cardiac arrests that are caused by VF begin with a run of sustained or nonsustained VT, which then degenerates into VF.

Sudden unexpected loss of effective circulation may be separated into "arrhythmic events" and "circulatory failure." Arrhythmic events are characterized by a high likelihood of patients being awake and active immediately prior to the event, are dominated by VF as the electrical mechanism, and have a short duration of terminal illness (<1 h). In contrast, circulatory failure deaths occur in patients who are inactive or comatose, have a higher incidence of asystole than VF, have a tendency to a longer duration of terminal illness, and are dominated by noncardiac events preceding the terminal illness.

The onset of cardiac arrest may be characterized by typical symptoms of an acute cardiac event, such as prolonged angina or the pain of onset of MI, acute dyspnea or orthopnea, or the sudden onset of palpitations, sustained tachycardia, or light-headedness. However, in many patients, the onset is precipitous, with minimal forewarning.

Cardiac arrest is, by definition, abrupt. Mentation may be impaired in patients with sustained VT during the onset of the terminal event. However, complete loss of consciousness is a *sine qua non* in cardiac arrest. Although rare spontaneous reversions occur, it is usual that cardiac arrest progresses to death within minutes (i.e., SCD has occurred) if active interventions are not undertaken promptly.

The probability of achieving successful resuscitation from cardiac arrest is related to the interval from onset to institution of resuscitative efforts, the setting in which the event occurs, the mechanism (VF, VT, pulseless electrical activity, asystole), and the clinical status of the patient prior to the cardiac arrest. Those settings in which it is possible to institute prompt cardiopulmonary resuscitation (CPR) provide a better chance of a successful outcome. However, the outcome in intensive care units and other in-hospital environments is heavily influenced by the patient's preceding clinical status. The immediate outcome is good for cardiac arrest occurring in the intensive care unit in the presence of an acute cardiac event or transient metabolic disturbance, but the outcome for patients with far-advanced chronic cardiac disease or advanced noncardiac diseases (e.g., renal failure, pneumonia, sepsis, diabetes, cancer) is not much more successful in hospital than in the out-of-hospital setting.

The success rate for initial resuscitation and survival to hospital discharge after an out-of-hospital cardiac arrest depends in part on the mechanism of the event. When the mechanism is VT, the outcome is best; VF is the next most successful; and asystole and pulseless electrical activity generate dismal outcome statistics (Fig. 39-1). Advanced age also influences adversely the chances of successful resuscitation.

Progression to biologic death is a function of the mechanism of cardiac arrest and the length of the delay before interventions. VF or asystole without CPR within the first 4 to 6 min has a poor outcome, and there are few survivors among patients who had no life support activities for the first 8 min after onset. Outcome statistics are improved by lay bystander intervention (basic life support—see below) prior to definitive interventions (advanced life support—defibrillation) and even more by early defibrillation. In regard to the latter, the notion that deployment of automatic external defibrillators in communities

(e.g., police vehicles, large buildings, stadiums, etc.) will result in improved survival is currently being evaluated.

Death during the hospitalization after a successfully resuscitated cardiac arrest relates closely to the severity of central nervous system injury. Anoxic encephalopathy and infections subsequent to prolonged respirator dependence account for 60% of the deaths. Another 30% occur as a consequence of low cardiac output states that fail to respond to interventions. Recurrent arrhythmias are the least common cause of death, accounting for only 10% of in-hospital deaths.

In the setting of acute MI, it is important to distinguish between primary and secondary cardiac arrests. *Primary* cardiac arrests refer to those that occur in the absence of hemodynamic instability, and *secondary* cardiac arrests are those that occur in patients in whom abnormal hemodynamics dominate the clinical picture before cardiac arrest. The success rate for immediate resuscitation in primary cardiac arrest during acute MI in a monitored setting should approach 100%. In contrast, as many as 70% of patients with secondary cardiac arrest succumb immediately or during the same hospitalization.

IDENTIFICATION OF PATIENTS AT RISK FOR SUDDEN CARDIAC DEATH   Primary prevention of cardiac arrest depends on the ability to identify individual patients at high risk. One must view the problem in the context of the total number of events and the population pools from which they are derived. The annual incidence of SCD among an unselected adult population is 1 to 2 per 1000 population (Fig. 39-2A), largely reflecting the prevalence of those coronary heart disease patients among whom SCD is the first clinically recognized manifestation (20 to 25% of first coronary events are SCD). The incidence (percent per year) increases progressively with the addition of identified coronary risk factors to populations free of prior coronary events. The most powerful factors are age, elevated blood pressure, LV hypertrophy, cigarette smoking, elevated serum cholesterol level, obesity, and nonspecific electrocardiographic abnormalities. These coronary risk factors are not specific for SCD but rather represent increasing risk for all coronary deaths. The proportion of coronary deaths that are sudden remains at approximately 50% in all risk categories. Despite the marked *relative* increased risk of SCD with addition of multiple risk factors (from 1 to 2 per 1000 population per year in an unselected population to as much as 50 to 60 per 1000 in subgroups having multiple risk factors for coronary artery disease), the *absolute* incidence remains relatively low when viewed as the relationship between the number of individuals who have a preventive intervention and the number of events that can be prevented. Specifically, a 50% reduction in annual SCD risk would be a huge *relative* decrease but would require an intervention in up to 200 unselected individuals to prevent one sudden death. These figures highlight the importance of primary prevention of coronary heart disease. Control of coronary risk factors may be the only practical method to prevent SCD in major segments of the population, because of the paradox that the majority of events occur in the large unselected subgroups rather than in the specific high-risk subgroups (compare "Events/Year" with "Percent/Year" in Fig. 39-2A). Under most conditions of higher level of risk, particularly those indexed to a recent major cardiovascular event (e.g., MI, recent onset of heart failure, survival after out-of-hospital cardiac arrest), the highest risk of sudden death occurs within the initial 6 to 18 months and then decreases toward baseline risk of the underlying disease (Fig. 39-2B). Accordingly, preventive interventions are most likely to be effective when initiated early.

For patients with acute or prior clinical manifestations of coronary heart disease, high-risk subgroups having a much higher ratio of SCD risk to population base can be identified. The acute, convalescent, and chronic phases of MI provide large population subsets with more highly focused risk (Chap. 243). The potential risk of cardiac arrest from the onset through the first 72 h after acute MI (the acute phase) may be as high as 15 to 20%. The highest risk of SCD in relation to MI is found in the subgroup that has experienced sustained VT or VF during the convalescent phase (3 days to 8 weeks) after MI. A greater than 50% mortality in 6 to 12 months has been observed among these patients, when managed with conservative medical therapy, and

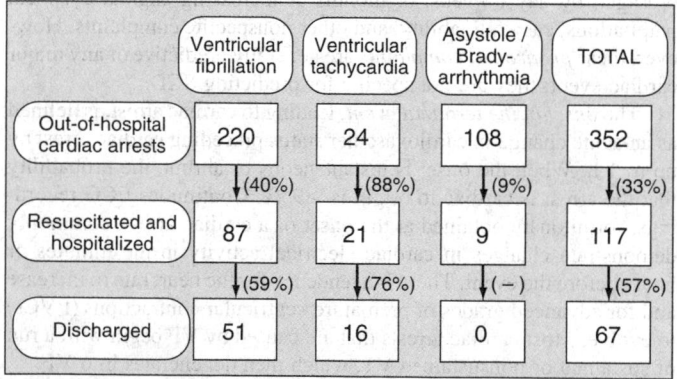

	Ventricular fibrillation	Ventricular tachycardia	Asystole / Brady-arrhythmia	TOTAL
Out-of-hospital cardiac arrests	220	24	108	352
	↓(40%)	↓(88%)	↓(9%)	↓(33%)
Resuscitated and hospitalized	87	21	9	117
	↓(59%)	↓(76%)	↓(−)	↓(57%)
Discharged	51	16	0	67

FIGURE 39-1   Initial electrophysiologic mechanisms recorded during out-of-hospital cardiac arrest. The figures highlighted by the boxes indicate the number of patients in each of three mechanism categories (ventricular fibrillation, ventricular tachycardia, and bradyarrhythmia/asystole). In each category, the data indicate the number of prehospital cardiac arrests (*top*), the number of patients successfully resuscitated in the field and transferred to the hospital alive (*middle*), and the number of patients who survived to be discharged from hospital (*bottom*). The percentages in parentheses indicate survivals between each level of care for each category. (*Modified from RJ Myerburg et al: Clinical, electrophysiologic, and hemodynamic profile of patients resuscitated from prehospital cardiac arrest. Am J Med 68:568, 1980, with permission.*)

A

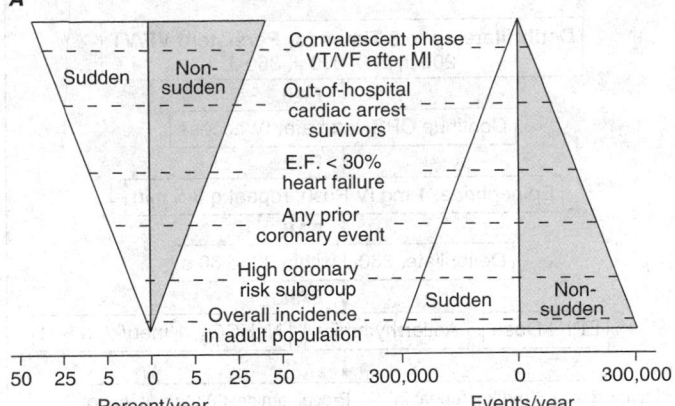

B

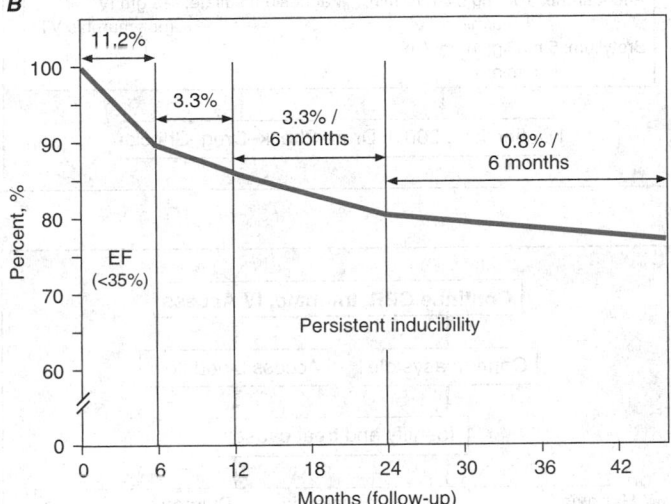

FIGURE 39-2 *A.* Incidence of sudden and nonsudden cardiac deaths in population subgroups, and the relation of total number of events per year to incidence figures. Approximations of subgroup incidence figures, and the related population pool from which they are derived, are presented. Approximately 50% of all cardiac deaths are sudden and unexpected. The incidence triangle on the left ("Percent/Year") indicates the approximate percentage of sudden and nonsudden deaths in each of the population subgroups indicated, ranging from the lowest percentage in unselected adult populations (0.1 to 2% per year) to the highest percentage in patients with VT or VF during convalescence after an MI (approximately 50% per year). The triangle on the right indicates the total number of events per year in each of these groups, to reflect incidence in context with the size of the population subgroups. The highest risk categories identify the smallest number of total annual events, and the lowest incidence category accounts for the largest number of events per year. (EF, ejection fraction; VT, ventricular tachycardia; VF, ventricular fibrillation; MI, myocardial infarction.) *B.* Time dependence of risk among survivors of out-of-hospital cardiac arrest. Recurrence risk is highest in the first 6 months of the index event. Survival is expressed as a percentage. High risk is best predicted initially by an ejection fraction ≤ 35% during the first 6 months, and subsequently persistent inducibility of VT during electrophysiologic testing becomes an added major risk. *n* = 101 at *t* = 0. [*After T Furukawa et al, in RJ Myerburg et al, Circulation 85(Suppl 1):2, 1992. Reproduced with permission of the American Heart Association.*]

at least 50% of the deaths are sudden. Aggressive intervention techniques may reduce this incidence.

After the acute phase of MI, long-term risk for total mortality and SCD are predicted by a number of factors. The most important for both SCD and non-SCD is the extent of myocardial damage sustained during the acute event. This is measured by the degree of reduction in the ejection fraction (EF), functional capacity, and/or the occurrence of heart failure. Increasing *frequency* of postinfarction PVCs, with a plateau above the range of 10 to 30 PVCs per hour on 24-h ambulatory

monitor recordings, also indicates increased risk, but advanced *forms* (salvos, nonsustained VT) may be more powerful predictors. PVCs interact strongly with decreased left ventricular EF. The combination of frequent PVCs, salvos or nonsustained VT, and an EF ≤ 35% identifies patients who have an annual risk of greater than 20%. The risk falls off sharply with decreasing PVC frequency and the absence of advanced forms, as well as with higher EF. Despite the risk implications of postinfarction PVCs, improved outcome as a result of PVC suppression has not been demonstrated (Chap. 230).

The extent of underlying disease due to any cause and/or prior clinical expression of risk of SCD (i.e., survival after out-of-hospital cardiac arrest not associated with acute MI) identify patients at very high risk for subsequent (recurrent) cardiac arrest. Survival after out-of-hospital cardiac arrest predicts up to a 30% 1-year recurrent cardiac arrest rate in the absence of specific interventions (see below).

A general rule is that the risk of SCD is approximately one-half the total cardiovascular mortality rate. As shown in Fig. 39-2*A*, the very high risk subgroups provide more focused population fractions ("Percent/Year") for predicting cardiac arrest or SCD; but the impact on the overall population, indicated by the absolute number of preventable events ("Events/Year"), is considerably smaller. The requirements for achieving a major population impact are effective prevention of the underlying diseases and/or new epidemiologic probes that will allow better resolution of subgroups within large general populations.

TREATMENT   The individual who collapses suddenly is managed in four stages: (1) the initial response and basic life support; (2) advanced life support; (3) postresuscitation care; and (4) long-term management. The initial response and basic life support can be carried out by physicians, nurses, paramedical personnel, and trained lay persons. There is a requirement for increasingly specialized skills as the patient moves through the stages of advanced life support, postresuscitation care, and long-term management.

Initial Response and Basic Life Support   The initial response will confirm whether a sudden collapse is indeed due to a cardiac arrest. Observations for respiratory movements, skin color, and the presence or absence of pulses in the carotid or femoral arteries will promptly determine whether a life-threatening cardiac arrest has occurred. As soon as a cardiac arrest is suspected or confirmed, contacting an emergency rescue system (e.g., 911) should be the immediate priority.

Agonal respiratory movements may persist for a short time after the onset of cardiac arrest, but it is important to observe for severe stridor with a persistent pulse as a clue to aspiration of a foreign body or food. If this is suspected, a Heimlich maneuver (see below) may dislodge the obstructing body. A precordial blow, or "thump," delivered firmly by the clenched fist to the junction of the middle and lower third of the sternum may occasionally revert VT or VF, but there is concern about converting VT *to* VF. Therefore, it has been recommended to use precordial thumps as an advanced life support technique when monitoring and defibrillation are available. This conservative application of the technique remains controversial.

The third action during the initial response is to clear the airway. The head is tilted back and chin lifted so that the oropharynx can be explored to clear the airway. Dentures or foreign bodies are removed, and the Heimlich maneuver is performed if there is reason to suspect that a foreign body is lodged in the oropharynx. If respiratory arrest precipitating cardiac arrest is suspected, a second precordial thump is delivered after the airway is cleared.

Basic life support, more popularly known as CPR, is intended to maintain organ perfusion until definitive interventions can be instituted. The elements of CPR are the maintenance of ventilation of the lungs and compression of the chest. Mouth-to-mouth respiration may be used if no specific rescue equipment is immediately available (e.g., plastic oropharyngeal airways, esophageal obturators, masked Ambu bag). Conventional ventilation techniques during CPR require the lungs to be inflated 10 to 12 times per minute, i.e., once every fifth chest compression when two persons are performing the resuscitation and twice in succession every 15 chest compressions when one person is carrying out both ventilation and chest wall compression.

Chest compression is based on the assumption that cardiac compression allows the heart to maintain a pump function by sequential filling and emptying of its chambers, with competent valves maintaining forward direction of flow. The palm of one hand is placed over the lower sternum, with the heel of the other resting on the dorsum of the lower hand. The sternum is depressed, with the arms remaining straight, at a rate of approximately 80 to 100 per minute. Sufficient force is applied to depress the sternum 3 to 5 cm, and relaxation is abrupt.

Advanced Life Support   Advanced life support is intended to achieve adequate ventilation, control cardiac arrhythmias, stabilize blood pressure and cardiac output, and restore organ perfusion. The activities carried out to achieve these goals include (1) intubation with an endotracheal tube, (2) defibrillation/cardioversion and/or pacing, and (3) insertion of an intravenous line. Ventilation with O_2 (room air if O_2 is not immediately available) may promptly reverse hypoxemia and acidosis. The speed with which defibrillation/cardioversion is carried out is an important element for successful resuscitation. When possible, immediate defibrillation should precede intubation and insertion of an intravenous line; CPR should be carried out while the defibrillator is being charged. As soon as a diagnosis of VT or VF is obtained, a 200-J shock should be delivered. Additional shocks at higher energies, up to a maximum of 360 J, are tried if the initial shock does not successfully abolish VT or VF. Epinephrine, 1 mg intravenously, is given after failed defibrillation, and attempts to defibrillate are repeated. The dose of epinephrine may be repeated after intervals of 3 to 5 min (see Fig. 39-3A).

If the patient is less than fully conscious upon reversion, or if two or three attempts fail, prompt intubation, ventilation, and arterial blood gas analysis should be carried out. Intravenous $NaHCO_3$, which was formerly used in large quantities, is no longer considered routinely necessary and may be dangerous in larger quantities. However, the patient who is persistently acidotic after successful defibrillation and intubation should be given 1 meq/kg $NaHCO_3$ initially and an additional 50% of the dose repeated every 10 to 15 min.

After initial unsuccessful defibrillation attempts, or with persistent electrical instability, a bolus of 1 mg/kg lidocaine is given intravenously (Chap. 243), and the dose is repeated in 2 min in those patients who have persistent ventricular arrhythmias or remain in VF. This is followed by a continuous infusion at a rate of 1 to 4 mg/min. If lidocaine fails to provide control, other antiarrhythmic therapies should be tried. For persistent, hemodynamically unstable ventricular arrhythmias, intravenous amiodarone has emerged as the treatment of choice (150 mg over 10 min, followed by 1 mg/min for up to 6 h, and 0.5 mg/min thereafter) (Fig. 39-3A). Intravenous procainamide (loading infusion of 100 mg/5 min to a total dose of 500 to 800 mg, followed by continuous infusion at 2 to 5 mg/min) may be tried for persisting, hemodynamically stable arrhythmias; or bretylium tosylate (loading dose 5 to 10 mg/kg in 5 min; maintenance dose 0.5 to 2 mg/min) may be tried as an alternative for unstable arrhythmias. Intravenous calcium gluconate is no longer considered safe or necessary for routine administration. It is used only in patients in whom acute hyperkalemia is known to be the triggering event for resistant VF, in the presence of known hypocalcemia, or in patients who have received toxic doses of calcium channel antagonists.

Cardiac arrest secondary to bradyarrhythmias or asystole is managed differently (Fig. 39-3B). The patient is promptly intubated, CPR is continued, and an attempt is made to control hypoxemia and acidosis. Epinephrine and/or atropine are given intravenously or by an intracardiac route. External pacing devices are now available to attempt to establish a regular rhythm, but the prognosis is generally very poor in this form of cardiac arrest, even with successful electrical pac-

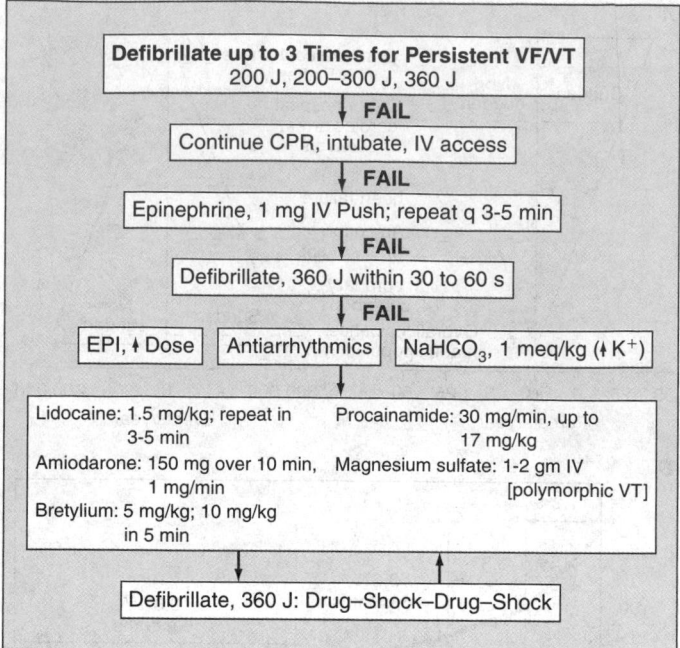

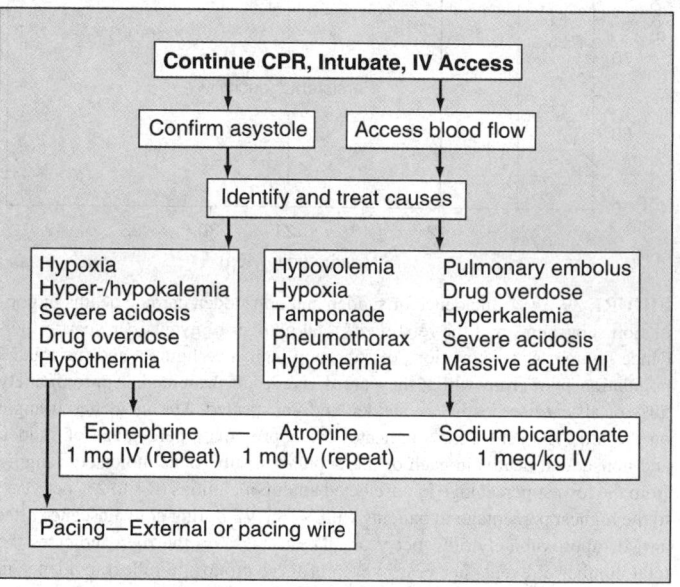

FIGURE 39-3   Management of cardiac arrest. *A.* The algorithm of ventricular fibrillation or hypotensive ventricular tachycardia begins with defibrillation attempts. If that fails, it is followed by epinephrine and then antiarrhythmic drugs. See text for details. *B.* The algorithms for bradyarrhythmia/asystole (*left*) or pulseless electrical activity (*right*) is dominated first by continued life support and a search for reversible causes. Subsequent therapy is nonspecific and accompanied by a low success rate. See text for details.

ing. Pulseless electrical activity (PEA) is treated similarly to bradyarrhythmias, but its outcome is also dismal. The one exception is bradyarrhythmic/asystolic cardiac arrest secondary to airway obstruction. This form of cardiac arrest may respond promptly to removal of foreign bodies by the Heimlich maneuver or, in hospitalized patients, by intubation and suctioning of obstructing secretions in the airway.

Postresuscitation Care   This phase of management is determined by the clinical setting of the cardiac arrest. *Primary* VF in acute MI (Chap. 243) is generally very responsive to life-support techniques and easily controlled after the initial event. Patients are maintained on a lidocaine infusion at the rate of 2 to 4 mg/min for 24 to 72 h after the event. In the in-hospital setting, respirator support is usually not necessary or is needed for only a short time, and hemodynamics stabilize promptly after defibrillation or cardioversion. In *secondary* VF in acute MI (those events in which hemodynamic abnormalities predispose to the potentially fatal arrhythmia), resuscitative efforts are less often successful, and in those patients who are successfully resuscitated, the recurrence rate is high. The clinical picture and outcome are dominated by hemodynamic instability and the ability to control hemodynamic dysfunction. Bradyarrhythmias, asystole, and pulseless electrical activity are commonly secondary events in hemodynamically unstable patients.

The outcome after in-hospital cardiac arrest associated with *noncardiac* diseases is poor, and in the few successfully resuscitated patients, the postresuscitation course is dominated by the nature of the underlying disease. Patients with cancer, renal failure, acute central nervous system disease, and uncontrolled infections, as a group, have a survival rate of less than 10% after in-hospital cardiac arrest. Some major exceptions are patients with transient airway obstruction, electrolyte disturbances, proarrhythmic effects of drugs, and severe metabolic abnormalities, most of whom may have an excellent chance of survival if they can be resuscitated promptly and maintained while the transient abnormalities are being corrected.

Long-Term Management after Survival of Out-of-Hospital Cardiac Arrest   Patients who do not suffer irreversible injury of the central nervous system and who achieve hemodynamic stability should have extensive diagnostic and therapeutic testing to guide long-term management. This aggressive approach is driven by the fact that statistics from the 1970s indicated survival after out-of-hospital cardiac arrest was followed by a 30% recurrent cardiac arrest rate at 1 year, 45% at 2 years, and a total mortality rate of almost 60% at 2 years. Historical comparisons suggest that these dismal statistics may be significantly improved by newer interventions, but the magnitude of the improvement is unknown because of the lack of concurrently controlled intervention studies.

Among those patients in whom an acute transmural MI is the cause of out-of-hospital cardiac arrest, the management is the same as in any other patient who suffers cardiac arrest during the acute phase of a documented MI (Chap. 243). For almost all other categories of patients, however, extensive diagnostic studies are carried out to determine etiology, functional impairment, and electrophysiologic instability as guides to future management. In general, patients who have out-of-hospital cardiac arrest due to chronic ischemic heart disease, without an acute MI, are evaluated to determine whether transient ischemia or chronic electrophysiologic instability was the more likely cause of the event. If there is reason to suspect an ischemic mechanism, coronary revascularization by angioplasty or bypass surgery, plus drugs (most commonly beta blockers), are used to reduce ischemic burden.

Electrophysiologic instability has been identified by the use of programmed electrical stimulation to determine whether sustained VT or VF can be induced (Chap. 230). If so, this information can be used as a baseline against which to evaluate drug efficacy for prevention of inducibility. The rationale for this approach is the assumption that suppression of inducibility predicts long-term benefit by the drug that achieves such suppression. For patients for whom successful drug therapy could not be identified by this technique, insertion of an implantable cardioverter-defibrillator (ICD), antiarrhythmic surgery (e.g., coronary bypass surgery, aneurysmectomy, cryoablation), or empiric amiodarone therapy have been recommended (Chap. 230). Primary surgical success, defined as surviving the procedure and reverting to a noninducible status without drug therapy, is better than 90% when patients are selected for ability to be mapped in the operating room. However, only a small fraction of patients meet the criteria. In addition, VT/VF *cannot* be induced in a number of survivors of cardiac arrest (30 to 50%), and inducible arrhythmias can be suppressed by drugs in no more than 20 to 30% of those whose arrhythmias can be induced. Because of these limitations of drug therapy and surgical approaches, ICD therapy has evolved into the most commonly used strategy for cardiac arrest survivors. ICDs have long been recognized to have very good success rates for sensing and reverting life-threatening arrhythmias, but improvement in long-term total survival outcomes remained lacking until a number of studies solidified the benefit of ICD therapy for specific subgroups. After empiric amiodarone therapy had been suggested to be as good as, or better than, conventional antiarrhythmic drug therapy for survivors of cardiac arrest, ICDs were demonstrated to be superior to amiodarone. Moreover, ICDs were also found to be superior for high risk patients with VT after myocardial infarction.

BIBLIOGRAPHY

AKHTAR M et al: Implantable cardioverter-defibrillator therapy for prevention of sudden cardiac death. Cardiol Clin 11:97, 1993

CUMMINS RO et al: Improving survival from sudden cardiac arrest: The "chain of survival" concept. Circulation 83:1832, 1991

EMERGENCY CARDIAC CARE COMMITTEE AND SUBCOMMITTEES, AMERICAN HEART ASSOCIATION: Guidelines for cardiopulmonary resuscitation and emergency cardiac care. JAMA 268:2172, 1992

EWY GA, ORNATO JP: Emergency Cardiac Care Task Force 1: Cardiac arrest. J Am Coll Cardiol 35:832, 2000

JOSLYN et al: Survival from out-of-hospital cardiac arrest: Effects of patient age and presence of 911 Emergency Medical Services phone access. Am J Emerg Med 11:200, 1993

KANNEL WB, SCHATZKIN A: Sudden death: Lessons from subsets in population studies. J Am Coll Cardiol 5(Suppl 6):141B, 1985

MYERBURG RJ, CASTELLANOS A: Cardiac arrest and sudden cardiac death, in *Heart Disease*, 6th ed, E Braunwald et al (eds). Philadelphia, Saunders, 2001

MYERBURG RJ, CASTELLANOS A et al: Epidemiology, transient risk, and intervention assessment. Ann Intern Med 119:1187, 1993

ORNATO JP: Use of adrenergic agonists during CPR in adults. Ann Emerg Med 22:411, 1993

WILBER DJ et al: Out-of-hospital cardiac arrest: Use of electrophysiologic testing in the prediction of long-term outcome. N Engl J Med 318:19, 1988

Section 6
ALTERATIONS IN GASTROINTESTINAL FUNCTION

40   *Raj K. Goyal*

DYSPHAGIA

Dysphagia is defined as a sensation of "sticking" or obstruction of the passage of food through the mouth, pharynx, or esophagus. It should be distinguished from other symptoms related to swallowing. *Aphagia* signifies complete esophageal obstruction, which is usually due to bolus impaction and represents a medical emergency. *Difficulty in initiating a swallow* occurs in disorders of the voluntary phase of swallowing. However, once initiated, swallowing is completed normally. *Odynophagia* means painful swallowing. Frequently, odynophagia and dysphagia occur together. *Globus pharyngeus* is the sensation of a lump lodged in the throat. However, no difficulty is encountered when swallowing is performed. *Misdirection of food*, resulting in nasal regurgitation and laryngeal and pulmonary aspiration of food during swallowing, is characteristic of oropharyngeal dysphagia. *Phagophobia*, meaning fear of swallowing, and *refusal to swallow* may occur in hysteria, rabies, tetanus, and pharyngeal paralysis due to fear of aspiration. Painful inflammatory lesions that cause odynophagia may also cause refusal to swallow. Some patients may feel the food as it goes down the esophagus. This esophageal sensitivity is not associated with either food sticking or obstruction, however. Similarly, the *feeling of fullness in the epigastrium* that occurs after a meal or after swallowing air should not be confused with dysphagia.

PHYSIOLOGY OF SWALLOWING   The process of swallowing begins with a voluntary (oral) phase during which a bolus of food is pushed into the pharynx by the contraction of the tongue. The bolus then activates oropharyngeal sensory receptors that initiate the involuntary (pharyngeal and esophageal) phase, or deglutition reflex. The deglutition reflex is a complex series of events and serves both to propel food through the pharynx and the esophagus and to prevent its entry into the airway. When the bolus is propelled backward by the tongue, the larynx moves forward and the upper esophageal sphincter opens. As the bolus moves into the pharynx, contraction of the superior pharyngeal constrictor against the contracted soft palate initiates a peristaltic contraction that proceeds rapidly downward to move the bolus through the pharynx and the esophagus. The lower esophageal sphincter opens as the food enters the esophagus and remains open until the peristaltic contraction has swept the bolus into the stomach. Peristaltic contraction in response to a swallow is called *primary peristalsis*. It involves inhibition followed by sequential contraction of muscles along the entire swallowing passage. The inhibition that precedes the peristaltic contraction is called *deglutitive inhibition*. Local distention of the esophagus from food activates intramural reflexes in the smooth muscle and results in *secondary peristalsis*, which is limited to the thoracic esophagus. *Tertiary contractions* are nonperistaltic because they occur simultaneously over a long segment of the esophagus. Tertiary contractions may occur in response to a swallow or esophageal distention, or they may occur spontaneously.

PATHOPHYSIOLOGY OF DYSPHAGIA   The normal transport of an ingested bolus through the swallowing passage depends on the size of the ingested bolus; the luminal diameter of the swallowing passage; the force of peristaltic contraction; and deglutitive inhibition, including normal relaxation of upper and lower esophageal sphincters during swallowing. Dysphagia caused by a large bolus or luminal narrowing is called *mechanical dysphagia*, whereas dysphagia due to weakness of peristaltic contractions or to impaired deglutitive inhibition causing nonperistaltic contractions and impaired sphincter relaxation is called *motor dysphagia*.

Mechanical Dysphagia   Mechanical dysphagia can be caused by a very large food bolus, intrinsic narrowing, or extrinsic compression of the lumen. In an adult, the esophageal lumen can distend up to 4 cm in diameter. When the esophagus cannot dilate beyond 2.5 cm in diameter, dysphagia to normal solid food can occur. Dysphagia is always present when the esophagus cannot distend beyond 1.3 cm. Circumferential lesions produce dysphagia more consistently than do lesions that involve only a portion of circumferences of the esophageal wall, as uninvolved segments retain their distensibility. The causes of mechanical dysphagia are listed in Table 40-1. Common causes include carcinoma, peptic and other benign strictures, and lower esophageal ring.

Motor Dysphagia   Motor dysphagia may result from difficulty in initiating a swallow or from abnormalities in peristalsis and deglutitive inhibition due to diseases of the esophageal striated or smooth muscle.

Diseases of the striated muscle involve the pharynx, upper esophageal sphincter, and cervical esophagus. The striated muscle is innervated by a somatic component of the vagus with cell bodies of the lower motor neurons located in the nucleus ambiguus. These neurons are cholinergic and excitatory and are the sole determinant of the muscle activity. Peristalsis in the striated muscle segment is due to sequential central activation of neurons innervating muscles at different levels along the esophagus. Motor dysphagia of the pharynx results from neuromuscular disorders causing muscle paralysis, simultaneous nonperistaltic contraction, or loss of opening of the upper esophageal sphincter. Loss of opening of the upper sphincter is caused by paralysis of geniohyoid and other suprahyoid muscles or loss of deglutitive inhibition of the cricopharyngeus muscle. Because each side of the pharynx is innervated by ipsilateral nerves, a unilateral lesion of motor neurons leads to unilateral pharyngeal paralysis. Although lesions of striated muscle also involve the cervical part of the esophagus, the clinical manifestations of pharyngeal dysfunction usually overshadow those due to esophageal involvement.

Diseases of the smooth-muscle segment involve the thoracic part of the esophagus and the lower esophageal sphincter. The smooth muscle is innervated by the parasympathetic component of the vagal preganglionic fibers and postganglionic neurons in the myenteric ganglia. The vagal pathway consists of parallel excitatory and inhibitory pathways that use acetylcholine and nitric oxide as neurotransmitters, respectively. The activation of inhibitory nerves causes inhibition that is followed by rebound contraction. These pathways are involved in the resting tone of the lower esophageal sphincter as well as swallow-induced lower esophageal sphincter opening and inhibition followed by peristaltic contractions in the esophageal body. Dysphagia results when the peristaltic contractions are weak or nonperistaltic or when the lower sphincter fails to relax normally. Loss of contractile power occurs due to muscle weakness, as in scleroderma. The nonperistaltic contractions and impaired relaxation of the lower esophageal sphincter result from a defect in inhibitory vagal innervation and account for dysphagia in achalasia.

The causes of motor dysphagia are also listed in Table 40-1. Important causes are pharyngeal paralysis, cricopharyngeal achalasia, scleroderma of the esophagus, achalasia, and diffuse esophageal spasm and related motor disorders.

Approach to the Patient

History   The history can provide a presumptive diagnosis in over 80% of patients. The type of food causing dysphagia provides useful information. Difficulty only with solids implies mechanical dysphagia with a lumen that is not severely narrowed. In advanced obstruction, dysphagia occurs with liquids as well as solids. In contrast, motor dysphagia due to achalasia and diffuse esophageal spasm is equally affected by solids and liquids from the very onset. Patients with scleroderma have dysphagia to solids that is unrelated to posture and to liquids while recumbent but not upright. When peptic stricture develops in patients with scleroderma, dysphagia becomes more persistent.

The duration and course of dysphagia are helpful in diagnosis. Transient dysphagia may be due to an inflammatory process. Progressive dysphagia lasting a few weeks to a few months is suggestive of carcinoma of the esophagus. Episodic dysphagia to solids lasting several years indicates a benign disease characteristic of a lower esophageal ring.

The site of dysphagia described by the patient helps to determine the site of esophageal obstruction; the lesion is at or below the perceived location of dysphagia.

Associated symptoms provide important diagnostic clues. Nasal regurgitation and tracheobronchial aspiration with swallowing are hallmarks of pharyngeal paralysis or a tracheoesophageal fistula. Tracheobronchial aspiration unrelated to swallowing may be secondary to achalasia, Zenker's diverticulum, or gastroesophageal reflux.

Severe weight loss that is out of proportion to the degree of dysphagia is highly suggestive of carcinoma. When hoarseness precedes dysphagia, the primary lesion is usually in the larynx. Hoarseness following dysphagia may suggest involvement of the recurrent laryngeal nerve by extension of esophageal carcinoma. Sometimes hoarseness may be due to laryngitis secondary to gastroesophageal reflux. Association of laryngeal symptoms and dysphagia also occurs in various neuromuscular disorders. Hiccups may rarely occur with a lesion in

Table 40-1 Causes of Dysphagia

MECHANICAL DYSPHAGIA	MOTOR (NEUROMUSCULAR) DYSPHAGIA

I. Luminal
  A. Large bolus
  B. Foreign body
II. Intrinsic narrowing
  A. Inflammatory condition causing edema and swelling
    1. Stomatitis
    2. Pharyngitis, epiglottitis
    3. Esophagitis
      a. Viral (herpes simplex, varicella-zoster, cytomegalovirus)
      b. Bacterial
      c. Fungal (candidal)
      d. Mucocutaneous bullous diseases
      e. Caustic, chemical, thermal injury
  B. Webs and rings
    1. Pharyngeal (Plummer-Vinson syndrome)
    2. Esophageal (congenital, inflammatory)
    3. Lower esophageal mucosal ring (Schatzki ring)
  C. Benign strictures
    1. Peptic
    2. Caustic and pill-induced
    3. Inflammatory (Crohn's disease, candidal, mucocutaneous lesions)
    4. Ischemic
    5. Postoperative, postirradiation
    6. Congenital
  D. Malignant tumors
    1. Primary carcinoma
      a. Squamous cell carcinoma
      b. Adenocarcinoma
      c. Carcinosarcoma
      d. Pseudosarcoma
      e. Lymphoma
      f. Melanoma
      g. Kaposi's sarcoma
    2. Metastatic carcinoma
  E. Benign tumors
    1. Leiomyoma
    2. Lipoma
    3. Angioma
    4. Inflammatory fibroid polyp
    5. Epithelial papilloma
III. Extrinsic compression
  A. Cervical spondylitis
  B. Vertebral osteophytes
  C. Retropharyngeal abscess and masses
  D. Enlarged thyroid gland
  E. Zenker's diverticulum
  F. Vascular compression
    1. Aberrant right subclavian artery
    2. Right-sided aorta
    3. Left atrial enlargement
    4. Aortic aneurysm
  G. Posterior mediastinal masses
  H. Pancreatic tumor, pancreatitis
  I. Postvagotomy hematoma and fibrosis
	I. Difficulty in initiating swallowing reflex
	  A. Paralysis of the tongue
	  B. Oropharyngeal anesthesia
	  C. Lack of saliva (e.g., Sjögren's syndrome)
	  D. Lesions of sensory components of vagus and glossopharyngeal nerves
	  E. Lesions of swallowing center
	II. Disorders of pharyngeal and esophageal striated muscle
	  A. Muscle weakness
	    1. Lower motor neuron lesion (bulbar paralysis)
	      a. Cerebrovascular accident
	      b. Motor neuron disease
	      c. Poliomyelitis, postpolio syndrome
	      d. Polyneuritis
	      e. Amyotrophic lateral sclerosis
	      f. Familial dysautonomia
	    2. Neuromuscular
	      a. Myasthenia gravis
	    3. Muscle disorders
	      a. Polymyositis
	      b. Dermatomyositis
	      c. Myopathies (myotonic dystrophy, oculopharyngeal myopathy)
	  B. Nonperistaltic contractions or impaired deglutitive inhibition
	    1. Pharynx and upper esophagus
	      a. Rabies
	      b. Tetanus
	      c. Extrapyramidal tract disease
	      d. Upper motor neuron lesions (pseudobulbar paralysis)
	    2. Upper esophageal sphincter (UES)
	      a. Paralysis of suprahyoid muscles (causes same as paralysis of pharyngeal musculature)
	      b. Cricopharyngeal achalasia
	III. Disorders of esophageal smooth muscle
	  A. Paralysis of esophageal body causing weak contractions
	    1. Scleroderma and related collagen-vascular diseases
	    2. Hollow visceral myopathy
	    3. Myotonic dystrophy
	    4. Metabolic neuromyopathy (amyloid, alcohol?, diabetes?)
	    5. Achalasia (classical)
	  B. Nonperistaltic contractions or impaired deglutitive inhibition
	    1. Esophageal body
	      a. Diffuse esophageal spasm
	      b. Achalasia (vigorous)
	      c. Variants of diffuse esophageal spasm
	    2. Lower esophageal sphincter
	      a. Achalasia
	        (1) Primary
	        (2) Secondary
	          (a) Chagas' disease
	          (b) Carcinoma
	          (c) Lymphoma
	          (d) Neuropathic intestinal pseudoobstruction syndrome
	          (e) Toxins and drugs
	      b. Lower esophageal muscular (contractile) ring

the distal portion of the esophagus. Unilateral wheezing with dysphagia indicates a mediastinal mass involving the esophagus and a large bronchus.

Chest pain with dysphagia occurs in diffuse esophageal spasm and related motor disorders. Chest pain resembling diffuse esophageal spasms may occur in esophageal obstruction due to a large bolus. A prolonged history of heartburn and reflux preceding dysphagia indicates peptic stricture. A history of prolonged nasogastric intubation, ingestion of caustic agents, ingestion of pills without water, previous radiation therapy, or associated mucocutaneous diseases may provide the cause of esophageal stricture. If odynophagia is present, candidal or herpes esophagitis or pill-induced esophagitis should be suspected.

In patients with AIDS or other immunodeficiency states, esophagitis due to opportunistic infections such as *Candida*, herpes simplex virus, or cytomegalovirus and tumors such as Kaposi's sarcoma and lymphoma should be suspected.

Physical Examination Physical examination is important in motor dysphagia due to skeletal muscle, neurologic, and oropharyngeal diseases. Signs of bulbar or pseudobulbar palsy, including dysarthria, dysphonia, ptosis, tongue atrophy, and hyperactive jaw jerk, in addition to evidence of generalized neuromuscular disease, should be sought. The neck should be examined for thyromegaly or a spinal abnormality. A careful inspection of the mouth and pharynx should disclose lesions that may interfere with passage of food because of pain or obstruction. Changes in the skin and extremities may suggest a diagnosis of scleroderma and other collagen-vascular diseases or mucocutaneous diseases such as pemphigoid or epidermolysis bullosa, which may involve the esophagus. Cancer spread to lymph nodes and liver may be evident. Pulmonary complications of acute aspiration pneumonia or chronic aspiration may be present.

Diagnostic Procedures Dysphagia is nearly always a symptom of organic disease rather than a functional compaint. If oropharyngeal dysphagia is suspected, videofluoroscopy of oropharyngeal swallowing should be obtained. If mechanical dysphagia is suspected on clinical history, barium swallow, esophagogastroscopy and endoscopic biopsies are the diagnostic procedures of choice. Barium swallow and esophageal motility studies are diagnostic tests for motor dysphagia. Esophagogastroscopy may be needed in patients with motor dysphagia to exclude an associated structural abnormality (Chap. 284).

BIBLIOGRAPHY

GOYAL RK, SIVARAO DV: Functional anatomy and physiology of swallowing and esophageal motility, in *The Esophagus*, 3d ed, DO Castell, JE Richter (eds). Philadelphia, Lippincott Williams &Wilkins, 1999, pp 1–31

SPECHLER SJ: American Gastroenterological Association medical position statement on treatment of patients with dysphagia caused by benign disorders of the distal esophagus. Gastroenterology 117:229, 1999

————: American Gastroenterological Association technical review on treatment of patients with dysphagia caused by benign disorders of the distal esophagus. Gastroenterology 117:233, 1999

41   *William L. Hasler*

NAUSEA, VOMITING, AND INDIGESTION

Nausea is the subjective feeling of a need to vomit. Vomiting (emesis) is the oral expulsion of upper gastrointestinal contents resulting from contractions of gut and thoracoabdominal wall musculature. *Vomiting* is contrasted with regurgitation, the effortless passage of gastric contents into the mouth. *Rumination* is the repeated regurgitation of stomach contents, which are often rechewed and then reswallowed. In contrast to vomiting, these phenomena often exhibit some volitional control. *Indigestion* is a nonspecific term that encompasses a variety of upper abdominal complaints including nausea, vomiting, heartburn, regurgitation, and dyspepsia (upper abdominal discomfort or pain). Individuals with ulcer-like dyspepsia report epigastric burning or gnawing discomfort. Dysmotility-like dyspepsia is characterized by postprandial fullness, bloating, eructation (belching), anorexia (loss of appetite), and early satiety (an inability to complete a meal due to premature fullness).

NAUSEA AND VOMITING

MECHANISMS   Vomiting is coordinated by the brain stem and is effected by neuromuscular responses in the gut, pharynx, and thoracoabdominal wall. The mechanisms underlying nausea are poorly understood. Because nausea requires conscious perception, the sensation is probably mediated by the cerebral cortex. Electroencephalographic studies show activation of temporofrontal cortical regions with induction of nausea.

Coordination of Emesis   Animal studies suggested that vomiting was coordinated by a single locus in the medullary reticular formation. However, further work has shown that no one "vomiting center" exists and that several brain stem nuclei initiate emesis, including the nucleus tractus solitarius; the dorsal vagal and phrenic nuclei; medullary nuclei that regulate respiration; and nuclei that control pharyngeal, facial, and tongue movements. The neurotransmitters involved in coordinating emesis are uncertain; however, neurokinin NK_1, serotonin, and vasopressin pathways are postulated.

Somatic and visceral muscles exhibit stereotypic responses during emesis. Inspiratory thoracic and abdominal wall muscles contract, producing high intrathoracic and intraabdominal pressures that facilitate expulsion of gastric contents. The gastric cardia herniates across the diaphragm, and the larynx moves upward to promote oral propulsion of the vomitus. Under normal conditions, distally migrating upper gut contractions are regulated by an electrical phenomenon, the slow wave, which cycles at 3 cycles per minute in the stomach and 11 cycles per minute in the duodenum. With emesis, slow waves are replaced by orally propagating spike activity, which induces retrograde contractions that assist in the oral expulsion of small intestinal contents.

Activators of Emesis   Emetic stimuli act at several anatomic sites. Emesis provoked by noxious thoughts or smells originates in the cerebral cortex, whereas cranial nerves mediate vomiting after gag reflex activation. Motion sickness and inner ear disorders act on the labyrinthine apparatus, while gastric irritants and emetogenic anticancer agents such as cisplatin stimulate gastroduodenal vagal afferent nerves. Nongastric visceral afferents are activated by small intestinal and colonic obstruction and mesenteric ischemia. The area postrema, a medullary nucleus, responds to bloodborne emetic stimuli and is termed the *chemoreceptor trigger zone*. Many emetic drugs act on the area postrema as do bacterial toxins and metabolic disorders such as uremia, hypoxia, and ketoacidosis.

Neurotransmitters that mediate induction of vomiting are selective for these anatomic sites. Labyrinthine disorders stimulate vestibular cholinergic muscarinic M_1 and histaminergic H_1 receptors, whereas gastroduodenal vagal afferent stimuli activate serotonin 5-HT_3 receptors. The area postrema is richly served by nerve fibers acting on diverse receptor subtypes including 5-HT_3, M_1, H_1, and dopamine D_2. Optimal pharmacologic management of the patient with vomiting requires an understanding of these pathways.

DIFFERENTIAL DIAGNOSIS   Nausea and vomiting are caused by conditions within and outside the gut as well as by drugs and circulating toxins (Table 41-1).

Intraperitoneal Disorders   Visceral obstruction and inflammation of hollow and solid viscera may produce vomiting as the main symptom. Gastric obstruction results from ulcer disease and malignancy, whereas small bowel and colonic obstructions occur as a consequence of adhesions, benign or malignant tumors, volvulus, intussusception, or inflammatory diseases such as Crohn's disease. The superior mesenteric artery syndrome, occurring after weight loss or prolonged bed rest, results when the duodenum is compressed by the overlying superior mesenteric artery. Abdominal irradiation evokes emesis by impairing intestinal contractile function and by inducing strictures. Biliary colic causes nausea likely by action on visceral afferent nerves. Vomiting with pancreatitis, cholecystitis, and appendicitis is due to localized visceral irritation and induction of ileus. Enteric infections with viruses or bacteria such as *Staphylococcus aureus* and *Bacillus cereus* are among the most common causes of acute vomiting, especially in children. Opportunistic infections such as cytomegalovirus or herpes simplex induce emesis in immunocompromised individuals.

Disorders of gastrointestinal motor function also commonly cause nausea and vomiting. Gastroparesis is defined as a delay in emptying of food from the stomach and occurs after vagotomy for peptic ulcer, with pancreatic adenocarcinoma, or in systemic diseases such as diabetes, scleroderma, and amyloidosis. Idiopathic gastroparesis develops in the absence of systemic illness and may follow a viral prodrome suggesting an infectious etiology. Intestinal pseudoobstruction is characterized by disruption of intestinal and colonic motor activity and leads to intestinal retention of food residue and secretions, bacterial overgrowth, nutrient malabsorption, and development of nausea, vomiting, bloating, pain, and alteration of bowel pattern. Intestinal pseudoobstruction may be idiopathic, may be inherited as a familial visceral myopathy or neuropathy, or may result from systemic disease or be a paraneoplastic consequence of malignancy (especially small cell lung carcinoma).

Extraperitoneal Disorders   Myocardial infarction and congestive heart failure are cardiac causes of nausea and vomiting. Nausea and vomiting occur after 25% of surgical operations, both within and outside the peritoneum. Postoperative emesis is more common after laparotomy and orthopedic surgery than after laparoscopy and is more prevalent in women. Increased intracranial pressure from tumors, bleeding, abscess, or obstruction to cerebrospinal fluid outflow produces prominent vomiting with or without concurrent nausea. Motion sickness, labyrinthitis, and Ménière's disease evoke symptoms via labyrinthine pathways. Cyclic vomiting syndrome is a rare disorder of unknown etiology that produces episodes of intractable nausea and vomiting, usually in children. The syndrome shows a strong association with migraine headaches, suggesting that some cases may be migraine variants. Patients with psychiatric illnesses, including anorexia nervosa, bulimia nervosa, and depression, may report significant nausea. Psychogenic vomiting occurs most commonly in women with other emotional problems.

Table 41-1 Causes of Nausea and Vomiting

Intraperitoneal	Extraperitoneal	Medications/Metabolic Disorders
Obstructing disorders	Cardiopulmonary disease	Drugs
Pyloric obstruction	Cardiomyopathy	Cancer chemotherapy
Small bowel obstruction	Myocardial infarction	Antibiotics
Colonic obstruction	Labyrinthine disease	Cardiac antiarrhythmics
Superior mesenteric artery syndrome	Motion sickness	Digoxin
Enteric infections	Labyrinthitis	Oral hypoglycemics
Viral	Malignancy	Oral contraceptives
Bacterial	Intracerebral disorders	Endocrine/metabolic disease
Inflammatory diseases	Malignancy	Pregnancy
Cholecystitis	Hemorrhage	Uremia
Pancreatitis	Abscess	Ketoacidosis
Appendicitis	Hydrocephalus	Thyroid and parathyroid disease
Hepatitis	Psychiatric illness	Adrenal insufficiency
Impaired motor function	Anorexia and bulimia nervosa	Toxins
Gastroparesis	Depression	Liver failure
Intestinal pseudoobstruction	Psychogenic vomiting	Ethanol
Functional dyspepsia	Postoperative vomiting	
Gastroesophageal reflux	Cyclic vomiting syndrome	
Biliary colic		
Abdominal irradiation		

Medications and Metabolic Disorders Drugs are frequent causes of vomiting and may act on the stomach (analgesics, erythromycin) or area postrema (digoxin, opiates, anti-Parkinsonian drugs). Agents that cause emesis include antibiotics, antiarrhythmics, antihypertensives, oral hypoglycemics, and contraceptives. Cancer chemotherapy causes vomiting that is acute (within hours of administration), delayed (after 1 or more days), or anticipatory. Acute emesis resulting from highly emetogenic agents such as cisplatin is mediated by 5-HT$_3$ pathways, whereas delayed emesis is independent of 5-HT$_3$. Anticipatory nausea often responds better to anxiolytic therapy than to antiemetics.

Metabolic disorders are in the differential diagnosis in certain settings. Pregnancy is the most prevalent endocrinologic cause of nausea, occurring in 70% of women in the first trimester. Hyperemesis gravidarum is a severe form of nausea of pregnancy that can produce significant fluid loss and electrolyte disturbances. Uremia, ketoacidosis, adrenal insufficiency, as well as parathyroid and thyroid disease are other metabolic causes of emesis.

Circulating toxins evoke symptoms through effects on the area postrema. Endogenous toxins are generated in fulminant liver failure, whereas exogenous enterotoxins may be produced by enteric bacterial infection. Ethanol intoxication is a common toxic cause of nausea and vomiting.

Approach to the Patient

History and Physical Examination The history helps determine the etiology of unexplained nausea and vomiting. Drugs and toxins often cause acute symptoms, while established illnesses evoke chronic complaints. Vomiting within 1 h of eating characterizes pyloric obstruction, whereas emesis in the late postprandial period is reported with intestinal obstruction. Gastroparesis can produce nausea within minutes of food consumption but, in severe cases, leads to vomiting of meal residue ingested hours or days previously. Blood in the vomitus raises suspicion of an ulcer or malignancy; feculent emesis is noted with distal intestinal or colonic obstruction. Bilious vomiting excludes gastric obstruction, whereas emesis of undigested food is consistent with a pharyngoesophageal process such as Zenker's diverticulum or achalasia. Relief of abdominal pain by emesis characterizes small bowel obstruction, but vomiting has no effect on pancreatitis or cholecystitis pain. Pronounced weight loss raises concern about malignancy or obstruction. Fevers suggest inflammation, while an intracranial source is considered if there are headaches or visual field changes. Vertigo or tinnitus indicate labyrinthine disease.

The physical examination complements the history. Abdominal auscultation may reveal absent bowel sounds with ileus. High-pitched rushes suggest bowel obstruction, while a succession splash on abrupt lateral movement of the patient is found with gastroparesis or pyloric obstruction. Tenderness or involuntary guarding raises suspicion of inflammation, whereas fecal blood suggests mucosal injury from ulcer, ischemia, or tumor. Neurologic etiologies present with papilledema, visual field loss, or focal neural abnormalities. Neoplasm is suggested by palpable masses or adenopathy.

The history and examination can characterize complications of emesis. Reports of lightheadedness with demonstration of orthostatic hypotension and reduced skin turgor indicate intravascular fluid loss. Hematemesis, especially with repeated vomiting, suggests a Mallory-Weiss tear of the gastroesophageal junction, while pulmonary abnormalities raise concern for aspiration of vomitus.

Diagnostic Testing With intractable symptoms or an elusive diagnosis, selected diagnostic tests can direct clinical management. Electrolyte replenishment is indicated if hypokalemia or metabolic alkalosis is found. Detection of iron-deficiency anemia mandates a search for mucosal injury. Pancreaticobiliary disease is suggested by abnormal pancreatic enzymes or liver biochemistries, whereas endocrinologic or rheumatologic etiologies are diagnosed by specific hormone or serologic testing. If lumenal obstruction is considered, supine and upright abdominal radiographs may show intestinal air-fluid levels with reduced colonic air. Ileus is characterized by diffusely dilated air-filled bowel loops.

If initial testing is unrevealing, additional anatomic studies may be indicated. Upper endoscopy detects ulcer disease or gastroesophageal malignancy, and small bowel barium radiography diagnoses partial small bowel obstruction. Colonoscopy or barium enema can detect colonic obstruction. Ultrasound or computed tomography of the abdomen defines intraperitoneal inflammatory processes, while computed tomography or magnetic resonance imaging of the head can delineate intracranial sources of nausea and vomiting.

Gastrointestinal motility testing may detect a functional gastrointestinal disorder responsible for symptoms when investigation of anatomic abnormalities is negative. Gastroparesis is most commonly diagnosed with gastric scintigraphy, by which emptying of a radiolabeled meal is measured. A noninvasive means of quantitating gastric slow wave activity with cutaneous electrodes placed over the stomach, electrogastrography, has been proposed as an alternate means of diagnosing abnormal gastric emptying. With intestinal pseudoobstruction, small bowel barium radiography often suggests the diagnosis. Manometry of the small intestine may provide confirmation of the diagnosis as well as complementary information by characterizing the motor abnormality as neuropathic or myopathic based on contractile patterns. Such investigation can obviate the need for open biopsy of the intestine to evaluate for smooth muscle or neuronal degeneration.

℞ **TREATMENT** **General Principles** Therapy of vomiting is tailored to the underlying disease, with the medical or surgical correction of abnormalities if possible. Hospitalization is considered for severe dehydration, especially if oral fluid replenishment cannot be sustained. Once oral intake is tolerated, nutrients are restarted as liquids that are low in fat, as lipids delay gastric emptying. Foods high in indigestible residues are avoided because these also prolong gastric retention.

Antiemetic Medications Drugs that act on the central nervous system serve as antiemetic agents (Table 41-2). Antihistamines such as meclizine and dimenhydrinate and anticholinergic drugs such as scopolamine act on labyrinthine-activated pathways and are useful in the treatment of motion sickness and inner ear disorders. Phenothiazine and butyrophenone dopamine D_2 antagonists are used to treat emesis evoked by area postrema stimuli and are effective for many medication, toxic, and metabolic etiologies. Dopamine antagonists freely cross the blood-brain barrier and may cause anxiety, dystonic reactions, hyperprolactinemic effects (galactorrhea and sexual dysfunction), and irreversible tardive dyskinesia.

Other drug classes have antiemetic properties. Serotonin $5\text{-}HT_3$ antagonists such as ondansetron and granisetron are useful in the treatment of postoperative vomiting and after radiation therapy but are mainly used to prevent cancer chemotherapy-induced emesis. The usefulness of $5\text{-}HT_3$ antagonists to control other causes of refractory emesis is less well established. Antidepressant drugs are established therapeutic options for patients with functional bowel disorders such as irritable bowel syndrome. Low-dose tricyclic antidepressants provide moderate symptomatic benefit in patients with unexplained nausea of a functional nature.

Gastrointestinal Motor Stimulants Drugs that stimulate gastric emptying are indicated for gastroparesis (Table 41-2). Cisapride, a serotonin $5\text{-}HT_4$ agonist that stimulates cholinergic nerves in the stomach, has become the preferred drug for outpatient management of gas-troparesis. The drug is well tolerated but exhibits very rare drug interactions with selected antibiotics, antifungals, and other agents that predispose to fatal cardiac arrhythmias. Metoclopramide, a combined $5\text{-}HT_4$ agonist and D_2 antagonist, is efficacious in the treatment of gastroparesis, but anti-dopaminergic side effects limit its use in 20% of patients. Erythromycin, a macrolide antibiotic, potently increases gastroduodenal motility by action on receptors for motilin, an endogenous stimulant of fasting motor activity. Erythromycin may be most useful when given intravenously to inpatients with refractory gastroparesis; however, oral forms of the drug also have some effect. Domperidone, a D_2 antagonist not available in the United States, has prokinetic and antiemetic effects but does not cross into most other brain regions; thus, anxiety and dystonic reactions are rare. The main side effects of domperidone are induction of hyperprolactinemia through effects on pituitary regions served by a porous blood-brain barrier.

Patients with refractory upper gut motility disorders pose significant therapeutic challenges. Liquid suspensions of prokinetic drugs may be beneficial inasmuch as liquids empty from the stomach more rapidly than pills. Metoclopramide can be administered subcutaneously in patients who do not respond to oral drugs. Intestinal pseudoobstruction may respond to the somatostatin analogue octreotide, which induces propagative small intestinal motor complexes. Placement of a feeding jejunostomy reduces hospitalizations and improves overall health in some patients with gastroparesis who do not respond to drug therapy. Surgical options are limited for refractory cases, but postvagotomy gastroparesis may improve with near-total resection of the stomach. Electrical pacing of the stomach may also be useful.

Selected Clinical Settings Cancer chemotherapeutic agents such as cisplatin are intensely emetogenic. Given prophylactically, $5\text{-}HT_3$ antagonists prevent chemotherapy-induced acute vomiting in most cases (Table 41-2). Optimal antiemetic effects often are obtained with a $5\text{-}HT_3$ antagonist in combination with a glucocorticoid. In high doses, metoclopramide is effective in controlling chemotherapy-evoked emesis, whereas benzodiazepines such as lorazepam are most useful in reducing anticipatory nausea and vomiting. In contrast, delayed emesis 1 to 5 days after chemotherapy is more refractory to treatment. Agents that act as neurokinin NK_1 antagonists in the brain stem may be potent antiemetic and antinausea drugs during both the acute and the delayed periods after chemotherapy. Cannabinoids such as tetrahydrocannabinol have been advocated for cancer-associated emesis, but these drugs produce significant side effects and are no more effective than antidopaminergic agents.

The clinician should exercise caution in the management of the patient with nausea of pregnancy. Studies of the teratogenic effects of available antiemetic agents have provided conflicting results. Few controlled trials have been performed in the nausea of pregnancy, although antihistamines such as meclizine and antidopaminergics such as prochlorperazine are more efficacious than placebo. As a consequence, alternative therapies such as pyridoxine or ginger have been recommended.

INDIGESTION

MECHANISMS Most patients with indigestion have symptoms of a functional nature that result from gastroesophageal

Table 41-2 Treatment of Nausea and Vomiting

Treatment	Mechanism	Examples	Clinical Indications
Antiemetic agents	Antihistaminergic	Dimenhydrinate, meclizine	Motion sickness, inner ear disease
	Anticholinergic	Scopolamine	Motion sickness, inner ear disease
	Antidopaminergic	Prochlorperazine, droperidol	Medication-, toxin-, or metabolic-induced emesis
	$5\text{-}HT_3$ antagonist	Ondansetron, granisetron	Chemotherapy- and radiation-induced emesis, postoperative emesis
	Tricyclic antidepressant	Amitriptyline, nortriptyline	Functional nausea
Prokinetic agents	$5\text{-}HT_4$ agonist	Cisapride	Gastroparesis functional dyspepsia, gastroesophageal reflux disease, intestinal pseudoobstruction
	$5\text{-}HT_4$ agonist and antidopaminergic	Metoclopramide	Gastroparesis, functional dyspepsia
	Motilin agonist	Erythromycin	Gastroparesis, ? Intestinal pseudoobstruction
	Peripheral antidopaminergic	Domperidone	Gastroparesis, functional dyspepsia
	Somatostatin analogue	Octreotide	Intestinal pseudoobstruction
Special settings	Benzodiazepines	Lorazepam	Anticipatory nausea and vomiting with chemotherapy
	Glucocorticoids	Methylprednisolone, dexamethasone	Chemotherapy-induced emesis
	Cannabinoids	Tetrahydrocannabinol	?Chemotherapy-induced emesis

acid reflux or from gastric abnormalities including dysfunctional motor activity and afferent hypersensitivity; these symptoms comprise the syndrome functional dyspepsia. Some cases are a consequence of a more serious organic illness.

Gastroesophageal Acid Reflux   Acid reflux results from selected physiologic defects. In scleroderma and pregnancy, lower esophageal sphincter (LES) tone is low, but most patients with acid reflux have normal LES pressures. Many individuals show frequent transient LES relaxations during which acid bathes the esophagus. The role of hiatal hernias is controversial—although most reflux patients exhibit hiatal hernias, most individuals with hiatal hernias do not have excess heartburn.

Gastric Motor Dysfunction   Disturbed gastric motility is purported to cause acid reflux in some patients with indigestion. Delayed gastric emptying also is found in 25 to 50% of individuals with functional dyspepsia. The relation of these defects to symptom induction is uncertain as many studies show poor correlation between symptom severity and the degree of motor dysfunction. Abnormal gastric fundic relaxation may cause dyspeptic symptoms such as bloating, fullness, nausea, and early satiety.

Visceral Afferent Hypersensitivity   Disturbed gastric sensory function also may cause functional dyspepsia. Visceral afferent hypersensitivity was first demonstrated in patients with irritable bowel syndrome who had heightened perception of rectal balloon inflation without changes in rectal compliance. Patients with dyspepsia may experience discomfort with fundic distention to lower pressures than healthy control subjects.

Other Factors   *Helicobacter pylori* has a clear etiologic role in peptic ulcer disease, but ulcers cause only a minority of cases of dyspepsia. The importance of *H. pylori* in the genesis of functional dyspepsia is controversial, but most investigators believe it is of minor importance. Analgesics cause dyspepsia; nitrates, calcium channel blockers, theophylline, and progesterone promote acid reflux. Other exogenous factors that induce acid reflux include ethanol, tobacco, and caffeine via LES relaxation. Finally, functional dyspepsia is exacerbated by stress, suggesting a pathogenic role for psychological factors.

DIFFERENTIAL DIAGNOSIS   Functional Causes   Gastroesophageal reflux disease (GERD) is prevalent in Western society. Heartburn is reported once monthly by 40% of Americans and daily by 7%. Functional dyspepsia, defined as ≥3 months of dyspepsia without an organic cause, also is common. Nearly 25% of the populace has abdominal discomfort at least six times yearly, consistent with functional dyspepsia, but only 10 to 20% consult physicians. The clinician must distinguish these illnesses, which have a benign course, from conditions that have deleterious consequences.

Ulcer Disease   In most cases of GERD, the esophagus is not damaged. However, 5% of patients develop esophageal ulcers, and some form esophageal strictures. Functional dyspepsia is the cause of symptoms in 60% of individuals with dyspepsia. However, 15 to 25% of cases stem from ulcers of the stomach or duodenum. The most common causes of ulcer disease are gastric infection with *H. pylori* and use of nonsteroidal anti-inflammatory drugs. Other rare causes of gastroduodenal ulcer include Crohn's disease and Zollinger-Ellison syndrome, a condition resulting from gastrin overproduction by an endocrine tumor (Chap. 285).

Malignancy   Patients with dyspepsia often seek care because of fear of cancer. However, <2% of cases result from gastroesophageal malignancy. Esophageal squamous cell carcinoma occurs most often in those patients with histories of tobacco or ethanol intake. Other risk factors include prior caustic ingestion, achalasia, and the hereditary disorder tylosis. Esophageal adenocarcinoma usually complicates long-standing acid reflux. Eight to 20% of patients with GERD exhibit glandular mucosal metaplasia of the squamous epithelium in the lower esophagus, termed *Barrett's metaplasia*. This condition predisposes to esophageal adenocarcinoma. Gastric malignancies include adenocarcinoma, which is more prevalent in certain Asian societies, and lymphoma (see Chap. 90).

Other Causes   Alkaline reflux esophagitis produces GERD-like symptoms in patients who have had surgery for peptic ulcer disease. Opportunistic fungal or viral esophageal infections may produce heartburn or chest discomfort but more often cause painful swallowing. Although biliary colic is in the differential diagnosis of dyspepsia, most patients with true biliary colic report discrete episodes of right upper quadrant or epigastric pain rather than chronic burning discomfort, nausea, and bloating. Lactose intolerance resulting from intestinal lactase deficiency produces gas, bloating, discomfort, and diarrhea. Lactase deficiency occurs in 15% of Caucasians of northern European descent but is more common in African Americans and Asians. Pancreatic disease (chronic pancreatitis and malignancy), hepatocellular carcinoma, celiac sprue, Ménétrier's disease, infiltrative diseases (sarcoidosis and eosinophilic gastroenteritis), mesenteric ischemia, thyroid and parathyroid disease, and abdominal wall strain cause dyspepsia. Extraperitoneal etiologies of indigestion include congestive heart failure and tuberculosis.

Approach to the Patient

History and Physical Examination   GERD classically produces heartburn, a substernal warmth beginning in the epigastrium that moves toward the neck. Heartburn often is exacerbated by meals and may awaken the patient. Associated symptoms include regurgitation of acid and water brash, the reflex release of salty salivary secretions into the mouth. Atypical symptoms include pharyngitis, asthma, cough, bronchitis, hoarseness, and chest pain that mimics angina. Some patients with acid reflux on esophageal pH testing do not report heartburn and instead note abdominal pain or other symptoms.

Individuals with ulcer-like dyspepsia have epigastric gnawing or burning that is relieved by meals or acid suppression. Dysmotility-like dyspepsia is a fullness or pain that is aggravated by eating and associated with nausea, bloating, eructation, and early satiety. There is overlap among the different dyspepsia subclasses and with other functional disorders such as irritable bowel syndrome.

The physical examination of individuals with functional causes of indigestion is usually normal. In atypical GERD, pharyngeal erythema and wheezing over the lung fields may be present. Poor dentition may occur with prolonged acid regurgitation. Patients with functional dyspepsia may have epigastric tenderness or abdominal distension.

Discrimination between functional and organic causes of indigestion mandates exclusion of selected historical and examination features. Odynophagia suggests esophageal infection, while dysphagia promotes concern about a benign or malignant esophageal blockage. Other features that raise alarm include unexplained weight loss, recurrent vomiting with evidence of dehydration, occult or gross gastrointestinal bleeding, and a palpable mass or adenopathy.

Diagnostic Testing   Because indigestion is prevalent in the community and because most cases result from functional illness, a general principle of diagnostic testing is to perform only limited and directed testing of selected individuals.

Once alarm factors are excluded, patients with typical GERD do not need further evaluation and are treated empirically. Upper endoscopy is indicated to exclude mucosal injury in patients with atypical symptoms, symptoms unresponsive to acid-suppressing drugs, or alarm factors. In patients with >5 years of heartburn, endoscopy is performed to screen for Barrett's metaplasia. Upper gastrointestinal barium radiography has a slightly higher sensitivity for detecting strictures and rings than endoscopy; however, benign esophageal obstructions may be dilated with an endoscopic approach. Ambulatory esophageal pH testing is considered for atypical symptoms such as unexplained chest pain and for the symptoms that are unresponsive to appropriate medications. Esophageal manometry is most commonly ordered when surgical treatment of GERD is considered. A low LES pressure may predict failure with drug therapy and identify patients who may require surgery. The demonstration of disordered esophageal body peristalsis may affect the decision to operate or modify the type of operation chosen. Manometry with provocative testing may clarify the diagnosis in patients with atypical symptoms. Blinded perfusion of saline and then acid into the esophagus, known as the Bernstein test, can delineate whether unexplained chest discomfort results from acid reflux.

The approach to unexplained dyspepsia is dependent on the patient's age, symptom profile, and findings on examination. In individuals <45 years of age without alarm factors, blood serology for *H. pylori* is obtained to exclude the organism as a cause of ulcer disease. Upper endoscopy in this patient subset is reserved for those who fail to respond to treatment of *H. pylori*-positive or -negative dyspepsia. Upper endoscopy is performed as the initial diagnostic test in any individual with alarm factors or in patients >45 years of age because of the elevated risk of gastroesophageal malignancy with advancing age.

Further testing is indicated only if other factors are present. If there is blood loss, a blood count is obtained to exclude anemia. Thyroid chemistries or calcium levels screen for metabolic disease. With suspected pancreaticobiliary causes, blood is obtained for amylase, lipase, and liver chemistry determination. If biochemical abnormalities are found, abdominal ultrasound or computed tomography may give important information. Patients with dysmotility-like dyspepsia may selectively exhibit delayed gastric emptying; thus, gastric scintigraphy can be considered when drug treatment fails. Hydrogen breath testing after lactose ingestion may be performed for suspected lactase deficiency.

℞ **TREATMENT** **General Principles** In mild dyspepsia, reassurance that a careful evaluation revealed no serious organic disease may be the only intervention required. Drugs that cause acid reflux or dyspepsia should be stopped if possible. Patients with GERD should limit ethanol, caffeine, chocolate, and tobacco use because of their effects on the LES. Other measures with efficacy in GERD include ingestion of a low-fat diet, avoidance of snacks before bedtime, and elevation of the head of the bed.

Specific therapy for organic diseases should be offered when possible. In disorders such as biliary colic, surgery is appropriate; whereas lactase deficiency and celiac sprue respond to special diets. Some illnesses such as peptic ulcer disease require specific medical regimens to effect cure. However, as most patients present with functional causes of indigestion, medications that reduce gastric acid, stimulate upper gut motility, or blunt gastric sensitivity are indicated.

Acid Suppressing or Neutralizing Medications Drugs that reduce or neutralize gastric acid are the most prescribed agents for GERD. Histamine H_2 receptor antagonists such as cimetidine, ranitidine, famotidine, and nizatidine are useful in the treatment of mild to moderate GERD. For uncomplicated heartburn, H_2 receptor antagonists are given for 4 weeks before endoscopy is considered. For severe symptoms or for many cases of erosive or ulcerative esophagitis, proton pump inhibitors such as omeprazole and lansoprazole are needed. These drugs, which inhibit gastric H^+, K^+-ATPase, are more potent than H_2 receptor antagonists. Liquid antacids are useful for short-term control of mild GERD but are less effective for severe disease unless given at high doses that produce side effects (diarrhea with magnesium-containing agents and constipation with aluminum-containing agents). Sucralfate is a salt of aluminum hydroxide and sucrose octasulfate and buffers acid and binds pepsin and bile salts. Its efficacy in GERD and functional dyspepsia is unproven.

Acid suppressing drugs are advocated for first-line therapy of *H. pylori* negative dyspepsia, especially with ulcer-like symptoms. Ranitidine is of benefit in the treatment of functional dyspepsia versus placebo. In young patients without alarm symptoms, a 4-week trial of an H_2 receptor antagonist or proton pump inhibitor is given. Endoscopy is performed only if symptoms do not improve.

***Helicobacter pylori* Eradication** Regimens to eradicate *H. pylori* are recommended for young patients with dyspepsia without alarm symptoms in whom the bacterium has been detected by serology. Several drug combinations show efficacy, but most include 10 to 14 days of a proton pump inhibitor or bismuth subsalicylate in concert with two antibiotics. If symptoms resolve, no further intervention is required. Most patients who respond to this "treatment-first" approach have underlying ulcer disease. The usefulness of *Helicobacter* eradication in patients with functional dyspepsia is unproven, but evidence suggests that <15% of cases relate to *H. pylori*. No evidence demonstrates that *H. pylori* eradication is useful in the treatment of GERD.

Gastrointestinal Motor Stimulants Cisapride is superior to placebo in treating GERD and can be prescribed as sole therapy or as an adjunct to an acid-suppressing drug. Other motor stimulants such as metoclopramide, erythromycin, and domperidone are of limited use in the treatment of GERD.

Prokinetic agents are frequently used for treatment of functional dyspepsia. Cisapride and domperidone relieve symptoms more effectively than placebo. In general, these drugs are more potent than acid-reducing agents in the treatment of functional dyspepsia and may be given instead of acid suppressants as the initial empirical treatment of young patients with dyspepsia without alarm symptoms who are not infected with *H. pylori*. Patients with dysmotility-like dyspepsia may respond preferentially to motor-stimulating drugs.

Other Options In patients with GERD who do not respond to drug therapy, antireflux surgery may be offered. Operations include the Nissen fundoplication, in which the proximal stomach is wrapped completely around the LES to increase LES pressure, and the Belsey procedure, in which the wrap encircles 270° of the circumference of the LES. The latter is selected if esophageal peristalsis is suboptimal when a 360° wrap might cause dysphagia. Fundoplications can be performed laparoscopically, thereby reducing the morbidity and the postoperative recuperation period.

Some patients with functional dyspepsia do not respond to acid suppressants or prokinetic drugs but may respond to low-dose tricyclic antidepressant therapy. The mechanism of action of these agents in functional dyspepsia is unknown but may involve blunting of visceral pain processing in the brain. Gas and bloating may be the most troubling symptoms in some patients with indigestion and can be difficult to treat. Successes with dietary exclusion of gas-producing foods such as legumes and use of the surface-active compound simethicone or the gas-absorptive agent activated charcoal have been reported. Psychological treatments have been proposed for functional dyspepsia; however, convincing data on their efficacy are lacking.

BIBLIOGRAPHY

BLUM AL et al: Lack of effect of treating *Helicobacter pylori* infection in patients with nonulcer dyspepsia. Omeprazole plus clarithromycin and amoxicillin effect one year after treatment (OCAY) study group. N Engl J Med 339:1928, 1998

CAMILLERI M et al: Measurement of gastrointestinal motility in the GI laboratory. Gastroenterology 115:747, 1998

DEVAULT KR, CASTELL DO: Guidelines for the diagnosis and treatment of gastroesophageal reflux disease. Practice Parameters Committee of the American College of Gastroenterology. Arch Intern Med 155:2165, 1995

FINNEY JS et al: Meta-analysis of antisecretory and gastrokinetic compounds in functional dyspepsia. J Clin Gastroenterol 26:312, 1998

JANTUNEN IT et al: An overview of randomised studies comparing 5-HT₃ receptor antagonists to conventional anti-emetics in the prophylaxis of acute chemotherapy-induced vomiting. Eur J Cancer 33:66, 1997

LACROIX R et al: Nausea and vomiting during pregnancy. Am J Obstet Gynecol 182:931, 2000

MITCHELSON F: Pharmacological agents affecting emesis: A review (part I). Drugs 43:295, 1992

PRAKASH C et al: Tricyclic antidepressants for functional nausea and vomiting: Clinical outcome in 37 patients. Dig Dis Sci 43:1951, 1998

RICHTER JE: Typical and atypical presentations of gastroesophageal reflux disease. The role of esophageal testing in the diagnosis and management. Gastroenterol Clin North Am 25:75, 1996

TALLEY NJ et al: AGA technical review: Evaluation of dyspepsia. Gastroenterology 114:582, 1998

DIARRHEA AND CONSTIPATION

Diarrhea and constipation are exceedingly common and together exact an enormous toll in terms of morbidity, loss of work productivity, and consumption of medical resources. Worldwide, more than one billion people suffer one or more episodes of acute diarrhea each year. Among the 100 million persons affected annually by acute diarrhea in the United States, nearly half must restrict activities, 10% consult physicians, 250,000 require hospitalization, and roughly 3000 die (primarily the elderly). The economic burden to society is estimated at more than $20 billion. Because of poor sanitation and more limited access to health care, acute infectious diarrhea remains one of the most common causes of mortality in developing countries, particularly among children, accounting for 5 to 8 million deaths per year. Population statistics on chronic diarrhea and constipation are more uncertain, perhaps due to variable definitions and reporting, but the frequency of these conditions is also high. Based on United States population surveys, prevalence rates for chronic diarrhea range from 2 to 7% and for chronic constipation from 3 to 17%. Diarrhea and constipation are among the most common patient complaints faced by internists and primary care physicians, and they account for nearly 50% of referrals to gastroenterologists.

Although diarrhea and constipation may present as mere nuisance symptoms at one extreme, they can be severe or life-threatening at the other. Even mild symptoms may signal a serious underlying gastrointestinal lesion, like colorectal cancer, or systemic disorder, like thyroid disease. Given the heterogeneous causes and potential severity of these common complaints, it is imperative for clinicians to appreciate the pathophysiology, etiologic classification, diagnostic strategies, and therapeutic principles of diarrhea and constipation so that rational and cost-effective care can be delivered.

NORMAL PHYSIOLOGY

The human small intestine and colon perform important functions including the secretion and absorption of water and electrolytes, the storage and subsequent transport of intraluminal contents aborally, and the salvage of some nutrients after bacterial metabolism of carbohydrate that are not absorbed in the small intestine. The main motor functions are summarized in Table 42-1. Alterations in fluid and electrolyte handling contribute significantly to diarrhea. Alterations in motor and sensory functions of the human colon result in highly prevalent syndromes such as irritable bowel syndrome, chronic diarrhea, and chronic constipation.

NEURAL CONTROL The small intestine and colon have intrinsic and extrinsic innervation. The *intrinsic innervation* also called the enteric nervous system, comprises myenteric, submucosal, and mucosal neuronal layers. The function of these layers is modulated by interneurons through the actions of neurotransmitter amines or peptides, including acetylcholine, opioids, norepinephrine, serotonin, ATP, and nitric oxide. The myenteric plexus regulates smooth muscle function, and the submucosal plexus affects secretion and absorption.

Table 42-1 Normal Gastrointestinal Motility: Functions at Different Anatomic Levels

Stomach and small bowel	Colon: Irregular mixing, absorption,
Synchronized MMCs in fasting	transit
Accommodation, trituration, mixing, transit	Ascending, transverse: reservoirs
Stomach, ~3 h	Descending: conduit
Small bowel, ~3 h	Sigmoid/rectum: volitional reservoir
Ileal reservoir empties boluses	

NOTE: MMC, migrating motor complex.

The *extrinsic innervations* of the small intestine and colon are part of the autonomic nervous system and also modulate both motor and secretory functions. The parasympathetic nerve supply conveys both visceral sensory as well as excitatory pathways to the motor components of the colon. Parasympathetic fibers via the vagus nerve reach the small intestine and proximal colon along the branches of the superior mesenteric artery. The distal colon is supplied by sacral parasympathetic nerves (S_{2-4}) via the pelvic plexus; these fibers course through the wall of the colon as ascending intracolonic fibers as far as, and in some instances including, the proximal colon. The chief excitatory neurotransmitters controlling motor function are acetylcholine and the tachykinins, such as substance P. The sympathetic nerve supply modulates motor functions and reaches the small intestine and colon alongside the arterial arcades of the superior and inferior mesenteric vessels. Sympathetic input to the gut is generally excitatory to sphincters and inhibitory to nonsphincteric muscle. Visceral afferents convey sensation from the gut to the central nervous system; initially, they course along sympathetic fibers, but as they approach the spinal cord they separate, have cell bodies in the dorsal root ganglion, and enter the dorsal horn of the spinal cord. Afferent signals are conveyed to the brain along the lateral spinothalamic tract and the nociceptive dorsal column pathway and are then perceived. Other afferent fibers synapse in the prevertebral ganglia and reflexly modulate intestinal motility.

INTESTINAL FLUID ABSORPTION AND SECRETION On an average day, 9 L of fluid enters the gastrointestinal tract; approximately 1 L of residual fluid reaches the colon; the stool excretion of fluid constitutes about 0.2 L/d. The colon has a large capacitance and functional reserve and may recover up to four times its usual volume of 0.8 L/d, provided the rate of flow permits reabsorption to occur. Thus, the colon can partially compensate for intestinal absorptive or secretory disorders.

In the colon, sodium absorption is predominantly electrogenic, and uptake takes place at the apical membrane; it is also compensated by the pumping out functions of the basolateral sodium pump. A variety of neural and non-neural mediators regulate colonic fluid and electrolyte balance, including cholinergic, adrenergic and serotonergic mediators. Angiotensin and aldosterone also influence colonic absorption, reflecting the common embryologic development of the distal colonic epithelium and the renal tubules.

ILEOCOLONIC STORAGE AND SALVAGE The distal ileum acts as a reservoir, emptying intermittently by bolus movements. This action allows time for salvage of fluids, electrolytes, and nutrients. Segmentation by haustra compartmentalizes the colon and facilitates mixing, retention of residue, and formation of solid stools. In health, the ascending and transverse regions of colon function as reservoirs (average transit, 15 h), and the descending colon acts as a conduit (average transit, 3 h). The colon is efficient at conserving sodium and water, a function that is particularly important in sodium-depleted patients in whom the small intestine alone is unable to maintain sodium balance. Diarrhea or constipation may result from alteration in the reservoir function of the proximal colon, or the propulsive function of the left colon. Constipation may also result from disturbances of the rectal or sigmoid reservoir, typically as a result of dysfunction of the pelvic floor or the coordination of defecation.

SMALL INTESTINAL MOTILITY During fasting, the motility of the small intestine is characterized by a cyclical event called the migrating motor complex (MMC), which serves to clear nondigestible residue from the small intestine. This organized, propagated series of contractions lasts on average 4 min, occurs every 60 to 90 min, and usually involves the entire small intestine. After food ingestion, the small intestine produces irregular, mixing contractions of relatively low amplitude, except in the distal ileum where more powerful contractions occur intermittently and empty the ileum by bolus transfers.

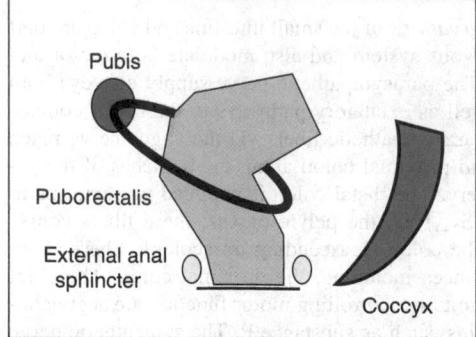

Resting

Pubis

Puborectalis

External anal sphincter

Coccyx

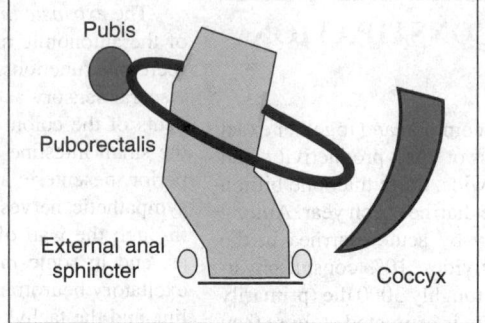

Straining

Pubis

Puborectalis

External anal sphincter

Coccyx

Continence requires
Contraction of puborectalis
Maintenance of anorectal angle
Normal rectal sensation
Contraction of sphincter

Defecation requires
Relaxation of puborectalis
Straightening of anorectal angle
Relaxation of sphincter

FIGURE 42-1 Mechanisms involved in continence and defecation. Note the importance of pelvic floor and anal sphincter functions.

COLONIC MOTILITY AND TONE The small intestinal MMC only rarely continues into the colon. However, short duration or phasic contractions mix colonic contents, and high amplitude propagated contractions (HAPCs) are sometimes associated with mass movements through the colon and occur approximately five times per day, usually on awakening in the morning and postprandially. Increased frequency of HAPCs may result in diarrhea. The predominant phasic contractions are irregular and nonpropagated and serve as a "mixing" function.

Colonic tone refers to the background contractility upon which phasic contractile activity (typically contractions lasting less than 15 s) is superimposed. It is an important cofactor in the colon's capacitance (volume accommodation) and sensation.

COLONIC MOTILITY AFTER MEAL INGESTION After meal ingestion, colonic phasic and tonic contractility increase for a period of approximately 2 h. The initial phase (about 10 min) is mediated by the vagus nerve in response to mechanical distention of the stomach. The subsequent response of the colon requires caloric stimulation and is at least in part mediated by hormones, e.g., gastrin and serotonin.

DEFECATION Tonic contraction of the puborectalis muscle, which forms a sling around the rectoanal junction, is important to maintain continence; during defecation, sacral parasympathetic nerves relax this muscle, facilitating the straightening of the rectoanal angle (Fig. 42-1). Distention of the rectum results in transient relaxation of the internal anal sphincter via intrinsic and reflex sympathetic innervation. As sigmoid and rectal contractions increase the pressure within the rectum, the rectosigmoid angle opens by more than 15°. Voluntary relaxation of the external anal sphincter (striated muscle innervated by the pudendal nerve) permits the evacuation of feces; this evacuation process can be augmented by an increase in intraabdominal pressure created by the Valsalva maneuver.

DIARRHEA

DEFINITION Diarrhea is loosely defined as passage of abnormally liquid or unformed stools at an increased frequency. For adults on a typical Western diet, stool weight exceeding 200 g/d can generally be considered diarrheal. Because of the fundamental importance of duration to diagnostic considerations, diarrhea may be further defined as *acute* if <2 weeks, *persistent* if 2 to 4 weeks, and *chronic* if >4 weeks in duration.

Two common conditions, usually associated with the passage of stool totaling <200 g/d, must be distinguished from diarrhea, as diagnostic and therapeutic algorithms differ. *Pseudodiarrhea*, or the fre-

quent passage of small volumes of stool, often is associated with rectal urgency and accompanies the irritable bowel syndrome or anorectal disorders like proctitis. *Fecal incontinence* is the involuntary discharge of rectal contents and is most often caused by neuromuscular disorders or structural anorectal problems. Diarrhea and urgency, especially if severe, may aggravate or cause incontinence. Pseudodiarrhea and fecal incontinence occur at prevalence rates comparable to or higher than that of chronic diarrhea and should always be considered in patients complaining of "diarrhea." A careful history and physical examination generally allow these conditions to be discriminated from true diarrhea.

ACUTE DIARRHEA More than 90% of cases of acute diarrhea are caused by infectious agents; these cases are often accompanied by vomiting, fever, and abdominal pain. The remaining 10% or so are caused by medications, toxic ingestions, ischemia, and other conditions.

Infectious Agents Most infectious diarrheas are acquired by fecal-oral transmission via direct personal contact or, more commonly, via ingestion of food or water contaminated with pathogens from human or animal feces. In the immunologically competent person, the resident fecal microflora, containing more than 500 taxonomically distinct species, are rarely the source of diarrhea and may actually play a role in suppressing the growth of ingested pathogens. Acute infection or injury occurs when the ingested agent overwhelms the host's mucosal immune and nonimmune (gastric acid, digestive enzymes, mucus secretion, peristalsis, and suppressive resident flora) defenses. Established clinical associations with specific enteropathogens may offer diagnostic clues.

In the United States, high risk groups are recognized:

1. *Travelers.* Nearly 40% of tourists to endemic regions of Latin America, Africa, and Asia develop so-called traveler's diarrhea, most commonly due to enterotoxigenic *Escherichia coli* as well as to *Campylobacter, Shigella,* and *Salmonella*. Visitors to Russia (especially St. Petersburg) may have increased risk of *Giardia*-associated diarrhea; visitors to Nepal may acquire *Cyclospora*. Campers, backpackers, and swimmers in wilderness areas may become infected with *Giardia*.

2. *Consumers of certain foods.* Diarrhea closely following food consumption at a picnic, banquet, or restaurant may suggest infection with *Salmonella, Campylobacter,* or *Shigella* from chicken; enterohemorrhagic *E. coli* (O157:H7) from undercooked hamburger; *Bacillus aureus* from fried rice; *Staphylococcus aureus* or *Salmonella* from mayonnaise or creams; *Salmonella* from eggs; and *Vibrio* species, *Salmonella*, or acute hepatitis A or B from seafood, especially if raw.

3. *Immunodeficient persons.* Individuals at risk for diarrhea include those with either primary immunodeficiency (e.g., IgA deficiency, common variable hypogammaglobulinemia, chronic granulomatous disease) or the much more common secondary immunodeficiency states (e.g., AIDS, senescence, pharmacologic suppression). Common enteropathogens often cause a more severe and protracted diarrheal illness; and, particularly in persons with AIDS, opportunistic infections, such as by *Mycobacterium* species, certain viruses (cytomegalovirus, adenovirus, and herpes simplex), and protozoa (*Cryptosporidium, Isospora belli,* Microsporidia, and *Blastocystis hominis*) may also play a role (Chap. 309). In patients with AIDS, agents transmitted venereally per rectum (e.g., *Neisseria gonorrhoeae, Treponema pallidum, Chlamydia*) may contribute to proctocolitis.

4. *Daycare participants and their family members.* Infections with *Shigella, Giardia, Cryptosporidium,* rotavirus, and other agents are very common and should be considered.

5. *Institutionalized persons.* Infectious diarrhea is one of the most frequent categories of nosocomial infections in many hospitals and long-term care facilities; the causes are a variety of microorganisms but most commonly *Clostridium difficile.*

The pathophysiology underlying acute diarrhea by infectious agents produces specific clinical features that may also be helpful in diagnosis (Table 42-2). Profuse watery diarrhea secondary to small bowel hypersecretion occurs with ingestion of preformed bacterial toxins, enterotoxin-producing bacteria, and enteroadherent pathogens. Diarrhea associated with marked vomiting and minimal or no fever may occur abruptly within a few hours after ingestion of the former two types; vomiting is usually less, and abdominal cramping or bloating is greater; fever is higher with the latter. Cytotoxin-producing and invasive microorganisms all cause high fever and abdominal pain. Invasive bacteria and *Entamoeba histolytica* often cause bloody diarrhea (referred to as *dysentery*). *Yersinia* invades the terminal ileal and proximal colon mucosa and may cause especially severe abdominal pain with tenderness mimicking acute appendicitis.

Finally, infectious diarrhea may be associated with systemic manifestations. Reiter's syndrome (arthritis, urethritis, and conjunctivitis) may accompany or follow infections by *Salmonella, Campylobacter, Shigella,* and *Yersinia.* Yersiniosis may also lead to an autoimmune-type thyroiditis, pericarditis, and glomerulonephritis. Both enterohemorrhagic *E. coli* (O157:H7) and *Shigella* can lead to the *hemolytic-uremic syndrome* with an attendant high mortality rate. Acute diarrhea can also be a major symptom of several systemic infections including *viral hepatitis, listeriosis, legionellosis,* and *toxic shock syndrome.*

Other Causes Side effects from medications are probably the most common noninfectious cause of acute diarrhea, and etiology may be suggested by a temporal association between use and symptom onset. Although innumerable medications may produce diarrhea, some of the more frequently incriminated include antibiotics, cardiac antidysrhythmics, antihypertensives, nonsteroidal anti-inflammatory drugs, certain antidepressants, chemotherapeutic agents, bronchodilators, antacids, and laxatives. Occlusive or nonocclusive *ischemic colitis* typically occurs in persons older than 50 years of age, often presents as acute lower abdominal pain preceding watery, then bloody diarrhea, and generally results in acute inflammatory changes in the sigmoid or left colon while sparing the rectum. Acute diarrhea may accompany colonic *diverticulitis* and *graft-versus-host disease.* Acute diarrhea, often associated with systemic compromise, can follow ingestion of toxins including organophosphate insecticides, amanita and other mushrooms, arsenic, and preformed environmental toxins in seafoods, like ciguatera and scombroid. The conditions causing chronic

Table 42-2 Association between Pathobiology of Causative Agents and Clinical Features in Acute Infectious Diarrhea

Pathobiology/Agents	Incubation Period	Vomiting	Abdominal Pain	Fever	Diarrhea
Toxin producers					
Preformed toxin					
Bacillus cereus, Staphylococcus aureus, Clostridium perfringens	1–8 h 8–24 h	3–4+	1–2+	0–1+	3–4+, watery
Enterotoxin					
Vibrio cholerae, enterotoxigenic *Escheria coli, Klebsiella pneumoniae, Aeromonas* species	8–72 h	2–4+	1–2+	0–1+	3–4+, watery
Enteroadherent					
Enteropathogenic and enteroadherent, *E. coli, Giardia* organisms, cryptosporidiosis, helminths	1–8 d	0–1+	1–3+	1–2+	1–2+, watery
Cytotoxin-producers					
Clostridium difficile	1–3 d	0–1+	3–4+	1–2+	1–3+, usually watery, occasionally bloody
Hemorrhagic *E. coli*	12–72 h	0–1+	3–4+	1–2+	1–3+, initially watery, quickly bloody
Invasive organisms					
Minimal inflammation					
Rotavirus and Norwalk agent	1–3 d	1–2+	2–3+	3–4+	1–3+, watery
Variable inflammation					
Salmonella, Campylobacter, and *Aeromonas* species, *Vibrio parahaemolyticus, Yersinia*	12 h–11 d	0–3+	2–4+	3–4+	1–4+, watery or bloody
Severe inflammation					
Shigella species, enteroinvasive *E. coli, Entamoeba histolytica*	12 h–8 d	0–1+	3–4+	3–4+	1–2+, bloody

SOURCE: Adapted from DW Powell, in T Yamada (ed): *Textbook of Gastroenterology,* 2d ed. Philadelphia, Lippincott, 1995; and DR Syndman, in SL Gorbach (ed): *Infectious Diarrhea.* London, Blackwell, 1986.

diarrhea can also be confused with acute diarrhea early in their course. This confusion may occur with inflammatory bowel disease and some of the other inflammatory chronic diarrheas that may have an abrupt rather than insidious onset and exhibit features that mimic infection.

Approach to the Patient

The decision to evaluate acute diarrhea depends on its severity and duration and on various host factors (Fig. 42-2). Most episodes of acute diarrhea are mild and self-limited, and they do not justify the cost and potential morbidity of diagnostic or pharmacologic interventions. Indications for evaluation include profuse diarrhea with dehydration, grossly bloody stools, fever ≥38.5° C, duration >48 h without improvement, new community outbreaks, associated severe abdominal pain in patients older than 50 years of age, and elderly (≥70 years) or immunocompromised patients. In some patients with moderately severe febrile diarrhea with fecal leukocytes (or increased fecal levels of the leukocyte proteins lactoferrin or calprotectin) present or with dysentery, a diagnostic evaluation might be eschewed in favor of an empiric antibiotic trial (see below).

The cornerstone of diagnosis in those suspected of severe acute infectious diarrhea is microbiologic analysis of the stool. Workup includes cultures for bacterial and viral pathogens, direct inspection for ova and parasites, and immunoassays for certain bacterial toxins (*C. difficile*), viral antigens (rotavirus), and protozoal antigens (*Giardia,*

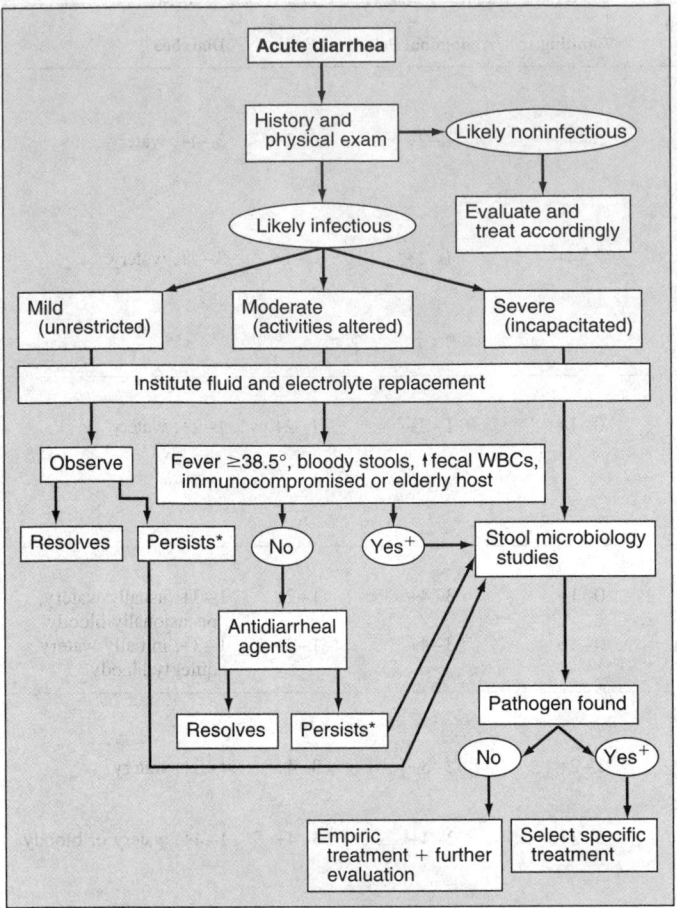

*Consider empiric Rx with metronidazole before eval;
†Consider empiric Rx with quinolone before eval.

FIGURE 42-2 Algorithm for the management of acute diarrhea. Consider empiric Rx before evaluation with (*) metronidazole and (†) with quinolone.

E. histolytica). The aforementioned clinical and epidemiologic associations may assist in focusing the evaluation. If a particular pathogen or set of possible pathogens is so implicated, then either the whole panel of routine studies may not be necessary or, in some instances, special cultures may be appropriate as for enterohemorrhagic and other types of *E. coli*, *Vibrio* species, and *Yersinia*. Molecular diagnosis of pathogens in stool can be made by identification of unique DNA sequences; and evolving microarray technologies could lead to a more rapid, sensitive, specific, and cost-effective diagnostic approach in the future.

Persistent diarrhea is commonly due to *Giardia*, but additional causative organisms that should be considered include *C. difficile* (especially if antibiotics had been administered), *E. histolytica*, *Cryptosporidium*, *Campylobacter*, and others. If stool studies are unrevealing, then flexible sigmoidoscopy with biopsies and upper endoscopy with duodenal aspirates and biopsies may be indicated.

Structural examination by sigmoidoscopy, colonoscopy, or abdominal CT scanning (or other imaging approaches) may be appropriate in patients with uncharacterized persistent diarrhea to exclude inflammatory bowel disease, or as an initial approach in patients with suspected noninfectious acute diarrhea such as might be caused by ischemic colitis, diverticulitis, or partial bowel obstruction.

℞ TREATMENT Fluid and electrolyte replacement are of central importance to all forms of acute diarrhea. Fluid replacement alone may suffice for mild cases. Oral sugar-electrolyte solutions (sport drinks or designed formulations) should be instituted promptly with

severe diarrhea to limit dehydration, which is the major cause of death. Profoundly dehydrated patients, especially infants and the elderly, require intravenous rehydration.

In moderately severe nonfebrile and nonbloody diarrhea, antimotility antisecretory agents like loperamide can be useful adjuncts to control symptoms. Such agents should be avoided with febrile dysentery, which may be exacerbated or prolonged by them. Bismuth subsalicylate may reduce symptoms of vomiting and diarrhea but should not be used to treat immunocompromised patients because of the risk of bismuth encephalopathy.

Judicious use of antibiotics is appropriate in selected instances of acute diarrhea and may reduce its severity and duration (Fig. 42-2). Many physicians treat moderately to severely ill patients with febrile dysentery empirically without diagnostic evaluation using a quinolone, such as ciprofloxacin (500 mg bid for 3 to 5 d). Empiric treatment can also be considered for suspected giardiasis with metronidazole (250 mg qid for 7d). Selection of antibiotics and dosage regimens is otherwise dictated by specific pathogens and conditions found (Chaps. 131, 153, 156–162). Antibiotic coverage is indicated whether or not a causative organism is discovered in patients that are immunocompromised, have mechanical heart valves or recent vascular grafts, or are elderly. Antibiotic prophylaxis is indicated for certain patients traveling to high-risk countries in whom the likelihood or seriousness of acquired diarrhea would be especially high, including those with immunocompromise, inflammatory bowel disease, or gastric achlorhydria. Use of trimethoprim/sulfamethoxazole or ciprofloxacin may reduce bacterial diarrhea in such travelers by 90%.

CHRONIC DIARRHEA Diarrhea lasting more than 4 weeks warrants evaluation to exclude serious underlying pathology. In contrast to acute diarrhea, most of the many causes of chronic diarrhea are noninfectious. The classification of chronic diarrhea by pathophysiologic mechanism facilitates a rational approach to management (Table 42-3).

Secretory Causes Secretory diarrheas are due to derangements in fluid and electrolyte transport across the enterocolic mucosa. They are characterized clinically by watery, large-volume fecal outputs that are typically painless and persist with fasting. Because there is no malabsorbed solute, stool osmolality is accounted for by normal endogenous electrolytes with no fecal osmotic gap.

Medications Side effects from regular ingestion of drugs and toxins are the most common secretory causes of chronic diarrhea. Hundreds of prescription and over-the-counter medications (see "Other Causes of Acute Diarrhea," above) may produce unwanted diarrhea. Surreptitious or habitual use of stimulant laxatives [e.g., senna, cascara, bisacodyl, ricinoleic acid (castor oil)] must also be considered. Chronic ethanol consumption may cause a secretory-type diarrhea due to enterocyte injury with impaired sodium and water absorption as well as to rapid transit and other alterations. Inadvertent ingestion of certain environmental toxins (e.g., arsenic) may lead to chronic rather than acute forms of diarrhea. Certain bacterial infections may occasionally persist and be associated with a secretory-type diarrhea.

Bowel resection, mucosal disease, or enterocolic fistula These conditions may result in a secretory-type diarrhea because of inadequate surface for resorption of secreted fluids and electrolytes. Unlike other secretory diarrheas, this subset of conditions tends to worsen with eating. With disease (e.g., Crohn's ileitis) or resection of <100 cm of terminal ileum, dihydroxy bile acids may escape absorption and stimulate colonic secretion (cholorrheic diarrhea). This mechanism may contribute to so-called *idiopathic secretory diarrhea*, in which bile acids are functionally malabsorbed from a normal-appearing terminal ileum. Partial bowel obstruction, ostomy stricture, or fecal impaction may paradoxically lead to increased fecal output due to hypersecretion.

Hormones Although uncommon, the classic examples of secretory diarrhea are those mediated by hormones. *Metastatic gastrointestinal carcinoid tumors* or, rarely, *primary bronchial carcinoids* may

Table 42-3 Major Causes of Chronic Diarrhea According to Predominant Pathophysiologic Mechanism

Secretory causes
  Exogenous stimulant laxatives
  Chronic ethanol ingestion
  Other drugs and toxins
  Endogenous laxatives (dihydroxy bile acids)
  Idiopathic secretory diarrhea
  Certain bacterial infections
  Bowel resection, disease, or fistula (↓ absorption)
  Partial bowel obstruction or fecal impaction
  Hormone-producing tumors (carcinoid, vipoma, medullary cancer of thyroid, mastocytosis, gastrinoma, colorectal villous adenoma)
  Addison's disease
  Congenital electrolyte absorption defects
Osmotic causes
  Osmotic laxatives (Mg^{2+}, PO_4^{3-}, SO_4^{2-})
  Lactase and other disaccharide deficiencies
  Nonabsorbable carbohydrates (sorbitol, lactulose, polyethylene glycol)
Steatorrheal causes
  Intraluminal maldigestion (pancreatic exocrine insufficiency, bacterial overgrowth, liver disease)
  Mucosal malabsorption (celiac sprue, Whipple's disease, infections, abetalipoproteinemia, ischemia)
  Postmucosal obstruction (1° or 2° lymphatic obstruction)

Inflammatory causes
  Idiopathic inflammatory bowel disease (Crohn's chronic ulcerative colitis)
  Microscopic and collagenous colitis
  Immune-related mucosal disease (1° or 2° immunodeficiencies, food allergy, eosinophilic gastroenteritis, graft-vs-host disease)
  Infections (invasive bacteria, viruses, and parasites)
  Radiation injury
  Gastrointestinal malignancies
Dysmotile causes
  Visceral neuromyopathies
  Hyperthyroidism
  Drugs (prokinetic agents)
Factitial causes
  Munchausen
  Bulimia

produce watery diarrhea alone or as part of the carcinoid syndrome that comprises episodic flushing, wheezing, dyspnea, and right-sided valvular heart disease. Diarrhea is due to the release into the circulation of potent intestinal secretagogues including serotonin, histamine, prostaglandins, and various kinins. Pellagra-like skin lesions may rarely occur as the result of serotonin overproduction with niacin depletion. *Gastrinoma*, one of the most common neuroendocrine tumors, most typically presents with refractory peptic ulcers, but diarrhea occurs in up to one-third of cases and may be the only clinical manifestation in 10%. While various secretagogues released with gastrin may play a role, the diarrhea most often results from fat maldigestion owing to pancreatic enzyme inactivation by low intraduodenal pH. The watery diarrhea hypokalemia achlorhydria (WDHA) syndrome, also called *pancreatic cholera*, is due to a non-β cell pancreatic adenoma, referred to as a VIPoma, that secretes vasoactive intestinal peptide (VIP) and a host of other peptide hormones including pancreatic polypeptide, secretin, gastrin, gastrin-inhibitory polypeptide, neurotensin, calcitonin, and prostaglandins. The secretory diarrhea is often massive with stool volumes >3 L/d; daily volumes as high as 20 L have been reported. Life-threatening dehydration, neuromuscular dysfunction from associated hypokalemia, hypomagnesemia, or hypercalcemia, flushing, and hyperglycemia may accompany vipoma. *Medullary carcinoma of the thyroid* may present with watery diarrhea caused by calcitonin, other secretory peptides, or prostaglandins. This tumor occurs sporadically or, in 25 to 50% of cases, as a feature of multiple endocrine neoplasia type IIa with pheochromocytomas and hyperparathyroidism. Prominent diarrhea is often associated with metastatic disease and poor prognosis. *Systemic mastocytosis*, which may be associated with the skin lesion urticaria pigmentosa, may cause diarrhea that is either secretory and mediated by histamine, or inflammatory and due

to intestinal filtration by mast cells. Large *colorectal villous adenomas* may rarely be associated with a secretory diarrhea that may cause hypokalemia, can be inhibited by NSAIDs, and is apparently mediated by prostaglandins.

Congenital defects in ion absorption   Rarely, these defects cause watery diarrhea from birth and include defective Cl^-/HCO_3^- exchange (*congenital chloridorrhea*) with alkalosis and defective Na^+/H^+ exchange with acidosis. Some hormone deficiencies may be associated with watery diarrhea, such as occurs with adrenocortical insufficiency (Addison's disease) that may be accompanied by hyperpigmentation.

Osmotic Causes   Osmotic diarrhea occurs when ingested, poorly absorbable, osmotically active solutes draw enough fluid lumenward to exceed the resorptive capacity of the colon. Fecal water output increases in proportion to such a solute load. Osmotic diarrhea characteristically ceases with fasting or with discontinued oral intake of the offending agent.

Osmotic laxatives   Ingestion of magnesium-containing antacids, health supplements, or laxatives may induce osmotic diarrhea typified by a stool osmotic gap: 2([Na] + [K]) ≪290 mosm/kg. Anionic laxatives containing sulfates or phosphates produce osmotic diarrhea without an osmotic gap, as sodium accompanies the anionic solutes; direct measurement of stool sulfates and phosphates may be necessary to confirm the cause of diarrhea.

Carbohydrate malabsorption   Carbohydrate malabsorption due to acquired or congenital defects in brush-border disaccharidases and other enzymes leads to osmotic diarrhea with a low pH. One of the most common causes of chronic diarrhea in adults is *lactase deficiency*, which affects three-fourths of non-Caucasians worldwide and 5 to 30% of persons in the United States; most learn to avoid milk products without an intervention. Some sugars, such as sorbitol, are universally malabsorbed, and diarrhea ensues with ingestion of ample medications, gum, or candies sweetened with these nonabsorbable sugars. Lactulose, used to acidify stools in patients with hepatic failure, also causes diarrhea on this basis.

Steatorrheal Causes   Fat malabsorption may lead to greasy, foul-smelling, difficult-to-flush diarrhea often associated with weight loss and nutritional deficiencies due to concomitant malabsorption of amino acids and vitamins. Increased fecal output is caused by the osmotic effects of fatty acids, especially after bacterial hydroxylation, and, to a lesser extent, by the burden of neutral fat. Quantitatively, steatorrhea is defined as stool fat exceeding the normal 7 g/d; daily fecal fat averages 15 to 25 g with small intestinal diseases and often exceeds 40 g with pancreatic exocrine insufficiency. Intraluminal maldigestion, mucosal malabsorption, or lymphatic obstruction may produce steatorrhea.

Intraluminal maldigestion   This condition most commonly results from pancreatic exocrine insufficiency, which occurs when >90% of pancreatic secretory function is lost. *Chronic pancreatitis*, usually a sequela of ethanol abuse, most frequently causes pancreatic insufficiency. Other causes include *cystic fibrosis, pancreatic duct obstruction*, and rarely, *somatostatinoma*. Bacterial overgrowth in the small intestine may deconjugate bile acids and alter micelle formation that impair fat digestion; it occurs with stasis from a blind-loop, small bowel diverticulum, or dysmotility and is especially likely in the elderly. Finally, cirrhosis or biliary obstruction may lead to mild steatorrhea due to deficient intraluminal bile acid concentration.

Mucosal malabsorption   Mucosal malabsorption occurs from a variety of enteropathies, but most prototypically and perhaps most commonly from *celiac sprue*. This gluten-sensitive enteropathy characterized by villous atrophy and crypt hyperplasia in the proximal small bowel often presents with fatty diarrhea associated with multiple nutritional deficiencies of varying severity and affects all ages. *Tropical sprue* may produce a similar histologic and clinical syndrome, but it occurs in residents of or travelers to tropical climates; its often abrupt onset and response to antibiotics suggest an infectious etiology. *Whipple's disease*, due to the actinomycete *Treponema whippleii* and histiocytic infiltration of the small bowel mucosa, is a less common cause of steatorrhea that most typically occurs in young or middle-aged men; it is frequently associated with arthralgias, fever, lymphadenopathy, and extreme fatigue and may affect the central nervous system and endocardium. A similar clinical and histologic picture results from *Mycobacterium avium intracellulare* infection in patients with AIDS. *Abetalipoproteinemia* is a rare defect of chylomicron formation and fat malabsorption in children associated with acanthocytic erythrocytes, ataxia, and retinitis pigmentosa. Several other conditions may cause mucosal malabsorption including infections, especially with protozoa like *Giardia*, numerous medications (e.g., colchicine, cholestyramine, neomycin), and chronic ischemia.

Postmucosal lymphatic obstruction   The pathophysiology of this condition, which is due to the rare *congenital intestinal lymphangiectasia* or to *acquired lymphatic obstruction* secondary to trauma, tumor, or infection, leads to the unique constellation of fat malabsorption with enteric losses of protein (often causing edema) and lymphocytes (with resultant lymphocytopenia) that enter the portal circulation directly. Carbohydrate and amino acid absorption are preserved.

Inflammatory Causes   Inflammatory diarrheas are generally accompanied by pain, fever, bleeding, or other manifestations of inflammation. The mechanism of diarrhea may not only be exudation but, depending on lesion site, may include fat malabsorption, disrupted fluid/electrolyte absorption, and hypersecretion or hypermotility from release of cytokines and other inflammatory mediators. The unifying feature on stool analysis is the presence of leukocytes or leukocyte-derived proteins such as calprotectin. With severe inflammation, exudative protein loss can lead to anasarca (generalized edema). Any middle-aged or older person with chronic inflammatory-type diarrhea, especially with blood, should be carefully evaluated to exclude a colorectal or large enteric tumor.

Idiopathic inflammatory bowel disease   The illnesses in this category, which include *Crohn's disease* and *chronic ulcerative colitis*, are among the most common organic causes of chronic diarrhea in adults and range in severity from mild to fulminant and life threatening. They may be associated with uveitis, polyarthralgias, cholestatic liver disease (primary sclerosing cholangitis), and various skin lesions (erythema nodosum, pyoderma gangrenosum). *Microscopic colitis*, including *collagenous colitis*, is an increasingly recognized cause of chronic watery diarrhea; biopsy of a normal appearing colorectum is required for histologic diagnosis.

Primary or secondary forms of immunodeficiency   Immunodeficiency may lead to prolonged infectious diarrhea. With common, variable *hypogammaglobulinemia*, diarrhea is particularly prevalent and often the result of giardiasis.

Eosinophilic gastroenteritis   Eosinophil infiltration of the mucosa, muscularis, or serosa at any level of the gastrointestinal tract may cause diarrhea, pain, vomiting, or ascites. Affected patients often have an atopic history, Charcot-Leyden crystals due to extruded eosinophil contents may be seen on microscopic inspection of stool, and peripheral eosinophilia is present in 50 to 75% of patients. While hypersensitivity to certain foods occurs in adults, true food allergy causing chronic diarrhea is rare.

Other causes   Chronic inflammatory diarrhea may be caused by *radiation enterocolitis, chronic graft-versus-host disease, Behcet's syndrome*, and *Cronkite-Canada syndrome*, among others.

Dysmotile Causes   Rapid transit may accompany many diarrheas as a secondary or contributing phenomenon, but primary dysmotility is an unusual etiology of true diarrhea. Stool features often suggest a secretory diarrhea, but mild steatorrhea up to 14 g of fat per day can be produced by maldigestion from rapid transit alone. *Hyperthyroidism, carcinoid syndrome*, and certain drugs (e.g., prostaglandins, prokinetic agents) may produce hypermotility with resultant diarrhea. Primary visceral neuromyopathies or idiopathic acquired intestinal pseudo-obstruction may lead to stasis with secondary bacterial overgrowth causing diarrhea. *Diabetic diarrhea*, often accompanied by peripheral and generalized autonomic neuropathies, may occur in part because of intestinal dysmotility.

The exceedingly common *irritable bowel syndrome* (10% point prevalence, 1 to 2% per year incidence) is characterized by disturbed intestinal and colonic motor and sensory responses to various stimuli. Symptoms of stool frequency typically cease at night, alternate with periods of constipation, are accompanied by abdominal pain relieved with defecation, and rarely result in weight loss or true diarrhea.

Factitial Causes   Factitial diarrhea accounts for up to 15% of unexplained diarrheas referred to tertiary care centers. Either as a form of *Munchausen syndrome* (deception or self-injury for secondary gain) or *bulimia*, some patients covertly self-administer laxatives alone or in combination with other medications (e.g., diuretics) or surreptitiously add water or urine to stool sent for analysis. Such patients are typically women, often with histories of psychiatric illness and disproportionately from careers in health care. Hypotension and hypokalemia are common co-presenting features. Such patients often deny this possibility when confronted, but they do benefit from psychiatric counseling when they acknowledge their behavior.

Approach to the Patient

The laboratory tools available to evaluate the very common problem of chronic diarrhea are extensive, and many are costly and invasive. As such, the diagnostic evaluation must be rationally directed by a careful history and physical examination, and simple triage tests are often warranted before complex investigations are launched (Fig. 42-3). The history, physical examination, and routine blood studies should attempt to characterize the mechanism of diarrhea, identify diagnostically helpful associations, and assess the patient's fluid/electrolyte and nutritional status. Patients should be questioned about the onset, duration, pattern, aggravants (especially diet), relieving factors, and stool characteristics of their diarrhea. The presence or absence of fecal incontinence, fever, weight loss, pain, certain exposures (travel, medications, contacts with diarrhea), and common extraintestinal manifestations (skin changes, arthralgias, oral aphtha) should be noted. Physical findings may offer clues such as a thyroid mass, wheezing, heart murmurs, edema, hepatomegaly, abdominal masses, lymphadenopathy, mucocutaneous abnormalities, perianal fistulae, or anal sphincter laxity. Peripheral blood counts may reveal leukocytosis that suggests inflammation; anemia that reflects blood loss or nutritional deficiencies; or eosinophilia that may occur with parasitoses, neoplasia, collagen-vascular disease, allergy, or eosinophilic gastroenteritis. Blood chemistries may demonstrate electrolyte, hepatic, or other metabolic disturbances.

A therapeutic trial is often appropriate, definitive, and highly cost-effective when a specific diagnosis is suggested on the initial physician encounter. For example, chronic watery diarrhea, which ceases with fasting in an otherwise healthy young adult, may justify a trial of a lactose-restricted diet; bloating and diarrhea persisting since a mountain backpacking trip may warrant a trial of metronidazole for likely giardiasis; and postprandial diarrhea persisting since an ileal resection might be treated with cholestyramine before further evaluation. Persistent symptoms require additional investigation.

Certain diagnoses may be suggested on the initial encounter, e.g., idiopathic inflammatory bowel disease; however, additional focused evaluations may be necessary to confirm the diagnosis and characterize the severity or extent of disease so that treatment can be best guided. Patients suspected of having irritable bowel syndrome should be initially evaluated with proctosigmoidoscopy and mucosal biopsies; those with normal findings might be reassured and, as indicated, treated empirically with antispasmodics, antidiarrheals, bulk agents, anxiolytes, or antidepressants. Any patient who presents with chronic diarrhea and hematochezia should be evaluated with stool microbiologic studies and colonoscopy.

In an estimated two-thirds of cases, the cause for chronic diarrhea remains unclear after the initial encounter, and further testing is required. Quantitative stool collection and analyses can yield important objective data that may establish a diagnosis or characterize the type of diarrhea as a triage for focused additional studies (Fig. 42-3). If stool weight exceeds 200 g/d, additional stool analyses should be performed that might include electrolyte concentration, pH, occult blood testing, leukocyte inspection (or leukocyte protein assay), fat quantitation, and laxative screens.

For secretory diarrheas (watery, normal osmotic gap), possible medication-related side effects or surreptitious laxative use should be reconsidered. Microbiologic studies should be done including fecal bacterial cultures (including media for *Aeromonas* and *Pleisiomonas*), inspection for ova and parasites, and *Giardia* antigen assay (the most sensitive test for giardiasis). Small bowel bacterial overgrowth can be excluded by intestinal aspirates with quantitative cultures or with glucose or xylose breath tests involving measurement of breath hydrogen or other metabolite (e.g., $^{14}CO_2$). However, interpretation of these breath tests may be confounded by disturbances of intestinal transit. When suggested by history or other findings, screens for peptide hormones should be pursued (e.g., serum gastrin, VIP, calcitonin, and thyroid hormone/thyroid stimulating hormone, or urinary 5-hydroxyindolacetic acid and histamine). Upper endoscopy and colonoscopy with biopsies and small bowel barium x-rays are helpful to rule out structural or occult inflammatory disease.

Further evaluation of osmotic diarrhea should include tests for lactose intolerance and magnesium ingestion, the two most common causes. Low fecal pH suggests carbohydrate malabsorption; lactose malabsorption can be confirmed by lactose breath testing or by a therapeutic trial with lactose exclusion and observation of the effect of lactose challenge (e.g., a quart of milk). Lactase determination on small bowel biopsy is generally not available. If fecal Mg^{2+} or laxative levels are elevated, then inadvertent or surreptitious ingestion should be considered and psychiatric help should be sought.

For those with proven fatty diarrhea, endoscopy with small bowel biopsy (including aspiration for *Giardia* and quantitative cultures) should be performed; if this procedure is unrevealing, a small bowel radiograph is often an appropriate next step. If small bowel studies are negative or if pancreatic disease is suspected, pancreatic exocrine insufficiency should be excluded with direct tests, such as the secretin-cholecystokinin stimulation test, or by indirect tests, such as assay of fecal chymotrypsin activity or a bentiromide test.

Chronic inflammatory-type diarrheas should be suspected by the presence of blood or leukocytes in the stool. Such findings warrant stool cultures, inspection for ova and parasites, *C. difficile* toxin assay, colonoscopy with biopsies, and if indicated, small bowel oral contrast studies.

TREATMENT   Treatment of chronic diarrhea depends on the specific etiology and may be curative, suppressive, or empiric. If the cause can be eradicated, treatment is curative as with resection of a colorectal cancer, antibiotic administration for Whipple's disease, or discontinuation of an offending drug. For many chronic conditions, diarrhea can be controlled by suppression of the underlying mechanism. Examples include elimination of dietary lactose for lactase deficiency or gluten for celiac sprue, use of glucocorticoids or other anti-inflammatory agents for idiopathic inflammatory bowel diseases, adsorptive agents such as cholestyramine for ileal bile acid malabsorption, proton pump inhibitors such as omeprazole for the gastric hypersecretion of gastrinomas, somatostatin analogues such as octreotide for malignant carcinoid, prostaglandin inhibitors such as indomethacin for medullary carcinoma of the thyroid, and pancreatic enzyme replacement for pancreatic insufficiency. When the specific cause or mechanism of chronic diarrhea evades diagnosis, empiric therapy may be beneficial. Mild opiates such as diphenoxylate or loperamide are often helpful in mild or moderate watery diarrhea. For those with more severe diarrhea, codeine or tincture of opium may be beneficial. Such antimotility agents should be avoided with inflammatory bowel disease, as toxic megacolon may be precipitated. Clonidine, an α_2-adrenergic agonist, may allow control of diabetic diarrhea. For all patients with chronic diarrhea, fluid and electrolyte repletion is an important component of management (see "Acute Diarrhea," above). Replacement of fat-soluble vitamins may also be necessary in patients with chronic steatorrhea.

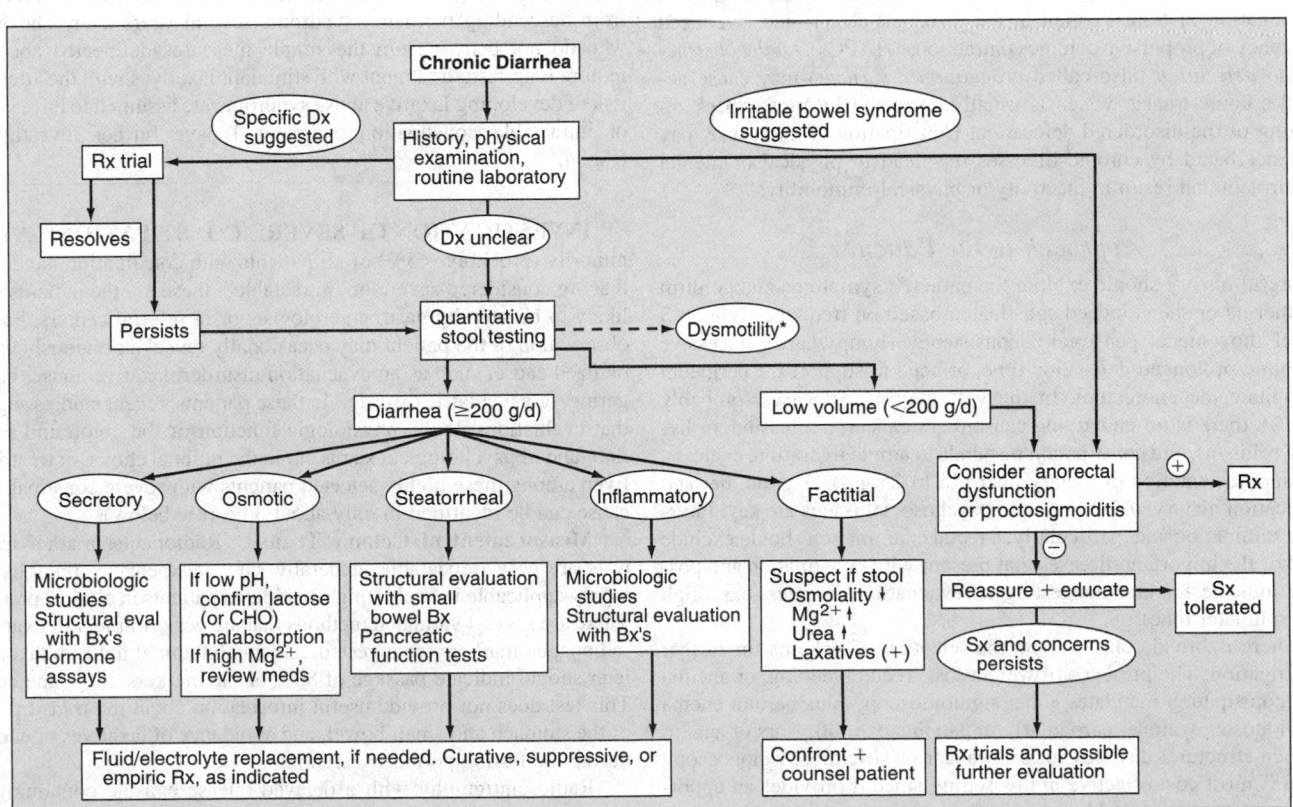

FIGURE 42-3   Algorithm for the management of chronic diarrhea.* Dysmotility presents variable stool profile.

CONSTIPATION

DEFINITION   Constipation is a common complaint in clinical practice and usually refers to persistent, difficult, infrequent, or seemingly incomplete defecation. Because of the wide range of normal bowel habits, constipation is difficult to define precisely. Most persons have at least three bowel movements per week; however, stool frequency alone is not a sufficient criterion for the diagnosis of constipation because many constipated patients describe a normal frequency of defecation but subjective complaints of excessive straining, hard stools, lower abdominal fullness, and a sense of incomplete evacuation. The individual patient's symptoms must be analyzed in detail to ascertain what is meant by "constipation" or "difficulty" with defecation.

Stool form and consistency are well correlated with the time elapsed from the preceding defecation. Hard, pellety stools occur with slow transit, while loose watery stools are associated with rapid transit. Small, pellety stools are more difficult to expel than large ones.

The perception of hard stools or excessive straining is more difficult to assess objectively, and the need for enemas or digital disimpaction is a clinically useful way to corroborate the patient's perceptions of difficult defecation.

Psychosocial factors may also be important. A person whose parents attached great importance to daily defecation will become greatly concerned when he or she misses a daily bowel movement; some children withhold stool to gain attention; and some adults are simply too busy or too embarrassed to interrupt their work when the call to have a bowel movement is sensed.

CAUSES   Pathophysiologically, chronic constipation generally results from inadequate fiber intake or from disordered colonic transit or anorectal function as a result of a neurogastroenterologic disturbance, certain drugs, or in association with a large number of systemic diseases that affect the gastroinestinal tract (Table 42-4). Constipation of recent onset may be a symptom of significant organic disease such as tumor or stricture. In *idiopathic constipation*, a subset of patients exhibit delayed emptying of the ascending and transverse colon with prolongation of transit (often in the proximal colon) and a reduced frequency of propulsive colonic contractions (HAPCs). *Outlet obstruction to defecation* (also called *evacuation disorders*) may cause delayed colonic transit, which is usually corrected by biofeedback retraining of the disordered defecation. Constipation of any cause may be exacerbated by chronic illnesses that lead to physical or mental impairment and result in inactivity or physical immobility.

Approach to the Patient

A careful history should explore the patient's symptoms and confirm whether he or she is indeed constipated based on frequency (e.g., <3 bowel movements per week), consistency (lumpy/hard), excessive straining, prolonged defecation time, or need to support the perineum or digitate the anorectum. In the vast majority of cases (probably >90%), there is no underlying cause (e.g., cancer, depression, or hypothyroidism), and constipation responds to ample hydration, exercise, and supplementation of dietary fiber (15 to 25 g/d). A good diet and medication history and attention to psychosocial issues are key. Physical examination and, particularly, a rectal examination should exclude most of the important diseases that present with constipation and possibly indicate features suggesting an evacuation disorder (e.g., high anal sphincter tone).

There is broad consensus on the selection of patients for further investigation. The presence of weight loss, rectal bleeding, or anemia with constipation mandates either sigmoidoscopy plus barium enema or colonoscopy alone, particularly in patients over 40 years of age, to exclude structural diseases such as cancer or strictures. Colonoscopy alone is most cost effective in this setting since it provides an opportunity to biopsy mucosal lesions, perform polypectomy, or dilate strictures. Barium enema has advantages over colonoscopy in the patient

Table 42-4   Causes of Constipation in Adults

Types of Constipation and Causes	Examples
Recent Onset	
Colonic obstruction	Neoplasm: stricture: ischemic, diverticular, inflammatory
Anal sphincter spasm	Anal fissure, painful hemorrhoids
Medications	
Chronic	
Irritable bowel syndrome	Constipation–predominant, alternating
Medications	Ca^{2+} blockers, antidepressants
Colonic pseudo-obstruction	Slow transit constipation, megacolon (rare Hirschsprung's, Chagas)
Disorders of rectal evacuation	Pelvic floor dysfunction, anismus, descending perineum syndrome, rectal mucosal prolapse, rectocele
Endocrinopathies	Hypothyroidism, hypercalcemia, pregnancy
Psychiatric disorders	Depression, eating disorders, drugs
Neurologic disease	Parkinsonism, multiple sclerosis, spinal cord injury
Generalized muscle disease	Progressive systemic sclerosis

with isolated constipation, since it is less costly and identifies colonic dilatation and all significant mucosal lesions or strictures that are likely to present with constipation. Melanosis coli, or pigmentation of the colon mucosa, indicates the use of anthraquinone laxatives such as cascara or senna; however, this is usually apparent from a careful history. An unexpected disorder such as megacolon or cathartic colon may also be detected by colonic radiographs. Measurement of serum calcium and thyroid stimulating hormone levels will identify rare patients with metabolic disorders.

Patients with more troublesome constipation may not respond to fiber alone and may be helped by a bowel training regimen: taking an osmotic laxative and evacuating with enema or glycerine suppository as needed. After breakfast, a distraction-free 15 to 20 min on the toilet without straining is encouraged. Excessive straining may lead to development of hemorrhoids, and, if there is weakness of the pelvic floor or injury to the pudendal nerve, may result in obstructed defecation from descending perineum syndrome several years later. Those few who do not benefit from the simple measures delineated above or require long-term treatment with stimulant laxatives with the attendant risk of developing laxative abuse syndrome are assumed to have severe or intractable constipation and should have further investigation (Fig. 42-4).

INVESTIGATION OF SEVERE CONSTIPATION   A small minority (probably <5%) of all patients with constipation have cases that are considered severe or "intractable"; these are the patients most likely to be seen by gastroenterologists or in referral centers. Further observation of the patient may occasionally reveal a previously unrecognized cause, such as an evacuation disorder, laxative abuse, malingering, or psychiatric disorder. In these patients, recent studies suggest that evaluations of the physiologic function of the colon and pelvic floor and of psychological status aid in the rational choice of treatment. Even among these highly selected patients with severe constipation, a cause can be identified in only about 30% (see below).

Measurement of Colonic Transit   Radiopaque marker transit tests are easy, repeatable, generally safe, inexpensive, reliable, and highly applicable in evaluating constipated patients in clinical practice. There are several validated methods that are very simple. For example, radiopaque markers are ingested, and an abdominal flat film taken 5 d later should indicate passage of 80% of the markers out of the colon. This test does not provide useful information about the transit profile of the stomach and small bowel, and avoidance of laxatives or enemas during the testing period is essential.

Radioscintigraphy with a delayed-release capsule containing radiolabeled particles has been used to noninvasively characterize normal, accelerated, or delayed colonic function over 24 to 48 h with low

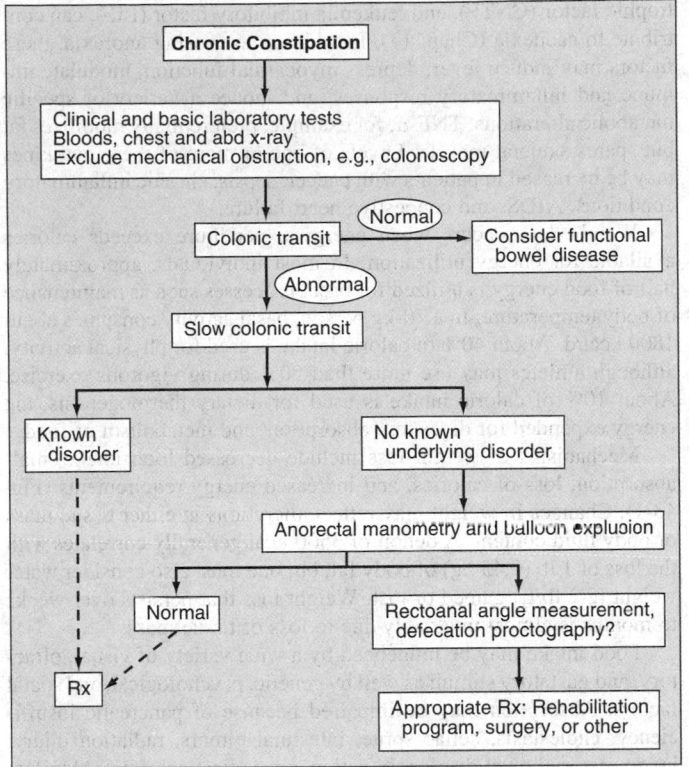

FIGURE 42-4 Algorithm for the management of constipation.

radiation exposure. This approach simultaneously assesses gastric, small bowel, and colonic transit. The disadvantages are the greater cost and the need for specific materials prepared in a nuclear medicine laboratory.

Anorectal and Pelvic Floor Tests Pelvic floor dysfunction is suggested by the inability to evacuate the rectum, a feeling of persistent rectal fullness, rectal pain, the need to extract stool from the rectum digitally, application of pressure on the posterior wall of the vagina, support of the perineum during straining, and excessive straining. These significant symptoms should be contrasted with the sense of incomplete rectal evacuation, which is common in irritable bowel syndrome.

Patients with clinically suspected obstruction of defecation should also be evaluated by a psychologist to identify eating disorders or a "need to control," to provide stress management or relaxation training, and to identify depression.

A simple clinical test in the office to document a nonrelaxing puborectalis muscle is to have the patient strain to expel the index finger during a digital rectal exam. Motion of the puborectalis posteriorly during straining indicates proper coordination of the pelvic floor muscles.

Measurement of perineal descent is relatively easy to gauge clinically by placing the patient in the left decubitus position and watching the perineum to assess either paucity or lack of descent (<1.5 cm, a sign of pelvic floor dysfunction) or perineal ballooning during straining relative to bony landmarks (>4 cm, suggesting excessive perineal descent).

A useful overall test of evacuation is the balloon expulsion test. A urinary catheter is placed in the rectum, the balloon is inflated to 50 ml with water, and a determination is made about whether the patient can expel it while seated on a toilet or in the left lateral decubitus position. In the lateral position, the weight needed to facilitate expulsion of the balloon (normal, 0 to 200 g) is determined.

Anorectal manometry is not often contributory in the evaluation of patients presenting with severe constipation, except when an excessively high resting or squeeze anal sphincter tone suggests anismus (anal sphincter spasm). This test also identifies rare syndromes, such

as adult Hirschsprung's disease, by the absence of the rectoanal inhibitory reflex or the presence of occult incontinence.

Defecography (a dynamic barium enema including lateral views obtained during barium expulsion) reveals "soft abnormalities" in many patients; the most relevant findings are the measured changes in rectoanal angle, anatomic defects of the rectum, and enteroceles or rectoceles. In a very small proportion of patients, significant anatomic defects associated with intractable constipation respond best to surgical treatment. These defects include severe intussusception with complete outlet obstruction due to funnel-shaped plugging at the anal canal or an extremely large rectocele that is preferentially filled during attempts at defecation instead of expulsion of the barium through the anus. In summary, defecography requires an interested and experienced radiologist, and abnormalities are not pathognomonic for pelvic floor dysfunction. More commonly, outlet obstruction results from a nonrelaxing puborectalis muscle, which impedes rectal emptying, rather than from defects identified by defecography.

Dynamic imaging studies such as proctography during defecation or scintigraphic expulsion of artificial stool help measure perineal descent and the rectoanal angle during rest, squeezing and straining, and scintigraphic expulsion quantitates the amount of "artificial stool" emptied. Failure of the rectoanal angle to increase significantly ($\sim 15°$) during straining confirms pelvic floor dysfunction.

Neurologic testing (EMG) is more helpful in the evaluation of patients with incontinence than of those with symptoms suggesting obstructed defecation. The absence of neurologic signs in the lower extremities suggests that any documented denervation of the puborectalis results from pelvic (e.g., obstetric) injury or from stretching of the pudendal nerve by chronic, long-standing straining.

Ultrasonography identifies sphincter or rectal wall defects and may help select patients for surgical correction. Spinal-evoked responses during electrical rectal stimulation or stimulation of external anal sphincter contraction by applying magnetic stimulation over the lumbosacral cord identify patients with limited sacral neuropathies with sufficient residual nerve conduction to attempt biofeedback training.

In summary, a balloon expulsion test is an important screening test for anorectal dysfunction. If positive, an anatomic evaluation of the rectum or anal sphincters and an assessment of pelvic floor relaxation are the tools for evaluating patients in whom obstructed defecation is suspected.

TREATMENT After the cause of constipation is characterized, a treatment decision can be made. Slow transit constipation requires aggressive medical or surgical treatment; anismus or pelvic floor dysfunction usually responds to biofeedback management (Fig. 42-4). However, only about 30% of patients with severe constipation are found to have such a physiologic disorder.

Patients with slow transit constipation are treated with bulk, osmotic, and stimulant laxatives, including fiber, psyllium, milk of magnesia, lactulose, polyethylene glycol (colonic lavage solution), and bisacodyl. If a 2- to 3-month trial of medical therapy fails and patients continue to have documented slow transit constipation unassociated with obstructed defecation, colectomy with ileorectostomy is indicated. The decision to resort to surgery is facilitated in the presence of megacolon and megarectum. The complications after surgery include small bowel obstruction (11%) and fecal soiling, particularly at night during the first postoperative year.

Patients who have a combined disorder should pursue pelvic floor retraining (biofeedback and muscle relaxation), psychological counseling, and dietetic advice first, followed by colectomy and ileorectostomy if colonic transit studies do not normalize with biofeedback alone. In patients with pelvic floor dysfunction alone, biofeedback training has a 70 to 80% success rate, measured by the acquisition of comfortable stool habits. Attempts to manage pelvic floor dysfunction with operations (internal anal sphincter or puborectalis muscle division) have achieved only mediocre success and have been largely abandoned.

BIBLIOGRAPHY

AMERICAN GASTROENTEROLOGICAL ASSOCIATION MEDICAL POSITION STATEMENT. Guidelines for the evaluation and management of chronic diarrhea. Gastroenterology 116:1461, 1991

CAMILLERI M et al: Clinical management of intractable constipation. Ann Intern Med 121:520, 1994

DUPONT HL and PRACTICE PARAMETERS COMMITTEE OF THE AMERICAN COLLEGE OF GASTROENTEROLOGY: Guidelines on acute infectious diarrhea in adults. Am J Gastroenterol 92:1962, 1997

FINE KD, SCHILLER LR: AGA technical review on the evaluation and management of chronic diarrhea. Gastroenterology 116:1461, 1999

LOCKE GR: The epidemiology of functional gastrointestinal disorders in North America. Gastroenterol Clin North Am 25:1, 1996

PROANO M et al: Transit of solids through the human colon: regional quantification in the unprepared bowel. Am J Physiol 1990;258:G856-62.

ROHNER P et al: Etiological agents of infectious diarrhea: Implications for requests for microbial culture. J Clin Microbiol 35:1427, 1997

SUAREZ FL et al: Bismuth subsalicylate markedly decreases hydrogen sulfide release in the human colon. Gastroenterology 114:923, 1998

SURRENTI E et al: Audit of constipation in a tertiary-referral gastroenterology practice. Am J Gastroenterol 90:1471, 1995

43   Carol M. Reife

WEIGHT LOSS

Significant unintentional weight loss in a previously healthy individual is often a harbinger of underlying systemic disease. During the routine medical history, therefore, inquiry should always be made about changes in weight; loss of 5% of body weight over 6 to 12 months should prompt further evaluation.

PHYSIOLOGY OF WEIGHT REGULATION   The normal individual maintains weight at a remarkably stable "set point," given the wide variation in daily caloric intake and level of activity. Because of the physiologic importance of maintaining energy stores, voluntary weight loss is difficult to achieve and sustain.

Appetite and metabolism are regulated by an intricate network of neural and hormonal factors. The hypothalamic feeding and satiety centers play a central role in these processes (Chap. 77). Neuropeptides, like corticotropin-releasing hormone (CRH), α-melanocyte stimulating hormone (α-MSH), and cocaine and amphetamine-related transcript (CART) induce anorexia by acting centrally on satiety centers. Epinephrine and norepinephrine cause a decrease in food intake and an increase in metabolic rate (Chap. 72). Amphetamines and related drugs used to suppress appetite act by releasing norepinephrine in the central nervous system. The gastrointestinal peptides glucagon, somatostatin, and particularly cholecystokinin induce a decrease in food intake by acting through a vagal mechanism to signal satiety. Hypoglycemia decreases levels of insulin which reduces glucose utilization and inhibits activity of the satiety center.

Leptin plays a central role in the long-term maintenance of weight homeostasis (Chap. 77). Leptin is produced by adipose tissue and acts on the hypothalamus to decrease food intake and increase energy expenditure. It suppresses expression of hypothalamic neuropeptide Y, a potent appetite stimulatory peptide. In parallel, leptin increases the expression of α-MSH, which decreases appetite by acting on the MC4R melanocortin receptor. Thus, leptin activates a series of downstream neural pathways that alter food-seeking behavior and metabolism. However, leptin deficiency, which occurs in conjunction with the loss adipose tissue, stimulates appetite and induces other adaptive responses including inhibition of hypothalamic thyrotropin releasing hormone (TRH) and gonadotropin releasing hormone (GnRH).

A variety of cytokines, including tumor necrosis factor α (TNF-α), interleukin (IL) (IL-6), IL-1, interferon γ (IFN-γ), ciliary neuro-trophic factor (CNTF), and leukemia inhibitory factor (LIF), can contribute to cachexia (Chap. 17). In addition to causing anorexia, these factors may induce fever, depress myocardial function, modulate immune and inflammatory responses, and induce a variety of specific metabolic alterations. TNF-α, for example, preferentially mobilizes fat but spares skeletal muscle. Levels of one or more of these cytokines may be increased in patients with cancer, sepsis, chronic inflammatory conditions, AIDS, and congestive heart failure.

Weight loss occurs when energy expenditure exceeds calories available for energy utilization. In most individuals, approximately half of food energy is utilized for basal processes such as maintenance of body temperature. In a 70-kg person, basal activity consumes about 1800 kcal/d. About 40% of caloric intake is used for physical activity, although athletes may use more than 50% during vigorous exercise. About 10% of caloric intake is used for dietary thermogenesis, the energy expended for digestion, absorption, and metabolism of food.

Mechanisms of weight loss include decreased food intake, malabsorption, loss of calories, and increased energy requirements (Fig. 43-1). Changes in weight may reflect alterations in either tissue mass or body fluid content. A deficit of 3500 kcal generally correlates with the loss of 1 lb (0.45 kg) of body fat, but one must also consider water weight (2.2 lb/L) gained or lost. Weight loss that persists over weeks to months is almost invariably due to loss of tissue mass.

Food intake may be influenced by a wide variety of visual, olfactory, and gustatory stimuli as well by genetic, psychological, and social factors. Absorption may be impaired because of pancreatic insufficiency, cholestasis, celiac sprue, intestinal tumors, radiation injury, inflammatory bowel disease, infection, or medication effect. Manifestations of these disease processes may be suggested by changes in stool frequency and consistency. Calories also may be lost due to vomiting or diarrhea, glucosuria in diabetes mellitus, or fistulous drainage. Resting energy expenditure decreases with age and can be affected by thyroid status. Beginning at about age 60, body weight declines by an average of 0.5% per year. Body composition is also affected by aging; adipose tissue increases and lean muscle mass decreases with age.

SIGNIFICANCE OF WEIGHT LOSS   Unintentional weight loss, especially in the elderly, is not uncommon and is associated with increased morbidity and mortality rates, even after comorbid conditions have been taken into account. Prospective studies indicate that significant involuntary weight loss is associated with a mortality rate of 25% over the next 18 months. Retrospective studies of significant weight loss in the elderly document mortality rates of 9 to 38% over a 2- to 3-year period.

Cancer patients with weight loss have decreased performance status, response to chemotherapy, and median survival (Chap. 79).

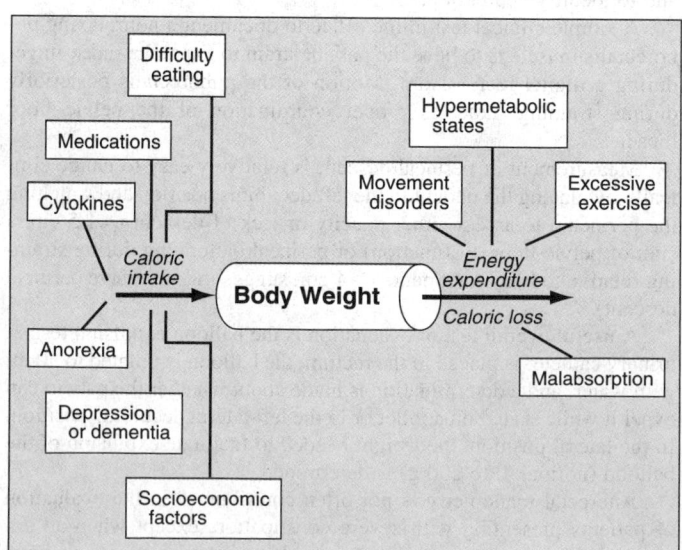

FIGURE 43-1   Energy balance and pathophysiology of weight loss.

Marked degrees of weight loss also predispose to infection. Patients undergoing elective surgery, who have lost more than 10 lb (4.5 kg) in 6 months, have higher surgical mortality rates. Vitamin and nutrient deficiencies also can accompany significant weight loss (Chap. 74).

CAUSES OF WEIGHT LOSS The list of possible causes of weight loss is extensive (Table 43-1). In the elderly, the most common causes of weight loss are depression, cancer, and benign gastrointestinal disease. Lung and gastrointestinal cancer are the most common malignancies in patients presenting with weight loss. In younger individuals, diabetes mellitus, hyperthyroidism, psychiatric disturbances including eating disorders, and infection, especially with HIV, should be considered.

The cause of involuntary weight loss is rarely occult. Careful history and physical examination, in association with directed diagnostic testing, will identify the cause of weight loss in 75% of patients. The etiology of weight loss will not be found in the remaining patients, despite extensive testing. Patients with negative evaluations tend to have lower mortality rates than those found to have organic disease.

Patients with medical causes of weight loss usually have signs or symptoms that suggest involvement of a particular organ system. Gastrointestinal tumors, including those of the pancreas and liver, may affect food intake early in the course of illness, causing weight loss before other symptoms are apparent. Lung cancer may present with post-obstructive pneumonia, dyspnea, or cough and hemoptysis; however, it may be silent and should be considered even in those without a history of cigarette smoking. Depression and isolation can cause profound weight loss, especially in the elderly. Chronic pulmonary disease and congestive heart failure can produce anorexia and may also increase resting energy expenditure. Weight loss may be the presenting sign of infectious diseases such as HIV infection, tuberculosis, endocarditis, and fungal and parasitic infections. Hyperthyroidism or pheochromocytoma increase metabolism; elderly patients with apathetic hyperthyroidism may present with weight loss alone. New onset diabetes mellitus is often accompanied by weight loss, reflecting glucosuria and loss of the anabolic actions of insulin. Adrenal insufficiency may be suggested by increased pigmentation, hyponatremia, and hyperkalemia.

Table 43-1 Causes of Weight Loss

Cancer	Medications
Endocrine and metabolic causes	Antibiotics
Hyperthyroidism	Nonsteroidal anti-inflammatory drugs
Diabetes mellitus	Serotonin reuptake inhibitors
Pheochromocytoma	Metformin
Adrenal insufficiency	Levodopa
Gastrointestinal disorders	ACE inhibitors
Malabsorption	Other drugs
Obstruction	Disorders of the mouth and teeth
Pernicious anemia	Age-related factors
Cardiac disorders	Physiologic changes
Chronic ischemia	Decreased taste and smell
Chronic congestive heart failure	Functional disabilities
Respiratory disorders	Neurologic causes
Emphysema	Stroke
Chronic obstructive pulmonary disease	Parkinson's disease
Renal insufficiency	Neuromuscular disorders
Rheumatologic disease	Dementia
Infections	Social Causes
HIV	Isolation
Tuberculosis	Economic hardship
Parasitic infection	Psychiatric and behavioral causes
Subacute bacterial endocarditis	Depression
	Anxiety
	Bereavement
	Alcoholism
	Eating disorders
	Increased activity or exercise
	Idiopathic

Table 43-2 Screening Tests for Evaluation of Involuntary Weight Loss

Initial testing	Additional testing
CBC	HIV test
Electrolytes, calcium, glucose	Upper and/or lower gastrointestinal endoscopy
Renal and liver function tests	
Urinalysis	Abdominal CT scan or MRI
TSH	Chest CT scan
Chest x-ray	
Recommended cancer screening	

Approach to the Patient

Before extensive evaluation is undertaken, it is important to confirm that weight loss has occurred. Almost half of patients who claim significant weight loss have no actual change in weight when it is measured objectively. If weight loss is present, efforts should be made to determine the time interval over which it has occurred. In the absence of documentation, changes in belt notch size or the fit of clothing may help confirm loss of weight. Not infrequently, patients who have actually sustained significant weight loss are unaware that it has occurred. Routine documentation of weight during office visits is therefore important.

The review of systems should focus on signs or symptoms that are associated with disorders that commonly cause weight loss. These include fever, pain, shortness of breath or cough, palpitations, changes in pattern of urination, and evidence of neurologic disease. Gastrointestinal disturbances, including difficulty eating, dysphagia, anorexia, nausea, and change in bowel habits, should be sought. Use of cigarettes, alcohol, and all medications should be reviewed, and patients should be questioned about previous illness or surgery as well as diseases in family members. Risk factors for HIV infection should be assessed. Signs of depression, evidence of dementia, and social factors, including financial issues that might affect food intake, should be considered.

Physical examination should begin with weight determination and documentation of vital signs. The skin should be examined for pallor, jaundice, turgor, scars from prior surgery, and stigmata of systemic disease. The search for oral thrush or dental disease, thyroid gland enlargement, adenopathy, and respiratory or cardiac abnormalities and a detailed examination of the abdomen often lead to clues for further evaluation. Rectal examination, including prostate exam and testing of stool for occult blood, should be performed in men; and all women should have a pelvic examination, even if they have had a hysterectomy. Neurologic examination should include mental status assessment and screening for depression.

Laboratory testing should confirm or exclude possible diagnoses elicited from the history and physical examination (Table 43-2). An initial phase of testing should include a complete blood count with differential, serum chemistry tests including glucose, electrolytes, renal and liver tests, calcium, thyroid stimulating hormone (TSH), urinalysis, and chest x-ray. Patients at risk for HIV infection should have HIV antibody testing. In all cases, recommended cancer screening tests appropriate for the gender and age group, such as mammograms and Pap smears, should be updated (Chap. 80). If gastrointestinal signs or symptoms are present, upper and/or lower endoscopy and abdominal imaging with either computed tomography (CT) or magnetic resonance imaging (MRI) have a relatively high yield, consistent with the high prevalence of gastrointestinal disorders in patients with weight loss. If an etiology of weight loss is not found, careful clinical follow-up, rather than persistent undirected testing, is reasonable.

BIBLIOGRAPHY

FISCHER J, JOHNSON MA: Low body weight and weight loss in the aged. J Am Diet Assoc 90:1697, 1990

FLIER JS, MARATOS-FLIER E: Obesity and the hypothalamus: Novel peptides for new pathways. Cell 92:437, 1998

GAZEWOOD JD, MEHR DR: Diagnosis and management of weight loss in the elderly. J Fam Pract 47:19, 1998

MARTON KI et al: Involuntary weight loss: Diagnostic and prognostic significance. Ann Intern Med 95:568, 1981

RABINOVITZ M et al: Unintentional weight loss: A retrospective analysis of 154 cases. Arch Intern Med 146:186, 1986

REIFE CM: Involuntary weight loss. Med Clin North Am 79:299, 1995

THOMPSON MP, MORRIS LK: Unexplained weight loss in the ambulatory elderly. J Am Geriatr Soc 39:497, 1991

WALLACE JI et al: Involuntary weight loss in older outpatients: incidence and clinical significance. J Am Geriatr Soc 43:329, 1995

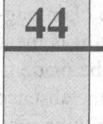

44   *Loren Laine*

GASTROINTESTINAL BLEEDING

Bleeding from the gastrointestinal (GI) tract may present in 5 ways. *Hematemesis* is vomitus of red blood or "coffee-grounds" material. *Melena* is black, tarry, foul-smelling stool. *Hematochezia* is the passage of bright red or maroon blood from the rectum. *Occult GI bleeding (GIB)* may be identified in the absence of overt bleeding by special examination of the stool (e.g., guaiac testing). Finally, patients may present only with *symptoms of blood loss or anemia* such as light-headedness, syncope, angina, or dyspnea.

SOURCES OF GASTROINTESTINAL BLEEDING

UPPER GASTROINTESTINAL SOURCES OF BLEEDING (Table 44-1) The annual incidence of hospital admissions for upper GIB (UGIB) in the United States and Europe is approximately 0.1%, with a mortality rate of ~10%. Patients rarely die from exsanguination; rather, they die due to decompensation from other underlying illnesses. The mortality rate for patients under 60 years of age in the absence of malignancy or organ failure is <1%.

Peptic ulcers are the most common cause of UGIB, accounting for about 50% of cases. Mallory-Weiss tears account for 5 to 15% of cases. The proportion of patients bleeding from varices varies widely from ~5 to 30%, depending on the population. Hemorrhagic or erosive gastropathy [e.g., due to nonsteroidal anti-inflammatory drugs (NSAIDs) or alcohol] and erosive esophagitis often cause mild UGIB, but major bleeding is rare.

Peptic Ulcers Clinical features that predict poorer outcome include hemodynamic instability, the number of units of blood transfused, red blood in the emesis and the stool, increasing age, and the presence of concurrent illness. Characteristics of the ulcer at endoscopy also provide important prognostic information. One-third of patients with active bleeding or a non-bleeding visible vessel have further bleeding that requires urgent surgery if they are treated conservatively.

Table 44-1   Sources of Bleeding in Patients Hospitalized for Acute UGIB

Sources of Bleeding	Proportion of Patients (%)
Ulcers	35–62
Varices	4–31
Mallory-Weiss tears	4–13
Gastroduodenal erosions	3–11
Erosive esophagitis	2–8
Malignancy	1–4
No source identified	7–25

SOURCE: Data from Rockall et al; GF Longstreth: Am J Gastroenterol 90:206, 1995; EM Vreeburg et al: Am J Gastroenterol 92:236, 1997; and L Laine: West J Med 155:274, 1991.

These patients clearly benefit from endoscopic therapy with bipolar electrocoagulation, heater probe, or injection therapy (e.g., absolute alcohol, 1:10,000 epinephrine), with reductions in bleeding, hospital stay, mortality rate, and costs. In contrast, patients with clean-based ulcers have rates of recurrent bleeding approaching zero. If there is no other reason for hospitalization, such patients may be discharged on the first hospital day, following stabilization. Patients without clear-based ulcers should usually remain in the hospital for 3 days, since most episodes of recurrent bleeding occur within 3 days.

Various pharmacologic agents have been assessed in the past for the treatment of ulcer bleeding without clearcut benefit. However, in recent controlled trials in Europe and Asia, high-dose intravenous omeprazole used to raise intragastric pH to 6 to 7 and enhance clot stability decreased further bleeding (but not mortality), even after the use of appropriate endoscopic therapy.

Approximately one-third of patients with a bleeding ulcer will rebleed within the next 1 to 2 years. Prevention of recurrent bleeding focuses on the three main factors in ulcer pathogenesis, *Helicobacter pylori*, NSAIDs, and acid. Eradication of *H. pylori* in patients with bleeding ulcers dramatically decreases rates of rebleeding to < 5%. If a bleeding ulcer develops in a patient taking NSAIDs, the NSAIDs should be discontinued if possible. If NSAIDs must be continued, initial treatment should be with a proton pump inhibitor, and subsequent prophylactic therapy with a proton pump inhibitor or misoprostol should be continued as long as the patient is taking NSAIDs. Changing from a standard NSAID to a COX-2-specific inhibitor should markedly lower the risk of recurrent UGIB. Patients with bleeding ulcers unrelated to *H. pylori* or NSAIDs should remain on full-dose antisecretory therapy indefinitely. →*Peptic ulcers are discussed in Chap. 285.*

Mallory-Weiss Tears The classic history is vomiting, retching, or coughing preceding hematemesis, especially in an alcoholic patient. Bleeding from these tears, which are usually on the gastric side of the gastroesophageal junction, stops spontaneously in 80 to 90% of patients and recurs in only 0 to 5%. Endoscopic therapy is effective for actively bleeding Mallory-Weiss tears. Angiographic therapy with intra-arterial infusion of vasopressin or embolization also may be useful. Rarely, operative therapy with oversewing of the tear may be required. →*Mallory-Weiss tears are discussed in Chap. 284.*

Esophageal Varices Patients with UGIB and clinical evidence suggesting the possibility of liver disease should undergo early endoscopy to determine if varices are the sources of bleeding, because patients with variceal hemorrhage have poorer outcomes than patients with other sources of UGIB. Endoscopic therapy at this time decreases further bleeding, and repeated sessions with endoscopic therapy to eradicate esophageal varices significantly reduces rebleeding and mortality. Endoscopic ligation therapy is the endoscopic therapy of choice for esophageal varices because it has less rebleeding, a lower mortality rate, fewer local complications, and requires fewer treatment sessions to achieve variceal eradication as compared to sclerotherapy.

Acute treatment with octreotide (50 μg bolus and 50 μg/h intravenous infusion for 2 to 5 days) or somatostatin may help in the control of acute bleeding, and these agents have replaced vasopressin as the medical therapy of choice for acute variceal bleeding. Over the long term, treatment with nonselective beta blockers (e.g., propranolol) has also been shown to decrease recurrent bleeding from esophageal varices. These agents commonly are given along with chronic endoscopic therapy.

In patients who have persistent or recurrent bleeding despite endoscopic and medical therapy, more invasive therapy is warranted. Transjugular intrahepatic portosystemic shunt (TIPS) decreases rebleeding more effectively than endoscopic therapy, although hepatic encephalopathy is more common and the mortality rates are comparable. Most patients with TIPS have shunt stenosis within 1 to 2 years and require re-instrumentation. Therefore, TIPS is most appropriate for patients with more severe liver disease and those in whom transplant is anticipated. Patients with milder, well-compensated cirrhosis probably should undergo decompressive surgery (e.g., distal spleno-renal shunt).

Portal hypertension is also responsible for bleeding from gastric varices, ectopic varices in the small and large intestine, and portal hypertensive gastropathy and enterocolopathy.

Hemorrhagic and Erosive Gastropathy ("Gastritis") Hemorrhagic and erosive gastropathy or gastritis refers to endoscopically visualized subepithelial hemorrhages and erosions. These are mucosal lesions and thus do not cause major bleeding. They develop in various clinical settings, the most important of which are ingestion of NSAIDs, alcohol, and stress. Half of patients who chronically ingest NSAIDs have erosions (15 to 30% have ulcers), while up to 20% of actively drinking alcoholic patients with symptoms of UGIB have evidence of subepithelial hemorrhages or erosions.

Stress-related gastric mucosal injury occurs only in extremely sick patients: those who have experienced serious trauma, major surgery, burns covering more than one-third of the body surface area, major intracranial disease, and severe medical illness (ventilator dependency, coagulopathy). Significant bleeding probably does not develop unless ulceration occurs. The mortality rate in these patients is quite high because of their serious underlying illnesses.

The incidence of bleeding from stress-related gastric mucosal injury or ulceration has decreased dramatically in recent years, most likely due to better care of critically ill patients. Pharmacologic prophylaxis for bleeding may be considered in the high-risk patients mentioned above. The best clinical data suggest that intravenous H_2-receptor antagonist therapy is the treatment of choice, although sucralfate also is effective. Prophylactic therapy decreases bleeding, but it does not lower the mortality rate.

Other Causes Other, less frequent causes of UGIB include erosive duodenitis, neoplasms, aortoenteric fistulas, vascular lesions [including hereditary hemorrhagic telengectasias (Osler-Weber-Rendu) and gastric antral vascular ectasia ("watermelon stomach")], Dieulafoy's lesion (in which an aberrant vessel in the mucosa bleeds from a pinpoint mucosal defect), prolapse gastropathy (prolapse of proximal stomach into esophagus with retching, especially in alcoholics), and hemobilia and hemosuccus pancreaticus (bleeding from the bile duct or pancreatic duct).

SMALL INTESTINAL SOURCES OF BLEEDING Small intestinal sources of bleeding (bleeding from sites beyond the reach of the standard upper endoscope) are difficult to diagnose and are responsible for the majority of cases of obscure GIB. Fortunately, small intestinal bleeding is uncommon. The most common causes are vascular ectasias and tumors (e.g., adenocarcinoma, leiomyoma, lymphoma, benign polyps, carcinoid, metastases, and lipoma). Other less common causes include Crohn's disease, infection, ischemia, vasculitis, small bowel varices, diverticula, Meckel's diverticula, duplication cysts, and intussusception. NSAIDs induce small intestinal erosions and ulcers and may be a relatively common cause of chronic, obscure GIB.

Meckel's diverticulum is the most common cause of significant lower GIB (LGIB) in children, decreasing in frequency as a cause of bleeding with age. In adults younger than 40 to 50 years, small bowel tumors often account for obscure GIB, while in patients older than 50 to 60 years, vascular ectasias are usually responsible.

Vascular ectasias should be treated with endoscopic therapy if possible. Surgical therapy can be used for vascular ectasias isolated to a segment of the small intestine when endoscopic therapy is unsuccessful; estrogen/progesterone compounds may also be tried. Isolated lesions, such as tumors, diverticula, or duplications, generally are treated with surgical resection.

COLONIC SOURCES OF BLEEDING The incidence of hospitalizations for LGIB is about one-fifth that for UGIB. Hemorrhoids are probably the most common cause of LGIB; anal fissures also cause minor bleeding and pain. If these local anal processes, which rarely require hospitalization, are excluded, the most common causes of LGIB in adults are diverticula, vascular ectasias (especially in the proximal colon of patients > 70 years), neoplasms (adenomatous polyps and adenocarcinoma), and colitis—most commonly infectious or idiopathic inflammatory bowel disease, but occasionally ischemic or radiation-induced. Uncommon causes include post-polypectomy bleeding, solitary rectal ulcer syndrome, NSAID-induced ulcers or colitis, other neoplasms, trauma, ectopic varices (most commonly rectal), lymphoid nodular hyperplasia, vasculitis, and aortocolic fistulas. In children and adolescents, the most common colonic causes of significant GIB are inflammatory bowel disease and juvenile polyps.

Diverticular bleeding is abrupt in onset, usually painless, sometimes massive, and often from the right colon; minor and occult bleeding is not characteristic. Clinical reports suggest that bleeding colonic diverticula stop bleeding spontaneously in approximately 80% of patients, and rebleed in 20 to 25% of patients. Intraarterial vasopressin may halt the bleeding, at least temporarily. If bleeding persists or recurs, segmental surgical resection is indicated.

Bleeding from right colonic vascular ectasias in the elderly may be overt or occult; it tends to be chronic and only occasionally is hemodynamically significant. Endoscopic hemostatic therapy may be useful in the treatment of vascular ectasias, as well as discrete bleeding ulcers and post-polypectomy bleeding, while endoscopic polypectomy, if possible, is used for bleeding colonic polyps. Surgical therapy is generally required for major, persistent, or recurrent bleeding from the wide variety of colonic sources of GIB that cannot be treated medically or endoscopically.

Approach to the Patient

Measurement of the heart rate and blood pressure is the best way to assess a patient with GIB. Clinically significant bleeding leads to postural changes in heart rate or blood pressure, tachycardia, and, finally, recumbent hypotension. Patients also may have a vasovagal reaction with bradycardia during bleeding episodes.

In contrast, the hemoglobin does not fall immediately with acute GIB, due to proportionate reductions in plasma and red cell volumes (i.e., "people bleed whole blood"). Thus, hemoglobin may be normal or only minimally decreased at the initial presentation of a severe bleeding episode. As extravascular fluid enters the vascular space to restore volume, the hemoglobin falls, but this process may take up to 72 h. Patients with slow, chronic GIB may have very low hemoglobin values despite normal blood pressure and heart rate. With the development of iron deficiency anemia, the mean corpuscular volume will be low and red blood cell distribution width will be increased.

Differentiation of Upper from Lower GIB Hematemesis indicates an upper GI source of bleeding (above the ligament of Treitz). Melena indicates that blood has been present in the GI tract for at least 14 h. Thus, the more proximal the bleeding site, the more likely melena will occur. Hematochezia usually represents a lower GI source of bleeding, although an upper GI lesion may bleed so rapidly that blood does not remain in the bowel long enough for melena to develop. When hematochezia is the presenting symptom of UGIB, it is associated with hemodynamic instability and dropping hemoglobin. Bleeding lesions of the small bowel may present as melena or hematochezia.

A non-bloody nasogastric aspirate may be seen in up to 16% of patients with UGIB—usually from a duodenal source. Even a bile-stained appearance does not exclude a bleeding post-pyloric lesion since reports of bile in the aspirate are incorrect in about 50% of cases. Testing of aspirates that are not grossly bloody for occult blood is of no clinical value. Other clues to UGIB include hyperactive bowel sounds and an elevated BUN (due to volume depletion and absorbed blood proteins).

Diagnostic Evaluation of the Patient with GIB • *Upper GIB* (Fig. 44-1) The history and physical exam seldom are diagnostic of the source of GIB. Upper endoscopy is the test of choice in patients

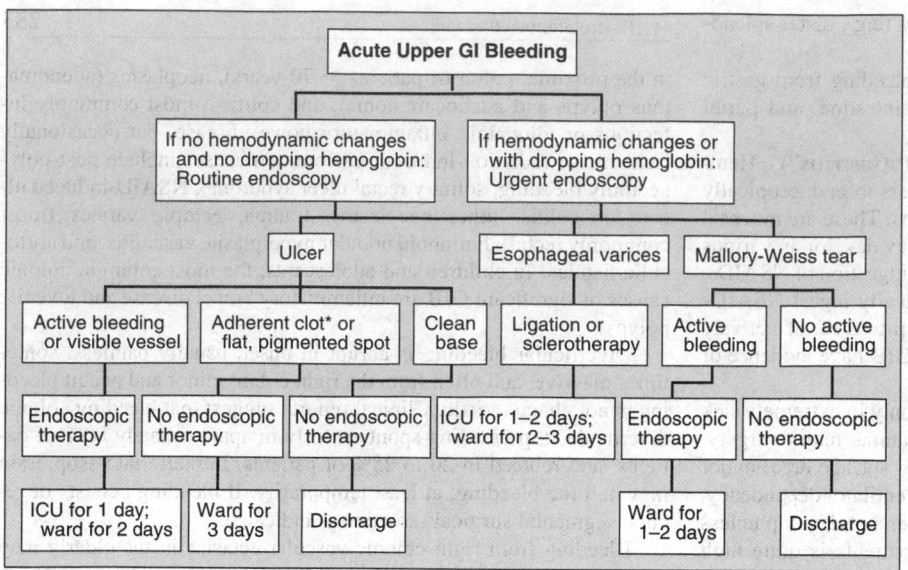

FIGURE 44-1 Suggested algorithm for patients with acute UGIB. Recommendations on level of care and time of discharge assume patient is stabilized without further bleeding or other concomitant medical problems. Upper GI endoscopy is the major diagnostic and therapeutic tool. *Some authors suggest endoscopic therapy for adherent clots.

with UGIB, and should be performed urgently in patients with hemodynamic instability (hypotension, tachycardia, or postural changes in heart rate or blood pressure). Early routine endoscopy is also beneficial in cases of milder bleeding for management decisions. Patients with major bleeding and high risk endoscopic findings (varices, ulcers with active bleeding or a visible vessel) benefit from endoscopic hemostatic therapy, while patients with low-risk lesions (e.g., clean based ulcers, non-bleeding Mallory-Weiss tears, erosive or hemorrhagic gastropathy) who have stable vital signs and hemoglobin, and no other medical problems, can be discharged home.

Lower GIB (Fig. 44-2) Patients with presumed LGIB may undergo early sigmoidoscopy for the detection of obvious, low-lying lesions. However, the procedure is difficult with brisk bleeding, and it often is impossible to identify the area of bleeding. Sigmoidoscopy

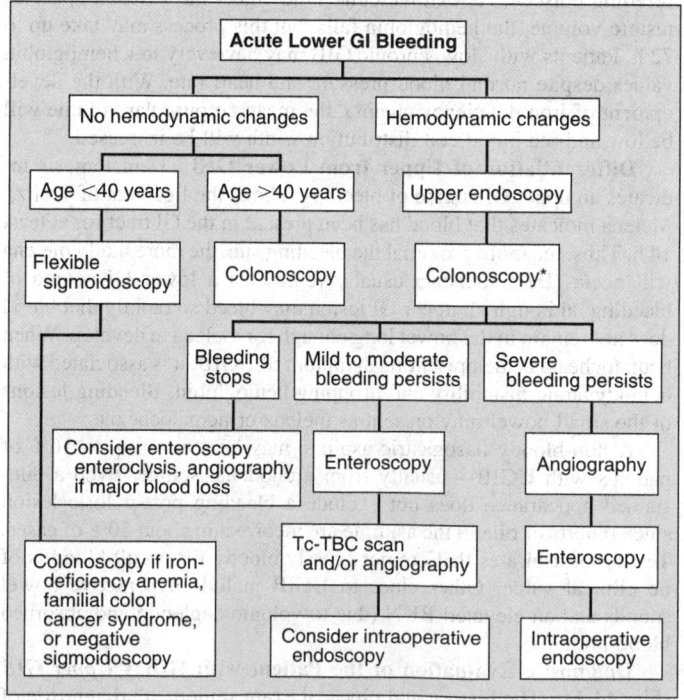

FIGURE 44-2 Suggested algorithm for patients with acute LGIB. *If massive bleeding does not allow time for colonic lavage, proceed to angiography.

is useful primarily in patients < 40 years with relatively minor bleeding. Patients with hematochezia and hemodynamic instability should have upper endoscopy to rule out an upper GI source before evaluation of the lower GI tract.

Colonoscopy after an oral lavage solution is the procedure of choice in patients with LGIB unless bleeding is too massive or unless sigmoidoscopy has disclosed an obvious actively bleeding lesion. ^{99M}Tc-labeled red cell scan allows repeated imaging for up to 24 h and may identify the general location of bleeding. However, radionuclide scans should be interpreted with caution because results are highly variable. In active LGIB, angiography can detect the site of bleeding (extravasation of contrast into the gut) and permits treatment with intraarterial infusion of vasopressin or embolization. Even after bleeding has stopped, angiography may identify lesions with abnormal vasculature such as vascular ectasias or tumors.

GIB of obscure origin Obscure GIB is defined as recurrent acute or chronic bleeding for which no source has been identified by routine endoscopic and contrast studies. Push enteroscopy, with a specially designed enteroscope or a pediatric colonoscope to inspect the entire duodenum and part of the jejunum, is generally the next step. Push enteroscopy may identify probable bleeding sites in 20 to 40% of patients with obscure GIB. If enteroscopy is negative or unavailable, a specialized radiographic examination of the small bowel (e.g., enteroclysis) should be performed.

Patients with recurrent bleeding who require transfusions or repeated hospitalizations warrant further investigations. ^{99M}Tc-labeled red blood cell scintigraphy should be employed. Angiography is useful even if bleeding has subsided, since it may disclose vascular anomalies or tumor vessels. ^{99M}Tc-pertechnetate scintigraphy for diagnosis of Meckel's diverticulum should be done, especially in the evaluation of young patients with LGIB. When all tests are unrevealing, intraoperative endoscopy is indicated in patients with severe recurrent or persistent bleeding requiring repeated transfusions.

Occult GIB Occult GIB is manifested by either a positive test for fecal occult blood or iron deficiency anemia. Unless a patient has upper GI symptoms, evaluation of occult bleeding generally should begin with colonoscopy, particularly in patients older than 40 years. If evaluation of the colon is negative, some perform upper endoscopy only if iron deficiency anemia or upper GI symptoms are present, while others recommend upper endoscopy in all patients since up to 25 to 40% of these patients have some abnormality noted on upper endoscopy. If standard endoscopic tests are unrevealing, enteroscopy and/or enteroclysis may be considered in patients with iron-deficiency anemia.

BIBLIOGRAPHY

COOK DJ et al: Endoscopic therapy for acute non-variceal upper gastrointestinal hemorrhage—a meta-analysis. Gastroenterology 102:139, 1992

———— et al: A comparison of sucralfate and ranitidine for the prevention of upper gastrointestinal bleeding in patients requiring mechanical ventilation. N Engl J Med 338:791, 1998.

LAINE L, PETERSON WL: Bleeding peptic ulcer. N Engl J Med 331:717, 1994

MOLONEY M, WILKINSON M: Early administration of somatostatin and efficacy of sclerotherapy in acute oesophageal bleeds: The European Acute Bleeding Oesophageal Variceal Episodes (ABOVE) randomised trial. Gastrointest Endosc 51:372, 2000

ROCKALL TA et al: Incidence of and mortality from acute upper gastrointestinal haemorrhage in the United Kingdom. BMJ 311:222, 1995

ROCKEY DC: Occult gastrointestinal bleeding. N Engl J Med 341:38, 1999

45

Daniel S. Pratt, Marshall M. Kaplan

JAUNDICE

ALT	alanine aminotransferase	MRCP	magnetic resonance
AST	aspartate aminotransferase		cholangiopancreatography
CMV	cytomegalovirus	PSC	primary sclerosing cholangitis
CT	computed tomography	TPN	total parenteral nutrition
EBV	Epstein-Barr virus	UDP	uridine-diphosphate
ERCP	endoscopic retrograde		
cholangiopancreatography			

Jaundice, or icterus, is a yellowish discoloration of tissue resulting from the deposition of bilirubin. Tissue deposition of bilirubin occurs only in the presence of serum hyperbilirubinemia and is a sign of either liver disease or, less often, a hemolytic disorder. The degree of serum bilirubin elevation can be estimated by physical examination. Slight increases in serum bilirubin are best detected by examining the sclerae which have a particular affinity for bilirubin due to their high elastin content. The presence of scleral icterus indicates a serum bilirubin of at least 3.0 mg/dL. The ability to detect scleral icterus is made more difficult if the examining room has fluorescent lighting. If the examiner suspects scleral icterus, a second place to examine is underneath the tongue. As serum bilirubin levels rise, the skin will eventually become yellow in light-skinned patients and even green if the process is long-standing; the green color is produced by oxidation of bilirubin to biliverdin.

The differential diagnosis for yellowing of the skin is limited. In addition to jaundice, it includes carotenoderma, the use of the drug quinacrine, and excessive exposure to phenols. Carotenoderma is the yellow color imparted to the skin by the presence of carotene; it occurs in healthy individuals who ingest excessive amounts of vegetables and fruits that contain carotene, such as carrots, leafy vegetables, squash, peaches, and oranges. Unlike jaundice, where the yellow coloration of the skin is uniformly distributed over the body, in carotenoderma the pigment is concentrated on the palms, soles, forehead, and nasolabial folds. Carotenoderma can be distinguished from jaundice by the sparing of the sclerae. Quinacrine causes a yellow discoloration of the skin in 4 to 37% of patients treated with it. Unlike carotene, quinacrine can cause discoloration of the sclerae.

Another sensitive indicator of increased serum bilirubin is darkening of the urine, which is due to the renal excretion of conjugated bilirubin. Patients often describe their urine as tea or cola colored. Bilirubinuria indicates an elevation of the direct serum bilirubin fraction and therefore the presence of liver disease.

Increased serum bilirubin levels occur when an imbalance exists between bilirubin production and clearance. A logical evaluation of the patient who is jaundiced requires an understanding of bilirubin production and metabolism.

PRODUCTION AND METABOLISM OF BILIRUBIN (See also Chap. 294) Bilirubin, a tetrapyrrole pigment, is a breakdown product of heme (ferroprotoporphyrin IX). About 70 to 80% of the 250 to 300 mg of bilirubin produced each day is derived from the breakdown of hemoglobin in senescent red blood cells. The remainder comes from prematurely destroyed erythroid cells in bone marrow and from the turnover of hemoproteins such as myoglobin and cryto-chromes found in tissues throughout the body.

The formation of bilirubin occurs in reticuloendothelial cells, primarily in the spleen and liver. The first reaction, catalyzed by the enzyme heme oxygenase, oxidatively cleaves the α bridge of the porphyrin group and opens the heme ring. The end products of this reaction are biliverdin, carbon monoxide, and iron. The second reaction, catalyzed by the cytosolic enzyme biliverdin reductase, reduces the central methylene bridge of biliverdin and converts it to bilirubin. Bilirubin formed in the reticuloendothelial cells is virtually insoluble in water. To be transported in blood, it must be solubilized. This is ac-complished by its reversible, noncovalent binding to albumin. Unconjugated bilirubin bound to albumin is transported to the liver, where it, but not the albumin, is taken up by hepatocytes via a process that at least partly involves carrier-mediated membrane transport.

In the cytosol of the hepatocyte, unconjugated bilirubin is coupled predominantly to the protein ligandin (formerly called the Y protein). Ligandin was initially thought to be a transport protein facilitating the movement of bilirubin from the sinusodial membrane to the endoplasmic reticulum. It is now thought to slow the cytosolic diffusion of bilirubin and to reduce its efflux back into serum. In the endoplasmic reticulum, bilirubin is solubilized by conjugation to glucuronic acid, forming bilirubin monoglucuronide and diglucuronide. The conjugation of glucuronic acid to bilirubin is catalyzed by bilirubin uridine-diphosphate (UDP) glucuronosyltransferase.

The now hydrophilic bilirubin conjugates diffuse from the endoplasmic reticulum to the canalicular membrane, where bilirubin monoglucuronide and diglucuronide are actively transported into canalicular bile by an energy-dependent mechanism involving the multiple organic ion transport protein/multiple drug resistance protein. The conjugated bilirubin excreted into bile drains into the duodenum and passes unchanged through the proximal small bowel. Conjugated bilirubin is not taken up by the intestinal mucosa. When the conjugated bilirubin reaches the distal ileum and colon, it is hydrolyzed to unconjugated bilirubin by bacterial β-glucuronidases. The unconjugated bilirubin is reduced by normal gut bacteria to form a group of colorless tetrapyrroles called urobilinogens. About 80 to 90% of these products are excreted in feces, either unchanged or oxidized to orange derivatives called urobilins. The remaining 10 to 20% of the urobilinogens are passively absorbed, enter the portal venous blood, and are re-excreted by the liver. A small fraction (usually less than 3 mg/dL) escapes hepatic uptake, filters across the renal glomerulus, and is excreted in urine.

MEASUREMENT OF SERUM BILIRUBIN The terms direct- and indirect-reacting bilirubin are based on the original van den Bergh reaction. This assay, or a variation of it, is still used in most clinical chemistry laboratories to determine the serum bilirubin level. In this assay, bilirubin is exposed to diazotized sulfanilic acid, splitting into two relatively stable dipyrrylmethene azopigments that absorb maximally at 540 nm, allowing for photometric analysis. The direct fraction is that which reacts with diazotized sulfanilic acid in the absence of an accelerator substance such as alcohol. The direct fraction provides an approximate determination of the conjugated bilirubin in serum. The total serum bilirubin is the amount that reacts after the addition of alcohol. The indirect fraction is the difference between the total and the direct bilirubin and provides an estimate of the unconjugated bilirubin in serum.

With the van den Bergh method, the normal serum bilirubin concentration usually is <1 mg/dL (17 μmol/L). Up to 30%, or 0.3 mg/dL (5.1 μmol/L), of the total may be direct-reacting (conjugated) bilirubin. Total serum bilirubin concentrations are between 0.2 and 0.9 mg/dL in 95% of a normal population.

Several new techniques, although less convenient to perform, have added considerably to our understanding of bilirubin metabolism. First, they demonstrate that in normal people or those with Gilbert's syndrome, almost 100% of the serum bilirubin is unconjugated; less than 3% is monoconjugated bilirubin. Second, in jaundiced patients with hepatobiliary disease, the total serum bilirubin concentration measured by these new, more accurate methods is lower than the values found with diazo methods. This suggests that there are diazo-positive compounds distinct from bilirubin in the serum of patients with hepatobiliary disease. Third, these studies indicate that in jaundiced patients with hepatobiliary disease, monoglucuronides of bilirubin predominate over the diglucuronides. Fourth, part of the direct-reacting bilirubin fraction includes conjugated bilirubin that is covalently linked to albumin. This albumin-linked bilirubin fraction (*delta fraction* or *biliprotein*) represents an important fraction of total

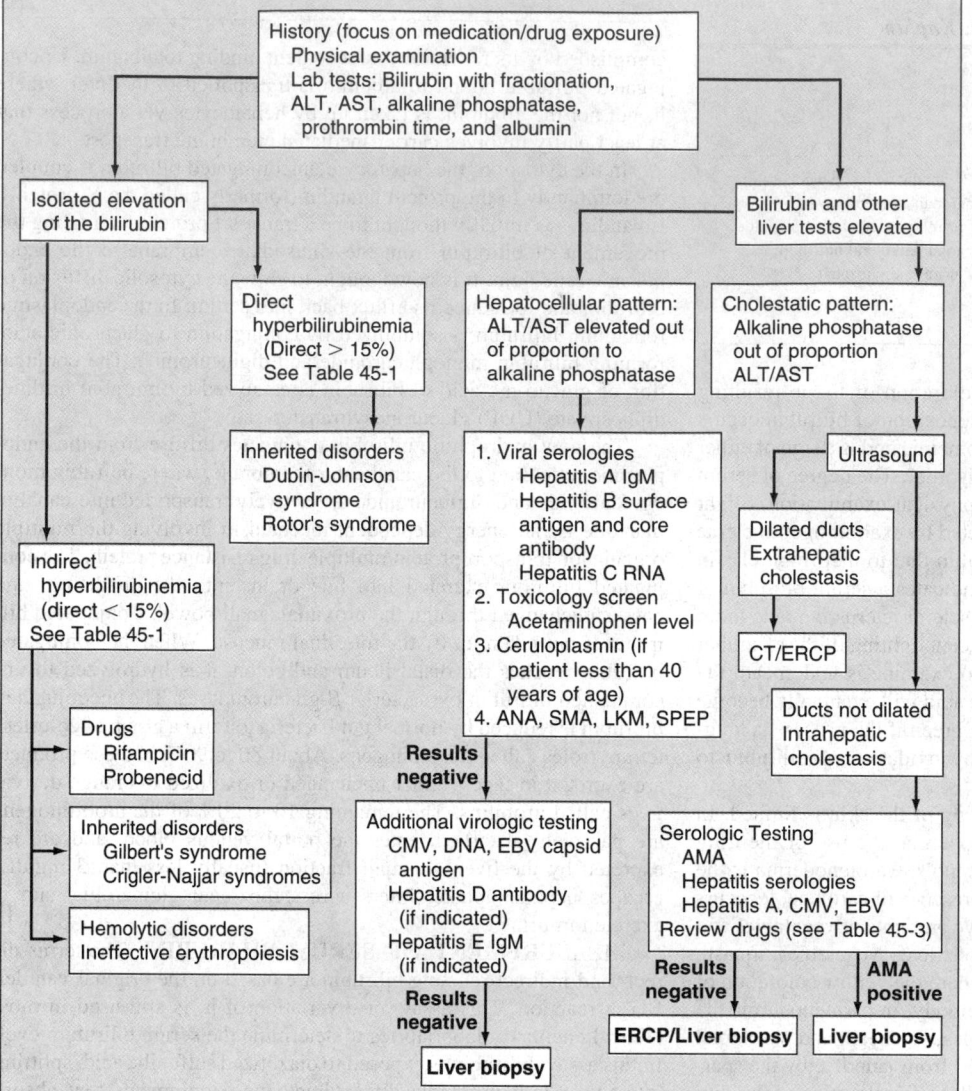

FIGURE 45-1 Evaluation of the patient with jaundice. ERCP, endoscopic retrograde cholangiopancreatography; CT, computed tomography; ALT, alanine aminotransferase; AST, aspartate aminotransferase; SMA, smooth muscle antibody; AMA, antimitochondrial antibody; LKM, liver-kidney microsomal antibody; SPEP, serum protein electrophoresis; CMV, cytomegalovirus; EBV, Epstein-Barr virus.

serum bilirubin in patients with cholestasis and hepatobiliary disorders. Albumin-bound conjugated bilirubin is formed in serum when hepatic excretion of bilirubin glucuronides is impaired and the glucuronides are present in serum in increasing amounts. By virtue of its tight binding to albumin, the clearance rate of albumin-bound bilirubin from serum approximates the half-life of albumin, 12 to 14 days, rather than the short half-life of bilirubin, about 4 h.

The prolonged half-life of albumin-bound conjugated bilirubin explains two previously unexplained enigmas in jaundiced patients with liver disease: (1) that some patients with conjugated hyperbilirubinemia do not exhibit bilirubinuria during the recovery phase of their disease because the bilirubin is bound to albumin and therefore not filtered by the renal glomeruli and (2) that the elevated serum bilirubin level declines more slowly than expected in some patients who otherwise appear to be recovering satisfactorily. Late in the recovery phase of hepatobiliary disorders, all the conjugated bilirubin may be in the albumin-linked form. Its value in serum falls slowly because of the long half-life of albumin.

MEASUREMENT OF URINE BILIRUBIN Unconjugated bilirubin is always bound to albumin in the serum, is not filtered by the kidney, and is not found in the urine. Conjugated bilirubin is filtered at the glomerulus and the majority is reabsorbed by the proximal tubules; a small fraction is excreted in the urine. Any bilirubin found

in the urine is conjugated bilirubin. The presence of bilirubinuria implies the presence of liver disease. A urine dipstick test (Ictotest) gives the same information as fractionation of the serum bilirubin. This test is very accurate. A false-negative test is possible in patients with prolonged cholestasis due to the predominance of conjugated bilirubin covalently bound to albumin.

THE EVALUATION OF JAUNDICE The bilirubin present in serum represents a balance between input from production of bilirubin and hepatic/biliary removal of the pigment. Hyperbilirubinemia may result from (1) overproduction of bilirubin; (2) impaired uptake, conjugation, or excretion of bilirubin; or (3) regurgitation of unconjugated or conjugated bilirubin from damaged hepatocytes or bile ducts. An increase in unconjugated bilirubin in serum results from either overproduction, impairment of uptake, or conjugation of bilirubin. An increase in conjugated bilirubin is due to decreased excretion into the bile ductules or backward leakage of the pigment. The initial steps in evaluating the patient with jaundice are to determine (1) whether the hyperbilirubinemia is predominantly conjugated or unconjugated in nature, and (2) whether other biochemical liver tests are abnormal. The thoughtful interpretation of limited data will allow for a rational evaluation of the patient (Fig. 45-1). This discussion will focus solely on the evaluation of the adult patient with jaundice.

ISOLATED ELEVATION OF SERUM BILIRUBIN Unconjugated Hyperbilirubinemia The differential diagnosis of an isolated unconjugated hyperbilirubinemia is limited (Table 45-1). The critical determination is whether the patient is suffering from

a hemolytic process resulting in an overproduction of bilirubin (hemolytic disorders and ineffective erythropoiesis) or from impaired hepatic uptake/conjugation of bilirubin (drug effect or genetic disorders).

Hemolytic disorders that cause excessive heme production may be either inherited or acquired. Inherited disorders include spherocytosis, sickle cell anemia, and deficiency of red cell enzymes such as pyruvate kinase and glucose-6-phosphate dehydrogenase. In these conditions, the serum bilirubin rarely exceeds 5 mg/dL. Higher levels may occur when there is coexistent renal or hepatocellular dysfunction, or in acute hemolysis such as a sickle cell crisis. In evaluating jaundice in patients with chronic hemolysis, it is important to remember the high incidence of pigmented (calcium bilirubinate) gallstones found in these patients, which increases the likelihood of choledocholithiasis as an alternative explanation for hyperbilirubinemia.

Acquired hemolytic disorders include microangiopathic hemolytic anemia (e.g., hemolytic-uremic syndrome), paroxysmal nocturnal hemoglobinuria, and immune hemolysis. Ineffective erythropoiesis occurs in cobalamin, folate, and iron deficiencies.

In the absence of hemolysis, the physician should consider a problem with the hepatic uptake or conjugation of bilirubin. Certain drugs, including rifampicin and probenecid, may cause unconjugated hyperbilirubinemia by diminishing hepatic uptake of bilirubin. Impaired bilirubin conjugation occurs in three genetic conditions: *Crigler-Najjar*

Table 45-1 Causes of Isolated Hyperbilirubinemia

I. Indirect hyperbilirubinemia
  A. Hemolytic disorders
    1. Inherited
      a. Spherocytosis, elliptocytosis
        Glucose-6-phosphate dehydrogenase and pyruvate kinase deficiencies
      b. Sickle cell anemia
    2. Acquired
      a. Microangiopathic hemolytic anemias
      b. Paroxysmal nocturnal hemoglobinuria
      c. Immune hemolysis
  B. Ineffective erythropoiesis
    1. Cobalamin, folate, and iron deficiencies
  C. Drugs
    1. Rifampicin, probenecid, ribavirin
  D. Inherited conditions
    1. Crigler-Najjar types I and II
    2. Gilbert's syndrome
II. Direct hyperbilirubinemia
  A. Inherited conditions
    1. Dubin-Johnson syndrome
    2. Rotor's syndrome

syndrome, types I and II, and *Gilbert's syndrome. Crigler-Najjar type I* is an exceptionally rare condition found in neonates and characterized by severe jaundice (bilirubin > 20 mg/dL) and neurologic impairment due to kernicterus, frequently leading to death in infancy or childhood. These patients have a complete absence of bilirubin UDP glucuronosyltransferase activity, usually due to mutations in the critical 3′ domain of the UDP glucuronosyltransferase gene, and are totally unable to conjugate, hence cannot excrete bilirubin. The only effective treatment is orthotopic liver transplantation. Use of gene therapy and allogeneic hepatocyte infusion are experimental approaches of future promise for this devastating disease.

Crigler-Najjar type II is somewhat more common than type I. Patients live into adulthood with serum bilirubin levels that range from 6 to 25 mg/dL. In these patients, mutations in the bilirubin UDP glucuronosyltransferase gene cause reduced but not completely absent activity of the enzyme. Bilirubin UDP glucuronosyltransferase activity can be induced by the administration of phenobarbital, which can reduce serum bilirubin levels in these patients. Despite marked jaundice, these patients usually survive into adulthood, although they may be susceptible to kernicterus under the stress of intercurrent illness or surgery.

Gilbert's syndrome is also marked by the impaired conjugation of bilirubin due to reduced bilirubin UDP glucuronosyltransferase activity. Molecular analyses show that Gilbert's syndrome is due to reduced expression of UDP glucuronosyltransferase activity caused by lengthening of the TATAA box from A(TA)$_6$ TAA to A(TA)$_7$ TAA in the promoter element of the gene. This results in mild unconjugated hyperbilirubinemia with serum levels almost always less than 6 mg/dL. The serum levels may fluctuate and jaundice is often identified only during periods of fasting. Unlike both Crigler-Najjar syndromes, Gilbert's syndrome is very common. The reported incidence is 3 to 7% of the population with males predominating over females by a ratio of 2–7:1.

Conjugated Hyperbilirubinemia Elevated conjugated hyperbilirubinemia is found in two rare inherited conditions: *Dubin-Johnson syndrome* and *Rotor's syndrome* (Table 45-1). Patients with both conditions present with asymptomatic jaundice, typically in the second generation of life. The defect in Dubin-Johnson syndrome is a point mutation in the gene for the canalicular multispecific organic anion transporter. These patients have altered excretion of bilirubin into the bile ducts. Rotor's syndrome seems to be a problem with the hepatic storage of bilirubin. Differentiating between these syndromes is possible, but clinically unnecessary, due to their benign nature.

ELEVATION OF SERUM BILIRUBIN WITH OTHER LIVER TEST ABNORMALITIES The remainder of this chapter will focus on the evaluation of the patient with a conjugated hyperbilirubinemia in the setting of other liver test abnormalities. This group of patients can be divided into those with a primary hepatocellular process and those with intra- or extrahepatic cholestasis. Being able to make this differentiation will guide the physician's evaluation (Fig. 45-1). This differentiation is made on the basis of the history and physical examination as well as the pattern of liver test abnormalities.

History A complete medical history is perhaps the single most important part of the evaluation of the patient with unexplained jaundice. Important considerations include the use of or exposure to any chemical or medication, either physician-prescribed or over-the-counter, such as herbal and vitamin preparations and other drugs such as anabolic steroids. The patient should be carefully questioned about possible parenteral exposures, including transfusions, intravenous and intranasal drug use, tattoos, and sexual activity. Other important questions include recent travel history, exposure to people with jaundice, exposure to possibly contaminated foods, occupational exposure to hepatotoxins, alcohol consumption, the duration of jaundice, and the presence of any accompanying symptoms such as arthralgias, myalgias, rash, anorexia, weight loss, abdominal pain, fever, pruritis, and changes in the urine and stool. While none of these latter symptoms are specific for any one condition, they can suggest a particular diagnosis. A history of arthralgias and myalgias predating jaundice suggests hepatitis, either viral or drug-related. Jaundice associated with the sudden onset of severe right upper quadrant pain and shaking chills suggests choledocholithiasis and ascending cholangitis.

Physical Examination The general assessment should include assessment of the patient's nutritional status. Temporal and proximal muscle wasting suggests longstanding diseases such as pancreatic cancer or cirrhosis. Stigmata of chronic liver disease, including spider nevi, palmar erythema, gynecomastia, caput medusae, Dupuytren's contractures, parotid gland enlargement, and testicular atrophy are commonly seen in advanced alcoholic (Laennec's) cirrhosis and occasionally in other types of cirrhosis. An enlarged left supraclavicular node (Virchow's node) or periumbilical nodule (Sister Mary Joseph's nodule) suggest an abdominal malignancy. Jugular venous distention, a sign of right-sided heart failure, suggests hepatic congestion. Right pleural effusion, in the absence of clinically apparent ascites, may be seen in advanced cirrhosis.

The abdominal examination should focus on the size and consistency of the liver, whether the spleen is palpable and hence enlarged, and whether there is ascites present. Patients with cirrhosis may have an enlarged left lobe of the liver which is felt below the xiphoid and an enlarged spleen. A grossly enlarged nodular liver or an obvious abdominal mass suggests malignancy. An enlarged tender liver could be viral or alcoholic hepatitis or, less often, an acutely congested liver secondary to right-sided heart failure. Severe right upper quadrant tenderness with respiratory arrest on inspiration (Murphy's sign) suggests cholecystitis or, occasionally, ascending cholangitis. Ascites in the presence of jaundice suggests either cirrhosis or malignancy with peritoneal spread.

Laboratory Tests When the physician encounters a patient with unexplained jaundice, there are a battery of tests that are helpful in the initial evaluation. These include total and direct serum bilirubin with fractionation, aminotransferases, alkaline phosphatase, albumin, and prothrombin time tests. Enzyme tests [alanine aminotransferase (ALT), aspartate aminotransferase (AST), and alkaline phosphatase] are helpful in differentiating between a hepatocellular process and a cholestatic process (see Table 293-1 and Fig. 45-1), a critical step in determining what additional workup is indicated. Patients with a hepatocellular process generally have a disproportionate rise in the aminotransferases compared to the alkaline phosphatase. Patients with a cholestatic process have a disproportionate rise in the alkaline phosphatase compared to the aminotransferases. The bilirubin can be prominently elevated in both hepatocellular and cholestatic conditions and therefore is not necessarily helpful in differentiating between the two.

In addition to the enzyme tests, all jaundiced patients should have additional blood tests, specifically an albumin and a prothrombin time, to assess liver function. A low albumin suggests a chronic process such as cirrhosis or cancer. A normal albumin is suggestive of a more acute process such as viral hepatitis or choledocholithiasis. An elevated prothrombin time indicates either vitamin K deficiency due to prolonged jaundice and malabsorption of vitamin K or significant hepatocellular dysfunction. The failure of the prothrombin time to correct with parenteral administration of vitamin K indicates severe hepatocellular injury.

The results of the bilirubin, enzyme, albumin, and prothrombin time tests will usually indicate whether a jaundiced patient has a hepatocellular or a cholestatic disease. The causes and evaluation of each of these is quite different.

Hepatocellular Conditions   Hepatocellular diseases that can cause jaundice include viral hepatitis, drug or environmental toxicity, alcohol, and end-stage cirrhosis from any cause (Table 45-2). Wilson's disease should be considered in young adults. Autoimmune hepatitis is typically seen in young to middle-aged women, but may affect men and women of any age. Alcoholic hepatitis can be differentiated from viral and toxin-related hepatitis by the pattern of the aminotransferases. Patients with alcoholic hepatitis typically have an AST:ALT ratio of at least 2:1. The AST rarely exceeds 300 U/L. Patients with acute viral hepatitis and toxin-related injury severe enough to produce jaundice typically have aminotransferases greater than 500 U/L, with the ALT greater than or equal to the AST. The degree of aminotransferase elevation can occasionally help in differentiating between hepatocellular and cholestatic processes. While ALT and AST values less than 8 times normal may be seen in either hepatocellular or cholestatic liver disease, values 25 times normal or higher are seen primarily in acute hepatocellular diseases. Patients with jaundice from cirrhosis can have normal or only slight elevations of the aminotransferases.

When the physician determines that the patient has a hepatocellular disease, appropriate testing for acute viral hepatitis includes a hepatitis A IgM antibody, a hepatitis B surface antigen and core IgM antibody, and a hepatitis C viral RNA test. It can take many weeks for the hepatitis C antibody to become detectable, making it an unreliable test if acute hepatitis C is suspected. Depending on circumstances, studies for hepatitis D, E, Epstein-Barr virus (EBV), and cytomegalovirus (CMV) may be indicated. Ceruloplasmin is the initial screening test for Wilson's disease. Testing for autoimmune hepatitis usually includes an antinuclear antibody and measurement of specific immunoglobulins.

Drug-induced hepatocellular injury can be classified either as predictable or unpredictable. Predictable drug reactions are dose-dependent and affect all patients who ingest a toxic dose of the drug in question. The classic example is acetaminophen hepatotoxicity. Unpredictable or idiosyncratic drug reactions are not dose-dependent and occur in a minority of patients. A great number of drugs can cause

Table 45-2   Hepatocellular Conditions That May Produce Jaundice

Viral hepatitis
  Hepatitis A, B, C, D, and E
  Epstein-Barr virus
  Cytomegalovirus
  Herpes simplex
Alcohol
Drug toxicity
  Predictable, dose-dependent, e.g., acetaminophen
  Unpredictable, idosyncratic, e.g., isoniazid
Environmental toxins
  Vinyl chloride
  Jamaica bush tea—pyrrolizidine alkaloids
  Wild mushrooms—Amanita phalloides or verna
Wilson's disease
Autoimmune hepatitis

idiosyncratic hepatic injury. Environmental toxins are also an important cause of hepatocellular injury. Examples include industrial chemicals such as vinyl chloride, herbal preparations containing pyrrolizidine alkaloids (Jamaica bush tea), and the mushrooms Amanita phalloides or verna containing highly hepatotoxic amatoxins.

Cholestatic Conditions   When the pattern of the liver tests suggests a cholestatic disorder, the next step is to determine whether it is intra- or extrahepatic cholestasis (Fig. 45-1). Distinguishing intrahepatic from extrahepatic cholestasis may be difficult. History, physical examination, and laboratory tests are often not helpful. The next appropriate test is an ultrasound. The ultrasound is inexpensive, does not expose the patient to ionizing radiation, and can detect dilation of the intra- and extrahepatic biliary tree with a high degree of sensitivity and specificity. The absence of biliary dilatation suggests intrahepatic cholestasis, while the presence of biliary dilatation indicates extrahepatic cholestasis. False-negative results occur in patients with partial obstruction of the common bile duct or in patients with cirrhosis or primary sclerosing cholangitis (PSC) where scarring prevents the intrahepatic ducts from dilating.

Although ultrasonography may indicate extrahepatic cholestasis, it rarely identifies the site or cause of obstruction. The distal common bile duct is a particularly difficult area to visualize by ultrasound because of overlying bowel gas. Appropriate next tests include computed tomography (CT) and endoscopic retrograde cholangiopancreatography (ERCP). CT scanning is better than ultrasonography for assessing the head of the pancreas and for identifying choledocholithiasis in the distal common bile duct, particularly when the ducts are not dilated. ERCP is the gold standard for identifying choledocholithiasis. It is performed by introducing a side-viewing endoscope perorally into the duodenum. The ampulla of Vater is visualized and a catheter is advanced through the ampulla. Injection of dye allows for the visualization of the common bile duct and the pancreatic duct. The success rate for cannulation of the common bile duct ranges from 80 to 95%, depending on the operator's experience. Beyond its diagnostic capabilities, ERCP allows for therapeutic interventions, including the removal of common bile duct stones and the placement of stents. In patients in whom ERCP is unsuccessful, transhepatic cholangiography can provide the same information. Magnetic resonance cholangiopancreatography (MRCP) is a rapidly developing, noninvasive technique for imaging the bile and pancreatic ducts; this may replace ERCP as the initial diagnostic test in cases where the need for intervention is felt to be small.

In patients with apparent *intrahepatic cholestasis*, the diagnosis is often made by serologic testing in combination with percutaneous liver biopsy. The list of possible causes of intrahepatic cholestasis is long and varied (Table 45-3). A number of conditions that typically cause a hepatocellular pattern of injury can also present as a cholestatic variant. Both hepatitis B and C can cause a cholestatic hepatitis (fibrosing cholestatic hepatitis) that has histologic features that mimic large duct obstruction. This disease variant has been reported in patients who have undergone solid organ transplantation. Hepatitis A, alcoholic hepatitis, EBV, and CMV may also present as cholestatic liver disease.

Drugs may cause intrahepatic cholestasis, a variant of drug-induced hepatitis. Drug-induced cholestasis is usually reversible after eliminating the offending drug, although it may take many months for cholestasis to resolve. Drugs most commonly associated with cholestasis are the anabolic and contraceptive steroids. Cholestatic hepatitis has been reported with chlorpromazine, imipramine, tolbutamide, sulindac, cimetidine, and erythromycin estolate. It also occurs in patients taking trimethoprim, sulfamethoxazole, and penicillin-based antibiotics such as ampicillin, dicloxacillin, and clavulinic acid. Rarely, cholestasis may be chronic and associated with progressive fibrosis despite early discontinuation of the drug. Chronic cholestasis has been associated with chlorpromazine and prochlorperazine.

Primary biliary cirrhosis is a disease predominantly of middle-aged women in which there is a progressive destruction of interlobular bile ducts. The diagnosis is made by the presence of the antimitochondrial antibody that is found in 95% of patients. *Primary sclerosing*

Table 45-3 Cholestatic Conditions That May Produce Jaundice

I. Intrahepatic
  A. Viral hepatitis
    1. Fibrosing cholestatic hepatitis—hepatitis B and C
    2. Hepatitis A, Epstein-Barr virus, cytomegalovirus
  B. Alcoholic hepatitis
  C. Drug toxicity
    1. Pure cholestasis—anabolic and contraceptive steroids
    2. Cholestatic hepatitis—chlorpromazine, erythromycin estolate
    3. Chronic cholestasis—chlorpromazine and prochlorperazine
  D. Primary biliary cirrhosis
  E. Primary sclerosing cholangitis
  F. Vanishing bile duct syndrome
    1. Chronic rejection of liver tranplants
    2. Sarcoidosis
    3. Drugs
  G. Inherited
    1. Benign recurrent cholestasis
  H. Cholestasis of pregnancy
  I. Total parenteral nutrition
  J. Nonhepatobiliary sepsis
  K. Benign postoperative cholestasis
  L. Paraneoplastic syndrome
  M. Venooclusive disease
  N. Graft-versus-host disease
II. Extrahepatic
  A. Malignant
    1. Cholangiocarcinoma
    2. Pancreatic cancer
    3. Gallbladder cancer
    4. Ampullary cancer
    5. Malignant involvement of the porta hepatis lymph nodes
  B. Benign
    1. Choledocholithiasis
    2. Primary sclerosing cholangitis
    3. Chronic pancreatitis
    4. AIDS cholangiopathy

cholangitis (PSC) is characterized by the destruction and fibrosis of larger bile ducts. The disease may involve only the intrahepatic ducts and present as intrahepatic cholestasis. However, in 65% of patients with PSC, both intra- and extrahepatic ducts are involved. The diagnosis of PSC is made by ERCP. The pathognomonic findings are multiple strictures of bile ducts with dilatations proximal to the strictures. Approximately 75% of patients with PSC have inflammatory bowel disease.

The *vanishing bile duct syndrome* and *adult bile ductopenia* are rare conditions in which there are a decreased number of bile ducts seen in liver biopsy specimens. The histologic picture is similar to that found in primary biliary cirrhosis. This picture is seen in patients who develop chronic rejection after liver transplantation and in those who develop graft-versus-host disease after bone marrow transplantation. Vanishing bile duct syndrome also occurs in rare cases of sarcoidosis, in patients taking certain drugs including chlorpromazine, and idiopathically. There are also familial forms of intrahepatic cholestasis, including the *familial intrahepatic cholestatic syndromes, I-III*. Benign recurrent cholestasis is an autosomal recessive disease that appears to be due to mutations in a P type ATPase, which probably acts as a bile acid transporter. The disease is marked by recurrent episodes of jaundice and pruritis; the episodes are self-limited but can be debilitating. *Cholestasis of pregnancy* occurs in the second and third trimesters and resolves after delivery. Its cause is unknown, but the condition is probably inherited and cholestasis can be triggered by estrogen administration.

Other causes of intrahepatic cholestasis include total parenteral nutrition (TPN), nonhepatobiliary sepsis, benign postoperative chole-

stasis, and a paraneoplastic syndrome associated with a number of different malignancies, including Hodgkin's disease, medullary thyroid cancer, hypernephroma, renal sarcoma, T cell lymphoma, prostate cancer, and several GI malignancies. In patients developing cholestasis in the intensive care unit, the major considerations should be sepsis, shock liver, and TPN jaundice. Jaundice occurring after bone marrow transplantation is most likely due to venoocclusive disease or graft-versus-host disease.

Causes of *extrahepatic cholestasis* can be split into malignant and benign (Table 45-3). Malignant causes include pancreatic, gallbladder, ampullary, and cholangiocarcinoma. The latter is most commonly associated with PSC and is exceptionally difficult to diagnose because its appearance is often identical to PSC. Pancreatic and gallbladder tumors, as well as cholangiocarcinoma, are rarely resectable and have poor prognoses. Ampullary carcinoma has the highest surgical cure rate of all the tumors that present as painless jaundice. Hilar lymphadenopathy due to metastases from other cancers may cause obstruction of the extrahepatic biliary tree.

Choledocholithiasis is the most common cause of extrahepatic cholestasis. The clinical presentation can range from mild right upper quadrant discomfort with only minimal elevations of the enzyme tests to ascending cholangitis with jaundice, sepsis, and circulatory collapse. PSC may occur with clinically important strictures limited to the extrahepatic biliary tree. In cases where there is a dominant stricture, patients can be effectively managed with serial endoscopic dilatations. Chronic pancreatitis rarely causes strictures of the distal common bile duct, where it passes through the head of the pancreas. AIDS cholangiopathy is a condition, usually due to infection of the bile duct epithelium with CMV or cryptosporidium, which has a cholangiographic appearance similar to PSC. These patients usually present with greatly elevated serum alkaline phosphatase levels, mean of 800 IU/L, but the bilirubin is often near normal. These patients do not typically present with jaundice.

SUMMARY The goal of this chapter is not to provide an encyclopedic review of all of the conditions that can cause jaundice. Rather, it is intended to provide a framework that helps a physician to evaluate the patient with jaundice in a logical way (Fig. 45-1).

Simply stated, the initial step is to obtain appropriate blood tests to determine if the patient has an isolated elevation of serum bilirubin. If so, is the bilirubin elevation due to an increased unconjugated or conjugated fraction? If the hyperbilirubinemia is accompanied by other liver test abnormalities, is the disorder hepatocellular or cholestatic? If cholestatic, is it intra- or extrahepatic? All of these questions can be answered with a thoughtful history, physical examination, and interpretation of laboratory and radiologic tests and procedures.

BIBLIOGRAPHY

BERG CL et al: Bilirubin metabolism and the pathophysiology of jaundice, in *Schiff's Diseases of the Liver*, 8th ed, ER Schiff et al (eds). Philadelphia, Lippincott, 1999

BERK PD, NOYER C (eds): Bilirubin metabolism and the hereditary hyperbilirubinemias. Semin Liv Dis 14:321, 1994

BLANCKAERT N, FEVERY J: Physiology and pathophysiology of bilirubin metabolism, in *Hepatology: A Textbook of Liver Disease*, 3d ed, D Zakin, TD Boyer (eds). Philadelphia, Saunders, 1997

FOX IJ et al: Treatment of the Crigler-Najjar syndrome type I with hepatocyte transplantation. N Engl J Med 338:1422, 1998

PRATT DS, KAPLAN MM: Laboratory tests, in *Schiff's Diseases of the Liver*, 8th ed, ER Schiff et al (eds). Philadelphia, Lippincott, 1999

TRAUNER M et al: Molecular pathogenesis of cholestasis. N Engl J Med 339:1217, 1998

WEISS JS et al: The clinical importance of a protein-bound fraction of serum bilirubin in patients with hyperbilirubinemia. N Engl J Med 309:147, 1983

ZIMMERMAN HJ: *Hepatoxicity: The Adverse Effects of Drugs and Other Chemicals on the Liver*, 2d ed. Philadelphia, Lippincott Williams & Wilkins, 1999

46   *Robert M. Glickman*

ABDOMINAL SWELLING AND ASCITES

ABDOMINAL SWELLING Abdominal swelling or distention is a common problem in clinical medicine and may be the initial manifestation of a systemic disease or of otherwise unsuspected abdominal disease. *Subjective* abdominal enlargement, often described as a sensation of fullness or bloating, is usually transient and is often related to a functional gastrointestinal disorder when it is not accompanied by objective physical findings of increased abdominal girth or local swelling. *Obesity* and lumbar lordosis, which may be associated with prominence of the abdomen, may usually be distinguished from true increases in the volume of the peritoneal cavity by history and careful physical examination.

Clinical History Abdominal swelling may first be noticed by the patient because of a progressive increase in belt or clothing size, the appearance of abdominal or inguinal hernias, or the development of a localized swelling. Often, considerable abdominal enlargement has gone unnoticed for weeks or months, either because of coexistent obesity or because the ascites formation has been insidious, without pain or localizing symptoms. Progressive abdominal distention may be associated with a sensation of "pulling" or "stretching" of the flanks or groins and vague low back pain. Localized pain usually results from involvement of an abdominal organ (e.g., a passively congested liver, large spleen, or colonic tumor). Pain is uncommon in cirrhosis with ascites, and when it is present, pancreatitis, hepatocellular carcinoma, or peritonitis should be considered. Tense ascites or abdominal tumors may produce increased intraabdominal pressure, resulting in indigestion and heartburn due to gastroesophageal reflux or dyspnea, orthopnea, and tachypnea from elevation of the diaphragm. A coexistent pleural effusion, more commonly on the right, presumably due to leakage of ascitic fluid through lymphatic channels in the diaphragm, also may contribute to respiratory embarrassment. The patient with diffuse abdominal swelling should be questioned about increased alcohol intake, a prior episode of jaundice or hematuria, or a change in bowel habits. Such historic information may provide the clues that will lead one to suspect an occult cirrhosis, a colonic tumor with peritoneal seeding, congestive heart failure, or nephrosis.

Physical Examination A carefully executed general physical examination can yield valuable clues concerning the etiology of abdominal swelling. Thus palmar erythema and spider angiomas suggest an underlying cirrhosis, while supraclavicular adenopathy (Virchow's node) should raise the question of an underlying gastrointestinal malignancy.

Inspection of the abdomen is important. By noting the abdominal contour, one may be able to distinguish localized from generalized swelling. The tensely distended abdomen with tightly stretched skin, bulging flanks, and everted umbilicus is characteristic of ascites. A prominent abdominal venous pattern with the direction of flow away from the umbilicus often is a reflection of portal hypertension; venous collaterals with flow from the lower part of the abdomen toward the umbilicus suggest obstruction of the inferior vena cava; flow downward toward the umbilicus suggests superior vena cava obstruction. "Doming" of the abdomen with visible ridges from underlying intestinal loops is usually due to intestinal obstruction or distention. An epigastric mass, with evident peristalsis proceeding from left to right, usually indicates underlying pyloric obstruction. A liver with metastatic deposits may be visible as a nodular right upper quadrant mass moving with respiration.

Auscultation may reveal the high-pitched, rushing sounds of early intestinal obstruction or a succussion sound due to increased fluid and gas in a dilated hollow viscus. Careful auscultation over an enlarged liver occasionally reveals the harsh bruit of a vascular tumor, especially a hepatocellular carcinoma, or the leathery friction rub of a surface nodule. A venous hum at the umbilicus may signify portal hypertension and an increased collateral blood flow around the liver. A fluid wave and flank dullness that shifts with change in position of the patient are important signs that indicate the presence of peritoneal fluid. In obese patients, small amounts of fluid may be difficult to demonstrate; on occasion, the fluid may be detected by abdominal percussion with patients on their hands and knees. Small amounts of ascites often can only be detected by ultrasound examination of the abdomen, which can detect as little as 100 mL of fluid. Careful percussion should serve to distinguish generalized abdominal enlargement from localized swelling due to an enlarged uterus, ovarian cyst, or distended bladder. Percussion also can outline an abnormally small or large liver. Loss of normal liver dullness may result from massive hepatic necrosis; it also may be a clue to free gas in the peritoneal cavity, as from perforation of a hollow viscus.

Palpation is often difficult with massive ascites, and ballottement of overlying fluid may be the only method of palpating the liver or spleen. A slightly enlarged spleen in association with ascites may be the only evidence of an occult cirrhosis. When there is evidence of portal hypertension, a soft liver suggests that obstruction to portal flow is extrahepatic; a firm liver suggests cirrhosis as the likely cause of the portal hypertension. A very hard or nodular liver is a clue that the liver is infiltrated with tumor, and when accompanied by ascites, it suggests that the latter is due to peritoneal seeding. The presence of a hard periumbilical nodule (Sister Mary Joseph's nodule) suggests metastatic disease from a pelvic or gastrointestinal primary tumor. A pulsatile liver and ascites may be found in tricuspid insufficiency.

An attempt should be made to determine whether a mass is solid or cystic, smooth or irregular, and whether it moves with respiration. The liver, spleen, and gallbladder should descend with respiration unless they are fixed by adhesions or extension of tumor beyond the organ. A fixed mass not descending with respiration may indicate that it is retroperitoneal. Tenderness, especially if localized, may indicate an inflammatory process such as an abscess; it also may be due to stretching of the visceral peritoneum or tumor necrosis. Rectal and pelvic examinations are mandatory; they may reveal otherwise undetected masses due to tumor or infection.

Radiographic and laboratory examinations are essential for confirming or extending the impressions gained on physical examination. Upright and recumbent films of the abdomen may demonstrate the dilated loops of intestine with fluid levels characteristic of intestinal obstruction or the diffuse abdominal haziness and loss of psoas margins suggestive of ascites. Ultrasonography is often of value in detecting ascites, determining the presence of a mass, or evaluating the size of the liver and spleen. Computed tomography (CT) scanning provides similar information. CT scanning is often necessary to visualize the retroperitoneum, pancreas, and lymph nodes. A plain film of the abdomen may reveal the distended colon of otherwise unsuspected ulcerative colitis and give valuable information as to the size of the liver and spleen. An irregular and elevated right side of the diaphragm may be a clue to a liver abscess or hepatocellular carcinoma. Studies of the gastrointestinal tract with barium or other contrast media are usually necessary in the search for a primary tumor.

ASCITES The evaluation of a patient with ascites requires that the cause of the ascites be established. In most cases ascites appears as part of a well-recognized illness, that is, cirrhosis, congestive heart failure, nephrosis, or disseminated carcinomatosis. In these situations, the physician should determine that the development of ascites is indeed a consequence of the basic underlying disease and not due to the presence of a separate or related disease process. This distinction is necessary even when the cause of ascites seems obvious. For example, when the patient with compensated cirrhosis and minimal ascites develops progressive ascites that is increasingly difficult to control with sodium restriction or diuretics, the temptation is to attribute the worsening of the clinical picture to progressive liver disease. However, an occult hepatocellular carcinoma, portal vein thrombosis, spontaneous

decompensation. The disappointingly low success in diagnosing tuberculous peritonitis or hepatocullar carcinoma in the patient with cirrhosis and ascites reflects the too-low index of suspicion for the development of such superimposed conditions. Similarly, the patient with congestive heart failure may develop ascites from a disseminated carcinoma with peritoneal seeding.

Diagnostic paracentesis (50 to 100 mL) should be part of the routine evaluation of the patient with ascites. The fluid should be examined for its gross appearance; protein content, cell count, and differential cell count should be determined; and Gram's and acid-fast stains and culture should be performed. Cytologic and cell-block examination may disclose an otherwise unsuspected carcinoma. Table 46-1 presents some of the features of ascitic fluid typically found in various disease states. In some disorders, such as cirrhosis, the fluid has the characteristics of a transudate (<25 g protein per liter and a specific gravity of <1.016); in others, such as peritonitis, the features are those of an exudate. Rather than the total protein content of ascites, many authors prefer the use of a *serum-ascites albumin gradient (SAG)* to characterize ascites. The gradient correlates directly with portal pressure. A gradient >1.1 g/dL (high gradient) is characteristic of uncomplicated cirrhotic ascites and differentiates ascites due to portal hypertension from ascites not due to portal hypertension >95% of the time. A gradient <1.1 g/dL (low gradient) suggests that the ascites is not due to portal hypertension with >95% accuracy and mandates a search for other causes (Table 46-1). Although there is variability of the ascitic fluid in any given disease state, some features are sufficiently characteristic to suggest certain diagnostic possibilities. For example, blood-stained fluid with >25 g protein per liter is unusual in uncomplicated cirrhosis but is consistent with tuberculous peritonitis or neoplasm. Cloudy fluid with a predominance of polymorphonuclear cells and a positive Gram's stain are characteristic of bacterial peritonitis; if most cells are lymphocytes, tuberculosis should be suspected. The complete examination of each fluid is most important, for occasionally only one finding may be abnormal. For example, if the fluid is a typical transudate but contains >250 white blood cells per microliter, the finding should be recognized as atypical for cirrhosis and should warrant a search for tumor or infection. This is especially true in the evaluation of cirrhotic ascites where occult peritoneal infection may be present with only minor elevations in the white blood cell count of the peritoneal fluid (300 to 500 cells per microliter). Since Gram's stain of the fluid may be negative in a high proportion of such cases, careful culture of the peritoneal fluid is mandatory. Bedside innoculation of blood culture flasks with ascitic fluid results in a dramatically increased incidence of positive cultures when bacterial infection is present (90 versus 40% positivity with conventional cultures done by the laboratory). Direct visualization of the peritoneum (laparoscopy) may disclose peritoneal deposits of tumor, tuberculosis, or metastatic disease of the liver. Biopsies are taken under direct vision, often adding to the diagnostic accuracy of the procedure.

Chylous ascites refers to a turbid, milky, or creamy peritoneal fluid due to the presence of thoracic or intestinal lymph. Such a fluid shows Sudan-staining fat globules microscopically and an increased triglyceride content by chemical examination. Opaque milky fluid usually has a triglyceride concentration of >1000 mg/dL. A turbid fluid due to leukocytes or tumor cells may be confused with chylous fluid (pseudochylous), and it is often helpful to carry out alkalinization and ether extraction of the specimen. Alkali tend to dissolve cellular proteins and thereby reduce turbidity; ether extraction leads to clearing if the turbidity of the fluid is due to lipid. Chylous ascites is most often the result of lymphatic obstruction from trauma, tumor, tuberculosis, filariasis (Chap. 221), or congenital abnormalities. It also may be seen in the nephrotic syndrome.

Rarely, ascitic fluid may be *mucinous* in character, suggesting either pseudomyxoma peritonei (Chap. 289) or rarely a colloid carcinoma of the stomach or colon with peritoneal implants.

On occasion, ascites may develop as a seemingly isolated finding in the absence of a clinically evident underlying disease. Then, a care-

Table 46-1 Characteristics of Ascitic Fluid in Various Disease States

Condition	Gross Appearance	Protein, g/dL	Serum-Ascites Albumin Gradient, g/dL	Cell Count Red Blood Cells, >10,000/μL	Cell Count White Blood Cells, per μL	Other Tests
Cirrhosis	Straw-colored or bile-stained	<25 (95%)	>1.1	1%	<250 (90%);[a] predominantly mesothelial	
Neoplasm	Straw-colored, hemorrhagic, mucinous, or chylous	>25 (75%)	<1.1	20%	>1000 (50%); variable cell types	Cytology, cell block, peritoneal biopsy
Tuberculous peritonitis	Clear, turbid, hemorrhagic, chylous	>25 (50%)	<1.1	7%	>1000 (70%); usually >70% lymphocytes	Peritoneal biopsy, stain and culture for acid-fast bacilli
Pyogenic peritonitis	Turbid or purulent	If purulent, >25	<1.1	Unusual	Predominantly polymorphonuclear leukocytes	Positive Gram's stain, culture
Congestive heart failure	Straw-colored	Variable, 15–53	>1.1	10%	<1000 (90%); usually mesothelial, mononuclear	
Nephrosis	Straw-colored or chylous	<25 (100%)	<1.1	Unusual	<250; mesothelial, mononuclear	If chylous, ether extraction, Sudan staining
Pancreatic ascites (pancreatitis, pseudocyst)	Turbid, hemorrhagic, or chylous	Variable, often >25	<1.1	Variable, may be blood-stained	Variable	Increased amylase in ascitic fluid and serum

[a] Because the conditions of examining fluid and selecting patients were not identical in each series, the percentage figures (in parentheses) should be taken as an indication of the order of magnitude rather than as the precise incidence of any abnormal finding.

ful analysis of ascitic fluid may indicate the direction the evaluation should take. A useful framework for the workup starts with an analysis of whether the fluid is classified as a high (transudate) or low (exudate) gradient fluid. *High gradient (transudative) ascites* of unclear etiology is most often due to occult cirrhosis, right-sided venous hypertension raising hepatic sinusoidal pressure, or hypoalbuminemic states such as nephrosis or protein-losing enteropathy. Cirrhosis with well-preserved liver function (normal albumin) resulting in ascites invariably is associated with significant portal hypertension (Chap. 298). Evaluation should include liver function tests, liver-spleen scan, or other hepatic imaging procedure (i.e., CT or ultrasound) to detect nodular changes in the liver or a colloid shift of isotope to suggest portal hypertension. On occasion, a wedged hepatic venous pressure can be useful to document portal hypertension. Finally, if clinically indicated, a liver biopsy will confirm the diagnosis of cirrhosis and perhaps suggest its etiology. Other etiologies may result in hepatic venous congestion and resultant ascites. Right-sided cardiac valvular disease and particularly constrictive pericarditis should raise a high index of suspicion and may require cardiac imaging and cardiac catheterization for definitive diagnosis. Hepatic vein thrombosis is evaluated by visualizing the hepatic veins with imaging techniques (Doppler ultrasound, angiography, CT scans, magnetic resonance imaging) to demonstrate obliteration, thrombosis, or obstruction by tumor. Uncommonly, transudative ascites may be associated with benign tumors of the ovary, particularly fibroma (Meigs' syndrome) with ascites and hydrothorax.

Low gradient (exudative) ascites should initiate an evaluation for primary peritoneal processes, most importantly infection and tumor. Routine bacteriologic culture of ascitic fluid often yields a specific organism causing infectious peritonitis. Tuberculous peritonitis (Table 46-1) is best diagnosed by peritoneal biopsy, either percutaneously or via laparoscopy. Histologic examination invariably shows granulomata that may contain acid-fast bacilli. Since cultures of peritoneal fluid and biopsies for tuberculosis may require 6 weeks, characteristic histology with appropriate stains allows antituberculosis therapy to be started promptly. Similarly, the diagnosis of peritoneal seeding by tumor can usually be made by cytologic analysis of peritoneal fluid or by peritoneal biopsy if cytology is negative. Appropriate diagnostic studies can then be undertaken to determine the nature and site of the primary tumor. Pancreatic ascites (Table 46-1) is invariably associated with an extravasation of pancreatic fluid from the pancreatic ductal system, most commonly from a leaking pseudocyst. Ultrasound or CT examination of the pancreas followed by visualization of the pancreatic duct by direct cannulation [viz., endoscopic retrograde cholangiopancreatography (ERCP)] usually discloses the site of leakage and permits resective surgery to be carried out.

An analysis of the physiologic and metabolic factors involved in the production of ascites (detailed in Chap. 298), coupled with a complete evaluation of the nature of the ascitic fluid, invariably discloses the etiology of the ascites and permits appropriate therapy to be instituted.

ACKNOWLEDGMENT
Dr. Kurt J. Isselbacher was the co-author of this chapter in previous editions.

BIBLIOGRAPHY

LIPSKY MS, STERNBACH MR: Evaluation and initial management of patients with ascites. Am Fam Physician 54:1327, 1996

McHUTCHISON JG: Differential diagnosis of ascites. Semin Liver Dis 17:191, 1997

PARSONS SL et al: Malignant ascites. Br J Surg 83:6, 1996

PINTO PC et al: Large volume paracentesis in nonedematous patients with tense ascites: Its effect on intravascular volume. Hepatology 8:207, 1988

RECTOR WG JR, REYNOLDS TB: Superiority of the serum: ascites albumin difference over the ascites total protein concentration in separation of "transudative" and "exudative" ascites. Am J Med 77:83, 1988

RUNYON BA: Management of adult patients with ascites caused by cirrhosis. Hepatology 27:264, 1998

——— et al: The serum-ascites albumin gradient in the differential diagnosis of ascites. Ann Intern Med 117:215, 1992

Section 7
ALTERATIONS IN RENAL AND URINARY TRACT FUNCTION

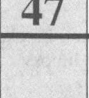
47

Bradley M. Denker, Barry M. Brenner

AZOTEMIA AND URINARY ABNORMALITIES

Body homeostasis is maintained predominantly through the cellular processes that together comprise normal kidney function. Disturbances to any of these functions can lead to a constellation of abnormalities that may be detrimental to survival. The clinical manifestations of these diseases will depend upon the pathophysiology of the renal injury and will often be initially identified as a complex of symptoms, abnormal physical findings, and laboratory changes that will allow the identification of specific syndromes. These renal syndromes (summarized in Table 47-1) may arise as the consequence of a systemic illness or can occur as a primary renal disease. Nephrologic syndromes usually consist of several elements that reflect the underlying pathologic processes and the duration of the disease and typically include one or more of the following features: (1) disturbances in urine volume (oliguria, anuria, polyuria); (2) abnormalities of urine sediment [red blood cells (RBC); white blood cells, casts, and crystals]; (3) abnormal excretion of serum proteins (proteinuria); (4) reduction in glomerular filtration rate (GFR) (azotemia); (5) presence of hypertension and/or expanded total body volume (edema); (6) electrolyte abnormalities, or (7) in some syndromes, fever/pain. The combination of these findings should permit identification of one of the major nephrologic syndromes (Table 47-1) and will allow the differential diagnoses to be narrowed and the appropriate diagnostic evaluation and therapeutic course to be determined. Each of these syndromes and their associated diseases are discussed in more detail in subsequent chapters. This chapter will focus on several aspects of renal abnormalities that are critically important to distinguishing these processes: (1) reduction in GFR leading to azotemia, (2) alterations of the urinary sediment and/or protein excretion, and (3) abnormalities of urinary volume.

AZOTEMIA

ASSESSMENT OF GLOMERULAR FILTRATION RATE
Monitoring the GFR is important in both the hospital and outpatient settings, and several different methodologies are available (discussed below). In most acute clinical circumstances a measured GFR is not available, and it is necessary to estimate the GFR from the serum creatinine level in order to provide appropriate doses of drugs that are excreted into the urine. Serum creatinine is the most widely used marker for GFR and is related directly to the urine creatinine excretion and inversely to the serum creatinine (U_{Cr}/P_{Cr}). Based upon this relationship and some important caveats (discussed below), the GFR will fall proportionally with the increase in P_{Cr}. Failure to account for GFR

Table 47-1 Initial Clinical and Laboratory Data Base for Defining Major Syndromes in Nephrology

Syndromes	Important Clues to Diagnosis	Findings That Are Common	Location of Discussion of Diseases Causing Syndrome
Acute or rapidly progressive renal failure	Anuria Oliguria Documented recent decline in GFR	Hypertension, hematuria Proteinuria, pyuria Casts, edema	Chaps. 269, 274, 277, 281
Acute nephritis	Hematuria, RBC casts Azotemia, oliguria Edema, hypertension	Proteinuria Pyuria Circulatory congestion	Chaps. 273, 274, 275
Chronic renal failure	Azotemia for >3 months Prolonged symptoms or signs of uremia Symptoms or signs of renal osteodystrophy Kidneys reduced in size bilaterally Broad casts in urinary sediment	Hematuria, proteinuria Casts, oliguria Polyuria, nocturia Edema, hypertension Electrolyte disorders	Chaps. 268, 270
Nephrotic syndrome	Proteinuria >3.5 g per 1.73 m² per 24 h Hypoalbuminemia Hyperlipidemia Lipiduria	Casts Edema	Chap. 274
Asymptomatic urinary abnormalities	Hematuria Proteinuria (below nephrotic range) Sterile pyuria, casts		Chap. 274
Urinary tract infection	Bacteriuria >10⁵ colonies per milliliter Other infectious agent documented in urine Pyuria, leukocyte casts Frequency, urgency Bladder tenderness, flank tenderness	Hematuria Mild azotemia Mild proteinuria Fever	Chap. 280
Renal tubule defects	Electrolyte disorders Polyuria, nocturia Symptoms or signs of renal osteodystrophy Large kidneys Renal transport defects	Hematuria "Tubular" proteinuria Enuresis	Chaps. 276, 277
Hypertension	Systolic/diastolic hypertension	Proteinuria Casts Azotemia	Chaps. 35, 246, 278
Nephrolithiasis	Previous history of stone passage or removal Previous history of stone seen by x-ray Renal colic	Hematuria Pyuria Frequency, urgency	Chap. 279
Urinary tract obstruction	Azotemia, oliguria, anuria Polyuria, nocturia, urinary retention Slowing of urinary stream Large prostate, large kidneys Flank tenderness, full bladder after voiding	Hematuria Pyuria Enuresis, dysuria	Chap. 281

reductions in drug dosing can lead to significant morbidity and mortality from drug toxicities (e.g., digoxin, aminoglycosides). In the outpatient setting, serial determinations of GFR are helpful for following the progression of chronic renal insufficiency, but again, the serum creatinine is often used as a surrogate for GFR (although much less accurate; see below). In patients with chronic progressive renal insufficiency there is an approximately linear relationship between $1/P_{Cr}$ and time. The slope of this line will remain constant for an individual patient, and when values are obtained that do not fall on this line, an investigation for a superimposed acute process (e.g., volume depletion, drug reaction) should be initiated. It should be emphasized that the signs and symptoms of uremia will develop at significantly different levels of serum creatinine depending upon the patient (size, age, and sex), the underlying renal disease, existence of concurrent diseases, and true GFR. In general, patients do not develop symptomatic uremia until renal insufficiency is usually quite severe (GFR < 15 mL/min) and in some patients it does not occur until the GFR < 5 mL/min.

A reduced GFR leads to retention of nitrogenous waste products (azotemia) such as serum urea nitrogen and creatinine. Azotemia may result from reduced renal perfusion, intrinsic renal disease, or postrenal processes (ureteral obstruction; see below and Fig. 47-1). Precise determination of GFR is problematic as both commonly used markers (urea and creatinine) have characteristics that affect their accuracy as markers of clearance. Urea clearance is generally an underestimate of GFR because of tubule urea reabsorption and may be as low as one-half of GFR measured by other techniques.

Creatinine is a small, freely filtered solute that varies little from day to day (since it is derived from muscle metabolism of creatine).

However, serum creatinine can increase acutely from dietary ingestion of cooked meat. Creatinine can be secreted by the proximal tubule through an organic cation pathway. There are many clinical settings where a creatinine clearance is not available, and decisions concerning drug dosing must be made based on the serum creatinine. A formula that allows an estimate of creatinine clearance in men that accounts for age-related decreases in GFR, body weight, and sex has been derived by Cockcroft-Gault:

$$\text{Creatinine clearance (mL/min)} = \frac{(140 - \text{age}) \times \text{lean body weight (kg)}}{\text{plasma creatinine (mg/dL)} \times 72}$$

This value should be multiplied 0.85 for women, since a lower fraction of the body weight is composed of muscle. The gradual loss of muscle from chronic illness, chronic use of glucocorticoids, or malnutrition can mask significant changes in GFR with small or imperceptible changes in serum creatinine. More accurate determinations of GFR are available using inulin clearance or radionuclide-labeled markers such as ¹²⁵I-iothalamate or EDTA. These methods are highly accurate due to precise quantitation and the absence of any renal reabsorption/secretion and should be used to follow GFR in patients in whom creatinine is not likely to be a reliable indicator (patients with decreased muscle mass secondary to age, malnutrition, concurrent illnesses).

Approach to the Patient

Once it has been established that GFR is reduced, the physician must decide if this represents acute or chronic renal failure. The clinical

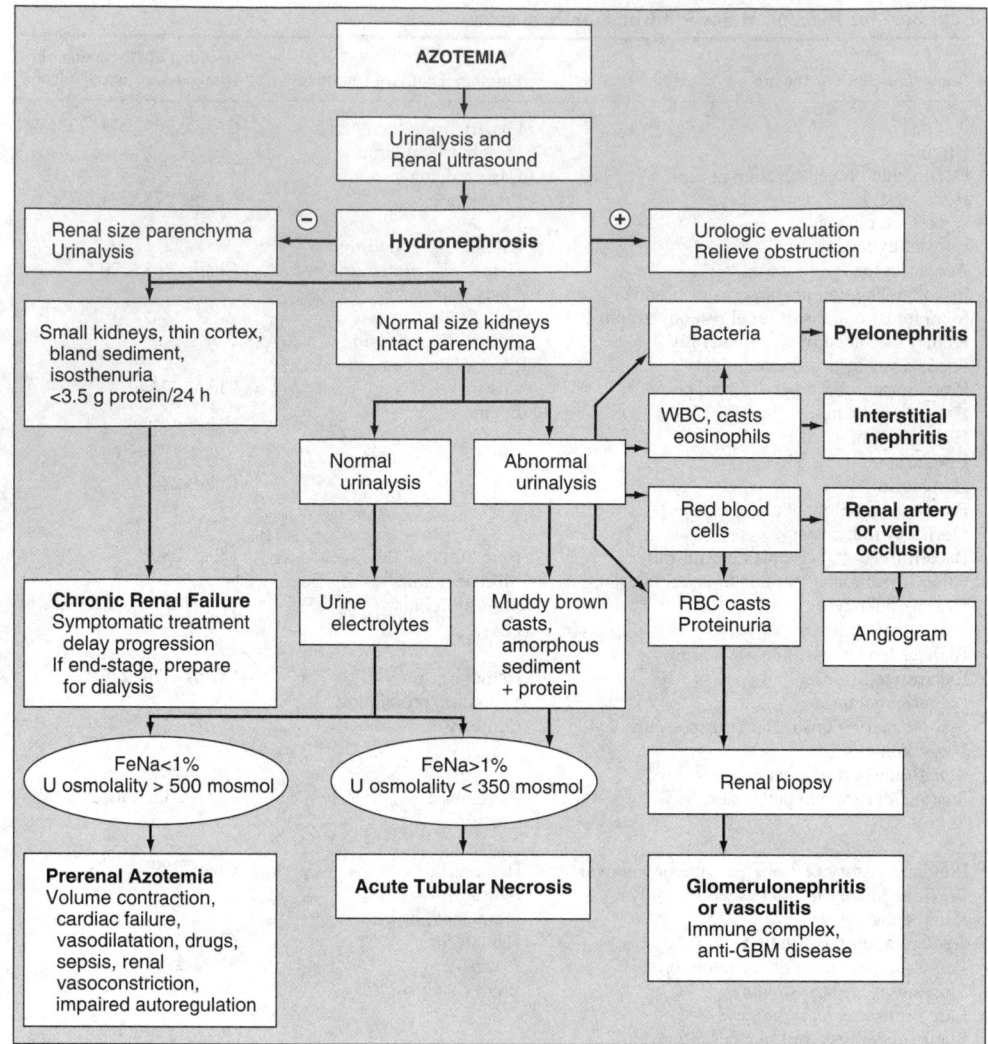

FIGURE 47-1 Approach to the patient with azotemia. (WBC, white blood cell; RBC, red blood cell; GBM, glomerular basement membrane.)

situation, history, and laboratory data often make this an easy distinction. However, the laboratory abnormalities characteristic of chronic renal failure, including anemia, hypocalcemia, and hyperphosphatemia, are often also present in patients presenting with acute renal failure. Radiographic evidence of renal osteodystrophy (Chap. 270) would be seen only in chronic renal failure but is a very late finding, and these patients are usually on dialysis. The urinalysis and renal ultrasound can occasionally facilitate distinguishing acute from chronic renal failure. An approach to the evaluation of azotemic patients is shown in Fig. 47-1. Patients with advanced chronic renal insufficiency often have some proteinuria, nonconcentrated urine (isosthenuria), and small kidneys on ultrasound characterized by increased echogenicity and cortical thinning. Treatment should be directed toward slowing the progression of renal disease and providing symptomatic relief for edema, acidosis, anemia, and hyperphosphatemia, as discussed in Chap. 270. Acute renal failure (Chap. 269) can result from processes affecting renal blood flow (prerenal azotemia), intrinsic renal diseases (affecting vessels, glomeruli, or tubules), or postrenal processes (obstruction to urine flow in ureters, bladder, or urethra) (Chap. 281).

Prerenal Failure Decreased renal perfusion accounts for 40 to 80% of acute renal failure and, if appropriately treated, is readily reversible. The etiologies of prerenal azotemia include any cause of decreased circulating blood volume including volume loss (gastrointestinal hemorrhage, burns, diarrhea, diuretics), volume sequestration (pancreatitis, peritonitis, rhabdomyolysis), or decreased effective circulating volume (cardiogenic shock, sepsis). Renal perfusion can also

be affected by reductions in cardiac output from peripheral vasodilatation (sepsis, drugs) or profound renal vasoconstriction [severe heart failure, hepatorenal syndrome, drugs (such as nonsteroidal anti-inflammatory drugs (NSAIDs)]. True, or "effective," hypovolemia leads to a fall in mean arterial pressure, which in turn triggers a series of neural and humoral responses that include activation of the sympathetic nervous and renin-angiotensin-aldosterone systems and ADH release. GFR is maintained by prostaglandin-mediated relaxation of afferent arterioles and angiotensin II–mediated constriction of efferent arterioles. Once the mean arterial pressure falls below 80 mmHg, there is a steep decline in GFR.

Blockade of prostaglandin production by NSAIDs can result in severe vasoconstriction and acute renal failure under these circumstances. Angiotensin-converting enzyme (ACE) inhibitors decrease efferent arteriolar tone and can decrease glomerular capillary perfusion pressure. Patients on NSAIDs and/or ACE inhibitors are most susceptible to hemodynamically mediated acute renal failure when blood volume is reduced for any reason. Patients with renal artery stenosis are dependent upon efferent arteriolar vasoconstriction for maintenance of glomerular filtration pressure and are particularly susceptible to precipitous decline in GFR when given ACE inhibitors.

Prolonged renal hypoperfusion can lead to acute tubular necrosis (ATN; an intrinsic renal disease discussed below). The urinalysis and urinary electrolytes can be useful in distinguishing prerenal azotemia from ATN (Table 47-2). The urine of patients with prerenal azotemia can be predicted from the stimulatory actions of norepinephrine, angiotensin II, ADH, and low tubule fluid flow on salt and water reabsorption from the urine. In prerenal conditions the tubules are intact, leading to a concentrated urine (>500 mosm), avid Na retention (urine Na concentration <20 mM/L; fractional excretion of Na <1%), and U_{Cr}/P_{Cr} > 40 (Table 47-2). The prerenal urine sediment is usually normal or has occasional hyaline and granular casts, while the sediment of ATN is usually filled with cellular debris and muddy brown granular casts.

Intrinsic Renal Disease When prerenal and postrenal azotemia have been excluded as etiologies of renal failure, an intrinsic parenchymal renal disease is present. Intrinsic renal disease can arise from processes involving large renal vessels, microvasculature and glomeruli, or tubulointerstitium. Ischemic and toxic ATN account for about 90% of acute intrinsic renal failure. As outlined in Fig. 47-1, the clinical setting and urinalysis are helpful in separating the possible etiologies of acute intrinsic renal failure. Prerenal azotemia and ATN are part of a spectrum of renal hypoperfusion; evidence of structural tubule injury is present in ATN, whereas prompt reversibility occurs with prerenal azotemia upon restoration of adequate renal perfusion. Thus, ATN can often be distinguished from prerenal azotemia by urinalysis and urine electrolyte composition (Table 47-2 and Fig. 47-1). Ischemic ATN is observed most frequently in patients who have undergone ma-

Table 47-2 Laboratory Findings in Acute Renal Failure

Index	Prerenal Azotemia	Oliguric Acute Renal Failure
BUN/P_{Cr} Ratio	>20:1	10–15:1
Urine sodium (U_{Na}), meq/L	<20	>40
Urine osmolality, mosmol/L H_2O	>500	<350
Fractional excretion of sodium	<1%	>2%
$FE_{Na} = \dfrac{U_{Na} \times P_{Cr} \times 100}{P_{Na} \times U_{Cr}}$		
Urine/plasma creatinine (U_{Cr}/P_{Cr})	>40	<20

NOTE: BUN, Blood urea nitrogen; P_{Cr}, plasma creatinine; U_{Na}, urine sodium concentration; P_{Na}, plasma sodium concentration; U_{Cr}, urine creatinine concentration.

jor surgery, trauma, severe hypovolemia, overwhelming sepsis, or extensive burns. Nephrotoxic ATN complicates the administration of many common medications, usually by inducing a combination of intrarenal vasoconstriction, direct tubule toxicity, and/or tubular obstruction. The kidney is vulnerable to toxic injury by virtue of its rich blood supply (25% of cardiac output) and its ability to concentrate and metabolize toxins. A diligent search for hypotension and nephrotoxins will usually uncover the specific etiology of ATN. Discontinuation of nephrotoxins and stabilizing blood pressure will often suffice without the need for dialysis while the tubules recover. →*An extensive list of potential drugs and toxins implicated in ATN can be found in Chap. 269.*

Processes that involve the tubules and interstitium can lead to acute renal failure. These include drug-induced interstitial nephritis (especially antibiotics, NSAIDs, and diuretics), severe infections (both bacterial and viral), systemic diseases (e.g., systemic lupus erythematosus), or infiltrative disorders (e.g., sarcoid, lymphoma, or leukemia). A list of drugs associated with allergic interstitial nephritis can be found in Chap. 277. The urinalysis usually shows mild to moderate proteinuria, hematuria, and pyuria (approximately 75% of cases) and occasionally white blood cell casts. The finding of RBC casts in interstitial nephritis has been reported but should prompt a search for glomerular diseases. Occasionally renal biopsy will be needed to distinguish among these possibilities. The finding of eosinophils in the urine is suggestive of allergic interstitial nephritis and is optimally observed by using a Hansel stain. The absence of eosinophiluria, however, does not exclude the possibility of acute interstitial nephritis.

Occlusion of large renal vessels including arteries and veins is an uncommon cause of acute renal failure. A significant reduction in GFR by this mechanism suggests bilateral processes or a unilateral process in a patient with a single functioning kidney. Renal arteries can be occluded with atheroemboli, thromboemboli, in situ thrombosis, aortic dissection, or vasculitis. Atheroembolic renal failure can occur spontaneously but is most often associated with recent aortic instrumentation. The emboli are cholesterol-rich and lodge in medium and small renal arteries leading to an eosinophil-rich inflammatory reaction. Atheroembolic acute renal failure often has a normal urinalysis but may contain eosinophils and casts. The diagnosis can be confirmed by renal biopsy, but this is often unnecessary when other stigmata of atheroemboli are present (livedo reticularis, distal peripheral infarcts, eosinophilia). Renal artery thrombosis may lead to mild proteinuria and hematuria, whereas renal vein thrombosis typically induces heavy proteinuria and hematuria. →*These vascular catastrophes often require angiography for confirmation and are discussed in Chap. 278.*

Diseases of glomeruli (glomerulonephritis or vasculitis) and the renal microvasculature (hemolytic uremic syndromes, thrombotic thrombocytopenic purpura, or malignant hypertension) usually present with various combinations of glomerular injury: proteinuria, hematuria, reduced GFR, and alterations of Na excretion leading to hypertension, edema, and circulatory congestion (acute nephritic syndrome). These findings may occur as primary renal diseases or as renal manifestations of systemic diseases. The clinical setting and other laboratory data will help distinguish primary renal from systemic diseases. The finding of RBC casts in the urine is an indication for early renal

biopsy (Fig. 47-1) as the pathologic pattern has important implications for diagnosis, prognosis, and treatment. Hematuria without RBC casts can also be an indication of glomerular disease, and this evaluation is summarized in Fig. 47-2. →*A detailed discussion of glomerulonephritis and diseases of the microvasculature can be found in Chap. 274.*

Postrenal Azotemia Urinary tract obstruction accounts for fewer than 5% of cases of acute renal failure, but it is usually reversible and must be ruled out early in the evaluation (Fig. 47-1). Since a single kidney is capable of adequate clearance, acute renal failure from obstruction requires obstruction at the urethra or bladder outlet, bilateral ureteral obstruction, or unilateral obstruction in a patient with a single functioning kidney. Obstruction is usually diagnosed by the presence of ureteral dilatation on renal ultrasound. However, early in the course of obstruction or if the ureters are unable to dilate (such as encasement by pelvic tumors), the ultrasound examination may be negative. →*The specific urologic conditions that cause obstruction are discussed in Chap. 281.*

Oliguria and Anuria *Oliguria* refers to a 24-h urine output of <500 mL, and *anuria* is the complete absence of urine formation. Anuria can be caused by total urinary tract obstruction, total renal artery or vein occlusion, and shock (manifested by severe hypotension and intense renal vasoconstriction). Cortical necrosis, ATN, and rapidly progressive glomerulonephritis can occasionally cause anuria. Oliguria can accompany any cause of acute renal failure and carries a more serious prognosis for renal recovery in all conditions except prerenal azotemia. *Nonoliguria* refers to urine output in excess of

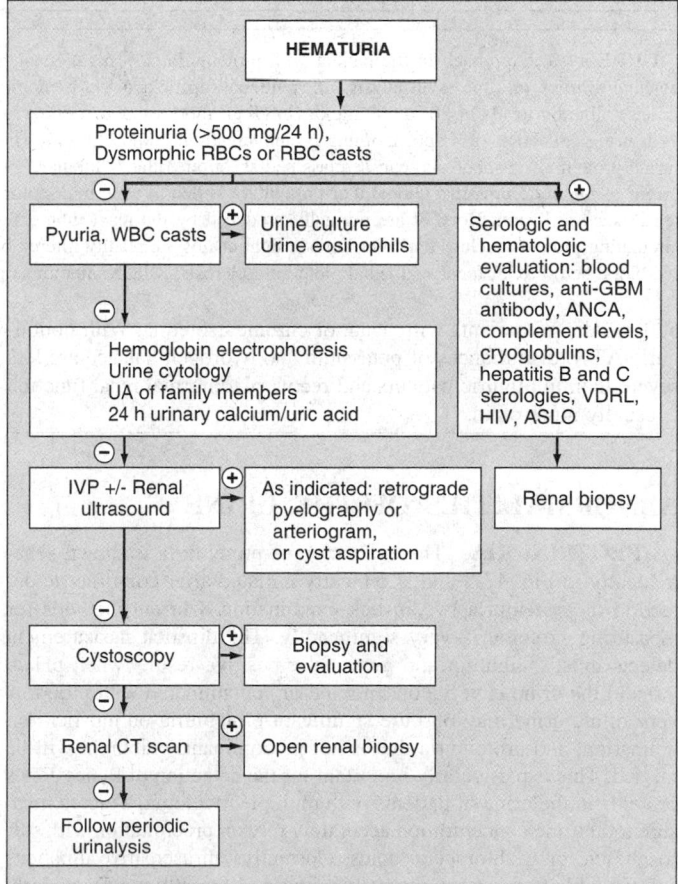

FIGURE 47-2 Approach to the patient with hematuria. (RBC, red blood cell; WBC, white blood cell; GBM, glomerular basement membrane; ANCA, antineutrophil cytoplasmic antibody; VDRL, venereal disease research laboratory; ASLO, antistreptolysin O; UA, urinalysis; IVP, intravenous pyelography; CT, computed tomography.)

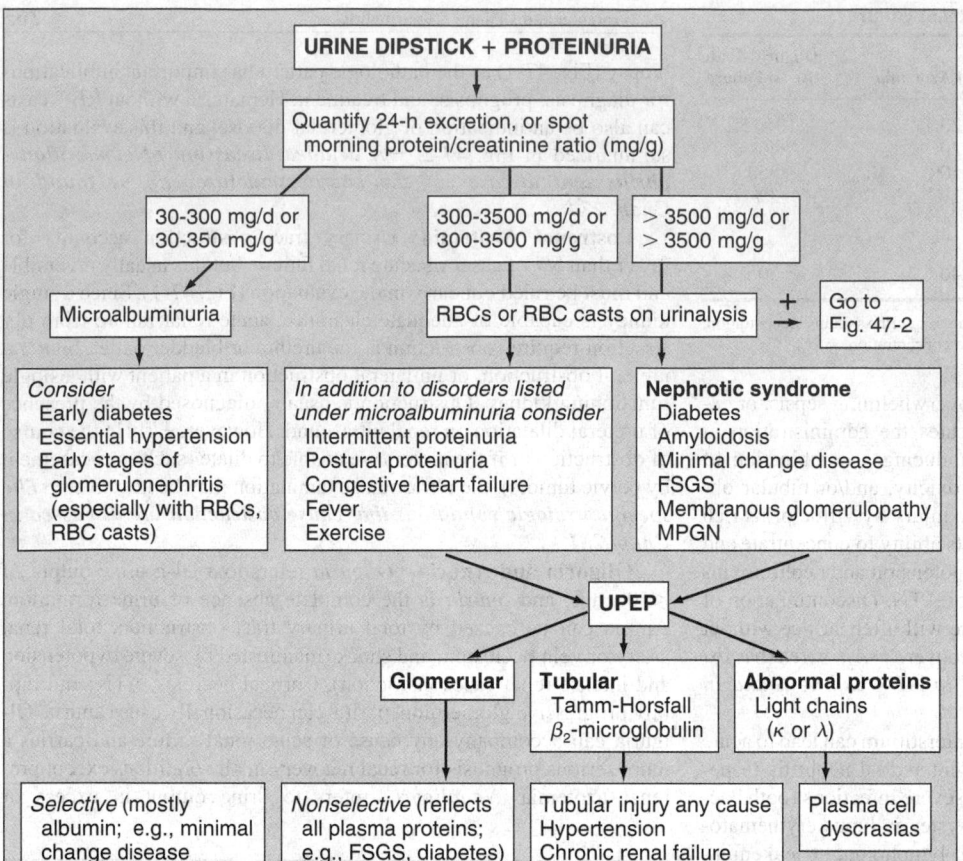

FIGURE 47-3 Approach to the patient with proteinuria. Investigation of proteinuria is often initiated by a positive dipstick on routine urinalysis. Conventional dipsticks detect predominantly albumin and cannot detect urinary albumin levels of 30 to 300 mg/d. However, more exact determination of proteinuria should employ a 24-h urine collection or a spot morning protein/creatinine ration (mg/g). The pattern of proteinuria on UPEP (urine protein electrophoresis) can be classified as "glomerular," "tubular," or "abnormal" depending upon the origin of the urine proteins. Glomerular proteinuria is due to abnormal glomerular permeability. "Tubular proteins" such as Tamm-Horsfall are normally produced by the renal tubule and shed into the urine. Abnormal circulating proteins such as kappa or lambda light chains are readily filtered because of their small size. (RBC, red blood cell; FSGS, focal segmental glomerulosclerosis; MPGN, membranoproliferative glomerulonephritis.)

500 mL/day in patients with acute or chronic azotemia. With nonoliguric ATN, disturbances of potassium and hydrogen balance are less severe than in oliguric patients and recovery to normal renal function is usually more rapid.

ABNORMALITIES OF THE URINE

PROTEINURIA The evaluation of proteinuria is shown schematically in Fig. 47-3 and is typically initiated after colorimetric detection of proteinuria by dipstick examination. Current methods for measuring proteinuria vary significantly. The dipstick measurement detects mostly albumin and gives false-positive results when pH > 7.0 and the urine is very concentrated or contaminated with blood. A very dilute urine may obscure significant proteinuria on dipstick examination, and proteinuria that is not predominantly albumin will be missed. This is particularly important for the detection of Bence Jones proteins in the urine of patients with multiple myeloma. Tests to measure total urine concentration accurately rely on precipitation with sulfosalicylic or trichloracetic acids. Currently, ultrasensitive dipsticks are available to measure microalbuminuria (30 to 300 mg/d), an early marker of glomerular disease that has been shown to predict glomerular injury in early diabetic nephropathy (Fig. 47-3).

The magnitude of proteinuria and the protein composition in the urine depend upon the mechanism of renal injury leading to protein losses. Large amounts of plasma proteins normally course through the glomerular capillaries but do not enter the urinary space. Both charge and size selectivity prevent virtually all of albumin, globulin, and other large-molecular-weight proteins from crossing the glomerular wall. However, if this barrier is disrupted, there can be leakage of plasma proteins into the urine (glomerular proteinuria; Fig. 47-3). Smaller proteins (<20 kDa) are freely filtered but are readily reabsorbed by the proximal tubule. Normal individuals excrete less than 150 mg/d of total protein and only about 30 mg/d of albumin. The remainder of the protein in the urine is secreted by the tubules (Tamm-Horsfall, IgA, and urokinase) or represents small amounts of filtered β_2-microglobulin, apoproteins, enzymes, and peptide hormones. Another mechanism of proteinuria occurs when there is excessive production of an abnormal protein that exceeds the capacity of the tubule for reabsorption. This most commonly occurs with plasma cell dyscrasias such as multiple myeloma and lymphomas that are associated with monoclonal production of immunoglobulin light chains.

The normal glomerular endothelial cell forms a barrier penetrated by pores of about 100 nm that holds back cells and other particles but offers little impediment to passage of most proteins. The glomerular basement membrane traps most large proteins (>100 kDa), while the foot processes of epithelial cells (podocytes) cover the urinary side of the glomerular basement membrane and produce a series of narrow channels (slit diaphragms) to allow molecular passage of small solutes and water (Fig. 47-4). The channels are coated with anionic glycoproteins that are rich in glutamate, aspartate, and sialic acid, which are negatively charged at physiologic pH. This negatively charged barrier impedes the passage of anionic molecules such as albumin. Some glomerular diseases, such as minimal change disease, cause fusion of glomerular epithelial cell foot processes, resulting in predominantly "selective" (Fig. 47-3) loss of albumin. Other glomerular diseases can present with disruption of the basement membrane and slit diaphragms (e.g., by immune complex deposition), resulting in large amounts of protein losses that include albumin and other plasma proteins. The fusion of foot processes causes increased pressure across the capillary basement membrane, resulting in areas with larger pore sizes. The combination of increased pressure and larger pores results in significant proteinuria ("nonselective"; Fig. 47-3).

When the total daily excretion of protein exceeds 3.5 g, there is often associated hypoalbuminemia, hyperlipidemia, and edema (nephrotic syndrome; Table 47-1). However, total daily urinary protein excretion greater than 3.5 g can occur without the other features of the nephrotic syndrome in a variety of other renal diseases (Fig. 47-3). Plasma cell dyscrasias (multiple myeloma) can be associated with large amounts of excreted light chains in the urine, which may not be detected by dipstick (which detects mostly albumin). The light chains produced from these disorders are filtered by the glomerulus and overwhelm the reabsorptive capacity of the proximal tubule. A sulfosalicylic acid precipitate that is out of proportion to the dipstick estimate is suggestive of light chains (Bence Jones protein), and light chains typically redissolve upon warming of the precipitate. Renal failure

Urinary Space

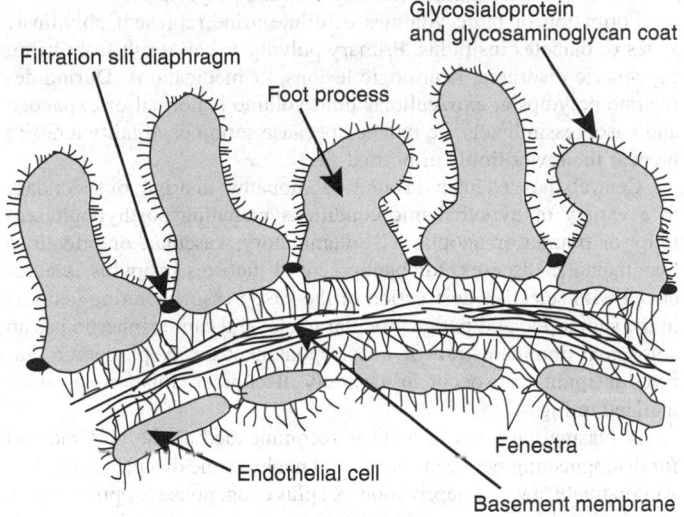

FIGURE 47-4 Diagram showing normal structures separating the capillary lumen and urinary space in the glomerulus. In the process of glomerular filtration, an ultrafiltrate of plasma traverses the capillary wall through endothelial fenestrae, basement membrane, and filtration slit diaphragms (now known to contain the protein nephrin). Proteins are restricted from access to the urinary space by the filtration slit diaphragm and by negatively charged glycosialoproteins and glycosaminoglycans, which coat the glomerular epithelial cell foot processes as well as glomerular endothelial cells lining the capillary lumen.

from these disorders occurs through a variety of mechanisms including tubule obstruction (cast nephropathy) and light chain deposition (Chap. 275).

Hypoalbuminemia in nephrotic syndrome occurs through excessive urinary losses, increased renal catabolism, and inadequate hepatic synthesis. The resulting decrease in plasma oncotic pressure contributes to edema formation by altering the Starling forces and favoring fluid movement from capillaries to interstitium. The resulting homeostatic mechanisms designed to correct the decrease in effective intravascular volume contribute to edema formation in some patients. These mechanisms include activation of the renin-angiotensin system, antidiuretic hormone, and the sympathetic nervous system, which contribute to excessive renal salt and water reabsorption and can contribute to unrelenting edema.

The severity of edema correlates with the degree of hypoalbuminemia and is modified by other factors such as heart disease or peripheral vascular disease. The diminished plasma oncotic pressure and urinary losses of regulatory proteins appear to stimulate hepatic lipoprotein synthesis. The resulting hyperlipidemia results in lipid bodies (fatty casts, oval fat bodies) in the urine. Other proteins are lost in the urine, leading to a variety of metabolic disturbances. These include thyroxine-binding globulin, cholecalciferol-binding protein, transferrin, and metal-binding proteins. A hypercoagulable state frequently accompanies severe nephrotic syndrome due to urinary losses of antithrombin III, reduced serum levels of proteins S and C, hyperfibrinogenemia, and enhanced platelet aggregation. Some patients develop severe IgG deficiency with resulting defects in immunity. Many diseases (some listed in Fig. 47-3) and drugs can cause the nephrotic syndrome, and a complete list can be found in Chap. 274.

HEMATURIA, PYURIA, AND CASTS Isolated hematuria without proteinuria, other cells, or casts is often indicative of bleeding from the urinary tract. Normal red blood cell excretion is up to 2 million RBCs per day. Hematuria is defined as two to five RBCs per high-power field (HPF) and can be detected by dipstick. Common causes of isolated hematuria include stones, neoplasms, tuberculosis, trauma, and prostatitis. Gross hematuria with blood clots is almost never indicative of glomerular bleeding; rather, it suggests a postrenal

source in the urinary collecting system. Evaluation of patients presenting with microscopic hematuria is outlined in Fig. 47-2. A single urinalysis with hematuria is common and can result from menstruation, viral illness, allergy, exercise, or mild trauma. Annual urinalysis of servicemen over a 10-year period showed an incidence of 38%. However, persistent or significant hematuria (>three RBCs/HPF on three urinalyses, or single urinalysis with >100 RBCs, or gross hematuria) identified significant renal or urologic lesions in 9.1% of over 1000 patients. Even patients who are chronically anticoagulated should be investigated as outlined in Fig. 47-2. The suspicion for urogenital neoplasms in patients with isolated painless hematuria (nondysmorphic RBCs) increases with age. Neoplasms are rare in the pediatric population, and isolated hematuria is more likely to be "idiopathic" or associated with a congenital anomaly. Hematuria with pyuria and bacteriuria is typical of infection and should be treated with antibiotics after appropriate cultures. Acute cystitis or urethritis in women can cause gross hematuria. Hypercalciuria and hyperuricosuria are also risk factors for unexplained isolated hematuria in both children and adults. In some of these patients (50 to 60%), reducing calcium and uric acid excretion through dietary interventions can eliminate the microscopic hematuria.

Isolated microscopic hematuria can be a manifestation of glomerular diseases. The RBCs of glomerular origin are often dysmorphic when examined by phase-contrast microscopy. Irregular shapes of RBCs may also occur due to pH and osmolarity changes found in the distal tubule. There is, however, significant observer variability in detecting dysmorphic RBCs, especially if a phase-contrast microscope is not available. The most common etiologies of isolated glomerular hematuria are IgA nephropathy, hereditary nephritis, and thin basement membrane disease. IgA nephropathy and hereditary nephritis can have episodic gross hematuria. A family history of renal failure is often present in patients with hereditary nephritis, and patients with thin basement membrane disease often have other family members with microscopic hematuria. A renal biopsy is needed for the definitive diagnosis of these disorders, which are discussed in more detail in Chap. 275. Hematuria with dysmorphic RBCs, RBC casts, and protein excretion >500 mg/d is virtually diagnostic of glomerulonephritis. RBC casts form as RBCs that enter the tubular fluid become trapped in a cylindrical mold of gelled Tamm-Horsfall protein. Even in the absence of azotemia, these patients should undergo serologic evaluation and renal biopsy as outlined in Fig. 47-2.

Isolated pyuria is unusual since inflammatory reactions in the kidney or collecting system are also associated with hematuria. The presence of bacteria suggests infection, and white blood cell casts with bacteria are indicative of pyelonephritis. White blood cells and/or white blood cell casts may also be seen in tubulointerstitial processes such as interstitial nephritis, systemic lupus erythematosus, and transplant rejection. In chronic renal diseases, degenerated cellular casts called *waxy casts* can be seen in the urine. *Broad casts* are thought to arise in the dilated tubules of enlarged nephrons that have undergone compensatory hypertrophy in response to reduced renal mass (i.e., chronic renal failure). A mixture of broad casts typically seen with chronic renal failure together with cellular casts and RBCs may be seen in smoldering processes such as chronic glomerulonephritis with active glomerulitis.

ABNORMALITIES OF URINE VOLUME

The volume of urine produced varies depending upon the fluid intake, renal function, and physiologic demands of the individual. See "Azotemia," above, for discussion of decreased (oliguria) or absent urine production (anuria). →*The physiology of water formation and renal water conservation are discussed in Chap. 268.*

POLYURIA By history, it is often difficult for patients to distinguish urinary frequency (often of small volumes) from polyuria, and a 24-h urine collection is needed for evaluation (Fig. 47-5). It is

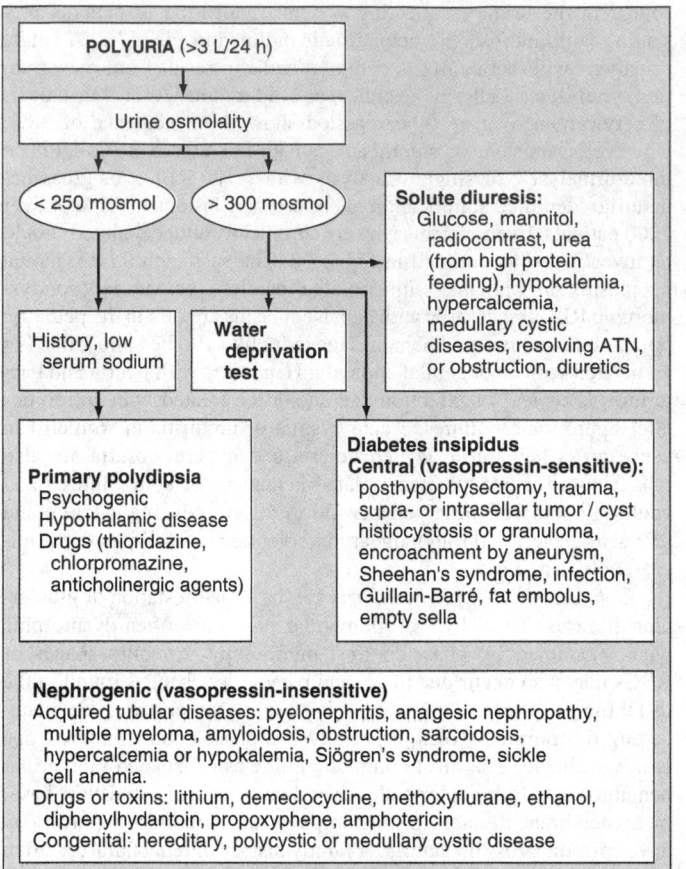

FIGURE 47-5 Approach to the patient with polyuria. (Osm, osmolality; ATN, acute tubular necrosis.)

necessary to determine if the polyuria represents a solute or water diuresis and if the diuresis is appropriate for the clinical circumstances. The average person excretes between 600 and 800 mosmol of solutes per day, primarily as urea and electrolytes. The urine osmolality can help distinguish a solute from water diuresis. If the urine output is >3 L/d (arbitrarily defined as polyuria) and the urine is dilute (<250 mosmol/L), then total mosmol excretion is normal and a water diuresis is present. This circumstance could arise from polydipsia, inadequate secretion of vasopressin (central diabetes insipidus), or failure of renal tubules to respond to vasopressin (nephrogenic diabetes insipidus). If the urine volume is >3 L/d and urine osmolality is >300 mosmol/L, then a solute diuresis is clearly present and a search for the responsible solute(s) is mandatory.

Excessive filtration of a poorly reabsorbed solute such as glucose, mannitol, or urea can depress reabsorption of NaCl and water in the proximal tubule and lead to enhanced excretion in the urine. Poorly controlled diabetes mellitus is the most common cause of a solute diuresis, leading to volume depletion and serum hypertonicity. Since the urine Na concentration is less than that of blood, more water than Na is lost, causing hypernatremia and hypertonicity. Common iatrogenic solute diuresis occurs from mannitol administration, radiocontrast media, and high-protein feedings (enterally or parenterally), leading to increased urea production and excretion. Less commonly, excessive Na loss may occur from cystic renal diseases, Bartter's syndrome, or during the course of a tubulointerstitial process (such as resolving ATN). In these so-called salt-wasting disorders, the tubule damage results in direct impairment of Na reabsorption and indirectly reduces the responsiveness of the tubule to aldosterone. Usually, the Na losses are mild, and the obligatory urine output is less than 2 L/d

(resolving ATN and postobstructive diuresis are exceptions and may be associated with significant natriuresis and polyuria.)

Formation of large volumes of dilute urine represent polydipsic states or diabetes insipidus. Primary polydipsia can result from habit, psychiatric disorders, neurologic lesions, or medications. During deliberate polydipsia, extracellular fluid volume is normal or expanded and vasopressin levels are reduced because serum osmolality tends to be near the lower limits of normal.

Central diabetes insipidus may be idiopathic in origin or secondary to a variety of hypothalamic conditions including posthypophysectomy or trauma or neoplastic, inflammatory, vascular, or infectious hypothalamic diseases. Idiopathic central diabetes insipidus is associated with selective destruction of the vasopressin-secreting neurons in the supraoptic and paraventricular nuclei and can be inherited as an autosomal dominant trait or occur spontaneously. Nephrogenic diabetes insipidus can occur in a variety of clinical situations as summarized in Fig. 47-5.

A plasma vasopressin level is recommended as the best method for distinguishing between central and nephrogenic diabetes insipidus. Alternatively, a water deprivation test plus exogenous vasopressin may also distinguish primary polydipsia from central and nephrogenic diabetes insipidus. *→For a detailed discussion, see Chap. 329.*

BIBLIOGRAPHY

ANDERSON S et al: Renal and systemic manifestations of glomerular disease, in *Brenner & Rector's The Kidney*, 6th ed, BM Brenner (ed). Philadelphia, Saunders, 2000, pp 1871–1900.

BERL T, ROBERTSON GL: Pathophysiology of water metabolism, in *Brenner & Rector's The Kidney*, 6th ed, BM Brenner (ed). Philadelphia, Saunders, 2000, pp 66–924

BICHET DG: Nephrogenic diabetes insipidus. Am J Med 105(5):431, 1998

GROSSFELD GD, CARROLL PR: Evaluation of asymptomatic microscopic hematuria. Urol Clin North Am 25(4):661, 1998

KASISKE BL, KEANE WF: Laboratory assessment of renal disease: Clearance, urinalysis and renal biopsy, in *Brenner & Rector's The Kidney*, 6th ed, BM Brenner (ed). Philadelphia, Saunders, 2000, pp 129–1170

KESTILA M et al: Positively cloned gene for a novel glomerular protein—nephrin—is mutated in congenital nephrotic syndrome. Mol Cell 1(4):575, 1998

MARIANI AJ et al: The significance of adult hematuria: 1000 hematuria evaluations including a risk-benefit and cost-effectiveness analysis. J Urol 141:350, 1989

NOLAN CR, ANDERSON RJ: Hospital-acquired acute renal failure. J Am Soc Nephrol 9: 710, 1998

48   *Philippe E. Zimmern, John D. McConnell*

INCONTINENCE AND LOWER URINARY TRACT SYMPTOMS

PHYSIOLOGY OF VOIDING

Normal bladder filling depends on unique elastic properties of the bladder wall that allow it to increase in volume at a pressure lower than that of the bladder neck and urethra (otherwise incontinence would occur). Despite provocative maneuvers such as coughing, voluntary bladder contractions do not occur. Emptying is dependent on the integrity of a complex neuromuscular network that causes relaxation of the urethral sphincter a few milliseconds before the onset of the detrusor (bladder muscle) contraction. With normal, sustained detrusor contraction, the bladder empties completely. A bladder that can fill and empty in this manner has a normal detrusor muscle and is described as *stable* according to conventional terminology.

Since the voluntary control of micturition depends on the neural connections between the cerebral cortex and the brainstem, disruption of these pathways (brain tumor, stroke, head trauma, Parkinson's disease) impairs the ability to suppress and control bladder contractions.

A bladder contraction without voluntary effort characterizes an unstable bladder. Bladder or detrusor instability of neurologic origin is termed *detrusor hyperreflexia*. Conversely, the detrusor muscle that cannot contract during voiding is called *noncontractile*; underactivity of the detrusor due to a lesion of the sacral cord or pelvic nerves is termed *detrusor areflexia*.

Contrary to common belief, the center that controls normal micturition is not in the spinal cord but in the brainstem. Proper coordination (*synergia*) between the detrusor and urethral sphincters requires an intact neural (autonomic and somatic nervous systems) communication between bladder and urethra. Injury to the upper spinal cord, for example, can cause dyssynergia between bladder and urethra that results in urge incontinence, residual urine retention, bladder wall changes (trabeculation and fibrosis), and possibly renal insufficiency.

A simple way to classify voiding dysfunction is to determine whether it is primarily a *storage failure* or an *emptying failure* by asking two questions:

Is the voiding dysfunction due to the bladder or outlet (bladder neck or urethra) (failure to store)?
Is there neurologic dysfunction (failure to empty)?

Bladder storage and emptying problems may coexist in the same individual and can cause similar lower urinary tract symptoms (LUTS).

LOWER URINARY TRACT SYMPTOMS IN MEN The most common cause of LUTS in men of middle age and older is prostatic hyperplasia, which causes obstruction to urine flow by encroachment on the urethral lumen (Chap. 95). Histologically, 50 to 80% of the prostatic volume is composed of stromal tissue (smooth muscle), while the remainder is glandular. The transitional zone, which is responsible for benign prostatic growth, comprises 10 to 15% of the prostate at the end of puberty but increases in volume after age 40. However, prostatic enlargement is not always accompanied by symptoms because the direction of growth can be outward, so that little change may occur in urine flow. Alternatively, men with early histologic evidence of prostatic hyperplasia can experience significant voiding symptoms. In this circumstance, increased tone of the prostatic smooth muscle and enhanced prostatic tension within a nondistensible capsule can cause obstruction.

In response to obstruction, the bladder smooth-muscle cells hypertrophy to generate the higher pressures necessary for voiding, and the increase in bladder muscle mass leads to reduced elasticity, or compliance, and decreased bladder capacity. Detrusor dysfunction from bladder outlet obstruction can cause any combination of the LUTS described above. When the obstruction progresses, infiltration of extracellular matrix between the smooth-muscle bundles of the bladder wall can result in a hypocontractile or acontractile bladder (bladder failure).

Other complications such as urinary tract infections or bladder stones secondary to the large postvoid residuals (stasis) and upper tract damage (hydronephrosis, reflux) can develop during the course of the obstructive process. Although prostatic hyperplasia is the most common cause of bladder outlet obstruction in men, other sources of obstruction include prostate cancer, urethral stricture, and lack of proper sphincteric relaxation (neurologic cause). Nonobstructive causes of LUTS include diabetic neuropathy, which can affect the parasympathetic nerves of the bladder. Decreased sensation of bladder fullness leads to incomplete emptying and overdistention of the bladder and, in turn, to increased frequency and nocturia due to bladder overflow; these symptoms are frequently made worse by the polydipsia/polyuria of diabetes mellitus. At times, storage symptoms can be caused by other neurologic causes such as stroke, multiple sclerosis, or Parkinson's disease.

The International Prostate Symptom Score (IPSS) is used to assess the severity of LUTS:

Decreased force of stream—over the past month how often have you had a weak urinary stream?

Intermittency—over the past month how often have you found you stopped and started again several times when urinating?
Incomplete emptying—over the past month how often have you had a sensation of not emptying your bladder completely after finishing urination?
Straining—over the past month how often have you had to push or strain to begin urination?

The IPSS also assesses the impact of storage symptoms:

Frequency—over the past month how often have you had to urinate again within 2 h after urinating?
Urgency—over the past month how often have you found it difficult to postpone urination?
Nocturia—over the past month how many times did you typically get up to urinate between going to bed and getting up in the morning? (Range: none to five or more times.)

Except for nocturia, the answers range from 0 (not at all) to 5 (almost always). A total score of <8 indicates minimal voiding dysfunction; a total score of ≥13 is usually required to enroll patients in drug studies for the management of benign prostatic hyperplasia (BPH); and symptom scores >23 suggest significant bladder outlet obstruction. Because similar symptoms can result from neurologic causes, the IPSS questionnaire cannot be used to make the diagnosis of prostatic hyperplasia but is useful only as an index of severity and of the response to treatment.

LOWER URINARY TRACT SYMPTOMS IN WOMEN Urethral obstruction is an uncommon cause of LUTS in women. A careful bimanual examination and passage of a urethral catheter are sufficient to exclude urethral stenosis, which is usually secondary to prior instrumentation or operative procedures, and urethral cancer. Urinary tract infection (cystitis) is more prevalent in women and must be excluded by urinalysis. Multiple sclerosis should be considered in middle-aged women presenting with frequency, urgency, or incontinence. In addition to many of the same disorders that produce voiding symptoms in men, estrogen deficiency, frequency-urgency syndrome, and interstitial cystitis (IC) with minimal pain must be considered. Cystocele and pelvic prolapse can cause urinary frequency secondary to impairment of bladder emptying.

EVALUATION Men and women with LUTS and concomitant neurologic disease should undergo a complete urodynamic evaluation. In the absence of neurologic disease, men with LUTS most commonly have prostatic hyperplasia. However, it is necessary to exclude prostate cancer, especially if there is a positive family history, an abnormal prostate examination, or an elevated level of prostate-specific antigen (PSA). In both sexes bladder cancer can also cause storage symptoms and is suggested by microscopic hematuria and/or abnormal urine cytology. Usually, a detailed genitourinary history, a symptom assessment, a careful neurologic examination including rectal examination and assessment of the bulbocavernosus reflex, measurements of urine flow and postvoid residual urine volume (by bladder ultrasound), and limited laboratory evaluation (urinalysis, urine culture, PSA levels, urine cytology, urea/creatinine levels, as indicated) should be sufficient to direct therapy. More complex investigations of the lower urinary tract (cystoscopy, voiding cystography, urodynamics) and upper urinary tract (pyelogram or ultrasonography) are sometimes indicated. →*For therapy of BPH, see Chap. 95.*

INCONTINENCE

Incontinence is a condition where involuntary loss of urine is objectively demonstrated and is a social or hygienic problem. A common variant, *stress incontinence*, denotes involuntary loss of urine with physical exercise (coughing, sneezing, sports, sexual activity). *Urge incontinence* is an involuntary loss of urine associated with a strong desire to void, and *overflow incontinence* is an involuntary loss of urine when the elevation of intravesical pressure with bladder overfilling or distention exceeds the maximal urethral pressure. Loss of urine through channels other than the urethra is rare (ectopic ureter, fistulae) but causes total or continuous incontinence.

INCONTINENCE IN WOMEN   Among noninstitutionalized women 60 years of age and older, 25 to 30% have urinary incontinence daily or weekly, and approximately half of institutionalized women are incontinent more than once a day. The annual cost of caring for incontinent persons is very high and, if not well managed, can be associated with complications such as decubitus ulcers.

Stress urinary incontinence (SUI) is secondary to urethral hypermobility or, less commonly (<10%), to intrinsic sphincteric deficiency (ISD). In the continent woman the bladder neck and proximal urethra are supported by the anterior vaginal wall and its lateral attachment to the levator muscles. Anterior vaginal wall relaxation causes urethral hypermobility, usually due to aging and/or estrogen deficiency or a prior traumatic delivery or pelvic surgery. Paradoxically, women can have clinical evidence of urethral hypermobility but no stress urinary incontinence.

Some women have an anatomically normal urethra and bladder neck but still have SUI due to damage to the internal sphincter (fixed, rigid, or "pipestem" urethra), due to prior anti-incontinence surgery, pelvic radiation or trauma, or neurologic disorders that cause denervation of the urethra. Urethral hypermobility and ISD can coexist in some patients and cause persistence (or rapid recurrence) of incontinence after a simple bladder neck suspension procedure that fixes the hypermobility but leaves the sphincter untreated.

Urge incontinence can be present alone or in association with SUI (mixed incontinence). The cause of the unsuppressible or uninhibited bladder contractions is usually idiopathic, but bacterial cystitis, bladder tumor, bladder outlet obstruction, and neurogenic bladder must be excluded. Overflow incontinence is due either to bladder outlet obstruction (rare in women), an acontractile bladder (diabetic neuropathy, multiple sclerosis), excessive smooth-muscle relaxation from drugs (anticholinergic medications), or psychogenic retention.

INCONTINENCE IN MEN   In men incontinence is less common than obstruction, but urgency and urge incontinence can occur as the result of bladder outlet obstruction (as from prostatic hyperplasia) that impairs detrusor smooth-muscle function and leads to detrusor instability. Men with neurogenic bladders (diabetic neuropathy, multiple sclerosis, Parkinson's disease, stroke) can develop urge incontinence. Other causes such as bacterial cystitis or bladder tumor must be excluded. SUI in men is usually the result of distal sphincteric damage, for example, as the result of radical prostatectomy for prostate cancer.

INCONTINENCE IN THE ELDERLY   Transient urinary incontinence is common in the elderly. A mnemonic devised by Resnick delineates its numerous causes, namely *d*elirium, *i*nfection, *a*trophic urethritis, *p*harmacologic, *p*sychological, *e*xcessive urine output (hyperglycemia, congestive heart failure), *r*estricted mobility, and *s*tool impaction (DIAPPERS). Urge incontinence is the next most common disorder in this age group and is attributed to the progressive loss of the modulating influence of the frontal lobes of the cortex on the micturition center in the brainstem.

EVALUATION   The evaluation of urinary incontinence in women should include history and quality-of-life assessment, voiding diary, physical examination including pelvic examination, urinalysis and urine culture, and measurement of postvoid residual urine volume. For patients with an unclear history or after prior pelvic or anti-incontinence procedures, evaluation may include cystoscopy, urodynamic evaluation, and imaging studies (lower and/or upper urinary tract). The history should define the onset, duration, evolution, and triggering events of leakage. Prior treatments with medications, frequent voiding schedules, and exercise regimens should be noted. Severity of incontinence is denoted by recording the type and number of pads used per day or at night and how the incontinence affects daily activities (incontinence-impact questionnaire). The amount and type of fluid consumed, sexual history (hormonal status, deliveries, venereal diseases), gastrointestinal function (fecal incontinence, constipation), and past urologic history (bed-wetting, surgeries) must also be documented. The physical examination should place special emphasis on the abdominal, genital, pelvic (associated prolapses), and neurologic systems. SUI must be demonstrated by asking the patient to cough, strain, or even stand or squat. While leakage during a cough confirms SUI, leakage after a cough is due to bladder instability (stress-induced instability). SUI in the absence of urethral hypermobility raises the suspicion of a sphincteric defect. More complex testing is needed to determine whether the urethral anatomy is normal (evaluation of urethral mobility, lateral view of the urethra on the voiding cystourethrogram, cystoscopy), whether urethral function is normal with adequate closure (leak point pressure, urethral profilometry, videourodynamics), or whether bladder function is normal (bladder volume based on home diary, filling cystometrogram).

$\boxed{R_x}$ **TREATMENT**   Mild stress incontinence can be treated nonoperatively with medications, estrogen replacement, or biofeedback techniques. Modalities such as urethral plugs and anterior vaginal wall prostheses are under investigation. Moderate to severe stress incontinence responds to surgical procedures aimed at supporting the anterior vaginal wall (vaginal, laparoscopic, or abdominal operations) or enhancing urethral closure when stress incontinence is secondary to internal sphincter deficiency (periurethral injection of fat or collagen, autologous or cadaveric fascial sling, synthetic sling, or insertion of an artificial urinary sphincter).

Urge incontinence responds to the management of its cause. When it is due to neurogenic or idiopathic causes, anticholinergic agents are partially effective, although side effects such as mouth dryness, blurring of vision, or constipation can limit their usefulness. Better tolerated medications are now available including slow-release oxybutinin (Ditropan XL), which is administered as 5- to 10-mg tablets once daily, and the more specific antimuscarinic agent, tolterodine (Detrol), which is usually given as 2 mg orally twice daily. Fluid restriction (which must be undertaken only with great caution) and bladder retraining with biofeedback may also be helpful. More aggressive intervention with bladder augmentation or urinary diversion are seldom necessary in the absence of neurologic disease.

BLADDER PAIN

Painful bladder disease is a general term for any bladder pathology that causes suprapubic, urethral, or pelvic pain. IC is the most common cause of bladder pain, but endometriosis, bacterial cystitis, and outlet obstruction that causes bladder instability can mimic the symptoms of IC.

INTERSTITIAL CYSTITIS   IC is a severe, chronic bladder disorder that causes frequency, nocturia, and suprapubic pain. The disorder usually affects women and is rare in blacks. Routine urine culture is uniformly negative, and the symptoms do not respond to antibiotic therapy. The etiology is probably multifactorial (Table 48-1). Current hypotheses as to etiology include autoimmune reaction against bladder antigens, deficiency in the glycosaminoglycan layer of the bladder surface allowing presumed toxins to penetrate the mucosa, mast cell infiltration and activation leading to the histamine release, and local bladder wall damage from bacteria.

The National Institutes of Health has established a series of criteria to define IC clinically (Table 48-2). The diagnosis is one of exclusion—infection, radiation cystitis, urethral diverticula, herpes simplex, and malignancy must be excluded. Cystoscopy under anesthesia may be used for the following: (1) reveal glomerulations (submucosal vascular anomalies) or the infrequent Hunner's ulcer suggestive of IC; (2) make it possible to estimate bladder capacity (an important guide to treatment); (3) allow biopsy of the bladder wall when indicated; and (4) by bladder filling, sometimes provide therapeutic benefit with a

Table 48-1 Consensus Criteria for Diagnosis of Interstitial Cystitis

Automatic Exclusions
Less than 18 years old
Benign or malignant bladder tumors
Radiation cystitis
Bacterial cystitis
Vaginitis
Cyclophosphamide cystitis
Symptomatic urethral diverticulum
Uterine, cervical, vaginal, or urethral cancers
Active herpes
Bladder or lower urethral calculi
Waking frequency less than five times in 12 h
Nocturia less than twice nightly
Symptoms relieved by antibiotics, urinary antiseptics, urinary analgesics
  (e.g., phenazopyridine hydrochloride)
Duration less than 12 months
Involuntary bladder contractions (urodynamics)
Capacity greater than 400 mL, absence of sensory urgency
Automatic Inclusions
Hunner's ulcer
Positive Factors
Pain on bladder filling relieved by emptying
Pain (suprapubic, pelvic, urethral, vaginal, or perineal)
Glomerulations after hydrodistention on cystoscopy

Table 48-2 Possible Causes of Interstitial Cystitis

Infection	Allergic/immune/autoimmune
Fastidious bacteria	causes
Latent viruses	Neurogenic disturbances
Dysfunctional bladder epithelium	Bladder mastocytosis
Defective glycosaminoglycan layer	Psychosomatic
Abnormal intercellular junctions	Others
Toxic substances in urine	Food intolerance
	Endocrine causes

---

reduction in pain level and urinary frequency up to 6 months or rarely longer.

EVALUATION Chronic urinary frequency and bladder pain affect the quality of life to an extreme degree, though most patients experience a waxing and waning evolution; only 10% of patients have a consistent progression in symptoms. Evaluation should include a detailed history; physical examination designed to exclude neurologic and gynecologic pathology; voiding cystogram to exclude urethral defects; and urodynamic testing to eliminate a neurogenic bladder, bladder instability, or outlet obstruction and to document sensory instability. Referral to specialists may be indicated to exclude adnexal pathology, endometriosis, or bowel dysfunction or to utilize modern pain management techniques to prevent drug addiction.

℞ **TREATMENT** Empirical treatments that have been used include oral medications (amitriptyline, hydroxyzine, pentosanpolysulfate) and intravesical agents (dimethyl sulfoxide, chlorpactin, heparin). These measures may improve the urinary symptoms and occasionally reduce pain but do not modify the long-term course. Surgical intervention (augmentation cystoplasty, urinary diversion) is indicated in fewer than 5% of cases because this is a non-life-threatening, chronic disease with occasional spontaneous remissions. "Last-resort" interventions such as removal of the bladder and urethra are not a guarantee of success because some patients continue to experience pelvic pain afterwards.

BIBLIOGRAPHY

BARRY MJ et al: The American Urological Association symptom index for benign prostatic hyperplasia. The measurement committee of the American Urological Association. J Urol 148:1549, 1992

CHAI TB, STEERS WD: Neurophysiology of micturition and continence. Urol Clin North Am 23:221, 1996

DUPONT MC et al: Diagnosis of stress urinary incontinence. An overview. Urol Clin North Am 23:407, 1996

HAAB F et al: Female stress urinary incontinence due to intrinsic sphincteric deficiency: Recognition and management. J Urol 156:3, 1996

HOLTGREWE HL: The evaluation and management of the adult male with lower urinary tract symptoms. Urology 51(Suppl):1, 1998

LEACH GE et al: Female stress urinary incontinence: Clinical Guidelines Panel summary report on surgical management of female stress urinary incontinence. J Urol 158:875, 1997

RESNICK N: Geriatric incontinence. Urol Clin North Am 23:55, 1996

SIMON LJ et al: The Interstitial Cystitis Data Base Study: Concepts and preliminary baseline descriptive statistics. Urology 49(Suppl 5A):64, 1997

WALSH PC et al (eds): Campbell's Urology, 7th ed. Philadelphia, Saunders, 1998

---

49 *Gary G. Singer, Barry M. Brenner*

FLUID AND ELECTROLYTE DISTURBANCES

ACE	angiotensin-converting enzyme	NSAIDs	nonsteroidal anti-inflammatory drugs
AVP	arginine vasopressin		
BUN	blood urea nitrogen	ODS	osmotic demyelination syndrome
CCD	cortical collecting duct		
CDI	central diabetes insipidus	RBCs	red blood cells
ECF	extracellular fluid	RTA	renal tubular acidosis
GFR	glomerular filtration rate	SIADH	syndrome of inappropriate antidiuretic hormone secretion
11β-HSDH	11β-hydroxysteroid dehydrogenase		
ICF	intracellular fluid	TEPD	transepithelial potential difference
MCD	medullary collecting duct	TTKG	transtubular K^+ concentration gradient
NDI	nephrogenic diabetes insipidus		

SODIUM AND WATER

COMPOSITION OF BODY FLUIDS Water is the most abundant constituent in the body, comprising approximately 50% of body weight in women and 60% in men. This difference is attributable to differences in the relative proportions of adipose tissue in men and women. Total body water is distributed in two major compartments—55 to 75% is intracellular [intracellular fluid (ICF)], and 25 to 45% is extracellular [extracellular fluid (ECF)]. The ECF is further subdivided into intravascular (plasma water) and extravascular (interstitial) spaces in a ratio of 1:3.

The solute or particle concentration of a fluid is known as its *osmolality* and is expressed as milliosmoles per kilogram of water (mosmol/kg). Water crosses cell membranes to achieve osmotic equilibrium (ECF osmolality = ICF osmolality). The extracellular and intracellular solutes or osmoles are markedly different due to disparities in permeability and the presence of transporters and active pumps. The major ECF particles are Na^+ and its accompanying anions Cl^- and HCO_3^-, whereas K^+ and organic phosphate esters (ATP, creatine phosphate, and phospholipids) are the predominant ICF osmoles. Solutes that are restricted to the ECF or the ICF determine the *effective osmolality* (or *tonicity*) of that compartment. Since Na^+ is largely restricted to the extracellular compartment, total body Na^+ content is a reflection of ECF volume. Likewise, K^+ and its attendant anions are predominantly limited to the ICF and are necessary for normal cell function. Therefore, the number of intracellular particles is relatively constant, and a change in ICF osmolality is usually due to a change in ICF water content. However, in certain situations, brain cells can vary the number of intracellular solutes in order to defend against large water shifts. This process of *osmotic adaptation* is important in the defense of cell volume and occurs in chronic hyponatremia and hypernatremia. This response is mediated initially by transcellular shifts of K^+ and Na^+, followed by synthesis, import, or export of organic solutes (so-called osmolytes) such as inositol, betaine, and glutamine.

During chronic hyponatremia, brain cells lose solutes, thereby defending cell volume and diminishing neurologic symptoms. The converse occurs during chronic hypernatremia. Certain solutes, such as urea, do not contribute to water shift across cell membranes and are known as *ineffective osmoles*.

Fluid movement between the intravascular and interstitial spaces occurs across the capillary wall and is determined by the Starling forces—capillary hydraulic pressure and colloid osmotic pressure. The transcapillary hydraulic pressure gradient exceeds the corresponding oncotic pressure gradient, thereby favoring the movement of plasma ultrafiltrate into the extravascular space. The return of fluid into the intravascular compartment occurs via lymphatic flow.

WATER BALANCE   (See also Chap. 268)   The normal plasma osmolality is 275 to 290 mosmol/kg and is kept within a narrow range by mechanisms capable of sensing a 1 to 2% change in tonicity. To maintain a steady state, water intake must equal water excretion. Disorders of water homeostasis result in hypo- or hypernatremia. Normal individuals have an obligate water loss consisting of urine, stool, and evaporation from the skin and respiratory tract. Gastrointestinal excretion is usually a minor component of total water output, except in patients with vomiting, diarrhea, or high enterostomy output states. Evaporative or insensitive water losses are important in the regulation of core body temperature. Obligatory renal water loss is mandated by the minimum solute excretion required to maintain a steady state. Normally, about 600 mosmols must be excreted per day, and since the maximal urine osmolality is 1200 mosmol/kg a minimum urine output of 500 mL/d is required for neutral solute balance.

Water Intake   The primary stimulus for water ingestion is *thirst*, mediated either by an increase in effective osmolality or a decrease in ECF volume or blood pressure. *Osmoreceptors*, located in the anterolateral hypothalamus, are stimulated by a rise in tonicity. Ineffective osmoles, such as urea and glucose, do not play a role in stimulating thirst. The average osmotic threshold for thirst is approximately 295 mosmol/kg and varies among individuals. Under normal circumstances, daily water intake exceeds physiologic requirements.

Water Excretion   In contrast to the ingestion of water, its excretion is tightly regulated by physiologic factors. The principal determinant of renal water excretion is *arginine vasopressin* (AVP; formerly antidiuretic hormone), a polypeptide synthesized in the supraoptic and paraventricular nuclei of the hypothalamus and secreted by the posterior pituitary gland. The binding of AVP to V_2 receptors on the basolateral membrane of principal cells in the collecting duct activates adenylyl cyclase and initiates a sequence of events that leads to the insertion of water channels into the luminal membrane. These water channels that are specifically activated by AVP are encoded by the *aquaporin-2 gene* (Chap. 329). The net effect is passive water reabsorption along an osmotic gradient from the lumen of the collecting duct to the hypertonic medullary interstitium. The major stimulus for AVP secretion is hypertonicity. Since the major ECF solutes are Na+ salts, effective osmolality is primarily determined by the plasma Na+ concentration. An increase or decrease in tonicity is sensed by hypothalamic osmoreceptors as a decrease or increase in cell volume, respectively, leading to enhancement or suppression of AVP secretion. The osmotic threshold for AVP release is 280 to 290 mosmol/kg, and the system is sufficiently sensitive that plasma osmolality varies by no more than 1 to 2%.

Nonosmotic factors that regulate AVP secretion include *effective circulating* (arterial) *volume*, nausea, pain, stress, hypoglycemia, pregnancy, and numerous drugs. The hemodynamic response is mediated by baroreceptors in the carotid sinus. The sensitivity of these receptors is significantly lower than that of the osmoreceptors. In fact, depletion of blood volume sufficient to result in a decreased mean arterial pressure is necessary to stimulate AVP release, whereas small changes in effective circulating volume have little effect. In the setting of hypovolemia, the osmotic regulation of AVP remains intact. However, the osmotic threshold, or set point, for AVP release is decreased, and the sensitivity is increased.

To maintain homeostasis and a normal plasma Na+ concentration, the ingestion of solute-free water must eventually lead to the loss of the same volume of electrolyte-free water. Three steps are required for the kidney to excrete a water load: (1) filtration and delivery of water (and electrolytes) to the diluting sites of the nephron; (2) active reabsorption of Na+ and Cl- without water in the thick ascending limb of the loop of Henle and, to a lesser extent, in the distal nephron; and (3) maintenance of a dilute urine due to impermeability of the collecting duct to water in the absence of AVP. Abnormalities of any of these steps can result in impaired free water excretion, and eventual hyponatremia.

SODIUM BALANCE   Sodium is actively pumped out of cells by the Na+,K+-ATPase pump. As a result, 85 to 90% of all Na+ is extracellular, and the ECF volume is a reflection of total body Na+ content. Normal volume regulatory mechanisms ensure that Na+ loss balances Na+ gain. If this does not occur, conditions of Na+ excess or deficit ensue and are manifest as edematous or hypovolemic states, respectively. It is important to distinguish between disorders of osmoregulation and disorders of volume regulation since water and Na+ balance are regulated independently. Changes in Na+ concentration generally reflect disturbed water homeostasis, whereas alterations in Na+ content are manifest as ECF volume contraction or expansion and imply abnormal Na+ balance.

Sodium Intake   Individuals eating a typical western diet consume approximately 150 mmol of NaCl daily. This normally exceeds basal requirements. As noted above, sodium is the principal extracellular cation. Therefore, dietary intake of Na+ results in ECF volume expansion, which in turn promotes enhanced renal Na+ excretion to maintain steady state Na+ balance.

Sodium Excretion   (See also Chap. 268)   The regulation of Na+ excretion is multifactorial and is the major determinant of Na+ balance. A Na+ deficit or excess is manifest as a decreased or increased effective circulating volume, respectively. Changes in effective circulating volume tend to lead to parallel changes in glomerular filtration rate (GFR). However, tubule Na+ reabsorption, and not GFR, is the major regulatory mechanism controlling Na+ excretion. Almost two-thirds of filtered Na+ is reabsorbed in the proximal convoluted tubule—this process is electroneutral and isoosmotic. Further reabsorption (25 to 30%) occurs in the thick ascending limb of the loop of Henle via the apical *Na+-K+-2Cl- cotransporter*—this is an active process and is also electroneutral. Distal convoluted tubule reabsorption of Na+ (5%) is mediated by the *thiazide-sensitive Na+-Cl- cotransporter*. Final Na+ reabsorption occurs in the cortical and medullary collecting ducts, the amount excreted being reasonably equivalent to the amount ingested per day (Chap. 268).

HYPOVOLEMIA

ETIOLOGY   True volume depletion, or hypovolemia, generally refers to a state of combined salt and water loss exceeding intake, leading to ECF volume contraction. The loss of Na+ may be renal or extrarenal (Table 49-1).

Renal   Many conditions are associated with excessive urinary NaCl and water losses, including diuretics. Pharmacologic diuretics inhibit specific pathways of Na+ reabsorption along the nephron with a consequent increase in urinary Na+ excretion. Enhanced filtration of non-reabsorbed solutes, such as glucose or urea, can also impair tubular reabsorption of Na+ and water, leading to an osmotic or solute diuresis. This often occurs in poorly controlled diabetes mellitus and in patients receiving high-protein hyperalimentation. Mannitol is a diuretic that produces an osmotic diuresis because the renal tubule is impermeable to mannitol. Many tubule and interstitial renal disorders are associated with Na+ wasting. Excessive renal losses of Na+ and water may also occur during the diuretic phase of acute tubular necrosis (Chap. 269) and following the relief of bilateral urinary tract ob-

I. ECF volume contracted
  A. Extrarenal Na$^+$ loss
     1. Gastrointestinal
        (vomiting, nasogastric suction, drainage, fistula, diarrhea)
     2. Skin/respiratory
        (insensible losses, sweat, burns)
     3. Hemorrhage
  B. Renal Na$^+$ and water loss
     1. Diuretics
     2. Osmotic diuresis
     3. Hypoaldosteronism
     4. Salt-wasting nephropathies
  C. Renal water loss
     1. Diabetes insipidus (central or nephrogenic)
II. ECF volume normal or expanded
  A. Decreased cardiac output
     1. Myocardial, valvular, or pericardial disease
  B. Redistribution
     1. Hypoalbuminemia
        (hepatic cirrhosis, nephrotic syndrome)
     2. Capillary leak
        (acute pancreatitis, ischemic bowel, rhabdomyolysis)
  C. Increased venous capacitance
     1. Sepsis

NOTE: ECF, extracellular fluid.

struction. The natriuresis and water diuresis associated with these two conditions are often short-lived and an appropriate response to a state of ECF volume expansion that ensued as a result of prior oliguria. However, ongoing losses in the absence of adequate replacement fluids may eventually lead to a state of hypovolemia. Chronic renal insufficiency is associated with a diminished ability to regulate renal salt and water excretion appropriately (Chap. 270). Therefore, patients with a GFR of less than 25 mL/min have an obligatory renal Na$^+$ loss that may result in progressive ECF volume depletion if Na$^+$ intake is restricted. Finally, mineralocorticoid deficiency (hypoaldosteronism) causes salt wasting in the presence of normal intrinsic renal function.

Massive renal water excretion can also lead to hypovolemia. The ECF volume contraction is usually less severe since two-thirds of the volume lost is intracellular. Conditions associated with excessive urinary water loss include *central diabetes insipidus* (CDI) and *nephrogenic diabetes insipidus* (NDI). These two disorders are due to impaired secretion of and renal unresponsiveness to AVP, respectively, and are discussed below.

Extrarenal   Nonrenal causes of hypovolemia include fluid loss from the gastrointestinal tract, skin, and respiratory system and third space accumulations (burns, pancreatitis, peritonitis). Approximately 9 L of fluid enters the gastrointestinal tract daily, 2 L by ingestion and 7 L by secretion. Almost 98% of this volume is reabsorbed so that fecal fluid loss is only 100 to 200 mL/d. Impaired gastrointestinal reabsorption or enhanced secretion leads to volume depletion. Since gastric secretions have a low pH (high H$^+$ concentration) and biliary, pancreatic, and intestinal secretions are alkaline (high HCO$_3^-$ concentration), vomiting and diarrhea are often accompanied by metabolic alkalosis and acidosis, respectively.

Water evaporation from the skin and respiratory tract contributes to thermoregulation. These *insensible losses* amount to 500 mL/d. During febrile illnesses, prolonged heat exposure, or exercise, increased salt and water loss from skin, in the form of sweat, can be significant and lead to volume depletion. The Na$^+$ concentration of sweat is normally 20 to 50 mmol/L and decreases with profuse sweating due to the action of aldosterone. Since sweat is hypotonic, the loss of water exceeds that of Na$^+$. The water deficit is minimized by enhanced thirst. Nevertheless, ongoing Na$^+$ loss is manifest as hypovolemia. Enhanced evaporative water loss from the respiratory tract may be associated with hyperventilation, especially in mechanically ventilated febrile patients.

Certain conditions lead to fluid sequestration in a *third space*. This compartment is extracellular but is not in equilibrium with either the ECF or the ICF. The fluid is effectively lost from the ECF and can result in hypovolemia. Examples include the bowel lumen in gastrointestinal obstruction, subcutaneous tissues in severe burns, retroperitoneal space in acute pancreatitis, and peritoneal cavity in peritonitis. Finally, severe hemorrhage from any source can result in volume depletion.

PATHOPHYSIOLOGY   ECF volume contraction is manifest as a decreased plasma volume and hypotension. Hypotension is due to decreased venous return (preload) and diminished cardiac output; it triggers baroreceptors in the carotid sinus and aortic arch and leads to activation of the sympathetic nervous system and the renin-angiotensin system. The net effect is to maintain mean arterial pressure and cerebral and coronary perfusion. In contrast to the cardiovascular response, the renal response is aimed at restoring the ECF volume by decreasing the GFR and filtered load of Na$^+$ and, most importantly, by promoting tubular reabsorption of Na$^+$. Increased sympathetic tone increases proximal tubular Na$^+$ reabsorption and decreases GFR by causing preferential afferent arteriolar vasoconstriction. Sodium is also reabsorbed in the proximal convoluted tubule in response to increased angiotensin II and altered peritubular capillary hemodynamics (decreased hydraulic and increased oncotic pressure). Enhanced reabsorption of Na$^+$ by the collecting duct is an important component of the renal adaptation to ECF volume contraction. This occurs in response to increased *aldosterone* and AVP secretion, and suppressed *atrial natriuretic peptide* secretion.

CLINICAL FEATURES   A careful history is often helpful in determining the etiology of ECF volume contraction (e.g., vomiting, diarrhea, polyuria, diaphoresis). Most symptoms are nonspecific and secondary to electrolyte imbalances and tissue hypoperfusion and include fatigue, weakness, muscle cramps, thirst, and postural dizziness. More severe degrees of volume contraction can lead to end-organ ischemia manifest as oliguria, cyanosis, abdominal and chest pain, and confusion or obtundation. Diminished skin turgor and dry oral mucous membranes are poor markers of decreased interstitial fluid. Signs of intravascular volume contraction include decreased jugular venous pressure, postural hypotension, and postural tachycardia. Larger and more acute fluid losses lead to hypovolemic shock, manifest as hypotension, tachycardia, peripheral vasoconstriction, and hypoperfusion—cyanosis, cold and clammy extremities, oliguria, and altered mental status.

DIAGNOSIS   A thorough history and physical examination are generally sufficient to diagnose the etiology of hypovolemia. Laboratory data usually confirm and support the clinical diagnosis. The blood urea nitrogen (BUN) and plasma creatinine concentrations tend to be elevated, reflecting a decreased GFR. Normally, the BUN:creatinine ratio is about 10:1. However, in *prerenal azotemia*, hypovolemia leads to increased urea reabsorption and a proportionately greater elevation in BUN than plasma creatinine, and a BUN:creatinine ratio of 20:1 or higher. An increased BUN (relative to creatinine) may also be due to increased urea production that occurs with hyperalimentation (high-protein), glucocorticoid therapy, and gastrointestinal bleeding.

Volume depletion may be associated with hyponatremia, hypernatremia, or a normal plasma Na$^+$ concentration, depending on the tonicity of the fluid lost, the presence of thirst, and the access to water. Hypokalemia is common in settings of increased renal or gastrointestinal K$^+$ loss, and hyperkalemia occurs in renal failure, adrenal insufficiency, and certain types of metabolic acidosis. Metabolic alkalosis occurs with diuretic-induced hypovolemia and in cases of vomiting or nasogastric suction. In contrast, metabolic acidosis is associated with renal failure, tubulointerstitial disorders, adrenal insufficiency, diarrhea, diabetic ketoacidosis, and lactic acidosis. Since albumin and erythrocytes are confined to the intravascular compartment, ECF volume contraction often leads to a relative elevation in hematocrit (hemoconcentration) and plasma albumin concentration.

The appropriate response to hypovolemia is enhanced renal Na^+ and water reabsorption, which is reflected in the urine composition. Therefore, the urine Na^+ concentration should usually be less than 20 mmol/L except in conditions associated with impaired Na^+ reabsorption, as in acute tubular necrosis (Chap. 269). Another exception is hypovolemia due to vomiting, since the associated metabolic alkalosis and increased filtered HCO_3^- impair proximal Na^+ reabsorption. In this case, the urine Cl^- is low (<20 mmol/L). The urine osmolality and specific gravity in hypovolemic subjects are generally greater than 450 mosmol/kg and 1.015, respectively, reflecting the presence of enhanced AVP secretion. However, in hypovolemia due to diabetes insipidus, urine osmolality and specific gravity are indicative of inappropriately dilute urine.

℞ **TREATMENT**   The therapeutic goals are to restore normovolemia with fluid similar in composition to that lost and to replace ongoing losses. Symptoms and signs, including weight loss, can help estimate the degree of volume contraction and should also be monitored to assess response to treatment. Mild volume contraction can usually be corrected via the oral route. More severe hypovolemia requires intravenous therapy. Isotonic or normal saline (0.9% NaCl or 154 mmol/L Na^+) is the solution of choice in normonatremic and mildly hyponatremic individuals and should be administered initially in patients with hypotension or shock. Severe hyponatremia may require hypertonic saline (3.0% NaCl or 513 mmol/L Na^+). Hypernatremia reflects a proportionally greater deficit of water than Na^+, and its correction will therefore require a hypotonic solution such as half-normal saline (0.45% NaCl or 77 mmol/L Na^+) or 5% dextrose in water. Patients with significant hemorrhage, anemia, or intravascular volume depletion may require blood transfusion or colloid-containing solutions (albumin, dextran). Hypokalemia may be present initially or may ensue as a result of increased urinary K^+ excretion; it should be corrected by adding appropriate amounts of KCl to replacement solutions.

HYPONATREMIA

ETIOLOGY   A plasma Na^+ concentration less than 135 mmol/L usually reflects a hypotonic state. However, plasma osmolality may be normal or increased in some cases of hyponatremia, referred to as *pseudohyponatremia*. Plasma is 93% water, the remaining 7% consisting of plasma proteins and lipids. Since Na^+ ions are dissolved in plasma water, increasing the nonaqueous phase artificially lowers the Na^+ concentration measured per liter of plasma (except when Na^+-sensitive glass electrodes are used). The plasma osmolality and the Na^+ concentration remain normal. This type of hyponatremia has little clinical significance, except to ascertain the cause of the hyperproteinemia or hyperlipidemia. Isotonic or slightly hypotonic hyponatremia may complicate transurethral resection of the prostate or bladder because large volumes of isoosmotic (mannitol) or hypoosmotic (sorbital or glycine) bladder irrigation solution can be absorbed and result in a dilutional hyponatremia. The metabolism of sorbitol and glycine to CO_2 and water may lead to hypotonicity if the accumulated fluid and solutes are not rapidly excreted. Hypertonic hyponatremia is usually due to hyperglycemia or, occasionally, intravenous administration of mannitol. Relative insulin deficiency causes myocytes to become impermeable to glucose. Therefore, during poorly controlled diabetes mellitus, glucose is an effective osmole and draws water from muscle cells, resulting in hyponatremia. Plasma Na^+ concentration falls by 1.4 mmol/L for every 100 mg/dL rise in the plasma glucose concentration.

Most causes of hyponatremia are associated with a low plasma osmolality (Table 49-2). In general, hypotonic hyponatremia is due either to a primary water gain (and secondary Na^+ loss) or a primary Na^+ loss (and secondary water gain). In the absence of water intake or

Table 49-2   Causes of Hyponatremia

I. Pseudohyponatremia
   A. Normal plasma osmolality
      1. Hyperlipidemia
      2. Hyperproteinemia
      3. Posttransurethral resection of prostate/bladder tumor
   B. Increased plasma osmolality
      1. Hyperglycemia
      2. Mannitol
II. Hypoosmolal hyponatremia
   A. Primary Na^+ loss (secondary water gain)
      1. Integumentary loss: sweating, burns
      2. Gastrointestinal loss: vomiting, tube drainage, fistula, obstruction, diarrhea
      3. Renal loss: diuretics, osmotic diuresis, hypoaldosteronism, salt-wasting nephropathy, postobstructive diuresis, nonoliguric acute tubular necrosis
   B. Primary water gain (secondary Na^+ loss)
      1. Primary polydipsia
      2. Decreased solute intake (e.g., beer potomania)
      3. AVP release due to pain, nausea, drugs
      4. Syndrome of inappropriate AVP secretion
      5. Glucocorticoid deficiency
      6. Hypothyroidism
      7. Chronic renal insufficiency
   C. Primary Na^+ gain (exceeded by secondary water gain)
      1. Heart failure
      2. Hepatic cirrhosis
      3. Nephrotic syndrome

hypotonic fluid replacement, hyponatremia is usually associated with hypovolemic shock due to a profound sodium deficit and transcellular water shift. Contraction of the ECF volume stimulates thirst and AVP secretion. The increased water ingestion and impaired renal excretion result in hyponatremia. It is important to note that *diuretic-induced hyponatremia* is almost always due to thiazide diuretics. Loop diuretics decrease the tonicity of the medullary interstitium and impair maximal urinary concentrating capacity. This limits the ability of AVP to promote water retention. In contrast, thiazide diuretics lead to Na^+ and K^+ depletion, and AVP-mediated water retention. In the presence of a large K^+ deficit, transcellular ion exchange (K^+ exits and Na^+ enters cells) may contribute to hyponatremia. Hyponatremia can also occur by a process of *desalination*. This occurs when the urine tonicity (the sum of the concentrations of Na^+ and K^+) exceeds that of administered intravenous fluids (including isotonic saline). This accounts for some cases of acute postoperative hyponatremia and cerebral salt wasting after neurosurgery.

Hyponatremia in the setting of ECF volume expansion is usually associated with edematous states, such as congestive heart failure, hepatic cirrhosis, and the nephrotic syndrome. These disorders all have in common a decreased effective circulating arterial volume, leading to increased thirst and increased AVP levels. Additional factors impairing the excretion of solute-free water include a reduced GFR, decreased delivery of ultrafiltrate to the diluting site (due to increased proximal fractional reabsorption of Na^+ and water), and diuretic therapy. The degree of hyponatremia often correlates with the severity of the underlying condition and is an important prognostic factor. Oliguric acute and chronic renal failure may be associated with hyponatremia if water intake exceeds the ability to excrete equivalent volumes.

Hyponatremia in the absence of ECF volume contraction, decreased effective circulating arterial volume, or renal insufficiency is usually due to increased AVP secretion resulting in impaired water excretion. Ingestion or administration of water is also required since high levels of AVP alone are usually insufficient to produce hyponatremia. This disorder, commonly termed the *syndrome of inappropriate antidiuretic hormone secretion* (SIADH), is the most common cause of normovolemic hyponatremia and is due to the nonphysiologic release of AVP from the posterior pituitary or an ectopic source (Chap. 329). Renal free water excretion is impaired while the regulation of

Na⁺ balance is unaffected. The most common causes of SIADH include neuropsychiatric and pulmonary diseases, malignant tumors, major surgery (postoperative pain), and pharmacologic agents. Severe pain and nausea are physiologic stimuli of AVP secretion; these stimuli are inappropriate in the absence of hypovolemia or hyperosmolality. A variety of central nervous system disorders may be associated with SIADH, such as meningitis, encephalitis, hemorrhage, stroke, psychosis, primary and metastatic tumors, and acute porphyria. Pneumonia, empyema, tuberculosis, and acute respiratory failure can be complicated by hyponatremia secondary to SIADH. Hypoxemia, hypercarbia, and positive-pressure ventilation are all nonosmotic stimuli for AVP release. Various tumors, notably oat cell carcinoma of the lung, have been demonstrated to secrete AVP ectopically. Many drugs either stimulate AVP release or potentiate its actions on the kidney. The pattern of AVP secretion can be used to classify SIADH into four subtypes: (1) erratic autonomous AVP secretion (ectopic production); (2) normal regulation of AVP release around a lower osmolality set point or *reset osmostat* (cachexia, malnutrition); (3) normal AVP response to hypertonicity with failure to suppress completely at low osmolality (incomplete pituitary stalk section); and (4) normal AVP secretion with increased sensitivity to its actions or secretion of some other antidiuretic factor (rare).

Hormonal excess or deficiency may cause hyponatremia. Adrenal insufficiency (Chap. 331) and hypothyroidism (Chap. 330) may present with hyponatremia and should not be confused with SIADH. Although decreased mineralocorticoids may contribute to the hyponatremia of adrenal insufficiency, it is the cortisol deficiency that leads to hypersecretion of AVP both indirectly (secondary to volume depletion) and directly (cosecreted with corticotropin-releasing factor). The mechanisms by which hypothyroidism leads to hyponatremia include decreased cardiac output and GFR and increased AVP secretion in response to hemodynamic stimuli.

Finally, hyponatremia may occur in the absence of AVP or renal failure if the kidney is unable to excrete the dietary water load. In psychogenic or primary polydipsia, compulsive water consumption may overwhelm the normally large renal excretory capacity of 12 L/d (Chap. 329). These patients often have psychiatric illnesses and may be taking medications, such as phenothiazines, that enhance the sensation of thirst by causing a dry mouth. The maximal urine output is a function of the minimum urine osmolality achievable and the mandatory solute excretion. Metabolism of a normal diet generates about 600 mosmol/d, and the minimum urine osmolality in humans is 50 mosmol/kg. Therefore, the maximum daily urine output will be about 12 L (600 ÷ 50 = 12). A solute excretion rate of greater than ~750 mosmol/d is, by definition, an *osmotic diuresis*. A low-protein diet may yield as few as 250 mosmol/d, which translates into a maximal urine output of 5 L/d at a minimum urine tonicity of 50 mosmol/kg. Beer drinkers typically have a poor dietary intake of protein and electrolytes and consume large volumes (of beer), which may exceed the renal excretory capacity and result in hyponatremia. This phenomenon is referred to as *beer potomania*.

CLINICAL FEATURES The clinical manifestations of hyponatremia are related to osmotic water shift leading to increased ICF volume, specifically brain cell swelling or cerebral edema. Therefore, the symptoms are primarily neurologic, and their severity is dependent on the rapidity of onset and absolute decrease in plasma Na⁺ concentration. Patients may be asymptomatic or complain of nausea and malaise. As the plasma Na⁺ concentration falls, the symptoms progress to include headache, lethargy, confusion, and obtundation. Stupor, seizures, and coma do not usually occur unless the plasma Na⁺ concentration falls acutely below 120 mmol/L or decreases rapidly. As described above, adaptive mechanisms designed to protect cell volume occur in chronic hyponatremia. Loss of Na⁺ and K⁺, followed by organic osmolytes, from brain cells decreases brain swelling due to secondary transcellular water shifts (from ICF to ECF). The net effect is to minimize cerebral edema and its symptoms. Hospitalized patients with hyponatremia have an increased mortality rate compared to normonatremic control subjects. However, the excess mortality is usually

attributed to the underlying disorder rather than the electrolyte disturbance.

DIAGNOSIS Hyponatremia is not a disease but a manifestation of a variety of disorders. The underlying cause can often be ascertained from an accurate history and physical examination, including an assessment of ECF volume status and effective circulating arterial volume. The differential diagnosis of hyponatremia, an expanded ECF volume, and decreased effective circulating volume includes congestive heart failure, hepatic cirrhosis, and the nephrotic syndrome. Hypothyroidism and adrenal insufficiency tend to present with a near-normal ECF volume and decreased effective circulating arterial volume. All of these diseases have characteristic signs and symptoms. Patients with SIADH are usually euvolemic.

Four laboratory findings often provide useful information and can narrow the differential diagnosis of hyponatremia: (1) the plasma osmolality, (2) the urine osmolality, (3) the urine Na⁺ concentration, and (4) the urine K⁺ concentration. Since ECF tonicity is determined primarily by the Na⁺ concentration, most patients with hyponatremia have a decreased plasma osmolality. If the plasma osmolality is not low, pseudohyponatremia must be ruled out. The appropriate renal response to hypoosmolality is to excrete the maximum volume of dilute urine, i.e., urine osmolality and specific gravity of less than 100 mosmol/kg and 1.003, respectively. This occurs in patients with primary polydipsia. If this is not present, it suggests impaired free water excretion due to the action of AVP on the kidney. The secretion of AVP may be a physiologic response to hemodynamic stimuli or it may be inappropriate in the presence of hyponatremia and euvolemia. Since Na⁺ is the major ECF cation and is largely restricted to this compartment, ECF volume contraction represents a deficit in total body Na⁺ content. Therefore, volume depletion in patients with normal underlying renal function results in enhanced tubule Na⁺ reabsorption and a urine Na⁺ concentration less than 20 mmol/L. The finding of a urine Na⁺ concentration greater than 20 mmol/L in hypovolemic hyponatremia implies a salt-wasting nephropathy, diuretic therapy, hypoaldosteronism, or occasionally vomiting. Both the urine osmolality and the urine Na⁺ concentration can be followed serially when assessing response to therapy.

SIADH is characterized by hypoosmotic hyponatremia in the setting of an inappropriately concentrated urine (urine osmolality greater than 100 mosmol/kg). Patients are typically normovolemic and have normal Na⁺ balance. They tend to be mildly volume expanded secondary to water retention and have a urine Na⁺ excretion rate equal to intake (urine Na⁺ concentration usually greater than 40 mmol/L). By definition, they have normal renal, adrenal, and thyroid function and usually have normal K⁺ and acid-base balance. SIADH is often associated with hypouricemia due to the uricosuric state induced by volume expansion. In contrast, hypovolemic patients tend to be hyperuricemic secondary to increased proximal urate reabsorption.

CLINICAL APPROACH See Fig. 49-1.

Ⓡ **TREATMENT** The goals of therapy are twofold: (1) to raise the plasma Na⁺ concentration by restricting water intake and promoting water loss; and (2) to correct the underlying disorder. Mild asymptomatic hyponatremia is generally of little clinical significance and requires no treatment. The management of asymptomatic hyponatremia associated with ECF volume contaction should include Na⁺ repletion, generally in the form of isotonic saline. The direct effect of the administered NaCl on the plasma Na⁺ concentration is trivial. However, restoration of euvolemia removes the hemodynamic stimulus for AVP release, allowing the excess free water to be excreted. The hyponatremia associated with edematous states tends to reflect the severity of the underlying disease and is usually asymptomatic. These patients have increased total body water that exceeds the increase in total body Na⁺ content. Treatment should include restriction of Na⁺ and water intake, correction of hypokalemia, and promotion of water loss in excess of Na⁺. The latter may require the use of loop diuretics

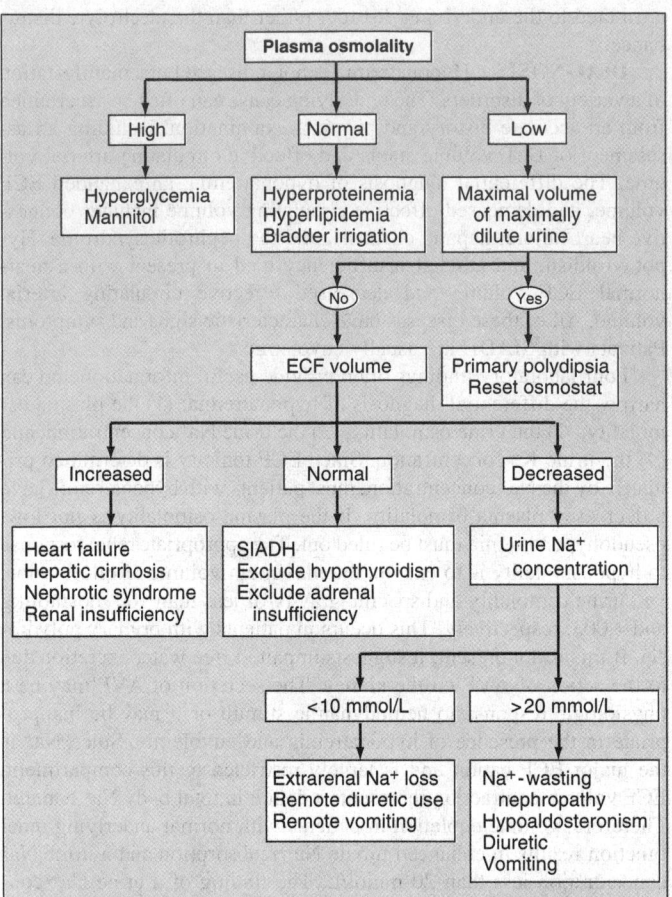

FIGURE 49-1 Algorithm depicting clinical approach to hyponatremia. ECF, extracellular fluid; SIADH, syndrome of inappropriate antidiuretic hormone secretion.

with replacement of a proportion of the urinary Na⁺ loss to ensure net free water excretion. Dietary water restriction should be less than the urine output. Correction of the K⁺ deficit may raise the plasma Na⁺ concentration by favoring a shift of Na⁺ out of cells as K⁺ moves in. Water restriction is also a component of the therapeutic approach to hyponatremia associated with primary polydipsia, renal failure, and SIADH (Chap. 329).

The rate of correction of hyponatremia depends on the absence or presence of neurologic dysfunction. This, in turn, is related to the rapidity of onset and magnitude of the fall in plasma Na⁺ concentration. In asymptomatic patients, the plasma Na⁺ concentration should be raised by no more than 0.5 to 1.0 mmol/L per hour and by less than 10 to 12 mmol/L over the first 24 h. Acute or severe hyponatremia (plasma Na⁺ concentration <110 to 115 mmol/L) tends to present with altered mental status and/or seizures and requires more rapid correction. Severe symptomatic hyponatremia should be treated with hypertonic saline, and the plasma Na⁺ concentration should be raised by 1 to 2 mmol/L per hour for the first 3 to 4 h or until the seizures subside. Once again, the plasma Na⁺ concentration should probably be raised by no more than 12 mmol/L during the first 24 h. The quantity of Na⁺ required to increase the plasma Na⁺ concentration by a given amount can be estimated by multiplying the deficit in plasma Na⁺ concentration by the total body water. Under normal conditions, total body water is 50 or 60% of lean body weight in women or men, respectively. Therefore, to raise the plasma Na⁺ concentration from 105 to 115 mmol/L in a 70-kg man requires 420 mmol [(115 − 105) × 70 × 0.6] of Na⁺. The risk of correcting hyponatremia too rapidly is the development of the *osmotic demyelination syndrome* (ODS). This is a neurologic disorder characterized by flaccid paralysis, dysarthria, and dys-

phagia. The diagnosis is usually suspected clinically and can be confirmed by appropriate neuroimaging studies. There is no specific treatment for the disorder, which is associated with significant morbidity and mortality. Patients with chronic hyponatremia are most susceptible to the development of ODS, since their brain cell volume has returned to near normal as a result of the osmotic adaptive mechanisms described above. Therefore, administration of hypertonic saline to these individuals can cause sudden osmotic shrinkage of brain cells. In addition to rapid or overcorrection of hyponatremia, risk factors for ODS include prior cerebral anoxic injury, hypokalemia, and malnutrition, especially secondary to alcoholism. Water restriction in primary polydipsia and intravenous saline therapy in ECF volume–contracted patients may also lead to overly rapid correction of hyponatremia as a result of AVP suppression and a brisk water diuresis. This can be prevented by administration of water or use of an AVP analogue to slow down the rate of free water excretion. →*For further discussion, see Chap. 329.*

HYPERNATREMIA

ETIOLOGY Hypernatremia is defined as a plasma Na⁺ concentration greater than 145 mmol/L. Since Na⁺ and its accompanying anions are the major effective ECF osmoles, hypernatremia is a state of hyperosmolality. As a result of the fixed number of ICF particles, maintenance of osmotic equilibrium in hypernatremia results in ICF volume contraction. Hypernatremia may be due to primary Na⁺ gain or water deficit. The two components of an appropriate response to hypernatremia are increased water intake stimulated by thirst and the excretion of the minimum volume of maximally concentrated urine reflecting AVP secretion in response to an osmotic stimulus.

In practice, the majority of cases of hypernatremia result from the loss of water. Since water is distributed between the ICF and the ECF in a 2:1 ratio, a given amount of solute-free water loss will result in a twofold greater reduction in the ICF compartment than the ECF compartment. For example, consider three scenarios: the loss of 1 L of water, isotonic NaCl, or half-isotonic NaCl. If 1 L of water is lost, the ICF volume will decrease by 667 mL, whereas the ECF volume will fall by only 333 mL. Due to the fact that Na⁺ is largely restricted to the ECF, this compartment will decrease by 1 L if the fluid lost is isoosmotic. One liter of half-isotonic NaCl is equivalent to 500 mL of water (one-third ECF, two-thirds ICF) plus 500 mL of isotonic saline (all ECF). Therefore, the loss of 1 L of half-isotonic saline decreases the ECF and ICF volumes by 667 mL and 333 mL, respectively.

The degree of hyperosmolality is typically mild unless the thirst mechanism is abnormal or access to water is limited. The latter occurs in infants, the physically handicapped, patients with impaired mental status, in the postoperative state, and in intubated patients in the intensive care unit. On rare occasions, impaired thirst may be due to *primary hypodipsia*. This usually occurs as a result of damage to the hypothalamic osmoreceptors that control thirst and tends to be associated with abnormal osmotic regulation of AVP secretion. Primary hypodipsia may be due to a variety of pathologic changes including granulomatous disease, vascular occlusion, and tumors. A subset of hypodipsic hypernatremia, referred to as *essential hypernatremia*, does not respond to forced water intake. This appears to be due to a specific osmoreceptor defect resulting in nonosmotic regulation of AVP release. Thus, the hemodynamic effects of water loading lead to AVP suppression and excretion of dilute urine.

The source of free water loss is either renal or extrarenal. Nonrenal loss of water may be due to evaporation from the skin and respiratory tract (insensible losses) or loss from the gastrointestinal tract. Insensible losses are increased with fever, exercise, heat exposure, and severe burns and in mechanically ventilated patients. Furthermore, the Na⁺ concentration of sweat decreases with profuse perspiration, thereby increasing solute-free water loss. Diarrhea is the most common gastrointestinal cause of hypernatremia. Specifically, osmotic diarrheas (induced by lactulose, sorbitol, or malabsorption of carbohydrate) and viral gastroenteritides result in water loss exceeding that of

Na⁺ and K⁺. In contrast, secretory diarrheas (e.g., cholera, carcinoid, VIPoma) have a fecal osmolality (twice the sum of the concentrations of Na⁺ and K⁺) similar to that of plasma and present with ECF volume contraction and a normal plasma Na⁺ concentration or hyponatremia.

Renal water loss is the most common cause of hypernatremia and is due to drug-induced or osmotic diuresis or diabetes insipidus (Chap. 329). Loop diuretics interfere with the countercurrent mechanism and produce an isoosmotic solute diuresis. This results in a decreased medullary interstitial tonicity and impaired renal concentrating ability. The presence of non-reabsorbed organic solutes in the tubule lumen impairs the osmotic reabsorption of water. This leads to water loss in excess of Na⁺ and K⁺, known as an osmotic diuresis. The most frequent cause of an osmotic diuresis is hyperglycemia and glucosuria in poorly controlled diabetes mellitus. Intravenous administration of mannitol and increased endogenous production of urea (high-protein diet) can also result in an osmotic diuresis. Hypernatremia secondary to nonosmotic urinary water loss is usually due to: (1) CDI or neurogenic diabetes insipidus characterized by impaired AVP secretion, or (2) NDI resulting from end-organ (renal) resistance to the actions of AVP. The most common cause of CDI is destruction of the neurohypophysis. This may occur as a result of trauma, neurosurgery, granulomatous disease, neoplasms, vascular accidents, or infection. In many cases, CDI is idiopathic and may occasionally be hereditary. The familial form of the disease is inherited in an autosomal dominant fashion and has been attributed to mutations in the propressophysin (AVP precursor) gene. NDI may be either inherited or acquired. Congenital NDI is an X-linked recessive trait due to mutations in the V_2 receptor gene. Mutations in the autosomal aquaporin-2 gene may also result in NDI. The aquaporin-2 gene encodes the water channel protein whose membrane insertion is stimulated by AVP. The causes of sporadic NDI are numerous and include drugs (especially lithium), hypercalcemia, hypokalemia, and conditions that impair medullary hypertonicity (e.g., papillary necrosis or osmotic diuresis). Pregnant women, in the second or third trimester, may develop NDI as a result of excessive elaboration of vasopressinase by the placenta.

Finally, although infrequent, a primary Na⁺ gain may cause hypernatremia. For example, inadvertent administration of hypertonic NaCl or NaHCO₃ or replacing sugar with salt in infant formula can produce this complication.

CLINICAL FEATURES As a consequence of hypertonicity, water shifts out of cells, leading to a contracted ICF volume. A decreased brain cell volume is associated with an increased risk of subarachnoid or intracerebral hemorrhage. Hence, the major symptoms of hypernatremia are neurologic and include altered mental status, weakness, neuromuscular irritability, focal neurologic deficits, and occasionally coma or seizures. Patients may also complain of polyuria or thirst. For unknown reasons, patients with polydipsia from CDI tend to prefer ice-cold water. The signs and symptoms of volume depletion are often present in patients with a history of excessive sweating, diarrhea, or an osmotic diuresis. The mortality rate associated with a plasma Na⁺ concentration greater than 180 mmol/L is very high. As with hyponatremia, the severity of the clinical manifestations is related to the acuity and magnitude of the rise in plasma Na⁺ concentration. Chronic hypernatremia is generally less symptomatic as a result of adaptive mechanisms designed to defend cell volume. Brain cells initially take up Na⁺ and K⁺ salts, later followed by accumulation of organic osmolytes such as inositol. This serves to restore the brain ICF volume towards normal.

DIAGNOSIS A complete history and physical examination will often provide clues as to the underlying cause of hypernatremia. Relevant symptoms and signs include the absence or presence of thirst, diaphoresis, diarrhea, polyuria, and the features of ECF volume contraction. The history should include a list of current and recent medications, and the physical examination is incomplete without a thorough mental status and neurologic assessment. Measurement of urine volume and osmolality are essential in the evaluation of hyperosmolality. The appropriate renal response to hypernatremia is the excretion of the minimum volume (500 mL/d) of maximally concentrated urine

(urine osmolality >800 mosmol/kg). These findings suggest extrarenal or remote renal water loss or administration of hypertonic Na⁺ salt solutions. The presence of a primary Na⁺ excess can be confirmed by the presence of ECF volume expansion and natriuresis (urine Na⁺ concentration usually >100 mmol/L). Many causes of hypernatremia are associated with polyuria and a submaximal urine osmolality. The product of the urine volume and osmolality, i.e., the solute excretion rate, is helpful in determining the basis of the polyuria (see above). To maintain a steady state, total solute excretion must equal solute production. As stated above, individuals eating a normal diet generate ~600 mosmol/d. Therefore, daily solute excretion in excess of 750 mosmol defines an osmotic diuresis. This can be confirmed by measuring the urine glucose and urea. In general, both CDI and NDI present with polyuria and hypotonic urine (urine osmolality <250 mosmol/kg). The degree of hypernatremia is usually mild unless there is an associated thirst abnormality. The clinical history, physical examination, and pertinent laboratory data can often rule out causes of acquired NDI. CDI and NDI can generally be distinguished by administering the AVP analogue desmopressin (10 μg intranasally) after careful water restriction. The urine osmolality should increase by at least 50% in CDI and will not change in NDI. Unfortunately, the diagnosis may sometimes be difficult due to partial defects in AVP secretion and action.

CLINICAL APPROACH See Fig. 49-2.

℞ TREATMENT The therapeutic goals are to stop ongoing water loss by treating the underlying cause and to correct the water deficit. The ECF volume should be restored in hypovolemic patients. The quantity of water required to correct the deficit can be calculated from the following equation:

$$\text{Water deficit} = \frac{\text{plasma Na}^+ \text{ concentration} - 140}{140} \times \text{total body water}$$

In hypernatremia due to water loss, total body water is approxi-

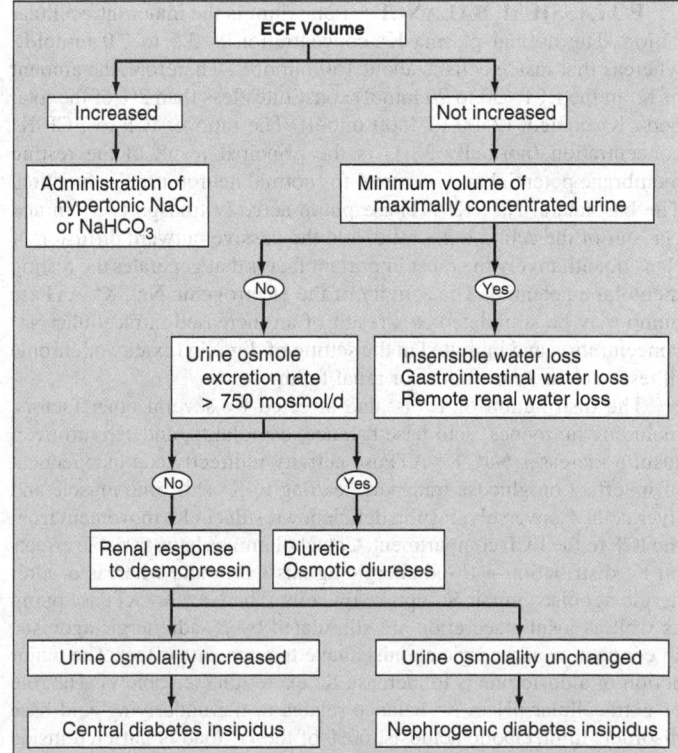

FIGURE 49-2 Algorithm depicting clinical approach to hypernatremia.

mately 50 and 40% of lean body weight in men and women, respectively. For example, a 50-kg woman with a plasma Na^+ concentration of 160 mmol/L has an estimated free water deficit of 2.9 L $\{[(160 - 140) \div 140] \times (0.4 \times 50)\}$. As in hyponatremia, rapid correction of hypernatremia is potentially dangerous. In this case, a sudden decrease in osmolality could potentially cause a rapid shift of water into cells that have undergone osmotic adaptation. This would result in swollen brain cells and increase the risk of seizures or permanent neurologic damage. Therefore, the water deficit should be corrected slowly over at least 48 to 72 h. When calculating the rate of water replacement, ongoing losses should be taken into account, and the plasma Na^+ concentration should be lowered by 0.5 mmol/L per hour and by no more than 12 mmol/L over the first 24 h. The safest route of administration of water is by mouth or via a nasogastric tube (or other feeding tube). Alternatively, 5% dextrose in water or half-isotonic saline can be given intravenously. The appropriate treatment of CDI consists of administering desmopressin intranasally (Chap. 329). Other options for decreasing urine output include a low-salt diet in combination with low-dose thiazide diuretic therapy. In some patients with partial CDI, drugs that either stimulate AVP secretion or enhance its action on the kidney have been useful. These include chlorpropamide, clofibrate, carbamazepine, andnonsteroidal anti-inflammatory drugs (NSAIDs). The concentrating defect in NDI may be reversible by treating the underlying disorder or eliminating the offending drug. Symptomatic polyuria due to NDI can be treated with a low-Na^+ diet and thiazide diuretics as described above. This induces mild volume depletion, which leads to enhanced proximal reabsorption of salt and water and decreased delivery to the site of action of AVP, the collecting duct. By impairing renal prostaglandin synthesis, NSAIDs potentiate AVP action and thereby increase urine osmolality and decrease urine volume. Amiloride may be useful in patients with NDI who need to be on lithium. The nephrotoxicity of lithium requires the drug to be taken up into collecting duct cells via the amiloride-sensitive Na^+ channel.

POTASSIUM

POTASSIUM BALANCE Potassium is the major intracellular cation. The normal plasma K^+ concentration is 3.5 to 5.0 mmol/L, whereas that inside cells is about 150 mmol/L. Therefore, the amount of K^+ in the ECF (30 to 70 mmol) constitutes less than 2% of the total body K^+ content (2500 to 4500 mmol). The ratio of ICF to ECF K^+ concentration (normally 38:1) is the principal result of the resting membrane potential and is crucial for normal neuromuscular function. The basolateral Na^+, K^+-ATPase pump actively transports K^+ in and Na^+ out of the cell in a 2:3 ratio, and the passive outward diffusion of K^+ is quantitatively the most important factor that generates the resting membrane potential. The activity of the electrogenic Na^+, K^+-ATPase pump may be stimulated as a result of an increased intracellular Na^+ concentration and inhibited in the setting of digoxin toxicity or chronic illness such as heart failure or renal failure.

The distribution of K^+ is also affected by several other factors, including hormones, acid-base balance, osmolality, and cell turnover. Insulin increases Na^+, K^+-ATPase activity indirectly and independent of its effect on glucose transport, leading to K^+ shift into muscle and liver cells. Conversely, insulin deficiency results in K^+ movement from the ICF to the ECF compartment. Catecholamines have variable effects on K^+ distribution—β_2-adrenergic agonists promote whereas α-adrenergic agonists impair K^+ uptake by cells. The Na^+, K^+-ATPase pump as well as insulin secretion are stimulated by β_2-adrenergic agonists. In contrast, α-adrenergic agonists have the opposite effect. The major action of aldosterone is to increase K^+ excretion (see below). The role of extracellular pH in K^+ balance relates to the underlying acid-base disorder. In metabolic acidosis, 60% of the H^+ load is buffered inside cells. To maintain electroneutrality, the H^+ ion must either be accompanied by an anion or exchanged for intracellular K^+ (leading to hy-

perkalemia). Organic acidoses are not usually associated with a pH-related K^+ shift, since anions such as lactate and β-hydroxybutyrate can be readily taken up by the cell. The converse, movement of K^+ into cells, may be seen with metabolic alkalosis. However, this is less important due to diminished intracellular buffering. Primary respiratory disturbances in acid-base balance result in minimal transcellular K^+ shifts. In hyperosmolal states, K^+ diffuses out of cells along with water due to *solvent drag*. The concentration gradient favoring K^+ movement out of cells is also increased as a result of ICF water loss. Tissue destruction or breakdown results in the release of intracellular K^+, whereas the production of new cells shifts K^+ out of the ECF. Finally, moderate to severe exercise may be associated with K^+ release from muscle, leading to glycogenolysis and local vasodilatation. This is usually transient but may affect the plasma K^+ concentration if patients repeatedly clench and unclench their fist prior to venipuncture.

The K^+ intake of individuals on an average western diet is 40 to 120 mmol/d or approximately 1 mmol/kg per day, 90% of which is absorbed by the gastrointestinal tract. Maintenance of the steady state necessitates matching K^+ ingestion with excretion. Initially, extrarenal adaptive mechanisms, followed later by urinary excretion, prevent a doubling of the plasma K^+ concentration that would occur if the dietary K^+ load remained in the ECF compartment. Immediately following a meal, most of the absorbed K^+ enters cells as a result of the initial elevation in the plasma K^+ concentration and facilitated by insulin release and basal catecholamine levels. Eventually, however, the excess K^+ is excreted in the urine (see below). The regulation of gastrointestinal K^+ handling is not well understood. The amount of K^+ lost in the stool can increase from 10 to 50 or 60% (of dietary intake) in chronic renal insufficiency. In addition, colonic secretion of K^+ is stimulated in patients with large volumes of diarrhea, resulting in potentially severe K^+ depletion.

POTASSIUM EXCRETION (See also Chap. 268) Renal excretion is the major route of elimination of dietary and other sources of excess K^+. The filtered load of K^+ (GFR $\times$ plasma K^+ concentration = 180 L/d $\times$ 4 mmol/L = 720 mmol/d) is 10- to 20-fold greater than the ECF K^+ content. Some 90% of filtered K^+ is reabsorbed by the proximal convoluted tubule and loop of Henle. Proximally, K^+ is reabsorbed passively with Na^+ and water, whereas the luminal Na^+-K^+-$2Cl^-$ cotransporter mediates K^+ uptake in the thick ascending limb of the loop of Henle. Therefore, K^+ delivery to the distal nephron [distal convoluted tubule and cortical collecting duct (CCD)] approximates dietary intake. Net distal K^+ secretion or reabsorption occurs in the setting of K^+ excess or depletion, respectively. The cell responsible for K^+ secretion in the late distal convoluted tubule (or connecting tubule) and CCD is the principal cell. Virtually all regulation of renal K^+ excretion and total body K^+ balance occurs in the distal nephron. The driving force for K^+ secretion is a favorable electrochemical gradient across the luminal membrane of the principal cell. As a result of the action of the basolateral Na^+, K^+-ATPase pump, the intracellular K^+ concentration far exceeds that of the fluid in the lumen of the CCD. The electrical gradient is created by electrogenic Na^+ reabsorption leading to a lumen-negative transepithelial potential difference (TEPD), favoring K^+ secretion. The generation of a lumen-negative TEPD depends on the relative rates of reabsorption of Na^+ and its accompanying anion (primarily Cl^-). Equimolar reabsorption of Na^+ and Cl^- at equivalent rates is electroneutral, whereas reabsorption of Na^+ in excess of Cl^- is electrogenic. The cellular uptake of Na^+ by the principal cell occurs via an apical Na^+ channel and is driven by a low intracellular Na^+ concentration relative to that in the lumen of the CCD. The mechanism and regulation of distal nephron Cl^- transport is less clear. Obviously, factors that impact on either Na^+ or Cl^- reabsorption by the principal cell will influence the TEPD. Potassium secretion is regulated by two physiologic stimuli—aldosterone and hyperkalemia. Aldosterone is secreted by the zona glomerulosa cells of the adrenal cortex in response to high renin and angiotensin II or hyperkalemia. The actions of aldosterone on the principal cell include enhanced apical membrane Na^+ conductivity, stimulation of the basolateral Na^+, K^+-ATPase, and increased luminal K^+ channels. The plasma K^+ concentration, independent of aldosterone, can directly affect K^+ secretion. In addition to the K^+ concentration in the lumen of the CCD, renal K^+ loss depends on the urine flow rate, a function of daily solute excretion (see above). Since excretion is equal to the product of concentration and volume, increased distal flow rate can significantly enhance urinary K^+ output. Finally, in severe K^+ depletion, secretion of K^+ is reduced and reabsorption, via apical H^+, K^+-ATPase pumps in cortical and medullary collecting ducts, is upregulated.

HYPOKALEMIA

ETIOLOGY (See Table 49-3) Hypokalemia, defined as a plasma K^+ concentration < 3.5 mmol/L, may result from one (or more) of the following: decreased net intake, shift into cells, or increased net loss. Diminished intake is seldom the sole cause of K^+ depletion since urinary excretion can be effectively decreased to less than 15 mmol/d as a result of net K^+ reabsorption in the distal nephron. With the exception of the urban poor and certain cultural groups, the amount of K^+ in the diet almost always exceeds that excreted in the urine. However, dietary K^+ restriction may exacerbate the hypokalemia secondary to increased gastrointestinal or renal loss. An unusual cause of decreased K^+ intake is ingestion of clay (geophagia), which binds dietary K^+ and iron. This custom was previously common among African Americans in the American South.

Redistribution into Cells Movement of K^+ into cells may transiently decrease the plasma K^+ concentration without altering total body K^+ content. For any given cause, the magnitude of the change is relatively small, often less than 1 mmol/L. However, a combination of factors may lead to a significant fall in the plasma K^+ concentration and may amplify the hypokalemia due to K^+ wasting. Alkalosis, especially that due to a primary increase in plasma HCO_3^- (metabolic alkalosis), is often associated with hypokalemia. This occurs as a result

Table 49-3 Causes of Hypokalemia

I. Decreased intake
  A. Starvation
  B. Clay ingestion
II. Redistribution into cells
  A. Acid-base
    1. Metabolic alkalosis
  B. Hormonal
    1. Insulin
    2. β_2-Adrenergic agonists (endogenous or exogenous)
    3. α-Adrenergic antagonists
  C. Anabolic state
    1. Vitamin B_{12} or folic acid (red blood cell production)
    2. Granulocyte-macrophage colony stimulating factor (white blood cell production)
    3. Total parenteral nutrition
  D. Other
    1. Pseudohypokalemia
    2. Hypothermia
    3. Hypokalemic periodic paralysis
    4. Barium toxicity
III. Increased loss
  A. Nonrenal
    1. Gastrointestinal loss (diarrhea)
    2. Integumentary loss (sweat)
  B. Renal
    1. Increased distal flow: diuretics, osmotic diuresis, salt-wasting nephropathies
    2. Increased secretion of potassium
      a. Mineralocorticoid excess: primary hyperaldosteronism, secondary hyperaldosteronism (malignant hypertension, renin-secreting tumors, renal artery stenosis, hypovolemia), apparent mineralocorticoid excess (licorice, chewing tobacco, carbenoxolone), congenital adrenal hyperplasia, Cushing's syndrome, Bartter's syndrome
      b. Distal delivery of non-reabsorbed anions: vomiting, nasogastric suction, proximal (type 2) renal tubular acidosis, diabetic ketoacidosis, glue-sniffing (toluene abuse), penicillin derivatives
      c. Other: amphotericin B, Liddle's syndrome, hypomagnesemia

of K^+ redistribution as well as excessive renal K^+ loss. Treatment of diabetic ketoacidosis with insulin may lead to hypokalemia due to stimulation of the Na^+-H^+ antiporter and (secondarily) the Na^+, K^+-ATPase pump. Furthermore, uncontrolled hyperglycemia often leads to K^+ depletion from an osmotic diuresis (see below). Stress-induced catecholamine release and administration of β_2-adrenergic agonists directly induce cellular uptake of K^+ and promote insulin secretion by pancreatic islet β cells. *Hypokalemic periodic paralysis* is a rare condition characterized by recurrent episodic weakness or paralysis (Chap. 381). Since K^+ is the major ICF cation, anabolic states can potentially result in hypokalemia due to a K^+ shift into cells. This may occur following rapid cell growth seen in patients with pernicious anemia treated with vitamin B_{12} or with neutropenia after treatment with granulocyte-macrophage colony stimulating factor. Massive transfusion with thawed washed red blood cells (RBCs) could cause hypokalemia since frozen RBCs lose up to half of their K^+ during storage.

Nonrenal Loss of Potassium Excessive sweating may result in K^+ depletion from increased integumentary and renal K^+ loss. Hyperaldosteronism, secondary to ECF volume contraction, enhances K^+ excretion in the urine (Chap. 331). Normally, K^+ lost in the stool amounts to 5 to 10 mmol/d in a volume of 100 to 200 mL. Hypokalemia subsequent to increased gastrointestinal loss can occur in patients with profuse diarrhea (usually secretory), villous adenomas, VIPomas, or laxative abuse. However, the loss of gastric secretions does not account for the moderate to severe K^+ depletion often associated with vomiting or nasogastric suction. Since the K^+ concentration of gastric fluid is 5 to 10 mmol/L, it would take 30 to 80 L of vomitus to achieve a K^+ deficit of 300 to 400 mmol typically seen in these patients. In fact, the hypokalemia is primarily due to increased renal K^+ excretion. Loss of gastric contents results in volume depletion and metabolic alkalosis, both of which promote kaliuresis. Hypovolemia stimulates aldosterone release, which augments K^+ secretion by the principal cells. In addition, the filtered load of HCO_3^- exceeds the reabsorptive capacity of the proximal convoluted tubule, thereby increasing distal delivery of $NaHCO_3$, which enhances the electrochemical gradient favoring K^+ loss in the urine.

Renal Loss of Potassium In general, most cases of chronic hypokalemia are due to renal K^+ wasting. This may be due to factors that increase the K^+ concentration in the lumen of the CCD or augment distal flow rate. As described above, distal nephron K^+ secretion is driven by a lumen-negative TEPD, affected by aldosterone and the relative rates of reabsorption of Na^+ and its accompanying anion(s). Mineralocorticoid excess commonly results in hypokalemia (Chap. 331). *Primary hyperaldosteronism* is due to dysregulated aldosterone secretion by an adrenal adenoma (Conn's syndrome) or carcinoma or to adrenocortical hyperplasia. In a rare subset of patients, the disorder is familial (autosomal dominant) and aldosterone levels can be suppressed by administering low doses of exogenous glucocorticoid. The molecular defect responsible for *glucocorticoid-remediable hyperaldosteronism* is a rearranged gene (due to a chromosomal crossover), containing the 5′-regulatory region of the 11β-hydroxylase gene and the coding sequence of the aldosterone synthase gene. Consequently, mineralocorticoid is synthesized in the zona fasciculata and regulated by corticotropin. A number of conditions associated with hyperreninemia result in secondary hyperaldosteronism and renal K^+ wasting. High renin levels are commonly seen in both renovascular and malignant hypertension. Renin-secreting tumors of the juxtaglomerular apparatus are a rare cause of hypokalemia. Other tumors that have been reported to produce renin include renal cell carcinoma, ovarian carcinoma, and Wilms' tumor. Hyperreninemia may also occur secondary to decreased effective circulating arterial volume.

In the absence of elevated renin or aldosterone levels, enhanced distal nephron secretion of K^+ may result from increased production of non-aldosterone mineralocorticoids in *congenital adrenal hyperplasia* (Chap. 331). Glucocorticoid-stimulated kaliuresis does not normally occur due to the conversion of cortisol to cortisone by 11β-

hydroxysteroid dehydrogenase (11β-HSDH). Therefore, 11β-HSDH deficiency or suppression allows cortisol to bind to the aldosterone receptor and leads to the *syndrome of apparent mineralocorticoid excess*. Drugs that inhibit the activity of 11β-HSDH include glycyrrhetinic acid, present in licorice, chewing tobacco, and carbenoxolone. The presentation of Cushing's syndrome may include hypokalemia if the capacity of 11β-HSDH to inactivate cortisol is overwhelmed by persistently elevated glucocorticoid levels.

Liddle's syndrome is a rare familial (autosomal dominant) disease characterized by hypertension, hypokalemic metabolic alkalosis, renal K^+ wasting, and suppressed renin and aldosterone secretion (Chap. 331). Increased distal delivery of Na^+ with a non-reabsorbable anion (not Cl^-) enhances the lumen-negative TEPD and K^+ secretion. Classically, this is seen with *proximal (type 2) renal tubular acidosis* (RTA) and vomiting, associated with bicarbonaturia. Diabetic keto-acidosis and toluene abuse (glue-sniffing) can lead to increased delivery of β-hydroxybutyrate and hippurate, respectively, to the CCD and to renal K^+ loss. High doses of penicillin derivatives administered to volume-depleted patients may likewise promote renal K^+ secretion as well as an osmotic diuresis. *Classic distal (type 1) RTA* is associated with hypokalemia due to increased renal K^+ loss, the mechanism of which is uncertain. Amphotericin B causes hypokalemia due to increased distal nephron permeability to Na^+ and K^+ and to renal K^+ wasting.

Bartter's syndrome is a disorder characterized by hypokalemia, metabolic alkalosis, hyperreninemic hyperaldosteronism secondary to ECF volume contraction, and juxtaglomerular apparatus hyperplasia (Chap. 331). Finally, diuretic use and abuse are common causes of K^+ depletion. Carbonic anhydrase inhibitors, loop diuretics, and thiazides are all kaliuretic. The degree of hypokalemia tends to be greater with long-acting agents and is dose-dependent. Increased renal K^+ excretion is due primarily to increased distal solute delivery and secondary hyperaldosteronism (due to volume depletion).

CLINICAL FEATURES   The clinical manifestations of K^+ depletion vary greatly between individual patients, and their severity depends on the degree of hypokalemia. Symptoms seldom occur unless the plasma K^+ concentration is less than 3 mmol/L. Fatigue, myalgia, and muscular weakness of the lower extremities are common complaints and are due to a lower (more negative) resting membrane potential. More severe hypokalemia may lead to progressive weakness, hypoventilation (due to respiratory muscle involvement), and eventually complete paralysis. Impaired muscle metabolism and the blunted hyperemic response to exercise associated with profound K^+ depletion increase the risk of rhabdomyolysis. Smooth-muscle function may also be affected and manifest as paralytic ileus.

The electrocardiographic changes of hypokalemia (Fig. 226-19) are due to delayed ventricular repolarization and do not correlate well with the plasma K^+ concentration. Early changes include flattening or inversion of the T wave, a prominent U wave, ST-segment depression, and a prolonged QU interval. Severe K^+ depletion may result in a prolonged PR interval, decreased voltage and widening of the QRS complex, and an increased risk of ventricular arrhythmias, especially in patients with myocardial ischemia or left ventricular hypertrophy. Hypokalemia may also predispose to digitalis toxicity. Epidemiologic studies have linked a low-K^+ diet with an increased prevalence of hypertension, particularly among African Americans. Furthermore, in patients with essential hypertension, systemic blood pressure may be lowered by K^+ supplementation. The mechanism of the hypertensive effect of K^+ depletion is not certain but may relate to enhanced distal NaCl reabsorption.

Hypokalemia is often associated with acid-base disturbances related to the underlying disorder. In addition, K^+ depletion results in intracellular acidification and an increase in net acid excretion or new HCO_3^- production. This is a consequence of enhanced proximal HCO_3^- reabsorption, increased renal ammoniagenesis, and increased distal H^+ secretion. This contributes to the generation of metabolic

alkalosis frequently present in hypokalemic patients. NDI (see above) is not uncommonly seen in K^+ depletion and is manifest as polydipsia and polyuria. Glucose intolerance may also occur with hypokalemia and has been attributed to either impaired insulin secretion or peripheral insulin resistance.

DIAGNOSIS   In most cases, the etiology of K^+ depletion can be determined by a careful history. Diuretic and laxative abuse as well as surreptitious vomiting may be difficult to identify but should be excluded. Rarely, patients with a marked leukocytosis (e.g., acute myeloid leukemia) and normokalemia may have a low measured plasma K^+ concentration due to white blood cell uptake of K^+ at room temperature. This *pseudohypokalemia* can be avoided by storing the blood sample on ice or rapidly separating the plasma (or serum) from the cells. After eliminating decreased intake and intracellular shift as potential causes of hypokalemia, examination of the renal response can help to clarify the source of K^+ loss. The appropriate response to K^+ depletion is to excrete less than 15 mmol/d of K^+ in the urine, due to increased reabsorption and decreased distal secretion. Hypokalemia with minimal renal K^+ excretion suggests that K^+ was lost via the skin or gastrointestinal tract or that there is a remote history of vomiting or diuretic use. As described above, renal K^+ wasting may be due to factors that either increase the K^+ concentration in the CCD or increase the distal flow rate (or both). The ECF volume status, blood pressure, and associated acid-base disorder may help to differentiate the causes of excessive renal K^+ loss. A rapid and simple test designed to evaluate the driving force for net K^+ secretion is the *transtubular K^+ concentration gradient* (TTKG). The TTKG is the ratio of the K^+ concentration in the lumen of the CCD ($[K^+]_{CCD}$) to that in peritubular capillaries or plasma ($[K^+]_P$). The validity of this measurement depends on three assumptions: (1) few solutes are reabsorbed in the medullary collecting duct (MCD), (2) K^+ is neither secreted nor reabsorbed in the MCD, and (3) the osmolality of the fluid in the terminal CCD is known. Significant reabsorption or secretion of K^+ in the MCD seldom occurs, except in profound K^+ depletion or excess, respectively. When AVP is acting ($OSM_U \geq OSM_P$), the osmolality in the terminal CCD is the same as that of plasma, and the K^+ concentration in the lumen of the distal nephron can be estimated by dividing the urine K^+ concentration ($[K^+]_U$) by the ratio of the urine to plasma osmolality (OSM_U/OSM_P):

$$[K^+]_{CCD} = [K^+]_U \div (OSM_U/OSM_P)$$

$$\text{TTKG} = \frac{[K^+]_{CCD}}{[K^+]_P} = \frac{[K^+]_U \div (OSM_U/OSM_P)}{[K^+]_P}$$

Hypokalemia with a TTKG greater than 4 suggests renal K^+ loss due to increased distal K^+ secretion. Plasma renin and aldosterone levels are often helpful in differentiating the various causes of hyperaldosteronism. Bicarbonaturia and the presence of other non-reabsorbed anions also increase the TTKG and lead to renal K^+-wasting.

CLINICAL APPROACH   See Fig. 49-3.

TREATMENT   The therapeutic goals are to correct the K^+ deficit and to minimize ongoing losses. With the exception of periodic paralysis, hypokalemia resulting from transcellular shifts rarely requires intravenous K^+ supplementation, which can lead to rebound hyperkalemia. It is generally safer to correct hypokalemia via the oral route. The degree of K^+ depletion does not correlate well with the plasma K^+ concentration. A decrement of 1 mmol/L in the plasma K^+ concentration (from 4.0 to 3.0 mmol/L) may represent a total body K^+ deficit of 200 to 400 mmol, and patients with plasma levels under 3.0 mmol/L often require in excess of 600 mmol of K^+ to correct the deficit. Furthermore, factors promoting K^+ shift out of cells (e.g., insulin deficiency in diabetic ketoacidosis) may result in underestimation of the K^+ deficit. Therefore, the plasma K^+ concentration should be monitored frequently when assessing the response to treatment. Potassium chloride is usually the preparation of choice and will promote more rapid correction of hypokalemia and metabolic alkalosis. Potas-

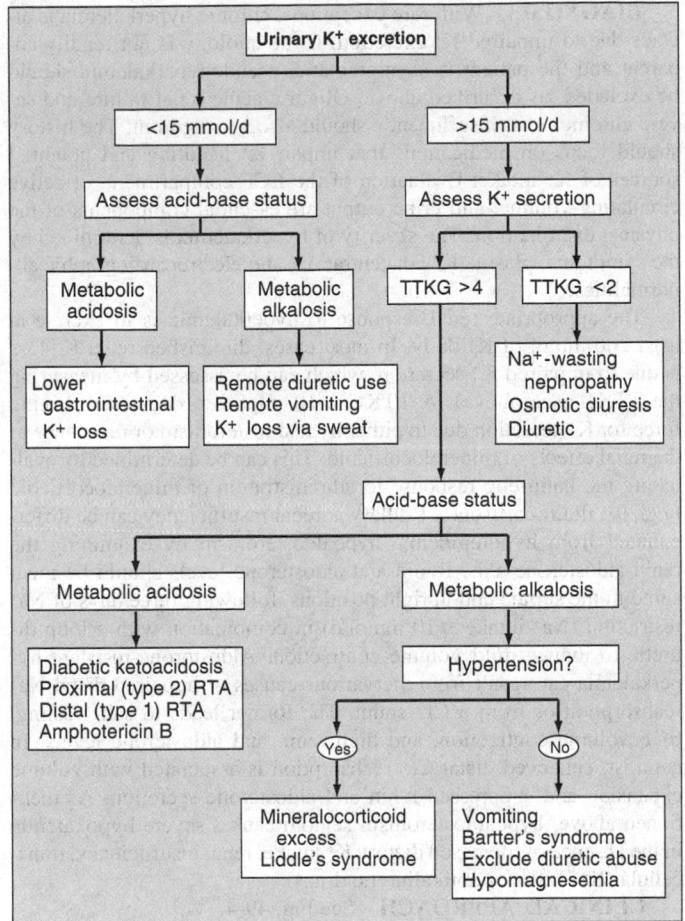

FIGURE 49-3 Algorithm depicting clinical approach to hypokalemia. TTKG, transtubular K$^+$ concentration gradient; RTA, renal tubular acidosis.

sium bicarbonate and citrate (metabolized to HCO_3^-) tend to alkalinize the patient and would be more appropriate for hypokalemia associated with chronic diarrhea or RTA.

Patients with severe hypokalemia or those unable to take anything by mouth require intravenous replacement therapy with KCl. The maximum concentration of administered K$^+$ should be no more than 40 mmol/L via a peripheral vein or 60 mmol/L via a central vein. The rate of infusion should not exceed 20 mmol/h unless paralysis or malignant ventricular arrhythmias are present. Ideally, KCl should be mixed in normal saline since dextrose solutions may initially exacerbate hypokalemia due to insulin-mediated movement of K$^+$ into cells. Rapid intravenous administration of K$^+$ should be used judiciously and requires close observation of the clinical manifestations of hypokalemia (electrocardiogram and neuromuscular examination).

HYPERKALEMIA

ETIOLOGY   Hyperkalemia, defined as a plasma K$^+$ concentration >5.0 mmol/L, occurs as a result of either K$^+$ release from cells or decreased renal loss. Increased K$^+$ intake is rarely the sole cause of hyperkalemia since the phenomenon of *potassium adaptation* ensures rapid K$^+$ excretion in response to increases in dietary consumption. Iatrogenic hyperkalemia may result from overzealous parenteral K$^+$ replacement or in patients with renal insufficiency. *Pseudohyperkalemia* represents an artificially elevated plasma K$^+$ concentration due to K$^+$ movement out of cells immediately prior to or following venipuncture. Contributing factors include prolonged use of a tourniquet with or without repeated fist clenching, hemolysis, and marked leukocytosis or thrombocytosis. The latter two result in an elevated serum K$^+$ concentration due to release of intracellular K$^+$ following clot formation. Pseudohyperkalemia should be suspected in an otherwise

asymptomatic patient with no obvious underlying cause. If proper venipuncture technique is used and a plasma (not serum) K$^+$ concentration is measured, it should be normal. Intravascular hemolysis, tumor lysis syndrome, and rhabdomyolysis all lead to K$^+$ release from cells as a result of tissue breakdown. Metabolic acidoses, with the exception of those due to the accumulation of organic anions, can be associated with mild hyperkalemia resulting from intracellular buffering of H$^+$ (see above). As previously described (p. 278), insulin deficiency and hypertonicity (e.g., hyperglycemia) promote K$^+$ shift from the ICF to the ECF. The severity of exercise-induced hyperkalemia is related to the degree of exertion. It is due to release of K$^+$ from muscles and is usually rapidly reversible, often associated with rebound hypokalemia. Treatment with beta blockers rarely causes hyperkalemia but may contribute to the elevation in plasma K$^+$ concentration seen with other conditions. *Hyperkalemic periodic paralysis* (Chap. 381) is a rare autosomal dominant disorder characterized by episodic weakness or paralysis, precipitated by stimuli that normally lead to mild hyperkalemia (e.g., exercise). The genetic defect appears to be a single amino acid substitution due to a mutation in the gene for the skeletal muscle Na$^+$ channel. Hyperkalemia may occur with severe digitalis toxicity due to inhibition of the Na$^+$, K$^+$-ATPase pump. Depolarizing muscle relaxants such as succinylcholine can increase the plasma K$^+$ concentration, especially in patients with massive trauma, burns, or neuromuscular disease.

Chronic hyperkalemia is virtually always associated with decreased renal K$^+$ excretion due to either impaired secretion or diminished distal solute delivery (Table 49-4). The latter is seldom the only cause of impaired K$^+$ excretion but may significantly contribute to hyperkalemia in protein-malnourished (low urea excretion) and ECF volume–contracted (decreased distal NaCl delivery) patients. Decreased K$^+$ secretion by the principal cells results from either impaired Na$^+$ reabsorption or increased Cl$^-$ reabsorption, both of which give rise to a diminished (less lumen-negative) TEPD in the CCD. *Hyporeninemic hypoaldosteronism* is a syndrome characterized by euvolemia or ECF volume expansion and suppressed renin and aldosterone levels (Chaps. 331 and 333). This disorder is commonly seen in mild renal insufficiency, diabetic nephropathy, or chronic tubulointerstitial disease. Patients frequently have an impaired kaliuretic response to exogenous mineralocorticoid administration, suggesting that enhanced distal Cl$^-$ reabsorption (electroneutral Na$^+$ reabsorption) may account for many of the findings of hyporeninemic hypoaldosteronism. NSAIDs inhibit renin secretion and the synthesis of vasodilatory renal prostaglandins. The resultant decrease in GFR and K$^+$ secretion is often manifest as hyperkalemia. As a rule, the degree of hyperkalemia due to hypoaldosteronism is mild in the absence of increased K$^+$ intake or renal dysfunction. Angiotensin-converting enzyme (ACE) inhibitors block the conversion of angiotensin I to angiotensin II, resulting in

Table 49-4   Causes of Hyperkalemia

I. Renal failure
II. Decreased distal flow (i.e., decreased effective circulating arterial volume)
III. Decreased K$^+$ secretion
  A. Impaired Na$^+$ reabsorption
    1. Primary hypoaldosteronism: adrenal insufficiency, adrenal enzyme deficiency (21-hydroxylase, 3β-hydroxysteroid dehydrogenase, corticosterone methyl oxidase)
    2. Secondary hypoaldosteronism: hyporeninemia, drugs (ACE inhibitors, NSAIDs, heparin)
    3. Resistance to aldosterone: pseudohypoaldosteronism, tubulointerstitial disease, drugs (K$^+$-sparing diuretics, trimethoprim, pentamidine)
  B. Enhanced Cl$^-$ reabsorption (chloride shunt)
    1. Gordon's syndrome
    2. Cyclosporine

NOTE: ACE, angiotensin-converting enzyme; NSAIDs, nonsteroidal anti-inflammatory drugs.

impaired aldosterone release. Patients at increased risk of ACE inhibitor–induced hyperkalemia include those with diabetes mellitus, renal insufficiency, decreased effective circulating arterial volume, bilateral renal artery stenosis, or concurrent use of K⁺-sparing diuretics or NSAIDs.

Decreased aldosterone synthesis may be due to *primary adrenal insufficiency* (Addison's disease) or congenital adrenal enzyme deficiency (Chap. 331). Heparin (including low-molecular-weight heparin) inhibits production of aldosterone by the cells of the zona glomerulosa and can lead to severe hyperkalemia in a subset of patients with underlying renal disease; diabetes mellitus; or those receiving K⁺-sparing diuretics, ACE inhibitors, or NSAIDs. *Pseudohypoaldosteronism* is a rare familial disorder characterized by hyperkalemia, metabolic acidosis, renal Na⁺ wasting, hypotension, high renin and aldosterone levels, and end-organ resistance to aldosterone. The gene encoding the mineralocorticoid receptor is normal in these patients, and the electrolyte abnormalities can be reversed with suprapharmacologic doses of an exogenous mineralocorticoid (e.g., 9α-fludrocortisone) or an inhibitor of 11β-HSDH (e.g., carbenoxolone). The kaliuretic response to aldosterone is impaired by K⁺-sparing diuretics. Spironolactone is a competitive mineralocorticoid antagonist, whereas amiloride and triamterene block the apical Na⁺ channel of the principal cell. Two other drugs that impair K⁺ secretion by blocking distal nephron Na⁺ reabsorption are trimethoprim and pentamidine. These antimicrobial agents may contribute to the hyperkalemia often seen in patients infected with HIV who are being treated for *Pneumocystis carinii* pneumonia.

Hyperkalemia frequently complicates acute oliguric renal failure due to increased K⁺ release from cells (acidosis, catabolism) and decreased excretion. Increased distal flow rate and K⁺ secretion per nephron compensate for decreased renal mass in chronic renal insufficiency. However, these adaptive mechanisms eventually fail to maintain K⁺ balance when the GFR falls below 10 to 15 mL/min or oliguria ensues. Otherwise asymptomatic urinary tract obstruction is an often overlooked cause of hyperkalemia. Other nephropathies associated with impaired K⁺ excretion include drug-induced interstitial nephritis, lupus nephritis, sickle cell disease, and diabetic nephropathy.

Gordon's syndrome is a rare condition characterized by hyperkalemia, metabolic acidosis, and a normal GFR. These patients are usually volume-expanded with suppressed renin and aldosterone levels as well as refractory to the kaliuretic effect of exogenous mineralocorticoids. It has been suggested that these findings could all be accounted for by increased distal Cl⁻ reabsorption (electroneutral Na⁺ reabsorption), also referred to as a *Cl⁻ shunt*. A similar mechanism may be partially responsible for the hyperkalemia associated with cyclosporine nephrotoxicity. *Hyperkalemic distal (type 4) RTA* may be due to either hypoaldosteronism or a Cl⁻ shunt (aldosterone-resistant).

CLINICAL FEATURES Since the resting membrane potential is related to the ratio of the ICF to ECF K⁺ concentration, hyperkalemia partially depolarizes the cell membrane. Prolonged depolarization impairs membrane excitability and is manifest as weakness, which may progress to flaccid paralysis and hypoventilation if the respiratory muscles are involved. Hyperkalemia also inhibits renal ammoniagenesis and reabsorption of NH_4^+ in the thick ascending limb of the loop of Henle. Thus, net acid excretion is impaired and results in metabolic acidosis, which may further exacerbate the hyperkalemia due to K⁺ movement out of cells.

The most serious effect of hyperkalemia is cardiac toxicity, which does not correlate well with the plasma K⁺ concentration. The earliest electrocardiographic changes include increased T-wave amplitude, or peaked T waves. More severe degrees of hyperkalemia result in a prolonged PR interval and QRS duration, atrioventricular conduction delay, and loss of P waves. Progressive widening of the QRS complex and merging with the T wave produces a sinewave pattern. The terminal event is usually ventricular fibrillation or asystole.

DIAGNOSIS With rare exceptions, chronic hyperkalemia is always due to impaired K⁺ excretion. If the etiology is not readily apparent and the patient is asymptomatic, pseudohyperkalemia should be excluded, as described above. Oliguric acute renal failure and severe chronic renal insufficiency should also be ruled out. The history should focus on medications that impair K⁺ handling and potential sources of K⁺ intake. Evaluation of the ECF compartment, effective circulating volume, and urine output are essential components of the physical examination. The severity of hyperkalemia is determined by the symptoms, plasma K⁺ concentration, and electrocardiographic abnormalities.

The appropriate renal response to hyperkalemia is to excrete at least 200 mmol of K⁺ daily. In most cases, diminished renal K⁺ loss is due to impaired K⁺ secretion, which can be assessed by measuring the TTKG (see above). A TTKG <10 implies a decreased driving force for K⁺ secretion due to either hypoaldosteronism or resistance to the renal effects of mineralocorticoid. This can be determined by evaluating the kaliuretic response to administration of mineralocorticoid (e.g., 9α-fludrocortisone). Primary adrenal insufficiency can be differentiated from hyporeninemic hypoaldosteronism by examining the renin-aldosterone axis. Renin and aldosterone levels should be measured in the supine and upright positions, following three days of Na⁺ restriction (Na⁺ intake <10 mmol/d) in combination with a loop diuretic to induce mild volume contraction. Aldosterone-resistant hyperkalemia can result from the various causes of impaired distal Na⁺ reabsorption or from a Cl⁻ shunt. The former leads to salt wasting, ECF volume contraction, and high renin and aldosterone levels. In contrast, enhanced distal Cl⁻ reabsorption is associated with volume expansion and suppressed renin and aldosterone secretion. As mentioned above, hypoaldosteronism seldom causes severe hypokalemia in the absence of increased dietary K⁺ intake, renal insufficiency, transcellular K⁺ shifts, or antikaliuretic drugs.

CLINICAL APPROACH See Fig. 49-4.

℞ TREATMENT The approach to therapy depends on the degree of hyperkalemia as determined by the plasma K⁺ concentration, associated muscular weakness, and changes on the electrocardiogram. Potentially fatal hyperkalemia rarely occurs unless the plasma K⁺ concentration exceeds 7.5 mmol/L and is usually associated with profound weakness and absent P waves, QRS widening, or ventricular arrhythmias on the electrocardiogram.

Severe hyperkalemia requires emergent treatment directed at minimizing membrane depolarization, shifting K⁺ into cells, and promoting K⁺ loss. In addition, exogenous K⁺ intake and antikaliuretic drugs should be discontinued. Administration of calcium gluconate decreases membrane excitability. The usual dose is 10 mL of a 10% solution infused over 2 to 3 min. The effect begins within minutes but is short-lived (30 to 60 min), and the dose can be repeated if no change in the electrocardiogram is seen after 5 to 10 min. Insulin causes K⁺ to shift into cells by mechanisms described previously and will temporarily lower the plasma K⁺ concentration. Although glucose alone will stimulate insulin release from normal pancreatic β cells, a more rapid response generally occurs when exogenous insulin is administered (with glucose to prevent hypoglycemia). A commonly recommended combination is 10 to 20 units of regular insulin and 25 to 50 g of glucose. Obviously, hyperglycemic patients should not be given glucose. If effective, the plasma K⁺ concentration will fall by 0.5 to 1.5 mmol/L in 15 to 30 min and the effect will last for several hours. Alkali therapy with intravenous $NaHCO_3$ can also shift K⁺ into cells. This is safest when administered as an isotonic solution of 3 ampules per liter (134 mmol/L $NaHCO_3$) and ideally should be reserved for severe hyperkalemia associated with metabolic acidosis. Patients with end-stage renal disease seldom respond to this intervention and may not tolerate the Na⁺ load and resultant volume expansion. When administered parenterally or in nebulized form, $β_2$-adrenergic agonists promote cellular uptake of K⁺ (see above). The onset of action is 30 min, lowering the plasma K⁺ concentration by 0.5 to 1.5 mmol/L, and the effect lasts 2 to 4 h.

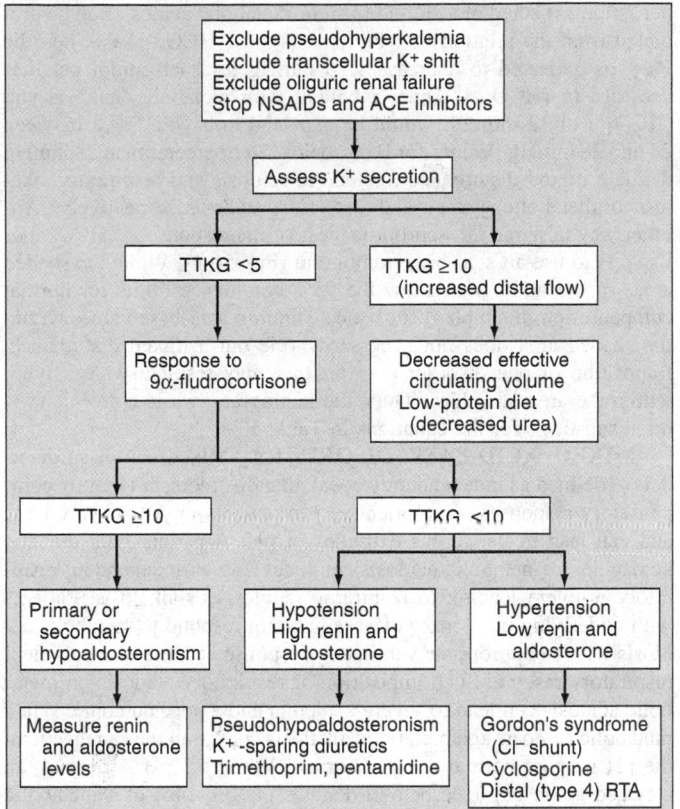

FIGURE 49-4 Algorithm depicting clinical approach to hyperkalemia. NSAID, nonsteroidal anti-inflammatory drug; ACE, angiotensin-converting enzyme; RTA, renal tubular acidosis; TTKG, transtubular K⁺ concentration gradient.

Removal of K⁺ can be achieved using diuretics, cation-exchange resin, or dialysis. Loop and thiazide diuretics, often in combination, may enhance K⁺ excretion if renal function is adequate. Sodium polystyrene sulfonate is a cation-exchange resin that promotes the exchange of Na⁺ for K⁺ in the gastrointestinal tract. Each gram binds 1 mmol of K⁺ and releases 2 to 3 mmol of Na⁺. When given by mouth, the usual dose is 25 to 50 g mixed with 100 mL of 20% sorbitol to prevent constipation. This will generally lower the plasma K⁺ concentration by 0.5 to 1.0 mmol/L within 1 to 2 h and last for 4 to 6 h. Sodium polystyrene sulfonate can also be administered as a retention enema consisting of 50 g of resin and 50 mL of 70% sorbitol mixed in 150 mL of tap water. The sorbitol should be omitted from the enema in postoperative patients due to the increased incidence of sorbitol-induced colonic necrosis, especially following renal transplantation. The most rapid and effective way of lowering the plasma K⁺ concentration is hemodialysis. This should be reserved for patients with renal failure and those with severe life-threatening hyperkalemia unresponsive to more conservative measures. Peritoneal dialysis also removes K⁺ but is only 15 to 20% as effective as hemodialysis. Finally, the underlying cause of the hyperkalemia should be treated. This may involve dietary modification, correction of metabolic acidosis, cautious volume expansion, and administration of exogenous mineralocorticoid.

BIBLIOGRAPHY

SODIUM AND WATER

ABRAHAM WT, SCHRIER RW: Body fluid volume regulation in health and disease. Adv Intern Med 39:23, 1994

BERL T, ROBERTSON GL: Pathophysiology of water metabolism, in *Brenner & Rector's The Kidney*, 6th ed, BM Brenner (ed). Philadelphia, Saunders, 2000, pp 866–924

FUJIWARA TM et al: Molecular biology of diabetes insipidus. Ann Rev Med 46:331, 1995

GINES P et al: Vasopressin in pathophysiological states. Semin Nephrol 14:384, 1994

GOLDSZMIDT MA, ILIESCU EA: DDAVP to prevent rapid correction in hyponatremia. Clin Nephrol 53:226, 2000

GULLANS SR, VERBALIS JG: Control of brain volume during hyperosmolar and hypoosmolar conditions. Ann Rev Med 44:289, 1993

KNEPPER MA et al: Role of aquaporins in water balance. Curr Opin Nephrol Hypertens 6:367, 1997

KUMAR S, BERL T: Sodium. Lancet 352:220, 1998

MCKENNA K, THOMPSON C: Osmoregulation in clinical disorders of thirst appreciation. Clin Endocrinol 49:139, 1998

STERNS RH et al: Neurologic sequelae after treatment of severe hyponatremia: A multicenter perspective. J Am Soc Nephrol 4:1522, 1994

VERBALIS JG: Adaptation to acute and chronic hyponatremia: Implications for symptomatology, diagnosis, and therapy. Semin Nephrol 18:3, 1998

POTASSIUM

DEFRONZO RA, SMITH JD: Clinical disorders of hyperkalemia, in *Clinical Disorders of Fluid and Electrolyte Metabolism*, 5th ed, RG Narins (ed). New York, McGraw-Hill, 1994, pp 697–754

FIELD MJ et al: Regulation of renal potassium metabolism, in *Clinical Disorders of Fluid and Electrolyte Metabolism*, 5th ed, RG Narins (ed). New York, McGraw-Hill, 1994, pp 147–174

HALPERIN ML, KAMEL KS: Potassium. Lancet 352:135, 1998

KUPIN WL, NARINS RG: The hyperkalemia of renal failure: Pathophysiology, diagnosis, and therapy. Contrib Nephrol 102:1, 1993

SCHEINMAN SJ et al: Genetic disorders of renal electrolyte transport. N Engl J Med 340:1177, 1999

WHITE PC: Disorders of aldosterone biosynthesis and action. N Engl J Med 331:250, 1994

WINGO CS, WEINER ID: Disorders of potassium balance, in *Brenner & Rector's The Kidney*, 6th ed, BM Brenner (ed). Philadelphia, Saunders, 2000, pp 998–1035

50 *Thomas D. DuBose, Jr.*

ACIDOSIS AND ALKALOSIS

NORMAL ACID-BASE HOMEOSTASIS

Systemic arterial pH is maintained between 7.35 and 7.45 by extracellular and intracellular chemical buffering together with respiratory and renal regulatory mechanisms. The control of arterial CO_2 tension (Pa_{CO_2}) by the central nervous system and respiratory systems and the control of the plasma bicarbonate by the kidneys stabilize the arterial pH by excretion or retention of acid or alkali. The metabolic and respiratory components that regulate systemic pH are described by the Henderson-Hasselbalch equation:

$$pH = 6.1 + \log \frac{HCO_3^-}{Pa_{CO_2} \times 0.0301}$$

Under most circumstances, CO_2 production and excretion are matched, and the usual steady-state Pa_{CO_2} is maintained at 40 mmHg. Underexcretion of CO_2 produces hypercapnia, and overexcretion causes hypocapnia. Nevertheless, production and excretion are again matched at a new steady-state Pa_{CO_2}. Therefore, the Pa_{CO_2} is regulated primarily by neural respiratory factors (Chap. 263) and is not subject to regulation by the rate of CO_2 production. Hypercapnia is usually the result of hypoventilation rather than of increased CO_2 production. Increases or decreases in Pa_{CO_2} represent derangements of neural respiratory control or are due to compensatory changes in response to a primary alteration in the plasma [HCO_3^-].

Primary changes in Pa_{CO_2} can cause acidosis or alkalosis, depending on whether Pa_{CO_2} is above or below the normal value of 40 mmHg (respiratory acidosis or alkalosis, respectively). Primary alteration of Pa_{CO_2} evokes cellular buffering and renal adaptation, a slow process that becomes more efficient with time. A primary change in the plasma [HCO_3^-] as a result of metabolic or renal factors results in compensatory changes in ventilation that blunt the changes in blood pH that would occur otherwise. Such respiratory alterations are referred to as *secondary*, or compensatory, changes, since they occur in response to primary metabolic changes.

The kidneys regulate plasma [HCO_3^-] through three main processes: (1) "reabsorption" of filtered HCO_3^-, (2) formation of titratable acid, and (3) excretion of NH_4^+ in the urine. The kidney filters approximately 4000 mmol of HCO_3^- per day. To reabsorb the filtered load of HCO_3^-, the renal tubules must therefore secrete 4000 mmol of hydrogen ions. Between 80 and 90% of HCO_3^- is reabsorbed in the proximal tubule. The distal nephron reabsorbs the remainder and secretes protons, as generated from metabolism, to defend systemic pH. While this quantity of protons, 40 to 60 mmol/d, is small, it must be secreted to prevent chronic positive H^+ balance and metabolic acidosis. This quantity of secreted protons is represented in the urine as titratable acid and NH_4^+. Metabolic acidosis in the face of normal renal function increases NH_4^+ production and excretion. NH_4^+ production and excretion are impaired in chronic renal failure, hyperkalemia, and renal tubular acidosis.

In sum, these regulatory responses, including chemical buffering, the regulation of Pa_{CO_2} by the respiratory system, and of [HCO_3^-] by the kidneys, act in concert to maintain a systemic arterial pH between 7.35 and 7.45.

DIAGNOSIS OF GENERAL TYPES OF DISTURBANCES

The most common clinical disturbances are simple acid-base disorders, i.e., metabolic acidosis or alkalosis or respiratory acidosis or alkalosis. Since compensation is not complete, the pH is abnormal in simple disturbances. More complicated clinical situations can give rise to mixed acid-base disturbances.

SIMPLE ACID-BASE DISORDERS Primary respiratory disturbances (primary changes in Pa_{CO_2}) invoke compensatory metabolic responses (secondary changes in [HCO_3^-]), and primary metabolic disturbances elicit predictable compensatory respiratory responses. Physiologic compensation can be predicted from the relationships displayed in Table 50-1. Primary changes in Pa_{CO_2} or [HCO_3^-] alter systemic pH and cause acidosis or alkalosis. To illustrate, metabolic acidosis due to an increase in endogenous acids (e.g., ketoacidosis) lowers extracellular fluid [HCO_3^-] and decreases extracellular pH. This stimulates the medullary chemoreceptors to increase ventilation and to return the ratio of [HCO_3^-] to Pa_{CO_2}, and thus pH, toward normal, although not to normal. The degree of respiratory compensation expected in a simple form of metabolic acidosis can be predicted from the relationship: $Pa_{CO_2} = (1.5 \times [HCO_3^-]) + 8$, i.e., the Pa_{CO_2} is expected to decrease 1.25 mmHg for each mmol per liter decrease in [HCO_3^-]. Thus, a patient with metabolic acidosis and [HCO_3^-] of 12 mmol/L would be expected to have a Pa_{CO_2} between 24 and 28 mmHg. Values for Pa_{CO_2} below 24 or greater than 28 mmHg define a mixed disturbance (metabolic acidosis and respiratory alkalosis or metabolic acidosis and respiratory acidosis, respectively). Another way to judge the appropriateness of the response in [HCO_3^-] or Pa_{CO_2} is to use an acid-base nomogram (Fig. 50-1). While the shaded areas of the nomogram show the 95% confidence limits for normal compensation in simple disturbances, finding acid-base values within the shaded area does not necessarily rule out a mixed disturbance. Imposition of one disorder over another may result in values lying within the area of a third. Thus, the nomogram, while convenient, is not a substitute for the equations in Table 50-1.

MIXED ACID-BASE DISORDERS Mixed acid-base disorders—defined as independently coexisting disorders, not merely compensatory responses—are often seen in patients in critical care units and can lead to dangerous extremes of pH. A patient with diabetic ketoacidosis (metabolic acidosis) may develop an independent respiratory problem leading to respiratory acidosis or alkalosis. Patients with underlying pulmonary disease may not respond to metabolic acidosis with an appropriate ventilatory response because of insufficient respiratory reserve. Such imposition of respiratory acidosis on metabolic acidosis can lead to severe acidemia and a poor outcome. When metabolic acidosis and metabolic alkalosis coexist in the same patient, the pH may be normal or near normal. When the pH is normal, an elevated anion gap (see below) denotes the presence of a metabolic acidosis. A diabetic patient with ketoacidosis may have renal dysfunction resulting in simultaneous metabolic acidosis. Patients who have ingested an overdose of drug combinations such as sedatives and salicylates may have mixed disturbances as a result of the acid-base response to the individual drugs (metabolic acidosis mixed with respiratory acidosis or respiratory alkalosis, respectively). Even more complex are triple acid-base disturbances. For example, patients with metabolic acidosis due to alcoholic ketoacidosis may develop metabolic alkalosis due to vomiting and superimposed respiratory alkalosis due to the hyperventilation of hepatic dysfunction or alcohol withdrawal.

DIAGNOSIS OF ACID-BASE DISORDERS Care should be taken when measuring blood gases to obtain the arterial blood sample without using excessive heparin. In the determination of arterial blood gases by the clinical laboratory, both pH and Pa_{CO_2} are measured, and the [HCO_3^-] is calculated from the Henderson-Hasselbalch equation. This calculated value should be compared with the measured [HCO_3^-] (total CO_2) on the electrolyte panel. These two values should agree within 2 mmol/L. If they do not, the values may not have been drawn simultaneously, a laboratory error may be present, or an error could have been made in calculating the [HCO_3^-]. After verifying the blood acid-base values, one can then identify the precise acid-base disorder.

The most common causes of acid-base disorders should be kept in mind while probing the history for clues about the etiology. For example, established chronic renal failure is expected to cause a metabolic acidosis, and chronic vomiting frequently causes metabolic alkalosis. Patients with pneumonia, sepsis, or cardiac failure frequently have respiratory alkalosis, and patients with chronic obstructive pulmonary disease or a sedative drug overdose often display a respiratory acidosis. The drug history is important since loop or thiazide diuretics may cause metabolic alkalosis, and the carbonic anhydrase inhibitor, acetazolamide, can result in metabolic acidosis.

Blood for electrolytes and arterial blood gases should be drawn simultaneously prior to therapy, since an increase in [HCO_3^-] occurs with metabolic alkalosis and respiratory acidosis. Conversely, a decrease in [HCO_3^-] occurs in metabolic acidosis and respiratory alkalosis.

Table 50-1 Prediction of Compensatory Responses on Simple Acid-Base Disturbances

Disorder	Prediction of Compensation
Metabolic acidosis	$Pa_{CO_2} = (1.5 \times HCO_3^-) + 8$
	or
	Pa_{CO_2} will ↓ 1.25 mmHg per mmol/L ↓ in [HCO_3^-]
	or
	$Pa_{CO_2} = [HCO_3^-] + 15$
Metabolic alkalosis	Pa_{CO_2} will ↑ 0.75 mmHg per mmol/L ↑ in [HCO_3^-]
	or
	Pa_{CO_2} will ↑ 6 mmHg per 10-mmol/L ↑ in [HCO_3^-]
	or
	$Pa_{CO_2} = [HCO_3^-] + 15$
Respiratory alkalosis	
Acute	[HCO_3^-] will ↓ 2 mmol/L per 10-mmHg ↓ in Pa_{CO_2}
Chronic	[HCO_3^-] will ↓ 4 mmol/L per 10-mmHg ↓ in Pa_{CO_2}
Respiratory acidosis	
Acute	[HCO_3^-] will ↑ 1 mmol/L per 10-mmHg ↑ in Pa_{CO_2}
Chronic	[HCO_3^-] will ↓ 4 mmol/L per 10-mmHg ↑ in Pa_{CO_2}

Metabolic acidosis leads to hyperkalemia as a result of cellular shifts in which H^+ is exchanged for K^+ or Na^+. For each decrease in blood pH of 0.10, the plasma $[K^+]$ should rise by 0.6 mmol/L. This relationship is not invariable. Diabetic ketoacidosis, lactic acidosis, diarrhea, and renal tubular acidosis (RTA) are often associated with potassium depletion because of urinary K^+ wasting.

Anion Gap All evaluations of acid-base disorders should include a simple calculation of the anion gap (AG); it represents those unmeasured anions in plasma (normally 10 to 12 mmol/L) and is calculated as follows: $AG = Na^+ - (Cl^- + HCO_3^-)$. The unmeasured anions include anionic proteins, phosphate, sulfate, and organic anions. When acid anions, such as acetoacetate and lactate, accumulate in extracellular fluid, the AG increases, causing a high-AG acidosis. An increase in the AG is most often due to an increase in unmeasured anions and less commonly is due to a decrease in unmeasured cations (calcium, magnesium, potassium). In addition, the AG may increase with an increase in anionic albumin, either because of increased albumin concentration or alkalosis, which alters albumin charge. A decrease in the AG can be due to: (1) an increase in unmeasured cations; (2) the addition to the blood of abnormal cations, such as lithium (lithium intoxication) or cationic immunoglobulins (plasma cell dyscrasias); (3) a reduction in the major plasma anion albumin concentration (nephrotic syndrome); (4) a decrease in the effective anionic charge on albumin by acidosis; or (5) hyperviscosity and severe hyperlipidemia, which can lead to an underestimation of sodium and chloride concentrations.

In the face of a normal serum albumin, a high AG is usually due to non-chloride-containing acids that contain inorganic (phosphate, sulfate), organic (ketoacids, lactate, uremic organic anions), exogenous (salicylate or ingested toxins with organic acid production), or unidentified anions. By definition, therefore, a high-AG acidosis has two identifying features: a low $[HCO_3^-]$ and an elevated AG. The latter is present even if an additional acid-base disorder is superimposed to modify the $[HCO_3^-]$ independently. Simultaneous metabolic acidosis of the high-AG variety plus either chronic respiratory acidosis or metabolic alkalosis represents such a situation in which $[HCO_3^-]$ may be normal or even high. However, the AG is elevated, and $[Cl^-]$ is depressed.

Similarly, normal values for $[HCO_3^-]$, Pa_{CO_2}, and pH do not ensure the absence of an acid-base disturbance. For instance, an alcoholic who has been vomiting may develop a metabolic alkalosis with a pH of 7.55, Pa_{CO_2} of 48 mmHg, $[HCO_3^-]$ of 40 mmol/L, $[Na^+]$ of 135, $[Cl^-]$ of 80, and $[K^+]$ of 2.8. If such a patient were then to develop a superimposed alcoholic ketoacidosis with a β-hydroxybutyrate concentration of 15 mM, arterial pH would fall to 7.40, $[HCO_3^-]$ to 25 mmol/L, and the Pa_{CO_2} to 40 mmHg. Although these blood gases are normal, the AG is elevated at 30 mmol/L, indicating a mixed metabolic alkalosis and metabolic acidosis.

METABOLIC ACIDOSIS

Metabolic acidosis can occur because of an increase in endogenous acid production (such as lactate and ketoacids), loss of bicarbonate (as in diarrhea), or accumulation of endogenous acids (as in renal failure). Metabolic acidosis has profound effects on the respiratory, cardiac, and nervous systems. The fall in blood pH is accompanied by a char-

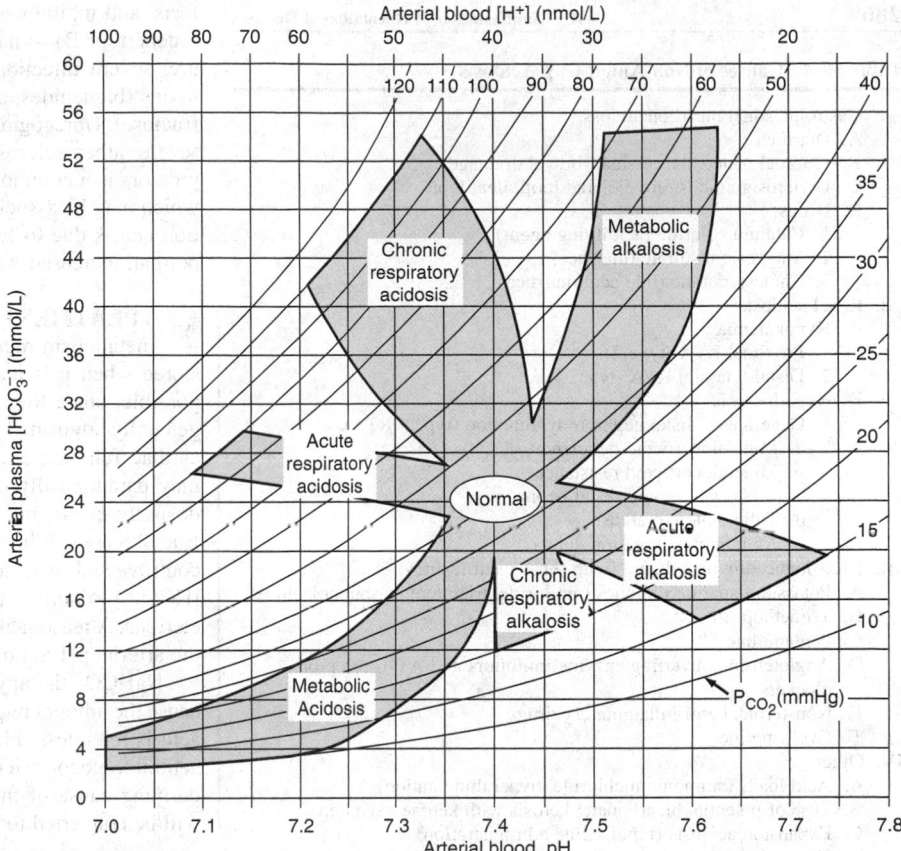

FIGURE 50-1 Acid-base nomogram. Shown are the 90% confidence limits of the normal respiratory and metabolic compensations for primary acid-base disturbances. (*From DuBose*, used with permission.)

acteristic increase in ventilation, especially the tidal volume (Kussmaul respiration). Intrinsic cardiac contractility may be depressed, but inotropic function can be normal because of catecholamine release. Both peripheral arterial vasodilation and central venoconstriction can be present; the decrease in central and pulmonary vascular compliance predisposes to pulmonary edema with even minimal volume overload. Central nervous system function is depressed, with headache, lethargy, stupor, and, in some cases, even coma. Glucose intolerance may also occur.

There are two major categories of clinical metabolic acidosis: high-AG and normal-AG, or hyperchloremic acidosis (Table 50-2 and Table 50-3).

TREATMENT Treatment of metabolic acidosis with alkali should be reserved for severe acidemia except when the patient has no "potential HCO_3^-" in plasma. Potential $[HCO_3^-]$ can be estimated from the increment (Δ) in the anion gap ($\Delta AG =$ patient's $AG - 10$). It must be determined if the acid anion in plasma is metabolizable (i.e., β-hydroxybutyrate, acetoacetate, and lactate) or nonmetabolizable (anions that accumulate in chronic renal failure and after toxin ingestion). The latter requires return of renal function to replenish the $[HCO_3^-]$ deficit, a slow and often unpredictable process. Consequently, patients with a normal AG acidosis (hyperchloremic acidosis), a slightly elevated AG (mixed hyperchloremic and AG acidosis), or an AG attributable to a nonmetabolizable anion in the

Table 50-2 Causes of High-Anion-Gap Metabolic Acidosis

Lactic acidosis	Toxins
Ketoacidosis	Ethylene glycol
Diabetic	Methanol
Alcoholic	Salicylates
Starvation	Renal failure (acute and chronic)

Table 50-3 Causes of Non-Anion-Gap Acidosis

I. Gastrointestinal bicarbonate loss
  A. Diarrhea
  B. External pancreatic or small-bowel drainage
  C. Ureterosigmoidostomy, jejunal loop, ileal loop
  D. Drugs
    1. Calcium chloride (acidifying agent)
    2. Magnesium sulfate (diarrhea)
    3. Cholestyramine (bile acid diarrhea)
II. Renal acidosis
  A. Hypokalemia
    1. Proximal RTA (type 2)
    2. Distal (classic) RTA (type 1)
  B. Hyperkalemia
    1. Generalized distal nephron dysfunction (type 4 RTA)
      a. Mineralocorticoid deficiency
      b. Mineralocorticoid resistance
      c. ↓ Na$^+$ delivery to distal nephron
      d. Tubulointerstitial disease
      e. Ammonium excretion defect
III. Drug-induced hyperkalemia (with renal insufficiency)
  A. Potassium-sparing diuretics (amiloride, triamterene, spironolactone)
  B. Trimethoprim
  C. Pentamidine
  D. Angiotensin-converting enzyme inhibitors and AT-II receptor blockers
  E. Nonsteroidal anti-inflammatory drugs
  F. Cyclosporine
IV. Other
  A. Acid loads (ammonium chloride, hyperalimentation)
  B. Loss of potential bicarbonate: ketosis with ketone excretion
  C. Expansion acidosis (rapid saline administration)
  D. Hippurate
  E. Cation exchange resins

NOTE: RTA, renal tubular acidosis; AT-II, angiotensin-II receptor blockers.

face of renal failure should receive alkali therapy, either orally (NaHCO$_3$ or Shohl's solution) or intravenously (NaHCO$_3$), in an amount necessary to slowly increase the plasma [HCO$_3^-$] into the 20 to 22 mmol/L range.

Controversy exists, however, in regard to the use of alkali in patients with a pure AG acidosis owing to accumulation of a metabolizable organic acid anion (ketoacidosis or lactic acidosis). In general, severe acidosis (pH < 7.20) warrants the intravenous administration of 50 to 100 meq of NaHCO$_3$, over 30 to 45 min, during the initial 1 to 2 h of therapy. Provision of such modest quantities of alkali in this situation seems to provide an added measure of safety, but it is essential to monitor plasma electrolytes during the course of therapy, since the [K$^+$] may decline as pH rises. The goal is to increase the [HCO$_3^-$] to 10 meq/L and the pH to 7.25, not to increase these values to normal.

HIGH-ANION-GAP ACIDOSES There are four principal causes of a high-AG acidosis: (1) lactic acidosis, (2) ketoacidosis, (3) ingested toxins (Table 50-2), and (4) acute and chronic renal failure. Initial screening to differentiate the high-AG acidoses should include: (1) a probe of the history for evidence of drug and toxin ingestion and measurement of arterial blood gas to detect coexistent respiratory alkalosis (salicylates); (2) determination of whether diabetes mellitus is present (diabetic ketoacidosis); (3) a search for evidence of alcoholism or increased levels of β-hydroxybutyrate (alcoholic ketoacidosis); (4) observation for clinical signs of uremia and determination of the blood urea nitrogen (BUN) and creatinine (uremic acidosis); (5) inspection of the urine for oxalate crystals (ethylene glycol); and (6) recognition of the numerous clinical settings in which lactate levels may be increased (hypotension, shock, cardiac failure, leukemia, cancer, and drug or toxin ingestion).

Lactic Acidosis An increase in plasma L-lactate may be secondary to poor tissue perfusion (type A)—circulatory insufficiency (shock, circulatory failure), severe anemia, mitochondrial enzyme de-

fects, and inhibitors (carbon monoxide, cyanide)—or to aerobic disorders (type B)—malignancies, diabetes mellitus, renal or hepatic failure, severe infections (cholera, malaria), seizures, AIDS, or drugs/toxins (biguanides, ethanol, methanol, isoniazid, AZT analogues, and fructose). Unrecognized bowel ischemia or infarction in a patient with severe atherosclerosis or cardiac decompensation receiving vasopressors is a common cause of lactic acidosis. D-Lactic acid acidosis, which may be associated with jejunoileal bypass or intestinal obstruction and is due to formation of D-lactate by gut bacteria, may cause both an increased AG and hyperchloremia.

TREATMENT The underlying condition that disrupts lactate metabolism must first be corrected; tissue perfusion must be restored when it is inadequate. Vasoconstrictors should be avoided, if possible, since they may worsen tissue perfusion. Alkali therapy is generally advocated for acute, severe acidemia (pH < 7.1) to improve cardiac function and lactate utilization. However, NaHCO$_3$ therapy may paradoxically depress cardiac performance and exacerbate acidosis by enhancing lactate production (HCO$_3^-$ stimulates phosphofructokinase). While the use of alkali in moderate lactic acidosis is controversial, it is generally agreed that attempts to return the pH or [HCO$_3^-$] to normal by administration of exogenous NaHCO$_3$ are deleterious. A reasonable approach is to infuse sufficient NaHCO$_3$ to raise the arterial pH to no more than 7.2 over 30 to 40 min.

NaHCO$_3$ therapy can cause fluid overload and hypertension because the amount required can be massive when accumulation of lactic acid is relentless. Fluid administration is poorly tolerated because of central venoconstriction, especially in the oliguric patient. If the underlying cause of the lactic acidosis can be remedied, blood lactate will be converted to HCO$_3^-$ and may result in an overshoot alkalosis.

Ketoacidosis • *Diabetic ketoacidosis* This condition is caused by increased fatty acid metabolism and the accumulation of ketoacids (acetoacetate and β-hydroxybutyrate). Diabetic ketoacidosis usually occurs in insulin-dependent diabetes mellitus in association with cessation of insulin or an intercurrent illness, such as an infection, gastroenteritis, pancreatitis, or myocardial infarction, which increases insulin requirements temporarily and acutely. The accumulation of ketoacids accounts for the increment in the AG and is accompanied most often by hyperglycemia [glucose > 17 mmol/L (300 mg/dL)]. It should be noted that since insulin prevents production of ketones, bicarbonate therapy is rarely needed except with extreme acidemia (pH < 7.1), and then in only limited amounts (see "Treatment" for lactic acidosis). →*The management of this condition is described in Chap. 333.*

Alcoholic ketoacidosis Chronic alcoholics can develop ketoacidosis when alcohol consumption is abruptly curtailed; it is usually associated with binge drinking, vomiting, abdominal pain, starvation, and volume depletion. The glucose concentration is low or normal, and acidosis may be severe because of elevated ketones, predominantly β-hydroxybutyrate. Mild lactic acidosis may coexist because of alteration in the redox state. The nitroprusside ketone reaction (Acetest) can detect acetoacetic acid but not β-hydroxybutyrate, so that the degree of ketosis and ketonuria can be underestimated. Typically, insulin levels are low, and concentrations of triglyceride, cortisol, glucagon, and growth hormone are increased.

TREATMENT Extracellular fluid deficits should be repleted by intravenous administration of saline and glucose (5% dextrose in 0.9% NaCl). Hypophosphatemia, hypokalemia, and hypomagnesemia may coexist and should be corrected. Hypophosphatemia usually emerges 12 to 24 h after admission, may be exacerbated by glucose infusion, and, if severe, may induce rhabdomyolysis. Upper gastrointestinal hemorrhage, pancreatitis, and pneumonia may accompany this disorder.

Drug- and Toxin-Induced Acidosis • *Salicylates* (See also Chap. 396) Salicylate intoxication in adults usually causes respiratory alkalosis, mixed metabolic acidosis–respiratory alkalosis, or a pure high-AG metabolic acidosis. In the latter example, which is less common, only a portion of the AG is due to the salicylates. Lactic acid production is also often increased.

℞ **TREATMENT** This should begin with vigorous gastric lavage with isotonic saline (not NaHCO₃) followed by administration of activated charcoal. In the acidotic patient, to facilitate removal of salicylate, intravenous NaHCO₃ is administered in amounts adequate to alkalinize the urine and to maintain urine output (urine pH > 7.5). While this form of therapy is straightforward in acidotic patients, a coexisting respiratory alkalosis may make this approach hazardous. Acetazolamide may be administered when an alkaline diuresis cannot be achieved, but this drug can cause systemic metabolic acidosis if HCO₃⁻ is not replaced. Hypokalemia may occur with an alkaline diuresis from NaHCO₃ and should be treated promptly and aggressively. Glucose-containing fluids should be administered because of the danger of hypoglycemia. Excessive insensible fluid losses may cause severe volume depletion and hypernatremia. If renal failure prevents rapid clearance of salicylate, hemodialysis can be performed against a bicarbonate dialysate.

Alcohols Under most physiologic conditions, sodium, urea, and glucose generate the osmotic pressure of blood. Plasma osmolality is calculated according to the following expression: $P_{osm} = 2Na^+ + Glu + BUN$ (all in mmol/L), or, using conventional laboratory values in which glucose and BUN are expressed in milligrams per deciliter: $P_{osm} = 2Na^+ + Glu/18 + BUN/2.8$. The calculated and determined osmolality should agree within 10 to 15 mmol/kg H₂O. When the measured osmolality exceeds the calculated osmolality by more than 15 to 20 mmol/kg H₂O, one of two circumstances prevails. Either the serum sodium is spuriously low, as with hyperlipidemia or hyperproteinemia (pseudohyponatremia), or osmolytes other than sodium salts, glucose, or urea have accumulated in plasma. Examples include mannitol, radiocontrast media, isopropyl alcohol, ethylene glycol, ethanol, methanol, and acetone. In this situation, the difference between the calculated osmolality and the measured osmolality (*osmolar gap*) is proportional to the concentration of the unmeasured solute. With an appropriate clinical history and index of suspicion, identification of an osmolar gap is helpful in identifying the presence of poison-associated AG acidosis.

Ethylene glycol (See also Chap. 396) Ingestion of ethylene glycol (commonly used in antifreeze) leads to a metabolic acidosis and severe damage to the central nervous system, heart, lungs, and kidneys. The increased AG and osmolar gap are attributable to ethylene glycol and its metabolites, oxalic acid, glycolic acid, and other organic acids. Lactic acid production increases secondary to inhibition of the tricarboxylic acid cycle and altered intracellular redox state. Diagnosis is facilitated by recognizing oxalate crystals in the urine, the presence of an osmolar gap in serum, and a high-AG acidosis. Treatment should not be delayed while awaiting measurement of ethylene glycol levels in this setting.

℞ **TREATMENT** This includes the prompt institution of a saline or osmotic diuresis, thiamine and pyridoxine supplements, fomepizole or ethanol, and hemodialysis. The intravenous administration of the new alcohol dehydrogenase inhibitor, fomepizole (4-methylpyrazole; 7 mg/kg as a loading dose), or ethanol intravenously to achieve a level of 22 mmol/L (100 mg/dL) serves to lessen toxicity because they compete with ethylene glycol for metabolism by alcohol dehydrogenase. Fomepizole, although expensive, offers the advantages of a predictable decline in ethylene glycol levels without the adverse effects, such as excessive obtundation, associated with ethyl alcohol infusion.

Methanol (See also Chap. 396) The ingestion of methanol (wood alcohol) causes metabolic acidosis, and its metabolites formaldehyde and formic acid cause severe optic nerve and cental nervous system

damage. Lactic acid, ketoacids, and other unidentified organic acids may contribute to the acidosis. Due to its low molecular weight (32 Da), an osmolar gap is usually present.

℞ **TREATMENT** This is similar to that for ethylene glycol intoxication, including general supportive measures, fomepizole or ethanol administration, and hemodialysis.

Renal Failure (See also Chaps. 269 and 270) The hyperchloremic acidosis of moderate renal insufficiency is eventually converted to the high-AG acidosis of advanced renal failure. Poor filtration and reabsorption of organic anions contribute to the pathogenesis. As renal disease progresses, the number of functioning nephrons eventually becomes insufficient to keep pace with net acid production. Uremic acidosis is characterized, therefore, by a reduced rate of NH₄⁺ production and excretion, primarily due to decreased renal mass. [HCO₃⁻] rarely falls below 15 mmol/L, and the AG rarely exceeds 20 mmol/L. The acid retained in chronic renal disease is buffered by alkaline salts from bone. Despite significant retention of acid (up to 20 mmol/d), the serum [HCO₃⁻] does not decrease further, indicating participation of buffers outside the extracellular compartment. Chronic metabolic acidosis results in significant loss of bone mass due to reduction in bone calcium carbonate. Chronic acidosis also increases urinary calcium excretion, proportional to cumulative acid retention.

℞ **TREATMENT** Both uremic acidosis and the hyperchloremic acidosis of renal failure require oral alkali replacement to maintain the [HCO₃⁻] between 20 and 24 mmol/L. This can be accomplished with relatively modest amounts of alkali (1.0 to 1.5 mmol/kg body weight per day). It is assumed that alkali replacement prevents the harmful effects of H⁺ balance on bone and prevents or retards muscle catabolism. Sodium citrate (Shohl's solution) or NaHCO₃ tablets are equally effective alkalinizing salts. Citrate enhances the absorption of aluminum from the gastrointestinal tract and should never be given together with aluminum-containing antacids because of the risk of aluminum intoxication. When hyperkalemia is present, furosemide (60 to 80 mg/d) should be added.

HYPERCHLOREMIC METABOLIC ACIDOSES Alkali can be lost from the gastrointestinal tract in diarrhea or from the kidneys (renal tubular acidosis, RTA). In these disorders (Table 50-3), reciprocal changes in [Cl⁻] and [HCO₃⁻] result in a normal AG. In pure hyperchloremic acidosis, therefore, the increase in [Cl⁻] above the normal value approximates the decrease in [HCO₃⁻]. The absence of such a relationship suggests a mixed disturbance.

In diarrhea, stools contain a higher [HCO₃⁻] and decomposed HCO₃⁻ than plasma so that metabolic acidosis develops along with volume depletion. Instead of an acid urine pH (as anticipated with systemic acidosis), urine pH is usually around 6 because metabolic acidosis and hypokalemia increase renal synthesis and excretion of NH₄⁺, thus providing a urinary buffer that increases urine pH. Metabolic acidosis due to gastrointestinal losses with a high urine pH can be differentiated from RTA (Chap. 276) because urinary NH₄⁺ excretion is typically low in RTA and high with diarrhea. Urinary NH₄⁺ levels can be estimated by calculating the urine anion gap (UAG): $UAG = [Na^+ + K^+]_u - [Cl^-]_u$. When $[Cl^-]_u > [Na^+ + K^+]$, the urine ammonium level is appropriately increased, suggesting an extrarenal cause of the acidosis.

Loss of functioning renal parenchyma by progressive renal disease leads to hyperchloremic acidosis when the glomerular filtration rate (GFR) is between 20 and 50 mL/min and to uremic acidosis with a high AG when the GFR falls to <20 mL/min. Such a progression occurs commonly with tubulointerstitial forms of renal disease, but hyperchloremic metabolic acidosis can persist with advanced glomerular disease. In advanced renal failure, ammoniagenesis is reduced in proportion to the loss of functional renal mass, and ammonium accumulation and trapping in the outer medullary collecting tubule may also be impaired. Because of adaptive increases in K^+ secretion by the collecting duct and colon, the acidosis of chronic renal insufficiency is typically normokalemic.

Proximal RTA (type 2 RTA) is most often due to generalized proximal tubular dysfunction manifested by glycosuria, generalized aminoaciduria, and phosphaturia (Fanconi syndrome). With a low plasma [HCO_3^-], the urine pH is acid (pH < 5.5). The fractional excretion of [HCO_3^-] may exceed 10 to 15% when the serum $HCO_3^- >$ 20 mmol/L. Since HCO_3^- is not reabsorbed normally in the proximal tubule, therapy with $NaHCO_3$ will enhance renal potassium wasting and hypokalemia.

The typical findings in classic distal RTA (type 1 RTA) (Chap. 276) include hypokalemia, hyperchloremic acidosis, low urinary NH_4^+ excretion (positive UAG, low urine [NH_4^+]), and inappropriately high urine pH (pH > 5.5). Such patients are unable to acidify the urine below a pH of 5.5. Most patients have hypocitraturia and hypercalciuria, so that nephrolithiasis, nephrocalcinosis, and bone disease are common. In type 4 RTA, hyperkalemia is disproportionate to the reduction in GFR because of coexisting dysfunction of potassium and acid secretion. Urinary ammonium excretion is invariably depressed, and renal function may be compromised, for example, due to diabetic nephropathy, amyloidosis, or tubulointerstital disease. →*See Chap. 276 for the pathophysiology, diagnosis, and treatment of RTA.*

Hyporeninemic Hypoaldosteronism (See also Chap. 331) This condition typically causes hyperchloremic metabolic acidosis, most commonly in older adults with diabetes mellitus or tubulointerstitial disease and renal insufficiency. Patients usually have mild to moderate renal insufficiency and acidosis, with elevation in serum [K^+] (5.2 to 6.0 mmol/L), concurrent hypertension, and congestive heart failure. Both the metabolic acidosis and the hyperkalemia are out of proportion to impairment in GFR. Nonsteroidal anti-inflammatory drugs—trimethoprim, pentamidine, and ACE-inhibitors—can also cause hyperkalemia with hyperchloremic metabolic acidosis in patients with renal insufficiency (Table 50-3).

METABOLIC ALKALOSIS

Metabolic alkalosis is manifested by an elevated arterial pH, an increase in the serum [HCO_3^-], and an increase in Pa_{CO_2} as a result of compensatory alveolar hypoventilation. It is often accompanied by hypochloremia and hypokalemia. The patient with a high [HCO_3^-] and a low [Cl^-] has either metabolic alkalosis or chronic respiratory acidosis. As shown in Table 50-1, the Pa_{CO_2} increases 6 mmHg for each 10-mmol/L increase in the [HCO_3^-] above normal. Stated differently, in the range of [HCO_3^-] from 10 to 40 mmol/L, the predicted Pa_{CO_2} is approximately equal to the [HCO_3^-] + 15. The arterial pH establishes the diagnosis, since it is increased in metabolic alkalosis and decreased or normal in respiratory acidosis. Metabolic alkalosis frequently occurs in association with other disorders such as respiratory acidosis or alkalosis or metabolic acidosis.

PATHOGENESIS Metabolic alkalosis occurs as a result of net gain of [HCO_3^-] or loss of nonvolatile acid (usually HCl by vomiting) from the extracellular fluid. Since it is unusual for alkali to be added to the body, the disorder involves a generative stage, in which the loss of acid usually causes alkalosis, and a maintenance stage, in which the kidneys fail to compensate by excreting HCO_3^- because of volume contraction, a low GFR, or depletion of Cl^- or K^+.

Under normal circumstances, the kidneys have an impressive capacity to excrete HCO_3^-. Continuation of metabolic alkalosis represents a failure of the kidneys to eliminate HCO_3^- in the usual manner. For HCO_3^- to be added to the extracellular fluid, it must be administered exogenously or synthesized endogenously, in part or entirely by the kidneys. The kidneys will retain, rather than excrete, the excess alkali and maintain the alkalosis if (1) volume deficiency, chloride deficiency, and K^+ deficiency exist in combination with a reduced

GFR, which augments distal tubule H^+ secretion; or (2) hypokalemia exists because of autonomous hyperaldosteronism. In the first example, alkalosis is corrected by administration of NaCl and KCl, while in the latter it is necessary to repair the alkalosis by pharmacologic or surgical intervention, not with saline administration.

DIFFERENTIAL DIAGNOSIS To establish the cause of metabolic alkalosis (Table 50-4), it is necessary to assess the status of the extracellular fluid volume (ECFV), the recumbent and upright blood pressure, the serum [K^+], and the renin-aldosterone system. For example, the presence of chronic hypertension and chronic hypokalemia in an alkalotic patient suggests either mineralocorticoid excess or that the hypertensive patient is receiving diuretics. Low plasma renin activity and normal urine [Na^+] and [Cl^-] in a patient who is not taking diuretics indicate a primary mineralocorticoid excess syndrome. The combination of hypokalemia and alkalosis in a normotensive, nonedematous patient can be due to Bartter's or Gitelman's syndrome, magnesium deficiency, vomiting, exogenous alkali, or diuretic ingestion. Determination of urine electrolytes (especially the urine [Cl^-]) and screening of the urine for diuretics may be helpful. If the urine is alkaline, with an elevated [Na^+] and [K^+] but low [Cl^-], the diagnosis is usually either vomiting (overt or surreptitious) or alkali ingestion.

Table 50-4   Causes of Metabolic Alkalosis

I. Exogenous HCO_3^- loads
  A. Acute alkali administration
  B. Milk-alkali syndrome
II. Effective ECFV contraction, normotension, K^+ deficiency, and secondary hyperreninemic hyperaldosteronism
  A. Gastrointestinal origin
    1. Vomiting
    2. Gastric aspiration
    3. Congenital chloridorrhea
    4. Villous adenoma
    5. Combined administration of sodium polystyrene sulfonate (Kayexalate) and aluminum hydroxide
  B. Renal origin
    1. Diuretics
    2. Edematous states
    3. Posthypercapnic state
    4. Hypercalcemia/hypoparathyroidism
    5. Recovery from lactic acidosis or ketoacidosis
    6. Nonreabsorbable anions including penicillin, carbenicillin
    7. Mg^{2+} deficiency
    8. K^+ depletion
    9. Bartter's syndrome (loss of function mutations in TALH)
    10. Gitelman's syndrome (loss of function mutation in Na^+-Cl^- cotransporter in DCT)
III. ECFV expansion, hypertension, K^+ deficiency, and mineralocorticoid excess
  A. High renin
    1. Renal artery stenosis
    2. Accelerated hypertension
    3. Renin-secreting tumor
    4. Estrogen therapy
  B. Low renin
    1. Primary aldosteronism
      a. Adenoma
      b. Hyperplasia
      c. Carcinoma
    2. Adrenal enzyme defects
      a. 11β-Hydroxylase deficiency
      b. 17α-Hydroxylase deficiency
    3. Cushing's syndrome or disease
    4. Other
      a. Licorice
      b. Carbenoxolone
      c. Chewer's tobacco
      d. Lydia Pincham tablets
IV. Gain of function mutation of renal sodium channel with ECFV expansion, hypertension, K^+ deficiency, and hyporeninemic-hypoaldosteronism
  A. Liddle's syndrome

NOTE: ECFV, extracellular fluid volume; TALH, thick ascending limb of Henle's loop; DCT, distal convoluted tubule.

If the urine is relatively acid and has low concentrations of Na^+, K^+, and Cl^-, the most likely possibilities are prior vomiting, the posthypercapnic state, or prior diuretic ingestion. If, on the other hand, neither the urine sodium, potassium, nor chloride concentrations are depressed, magnesium deficiency, Bartter's or Gitelman's syndrome, or current diuretic ingestion should be considered. Bartter's syndrome is distinguished from Gitelman's syndrome because of hypocalciuria and hypomagnesemia in the latter disorder. The genetic and molecular basis of these two disorders has been elucidated recently (Chap. 276).

Alkali Administration Chronic administration of alkali to individuals with normal renal function rarely, if ever causes alkalosis. However, in patients with coexistent hemodynamic disturbances, alkalosis can develop because the normal capacity to excrete HCO_3^- may be exceeded or there may be enhanced reabsorption of HCO_3^-. Such patients include those who receive oral or intravenous HCO_3^-, acetate loads (parenteral hyperalimentation solutions), citrate loads (transfusions), or antacids plus cation-exchange resins (aluminum hydroxide and sodium polystyrene sulfonate).

METABOLIC ALKALOSIS ASSOCIATED WITH ECFV CONTRACTION, K^+ DEPLETION, AND SECONDARY HYPERRENINEMIC HYPERALDOSTERONISM **Gastrointestinal Origin** Gastrointestinal loss of H^+ from vomiting or gastric aspiration results in retention of HCO_3^-. The loss of fluid and NaCl in vomitus or nasogastric suction results in contraction of the ECFV and an increase in the secretion of renin and aldosterone. Volume contraction causes a reduction in GFR and an enhanced capacity of the renal tubule to reabsorb HCO_3^-. During active vomiting, there is continued addition of HCO_3^- to plasma in exchange for Cl^-, and the plasma [HCO_3^-] exceeds the reabsorptive capacity of the proximal tubule. The excess $NaHCO_3$ reaches the distal tubule, where secretion is enhanced by an aldosterone and the delivery of the poorly reabsorbed anion, HCO_3^-. Because of contraction of the ECFV and hypochloremia, Cl^- is avidly conserved by the kidney. Correction of the contracted ECFV with NaCl and repair of K^+ deficits corrects the acid-base disorder.

Renal Origin • *Diuretics* (See also Chap. 232) Drugs that induce chloruresis, such as thiazides and loop diuretics (furosemide, bumetanide, torsemide, and ethracrynic acid), acutely diminish the ECFV without altering the total body bicarbonate content. The serum [HCO_3^-] increases. The chronic administration of diuretics tends to generate an alkalosis by increasing distal salt delivery, so that K^+ and H^+ secretion are stimulated. The alkalosis is maintained by persistence of the contraction of the ECFV, secondary hyperaldosteronism, K^+ deficiency, and the direct effect of the diuretic (as long as diuretic administration continues). Repair of the alkalosis is achieved by providing isotonic saline to correct the ECFV deficit.

Bartter's syndrome and Gitelman's syndrome See Chap. 276.

Nonreabsorbable anions and magnesium deficiency Administration of large quantities of nonreabsorbable anions, such as penicillin or carbenicillin, can enhance distal acidification and K^+ secretion by increasing the transepithelial potential difference (lumen negative). Mg^{2+} deficiency results in hypokalemic alkalosis by enhancing distal acidification through stimulation of renin and hence aldosterone secretion.

Potassium depletion Chronic K^+ depletion may cause metabolic alkalosis by increasing urinary acid excretion. Both NH_4^+ production and absorption are enhanced and HCO_3^- reabsorption is stimulated. Chronic K^+ deficiency upregulates the renal H^+, K^+-ATPase to increase K^+ absorption at the expense of enhanced H^+ secretion. Alkalosis associated with severe K^+ depletion is resistant to salt administration, but repair of the K^+ deficiency corrects the alkalosis.

After treatment of lactic acidosis or ketoacidosis When an underlying stimulus for the generation of lactic acid or ketoacid is removed rapidly, as with repair of circulatory insufficiency or with insulin therapy, the lactate or ketones are metabolized to yield an equivalent amount of HCO_3^-. Other sources of new HCO_3^- are additive with the original amount generated by organic anion metabolism to create a surfeit of HCO_3^-. Such sources include (1) new HCO_3^- added to the blood by the kidneys as a result of enhanced acid excretion

during the preexisting period of acidosis, and (2) alkali therapy during the treatment phase of the acidosis. Acidosis-induced contraction of the ECFV and K^+ deficiency act to sustain the alkalosis.

Posthypercapnia Prolonged CO_2 retention with chronic respiratory acidosis enhances renal HCO_3^- absorption and the generation of new HCO_3^- (increased net acid excretion). If the Pa_{CO_2} is returned to normal, metabolic alkalosis results from the persistently elevated [HCO_3^-]. Alkalosis develops if the elevated Pa_{CO_2} is abruptly returned toward normal by a change in mechanically controlled ventilation. Associated ECFV contraction does not allow complete repair of the alkalosis by correction of the Pa_{CO_2} alone, and alkalosis persists until Cl^- supplementation is provided.

METABOLIC ALKALOSIS ASSOCIATED WITH ECFV EXPANSION, HYPERTENSION, AND HYPERALDOSTERONISM Mineralocorticoid administration or excess production [primary aldosteronism of Cushing's syndrome and adrenal cortical enzyme defects (Chap. 331)] increases net acid excretion and may result in metabolic alkalosis, which may be worsened by associated K^+ deficiency. ECFV expansion from salt retention causes hypertension and antagonizes the reduction in GFR and/or increases tubule acidification induced by aldosterone and by K^+ deficiency. The kaliuresis persists and causes continued K^+ depletion with polydipsia, inability to concentrate the urine, and polyuria. Increased aldosterone levels may be the result of autonomous primary adrenal overproduction or of secondary aldosterone release due to renal overproduction of renin. In both situations, the normal feedback of ECFV on net aldosterone production is disrupted, and hypertension from volume retention can result.

Liddle's syndrome (Chap. 276) results from increased activity of collecting duct Na^+ channel (ENaC) and is a rare inherited disorder associated with hypertension due to volume expansion manifested as hypokalemic alkalosis and normal aldosterone levels.

Symptoms With metabolic alkalosis, changes in central and peripheral nervous system function are similar to those of hypocalcemia (Chap. 340); symptoms include mental confusion, obtundation, and a predisposition to seizures, paresthesia, muscular cramping, tetany, aggravation of arrhythmias, and hypoxemia in chronic obstructive pulmonary disease. Related electrolyte abnormalities include hypokalemia and hypophosphatemia.

℞ **TREATMENT** This is primarily directed at correcting the underlying stimulus for HCO_3^- generation. If primary aldosteronism is present, correction of the underlying cause will reverse the alkalosis. [H^+] loss by the stomach or kidneys can be mitigated by the use of H_2 receptor blockers, H^+, K^+-ATPase inhibitors, or the discontinuation of diuretics. The second aspect of treatment is to remove the factors that sustain HCO_3^- reabsorption, such as ECFV contraction or K^+ deficiency. Although K^+ deficits should be repaired, NaCl therapy is usually sufficient to reverse the alkalosis if ECFV contraction is present, as indicated by a low urine [Cl^-].

If associated conditions preclude infusion of saline, renal HCO_3^- loss can be accelerated by administration of acetazolamide, a carbonic anhydrase inhibitor, which is usually effective in patients with adequate renal function but can worsen K^+ losses. Dilute hydrochloric acid (0.1 N HCl) is also effective but can cause hemolysis. Alternatively, acidification can also be achieved with oral NH_4Cl, which should be avoided in the presence of liver disease. Hemodialysis against a dialysate low in [HCO_3^-] and high in [Cl^-] can be effective when renal function is impaired.

RESPIRATORY ACIDOSIS

Respiratory acidosis can be due to severe pulmonary disease, respiratory muscle fatigue, or abnormalities in ventilatory control and is recognized by an increase in Pa_{CO_2} and decrease in pH (Table 50-5). In acute respiratory acidosis, there is an immediate compensatory el-

Table 50-5   Respiratory Acid-Base Disorders

I. Alkalosis	II. Acidosis
A. Central nervous system stimulation	A. Central
1. Pain	1. Drugs (anesthetics, morphine, sedatives)
2. Anxiety, psychosis	2. Stroke
3. Fever	3. Infection
4. Cerebrovascular accident	B. Airway
5. Meningitis, encephalitis	1. Obstruction
6. Tumor	2. Asthma
7. Trauma	C. Parenchyma
B. Hypoxemia or Tissue hypoxia	1. Emphysema
1. High altitude, $\downarrow$ Pa_{CO_2}	2. Pneumoconiosis
2. Pneumonia, pulmonary edema	3. Bronchitis
3. Aspiration	4. Adult respiratory distress syndrome
4. Severe anemia	5. Barotrauma
C. Drugs or hormones	D. Neuromuscular
1. Pregnancy, progesterone	1. Poliomyelitis
2. Salicylates	2. Kyphoscoliosis
3. Nikethamide	3. Myasthenia
D. Stimulation of chest receptors	4. Muscular dystrophies
1. Hemothorax	E. Miscellaneous
2. Flail chest	1. Obesity
3. Cardiac failure	2. Hypoventilation
4. Pulmonary embolism	3. Permissive hypercapnia
E. Miscellaneous	
1. Septicemia	
2. Hepatic failure	
3. Mechanical hyperventilation	
4. Heat exposure	
5. Recovery from metabolic acidosis	

evation (due to cellular buffering mechanisms) in HCO_3^-, which increases 1 mmol/L for every 10-mmHg increase in Pa_{CO_2}. In chronic respiratory acidosis (24 h), renal adaptation increases the $[HCO_3^-]$ by 4 mmol/L for every 10-mmHg increase in Pa_{CO_2}. The serum HCO_3^- usually does not increase above 38 mmol/L.

The clinical features vary according to the severity and duration of the respiratory acidosis, the underlying disease, and whether there is accompanying hypoxemia. A rapid increase in Pa_{CO_2} may cause anxiety, dyspnea, confusion, psychosis, and hallucinations and may progress to coma. Lesser degrees of dysfunction in chronic hypercapnia include sleep disturbances, loss of memory, daytime somnolence, personality changes, impairment of coordination, and motor disturbances such as tremor, myoclonic jerks, and asterixis. Headaches and other signs that mimic raised intracranial pressure, such as papilledema, abnormal reflexes, and focal muscle weakness, are due to vasoconstriction secondary to loss of the vasodilator effects of CO_2.

Depression of the respiratory center by a variety of drugs, injury, or disease can produce respiratory acidosis. This may occur acutely with general anesthetics, sedatives, and head trauma or chronically with sedatives, alcohol, intracranial tumors, and the syndromes of sleep-disordered breathing, including the primary alveolar and obesity-hypoventilation syndromes (Chaps. 263 and 264). Abnormalities or disease in the motor neurons, neuromuscular junction, and skeletal muscle can cause hypoventilation via respiratory muscle fatigue. Mechanical ventilation, when not properly adjusted and supervised, may result in respiratory acidosis, particularly if CO_2 production suddenly rises (because of fever, agitation, sepsis, or overfeeding) or alveolar ventilation falls because of worsening pulmonary function. High levels of positive end-expiratory pressure in the presence of reduced cardiac output may cause hypercapnia as a result of large increases in alveolar dead space (Chap. 266). Permissive hypercapnia is being used with increasing frequency because of studies suggesting lower mortality rates than with conventional mechanical ventilation, especially with severe central nervous system or heart disease. Although the potential

beneficial effects of permissive hypercapnia may be mitigated by correction of the acidemia, it seems prudent, nevertheless, to keep the pH in the range of 7.2 to 7.3 by administration of $NaHCO_3$.

Acute hypercapnia follows sudden occlusion of the upper airway or generalized bronchospasm as in severe asthma, anaphylaxis, inhalational burn, or toxin injury. Chronic hypercapnia and respiratory acidosis occur in end-stage obstructive lung disease. Restrictive disorders involving both the chest wall and the lungs can cause respiratory acidosis because the high metabolic cost of respiration causes ventilatory muscle fatigue. Advanced stages of intrapulmonary and extrapulmonary restrictive defects present as chronic respiratory acidosis.

The diagnosis of respiratory acidosis requires, by definition, the measurement of Pa_{CO_2} and arterial pH. A detailed history and physical examination often indicate the cause. Pulmonary function studies (Chap. 250), including spirometry, diffusion capacity for carbon monoxide, lung volumes, and arterial Pa_{CO_2} and O_2 saturation, usually make it possible to determine if respiratory acidosis is secondary to lung disease. The workup for nonpulmonary causes should include a detailed drug history, measurement of hematocrit, and assessment of upper airway, chest wall, pleura, and neuromuscular function.

TREATMENT   The management of respiratory acidosis depends on its severity and rate of onset. Acute respiratory acidosis can be life-threatening, and measures to reverse the underlying cause should be undertaken simultaneously with restoration of adequate alveolar ventilation. This may necessitate tracheal intubation and assisted mechanical ventilation. Oxygen administration should be titrated carefully in patients with severe obstructive pulmonary disease and chronic CO_2 retention who are breathing spontaneously (Chap. 258). When oxygen is used injudiciously, these patients may experience progression of the respiratory acidosis. Aggressive and rapid correction of hypercapnia should be avoided, because the falling Pa_{CO_2} may provoke the same complications noted with acute respiratory alkalosis (i.e., cardiac arrhythmias, reduced cerebral perfusion, and seizures). The Pa_{CO_2} should be lowered gradually in chronic respiratory acidosis, aiming to restore the Pa_{CO_2} to baseline levels and to provide sufficient Cl^- and K^+ to enhance the renal excretion of HCO_3^-.

Chronic respiratory acidosis is frequently difficult to correct, but measures aimed at improving lung function (Chap. 258) can help some patients and forestall further deterioration in most.

RESPIRATORY ALKALOSIS

Alveolar hyperventilation decreases Pa_{CO_2} and increases the HCO_3^-/Pa_{CO_2} ratio, thus increasing pH (Table 50-5). Nonbicarbonate cellular buffers respond by consuming HCO_3^-. Hypocapnia develops when a sufficiently strong ventilatory stimulus causes CO_2 output in the lungs to exceed its metabolic production by tissues. Plasma pH and $[HCO_3^-]$ appear to vary proportionately with Pa_{CO_2} over a range from 40 to 15 mmHg. The relationship between arterial $[H^+]$ concentration and Pa_{CO_2} is about 0.7 mmol/L per mmHg (or 0.01 pH unit/mmHg), and that for plasma $[HCO_3^-]$ is 0.2 mmol/L per mmHg. Hypocapnia sustained longer than 2 to 6 h is further compensated by a decrease in renal ammonium and titrable acid excretion and a reduction in filtered HCO_3^- reabsorption. Full renal adaptation to respiratory alkalosis may take several days and requires normal volume status and renal function. The kidneys appear to respond directly to the lowered Pa_{CO_2} rather than to alkalosis per se. In chronic respiratory alkalosis a 1-mmHg fall in Pa_{CO_2} causes a 0.4- to 0.5-mmol/L drop in $[HCO_3^-]$ and a 0.3-mmol/L fall (or 0.003 rise in pH) in $[H^+]$.

The effects of respiratory alkalosis vary according to duration and severity but are primarily those of the underlying disease. Reduced cerebral blood flow as a consequence of a rapid decline in Pa_{CO_2} may cause dizziness, mental confusion, and seizures, even in the absence of hypoxemia. The cardiovascular effects of acute hypocapnia in the conscious human are generally minimal, but in the anesthetized or mechanically ventilated patient, cardiac output and blood pressure may fall because of the depressant effects of anesthesia and positive-pressure ventilation on heart rate, systemic resistance, and venous return. Cardiac arrhythmias may occur in patients with heart disease as a result of changes in oxygen unloading by blood from a left shift in the hemoglobin-oxygen dissociation curve (Bohr effect). Acute respiratory alkalosis causes intracellular shifts of Na^+, K^+, and PO_4^- and reduces free $[Ca^{2+}]$ by increasing the protein-bound fraction. Hypocapnia-induced hypokalemia is usually minor.

Chronic respiratory alkalosis is the most common acid-base disturbance in critically ill patients and, when severe, portends a poor prognosis. Many cardiopulmonary disorders manifest respiratory alkalosis in their early to intermediate stages, and the finding of normocapnia and hypoxemia in a patient with hyperventilation may herald the onset of rapid respiratory failure and should prompt an assessment to determine if the patient is becoming fatigued. Respiratory alkalosis is common during mechanical ventilation.

The hyperventilation syndrome may be disabling. Paresthesia, circumoral numbness, chest wall tightness or pain, dizziness, inability to take an adequate breath, and, rarely, tetany may themselves be sufficiently stressful to perpetuate the disorder. Arterial blood-gas analysis demonstrates an acute or chronic respiratory alkalosis, often with hypocapnia in the range of 15 to 30 mmHg and no hypoxemia. Central nervous system diseases or injury can produce several patterns of hyperventilation and sustained Pa_{CO_2} levels of 20 to 30 mmHg. Hyperthyroidism, high caloric loads, and exercise raise the basal metabolic rate, but ventilation usually rises in proportion so that arterial blood gases are unchanged and respiratory alkalosis does not develop. Salicylates are the most common cause of drug-induced respiratory alkalosis as a result of direct stimulation of the medullary chemoreceptor (Chap. 396). The methylxanthines, theophylline, and aminophylline stimulate ventilation and increase the ventilatory response to CO_2. Progesterone increases ventilation and lowers arterial Pa_{CO_2} by as much as 5 to 10 mmHg. Therefore, chronic respiratory alkalosis is a common feature of pregnancy. Respiratory alkalosis is also prominent in liver failure, and the severity correlates with the degree of hepatic insufficiency. Respiratory alkalosis is often an early finding in gram-negative septicemia, before fever, hypoxemia, or hypotension develop.

The diagnosis of respiratory alkalosis depends on measurement of arterial pH and Pa_{CO_2}. The plasma $[K^+]$ is often reduced and the

$[Cl^-]$ increased. In the acute phase, respiratory alkalosis is not associated with increased renal HCO_3^- excretion, but within hours net acid excretion is reduced. In general, the HCO_3^- concentration falls by 2.0 mmol/L for each 10-mmHg decrease in Pa_{CO_2}. Chronic hypocapnia reduces the serum $[HCO_3^-]$ by 5.0 mmol/L for each 10-mmHg decrease in Pa_{CO_2}. It is unusual to observe a plasma $HCO_3^- < 12$ mmol/L as a result of a pure respiratory alkalosis.

When a diagnosis of respiratory alkalosis is made, its cause should be investigated. The diagnosis of hyperventilation syndrome is made by exclusion. In difficult cases, it may be important to rule out other conditions such as pulmonary embolism, coronary artery disease, and hyperthyroidism.

℞ **TREATMENT** The management of respiratory alkalosis is directed toward alleviation of the underlying disorder. If respiratory alkalosis complicates ventilator management, changes in dead space, tidal volume, and frequency can minimize the hypocapnia. Patients with the hyperventilation syndrome may benefit from reassurance, rebreathing from a paper bag during symptomatic attacks, and attention to underlying psychological stress. Antidepressants and sedatives are not recommended. β-Adrenergic blockers may ameliorate peripheral manifestations of the hyperadrenergic state.

BIBLIOGRAPHY

ALPERN RJ et al: Metabolic alkalosis, in *The Kidney: Physiology and Pathophysiology*, 2d ed, DW Seldin, G Giebisch (eds). New York, Raven, 1992, pp 2733–2758

DuBose TD Jr: Acid-base disorders, in *Brenner and Rector's The Kidney*, 6th ed, BM Brenner (ed). Philadelphia, Saunders, 2000, pp 925–997

———, ALPERN RJ: Renal tubular acidosis, in *The Metabolic and Molecular Bases of Inherited Disease*, 8th ed, CR Scriver et al (eds). New York, McGraw-Hill, 2001

FALL PJ: A stepwise approach to acid-base disorders: Practical patient evaluation for metabolic acidosis and other conditions. Postgrad Med 107:249–50, 253–4, 257–8, 2000

GALLA JH: Metabolic alkalosis. J Am Soc Nephrol 11:369, 2000

MADIAS NE, COHEN JJ: Respiratory alkalosis and acidosis, in *The Kidney: Physiology and Pathophysiology*, 2d ed, DW Seldin, G Giebisch (eds). New York, Raven, 1992, pp 2733–2758

Section 8
ALTERATIONS IN SEXUAL FUNCTION AND REPRODUCTION

51 *Kevin T. McVary*

ERECTILE DYSFUNCTION

Erectile dysfunction (ED) affects 10 to 25% of middle-aged and elderly men. Demographic changes, the popularity of newer treatments, and greater acceptance of ED by patients and society have led to increased diagnosis and associated health care expenditures for the management of this common disorder. Impairment of erectile function has a profound impact on the well-being of affected men. Because many patients are reluctant to initiate discussion of sexual function, the physician should address this topic directly to elicit a history of ED.

PHYSIOLOGIC CONTROL OF ERECTION AND MALE SEXUAL FUNCTION

Normal male sexual function requires (1) an intact libido, (2) the ability to achieve and maintain penile erection, (3) ejaculation, and (4) detumescence. *Libido* refers to sexual desire and is influenced by

a variety of visual, olfactory, tactile, auditory, imaginative and hormonal stimuli. Sex steroids, particularly testosterone, act to increase libido. Libido can be diminished by hormonal or psychiatric disorders or by medications.

The major anatomic structures of the penis that are involved in erectile function include the three corpora, which consist of the paired cavernosa and a single spongiosum that encloses the urethra. A collagenous sheath, called the *tunica albuginea*, individually surrounds each corpora. The micro-architecture of the corpora is composed of a mass of smooth muscle (trabecula) which contains a network of endothelial-lined vessels (lacunar spaces).

Penile tumescence leading to erection depends on the increased flow of blood into the lacunar network after complete relaxation of the arteries and corporal smooth muscle. Subsequent compression of the trabecular smooth muscle against the fibroelastic tunica albuginea causes a passive closure of the emissary veins and accumulation of blood in the corpora. In the presence of a full erection and a competent valve mechanism, the corpora become noncompressible cylinders from which blood does not escape.

The central nervous system exerts an important influence by either stimulating or antagonizing spinal pathways that mediate erectile function and ejaculation. The erectile response is mediated by a combination of central (psychogenic) and peripheral (reflexogenic) innervation. Sensory nerves that originate from receptors in the penile skin and glans converge to form the dorsal nerve of the penis, which travels to the S2-S4 dorsal root ganglia via the pudendal nerve. Parasympathetic nerve fibers to the penis arise from neurons in the intermediolateral columns of S2-S4 sacral spinal segments. Sympathetic innervation originates from the T-11 to the L-2 spinal segments and descends through the hypogastric plexus.

Neural input to smooth muscle tone is crucial to the initiation and maintenance of an erection. There is also an intricate interaction between the corporal smooth muscle cell and its overlying endothelial cell lining (Fig. 51-1A). Nitric oxide, which induces vascular relaxation, promotes erection and is opposed by endothelin-1 (ET-1), which mediates vascular contraction. Nitric oxide is synthesized from L-arginine by nitric oxide synthase, and is released from the nonadrenergic, noncholinergic (NANC) autonomic nerve supply to act postjunctionally on smooth muscle cells. Nitric oxide increases the production of cyclic 3',5'-guanosine monophosphate (cyclic GMP), which interacts with protein kinase G and decreases intracellular calcium, causing relaxation of the smooth muscle (Fig. 51-1B). Cyclic GMP is gradually broken down by phosphodiesterase type 5 (PDE-5). Inhibitors of PDE-5, such as the oral medication sildenafil, maintain erections by reducing the breakdown of cyclic GMP. However, if nitric oxide is not produced at some level, the addition of PDE-5 inhibitor is not effective, as the drug facilitates but does not initiate the initial enzyme cascade. In addition to nitric oxide, vasoactive prostaglandins (PGE₁, PGF₂ₐ) are synthesized within the cavernosal tissue and increase cyclic AMP levels, also leading to relaxation of cavernosal smooth muscle cells.

Ejaculation is stimulated by the sympathetic nervous system, which results in contraction of the epididymis, vas deferens, seminal vesicles, and prostate, causing seminal fluid to enter the urethra. Seminal fluid emission is followed by rhythmic contractions of the bulbocavernosus and ischiocavernosus muscles, leading to ejaculation. *Premature ejaculation* is usually related to anxiety or a learned behavior and is amenable to behavioral therapy or treatment with medications such as selective serotonin reuptake inhibitors (SSRIs). *Retrograde ejaculation* results when the internal urethral sphincter does not close, and it may occur in men with diabetes or after surgery involving the bladder neck.

Detumescence is mediated by released norepinephrine from the sympathetic nerves, release of endothelin from the vascular surface, and contraction of smooth muscle induced by activation of postsynaptic α-adrenergic receptors. These events increase venous outflow and restore the flaccid state. Venous leak can cause premature detumescence and is thought to be caused by insufficient relaxation of the corporal smooth muscle rather than a specific anatomic defect. *Priapism* refers to a persistent and painful erection and may be associated with sickle cell anemia, hypercoagulable states, spinal cord injury, or injection of vasodilator agents into the penis.

ERECTILE DYSFUNCTION

EPIDEMIOLOGY   In the Massachusetts Male Aging Study (MMAS), a community-based survey of men between the ages of 40 and 70, 52% of responders reported some degree of ED. Complete ED occurred in 10% of respondents, moderate ED occurred in 25%, and minimal ED in 17%. The incidence of moderate or severe ED more than doubled between the ages of 40 and 70. In the National Health and Social Life Survey (NHSLS), which was a nationally representative sample of men and women age 18 to 59 years, 10% of men reported being unable to maintain an erection (corresponding to the proportion of men in the MMAS reporting severe ED). Incidence was highest among men in the 50 to 59 age group (21%) and among men who were poor (14%), divorced (14%), and less educated (13%).

The incidence of ED is also higher among men with certain medical disorders. In the MMAS, ED correlated with the presence of diabetes mellitus, heart disease, hypertension, and decreased HDL levels. Medications used to treat diabetes or cardiovascular disease are additional risk factors (see below). There is a higher incidence of ED among men who have undergone radiation or surgery for cancer of the prostate and in those with a lower spinal cord injury. Psychological causes of ED include depression and anger. The NHSLS found a higher incidence of ED among men who reported fair-to-poor health or experienced stress from unemployment or other causes. ED is not considered a normal part of the aging process. Nonetheless, it is associated with certain physiologic and psychological changes related to age.

PATHOPHYSIOLOGY   ED may result from three basic mechanisms: (1) failure to initiate (psychogenic, endocrinologic, or neurogenic); (2) failure to fill (arteriogenic); or (3) failure to store (venoocclusive dysfunction) adequate blood volume within the lacunar network. The inability to initiate an erection may have psychogenic, endocrinologic, or neurogenic etiologies. These categories are not mutually exclusive, and multiple factors contribute to ED in many patients. For example, diminished filling pressure can lead secondarily to venous leak. Psychogenic factor frequently co-exist with other etiologic factors and should be considered in all cases. Diabetic, atherosclerotic, and drug-related causes account for >80% of cases of ED in older men.

Vasculogenic   The most frequent organic cause of ED is a disturbance of blood flow to and from the penis. Atherosclerotic or traumatic arterial disease can decrease flow to the lacunar spaces, resulting in decreased rigidity and an increased time to full erection. Excessive

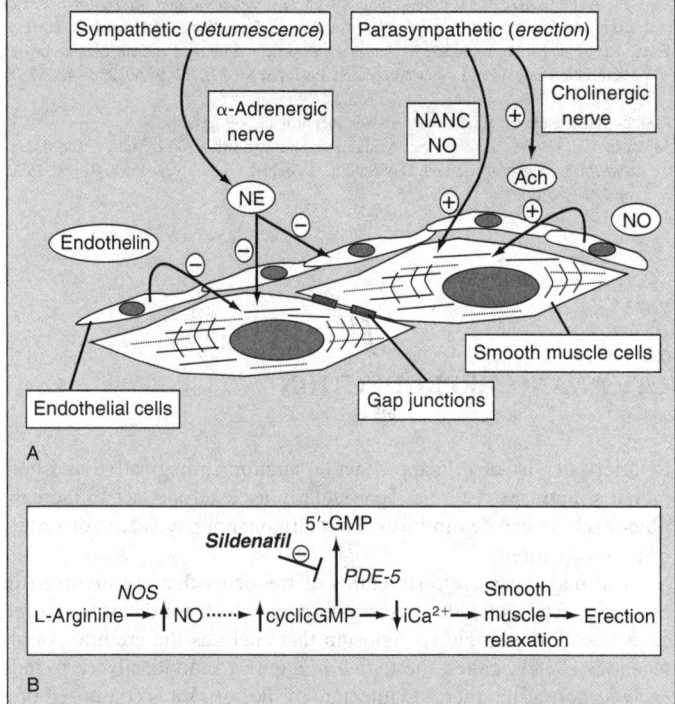

FIGURE 51-1   Pathways that control erection and detumescence. *A.* Erection is mediated by cholinergic parasympathetic pathways, and nonadrenergic, noncholinergic (NANC) pathways, which release nitric oxide (NO). Endothelial cells also release NO, which induces vascular smooth muscle cell relaxation, allowing enhanced blood flow, and leading to erection. Detumescence is mediated by sympathetic pathways that release norepinephrine and stimulate α-adrenergic pathways, leading to contraction of vascular smooth muscle cells. Endothelin, released from endothelial cells, also induces contraction. *B.* Biochemical pathways of NO synthesis and action. Sildenafil enhances erectile function by inhibiting phosphodiesterase type 5 (PDE-5), thereby maintaining high levels of cyclic 3',5'-guanosine monophosphate (cyclic GMP). NOS, nitric oxide synthase; iCa²⁺, intracellular calcium.

outflow through the veins, despite adequate inflow, may also contribute to ED. In this case, the achieved perfusion pressures cannot compensate for the unrestricted outflow needed to ensure adequate erection. This situation may be due to insufficient relaxation of trabecular smooth muscle and may occur in anxious individuals with excessive adrenergic tone or in those with damaged parasympathetic outflow. Structural alterations to the fibroelastic components of the corpora may cause a loss of compliance and an inability to compress the tunical veins. This condition may result from aging, increased cross-leaking of collagen fibers induced by nonenzymatic glycosylation, hypoxia, or altered synthesis of collagen associated with hypercholesterolemia. Fibroelastic structures can also be damaged by surgery, radiation, or trauma to the penis.

Neurogenic Disorders that affect the sacral spinal cord or the autonomic fibers to the penis preclude nervous system relaxation of penile smooth muscle, thus leading to ED. In patients with spinal cord injury, the degree of ED depends on the completeness and level of the lesion. Patients with incomplete lesions or injuries to the upper part of the spinal cord are more likely to retain erectile capabilities than those with complete lesions or injuries to the lower part. Although 75% of patients with spinal cord injuries have some erectile capability, only 25% have erections sufficient for penetration. Other neurologic disorders commonly associated with ED include multiple sclerosis and peripheral neuropathy. The latter is often due to either diabetes or alcoholism. Pelvic surgery may cause ED through disruption of the autonomic nerve supply.

Endocrinologic Androgens increase libido, but their exact role in erectile function remains unclear. Individuals with castrate levels of testosterone can achieve erections from visual or sexual stimuli. Nonetheless, normal levels of testosterone appear to be important for erectile function, particularly in older males. Androgen replacement therapy can improve depressed erectile function when it is secondary to hypogonadism; it is not useful for ED when endogenous testosterone levels are normal. Increased prolactin may decrease libido by suppressing gonadotropin-releasing hormone (GnRH), and it also leads to decreased testosterone levels. Treatment of hyperprolactinemia with dopamine agonists can restore libido and testosterone.

Diabetic ED occurs in 35 to 75% of men with diabetes mellitus. Pathologic mechanisms are primarily related to diabetes-associated vascular and neurologic complications. Diabetic macrovascular complications are mainly related to age, whereas microvascular complications correlate with the duration of diabetes and the degree of glycemic control (Chap. 333). Individuals with diabetes also have reduced amounts of nitric oxide synthase in both endothelial and neural tissues.

Psychogenic Two mechanisms contribute to the inhibition of erections in psychogenic ED. First, psychogenic stimuli to the sacral cord may inhibit reflexogenic responses, thereby blocking activation of vasodilator outflow to the penis. Second, excess sympathetic stimulation in an anxious man may increase penile smooth muscle tone. The most common causes of psychogenic ED are performance anxiety, depression, relationship conflict, loss of attraction, sexual inhibition, conflicts over sexual preference, sexual abuse in childhood, and fear of pregnancy or sexually transmitted disease. Almost all patients with ED, even when it has a clear-cut organic basis, develop a psychogenic component as a reaction to ED.

Medication-Related Medication-induced ED (Table 51-1) is estimated to occur in 25% of men seen in general medical outpatient clinics. Among the antihypertensive agents, the thiazide diuretics and beta blockers have been implicated most frequently. Calcium channel blockers and angiotensin-converting enzyme inhibitors are less frequently cited. These drugs may act directly at the corporal level (e.g., calcium channel blockers) or indirectly by reducing pelvic blood pressure, which is important in the development of penile rigidity. Alpha adrenergic blockers are less likely to cause ED. Estrogens, GnRH agonists, H_2 antagonists, and spironolactone cause ED by suppressing gonadotropin production or by blocking androgen action. Antidepressant and antipsychotic agents—particularly neuroleptics, tricyclics, and SSRIs—are associated with erectile, ejaculatory, orgasmic, and

Table 51-1 Drugs Associated with Erectile Dysfunction

Classification	Drugs
Diuretics	Thiazides
	Spironolactone
Antihypertensives	Calcium channel blockers
	Methyldopa
	Clonidine
	Reserpine
	β-Blockers
	Guanethidine
Cardiac/anti-hyperlipidemics	Digoxin
	Gemfibrozil
	Clofibrate
Antidepressants	Selective serotonin reuptake inhibitors
	Tricyclic antidepressants
	Lithium
	Monoamine oxidase inhibitors
Tranquilizers	Butyrophenones
	Phenothiazines
H_2 antagonists	Ranitidine
	Cimetidine
Hormones	Progesterone
	Estrogens
	Corticosteroids
	GnRH agonists
	5α-Reductase inhibitors
	Cyproterone acetate
Cytotoxic agents	Cyclophosphamide
	Methotrexate
	Roferon-A
Anticholinergics	Disopyramide
	Anticonvulsants
Recreational	Ethanol
	Cocaine
	Marijuana

sexual desire difficulties. Digoxin induces ED via blockade of the Na^+,K^+-ATPase pump, resulting in a net increase in intracellular calcium and increased corporal smooth muscle tone.

Although many medications can cause ED, patients frequently have concomitant risk factors that confound the clinical picture. If there is a strong association between the institution of a drug and the onset of ED, alternative medications should be considered. Otherwise, it is often practical to treat the ED without attempting multiple changes in medications, as it may be difficult to establish a causal role for the drug.

CLINICAL EVALUATION A good physician-patient relationship helps to unravel the possible causes of ED, many of which require discussion of personal and sometimes embarrassing topics. For this reason, a primary care provider is often ideally suited to initiate the evaluation. A complete medical and sexual history should be taken in an effort to assess whether the cause of ED is organic, psychogenic, or multifactorial (Fig. 51-2). Initial questions should focus on the onset of symptoms, the presence and duration of partial erections, and the progression of ED. A history of nocturnal or early morning erections is useful for distinguishing physiologic from psychogenic ED. Nocturnal erections occur during rapid eye movement (REM) sleep and require intact neurologic and circulatory systems. Organic causes of ED are generally characterized by a gradual and persistent change in rigidity or the inability to sustain nocturnal, coital, or self-stimulated erections. The patient should also be questioned about the presence of penile curvature or pain with coitus. It is also important to address libido, as decreased sexual drive and ED are sometimes the earliest signs of endocrine abnormalities (e.g., increased prolactin, decreased testosterone levels). It is useful to ask whether the problem is confined to coitus with one or other partners; ED arises not uncommonly in association with new or extramarital sexual relationships. Situational ED, as opposed to consistent ED, suggests psychogenic causes. Ejac-

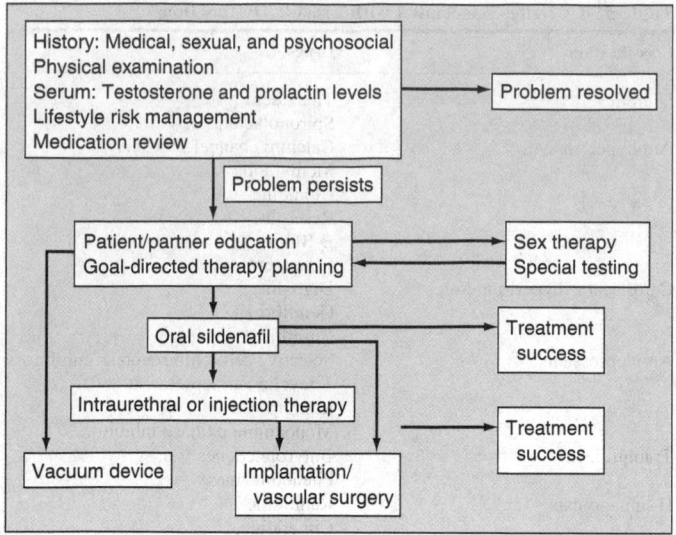

FIGURE 51-2   Algorithm for the evaluation and management of patients with ED.

ulation is much less commonly affected than erection, but questions should be asked about whether ejaculation is normal, premature, delayed, or absent. Relevant risk factors should be identified, such as diabetes mellitus, coronary artery disease, lipid disorders, hypertension, peripheral vascular disease, smoking, alcoholism, and endocrine or neurologic disorders. The patient's surgical history should be explored with an emphasis on bowel, bladder, prostate, or vascular procedures. A complete drug history is also important, as medications constitute a major source of reversible ED. Social changes that may precipitate ED are also crucial to the evaluation, including health worries, spousal death, divorce, relationship difficulties, and financial concerns.

The physical examination is an essential element in the assessment of ED. Signs of hypertension as well as evidence of thyroid, hepatic, hematologic, cardiovascular, or renal diseases should be sought. An assessment should be made of the endocrine and vascular systems, the external genitalia, and the prostate gland. The penis should be carefully palpated along the corpora to detect fibrotic plaques. Reduced testicular size and loss of secondary sexual characteristics are suggestive of hypogonadism. Neurologic examination should include assessment of anal sphincter tone, the bulbocavernosus reflex, and testing for peripheral neuropathy.

Selected laboratory testing is recommended in all cases. Although hyperprolactinemia is uncommon, a serum prolactin level should be measured, as decreased libido and/or erectile dysfunction may be the presenting symptoms of a prolactinoma or other mass lesions of the sella (Chap. 328). The serum testosterone level should be measured and, if low, gonadotropins should be measured to determine whether hypogonadism is primary (testicular) or secondary (hypothalamic-pituitary) in origin (Chap. 335). Serum chemistries, CBC, and lipid profiles may be of value, if not performed recently, as they can yield evidence of anemia, diabetes, hyperlipidemia, or other systemic diseases associated with ED. Determination of serum PSA should be conducted according to recommended clinical guidelines (Chap. 95).

Additional diagnostic testing is rarely necessary in the evaluation of ED. However, in selected patients, specialized testing may provide insight into pathologic mechanisms of ED and aid in the selection of treatment options. Optional specialized testing includes: (1) studies of nocturnal penile tumescence and rigidity; (2) vascular testing (in-office injection of vasoactive substances, penile Doppler ultrasound, penile angiography, dynamic infusion cavernosography/cavernosometry); (3) neurologic testing (biothesiometry-graded vibratory perception; somatosensory evoked potentials); and (4) psychological diagnostic tests. The information potentially gained from these procedures must be balanced against their invasiveness and cost.

℞   TREATMENT   Patient Education   Patient and partner education is essential in the treatment of ED. In goal-directed therapy, education facilitates understanding of the disease, results of the tests, and selection of treatment. Discussion of treatment options helps to clarify how treatment is best offered, and to stratify first- and second-line therapies. Patients with high-risk lifestyle issues, such as smoking, alcohol abuse, or recreational drug use, should be counseled on the role these factors play in the development of ED.

Oral Agents   Sildenafil is the only approved and effective oral agent for the treatment of ED. Sildenafil has markedly improved the management of ED because it is effective for the treatment of a broad range of causes of ED, including psychogenic, diabetic, vasculogenic, post-radical prostatectomy (nerve-sparing procedures), and spinal cord injury. Sildenafil is a selective and potent inhibitor of PDE-5, the predominant phosphodiesterase isoform found in the penis. It is administered in doses of 25, 50, or 100 mg, and enhances erections after sexual stimulation. The onset of action is approximately 60 to 90 min. Reduced initial doses should be considered for patients who are elderly, have renal insufficiency, or are taking medications that inhibit the CYP3A4 metabolic pathway in the liver (e.g., erythromycin, cimetidine, ketoconazole, and, possibly, itraconazole and mibefradil), as they may increase the serum concentration of sildenafil. The drug does not affect ejaculation, orgasm, or sexual drive. Side effects associated with sildenafil include headaches (19%), facial flushing (9%), dyspepsia (6%) and nasal congestion (4%). Approximately 7% of men may experience transient altered color vision (blue halo effect). Sildenafil is contraindicated in men receiving nitrate therapy for cardiovascular disease, including agents delivered by oral, sublingual, transnasal, or topical routes. These agents can potentiate its hypotensive effect and may result in profound shock. Likewise, amyl/butyl nitrates (poppers) may have a fatal synergistic effect on blood pressure. Sildenafil should also be avoided in patients with congestive heart failure and cardiomyopathy because of the risk of vascular collapse. Because sexual activity leads to an increase in physiologic expenditure [5 to 6 metabolic equivalents (METS)], physicians have been advised to exercise caution in prescribing any drug for sexual activity to those with active coronary disease, heart failure, borderline hypotension, hypovolemia, and to those on complex antihypertensive regimens.

Androgen Therapy   Testosterone replacement is used to treat both primary and secondary causes of hypogonadism (Chap. 335). Androgen supplementation in the setting of normal testosterone is rarely efficacious and is discouraged. Methods of androgen replacement include parenteral administration of long-acting testosterone esters (enanthate and cypionate), oral preparations (17 α-alkylated derivatives), and transdermal patches (Chap. 335). The long-acting 17 β-hydroxy esters of testosterone are the safest, most cost-effective, and practical preparations available. The administration of 200 to 300 mg intramuscularly every 2 to 3 weeks provides a practical option but is far from an ideal physiologic replacement. Oral androgen preparations have the potential for hepatotoxicity and should be avoided. Transdermal delivery of testosterone more closely mimics physiologic testosterone levels, but it is unclear whether this translates into improved sexual function. Because testosterone gradually decreases into the hypogonadal range by 24 hours, patches need to replaced daily. Testosterone therapy is contraindicated in men with androgen-sensitive cancers and may be inappropriate for men with bladder neck obstruction. It is generally advisable to measure PSA before giving androgen. Hepatic function should be tested before and during testosterone therapy.

Vacuum Constriction Devices   Vacuum constriction devices (VCD) are a well-established, noninvasive therapy. They are a reasonable treatment alternative for select patients who cannot take sildenafil or do not desire other interventions. VCD draw venous blood into the penis and use a constriction ring to restrict venous return and maintain tumescence. Adverse events with VCD include pain, numbness, bruising, and altered ejaculation. Additionally, many patients complain that

Intraurethral Alprostadil If a patient fails to respond to oral agents, a reasonable next choice is intraurethral or self-injection or vasoactive substances. Intraurethral prostaglandin E$_1$ (alprostadil), in the form of a semisolid pellet (doses of 125 to 1000 μg), is delivered with an applicator. Approximately 65% of men receiving intraurethral alprostadil respond with an erection when tested in the office, but only 50% of those achieve successful coitus at home. Intraurethral insertion is associated with a markedly reduced incidence of priapism in comparison to intracavernosal injection.

Intracavernosal Self-Injection Injection of synthetic formulations of alprostadil is effective in 70 to 80% of patients with ED, but discontinuation rates are high because of the invasive nature of administration. Doses range between 1 and 40 μg. Injection therapy is contraindicated in men with a history of hypersensitivity to the drug and in men at risk for priapism (hypercoagulable states, sickle cell disease). Side effects include local adverse events, prolonged erections, pain, and fibrosis with chronic use. Various combinations of alprostadil, phentolamine, and/or papaverine are sometimes used.

Surgery A less frequently used form of therapy for ED involves the surgical implantation of a semi-rigid or inflatable penile prosthesis. These surgical treatments are invasive, associated with potential complications, and generally reserved for treatment of refractory ED. Despite their high cost and invasiveness, penile prostheses are associated with high rates of patient satisfaction.

Sex Therapy A course of sex therapy may be useful for addressing specific interpersonal factors that may affect sexual functioning. Sex therapy generally consists of in-session discussion and at-home exercises specific to the person and the relationship. It is preferable if therapy includes both partners, provided the patient is involved in an ongoing relationship.

BIBLIOGRAPHY

ABRAMOWICZ M et al: Drugs that cause sexual dysfunction. Med Let 29:65, 1987

BURNETT AL et al: Nitric oxide: A physiologic mediator of penile erection. Science 257:401, 1992

FELDMAN HA et al: Impotence and its medical and psychosocial correlates: Results of the Massachusetts Male Aging Study. J Urol 151:54, 1994

GOLDSTEIN I et al: Oral sildenafil in the treatment of erectile impotence. N Engl J Med 338:1397, 1998

KWAN M et al: The nature of androgen action on male sexuality: A combined laboratory–self-report study on hypogonadal men. J Clin Endocrinol Metab 57:557, 1983

LAUMANN AO et al: Sexual dysfunction in the United States. JAMA 81:553, 1999

LEVY A et al: Non-surgical management of erectile dysfunction. Clin Endocrinol (oxf) 52:253, 2000

LUE TF: Drug therapy: Erectile dysfunction. N Engl J Med 342:1802, 2000

NIH CONSENSUS CONFERENCE ON IMPOTENCE: JAMA 270:83, 1993

PADMA-NATHAN H et al: Treatment of men with erectile dysfunction with transurethral alprostadil. N Engl J Med 336:1, 1997

SAENZ DE TEJADA I et al: Impaired neurogenic and endothelium-mediated relaxation of penile smooth muscle from diabetic men with impotence. N Engl J Med 320:1025, 1989

52

Bruce R. Carr, Karen D. Bradshaw

DISTURBANCES OF MENSTRUATION AND OTHER COMMON GYNECOLOGIC COMPLAINTS IN WOMEN

Complaints related to the female reproductive tract can be categorized as disorders of menstruation, pelvic pain, disturbances in sexual function, or infertility. However, a single disorder, e.g., leiomyoma of the uterus, can present with symptoms referable to any one or more of these categories. Furthermore, sexual dysfunction can interdigitate with other problems in several ways. On the one hand, in women with

complaints related to other reproductive tract functions, the underlying problem may actually be severe sexual dysfunction or marital conflict. Alternatively, women with severe organic disorders of the pelvis, e.g., pelvic inflammatory disease or endometriosis, may present with sexual dysfunction such as dyspareunia that in fact is only a minor manifestation of the underlying disease.

Since normal reproductive function depends on the integrated action of the central nervous system, the endocrine glands, and the reproductive organs, menstrual cycle abnormalities, sexual dysfunction, and infertility may be the result of systemic and psychological disorders as well as of primary defects in the endocrine and reproductive organs. The endocrine and physiologic control—normal and abnormal—of puberty, reproductive life, and menopause are discussed in Chap. 336. The focus of this chapter is on the initial evaluation of women with disturbances of the reproductive tract.

DISTURBANCES IN MENSTRUATION Disorders of menstruation can be divided into abnormal uterine bleeding and amenorrhea.

Abnormal Uterine Bleeding The menstrual cycle is defined as the interval between the onset of one bleeding episode and the onset of the next. In normal women the cycle averages 28 ± 3 days, the mean duration of menstrual flow is 4 ± 2 days, and the average blood loss is 35 to 80 mL. Between menarche and menopause most women experience one or more episodes of abnormal uterine bleeding, here defined as any bleeding pattern outside the normal ranges of frequency, duration, and/or amount of blood loss. The decision to evaluate a patient depends on the severity and frequency of the abnormal bleeding pattern.

When vaginal bleeding occurs, it should first be determined whether the blood is derived from the uterine endometrium. Rectal, bladder, cervical, and vaginal sources of bleeding must be excluded. Once the bleeding is established to be uterine in origin, a pregnancy-related disorder (such as threatened or incomplete abortion or ectopic pregnancy) must be ruled out by physical examination and appropriate laboratory tests. It should also be remembered that uterine bleeding may also be the initial or principal manifestation of a generalized bleeding diathesis. The remaining causes of abnormal uterine bleeding can be divided into those associated with ovulatory or anovulatory cycles.

Ovulatory cycles Menstrual bleeding with ovulatory cycles is spontaneous, regular in onset, predictable in duration and amount of flow, and frequently associated with discomfort; it is the consequence of progesterone withdrawal at the end of the luteal (postovulatory) phase and requires prior estrogen priming of the endometrium during the follicular (preovulatory) phase of the cycle. When deviations from an established pattern of menstrual flow occur but the cycles are still regular, the usual cause is disease of the outflow tract. For example, regular, prolonged, excessive bleeding episodes can result from abnormalities of the uterus such as submucous leiomyomas, adenomyosis, or endometrial polyps. On the other hand, cyclic, predictable menstruation characterized by spotting or light bleeding suggests obstruction of the outflow tract as with uterine synechiae or scarring of the cervix. Intermittent bleeding between cyclic ovulatory menses is often due to cervical or endometrial lesions.

Anovulatory cycles Uterine bleeding that is irregular in occurrence, unpredictable as to amount and duration of flow, and usually painless is called *dysfunctional or anovulatory uterine bleeding*. This type of bleeding is the result of a failure of normal follicular maturation with consequent anovulation and may be either transient or chronic. Transient disruption of ovulatory cycles occurs most often in the early menarcheal years, during the perimenopausal period, or as the consequence of a variety of stresses and intercurrent illnesses. Persistent dysfunctional uterine bleeding during the reproductive years can occur in several organic diseases that affect ovarian function and is most often due to estrogen breakthrough bleeding. Estrogen breakthrough bleeding occurs when estrogen stimulation of the endometrium is continuous and is not interrupted by cyclic progesterone withdrawal, as can occur in polycystic ovarian disease.

Amenorrhea *Amenorrhea* is defined either as failure of menarche by age 16, regardless of the presence or absence of secondary sexual characteristics, or as the absence of menstruation for 6 months in a woman with previous periodic menses. Amenorrhea in a woman who has never menstruated is termed *primary amenorrhea*; cessation of menses is termed *secondary amenorrhea*. Because some disorders can cause both primary and secondary amenorrhea, we prefer a functional classification based on the nature of the underlying defect, namely, anatomic defects of the outflow tract (uterus, cervix, or vagina), ovarian failure, and chronic anovulation.

Anatomic defects of the outflow tract include congenital defects of the vagina, imperforate hymen, transverse vaginal septa, cervical stenosis, intrauterine adhesions (synechiae), absence of the vagina or uterus, and uterine maldevelopment. The diagnosis of an anatomic defect is usually made by physical examination but may be confirmed by demonstrating failure of bleeding following administration of estrogen plus a progestogen for 21 days. Pelvic ultrasonography, magnetic resonance imaging, hysterosalpingogram, or hysteroscopy may be helpful in defining the defect.

Causes of *ovarian failure* include gonadal dysgenesis, deficiency of 17α-hydroxylase, resistant ovary syndrome, and premature ovarian failure. Ovarian failure encompasses disorders in which the ovary is deficient in germ cells and those in which the germ cells are resistant to follicle-stimulating hormone (FSH). The diagnosis of ovarian failure as the cause of amenorrhea is confirmed by an elevated plasma FSH level.

Women with *chronic anovulation* fail to ovulate spontaneously but have the capability of ovulating with appropriate therapy. In some women with chronic anovulation, total estrogen production is adequate, but it is not secreted in a cyclic fashion. In others, estrogen production is deficient.

Women who have adequate estrogen production and demonstrate withdrawal bleeding after progestogen challenge often have polycystic ovarian disease (see Fig. 336-8). Other causes include hormone-secreting ovarian and adrenal tumors. Women with deficient or absent estrogen production, and therefore with absence of withdrawal bleeding after progestogen administration, usually have hypogonadotropic hypogonadism due to organic or functional disorders of the pituitary or central nervous system such as brain tumors, pituitary tumors (especially prolactin-secreting adenomas), primary hypopituitarism, or Sheehan's syndrome.

PELVIC PAIN Pelvic pain may originate in the pelvis or be referred from another region of the body. A pelvic source is suggested by the history (e.g., dysmenorrhea and dyspareunia) and physical findings, but a high index of suspicion must be entertained for extrapelvic disorders that refer to the pelvis, such as appendicitis, diverticulitis, cholecystitis, intestinal obstruction, and urinary tract infections (Chap. 14).

"Physiologic" Pelvic Pain • *Pain associated with ovulation* ("*mittelschmerz*") Many women experience low abdominal discomfort with ovulation, typically a dull aching pain at midcycle in one lower quadrant lasting from minutes to hours. It is rarely severe or incapacitating. The pain may result from peritoneal irritation by follicular fluid released into the peritoneal cavity at ovulation. The onset at midcycle and short duration of pain suggest this diagnosis.

Premenstrual or menstrual pain In normal ovulatory women, somatic symptoms during the few days prior to menses may be insignificant or disabling. Such symptoms include edema, breast engorgement, and abdominal bloating or discomfort. A symptom complex of cyclic irritability, depression, and lethargy is known as the *premenstrual syndrome* (PMS). PMS appears to be caused by changes in gonadal steroid levels. Although there is no consensus about therapy, randomized, controlled trials suggest significant improvement with the daily use of serotonin-reuptake inhibitors.

Severe or incapacitating uterine cramping during ovulatory menses and in the absence of demonstrable disorders of the pelvis is termed *primary dysmenorrhea*. Primary dysmenorrhea is caused by prostaglandin-induced uterine ischemia and is treated with prostaglandin synthetase inhibitors and/or oral contraceptive agents.

Pelvic Pain due to Organic Causes Severe dysmenorrhea associated with disease of the pelvis is termed *secondary dysmenorrhea*. Organic causes of pelvic pain can be classified as (1) uterine, (2) adnexal, (3) vulvar or vaginal, and (4) pregnancy-associated.

Uterine pain Pain of uterine etiology is often chronic and continuous and increases in intensity during menstruation and intercourse. Causes include leiomyomas of the uterus (particularly submucous and degenerating leiomyomas), adenomyosis, and cervical stenosis. Infections of the uterus associated with intrauterine manipulation following dilatation and curettage or with the insertion of intrauterine devices can also cause pelvic pain (Chap. 336). Pelvic pain due to endometrial or cervical cancer is usually a late manifestation (Chap. 336).

Adnexal pain The most common cause of pain in the adnexae (fallopian tubes and ovaries) is infection (Chap. 133). Acute salpingo-oophoritis presents as low abdominal pain, fever, and chills; begins a few days after a menstrual period; and is usually due to chlamydial or gonococcal disease with or without a superimposed pyogenic infection. Chronic pelvic inflammatory disease results from either a single episode or multiple episodes of infection and may present as infertility associated with chronic pelvic pain that increases in intensity with menses and intercourse. On physical examination, cervical motion tenderness, adnexal tenderness, and adnexal thickening and/or masses may be present. Pelvic inflammatory disease may become a surgical emergency if peritonitis results from rupture of a tuboovarian abscess. Ovarian cysts or neoplasms may cause pelvic pain that becomes more severe with torsion or rupture of the mass, and ectopic pregnancy must be considered in the differential diagnosis (see below). Endometriosis involving fallopian tubes, ovaries, or peritoneum may cause both chronic low abdominal pain and infertility; the magnitude of tissue involvement does not always correlate with the severity of symptoms. Endometriosis pain typically increases with menstruation and, if the posterior ligaments of the uterus are involved, with intercourse.

Vulvar or vaginal pain Pain in these areas is most often due to infectious vaginitis caused by *Monilia*, *Trichomonas*, or bacteria and is characteristically associated with vaginal discharge and pruritus. Herpetic vulvitis, other dermatologic conditions of the vulva, condyloma acuminatum, and cysts or abscesses of Bartholin's glands may also cause vulvar pain.

Pregnancy-associated disorders Pregnancy must be considered in the differential diagnosis of pelvic pain during the reproductive years. Threatened abortion or incomplete abortion often presents with uterine cramping, bleeding, or passage of tissue following a period of amenorrhea. Ectopic pregnancy may be insidious in presentation or result in abrupt intraperitoneal hemorrhage and maternal death.

Evaluation of Pelvic Pain The evaluation of pelvic pain requires a careful history and pelvic examination. This often leads to the correct diagnosis and institution of appropriate treatment. If the pain is severe and the diagnosis is unclear, the workup should follow that outlined for the acute abdomen (Chap. 14). A culdocentesis may be indicated if a ruptured ectopic pregnancy is suspected. If there is a question of an adnexal mass or if the patient is so obese as to preclude a thorough pelvic examination, abdominal or vaginal sonography may be useful. Serial human chorionic gonadotropin (hCG) measurements may help in establishing a diagnosis of tubal pregnancy and are useful in determining if an intrauterine pregnancy is viable. Finally, diagnostic laparoscopy and laparotomy may be indicated with pain of undetermined etiology.

SEXUAL DYSFUNCTION Some women with sexual dysfunction describe minor complaints related to the reproductive tract as a means of bringing sexual problems to the attention of the physician. Alternatively, sexual dysfunction may be thought to be the cause of low abdominal discomfort or dyspareunia when the actual etiology is organic. However, more and more women seek medical advice because of sexual problems that interface in provenance between medicine, psychiatry, and sociology.

The normal sexual response begins with sexual arousal, which causes genital vasocongestion that results in vaginal lubrication in preparation for intromission. The lubrication is due to the formation of a transudate in the vagina and in conjunction with genital congestion produces the so-called orgasmic platform prior to orgasm. Sexual stimuli (visual, tactile, auditory, and olfactory) as well as healthy vaginal tissue are prerequisites for genital vasocongestion and vaginal lubrication. During the second stage of the sexual response, involuntary contractions of the muscles of the pelvis result in a pleasurable cortical sensory phenomenon known as orgasm. Direct or indirect stimulation of the clitoris is important in the production of the female orgasm. In simple terms, sexual dysfunction can be due to interference with the arousal or orgasmic phases of the sexual response. Either disorder can be due to an organic or functional cause or both.

Illnesses that impair neurologic function such as diabetes mellitus or multiple sclerosis can prevent normal sexual arousal. Local pelvic diseases such as vaginitis, endometriosis, and salpingo-oophoritis may preclude normal sexual response because of resulting dyspareunia. Debilitating systemic diseases such as cancer and cardiovascular diseases may inhibit normal sexual response indirectly.

More commonly, failure of a normal sexual response is due to psychological factors that impair sexual arousal. Such problems include misinformation, e.g., the perception of sexual satisfaction as bad, or feelings of guilt about previous psychologically traumatic events such as incest, rape, or unwanted pregnancy. In addition, women who have had previous hysterectomy or mastectomy may perceive themselves as "incomplete." Stresses such as anxiety, depression, fatigue, and marital or interpersonal conflicts may lead to failure of the vasocongestive response and prevent normal vaginal lubrication. Women with such experiences may be unable to achieve normal sexual response unless they receive professional counseling. Such problems are approached by attempting to identify and reduce the causative stresses.

Failure to achieve orgasm is a specific form of sexual dysfunction. In the absence of orgasm many women enjoy sexual encounters to variable degrees because of the pleasure derived from closeness in a cherished relationship, particularly with a loving partner. However, for other women sexual relations with rare or absent orgasms are frustrating and unsatisfying. In many instances, failure of orgasm is due to insufficient clitoral stimulation and may be rectified by appropriate counseling and patient education.

A specific entity, "vaginismus," painful, involuntary contractions of the musculature surrounding the entrance to the vagina, is a rare cause of dyspareunia. It is a conditioned response to a previous real or imagined frightening or traumatic sexual experience. Treatment is directed to elimination of the conditioned response by progressive vaginal dilation by the patient in conjunction with marital therapy.

REPRODUCTION Infertility is discussed in detail in Chap. 54. The approach to infertile couples always involves evaluation of both the man and woman. The history should address the frequency of intercourse, the sexual responses of both, the use of contraceptives or lubricants, prior pregnancies, interval to conception and outcome of pregnancy, previous or past medical illnesses, and all medications taken.

Male-associated factors account for a third of infertility problems. Therefore, one of the first procedures in the workup of infertile couples should be a semen analysis. The initial evaluation of the woman includes documentation of normal ovulatory cycles. A history of regular, cyclic, predictable, spontaneous menses usually indicates ovulatory cycles, which may be confirmed by basal body temperature graphs, properly timed endometrial biopsies, or plasma progesterone measurements during the luteal phase of the cycle. Also, the diagnosis of luteal-phase dysfunction (low progesterone secretion during the luteal phase) can be established by these methods. Transvaginal ultrasonography is useful for evaluating follicular development.

The most common cause of infertility in women is tubal disease, usually due to infection (pelvic inflammatory disease) or endometriosis. Tubal disease can be evaluated by obtaining a hysterosalpingogram or by diagnostic laparoscopy. Tubal diseases can usually be treated by laparoscopic tuboplasty and lysis of adhesions.

In many instances of infertility, it is now possible to use assisted reproductive technologies including in vitro fertilization and embryo transfer, gamete intrafallopian tube transfer, transfer of cryopreserved ova and embryos, donor oocytes or donor sperm, and ovarian hyperstimulation with clomiphene citrate or gonadotropins followed by intrauterine insemination.

The desire for contraception is also a frequent cause for women to seek medical treatment or evaluation. The most widely used methods for fertility control include (1) rhythm and withdrawal techniques, (2) barrier methods, (3) intrauterine devices, (4) oral steroid contraceptives, (5) sterilization, and (6) abortion. →*These methods and their complications are discussed in Chap. 54.*

BIBLIOGRAPHY

CARR BR, BLACKWELL RE: *Textbook of Reproductive Medicine*, 2d ed. Stamford, CT, Appleton & Lange, 1998
CUNNINGHAM FG et al: *Williams Obstetrics*, 20th ed. Stamford, CT, Appleton & Lange, 1998
FORDNEY DS: Dyspareunia and vaginismus. Clin Obstet Gynecol 21:205, 1978
HERBST AL et al: *Comprehensive Gynecology*, 2d ed. St. Louis, Mosby, 1992
HAMMOND DC: Screening for sexual dysfunction. Clin Obstet Gynecol 27:732, 1984
HATCHER RA et al: *Contraceptive Technology*, 17th ed. New York, Ardent Media, 1998
MASTERS W, JOHNSON V: *Human Sexual Response*. Boston, Little, Brown, 1966
ROSEN RJ et al: Prevention of sexual dysfunction in women. J Sex Med Ther 19:171, 1993
SCHMIDT PJ et al: Differential behavioral effects of gonadal steroids in women with and in those without premenstrual syndrome. N Engl J Med 338:209, 1998
SEIPPEL L, BÄCKSTRÖM T: Luteal-phase estradiol relates to symptom severity in patients with premenstrual syndrome. J Clin Endocrinol Metab 83:1988, 1998
SPEROFF L et al: *Clinical Gynecologic Endocrinology and Infertility*, 5th ed. Baltimore, Williams & Wilkins, 1994

53 *David A. Ehrmann*

HIRSUTISM AND VIRILIZATION

Hirsutism, defined as excessive male-pattern hair growth, affects approximately 10% of women of reproductive age. Hirsutism may be mild, essentially representing a variation of normal hair growth, or rarely it may be the harbinger of a serious underlying condition. It is often idiopathic but may be caused by several conditions associated with androgen excess, such as polycystic ovarian syndrome (PCOS) or congenital adrenal hyperplasia (CAH) (Table 53-1). Cutaneous manifestations commonly associated with hirsutism include acne and male-pattern balding (androgenic alopecia). *Virilization*, on the other hand, refers to the state in which androgen levels are sufficiently high to cause additional signs and symptoms such as deepening of the voice, breast atrophy, increased muscle bulk, clitoromegaly, and increased libido; virilization is an ominous sign that suggests the possibility of an ovarian or adrenal neoplasm.

HAIR FOLLICLE GROWTH AND DIFFERENTIATION Hair can be categorized as either *vellus* (fine, soft, and not pigmented) or *terminal* (long, coarse, and pigmented). The number of hair follicles does not change over an individual's lifetime, but the follicle size and type of hair can change in response to numerous factors, particularly androgens. Androgens are necessary for terminal hair and sebaceous gland development and mediate differentiation of pilosebaceous units (PSUs) into either a terminal hair follicle or a sebaceous gland. In the former case, androgens transform the vellus hair into a terminal hair; in the latter, the sebaceous component proliferates and the hair remains vellus.

There are three phases in the cycle of hair growth: (1) *anagen*

Table 53-1   Causes of Hirsutism

Gonadal hyperandrogenism
  Ovarian hyperandrogenism
  Polycystic ovary syndrome/functional ovarian hyperandrogenism
  Ovarian steroidogenic blocks
  Syndromes of extreme insulin resistance
  Ovarian neoplasms
Adrenal hyperandrogenism
  Premature adrenarche
  Functional adrenal hyperandrogenism
  Congenital adrenal hyperplasia (nonclassic and classic)
  Abnormal cortisol action/metabolism
  Adrenal neoplasms
Other endocrine disorders
  Cushing's syndrome
  Hyperprolactinemia
  Acromegaly
Peripheral androgen overproduction
  Obesity
  Idiopathic
Pregnancy-related hyperandrogenism
  Hyperreactio luteinalis
  Thecoma of pregnancy
Drugs
  Androgens
  Oral contraceptives containing androgenic progestins
Drugs associated with hypertrichosis
  Minoxidil
  Phenytoin
  Diazoxide
  Cyclosporine
True hermaphroditism

(growth phase), (2) *catagen* (involution phase), and (3) *telogen* (rest phase). Depending on the body site, hormonal regulation may play an important role in the hair growth cycle. For example, the eyebrows, eyelashes, and vellus hairs are androgen-insensitive, whereas the axillary and pubic areas are sensitive to low doses of androgens. Hair growth on the face, chest, upper abdomen, and back requires greater levels of androgens and is therefore more characteristic of the pattern typically seen in males. Androgen excess in women leads to increased hair growth in most androgen-sensitive sites but will manifest with loss of hair in the scalp region, in part by reducing the time hairs spend in anagen phase.

Although androgen excess underlies most cases of hirsutism, there is only a modest correlation between androgen levels and the quantity of hair growth. This is due to the fact that hair growth from the follicle depends on local factors and variability in end-organ sensitivity, as well as circulating androgen concentrations. Genetic factors and ethnic background also influence hair growth. In general, dark-haired individuals tend to be more hirsute than blonde or fair individuals. Asians and Native Americans have relatively sparse hair in regions sensitive to high androgen levels, whereas people of Mediterranean descent are more hirsute. For these reasons, family history and ethnic background are important considerations when assessing the etiology and severity of hirsutism.

CLINICAL ASSESSMENT   Historic elements relevant to the assessment of hirsutism include the age of onset and rate of progression of hair growth and associated symptoms or signs (e.g., acne). Depending on the cause, excess hair growth is typically first noted during the second and third decades. The growth is usually slow but progressive. Sudden development and rapid progression of hirsutism suggests the possibility of an androgen-secreting neoplasm, in which case findings of virilization may also be present.

The age of onset of menstrual cycles (menarche) and the pattern of the menstrual cycle should be ascertained; irregular cycles from the time of menarche onward are more likely to result from ovarian rather than adrenal androgen excess. Associated symptoms such as galactor-

rhea should prompt evaluation for hyperprolactinemia (Chap. 328) and possibly hypothyroidism (Chap. 330). Hypertension, striae, easy bruising, centripetal weight gain, and weakness suggest hypercortisolism (Cushing's syndrome; Chap. 331). Rarely, patients with growth hormone excess (i.e., acromegaly) will present with hirsutism. Use of medications such as phenytoin, minoxidil, or cyclosporine may be associated with androgen-independent causes of excess hair growth (i.e., hypertrichosis). A family history of infertility and/or hirsutism may indicate disorders such as nonclassic congenital adrenal hyperplasia (CAH), a disorder particularly common in Ashkenazi Jews, among others (Chap. 331).

Physical examination should include measurement of height, weight, and calculation of body mass index (BMI). A BMI >25 kg/m² is indicative of excess weight for height, and values >30 kg/m² are often seen in association with hirsutism. Notation should be made of blood pressure. Cutaneous signs sometimes associated with androgen excess and insulin resistance include acanthosis nigricans and skin tags.

An objective clinical assessment of hair distribution and quantity is central to the evaluation in any woman presenting with hirsutism. This assessment permits the distinction between hirsutism and hypertrichosis and provides a baseline reference point to gauge the response to treatment. *Hypertrichosis* refers to the excessive growth of androgen-independent hair which is vellus, prominent in nonsexual areas, and most commonly familial or caused by metabolic disorders (e.g., thyroid disturbances, anorexia nervosa) or medications (e.g., phenytoin, minoxidil or cyclosporine).

A simple and commonly used method to grade hair growth is the modified scale of Ferriman and Gallwey (Fig. 53-1), where each of nine androgen-sensitive sites is graded from 0 to 4. Approximately 95% of Caucasian women have a score below 8 on this scale; thus, it is normal for most women to have some hair growth in androgen-sensitive sites. Scores above 8 suggest an excess of androgen-mediated hair growth, a finding that should be assessed further by hormonal evaluation (see below). In racial/ethnic groups that are less likely to manifest hirsutism (e.g., Asian women), additional cutaneous evidence of androgen excess should be sought, including pustular acne or thinning hair.

HORMONAL EVALUATION   Androgens are secreted by both the ovaries and adrenal glands in response to their respective tropic hormones, luteinizing hormone (LH) and adrenocorticotropic hormone (ACTH). The principal circulating steroids involved in the etiology of hirsutism are androstenedione, dehydroepiandrosterone (DHEA) and its sulfated form (DHEAS), and testosterone. The ovaries and adrenal glands normally contribute about equally to testosterone production. Further, approximately half of the total testosterone originates from direct glandular secretion, and the remainder is derived from the peripheral conversion of androstenedione and DHEA (Chap. 335).

Although it is the most important circulating androgen, testosterone is, in effect, the penultimate androgen in mediating hirsutism; it is converted to the more potent dihydrotestosterone (DHT) by the enzyme 5α-reductase, which is located in the pilosebaceous unit. DHT has a higher affinity for, and slower dissociation from, the androgen receptor. The local production of DHT allows it to serve as the primary mediator of androgen action at the level of the pilosebaceous unit. There are two isoenzymes of 5α-reductase: type 2 is found in the prostate gland and in hair follicles, whereas type 1 is primarily found in sebaceous glands.

One approach to testing for hyperandrogenemia is depicted in Fig. 53-2. This involves measuring blood levels of testosterone and DHEAS. It is also important to measure the level of free (or unbound) testosterone, because it is the fraction of testosterone that is not bound to its carrier protein, sex-hormone binding globulin (SHBG), that is biologically available. Hyperinsulinemia and/or androgen excess decrease hepatic production of SHBG, often resulting in levels of total testosterone within the high-normal range at a time when the free hormone is substantially elevated. Because adrenal androgens are readily

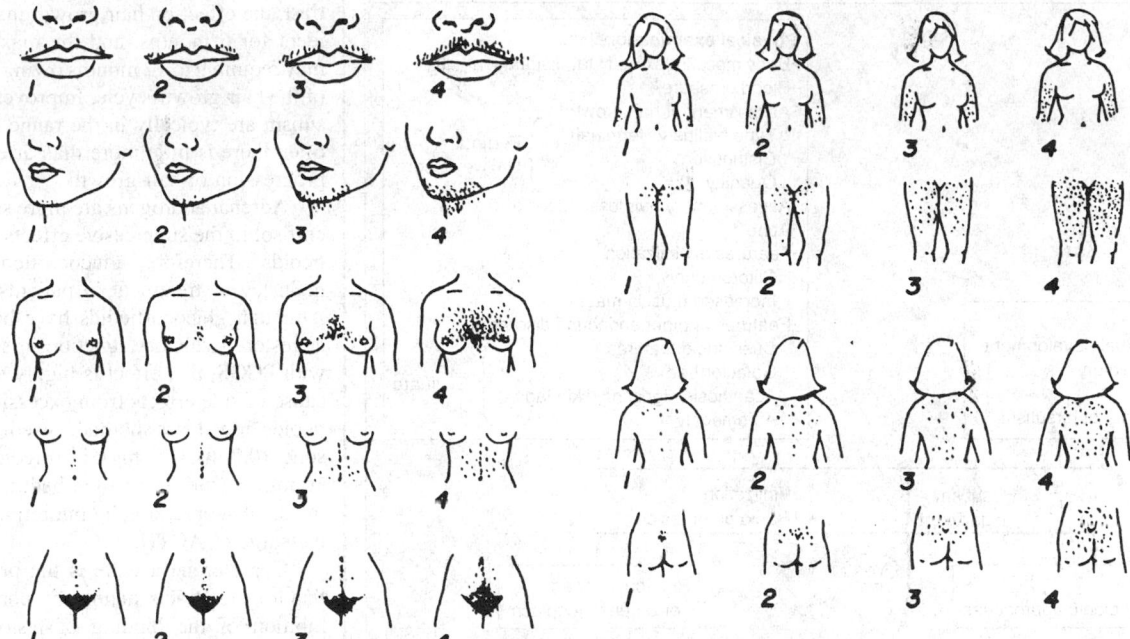

FIGURE 53-1 Hirsutism scoring scale of Ferriman and Gallwey. The nine body areas possessing androgen-sensitive areas are graded from 0 (no terminal hair) to 4 (frankly virile) to obtain a total score. A normal hirsutism score is less than 8. (*Reproduced from Ehrmann et al., 2000.*)

suppressed by low doses of glucocorticoids, the dexamethasone androgen-suppression test may broadly distinguish ovarian from adrenal androgen overproduction. A blood sample is obtained before and after administering dexamethasone (0.5 mg orally every 6 h for 4 days). An adrenal source is suggested by suppression of plasma free testosterone into the normal range; incomplete suppression suggests ovarian androgen excess.

A baseline plasma total testosterone level >12 nmol/L (>3.5 ng/mL) usually indicates a virilizing tumor, whereas a level >7 nmol/L (>2 ng/mL) is suggestive. A basal DHEAS level >18.5 μmol/L (>7000 μg/L) suggests an adrenal tumor. Although DHEAS has been proposed as a "marker" of predominant adrenal androgen excess, it is not unusual to find modest elevations in DHEAS among women with PCOS. Computed tomography (CT) or magnetic resonance imaging (MRI) should be used to localize an adrenal mass, and ultrasound will usually suffice to identify an ovarian mass, if clinical evaluation and hormonal levels suggest these possibilities.

PCOS is the most common cause of ovarian androgen excess (Chap. 336). However, the increased ratio of LH to follicle-stimulating hormone that is often seen in carefully studied patients with PCOS may not be exhibited in up to half of these women due to the pulsatility of gonadotropins. If performed, ultrasound shows enlarged ovaries and/or increased stroma in many women with PCOS. However, polycystic ovaries may also be found in women without clinical or laboratory features of PCOS. Therefore, polycystic ovaries are a relatively insensitive and nonspecific finding for the diagnosis of ovarian hyperandrogenism. Though it is not widely used, gonadotropin-releasing hormone agonist testing can be used to make a specific diagnosis of ovarian hyperandrogenism. A peak 17-hydroxyprogesterone level ≥7.8 nmol/L (≥2.6 μg/L), after the administration of 100 μg nafarelin (or 10 μg/kg leuprolide) subcutaneously, is virtually diagnostic of ovarian hyperandrogenism.

Nonclassic CAH is most commonly due to 21-hydroxylase deficiency but can also be caused by autosomal recessive defects in other steroidogenic enzymes necessary for adrenal corticosteroid synthesis (Chap. 331). Because of the enzyme defect, the adrenal gland cannot secrete glucocorticoids efficiently (especially cortisol). This results in diminished negative feedback inhibition of ACTH, leading to compensatory hyperplasia of the adrenal cortex and accumulation of steroid precursors proximal to the enzyme defect. These precursors are subsequently converted to androgen.

Deficiency of 21-hydroxylase can be reliably excluded by determining a morning 17-hydroxyprogesterone level <6 nmol/L (<2 μg/L) (drawn in the follicular phase). Alternatively, 21-hydroxylase deficiency can be diagnosed by measurement of 17-hydroxyprogesterone 1 h after administration of 250 μg of synthetic ACTH (cosyntropin) intravenously. Measurement after ACTH is slightly more cumbersome, though the results obtained in this manner are highly reproducible and can be compared to published nomograms.

℞ TREATMENT Treatment of hirsutism may be accomplished pharmacologically and by mechanical means of hair removal. Nonpharmacologic treatments should be considered in all patients, either as the only treatment or as an adjunct to drug therapy.

Nonpharmacologic treatments include (1) bleaching; (2) depilatory (removal from the skin surface) such as shaving and chemical treatments; or (3) epilatory (removal of the hair including the root) such as plucking, waxing, electrolysis, and laser therapy. Despite perceptions to the contrary, shaving does not increase the rate or density of hair growth. Chemical depilatory treatments may be useful for mild hirsutism that affects only limited skin areas, though they can cause skin irritation. Wax treatment removes hair temporarily but is uncomfortable. Electrolysis is effective for more permanent hair removal, particularly in the hands of a skilled electrologist. Laser phototherapy appears to be efficacious for hair removal. It delays hair regrowth and causes permanent hair removal in some patients. The long-term effects and complications associated with laser treatment are being evaluated.

Pharmacologic therapy for androgen excess is directed at interrupting one or more of the steps in the pathway leading to its expression: (1) suppression of adrenal and/or ovarian androgen production; (2) enhancement of androgen-binding to plasma-binding proteins, particularly SHBG; (3) impairment of the peripheral conversion of androgen precursors to active androgen; and (4) inhibition of androgen action at the target tissue level. Attenuation of hair growth is typically not evident until 4 to 6 months after initiation of medical treatment and, in most cases, leads to a modest reduction in hair growth.

Combination estrogen-progestin therapy, in the form of an oral contraceptive, is usually the first-line endocrine treatment for hirsutism and acne, after cosmetic and dermatologic management. The estrogenic component of most oral contraceptives currently in use is either ethinyl estradiol or mestranol. The suppression of LH leads to reduced

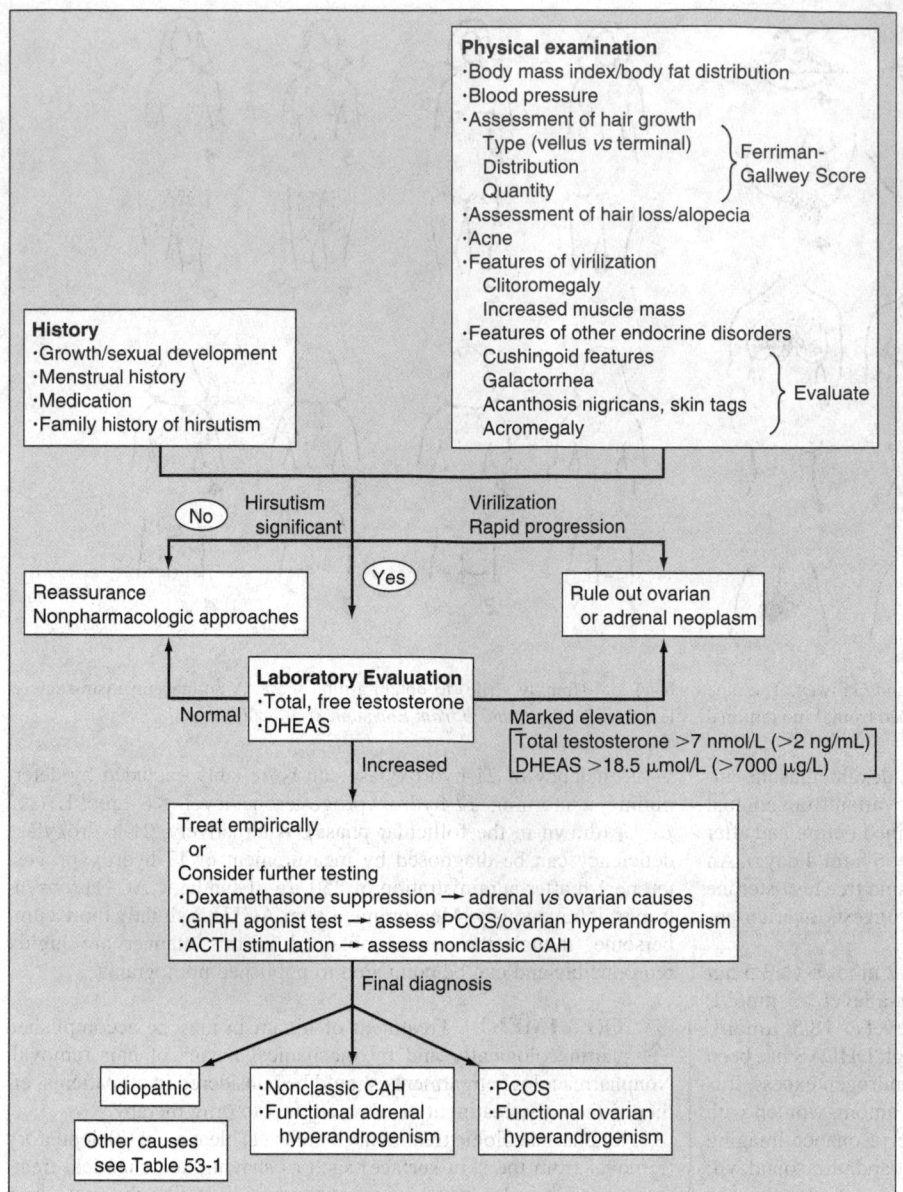

FIGURE 53-2 Algorithm for the evaluation and differential diagnosis of hirsutism. ACTH, adrenocorticotropic hormone; CAH, congenital adrenal hyperplasia; DHEAS, sulfated form of dehydroepiandrosterone; GnRH, gonadotropin-releasing hormone; PCOS, polycystic ovarian syndrome.

trast, the effect on hair growth may not be evident for 6 months, and the maximum effect may require 9 to 12 months owing to the length of the hair growth cycle. Improvements in hirsutism are typically in the range of 20%, and often there is little more than arrest of further progression of hair growth.

Adrenal androgens are more sensitive than cortisol to the suppressive effects of glucocorticoids. Therefore, glucocorticoids are the mainstay of treatment in patients with CAH. Although glucocorticoids have been reported to restore ovulatory function in some women with PCOS, this effect is highly variable. Because of side effects from excessive glucocorticoids, low doses should be used. Dexamethasone (0.2 to 0.5 mg) or prednisone (5 to 10 mg) should be given at bedtime to achieve maximal suppression by inhibiting the nocturnal surge of ACTH.

Cyproterone acetate is the prototypic antiandrogen. It acts mainly by competitive inhibition of the binding of testosterone and DHT to the androgen receptor. In addition, it may act to enhance the metabolic clearance of testosterone by inducing hepatic enzymes. Although not available for use in the United States, cyproterone acetate is widely used in Canada, Mexico, and Europe. Cyproterone (50 to 100 mg) is given on days 1 to 15 and ethinyl estradiol (50 μg) is given on days 5 to 26 of the menstrual cycle. Side effects of cyproterone acetate include irregular uterine bleeding, nausea, headache, fatigue, weight gain, and decreased libido.

Spironolactone, usually used as a mineralocorticoid antagonist, is also a weak antiandrogen. It is almost as effective as cyproterone acetate when used at high enough doses (100 to 200 mg daily). Patients should be monitored intermittently for hyperkalemia or hypotension, though these side effects are uncommon. Pregnancy should be avoided because of the risk of feminization of a male fetus. Spironolactone can also cause menstrual irregularity. It is often used in combination with an oral contraceptive, which helps in prevention of pregnancy and suppression of ovarian androgen production.

production of ovarian androgens. The reduced androgen levels also result in a dose-related increase in SHBG, thereby lowering the fraction of unbound plasma testosterone. Combination therapy has also been demonstrated to decrease DHEAS, perhaps by reducing ACTH levels. Estrogens also have a direct, dose-dependent suppressive effect on sebaceous cell function.

The choice of a specific oral contraceptive should be predicated on the progestational component, as progestins vary in their suppressive effect on SHBG levels and in their androgenic potential. Ethynodiol diacetate has relatively low androgenic potential, whereas progestins such as norgestrel and levonorgestrel are particularly androgenic, as judged from their attenuation of the estrogen-induced increase in SHBG. Norgestimate exemplifies the newer generation of progestins that are virtually nonandrogenic. Oral contraceptives are contraindicated in women with a history of thromboembolic disease or in women with breast cancer or other estrogen-dependent cancers (Chap. 336). There is a relative contraindication to the use of oral contraceptives in smokers or in those with hypertension or a history of migraine headaches. In most trials, estrogen-progestin therapy alone improves the extent of acne by a maximum of 50 to 70%. In con-

Flutamide is a potent nonsteroidal antiandrogen that is effective in treating hirsutism, but concerns about the induction of hepatocellular dysfunction have limited its use. Finasteride is a competitive inhibitor of 5α-reductase type 2. Beneficial effects on hirsutism have been reported, but the prominence of 5α-reductase type 1 in the pilosebaceous unit appears to account for its limited efficacy. Finasteride would also be expected to impair sexual differentiation in a male fetus, and thus it should be used in women who may become pregnant.

A prospective, randomized trial comparing low-dose flutamide, finasteride, and combination cyproterone acetate–ethinyl estradiol demonstrated relative superiority of flutamide and cyproterone acetate–ethinyl estradiol in the treatment of hirsutism. Ultimately, the choice of any specific agent(s) must be tailored to the unique needs of the patient being treated. As noted previously, pharmacologic treatments for hirsutism should be used in conjunction with nonpharmacologic approaches. Patients should be reminded about the relatively slow and usually modest responses to pharmacologic treatment. It is also helpful to review the pattern of female hair distribution in the normal population to dispel unrealistic expectations.

BIBLIOGRAPHY

DIERICKX C et al: A clinical overview of hair removal using lasers and light sources. Dermatol Clin 17:357, 1999

EHRMANN DA, ROSENFIELD RL: Clinical review: An endocrinologic approach to the patient with hirsutism. J Clin Endocrinol Metab 71:1, 1990

———— et al: Polycystic ovary syndrome as a form of functional ovarian hyperandrogenism due to dysregulation of androgen secretion. Endocr Rev 16:322, 1995

———— et al: Hyperandrogenism, hirsutism, and polycystic ovarian syndrome, in *Endocrinology*, 4th ed, LJ DeGroot et al (eds). Philadelphia, Saunders, 2000, chap 160

PAUS R, COTSARELIS G: The biology of hair follicles. N Engl J Med 341:491, 1999

RITTMASTER RS: Antiandrogen treatment of polycystic ovary syndrome. Endocrinol Metab Clin North Am 28:409, 1999

VENTUROLI S et al: A prospective randomized trial comparing low dose flutamide, finasteride, ketoconazole, and cyproterone acetate–estrogen regimens in the treatment of hirsutism. J Clin Endocrinol Metab 84:1304, 1999

54	*Janet E. Hall*

INFERTILITY AND FERTILITY CONTROL

FDA	Food and Drug Administration	IUI	intrauterine insemination
FSH	follicle-stimulating hormone	IVF	in vitro fertilization
GnRH	gonadotropin-releasing hormone	LH	luteinizing hormone
hCG	human chorionic gonadotropin	PCOS	polycystic ovarian syndrome
ICSI	intracytoplasmic sperm injection	STDs	sexually transmitted diseases
IUD	intrauterine device		

The concept of reproductive choice is now firmly entrenched in developed countries and has dramatically altered reproductive behavior. The availability of effective contraceptive methods prevents unintended pregnancies and gives women the option of pursuing educational and career opportunities without interruption. Population control also has important economic and social implications. Infertility, on the other hand, can be accompanied by substantial stress and disappointment. Fortunately, the ability to diagnose and to treat various causes of infertility now provides an array of effective new approaches to this condition.

INFERTILITY

DEFINITION AND PREVALENCE *Infertility* is defined as the inability to conceive after 12 months of unprotected sexual intercourse. In a study of 5574 English and American women who ultimately conceived, pregnancy occurred in 50% within 3 months, 72% within 6 months, and 85% within 12 months. These findings are consistent with predictions based on *fecundability*, the probability of achieving pregnancy in one menstrual cycle (approximately 20 to 25% in healthy young couples). Assuming a fecundability of 0.25, 98% of couples should conceive within 13 months. Based on this definition, the National Survey of Family Growth reports a 14% rate of infertility in the United States in married women aged 15 to 44. The infertility rate has remained relatively stable over the past 30 years, although the proportion of couples without children has risen, reflecting a trend to delay childbearing. This trend has important implications because of an age-related decrease in fecundability, which begins at age 35, and decreases markedly after age 40.

CAUSES OF INFERTILITY There is a spectrum of infertility, ranging from reduced conception rates or the need for medical intervention to irreversible causes of infertility (*sterility*). Infertility can be attributed primarily to male factors in 25%, female factors in 58%, and is unexplained in about 17% of couples (Fig. 54-1). Not uncommonly, both male and female factors contribute to infertility.

————————— *Approach to the Patient* —————————

Initial Evaluation In all couples presenting with infertility, the initial evaluation includes discussion of the appropriate timing of in-tercourse and a description of the range of investigations that may be required. A brief description of infertility treatment options, including adoption, should be reviewed. Initial investigations are focused on determining whether the primary cause of the infertility is male, female, or both. These investigations include a semen analysis in the male, confirmation of ovulation in the female, and, in the majority of situations, documentation of tubal patency in the female. Although frequently used in the past, recent studies have not supported the efficacy of postcoital testing of sperm interaction with cervical mucus as a routine component of initial testing. Strategies for further evaluation are described below and in Chaps. 335 and 336. In some cases, after an extensive workup excluding all male and female factors, a specific cause cannot be identified and infertility may ultimately be classified as unexplained.

Psychological Aspects of Infertility Infertility is invariably associated with psychological stress related not only to the diagnostic and therapeutic procedures themselves but also to repeated cycles of hope and loss associated with each new procedure or cycle of treatment that does not result in the birth of a child. These feelings are often combined with a sense of isolation from friends and family. Counseling and stress-management techniques should be introduced early in the evaluation of infertility. In addition to the psychological benefits of stress management, it is possible that stress contributes to infertility in some couples (e.g., impaired ovulation). Importantly, infertility and its treatment do not appear to be associated with long-term psychological sequelae.

Female Causes Abnormalities in menstrual function constitute the most common cause of female infertility. These disorders, which include ovulatory dysfunction and abnormalities of the uterus or outflow tract, may present as amenorrhea (absence of menses) or as irregular or short menstrual cycles. A careful history and physical examination and a limited number of laboratory tests will help to determine whether the abnormality is: (1) hypothalamic or pituitary [low follicle-stimulating hormone (FSH), luteinizing hormone (LH), and estradiol with or without an increase in prolactin]; (2) polycystic ovarian syndrome (PCOS; irregular cycles and hyperandrogenism in the absence of other causes of androgen excess); (3) ovarian (low estradiol with increased FSH); or (4) uterine or outflow tract abnormality. The frequency of these diagnoses depends on whether the amenorrhea is primary or occurs after normal puberty and menarche (Fig. 54-1). →*The approach to further evaluation of these disorders is described in detail in Chap. 52.*

Ovulatory dysfunction In women with a history of regular menstrual cycles, *evidence of ovulation* should be sought by using urinary ovulation predictor kits (they reflect the preovulatory gonadotropin surge but do not confirm ovulation), basal body temperature charts, or a mid-luteal phase progesterone level. The mid-luteal phase progesterone increase (usually >3 ng/mL) confirms ovulation and corpus luteum function and is responsible for the rise in basal body temperature [0.3°C (>0.6°F) for 10 days]. An endometrial biopsy to exclude luteal phase insufficiency is no longer considered an essential part of the infertility workup for most patients. Even in the presence of ovulatory cycles, evaluation of *ovarian reserve* is recommended for women over 35 by measurement of FSH on day 3 of the cycle or in response to clomiphene, an estrogen antagonist (see below). An FSH level <10 IU/mL on cycle day 3 predicts adequate ovarian oocyte reserve. Inhibin B, an ovarian hormone that selectively suppresses FSH, is being investigated as an additional marker of ovarian reserve.

Tubal disease This may result from pelvic inflammatory disease (PID), appendicitis, endometriosis, pelvic adhesions, tubal surgery, and previous use of an intrauterine device (IUD). However, a cause is not identified in up to 50% of patients with documented tubal factor infertility. Because of the high prevalence of tubal disease, testing should occur early in the majority of couples with infertility. Subclinical infections with *Chlamydia trachomatis* may be an underdiagnosed cause of tubal infertility and requires the treatment of both partners.

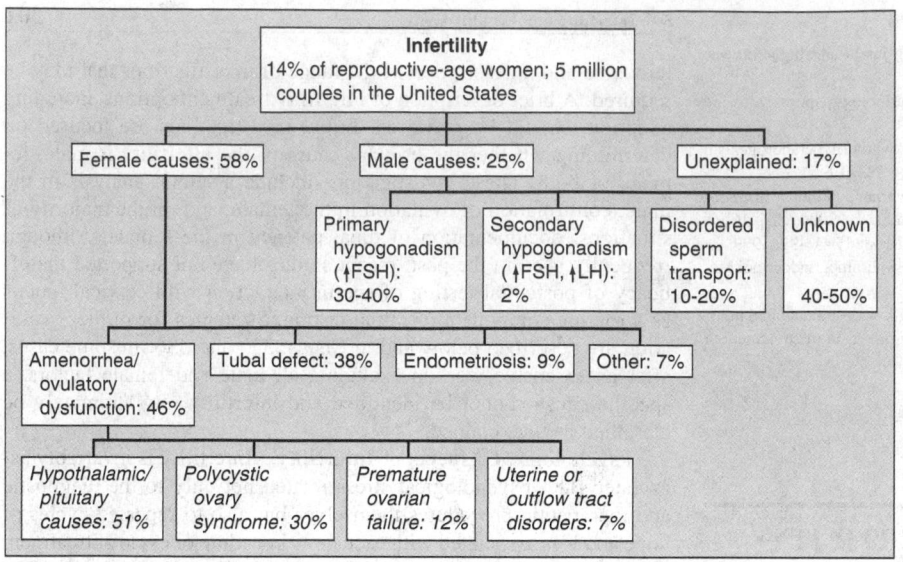

FIGURE 54-1 Causes of infertility. FSH, follicle-stimulating hormone; LH, luteinizing hormone.

A hysterosalpingogram (HSG) is the most common screening test and will determine the presence of tubal patency and identify potential abnormalities of the uterine cavity.

Endometriosis Endometriosis is defined as the presence of endometrial glands or stroma outside the endometrial cavity and uterine musculature. Its presence is suggested by a history of dyspareunia (painful intercourse), worsening dysmenorrhea that often begins before menses, or by a thickened rectovaginal septum or deviation of the cervix on pelvic examination. The pathogenesis of the infertility associated with endometriosis is unclear but may involve indirect effects on the normal endometrium as well as the direct effects of adhesions in advanced disease. Endometriosis is often clinically silent, however, and can only be excluded definitively by laparoscopy.

Male Causes Known causes of male infertility include primary testicular disease, disorders of sperm transport, and hypothalamic-pituitary disease resulting in secondary hypogonadism. However, the etiology is not ascertained in up to half of men with suspected male factor infertility (Fig. 54-1). The key initial diagnostic test is a *semen analysis.* Although 95% confidence limits can be used to define normal semen parameters, data relating sperm counts to fecundability are more useful. Such studies suggest that sperm counts of <20 million/mL, with a motility of less than 40%, are associated with an increased risk of infertility. Analysis of sperm morphology is less well validated, but >40% normal forms are usually present in fertile men. Successful in vitro fertilization (IVF) can usually be accomplished with >14% normal forms (using strict Kruger criteria), whereas low fertilization is seen with <4% normal forms. Other tests such as the hamster egg penetration test and the zona-binding assay are not of proven value.

Testosterone levels should be measured if the sperm count is low on repeated examination or if there is clinical evidence of hypogonadism. A low testosterone level may result from *primary gonadal deficiency*; in this condition, levels of LH and FSH will be elevated. Less commonly, low testosterone and decreased spermatogenesis result from hypothalamic or pituitary disease, in which case the LH and FSH levels will be low (Chap. 335).

Abnormalities of spermatogenesis may have a genetic component. Y chromosome microdeletions and substitutions are increasingly recognized as a cause of *azoospermia* (absence of sperm) or *oligospermia* (low sperm count). Microdeletions (Yq6 region) have also been identified in a subset of men with elevated FSH levels or otherwise idiopathic infertility. Several candidate genes have been identified including *DAZ* (deleted in azoospermia) and *YRRM* (Y chromosome RNA recognition motif).

Acquired disorders of the testes are often associated with impaired spermatogenesis with relatively preserved Leydig cell function; thus,

testosterone levels may be normal. Such abnormalities include viral orchitis (especially mumps) and other infectious causes such as tuberculosis or sexually transmitted diseases (STDs), chemotherapy (especially the alkylating agents cyclophosphamide and chlorambucil), ionizing radiation, and drugs that may impair fertility directly or through inhibition of testicular androgen production or action. Anabolic androgen abuse should be considered in a well-androgenized man with low gonadotropins and testosterone but a suppressed sperm count. Prolonged elevation of testicular temperature may impair spermatogenesis, e.g., after an acute febrile illness or in association with varicocele. A potential role for environmental toxins as a cause of impaired spermatogenesis has been suggested based on an apparent decrease in sperm counts over the past several decades, but a direct cause-and-effect relationship has not been established.

Secondary hypogonadism Low gonadotropin levels, associated with low testosterone, may signal the presence of a pituitary macroadenoma or hypothalamic tumor (in both cases prolactin levels may be elevated; Chap. 328) or may be the first presentation of hemochromatosis (Chap. 345) or other systemic illness. Recent studies have identified several genetic causes of gonadotropin-releasing hormone (GnRH) deficiency (*KAL* and *DAX-1*), as well as mutations that lead to isolated gonadotropin deficiency (GnRH receptor, LHβ, FSHβ mutations) (Chap. 328).

Disordered sperm transport Patients with low sperm counts and normal hormonal levels may be found to have obstructive abnormalities of the vas deferens or epididymus. The most common causes of vas deferens obstruction are previous vasectomy or accidental ligation during inguinal surgery. Patency rates with microsurgical reversal techniques are high in the first 3 years after vasectomy but decrease markedly thereafter. Congenital absence of the vas deferens can be diagnosed by a deficiency of fructose in the ejaculate and is often associated with an abnormality of the cystic fibrosis transmembrane regulator (*CFTR*) gene. Young's syndrome, characterized by inspissated secretions, can also preclude normal sperm transport.

TREATMENT The treatment of infertility should be tailored to the problems unique to each couple (Table 54-1). In many situations, including unexplained infertility, mild to moderate endometriosis, and/or borderline semen parameters, a stepwise approach to infertility is optimal, beginning with low-risk interventions and moving to more invasive, higher risk interventions only if necessary. After determination of all infertility factors and their correction, if possible, this approach might include, in increasing order of complexity: (1) expectant management, (2) clomiphene citrate (see below) with or without intrauterine insemination (IUI), (3) gonadotropins with or without IUI, and (4) IVF. The time used to complete the evaluation, correction, and expectant management can be longer in women <30, but this process should be advanced rapidly in women >35. In some situations expectant management will not be appropriate.

Ovulatory Dysfunction Treatment of ovulatory dysfunction should first be directed at identification of the etiology of the disorder to allow specific management when possible. Dopamine agonists, for example, may be indicated in patients with hyperprolactinemia (Chap. 328); lifestyle modification may be successful in women with low body weight or a history of intensive exercise (Chap. 78).

Pulsatile GnRH is highly effective for restoring ovulation in patients with hypothalamic amenorrhea. When administered subcutaneously by an automated pump at a physiologic dose and frequency, pulsatile GnRH induces normal LH and FSH dynamics. Direct comparisons between pulsatile GnRH and gonadotropin treatment for ovulation induction indicate similar pregnancy rates; pulsatile GnRH is associated with lower rates of multiple gestation and virtually no risk of ovarian hyperstimulation.

Clomiphene citrate is a nonsteroidal estrogen antagonist that increases FSH and LH levels by blocking estrogen negative feedback at the hypothalamus. The efficacy of clomiphene for ovulation induction is highly dependent on patient selection. It induces ovulation in ~60% of women with PCOS and is the initial treatment of choice in these patients. The starting dose is 50 mg daily for 5 days beginning on day 5 of a spontaneous cycle or after a progestin-induced withdrawal bleed. The dose can be increased to 150 mg, if necessary, in subsequent cycles, and human chorionic gonadotropin (hCG) can be added as the ovulatory stimulus. In women with PCOS, the use of insulin-sensitizing agents, such as metformin appears to be particularly effective in combination with clomiphene.

Gonadotropins are highly effective for ovulation induction in women with hypogonadotropic hypogonadism and PCOS. Gonadotropins are also used to induce multiple follicular recruitment in unexplained infertility and in older reproductive-aged women, particularly in conjunction with IUI. Disadvantages include a significant risk of multiple gestation and the risk of ovarian hyperstimulation, a side effect that is more common in women with PCOS. However, careful monitoring and a conservative approach to ovarian stimulation reduce these risks; gonadotropin stimulation is an effective and safe treatment when applied by experienced practitioners. Currently available gonadotropins include urinary preparations of LH and FSH, highly purified FSH, and recombinant FSH. Though FSH is the key component, there is growing data that the addition of some LH (or hCG) may improve results, particularly in hypogonadotropic patients.

None of these methods are effective in women with premature ovarian failure in whom donor oocyte or adoption are the methods of choice.

Tubal Disease   If hysterosalpingography suggests a tubal or uterine cavity abnormality, or if a patient is ≥35 at the time of initial evaluation, laparoscopy with tubal lavage is recommended, often with a hysteroscopy. Although tubal reconstruction may be attempted if tubal disease is identified, it is generally being replaced by the use of IVF, as these patients are at increased risk of developing an ectopic pregnancy.

Endometriosis   Though 60% of women with minimal or mild endometriosis may conceive within 1 year without treatment, laparoscopic resection or ablation appear to improve conception rates. Medical management of advanced stages of endometriosis is widely used for symptom control but has not been shown to enhance fertility (Chap. 336). In moderate to severe endometriosis, conservative surgery is associated with pregnancy rates of 50 and 39% respectively, compared with rates of 25 and 5% with expectant management alone. In some patients, IVF may be the treatment of choice.

Male Factor Infertility   The treatment options for male factor infertility have expanded greatly in recent years. Secondary hypogonadism is highly amenable to treatment with pulsatile GnRH or gonadotropins (Chap. 335). In vitro techniques have provided new opportunities for patients with primary testicular failure and disorders of sperm transport. Choice of initial treatment options depends on sperm concentration and motility. Expectant management should be attempted initially in men with mild male factor infertility (sperm count of 15 to 20 × 10^6/mL and normal motility). Moderate male factor infertility (10 to 15 × 10^6/mL and 20 to 40% motility) should begin with IUI alone or in combination with treatment of the female partner with clomiphene or gonadotropins, but it may require IVF with or without intracytoplasmic sperm injection (ICSI). For men with a severe defect (sperm count of <10 × 10^6/mL, 10% motility), IVF with ICSI or donor sperm should be used.

Assisted Reproductive Technologies   The development of assisted reproductive technologies (ART) has dramatically altered the treatment of male and female infertility. IVF is indicated for patients with many causes of infertility that have not been successfully managed with more conservative approaches. IVF or ICSI is often the treatment of choice in couples with a significant male factor or tubal disease, whereas IVF using donor oocytes is used in patients with premature ovarian failure and in women of advanced reproductive age. Success rates depend on the age of the woman and the cause of the infertility and are generally 18 to 24% per cycle when initiated in women <40. In women >40, there is a marked decrease in both the number of oocytes retrieved and their ability to be fertilized. Though often effective, IVF is expensive and requires careful monitoring of ovulation induction and invasive techniques including the aspiration of multiple follicles. IVF is associated with a significant risk of multiple gestation (29% twins, 7% triplets, and 0.6% higher order multiples). More recently developed blastocyst transfer protocols decrease the number of transfers but increase pregnancy rates.

CONTRACEPTION

Though various forms of contraception are widely available, approximately 30% of births in the United States are the result of unintended pregnancy. Teenage pregnancies continue to represent a serious public health problem in the United States, with >1 million unintended pregnancies each year—a significantly greater incidence than in other industrialized nations (Chap. 8).

Contraceptive methods are widely used (Table 54-2). Only 15% of couples report having unprotected sexual intercourse in the past 3 months. A reversible form of contraception is used by >50% of couples. Sterilization (in either the male or female) has been employed as a permanent form of contraception by about 25% of couples. Preg-

Table 54-1   Treatment Approaches for Various Causes of Infertility

	Surgery	Clomiphene	Gonadotropins	Pulsatile GnRH	IUI	Donor Sperm	IVF	ICSI	Donor Egg
FEMALE									
Ovulatory dysfunction									
Hypothalamic-pituitary			✔	✔					
Polycystic ovary syndrome		✔	✔	✔					
Premature ovarian failure									✔
Tubal disease	✔						✔		
Endometriosis	✔	✔	✔		✔		✔		
MALE									
Primary hypogonadism						✔	✔	✔	
Secondary hypogonadism			✔						
Disorders of sperm transport	✔						✔	✔	
Unexplained		✔	✔		✔		✔		

NOTE: GnRH, gonadotropin-releasing hormone; IUI, intrauterine insemination; IVF, in vitro fertilization; ICSI, intracytoplasmic sperm injection.

Table 54-2 Effectiveness of Different Forms of Contraception

Method of Contraception	Theoretical Effectiveness[a]	Actual Effectiveness[a]	Percent Continuing Use at 1 year[b]	Contraceptive Methods used by U.S. women[c]
Barrier methods				
Condoms	98	88	63	19
Diaphragm	94	82	58	2
Cervical cap	94	82	50	<1
Spermacides	97	79	43	1
Sterilization				
Male	99.9	99.9	100	10
Female	99.8	99.6	100	15
Intrauterine device				1
Copper T380	99	97	78	
Progestasert	98	97	81	
Oral contraceptive pill			72	26
Combination	99.9	97		
Progestin only	99.5	97		
Long-acting progestins				
Depo-Provera	99.7	99.7	70	<1
Norplant	99.96	99.96	85	1

[a] Adapted from Trussel J et al, Obstet Gynecol 76:558, 1990.
[b] Adapted from Contraceptive Technology Update. Contraceptive Technology, Feb. 1996, vol 17, No 1, pp 13–24.
[c] Adapted from 1995 Ortho Birth Control Survey. Raritan, NJ, Ortho Pharmaceutical, 1996. 20% used no method, 5% used other.

nancy termination is relatively safe when directed by health care professionals but is rarely the option of choice.

No single contraceptive method is ideal, although all are safer than carrying a pregnancy to term. The effectiveness of a given method of contraception is dependent on the efficacy of the method itself, compliance, and appropriate use. Knowledge of the advantages and disadvantages of each contraceptive is essential for counseling an individual about the methods that are safest and most consistent with his or her lifestyle. Discrepancies between theoretical and actual effectiveness emphasize the importance of patient education and compliance when considering various forms of contraception (Table 54-2).

BARRIER METHODS Barrier contraceptives, such as condoms, diaphragms, cervical caps, and spermicides, are easily available, reversible, and have fewer side effects than hormonal methods. However, their effectiveness is highly dependent on compliance and proper use (Table 54-2). A major advantage of barrier contraceptives is the protection provided against STDs (Chap. 132). Consistent use is associated with a decreased risk of gonorrhea, nongonococcal urethritis, and genital herpes, probably due in part to the concomitant use of spermicides. Condom use also reduces the transmission of HIV infection. Natural membrane condoms may be less effective than latex condoms, and petroleum-based lubricants can degrade condoms and decrease their efficacy for preventing HIV infection. A highly effective female condom, which also provides protection against STDs, was approved in 1994 but has not achieved widespread use.

STERILIZATION Sterilization is the method of birth control most frequently chosen by fertile men and multiparous women >30 (Table 54-2). Sterilization refers to a procedure that prevents fertilization by surgical interruption of the fallopian tubes in women or the vas deferens in men. Although tubal ligation and vasectomy are potentially reversible, these procedures should be considered permanent and should not be undertaken without careful patient counseling.

Several methods of *tubal ligation* have been developed, all of which are highly effective with a 10-year cumulative pregnancy rate of 1.85 per 100 women. However, when pregnancy does occur, the risk of ectopic pregnancy may be as high as 30%. The success rate of tubal reanastomosis depends on the method used—the clip, silastic band, and modified Pomeroy procedures are easier to reverse than the Irving, Uchida, and electrocoagulation methods. Even after successful

reversal, the risk of ectopic pregnancy remains great. In addition to prevention of pregnancy, tubal ligation reduces the risk of ovarian cancer, possibly by limiting the upward migration of potential carcinogens.

Vasectomy is an outpatient surgical procedure that has little risk and is highly effective. The development of azoospermia may be delayed for 2 to 6 months, and other forms of contraception must be used until two sperm-free ejaculations provide proof of sterility. Reanastomosis may restore fertility in 30 to 50% of men, but the success rate appears to decline with time after vasectomy and may be influenced by nonmechanical factors such as the development of anti-sperm antibodies.

INTRAUTERINE DEVICES IUDs inhibit pregnancy primarily through a spermicidal effect caused by a sterile inflammatory reaction produced by the presence of a foreign body in the uterine cavity. There may also be effects on cervical mucus sperm transport through the oviduct. IUDs provide a high level of efficacy in the absence of systemic metabolic effects. An additional advantage is that ongoing motivation is not required to ensure efficacy once the device has been placed. However, only 1% of women in the United States use this method compared to a utilization rate of 15 to 30% in much of Europe and Canada. This relatively low utilization rate continues despite evidence that the newer devices are not associated with increased rates of pelvic infection and infertility, as occurred with earlier devices. Screening for STD should be performed prior to insertion, and an IUD should not be used in women at high risk for development of STD or in women at high risk for bacterial endocarditis. In addition, the IUD may not be effective in women with uterine leiomyomas because they alter the size or shape of the uterine cavity. IUD use is associated with increased menstrual blood flow, although this is less pronounced with the progesterone-releasing IUD than the copper-containing device.

HORMONAL METHODS No male hormonal contraceptive methods are currently approved in the United States. However, hormonal methods of male contraception, including GnRH-mediated suppression of the hypothalamic-pituitary-gonadal axis in combination with testosterone replacement, are under investigation.

Oral Contraceptive Pills Because of their ease of use and efficacy, oral contraceptive pills are the most widely used form of hormonal contraception. They act by suppressing ovulation, changing cervical mucus, and altering the endometrium. The current formulations are made from synthetic estrogens and progestins. The estrogen component of the pill consists of ethinyl estradiol or mestranol, which is metabolized to ethinyl estradiol. Multiple synthetic progestins are used. Norethindrone and its derivatives are used in many formulations. Low-dose norgestimate and third-generation progestins (desogestrel, gestodene) have a less androgenic profile; levonorgestrel appears to be the most androgenic of the progestins and should be avoided in patients with hyperandrogenic symptoms. The three major formulations of oral contraceptives include: (1) fixed-dose estrogen-progestin combination, (2) phasic estrogen-progestin combination, and (3) progestin only. Each of these formulations is administered daily for 3 weeks followed by a week of no medication during which menstrual bleeding generally occurs.

Current doses of ethinyl estradiol range from 20 to 50 μg. However, indications for the 50-μg dose are rare, and the majority of formulations contain 35 μg of ethinyl estradiol. The reduced estrogen and progesterone content in the second- and third-generation pills has decreased both side effects and risks associated with oral contraceptive use. At the currently used doses, patients must be cautioned not to miss pills due to the potential for ovulation. Side effects, including break-through bleeding, amenorrhea, and weight gain, are often responsive to a change in formulation. There is no evidence that low-dose oral contraceptives increase the risk of cardiovascular disease in women <30 or in nonsmoking women without additional risk factors. However, the risk of myocardial infarction and stroke in women who smoke is increased by the use of oral contraceptives. The risk of developing hypertension is increased somewhat, even with the low-dose preparations. An increased risk of venous thromboembolism occurs with all oral contraceptives and may be even greater with the third-generation preparations. The factor V Leiden mutation and other thrombophilic disorders (Chap. 117) are important risk factors for venous thrombosis during oral contraceptive therapy. However, biochemical or genetic screening for these disorders before starting oral contraceptives is not cost-effective at present. In most studies, oral contraceptive use has not been shown to increase the risk of breast cancer, but there is a slight increase in the risk of cervical cancer. Risks for endometrial and ovarian cancer are decreased in oral contraceptive users.

Previous thromboembolic events or stroke are absolute contraindications for the use of oral contraceptive pills. A history of hormone-dependent tumors and liver disease are also contraindications. Oral contraceptive pills should not be given in pregnancy or in women with undiagnosed uterine bleeding or amenorrhea.

The microdose progestin-only minipill is less effective as a contraceptive, having a pregnancy rate of 2 to 7 per 100 women-years. However, it may be appropriate for women with cardiovascular disease or for women who cannot tolerate synthetic estrogens.

Injectable Contraceptives   Depot medroxyprogesterone acetate (Depo-Provera) and Norplant (Table 54-2) act primarily by inhibiting ovulation and causing changes in the endometrium and cervical mucus that result in decreased implantation and sperm transport. Depo-Provera is effective for 3 months, but return of fertility after discontinuation may be delayed for up to 12 to 18 months. Norplant requires surgical insertion but is effective for up to 5 years afer insertion; fertility is possible shortly after its removal. The U.S. Food and Drug Administration (FDA) has recently approved the use of covered rods in addition to the capsules. Amenorrhea, irregular bleeding, and weight gain are the most common adverse effects associated with both injectable forms of contraception. An injectable progestin/estrogen combination con-

traceptive will be available soon. It requires monthly injection, but irregular bleeding and weight gain are less common. A major advantage of the injectable progestin-based contraceptives is the apparent lack of increased arterial and venous thromboembolic events.

POSTCOITAL CONTRACEPTION   Postcoital contraceptive methods prevent implantation or cause regression of the corpus luteum and are highly efficacious if used appropriately. Although postcoital contraception is not specifically licensed for use in the United States, an FDA notice published in 1997 indicated that certain oral contraceptive pills could be used within 72 h of unprotected intercourse [Ovral (2 tablets 12 h apart) and Lo/Ovral (4 tablets 12 h apart)]. The Preven Emergency Contraceptive Kit contains four combination tablets (50 mg ethinyl estradiol and 0.25 mg levonorgestrel) and a pregnancy kit to rule out pregnancy before taking the pills. Side effects are common with these high doses of hormones and include nausea, vomiting, and breast soreness. Recent studies suggest that 600 mg mifepristone (RU486), a progesterone receptor antagonist, may be equally as effective or more effective than hormonal regimens, with fewer side effects. Mifepristone is not currently available in the United States.

BIBLIOGRAPHY

ABMA JC et al and the National Center for Health Statistics: Fertility, family planning, and women's health: New data from the 1995 Survey of Family Growth. Vital Statistics: Series 23, No. 10

BARBIERI RL: Assisted reproduction, in *Reproductive Endocrinology: Physiology, Pathophysiology and Clinical Management*, SSc Yen, RB Jaffe, RL Barbieri (eds). Philadelphia, Saunders, pp 594–621, 1999

———— et al: The safety of third-generation oral contraceptives. J Clin Endocrinol Metab 84:1822, 1999

BHASIN S et al: Y-chromosome microdeletions and male infertility. Ann Intern Med 29: 261, 1997

COLLINS JA: Unexplained infertility, in *Infertility: Evaluation and Treatment*, WR Keye et al (eds). Philadelphia, Saunders, 1995, pp 249–262

GLASIER A: Emergency postcoital contraception. N Engl J Med 337:1058, 1997

TRUSSELL J, VAUGHAN B: Contraceptive failure, method-related discontinuation and resumption of use: Results from the 1995 National Survey of Family Growth. Fam Plann Perspect 31:64, 1999

WANG C, SWERDLOFF R: Medical treatment of male infertility, in *Infertility: Evaluation and Treatment*, WR Keye et al (eds). Philadelphia, Saunders, 1995, pp 143–150

Section 9
ALTERATIONS IN THE SKIN

55   *Thomas J. Lawley, Kim B. Yancey*

APPROACH TO THE PATIENT WITH A SKIN DISORDER

The challenge of examining the skin lies in distinguishing normal from abnormal, significant findings from trivial ones, and in integrating pertinent signs and symptoms into an appropriate differential diagnosis. The fact that the largest organ in the body is visible is both an advantage and a disadvantage to those who examine it. It is advantageous because no special instrumentation, other than a magnifying glass, is necessary and because the skin can be biopsied with little morbidity. However, the casual observer can be overwhelmed by a variety of stimuli and overlook important, subtle signs of skin or systemic disease. For instance, the sometimes minor differences in color and shape that distinguish a malignant melanoma **(see Plate IIC-30)** from a benign pigmented nevus **(see Plate IIC-28)** can be difficult to recognize. To aid in the interpretation of skin lesions, a variety of descriptive

terms have been developed to characterize cutaneous lesions (Tables 55-1 and 55-2 and Fig. 55-1) and to formulate a differential diagnosis (Table 55-3). For instance, the finding of large numbers of scaling papules, usually indicative of a primary skin disease, places the patient in a different diagnostic category than would hemorrhagic papules, which may indicate vasculitis or sepsis **(see Plates IIE-71 and IID-44, respectively)**. It is important to differentiate primary skin lesions from secondary skin changes. If the examiner focuses on linear erosions overlying an area of erythema and scaling, he or she may incorrectly assume that the erosion is the primary lesion and the redness and scale are secondary, while the correct interpretation would be that the patient has a pruritic eczematous dermatitis and the erosions have been caused by scratching.

Approach to the Patient

In examining the skin it is usually advisable to assess the patient before taking a history. This way, the entire cutaneous surface is sure to be evaluated, and objective findings can be integrated with relevant historic data. Four basic features of any cutaneous lesion must be noted

Table 55-1　Descriptions of Primary Skin Lesions

Macule: A flat, colored lesion, <2 cm in diameter, not raised above the surface of the surrounding skin. A "freckle," or ephelid, is a prototype pigmented macule.

Patch: A large (>2 cm), flat lesion with a color different from the surrounding skin. This differs from a macule only in size.

Papule: A small, solid lesion, <1 cm in diameter, raised above the surface of the surrounding skin and hence palpable (e.g., a closed comedone, or whitehead, in acne).

Nodule: A larger (1–5 cm), firm lesion raised above the surface of the surrounding skin. This differs from a papule only in size (e.g., dermal nevus).

Tumor: A solid, raised growth >5 cm in diameter.

Plaque: A large (>1 cm), flat-topped, raised lesion; edges may either be distinct (e.g., in psoriasis) or gradually blend with surrounding skin (e.g., in eczematous dermatitis).

Vesicle: A small, fluid-filled lesion, <1 cm in diameter, raised above the plane of surrounding skin. Fluid is often visible, and the lesions are often translucent [e.g., vesicles in allergic contact dermatitis caused by *Toxicodendron* (poison ivy)].

Pustule: A vesicle filled with leukocytes. Note: The presence of pustules does not necessarily signify the existence of an infection.

Bulla: A fluid-filled, raised, often translucent lesion >1 cm in diameter.

Cyst: A soft, raised, encapsulated lesion filled with semisolid or liquid contents.

Wheal: A raised, erythematous papule or plaque, usually representing short-lived dermal edema.

Telangiectasia: Dilated, superficial blood vessels.

Table 55-2　Common Dermatologic Terms

Lichenification: A distinctive thickening of the skin that is characterized by accentuated skin-fold markings and that feels thick and firm on palpation.

Crust: Dried exudate of body fluids that may be either yellow (serous exudate) or red (hemorrhagic exudate).

Milia: Small, firm, white papules that are filled with keratin (and may in part resemble pustules).

Erosion: Loss of epidermis without an associated loss of dermis.

Ulcer: Loss of epidermis and at least a portion of the underlying dermis.

Excoriations: Linear, angular erosions that may be covered by crust and are caused by scratching.

Atrophy: An acquired loss of substance. In the skin, this may appear as a depression with intact epidermis (i.e., loss of dermal or subcutaneous tissue) or as sites of shiny, delicate, wrinkled lesions (i.e., epidermal atrophy).

Scar: A change in the skin secondary to trauma or inflammation. Sites may be erythematous, hypopigmented, or hypertrophic depending on their age or character. Sites on hair-bearing areas may be characterized by destruction of hair follicles.

Pruritus: A sensation that elicits the desire to scratch. Pruritus is often the predominant symptom of inflammatory skin diseases (e.g., atopic dermatitis, allergic contact dermatitis); it is also commonly associated with xerosis and aged skin. Systemic conditions that can be associated with pruritis include chronic renal disease, cholestasis, pregnancy, malignancy, polycythemia vera, and delusions of parasitosis.

and considered in the examination of skin: the distribution of the eruption, the type(s) of primary lesion, the shape of individual lesions, and the arrangement of the lesions. In the initial examination it is important that the patient be disrobed as completely as possible. This will minimize chances of missing important individual skin lesions and make it possible to assess the distribution of the eruption accurately. The patient should first be viewed from a distance of about 1.5 to 2 m (4 to 6 ft) so that the general character of the skin and the distribution of lesions can be evaluated. Indeed, distribution of lesions often correlates highly with diagnosis (Fig. 55-2). For example, a hospitalized patient with a generalized erythematous exanthem is more likely to have a drug eruption than is a patient with a similar rash limited to the sun-exposed portions of the face. The presence or absence of lesions on mucosal surfaces should also be determined. Once the distribution of the lesions has been established, the nature of the primary lesion must be determined. Thus, when lesions are distributed on elbows, knees, and scalp, the most likely possibility based solely on distribution is psoriasis or dermatitis herpetiformis **(see Plates IIA-3 and IIE-68, respectively)**. The primary lesion in psoriasis is a scaly papule that soon forms erythematous plaques covered with a white scale, whereas that of dermatitis herpetiformis is an urticarial papule that quickly becomes a small vesicle. In this manner, identification of the primary lesion directs the examiner toward the proper diagnosis. Secondary changes in skin can also be quite helpful. For example, scale represents excessive epidermis, while crust is the result of an inadequate or discontinuous epithelial cell layer. Palpation of skin lesions can also yield insight into the character of an eruption. Thus red papules on the lower extremities that blanch with pressure can be a manifestation of many different diseases, but hemorrhagic red papules that do not blanch with pressure indicate palpable purpura characteristic of necrotizing vasculitis **(see Plate IIE-71)**.

The shape of lesions is also an important feature. Flat, round, erythematous papules and plaques are common in many cutaneous diseases. However, target-shaped lesions that consist in part of erythematous plaques are specific for erythema multiforme **(see Plate IIE-67)**. In the same way, the arrangement of individual lesions is important. Erythematous papules and vesicles can occur in many conditions, but their arrangement in a specific linear array suggests an external etiology such as allergic contact **(see Plate IIA-8)** or primary irritant dermatitis. In contrast, lesions with a generalized arrangement are common and suggest a systemic etiology.

As in other branches of medicine, a complete history should be obtained to emphasize the following features:

1. Evolution of lesions
   a. Site of onset
   b. Manner in which eruption progressed or spread
   c. Duration
   d. Periods of resolution or improvement in chronic eruptions
2. Symptoms associated with the eruption
   a. Itching, burning, pain, numbness
   b. What, if anything, has relieved symptoms
   c. Time of day when symptoms are most severe
3. Current or recent medications (prescribed as well as over-the-counter)
4. Associated systemic symptoms (e.g., malaise, fever, arthralgias)
5. Ongoing or previous illnesses
6. History of allergies
7. Presence of photosensitivity
8. Review of systems

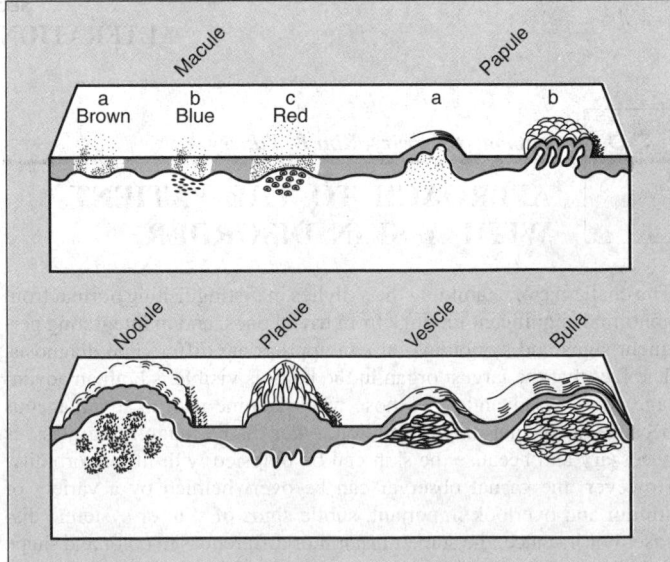

FIGURE 55-1 A schematic representation of several common primary skin lesions (see Table 55-1).

Table 55-3 Selected Common Dermatologic Conditions[a]

Diagnosis	Common Distribution	Usual Morphology	Diagnosis	Common Distribution	Usual Morphology
Acne vulgaris	Face, upper back	Open and closed comedones, erythematous papules, pustules, cysts	Seborrheic keratosis	Trunk, face	Brown plaques with adherent, greasy scale; "stuck on" appearance
Rosacea	Blush area of cheeks, nose, forehead, chin	Erythema, telangiectasias, papules, pustules	Folliculitis	Any hair-bearing area	Follicular pustules
Seborrheic dermatitis	Scalp, eyebrows, perinasal	Erythema with greasy yellow-brown scale	Impetigo	Anywhere	Papules, vesicles, pustules, often with honey-colored crusts
Atopic dermatitis	Antecubital and popliteal fossae; may be widespread	Patches and plaques of erythema, scaling, and lichenification; pruritus	Herpes simplex	Lips, genitalia	Grouped vesicles progressing to crusted erosions
Stasis dermatitis	Ankles, lower legs	Patches of erythema and scaling on background of hyperpigmentation associated with signs of venous insufficiency	Herpes zoster	Dermatomal, usually trunk but may be anywhere	Vesicles limited to a dermatome (often painful)
Dyshidrotic eczema	Palms, soles, sides of fingers and toes	Deep vesicles	Varicella	Face, trunk, relative sparing of extremities	Lesions arise in crops and quickly progress from erythematous macules to papules to vesicles to pustules to crusts
Allergic contact dermatitis	Anywhere	Localized erythema, vesicles, scale, and pruritus, e.g., fingers, earlobes—nickel; dorsal aspect of foot—shoe dermatitis; exposed surfaces—poison ivy dermatitis; etc.	Pityriasis rosea	Trunk (Christmas tree pattern) herald patch followed by multiple smaller lesions	Symmetric erythematous patches with a collarette of trailing scale
Psoriasis	Elbows, knees, scalp, lower back, fingernails (may be generalized)	Papules and plaques covered with silvery scale; nails have pits	Tinea versicolor	Chest, back, abdomen, proximal extremities	Scaly hyper- or hypopigmented macules
Lichen planus	Wrists, ankles, mouth (may be widespread)	Violaceous flat-topped papules and plaques	Candidiasis	Groin, beneath breasts, vagina, oral cavity	Erythematous macerated areas with satellite pustules; white, friable patches on mucous membranes
Keratosis pilaris	Extensor surfaces of arms and thighs, buttocks	Keratotic follicular papules with surrounding erythema	Dermatophytosis	Feet, groin, beard, or scalp	Varies with site, e.g., tinea corporis—scaly annular patch
Melasma	Forehead, cheeks, temples, upper lip	Tan to brown patches	Scabies	Groin, axillae, between fingers and toes, beneath breasts	Excoriated papules, burrows, pruritus
Vitiligo	Periorificial, trunk, extensor surfaces of extremities, flexor wrists, axillae	Chalk-white macules	Insect bites	Anywhere	Erythematous papules with central puncta
			Cherry angioma	Trunk	Red, blood-filled papules
Actinic keratosis	Sun-exposed areas	Skin-colored or red-brown macule or papule with dry, rough, adherent scale	Keloid	Anywhere (site of previous injury)	Firm tumor, pink, purple, or brown
			Dermatofibroma	Anywhere	Firm red to brown nodule that shows dimpling of overlying skin with lateral compression
Basal cell carcinoma	Face	Papule with pearly, telangiectatic border on sun-damaged skin	Acrochordons (skin tags)	Groin, axilla, neck	Fleshy papules
			Urticaria	Anywhere	Wheals, sometimes with surrounding flare, pruritus
Squamous cell carcinoma	Face, especially lower lip, ears	Indurated and possibly hyperkaratotic lesions often showing ulceration and/or crusting	Transient acantholytic dermatosis	Trunk, especially anterior chest	Erythematous papules
			Xerosis	Extensor extremities, especially legs	Dry, erythematous, scaling patches, pruritus

[a] See Color Plates for specific examples and additional information.

DIAGNOSTIC TECHNIQUES Many skin diseases can be diagnosed on gross clinical appearance, but sometimes relatively simple diagnostic procedures can yield valuable information. In most instances, they can be performed at the bedside with a minimum of equipment.

Skin Biopsy A skin biopsy is a straightforward minor surgical procedure; however, it is important to biopsy the anatomic site most likely to yield diagnostic findings. This decision may require expertise in skin diseases and knowledge of superficial anatomic structures in selected areas of the body. In this procedure, a small area of skin is anesthetized with 1% lidocaine with or without epinephrine. The skin lesion in question can be excised with a scalpel or removed by punch biopsy. In the latter technique, a punch is pressed against the surface of the skin and rotated with downward pressure until it penetrates to the subcutaneous tissue. The circular biopsy is then lifted with forceps, and the bottom is cut with iris scissors. Biopsy sites may or may not need suture closure, depending on size and location.

KOH Preparation A potassium hydroxide (KOH) preparation is performed on scaling skin lesions when a fungal etiology is suspected. The edge of such a lesion is scraped gently with a scalpel blade, and the removed scale is collected on a glass microscope slide and treated with 1 to 2 drops of a solution of 10 to 20% KOH. KOH dissolves keratin and allows easier visualization of fungal elements. Brief heating of the slide accelerates dissolution of keratin. When the preparation is viewed under the microscope, the refractile hyphae will be seen more easily when the light intensity is reduced. This technique can be utilized to identify hyphae in dermatophyte infections (**see Plate IID-51**), pseudohyphae and budding yeast in *Candida* infections (**see Plate IID-43**), and fragmented hyphae and spores in tinea versicolor. The same sampling technique

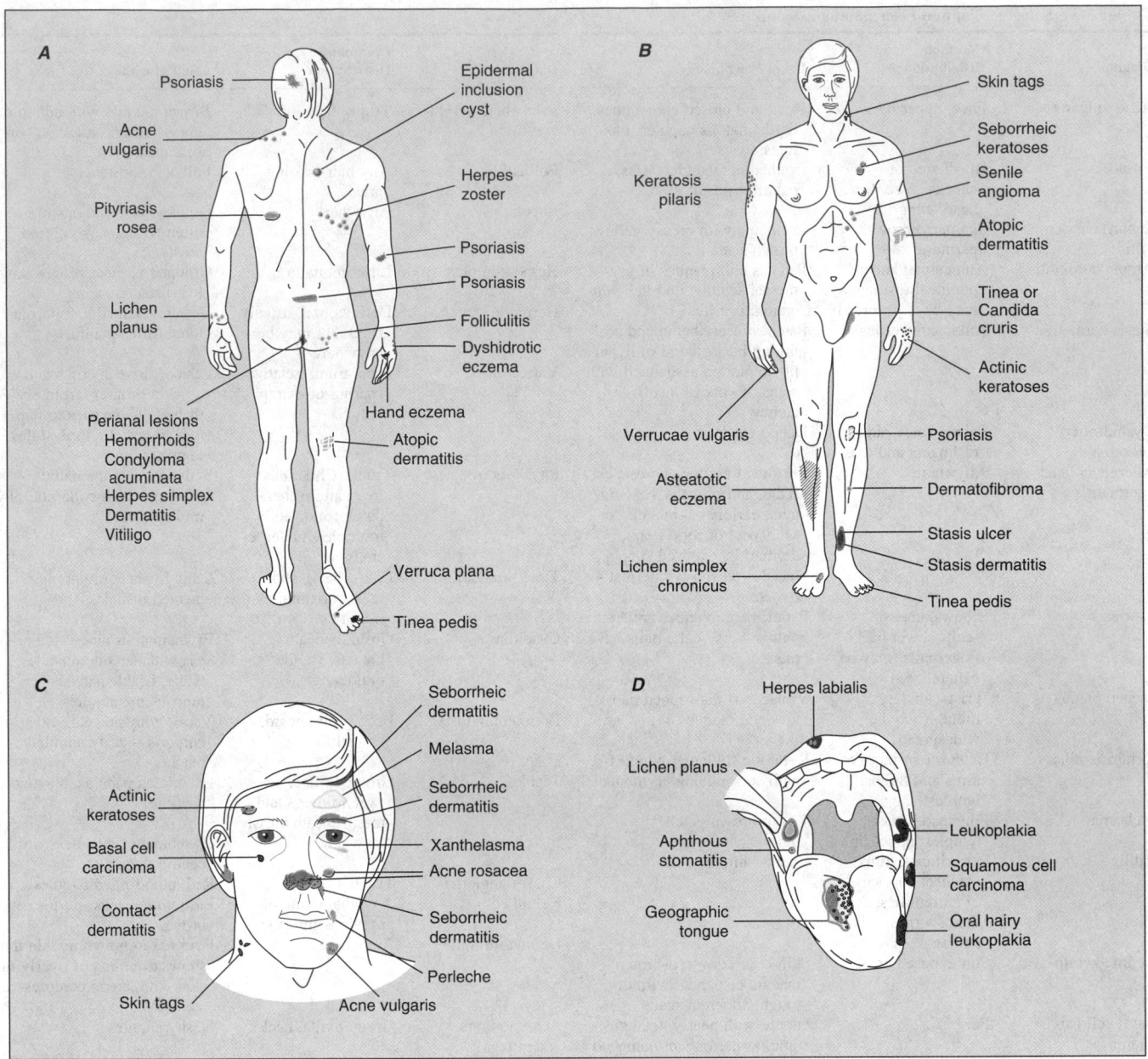

FIGURE 55-2 *A–D*. The distribution of some common dermatologic diseases and lesions.

can be used to obtain scale for culture of selected pathogenic organisms.

Tzanck Smear A Tzanck smear is a cytologic technique most often used in the diagnosis of herpesvirus infections [simplex or varicella-zoster (**see Plates IID-36 and IID-37**)]. An early vesicle, not a pustule or crusted lesion, is unroofed, and the base of the lesion is scraped gently with a scalpel blade. The material is placed on a glass slide, air-dried, and stained with Giemsa or Wright's stain. Multinucleated giant cells suggest the presence of herpes, but culture or immunofluorescence testing must be performed to identify the specific virus.

Diascopy Diascopy is designed to assess whether a skin lesion will blanch with pressure as, for example, in determining whether a red lesion is hemorrhagic or simply blood-filled. For instance, a hemangioma (**see Plate IIA-17**) will blanch with pressure, whereas a purpuric lesion caused by necrotizing vasculitis (**see Plate IIE-71**) will not. Diascopy is performed by pressing a microscope slide or magnifying lens against a specified lesion and noting the amount of blanching that occurs. Granulomas often have an "apple jelly" appearance on diascopy.

Wood's Light A Wood's lamp generates 360-nm ultraviolet (or "black") light that can be used to aid the evaluation of certain skin disorders. For example, a Wood's lamp will cause erythrasma (a superficial, intertriginous infection caused by *Corynebacterium minutissimum*) to show a characteristic coral red color, and wounds colonized by *Pseudomonas* to appear pale blue. Tinea capitis caused by certain dermatophytes such as *Microsporum canis* or *M. audouini* exhibits a yellow fluorescence. Pigmented lesions of the epidermis such as freckles are accentuated, while dermal pigment such as postinflammatory hyperpigmentation fades under a Wood's light. Vitiligo (**see Plate IIA-11**) appears totally white under a Wood's lamp, and previously unsuspected areas of involvement often become apparent. A Wood's lamp may also aid in the demonstration of tinea versicolor and in recognition of ash leaf spots in patients with tuberous sclerosis.

Patch Tests Patch testing is designed to document sensitivity to a specific antigen. In this procedure, a battery of suspected allergens is applied to the patient's back under occlusive dressings and allowed to remain in contact with the skin for 48 h. The dressings are removed, and the area is examined for evidence of delayed hypersensitivity reactions (e.g., erythema, edema, or papulovesicles). This test is best performed by physicians with special expertise in patch testing and is often helpful in the evaluation of patients with chronic dermatitis.

BIBLIOGRAPHY

ARNDT KA et al (eds): *Cutaneous Medicine and Surgery, An Integrated Program in Dermatology.* Philadelphia, Saunders, 1996

CHAMPION RH et al (eds): *Textbook of Dermatology,* 6th ed. Oxford, Blackwell Scientific, 1999

FREEDBERG IM et al (eds): *Fitzpatrick's Dermatology in General Medicine,* 5th ed. New York, McGraw-Hill, 1999

56 *Robert A. Swerlick, Thomas J. Lawley*

ECZEMA, PSORIASIS, CUTANEOUS INFECTIONS, ACNE, AND OTHER COMMON SKIN DISORDERS

ECZEMA AND DERMATITIS

Eczema, or dermatitis, is a reaction pattern that presents with variable clinical and histologic findings and is the final common expression for a number of disorders, including atopic dermatitis, allergic contact and irritant contact dermatitis, dyshidrotic eczema, nummular eczema, lichen simplex chronicus, asteatotic eczema, and seborrheic dermatitis. Primary lesions may include papules, erythematous macules, and vesicles, which can coalesce to form patches and plaques. In severe eczema, secondary lesions from infection or excoriation, marked by weeping and crusting, may predominate. Long-standing dermatitis is often dry and is characterized by thickened, scaling skin (*lichenification*).

ATOPIC DERMATITIS Atopic dermatitis (AD) is the cutaneous expression of the atopic state, characterized by a family history of asthma, hay fever, or dermatitis in up to 70% of patients. The criteria for the diagnosis of atopic eczema are shown in Table 56-1. The prevalence of atopic dermatitis is increasing worldwide, with a point prevalence in Norwegian school children as high as 23%.

The etiology of AD is only partially defined. There is a clear genetic predisposition. When both parents are affected by AD, over 80% of their children manifest the disease. When only one parent is affected, the prevalence drops to slightly over 50%. A number of genes have been tentatively linked to AD including genes coding for IgE, the high-affinity IgE receptor, mast cell tryptase, and interleukin (IL) 4. Patients with AD may display a variety of immunoregulatory abnormalities including increased IgE synthesis; increased specific IgE to foods, aeroallergens, bacteria, and bacterial products; increased expression of CD23 (low-affinity IgE receptor) on monocytes and B cells; impaired delayed type hypersensitivity reactions; and increased type II and decreased type I cytokine responses.

The clinical presentation often varies with age. Half of patients with AD present within the first year of life, and 80% present by 5 years of age. Some 80% ultimately coexpress allergic rhinitis or asthma later in life. The infantile pattern is characterized by weeping inflammatory patches and crusted plaques that occur on the face, neck, extensor surfaces, and groin. The childhood and adolescent pattern is

Table 56-1 Clinical Criteria for the Diagnosis of Atopic Dermatitis

1. Pruritus and scratching
2. Course marked by exacerbations and remissions
3. Lesions typical of eczematous dermatitis
4. Personal or family history of atopy (asthma, allergic rhinitis, food allergies, or eczema)
5. Clinical course lasting longer than 6 weeks

marked by dermatitis of flexural skin, particularly in the antecubital and popliteal fossae (**see Plate IIA-4**). AD may resolve spontaneously in adults, but the dermatitis will persist into adult life in over half of individuals affected as children. The distribution of lesions may be similar to those seen in childhood. However, adults affected with AD frequently have localized disease, manifesting as hand eczema or lichen simplex chronicus (see below).

Pruritus is a prominent characteristic of AD, and many of the cutaneous findings in affected patients are secondary to rubbing and scratching. Other cutaneous stigmata of AD are perioral pallor, an extra fold of skin beneath the lower eyelid (Dennie's line), increased palmar markings, and increased incidence of cutaneous infections, particularly with *Staphylococcus aureus*. Atopic individuals often have dry itchy skin, abnormalities in cutaneous vascular responses, and, in some instances, elevations in serum IgE.

Histologic examinaton of the skin affected by AD may demonstrate features of acute or chronic dermatitis. Immunopathology shows activated, memory T helper cells, which express the cutaneous lymphocyte antigen, the ligand for the inducible endothelial cell adhesion molecule E-selectin. AD skin lesions may also demonstrate IgE-bearing CD1a+ positive Langerhans cells, and these cells have been implicated in AD disease pathophysiology through mediation of hypersensitivity responses to environmental antigens.

TREATMENT Therapy of AD should be based on avoidance of cutaneous irritants, adequate cutaneous hydration, judicious use of low- or midpotency topical glucocorticoids, and prompt treatment of secondarily infected skin lesions. Patients should be instructed to bathe using warm, but not hot, water and to limit their use of soap. Immediately after bathing while the skin is still moist, the skin should be lubricated with a low- or midpotency topical glucocorticoid in a cream or ointment base. Potent fluorinated topical glucocorticoids should not be used on the face or intertriginous areas. It takes a minimum of 30 g of glucocorticoid ointment to cover the entire body surface of an average adult.

Crusted and weeping skin lesions should be treated with systemic antibiotics with activity against *S. aureus* since secondary infection often exacerbates eczema. The frequency of macrolide-resistant organisms makes the use of penicillinase-resistant penicillins or cephalosporins preferable. Dicloxacillin or cephalexin (250 mg four times daily for 7 to 10 days) is generally adequate to decrease heavy colonization. As an adjunct, the use of triclosan-containing antibacterial washes and intermittent nasal mupirocin may be useful as prophylactic measures. The role of dietary allergens in atopic dermatitis is controversial, and there is little evidence that they play any role outside of infancy.

Control of pruritus is essential for treatment, since AD often represents "an itch that rashes." Antihistamines are useful to control the pruritus, but sedation may limit their usefulness. Unlike their effects in urticaria, nonsedating antihistamines are of little use since the effectiveness of antihistamines in the treatment of pruritus associated with AD is primarily related to their sedative effects as opposed to any specific action on histamine-mediated pathways.

Treatment with systemic glucocorticoids should be limited to severe exacerbations unresponsive to conservative topical therapy. In the patient with chronic AD, therapy with systemic glucocorticoids will generally clear the skin only briefly, but cessation of the systemic therapy will invariably be accompanied by return, if not worsening, of the dermatitis. Patients who do not respond to conventional therapies should be considered for patch testing to rule out allergic contact dermatitis. Immunotherapy with aeroallergens has not proven useful in AD, unlike its effect in allergic rhinitis and extrinsic asthma.

CONTACT DERMATITIS Contact dermatitis is an inflammatory process in skin caused by an exogenous agent or agents that directly or indirectly injure the skin. This injury may be caused by an inherent characteristic of a compound—irritant contact dermatitis (ICD). An example of ICD would be dermatitis induced by a concentrated acid or base. Agents that cause allergic contact dermatitis (ACD) induce an antigen-specific immune response. The clinical lesions of contact dermatitis may be acute (wet and edematous) or chronic (dry, thickened, and scaly), depending on the persistence of the insult (see Plate IIA-8). The most common presentation of contact dermatitis is hand eczema, and it is frequently related to occupational exposures. Occupation-related contact dermatitis represents a significant proportion of occupation-induced injury, affecting over 60,000 persons annually.

ICD is generally strictly demarcated and often localized to areas of thin skin (eyelids, intertriginous areas) or to areas where the irritant was occluded. Lesions may range from minimal skin erythema to areas of marked edema, vesicles, and ulcers. Chronic low-grade irritant dermatitis is the most common type of ICD and the most common area of involvement is the hands (see below). The most common irritants encountered are chronic wet work, soaps, and detergents. Treatment should be directed to avoidance of irritants and use of protective gloves or clothing.

ACD is a manifestation of delayed type hypersensitivity mediated by memory T lymphocytes in the skin. The most common cause of ACD is exposure to plants, specifically to members of the family Anacardiaceae; including the genera *Toxicodendrun, Anacardium, Gluta, Mangifera,* and *Semecarpus.* Poison ivy, poison oak, and poison sumac are members of the genus *Toxicodendron* and cause an allergic reaction marked by erythema, vesiculation, and severe pruritus. The eruption is often linear, corresponding to areas where plants have touched the skin. However, other allergens may be more difficult to identify, especially if the exposure is chronic and the skin becomes thickened and scaly. The sensitizing antigen common to these plants is urushiol, an oleoresin containing the active ingredient pentadecyl-catechol. The oleoresin may adhere to skin, clothing, tools, and pets, and contaminated articles may cause dermatitis even after prolonged storage. Blister fluid does not contain urushiol and is not capable of inducing skin eruption in exposed subjects.

℞ **TREATMENT**   If ACD is suspected and an offending agent is identified and removed, the eruption will resolve. Usually, treatment with high-potency fluorinated topical glucocorticoids is enough to relieve symptoms while the ACD runs its course. For those patients who require systemic therapy, a tapering course over 2 to 3 weeks given as single morning doses is the preferred method.

Identification of a contact allergen can be a difficult and time-consuming task. Patients with dermatitis unresponsive to conventional therapy or with an unusual and patterned distribution should be suspected of having ACD. They should be questioned carefully regarding occupational exposures, topical medicaments, and oral medications. Common sensitizers include preservatives in topical preparations, nickel sulfate, potassium dichromate, thimerosal in ocular preparations, neomycin sulfate, fragrances, formaldehyde, and rubber-curing agents. Patch testing is helpful in identifying these agents, but should not be attempted on patients with widespread active dermatitis or on those taking systemic glucocorticoids.

HAND ECZEMA   Hand eczema is a very common, chronic skin disorder. It represents a large proportion of occupation-associated skin disease. It may be associated with other cutaneous disorders such as atopic dermatitis or may occur by itself. Similar to other forms of dermatitis, both exogenous and endogenous factors play important roles in the expression of hand dermatitis. Chronic, excessive exposure to water and detergents may initiate or aggravate this disorder. It may present with dryness and cracking of the skin of the hands as well as with variable amounts of erythema and edema. Often, the dermatitis will begin under rings where water and irritants are trapped. A variant

of hand dermatitis, dyshidrotic eczema, presents with multiple, intensely pruritic, small papules and vesicles occurring on the thenar and hypothenar eminences and the sides of the fingers (see Plate IA-5). Lesions tend to occur in crops that slowly form crusts and heal.

The evaluation of a patient with hand eczema should include an assessment of potential occupation-associated exposures. Predominant involvement of the dorsal surface of the hands with sparing of the palmar surface suggests a possible contact dermatitis. The history should be directed to identifying possible irritant or allergen exposures. The use of rubber gloves to protect dermatitic skin is sometimes associated with the development of delayed type hypersensitivity reactions to agents used for cross-linking rubber. Such reactions can be detected by patch testing. Less commonly, patients may manifest hand dermatitis as a consequence of developing immediate type hypersensitivity reactions to latex. These are of particular concern since these patients are at risk for anaphylactic reactions. The most sensitive method of detection is the use of scratch testing with latex extract. However, this should be done with extreme caution only in a setting where an anaphylactic reaction can be treated. A latex radioallergosorbent test is available but is only about 60% sensitive.

℞ **TREATMENT**   Therapy of hand dermatitis is directed toward avoidance of irritants, identification of possible contact allergens, treatment of coexistent infection, and application of topical glucocorticoids. Whenever possible, the hands should be protected by gloves, preferably vinyl. Most patients can be treated with cool moist compresses (dressings) to dry and debride acute inflammatory lesions and to decrease swelling, followed by application of a mid- to high-potency topical glucocorticoid in a cream or ointment base. As with atopic dermatitis, treatment of secondary infection by staphylococci or streptococci is essential for good control. Additionally, patients with hand dermatitis should be examined for dermatophyte infection by KOH preparation and culture (see below).

NUMMULAR ECZEMA   Nummular eczema is characterized by circular or oval "coinlike" lesions. Initially, this eruption consists of small edematous papules that become crusted and scaly. The most common locations are on the trunk or the extensor surfaces of the extremities, particularly on the pretibial areas or dorsum of the hands. It occurs more frequently in men and is most commonly seen in middle age. The etiology of nummular eczema is unknown. Whether nummular eczema represents a variant of atopic eczema is controversial. The treatment of nummular eczema is similar to that for other forms of dermatitis.

LICHEN SIMPLEX CHRONICUS   Lichen simplex chronicus may represent the end stage of a variety of pruritic and eczematous disorders. It consists of a well-circumscribed plaque or plaques with lichenified or thickened skin due to chronic scratching or rubbing. Common areas involved include the posterior nuchal region, dorsum of the feet, or ankles. Treatment of lichen simplex chronicus centers around breaking the cycle of chronic itching and scratching, which often occur during sleep. High-potency topical glucocorticoids are helpful in alleviating pruritus in most cases, but in recalcitrant cases, application of topical glucocorticoids under occlusion or intralesional injection of glucocorticoids may be required. Oral antihistamines such as hydroxyzine (10 to 50 mg every 6 h) or tricyclic antidepressants with antihistaminic activity such as doxepin (10 to 25 mg at bedtime) are useful as antipruritics primarily due to their sedating action, and are particularly useful at bedtime (see above). Patients need to be counseled regarding driving or operating heavy equipment after taking these medications due to their potentially potent sedative activity.

ASTEATOTIC ECZEMA   Asteatotic eczema, also known as xerotic eczema or "winter itch," is a mildly inflammatory variant of dermatitis that develops most commonly on the lower legs of elderly individuals during dry times of year. Fine cracks, with or without erythema, characteristically develop on the anterior surface of the lower extremities. Pruritus is variable. Asteatotic eczema responds well to avoidance of irritants, rehydration of the skin, and application of topical emollients.

STASIS DERMATITIS AND STASIS ULCERATION

Stasis dermatitis develops on the lower extremities secondary to venous incompetence and chronic edema. Early findings in stasis dermatitis consist of mild erythema and scaling associated with pruritus. The typical initial site of involvement is the medial aspect of the ankle, often over a distended vein (see Plate IIA-7). As the disorder progresses, the dermatitis becomes progressively pigmented, due to chronic erythrocyte extravasation leading to cutaneous hemosiderin deposition. As with other forms of dermatitis, stasis dermatitis may become acutely inflamed, with crusting and exudate. Chronic stasis dermatitis is often associated with dermal fibrosis that is recognized clinically as brawny edema of the skin. Stasis dermatitis is often complicated by secondary infection and contact dermatitis. Severe stasis dermatitis may precede the development of stasis ulcers.

R̲x̲ **TREATMENT** Avoidance of irritants and use of emollients and/or midpotency topical glucocorticoids are the cornerstones of therapy for stasis dermatitis. Control of chronic edema is important to prevent leg ulcers. Patients should be encouraged to elevate the affected extremity when sitting. A compression stocking with a gradient of at least 30 to 40 mmHg is most effective for edema control and is much more effective for preventing chronic edema than is antiembolism hose.

Stasis ulcers are difficult to treat, and resolution of these lesions is slow even under the best of circumstances. It is extremely important to elevate the affected limb as much as possible. The ulcer should be kept clear of necrotic material by gentle debridement and covered with a semipermeable dressing under pressure. Glucocorticoids should not be applied to ulcers, since they may retard healing. Secondarily infected lesions should be treated with appropriate oral antibiotics, but it should be noted that all ulcers will become colonized with bacteria, and the purpose of antibiotic therapy should not be to clear all bacterial growth. Some ulcers may take months to heal or require skin grafting.

SEBORRHEIC DERMATITIS Seborrheic dermatitis is a common, chronic disorder, characterized by greasy scales overlying erythematous patches or plaques. The most common location is in the scalp where it may be recognized as severe dandruff. On the face, seborrheic dermatitis affects the eyebrows, eyelids, glabella, nasolabial fold, or ears (see Plate IIA-6). Scaling within the external ear is often mistaken for a chronic fungal infection (otomycosis), and postauricular dermatitis often becomes macerated and tender. Additionally, seborrheic dermatitis may develop in the central chest, axilla, groin, submammary folds, and gluteal cleft. Rarely, it may cause a widespread generalized dermatitis. Seborrheic dermatitis is usually symptomatic, with patients complaining of itching or burning.

Seborrheic dermatitis may be evident within the first few weeks

of life, and within this context it occurs in the scalp ("cradle cap"), face, or groin. It is rarely seen in children beyond infancy but becomes evident again during adult life. Although it is frequently seen in patients with Parkinson's disease, in those who have had cerebrovascular accidents, and in those with human immunodeficiency virus (HIV) infection, the overwhelming majority of individuals with seborrheic dermatitis have no underlying disorder.

R̲x̲ **TREATMENT** Treatment with low-potency topical glucocorticoids in conjunction with shampoos containing coal tar and/or salicylic acid is generally sufficient to control activity of this disorder. High-potency topical glucocorticoid solutions (betamethasone or fluocinonide) are effective for control of scalp involvement. Fluorinated topical glucocorticoids should not be used on the face since this is often associated with the development of rebound worsening and steroid-induced rosacea or atrophy.

PAPULOSQUAMOUS DISORDERS (Table 56-2)

PSORIASIS Psoriasis is one of the most common dermatologic diseases, affecting up to 1 to 2% of the world's population. It is a chronic inflammatory skin disorder clinically characterized by erythematous, sharply demarcated papules and rounded plaques, covered by silvery micaceous scale. The skin lesions of psoriasis are variably pruritic. Traumatized areas often develop lesions of psoriasis (Koebner or isomorphic phenomenon). Additionally, other external factors may exacerbate psoriasis including infections, stress, and medications (lithium, beta blockers, and antimalarials).

The most common variety of psoriasis is called *plaque type*. Patients with plaque-type psoriasis will have stable, slowly growing plaques, which remain basically unchanged for long periods of time. The most common areas for plaque psoriasis to occur are the elbows, knees, gluteal cleft, and the scalp. Involvement tends to be symmetric. *Inverse psoriasis* affects the intertriginous regions including the axilla, groin, submammary region, and navel, it also tends to affect the scalp, palms, and soles. The individual lesions are sharply demarcated plaques (see Plate IIA-3) but may be moist due to their location. Plaque psoriasis generally develops slowly and runs an indolent course. It rarely remits spontaneously.

Eruptive psoriasis (guttate psoriasis) is most common in children and young adults. It develops acutely in individuals without psoriasis or in those with chronic plaque psoriasis. Patients present with many small erythematous, scaling papules, frequently after upper respiratory tract infection with β-hemolytic streptococci. The differential diagnosis should include pityriasis rosea and secondary syphilis. Patients with psoriasis may also develop pustular lesions. These may be localized to the palms and soles or may be generalized and associated with fever, malaise, diarrhea, and arthralgias.

Table 56-2 Papulosquamous Disorders

	Clinical Features	Other Notable Features	Histologic Features
Psoriasis	Sharply demarcated, erythematous plaques with mica-like scale; predominantly elbows, knees, and scalp; atypical forms may localize to intertriginous areas; eruptive forms may be associated with infection (Reiter's syndrome)	May be aggravated by certain drugs, infection; severe forms seen associated with HIV	Acanthosis, vascular proliferation
Lichen planus	Purple polygonal papules marked by severe pruritus; lacy white markings, especially associated with mucous membrane lesions	Certain drugs may induce: thiazides, antimalarial drugs	Interface dermatitis
Pityriasis rosea	Rash often preceded by herald patch; oval to round plaques with trailing scale; most often affects the trunk, and eruption lines up in skin folds give a "fir tree"-like appearance; generally spares palms and soles	Variable pruritus; self-limited resolving in 2–8 weeks; may be imitated by secondary syphilis	Pathologic features often nonspecific
Dermatophytosis	Polymorphous appearance depending on dermatophyte, body site, and host response; sharply defined to ill-demarcated scaly plaques with or without inflammation; may be associated with hair loss	KOH preparation may show branching hyphae; culture helpful	Hyphae and neutrophils in stratum corneum

About half of all patients with psoriasis have fingernail involvement, appearing as punctate pitting, nail thickening, or subungual hyperkeratosis. About 5 to 10% of patients with psoriasis have associated joint complaints, and these are most often found in patients with fingernail involvement. Although some have the coincident occurrence of classic rheumatoid arthritis (Chap. 312), many have joint disease that falls into one of three types associated with psoriasis: (1) asymmetric inflammatory arthritis most commonly involving the distal and proximal interphalangeal joints and less commonly the knees, hips, ankles, and wrists; (2) a seronegative rheumatoid arthritis–like disease; a significant portion of these patients go on to develop a severe destructive arthritis; or (3) disease limited to the spine (psoriatic spondylitis).

The etiology of psoriasis is still poorly understood. There is clearly a genetic component to psoriasis. Over 50% of patients with psoriasis report a positive family history, and a 65 to 72% concordance among monozygotic twins has been reported in twin studies. Psoriasis has been linked to HLA-Cw6 and, to a lesser extent, to HLA-DR7. Evidence has accumulated clearly indicating a role for T cells in the pathophysiology of psoriasis. Stimulation of immune function with cytokines such as IL-2 has been associated with abrupt worsening of preexisting psoriasis, and bone marrow transplantation has resulted in clearance of disease. Psoriatic lesions are characterized by infiltration of skin with activated memory T cells, with CD8+ cells predominating in the epidermis. Agents that inhibit activated T cell function are often effective for the treatment of severe psoriasis. Presumably, cytokines from activated T cells elaborate growth factors that stimulate keratinocyte hyperproliferation.

℞ **TREATMENT**   Treatment of psoriasis depends on the type, location, and extent of disease. All patients should be instructed to avoid excess drying or irritation of their skin and to maintain adequate cutaneous hydration. Most patients with localized plaque-type psoriasis can be managed with midpotency topical glucocorticoids, although their long-term use is often accompanied by loss of effectiveness (tachyphylaxis). Crude coal tar (1 to 5% in an ointment base) is an old but useful method of treatment in conjunction with ultraviolet light therapy. A topical vitamin D analogue (calcipitriol) is also efficacious in the treatment of psoriasis.

Ultraviolet light is an effective therapy for patients with widespread psoriasis. The ultraviolet B (UV-B) spectrum is effective alone, or may be combined with coal tar (Goeckerman regimen) or anthralin (Ingram regimen). Natural sunlight or an artificial light source can be used. The combination of the ultraviolet A (UV-A) spectrum with either oral or topical psoralens (PUVA) is also extremely effective for the treatment of psoriasis, but long-term use may be associated with an increased incidence of squamous cell cancer and melanoma of the skin.

Various other agents can be used for widespread psoriatic disease.

Methotrexate is an effective agent, especially in patients with associated psoriatic arthritis. Liver toxicity from long-term use limits its use to patients with widespread disease not responsive to less aggressive modalities. The synthetic retinoid, acetretin, has been shown to be effective in some patients with severe psoriasis but is a potent teratogen, thus limiting its use in women with childbearing potential. The evidence implicating psoriasis as a T cell–mediated disorder has created a new perspective relating to the treatment of psoriasis. Based on this presumed disease mechanism, immunomodulatory therapy utilizing cyclosporine has proven to be highly effective in selected patients with severe, crippling, and potentially life-threatening disease.

LICHEN PLANUS   Lichen planus (LP) is a papulosquamous disorder in which the primary lesions are pruritic, polygonal, flat-topped, violaceous papules. Close examination of the surface of these papules often reveals a network of gray lines (Wickham's striae). The skin lesions may occur anywhere but have a predilection for the wrists, shins, lower back, and genitalia **(see Plate IIA-9)**. Involvement of the scalp may lead to hair loss. LP commonly involves mucous membranes, particularly the buccal mucosa, where it can present as a white netlike eruption. Its etiology is unknown, but cutaneous eruptions clinically resembling LP have been observed after administration of numerous drugs, including diuretics, gold, antimalarials, penicillamine, and phenothiazines, and in patients with skin lesions of chronic graft-versus-host disease. Additionally, LP associated with abnormal liver function has been correlated with viral hepatitis, particularly hepatitis C infection. The course of LP is variable, but most patients have spontaneous remissions 6 months to 2 years after the onset of disease. Topical glucocorticoids are the mainstay of therapy.

PITYRIASIS ROSEA   Pityriasis rosea (PR) is a papulosquamous eruption of unknown etiology that occurs more commonly in the spring and fall. Its first manifestation is the development of a 2- to 6-cm annular lesion (the herald patch). This is followed in a few days to a few weeks by the appearance of many smaller annular or papular lesions with a predilection to occur on the trunk **(see Plate IIA-13)**. The lesions are generally oval, with their long axis parallel to the skin-fold lines. Individual lesions may range in color from red to brown and have a trailing scale. PR shares many clinical features with the eruption of secondary syphilis, but palm and sole lesions are extremely rare in PR and common in secondary syphilis. The eruption tends to be moderately pruritic and lasts 3 to 8 weeks. Treatment is generally directed at alleviating pruritus and consists of oral antihistamines, midpotency topical glucocorticoids, and, in some cases, the use of UV-B phototherapy.

CUTANEOUS INFECTIONS (Table 56-3)

IMPETIGO AND ECTHYMA   Impetigo is a common superficial bacterial infection of skin caused by group A β-hemolytic streptococci (Chap. 140) or *S. aureus* (Chap. 139). The primary lesion is a

Table 56-3   Common Skin Infections

	Clinical Features	Etiologic Agent	Treatment
Impetigo	Honey-colored crusted papules, plaques, or bullae	Group A *Streptococcus* and *Staphylococcus aureus*	Systemic or topical anti-staphylococcal antitibiotics
Dermatophytosis	Inflammatory or noninflammatory annular scaly plaques; may have hair loss; groin involvement spares scrotum; hyphae on KOH preparation	*Trichophyton, Epidermophyton,* or *Microsporum* sp.	Topical azoles, systemic griseofulvin, or azoles
Candidiasis	Inflammatory papules and plaques with satellite pustules, frequently in intertriginous areas; may involve scrotum; pseudohyphae on KOH preparation	*Candida albicans* and other *Candida* species	Topical nystatin or azoles; systemic azoles for resistant disease
Tinea versicolor	Hyperpigmented or hypopigmented scaly patches on the trunk; characteristic mixture of hyphae and spores on KOH preparation ("spaghetti and meatballs")	KOH preparation may show branching hyphae; culture helpful	Topical selenium sulfide lotion or azoles

superficial pustule that ruptures and forms a characteristic yellow-brown honey-colored crust (see Plate IID-38). Lesions caused by staphylococci may be tense, clear bullae, and this less common form of the disease is called *bullous impetigo*. Lesions may occur on normal skin or in areas already affected by another skin disease. Ecthyma is a variant of impetigo that generally occurs on the lower extremities and causes punched-out ulcerative lesions. Treatment of both ecthyma and impetigo involves gentle debridement of adherent crusts, which is facilitated by the use of soaks and topical antibiotics, in conjunction with appropriate oral antibiotics.

ERYSIPELAS AND CELLULITIS See Chap. 128

DERMATOPHYTOSIS Dermatophytes are fungi that infect skin, hair, and nails and include members of the genera *Trichophyton*, *Microsporum*, and *Epidermophyton*. Infection of the foot (tinea pedis) is most common and is often chronic; it is characterized by variable erythema and edema, scaling, pruritus, and occasionally vesiculation. Involvement may be widespread or localized, but almost invariably the web space between the fourth and fifth toes is affected. Infection of the nails (tinea unguium) occurs in many patients with tinea pedis and is characterized by opacified, thickened nails and subungual debris. The groin is the next most commonly involved area (tinea cruris), with males affected much more often than females. It presents as a scaling erythematous eruption that spares the scrotum. Microscopic examination of either untreated tinea pedis or tinea cruris scale after digestion with KOH preparation will generally demonstrate hyphae.

Dermatophyte infection of the scalp (tinea capitis) has returned in epidemic proportions, particularly affecting inner city children. The predominant organism is *T. tonsurans*. This organism can produce an inflammatory or relatively noninflammatory infection that may present with either well-defined or irregular, diffuse areas of mild scaling and hair loss. Tinea corporis, or infection on non-hair-bearing skin, may have a variable appearance, depending on the extent of the associated inflammatory reaction (see Plate IID-51). It may have the typical annular appearance of "ringworm" or appear as deep inflammatory nodules (on the scalp known as a *kerion*) or granulomas. KOH examination of scale or hair from patients with tinea capitis or inflammatory tinea corporis often does not reveal hyphae, and diagnosis may require culture or biopsy.

℞ **TREATMENT** Both topical and systemic therapies may be used to treat dermatophyte infection. Treatment depends on the site involved and the type of infection. Topical therapy is generally effective for uncomplicated tinea corporis, tinea cruris, and limited tinea pedis. It is not effective as monotherapy for tinea capitis or tinea unguium. Topical imidazoles (miconazole, ketoconazole, econazole, clotrimazole, oxiconazole, and sulconazole), triazoles (terconazole), and allylamines (terbinafine and naftifine) may all be effective topical therapies for dermatophyte infections. Haloprogin, undecylic acid, ciclopirox-olamine, and tolnaftate are also effective, but nystatin is not active against dermatophytes. Treatment should continue until the patient is clear of infection by clinical examination and culture. Tinea pedis often requires longer treatment courses and is associated with a high relapse rate.

Griseofulvin is the drug of choice for dermatophyte infections requiring systemic therapy. A daily dose of 500 mg of microsized or 350 mg of ultramicrosized griseofulvin administered with a fatty meal is an adequate dose for most dermatophyte infections. The duration of therapy may be as short as 2 weeks for uncomplicated tinea corporis but may be as long as 6 to 12 months for nail infections. The most common side effects of griseofulvin are gastrointestinal distress and headache. Dermatophyte infection of hair-bearing areas (e.g., tinea capitis) requires systemic antifungal therapy. The usual adult dose of griseofulvin is 1 g of microsized or 0.5 g of ultramicrosized given daily, and treatment should be continued for 6 to 8 weeks. Children should be treated with 15 to 20 mg/kg as a single daily dose given with a fatty meal. The adjunctive use of topical antifungal agents in addition to systemic therapy may be useful, but topical therapy alone

is not adequate. Markedly inflammatory tinea capitis may result in scarring and hair loss, and systemic or topical glucocorticoids may be helpful in preventing this sequela. Recent studies in children have also suggested that both itraconazole (3 to 5 mg/kg for 6 to 10 weeks) and terbinafine (125 mg/d for 6 weeks) may be effective treatments for tinea capitis.

Until recently, griseofulvin was the recommended therapy for dermatophyte infection of the nails. However, despite prolonged treatment, cure rates were poor. Itraconazole given as either continuous daily therapy (200 mg/d for 3 months) or pulses (200 mg twice daily for 1 week per month for 3 consecutive months) has been shown to be a safe and effective therapy. Itraconazole has the potential for interactions with other drugs requiring the P450 enzyme system for metabolism. Similarly, terbinafine (250 mg/d for 3 months) has shown similar cure rates. Only limited data are available on the dosing and effectiveness of the newer antifungal agents in tinea corporis, tinea cruris, and uncomplicated tinea pedis.

TINEA VERSICOLOR Tinea versicolor is caused by a non-dermatophyte dimorphic fungus that is a normal inhabitant of the skin. As the yeast form *Pityrosporum orbiculare*, it generally does not cause disease (except for folliculitis in certain individuals). However, in some individuals, it converts to the hyphal form and causes characteristic lesions. The expression of infection is promoted by heat and humidity. The typical lesions consist of oval scaly macules, papules, and patches concentrated on the chest, shoulders, and back but only rarely on the face or distal extremities. On dark skin, they often appear as hypopigmented areas, while on light skin, they are slightly hyperpigmented. In some darkly pigmented individuals, they may only appear as scaling patches. A KOH preparation from scaling lesions will demonstrate a confluence of short hyphae and round spores (so-called spaghetti and meatballs). Solutions containing sulfur, salicylic acid, or selenium sulfide will clear the infection if used daily for a week and then intermittently thereafter. Treatment with a single 400-mg dose of ketoconazole is also effective.

CANDIDIASIS Candidiasis is a fungal infection caused by a related group of yeasts, whose manifestations may be localized to the skin, or rarely, may be systemic and life-threatening. The causative organism is usually *Candida albicans*, but may also be *C. tropicalis*, *C. parapsilosis*, or *C. krusei*. These organisms are normal saprophytic inhabitants of the gastrointestinal tract but may overgrow (usually due to broad-spectrum antibiotic therapy) and cause disease at a number of cutaneous sites. Other predisposing factors include diabetes mellitus, chronic intertrigo, oral contraceptive use, and cellular immune deficiency. Candidiasis is a very common infection in HIV-infected individuals (Chap. 309). The oral cavity is commonly involved. Lesions may occur on the tongue or buccal mucosa (thrush) and appear as white plaques (see Plate IID-43). Microscopic examination of scrapings demonstrate both pseudohyphae and yeast forms. Fissured, macerated lesions at the corners of the mouth (perlèche) are often seen in individuals with poorly fitting dentures and may also be associated with candidal infection. Additionally, candidal infections have an affinity for sites that are chronically wet and macerated and may occur around nails (onycholysis and paronychia) and in intertriginous areas. Intertriginous lesions are characteristically edematous, erythematous, and scaly, with scattered "satellite pustules." In males, there is often involvement of the penis and scrotum as well as the inner aspect of the thighs. In contrast to dermatophyte infections, candidal infections are frequently accompanied by a marked inflammatory response. Diagnosis of candidal infection is based upon the clinical pattern and demonstration of yeast on KOH preparation, or culture.

℞ **TREATMENT** Treatment routinely involves removing any predisposing factors such as antibiotic therapy or chronic wetness and the use of appropriate topical or systemic antifungal therapy. Effective topical agents include nystatin or topical azoles (miconazole, clotrimazole, econazole, or ketoconazole). These agents are generally effective in clearing mucous membrane or glabrous skin involvement in nonimmunosuppressed patients. The associated inflammatory response that often accompanies candidal infection on glabrous skin should be treated with a mild glucocorticoid lotion or cream (2.5% hydrocortisone). Systemic therapy is generally reserved for immunosuppressed patients or individuals with chronic or recurrent disease who fail to respond to or tolerate appropriate topical therapy. Vulvovaginal candidiasis may respond to treatment with a single dose of fluconazole (150 mg). Chronic recurrent oral or vaginal candidiasis may be treated with weekly to monthly oral fluconazole (150 to 200 mg) in conjunction with topical therapy.

WARTS   Warts are cutaneous neoplasms that are caused by papilloma viruses. Over 50 different human papilloma viruses (HPV) have been described, and this number will almost certainly continue to grow. Typical verruca vulgaris lesions are sessile, dome-shaped, usually about a centimeter in diameter, and their surface is made up of many small filamentous projections. The HPV that cause typical verruca vulgaris also cause typical plantar warts, flat warts (or verruca plana), and filiform warts in intertriginous areas. Plantar warts are endophytic and are covered by thick keratin. Paring of the wart will generally demonstrate a central core of keratinized debris and punctate bleeding points. Filiform warts are most commonly seen on the face, neck, and skin folds and present as papillomatous lesions on a narrow base. Flat warts are only slightly elevated and have a velvety, nonverrucous surface. They have a propensity for the face, arms, and legs and are often spread by shaving.

Multiple HPV types have been associated with genital tract lesions. They generally begin as small papillomas that may grow to form large fungating lesions. In women, they may involve either the labia, perineum, or perianal skin. Additionally, the mucosa of the vagina, urethra, and anus can be involved, as well as the cervical epithelium. In men, the lesions often occur initially in the coronal sulcus, but may be seen on the shaft of the penis, the scrotum, perianal skin, or in the urethra.

Within the past decade, appreciable evidence has accumulated that suggests HPV plays a role in the development of neoplasia of the uterine cervix and external genitalia (Chap. 97). HPV types 16 and 18 have been most intensely studied, while recent evidence also implicates other types. Lesions may initially appear as small, flat, velvety, hyperpigmented papules occurring on the genitalia or perianal skin. Histologic examination of biopsies from affected sites may reveal changes associated with typical warts and/or features typical of intraepidermal carcinoma (Bowen's disease). Squamous cell carcinomas associated with HPV infections have also been observed in extragenital skin (Chap. 86). This is most commonly seen in patients immunosuppressed after organ transplantation.

℞ TREATMENT   There are many modalities available to treat warts, but no single therapy is universally effective. Factors that influence the choice of therapy include the location of the wart, extent of disease, the age and immunologic status of the patient, and the patient's desire for therapy. Perhaps the most useful and convenient method for treating warts in almost any location is cryotherapy with liquid nitrogen. Equally effective, but requiring much more patient compliance, is the use of keratolytic agents such as salicylic acid plasters or combinations of lactic acid and salicylic acid. For genital warts, application of podophyllin solution is moderately effective but may be associated with marked local reactions in certain individuals. Dilute preparations of purified podophyllin permit physician-directed by patient-applied use, facilitating treatment of mucosal warts. Topical imiquimod, a potent inducer of local cytokine release, has also been approved for use in genital warts. Other topical agents that are used include trichloracetic acid or cantharidin. Electrodessication and curettage or CO_2 laser excision are also effective therapies but require local anesthesia. Recurrence of warts appears to be common to all

these modalities because viral genomic material is present in normal-appearing skin adjacent to the clinical lesions.

Treatment of warts should be tempered by the observation that an overwhelming majority of warts in normal individuals resolve spontaneously within 1 to 2 years. Also, only an extremely small proportion of warts is associated with neoplasia, and those are almost exclusively located on the genitalia or perianal skin.

HERPES SIMPLEX   →*See Chap. 182*
HERPES ZOSTER   →*See Chap. 183*

ACNE

ACNE VULGARIS   Acne vulgaris is a self-limited disorder primarily of teenagers and young adults, although perhaps 10 to 20% of adults may continue to experience some form of the disorder. The permissive factor for the expression of the disease in adolescence is the increase in sebum release by sebaceous glands after puberty. Small cysts, called *comedones*, form in hair follicles due to blockage of the follicular orifice by retention of sebum and keratinous material. The activity of lipophilic yeast (*Pityrosporum orbiculare*) and bacteria (*Proprionobacterium acnes*) within the comedones releases free fatty acids from sebum, causes inflammation within the cyst, and results in rupture of the cyst wall. An inflammatory foreign-body reaction develops as a result of extrusion of oily and keratinous debris from the cyst.

The clinical hallmark of acne vulgaris is the comedone, which may be closed (whitehead) or open (blackhead). Closed comedones appear as 1- to 2-mm pebbly white papules, which are accentuated when the skin is stretched. They are the precursors of inflammatory lesions of acne vulgaris. The contents of closed comedones are not easily expressed. Open comedones, which rarely result in inflammatory acne lesions, have a large dilated follicular orifice and are filled with easily expressible oxidized, darkened, oily debris. Comedones are usually accompanied by inflammatory lesions: papules, pustules, or nodules.

The earliest lesions seen in early adolescence are generally mildly inflamed or noninflammatory comedones on the forehead. Subsequently, more typical inflammatory lesions develop on the cheeks, nose, and chin **(see Plate IIA-1)**. The most common location for acne is the face, but involvement of the chest and back is not uncommon. Most disease remains mild and does not lead to scarring. However, a small number of patients develop large inflammatory cysts and nodules, which may drain and result in significant scarring.

Exogenous and endogenous factors can alter the expression of acne vulgaris. Friction and trauma may rupture preexisting microcomedones and elicit inflammatory acne lesions. This is commonly seen with headbands or chin straps of athletic helmets. Application of comedogenic topical agents in cosmetics or hair preparations or chronic topical exposure to certain industrial compounds that are comedogenic may elicit or aggravate acne. Glucocorticoids, applied topically or administered systemically in high doses, may also elicit acne. Other systemic medications such as lithium, isoniazid, halogens, phenytoin, and phenobarbital may produce acneiform eruptions, or aggravate preexisting acne.

℞ TREATMENT   Treatment of acne vulgaris is directed toward elimination of comedones by normalization of follicular keratinization, decreasing sebaceous gland activity, decreasing the population of lipophilic bacteria and yeast, and decreasing inflammation. Acne vulgaris may be treated with either local or systemic medications. Minimal to moderate, pauci-inflammatory disease may respond adequately to local therapy alone. Although areas affected with acne should be kept clean, there is little evidence to suggest that removal of surface oils plays an important role in therapy. Overly vigorous scrubbing may aggravate acne due to mechanical rupture of comedones. Topical agents such as retinoic acid, benzoyl peroxide, or salicylic acid may alter the pattern of epidermal desquamation, preventing the formation of comedones and aiding in the resolution of preexisting cysts. Topical antibacterial agents such as benzoyl peroxide, azelaic acid, topical erythromycin (with or without zinc), clindamycin, or tetracycline are also useful adjuncts to therapy.

Patients with moderate to severe acne with a prominent inflammatory component will benefit from the addition of systemic therapy. Oral tetracyclines or erythromycin in doses of 250 to 1000 mg/d will decrease follicular colonization with some of the lipophilic organisms. They also appear to have an anti-inflammatory effect independent of their antibacterial effect. Female patients who do not respond to oral antibiotics may benefit from hormonal therapy. Women placed on oral contraceptives containing ethinyl estradiol and norgestimate have demonstrated improvement in their acne when compared to a placebo control.

Severe nodulocystic acne not responsive to oral antibiotics, hormonal therapy, or topical therapy may be treated with the synthetic retinoid isotretinoin. It is used at doses of 0.5 to 2.0 mg/kg as a single daily dose for 15 to 20 weeks. The use of this drug is limited by its teratogenicity, and female patients must be screened for pregnancy prior to initiating therapy, maintain a method of birth control during therapy, and be screened for pregnancy during treatment. Patients receiving this medication develop extremely dry skin and cheilitis and must be followed for development of hypertriglyceridemia.

ACNE ROSACEA   Acne rosacea is an inflammatory disorder predominantly affecting the central face. It is seen almost exclusively in adults, only rarely affecting patients under 30 years of age. Rosacea is seen more often in women, but those most severely affected are men. It is characterized by the presence of erythema, telangiectases, and superficial pustules **(see Plate IIA-2)**, but is not associated with the presence of comedones. Rosacea only rarely involves the chest or back.

There is a relationship between the tendency for pronounced facial flushing and the subsequent development of acne rosacea. Often, individuals with rosacea initially demonstrate a pronounced flushing reaction. This may be in response to heat, emotional stimuli, alcohol, hot drinks, or spicy foods. As the disease progresses, the flush persists longer and longer and may eventually become permanent. Papules, pustules, and telangiectases can become superimposed on the persistent flush. Rosacea of very long standing may lead to connective tissue overgrowth, particularly of the nose (rhinophyma). Rosacea may also be complicated by various inflammatory disorders of the eye, including keratitis, blepharitis, iritis, and recurrent chalazion. These ocular problems are potentially sight-threatening and warrant ophthalmologic evaluation.

℞ **TREATMENT**   Acne rosacea can generally be treated effectively with oral tetracycline in doses ranging from 250 to 1000 mg/d. Topical metronidazole or sodium sulfacetamide has also been shown to be effective. In addition, the use of low-potency, nonfluorinated topical glucocorticoids, particularly after cool soaks, is helpful in alleviating facial erythema. Fluorinated topical glucocorticoids should be avoided since chronic use of these preparations may actually elicit rosacea. Topical therapy is not effective treatment for ocular disease.

BIBLIOGRAPHY

ARNDT KA et al (eds): *Cutaneous Medicine and Surgery: An Integrated Program in Dermatology*. Philadelphia, Saunders, 1996

BATA-CSORGO Z et al: Intralesional T-lymphocyte activation as a mediator of psoriatic epidermal hyperplasia. J Invest Dermatol 105:89S, 1995

BOS JD, DERIE MA: The pathogenesis of psoriasis: Immunological facts and speculations. Immunol Today 20:40, 1999

COHEN DE: Occupational dermatoses, in *Handbook of Occupational Safety and Health*, 2d ed, LJ DiBerardinis (ed). New York, Wiley, 1999, p 697

FREEDBURG IM et al (eds): *Fitzpatrick's Dermatology in General Medicine*, 5th ed. New York, McGraw-Hill, 1999

GOTTLIEB SL et al: Response of psoriasis to a lymphocyte-selective toxin (DAB389 IL-2) suggests a primary immune, but not keratinocyte, pathogenic basis. Nat Med 1:442, 1995

HANAFIN JM et al: Recombinant interferon gamma therapy for atopic dermatitis. J Am Acad Dermatol 28:189, 1993

PETO R, ZUR HAUSEN H: *Viral Etiology of Cervical Cancer. Banbury Report*. Cold Spring Harbor, NY, Cold Spring Harbor Laboratory, 1986

57 Jean L. Bolognia, Irwin M. Braverman

SKIN MANIFESTATIONS OF INTERNAL DISEASE

ACE angiotensin-converting enzyme	MEN multiple endocrine neoplasia
AV arteriovenous	MSH melanocyte-stimulating hormone
BCEs basal cell epitheliomas	
CALM café au lait macules	NAME *n*evus, *a*trial myxoma, *m*yxoid neurofibroma, and *e*phelides (freckles) syndrome
CNS central nervous system	
CREST *c*alcinosis cutis, *R*aynaud's phenomenon, *e*sophageal dysmotility, *s*clerodactyly, and *t*elangiectasia	
	NF neurofibromatosis
CTCL cutaneous T cell lymphoma	NSAIDs nonsteroidal anti-inflammatory drugs
DIC disseminated intravascular coagulation	OCA oculocutaneous albinism
	PAN polyarteritis nodosa
DM dermatomyositis	PCR polymerase chain reaction
EED erythema elevatum diutinum	PCT porphyria cutanea tarda
EM erythema multiforme	PMLE polymorphous light eruption
JRA juvenile rheumatoid arthritis	POEMS *p*olyneuropathy; *o*rganomegaly (liver, spleen, lymph nodes); *e*ndocrinopathies (impotence, gynecomastia); *M*-protein; and *s*kin changes
LAMB *l*entigines, *a*trial myxomas, *m*ucocutaneous myxomas, and *b*lue nevi	
LCV leukocytoclastic vasculitis	
LEOPARD *l*entigines; *E*CG abnormalities, primarily conduction defects, *o*cular hypertelorism; *p*ulmonary stenosis and subaortic valvular stenosis; *a*bnormal genitalia (cryptorchidism, hypospadias); *r*etardation of growth; and *d*eafness (sensorineural)	PVA poikiloderma vasculare atrophicans
	PXE pseudoxanthoma elasticum
	SSSS staphylococcal scalded-skin syndrome
	TEN toxic epidermal necrolysis
	TSS toxic shock syndrome

It is now a generally accepted concept in medicine that the skin can show signs of internal disease. Therefore, in textbooks of medicine one finds a chapter describing in detail the major systemic disorders that can be identified by cutaneous signs. The underlying assumption of such a chapter is that the clinician has been able to identify the disorder in the patient and needs only to read about it in the textbook. In reality, concise differential diagnoses and the identification of these disorders are actually difficult for the nondermatologist because he or she is not well versed in the recognition of cutaneous lesions or their spectrum of presentations. Therefore, the authors of this chapter have decided to cover this particular topic of cutaneous medicine not by discussing individual disorders but by describing and discussing the various presenting clinical signs and symptoms that indicate the presence of these disorders. Concise differential diagnoses will be generated in which the significant diseases will be briefly discussed and distinguished from the more common disorders that have no significance for internal diseases. The latter disorders are reviewed in table form and always need to be excluded when considering the former. For a detailed description of individual diseases, the reader should consult a dermatologic text.

PAPULOSQUAMOUS SKIN LESIONS (Table 57-1)   When an eruption is characterized by elevated lesions, papules (<1 cm) or plaques (>1 cm), in association with scale, it is referred to as *papulosquamous*. The most common papulosquamous diseases—*psoriasis, tinea, pityriasis rosea,* and *lichen planus*—are primary cutaneous disorders (Chap. 56). When psoriatic lesions are accompanied by arthritis, the possibility of psoriatic arthritis or *Reiter's disease* should be considered. A history of oral ulcers, conjunctivitis, uveitis, and/or urethritis points to the latter diagnosis. In *guttate psoriasis* there is an acute onset of small, widely scattered, uniform lesions, often in association with a streptococcal infection. Lithium, beta blockers, HIV infection, and a rapid taper of systemic glucocorticoids are also known to exacerbate psoriasis.

Whenever the diagnosis of pityriasis rosea or lichen planus is made, it is important to review the patient's medications because the

Table 57-1   Selected Causes of Papulosquamous Skin Lesions

1. Primary cutaneous disorders
   a. Psoriasis[a]
   b. Tinea[a]
   c. Pityriasis rosea[a]
   d. Lichen planus[a]
   e. Parapsoriasis
   f. Bowen's disease (squamous cell carcinoma in situ)[b]
2. Drugs
3. Systemic diseases
   a. Lupus erythematosus[c]
   b. Cutaneous T cell lymphoma
   c. Secondary syphilis
   d. Reiter's disease
   e. Sarcoidosis[d]

[a] Discussed in detail in Chap. 56.
[b] Associated with chronic sun exposure and exposure to arsenic.
[c] See also "Red Lesions" in "Papulonodular Skin Lesions."
[d] See also "Red-Brown Lesions" in "Papulonodular Skin Lesions."

Table 57-2   Causes of Erythroderma

1. Primary cutaneous disorders
   a. Psoriasis[a]
   b. Dermatitis (atopic, stasis, contact, seborrheic)[a]
   c. Pityriasis rubra pilaris
2. Drugs
3. Systemic diseases
   a. Cutaneous T cell lymphoma
   b. Lymphoma
4. Idiopathic

[a] Discussed in detail in Chap. 56.

eruption can be treated by simply discontinuing the offending agent. Pityriasis rosea–like drug eruptions are seen most commonly with beta blockers, angiotensin-converting enzyme (ACE) inhibitors, gold, and metronidazole, while the drugs that can produce a lichenoid eruption include gold, antimalarials, thiazides, quinidine, phenothiazines, sulfonylureas, and ACE inhibitors. Lichen planus–like lesions are also observed in chronic graft-versus-host disease.

Parapsoriasis is an intermediate disease, for it can remain solely as a primary cutaneous disease or it can progress to cutaneous T cell lymphoma (CTCL) after a latency period of as long as 40 years. There are several forms of parapsoriasis, including small plaque (0.5 to 5 cm), large plaque (>6 cm), and retiform. The lesions of both small plaque and large plaque parapsoriasis are thin and salmon-pink in color with fine white scale. In small plaque forms, the lesions are commonly on the trunk but can be widely scattered. In large plaque forms, the most common location is the "girdle" area, and fine wrinkling secondary to epidermal atrophy is often seen. Retiform parapsoriasis forms a netlike pattern, and the individual papules are red-brown and flat-topped. The latter two forms of parapsoriasis, large plaque and retiform, can progress to CTCL.

A clue to the development of *CTCL* within lesions of large plaque or retiform parapsoriasis is an increase in the palpable component of the plaque (increased infiltration). In its early stages, CTCL may be confused with ezcema or psoriasis, but it often fails to respond to the appropriate therapy for those inflammatory diseases. The diagnosis of CTCL is established by skin biopsy in which collections of atypical T lymphocytes are found in the epidermis and dermis. As the disease progresses, cutaneous tumors and lymph node involvement may appear.

In *secondary syphilis* there are scattered red-brown papules with thin scale. The eruption often involves the palms and soles and can resemble pityriasis rosea. Associated findings are helpful in making the diagnosis and include annular plaques on the face, nonscarring alopecia, condyloma lata (broad-based and moist), and mucous patches as well as lymphadenopathy, malaise, fever, headache, and myalgias. The interval between the primary chancre and the secondary stage is usually 4 to 8 weeks, and spontaneous resolution without appropriate therapy is seen.

ERYTHRODERMA (Table 57-2) *Erythroderma* is the term used when the majority of the skin surface is erythematous (red in color). There may be associated scale, erosions, or pustules as well as shedding of the hair and nails. Potential systemic manifestations include fever, chills, hypothermia, reactive lymphadenopathy, peripheral edema, hypoalbuminemia, and high-output cardiac failure. The major etiologies of erythroderma are (1) *cutaneous diseases* such as psoriasis and dermatitis (Table 57-3); (2) *drugs*; (3) *systemic diseases*, most commonly CTCL; and (4) *idiopathic*. In the first three groups, the

location and description of the initial lesions, prior to the development of the erythroderma, aid in the diagnosis. For example, a history of red scaly plaques on the elbows and knees would point to psoriasis. It is also important to examine the skin carefully for a migration of the erythema and associated secondary changes such as pustules or erosions. Migratory waves of erythema studded with superficial pustules are seen in *pustular psoriasis*.

Drug-induced erythroderma (exfoliative dermatitis) may begin as a morbilliform eruption (Chap. 59) or may arise as diffuse erythema. Fever and peripheral eosinophilia often accompany the eruption, and occasionally there is an associated allergic interstitial nephritis. A number of drugs can produce an erythroderma, including penicillins, sulfonamides, carbamazepine, phenytoin, gold, allopurinol, and captopril. While reactions to anticonvulsants can lead to a pseudolymphoma syndrome, reactions to allopurinol may be accompanied by hepatitis, gastrointestinal bleeding, and nephropathy.

The most common malignancy that is associated with erythroderma is CTCL; in some series, up to 25% of the cases of erythroderma were due to CTCL. The patient may progress from isolated plaques and tumors, but more commonly the erythroderma is present throughout the course of the disease (Sézary syndrome). In the Sézary syndrome, there are circulating atypical T lymphocytes, pruritus, and lymphadenopathy. In cases of erythroderma where there is no apparent cause (idiopathic), longitudinal follow-up is mandatory to monitor for the possible development of CTCL. There have been isolated case reports of erythroderma secondary to some solid tumors—lung, liver, prostate, thyroid, and colon—but it is usually in a late stage of the disease.

ALOPECIA (Table 57-4)   The two major forms of alopecia are scarring and nonscarring. In *scarring alopecia* there is associated fibrosis, inflammation, and loss of hair follicles. A smooth scalp with a decreased number of follicular openings is usually observed clinically, but in some cases the changes are seen only in biopsy specimens from the affected areas. In *nonscarring alopecia* the hair shafts are gone, but the hair follicles are preserved, explaining the reversible nature of nonscarring alopecia.

Primary cutaneous disorders are the most common causes of nonscarring alopecia and they include *telogen effluvium, androgenetic alopecia, alopecia areata, tinea capitis*, and *traumatic alopecia* (Table 57-5). In women with androgenetic alopecia, an elevation in circulating levels of androgens may be seen as a result of ovarian or adrenal gland dysfunction. When there are signs of virilization, such as a deepened voice and enlarged clitoris, the possibility of an ovarian or adrenal gland tumor should be considered.

Exposure to various *drugs* can also cause diffuse hair loss, usually by inducing a telogen effluvium. An exception is the anagen effluvium observed with antimitotic agents such as daunorubicin. Alopecia is a side effect of the following drugs: warfarin, heparin, propylthiouracil, carbimazole, vitamin A, isotretinoin, acetretin, lithium, beta blockers, colchicine, and amphetamines. Fortunately, spontaneous regrowth usually follows discontinuation of the offending agent.

Less commonly, nonscarring alopecia is associated with *lupus erythematosus* and *secondary syphilis*. In systemic lupus there are two forms of alopecia—one is scarring secondary to discoid lesions (see below) and the other is nonscarring. The latter form may be diffuse

Table 57-3   Erythroderma (Primary Cutaneous Disorders)

	Initial Lesions	Location of Initial Lesions	Other Findings	Diagnostic Aids	Treatment
Psoriasis[a]	Pink-red, silvery scale, sharply demarcated	Elbows, knees, scalp, presacral area	Nail dystrophy, arthritis, pustules	Skin biopsy	Oral retinoid ± PUVA; UV-B; methotrexate; cyclosporine
Dermatitis[a]					
Atopic	Acute: Erythema, fine scale, crust, indistinct borders Chronic: Lichenification (increased skin markings)	Antecubital and popliteal fossae, neck, hands	Pruritus Family history of atopy, including asthma, allergic rhinitis or conjunctivitis, and atopic dermatitis Rule out secondary infection with *S. aureus* Rule out superimposed irritant contact dermatitis	Skin biopsy	Topical glucocorticoids, tar, and antipruritics; oral antihistamines; open wet dressings; UV-B + UV-A; PUVA; oral/IM glucocorticoids Topical or oral antibiotics
Stasis	Erythema, crusting, excoriations	Lower extremities	Pruritus, lower extremity edema History of venous ulcers, thrombophlebitis, and/or cellulitis Rule out cellulitis Rule out superimposed contact dermatitis, e.g., topical neomycin	Skin biopsy	Topical glucocorticoids; open wet dressings; leg elevation; pressure stockings
Contact	Local: Erythema, crusting, vesicles, and bullae	Depends on offending agent	Irritant—onset often within hours Allergic—delayed-type hypersensitivity; lag time of 48 h	Patch testing	Remove irritant or allergen; topical glucocorticoids; oral antihistamines; oral/IM glucocorticoids
	Systemic: Erythema, fine scale, crust	Generalized	Patient has history of allergic contact dermatitis to topical agent and then receives systemic medication that is structurally related, e.g., ethylenediamine (topical) aminophylline (IV)	Patch testing	Same as local
Seborrheic	Pink-red, greasy scale	Scalp, nasolabial folds, eyebrows, intertriginous zones	Flares with stress, HIV infection Associated with Parkinson's disease	Skin biopsy	Topical glucocorticoids and imidazoles
Pityriasis rubra pilaris	Orange-red, perifollicular papules	Generalized, but characteristic "skip" areas of normal skin	Wax-like keratoderma Rule out cutaneous T cell lymphoma	Skin biopsy	Isotretinoin or acetretin; methotrexate

[a] Discussed in detail in Chap. 56.

NOTE: PUVA, *p*soralens + *u*ltraviolet *A* irradiation; UV-B, *u*ltraviolet *B*; UV-A, *u*ltraviolet *A*; IM, intramuscular; IV, intravenous.

Table 57-4   Causes of Alopecia

I. Nonscarring alopecia	II. Scarring alopecia

A. Primary cutaneous disorders
  1. Telogen effluvium
  2. Androgenetic alopecia
  3. Alopecia areata
  4. Tinea capitis
  5. Traumatic alopecia
B. Drugs
C. Systemic diseases
  1. Lupus erythematosus
  2. Secondary syphilis
  3. Hypothyroidism
  4. Hyperthyroidism
  5. Hypopituitarism
  6. Deficiencies of protein, iron, biotin, and zinc
  7. HIV infection
	A. Primary cutaneous disorders
	  1. Cutaneous lupus
	  2. Lichen planus
	  3. Folliculitis decalvans
	  4. Linear scleroderma (morphea)
	  5. Traumatic alopecia[a]
	B. Systemic diseases
	  1. Lupus erythematosus
	  2. Sarcoidosis
	  3. Cutaneous metastases

[a] Also referred to as follicular degeneration.

and involve the entire scalp, or it may localized to the frontal scalp and result in multiple short hairs ("lupus hairs"). Scattered, poorly circumscribed patches of alopecia with a "moth-eaten" appearance are a manifestation of the secondary stage of syphilis. Diffuse thinning of the hair is also associated with hypothyroidism, hyperthyroidism, and HIV infection (Table 57-4).

Scarring alopecia is more frequently the result of a primary cutaneous disorder such as *lichen planus, folliculitis decalvans, cutaneous lupus,* or *linear scleroderma (morphea)* than it is a sign of systemic disease. Although the scarring lesions of *discoid lupus* can be seen in patients with systemic lupus, in the majority of cases the disease process is limited to the skin. Less common causes of scarring alopecia include *sarcoidosis* (see "Papulonodular Skin Lesions") and cutaneous *metastases.*

In the early phases of discoid lupus, lichen planus, and folliculitis decalvans, there are circumscribed areas of alopecia. Fibrosis and subsequent loss of follicles are observed primarily in the center of the individual lesions, while the inflammatory process is most prominent at the periphery. The areas of active inflammation in discoid lupus are

Table 57-5 Nonscarring Alopecia (Primary Cutaneous Disorders)

	Clinical Characteristics	Pathogenesis	Treatment
Telogen effluvium	Diffuse shedding of normal hairs Follows either major stress (high fever, severe infection) or change in hormones (post partum) Reversible without treatment	Stress causes the normally asynchronous growth cycles of individual hairs to become synchronous; therefore, large numbers of growing (anagen) hairs simultaneously enter the dying (telogen) phase	Observation; discontinue any drugs that have alopecia as a side effect; must exclude underlying metabolic causes, e.g., hypothyroidism, hyperthyroidism
Androgenetic alopecia	Miniaturization of hairs along the midline of the scalp Recession of the anterior scalp line in men and some women	Increased sensitivity of affected hairs to the effects of testosterone Increased levels of circulating androgens (ovarian or adrenal source in women)	If no evidence of hyperandrogen state, then topical minoxidil ± tretinoin; finasteride[a]; hair transplant
Alopecia areata	Well-circumscribed, circular areas of hair loss, 2–5 cm in diameter In extensive cases, coalescence of lesions and/or involvement of other hair-bearing surfaces of the body Pitting of the nails	The germinative zones of the hair follicles are surrounded by T lymphocytes Occasional associated diseases: hyperthyroidism, hypothyroidism, vitiligo, Down's syndrome	Topical anthralin; intralesional glucocorticoids; topical contact sensitizers
Tinea	Varies from scaling with minimal hair loss to discrete patches with "black dots" (broken hairs) to boggy plaque with pustules (kerion)	Invasion of hairs by dermatophytes, most commonly *Trichophyton tonsurans*	Oral griseofulvin plus 2.5% selenium sulfide or ketoconazole shampoo; examine family members
Traumatic alopecia	Broken hairs Irregular outline	Traction with curlers, rubber bands, braiding Exposure to heat or chemicals Mechanical pulling (trichotillomania)	Discontinuation of offending hair style or chemical treatments; trichotillomania may require hair clipping and observation of shaved hairs or biopsy for diagnosis, followed by psychotherapy

[a] To date, FDA-approved for men.

Table 57-6 Causes of Figurate Skin Lesions

I. Primary cutaneous disorders
  A. Tinea
  B. Urticaria
  C. Erythema annulare centrifugum
  D. Granuloma annulare
  E. Psoriasis
II. Systemic diseases
  A. Migratory
    1. Erythema migrans
    2. Erythema gyratum repens
    3. Erythema marginatum
    4. Pustular psoriasis
    5. Necrolytic migratory erythema (glucagonoma syndrome)[a]
  B. Nonmigratory
    1. Sarcoidosis
    2. Subacute lupus erythematosus
    3. Secondary syphilis
    4. Cutaneous T cell lymphoma (e.g., mycosis fungoides)

[a] Migratory erythema with erosions; favors lower extremities and girdle area.

erythematous with scale, whereas the areas of previous inflammation are often hypopigmented with a rim of hyperpigmentation. In lichen planus the peripheral perifollicular macules are usually violet-colored. Complete examination of the skin and oral mucosa combined with a biopsy and direct immunofluorescence microscopy will aid in distinguishing these two entities. The peripheral active lesions in folliculitis decalvans are perifollicular pustules; these patients can develop a reactive arthritis.

FIGURATE SKIN LESIONS (Table 57-6) In *figurate* eruptions, the lesions form rings and arcs that are usually erythematous but can be flesh-colored to brown. Most commonly, they are due to primary cutaneous diseases such as *tinea, urticaria, erythema annulare centrifugum*, and *granuloma annulare* (Chaps. 56 and 58). An underlying systemic illness is found in a second, less common group of migratory annular erythemas. It includes *erythema gyratum repens, erythema migrans, erythema marginatum*, and *necrolytic migratory erythema*.

In erythema gyratum repens, one sees hundreds of mobile concentric arcs and wavefronts that resemble the grain in wood. A search for an underlying malignancy is mandatory in a patient with this eruption. Erythema migrans is the cutaneous manifestation of Lyme disease, which is caused by the spirochete *Borrelia burgdorferi*. In the initial stage (3 to 30 days after tick bite), a single annular lesion is usually seen, which can expand to ≥10 cm in diameter. Within several days, approximately half the patients develop multiple smaller erythematous lesions at sites distant from the bite. Associated symptoms include fever, headache, photophobia, myalgias, arthralgias, and malar rash. Erythema marginatum is seen in patients with rheumatic fever, primarily on the trunk. Lesions are pink-red in color, flat to mildly elevated, and transient.

There are additional cutaneous diseases that present as annular eruptions but lack an obvious migratory component. Examples include *CTCL, annular cutaneous lupus*, also referred to as *subacute lupus*, *secondary syphilis*, and *sarcoidosis* (see "Papulonodular Skin Lesions").

ACNE (Table 57-7) *Acne vulgaris* and *acne rosacea* are the two major forms of acne (Chap. 56). Estrogens decrease sebaceous gland activity, whereas androgens enhance sebum production. Therefore,

Table 57-7 Causes of Acneiform Eruptions

I. Primary cutaneous disorders
  A. Acne vulgaris
  B. Acne rosacea
II. Drugs
III. Systemic diseases
  A. Increased androgen production
    1. Adrenal origin, e.g., Cushing's disease, 21-hydroxylase deficiency
    2. Ovarian origin, e.g., polycystic ovary disease
  B. Cryptococcosis, disseminated
  C. Dimorphic fungi
  D. Behçet's disease

acne vulgaris in an adult, especially if it is of recent onset, may be a reflection of increased levels of circulating *androgens*. Dysfunction of the ovary or adrenal gland, e.g., polycystic ovary disease or Cushing's syndrome, can lead to the hormonal imbalance. Examination of the patient for signs such as hirsutism, androgenetic alopecia, hypertension, and redistribution of subcutaneous fat will aid in the diagnosis.

Exacerbations of acne vulgaris follow the ingestion of several *drugs*, such as anabolic steroids, glucocorticoids, lithium, and iodides as well as the application of oil-containing compounds. Acne-like lesions can be seen in patients with Behçet's disease (see "Ulcers"), and in immunocompromised hosts, disseminated fungal infections (e.g., cryptococcosis) may present as an acneiform eruption.

Patients with the carcinoid syndrome have episodes of flushing of the head, neck, and sometimes the trunk. Resultant skin changes of the face, in particular telangiectasias, may mimic the clinical appearance of acne rosacea.

PUSTULAR LESIONS *Acneiform eruptions* (see "Acne") and *folliculitis* represent the most common pustular dermatoses. An important consideration in the evaluation of perifollicular pustules is a determination of the associated pathogen, e.g., normal flora, *Staphylococcus aureus*, *Pityrosporum*. Noninfectious forms of folliculitis include HIV-associated eosinophilic folliculitis and folliculitis secondary to drugs such as glucocorticoids and lithium. Administration of high-dose oral glucocorticoids can result in a widespread eruption of perifollicular pustules on the trunk, characterized by lesions in the same stage of development. With regard to underlying systemic diseases, pustules are a characteristic component of pustular psoriasis and can be seen in septic emboli of bacterial or fungal origin (see "Purpura").

TELANGIECTASIAS (Table 57-8)   In order to distinguish the various types of telangiectasias, it is important to examine the shape and configuration of the dilated blood vessels. *Linear telangiectasias* are seen on the face of patients with *actinically damaged skin* and *acne rosacea* and they are found on the legs of patients with *venous hypertension* and *essential telangiectasia*. Patients with an unusual form of *mastocytosis* (telangiectasia macularis eruptiva perstans), the *carcinoid* syndrome (see "Acne"), and *ataxia-telangiectasia* also have linear telangiectasias. In ataxia-telangiectasia, linear telangiectasias appear on the bulbar conjunctiva during childhood. Eventually, there is involvement of the ears, eyelids, cheeks, and/or flexural areas such as the antecubital and popliteal fossae. Lastly, linear telangiectasias are found in areas of cutaneous inflammation. For example, lesions of discoid lupus frequently have telangiectasias within them.

Poikiloderma is a term used to describe a patch of skin with (1) reticulated hypo- and hyperpigmentation, (2) wrinkling secondary to epidermal atrophy, and (3) telangiectasias. Poikiloderma does not imply a single disease entity—it is seen in skin damaged by *ionizing*

radiation, in the disorders *poikiloderma vasculare atrophicans* (PVA) and *xeroderma pigmentosum*, as well as in patients with connective-tissue diseases, primarily *dermatomyositis* (DM). PVA is a precursor lesion of CTCL, and the areas of poikiloderma usually begin in the flexural areas of the axillae and groin.

In *scleroderma*, the dilated blood vessels have a unique configuration and are known as *mat telangiectasias*. The lesions are broad macules that usually measure 2 to 7 mm in diameter but occasionally are larger. Mats have a polygonal or oval shape, and their erythematous color may be uniform or the result of delicate telangiectasias. The most common locations for mat telangiectasias are the face, oral mucosa, and hands—peripheral sites that are prone to intermittent ischemia. The CREST (*c*alcinosis cutis, *R*aynaud's phenomenon, *e*sophageal dysmotility, *s*clerodactyly, and *t*elangiectasia) variant of scleroderma (Chap. 313) is associated with a chronic course and anticentromere antibodies. Mat telangiectasias are an important clue to the diagnosis of the CREST syndrome as well as systemic scleroderma, for they may be the only cutaneous finding.

Periungual telangiectasias are pathognomonic signs of the three major connective tissue diseases—*lupus erythematosus*, *scleroderma*, and *DM*. They are easily visualized by the naked eye and occur in at least two-thirds of these patients. In both DM and lupus there is associated nailfold erythema, and in DM the erythema is often accompanied by "ragged" cuticles and fingertip tenderness. Under 10× magnification, the blood vessels in the nailfolds of lupus patients are tortuous and resemble "glomeruli," whereas in scleroderma and DM there is a loss of capillary loops and those that remain are markedly dilated.

In *hereditary hemorrhagic telangiectasia* (Osler-Rendu-Weber disease), the lesions usually appear during adulthood and are most commonly seen on the mucous membranes, face, and distal extremities, including under the nails. They represent arteriovenous (AV) malformations of the dermal microvasculature, are dark red in color, and are usually slightly elevated. When the skin is stretched over an individual lesion, an eccentric punctum with radiating legs is seen. Although the degree of systemic involvement varies in this autosomal dominant disease (due to mutations in either the endoglin or activin receptor–like kinase gene), the major symptoms are recurrent epistaxis and gastrointestinal bleeding. The fact that these mucosal telangiectasias are actually AV communications helps to explain their tendency to bleed.

HYPOPIGMENTATION (Table 57-9)   Disorders of hypopigmentation are classified as either diffuse or localized. The classic ex-

Table 57-8   Causes of Telangiectasias

I. Primary cutaneous disorders	II. Systemic diseases
A. Linear	A. Linear
1. Acne rosacea	1. Carcinoid
2. Actinically damaged skin	2. Ataxia-telangiectasia
3. Venous hypertension	3. Mastocytosis
4. Essential telangiectasia	B. Poikiloderma
B. Poikiloderma	1. Dermatomyositis
1. Ionizing radiation	2. Xeroderma pigmentosum
2. Poikiloderma vasculare	3. Cutaneous T cell
atrophicans	lymphoma
C. Spider angioma	C. Mat
1. Idiopathic	1. Scleroderma
2. Pregnancy	D. Periungual
	1. Lupus erythematosus
	2. Scleroderma
	3. Dermatomyositis
	E. Papular
	1. Hereditary hemorrhagic
	telangiectasia
	F. Spider angioma
	1. Cirrhosis

Table 57-9   Causes of Hypopigmentation

I. Primary cutaneous disorders	II. Systemic diseases
A. Diffuse	A. Diffuse
1. Generalized vitiligo	1. Oculocutaneous albinism
B. Localized	a. Hermansky-Pudlak
1. Idiopathic guttate	syndrome[a]
hypomelanosis	b. Chédiak–Higashi
2. Postinflammatory[b]	syndrome[b]
3. Tinea (pityriasis)	B. Localized
versicolor	1. Vogt-Koyanagi-Harada
4. Vitiligo	2. Scleroderma
5. Chemical leukoderma	3. Melanoma-associated
6. Nevus depigmentosus	leukoderma
7. Piebaldism	4. Tuberous sclerosis
	5. Hypomelanosis of
	Ito/mosaicism
	6. Sarcoidosis
	7. Tuberculoid and indeterminate
	leprosy
	8. Cutaneous T cell lymphoma

[a] Platelet storage defect and restrictive lung disease secondary to deposits of ceroid-like material.
[b] Giant lysosomal granules and recurrent infections.

ample of *diffuse hypopigmentation* is *oculocutaneous albinism* (OCA). The most common forms are due to mutations in the tyrosinase gene (type I) or the *P* gene (type II); patients with type IA OCA have a total lack of enzyme activity. At birth, different forms of OCA can appear similar—white hair, gray-blue eyes, and pink-white skin. However, the patients with no tyrosinase activity maintain this phenotype, whereas those with decreased activity or *P* gene mutations will acquire some pigmentation of the eyes, hair, and skin as they age. The degree of pigment formation is also a function of racial background, and the pigmentary dilution is readily apparent when patients are compared to their first-degree relatives.

The ocular findings in OCA correlate with the degree of hypopigmentation and include decreased visual acuity, nystagmus, photophobia, and monocular vision. Generalized vitiligo, phenylketonuria, and homocystinuria are other unusual causes of diffuse pigmentary dilution. In generalized vitiligo, melanocytes are not found in affected skin, whereas in OCA they are present but have decreased activity. Appropriate laboratory tests exclude the other disorders of metabolism.

The differential diagnosis of *localized hypomelanosis* includes the following primary cutaneous disorders: *idiopathic guttate hypomelanosis, postinflammatory hypopigmentation, tinea (pityriasis) versicolor, vitiligo, chemical leukoderma, nevus depigmentosus* (see below), and *piebaldism* (Table 57-9). In this group of diseases, the areas of involvement are macules or patches with a decrease or absence of pigmentation. Patients with vitiligo also have an increased incidence of several autoimmune disorders, including hypothyroidism, Graves' disease, pernicious anemia, Addison's disease, uveitis, alopecia areata, chronic mucocutaneous candidiasis, and the polyglandular autoimmune syndromes (types I and II). Diseases of the thyroid gland are the most frequently associated disorders, occurring in up to 30% of patients with vitiligo. Circulating autoantibodies are often found, and the most common ones are antithyroglobulin, antimicrosomal, and antiparietal cell antibodies.

There are three systemic diseases that should be considered in a patient with skin findings suggestive of vitiligo—*Vogt-Koyanagi-Harada syndrome, scleroderma*, and *melanoma-associated leukoderma*. A history of aseptic meningitis, nontraumatic uveitis, tinnitus, hearing loss, and/or dysacousis points to the diagnosis of the Vogt-Koyanagi-Harada syndrome. In these patients, the face and scalp are the most common locations of pigment loss. The vitiligo-like leukoderma seen in patients with scleroderma has a clinical resemblance to idiopathic vitiligo that has begun to repigment as a result of treatment; that is, perifollicular macules of normal pigmentation are seen within areas of depigmentation. The basis of this leukoderma is unknown; there is no evidence of inflammation in areas of involvement, but it can resolve if the underlying connective tissue disease becomes inactive. In contrast to idiopathic vitiligo, melanoma-associated leukoderma often begins on the trunk, and its appearance should prompt a search for metastatic disease. The possibility exists that the destruction of normal melanocytes is the result of an immune response against malignant melanocytes.

There are two systemic disorders that may have the cutaneous findings of piebaldism (Table 57-10). They are *Hirschsprung's disease* and *Waardenburg's syndrome*. A possible explanation for both disorders is an abnormal embryonic migration or survival of two neural crest–derived elements, one of them being melanocytes and the other myenteric ganglion cells (Hirschsprung's disease) or auditory nerve cells (Waardenburg's syndrome). The latter syndrome is characterized by congenital sensorineural hearing loss, dystopia canthorum (lateral displacement of the inner canthi but normal interpupillary distance), heterochromic irises, and a broad nasal root, in addition to the piebaldism. Patients with Waardenburg's syndrome have been shown to have mutations in two genes that encode DNA-binding proteins, *PAX-3* and *MITF*, while patients with Hirschsprung's disease and white spotting have mutations in one of three genes—endothelin 3, endothelin B receptor, and *SOX-10*.

In *tuberous sclerosis*, the earliest cutaneous sign is an ash leaf spot. These lesions are often present at birth and are usually multiple; however, detection may require Wood's lamp examination, especially in fair-skinned individuals. The pigment within them is reduced but not absent. The average size is 1 to 3 cm, and the common shapes are polygonal and lance-ovate. Examination of the patient for additional cutaneous signs such as adenoma sebaceum (multiple angiofibromas of the face), ungual and gingival fibromas, fibrous plaques of the forehead, and connective tissue nevi (shagreen patches) is recommended. It is important to remember that an ash leaf spot on the scalp will result in *poliosis*, which is a circumscribed patch of gray-white hair. Internal manifestations include seizures, mental retardation, central nervous system (CNS) and retinal hamartomas, renal angiomyolipomas, and cardiac rhabdomyomas. The latter can be detected in up to 60% of children (<18 years) with tuberous sclerosis by echocardiography.

Nevus depigmentosus is a stable, well-circumscribed hypomelanosis that is present at birth. There is usually a single circular or rectangular lesion, but occasionally the nevus has a dermatomal or whorled pattern. It is important to distinguish this more common entity from ash leaf spots especially when there are multiple lesions. In *hypomelanosis of Ito*, swirls and streaks of hypopigmentation run parallel to one another in a pattern that resembles a marble cake. Lesions may progress or regress with time, and in up to a third of patients, associated abnormalities are found including in the musculoskeletal system (asymmetry), the CNS (seizures and mental retardation), and the eyes (strabismus and hypertelorism). Chromosomal mosaicism has been detected in these patients; this lends support to the hypothesis that the pattern is the result of the migration of two clones of primordial melanocytes, each with a different pigment potential.

Localized areas of decreased pigmentation are commonly seen as a result of cutaneous inflammation (Table 57-10) and have been observed in the skin overlying active lesions of sarcoidosis (see "Papulonodular Skin Lesions") as well as in CTCL. Cutaneous infections also present as disorders of hypopigmentation, and in *tuberculoid leprosy* there are a few asymmetric patches of hypomelanosis that have associated anesthesia, anhidrosis, and alopecia. Biopsy specimens of the palpable border show dermal granulomas that lack *Mycobacterium leprae* organisms.

HYPERPIGMENTATION (Table 57-11) Disorders of hyperpigmentation are also divided into two groups—localized and diffuse. The *localized* forms are due to an epidermal alteration, a proliferation of melanocytes, or an increase in pigment production. Both seborrheic keratoses and acanthosis nigricans belong to the first group. *Seborrheic keratoses* are common lesions, but in one clinical setting they are a sign of systemic disease, and that setting is the sudden appearance of multiple lesions, often with an inflammatory base and in association with acrochordons (skin tags) and acanthosis nigricans. This is termed the *sign of Leser-Trélat* and signifies an internal malignancy. *Acanthosis nigricans* can also be a reflection of an internal malignancy, most commonly of the gastrointestinal tract, and it appears as velvety hyperpigmentation, primarily in flexural areas. In the majority of patients, acanthosis nigricans is associated with obesity, but it may be a reflection of an endocrinopathy such as acromegaly, Cushing's syndrome, the Stein-Leventhal syndrome, or insulin-resistant diabetes mellitus (type A, type B, and lipoatrophic forms).

A proliferation of melanocytes results in the following pigmented lesions: *lentigo, melanocytic nevus*, and *melanoma* (Chap. 86). In an adult, the majority of lentigines are related to sun exposure, which explains their distribution. However, in the Peutz-Jeghers and LEOPARD [*l*entigines; *E*CG abnormalities, primarily conduction defects, *o*cular hypertelorism; *p*ulmonary stenosis and subaortic valvular stenosis; *a*bnormal genitalia (cryptorchidism, hypospadias); *r*etardation of growth; and *d*eafness (sensorineural)] syndromes, lentigines do serve as a clue to systemic disease. In the multiple lentigines or *LEOPARD syndrome*, hundreds of lentigines develop during childhood and are scattered over the entire surface of the body. The lentigines in patients with *Peutz-Jeghers syndrome* are located primarily around the nose and mouth, on the hands and feet, and within the oral cavity.

Table 57-10 Hypopigmentation (Primary Cutaneous Disorders, Localized)

	Clinical Characteristics	Wood's Lamp Examination (UV-A; Peak = 365 nm)	Skin Biopsy Specimen	Pathogenesis	Treatment
Idiopathic guttate hypomelanosis	Common; acquired; 1 to 4 mm in diameter Shins and extensor forearms	Less enhancement than vitiligo	Abrupt decrease in epidermal melanin content	Possible somatic mutations as a reflection of aging; UV exposure	None
Postinflammatory hypopigmentation	Can develop within active lesions, as in subacute lupus, or after the lesion fades, as in dermatitis	Depends on particular disease Usually less enhancement than in vitiligo	Type of inflammatory infiltrate depends on specific disease	Block in transfer of melanin from melanocytes to keratinocytes could be secondary to edema or decrease in contact time Destruction of melanocytes if inflammatory cells attack basal layer	Treat underlying inflammatory disease
Tinea (pityriasis) versicolor	Common disorder Upper trunk and neck Shawl-like distribution Young adults Macules have fine white scale when scratched	Golden fluorescence	Hyphae and budding yeast in stratum corneum	Invasion of stratum corneum by the yeast *Pityrosporum* Yeast is lipophilic and produces C_9 and C_{11} dicarboxylic acids which in vitro inhibit tyrosinase	Selenium sulfide 2.5%; topical imidazoles; oral imidazoles or triazoles
Vitiligo	Acquired; progressive Symmetric areas of complete pigment loss Periorificial—around mouth, nose, eyes, nipples, umbilicus, anus Other areas—flexor wrists, extensor distal extremities Segmental form is less common—unilateral, dermatomal-like	More apparent Chalk-white	Absence of melanocytes Mild inflammation	Possible autoimmune phenomenon that results in destruction of melanocytes—humoral and/or cellular Alternative hypothesis is self-destruction of melanocytes and circulating antibodies or cytotoxic T cells as a secondary phenomenon	Topical glucocorticoids; PUVA; UV-B; transplants; depigmentation if widespread
Chemical leukoderma	Similar appearance to vitiligo Often begins on hands Satellite lesions in areas not exposed to chemicals	More apparent Chalk-white	Decreased number or absence of melanocytes	Exposure to chemicals that selectively destroy melanocytes, in particular, phenols and catechols (germicides; adhesives) Release of cellular antigens and activation of circulating lymphocytes may explain satellite phenomenon	Avoid exposure to offending agent, then treat as vitiligo
Piebaldism	Autosomal dominant Congenital, stable White forelock Areas of hypomelanosis contain normally pigmented and hyperpigmented macules of various sizes Symmetric involvement of central forehead, ventral trunk, and mid regions of upper and lower extremities	Enhancement of leukoderma and hyperpigmented macules	Hypomelanotic areas—few to no melanocytes	Defect in migration of melanoblasts from neural crest to ventral skin or failure of melanoblasts to survive or differentiate in these areas Mutations within the c-*kit* proto-oncogene that encodes the tyrosine kinase receptor for mast/stem cell growth factor	None; occasionally transplants

NOTE: PUVA, *p*soralens + *u*ltraviolet *A* irradiation; UV-B, *u*ltraviolet B.

While the pigmented macules on the face may fade with age, the oral lesions persist. However, similar intraoral lesions are also seen in Addison's disease and as a normal finding in darkly pigmented individuals. Patients with this autosomal dominant syndrome (due to mutations in a novel serine threonine kinase gene) have multiple benign polyps of the gastrointestinal tract, testicular tumors, and an increased risk of developing gastrointestinal (primarily colon), breast, and gynecologic cancers.

Lentigines are also seen in association with cardiac myxomas and have been described in two syndromes whose findings overlap: *LAMB* (*l*entigines, *a*trial myxomas, *m*ucocutaneous myxomas, and *b*lue nevi) *syndrome* and *NAME* [*n*evus, *a*trial myxoma, *m*yxoid neurofibroma, and *e*phelides (freckles)] *syndrome*. These patients can also have evidence of endocrine overactivity in the form of Cushing's syndrome, acromegaly, or sexual precocity.

The third type of localized hyperpigmentation is due to a local increase in pigment production, and it includes *ephelides* and café au lait macules (CALM). The latter are most commonly associated with two disorders—neurofibromatosis (NF) and McCune-Albright syndrome. *CALM* are flat, uniformly light brown in color, and can vary in size from 0.5 to 12 cm. Approximately 80% of adult patients with *type I NF* will have six or more CALM measuring 1.5 cm or greater in diameter. Additional findings are discussed in the section on neurofibromas (see "Papulonodular Skin Lesions"). In comparison with NF, the CALM in patients with *McCune-Albright syndrome* [polyostotic fibrous dysplasia with precocious puberty in females due to

Table 57-11   Causes of Hyperpigmentation

I. Primary cutaneous disorders
  A. Localized
    1. Epidermal alteration
      a. Seborrheic keratosis
      b. Acanthosis nigricans (obesity)
      c. Pigmented actinic keratosis
    2. Proliferation of melanocytes
      a. Lentigo
      b. Nevus
      c. Melanoma
    3. Increased pigment production
      a. Ephelides (freckles)
      b. Café au lait macule
  B. Localized and diffuse
    1. Drugs
II. Systemic diseases
  A. Localized
    1. Epidermal alteration
      a. Seborrheic keratoses (sign of Leser-Trélat)
      b. Acanthosis nigricans (endocrine disorders, paraneoplastic)
    2. Proliferation of melanocytes
      a. Lentigines (Peutz-Jeghers and LEOPARD syndromes; xeroderma pigmentosum)
      b. Nevi [Carney complex (LAMB and NAME syndromes)][a]
    3. Increased pigment production
      a. Café au lait macules (neurofibromatosis, McCune-Albright syndrome[b])
      b. Urticaria pigmentosa[c]
    4. Dermal pigmentation
      a. Incontinentia pigmenti
      b. Dyskeratosis congenita
  B. Diffuse
    1. Endocrinopathies
      a. Addison's disease
      b. Nelson syndrome
      c. Ectopic ACTH syndrome
    2. Metabolic
      a. Porphyria cutanea tarda
      b. Hemochromatosis
      c. Vitamin B_{12}, folate deficiency
      d. Pellagra
      e. Malabsorption, Whipple's disease
    3. Melanosis secondary to metastatic melanoma
    4. Autoimmune
      a. Biliary cirrhosis
      b. Scleroderma
      c. POEMS syndrome
      d. Eosinophilia-myalgia syndrome
    5. Drugs and metals

[a] Also lentigines.
[b] Polyostotic fibrous dysplasia.
[c] See also "Papulonodular Skin Lesions."

mosaicism for an activating mutation in a G protein ($G_s\alpha$) gene] are usually larger, more irregular in outline, and tend to respect the midline. CALM have also been associated with pulmonary stenosis (Watson syndrome), tuberous sclerosis, the LEOPARD syndrome, and ataxia telangiectasia, but a few such lesions can be found in normal individuals.

In incontinentia pigmenti, dyskeratosis congenita, and bleomycin pigmentation, the areas of localized hyperpigmentation form a pattern—swirled in the first, reticulated in the second, and flagellate in the third. Patients with the X-linked dominant disorder *incontinentia pigmenti* can have linear blisters and verrucous papules during infancy. During childhood, parallel swirls and streaks of hyperpigmentation appear on the trunk, and occasionally streaks of hypopigmentation appear on the extremities. Associated findings include seizures, mental retardation, retinal vascular abnormalities, and delayed or impaired dentition. Biopsy specimens of the streaks will show pigment within dermal macrophages ("incontinent pigment"). In *dyskeratosis congenita*, atrophic reticulated hyperpigmentation is seen on the neck, thighs,

and trunk and is accompanied by nail dystrophy, pancytopenia, and leukoplakia of the oral and anal mucosa. The latter often develops into squamous cell carcinoma. In addition to the flagellate pigmentation (linear streaks) on the trunk, patients receiving bleomycin often have hyperpigmentation on the elbows, knees, and small joints of the hand.

Localized hyperpigmentation is seen as a side effect of several other *systemic medications*, including those that produce fixed drug reactions [phenolphthalein, nonsteroidal anti-inflammatory drugs (NSAIDs), sulfonamides, and barbiturates] and those that can complex with melanin (antimalarials). Fixed drug eruptions recur in the same location as circular areas of erythema that can become bullous and then resolve as brown macules. The eruption usually appears within hours of administration of the offending agent, and common locations include the genitalia, extremities, and perioral region. Chloroquine and hydroxychloroquine produce gray-brown to blue-black discoloration of the shins, hard palate, and face, while blue macules can be seen on the lower extremities and in sites of inflammation with prolonged minocycline administration. Estrogen in oral contraceptives can induce melasma—symmetric brown patches on the face, especially the cheeks, upper lip, and forehead. Similar changes are seen in pregnancy, in patients receiving hydantoin, and in the adult form of Gaucher's disease. In the latter group there is also hyperpigmentation of the distal lower extremities.

In the *diffuse* forms of hyperpigmentation, the darkening of the skin may be of equal intensity over the entire body or may be accentuated in sun-exposed areas. The causes of diffuse hyperpigmentation can be divided into four groups—endocrine, metabolic, autoimmune, and drugs. The endocrinopathies that frequently have associated hyperpigmentation include *Addison's disease, Nelson syndrome*, and *ectopic ACTH syndrome*. In these diseases, the increased pigmentation is diffuse but is accentuated in the palmar creases, sites of friction, scars, and the oral mucosa. An overproduction of the pituitary hormones α-MSH (melanocyte-stimulating hormone) and ACTH can lead to an increase in melanocyte activity. These peptides are products of the proopiomelanocortin gene and exhibit homology; e.g., α-MSH and ACTH share 13 amino acids. A minority of the patients with Cushing's disease or hyperthyroidism have generalized hyperpigmentation.

The metabolic causes of hyperpigmentation include *porphyria cutanea tarda* (PCT), *hemochromatosis, vitamin B_{12} deficiency, folic acid deficiency, pellagra, malabsorption*, and *Whipple's disease*. In patients with PCT (see "Vesicles/Bullae"), the skin darkening is seen in sun-exposed areas and is a reflection of the photoreactive properties of porphyrins. The increased level of iron in the skin of patients with hemochromatosis stimulates melanin pigment production and leads to the classic bronze color. Patients with pellagra have a brown discoloration of the skin, especially in sun-exposed areas, as a result of nicotinic acid (niacin) deficiency. In the areas of increased pigmentation, there is a thin varnish-like scale. These changes are also seen in patients who are vitamin B_6 deficient, have functioning carcinoid tumors (increased consumption of niacin), or take isoniazid. Approximately 50% of the patients with Whipple's disease have an associated generalized hyperpigmentation in association with diarrhea, weight loss, arthritis, and lymphadenopathy. A diffuse slate-blue color is seen in patients with melanosis secondary to metastatic melanoma. Although there is a debate as to whether the color is due to single-cell metastases in the dermis or to a widespread deposition of melanin resulting from the high concentration of circulating melanin precursors, there is more evidence to support the latter.

Of the autoimmune diseases associated with diffuse hyperpigmentation, *biliary cirrhosis* and *scleroderma* are the most common, and occasionally, both disorders are seen in the same patient. The skin is dark brown in color, especially in sun-exposed areas. In biliary cirrhosis the hyperpigmentation is accompanied by pruritus, jaundice, and xanthomas, whereas in scleroderma it is accompanied by sclerosis of the extremities, face, and, less commonly, the trunk. Additional clues to the diagnosis of scleroderma are telangiectasias, calcinosis cutis, Raynaud's phenomenon, and distal ulcerations (see "Telangiectasias"). The differential diagnosis of cutaneous sclerosis with hyperpigmentation includes the POEMS [*polyneuropathy*; *organomegaly* (liver, spleen, lymph nodes); *endocrinopathies* (impotence, gynecomastia); *M*-protein; and *skin changes*] syndrome. The skin changes include hyperpigmentation, skin thickening, hypertrichosis, and angiomas.

In the late 1980s, an epidemic of the eosinophilia-myalgia syndrome was described that was presumably due to contaminated L-tryptophan preparations. In addition to maculopapular eruptions and alopecia, large areas of scleroderma-like induration were observed with overlying hyperpigmentation.

Diffuse hyperpigmentation that is due to *drugs* or *metals* can result from one of several mechanisms—induction of melanin pigment formation, complexing of the drug or its metabolites to melanin, and deposits of the drug in the dermis. Busulfan, cyclophosphamide, long-term, high-dose ACTH, and inorganic arsenic induce pigment production. Complexes containing melanin or hemosiderin plus the drug or its metabolites are seen in patients receiving chlorpromazine and minocycline. The sun-exposed skin as well as the conjunctivae of patients on long-term, high-dose chlorpromazine can become blue-gray in color. Patients taking minocycline may develop a diffuse blue-gray, muddy appearance in sun-exposed areas in addition to pigmentation of the mucous membranes, teeth, nails, bones, and thyroid. Administration of amiodarone can result in both a phototoxic eruption (exaggerated sunburn) and/or a brown or blue-gray discoloration of sun-exposed skin. Biopsy specimens of the latter show yellow-brown granules in dermal macrophages, which represent intralysosomal accumulations of lipids, amiodarone, and its metabolites. Actual deposits of a particular drug or metal in the skin are seen with silver (argyria), where the skin appears blue-gray in color; gold (chrysiasis), where the skin has a brown to blue-gray color; and clofazimine, where the skin appears reddish brown. The associated hyperpigmentation is accentuated in sun-exposed areas, and discoloration of the eye is seen with gold (sclerae) and clofazimine (conjunctivae).

VESICLES/BULLAE (Table 57-12) Depending on their size, cutaneous blisters are referred to as *vesicles* (<0.5 cm) or *bullae* (>0.5 cm). The primary blistering disorders include *pemphigus vulgaris, pemphigus foliaceus, pemphigus erythematosus, paraneoplastic pemphigus, bullous pemphigoid, herpes gestationis, cicatricial pemphigoid, epidermolysis bullosa acquisita, linear IgA disease,* and *dermatitis herpetiformis* (Chap. 58).

Vesicles and bullae are also seen in *contact dermatitis*, both allergic and irritant forms (Chap. 56). When there is a linear arrangement of vesicular lesions, an exogenous cause should be suspected. Bullous disease secondary to the ingestion of drugs can take one of several forms, including phototoxic eruptions, isolated bullae, toxic epidermal necrolysis, and erythema multiforme (Chap. 59). Clinically, phototoxic eruptions resemble an exaggerated sunburn with diffuse erythema and bullae in sun-exposed areas. The most commonly associated drugs are thiazides, doxycycline, sulfonamides, NSAIDs, and psoralens. The development of a phototoxic eruption is dependent on the doses of both the drug and UV-A irradiation.

Toxic epidermal necrolysis (TEN) is characterized by bullae that arise on widespread areas of erythema and then slough. This results in large areas of denuded skin. The associated morbidity, such as sepsis, and mortality are relatively high and are a function of the extent of epidermal necrosis. In addition, these patients may also have involvement of the mucous membranes and intestinal tract. Drugs are the primary cause of TEN, and the most common offenders are phenytoin, barbiturates, sulfonamides, penicillins, and NSAIDs. Severe acute graft-versus-host disease (grade 4) also can resemble TEN.

In *erythema multiforme* (EM), the primary lesions are pink-red macules and edematous papules, the centers of which may become vesicular. The clue to the diagnosis of EM, as opposed to a drug-induced morbilliform exanthem, is the development of a "dusky" violet color or petechiae in the center of the lesions. Target or iris lesions are also characteristic of EM and arise as a result of active centers and borders in combination with centrifugal spread. However, iris lesions need not be present to make the diagnosis of EM. Preferred sites of involvement include the distal extremities and mucous membranes (oral, nasal, ocular, and genital). Hemorrhagic crusts of the lips are characteristic of EM as well as herpes simplex, pemphigus vulgaris, and paraneoplastic pemphigus. Fever, malaise, myalgias, sore throat, and cough may precede or accompany the eruption. The lesions of EM usually resolve over 3 to 6 weeks but may be recurrent.

Drugs can induce EM, in particular sulfonamides, phenytoin, barbiturates, penicillins, and carbamazepine, but they do not cause the majority of cases, especially in young adults. Infections with herpes simplex are the most common cause of EM in this age group, and the lesions appear 7 to 12 days after the viral eruption. Other infectious agents associated with EM include *Mycoplasma pneumoniae*, dimorphic fungi, and several viruses (echovirus, coxsackievirus, Epstein-Barr, and influenza). EM can also follow vaccinations with BCG, poliomyelitis, or vaccinia viruses; radiation therapy; and exposure to environmental toxins.

In addition to primary blistering disorders and hypersensitivity reactions, bacterial and viral infections can lead to vesicles and bullae. The most common infectious agents are herpes simplex (Chap. 182), herpes varicella-zoster (Chap. 183), and staphylococci (Chap. 139).

Staphylococcal scalded-skin syndrome (SSSS) and *bullous impetigo* are two blistering disorders associated with staphylococcal (phage group II) infection. In SSSS, the initial findings are redness and tenderness of the central face, neck, trunk, and intertriginous zones. This is followed by short-lived flaccid bullae and a slough or exfoliation of the superficial epidermis. Crusted areas then develop, characteristically around the mouth. SSSS is distinguished from TEN by the following features: younger age group, more superficial site of blister formation, no oral lesions, shorter course, less morbidity and mortality, and an association with staphylococcal exfoliative toxin ("exfoliatin"), not drugs. A rapid diagnosis of SSSS versus TEN can be made by a frozen section of the blister roof or exfoliative cytology of the blister contents. In SSSS the site of staphylococcal infection is usually extracutaneous (conjunctivitis, rhinorrhea, otitis media, pharyngitis, tonsillitis), and the cutaneous lesions are sterile, whereas in bullous impetigo the skin lesions are the site of infection. Impetigo is more localized than SSSS

Table 57-12 Causes of Vesicles/Bullae

I. Primary cutaneous diseases
  A. Primary blistering diseases (autoimmune)
    1. Pemphigus[a]
    2. Bullous pemphigoid[b]
    3. Herpes gestationis[b]
    4. Cicatricial pemphigoid[b]
    5. Dermatitis herpetiformis[b,c]
    6. Linear IgA disease[b]
    7. Epidermolysis bullosa acquisita[b,d]
  B. Secondary blistering diseases
    1. Contact[a]
    2. Erythema multiforme[a,b]
    3. Toxic epidermal necrolysis[b]
  C. Infections
    1. Varicella/zoster[a,e]
    2. Herpes simplex[a,e]
    3. Enteroviruses, e.g., hand-foot-and-mouth disease
    4. Staphylococcal scalded-skin syndrome[a,f]
    5. Bullous impetigo[a]

II. Systemic diseases
  A. Autoimmune
    1. Paraneoplastic pemphigus[a]
  B. Infections
    1. Cutaneous emboli[b]
  C. Metabolic
    1. Diabetic bullae[a,b]
    2. Porphyria cutanea tarda[b]
    3. Porphyria variegata[b]
    4. Pseudoporphyria[b]
    5. Bullous dermatosis of hemodialysis[b]
  D. Ischemia
    1. Coma bullae

[a] Intraepidermal.
[b] Subepidermal.
[c] Associated with gluten enteropathy.
[d] Associated with inflammatory bowel disease.
[e] Also systemic.
[f] In adults, associated with renal failure and immunocompromised state.

and usually presents with honey-colored crusts. Occasionally, superficial purulent blisters also form. *Cutaneous emboli* from gram-negative infections may present as isolated bullae, but the base of the lesion is purpuric or necrotic, and it may develop into an ulcer (see "Purpura").

Several metabolic disorders are associated with blister formation, including diabetes mellitus, renal failure, and porphyria. Local hypoxia secondary to decreased cutaneous blood flow can also produce blisters, which explains the presence of bullae over pressure points in comatose patients (coma bullae). In *diabetes mellitus*, tense bullae with clear viscous fluid arise on normal skin. The lesions can be as large as 6 cm in diameter and are located on the distal extremities. There are several types of porphyria, but the most common form with cutaneous findings is *PCT*. In sun-exposed areas (primarily the face and hands), the skin is very fragile, and trauma leads to erosions and tense vesicles. These lesions then heal with scarring and formation of milia; the latter are firm, 2- to 3-mm white or yellow papules that represent epidermoid inclusion cysts. Associated findings can include hypertrichosis of the lateral malar region (males) or face (females) and, in sun-exposed areas, hyperpigmentation and firm sclerotic plaques. An elevated level of urinary uroporphyrins confirms the diagnosis and is due to a decrease in uroporphyrinogen decarboxylase activity. Precipitating agents include alcohol, iron, chlorinated hydrocarbons, and hepatitis C infection.

The differential diagnosis of PCT includes (1) *porphyria variegata*—the skin signs of PCT plus the systemic findings of acute intermittent porphyria; it has a diagnostic plasma porphyrin fluorescence emission at 626 nm; (2) *drug-induced bullous photosensitivity* (pseudoporphyria)—the clinical and histologic findings are similar to PCT, but porphyrins are normal; etiologic agents include naproxen, furosemide, tetracycline, and nalidixic acid; (3) *bullous dermatosis of hemodialysis*—the same appearance as PCT, but porphyrins are usually normal or occasionally borderline elevated; patients have chronic renal failure and are on hemodialysis; (4) PCT associated with hepatomas, hepatic carcinomas, and hemodialysis; and (5) *epidermolysis bullosa acquisita* (Chap. 58).

EXANTHEMS (Table 57-13)   Exanthems are characterized by an acute generalized eruption. The two most common presentations are erythematous macules and papules (morbilliform) and confluent blanching erythema (scarlatiniform). *Morbilliform* eruptions are usually due to either *drugs* or *viral infections*. For example, up to 5% of the patients receiving penicillins, sulfonamides, phenytoin, or gold will develop a maculopapular eruption. Accompanying signs may include pruritus, fever, eosinophilia, and transient lymphadenopathy. Similar maculopapular eruptions are seen in the classic childhood viral exanthems, including (1) *rubeola* (measles)—a prodrome of coryza, cough, and conjunctivitis followed by Koplik's spots on the buccal mucosa;

Table 57-13   Causes of Exanthems

I. Morbilliform
  A. Drugs
  B. Viral
    1. Rubeola (measles)
    2. Rubella
    3. Erythema infectiosum
    4. Epstein-Barr, echovirus, coxsackievirus, and adenovirus
    5. Early HIV
  C. Bacterial
    1. Typhoid fever
    2. Early secondary syphilis
    3. Early *Rickettsia*
    4. Early meningococcus
  D. Acute graft-versus-host disease
  E. Kawasaki's disease
II. Scarlatiniform
  A. Scarlet fever
  B. Toxic shock syndrome
  C. Kawasaki's disease

the eruption begins behind the ears, at the hairline, and on the forehead and then spreads down the body, often becoming confluent; (2) *rubella*—it begins on the forehead and face and then spreads down the body; it resolves in the same order and is associated with retroauricular and suboccipital lymphadenopathy; and (3) *erythema infectiosum* (fifth disease)—erythema of the cheeks is followed by a reticulated pattern on extremities; it is secondary to a parvovirus B19 infection, and an associated arthritis is seen in adults.

Both measles and rubella are seen in unvaccinated young adults, and an atypical form of measles is seen in adults immunized with either killed measles vaccine or killed vaccine followed in time by live vaccine. In contrast to classic measles, the eruption of atypical measles begins on the palms, soles, wrists, and knuckles, and the lesions may become purpuric. The patient with atypical measles can have pulmonary involvement and be quite ill. Rubelliform and roseoliform eruptions are also associated with *Epstein-Barr virus* (5 to 15% of patients), *echovirus*, *coxsackievirus*, and *adenovirus* infections. Detection of specific IgM antibodies or fourfold elevations in IgG antibodies allows the proper diagnosis. Occasionally, a maculopapular eruption is the result of a drug-viral interaction. For example, about 95% of the patients with infectious mononucleosis who are given ampicillin will develop a rash.

Of note, early in the course of infections with *Rickettsia* and *meningococcus*, prior to the development of purpura, the lesions may be erythematous macules and papules. This is also the case in chickenpox prior to the development of vesicles. Maculopapular eruptions are associated with early *HIV infection*, early secondary *syphilis*, *typhoid fever*, and *acute graft-versus-host disease*. In the last, lesions frequently begin on the palms and soles; the macular rose spots of typhoid fever involve primarily the anterior trunk.

The prototypic *scarlatiniform* eruption is seen in *scarlet fever* and is due to an erythrotoxin produced by group A β-hemolytic streptococcal infections, most commonly pharyngitis. This eruption is characterized by diffuse erythema, which begins on the neck and upper trunk, and red perifollicular puncta. Additional findings include a white strawberry tongue (white coating with red papillae) followed by a red strawberry tongue (red tongue with red papillae); petechiae of the palate; a facial flush with circumoral pallor; linear petechiae in the antecubital fossae; and desquamation of the involved skin, palms, and soles 5 to 20 days after onset of the eruption. A similar desquamation of the palms and soles is seen in toxic shock syndrome, Kawasaki's disease, and after severe febrile illnesses. Certain strains of staphylococci also produce an erythrotoxin that leads to the same clinical findings as in streptococcal scarlet fever, except that the antistreptolysin O titers are not elevated.

In *toxic shock syndrome* (TSS), staphylococcal (phage group I) infections produce an exotoxin (TSST-1) that causes the fever and rash, as well as enterotoxins. Initially, the majority of cases were reported in menstruating women who were using tampons. However, other sites of infection, including wounds and vaginitis, may produce TSS. The diagnosis of TSS is based on clinical criteria (Chap. 139), and three of these involve mucocutaneous sites. The clinical criteria are (1) fever; (2) diffuse erythema of the skin; (3) desquamation of the palms and soles 1 to 2 weeks after onset of illness; (4) hypotension; and (5) involvement of three or more organ systems, including the gastrointestinal tract, muscles, kidney, liver, CNS, hematologic (thrombocytopenia), and mucous membranes. The latter is characterized as hyperemia of the vagina, oropharynx, or conjunctivae. Similar systemic findings have been described in *streptococcal toxic shock–like syndrome* (Chap. 140), and although an exanthem is seen less often than in TSS due to a staphylococcal infection, the underlying infection is often in the soft tissue.

The cutaneous eruption in *Kawasaki's disease* (mucocutaneous lymph node syndrome) (Chap. 317) is polymorphous, but the two most common forms are morbilliform and scarlatiniform. The majority of cases are seen in children less than 5 years of age, but adult cases have been reported. The diagnosis is based on a fever lasting more than 5 days plus four of the five following criteria: (1) bilateral conjunctival

Table 57-14 Causes of Urticaria

I. Primary cutaneous disorders
  A. Acute and chronic urticaria
  B. Physical urticaria
    1. Dermatographism
    2. Solar urticaria[a]
    3. Cold urticaria[a]
    4. Cholinergic urticaria[a]
  C. Angioedema (hereditary and acquired)[a]
II. Systemic diseases
  A. Urticarial vasculitis
  B. Hepatitis B or C infection
  C. Serum sickness
  D. Angioedema (hereditary and acquired)

[a] Also systemic.

injection; (2) exanthem; (3) cervical lymphadenopathy, usually unilateral; (4) erythema and edema of the hands and feet followed by desquamation; and (5) diffuse erythema of the oropharynx, red strawberry tongue, and erosions with crusting on the lips. This clinical picture can resemble TSS and scarlet fever, but clues to the diagnosis of Kawasaki's disease are the cervical lymphadenopathy, lip erosions, and increased platelets. The most serious associated systemic finding in this disease is coronary aneurysm secondary to arteritis. Aneurysms may lead to sudden death, primarily within the first 30 days of the illness. Scarlatiniform eruptions are also seen in the early phase of SSSS (see "Vesicles/Bullae") and as reactions to drugs.

URTICARIA (Table 57-14) *Urticaria* (hives) are transient lesions that are composed of a central wheal surrounded by an erythematous halo. Individual lesions are round, oval, or figurate and are often pruritic. *Acute* and *chronic* urticaria have a wide variety of allergic etiologies. Less common systemic causes of urticaria are mastocytosis (urticaria pigmentosa), hyperthyroidism, malignancy, and juvenile rheumatoid arthritis (JRA). In JRA, the lesions coincide with the fever spike and are transient but not migratory as in erythema marginatum.

The common *physical urticarias* include dermographism, solar urticaria, cold urticaria, and cholinergic urticaria. Patients with *dermographism* exhibit linear wheals following minor pressure or scratching of the skin. It is a common disorder, affecting approximately 5% of the population. *Solar urticaria* characteristically occur within minutes of sun exposure and are a skin sign of one systemic disease—erythropoietic protoporphyria. In addition to the urticaria, these patients have subtle pitted scarring of the nose and hands. *Cold urticaria* are precipitated by exposure to the cold, and therefore exposed areas are usually affected. In some cases, the disease is associated with abnormal circulating proteins—more commonly cryoglobulins and less commonly cryofibrinogens and cold agglutinins. Additional systemic symptoms include wheezing and syncope, thus explaining the need for these patients to avoid swimming in cold water. *Cholinergic urticaria* are precipitated by heat, exercise, or emotion and are characterized by small wheals with relatively large flares. They are occasionally associated with wheezing.

Whereas urticaria are the result of dermal edema, subcutaneous edema leads to the clinical picture of *angioedema*. Sites of involvement include the eyelids, lips, tongue, larynx, and gastrointestinal tract as well as the subcutaneous tissue. Angioedema occurs alone or in combination with urticaria, including urticarial vasculitis and the physical urticarias. Both acquired and hereditary (autosomal dominant) forms of angioedema occur (Chap. 310), and in the latter, urticaria is rarely seen.

Urticarial vasculitis is an immune complex disease that may be confused with simple urticaria. In contrast to simple urticaria, individual lesions tend to last longer than 24 h and usually develop central petechiae that can be observed even after the urticarial phase has resolved. The patient may also complain of burning rather than pruritus. On biopsy, there is a leukocytoclastic vasculitis of the small blood vessels. Although many cases of urticarial vasculitis are idiopathic in origin, it can be a reflection of an underlying systemic illness such as lupus erythematosus, Sjögren's syndrome, or hereditary complement deficiency. There is a spectrum of urticarial vasculitis that ranges from purely cutaneous to multisystem involvement. The most common systemic signs and symptoms are arthralgias and/or arthritis, nephritis, and crampy abdominal pain, with asthma and chronic obstructive lung disease seen less often. Hypocomplementemia occurs in one- to two-thirds of patients, even in the idiopathic cases. Urticarial vasculitis can also be seen in patients with *hepatitis B* and *hepatitis C* infections, *serum sickness*, and *serum sickness–like illnesses*.

PAPULONODULAR SKIN LESIONS (Table 57-15) In the *papulonodular diseases*, the lesions are elevated above the surface of the skin and may coalesce to form plaques. The location, consistency, and color of the lesions are the keys to their diagnosis; this section is organized on the basis of color.

White Lesions In *calcinosis cutis* there are firm white to white-yellow papules with an irregular surface. When the contents are dis-

Table 57-15 Papulonodular Skin Lesions According to Color Groups

I. White
  A. Calcinosis cutis
II. Skin-colored
  A. Rheumatoid nodules
  B. Neurofibromas (von Recklinghausen's disease)
  C. Angiofibromas (tuberous sclerosis, MEN syndrome, type 1)
  D. Neuromas (MEN syndrome, type 2b)
  E. Adnexal tumors
    1. Basal cell epitheliomas (basal cell nevus syndrome)
    2. Tricholemmomas (Cowden disease)
  F. Osteomas (Gardner syndrome)
  G. Primary cutaneous disorders
    1. Epidermal inclusion cysts
    2. Lipomas
III. Pink/translucent[a]
  A. Amyloidosis
  B. Papular mucinosis
IV. Yellow
  A. Xanthomas
  B. Tophi
  C. Necrobiosis lipoidica
  D. Pseudoxanthoma elasticum
  E. Sebaceous adenomas (Torre syndrome)
V. Red[a]
  A. Papules
    1. Angiokeratomas (Fabry's disease)
    2. Bacillary angiomatosis (primarily in AIDS)
  B. Papules/plaques
    1. Cutaneous lupus
    2. Lymphoma cutis
    3. Leukemia cutis
  C. Nodules
    1. Panniculitis
    2. Cutaneous polyarteritis nodosa
    3. Systemic vasculitis
  D. Primary cutaneous disorders
    1. Arthropod bites
    2. Cherry hemangiomas
    3. Infections, e.g., erysipelas, sporotrichosis
    4. Polymorphous light eruption
    5. Lymphocytoma cutis (pseudolymphoma)
VI. Red-brown[a]
  A. Sarcoidosis
  B. Sweet's syndrome
  C. Urticaria pigmentosa
  D. Erythema elevatum diutinum (chronic leukocytoclastic vasculitis)
  E. Lupus vulgaris
VII. Blue[a]
  A. Venous malformations (blue rubber bleb syndrome)
  B. Primary cutaneous disorders
    1. Venous lake
    2. Blue nevus
VIII. Violaceous
  A. Lupus pernio (sarcoidosis)
  B. Lymphoma cutis
  C. Cutaneous lupus
IX. Purple
  A. Kaposi's sarcoma
  B. Angiosarcoma
  C. Palpable purpura
X. Brown-black[b]
XI. Any color
  A. Metastases

[a] May have darker hue in more darkly pigmented individuals.
[b] See also "Hyperpigmentation."
NOTE: MEN, multiple endocrine neoplasia.

charged, a chalky white material is seen. *Dystrophic* calcification is seen at sites of previous inflammation or damage to the skin. It develops in acne scars as well as on the distal extremities of patients with scleroderma and in the subcutaneous tissue and intermuscular fascial planes in DM. The latter is more extensive and is more commonly seen in children. An elevated calcium phosphate product, as in secondary hyperparathyroidism, can lead to nodules of *metastatic* calcinosis cutis, which tend to be subcutaneous and periarticular. This form is often accompanied by calcification of muscular arteries and subsequent ischemic necrosis (calciphylaxis).

Skin-Colored Lesions   There are several types of skin-colored lesions, including epidermoid inclusion cysts, lipomas, rheumatoid nodules, neurofibromas, angiofibromas, neuromas, and adnexal tumors such as tricholemmomas. Both *epidermoid inclusion cysts* and *lipomas* are very common mobile subcutaneous nodules—the former are rubbery and compressible and drain cheeselike material (sebum and keratin) if incised. Lipomas are firm and somewhat lobulated on palpation. When extensive facial epidermoid inclusion cysts develop in childhood or there is a family history of such lesions, the patient should be examined for other signs of Gardner syndrome, including osteomas and desmoid tumors. *Rheumatoid nodules* are firm, 0.5- to 4-cm nodules that tend to localize around pressure points, especially the elbows. They are seen in approximately 20% of patients with rheumatoid arthritis and 6% of patients with Still's disease. Biopsies of the nodules show palisading granulomas. Similar lesions that are smaller and shorter-lived are seen in rheumatic fever.

Neurofibromas (benign Schwann cell tumors) are soft papules or nodules that exhibit the "button-hole" sign, that is, they invaginate into the skin with pressure in a manner similar to a hernia. Single lesions are seen in normal individuals, but multiple neurofibromas, usually in combination with six or more CALM measuring >1.5 cm (see "Hyperpigmentation") and multiple Lisch nodules, are seen in von Recklinghausen's disease (NF type I). Lisch nodules are 1-mm yellow-brown spots within the iris that are best observed with slit-lamp examination. Additional manifestations include axillary freckling and peripheral and CNS tumors (Chap. 370). In some patients the neurofibromas are localized and unilateral, whereas in others they are limited to the CNS.

Angiofibromas are firm, pink to skin-colored papules that measure from 3 mm to several centimeters in diameter. When they are located on the central cheeks (adenoma sebaceum) or multiple fibromas are seen around the nails, the patient has tuberous sclerosis. It is an autosomal disorder due to mutations in two different genes, and the associated findings are discussed in the section on ash leaf spots as well as in Chap. 370. Multiple facial angiofibromas have also been observed in patients with multiple endocrine neoplasia (MEN) syndrome, type 1.

Neuromas (benign proliferations of nerve fibers) are also firm, skin-colored papules. They are more commonly found at sites of amputation and as rudimentary supernumerary digits. However, when there are multiple neuromas on the eyelids, lips, distal tongue, and/or oral mucosa, the patient should be investigated for other signs of the MEN syndrome, type 2b. Associated findings include marfanoid habitus, protuberant lips, intestinal ganglioneuromas, and medullary thyroid carcinoma (>75% of patients; Chap. 339).

Adnexal tumors are derived from pluripotential cells of the epidermis that can differentiate toward hair, sebaceous, apocrine, or eccrine glands or remain undifferentiated. *Basal cell epitheliomas* (BCEs) are examples of adnexal tumors that have little or no evidence of differentiation. Clinically, they are translucent papules with rolled borders, telangiectasias, and central erosion. BCEs commonly arise in sun-damaged skin of the head and neck. When a patient has multiple BCEs, especially prior to age 30, the possibility of the basal cell nevus syndrome should be raised. It is inherited as an autosomal dominant trait and is associated with jaw cysts, palmar and plantar pits, frontal bossing, medulloblastomas and calcification of the falx cerebri and diaphragma sellae. *Tricholemmomas* are also skin-colored adnexal tumors but differentiate toward hair follicles and can have a wartlike appearance. The presence of multiple tricholemmomas on the face and cobblestoning of the oral mucosa points to the diagnosis of Cowden's disease (multiple hamartoma syndrome) due to mutations in the *PTEN* gene. Internal organ involvement (in decreasing order of frequency) includes fibrocystic disease and carcinoma of the breast, adenomas and carcinomas of the thyroid, and gastrointestinal polyposis. Keratoses of the palms, soles, and dorsa of the hands are also seen.

Pink Lesions   The cutaneous lesions associated with primary systemic *amyloidosis* are pink in color and translucent. Common locations are the face, especially the periorbital and perioral regions, and flexural areas. On biopsy, homogeneous deposits of amyloid are seen in the dermis and in the walls of blood vessels; the latter lead to an increase in vessel wall fragility. As a result, petechiae and purpura develop in clinically normal skin as well as in lesional skin following minor trauma, hence the term "pinch purpura." Amyloid deposits are also seen in the striated muscle of the tongue and result in macroglossia.

Even though specific mucocutaneous lesions are rarely seen in secondary amyloidosis and are present in only about 30% of the patients with primary amyloidosis, a rapid diagnosis of systemic amyloidosis can be made by an examination of abdominal subcutaneous fat. By special staining, deposits are seen around blood vessels or individual fat cells in 40 to 50% of patients. There are also three forms of amyloidosis that are limited to the skin and that should not be construed as cutaneous lesions of systemic amyloidosis. They are macular amyloidosis (upper back), lichenoid amyloidosis (usually lower extremities), and nodular amyloidosis. In macular and lichenoid amyloidosis, the deposits are composed of altered epidermal keratin. Recently, macular and lichenoid amyloidosis have been associated with MEN syndrome, type 2a.

Patients with *multicentric reticulohistiocytosis* also have pink-colored papules and nodules on the face and mucous membranes as well as on the extensor surface of the hands and forearms. They have a polyarthritis that can mimic rheumatoid arthritis clinically. On histologic examination, the papules have characteristic giant cells that are not seen in biopsies of rheumatoid nodules. Pink to skin-colored papules that are firm, 2 to 5 mm in diameter, and often in a linear arrangement are seen in patients with *papular mucinosis*. This disease is also referred to as *lichen myxedematosus* or *scleromyxedema*. The latter name comes from the brawny induration of the face and extremities that may accompany the papular eruption. Biopsy specimens of the papules show localized mucin deposition, and serum protein electrophoresis demonstrates a monoclonal spike of IgG, usually with a λ light chain.

Yellow Lesions   Several systemic disorders are characterized by yellow-colored cutaneous papules or plaques—hyperlipidemia (xanthomas), gout (tophi), diabetes (necrobiosis lipoidica), pseudoxanthoma elasticum, and Torre syndrome (sebaceous tumors). Eruptive xanthomas are the most common form of *xanthomas*, and are associated with hypertriglyceridemia (types I, III, IV, and V). Crops of yellow papules with erythematous halos occur primarily on the extensor surfaces of the extremities and the buttocks, and they spontaneously involute with a fall in serum triglycerides. Increased β-lipoproteins (primarily types II and III) result in one or more of the following types of xanthoma: xanthelasma, tendon xanthomas, and plane xanthomas. Xanthelasma are found on the eyelids, whereas tendon xanthomas are frequently associated with the Achilles and extensor finger tendons; plane xanthomas are flat and favor the palmar creases, face, upper trunk, and scars. Tuberous xanthomas are frequently associated with hypertriglyceridemia, but they are also seen in patients with hypercholesterolemia (type II) and are found most frequently over the large joints or hand. Biopsy specimens of xanthomas show collections of lipid-containing macrophages (foam cells).

Patients with several disorders, including biliary cirrhosis, can have a secondary form of hyperlipidemia with associated tuberous and planar xanthomas. However, patients with myeloma have *normoli-*

pemic flat xanthomas. This latter form of xanthoma may be ≥12 cm in diameter and is most frequently seen on the upper trunk or side of the neck. It is also important to note that the most common setting for eruptive xanthomas is uncontrolled diabetes mellitus. The least specific sign for hyperlipidemia is xanthelasma, because at least 50% of the patients with this finding have normal lipid profiles.

In *tophaceous gout* there are deposits of monosodium urate in the skin around the joints, particularly those of the hands and feet. Additional sites of *tophi* formation include the helix of the ear and the olecranon and prepatellar bursae. The lesions are firm, yellow in color, and occasionally discharge a chalky material. Their size varies from 1 mm to 7 cm, and the diagnosis can be established by polarization of the aspirated contents of a lesion. Lesions of *necrobiosis lipoidica* are found primarily on the shins (90%), and patients can have diabetes mellitus or develop it subsequently. Characteristic findings include a central yellow color, atrophy (transparency), telangiectasias, and an erythematous border. Ulcerations can also develop within the plaques. Biopsy specimens show necrobiosis of collagen, granulomatous inflammation, and obliterative endarteritis.

In *pseudoxanthoma elasticum* (PXE) there is an abnormal deposition of calcium on the elastic fibers of the skin, eye, and blood vessels. In the skin, the flexural areas such as the neck, axillae, antecubital fossae, and inguinal area are the primary sites of involvement. Yellow papules coalesce to form reticulated plaques that have an appearance similar to that of plucked chicken skin. In severely affected skin, hanging, redundant folds develop. Some patients have a more subtle macular form of the disease, and careful inspection is required. Biopsy specimens of involved skin show swollen and irregularly clumped elastic fibers with deposits of calcium. In the eye, the calcium deposits in Bruch's membrane lead to angioid streaks and choroiditis; in the arteries of the heart, kidney, gastrointestinal tract, and extremities, the deposits lead to angina, hypertension, gastrointestinal bleeding, and claudication, respectively. Long-term administration of D-penicillamine can lead to PXE-like skin changes as well as elastic fiber alterations in internal organs.

Adnexal tumors that have differentiated toward sebaceous glands include sebaceous adenoma, sebaceous epithelioma, sebaceous carcinoma, and sebaceous hyperplasia. Except for sebaceous hyperplasia, which is commonly seen on the face, these tumors are fairly rare. Patients with Torre syndrome have *sebaceous adenomas*, and in the majority of cases there are multiple such tumors. These patients can also have sebaceous carcinomas and sebaceous hyperplasia as well as keratoacanthomas. The internal manifestations of Torre syndrome include *multiple* carcinomas of the gastrointestinal tract (primarily colon) as well as cancers of the larynx, genitourinary tract, and endometrium. Some patients also have a strong family history of cancer.

Red Lesions Cutaneous lesions that are red in color have a wide variety of etiologies; in an attempt to simplify their identification, they will be subdivided into papules, papules/plaques, and subcutaneous nodules. Common red papules include *arthropod bites* and *cherry hemangiomas*; the latter are small, bright-red, dome-shaped papules that represent benign proliferation of capillaries. In patients with AIDS, the development of multiple red hemangioma-like lesions points to bacillary angiomatosis, and biopsy specimens show clusters of bacilli that stain positive with the Warthin-Starry stain; the pathogens have been identified as *Bartonella henselae* and *B. quintana*. Disseminated visceral disease is seen primarily in immunocompromised hosts but can occur in immunocompetent individuals.

Multiple *angiokeratomas* are seen in Fabry's disease, an X-linked recessive lysosomal storage disease that is due to a deficiency of α-galactosidase A. The lesions are red to red-blue in color and can be quite small in size (1 to 3 mm), with the most common location being the lower trunk. Associated findings include chronic renal failure, peripheral neuropathy, and corneal opacities (cornea verticillata). Electron photomicrographs of angiokeratomas and clinically normal skin demonstrate lamellar lipid deposits in fibroblasts, pericytes, and endothelial cells that are diagnostic of this disease. Widespread acute

eruptions of erythematous papules are discussed in the section on exanthems.

There are several infectious diseases that present as erythematous papules or nodules in a sporotrichoid pattern, that is, in a linear arrangement along the lymphatic channels. The two most common etiologies are *Sporothrix schenckii* (sporotrichosis) and *M. marinum* (atypical mycobacteria). The organisms are introduced as a result of trauma, and a primary inoculation site is often seen in addition to the lymphatic nodules. Additional causes include *Nocardia, Leishmania,* and other dimorphic fungi; culture of lesional tissue will aid in the diagnosis.

The diseases that are characterized by erythematous plaques with scale are reviewed in the papulosquamous section, and the various forms of dermatitis are discussed in the section on erythroderma. Additional disorders in the differential diagnosis of red papules/plaques include *erysipelas, polymorphous light eruption* (PMLE), *lymphocytoma cutis, cutaneous lupus, lymphoma cutis,* and *leukemia cutis.* The first three diseases represent primary cutaneous disorders. PMLE is characterized by erythematous papules and plaques in a primarily sun-exposed distribution—dorsum of the hand, extensor forearm, and face. Lesions follow exposure to UV-B and/or UV-A, and in northern latitudes PMLE is most severe in the late spring and early summer. A process referred to as "hardening" occurs with continued UV exposure, and the eruption fades, but in temperate climates it will recur in the spring. PMLE must be differentiated from cutaneous lupus, and this is accomplished by histologic examination and direct immunofluorescence of the lesions. Lymphocytoma cutis (pseudolymphoma) is a *benign* polyclonal proliferation of lymphocytes in the skin that presents as infiltrated pink-red to red-purple papules and plaques; it must be distinguished from lymphoma cutis.

Several types of red plaques are seen in patients with systemic *lupus,* including (1) erythematous urticarial plaques across the cheeks and nose in the classic butterfly rash; (2) erythematous discoid lesions with fine or "carpet-tack" scale, telangiectasias, central hypopigmentation, peripheral hyperpigmentation, follicular plugging, and atrophy located on the face, scalp, external ears, arms, and upper trunk; and (3) psoriasiform or annular lesions of subacute lupus with hypopigmented centers located on the face, extensor arms, and upper trunk. Additional cutaneous findings include (1) a violaceous flush on the face and V of the neck; (2) urticarial vasculitis (see "Urticaria"); (3) lupus panniculitis (see below); (4) diffuse alopecia; (5) alopecia secondary to discoid lesions; (6) periungual telangiectasias and erythema; (7) erythema multiforme–like lesions that may become bullous; and (8) distal ulcerations secondary to Raynaud's phenomenon, vasculitis, or livedoid vasculitis. Patients with only discoid lesions usually have the form of lupus that is limited to the skin. However, 2 to 10% of these patients eventually develop systemic lupus. Direct immunofluorescence of involved skin shows deposits of IgG or IgM and C3 in a granular distribution along the dermal-epidermal junction.

In *lymphoma cutis* there is a proliferation of malignant lymphocytes or histiocytes in the skin, and the clinical appearance resembles that of lymphocytoma cutis—infiltrated pink-red to red-purple papules and plaques. Lymphoma cutis can occur anywhere on the surface of the skin, whereas the sites of predilection for lymphocytomas include the malar ridge, tip of the nose, and earlobes. Patients with non-Hodgkin's lymphomas have specific cutaneous lesions more often than those with Hodgkin's disease, and occasionally, the skin nodules precede the development of extracutaneous non-Hodgkin's lymphoma or represent the only site of involvement. Arcuate lesions are sometimes seen in lymphoma and lymphocytoma cutis as well as in CTCL. *Leukemia cutis* has the same appearance as lymphoma cutis, and specific lesions are seen more commonly in monocytic leukemias than in lymphocytic or granulocytic leukemias. Cutaneous chloromas (granulocytic sarcomas) may precede the appearance of circulating blasts in acute nonlymphocytic leukemia and, as such, represent a form of aleukemic leukemia cutis.

Common causes of erythematous subcutaneous nodules include inflamed epidermoid inclusion cysts, acne cysts, and furuncles. *Panniculitis*, an inflammation of the fat, also presents as subcutaneous nodules and is frequently a sign of systemic disease. There are several forms of panniculitis, including erythema nodosum, erythema induratum, lupus profundus, lipomembranous lipodermatosclerosis, α_1-antitrypsin deficiency, facticial, and fat necrosis secondary to pancreatic disease. Except for erythema nodosum, these lesions may break down and ulcerate or heal with a scar. The shin is the most common location for the nodules of erythema nodosum, whereas the calf is the most common location for lesions of erythema induratum. In erythema nodosum the nodules are initially red but then develop a blue color as they resolve. Patients with erythema nodosum but no underlying systemic illness can still have fever, malaise, leukocytosis, arthralgias, and/or arthritis. However, the possibility of an underlying illness should be excluded, and the most common associations are streptococcal infections, upper respiratory infections, sarcoidosis, and inflammatory bowel disease. The less common associations include tuberculosis, histoplasmosis, coccidioidomycosis, psittacosis, drugs (oral contraceptives, sulfonamides, aspartame, bromides, iodides), cat-scratch fever, and infections with *Yersinia*, *Salmonella*, and *Chlamydia*.

In some patients, erythema induratum/nodular vasculitis is an idiopathic disease; however, in approximately 25 to 70% of patients, polymerase chain reaction (PCR) analysis will demonstrate *M. tuberculosis* complex DNA. The lesions of lupus profundus are found primarily on the upper arms and buttocks (sites of abundant fat) and are seen in both the cutaneous and systemic forms of lupus. The overlying skin may be normal, erythematous, or have the changes of discoid lupus. The subcutaneous fat necrosis that is associated with pancreatic disease is presumably secondary to circulating lipases and is seen in patients with pancreatic carcinoma as well as in patients with acute and chronic pancreatitis. In this disorder there may be an associated arthritis, fever, and inflammation of visceral fat. Histologic examination of deep incisional biopsy specimens will aid in the diagnosis of the particular type of panniculitis.

Subcutaneous erythematous nodules are also seen in *cutaneous polyarteritis nodosa* (PAN) and as a manifestation of *systemic vasculitis*, e.g., systemic PAN, allergic granulomatosis, or Wegener's granulomatosis (Chap. 317). Cutaneous PAN presents with painful subcutaneous nodules and ulcers within a red-purple, netlike pattern of livedo reticularis. The latter is due to slowed blood flow through the superficial horizontal venous plexus. The majority of lesions are found on the lower extremity, and while arthralgias and myalgias may accompany cutaneous PAN, there is no evidence of systemic involvement. In both the cutaneous and systemic forms of vasculitis, skin biopsy specimens of the associated nodules will show the changes characteristic of a vasculitis; the size of the vessel involved will depend on the particular disease.

Red-Brown Lesions   The cutaneous lesions in *sarcoidosis* (Chap. 318) are classically red to red-brown in color, and with diascopy (pressure with a glass slide) a yellow-brown residual color is observed that is secondary to the granulomatous infiltrate. The waxy papules and plaques may be found anywhere on the skin, but the face is the most common location. Usually there are no surface changes, but occasionally the lesions will have scale. Biopsy specimens of the papules show "naked" granulomas in the dermis, i.e., granulomas surrounded by a minimal number of lymphocytes. Other cutaneous findings in sarcoidosis include annular lesions with an atrophic or scaly center, papules within scars, hypopigmented macules and papules, alopecia, acquired ichthyosis, erythema nodosum, and lupus pernio (see below). Additional physical findings are peripheral lymphadenopathy and parotid and lacrimal gland enlargement. When there is cutaneous involvement of the hands, radiographs will often show lytic lesions in the underlying bone.

The differential diagnosis of sarcoidosis includes foreign-body granulomas produced by chemicals such as beryllium and zirconium, late secondary syphilis, and *lupus vulgaris*. Lupus vulgaris is a form of cutaneous tuberculosis that is seen in previously infected and sensitized individuals. There is often underlying active tuberculosis elsewhere, usually in the lungs or lymph nodes. At least 90% of the lesions occur in the head and neck area and are red-brown plaques with a yellow-brown color on diascopy. Secondary scarring and squamous cell carcinomas can develop within the plaques. Cultures or PCR analysis of the lesions should be done because it is rare for the acid-fast stain to show bacilli within the dermal granulomas.

Sweet's syndrome is characterized by red to red-brown plaques and nodules that are frequently painful and occur primarily on the head, neck, and upper extremities. The patients also have fever, neutrophilia, and a dense dermal infiltrate of neutrophils in the lesions. In approximately 10% of the patients there is an associated malignancy, most commonly acute nonlymphocytic leukemia. Sweet's syndrome has also been reported with lymphoma, chronic leukemia, myeloma, myelodysplastic syndromes, and solid tumors (primarily of the genitourinary tract). The differential diagnosis includes neutrophilic eccrine hidradenitis and atypical forms of pyoderma gangrenosum. Extracutaneous sites of involvement include joints, muscles, eye, kidney (proteinuria, occasionally glomerulonephritis), and lung (neutrophilic infiltrates). The idiopathic form of Sweet's syndrome is seen more often in women, following a respiratory tract infection.

A generalized distribution of red-brown macules and papules is seen in the form of mastocytosis known as *urticaria pigmentosa* (Chap. 310). Each lesion represents a collection of mast cells in the dermis, with hyperpigmentation of the overlying epidermis. Stimuli such as rubbing cause these mast cells to degranulate, and this leads to the formation of localized urticaria (Darier's sign). Additional symptoms can result from mast cell degranulation and include headache, flushing, diarrhea, and pruritus. Mast cells also infiltrate various organs such as the liver, spleen, and gastrointestinal tract in up to 30 to 50% of patients with urticaria pigmentosa, and accumulations of mast cells in the bones may produce either osteosclerotic or osteolytic shadows on radiographs. In the majority of these patients, however, the internal involvement remains fairly static. A subtype of chronic leukocytoclastic vasculitis, *erythema elevatum diutinum* (EED), also presents with papules that are red-brown in color. The papules coalesce into plaques on the extensor surfaces of knees, elbows, and the small joints of the hand. Flares of EED have been associated with streptococcal infections.

Blue Lesions   Lesions that are blue in color are the result of either vascular ectasias and tumors or melanin pigment in the dermis. *Venous lakes* (ectasias) are compressible dark-blue lesions that are found commonly in the head and neck region. *Venous malformations* are also compressible blue papules and nodules that can occur anywhere on the body, including the oral mucosa. When they are multiple rather than single congenital lesions, the patient may have the blue rubber bleb syndrome or Mafucci's syndrome. Patients with the blue rubber bleb syndrome also have vascular anomalies of the gastrointestinal tract that may bleed, whereas patients with Mafucci's syndrome have associated dyschondroplasia and osteochondromas. *Blue nevi* (moles) are seen when there are collections of pigment-producing nevus cells in the dermis. These benign papular lesions are dome-shaped and occur most commonly on the dorsum of the hand or foot.

Violaceous Lesions   Violaceous papules and plaques are seen in *lupus pernio*, *lymphoma cutis*, and *cutaneous lupus*. Lupus pernio is a particular type of sarcoidosis that involves the tip of the nose and the earlobes, with lesions that are violaceous in color rather than red-brown. This form of sarcoidosis is associated with involvement of the upper respiratory tract. The plaques of lymphoma cutis and cutaneous lupus may be red or violaceous in color and were discussed above.

Purple Lesions   Purple-colored papules and plaques are seen in vascular tumors, such as *Kaposi's sarcoma* (Chap. 309) and *angiosarcoma*, and when there is extravasation of red blood cells into the skin in association with inflammation, as in *palpable purpura* (see "Purpura"). Patients with congenital or acquired AV fistulas and venous hypertension can develop purple papules on the lower extremities that can resemble Kaposi's sarcoma clinically and histologically; this condition is referred to as pseudo-Kaposi sarcoma (acral angiodermatitis). Angiosarcoma is found most commonly on the scalp and face of elderly patients or within areas of chronic lymphedema and presents as purple papules and plaques. In the head and neck region the tumor often extends beyond the clinically defined borders and may be accompanied by facial edema.

Brown and Black Lesions Brown- and black-colored papules are reviewed in "Hyperpigmentation."

Cutaneous Metastases These are discussed last because they can have a wide range of colors. Most commonly they present as either firm, skin-colored subcutaneous nodules or firm, red to red-brown papulonodules. The lesions of lymphoma cutis range from pink-red to plum in color, whereas metastatic melanoma can be pink, blue, or black in color. Cutaneous metastases develop from hematogenous or lymphatic spread and are most often due to the following primary carcinomas: in men, lung, colon, melanoma, and oral cavity; and in women, breast, colon, and lung. These metastatic lesions may be the initial presentation of the carcinoma, especially when the primary site is the lung, kidney, or ovary.

PURPURA (Table 57-16) *Purpura* are seen when there is an extravasation of red blood cells into the dermis, and as a result, the lesions do not blanch with pressure. This is in contrast to those erythematous or violet-colored lesions that are due to localized vasodilatation—they do blanch with pressure. Purpura ($\geq$3 mm) and petechiae ($\leq$2 mm) are divided into two major groups, palpable and nonpalpable. The most frequent causes of *nonpalpable* petechiae and purpura are primary cutaneous disorders such as *trauma*, *solar purpura*, and *capillaritis*. Less common causes are *steroid purpura* and *livedoid vasculitis* (see "Ulcers"). Solar purpura are seen primarily on the extensor forearms, while glucocorticoid purpura secondary to potent topical steroids or endogenous or exogenous Cushing's syndrome can be more widespread. In both cases there is alteration of the supporting connective tissue that surrounds the dermal blood vessels. In contrast, the petechiae that result from capillaritis are found primarily on the lower extremities. In capillaritis there is an extravasation of erythrocytes as a result of perivascular lymphocytic inflammation. The petechiae are bright red, 1 to 2 mm in size, and scattered within annular or coin-shaped yellow-brown macules. The yellow-brown color is caused by hemosiderin deposits within the dermis.

Systemic causes of nonpalpable purpura fall into several categories, and those secondary to clotting disturbances and vascular fragility will be discussed first. The former group includes *thrombocytopenia* (Chap. 116), *abnormal platelet function* as is seen in uremia, and *clotting factor defects*. The initial site of presentation for thrombocytopenia-induced petechiae is the distal lower extremity. Capillary fragility leads to nonpalpable purpura in patients with systemic *amyloidosis* (see "Papulonodular Skin Lesions"), disorders of collagen production such as *Ehlers-Danlos syndrome*, and *scurvy*. In scurvy there are flattened corkscrew hairs with surrounding hemorrhage on the lower extremities, in addition to gingivitis. Vitamin C is a cofactor for lysyl hydroxylase, an enzyme involved in the posttranslational modification of procollagen that is necessary for cross-link formation.

In contrast to the previous group of disorders, the purpura seen in the following group of diseases are associated with thrombi formation within vessels. It is important to note that these thrombi are demonstrable in skin biopsy specimens. This group of disorders includes disseminated intravascular coagulation (DIC), monoclonal cryoglobulinemia, thrombotic thrombocytopenic purpura, and reactions to warfarin. DIC is triggered by several types of infection (gram-negative, gram-positive, viral, and rickettsial) as well as by tissue injury and neoplasms. Widespread purpura and hemorrhagic infarcts of the distal extremities are seen. Similar lesions are found in purpura fulminans, which is a form of DIC associated with fever and hypotension that occurs more commonly in children following an infectious illness such as varicella, scarlet fever, or an upper respiratory tract infection. In both disorders, hemorrhagic bullae can develop in involved skin.

Monoclonal cryoglobulinemia is associated with multiple myeloma, Waldenström's macroglobulinemia, lymphocytic leukemia, and lymphoma. Purpura, primarily of the lower extremities, and hemorrhagic infarcts of the fingers and toes are seen in these patients. Exacerbations of disease activity can follow cold exposure or an increase in serum viscosity. Biopsy specimens show precipitates of the cryoglobulin within dermal vessels. Similar deposits have been found in the lung, brain, and renal glomeruli. Patients with *thrombotic thrombocytopenic purpura* can also have hemorrhagic infarcts as a result of intravascular thromboses. Additional signs include thrombocytopenic purpura, fever, and microangiopathic hemolytic anemia (Chap. 108).

Administration of *warfarin* can result in painful areas of erythema that become purpuric and then necrotic with an adherent black eschar. This reaction is seen more often in women and in areas with abundant subcutaneous fat—breasts, abdomen, buttocks, thighs, and calves. The erythema and purpura develop between the third and tenth day of therapy, most likely as a result of a transient imbalance in the levels of anticoagulant and procoagulant vitamin K–dependent factors. Continued therapy does not exacerbate preexisting lesions, and patients with an inherited or acquired deficiency of protein C are at increased risk for this particular reaction as well as for purpura fulminans.

Purpura secondary to *cholesterol emboli* are usually seen on the lower extremities of patients with atherosclerotic vascular disease. They often follow anticoagulant therapy or an invasive vascular procedure such as an arteriogram but also occur spontaneously from disintegration of atheromatous plaques. Associated findings include livedo reticularis, gangrene, cyanosis, subcutaneous nodules, and ischemic ulcerations. Multiple step sections of the biopsy specimen may be necessary to demonstrate the cholesterol clefts with the vessels. Petechiae are also an important sign of *fat embolism* and occur primarily on the upper body 2 to 3 days after a major injury. By using special fixatives, the emboli can be demonstrated in biopsy specimens of the petechiae. Emboli of tumor or thrombus are seen in patients with atrial myxomas and marantic endocarditis.

In the *Gardner-Diamond syndrome* (autoerythrocyte sensitivity), female patients develop large ecchymoses within areas of painful, warm erythema. An episode of significant trauma frequently precedes the onset of this syndrome. Intradermal injections of autologous erythrocytes or phosphatidyl serine derived from the red cell membrane can

Table 57-16 Causes of Purpura

I. Primary cutaneous disorders	c. Thrombotic thrombocytopenic purpura
A. Nonpalpable	
1. Trauma	d. Warfarin reaction
2. Solar purpura	4. Emboli
3. Steroid purpura	a. Cholesterol
4. Capillaritis	b. Fat
5. Livedoid vasculitis[a]	5. Possible immune complex
II. Systemic diseases	a. Gardner-Diamond syndrome (autoerythrocyte sensitivity)
A. Nonpalpable	
1. Clotting disturbances	b. Waldenström's hypergammaglobulinemic purpura
a. Thrombocytopenia (including ITP)	B. Palpable
b. Abnormal platelet function	1. Vasculitis
c. Clotting factor defects	a. Leukocytoclastic vasculitis
2. Vascular fragility	b. Polyarteritis nodosa
a. Amyloidosis	2. Emboli[b]
b. Ehlers-Danlos syndrome	a. Acute meningococcemia
c. Scurvy	b. Disseminated gonococcal infection
3. Thrombi	c. Rocky Mountain spotted fever
a. Disseminated intravascular coagulation	d. Ecthyma gangrenosum
b. Monoclonal cryoglobulinemia	

[a] Also associated with systemic diseases.
[b] Bacterial, fungal, or parasitic.
NOTE: ITP, idiopathic thrombocytopenic purpura.

reproduce the lesions in some patients; however, there are instances where a reaction is seen at an injection site of the forearm but not in the midback region. The latter has led some observers to view Gardner-Diamond syndrome as a cutaneous manifestation of severe emotional stress. *Waldenström's hypergammaglobulinemic purpura* is a chronic disorder characterized by petechiae on the lower extremities. There are circulating complexes of IgG–anti-IgG molecules, and exacerbations are associated with prolonged standing or walking.

Palpable purpura are further subdivided into vasculitic and embolic. In the group of vasculitic disorders, *leukocytoclastic vasculitis* (LCV), also known as *allergic vasculitis*, is the one most commonly associated with palpable purpura (Chap. 317). *Henoch-Schönlein purpura* is a subtype of acute LCV that is seen primarily in children and adolescents following an upper respiratory infection. The majority of lesions are found on the lower extremities and buttocks. Systemic manifestations include fever, arthralgias (primarily of the knees and ankles), abdominal pain, gastrointestinal bleeding, and nephritis. Direct immunofluorescence examination shows deposits of IgA within dermal blood vessel walls. In *polyarteritis nodosa*, specific cutaneous lesions result from a vasculitis of arterial vessels rather than postcapillary venules as in LCV. The arteritis leads to ischemia of the skin, and this explains the irregular outline of the purpura (see below).

Several types of infectious emboli can give rise to palpable purpura. These embolic lesions are usually *irregular* in outline as opposed to the lesions of leukocytoclastic vasculitis, which are *circular* in outline. The irregular outline is indicative of a cutaneous infarct, and the size corresponds to the area of skin that received its blood supply from that particular arteriole or artery. The palpable purpura in LCV are circular because the erythrocytes simply diffuse out evenly from the postcapillary venules as a result of inflammation. Infectious emboli are most commonly due to gram-negative cocci (meningococcus, gonococcus), gram-negative rods (Enterobacteriaceae), and gram-positive cocci (staphylococcus). Additional causes include *Rickettsia* and, in immunocompromised patients, *Candida* and opportunistic fungi.

The embolic lesions in *acute meningococcemia* are found primarily on the trunk, lower extremities, and sites of pressure, and a gunmetal-gray color often develops within them. Their size varies from 1 mm to several centimeters, and the organisms can be cultured from the lesions. Associated findings include a preceding upper respiratory tract infection, fever, meningitis, DIC, and, in some patients, a deficiency of the terminal components of complement. In *disseminated gonococcal infection* (arthritis-dermatitis syndrome), a small number of papules and vesicopustules with central purpura or hemorrhagic necrosis are found over the joints of the distal extremities. Additional symptoms include arthralgias, tenosynovitis, and fever. To establish the diagnosis, a Gram stain of these lesions should be performed. *Rocky mountain spotted fever* is a tick-borne disease that is caused by *R. rickettsii*. A several-day history of fever, chills, severe headache, and photophobia precedes the onset of the cutaneous eruption. The initial lesions are erythematous macules and papules on the wrists, ankles, palms, and soles. With time, the lesions spread centripetally and become purpuric.

Lesions of *ecthyma gangrenosum* begin as edematous, erythematous papules or plaques and then develop central purpura and necrosis. Bullae formation also occurs in these lesions, and they are frequently found in the girdle region. The organism that is classically associated with ecthyma gangrenosum is *Pseudomonas aeruginosa*, but other gram-negative rods such as *Klebsiella*, *Escherichia coli*, and *Serratia* can produce similar lesions. In immunocompromised hosts, the list of potential pathogens is expanded to include *Candida* and opportunistic fungi.

ULCERS The approach to the patient with a cutaneous ulcer, is outlined in Table 57-17. →*Peripheral vascular diseases of the extremities are reviewed in Chap. 248, as is Raynaud's phenomenon.*

Livedoid vasculitis (atrophie blanche) represents a combination of a vasculopathy with intravascular thrombosis. Purpuric lesions and

Table 57-17 Causes of Cutaneous Ulcers

I. Primary cutaneous disorders
  A. Peripheral vascular disease (Chap. 248)
    1. Venous
    2. Arterial
  B. Livedoid vasculitis[a]
  C. Squamous cell carcinoma, e.g., within scars
  D. Infections, e.g., ecthyma caused by *Streptococcus* (Chap. 140)
II. Systemic diseases
  A. Lower legs
    1. Leukocytoclastic vasculitis[b]
    2. Hemoglobinopathies (Chap. 106)
    3. Cryoglobulinemia,[b] cryofibrinogenemia
    4. Cholesterol emboli[b]
    5. Necrobiosis lipoidica[c]
    6. Antiphospholipid syndrome (Chap. 117)
    7. Neuropathic[d] (Chap. 333)
  B. Hands and feet
    1. Raynaud's phenomenon (Chap. 248)
  C. Generalized
    1. Pyoderma gangrenosum
    2. Calciphylaxis (Chap. 341)
    3. Infections, e.g., dimorphic fungi, chronic herpes varicella–zoster
    4. Lymphoma
  D. Mucosal
    1. Behçet's syndrome (Chap. 316)
    2. Erythema multiforme
    3. Primary blistering disorders (Chap. 58)
    4. Lupus erythematosus
    5. Inflammatory bowel disease

---

[a] Also associated with systemic diseases.
[b] Reviewed in section on "Purpura."
[c] Reviewed in section on "Papulonodular Skin Lesions."
[d] Favors plantar surface of the foot.

---

livedo reticularis are found in association with painful ulcerations of the lower extremities. These ulcers are often slow to heal, but when they do, irregularly shaped white scars are formed. The majority of cases are secondary to venous hypertension, but possible underlying illnesses include cryofibrinogenemia and disorders of hypercoagulability, e.g., the antiphospholipid syndrome (Chap. 117).

In *pyoderma gangrenosum*, the border of the ulcers has a characteristic appearance of an undermined necrotic bluish edge and a peripheral erythematous halo. The ulcers often begin as pustules that then expand rather rapidly to a size as large as 20 cm. Although these lesions are most commonly found on the lower extremities, they can arise anywhere on the surface of the body, including sites of trauma (pathergy). An estimated 30 to 50% of cases are idiopathic, and the most common associated disorders are ulcerative colitis and Crohn's disease. Less commonly, it is associated with chronic active hepatitis, seropositive rheumatoid arthritis, acute and chronic granulocytic leukemia, polycythemia vera, and myeloma. Additional findings in these patients, even those with idiopathic disease, are cutaneous anergy and a benign monoclonal gammopathy. Because the histology of pyoderma gangrenosum is nonspecific, the diagnosis is made clinically by excluding less common causes of similar-appearing ulcers such as necrotizing vasculitis, Meleney's ulcer (synergistic infection at a site of trauma or surgery), dimorphic fungi, cutaneous amebiasis, spider bites, and facticial. In the myeloproliferative disorders, the ulcers may be more superficial with a pustulobullous border, and these lesions provide a connection between classic pyoderma gangrenosum and acute febrile neutrophilic dermatosis (Sweet's syndrome).

FEVER AND RASH The major considerations in a patient with a fever and a rash are inflammatory diseases versus infectious diseases. In the hospital setting, the most common scenario is a patient who has a drug rash plus a fever secondary to an underlying infection. However, it should be emphasized that a drug reaction can lead to both a cutaneous eruption and a fever ("drug fever"). Additional inflammatory diseases that are often associated with a fever include pustular psoriasis, erythroderma, and Sweet's syndrome. Lyme disease, secondary syphilis, and viral and bacterial exanthems (see "Exanthems") are examples of infectious diseases that produce a rash and a fever. Lastly, it is important to determine whether or not the cutaneous lesions represent septic emboli (see "Purpura"). Such lesions usually have evidence of ischemia in the form of purpura, necrosis, or impending necrosis (gunmetal-gray color). In the patient with thrombocytopenia, however, purpura can be seen in inflammatory reactions such as morbilliform drug eruptions and infectious lesions.

BIBLIOGRAPHY

ARNDT KA et al: *Cutaneous Medicine and Surgery*. Philadelphia, Saunders, 1996

BRAVERMAN IM: *Skin Signs of Systemic Disease*, 3d ed. Philadelphia, Saunders, 1998

CALLEN JP: *Dermatology Clinics*, vol 8, no 2: *Skin Signs of Internal Disease II*. Philadelphia, Saunders, 1990

———, JORIZZO JL: *Dermatology Clinics*, vol 7, no 3: *Skin Signs of Internal Disease*. Philadelphia, Saunders, 1989

CHAMPION RH et al (eds): *Textbook of Dermatology*, 6th ed. Oxford, Blackwell Scientific, 1998

ELDER D et al: *Lever's Histopathology of the Skin*, 8th ed. Philadelphia, Lippincott, 1997

LITT JZ, PAWLAK WA JR: *Drug Eruption Reference Manual 1999*. New York, Parthenon, 1999

SYBERT VP: *Genetic Skin Disorders*. New York, Oxford University Press, 1997

ZURCHER K, KREBS A: *Cutaneous Drug Reactions*, 2d ed. Basel, Karger, 1992

58 *Kim B. Yancey, Thomas J. Lawley*

IMMUNOLOGICALLY MEDIATED SKIN DISEASES

BP bullous pemphigoid	PF pemphigus foliaceus
BPAG bullous pemphigoid antigen	PG pemphigoid gestationis
CP cicatricial pemphigoid	PNP paraneoplastic pemphigus
DH dermatitis herpetiformis	PV pemphigus vulgaris
DLE discoid lupus erythematosus	SCLE subacute cutaneous lupus erythematosus
EBA epidermolysis bullosa acquisita	SLE systemic lupus erythematosus
LE lupus erythematosus	

A number of immunologically mediated skin diseases and cutaneous manifestations of immunologically mediated systemic disorders are now recognized as distinct entities with relatively consistent clinical, histologic, and immunopathologic findings. Many of these disorders are due to autoimmune mechanisms. Clinically, they are characterized by morbidity (pain, pruritus, disfigurement) and in some instances by mortality (largely due to loss of epidermal barrier function and/or secondary infection). The major features of the more common immunologically mediated skin diseases are summarized in this chapter (Table 58-1).

PEMPHIGUS VULGARIS Pemphigus vulgaris (PV) is a blistering skin disease seen predominantly in elderly patients. Patients with PV have an increased incidence of the HLA-DR4 and -DRw6 serologically defined haplotypes. This disorder is characterized by the loss of cohesion between epidermal cells (a process termed *acantholysis*) with the resultant formation of intraepidermal blisters. Clinical lesions of PV typically consist of flaccid blisters on either normal-appearing or erythematous skin. These blisters rupture easily, leaving denuded areas that may crust and enlarge peripherally **(Plate IIE-69)**. Substantial portions of the body surface may be denuded in severe cases. Manual pressure to the skin of these patients may elicit the separation of the epidermis (Nikolsky's sign). This finding, while characteristic of PV, is not specific to this disorder and is also seen in toxic epidermal necrolysis, Stevens-Johnson syndrome, and a few other skin diseases. Lesions in PV typically present on the oral mucosa, scalp, face, neck, axilla, and trunk. In half or more of patients, lesions begin in the mouth; approximately 90% of patients have oromucosal involvement at some time during the course of their disease. Involvement of other mucosal surfaces (e.g., pharyngeal, laryngeal, esophageal, con-

junctival, vulval, or rectal) can occur in severe disease. Pruritus may be a feature of early pemphigus lesions; extensive denudation may be associated with severe pain. Lesions usually heal without scarring, except at sites complicated by secondary infection or mechanically induced dermal wounds. Nonetheless, postinflammatory hyperpigmentation is usually present at sites of healed lesions for some time.

Biopsies of early lesions demonstrate intraepidermal vesicle formation secondary to loss of cohesion between epidermal cells (i.e., acantholytic blisters). Blister cavities contain acantholytic epidermal cells, which appear as round homogeneous cells containing hyperchromatic nuclei. Basal keratinocytes remain attached to the epidermal basement membrane, hence blister formation is within the suprabasal portion of the epidermis. Lesional skin may contain focal collections of intraepidermal eosinophils within blister cavities; dermal alterations are slight, often limited to an eosinophil-predominant leukocytic infiltrate. Direct immunofluorescence microscopy of lesional or intact patient skin shows deposits of IgG on the surface of keratinocytes; in contrast, deposits of complement components are typically found in lesional but not uninvolved skin. Deposits of IgG on keratinocytes are derived from circulating autoantibodies directed against cell-surface antigens. Circulating autoantibodies can be demonstrated in 80 to 90% of PV patients by indirect immunofluorescence microscopy; monkey esophagus is the optimal substrate for demonstration of these autoantibodies. Patients with PV have IgG autoantibodies directed against desmogleins (Dsgs), transmembrane desmosomal glycoproteins that belong to the cadherin supergene family of calcium-dependent adhesion molecules. While Dsg3 is specifically recognized by PV autoantibodies, approximately 50% of PV sera also contain IgG against Dsg1. Most patients with early PV and only mucosal involvement have only anti-Dsg3 autoantibodies, whereas most patients with advanced disease (i.e., involvement of skin and mucosa) have both anti-Dsg3 and anti-Dsg1 autoantibodies. Recent studies have shown that the anti-Dsg autoantibody profile in these patients' sera as well as the tissue distribution of Dsg3 and Dsg1 determine the site of blister formation in patients with pemphigus. Experimental studies have also shown that these autoantibodies are pathogenic (i.e., responsible for blister formation) and that their titer correlates with disease activity.

PV can be life-threatening. Prior to the availability of glucocorticoids, the mortality ranged from 60 to 90%; the current mortality is approximately 5%. Common causes of morbidity and mortality are infection and complications of treatment with glucocorticoids. Bad prognostic factors include advanced age, widespread involvement, and the requirement for high doses of glucocorticoids (with or without other immunosuppressive agents) for control of disease. The course of PV in individual patients is variable and difficult to predict. Some patients achieve remission (40% of patients in some series), but others may require long-term treatment or succumb to complications of their disease or its treatment. The mainstay of treatment is systemic glucocorticoids. Patients with moderate to severe disease are usually started on prednisone, 60 to 80 mg/d. If new lesions continue to appear after 1 to 2 weeks of treatment, the dose should be increased. Many regimens combine an immunosuppressive agent with systemic glucocorticoids for control of PV. The two most frequently used are either azathioprine (1 mg/kg per day) or cyclophosphamide (1 mg/kg per day). It is important to bring severe or progressive disease under control quickly to lessen the severity and/or duration of this disorder.

PEMPHIGUS FOLIACEUS Pemphigus foliaceus (PF) is distinguished from PV by several features. In PF, acantholytic blisters are located high within the epidermis, usually just beneath the stratum corneum. Hence PF is a more superficial blistering disease than PV. The distribution of lesions in the two disorders is much the same, except that in PF mucous membrane lesions are very rare. Patients with PF rarely demonstrate intact blisters but rather exhibit shallow erosions associated with erythema, scale, and crust formation. Mild cases of PF resemble severe seborrheic dermatitis; severe PF may cause extensive exfoliation. Sun exposure (ultraviolet irradiation) may

Table 58-1 Immunologically Mediated Blistering Diseases

Disease	Clinical	Histology	Immunopathology	Autoantigens[a]
Pemphigus foliaceus	Crusts and shallow erosions on scalp, central face, upper chest, and back	Acantholytic blister formed in superficial layer of epidermis	Cell surface deposits of IgG on keratinocytes	Dsg1
Pemphigus vulgaris	Flaccid blisters, denuded skin, oromucosal lesions	Acantholytic blister formed in suprabasal layer of epidermis	Cell surface deposits of IgG on keratinocytes	Dsg3 (plus Dsg1 in some patients)
Bullous pemphigoid	Large tense blisters on flexor surfaces, oral mucosal blisters and erosions	Blister formed in subepidermal region, usually eosinophil rich	Linear band of IgG and/or C3 in epidermal BMZ[a]	BPAG1, BPAG2
Pemphigoid gestationis	Pruritic, urticarial plaques, rimmed by vesicles and bullae on the trunk and extremities	Teardrop-shaped, subepidermal blisters in dermal papillae; eosinophil-rich infiltrate	Linear band of C3 in epidermal BMZ	BPAG2 (plus BPAG1 in some patients)
Linear IgA disease	Pruritic small papules on extensor surfaces; occasionally larger, arciform blisters	Subepidermal blister with neutrophils in dermal papillae	Linear band of IgA in epidermal BMZ	BPAG2 (see text for specific details)
Cicatricial pemphigoid	Erosive and/or blistering lesions of mucous membranes and possibly the skin; scarring of some sites	Subepidermal blister that may or may not include an inflammatory infiltrate	Linear band of IgG, IgA, and/or C3 in epidermal BMZ	BPAG2, laminin 5, or others
Epidermolysis bullosa acquisita	Blisters, erosions, scars, and milia on sites exposed to trauma; widespread, inflammatory, tense blisters may be seen initially	Subepidermal blister that may or may not include an inflammatory infiltrate	Linear band of IgG and/or C3 in epidermal BMZ	Type VII collagen
Dermatitis herpetiformis	Extremely pruritic small papules and vesicles on elbows, knees, buttocks, and posterior neck	Subepidermal blister with neutrophils in dermal papillae	Granular deposits of IgA in dermal papillae	

[a] Autoantigens bound by these patients' autoantibodies are defined as follows: Dsg1, desmoglein 1; Dsg3, desmoglein 3; BPAG1, bullous pemphigoid antigen 1; BPAG2, bullous pemphigoid antigen 2; BMZ, basement membrane zone.

be an aggravating factor. A blistering skin disease endemic to south central Brazil known as *fogo selvagem*, or *Brazilian pemphigus*, is clinically, histologically, and immunopathologically indistinguishable from PF.

Patients with PF have immunopathologic features in common with PV. Specifically, direct immunofluorescence microscopy of perilesional skin demonstrates IgG on the surface of keratinocytes. As in PV, patients with PF frequently have circulating IgG autoantibodies against keratinocyte cell surface antigens. Guinea pig esophagus is the optimal substrate for indirect immunofluorescence microscopy studies of sera from patients with PF. In PF, autoantibodies are directed against Dsg1, a 160-kDa desmosomal cadherin. As noted for PV, the autoantibody profile in patients with PF (i.e., anti-Dsg1) and the normal tissue distribution of this autoantigen (i.e., low expression in oral mucosa) is thought to account for the distribution of lesions in this disease.

Although pemphigus has been associated with several autoimmune diseases, its association with thymoma and/or myasthenia gravis is particularly notable. To date, more than 30 cases of thymoma and/or myasthenia gravis have been reported in association with pemphigus, usually with PF. Patients may also develop pemphigus as a consequence of drug exposure. The most frequently implicated agent is penicillamine; other offenders include captopril, rifampin, piroxicam, penicillin, and phenobarbital. Drug-induced pemphigus usually resembles PF rather than PV; autoantibodies in these patients have the same antigenic specificity as they do in other pemphigus patients. In most patients, lesions resolve following discontinuation of the drug; however, some patients require treatment with systemic glucocorticoids and/or immunosuppressive agents.

PF is generally a far less severe disease than PV and carries a better prognosis. Localized disease can be treated conservatively with topical or intralesional glucocorticoids; more active cases can usually be controlled with systemic glucocorticoids.

PARANEOPLASTIC PEMPHIGUS Paraneoplastic pemphigus (PNP) is an autoimmune acantholytic mucocutaneous disease associated with an occult or confirmed neoplasm. Patients with PNP typically show painful mucosal erosive lesions in association with pruritic papulosquamous eruptions that often progress to blisters. Palm and sole involvement is common in these patients and raises the possibility that prior reports of neoplasia-associated erythema multiforme actually may have represented unrecognized cases of PNP. Biopsies of lesional skin from these patients show varying combinations of acantholysis, keratinocyte necrosis, and vacuolar-interface dermatitis. Direct immunofluorescence microscopy of patient skin shows deposits of IgG and complement on the surface of keratinocytes and (variably) similar immunoreactants in the epidermal basement membrane zone. Patients with PNP have IgG autoantibodies against cytoplasmic proteins that are members of the plakin family (e.g., desmoplakins I and II, bullous pemphigoid antigen 1, envoplakin, periplakin, and plectin) and cell-surface proteins that are members of the cadherin family (e.g., Dsg3 and Dsg1). Because immunoadsorption of anti-Dsg3 IgG is sufficient to eliminate the ability of PNP sera to induce blisters in an experimental passive transfer animal model, these particular autoantibodies are thought to play a key pathogenic role in blister formation in these patients.

Although PNP is generally resistant to conventional therapies (i.e., those used to treat PV), patients may improve (or even remit) following resection of underlying neoplasms. The predominant neoplasms associated with this disorder are non-Hodgkin's lymphoma, chronic lymphocytic leukemia, Castleman's disease, thymoma, and spindle cell tumors.

BULLOUS PEMPHIGOID Bullous pemphigoid (BP) is an autoimmune subepidermal blistering disease usually seen in the elderly. Lesions typically consist of tense blisters on either normal-appearing or erythematous skin **(Plate IIE-72)**. The lesions are usually distributed over the lower abdomen, groin, and flexor surface of the extremities; oral mucosal lesions are found in 10 to 40% of patients. Pruritus may be nonexistent or severe. As lesions evolve, tense blisters tend to rupture and be replaced by flaccid lesions or erosions with or without surmounting crust. Nontraumatized blisters heal without scarring. The major histocompatibility complex class II allele HLA-DQβ1*0301 is prevalent in patients with BP. Despite isolated reports, several studies have shown that patients with BP do not have an increased incidence of malignancy in comparison with appropriately age- and sex-matched controls.

While biopsies of early lesional skin demonstrate subepidermal blisters, the histologic features depend on the character of the particular lesion. Lesions on normal-appearing skin generally show a sparse perivascular leukocytic infiltrate with some eosinophils; conversely, biopsies of inflammatory lesions typically show an eosinophil-rich infiltrate within the papillary dermis at sites of vesicle formation and in perivascular areas. In addition to eosinophils, cell-rich lesions also contain mononuclear cells and neutrophils. It is not always possible to distinguish BP from other subepidermal blistering diseases by routine histologic techniques.

Immunopathologic studies have broadened our understanding of this disease and aided its diagnosis. Direct immunofluorescence microscopy of normal-appearing perilesional skin shows linear deposits of IgG and/or C3 in the epidermal basement membrane. The sera of approximately 70% of these patients contain circulating IgG autoantibodies that bind the epidermal basement membrane of normal human skin in indirect immunofluorescence microscopy. An even higher percentage of patients shows reactivity to the epidermal side of 1 M NaCl split skin [an alternative immunofluorescence microscopy test substrate that is commonly used to distinguish circulating IgG anti-basement membrane autoantibodies in patients with BP from those in patients with similar, yet different, subepidermal blistering diseases (e.g., epidermolysis bullosa acquisita, see below)]. No correlation exists between the titer of these autoantibodies and disease activity. In BP, circulating autoantibodies recognize 230- and (in approximately 70% of BP patients) 180-kDa hemidesmosome-associated proteins in basal keratinocytes [i.e., bullous pemphigoid antigen (BPAG)1 and BPAG2, respectively]. Autoantibodies are thought to develop against these antigens (more specifically, initially against BPAG2), deposit in situ, and activate complement that subsequently produces dermal mast cell degranulation and granulocyte-rich infiltrates that cause tissue damage and blister formation.

BP may persist for months to years, with exacerbations or remissions. Although extensive involvement may result in widespread erosions and compromise cutaneous integrity, the mortality rate is low even in the absence of treatment. Nonetheless, deaths may occur in elderly and/or debilitated patients. The mainstay of treatment is systemic glucocorticoids. Patients with local or minimal disease can sometimes be controlled with topical glucocorticoids alone; patients with more extensive lesions generally respond to systemic glucocorticoids either alone or in combination with immunosuppressive agents. Patients will usually respond to prednisone, 40 to 60 mg/d. In some instances, azathioprine (1 mg/kg per day) or cyclophosphamide (1 mg/ kg per day) are necessary adjuncts.

PEMPHIGOID GESTATIONIS Pemphigoid gestationis (PG), also known as herpes gestationis, is a rare, nonviral, subepidermal blistering disease of pregnancy and the puerperium. PG may begin during any trimester of pregnancy or present shortly after delivery. Lesions are usually distributed over the abdomen, trunk, and extremities; mucous membrane lesions are rare. Skin lesions in these patients may be quite polymorphic and consist of erythematous urticarial papules and plaques, vesiculopapules, and/or frank bullae. Lesions are almost always very pruritic. Severe exacerbations of PG frequently occur after delivery, typically within 24 to 48 h. PG tends to recur in subsequent pregnancies, often beginning earlier during such gestations. Brief flare-ups of disease may occur with resumption of menses and may develop in patients later exposed to oral contraceptives. Occasionally, infants of affected mothers demonstrate transient skin lesions.

Biopsies of early lesional skin show teardrop-shaped subepidermal vesicles forming in dermal papillae in association with an eosinophil-rich leukocytic infiltrate. Differentiation of PG from other subepidermal bullous diseases by light microscopy is often difficult. However, direct immunofluorescence microscopy of perilesional skin from PG patients reveals the immunopathologic hallmark of this disorder—linear deposits of C3 in the epidermal basement membrane zone. These deposits develop as a consequence of complement activation produced by low titer IgG anti-basement membrane zone autoantibodies. Recent studies have shown that the majority of PG sera contain autoantibodies that recognize BPAG2, the same 180-kDa hemidesmosome-associated protein that is targeted by autoantibodies in roughly 70% of patients with BP—a subepidermal bullous disease that resembles PG morphologically, histologically, and immunopathologically.

The goals of therapy in patients with PG are to prevent the development of new lesions, relieve intense pruritus, and care for erosions at sites of blister formation. Most patients require treatment with moderate doses of daily glucocorticoids (i.e., 20 to 40 mg of prednisone) at some point in their course. Mild cases (or brief flare-ups) may be controlled by vigorous use of potent topical glucocorticoids. Although PG was once thought to be associated with an increased risk of fetal morbidity and mortality, the best evidence now suggests that these infants may only be at increased risk of being slightly premature or "small for dates." Current evidence suggests that there is no difference in the incidence of uncomplicated live births in PG patients treated with systemic glucocorticoids and in those managed more conservatively. If systemic glucocorticoids are administered, newborns are at risk for development of reversible adrenal insufficiency.

DERMATITIS HERPETIFORMIS Dermatitis herpetiformis (DH) is an intensely pruritic, papulovesicular skin disease characterized by lesions symmetrically distributed over extensor surfaces (i.e., elbows, knees, buttocks, back, scalp, and posterior neck) (**Plate IIE-68**). The primary lesion in this disorder is a papule, papulovesicle, or urticarial plaque. Because pruritus is prominent, patients may present with excoriations and crusted papules but no observable primary lesions. Patients sometimes report that their pruritus has a distinctive burning or stinging component; the onset of such local symptoms reliably heralds the development of distinct clinical lesions 12 to 24 h later. Almost all DH patients have an associated, usually subclinical, gluten-sensitive enteropathy (Chap. 286), and more than 90% express the HLA-B8/DRw3 and HLA-DQw2 haplotypes. DH may present at any age, including childhood; onset in the second to fourth decades is most common. The disease is typically chronic.

Biopsy of early lesional skin reveals neutrophil-rich infiltrates within dermal papillae. Neutrophils, fibrin, edema, and microvesicle formation at these sites are characteristic of early disease. Older lesions may demonstrate nonspecific features of a subepidermal bulla or an excoriated papule. Because the clinical and histologic features of this disease can be variable and resemble other subepidermal blistering disorders, the diagnosis is confirmed by direct immunofluorescence microscopy of normal-appearing perilesional skin. Such studies demonstrate granular deposits of IgA (with or without complement components) in the papillary dermis and along the epidermal basement membrane zone. IgA deposits in the skin are unaffected by control of disease with medication; however, these immunoreactants may diminish in intensity or disappear in patients maintained for long periods on a strict gluten-free diet (see below). Patients with granular deposits of IgA in their epidermal basement membrane zone typically do not have circulating IgA anti-basement membrane autoantibodies and should be distinguished from individuals with linear IgA deposits at this site (see below).

Although most DH patients do not report overt gastrointestinal symptoms or laboratory evidence of malabsorption, biopsies of small bowel usually reveal blunting of intestinal villi and a lymphocytic infiltrate in the lamina propria. As is true for patients with celiac disease, this gastrointestinal abnormality can be reversed by a gluten-free diet. Moreover, if maintained, this diet alone may control the skin disease and eventuate in clearance of IgA deposits from these patients' epidermal basement membrane zone. Subsequent gluten exposure in such patients alters the morphology of their small bowel, elicits a flare-up of their skin disease, and is associated with the reappearance of IgA in their epidermal basement membrane zone. Additional evidence that DH develops as a consequence of dietary gluten exposure is the demonstration of IgA anti-endomysial antibodies in these patients' sera (as found in the sera of patients with ordinary gluten-sensitive enteropathy). Recent studies have shown that such autoantibodies are directed against tissue transglutaminase. Patients with DH also have an increased incidence of thyroid abnormalities, achlorhydria, atrophic gastritis, and antigastric parietal cell antibodies. These associations likely relate to the high frequency of the HLA-B8/DRw3 haplotype in these patients, since this marker is commonly linked to autoimmune disorders. The mainstay of treatment of DH is dapsone, a sulfone. Patients respond rapidly (24 to 48 h) to dapsone but require careful pretreatment evaluation and close follow-up to ensure that complications are avoided or controlled. All patients on more than 100 mg/d dapsone will have some hemolysis and methemoglobinemia. These are expected pharmacologic side effects of this agent. Gluten restriction can control DH and lessen dapsone requirements; this diet must rigidly exclude gluten to be of maximal benefit. Many months of dietary restriction may be necessary before a beneficial result is achieved. Good dietary counselling by a trained dietitian is essential.

LINEAR IgA DISEASE Linear IgA disease, once considered a variant form of dermatitis herpetiformis, is actually a separate and distinct entity. Clinically, these patients may resemble patients with typical cases of DH, BP, or other subepidermal blistering diseases. Lesions typically consist of papulovesicles, bullae, and/or urticarial plaques, predominantly on extensor (as seen in "classic" DH), central, or flexural sites. Oral mucosal involvement occurs in some patients. Severe pruritus resembles that in patients with DH. Patients with linear IgA disease do not have an increased frequency of the HLA-B8/DRw3 haplotype or an associated enteropathy and hence are not candidates for a gluten-free diet.

The histologic alterations in early lesions may be virtually indistinguishable from those in DH. However, direct immunofluorescence microscopy of normal-appearing perilesional skin reveals linear deposits of IgA (and often C3) in the epidermal basement membrane zone. Most patients with linear IgA disease demonstrate circulating IgA anti-basement membrane autoantibodies against epitopes in the extracellular domain of BPAG2, a transmembrane protein found in hemidesmosomes of basal keratinocytes. These patients generally respond to treatment with dapsone, 50 to 150 mg/d.

EPIDERMOLYSIS BULLOSA ACQUISITA EBA is a rare, noninherited, polymorphic, subepidermal blistering disease. (The inherited form is discussed in Chap. 351.) Patients with classic or noninflammatory EBA have blisters on noninflamed skin, atrophic scars, milia, nail dystrophy, and oral lesions. Because lesions generally occur at sites exposed to minor trauma, classic EBA is considered to be a mechanobullous disease. Other patients with EBA have widespread inflammatory, scarring, bullous lesions and oromucosal involvement that resembles severe BP. Some patients present with an inflammatory bullous disease that evolves into the classic noninflammatory form of this disorder. In general, EBA is chronic; associations with multiple myeloma, amyloidosis, inflammatory bowel disease, and diabetes mellitus have been reported. The HLA-DR2 haplotype is found with increased frequency in these patients.

The histology of lesional skin varies depending on the character of the lesion being studied. Noninflammatory bullae show subepidermal blisters with a sparse leukocytic infiltrate and resemble those in patients with porphyria cutanea tarda. Inflammatory lesions consist of a subepidermal blister and neutrophil-rich leukocytic infiltrates in the superficial dermis. EBA patients have continuous deposits of IgG (and frequently C3 as well as other complement components) in a linear

pattern within the epidermal basement membrane zone. Ultrastructurally, these immunoreactants are found in the sublamina densa region in association with anchoring fibrils, wheat stack–like structures that extend from the lamina densa into the underlying papillary dermis. Approximately 25 to 50% of EBA patients have circulating IgG anti-basement membrane autoantibodies directed against type VII collagen—the collagen species that comprises anchoring fibrils. Such IgG autoantibodies bind the dermal side of 1 M NaCl split skin (in contrast to IgG autoantibodies in patients with BP that bind either epidermal or both sides of this indirect immunofluorescence microscopy test substrate).

Treatment of EBA is generally unsatisfactory. Some patients with inflammatory EBA may respond to systemic glucocorticoids, either alone or in combination with immunosuppressive agents. Other patients (especially those with neutrophil-rich inflammatory lesions) may respond to dapsone. The chronic, noninflammatory form of this disease is largely resistant to treatment, although some patients may respond to cyclosporine.

CICATRICIAL PEMPHIGOID Cicatricial pemphigoid (CP) is a rare, acquired, subepithelial blistering disease characterized by erosive lesions of mucous membranes and skin that result in scarring of at least some sites of involvement. Immunopathologically, perilesional mucosa and skin of patients with CP demonstrate in situ deposits of immunoreactants in epithelial basement membranes. Common sites of involvement include the oral mucosa (especially the gingiva) and conjunctiva; other sites that may be affected include the nasopharyngeal, laryngeal, esophageal, urogenital, and rectal mucosa. Skin lesions (present in about one-third of patients) tend to predominate on the scalp, face, and upper trunk and generally consist of a few scattered erosions or tense blisters on an erythematous or urticarial base. CP is typically a chronic and progressive disorder. Serious complications may arise as a consequence of ocular, laryngeal, esophageal, or urogenital lesions. Erosive conjunctivitis may result in shortened fornices, symblephara, ankyloblepharon, entropion, corneal opacities, and (in severe cases) blindness. Similarly, erosive lesions of the larynx may cause hoarseness, pain, and tissue loss that if unrecognized and untreated may eventuate in complete destruction of the airway. Esophageal lesions may result in stenosis and/or strictures that may place patients at risk for aspiration. Strictures may also complicate urogenital involvement.

Biopsies of lesional tissue generally demonstrate subepithelial vesiculobullae and a mononuclear leukocytic infiltrate. Neutrophils and eosinophils may be seen in biopsies of early lesions; older lesions may demonstrate a scant leukocytic infiltrate and fibrosis. Direct immunofluorescence microscopy of perilesional tissue typically demonstrates deposits of IgG, IgA, and/or C3 in these patients' epithelial basement membranes. Because many of these patients show no evidence of circulating anti-basement membrane autoantibodies, testing of perilesional skin is important diagnostically. Although CP was once thought to be a single nosologic entity, it is now largely regarded as a disease phenotype that may develop as a consequence of an autoimmune reaction against a variety of different molecules in epithelial basement membranes (e.g., BPAG2, laminin 5, type VII collagen, and other antigens yet to be completely defined). Treatment of CP is largely dependent upon sites of involvement. Due to potentially severe complications, ocular, laryngeal, esophageal, and/or urogenital involvement require aggressive systemic treatment with dapsone, prednisone, or the latter in combination with another immunosuppressive agent (e.g., azathioprine or cyclophosphamide). Less threatening forms of the disease may be managed with topical or intralesional glucocorticoids.

AUTOIMMUNE SYSTEMIC DISEASES WITH PROMINENT CUTANEOUS FEATURES

DERMATOMYOSITIS The cutaneous manifestations of dermatomyositis (Chap. 382) are often distinctive but at times may resemble those of systemic lupus erythematosus (SLE) (Chap. 311), scleroderma (Chap. 313), or other overlapping connective tissue diseases (Chap. 313). The extent and severity of cutaneous disease may or may not correlate with the extent and severity of the myositis. Patients with severe muscle involvement may have relatively minor skin changes, whereas patients with marked skin involvement may have mild muscle disease. The cutaneous manifestations of dermatomyositis are similar whether the disease appears in childhood or old age, except that calcification of subcutaneous tissue is a common late sequela in childhood dermatomyositis.

The cutaneous signs of dermatomyositis may precede or follow the development of myositis by weeks to years. Cases lacking muscle involvement (i.e., dermatomyositis sine myositis) have also been reported. The most common manifestation is a purple-red discoloration of the upper eyelids, sometimes associated with scaling ("heliotrope" erythema; **Plate IIE-63**) and periorbital edema. Erythema on the cheeks and nose in a "butterfly" distribution may resemble the eruption in SLE. Erythematous or violaceous scaling patches are common on the upper anterior chest, posterior neck, scalp, and the extensor surfaces of the arms, legs, and hands. Erythema and scaling may be particularly prominent over the elbows, knees, and the dorsal interphalangeal joints. Approximately one-third of patients have violaceous, flat-topped papules over the dorsal interphalangeal joints that are pathognomonic of dermatomyositis (Gottron's sign or Gottron's papules; **Plate IIE-65**). These lesions can be contrasted with the erythema and scaling on the dorsum of the fingers in some patients with SLE, which spares the skin over the interphalangeal joints. Periungual telangiectasia may be prominent, and a lacy or reticulated erythema may be associated with fine scaling on the extensor surfaces of the thighs and upper arms. Other patients, particularly those with long-standing disease, develop areas of hypopigmentation, hyperpigmentation, mild atrophy, and telangiectasia known as *poikiloderma vasculare atrophicans*. Poikiloderma is rare in both SLE and scleroderma and thus can serve as a clinical sign that distinguishes dermatomyositis from these two diseases. Cutaneous changes may be similar in scleroderma and dermatomyositis and may include thickening and binding down of the skin of the hands (sclerodactyly) as well as Raynaud's phenomenon. However, the presence of severe muscle disease, Gottron's papules, heliotrope erythema, and poikiloderma serve to distinguish patients with dermatomyositis. Skin biopsy of erythematous, scaling lesions of dermatomyositis may reveal only mild nonspecific inflammation but sometimes may show changes indistinguishable from those found in SLE, including epidermal atrophy, hydropic degeneration of basal keratinocytes, edema of the upper dermis, and a mild mononuclear cell infiltrate. Direct immunofluorescence microscopy of lesional skin is usually negative, although granular deposits of immunoglobulin(s) and complement in the epidermal basement membrane zone have been described in some patients. Treatment should be directed at the systemic disease. In the few instances where adjunctive cutaneous therapy is desirable, topical glucocorticoids are sometimes useful. These patients should avoid exposure to ultraviolet irradiation and use photoprotective measures such as sunscreens.

LUPUS ERYTHEMATOSUS The cutaneous manifestations of lupus erythematosus (LE) (Chap. 311) can be divided into acute, subacute, and chronic (i.e., discoid LE) types. *Acute cutaneous LE* is characterized by erythema of the nose and malar eminences in a "butterfly" distribution **(Plate IIE-61)**. The erythema is often sudden in onset, accompanied by edema and fine scale, and correlated with systemic involvement. Patients may have widespread involvement of the face as well as erythema and scaling of the extensor surfaces of the extremities and upper chest. These acute lesions, while sometimes evanescent, usually last for days and are often associated with exacerbations of systemic disease. Skin biopsy of acute lesions may show only a sparse dermal infiltrate of mononuclear cells and dermal edema. In some instances, cellular infiltrates around blood vessels and hair follicles are notable, as is hydropic degeneration of basal cells of the epidermis. Direct immunofluorescence microscopy of lesional skin frequently reveals deposits of immunoglobulin(s) and complement in the epidermal basement membrane zone. Treatment is aimed at control

of systemic disease; photoprotection in this, as well as in other forms of LE, is very important.

Subacute cutaneous lupus erythematosus (SCLE) is characterized by a widespread photosensitive, nonscarring eruption. About half of these patients have SLE in which severe renal and central nervous system involvement is uncommon. SCLE may present as a papulosquamous eruption that resembles psoriasis or annular lesions that resemble those seen in erythema multiforme. In the papulosquamous form, discrete erythematous papules arise on the back, chest, shoulders, extensor surfaces of the arms, and the dorsum of the hands; lesions are uncommon on the face, flexor surfaces of the arms, and below the waist. The slightly scaling papules tend to merge into large plaques, some with a reticulate appearance. The annular form involves the same areas and presents with erythematous papules that evolve into oval, circular, or polycyclic lesions. The lesions of SCLE are more widespread but have less tendency for scarring than do lesions of discoid LE. Skin biopsy reveals a dense mononuclear cell infiltrate around hair follicles and blood vessels in the superficial dermis, combined with hydropic degeneration of basal cells in the epidermis. Direct immunofluorescence microscopy of lesional skin reveals deposits of immunoglobulin(s) in the epidermal basement membrane zone in about half these cases. A particulate pattern of IgG deposition around basal keratinocytes has recently been associated with SCLE. Most SCLE patients have anti-Ro antibodies. Local therapy is usually unsuccessful, and most patients require treatment with aminoquinoline antimalarials. Low-dose therapy with oral glucocorticoids is sometimes necessary; photoprotective measures against both ultraviolet B and A wavelengths are very important.

Discoid lupus erythematosus (DLE) is characterized by discrete lesions, most often on the face, scalp, or external ears. The lesions are erythematous papules or plaques with a thick, adherent scale that occludes hair follicles (follicular plugging). When the scale is removed, its underside will show small excrescences that correlate with the openings of hair follicles and is termed a "carpet tack" appearance. This finding is relatively specific for DLE. Long-standing lesions develop central atrophy, scarring, and hypopigmentation but frequently have erythematous, sometimes raised borders at the periphery **(Plate IIE-62)**. These lesions persist for years and tend to expand slowly. Only 5 to 10% of patients with DLE meet the American Rheumatism Association criteria for SLE. However, typical discoid lesions are frequently seen in patients with SLE. Biopsy of DLE lesions shows hyperkeratosis, follicular plugging, and atrophy of the epidermis. The dermal-epidermal junction reveals hydropic degeneration of basal keratinocytes, and a mononuclear cell infiltrate surrounding hair follicles and blood vessels. Direct immunofluorescence microscopy demonstrates immunoglobulin(s) and complement deposits at the basement membrane zone in about 90% of cases. Treatment is focused on control of local cutaneous disease and consists mainly of photoprotection and topical or intralesional glucocorticoids. If local therapy is ineffective, use of aminoquinoline antimalarials may be indicated.

SCLERODERMA AND MORPHEA The skin changes of scleroderma (Chap. 313) usually begin on the hands, feet, and face, with episodes of recurrent nonpitting edema. Sclerosis of the skin begins distally on the fingers (sclerodactyly) and spreads proximally, usually accompanied by resorption of bone of the fingertips, which may have punched out ulcers, stellate scars, or areas of hemorrhage **(Plate IIE-66)**. The fingers may actually shrink in size and become sausage-shaped, and since the fingernails are usually unaffected, the nails may curve over the end of the fingertips. Periungual telangiectasias are usually present, but periungual erythema is rare. In advanced cases, the extremities show contractures and calcinosis cutis. Face involvement includes a smooth, unwrinkled brow, taut skin over the nose, shrinkage of tissue around the mouth, and perioral radial furrowing **(Plate IIE-64)**. Matlike telangiectasias are often present, particularly on the face and hands. Involved skin feels indurated, smooth, and bound to underlying structures; hyperpigmentation and hypopigmentation are also often present. Raynaud's phenomenon, i.e., cold-induced blanching, cyanosis, and reactive hyperemia, is present in almost all patients and can precede development of scleroderma by many years. The combination of calcinosis cutis, Raynaud's phenomenon, esophageal dysmotility, sclerodactyly, and telangiectasia has been termed the *CREST syndrome*. Anticentromere antibodies have been reported in a very high percentage of patients with the CREST syndrome but in only a small minority of patients with scleroderma. Skin biopsy reveals thickening of the dermis and homogenization of collagen bundles. Direct immunofluorescence microscopy of lesional skin is usually negative.

Morphea, which has been called *localized scleroderma*, is characterized by localized thickening and sclerosis of skin, usually affecting young adults or children. Morphea begins as erythematous or flesh-colored plaques that become sclerotic, develop central hypopigmentation, and demonstrate an erythematous border. In most cases, patients have one or a few lesions, and the disease is termed *localized morphea*. In some patients, widespread cutaneous lesions may occur, without systemic involvement. This form is called *generalized morphea*. Most patients with morphea do not have autoantibodies. Skin biopsy of morphea is indistinguishable from that of scleroderma. Linear scleroderma is a limited form of disease that presents in a linear, bandlike distribution and tends to involve deep as well as superficial layers of skin. Scleroderma and morphea are usually quite resistant to therapy. For this reason, physical therapy to prevent joint contractures and to maintain function is employed and is often helpful.

Diffuse fasciitis with eosinophilia is a clinical entity that can sometimes be confused with scleroderma. There is usually the sudden onset of swelling, induration, and erythema of the extremities frequently following significant physical exertion. The proximal portions of extremities (arms, forearms, thighs, legs) are more often involved than are the hands and feet. While the skin is indurated, it is usually not bound down as in scleroderma; contractures may occur early secondary to fascial involvement. The latter may also cause muscle groups to be separated (i.e., the "groove sign") and veins to appear depressed (i.e., sunken veins). These skin findings are accompanied by peripheral blood eosinophilia, increased erythrocyte sedimentation rate, and sometimes hypergammaglobulinemia. Deep biopsy of affected areas of skin reveals inflammation and thickening of the deep fascia overlying muscle. An inflammatory infiltrate composed of eosinophils and mononuclear cells is usually found. Patients with eosinophilic fasciitis appear to be at increased risk to develop bone marrow failure or other hematologic abnormalities. While the ultimate course of eosinophilic fasciitis is uncertain, many patients respond favorably to treatment with prednisone in doses ranging from 40 to 60 mg/d.

The *eosinophilia-myalgia syndrome*, a disorder reported in epidemic numbers in 1989 and linked to ingestion of L-tryptophan manufactured by a single company in Japan, is a multisystem disorder characterized by debilitating myalgias and absolute eosinophilia in association with varying combinations of arthralgias, pulmonary symptoms, and peripheral edema. In a later phase (i.e., 3 to 6 months after initial symptoms), these patients often develop localized sclerodermatous skin changes, weight loss, and/or neuropathy (Chap. 313). The precise cause of this syndrome, which may resemble other sclerotic skin conditions, is unknown. However, the implicated lots of L-tryptophan contained the contaminant 1,1-ethylidene bis[tryptophan]. This contaminant may be pathogenic or a marker for another substance that provokes the disorder.

BIBLIOGRAPHY

AMAGAI M: Pemphigus: Autoimmunity to epidermal cell adhesion molecules. Adv Dermatol 11:319, 1996

—— et al: Antibodies against desmoglein 3 (pemphigus vulgaris antigen) are present in sera from patients with paraneoplastic pemphigus and cause acantholysis in vivo in neonatal mice. J Clin Invest 102:775, 1998

ANHALT GJ et al: Paraneoplastic pemphigus: An autoimmune mucocutaneous disease associated with neoplasia. N Engl J Med 323:1729, 1990

BRAVERMAN IM: Connective tissue diseases, in *Skin Signs of Systemic Disease*, 3d ed. Philadelphia, Saunders, 1998

FINE JD: Management of acquired bullous skin disease. N Engl J Med 333:1475, 1995

HALL RP: Dermatitis herpetiformis. J Invest Dermatol 99:873, 1992

LIU Z et al: A passive transfer model of the organ-specific autoimmune disease, bullous pemphigoid, using antibodies generated against the hemidesmosomal antigen, BP180. J Clin Invest 92:2480, 1993

MAHONEY MG et al: Explanations for the clinical and microscopic localization of lesions in pemphigus foliaceus and vulgaris. J Clin Invest 103:461, 1999

STANLEY JR: Cell adhesion molecules as targets of autoantibodies in pemphigus and pemphigoid, bullous diseases due to defective epidermal cell adhesion. Adv Immunol 53:291, 1992

YANCEY KB: Adhesion molecules. II: Interactions of keratinocytes with epidermal basement membrane. J Invest Dermatol 104:1008, 1995

| **59** | *Robert S. Stern, Olivier M. Chosidow, Bruce U. Wintroub* |

CUTANEOUS DRUG REACTIONS

Cutaneous reactions are among the most frequent adverse reactions to drugs. Prompt recognition of these reactions, drug withdrawal, and appropriate therapeutic interventions can minimize toxicity. This chapter focuses on adverse cutaneous reactions to drugs other than topical agents and reviews the incidence, patterns, and pathogenesis of cutaneous reactions to drugs and other therapeutic agents.

USE OF PRESCRIPTION DRUGS IN THE UNITED STATES More than 1.5 billion prescriptions for 60,000 drug products, which include over 2000 different active agents, are dispensed each year in the United States. Hospital inpatients alone annually receive about 120 million courses of drug therapy, and half of adult Americans receive prescription drugs on a regular outpatient basis. Many additional patients use over-the-counter medicines that may cause adverse cutaneous reactions.

INCIDENCE OF CUTANEOUS REACTIONS Although adverse drug reactions are common, it is difficult to ascertain their incidence, seriousness, and ultimate health effects. Available information comes from evaluations of hospitalized patients, epidemiologic surveys, premarketing studies, and voluntary reporting, most notably to the U.S. Food and Drug Administration's Medwatch System. None of these efforts provides comprehensive comparable data on the risk of cutaneous reactions associated with most medicines.

In one study about 2% of medical inpatients had skin reactions consisting of rash, urticaria, or pruritus during hospitalization. The overall reaction rate per course of drug therapy was about 3:1000. Among inpatients, penicillins, sulfonamides, and blood products accounted for two-thirds of cutaneous reactions. Among outpatients, reaction rates for many antibiotics were comparable to those observed in inpatients. Fluoroquinolones are notable causes of cutaneous reactions not observed in earlier studies. Reaction rates for selected commonly used antibiotics are summarized in Table 59-1. Most cutaneous reactions occur within 2 weeks of exposure to a drug. The risk of

Table 59-1 Rates (per 1000 Recipients) of Skin Reactions to Selected Medications

Drug	Reaction Rate
Trimethoprim-sulfamethoxazole	21
Fluoroquinolones	5
Amoxicillin (Augmentin)	12
Other penicillins	11
Tetracyclines	5
Macrolides	6

SOURCE: Adapted from van der Linden et al.

allergic reactions does not vary greatly with age or sex. Among outpatients, the risk of a reaction to an antibiotic was comparable for first and subsequent courses of a given drug.

The distribution of morphologic patterns of drug eruptions cared for within a Finnish hospital dermatology department with a special interest in fixed drug eruptions included exanthematous reactions (32%), urticaria and/or angioedema (20%), fixed drug eruptions (34%), erythema multiforme (2%), Stevens-Johnson syndrome (SJS; 1%), exfoliative dermatitis (1%), and photosensitivity reactions (3%). Other studies suggest that about 80% of all cutaneous reactions are morbilliform or erythematous, 10 to 15% are urticaria or angioedema, and all other types of reactions are relatively rare.

The relative risk of SJS and toxic epidermal necrolysis (TEN), perhaps the most important severe cutaneous reactions, has been quantified in an international case control study and case series. Sulfonamide antibiotics, allopurinol, amine antiepileptic drugs (phenytoin and carbamazepine), and lamotrigine (a new antiepileptic) are associated with the highest risk of these reactions.

PATHOGENESIS OF DRUG REACTIONS

Untoward cutaneous responses to drugs can arise as a result of immunologic or nonimmunologic mechanisms. Immunologic reactions require activation of host immunologic pathways and are designated *drug allergy*. Drug reactions occurring through nonimmunologic mechanisms may be due to activation of effector pathways, overdosage, cumulative toxicity, side effects, ecologic disturbance, interactions between drugs, metabolic alterations, exacerbation of preexisting dermatologic conditions, or inherited protein or enzyme deficiencies. It is often not possible to specify the responsible drug or pathogenic mechanism because the skin responds to a variety of stimuli through a limited number of reaction patterns. The mechanism of many drug reactions is unknown.

IMMUNOLOGIC DRUG REACTIONS Drugs frequently elicit an immune response, but only a small number of individuals experience clinical hypersensitivity reactions. For example, most patients exposed to penicillin develop demonstrable antibodies to penicillin but do not manifest drug reactions when exposed to penicillin. Multiple factors determine the capacity of a drug to elicit an immune response, including the molecular characteristics of the drug and host effects.

Increases in *molecular* size and complexity are associated with increased immunogenicity, and macromolecular drugs such as protein or peptide hormones are highly antigenic. Most drugs are small organic molecules <1000 Da in size, and the capacity of such small molecules to elicit an immune response depends on their ability to act as haptens, i.e., to form stable, usually covalent, bonds with tissue macromolecules, an extremely rare event.

Route of administration of a drug or simple chemical can influence the nature of the *host* immune response. For example, topical application of antigens tends to induce delayed hypersensitivity, and exposure to antigens via oral or nasal cavities stimulates production of secretory immunoglobins, IgA and IgE, and occasionally IgM. Frequency of sensitization through intravenous administration of drugs varies, but anaphylaxis is a more likely consequence with this route of exposure than following oral administration.

The degree of drug exposure and individual variability in absorption and metabolism of a given agent may alter immunogenic load. The variable degree of in vivo acetylation of hydralazine provides a clinical example of this phenomenon. Hydralazine produces a lupus-like syndrome associated with antinuclear antibody formation more frequently in patients who acetylate the drug slowly. Frequent high-dose and interrupted courses of therapy are also important risk factors for development of drug allergy.

Pathogenesis of Allergic Drug Reactions • *IgE-Dependent Reactions* IgE-dependent drug reactions are usually manifest in the skin and gastrointestinal, respiratory, and cardiovascular systems

(Chap. 310). Primary symptoms and signs include pruritus, urticaria, nausea, vomiting, cramps, bronchospasm, and laryngeal edema and, on occasion, anaphylactic shock with hypotension and death. Immediate reactions may occur within minutes of drug exposure, and accelerated reactions occur hours or days after drug administration. Accelerated reactions are usually urticarial and may include laryngeal edema. Penicillin and related drugs are the most frequent causes of IgE-dependent reactions. Release of chemical mediators such as histamine, adenosine, leukotrienes, prostaglandins, platelet-activating factor, enzymes, and proteoglycans from sensitized tissue, mast cells, or circulating basophilic leukocytes results in vasodilation and edema. Release is triggered when polyvalent drug protein conjugates crosslink IgE molecules fixed to sensitized cells. The clinical manifestations are determined by interaction of the released chemical mediator with its target organ, i.e., skin, respiratory, gastrointestinal, and/or cardiovascular systems. Certain routes of administration favor different clinical patterns (i.e., oral route: gastrointestinal effects; intravenous route: circulatory effects).

Immune-complex–dependent reactions Serum sickness is produced by circulating immune complexes and is characterized by fever, arthritis, nephritis, neuritis, edema, and an urticarial, papular, or purpuric rash (Chap. 317). The syndrome requires an antigen that remains in the circulation for prolonged periods so that when antibody is synthesized, circulating antigen-antibody complexes are formed. Serum sickness was first described following administration of foreign sera, but drugs are now the usual cause. Drugs that produce serum sickness include the penicillins, sulfonamides, thiouracils, cholecystographic dyes, phenytoin, aminosalicylic acid, heparin, and antilymphocyte globulin. Cephalosporin administration in febrile children is associated with a high risk of a clinically similar reaction, but the mechanism of this reaction is unknown. In classic serum sickness, symptoms develop 6 days or more after exposure to a drug, the latent period representing the time needed to synthesize antibody. The antibodies responsible for immune-complex–dependent drug reactions are largely of the IgG or IgM class. Vasculitis, a relatively rare cutaneous complication of drugs, may also be a result of immune complex deposition (Chap. 317).

Cytotoxicity and delayed hypersensitivity Cytotoxicity and delayed hypersensitivity mechanisms may be important in the etiology of morbilliform exanthema, hypersensitivity syndrome, SJS, or TEN, but this is not proven. Systemic manifestations occur frequently. The nature of the antigen leading to cytotoxic reactions is unknown, but it is likely that different T lymphocyte populations are activated. T_H1 type cells will lead to the production of interleukin (IL)-2 and interferon (IFN)-γ and subsequent activation of cytotoxic T cells. In early lesions of morbilliform exanthema or TEN, histopathologic studies have shown expression of HLA-DR and intercellular adhesion molecule (ICAM-1) by keratinocytes, CD4 cells (in the dermis), and CD8 T cells (in the epidermis) and apoptosis of keratinocytes (facilitated by tumor necrosis factor α secretion and *fas*-ligand expression). T_H2 type cells produce cytokines such as IL-5, which may be involved in hypersensitivity syndrome (see below).

NONIMMUNOLOGIC DRUG REACTIONS Nonimmunologic mechanisms are responsible for the majority of drug reactions; however, only the most important mechanisms will be discussed.

Nonimmunologic Activation of Effector Pathways Drug reactions may result from nonimmunologic activation of effector pathways by three mechanisms: First, drugs may release mediators directly from mast cells and basophils and present as anaphylaxis, urticaria, and/or angioedema. Urticarial anaphylactic reactions induced by opiates, polymyxin B, tubocurarine, radiocontrast media, and dextrans may occur by this mechanism. Second, drugs may activate complement in the absence of antibody. This is an additional mechanism through which radiocontrast media may act. Third, drugs such as aspirin and other nonsteroidal anti-inflammatory agents (NSAIDs) may alter pathways of arachidonic acid metabolism and induce urticaria.

Phototoxicity Phototoxic reactions may be drug-induced or may occur in metabolic disorders in which a photosensitizing chemical is overproduced. A phototoxic reaction occurs when enough chromophore (drug or metabolic product) absorbs sufficient radiation to cause a reaction or interaction with target tissue. Drug-induced phototoxic reactions can occur on first exposure. The incidence of phototoxicity is a direct function of the concentration of sensitizer and the amount of light of the appropriate wavelengths. At least three distinct photochemical mechanisms have been described: (1) the reaction between the excited state of a phototoxic molecule and a biologic target may cause formation of a covalent photoaddition product, (2) the phototoxic molecule may form stable photoproducts that are toxic to biologic substrates, and (3) radiation of a phototoxic molecule may result in transfer of energy to oxygen molecules and cause formation of toxic oxygen species, such as singlet oxygen superoxide anion, or hydroxyl radicals. Interaction of these reactive species with biologic targets produces photooxidized molecules. Phototoxic injury is usually manifest as a sunburn-like reaction.

Exacerbation of Preexisting Diseases A variety of agents can exacerbate preexisting diseases. For example, lithium can exacerbate acne and psoriasis in a dose-dependent manner. Beta-blocking agents and IFN-α may induce psoriasis. Withdrawal of glucocorticoids can exacerbate psoriasis or atopic dermatitis.

Inherited Enzyme or Protein Deficiencies Specific genetically determined defects in the ability of an individual to detoxify toxic reactive drug metabolites may predispose such individuals to the development of severe drug reactions, especially hypersensitivity syndrome, and perhaps TEN associated with use of sulfonamides and anticonvulsants.

Alterations of Immunologic Status Alterations in patients' immunologic status may also modify the risk of cutaneous reactions. Bone marrow transplant patients, HIV-infected persons, and persons with Epstein-Barr virus infection are at higher risk of developing cutaneous reactions to drugs. Skin reactions to trimethoprim-sulfamethoxazole are seen in about a third of HIV-infected users of this drug, but desensitization can be accomplished. Dapsone, trimethoprim alone, and amoxicillin-clavulanate are also frequent causes of drug eruptions in HIV-infected patients. The advent of highly active antiretroviral therapy (HAART) may have decreased the risk of cutaneous reactions in HIV patients (Chap. 309).

A CLINICAL CLASSIFICATION OF CUTANEOUS DRUG REACTIONS

URTICARIA/ANGIOEDEMA *Urticaria* is a skin reaction characterized by pruritic, red wheals. Lesions may vary from a small point to a large area. Individual lesions rarely last more than 24 h. When deep dermal and subcutaneous tissues are also swollen, this reaction is known as *angioedema*. Angioedema may involve mucous membranes and may be part of a life-threatening anaphylactic reaction. Urticarial lesions, along with pruritus and morbilliform (or maculopapular) eruptions, are among the most frequent types of cutaneous reactions to drugs.

Drug-induced urticaria may be caused by three mechanisms: an IgE-dependent mechanism, circulating immune complexes (serum sickness), and nonimmunologic activation of effector pathways. IgE-dependent urticarial reactions usually occur within 36 h but can occur within minutes. Reactions occurring within minutes to hours of drug exposure are termed *immediate reactions*, whereas those that occur 12 to 36 h after drug exposure are designated *accelerated reactions*. Immune-complex–induced urticaria associated with serum sickness usually occurs from 6 to 12 days after first exposure. In this syndrome, the urticarial eruption may be accompanied by fever, hematuria, arthralgias, hepatic dysfunction, and neurologic symptoms.

Certain drugs, such as NSAIDs, angiotensin-converting enzyme (ACE) inhibitors, and radiographic dyes, may induce urticarial reactions, angioedema, and anaphylaxis in the absence of drug-specific antibody. Although ACE inhibitors, aspirin, penicillin, and blood products are the most frequent causes of urticarial eruptions, urticaria has been observed in association with nearly all drugs. Drugs also may cause chronic urticaria, which lasts more than 6 weeks. Aspirin frequently exacerbates this problem.

The treatment of urticaria or angioedema depends on the severity of the reaction and the rate at which it is evolving. In severe cases, especially with respiratory or cardiovascular compromise, epinephrine is the mainstay of therapy, but its effect is reduced in patients using beta blockers. For more seriously affected patients, treatment with systemic glucocorticoids, sometimes intravenously administered, are helpful. In addition to drug withdrawal, for patients with only cutaneous symptoms and without symptoms of angioedema or anaphylaxis, oral antihistamines are usually sufficient.

PHOTOSENSITIVITY ERUPTIONS Photosensitivity eruptions are usually most marked in sun-exposed areas but may extend to sun-protected areas. Phototoxic reactions are more common with some drugs. Photoallergic reactions to systemically administered drugs are very rare. Phototoxic reactions usually resemble sunburn and can occur with the first exposure to a drug. Their severity depends on the tissue level of the drug, the extent of exposure to light, and the efficiency of the photosensitizer (Chap. 60).

Orally administered phototoxic drugs include many fluoroquinolones, chlorpromazine, tetracycline, thiazides, and at least two NSAIDs (benoxaprofen and piroxicam). The majority of the common phototoxic drugs have action spectrums in the long-wave ultraviolet A (UV-A) range. Phototoxic reactions abate with removal of either the drug or ultraviolet radiation. Because UV-A and visible light, which trigger these reactions, are not easily absorbed by nonopaque sunscreens and are transmitted through window glass, these reactions may be difficult to block.

Photosensitivity reactions are treated by avoiding exposure to ultraviolet light (sunlight) and treating the reaction as one would a sunburn. Rarely, individuals develop persistent reactivity to light, necessitating long-term avoidance of sun exposure.

PIGMENTATION CHANGES Drugs may cause a variety of pigmentary changes in the skin. Some drugs stimulate melanocytic activity and increase pigmentation. Drug deposition can also lead to pigmentation; this phenomenon occurs with heavy metals. Phenothiazines may be deposited in the skin and cause a slate-gray color. Antimalarial drugs may cause a slate-gray or yellow pigmentation. Long term minocycline use may cause slate-gray hyperpigmentation, especially in areas of chronic inflammation. Inorganic arsenic, once used to treat psoriasis, is associated with diffuse macular pigmentation. Other heavy metals that cause pigmentary changes include silver, gold, bismuth, and mercury. Long-term use of phenytoin can produce a chloasma-like pigmentation in women. Certain cytostatic agents can also cause pigmentary changes. Histologic examination is often diagnostic for drug deposition diseases.

Zidovudine (AZT) is a frequent cause of pigmentation, especially of the nails (Chap. 309). Nicotinic acid in large doses may cause brown pigmentation, and oral contraceptives may produce chloasma. In addition, amiodarone may cause violaceous hyperpigmentation that is increased in sun-exposed skin. Drugs such as heavy metals, copper antimalarial and arsenical agents, and ACTH also may discolor oral mucosa.

VASCULITIS Cutaneous necrotizing vasculitis often presents as palpable purpuric lesions that may be generalized or limited to the lower extremities or other dependent areas (Chap. 317). Urticarial lesions, ulcers, and hemorrhagic blisters also occur. Vasculitis may involve other organs, including the liver, kidney, brain, and joints. Drugs are only one cause of vasculitis, with infection and collagen vascular disease responsible for the majority of cases.

Propylthiouracil induces a cutaneous vasculitis that is accompanied by leukopenia and splenomegaly. Direct immunofluorescent

HYPERSENSITIVITY SYNDROME Initially described with phenytoin, hypersensitivity syndrome presents as an erythematous eruption that may become purpuric and is accompanied by many of the following features: fever, facial and periorbital edema, tender generalized lymphadenopathy, leukocytosis (often with atypical lymphocytes and eosinophils), hepatitis, and sometimes nephritis or pneumonitis. The cutaneous reaction usually begins 1 to 6 weeks after phenytoin is begun and usually resolves with drug cessation, but symptoms, especially hepatitis, may persist. The eruption recurs with rechallenge, and cross-reactions among aromatic anticonvulsants, including phenytoin, carbamazepine, and barbiturates, are frequent. With phenytoin, an increased risk of this syndrome is associated with an inherited deficiency of epoxide hydrolase, an enzyme required for metabolism of a toxic intermediate arene oxide that is formed during metabolism of phenytoin by the cytochrome P450 system. Other drugs causing this syndrome include lamotrigine, dapsone, allopurinol, sulfonamides, minocycline, and sulfones. Systemic glucocorticoids (prednisone, 0.5 to 1.0 mg/kg) seem to reduce symptoms. Mortality as high as 10% has been reported.

WARFARIN NECROSIS OF THE SKIN This rare reaction occurs usually between the third and tenth days of therapy with warfarin derivatives, usually in women. Lesions are sharply demarcated, erythematous, indurated, and purpuric and may resolve or progress to form large, irregular, hemorrhagic bullae with eventual necrosis and slow-healing eschar formation.

Development of the syndrome is unrelated to drug dose or underlying condition. Favored sites are breasts, thighs, and buttocks. The course is not altered by discontinuation of the drug after onset of the eruption. Similar reactions have been associated with heparin. Warfarin reactions are associated with protein C deficiency. Protein C is a vitamin K–dependent protein with a shorter half-life than other clotting proteins and is in part responsible for control of fibrinolysis. Since warfarin inhibits synthesis of vitamin K–dependent coagulation factors, warfarin anticoagulation in heterozygotes for protein C deficiency causes a precipitous fall in circulating levels of protein C, permitting hypercoagulability and thrombosis in the cutaneous microvasculature, with consequent areas of necrosis. Heparin-induced necrosis may have clinically similar features but is probably due to heparin-induced platelet aggregation with subsequent occlusion of blood vessels.

Warfarin-induced cutaneous necrosis is treated with vitamin K and heparin. Vitamin K reverses the effects of warfarin, and heparin acts as an anticoagulant. Treatment with protein C concentrates may also be helpful in individuals with deficiencies of protein C, the predisposing factor for development of these reactions.

MORBILLIFORM REACTIONS Morbilliform or maculopapular eruptions are the most common of all drug-induced reactions, often start on the trunk or areas of pressure or trauma, and consist of erythematous macules and papules that are frequently symmetric and may become confluent. Involvement of mucous membranes, palms, and soles is variable; the eruption may be associated with moderate to severe pruritus and fever.

The pathogenesis is unclear. A hypersensitivity mechanism has been suggested, although these reactions do not always recur following drug rechallenge. Diagnosis is rarely assisted by laboratory or patch testing; differentiation from viral exanthem is the principal differential diagnostic consideration. Unless the suspect drug is essential it should be discontinued. Occasionally these eruptions may decrease or fade with continued use of the responsible drug.

Morbilliform reactions usually develop within 1 week of initiation of therapy and last 1 to 2 weeks; however, reactions to some drugs, especially penicillin and drugs with long half-lives, may begin more than 2 weeks after therapy has begun and last as long as 2 weeks after therapy has ceased.

Morbilliform eruptions are usually treated by discontinuing the suspect medications symptomatically. Oral antihistamines, emollients, and soothing baths are useful for treatment of pruritus. Short courses of potent topical glucocorticoids can reduce inflammation and symptoms and are probably helpful. The beneficial effect of systemic glucocorticoids relative to risk is less clear.

FIXED DRUG REACTIONS These reactions are characterized by one or more sharply demarcated, erythematous lesions in which hyperpigmentation results after resolution of the acute inflammation; with rechallenge, the lesion recurs in the same (i.e., "fixed") location. Lesions often involve the lips, hands, legs, face, genitalia, and oral mucosa and cause burning. Most patients have multiple lesions. Patch testing is useful to establish the etiology. Fixed drug eruptions have been associated with phenolphthalein, sulfonamides, tetracyclines, phenylbutazone, NSAIDs, and barbiturates. Although cross-sensitivity appears to occur between different tetracycline compounds, cross-sensitivity was not elicited when different sulfonamide compounds were administered to patients as part of provocation testing.

LICHENOID DRUG ERUPTIONS A lichenoid cutaneous reaction, clinically and morphologically indistinguishable from lichen planus, is associated with a variety of drugs and chemicals. Eosinophils are more common when the reaction is drug-induced. Gold and antimalarials are most often associated with this eruption. Antihypertensive agents, including beta blockers and captopril, have also been reported to cause lichenoid reactions.

BULLOUS ERUPTIONS Blisters accompany a wide variety of cutaneous reactions, including fixed drug eruptions, severe morbilliform eruptions in dependent areas of the body, and phototoxic reactions. SJS and TEN are the most serious and important bullous reactions to drugs. Nalidixic acid and furosemide cause blistering eruptions indistinguishable from the primary bullous diseases. A pemphigus foliaceus–like eruption is seen with penicillamine.

PUSTULAR ERUPTIONS Acute generalized exanthematous pustulosis is often associated with exposure to drugs, most notably antibiotics. Usually beginning on the face or intertriginous areas, small nonfollicular pustules overlying erythematous and edematous skin may coalesce and lead to superficial ulceration. Fever is present and differentiating this eruption from TEN in its initial stages may be difficult. Acute generalized exanthematous pustulosis often begins within a few days of initiating drug treatment.

ERYTHEMA MULTIFORME Erythema multiforme is an acute, self-limited inflammatory disorder of skin and mucous membranes characterized by distinctive iris or target lesions, usually acrally distributed and often associated with sore throat, mucosal lesions, and malaise. Classic erythema multiforme usually has nondrug causes, most commonly herpes simplex infection, and must be differentiated from true SJS, which is usually drug related.

STEVENS-JOHNSON SYNDROME SJS is a blistering disorder that is usually more severe than erythema multiforme. Initial presentation is often a sore throat, malaise, and fever. Within a few days, in addition to erosions of multiple mucous membranes, small blisters developing on dusky or purpuric macules or atypical target lesions characterize this eruption. Total percent of body surface area blistering and eventual detachment is less than 10%. Overlap SJS/TEN shares characteristics of both SJS and TEN, with 10 to 30% of body surface area exhibiting epidermal detachment.

TOXIC EPIDERMAL NECROLYSIS TEN is the most serious cutaneous drug reaction and may be fatal. Drugs are usually the cause of TEN. Onset is generally acute and is characterized by fever >39°C (102.2°F), blisters or ulcers of multiple mucous membranes, malaise, and epidermal necrosis involving >30% of body surface area. Intestinal and pulmonary involvement is associated with a poor prognosis, as is a greater extent of epidermal detachment and older age. About 30% of affected persons die. Many treatments affecting immune response or cytokines (thalidomide) or apoptosis (intravenous immunoglobulin) have been advocated, but none have been shown to be efficacious in well-controlled trials. In spite of its theoretical potential benefits, thalidomide therapy increases TEN-associated mortality. Supportive treatment in burn units is helpful in reducing morbidity and mortality.

DRUGS OF SPECIAL INTEREST

PENICILLIN   The incidence of cutaneous reactions to penicillin is about 1%. About 85% of cutaneous reactions to penicillin are morbilliform, and about 10% are urticaria or angioedema.

IgG, IgM, and IgE antibodies can be produced; IgG and IgM antipenicillin antibodies play a role in the development of hemolytic anemia, whereas anaphylaxis and serum sickness appear to be due to IgE antibodies in serum.

In patients with suspected IgE-mediated reactions to penicillin for whom future treatment is anticipated, accurate tests for sensitization are available. Current practice is to perform skin testing with a commercially available penicilloyl determinant preparation (Pre-pen, Kremers-Urban) and with fresh penicillin and, if possible, with another source of minor (nonpenicilloyl) determinants such as aged or base-treated penicillin. Antibodies to minor determinants are common in patients experiencing anaphylaxis, but testing with major determinants alone detects most patients at risk for anaphylaxis.

About one-fourth of patients with positive history of penicillin allergy have a positive skin test, while 6% (3 to 10%) with no history of penicillin sensitivity demonstrate a positive skin response to penicillin. Administering penicillin to those patients with a positive skin test produces reactions in a high proportion (50 to 100%); conversely, only a few patients (0.5%) with a negative skin test react to the drug, and reactions tend to be mild and to occur late. Since a false-negative skin test may occur during or just after an acute reaction, testing should be performed either prospectively or several months after a suspected reaction. As many as 80% of patients lose anaphylactic sensitivity and IgE antibody after several years. Radioallergosorbent tests and other in vitro tests offer no advantage over properly performed skin testing. Some cross-reactivity between penicillin and nonpenicillin β-lactam antibiotics (e.g., cephalosporins) occurs, but the majority of penicillin-allergic patients will tolerate cephalosporins. Persons who have negative skin tests to penicillin rarely develop reactions to cephalosporins.

In the face of a positive clinical history of penicillin reaction, another drug should be chosen. If this is not feasible or prudent (e.g., in a pregnant patient with syphilis or with enterococcal endocarditis), skin testing with penicillin is warranted. If skin tests are negative, cautious administration of penicillin is acceptable, although some recommend desensitization of such patients if the reaction was likely to be IgE-mediated. In those with positive skin tests, desensitization is mandatory if therapeutic use of β-lactam antibiotics is to be undertaken. Various protocols are available, including oral and parenteral approaches. Oral desensitization appears to have lower risk of serious anaphylactic reactions during desensitization. However, desensitization carries the risk of anaphylaxis regardless of how it is performed. After desensitization, many patients experience non-life-threatening IgE-mediated untoward reactions to penicillin during their course of therapy. Desensitization is not effective in those with exfoliative dermatitis or morbilliform reactions due to penicillin.

NONSTEROIDAL   ANTI-INFLAMMATORY   DRUGS   NSAIDs, including aspirin and indomethacin (indometacin), cause two broad categories of allergic-like symptoms in susceptible individuals: (1) approximately 1% of persons experience urticaria or angioedema, and (2) about half as many (0.5%) experience rhinosinusitis and asthma; however, about 10% of adults with asthma and one-third of individuals with nasal polyposis and sinusitis may respond adversely to aspirin.

Urticaria/angioedema may be delayed up to 24 h and may occur at any age. The rhinosinusitis-asthma syndrome generally develops within 1 h of drug administration. In young patients, the reaction pattern often begins as watery rhinorrhea, which can be complicated by nasal and sinus infection, and polyposis, bloody discharge, and nasal eosinophilia. In many individuals with this syndrome, asthma that can be life-threatening eventually ensues whenever NSAIDs are subsequently ingested, and symptoms may persist despite avoidance of these drugs. Proof of the association of symptoms and NSAID use requires either clear-cut history of symptoms following drug ingestion or an oral challenge. For the latter to be performed with relative safety, (1) asthma must be under good control, (2) the procedure must be conducted in a hospital setting by experienced personnel capable of recognizing and treating acute respiratory responses, and (3) the challenge should begin with very low doses (i.e., not >30 mg) of aspirin and increase every 1 to 2 h in doubling doses as tolerated to 650 mg.

While cross-reactivity between NSAIDs is common, it is not immunologic, and patients who are sensitive to NSAIDs cannot be identified by assessment of IgE antibody to aspirin, lymphocyte sensitization, or in vitro immunologic testing.

RADIOCONTRAST MEDIA   Large numbers of patients are exposed to radiocontrast agents. High-osmolality radiocontrast media are about five times more likely to induce urticaria (1%) or anaphylaxis than newer low-osmolality media. Severe reactions are rare with either type of contrast media. About one-third of those with mild reactions to previous exposure rereact on reexposure. In most cases, these reactions are probably not immunologic. Pretreatment with prednisone and diphenhydramine reduces reaction rates. Persons with a reaction to a high-osmolality contrast media should be given low-osmolality media if later contrast studies are required.

ANTICONVULSANTS   Of the anticonvulsants, the single orally administered agent with the highest risk of severe adverse cutaneous reactions is the antiseizure medicine lamotrigine. Older anticonvulsants, including phenytoin and carbamazepine, are also associated with many types of severe reactions and a high incidence of less severe reactions, particularly in children. In addition to SJS, TEN, and the hypersensitivity syndrome discussed above, the aromatic anticonvulsants can induce a pseudolymphoma syndrome and induce gingival hyperplasia.

SULFONAMIDES   Sulfonamides have perhaps the highest risk of causing cutaneous eruptions and are the drugs most frequently implicated in SJS and TEN. The combination of sulfamethoxazole and trimethoprim frequently induces adverse cutaneous reactions in patients with AIDS (Chap. 309). Desensitization is often successful in AIDS patients with morbilliform eruptions but is a high-risk procedure in AIDS patients who manifest erythroderma, fever, or a bullous reaction in response to their earlier sulfonamide exposure.

AGENTS USED IN CANCER CHEMOTHERAPY   Since many agents used in cancer chemotherapy inhibit cell division, rapidly proliferating elements of the skin, including hair, mucous membranes, and appendages, are sensitive to their effects; as a result, stomatitis and alopecia are among the most frequent dose-dependent side effects of chemotherapy. Onychodystrophy (dystrophic changes in nails) is also seen with bleomycin, hydroxyurea (hydroxycarbamide), and 5-fluorouracil. Sterile cellulitis and phlebitis and ulceration of pressure areas occur with many of these agents. Urticaria, angioedema, exfoliative dermatitis, and erythema of the palms and soles have also been seen, as has local and diffuse hyperpigmentation.

GLUCOCORTICOIDS   Both systemic and topical glucocorticoids cause a variety of skin changes, including acneiform eruptions, atrophy, striae, and other stigmata of Cushing's syndrome, and in sufficiently high doses can retard wound healing. Patients using glucocorticoids are at higher risk for bacterial, yeast, and fungal skin infections that may be misinterpreted as drug eruptions but are instead drug side effects.

CYTOKINE THERAPY   Alopecia is a common complication of IFN-α. Induction or exacerbation of various immune-mediated disorders (psoriasis, lichen planus, lupus erythematosus) has been also reported with this agent. IFN-β injection has been associated with local necrosis of the skin. Granulocyte colony stimulating factor may induce various neutrophilic dermatosis, including Sweet's syndrome, pyo-

Table 59-2 Clinical and Laboratory Findings Associated with More Serious Drug-Induced Cutaneous Clinical Findings

Cutaneous
  Confluent erythema
  Facial edema or central facial involvement
  Skin pain
  Palpable purpura
  Skin necrosis
  Blisters or epidermal detachment
  Positive Nikolsky's sign
  Mucous membrane erosions
  Urticaria
  Swelling of tongue

General
  High fever [temperature >40°C (>104°F)]
  Enlarged lymph nodes
  Arthralgias or arthritis
  Shortness of breath, wheezing, hypotension

Laboratory results
  Eosinophil count >1000/μL
  Lymphocytosis with atypical lymphocytes
  Abnormal liver function tests

SOURCE: Adapted from Roujeau and Stern.

derma gangrenosum, neutrophilic eccrine hidradenitis, and vasculitis, and can exacerbate psoriasis.

IL-2 is associated with frequent cutaneous reactions including exanthema, facial edema, xerosis, and pruritus. Cases of pemphigus vulgaris, linear IgA disease, psoriasis, and vitiligo have also been described in association with this drug.

ANTIMALARIAL AGENTS Antimalarial agents are used as therapy for several skin diseases, including the skin manifestations of lupus and polymorphous light eruption, but they can also induce cutaneous reactions. Although also used to treat porphyria cutanea tarda at low doses, in patients with asymptomatic porphyria cutanea tarda, higher doses of chloroquine increase porphyrin levels to such an extent that they may exacerbate the disease.

Pigmentation disturbances, including black pigmentation of the face, mucous membranes, and pretibial and subungual areas, occur with antimalarials. Quinacrine (mepacrine) causes generalized, cutaneous yellow discoloration.

GOLD Chrysotherapy has been associated with a variety of dose-related dermatologic reactions (including maculopapular eruptions), which can develop as long as 2 years after initiation of therapy and require months to resolve. Erythema nodosum, psoriasiform dermatitis, vaginal pruritus, eruptions similar to those of pityriasis rosea, hyperpigmentation, and lichenoid eruptions resembling those seen with antimalarial agents have been reported. After a cutaneous reaction, it is sometimes possible to reinstitute gold therapy at lower doses without recurrence of the dermatitis.

DIAGNOSIS OF DRUG REACTIONS

Possible causes of an adverse reaction can be assessed as definite, probable, possible, or unlikely based on six variables: (1) previous experience with the drug in the general population, (2) alternative etiologic candidates, (3) timing of events, (4) drug levels or evidence of

Table 59-3 Clinical Features of Selected Severe Cutaneous Reactions Often Induced by Drugs

Diagnosis	Mucosal Lesions	Typical Skin Lesions	Frequent Signs and Symptoms	Alternative Causes not Related to Drugs
Stevens-Johnson syndrome	Erosions usually at ≥two sites	Small blisters on dusky purpuric macules or atypical targets; rare areas of confluence; detachment ≤10% of body surface area	10–30% of cases involve fever	Postinfectious erythema multiforme major (especially in the case of infection with herpes simplex or mycoplasma)
Toxic epidermal necrolysis[a]	Erosions usually at ≥two sites	Individual lesions like those seen in Stevens-Johnson syndrome; confluent erythema; outer layer of epidermis separates readily from basal layer with lateral pressure; large sheet of necrotic epidermis; total detachment of >30% of body surface area	Nearly all cases involve fever, "acute skin failure," leukopenia	
Hypersensitivity syndrome	Infrequent	Severe exanthematous rash (may become purpuric), exfoliative dermatitis	30–50% of cases involve fever, lymphadenopathy, hepatitis, nephritis, carditis, eosinophilia, atypical lymphocytes	Cutaneous lymphoma
Acute generalized exanthematous pustulosis	About 50% erosions mouth, tongue	Initially nonfollicular small pustules overlying edematous erythema, sometimes leading to superficial ulcers	Fever, burning, pruritus, facial swelling, leukocytosis, hypocalcemia	Infection
Serum sickness or reactions resembling serum sickness	Absent	Morbilliform lesions, sometimes with urticaria	Fever, arthralgias	Infection
Anticoagulant-induced necrosis	Infrequent	Erythema then purpura and necrosis, especially of fatty areas	Pain in affected areas	Disseminated intravascular coagulopathy, septicemia
Angioedema	Often involved	Urticaria or swelling of central part of face	Respiratory distress, cardiovascular collapse	Insect stings, foods

[a] Overlap of Stevens-Johnson syndrome and toxic epidermal necrolysis with features of both and attachment of 10 to 30% of body surface area may occur.

SOURCE: Adapted from Roujeau and Stern.

overdose, (5) patient reaction to drug discontinuation, and (6) patient reaction to rechallenge.

PREVIOUS EXPERIENCE Tables of relative reaction rates are available and are useful to assess the likelihood that a given drug is responsible for a given cutaneous reaction. The specific morphologic pattern of a drug reaction, however, may modify these reaction rates by increasing or decreasing the likelihood that a given drug is responsible for a given reaction. For example, since fixed eruptions due to drugs are more often seen with barbiturates than with penicillin, a fixed drug reaction in a patient taking both types of agents is more likely to be due to the barbiturate, even though penicillins have a higher overall drug reaction rate.

ALTERNATIVE ETIOLOGIC CANDIDATES A cutaneous eruption may be due to exacerbation of preexisting disease or to development of new disease unrelated to drugs. For example, a patient with psoriasis may have a flare-up of disease coincidental with administration of penicillin for streptococcal infection; in this case, infection is a more likely cause for the flare-up than drug reaction.

TIMING OF EVENTS Most drug reactions of the skin occur within 1 to 2 weeks of initiation of therapy. Hypersensitivity syndrome may occur later (up to 8 weeks) after initiating drug therapy. Fixed drug reactions and generalized exanthematous pustulosis often occur earlier (within 48 h), as do reactions of all types in persons with prior sensitization to that drug or a cross-sensitizing agent.

DRUG LEVELS Some cutaneous reactions are dependent on dosage or cumulative toxicity. For example, lichenoid dermatoses due to gold administration appear more often in patients taking high doses.

DISCONTINUATION Most adverse cutaneous reactions to drugs remit with discontinuation of the suspected agent. A reaction is considered unlikely to be drug-related if improvement occurs while the drug is continued or if a patient fails to improve after stopping the drug and appropriate therapy.

RECHALLENGE Rechallenge provides the most definitive information concerning adverse cutaneous reactions to drugs, since a reaction failing to recur on rechallenge with a drug is unlikely to be due to that agent. Rechallenge is usually impractical, however, because the need to ensure patient safety and comfort outweighs the value of the possible information derived from rechallenge.

Of special importance is the rapid recognition of reactions that may become serious or life-threatening. Table 59-2 lists clinical and laboratory features that, if present, suggest the reaction may be serious. Table 59-3 provides key features of the most serious adverse cutaneous reactions.

DIAGNOSIS OF DRUG ALLERGY

Tests for IgE responses include in vivo and in vitro methods, but such tests are available for only a limited number of drugs, including penicillins and cephalosporins, some peptide and protein drugs (insulin, xenogeneic sera), and some agents used for general anesthesia. In vivo testing is accomplished by prick puncture and/or by intradermal skin testing. A wheal-and-flare response 2×2 mm greater than that seen with a saline control within 20 min is considered indicative of IgE-mediated mast cell degranulation, provided (1) the patient is not dermographic, (2) the drug does not nonspecifically degranulate mast cells, (3) the drug concentration is not high enough to be irritating, and (4) the buffer itself does not cause wheal-and-flare responses.

Skin testing with major and minor determinants of penicillins or cephalosporins has proved useful for identifying patients at risk of anaphylactic reactions to these agents. However, skin tests themselves carry a small risk of anaphylaxis. Negative skin tests do not rule out IgE-mediated reactivity, and the risk of anaphylaxis in response to penicillin administration in patients with negative skin tests is about 1%; about two-thirds of patients with a positive skin test and history of a previous adverse reaction to penicillin experience an allergic response on rechallenge. Skin tests may be negative in allergic patients receiving antihistamines or in those whose allergy is to determinants not present in the test reagent. Although less well studied, similar techniques can identify patients who are sensitive to protein drugs and to agents such as gallamine and succinylcholine. Most other drugs are small molecules, and skin testing with them is unreliable.

There are no generally available and reliable tests for assessing causality of non-IgE-mediated reactions, except possibly patch tests for assessment of fixed drug reactions. Therefore, diagnosis usually relies on clinical factors rather than test results.

BIBLIOGRAPHY

BASTUJI-GARIN S et al: Clinical classification of cases of toxic epidermal necrolysis, Stevens-Johnson syndrome, and erythema multiforme. Arch Dermatol 129:92, 1993

BIGBY M et al: Drug-induced cutaneous reactions. A report from the Boston Collaborative Drug Surveillance Program on 15,438 consecutive inpatients, 1975–1982. JAMA 256:3358, 1986

COOPMAN SA et al: Cutaneous disease and drug reactions in HIV infection. N Engl J Med 328:1670, 1993

ROUJEAU JC, STERN RS: Severe adverse cutaneous reactions to drugs. N Engl J Med 331: 1272, 1994

—— et al: Medication use and the risk of Stevens-Johnson syndrome or toxic epidermal necrolysis. N Engl J Med 333:1600, 1995

SCHLIENGER RG et al: Lamotrigine-associated anticonvulsant hypersensitivity syndrome. Neurology 51:1172, 1998

VAN DER LINDEN PD et al: Skin reactions to antibacterial agents in general practice. J Clin Epidemiol 51:703, 1998

VIARD I et al: Inhibition of toxic epidermal necrolysis by blockade of CD95 with human intravenous immunoglobulin. Science 282:490, 1998

---

60   *David R. Bickers*

PHOTOSENSITIVITY AND OTHER REACTIONS TO LIGHT

SOLAR RADIATION Sunlight is the most visible and obvious source of comfort in the environment. This natural proclivity for the sun has the beneficial results of warmth and vitamin D synthesis but also can produce pathologic consequences. Few effects of sun exposure beyond those affecting the skin have been identified, but cutaneous exposure to sunlight can evoke immunosuppressive responses and genetic changes that may be relevant to the pathogenesis of nonmelanoma skin cancer and perhaps infections such as herpes simplex.

The sun's energy encompasses a broad range from ultrashort highly energetic ionizing radiation (10^{-2} μm) to ultralong radiowaves of very low photon energy (10^7 μm). Thus, the emission spectrum ranges over nine orders of magnitude, but that reaching the earth's surface is narrow and is limited to components of the ultraviolet (UV), visible light, and portions of the infrared. The cutoff at the short end of the UV is at approximately 290 nm, because stratospheric ozone is formed by ionizing radiation of wavelengths less than 100 nm and absorbs solar energy between 120 and 310 nm, thereby preventing penetration to the earth's surface of the shorter, more energetic, potentially more harmful wavelengths of solar radiation. Indeed, concern about destruction of the ozone layer by chlorofluorocarbons released into the atmosphere has led to international agreements to reduce production of these chemicals.

Measurements of solar flux indicate that there is a twentyfold regional variation in the amount of energy at 300 nm that reaches the earth's surface. This variability relates to seasonal effects, the path of sunlight transmission through ozone and air, the altitude (4% increase for each 300 m of elevation), the latitude (increasing intensity with decreasing latitude), and the amount of cloud cover, fog, and pollution.

The major components of the photobiologic action spectrum include the UV and visible wavelengths between 290 and 700 nm. In addition, the wavelengths beyond 700 nm in the infrared primarily evoke heat, but warming of the skin may enhance biologic responses to wavelengths in the UV and visible spectrum.

The UV spectrum is arbitrarily divided into three major segments: C, B, and A. This includes the wavelengths between 10 and 400 nm. Ultraviolet C (UV-C) consists of wavelengths between 10 and 290 nm and does not reach the earth because of its absorption by stratospheric ozone. These wavelengths are not a cause of photosensitivity except in occupational settings where artificial sources of this energy are employed—e.g., for germicidal effects. Ultraviolet B (UV-B) consists of wavelengths between 290 and 320 nm. This portion of the photobiologic action spectrum is the most efficient in producing redness or erythema in human skin and hence is sometimes known as the "sunburn spectrum." Ultraviolet A (UV-A) represents those wavelengths between 320 and 400 nm and is approximately 1000-fold less efficient in producing skin hyperemia than is UV-B. The UV-A has also been divided into two parts known as UV-A 1 (340 to 400 nm) and UV-A 2 (320 to 340 nm).

The visible wavelengths between 400 and 700 nm include the familiar white light which when directed through a prism can be shown to consist of various colors including violet, indigo, blue, green, yellow, orange, and red. The energy possessed by photons in the visible spectrum is not capable of damaging human skin in the absence of a photosensitizing chemical. The absorption of energy is critical to the development of photosensitivity. Thus the *absorption spectrum* of a molecule is defined as the range of wavelengths absorbed by it, whereas the *action spectrum* for an effect of incident radiation is defined as the range of wavelengths that evoke the response.

Photosensitivity occurs when a photon-absorbing chemical (chromophore) present in the skin absorbs incident energy, becomes excited, and transfers the absorbed energy to various structures or to oxygen. The absorbed energy must be dissipated by processes including heat, fluorescence, and phosphorescence. It is important to emphasize that absorption spectra and action spectra need not be superimposable, but there must be overlap at some point to produce photosensitization.

STRUCTURE AND FUNCTION OF SKIN The skin's exposure to sunlight permits the absorption of some wavelengths and the transmission of others. Essentially, human skin is a sandwich of two distinctive compartments, the epidermis and dermis, separated by a basement membrane. The outer epidermis is a stratified squamous epithelium comprising the surface stratum corneum (a protein- and lipid-rich compact membrane), the stratum granulosum, stratum spinosum, and the basal cell layer. The basal cell layer contains a heterogeneous population of cells, a subset of which migrate upward in the process of terminal differentiation that results in the expression of specific keratin genes and the formation of the stratum corneum. Epidermal cells include resident keratinocytes and melanocytes and immigrant cells, including the immunologically active Langerhans cells, lymphocytes, polymorphonuclear leukocytes, monocytes, and macrophages, making the epidermis a major component of the immune system. Branches of sensory nerve endings also reach into this compartment.

The second major component of skin is the dermis, which is relatively large and less densely populated with cells that include fibroblasts, endothelial cells within dermal vessels, and mast cells. Tissue macrophages and sparsely distributed inflammatory cells are also present. All these cells exist within an extracellular matrix of collagen, elastin, and glycosaminoglycans. In contrast to the epidermis, rich vascularization of the dermis allows it to play an important role in temperature regulation and in inflammatory responses to skin injury.

UV RADIATION (UVR) AND SKIN The epidermis and the dermis contain several chromophores capable of interacting with incident solar energy. These interactions include reflection, refraction, absorption, and transmission. The stratum corneum is a major impediment to the transmission of UV-B, and less than 10% of incident wavelengths in this region penetrate the basement membrane. Approximately 3% of radiation below 300 nm, 20% of radiation below 360 nm, and 33% of short visible radiation reaches the basal cell layer in untanned human skin. Proteins and nucleic acids absorb intensely in the short UV-B. In contrast, UV-A 1 and 2 penetrate the epidermis efficiently to reach the dermis, where they likely produce changes in

structural and matrix proteins that contribute to the aged appearance of chronically sun-exposed skin, particularly in individuals of light complexion.

One of the consequences of UV-B absorption by DNA is the production of pyrimidine dimers. These structural changes can be repaired by mechanisms that result in their recognition and excision, and the reestablishment of normal base sequences. The efficient repair of these structural aberrations is crucial, since individuals with defective DNA repair are at high risk for the development of cutaneous cancer. For example, patients with xeroderma pigmentosum, an autosomal recessive disorder, are characterized by variably decreased repair of UV-induced photoproducts, and their skin may develop the xerotic appearance of photoaging as well as basal cell and squamous cell carcinomas and melanoma in the first two decades of life. Studies in mice using knockout gene technology have verified the importance of genes regulating these repair pathways in preventing the development of UV-induced cancer.

Cutaneous Optics and Chromophores Chromophores are endogenous or exogenous chemical components that can absorb physical energy. Endogenous chromophores of skin are of two types: (1) chemicals that are normally present, including nucleic acids, proteins, lipids, and 7-dehydrocholesterol, the precursor of vitamin D; and (2) chemicals, such as porphyrins, synthesized elsewhere in the body that circulate in the bloodstream and diffuse into the skin. Normally, only trace amounts of porphyrins are present in the skin, but in the diseases known as the porphyrias, increased amounts are released into the circulation and are transported to the skin, where they absorb incident energy both in the Soret band around 400 nm (short visible) and to a lesser extent in the red portion of the visible spectrum (580 to 660 nm). This results in structural damage to the skin that may be manifest as erythema, edema, urticaria, or blister formation (Chap. 346).

Acute Effects of Sun Exposure The immediate cutaneous consequences of sun exposure include sunburn and vitamin D synthesis.

Sunburn This very common affliction of human skin is caused by exposure to UVR. Generally speaking, the individual's ability to tolerate sunlight is inversely proportional to his or her melanin pigmentation. Melanin is a complex polymer of tyrosine that functions as an efficient neutral-density filter with broad absorbance within the UV portion of the solar spectrum. Melanin is synthesized in specialized epidermal dendritic cells termed *melanocytes* and is packaged into *melanosomes* that are transferred via dendritic processes into *keratinocytes*, where they provide photoprotection. Sun-induced melanogenesis is a consequence of increased tyrosinase activity in melanocytes that in turn may be due to a combination of eicosanoid and endothelin-1 release. Tolerance of sun exposure is a function of the efficiency of the epidermal-melanin unit and can usually be ascertained by asking an individual two questions: (1) Do you burn after sun exposure? and (2) Do you tan after sun exposure? By the answers to these questions, it is usually possible to divide the population into six skin types varying from type I (always burn, never tan) to type VI (never burn, always tan) (Table 60-1).

There are two general theories about the pathogenesis of the sunburn response. First, the lag phase in time between skin exposure and the development of visible redness (usually 4 to 12 h) suggests an epidermal chromophore that causes delayed production and/or release

Table 60-1 Skin Type and Sunburn Sensitivity

Type	Description
I	Always burn, never tan
II	Always burn, sometimes tan
III	Sometimes burn, sometimes tan
IV	Sometimes burn, always tan
V	Never burn, sometimes tan
VI	Never burn, always tan

of vasoactive mediator(s), or cytokines, that diffuse to the dermal vasculature to evoke vasodilatation. Indeed, UVR stimulates the release of numerous proinflammatory cytokines and nitric oxide by keratinocytes. Second, it is possible that the small amount of incident UV-B radiation (10% or less) that penetrates to the dermis can be absorbed directly by endothelial cells in the vasculature, thereby resulting in vasodilatation. The issue remains unresolved.

The action spectrum for sunburn erythema includes the UV-B and UV-A regions. Photons in the shorter UV-B are at least 1000-fold more efficient than photons in the longer UV-B and the UV-A in evoking the response. However, UV-A may contribute to sunburn erythema at midday when much more UV-A than UV-B is present.

The mechanism of injury remains poorly defined, but the action spectrum for UV-B erythema closely resembles the absorption spectrum for DNA after adjusting for the absorbance of incident energy by the stratum corneum. Apoptotic keratinocytes (so-called sunburn cells) are visible histologically within an hour of exposure and are maximal within 24 h. UV-A is less effective than UV-B in producing sunburn cells. Mast cells may release inflammatory mediators after exposure to UV-B and UV-A. For example, erythema doses of both UV-B and UV-A increase histamine levels in experimentally induced suction blisters of human skin that return to normal after 24 h (before visible erythema has subsided). Prostaglandin E_2 increases to approximately 150% of control levels after 24 h and then diminishes. Since prostaglandins evoke both pain and redness when injected intradermally, their presence in suction blisters after UV-B exposure suggests a role in UV-B erythema. Age-related declines occur in the amount of inflammatory mediators detectable in human skin after UV-B irradiation. UV-A erythema results in few epidermal sunburn cells, but vascular endothelial injury is greater than with UV-B. In addition, there are increased levels of arachidonic acid and of prostaglandins D_2, E_2, and I_2 that peak within 5 to 9 h and then subside before peak redness occurs. Despite evidence for the role of prostaglandins in both UV-B- and UV-A-irradiated skin, administration of nonsteroidal anti-inflammatory drugs is more effective in reducing erythema evoked by UV-B than by UV-A. UV-B also induces cutaneous matrix-degrading metalloproteinases within hours of exposure.

Vitamin D photochemistry   Cutaneous exposure to UV-B causes photolysis of epidermal previtamin D_3 (7-dehydrocholesterol) to previtamin D_3, which then undergoes a temperature-dependent isomerization to form the stable hormone vitamin D_3. This compound then diffuses to the dermal vasculature and circulates systemically where it is converted to the functional hormone 1,25-dihydroxy vitamin D_3 [1,25(OH)$_2$D$_3$]. Vitamin D metabolites from the circulation or those produced in the skin itself can augment epidermal differentiation signaling. Aging substantially decreases the ability of human skin to produce vitamin D_3. This, coupled with the widespread use of sunscreens that filter out UV-B, has led to concern that vitamin D deficiency may become a significant clinical problem in the elderly. Indeed, studies have shown that the use of sunscreens can diminish the production of vitamin D_3 in human skin.

Chronic Effects of Sun Exposure: Nonmalignant   The clinical features of photodamaged sun-exposed skin consist of wrinkling, blotchiness, telangiectasia, and a roughened, irregular, "weather-beaten" appearance. Whether these changes, which some refer to as *photoaging* or *dermatoheliosis*, represent accelerated chronologic aging or a separate and distinct process is not clear.

Within chronically sun-exposed epidermis, there is thickening (acanthosis) and morphologic heterogeneity within the basal cell layer. Higher but irregular melanosome content may be present in some keratinocytes, indicating prolonged residence of the cells in the basal cell layer. These structural changes may help to explain the leathery texture and the blotchy discoloration of sun-damaged skin.

The dermis is the major site for sun-associated chronic damage, manifest as a massive increase in thickened irregular masses of tangled elastic fibers resulting from enhanced expression of elastin genes. Collagen fibers are also abnormally clumped in the deeper dermis. Fibroblasts are increased in number and show morphologic signs suggesting activation. Degraded mast cells may be present in the dermis, the relevance of which remains unclear.

These morphologic changes, both gross and microscopic, are features of chronically sun-exposed skin. The chromophore(s), the action spectra, and the specific biochemical events orchestrating these changes are unknown.

Chronic Effects of Sun Exposure: Malignant   One of the major known consequences of chronic skin exposure to sunlight is nonmelanoma skin cancer. The two types of nonmelanoma skin cancer are basal cell and squamous cell carcinoma (Chap. 86). There are three major steps for cancer induction: initiation, promotion, and progression. Chronic exposure of animal skin to artificial light sources that mimic solar UVR results in *initiation*, a step whereby structural (mutagenic) changes in DNA evoke an irreversible alteration in the target cell (keratinocyte) that begins the tumorigenic process. Exposure to a tumor initiator is believed to be a necessary but not sufficient step in the malignant process, since initiated skin cells not exposed to tumor promoters do not generally develop tumors. The second stage in tumor development is *promotion*, a multistep process whereby initiated cells are exposed to chemical and physical agents that evoke epigenetic changes that culminate in the clonal expansion of initiated cells and cause the development, over a period of weeks to months, of benign growths known as *papillomas*. Again, using transgenic animals, the importance of UV effects on the expression of additional oncogenes such as *fos* and *jun* in developing papillomas has been demonstrated. UV-B is a *complete carcinogen*, meaning that it can function as both an initiator and a promoter, leading to tumor induction. *Incomplete carcinogens* can initiate tumorigenesis but require additional skin exposure to tumor promoters to elicit tumors. The prototype tumor promoter is the phorbol ester 12-*O*-tetradecanoyl phorbol-13-acetate. Tumor promotion usually requires multiple exposures over time to evoke a neoplasm.

The final step in the malignant process is the conversion of benign precursors into malignant lesions, a process thought to require additional genetic alterations in already transformed cells. Indeed, *ras* gene mutations have been detected in a minority of human nonmelanoma skin cancers. Mutations of the tumor suppressor gene p53 also occur in sun-damaged human skin.

Sun exposure causes nonmelanoma and melanoma cancers of the skin, although the evidence is far more direct for its role in nonmelanoma (basal cell and squamous cell carcinoma) than in melanoma. Approximately 80% of nonmelanoma skin cancers develop on exposed body area, including the face, the neck, and the hands. Men of fair complexion who work outdoors are twice as likely as women to develop these types of cancers. Whites of darker complexions (e.g., Hispanics) have one-tenth the risk of developing such cancers as do light-skinned individuals. Blacks are at lowest risk for all forms of skin cancer. Between 600,000 and 800,000 individuals in the United States develop nonmelanoma skin cancer annually, and the lifetime risk for a white individual to develop such a neoplasm is estimated at approximately 15%. A consensus exists that the incidence of nonmelanoma skin cancer in the population is rising, for reasons that are unclear.

The relationship of sun exposure to melanoma is less clear-cut, but suggestive evidence supports an association. Melanomas occasionally develop by the teenage years, indicating that the latent period for tumor growth is less than that of nonmelanoma skin cancer. Melanomas are among the most rapidly increasing of all human malignancies (Chap. 86). Epidemiologic studies of immigrants of similar ethnic stock indicate that individuals born in one area or who migrated to the same locale before age 10 have higher age-specific melanoma rates than individuals arriving later. It is thus reasonable to conclude that life in a sunny climate from birth or early childhood increases the risk of melanoma. In general, risk does not correlate with cumulative sun exposure but may relate to sequelae of sun exposure in childhood. Thus, a blistering sunburn is associated with a doubling of melanoma risk at the site of the reaction.

Immunologic Effects Exposure to solar radiation influences both local and systemic immune responses. UV-B appears to be most efficient in altering immune responses, likely related to the capacity of such energy to affect antigen presentation in skin by interacting with epidermal Langerhans cells. These bone marrow–derived dendritic cells possess surface markers characteristic of monocytes and macrophages. Following skin exposure to erythema doses of UV-B, Langerhans cells undergo both morphologic and functional changes that result in decreased contact allergic responses when haptens are applied to the irradiated site. This diminished capacity for sensitization is due to the induction of antigen-specific suppressor T lymphocytes. Indeed, while the immunosuppressive effect of irradiation is limited to haptens applied to the irradiated site, the net result is systemic immune suppression to that antigen because of the induction of suppressor T cells.

Higher doses of radiation evoke diminished immunologic responses to antigens introduced either epicutaneously or intracutaneously at sites distant from the irradiated site. These suppressed responses are also associated with the induction of antigen-specific suppressor T lymphocytes and may be mediated by as yet undefined factors that are released from epidermal cells at the irradiated site. The implications of this generalized immune suppression in terms of altered susceptibility to cutaneous cancer or to infection remain to be defined.

It is known that UV-induced tumors in murine skin are antigenic and are rapidly rejected when transplanted into normal syngeneic animals. If the tumors are transplanted into animals previously exposed to subcarcinogenic doses of UV-B, they are not rejected and instead grow progressively in the recipients. This failure of irradiated animals to reject the transplanted tumors is due to the development of T suppressor cells that prevent the rejection response. While the mechanism of suppression of tumor rejection is unknown, such a response might be a critical determinant of cancer risk in human skin.

PHOTOSENSITIVITY DISEASES The diagnosis of photosensitivity requires a careful history to define the duration of the signs and symptoms, the length of time between exposure to sunlight and the development of subjective complaints, and visible changes in the skin. The age of onset also can be a helpful clue; for example, the acute photosensitivity of erythropoietic protoporphyria almost always begins in childhood, whereas the chronic photosensitivity of porphyria cutanea tarda typically begins in the fourth and fifth decades. A history of exposure to topical and systemic drugs and chemicals may provide important information. Many classes of drugs can cause photosensitivity on the basis of either phototoxicity or photoallergy. Fragrances such as musk ambrette that were previously present in numerous cosmetic products are also potent photosensitizers.

Examination of the skin may also offer important clues. Anatomic areas that are naturally protected from direct sunlight such as the hairy scalp, the upper eyelids, the retroauricular areas, and the infranasal and submental regions may be spared, whereas exposed areas show characteristic features of the pathologic process. These anatomic localization patterns are often helpful but not infallible in making the diagnosis. For example, airborne contact sensitizers that are blown onto the skin may produce dermatitis that can be difficult to distinguish from photosensitivity, despite the fact that such material may trigger skin reactivity in areas shielded from direct sunlight.

Many dermatologic conditions may be caused or aggravated by light (Table 60-2). The role of light in evoking these responses may be dependent on genetic abnormalities ranging from well-described defects in DNA repair that occur in xeroderma pigmentosum to the inherited abnormalities in heme synthesis that characterize the porphyrias. In certain photosensitivity diseases, the chromophore has been identified, whereas in the majority, the energy-absorbing agent is unknown.

Polymorphous Light Eruption After sunburn, the most common type of photosensitivity disease is *polymorphous light eruption*, the mechanism of which is unknown. Many affected individuals never seek medical attention because the condition is often transient, becoming manifest each spring with initial sun exposure but then subsiding spontaneously with continuing exposure, a phenomenon known as "hardening." The major manifestations of polymorphous light eruption include pruritic (often intensely so) erythematous papules that may coalesce into plaques on exposed areas of the face and arms or other areas as well, making the distribution spotty and uneven.

The diagnosis can be confirmed by skin biopsy and by performing phototest procedures in which skin is exposed to multiple erythema doses of UV-A and UV-B. The action spectrum for polymorphous light eruption is usually within these portions of the solar spectrum.

Treatment of this disease includes the induction of hardening by the cautious administration of UV light, either alone or in combination with photosensitizers such as the psoralens (see below).

Phototoxicity and Photoallergy These photosensitivity disorders are related to the topical or systemic administration of drugs and other chemicals. Both reactions require the absorption of energy by a drug or chemical resulting in the production of an excited-state photosensitizer that can transfer its absorbed energy to a bystander molecule or to molecular oxygen, thereby generating tissue-destructive chemical species.

Phototoxicity is a nonimmunologic reaction caused by drugs and chemicals, a few of which are listed in Table 60-3. The usual clinical manifestations include erythema resembling a sunburn that quickly desquamates or "peels" within several days. In addition, edema, vesicles, and bullae may occur.

Photoallergy is distinct in that the immune system participates in the pathologic process. The excited-state photosensitizer may create

Table 60-2 Classification of Photosensitivity Diseases

Type	Disease
Genetic	Erythropoietic porphyria
	Erythropoietic protoporphyria
	Porphyria cutanea tarda—familial
	Variegate porphyria
	Hepatoerythropoietic porphyria
	Albinism
	Xeroderma pigmentosum
	Rothmund-Thompson disease
	Bloom syndrome
	Cockayne's disease
	Phenylketonuria
Metabolic	Porphyria cutanea tarda—sporadic
	Hartnup disease
	Kwashiorkor
	Pellagra
	Carcinoid syndrome
	Pseudoporphyria
Phototoxic	
Internal	Drugs
External	Drugs, plants, food
Photoallergic	
Immediate	Solar urticaria
Delayed	Drug photoallergy
	Persistent light reaction/chronic actinic dermatitis
Neoplastic and	Photoaging
degenerative	Actinic keratosis
	Melanoma and nonmelanoma skin cancer
Idiopathic	Polymorphous light eruption
	Hydroa aestivale
	Actinic reticuloid
Photoaggravated	Lupus erythematosus
	Systemic
	Subacute cutaneous
	Dermatomyositis
	Pemphigus foliaceus
	Herpes simplex
	Lichen planus actinicus
	Acne vulgaris (aestivale)
	Transient acantholytic dermatosis

Table 60-3   Phototoxic Drugs and Chemicals

	Topical	Systemic
Coal Tar Derivatives		
Acridine	+	
Anthracene	+	
Phenanthrene	+	
Drugs		
Amiodarone		+
Dacarbazine		+
Fluoroquinolones		+
5-Fluorouracil	+	+
Furosemide		+
Nalidixic acid		+
Phenothiazines		+
Psoralens	+	+
Retinoids	+/−	+
Sulfonamides		+
Sulfonylureas		+
Tetracyclines		+
Thiazides		+
Vinblastine		+
Dyes		
Anthraquinone		+
Eosin		+
Methylene blue		+
Rose bengal		+

highly unstable haptenic free radicals that bind covalently to macromolecules to form a functional antigen capable of evoking a delayed hypersensitivity response. Some of the drugs and chemicals that produce photoallergy are listed in Table 60-4. The clinical manifestations typically differ from those of phototoxicity in that an intensely pruritic eczematous dermatitis tends to predominate and evolves into lichenified, thickened, "leathery" changes in sun-exposed areas. A small subset (perhaps 5 to 10%) of patients with photoallergy may develop a persistent exquisite hypersensitivity to light even when the offending drug or chemical is identified and eliminated. Known as *persistent light reaction*, this may be incapacitating for years. Some have used the term *chronic actinic dermatitis* to encompass these chronic hyperresponsive states.

Table 60-4   Photoallergic Drugs and Chemicals

	Topical	Systemic
Antibiotics		
Sulfonamides		+
Antifungals		
Fenticlor	+	
Jadit	+	
Multifungin	+	
Diuretics		
Thiazides		+
Fragrances		
Musk ambrette	+	
6-Methylcoumarin	+	
Plant oleoresins	+	
Halogenated salicylanilides		
Bithionol	+	
Tetrachlorosalicylanilide	+	
Tribromosalicylanilide	+	
Nonsteroidal antiinflammatory agents		
Piroxicam	+	
Phenothiazines		
Chlorpromazine	+	
Promethazine	+	
Sulfonylureas		+
Sunscreens		
p-Aminobenzoic acid and esters	+	
Whitening Agents		
Stilbenes	+	

Diagnostic confirmation of phototoxicity and photoallergy often can be obtained using phototest procedures. In patients with suspected phototoxicity, determination of the minimal erythema dose (MED) while the patient is exposed to a suspected agent and then repeating the MED after discontinuation of the agent may provide a clue to the causative drug or chemical. Photopatch testing can be performed to confirm the diagnosis of photoallergy. This is a simple variant of ordinary patch testing in which a series of known photoallergens is applied to the skin in duplicate and one set is irradiated with a suberythema dose of UV-A. Development of eczematous changes at sites exposed to sensitizer and light is a positive result. The characteristic abnormality in patients with persistent light reaction is a diminished threshold to erythema evoked by UV-B. Patients with chronic actinic dermatitis may have a broad spectrum of UV hyperresponsiveness.

The management of drug photosensitivity is first and foremost to eliminate exposure to the chemical agents responsible for the reaction and to minimize sun exposure. The acute symptoms of phototoxicity may be ameliorated by cool, moist compresses, topical glucocorticoids, and systemically administered nonsteroidal antiinflammatory agents. In severely affected individuals, a rapidly tapered course of systemic glucocorticoids may be useful. Judicious use of analgesics may be necessary.

Photoallergic reactions require a similar management approach. Furthermore, individuals suffering from persistent light reactivity must be meticulously protected against light exposure. In selected patients in whom chronic systemic high-dose glucocorticoids pose unacceptable risks, it may be necessary to employ cytotoxic agents such as azathioprine or cyclophosphamide.

Porphyria   The porphyrias (Chap. 346) are a group of diseases that have in common various derangements in the synthesis of heme. Heme is an iron-chelated tetrapyrrole or porphyrin, and the nonmetal chelated porphyrins are potent photosensitizers that absorb light intensely in both the short (400 to 410 nm) and the long (580 to 650 nm) portions of the visible spectrum.

Heme cannot be reutilized and must be continuously synthesized, and the two body compartments with the largest capacity for its production are the bone marrow and the liver. Accordingly, the porphyrias originate in one or the other of these organs, with the end result of excessive endogenous production of potent photosensitizing porphyrins. The porphyrins circulate in the bloodstream and diffuse into the skin, where they absorb solar energy, become photoexcited, and evoke cutaneous photosensitivity. The mechanism of porphyrin photosensitization is known to be photodynamic or oxygen-dependent and is mediated by reactive oxygen species such as superoxide anions.

Porphyria cutanea tarda is the most common type of human porphyria and is associated with decreased activity of the enzyme uroporphyrinogen decarboxylase associated with a number of gene mutations. There are two basic types of porphyria cutanea tarda: the sporadic or acquired type, generally seen in individuals ingesting ethanol or receiving estrogens; and the inherited type, in which there is autosomal dominant transmission of deficient enzyme activity. Both forms are associated with increased hepatic iron stores.

In both types of porphyria cutanea tarda, the predominant feature is a chronic photosensitivity characterized by increased fragility of sun-exposed skin, particularly areas subject to repeated trauma such as the dorsa of the hands, the forearms, the face, and the ears. The predominant skin lesions are vesicles and bullae that rupture, producing moist erosions, often with a hemorrhagic base, that heal slowly with crusting and purplish discoloration of the affected skin. Hypertrichosis, mottled pigmentary change, and scleroderma-like induration are associated features. Biochemical confirmation of the diagnosis can be obtained by measurement of urinary porphyrin excretion, plasma porphyrin assay, and by assay of erythrocyte and/or hepatic uroporphyrinogen decarboxylase. Multiple mutations of the uroporphyrinogen decarboxylase gene have been identified in human populations, including exon skipping and base substitutions.

Treatment consists of repeated phlebotomies to diminish the excessive hepatic iron stores and/or intermittent low doses of the antimalarial drugs chloroquine and hydroxychloroquine. Long-term remission of the disease can be achieved if the patient eliminates exposure to porphyrinogenic agents.

Erythropoietic protoporphyria originates in the bone marrow and is due to a decrease in the mitochondrial enzyme ferrochelatase secondary to numerous gene mutations. The major clinical features include an acute photosensitivity characterized by subjective burning and stinging of exposed skin that often develops during or just after exposure. There may be associated skin swelling and, after repeated episodes, a waxlike scarring.

The diagnosis is confirmed by demonstration of measurement of free elevated erythrocyte protoporphyrin. Detection of increased plasma protoporphyrin helps to differentiate lead poisoning and iron-deficiency anemia, in both of which elevated erythrocyte protoporphyrin occurs in the absence of cutaneous photosensitivity and of elevated plasma protoporphyrin.

Treatment consists of reducing sun exposure and the oral administration of the carotenoid β-carotene, which is an effective scavenger of free radicals. This drug increases tolerance to sun exposure in many affected individuals, although it has no effect on deficient ferrochelatase.

An algorithm for the approach to a patient with photosensitivity is illustrated in Fig. 60-1.

PHOTOPROTECTION   Since photosensitivity of the skin results from exposure to sunlight, it follows that avoidance of the sun would eliminate these disorders. Unfortunately, social pressures make this an impractical alternative for most individuals, and this has led to a search for better approaches to photoprotection.

Natural photoprotection is provided by structural proteins in the epidermis, particularly keratins and melanin. The amount of melanin and its distribution in cells is genetically regulated, and individuals of darker complexion (skin types IV to VI) are at decreased risk for the development of cutaneous malignancy.

Other forms of photoprotection include clothing and sunscreens. Clothing constructed of tightly woven sun-protective fabrics, irrespective of color, affords substantial protection. Wide-brimmed hats, long sleeves, and trousers all reduce direct exposure. Sunscreens are of two major types—chemical and physical. Chemical sunscreens are chromophores that absorb energy in the UV-B and/or UV-A regions, thereby diminishing photon absorption by the skin (Table 60-5). Sunscreens are rated for their photoprotective effect by their *sun protective factor* (SPF). The SPF is simply a ratio of the time required to produce sunburn erythema with and without sunscreen application. SPF ratings of 15 or higher provide effective protection against UV-B and, to a lesser extent, UV-A. The major categories of chemical sunscreens include *p*-aminobenzoic acid and its esters, benzophenones, anthranilates, cinnamates, and salicylates. Physical sunscreens are light-opaque mixtures containing metal particles such as titanium oxide and zinc oxide that scatter light, thereby reducing photon absorption by the skin.

In addition to light absorption, a critical determinant of the photoprotective effect of sunscreens is their ability to remain on the skin, a property known as *substantivity*. In general, the *p*-aminobenzoic acid esters formulated in moisturizing vehicles provide the greatest substantivity.

Photoprotection can also be achieved by limiting the time of exposure during the day. Since the majority of an individual's total lifetime sun exposure may occur by the age of 18, it is important to educate parents and young children about the hazards of sunlight. Simply eliminating exposure at midday will substantially reduce lifetime UV-B exposure.

PHOTOTHERAPY AND PHOTOCHEMOTHERAPY   UVR can also be used therapeutically. The administration of UV-B alone or in combination with topically applied agents can induce remissions of psoriasis and atopic dermatitis.

Photochemotherapy in which topically applied or systemically administered *psoralens* are combined with UV-A (PUVA) is also effective in treating psoriasis and in the early stages of cutaneous T cell

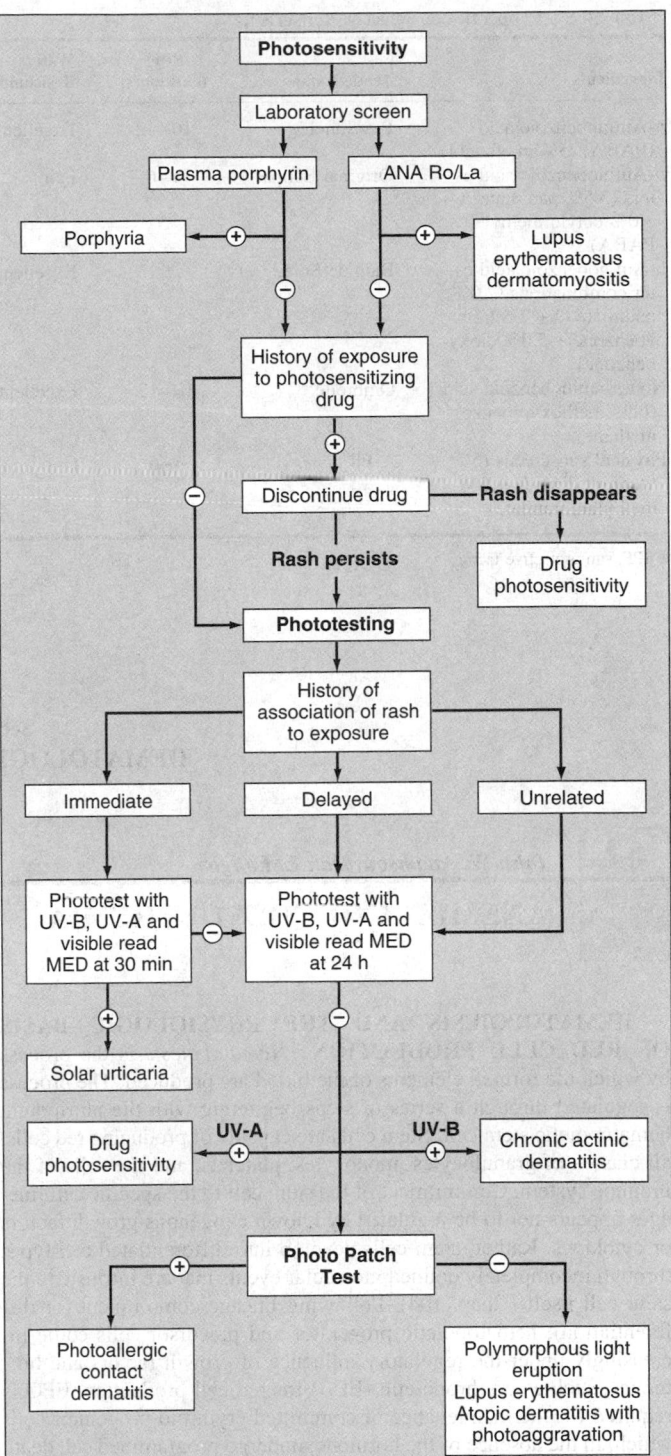

FIGURE 60-1   An algorithm for the diagnosis of a patient with photosensitivity.

lymphoma and vitiligo. Psoralens are tricyclic furocoumarins that, when intercalated into DNA and exposed to UV-A, form adducts with pyrimidine bases and eventually form DNA cross-links. These structural changes are thought to decrease DNA synthesis and relate to improvement that occurs in psoriasis. The reason that PUVA photochemotherapy is effective in cutaneous T cell lymphoma is not clear.

In addition to its effects on DNA, PUVA photochemotherapy also stimulates melanin synthesis, and this provides the rationale for its use in the depigmenting disease vitiligo. Oral 8-methoxypsoralen and UV-A appear to be most effective in this regard, but as many as 100 treat-

Table 60-5   Properties of Selected Sunscreens

Ingredients	Trade Names	SPF[a] (Outdoors)	Water Resistance
p-Aminobenzoic acid (PABA) (5% in ethanol)	Pre-Sun-15	10–12	Excellent
p-Aminobenzoic acid esters (3.5% padimate A + 3.0% octyldimethyl PABA)	Original Eclipse	4–6	Fair
p-Aminobenzoic acid ester combinations (7.0% padimate O + 2.5% oxybenzone + 5.0% dioxybenzone)	Bain de Soleil	9	Excellent
Non-p-aminobenzoic acid (butylmethoxydibenzoyl methane)	Ombrelle	10–12	Excellent
Physical sunscreens (5% titanium dioxide + 5% methylanthranilate)	A-Fil	4–6	Good

[a] SPF, sun protective factor.

ments extending over 12 to 18 months may be required to promote satisfactory repigmentation.

The major side effects of UV-B phototherapy and PUVA photochemotherapy are due to the cumulative effects of photon absorption and include skin dryness, actinic keratoses, and an increased risk of nonmelanoma skin cancer. Despite these risks, the therapeutic index of these modalities is quite acceptable.

BIBLIOGRAPHY

FISHER GJ et al: Molecular basis of sun-induced premature skin aging and retinoid antagonism. Nature 379:335, 1996

GILCHREST BA et al: Mechanisms of ultraviolet light-induced pigmentation. Photochem Photobiol 63:1, 1996

GOULD JW et al: Cutaneous photosensitivity diseases induced by exogenous agents. J Am Acad Dermatol 33:551, 1995

HARBER LC, BICKERS DR: *Photosensitivity Diseases*, 2d ed. Toronto, Decker, 1989

HONIGSMANN H, STINGL G: *Therapeutic Photomedicine*. Basel, Karger, 1986

MAGNUS IA: *Dermatological Photobiology*. Oxford, Blackwell, 1976

PATHAK MA et al: Sun-protective agents: Formulations, effects, and side effects in *Dermatology in General Medicine*, 5th ed, IM Freedberg et al (eds). New York, McGraw-Hill, 1999, Chap. 248

ZIEGLER A et al: Sunburn and p53 in the onset of skin cancer. Nature 372:773, 1994

Section 10
HEMATOLOGIC ALTERATIONS

61

John W. Adamson, Dan L. Longo

ANEMIA AND POLYCYTHEMIA

HEMATOPOIESIS AND THE PHYSIOLOGIC BASIS OF RED CELL PRODUCTION *Hematopoiesis* is the process by which the formed elements of the blood are produced. The process is regulated through a series of steps beginning with the pluripotent hematopoietic stem cell. Stem cells are capable of producing red cells, all classes of granulocytes, monocytes, platelets, and the cells of the immune system. Commitment of the stem cell to the specific cell lineages appears not to be regulated by known exogenous growth factors or cytokines. Rather, stem cells develop into differentiated cell types through incompletely defined molecular events that are intrinsic to the stem cell itself (Chap. 104). Following lineage commitment (or differentiation), hematopoietic progenitor and precursor cells come increasingly under the regulatory influence of growth factors and hormones, such as erythropoietin (EPO) for red cell production. EPO is required for the maintenance of committed erythroid progenitor cells which, in the absence of the hormone, undergo programmed cell death (*apoptosis*). The regulated process of red cell production is *erythropoiesis*, and its key elements are illustrated in Fig. 61-1.

In the bone marrow, the first morphologically recognizable erythroid precursor is the pronormoblast. This cell can undergo 4 to 5 cell divisions that result in the production of 16 to 32 mature red cells. With increased EPO production, or the administration of EPO as a drug, early progenitor cell numbers are amplified and, in turn, give rise to increased numbers of erythrocytes. The regulation of EPO production itself is linked to O_2 transport.

In mammals, O_2 is transported to tissues bound to the hemoglobin contained within circulating red cells. The mature red cell is $8\mu m$ in diameter, anucleate, discoid in shape, and extremely pliable in order for it to traverse the microcirculation successfully; its membrane integrity is maintained by the intracellular generation of ATP. Normal

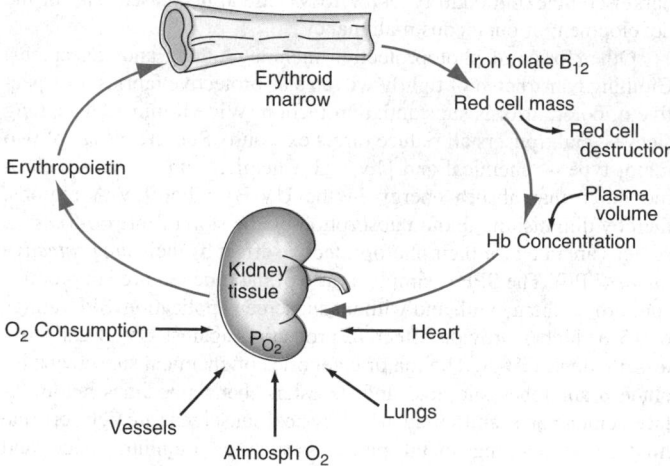

FIGURE 61-1 The physiologic regulation of red cell production by tissue oxygen tension. Hb, hemoglobin.

red cell production results in the daily replacement of 0.8 to 1% of all circulating red cells in the body. The average red cell lives 100 to 120 days. The machinery responsible for red cell production is called the *erythron*. The erythron is a dynamic organ made up of a rapidly proliferating pool of marrow erythroid precursor cells and a large mass of mature circulating red blood cells. The size of the red cell mass reflects the balance of red cell production and destruction. The physiologic basis of red cell production and destruction provides an understanding of the mechanisms that can lead to anemia.

The physiologic regulator of red cell production, the glycoprotein hormone EPO, is produced and released by peritubular capillary lining cells within the kidney. These cells are highly specialized epithelial-like cells. A small amount of EPO is produced by hepatocytes. The fundamental stimulus for EPO production is the availability of O_2 for tissue metabolic needs. Impaired O_2 delivery to the kidney can result from a decreased red cell mass (*anemia*), impaired O_2 loading of the

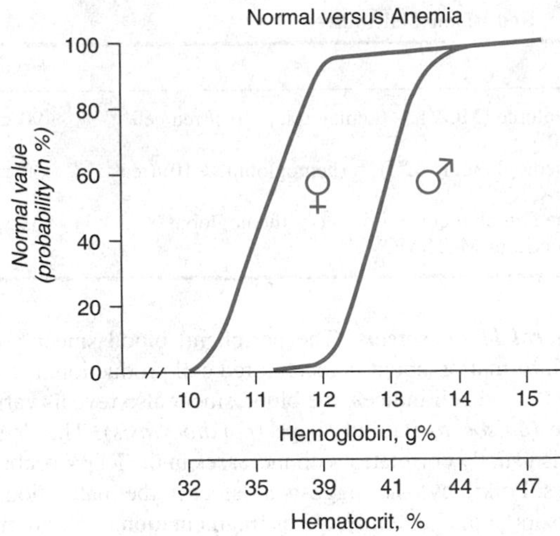

Normal versus Anemia

FIGURE 61-2 The probability that a particular hemoglobin or hematocrit value is abnormal is different in men and women.

hemoglobin molecule (*hypoxemia*), or, rarely, impaired blood flow to the kidney (renal artery stenosis). EPO governs the day-to-day production of red cells, and ambient levels of the hormone can be measured in the plasma by sensitive immunoassays—the normal level being 10 to 25 U/L. When the hemoglobin concentration falls below 100 to 120 g/L (10 to 12 g/dL), plasma EPO levels increase logarithmically in inverse proportion to the severity of the anemia. In circulation, EPO has a half-clearance time of 6 to 9 h. EPO acts by binding to specific receptors on the surface of marrow erythroid precursors, inducing them to proliferate and to mature. Under the stimulus of EPO, red blood cell production can increase four- to fivefold within a 1- to 2-week period but only in the presence of adequate nutrients, especially iron. The functional capacity of the erythron, therefore, requires normal renal production of EPO, a functioning erythroid marrow, and an adequate supply of substrates for hemoglobin synthesis. A defect in any of these key components can lead to anemia. Generally, anemia is recognized in the laboratory when a patient's hemoglobin level or hematocrit is reduced below an expected value (the normal range). The likelihood and severity of anemia are defined based on the deviation of the patient's hemoglobin/hematocrit from values expected for age- and sex-matched normal subjects. The lower ranges of distribution of hemoglobin/hematocrit values for adult males and females are shown in Fig. 61-2. The hemoglobin concentration in adults has a Gaussian distribution. The mean hematocrit value for adult males is 47% (± SD 7) and that for adult females is 42% (± 5). Any individual hematocrit or hemoglobin value carries with it a likelihood of associated anemia. Thus, a hematocrit of ≤39% in an adult male or <35% in an adult female has only about a 25% chance of being normal. Suspected low hemoglobin or hematocrit values are more easily interpreted if there are historic values for the same patient for comparison.

The critical elements of erythropoiesis—EPO production, iron availability, the proliferative capacity of the bone marrow, and effective maturation of red cell precursors—are used for the initial classification of anemia (see "Definition and Classification, below).

ANEMIA

CLINICAL PRESENTATION OF ANEMIA   Signs and Symptoms   Anemia is most often recognized by abnormal screening laboratory tests. Patients only occasionally present with advanced anemia and its attendant signs and symptoms. Acute anemia is nearly always due to blood loss or hemolysis. In fact, with acute blood loss, hypovolemia dominates the clinical picture and the hematocrit and hemoglobin levels do not reflect the volume of blood lost. Signs of vascular instability dominate with acute losses of 10 to 15% of the total blood volume. In such patients, the issue is not anemia but hy-

potension and decreased organ perfusion. When >30% of the blood volume is lost suddenly, patients are unable to compensate with the usual mechanisms of vascular contraction and changes in regional blood flow. The patient prefers to remain supine and will show postural hypotension and tachycardia if upright. If the volume of blood lost is >40% (i.e., >2 L in the average-sized adult), signs of hypovolemic shock including confusion, air hunger, diaphoresis, hypotension, and tachycardia appear (Chap. 108). Such patients have significant deficits in vital organ perfusion and require immediate volume replacement. With mild blood loss, enhanced O_2 delivery is achieved through changes in the O_2-hemoglobin dissociation curve mediated by a decreased pH or increased CO_2 (*Bohr effect*).

With acute hemolytic disease, the signs and symptoms depend on the mechanism that leads to red cell destruction. Intravascular hemolysis with release of free hemoglobin may be associated with acute back pain, free hemoglobin in the plasma and urine, and renal failure. Symptoms associated with more chronic or progressive anemia depend on the age of the patient and the adequacy of blood supply to critical organs. Symptoms associated with moderate anemia include fatigue, loss of stamina, breathlessness, and tachycardia (particularly with physical exertion). However, because of the intrinsic compensatory mechanisms that govern the O_2-hemoglobin dissociation curve, the gradual onset of anemia—particularly in young patients—may not be associated with signs or symptoms until the anemia is severe [hemoglobin <70 to 80 g/L (7 to 8 g/dL)]. When anemia develops over a period of days or weeks, the total blood volume is normal to slightly increased and changes in cardiac output and regional blood flow help compensate for the overall loss in O_2-carrying capacity. Changes in the position of the O_2-hemoglobin dissociation curve account for some of the compensatory response to anemia. With chronic anemia, intracellular levels of 2,3-bisphosphoglycerate (BPG) rise, shifting the dissociation curve to the right and facilitating O_2 unloading. This compensatory mechanism can only maintain normal tissue O_2 delivery in the face of a 20 to 30 g/L (2 to 3 g/dL) deficit in hemoglobin concentration. Finally, further protection of O_2 delivery to vital organs is achieved by the shunting of blood away from organs that are relatively rich in blood supply, particularly the kidney, gut, and skin.

Certain disorders are commonly associated with anemia. Chronic inflammatory states (e.g., infection, rheumatoid arthritis) are associated with mild to moderate anemia, whereas lymphoproliferative disorders, such as chronic lymphocytic leukemia and certain other B cell neoplasms, may be associated with autoimmune hemolysis.

Approach to the Patient

The evaluation of the patient with anemia requires a careful history and physical examination. Historic information that may be useful includes exposure to certain toxic agents or drugs and symptoms related to other disorders commonly associated with anemia. These include symptoms and signs such as bleeding, fatigue, malaise, fever, weight loss, night sweats, and other systemic symptoms. Clues to the mechanisms of anemia may be provided on physical examination by findings of infection, blood in the stool, lymphadenopathy, splenomegaly, or petechiae. Splenomegaly and lymphadenopathy suggest an underlying lymphoproliferative disease, while petechiae suggest platelet dysfunction. If it is uncertain whether a mild anemia represents an extreme normal value or an abnormal finding, past laboratory measurements may be helpful. Nutritional history related to drugs or alcohol intake and family history of anemia should always be assessed. Certain geographic backgrounds and ethnic origins are associated with an increased likelihood of an inherited disorder of the hemoglobin molecule or intermediary metabolism. Glucose-6-phosphate dehydrogenase deficiency and certain hemoglobinopathies are seen more commonly in those of middle-Eastern or African origin.

In the anemic patient, physical examination may demonstrate a forceful heartbeat, strong peripheral pulses, and a systolic "flow" murmur. The skin and mucous membranes may be pale if the hemoglobin is <80 to 100 g/L (8 to 10 g/dL). This part of the physical examination should focus on areas where vessels are close to the surface such as the mucous membranes, nail beds, and palmar creases. If the palmar creases are lighter in color than the surrounding skin when the hand is hyperextended, the hemoglobin level is usually <80 g/L (8 g/dL).

Laboratory Evaluation   Table 61-1 lists the tests used in the initial workup of anemia. A routine complete blood count (CBC) is required as part of the evaluation and includes the hemoglobin, hematocrit, and red cell indices: the mean cell volume (MCV) in femtoliters, mean cell hemoglobin (MCH) in picograms per cell, and mean concentration of hemoglobin per volume of red cells (MCHC) in grams per liter (non-SI: grams per deciliter). The red cell indices are calculated as shown in Table 61-2, and the normal variations in the CBC with age are shown in Table A-7. A number of physiologic factors affect the normal CBC values including age, gender, pregnancy, smoking, and altitude. High-normal hemoglobin values may be seen in men and women who live at altitude or smoke heavily. The elevations in smokers reflect normal compensation due to the displacement of O_2 by CO in hemoglobin binding. Other important information is provided by the reticulocyte count and measurements of iron supply including the *serum iron*, the *total iron-binding capacity* (TIBC; an indirect measure of the transferrin level), and *serum ferritin*. Marked alterations in the red cell indices usually reflect disorders of maturation or iron deficiency. Clinical laboratories also provide a description of both the red and white cells, a white cell differential count, and the platelet count. In patients with severe anemia and abnormalities in red blood cell morphology, a bone marrow aspirate or biopsy may be important to assist in the diagnosis. Other tests of value in the diagnosis of specific anemias are discussed in chapters on specific disease states.

The components of the CBC also help in the classification of anemia. *Microcytosis* is reflected by a lower than normal MCV (<80), whereas high values (>100) reflect *macrocytosis*. The MCH and MCHC reflect defects in hemoglobin synthesis (*hypochromia*). Automated cell counters describe the red cell volume distribution width (RDW). The MCV (representing the peak of the distribution curve) is insensitive to the appearance of small populations of macrocytes or microcytes. An experienced laboratory technician will be able to identify minor populations of large or small cells or hypochromic cells before the red cell indices change.

Table 61-1   Laboratory Tests in Anemia Diagnosis

I. Complete blood count (CBC)
  A. Red blood cell count
    1. Hemoglobin
    2. Hematocrit
  B. Red blood cell indices
    1. Mean cell volume (MCV)
    2. Mean cell hemoglobin (MCH)
    3. Mean cell hemoglobin concentration (MCHC)
    4. Red cell distribution width (RDW)
  C. White blood cell count
    1. Cell differential
    2. Nuclear segmentation of neutrophils
  D. Platelet count
  E. Cell morphology
    1. Cell size
    2. Hemoglobin content
    3. Anisocytosis
    4. Poikilocytosis
    5. Polychromasia
II. Reticulocyte count
III. Iron supply studies
  A. Serum iron
  B. Total iron-binding capacity
  C. Serum ferritin, marrow iron stain
IV. Marrow examination
  A. Aspirate
    1. E/G ratio[a]
    2. Cell morphology
    3. Iron stain
  B. Biopsy
    1. Cellularity
    2. Morphology

[a] E/G ratio, ratio of erythroid to granulocytic precursors.

Table 61-2   Red Blood Cell Indices

Index	Normal Value
Mean cell volume (MCV) = (hematocrit × 10)/(red cell count × 10⁶)	90 ± 8 fL
Mean cell hemoglobin (MCH) = (hemoglobin × 10)/(red cell count × 10⁶)	30 ± 3 pg
Mean cell hemoglobin concentration = (hemoglobin × 10)/hematocrit, or MCH/MCV	33 ± 2%

Peripheral blood smear   The peripheral blood smear provides important information about defects in red cell production. As a complement to the red cell indices, the blood smear also reveals variations in cell size (*anisocytosis*) and shape (*poikilocytosis*). The degree of anisocytosis usually correlates with increases in the RDW or the range of cell sizes. Poikilocytosis suggests a defect in the maturation of red cell precursors in the bone marrow or fragmentation of circulating red cells. The blood smear may also reveal *polychromasia*—red cells that are slightly larger than normal and grayish blue in color on the Wright-Giemsa stain. These cells are reticulocytes that have been prematurely released from the bone marrow, and their color represents residual amounts of ribosomal RNA. These cells appear in circulation in response to EPO stimulation or to architectural damage of the bone marrow (fibrosis, infiltration of the marrow by malignant cells, etc.) that results in their disordered release from the marrow. The appearance of nucleated red cells, Howell-Jolly bodies, target cells, sickle cells, and others may provide clues to specific disorders (**see Plates V-2, 3, 8, 9, 16, 21, 24, 26–28, 39**).

Reticulocyte count   An accurate reticulocyte count is key to the initial classification of anemia. Normally, reticulocytes are red cells that have been recently released from the bone marrow. They are identified by staining with a supravital dye that precipitates the residual ribosomal RNA. These precipitates appear as blue or black punctate spots. This residual RNA is metabolized over the first 24 to 36 h of the reticulocyte's lifespan in circulation. Normally, the reticulocyte count ranges from 1 to 2% and reflects the daily replacement of 0.8 to 1.0% of the circulating red cell population. A correctly interpreted reticulocyte count provides a reliable measure of red cell production.

In the initial classification of anemia, the patient's reticulocyte count is compared with the expected reticulocyte response. In general, if the EPO and erythroid marrow responses to moderate anemia [hemoglobin <100 g/L (10 g/dL)] are intact, the red cell production rate increases to two to three times normal within 10 days following the onset of anemia. In the face of established anemia, a reticulocyte response less than two to three times normal indicates an inadequate marrow response.

In order to use the reticulocyte count to estimate marrow response, two corrections are necessary. The first correction adjusts the reticulocyte count based on the reduced number of circulating red cells. With anemia, the percentage of reticulocytes may be increased while the absolute number is unchanged. To correct for this effect, the reticulocyte percentage is multiplied by the ratio of the patient's hemoglobin or hematocrit to the expected hemoglobin/hematocrit for the age and gender of the patient (Table 61-3). This provides an estimate of the

Table 61-3   Calculation of Reticulocyte Production Index

Correction #1 for anemia:
  This correction produces the absolute reticulocyte count
  In a person whose reticulocyte count is 9%, hemoglobin 7.5 g/dL, hematocrit 23%, absolute reticulocyte count = 9 × (7.5/15)[or ×(23/45)] = 4.5%
Correction #2 for longer life of prematurely released reticulocytes in the blood:
  This correction produces the reticulocyte production index
  In a person whose reticulocyte count is 9%, hemoglobin 7.5 gm/dL, hematocrit 23%, reticulocyte production index

$$= 9 \times \frac{(7.5/15)(\text{hemoglobin correction})}{2 \; (\text{maturation time correction})} = 2.25$$

absolute reticulocyte count. In order to convert the corrected reticulocyte count to an index of marrow production, a further correction is required, depending on whether some of the reticulocytes in circulation have been released from the marrow prematurely. For this second correction, the peripheral blood smear is examined to see if there are polychromatophilic macrocytes present. These cells, representing prematurely released reticulocytes, are referred to as "shift" cells, and the relationship between the degree of shift (and the necessary shift correction factor) is shown in Fig. 61-3. The correction is necessary because these prematurely released cells survive as reticulocytes in circulation for >1 day, thereby providing a falsely high estimate of daily red cell production. If polychromasia is increased, the reticulocyte count, already corrected for anemia, should be divided again by a factor of 2 to account for the prolonged reticulocyte maturation time. The second correction factor varies from 1 to 3 depending upon the severity of anemia. In general, a correction of 2 is commonly used. An appropriate correction is shown in Table 61-3. If polychromatophilic cells are not seen on the blood smear, the second correction is not required. The now doubly corrected reticulocyte count is the *reticulocyte production index*, and it provides an estimate of marrow production relative to normal.

Premature release of reticulocytes is normally due to increased EPO stimulation. However, if the integrity of the bone marrow release process is lost through tumor infiltration, fibrosis, or other disorders, the appearance of nucleated red cells or polychromatophilic macrocytes should still invoke the second reticulocyte correction. The shift correction should always be applied to a patient with anemia and a very high reticulocyte count to provide a true index of effective red cell production. Patients with severe chronic hemolytic anemia may increase red cell production as much as six- to sevenfold. This measure alone, therefore, confirms the fact that the patient has an appropriate EPO response, a normally functioning bone marrow, and sufficient iron available to meet the demands for new red cell formation. If the reticulocyte production index is <2 in the face of established anemia, a defect in erythroid marrow proliferation or maturation must be present.

Tests of iron supply and storage The laboratory measurements that reflect the availability of iron for hemoglobin synthesis include the serum iron, the TIBC, and the percent transferrin saturation. The percent transferrin saturation is derived by dividing the serum iron level ($\times$ 100) by the TIBC. The normal serum iron ranges from 9 to 27 μmol/L (50 to 150 μg/dL), while the normal TIBC is 54 to 64 μmol/L (300 to 360 μg/dL); the transferrin saturation ranges from 25 to 50%. A diurnal variation in the serum iron leads to a variation in the percent transferrin saturation. The serum ferritin is used to evaluate total-body iron stores. Adult males have serum ferritin levels that average about 100 μg/L, corresponding to iron stores of about 1 g. Adult females have lower serum ferritin levels averaging 30 μg/L, reflecting lower iron stores. A serum ferritin level of 10 to 15 μg/L represents depletion of body iron stores. However, ferritin is also an acute-phase reactant and, in the presence of acute or chronic inflammation, may rise severalfold above baseline levels. As a rule, a serum ferritin >200 μg/L means there is at least some iron in tissue stores.

Bone marrow examination A bone marrow aspirate and smear or a needle biopsy may be useful in the diagnosis of a marrow disorder such as myelofibrosis, a red cell maturation defect, or an infiltrative disease (**Plates V-5, 13–15, 19, 29, 33**). The increase or decrease of one cell lineage (myeloid vs. erythroid) compared to another is obtained by a differential count of nucleated cells in a bone marrow smear [the erythroid/granulocytic (E/G) ratio]. A patient with a hypoproliferative anemia (see below) and a reticulocyte production index <2 will demonstrate an E/G ratio of 1:2 or 1:3. In contrast, patients with hemolytic disease and a production index >3 will have an E/G ratio of at least 1:1. Maturation disorders are identified from the discrepancy between a high E/G ratio and a low reticulocyte production index (see below). Either the marrow smear or biopsy can be stained for the presence of iron stores or iron in developing red cells. The storage iron is in the form of *ferritin* or *hemosiderin*. On carefully prepared bone marrow smears, small ferritin granules can normally be seen in 10 to 20% of developing erythroblasts. Such cells are called *sideroblasts*.

Other laboratory measurements Additional laboratory tests may be of value in confirming specific diagnoses. →*For details of these tests and how they are applied in individual disorders, see Chaps. 105 to 109.*

DEFINITION AND CLASSIFICATION OF ANEMIA

Initial Classification of Anemia Classifying an anemia according to the functional defect in red cell production helps organize the subsequent use of laboratory studies. The three major classes of anemia are: (1) marrow production defects (*hypoproliferation*), (2) red cell maturation defects (*ineffective erythropoiesis*), and (3) decreased red cell survival (*blood loss/hemolysis*). This functional classification of anemia then guides the selection of specific clinical and laboratory studies designed to complete the differential diagnosis and to plan appropriate therapy. The classification is shown in Fig. 61-4. A hypoproliferative anemia is typically seen with a low reticulocyte production index together with little or no change in red cell morphology (a normocytic, normochromic anemia) (Chap. 105). Maturation disorders typically have a slight to moderately elevated reticulocyte production index that is accompanied by either macrocytic (Chap. 107) or microcytic (Chaps. 105, 106) red cell indices. Increased red blood cell destruction secondary to hemolysis results in an increase in the reticulocyte production index to at least three times normal (Chap. 108), provided sufficient iron is available for hemoglobin synthesis. Hemorrhagic anemia does not typically result in production indices of more than 2.5 times normal because of the limitations placed on expansion of the erythroid marrow by iron availability.

In the first branch point of the classification of anemia, a reticulocyte production index >2.5 indicates that hemolysis is most likely. A reticulocyte production index of <2 indicates either a hypoproliferative anemia or maturation disorder. The latter two possibilities can often be distinguished by the red cell indices, by examination of the peripheral blood smear, or by a marrow examination. If the red cell indices are normal, the anemia is almost certainly hypoproliferative in nature. Maturation disorders are characterized by ineffective red cell production and a low reticulocyte production index with bizarre red cell shapes—macrocytes or hypochromic microcytes on the peripheral blood smear. With a hypoproliferative anemia, no erythroid hyperpla-

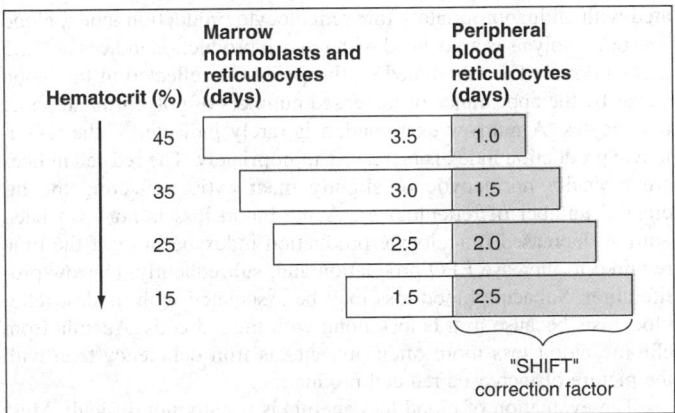

Hematocrit (%)	Marrow normoblasts and reticulocytes (days)	Peripheral blood reticulocytes (days)
45	3.5	1.0
35	3.0	1.5
25	2.5	2.0
15	1.5	2.5

"SHIFT" correction factor

FIGURE 61-3 Correction of reticulocyte count based upon level of anemia and the circulatory life span of prematurely released reticulocytes. Erythroid cells take about 4.5 days to mature. At normal hematocrit levels, they are released to the circulation with about 1 day left as reticulocytes. However, with different levels of anemia, erythroid cells are released from the marrow prematurely. Most patients come to clinical attention with hematocrits in the mid-20s and thus, a correction factor of 2 is commonly used because the observed reticulocytes will live for 2 days in the circulation before losing their RNA.

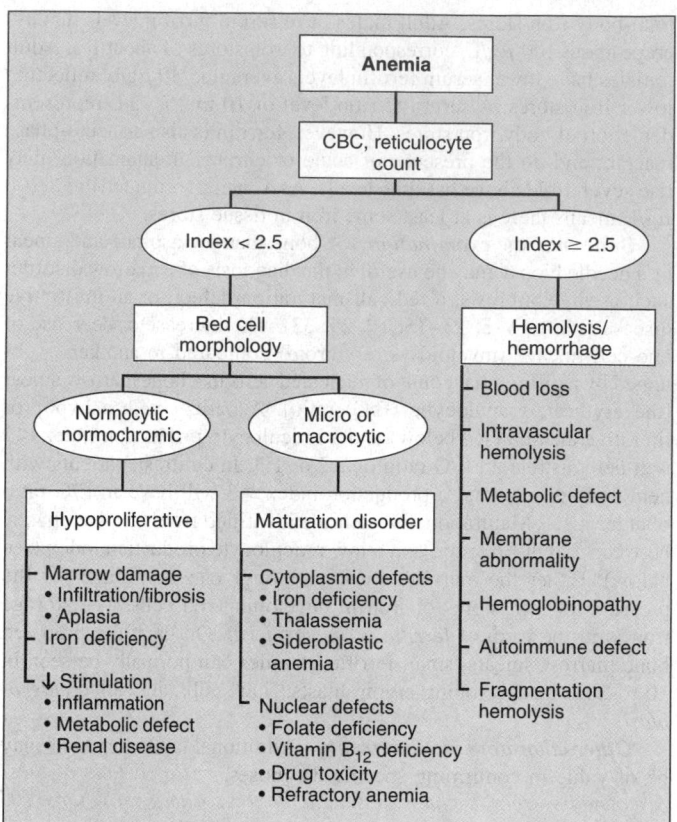

FIGURE 61-4 The physiologic classification of anemia. CBC, complete blood count.

sia is noted in the marrow, whereas patients with ineffective red cell production have erythroid hyperplasia and an E/G ratio ≥1:1.

Hypoproliferative Anemias   At least 75% of all cases of anemia are hypoproliferative in nature. A hypoproliferative anemia reflects absolute or relative marrow failure in which the erythroid marrow has not proliferated appropriately for the degree of anemia. The majority of hypoproliferative anemias are due to mild to moderate iron deficiency or inflammation. A hypoproliferative anemia can result from marrow damage, iron deficiency, or inadequate EPO stimulation. The last may reflect impaired renal function, suppression of EPO production by inflammatory cytokines such as interleukin 1, or reduced tissue needs for O_2 from metabolic disease such as hypothyroidism. Only occasionally is the marrow unable to produce red cells at a normal rate, and this is most prevalent in patients with renal failure. In general, hypoproliferative anemias are characterized by normocytic, normochromic red cells, although microcytic, hypochromic cells may be observed with mild iron deficiency or long-standing chronic inflammatory disease. The key laboratory tests in distinguishing between the various forms of hypoproliferative anemia include the serum iron and iron-binding capacity, evaluation of renal and thyroid function, a marrow biopsy or aspirate to detect marrow damage or infiltrative disease, and serum ferritin to assess iron stores. Occasionally, an iron stain of the marrow will be needed to determine the pattern of iron distribution. Patients with the anemia of acute or chronic inflammation show a distinctive pattern of serum iron (low), TIBC (normal or low), percent transferrin saturation (low), and serum ferritin (normal or high). A distinct pattern of results is noted in mild to moderate iron deficiency (low serum iron, high TIBC, low percent transferrin saturation, low serum ferritin) (Chap. 105). Marrow damage by a drug, infiltrative disease such as leukemia or lymphoma, or marrow aplasia can usually be diagnosed from the peripheral blood and bone marrow morphology. With infiltrative disease or fibrosis, a marrow biopsy will likely be required.

Maturation Disorders   The presence of anemia with an inappropriately low reticulocyte production index, macro- or microcytosis on smear, and abnormal red cell indices suggests a maturation disorder. Maturation disorders are divided into two categories: nuclear maturation defects, associated with macrocytosis and abnormal marrow development, and cytoplasmic maturation defects, associated with microcytosis and hypochromia usually from defects in hemoglobin production. The low reticulocyte production index is a reflection of the ineffective erythropoiesis that results from the destruction within the marrow of developing erythroblasts. Marrow morphology shows an E/G ratio of ≥ 1:1, diagnostic of erythroid hyperplasia.

Nuclear maturation defects result from vitamin B_{12} or folic acid deficiency, drug damage, or myelodysplasia. Drugs that interfere with cellular DNA metabolism, such as methotrexate or alkylating agents, can produce a nuclear maturation defect. Alcohol, alone, is also capable of producing macrocytosis and a variable degree of anemia, but this is usually associated with coincident folic acid deficiency. Measurements of folic acid and vitamin B_{12} are key not only in identifying the specific vitamin deficiency but also because they reflect different pathogenetic mechanisms.

Cytoplasmic maturation defects result from severe iron deficiency or abnormalities in globin or heme synthesis. Iron deficiency occupies an unusual position in the classification of anemia. If the iron-deficiency anemia is mild to moderate, erythroid marrow proliferation is decreased and the anemia is classified as hypoproliferative. However, if the anemia is severe and prolonged, the erythroid marrow will become hyperplastic despite the inadequate iron supply, and the anemia will be classified as ineffective erythropoiesis with a cytoplasmic maturation defect. In either case, a reduced reticulocyte production index, microcytosis, and a classic pattern of iron values make the diagnosis clear and easily distinguish iron deficiency from other cytoplasmic maturation defects such as the thalassemias. Defects in heme synthesis, in contrast to globin synthesis, are less common and may be acquired or inherited (Chap. 346). Acquired abnormalities are usually associated with myelodysplasia, may lead to either a macro- or microcytic anemia, and are frequently associated with mitochondrial iron loading. In these cases, iron is taken up by the mitochondria of the developing erythroid cell but not incorporated into heme. The iron-encrusted mitochondria surround the nucleus of the erythroid cell, forming a ring. Based on the distinctive finding of so-called ringed sideroblasts on the marrow iron stain (**see Plate V-37**), patients are diagnosed as having a sideroblastic anemia—almost always reflecting myelodysplasia. Again, studies of iron parameters are helpful in the differential diagnosis and management of these patients.

Blood Loss/Hemolytic Anemia   In contrast to anemias associated with an inappropriately low reticulocyte production index, blood loss or hemolysis is associated with red cell production indices of ≥2.5 times normal. The stimulated erythropoiesis is reflected in the blood smear by the appearance of increased numbers of polychromatophilic macrocytes. A marrow examination is rarely indicated if the reticulocyte production index is increased appropriately. The red cell indices are typically normocytic or slightly macrocytic, reflecting the increased number of reticulocytes. Acute blood loss is not associated with an increased reticulocyte production index because of the time required to increase EPO production and, subsequently, marrow proliferation. Subacute blood loss may be associated with modest reticulocytosis because iron is lost along with the red cells. Anemia from chronic blood loss more often presents as iron deficiency than with the picture of increased red cell production.

The evaluation of blood loss anemia is usually not difficult. Most problems arise when a patient presents with an increased red cell production index from an episode of acute blood loss that went unrecognized. The cause of the anemia and increased red cell production may not be obvious. The confirmation of a recovering state may require observations over a period of 2 to 3 weeks, during which the hemoglobin concentration will be seen to rise and the reticulocyte production index fall.

Hemolytic disease, while dramatic, is among the least common forms of anemia. The ability to sustain a high reticulocyte production index reflects the ability of the erythroid marrow to compensate for hemolysis and the efficient recycling of iron from the destroyed red cells to support new hemoglobin synthesis. The level of response will depend on the severity of the anemia and the nature of the underlying disease process.

Hemolytic anemias present in different ways. Some appear suddenly as an acute, self-limited episode of intravascular or extravascular hemolysis, a presentation pattern often seen in patients with autoimmune hemolysis or with inherited defects of the Embden-Myerhof pathway or the glutathione reductase pathway. Patients with inherited disorders of the hemoglobin molecule or red cell membrane generally have a lifelong clinical history typical of the disease process. Those with chronic hemolytic disease, such as hereditary spherocytosis, may actually present not with anemia but with a complication stemming from the prolonged increase in red cell destruction such as aplastic crisis, symptomatic bilirubin gallstones, or splenomegaly.

The differential diagnosis of an acute or chronic hemolytic event requires the careful integration of family history, pattern of clinical presentation, and a number of highly specific laboratory studies (Chap. 108). Some of the more common congenital hemolytic anemias may be identified from the red cell morphology, a routine laboratory test such as hemoglobin electrophoresis, or a screen for red cell enzymes. Acquired defects in red cell survival are often immunologically mediated and require the immunoglobulin test or a cold agglutinin titer to detect the presence of hemolytic antibodies or complement-mediated red cell destruction.

℞ **TREATMENT** An overriding principle is to not initiate treatment of mild to moderate anemia without a specific diagnosis. Rarely, in the acute setting, anemia may be so severe that red cell transfusions are required before a specific diagnosis is made. Whether the anemia is of acute or gradual onset, the selection of the appropriate treatment is determined by the documented cause(s) of the anemia. Often, the cause of the anemia may be multifactorial. For example, a patient with severe rheumatoid arthritis who has been taking anti-inflammatory drugs may have a hypoproliferative anemia associated with chronic inflammation as well as chronic blood loss associated with intermittent gastrointestinal bleeding. In every circumstance, it is important to evaluate the patient's iron status fully before and during the treatment of any anemia. →*Transfusion is discussed in Chap. 114; iron therapy is discussed in Chap. 105; treatment of megaloblastic anemia is discussed in Chap. 107; treatment of other entities is discussed in their respective chapters (sickle cell anemia, Chap. 106; hemolytic anemias, Chap. 108; aplastic anemia and myelodysplasia, Chap. 109).*

Therapeutic options for the treatment of anemias have expanded dramatically during the past 25 years. Blood component therapy is available and safe. Recombinant EPO as an adjunct to anemia management has transformed the lives of patients with chronic renal failure on dialysis. Improvements in the management of sickle cell crises and sickle cell anemia have also occurred. Eventually, patients with inherited disorders of globin synthesis or mutations in the globin gene, such as sickle cell disease, may benefit from the successful introduction of targeted genetic therapy (Chap. 69).

POLYCYTHEMIA

Polycythemia is defined as an increase in circulating red blood cells above normal. This increase may be real or only apparent (spurious or relative) because of a decrease in plasma volume. The term *erythrocytosis* may be used interchangeably with polycythemia, but some draw a distinction between them; erythrocytosis implies documentation of increased red cell mass, whereas polycythemia refers to any increase in red cells. Often patients with polycythemia are detected through an incidental finding of elevated hemoglobin or hematocrit levels. Concern that the hemoglobin level may be abnormally high is usually triggered at 170 g/L (17 g/dL) for men and 150 g/L (15 g/dL)

for women. Hematocrit levels >50% in men or >45% in women may be abnormal. Hematocrits >60% in men and >55% in women are almost invariably associated with increased red cell mass.

Historic features useful in the differential diagnosis include smoking history; living at high altitude; or a history of congenital heart disease, peptic ulcer disease, sleep-apnea, chronic lung disease, or renal disease.

Patients with polycythemia may be asymptomatic or experience symptoms related to the increased red cell mass or an underlying disease process that leads to increased red cell production. The dominant symptoms from increased red cell mass are thrombotic (both venous and arterial), because the blood viscosity increases logarithmically at hematocrits >55%. Manifestations range from digital ischemia to Budd-Chiari syndrome with hepatic vein thrombosis. Abdominal thromboses are particularly common. Neurologic symptoms such as vertigo, tinnitus, headache, and visual disturbances may occur. Hypertension is often present. Patients with *polycythemia vera* may have aquagenic pruritus and symptoms related to hepatosplenomegaly. Patients may have easy bruising, epistaxis, or bleeding from the gastrointestinal tract. Patients with hypoxemia may develop cyanosis on minimal exertion or have headache, impaired mental acuity, and fatigue.

The physical examination usually reveals a ruddy complexion. Splenomegaly favors polycythemia vera as the diagnosis (Chap. 110). The presence of cyanosis or evidence of a right-to-left shunt suggests congenital heart disease presenting in the adult, particularly tetralogy of Fallot or Eisenmenger syndrome (Chap. 234). Increased blood viscosity raises pulmonary artery pressure; hypoxemia can lead to increased pulmonary vascular resistance. Together these factors can produce cor pulmonale.

Polycythemia can be spurious (related to a decrease in plasma volume; Gaisbock's syndrome), primary, or secondary in origin. The secondary causes are all associated with increases in EPO levels: either a physiologically adapted appropriate elevation based upon tissue hypoxia (lung disease, high altitude, CO poisoning, high-affinity hemoglobinopathy) or an abnormal overproduction (renal disease, tumors with ectopic EPO production). A rare familial form of polycythemia is associated with normal EPO levels but mutations producing hyperresponsive EPO receptors.

Approach to the Patient

As shown in Fig. 61-5, the first step is to document the presence of an increased red cell mass using the principle of isotope dilution by administering ^{51}Cr-labeled autologous red blood cells to the patient and sampling blood radioactivity over a 2-h period. If the red cell mass is normal (<36 mL/kg in men, <32 mL/kg in women), the patient has spurious polycythemia. If the red cell mass is increased (>36 mL/kg in men, >32 mL/kg in women), serum EPO levels should be measured. If EPO levels are low or absent, the patient most likely has polycythemia vera. Ancillary tests that support this diagnosis include elevated white blood cell count, increased absolute basophil count, thrombocytosis, elevated leukocyte alkaline phosphatase levels, and elevated serum vitamin B_{12} and vitamin B_{12}-binding protein levels.

If serum EPO levels are elevated, one attempts to distinguish whether the elevation is a physiologic response to hypoxia or is related to autonomous production. Patients with low arterial O_2 saturation (<92%) should be further evaluated for the presence of heart or lung disease, if they are not living at high altitude. Patients with normal O_2 saturation who are smokers may have elevated EPO levels because of CO displacement of O_2. If carboxyhemoglobin (COHb) levels are high, the diagnosis is smoker's polycythemia. Such patients should be urged to stop smoking. Those who cannot stop smoking require phlebotomy to control their polycythemia. Patients with normal O_2 saturation who do not smoke either have an abnormal hemoglobin that does not deliver O_2 to the tissues (evaluated by finding elevated O_2-hemoglobin

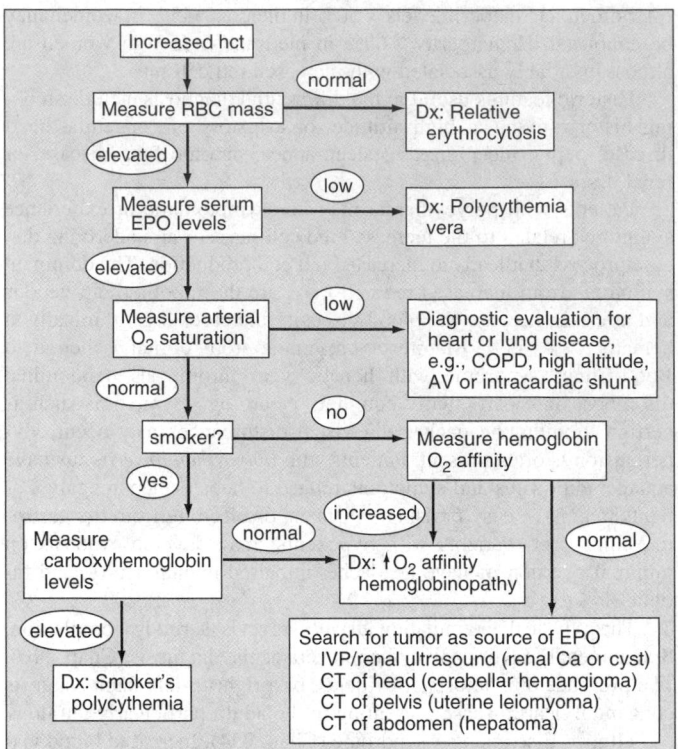

FIGURE 61-5 An approach to diagnosing patients with polycythemia. RBC, red blood cell; EPO, erythropoietin; COPD, chronic obstructive pulmonary disease; AV, atrioventricular; IVP, intravenous pyelogram; CT, computed tomography.

affinity) or have a source of EPO production that is not responding to the normal feedback inhibition. Further workup is dictated by the differential diagnosis of EPO-producing neoplasms. Hepatoma, uterine leiomyoma, and renal disease or cysts are all detectable with abdominopelvic computed tomography scans. Cerebellar hemangiomas may produce EPO, but they nearly always present with localizing neurologic signs and symptoms rather than polycythemia-related symptoms.

ACKNOWLEDGMENT
Dr. Robert S. Hillman wrote this chapter in the 14th edition, and elements of his chapter were retained here.

BIBLIOGRAPHY

HILLMAN RS, AULT KA: *Hematology in Clinical Practice.* New York, McGraw-Hill, 1998

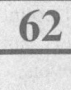

62   *Robert I. Handin*

BLEEDING AND THROMBOSIS

Hemorrhage, intravascular thrombosis, and embolism are common clinical manifestations of many diseases. The normal hemostatic system limits blood loss by precisely regulated interactions between components of the vessel wall, blood platelets, and plasma proteins. However, when disease or trauma damages large arteries and veins, excessive bleeding may occur, despite a normal hemostatic system. Less frequently, hemorrhage is caused by an inherited or acquired disorder of the hemostatic machinery itself. A large number of such bleeding disorders have been identified.

In addition, unregulated activation of the hemostatic system may cause thrombosis and embolism, which can reduce blood flow to critical organs such as the brain and myocardium. Although we understand less about the pathophysiology of thrombosis than of hemostatic failure, certain patient groups have been identified that are particularly prone to thrombosis and embolism. These include patients who (1) are immobilized after surgery, (2) have chronic congestive heart failure, (3) have atherosclerotic vascular disease, (4) have a malignancy, or (5) are pregnant. Most of these "thrombosis-prone" patients have inherited or acquired "hypercoagulable" or "prethrombotic" disorders.

Certain information in the patient's history, such as the mode of onset and sites of bleeding, a family bleeding tendency, and a record of drug ingestion, helps establish the correct diagnosis. Physical examination can identify bleeding in the skin or joint deformities due to previous hemarthroses. Ultimately, however, bleeding disorders are diagnosed by laboratory tests. General screening tests are used first, to document a systemic disorder, and are then supplemented by specific tests of coagulation protein or platelet function to arrive at an accurate diagnosis.

The hypercoagulable or prethrombotic patient can also be identified by a careful history. Three important clues to this diagnosis are: (1) repeated episodes of thromboembolism without an obvious predisposing condition, (2) a family history of thrombosis, and (3) well-documented thromboembolism in adolescents and young adults. All of the known inherited prethrombotic disorders can be diagnosed with specific immunologic, functional, and, in some cases, genetic tests.

NORMAL HEMOSTASIS

Accurate diagnosis and treatment of patients with either bleeding or thrombosis require knowledge of the pathophysiology of hemostasis. The process can be divided into primary and secondary components and is initiated when trauma, surgery, or disease disrupts the vascular endothelial lining and blood is exposed to subendothelial connective tissue. *Primary hemostasis* is the name given to the process of platelet plug formation at sites of injury. It occurs within seconds of injury and is of prime importance in stopping blood loss from capillaries, small arterioles, and venules (Fig. 62-1). *Secondary hemostasis* consists of the reactions of the plasma coagulation system that result in fibrin formation. It requires several minutes for completion. The fibrin strands that are produced strengthen the primary hemostatic plug. This

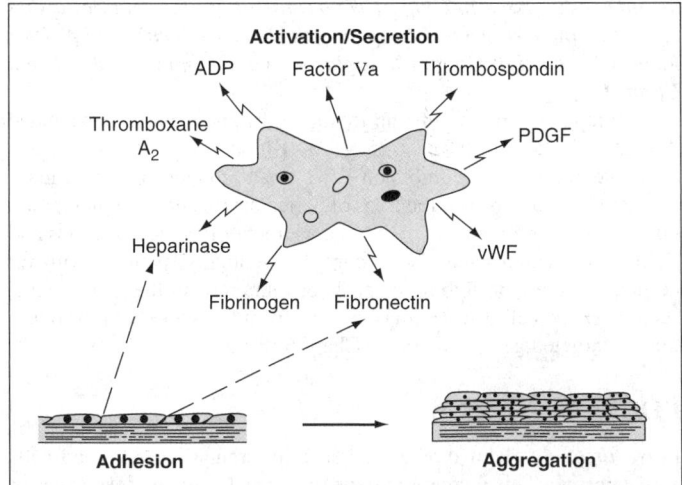

FIGURE 62-1 Schematic presentation of the major events in primary hemostasis. The first event is platelet adhesion, the interaction of platelets with a nonplatelet surface such as vascular subendothelium. This is followed by platelet activation and secretion. Some of the products secreted by platelets are depicted. Abbreviations: ADP, adenosine diphosphate; PDGF, platelet-derived growth factor; vWF, von Willebrand factor. The final event is the binding of activated platelets to the adherent monolayer in the process of platelet aggregation.

reaction is particularly important in larger vessels and prevents bleeding from recurring hours or days after the injury. Although presented here as separate events, primary and secondary hemostasis are closely linked. For example, activated platelets accelerate plasma coagulation, and products of the plasma coagulation reaction, such as thrombin, induce platelet activation.

Effective primary hemostasis requires three critical events—platelet adhesion, granule release, and platelet aggregation. Within a few seconds of injury, platelets adhere to collagen fibrils in vascular subendothelium via a specific platelet collagen receptor, glycoprotein Ia/IIa, which is a member of the integrin family. As shown in Fig. 62-2, this interaction is stabilized by the von Willebrand factor, an adhesive glycoprotein that allows platelets to remain attached to the vessel wall despite the high shear forces generated within the vascular lumen. The von Willebrand factor accomplishes this task by forming a link between a platelet receptor site on glycoprotein Ib/IX and subendothelial collagen fibrils. The adherent platelets then release preformed granule constituents and generate de novo mediators like those depicted in Fig. 62-1.

As in other cells, platelet activation and secretion are regulated by changes in the level of cyclic nucleotides, the influx of calcium, hydrolysis of membrane phospholipids, and phosphorylation of critical intracellular proteins. The relevant pathways are depicted in Figs. 62-3 and 62-4. The binding of agonists such as epinephrine, collagen, or thrombin to platelet surface receptors activates two membrane enzymes—phospholipase C and phospholipase A₂. These enzymes catalyze the release of arachidonic acid from two of the major membrane phospholipids, phosphatidylinositol and phosphatidylcholine. Initially, a small quantity of the released arachidonic acid is converted to thromboxane A₂ (TXA₂), which, in turn, can activate phospholipase C. The formation of TXA₂ from arachidonic acid is mediated by the enzyme cyclooxygenase (Fig. 62-3). This enzyme is inhibited by aspirin and nonsteroidal anti-inflammatory drugs. Inhibition of TXA₂ synthesis is a cause of mild bleeding in some patients and is the same way some antithrombotic drugs work.

Hydrolysis of the membrane phospholipid phosphatidylinositol 4,5-bisphosphate produces diacylglycerol (DAG) and inositol triphosphate (IP₃), both of which play critical roles in platelet metabolism. IP₃ mediates the movement of calcium into the platelet cytosol and stimulates the phosphorylation of myosin light chains. The latter interact with actin to facilitate granule movement and platelet shape change. DAG activates protein kinase C, which, in turn, phosphorylates several substrates, including myosin light chain kinase and a 47-

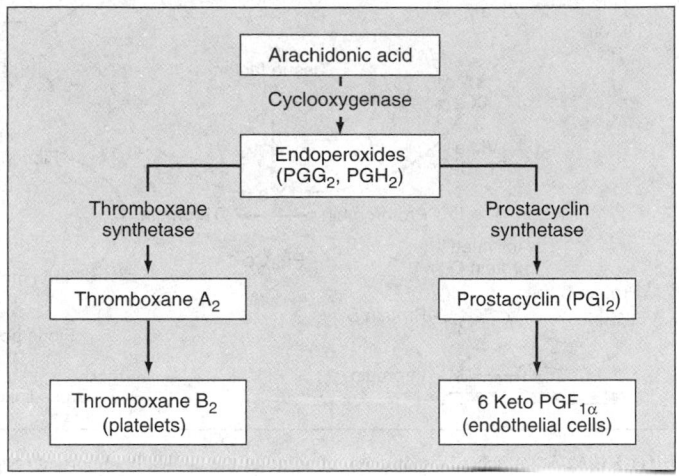

FIGURE 62-3 Generation of thromboxane A₂ in platelets and prostacyclin (PGI₂) in endothelial cells.

kDa protein (plekstrin). Phosphorylation of these or other proteins may regulate platelet granule secretion.

A finely balanced mechanism controls the rate and extent of platelet activation (Fig. 62-3). TXA₂, a platelet product of arachidonic acid, stimulates platelet activation and secretion. In contrast, prostacyclin, an endothelial cell product of arachidonic acid metabolism, inhibits platelet activation by raising intraplatelet levels of cyclic adenosine monophosphate.

Following activation, platelets secrete their granule contents into

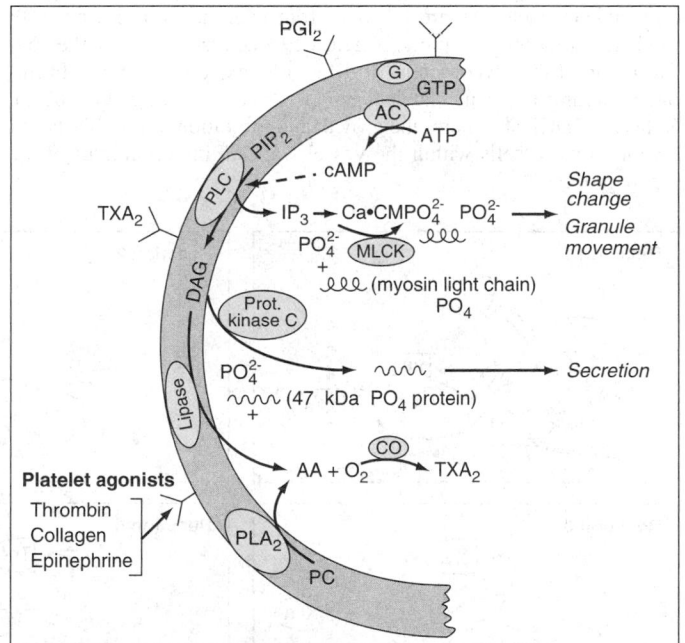

FIGURE 62-4 The biochemical basis of platelet activation and secretion. Binding of agonists such as thrombin, epinephrine, or collagen sets in motion a chain of events that hydrolyzes membrane phospholipids, inhibits adenylate cyclase, mobilizes intracellular calcium, and phosphorylates critical intracellular proteins. The net result is shape change, movement of granules to the canalicular system, generation of mediators such as thromboxane A₂, and granule secretion. Abbreviations: AC, adenylate cyclase; G, guanine nucleotide–binding protein; PIP₂, phosphatidylinositol 4,5-bisphosphate; PLC, phospholipase C; DAG, diacylglycerol; PLA₂, phospholipase A₂; PC, phosphatidylcholine; AA, arachidonic acid; CO, cyclooxygenase; O₂, oxygen; IP₃, inositol triphosphate; cAMP, cyclic AMP; Ca-CM, calcium calmodulin complex; MLCK, myosin light chain kinase.

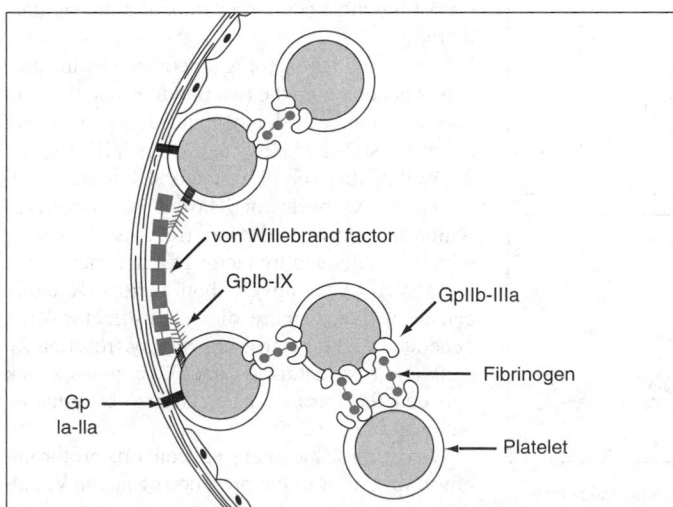

FIGURE 62-2 The molecular basis of platelet adhesion and aggregation. Adhesion of platelets to vascular subendothelium is facilitated by von Willebrand factor, which forms a bridge between collagen fibrils in the vessel wall and receptors on platelet glycoprotein Ib/IX (GpIb–IX). In a similar manner, platelet aggregation is mediated by fibrinogen, which links adjacent platelets via receptors on the platelet glycoprotein IIb and IIIa complex (GpIIb–IIIa).

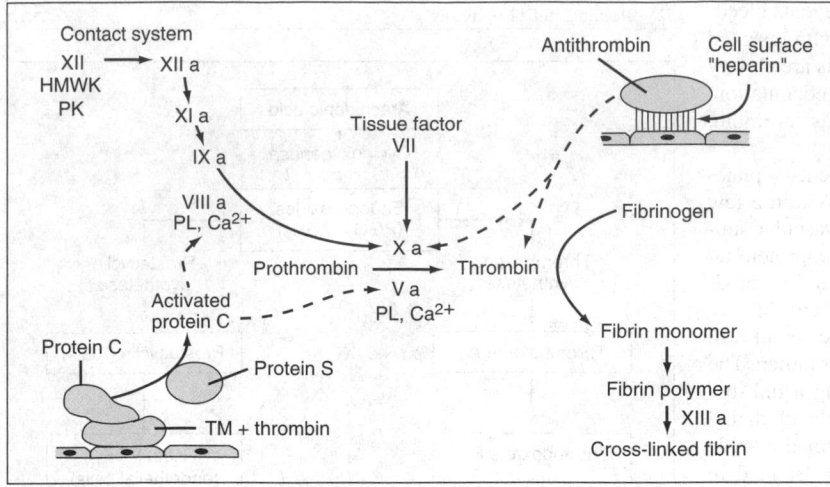

FIGURE 62-5 A schematic diagram of some of the clinically important coagulation reactions. The unactivated or precursor proteins are indicated by roman numerals, and the active form by the addition of a lowercase "a"—a standard convention. Other abbreviations: HMWK, high-molecular-weight kininogen; PK, prekallikrein; PL, phospholipid; TM, thrombomodulin; Ca^{2+}, calcium. There are two independent activation pathways, the contact system and the tissue factor–mediated or extrinsic system. They merge at the point of factor X activation and lead to the generation of thrombin, which converts fibrinogen into fibrin. These reactions are regulated by antithrombin, which forms complexes with all of the coagulation protein serine proteases except factor VII, and by the protein C–protein S system, which inactivates factors V and VIII.

plasma. Endoglycosidases and a heparin-cleaving enzyme are released from lysosomes; calcium, serotonin, and adenosine diphosphate (ADP) are released from the dense granules; and several proteins, including the von Willebrand factor, fibronectin, thrombospondin, the platelet-derived growth factor (PDGF), and a heparin-neutralizing protein (platelet factor 4), are released from α granules. Released ADP binds to purinergic receptors, which, when activated, change the conformation of the glycoprotein IIb/IIIa complex so that it binds fibrinogen, linking adjacent platelets into a hemostatic plug (Fig. 62-2). Released PDGF stimulates the growth and migration of fibroblasts and smooth-muscle cells within the vessel wall, an important part of the repair process.

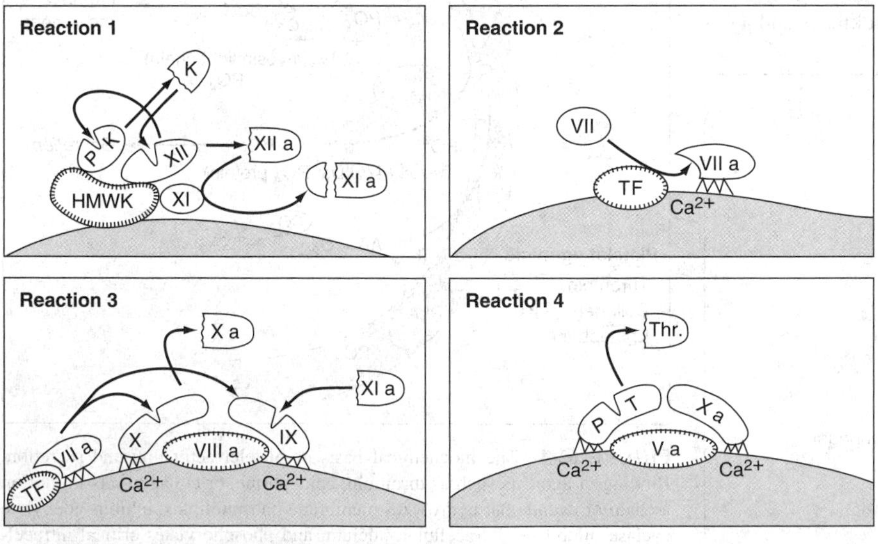

As the primary hemostatic plug is being formed, plasma coagulation proteins are activated to initiate secondary hemostasis. An overall picture of the coagulation scheme, including the role of various inhibitors, is shown in Fig. 62-5. The coagulation pathway can be broken down into a series of reactions (Fig. 62-6) that culminate in the production of enough thrombin to convert a small amount of plasma fibrinogen to fibrin. Each of the reactions requires the formation of a surface-bound complex and the conversion of inactive precursor proteins into active proteases by limited proteolysis, and each is regulated by both plasma and cellular cofactors and calcium.

In *reaction 1*, the intrinsic or contact phase of coagulation, three plasma proteins, Hageman factor (factor XII), high-molecular-weight kininogen (HMWK), and prekallikrein (PK), form a complex on vascular subendothelial collagen. After binding to HMWK, factor XII is slowly converted to an active protease (XIIa), which then activates PK to kallikrein and factor XI to XIa. Kallikrein accelerates the conversion of XII to XIIa, while XIa participates in subsequent coagulation reactions. An alternative mechanism for the activation of factor XI may exist, as patients who are deficient in either factor XII, HMWK, or PK have apparently normal hemostasis and no clinical bleeding.

Reaction 2 provides a second pathway to initiate coagulation by activating factor VII to a protease. In this extrinsic or tissue-factor-dependent pathway, a complex is formed between factor VII, calcium, and tissue factor, a ubiquitous lipoprotein present in cellular membranes and exposed by cellular injury. The tissue factor–VII pathway is continuously active and makes a major contribution to basal coagulation. Factor VII and three other coagulation proteins—factors II (prothrombin), IX, and X—require calcium and vitamin K for biologic activity. These proteins are synthesized in the liver, where a vitamin K–dependent carboxylase catalyzes a unique posttranslational modification that adds a second carboxyl group to certain glutamic acid residues. Pairs of these di-γ-carboxyglutamic acid (Gla) residues bind calcium, which alters protein comformation for binding to phospholipid surfaces and confers biologic activity. Inhibition of this modification by vitamin K antagonists (e.g., warfarin) is the basis of one of the most common forms of anticoagulant therapy.

In *reaction 3*, factor X is activated by the proteases generated in the two previous reactions. In one reaction, a calcium- and lipid-dependent complex is formed between factors VIII, IX, and X. Within this complex, factor IX is first converted to IXa by factor XIa that was generated within the intrinsic pathway (reaction 1). Factor X is then activated by factor IXa in concert with factor VIII. Alternatively, both factors IX and X can be activated more directly by factor VIIa, generated via the extrinsic pathway (reaction 2). Activation of factors IX and X provides a link between the intrinsic and extrinsic coagulation pathways (Fig. 62-5).

Reaction 4, the final step, converts prothrombin to thrombin in the presence of factor V, calcium, and phospholipid. Although prothrombin conversion can take place on various natural and artificial phospholipid-rich surfaces, it proceeds several thousand times faster on the surface of activated platelets or endothelial cells. Thrombin has multiple functions in hemostasis. Although its principal role in hemostasis is the conversion

FIGURE 62-6 The major coagulation reactions are subdivided and depicted in schematic form to emphasize their similarity. They all rely on the formation of surface-bound enzyme-cofactor complexes. Abbreviations: PK, prekallikrein; K, kallikrein; HMWK, high-molecular-weight kininogen; TF, tissue factor; Ca^{2+}, calcium; PT, prothrombin; Thr, thrombin. By convention, other coagulation factors are indicated by roman numerals, with a lowercase "a" appended to indicate their active form. The ^^^ is used to indicate the Gla (di-γ-carboxyglutamic acid)–containing domains of factors VII, IX, X, Xa, and PT, which bind calcium and phospholipid. Hatching is used to indicate proteins that adhere to surfaces by hydrophobic interaction.

of fibrinogen to fibrin, it also activates factors V, VIII, and XIII and stimulates platelet aggregation and secretion. Following the release of fibrinopeptides A and B from the α and β chains of fibrinogen, the modified molecule, now called *fibrin monomer*, polymerizes into an insoluble gel. The fibrin polymer is then stabilized by the cross-linking of individual chains by factor XIIIa, a plasma transglutaminase (Fig. 62-5).

Although the classic view of coagulation had clinical utility, it left several important questions unanswered: (1) Why does factor XII deficiency dramatically prolong partial thromboplastin time (PTT) but not cause bleeding? (2) Why is there heterogeneity in the bleeding symptoms of patients with factor XI deficiency? (3) Why do deficiencies in factors VIII or IX produce such dramatic bleeding even though the "extrinsic" pathway remains intact? Activation of factors IX and X by the tissue factor–VIIa complex is thought to play a major role in the initiation of hemostasis. Once coagulation is initiated by this interaction, the tissue factor pathway inhibitor (TFPI) blocks the pathway, and elements of the intrinsic pathway, particularly factors VIII and IX, become the dominant regulators of thrombin generation. This step in the pathway explains why factor XII–deficient patients are asymptomatic and why factor XI–deficient patients have only a mild to moderate bleeding diathesis (Fig. 62-7).

Clot lysis and vessel repair begin immediately after the formation of the definitive hemostatic plug. Three potential activators of the fibrinolytic system are: Hageman factor fragments, urinary plasminogen activator (uPA) or urokinase, and tissue plasminogen activator (tPA). The principal physiologic activators, tPA and uPA, diffuse from endothelial cells and convert plasminogen, adsorbed to the fibrin clot, into plasmin (Fig. 62-8). Plasmin then degrades fibrin polymer into small fragments, which are cleared by the monocyte-macrophage scavenger system. Although plasmin can also degrade fibrinogen, the reaction remains localized because (1) tPA and some forms of uPA activate plasminogen more effectively when it is adsorbed to fibrin clots; (2) any plasmin that enters the circulation is rapidly bound and neutralized by the α_2 plasmin inhibitor (patients who lack this factor have unchecked fibrinolysis and bleed); and (3) endothelial cells release a plasminogen activator inhibitor (PAI-1), which blocks the action of tPA.

Only a small quantity of each coagulation enzyme is converted to its active form. As a consequence, the hemostatic plug does not propagate beyond the site of injury. Precise regulation is important, since each milliliter of blood contains enough clotting potential to clot all the fibrinogen in the body in 10 to 15 s. Blood fluidity is maintained

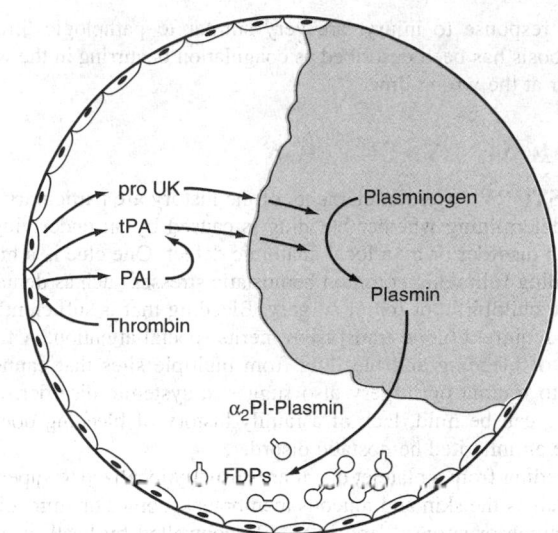

FIGURE 62-8 A schematic diagram of the fibrinolytic pathway. Tissue plasminogen activator (tPA) is released from endothelial cells, enters the fibrin clot, and activates plasminogen to plasmin. Any free plasmin is complexed with α_2 plasmin inhibitor (α_2PI). Fibrin is degraded to low-molecular-weight fragments, fibrin degradation products (FDPs).

by the flow of blood, the adsorption of coagulation factors to surfaces and their trapping in the emerging clot, and by multiple inhibitors in plasma. Antithrombin, proteins C and S, and TFPI are important inhibitors that maintain blood fluidity.

These inhibitors have distinct modes of action. Antithrombin forms complexes with all serine protease coagulation factors except factor VII (Fig. 62-5). Rates of complex formation are accelerated by heparin and heparin-like molecules on the surface of the endothelial cells. Heparin's ability to accelerate antithrombin activity is the basis for its anticoagulant action. Protein C is converted to an active protease by thrombin after it is bound to an endothelial cell protein called *thrombomodulin*. Activated protein C then inactivates the two plasma cofactors V and VIII by limited proteolysis, which slows down two critical coagulation reactions. Protein C may also stimulate the release of tPA from endothelial cells. The inhibitory function of protein C is enhanced by protein S. Reduced levels of antithrombin or proteins C and S, or dysfunctional forms of these molecules, result in a hypercoagulable or prethrombotic state. In addition, a particularly common heritable defect associated with a hypercoagulable state is the presence of a form of factor V (factor V Leiden) that is resistant to protein C inhibition. Between 20 and 50% of patients with unexplained venous thromboembolism have this defect.

Blood coagulation is not uniform throughout the body. The composition of the blood clot varies with the site of injury. Hemostatic plugs or thrombi that form in veins where blood flow is slow are rich in fibrin and trapped red blood cells and contain relatively few platelets. They are often called *red thrombi* because of their appearance in surgical and pathologic specimens. The friable ends of these red thrombi, which most often form in leg veins, can break off and embolize to the pulmonary circulation. Conversely, clots that form in arteries under conditions of high flow are predominantly composed of platelets and have little fibrin. These *white thrombi* may readily dislodge from the arterial wall and embolize to distant sites, causing temporary or permanent ischemia. These clots are a particularly common cause of embolism in the cerebral and retinal circulation, where they may lead to transient neurologic dysfunction (transient ischemic attacks), including temporary monocular blindness (amaurosis fugax), or to strokes. In addition, most episodes of myocardial infarction are due to thrombi that form after the rupture of atherosclerotic plaques within diseased coronary arteries. Hemostatic plugs, which are a phys-

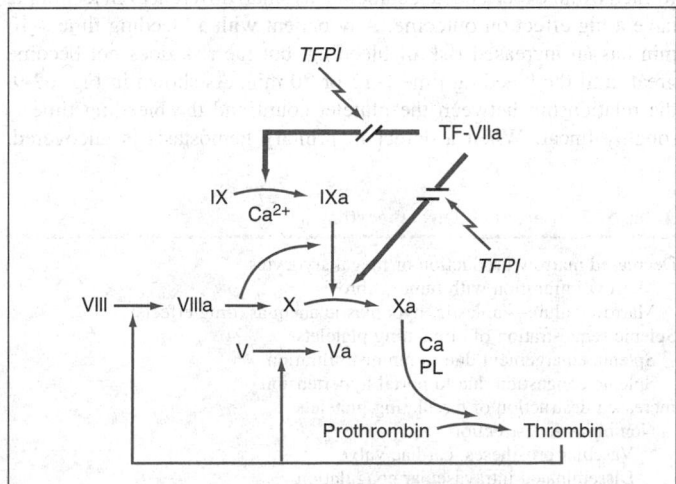

FIGURE 62-7 The contribution of the tissue factor–VIIa complex (TF-VIIa) and tissue factor pathway inhibitor (TFPI) to coagulation. Initial activation of factor IX by TF-VIIa compensates for deficiencies in the early factors, e.g., factors XII and XI. The subsequent inhibition of TF-VIIa by TFPI makes sustained activation of factor X by IXa and VIIIa critical for normal hemostasis. PL, phospholipid.

iologic response to injury, are very similar to pathologic thrombi. Thrombosis has been described as coagulation occurring in the wrong place or at the wrong time.

CLINICAL EVALUATION

HISTORY Certain elements of the history are particularly useful in determining whether bleeding is caused by an underlying hemostatic disorder or by a local anatomic defect. One clue is a history of bleeding following common hemostatic stresses such as dental extraction, childbirth, or minor surgery. Bleeding that is sufficiently severe to require a blood transfusion merits special attention. A family history of bleeding and bleeding from multiple sites that cannot be linked to trauma or surgery also suggest a systemic disorder. Since bleeding can be mild, lack of a family history of bleeding does not exclude an inherited hemostatic disorder.

Bleeding from a platelet disorder is usually localized to superficial sites such as the skin and mucous membranes, comes on immediately after trauma or surgery, and is readily controlled by local measures (Table 62-1). In contrast, bleeding from secondary hemostatic or plasma coagulation defects occurs hours or days after injury and is unaffected by local therapy. Such bleeding most often occurs in deep subcutaneous tissues, muscles, joints, or body cavities. A careful and thorough history may establish the presence of a hemostatic disorder and guide initial laboratory testing.

PHYSICAL EXAMINATION The most common site to observe bleeding is in the skin and mucous membranes. Collections of blood in the skin are called *purpura* and may be subdivided on the basis of the site of bleeding in the skin. Small pinpoint hemorrhages into the dermis due to the leakage of red cells through capillaries are called *petechiae* and are characteristic of platelet disorders—in particular, severe thrombocytopenia. Larger subcutaneous collections of blood due to leakage of blood from small arterioles and venules are called *ecchymoses* (common bruises) or, if somewhat deeper and palpable, *hematomas*. They are also common in patients with platelet defects and result from minor trauma. Dilated capillaries, or *telangiectasia*, may cause bleeding without any hemostatic defect. In addition, the loss of connective tissue support for capillaries and small veins that accompanies aging increases the fragility of superficial vessels, such as those on the dorsum of the hand, leading to extravasation of blood into subcutaneous tissue—*senile purpura*. Menorrhagia is sometimes a serious problem in women with severe thrombocytopenia or platelet dysfunction. Some patients with primary hemostatic defects, especially von Willebrand's disease, may have recurrent gastrointestinal hemorrhage, often associated with angiodysplasia, a common vascular malformation in the gastrointestinal tract.

Bleeding into body cavities, the retroperitoneum, or joints is a common manifestation of plasma coagulation defects. Repeated joint bleeding may cause synovial thickening, chronic inflammation, and fluid collections and may erode articular cartilage and lead to chronic joint deformity and limited mobility. Such deformities are particularly common in deficiencies of factors VIII and IX, the two sex-linked coagulation disorders referred to as the *hemophilias*. For unclear reasons, hemarthroses are much less common in patients with other plasma coagulation defects. Blood collections in various body cavities or soft tissues can cause secondary necrosis of tissues or nerve compression. Retroperitoneal hematomas can cause femoral nerve compression, and large collections of poorly coagulated blood in soft tissues occasionally mimic malignant growths—the pseudotumor syndrome. Two of the most life-threatening sites of bleeding are in the oropharynx, where bleeding can compromise the airway, and in the central nervous system. Intracerebral hemorrhage is one of the leading causes of death in patients with severe coagulation disorders. Because of their need for plasma and factor concentrates derived from multiple donors, many patients with hemophilia were infected with HIV before effective testing of donors was in place.

LABORATORY TESTS The most important screening tests of the primary hemostatic system are (1) a *bleeding time* (a sensitive measure of platelet function), and (2) a *platelet count*. The latter correlates well with the propensity to bleed. The normal platelet count is 150,000 to 450,000/μL of blood. As long as the count is >100,000/μL, patients are usually not symptomatic and the bleeding time remains normal. Platelet counts of 50,000 to 100,000/μL cause mild prolongation of the bleeding time; bleeding occurs only from severe trauma or other stress. Patients with platelet counts <50,000/μL have easy bruising, manifested by skin purpura after minor trauma and bleeding after mucous membrane surgery. Patients with a platelet count <20,000/μL have an appreciable incidence of spontaneous bleeding, usually have petechiae, and may have intracranial or other spontaneous internal bleeding. The major causes of thrombocytopenia are outlined in Table 62-2.

Patients with qualitative platelet abnormalities have a normal platelet count and a prolonged bleeding time (Table 62-3). The bleeding time is ascertained by making a small, superficial skin incision and timing the duration of blood flow from the wounded area. By careful standardization, bleeding time is a reliable and sensitive test of platelet function. A template or an automated scalpel controls the length and depth of the incision (usually 1 mm deep by 9 mm long), and a sphygmomanometer inflated to 40 mmHg distends the capillary bed of the forearm uniformly. The bleeding time test must be performed by an experienced technician, as small differences in technique have a big effect on outcome. Any patient with a bleeding time >10 min has an increased risk of bleeding, but the risk does not become great until the bleeding time >15 or 20 min. As shown in Fig. 62-9, the relationship between the platelet count and the bleeding time is roughly linear. When a defect in primary hemostasis is uncovered,

---

Table 62-1 Differences in the Clinical Manifestations of Disorders of Primary and Secondary Hemostasis

Manifestations	Defects of Primary Hemostasis (Platelet Defects)	Defects of Secondary Hemostasis (Plasma Protein Defects)
Onset of bleeding after trauma	Immediate	Delayed—hours or days
Sites of bleeding	Superficial—skin, mucous membranes, nose, gastrointestinal and genitourinary tracts	Deep—joints, muscle, retroperitoneum
Physical findings	Petechiae, ecchymoses	Hematomas, hemarthroses
Family history	Autosomal dominant	Autosomal or X-linked recessive
Response to therapy	Immediate; local measures effective	Requires sustained systemic therapy

---

Table 62-2 Causes of Thrombocytopenia

Decreased marrow production of megakaryocytes
  Marrow infiltration with tumor, fibrosis
  Marrow failure—aplastic, hypoplastic anemias, drug effects
Splenic sequestration of circulating platelets
  Splenic enlargement due to tumor infiltration
  Splenic congestion due to portal hypertension
Increased destruction of circulating platelets
  Nonimmune destruction
    Vascular prostheses, cardiac valves
    Disseminated intravascular coagulation
    Sepsis
    Vasculitis
  Immune destruction
    Autoantibodies to platelet antigens
    Drug-associated antibodies
    Circulating immune complexes (systemic lupus erythematosus, viral agents, bacterial sepsis)

Table 62-3   Primary Hemostatic (Platelet) Disorders

Defects of platelet adhesion
    von Willebrand's disease
    Bernard-Soulier syndrome (absence or dysfunction of GpIb/IX)
Defects of platelet aggregation
    Glanzmann's thrombasthenia (absence or dysfunction of GpIIb/IIIa)
Defects of platelet release
    Decreased cyclooxygenase activity
        Drug-induced—aspirin, nonsteroidal anti-inflammatory agents
        Congenital
    Granule storage pool defects
        Congenital
        Acquired
    Uremia
    Platelet coating (e.g., penicillin or paraproteins)
Defect of platelet coagulant activity
    Scott's syndrome

ABBREVIATION: Gp, glycoprotein.

specialized testing is needed to determine the cause of the platelet dysfunction (Table 62-3). A precise diagnosis is important in determining the proper treatment. Occasional patients with a strong history of bleeding, particularly those with mild von Willebrand's disease, may have a normal bleeding time when initially tested, owing to cyclical variations in the level of the von Willebrand factor. Repeated testing may be necessary to establish an accurate diagnosis. Bleeding time is not an effective screening test for preoperative patients.

Plasma coagulation function is readily assessed with the PTT, prothrombin time (PT), thrombin time (TT), and quantitative fibrinogen determination (Fig. 62-5, Table 62-4). The PTT screens the intrinsic limb of the coagulation system and tests for the adequacy of factors XII, HMWK, PK, XI, IX, and VIII. The PT screens the extrinsic or tissue factor–dependent pathway. Both tests also evaluate the common coagulation pathway involving all the reactions that occur after the activation of factor X. Prolongation of the PT and PTT that does not resolve after the addition of normal plasma suggests a coagulation inhibitor. A specific test for the conversion of fibrinogen to fibrin is needed when both the PTT and PT are prolonged—either a TT or a clottable fibrinogen level can be employed. When abnormalities are noted in any of the screening tests, more specific coagulation factor assays can be ordered to determine the nature of the defect.

Several rare coagulation abnormalities that may be missed as they do not affect these screening tests: factor XIII deficiency, α_2 plasmin inhibitor deficiency, PAI-1 deficiency (PAI-1 is the major inhibitor of plasminogen activators), and Scott's syndrome, a platelet coagulant defect. A test for factor XIII–dependent fibrin cross-linking, such as clot solubility in 5 M urea, should be ordered when the PT and PTT

Table 62-4   Relationship between Secondary Hemostatic Disorders and Coagulation Test Abnormalities

Prolonged partial thromboplastin time (PTT)
    No clinical bleeding—factors XII, HMWK, PK
    Mild or rare bleeding—factor XI
    Frequent, severe bleeding—factors VIII and IX
Prolonged prothrombin time (PT)
    Factor VII deficiency
    Vitamin K deficiency—early
    Warfarin anticoagulant ingestion
Prolonged PTT and PT
    Factor II, V, or X deficiency
    Vitamin K deficiency—late
    Warfarin anticoagulant ingestion
Prolonged thrombin time (TT)
    Mild or rare bleeding—afibrinogenemia
    Frequent, severe bleeding—dysfibrinogenemia
    Heparin-like inhibitors or heparin administration
Prolonged PT and/or PTT not corrected with normal plasma
    Specific or nonspecific inhibitor syndromes
Clot solubility in 5 M urea
    Factor XIII deficiency
    Inhibitors or defective cross-linking
Rapid clot lysis
    α_2 plasmin inhibitor

ABBREVIATIONS: HMWK, high-molecular-weight kininogen; PK, prekallikrein.

are both normal but the history of bleeding is strong. The fibrinolytic system can be assessed by measuring the rate of clot lysis with the euglobulin lysis or whole blood clot lysis tests and by measuring the levels of α_2 plasmin inhibitor and PAI-1. Scott's syndrome can be detected by measuring the serum PT, which assesses the amount of residual prothrombin.

Conditions associated with thrombosis are listed in Table 62-5. Patients suspected of having a hypercoagulable or prethrombotic disorder on the basis of clinical information should be tested with specific

Table 62-5   Thrombotic Disorders

Inherited
    Defective inhibition of coagulation factors
        Factor V Leiden (resistant to inhibition by activated protein C)
        Antithrombin III deficiency
        Protein C deficiency
        Protein S deficiency
        Prothrombin gene mutation (G40210A)
    Impaired clot lysis
        Dysfibrinogenemia
        Plasminogen deficiency
        tPA deficiency
        PAI-1 excess
    Uncertain mechanism
        Homocystinuria - ? endothelial damage
Acquired
    Diseases or syndromes
        Lupus anticoagulant/anticardiolipin antibody syndrome
        Malignancy
        Myeloproliferative disorder
        Thrombotic thrombocytopenic purpura
        Estrogen treatment
        Hyperlipidemia
        Diabetes mellitus
        Hyperviscosity
        Nephrotic syndrome
        Congestive heart failure
        Paroxysmal nocturnal hemoglobinuria
    Physiologic states
        Pregnancy (especially postpartum)
        Obesity
        Postoperative state
        Immobilization
        Old age

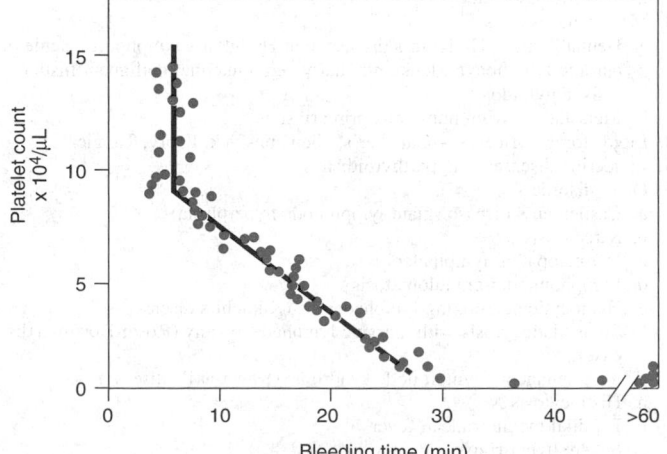

FIGURE 62-9 The relationship between the platelet count and the bleeding time. (*From LA Harker, Hemostasis Manual, 2d ed. Philadelphia, FA Davis Company, 1974.*)

assays to screen for the known defects. Currently available tests can identify 50 to 60% of the cases of familial or recurrent venous thrombosis.

Inhibitor syndromes or circulating anticoagulants are usually due to antibodies that impair coagulation factor activity. They are an infrequent cause of bleeding and require specialized diagnostic testing. Inhibitors are likely when screening test abnormalities cannot be reversed by adding normal plasma to patient plasma. Antibodies against specific coagulation factors may develop in (1) postpartum women, (2) patients with autoimmune disorders such as systemic lupus erythematosus, (3) patients taking drugs such as penicillin and streptomycin, and (4) otherwise healthy elderly individuals. In addition, between 10 to 20% of patients with severe hemophilia who have received multiple plasma infusions develop inhibitory antibodies. Some patients, especially those with systemic lupus erythematosus, may also have a nonspecific form of anticoagulant antibody that interferes with phospholipid binding of coagulation factors and prolongs the PT and PTT but does not cause clinical bleeding. The presence of the lupus anticoagulant may increase the risk of thromboembolism and may cause placental infarction, recurrent midtrimester abortion, and venous and arterial thrombosis. The lupus-like anticoagulant is one manifestation of the anticardiolipin antibody syndrome. Patients may have anticardiolipin antibodies that do not prolong the PTT, but patients are still at risk from thrombosis. Occasionally, patients develop inhibitors that are not antibodies. For example, several patients with clinical bleeding have been found to have circulating mucopolysaccharides that have heparin-like activity.

BIBLIOGRAPHY

Berting RM: Introduction: Hypercoagulable states. Sem Hematol 34:167, 1997

Colman RW et al (eds): *Hemostasis and Thrombosis: Basic Principles and Clinical Practice*, 4th ed. Philadelphia, Lippincott, 1996

Handin RI: Diseases of the platelet and vessel wall, in *Hematology of Infancy and Childhood*, 5th ed., DG Nathan et al (eds). Philadelphia, Saunders, 1997, pp 1511–1530

——— et al (eds): *Blood: Principles and Practice of Hematology and Hematologic Oncology*, 4th ed. Philadelphia, Lippincott, 1994

Mann KC: Biochemistry and physiology of blood coagulation. Thromb Haemost 82:165, 1999

63   *Patrick H. Henry, Dan L. Longo*

ENLARGEMENT OF LYMPH NODES AND SPLEEN

This chapter is intended to serve as a guide to the evaluation of patients who present with enlargement of the lymph nodes (*lymphadenopathy*) or the spleen (*splenomegaly*). Lymphadenopathy is a rather common clinical finding in primary care settings, whereas palpable splenomegaly is less so.

LYMPHADENOPATHY

Lymphadenopathy may be an incidental finding in patients being examined for various reasons or it may be a presenting sign or symptom of the patient's illness. The physician must eventually decide whether the lymphadenopathy is a normal finding or one that requires further study, up to and including biopsy. Soft, flat, submandibular nodes (<1 cm) are often palpable in healthy children and young adults, and healthy adults may have palpable inguinal nodes of up to 2 cm, which are considered normal. Further evaluation of these normal nodes is not warranted. In contrast, if the physician believes the node(s) to be abnormal, then pursuit of a more precise diagnosis is needed.

Lymphadenopathy may be a primary or secondary manifestation of numerous disorders, as shown in Table 63-1. Many of these disorders are infrequent causes of lymphadenopathy. Analysis of lymphadenopathy in primary care practice has shown that more than two-thirds of patients have nonspecific causes or upper respiratory illnesses (viral or bacterial), and fewer than 1% have a malignancy. In one study, researchers reported that 186 of 220 patients (84%) referred for evaluation of lymphadenopathy had a "benign" diagnosis. The remaining 34 patients (16%) had a malignancy (lymphoma or metastatic adenocarcinoma). Sixty-three percent (112) of the 186 patients with benign lymphadenopathy had a nonspecific or reactive etiology (no causative agent found), and the remainder had a specific cause demonstrated, most commonly infectious mononucleosis, toxoplasmosis, or tuberculosis. Thus, the vast majority of patients with lymphadenopathy will have a nonspecific etiology requiring few diagnostic tests.

Clinical Assessment   The physician will be aided in the pursuit of an explanation for the lymphadenopathy by a careful medical history, physical examination, selected laboratory tests, and perhaps an excisional lymph node biopsy.

The *medical history* should reveal the setting in which lymphadenopathy is occurring. Symptoms such as sore throat, cough, fever,

Table 63-1   Diseases Associated with Lymphadenopathy

1. Infectious diseases
   a. Viral—infectious mononucleosis syndromes (EBV, CMV), infectious hepatitis, herpes simplex, herpesvirus-6, varicella-zoster virus, rubella, measles, adenovirus, HIV, epidemic keratoconjunctivitis, vaccinia, herpesvirus-8
   b. Bacterial—streptococci, staphylococci, cat-scratch disease, brucellosis, tularemia, plague, chancroid, melioidosis, glanders, tuberculosis, atypical mycobacterial infection, primary and secondary syphilis, diphtheria, leprosy
   c. Fungal—histoplasmosis, coccidioidomycosis, paracoccidioidomycosis
   d. Chlamydial—lymphogranuloma venereum, trachoma
   e. Parasitic—toxoplasmosis, leishmaniasis, trypanosomiasis, filariasis
   f. Rickettsial—scrub typhus, rickettsialpox
2. Immunologic diseases
   a. Rheumatoid arthritis
   b. Juvenile rheumatoid arthritis
   c. Mixed connective tissue disease
   d. Systemic lupus erythematosus
   e. Dermatomyositis
   f. Sjögren's syndrome
   g. Serum sickness
   h. Drug hypersensitivity—diphenylhydantoin, hydralazine, allopurinol, primidone, gold, carbamazepine, etc.
   i. Angioimmunoblastic lymphadenopathy
   j. Primary biliary cirrhosis
   k. Graft-vs.-host disease
   l. Silicone-associated
3. Malignant diseases
   a. Hematologic—Hodgkin's disease, non-Hodgkin's lymphomas, acute or chronic lymphocytic leukemia, hairy cell leukemia, malignant histiocytosis, amyloidosis
   b. Metastatic—from numerous primary sites
4. Lipid storage diseases—Gaucher's, Niemann-Pick, Fabry, Tangier
5. Endocrine diseases—hyperthyroidism
6. Other disorders
   a. Castleman's disease (giant lymph node hyperplasia)
   b. Sarcoidosis
   c. Dermatopathic lymphadenitis
   d. Lymphomatoid granulomatosis
   e. Histiocytic necrotizing lymphadenitis (Kikuchi's disease)
   f. Sinus histiocytosis with massive lymphadenopathy (Rosai-Dorfman disease)
   g. Mucocutaneous lymph node syndrome (Kawasaki's disease)
   h. Histiocytosis X
   i. Familial mediterranean fever
   j. Severe hypertriglyceridemia
   k. Vascular transformation of sinuses
   l. Inflammatory pseudotumor of lymph node

NOTE: EBV, Epstein-Barr virus; CMV, cytomegalovirus.

night sweats, fatigue, weight loss, or pain in the nodes should be sought. The patient's age, sex, occupation, exposure to pets, sexual behavior, and use of drugs such as diphenylhydantoin are other important historic points. For example, children and young adults usually have benign (i.e., nonmalignant) disorders, such as viral or bacterial upper respiratory infections, infectious mononucleosis, toxoplasmosis, and, in some countries, tuberculosis, which account for the observed lymphadenopathy. In contrast, after age 50 the incidence of malignant disorders increases and that of benign disorders decreases.

The *physical examination* can provide useful clues such as the extent of lymphadenopathy (localized or generalized), size of nodes, texture, presence or absence of nodal tenderness, signs of inflammation over the node, skin lesions, and splenomegaly. A thorough ear, nose, and throat (ENT) examination is indicated in adult patients with cervical adenopathy and a history of tobacco use. Localized or regional adenopathy implies involvement of a single anatomic area. Generalized adenopathy has been defined as involvement of three or more noncontiguous lymph node areas. Many of the causes of lymphadenopathy (Table 63-1) can produce localized *or* generalized adenopathy, so this distinction is of limited utility in the differential diagnosis. Nevertheless, generalized lymphadenopathy is frequently associated with nonmalignant disorders such as infectious mononucleosis [Epstein-Barr virus (EBV) or cytomegalovirus (CMV)], toxoplasmosis, AIDS, other viral infections, systemic lupus erythematosus (SLE), and mixed connective tissue disease. Acute and chronic lymphocytic leukemias and malignant lymphomas also produce generalized adenopathy in adults.

The site of localized or regional adenopathy may provide a useful clue about the cause. Occipital adenopathy often reflects an infection of the scalp, and preauricular adenopathy accompanies conjunctival infections and cat-scratch disease. The most frequent site of regional adenopathy is the neck, and most of the causes are benign—upper respiratory infections, oral and dental lesions, infectious mononucleosis, other viral illnesses. The chief malignant causes include metastatic cancer from head and neck, breast, lung, and thyroid primaries. Enlargement of supraclavicular and scalene nodes is always abnormal. Because these nodes drain regions of the lung and retroperitoneal space, they can reflect either lymphomas, other cancers, or infectious processes arising in these areas. Virchow's node is an enlarged left supraclavicular node infiltrated with metastatic cancer from a gastrointestinal primary. Metastases to supraclavicular nodes also occur from lung, breast, testis, or ovarian cancers. Tuberculosis, sarcoidosis, and toxoplasmosis are nonneoplastic causes of supraclavicular adenopathy. Axillary adenopathy is usually due to injuries or localized infections of the ipsilateral upper extremity. Malignant causes include melanoma or lymphoma and, in women, breast cancer. Inguinal lymphadenopathy is usually secondary to infections or trauma of the lower extremities and may accompany sexually transmitted diseases such as lymphogranuloma venereum, primary syphilis, genital herpes, or chancroid. These nodes may also be involved by lymphomas and metastatic cancer from primary lesions of the rectum, genitalia, or lower extremities (melanoma).

The size and texture of the lymph node(s) and the presence of pain are useful parameters in evaluating a patient with lymphadenopathy. Nodes <1.0 cm² in area (1.0 × 1.0 cm or less) are almost always secondary to benign, nonspecific reactive causes. In one retrospective analysis of younger patients (9 to 25 years) who had a lymph node biopsy, a maximum diameter of >2 cm served as one discriminant for predicting that the biopsy would reveal malignant or granulomatous disease. Another study showed that a lymph node size of 2.25 cm² (1.5 cm × 1.5 cm) was the best discriminating limit for distinguishing malignant or granulomatous lymphadenopathy from other causes of lymphadenopathy. Patients with node(s) ≤1.0 cm² should be observed after excluding infectious mononucleosis and/or toxoplasmosis unless there are symptoms and signs of an underlying systemic illness.

The texture of lymph nodes may be described as soft, firm, rubbery, hard, discrete, matted, tender, movable, or fixed. Tenderness is found when the capsule is stretched during rapid enlargement, usually secondary to an inflammatory process. Some malignant diseases such as acute leukemia may produce rapid enlargement and pain in the nodes. Nodes involved by lymphoma tend to be large, discrete, symmetric, rubbery, firm, mobile, and nontender. Nodes containing metastatic cancer are often hard, nontender, and nonmovable because of fixation to surrounding tissues. The coexistence of splenomegaly in the patient with lymphadenopathy implies a systemic illness such as infectious mononucleosis, lymphoma, acute or chronic leukemia, SLE, sarcoidosis, toxoplasmosis, cat-scratch disease, or other less common hematologic disorders. The patient's story should provide helpful clues about the underlying systemic illness.

Nonsuperficial presentations (thoracic or abdominal) of adenopathy are usually detected as the result of a symptom-directed diagnostic workup. Thoracic adenopathy may be detected by routine chest roentgenography or during the workup for superficial adenopathy. It may also be found because the patient complains of a cough or wheezing from airway compression; hoarseness from recurrent laryngeal nerve involvement; dysphagia from esophageal compression; or swelling of the neck, face, or arms secondary to compression of the superior vena cava or subclavian vein. The differential diagnosis of mediastinal and hilar adenopathy includes primary lung disorders and systemic illnesses that characteristically involve mediastinal or hilar nodes. In the young, mediastinal adenopathy is associated with infectious mononucleosis and sarcoidosis. In endemic regions, histoplasmosis can cause unilateral paratracheal lymph node involvement that mimics lymphoma. Tuberculosis can also cause unilateral adenopathy. In older patients, the differential diagnosis includes primary lung cancer (especially among smokers), lymphomas, metastatic carcinoma (usually lung), tuberculosis, fungal infection, and sarcoidosis.

Enlarged intraabdominal or retroperitoneal nodes are usually malignant. Although tuberculosis may present as mesenteric lymphadenitis, these masses usually contain lymphomas or, in young men, germ cell tumors.

Laboratory Investigation   The laboratory investigation of patients with lymphadenopathy must be tailored to elucidate the etiology suspected from the patient's history and physical findings. One study from a family practice clinic evaluated 249 younger patients with "enlarged lymph nodes, not infected" or "lymphadenitis." No laboratory studies were obtained in 51%. When studies were performed, the most common were a complete blood count (33%), throat culture (16%), chest x-ray (12%), or monospot test (10%). Only eight patients (3%) had a node biopsy, and half of those were normal or reactive. The complete blood count can provide useful data for the diagnosis of acute or chronic leukemias, EBV or CMV mononucleosis, lymphoma with a leukemic component, pyogenic infections, or immune cytopenias in illnesses such as SLE. Serologic studies may demonstrate antibodies specific to components of EBV, CMV, HIV, and other viruses; *Toxoplasma gondii*; *Brucella*; etc. If SLE is suspected, then antinuclear and anti-DNA antibody studies are warranted.

The chest x-ray is usually negative, but the presence of a pulmonary infiltrate or mediastinal lymphadenopathy would suggest tuberculosis, histoplasmosis, sarcoidosis, lymphoma, primary lung cancer, or metastatic cancer and demands further investigation.

A variety of imaging techniques [computed tomography (CT), magnetic resonance imaging (MRI), ultrasound, color Doppler ultrasonography] have been employed to differentiate benign from malignant lymph nodes, especially in patients with head and neck cancer. CT and MRI are comparably accurate (65 to 90%) in the diagnosis of metastases to cervical lymph nodes. Ultrasonography has been used to determine the long (L) axis, short (S) axis, and a ratio of long to short axis in cervical nodes. An L/S ratio of <2.0 has a sensitivity and a specificity of 95% for distinguishing benign and malignant nodes in patients with head and neck cancer. This ratio has greater specificity and sensitivity than palpation or measurement of either the long or the short axis alone.

The indications for lymph node biopsy are imprecise, yet it is a valuable diagnostic tool. The decision to biopsy may be made early in a patient's evaluation or delayed for up to 2 weeks. Prompt biopsy should occur if the patient's history and physical findings suggest a malignancy; examples include a solitary, hard, nontender cervical node in an older patient who is a chronic user of tobacco; supraclavicular adenopathy; and solitary or generalized adenopathy that is firm, movable, and suggestive of lymphoma. If a primary head and neck cancer is suspected as the basis of a solitary, hard cervical node, then a careful ENT examination should be performed. Any mucosal lesion that is suspicious for a primary neoplastic process should be biopsied first. If no mucosal lesion is detected, an excisional biopsy of the largest node should be performed. Fine-needle aspiration should not be performed as the first diagnostic procedure. Most diagnoses require more tissue than such aspiration can provide and it often delays a definitive diagnosis. Fine-needle aspiration should be reserved for thyroid nodules and for confirmation of relapse in patients whose primary diagnosis is known. If the primary physician is uncertain about whether to proceed to biopsy, consultation with a hematologist or medical oncologist should be helpful. In primary care practices, fewer than 5% of lymphadenopathy patients will require a biopsy. That percentage will be considerably larger in referral practices, i.e., hematology, oncology, or otolaryngology (ENT).

Two groups have reported algorithms that they claim will identify more precisely those lymphadenopathy patients who should have a biopsy. Both reports were retrospective analyses in referral practices. The first study involved patients 9 to 25 years of age who had a node biopsy performed. Three variables were identified that predicted those young patients with peripheral lymphadenopathy who should undergo biopsy; lymph node size >2 cm in diameter and abnormal chest x-ray had positive predictive value, whereas recent ENT symptoms had negative predictive values. The second study evaluated 220 lymphadenopathy patients in a hematology unit and identified five variables [lymph node size, location (supraclavicular or non-supraclavicular), age (>40 years or <40 years), texture (nonhard or hard), and tenderness] that were utilized in a mathematical model to identify those patients requiring a biopsy. Positive predictive value was found for age >40 years, supraclavicular location, node size >2.25 cm^2, hard texture, and lack of pain or tenderness. Negative predictive value was evident for age <40 years, node size <1.0 cm^2, nonhard texture, and tender or painful nodes. Ninety-one percent of those who required biopsy were correctly classified by this model. Since both of these studies were retrospective analyses and one was limited to young patients, it is not known how useful these models would be if applied prospectively in a primary care setting.

Most lymphadenopathy patients do not require a biopsy, and at least half require no laboratory studies. If the patient's history and physical findings point to a benign cause for lymphadenopathy, then careful follow-up at a 2- to 4-week interval can be employed. The patient should be instructed to return for reevaluation if the node(s) increase in size. Antibiotics are not indicated for lymphadenopathy unless there is strong evidence of a bacterial infection. Glucocorticoids should not be used to treat lymphadenopathy because their lympholytic effect obscures some diagnoses (lymphoma, leukemia, Castleman's disease) and they contribute to delayed healing or activation of underlying infections. An exception to this statement is the life-threatening pharyngeal obstruction by enlarged lymphoid tissue in Waldeyer's ring that is occasionally seen in infectious mononucleosis.

SPLENOMEGALY

STRUCTURE AND FUNCTION OF THE SPLEEN The spleen is a reticuloendothelial organ that has its embryologic origin in the dorsal mesogastrium at about 5 weeks' gestation. It arises in a series of hillocks, migrates to its normal adult location in the left upper quadrant (LUQ), and is attached to the stomach via the gastrolienal

ligament and to the kidney via the lienorenal ligament. When the hillocks fail to unify into a single tissue mass, accessory spleens may develop in around 20% of persons. The function of the spleen has been elusive. Galen believed it was the source of "black bile" or melancholia, and the word *hypochondria* (literally, beneath the ribs) and the idiom "to vent one's spleen" attest to the beliefs that the spleen had an important influence on the psyche and emotions. In humans, its normal physiologic roles seem to be the following:

1. Maintenance of quality control over erythrocytes in the red pulp by removal of senescent and defective red blood cells. The spleen accomplishes this function through a unique organization of its parenchyma and vasculature (Fig. 63-1).
2. Synthesis of antibodies in the white pulp.
3. The removal of antibody-coated bacteria and antibody-coated blood cells from the circulation.

An increase in these normal functions may result in splenomegaly.

The spleen is composed of red pulp and white pulp, which are Malpighi's terms for the red blood–filled sinuses and reticuloendothelial cell–lined cords and the white lymphoid follicles arrayed within the red pulp matrix. The spleen is in the portal circulation. The reason for this is unknown but may relate to the fact that lower blood pressure

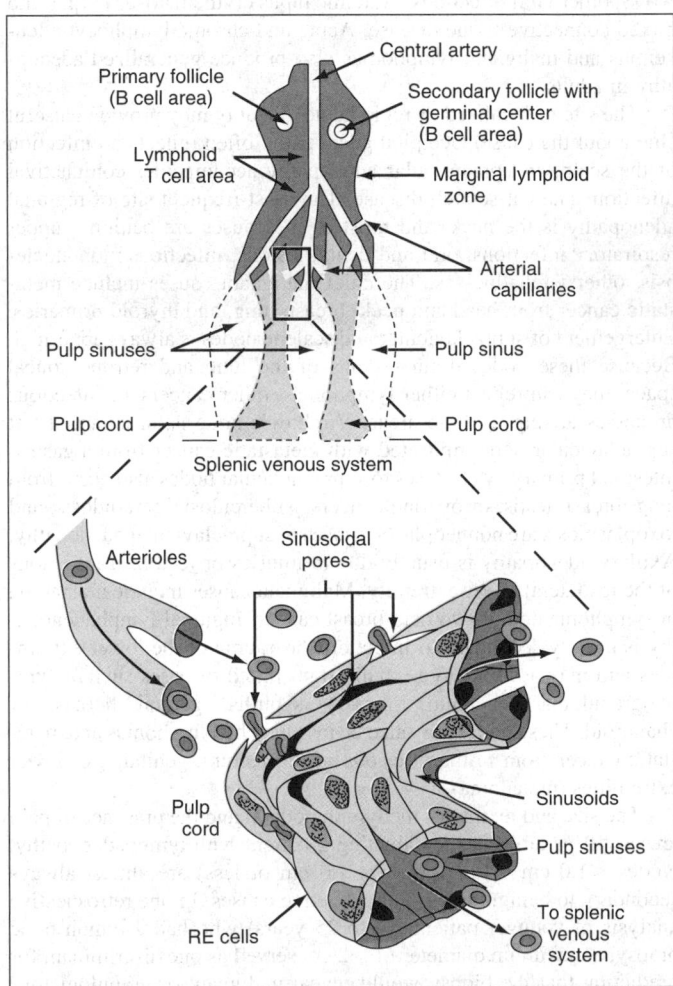

FIGURE 63-1   Schematic spleen structure. The spleen comprises many units of red and white pulp centered around small branches of the splenic artery, called central arteries. White pulp is lymphoid in nature and contains B cell follicles, a marginal zone around the follicles, and T cell–rich areas sheathing arterioles. The red pulp areas include pulp sinuses and pulp cords. The cords are dead ends. In order to regain access to the circulation, red blood cells must traverse tiny openings in the sinusoidal lining. Stiff, damaged, or old red cells cannot enter the sinuses. (*Bottom portion of figure from RS Hillman, KA Ault: Hematology in Clinical Practice. New York, McGraw-Hill, 1995.*)

allows less rapid flow and minimizes damage to normal erythrocytes. Blood flows into the spleen at a rate of about 150 mL/min through the splenic artery, which ultimately ramifies into central arterioles. Some blood goes from the arterioles to capillaries and then to splenic veins and out of the spleen, but the majority of blood from central arterioles flows into the macrophage-lined sinuses and cords. The blood entering the sinuses reenters the circulation through the splenic venules, but the blood entering the cords is subjected to an inspection of sorts. In order to return to the circulation, the blood cells in the cords must squeeze through slits in the cord lining to enter the sinuses that lead to the venules. Old and damaged erythrocytes are less deformable and are retained in the cords, where they are destroyed and their components recycled. Red cell inclusion bodies such as parasites, nuclear residua (Howell-Jolly bodies), or denatured hemoglobin (Heinz bodies) are pinched off in the process of passing through the slits, a process called *pitting*. The culling of dead and damaged cells and the pitting of cells with inclusions appear to occur without significant delay since the blood transit time through the spleen is only slightly slower than in other organs.

The spleen is also capable of assisting the host in adapting to its hostile environment. It has at least three adaptational functions: (1) clearance of bacteria and particulates from the blood, (2) the generation of immune responses to certain invading pathogens, and (3) the generation of cellular components of the blood under circumstances in which the marrow is unable to meet the needs (i.e., extramedullary hematopoiesis). The latter adaptation is a recapitulation of the blood-forming function the spleen plays during gestation. In some animals, the spleen also serves a role in the vascular adaptation to stress because it stores red blood cells (often hemoconcentrated to higher hematocrits than normal) under normal circumstances and contracts under the influence of β-adrenergic stimulation to provide the animal with an autotransfusion and improved oxygen-carrying capacity. However, the normal human spleen does not sequester or store red blood cells and does not contract in response to sympathetic stimuli. The normal human spleen contains approximately one-third of the total body platelets and a significant number of marginated neutrophils. These sequestered cells are available when needed to respond to bleeding or infection.

Approach to the Patient

Clinical Assessment The most common *symptoms* produced by diseases involving the spleen are pain and a heavy sensation in the LUQ. Massive splenomegaly may cause early satiety. Pain may result from acute swelling of the spleen with stretching of the capsule, infarction, or inflammation of the capsule. For many years, it was believed that splenic infarction was clinically silent, which at times is true. However, Soma Weiss, in his classic 1942 report of the self-observations by a Harvard medical student on the clinical course of subacute bacterial endocarditis, documented that severe LUQ and pleuritic chest pain may accompany thromboembolic occlusion of splenic blood flow. Vascular occlusion, with infarction and pain, is commonly seen in children with sickle cell crises. Rupture of the spleen, either from trauma or infiltrative disease that breaks the capsule, may result in intraperitoneal bleeding, shock, and death. The rupture itself may be painless.

A palpable spleen is the major *physical sign* produced by diseases affecting the spleen and suggests enlargement of the organ. The normal spleen is said to weigh less than 250 g, decreases in size with age, normally lies entirely within the rib cage, has a maximum cephalocaudad diameter of 13 cm by ultrasonography or maximum length of 12 cm and/or width of 7 cm by radionuclide scan, and is usually not palpable. However, a palpable spleen was found in 3% of 2200 asymptomatic, male, freshman college students. Follow-up at 3 years revealed that 30% of those students still had a palpable spleen without any increase in disease prevalence. Ten-year follow-up found no evidence for lymphoid malignancies. Furthermore, in some tropical countries (e.g., New Guinea) the incidence of splenomegaly may reach 60%. Thus, the presence of a palpable spleen does not always equate

with presence of disease. Even when disease is present, splenomegaly may not reflect the primary disease, but rather a reaction to it. For example, in patients with Hodgkin's disease, only two-thirds of the palpable spleens show involvement by the cancer.

Physical examination of the spleen utilizes primarily the techniques of palpation and percussion. Inspection may reveal a fullness in the LUQ that descends on inspiration, a finding associated with a massively enlarged spleen. Auscultation may reveal a venous hum or a friction rub.

Palpation can be accomplished by bimanual palpation, ballotment, and palpation from above (Middleton maneuver). For bimanual palpation, which is at least as reliable as the other techniques, the patient is supine with flexed knees. The examiner's left hand is placed on the lower rib cage and pulls the skin toward the costal margin, allowing the fingertips of the right hand to feel the tip of the spleen as it descends while the patient inspires slowly, smoothly, and deeply. Palpation is begun with the right hand in the left lower quadrant with gradual movement toward the left costal margin, thereby identifying the lower edge of a massively enlarged spleen. When the spleen tip is felt, the finding is recorded as centimeters below the left costal margin at some arbitrary point, i.e., 10 to 15 cm, from the midpoint of the umbilicus or the xiphisternal junction. This allows other examiners to compare findings or the initial examiner to determine changes in size over time. Bimanual palpation in the right lateral decubitus position adds nothing to the supine examination.

Percussion for splenic dullness is accomplished with any of three techniques described by Nixon, Castell, or Barkun:

1. *Nixon's method*: The patient is placed on the right side so that the spleen lies above the colon and stomach. Percussion begins at the lower level of pulmonary resonance in the posterior axillary line and proceeds diagonally along a perpendicular line toward the lower midanterior costal margin. The upper border of dullness is normally 6 to 8 cm above the costal margin. Dullness greater than 8 cm in an adult is presumed to indicate splenic enlargement.

2. *Castell's method*: With the patient supine, percussion in the lowest intercostal space in the anterior axillary line (8th or 9th) produces a resonant note if the spleen is normal in size. This is true during expiration or full inspiration. A dull percussion note on full inspiration suggests splenomegaly.

3. *Percussion of Traube's semilunar space*: The borders of Traube's space are the sixth rib superiorly, the left midaxillary line laterally, and the left costal margin inferiorly. The patient is supine with the left arm slightly abducted. During normal breathing, this space is percussed from medial to lateral margins, yielding a normal resonant sound. A dull percussion note suggests splenomegaly.

Studies comparing methods of percussion and palpation with a standard of ultrasonography or scintigraphy have revealed sensitivity of 56 to 71% for palpation and 59 to 82% for percussion. Reproducibility among examiners is better for palpation than percussion. Both techniques are less reliable in obese patients or patients who have just eaten. Thus, the physical examination techniques of palpation and percussion are imprecise at best. It has been suggested that the examiner perform percussion first and, if positive, proceed to palpation; if the spleen is palpable, then one can be reasonably confident that splenomegaly exists. However, not all LUQ masses are enlarged spleens; gastric or colon tumors and pancreatic or renal cysts or tumors can mimic splenomegaly.

The presence of an enlarged spleen can be more precisely determined, if necessary, by liver-spleen radionuclide scan, CT, MRI, or ultrasonography. The latter technique is the current procedure of choice for routine assessment of spleen size (normal = a maximum cephalocaudad diameter of 13 cm) because it has high sensitivity and specificity and is safe, noninvasive, quick, mobile, and less costly. Nuclear medicine scans are accurate, sensitive, and reliable but are costly, require greater time to generate data, and utilize immobile equipment. They have the advantage of demonstrating accessory

Table 63-2   Diseases Associated with Splenomegaly Grouped by Pathogenic Mechanism

ENLARGEMENT DUE TO INCREASED DEMAND FOR SPLENIC FUNCTION

Reticuloendothelial system hyperplasia (for removal of defective erythrocytes)
　Spherocytosis
　Early sickle cell anemia
　Ovalocytosis
　Thalassemia major
　Hemoglobinopathies
　Paroxysmal nocturnal hemoglobinuria
　Nutritional anemias
Immune hyperplasia
　Response to infection (viral, bacterial, fungal, parasitic)
　　Infectious mononucleosis
　　AIDS
　　Viral hepatitis
　　Cytomegalovirus
　　Subacute bacterial endocarditis
　　Bacterial septicemia
　　Congenital syphilis
　　Splenic abscess
　　Tuberculosis
　　Histoplasmosis
　　Malaria
　　Leishmaniasis
　　Trypanosomiasis
　　Ehrlichiosis
　Disordered immunoregulation
　　Rheumatoid arthritis (Felty's syndrome)
　　Systemic lupus erythematosus
　　Collagen vascular diseases
　　Serum sickness
　　Immune hemolytic anemias
　　Immune thrombocytopenias
　　Immune neutropenias
　　Drug reactions
　　Angioimmunoblastic lymphadenopathy
　　Sarcoidosis
　　Thyrotoxicosis (benign lymphoid hypertrophy)
　　Interleukin-2 therapy
Extramedullary hematopoiesis
　Myelofibrosis
　Marrow damage by toxins, radiation, strontium
　Marrow infiltration by tumors, leukemias, Gaucher's disease

ENLARGEMENT DUE TO ABNORMAL SPLENIC OR PORTAL BLOOD FLOW

Cirrhosis
Hepatic vein obstruction
Portal vein obstruction, intrahepatic or extrahepatic
Cavernous transformation of the portal vein
Splenic vein obstruction
Splenic artery aneurysm
Hepatic schistosomiasis
Congestive heart failure
Hepatic echinococcosis
Portal hypertension (any cause including the above): "Banti's disease"

INFILTRATION OF THE SPLEEN

Intracellular or extracellular depositions
　Amyloidosis
　Gaucher's disease
　Niemann-Pick disease
　Tangier disease
　Hurler's syndrome and other mucopolysaccharidoses
　Hyperlipidemias
Benign and malignant cellular infiltrations
　Leukemias (acute, chronic, lymphoid, myeloid, monocytic)
　Lymphomas
　Hodgkin's disease
　Myeloproliferative syndromes (e.g., polycythemia vera)
　Angiosarcomas
　Metastatic tumors (melanoma is most common)
　Eosinophilic granuloma
　Histiocytosis X
　Hamartomas
　Hemangiomas, fibromas, lymphangiomas
　Splenic cysts

UNKNOWN ETIOLOGY

Idiopathic splenomegaly
Berylliosis
Iron-deficiency anemia

The differential diagnostic possibilities are much fewer when the spleen is "massively enlarged," that is, it is palpable more than 8 cm below the left costal margin or its drained weight is ≥1000 g (Table 63-3). The vast majority of such patients will have non-Hodgkin's lymphoma, chronic lymphocytic leukemia, hairy cell leukemia, chronic myelogenous leukemia, myelofibrosis with myeloid metaplasia, or polycythemia vera.

Laboratory Assessment　The major laboratory abnormalities accompanying splenomegaly are determined by the underlying systemic illness. Erythrocyte counts may be normal, decreased (thalassemia major syndromes, SLE, cirrhosis with portal hypertension), or increased (polycythemia vera). Granulocyte counts may be normal, decreased (Felty's syndrome, congestive splenomegaly, leukemias), or increased (infections or inflammatory disease, myeloproliferative disorders). Similarly, the platelet count may be normal, decreased when there is enhanced sequestration or destruction of platelets in an enlarged spleen (congestive splenomegaly, Gaucher's disease, immune thrombocytopenia), or increased in the myeloproliferative disorders such as polycythemia vera.

The complete blood count may reveal cytopenia of one or more blood cell types, which should suggest *hypersplenism*. This condition is characterized by splenomegaly, cytopenia(s), normal or hyperplastic bone marrow, and a response to splenectomy. The latter characteristic is less precise because reversal of cytopenia, particularly granulocytopenia, is sometimes not sustained after splenectomy. The cytopenias result from increased destruction of the cellular elements secondary to reduced flow of blood through enlarged and congested cords (congestive splenomegaly) or to immune-mediated mechanisms. In hypersplenism, various cell types usually have normal morphology on the peripheral blood smear, although the red cells may be spherocytic due to loss of surface area during their longer transit through the enlarged spleen. The increased marrow production of red cells should be reflected as an increased reticulocyte production index, although the value may be less than expected due to increased sequestration of reticulocytes in the spleen.

The need for additional laboratory studies is dictated by the differential diagnosis of the underlying illness of which splenomegaly is a manifestation.

splenic tissue. CT and MRI provide accurate determination of spleen size, but the equipment is immobile and the procedures are expensive. MRI appears to offer no advantage over CT. Changes in spleen structure such as mass lesions, infarcts, inhomogeneous infiltrates, and cysts are more readily assessed by CT, MRI, or ultrasonography. None of these techniques is very reliable in the detection of patchy infiltration (e.g., Hodgkin's disease).

Differential Diagnosis　Many of the diseases associated with splenomegaly are listed in Table 63-2. They are grouped according to the presumed basic mechanisms responsible for organ enlargement:

1. Hyperplasia or hypertrophy related to a particular splenic function such as reticuloendothelial hyperplasia (work hypertrophy) in diseases such as hereditary spherocytosis or thalassemia syndromes that require removal of large numbers of defective red blood cells; immune hyperplasia in response to systemic infection (infectious mononucleosis, subacute bacterial endocarditis) or to immunologic diseases (immune thrombocytopenia, SLE, Felty's syndrome).

2. Passive congestion due to decreased blood flow from the spleen in conditions that produce portal hypertension (cirrhosis, Budd-Chiari syndrome, congestive heart failure).

3. Infiltrative diseases of the spleen (lymphomas, metastatic cancer, amyloidosis, Gaucher's disease, myeloproliferative disorders with extramedullary hematopoiesis).

Table 63-3   Diseases Associated with Massive Splenomegaly*[a]*

Chronic myelogenous leukemia	Gaucher's disease
Lymphomas	Chronic lymphocytic leukemia
Hairy cell leukemia	Sarcoidosis
Myelofibrosis with myeloid metaplasia	Autoimmune hemolytic anemia
Polycythemia vera	Diffuse splenic hemangiomatosis

[a] The spleen extends greater than 8 cm below left costal margin and/or weighs more than 1000 g.

Splenectomy is infrequently performed for diagnostic purposes, especially in the absence of clinical illness or other diagnostic tests that suggest underlying disease. More often splenectomy is performed for staging the extent of disease in patients with Hodgkin's disease, for symptom control in patients with massive splenomegaly, for disease control in patients with traumatic splenic rupture, or for correction of cytopenias in patients with hypersplenism or immune-mediated destruction of one or more cellular blood elements. Splenectomy is necessary for routine staging of patients with Hodgkin's disease only in those with clinical stage I or II disease in whom radiation therapy alone is contemplated as the treatment. Noninvasive staging of the spleen in Hodgkin's disease is not a sufficiently reliable basis for treatment decisions because one-third of normal-sized spleens will be involved with Hodgkin's disease and one-third of enlarged spleens will be tumor-free. Although splenectomy in chronic myelogenous leukemia does not affect the natural history of disease, removal of the massive spleen usually makes patients significantly more comfortable and simplifies their management by significantly reducing transfusion requirements. Splenectomy is an effective secondary or tertiary treatment for two chronic B cell leukemias, hairy cell leukemia and prolymphocytic leukemia, and for the very rare splenic mantle cell or marginal zone lymphoma. Splenectomy in these diseases may be associated with significant tumor regression in bone marrow and other sites of disease. Similar regressions of systemic disease have been noted after splenic irradiation in some types of lymphoproliferative disease, especially chronic lymphocytic leukemia and prolymphocytic leukemia. This has been termed the *abscopal effect*. Such systemic tumor responses to local therapy directed at the spleen suggest that there may be some hormone or growth factor produced by the spleen that affects tumor cell proliferation, but this conjecture is not yet substantiated. The most common indication for splenectomy is traumatic or iatrogenic splenic rupture. In a fraction of patients with splenic rupture, peritoneal seeding of splenic fragments can lead to splenosis—the presence of multiple rests of spleen tissue not connected to the portal circulation. This ectopic spleen tissue may cause pain or gastrointestinal obstruction, as in endometriosis. A large number of hematologic, immunologic, and congestive causes of splenomegaly can lead to destruction of one or more cellular blood elements. In the majority of such cases, splenectomy can correct the cytopenias, particularly anemia and thrombocytopenia. Perhaps the only contraindication to splenectomy is the presence of marrow failure, in which the enlarged spleen is the only source of hematopoietic tissue.

The absence of the spleen has minimal long-term effects on the hematologic profile. In the immediate postsplenectomy period, there may be some leukocytosis (up to 25,000/μL) and thrombocytosis (up to $1 \times 10^6/\mu$L), but within 2 to 3 weeks, blood cell counts and survival of each cell lineage are usually normal. The chronic manifestations of splenectomy are marked variation in size and shape of erythrocytes (anisocytosis, poikilocytosis) and the presence of Howell-Jolly bodies (nuclear remnants), Heinz bodies (denatured hemoglobin), basophilic stippling, and an occasional nucleated erythrocyte in the peripheral blood. When such erythrocyte abnormalities appear in a patient whose spleen has not been removed, one should suspect splenic infiltration by tumor that has interfered with its normal culling and pitting function.

The most serious consequence of splenectomy is increased susceptibility to bacterial infections, particularly those with capsules such as *Streptococcus pneumoniae*, *Haemophilus influenzae*, and some gram-negative enteric organisms. Patients under age 20 years are particularly susceptible to overwhelming sepsis with *S. pneumoniae*, and the overall actuarial risk of sepsis in patients who have had their spleens removed is about 7% in 10 years. The case-fatality rate for pneumococcal sepsis in splenectomized patients is 50 to 80%. About

25% of patients without spleens will develop a serious infection at some time in their life. The frequency is highest within the first 3 years after splenectomy. About 15% of the infections are polymicrobial, and lung, skin, and blood are the most common sites. No increased risk of viral infection has been noted in patients who have no spleen. The susceptibility to bacterial infections relates to the inability to remove opsonized bacteria from the bloodstream and a defect in making antibodies to T cell–independent antigens such as the polysaccharide components of bacterial capsules. Pneumococcal vaccine (23-valent polysaccharide vaccine) should be administered to all patients 2 weeks before elective splenectomy. The Advisory Committee on Immunization Practices recommends that even splenectomized patients receive pneumococcal vaccine with a repeat vaccination 5 years later. Efficacy has not been proven in this setting, and the recommendation discounts the possibility that administration of the vaccine may actually lower the titer of specific pneumococcal antibodies. A more effective pneumococcal vaccine that involves T cells in the response is in development. The vaccine to *H. influenzae* should also be given to patients in whom elective splenectomy is planned. No other vaccines are routinely recommended in this setting.

Splenectomized patients should be educated to consider any unexplained fever as a medical emergency. Prompt medical attention with evaluation and treatment of suspected bacteremia may be life-saving. Routine chemoprophylaxis with oral penicillin can result in the emergence of drug-resistant strains and is not recommended.

In addition to an increased susceptibility to bacterial infections, splenectomized patients are also more susceptible to the parasitic disease babesiosis. The splenectomized patient should avoid areas where the parasite *Babesia* is endemic (e.g., Cape Cod, MA).

Surgical removal of the spleen is an obvious cause of *hyposplenism*. Patients with sickle cell disease often suffer from autosplenectomy as a result of splenic destruction by the numerous infarcts associated with sickle cell crises during childhood. Indeed, the presence of a palpable spleen in a patient with sickle cell disease after age 5 suggests a coexisting hemoglobinopathy, e.g., thalassemia or hemoglobin C. In addition, patients who receive splenic irradiation for a neoplastic or autoimmune disease are also functionally hyposplenic. The term *hyposplenism* is preferred to *asplenism* in referring to the physiologic consequences of splenectomy because asplenia is a rare, specific, and fatal congenital abnormality in which there is a failure of the left side of the coelomic cavity (which includes the splenic anlagen) to develop normally. Infants with asplenia have no spleens, but that is the least of their problems. The right side of the developing embryo is duplicated on the left so there is liver where the spleen should be, there are two right lungs, and the heart comprises two right atria and two right ventricles.

BIBLIOGRAPHY

BARKUN AN et al: The bedside assessment of splenic enlargement. Am J Med 91:512, 1991

GRAVES SA et al: Does this patient have splenomegaly? JAMA 270:2218, 1993

KAJI A et al: Imaging of cervical adenopathy. Semin Ultrasound CT MRI 18:220, 1997

MCINTYRE OR, EBAUGH FG JR: Palpable spleens: Ten year follow-up. Ann Intern Med 90:130, 1979

PANGALIS GA et al: Clinical approach to lymphadenopathy. Semin Oncol 20:570, 1993

PREVENTION OF PNEUMOCOCCAL DISEASE: Recommendations of the Advisory Committee on Immunization Practices. MMWR 46(RR-8):1, 1997

SLAP GB et al: Validation of a model to identify young patients for lymph node biopsy. JAMA 255:2768, 1986

STEINKAMP HJ et al: Cervical lymphadenopathy: Ratio of long- to short-axis diameter as a predictor of malignancy. Br J Radiol 68:266, 1995

WILLIAMSON HA JR: Lymphadenopathy in a family practice: A descriptive study of 240 cases. J Fam Pract 20:449, 1985

64   *Steven M. Holland, John I. Gallin*

DISORDERS OF GRANULOCYTES AND MONOCYTES

Leukocytes are the major cells comprising inflammatory and immune responses and include neutrophils, T and B lymphocytes, natural killer (NK) cells, monocytes, eosinophils, and basophils. These cells have specific functions, such as antibody production by B lymphocytes or destruction of bacteria by neutrophils, but in no single infectious disease is the exact role of the cell types completely established. Thus, whereas neutrophils are classically thought to be critical to host defense against bacteria, they may also play important roles in defense against viral infections.

The blood delivers leukocytes to the various tissues from the bone marrow, where they are produced. Normal blood leukocyte counts are given in the Appendix (Tables A-7 and A-8). The various leukocytes are derived from a common stem cell in the bone marrow. Three-fourths of the nucleated cells of bone marrow are committed to the production of leukocytes. Leukocyte maturation in the marrow is under the regulatory control of a number of different factors, known as colony stimulating factors and interleukins (Chap. 104). Because an alteration in the number and type of leukocytes is often associated with disease processes, total white blood count (WBC) (cells per microliter) and differential counts are informative. The lymphocytes and basophils are discussed in Chaps. 305 and 310, respectively. This chapter focuses on the neutrophils, monocytes, and eosinophils.

NEUTROPHILS

MATURATION Important events in neutrophil life are summarized in Fig. 64-1. In normal humans, neutrophils are produced only in the bone marrow. The minimum number of stem cells necessary to support hematopoiesis is estimated to be 400 to 500. Human blood monocytes, tissue macrophages, and stromal cells produce colony stimulating factors, hormones required for the growth of monocytes and neutrophils in the bone marrow. The hematopoietic system not only produces enough neutrophils ($\sim 1.3 \times 10^{11}$ cells per 80-kg person

per day) to carry out physiologic functions but also has a large reserve stored in the marrow which can be mobilized in response to inflammation or infection. An increase in the number of blood neutrophils is called neutrophilia, and the presence of immature cells is termed a shift to the left. A decrease in the number of blood neutrophils is called neutropenia.

Neutrophils and monocytes evolve from pluripotent stem cells under the influence of cytokines and colony stimulating factors (Fig. 64-2). The proliferation phase through the metamyelocyte takes about 1 week, while the maturation phase from metamyelocyte to mature neutrophil takes another week. The myeloblast is the first recognizable precursor cell and is followed by the *promyelocyte* (**Plate V-23**). The promyelocyte evolves when the classic lysosomal granules, called the *primary* or *azurophil granules*, are produced. The primary granules contain hydrolases, elastase, myeloperoxidase, cationic proteins, and bactericidal/permeability-increasing protein, which is important for killing gram-negative bacteria. Azurophil granules also contain *defensins*, a family of cysteine-rich polypeptides with broad antimicrobial activity against bacteria, fungi, and certain enveloped viruses. The promyelocyte divides to produce the *myelocyte*, a cell responsible for the synthesis of the *specific* or *secondary granules* which contain unique (specific) constituents such as lactoferrin, vitamin B_{12}–binding proteins, membrane components of the nicotinamide-adenine dinucleotide phosphate (NADPH) oxidase required for hydrogen peroxide production, histaminase, and receptors for certain chemoattractants and adherence-promoting factors (CR3) as well as receptors for the basement membrane component, laminin. The secondary granules do not contain acid hydrolases and therefore are not classic lysosomes. Packaging of secondary granule contents during myelopoiesis is controlled by CCAAT/enhancer binding protein-ε. Secondary granule contents are readily released extracellularly, and their mobilization is important in modulating inflammation. During the final stages of maturation no cell division occurs, and the cell passes through the *metamyelocyte* stage and then to the *band* neutrophil with a sausage-shaped nucleus (**Plate V-35**). As the band cell matures, the nucleus assumes a lobulated configuration. The nucleus of neutrophils normally contains up to four segments. Excessive segmentation (more than five nuclear lobes) may be a manifestation of folate or vitamin B_{12} deficiency (**Plate V-38**). The Pelger-Hüet anomaly (**Plate V-34B**), an infrequent dominant benign inherited trait, results in neutrophils with distinctive bilobed nuclei that must be distinguished from band forms.

The physiologic role of the multilobed nucleus of neutrophils is unknown, but it may allow great deformation of neutrophils during migration into tissues at sites of inflammation.

In severe acute bacterial infection, prominent neutrophil cytoplasmic granules called *toxic granulations* are occasionally seen (**Plate V-11**). Toxic granulations are immature or abnormally staining azurophil granules. Cytoplasmic inclusions, also called *Döhle bodies* (**Plate V-35**), can be seen during infection and are fragments of ribosome-rich endoplasmic reticulum. Large neutrophil vacuoles are often present in acute bacterial infection and probably represent pinocytosed (internalized) membrane.

Neutrophils are heterogeneous in function. Monoclonal antibodies have been developed that recognize only a subset of mature neutrophils. The meaning of neutrophil heterogeneity is not known.

MARROW RELEASE AND CIRCULATING COMPARTMENTS Specific signals, including interleukin (IL) 1, tumor necrosis factor-α (TNF-α), the colony stimulating factors, complement fragment C3e, and perhaps other cytokines mobilize leukocytes

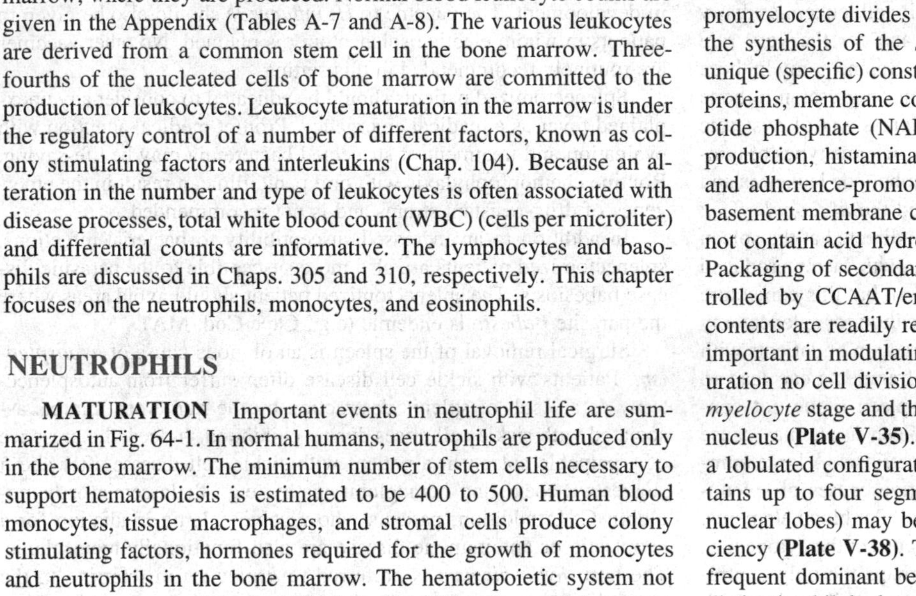

FIGURE 64-1 Schematic events in neutrophil production, recruitment, and inflammation. The four cardinal signs of inflammation (rubor, tumor, calor, dolor) are indicated as are the interactions of neutrophils with other cells and cytokines. PMN, polymorphonuclear leukocytes; G-CSF, granulocyte colony stimulating factor; IL, interleukin; TNF-α, tumor necrosis factor.

from the bone marrow and deliver them to the blood in an unstimulated state. Under normal conditions, about 90% of the neutrophil pool is in the bone marrow, 2 to 3% in the circulation, and the remainder in the tissues (Fig. 64-3).

The circulating pool exists in two dynamic compartments: one freely flowing and one marginated. The freely flowing pool is about one-half the neutrophils in the basal state and is composed of those cells that are in the blood and not in contact with the endothelium. Marginated leukocytes are those that are in close physical contact with the endothelium (Fig. 64-4). In the pulmonary circulation, where an extensive capillary bed (~1000 capillaries per alveolus) exists, margination occurs because the capillaries are about the same size as a mature neutrophil. Therefore, neutrophil fluidity and deformability are necessary to make the transit through the pulmonary bed. Increased neutrophil rigidity and decreased deformability lead to augmented neutrophil trapping and margination in the lung. In contrast, in the systemic postcapillary venules, margination is mediated by the interaction of specific cell-surface molecules. *Selectins* are glycoproteins expressed on neutrophils and endothelial cells, among others, that cause a low-affinity interaction, resulting in "rolling" of the neutrophil along the endothelial surface. On neutrophils, the molecule L-selectin [cluster determinant (CD) 62L] binds to glycosylated proteins on endothelial cells [e.g., glycosylation-dependent cell adhesion molecule (GlyCAM1) and CD34]. Glycoproteins on neutrophils, most importantly sialyl-Lewis^x (SLe^x, CD15s), are targets for binding of selectins expressed on endothelial cells [E-selectin (CD62E) and P-selectin (CD62P)] and other leukocytes. In response to chemotactic stimuli from injured tissues (e.g., complement product C5a, leukotriene B$_4$, IL-8) or bacterial products [e.g., N-formylmethionyl-leucylphenylalanine (f-metleuphe)], neutrophil adhesiveness increases, and the cells "stick" to the endothelium through *integrins*. The integrins are leukocyte glycoproteins that exist as complexes of a common CD18 β-chain with CD11a (LFA-1), CD11b (also called either Mac-1, CR3, or the C3bi receptor), and CD11c (p150,95). CD11a/CD18 and CD11b/CD18 bind to specific endothelial receptors [intercellular adhesion molecules (ICAM) 1 and 2].

On cell stimulation, L-selectin is shed; receptors for chemoattractants and opsonins are mobilized; the phagocytes orient toward the chemoattractant source in the extravascular space, increase their motile activity (chemokinesis), and migrate directionally (chemotaxis) into tissues. The process of migration into tissues is called *diapedesis* and involves the crawling of neutrophils between postcapillary endothelial cells that open junctions between adjacent cells to permit leukocyte passage. Diapedesis involves platelet/endothelial cell adhesion molecule (PECAM) 1 (CD31), which is expressed on both the emigrating leukocyte and the endothelial cells. The endothelial responses (increased blood flow from increased vasodilation and permeability) are mediated by anaphylatoxins (e.g., C3a and C5a) as well as vasodilators such as histamine, bradykinin, serotonin, nitric oxide, vascular endothelial growth factor (VEGF), and prostaglandins E and I. Cytokines regulate some of these processes [e.g., TNF-α induction of VEGF, interferon (IFN) γ inhibition of prostaglandin E].

In the healthy adult, most neutrophils leave the body by migration through the mucous membrane of the gastrointestinal tract. Normally, neutrophils spend a short time in the circulation (half-life, 6 to 7 h).

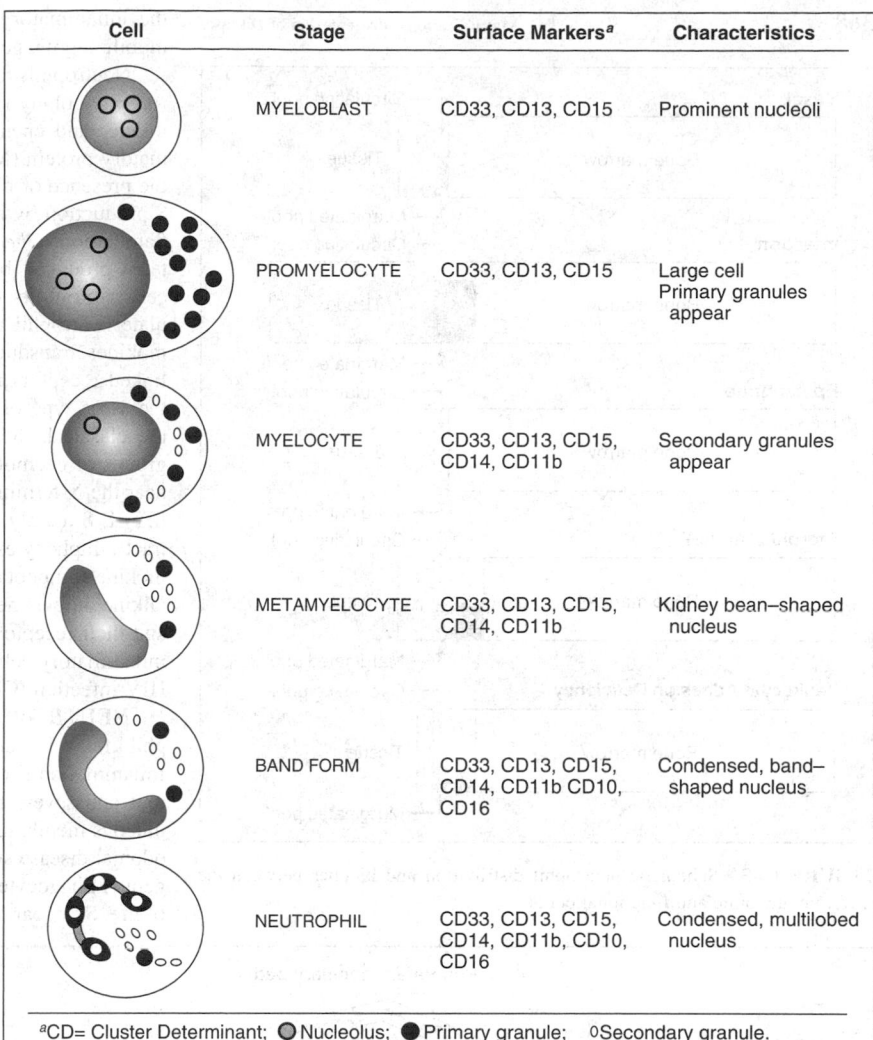

Cell	Stage	Surface Markers[a]	Characteristics
	MYELOBLAST	CD33, CD13, CD15	Prominent nucleoli
	PROMYELOCYTE	CD33, CD13, CD15	Large cell Primary granules appear
	MYELOCYTE	CD33, CD13, CD15, CD14, CD11b	Secondary granules appear
	METAMYELOCYTE	CD33, CD13, CD15, CD14, CD11b	Kidney bean–shaped nucleus
	BAND FORM	CD33, CD13, CD15, CD14, CD11b CD10, CD16	Condensed, band–shaped nucleus
	NEUTROPHIL	CD33, CD13, CD15, CD14, CD11b, CD10, CD16	Condensed, multilobed nucleus

[a]CD= Cluster Determinant; ⦿ Nucleolus; ● Primary granule; ○ Secondary granule.

FIGURE 64-2 Stages of neutrophil development are schematically shown. G-CSF and GM-CSF are critical to this process. Identifying cellular characteristics and specific cell-surface markers are listed for each maturational stage.

Senescent neutrophils are cleared from the circulation by macrophages in the lung and spleen. Once in the tissues, neutrophils release enzymes, such as collagenase and elastase, that help establish abscess cavities. Neutrophils ingest pathogenic materials that have been opsonized by IgG and C3b. Fibronectin and the tetrapeptide tuftsin facilitate phagocytosis.

With phagocytosis comes a burst of oxygen consumption and activation of the hexose-monophosphate shunt. A membrane-associated NADPH oxidase, consisting of membrane and cytosolic components, is assembled and catalyzes the reduction of oxygen to superoxide anion, which is then converted to hydrogen peroxide and other toxic oxygen products (e.g., hydroxyl radical). Hydrogen peroxide + chloride + neutrophil myeloperoxidase generates hypochlorous acid (bleach), hypochlorite, and chlorine. These products oxidize and halogenate microorganisms and tumor cells and, when uncontrolled, can damage host tissue. Strongly cationic proteins, defensins, and probably nitric oxide also participate in microbial killing. Other enzymes, such as lysozyme and acid proteases, help digest microbial debris. After 1 to 4 days in tissues neutrophils die. The apoptosis of neutrophils is also cytokine regulated; granulocyte colony stimulating factor (G-CSF) and IFN-γ prevent their death. Under certain conditions, such as in delayed-type hypersensitivity, monocyte accumulation occurs within 6 to 12 h of initiation of inflammation. Neutrophils, monocytes, microorganisms in various states of digestion, and altered local tissue cells make up the inflammatory exudate, pus. Myeloperoxidase confers the characteristic green color to pus and may participate in turning off

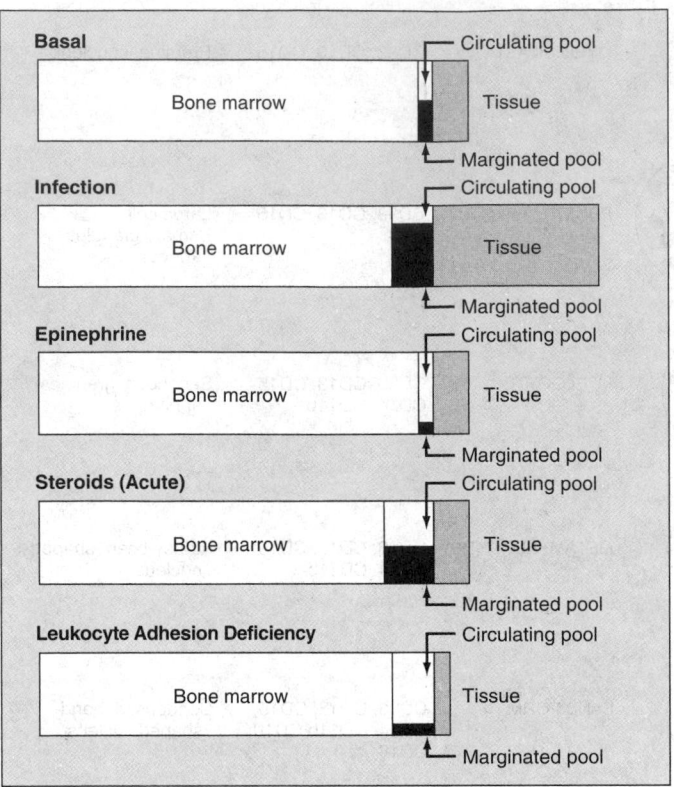

FIGURE 64-3 Schematic neutrophil distribution and kinetics between the different anatomic and functional pools.

the inflammatory process by inactivating chemoattractants and immobilizing phagocytic cells.

Neutrophils respond to certain cytokines [IFN-γ, granulocyte-macrophage colony stimulating factor (GM-CSF), IL-8] and produce cytokines and chemotactic signals [TNF-α, IL-8, macrophage inflammatory protein (MIP) 1] that modulate the inflammatory response. In the presence of fibrinogen, f-metleuphe or leukotriene B$_4$ induces IL-8 production by neutrophils, providing autocrine amplification of inflammation. *Chemokines* (*chemo*attractant cyto*kines*) are small proteins produced by many different cell types, including endothelial cells, fibroblasts, epithelial cells, neutrophils, and monocytes, that regulate neutrophil and monocyte recruitment and activation. The chemokines transduce their signals through heterotrimeric G protein–linked receptors that have seven cell membrane–spanning domains, the same type of cell-surface receptor that mediates the response to the classical chemoattractants *N*-f-metleuphe and C5a. Four major groups of chemokines are recognized based on the cysteine structure near the N terminus: C, CC, CXC, and CXXXC. The CXC cytokines like IL-8 mainly attract neutrophils; CC chemokines like MIP-1α attract lymphocytes, monocytes, eosinophils, and basophils; the C chemokine lymphotactin is T cell tropic; the CXXXC chemokine fractalkine attracts neutrophils, monocytes, and T cells. These molecules and their receptors not only regulate the trafficking and activation of inflammatory cells, but chemokine receptors serve as co-receptors for HIV infection (Chap. 309).

NEUTROPHIL ABNORMALITIES A defect in the neutrophil life cycle can lead to dysfunction and compromised host defenses. Inflammation is often depressed, and the clinical result is often recurrent and severe bacterial and fungal infections. Aphthous ulcers of mucous membranes (gray ulcers without pus) and gingivitis and periodontal disease suggest a phagocytic cell disorder. Patients with congenital phagocyte defects can have infections within the first few days of life. Skin, ear, upper and lower respiratory tract, and bone infections are common. Sepsis and meningitis are rare. In some disorders the frequency of infection is variable, and patients can go for months or even years without major infection. Aggressive management of these congenital diseases has extended the life span of patients beyond 30 years.

Neutropenia The consequences of absent neutrophils are dramatic. Susceptibility to infectious diseases increases sharply when neutrophil counts fall below 1000 cells/μL. When the absolute neutrophil count (ANC; band forms and mature neutrophils combined) falls below 500 cells/μL, control of endogenous microbial flora (e.g., mouth, gut) is impaired; when the ANC is < 200/μL, the inflammatory process is absent. Neutropenia can be due to depressed production, increased peripheral destruction, or excessive peripheral pooling. A falling neutrophil count or a significant decrease in the number of neutrophils below steady state levels, together with a failure to increase neutrophil counts in the setting of infection or other challenge, requires investigation. Acute neutropenia, such as that caused by cancer chemotherapy, is more likely to be associated with increased risk of infection than neutropenia of long duration (months to years) that reverses in response to

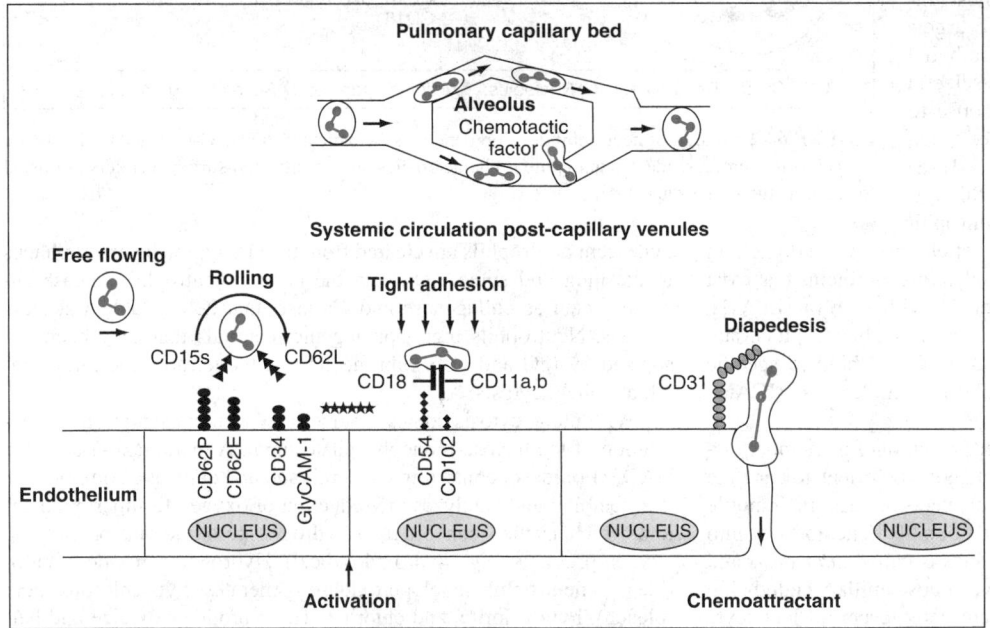

FIGURE 64-4 Neutrophil travel through the pulmonary capillaries is dependent on neutrophil deformability. Neutrophil rigidity (e.g., caused by C5a) enhances pulmonary trapping and response to pulmonary pathogens in a way that is not so dependent upon cell-surface receptors. Intraalveolar chemotactic factors, such as those caused by certain bacteria (e.g., *Streptococcus pneumoniae*) lead to diapedesis of neutrophils from the pulmonary capillaries into the alveolar space. Neutrophil interaction with the endothelium of the systemic postcapillary venules is dependent on molecules of attachment. The neutrophil "rolls" along the endothelium using selectins: neutrophil CD15s (sialyl-Lewis^x) binds to CD62E (E-selectin) and CD62P (P-selectin) on endothelial cells; CD62L (L-selectin) on neutrophils binds to CD34 and other molecules (e.g., GlyCAM-1) expressed on endothelium. Chemokines or other activation factors stimulate integrin-mediated "tight adhesion": CD11a/CD18 (LFA-1) and CD11b/CD18 (Mac-1, CR3) bind to CD54 (ICAM-1) and CD102(ICAM-2) on the endothelium. Diapedesis occurs between endothelial cells: CD31 (PECAM-1) expressed by the emigrating neutrophil interacts with CD31 expressed at the endothelial cell-cell junction.

infection or carefully controlled administration of endotoxin (see "Laboratory Diagnosis," below).

64 Disorders of Granulocytes and Monocytes **369**

Some causes of inherited and acquired neutropenia are listed in Table 64-1. The most common neutropenias are iatrogenic, resulting from the use of cytotoxic or immunosuppressive therapies for malignancy or control of autoimmune disorders. These drugs cause neutropenia because they result in decreased production of rapidly growing progenitor (stem) cells of the marrow. Certain antibiotics such as chloramphenicol, trimethoprim-sulfamethoxazole, flucytosine, vidarabine, and the antiretroviral drug zidovudine may cause neutropenia by inhibiting proliferation of myeloid precursors. The marrow suppression is generally dose-related and dependent on continued administration of the drug. Recombinant human G-CSF reverses this form of neutropenia.

Another important mechanism for iatrogenic neutropenia is the effect of drugs that serve as immune haptens and sensitize neutrophils or neutrophil precursors to immune-mediated peripheral destruction. This form of drug-induced neutropenia can be seen within 7 days of exposure to the drug; with previous drug exposure, resulting in pre-existing antibodies, neutropenia may occur a few hours after administration of the drug. Although any drug can cause this form of neutropenia, the most frequent causes are commonly used antibiotics, such as sulfa-containing compounds, penicillins, and cephalosporins. Fever and eosinophilia also may be associated drug reactions, but often these signs are not present. Drug-induced neutropenia can be severe, but discontinuation of the sensitizing drug is sufficient for recovery, which is usually seen within 5 to 7 days and is complete by 10 days. Readministration of the sensitizing drug should be avoided, since abrupt neutropenia often will result. For this reason, diagnostic challenge should be avoided.

Autoimmune neutropenias caused by circulating antineutrophil antibodies are another form of acquired neutropenia that results in increased destruction of neutrophils. Acquired neutropenia also may be seen with viral infections, including infection with HIV. Acquired neutropenia may be cyclic in nature, occurring at intervals of several weeks. Acquired cyclic or stable neutropenia may be associated with an expansion of large granular lymphocytes (LGL), which may be T cells, NK cells, or NK-like cells. Patients with LGL lymphocytosis may have moderate blood and bone marrow lymphocytosis, neutropenia, polyclonal hypergammaglobulinemia, splenomegaly, rheumatoid arthritis, and absence of lymphadenopathy. Such patients may have a chronic and relatively stable course. Recurrent bacterial infections are frequent. Benign and malignant forms of this syndrome oc-

cur. In some patients, a spontaneous regression has occurred even after 11 years, suggesting an immunoregulatory defect as the basis for at least one form of the disorder. Glucocorticoids, cyclosporine, IFN-α, and nucleosides such as 2-chlorodeoxyadenosine each have induced remission.

Hereditary Neutropenias Hereditary neutropenias are rare and may manifest in early childhood as a profound constant neutropenia or agranulocytosis. Congenital forms of neutropenia include Kostmann's syndrome (neutrophil count $<100/\mu L$), which is often fatal; more benign chronic idiopathic neutropenia (neutrophil count of 300 to $1500/\mu L$); the cartilage-hair hypoplasia syndrome; Shwachman's syndrome associated with pancreatic insufficiency; myelokathexis, a congenital disorder characterized by neutrophil degeneration, hypersegmentation, and myeloid hyperplasia in the marrow associated with decreased expression of bcl-X_L in myeloid precursors and accelerated apoptosis; and neutropenias associated with other immune defects (X-linked agammaglobulinemia, ataxia telangiectasia, IgA deficiency). Mutations in the G-CSF receptor on chromosome 1 associated with poor response to G-CSF can occur with severe congenital neutropenia and predispose to myeloid malignancy. Hereditary cyclic neutropenia, an autosomal dominant trait, may occur in infancy and is characterized by a remarkably regular 3-week cycle. Hereditary cyclic neutropenia actually is cyclic hematopoiesis, due to mutations in the neutrophil elastase gene. Glucocorticoids and G-CSF blunt the cycling in some patients.

Maternal factors can be associated with neutropenia in the newborn. Transplacental transfer of IgG directed against antigens on fetal neutrophils can result in peripheral destruction. Drugs (e.g., thiazides) ingested during pregnancy can cause neutropenia in the newborn by either depressed production or peripheral destruction.

The presence of immunoglobulin directed toward neutrophils is seen in Felty's syndrome—a triad of rheumatoid arthritis, splenomegaly, and neutropenia (Chap. 312). Patients with Felty's syndrome who respond to splenectomy with an increase in their neutrophil count also have lower postoperative serum neutrophil-binding IgG. Some of these patients have neutropenia associated with an increased number of LGL. Splenomegaly with peripheral trapping and destruction of neutrophils is also seen in lysosomal storage diseases and in portal hypertension.

Neutrophilia Neutrophilia results from increased neutrophil production, increased marrow release, or defective margination (Table 64-2). The most important acute cause of neutrophilia is infection.

Table 64-1 Causes of Neutropenia

Decreased Production
Drug-induced—alkylating agents (nitrogen mustard, busulfan, chlorambucil, cyclophosphamide); antimetabolites (methotrexate, 6-mercaptopurine, 5-flucytosine); noncytotoxic agents [antibiotics (chloramphenicol, penicillins, sulfonamides), phenothiazines, tranquilizers (meprobamate), anticonvulsants (carbamazepine), antipsychotics (clozapine), certain diuretics, anti-inflammatory agents, antithyroid drugs, many others]
Hematologic diseases—idiopathic, cyclic neutropenia, Chédiak-Higashi syndrome, aplastic anemia, infantile genetic disorders (see text)
Tumor invasion, myelofibrosis
Nutritional deficiency—vitamin B_{12}, folate (especially alcoholics)
Infection—tuberculosis, typhoid fever, brucellosis, tularemia, measles, infectious mononucleosis, malaria, viral hepatitis, leishmaniasis, AIDS
Peripheral Destruction
Antineutrophil antibodies and/or splenic or lung (alveolar macrophage) trapping
Autoimmune disorders—Felty's syndrome, rheumatoid arthritis, lupus erythematosus
Drugs as haptens—aminopyrine, α-methyl dopa, phenylbutazone, mercurial diuretics, some phenothiazines
Wegener's granulomatosis
Peripheral Pooling (Transient Neutropenia)
Overwhelming bacterial infection (acute endotoxemia)
Hemodialysis
Cardiopulmonary bypass

Table 64-2 Causes of Neutrophilia

Increased Production
  Idiopathic
  Drug-induced—glucocorticoids
  Infection—bacterial, fungal, rarely viral
  Inflammation—thermal injury, tissue necrosis, myocardial and pulmonary infarction, hypersensitivity states, collagen vascular diseases
  Myeloproliferative diseases—myelocytic leukemia, myeloid metaplasia, polycythemia vera
Increased Marrow Release
  Glucocorticoids
  Acute infection (endotoxin)
  Inflammation—thermal injury
Defective Margination
  Drugs—epinephrine, glucocorticoids, nonsteroidal anti-inflammatory agents
  Stress, excitement, vigorous exercise
  Leukocyte adhesion deficiency type 1 (integrin β chain, CD18); leukocyte adhesion deficiency type 2 (selectin ligand, CD15s, sialyl-Lewis^x)
Miscellaneous
  Metabolic disorders—ketoacidosis, acute renal failure, eclampsia, acute poisoning
  Drugs—lithium
  Other—metastatic carcinoma, acute hemorrhage or hemolysis

Table 64-3 Types of Granulocyte and Monocyte Disorders

Function	Cause of Indicated Dysfunction		
	Drug-Induced	Acquired	Inherited
Adherence-aggregation	Aspirin, colchicine, alcohol, glucocorticoids, ibuprofen, piroxicam	Neonatal state, hemodialysis	Leukoctye adhesion deficiency types 1 and 2
Deformability		Leukemia, neonatal state, diabetes mellitus, immature neutrophils	
Chemokinesis-chemotaxis	Glucocorticoids (high dose), auranofin, colchicine (weak effect), phenylbutazone, naproxen, indomethacin, interleukin 2	Thermal injury, malignancy, malnutrition, periodontal disease, neonatal state, systemic lupus erythematosus, rheumatoid arthritis, diabetes mellitus, sepsis, influenza virus infection, herpes simplex virus infection, acrodermatitis enteropathica, AIDS	Chédiak-Higashi syndrome, neutrophil-specific granule deficiency, hyper IgE–recurrent infection (Job's) syndrome (in some patients), Down syndrome, α-mannosidase deficiency, severe combined immunodeficiency, Wiskott-Aldrich syndrome
Microbicidal activity	Colchicine, cyclophosphamide, glucocorticoids (high dose)	Leukemia, aplastic anemia, certain neutropenias, tuftsin deficiency, thermal injury, sepsis, neonatal state, diabetes mellitus, malnutrition, AIDS	Chédiak-Higashi syndrome, neutrophil-specific granule deficiency, chronic granulomatous disease, interferon γ receptor deficiency, IL-12 receptor deficiency, IL-12 deficiency

Neutrophilia from acute infection represents both increased production and increased marrow release. Increased production is also associated with chronic inflammation and certain myeloproliferative diseases. Increased marrow release and mobilization of the marginated leukocyte pool are induced by glucocorticoids. Release of epinephrine, as with vigorous exercise, excitement, or stress, will demarginate neutrophils in the spleen and lungs and double the neutrophil count in minutes. Leukocytosis with cell counts of 10,000 to 25,000/μL occurs in response to infection and other forms of acute inflammation and results from both release of the marginated pool and mobilization of marrow reserves. Persistent neutrophilia with cell counts of 30,000 to 50,000/μL or higher is called a *leukemoid reaction*, a term often used to distinguish this degree of neutrophilia from leukemia. In a leukemoid reaction, the circulating neutrophils are usually mature and not clonally derived.

Abnormal Neutrophil Function Inherited and acquired abnormalities of phagocyte function are listed in Table 64-3. The resulting diseases are best considered in terms of the functional defects of adherence, chemotaxis, and microbicidal activity. The distinguishing features of the important inherited disorders of phagocyte function are shown in Table 64-4.

Disorders of adhesion Two types of leukocyte adhesion deficiency (LAD) have been described. Both are autosomal recessive traits and result in the inability of neutrophils to exit the circulation to sites of infection, leading to leukocytosis and increased susceptibility to infection (Fig. 64-4). Patients with LAD 1 have mutations in CD18, the common component of the integrins LFA-1, Mac-1, and p150,95, leading to a defect in tight adhesion between neutrophils and the endothelium. The heterodimer formed by CD18/CD11b (Mac-1) is also the receptor for the complement-derived opsonin C3bi (CR3). The CD18 gene is located on distal chromosome 21q. Variable expression of the defect determines the severity of clinical disease. Complete lack of expression of the leukocyte adhesion proteins results in the severe phenotype in which inflammatory cytokines do not increase the expression of leukocyte adhesion proteins on neutrophils or activated T and B cells. Neutrophils (and monocytes) from patients with LAD 1

adhere poorly to endothelial cells and protein-coated surfaces and exhibit defective spreading, aggregation, and chemotaxis. Patients with LAD 1 have recurrent bacterial and fungal infections involving skin, oral and genital mucosa, and respiratory and intestinal tracts; persistent leukocytosis (neutrophil counts of 15,000 to 20,000/μL) because cells do not marginate; and, in severe cases, a history of delayed separation of the umbilical stump. Infections, especially of the skin, may become necrotic with progressively enlarging borders, slow healing, and development of dysplastic scars. The most common bacteria are *Staphylococcus aureus* and enteric gram-negative bacteria. LAD 2 is caused by an abnormality of SLe^x(CD15s), the ligand on neutrophils that interacts with selectins on endothelial cells.

Disorders of neutrophil granules The most common neutrophil defect is *myeloperoxidase deficiency*, a primary granule defect inherited as an autosomal recessive trait; the incidence is ~1 in 2000 persons. Isolated myeloperoxidase deficiency is not associated with clinically compromised defenses, because other defense systems such as hydrogen peroxide generation are amplified. Microbicidal activity of neutrophils is delayed but not absent. Myeloperoxidase deficiency may make other acquired host defense defects more serious. An acquired form of myeloperoxidase deficiency occurs in myelomonocytic leukemia and acute myeloid leukemia.

Chédiak-Higashi syndrome (CHS) is a rare disease with autosomal recessive inheritance due to defects in the lysosomal transport protein LYST, encoded by the gene *CHS1* at 1q42. This protein is required for normal packaging and disbursement of granules. Neutrophils (and all cells containing lysosomes) from patients with CHS characteristically have large granules **(Plate V-34A)**. Patients with CHS have an increased number of infections resulting from many agents. CHS neutrophils and monocytes have impaired chemotaxis and abnormal rates of microbial killing due to slow rates of fusion of the lysosomal granules with phagosomes. NK cell function is also impaired.

Specific granule deficiency is a rare autosomal recessive disease in which the production of secondary granules and their contents, as well as primary granule component defensins, is defective. The defect in bacterial killing leads to severe bacterial infections. One type of specific granule deficiency is due to a mutation in the CCAAT/enhancer binding protein-ε, a regulator of expression of granule components.

Chronic granulomatous disease Chronic granulomatous disease (CGD) is a group of disorders of granulocyte and monocyte oxidative metabolism. Although CGD is rare, with an incidence of 1 in 200,000 individuals, it is an important model of defective neutrophil oxidative metabolism. Most often CGD is inherited as an X-linked recessive trait; 30% of patients inherit the disease in an autosomal recessive pattern. Mutations in the genes for the four proteins that assemble at the plasma membrane account for all patients with CGD. Two proteins (a 91-kDa protein, abnormal in X-linked CGD, and a 22-kDa protein, absent in one form of autosomal recessive CGD) form the heterodimer cytochrome b-558 in the plasma membrane. Two other proteins (47 and 67 kDa, abnormal in the other autosomal recessive forms of CGD) are cytoplasmic in origin and interact with the cytochrome after cell activation to form NADPH oxidase, required for hydrogen peroxide production. Leukocytes from patients with CGD have severely diminished hydrogen peroxide production. The genes involved in each of the defects have been cloned and sequenced and the chromosome locations identified. Patients with CGD characteristically have increased numbers of infections due to catalase-positive microorganisms (organisms that destroy their own hydrogen peroxide). When patients with CGD become infected, they often have extensive inflammatory reactions, and lymph node suppuration is common despite the administration of appropriate antibiotics. Aphthous ulcers and chronic inflammation of the nares are often present. Granulomas are frequent and can obstruct the gastrointestinal or genitourinary tracts. The excessive inflammation probably reflects failure to degrade chemoattractants and antigens, leading to persistent neutrophil accumulation. Impaired killing of intracellular microorganisms by macrophages may lead to persistent cell-mediated immunity and granuloma formation.

MONONUCLEAR PHAGOCYTES

The mononuclear phagocyte system is composed of monoblasts, promonocytes, and monocytes in addition to the structurally diverse tissue macrophages that make up what was previously referred to as the reticuloendothelial system. Macrophages are long-lived phagocytic cells capable of many of the functions of neutrophils. They are also secretory cells that participate in many immunologic and inflammatory processes distinct from neutrophils. Monocytes leave the circulation by diapedesis more slowly than neutrophils and have a half-life in the blood of 12 to 24 h.

After blood monocytes arrive in the tissues, they differentiate into macrophages ("big eaters") with specialized functions suited for specific anatomic locations. Macrophages are particularly abundant in capillary walls of the lung, spleen, liver, and bone marrow, where they function to remove microorganisms and other noxious elements from the blood. Alveolar macrophages, liver Kupffer cells, splenic macrophages, peritoneal macrophages, bone marrow macrophages, lymphatic macrophages, brain microglial cells, and dendritic macrophages all have specialized functions. Macrophage-secreted products include lysozyme, neutral proteases, acid hydrolases, arginase, complement components, enzyme inhibitors (plasmin, α_2-macroglobulin), binding proteins (transferrin, fibronectin, transcobalamin II), nucleosides, and cyto-

Table 64-4 Inherited Disorders of Phagocyte Function: Differential Features

Clinical Manifestations	Cellular or Molecular Defects	Diagnosis
CHRONIC GRANULOMATOUS DISEASES OF CHILDHOOD (70% X-LINKED, 30% AUTOSOMAL RECESSIVE)		
Severe infections of skin, ears, lungs, liver, and bone with catalase-positive microorganisms such as *S. aureus*, *Burkholderia cepacia*, *Aspergillus* spp., *Chromobacterium violaceum*; often hard to culture organism; excessive inflammation with granulomas, frequent lymph node suppuration; granulomas can obstruct GI or GU tracts; gingivitis, aphthous ulcers, seborrheic dermatitis	No respiratory burst due to the lack of one of four NADPH oxidase subunits in neutrophils, monocytes, and eosinophils	NBT test; no superoxide and H$_2$O$_2$ production by neutrophils; no chemiluminescence; immunoblot for NADPH oxidase components
CHÉDIAK-HIGASHI SYNDROME (AUTOSOMAL RECESSIVE)		
Recurrent pyogenic infections, especially with *S. aureus*; many patients get lymphoma-like illness during adolescence; periodontal disease; partial oculocutaneous albinism, nystagmus, progressive peripheral neuropathy, mental retardation in some patients	Reduced chemotaxis and phagolysosome fusion, increased respiratory burst activity, defective egress from marrow, abnormal skin window	Giant primary granules in neutrophils and other granule-bearing cells (Wright's stain)
SPECIFIC GRANULE DEFICIENCY (AUTOSOMAL RECESSIVE?)		
Recurrent infections of skin, ears, and sinopulmonary tract; delayed wound healing; decreased inflammation; bleeding diathesis	Abnormal chemotaxis, impaired respiratory burst and bacterial killing, failure to upregulate chemotactic and adhesion receptors with stimulation, defect in transcription of granule proteins	Lack of secondary (specific) granules in neutrophils (Wright's stain), no neutrophil-specific granule contents (i.e., lactoferrin), no defensins, platelet α granule abnormality
MYELOPEROXIDASE DEFICIENCY (AUTOSOMAL RECESSIVE)		
Clinically normal except in patients with underlying disease such as diabetes mellitus; then candidiasis or other fungal infections	No myeloperoxidase due to pre- and post-translational defects	No peroxidase in neutrophils
LEUKOCYTE ADHESION DEFICIENCY (AUTOSOMAL RECESSIVE)		
Type 1: Delayed separation of umbilical cord, sustained neutrophilia, recurrent infections of skin and mucosa, gingivitis, periodontal disease	Impaired phagocyte adherence, aggregation, spreading, chemotaxis, phagocytosis of C3bi-coated particles; defective production of CD18 subunit common to leukocyte integrins	Reduced phagocyte surface expression of the CD18-containing integrins with monoclonal antibodies against LFA-1 (CD18/CD11a), Mac-1 or CR3 (CD18/CD11b), p150,95 (CD18/CD11c)
Type 2: Severe mental retardation, short stature, Bombay (hh) blood phenotype, recurrent infections, neutrophilia	Impaired phagocyte rolling along endothelium	Reduced phagocyte surface expression of Sialyl-Lewis^x, with monoclonal antibodies against CD15s
HYPER IGE–RECURRENT INFECTION SYNDROME (AUTOSOMAL DOMINANT) (JOB'S SYNDROME)		
Eczematoid or pruritic dermatitis, "cold" skin abscesses, recurrent pneumonias with *S. aureus* with bronchopleural fistulas and cyst formation, mild eosinophilia, mucocutaneous candidiasis, atopy, characteristic facies, restrictive lung disease, scoliosis delayed primary dental decidiation	Reduced chemotaxis in some patients, reduced suppressor T cell activity	Clinical features, serum IgE > 2000 IU/mL, high serum anti-*S. aureus* IgE, low or no serum and salivary anti-*S. aureus* IgA
MYCOBACTERIA SUSCEPTIBILITY (AUTOSOMAL DOMINANT AND RECESSIVE FORMS)		
Severe local or disseminated infections with bacilli Calmette-Gutrin, nontuberculous mycobacteria, salmonella, historiasmosis, poor granuloma formation	Inability to kill intracellular organisms due to low IFN-γ production; mutations in IFN-γ receptors, IL-12 receptor, IL-12 p40	Low or very high levels of IFN-γ receptor 1; functional assays of cytokine production and response

kines (TNF-α; IL-1, -8, -12, and -18). IL-1 (Chaps. 17 and 305) has many functions, including initiating fever in the hypothalamus, mobilizing leukocytes from the bone marrow, activating lymphocytes and neutrophils. TNF-α is a pyrogen that duplicates many of the actions of IL-1 and plays an important role in the pathogenesis of gram-negative shock (Chap. 124). TNF-α stimulates production of hydrogen peroxide and related toxic oxygen species by macrophages and neutrophils. In addition, TNF-α induces catabolic changes that contribute to the profound wasting (cachexia) associated with many chronic diseases.

Other macrophage-secreted products include reactive oxygen and nitrogen metabolites, bioactive lipids (arachidonic acid metabolites and platelet-activating factors), chemokines, colony stimulating factors, and factors stimulating fibroblast and vessel proliferation. Macrophages help regulate the replication of lymphocytes and participate in the killing of tumors, viruses, and certain bacteria (*Mycobacterium tuberculosis* and *Listeria monocytogenes*). Macrophages are key effector cells in the elimination of intracellular microorganisms. Their ability to fuse to form giant cells that coalesce into granulomas in response to some inflammatory stimuli is important in the elimination of intracellular microbes and is under the control of IFN-γ. Nitric oxide induced by IFN-γ is an important effector against intracellular parasites including tuberculosis and *Leishmania*.

Macrophages play an important role in the immune response (Chap. 305). They process and present antigen to lymphocytes and secrete cytokines that modulate and direct lymphocyte development and function. Macrophages participate in autoimmune phenomena by removing immune complexes and other substances from the circulation. Polymorphisms in macrophage receptors for immunoglobulin (FcγRII) determine suceptibility to some infections and autoimmune diseases. In wound healing, they dispose of senescent cells, and they contribute to atheroma development. Macrophage elastase mediates development of emphysema from cigarette smoking.

DISORDERS OF THE MONONUCLEAR PHAGOCYTE SYSTEM Many disorders of neutrophils extend to mononuclear phagocytes. Thus, drugs that suppress neutrophil production in the bone marrow can cause monocytopenia. Transient monocytopenia occurs after stress or glucocorticoid administration. Monocytosis is associated with tuberculosis, brucellosis, subacute bacterial endocarditis, Rocky Mountain spotted fever, malaria, and visceral leishmaniasis (kala azar). Monocytosis also occurs with malignancies, leukemias, myeloproliferative syndromes, hemolytic anemias, chronic idiopathic neutropenias, and granulomatous diseases such as sarcoidosis, regional enteritis, and some collagen vascular diseases. Patients with LAD, hyperimmunoglobulin E–recurrent infection (Job's) syndrome, CHS, and CGD all have defects in the mononuclear phagocyte system.

Monocyte cytokine production is impaired in some patients with disseminated nontuberculous mycobacterial infection who are not infected with HIV. Genetic defects in IFN-γ receptors 1 and 2 impair monocyte killing of intracellular parasites, as do lesions in the potent IFN-γ inducer, IL-12 and its receptor (Fig. 64-5).

Certain viral infections impair mononuclear phagocyte function. For example, influenza virus infection causes abnormal monocyte chemotaxis. Mononuclear phagocytes can be infected by HIV using CCR5, the chemokine receptor that acts as a coreceptor with CD4 for HIV. T lymphocytes produce IFN-γ, which induces FcR expression and phagocytosis and stimulates hydrogen peroxide production by mononuclear phagocytes and neutrophils. In certain diseases, such as AIDS, IFN-γ production may be deficient, while in other diseases, such as T cell lymphomas, excessive release of IFN-γ may be associated with erythrophagocytosis by splenic macrophages.

Monocytopenia occurs with acute infections, with stress, and after treatment with glucocorticoids. Monocytopenia also occurs in aplastic anemia, hairy cell leukemia, acute myeloid leukemia, and as a direct result of myelotoxic drugs.

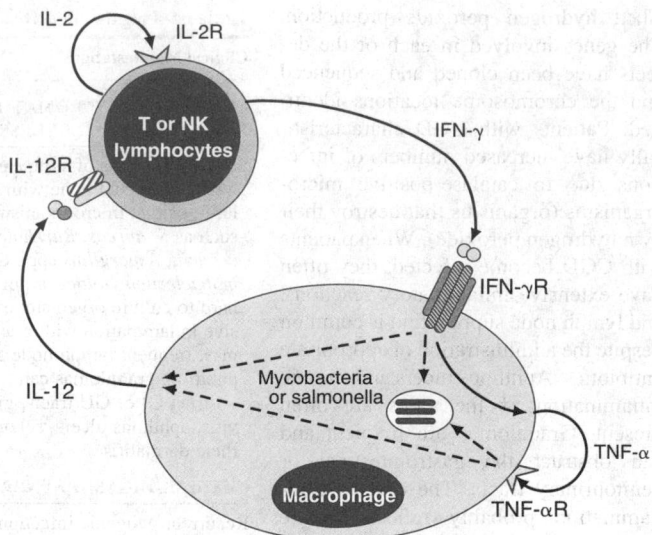

FIGURE 64-5 Lymphocyte-macrophage interactions underlying resistance to mycobacteria and other intracellular parasites such as Salmonella. Mycobacteria infect macrophages, leading to the production of IL-12, which activates T or NK cells through its receptor, leading to production of IL-1 and IFN-γ. IFN-γ acts through its receptor on macrophages to upregulate TNF-α and IL-12 and kill intracellular parasites. Mutant forms of the cytokines and receptors shown in large type have been found in severe cases of nontuberculous mycobacterial infection and salmonellosis.

EOSINOPHILS

Eosinophils and neutrophils share similar morphology, many lysosomal constituents, phagocytic capacity, and oxidative metabolism. Eosinophils express a specific chemoattractant receptor and respond to a specific chemokine, eotaxin. Little is known about the role of eosinophils. Eosinophils are much longer lived than neutrophils, and unlike neutrophils, tissue eosinophils can recirculate. During most infections, eosinophils are not important. However, in invasive helminthic infections, such as hookworm, schistosomiasis, strongyloidiasis, toxocariasis, trichinosis, filariasis, echinococcosis, and cysticercosis, the eosinophil plays a central role in host defense. Eosinophils are associated with bronchial asthma, cutaneous allergic reactions, and other hypersensitivity states.

The distinctive feature of the red-staining (Wright's stain) eosinophil granules is its crystalline core consisting of an arginine-rich protein (major basic protein) with histaminase activity, important in host defense against parasites. Eosinophil granules also contain a unique eosinophil peroxidase that catalyzes the oxidation of many substances by hydrogen peroxide and may facilitate killing of microorganisms.

Eosinophil peroxidase, in the presence of hydrogen peroxide and halide, initiates mast cell secretion in vitro and thereby promotes inflammation. Eosinophils contain cationic proteins, some of which bind to heparin and reduce its anticoagulant activity. Eosinophil-derived neurotoxin and eosinophil cationic protein are ribonucleases that can kill respiratory syncytial virus. Eosinophil cytoplasm contains Charcot-Leyden crystal protein, a hexagonal bipyramidal crystal first observed in a patient with leukemia and then in sputum of patients with asthma; this protein is lysophospholipase and may function to detoxify certain lysophospholipids.

Several factors enhance the eosinophil's function in host defense. T cell–derived factors enhance the ability of eosinophils to kill parasites. Mast cell–derived eosinophil chemotactic factor of anaphylaxis (ECFa) increases the number of eosinophil complement receptors and enhances eosinophil killing of parasites. Eosinophil colony stimulating factors (e.g., IL-5) produced by macrophages increase eosinophil production in the bone marrow and activate eosinophils to kill parasites.

EOSINOPHILIA Eosinophilia is the presence of >500 eosinophils per microliter of blood and is common in many settings besides parasite infection. Significant tissue eosinophilia can occur without an elevated blood count. The most common cause of eosinophilia is allergic reactions to drugs (iodides, aspirin, sulfonamides, nitrofurantoin, penicillins, and cephalosporins). Allergies such as hay fever, asthma, eczema, serum sickness, allergic vasculitis, and pemphigus are associated with eosinophilia. Eosinophilia also occurs in collagen vascular diseases (e.g., rheumatoid arthritis, eosinophilic fasciitis, allergic angiitis, and periarteritis nodosa) and malignancies (e.g., Hodgkin's disease; mycosis fungoides; chronic myelogenous leukemia; and cancer of the lung, stomach, pancreas, ovary, or uterus), as well as in Job's syndrome and CGD. Eosinophilia commonly is present in the helminthic infections. IL-5 is the dominant eosinophil growth factor. Therapeutic administration of the cytokines IL-2 and GM-CSF frequently leads to transient eosinophilia. The most dramatic hypereosinophilic syndromes are Loeffler's syndrome, tropical pulmonary eosinophilia, Loeffler's endocarditis, eosinophilic leukemia, and idiopathic hypereosinophilic syndrome (50,000 to 100,000/μL).

The idiopathic hypereosinophilic syndrome represents a heterogeneous group of disorders with the common feature of prolonged eosinophilia of unknown cause and organ system dysfunction, including the heart, central nervous system, kidneys, lungs, gastrointestinal tract, and skin. The bone marrow is involved in all affected individuals, but the most severe complications involve the heart and central nervous system. Clinical manifestations and organ dysfunction are highly variable. Eosinophils are found in the involved tissues and likely cause tissue damage by local deposition of toxic eosinophil proteins such as eosinophil cationic protein and major basic protein. In the heart, the pathologic changes lead to thrombosis, endocardial fibrosis, and restrictive endomyocardiopathy. The damage to tissues in other organ systems is similar. The mechanism for the hypereosinophilia is not known. Glucocorticoids usually induce remission. In patients who do not respond to glucocorticoids, a cytotoxic agent such as hydroxyurea has been used successfully to lower the peripheral blood eosinophil counts and to improve markedly the prognosis. IFN-α also is effective in some patients, including those unresponsive to hydroxyurea. Aggressive medical and surgical approaches are used to manage patients with cardiovascular complications.

The *eosinophilia-myalgia syndrome* is a multisystem disease with prominent cutaneous, hematologic, and visceral manifestations that frequently evolves into a chronic course and can occasionally be fatal. The syndrome is characterized by eosinophilia (eosinophil count >1000/μL) and generalized disabling myalgias without other recognized causes. Eosinophil fasciitis, pneumonitis, and myocarditis; neuropathy culminating in respiratory failure; and encephalopathy may occur. The disease is caused by ingesting contaminants in L-tryptophan–containing products. Eosinophils, lymphocytes, macrophages, and fibroblasts accumulate in the affected tissues, but their role in pathogenesis is unclear. Activation of eosinophils and fibroblasts and the deposition of eosinophil-derived toxic proteins in affected tissues may contribute. IL-5 and transforming growth factor β have been implicated as potential mediators. Treatment is withdrawal of L-tryptophan–containing products and the administration of glucocorticoids. Most patients recover fully, remain stable, or show slow recovery; but the disease can be fatal in up to 5% of patients.

EOSINOPENIA Eosinopenia occurs with stress, such as acute bacterial infection, and after treatment with glucocorticoids. The mechanism of eosinopenia of acute bacterial infection is unknown but is independent of endogenous glucocorticoids, since it occurs in animals after total adrenalectomy. There is no known adverse effect of eosinopenia.

HYPERIMMUNOGLOBULIN E-RECURRENT INFECTION SYNDROME

The hyperimmunoglobulin E–recurrent infection (HIE) syndrome or *Job's syndrome* is a rare multisystem disease in which the immune system, bone, teeth, lung and skin are affected. Abnormal chemotaxis

is a variable feature. The molecular basis for this syndrome is not known, but some cases show autosomal dominant transmission with linkage to 4q. Patients with this syndrome have characteristic facies with broad nose, kyphoscoliosis and osteoporosis, and eczema. The primary teeth erupt normally but do not deciduate, often requiring extraction. Patients develop recurrent sinopulmonary and cutaneous infections that tend to be much less inflamed than appropriate for the degree of infection and have been referred to as "cold abscesses." A high degree of suspicion is required to diagnose infections in these patients, who may appear well despite extensive disease. The cold abscesses have been considered a reflection of impaired chemotaxis with too few phagocytes arriving too late, perhaps due to a lymphocyte factor inhibiting chemotaxis. However, the chemotactic defect in these patients is variable, and the fundamental basis for the impaired defenses is complex and poorly defined.

LABORATORY DIAGNOSIS AND MANAGEMENT

Initial studies of WBC and differential and often a bone marrow examination are followed by assessment of bone marrow reserves (steroid challenge test), marginated circulating pool of cells (epinephrine challenge test), and marginating ability (endotoxin challenge test) (Fig. 64-3). In vivo assessment of inflammation is possible with a Rebuck skin window test or an in vivo blister assay, which measures the ability of leukocytes and inflammatory mediators to accumulate locally in the skin. In vitro tests of phagocyte aggregation, adherence, chemotaxis, phagocytosis, degranulation, and microbicidal activity (for *S. aureus*) may help pinpoint cellular or humoral lesions. Deficiencies of oxidative metabolism are detected with the nitroblue tetrazolium (NBT) dye test, which is based on the ability of products of oxidative metabolism to reduce yellow, soluble NBT to blue-black formazan, an insoluble material that can be seen microscopically. Studies of superoxide and hydrogen peroxide production may further define neutrophil oxidative function.

Patients with leukopenias or leukocyte dysfunction often have delayed inflammatory responses. Therefore, clinical manifestations may be minimal despite overwhelming infection, and unusual infections must always be suspected. Early signs of infection demand prompt, aggressive culturing for microorganisms, use of antibiotics, and surgical drainage of abscesses. Prolonged antibiotics are often required. In patients with CGD, prophylactic antibiotics (trimethoprim-sulfamethoxazole) diminish the frequency of life-threatening infections. Short courses of glucocorticoids may relieve gastrointestinal or genitourinary tract obstruction by granulomas in patients with CGD. Recombinant human IFN-γ, which nonspecifically stimulates phagocytic cell function, reduces the frequency of infections in patients with CGD by 70% and reduces the severity of infection. This effect of IFN-γ in CGD is additive to the effect of prophylactic antibiotics. The recommended dose is 50 μg/m² subcutaneously three times weekly. IFN-γ also has been used successfully in the treatment of leprosy, nontuberculous mycobacteria, and visceral leishmaniasis.

Rigorous oral hygiene reduces but does not eliminate the discomfort of gingivitis, periodontal disease, and aphthous ulcers; chlorhexidine mouthwash and tooth brushing with a hydrogen peroxide–sodium bicarbonate paste helps many patients. Oral antifungal agents (fluconazole) have reduced mucocutaneous candidiasis in patients with Job's syndrome. Androgens, glucocorticoids, lithium, and immunosuppressive therapy have been used to restore myelopoiesis in patients with neutropenia due to impaired production. Recombinant G-CSF is useful in the management of certain forms of neutropenia due to depressed neutrophil production, especially that related to cancer chemotherapy. Patients with chronic neutropenia with evidence of a good bone marrow reserve need not receive prophylactic antibiotics.

Patients with constant or cyclic neutrophil counts <500/μL may benefit from prophylactic antibiotics and G-CSF during periods of neutropenia. Oral trimethoprim-sulfamethoxazole (160/800 mg) twice daily can prevent infection. Increased numbers of fungal infections are not seen in patients with CGD on this regimen. Oral quinolones such as norfloxacin and ciprofloxacin are alternatives.

In the setting of cytotoxic chemotherapy with severe, persistent neutropenia, trimethoprim-sulfamethoxazole prevents *Pneumocystis carinii* pneumonia. These patients, and patients with phagocytic cell dysfunction, should avoid heavy exposure to airborne soil, dust, or decaying matter (mulch, manure), which are often rich in spores of *Aspergillus* or other fungi. Restriction of activities or social contact has no proven role in reducing risk of infection.

Cure of some congenital phagocyte defects is possible by bone marrow transplantation (Chap. 115). However, complications of bone marrow transplantation are still serious, and with rigorous medical care many patients with phagocytic disorders can go for years without a life-threatening infection. The identification of specific gene defects in patients with LAD 1 and CGD has led to gene therapy trials in a number of genetic white cell disorders.

BIBLIOGRAPHY

GRIMBACHER B et al: Hyper-IgE syndrome with recurrent infections—an autosomal dominant multisystem disorder. N Engl J Med 340:692, 1999

HOLLAND SM et al: Abnormal regulation of interferon-γ, interleukin-12, and tumor necrosis factor-α in human interferon-γ receptor 1 deficiency. J Infect Dis 178:1095, 1998

HOLLAND SM, GALLIN JI: Disorders of phagocytic cells, in *Inflammation: Basic Principles and Clinical Correlates*, 3d ed. JI Gallin, R Snyderman (eds). Philadelphia, Lippincott-Williams & Wilkins, 1999

HUNTER MG, AVALOS BR: Deletion of a critical internalization domain in the G-CSF receptor in acute myelogenous leukemia preceded by severe congenital neutropenia. Blood 93:440, 1999

LEKSTROM-HIMES JA et al: Neutrophil-specific granule deficiency results from a novel mutation with loss of function of the transcription factor CCAAT/enhancer binding protein-ε. J Exp Med 189:1847, 1999

LOCATI M, MURPHY PM: Chemokines and chemokine receptors: Biology and clinical relevance in inflammation and AIDS. Annu Rev Med 50:425, 1999

NEUFELD G et al: Vascular endothelial growth factor (VEGF) and its receptors. FASEB J 13:9, 1999

ROSENBERG HF: The eosinophil ribonucleases. Cell Mol Life Sci 54:795, 1998

SEMENZATO G et al: The lymphoproliferative disease of granular lymphocytes: Updated criteria for diagnosis. Blood 89:256, 1997

WINKELSTEIN JA et al: Chronic granulomatous disease: Report on a national registry of 368 patients. Medicine (Baltimore) 79:155, 2000

NOBEL PRIZE IN PHYSIOLOGY OR MEDICINE, 1990

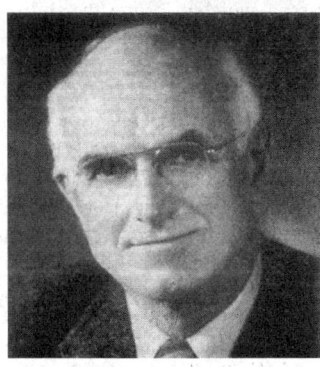

Joseph Edward Murray was born April 1, 1919, in Milford, Massachusetts, the third child of William and Mary Murray. After high school he attended the College of Holy Cross, then entered Harvard Medical School. He received his medical degree in 1943. After an internship in surgery at the Peter Bent Brigham Hospital, Murray entered the military and was assigned to Valley Forge General Hospital where there were many badly burned World War II patients. He was there from 1944 to 1947 and during that time developed substantial expertise in both grafting and plastic surgery. After discharge he completed his residency in surgery at the Peter Bent Brigham and New York Hospitals. He then became director of the laboratory for surgical research at Harvard Medical School. In 1951 at Harvard, David Hume began a series of nine renal transplants into the thighs of recipients, but they were all ultimately rejected. During his surgical residency, Murray had carried out numerous renal autografts in dogs and concluded that transplants could function normally if the immunologic barrier could be overcome. The opportunity to test this theory in patients occurred with an end-stage renal patient who had a twin brother. The kidney transplant from the twin brother was a resounding success. The patient married his recovery room nurse, fathered two children, and lived more than seven years with the transplanted kidney.

In 1961 the Brigham team began using immunosuppressive drugs to perform kidney transplants in non-twins. The results by 1965 were 80% allograft survival at 1 year and 65% unrelated cadaveric graft survival at 1 year. Murray subsequently returned to plastic surgery with a specialty in the repair of facial defects in children. His contribution of successfully transplanting the first organ in a human was a seminal event that launched the era of organ transplantation. For this contribution he shared the Nobel Prize in Physiology or Medicine in 1990 with Donnall Thomas.

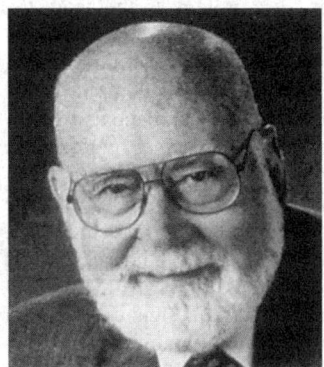

Edward Donnall Thomas was born March 15, 1920, in Mart, Texas. Thomas received his B.A. degree at the University of Texas, where he met and married his wife, Dorothy. He then attended Harvard Medical School and on graduation had his internship at the Peter Bent Brigham Hospital. This was the same time at the Brigham when Murray had been successful in transplanting kidneys. This led Thomas to believe that bone marrow tissue could also be transplanted to treat patients with aplastic anemia. Thomas then joined the staff at Mary Bassett Hospital in Cooperstown, New York, where, in collaboration with Dr. Joseph Ferrabee, Thomas showed that dogs could survive otherwise fatal radiation if their own marrow had been previously harvested and then returned to the animals following radiation. The ability to store bone marrow without loss of vitality was a major breakthrough. However, bone marrow from other animals, that is, an allogeneic graft, was not successful. Thomas and Ferrabee then treated a twin suffering from leukemia with supralethal radiation, followed by marrow infusion from the twin sibling. The use of the antimetabolite methotrexate and the availability of histocompatibility typing then allowed for non-twin allogeneic bone marrow transplantation. In March 1967 Thomas moved to the University of Washington, and in March 1969 the Thomas team performed the first bone marrow infusion from a matched brother donor to his sister who was dying of leukemia; 20 years later the woman was still in good health. In 1974 Thomas became director of medical oncology at the Fred Hutchinson Cancer Research Center, which, with his leadership, became the largest bone marrow transplant center in the world and the training site for the majority of individuals who started bone marrow transplant units worldwide. The "biological force," which was supposed to prevent tissue and organ transplant, had thus been overcome. In 1990 Murray and Thomas were rewarded as pioneers in the area of transplantation with the Nobel Prize.

REFERENCES

1. Magill FN (ed): *Nobel Prize Winners: Physiology or Medicine*, vol 3. Pasadena, Salem Press, 1993

2. Schrier RW: *A Salute to Nobel Laureates in Physiology and Medicine*, Proceedings of the Association of American Physicians. 108(1): Jan 1996

Robert W. Schrier, MD

65   J. Larry Jameson, Peter Kopp

PRINCIPLES OF HUMAN GENETICS

ACTH adrenocorticotropic hormone	RFLPs restriction fragment length
BACs bacterial artificial	polymorphisms
chromosomes	RT reverse transcriptase
CREB cyclic AMP response element	SNPs single nucleotide
binding	polymorphisms
HGP Human Genome Project	STRs short tandem repeats
HNPCC hereditary nonpolyposis	VNTRs variable number of tandem
colon cancer	repeats
MEN multiple endocrine neoplasia	YACs yeast artificial chromosomes
PCR polymerase chain reaction	

IMPACT OF GENETICS ON MEDICAL PRACTICE

New insights into the genetic basis of disease are being generated at an ever-increasing rate. This explosion of information was ignited by technological advances, such as the polymerase chain reaction (PCR) and automated DNA sequencing, and is fueled by rapid progress in the Human Genome Project (HGP). Although its promise is great, the integration of genetics into the everyday practice of medicine remains challenging. To date, the most significant impact of genetics has been to enhance our understanding of disease etiology and pathogenesis. In the near term, we can expect an even greater role for genetics in the diagnosis, prevention, and treatment of disease (Chaps. 68 and 69).

Genetic disorders are more common than generally appreciated. It is estimated, for example, that 3% of pregnancies result in a child with a genetic disease or birth defect. About 10% of all pediatric and adult hospitalization admissions involve genetic diseases. This number would increase substantially if one included complex, multifactorial genetic diseases, such as diabetes or cardiovascular disease. The prevalence of genetic diseases, combined with their severity and chronic nature, imposes a great financial, social, and emotional burden on society.

Genetics has historically focused on chromosomal and metabolic disorders, reflecting the long-standing availability of techniques to diagnose these conditions. For example, conditions such as trisomy 21 (Down syndrome) or monosomy X (Turner syndrome) can be diagnosed using cytogenetics (Chap. 66). Likewise, many metabolic disorders (e.g., phenylketonuria, familial hypercholesterolemia) have been diagnosed using biochemical analyses. Recent advances in DNA diagnostics have extended the field of genetics to include virtually all medical specialties. In cardiology, for example, the molecular basis of inherited cardiomyopathies and ion channel defects that predispose to arrhythmias is being defined (Chaps. 230 and 238). In neurology, genetics has unmasked the pathophysiology of a startling number of neurodegenerative disorders (Chap. 359). Hematology has evolved dramatically, from its incipient genetic descriptions of hemoglobinopathies to the current understanding of the molecular basis of red cell membrane defects, clotting disorders, and thrombotic disorders (Chaps. 106 and 117). It is now abundantly clear that neoplasia and the acquisition of metastatic potential can be described in genetic terms (Chaps. 81, 82, and 83).

New concepts derived from genetic studies can sometimes clarify topics that were previously opaque. For example, although many different genetic defects can cause peripheral neuropathies, disruption of the normal folding of the myelin sheaths is frequently a common final

pathway (Chap. 379). Several genetic causes of obesity appear to converge on a physiologic pathway that involves products of the proopiomelanocortin polypeptide and the MC4R receptor, thus identifying a key mechanism for appetite control (Chap. 77). A similar situation is emerging for genetically distinct forms of Alzheimer disease, several of which lead to the formation of neurofibrillary tangles (Chap. 362). Increasingly, the identification of defective genes can pinpoint cellular pathways involved in key physiologic processes. Examples include identification of the cystic fibrosis conductance regulator (*CFTR*) gene, the Duchenne's muscular dystrophy (*DMD*) gene, which encodes dystrophin, and the fibroblast growth factor receptor-3 (*FGFR3*) gene, which is responsible for achondroplastic dwarfism. Similarly, transgenic and gene "knockout" models can help to unravel the physiologic function of genes. Genetic approaches have proven invaluable for the detection of infectious pathogens and are used clinically to identify agents that are difficult to culture such as mycobacteria, viruses, and parasites (Chap. 121). In many cases, molecular genetics has improved the feasibility and accuracy of diagnostic testing, enhanced our understanding of pathophysiology, and is beginning to open new avenues for therapy, including gene therapy (Chap. 69).

It is increasingly apparent that genetic background plays some role in virtually every medical condition. This is particularly true when one considers disease susceptibility, the interaction of genetic background with the environment, host responses to illness and to pharmaceutical agents, or the metabolism of drugs. Although genetics has traditionally been viewed through the window of relatively rare single-gene diseases, many disorders such as hypertension, asthma, diabetes, susceptibility to cardiovascular disease, and mental illness are also affected by genetic background, as often evident from a patient's family history. These complex genetic traits involve the contributions of many different genes, as well as environmental factors that can modify disease risk (Chap. 68).

The astounding rate at which new genetic information is being generated creates a major challenge for physicians and other health care providers. The terminology and techniques used for discovery evolve continuously. Much genetic information presently resides in computer databases or is being published in basic science journals. The ongoing development of bioinformatics promises to simplify this seemingly daunting onslaught of new information. It is now possible, for example, to search for genetic testing centers through a web site (www.genlink.wustl.edu) that can be accessed conveniently by organ system, disease state, or gene. Monogenic disorders are summarized in a large, continuously evolving compendium, referred to as the *Online Mendelian Inheritance in Man* (OMIM; www.ncbi.nlm.nih.gov/omim/). These and other databases (www.genebank.com) will expand rapidly in conjunction with advances in the HGP.

CHROMOSOMES AND DNA REPLICATION

ORGANIZATION OF DNA INTO CHROMOSOMES
Size of the Human Genome   The human genome is divided into 23 different chromosomes, including 22 autosomes (numbered 1 to 22) and the X and Y sex chromosomes. Adult cells are diploid, meaning they contain two homologous sets of 22 autosomes and a pair of sex chromosomes. Females have two X chromosomes (XX), whereas males have one X and one Y chromosome (XY). As a consequence of meiosis, germ cells (sperm or oocytes) are haploid and contain one set of 22 autosomes and one of the sex chromosomes. At the time of fertilization, the diploid genome is reconstituted by pairing of the homologous chromosomes from the mother and father. With each cell division (mitosis), chromosomes are replicated, paired, segregated, and divided into two daughter cells (Chap. 66).

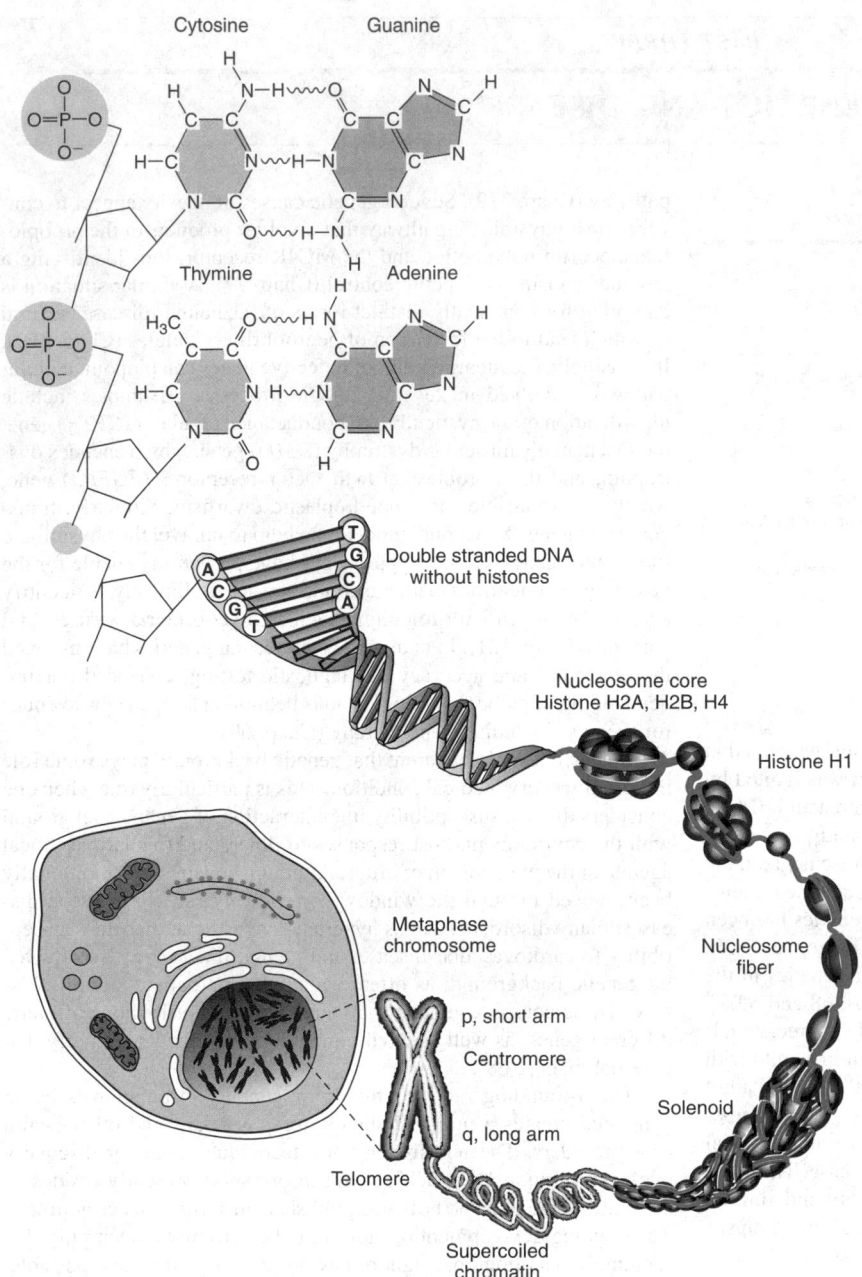

Cytosine   Guanine

Thymine   Adenine

Double stranded DNA
without histones

Nucleosome core
Histone H2A, H2B, H4

Histone H1

Metaphase
chromosome

Nucleosome
fiber

p, short arm

Centromere

Solenoid

q, long arm

Telomere

Supercoiled
chromatin

FIGURE 65-1 Structure of chromatin and chromosomes. Chromatin is composed of double-stranded DNA that is wrapped around histone and nonhistone proteins forming nucleosomes. The nucleosomes are further organized into solenoid structures. Chromosomes assume their characteristic structure, with short (p) and long (q) arms at the metaphase stage of the cell cycle.

genes are about this size, the range is quite broad. For example, some genes are only a few hundred bp, whereas others, like the *DMD* gene, are extraordinarily large (2 million bp).

Structure of DNA Each gene is composed of a linear polymer of DNA. DNA is a double-stranded helix composed of four different bases: adenine (A), thymidine (T), guanine (G), and cytosine (C). Adenine is paired to thymidine, and guanine is paired to cytosine, by hydrogen bond interactions that span the double helix. DNA has several remarkable features that make it ideal for the transmission of genetic information. It is relatively stable, at least in comparison to RNA or proteins. The double-stranded nature of DNA and its feature of strict base-pair complementarity permit faithful replication during cell division. As described below, complementarity also allows the transmission of genetic information from DNA → RNA → protein (Fig. 65-2). Messenger RNA (mRNA) is encoded by the so-called sense strand of the DNA double helix and is translated into proteins by ribosomes.

The presence of four different bases provides surprising genetic diversity. In the protein-coding regions of genes, the DNA bases are arranged into codons, a triplet of bases that specifies a particular amino acid. It is possible to arrange the four bases into 64 different triplet codons (4^3). Each codon specifies 1 of the 20 different amino acids, or a regulatory signal, such as stop translation. Because there are more codons than amino acids, the genetic code is degenerate; that is, most amino acids can be specified by several different codons. By arranging the codons in different combinations and in various lengths, it is possible to generate the tremendous diversity of primary protein structure.

REPLICATION OF DNA AND MITOSIS
Genetic information in DNA is transmitted to daughter cells under two different circumstances: (1) somatic cells divide by mitosis, allowing the diploid ($2n$) genome to replicate itself completely in conjunction with cell division; and (2) germ cells (sperm and ova) undergo meiosis, a process that enables the reduction of the diploid ($2n$) set of chromosomes to the haploid state ($1n$) (Chap. 66).

Prior to mitosis, cells exit the resting, or G_0 state, and enter the cell cycle (Chap. 82). After traversing a critical checkpoint in G_1, cells undergo DNA synthesis (S phase), during which the DNA in each chromosome is replicated, yielding two pairs of sister chromatids ($2n → 4n$). The process of DNA synthesis requires stringent fidelity in order to avoid transmitting errors to subsequent generations of cells. Genetic abnormalities of DNA mismatch/repair include xeroderma pigmentosum, Bloom syndrome, ataxia telangiectasia, and hereditary nonpolyposis colon cancer (HNPCC), among others. Many of these disorders strongly redispose to neoplasia because of the rapid acquisition of additional mutations (Chap. 81). After completion of DNA synthesis, cells enter G_2 and progress through a second checkpoint before entering mitosis. At this stage, the chromosomes condense and are aligned along the equatorial plate at metaphase. The two identical sister chromatids, held together at the centromere, divide and migrate to opposite poles of the cell (Fig. 66-3). After formation of a nuclear membrane around the two separated sets of chromatids, the cell divides and two daughter cells are formed, thus restoring the diploid ($2n$) state.

ASSORTMENT AND SEGREGATION OF GENES DURING MEIOSIS Meiosis occurs only in germ cells of the gonads. It shares certain features with mitosis but involves two distinct steps of

The genome is estimated to contain about 100,000 genes that are divided among the 23 chromosomes. A *gene* is a functional unit that is regulated by transcription (see below) and encodes a product, either RNA or protein, that exerts activity within the cell. Historically, genes were identified because they conferred specific traits that are transmitted from one generation to the next.

Human DNA is estimated to consist of about 3 billion base pairs (bp) of DNA per haploid genome. DNA length is normally measured in units of 1000 bp (kilobases, kb) or 1,000,000 bp (megabases, Mb). Not all DNA encodes genes. In fact, genes account for only about 10 to 15% of DNA. Much of the remaining DNA consists of highly repetitive sequences, the function of which is poorly understood. These repetitive DNA regions, along with nonrepetitive sequences that do not encode genes, may serve a structural role in the packaging of DNA into chromatin (DNA bound to histone proteins) and chromosomes (Fig. 65-1). If only 10% of DNA is expressed and there are 100,000 genes, the average gene would be about 3 kb in length. Although many

cell division that reduce the chromosome number to the haploid state. In addition, there is active recombination that generates genetic diversity. During the first cell division, two sister chromatids ($2n \rightarrow 4n$) are formed for each chromosome pair and there is an exchange of DNA between homologous paternal and maternal chromosomes. This process involves the formation of *chiasmata*, structures that correspond to the DNA segments that cross over between the maternal and paternal homologues (Fig. 65-3). Usually there is at least one crossover on each chromosomal arm; recombination occurs more frequently in female meiosis than in male meiosis. Subsequently, the chromosomes segregate randomly. Because there are 23 chromosomes, there exist 2^{23} (>8 million) possible combinations of chromosomes. Together with the genetic exchanges that occur during recombination, chromosomal segregation generates tremendous diversity, and each gamete is genetically unique. The process of recombination, and the independent segregation of chromosomes, provide the foundation for performing linkage analyses, whereby one attempts to correlate the inheritance of certain chromosomal regions (or linked genes) with the presence of a disease or genetic trait (see below).

After the first meiotic division, which results in two daughter cells ($2n$), the two chromatids of each chromosome separate during a second meiotic division to yield four gametes with a haploid state ($1n$). When the egg is fertilized by sperm, the two haploid sets are combined, thereby restoring the diploid state ($2n$) in the zygote.

REGULATION OF GENE EXPRESSION

Mechanisms that regulate gene expression play a critical role in the function of genes. The new field of *functional genomics* is based on the concept that understanding gene regulation and function will provide a better understanding of physiology and offer novel therapeutic opportunities. The transcription of genes is controlled primarily by *transcription factors* that bind to DNA sequences in the regulatory regions of genes. As described below, mutations in transcription factors cause an unexpectedly large number of genetic disorders. Gene expression is also influenced by *epigenetic events*, such as X-inactivation and imprinting, processes in which DNA methylation is associated with the silencing (i.e., suppression) of expression. Several genetic disorders, such as Prader-Willi syndrome (neonatal hypotonia, developmental delay, obesity, short stature, and hypogonadism) and Albright hereditary osteodystrophy (resistance to parathyroid hormone, short stature, brachydactyly, resistance to other hormones in certain subtypes), exhibit the consequences of genomic imprinting. Most studies of gene expression have focused on the regulatory DNA elements of genes that control transcription. However, it should be emphasized that gene expression requires a series of steps including mRNA processing, protein translation, and posttranslational modifications, all of which are actively regulated (Fig. 65-2).

STRUCTURE OF GENES A gene product is usually a protein but can occasionally consist of RNA that is not translated. *Exons* refer to the portion of genes that are eventually spliced together to form mRNA. *Introns* refer to the spacing regions between the exons that are spliced out of precursor RNAs during RNA processing (Fig. 65-2).

The gene locus also includes regions that are necessary to control

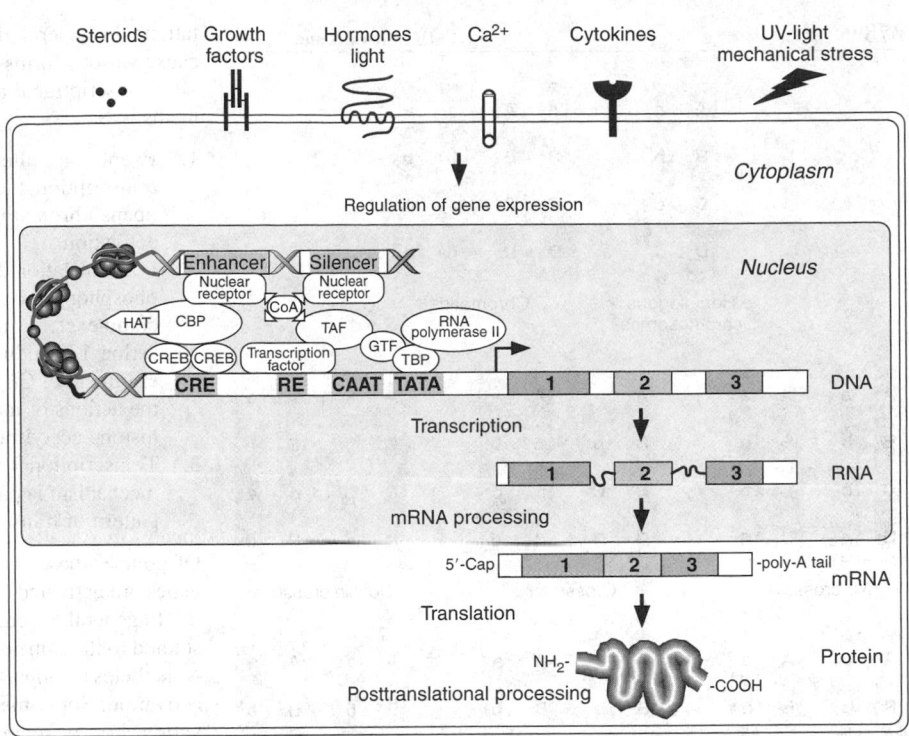

FIGURE 65-2 Flow of genetic information. Multiple extracellular signals activate intracellular signal cascades that result in altered regulation of gene expression through the interaction of transcription factors with regulatory regions of genes. RNA polymerase transcribes DNA into RNA that is processed to mRNA by excision of intronic sequences. The mRNA is translated into a polypeptide chain to form the mature protein after undergoing posttranslational processing. HAT, histone acetyl transferase; CBP, CREB-binding protein; CREB, cyclic AMP response element binding protein; CRE, cyclic AMP responsive element; CoA, Co activator; TAF, TBP-associated factors; GTF, general transcription factors; TBP, TATA-binding protein; TATA, TATA box; RE, response element; NH$_2$, aminoterminus; COOH, carboxyterminus.

its expression. The regulatory regions most commonly involve sequences upstream (5′) of the transcription start site, although there are also examples of control elements within introns or downstream of the coding regions of a gene. The upstream regulatory regions are also referred to as the *promoter*. The minimal promoter usually consists of a TATA box (which binds TATA-binding protein, TBP) and initiator sequences that enhance the formation of an active transcription complex. Transcriptional termination signals reside downstream, or 3′, of a gene. Specific sequences, such as the AAUAAA sequence at the 3′ end of the mRNA, designate the site for polyadenylation (poly-A tail), a process that influences mRNA transport to the cytoplasm, stability, and translation efficiency. A rigorous test of the regulatory region boundaries involves expressing a gene in a transgenic animal to determine whether the isolated DNA flanking sequences are sufficient to recapitulate the normal developmental, tissue-specific, and signal-responsive features of the endogenous gene. This has been accomplished for only a few genes; there are many examples in which large genomic fragments only partially reconstitute normal gene regulation in vivo, implying the presence of distant regulatory sequences. This approach is critical to our understanding of mechanisms that regulate genes and is also relevant for gene therapy strategies that require normal gene regulation (Chap. 69).

As genes are dissected with greater resolution, the number of DNA sequences and transcription factors that regulate transcription is much greater than originally anticipated. Most genes contain at least 15 to 20 discrete regulatory elements within 300 bp of the transcription start site. This densely packed promoter region often contains binding sites for ubiquitous transcription factors such as CAAT box/enhancer binding protein (C/EBP), cyclic AMP response element binding (CREB) protein, selective promoter factor 1 (Sp-1), or activator protein 1 (AP-1). However, factors involved in cell-specific expression may also bind to these sequences. For example, basic helix-loop-helix (bHLH) proteins bind to E-boxes in the promoters of myogenic genes, and ste-

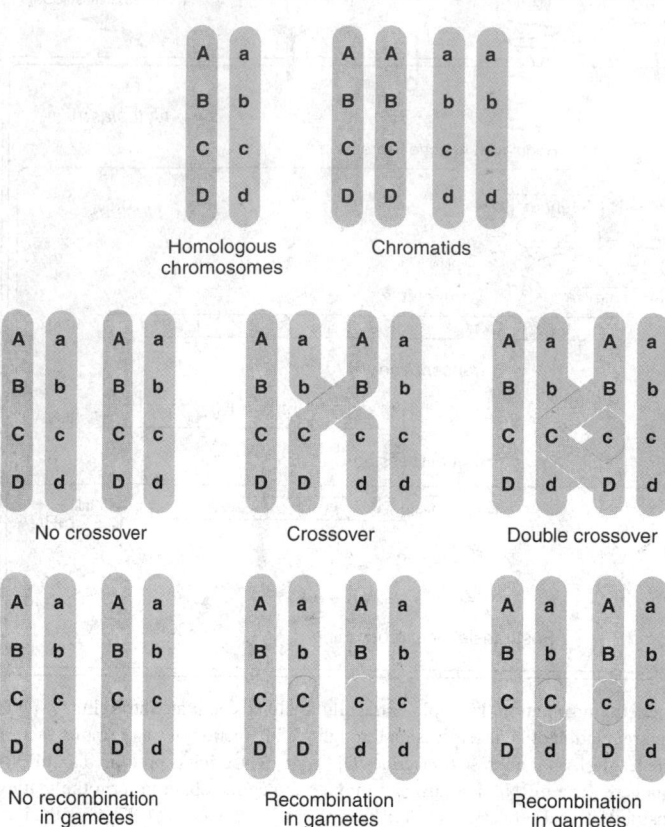

FIGURE 65-3 Crossing-over and genetic recombination. During chiasma formation, either of the two sister chromatids on one chromosome pairs with one of the chromatids of the homologous chromosome. Genetic recombination occurs through crossing-over and results in recombinant and nonrecombinant chromosome segments in the gametes. Together with the random segregation of the maternal and paternal chromosomes, recombination contributes to genetic diversity and forms the basis of the concept of linkage.

roidogenic factor 1 (SF-1) binds to a specific recognition site in the regulatory region of multiple steroidogenic enzyme genes. Key regulatory elements may also reside at some distance from the proximal promoter. The globin and the immunoglobulin genes, for example, contain *locus control regions* that are several kilobases away from the structural sequences of the gene. Specific groups of transcription factors that bind to these promoter and enhancer sequences provide a combinatorial code for regulating transcription. In this manner, relatively ubiquitous factors interact with more restricted factors to allow each gene to be expressed and regulated in a unique manner. As described below, the transcription factors that bind to DNA actually represent only the first level of regulatory control. Other proteins—*coactivators* and *corepressors*—interact with the DNA-binding transcription factors to generate large regulatory complexes. These complexes are subject to control by numerous cell-signaling pathways, including phosphorylation and acetylation. Ultimately, the recruited transcription factors interact with, and stabilize, components of the basal transcription complex that assembles at the site of the TATA box and initiator region. This basal transcription factor complex consists of >30 different proteins. Gene transcription occurs when RNA polymerase begins to synthesize RNA from the DNA template.

TRANSCRIPTIONAL ACTIVATION AND REPRESSION Every gene is controlled uniquely, whether in its spatial or temporal pattern of expression or in its response to extracellular signals. It is estimated that transcription factors account for about 30% of expressed genes. A growing number of identified genetic diseases involve transcription factors (Table 65-1). The MODY (maturity-onset diabetes of the young) disorders are representative of this group of diseases; mu-

tations in several different islet cell–specific transcription factors cause various forms of MODY (Chap. 333).

Transcriptional activation can be divided into three main mechanisms:

1. Events that alter chromatin structure can enhance the access of transcription factors to DNA. For example, histone acetylation opens chromatin structure and is correlated with transcriptional activation.
2. Posttranslational modifications of transcription factors, such as phosphorylation, can induce the assembly of active transcription complexes. As an example, phosphorylation of CREB protein on serine 133 induces a conformational change that allows the recruitment of CREB-binding protein (CBP), a factor that integrates the actions of many transcription factors, including proteins, with histone acetyltransferase activity.
3. Transcriptional activators can displace a repressor protein. This mechanism is particularly common during development when the pattern of transcription factor expression changes dynamically.

Of course, these mechanisms are not mutually exclusive, and most genes are activated by some combination of these events.

In general, mechanisms of transcriptional repression have not been studied to the same extent as mechanisms of transcriptional activation. Nonetheless, suppression of gene expression is as important as gene activation. Some mechanisms of repression are the corollary of activation. For example, repression is often associated with histone deacetylation or protein dephosphorylation. For nuclear hormone receptors, transcriptional silencing involves the recruitment of repression complexes that contain histone deacetylase activity. Aberrant expression of repressor proteins is sometimes associated with neoplasia. The t(15;17) chromosomal translocation that occurs in promyelocytic leukemia fuses the *PML* gene to a portion of the retinoic acid receptor α (*RAR α*) gene (Table 65-1). This event causes unregulated transcriptional repression in a manner that precludes normal cellular differentiation. The addition of the RAR ligand, retinoic acid, activates the receptor, thereby relieving repression and allowing cells to differentiate and ultimately undergo apoptosis. This mechanism has therapeutic importance as the addition of retinoic acid to treatment regimens induces a higher remission rate in patients with promyelocytic leukemia (Chap. 111).

CLONING AND SEQUENCING DNA

Since the mid-1970s, eight Nobel prizes have been awarded for research that led, directly or indirectly, to major methodological advances as well as to profound insights into genetics. Examples include the discoveries of reverse transcriptase, restriction enzymes, plasmid cloning vectors, DNA sequencing, and PCR. A description of recombinant DNA techniques, the methodology used for the manipulation, analysis, and characterization of DNA segments, is beyond the scope of this chapter. As these methods are widely used in genetics and molecular diagnostics, however, it is useful to review briefly some of the fundamental principles of cloning and DNA sequencing.

CLONING OF GENES *Cloning* refers to the creation of a recombinant DNA molecule that can be propagated indefinitely. The ability to clone genes and cDNAs therefore provides a permanent and renewable source of these reagents. Cloning is essential for DNA sequencing, nucleic acid hybridization studies, expression of recombinant proteins, and other recombinant DNA procedures.

The cloning of DNA involves the insertion of a DNA fragment into a cloning vector, followed by the propagation of the recombinant DNA in a host cell. The most straightforward cloning strategy involves inserting a DNA fragment into bacterial plasmids. Plasmids are small, autonomously replicating, circular DNA molecules that propagate separately from the chromosome in bacterial cells. The process of DNA insertion relies heavily on the use of restriction enzymes, which cleave DNA at highly specific sequences (usually 4 to 6 bp in length). Restriction enzymes generate complementary, cohesive sequences at the ends of the DNA fragment, which allow them to be efficiently ligated to the plasmid vector. Because plasmids contain genes that confer resistance to antibiotics, their presence in the host cell can be used for selection and DNA amplification.

A variety of vectors and appropriate hosts are now used for cloning (Table 65-2). Many of these are used for creating *libraries*, a term that refers to a collection of DNA clones. A genomic library represents an array of clones derived from genomic DNA. These overlapping DNA fragments represent the entire genome and can ultimately be arranged according to their linear order. Genomic libraries are propagated using a variety of vectors, such as lambda (λ) phage, cosmids, bacterial artificial chromosomes (BACs), and yeast artificial chromosomes (YACs). Phage libraries have been used extensively to isolate specific genes. Cosmids, BACs, and YACs are particularly useful for studying large genes and for defining the order of genes along the chromosomes (Fig. 65-4). cDNA libraries reflect clones derived from mRNA, typically from a particular tissue source. Thus, a cDNA library from the heart contains copies of mRNA expressed specifically in cardiac myocytes, in addition to those that are expressed ubiquitously. For this reason, a heart cDNA library will be enriched with cardiac-specific gene products and will differ from cDNA libraries generated from liver or pituitary mRNAs. As an example of the complexity of a genomic library, consider that the human genome contains 3×10^9 bp and the average genomic insert in a λ phage library is about 10^4 bp. Therefore, it requires at least 3×10^5 clones to represent all of the genomic DNA. Specific clones are isolated from the several hundred thousand clones by using DNA hybridization.

With completion of the HGP, all human genes have been cloned and sequenced. As a result, many of these cloning procedures will be unnecessary or greatly facilitated by the extensive information concerning DNA markers and the sequence of DNA (see below).

NUCLEIC ACID HYBRIDIZATION

Nucleic acid *hybridization* is a fundamental principle in molecular biology that takes advantage of the fact that the two complementary strands of nucleic acids bind, or *hybridize*, to one another with very high specificity. The goal of hybridization is to detect specific nucleic acid (DNA or RNA) sequences in a complex background of other sequences. This technique is used for Southern blotting, northern blotting, and for screening libraries (see above). Further adaptation of hybridization techniques has led to the development of microarray DNA chips.

Southern Blot Southern blotting is used to analyze whether genes have been deleted or rearranged. It is also used to detect restriction fragment length polymorphisms (RFLPs). Genomic DNA is digested with restriction endonucleases and separated by gel electrophoresis. Individual fragments can then be transferred to

Table 65-1 Examples of Diseases Caused by Transcription Factor Mutations and Rearrangements

Transcription Factor Class	Disorder
Nuclear receptors	
Androgen receptor	Complete or partial androgen insensitivity
	Spinobulbar muscular atrophy
Estrogen receptor	Unfused epiphyses, osteopenia, impaired fertility
	Amplified coactivators in breast cancer
Glucocorticoid receptor	Elevated cortisol without signs of hypercortisolism; increased mineralocorticoids and androgens
Thyroid hormone receptor β	Thyroid hormone resistance
Vitamin D receptor	Vitamin D–resistant rickets type II
AHC (DAX1)	Adrenal hypoplasia congenita
DAX1	Dosage-sensitive sex reversal
SF-1	Adrenal and gonadal deficiency
Zinc finger proteins	
WT1	WAGR syndrome: Wilm's tumor, aniridia, genitourinary malformations, mental retardation
	Denys-Drash syndrome: Wilm's tumor, renal dysgenesis and failure, gonadoblastomas
GLI-3	Greig cephalopolysyndactyly; polydactyly
Paired homeodomain (PAX) proteins	
PAX-2	Colobomas, renal hypoplasia
PAX-3	Waardenburg syndrome types 1 and 3
PAX-6	Aniridia, anophthalmia; autosomal dominant keratitis; Peter's anomaly: malformations of anterior chamber
Basic helix-loop-helix (bHLH) proteins	
MITF	Waardenburg syndrome type 2A
TWIST	Saethre-Chotzen syndrome: craniosynostosis, cleft palate, conductive deafness
Homeodomain proteins	
MSX1 (HOX7.1)	Tooth agenesis
MSX2 (HOX8.1)	Craniosynostosis
HOXD13	Synpolydactyly
RIEG	Rieger syndrome: craniofacial malformations, microcornea, pupillary distortion, dental abnormalities
IPF-1	Maturity-onset of diabetes mellitus type 4; pancreatic agenesis, diabetes mellitus type 2
High-mobility group (HMG) proteins	
SRY	Sex reversal
SOX-9	Campomelic dysplasia, sex reversal
Forkhead transcription factors	
HNF-4α	Maturity-onset of diabetes mellitus type 1
HNF-1α	Maturity-onset of diabetes mellitus type 3
HNF-1β	Maturity-onset of diabetes mellitus type 5
TITF2/FKHL15	Congenital hypothyroidism, cleft palate, spiky hair
POU homeodomain proteins	
POUF1 (PIT1)	Combined pituitary hormone deficiency (GH, PRL, TSH)
POU3F4/BRN4	X-linked deafness DFN3, stapes fusion
Coactivators	
CREB binding protein (CBP)	Rubenstein-Taybi syndrome
General transcription factors	
TFIIH subunits	Xeroderma pigmentosum; Cochayne syndrome; trichothiodystrophy
Cell cycle control proteins	
Rb	Retinoblastoma, other cancers
p53	Li-Fraumeni syndrome, other cancers
Transcription elongation factor	
VHL	von-Hippel–Lindau syndrome, pheochromocytoma
Chimeric proteins	
FUS—CHOP (transcription factor—b-Zip)	Mixed liposarcomas
PAX3 or 7—FKHR (paired box homeodomain—forkhead)	Alveolar rhabdomyosarcomas
EWS—ATF-1 (b-Zip)	Ewing's sarcoma
E2A—PBX1 (bHLH—homeodomain)	Acute lymphoblastic leukemia
MLL—ELL (transcription elongation)	Acute myeloid leukemia
PML—RAR (retinoid action)	Acute promyelocytic leukemia
PDGFR—ETS	Chronic myelogenous leukemia
TCR—TAL-1,2 (twist)	T cell leukemia
Ig-MYC (bHLH)	Lymphomas, leukemia

NOTE: Selected abbreviations include: AHC, adrenal hypoplasia congenita; DAX-1, dosage-sensitive sex-reversal adrenal hypoplasia congenita (critical region on the X chromosome); GLI, amplified in glioblastoma; SRY, sex-determining region Y; SOX, SRY box; HNF, hepatocyte nuclear factor; CREB, cAMP responsive element binding protein; VHL, Von Hippel–Lindau; FUS, fusion; EWS, Ewing's sarcoma; CHOP, C/EBP homologous protein; PBX, pre-B cell leukemia; MLL, mixed lineage leukemia; ELL, elongation factor homologous to MLL; PML, promyelocytic leukemia; RAR, retinoic acid receptor; PDGFR, platelet-derived growth factor receptor; TCR, T cell receptor; TAL, T cell acute leukemia.

Table 65-2   Commonly Used Vectors for Cloning of DNA

Vector	DNA Insert in kb	Host
Yeast artificial chromosome (YAC)	1000	*Saccharomyces cerevisiae*
Bacterial artificial chromosome (BAC)	250	*Escherichia coli*
P1 artificial chromosomes (PAC)	150	*E. coli*
Cosmid	35	*E. coli*
λ phage	15	*E. coli*
Plasmid	10	*E. coli*

NOTE: kb, kilobases.

a membrane and detected after hybridization with specific radioactive DNA probes. Because single base-pair mismatches can disrupt the hybridization of short DNA probes (oligonucleotides), a variation of the Southern blot, termed *oligonucleotide-specific hybridization* (OSH), uses short oligonucleotides to distinguish normal from mutant genes.

Northern Blot   Northern blots are used to analyze patterns and levels of gene expression in different tissues. In a northern blot, mRNA is separated on a gel and transferred to a membrane, and specific transcripts are detected using radiolabeled DNA as a probe. This technique is rapidly being supplanted by more sensitive and comprehensive methods such as reverse transcriptase (RT)–PCR and gene expression arrays on DNA chips (see below).

Microarray Technology   A rapidly evolving approach to genome-scale studies consists of *microarrays*, or *DNA chips*. These approaches consist of thousands of synthetic nucleic acid sequences aligned on thin glass or silicon surfaces. Fluorescently labeled test sample DNA or RNA is hybridized to the chip, and a computerized scanner detects sequence matches. Microarrays allow the detection of variations in DNA sequence and are used for mutational analysis and genotyping. Alternatively, the expression pattern of large numbers of mRNA transcripts can be determined by hybridization of RNA samples to cDNA or genomic microarrays. This method has tremendous potential in the era of functional genomics. As one example, microarrays can be used to develop genetic fingerprints of different types of lymphomas, providing information useful for classification, pathophysiology, prognosis, and treatment.

THE POLYMERASE CHAIN REACTION   The PCR, introduced in 1985, has revolutionized the way DNA analyses are performed and has become a cornerstone of molecular biology and genetic analysis. In essence, PCR provides a rapid way of cloning (amplifying) specific DNA fragments in vitro (Fig. 65-5). Exquisite specificity is conferred by the use of PCR primers, which are designed for a given DNA sequence. The geometric amplification of the DNA after multiple cycles yields remarkable sensitivity. As a result, PCR can be used to amplify DNA from very small samples, including single cells. These properties also allow DNA amplification from a variety of tissue sources including blood samples, biopsies, surgical or autopsy specimens, or cells from hair or saliva. PCR can also be used to study mRNA. In this case, the enzyme RT is first used to convert the RNA to DNA, which can then be amplified by PCR. This procedure, commonly known as *RT-PCR*, is useful as a quantitative measure of gene expression.

PCR provides a key component of molecular diagnostics. It provides a strategy for the rapid amplification of DNA (or mRNA) to search for mutations by a wide array of techniques, including DNA sequencing. PCR is also used for the amplification of highly polymorphic di- or trinucleotide repeat sequences, which allow various polymorphic alleles to be traced in genetic linkage or association studies. PCR is increasingly used to diagnose various microbial pathogens (Chap. 121).

DNA SEQUENCING   DNA sequencing is now an automated procedure. Although many protocols exist, the most commonly used strategy is based on the Sanger method in which dideoxynucleotides are used to randomly terminate DNA polymerization at each of the four bases (A,G,T,C). After separating the array of terminated DNA fragments using high-resolution gel or capillary electrophoresis, it is

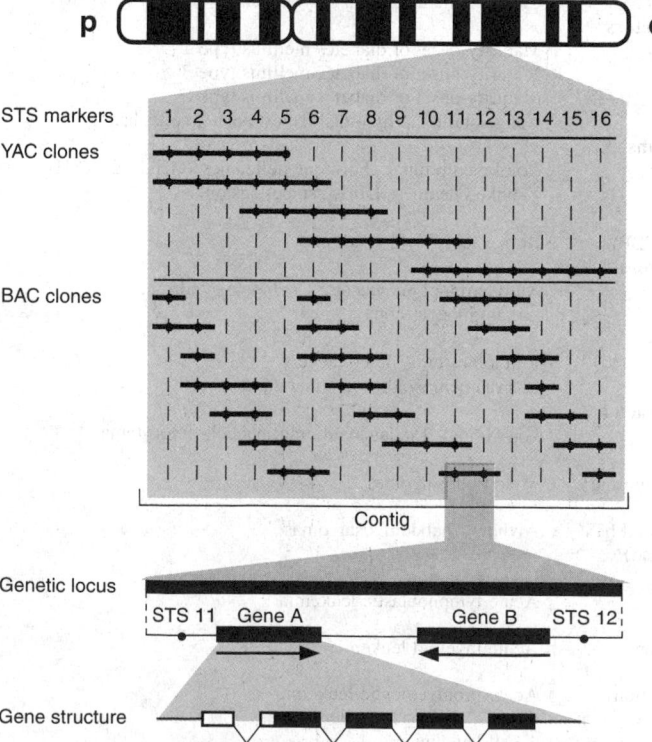

FIGURE 65-4   Overlapping genomic clones. A chromosomal region can be mapped after the cloning of DNA fragments into vectors, such as yeast artificial chromosomes (YAC) or bacterial artificial chromosomes (BAC). Sequenced-tag sites (STS) allow each clone to be characterized, and the order of clones can be determined based on overlapping sequences. A series of overlapping clones is called a contig.

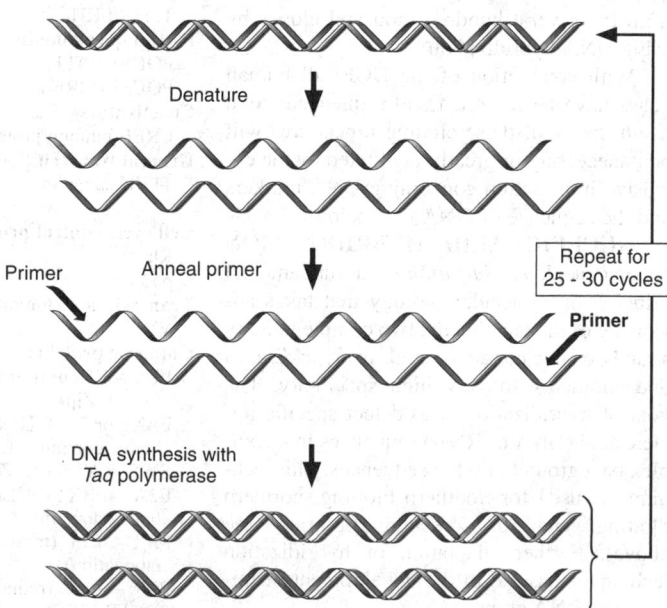

FIGURE 65-5   Polymerase chain reaction. The polymerase chain reaction (PCR) generates multiple copies of a DNA segment. After denaturing the double-stranded (ds) DNA, complementary synthetic oligonucleotide primers of about 20 bp are annealed on each side of the fragment of interest. A heat-stable polymerase then extends the oligonucleotides and synthesizes the complementary strand. This cycle is repeated 25 to 30 times. The number of DNA amplified DNA segments is thus doubled after every PCR cycle.

possible to deduce the DNA sequence by examining the progression of fragment lengths generated in each of the four nucleotide reactions. The use of fluorescently labeled dideoxynucleotides allows automated detection of the different bases and direct computer analysis of the DNA sequence. Efforts are underway to develop faster, more cost-effective DNA sequencing technologies. These include the use of mass spectrometry; detection of fluorescently labeled bases in flow cytometry; direct reading of the DNA sequence by scanning, tunneling, or atomic force microscopy; and sequence analysis using DNA chips.

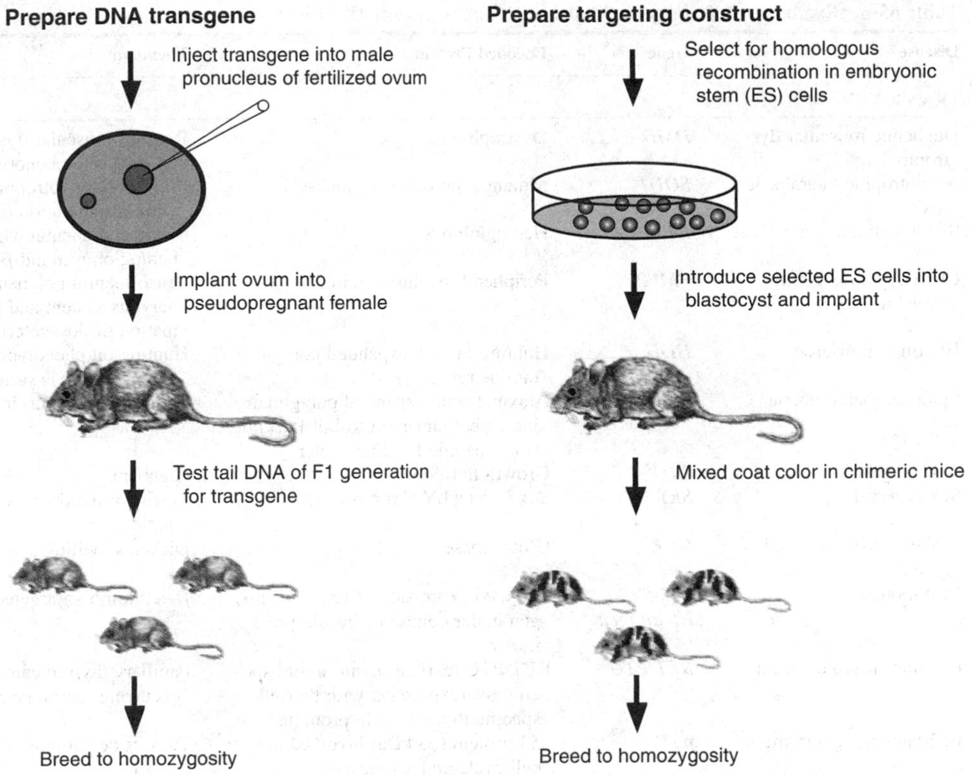

TRANSGENIC MICE AS MODELS OF GENETIC DISEASE

Several organisms have been studied extensively as genetic models, including *Mus musculus* (mouse), *Drosophila melanogaster* (fruit fly), *Caenorhabditis elegans* (nematode), *Saccharomyces cerevisiae* (baker's yeast), and *Eschericia coli* (colonic bacterium). The ability to use these evolutionarily distant organisms as genetic models that are relevant to human physiology reflects a surprising conservation of genetic pathways and gene function. Transgenic mouse models have been particularly valuable, because many human and mouse genes exhibit similar structure and function and because manipulation of the mouse genome is relatively straightforward compared to those of other mammalian species.

Transgenic strategies in mice can be divided into two main approaches: (1) overexpression of a gene by random insertion into the genome, and (2) deletion or targeted mutagenesis of a gene by homologous recombination with the native endogenous gene (Fig. 65-6). Many variations of these basic approaches now exist that allow genes to be expressed in specific cell types, at different times during development, or at varying levels. Consequently, transgenic technology has emerged as a powerful strategy for defining the physiologic effects of deleting or overexpressing a gene, as well as providing unique genetic models for dissecting pathophysiology or testing therapies.

Examples of transgenic models relevant to human genetic disorders are listed in Table 65-3. Transgenic overexpression of genes is useful for studying disorders that are sensitive to gene dosage. Overexpression of *PMP22*, for example, mimics a common duplication of this gene in type IA Charcot-Marie-Tooth disease (Chap. 379). Duplication of the *PMP22* gene results in high levels of expression of peripheral myelin protein 22, and this dosage effect is responsible for the demyelinating neuropathy. Expression of the Y chromosome–specific gene, *SRY*, in XX females demonstrates that *SRY* is sufficient to induce the formation of testes. This finding confirms the pathogenic role of *SRY* translocations to the X chromosome in sex-reversed XX females. Huntington disease is an autosomal dominant disorder caused by expansion of a CAG trinucleotide repeat that encodes a polyglutamine tract. Targeted deletion of the Huntington disease (*HD*) gene does not induce the neurologic disorder. On the other hand, transgenic expression of the entire gene or of the first exon containing the expanded polyGlu repeat is sufficient to cause many features of the neurologic disorder, indicating a gain-of-function property for the ex-

panded polyGlu-containing protein. Transgenic strategies can also be used as a precursor to gene therapy. Expression of dystrophin, the protein that is deleted in Duchenne muscular dystrophy, partially corrects the disorder in a mouse model of Duchenne's. Targeted expression of oncogenes has been valuable to study mechanisms of neoplasia and to generate immortalized cell lines. For example, expression of the simian virus 40 (SV40) large T antigen under the direction of the insulin promoter induces the formation of islet cell tumors.

Targeted deletion mutagenesis, commonly known as *gene knockout*, is performed using a targeting vector that carries a mutant version of the gene. After homologous recombination in embryonic stem (ES) cells, chimeric animals are produced by injection of ES cells into blastocysts. Subsequently, animals are bred to be heterozygous or homozygous for the mutation. In addition to their use in examining gene function, gene knockouts provide valuable animal models for many loss-of-function mutations. A variation of this strategy is to use cre recombinase to induce genetic recombination in vivo. Cre recombinase will delete genes that have been flanked by its recognition sequences, called *loxP* sites. One advantage to this approach is that transgenic expression of cre in specific tissues can be used to delete a gene in a tissue-specific or developmentally staged manner. This is particularly useful for genes that would be lethal if deleted universally or during early development.

The list of genes that have been knocked out in mice is already very large. Many of these knockouts do not have an apparent phenotype, either because of redundant functions of the other genes or because the phenotype is subtle. For example, deletion of the hypoxanthine phosphoribosyltransferase (HPRT) gene (*Hprt*) does not cause characteristic features of Lesch-Nyhan syndrome in mice because of their reliance on adenine phosphoribosyltransferase (APRT) in the purine salvage pathway. The administration of an APRT inhibitor to HPRT-deficient mice, however, results in the typical self-injurious be-

---

Prepare DNA transgene

Inject transgene into male pronucleus of fertilized ovum

Implant ovum into pseudopregnant female

Test tail DNA of F1 generation for transgene

Breed to homozygosity

Prepare targeting construct

Select for homologous recombination in embryonic stem (ES) cells

Introduce selected ES cells into blastocyst and implant

Mixed coat color in chimeric mice

Breed to homozygosity

FIGURE 65-6 Transgenic mouse models. *Left.* Transgenic mice are generated by pronuclear injection of foreign DNA into fertilized mouse oocytes and subsequent transfer into the oviduct of pseudopregnant foster mothers. *Right.* For targeted mutagenesis (gene knockout/knockin), embryonic stem (ES) cells are transfected with the targeted (mutagenized) transgene. The transgene undergoes homologous recombination with the wild-type gene. After selection, positive ES cells are introduced into blastocysts and implanted into foster mothers. Chimeric mice can be identified based on the mixed coat color of the offspring. Heterozygous mice are bred to obtain mice homozygous for the mutant allele.

Table 65-3 Examples of Transgenic Models of Human Genetic Disorders[a]

Disease	Gene	Encoded Protein	Phenotype
TRANSGENIC MODELS			
Duchenne muscular dystrophy	DMD	Dystrophin	Rescues muscular dystrophy in the *mdx* mouse, a natural mutant with a DMD-like phenotype
Amyotrophic lateral sclerosis	SOD1	Mutant superoxide dismutase 1	Similar to amyotrophic lateral sclerosis: motor neuron degeneration with accumulation of mutant SOD in perikarya and neurons
Sickle cell anemia	HBB	Hemoglobin S	Sickle cell anemia when in the genetic background of deleted normal hemoglobin α and β genes
Charcot-Marie-Tooth type 1A	PMP22	Peripheral myelin protein 22	Sensorineural polyneuropathy with demyelination in the peripheral nervous system and progressive weakness of the hind legs; confirmation of dosage effect of *PMP22* duplication
Huntington disease	HDH	Huntingtin with expanded polyglutamine repeat	Huntington phenotype; demonstration that expansion of the polyglutamine repeat is sufficient to induce neurologic abnormalities
Spinocerebellar ataxia	SCA1	Ataxin 1 with expanded polyglutamine repeat under control of Purkinje cell–specific Pcp2 promoter	Ataxia, loss of Purkinje cells, glial proliferation
Acromegaly	GH	Growth hormone	Giantism
Sex-reversal	SRY	Sex-reversal Y chromosome	Testis formation in XX females, confirming role of SRY in testis formation
Diabetes mellitus MODY type 2	GCK	Glucokinase	Diabetes mellitus
Insulinoma	INS-SV40 LT antigen	Targeted expression of large T antigen under control of insulin promoter	β-cell tumors; targeted oncogenesis with viral antigen
Papillary thyroid cancer	RET/PTC	RET/PTC rearrangement; tissue-specific overexpression with thyroid-specific thyroglobulin promoter	Papillary thyroid carcinoma; targeted oncogenesis using a naturally occurring rearrangement
Li-Fraumeni syndrome	p53	p53 protein (53 kDa) involved in cell cycle and apoptosis	Tumors developing at very early age with 100% penetrance
Cystic fibrosis	CFTR	Cystic fibrosis transmembrane conductance regulator	Similar to cystic fibrosis: defect in chloride transport; alterations in lung, intestinal system, pancreas; and premature death
Hemochromatosis	HFE	HFE hemochromatosis protein	Elevated plasma iron and transferrin saturation, increased hepatic iron concentration
Hemophilia A	Factor VIII	Factor VIII	Absent factor VIII; prolonged bleeding
Familial polyposis coli	APC	APC tumor suppressor protein	Intestinal polyps
Xeroderma pigmentosa	XPC XPA	Xeroderma pigmentosum C Xeroderma pigmentosum A	High susceptibility for chemical and UV light–induced skin cancer
Ataxia telangiectasia	ATM	ATM kinase (cell cycle regulator)	Growth retardation, neurologic dysfunction, infertility, defective T cell maturation, sensitivity to γ-irradiation, lymphomas
Apparent mineralocorticoid excess	HSD11B2	11β-Hydroxysteroid dehydrogenase 2	Hypertension, hypokalemia, low plasma renin activity, low aldosterone, decreased conversion of cortisol to cortisone
Glycogen storage disease type II (Pompe's disease)	GAA	Acid α-glucosidase	Accumulation of glycogen in cardiac and skeletal muscle lysosomes, muscle weakness
Obesity	MC4R	Melanocortin 4 receptor	Maturity onset of obesity, hyperphagia, hyperinsulinemia
Neurofibromatosis type 1	NF1/p53	Neurofibromin (tumor suppressor)	No tumors in +/− mice; neurofibromas in *Nf1* −/− mice and soft tissue sarcomas in *Nf1/p53* −/− mice
Lipoid congenital adrenal hyperplasia	StAR	Steroidogenic acute regulatory protein	Female external genitalia in males and females, death due to adrenocortical insufficiency, defects in adrenal steroids, lipid deposits in adrenal cortex
Atherosclerosis	APOE	Apolipoprotein E	Atherosclerosis, increase of VLDL and LDL, decreased efflux of LDL from macrophages
Familial hypercholesteronemia	LDLR	LDL receptor	Increased LDL and VLDL cholesterol levels, atherosclerosis, xanthomas
Prader-Willi syndrome	NDN	Necdin	Neonatal respiratory distress and lethality in mice carrying paternally inherited *Ndn* deletion
Polycystic kidney disease	Pkd1	PKD1 protein (protein-protein adhesion in extracellular compartment)	Pancreatic ductal cysts, massive renal cysts, perinatal lethality
TARGETED MUTAGENESIS: GENE KNOCK-IN			
Osteogenesis imperfecta	Col1a1	Collagen 1	Osteogenesis imperfecta type 4 with variability in phenotype
Gaucher disease	GD1	Glucocerebrosidase	Glucosylceramide accumulation in brain and liver; premature death
Acute lymphoblastic leukemia	BCL-ABL	Reciprocal translocation of BCL and ABL	Transgenic model using a tetracycline-responsive promoter for BCL-ABL expression

[a] A comprehensive list of transgenic mouse models and spontaneous mouse mutants can be found at the Jackson laboratory (www.jax.org/tbase). This site contains numerous links to other databases with murine and other mammalian transgenic models.
NOTE: LDL, low-density lipoprotein; VLDL, very low density lipoprotein.

havior seen in patients with Lesch-Nyhan syndrome. The phenotypes of some knockouts are quite different from their human disease counterparts. For example, deletion of the retinoblastoma (*Rb*) gene does not lead to retinoblastoma or other tumors that characterize the human syndrome. These examples underscore the fact that the functions of genes, and their interactions with genetic background and the environment, cannot be assumed to be identical in mice and humans. On the other hand, the deletion of many genes provides a remarkably

In addition to transgenic animal models, naturally occurring mu-tations in mice and other species continue to provide fundamental insights into human disease. A compendium of natural and transgenic animal models is provided in continuously evolving databases (Online Mendelian Inheritance in Animals OMIA: www.angis.su.oz.au/Data-bases/BIRX/omia/; The Jackson Library: www.jax.org/).

Human pluripotential *stem cells* have recently been developed, and, consistent with their potential for self-renewal, these cell lines express high levels of telomerase, an enzyme that is essential for al-lowing repeated replication of the ends of eukaryotic chromosomes. Although much remains to be learned about the properties of pluri-potential stem cells, they may prove useful for transplantation, drug testing, or for other purposes.

THE HUMAN GENOME PROJECT

The HGP was initiated in the mid-1980s as an ambitious effort to characterize the human genome, culminating in a complete DNA se-quence. In the United States, the National Institutes of Health (NIH) and the Department of Energy (DOE) officially launched the genome project in 1990; the project has evolved as an international effort and has also included important contributions from the private sector. The main goals include: (1) creation of genetic maps, (2) development of physical maps, and (3) determination of the complete human DNA sequence.

Some analogies help in appreciating the scope of the HGP. The 23 pairs of human chromosomes are thought to encode approximately 100,000 genes. The total length of DNA is about 3 billion bp, which is nearly 1000-fold greater than the *E. coli* genome. If the human DNA sequence were printed out, it would correspond to about 120 volumes of *Harrison's Principles of Internal Medicine*.

THE GENETIC MAP Given the size and complexity of the human genome, genetic maps have been developed to provide orien-tation and to delimit where a gene of interest may be located. A *genetic map* describes the order of genes and defines the position of a gene relative to other loci on the same chromosome. It is constructed by assessing how frequently two markers are inherited together by linkage studies. Distances of the genetic map are expressed in recombination units, or centimorgans (cM). One cM corresponds to a recombination frequency of 1% between two polymorphic markers; 1 cM corresponds to approximately 1 Mb of DNA (Fig. 65-3). Any polymorphic se-quence variation can be useful for mapping purposes. Examples of polymorphic markers include variable number of tandem repeats (VNTRs), RFLPs, microsatellite repeats, and single nucleotide poly-morphisms (SNPs); the latter two methods are now used predomi-nantly because of the high density of markers and because they are amenable to automated procedures.

The current genetic map exists at about 1 cM resolution. A goal for the near term is to add about 100,000 SNPs to these maps. This would provide 1 SNP approximately every 100,000 bp. The addition of SNPs will facilitate automation using DNA chips and will enhance the ability to perform linkage studies of complex genetic diseases.

THE PHYSICAL MAP Cytogenetics and chromosomal banding techniques provide a relatively low-resolution microscopic view of genetic loci. Physical maps indicate the position of a locus or gene in absolute values. Sequence-tagged sites (STSs) are used as a standard unit for physical mapping and serve as sequence-specific landmarks for arranging overlapping cloned fragments in the same order as they occur in the genome. These overlapping clones, usually in YACs or BACs, allow the characterization of contiguous DNA se-quences, commonly referred to as *contigs* (Fig. 65-4). The STSs con-sist of 200 to 500 bp, which can be retrieved from computer databases; >50,000 STSs have been mapped. The goal of achieving a high-resolution physical map of the human genome has essentially been achieved as all of the genome has been cloned into overlapping

fragments. The highest resolution physical map will provide the com-plete DNA sequence of each chromosome in the human genome.

STATUS OF DNA SEQUENCING The primary focus of the genome project is to obtain DNA sequence for the entire human ge-nome as well as model organisms. The sequences of *E. coli* and many other bacteria, *S. cerevisiae*, *C. elegans*, and *D. melanogaster* have already been completed. Sequencing of the laboratory mouse genome is in progress. Although the prospect of determining the complete se-quence of the human genome was a daunting prospect several years ago, technical advances in DNA sequencing and bioinformatics have led to the completion of a draft human sequence in June 2000, well in advance of the original goal of the year 2003. The current standard is to achieve 99.99% (1 error in 10,000 bp) accuracy. This level of ac-curacy is important for many reasons, including efforts to determine the degree of DNA sequence variation in the population. Comparisons of the DNA sequence from multiple individuals or populations will allow assessments of genetic variance in the human population. An-other goal is to develop a complete set of full-length human cDNAs and to define their locations on the physical map.

ETHICAL ISSUES Implicit in the HGP is the idea and hope that identifying disease-causing genes can lead to improvements in diagnosis, prognosis, and treatment. It is estimated that most individ-uals harbor several serious recessive genes. However, completion of the human genome sequence, determination of the association of ge-netic defects with disease, and studies of genetic variation raise many new issues with implications for the individual and mankind. The con-troversies concerning the cloning of mammals and the establishment of human embryonic stem cells underscore the relevance of these ques-tions. Moreover, the information gleaned from genotypic results can have quite different impacts, depending on the availability of strategies to modify the course of disease. For example, the identification of mutations that cause multiple endocrine neoplasia (MEN) type 2 or hemochromatosis allows specific interventions for affected family members. On the other hand, at present the identification of an Alz-heimer or Huntington disease gene does not alter therapy. Genetic test results can generate anxiety in affected individuals and family mem-bers, and there is the possibility of discrimination on the basis of the test results. Most genetic disorders are likely to fall into an interme-diate category where the opportunity for prevention or treatment is significant but limited (Chap. 68). For these reasons, the scientific components of the HGP have been paralleled by efforts to examine ethical and legal implications as new issues arise.

Many issues raised by the genome project are familiar, in principle, to medical practitioners. For example, an asymptomatic patient with increased low-density lipoprotein (LDL) cholesterol, high blood pres-sure, or a strong family history of early myocardial infarction, is known to be at increased risk of coronary heart disease. In such cases, it is clear that the identification of risk factors and an appropriate in-tervention are beneficial. Likewise, patients with phenylketonuria, cys-tic fibrosis, or sickle cell anemia are often identified as having a genetic disease early in life. These precedents can be helpful for adapting policies that relate to genetic information. We can anticipate similar efforts, whether based on genotypes or other markers of genetic pre-disposition, to be applied to many disorders. One confounding aspect of the rapid expansion of information is that our ability to make clinical predictions often lags behind genetic advances. For example, when genes that predispose to breast cancer, such as *BRCA1*, are described, they generate tremendous public interest in the potential to predict disease, but many years of clinical research are still required to rig-orously establish genotype and phenotype correlations.

Whether related to informed consent, participation in research, or the management of a genetic disorder that affects an individual or their families, there is a great need for more information about fundamental principles of genetics. The pervasive nature of the role of genetics in medicine makes it imperative for physicians and other health care pro-fessionals to become more informed about genetics and to provide advice and counseling in conjunction with trained genetic counselors (Chap. 68). The application of screening and prevention strategies will therefore require intensive patient and physician education, changes in health care financing, and legislation to protect patient's rights.

TRANSMISSION OF GENETIC DISEASE

ORIGINS AND TYPES OF MUTATIONS   A *mutation* can be defined as any change in the primary nucleotide sequence of DNA regardless of its functional consequences. Some mutations may be lethal, others are less deleterious, and some may confer an evolutionary advantage. Mutations can occur in the germline (sperm or oocytes); these can be transmitted to progeny. Alternatively, mutations can occur during embryogenesis or in somatic tissues. Mutations that occur during development lead to *mosaicism*, a situation in which tissues are composed of cells with different genetic constitutions. If the germline is mosaic, a mutation can be transmitted to some progeny but not others, which sometimes leads to confusion in assessing the pattern of inheritance. Somatic mutations that do not affect cell survival can sometimes be detected because of variable phenotypic effects in tissues (e.g., pigmented lesions in McCune-Albright syndrome). Other somatic mutations are associated with neoplasia because they confer a growth advantage to cells. Epigenetic events such as altered DNA methylation may also influence gene expression. With the exception of triplet nucleotide repeats, which can expand (see below), mutations are usually stable.

Mutations are structurally diverse—they can involve the entire genome, as in triploidy (one extra set of chromosomes), or gross numerical or structural alterations in chromosomes or individual genes (Chap. 66). Large deletions may affect a portion of a gene or an entire gene, or, if several genes are involved, they may lead to a *contiguous gene syndrome*. Unequal crossing-over between homologous genes can result in fusion gene mutations, as illustrated by color blindness (Chap. 28). Mutations involving single nucleotides are referred to as *point mutations*. Substitutions are called *transitions* if a purine is replaced by another purine base (A ↔ G) or if a pyrimidine is replaced by another pyrimidine (C ↔ T). Changes from a purine to a pyrimidine, or vice versa, are referred to as *transversions*. If the DNA sequence change occurs in a coding region and alters an amino acid, it is called a *missense mutation*. Depending on the functional consequences of such a missense mutation, amino acid substitutions in different regions of the protein can lead to distinct phenotypes. *Polymorphisms* are sequence variations that have a frequency of at least 1%. Usually, they do not result in a perceptible phenotype. Often they consist of single base-pair substitutions that do not alter the protein coding sequence because of the degenerate nature of the genetic code, although it is possible that some might alter mRNA stability, translation, or the amino acid sequence. These types of silent base substitutions and SNPs are encountered frequently during genetic testing and must be distinguished from true mutations that alter protein expression or function. Small nucleotide deletions or insertions cause a shift of the codon reading frame. Most commonly, reading frame alterations result in an abnormal protein segment of variable length before termination of translation occurs at a stop codon (*nonsense mutation*). Mutations in intronic sequences or in exon junctions may destroy or create splice donor or splice acceptor sites. Mutations may also be found in the regulatory sequences of genes, resulting in reduced gene transcription.

Mutation Rates   As noted before, mutations represent an important cause of genetic diversity as well as disease. Mutation rates are difficult to determine in humans because many mutations are silent and because testing is often not adequate to detect the phenotypic consequences. Mutation rates vary in different genes but are estimated to occur at a rate of about 10^{-10}/bp per cell division. Germline mutation rates (as opposed to somatic mutations) are relevant in the transmission of genetic disease. Because the population of oocytes is established

very early in development, only about 20 cell divisions are required for completed oogenesis, whereas spermatogenesis involves about 30 divisions by the time of puberty and 20 cell divisions each year thereafter. Consequently, the probability of acquiring new point mutations is much greater in the male germline than the female germline, in which rates of aneuploidy are increased (Chap. 66). Thus, the incidence of new point mutations in spermatogonia increases with paternal age (e.g., achondrodysplasia, Marfan syndrome, neurofibromatosis). It is estimated that about 1 in 10 sperm carries a new deleterious mutation. The rates for new mutations are calculated most readily for autosomal dominant and X-linked disorders and are ~10^{-5} to 10^{-6}/locus per generation. Because most monogenic diseases are relatively rare, new mutations account for a significant fraction of cases. This is important in the context of genetic counseling, as a new mutation can be transmitted to the affected individual but does not necessarily imply that the parents are at risk to transmit the disease to other children. An exception to this is when the new mutation occurs early in germline development, leading to *gonadal mosaicism*.

Unequal Crossing-Over   Normally, DNA recombination in germ cells occurs with remarkable fidelity to maintain the precise junction sites for the exchanged DNA sequences (Fig. 65-2). However, mispairing of homologous sequences leads to unequal crossover, with gene duplication on one of the chromosomes and gene deletion on the other chromosome. A significant fraction of growth hormone (*GH*) gene deletions, for example, involve unequal crossing-over (Chap. 328). The *GH* gene is a member of a large gene cluster that includes a growth hormone variant gene as well as several structurally related chorionic somatomammotropin genes and pseudogenes (highly homologous but functionally inactive relatives of a normal gene). Because such gene clusters contain multiple homologous DNA sequences arranged in tandem, they are particularly prone to undergo recombination and, consequently, gene duplication or deletion. On the other hand, duplication of the *PMP22* gene as a result of unequal crossing-over results in increased gene dosage and type IA Charcot-Marie-Tooth disease (Chap. 379). Unequal crossing-over resulting in deletion of *PMP22* results in a distinct neuropathy called *hereditary liability to pressure palsy* (Chap. 379).

Glucocorticoid-remediable aldosteronism (GRA) is caused by a rearrangement involving the genes that encode aldosterone synthase (*CYP11B2*) and steroid 11β-hydroxylase (*CYP11B1*), normally arranged in tandem on chromosome 8q. These two genes are 95% identical, predisposing to gene duplication and deletion by unequal crossing-over. The rearranged gene product contains the regulatory regions of 11β-hydroxylase fused to the coding sequence of aldosterone synthetase. Consequently, the latter enzyme is expressed in the adrenocorticotropic hormone (ACTH)-dependent zone of the adrenal gland, resulting in overproduction of mineralocorticoids and hypertension (Chap. 331).

Gene conversion refers to a nonreciprocal exchange of homologous genetic information; it is probably more common than generally recognized. In human genetics, gene conversion has been used to explain how an internal portion of a gene is replaced by a homologous segment copied from another allele or locus; these genetic alterations may range from a few nucleotides to a few thousand nucleotides. As a result of gene conversion, it is possible for short DNA segments of two chromosomes to be identical, even though these sequences are distinct in the parents. A practical consequence of this phenomenon is that nucleotide substitutions can occur during gene conversion between related genes, often altering the function of the gene. In disease states, gene conversion often involves intergenic exchange of DNA between a gene and a related pseudogene. For example, the 21-hydroxylase gene (*CYP21A*) is adjacent to a nonfunctional pseudogene. Many of the nucleotide substitutions that are found in the *CYP21A* gene in patients with congenital adrenal hyperplasia correspond to sequences that are present in the pseudogene, suggesting gene conversion as a mechanism of mutagenesis. In addition, mitotic gene conversion has been suggested as a mechanism to explain revertant mosaicism in which an inherited mutation is "corrected" in certain cells. For example, patients with autosomal recessive generalized atrophic benign epidermolysis bullosa have acquired reverse mutations in one of the two mutated *COL17A1* alleles, leading to clinically unaffected patches of skin.

Insertions and Deletions Though many instances of insertions and deletions occur as a consequence of unequal crossing-over, there is also evidence for internal duplication, inversion, or deletion of DNA sequences. The fact that certain deletions or insertions appear to occur repeatedly as independent events suggests that specific regions within the DNA sequence predispose to these errors. For example, certain regions of the *DMD* gene appear to be hot spots for deletions.

Errors in DNA Repair Because mutations caused by defects in DNA repair accumulate as somatic cells divide, these types of mutations are particularly important in the context of neoplastic disorders (Chap. 82). Several genetic disorders involving DNA repair enzymes underscore their importance. Patients with xeroderma pigmentosum have defects in DNA damage recognition or in the nucleotide excision and repair pathway (Chap. 86). Exposed skin is dry and pigmented and is extraordinarily sensitive to the mutagenic effects of ultraviolet irradiation. More than 10 different genes have been shown to cause the different forms of xeroderma pigmentosum. This finding is consistent with the earlier classification of this disease into different complementation groups (Table 65-4) in which normal function is rescued by the fusion of cells derived from two different forms of xeroderma pigmentosum.

Ataxia telangiectasia causes large telangiectatic lesions of the face, cerebellar ataxia, immunologic defects, and hypersensitivity to ionizing radiation (Chap. 364). The discovery of the ataxia telangiectasia mutated (*ATM*) gene reveals that it is homologous to genes involved in DNA repair and control of cell cycle checkpoints. Mutations in the *ATM* gene give rise to defects in meiosis as well as increasing susceptibility to damage from ionizing radiation. Fanconi's anemia is also associated with an increased risk of multiple acquired genetic abnormalities. It is characterized by diverse congenital anomalies and a strong predisposition to develop aplastic anemia and acute myelogenous leukemia (Chap. 111). Cells from these patients are susceptible to chromosomal breaks caused by a defect in genetic recombination. At least eight different complementation groups have been identified, and several loci and genes associated with Fanconi's anemia have been mapped or cloned (Table 65-4).

HNPCC is caused by mutations in one of several different mismatch repair (MMR) genes including MutS homologue 2 (*MSH2*) and MutL homologue 1 (*MLH1*) (Chap. 90). These enzymes are involved in the detection of nucleotide mismatches and in the recognition of slipped-strand trinucleotide repeats. Germline mutations in these genes lead to microsatellite instability and a high mutation rate in colon cancer. This syndrome is characterized by autosomal dominant trans-

mission of colon cancer, young age (<50 years) of presentation, predisposition to lesions in the proximal large bowel, and associated malignancies such as uterine cancer and ovarian cancer. Genetic screening tests for this disorder are now being used for families considered to be at risk (Chap. 68). Recognition of HNPCC allows early screening with colonoscopy and the implementation of prevention strategies using nonsteroidal anti-inflammatory drugs.

CpG and Dipyrimidine Sequences Certain DNA sequences are particularly susceptible to mutagenesis. Successive pyrimidine residues (e.g., T-T or C-C) are subject to the formation of ultraviolet light–induced photoadducts. If these pyrimidine dimers are not repaired by the nucleotide excision repair pathway, mutations will be introduced after DNA synthesis. The dinucleotide C-G, or CpG, is also a hot spot for a specific type of mutation. In this case, methylation of the cytosine is associated with an enhanced rate of deamination to uracil, which is then replaced with thymine. This C → T transition (or G → A on the opposite strand) accounts for at least one-third of point mutations associated with polymorphisms and mutations. Many of the *MSH2* mutations in HNPCC, for example, involve CpG sequences.

Table 65-4 Selected Examples of Locus Heterogeneity

Phenotype	Gene/Locus	Chromosomal Location	Protein
Hypertrophic cardiomyopathy			
CMH1	*MYH7*	14q12	Myosin heavy chain β
CMH2	*TNNT2*	1q2	Troponin-T2
CMH3	*TPM1*	15q22.1	Tropomyosin α
CMH4	*MYBPC3*	11p11q	Myosin binding protein C
Osteogenesis imperfecta			
Type 1	*COL1A1*	17q21.31-q22.05	Collagen α₁
Type 2	*COL1A2*	7q22.1	Collagen α₂
Retinitis pigmentosa			
RP1	*ORP1*	8q11-13	Oxygen-regulated photoreceptor ORP1
RP2	*RP2*	Xp11.3	RP2
RP3	*RP3*	Xp21.1	Retinitis pigmentosa GTPase regulator
Numerous other syndromic and nonsyndromic forms of RP			
Tuberous sclerosis			
TSC1	*TSC1*	9q34	Hamartin
TSC2	*TSC2*	16p13.3	Tuberin
Familial Alzheimer disease			
AD1	*APP*	21q21.3-22.05	Amyloid precursor protein
AD2 (modifying gene)	*APOE*	19q13.2	Apolipoprotein E
AD3	*PSEN1*	14q24.3	Presenilin 1
AD4	*PSEN2*	1q31-42	Presenilin 2
Familial breast cancer			
BRCA1	*BRCA1*	17q21	BRCA1 (RNA polymerase II component)
BRCA2	*BRCA2*	13q12.3	BRCA2
Xeroderma pigmentosum			
XP1	*XPA*	9q22.3	XPA
XP	*XPCC*	3p25	XPCC nucleotide excision repair protein
XP4	*ERCC2*	19q13.2-13.3	ERCC2 DNA repair protein
Fanconi anemia			
FANCA	*FAA*	16q24.3	FAA protein
FANCA	*FAB* locus	?	?
FANCC	*FAC*	9q22.3	FAC protein
FANCD	*FAD* locus	3p26-22	?
FANCE	*FAE* locus	6p22-21	?
FANCF	*FAF*	11p15	FAF/ROM
FANCG	*FAG*	9p13	FAG/XRCC9
FANCH	*FAH* locus	?	?
Polycystic kidney disease			
PKD1	*PKD1*	16p13.3-13.12	Polycystin 1
PKD2	*PKD2*	4q21-23	Polycystin 2

Certain types of mutations (C → T or G → A) are relatively common. Moreover, the redundant nature of the genetic code results in overrepresentation of certain amino acid substitutions. For example, arginine codons are most likely to be converted to cysteine, tryptophan, or a stop codon when a C → T transition occurs, and to histidine or glutamine when a G → A transition occurs.

Unstable DNA Sequences *Trinucleotide repeats* may be unstable and expand beyond a critical number. Mechanistically, the expansion is thought to be caused by unequal recombination and slipped mispairing. A premutation represents a small increase in trinucleotide copy number. In subsequent generations, the expanded repeat may increase further in length and result in an increasingly severe phenotype, a process called *dynamic mutation* (see below for discussion of anticipation). Trinucleotide expansion was first recognized as a cause of the fragile X syndrome, one of the most common causes of mental retardation (Chap. 359). Other disorders arising from a similar mechanism include Huntington disease (Chap. 362), X-linked spinobulbar muscular atrophy (Chap. 365), and myotonic dystrophy (Chap. 383) (Tables 65-5 and 65-6). Malignant cells are also characterized by genetic instability, indicating a breakdown in mechanisms that regulate DNA repair and the cell cycle.

FUNCTIONAL CONSEQUENCES OF MUTATIONS Functionally, mutations can be broadly classified as gain-of-function and loss-of-function mutations. Gain-of-function mutations are typically dominant; that is, they result in phenotypic alterations when a single allele is affected. Inactivating mutations are usually recessive, and an affected individual is homozygous or compound heterozygous (i.e., carrying two different mutant alleles) for the disease-causing mutations. Alternatively, mutation in a single allele can result in *haploinsufficiency*, a situation in which one normal allele is not sufficient for a normal phenotype. This phenomenon applies, for example, to expression of rate-limiting en-

Table 65-5   Selected Monogenic Disorders for Which Genetic Testing Is Available

Disorder	Inheritance[a]	Gene[b]	Chapters
Oncology			
Hereditary nonpolyposis colon cancer	AD	*MSH2, MLH1*	81, 90
Familial adenomatous polyposis	AD	*APC*	81, 90
Familial breast cancer	AD	*BRCA1, BRCA2*	81, 89, 97
Basal cell nevus	AD	*PTCH*	57, 81, 89
Li-Fraumeni syndrome	AD	*P53*	81, 88, 89, 98
Von Hippel–Lindau syndrome	AD	*VHL*	81, 94, 332, 370
Retinoblastoma	AD	*RB*	81, 359
Familial malignant melanoma	AD	*CDKN2A*	81, 86
Multiple endocrine neoplasia type 1	AD	*MEN1*	81, 93, 339, 341
Multiple endocrine neoplasia type 2	AD	*RET*	81, 93, 339, 341
Ataxia telangiectasia	AR	*ATM*	57, 81, 308, 364
Hematology			
Spherocytosis	AD	*SPTB, SLC4A1, ANK1, EPB42*	108
von Willebrand's disease	AD	*VWF*	62, 116
Antithrombin III	AD	*AT*	62, 117
Factor V Leiden	AD	*F5*	62, 117, 261, 361
Sickle cell disease	AR	*HBB*	106
α Thalassemia	AR	*HBA2* and others	106
β Thalassemia	AR	*HBB* and others	106
Familial Mediterranean fever	AR	*MEFV*	289
Hemophilia A	XL	*F8C*	117
Hemophilia B	XL	*F9*	117
Glucose-6-phosphate dehydrogenase deficiency	XL	*G6PD*	71, 108
Cardiovascular			
Hypertrophic obstructive cardiomyopathy	AD	*MYH7, MYBPC3, TNNT2, TPM1*	238
Long QT syndrome	AD	*KCNQ1, KCNH2, SCN5A*	230
Pulmonary			
Cystic fibrosis	AR	*CFTR*	257, 304
α₁ Antitrypsin deficiency	AR	*PI*	258, 300
Nephrology			
Polycystic kidney disease	AD	*PKD1, PKD2*	276
Nephrogenic diabetes insipidus	XL/AR	*AVPR2, AQP2*	49, 329
Gastrointestinal			
Hereditary hemorrhagic telangiectasia	AD	*ENG*	44
Peutz-Jegher syndrome	AD	*STK11*	90
Wilson's disease	AR	*ATP7B*	300, 348
Hemochromatosis	AR	*HFE*	345
Bone/Connective tissue			
Achondroplasia	AD	*FGFR3*	343
Crouzon syndrome	AD	*FGFR2*	343
Marfan syndrome	AD	*FBN1*	234, 351
Osteogenesis imperfecta	AD	*COL1A1, COL1A2*	351
Ehlers-Danlos syndrome	AD	Multiple genes	351
Amyloidosis	AD	*TTR*	238, 319
Menkes syndrome	XL	*ATP7A*	351, 359
Endocrinology			
Maturity-onset diabetes of the young	AD	Multiple genes	333
Neurohypophyseal diabetes insipidus	AD	*AVP*	49, 329
Thyroid hormone resistance	AD	*THRB*	330
Male-limited precocious puberty	AD	*LHCGR*	338
Congenital adrenal hyperplasia	AR	*CYP21*	53, 331, 338
Obesity	AR	*MC4R, LEPR, LEP, POMC*	77
Androgen insensitivity	XL	*AR*	338
Male-to-female sex reversal	YL	*SRY*	338
Metabolism			
Familial hypercholesterolemia	AD	*LDLR*	241, 344
Glycogen storage disease type I–VIII	AR	Multiple genes	350
Tay-Sachs disease	AR	*HEXA*	349, 359
Gaucher disease	AR	*GBA*	349
Mucopolysaccharidosis type I–VII	AR	Multiple genes	349
Phenylketonuria	AR	*PAH*	352
Pseudocholinesterase deficiency	AR	*BCHE*	71, 72
Niemann-Pick disease	AR	*SMPD1, NPC1*	349

(continued)

Table 65-5 Selected Monogenic Disorders for Which Genetic Testing is Available—(continued)

Disorder	Inheritance[a]	Gene[b]	Chapters
Neurologic			
Huntington disease	AD	HD	359, 362
Neurofibromatosis type I and II	AD	NF1, NF2	81, 359, 370
Familial Parkinson disease	AD	SNCA, PARK2	359, 364
Spinocerebellar ataxia type 1–12	AD	Multiple genes	359, 364
Amyotrophic lateral sclerosis	AD	SOD1	359, 365
Tuberous sclerosis type 1 and 2	AD	TSC1, TSC2	359, 370
Familial Alzheimer disease	AD	PSEN1, PSEN2, APP, APOE	359, 362
Malignant hyperthermia	AD	RYR1	17, 381, 359
Familial fatal insomnia	AD	PRNP	27, 359, 373
Charcot-Marie-Tooth disease	AD	Multiple genes	359, 377
Hyperkalemic periodic paralysis	AD	SCN4A	49, 359, 381
Hypokalemic periodic paralysis	AD	CACNA1S	49, 359, 381
Friedreich ataxia	AR	FRDA1	359, 364
Duchenne and Becker muscular dystrophy	XL	DMD	238, 359, 381
Fragile X syndrome	XL	FMR1, FRAXE	359
Adrenoleukodystrophy	XL	ALD	331, 359
Spinobulbar muscular atrophy	XL	AR	359, 364

[a] For many disorders, several different types of inheritance have been described. The most common form of transmission is listed. Additional information on these disorders, including specific mutations, can be found on-line at the Human Genome Mutation Database (HGMD) www.uwcm.ac.uk, or in the On-line Mendelian Inheritance in Man (OMIM) catalogue www.ncbi.nlm.nih.gov/Omim. An overview of available genetic tests and laboratories can be found at www.genetests.org.

[b] Only some of the genes associated with these disorders have been listed. In some instances, there is genetic heterogeneity.

NOTE: AD, autosomal dominant; AR, autosomal recessive; XL, X-linked; YL, Y-linked.

zymes in heme synthesis that cause porphyrias (Chap. 346). An increase in dosage of a gene product may also result in disease, as illustrated by the duplication of the *DAX1* gene in dosage-sensitive sex-reversal (Chap. 338). Mutation in a single allele can also result in loss of function due to a dominant-negative effect. In this case, the mutated allele interferes with the function of the normal gene product by one of several different mechanisms: (1) a mutant protein may interfere with the function of a multimeric protein complex, as illustrated by mutations in type 1 collagen (*COL1A1, COL1A2*) genes in osteogenesis imperfecta (Chap. 351); (2) a mutant protein may occupy binding sites on proteins or promoter response elements, as illustrated by thyroid hormone resistance, a disorder in which inactivated thyroid hormone receptor binds to target genes and functions as an antagonist of normal receptors (Chap. 330); or (3) a mutant protein can be cytotoxic as in α_1 antitrypsin deficiency (Chap. 258) or autosomal dominant neurohypophyseal diabetes insipidus (Chap. 329), in which the abnormally folded proteins are trapped within the endoplasmic reticulum and ultimately cause cellular damage.

GENOTYPE AND PHENOTYPE Alleles, Genotypes, and Haplotypes An observed trait is referred to as a *phenotype*; the genetic information defining the phenotype is called the *genotype*. Alternative forms of a gene or a genetic marker are referred to as alleles. Alleles may be polymorphic variants of nucleic acids that have no apparent effect on gene expression or function. In other instances, these variants may have subtle effects on gene expression, thereby conferring the adaptive advantages associated with genetic diversity. On the other hand, allelic variants may reflect mutations in a gene that clearly alter its function. The common Glu → Val sickle cell mutation (E6V) in the β-globin gene and the ΔF508 deletion of phenylalanine (F) in the *CFTR* gene are examples of allelic variants of these genes. Because each individual has two copies of each chromosome (one inherited from the mother and one inherited from the father), he or she can only have two alleles at a given locus. However, there can be many different alleles in the population. The normal or common allele is usually referred to as *wild type*. When alleles at a given locus are identical, the individual is *homozygous*. Inheriting such identical copies of a mutant allele occurs in many autosomal recessive disorders, particularly in circumstances of consanguinity. If the alleles are different, the individual is *heterozygous* at this locus. If two different mutant alleles are inherited at a given locus, the individual is said to be a *compound heterozygote*. *Hemizygous* is used to describe males with a mutation in an X chromosomal gene, or a female with a loss of one X chromosomal locus.

Genotypes describe the specific alleles at a particular locus. For example, there are three common alleles (E2, E3, E4) of the apolipoprotein E (*APOE*) gene. The genotype of an individual can therefore be described as *APOE3/4* or *APOE4/4* or any other variant. These designations indicate which alleles are present on the two chromosomes in the *APOE* gene at locus 19q13.2. In other cases, the genotype might be assigned arbitrary numbers (e.g., 1/2) or letters (e.g., B/b) to distinguish different alleles.

A *haplotype* refers to a group of alleles that are closely linked

Table 65-6 Selected Trinucleotide Repeat Disorders

Disease	Locus	Repeat	Triplet Length Normal	Triplet Length Disease	Inheritance	Gene Product
X-chromosomal spinobulbar muscular atrophy (SBMA)	Xq11-q12	CAG	11–34	40–62	XR	Androgen receptor
Fragile X-syndrome (FRAXA)	Xq27.3	CGG	6–50	200–300	XR	FMR-1 protein
Fragile X-syndrome (FRAXE)	Xq28	GCC	6–25	>200	XR	FMR-2 protein
Dystrophia myotonica (DM)	19q13.2-q13.3	CTG	5–30	200–1000	AD, variable penetrance	Myotonin protein kinase
Huntington disease (HD)	4p16.3	CAG	11–34	37–121	AD	Huntingtin
Spinocerebellar ataxia type 1 (SCA1)	6p21.3-21.2	CAG	19–36	39–83	AD	Ataxin 1
Spinocerebellar ataxia type 2 (SCA2)	12q24.1	CAG	15–31	34–400	AD	Ataxin 2
Spinocerebellar ataxia type 3 (SCA3); Machado Joseph disease (MD)	14q21	CAG	13–36	55–86	AD	SC3/MJD1
Spinocerebellar ataxia type 6 (SCA6, CACNAIA)	19p13.1-13.2	CAG	4–16	20–33	AD	Alpha 1A voltage-dependent calcium channel
Spinocerebellar ataxia type 7 (SCA7)	3p21.1-p12	CAG	4–19	37->300	AD	Ataxin 7
Spinocerebellar ataxia type 8 (SCA8)	13q21	CTG	16–34	100–250	AD	?
Spinocerebellar ataxia type 12 (SCA12)	5q31	CAG	6–26	66–78	AD	Protein phosphatase 2A
Dentorubral pallidoluysiane atrophy (DRPLA)	12p	CAG	7–23	49–75	AD	Atrophin
Friedereich ataxia (FRDA1)	9q13-21	GAA	7–22	200–900	AR	Frataxin

NOTE: AD, autosomal dominant; AR, autosomal recessive; XR, X-linked recessive.

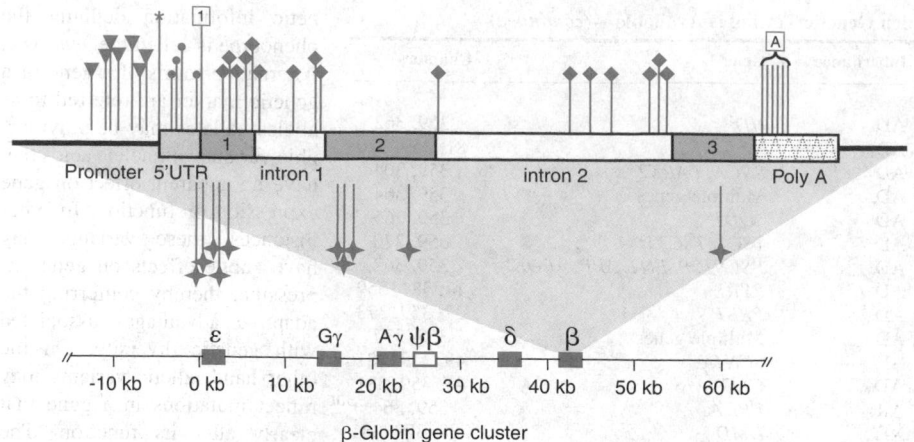

FIGURE 65-7 Point mutations causing β-thalassemia as example of allelic heterogeneity. The β-globin gene is located in the globin gene cluster. Point mutations can be located in the promoter, the CAP site, the 5'-untranslated region, the initiation codon, each of the three exons, the introns, or the polyadenylation signal. Many mutations introduce missense or nonsense mutations, whereas others cause defective RNA splicing. Not shown here are deletion mutations of the β-globin gene or larger deletions of the globin locus that can also result in thalassemia. ▼, Promoter mutations; *, CAP site; ●, 5′UTR; [1], Initiation codon; ◆, Defective RNA processing; ✦, Missense and nonsense mutations; [A], Poly A signal.

together at a genomic locus. Haplotypes are useful for tracking the transmission of genomic segments within families and for detecting evidence of genetic recombination, if the crossover event occurs between the alleles (Fig. 65-3). As an example, various alleles at the histocompatibility locus antigen (HLA) on chromosome 6p are used to establish haplotypes associated with certain disease states. For example, 21-hydroxylase deficiency, complement deficiency, and hemochromatosis are each associated with specific HLA haplotypes. It is now recognized that these genes lie in close vicinity to the HLA locus, which explains why HLA associations were identified even before the disease genes were cloned and localized. In other cases, specific HLA associations with diseases such as ankylosing spondylitis (HLA-B27) or type 1 diabetes mellitus (HLA-DR4) reflect the role of specific HLA allelic variants in susceptibility to these autoimmune diseases.

Allelic Heterogeneity *Allelic heterogeneity* refers to the fact that different mutations in the same genetic locus can cause an identical or similar phenotype. For example, many different mutations of the β-globin locus can cause β-thalassemia (Fig. 65-7). In essence, allelic heterogeneity reflects the fact that many different mutations are capable of altering protein structure and function. For this reason, maps of inactivating mutations in genes usually show a near-random distribution. Exceptions include: (1) a founder effect, in which a particular mutation that does not affect reproductive capacity can be traced to a single individual; (2) "hot spots" for mutations, in which the nature of the DNA sequence predisposes to a recurring mutation; and (3) localization of mutations to certain domains that are particularly critical for protein function. Allelic heterogeneity creates a practical problem for genetic testing because one must often examine the entire genetic locus for mutations, as these can differ in each patient.

Phenotypic Heterogeneity *Phenotypic heterogeneity* occurs when more than one phenotype is caused by allelic mutations (e.g., different mutations in the same gene). For example, mutations in the *myosin VIIIA* gene can result in four distinct clinical disorders: (1) autosomal recessive deafness DFNB2, (2) autosomal dominant nonsyndromic deafness DFNA11, (3) Usher 1B syndrome [congenital deafness, retinitis pigmentosa (**Plate IV-14**)], and (4) an atypical variant of Usher's syndrome. Similarly, identical mutations in the *FGFR2* gene can result in very distinct phenotypes: Crouzon syndrome (craniofacial synostosis), or Pfeiffer syndrome (acrocephalopolysyndactyly).

Locus or Nonallelic Heterogeneity and Phenocopies *Nonallelic or locus heterogeneity* refers to the situation in which a similar disease phenotype results from mutations at different genetic loci (Ta-

ble 65-4). This often occurs when more than one gene product produces different subunits of an interacting complex or when different genes are involved in the same genetic cascade or physiologic pathway. For example, osteogenesis imperfecta can arise from mutations in two different procollagen genes (*COL1A1* or *COL1A2*) that are located on different chromosomes (Chap. 351). The effects of inactivating mutations in these two genes are similar because the protein products comprise different subunits of the helical collagen fiber. Similarly, muscular dystrophy syndromes can be caused by mutations in various genes, consistent with the fact that it can be transmitted in an X-linked (Duchenne or Becker), autosomal dominant (limb-girdle muscular dystrophy type 1), or autosomal recessive (limb-girdle muscular dystrophy type 2) manner (Chap. 383). Mutations in the X-linked *DMD* gene, which encodes dystrophin, are the most common cause of muscular dystrophy. This feature reflects the large size of the gene as well as the fact that the phenotype is expressed in hemizygous males because they only have a single copy of the X chromosome. Dystrophin is associated with a large group of additional proteins that form the membrane-associated cytoskeleton in muscle. Mutations in several components of this protein complex can also cause muscular dystrophy syndromes. Although the phenotypic features of some of these disorders are distinct, the phenotypic spectrum caused by mutations in different genes overlaps, thereby leading to nonallelic heterogeneity. It should be noted that mutations in dystrophin also cause allelic heterogeneity. For example, mutations in the *DMD* gene can cause either Duchenne or the less severe Becker muscular dystrophy, depending on the severity of the protein defect.

Recognition of nonallelic heterogeneity is important for several reasons: (1) the ability to identify disease loci in linkage studies is reduced by including patients with similar phenotypes but different genetic disorders; (2) genetic testing is more complex because several different genes need to be considered along with the possibility of different mutations in each of the candidate genes; and (3) novel information is gained about how genes or proteins interact, providing unique insights into molecular physiology.

Phenocopies refer to circumstances in which nongenetic conditions mimic a genetic disorder. For example, features of toxin- or drug-induced neurologic syndromes can resemble those seen in Huntington disease, and vascular causes of dementia share phenotypic features with familial forms of Alzheimer dementia (Chap. 362). Children born with activating mutations of the thyroid-stimulating hormone receptor (TSH-R) exhibit goiter and thyrotoxicosis similar to that seen in neonatal Graves' disease, which is caused by the transfer of maternal autoantibodies to the fetus (Chap. 330). As in nonallelic heterogeneity, the presence of phenocopies has the potential to confound linkage studies and genetic testing. Patient history and subtle differences in phenotype can often provide clues that distinguish these disorders from related genetic conditions.

Variable Expressivity and Incomplete Penetrance It is not uncommon for the same genetic mutation to cause a phenotypic spectrum illustrating the phenomenon of *variable expressivity*. This may include different manifestations of a complex disorder (e.g., MEN), the severity of the disorder (e.g., sickle cell anemia), or the age of disease onset (e.g., Alzheimer dementia). MEN-1 illustrates several of these features. Families with this autosomal dominant disorder develop tumors of the parathyroid gland, endocrine pancreas, and the pituitary gland (Chap. 339). However, the pattern of tumors in the different glands, the age at which tumors develop, and the types of hormones produced vary among affected individuals, even within a given family.

In this example, the phenotypic variability arises, in part, because of the requirement for a second mutation in the normal copy of the *MEN1* gene, as well as the large array of different cell types that are susceptible to the effects of *MEN1* gene mutations. In part, variable expression reflects the influence of other genes, or genetic background, on the effects of a particular mutation. Even in identical twins, in whom the genetic constitution is the same, one can occasionally see variable expression of a genetic disease.

Interactions with the environment can also influence the course of a disease. For example, the manifestations and severity of hemochromatosis can be influenced by iron intake (Chap. 345), and the course of phenylketonuria is affected by exposure to phenylalanine in the diet (Chap. 352). Other metabolic disorders, such as hyperlipidemias and porphyria, also fall into this category. Many mechanisms, including genetic effects and environmental influences, can therefore lead to variable expressivity. In genetic counseling, it is particularly important to recognize this variability, as one cannot always predict the course of disease, even when the mutation is known.

Penetrance is the probability of expressing the phenotype given a defined genotype; it can be complete or incomplete. For example, hypertrophic obstructive cardiomyopathy (HOCM) caused by mutations in the *myosin heavy chain β* gene is a dominant disorder with clinical features in only a subset of patients who carry the mutation (Chap. 238). Patients who have the mutation but no evidence of the disease can still transmit the disorder to subsequent generations. In this situation, the disorder is said to be *nonpenetrant* or *incompletely penetrant*. This classification depends to some degree on the criteria and techniques used for diagnosis. For disorders such as Huntington disease or familial amyotrophic lateral sclerosis, which present late in life, the rate of penetrance is influenced by the age at which the clinical assessment is performed. *Imprinting* can also modify the penetrance of a disease (see below). For example, in patients with Albright hereditary osteodystrophy, mutations in the Gsα subunit (*GNAS1* gene) are expressed clinically only in individuals who inherit the mutation from their mother (Chap. 343).

Sex-Influenced Phenotypes Certain mutations affect males and females quite differently. In some instances, this is because the gene resides on the X or Y sex chromosomes (X-linked disorders and Y-linked disorders). As a result, the phenotype of mutated X-linked genes will be expressed fully in males but variably in heterozygous females, depending on the degree of X-inactivation and the function of the gene. For example, most heterozygous female carriers of factor VIII deficiency (hemophilia A) are asymptomatic because sufficient factor VIII is produced to prevent a defect in coagulation (Chap. 117). On the other hand, some females heterozygous for the X-linked lipid storage defect caused by α-galactosidase A deficiency (Fabry disease) experience mild manifestations of painful neuropathy, as well as other features of the disease (Chap. 349). Because only males have a Y chromosome, mutations in genes such as *SRY* (which causes male-to-female sex-reversal) or *DAZ* (which causes abnormalities of spermatogenesis) are unique to males (Chap. 338).

Other diseases are expressed in a sex-limited manner because of the differential function of the gene product in males and females. Activating mutations in the luteinizing hormone receptor cause dominant male-limited precocious puberty in boys (Chap. 335). The phenotype is unique to males because activation of the receptor induces testosterone production in the testis, whereas it is functionally silent in the immature ovary. Homozygous inactivating mutations of the follicle-stimulating hormone (FSH) receptor cause primary ovarian failure in females because the follicles do not develop in the absence of FSH action. In contrast, affected males have a more subtle phenotype, because testosterone production is preserved (allowing sexual maturation) and spermatogenesis is only partially impaired (Chap. 335). In congenital adrenal hyperplasia, most commonly caused by 21-hydroxylase deficiency, cortisol production is impaired and ACTH stimulation of the adrenal gland leads to increased production of androgenic precursors (Chap. 331). In females, the increased androgen level causes ambiguous genitalia, which can be recognized at the time of birth. In males, the diagnosis may be made on the basis of adrenal insufficiency at birth, because the increased adrenal androgen level does not alter sexual differentiation, or later in childhood, because of the development of precocious puberty. Hemochromatosis is more common in males than in females, presumably because of differences in dietary iron intake and losses associated with menstruation and pregnancy in females (Chap. 345).

GENETIC LINKAGE *Genetic linkage* refers to the fact that genes are physically connected, or linked, to one another along the chromosomes. Two fundamental principles are essential for understanding the concept of a genetic linkage: (1) When two genes are close together on a chromosome, they are usually transmitted together, unless a recombination event separates them (Fig. 65-3); and (2) the odds of a crossover, or recombination event, between two linked genes is proportional to the distance that separates them. Thus, genes that are further apart are more likely to undergo a recombination event than genes that are very close together. Linkage is used in genetic counseling to predict the odds of disease gene transmission.

Polymorphisms are essential for linkage studies because they provide a means to distinguish the maternal and paternal chromosomes in an individual. On average, 1 out of every 1000 bp varies from one person to the next. Although this degree of variation seems low (99.9% identical), it means that >3 million sequence differences exist between any two unrelated individuals. This sequence variation usually has no significant functional consequence and provides much of the basis for variation in genetic traits. Although many of these sequence variations are SNPs, other variants include VNTRs or short tandem repeats (STRs). In VNTRs and STRs, the number of times a sequence is repeated is highly variable in the population. Consequently, the probability that sequences will differ on the two homologous chromosomes is high (often >70 to 90%). Most STRs, also called *polymorphic microsatellite markers*, consist of di-, tri-, or tetranucleotide repeats that can be measured readily using PCR and primers that reside on either side of the repeat sequences (Fig. 65-8). Many other methods for analyzing polymorphic variation are also available. Historically, RFLPs were used to detect sequence variations that caused changes in the recognition sites for restriction enzymes. This procedure has been largely replaced by the use of STRs. Analyses of SNPs, using DNA chips, provide a promising means for rapid analysis of genetic variation and linkage.

In order to identify a chromosomal locus that segregates with a disease, it is necessary to determine the genotype or haplotype of DNA samples from one or several pedigrees. One can then assess whether certain marker alleles cosegregate with the disease. Markers that are closest to the disease gene are less likely to undergo recombination events and therefore receive a higher linkage score. Linkage is expressed as a lod (logarithm of odds) score—the ratio of the probability that the disease and marker loci are linked rather than unlinked. Lod scores of +3 (1000:1) are generally accepted as supporting linkage, whereas a score of −2 is consistent with the absence of linkage.

An example of the use of linkage analysis is shown in Fig. 65-8. In this case, the gene for the autosomal dominant disorder, MEN-1, is known to be located on chromosome 11q13. Using positional cloning, the *MEN1* gene was identified and shown to encode menin, the function of which is poorly understood. However, the transmission of the disorder suggests that menin acts like a tumor-suppressor gene. Affected individuals inherit a mutant form of the *MEN1* gene, predisposing them to certain types of tumors (parathyroid, pituitary, pancreatic islet) (Chap. 339). In the tissues that develop a tumor, a "second hit" occurs in the normal copy of the *MEN1* gene. This somatic mutation may be a point mutation, a microdeletion, or loss of a chromosomal fragment (detected as loss of heterozygosity, LOH). Within a given family, linkage to the *MEN1* gene locus can be assessed without necessarily knowing the specific mutation in the *MEN1* gene. Using polymorphic STRs that are close to the *MEN1* gene, one can assess transmission of the different *MEN1* alleles and compare this pattern

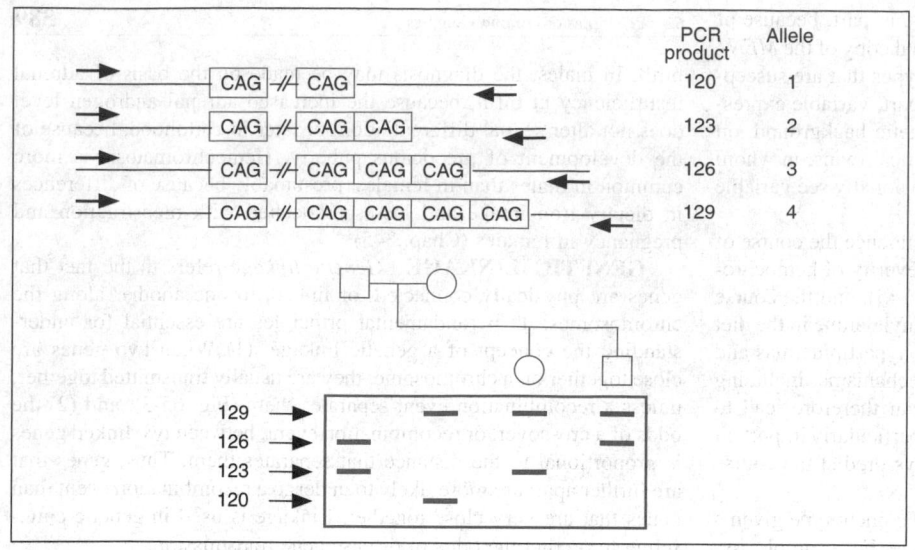

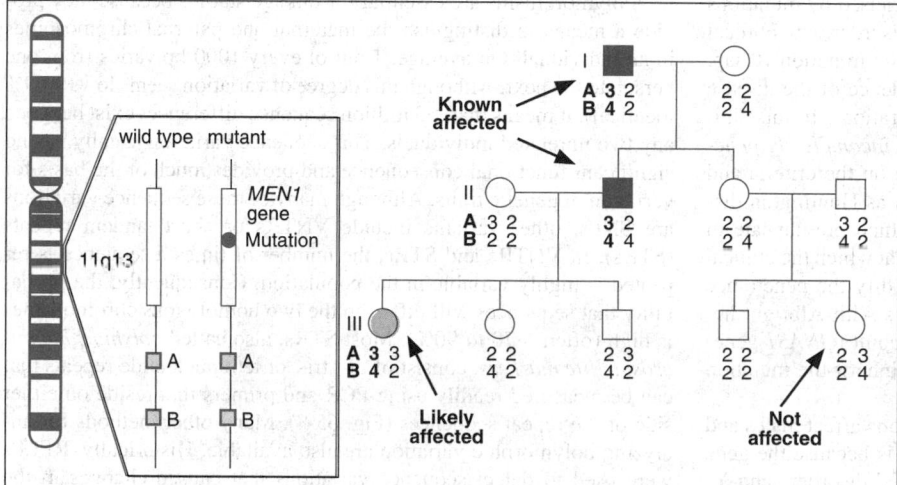

FIGURE 65-8 CAG repeat length and linkage analysis in multiple endocrine neoplasia type 1. *Upper panel.* Detection of different alleles using polymorphic microsatellite markers. The example depicts a CAG trinucleotide repeat. PCR with primers flanking the polymorphic region results in products of variable length, depending on the number of CAG repeats. After characterization of the alleles in the parents, transmission of the paternal and maternal alleles can be determined. *Lower panel.* Genotype analysis using microsatellite markers in a family with multiple endocrine neoplasia type 1. Two microsatellite markers, A and B, are located in close proximity to the *MEN1* gene on chromosome 11q13. For each individual, the A and B alleles have been determined. Based on this analysis, the genotype A3,B4 is linked to the disease because it occurs in the two affected individuals I-1 and II-1 but not in unaffected siblings. Because the disease allele is linked to A3,B4 within the affected family, it is likely that the individual III-1 is a carrier of the mutated *MEN1* gene. Although III-5 also has the A3,B4 genotype, she has inherited the allele from her unaffected father (III-4), who is not related to the original family. The A3,B4 genotype is only associated with MEN-1 in the original family, but not in the general population. Therefore, individual III-5 is not at risk for developing the disease.

to development of the disorder to determine which allele is associated with risk of MEN-1. In the pedigree shown, the affected grandfather in generation I carries alleles 3 and 4 on the chromosome with the mutated *MEN1* gene and alleles 2 and 2 on his other chromosome 11. Consistent with linkage of the 3/4 genotype to the *MEN1* locus, his son in generation II is affected, whereas his daughter (who inherits the 2/2 genotype from her father) is unaffected. In the third generation, transmission of the 3/4 genotype indicates risk of developing MEN-1, assuming that no genetic recombination between the 3/4 alleles and the *MEN1* gene has occurred. After a specific mutation in the *MEN1* gene is identified within a family, it is possible to track transmission of the mutation itself, thereby eliminating uncertainty caused by recombination.

CHROMOSOMAL DISORDERS Chromosomal or cytogenetic disorders are caused by numerical or structural aberrations in chromosomes. Deviations in chromosome number are common causes of abortions, developmental disorders, and malformations. →*For discussion of disorders of chromosome number and structure, see Chap. 66.*

Contiguous Gene Syndromes Large deletions or duplications may affect a portion of a gene, an entire gene, or, if several genes are involved, cause a *contiguous gene syndrome*. Syndromes associated with chromosomal deletions or duplications have a wide phenotypic spectrum that is dependent on the number of involved gene loci. For example, the cri-du-chat syndrome, one of the most common deletion disorders, is associated with deletions on the short arm of chromosome 5 that vary in size from extremely small deletions within 5p15.2 to the loss of the entire short arm. Because of the variable size of the involved deletions, the phenotype encompasses a spectrum that ranges from severe mental retardation and microcephaly to an isolated catlike cry without morphologic or mental abnormalities.

Contiguous gene syndromes have been useful for identifying the location of new disease-causing genes. Because of the variable size of gene deletions in different patients, a systemic comparison of phenotypes and locations of deletion breakpoints allows positions of particular genes to be mapped within the critical genomic region.

MONOGENIC MENDELIAN DISORDERS Monogenic human diseases are frequently referred to as *Mendelian disorders* because they obey the principles of genetic transmission originally set forth in Gregor Mendel's classic work. The mode of inheritance for a given phenotypic trait or disease is determined by pedigree analysis. All affected and unaffected individuals in the family are recorded in a pedigree using standard symbols (Fig. 65-9). The principles of allelic segregation, and the transmission of alleles from parents to children, are illustrated in Fig. 65-10. One dominant (A) allele and one recessive (a) allele can display three Mendelian modes of inheritance: autosomal dominant, autosomal recessive, and X-chromosomal. About 65% of human monogenic disorders are autosomal dominant, 25% are autosomal recessive, and 5% are X-linked (Table 65-5). Genetic testing is now available for many of these disorders and plays an increasingly important role in clinical medicine.

Autosomal Dominant Disorders Autosomal dominant disorders assume particular relevance because mutations in a single allele are sufficient to cause the disease. In contrast to recessive disorders, in which disease pathogenesis is relatively straightforward because there is loss of gene function, in dominant disorders there are various disease mechanisms, many of which are unique to the function of the genetic pathway involved.

In autosomal dominant disorders, individuals are affected in successive generations; the disease does not occur in the offspring of unaffected individuals. Males and females are affected with equal frequency because the defective gene resides on one of the 22 autosomes (Fig. 65-11A). Autosomal dominant mutations alter one of the two alleles at a given locus. Because the alleles segregate randomly at meiosis, the probability that an offspring will be affected is 50%. Un-

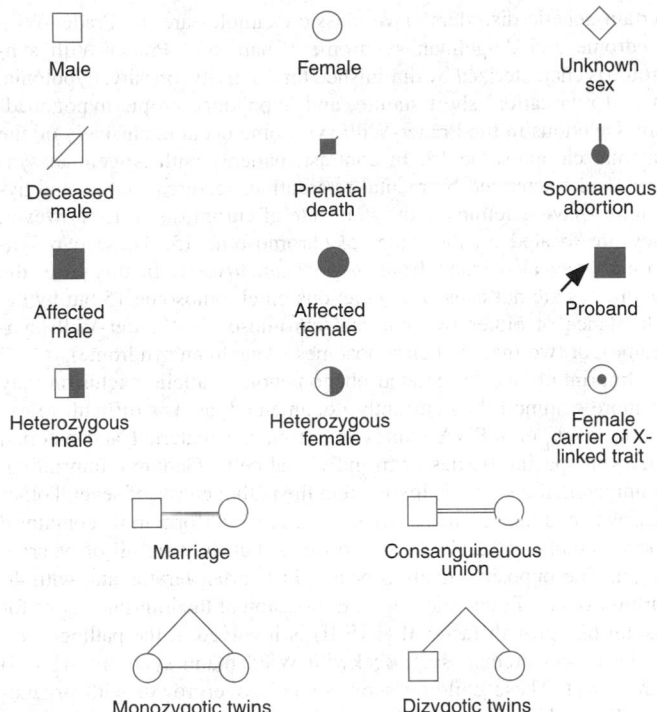

Male Female Unknown sex

Deceased male Prenatal death Spontaneous abortion

Affected male Affected female Proband

Heterozygous male Heterozygous female Female carrier of X-linked trait

Marriage Consanguineuous union

Monozygotic twins Dizygotic twins

FIGURE 65-9 Symbols used in pedigree analysis.

less there is a new germline mutation, an affected individual has an affected parent. Children with a normal genotype do not transmit the disorder. Due to differences in penetrance or expressivity (see above), the clinical manifestations of autosomal dominant disorders may be variable. Because of these variations, it is sometimes challenging to determine the pattern of inheritance.

It should be recognized, however, that some individuals acquire a mutated gene from an unaffected parent. De novo germline mutations occur more frequently during later cell divisions in gametogenesis, explaining why siblings are rarely affected. As noted before, new germline mutations occur more frequently in fathers of advanced age. For example, the average age of fathers with new germline mutations that cause Marfan's syndrome is approximately 37 years, whereas fathers who transmit the disease by inheritance have an average age of about 30 years.

Autosomal Recessive Disorders The clinical expression of autosomal recessive disorders is more uniform than in autosomal dominant disorders. Most mutated alleles lead to a complete or partial loss of function. They frequently involve enzymes in metabolic pathways, receptors, or proteins in signaling cascades. Though most recessive disorders are rare, the relatively high frequency of certain recessive disorders, such as sickle cell anemia, cystic fibrosis, and thalassemia, is partially explained by a selective biologic advantage for the heterozygous state (see below).

In an autosomal recessive disease, the affected individual, who can be of either sex, is a homozygote or compound heterozygote for a

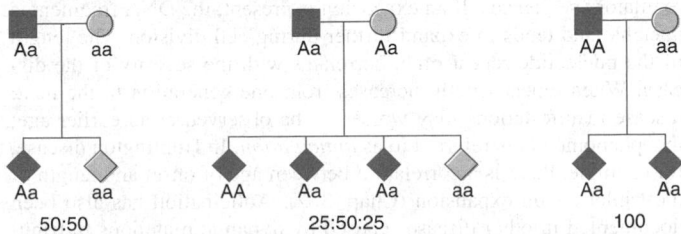

FIGURE 65-10 Segregation of alleles. Segregation of genotypes in the offspring of parents with one dominant (A) and one recessive (a) allele. The distribution of the parental alleles to their offspring depends on the combination present in the parents.

single-gene defect. With a few important exceptions, autosomal recessive diseases are rare and often occur in the context of parental consanguinity. Though heterozygous carriers of a defective allele are usually clinically normal, they may display subtle differences in phenotype that only become apparent with more precise testing or in the context of certain environmental influences. In sickle cell anemia, for example, heterozygotes are normally asymptomatic. However, in situations of dehydration or diminished oxygen pressure, sickle cell crises can also occur in heterozygotes (Chap. 106).

In most instances, an affected individual is the offspring of heterozygous parents. In this situation, there is a 25% chance that the offspring will have a normal genotype, a 50% probability of a heterozygous state, and a 25% risk of homozygosity for the recessive alleles (Fig. 65-11B). In the case of one unaffected heterozygous and one affected homozygous parent, the probability of disease increases to 50% for each child. In this instance, the pedigree analysis mimics an autosomal dominant mode of inheritance (*pseudodominance*). In contrast to autosomal dominant disorders, new mutations in recessive alleles are rarely manifest because they usually result in an asymptomatic carrier state.

X-Linked Disorders Males have only one X chromosome; consequently, a daughter always inherits her father's X chromosome in addition to one of her mother's two X chromosomes. A son inherits the Y chromosome from his father and one maternal X chromosome. Thus, the characteristic features of X-linked inheritance are (1) the absence of father-to-son transmission, and (2) the fact that all daughters of an affected male are obligate carriers of the mutant allele (Fig. 65-11C). The risk of developing disease due to a mutant X-chromosomal gene differs in the two sexes. Because males have only one X chromosome, they are hemizygous for the mutant allele; thus, they are more likely to develop the mutant phenotype, regardless of whether

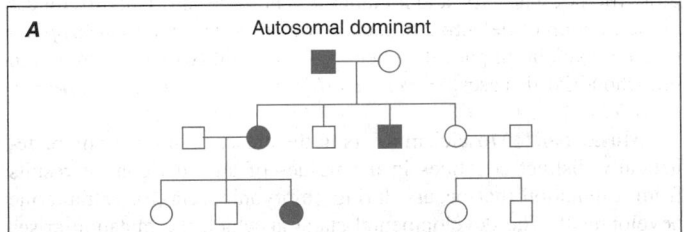

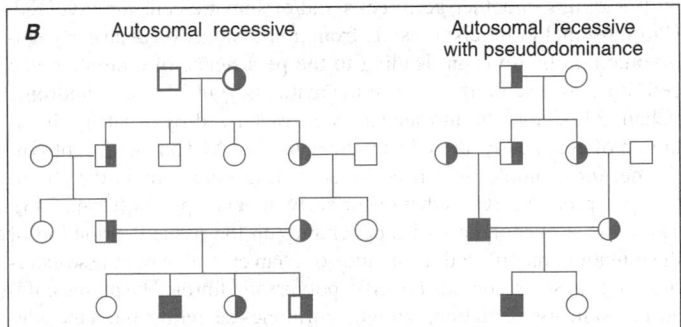

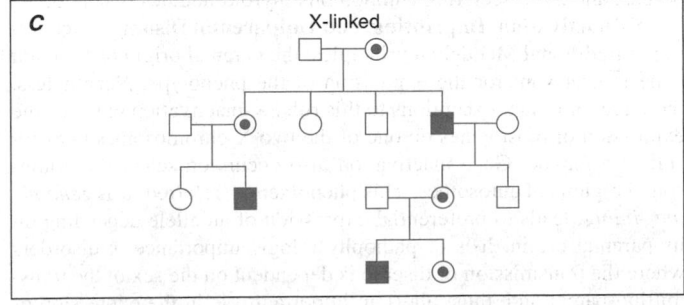

FIGURE 65-11 Dominant, recessive, and X-linked inheritance.

the mutation is dominant or recessive. A female may be either heterozygous or homozygous for the mutant allele, which may be dominant or recessive. The terms *X-linked dominant* or *X-linked recessive* are therefore only applicable to expression of the mutant phenotype in women. In addition, the expression of X-chromosomal genes is influenced by X chromosome inactivation (see below).

Y-Linked Disorders   Only a few genes are known on the Y chromosome. One such gene, the sex-region determining Y factor (*SRY*), or testis-determining factor (*TDF*), is crucial for normal male development. Normally there is infrequent exchange of sequences on the Y chromosome with the X chromosome. Because the *SRY* region is closely adjacent to the pseudoautosomal region, a chromosomal segment on the X and Y chromosomes with a high degree of homology, a crossing-over occasionally involves the *SRY* region. Translocations can result in XY females with the Y chromosome lacking the *SRY* gene or XX males harboring the *SRY* gene on one of the X chromosomes (Chap. 338). Point mutations in the *SRY* gene may also result in individuals with an XY genotype and an incomplete female phenotype. Most of these mutations occur de novo. Men with oligospermia/azoospermia frequently have microdeletions on the long arm of the Y chromosome that involve one or more of the azoospermia factor (*AZF*) genes.

EXCEPTIONS TO SIMPLE MENDELIAN INHERITANCE PATTERNS Mitochondrial Disorders   Each mitochondrion contains several copies of a circular chromosome. Mitochondrial DNA predominantly encodes transfer RNAs and proteins that are components of the respiratory chain involved in oxidative phosphorylation and ATP generation. The mitochondrial genome is inherited through the maternal line because sperm does not contribute significant cytoplasmic components to the zygote. All children from an affected mother will inherit the disease, but it will not be transmitted from an affected father to his children. During cell replication, the proportion of wild-type and mutant mitochondria can drift; differences in the fraction of defective mitochondria are referred to as *heteroplasmia* and explain, in part, the phenotypic variability that is common in mitochondrial diseases. →*For detailed discussion of mitochondrial disorders, see Chap. 67.*

Mosaicism   Mosaicism refers to the presence of two or more genetically distinct cell lines in the tissues of an individual. It results from a mutation that occurs during embryonic, fetal, or extrauterine development. The developmental stage at which the mutation arises will determine whether germ cells and/or somatic cells are involved. Chromosomal mosaicism results from non-disjunction at an early embryonic mitotic division, leading to the persistence of more than one cell line, as exemplified by some patients with Turner syndrome (Chap. 338). Somatic mosaicism is characterized by a patchy distribution of genetically altered somatic cells. The McCune-Albright syndrome, for example, is caused by activating mutations in the stimulatory G protein α ($G_s\alpha$) that occur early in development (Chap. 343). The clinical phenotype varies depending on the tissue distribution of the mutation; manifestations include ovarian cysts that secrete sex steroids and cause precocious puberty, polyostotic fibrous dysplasia, café-au-lait skin pigmentation, growth hormone–secreting pituitary adenomas, and hypersecreting autonomous thyroid nodules (Chap. 336).

X-Inactivation, Imprinting, and Uniparental Disomy   According to traditional Mendelian principles, the parental origin of a mutant gene is irrelevant for the expression of the phenotype. Nonetheless, there are important exceptions to this rule. X-inactivation prevents the expression of most genes on one of the two X-chromosomes in every cell of a female. Gene inactivation also occurs on selected chromosomal regions of autosomes. This phenomenon, referred to as *genomic imprinting*, leads to preferential expression of an allele depending on its parental origin. It is of pathophysiologic importance in disorders where the transmission of disease is dependent on the sex of the transmitting parent and, thus, plays an important role in the expression of

certain genetic disorders. Two classic examples are the Prader-Willi syndrome and Angelman syndrome (Chap. 66). Prader-Willi syndrome is characterized by diminished fetal activity, obesity, hypotonia, mental retardation, short stature, and hypogonadotropic hypogonadism. Deletions in the Prader-Willi syndrome occur exclusively on the paternal chromosome 15. In contrast, patients with Angelman syndrome, characterized by mental retardation, seizures, ataxia, and hypotonia, have deletions at the same site of chromosome 15; however, they are located on the maternal chromosome 15. These two syndromes may also result from *uniparental disomy*. In this case, the syndromes are not caused by deletions on chromosome 15 but by the inheritance of either two paternal chromosomes (Prader-Willi syndrome), or two maternal chromosomes (Angelman syndrome).

Imprinting and the related phenomenon of allelic exclusion may be more common than currently documented, as it is difficult to examine levels of mRNA expression from the maternal and paternal alleles in specific tissues or in individual cells. Genomic imprinting, or uniparental disomy, is involved in the pathogenesis of several other disorders and malignancies (Chap. 66). Hydatidiform mole contains a normal number of diploid chromosomes, but they are all of paternal origin. The opposite situation occurs in ovarian teratomata, with 46 chromosomes of maternal origin. Expression of the imprinted gene for insulin-like growth factor II (IGF-II) is involved in the pathogenesis of the cancer-predisposing Beckwith-Wiedemann syndrome (BWS) (Chap. 81). These children show somatic overgrowth with organomegalies and hemihypertrophy, and they have an increased risk of embryonal malignancies such as Wilm's tumor. Normally only the paternally derived copy of the *IGF-II* gene is active and the maternal copy is inactive. Imprinting of the *IGF-II* gene is regulated by *H19*, which encodes an RNA transcript that is not translated into protein. Disruption or lack of *H19* methylation leads to a relaxation of *IGF-II* imprinting and expression of both alleles. Heritable changes in gene expression not associated with DNA sequence alterations are referred to as *epigenetic effects*; these changes are increasingly recognized to play a role in human diseases and possibly in aging as well (Chap. 9).

Somatic Mutations   In many cancer syndromes, there is an inherited predisposition to tumor formation. However, the neoplastic process requires the acquisition of additional somatic mutations (Chap. 81). In retinoblastoma, the tumor develops when both copies of the retinoblastoma (*RB*) gene are inactivated through two somatic events (sporadic retinoblastoma) or through a somatic loss of the normal allele in an individual with a hereditary defect in the other allele (hereditary retinoblastoma). This "two-hit" model applies to other inherited cancer syndromes such as MEN-1 (Chap. 339) and neurofibromatosis type 2 (Chap. 370). The defective allele is transmitted in a dominant pattern, though tumorigenesis results from a recessive loss of the tumor suppressor gene in an affected tissue. In other instances, the development of cancer typically requires somatic defects in multiple genes, a process termed *multistep carcinogenesis* (Chap. 82).

Nucleotide Repeat Expansion Disorders   Several diseases are associated with an increase in the number of nucleotide repeats above a certain threshold (Table 65-6). The repeats are sometimes located within the coding region of the genes, as in Huntington disease or the X-linked form of spinal and bulbar muscular atrophy (SBMA, Kennedy syndrome). In other instances, the repeats probably alter gene regulatory sequences. If an expansion is present, the DNA fragment is unstable and tends to expand further during cell division. The length of the nucleotide repeat often correlates with the severity of the disease. When repeat length increases from one generation to the next, disease manifestations may worsen or be observed at an earlier age; this phenomenon is referred to as *anticipation*. In Huntington disease, for example, there is a correlation between age of onset and length of the triplet codon expansion (Chap. 362). Anticipation has also been documented in other diseases caused by dynamic mutations in trinucleotide repeats (Table 65-6). The repeat number may also vary in a tissue-specific manner. In myotonic dystrophy, the CTG repeat may be tenfold greater in muscle tissue than in lymphocytes (Chap. 383).

POPULATION GENETICS AND AS-SOCIATION STUDIES **Overview of Population Genetics** In population genetics, the focus changes from alterations in an individual's genome to the distribution pattern of different genotypes of alleles in the population. In a case where there are only two alleles, A and a, the frequency of the genotypes will be $p^2 + 2pq + q^2 = 1$, with p^2 corresponding to the frequency of AA, $2pq$ to the frequency of Aa, and q^2 to aa. When the frequency of an allele is known, the frequency of the genotype can be calculated. Alternatively, one can determine an allele frequency, if the genotype frequency has been determined.

Allele frequencies vary among ethnic groups and geographical regions. For example, heterozygous mutations in the *CFTR* gene are relatively common in populations of European origin but are rare in the African population. Allele frequencies may vary because certain allelic variants confer a selective advantage. For example, heterozygotes for the sickle cell mutation, which is particularly common in West Africa, are more resistant to malarial infection because the erythrocytes of heterozygotes provide a less favorable environment for *Plasmodium* parasites. Though homozygosity for the sickle cell gene is associated with severe anemia and sickle crises (Chap. 106), heterozygotes have a higher probability of survival because of the reduced morbidity and mortality from malaria; this phenomenon has led to an increased frequency of the mutant allele. Recessive conditions are more prevalent in geographically isolated populations because of the more restricted gene pool.

Allelic Association and Linkage Disequilibrium There are two primary strategies for mapping genes that cause or increase susceptibility to human disease: (1) classic linkage can be performed based on a known genetic model (see above) or, when the model is unknown, by studying pairs of affected relatives; or (2) disease genes can be mapped using allelic association studies (Table 65-7). *Allelic association* refers to a situation in which the frequency of an allele is significantly increased or decreased in a particular disease. Linkage and association differ in several aspects. Genetic linkage is demonstrable in families or sibships. Association studies, on the other hand, compare a population of affected individuals with a control population. Association studies can be performed as case-control studies that include unrelated affected individuals and matched controls, or as family-based studies that compare the frequencies of alleles transmitted or not transmitted to affected children.

Allelic association studies are particularly useful for identifying susceptibility genes in complex diseases. When alleles at two loci occur more frequently in combination than would be predicted (based on known allele frequencies and recombination fractions), they are said to be in *linkage disequilibrium*. In Fig. 65-12, a mutation, Z, has occurred at a susceptibility locus where the normal allele is Y. The mutation is in close proximity to a genetic polymorphism with allele A or B. With time, the chromosomes carrying the A and Z alleles accumulate and represent 10% of the chromosomes in the population. The fact that the disease susceptibility gene, Z, is found preferentially, or exclusively, in association with the A allele illustrates linkage disequilibrium. Though not all chromosomes carrying the A allele carry the disease gene, the A allele is associated with an increased risk because of its possible association with the Z allele. This model implies that it may be possible in the future to identify Z directly to provide a more accurate prediction of disease susceptibility. Evidence for linkage disequilibrium can be helpful in mapping disease genes because it suggests that the two loci, in this case A and Z, are tightly linked.

Table 65-7 Genetic Approaches for Identifying Disease Genes

Method	Indications and Advantages	Limitations
Linkage analysis	Analysis of monogenic traits Suitable for genome scan Control population not required Useful for multifactorial disorders in isolated populations	Difficult to collect large informative pedigrees Difficult to obtain sufficient statistical power for complex traits
Allele-sharing methods Affected sib and relative pair analyses Sib pair analysis	Suitable for identification of susceptibility genes in polygenic and multifactorial disorders Suitable for genome scan Control population not required if allele frequencies are known Statistical power can be increased by including parents and relatives	Difficult to collect sufficient number of subjects Difficult to obtain sufficient statistical power for complex traits
Association studies Case-control studies Linkage disequilibrium Transmission distortion test	Suitable for identification of susceptibility genes in polygenic and multifactorial disorders Suitable for testing specific allelic variants of known candidate loci Does not necessarily need relatives	Requires large sample size and matched control population False-positive results in the absence of suitable control population

POLYGENIC DISEASE AND COMPLEX GENETIC TRAITS **Approach to Polygenic and Multifactorial Disease** The expression of many common diseases such as cardiovascular disease, hypertension, diabetes, asthma, psychiatric disorders, and certain cancers is determined by genetic background, environmental factors, and lifestyle (Table 65-8). A trait is called *polygenic* if multiple genes are thought to contribute to the phenotype or *multifactorial* if multiple genes are assumed to interact with environmental factors. Genetic models for complex traits need to account for genetic heterogeneity and interactions with other genes and the environment. Complex genetic traits may be influenced by modifying genes that are not linked to the main gene involved in the pathogenesis of the trait. This type of gene-gene interaction, or *epistasis*, plays an important role in polygenic traits that require the simultaneous presence of variations in multiple genes in order to result in a pathologic phenotype. Gene-environment interactions are relevant for many monogenic and polygenic disorders. In phenylketonuria, the phenotypic expression of the disease depends not only on the presence of the mutation in the phenylalanine hydroxylase gene but also on the exposure to the amino acid phenylalanine (Chap. 352). Another example is type 2 diabetes

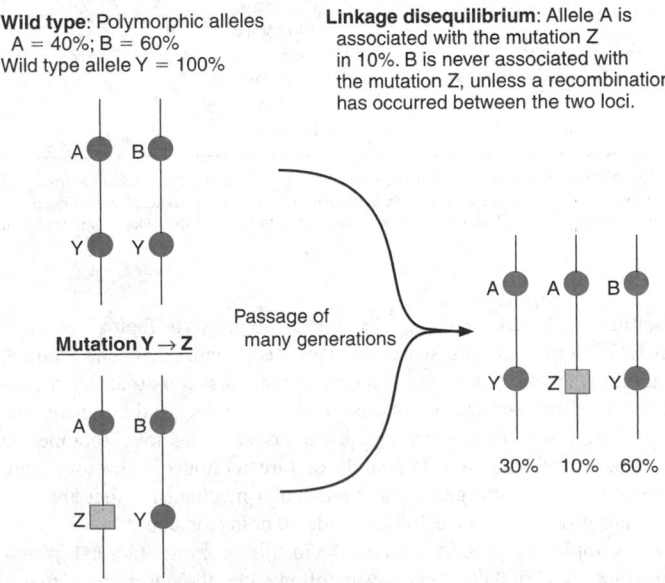

Wild type: Polymorphic alleles
A = 40%; B = 60%
Wild type allele Y = 100%

Linkage disequilibrium: Allele A is associated with the mutation Z in 10%. B is never associated with the mutation Z, unless a recombination has occurred between the two loci.

Mutation Y → Z

Passage of many generations

30%   10%   60%

FIGURE 65-12 Linkage disequilibrium.

Table 65-8   Selected Multifactorial and Polygenic Disorders

Disorder	Genes or Susceptibility Loci[a]	Chromosomal Location	Other Factors
Diabetes mellitus type 1	HLA-DQB1,-DRB1 (IDDM1)	6p21	Viral infections
	Insulin VNTR (IDDM2)	11p15	Autoimmunity
	Cytotoxic T lymphocyte–associated 4 (CTLA-4, IDDM12)	2q33	
	IGF binding protein 2, -5 (IDDM13)	2q34	
	Glucokinase	7p15.1-15.3	
Diabetes mellitus type 2	Insulin promoter factor 1 (IPF1)	13q12.1	Diet
	Insulin receptor substrate (IRS-1)	2q36	Energy expenditure
	Peroxisome proliferator receptor γ	3p25	Obesity
	Sulfonylurea receptor	11p15.1	
	Amylin	12p12.3-p12.1	
	Phosphoenolpyruvate carboxykinase 1 (PEPCK1)	20q13.31	
	Hepatocyte nuclear factor 1α (HNF1A)	12q24.2	
	Cholecystokinin receptor B	11p15.5-p15.4	
	Growth hormone	17q22-q24	
	Ras-related associated with diabetes (RRAD)	16q22	
	Apolipoprotein A2	1q21-q23	
Hypertension	Angiotensinogen	1q42-43	Salt intake
	Angiotensin-converting enzyme	17q23	
	Angiotensin receptor 1	3q21-25	
	G-protein subunit 3	12p13	
	Hypertension susceptibility locus 1 (HYT1)	17q	
	Hypertension susceptibility locus 2 (HYT2)	15q	
Coronary artery disease— atherosclerosis	Low-density lipoprotein receptor	19p13.2-p13.1	Diet
	Apolipoprotein E4	19q13.2	Exercise
	Apolipoprotein (a)	6q27	Smoking
	Homocysteine	Unknown	Diabetes
	Plasminogen-activator inhibitor	7q21.3-q22	Hypertension
			Hormones
			Infection of endothelial cells
Asthma—bronchial hyperreactivity	IgE receptor	11q13	Allergens
	5q31 locus	5q32-33	Pollution
	MHC locus	6p21	
	Interleukin receptor	Xq28	
Manic-depressive psychosis	Xq26 locus	Xq26	Familial and social environment
	18p locus	18p	
	4p locus	4p	
	21q locus	21q	
	18q locus	18q	
Psoriasis	HLA-Cw6,-DR7,-B13,-Bw57, and others	6p21	Environmental stimuli
	17q locus	17q	
	16q locus	16q	
	20p locus	20p	
Systemic lupus erythematosus	HLA-DR2,-DR3	6p21	Hormones
	C4 deficiency	6p21.3	Unspecified environmental stimuli
	1q locus	1q41-q42	

[a] The relative importance of the listed susceptibility genes and loci is in part controversial among different studies, and positive associations may vary among different populations. Additional genes and loci have been associated with most of the disorders included in this table.

NOTE: IGF, insulin-like growth factor; MHC, major histocompatibility complex; VNTR, variable number of tandem repeats.

mellitus, in which genetic, nutritional, and lifestyle factors are intimately interrelated in disease pathogenesis (Chap. 333). The identification of genetic variations and environmental factors that either predispose or protect against disease is essential for predicting disease risk, designing preventive strategies, and developing novel therapeutic approaches (Chap. 68). The study of rare monogenic diseases may provide insights into genetic and molecular mechanisms that are subsequently of importance for the understanding of complex diseases. For example, the identification of the insulin promoter factor 1 in maturity-onset of diabetes type 4 was followed by the observation that it also plays a role in the pathogenesis of diabetes mellitus type 2 (Tables 65-1 and -8).

394

Approach to the Patient

Identifying the Disease-Causing Gene   *Genomic medicine* aims to enhance the quality of medical care through the use genotypic analysis (DNA testing) to identify genetic predisposition to disease, to select more specific pharmacotherapy, and to design individualized medical care based on genotype. Genotype can be deduced by analysis of protein (e.g., hemoglobin, apoprotein E), mRNA, or DNA. However, technological advances have made DNA analysis particularly useful because it can be readily applied to all but the largest genes (Fig. 65-13).

DNA testing is performed by mutational analysis or linkage studies in individuals at risk for a genetic disorder known to be present in a family. Mass screening programs require tests of high sensitivity and specificity to be cost-effective. Prerequisites for the success of genetic screening programs include the following: that the disorder is potentially serious; that it can be influenced at a presymptomatic stage by changes in behavior, diet, and/or pharmaceutical manipulations; and that the screening does not result in any harm or discrimination. Screening in Jewish populations for the autosomal recessive neurodegenerative storage disease Tay-Sachs has reduced the number of affected individuals. In contrast, screening for sickle cell trait/disease in African Americans has led to unanticipated problems of discrimination by health insurers and employers. Mass screening programs harbor additional potential problems. For example, screening for the most common genetic alteration in cystic fibrosis, the ΔF508 mutation with a frequency of ~70% in northern Europe, is feasible and seems to be effective. One has to keep in mind, however, that there is pronounced allelic heterogeneity and that the disease can be caused by >600 other mutations. The search for these less common mutations would substantially increase costs but not the effectiveness of the screening program as a whole. Occupational screening programs aim to detect individuals with increased risk for certain professional activities (e.g., α_1 antitrypsin deficiency and smoke or dust exposure).

Mutational analyses DNA sequence analysis is increasingly used as a diagnostic tool and significantly enhanced diagnostic accuracy. It is used for determining carrier status and for prenatal testing in monogenic disorders (Table 65-5). Certain cancer susceptibility genes, such as *BRCA1* and *BRCA2*, may identify individuals with an increased risk for the development of malignancies. The detection of mutations is an important diagnostic and prognostic tool in leukemias and lymphomas. The demonstration of the presence or absence of mutations is also relevant for the rapidly evolving field of pharmacogenetics, including the identification of differences in drug treatment response or metabolism as a function of genetic background.

A general algorithm for the approach to mutational analysis is outlined in Fig. 65-13. The importance of a detailed clinical phenotype

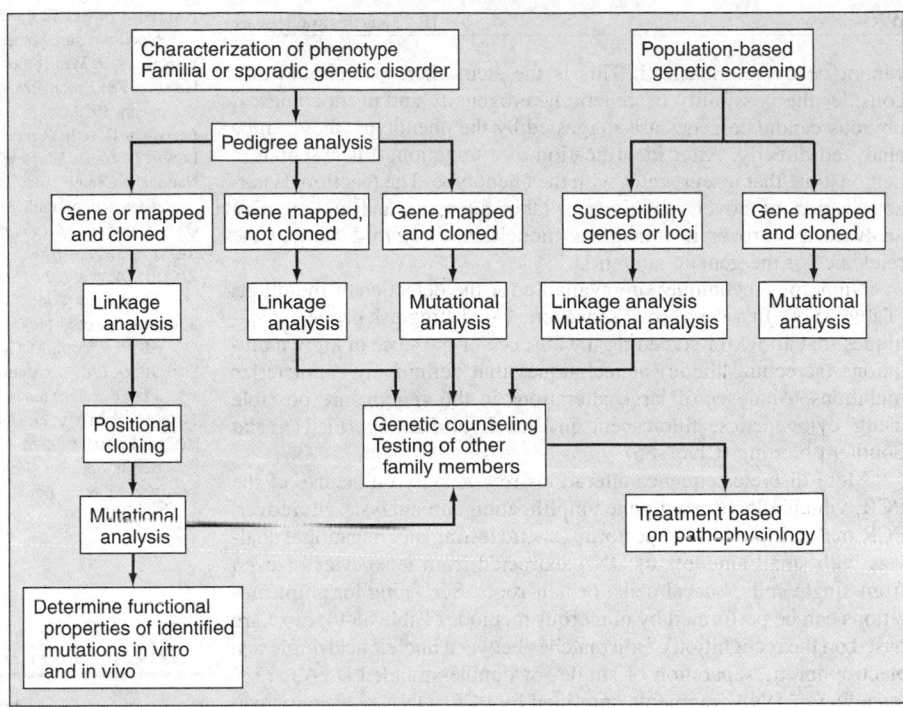

FIGURE 65-13 Approach to genetic disease.

Table 65-9 Methods Used for the Detection of Mutations

Method	Principle	Type of Mutation Detected
Cytogenic analysis	Unique visual appearance of various chromosomes	Numerical or structural abnormalities in chromosomes
Fluorescent in situ hybridization (FISH)	Hybridization to chromosomes with fluorescently labeled probes	Numerical or structural abnormalities in chromosomes
Southern blot	Hybridization with genomic probe or cDNA probe after digestion of high molecular DNA	Large deletion, insertion, rearrangement, expansions of triplet repeat, amplification
Polymerase chain reaction (PCR)	Amplification of DNA segment	Expansion of triplet repeats, variable number of tandem repeats (VNTR), gene rearrangements, translocations; prepare DNA for other mutation methods
Reverse transcriptase PCR (RT-PCR)	Reverse transcription, amplification of DNA segment → absence or reduction of mRNA transcription	Analyzed expressed mRNA (cDNA) sequence; detect loss of expression
DNA sequencing	Direct sequencing of PCR products. Sequencing of DNA segments cloned into plasmid vectors	Point mutations, small deletions and insertions
Single-strand conformational polymorphism (SSCP)	PCR of DNA segment: Mutations result in conformational change and altered mobility	Point mutations, small deletions and insertions
Denaturing gradient gel electrophoresis (DGGE)	PCR of DNA segment: Mutations result in conformational change and altered mobility	Point mutations, small deletions and insertions
RNAse cleavage	Cleavage of mismatch between mutated and wild-type sequence	Point mutations, small deletions and insertions
Restriction fragment length polymorphism (RFLP)	Detection of altered restriction pattern of genomic DNA (Southern blot) or PCR products	Point mutations, small deletions and insertions
Oligonucleotide specific hybridization (OSH)	Hybridization of PCR products to wild-type or mutated oligonucleotides immobilized on chips or slides	Point mutations, small deletions and insertions
Microarrays	Hybridization of PCR products to wild-type or mutated oligonucleotides	Point mutations, small deletions and insertions
Protein truncation test (PTT)	Transcription/translation of cDNA isolated from tissue sample	Mutations leading to premature truncations

cannot be overemphasized. This is the step where one should also consider the possibility of genetic heterogeneity and phenocopies. If obvious candidate genes are suggested by the phenotype, they can be analyzed directly. After identification of a mutation, it is essential to demonstrate that it segregates with the phenotype. The functional characterization of novel mutations is labor-intensive and may require analyses in vitro or in transgenic models in order to document the relevance of the genetic alteration.

Numerous techniques are available for the detection of mutations (Table 65-9). In a very broad sense, one can distinguish between techniques that allow for screening the absence or presence of known mutations (screening mode) or techniques that definitively characterize mutations. Analyses of large alterations in the genome are possible using cytogenetics, fluorescent in situ hybridization (FISH), and Southern blotting (Chap. 66).

More discrete sequence alterations rely heavily on the use of the PCR, which allows rapid gene amplification and analysis. Moreover, PCR makes it possible to perform genetic testing and mutational analysis with small amounts of DNA extracted from leukocytes or even from single cells, buccal cells, or hair roots. Screening for point mutations can be performed by numerous methods (Table 65-9); most are based on the recognition of mismatches between nucleic acid duplexes, electrophoretic separation of single- or double-stranded DNA, or sequencing of DNA fragments amplified by PCR. DNA sequencing can be performed directly on PCR products or on fragments cloned into plasmid vectors amplified in bacterial host cells.

RT-PCR may be useful to detect absent or reduced levels of mRNA expression due to a mutated allele. Protein truncation tests (PTT) can be used to detect the broad array of mutations that result in premature termination of a polypeptide during its synthesis. The isolated cDNA is transcribed and translated in vitro, and the proteins are analyzed by gel electrophoresis. Comparison of electrophoretic mobility with the wild-type protein allows detection of truncated mutants.

The majority of traditional diagnostic methods are gel-based. Novel technologies for the analysis of mutations, genetic mapping, and mRNA expression profiles are in rapid development. DNA chip technologies allow hybridization of DNA or RNA to hundreds of thousands of probes simultaneously. Microarrays are being used clinically for mutational analysis of several human disease genes, as well as for the identification of viral sequence variations. Together with the knowledge gained from the HGP, these technologies provide the foundation to expand from a focus on single genes to analyses at the scale of the genome.

ACKNOWLEDGMENTS

This chapter reflects the cumulative contributions of many past contributors to Harrison's Principles of Internal Medicine. Most recently, this includes Dr. Joseph L. Goldstein, Dr. Michael S. Brown, Dr. Andrea Ballabio, and Dr. Arthur L. Beaudet.

BIBLIOGRAPHY

ALBERTS B et al (eds): *Molecular Biology of the Cell*, 3d ed. New York, Garland, 1995
BRENT R: Genomic biology. Cell 100(1):169, 2000
BROWN PO, BOTSTEIN D: Exploring the new world of the genome with DNA microarrays. Nat Genet Suppl 21:33, 1999
BURLEY SK et al: Structural genomics: Beyond the Human Genome Project. Nat Genet 23:151, 1999
COLLINS FS et al: New goals for the U.S. human genome project: 1998–2003. Science 282:682, 1998
CONNOR JM, FERGUSON-SMITH M (eds): *Essential Medical Genetics*. Oxford, Blackwell Scientific, 1993
COTTON RGH, KAZAZIAN HH JR: The HUGO mutation database initiative: Issues, databases, and perspectives for the new millenium. Hum Mutat 15(1):1, 2000
DARNELL J et al (eds): *Molecular Cell Biology*, 3d ed. New York, Scientific American, 1995
Ethical, Legal, and Social Implications of Biotechnology. www.ncgr.org/gpi/
GELEHERTER TD et al (eds): *Principles of Medical Genetics*, 2d ed. Philadelphia, Lippincott, 1998
HAINES JL, PERICAK-VANCE MA (eds): Approaches to gene mapping in complex human diseases. New York, Wiley-Liss, 1998
HALUSKA MK et al: Patterns of single-nucleotide polymorphisms in candidate genes for blood-pressure homeostasis. Nat Genet 22:239, 1999
HANAKAN D, WEINBERG RA: The hallmarks of cancer. Cell 100(1):57, 2000
HARPER PS: *Practical Genetic Counseling*, 5th ed. Stoneham, MA, Butterworth-Heinemann, 1998
JAMESON JL (ed): *Principles of Molecular Medicine*. Totowa, NJ, Humana, 1998
LEWIN B: *Genes VI*. New York, Oxford, 1997
National Center for Biotechnology Information (GenBank, Medline, OMIM). www.ncbi.nlm.nih.gov
OTT J: *Analysis of Human Genetic Linkage*. Baltimore, John Hopkins, 1991
READ AP, STRACHAN T: *Human Molecular Genetics*. New York, Wiley, 1997
RIMOIN DL et al (eds): *Emery and Rimoin's Principles and Practice of Medical Genetics*, 3d ed. New York, Churchill Livingstone, 1996
SCRIVER CR et al (eds): *The Metabolic and Molecular Bases of Inherited Disease*, 8th ed. New York, McGraw-Hill, 2000
SOUTHERN EM: DNA chips: Analyzing sequence by hybridization to oligonucleotides on a large scale. Trends Genet 12:110, 1996
THOMPSON MW et al: *Genetics in Medicine*. Philadelphia, Saunders, 1993
VOGEL F, MOTULSKY AG (eds): *Human Genetics: Problems and Approaches*, 3d ed. Berlin, Springer, 1996
WRIGHT AF et al: Population choice in mapping genes for complex diseases. Nat Genet 23:397, 1999

66   *Terry Hassold, Stuart Schwartz*

CHROMOSOME DISORDERS

AS Angelman syndrome	MDS Miller-Dieker syndrome
BACs bacterial artificial chromosomes	PUBS percutaneous umbilical blood sampling
CML chronic myelogenous leukemia	PWS Prader-Willi syndrome
CMT1A Charcot-Marie-Tooth type 1A	UPD uniparental disomy
CVS chorionic villus sampling	VCF velocardiofacial syndrome
FISH fluorescence in situ hybridization	WAGR Wilms' tumor–aniridia complex
	YACs yeast artificial chromosomes

In humans, the normal diploid number of chromosomes is 46, consisting of 22 pairs of autosomal chromosomes (numbered 1 to 22 in decreasing size) and one pair of sex chromosomes (XX in females and XY in males). The genome is estimated to contain between 80,000 and 100,000 genes, with the smallest autosome housing between 500 and 1000 genes. Not surprisingly, duplications or deletions of even small chromosome segments have profound consequences on normal gene expression.

Deviations in the number or structure of the 46 human chromosomes are astonishingly common, despite severe deleterious consequences. Chromosomal disorders occur in an estimated 10 to 25% of all pregnancies. They are the leading cause of fetal loss and, among pregnancies surviving to term, the leading known cause of birth defects and mental retardation.

In recent years, the practice of cytogenetics has shifted from conventional cytogenetic methodology to a union of cytogenetic and molecular techniques. Formerly the province of research laboratories, *fluorescence in situ hybridization* (FISH) and related molecular cytogenetic technologies have been incorporated into everyday practice in clinical laboratories. As a result, there is an increased appreciation of the importance of "subtle" constitutional cytogenetic abnormalities, such as microdeletions and imprinting disorders, as well as previously recognized translocations and disorders of chromosome number.

VISUALIZING CHROMOSOMES

CONVENTIONAL CYTOGENETIC ANALYSIS   In theory, chromosome preparations can be obtained from any actively dividing tissue by causing the cells to arrest in metaphase, the stage of the cell cycle at which chromosomes are maximally condensed. In practice, only a small number of tissues are used for routine chromosome analysis: amniocytes or chorionic villi for prenatal testing; and blood, bone marrow, or skin fibroblasts for postnatal studies. Samples of blood, bone marrow, and chorionic villi can be processed using short-term culture techniques that yield results in 1 to 3 days. Analysis of other tissue types typically involves long-term tissue culture, requiring 1 to 3 weeks of processing before cytogenetic analysis is possible.

Regardless of the culturing technique, cells are processed to recover chromosomes at metaphase or prometaphase and treated chemically or enzymatically to reveal chromosome "bands" (Fig. 66-1). Analysis of the number of chromosomes in the cell, and the distribution of bands on individual chromosomes, allows the identification of numerical or structural abnormalities. This strategy is useful for characterizing the normal chromosome complement and determining the incidence and types of major chromosome abnormalities.

Chromosomes are complex structures, consisting of the DNA double helix and chromosome-associated proteins. As for virtually all organisms, each human chromosome contains two specialized structures: a centromere and two telomeres. The *centromere*, or primary constriction, divides the chromosome into short (p) and long (q) arms and is responsible for the segregation of chromosomes during cell division. The *telomeres*, or chromosome ends, "cap" the p and q arms and are important for allowing DNA replication at the ends of the chromosomes. Prior to DNA replication, each chromosome consists of a single chromatid copy of the DNA double helix. After DNA replication and continuing until the time of cell division (including metaphase, when chromosomes are typically visualized), each chromosome consists of two identical sister chromatids (Fig. 66-1).

MOLECULAR CYTOGENETICS The introduction of FISH methodologies in the late 1980s revolutionized the field of cytogenetics. In principle, FISH is similar to other DNA-DNA hybridization methodologies. The labeled probe DNA and the target DNA (usually metaphase chromosomes) are denatured to become single-stranded and are hybridized together. The probe is labeled with a hapten, such as biotin or digoxigenin, to allow detection with a fluorophore (e.g., FITC or rhodamine). Alternatively, many probes are already labeled with fluorophores and thus can be detected directly. After the hybridization step, the specimen is counter-stained and the preparations are visualized with a fluorescence microscope.

Types of FISH Probes A variety of probes are available for use with FISH, including chromosome-specific paints (chromosome libraries), repetitive probes, and single-copy probes. Chromosome libraries were developed initially from flow-sorted individual chromosomes and more recently from monochromosomal human-rodent hybrids. These probes hybridize to sequences that span the entirety of the chromosome from which they are derived and, as a result, they can be used to "paint" individual chromosomes (Fig. 66-2).

Repetitive probes recognize amplified DNA sequences present in chromosomes. The most common are α-satellite DNA probes that are complementary to DNA sequences found at the centromeric regions of all human chromosomes. There are also α-satellite probes that hybridize to the centromeric regions of specific chromosomes (Fig. 66-2).

A vast number of *single-copy probes* are now available, both commercially and as a result of the human genome project. These probes can be as small as 1 kb, though normally they are packaged in cosmids (40 kb), bacterial artificial chromosomes (BACs) or P1 clones (100 to 200 kb), or yeast artificial chromosomes (YACs) (1 to 2 Mb). With the advent of the National Cancer Institute BAC initiative, these large DNA fragments will be placed at 1-Mb intervals on every chromosome, each of which can be used for FISH hybridization. Probes for a variety of microdeletion syndromes and for subtelomeric regions of individual chromosomes are commercially available (Fig. 66-2).

Applications of FISH The majority of FISH applications involve hybridization of one or two probes of interest as an adjunctive procedure to conventional chromosomal banding techniques. In this

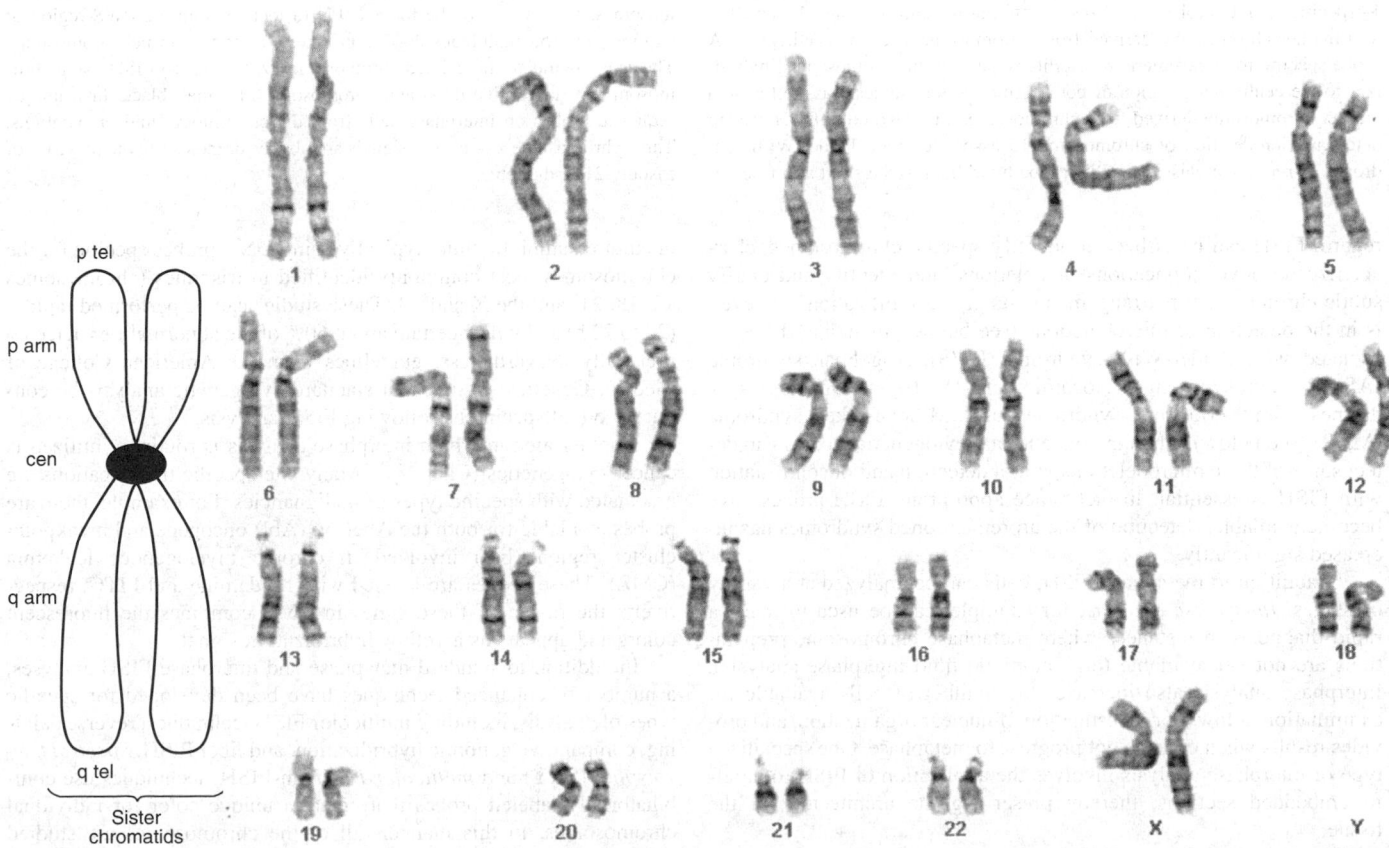

FIGURE 66-1 *A.* An idealized human chromosome, showing the centromere (cen), long (q) and short (p) arms, and telomeres (tel). *B.* A G-banded human karyotype from a normal (46,XX) female.

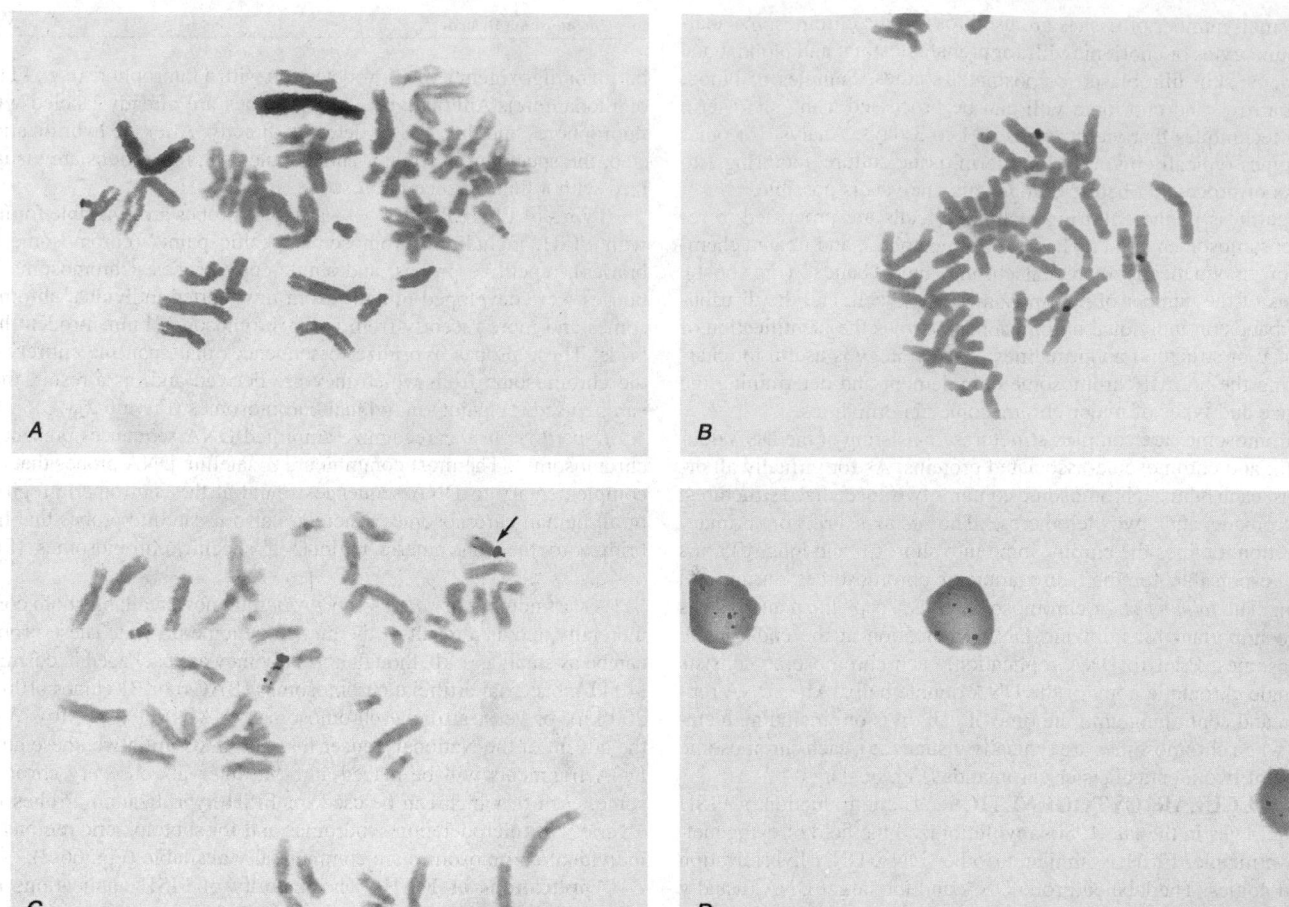

FIGURE 66-2 Examples of different applications of fluorescence in situ hybridization (FISH) to metaphase or interphase preparations. *A.* A chromosome 1–specific "paint" probe hybridizes to both normal chromosomes 1 as well as to a marker chromosome derived from chromosome 1. *B.* A repetitive DNA probe specific for centromeric α-satellite sequences on chromosome 1 hybridizes to the centromeric region of both normal chromosomes 1 as well as to a marker chromosome derived from chromosome 1. *C.* Two-color FISH used to detect a microdeletion of chromosome 15 associated with Prader-Willi syndrome. A repetitive classic satellite probe hybridizes to the short arm of chromosome 15 (large blue dots) and a probe for PML (a locus on the distal portion of chromosome 15, visualized as small black dots) are observed on both chromosomes. However, a probe for SNRPN (a locus within the PWS region of chromosome 15, small black dots) hybridizes only to the normal chromosome. The arrow points to the deleted chromosome. *D.* Interphase FISH using chromosome 13 (large blue dots) and chromosome 21 (small black dots) unique sequence probes on interphase cells from direct amniotic fluid preparations. Three chromosome 21-specific signals are observed, indicating the presence of trisomy 21 in the fetus.

regard, FISH can be utilized to identify specific chromosomes, characterize de novo duplications or deletions, and identify and clarify subtle chromosomal rearrangements. Its greatest utilization, however, is in the detection of microdeletions (see below), including those associated with Prader-Willi syndrome (PWS), Angelman syndrome (AS), William syndrome, velocardiofacial (VCF) and DiGeorge syndromes, Smith-Magenis syndrome, and Miller-Dieker syndrome (MDS) (see below). Though conventional cytogenetic studies can detect some of these microdeletions, initial detection and/or confirmation with FISH is essential. In fact, since appropriate FISH probes have become available, detection of the aforementioned syndromes has increased significantly.

In addition to metaphase FISH, cells can be analyzed at a variety of stages. *Interphase analysis*, for example, can be used to make a rapid diagnosis in instances where metaphase chromosome preparations are not yet available (e.g., amniotic fluid interphase analysis). Interphase analysis also increases the number of cells available for examination, allows for investigation of nuclear organization, and provides results when cells do not progress to metaphase. One specialized type of interphase analysis involves the application of FISH to paraffin-embedded sections, thereby preserving the architecture of the tissue.

The use of interphase FISH has increased recently, especially for analyses of amniocentesis samples. These studies are performed on uncultured amniotic fluid, typically using DNA probes specific for the chromosomes most commonly identified in trisomies (chromosomes 13, 18, 21, and the X and Y). These studies can be performed rapidly (24 to 72 h) and will ascertain about 60% of the abnormalities detected prenatally. Nevertheless, guidelines from the American College of Medical Genetics suggest that standard cytogenetic analysis be conducted on all specimens following FISH analysis.

Another area in which interphase analysis is routinely utilized is cancer cytogenetics (Chap. 81). Many site-specific translocations are associated with specific types of malignancies. For example, there are probes available for both the Abelson (Abl) oncogene and breakpoint cluster region (bcr) involved in chronic myelogenous leukemia (CML). These probes are labeled with rhodamine and FITC, respectively; the fusion of these genes in CML combines the fluorescent colors and appears as a yellow hybridization signal.

In addition to standard metaphase and interphase FISH analyses, a number of enhanced techniques have been developed for specific types of analysis, including multicolor FISH techniques, reverse painting, comparative genomic hybridization, and fiber FISH. *Spectral karyotyping* (SKY) and *multicolor FISH* (m-FISH) techniques use combinatorially labeled probes that create a unique color for individual chromosomes. In this manner, all of the chromosomes are studied simultaneously, and computer software is used to generate "pseudocolors" for the individual chromosomes. This technology is useful in the identification of unknown chromosome material (such as markers of duplications) but is most commonly used with the complex rearrangements seen in cancer specimens.

Reverse painting is accomplished by either flow-sorting a chromosome of interest or scraping the chromosome off a slide. The DNA from this chromosome (or portion of a chromosome) is extracted, amplified, labeled, and used as a FISH probe. This probe is then hybridized to a normal metaphase chromosome to identify the origin of the DNA of interest. It is also utilized to identify marker chromosomes or chromosome duplications of unknown origin.

Comparative genomic hybridization (CGH) is a method that can be used when only DNA is available from a specimen of interest. The entire DNA specimen from the sample of interest is labeled in one color (e.g., green), and the normal control DNA specimen in another color (e.g., red). These are mixed in equal amounts and hybridized to normal metaphase chromosomes. The red-to-green ratio is analyzed by a computer program, which determines where the DNA of interest may have gains or loss of material. This technique is useful in the analysis of tumors, particularly in those cases where cytogenetic analysis is not possible.

Fiber FISH is a technique in which chromosomes are mechanically stretched, using one of a variety of different methods. Fiber FISH provides a higher resolution of analysis than conventional FISH and more precise information on the chromosomal localization of a specific probe.

CYTOGENETIC TESTING IN PRENATAL DIAGNOSIS

(See also Chap. 68)   The vast majority of prenatal diagnostic studies are performed to rule out a chromosomal abnormality, but cells may also be propagated for biochemical studies or molecular analyses of DNA. Three procedures are used to obtain samples for prenatal diagnosis: amniocentesis, chorionic villus sampling (CVS), and fetal blood sampling. *Amniocentesis* is the most commonly used procedure and is routinely performed at 15 to 17 weeks of gestation. On some occasions, early amniocentesis at 12 to 14 weeks is done to expedite results, though less fluid is obtained at this time. Early amniocentesis carries a greater risk of spontaneous abortion or fetal injury but provides results at an earlier stage of pregnancy.

The vast majority of amniocentesis are performed in the context of advanced maternal age, the best-known correlate of trisomy (see below). Additional reasons for referral for amniocentesis include an abnormal "triple-marker assay" and/or detection of ultrasound abnormalities. In the triple-marker assay, levels of human chorionic gonadotropin, α fetoprotein, and unconjugated estriol in the maternal serum are quantified and used to adjust the maternal age-predicted risk of a trisomy 21 or trisomy 18 fetus. Specific ultrasound abnormalities, when detected at mid-trimester, can also be associated with chromosomal defects. When a nonspecific ultrasound abnormality is present, the estimated risk of a chromosomal defect is approximately 16%. Associations of chromosomal abnormalities and specific types of abnormal ultrasound findings are listed in Table 66-1.

Chorionic villus sampling is the second most common procedure for genetic prenatal diagnosis. Because this procedure is routinely performed at about 8 to 10 weeks of gestation, it allows for an earlier detection of abnormalities and a safer pregnancy termination, if desired. CVS is a relatively safe procedure (spontaneous abortions < 0.5

to 1%). Because there is an increased association of limb defects when the procedure is performed later (≥ 11 weeks of gestation), CVS is applicable during a very narrow window of time of gestation. CVS involves the use of a catheter inserted transvaginally; approximately 25 mg of villi are aspirated from the chorion frondosum (the fetal portion of the placenta). Care must be taken not to obtain villi from the maternal portion from the placenta to avoid compromising the analysis. The majority of the sample (the mesenchymal cells from the CVS sample) is enzymatically digested and cultured in a fashion similar to amniotic fluid cells. However, cells in the outer layer of the villi—the cytotrophoblasts—are actively dividing and can be analyzed directly. Therefore, by adding colchicine directly to these cells, a result can be obtained within 24 to 48 h. Findings from these procedures should be confirmed by analyses of cultured mesenchymal cells, as they are more reliably derived from the fetus.

Percutaneous umbilical blood sampling (PUBS) is a method for obtaining fetal blood during the second and third trimesters of pregnancy. It allows for acquisition of a blood sample, which can be used for cytogenetic studies; results can be obtained within 48 h of sampling. PUBS is carried out under ultrasound guidance. It is usually performed when ultrasound abnormalities are detected late in the second trimester. PUBS is also used when cytogenetic results from amniocentesis need clarification, such as the detection of mosaicism.

CHROMOSOME ABNORMALITIES

CHROMOSOMES IN CELL DIVISION   To understand the etiology of chromosome abnormalities, it is important to review the movement of chromosomes during cell division. In somatic tissues, chromosomes are replicated during the S-phase of the cell cycle, so that each replicated chromosome consists of two identical sister chromatids (Fig. 66-1). When the cell enters mitosis, each of the 46 chromosomes align on the metaphase plate, with the centromeres cooriented toward opposite spindle poles (Fig. 66-3). At anaphase the sister chromatids separate, with each of the daughter cells receiving one sister chromatid from each of the 46 chromosomes.

Chromosome segregation is more complicated in germ cell division, since the number of chromosomes must be reduced from 46 to 23 in the mature sperm and eggs. This is accomplished by two rounds of division—meiosis I and meiosis II (Fig. 66-3). In meiosis I, homologous chromosomes become paired and exchange genetic material, then align on the metaphase plate, and finally separate from one another. Thus, by the end of meiosis I, only 23 of the original 46 chromosomes are represented in each of the two daughter cells. Meiosis II quickly follows meiosis I and is essentially a "haploid mitosis," involving separation of the sister chromatids in each of the 23 chromosomes.

Although the fundamentals of meiosis are the same in males and females, there are important distinctions, particularly in the timing of the meiotic divisions. In males, meiosis begins with puberty and continues throughout the individual's lifetime. In females, meiosis begins prenatally, with oocytes proceeding through the first stages of meiosis I but arresting at mid-prophase. At the time of birth, the first meiotic division is suspended in oocytes. Only after ovulation many years later do oocytes complete meiosis I and proceed to the metaphase stage of meiosis II; if fertilized, the oocyte then completes the second meiotic division. Thus, in females, the first meiotic division takes at least 10 to 15 years, and possibly as many as 40 to 45 years, to complete. Maternal age-related increases in the incidence of trisomy are likely the consequence of this protracted process of cell division.

INCIDENCE AND TYPES OF CHROMOSOME ABNORMALITIES   Errors in meiosis, or in early cleavage divisions, occur with extraordinary frequency. At least 10 to 25% of all pregnancies, for example, involve chromosomally abnormal conceptions. A large proportion of these terminate in the earliest stages of pregnancy. Nevertheless, even among clinically recognized pregnancies, nearly 10%

Table 66-1   Frequency of Chromosome Abnormalities, Identified on the Basis of Abnormal Ultrasound Findings

Ultrasound Finding	Chromosomal Abnormalities (Frequency)	
	Average, %	Range in Different Studies, %
Abnormal ultrasound (nonspecific)	16	13–35
Omphalocele	39	26–54
Cystic hygroma	68	46–78
Congenital heart disease	30	8–40
Choroid plexus cyst	5	4–10

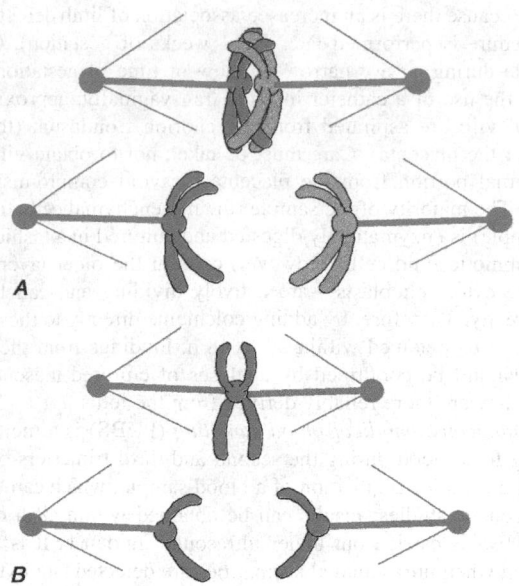

FIGURE 66-3 Chromosome segregation in meiosis. *A.* In meiosis I (MI), each of the 23 pairs of chromosomes finds its "partner," or homologue, and exchanges genetic material (recombines) with it. At metaphase, each homologous pair aligns on the equatorial plate; at anaphase, each member of the homologous pair segregates from its partner. Thus, at the end of MI, each daughter cell contains 23 chromosomes, with each chromosome consisting of two sister chromatids. *B.* In meiosis II (MII), each chromosome aligns on the metaphase plate, and at anaphase, each of the two sister chromatids divide from one another. Thus, at the end of MII, each daughter cell (e.g., the oocyte or spermatocyte) contains 23 chromosomes, with each chromosome consisting of one sister chromatid.

In mitosis, the chromosomes behave exactly as they do in MII, except that somatically dividing cells contain 46 chromosomes, not the 23 that are present in the MII cell.

of fetuses are chromosomally unbalanced. The occurrence of different classes of chromosome abnormalities are summarized in Table 66-2 for the three types of clinically recognized pregnancies: spontaneous abortions, stillbirths, and livebirths. The commonest abnormalities are numerical, involving fetuses with additional (*trisomy*) or missing (*monosomy*) chromosomes or those with one (*triploidy*) or two (*tetraploidy*) additional sets of chromosomes. Structural chromosome abnormalities are much less common, although several of the most important clinical chromosomal disorders involve structural rearrangements (see below).

By far the most common abnormality is trisomy, which is identified in approximately 25% of spontaneous abortions and 0.3% of newborns. Trisomies for all chromosomes have now been identified in embryos or fetuses, but there is considerable variation in frequency for various chromosomes. For example, trisomy 16 is extraordinarily common, accounting for about one-third of all trisomies in spontaneous abortions, whereas trisomies 1, 5, 11, and 19 have been identified less often. Available evidence suggests two reasons for this variation: (1) some chromosomes (e.g., chromosome 16) are more likely to segregate abnormally or undergo nondisjunction during meiosis than others; and (2) the potential for development varies widely among different trisomic conditions, with some being eliminated very early in gestation, others surviving to the time of clinical pregnancy recognition, and some (e.g., trisomies 13, 18, and 21 and sex chromosome trisomies) being compatible with survival to term.

CHROMOSOMAL SYNDROMES While most chromosomally abnormal conceptions perish in utero (Table 66-2), several conditions are compatible with survival to term. The best-characterized of these are numerical abnormalities involving loss or gain of individual

chromosomes and abnormalities resulting from unbalanced translocations. FISH and other molecular studies have led to the identification of two "new" types of chromosome abnormalities, commonly referred to as *microdeletion syndromes* and *imprinting syndromes*.

Numerical Abnormalities Virtually all types of numerical abnormalities are eliminated prenatally, so that only those involving small, gene-poor autosomes or the sex chromosomes are identified with any frequency among live-borns. Clinically, the most important of these is *trisomy 21*, the most frequent cause of Down syndrome. Depending on the maternal age structure of the population and the utilization of prenatal testing, the incidence of trisomy 21 ranges from 1/600 to 1/1000 live births, making it the most common chromosome abnormality in live-born individuals. Like most trisomies, the incidence of trisomy 21 is highly correlated with maternal age, increasing from about 1/1500 live births for women 20 years of age to 1/30 for women 45 years of age and older.

In addition to trisomy 21, only two other autosomal trisomies, 13 and 18, occur with any frequency in livebirths. Incidence rates for trisomies 13 and 18 in live births are 1/20,000 and 1/10,000 respectively. Unlike trisomy 21, which is associated with near-normal life expectancy, both trisomies 13 and 18 are associated with death in infancy, typically occurring during the first year of life.

Three sex chromosome trisomies—the 47,XXX, 47,XXY (*Klinefelter syndrome*), and 47,XYY conditions—are quite common, with each occurring in about 1/2000 newborns. Of all the trisomic conditions, these three have the fewest phenotypic complications. In fact, with the exception of infertility in Klinefelter syndrome (Chap. 335), it is likely that most individuals with such trisomic conditions would go undetected. The additional chromosome in the 47,XYY condition is small and contains only a few genes. Most Y-linked genes are involved in testicular development or spermatogenesis. Thus, dosage imbalance of Y-linked genes has relatively little effect on other developmental processes. The 47,XYY genotype is associated with increased height. Its role in antisocial behavior, postulated initially because of an increased prevalence among some penalized populations, is unclear.

For the 47,XXX and 47,XXY conditions, the situation is different—the X chromosome contains over 1000 genes, many of them essential for normal development. How, then, are 47,XXX and 47,XXY individuals spared from the catastrophic consequences of dosage imbalance? The answer lies in the biology of X chromosome gene expression. In normal females, one of the X chromosomes is inactivated in somatic cells. The inactivation of the paternal or maternal X chromosome occurs randomly in each somatic cell and thereby serves as a mechanism of dosage compensation, ensuring that males and females have equal expression of most X-linked genes. The inactivation process occurs at the blastocyst stage of development; prior to this time both X chromosomes are active. In addition, the rules for inactivation are different for germ cells than for somatic cells: in female germ cells both X chromosomes remain active, whereas in male germ cells the X chromosome is inactivated. In addition, not all X-linked genes are inactivated. Some genes on the X chromosome "escape" the inactivating mechanism and are expressed from both X chromosomes. In disorders such as Klinefelter syndrome, some genes may be expressed from both X chromosomes, resulting in phenotypic abnormalities. Individuals with Klinefelter syndrome have small testes, hyalinized seminiferous tubules, and azoospermia or severe oligospermia (Chap. 335). Testosterone levels are variably reduced, and often there is gynecomastia and eunuchoidal body proportions. Antisocial behavior and mild mental deficiency are seen in some individuals. Females with the 47,XXX genotype are more likely to have mild mental deficiency and may be subfertile. Despite these features, sex chromosome trisomies impart relatively minor phenotypic complications in comparison to aneuploidies that involve autosomal chromosomes.

As a rule, monosomic conditions are incompatible with fetal development and, consequently, autosomal monosomies are only rarely identified in spontaneous abortions and are not found among live-born individuals. In fact, the only monosomy compatible with live birth is the 45,X condition, which causes *Turner syndrome*. The 45,X chromosome constitution occurs with surprisingly high frequency, being present in at least 1 to 2% of all pregnancies. More than 99% of all 45,X conceptions are spontaneously aborted. Thus, live-born individuals with a 45,X chromosome constitution represent a rare group of survivors. The 45,X phenotype is mild, presumably because the second copy of many X chromosomal genes is normally inactivated. Nonetheless, Turner syndrome causes gonadal dysgenesis, resulting in infertility and failure to undergo secondary sexual development. Other prominent features are more variable and include short stature, webbing of the neck, and shield-shaped chest; lymphedema; increased carrying angle at the elbow, cardiovascular and renal abnormalities; and a propensity to hypertension, glucose intolerance, and autoimmune thyroid disease (Chap. 336). Several other structural abnormalities of the X chromosome such as partial deletions, isochromosome X, or ring chromosomes can cause Turner syndrome. Mosaicism, including 45,X/45,XX, 45X/45,XXX, 45,X/45,XY, and others, also occurs (see below) and contributes to the phenotypic spectrum seen in Turner syndrome.

Because numerical abnormalities originate in meiosis (Table 66-3), affected individuals have missing or extra chromosomes in all cells. In a small proportion of cases, though, a mitotic nondisjunctional event occurs at an early stage in an individual with an initially normal chromosome constitution. Alternatively, a "normalizing" mitotic nondisjunctional event may result in a normal chromosome complement in some cells of an embryo. In either case, the embryo is a *mosaic*, with some cells bearing a normal chromosome constitution and others an aneuploid number of chromosomes. The phenotypic consequences are difficult to predict because they depend on the timing of nondisjunction and the distribution of normal and abnormal cells in different tissues. Nevertheless, mosaicism may lead to clinical abnormalities indistinguishable from those of nonmosaic individuals; for example, nearly 5% of all cases of Down syndrome involve individuals with mosaic trisomy 21, and about 15% of individuals with Turner syndrome are mosaic for various sex chromosomal constitutions as described above.

The Origin and Etiology of Numerical Abnormalities Over the past decade, a number of studies have used DNA polymorphisms to investigate the origin of different types of chromosome abnormalities (Fig. 66-4). The most thoroughly investigated types have been numerical abnormalities (Table 66-3). Sex chromosome monosomy usually results from loss of the paternal sex chromosome. This is the case regardless of whether the conception is live-born or spontaneously aborted, indicating that the parental origin of the abnormality does not affect its likelihood of surviving to term.

Trisomies show remarkable variation in parental origin. For example, paternal nondisjunction is responsible for nearly 50% of 47,XXY but only 5 to 10% of cases of trisomies 13, 14, 15, 21, and 22; it is rarely, if ever, the source of the additional chromosome in trisomy 16. Similarly, there is considerable variability in the meiotic stage of origin. For example, among maternally derived trisomies, all cases of trisomy 16 may be due to meiosis I errors, whereas for trisomy 21, one-third of cases are associated with meiosis II errors, and for trisomy 18, the majority of cases are apparently due to meiosis II nondisjunction. In spite of this variation in parental and meiotic origin, nondisjunction at maternal meiosis I appears to be the most common source of trisomy.

Molecular studies have also begun to shed light on the molecular mechanisms underlying nondisjunction, the source of trisomy and monosomy. Most, if not all, trisomies are associated with alterations in genetic recombination. This is the process by which chromosomes exchange genetic material during the first of the two meiotic divisions. In other organisms, the physical connections, or chiasmata, associated with recombination are known to hold chromosomes together at meiosis I. This mechanism is now known to be true for humans as well. Nondisjunction at meiosis I is linked to a reduced extent of crossing-over, with some cases involving outright failure of recombination between the homologous chromosomes, and others associated with distally placed exchanges. Unexpectedly—since recombination occurs at meiosis I—maternal meiosis II errors involving chromosome 21 may also be linked to altered recombination. In this instance, though, the effect involves increased—not decreased—recombination, especially in proximal 21q. Presumably, this indicates that errors scored as arising at meiosis II are, in fact, precipitated by events occurring at meiosis I.

Maternal Age and Trisomy The association between increasing maternal age and trisomy is arguably the most important etiologic factor in congenital chromosomal disorders. Among women under the age of 25, approximately 2% of all clinically recognized pregnancies are trisomic; by the age of 36, however, this figure increases to 10% and by the age of 42, to >33% (Fig. 66-5). This association between maternal age and trisomy is exerted without respect to race, geography, or socioeconomic factors and likely affects segregation of all chromosomes.

Despite the importance of increasing age, almost nothing is known about the mechanism by which aging leads to abnormal chromosomal segregation. As noted above, it is thought to originate in maternal meiosis I owing to the protracted time to completion (often ≥40 years) in females. As noted above, alterations in genetic recombination may

Table 66-2 Frequency and Distribution of Chromosome Abnormalities in Different Types of Clinically Recognizable Pregnancies

Chromosome Abnormality	Frequency of Abnormality			Probability of Surviving to Term, %
	Spontaneous Abortion	Stillbirth	Livebirth	
Trisomy, all	25.1	4.0	0.3	5
+13, 18, 21	4.5	2.7	0.14	15
+16	7.5	—	—	0
Sex chromosome monosomy (45,X)	8.7	0.1	0.01	1
Triploidy	6.4	0.2	—	0
Tetraploidy	2.4	—	—	0
Structural abnormality	2.0	0.8	0.3	45
Total abnormalities	50.0	5.1	0.6	5

Table 66-3 Studies of the Parent and Meiotic/Mitotic Stage of Origin of Human Trisomies and Sex Chromosome Monosomy

	Origin, %				
	Paternal		Maternal		
	I	II	I	II	Mitotic
TRISOMY					
2	28	—	54	13	6
7	—	—	17	26	57
15	—	15	76	9	—
16	—	1	96	3	—
18	—	—	33	56	11
21	3	5	67	22	2
22	3	—	94	3	—
XXY	46	—	38	14	3
XXX	—	6	60	16	18
MONOSOMY					
X[a]	80		20		

[a] Results pertain to nonmosaic 45,X individuals.

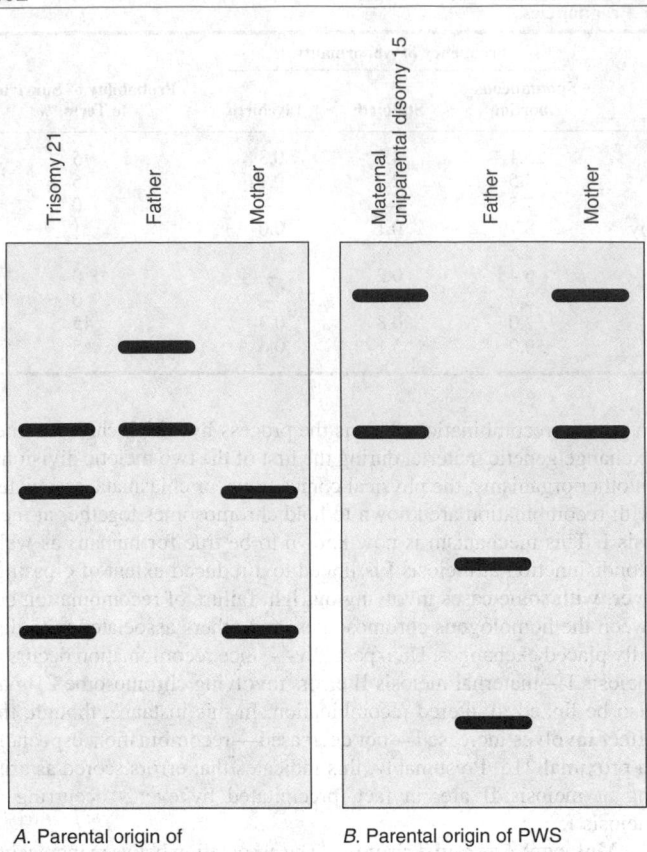

A. Parental origin of
   trisomy 21

B. Parental origin of PWS

FIGURE 66-4 Use of DNA technology to determine the origin of chromosome abnormalities. *A.* Analysis of a chromosome 21–specific DNA polymorphism demonstrates that the trisomic individual received two chromosomes 21 from his mother and one from his father; thus, the extra chromosome 21 resulted from an error in oogenesis. *B.* Inheritance of a chromosome 15–specific DNA polymorphism in an individual with Prader-Willi syndrome (PWS). The affected individual has received two maternal, but no paternal, chromosomes 15; thus, the individual is said to have maternal uniparental disomy 15, a common cause of PWS.

explain age-related trisomy. In trisomy 21, for example, recombination patterns appear to be similarly altered in younger and older mothers of trisomic conceptions. With this in mind, it has been suggested that two distinct steps, or "hits," may be involved in maternal age-related nondisjunction. The first hit, which is age-independent, involves the establishment of a "vulnerable" recombination configuration in the fetal oocyte; the second hit, which is age-dependent, involves abnormal processing of the vulnerable bivalent structure at metaphase I. If this model is correct, it means that the nondisjunctional process is the same in younger and older women, but it occurs more frequently with aging, possibly because of age-dependent degradation of cell cycle proteins or meiotic proteins responsible for maintaining sister chromatid cohesion.

Structural Chromosome Abnormalities Structural rearrangements involve breakage and reunion of chromosomes. Although less common than numerical abnormalities, they present additional challenges from a genetic counseling standpoint. This is because structural abnormalities, unlike numerical abnormalities, can be present in "balanced" form in clinically normal individuals but transmitted in "unbalanced" form to progeny, thereby resulting in a hereditary form of chromosome abnormality.

Rearrangements may involve exchanges of material between different chromosomes (*translocations*) or loss, gain, or rearrangements of individual chromosomes (e.g., *deletions, duplications, inversions,*

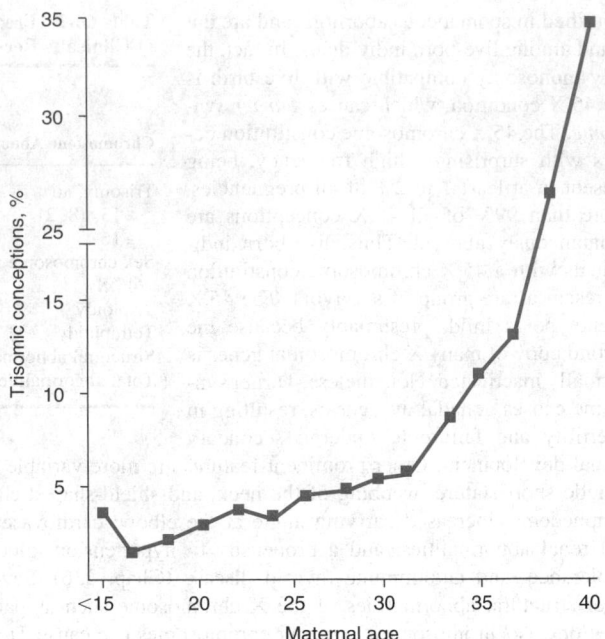

FIGURE 66-5 Estimated maternal age–adjusted rates of trisomy among all clinically recognized pregnancies (e.g., spontaneous abortions, stillbirths, and livebirths). Among women in their forties, over 25% of all pregnancies are estimated to involve a trisomic conception; the vast majority of these spontaneously abort, with only trisomies 13, 18, and 21 and sex chromosome trisomies surviving to term with any appreciable frequency.

rings or *isochromosomes*). Of particular clinical importance are translocations, which involve two basic types: Robertsonian and reciprocal. *Robertsonian rearrangements* are a special class of translocation, in which the long arms of two acrocentric chromosomes (chromosomes 13, 14, 15, 21, and 22) join together, generating a fusion chromosome that contains virtually all of the genetic material of the original two chromosomes. If the Robertsonian translocation is present in unbalanced form, a monosomic or trisomic conception ensues. For example, approximately 3% of cases of Down syndrome are attributable to unbalanced Robertsonian translocations, most often involving chromosomes 14 and 21. In this instance, the affected individual has 46 chromosomes, including one structurally normal chromosome 14, two structurally normal chromosomes 21, and one fusion 14/21 chromosome. This effect leads to a normal diploid dosage for chromosome 14 and to a triplication of chromosome 21, thus resulting in Down syndrome. Similarly, a small proportion of individuals with trisomy 13 syndrome are clinically affected because of an unbalanced Robertsonian translocation.

Reciprocal translocations involve exchanges between any two chromosomes. In this circumstance, the phenotypic consequences associated with unbalanced translocations depend on the location of the breakpoints, which dictate the amount of material that has been "exchanged" between the two chromosomes. Because most reciprocal translocations involve unique sets of breakpoints, it is difficult to predict the phenotypic consequences in any one situation. In general, severity is determined by the amount of excess or missing chromosome material in individuals with unbalanced translocations.

In addition to rearrangements between chromosomes, there are several examples of intrachromosome structural abnormalities. The most common and deleterious of these involve loss of chromosome material due to deletions. The two best-characterized deletion syndromes, *Wolf-Hirschhorn syndrome* and *cri-du-chat syndrome*, result from loss of relatively small chromosomal segments on chromosomes 4p and 5p, respectively. Nonetheless, each is associated with multiple congenital anomalies, developmental delays, profound retardation, and reduced lifespan.

Microdeletion Syndromes The term *contiguous gene syndromes* refers to genetic disorders that mimic a combination of single gene disorders. They result from the deletion of a small number of tightly clustered genes. Because they are usually too small to be detected cytogenetically, they are termed *microdeletions*. The application of molecular techniques has led to the identification of at least 18 of these microdeletion syndromes (Table 66-4). Some of the more common ones include the Wilms' tumor–aniridia complex (WAGR), MDS, and VCF syndrome. *WAGR* is characterized by mental retardation and involvement of multiple organs, including kidney (Wilm's tumor), eye (aniridia), and the genitourinary system. The cytogenetic abnormality involves a deletion of part of the short arm of chromosome 11 (11p13), which typically is detectable on well-banded chromosome preparations. In *MDS*, a disorder characterized by mental retardation, dysmorphic faces, and lissencephaly, the deletion involves chromosome 17 (17p13). Using FISH, 17p deletions have been detected in >90% of MDS patients as well as in 20% of cases of isolated lissencephaly.

Deletions involving the long arm of chromosome 22 (22q11) are the most common microdeletions identified to date, present in approximately 1/3000 newborns. VCF syndrome, the most commonly associated syndrome, consists of learning disabilities or mild mental retardation, palatal defects, a hypoplastic aloe nasi and long nose, and congenital heart defects (conotruncal defect). Some individuals with 22q11 deletion are more severely affected and present with *DiGeorge syndrome*, which involves abnormalities in the development of the third and fourth branchial arches leading to thymic hypoplasia, parathyroid hypoplasia, and conotruncal heart defects. In approximately 30% of these cases, a deletion at 22q11 can be detected with high-resolution banding; by combing conventional cytogenetics, FISH, and molecular detection techniques (i.e., Southern blotting or polymerase chain reaction analyses), these rates improve to >90%. Additional studies have demonstrated a surprisingly high frequency of 22q11 deletions in individuals with nonsyndromic conotruncal defects. Approximately 10% of individuals with a 22q11 deletion inherited it from a parent with a similar deletion.

Smith-Magenis syndrome involves a microdeletion localized to the short arm of chromosome 17 (17p11.2). Affected individuals have mental retardation, dysmorphic facial features, delayed speech, peripheral neuropathy, and behavior abnormalities. Most of these deletions can be detected with cytogenetic analysis, although FISH is available to confirm these findings. In contrast, *William syndrome*, a chromosome 7 (7q11.23) microdeletion, cannot be diagnosed with standard or high-resolution analysis; it is only detectable utilizing FISH or other molecular methods. William syndrome involves a deletion of the elastin gene and is characterized by mental retardation, dysmorphic features, a gregarious personality, premature aging, and congenital heart disease (usually supravalvular aortic stenosis).

In addition to microdeletion syndromes, there is now at least one well-described microduplication syndrome, Charcot-Marie-Tooth type 1A (CMT1A). This is a nerve conduction disease previously though to be transmitted as a simple autosomal dominant disorder. Recent molecular studies have demonstrated that affected individuals are heterozygous for duplication of a small region of chromosome 17 (17p11.2-12). Although it is not yet clear why increased gene dosage

Table 66-4 Some Commonly Identified Microdeletion and Microduplication Syndromes

Syndrome	Cytogenetic Location	Principal Features	Imprinting Effects
Langer-Giedion syndrome	8q24.1 (del)	Sparse hair, bulbous nose, variable mental retardation	No
WAGR complex	11p13 (del)	Wilms' tumor, aniridia, genitourinary disorders, mental retardation	No
Beckwith-Wiedemann syndrome	11p15 (dup)	Macrosomia, macroglossia, omphalocoele	Yes, occasionally associated with "paternal uniparental disomy" (see text)
Retinoblastoma	13q14.11 (del)	Retinoblastoma due to homozygous loss of functional RB allele	No obvious effect, although abnormal RB allele more likely to be paternal
Prader-Willi syndrome	15q11-13 (del)	Obesity, hypogonadism, mental retardation	Yes; prototypic imprinting disorder (see text)
Angelman syndrome	15q11-13 (del)	Ataxic gait	With Prader-Willi syndrome, prototypic imprinting disorder (see text)
α-Thalassemia and mental retardation	16p13.3 (del)	α-thalassemia and mental retardation, due to deletion of distal 16p, including α-globin locus	No
Smith-Magenis syndrome	17p11.2 (del)	Brachycephaly, midface hypoplasia, mental retardation	No
Miller-Dieker syndrome	17p13 (del)	Dysmorphic facies, lissencephaly	No
Charcot-Marie-Tooth syndrome type 1A	17p11.2 (dup)	Progressive neuropathy due to microduplication	No
DiGeorge syndrome/velocardiofacial syndrome	22q11 (del)	Abnormalities of third and fourth branchial arches	No

would result in CMT1A, the inheritance pattern is explained by the fact that one-half of the offspring of affected individuals inherit the duplication-carrying chromosome.

Imprinting Disorders Two other microdeletion syndromes, PWS and AS, exhibit parent-of-origin, or "imprinting," effects. For many years, it has been known that cytogenetically detectable deletions of chromosome 15 occur in a proportion of patients with PWS, as well as in those with AS. This seemed curious, as the clinical manifestations of the two syndromes are very dissimilar. PWS is characterized by obesity, hypogonadism, and mild to moderate mental retardation, whereas AS is associated with microcephaly, ataxic gait, seizures, inappropriate laughter, and severe mental retardation. New insight into the pathogenesis of these disorders has been provided by the recognition that parental origin of the deletion determines which phenotype ensues: if the deletion is paternal, the result is PWS, whereas if the deletion is maternal, the result is AS (Fig. 66-2).

This scenario is complicated further by the recognition that not all individuals with PWS or AS carry the chromosome 15 deletion. For such individuals, it turns out that the parental origin of the chromosome 15 region is again the important determinant. In PWS, for example, nondeletion patients invariably have two maternal and no paternal chromosomes 15 [*maternal uniparental disomy* (UPD)], whereas for some nondeletion AS patients the reverse is true (*paternal UPD*). This indicates that at least some genes on chromosome 15 are differently expressed, depending on which parent contributed the chromosome. Additionally, this means that normal fetal development requires the presence of one maternal and one paternal copy of chromosome 15.

Approximately 70% of PWS cases are due to paternal deletions of

15q11-q13, whereas 25% are due to maternal uniparental disomy, and about 5% are caused by mutations in a chromosome 15 imprinting center. Though 75% of the AS cases are due to maternal deletions, only 2% are due to paternal uniparental disomy. The rest of the cases are presumed to be caused by imprinting mutations (5%) or mutations in the UBE3A gene, which is one of the genes associated with AS. The UPD cases are mostly caused by meiotic nondisjunction resulting in trisomy 15, subsequently followed by a normalizing mitotic non-disjunction event ("trisomy rescue") resulting in two normal chromosomes 15, both from the same parent. *UBE3A* is the only maternally imprinted gene known in the critical region of chromosome 15. However, several paternally imprinted genes, or expressed-sequence tags (ESTs), have been identified, including *ZNF127*, *IPW*, *SNRPN*, *SNURF*, *PAR1*, and *PAR5*.

Chromosomal regions that behave in the manner observed in PWS and AS are said to be *imprinted*. This phenomenon is involved in differential expression of certain genes on different chromosomes. Chromosome 11 must be one of these with an imprinted region, since it is known that a small proportion of individuals with the *Beckwith-Wiedemann overgrowth syndrome* have two paternal but no maternal copies of this chromosome.

ACQUIRED CHROMOSOME ABNORMALITIES IN CANCER

In addition to the constitutional cytogenetic chromosomal abnormalities that are present at birth, somatic chromosomal changes can be acquired later in life and are often associated with malignant conditions. As with constitutional abnormalities, somatic changes can include the net loss of chromosomal material (due to a deletion or loss of a chromosome), net gain of material (duplication or gain of a chromosome), and relocation of DNA sequences (translocation). These chromosomal changes are intertwined with the three major categories of cancer genes: (1) *tumor-suppressor genes* that inhibit cell proliferation may be deleted; (2) *oncogenes* that activate cell proliferation may be activated by duplication, amplification, or translocation; and (3) *DNA repair genes* may also be deleted from somatic cells, thereby predisposing to the accumulation of additional DNA damage. Cytogenetic changes have been particularly well studied in (1) leukemias, e.g., Philadelphia chromosome translocation in CML[t(9;22)(q34.1; q11.2)]); and (2) lymphomas, e.g., translocations of MYC in Burkitt's [t(8;14)(q24;q32)]. These and other translocations are useful for diagnosis, classification, and prognosis. Analyses of cytogenetic changes are also proving useful in certain solid tumors. For example, a complex karyotype with Wilms' tumor, diploidy in medulloblastoma, and Her-2/neu amplification in breast cancer are poor prognostic signs. The genetic basis of malignancy, including the role of germline and somatic chromosomal alterations, is discussed further in Chap. 81.

BIBLIOGRAPHY

GELEHRTER TD et al (eds): *Principles of Medical Genetics*, 2d ed. Baltimore, Williams & Wilkins, 1998

GERSEN SL, KEAGLE MB (eds): *The Principles of Clinical Cytogenetics*. Totowa, NJ, Humana, 1999

JAMESON JL (ed): *Principles of Molecular Medicine*. Totowa, NJ, Humana, 1998

MITLEMAN F: *Catalog of Chromosome Aberrations in Cancer*, 6th ed. New York, Wiley, 1998

NICHOLLS RD et al: Imprinting in Prader-Willi and Angelman syndromes. Trends Genet 14:194, 1998

RIMOIN DL et al (eds): *Emery and Rimoin's Principles and Practice of Medical Genetics*, 3d ed. New York, Churchill Livingstone, 1996

SCRIVER CR et al (eds): *The Metabolic and Molecular Bases of Inherited Disease*, 8th ed. New York, McGraw-Hill, 2001

STUMM M et al: Molecular cytogenetic techniques for the diagnosis of chromosomal abnormalities in childhood disease. Eur J Pediatr 158:531, 1999

Donald R. Johns

DISEASES CAUSED BY GENETIC DEFECTS OF MITOCHONDRIA

Mitochondrial defects play a role in several metabolic and neurodegenerative diseases as well as aging. Mitochondrial disorders have protean clinical manifestations, reflecting the fact that nearly all organ systems utilize oxidative metabolism. Clinical features often involve tissues with high energy requirements such as the central and peripheral nervous systems, the eye, muscle, kidney, and endocrine organs. The age and mode of onset and clinical course of mitochondrial diseases range widely as a result of the unusual mechanisms of mitochondrial DNA (mtDNA) replication, which is distinct from that of the nuclear genome. A maternal mode of inheritance is characteristic of many mitochondrial diseases because mtDNA is transmitted by the oocyte. Hundreds of different mtDNA mutations have been described since the first mutation was described in 1988.

STRUCTURE AND FUNCTION OF MITOCHONDRIAL DNA   Most cells contain several hundred mitochondria, though the number varies depending on the energy requirements and function of a tissue. Mitochondria are the only cellular organelles that contain their own extrachromosomal DNA. Human mtDNA is a small (16,569 bp) double-stranded, circular molecule that encodes 13 protein subunits of 4 different oxidative phosphorylation biochemical complexes. mtDNA also encodes the 24 structural RNAs (2 ribosomal RNAs and 22 transfer RNAs) required for the intramitochondrial translation of these proteins. The noncoding D (displacement)-loop is a regulatory region that controls transcription and replication. mtDNA mutations are found in each type of mitochondrial gene (Fig. 67-1).

Mitochondria probably evolved from independent organisms that became endosymbiotically incorporated into the cell. As a result, mitochondria replicate, transcribe, and translate their DNA independently of nuclear DNA. However, cellular and mitochondrial function are interdependent. Nuclear DNA-encoded proteins are also involved in oxidative phosphorylation, and the myriad macromolecular compounds required for mitochondrial structure and function (e.g., mtDNA replication, transcription, and translation) are imported from the cytoplasm into the mitochondria.

Oxidative phosphorylation and the generation of adenosine triphosphate (ATP) for energy-requiring cellular processes are the central functions of mitochondria. Alterations in mitochondrial function lead to disease pathogenesis by three main mechanisms: (1) reduction of ATP supply when mutations impair oxidative phosphorylation; (2) generation of reactive oxygen species such as H_2O_2 and OH· free radicals that can damage DNA, proteins, or lipids; and (3) execution of the apoptosis pathway when mitochondria release cell death–promoting factors including caspases, cytochrome c, and apoptosis-inducing factor.

Several unique features of mtDNA render it vulnerable to mutations and contribute to its role in disease. For example, mtDNA has no introns (a random mutation will therefore usually strike a coding DNA sequence) or protective histones, and it has an imperfect DNA repair system and is exposed to oxygen free radicals generated by oxidative phosphorylation. mtDNA is estimated to mutate 10 times more rapidly than nuclear DNA. Importantly, mtDNA is strictly *maternally inherited* and does not recombine, and mtDNA mutations sequentially accumulate along maternal lineages. These properties have made mtDNA sequence variation an invaluable tool for evolutionary biologists and forensic scientists.

Each mitochondrion contains 2 to 10 mtDNA molecules, and each cell contains multiple mitochondria (*polyplasmy*). Population genetic principles, as opposed to Mendelian genetics, govern mitochondrial genetics. When a new mtDNA mutation arises, cells initially harbor copies of both normal and mutant DNA sequences—a condition

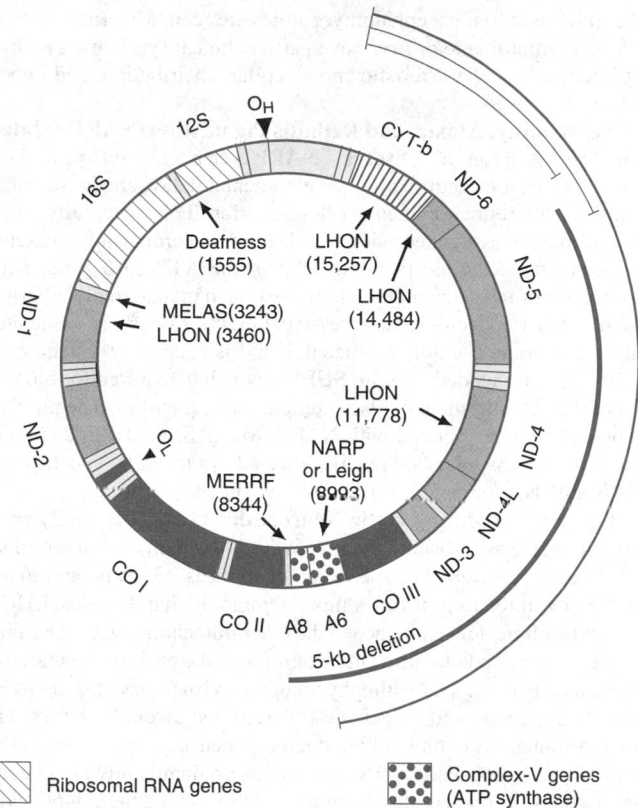

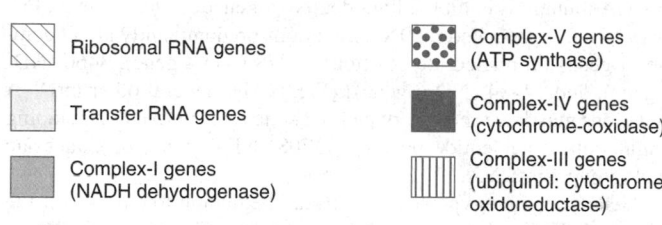

FIGURE 67-1 Schematic diagram of human mitochondrial DNA and the most prominent pathogenetic mutations. Point mutations in structural and protein-coding genes are indicated inside the circle, with the clinical phenotype and the nucleotide position of the mutation. The thick arc indicates the position of the most common single deletion, which is 5 kb in length, and the thin arcs outside the circle indicate the multiple deletions. MERRF, myoclonic epilepsy with ragged red fibers; MELAS, the syndrome of mitochondrial encephalomyopathy, lactic acidosis, and strokelike episodes; LHON, Leber's hereditary optic neuropathy; NARP, neuropathy, ataxia, and retinitis pigmentosa; Leigh, maternally inherited Leigh's disease. *(Adapted from Johns, with permission.)*

known as *heteroplasmy*—which allows an otherwise lethal mutation to persist and cause disease. The presence of either completely normal or completely mutant mtDNA is known as *homoplasmy*. During cell division, mitchondria are unevenly partitioned to the daughter cells through the process of *replicative segregation*; consequently, the proportion of mutant and normal mtDNA molecules can drift. Selection pressures apply at the molecular, cellular, and organismal levels. The critical proportion of mutant mtDNA required for deleterious phenotypic expression is known as the *threshold effect*. It varies among individuals, among organ systems, and within a given tissue, depending on the delicate balance of oxidative supply and demand. These features of mtDNA segregation, combined with the uneven transmission of mitochondria to daughter cells during cell division, form much of the basis for the phenotypic diversity seen in mitochondrial diseases.

MITOCHONDRIAL DNA MUTATIONS mtDNA mutations that cause a severe, lethal impairment of oxidative phosphorylation—such as gross structural defects or point mutations in structural RNAs—are only viable if heteroplasmic. In contrast, the majority of the milder, missense mtDNA mutations in protein-coding genes are homoplasmic. mtDNA point mutations have been found in each type of mtDNA gene, but tRNA mutations predominate in severe, multisystemic mitochondrial encephalomyopathy phenotypes; protein-coding gene mutations predominate in Leber's hereditary optic neuropathy (LHON). A point mutation in the 12S ribosomal RNA gene is associated with both spontaneous and aminoglycoside-associated sensorineural deafness (Fig. 67-1).

A definitive cause-and-effect relationship between a mtDNA mutation and a clinical phenotype can be difficult to establish for several reasons: (1) mtDNA is highly polymorphic, (2) different mutations can be associated with the same phenotype or the same mutation can be associated with different phenotypes, and (3) epigenetic factors can affect clinical manifestations.

CLASSIC MITOCHONDRIAL ENCEPHALOMYOPATHY PHENOTYPES Many diseases were provisionally classified as mitochondrial disorders on the basis of abnormal mitochondrial morphology, biochemistry, or a pattern of maternal inheritance. Disease-associated mtDNA mutations are now an important diagnostic criterion. Though each classic mitochondrial encephalomyopathy phenotype has distinctive clinical features (Table 67-1), each also shares many clinical and laboratory features (Tables 67-2 and 67-3).

Mitochondrial Myopathy Mitochondrial myopathy is characterized by fixed proximal weakness with marked exercise intolerance. Fatigability and poor stamina are prominent clinical features, but a mitochondrial etiology is often considered in the context of other neurologic, somatic, or laboratory features. Frank rhabdomyolysis is rare. Electromyography documents a nonirritative myopathy, and serum creatine kinase is usually normal or slightly elevated. Skeletal muscle biopsy shows abnormal proliferating mitochondria and "ragged red fibers," a histologic hallmark of the severe biochemical defects in oxidative phosphorylation. Large mtDNA deletions and a variety of mtDNA point mutations occur in mitochondrial myopathy.

Chronic Progressive External Ophthalmoplegia (CPEO) Ptosis, ophthalmoplegia, and limb myopathy characterize CPEO. Additional clinical features (Table 67-2) may also occur along with the laboratory abnormalities characteristic of mitochondrial disorders (Table 67-3). Patients with CPEO have abnormal skeletal muscle biopsies, with ragged red fibers and ultrastructural changes. Additional somatic and central nervous system findings in conjunction with CPEO are known as the "CPEO-plus" syndromes. Kearns-Sayre syndrome is a subset of CPEO-plus that begins before age 20 and is characterized by CPEO and atypical pigmentary retinopathy; ancillary features include elevated cerebrospinal fluid protein, ataxia, or heart block.

Most patients with CPEO have large, single deletions in mtDNA that can be reliably detected by molecular genetic methods. However, skeletal muscle is required as the source of DNA because almost all single mtDNA deletions occur sporadically. The presence of pigmentary retinopathy is strongly predictive of a deletion. The mechanism of DNA deletion is unknown, though recombination or slippage during replication is plausible. The junctions of most deletions contain directly repeated sequences, including a 13-nucleotide direct repeat "hot spot" that accounts for about 25% of all deletions. Approximately half of all deletions are bound by other direct repeats; one-quarter have no apparent direct repeat. A few patients have partially duplicated

Table 67-1 Cardinal Neurologic Manifestations of Mitochondrial Diseases

Disease	Neurologic Manifestation
Chronic progressive external ophthalmoplegia	Ophthalmoplegia
Mitochondrial myopathy	Myopathy
Mitochondrial encephalomyopathy, lactic acidosis, and strokelike episodes	Strokelike episodes
Myoclonic epilepsy with ragged red fibers	Myoclonus, epilepsy
Neuropathy, ataxia, and retinitis pigmentosa	Neuropathy, ataxia, retinitis pigmentosa
Leber's hereditary optic neuropathy	Optic neuropathy

Table 67-2 Clinical Features of Mitochondrial Diseases

Neurologic manifestations	Systemic manifestations
Sensorineural hearing loss	Cardiac conduction defects
Myopathy with fatigability	Cardiomyopathy
Peripheral neuropathy	Diabetes mellitus
Myoclonus	Pseudohypoparathyroidism
Myelopathy	Short stature
Ataxia	Pigmentary retinopathy
Seizures	Lactic acidosis
Dementia	Fanconi's proximal nephron dysfunction
Vascular headache	Glomerulopathy
	Hepatic dysfunction
	Intestinal pseudo-obstruction
	Lipomas
	Pancytopenia, sideroblastic anemia
	Psychiatric disease (depression)

mtDNA molecules. A point mutation at nucleotide position 3243 has been found in many patients who lack a mtDNA deletion or duplication.

Autosomally Transmitted Multiple Mitochondrial DNA Deletions Several families with clinical variants of CPEO have been found to harbor multiple mtDNA deletions in skeletal muscle. The autosomal inheritance of multiple mtDNA deletions implies a primary defect in a nuclear DNA gene that has secondary qualitative effects on mtDNA. Multiple mtDNA deletions can be transmitted in either an autosomal dominant or autosomal recessive mode or can occur as somatic mutations.

Thymidine phosphorylase was the first nuclear-encoded gene shown to influence the regulation and function of normal mtDNA in a trans-acting manner. Mutations in thymidine phosphorylase cause an autosomal recessive disease known as *myoneurogastrointestinal encephalomyopathy* (MNGIE). Several different nuclear loci have been linked to the autosomal dominant forms of CPEO. Tissue-specific, autosomally transmitted depletion of mtDNA represents a quantitative mtDNA defect caused by an intergenomic communication error.

Mitochondrial Encephalomyopathy, Lactic Acidosis, and Strokelike Episodes (MELAS) This syndrome is characterized by strokelike events that cause subacute brain dysfunction, cerebral structural changes, seizures, and several other common clinical and laboratory features (Tables 67-2, 67-3). Maternal inheritance of the MELAS syndrome may be obscured because of mild clinical features in relatives. A point mutation at nucleotide 3243 in the tRNA$^{Leu(UUR)}$ gene accounts for 80% of MELAS cases. However, the clinical features of the 3243 mtDNA mutation are pleiomorphic; it is also associated with nondeletion CPEO, myopathy, deafness, diabetes, and dystonia.

Myoclonic Epilepsy with Ragged Red Fibers (MERRF) Syndrome The MERRF syndrome consists of myoclonus, seizures, cerebellar ataxia, and mitochondrial myopathy. Pathogenetic mutations have been demonstrated at nucleotide positions 8344 and 8356 in the tRNA^{Lys} gene. Neurologic and laboratory features common to

Table 67-3 Laboratory Findings in Mitochondrial Diseases

Ragged red fibers and COX-negative fibers on skeletal muscle biopsy
Elevated serum and cerebrospinal fluid lactate concentration
Myopathic potentials on electromyography
Axonal or demyelinating peripheral neuropathy on nerve conduction studies
Sensorineural hearing loss on audiogram
Abnormal glucose tolerance test or elevated hemoglobin A$_{1c}$
Cardiac conduction defects
Basal ganglia calcification or focal abnormalities on MRI
Altered phosphorus magnetic resonance spectroscopy
Defects in oxidative phosphorylation on biochemical studies
Molecular genetic demonstration of mtDNA mutations

NOTE: COX, cytochrome c oxidase; MRI, magnetic resonance imaging.

other mitochondrial encephalomyopathies are seen. Maternal relatives may be asymptomatic or may have partial clinical syndromes, including lipomas in a characteristic "horse-collar" distribution, and hypertension.

Neuropathy, Ataxia, and Retinitis Pigmentosa (NARP)/Maternally Inherited Leigh's Disease NARP is characterized by proximal weakness, sensory neuropathy, developmental delay, ataxia, seizures, dementia, and retinal pigmentary degeneration. This maternally inherited disorder is associated with two different heteroplasmic missense mutations at nucleotide position 8993 in the ATPase 6 gene. High proportions of the same mutations are also seen in maternally inherited Leigh's disease. Autosomal recessive Leigh's disease is associated with cytochrome c oxidase deficiency and is caused by a deficiency of the nuclear-encoded protein, SURF1, which is required for biogenesis of the cytochrome c oxidase complex (complex IV). The mtDNA point mutations associated with NARP, MELAS, MERRF, and other mitochondrial disorders are readily detected by molecular genetic analysis of mtDNA extracted from muscle or blood.

Leber's Hereditary Optic Neuropathy LHON typically presents with painless, subacute, bilateral visual loss with central scotomas and dyschromatopsia. The mean age of onset is 23 years, and males are affected three to four times more commonly than females. LHON bears little clinical resemblance to the other mitochondrial disease phenotypes. It was first classified in this group on the basis of the maternal inheritance pattern. The pathophysiology of visual loss appears to involve both genetic and epigenetic (tobacco and alcohol) factors. The mtDNA mutations exhibit a high degree of genetic heterogeneity. Primary LHON-associated mtDNA mutations predominantly affect complex I genes [at nucleotide positions 11778 (ND-4 gene), 3460 (ND-1 gene), and 14484 (ND-6 gene)] (Fig. 67-1). Several other mtDNA mutations may have secondary pathogenetic roles in LHON, including a mutation at nucleotide position 13708 (ND-5 gene) of Caucasian haplogroup J mtDNA.

Genotype-phenotype correlations are beginning to emerge for the primary LHON-associated mtDNA mutations. The prognosis for visual recovery, for example, varies nearly ten-fold depending on the mutation. mtDNA mutations that cause LHON plus dystonia have also been described.

ORGAN SYSTEM MANIFESTATIONS OF MITOCHONDRIAL DISEASE Because virtually all tissues of the body depend, to some extent, on oxidative metabolism, patients with mitochondrial disease can present to many specialists in medicine. The somatic manifestations listed in Table 67-2, first noted in association with the classic mitochondrial diseases, may be the dominant or initial clinical symptom or may be important comorbid features.

The ophthalmologic manifestations of mtDNA mutations are prominent, with involvement of virtually the entire visual axis from the lids, cornea, and extraocular muscles to the occipital cortex. The cardinal eye findings include ophthalmoplegia, optic neuropathy, and pigmentary retinopathy. Cardiovascular manifestations include dilated and hypertrophic cardiomyopathy, conduction disease and heart block, Wolff-Parkinson-White syndrome, and hypertension. The prevalence of diabetes mellitus is higher than expected in patients with mitochondrial encephalomyopathies, and it occurs in association with a variety of mtDNA mutations. Diabetes mellitus has been linked with the 3243 mtDNA point mutation, usually, but not exclusively, in association with sensorineural hearing loss.

ROLE OF MITOCHONDRIAL DNA MUTATIONS IN PREVALENT DISEASES The role of mtDNA mutations in common, socioeconomically significant diseases is under active investigation. The genetic basis of many prevalent diseases is complex and does not follow simple, single-gene Mendelian inheritance (Chap. 65). Mitochondrial diseases, such as LHON and aminoglycoside-induced deafness, illustrate the potential for complex pathophysiologic interactions between genetic and epigenetic factors. As a result of these interactions, mtDNA mutations may be involved in subsets of common diseases, such as diabetes mellitus, in which the maternal inheritance pattern is not obvious.

The tissue-specific accumulation of somatic (noninherited) mtDNA mutations is likely relevant to some late-onset degenerative disorders, such as Alzheimer's disease and Parkinson's disease. It has been shown, for example, that as people age, mtDNA mutations accumulate in tissues, including some postmitotic tissues such as the basal ganglia and cerebral cortex. The high mutations rate and poor repair capacity of mtDNA contribute to the buildup of mtDNA mutations in postmitotic tissues or those with a slower turnover rate. Oxidative damage, as occurs with repeated episodes of ischemia and reperfusion, markedly increases the accumulation of mtDNA mutations. Environmental factors may also affect mtDNA. The anti-retroviral drug azidothymidine depletes muscle mtDNA and causes an acquired mitochondrial myopathy. Cumulative, age-dependent mitochondrial dysfunction, mediated to a significant degree by oxidative damage to mtDNA and other mitochondrial macromolecules, may be a major contributor to aging.

The unequivocal establishment of the diagnosis of a mitochondrial disease by molecular genetic methods is a prerequisite for proper genetic counseling and ultimately treatment.

BIBLIOGRAPHY

BEAL MF et al: Do defects in mitochondrial energy metabolism underlie the pathology of neurodegenerative disease? Trends Neurosci 16:125, 1993

JOHNS DR: Mitochondrial DNA and disease. N Engl J Med 333:638, 1995

SHIGENAGA MK et al: Oxidative damage and mitochondrial decay in aging. Proc Natl Acad Sci USA 91:10771, 1994

SIMON DK, JOHNS DR: Mitochondrial disorders: Clinical and genetic features. Annu Rev Med 50:111, 1999

WALLACE DC: Mitochondrial diseases in man and mouse. Science 283:1482, 1999

ZEVIANI M et al: Mitochondrial disorders. Medicine (Baltimore) 77:59, 1998

68 *Susan Miesfeldt, J. Larry Jameson*

SCREENING, COUNSELING, AND PREVENTION OF GENETIC DISORDERS

IMPLICATIONS OF MOLECULAR GENETICS FOR INTERNAL MEDICINE

Approximately 1 in 50 children is born with a serious congenital abnormality or mental handicap. It is known that each of us harbors mutations in several genes that can potentially lead to serious diseases. The field of medical genetics has traditionally focused on chromosomal abnormalities (Chap. 66) and Mendelian disorders (Chap. 65). However, there is genetic susceptibility to many common adult-onset diseases including atherosclerosis, hypertension, autoimmune diseases, diabetes mellitus, Alzheimer disease, psychiatric disorders, and many forms of cancer. Genetic contributions to these common disorders involve more than the ultimate expression of a disease; these genes can also influence the severity of infirmity, response to treatment, and progression of disease.

The primary care clinician is now faced with the role of recognizing and counseling patients at risk for a large number of genetically influenced illnesses. This role reflects the advances in genetic medicine that are changing the way diseases are classified, enhancing our understanding of pathophysiology, providing practical information concerning drug metabolism and therapeutic responses, and promising to allow individualized screening and health care management programs. In view of these changes, the physician must integrate personal medical history, family history, and diagnostic molecular testing into the overall care of individual patients and their families. In addition, the internist has an important role in educating patients about the indications, benefits, risks, and limitations of genetic testing in the management of diverse diseases. This is a formidable task as scientific advances in genetic medicine, and media attention to these advances, have outpaced the translation into standards of clinical care.

PRENATAL AND NEWBORN GENETIC SCREENING AND TESTING

During pregnancy and in the newborn period, genetic screening and testing are both used to detect genetic disorders (Table 68-1). *Genetic screening* refers to the search for a genetic disorder in the entire population or in a high-risk population. Screening techniques must be cost-effective, have a high positive predictive value, and should yield information that leads to disease prevention or a useful therapeutic intervention. Examples of screening tests include maternal serum markers used to detect increased risk of Down syndrome, postnatal tests for phenylketonuria, and cholesterol levels in children used to identify individuals at risk for familial hyperlipidemias. Thus, genetic screening tests do not necessarily imply DNA- or chromosome-based tests. Instead, many such tests use a surrogate biochemical marker or phenotypic feature of the underlying genetic disorder. Determination of which genetic disorders should be screened routinely depends on disease frequency, the severity of the disorder, cost of screening, and whether treatment interventions can alter the course of the disease.

Genetic testing, on the other hand, is used in an individual suspected to have a disease based on physical features, family history, or biochemical findings. Genetic testing can include the following: (1) diagnostic testing as for hemochromatosis, (2) predictive testing as for breast cancer predisposition, (3) carrier testing as for muscular dystrophy, and (4) prenatal testing as for β-thalassemia when both parents are carriers.

Depending on the disorder(s) under consideration, several different techniques are currently used for genetic screening during pregnancy. For instance, first-trimester screening for Down syndrome is performed using measurements of maternal serum pregnancy-associated plasma protein A and the free β subunit of human chorionic gonadotropin in combination with ultrasonographic measurement of nuchal translucency (at 10 to 14 weeks of gestation). Second-trimester maternal serum screening includes measurements of human chorionic gonadotropin, unconjugated estriol, α-fetoprotein, and inhibin that, in combination, increase the sensitivity of Down syndrome detection (Chap. 66). Increased α-fetoprotein levels are also associated with open neural tube defects.

Amniocentesis or *chorionic villus sampling* (CVS) is used to isolate fetal cells for chromosomal analysis or to test for specific genetic abnormalities. Amniocentesis is typically performed during the early second trimester (14 to 16 weeks' gestational age). CVS can be performed earlier (8 to 10 weeks' gestational age) and involves transcervical or transabdominal biopsy of fetal trophoblastic tissue. CVS is associated with a somewhat greater risk of spontaneous abortion (<0.5 to 1%) than amniocentesis (<0.5%) but allows for elective abortion

Table 68-1 Examples of Screening Tests for Genetic Disorders in the Newborn[a]

Disorder	Inheritance	Incidence[b]
Phenylketonuria	AR	1/10,000
Hypothyroidism	Sporadic or AR	1/4000
Galactosemia	AR	1/40,000
Maple syrup urine disease	AR	1/200,000
Homocystinuria	AR	1/200,000
Biotinidase deficiency	AR	1/100,000
Cystic fibrosis	AR	1/2000
Adrenal hyperplasia	AR	1/10,000
Hemoglobinopathy	AR	1/2500

[a] The panel of prenatal screening tests varies in different states and in different countries; additional information on screening tests is available online at: www.aap.org/policy.

[b] AR, autosomal recessive.

earlier during pregnancy. Ultrasonography is used to analyze the fetus directly at different stages of development. Preimplantation molecular diagnostic testing is now possible by isolating single cells from the 8- to 10-cell embryo. The polymerase chain reaction (PCR) is then used to test for selected single-gene disorders such as Tay-Sachs disease, cystic fibrosis, or sickle cell anemia. This testing strategy requires in vitro fertilization but has the advantage that affected embryos are not implanted.

It should be remembered that prenatal genetic testing focuses on chromosomal abnormalities (Chap. 66), along with specific genetic disorders for which there is increased risk of parental transmission. There is no guarantee that a child will be free of birth defects or other genetic disorders not included among the diagnostic tests.

The genetic counseling process should begin before prenatal testing and should include: (1) a description of the test, (2) the types of disorders that will be screened, (3) the limitations of the screening, (4) an exploration of what the parents will do with the information, and (5) an indication of when the results will be available. If a genetic disorder is identified, the full repertoire of genetic counseling skills is required (see below). The nature of the genetic disease needs to be reviewed with the parents, often on separate occasions. The counselor should also discuss the kinds of physical and emotional challenges that a genetic disease might pose for the affected individual and the family. Written information should be provided, if available. Ultimately, the parents must reach a decision to continue or terminate the pregnancy. If pregnancy is terminated, counseling should continue after the procedure. If pregnancy is continued, counseling should continue to address the medical needs of the affected fetus or child, as well as to help the family meet any challenges presented by the genetic disorder.

At the time of birth, all newborns undergo a complete physical examination to detect gross developmental abnormalities. Within 24 to 72 h of birth, blood samples from newborns are sent to a state-designated laboratory to screen for selected diseases, such as congenital hypothyroidism and a variety of inherited metabolic disorders (Table 68-1). This program represents a clear example of the benefits of selected genetic screening. The early diagnosis of phenylketonuria, for example, permits parents to introduce a phenylalanine-free diet before the development of severe neurologic sequelae (Chap. 352).

COMMON ADULT-ONSET GENETIC DISORDERS

MULTIFACTORIAL INHERITANCE   The risk for many adult-onset disorders reflects the additive effects of genetic factors at multiple loci that may function independently—or in combination—with other genes or environmental factors. Our understanding of the genetic basis of these disorders is incomplete, despite the clear recognition of genetic susceptibility. In type 2 diabetes mellitus, for example, the concordance rate in monozygotic twins ranges between 50 to 90%. Diabetes or impaired glucose tolerance occurs in 40% of siblings and in 30% of the offspring of an affected individual. Despite the fact that diabetes affects 5% of the population and exhibits a high degree of heritability, there are only a few examples of genetic mutations that might account for the familial nature of the disease (most of which are rare). They include certain mitochondrial DNA disorders (Chap. 67), mutations in a cascade of genes that control pancreatic islet cell development and function (*HNF4α, HNF1α, IPF1*), insulin receptor mutations, and others (Chap. 333). Obesity and other factors that contribute to insulin resistance also represent important risk factors for type 2 diabetes. Current models for the genetic basis of type 2 diabetes propose the involvement of more than a dozen genes: some genes influence pancreatic islet development or function; others likely modulate glucose-sensing; and an important group determine insulin sensitivity, either directly by affecting insulin signaling or indirectly by regulating body weight or composition. Superimposed on this ge-

netic background are environmental influences such as diet, exercise, pregnancy, and medications.

Identifying these susceptibility genes is a formidable task. Nonetheless, a reasonable goal for this type of disease is to identify genes that increase (or decrease) disease risk by a factor of two or more. For common diseases such as diabetes or heart disease, this level of risk has important implications for health. Much the same way that cholesterol is currently used as a biochemical marker of cardiovascular risk, we can anticipate the development of genetic panels with similar predictive power. Genetic tests for a large number of genetic disorders are now available; a web site (www.genetests.org) lists various laboratories that perform specific tests. The advent of DNA-sequencing chips represents an important technical advance that promises to make large-scale testing more feasible (Chap. 65). The decision whether or not to perform a genetic test for a particular inherited adult-onset disorder, such as hemochromatosis, multiple endocrine neoplasia (MEN) type 1, prolonged QT syndrome, or Huntington disease, is complex; it depends on the clinical features of the disorder, the desires of the patient and family, and whether the results of genetic testing will alter medical decision-making or treatment (see below).

THE FAMILY HISTORY   Pending additional advances in genetic testing, the key to determining the inherited risk for common adult-onset diseases still rests in the collection and interpretation of a detailed personal and family medical history in conjunction with a directed physical examination. For example, a history of multiple family members with early-onset coronary artery diseases, glucose intolerance, and hypertension should suggest increased risk for genetic, and perhaps environmental, predisposition to insulin resistance (Chap. 333). Individual patients with this family history should be monitored for the possible development of hypertension, diabetes, and hyperlipidemia. They should be counseled about the importance of avoiding additional risk factors such as obesity and cigarette smoking.

Family history, recorded in the form of a pedigree, greatly assists the assessment of risk in the individual patient. At a minimum, pedigrees should convey health-related data on all first-degree relatives and selected second-degree relatives, including grandparents. When pedigrees appear to suggest an inherited disease, they should be extended to include additional family members. The determination of risk for an asymptomatic individual will vary depending on the size of the pedigree, the number of unaffected relatives, and the types of diagnoses within the family. For example, a woman with two first-degree relatives with breast cancer is more at risk if she has a total of three female first-degree relatives than if she has a total of eight female first-degree relatives. Additional variables that factor into the assessment of risk—and should be documented in the pedigree—include the age at diagnosis of each affected family member, present age of all family members, and the presence or absence of nonhereditary risk factors among those affected with diseases.

When assessing the personal and family history, the physician should be alert to a younger age of disease onset than is usually seen in the general population. A 30-year-old with acute myocardial infarction should be considered at risk for a hereditary trait, even if there is no family history of premature coronary artery disease (Chap. 241). The absence of the nonhereditary risk factors typically associated with a disease also raises the prospect of genetic risk factors. A personal or family history of deep vein thrombosis, in the absence of known nongenetic risk factors, might suggest a hereditary thrombotic disorder (Chap. 117). The physical examination may also provide important clues concerning the risk for a specific inherited disorder. A patient with xanthomas at a young age should prompt consideration of familial hypercholesterolemia. Some adult-onset disease-causing mutations are more prevalent in certain ethnic groups. For instance, >2% of the Ashkenazi population carry one of three specific mutations in the *BRCA1* or *BRCA2* genes. The prevalence of the factor V Leiden allele ranges from 3 to 7% in Caucasians but is much less common in Africans or Asians.

Recall of family history is often inaccurate. This is especially so when the history is remote and as families become more dispersed. It can be helpful to ask patients to fill out family history forms before or after their visits, as this provides them with an opportunity to contact relatives. Attempts should be made to confirm the illnesses reported in the family history before making management decisions. This process is often labor-intensive and ideally involves interviews of additional family members or reviewing medical records, autopsy reports, and death certificates.

Nongenetic factors associated with disease risk should also be reviewed in full, including occupation, diet, living conditions, and social habits. For example, patients at hereditary risk for heart disease should be questioned about tobacco use, diet, exercise, and lipid levels. Patients should also be asked about their health screening and prevention behaviors. These nonhereditary factors contribute to the assessment of overall risk and represent an important focus for disease prevention.

Although many inherited disorders will be suggested by the clustering of relatives with the same or related conditions, it is important to note that *disease penetrance* is incomplete for most multifactorial genetic disorders. As a result, the pedigree obtained in such families may not exhibit a clear Mendelian pattern of inheritance, as not all family members carrying the disease-associated alleles will manifest disease. Furthermore, genes associated with some of these disorders often exhibit *variable expression* of disease. For example, the breast cancer–associated gene, *BRCA1*, can predispose to several different malignancies in the same family, including cancers of the breast, ovary, and prostate (Chap. 81). For common diseases such as breast cancer, some family members without the disease-causing mutation may also develop breast cancer, representing another confounding variable in the pedigree analysis.

Some of the aforementioned features of the family history are illustrated in Fig. 68-1. The proband, a 36-year-old woman, has a strong history of breast and ovarian cancer on the paternal side of her family. The early age of onset, as well as the co-occurrence of breast and ovarian cancer in this family, suggests the possibility of an inherited mutation in *BRCA1* or *BRCA2*. It is unclear though—without genetic testing—whether her father inherited such a mutation and transmitted it to her. After appropriate genetic counseling of the proband and her family, one approach to DNA analysis in this family is to test the potentially affected 42-year-old living cousin (IV-4) for the presence of a *BRCA1* or *BRCA2* mutation. If a mutation is found, then it is possible to test for this particular alteration in the proband and other family members, if they so desire. In the example shown, if the pro-

band's father has inherited the *BRCA1* mutation, there is a 50:50 probability that the mutation has been transmitted to her. Genetic testing can be used to establish the absence or presence of this particular risk factor.

GENETIC TESTING FOR ADULT-ONSET DISORDERS

A critical first step before initiating genetic testing is to assure that the correct clinical diagnosis has been made, whether based on family history, characteristic physical findings, or biochemical testing. Careful clinical assessment will prevent unnecessary testing and will direct testing towards the most probable candidate genes. Many disorders exhibit the feature of *locus heterogeneity*, which refers to the fact that mutations in different genes can cause phenotypically similar disorders. For example, osteogenesis imperfecta (Chap. 351), muscular dystrophy (Chap. 383), homocystinuria (Chap. 352), and hereditary predisposition to colon cancer (Chap. 90) or breast cancer (Chap. 89) can each be caused by mutations in distinct genes. The pattern of disease transmission, clinical course, and treatment may differ significantly, depending on which gene is affected. In these cases, the choice of which genes to test is often determined by unique clinical features, the relative prevalence of mutations in various genes, or test availability.

Like all laboratory tests, there are limitations to the accuracy and interpretation of genetic tests. In addition to technical errors, genetic tests are often designed to detect only the most common mutations. In this case, a negative result must be qualified by the possibility that the individual may have a mutation that is not included in the test.

In addition to molecular testing for established disease, presymptomatic testing for susceptibility to chronic disease is being increasingly integrated into the practice of medicine. In most cases, however, the discovery of disease-associated genes has greatly outpaced studies that assess clinical outcomes and the impact of interventions. Until such outcomes-based studies are available, predictive molecular testing must be approached with caution and should be offered only to patients who have been adequately counseled and have provided informed consent (Fig. 68-2). In the majority of cases, presymptomatic testing should be offered only to individuals with a suggestive personal or family medical history or in the context of a clinical trial.

Molecular analysis is generally more informative if testing is initiated in a symptomatic family member, since the identification of a mutation can direct the testing of other at-risk family members (whether they are symptomatic or not). In the absence of additional familial or environmental risk factors, individuals who test negative for the mutation found in the affected family member can be informed that they are at general population risk for that particular disease. Furthermore, they can be reassured that they are not at risk for passing on the mutation to their children. On the other hand, asymptomatic family members who test positive for the known mutation must be informed that they are at increased risk for disease development and for transmitting the mutation to their children. Nevertheless, for most multifactorial genetic disorders, the test results cannot predict with confidence whether, or when, the disease will develop. For example, not everyone with the apolipoprotein E allele (ε4) will develop Alzheimer disease, and many individuals without this susceptibility gene can still develop the disorder (Chap. 362).

A negative test result is interpreted differently when no genetic mutation is found in a symptomatic family member. In this difficult circumstance, the test performed on a given gene may not detect all mutations in that gene (false negative) or the individual may have a mutation in a different disease-associated gene that was not tested.

Clinicians providing pretest counseling and education should assess the patient's emotional ability to cope with test results. Individuals who demonstrate signs and symptoms of psychiatric illness should have their emotional needs addressed before proceeding with molecular testing. Generally, genetic testing should not be offered at a time

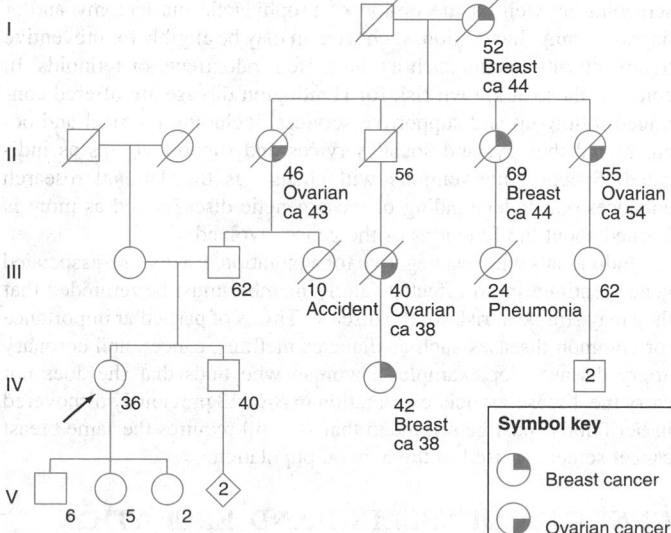

FIGURE 68-1 A 36-year-old woman (*arrow*) seeks consultation because of her family history of cancer. The patient expresses concern that the multiple cancers in her relatives imply an inherited predisposition to develop cancer. The family history is recorded and records of the patient's relatives confirm the reported diagnoses.

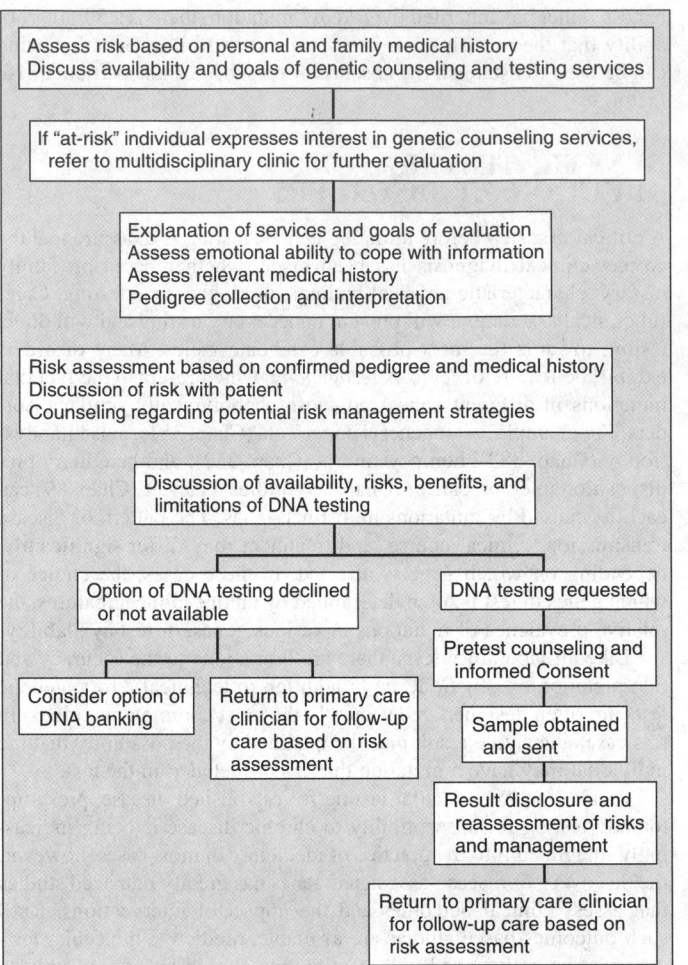

FIGURE 68-2 Algorithm for genetic counseling and testing.

should be offered in childhood for disorders that may be manifest early in life, especially when management options are available. For example, children at risk for familial adenomatous polyposis (FAP) may develop polyps as early as their teens, and progression to an invasive cancer can occur by their twenties. Likewise, children at risk for MEN type 2, which is caused by mutations in the *RET* proto-oncogene, may develop medullary thyroid cancer as early as 6 years of age, and the issue of prophylactic thyroidectomy should be addressed with the parents of children with documented mutations (Chap. 339).

INFORMED CONSENT When the issue of testing is addressed, patients should be strongly encouraged to involve other relatives in the decision-making process, as molecular diagnostics will likely have an impact on the entire family. Informed consent for molecular testing begins with detailed education and counseling. The patient must fully understand the risks, benefits, and limitations of undergoing the analysis. Informed consent should be in the form of a written document, drafted clearly and concisely in a language and format that is comprehensible to the patient, who should be made aware of the disposition of test results. Informed consent should also include a discussion of the mechanics of testing. Most molecular testing for hereditary disease involves DNA-based analysis of peripheral blood. In the majority of circumstances, test results should be given only to the individual, in person, and with a support person in the room.

Because molecular testing of an asymptomatic individual often allows prediction of future risk, the patient should understand any potential long-term medical, psychological, and social implications of this decision. In the United States, legislation affecting this area is still evolving, and it is important to explore with the patient the potential impact that test results may have on employment, future health, and life insurance coverage.

Patients should understand that alternatives to molecular analysis remain available if they decide not to proceed with this option. They should also be notified that testing is available in the future if they are not prepared to undergo analysis immediately. The option of DNA banking should be presented so that samples are readily available for future use by family members, if needed.

FOLLOW-UP CARE AFTER TESTING Depending on the nature of the genetic disorder, posttest interventions may include (1) cautious surveillance and appropriate health care screening, (2) specific medical interventions, (3) chemoprevention, (4) risk avoidance, and (5) referral to support services. For example, patients with known pathologic mutations in *BRCA1* or *BRCA2* are offered intensive screening as well as the option of prophylactic mastectomy and/or oophorectomy. In addition, such women may be eligible for preventive treatment with agents such as tamoxifen, raloxifene, or retinoids. In contrast, those at known risk for Huntington disease are offered continued follow-up and supportive services, including physical and occupational therapy, and social services and support groups as indicated. Specific interventions will change as translational research enhances our understanding of these genetic diseases and as more is learned about the functions of the genes involved.

Individuals who test negative for a mutation in a disease-associated gene identified in an affected family member must be reminded that they may still be at risk for the disease. This is of particular importance for common diseases such as diabetes mellitus, cancer, and coronary artery disease. For example, a woman who finds that she does not carry the disease-associated mutation in *BRCA2* previously discovered in her family must be reminded that she still requires the same breast cancer screening used in the general population.

of personal crisis or acute illness within the family. Patients will derive more benefit from test results if they are emotionally able to comprehend and absorb the information. It is important to assess patients' preconceived notions of their personal likelihood of disease in preparing pretest educational strategies. Often, patients harbor unwarranted fear or denial of their likelihood of genetic risk.

Genetic testing has the potential of affecting the way individual family members relate to one another, both negatively and positively. As a result, patients addressing the option of molecular testing must consider how test results might impact their relationships with relatives, spouses, and friends. In families with a known genetic mutation, those who test positive must address the impact of the disease on their present and future lifestyles; those who test negative may manifest survivor guilt. Family members are likely to differ in their emotional and social responses to the same information. Counseling should also address the potential consequences of test results on relationships with a spouse or child. Parents who are found to have a disease-associated mutation often express considerable anxiety and despair as they address the issue of risk to their children.

When a condition does not manifest until adulthood, clinicians will be faced with the question of whether at-risk children should be offered molecular testing and, if so, at what age. Several professional organizations have cautioned that genetic testing for adult-onset disorders should not be offered to children. Many of these conditions are not preventable and, consequently, such information can pose significant psychosocial risk. In addition, there is concern that testing during childhood violates a child's right to make an informed decision regarding testing upon reaching adulthood. On the other hand, testing

GENETIC COUNSELING AND EDUCATION

Genetic counseling should be distinguished from genetic testing and screening, even though genetic counselors are often involved in issues related to testing. Genetic counseling refers to *a communication process that deals with human problems associated with the occurrence or risk of a genetic disorder in a family.* Genetic risk assessment can be complex and often involves elements of uncertainty. Counseling therefore includes genetic education as well as psychosocial counseling. Genetic counselors may be called upon by other health care professionals (or by individual patients and families) to address a broad range of issues directly and indirectly involved with genetic disease (Table 68-2). The genetic counselor will do the following:

- Gather and document a detailed family history
- Educate the patient about general genetic principles related to disease risk, both for themselves and others in the family
- Assess and enhance the patient's ability to cope with the genetic information offered
- Discuss how nongenetic factors may relate to the ultimate expression of disease
- Address medical management issues
- Assist in determining the role of genetic testing for the individual and family
- Ensure that the patient is aware of the risks, benefits, and limitations of the various genetic testing options
- Refer the patient and other at-risk family members for additional medical and support services, if necessary.

The complexity of genetic counseling and the broad scope of genetic diseases are leading to the development of specialized, multidisciplinary clinics designed to provide broad-based support and medical care for those at risk and their family members. Such multidisciplinary teams are often composed of medical geneticists, specialist physicians, genetic counselors, nurses, psychologists, social workers, and biomedical ethicists who work together to consider difficult diagnostic, treatment, and testing decisions. Such a format also provides primary care physicians with invaluable support and assistance as they follow and treat at-risk patients.

The approach to genetic counseling has important ethical, social, and financial implications. Philosophies related to genetic counseling vary widely by country and center. In North American centers, for example, counseling is generally offered in a nondirective manner, wherein patients learn to understand how their values factor into a particular medical decision. Nondirective counseling is particularly appropriate when there are no data demonstrating a clear benefit associated with a particular intervention or when an intervention is considered experimental. For example, nondirective genetic counseling is employed when a person is deciding whether or not to undergo genetic testing for Huntington disease (Chap. 362). At this time, there is no clear benefit (in terms of medical outcome) to an at-risk individual undergoing genetic testing for this disease, as its course cannot be altered by therapeutic interventions. However, testing can have an important impact on such a person's perception of the future and his or her interpersonal relationships and plans for reproduction. Therefore, the decision to pursue testing rests on the individual's belief system and values. On the other hand, a more directive approach is appropriate when a condition can be treated. In a family with FAP (associated with mutations in the *APC* gene), colon cancer screening and prophylactic colectomy should be recommended for known *APC* mutation carriers. The counselor and clinician following this family must ensure that the at-risk individuals have access to the resources necessary to adhere to these recommendations.

Genetic education is central to an individual's ability to make an informed decision regarding testing options and treatment. Although genetic counselors represent one source of genetic education, other health care providers also need to contribute to patient education. Pa-

Table 68-2 Indications for Genetic Counseling

Advanced maternal (>35) or paternal (>50) age
Consanguinity
Previous history of a child with birth defects or a genetic disorder
Personal or family history suggestive of a genetic disorder
High-risk ethnic groups; known carriers of genetic mutations
Ultrasound or prenatal testing suggesting a genetic disorder

tients at risk for genetic disease should understand fundamental medical genetic principles and terminology relevant to their situation. This includes the concept of genes, how they are transmitted, and how they confer hereditary disease risk. An adequate knowledge of patterns of inheritance will allow patients to understand the probability of disease risk for themselves and other family members. It is also important to impart the concepts of disease penetrance and expression. For complex genetic disorders, asymptomatic patients should be advised that a positive test result does not always translate into future disease development. In addition, the role of nongenetic factors, such as environmental exposures, must be discussed in the context of multifactorial disease risk and disease prevention. Finally, patients should understand the natural history of the disease as well as the potential options for intervention, including screening, prevention, and—in certain circumstances—pharmacologic treatment or prophylactic surgery.

THERAPEUTIC INTERVENTIONS BASED ON GENETIC SUSCEPTIBILITY TO DISEASE

Specific treatments are now available for an increasing number of genetic disorders, whether identified through population-based screening or directed testing (Table 68-3). A number of metabolic disorders fall into this group. For example, the complications of phenylketonuria can be mitigated by recognizing the disease early and avoiding foods that contain phenylalanine (Chap. 352). Similar principles apply to maple syrup urine disease (Chap. 352) and galactosemia (Chap. 350). Children with 21-hydroxylase deficiency present with adrenal insufficiency, usually within the first few weeks of life (Chap. 331). Because of the block in cortisol synthesis, the adrenal steroid precursors are shunted into the androgen pathway, causing ambiguous genitalia in females and premature virilization in males. In this disorder, treatment with glucocorticoid and mineralocorticoid not only corrects the hormone deficits but is also required to suppress ACTH overproduction, which otherwise worsens virilization.

Although the strategies for therapeutic interventions are best developed for childhood genetic diseases, these principles are gradually making their way into the diagnosis and management of adult-onset disorders. Hereditary hemochromatosis illustrates many of the issues raised by the potential availability of genetic screening in the adult population. For instance, it is relatively common (approximately 1 in 200 individuals of northern European descent are homozygous), and its complications are potentially preventable through phlebotomy (Chap. 345). The recent identification of the *HFE* gene, mutations of which are associated with this syndrome, has sparked interest in the use of DNA-based testing for presymptomatic diagnosis of the disorder. However, up to one-third of individuals who are homozygous for the *HFE* mutation do not have evidence of iron overload. Consequently, in the absence of a positive family history, current recommendations are phenotypic screening for evidence of iron overload followed by genetic testing. Whether genetic screening for hemochromatosis will someday be coupled to assessment of phenotypic expression awaits further studies. In contrast to the issue of population screening, it is important to test and counsel other family members when the diagnosis of hemochromatosis has been made in a proband. Testing allows the physician to exclude family members who are not at risk. It also permits presymptomatic detection of iron overload and the institution of treatment (phlebotomy) before the development of organ damage.

Preventive measures and therapeutic interventions are not restricted to metabolic disorders. Identification of familial forms of long QT syndrome, associated with ventricular arrythmias, allows early electrocardiographic testing and the use of prophylactic antiarrythmic therapy (Chap. 230). Individuals with familial hypertrophic cardiomyopathy can be screened by ultrasound, treated with beta blockers or other drugs, and counseled about the importance of avoiding strenuous exercise and dehydration (Chap. 238). Likewise, individuals with Marfan syndrome can be treated with beta blockers and monitored for

Table 68-3 Examples of Interventions Based on Genetic Testing*

Genetic Disorders	Interventions	Chapter
Phenylketonuria	Avoid dietary phenylalanine	352
Homocystinuria	Treatment with folic acid, pyridoxine, and vitamin B$_{12}$	352
Hemochromatosis	Phlebotomy	345
Wilson's disease	D-Penicillamine treatment	348
Galactosemia	Avoid dietary galactose	350
Porphyrias	Avoid precipitants	346
Glucose-6-phosphate dehydrogenase deficiency	Avoid oxidant drugs	108
21-Hydroxylase deficiency	Glucocorticoid and mineralocorticoid treatment	331
Familial Mediterranean fever	Colchicine treatment	289
Malignant hyperthermia	Avoid precipitating anesthetics	17
α_1 Antitrypsin deficiency	Avoid smoking; avoid occupational and environmental toxins	258
Hypertrophic cardiomyopathy	Echocardiographic screening; early pharmacologic intervention	238
Long QT syndrome	Electrocardiographic screening and electrophysiologic testing; early pharmacologic intervention	230
Marfan syndrome	Echocardiographic screening; prophylactic beta blockers	247, 351
Factor V Leiden	Avoid thrombogenic risk factors and oral contraceptives	117
Hemophilia A	Factor VIII replacement	117
Hemophilia B	Factor IX replacement; possible gene therapy	117
Familial hypocalciuric hypercalcemia	Avoid parathyroidectomy	341
Kallmann syndrome	Induce puberty with hormone replacement	328
Neurohypophyseal diabetes insipidus	Replace vasopressin	329
Maturity onset diabetes of the young	Screen and treat for diabetes	333
Hereditary nonpolyposis colon cancer	Early colonoscopy screening	90
Familial adenomatous polyposis	Nonsteroidal anti-inflammatory drugs; early colonoscopy screening; colectomy	90
Familial breast cancer	Consider estrogen receptor antagonists; early screening by exams and mammography; consider prophylactic mastectomy; consider risk for additional types of cancers	89
Basal cell nevus syndrome	Avoid UV light; screening and biopsies	86
Familial melanoma	Avoid UV light; screening and biopsies	86
Multiple endocrine neoplasia type 2	Prophylactic thyroidectomy; screen for pheochromocytoma and hyperparathyroidism	339

See the Web site www.genetests.org for a compendium of available genetic tests.

the development of aortic aneurysms (Chap. 247). Individuals with α_1 antitrypsin deficiency can be strongly counseled to avoid cigarette smoking and exposure to environmental pulmonary and hepatotoxins. Various host genes influence the pathogenesis of certain infectious diseases in humans, including HIV (Chap. 309). The factor V Leiden allele increases risk of thrombosis (Chap. 62). Approximately 3% of the worldwide population is heterozygous for this mutation. Moreover, it is found in up to 25% of patients with recurrent deep venous thrombosis or pulmonary embolism. Women who are heterozygous or ho-

mozygous for this allele should therefore avoid the use of oral contraceptives and receive heparin prophylaxis after surgery or trauma.

The field of pharmacogenetics seeks to identify genes that alter drug metabolism or confer susceptibility to toxic drug reactions (Chap. 71). Examples include succinylcholine sensitivity, malignant hyperthermia, the porphyrias, and glucose-6-phosphase dehydrogenase (G6PD) deficiency.

As noted above, the identification of genes that increase the risk of specific types of neoplasia is rapidly changing the management of many cancers. Identifying family members with mutations that predispose to FAP or hereditary nonpolyposis colon cancer (HNPCC) can lead to recommendations of early screening by colonoscopy or prophylactic surgery (Chap. 90). Similar principles apply to familial forms of melanoma, basal cell carcinoma, and breast cancer. It should be recognized, however, that most cancers harbor several distinct genetic abnormalities by the time they acquire invasive or metastatic potential (Chaps. 81 and 82). Consequently, the major impact of genetic testing in these cases is to allow more intensive clinical screening, as it remains very challenging to predict disease penetrance or the clinical course of these diseases.

Although genetic diagnosis of these and other disorders is only beginning to be used in the clinical setting, susceptibility testing holds the promise of allowing earlier and more targeted interventions that can reduce the morbidity and mortality associated with these disorders. We can expect the availability of genetic tests to expand rapidly. A critical challenge for physicians and other health care providers is to keep pace with these advances in genetic medicine and to implement testing judiciously. Meeting this goal will enhance patient care through adequate counseling, directed testing, and appropriate interventions, with the ultimate objective being the reduction of morbidity and mortality from genetic diseases.

BIBLIOGRAPHY

BIESECKER BB, MARTEAU TM: Future of genetic counselling: An international perspective. Nat Genet 22:133, 1999

COUGHLIN SS: The intersection of genetics, public health, and preventative medicine. Am J Prev Med 16:89, 1999

FRASER FC: Genetic counseling. Am J Hum Genet 26:636, 1974

GELEHRTER TD et al: *Principles of Medical Genetics*, 2d ed. Baltimore, Williams & Wilkins, 1998

HARPER PS: *Practical Genetic Counselling*, 5th ed. Oxford, Butterworth Heinmann, 1998

MCKINNON WC et al: Predisposition genetic testing for late-onset disorders in adults: Position paper of the National Society of Genetic Counselors. JAMA 278:1217, 1997

MEHLMAN MJ, KODISH ED et al: The need for anonymous genetic counseling and testing. Am J Hum Genetic 58:393, 1996

ROSENDAAL FR: Risk factors for venous thrombosis: Prevalence, risk and interaction. Semin Hematol 34:171, 1997

STEPHENSON J: "Talking" genetics glossary (www.nhgri.nih.gov/DIR/VIP/Glossary/). JAMA 281: 600, 1999

THE AMERICAN SOCIETY OF HUMAN GENETICS: Report from the ASHG Information and Education Committee: Medical school core curriculum in genetics. Am J Hum Genet 56:535, 1995

———, THE AMERICAN COLLEGE OF MEDICAL GENETICS: Points to consider: Ethical, legal and psychosocial implications of genetic testing in children and adolescents. Am J Hum Genet 57:1233, 1995

69 *Mark A. Kay, David W. Russell*

GENE THERAPY

AAV	adeno-associated viruses	LTRs	long terminal repeats
ADA	adenosine deaminase	MLVs	murine leukemia viruses
CNS	central nervous system	RP	retinitis pigmentosa
CSF	colony stimulating factor	TK	thymidine kinase
IFNs	interferons	VEGF	vascular endothelial growth
ILs	interleukins		factor
LDL	low-density lipoprotein		

Gene therapy is generally defined as *the delivery of nucleic acids to alter or prevent a pathologic process.* Although initially considered primarily in the context of inherited monogenic disorders, gene therapy is now recognized as a potential treatment strategy for a wide range of acquired disorders, such as cancer, neurodegenerative diseases, and infections. Gene therapy has been used in several hundred protocols. Despite early hopes that gene therapy might be quickly incorporated into medical practice, it has yielded limited success to date and remains an investigational treatment. The technical challenges associated with gene therapy are formidable, but with steady progress in vector development, definitive therapeutic milestones may soon be realized for selected disorders.

GENERAL APPROACHES TO GENE THERAPY

FORMS OF GENE THERAPY   Gene therapy can be used, in principle, to modify all cells in the body, including the germ line. *Germ-line gene therapy* would allow transmission of the modified genetic information to the next generation and is not currently accepted as an appropriate therapeutic approach. For ethical reasons, opposition to germ-line gene therapy is likely to continue in the foreseeable future. *Somatic gene therapy* refers to modification of the somatic, differentiated cells of the body. It is used in an effort to correct inherited diseases such as cystic fibrosis and acquired disorders such as rheumatoid arthritis or malignancies.

Whole-organ transplantation (e.g., bone marrow, liver, and kidney) has been used for years as a strategy to replace the function of defective genes. The idea of using nonautologous cell transplantation has been revisited in the past few years, and with the advent of human embryonic stem cells, similar transplantation strategies are being considered for a variety of disorders once considered prime targets for gene therapy. Thus, the interface between gene therapy and *cell transplantation* is complementary.

The production of *genetically engineered proteins* is another area closely aligned with gene therapy. The cloning of human genes allows proteins to be produced in unlimited quantities and free of the potential contaminants associated with their purification from natural sources such as plasma. Moreover, recombinant DNA technology allows these proteins to be modified in ways that can enhance their therapeutic benefit. Examples of recombinant proteins are listed in Table 69-1. These include: (1) hormones such as insulin, growth hormone, and gonadotropins; (2) factors used to enhance blood cell production including erythropoietin, granulocyte colony stimulating factor (CSF), granulocyte-macrophage CSF, and thrombopoietin; (3) interferons (IFNs) and interleukins (ILs) used to treat a variety of autoimmune, infectious, and neoplastic diseases; (4) clotting factors VIII and IX; (5) thrombolytic agents such as tissue plasminogen activator or the antithrombotic agent hirudin; (6) recombinant antigens used for hepatitis B vaccines; and (7) humanized monoclonal antibodies used for immunosuppression or to treat specific types of malignancy. Although these recombinant proteins are an indirect form of gene therapy, they represent an important outgrowth of genetic medicine.

Long-Term versus Transient Gene Delivery Strategies for Gene Therapy   The goals of gene therapy vary depending on the nature of the disease being treated. For an inherited, monogenic disorder such as hemophilia, the goal is lifelong replacement of the missing gene product. Expression of the missing secreted clotting factor, even at modest levels, might ameliorate the disease or reduce the need for exogenous treatment. For other inherited disorders, such as sickle cell anemia, strategies for gene replacement are more demanding. In this case, there is a requirement for cell-specific and exquisitely regulated expression of the transferred gene, and one is still faced with endogenous expression of the mutant form of β-globin. Long-term gene delivery strategies typically involve direct modification of host chromosomal sequences, which allows normal inheritance and stability of the delivered gene.

A growing use of gene therapy involves transient gene expression

Table 69-1   Examples of Genetically Engineered Recombinant Proteins

Recombinant Proteins	Clinical Applications[a]
Hormones/growth factors	
Growth hormone	Growth hormone deficiency
Insulin-like growth factor 1	Growth disorders resistant to growth hormone
Insulin	Diabetes mellitus
Follicle-stimulating hormone	Ovulation induction
Luteinizing hormone	Ovulation induction
Thyroid-stimulating hormone	^{131}I scanning in thyroid cancer
Leptin	Obesity
Platelet-derived growth factor	Wound healing in diabetic ulcers
Blood cell stimulatory factors	
Erythropoietin	Anemia
Granulocyte CSF	Neutropenia
Granulocyte-macrophage CSF	Neutropenia
Thrombopoietin	Thrombocytopenia
Interleukin (IL) 11	Thrombocytopenia
Cytokines	
Interferon α-2a	Hepatitis C
Interferon β-1a	Multiple sclerosis
Interferon α-2b	Follicular lymphoma
IL-2	Renal cell carcinoma
IL-2 α receptor	Immunosuppression in renal transplantation
Soluble tumor necrosis factor α receptor	Rheumatoid arthritis
Clotting factors/anticoagulants	
Factor VIII	Hemophilia A
Factor IX	Hemophilia B
Tissue-plasminogen activator	Myocardial infarction, stroke, pulmonary embolus
Hirudin	Deep vein thrombosis
Enzymes	
Adenosine deaminase	Severe combined immune deficiency (SCID)
Glucocerebrosidase	Gaucher disease
Monoclonal antibodies	
Epidermal growth factor receptor	Breast cancer
IL-2α	Immunosuppression in renal transplantation
Tumor necrosis factor	Crohn's disease
GPIIb/IIIa receptor	Prevent platelet aggregation after angioplasty
CD20	Follicular lymphoma
Vaccines	
Hepatitis B antigen vaccine	Hepatitis B

[a] The efficacy and approval of some of these agents remain under investigation.
NOTE: CSF, colony stimulating factor.

to treat a variety of diseases (Table 69-2). Gene therapy is now being considered or used for (1) killing cancer cells; (2) providing chemoprotection to normal cells; (3) preventing coronary restenosis or enhancing vascularization; (4) providing DNA-based immunization (e.g., viral DNA), in which the injection of DNA results in antigen expression and generation of an immune response; and (5) impairing viral replication. In cancer therapy, for example, the requirements for long-term gene expression and the level of gene expression are not as stringent as for gene replacement. Rather, the challenge of many cancer-based gene therapies is to achieve highly efficient gene transfer into cancer cells without expression in surrounding normal cells.

EX VIVO VERSUS IN VIVO ADMINISTRATION OF GENE THERAPY   Gene therapy has been administered ex vivo for conditions in which cells can be readily harvested, manipulated in tissue culture, and then reintroduced into the patient. The ex vivo approach is potentially applicable to a variety of hematologic or immune deficiency disorders. For example, in adenosine deaminase (ADA) deficiency, the missing ADA gene has been integrated into the patient's T lymphocytes, which are then reintroduced after genetic manipulation. In familial hypercholesterolemia, an analogous approach has been

Table 69-2 Examples of Disorders Potentially Amenable to Gene Therapy

Disease	Gene Therapy Strategy
Inherited disorders	Gene addition
Cystic fibrosis	Express CFTR in pulmonary system and/or GI tract
Familial hypercholesterolemia	Express low-density lipoprotein receptor in liver
Hemophilias A and B	Express factor VIII or IX and secrete in circulation
Thalassemia	Express normal globin in red blood cells
Immunodeficiencies	Express mutant genes, such as adenosine deaminase
Metabolic disorders	Express missing enzymes or transporters
Duchenne's muscular dystrophy	Express mutant dystrophin protein in muscle cells
Retinitis pigmentosa (recessive)	Express normal protein in retina
	Gene correction
Lesch-Nyhan	Modify hypoxanthine phosphoribosyl transferase locus
Retinitis pigmentosa (dominant)	Correct missense mutation
Sickle cell disease	Correct β-globin mutation
Cystic fibrosis	Correct ΔF508 mutation in pulmonary system
Cardiovascular diseases	Modify vascular biology
Coronary artery restenosis	Block cell proliferation in vessel wall
Peripheral vascular disease	Induce angiogenesis
Hypertension	Express genes (e.g., tissue kallikrein) to induce vasodilation
Cancer	Multiples approaches
Many types	Express immunostimulants in or near malignant cells
	Express toxic genes in tumor cells (e.g., herpes simplex virus–TK)
	Express genes in normal cells to protect from chemotherapy
Infectious diseases	
Viral diseases	Express genes that block viral replication or function, including ribozymes, decoys, dominant negative proteins
Many	Express antigens as recombinant vaccines
Miscellaneous	
Rheumatoid arthritis	Express anti-inflammatory cytokines in joints
Parkinson's disease	Express genes required for L-dopa synthesis in striatum
Neurodegenerative disease	Express neurotrophic factors

NOTE: CFTR, cystic fibrous transmembrane regulator.

used for ex vivo treatment of hepatocytes. After surgical resection of liver tissue, the low-density lipoprotein (LDL) receptor gene is inserted into hepatocytes in cell culture, and the modified cells are infused back through the portal vein. Another form of ex vivo gene therapy involves the treatment of saphenous veins with oligonucleotides designed to block vascular smooth-muscle cell proliferation before using the tissue for coronary artery bypass graft.

In vivo approaches to gene therapy vary depending on the nature of the disease. In cystic fibrosis, an aerosol has been used to administer viral vectors to the lung. Factor IX expression has been achieved by introduction of the gene into muscle. Tumors have been injected directly with viral vectors expressing cytotoxic genes or immunotherapies. A major advantage of in vivo approaches is the potential to target cells that cannot easily be removed from the patient.

GENE TRANSFER VECTORS

A vector, or vehicle, is required to transfer a gene to an appropriate cell. When the goal is to add a gene (often called a *transgene*) to supply a function not present in the recipient cell, the vector typically contains DNA sequences encoding a therapeutic protein under the control of transcriptional regulatory elements necessary for gene expression (Fig. 69-1). The gene is expressed from an ectopic location as opposed to its normal chromosomal position. An alternative strategy is to correct mutant genes at their normal chromosomal location through *gene targeting*. Although this represents an ideal approach for many genetic diseases, it is far more technically demanding, and therapeutic gene-targeting efficiencies are difficult to achieve currently.

Two major classes of vectors are used for transferring nucleic acids into cells for the purposes of gene therapy: viral and nonviral vectors. *Viral vectors* have been genetically engineered so that the viruses transfer exogenous (therapeutic) nucleic acids into cells through a process called transduction. *Nonviral vectors* consist of nucleic acids that

are typically complexed with other chemicals to facilitate gene transfer. Although nonviral vectors offer improved safety by avoiding viral components, their gene transfer efficiencies are generally much lower than those of viral vectors. The major vector systems currently used in clinical trials or under development are summarized in Table 69-3.

Vectors that integrate into host chromosomes are considered ideal for lifelong gene expression, whereas episomal (unintegrated) vectors are preferred for transient gene delivery. The host range of a particular vector, in combination with the mode of delivery, will determine which cell types can be genetically modified. Also, it may be possible to alter the natural tropism of viral capsids or envelopes, as well as of nonviral vector complexes, to limit transduction to particular cell types. Transcriptional control elements, such as promoters and enhancers, can be used to regulate expression of the transgene. In some cases, the inclusion of special regulatory elements may allow gene expression to be controlled by the administration of pharmacologic agents that specifically switch the regulatory elements on or off. Many types of vectors, each exhibiting a unique set of properties, will ultimately be needed for safe and effective gene therapy of different diseases.

RETROVIRAL VECTORS Retroviral vectors based on murine leukemia viruses (MLVs) were the first vectors used in clinical gene transfer protocols and illustrate many of the principles of viral-mediated gene therapy. Typically, the vector genome consists of a transgene cassette placed between the two *cis*-acting long terminal repeats (LTRs) of the viral genome. Viral coding regions are removed from the vector genome to allow the insertion of the therapeutic gene and to prevent viral replication and toxicity to the host. The packaging capacity of MLV vectors is approximately 8 kb (including the LTRs), enough to accommodate most therapeutic cDNAs. The viral gene products needed for vector production and packaging are supplied by helper virus expression constructs.

The envelope protein of the virus interacts with specific cellular receptors to allow cellular entry of the core proteins and vector genome. After transduction, the vector gene integrates at random locations in host chromosomes and replicates with the host chromosome during cell proliferation, offering the potential for lifelong transgene expression. *Chromosomal integration* may also cause insertional mutagenesis, but no clinically relevant consequences of such events have been observed to date with replication-incompetent retroviral vectors.

Although MLV vectors are widely used, primarily because of their ability to integrate and simple production requirements, they still have significant disadvantages. Complement-mediated vector particle inactivation has largely limited their use to ex vivo applications. MLV vectors also require cell division for transduction because the vector genome can only enter the cell nucleus during mitosis, when the nuclear membrane breaks down. Since the majority of cells present in the human body are nondividing, this severely limits the potential uses of MLV-based vectors.

Promising new retroviral vectors are based on complex retroviruses (rather than the relatively simple oncoviruses such as MLV). Both lentiviral vectors and spumaviral vectors have broad host ranges, improved transduction of nondividing cells, and may function well in vivo. Although lentiviral vector production systems can be designed to eliminate the potential for replication-competent retrovirus contamination, and these vectors appear safe from a virologic standpoint, the

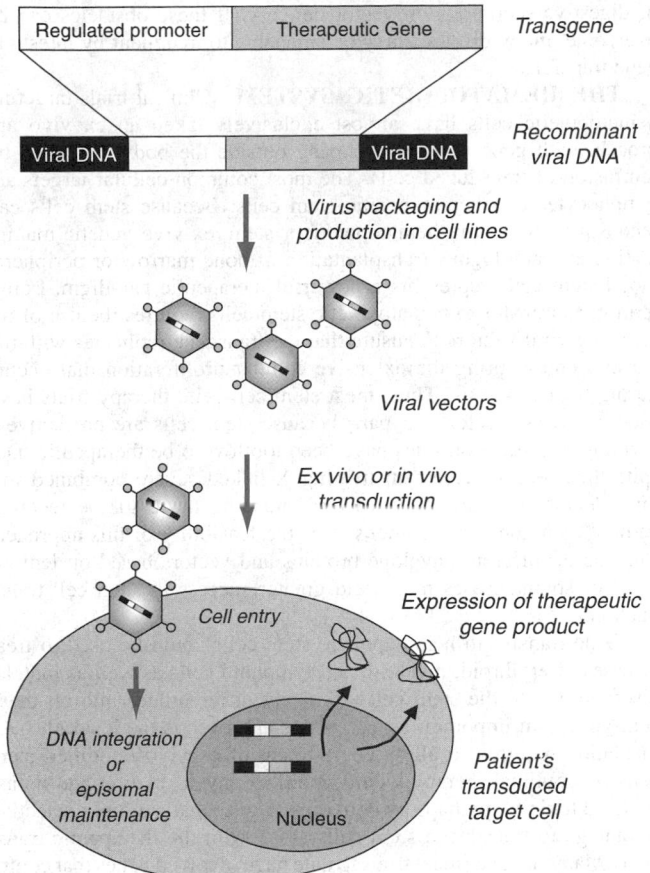

Regulated promoter | Therapeutic Gene — *Transgene*

Viral DNA | Viral DNA — *Recombinant viral DNA*

Virus packaging and production in cell lines

Viral vectors

Ex vivo or in vivo transduction

Cell entry

Expression of therapeutic gene product

DNA integration or episomal maintenance

Nucleus

Patient's transduced target cell

FIGURE 69-1 General design of viral vectors used for gene therapy.

stigma associated with vectors based on human pathogens such as HIV may limit their acceptance.

ADENOVIRAL VECTORS Adenoviral-mediated gene expression is not lifelong, making it well suited for applications that require transient gene expression. In contrast to retroviruses, which integrate into the host genome, the adenoviral vector genome remains *episomal*, or extrachromosomal. Adenoviral vectors typically are derived from serotypes 2 or 5 and contain double-stranded DNA genomes. Wild-type adenovirus encodes over 50 peptides on overlapping gene fragments from both DNA strands. Nonessential viral genes have been removed to make room for up to 8 kb of exogenous DNA. The vector containing the therapeutic transgene is amplified in a cell line that supplies viral proteins needed for replication and packaging. Recombinant adenoviruses can be generated at high titers in the range of 10^{13} to 10^{14} particles per milliliter, a feature that is important for efficient in vivo gene therapy.

In clinical practice, adenoviral vectors are limited by relatively short durations of expression (usually several weeks) and by the synthesis of remaining cytotoxic or antigenic viral proteins that can cause an acute inflammatory response and/or a robust cellular immune response. These features of the virus ap-

pear to have contributed to hepatic failure and death in an individual receiving adenoviral-based gene therapy for ornithine transcarbamylase deficiency. On the other hand, the inflammatory properties of adenoviruses may enhance their efficacy in cancer trials, as discussed below. Several methods that eliminate the remaining viral genes have been devised recently, and these "gutted" vectors appear to exhibit much reduced toxicity and inflammatory properties in comparison to previous generations of adenoviral vectors.

ADENO-ASSOCIATED VIRUS VECTORS Adeno-associated viruses (AAV) are parvoviruses that normally require a helper virus, such as adenovirus, to mediate a productive infection. A major limitation of the AAV vector is its relatively small packaging capacity, which restricts the size of exogenous DNA to about 4.5 kb. AAV vectors have been shown to transduce cells both through episomal transgene expression and by chromosomal integration. They can also be used to modify homologous chromosomal sequences through gene targeting, which is an important strategy for the correction of genetic mutations.

Since the AAV vector genome lacks viral coding sequences, the vector itself causes little immune or inflammatory response (except for the generation of neutralizing antibodies that may limit readministration). The vector particle can be delivered to many different organs [e.g., the central nervous system (CNS), liver, lung, and muscle] by in vivo administration, and AAV vectors have been found to transduce nondividing cells efficiently. Clinical trials using AAV for the treatment of cystic fibrosis and hemophilia are underway.

OTHER VIRAL VECTORS Many other viruses are under development as vector systems, such as herpesviruses, double-stranded RNA viruses, autonomous parvoviruses, and papovaviruses. Hybrid viral vectors that use components from more than one virus are also under development, offering the potential to combine the most desirable properties of different vectors. Ultimately, vectors will be developed that utilize both viral components and synthetic functions, allowing vectors to be custom designed.

NONVIRAL VECTORS Nonviral vectors usually consist of DNA complexes with lipids, carbohydrates, proteins, and/or other synthetic chemicals to facilitate delivery or increase vector stability. Gene delivery with naked DNA is also possible but is relatively inefficient.

Table 69-3 Properties of Vectors Used for Gene Therapy

Vector	Production	Cell Cycle Effects	Expression	Gene Status	Toxicity
Retrovirus (MLV-based)	Simple but low titers ~10^6 particles/mL	Mitosis required	Persistent	Integrated	Safe
Lentivirus	Can be concentrated to ~10^9 particles/mL	Cell division not always required	Persistent	Integrated	Untested
Adenovirus	Easily produced at titers up to 10^{13}–10^{14} particles/mL	Quiescent or dividing cells	Transient	Episomal	Initial vectors toxic; gutted vectors much improved
AAV	Difficult process, but high titers possible, ~10^{12} particles/mL	Quiescent or dividing cells, DNA synthesis sometimes beneficial	Persistent or transient	Integrated or episomal, often in concatamers	Safe
Nonviral	Highly concentrated	Quiescent or dividing cells	Transient	Episomal	Variable, based on type and dose

NOTE: MLV, murine leukemia virus; AAV, adeno-associated virus.

Nonviral vectors are desirable because they eliminate the risk of viral contamination and can be produced under more controlled conditions. Their major disadvantage is low gene transfer rates, at least in relation to most viral vector systems. Because the vectors do not integrate and the majority of DNA molecules that enter the cell are rapidly degraded, only transient gene expression is possible. Examples of applications that may be well suited to gene delivery with nonviral vectors include vaccination with specific antigen genes, ex vivo treatment of vessels used for coronary artery bypass graft, and perhaps transient immune modulation for the treatment of cancer.

Nonviral vectors composed of RNA or modified nucleotides may also prove useful, if problems associated with effective delivery can be addressed. For example, antisense oligonucleotides can be used to inhibit gene expression by pairing with complementary mRNA molecules. Antisense oligonucleotides might be used, for example, to block the expression of cell cycle proteins or cytokines. Oligonucleotides with binding sites for specific DNA- or RNA-binding proteins may be designed to function as decoys that inhibit protein function. Chimeric RNA/DNA oligonucleotides have been used to introduce specific genetic modifications through gene targeting. In animal studies, this novel approach has been shown to work efficiently in the liver, and it may be used soon for clinical trials of uridine diphosphate–glucuronosyltransferase deficiency.

GENE THERAPY FOR SELECTED DISEASE CATEGORIES

LIVER AND GASTROINTESTINAL TRACT The liver has been studied intensively as a target organ for gene therapy, in part because of the many genetic diseases amenable to gene replacement in hepatocytes. In addition, because of the regenerative capacity of the hepatocyte, integration of a vector offers the possibility of lifelong gene expression. The first hepatic gene therapy attempted in humans involved the ex vivo transplant of autologous hepatocytes transduced in culture by retroviral vectors encoding the LDL receptor as a treatment for familial hypercholesterolemia. Due to the low levels (nontherapeutic) of gene expression observed and the labor-intensive nature of the ex vivo transduction process, current strategies are geared towards in vivo gene transfer. MLV-based retroviral vectors require cell division for transduction of host cells. The use of growth factors (rather than partial hepatectomy) to stimulate hepatocellular replication can enhance the efficacy of MLV vectors. Alternative retroviral vectors based on lentiviruses may overcome these obstacles.

Adenovirus vectors are very effective at gene transfer into the liver, thus allowing for the transduction of a majority of hepatocytes. However, the early generations of these vectors exhibited dose-dependent toxicity, inflammation, and immunogenicity that limited the persistence of transgene expression. Adenoviral vectors devoid of all viral genes have been shown to transduce hepatocytes efficiently with reduced toxicity or immunogenicity. In rodents, transgene expression appears to be lifelong, but in nonhuman primates, expression declines by 90% over a 2-year period.

AAV vectors stably integrate their proviral DNA into hepatocytes in vivo with no apparent toxicity. This vector has been used in preclinical liver gene therapy studies to cure mice with hemophilia B and to partially correct the defect in dogs with hemophilia B. Hepatocyte gene transfer by AAV vectors is likely to be useful for treating a variety of metabolic diseases, such as urea cycle disorders, aminoacidopathies, disorders of carbohydrate metabolism, and lysosomal storage diseases. This strategy is particularly applicable when expression of the transgene in a relatively small percentage of hepatocytes is of therapeutic benefit.

The intestinal tract offers a large cell mass for gene therapy and is accessible by oral administration of vectors. Although a number of vectors have been tested in the gastrointestinal tract, major limitations still exist, such as the rapid turnover of the intestinal epithelial cells, the inability to target the stem or early progenitor cells, and the effects of digestive secretions on vector delivery. If these obstacles can be overcome, many diseases may be amenable to treatment by intestinal gene transfer.

THE HEMATOPOIETIC SYSTEM Clinical trials targeting hematopoietic cells have almost exclusively taken an ex vivo approach, with gene transfer occurring outside the body, followed by reinfusion of transduced cells. The most common cellular targets are lymphocytes and hematopoietic stem cells. Because stem cells can reconstitute the entire hematopoietic system, ex vivo genetic manipulation and autologous transplantation of bone marrow or peripheral blood stem cells represents a powerful therapeutic paradigm. Long-term gene transfer to hematopoietic stem cells requires the use of integrating viral vectors to ensure that the transgene replicates with the chromosomes during the extensive cellular proliferation that occurs during hematopoiesis. Thus, most stem cell gene therapy trials have used retroviral vectors. In part, because stem cells are not actively dividing, transduction rates have been too low to be therapeutic. Despite this, recent success in treating X-linked severe combined immunodeficiency with MLV vectors encoding the cytokine receptor gamma common chain demonstrates the feasibility of this approach. The use of different envelope proteins and vectors based on lentiviruses or spumaviruses may yield greater success in stem cell transduction.

Gene transfer to hematopoietic stem cells could be used to treat diseases of erythroid, myeloid, and lymphoid cells as well as platelet disorders (since the stem cell ultimately differentiates into all these cell types). An important aspect of this approach is the level of myeloablation required to allow engraftment of ex vivo–modified stem cells. An optimal therapy would minimize myeloablation and its associated toxicity, perhaps by delivering a gene that confers a selective advantage to transduced stem cells along with the therapeutic transgene. Many of the clinical trials to date have involved genes that confer increased resistance to chemotherapeutic agents used in treating cancer. An alternative strategy is to apply gene therapy to disorders in which expression is not required in all cells to prevent clinical disease. In chronic granulomatous disease, in which there is failure of granulocytes and monocytes to generate the hydrogen peroxide needed for bacterial killing, it may be feasible to achieve a threshold level of normal cells to respond to infections. Another major area of stem cell gene therapy research is the treatment of hemoglobinopathies with vectors expressing globin genes. Although clinical trials have not begun, these efforts have helped define the problems that must be solved for successful stem cell gene therapy, especially with regard to regulating transgene expression levels. Globin gene replacement is a daunting task, since the gene must be expressed at high levels in a select subset of erythroid cells, thus requiring the inclusion of a variety of transcriptional control elements in the vector (many of which have resulted in vector instability and low viral titers).

Lymphocyte gene transfer has the potential to treat genetic immunodeficiencies and to modulate immune functions. ADA deficiency was one of the first diseases to be treated with gene therapy and employed ex vivo transduction of lymphocytes. Although this early clinical trial represented an important milestone in gene therapy, the assessment of a therapeutic effect has been complicated by concomitant treatment with the ADA protein. Replacement of the ADA gene also confers a selective advantage to ADA-deficient lymphocytes, a property that would not be generally applicable to lymphocyte gene transfer. Still, as lymphocyte transduction protocols improve, many treatments may be developed with this cellular target, especially for acquired diseases. Genetic manipulations with antibody or cytokine genes offer a multitude of possible treatments for infectious and autoimmune diseases, as well as for cancer.

PULMONARY SYSTEM Gene therapy of the lung has concentrated primarily on treatments for cystic fibrosis. The gene for cystic fibrosis, *CFTR*, was cloned in 1989; by 1993 the first trials using adenovirus vectors were attempted in the nasal epithelium and airway. Though no clinical efficacy was demonstrated, these studies underscored the need to develop defined clinical endpoints for future trials. In addition to the adenovirus trials, clinical trials with nonviral liposome and AAV vectors also failed to demonstrate therapeutic effects. Difficulties encountered in pulmonary gene therapy include poor vector delivery due to respiratory secretions, lack of accessible vector receptors on the exposed cellular surface, transient transgene expression due to turnover of the respiratory epithelium, and vector-induced inflammation and pneumonitis. It also remains unclear which type of lung cells should be targeted with the *CFTR* gene to result in clinical benefit. As efficient and safe vectors for lung gene transfer are developed, treatments for acquired disorders such as chronic obstructive pulmonary disease may also be possible.

NERVOUS SYSTEM AND RETINA Gene transfer to the nervous system will be important for the treatment of many inherited and acquired neurologic diseases. Depending on the disorder, both glial cells and neurons may be appropriate cellular targets. Several vectors have been shown to transduce cells (including neurons) in animals after in vivo injection into the brain. Gene transfer is typically localized near the site of injection, a feature that is desirable for disorders such as Parkinson's disease, where transduction in the striatum could allow selective expression of genes involved in dopamine synthesis. Vector delivery throughout the nervous system will be more difficult to achieve, making gene therapy of global neurologic disorders problematic. The possibility of delivering neurotrophic factors to the CNS is a potential strategy for the treatment of neurodegenerative diseases, such as amyotrophic lateral sclerosis, and for facilitating recovery after spinal cord injury. Genetically modified stem cells have also been suggested as a strategy for the treatment of neurodegenerative disorders, but studies of these cells are at very early stages.

Retinitis pigmentosa (RP), a common cause of blindness from retinal degeneration, represents one class of disorders that stands to benefit from gene therapy. Though many different gene defects may cause RP, treatment of a form caused by mutation in the rod photoreceptor cGMP phosphodiesterase β-subunit gene has been studied in animal models by intraocular gene addition with adenovirus, lentivirus, and AAV vectors. In a different type of RP, progression of an autosomal dominant form of the disease was significantly slowed in a transgenic rat model using AAV vectors that express *ribozymes* (RNA enzymes) against the mutant mRNA. Ribozymes are catalytically active RNA molecules that specifically anneal to, and cleave, other RNA sequences, resulting in their selective degradation. This strategy may be useful for the treatment of other genetic diseases caused by dominant mutations. Viral vectors that express cytotoxic genes have been used to treat CNS tumors (see below).

MUSCULOSKELETAL SYSTEM Efficient gene transfer to myotubes through intramuscular injection has been demonstrated with adenoviral vectors, AAV vectors, and lentiviral vectors. In the case of AAV vectors, long-term transgene expression in muscles has been observed in several animal species. The treatment of the muscular dystrophies will require efficient delivery to multiple muscle groups throughout the body, and vector delivery to all the necessary locations remains a formidable task. In the case of Duchenne muscular dystrophy, the large size of the dystrophin cDNA also poses technical challenges in vector design. In contrast to primary diseases of muscle, success is more likely in muscle gene therapy trials aimed at the synthesis of secreted proteins, such as clotting factors. The large tissue mass and accessibility of muscle make it particularly attractive for these applications.

CARDIOVASCULAR SYSTEM The cardiovascular system (including the peripheral vasculature) has become an important target for gene therapy. Vascular wall gene delivery is being studied as a way to inhibit smooth-muscle cell proliferation and prevent restenosis. The transgenes used in this application are designed to interfere with the cell cycle or induce apoptosis in smooth-muscle cells. This approach is especially attractive if the vector can be delivered during angioplasty.

Other gene therapy strategies are used to promote the vascularization of tissues. There is some evidence for a therapeutic response in patients with critical limb ischemia due to poor peripheral vascularization who received intramuscular injection of naked DNA vectors encoding the vascular endothelial growth factor (VEGF) gene. Small amounts of the protein are secreted from the muscle, resulting in collateral vessel development that can reverse the ischemia. Patients who were expected to require limb amputation were spared this procedure after gene therapy. Similar clinical trials with the VEGF gene using nonviral and viral vectors are being studied in the context of myocardial ischemia.

CANCER Most of the gene therapy clinical trials to date have been aimed at the treatment of cancer. One approach uses gene therapy with cytokine or neoantigen genes to increase tumor immunogenicity. The vector is usually injected directly into the tumor, and there is some evidence that once the immune system is stimulated, nontransduced tumor cells may also be eliminated by the immune system. In melanoma, for example, cells have been genetically altered to express mismatched histocompatibility antigens or cytokines such as tumor necrosis factor, IFN-γ, or IL-2 in an effort to stimulate an immune response. Another approach involves the delivery of genes to tumor cells that convert a prodrug into a cytotoxic compound. Although several strategies are being developed, the most common involves the transfer of the herpes thymidine kinase (TK) gene. The TK enzyme converts gancyclovir into a thymidine analogue that interferes with DNA synthesis and causes cell death. The toxic effects also occur in adjacent nontransduced cells due to the uptake of the toxic analogue; this process is referred to as the *bystander effect*. Vectors designed to replace defective tumor-suppressor proteins with normal versions are being considered for cancer gene therapy, but it is difficult to envision success with this approach unless virtually all the tumor cells are genetically modified. Genes that control tumor growth when expressed in nontumor cells may also be effective in cancer gene therapy. The delivery of gene products that interfere with tumor angiogenesis best exemplifies this approach. Finally, lytic viral vectors that selectively replicate and kill malignant cells are being developed. One example is an adenovirus designed to replicate in cells deficient in p53, a tumor-suppressor protein that is mutated in many different cancers.

These and other related strategies have shown efficacy in animal models when tumor cells are transplanted into various anatomic locations. These models do not always emulate the natural processes that result in bonafide cancers, in part due to the tumor cells not being truly autologous in origin. Although there have been encouraging results in some of the clinical trials performed to date, efficacy has not been demonstrated definitively. In many cases the patient populations studied had advanced malignancies, and more informative results might be obtained at earlier disease stages. Still, cancer gene therapy has a promising future, and ongoing research involving tumor-specific antigens, angiogenesis, cell cycle control, and apoptosis are all likely to lead to new gene therapy approaches. Improvements in vector targeting of tumor cells and in the development of tumor-specific gene expression will also enhance future therapeutic approaches.

COAGULOPATHIES Inherited coagulopathies, especially hemophilia A and B, are promising areas of gene therapy research because even a low level of coagulation factor reconstitution can potentially benefit a patient with a severe phenotype. Although the liver is the major site of synthesis for factors VIII and IX, several other tissues may support factor synthesis and secretion into the bloodstream. AAV vectors, in particular, have shown prolonged therapeutic effects in animal models of hemophilia B when delivered to muscle or liver. Hemophilia A has been more difficult to treat, due to the larger cDNA (which approaches the packaging capacity of AAV vectors) and the requirement that expressing cells deliver the protein directly into the intravascular space. Other coagulopathies, such as factor X deficiency, are also good candidates for gene therapy. Various approaches to the treatment of hemophilia are currently in the early stages of clinical trials.

INFECTIOUS DISEASES Most infectious pathogens studied as targets for gene therapy are viral (particularly HIV), in part because they replicate inside human cells. One approach involves introducing inhibitory versions of essential viral proteins that disrupt the viral life cycle even in the presence of their normal counterparts (e.g., by disrupting the packaging of virions). Another strategy involves the expression of proteins, peptides, or even RNA transcripts that function as decoys by binding to other proteins required for viral replication and preventing them from acting on their normal viral target sites. The cellular proteins required for a pathogen's life cycle, such as receptor molecules used for viral entry, or specific proteins used for adherence of the pathogen, can also be manipulated through gene therapy; this tactic could also be applied to nonviral pathogens. Ribozymes can be engineered to cleave specific viral transcripts, thereby blocking expression of viral gene products or destroying viral genomes (in the case of RNA viruses). Because ribozymes can, in principle, be engineered to attack any RNA transcript, they are being considered as treatments for many different viral diseases. Clinical trials have begun using ribozymes to block HIV infection. Antisense oligonucleotides can also be used to interfere with viral or cellular nucleic acid sequences. Other gene therapy approaches that may be applied to infectious diseases include vaccination with specific antigens and manipulation of the immune system to enhance the clearance of pathogens.

SUMMARY

The gene can be thought of as a new pharmaceutical agent in the armamentarium used to treat disease. The availability of cloned genes has already yielded a large array of recombinant proteins for clinical use. The limited success of gene therapy to date is due primarily to difficulties inherent in the efficient and safe delivery of genes to their appropriate target cells. The field is still in its infancy, and many of the technical problems are likely to be solved by advances in vector design.

BIBLIOGRAPHY

AMADO RG, CHEN ISY: Lentiviral vectors—the promise of gene therapy within reach? Science 285:674, 1999

BLAESE M et al: T lymphocyte–directed gene therapy for ADA-SCID: Initial trial results after 4 years. Science 270:475, 1995

CAVAZZANA-CALVO M et al: Gene therapy of human severe combined immunodeficiency (SCID)-X1 disease. Science 288:669, 2000

FERRY N, HEARD JM: Liver-directed gene transfer vectors. Hum Gene Ther 9:1975, 1998

HALL SJ et al: The promise and reality of cancer gene therapy. Am J Hum Genet 61:785, 1997

HITT MM et al: Human adenovirus vectors for gene transfer into mammalian cells. Adv Pharmacol 40:137, 1997

KAY MA et al: Evidence for gene transfer and expression of blood coagulation factor IX in patients with severe hemophilia B treated with an AA vector. Nat Genet 24:257, 2000

MILLER AD: Development and applications of retroviral vectors, in *Retroviruses*, JM Coffin, SH Hughes, HE Varmus (eds). Cold Spring Harbor, NY, Cold Spring Harbor Laboratory, 1997, p 437

MORSY MA, CASKEY CT: Expanded-capacity adenoviral vectors—the helper dependent vectors. Mol Med Today 5:18, 1999

NABEL GJ: Immune recognition of malignancies: Relevance to immunotherapy. Cancer J Sci Am Suppl 1:S106, 1998

ORKIN SH, MOTULSKY AG: Report and recommendations of the panel to assess the NIH investment in research on gene therapy. www.nih.gov/news/panelrep.html

ROTH JA, CHRISTIANO RJ: Gene therapy for cancer: What have we done and where are we going? J Natl Cancer Inst 89:21, 1997

RUSSELL DW, KAY MA: Adeno-associated virus vectors and hematology. Blood 94:864, 1999

SVENSSON EC, SCHWARTZ LB: Gene therapy for vascular disease. Curr Opin Cardiol 13:369, 1998

NOBEL PRIZE IN PHYSIOLOGY OR MEDICINE, 1905

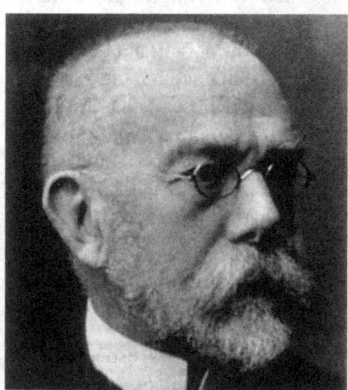

Robert Koch was born in Prussia on December 11, 1843. He was the third of thirteen children. He was a brilliant student, entering *Gymnasium* (German high school) at 8 years of age. He then matriculated into the University of Göttingen, where he studied medicine. In 1866 he graduated from medical school and started a general practice in Hamburg. His practice was interrupted by the Franco-German War. After discharge from the army, he became a public health physician in Wollstein, Germany. It was there that Koch launched his scientific career. He studied anthrax and developed techniques for the microscopy of bacteria. Earlier, Louis Pasteur had proposed the germ theory of disease, but leading pathologists, including Rudolph Virchow and Theodore Billroth, had rejected this possibility. It was Robert Koch's work on anthrax that convinced skeptics that microorganisms could cause infectious diseases. In 1880 Robert Koch moved to Berlin to become a member of the Imperial Health Office where he developed his culture plating technique, which is used basically unchanged today.

His real fame came in 1882 when he identified the tubercle bacillus as the cause of tuberculosis. Koch's postulates to incriminate microorganisms in causing an infectious disease are still the standard in microbiology. The organisms must be isolated and grown in pure culture from the infected tissue. The pure culture must then be shown to induce the disease experimentally and be recovered from the experimental animal. Koch accomplished all facets of this experimental design with tuberculosis by using a guinea pig model. He went on to

study cholera in Egypt and India. In Calcutta, Koch was able to isolate a pure culture of the cholera bacterium from autopsy specimens, which was morphologically the same comma bacillus as seen in Egyptian samples. In epidemiologic studies he demonstrated that cholera could be spread by contaminated water, a finding that led to control of the dreaded disease by water filtration. Koch then returned to the study of tuberculosis. He proposed that a glycerin extract of the tubercle bacilli, tuberculin, would lead to immunization against tuberculosis. Although patients with tuberculosis, but not healthy subjects, had a generalized and local reaction to tuberculin, immunity to tuberculosis was not achieved.

Koch's early warnings about the transmission of tuberculosis from human to human went largely unheeded. Eventually, however, measures were instituted around the world to prevent the spread of tuberculosis from infected individuals' sputum to other individuals. Koch was in Africa studying tropical diseases when he heard he had been awarded the 1905 Nobel Prize in Physiology or Medicine. He received the Nobel Prize for his contributions in tuberculosis, including identifying the causative agent and advocating public health measures to decrease the spread of the disease. Robert Koch, however, made many other important contributions and clearly deserves to be regarded as one of the founding fathers of the science of bacteriology.

REFERENCES

1. Magill FN (ed): *Nobel Prize Winners: Physiology or Medicine*, vol 1. Pasadena, Salem Press, 1993
2. Schrier RW: *A Salute to Nobel Laureates in Physiology and Medicine*, Proceedings of the Association of American Physicians 108(1): Jan 1996
3. Sourkes TL: *Nobel Prize Winners in Medicine and Physiology 1901–1965*. London, Abelard-Schuman, 1967

Robert W. Schrier, MD

70   *John A. Oates, Dan M. Roden, Grant R. Wilkinson*

PRINCIPLES OF DRUG THERAPY

Safe and effective drug therapy requires that drugs be delivered to their molecular targets in tissues at concentrations within the range that yields efficacy without toxicity. Variability in drug effects between individual patients can thus be attributed, in part, to differences in the processes that determine these concentrations, i.e., drug disposition involving absorption, distribution, and elimination. *Pharmacokinetics* provides a quantitative description of these processes, i.e., what the body does to the drug. In addition, variability in response may also reflect differences in the drug-target interaction that affect the concentration-related effects of the drug on the body, termed *pharmacodynamics*. This chapter reviews the principles of pharmacokinetics and pharmacodynamics and their application to optimizing therapeutic regimens.

CLINICAL PHARMACOKINETICS

PLASMA LEVELS AFTER A SINGLE DOSE   The levels of lidocaine in plasma following intravenous administration decline in two phases, as illustrated in Fig. 70-1; such a biphasic decline is typical for many drugs. Immediately after rapid injection, essentially all of the drug is in the plasma or central compartment, and the high initial plasma level reflects the confinement of the drug to this small volume. The drug is then transferred into an extravascular or peripheral compartment during a period called the *distribution phase*. For lidocaine, the distribution phase is virtually complete within 30 min. A phase of slower decline, the *equilibrium phase*, then occurs. During this phase, the drug levels in the plasma and in tissues change in parallel. Although this disposition profile is common to many drugs given intravenously, the characteristic parameters vary among drugs.

Distribution Phase   The pharmacologic effects during the distribution phase depend on whether the concentration of drug at the receptor site is similar to that in the plasma. If that is the case, the pharmacologic effects may be intense during this period because of the high initial levels in the plasma. For example, after a small bolus

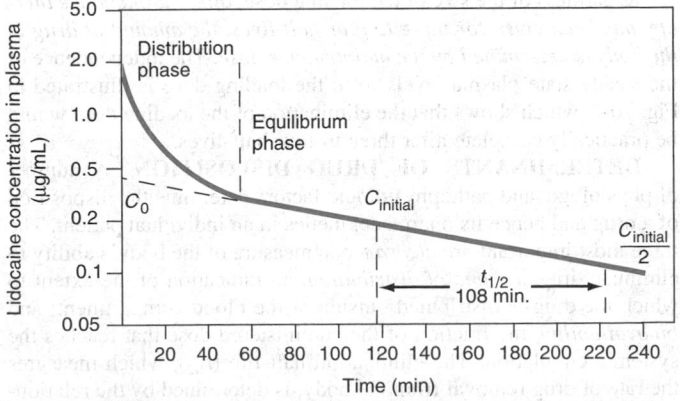

FIGURE 70-1   Concentrations of lidocaine in plasma following the administration of 50 mg intravenously. The half-life ($t_{1/2}$) of 108 min is computed as the time required for levels to fall from any given value during the equilibrium phase ($C_{initial}$) to one-half that level. C_0 is the hypothetical concentration of lidocaine in plasma at time zero if equilibrium had been achieved instantly.

dose (50 mg) of lidocaine, antiarrhythmic effects may be evident during the early distribution phase but will disappear as levels fall below those that are minimally effective, even before equilibrium between plasma and tissue is reached. Thus, a larger single dose or multiple small doses must be administered to achieve an effect that is sustained into the equilibrium phase. Toxicity resulting from high levels of some drugs during the distribution phase precludes administration of a single intravenous loading dose that will yield therapeutic levels during the equilibrium phase. For example, the administration of the entire loading dose of phenytoin as a single intravenous bolus can cause cardiovascular collapse due to the high levels during the distribution phase. If a loading dose of phenytoin is administered intravenously, it must be given slowly, e.g., at infusion rates of 25 to 50 mg/min. For similar reasons, the intravenous loading dose of many potent drugs that equilibrate rapidly with their receptors is either divided into fractional doses given at intervals or administered by infusion over a similar period.

A dose given orally results in lower plasma levels during the initial period than an intravenous bolus dose that delivers the same amount of drug to the systemic circulation. Because the drug is not absorbed instantly after oral administration and is delivered into the systemic circulation more slowly, much of it has been distributed by the time absorption is complete. Thus, procainamide, which is almost totally absorbed after oral administration, can be given orally as a single 750-mg loading dose with little risk of hypotension; in contrast, loading of this drug by the intravenous route is more safely accomplished by giving the dose in fractions of about 100 mg at 5-min intervals or by slow infusion to avoid hypotension during the distribution phase.

Some drugs are so predictably lethal when infused too rapidly that special precautions should be taken to prevent even the inadvertent occurrence. For example, solutions of potassium for intravenous administration in excess of 20 meq/L should be avoided in all but the most exceptional and carefully monitored circumstances. This minimizes the possibility of cardiac arrests, which can occur as a result of accidental increases in infusion rates of more concentrated solutions.

As these examples illustrate, excessively rapid administration of many drugs can lead to catastrophic consequences that result from high concentrations in the blood during the distribution phase.

In contrast, for some centrally active drugs, the higher concentration of drug during the distribution phase after intravenous administration is used to advantage. The use of midazolam for "IV sedation," for example, depends upon its rapid uptake by the brain during the distribution phase to produce sedation quickly, with subsequent egress from the brain during the redistribution of the drug as equilibrium is achieved.

Some drugs are distributed slowly to their sites of action during the distribution phase, i.e., concentration at the relevant receptor does not parallel that in plasma early after drug administration. For example, the level of digoxin at the receptor site (and the drug's pharmacologic effect) do not reflect plasma levels during the distribution phase. Digoxin is transported (or bound) to its cardiac receptors slowly by a process that proceeds throughout distribution. Thus, over the distribution phase of several hours, plasma levels fall while the level at the site of action and the pharmacologic effect increase. Only at the end of the distribution phase, when the drug has reached equilibrium with the receptor, does the concentration of digoxin in plasma reflect pharmacologic effect. For this reason, there should be a 6- to 8-h wait after administration before plasma levels of digoxin are measured as a guide to therapy.

Equilibrium Phase   After the concentration of drug in plasma has reached a dynamic equilibrium with that in the tissues, the levels in plasma and tissues fall in parallel as the drug is eliminated from the

Table 70-1   Amount of a Drug Dose Remaining in Body over Successive Half-Lives

No. of Elapsed Half-Lives	Amount of Dose Remaining in Body, %	Amount of Dose Eliminated, %
1	50.00	50.00
2	25.00	75.00
3	12.50	87.50
4	6.25	93.75
5	3.125	96.875

body. Thus, the equilibrium phase is also called the *elimination phase.* During this phase, drug concentrations measured in plasma can provide a useful index of drug levels in tissues.

Most drugs are eliminated as a first-order process. This means that the time required for the plasma level of the drug to fall to one-half the original value (the half-life, $t_{1/2}$) is the same regardless of the point on the plasma level curve at which measurement begins. Another characteristic of the first-order process is that a plot of the logarithm of the plasma concentration versus time is linear. From such a plot (Fig. 70-1), it can be seen that the half-life of lidocaine is 108 min. If the half-life is known, the amount of a dose remaining in the body at any time following administration of a single dose can be calculated. Table 70-1 shows how this amount changes over five successive half-lives.

From a clinical standpoint, elimination is essentially complete when it has reached about 90%. Therefore, for practical purposes, *a first-order elimination process reaches completion after three to four half-lives.*

DRUG ACCUMULATION—LOADING AND MAINTENANCE DOSES If a drug is given repeatedly at intervals shorter than the time required to eliminate a dose, both the amount of drug in the body and its pharmacologic effect increase with successive doses until they reach a plateau. Figure 70-2 shows the accumulation of digoxin administered in repeated maintenance doses (without a loading dose). Since the half-life of digoxin is about 1.6 days in a patient with normal renal function, 65% of a digoxin dose remains in the body at the end of 1 day. Thus, the second dose will raise the amount of digoxin in the body (and the average plasma level) to 165% of the level produced by the first dose. Each subsequent dose causes a further increase until a *steady state* is achieved. At that point, the drug dosing rate (bioavailable dose/dosage interval) is equal to the rate of elimination, with the fluctuation between peak and trough plasma levels remaining constant. If the rate of drug delivery is then altered, a new steady state will be attained. Continuous infusion of a drug at constant rate also results in progressive accumulation to a predictable steady state (Fig. 70-2). In this case, the steady-state plasma level (C_{ss}) is equivalent to the average between the peak and trough levels ($C_{avg,ss}$) produced by intermittent administration of the same amount of drug over the same period. For *all* drugs with first-order kinetics, the time required to achieve steady-state levels can be predicted from the half-life, because accumulation is a first-order process with a half-life identical to that for elimination. Thus, accumulation reaches 90% of steady-state levels at the end of three to four half-lives. This is true for either intermittent or continuous dosing (Fig. 70-2).

When a therapeutic effect is required urgently, simply administering the maintenance dose of a drug with a long half-life results in an unacceptable delay in reaching steady-state levels of the drug and its intended effect. The time required to achieve the desired pharmacologic effect may be shortened by the administration of a *loading dose*—the amount of drug that will bring the plasma concentration rapidly to the steady-state level. Therefore, if treatment with lidocaine ($t_{1/2} \sim 108$ min) were initiated by infusion at only the maintenance dose level, it would take about 4 to 8 h before the drug's maximal effect was achieved. Because ventricular arrhythmias may be life-threatening, it is not reasonable to wait that long to achieve an effective steady-state drug level. Accordingly, it would be appropriate to ad-

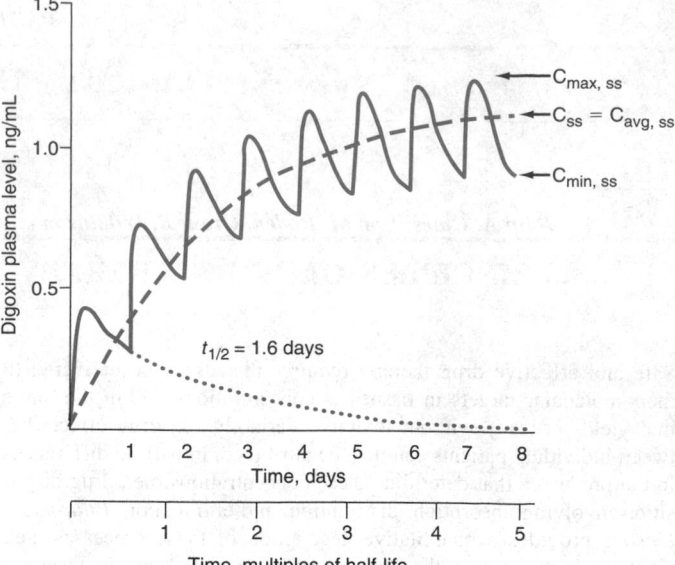

FIGURE 70-2   Time course of digoxin accumulation following repeated 0.25 mg/d oral maintenance dose administration (solid line), assuming bioavailability is about 85%. The smooth (dashed line) curve depicts the pattern of accumulation following administration of an equivalent dosing rate (150 ng/min) by continuous intravenous infusion. Note that accumulation and elimination are >90% complete after four half-lives and this is independent of the dosing regimen. Also, that steady state is proportional to the dosing rate (dose/dosing interval) and the ratio of bioavailability to clearance. The temporal relationships shown apply equally well to other drugs with linear pharmacokinetics and one-compartment distribution. For comparison, the plasma concentration-time curve if only the first dose were given is also shown (dotted line). $C_{max,ss}$, maximum plasma concentration at steady state; C_{avg}, average plasma concentration; C_{min}, minimal plasma concentration.

minister one or more loading doses at the onset of therapy, together with infusion at the rate of the maintenance dose.

Loading may be accomplished by the administration of a single loading dose or, if that would create a risk of toxicity, by the administration of the loading dose in a series of fractions of that dose over time. The latter approach is particularly appropriate for most drugs that have a low therapeutic index. A divided loading dose strategy or the administration of the loading dose in a slow intravenous infusion are particularly advisable when the drug is given intravenously. Thus, in the case of lidocaine, a common regimen is to administer an initial intravenous bolus of 1 mg/kg followed by up to three additional bolus injections of 0.5 mg/kg every 8 to 10 min as necessary, and a maintenance infusion of 2 mg/min.

Regardless of the size of the loading dose, *after maintenance therapy has been given for three to four half-lives, the amount of drug in the body is determined by the maintenance dose.* The independence of the steady state plasma levels from the loading dose is illustrated in Fig. 70-2, which shows that the elimination of the loading dose would be practically complete after three to four half-lives.

DETERMINANTS OF DRUG DISPOSITION A number of physiologic and pathophysiologic factors determine the disposition of a drug and hence its pharmacokinetics in an individual patient. The three most important are *clearance*, a measure of the body's ability to eliminate drug; *volume of distribution*, an indication of the extent to which the drug is distributed outside of the blood compartment; and *bioavailability*, the fraction of the administered dose that reaches the systemic circulation. The elimination half-life ($t_{1/2}$), which measures the rate of drug removal from the body, is determined by the relationship between the physiologically determined clearance and volume of distribution.

Clearance The majority of drugs are given over a prolonged period of time according to a multiple dosage regimen, e.g., x mg every y h. The clinical goal is to maintain the drug's steady-state concentration within the therapeutic range for the individual patient; if the level is too low, reduced efficacy results, whereas if it is too high, the likelihood of adverse effects increases.

Steady state is achieved when the rate of drug elimination equals the rate of drug delivery into the systemic circulation, which, if bioavailability is complete, corresponds to the rate at which the drug dose is administered:

$$\underset{\text{(amt/unit time)}}{\text{Dosing rate}} = \underset{\text{(vol/unit time)}}{Cl} \times \underset{\text{(amt/vol)}}{C_{ss}}$$

where Cl is clearance and C_{ss} is the steady-state concentration in plasma. Therefore, *at a given dosing rate the concentration of drug in plasma is completely dependent on its clearance.* If the drug is infused, the concentration remains constant so long as drug delivery continues; however, when the drug is given intermittently, the above relationship is expressed as:

$$\text{Dosing/dosage interval} = Cl \times C_{avg,ss}$$

where $C_{avg,ss}$ is the *average* value during the dosage interval and is equal to C_{ss} although the *actual* concentrations will be higher or lower at various points during this period. Thus, clearance determines the rate at which a drug should be administered in order to obtain a desired steady-state concentration; stated in a different fashion, steady-state drug levels can be modified either up or down by changing the dosage rate. *The clearance of the vast majority of drugs is constant over the therapeutic range of concentrations.*

Clearance is a measure of the rate at which the organs that eliminate drug from the body remove drug from the blood.

$$Cl = \text{Rate of elimination}/C$$

Accordingly, clearance reflects the volume of blood (or plasma) from which the drug would have to be removed per unit time to account for the elimination; it can be related to either total or unbound drug.

Drug elimination generally occurs as a result of metabolism and/or excretion in the liver, kidney, and possibly other organs. Clearance of drug from the body, therefore, reflects the overall contribution of each of these organs, as indicated by their individual rates of elimination normalized to the concentration of drug, and is additive.

$$Cl = Cl_{hepatic} + Cl_{renal} + Cl_{other}$$

Clearance of a drug is usually estimated following administration of an intravenous dose ($dose_{iv}$) and measurement of the resulting total area under the curve (AUC) for the blood or plasma concentration-time curve (AUC_{iv}) from zero to infinite time.

$$Cl = dose_{iv}/AUC_{iv}$$

Table 70-2 indicates the marked differences in plasma clearance for some commonly used drugs. Some drugs such as phenobarbital and valproic acid have relatively low values (<10 mL/min), whereas others such as procainamide and lidocaine have much larger clearances (>500 mL/min). Such differences mainly reflect different rate-limiting determinants such as blood flow through the organ(s) of clearance, the extent of binding of the drug to plasma proteins, and the efficiency of the clearance process to remove drug from tissue water by metabolism and/or excretion. The data in Table 70-2 also demonstrate that the relative contributions of the two major routes of elimination, i.e., renal and nonrenal, also vary according to the individual drug. In some cases, such as amikacin, digoxin, gentamicin, lithium, and tobramycin, excretion by the kidneys is predominant. However, with many other drugs (e.g., carbamezipine, lidocaine), nonrenal elimination, which usually reflects metabolism in the liver, is more important.

Volume of Distribution The relationship between the amount of drug in the body and the concentration of drug in the plasma provides a measure of the apparent volume of distribution:

$$\underset{\text{(vol)}}{V} = \text{amount of drug in the body} / \underset{\text{(amt)/(amt/vol)}}{C}$$

This volume does not, except in a limited number of special cases, reflect an identifiable physiologic volume but corresponds to the virtual volume of fluid that would be required to contain all of the drug in the body at the same concentration as in the plasma. In a typical 70-kg human, plasma volume is about 3 L, blood volume around 5.5 L, and extracellular water outside the vasculature is approximately 42 L. The volume of distribution of drugs that are extensively bound to plasma proteins but are not bound to tissue components approaches plasma volume. However, for most drugs, the volume of distribution is far greater than any physiologic space. For example, the volume of distribution of digoxin is about 700 L, which obviously exceeds total body volume. This simply indicates that digoxin is largely distributed outside the vascular system and hence the proportion of the drug present in the plasma compartment is low.

The volume of distribution may be estimated by back-extrapolation of the plasma concentration-time curve to zero time (C_0) (Fig.

Table 70-2 Pharmacokinetic Parameters (Mean ± Standard Deviation) and Plasma Therapeutic Ranges of Some Commonly Used Drugs

	Cl, mL/min	V, L	$t_{1/2}$, h	Oral F, %	Urinary Excretion, %	Plasma Binding, %	Effective Plasma Level, μg/mL	Toxic Plasma Level, μg/mL
Carbamazepine	90 ± 35	98 ± 28	15 ± 5	>70	<1	74 ± 3	4	10
Digoxin	133 ± 69[a]	658 ± 196	39 ± 13	70 ± 13	60 ± 11	25 ± 5	>0.8 ng/mL	2.0 ng/mL
Ethosuximide	13 ± 3	50 ± 11	45 ± 8	—	25 ± 15	0	40	100
Gentamicin	110 ± 35[a]	22 ± 7	53 ± 25	—	>90	<10	5	peak 10 trough 2
Lidocaine	644 ± 168	77 ± 18	1.8 ± 0.4	35 ± 11	2	70 ± 5	1.5	6
Lithium	24 ± 7	46 ± 11	22 ± 8	100	95 ± 15	0	0.5 meq/L	1.5meq/L
Midazolam	462 ± 126	77 ± 42	1.9 ± 0.6	44 ± 17	56 ± 26	95 ± 2	50	200
Phenobarbital	4.3 ± 0.9	38 ± 2	99 ± 18	100	24 ± 5	51 ± 3	10	30
Phenytoin	Dose-dependent	45 ± 8	6–24	90 ± 3	2 ± 8	89 ± 23	10	20
Primidone	38 ± 8	48 ± 13	15 ± 4	92 ± 18	48 ± 16	19	8	12
Procainamide	600 ± 200[b]	133 ± 21	3.0 ± 0.6	83 ± 16	67 ± 8	16 ± 5	3	14
Quinidine	329 ± 126	189 ± 84	6.2 ± 1.8	70–80	18 ± 3	87 ± 3	2	6
Tacrolimus	49 ± 19	62 ± 22	15 ± 7	16 ± 7	<1	75–99	15	25
Theophylline	45 ± 14	35 ± 11	9.0 ± 2.1	96 ± 8	18 ± 3	56 ± 4	5	20
Valproic acid	7.7 ± 14	15 ± 5	14 ± 3	100	1.8 ± 2.4	93 ± 1	30	100

[a] Dependent on renal function.
[b] Dependent on N-acetylator phenotype.

NOTE: Cl, clearance; V, volume of distribution; F, bioavailability.

70-1) and dividing this into the dose of drug administered intravenously.

$$V = dose_{iv}/C_0$$

When distribution of the drug is not instantaneous, a more useful volume estimate is based on the area under the plasma-concentration time curve (AUC) and the terminal elimination half-life of the drug $(t_{1/2})$.

$$V_{area} = \frac{dose_{iv} \times t_{1/2}}{0.693 \times AUC}$$

Extent and Rate of Bioavailability   After intravenous administration, all of the administered dose reaches the systemic circulation. In contrast, with all other routes of administration, such as oral, intramuscular, and subcutaneous, there is the potential for only a part of the dose to be absorbed; this fraction (F) is termed the drug's *bioavailability*. Lack of complete bioavailability may reflect the inability of the drug to be completely released from the dosage form or vehicle, chemical destruction at the site of administration, incomplete absorption into the vascular system, and metabolism and/or excretion during translocation of the drug from its site of administration to the systemic circulation. In the case of oral dosing, this would include the intestinal epithelium and the liver and lungs. Metabolism and/or excretion by the gastrointestinal tract (F_{GI}) and liver (F_L) are collectively referred to as the *first-pass effect*, since the resulting drug elimination only occurs during drug delivery to the systemic circulation. Loss of drug because of a first-pass effect thus requires that the dosing rate appropriately take into account bioavailability. For example, after oral drug administration:

$$F_{oral} \times dosing\ rate = Cl \times C_{avg,ss}$$

Bioavailability and the first-pass effect are important with respect to possible differences in drug responsiveness dependent on the route of administration. For example, glyceryl trinitrate has such a large oral first-pass effect ($>$99%) that systemic concentrations after an oral dose are negligible and no antianginal effect is present. Giving the drug by the sublingual or transdermal routes bypasses the splanchnic organs and allows essentially all of the drug to reach the systemic circulation. For drugs that are efficiently metabolized by the intestinal epithelium and/or liver, i.e., drugs with high extraction ratios in either of these organs, differences in the extent of the first-pass effect between individuals frequently explain variability in drug response. With propranolol, for example, the 15-fold variability in plasma concentrations after the same oral dose results from differences in the individual hepatic extraction ratios reflective of different levels of drug metabolizing activity.

Drug administration by nonintravenous routes involves an absorption process characterized by the plasma level increasing to a maximum value at some time after administration and then declining as the rate of drug elimination exceeds the rate of absorption. Thus, the peak concentration is lower and occurs later than after the same dose given by rapid intravenous injection. The rate of absorption can be an important consideration during the initial period after drug administration, especially for drugs with a narrow *therapeutic index*—the ratio of the toxic dose to the therapeutic dose. If absorption is too rapid, then the resulting high concentration may cause adverse effects not observed with a more slowly available formulation. At the other extreme, slow absorption is deliberately designed into "slow-release" or- "sustained-release" drug formulations in order to maintain plasma concentrations essentially constant during the dosage interval, because the drug's rate of elimination is offset by an equivalent rate of absorption controlled by formulation factors.

Half-Life   The organs of elimination can only clear drug from the blood. Thus, the rate at which drug is eliminated from the body is a function of both clearance and the extent to which drug is distributed outside of the vascular compartment. The fraction of total drug in the body that is eliminated in a given time is designated the *fractional elimination constant (k)*.

$$k = Cl/V$$

For example, if the volume of distribution is 10 L and clearance is 1 L/min, then one-tenth of the drug is eliminated per minute. If k is multiplied by the total amount of drug in the body, the actual rate of elimination at any given time can be determined:

Rate of elimination $= k \times$ amount in body $= k \times C \times V = Cl \times C$

This relationship, indicating that the rate of drug elimination is proportional to the drug concentration, describes a first-order, or monoexponential, process. With a few notable exceptions, the elimination of drugs used clinically is first-order.

Half-life $(t_{1/2})$ is the time that it takes for the plasma concentration or amount of drug in the body to decline by 50%. This parameter is related to k as follows:

$$t_{1/2} = 0.693/k$$

where 0.693 is the natural logarithm of $2(C_o/0.5\ C_o)$.
  Because

$$k = Cl/V$$

then

$$t_{1/2} = 0.693\ (V/Cl)$$

This is an important relationship since it indicates that the rate of drug elimination, reflected by $t_{1/2}$, is dependent on both the efficiency of drug removal (Cl) and the drug's volume of distribution (V). When V remains constant, $t_{1/2}$ is a reflection of clearance. Thus, $t_{1/2}$ is shortened when rifampin induces the enzymes responsible for a drug's hepatic clearance and is lengthened when a drug's renal clearance is impaired in renal failure. However, when there are concomitant alterations in V, as occurs for some drugs in cardiac failure, $t_{1/2}$ is not an accurate measure of Cl or drug dose.

DESIGNING DOSAGE REGIMENS   Most drugs are administered as part of long-term therapy involving multiple dosing, and it is critical that the dosage regimen be optimized to the individual patient. With some drugs, the desired response, e.g., coagulation or blood pressure, is readily measurable and an individualized dosage regimen can be developed with dosage titration. However, dosage changes should be conservative ($<$50% for drugs with a low therapeutic index) and not more frequent than every three to four half-lives. Other drugs have little dose-related toxicity so the therapeutic window is large, e.g., penicillins and β-adrenoceptor antagonists. In these situations, effective and prolonged drug effects may be obtained by a "maximal dose" strategy. It is also possible to use this strategy to extend the duration of action of a drug, especially one that is eliminated rapidly from the body. Thus, 75 mg of captopril will result in reduced blood pressure for up to 12 h, even though the elimination half-life of this angiotensin-converting enzyme (ACE) inhibitor is about 2 h; this is because the dose raises the concentration of drug in plasma many times higher than the threshold for its pharmacologic effect.

Determination of the Maintenance Dose   The relationship between the maintenance dose and the final steady-state concentration is

Maintenance dosing rate $= F \times$ dose/dosage interval $= Cl \times C_{avg,ss}$

Thus, steady-state concentrations can be predictably increased or decreased by appropriate modification of the maintenance dosing rate to achieve a desired target value:

$$C_{target} = C_{avg,ss} = \frac{F \times dose}{Cl \times dosing\ interval}$$

In most cases, this is best achieved by changing the drug dose but not the dosing interval, e.g., by giving 250 mg every 8 h instead of 200 mg every 8 h. However, this approach is acceptable only if the resulting maximum concentration is not toxic and the trough value does not fall below the minimum effective concentration for an undesirable period of time. Alternatively, the steady state may be changed by altering the frequency of intermittent dosing but not the size of each dose. In this case, the magnitude of the fluctuations around the average steady-state level will change—the shorter the dosing interval, the smaller the difference between peak and trough levels (Fig. 70-3).

The extent of fluctuation is determined by the relationship between the dosing interval and the drug's half-life. For example, if the dosing interval is equal to the drug's half-life, then the fluctuation would be twofold, which is usually a tolerable variation. If a longer dosing interval is used, then the difference between the maximum and minimum plasma levels will be greater (Fig. 70-3). Marked fluctuations increase the likelihood of increased concentration-dependent drug effects early during the dosing interval and possible ineffectiveness at the end of the period, even though the average steady-state drug concentration is the same as that following administration at the same dosing rate but at shorter intervals.

Determination of the Loading Dose The loading dose can be estimated if both the desired plasma level (C) and the apparent volume of distribution (V) are known:

$$Loading\ dose = C_{avg,ss} \times V$$

The loading amount required to achieve steady-state plasma levels can also be determined from the fraction of drug eliminated during the dosing interval and the maintenance dose. For example, if the fraction of digoxin eliminated daily is 35% and the planned maintenance dose is 0.25 mg daily, then the loading dose to achieve steady-state levels would be (100/35) times the maintenance dose, or approximately 0.75 mg. Thus,

$$Loading\ dose = \frac{100}{\%\ of\ drug\ eliminated\ per\ dosage\ interval} \times maintenance\ dose$$

NONLINEAR DRUG ELIMINATION The elimination of some drugs (e.g., phenytoin, salicylate, propafenone, and theophylline) does not follow first-order kinetics because the clearance of these drugs changes as levels in the body fall during elimination or change after alterations in dose. Such elimination is called *concentration-dependent* or *dose-dependent*. Accordingly, the time for the concentration to fall to one-half becomes less as plasma levels fall. (This halving time is not truly a half-life, because the term *half-life* applies to first-order kinetics and is a constant.) When a drug is eliminated by first-order kinetics, the plasma level at steady state is directly related to the amount of the maintenance dose, and a doubling of the dose should lead to doubling of the steady-state plasma level. However, for drugs with dose-dependent kinetics, an increase in the dose may be accompanied by a disproportionate increase in the plasma level. For example, a threefold increase in the dose of propafenone (from 300 mg to 900 mg daily) leads to a tenfold increase in the concentration of propafenone in plasma. Changes in dosage regimens for drugs with dose-dependent kinetics should always be accompanied by surveillance for adverse effects and by measurement of the concentration of the drug in plasma during the time of transition to the new steady-state, if this is feasible.

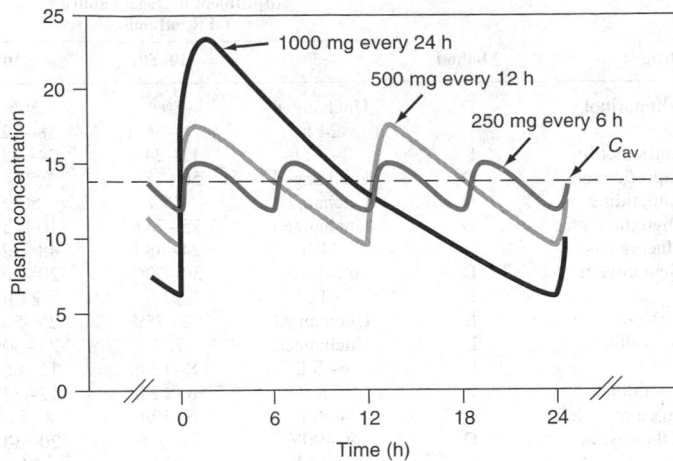

FIGURE 70-3 Plasma concentrations of a drug with an elimination half-life of 12 h during chronic therapy using different dosage regimens for a period sufficient to reach steady state. Proportionally reducing or increasing both the size of the maintenance dose and the interval between dosage changes the magnitude of the fluctuations in plasma levels but has no effect on the average steady-state (C_{av}) value, since this depends on the dosing rate (dose/dosing interval).

INDIVIDUALIZATION OF DRUG THERAPY

EFFECTS OF RENAL DISEASE Whether a drug's dosing rate needs to be modified in patients with renal dysfunction depends on whether the drug is primarily excreted through the kidneys and whether increased drug levels, secondary to impaired renal clearance, will be associated with adverse effects. If both of these factors are present, it is likely that with decreased renal clearance the drug will accumulate to a greater extent than in patients with normal renal function and toxicity will result. This is especially true for drugs with long half-lives and narrow therapeutic indexes (e.g., digoxin). In general, over 60 to 70% of the drug must be renally excreted for dosage modification to be necessary and then only when renal function is less than about 30 to 50% of normal.

The goal of any dosing rate adjustment is to modify the dosing schedule so that the drug's plasma concentration-time profile is as similar to the desired one as possible and that the steady state is reached in about the same time as in a patient with normal renal function. To obtain the desired profile, a modification may be made by decreasing the dose while maintaining the dosage interval, keeping the dose the same but increasing the dosing interval, or a combination of these two approaches.

A drug's renal clearance is proportional to creatinine's clearance (Cl_{CR}), which may be measured directly or estimated from the serum creatinine level (C_{CR}). In men:

$$Cl_{CR} = \frac{(140 - age) \times weight\ (kg)}{72 \times C_{CR}(mg/d\ L)}\ (mL/min)$$

For women, the estimate by the above equation should be multiplied by 0.85 to reflect their smaller muscle mass. It should also be noted that this equation is not valid for patients with severe renal insufficiency ($C_{CR} < 5$ mg/dL) or when renal function is changing rapidly. For simplicity, normal creatinine clearance is conveniently considered to be 100 mL/min. Thus, if the relative contributions of renal and nonrenal elimination to systemic clearance are known, an appropriate modification of the dose in a patient with a given level of insufficiency can be estimated. For example, if the fraction of drug excreted unchanged is 0.9 and creatinine clearance is reduced to 10% of normal, the dosing rate should be reduced to 19% of normal. This modification,

Table 70-3 Drug Dosing Rate Adjustment in Renal Failure

Drug	Method	Adjustment in Renal Failure GFR, mL/min >50	10–50	<10	Dosage Increase Needed in Dialysis[b]
Allopurinol	D	Unchanged	50%	30%	Yes
	I	24 h	24–36 h	48–72 h	
Carbenicillin	I	8–12 h	12–24 h	24–48 h	Yes
Ciprofloxacin	D	Unchanged	50–75%	50%	No
Cimetidine	D	Unchanged	75%	50%	No
Digoxin	D	Unchanged	25–75%	10–25%	No
Fluconazole	I	24 h	24–48 h	48–72 h	Yes
Gentamycin	D	60–90%	30–70%	20–30%	Yes
	I	8–12 h	12 h	24 h	
Lithium	D	Unchanged	50–75%	25–50%	Yes
Penicillin G	D	Unchanged	75%	25–50%	Yes
	I	6–8 h	8–12 h	12–66 h	
Primidone	I	8	8–12 h	12–24 h	Yes
Procainamide	I	4–6 h	6–12 h	8–24 h	Yes
Tobramycin	D	60–90%	30–70%	20–30%	Yes
	I	8–12 h	12 h	24 h	
Vancomycin	I	24–72 h	72–240 h	240 h	No

[a] D is a dosage method based on administering the indicated percentage of the usual maintenance dose at the usual dosage interval. I indicates a dosage interval extension method of adjusting the dosing rate where the values given are the dosage interval in hours at which the usual maintenance dose is administered.

[b] "Yes" indicates removal of enough drug by dialysis to require a dosage supplement to ensure adequate therapeutic drug concentrations. GFR, glomerular filtration rate

which in practice would be rounded to 20%, is based on the fact that nonrenal clearance is unchanged (10% of normal clearance); renal clearance is reduced from 90% to 9% of normal Cl; thus systemic clearance is reduced to $10 + 9 = 19$% of normal Cl.

In clinical practice today, most decisions involving dosing adjustment in patients with renal failure use published tables of recommended dosage reduction or dosing interval lengthening based on the level of renal function indicated by Cl_{CR}, or similar information provided in the drug "label" (Table 70-3). Such modifications are, however, rigorously based on pharmacokinetic principles and are best used when resulting plasma concentration data and clinical observation are used, as necessary, to further optimize therapy for the individual patient.

Often metabolites of the drug are pharmacologically active or cause toxicity, and renal insufficiency may result in their unanticipated accumulation. Meperidine, for example, is extensively metabolized, and renal failure has little effect on its plasma concentration; however, its metabolite, normeperidine, accumulates above its usual level when renal function is impaired. Because normeperidine has greater convulsant activity than meperidine, this accumulation probably accounts for the signs of central nervous system (CNS) excitation, such as irritability, twitching, and seizures, that appear when multiple doses of meperidine are administered to patients with renal disease.

EFFECTS OF LIVER DISEASE In contrast to the predictable decline in renal clearance of drugs in renal insufficiency, it is not possible to make a general prediction of the effect of liver disease on hepatic biotransformation of drugs (Chap. 292). Rather, the possible effects of hepatitis or cirrhosis range from impaired to increased drug clearance. Even in advanced hepatocellular disease, drug clearance is usually impaired only about two- to fivefold. The extent of such changes, however, cannot be predicted by the common tests of liver function. Consequently, even when it is suspected that drug elimination is altered in liver disease, there is no quantitative basis on which to adjust the dosage regimen other than assessment of clinical response and the concentration of the drug in plasma.

A drug's oral bioavailability may markedly increase in patients with liver disease. This is particularly the case for those drugs that normally are very well extracted by the liver and thus have a high first-pass effect. In addition, the presence of portacaval shunts may further reduce first-pass elimination and lead to higher drug concentrations reaching the systemic circulation, with the increased risk of adverse effects. For example, the oral availability for high first-pass drugs such as morphine, meperidine, midazolam, and nifedipine is almost doubled

in patients with cirrhosis, compared to those with normal liver function. The size of the oral dose of such drugs should, therefore, be reduced in such patients.

EFFECTS OF CIRCULATORY INSUFFICIENCY — CARDIAC FAILURE AND SHOCK Under conditions of decreased tissue perfusion, the cardiac output is redistributed to preserve blood flow to the heart and brain at the expense of other tissues (Chap. 38). As a result, the drug may be distributed into a smaller volume of distribution, higher drug concentrations will be present in the plasma, and the tissues that are best perfused will be exposed to these higher concentrations. If either the brain or heart is sensitive to the drug, an alteration in response will occur.

Furthermore, the decreased perfusion of the kidney and liver may impair drug clearance by these organs, directly or indirectly. Thus, in severe congestive heart failure, in hemorrhagic shock, and in cardiogenic shock, the response to the usual dose of drug may be excessive, and dosage modification may be necessary. For example, the clearance of lidocaine is reduced by about 50% in cardiac failure, and therapeutic plasma levels are achieved at infusion rates only about half those usually required. The volume of distribution of lidocaine is also reduced, meaning that the correct loading dose will be smaller than usual. Similar situations are thought to exist for procainamide, theophylline, and possibly quinidine. Unfortunately, predictors of these types of pharmacokinetic alterations are unavailable. Therefore, loading doses should be conservative, and continued therapy should be monitored closely, following clinical indicators of toxicity and plasma levels.

DISEASE-INDUCED CHANGES IN PLASMA BINDING Many drugs circulate in the plasma partly bound to plasma proteins. Since only the unbound (free) drug can distribute to the site of pharmacologic action, the therapeutic response should be related to the free rather than the total circulating plasma drug concentration. In most cases, the degree of binding is fairly constant across the therapeutic concentration range, so that the total drug levels in plasma can be used as a basis for adjusting dosage without resulting in significant error. However, conditions such as hypoalbuminemia, liver disease, and renal disease can decrease the extent of drug binding, particularly of acidic and neutral drugs so that at any total plasma level there is a greater concentration of free drug than usual and thus a risk of increased response and toxicity. By contrast, conditions that lead to an increased plasma concentration of the acute-phase reactant α_1-acid glycoprotein—such as myocardial infarction, surgery, neoplastic disease, rheumatoid arthritis, and burns—cause an increase in drug binding for the basic drugs, e.g., lidocaine and quinidine, that bind to this macromolecule, resulting in an opposite set of effects. The drugs for which changes in binding are important are those that are normally highly bound to plasma proteins (>90%), because a small alteration in the extent of binding produces a large change in the amount of unbound drug.

For many drugs, elimination and distribution are restricted largely to the unbound fraction, and so a decrease in binding leads to an increase in the clearance and distribution of the drug. The relative magnitudes of these changes are such that the net effect is a shortened half-life.

GENETIC DETERMINANTS OF THE RESPONSE TO DRUGS

Knowledge of the enzyme that catalyzes the predominant pathway of metabolism of a drug provides a basis for understanding the therapeutic consequences of variations in the genotype of that enzyme. For a number of the enzymes that metabolize drugs, there are differences (polymorphisms) in catalytic function that are genetically determined (Chap. 65). *A phenotypic trait or its corresponding gene is said to be polymorphic if there is more than one form of the trait or gene in the population.* Polymorphisms in the function of an enzyme are determined by allelic variants in its gene. Increasingly it is possible to individualize treatment based on analysis of the phenotype and/or genotype of the relevant drug-metabolizing enzyme.

Similarly, polymorphism in the receptor for a drug can determine variability in its pharmacologic effect. Genotyping those drug receptors for which polymorphisms influence response may also assist in individualizing drug therapy.

THIOPURINE S-METHYLTRANSFERASE (TPMT) The metabolism of azathioprine provides an example of the importance of genetic polymorphisms of enzymes. Azathioprine exerts its immunosuppressive action via an active metabolite, 6-mercaptopurine. Within target cells, the major pathway of inactivation of 6-mercaptopurine is by TPMT. Genetic polymorphisms in this enzyme lead to differences in inactivation of 6-mercaptopurine, with corresponding vast differences in the sensitivity of patients to the toxic and therapeutic effects of azathioprine. Homozygotes for alleles encoding inactive TPMT (0.3 to 1% of the population) predictably exhibit severe pancytopenia on standard doses of azathioprine. Heterozygotes for alleles encoding enzymes with deficient TPMT activity also experience more bone marrow suppression on "usual" doses. From a therapeutic standpoint it is likely that the bone marrow suppression in the heterozygotes has influenced the empiric determination of the "usual" dose range of azathioprine and that this results in undertreatment of some of the patients homozygous for the allele encoding a TPMT with full catalytic activity. To detect the TPMT deficient phenotype in patients anticipating therapy with azathioprine, the catalytic function of TPMT may be measured in red blood cells (if no blood or red cell transfusions have been given within 2 months). A high concordance of genotype with phenotype (~95%) suggests that analysis of genotype may be used to individualize dosing and therefore improve treatment with azathioprine (and 6-mercaptopurine) in the future.

ACETYLATION Isoniazid, hydralazine, sulfonamides, procainamide, and a number of other drugs are metabolized by acetylation of a hydrazino or amino group. This reaction is catalyzed by *N*-acetyl transferase-2 (NAT-2), an enzyme in the liver cytosol that transfers an acetyl group from acetyl coenzyme A to the drug. Individuals differ markedly in the rate at which drugs are acetylated, because of polymorphisms in the NAT-2 gene, resulting in a bimodal distribution of the population into "rapid acetylators" and "slow acetylators."

Acetylation phenotype can be determined by measuring the ratio of acetylated to nonacetylated forms of the probe drugs, dapsone, caffeine, or sulfamethazine, in plasma or urine following administration of a test dose of these acetylation substrates. Slow, intermediate, and rapid acetylators may be identified by these methods for phenotyping. It is also possible to identify slow acetylators by genotyping, using genomic DNA obtained from blood leukocytes.

METABOLISM BY CYTOCHROME P450 MONO-OXYGENASES In healthy individuals taking no other medications, the major determinant of the rate of metabolism of drugs by the cytochrome P450 monooxygenases is genetic. Hepatic endoplasmic reticulum contains a family of cytochrome P450 (CYP) isoforms with different substrate specificities. Many drugs undergo oxidative metabolism by more than one isoform, and the steady-state concentrations of such drugs in the plasma is a function of the sum of the activities of these and other metabolizing enzymes. When a drug is metabolized by multiple pathways, the catalytic activities of the participating enzymes are regulated by a number of genes, so that the clearance rates and steady-state concentrations of the drug tend to distribute unimodally within the population. The range of activity may differ markedly ($\geq$tenfold) between different individuals, as is the case for chlorpromazine, and there is no way to predict the rate before beginning therapy.

Certain metabolic pathways show a bimodal or trimodal distribu-

tion of activity, suggesting control by a single gene, and polymorphisms in these genes have been identified. Most individuals are extensive metabolizers (EM phenotype); a smaller group have a lower ability to metabolize the drug (or no ability at all) and are called poor metabolizers (PM phenotype). Heterozygotes for genes encoding the enzymes lacking catalytic activity may be intermediate metabolizers (IM phenotype). And patients with duplicate or multiple copies of the gene may exhibit ultrarapid metabolism. These polymorphisms are of greatest clinical relevance during administration of substrate drugs for which there are no major alternative routes of elimination. The clinical consequences of the PM phenotype will then depend on the resultant accumulation of the drug or occasionally on the absence of generation of active metabolites.

The cytochrome P450 isoform CYP2D6 is polymorphically distributed in the population, and about 8 to 10% of Caucasians are deficient in this enzyme. CYP2D6 represents the main metabolic pathway for a number of drugs, including antiarrhythmic agents (propafenone, flecainide), β-adrenoceptor blockers (timolol, metoprolol, and alprenolol), tricyclic antidepressants (nortriptyline, desipramine, imipramine, clomipramine), neuroleptic drugs (perphenazine, thioridazine, and possibly haloperidol), selective serotonin reuptake inhibitors (fluoxetine and paroxetine), and certain opiates, such as codeine and dextromethorphan. Thus, codeine has a much lower analgesic effect in PM patients because of impaired production of the active metabolite, morphine. Conversely, a patient with duplicate or multiple copies of CYP2D6 will exhibit an exaggerated response to codeine. Patients with the PM phenotype experience more pronounced systemic β-adrenoceptor blockade after the administration of timolol ophthalmic solution. The catalytic activity of CYP2D6 in humans may be assessed by using a test drug, debrisoquin, which is eliminated almost entirely via hydroxylation by CYP2D6. Individuals with the PM phenotype can be identified by genotyping for the alleles that encode proteins with loss of catalytic function. There are ethnic variations in the frequency of the PM phenotype, which occurs in 5 to 10% of Caucasians but with a lesser frequency in Asians (1 to 2%).

The isoform CYP2C19 also exhibits polymorphism; it was initially detected with the hydroxylation of mephenytoin, which is used as a probe drug for the function of this P450 isoform. This enzyme catalyzes the major metabolic pathway of omeprazole, proguanil, diazepam, and citalopram. The impact of the polymorphism in CYP2C19 on treatment outcome is clearly illustrated by omeprazole. The efficacy of omeprazole (20 mg in combination with amoxicillin) in eradicating *Helicobacter pylori* is markedly reduced in persons with the homozygous EM genotype (29% cured) as compared with 100% cure in those with homozygous PM genotype. This reflects the relative lack of effect of the recommended dose of omeprazole (20 mg) on gastric acid secretion and ulcer healing in patients with the CYP2C19 EM genotype. Certainly knowledge of a patient's CYP2C19 genotype would improve therapy with this proton pump inhibitor. Impaired hydroxylation of mephenytoin is present in only 3 to 5 percent of Caucasians, but the incidence is about 20 percent in individuals of Japanese and Chinese descent.

CYP2C9 catalyzes the major pathways of metabolism of warfarin and phenytoin. There are allelic variants of the gene for this enzyme that encode proteins with loss of catalytic function. These variant alleles are associated with requirement for a very low dose of warfarin, difficulties in initiating warfarin therapy, and an increased risk of bleeding complications. Similarly, high concentrations of phenytoin in plasma and resulting adverse effects of phenytoin occur in patients with loss of function alleles for CYP2C9.

Polymorphisms in drug-metabolizing ability may be associated with large differences in the disposition of a drug among individuals, especially when the involved pathway makes a major contribution to the elimination of the drug. For example, the clearance of mephenytoin given orally differs 100- to 200-fold between individuals of the EM and PM phenotypes. As a result, the peak plasma concentrations and bioavailability after oral administration are much higher, and the rate of drug elimination much lower, in PM than in EM individuals. In PM individuals, the result is excessive drug accumulation and exaggerated pharmacologic responses, including toxicity, when usual drug dosages are administered. Individualization of drug therapy is especially critical for drugs that exhibit polymorphic drug metabolism. The increasing availability of laboratory methods to identify the PM phenotype for NAT-2, CYP2D6, and CYP2C19 by genotyping should be useful for this purpose.

INTERINDIVIDUAL VARIABILITY IN THE MOLECULAR TARGETS WITH WHICH DRUGS INTERACT The increasing emphasis on identifying molecular mechanisms of disease (Chap. 65) has important consequences for further understanding a genetic basis for individual variability in drug actions. As molecular approaches identify the role of specific gene products in human physiology, polymorphisms that alter expression or function of those gene products are being recognized; it is estimated that such polymorphisms occur in 1 in 1000 bp in the human genome. These genes in turn, are now being recognized as the molecular targets with which available and new drugs interact to produce beneficial and adverse effects.

Genome-wide searches in families with premature Alzheimer's disease identified the *APOE* locus as linked to the disease (Chap. 362). Specifically, the *E4* allele of the *APOE* gene appears associated with a worse prognosis, and this is thought to relate to reduced expression of choline acetyl transferase. Further, a therapeutic response to the choline acetyl transferase inhibitor, tacrine, appears to be more common with the prognostically more benign *APOE2* or *APOE3* alleles. Multiple polymorphisms identified in the β_2-adrenergic receptor appear to be linked to specific phenotypes in asthma and congestive heart failure, diseases in which β_2-receptor function might be expected to determine prognosis. It has been suggested that polymorphisms in the β_2 receptor may be a determinant of response to inhaled β_2-receptor agonists.

The development of marked QT prolongation and the polymorphic ventricular tachycardia, *torsade de pointes* (Chap. 230), in response to certain action potential–prolonging drugs such as quinidine used to be characterized as an "idiosyncratic" response. Advances in understanding the molecular basis of normal cardiac repolarization have resulted in identification of genes encoding ion channel proteins, the molecules whose normal function results in physiologic cardiac repolarization. Mutations in these genes cause congenital arrhythmia syndromes, such as the long QT syndrome, and block of ion channels is a common mechanism whereby drugs prolong QT intervals. Patients with mutations in these genes that remain subclinical until challenge with drugs are now recognized. In summary, continuing efforts to unravel the molecular basis of disease are likely also to provide insights into determinants of the response to drug therapy.

DRUG USE IN THE ELDERLY (See also Chap. 9) Aging results in changes in organ function, especially of the organs involved in drug disposition, as well as alterations in body size and composition. Not surprisingly, therefore, pharmacokinetics are often different in elderly individuals than in younger adults. Also, elderly patients often have multiple diseases and may therefore be taking a large number of drugs. Consequently, drug interactions, as well as an increased vulnerability to morbidity and mortality, contribute to the higher incidence of adverse drug reactions in elderly patients. Increased sensitivity of target organs and impairment of physiologic control systems, such as those involved in the regulation of the circulation, may also be a factor. Accordingly, optimization of drug therapy in the elderly, particularly in frail patients, is often difficult, as a variety of factors (often poorly defined) accentuate the usual interindividual variability in drug response.

Although many individuals preserve good renal function into old age, elderly patients as a group have an increased likelihood of impaired renal excretion of drugs. Even in the absence of kidney disease, renal clearance is generally reduced by about 35 to 50% in elderly

patients. Dosage adjustments analogous to those in patients with renal dysfunction (see above) are therefore necessary for drugs that are eliminated mainly by the kidneys, such as digoxin, aminoglycosides, lithium, and other drugs listed in Table 70-3. In this regard, it is important to recognize that the reduced muscle mass of older individuals results in a reduced rate of creatinine production; thus, a normal serum creatinine concentration can be present even though creatinine clearance is impaired.

Aging also results in a decrease in the size of and blood flow to the liver and possibly in the activity of hepatic drug-metabolizing enzymes; accordingly, the hepatic clearance of some drugs is impaired in the elderly. Unfortunately, no consistent pattern of clinical application appears to be present. Moreover, the changes are often modest relative to other causes for interindividual variability in these patients. However, even a small reduction in hepatic extraction may significantly increase the oral bioavailability of drugs with a high first-pass effect, such as propranolol and labetalol.

Impaired clearance and/or increased distribution may cause the elimination half-life of a drug to increase with aging. Thus, if a dosage modification in an elderly patient is required, it is often possible to accomplish it by decreasing the frequency of drug administration, possibly along with a reduction in dose.

Even if the pharmacokinetics of a drug are not altered, an elderly patient may require a smaller dosage because of an increase in pharmacodynamic sensitivity. Examples include increased analgesic effects of opioids, increased sedation from benzodiazepines and other CNS depressants, and increased risk of bleeding while receiving anticoagulant therapy, even when clotting parameters are well controlled. Exaggerated responses to cardiovascular drugs are also common because of the impaired responsiveness of normal homeostatic mechanisms. Such age-related changes require close monitoring of the patient's clinical response and appropriate dosage titration. Accordingly, in the elderly, initial doses should be less than the usual adult dosage and should be increased slowly. The final therapeutic regimen should be as simple as possible, and the number of different drugs used should be kept as low as possible. Also, because interindividual variability in drug responsiveness is greater in geriatric patients than in younger adults, individualization of therapy is even more critical.

INTERACTIONS BETWEEN DRUGS

The effect of some drugs can be altered markedly by the administration of other agents. Such interactions can complicate therapy by adversely increasing or decreasing the action of a drug. Drug interactions must be considered in the differential diagnosis of unexpected responses to drugs, and it should be recognized that patients often come to the physician with a legacy of drugs acquired during previous medical experiences. A meticulous drug history will minimize such unknown elements. It should include examination of the patient's medications and, if necessary, calls to the pharmacist to identify prescriptions. It should also address the use agents not often volunteered on initial questioning, such as over-the-counter drugs, health food supplements, and topical agents such as eye drops.

There are two principal types of interactions between drugs. In *pharmacokinetic interactions*, the delivery of a drug to its site of action is altered, whereas in *pharmacodynamic interactions*, the responsiveness of the target organ or system is modified.

An index of the drug interactions discussed in this chapter is provided in Table 70-4. The table includes interactions that have verified significance in patients, plus a few that are so potentially dangerous that cognizance should be taken of the experimental data or case reports suggesting they occur.

I. PHARMACOKINETIC INTERACTIONS CAUSING DIMINISHED DRUG DELIVERY A. Impaired Gastrointestinal Absorption Examples include aluminum ions, present in antacids, which form insoluble chelates with the tetracyclines, preventing absorption of these drugs. Ferrous ions similarly block tetracycline absorption. Kaolin-pectin suspensions bind digoxin, and when these substances are administered together, digoxin absorption is reduced by about one-half. However, when kaolin-pectin is administered 2 h after digoxin, digoxin absorption is unaffected.

Ketoconazole is a weak base that dissolves well only at acidic pH. Histamine H_2 receptor antagonists, such as ranitidine and cimetidine, reduce gastric acidity and thus impair the dissolution and absorption of ketoconazole. By contrast, the absorption of fluconazole is not impaired by an increase in gastric pH.

B. Induction of Hepatic Drug-Metabolizing Enzymes When a drug is eliminated largely by metabolism, an increase in the rate of its metabolism reduces its availability to sites of action. Most drugs are metabolized largely in the liver because of this organ's large mass, high blood flow, and high concentration of drug metabolizing enzymes. The first step in the metabolism of many drugs is catalyzed by a group of cytochrome P450 mixed-function oxidases located in the endoplasmic reticulum (see "Metabolism by Cytochrome P450 Monooxygenases," above). These enzyme systems oxidize drug molecules by a variety of reactions, including aromatic hydroxylations, N-demethylations, O-demethylations, and sulfoxidations. The products of these reactions are usually more polar than the parent compound (and more readily excreted by the kidney).

The expression of some of the mixed-function oxidase (CYP) isoforms is regulated, and their content in the liver can be increased, by a number of drugs. Phenobarbital is the prototype of these inducers, and all the barbiturates in clinical use increase CYP enzyme activity. Induction with phenobarbital can occur with doses of as little as 60 mg daily. Mixed-function oxidases are also induced by rifampin, carbamazepine, phenytoin, and glutethimide and by smoking, exposure to chlorinated insecticides such as DDT, and chronic alcohol ingestion.

Phenobarbital, rifampin, and other inducers lower plasma levels of many drugs, including warfarin, quinidine, mexiletine, verapamil, ketoconazole, itraconazole, cyclosporine, dexamethasone, methylprednisolone, prednisolone (the active metabolite of prednisone), oral contraceptive steroids, methadone, metronidazole, and metyrapone. These interactions all have obvious clinical significance. In the case of the coumarin anticoagulants, the patient is placed at major risk if the appropriate level of anticoagulation is achieved when an inducer is also being administered and the inducer is later discontinued (for example, at discharge from the hospital). The plasma levels of the coumarin anticoagulant will rise as the induction effect wears off, leading to excessive anticoagulation. There is considerable variation among individuals in the extent to which drug metabolism can be induced.

C. Inhibition of Cellular Uptake or Binding The guanidinium antihypertensive agents guanethidine and guanadrel are transported to their site of action in adrenergic neurons by an energy-requiring membrane transport system for biogenic monoamines; the physiologic function of this system is reuptake of the adrenergic neurotransmitter. Inhibitors of norepinephrine uptake prevent the uptake of the guanidinium antihypertensive agents into adrenergic neurons and thereby block their pharmacologic effects. The tricyclic antidepressants are potent inhibitors of norepinephrine uptake. Consequently, concomitant administration of clinical doses of tricyclic antidepressants, including desipramine, protriptyline, nortriptyline, and amitriptyline, almost totally abolishes the antihypertensive effects of

Table 70-4 Drug Interaction Index

Drug	Section of Chapter Describing Interaction	Drug	Section of Chapter Describing Interaction
Allopurinol	IIA	6-Mercaptopurine	IIA
Amiloride	III	Methadone	IB
Amiodarone	IIA, IIB	Methotrexate	IIB
Amphetamine	IC	Methylprednisolone	IB, IIA
Antidepressants, tricyclic (desipramine, nortriptyline, imipramine, doxepin, protriptyline, amitriptyline)	IC	Metronidazole	IB, IIA
		Metyrapone	IB
		Mexiletine	IB
		Nicardipine	IIA
Aspirin	IIB, III	Nifedipine	IIA
Atorvastatin	IIA	Nitrates	III
Azathioprine	IIA	Nonsteroidal anti-inflammatory drugs	III
Barbiturates (class)	IB		
Carbamazepine	IB, IIA		
Chlorpromazine	IC, IIA	Oral contraceptive steroids	IB
Cholestyramine	IA		
Cimetidine	IA, IIA, IIB	Phenobarbital	IB
Cisapride	IIA	Phenylbutazone	IIA, IIB
Clofibrate	IIA	Phenytoin (diphenylhydantoin)	IB, IIA
Clonidine	IC		
Codeine	IIA	Piroxicam	III
Cotrimoxazole	IIA	Potassium	III
Cyclosporine	IB, IIA, IIB	Prednisone	IB
Dexamethasone	IB	Probenecid	IIB
Digoxin	IA, IIB	Procainamide	IIB
Diltiazem	IIA	Propranolol	III
Diuretics	III	Quinidine	IB, IIA, IIB, III
Ephedrine	IC	Ranitidine	IA, IIA
Erythromycin	IIA	Rifampin	IA, IB
Ethanol	IIA	Salicylate	IIB
Fluconazole	IIA	Sildenafil	III
Fluoxetine	IIA	Simvastatin	IIA
Guanadrel	IC	Spironolactone	III
Guanethidine	IC	Tetracycline	IA
Haloperidol	IIA	Theophylline	IIA
Indomethacin	III	Thiazide diuretics	III
Isoniazid	IIA	Tolbutamide	IIA
Itraconazole	IB, IIA, IIB	Triamterene	III
Kaolin-pectin	IA	Triazolam	IIA
Ketoconazole	IA, IB, IIA	Verapamil	IB, IIA, IIB
Lidocaine	IIA	Warfarin	IB, IIA, III
Lovastatin	IIA		

guanethidine and guanadrel. Although they are less potent inhibitors of norepinephrine uptake, doxepin and chlorpromazine produce dose-related antagonism of the action of the guanidinium antihypertensives.

The antihypertensive effect of clonidine is partially antagonized by tricyclic antidepressants. Clonidine lowers arterial pressure by reducing sympathetic outflow from the blood pressure–regulating centers in the hindbrain (Chap. 246). This central hypotensive action is antagonized by the tricyclic antidepressants.

II. PHARMACOKINETIC INTERACTIONS CAUSING INCREASED DRUG DELIVERY   A. Inhibition of Drug Metabolism If the active form of a drug is eliminated largely by biotransformation, inhibition of its metabolism leads to reduced clearance, prolonged half-life, and accumulation of the drug during maintenance therapy. Excessive accumulation due to inhibited metabolism can lead to adverse effects.

Cimetidine is a potent inhibitor of the oxidative metabolism of many drugs, including warfarin, quinidine, nifedipine, lidocaine, theophylline, and phenytoin. Adverse reactions, many of them severe, have resulted from the administration of these drugs in conjunction with cimetidine. Cimetidine is a more potent inhibitor of mixed-function oxidases than ranitidine, whereas ranitidine is more potent as a histamine H_2 receptor antagonist. Famotidine and nizatidine are not known to produce clinically appreciable inhibition of drug metabolism.

Knowledge of the CYP isoforms that catalyze the main pathway of metabolism of a drug provides a basis for predicting and understanding drug interactions. For example, the CYP3A subfamily of isoforms catalyzes the metabolism of many drugs for which blockage of metabolism results in toxicity. Drugs that depend on CYP3A as a major route of metabolism include cyclosporine, quinidine, lovastatin, simvastatin, atorvastatin, nifedipine, lidocaine, cisapride, erythromycin, methylprednisolone, carbamazepine, midazolam, and triazolam.

The antifungal agents ketoconazole and itraconazole are potent inhibitors of enzymes in the CYP3A family. When fluconazole levels are elevated as a result of higher doses and/or renal insufficiency, this drug can also inhibit CYP3A. The macrolide antibiotics erythromycin and clarithromycin inhibit CYP3A4 to a clinically significant extent, but azithromycin does not inhibit this enzyme. Some of the calcium antagonists, diltiazem, nicardipine, and verapamil can also inhibit CYP3A, as can some of its other substrates, such as cyclosporine.

Cyclosporine can cause serious toxicity when its metabolism is inhibited by erythromycin, ketoconazole, diltiazem, nicardipine, or verapamil. A serious complication of HMG-CoA reductase inhibitors is myopathy. Fortunately, this is infrequent except in the context of interactions of a subset of the HMG-CoA reductase inhibitors with other drugs, particularly those that inhibit CYP3A4. The disposition of lovastatin is reduced markedly by drugs that inhibit CYP3A4, causing increases in plasma levels by more than tenfold. As a consequence, lovastatin has produced severe myopathy with rhabdomyolysis when administered together with erythromycin or cyclosporine. Not all of the HMG-CoA reductase inhibitors are as dependent on CYP3A4 for disposition as is lovastatin. Blocking CYP3A4 causes moderate elevations of plasma levels of simvastatin and atorvastatin (increases of severalfold), whereas elevations of the levels of fluvastatin and cerivastatin are only slight. Pravastatin disposition and plasma levels are not altered by inhibitors of CYP3A4. Cisapride can cause polymorphic ventricular tachycardia (torsade de pointes) when its metabolism is blocked by inhibitors of CYP3A, such as ketoconazole, itraconazole, clarithromycin, and erythromycin.

Whenever an inhibitor of CYP3A4 is administered to a patient, the physician should be alert to the possibility of serious interactions with drugs that are metabolized by CYP3A.

The CYP2D6 isoform that catalyzes the polymorphic metabolism of debrisoquin is markedly inhibited by quinidine and is also blocked by a number of neuroleptic drugs, such as chlorpromazine and haloperidol, and by fluoxetine. The analgesic effect of codeine depends on its metabolism to morphine via CYP2D6 in individuals with the EM phenotype. Thus, quinidine reduces the analgesic efficacy of codeine in EMs. Since desipramine is cleared largely by metabolism via CYP2D6 in EMs, its levels are increased substantially by concurrent administration of quinidine, fluoxetine, or the neuroleptic drugs that inhibit CYP2D6.

Some drugs are inactivated by mechanisms other than the hepatic drug-metabolizing enzymes. Azathioprine is converted in the body to an active metabolite, 6-mercaptopurine, which in turn is oxidized by xanthine oxidase to 6-thiouric acid. When allopurinol, a potent inhibitor of xanthine oxidase, is administered concurrently with standard doses of azathioprine or 6-mercaptopurine, life-threatening toxicity (bone marrow suppression) can result.

Other drugs that inhibit biotransformation of pharmacologic compounds (with examples of drugs whose metabolism is blocked by the inhibitor listed in parenthesis) include:

- Amiodarone (warfarin, quinidine)
- Clofibrate (phenytoin, tolbutamide)
- Excessive ingestion of ethanol (warfarin)
- Isoniazid (phenytoin)
- Metronidazole, cotrimoxazole (warfarin)
- Phenylbutazone (warfarin, phenytoin, tolbutamide)

B.   Inhibition of Drug Transport   Specific molecules that transport drugs into and out of cells are increasingly recognized, and

inhibition of their function can be a major cause of clinically important drug interactions. The best studied to date is P-glycoprotein, originally isolated from tumor cells displaying resistance to multiple, structurally unrelated anticancer agents. The mechanism underlying this "multidrug resistance" phenomenon is P-glycoprotein-mediated pumping of anticancer agents out of cells, thereby inhibiting their anticancer effects. P-glycoprotein is also expressed in normal tissues (the luminal aspect of intestinal and renal tubular cells, the canalicular aspect of hepatocytes, the capillary endothelium of the blood-brain barrier), where it is responsible for efflux of not only antineoplastics but also digoxin and HIV protease inhibitors. Quinidine inhibits P-glycoprotein function in vitro, and it now seems apparent that the widely recognized doubling of plasma digoxin when quinidine is coadministered reflects this action in vivo, particularly since the effects of quinidine (increased digoxin bioavailability and reduced renal and hepatic secretion) occur at the sites of P-glycoprotein expression. Many other drugs also elevate digoxin concentrations (e.g., amiodarone, verapamil, cyclosporine, itraconazole, and erythromycin), and a similar mechanism seems likely. Reduced CNS penetration of multiple HIV protease inhibitors (with the attendant risk of facilitating a sanctuary site for the virus) appears attributable to P-glycoprotein-mediated exclusion of the drug from the CNS.

A number of drugs are secreted by the renal tubular transport systems for organic anions. Inhibition of this tubular transport system can cause excessive accumulation of a drug. Phenylbutazone, probenecid, and salicylates competitively inhibit this transport system. Salicylate, for example, reduces the renal clearance of methotrexate, an interaction that may lead to methotrexate toxicity. Renal tubular secretion contributes substantially to the elimination of penicillin, which can be inhibited by probenecid.

Inhibition of the tubular cation transport system by cimetidine impedes the renal clearance of procainamide and its active metabolite N-acetylprocainamide.

III.   PHARMACODYNAMIC AND OTHER INTERACTIONS BETWEEN DRUGS   Therapeutically useful interactions occur in which the effect of two drugs in combination is greater than the sum of their effects when used individually. Favorable drug combinations are described in specific therapeutic sections in this text, and this section focuses on interactions that create unwanted effects. Two drugs may act on separate components of a common process to yield effects greater than either has alone. For example, although small doses of aspirin (<1 g daily) do not alter the prothrombin time appreciably in patients who are receiving warfarin therapy, aspirin nevertheless increases the risk of bleeding in these patients because it inhibits platelet aggregation. Thus the combination of impaired functions of platelets and the clotting system, while useful for some therapeutic purposes, also increases the potential for hemorrhagic complications in patients receiving warfarin therapy.

Nonsteroidal antiinflammatory drugs (NSAIDs) cause gastric and duodenal ulcers, and, in patients treated with warfarin, the risk of bleeding from a peptic ulcer is increased almost threefold by concomitant use of a NSAID. This clearly is a serious drug interaction.

Indomethacin, piroxicam, and probably other NSAIDs antagonize the antihypertensive effects of β-adrenergic receptor blockers, diuretics, ACE inhibitors, and other drugs. The resulting elevation in blood pressure ranges from trivial to severe. Aspirin and sulindac, however, do not elevate the blood pressure in treated hypertensive patients.

Polymorphic ventricular tachycardia (torsade de pointes) during quinidine administration occurs much more frequently in patients receiving diuretics, probably owing to potassium and/or magnesium depletion.

The administration of supplemental potassium leads to more frequent and more severe hyperkalemia when potassium elimination is reduced by concurrent treatment with ACE inhibitors, spironolactone, amiloride, or triamterene.

The pharmacologic effects of sildenafil result from inhibition of the phosphodiesterase type 5 isoform that inactivates cyclic GMP in the vasculature. Nitroglycerin and related nitrates produce vasodilation by elevating cyclic GMP. Thus, coadministration of these nitrates with sildenafil will cause profound and potentially catastrophic hypotension.

CONCENTRATION OF DRUGS IN PLASMA AS A GUIDE TO THERAPY

In many cases, the plasma concentration of a drug is measured as a guide in the individualization of therapy. Genetic variation in elimination rates, interactions with other drugs, disease-induced alterations in elimination and distribution, and other factors combine to yield a wide range of plasma levels in patients given the same dose. Furthermore, the problem of noncompliance with prescribed regimens during continuing therapy is an endemic and elusive cause of therapeutic failure (see below). Clinical indicators assist in the titration of some drugs into the desired range, but no chemical determination is a substitute for careful observations of the response to treatment. However, the therapeutic and adverse effects are not precisely quantifiable for all drugs, and, in complex clinical situations, estimates of the action of a drug may be misleading. For example, previously existing neurologic disease may obscure the neurologic consequences of intoxication with phenytoin. Because clearance, half-life, accumulation, and steady-state plasma levels are difficult to predict, the measurement of plasma levels is often useful as a guide to the optimal dose. This is particularly true when there is a narrow range between the plasma levels yielding therapeutic and adverse effects. For drugs having such characteristics— e.g., digoxin, theophylline, lidocaine, aminoglycosides, cyclosporine, and anticonvulsants—dose optimization should involve modification of the standard dose on the basis of the pharmacokinetic principles described above. In certain instances, predictive nomograms and algorithms have been developed to facilitate the necessary modifications. However, the most flexible and accurate method for individualizing drug dosage appears to be a feedback approach using a small number of previously obtained plasma levels and Bayesian forecasting. In controlled studies, this type of computer-assisted dosing has been shown to improve patient care. However, the overall cost/benefit ratio of such methods in routine management still remains to be concusively demonstrated.

For drugs with a narrow therapeutic window that exhibit first-order elimination, then, dosage adjustments may be made on the assumption that the average, maximum, and minimum steady-state concentrations are related linearly to the dosing rate. Accordingly, the dose may be adjusted on the basis of the ratio between the desired and measured concentrations:

$$\frac{C_{ss} \text{ (desired)}}{C_{ss} \text{ (measured)}} = \frac{\text{dose (new)}}{\text{dose (previous)}}$$

For drugs that have dose-dependent kinetics (e.g., phenytoin and theophylline), plasma concentrations change disproportionately more than the alteration in the dosing rate. Not only should changes in dose be small to minimize the degree of unpredictability, but plasma concentration monitoring is also critical to ensure appropriate modification.

The variability among individual responses to given plasma levels must be recognized. This is illustrated by a hypothetical population concentration-response curve (Fig. 70-4) and its relationship to the therapeutic range or therapeutic window of desired plasma levels. The defined therapeutic window should include the levels at which the intended pharmacologic effect is achieved in most patients. However, a few persons, who are sensitive to the therapeutic effects, respond to lower levels, whereas others are refractory enough to require levels that may cause adverse effects. For example, a few patients with strong seizure foci require plasma levels of phenytoin exceeding 20 μg/mL to control seizures. Dosages to achieve this effect may be appropriate if tolerated.

As also illustrated in Fig. 70-4, some patients are prone to adverse

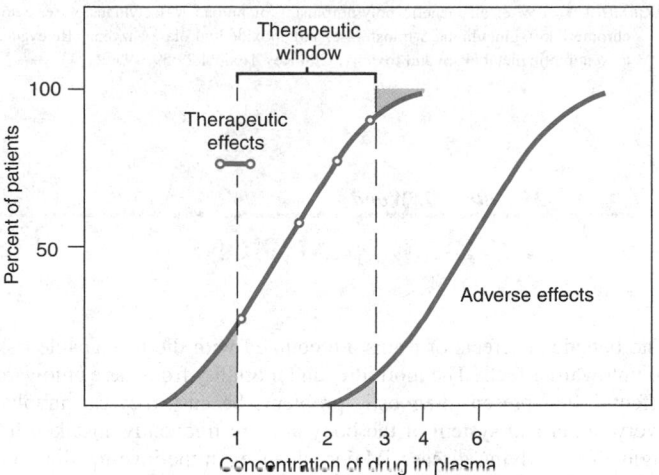

FIGURE 70-4 The cumulative percentage of patients responding to increasing levels of drug in plasma with both therapeutic and adverse effects. The therapeutic window defines the range of concentrations of drug that will achieve therapeutic effects in most patients with adverse effects in only a small percentage.

effects at levels that are tolerated by most of the population. Therefore, raising the plasma concentration of a drug to a level that has a high probability of being therapeutically effective may bring on unwanted actions in an occasional patient. Table 70-2 presents for a number of drugs the plasma concentrations that are associated with adverse and therapeutic effects in most patients. Use of this information according to the guidelines discussed should permit more effective and safer therapy for those patients who are not "average."

EFFECTIVE PARTICIPATION OF THE PATIENT IN THERAPY Measurement of the concentration of a drug in plasma is the most effective way to detect failure to take a drug. Such "noncompliance" is a frequent problem in the long-term treatment of diseases such as hypertension and epilepsy, occurring in 25% or more of patients in therapeutic environments in which no special effort is made to involve patients in the responsibility for their own health. Occasionally, noncompliance can be uncovered by sympathetic, nonincriminating questioning, but more often it is recognized only after determining that the concentration of drug in plasma is nil or is recurrently low. Because other factors can cause plasma levels to be lower than expected, comparison with levels obtained during inpatient treatment may be required to confirm that noncompliance has occurred. Once the physician is certain of noncompliance, a nonaccusatory discussion of the problem with the patient may clarify the reason for the noncompliance and serve as a basis for more effective cooperation on the part of the patient. Many approaches have been tried to help patients exercise more responsibility for their own treatment, most based on better communication regarding the nature of the disease and the chances of success or failure of the treatment. The patient is given a chance to discuss problems associated with treatment. The process may be improved by the involvement of nurses and other paramedical personnel. Minimizing the complexity of the regimen is helpful in terms of both the number of drugs and the frequency of administration. Educating patients to assume the principal role in their own health care requires a blend of the art and science of medicine.

BIBLIOGRAPHY

BENET LZ et al: Design and optimization of dosage regimens: Pharmacokinetic data, in *Goodman and Gilman's The Pharmacological Basis of Therapeutics*, 9th ed, JG Hardman et al (eds). New York, McGraw-Hill, 1995, Appendix II, p 1707

HOLFORD N (ed): *Clinical Pharmacokinetics—Drug Data Handbook*, 3d ed. Adis International, Auckland, New Zealand, 1998

REYNOLDS DJ, ARONSON JK: ABCs of monitoring drug therapy. Making the most of plasma drug concentration measurements. BMJ 306:48, 1993

WORMHOUDT LW et al: Genetic polymorphisms of human *N*-acetyltransferase, cytochrome P450, glutathione-*S*-transferase, and epoxide hydrolase enzymes: Relevance to xenobiotic metabolism and toxicity. Clin Rev Toxicol 29:59, 1999

71   *Alastair J. J. Wood*

ADVERSE REACTIONS TO DRUGS

The beneficial effects of drugs are coupled with the inescapable risk of untoward effects. The morbidity and mortality from these untoward effects often present diagnostic problems because they can involve every organ and system of the body and are frequently mistaken for signs of underlying disease. Major advances in the investigation, development, and regulation of drugs ensure in most instances that they are uniform, effective, and relatively safe and that their recognized hazards are publicized. However, prior to regulatory approval and marketing, new drugs are tested in relatively few patients who tend to be less sick and to have fewer concomitant diseases than those patients who subsequently receive the drug therapeutically. Because of the relatively small number of patients studied in clinical trials, and the selected nature of these patients, rare adverse effects may not be detected prior to a drug's approval, and physicians therefore need to be cautious in the prescription of new drugs and alert for the appearance of previously unrecognized adverse events.

The large number and variety of drugs available over the counter (OTC), herbal preparations, and by prescription, make it impossible for patient or physician to obtain or retain the knowledge necessary to use all drugs well. It is understandable, therefore, that many OTC drugs are used unwisely by the public and that restricted drugs may be prescribed incorrectly by physicians.

Most physicians use no more than 50 drug products in their practice, gaining familiarity with their effectiveness and safety. Most patients probably use only a limited number of OTC drugs. Nevertheless, many patients receive care and drug prescriptions from more than one physician, and in any 30-day period, many patients consume more than three different OTC drug products containing nine or more different chemical agents.

Some 25 to 50% of patients make errors in self-administration of prescribed medicines, and these errors can be responsible for adverse drug effects. Elderly patients are the group most likely to commit such errors, perhaps in part because they consume more medicines. One-third or more of patients also may not take their prescribed medications. Similarly, patients commit errors in taking OTC drugs by not reading or following the directions on the containers. Physicians must recognize that providing directions with prescriptions does not always guarantee compliance.

Every drug can produce untoward consequences, even when used according to standard or recommended methods of administration. When used incorrectly, the effectiveness may be reduced, and adverse reactions can be expected to occur more frequently. Also, the administration of several drugs concurrently may result in adverse drug interactions (Chap. 70). In the hospital, all drugs a patient is given should be under the control of a physician, and patient compliance is, in general, ensured. Errors may occur nevertheless—the wrong drug or dose may be given, or the drug may be given to the wrong patient—although improved drug distribution and administration systems have reduced this problem. On the other hand, there are no easy means for controlling how ambulatory patients take prescription or OTC drugs.

EPIDEMIOLOGY   Epidemiologic studies of adverse drug reactions have been helpful in evaluating the magnitude of the overall problem, in calculating the rate of reactions to individual drugs, and in characterizing some of the determinants of adverse drug effects.

Patients receive, on average, 10 different drugs during each hospitalization. The sicker the patient, the more drugs are given, and there is a corresponding increase in the likelihood of adverse drug reactions. When fewer than 6 different drugs are given to hospitalized patients, the probability of an adverse reaction is about 5%, but if more than 15 drugs are given, the probability is over 40%. Retrospective analyses of ambulatory patients have revealed adverse drug effects in 20%.

Thus, the magnitude of drug-induced disease is large. Of patients admitted to the medical and pediatric services of general hospitals, 2 to 5% are admitted because of illnesses attributed to drugs. The case/fatality ratio from drug-induced disease in hospitalized patients varies from 2 to 12%. Furthermore, some fetal or neonatal abnormalities are due to medicines taken by the mother during pregnancy or parturition.

A small group of widely used drugs accounts for a disproportionate number of reactions. Aspirin and other nonsteroidal anti-inflammatory drugs, analgesics, digoxin, anticoagulants, diuretics, antimicrobials, glucocorticoids, antineoplastics, and hypoglycemic agents account for 90% of reactions, although the drugs involved differ between ambulatory and hospitalized patients. Estimates of the cost of drug-related morbidity and mortality in the ambulatory setting range from $30 billion to $130 billion.

ADVERSE DRUG REACTIONS IN THE ELDERLY (See also Chap. 9)   The elderly as a group have a greater burden of disease and receive a greater number of medications than other persons. Thus, it is not surprising that adverse drug reactions occur frequently in elderly patients. The issue of whether an elderly individual is more likely to develop an adverse drug reaction than a young person with a similar number of concurrent diseases and taking the same number of drugs has not been answered unequivocally. However, in population surveys of the noninstitutionalized elderly, as many as 10% report having had at least one adverse drug reaction in the last year. The incidence appears to be even greater in hospitalized elderly patients. Although it is widely believed that the elderly are more sensitive to drugs than the young, that is not true for all drugs. For example, a consistent decrease in sensitivity to drugs acting at the β-adrenergic receptor has been demonstrated in the elderly. The consequences of adverse drug effects may differ in the elderly because of their greater likelihood of other disease. For example, use of long–half-life benzodiazepines is linked to the occurrence of hip fractures in elderly patients, perhaps reflecting both a risk of falls from these drugs and the increased incidence of osteoporosis in elderly patients. Even when a drug impairs function similarly in patients of different age groups, the poorer baseline function in elderly persons may put them at greater risk for an adverse drug reaction. When prescribing for an elderly patient, the possibility that hepatic or renal mechanisms of drug excretion may be impaired should be taken into account. Adverse drug effects in the elderly may be subtle and, as in all populations, the physician must be alert to the possibility that a patient's signs and symptoms reflect an adverse effect of medication.

ETIOLOGY   Most adverse drug reactions are preventable, and recent studies using a systems analysis approach suggest that the most common system failure associated with an adverse drug reaction is the failure to disseminate knowledge about drugs to individuals involved in prescribing and administering them. Most adverse reactions can be classified into two groups. The most frequent ones result from an exaggeration of a predicted pharmacologic action of the drug. Other adverse reactions ensue from toxic effects unrelated to the intended pharmacologic actions. The latter effects are often unpredictable, are frequently severe, and result from recognized as well as undiscovered mechanisms. Some mechanisms unrelated to the drug's primary pharmacologic activity may include direct cytotoxicity, initiation of abnormal immune responses, and perturbation of metabolic processes in individuals with genetic enzymatic defects. Further understanding of interindividual differences in the expression of the enzymes responsible for drug metabolism has contributed to the understanding of adverse drug reactions that previously were thought to be idiosyncratic (see below). Prior consideration of the factors known to modify drug action often make it possible to prevent adverse reactions of this type.

Genetic Variations in Drug Oxidation by Cytochromes   There is considerable interindividual variability in drug metabolism, resulting in variability in drug concentrations (Chap. 70). The majority of drugs are oxidized by cytochrome P450s (CYP) in the liver and gut. Some of these enzymes exhibit genetic polymorphisms resulting in enzymes with absent or reduced drug metabolizing activity, which may result in concentration-dependent toxicity. Conversely, where toxicity or pharmacologic effect is produced by a metabolite, individuals with low enzyme activity may have reduced drug effect whereas those with genetically determined increased enzyme activity will have increased drug effect. Examples of such polymorphically distributed oxidation enzymes include CYP2D6, CYP2C9, and CYP2C19.

The clinical consequences of the poor metabolizer phenotype are now becoming clearer and depend on the specific consequences of excessive drug concentrations. For example, the more potent (S) isomer of warfarin is metabolized by the polymorphically distributed enzyme CYP2C9, resulting in lower (S) warfarin clearance and higher concentrations in both heterozygotes and homozygotes for the allelic variants associated with reduced enzyme activity. Recently, the clinical consequences of this polymorphism have been demonstrated in patients followed in an anticoagulant clinic. Patients who were stabilized on warfarin doses of 1.5 mg/d or less had an increased frequency of the genotypes associated with low warfarin metabolism compared to either community controls or patients requiring higher doses of warfarin (Table 71-1). In addition, the group stabilized on low-dose warfarin had a greater incidence of initial over-anticoagulation and hemorrhage than the group on the higher dose. This serves as an example of how genetic variations of a cytochrome P450 enzyme alter the response to a drug.

The oral hypoglycemic glipizide is also metabolized by CYP2C9, and excessively low blood glucose concentrations occur after usual doses in genetic CYP2C9 poor metabolizers. Another oral hypoglycemic, phenformin, produced lactic acidosis in some patients. It is now recognized that phenformin is metabolized by another polymorphically distributed oxidative enzyme, CYP2D6. Patients who have genetically determined low activity of CYP2D6 may be at particular risk from phenformin-induced lactic acidosis.

Genotypically determined variability in drug toxicity may also occur with drugs metabolized by enzymes other than cytochrome P450s. Such toxicity can be severe with the clinical use of the antimetabolites azathioprine and 6-mercaptopurine (to which it is converted in vivo). The cytotoxic thioguanine nucleotides produced in vivo are detoxified by further metabolism by xanthine oxidase and thiopurine methyltransferase (TPMT). The latter enzyme shows a trimodal distribution (Fig. 71-1). In children receiving mercaptopurine for treatment of leukemia, low activity of this enzyme is associated with excessive myelosuppression, whereas children with high TPMT levels have a poor antileukemic response. Azathioprine is currently used as a disease-modifying agent in the treatment of rheumatoid arthritis. Individuals with mutant TPMT alleles that result in impaired metabolism devel-

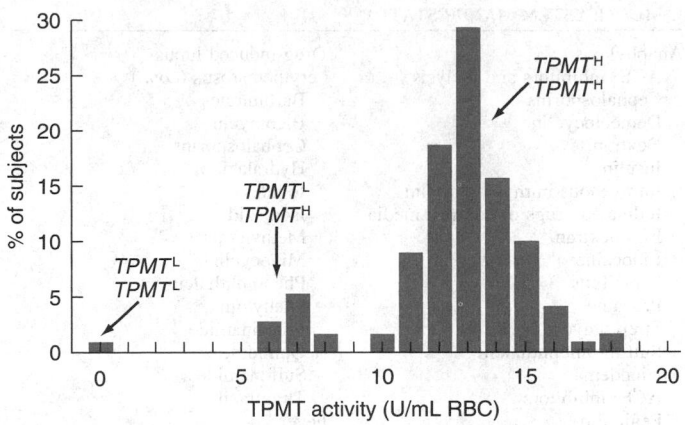

FIGURE 71-1   Thiopurine methyltransferase (TPMT) polymorphism: Frequency distribution of TPMT activity showing presumed genotype. *(From L Leonard: Lancet 336:225, 1990, with permission.)*

oped toxicity rapidly after beginning azathioprine and were uniformly unable to take the drug chronically. Thus the genotypic basis for drug toxicity is beginning to emerge.

Pharmacokinetic Bases for Adverse Reactions   *An abnormally high drug concentration at the receptor site* (site of action) owing to pharmacokinetic variability is the usual cause of these reactions (Chap. 70). For example, a reduction in the volume of distribution, in the rate of metabolism, or in the rate of excretion all result in higher than expected concentration of drug at the receptor site, with a consequent increase in the pharmacologic effect.

Alteration in the dose-response curve due to increased receptor sensitivity results in an increase in drug effect at a given drug concentration. An example is the excessive response of elderly persons to the anticoagulant warfarin at normal or lower than normal blood levels. Such alterations in the dose-response curve may reflect altered drug sensitivity due to receptor polymorphisms, which are now being recognized. One such example is the prolonged QT syndrome, which has both a genetic basis, in individuals with abnormal potassium channels involved in cardiac repolarization, and a pharmacologic basis in individuals who receive drugs known to prolong the QT interval. Such individuals may develop torsade de pointes (Chap. 230). A large number of drugs have now been identified that can produce this potentially lethal effect (Table 71-2; also www.dml.georgetown.edu/depts/ pharmacology/torsades.html).

The shape of the dose-response curve also determines the likelihood of adverse drug reactions. Drugs with a steep dose-response curve or a narrow therapeutic index (Chap. 70) are more likely to cause dose-related toxicity because a small increase in dose produces a large change in pharmacologic effect. An increase in the dose of drugs that exhibit nonlinear kinetics, such as phenytoin (Chap. 70), may produce a proportionately greater increase in the blood level, resulting in toxicity.

Concurrent administration of other drugs may affect pharmacokinetics or pharmacodynamics. Pharmacokinetics may be affected by alterations in bioavailability, protein binding, or the rate of metabolism or excretion. Pharmacodynamics may be altered by another drug that competes for the same receptor sites, that prevents the drug from reaching its site of action, or that antagonizes or enhances the drug's pharmacologic effect. Inhibition of the metabolism of one drug by another may occur when both drugs bind to the same CYP. Therefore, as the specific CYPs responsible for the metabolism of individual drugs become known, prediction of drug interactions is put on a more rational scientific basis. An important example of such a mechanism is the inhibition of terfenadine's metabolism by inhibitors of CYP3A, such as erythromycin and systemic antimycotics. Such inhibition has resulted in torsade de pointes and lethal cardiac arrhythmia (Chap. 70).

Table 71-1   Warfarin Dose and Genotype

Genotype, %	Distibution in Patients, %		Community, %
	<1.5 mg/d	>1.5 mg/d	
CYP2C9 *1/*1	19	62	60
*1/*2	33	17	20
*1/*3	28	19	17
*2/*3	14	0	2
*2/*2	6	2	0
*3/*3	0	0	1

NOTE: Warfarin dose and genotype. Distribution of CYP2D6 genotype in patients stabilized on warfarin doses of less than 1.5 mg/d and more than 1.5 mg/d compared to similar patients in the community, *1, *2, and *3 are the three genotypes. The genotype distribution in patients stabilized on > 1.5 mg/d is similar to that in the community population. However, patients stabilized on < 1.5 mg/d more frequently had genotypes other than *1/*1.

SOURCE: *Data from Aithal et al.*

Table 71-2 Clinical Manifestations of Adverse Reactions To Drugs

I. MULTISYSTEM MANIFESTATIONS

Anaphylaxis
  ACE[a] inhibitors and dialysis
  Cephalosporins
  Demeclocycline
  Dextran
  Insulin
  Intravenous immune globulin
  Iodinated drugs or contrast media
  Iron dextran
  Lidocaine
  Penicillins
  Procaine
  Streptomycin
  Sulfobromophthalein
Angioedema
  ACE[a] inhibitors
  Penicillin
  Rituximab
Drug-induced lupus erythematosus
  Acebutolol
  Asparaginase

Drug-induced lupus
  erythematosus (cont.)
  Barbiturates
  Bleomycin
  Cephalosporins
  Hydralazine
  Iodides
  Isoniazid
  Methyldopa
  Minocycline
  Phenolphthalein
  Phenytoin
  Procainamide
  Quinidine
  Sulfonamides
  Thiouracil
Fever
  Aminosalicylic acid
  Amphotericin B
  Antihistamines

Fever (cont.)
  Infliximab
  Interferon α
  Intravenous immune globulin
  Novobiocin
  Pamidronate
  Penicillins
  Streptokinase
Hyperpyrexia
  Antipsychotics
Increased susceptibility to infections
  Interferon α
Influenza-like reaction
  Interferon α
Neuroleptic malignant syndrome
  Antipsychotics
  Antidopaminergics
Serum sickness
  Aspirin
  β-lactams
  Penicillins

Serum sickness (cont.)
  Propylthiouracil
  Streptokinase
  Streptomycin
  Sulfonamides
Vasculitis
  Allopurinol
  Aminopenicillins
  Hydantoins
  Penicillin
  Propylthiouracil
  Sulfonamides
  Thiazides

II. ENDOCRINE MANIFESTATIONS

Addisonian-like syndrome
  Busulfan
  Etomidate
  Ketoconazole
Galactorrhea (may also cause
  amenorrhea)
  Domperidone
  Methyldopa
  Metoclopramide
  Phenothiazines
  Reserpine
  Tricyclic antidepressants
Gynecomastia
  Calcium channel antagonists
  Clomiphene
  Digitalis
  Estrogens
  Ethionamide
  Griseofulvin

Gynecomastia (cont.)
  Isoniazid
  Methyldopa
  Phenytoin
  Reserpine
  Spironolactone
  Testosterone
Sexual dysfunction
  Impaired ejaculation
    Bethanidine
    Debrisoquin
    Guanethidine
    Thioridazine
  Decreased libido and impotence
    Beta blockers
    Clonidine
    Diuretics
    HIV-protease inhibitors
    Lithium

Sexual dysfunction (cont.)
  Decreased libido and
    impotence (cont.)
    Major tranquilizers
    Methyldopa
    Oral contraceptives
    Sedatives
  Impairment of spermatogenesis or
    oogenesis
    Cytotoxic agents
  Priapism
    Trazodone
Thyroid dysfunction (disorders caus-
  ing abnormal results on thyroid
  function tests)
  Acetazolamide
  Amiodarone
  Bromsulfophthalein
  Chlorpropamide

Thyroid dysfunction (cont.)
  Clofibrate
  Colestipol and nicotinic acid
  Dimercaprol
  Gold salts
  Iodides
  Lithium
  Oral contraceptives
  Phenindione
  Phenothiazines (long-term)
  Phenylbutazone
  Phenytoin
  Sulfonamides
  Tolbutamide
Vaginal carcinoma
  Diethylstilbestrol (given to
    mother)

III. METABOLIC MANIFESTATIONS

Hyperbilirubinemia
  Novobiocin
  Rifampin
Hypercalcemia
  Antacids with absorbable alkali
  Calcitonin
  Thiazides
  Vitamin D
Hyperglycemia
  Asparaginase
  Chlorthalidone
  Diazoxide
  Encainide
  Ethacrynic acid
  Furosemide
  Glucocorticoids
  Growth hormone
  HIV-protease inhibitors
  Niacin
  Oral contraceptives
  Phenytoin
  Pentamidine
  Thiazides
Hypoglycemia
  ACE[a] inhibitors
  Insulin
  Octreotide
  Oral hypoglycemics
  Pentamidine
  Quinine

Hyperkalemia
  ACE[a] inhibitors
  Amiloride
  Cyclosporine
  Cytotoxics
  Digitalis overdose
  Heparin
  Lithium
  NSAIDs[b]
  Pentamidine
  Potassium preparations including
    salt substitute
  Potassium salts of drugs
  Spironolactone
  Succinylcholine
  Triamterene
  Trimethoprin
Hypokalemia
  Alkali-induced alkalosis
  Amphotericin B
  Carbenoxolone
  Corticosteroids
  Diuretics
  Gentamicin
  Insulin
  Laxatives (abused)
  Mineralocorticoids, some gluco-
    corticoids
  Osmotic diuretics
  Sympathomimetic agents

Hypokalemia (cont.)
  Tetracycline (degraded)
  Theophylline
  Vitamin B$_{12}$
Hyperuricemia
  Aspirin (low dose)
  Chlorthalidone
  Cyclosporine
  Cytotoxics
  Ethacrynic acid
  Fructose (IV)
  Furosemide
  Hyperalimentation
  Pyrazinamide
  Thiazides
Hyponatremia
  Dilutional:
    Antipsychotics
    Carbamazepine
    Chlorpropamide
    Cyclophosphamide
    Desmopressin
    Diuretics
    Intravenous immune globulin
    Octreotide
    Selective serotonin reuptake in-
      hibitors
    Vincristine

Hyponatremia (cont.)
  Salt-wasting:
    Diuretics
    Enemas
    Mannitol
Metabolic acidosis
  Acetazolamide
  Metformin
  Paraldehyde (degraded)
  Phenformin
  Salicylates
  Spironolactone
Porphyria exacerbation
  Barbiturates
  Chlordiazepoxide
  Chlorpropamide
  Estrogens
  Glutethimide
  Griseofulvin
  Meprobamate
  Oral contraceptives
  Phenytoin
  Rifampin
  Sulfonamides

(continued)

IV. DERMATOLOGIC MANIFESTATIONS

Acne
- Anabolic and androgenic steroids
- Bromides
- Glucocorticoids
- Iodides
- Isoniazid
- Oral contraceptives
- Troxidone

Alopecia
- Beta blockers
- Colchicine
- Cytotoxics
- Ethionamide
- Fluconazole
- Heparin
- Interferon
- Lithium
- Oral contraceptives (withdrawal)
- Retinoids

Eczema
- Captopril
- Cream and lotion preservatives
- Lanolin
- Topical antihistamines
- Topical antimicrobials
- Topical local anesthetics

Erythema multiforme or Stevens-Johnson syndrome/toxic epidermal necrolysis
- Allopurinol
- Aminopenicillins
- Barbiturates
- Carbamazepine
- Cephalosporins
- Chlorpropamide
- Codeine
- Ethosuximide
- Imidazoles

Erythema multiforme (cont.)
- Iodides
- Lamotrigine
- Nalidixic acid
- Penicillins
- Phenolphthalein
- Phenylbutazone
- Phenytoin
- Piroxicam
- Quinolones
- Salicylates
- Sulfonamides
- Sulfones
- Tetracyclines
- Thiazides
- Tocainide
- Valproic acid

Erythema nodosum
- Oral contraceptives
- Penicillins
- Sulfonamides

Exfoliative dermatitis
- Barbiturates
- Gold salts
- Penicillins
- Phenylbutazone
- Phenytoin
- Quinidine
- Sulfonamides

Fixed drug eruptions
- Barbiturates
- Captopril
- Foscarnet (penile ulceration)
- Phenolphthalein
- Phenylbutazone
- Quinine
- Salicylates
- Sulfonamides

Flushing
- Nicotinic acid
- Sildenafil

Hyperpigmentation
- Amiodarone
- Bleomycin
- Busulfan
- Chloroquine and other anti-malarials
- Corticotropin
- Cyclophosphamide
- Gold salts
- Minocycline
- Oral contraceptives
- Phenothiazines
- Vitamin A (hypervitaminosis A)

Hypertrichosis
- Cyclosporine
- Minoxidil
- Phenytoin

Leg ulcers
- Hydroxyurea

Lichenoid eruptions
- Aminosalicylic acid
- Antimalarials
- Chlorpropamide
- Gold salts
- Methyldopa
- Phenothiazines

Nail changes
- Penicillamine
- Retinoids
- Tetracyclines

Photodermatitis
- Captopril
- Chlordiazepoxide
- Furosemide

Photodermatitis (cont.)
- Griseofulvin
- NSAIDs[b]
- Oral contraceptives
- Phenothiazines
- Sulfonamides
- Sulfonylureas
- Tetracyclines, particularly deme-clocycline
- Thiazides

Purpura (see also thrombocytopenia)
- Aspirin
- Glucocorticoids

Rashes (nonspecific)
- Allopurinol
- Ampicillin
- Barbiturates
- Indapamide
- Methyldopa
- Phenytoin

Rash
- Infliximab

Raynaud's disease or digital necrosis
- Beta blockers
- Bleomycin
- Ergot alkaloids

Skin necrosis
- Warfarin

Urticaria
- Aspirin
- Barbiturates
- Captopril
- Enalapril
- Intravenous immune globulin
- Penicillins
- Sulfonamides

V. HEMATOLOGIC MANIFESTATIONS

Agranulocytosis (see also pancyto-penia)
- Aprindine
- Captopril
- Carbimazole
- Cefotaxime
- Chloramphenicol
- Clozapine
- Co-trimoxazole
- Cytotoxics
- Gold salts
- Indomethacin
- Methimazole
- Oxyphenbutazone
- Phenothiazines
- Phenylbutazone
- Propylthiouracil
- Sulfonamides
- Ticlopidine
- Tolbutamide
- Tricyclic antidepressants

Churg-Strauss syndrome
- Fluticasone propionate
- Montelukast
- Zafirlukast

Clotting and bleeding abnormalities/hypothrombinemia
- Cefamandole
- Cefoperazone
- Ketorolac
- Mezlocillin
- Moxalactam
- Piperacillin
- Valproic acid

Eosinophilia
- Aminosalicylic acid
- Chlorpropamide
- Erythromycin estolate

Eosinophilia (cont.)
- Imipramine
- L-Tryptophan
- Methotrexate
- Montelukast
- Nitrofurantoin
- Procarbazine
- Sulfonamides
- Zafirlukast

Hemolytic anemia
- Aminosalicylic acid
- Cephalosporins
- Chlorpromazine
- Dapsone
- Insulin
- Isoniazid
- Levodopa
- Mefenamic acid
- Melphalan
- Methyldopa
- Penicillins
- Phenacetin
- Procainamide
- Quinidine
- Rifampin
- Sulfonamides

Hemolytic anemia (in G6PD deficiency)
- Aminosalicylic acid
- Antimalarials, e.g., primaquine
- Aspirin
- Chloramphenicol
- Co-trimoxazole
- Dapsone
- Nalidixic acid
- Nitrofurantoin
- Phenacetin
- Probenecid

Hemolytic anemia (cont.)
- Procainamide
- Quinidine
- Sulfonamides
- Vitamin C
- Vitamin K

Leukocytosis
- Glucocorticoids
- Lithium

Lymphadenopathy
- Phenytoin
- Primidone

Megaloblastic anemia
- Co-trimoxazole
- Folate antagonists
- Nitrous oxide (repeated or pro-longed exposure)
- Oral contraceptives
- Phenobarbital
- Phenytoin
- Primidone
- Triamterene
- Trimethoprim

Pancytopenia (aplastic anemia)
- Carbamazepine
- Carbimazole
- Chloramphenicol
- Cytotoxics
- Felbamate
- Gold salts
- Mepacrine
- Mephenytoin
- Oxyphenbutazone
- Phenylbutazone
- Phenytoin
- Potassium perchlorate
- Quinacrine
- Sulfonamides

Pancytopenia (cont.)
- Thiouracils
- Ticlopidine
- Trimethadione
- Zidovudine (AZT)

Pure red cell aplasia
- Azathioprine
- Chlorpropamide
- Isoniazid
- Phenytoin

Thrombocytopenia (see also pancy-topenia)
- Acetazolamine
- Aspirin
- Carbamazepine
- Carbenicillin
- Chlorpropamide
- Chlorthalidone
- Co-trimoxazole
- Digitoxin
- Furosemide
- Gold salts
- Heparin
- Indomethacin
- Isoniazid
- Methyldopa
- Moxalactam
- Novobiocin
- Oxyphenbutazone
- Phenylbutazone
- Phenytoin and other hydantoins
- Quinidine
- Quinine
- Thiazides
- Ticarcillin

TTP[c]
- Ticlopidine

(continued)

VI. CARDIOVASCULAR MANIFESTATIONS

Acute chest pain (nonischemic)
  Bleomycin
Angina exacerbation
  Alpha blockers
  Beta-blocker withdrawal
  Ergotamine
  Excessive thyroxine
  Hydralazine
  Methysergide
  Minoxidil
  Nifedipine
  Oxytocin
  Sumatriptan
  Vasopressin
Arrhythmias (see also prolonged QT
  torsade de pointes)
  Adenosine
  Adriamycin
  Antiarrhythmic drugs
  Astemizole
  Atropine
  Anticholinesterases
  Beta blockers
  Cisapride
  Daunorubicin
  Digitalis
  Emetine
  Erythromycin
  Guanethidine
  Ketanserin
  Lithium
  Papaverine
  Pentamidine
  Phenothiazines, particularly thiori-
    dazine

Arrhythmias *(cont.)*
  Probucol
  Sympathomimetics
  Terfenadine
  Theophylline
  Thyroid hormone
  Tricyclic antidepressants
  Verapamil
AV block
  Clonidine
  Methyldopa
  Verapamil
Cardiomyopathy
  Adriamycin
  Daunorubicin
  Emetine
  Hydroxychloroquine
  Lithium
  Phenothiazines
  Sulfonamides
  Sympathomimetics
Fluid retention/congestive heart fail-
  ure/edema
  Beta blockers
  Calcium blockers
  Carbenoxolone
  Diazoxide
  Estrogens
  Growth hormone
  NSAIDs[b]
  Mannitol
  Minoxidil
  Phenylbutazone
  Steroids
  Verapamil

Hypotension (see also arrhythmias)
  Amiodarone (perioperative)
  Calcium channel blockers, e.g.,
    nifedipine
  Citrated blood
  Diuretics
  Interleukin 2
  Levodopa
  Morphine
  Nitroglycerin
  Phenothiazines
  Protamine
  Quinidine
  Sildenafil
Hypertension
  Clonidine withdrawal
  Corticotropin
  Cyclosporine
  Erythropoietin
  Glucocorticoids
  Monoamine oxidase inhibitors
    with sympathomimetics
  NSAIDs[b] (some)
  Oral contraceptives
  Sympathomimetics
  Tricyclic antidepressants with
    sympathomimetics
Pericarditis
  Emetine
  Hydralazine
  Methysergide
  Procainamide
Pericardial effusion
  Minoxidil

Prolonged QT interval/torsade de
pointes
  Amiodarone
  Amitriptyline
  Astemizole
  Bepridil
  Chlorpromazine
  Cisapride
  Clomipramine
  Desipramine
  Diphenylhydramine
  Disopyramide
  Doxepin
  Erythromycin
  Haloperidol
  Ibutilide
  Imipramine
  Maprotiline
  Pentamidine
  Probucol
  Procainamide
  Quinidine
  Risperidone
  Sotalol
  Terfenadine
  Trimethoprim-sulfamethoxazole
  Thioridazine
  Thiothixene
  Trifluoperazine
Thromboembolism
  Estrogen
  Oral contraceptives
Valvular heart disease
  Fenfluramine

VII. RESPIRATORY MANIFESTATIONS

Airway obstruction (bronchospasm,
  asthma; see also anaphylaxis)
  Adenosine
  Beta blockers
  Cephalosporins
  Cholinergic drugs
  NSAIDs,[b] e.g., aspirin, indo-
    methacin
  Penicillins
  Pentazocine
  Streptomycin
  Tartrazine (drugs with yellow
    dye)
Cough
  ACE[a] inhibitors

Nasal congestion
  Decongestant abuse
  Guanethidine
  Isoproterenol
  Oral contraceptives
  Reserpine
Pulmonary edema
  Contrast media
  Heroin
  Hydrochlorthiazide
  Interleukin 2
  Methadone
  Propoxyphene
Pulmonary hypertension
  Fenfluramine

Pulmonary infiltrates
  Acyclovir
  Amiodarone
  Azothioprine
  Bleomycin
  Busulfan
  Carmustine (BCNU)
  Chlorambucil
  Cyclophosphamide
  Gold
  Melphalan
  Methotrexate
  Methysergide
  Mitomycin C
  Nitrofurantoin

Pulmonary infiltrates *(cont.)*
  Procarbazine
  Sulfonamides
Respiratory depression
  Aminoglycosides
  Hypnotics
  Opiates
  Polymyxins
  Sedatives
  Trimethaphan

VIII. GASTROINTESTINAL MANIFESTATIONS

Cholestatic hepatitis
  Acetohexamide
  Anabolic steroids
  Androgens
  Chlorpropamide
  Clavulanic acid/amoxicillin
  Cyclosporine
  Erythromycin estolate
  Flucloxacillin
  Gold salts
  Methimazole
  Nitrofurantoin
  Oral contraceptives
  Phenothiazines
Constipation or ileus
  Aluminum hydroxide
  Barium sulfate
  Calcium carbonate

Constipation or ileus *(cont.)*
  Ferrous sulfate
  Ganglionic blockers
  Ion exchange resins
  Opiates
  Phenothiazines
  Tricyclic antidepressants
  Verapamil
Diarrhea or colitis
  Antibiotics (broad-spectrum)
  Clindamycin
  Cocaine
  Colchicine
  Digitalis
  Donepezil
  Guanethidine
  Lactose excipients
  Lincomycin

Diarrhea or colitis *(cont.)*
  Magnesium in antacids
  Methyldopa
  Misoprostol
  Oral contraceptives
  Purgatives
  Reserpine
  Ticlopidine
Diffuse hepatocellular damage
  Acetaminophen (paracetamol)
  Acebutolol
  Allopurinol
  Aminosalicylic acid
  Amiodarone
  Aprindine
  Bromfenae
  Carbenicillin
  Cyclophosphamide

Diffuse hepatocellular
damage *(cont.)*
  Dapsone
  Diclofenac
  Erythromycin estolate
  Ethionamide
  Felbamate
  Glyburide
  Halothane
  HMG-CoA reductase inhibitors
  Isoniazid
  Ketoconazole
  Labetalol
  Lovastatin
  Methimazole
  Methotrexate
  Methoxyflurane
  Methyldopa

(continued)

VIII. GASTROINTESTINAL MANIFESTATIONS (*cont.*)

Minocycline
Monamine oxidase inhibitors
Nefazodone
Niacin
Nifedipine
Nitrofura ntoin
Oxyphenisatin
Pemoline
Phenytoin and other hydantoins
Propoxyphene
Propylthiouracil
Pyridium
Quinidine
Quinolone antibiotics
Rifampin
Salicylates
Sodium valproate
Sulfonamides
Tacrine
Tetracyclines
Tolcapone
Trazodone
Troglitazone
Verapamil
Zidovudine (AZT)
Esophagitis
Alendronate
Fibrosing colonopathy and colonic
  stricture
Pancreatin

Gallstones/biliary pseudolithiasis
Ceftriaxone
Estrogens
Malabsorption
Aminosalicylic acid
Antibiotics (broad-spectrum)
Cholestyramine
Colchicine
Colestipol
Cytotoxic agents
Neomycin
Phenobarbital
Phenytoin
Primidone
Nausea or vomiting
Cytotoxic agents
Digitalis
Donepezil
Estrogens
Ferrous sulfate
Levodopa
Opiates
Potassium chloride
Tetracyclines
Theophylline
Oral conditions
Dental discoloration:
  Tetracycline
Dry mouth:
  Anticholinergics

Dry mouth: (*cont.*)
Brimonidine
Clonidine
Levodopa
Methyldopa
Tricyclic antidepressants
Gingival hyperplasia:
Calcium antagonists
Cyclosporine
Phenytoin
Salivary gland swelling:
Bethanidine
Bretylium
Clonidine
Guanethidine
Iodides
Phenylbutazone
Taste disturbances
Acetazolamide
Biguanides
Captopril
Griseofulvin
Lithium
Metronidazole
Penicillamine
Rifampin
Ulceration
Aspirin
Cytotoxic agents
Gentian violet

Ulceration (*cont.*)
Isoproterenol (sublingual)
Pancreatitis
Asparaginase
Azathioprine
Didanosine
Estrogens
Ethacrynic acid
Furosemide
Glucocorticoids
Mercaptopurine
Opiates
Oral contraceptives
Pentamidine
Sulfonamides
Thiazides
Valproic acid
Peptic ulceration or hemorrhage
Aspirin
Ethacrynic acid
Glucocorticoids
NSAIDs[b]
Reserpine (large doses)
Ulceration
Esophageal:
  Alendronate
Intestinal:
  Solid KCl preparations

IX. RENAL MANIFESTATIONS

Bladder dysfunction/incontinence
Anticholinergics
Disopyramide
Monoamine oxidase inhibitors
Prazosin
Terazosin
Tricyclic antidepressants
Calculi/crystaluria
Acetazolamide
Indinavir
Vitamin D
Concentrating defect with polyuria
  (or nephrogenic diabetes insipidus)
Demeclocycline
Lithium
Methoxyflurane
Vitamin D
Hemorrhage cystitis
Busulfan
Carmustine
Chlorambucil

Hemorrhage cystitis (*cont.*)
Cyclophosphamide
Extended-spectrum penicillins
Nitrogen mustard
Vincristine
Interstitial nephritis
Cephalosporins
Ciprofloxacin
Allopurinol
Furosemide
NSAIDs[b]
Penicillins, esp. methicillin
Phenindione
Rifampin
Sulfonamides
Thiazides
Nephropathies
Analgesics (e.g., phenacetin)
Nephrotic syndrome
Captopril
Gold salts

Nephrotic syndrome (*cont.*)
Ketoprofen
Penicillamine
Phenindione
Probenecid
Obstructive uropathy
Extrarenal:
  Methysergide
Intrarenal:
  Acyclovir
  Cytotoxic agents
  Methotrexate
  Metyrosine
Renal dysfunction
ACE inhibitors[a]
Cidofovir
Cyclosporine
NSAIDs[b]
Pentamidine
Tacrolimus
Triamterene

Renal tubular acidosis
Acetazolamide
Amphotericin B
Degraded tetracycline
Tubular necrosis
Aminoglycosides
Amphotericin B
Cephaloridine
Colistin
Cyclosporine
Intravenous immune globulin
Methoxyflurane
Polymyxins
Radioiodinated contrast medium
Sulfonamides
Tetracyclines

X. NEUROLOGIC MANIFESTATIONS

Aseptic meningitis
Intravenous immune globulin
NSAIDs
OKT3 antibodies
Antibiotics
CNS/vasculitis/cerebral hemorrhage
Cocaine
Phenylpropanolamine
Exacerbation of myasthenia
Aminoglycosides
D-Penicillamine
Polymyxins
Extrapyramidal effects
Butyrophenones, e.g., haloperidol
Levodopa
Methyldopa
Metoclopramide
Oral contraceptives
Phenothiazines
Reserpine
Tricyclic antidepressants

Headache
Bromides
Ergotamine (withdrawal)
Glyceryl trinitrate
Hydralazine
Indomethacin
Interferon α
Intravenous immune globulin
Sibutramine
Sildenafil
Peripheral neuropathy
Amiodarone
Chloramphenicol
Chloroquine
Chlorpropamide
Cisplatin
Clioquinol
Clofibrate
Demeclocycline
Disopyramide
Ethambutol

Peripheral neuropathy (*cont.*)
Ethionamide
Glutethimide
Hydralazine
Isoniazid
Methysergide
Metronidazole
Mustine
Nalidixic acid
Nitrofurantoin
Perhexiline
Phenelzine
Phenytoin
Polymyxin, colistin
Procarbazine
Streptomycin
Tolbutamide
Tricyclic antidepressants
Vincristine

Pseudotumor cerebri (or intracranial
  hypertension)
Amiodarone
Glucocorticoids, mineralocorti-
  coids
Vitamin A (hypervitaminosis A)
Oral contraceptives
Tetracyclines
Seizures
Amphetamines
Analeptics
Imipenem
Interferon α
Isoniazid
Lidocaine
Lithium
Nalidixic acid
Meperidine
Penicillins
Phenothiazines
Physostigmine

(*continued*)

X. NEUROLOGIC MANIFESTATIONS *(cont.)*

Seizures *(cont.)*	Sleep disorders	Stroke	Tremor
Theophylline	HMG-CoA reductase inhibitors	Cocaine	β-Adrenergic agonists
Tramadol	Lovastatin	Oral contraceptives	Cyclosporine
Tricyclic antidepressants			
Vincristine			

XI. OCULAR MANIFESTATIONS

Cataracts	Color vision alteration *(cont.)*	Glaucoma	Optic neuritis *(cont.)*
Busulfan	Thiazides	Ipratropium bromide	Phenothiazines
Chlorambucil	Troxidone	Mydriatics	Phenylbutazone
Glucocorticoids	Corneal edema	Sympathomimetics	Quinine
Phenothiazines	Oral contraceptives	Optic neuritis	Streptomycin
Color vision alteration	Corneal opacities	Aminosalicylic acid	Retinopathy
Barbiturates	Chloroquine	Amiodarone	Chloroquine
Digitalis	Indomethacin	Chloramphenicol	Phenothiazines
Methaqualone	Mepacrine	Clioquinol	Uveitis/iritis
Sildenafil	Vitamin D	Ethambutol	Cidofovir
Streptomycin	Eye pain	Isoniazid	
Sulfonamides	Nifedipine	Penicillamine	

XII. EAR MANIFESTATIONS

Deafness	Deafness *(cont.)*	Deafness *(cont.)*	
Aminoglycosides	Deferoxamine	Nortriptyline	
Aspirin	Erythromycin	Quinine	
Bleomycin	Ethacrynic acid	Vestibular disorders	
Chloroquine	Furosemide	Aminoglycosides	
Cidofovir	Interferon	Mustine	
Cisplatin	Mustine	Quinine	

XIII. MUSCULOSKELETAL MANIFESTATIONS

Arthralgias	Bone disorders *(cont.)*	Myopathy or myalgia *(cont.)*	Rhabdomyolysis
Growth hormone	Gout: see Hyperuricemia	Clofibrate	Gemfibrozil
Infiximab	Osteomalacia:	Glucocorticoids	HMG-CoA reductase inhibitors
Interferon α	Aluminum hydroxide	Growth hormone	Lovastatin
Avascular necrosis	Anticonvulsants	HMG-CoA reductase inhibitors	Tendon rupture
Glucocorticoids	Glutethimide	Infliximab	Quinolones
Bone disorders	Myopathy or myalgia	Interferon α	
Osteoporosis:	Amphotericin B	Oral contraceptives	
Glucocorticoids	Carbenoxolone	Zidovudine	
Heparin	Chloroquine		
Thyroxine	Cimetidine		

XIV. PSYCHIATRIC MANIFESTATIONS

Delirious or confusional states	Depression *(cont.)*	Hallucinatory states *(cont.)*	Schizophrenic-like or paranoid reactions *(cont.)*
Amantadine	Centrally acting antihypertensives	Meperidine	Glucocorticoids
Aminophylline	(reserpine, methyldopa,	Narcotics	Levodopa
Anticholinergics	clonidine)	Pentazocine	Lysergic acid
Antidepressants	Glucocorticoids	Tricyclic antidepressants	Monoamine oxidase inhibitors
Bromides	Isotretinoin	Hypomania, mania, or excited reactions	Tricyclic antidepressants
Cimetidine	Levodopa	Glucocorticoids	Sleep disturbances
Digitalis	Drowsiness	Levodopa	Anorexiants
Glucocorticoids	Antihistamines	Monoamine oxidase inhibitors	Levodopa
Isoniazid	Anxiolytic drugs	Sympathomimetics	Monoamine oxidase inhibitors
Levodopa	Brimonidine	Tricyclic antidepressants	Sympathomimetics
Methyldopa	Clonidine	Hypersexuality	
Penicillins	Major tranquilizers	Antiparkinsonian agents	
Phenothiazines	Methyldopa	Memory loss	
Ranitidine	Reserpine	Triazolam	
Sedatives and hypnotics	Tricyclic antidepressants	Schizophrenic-like or paranoid reactions	
Vigabatrin	Hallucinatory states	Amphetamines	
Depression	Amantadine	Bromides	
Amphetamine withdrawal	Beta blockers		
Beta blockers	Levodopa		

[a] ACE, angiotensin-converting enzyme.
[b] NSAID, nonsteroidal anti-inflammatory drug.
[c] TTP, thrombotic thrombocytopenic purpura.

TOXICITY UNRELATED TO A DRUG'S PRIMARY PHARMACOLOGIC ACTIVITY   Cytotoxic Reactions The understanding of so-called idiosyncratic reactions has greatly improved with the recognition that many of them are due to irreversible binding of a drug or its metabolites to tissue macromolecules by co-valent bonds. Some chemical carcinogens, such as the alkylating agents, combine directly with DNA. Usually, it is only after metabolic activation of a drug to reactive metabolites that covalent binding occurs. This activation usually occurs in the microsomal mixed-function oxidase system, the hepatic enzyme system responsible for the metabolism of many drugs (Chap. 70). During the course of drug metabolism, reactive metabolites may covalently bind to tissue macromolecules, causing tissue damage. Because of the reactive nature of these metabolites, covalent binding often occurs close to the site of production. Typically that is the liver, but the mixed-function oxidase system is found in other tissues as well.

An example of this type of adverse drug reaction is the hepatotoxicity associated with isoniazid. This drug is metabolized principally by acetylation to acetylisoniazid, which is then hydrolyzed to acetylhydrazine. The further metabolism of acetylhydrazine by the mixed-function oxidase system liberates reactive metabolites that covalently bind to hepatic macromolecules, causing hepatic necrosis. The administration of drugs known to increase the activity of the mixed-function oxidase system, such as phenobarbital or rifampin, together with isoniazid results in the production of increased amounts of reactive metabolites, increased covalent binding, and a greater risk of hepatic damage.

The hepatic necrosis produced by overdosage of acetaminophen is also caused by reactive metabolites. Normally these metabolites are detoxified by combining with hepatic glutathione. When glutathione becomes exhausted, the metabolites bind instead to hepatic protein, with resultant hepatocyte damage. The hepatic necrosis produced by the ingestion of acetaminophen can be prevented, or at least attenuated, by the administration of substances such as N-acetylcysteine that reduce the binding of electrophilic metabolites to hepatic proteins. The risk of hepatic necrosis is increased in patients receiving drugs such as phenobarbital that increase the rate of drug metabolism and the rate of production of toxic metabolite(s).

It is likely, though as yet not proved, that other idiosyncratic reactions are caused by the covalent binding of reactive metabolites to tissue macromolecules, resulting either in direct cytotoxicity or in the initiation of an immune response.

Immunologic Mechanisms Most pharmacologic agents are poor immunogens because they are small molecules with molecular weights of less than 2000. Stimulation of antibody synthesis or sensitization of lymphocytes by a drug or one of its metabolites usually requires in vivo activation and covalent linkage to protein, carbohydrate, or nucleic acid.

Drug stimulation of antibody production may mediate tissue injury by one of several mechanisms. The antibody may attack the drug when the drug is covalently attached to a cell, and thereby destroy the cell. This mechanism occurs in penicillin-induced hemolytic anemia. Antibody-drug-antigen complexes may be passively adsorbed by a bystander cell, which is then destroyed by activation of complement; this occurs in quinine- and quinidine-induced thrombocytopenia. Drugs or their reactive metabolites may alter a host tissue, rendering it antigenic and eliciting autoantibodies. For example, hydralazine and procainamide can chemically alter nuclear material, stimulating the formation of anti-nuclear antibodies and occasionally causing lupus erythematosus. Autoantibodies can be elicited by drugs that neither interact with the host antigen nor have any chemical similarity to the host tissue; for example, α-methyldopa frequently stimulates the formation of antibodies to host erythrocytes, yet the drug neither attaches to the erythrocyte nor shares any chemical similarities with the antigenic determinants on the erythrocyte.

Drug-induced pure red cell aplasia (Chap. 109) is due to an immune-based drug reaction. Red cell formation in bone marrow cultures can be inhibited by phenytoin and purified IgG obtained from a patient with pure red cell aplasia associated with phenytoin.

Serum sickness (Chap. 310) results from the deposition of circulating drug-antibody complexes on endothelial surfaces. Complement activation occurs, chemotactic factors are generated locally, and an inflammatory response develops at the site of complex entrapment. Arthralgias, urticaria, lymphadenopathy, glomerulonephritis, or cerebritis may result. Penicillin is the most common cause of serum sickness today. Many drugs, particularly antimicrobial agents, induce production of IgE, which binds to mast cell membranes. Contact with a drug antigen initiates a series of biochemical events in the mast cell and results in the release of mediators that can produce the urticaria, wheezing, flushing, rhinorrhea, and (occasionally) hypotension characteristic of anaphylaxis.

Drugs may also excite cell-mediated immune responses. Topically administered substances may interact with sulfhydryl or amino groups in the skin and react with sensitized lymphocytes to produce the rash characteristic of contact dermatitis. Other types of rashes may also result from the interaction of serum factors, drugs, and sensitized lymphocytes. The role of drug-activated lymphocytes in the immune mechanisms governing destruction of visceral tissue is unknown.

Toxicity Associated with Genetically Determined Enzymatic Defects In the porphyrias, drugs that increase the activity of enzymes proximal to the deficient enzyme in the biosynthetic pathway of porphyrins can increase the quantity of porphyrin precursors that accumulate proximal to the deficient enzyme (Chap. 346). These drugs are listed in Table 71-1.

Patients with a deficiency of glucose-6-phosphate dehydrogenase (G6PD) develop hemolytic anemia in response to primaquine and a number of other drugs (Table 71-1) that do not cause hemolysis in patients with adequate quantities of this enzyme (Chap. 108).

DIAGNOSIS The manifestations of drug-induced diseases frequently resemble those of other diseases, and a given set of manifestations may be produced by different and dissimilar drugs. Recognition of the role of a drug or drugs in an illness depends on appreciation of the possible adverse reactions to drugs in any disease, on identification of the temporal relationship between drug administration and development of the illness, and on familiarity with the common manifestations of the drugs. Many associations between particular drugs and specific reactions have been described, but there is always a "first time" for a novel association, and any drug should be suspected of causing an adverse effect if the clinical setting is appropriate.

Illness related to a drug's pharmacologic action is often more easily recognized than illness attributable to immune or other mechanisms. For example, side effects such as cardiac arrhythmias in patients receiving digitalis, hypoglycemia in patients given insulin, and bleeding in patients receiving anticoagulants are more readily related to a specific drug than are symptoms such as fever or rash, which may be caused by many drugs or by other factors.

Once an adverse reaction is suspected, discontinuance of the suspected drug followed by disappearance of the reaction is presumptive evidence of a drug-induced illness. Confirming evidence may be sought by cautiously reintroducing the drug and seeing if the reaction reappears. However, that should be done only if confirmation would be useful in the future management of the patient and if the attempt would not entail undue risk. With concentration-dependent adverse reactions, lowering the dosage may cause the reaction to disappear, and raising it may cause the reaction to reappear. When the reaction is thought to be allergic, however, readministration of the drug may be hazardous, since anaphylaxis may develop. Readministration is unwise under these conditions unless no alternative drugs are available and treatment is necessary.

If the patient is receiving many drugs when an adverse reaction is suspected, the drugs likeliest to be responsible can usually be identified. All drugs may be discontinued at once, or, if that is not practical, they should be discontinued one at a time, starting with the one that is most suspect, and the patient observed for signs of improvement. The time needed for a concentration-dependent adverse effect to disappear depends on the time required for the concentration to fall below the range associated with the adverse effect, and that, in turn, depends on the initial blood level and on the rate of elimination or metabolism of the drug. Adverse effects of drugs with long half-lives, such as phenobarbital, take a considerable time to disappear.

Drugs recognized as producing a number of reactions are listed in Table 71-1. This table includes both well-documented and some less well-documented reactions, focusing on those that are sufficiently important to require consideration. This information should be used to suggest the drug likely to be causing a reaction; the absence of a drug from the table does not mean that it cannot be responsible for the reaction, however.

Serum antibody has been demonstrated in some persons with drug allergies involving cellular blood elements, as in agranulocytosis, hemolytic anemia, and thrombocytopenia. For example, both quinine and quinidine can produce platelet agglutination in vitro in the presence of complement and the serum from a patient who has developed thrombocytopenia following use of this drug.

Eliciting a drug history from patients is important for diagnosis. Attention must be directed to OTC drugs and herbal preparations as well as to prescription drugs. Each type can be responsible for adverse drug effects, and adverse interactions may occur between OTC drugs and prescribed drugs. In addition, it is common for patients to be cared for by several physicians, and duplicative, additive, counteractive, or synergistic drug combinations may therefore be administered if the physicians are not aware of the patients' drug histories. Every physician should determine what drugs a patient has been taking, at least during the preceding 30 days, before prescribing any medications. A frequently overlooked source of additional drug exposure is topical therapy; for example, a patient complaining of bronchospasm may not mention that an ophthalmic beta blocker is being used unless specifically asked. A history of previous adverse drug effects in patients is common. Since these patients have shown a predisposition to drug-induced illnesses, such a history should dictate added caution in prescribing drugs.

Patients with biochemical abnormalities such as erythrocyte G6PD deficiency can be identified. Most patients with the G6PD defect are of African or Mediterranean descent. Drug-induced hemolytic crisis can be avoided by testing for the enzyme defect before administering drugs that could cause the reaction. Similarly, persons with an abnormal serum pseudocholinesterase level may have abnormally prolonged apnea when given succinylcholine.

GENERAL COMMENTS   No drug is completely without side effects, and a side effect in one patient may be the desired pharmacologic effect in another. Current drug regulations allow physicians to have considerable confidence in the purity, bioavailability, and effectiveness of the drugs they prescribe. However, physicians have to weigh potential toxicity against possible benefits. Toxicity that would be acceptable for an effective antineoplastic agent would not be permitted in an oral contraceptive, for example. Because of the necessarily small number of patients treated in premarketing studies, rare adverse reactions may not be identified, so the first responsibility for identifying and reporting these effects must rest with the practicing clinician through the use of the various national adverse reaction reporting systems, such as those operated by the Food and Drug Administration in the United States and the Committee on Safety of Medicines in Great Britain. The publication of a newly recognized adverse reaction can in a short time stimulate many similar such reports of reactions that previously had gone unrecognized.

The prevention of adverse drug reactions first involves a high index of suspicion that the development of a new symptom or sign may be drug-related. Reduction of the dose or discontinuation of the suspected agent usually clarifies the issue in concentration-dependent toxic reactions. Physicians should be familiar with the common adverse effects of the drugs they use and, when in doubt, should consult the literature.

BIBLIOGRAPHY

AITHAL GP et al: Association of polymorphisms in the cytochrome P450 CYP2C9 with warfarin dose requirement and risk of bleeding complications. Lancet 353:717, 1999

BLACK AJ et al: Thiopurine methyltransferase genotype predicts therapy-limiting severe toxicity from azathioprine. Ann Intern Med 129:716, 1998

DAVIES DM et al: *Textbook of Adverse Drug Reactions*, 5th ed. New York, Oxford University Press, 1998

FELDMANN U: Design and analysis of drug safety studies, with special reference to sporadic drug use and acute adverse reactions. J Clin Epidemiol 46:237, 1993

LAZAROU J et al: Incidence of adverse drug reactions in hospitalized patients: A meta-analysis of prospective studies. 279:1200, 1998

LENNARD I et al: Thiopurine drugs in the treatment of childhood leukemia: The activity influence of inherited thiopurine methyltransferase activity on drug metabolism and cytotoxicity. Br J Clin Pharmacol 44:445, 1997

ROUJEAU J-C, STERN RS: Severe adverse cutaneous reactions to drugs. N Engl J Med 331:1272, 1994

WOOD AJJ: The safety of new medicines: The importance of asking the right questions. JAMA 281:1753, 1999

——— et al: Making medicines safer: The need for an independent drug safety board. N Engl J Med 25:1851, 1998

72   *Lewis Landsberg, James B. Young*

PHYSIOLOGY AND PHARMACOLOGY OF THE AUTONOMIC NERVOUS SYSTEM

ACh	acetylcholine	IP$_3$	inositol-1,4,5-trisphosphate
AMP	adenosine monophosphate	MAO	monoamine oxidase
CNS	central nervous system	NE	norepinephrine
COMT	catechol-*O*-methyltransferase	NTS	nucleus of the solitary tract
DAG	1,2-diacylglycerol	PIP$_2$	phosphatidylinositol-4,5-bisphosphate
HDL	high-density lipoprotein		

FUNCTIONAL ORGANIZATION OF THE AUTONOMIC NERVOUS SYSTEM

The autonomic nervous system innervates vascular and visceral smooth muscle, exocrine and endocrine glands, and parenchymal cells throughout the various organ systems. Functioning below the conscious level, the autonomic nervous system responds rapidly and continuously to perturbations that threaten the constancy of the internal environment. The many functions governed by this system include the distribution of blood flow and the maintenance of tissue perfusion, the regulation of blood pressure, the regulation of the volume and composition of the extracellular fluid, the expenditure of metabolic energy and supply of substrate, and the control of visceral smooth muscle and glands.

ANATOMIC ORGANIZATION   The autonomic neurons, located in ganglia outside the central nervous system (CNS), give rise to the postganglionic autonomic nerves that innervate organs and tissues throughout the body (Fig. 72-1). The activity of autonomic nerves is regulated by central neurons responsive to diverse afferent inputs. After central integration of afferent information, autonomic outflow is adjusted to permit the functioning of the major organ systems in accordance with the needs of the organism as a whole. Connections between the cerebral cortex and the autonomic centers in the brainstem coordinate autonomic outflow with higher mental functions.

The Sympathetic and Parasympathetic Divisions   The preganglionic neurons of the parasympathetic nervous system leave the CNS in the third, seventh, ninth, and tenth cranial nerves and in the second and third sacral nerves, while the preganglionic neurons of the sympathetic nervous system exit the spinal cord between the first thoracic and the second lumbar segments (Fig. 72-1). Responses to sympathetic and parasympathetic stimulation are frequently antagonistic, as exemplified by their opposing effects on heart rate and gut motility. This antagonism reflects highly coordinated interactions within the CNS; the resultant changes in parasympathetic and sympathetic activity, often reciprocal, provide more precise control of autonomic responses

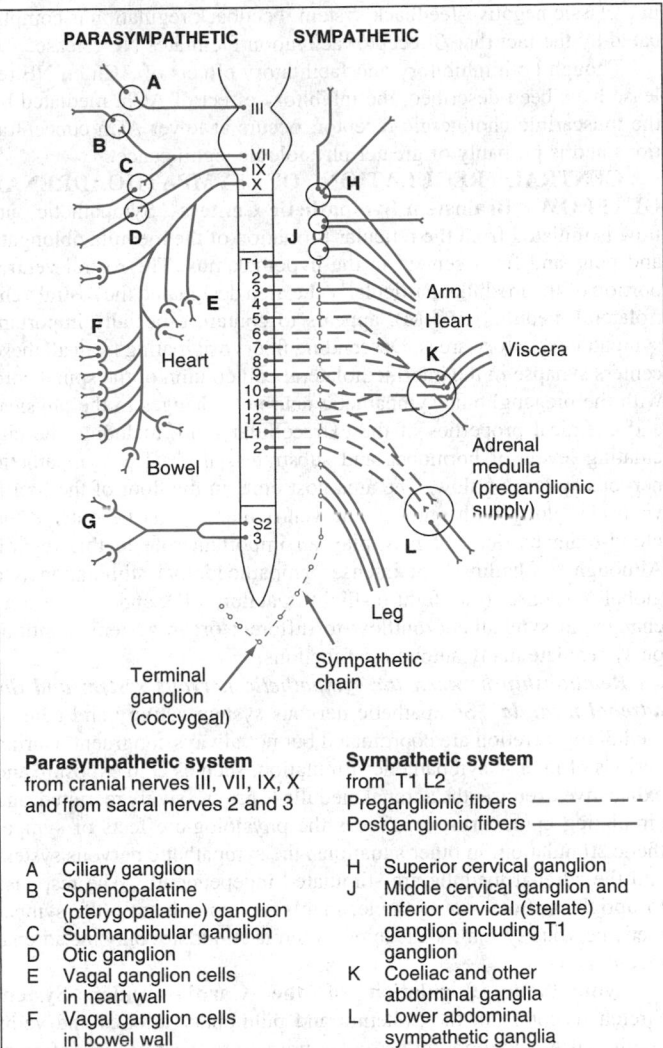

FIGURE 72-1 Schematic representation of the autonomic nervous system. *(From M. Moskowitz: Clin Endocrinol Metab 6:77, 1977.)*

Parasympathetic system
from cranial nerves III, VII, IX, X and from sacral nerves 2 and 3

Sympathetic system
from T1 L2
Preganglionic fibers — — — — —
Postganglionic fibers ——————

A	Ciliary ganglion	
B	Sphenopalatine (pterygopalatine) ganglion	
C	Submandibular ganglion	
D	Otic ganglion	
E	Vagal ganglion cells in heart wall	
F	Vagal ganglion cells in bowel wall	
G	Pelvic ganglia	
H	Superior cervical ganglion	
J	Middle cervical ganglion and inferior cervical (stellate) ganglion including T1 ganglion	
K	Coeliac and other abdominal ganglia	
L	Lower abdominal sympathetic ganglia	

than could be achieved by the modulation of a single system. Moreover, both sympathetic and parasympathetic portions of the autonomic nervous system are composed of multiple function-specific subdivisions. Neurons with the various subdivisions differ neurochemically and neurophysiologically and are controlled by distinct regions within the CNS. This specialization within sympathetic and parasympathetic divisions contributes to the precision and specificity of autonomic regulation.

Neurotransmitters *Acetylcholine* (ACh) is the preganglionic neurotransmitter for both divisions of the autonomic nervous system as well as the postganglionic neurotransmitter of the parasympathetic neurons. Nerves that release ACh are said to be cholinergic. *Norepinephrine* (NE) is the neurotransmitter of the postganglionic sympathetic neurons; these nerves are said to be adrenergic. Within the sympathetic outflow, postganglionic neurons innervating the eccrine sweat glands (and perhaps some blood vessels supplying skeletal muscle) are of the cholinergic type.

THE SYMPATHETIC NERVOUS SYSTEM AND ADRENAL MEDULLA

CATECHOLAMINES All three of the naturally occurring catecholamines, NE, *epinephrine* (E), and *dopamine*, function as neurotransmitters within the CNS. NE, the neurotransmitter of postgangli-

onic sympathetic nerve endings, exerts its effects locally, in the immediate vicinity of its release. Epinephrine, the circulating hormone of the adrenal medulla, influences processes throughout the body. A peripheral dopaminergic system also exists but has not been characterized in detail.

Biosynthesis (Fig. 72-2) Catecholamines are synthesized from the amino acid tyrosine, which is sequentially hydroxylated to form dihydroxyphenylalanine (dopa), decarboxylated to form dopamine, and hydroxylated on the β position of the side chain to form NE. The initial step, the hydroxylation of tyrosine, is rate-limiting and is regulated so that synthesis of dopa is coupled to NE release. This regulation is achieved by alterations in both the activity and the amount of tyrosine hydroxylase. In the adrenal medulla and in those central neurons utilizing epinephrine as neurotransmitter, NE is N-methylated to epinephrine by the enzyme phenylethanolamine-N-methyltransferase (PNMT).

Catecholamine Metabolism The major metabolic transformations of catecholamines involve O-methylation at the meta-hydroxyl group and oxidative deamination. O-Methylation is catalyzed by the enzyme catechol-O-methyltransferase (COMT), and oxidative deamination is promoted by monoamine oxidase (MAO). COMT in liver and kidney is important in the metabolism of circulating catecholamines. MAO, a mitochondrial enzyme present in most tissues, including nerve endings, has a lesser role in the metabolism of circulating catecholamines but is important in regulating the catecholamine stores within the peripheral sympathetic nerve endings. The metane-

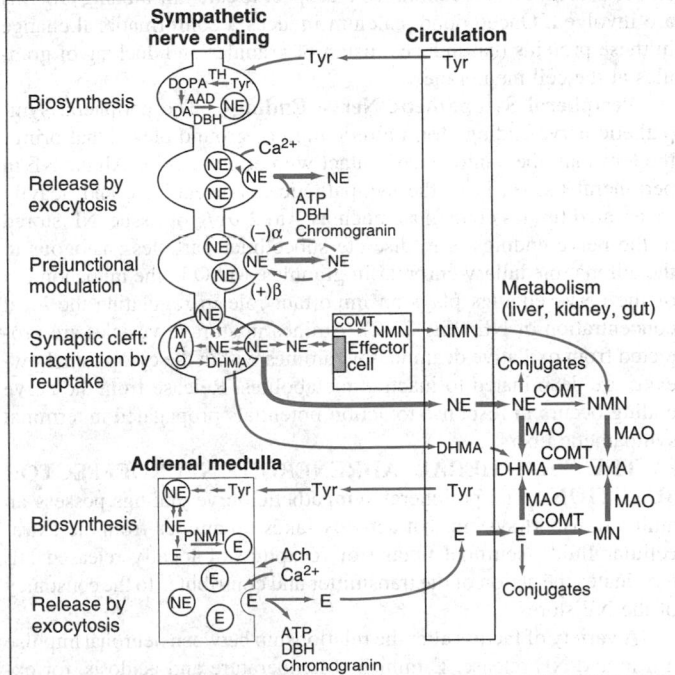

FIGURE 72-2 Catecholamine biosynthesis, release, and metabolism. Schematic representation of a peripheral sympathetic nerve ending is shown at the top; the bulbous areas on the terminal fiber represent varicosities identified by histochemical fluorescence techniques as areas of high neurotransmitter concentration. The processes of biosynthesis, release, modulation, and reuptake are shown sequentially for demonstration purposes only; in vivo they proceed concurrently. Adrenal medullary chromaffin cells are shown at the bottom of the diagram. (TH, tyrosine hydroxylase; AAD, aromatic-l-amino acid decarboxylase; DA, dopamine; DBH, dopamine-β-hydroxylase; NE, norepinephrine; PNMT, phenylethanolamine-N-methyltransferase; E, epinephrine; COMT, catechol-O-methyltransferase; NMN, normetanephrine; MAO, monoamine oxidase; DHMA, 3,4-dihydroxymandelic acid; VMA, 3-methoxy-4-hydroxymandelic acid.)

phrines and 3-methoxy-4-hydroxymandelic acid (vanilmandelic acid, VMA) are the major end products of E and NE metabolism. Homovanillic acid (HVA) is the end product of dopamine metabolism.

STORAGE AND RELEASE OF CATECHOLAMINES
In both the adrenal medulla and sympathetic nerve endings catecholamines are stored in subcellular vesicles and released by exocytosis. The large stores of catecholamines in these tissues provide an important physiologic reserve that maintains an adequate supply of catecholamines in the face of intense stimulation. A variety of substances may be stored along with catecholamines in sympathetic nerve endings and adrenal medulla and released with catecholamines during exocytosis. These substances, which may function as cotransmitters or neuromodulators, include peptides such as neuropeptide Y, substance P, and enkephalins; purines such as ATP and adenosine; and other amines such as serotonin. At the neuroeffector junction, coreleased neuromodulators modify the response to NE, while cotransmitters exert physiologic effects independent of those induced by NE.

Adrenal Medulla   The adrenal medullary chromaffin tissue in a pair of normal human adrenal glands weighs about 1 g and contains approximately 6 mg catecholamines, 85% of which is epinephrine.

Catecholamine secretion, stimulated by ACh from the preganglionic sympathetic nerves, occurs after calcium influx triggers fusion of the chromaffin granule membrane and cell membrane; obliteration of the cell membrane at the point of fusion and extrusion of the entire soluble contents of the granule into the extracellular space complete the process of exocytosis (Fig. 72-2). Although the molecular mechanisms involved in the exocytotic process are only partially understood, evidence has accumulated that specific calcium-binding proteins are involved. Once bound, calcium induces a conformational change in these proteins that induces fusion of granules and docking of granules at the cell membrane.

Peripheral Sympathetic Nerve Endings   The peripheral sympathetic nerve endings form a reticulum or ground plexus that brings the terminal fibers into close contact with effector cells. All the NE in peripheral tissues is in the sympathetic nerve endings, and heavily innervated tissues contain as much as 1 to 2 μg/g of tissue. NE stored in the nerve endings is in discrete subcellular particles analogous to the adrenal medullary chromaffin granules. MAO in the mitochondria of the nerve endings plays an important role in regulating the local concentration of NE (Fig. 72-2). Amines in storage vesicles are protected from oxidative deamination; amines within the cytoplasm, however, are deaminated to inactive metabolites. Release from the nerve ending occurs in response to action potentials propagated in terminal sympathetic fibers.

THE PERIPHERAL ADRENERGIC NEUROEFFECTOR JUNCTION
The peripheral sympathetic nerve endings possess an amine transport system that actively takes up amines from the extracellular fluid. Neuronal uptake or recapture of locally released NE terminates the action of the transmitter and contributes to the constancy of the NE stores.

A variety of factors alter the relationship between neuronal impulse traffic and NE release. Diminished temperature and acidosis, for example, both decrease the amount of NE released in response to sympathetic impulses. Several chemical mediators operate at the peripheral sympathetic nerve ending (referred to as *prejunctional* or *presynaptic sites*) to modify sympathetic neurotransmission by influencing the amount of NE released in response to nerve impulses. Prejunctional modulation may be either inhibitory or facilitatory. Certain modulators, such as catecholamines and ACh, may either inhibit or facilitate NE release, antagonistic effects that are mediated by different adrenergic or cholinergic receptors, respectively. Those compounds exerting an *inhibitory* effect on NE release at the prejunctional nerve ending include the following: catecholamines (α_2 receptor), ACh (muscarinic receptor), dopamine (D_2 receptor), histamine (H_2 receptor), serotonin, adenosine, enkephalins, and prostaglandins.

Catecholamines reduce NE release via prejunctional α receptors

in a classic negative-feedback system. Feedback regulation is complicated by the fact that β-receptor activation facilitates NE release.

Though both inhibitory and facilitatory effects of ACh on NE release have been described, the inhibitory effect of ACh, mediated by the muscarinic cholinergic receptor, occurs at lower ACh concentrations and is probably of greater physiologic significance.

CENTRAL REGULATION OF SYMPATHOADRENAL OUTFLOW
Brainstem Sympathetic Centers   Sympathetic outflow is initiated from the reticular formation of the medulla oblongata and pons and from centers in the hypothalamus. The rostral ventral portion of the medulla, particularly the area designated the rostral ventrolateral medulla (RVLM), appears to contain especially important sympathoexcitatory areas. Descending fibers originating from all these centers synapse in the intermediolateral cell column of the spinal cord with the preganglionic sympathetic neurons. Changes in the physical and chemical properties of the extracellular fluid, including the circulating levels of hormones and substrates, also affect sympathetic nervous system outflow. The area postrema, in the floor of the fourth ventricle, along with other circumventricular organs lie outside the blood-brain barrier and may play an important role in this regard. Although the hallmark of intense sympathoadrenal stimulation is a global response (the fight-or-flight reaction of Cannon), discrete changes in sympathetic outflow to different organ systems continuously regulate many autonomic functions.

Relationship between the sympathetic nervous system and the adrenal medulla   Sympathetic nervous system activity and adrenal medullary secretion are coordinated but not always congruent. During periods of intense sympathetic stimulation, such as cold exposure and exhaustive exercise, the adrenal medulla is progressively recruited, and circulating epinephrine reinforces the physiologic effects of sympathetic stimulation. In other situations, the sympathetic nervous system and the adrenal medulla are stimulated independently. The response to upright posture, for example, involves predominantly the sympathetic nervous system, while hypoglycemia stimulates only the adrenal medulla.

Sympathetic Regulation of the Cardiovascular System Stretch receptors in the systemic and pulmonary arteries and veins continuously monitor intravascular pressures; the resulting afferent impulses, after relay and integration in the brainstem, alter sympathetic activity in defense of blood pressure and blood flow to critical areas (Fig. 72-3).

Arterial baroreceptors   An increase in blood pressure stimulates receptors in the carotid sinus and aortic arch. The ensuing afferent impulses, after relay within the nucleus of the solitary tract (NTS) in the brainstem, suppress the brainstem sympathetic centers (Fig. 72-3). This baroreceptor reflex arc forms a negative-feedback loop in which a rise in arterial pressure results in the inhibition of central sympathetic outflow. A brainstem noradrenergic pathway interacts with the NTS to participate in suppression of sympathetic outflow. This noradrenergic inhibitory pathway is stimulated by centrally acting α-adrenergic agonists and may be involved in the action of certain antihypertensive drugs, such as clonidine, that potentiate the baroreceptor-mediated vasodepressor response (Chap. 246). In the opposite manner, when the blood pressure falls, decreased afferent impulses diminish central inhibition, resulting in an increase in sympathetic outflow and a rise in arterial pressure.

Central venous pressure   Receptors in the walls of the great veins and within the atria are also involved in the regulation of sympathetic outflow. Stimulation of these receptors by high venous pressure suppresses the brainstem sympathetic centers; when central venous pressure is low, sympathetic outflow increases. The central connections are poorly understood, but the afferent impulses are carried in the vagus (Fig. 72-3).

ASSESSMENT OF SYMPATHOADRENAL ACTIVITY
The clinical assessment of sympathoadrenal activity involves the measurement of catecholamines in plasma and of catecholamines and catecholamine metabolites in urine, and the assessment of sympathetic nerve impulse traffic by microneurography. Microneurography, util-

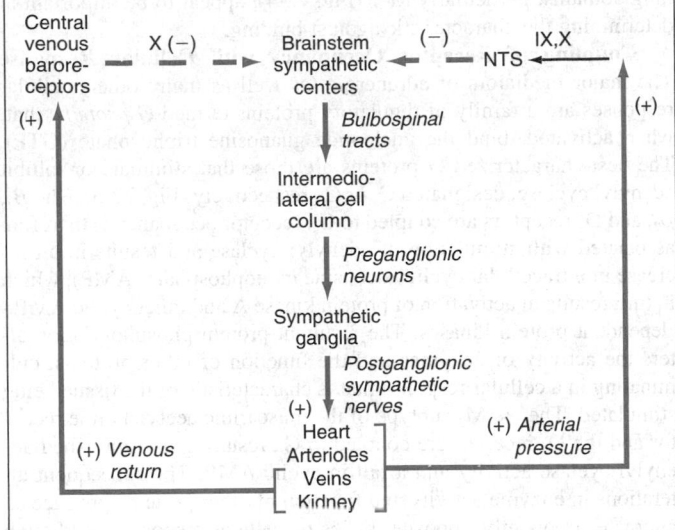

FIGURE 72-3 Sympathetic regulation of the circulation. Receptors in the venous and arterial circulations are stimulated by stretch, caused by an increase in pressure; afferent impulses from these receptors are carried to the central nervous system by the ninth (*IX*) and tenth (*X*) cranial nerves. The net result of these afferent impulses, after relay in the brainstem, is to inhibit central sympathetic outflow. The arterial baroreceptor reflex involves a relay in the nucleus of the tractus solitarius. (+, stimulation; −, inhibition.)

izing microelectrodes implanted in nerves supplying skeletal muscle (such as the peroneal nerve), is primarily a research tool. Quantitation of urinary catecholamines and metabolites is useful in the diagnosis of pheochromocytoma (Chap. 332).

Plasma Catecholamines Catecholamines in human plasma may be measured by radioenzymatic isotope derivative techniques or by high-performance liquid chromatography in conjunction with electrochemical detection. Plasma catecholamine measurements provide an index of sympathetic nervous system and adrenal medullary activity and have been widely used to assess sympathoadrenal activity in clinical investigation in human subjects. The usefulness of plasma catecholamine measurements, however, is compromised by factors that alter the relationship between the plasma concentration of catecholamines and the functional state of the sympathoadrenal system, and also by important regional differences in sympathetic outflow. Techniques utilizing tracer infusions of tritiated NE, which correct for changes in NE clearance when applied across a particular anatomic region, estimate regional sympathetic outflow with some precision and have helped to define differentiated sympathetic nervous system activity in the investigational setting. The clinical usefulness of plasma catecholamine levels remains limited to the evaluation of patients with autonomic insufficiency and, on occasion, patients with suspected pheochromocytoma (Chap. 332).

Basal plasma NE concentrations are in the range of 0.09 to 1.8 nmol/L (150 to 350 pg/mL); basal E levels are about 135 to 270 pmol/L (25 to 50 pg/mL). The half-time of disappearance of NE from the circulation is approximately 2 min. The plasma NE level is markedly affected by a variety of factors, including posture; accordingly, the conditions under which blood is obtained for assay must be controlled. By convention, basal plasma NE levels are those obtained through an indwelling intravenous line after the patient has rested supine in a relaxed environment for 30 min.

Plasma NE response to upright posture The predictable increase in circulating NE concentration during upright posture provides a convenient test of sympathetic nervous system function. Five minutes of quiet standing results in a two- to threefold increase in plasma NE level. A normal response requires an intact afferent system, appropriate CNS relays, and an intact peripheral sympathetic nervous system; a defect of any of these components reduces the increment in circulating NE.

Plasma E levels are also dependent on the physical and mental state of the subject. Change in plasma E with upright posture is usually small. Hypoglycemia, strenuous exercise, and various types of mental stress, however, can cause large increases in the plasma E level.

PERIPHERAL DOPAMINERGIC SYSTEM

In addition to its role as neurotransmitter in the CNS, dopamine functions as an inhibitory transmitter in the carotid body and the sympathetic ganglia. A distinct peripheral dopaminergic system is also believed to exist. Dopamine elicits a variety of responses not attributable to stimulation of classic adrenergic receptors; it relaxes the lower esophageal sphincter, delays gastric emptying, causes vasodilation in the renal and mesenteric arterial circulation, suppresses aldosterone secretion, directly stimulates renal sodium excretion, and suppresses NE release at sympathetic nerve terminals by a presynaptic inhibitory mechanism. The mediation of these dopaminergic effects in vivo is poorly understood. Dopamine does not appear to be a circulating hormone.

ADRENERGIC RECEPTORS

Catecholamines influence effector cells by interacting with specific surface *receptors* coupled to G proteins. Two major categories of response to catecholamines reflect the activation of two populations of adrenergic receptors, designated α and β. Both α and β receptors have been further divided into subtypes that serve different functions and are susceptible to differential stimulation and blockade.

α-ADRENERGIC RECEPTORS α-Adrenergic receptors mediate vasoconstriction, intestinal relaxation, and pupillary dilatation. Epinephrine and NE are approximately equipotent as α-receptor agonists. Distinct α_1- and α_2-receptor subtypes are also recognized. Originally the postsynaptic or postjunctional α-adrenergic receptors on effector cells were designated α_1, while the prejunctional α-adrenergic receptors on the sympathetic nerve endings were designated α_2. It is now recognized that nonneuronal (postsynaptic) processes are mediated by the α_2 receptor as well. The α_1 receptor mediates the classic α effects, including vasoconstriction; phenylephrine and methoxamine are selective α_1 agonists, and prazosin is a selective α_1 antagonist. The α_2 receptor mediates presynaptic inhibition of NE release from adrenergic nerves and other responses, including inhibition of ACh release from cholinergic nerves, inhibition of lipolysis in adipocytes, inhibition of insulin secretion, stimulation of platelet aggregation, and vasoconstriction in some vascular beds. Specific α_2 agonists include clonidine and α-methylnorepinephrine; these agents, the latter derived from α-methyldopa in vivo, exert an antihypertensive effect by interacting with α_2 receptors within the brainstem sympathetic centers that regulate blood pressure. Yohimbine is a specific α_2 antagonist.

β-ADRENERGIC RECEPTORS Physiologic events associated with β-adrenergic receptor responses include stimulation of heart rate and contractility, vasodilation, bronchodilation, and lipolysis. β-Receptor responses can also be divided into two types. The β_1 receptor responds equally to E and NE and mediates cardiac stimulation and lipolysis. The β_2 receptor is more responsive to E than to NE and mediates responses such as vasodilation and bronchodilation. Isoproterenol stimulates and propranolol blocks both β_1 and β_2 receptors. Other agonists and antagonists that have partial selectivity for the β_1 or β_2 receptors have been used therapeutically where the desired response involves predominantly one of the two subtypes.

Both pharmacologic and molecular genetic studies have demonstrated an additional distinct β_3-adrenergic receptor that subserves lipolysis in white and brown adipose tissue as well as the stimulation of heat production in brown adipose tissue. The human β_3-adrenergic receptor has been cloned, and a distinct polymorphism noted that may, in some populations, be associated with weight gain, insulin resistance, and type 2 diabetes mellitus. The β_3-adrenergic receptor has a much greater affinity for NE than E and, unlike the β_1 and β_2 receptors, does not undergo desensitization. Synthetic agonists for the β_3 receptor, currently under development, have a potential role in the treatment of obesity by increasing metabolic rate.

DOPAMINERGIC RECEPTORS Specific dopaminergic receptors, distinct from the classic α- and β-adrenergic receptors, are present in the CNS and peripheral nervous system and in several nonneural tissues. Two types of dopaminergic receptors serve different functions and have different second messengers. Dopamine is a potent agonist of both types of receptors; the action of dopamine is antagonized by phenothiazines and thioxanthenes. The D_1 receptor mediates vasodilation in the renal, mesenteric, coronary, and cerebral vascular beds. Fenoldopam is an agonist selective for the D_1 receptor. The D_2 receptor inhibits transmission in the sympathetic ganglia, inhibits NE release from sympathetic nerve endings by an effect on the presynaptic membrane (Fig. 72-2), inhibits prolactin release from the pituitary, and causes vomiting. Selective agonists of the D_2 receptor include bromocriptine, cabergoline, and apomorphine, while butyrophenones such as haloperidol (active within the CNS), domperidone (does not cross blood-brain barrier readily), and the benzamide sulpiride are relatively selective D_2 antagonists.

STRUCTURE AND FUNCTION OF ADRENERGIC RECEPTORS Adrenergic receptors belong to a superfamily of related membrane proteins, including the visual protein rhodopsin and the muscarinic acetylcholine receptors, that interacts with G proteins. These proteins share significant sequence homologies and, as deduced from the properties of the constituent amino acids, a similar topographic structure in the cell membrane. The postulated structure of this family of receptor proteins is shown schematically in Fig. 72-4. The characteristic features include seven membrane-spanning hydrophobic domains containing 20 to 28 amino acids each. The membrane-span-

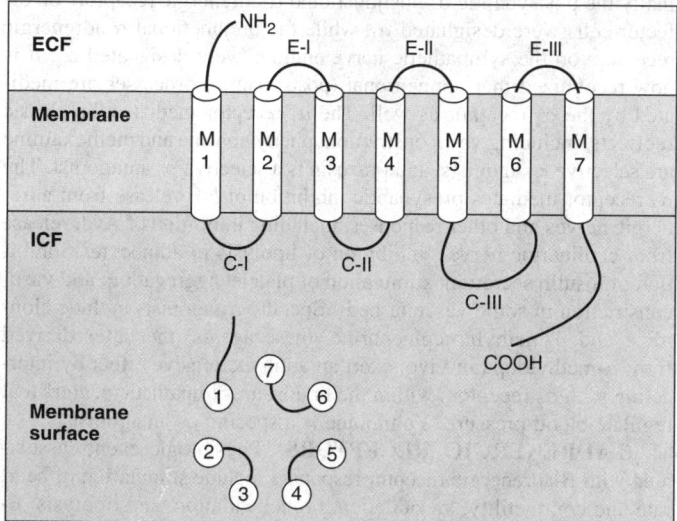

FIGURE 72-4 Proposed structure of adrenergic receptors as deduced from primary amino acid sequences. The single protein chain contains a hydrophilic N terminus (extracellular) and C terminus (intracellular) connected by seven lipophilic membrane-spanning regions (M-1 to M-7) which are interconnected by three extracellular loops (E-I to E-III) and three cytoplasmic loops (C-I to C-III). The β_1-, β_2-, α_1-, and α_2-adrenergic receptors have appreciable sequence homologies and are believed to fit the general structural model represented. Specificity of agonist binding may be conferred by the tertiary structure of several of the membrane-spanning domains while specificity of intracellular response may be related to the length and tertiary structure of the cytoplasmic loops and C terminus. The top portion of the figure is a longitudinal representation of the receptor protein in the cell membrane; shown below is a hypothetical, more compact arrangement seen from the membrane surface. (ECF, extracellular fluid; ICF, intracellular fluid.) *(From Landsberg and Young, 1998, with permission.)*

ning domains, particularly M-7 (Fig. 72-4), appear to be important in determining the characteristic agonist binding.

Coupling of Receptor Occupancy with Cellular Response The major mediators of adrenergic (as well as many other) cellular responses are a family of regulatory proteins termed *G proteins* that, when activated, bind the nucleotide guanosine triphosphate (GTP). The best-characterized G proteins are those that stimulate or inhibit adenylyl cyclase, designated G_s or G_i, respectively (Fig. 72-5). The β_1, β_2, and D_1 receptors are coupled to G_s; receptor occupancy is therefore associated with stimulation of adenylyl cyclase and results in an increase in intracellular cyclic adenosine monophosphate (AMP), which in turn results in activation of protein kinase A and other cyclic AMP–dependent protein kinases. The resultant protein phosphorylation alters the activity of enzymes and the function of other proteins, culminating in a cellular response that is characteristic of the tissue being stimulated. The α_2, M_2 subtype of the muscarinic acetylcholine receptor and the D_2 receptor are coupled to G_i, resulting in diminished adenylyl cyclase activity and a fall in cyclic AMP. The subsequent alterations in enzyme activity and function of other proteins produce an alternate, frequently opposite, series of cellular responses. Although many α_2 responses can be explained by inhibition of adenylyl cyclase, other mechanisms may be involved as well.

The α_1-adrenergic receptor (as well as the M_1 subtype of the acetylcholine receptor) is coupled to a different G protein that activates phospholipase C; this G protein has not been as well characterized but is sometimes designated G_q. Receptor occupancy in this system stimulates phospholipase C, which catalyzes the breakdown of membrane-bound phospholipids, particularly phosphatidylinositol-4,5-bisphosphate (PIP_2) with the production of inositol-1,4,5-trisphosphate (IP_3) and 1,2-diacylglycerol (DAG), both of which act as second messengers (Fig. 72-5). IP_3 rapidly mobilizes calcium from intracellular stores within the endoplasmic reticulum, producing an increase in free cytoplasmic calcium which by itself and via calcium-calmodulin–dependent protein kinases influences cellular processes appropriate to the stimulated cell. The transient rise in calcium induced by IP_3 from the intracellular stores is reinforced in the presence of continued agonist stimulation by alterations in membrane calcium flux that result eventually in net calcium uptake from the extracellular fluid by mechanisms that have been incompletely defined.

DAG, the other second messenger produced by the action of phospholipase C on PIP_2 (as well as other membrane phospholipids), remains associated with the cell membrane and activates protein kinase C, which has different substrates than the calcium-calmodulin kinases stimulated by IP_3. Protein phosphorylation stimulated by protein kinase C contributes to the tissue-specific response in ways that remain poorly understood. Increases in intracellular calcium also potentiate the activation of protein kinase C (Fig. 72-5).

REGULATION OF ADRENERGIC RECEPTORS Prolonged exposure to α- or β-adrenergic agonists decreases the number of corresponding adrenergic receptors on effector cells. Although the biochemical mechanisms involved are obscure, internalization of the β-adrenergic receptor within the cell occurs during agonist exposure in some systems, suggesting that internal translocation contributes to the decrease in receptor number under these circumstances.

Alteration in agonist concentration may also affect the affinity of the receptor for the agonist. Adrenergic receptors that utilize adenylyl cyclase for the second messenger (β receptors, α_2 receptors) exist in high- and low-affinity states; exposure to agonist diminishes the proportion of receptors in the high-affinity state. Such alterations in adrenergic receptors induced by adrenergic agonists are termed *homologous regulation*. Agonist-induced alterations in adrenergic-receptor density and affinity are believed to contribute to the diminished physiologic response that occurs after prolonged exposure of an effector tissue to adrenergic agonist, a phenomenon known as *tachyphylaxis* or *desensitization*.

Adrenergic receptors are also influenced by factors other than adrenergic agonists, so-called *heterologous regulation*. Enhanced α-adrenergic-receptor affinity, for example, may underlie the potentiation of α-adrenergic responses that occur in response to lowered environmental temperatures. Thyroid hormones potentiate β-receptor responses by alterations in β-receptor number and in the efficiency of coupling receptor occupancy with physiologic response. Estrogen and progesterone alter the sensitivity of the myometrium to catecholamines by effects on α-adrenergic receptors. Glucocorticoids may influence adrenergic function by antagonizing agonist-induced decreases in adrenergic receptors, thereby counteracting tachyphylaxis in response to intense adrenergic stimulation.

Alterations in sensitivity to catecholamines also occur as a consequence of postreceptor changes, although the latter remain poorly characterized.

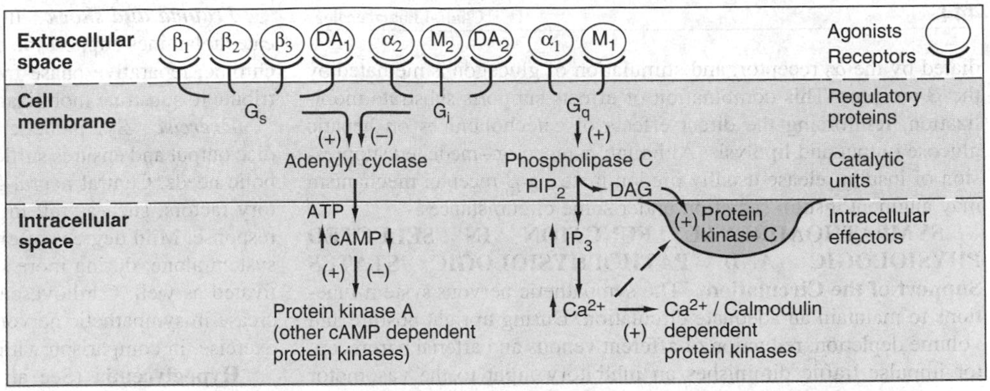

FIGURE 72-5 Interaction of autonomic agonists with membrane-bound regulatory proteins and cellular effector systems. The designations α and β refer to adrenergic receptors, DA refers to dopaminergic receptors, and M, to muscarinic receptors. G designates the GTP-associated regulatory protein which may have a stimulatory (s) or inhibitory (i) effect on adenylyl cyclase or may stimulate phospholipase C (q). [(+) designates stimulation; (−) designates inhibition; PIP_2, phosphatidylinositol-4,5-bisphosphate; DAG, 1,2-diacylglycerol; IP_3, inositol-1,4,5-trisphosphate. See text for details.]

PHYSIOLOGY OF THE SYMPATHOADRENAL SYSTEM

Catecholamines influence all of the major organ systems. The effects take place in seconds and may occur in anticipation of physiologic requirement. An increase in sympathoadrenal activity prior to strenuous exercise, for example, lessens the impact of exercise on the internal environment.

DIRECT EFFECTS OF CATECHOLAMINES **Cardiovascular System** Catecholamines stimulate vasoconstriction in the subcutaneous, mucosal, splanchnic, and renal vascular beds by α-receptor–mediated mechanisms. Although vasoconstriction was originally considered an α_1-receptor response, vascular tone appears to be more complexly regulated and, in many areas, involves α_2-mediated responses as well. The venous portion of the circulation, in particular, is endowed with α_2 receptors. Differential regulation of the two types of α receptors, under certain circumstances, contributes to an integrated physiologic response. Since vasoconstriction in the coronary and cerebral circulations is minimal, flow to these areas is maintained during sympathetic stimulation. Skeletal muscle vasculature contains β receptors sensitive to low circulating levels of epinephrine so that skeletal muscle blood flow is augmented during adrenal medullary activation.

The effects of catecholamines on the heart are mediated by β_1 receptors and include increase in heart rate, enhancement of cardiac contractility, and increase in conduction velocity. The increase in myocardial contractility is illustrated by a leftward and upward shift of the ventricular function curve (see Fig. 231-6) that relates cardiac work to ventricular diastolic fiber length; at any initial fiber length, catecholamines increase cardiac work. Catecholamines also enhance cardiac output by stimulating venoconstriction, enhancing venous return, and increasing the force of atrial contraction, thereby augmenting diastolic volume and hence fiber length. The acceleration of conduction in the junctional tissues results in a more synchronous, and hence more effective, ventricular contraction. Cardiac stimulation increases myocardial oxygen consumption, a major factor in the pathogenesis and treatment of myocardial ischemia.

Metabolism Catecholamines increase metabolic rate. In small mammals, mitochondrial respiration in brown adipose tissue is functionally uncoupled by NE. In a reaction unique to brown adipose tissue, NE stimulates the β_3-adrenergic receptor that activates a specific mitochondrial uncoupling protein that dissipates the proton gradient between the inner mitochondrial matrix and the cytoplasm, thereby uncoupling substrate utilization and ATP synthesis. In humans, a functional role for brown adipose tissue has not been established with certainty.

Substrate mobilization In a variety of tissues, catecholamines stimulate the breakdown of stored fuel with the production of substrate for local consumption; glycogenolysis in the heart, for example, provides substrate for immediate metabolism by the myocardium. Catecholamines also accelerate fuel mobilization in liver, adipose tissue, and skeletal muscle, liberating substrates (glucose, free fatty acids, lactate) into the circulation for use throughout the body.

Fluids and Electrolytes By a direct action on the renal tubule, NE stimulates sodium reabsorption, thereby defending extracellular fluid volume. Dopamine, in contrast, promotes sodium excretion. NE and E also promote cellular uptake of potassium.

Viscera Catecholamines affect visceral function by actions on smooth muscle and glandular epithelium. Urinary bladder and intestinal smooth muscle are relaxed while the corresponding sphincters are stimulated. Gallbladder emptying also involves sympathetic mechanisms. Catecholamine-mediated smooth-muscle contraction in the female aids ovulation and ovum transport along the fallopian tubes, and in the male provides propulsive force for the seminal fluid during ejaculation. Inhibitory α_2 receptors on cholinergic neurons within the gut contribute to intestinal relaxation. Catecholamines induce bronchodilation by a β_2-receptor mechanism.

INDIRECT EFFECTS OF CATECHOLAMINES The ultimate physiologic response induced by catecholamines involves changes in hormone secretion and in blood flow distribution, both of which support and amplify the direct effects of catecholamines.

Endocrine System Catecholamines influence the secretion of renin, insulin, glucagon, calcitonin, parathormone, thyroxine, gastrin, erythropoietin, progesterone, and, possibly, testosterone. Secretion of each of these hormones is governed by complex feedback loops. With the exception of thyroxine and the gonadal steroids, each is a polypeptide not under the direct control of the pituitary gland. Sympathoadrenal input into the secretion of these hormones provides a mechanism for regulation by the CNS and ensures a coordinated hormonal response in accord with the homeostatic needs of the organism.

Renin (See also Chap. 246) Sympathetic stimulation increases renin release by a direct β-receptor effect independent of vascular changes within the kidney. The renin response to volume depletion is sympathetically mediated and is initiated by a fall in central venous pressure. Since renin secretion activates the angiotensin-aldosterone system, angiotensin-induced vasoconstriction supports the direct effects of catecholamines on blood vessels, while aldosterone-mediated sodium reabsorption complements the direct increase in sodium reabsorption induced by sympathetic stimulation. β-receptor blocking agents suppress renin secretion.

Insulin and glucagon Stimulation of pancreatic sympathetic nerves or an elevation in circulating catecholamines suppresses insulin and increases glucagon release. Inhibition of insulin secretion is mediated by the α_2 receptor, and stimulation of glucagon is mediated by the β receptor. This combination of effects supports substrate mobilization, reinforcing the direct effects of catecholamines on hepatic glucose output and lipolysis. Although α-receptor–mediated suppression of insulin release usually predominates, a β-receptor mechanism may augment insulin secretion under some circumstances.

SYMPATHOADRENAL FUNCTION IN SELECTED PHYSIOLOGIC AND PATHOPHYSIOLOGIC STATES

Support of the Circulation The sympathetic nervous system functions to maintain an adequate circulation. During upright posture and volume depletion, reduction of afferent venous and arterial baroreceptor impulse traffic diminishes an inhibitory input to the vasomotor center, thereby increasing sympathetic activity (Fig. 72-3) and reducing efferent vagal tone. As a result, heart rate is increased, and cardiac output is diverted from the skin, subcutaneous tissues, mucosa, and viscera. Sympathetic stimulation of the kidney increases sodium reabsorption, and sympathetically mediated venoconstriction enhances venous return (Fig. 72-6). With pronounced hypotension, the adrenal medulla is recruited and epinephrine reinforces the effects of the sympathetic nervous system.

The intense sympathoadrenal stimulation that accompanies severe volume depletion may contribute to the development of ketoacidosis in alcoholics as well as to the ketoacidosis sometimes seen in association with hyperemesis gravidarum. Catecholamine-mediated suppression of insulin and stimulation of glucagon markedly potentiate ketogenesis in these disease states. Volume resuscitation and provision of adequate glucose promptly reverse the ketoacidosis in most cases.

Congestive heart failure The sympathetic nervous system also provides circulatory support during congestive heart failure (Chap. 232). Venoconstriction and sympathetic stimulation of the heart increase cardiac output while peripheral vasoconstriction directs blood flow to the heart and brain. The afferent signals are less clear than in simple volume depletion because the venous pressure is usually elevated. In severe heart failure, depletion of cardiac NE may impair the effectiveness of sympathetic circulatory support. On the other hand, the possibility has been raised that intense sympathetic stimulation may further impair cardiac function, suggesting possible benefit from β-adrenergic blockade. The use of beta blockers in the treatment of congestive heart failure, in fact, has increased in recent years.

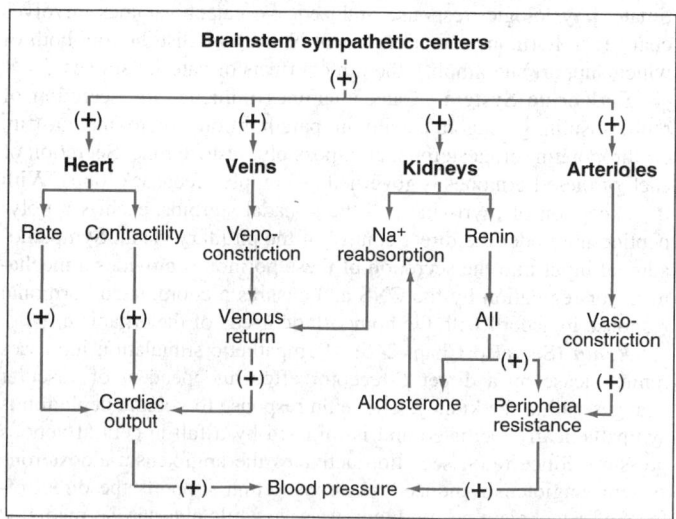

FIGURE 72-6 Sympathetic nervous system effects on blood pressure. Sympathetic stimulation (+) increases blood pressure by effects on the heart, the veins, the kidneys, and the arterioles. The net result of sympathetic stimulation is an increase in both cardiac output and peripheral resistance. AII, angiotensin II. *[From JB Young, L Landsberg, in P Sleight et al (eds), Scientific Foundations of Cardiology, London, Heinemann, 1981.]*

Trauma and shock In acute traumatic injury or shock, adrenal catecholamines support the circulation and mobilize substrates. In the chronic, reparative phase following injury, catecholamines also contribute to substrate mobilization and to the elevation in metabolic rate.

Exercise Sympathetic activation during exercise increases cardiac output and ensures sufficient substrate to meet the increased metabolic needs. Central neural factors, such as anticipation, and circulatory factors, such as fall in venous pressure, trigger the sympathetic response. Mild degrees of exercise stimulate the sympathetic nervous system alone; during more severe exertion the adrenal medulla is activated as well. Cardiovascular conditioning is associated with a decrease in sympathetic nervous system activity both at rest and during exercise, in comparison with the untrained state.

Hypoglycemia (See also Chap. 334) Hypoglycemia causes a marked increase in adrenal medullary epinephrine secretion. When glucose concentrations fall below overnight fasting levels, regulatory glucose-sensitive neurons in the CNS initiate a prompt increase in adrenal medullary secretion. The increase is especially intense at plasma glucose levels below 2.8 mmol/L (50 mg/dL), when plasma E levels increase 25 to 50 times above baseline, thereby increasing hepatic glucose output, providing alternative substrate in the form of free fatty acids, suppressing endogenous insulin release, and inhibiting insulin-mediated glucose utilization in muscle. Many clinical manifestations of hypoglycemia, such as tachycardia, palpitations, nervousness, tremor, and widened pulse pressure, are secondary to increased E secretion, and these manifestations constitute an "early warning" system in insulin-requiring diabetics. In patients with long-standing diabetes mellitus, however, the E response to hypoglycemia may be diminished or absent, leaving affected patients at greater risk to develop severe hypoglycemia.

Cold Exposure The sympathetic nervous system plays a critical role in the maintenance of normal body temperature during exposure to a cold environment. Receptors in the skin and CNS respond to a fall in temperature by activating hypothalamic and brainstem centers that increase sympathetic activity. Sympathetic stimulation leads to vasoconstriction in the superficial vascular beds, thereby diminishing heat loss. The sympathetic response involves a complex interaction between lowered environmental temperatures and α_2-adrenergic receptors. Acclimatization during chronic cold exposure increases the capacity for metabolic heat production in response to sympathetic stimulation.

Dietary Intake Fasting suppresses and overfeeding stimulates the sympathetic nervous system. The reduction in sympathetic activity during fasting or starvation contributes to the decrease in metabolic rate, bradycardia, and hypotension in these states. Enhanced sympathetic activity during periods of increased caloric intake contributes to the elevation in metabolic rate associated with a chronic increase in dietary intake.

Hypoxia Chronic hypoxia is associated with stimulation of the sympathoadrenal system, and some of the cardiovascular changes attendant to hypoxia are dependent on catecholamines.

Orthostatic Hypotension The maintenance of arterial pressure during upright posture depends on an adequate blood volume, an unimpaired venous return, and an intact sympathetic nervous system. Significant postural hypotension, therefore, often reflects extracellular fluid volume depletion or dysfunction of the circulatory reflexes. Diseases of the nervous system, such as tabes dorsalis, syringomyelia, or diabetes mellitus, may disrupt these sympathetic reflexes with resultant orthostatic hypotension. Although any antiadrenergic agent may impair the postural sympathetic response, orthostatic hypotension is most prominent with drugs that block neurotransmission within the ganglia or adrenergic neurons.

The term *idiopathic orthostatic hypotension* refers to a group of degenerative diseases involving either the pre- or postganglionic sympathetic neurons (Chaps. 21 and 365).

Treatment of orthostatic hypotension is usually unsatisfactory except in the mildest cases. There is no way of reestablishing the normal relationship between fall in venous return and sympathetic neuronal activation. Volume expansion with fludrocortisone and a liberal salt diet in conjunction with fitted stockings to the waist, as well as elevation of the head of the bed to avoid recumbency, will maintain plasma volume and venous return and frequently provide symptomatic improvement.

PHARMACOLOGY OF THE SYMPATHOADRENAL SYSTEM

A variety of therapeutic agents affect sympathetic nervous system function or interact with adrenergic receptors, making it possible to stimulate or suppress effects mediated by catecholamines with some degree of specificity (Table 72-1).

SYMPATHOMIMETIC AMINES Sympathomimetic amines may directly activate adrenergic receptors (direct acting) or release NE from the sympathetic nerve endings (indirect acting). Many agents have both direct and indirect effects.

Epinephrine and Norepinephrine The naturally occurring catecholamines act predominantly by the direct stimulation of adrenergic receptors. NE is employed to support the circulation and elevate the blood pressure in hypotensive states (Chap. 38). Peripheral vasoconstriction is the major effect, although cardiac stimulation occurs as well. Epinephrine, also employed as a pressor, has special usefulness in the treatment of allergic reactions, especially those associated with anaphylaxis. Epinephrine antagonizes the effects of histamine and other mediators on vascular and visceral smooth muscle and is useful in the treatment of bronchospasm.

Dopamine *Dopamine* is used in treating hypotension, shock (Chap. 38), and certain forms of heart failure (Chap. 232). At low infusion rates it exerts a positive inotropic effect both by a direct action on the cardiac β_1 receptors and by the indirect release of NE from sympathetic nerve endings in the heart. At low doses direct stimulation of dopaminergic receptors in the renal and mesenteric vasculature also results in vasodilation in the gut and kidney and facilitates sodium excretion. At

Table 72-1 Some Commonly Used Autonomic Drugs[a]

Agent	Indication	Dose and Route	Comment
ADRENERGIC AGONISTS[b]			
Epinephrine	Anaphylaxis	300–500 μg SC or IM (0.3–0.5 mL of 1/1000 solution of hydrochloride salt); 25–50 μg IV (slowly) every 5–15 min; titrate as needed	Nonselective α and β agonist; increases BP, heart rate Bronchodilation
Norepinephrine	Shock Hypotension	2–4 μg of NE base/min IV; titrate as needed	α and β_1 agonist Vasoconstriction predominates Extravasation causes tissue necrosis; infuse through IV cannula
Isoproterenol	Cardiogenic shock Bradyarrhythmias AV block	0.5–5.0 μg/min IV; titrate as needed	Nonselective β agonist Increases cardiac rate and contractility (β_1) Tachycardia limits usefulness
	Asthma	Inhalation	Dilates bronchi (β_2); cardiac stimulation also occurs
Dobutamine	Refractory CHF Cardiogenic shock	2.5–25 (μg/kg)/min IV	Selective β_1 agonist with greater effect on contractility than heart rate; a congener of dopamine but not a dopaminergic agonist
Phenylephrine	Hypotension	2–5 mg SC or IM 0.1–0.5 mg IV	Selective α_1 agonist; useful in antagonizing hypotension of spinal anesthesia
	Supraventricular tachycardia	150–800 μg slow IV push	Pressor effect induces vagotonic response; do not exceed 160 mmHg systolic BP
Terbutaline	Asthma	2.5–5.0 mg PO tid; 0.25–0.5 mg SC; inhalation every 4–5 h	Selective β_2 agonist; β_1 (cardiac) effects at higher doses (inhalation preferred route)
Bitolterol	Asthma	Inhalation every 4–6 h	Selective β_2 agonist
Salmeterol	Asthma	Inhalation bid	Selective β_2 agonist; long-acting agent for maintenance therapy
Albuterol	Asthma	2.0–4.0 mg PO tid or qid; 0.2 mg inhalation every 4–6 h	Selective β_2 agonist; β_1 effects (cardiac) at higher doses (inhalation preferred route)
Isoetharine	Asthma	Inhalation every 2–4 h	Selective β_2 agonist; some β_1 effects
Metaproterenol	Asthma	10–20 mg PO tid or qid; inhalation every 3–4 h	Selective β_2 agonist; some β_1 effects (inhalation preferred route)
Pirbuterol	Asthma	Inhalation every 4–6 h	Selective β_2 agonist; some β_1 effects
Ritodrine	Premature labor	50–350 μg/min IV	Selective β_2 agonist; hypokalemia, hyperglycemia, hypotension, cardiac stimulation may occur Neonatal hypoglycemia, hypocalcemia reported
DOPAMINERGIC AGONISTS			
Dopamine	Shock	2–5 (μg/kg)/min IV (dopaminergic range) 5–10 (μg/kg)/min IV (dopaminergic and beta range) 10–20 (μg/kg)/min IV (beta range) 20–50 (μg/kg)/min IV (alpha range)	Pharmacologic effects are dose dependent: renal and mesenteric vasodilation predominate at lower doses; cardiac stimulation and vasoconstriction develop as the dose is increased

(continued)

445

Table 72-1   Some Commonly Used Autonomic Drugs[a]—(continued)

Agent	Indication	Dose and Route	Comment
DOPAMINERGIC AGONISTS (cont.)			
Bromocriptine	Amenorrhea-galactorrhea	2.5 mg PO bid or tid	Selective agonist of D_2 receptor; inhibits prolactin secretion
	Acromegaly	5–15 mg PO tid or qid	Lowers growth hormone in a minority of patients with acromegaly
Cabergoline	Hyperprolactinemia	0.25–1.0 mg PO twice a week	Agonist at D_2 receptor; inhibits prolactin secretion
Fenoldopam	Hypertension, acute treatment	0.01–0.3 (μg/kg)/min infusion	Agonist at D_1 receptors
INHIBITORS OF CENTRAL SYMPATHETIC OUTFLOW			
Clonidine	Hypertension	0.1–0.6 mg PO bid	Selective α_2 agonist; potentiates central baroreceptor depressor reflex
			Abrupt discontinuation may result in withdrawal syndrome with rebound hypertension
Methyldopa	Hypertension	250–500 mg PO every 6–8 h	Metabolized by decarboxylation and β hydroxylation to α-methylnorepinephrine, a centrally active selective α_2 agonist
ADRENERGIC NEURON BLOCKING AGENTS			
Guanethidine	Hypertension	10–100 mg PO qd	Concentrated in sympathetic nerve endings; blocks release of NE in response to nerve impulses and depletes NE stores; prominent orthostatic hypotension
Bretylium	Ventricular fibrillation and tachycardia	150–300 mg IV 1–4 mg/min IV	In addition to blocking NE release, has direct effect on electrical properties of cardiac muscle
BETA-BLOCKING AGENTS[c]			
Propranolol	Hypertension	40–160 mg PO bid (or higher)	Lipophilic, nonselective Dosage highly variable
	Angina	10–40 mg PO tid or qid	
	Myocardial infarction	60–80 mg PO tid	Prolongs survival post MI
	Arrhythmias	10–30 mg PO tid or qid; 1–3 mg IV	
	Hypertrophic cardiomyopathy	20–40 mg PO tid or qid	
	Pheochromocytoma	10–20 mg PO tid or qid; 0.5–2.0 mg IV	After alpha blockade initiated
	Essential tremor	20–80 mg PO tid	
	Migraine	20–80 mg PO bid or tid	
	Hyperthyroidism	10–60 mg PO tid or qid	
Metoprolol	Hypertension	50–200 mg PO bid	Selective β_1 (cardiac), lipophilic
	Myocardial infarction	100 mg PO bid	Prolongs survival post MI
Nadolol	Hypertension	80–320 mg PO qd	Hydrophilic, nonselective; lengthen dosage interval with renal failure
	Angina	80–240 mg PO qd	
Timolol	Hypertension	10–30 mg PO bid	Lipophilic, nonselective
	Myocardial infarction	10 mg PO bid	Prolongs survival post MI
Atenolol	Hypertension	50–100 mg PO qd	Selective β_1, hydrophilic; lengthen dosage interval with renal failure
Pindolol	Hypertension	5–30 mg PO bid	Nonselective, lipophilic with partial agonist activity
	Angina	10 mg PO qid	
Acebutolol	Hypertension	200–800 mg qid	Selective β_1, hydrophilic, partial agonist activity
	Arrhythmias	200–600 mg bid	
Penbutolol	Hypertension	20–40 mg PO qd	Nonselective

(continued)

higher infusion rates interaction with α-adrenergic receptors results in vasoconstriction, an increase in peripheral resistance, and an elevation of blood pressure.

β-Receptor Agonists *Isoproterenol*, a direct-acting β-receptor agonist, stimulates the heart, decreases peripheral resistance, and relaxes bronchial smooth muscle. It raises the cardiac output and accelerates atrioventricular conduction while increasing the automaticity of ventricular pacemakers. Isoproterenol was formerly used in the treatment of heart block and bronchoconstriction. *Dobutamine*, a congener of dopamine with relative selectivity for the β_1 receptor and with a greater effect on myocardial contractility than on heart rate, is also used in the treatment of congestive heart failure, often in combination with vasodilators (Chap. 232). In conjunction with radionuclide imaging or echocardiographic assessment of wall motion, dobutamine, as well as other investigational congeners that have a relatively greater effect on heart rate, is used in the diagnosis of demand-induced myocardial ischemia.

Selective β_2-receptor agonists The cardiac stimulation caused by nonselective β agonists, such as isoproterenol or epinephrine, is occasionally dangerous when these agents are used in the treatment of bronchoconstriction (Chap. 252). Selective β_2 agonists, administered by inhalation for bronchoconstriction, include agents with an intermediate duration of action (*metaproterenol*, *albuterol*, *terbutaline*, *pirbuterol*, *isoetharine*, and *bitolterol*) and the newer long-acting agents (*salmeterol* and *formoterol*); these drugs improve the therapeutic ratio by achieving bronchial dilatation with less activation of the cardiovascular system (Chaps. 252 and 258). Although selectivity is relative and cardiac stimulation may occur with these agents at higher dose levels, inhaled agonists at the usual doses result in relatively little cardiac stimulation. Oral administration, which is no longer preferred, is associated with more systemic β-agonist effects. *Ritodrine*, another selective β_2 agonist, is used as a tocolytic agent (as is *terbutaline*) to relax the uterus and antagonize premature labor.

α-Adrenergic Agonists *Phenylephrine* and *methoxamine* are direct-acting α agonists that elevate blood pressure by increasing peripheral vasoconstriction. They are used primarily in the treatment of hypotension and paroxysmal supraventricular tachycardia (Chap. 230), in the latter case by increasing cardiac vagal tone through reflex baroreceptor stimulation. Phenylephrine and a related proprietary compound, *phenylpropanolamine*, are common constituents of decongestant medications (often combined with antihistamines) for the treatment of allergic rhinitis and upper respiratory infections.

Miscellaneous Sympathomimetic Amines with Mixed Actions *Ephedrine* has both direct β-receptor agonist properties and an indirect effect on sympathetic nerve endings, from which it releases NE, and is used primarily as a bronchodilator. *Sudephedrine*, a congener of ephedrine, is less potent at dilating bronchi and serves as a nasal decongestant. *Metaraminol* has both direct and indirect effects on sympathetic nerve endings and is employed in the treatment of hypotensive states.

Dopaminergic Agonists The D_2-receptor agonists, *bromocriptine* and *cabergoline*, are used to suppress prolactin secretion (Chap. 328). *Apomorphine*, another D_2-receptor agonist, is used to induce emesis. The D_1 receptor agonist, *fenoldapam*, has recently been approved for the short-term in-hospital treatment of severe hypertension.

ANTIADRENERGIC OR SYMPATHOLYTIC AGENTS (See also Chap. 246) **Agents Inhibiting Central Sympathetic Outflow** The antihypertensive agents *methyldopa*, *clonidine*, *guanabenz*, and *guanfacine* diminish central sympathetic outflow by stimulating a central α-adrenergic pathway ($α_2$ receptor) that diminishes vasomotor outflow. CNS side effects such as sedation are common. When administration of clonidine is stopped abruptly, a withdrawal syndrome characterized by rebound hyperactivity of the sympathetic nervous system can produce a state resembling the crises

Table 72-1   Some Commonly Used Autonomic Drugs[a]—*(continued)*

Agent	Indication	Dose and Route	Comment
BETA-BLOCKING AGENTS[c] (*cont.*)			
Betaxolol	Hypertension	15–20 mg PO qd	Selective $β_1$, hydrophilic
Carteolol	Hypertension	2.5–10 mg PO qd	Nonselective, partial agonist activity, hydrophilic; lengthen dosage interval with renal failure
Esmolol	Supraventricular tachycardia	50–200 ($μ$g/kg)/min IV after loading dose of 500 $μ$g/kg/min for 1 min	Selective $β_1$, very short duration of action
Sotalol	Arrythmias	80–320 mg bid	Nonselective, hydrophilic
Bisoprolol	Hypertension	5–20 mg qd	Selective $β_1$, lipophilic
Carvedilol	CHF	3.125–50 mg PO bid	Nonselective, $α_1$-blocking activity
	Hypertension	6.25–25 mg PO bid	
ALPHA-BLOCKING AGENTS			
Phenoxybenzamine	Pheochromocytoma	10–60 mg PO bid; titrate as needed	Noncompetitive, nonselective alpha blockade
Phentolamine	Pheochromocytoma	5 mg IV (after test dose of 0.5 mg)	Competitive, nonselective alpha blockade
Prazosin	Hypertension	1–5 mg PO bid or tid	Competitive, selective alpha$_1$ blockade
	CHF	2–7 mg PO qid	
Doxazosin	Hypertension Prostatism	1–16 mg PO qd	Competitive selective alpha$_1$ blockade, long duration of action
Terazosin	Hypertension Prostatism	1–5 mg PO qd	Competitive, selective alpha$_1$ blockade, long duration of action
Tamsulosin	Benign prostatic hypertrophy	0.4–0.8 PO qd	Selective $α_1$-blocking activity in prostate, predominantly $α_{1A}$
COMBINED ALPHA-BETA BLOCKING AGENT			
Labetalol	Hypertension	100–1200 mg PO bid; titrate slowly as needed; 20–80 mg IV (by increments up to 300 mg); 2 mg/min by IV infusion	Competitive α and β antagonist with relatively more activity against β receptors
DOPAMINERGIC ANTAGONIST[d]			
Metoclopramide	Diabetic gastroparesis	10–15 mg PO qid	Competitive dopaminergic antagonist with prominent cholinergic agonist activity
	Gastroesophageal reflex	10–15 mg PO qid	
	Antiemetic (cancer chemotherapy)	10 mg IV	
GANGLIONIC BLOCKING AGENT			
Trimethaphan	Hypertensive crisis (aortic dissection)	0.5–5 mg/min IV	Competitive ganglionic blocker; some direct vasodilating effects; inhibits parasympathetic as well as sympathetic nervous system
CHOLINERGIC AGENT			
Bethanechol	Urinary retention (nonobstructive)	10–20 mg PO tid or qid; 2.5 mg SC	M_2 receptor agonist
ANTICHOLINESTERASE AGENTS[e]			
Physostigmine	Central cholinergic blockade	1–2 mg IV (slow)	Tertiary amine; penetrates CNS well; may cause seizures; used to reverse central anticholinergic effects produced by overdose of atropine or tricyclic antidepressants
Edrophonium	Paroxysmal supraventricular tachycardia	5 mg IV (after 1.0-mg test dose)	Induces vagotonic response; rapid onset, short duration of action; effects reversed by atropine

(continued)

Table 72-1   Some Commonly Used Autonomic Drugs^a—(continued)

Agent	Indication	Dose and Route	Comment
CHOLINERGIC BLOCKING AGENTS^f			
Atropine	Bradycardia and hypotension	0.4–1.0 mg IV every 1–2 h	Competitive inhibition of M_1 and M_2 receptor; blocks hemodynamic changes associated with increased vagal tone
Ipratropium	Asthma Chronic obstructive pulmonary disease	500 mg by inhalation (nebulizer) tid or qid	Anticholinergic bronchodilator
Oxybutynin	Overactive bladder	5 mg PO bid or qid	Muscarinic receptor antagonist
Tolterodine	Overactive bladder	1–2 mg PO bid	Competitive muscarinic receptor antagonist

^{a} Consult complete prescribing information; doses for children are not given; only the more common indications and routes of administration are listed.

^{b} Dopaminergic agonists are listed separately although dopamine, at high doses, is an adrenergic agonist as well.

^{c} Clinical efficacy of most beta blockers appears similar for major indications. Not all beta blockers are FDA approved for all indications listed in the table. When beta-blocking agents are discontinued, gradual dosage reduction is recommended. Both beta$_1$ selective and nonselective agents have cardioprotective effects after myocardial infarction.

^{d} Neuroleptic and antipsychotic agents are also dopaminergic antagonists; these are not included in the table.

^{e} A major use of cholinesterase inhibitors is in myasthenia gravis (Chap. 380). These agents, quaternary amines that do not penetrate the CNS, are not included here.

^{f} A wide variety of synthetic atropine derivatives are available for the purpose of (1) diminishing GI tract motility and secretion and (2) increasing urinary bladder capacity. Their usefulness is limited by anticholinergic side effects. Some may be useful as adjuncts in the treatment of peptic ulcer disease.

NOTE: BP, blood pressure; NE; norepinephrine; AV, atrioventricular; CHF, congestive heart failure; MI, myocardial infarction; CNS, central nervous system; FDA, U.S. Food & Drug Administration; GI, gastrointestinal.

of patients with pheochromocytoma. *Opiates* also may exert a central sympatholytic effect; the sympathetic excitation of morphine withdrawal responds to clonidine and vice versa. *Propranolol* and *reserpine* may exert some sympatholytic effects at the level of the CNS.

Ganglionic Blocking Agents   Ganglionic transmission may be antagonized by drugs that block the (nicotinic) cholinergic synapse between the pre- and postganglionic autonomic nerves. These agents inhibit the parasympathetic as well as the sympathetic nervous system. Only *trimethaphan* is in general clinical use; its major application is in the treatment of hypertensive crises, particularly aortic dissection, when controlled hypotension and decreased myocardial contractility are desirable (Chap. 246).

Agents Acting at the Peripheral Sympathetic Nerve Endings   Adrenergic neuron-blocking agents depress the function of the peripheral sympathetic nerves by decreasing the amount of neurotransmitter released. *Guanethidine*, the prototype of this class of drugs, is concentrated in the sympathetic nerve endings by the amine-uptake mechanism. Within the terminal it blocks the release of NE in response to nerve impulses and eventually depletes the nerve of NE by displacing it from the intraneuronal storage granules. The drug was formerly useful in the management of severe hypertension, although orthostatic hypotension was a limiting side effect. *Bretylium*, an agent whose effects are similar to those of guanethidine, is employed in the treatment of ventricular fibrillation (Chap. 230). Both guanethidine and bretylium are antagonized by agents that affect the amine-uptake transport process such as sympathomimetic amines, tricyclic antidepressants, phenoxybenzamine, and phenothiazines. The antihypertensive action of guanethidine may be rapidly reversed by these drugs.

Reserpine depletes catecholamines from the peripheral sympathetic nerve endings, the brain, and the adrenal medulla. Its antihypertensive effect in humans is usually attributed to depletion of peripheral NE stores within sympathetic nerve endings. The sedation and occasionally morbid depression attending its use result from NE depletion within the CNS.

Adrenergic-Receptor Blocking Agents   Adrenergic blocking agents antagonize the effects of catecholamines at the level of the peripheral tissue.

α-Adrenergic-receptor blocking agents   *Phenoxybenzamine* and *phentolamine* are utilized principally in treating pheochromocytoma (Chap. 332). Phenoxybenzamine produces prolonged, noncompetitive alpha blockade, while phentolamine leads to reversible, competitive blockade. Because of its rapid action and short duration, phentolamine is commonly used in the treatment of acute hypertensive paroxysms secondary to catecholamine excess, such as occur with pheochromocytoma. Both phentolamine and phenoxybenzamine antagonize α_1 and α_2 receptors, although phenoxybenzamine is more potent at the α_1-receptor site. *Prazosin*, an α-adrenergic blocking agent with selectivity for the α_1 receptor, possesses properties that resemble those of primary vasodilators and has been used in the treatment of essential hypertension, as an afterload-reducing agent in congestive heart failure, and as an adjunct in the treatment of pheochromocytoma (Chap. 332). *Doxazosin* and *terazosin*, long-acting selective α_1 blockers, are more useful in the treatment of essential hypertension because of better dosing schedule and less orthostatic hypotension. These agents also lower triglyceride levels and raise high-density lipoprotein (HDL) cholesterol levels. These selective α_1 blockers, along with *tamsulosin* are useful in the symptomatic treatment of urinary outflow track obstruction and prostatism because they antagonize contraction of the sphincter at the bladder trigone and the prostate smooth muscle.

β-Adrenergic-receptor blocking agents   These drugs antagonize the effects of catecholamines on the heart and are useful in the treatment of angina pectoris, hypertension, and cardiac arrhythmias. The benefit of beta blockade in angina derives from the decrease in myocardial oxygen consumption following reduction in heart rate and myocardial contractility (Chap. 244). The hypotensive effect of beta blockade is not clearly understood (Chap. 246). Diminished cardiac output, decreased NE release at postganglionic sympathetic nerve endings, reduced renin secretion, and suppressed central sympathetic outflow are possible mechanisms. The efficacy of β-blocking agents in the treatment of arrhythmias depends on reduction of the rate of spontaneous depolarization of pacemaker cells in the sinus node and junctional pacemakers and on slowing conduction within the atria and atrioventricular node. Beta blockade is also effective in the symptomatic management of hyperthyroidism and the control of tachycardia and arrhythmias in patients with pheochromocytoma. β-adrenergic blocking agents are also useful in the treatment of migraine, essential tremor, idiopathic hypertrophic subaortic stenosis, and aortic dissection. Several trials have demonstrated that β-receptor blocking agents, administered long-term, diminish mortality following acute myocardial infarction. The mechanism of this cardioprotective effect may involve antiarrhythmic action, prevention of reinfarction, and reduction in infarct size (Chap. 243).

Pharmacologic properties of β-receptor blocking agents   Fourteen beta-blocking agents (atenolol, acebutolol, betaxolol, bisoprolol, carvedilol, carteolol, esmolol, metoprolol, nadolol, pindolol, penbutolol, propranolol, sotalol, and timolol) are available for use in the United States. Other agents (alprenolol, bevantolol, dilevalol, oxprenolol, etc.) are in use in other countries and investigational within the United States. The utility of these agents is derived predominantly from blockade of β-adrenergic receptors.

Although much has been written about other pharmacologic properties, including cardioselectivity, membrane-stabilizing (local anesthetic) effects, intrinsic sympathomimetic (partial-agonist) activity, and lipid solubility, the clinical significance of these additional properties is small. Local anesthetic properties are most prominent with propranolol; however, membrane stabilization probably does not contribute substantially to the clinical utility. The various beta blockers do differ in their water and lipid solubility. The lipophilic agents (propranolol, metoprolol, oxprenolol, bisoprolol, carvedilol) are readily absorbed from the gastrointestinal tract, metabolized by the liver, have large volumes of distribution, and penetrate the CNS well; the hydrophilic agents (acebutolol, atenolol, betaxolol, carteolol, nadolol, sotalol) are less readily absorbed, not extensively metabolized, and have relatively long plasma half-lives. As a consequence, the hydrophilic agents may be administered once per day. Hepatic failure may prolong the plasma half-life of the lipophilic agents, whereas renal failure may prolong the action of the hydrophilic group. The degree of lipid solubility, therefore, provides a basis for choice of a particular agent in patients with hepatic or renal insufficiency. Although the hydrophilic agents penetrate the CNS less well, CNS side effects (sedation, depression, hallucinations) are well described with the hydrophilic as well as with the lipophilic agents.

Some β-adrenergic blocking agents possess β-agonist activity. This has been referred to as "intrinsic sympathomimetic activity" (ISA). Agents with partial agonist activity (pindolol, alprenolol, acebutolol, carteolol, dilevalol, oxprenolol) cause little or no depression of resting heart rate (partial agonist effect) while blocking the increase in heart rate that occurs in response to exercise or the administration of a beta agonist such as isoproterenol. The presence of partial agonist activity may be useful when bradycardia limits treatment in patients with slow resting heart rates. Pindolol also produces mild vasodilation, perhaps in part related to peripheral β_2 stimulation. Agents with partial agonist activity cause less change in blood lipid levels than agents without agonist properties. On theoretical grounds, intrinsic sympathomimetic activity would be undesirable in the treatment of thyrotoxicosis, idiopathic hypertrophic subaortic stenosis, aortic dissection, and tachyarrhythmias.

Cardioselective (β_1) adrenergic-receptor blocking agents Propranolol, the prototype of the nonselective β-adrenergic blocking agent, induces a competitive blockade of both β_1 and β_2 receptors. Other nonselective beta-blocking agents include alprenolol, carteolol, dilevalol, nadolol, oxprenolol, penbutolol, pindolol, sotalol, timolol, and carvedilol. Metoprolol, esmolol, acebutolol, atenolol, and betaxolol possess relative selectivity for the β_1 receptor. Although β_1-(cardio-) selective agents have the theoretical advantage of producing less bronchoconstriction and less peripheral vasoconstriction, a clear-cut clinical advantage of the cardioselective agents has not been decisively demonstrated, since the β_1 selectivity is only relative. Bronchoconstriction may occur when β_1-selective agents are administered in full therapeutic doses.

Adverse effects of β-receptor blocking agents Aside from the effects on the CNS, most adverse reactions to beta-blocking agents are consequences of β-adrenergic blockade. These include the precipitation of heart failure in patients in whom cardiac compensation depends on enhanced sympathetic drive; the aggravation of bronchospasm in patients with asthma; predisposition to the development of hypoglycemia in insulin-requiring diabetics (blockade of catecholamine-mediated counterregulation and antagonism of the adrenergic warning signs of hypoglycemia); the development of hyperkalemia in diabetic or uremic patients with impaired potassium tolerance; the enhancement of coronary or peripheral arterial vasospasm; and elevation in triglycerides and depression of HDL levels. The lipid (and perhaps the peripheral vascular) effects are less (or absent) in agents with partial (β_2) agonist activity or alpha-blocking properties (carvedilol).

Miscellaneous adrenergic blocking agents Labetalol, approved for use in the United States as an antihypertensive agent, is a competitive antagonist of both α- and β-adrenergic receptors. Although labetalol induces relatively more β- than α-receptor blockade, fall in peripheral resistance may be marked following acute administration of the drug. Vasodilation may be mediated in part by a partial agonist effect on the β_2-adrenergic receptor; labetalol does not possess partial agonist activity for the β_1 (cardiac) receptor.

Metoclopramide is a dopaminergic antagonist with cholinergic agonist properties. It enhances gastric emptying, increases the tone of the lower esophageal sphincter, increases prolactin and aldosterone secretion, and antagonizes emesis induced by apomorphine. It is useful clinically in enhancing gastric emptying (in the absence of organic obstruction such as in diabetic gastroparesis), in antagonizing gastroesophageal reflux, and as an antiemetic during cancer chemotherapy.

THE PARASYMPATHETIC NERVOUS SYSTEM

ACETYLCHOLINE ACh serves as the neurotransmitter at all autonomic ganglia, at the postganglionic parasympathetic nerve endings, at the postganglionic sympathetic nerve endings innervating the eccrine sweat glands, and at the skeletal muscle end plate (neuromuscular junction). The enzyme choline acetyltransferase catalyzes the synthesis of ACh from acetyl coenzyme A (CoA) produced within the nerve ending and from choline, actively taken up from the extracellular fluid. Within the cholinergic nerve endings, ACh is stored in discrete synaptic vesicles and released in response to nerve impulses that depolarize the nerve terminals and increase calcium influx.

Cholinergic Receptors Different receptors for ACh exist on the postganglionic neurons within the autonomic ganglia and at the postjunctional autonomic effector sites. Those within the autonomic ganglia and adrenal medulla are stimulated predominantly by nicotine (*nicotinic receptors*) and those on autonomic effector cells by the alkaloid muscarine (*muscarinic receptors*). Ganglionic blocking agents antagonize the nicotinic receptors, while atropine blocks the muscarinic receptors. The muscarinic (M) receptor, furthermore, has been recently subdivided into additional types. The M_1 receptor is localized to the CNS and perhaps parasympathetic ganglia; the M_2 receptor is the nonneuronal muscarinic receptor on smooth muscle, cardiac muscle, and glandular epithelium. Bethanechol is a selective agonist of the M_2 receptor; pirenzepine, an investigational agent, is a selective antagonist of the M_1 receptor that markedly reduces gastric acid secretion. The M_2 receptor inhibits adenylyl cyclase and utilizes the regulatory G_i protein; the M_1 receptor interacts with G_q and stimulates phospholipase C (Fig. 72-5). The M_3 receptor, present on smooth muscle and secretory glands, is antagonized by atropine and utilizes phospholipase C, IP_3, and DAG as second messengers. Other subtypes have been identified by molecular biologic techniques but have not yet been fully characterized.

Acetylcholinesterase Hydrolysis of ACh by acetylcholinesterase inactivates the neurotransmitter at cholinergic synapses. This enzyme (also known as specific or true cholinesterase) is present within neurons and is distinct from butyrocholinesterase (serum cholinesterase or pseudocholinesterase). The latter enzyme is present in plasma and nonneuronal tissues and is not primarily involved in the termination of the effects of ACh at autonomic effector sites. The pharmacologic effects of anticholinesterase agents are due to inhibition of neuronal (true) acetylcholinesterase.

PHYSIOLOGY OF THE PARASYMPATHETIC NERVOUS SYSTEM The parasympathetic nervous system participates in the regulation of the cardiovascular system, the gastrointestinal tract, and the genitourinary system. Tissues such as liver, kidney, pancreas, and thyroid also receive parasympathetic innervation, suggesting a role for the parasympathetic nervous system in metabolic regulation as well, although cholinergic effects on metabolism are not well characterized.

Cardiovascular System Parasympathetic effects on the heart are mediated by the vagus nerve. ACh reduces the rate of spontaneous depolarization of the sinoatrial node and decreases heart rate. ACh also delays impulse conduction within the atrial musculature while shortening the effective refractory period, a combination of factors that may initiate or perpetuate atrial arrhythmias. At the atrioventricular node, ACh reduces conduction velocity, increases the effective refractory period, and thus diminishes the ventricular response during atrial flutter or fibrillation (Chap. 230). The decrease in inotropy induced by ACh is related to a prejunctional inhibitory effect on sympathetic nerve endings as well as to a direct inhibitory effect on the atrial myocardium. The ventricular myocardium is not much affected since innervation by cholinergic fibers is minimal. A direct cholinergic contribution to the regulation of peripheral resistance appears unlikely since parasympathetic innervation of the vasculature is not extensive. The parasympathetic nervous system, however, may influence peripheral resistance indirectly by inhibiting NE release from sympathetic nerves.

Gastrointestinal Tract   Parasympathetic innervation of the gut is via the vagus nerve and the pelvic sacral nerves. The parasympathetic nervous system increases the tone of gastrointestinal smooth muscle, enhances peristaltic activity, and relaxes the gastrointestinal sphincters. ACh stimulates exocrine secretion from the glandular epithelium and enhances the secretion of gastrin, secretin, and insulin.

Genitourinary and Respiratory Systems   Sacral parasympathetic nerves supply the urinary bladder and genitalia. ACh increases ureteral peristalsis, contracts the urinary detrusor muscle, and relaxes the trigone and sphincter, thereby playing a critical role in the coordination of urination. The respiratory tract is innervated with parasympathetic fibers derived from the vagus nerve. ACh increases tracheobronchial secretions and stimulates bronchial constriction.

PHARMACOLOGY OF THE PARASYMPATHETIC NERVOUS SYSTEM   Cholinergic Agonists   ACh itself has no therapeutic role because of its widespread effects and short duration of action. Congeners of ACh are less susceptible to hydrolysis by cholinesterase and have a narrower range of physiologic effects. Bethanechol, the only systemic cholinergic agonist in general use, stimulates gastrointestinal and genitourinary smooth muscle with minimal effect on the cardiovascular system. It is used in the treatment of urinary retention in the absence of outflow tract obstruction and, less commonly, in gastrointestinal disorders such as postvagotomy gastric atony. Pilocarpine and carbachol are topical cholinergic agonists used in the treatment of glaucoma.

Acetylcholinesterase Inhibitors   Cholinesterase inhibitors enhance the effects of parasympathetic stimulation by diminishing the inactivation of ACh. The therapeutic application of reversible cholinesterase inhibitors depends on the role of ACh as neurotransmitter at the skeletal muscle neuroeffector junction and within the CNS and includes the treatment of myasthenia gravis (Chap. 380), the termination of neuromuscular blockade following general anesthesia, and the reversal of intoxication by agents with a central anticholinergic action. Physostigmine, a tertiary amine, penetrates the CNS well, while related quaternary amines (neostigmine, pyridostigmine, ambenonium, and edrophonium) do not. Organophosphorous cholinesterase inhibitors produce irreversible cholinesterase blockade; these agents are used principally as insecticides and are primarily of toxicologic interest. With regard to the autonomic nervous system, cholinesterase inhibitors are of limited use in the treatment of intestinal and bladder smooth-muscle dysfunction such as occurs in paralytic ileus and atonic urinary bladder. Cholinesterase inhibitors induce a vagotonic response in the heart and may be useful in terminating attacks of paroxysmal supraventricular tachycardia (Chap. 230).

Cholinergic-Receptor Blocking Agents   *Atropine* blocks muscarinic cholinergic receptors, with little effect on cholinergic transmission at the autonomic ganglia and the neuromuscular junctions. Many of the CNS actions of atropine and atropine-like drugs are attributable to blockade of central muscarinic synapses. The related alkaloid, *scopolamine*, is similar to atropine but causes drowsiness, euphoria, and amnesia, effects that make it suitable as a preanesthetic medication.

Atropine increases heart rate and enhances atrioventricular conduction, actions that may be useful in combating the bradycardia or heart block associated with heightened vagal tone. In addition, atropine reverses cholinergically mediated bronchoconstriction and diminishes respiratory tract secretions. These effects contribute to its utility as a preanesthetic medication.

Atropine also decreases gastrointestinal tract motility and secretion. Although various derivatives and congeners of atropine (such as *propantheline, isopropamide,* and *glycopyrrolate*) have been advocated in patients with peptic ulcer or with diarrheal syndromes, the chronic use of such agents is limited by other manifestations of parasympathetic inhibition such as dry mouth and urinary retention. The investigational selective M_1 inhibitor pirenzepine inhibits gastric secretion at doses that have minimal anticholinergic effects at other sites; this agent may be useful in the treatment of peptic ulcer. Atropine and its congener *ipratropium*, when given by inhalation, cause bronchodilation and have been used experimentally in the treatment of asthma.

BIBLIOGRAPHY

ARNER P, HOFFSTEDT J: Adrenoceptor genes in human obesity. J Intern Med 245:667, 1999

CARON MG, LEFKOWITZ RJ: Catecholamine receptors: Structure, function and regulation. Recent Prog Horm Res 48:277, 1993

CHALMERS J, PILOWSKY P: Brainstem and bulbospinal neurotransmitter systems in the control of blood pressure. J Hypertens 9:675, 1991

ESLER M et al: Overflow of catecholamine neurotransmitters to the circulation: Source, fate, and functions. Physiol Rev 70:963, 1990

GRASSI G, ESLER M: How to assess sympathetic activity in humans. J Hypertens 17:719, 1999

JÄNIG W, MCLACHLAN EM: Specialized functional pathways are the building blocks of the autonomic nervous system. J Auton Nerv Syst 41:3, 1992

LAM YW: Clinical pharmacology of dopamine agonists. Pharmacotherapy 20:175, 2000

LOW PA: Autonomic nervous system function. J Clin Neurophysiol 10:14, 1993

NELSON H: β-Adrenergic bronchodilators. N Engl J Med 333:499, 1995

PITCHER JA et al: G protein–coupled receptor kinases. Annu Rev Biochem 67:653, 1998

RUFFOLO RR JR, HIEBLE JP: α-Adrenoceptors. Pharmacol Ther 61:1, 1994

STROSBERG AD: Structure and function of the β_3-adrenergic-receptor. Annu Rev Pharmacol Toxicol 37:421, 1997

YOUNG JB, LANDSBERG L: Catecholamines and the adrenal medulla, in *Williams' Textbook of Endocrinology,* 9th ed, JD Wilson et al (eds). Philadelphia, Saunders, 1998, p 665

73 | NUTRITIONAL REQUIREMENTS AND DIETARY ASSESSMENT

Johanna Dwyer

Nutrients are substances that are not synthesized in the body in sufficient amounts and therefore must be supplied by the diet. Nutrient requirements for groups of healthy persons have been thoroughly defined on the basis of experimental evidence. For good health we require energy-providing nutrients (protein, fat, and carbohydrate), vitamins, minerals, and water. Specific nutrient requirements include 9 essential amino acids, several fatty acids, 4 fat-soluble vitamins, 10 water-soluble vitamins, and choline. Several inorganic substances, including four minerals, seven trace minerals, three electrolytes, and the ultratrace elements, must also be supplied in the diet (Chap. 75).

The required amounts of the essential nutrients differ by age and physiologic state. Conditionally essential nutrients are not required in the diet but must be supplied to individuals who do not synthesize them in adequate amounts, such as those with genetic defects, those having pathologic states with nutritional implications, and developmentally immature infants (Chap. 74). Many organic phytochemicals and zoochemicals present in foods have various health effects. For example, dietary fiber has been shown to have beneficial effects on gastrointestinal function.

ESSENTIAL NUTRIENT REQUIREMENTS **Energy** For weight to remain stable, energy intake must match energy output (Chap. 77). The major categories of energy output are resting energy expenditure (REE) and physical activity; minor sources include the energy cost of metabolizing food (thermic effect of food or specific dynamic action) and shivering thermogenesis (e.g., cold-induced thermogenesis). The average energy intake is about 2800 kcal/d for American men and about 1800 kcal/d for American women, though these estimates vary with body size and activity level. Formulas for estimating REE are useful for assessing the energy needs of an individual whose weight is stable. Thus, for males, REE = 900 + 10w, and for females, REE = 700 + 7w, where w is weight in kg. The calculated REE is then adjusted for physical activity level by multiplying by 1.2 for sedentary, 1.4 for moderately active, or 1.8 for very active individuals. The final figure provides an estimate of total caloric needs in a state of energy balance.

Illness often alters energy needs. Unstressed hospitalized patients at bed rest usually require 1.2 times their REE, whereas those who are stressed, febrile, and catabolic require 1.5 to 2 times their REE (Chap. 74). Intestinal malabsorption may decrease net utilizable energy to as little as 25% of ingested energy and may necessitate feeding by parenteral routes (Chap. 76). Fever increases energy expenditure by 10 to 13% per degree Celsius above normal. Other diseases increase energy needs by varying amounts, such as burns (40 to 100%), trauma (40 to 100%), and hyperthyroidism (10 to 100%). Hypothyroidism and adrenal insufficiency decrease resting energy needs, but these alterations are corrected after adequate hormone replacement. In obese patients, weight reduction can be accomplished by reducing energy intakes by approximately 500 kcal/d to achieve a loss of 0.5 kg of fat per week, or 1000 kcal/d to lose 1 kg per week (Chap. 77).

Protein Dietary protein consists of both essential and nonessential amino acids that are required for protein synthesis, whereas certain amino acids can also be used for energy and gluconeogenesis (Chap. 334). The nine essential amino acids are histidine, isoleucine, leucine, lysine, methionine/cystine, phenylalanine/tyrosine, threonine, tryptophan, and valine. When energy intake is inadequate, protein intake must be increased, since ingested amino acids are diverted into pathways of glucose synthesis and oxidation. In extreme energy deprivation, protein-calorie malnutrition may ensue (Chaps. 74 and 76).

For adults, the recommended dietary allowance (RDA) for protein is about 0.6 g/kg desirable body weight per day, assuming that energy needs are met and that the protein is of relatively high biologic value. Current recommendations for a healthy diet call for at least 10 to 14% of calories from protein. Biologic value tends to be highest for animal proteins, followed by proteins from legumes (beans), cereals (rice, wheat, corn), and roots. Combinations of plant proteins that complement one another in biologic value or combinations of animal and plant proteins can increase biologic value and lower total protein requirements.

Protein needs increase during growth, pregnancy, lactation, and rehabilitation during treatment of malnutrition. The tolerance of dietary protein is decreased in renal insufficiency and liver failure. Normal protein intake can precipitate encephalopathy in patients with cirrhosis of the liver (Chap. 299) or worsen uremia in those with renal failure (Chap. 270).

Fat and Carbohydrate Fats are a concentrated source of energy and constitute on average 34% of calories in U.S. diets. However, for optimal health, fat intake should total no more than 30% of calories. Saturated fat and trans-fat should be limited to <10% of calories, and polyunsaturated fats to <10% of calories, with monounsaturated fats comprising the remainder of fat intake. At least 55% of total calories should be derived from carbohydrates. The brain requires about 100 g/d of glucose for fuel; other tissues use about 50 g/d. Over time, adaptations in carbohydrate needs are possible in hypocaloric states. For example, reduced insulin levels lead to adipose tissue breakdown and cause the body to burn more fatty acids. However, some tissues (e.g., brain and red blood cells) rely on glucose supplied either exogenously or from muscle proteolysis (Chap. 334).

Water For adults, 1 to 1.5 mL water per kcal of energy expenditure is sufficient under usual conditions to allow for normal variations in physical activity levels, sweating, and solute load of the diet. Water losses include 50 to 100 mL/d in the feces, 500 to 1000 mL/d by evaporation or exhalation, and, depending on the renal solute load, ≥1000 mL/d in the urine. If external losses increase, intakes must increase accordingly to avoid underhydration. Fever increases water losses by approximately 200 mL/d per °C; diarrheal losses vary but may be as great as 5 L/d in severe diarrhea. Heavy sweating and vomiting also increase water losses. When renal function is normal and solute intakes are adequate, the kidneys can adjust to increased water intake by excreting up to 18 L/d of excess water (Chap. 329). However, obligatory urine outputs can compromise hydration status when there is inadequate intake or when losses increase in disease or kidney damage.

Infants have high requirements for water because of their large ratio of surface area to volume, the limited capacity of the immature kidney to handle high renal solute loads, and their inability to communicate their thirst. Increased water needs during pregnancy are low, perhaps an additional 30 mL/d; but during lactation, milk production increases water requirements so that approximately 1000 mL/d of additional water is needed, or 1 mL for each mL of milk produced. Special attention must be paid to the water needs of the elderly, who have reduced total body water and blunted thirst sensation and may be taking diuretics.

Other Nutrients The vitamins and minerals required for health and the clinical disorders caused by vitamin deficiency or excess are discussed in Chap. 75.

451

DIETARY REFERENCE INTAKES, RECOMMENDED ALLOWANCES, AND TOLERANCES Fortunately, human life and well-being can be maintained within a fairly wide range for most nutrients. However, the capacity for adaptation is not infinite—too much, as well as too little, intake of a nutrient may have adverse effects or alter the health benefits conferred by another nutrient (Chap. 75). Therefore, benchmark recommendations on nutrient intakes have been developed to guide clinical practice. These quantitative estimates of nutrient intakes are collectively referred to as the *dietary reference intakes* (DRIs). The DRIs supplant the RDAs, the single reference values used in the United States since 1989. DRIs include the estimated average requirement (EAR) for nutrients, as well as three other reference values used for dietary planning for individuals: the RDAs, the adequate intake (AI), and the safe upper level (UL). The current RDAs and AIs are provided in Tables 73-1 and 73-2, respectively.

Estimated Average Requirement When florid dietary deficiency diseases such as rickets, scurvy, xerophthalmia, and protein-calorie malnutrition were common, nutrient adequacy was assumed by the absence of clinical signs of a dietary deficiency disease. Later, it was determined that biochemical and other changes were evident long before the clinical deficiency became apparent. Consequently, criteria of adequacy are chosen using such biologic markers when they are available. Current efforts focus on the amount of a nutrient that reduces the risk of chronic degenerative diseases. Priority is given to sensitive biochemical, physiologic, or behavioral tests that reflect early changes in regulatory processes or maintenance of body stores of nutrients.

The EAR is the amount of a nutrient estimated to be adequate for half of the healthy individuals of a specific age and sex. The types of evidence and criteria used to establish nutrient requirements vary by nutrient, age, and physiologic group. The EAR is not an effective estimate of nutrient adequacy in individuals because it is a median requirement for a group, and the variation around this number is considerable. As the EAR specifies, 50% of individuals in a group fall below the requirement and 50% fall above it. Thus, a person with a usual intake at the EAR has a 50% risk of an inadequate intake during the reporting period. For these reasons, other standards, described below, are more useful for clinical purposes.

Recommended Dietary Allowances The RDA is the average daily dietary intake level that meets the nutrient requirements of nearly all healthy persons of a specific sex, age, life stage, or physiologic condition (such as pregnancy or lactation). The RDA is commonly used as a nutrient-intake goal for planning diets of individuals.

The RDA is defined statistically as 2 standard deviations (SD) above the EAR to ensure that the needs of any given individual are met. The RDAs are used to formulate food guides such as the U.S. Department of Agriculture (USDA) Food Guide Pyramid for individuals, food exchange lists for therapeutic diet planning, and as a standard for describing the nutritional content of processed foods and nutrient supplements. The nutrient content in a food is stated by weight or as a percent of the daily value (DV), a varient of the RDA which, for an adult, represents the highest RDA for an adult consuming 2000 kcal/d.

The risk of dietary inadequacy increases as intakes fall further below the RDA. However, the RDA is an overly generous criterion for evaluating nutrient adequacy. For example, by definition the RDA exceeds the actual requirements of all but about 2 to 3% of the population. Therefore, many people whose intakes fall below the RDA may still be getting enough of the nutrient.

Adequate Intake It is not possible to set an RDA for some nutrients that do not have an established EAR. In this circumstance, the AI is based on observed, or experimentally determined, approximations of nutrient intakes in healthy people. In the DRIs established to date, AIs rather than RDAs are proposed for infants up to age 1, as well as for calcium, vitamin D, fluoride, pantothenic acid, biotin, and choline for persons of all ages.

Tolerable Upper Levels of Nutrient Intake Excessive nutrient intake can disturb body functions and cause acute, progressive, or permanent disabilities (Chap. 75). Some diseases of nutritional excess include fluorosis, hypervitaminosis A, hypervitaminosis D, and obesity. The tolerable UL is the highest level of chronic nutrient intake (usually daily) that is unlikely to pose a risk of adverse health effects for most of the population. An uncertainty factor is applied to ensure that even very sensitive persons would not experience adverse effects at the UL dose chosen. For many nutrients, data on the adverse effects of large amounts of the nutrient are unavailable or too limited establish a UL. Therefore, the lack of a UL does *not* mean that the risk of adverse

Table 73-1 Recommended Dietary Allowances[a]

Category	Age, Years, or Condition	Weight[b] kg	lb	Height[b] cm	in	Protein, g	Vitamin A, μg RE[c]	Vitamin E, mg α-TE[d]	Vitamin K, μg	Vitamin C, mg	Iron, mg	Zinc, mg	Iodine, μg	Selenium, μg
Infants	0.0–0.5	6	13	60	24	13	375	3	5	30	6	5	40	10
	0.5–1.0	9	20	71	28	14	375	4	10	35	10	5	50	15
Children	1–3	13	29	90	35	16	400	6	15	40	10	10	70	20
	4–6	20	44	112	44	24	500	7	20	45	10	10	90	20
	7–10	28	62	132	52	28	700	7	30	45	10	10	120	30
Males	11–14	45	99	157	62	45	1000	10	45	50	12	15	150	40
	15–18	66	145	176	69	59	1000	10	65	60	12	15	150	50
	19–24	72	160	177	70	58	1000	10	70	60	10	15	150	70
	25–50	79	174	176	70	63	1000	10	80	60	10	15	150	70
	51+	77	170	173	68	63	1000	10	80	60	10	15	150	70
Females	11–14	46	101	157	62	46	800	8	45	50	15	12	150	45
	15–18	55	120	163	64	44	800	8	55	60	15	12	150	50
	19–24	58	128	164	65	46	800	8	60	60	15	12	150	55
	25–50	63	138	163	64	50	800	8	65	60	15	12	150	55
	51+	65	143	160	63	50	800	8	65	60	10	12	150	55
Pregnant						60	800	10	65	70	30	15	175	65
Lactating	1st 6 months					65	1300	12	65	95	15	19	200	75
	2nd 6 months					62	1200	11	65	90	15	16	200	75

[a] This table does not include nutrients for which dietary reference intakes have recently been established. (See *Dietary Reference Intakes for Calcium, Phosphorus, Magnesium, Vitamin D, and Fluoride* and *Dietary Reference Intakes for Thiamin, Riboflavin, Niacin, Vitamin B₆, Folate, Vitamin B₁₂, Pantothenic Acid, Biotin, and Choline*. Washington DC, National Academy Press, 1997 and 1998, respectively.) The allowances, expressed as average daily intakes over time, are intended to provide for individual variations among most normal persons as they live in the United States under usual environmental stresses. Diets should be based on a variety of common foods in order to provide other nutrients for which human requirements have been less well defined.

[b] Weights and heights of Reference Adults are actual medians for the U.S. population of the designated age. The use of these figures does not imply that the height-to-weight ratios are ideal.

[c] Retinol equivalents. 1 retinol equivalent = 1 μg retinol or 6 μg β-carotene.

[d] α-Tocopherol equivalents. 1 mg d-α tocopherol = 1 α-TE.

SOURCE: Food and Nutrition Board, National Academy of Sciences–National Research Council Recommended Dietary Allowances, Revised 1989 (Abridged), reprinted with permission. Courtesy of the National Academy Press, Washington, DC.

effects from high intakes is nonexistent; caution is warranted in those who consume large amounts of such nutrients. Healthy individuals derive no established benefit from consuming nutrient levels above the RDA or AI. Individual nutrients in foods that most people eat rarely reach levels that exceed the UL. However, nutritional supplements provide more concentrated amounts of nutrients per dose and, as a result, pose a potential risk of toxicity. Nutrient supplements are labeled with "supplement facts" that express the amount of nutrient in absolute units or as the percent of the DV provided per recommended serving size. Those who use supplements should be advised that total nutrient consumption, including both food and supplements, should not exceed RDA levels.

FACTORS ALTERING NUTRIENT NEEDS The DRIs are affected by age, sex, rate of growth, pregnancy, lactation, physical activity, composition of diet, concomitant diseases, and drugs. When only slight differences exist between the requirements for nutrient sufficiency and excess, dietary planning becomes more difficult. Renal insufficiency provides one example in which protein intakes must be sufficient to maintain protein nutritional status, while avoiding exacerbation of uremic symptoms because of protein excess.

Physiologic Factors Growth, strenuous physical activity, pregnancy, and lactation increase needs for energy and several essential nutrients. Energy needs rise during pregnancy, due to the demands of fetal growth, and during lactation, because of the increased energy required for milk production. Energy needs decrease with loss of lean

body mass, the major determinant of REE. Because both health and physical activity tend to decline with age, energy needs in older persons, especially those over 70, tend to be less than those of younger persons.

Dietary Composition Dietary composition affects the biologic availability and utilization of nutrients. For example, the absorption of iron may be impaired by high amounts of calcium or lead; non-heme iron uptake may be impaired by the lack of ascorbic acid and amino acids in the meal. The absorption of calcium and magnesium is decreased by large amounts of phytates in the diet. Protein utilization by the body may be decreased when essential amino acids are not present in sufficient amounts. Animal foods, such as milk, eggs, and meat, have high biologic values with most of the needed amino acids present in adequate amounts. Plant proteins in corn (maize), soy, and wheat have lower biologic values and must be combined with other plant or animal proteins to achieve optimal utilization by the body.

Route of Administration The RDAs apply only to oral intakes. When nutrients are administered parenterally, similar values can sometimes be used for amino acids, carbohydrates, fats, sodium, chloride, potassium, and most of the vitamins, since their intestinal absorption is nearly 100% (Chap. 75). However, the oral bioavailability of most mineral elements may be only half that obtained by parenteral administration. For some nutrients that are not readily stored in the body, or

Table 73-2 Recommended Intakes for Individuals[a]

Life-Stage Group	Calcium, mg/d	Phos-phorus, mg/d	Mag-nesium, mg/d	Vita-min D, μg/d[bc]	Fluoride, mg/d	Thia-mine, mg/d	Ribo-flavin, mg/d	Niacin, mg/d[d]	Vitamin B₆, mg/d	Folate, μg/d[e]	Vita-min B₁₂, μg/d	Panto-thenic Acid, mg/d	Biotin, μg/d	Choline, mg/d[f]
Infants														
0–6 mo	210	100	30	5	0.01	0.2	0.3	2	0.1	65	0.4	1.7	5	125
7–12 mo	270	275	75	5	0.5	0.3	0.4	4	0.3	80	0.5	1.8	6	150
Children														
1–3 yr	500	**460**	**80**	5	0.7	**0.5**	**0.5**	**6**	**0.5**	**150**	**0.9**	2	8	200
4–8 yr	800	**500**	**130**	5	1	**0.6**	**0.6**	**8**	**0.6**	**200**	**1.2**	3	12	250
Males														
9–13 yr	1300	**1250**	**240**	5	2	**0.9**	**0.9**	**12**	**1.0**	**300**	**1.8**	4	20	375
14–18 yr	1300	**1250**	**410**	5	3	**1.2**	**1.3**	**16**	**1.3**	**400**	**2.4**	5	25	550
19–30 yr	1000	**700**	**400**	5	4	**1.2**	**1.3**	**16**	**1.3**	**400**	**2.4**	5	30	550
31–50 yr	1000	**700**	**420**	5	4	**1.2**	**1.3**	**16**	**1.3**	**400**	**2.4**	5	30	550
51–70 yr	1200	**700**	**420**	10	4	**1.2**	**1.3**	**16**	**1.7**	**400**	**2.4**[g]	5	30	550
>70 yr	1200	**700**	**420**	15	4	**1.2**	**1.3**	**16**	**1.7**	**400**	**2.4**[g]	5	30	550
Females														
9–13 yr	1300	**1250**	**240**	5	2	**0.9**	**0.9**	**12**	**1.0**	**300**	**1.8**	4	20	375
14–18 yr	1300	**1250**	**360**	5	3	**1.0**	**1.0**	**14**	**1.2**	**400**[h]	**2.4**	5	25	400
19–30 yr	1000	**700**	**310**	5	3	**1.1**	**1.1**	**14**	**1.3**	**400**[h]	**2.4**	5	30	425
31–50 yr	1000	**700**	**320**	5	3	**1.1**	**1.1**	**14**	**1.3**	**400**[h]	**2.4**	5	30	425
51–70 yr	1200	**700**	**320**	10	3	**1.1**	**1.1**	**14**	**1.5**	**400**	**2.4**[g]	5	30	425
>70 yr	1200	**700**	**320**	15	3	**1.1**	**1.1**	**14**	**1.5**	**400**	**2.4**[g]	5	30	425
Pregnancy														
≤18 yr	1300	**1250**	**400**	5	3	**1.4**	**1.4**	**18**	**1.6**	**600**[i]	**2.6**	6	30	450
19–30 yr	1000	**700**	**350**	5	3	**1.4**	**1.4**	**18**	**1.9**	**600**[i]	**2.6**	6	30	450
31–50 yr	1000	**700**	**360**	5	3	**1.4**	**1.4**	**18**	**1.9**	**600**[i]	**2.6**	6	30	450
Lactation														
≤18 yr	1300	**1250**	**360**	5	3	**1.5**	**1.6**	**17**	**2.0**	**500**	**2.8**	7	35	550
19–30 yr	1000	**700**	**310**	5	3	**1.5**	**1.6**	**17**	**2.0**	**500**	**2.8**	7	35	550
31–50 yr	1000	**700**	**320**	5	3	**1.5**	**1.6**	**17**	**2.0**	**500**	**2.8**	7	35	550

[a] This table presents recommended dietary allowances (RDAs) in bold type and adequate intakes (AIs) in ordinary type. RDAs and AIs may both be used as goals for individual intake. RDAs are set to meet the needs of almost all (97 to 98%) individuals in a group. For healthy breastfed infants, the AI is the mean intake. The AI for other life-stage and gender groups is believed to cover needs of all individuals in the group, but lack of data or uncertainty in the data prevent being able to specify with confidence the percentage of individuals covered by this intake.

[b] As cholecalciferol. 1 μg cholecalciferol = 40 IU vitamin D.

[c] In the absence of adequate exposure to sunlight.

[d] As niacin equivalents (NE). 1 mg of niacin = 60 mg of tryptophan; 0–6 months = preformed niacin (not NE).

[e] As dietary folate equivalents (DFE). 1 DFE = 1 μg food folate = 0.6 μg of folic acid from fortified food or as a supplement consumed with food = 0.5 μg of a supplement taken on an empty stomach.

[f] Although AIs have been set for choline, there are few data to assess whether a dietary

supply of choline is needed at all stages of the life cycle, and it may be that the choline requirement can be met by endogenous synthesis at some of these stages.

[g] Because 10 to 30% of older people may malabsorb food-bound B₁₂, it is advisable for those > 50 years to meet their RDA mainly by consuming foods fortified with B₁₂ or a supplement containing B₁₂.

[h] In view of evidence linking inadequate folate intake with neural tube defects in the fetus, it is recommended that all women capable of becoming pregnant consume 400 μg from supplements or fortified foods in addition to intake of food folate from a varied diet.

[i] It is assumed that women will continue consuming 400 μg from supplements or fortified food until their pregnancy is confirmed and they enter prenatal care, which ordinarily occurs after the end of the periconceptional period—the critical time for formation of the neural tube.

SOURCE: Food and Nutrition Board, Institute of Medicine—National Academy of Sciences Dietary Reference Intakes, 1999, reprinted with permission. Courtesy of the National Academy Press, Washington, DC.

Table 73-3 The USDA Food Guide Pyramid for Healthy Persons

Servings and Examples of Standard Portion Sizes	Lower: 1600 kcal	Moderate: about 2200 kcal	Higher: about 2800 kcal
Bread group			
1 slice bread; 1 oz. ready-to-eat cereal; ½ cup cooked cereal, rice, or pasta	6	9	22
Vegetable group			
1 cup raw leafy vegetables; ½ cup other vegetables, cooked or chopped raw; ¾ cup vegetable juice	3	4	5
Fruit group			
1 medium banana, apple, or orange; ½ cup chopped, cooked, or canned fruit; ¾ cup fruit juice	2	3	4
Milk group			
1 cup milk or yogurt, 1.5 oz natural cheese, 1 oz processed cheese	2–3[a]	2–3[a]	1–3[a]
Meat group			
2–3 oz cooked lean meat, poultry or fish; ½ cup cooked dry beans; 1 egg or 2 Tbsp. peanut butter count as 1 oz lean meat)	5	5	7
Total fat, g	53	73	93
Total added sugars, tsp	6	12	18

[a] Women who are pregnant or breastfeeding, teenagers, and young adults to age 24 need 3 servings.
SOURCE: US Department of Agriculture, Human Nutrition Information Service. *The Food Guide Pyramid*, Home and Garden Bulletin Number 252, US Department of Agriculture, Washington DC, August 1992.

cannot be stored in large amounts, timing of administration may also be important. For example, amino acids cannot be used for protein synthesis if they are not supplied together; instead they will be used for energy production.

Disease Specific dietary deficiency diseases include protein-calorie malnutrition; iron, iodine, and vitamin A deficiency; megaloblastic anemia due to vitamin B_{12} or folic acid deficiency; vitamin D deficiency rickets; and scurvy, beriberi, and pellagra (Chaps. 74 and 75). Each deficiency disease is characterized by imbalances at the cellular level between the supply of nutrients or energy and the body's nutritional needs for growth, maintenance, and other functions. Imbalances in nutrient intakes are recognized as risk factors for certain chronic degenerative diseases, such as saturated fat and cholesterol in coronary artery disease; sodium in hypertension; obesity in hormone-dependent endometrial, breast, and prostate cancers; and ethanol in alcoholism. Since the etiology and pathogenesis of these disorders are multifactorial, diet is only one of many risk factors. Osteoporosis, for example, is associated with calcium deficiency, as well as risk factors related to environment (e.g., smoking, sedentary lifestyle), physiology (e.g., estrogen deficiency), genetic determinants (e.g., defects in collagen metabolism), and drug use (chronic steroids) (Chap. 342).

DIETARY ASSESSMENT In clinical situations, nutritional assessment is an iterative process that involves: (1) screening for malnutrition, (2) assessing the diet and other data to establish either the absence or presence of malnutrition and its possible causes, and (3) planning for the most appropriate nutritional therapy. Some disease states affect the bioavailability, requirements, utilization, or excretion of specific nutrients. In these circumstances, specific measurements of various nutrients may be required to assure adequate replacement (Chap. 75).

Most health care facilities have a nutrition screening process in place for identifying possible malnutrition after hospital admission. Nutritional screening is required by the Joint Commission on Accreditation of Healthcare Organizations (JCAHO), but there are no universally recognized or validated standards, so techniques vary. The factors that are usually assessed include: abnormal weight for height or body mass index (e.g., BMI <19 or >25); reported weight change (involuntary loss or gain of >5 kg in past 6 months) (Chap. 43); diagnoses with known nutritional implications (metabolic disease, any disease affecting the gastrointestinal tract, alcoholism, and others); present therapeutic dietary prescription; chronic poor appetite; presence of chewing and swallowing problems or major food intolerances; need for assistance with preparing or shopping for food, eating, or other aspects of self care; and social isolation. Reassessment of

nutrition status should occur periodically in hospitalized patients—at least once every week.

A more complete dietary assessment is indicated for patients who exhibit a high risk of malnutrition on nutrition screening. The type of assessment varies based on the clinical setting, severity of the patient's illness, and stability of his or her condition.

Acute Care Settings In acute care settings, anorexia, various diseases, test procedures, and medications can compromise dietary intake. Under such circumstances, the goal is to identify and avoid inadequate intake and assure appropriate alimentation. Dietary assessment in acute care situations focuses on what patients are currently eating, whether they are able and willing to eat, and whether they experience any problems with eating. Dietary intake assessment is based on information from observed intakes; medical record; history; clinical examination; and anthropometric, biochemical, and functional status. The objective is to gather enough information to establish the likelihood of malnutrition due to poor dietary intake or other causes in order to determine whether nutritional therapy is indicated.

Simple observations may suffice to suggest inadequate oral intake. These include dietitians' and nurses' notes, the amount of food eaten on trays, frequent tests and procedures that are likely to cause meals to be skipped, nutritionally inadequate diet orders such as clear liquids or full liquids for more than a few days, fever, gastrointestinal distress, vomiting, diarrhea, or a comatose state. Patients with diseases or treatments that involve any part of the alimentary tract are at high nutritional risk. Acutely ill patients with diet-related diseases such as diabetes need assessment because an inappropriate diet may exacerbate these conditions and adversely affect other therapies. Abnormal biochemical values [serum albumin levels <35 g/L (<3.5 mg/dL); serum cholesterol levels <3.9 mmol/L (<150 mg/dL)] are nonspecific but may also indicate a need for further nutritional assessment.

Most therapeutic diets offered in hospitals are calculated to meet individual nutrient requirements and the RDA. Exceptions include clear liquids, some full liquid diets, and test diets, which are inadequate for several nutrients and should not be used, if possible, for more than 24 h. As much as half of the food served to hospitalized patients is not eaten, and so it cannot be assumed that the intakes of hospitalized patients are adequate. The dietary assessment should therefore compare how much and what food the patient has consumed with the diet that has been provided in the hospital. Major deviations in intakes of energy, protein, fluids, or other nutrients of special concern for the patient's illness should be noted and corrected.

Nutritional monitoring is especially important for patients who are very ill and who have extended lengths of stay. Patients who are fed by special enteral and parenteral routes also require special nutritional assessment and monitoring by physicians with training in nutrition support and/or dietitians with certification in nutrition support (Chap. 76).

Ambulatory Settings The aim of dietary assessment in the outpatient setting is to determine whether the patient's usual diet is a health risk in itself or if it contributes to existing chronic disease-related problems. It also provides the basis for planning a diet that fulfills therapeutic goals while ensuring patient compliance. The outpatient dietary assessment should review the adequacy of present and usual food intakes, including vitamin and mineral supplements, medications, and alcohol, as all of these may affect the patient's nutritional status. The dietary assessment should focus on the dietary constituents that are most likely to be involved or compromised by a specific diagnosis, as well as any comorbidities that are present. More than one day's intake should be reviewed to provide a better representation of the usual diet.

There are many ways to assess the adequacy of the patient's habitual diet. These include a food guide, a food exchange list, a diet history, or a food frequency questionnaire. A commonly used food guide for healthy persons is the USDA's food pyramid, which is useful as a basis for identifying inadequate intakes of essential nutrients, as well as likely excesses in fat, saturated fat, sodium, sugar, and alcohol (Table 73-3). The guide is calculated to provide approximately 1600 kcal for sedentary women and some older adults; 2200 kcal for most children, teenage girls, active women, and many sedentary men (women who are pregnant or breastfeeding may need somewhat more); and 2800 kcal for teenage boys, most active men, and some very active women. Results provide a rough guide to food groups that may be eaten either in excess of recommendations or in insufficient quantities. Respondents who follow ethnic or unusual dietary patterns may need extra instruction on how foods should be categorized, as well as the appropriate portion sizes that constitute a serving. The process of reviewing the guide with patients helps them transition to healthier dietary patterns. For those on therapeutic diets, assessment against food exchange lists may be useful. These include, for example, the American Diabetes Association food exchange lists for diabetes, or the American Dietetic Association food exchange lists for renal disease.

Nutritional Status Assessment Full nutritional status assessment is a complex, time-consuming, and expensive process that requires considerable expertise. Candidates include seriously ill patients and those at very high nutritional risk when the cause of malnutrition is still uncertain after initial clinical evaluation and dietary assessment. Full nutritional status assessment involves multiple dimensions, including documentation of dietary intake, anthropometric measurements, biochemical measurements of blood and urine, clinical examination, health history, and functional. →*For further discussion of Nutritional Assessment, see Chap. 74.*

BIBLIOGRAPHY

Committee on Micronutrient Deficiencies, Board on International Health, Food and Nutrition Board, Institute of Medicine: *Prevention of Micronutrient Deficiencies: Tools for Policymakers and Public Health Workers,* CP Howson et al (eds). Washington, National Academy Press, 1998

Food and Nutrition Board, Commission on Life Sciences, National Research Council: *Recommended Dietary Allowances,* 10th ed. Washington, National Academy Press, 1989

Owen OE et al: A reappraisal of caloric requirements in healthy women. Am J Clin Nutr 44:1, 1986

————: A reappraisal of the caloric requirements of men. Am J Clin Nutr 46:875, 1987

Sadler MJ et al (eds): *Encyclopedia of Human Nutrition.* San Diego, Academic Press, 1998

Shils ME et al (eds): *Modern Nutrition in Health and Disease,* 9th ed. Baltimore, Williams & Wilkins, 1999

Standing Committee on the Scientific Evaluation of Dietary Reference Intakes, Food and Nutrition Board, Institute of Medicine: *Dietary Reference Intakes for Calcium, Phosphorus, Magnesium, Vitamin D, and Fluoride.* Washington, National Academy Press, 1997

| 74 | *Charles H. Halsted* |

MALNUTRITION AND NUTRITIONAL ASSESSMENT

Malnutrition is a frequent and integral component of acute and chronic illness. When recognized by appropriate clinical assessment, malnutrition is found in >50% of all hospitalized adults. It contributes to increased in-hospital morbidity and mortality in both medical and surgical patients, and leads to more frequent hospital admissions among the elderly. Malnutrition results from various combinations of starvation, including inadequate intake or abnormal gastrointestinal assim-

ilation of the diet, the stress response to acute injury or chronic inflammation, and abnormal nutrient metabolism. Nutritional assessment should be considered an integral part of the clinical evaluation and be used as a basis for nutritional support in the overall therapeutic plan.

DEFINITIONS OF MALNUTRITION In the strict sense, the term *malnutrition* includes extremes of underweight and overweight. The current chapter, however, focuses on the evaluation of the undernourished patient who presents with diminished body protein and energy stores and micronutrient deficiencies.

To the practicing physician, both outpatients and inpatients should be considered at risk for malnutrition if they meet one or more of the following criteria: (1) unintentional loss of >10% of usual body weight in the preceding 3 months, (2) body weight <90% of ideal for height, or (3) body mass index (BMI; the weight in kilograms divided by the height in square meters) <18.5. With regard to varying levels of severity, body weight <90% of ideal for height represents risk of malnutrition, body weight <85% of ideal constitutes *malnutrition,* <70% of ideal represents *severe malnutrition,* and <60% of ideal is usually incompatible with survival.

Malnutrition may be endemic in regions of famine, and two forms of severe malnutrition are recognized under conditions of inadequate food supply or distribution: *marasmus* refers to generalized starvation with loss of body fat and protein, whereas *kwashiorkor* refers to selective protein malnutrition with edema and fatty liver. The latter form occurs following restriction of dietary protein among children in settings of recurrent diarrheal illness. These distinctions, however, seldom apply to malnourished patients in more developed societies. In this setting, features of combined protein-calorie malnutrition (PCM) are more commonly seen in the context of a wide variety of acute and chronic illnesses that lead to depletion of body fat, muscle wasting, multiple signs of micronutrient deficiencies, decubitus ulcers, and life-threatening infections. An overview of the evaluation of malnutrition in the sick adult is depicted in Fig. 74-1.

PATHOPHYSIOLOGY AND ETIOLOGIES OF MALNUTRITION In simple terms, patients lose weight when: (1) the intake or gastrointestinal assimilation of dietary calories is insufficient to meet normal energy expenditure; (2) the expenditure of body energy stores is greater than energy normally consumed and assimilated by the body; or (3) the metabolism of energy supplies, protein, and other nutrients is significantly impaired by the intrinsic disease process.

Body Composition As depicted in Fig. 74-2, the human body stores between 15 and 25% of its energy as fat (greater in women than men), which is available for the metabolism of endogenous fatty acids during starvation. The remaining fat-free mass (FFM) is composed of extracellular and intracellular water, the bony skeleton, glycogen, and skeletal and visceral protein. Aside from body fat, energy reserves are also provided by intracellular glycogen and protein, which, together with intracellular water, constitute the body cell mass (BCM). Thus, in addition to the enzymes that support the normal metabolic machinery of the body, the BCM provides reserve protein for energy production by gluconeogenesis during the stress response.

The Metabolic Response to Starvation and Stress The expenditure of body stores of energy (as fat, glycogen, and protein) is different during *starvation* (due to decreased intake and/or assimilation of the diet) and *stress* (due to excessive expenditure of energy and body protein). Consequently, these events affect body compartments differently. Starvation decreases the size of all body compartments, whereas stress reduces BCM, increases extracellular water, and has variable effects on body fat.

A normal 70-kg man stores fuel at about 15 kg as fat, 6 kg as protein, and 0.4 kg as glycogen. During a 24-h fast, energy needs are met by the consumption of liver glycogen stores and the conversion of up to 75 g of body protein to glucose (by gluconeogenesis). During prolonged starvation, metabolism is supported by stores of body fat (about 150 g/d), which provides fatty acid–derived ketones, and muscle protein (about 20 g/d), which is used for gluconeogenesis. Under

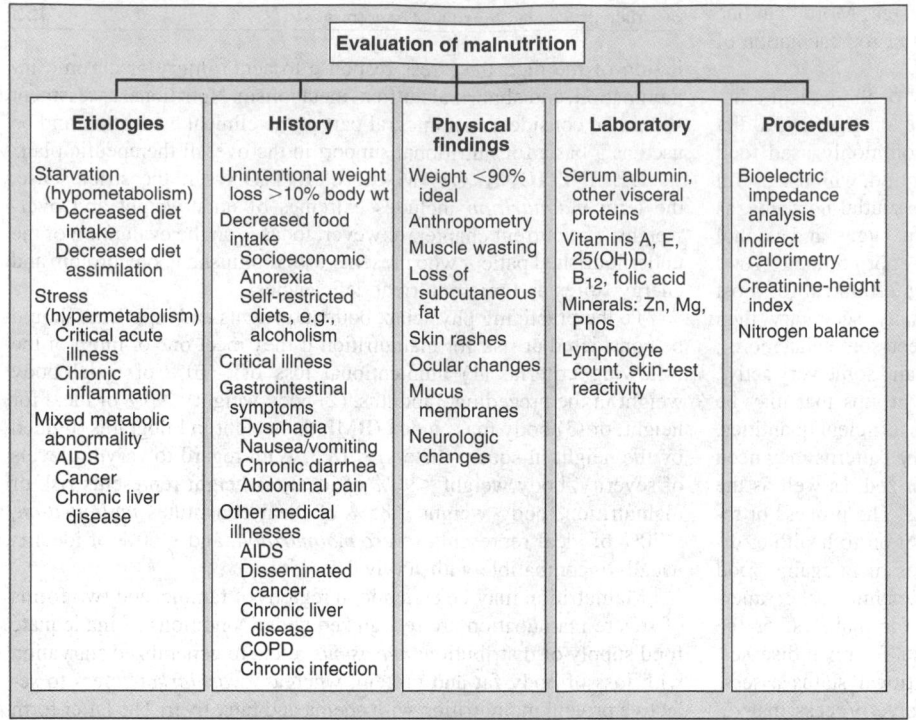

FIGURE 74-1 Conceptual framework for the nutritional assessment of sick patients. COPD, chronic obstructive pulmonary disease.

these conditions, total energy expenditure is decreased in order to conserve energy. While normal-weight individuals can sustain total fasting for about 2 months, obese individuals can fast for periods >12 months, depending on their fat stores.

The metabolic responses to the stress of acute critical illness (e.g., following accidental or surgical trauma or sepsis) significantly modify this sequence of events. In contrast to the hypometabolism, protein conservation, and reliance on body fat stores for energy needs during starvation, the acute stress response is characterized by hypermetabolism, in which the demands of accelerated energy expenditure are met by skeletal and visceral proteolysis to provide amino acid substrate for gluconeogenesis. Muscle proteolysis and gluconeogenesis are promoted by high levels of circulating catecholamines, glucagon, cortisol, and cytokines, including tumor necrosis factor (TNF) α and interleukins 1 and 6, in the setting of insulin resistance. When untreated, body protein catabolism is accelerated to 240 g/d, which is sufficient to deplete 50% of body protein stores within 3 weeks.

A more common clinical situation is the malnourished patient with

chronic illness in whom acute trauma or sepsis superimposes cytokine-mediated proteolysis with increased metabolic demands. If unchecked by appropriate therapy, the process of progressive PCM in such patients is associated with decreased cardiac and renal function, fluid retention, intestinal mucosal atrophy, loss of intracellular minerals (zinc, magnesium, and phosphorus), diminished cell-mediated immune functions, increased risk of infection, and eventual death (Fig. 74-3).

Etiologies of Malnutrition The causes of decreased dietary intake are diverse and include social and economic conditions, psychiatric diseases, neurodegenerative dementias, cytokine-mediated appetite suppression in chronic infections such as AIDS or in disseminated cancer, and self-limited food intake in abdominal pain syndromes (Table 74-1; Chap. 43). Given the central role of the gastrointestinal tract in the assimilation of nutrients, PCM is a predictable component of many chronic gastrointestinal diseases. These diseases promote starvation through decreased assimilation of the diet by: (1) blocking the transit of dietary constituents to the intestinal absorbing surface, (2) impairing normal processes of pancreatic or biliary digestion, or (3) preventing the intestinal mucosal transport of dietary constituents. Diseases that are characterized by increased catabolism of stored energy and protein include acute surgical or medical critical illness and acute or chronic inflammatory or infectious disorders affecting diverse organ systems. Other chronic diseases promote malnutrition through mixed mechanisms that contribute to abnormal nutrient metabolism. Both AIDS and disseminated malignancy, for example, cause progressive malnutrition through combinations of anorexia and futile cycles of fatty acid and glucose metabolism. Chronic obstructive pulmonary disease increases risk of malnutrition through the increased energy expenditure of labored respiration, chronic indolent bronchial infection, and the anorexic side effects of many bronchodilating drugs. Chronic liver disease is often

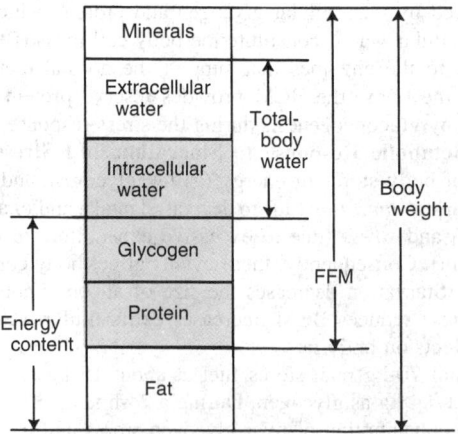

FIGURE 74-2 Schematic of body composition of a healthy subject. Body cell mass (BCM) is shown by shading as a composite of intracellular water, glycogen, and protein. FFM, fat-free mass. *(Adapted with permission from Heymsfield et al.)*

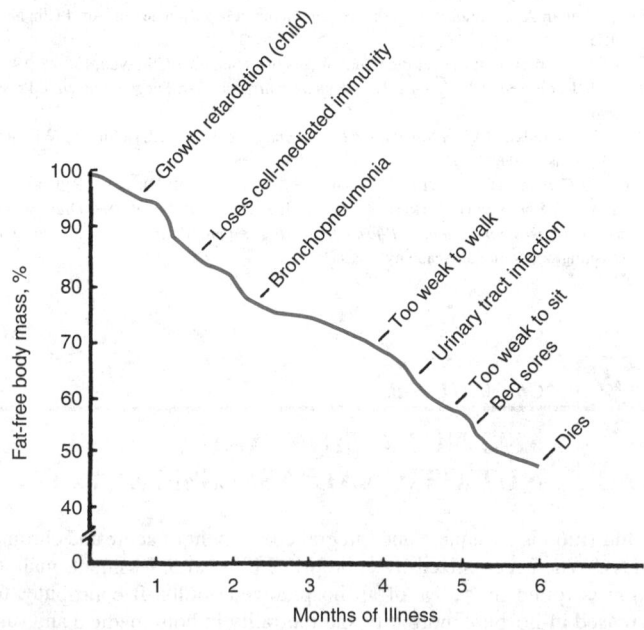

FIGURE 74-3 Hypothetical history of progressive protein-calorie malnutrition in a patient with wasting illness. *(Reproduced with permission from Heymsfield et al.)*

Table 74-1 Etiologies of Protein-Calorie Malnutrition

I. Starvation (hypometabolism with reliance on body fat stores)
   A. Decreased diet intake
      1. Social and economic: poverty, chronic alcoholism
      2. Psychiatric: anorexia nervosa, severe depression
      3. Neurodegenerative dementias of aging
      4. Anorexia associated with AIDS, disseminated cancer, renal failure
      5. Abdominal pain triggered by food intake: pancreatitis, intestinal ischemia
   B. Decreased assimilation of the diet
      1. Impaired transit of diet, e.g., benign or malignant esophageal, gastric, or intestinal obstruction
      2. Impaired digestion of diet, e.g., pancreatic insufficiency, short bowel syndrome
      3. Intestinal malabsorption of dietary constituents, e.g., celiac disease
II. Stress (hypermetabolism with reliance on protein stores for gluconeogenesis)
   A. Acute trauma, e.g., accident, burns, major surgery
   B. Acute sepsis
   C. Acute or chronic inflammation: pancreatitis, collagen diseases, chronic infectious disease, e.g., tuberculosis, AIDS opportunistic infections
III. Mixed mechanisms
   A. Futile metabolic cycles and anorexia, e.g., AIDS, disseminated cancer
   B. Increased energy demands, e.g., chronic obstructive pulmonary disease
   C. Abnormal metabolism and decreased biliary digestion, e.g., chronic liver disease
   D. Protein-losing enteropathy and chronic inflammation, e.g., Crohn's disease, ulcerative colitis

Table 74-2 The Patient History of Weight Loss and Malnutrition

Finding	Example/Interpretation
Involuntary diet restriction	Poverty due to inadequate income
Anorexia	Anorexia nervosa, severe depression, dementia, AIDS, cancer, chronic renal disease
Inadequate diet selection	Chronic alcoholism, fad diets, strict vegetarianism
Critical illness	Untreated stress response to trauma, burn, major surgery, sepsis
Gastrointestinal symptoms	
Dysphagia	Esophageal obstruction impairs diet transit
Nausea, vomiting	Gastric or intestinal obstruction impairs diet transit
Chronic diarrhea	Pancreatic, biliary, or intestinal mucosal disease impairs digestion and absorption Protein-losing enteropathy in inflammatory bowel disease
Chronic abdominal pain	Self-limited food intake reduces pain: e.g., pancreatitis, intestinal ischemia, inflammatory bowel disease
Other chronic medical diseases	Combinations of anorexia, increased energy demands, and abnormal nutrient metabolism: e.g., recurrent pancreatitis, AIDS, disseminated cancer, chronic liver disease, chronic obstructive pulmonary disease, chronic infectious illness

associated with PCM caused by the cumulative effects of anorexia; decreased biliary circulation; and abnormal lipid, carbohydrate, and protein metabolism. The chronic intestinal inflammation of Crohn's disease or ulcerative colitis accelerates fecal losses of protein, electrolytes, and zinc.

CLINICAL EVALUATION OF THE MALNOURISHED PATIENT

THE PATIENT HISTORY The clinical nutritional history should include diet and weight change, socioeconomic conditions, and symptoms unique to each clinical setting (Table 74-2). Social and economic conditions that may lead to poverty include inadequate income, homelessness, and activities that restrict real income and promote involuntary diet restriction, such as drug abuse or chronic alcoholism. Anorexia, or loss of appetite, is a feature of psychiatric disorders, such as anorexia nervosa and neurodegenerative dementia in the elderly. Many self-selected, inadequate diets may promote malnutrition. During binge drinking, chronic alcoholics typically substitute more than half their daily food calories with excessive amounts of ethanol, the metabolism of which consumes energy and promotes unbalanced metabolism of fat and carbohydrates. Other inadequate diets include unbalanced and commercially promoted formulas for rapid weight loss and strict vegetarianism, which may lead to selective deficiencies of specific nutrients such as vitamin B_{12} and iron.

Digestive diseases are major causes of malnutrition, both in the inpatient and outpatient settings. The malnourished patient with digestive disease may present with symptoms of: (1) dysphagia or recurrent vomiting due to benign or malignant esophageal or gastrointestinal obstruction; (2) chronic diarrhea due to abnormal pancreatic or biliary digestion, intestinal mucosal malabsorption, or protein-losing enteropathy; or (3) recurrent abdominal pain exacerbated by eating, as occurs in patients with chronic pancreatitis, inflammatory bowel disease, or intestinal ischemia.

On the general medical service, PCM is prevalent in patients with multiple chronic illnesses that are associated with anorexia, recurrent stress, and abnormal nutrient metabolism. In addition, PCM is comorbid with chronic recurrent pancreatitis, renal failure, chronic liver disease, chronic obstructive pulmonary disease, disseminated cancer, and chronic infections such as AIDS and tuberculosis. Depending on the severity of injury or illness, critically ill surgical and medical patients predictably develop stress-related PCM if increased nutritional needs are not met after 5 to 10 days.

THE PHYSICAL EXAMINATION A careful physical examination can both characterize and define the extent of malnutrition. Measurements of unclothed weight and height are essential for establishing the severity of malnutrition in all patients but may be confounded by the effects of fluid overload as a result of edema and ascites. The normal values for weight (in kg) and height (in cm) in men and women are provided in Table 74-3. These values can be adjusted by ±10% to account for variability in body frame.

Anthropometry Measurements of subcutaneous fat and skeletal muscle are important to determine the severity of PCM. Using specialized calipers and a tape measure, anthropometry estimates body fat from the thickness of the skin-fold of the posterior mid-upper arm. Anthropometric measurements in healthy and malnourished adults are shown in Table 74-4. Mid-arm muscle circumference is estimated from the equation:

Mid-arm muscle circumference
= mid-upper arm circumference − (π × triceps skin-fold thickness)
     (in cm)   (in cm)

The use of anthropometry is limited by the requirement for specialized calipers, the experience of the observer, and potential confounding effects of edema or dehydration.

Specific Physical Findings of Malnutrition During the conventional physical examination, the observant and experienced clinician can identify multiple and specific findings of PCM and its associated micronutrient deficiencies (Chap. 75). A variety of nutritional deficiencies can be identified by examination of the patient's general appearance, including skin, hair, nails, mucus membranes, and neurologic system (Table 74-5). Initially, a pinch of the posterior upper arm may reveal loss of subcutaneous fat in the malnourished patient. Hollowing of the temporal muscles, wasting of upper arms and thigh muscles, easily plucked hair, and peripheral edema are all consistent with protein deficiency. Examination of the skin may reveal the papular keratitis ("goose bump rash") of vitamin A deficiency, perifollicular

Table 74-3 Ideal Weight for Height

Men				Women			
Height[a]	Weight[a]	Height	Weight	Height	Weight	Height	Weight
145	51.9	166	64.0	140	44.9	161	56.9
146	52.4	167	64.6	141	45.4	162	57.6
147	52.9	168	65.2	142	45.9	163	58.3
148	53.5	169	65.9	143	46.4	164	58.9
149	54.0	170	66.6	144	47.0	165	59.5
150	54.5	171	67.3	145	47.5	166	60.1
151	55.0	172	68.0	146	48.0	167	60.7
152	55.6	173	68.7	147	48.6	168	61.4
153	56.1	174	69.4	148	49.2	169	62.1
154	56.6	175	70.1	149	49.8		
155	57.2	176	70.8	150	50.4		
156	57.9	177	71.6	151	51.0		
157	58.6	178	72.4	152	51.5		
158	59.3	179	73.3	153	52.0		
159	59.9	180	74.2	154	52.5		
160	60.5	181	75.0	155	53.1		
161	61.1	182	75.8	156	53.7		
162	61.7	183	76.5	157	54.3		
163	62.3	184	77.3	158	54.9		
164	62.9	185	78.1	159	55.5		
165	63.5	186	78.9	160	56.2		

[a] Values are expressed in cm for height and kg for weight. To obtain height in inches, divide by 2.54. To obtain weight in pounds, multiply by 2.2.

SOURCE: Adapted from Blackburn et al.

hemorrhages of vitamin C deficiency, ecchymoses of vitamin K deficiency, the "flaky paint" lower extremity rash of zinc deficiency, hyperpigmentation of skin-exposed areas from niacin deficiency, seborrhea of essential fatty acid deficiency, spooning of nails in iron deficiency, and transverse nail pigmentation in protein deficiency. The eye examination yields conjunctival pallor of anemia, pericorneal and corneal opacities of severe vitamin A deficiency ("Bitot spots"), and nystagmus and isolated ocular muscle paresis of thiamine deficiency. The oral examination may reveal angular stomatitis and cheilosis of either riboflavin or niacin deficiency; glossitis with smooth and red tongue of riboflavin, niacin, vitamin B_{12}, or pyridoxine deficiency; and hypertrophied bleeding gums of vitamin C deficiency. Examination of the neurologic system, particularly in the setting of chronic alcohol abuse, may detect memory loss with confabulation, a wide-based gait, and past pointing, which, together with ophthalmoplegia and peripheral neuropathy, constitute the Wernicke-Korsakoff syndrome of thiamine deficiency. Other neurologic causes of dementia include pellagra due to niacin and/or tryptophan deficiency. Additional causes of peripheral neuropathy include deficiencies of pyridoxine or vitamin E; loss of distal vibratory and position sense is characteristic of the subacute combined degeneration of vitamin B_{12} deficiency.

LABORATORY ASSESSMENT Selected use of laboratory tests, most of which are widely available, is essential for characterizing and quantifying malnutrition. Laboratory findings that are often attributed to chronic disease may, in actuality, reflect the response to PCM or selected micronutrient deficiencies in the setting of chronic illness.

Table 74-4 Anthropometric Measurements in Adults

% Standard	Men	Women	Interpretation
TRICEPS SKIN-FOLD, MM			
100	12.5	16.5	Adequate
50	6.0	8.0	Borderline
20	2.5	3.0	Severe depletion
MID-ARM MUSCLE CIRCUMFERENCE, CM			
100	25.5	23.0	Adequate
80	20.0	18.5	Borderline
60	15.0	14.0	Depletion
40	10.0	9.0	Severe depletion

SOURCE: Adapted from Morgan and Weinsier.

Serum Visceral Proteins Serum albumin, which has a 2- to 3-week half-life, is a highly sensitive but nonspecific measure of PCM. A normal serum albumin level in a well-hydrated patient is inconsistent with PCM. On the other hand, a low serum albumin level must be interpreted in its clinical context, since the concentration of albumin is decreased in the setting of increased plasma volume (as seen in acute trauma or sepsis and in chronic liver, renal, or cardiopulmonary failure). The acute stress of surgery, sepsis, or other acute inflammatory illness lowers the serum albumin level because of a combination of increased circulating extracellular volume and TNF-α-mediated inhibition of albumin synthesis. Hepatic albumin synthesis is inhibited in the setting of liver cirrhosis, AIDS, and disseminated cancer, whereas albumin loss from the body is accelerated in inflammatory bowel diseases, including ulcerative colitis, Crohn's disease, and radiation enteritis. Several shorter-lived visceral proteins can also be measured for estimation of the severity of PCM. These include transferrin (1-week half-life), prealbumin or retinol-binding protein complex (2-day half-life), and fibronectin (1-day half-life). However, like the serum albumin level, the circulating level of each of these proteins is affected by the changes in extracellular volume that occur in acute and chronic illnesses.

Vitamin and Mineral Assays Specific micronutrient deficiencies can be measured by a variety of serum and red blood cell assays, often utilizing high-performance liquid chromatography or enzyme or

Table 74-5 Physical Findings of Malnutrition

Finding	Deficiency/Interpretation
General appearance	
Weight loss	Malnutrition <90% of ideal body weight
	Severe <70% of ideal body weight
Decreased temporal and proximal extremity muscle mass	Decreased skeletal protein
Decreased skin-fold thickness by "pinch test"	Decreased body fat stores
Skin, nails, and hair	
Easily plucked hair	Protein
Easy bruising, perifollicular hemorrhages	Vitamin C
"Flaky paint" rash of lower extremities	Zinc
Coarse skin, "goose bumps"	Vitamin A
Hyperpigmentation of sun-exposed areas	Niacin, tryptophan
Spooning of nails	Iron
Eyes	
Conjunctival pallor	Anemia (nonspecific)
Bitot spot	Vitamin A
Ophthalmoplegia	Thiamine
Mouth and mucus membranes	
Nasolabial seborrhea	Essential fatty acids
Glossitis (smooth, red tongue) and/or cheilosis	Riboflavin, niacin, vitamin B_{12}, pyridoxine, folate
Diminished taste	Zinc
Neurologic system	
Disorientation	Niacin, phosphorus
Confabulation	Thiamine
Cerebellar gait, past pointing	Thiamine
Peripheral neuropathy	Thiamine, pyridoxine, vitamin E
Lost vibratory, position sense	Vitamin B_{12}

microbiologic assays (Chap. 75). Commonly available assays and their interpretations are listed in Table 74-6. PCM is typically associated with low serum levels of vitamin A, zinc, and magnesium. Abnormal digestion and absorption of dietary fat are associated with deficiencies of fat-soluble vitamins A, D, and E, whereas intestinal mucosal malabsorption (as in celiac disease) is commonly associated with additional deficiencies of iron and folic acid. Chronic alcoholism is frequently associated with thiamine, folate, vitamin A, and zinc deficiencies. Vitamin B_{12} deficiency due to achlorhydria occurs in up to 15% of elderly individuals as well as in those with pernicious anemia or with diseases involving the terminal ileum. As described in Chap. 105, both folate and vitamin B_{12} deficiencies are associated with elevations in plasma homocysteine; vitamin B_{12} deficiency can also elevate the plasma level of methylmalonic acid.

Assessment of Immune Function PCM is associated with atrophy of thymic-dependent lymphoid structures and reduced T cell–mediated immunity. Conversely, B cell–mediated production of immunoglobulins is usually unaffected. Total lymphocyte count (total white cell count × fraction as lymphocytes) is often $<1000/\mu L$ in PCM and may be accompanied by anergy to common skin test antigens. While sensitive for PCM, these measures of cell-mediated immunity are nonspecific and can be affected by other disorders such as acute or chronic infections, uremia, or immunosuppressive therapy.

SPECIALIZED PROCEDURES FOR NUTRITIONAL ASSESSMENT Several specialized procedures are used to assess energy and protein stores and energy expenditure in malnourished patients. These procedures may be employed during the initial nutritional assessment or may serve as an index of the efficacy of nutritional support during the treatment of malnourished patients.

Bioelectric Impedance Analysis Bioelectric impedance analysis (BIA) is a simplified and portable method for measurement of body fat, FFM, and total-body water. BIA is based on differences in the electric conductivity of a weak current between electrodes placed on the dorsal surfaces of the hands and feet. The measurement reflects differences in the impedance to electric current, which is greatest through fat and least through water. Lean body mass can be calculated as the difference between fat mass and body weight or as total-body water divided by 0.73.

Overall, BIA is most useful in assessing body fat and FFM in stable patients and in those who suffer from conditions leading to relative starvation. However, BIA can also be used to assess critically ill patients with decreased intracellular water space and BCM and expanded extracellular compartment size. Reduced BCM correlates inversely with increased metabolic rate. BIA may be confounded in AIDS patients receiving protease-inhibitor therapy, if they exhibit lipodystrophy with associated redistribution of interscapular, abdominal, and breast fat (Chap. 309).

Energy Expenditure Body weight and energy balance are sustained in health by the consumption of dietary calories in an amount equal to the daily expenditure of energy. Therefore, caloric needs can be determined from the estimated daily total energy expenditure (TEE), which is composed of basal or resting energy expenditure (REE, about 75% of total), the thermic expenditures of digestion (about 10% of total), and modest physical activity (about 15% of total). The REE is directly proportional to both the FFM and BCM and can be estimated in healthy people using the Harris and Benedict formula

Table 74-6 Commonly Available Vitamin and Mineral Assays

Vitamin/Mineral	Normal Range	Interpretation of Abnormal Result
Vitamin A	1.30–3.15 μmol/L (37–90 μg/dL)	Low value consistent with PCM, abnormal fat digestion or malabsorption, chronic liver disease. High value consistent with vitamin abuse; toxicity expressed as liver failure.
25(OH)D₃	25–150 nmol/L (10–60 ng/mL)	Low value consistent with abnormal fat digestion or absorption, primary rickets, chronic liver disease, osteomalacia. High value suggestive of vitamin toxicity expressed as calcinosis.
Vitamin E	12–35 μmol/L (0.5–1.5 mg/dL)	Low value consistent with abnormal fat digestion, chronic liver disease; expressed as peripheral neuropathy, tunnel vision.
Thiamine	6–60 pmol/L (0.2–2.0 μg/dL)	Low value seen in starvation, chronic alcoholism, malabsorption syndromes; expressed as Wernicke-Korsakoff syndrome, peripheral neuropathy, high-output cardiac failure.
Folate Serum	12–53 nmol/L (5–21 ng/mL)	Low levels in starvation, chronic alcoholism, intestinal malabsorption; expressed as macrocytic anemia, diarrhea, elevated homocysteine.
Red cell	>400 nmol/L (>160 ng/mL)	Same as above, but more stable and reflects tissue stores of folates.
Vitamin B₁₂	>104 pmol/L (>140 pg/mL)	Low level associated with gastric atrophy of aging, pernicious anemia; expressed as macrocytic anemia, neuropathy; elevated homocysteine and methylmalonic acid.
Zinc	10–21 mmol/L (65–140 μg/dL)	Low level in chronic diarrhea, PCM, alcoholic liver disease, inflammatory bowel disease, intestinal malabsorption; expressed as rash, delayed wound healing, decreased taste sensation.
Magnesium	0.72–0.99 mmol/L (1.8–2.4 mg/dL)	Low in chronic alcoholism, diabetes, intestinal malabsorption, PCM; expressed as hyperactive reflexes, hypocalcemia.
Phosphorus	0.81–1.43 mmol/L (2.5–4.4 mg/dL)	Low in starvation, chronic alcoholism, chronic diarrhea; expressed as confusion, disorientation.

NOTE: PCM, protein-calorie malnutrition.

on the basis of weight in kg (W), height in cm (H), and age in years (A):

$$REE \text{ (men)} = 66.473 + 13.751 \, (W) + 5.0033 \, (H) - 6.7550 \, (A) \text{ kcal/d}$$

$$REE \text{ (women)} = 655.0955 + 9.4634 \, (W) + 1.8496 \, (H) - 4.6756 \, (A) \text{ kcal/d}$$

A simplified bedside estimation for TEE in sick patients is 25 kcal/kg of body weight, to which is added 10% for digestion or metabolism of intravenous or enteral nutrition. In the acutely ill patient, one should include an additional 12.5% for each degree of fever over 37°C, as well as an additional multiplier commensurate with the severity of illness (e.g., 25% for general surgery, 50% for sepsis, and 100% for extensive third-degree burns).

While REE can be predicted by the Harris-Benedict equations in healthy persons, it is decreased in starvation because of hypometabolism. In contrast, REE is increased in the hypermetabolic stress that accompanies critical illness. REE and caloric requirements cannot be predicted in certain clinical conditions. These include the relatively starved, chronically ill patient admitted with a critical illness, the obese patient who develops a critical illness on the background of both increased body fat and FFM, or the patient with chronic liver disease accompanied by combinations of anorexia and ongoing hepatic inflammation. In these situations, REE can be measured accurately by the gas-exchange method of indirect calorimetry. In practice, indirect calorimetry is performed at the bedside using a mobile metabolic cart. This procedure is applicable to ventilator-independent and -dependent patients whose fractional intake of oxygen is less than 0.45. Because the goal is to reach an accurate approximation of the 24-h energy requirement, measurements must be taken at intervals during the day and must account for several variables, including food intake and activity. To calculate the energy cost of metabolism by indirect calorimetry, the volumes (V) of oxygen consumed and carbon dioxide produced are measured over a given period of time, according to the modified Weir equation where

$$REE = 3.9\ V_{O_2} + 1.1\ V_{CO_2}$$

Indirect calorimetry also provides the respiratory quotient (RQ), which is the ratio of carbon dioxide produced to oxygen consumed during the process of gas collection. The RQ decreases when fat is the predominant substrate for metabolism (as in starvation) and increases when the contribution of carbohydrate increases (as during stress with gluconeogenesis). In healthy individuals, the RQ usually falls between 0.80 and 0.90. A RQ <0.7 is consistent with active ketogenesis from endogenous fatty acid metabolism with limited generation of carbon dioxide. An RQ >1.0 indicates net lipogenesis, or the conversion of substrate carbohydrate to fat, a situation that occurs with overfeeding. Values that fall outside the range of 0.65 to 1.25 suggest an error in measurement technique.

Creatinine Excretion in the 24-h Urine Creatinine, the metabolic product of skeletal muscle creatine, is produced at a constant rate and in an amount directly proportional to skeletal muscle mass. With steady-state day-to-day renal function, each gram of creatinine in the 24-h urine collection represents 18.5 g of fat-free skeletal muscle. Since skeletal muscle is the major component of FFM and BCM, measurement of creatinine in the 24-h urine collection can be used as a relative measure of these body compartments during the initial assessment and/or during the course of nutritional support. The *creatinine coefficient* represents the amount of creatinine excreted per kilogram of body weight; it is equal to 23 mg/kg of ideal body weight in men and 18 mg/kg of ideal body weight in women. The *creatinine-height index* represents the ratio of the measured 24-h urine creatinine excretion to the value predicted by the creatinine coefficient for the patient's ideal body weight. These values can be calculated from estimation of the patient's ideal body weight (Table 74-3) or from tables that relate creatinine excretion to height in men and women (Table 74-7). In practice, the accuracy of the 24-h urine creatinine depends primarily on completeness of the urine collection. Together with variations due to fever and fluctuations in dietary intake, inaccuracies of urine collections may result in as much as 10% error in the quantitative 24-h urine creatinine measurement. The constancy of creatinine excretion depends on steady-state renal function, and unpredictable creatinine excretion may occur through feces or skin in patients with

serum creatinine levels >530 μmol/L (>6 mg/dL). The presence of ascites, however, apparently does not compromise the accuracy of the 24-h urine creatinine as a reflection of FFM or BCM in patients with chronic liver disease.

Urine Nitrogen Excretion and Nitrogen Balance Nitrogen balance provides an index of protein gain or loss: 1 g nitrogen is equivalent to 6.25 g protein. Nitrogen balance can be assessed by measuring the difference between nitrogen consumed through the mouth, enteral tube, or intravenous sources and nitrogen excreted in the urine, feces, and other intestinal sources. Protein requirements to achieve zero or positive balance are less in starvation states, where daily protein losses are minimized because of hypometabolism, than in clinical states of stress, where the catabolism of skeletal muscle is accelerated for gluconeogenesis. Accurate measurement of nitrogen balance requires complete measurement of nitrogen losses from all possible excretory routes. In most cases, total urine nitrogen can be calculated by dividing 24-h urinary urea nitrogen by 0.85 and assuming approximately 2 g/d for nitrogen losses in feces and sweat. On the other hand, when the clinical condition includes extensive diarrhea and/or protein losses from pancreatic or enterocutaneous fistulas, the accuracy of nitrogen balance requires measurement of total nitrogen by the modified Kjeldahl technique in both urine and enteric sources. Total nitrogen measurements are also advisable in patients with liver failure, where urinary ammonia becomes a major and alternative source of nitrogen.

INTEGRATED BEDSIDE NUTRITIONAL ASSESSMENT

Several different approaches have been developed in order to simplify the process of nutritional assessment by using selective measurements that relate malnutrition to the specific medical condition and the severity of the underlying disease process.

Subjective Global Assessment This approach incorporates historic and physical findings as a basis for nutrition assessment by the trained physician. Major components in the history include evaluation of the extent of recent weight loss, changes in dietary intake, presence of significant gastrointestinal symptoms persisting more than 2 weeks, alterations in functional status, and the metabolic demand of the patient's underlying disease. Emphasis in the physical examination is placed on findings of depletion of subcutaneous body fat; skeletal muscle wasting; typical changes in skin, mucus membranes, and neurologic examination; as well as the presence of edema. Integration of the historic and physical data permits ranking of patients according to the following categories: adequate nutrition, moderate malnutrition, or severe malnutrition. Though the developers of the subjective global assessment have reported good sensitivity and specificity, the approach is still quite dependent on the training and experience of the clinician.

Prognostic Nutritional Assessment Several paradigms have been developed to link different parameters of nutritional assessment with clinical prognosis. Each approach links specific features of malnutrition with certain measurements of cell-mediated immunity, since abnormal immune function is a common pathway for increased risk in the malnourished patient (Fig. 74-3). A surgical prognostic nutritional index predicts morbidity based on preoperative measurements of serum albumin, transferrin, triceps skin-fold thickness, and delayed hypersensitivity to skin-test antigens. Another PCM score was developed to link survival in alcoholic liver disease to both skin-fold and mid-arm muscle measurements; the creatinine-height index; values for serum albumin, transferrin, prealbumin, and retinol-binding protein; the total lymphocyte count; and the skin-test response to a series of antigens. The Maastricht index predicts survival in patients with serious gastrointestinal diseases on the basis of factors related to serum albumin, retinol-binding protein, lymphotyce count, and deviation from the patient's ideal body weight.

Table 74-7 Ideal 24-h Urine Creatinine Values

Men[a]		Women[b]	
Height, cm[c]	24-h Creatinine, mg	Height, cm	24-h Creatinine, mg
157.5	1288	147.3	830
160.0	1325	149.9	851
162.6	1359	152.4	875
165.1	1386	154.9	900
167.6	1426	157.5	925
170.2	1467	160.0	949
172.7	1513	162.6	977
175.3	1555	165.1	1006
177.8	1596	167.6	1044
180.3	1642	170.2	1076
182.9	1691	172.7	1109
185.4	1739	175.3	1141
188.0	1785	177.8	1174
190.5	1831	180.3	1206
193.0	1891	182.9	1240

[a] Creatinine coefficient for men is 23 mg/kg of ideal body weight.
[b] Creatinine coefficient for women is 18 mg/kg of ideal body weight.
[c] To obtain height in inches, divide by 2.54.
SOURCE: From Blackburn et al.

BIBLIOGRAPHY

BAKER JP et al: Nutritional assessment: A comparison of clinical judgment and objective measurements. N Engl J Med 306:969, 1982

BLACKBURN GL et al: Nutritional and metabolic assessment of the hospitalized patient. J Parenter Enteral Nutr 1:11, 1977

CAHILL GF: Starvation in man. N Engl J Med 282:668, 1970

HALSTED CH: Clinical nutrition education—relevance and role models. Am J Clin Nutr 67:192, 1998

HEYMSFIELD SB et al: Nutritional assessment of malnutrition by anthropomorphic methods, in *Modern Nutrition in Health and Disease*, 9th ed, ME Shils et al (eds). Philadelphia, Lea & Febiger, 1999, p 903

MENDENHALL C et al: Relationship of protein calorie malnutrition to alcoholic liver disease: A reexamination of data from two Veterans Administration Cooperative Studies. Alcohol Clin Exp Res 19:635, 1995

MORGAN SL, WEINSIER RL: *Fundamentals of Clinical Nutrition*. St. Louis, Mosby, 1998, p 167

MULLEN JL et al: Reduction of operative morbidity and mortality by combined preoperative and postoperative nutritional support. Ann Surg 192:604, 1980

NABER THJ et al: Prevalence of malnutrition in nonsurgical hospitalized patients and its association with disease complications. Am J Clin Nutr 66:1232, 1997

YANOVSKI SZ et al: Bioelectrical impedance analysis in body composition measurement: National Institutes of Health technology assessment conference statement. Am J Clin Nutr 64:524S, 1996

75   *Robert M. Russell*

VITAMIN AND TRACE MINERAL DEFICIENCY AND EXCESS

FAD	flavin adenine dinucleotide	NADP	NAD phosphate
FMN	flavin-mononucleotide	PLP	pyridoxal phosphate
HPLC	high-performance liquid chromatography	RDA	Recommended Dietary Allowance
LDL	low-density lipoprotein	RE	retinol equivalent
NAD	nicotinamide adenine dinucleotide	TPN	total parenteral nutrition
		VLDL	very low density lipoprotein

Vitamins and trace minerals are required constituents of the human diet since they are either inadequately synthesized or not synthesized in the human body. Only small amounts of these substances are needed for carrying out essential biochemical reactions (e.g., acting as coenzymes or prosthetic groups). Overt vitamin or trace mineral deficiencies are rare in western countries due to a plentiful, varied, and inexpensive food supply; however, multiple nutrient deficiencies may appear together in persons who are ill or alcoholic. Moreover, subclinical vitamin and trace mineral deficiencies, as diagnosed by laboratory testing, are quite common in the normal population—especially the geriatric population.

Body stores of vitamins and minerals vary tremendously. For example, vitamin B_{12} and vitamin A stores are large, and an adult may not become deficient for 1 or more years after being on a depleted diet. However, folate and thiamine may become depleted within weeks when eating a deficient diet. Therapeutic modalities can deplete essential nutrients from the body; for example, hemodialysis removes water-soluble vitamins, which must be replaced by supplementation.

There are several roles for vitamins and trace minerals in diseases: (1) deficiencies of vitamins and minerals may be caused by disease states such as malabsorption; (2) both deficiency and excess of vitamins and minerals can cause disease in and of themselves (e.g., vitamin A intoxication and liver disease); and (3) vitamins and minerals in high doses may be used as drugs (e.g., niacin for hypercholesterolemia). The hematologic-related vitamins and minerals (Chaps. 105, 107) are not considered in this chapter, nor are the bone-related vitamins and minerals (vitamin D, calcium, phosphorus; Chap. 340), as they are covered elsewhere.

VITAMINS

THIAMINE (VITAMIN B_1)   Thiamine was the first B vitamin to be identified and is therefore also referred to as vitamin B_1. Thiamine pyrophosphate, the coenzyme form of thiamine, is required for branched-chain amino acid metabolism and carbohydrate metabolism (Fig. 75-1). Thiamine functions in the decarboxylation of α-ketoacids, such as pyruvate α-ketoglutarate, and branched-chain amino acids and thus is a source of energy generation. In addition, thiamine pyrophosphate acts as a coenzyme for a transketolase reaction that mediates the conversion of hexose and pentose phosphates. It has also been postulated that thiamine plays a role in peripheral nerve conduction, although the exact chemical reactions underlying this function are unknown.

Absorption and Requirements   At high doses, thiamine is absorbed by a passive mechanism; at low doses, it is absorbed by a carrier-mediated, active transport system and becomes phosphorylated in the process. Once absorbed, thiamine circulates bound to plasma proteins (mainly albumin) and erythrocytes. Storage sites for thiamine include muscle, heart, liver, kidney, and brain, although muscle is the principal storage site. The total body store of thiamine, mainly in the form of thiamine pyrophosphate, is approximately 30 mg, and its biologic half-life ranges between 9 and 18 days.

Given the fact that thiamine is involved in carbohydrate metabolism and energy generation, the Recommended Dietary Allowance (RDA) for males has been adjusted upward to account for increased energy utilization. Experiments have shown that heavy athletic training also increases thiamine utilization slightly. The RDA for thiamine is 1.2 mg/d for males and 1.1 mg/d for females. The median intake of thiamine in the United States from food alone is 2 mg/d. There is a 10% increase in the need for thiamine in pregnancy, and a small further increase in lactating females.

Primary food sources for thiamine include yeast, pork, legumes, beef, whole grains, and nuts. Milled and polished rice contain little, if any, thiamine. Thiamine deficiency is therefore more common in cultures that rely heavily on a rice-based diet. The molecule is heat-sensitive and is destroyed at pH > 8. Tea, coffee (caffeinated and decaffeinated), raw fish, and shellfish contain thiamineases, which can destroy the vitamin. Thus, drinking large amounts of tea or coffee can theoretically lower thiamine body stores.

Deficiency   Most dietary deficiency of thiamine worldwide is the result of poor dietary intake. In western countries, the primary causes of thiamine deficiency are alcoholism and chronic illness, such as cancer. Alcohol is known to interfere directly with the absorption of thiamine and with the synthesis of thiamine pyrophosphate. Malnourished individuals with alcoholic liver disease are also at increased risk of thiamine deficiency because of diminished storage sites in liver and muscle. Thiamine should always be replenished when refeeding a patient with alcoholism, as carbohydrate repletion without adequate thiamine can precipitate acute thiamine deficiency.

Thiamine deficiency in its early stage induces anorexia, irritability, apathy, and generalized weakness. Prolonged thiamine deficiency causes beriberi, which is classically categorized as wet or dry, although there is considerable overlap. In either form of beriberi, patients may complain of pain and parathesia. *Wet beriberi* presents primarily with cardiovascular symptoms, due to impaired myocardial energy metabolism and dysautonomia, and can occur after 3 months of a thiamine-deficient diet. Patients present with an enlarged heart, tachycardia, high-output congestive heart failure, peripheral edema, and peripheral neuritis. Patients with *dry beriberi* present with a symmetric peripheral neuropathy of the motor and sensory systems with diminished reflexes. The neuropathy affects the legs most markedly, and patients have difficulty rising from a squatting position.

Alcoholic patients with chronic thiamine deficiency may also have central nervous system manifestations known as *Wernicke's encephalopathy*, consisting of horizontal nystagmus, ophthalmoplegia (due to weakness of one or more extraocular muscles), cerebellar ataxia, and mental impairment (Chap. 387). When there is an additional loss of memory and a confabulatory psychosis, the syndrome is known as *Wernicke-Korsakoff syndrome*. Although this syndrome is generally described in alcoholic patients, there may be a genetic predisposition to Wernicke-Korsakoff that involves a variant transketolase isozyme.

In severely malnourished infants 2 to 3 months old, thiamine de-

Vitamin	Active derivative or cofactor form	Principal function
Thiamine 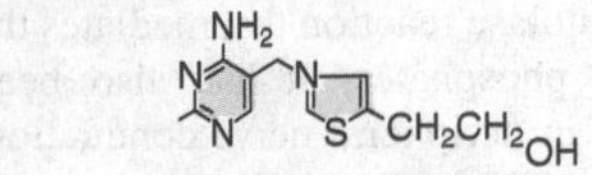 NH₂ ... N ... S ... CH₂CH₂OH	Thiamine pyrophosphatate	Coenzyme for cleavage of carbon-carbon bonds; amino acid and carbohydrate metabolism
Riboflavin 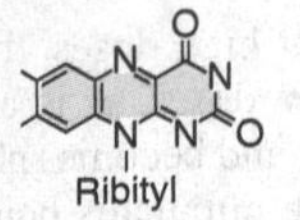 Ribityl	Flavin mononucleotide (FMN) and flavin adenine dinucleotide (FAD)	Cofactor for oxidation reduction reactions and covalently attached prosthetic groups for some enzymes
Niacin 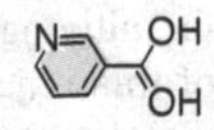 OH ... OH	Nicotanimide adenine dinucleotide phosphate (NADP) and nicotine adenine dinucleotide (NAD)	Coenzymes for oxidation and reduction reactions
Pyridoxine 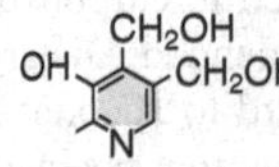 CH₂OH ... OH ... CH₂OH ... N	Pyridoxal phosphate	Cofactor for enzymes of amino acid metabolism
Ascorbic 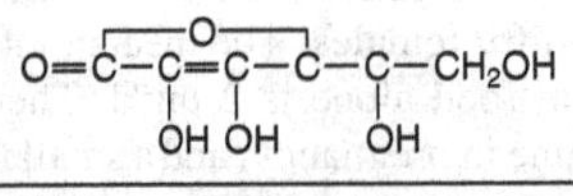 $O=C-C=C-C-C-CH_2OH$ ... OH OH ... OH	Ascorbic acid and dehydroascorbic acid	Participation as a redox ion in many biological oxidation and hydrogen transfer reactions
Vitamin A 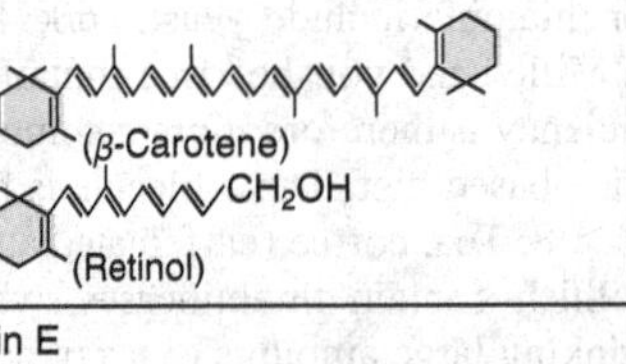 (β-Carotene) ... CH₂OH (Retinol)	Retinol, retinaldehyde, and retinoic acid	Formation of rhodopsin (vision) and glycoproteins (epithelial cell function); also regulates gene transcription
Vitamin E 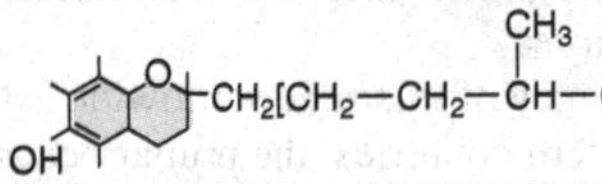 CH₃ ... O ... CH₂[CH₂—CH₂—CH—CH₂]₃H ... OH	Tocopherol and tocotrionols	Antioxidants
Vitamin K 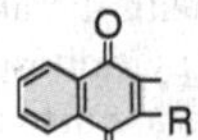 O ... R ... O	Napthoquinone	Cofactor for post-translation carboxylation of many proteins including essential clotting factors

FIGURE 75-1 The structures and principal functions of some of the vitamins associated with human disorders.

ficiency may occur precipitously with sudden cardiovascular failure and collapse, resulting in death within hours. In addition, infants with thiamine deficiency may present with features suggesting meningitis, including vomiting, nystagmus, and convulsions. An aphonic presentation has also been described in which there is extreme irritability and either a very hoarse cry or total inability to emit any noise whatsoever (a silent scream).

The laboratory diagnosis of thiamine deficiency is usually made by a functional enzymatic assay of transketolase activity measured before and after the addition of thiamine pyrophosphate. A >25% stimulation by the addition of thiamine pyrophosphate (an activity coefficient of 1.25) is taken as abnormal. Thiamine or the phosphorylated esters of thiamine in serum or blood can also be measured by high-performance liquid chromatography (HPLC) to detect deficiency. Moreover, a urinary level of thiamine <27 μg per gram of creatinine per day is abnormal. In measuring urinary excretion of thiamine, one should make sure the patient is not taking diuretics, which increase thiamine excretion.

℞ **TREATMENT** In acute thiamine deficiency with either cardiovascular or neurologic signs, 100 mg/d of thiamine should be given parenterally for 7 days, followed by 10 mg/d orally until there is complete recovery. Cardiovascular improvement occurs in ≤12 h, and ophthalmoplegic improvement occurs within 24 h. Other manifestations gradually clear, although psychosis in the Wernicke-Korsakoff syndrome may be permanent or persist for several months. Consistent with this, pathologic changes occur in the cortex, cerebellum, and mammillary bodies of the thalamus. Parenteral thiamine should be given prophylactically to all chronic alcoholic patients in the emergency room, or as soon as they are admitted, to prevent precipitation of thiamine deficiency after the provision of glucose-containing solutions.

Thiamine-responsive conditions requiring pharmacologic doses of thiamine include branched-chain ketoaciduria (maple sugar urine disease), subacute necrotizing encephalopathy due to thiamine dihydrophosphate deficiency in the brain (Leigh syndrome), thiamine-responsive lactic acidosis, and thiamine-responsive megaloblastic anemia associated with diabetes mellitus and deafness (Chap. 353). The gene for this recessive disorder, *SLC19A2*, encodes a thiamine transporter.

Toxicity Although anaphylaxis has been reported after high doses of thiamine, no adverse effects have been recorded from either food or supplements at high doses. Thiamine supplements may be bought over the counter in doses of up to 50 mg/d.

RIBOFLAVIN (VITAMIN B₂) Riboflavin is important for the metabolism of fat, carbohydrate, and protein, reflecting its role as a respiratory coenzyme and an electron donor. Riboflavin is esterified with phosphoric acid in the body to form two coenzymes, flavin-mononucleotide (FMN) and flavin adenine dinucleotide (FAD) which are involved in a variety of cellular oxidation-reduction processes. Enzymes that contain FAD or FMN as prosthetic groups are known as *flavoenzymes* (e.g., succinic acid dehydrogenase, monoamine oxidase, glutathione reductase). Riboflavin plays an important role in niacin metabolism, since flavoenzymes act as intermediaries in the oxidation of the reduced forms of nicotinamide adenine dinucleotide (NAD) and NAD phosphate (NADP).

Riboflavin is normally absorbed by active and carrier-mediated saturable mechanisms, whereas diffusion is the principal mechanism of absorption at high concentrations. Riboflavin phosphorylation takes place mainly in the wall of the small intestine. Both FMN and FAD are bound to immunoglobulins and albumin in the circulation, and both forms are stored to some degree in liver and muscle.

Although much is known about the chemical and enzymatic reactions of riboflavin, the clinical manifestations of riboflavin deficiency are nonspecific and similar to those of other B vitamin deficiencies. Further, riboflavin deficiency usually occurs in combination with other water-soluble vitamin deficiencies (Chap. 74). Riboflavin deficiency is manifested principally by lesions of the mucocutaneous surfaces of the mouth (angular stomatitis, cheilosis, atrophic glossitis, magenta tongue, pharyngitis) and skin (seborrhea, genital dermatitis). In addition to the mucocutaneous lesions, corneal vascularization, anemia, and personality changes have been described with riboflavin deficiency.

Deficiency and Excess Riboflavin deficiency is almost always due to dietary deficiency. The requirement for riboflavin is increased during pregnancy and lactation and possibly by heavy exercise. The use of phenothiazines and antibiotics also appears to increase the need for riboflavin. Milk, other dairy products, and enriched breads and cereals are the most important dietary sources of riboflavin in the United States, although lean meat, fish, eggs, broccoli, and legumes are also good sources. Riboflavin is extremely sensitive to light, and milk should be stored in containers that protect against photodegradation. In non-milk-drinking societies (e.g., Central America), the laboratory diagnosis of riboflavin deficiency is common. Laboratory diagnosis of riboflavin deficiency can be made by measurement of red blood cell or urinary riboflavin concentrations or by measurement of erythrocyte glutathione reductase activity, with and without added FAD. A stimulation (activity coefficient) of >1.4 is diagnostic of a deficient state. The RDA for riboflavin is 1.1 to 1.3 mg/d in adults, with slightly higher recommendations for lactating and pregnant women. Rare genetic defects of flavoprotein synthesis may require pharmacologic doses of riboflavin for treatment. Because the capacity of the gastrointestinal tract to absorb riboflavin is limited (~20 mg if given in one oral dose), riboflavin toxicity has not been described. Thus, the most recent revision of the RDAs did not set an upper limit for this nutrient.

NIACIN (VITAMIN B₃) The term *niacin* refers to nicotinic acid and nicotinamide and their biologically active derivatives. Nicotinic acid and nicotinamide serve as precursors of two coenzymes, NAD and NADP. These coenzymes are important in numerous oxidation and reduction reactions in the body. NAD and NADP serve as cofactors for dehydrogenases and are involved in the transfer of the hydride ion in many redox reactions. Thus, niacin is important in pentose, steroid, and fatty acid biosynthesis; glycolysis; protein metabolism; and the oxidation of fuels such as lactate, pyruvate, and alcohol. In addition, NAD and NADP are active in adenine diphosphate–ribose transfer reactions involved in DNA repair and calcium mobilization.

Absorption, Metabolism, and Requirements Nicotinic acid and nicotinamide are absorbed well from the stomach and small intestine. Both forms of niacin are absorbed by a sodium-dependent, facilitated diffusion mechanism at low doses, whereas passive diffusion occurs at high doses. Some storage of NAD takes place in the liver. The amino acid tryptophan can be converted to niacin with an efficiency of 60:1 by weight. Thus, the RDA for niacin is expressed in niacin equivalents. Greater conversion of tryptophan to niacin occurs in niacin-deficient states, pregnancy, and in women using oral contraceptives. However, a lower conversion efficiency occurs if a patient is vitamin B₆- or riboflavin-deficient. The drug isoniazid inhibits the conversion of tryptophan to niacin. The urinary excretion products of niacin include nicotinic acid and niacin oxide; however, the major urinary metabolites are 2-pyridone and 2-methyl nicotinamide, measurements of which are used in diagnosis of niacin deficiency.

The RDA for niacin is 16 niacin equivalents per day for men and 14 niacin equivalents for women. Median intakes of niacin in the United States considerably exceed these values. Diets that are corn-based can predispose to niacin deficiency due to the low tryptophan and niacin content. Niacin bioavailability is high from beans, milk, meat, and eggs; bioavailability from cereal grains is lower. Since flour is enriched with the "free" niacin (i.e., non-coenzyme form), bioavailability is excellent.

Deficiency Niacin deficiency causes *pellagra*, which is mostly found among people eating corn-based diets in parts of China, Africa, and India. Pellagra in North America is found mainly among alcoholics; in patients with congenital defects of intestinal and kidney absorption of tryptophan (Hartnup's disease; Chap. 352); and in patients with carcinoid syndrome (Chap. 93), in which there is increased conversion of tryptophan to serotonin. The early symptoms of pellagra include loss of appetite, generalized weakness and irritability, abdominal pain, and vomiting. Epithelial cell changes then ensue with stomatitis and bright-red glossitis, followed by a characteristic skin rash that is pigmented and scaling, particularly in skin areas exposed to sunlight. This rash is known as "Casal's necklace," when it rings the neck, and is seen in advanced cases. Vaginitis and esophagitis may also occur. Diarrhea (in part due to proctitis and in part due to malabsorption), depression, seizures, and dementia are also part of the pellagra syndrome—the four D's: *d*ermatitis, *d*iarrhea, and *d*ementia leading to *d*eath.

The diagnosis of niacin deficiency is based on low levels of the urinary metabolites 2-methyl nicotinamide and 2-pyridone. Treatment of pellagra consists of oral supplementation of 100 to 200 mg of nicotinamide or nicotinic acid three times daily for 5 days. High doses of nicotinic acid (≥3 g nicotinic acid per day) are used for the treatment of elevated cholesterol levels and in the treatment of types 2, 4, and 5 hyperlipidemias (Chap. 344).

Toxicity Prostaglandin-mediated flushing has been observed at daily doses as low as 50 mg of niacin when taken as a supplement or as therapy for hypertriglyceridemia. No toxicity has been seen from niacin derived from food sources. Flushing may be accompanied by skin dryness, itching, and headache. Premedication with aspirin may alleviate these symptoms. Nausea, vomiting, and abdominal pain also occur at similar doses of niacin. Hepatic toxicity is the most serious toxic reaction due to niacin and may present as jaundice with elevated AST and ALT levels. A few cases of fulminant hepatitis requiring liver transplantation have been reported at doses of 3 to 9 g/d. Other toxic reactions include glucose intolerance, macular edema, and macular cysts. It is not clear whether sustained-release forms of nicotinic acid are more toxic than regular forms. The upper limit for daily niacin intake has been set at 35 mg. However, this upper limit does not pertain to the therapeutic use of niacin.

PYRIDOXINE (VITAMIN B₆) Vitamin B₆ refers to a family of compounds including pyridoxine, pyridoxal, pyridoxamine, and their 5′-phosphate derivatives. 5′-Pyridoxal phosphate (PLP) is a cofactor for more than 100 enzymes involved in amino acid metabolism (e.g., 5′-PLP is a cofactor for the transulfuration enzymes involved in the conversion of homocysteine to cystathionine; Chap. 352). Vitamin B₆ is also involved in heme and neurotransmitter synthesis and in the metabolism of glycogen, lipids, steroids, sphingoid bases, and several vitamins, including the conversion of tryptophan to niacin.

Absorption and Metabolism Approximately 75% of vitamin B₆ is absorbed from a mixed diet by a nonsaturable, passive process. Much of dietary vitamin B₆ is in the phosphorylated form, and the phosphate must be removed by intestinal alkaline phosphatase before absorption takes place. Once absorbed, the vitamin becomes rephosphorylated in the liver, where the various forms can be interconverted. In the liver, PLP binds avidly to cellular proteins and albumin. Since these binding proteins protect it from phosphatase activity, tissue levels of PLP can become quite high with continuous supplementation. Sixty mg of vitamin B₆ is stored in the body, and much is in the form of PLP bound to phosphorylase A in muscle. The biologic half-life of vitamin B₆ is 25 days.

Dietary Sources Plants contain vitamin B₆ in the form of pyridoxine, whereas animal tissues contain PLP and pyridoxamine phosphate. The vitamin B₆ contained in plants is less bioavailable than that from animal tissues. All forms of vitamin B₆ are labile in alkaline conditions. Rich food sources of vitamin B₆ include legumes, nuts, wheat bran, and meat, although the vitamin is present in all food groups. The RDA for young adults (both males and females) has been set at 1.3 mg/d. For older adults, the RDA is slightly higher (1.5 mg/d for women, 1.7 mg/d for men).

Deficiency Symptoms of vitamin B₆ deficiency include seborrheic dermatitis, glossitis, stomatitis, and cheilosis, as frequently seen with other B vitamin deficiencies (Chap. 74). In addition, severe vitamin B₆ deficiency can lead to generalized weakness, irritability, peripheral neuropathy, abnormal electroencephalograms, and personality changes including depression and confusion. In infants, diarrhea, seizures, and anemia have been reported. Microcytic, hypochromic anemia is due to diminished hemoglobin synthesis, since the first enzyme involved in heme biosynthesis (amino-levulinate synthase) requires

PLP as a cofactor (Chap. 104). In some case reports, platelet dysfunction has also been reported. Since vitamin B_6 is necessary for the conversion of homocysteine to cystathionine, it is possible that chronic low-grade vitamin B_6 deficiency may result in hyperhomocystinemia and increased risk of cardiovascular disease (Chaps. 242 and 352).

Certain medications such as isoniazid, L-dopa, penicillamine, and cycloserine interact with PLP due to a reaction with carbonyl groups. Oral contraceptives have been reported to decrease vitamin B_6 status indicators, although the mechanism for this is uncertain. Alcoholism also decreases vitamin B_6 status due to poor diet, liver disease, and the fact that acetaldehyde can compete with PLP for protein binding, leading to increased degradation and excretion. The increased ratio of aspartate aminotransferase (AST or SGOT) to alanine aminotransferase (ALT or SGPT) seen in alcoholic liver disease reflects the relative vitamin B_6 dependence of ALT. Vitamin B_6 requirements are higher in preeclampsia, eclampsia, and hemodialysis. Vitamin B_6 dependency syndromes that require pharmacologic doses of vitamin B_6 are rare, but include cystathionine β-synthase deficiency, pyridoxine-responsive (primarily sideroblastic) anemias, and gyrate atrophy with chorioretinal degeneration due to decreased activity of the mitochondrial enzyme ornithine aminotransferase. In these situations, 100 to 200 mg/d of oral vitamin B_6 are required for treatment.

High doses of vitamin B_6 have been used to treat carpal tunnel syndrome, premenstrual tension, schizophrenia, autism, and diabetic neuropathy but have not been found to be effective.

The laboratory diagnosis of vitamin B_6 deficiency is generally made on the basis of low plasma PLP values (<20 nmol/L). Other measures of vitamin B_6 deficiency include low erythrocyte levels of PLP, low plasma pyridoxal, and low urinary levels of 4-pyridoxic acid. Treatment of vitamin B_6 deficiency is 50 mg/d; higher doses of 100 to 200 mg/d are given if vitamin B_6 deficiency is related to medication use. Vitamin B_6 should not be given with L-dopa, since the vitamin interferes with the action of this drug.

Toxicity The safe upper limit for vitamin B_6 has been set at 100 mg/d, although the lowest dose at which toxicity (sensory neuropathy) has been seen is 500 mg/d. No adverse effects have been associated with high intakes of vitamin B_6 from food sources only. When toxicity occurs, it causes a severe sensory neuropathy, leaving patients unable to walk. Some cases of photosensitivity and dermatitis have also been reported.

VITAMIN C Both ascorbic acid and its oxidized product dehydroascorbic acid are biologically active. Vitamin C participates in oxidation-reduction reactions and hydrogen ion transfer reactions. As an antioxidant, vitamin C donates electrons to quench reactive free radical and oxygen species. It also acts to regenerate other antioxidants such as vitamin E, flavonoids, and glutathione. Other actions of vitamin C include promotion of nonheme iron absorption, carnitine biosynthesis, and the conversion of dopamine to norepinephrine. Vitamin C is also important for connective tissue metabolism and cross-linking and is a component of many drug-metabolizing enzyme systems, particularly the mixed-function oxidase systems. As such, the vitamin participates in the synthesis of corticosteroids, aldosterone, and the metabolism of cholesterol. Vitamin C also participates in enzymatic reactions requiring a reduced metal, although the exact molecular basis for this role has not been delineated.

Absorption and Physiology Vitamin C is absorbed by an energy-dependent, saturable transport system, and a progressively smaller proportion of the vitamin is absorbed with increasing dose. Almost complete absorption of the vitamin occurs if <100 mg is administered in a single dose; however, only 50% or less is absorbed at doses >1 g. Enhanced degradation and fecal and urinary excretion of vitamin C occur at higher intake levels. High levels of the reduced form of vitamin C are contained in white blood cells, lens tissue, and brain. The maximum body pool in adult males is approximately 1500 mg, and 3% of this body pool is turned over each day, resulting in a half-life of approximately 18 days.

Dietary Sources and Requirements Good dietary sources of vitamin C include citrus fruits, green vegetables (especially broccoli), tomatoes, and potatoes. Appreciable amounts of vitamin C may be consumed as an antioxidant food additive, and the consumption of five servings of fruits and vegetables a day provides vitamin C in excess of the RDA of 60 mg/d for males and females. Moreover, approximately 40% of the U.S. population takes vitamin C as a dietary supplement. Vitamin C requirements are increased slightly to 70 mg in pregnancy and are increased further to 90 to 95 mg/d during lactation. Smoking, hemodialysis, and stress (e.g., infection, trauma) appear to increase vitamin C requirements. "Natural forms" of vitamin C are no more bioavailable than synthetic forms.

Deficiency Vitamin C deficiency causes scurvy; in the United States, this is seen primarily among poor and elderly people and alcoholics who consume <10 mg/d of vitamin C. Vitamin C deficiency has also been described among individuals consuming macrobiotic diets. Scurvy occurs when the body pool for vitamin C drops to <300 mg/d and plasma levels drop to <11 μmol/L. Symptoms of scurvy primarily reflect impaired formation of mature connective tissue and include bleeding into skin (petechiae, ecchymoses, perifollicular hemorrhages); inflamed and bleeding gums; and manifestations of bleeding into joints, the peritoneal cavity, pericardium, and the adrenal glands. Other generalized symptoms include weakness, fatigue, and depression. In children, vitamin C deficiency may cause impaired bone growth. Laboratory diagnosis of vitamin C deficiency is made on the basis of low plasma or leukocyte levels.

Administration of vitamin C (200 mg/d) results in marked improvement in the symptoms of scurvy in a matter of several days. High-dose vitamin C supplementation (e.g., 1 to 2 g/d) has been shown to slightly decrease the symptoms and duration of upper respiratory tract infections and to improve glycemic control. Vitamin C supplementation has also been reported to be useful in Chédiak-Higashi syndrome (Chap. 64) and osteogenesis imperfecta (Chap. 351). It has been claimed that foods high in vitamin C may lower the incidence of certain cancers, particularly esophageal and gastric cancers. If proven, this effect may be due to the fact that vitamin C can prevent the conversion of nitrites and secondary amines to carcinogenic nitrosomines. However, one intervention study from China did not show vitamin C to be protective. Other chronic diseases for which diets high in vitamin C have been reported to be protective include cardiovascular disease, stroke, and cataracts. However, these studies are correlational, and no large-scale intervention studies have been reported.

Toxicity Taking >2 g of vitamin C in a single dose may result in abdominal pain, diarrhea, and nausea; doses >3 g have been reported to elevate blood levels of alanine aminotransferase, lactic acid dehydrogenase, and uric acid. Since vitamin C may be metabolized to oxalate, it has been feared that chronic, high-dose vitamin C supplementation could result in an increased prevalence of kidney stones. However, this has not been borne out in several trials, except in individual patients with preexisting renal disease. Thus, it is reasonable to advise patients with a past history of kidney stones not to take large doses of vitamin C. There is also an unproven, but possible risk that chronic high doses of vitamin C could promote iron overload in patients taking supplemental iron. High doses of vitamin C can induce hemolysis in patients with glucose-6-phosphate dehydrogenase deficiency, and doses >1 g/d can cause false-negative guaiac reactions as well as interfering with tests for urinary glucose.

BIOTIN Biotin is a water-soluble vitamin with a bicyclic structure. The vitamin plays an important role in gluconeogenesis and fatty acid synthesis and serves as a CO_2 carrier on the surface of both cytosolic and mitochondrial carboxylase enzymes. The vitamin also functions in the catabolism of specific amino acids (e.g., leucine).

Biotin in food sources is bound to protein from which it must be cleaved in order to be absorbed. The enzyme biotinidase dissociates the vitamin and facilitates its subsequent transport. Excellent food sources of biotin include liver, soy, beans, yeast, and egg yolks, although egg white contains the protein avidin that strongly binds the vitamin and reduces its bioavailability. Biotin is contained in moderate amounts in legumes, nuts, mushrooms, cauliflower, and certain cereals. Although biotin is synthesized by intestinal bacteria, the relative importance of this source in humans is uncertain. The recommended intake of biotin for adults is 30 μg/d and 35 μg/d in lactating women.

Biotin deficiency has been induced by experimental feeding of egg white diets and in patients with short bowels who received biotin-free parenteral nutrition. In the adult, biotin deficiency results in mental changes (depression, hallucinations), paresthesia, anorexia, and nausea. A scaling, seborrheic, and erythematous rash may occur around the eyes, nose, and mouth as well as on the extremities. In infants, biotin deficiency presents as hypotonia, lethargy, and apathy. In addition, the infant may develop alopecia and a characteristic rash that includes the ears. Two types of inherited infantile biotin deficiency states have been described. Multiple carboxylase deficiency syndrome is an autosomal recessive disorder that is expressed during the first week of life and is characterized by severe metabolic ketoacidosis and dermatitis. Treatment requires pharmacologic doses of biotin, using up to 10 mg/d. Late-onset infantile biotin deficiency due to absorptive and transport defects occurs between 3 and 6 months with dermatitis, seizures, ataxia, hypotonia, and variable metabolic acidosis. The laboratory diagnosis of biotin deficiency can be established based on a decreased urinary concentration.

PANTOTHENIC ACID Pantothenic acid is a component of coenzyme A and phosphopantetheine, which are involved in fatty acid metabolism and the synthesis of cholesterol, steroid hormones, and all compounds formed from isoprenoid units. In addition, pantothenic acid is involved in the acetylation of proteins. Pantothenic acid is actively transported when given at low doses, but it is passively absorbed when given at high doses. The vitamin is excreted in the urine, and the laboratory diagnosis of deficiency is made on the basis of low urinary vitamin levels.

The vitamin is ubiquitous in the food supply. Liver, yeast, egg yolks, and vegetables are particularly good sources. The recommended adequate intake for adults is 5 mg/d. Human pantothenic acid deficiency has only been demonstrated in experimental feeding of diets low in pantothenic acid or by giving a specific pantothenic acid antagonist. The symptoms of pantothenic acid deficiency are nonspecific and include gastrointestinal disturbance, depression, muscle cramps, paresthesia, ataxia, and hypoglycemia. Pantothenic acid deficiency was thought to cause the burning feet syndrome seen in prisoners of war during World War II. No toxicity of this vitamin has been reported.

CHOLINE Choline is a precursor for acetylcholine, phospholipids, and betaine. Choline is necessary for the structural integrity of cell membranes, cholinergic neurotransmission, lipid and cholesterol metabolism, and transmembrane signaling. Recently, a recommended adequate intake was set at 550 mg/d for adult males and 425 mg/d for adult females. Choline is thought to be a "conditionally essential" nutrient, in that de novo synthesis occurs in the liver and is less than the vitamin's utilization only under certain stress conditions. Choline deficiency has occurred in patients receiving parenteral nutrition devoid of choline. Deficiency results in fatty liver and elevated transaminase levels. The diagnosis of choline deficiency is made on the basis of low plasma levels.

Toxicity from choline results in hypotension, cholinergic sweating, diarrhea, salivation, and a fishy body odor. The upper limit for choline has been set at 3.5 g/d. Therapeutically, choline has been suggested for patients with dementia and for patients at high risk of cardiovascular disease, due to its ability to lower cholesterol and homocysteine levels. However, such benefits have yet to be documented.

VITAMIN A *Vitamin A*, in the strictest sense, refers to retinol. However, the oxidized metabolites, retinaldehyde and retinoic acid, are also biologically active compounds. The term *retinoids* includes synthetic molecules that are chemically related to retinol. Retinaldehyde is the essential form of vitamin A that is required for normal vision, whereas retinoic acid is necessary for normal morphogenesis, growth, and cell differentiation. Retinoic acid does not function in vision and, in contrast to retinol, is not involved in reproduction. Vitamin A also plays a role in iron utilization, humoral immunity, T

cell–mediated immunity, natural killer cell activity, and phagocytosis. Vitamin A is commercially available in esterified forms (e.g., acetate, palmitate) since it is more stable as an ester.

There are over 600 carotenoids in nature, and approximately 50 of these can be metabolized to vitamin A. β-Carotene is the most prevalent carotenoid in the food supply that has provitamin A activity. Although the breakdown of β-carotene should theoretically yield two molecules of vitamin A, the conversion of carotenoids to vitamin A, in fact, is much less efficient. It is estimated that 6 μg or greater of dietary β-carotene is equivalent to 1 μg of retinol, whereas 12 μg or greater of other dietary provitamin A carotenoids (e.g., cryptoxanthin, α-carotene) is equivalent to 1 μg of retinol.

Absorption and Metabolism Approximately 80% of preformed vitamin A is absorbed from food, and absorption is via a carrier-mediated mechanism at low concentrations and passive diffusion at high concentrations. Approximately 15 to 30% of provitamin A carotenoids are absorbed passively from the diet, and the absorption becomes much less efficient at high dosage. The absorption of both vitamin A and carotenoids are partially dependent on an adequate bile concentration within the intestinal lumen for the formation of micelles. Once a provitamin A carotene is absorbed into the epithelial cell, a small proportion of it is split to form vitamin A. At higher doses of β-carotene, the conversion to vitamin A is less efficient, thereby preventing vitamin A toxicity. The absorption of both vitamin A and intact β-carotene is via the lymphatics after chylomicron formation.

Hepatic clearance of vitamin A in chylomicrons is efficient, and the liver contains approximately 90% of the vitamin A reserves. Approximately 10 to 40% of a vitamin A dose is oxidized or conjugated in the liver and excreted in urine or bile. Of a given dose of vitamin A, approximately 50% enters the liver storage pool. Storage of vitamin A takes place in the lipid storage (Ito) cell of the liver, which is also a collagen-producing cell. The liver secretes vitamin A in the form of retinol, which is bound to retinol-binding protein. Once this has occurred, the retinol-binding protein complex interacts with a second protein, transthryetin. This trimolecular complex functions to prevent vitamin A from being filtered by the kidney glomerulus, to protect the body against the toxicity of retinol and to allow retinol to be taken up by specific cell-surface receptors that recognize retinol-binding protein. A certain amount of vitamin A enters peripheral cells even if it is not bound to retinol-binding protein. After retinol is internalized by the cell, it becomes bound to a series of cellular retinol-binding proteins, which function as sequestering and transporting agents as well as coligands for enzymatic reactions. Certain cells also contain retinoic acid–binding proteins, which have the same sequestering functions as well as enabling retinoic acid metabolism.

11-*cis*-Retinaldehyde functions as a visual pigment chromophore to capture light. Rhodopsin is composed of the protein opsin and retinaldehyde and is contained in the rod cells, whereas iodopsin is contained in cones. When the dark-adapted retina is exposed to light, the 11-*cis*-retinaldehyde contained in rhodopsin isomerizes to an all-*trans* form. This conformational change causes dissociation from the opsin, resulting in a nerve impulse and a visual response. Once the retina returns to dim light conditions, rhodopsin is regenerated.

Retinoic acid is a ligand for certain nuclear receptors that act as transcription factors. Two families of receptors (RAR and RXR receptors) are active in retinoid-mediated gene transcription. Retinoid receptors regulate transcription by binding as dimeric complexes to specific DNA sites, the retinoic acid response elements, in target genes (Chap. 327). The receptors can either stimulate or repress gene expression in response to their ligands. RAR binds all-*trans* retinoic acid and 9-*cis* retinoic acid, whereas RXR binds only 9-*cis* retinoic acid.

The retinoid receptors play an important role in controlling cell proliferation and differentiation. Retinoic acid is useful in the treatment of promyeolcytic leukemia (Chap. 111). In this case, a gene rearrangement fuses the RAR to one of several other genes [e.g., t(15; 17)], causing an apparent block in cell differentiation. Treatment with retinoic acid activates the RAR, dissociating repressor complexes and leading to cell differentiation and more normal cell turnover. Retinoic acid is also used in the treatment of cystic acne because it inhibits keratinization, decreases sebum secretion, and possibly alters the inflammatory reaction (Chap. 56). RXRs dimerize with other nuclear receptors to function as coregulators of genes responsive to retinoids, thyroid hormone, and calcitriol. RXR agonists induce insulin sensitivity experimentally, perhaps because RXR is a cofactor for the peroxisome-proliferator-activated receptors (PPARs), which are targets for the thiazolidinedione drugs such as rosiglitazone and troglitazone (Chap. 333).

Dietary Sources The retinol equivalent (RE) is used to express the vitamin A value of food. One RE is defined as 1 μg of retinol (0.003491 mmol). In the past, 1 RE was considered to be equal to 6 μg of β-carotene, but additional studies indicate that 1 RE may, in fact, be equal to 12 to 20 μg of β-carotene from a dietary source. In older literature, vitamin A was often expressed in international units (IU), with 1 RE being equal to 3.33 IU of retinol and 12 IU of β-carotene, but these units are no longer in current medical or scientific use. The RDA for vitamin A is set at 1000 RE for adult males and 800 RE for adult females.

Liver and fish are excellent food sources for preformed vitamin A; vegetable sources of provitamin A carotenoids include dark-green and -colored fruits and vegetables. Diets consisting mainly of rice, wheat, maize, and tubers can produce vitamin A deficiency, as few carotenoids are contained in these foods. In areas where these foods are staples, children are particularly susceptible to vitamin A deficiency because neither breast nor cow's milk supplies enough vitamin A to prevent deficiency. Areas of the world where vitamin A deficiency is particularly prevalent include parts of Africa, South America, and Southeast Asia. Vitamin A deficiency occurs in more than 250,000 children each year, resulting in blindness and a 50% mortality rate within the year. In western countries, vitamin A deficiency is seen primarily among patients with diseases associated with fat malabsorption (e.g., celiac sprue, short-bowel syndrome). Concurrent zinc deficiency can interfere with the mobilization of vitamin A from liver stores as well as the synthesis of rhodopsin in the eye; thus vitamin A deficiency is exacerbated by concurrent zinc deficiency. Alcohol also interferes with the conversion of retinol to retinaldehyde in the eye by competing for alcohol (retinol) dehydrogenase. Drugs that interfere with the absorption of vitamin A include mineral oil, neomycin, and cholestyramine.

Deficiency Symptoms of vitamin A deficiency include hyperkeratotic skin lesions, night blindness (inability to see in dim light), dryness of the eyes, xerosis, and Bitôt spots, which are white patches of keratinized epithelium appearing on the sclera. Aggressive xerophthalmia can result in corneal ulceration. If untreated, proteolytic destruction and rupture of the cornea ensues with permanent blindness, although vitamin A treatment of patients with corneal ulcers can also result in blindness due to permanent corneal scarring. Children with vitamin A deficiency have increased mortality, primarily from infectious diseases, measles, respiratory diseases, and diarrhea. Extremely low birth weight infants (<1000 g) should be treated parenterally with 5000 IU (1500 μg or RE) of vitamin A three times a week for 4 weeks.

There are no specific deficiency signs or symptoms that result from carotenoid deficiency. However, dietary carotenoids have been suggested to protect against cataract formation, low-density lipoprotein (LDL) oxidation, and certain cancers. It was hoped that β-carotene would be an effective chemopreventive for cancer because numerous epidemiologic studies had shown that diets high in β-carotene were associated with lower incidences of cancers of the respiratory and digestive system. However, intervention studies using high doses of β-carotene actually resulted in more lung cancers than in placebo-treated groups. Non-provitamin A carotenoids, such as lutein and zeaxanthin, have been suggested to protect against macular degeneration. The non-provitamin A carotenoid lycopene has been suggested to protect against prostate cancer. However, the effectiveness of these agents has not been proven by intervention studies, and the mechanisms underlying these purported biologic actions are unknown.

The diagnosis of vitamin A deficiency is made by measurement of serum retinol (normal range, 30 to 65 μg/dL), tests of dark adaptation, impression cytology of the conjunctiva (decreased numbers of mucous-secreting cells), or measurement of body storage pools, either directly by liver biopsy or by isotopic dilution after administering a stable isotope of vitamin A.

Vitamin A deficiency with ocular changes should be treated by administering 100,000 IU (30 mg) of vitamin A intramuscularly, or 200,000 IU (60 mg) orally. In areas of endemic vitamin A deficiency, this is followed by vitamin A capsules of 200,000 IU at 6-month intervals. Vitamin A deficiency in patients with malabsorptive diseases, who have abnormal dark adaptation or symptoms of night blindness without ocular changes, should be treated for 1 month with 50,000 IU/d (15 mg/d) orally of a water micelle preparation of vitamin A. This is followed by lower maintenance doses with the exact amount determined by monitoring serum retinol.

Toxicity Acute toxicity of vitamin A was first noted in Arctic explorers after eating polar bear liver and has been seen after administration of 150 mg in adults or 100 mg in children. Acute toxicity is manifest by increased intracranial pressure, vertigo, diplopia, bulging fontanels in children, seizures, and exfoliative dermatitis; it may result in death. Chronic vitamin A intoxication has been seen in normal adults who ingest 50,000 IU/d (15 mg/d) of vitamin A for a period of several months and in children who ingest 20,000 IU/d (6 mg/d). Manifestations include dry skin, cheilosis, glossitis, vomiting, alopecia, bone pain, hypercalcemia, lymph node enlargement, hyperlipidemia, amenorrhea, and features of pseudotumor cerebri with increased intracranial pressure and papilledema. Liver fibrosis with portal hypertension and bone demineralization may also result from chronic vitamin A intoxication. When vitamin A is provided in excess of pregnant women, congenital malformations have included spontaneous abortions, craniofacial abnormalities, and valvular heart disease. In pregnancy, the daily dose of vitamin A should not exceed 10,000 IU (3 mg). Elderly individuals appear to be more prone to vitamin A intoxication, as are alcoholics and patients with liver disease. In fact acute hepatitis may precipitate vitamin A intoxication in patients who have extremely high vitamin A stores in the liver. It should be noted that the commercially available retinoid derivatives are also toxic, including 13-*cis*-retinoic acid, which has been associated with birth defects. As a result, contraception should be continued for a least 1 year, and possibly longer, in women who have taken 13-*cis* retinoic acid.

High doses of carotenoids do not result in toxic symptoms. However, carotenemia, which is characterized by a yellowing of the skin (creases of the palms and soles) but not the sclerae, may be seen after ingestion of >30 mg of β-carotene on a daily basis. Hypothyroid patients are particularly susceptible to the development of carotenemia due to impaired breakdown of carotene to vitamin A. Reduction of carotenes from the diet results in the disappearance of skin yellowing and carotenemia over a period of 30 to 60 days.

VITAMIN D (See Chap. 340).

VITAMIN E Vitamin E is a collective name for a group of tocopherols and tocotrionols, the latter having an unsaturated side-chain. There are eight naturally occurring plant compounds with vitamin E activity. RRR-α tocopherol is the most active, while synthetic stereoisomers of vitamin E are less biologically active. Vitamin E acts as a chain-breaking antioxidant and is an efficient pyroxyl radical scavenger, which protects LDLs and polyunsaturated fats in membranes from oxidation. A network of other antioxidants (e.g., vitamin C, glutathione) and enzymes maintains vitamin E in a reduced state. Vitamin E also inhibits prostaglandin synthesis and the activities of protein kinase C and phospholipase A$_2$.

Absorption and Metabolism Vitamin E is a fat-soluble vitamin and requires all the processes needed for micelle formation to be absorbed. About 15 to 40% is absorbed passively from a single physiologic dose, and there is less efficient absorption at high doses. Polyunsaturated fat may inhibit absorption. Vitamin E is taken up from chylomicrons by the liver, and an hepatic α tocopherol transport protein is involved in intracellular vitamin E transport and incorporation into very low density lipoprotein (VLDL). The transport protein has particular affinity for the RRR isomeric form of α tocopherol; thus this natural isomer has the most biologic activity. In the circulation, vitamin E is bound to all lipoprotein classes and becomes widely distributed in tissues, with fat and muscle being the most important storage depots. Vitamin E metabolites are mainly excreted in feces, although some are also excreted in urine.

Requirement The RDA for vitamin E is currently 10 mg for adults. Additional vitamin E is recommended during pregnancy (12 mg/d) and lactation (14 mg/d). Vitamin E is widely distributed in the food supply. The RRR-α isomers are particularly high in sunflower oil, safflower oil, and wheat germ oil; γ tocotrionols are notably present in soybean and corn oils. Vitamin E is also found in meats, nuts, and cereal grains, and small amounts are present in fruits and vegetables. Vitamin E pills containing doses of 50 to 1000 mg are ingested by a large fraction of the U.S. population. In the older literature, 1 IU of vitamin E is equal to 1 mg *all*-racemic α tocopherol acetate. Diets high in polyunsaturated fats may necessitate a slightly higher requirement for vitamin E.

Dietary deficiency of vitamin E does not exist. Vitamin E deficiency is seen only in severe and prolonged malabsorptive diseases, such as celiac disease, or after small-intestinal resection, leading to short-bowel syndrome. Children with cystic fibrosis or prolonged cholestasis may develop vitamin E deficiency characterized by areflexia and hemolytic anemia. Children with abetalipoproteinemia cannot absorb or transport vitamin E and become deficient quite rapidly. A familial form of isolated vitamin E deficiency also exists, which is due to a defect in the α tocopherol transport protein. Vitamin E deficiency causes axonal degeneration of the large myelinated axons and results in posterior column and spinocerebellar symptoms. Peripheral neuropathy is initially characterized by areflexia, with progression to an ataxic gait, and by decreased vibration and position sensations. Ophthalmoplegia, skeletal myopathy, and pigmented retinopathy may also be features of vitamin E deficiency. The laboratory diagnosis of vitamin E deficiency is made on the basis of low blood levels of α tocopherol (<5 μg/mL, or <0.8 mg of α tocopherol per gram of total lipids).

℞ TREATMENT Symptomatic vitamin E deficiency should be treated with 800 to 1200 mg of α tocopherol per day. Patients with abetalipoproteinemia may need as much as 5000 to 7000 mg/d. Children with symptomatic vitamin E deficiency should be treated with 400 mg/d orally of water-soluble esters; alternatively, 2 mg/kg per day may be administered intramuscularly. Vitamin E in high doses may protect against oxygen-induced retrolental fibroplasia and bronchopulmonary dysplasia in prematurity, as well as intraventricular hemorrhage of prematurity. Vitamin E has been suggested to increase sexual performance, to treat intermittent claudication, and to slow the aging process, but evidence for these properties is lacking. High doses (60 to 800 mg/d) of vitamin E have been shown in controlled trials to improve parameters of immune function, and there are two intervention studies showing that vitamin E at 400 to 800 mg/d may be protective against cardiovascular disease, possibly by inhibiting LDL oxidation. Also, supplemental intake of vitamin E (100 to 200 mg/d) has been associated with a decreased risk of cataracts.

Toxicity High doses of vitamin E (>800 mg/d) may reduce platelet aggregation and interfere with vitamin K metabolism and are therefore contraindicated in patients taking coumadin. Nausea, flatulence, and diarrhea have been reported at doses >1 g/d.

VITAMIN K There are two natural forms of vitamin K: vitamin K I, also known as *phylloquinone*, from vegetable and animal sources, and vitamin K II, or *menaquinone*, which is synthesized by bacterial flora and found in hepatic tissue. *Menadione*, or vitamin K III, is a chemically synthesized pro-vitamin that can be converted to menaquinone by the liver. Phylloquinone and menaquinones differ only in their lipophilic sidechains, and both are destroyed in an alkaline pH and by ultraviolet light.

Absorption and Physiology As with other fat-soluble vitamins, vitamin K absorption is dependent on normal pancreatic function and the presence of bile salts. Phylloquinones are absorbed by a saturable energy-dependent mechanism in the proximal small intestine, whereas menaquinones are absorbed by passive diffusion in the small intestine and colon. Approximately 100 μg of vitamin K is stored in the liver as well as in lung, bone marrow, kidneys, and adrenal glands. Most vitamin K circulates bound to VLDL, although it is also carried by LDL and high-density lipoprotein (HDL). The half-life of vitamin K is only 1½ days, despite the presence of a vitamin K regeneration cycle.

Vitamin K is necessary for the posttranslational carboxylation of glutamic acid, which is necessary for calcium binding to γ-carboxylated proteins such as prothrombin (factor II); factors VII, IX, and X; protein C; protein S; and proteins found in bone (bone gla, matrix gla protein, and osteocalcin). The importance of vitamin K for bone mineralization is not known. Warfarin-type drugs inhibit γ carboxylation by preventing the conversion of vitamin K to its active hydroquinone form. Vitamin E, at high doses, may act as a vitamin K antagonist.

Dietary Sources Vitamin K is found in green leafy vegetables such as kale and spinach, but appreciable amounts are also present in butter, margarine, liver, milk, ground beef, coffee, and pears. Vitamin K is present in vegetable oils and is particularly rich in olive oil and soybean oil. The recommended intake of vitamin K is 70 μg/d in adults. The average daily intake by Americans is estimated to be approximately 100 μg/d.

Deficiency The symptoms of vitamin K deficiency are due to hemorrhage, and newborns are particularly susceptible because of low fat stores, low breast milk levels of vitamin K, sterility of the infantile intestinal tract, liver immaturity, and poor placental transport. Intracranial bleeding, as well as gastrointestinal and skin bleeding, can be seen in vitamin K–deficient infants 1 to 7 days after birth. Thus, vitamin K (1 mg intramuscularly) is given prophylactically at the time of delivery.

Vitamin K deficiency in adults may be seen in patients with chronic small-intestinal disease (e.g., celiac disease, Crohn's disease), obstructed biliary tracts, or after small-bowel resection. Broad-spectrum antibiotic treatment can precipitate vitamin K deficiency by reducing gut bacteria, which synthesize menaquinones, as well as by inhibiting the metabolism of vitamin K. The diagnosis of vitamin K deficiency is usually made on the basis of an elevated prothrombin time or reduced clotting factors. Vitamin K may also be measured directly by HPLC. In addition, undercarboxylated prothrombin and low gla levels in urine are indicative of vitamin K deficiency. Vitamin K deficiency is treated using a parenteral dose of 10 mg. For patients with chronic malabsorption, 1 to 2 mg/d of vitamin K may be given orally, or 1 to 2 mg/week can be taken parenterally. Patients with liver disease may have an elevated prothrombin time because of liver cell destruction as well as vitamin K deficiency. If an elevated prothrombin time does not improve on vitamin K therapy, it can be assumed that it is not the result of vitamin K deficiency.

Toxicity Parenteral doses of the water-soluble vitamin K derivative (menadione) have been reported to cause hemolytic anemia and hypobilirubinemia in infants. Toxicity from dietary phylloquinones and menaquinones has not been described. High doses of vitamin K can impair the actions of oral anticoagulants.

TRACE MINERALS (See Table 75-1)

ZINC Zinc is an integral component of many metalloenzymes in the body; it is involved in the synthesis and stabilization of proteins,

Table 75-1 Deficiencies and Toxicities of Metals

Element	Deficiency	Toxicity

Zinc	Growth retardation, ↓ taste and smell, alopecia, dermatitis, diarrhea, immunologic dysfunction, failure to thrive, gonadal atrophy, impaired spermatogenesis, congenital malformations	General
		  Gastritis, sweating, fever, nausea, vomiting
		Occupational
		  Respiratory distress, pulmonary fibrosis

Copper	Anemia, growth retardation, defective keratinization and pigmentation of hair, hypothermia, degenerative changes in aortic elastin, osteopenia, mental deterioration, scurvy-like changes in skeleton	General Nausea, vomiting, diarrhea, hepatic failure, tremor, mental deterioration, hemolytic anemia, renal dysfunction

Selenium	Cardiomyopathy, congestive heart failure, striated muscle degeneration	General
		  Alopecia, nausea, vomiting, abnormal nails, emotional lability, peripheral neuropathy, lassitude, garlic odor to breath, dermatitis
		Occupational
		  Lung and nasal carcinomas, liver necrosis, pulmonary inflammation

Chromium	Impaired glucose tolerance	Occupational Renal failure, dermatitis, pulmonary cancer
Manganese	Bone demineralization, ataxia, convulsions, anemia	Occupational Encephalitis-like syndrome, Parkinson-like syndrome, psychosis, pneumoconiosis

DNA, and RNA and plays a structural role in ribosomes and membranes. Zinc is necessary for the binding of steroid hormone receptors and several other transcription factors to DNA and thereby plays an important role in the regulation of gene transcription. Zinc is absolutely required for normal spermatogenesis, fetal growth, and embryonic development.

Absorption and Physiology Zinc is absorbed in the small intestine by a carrier-mediated mechanism. The absorption of zinc from the diet is inhibited by dietary phytate, fiber, oxalate, iron, and copper, as well as by certain drugs including penicillamine, sodium valproate, and ethambutol. The RDA for zinc is 15 mg in males and 12 mg in females, with an additional 3 mg in pregnancy and 4 to 7 mg during lactation. Supplemental zinc is recommended for women taking ≥60 mg/d of iron during pregnancy.

Meat, shellfish, nuts, and legumes are good sources of bioavailable zinc, whereas zinc in grains is less available for absorption. Zinc is excreted mainly in the feces but also in urine and sweat. The body contains approximately 2 g of zinc, and high concentrations are found in liver, prostate, pancreas, bone, and brain (hippocampus and cerebral cortex), where the metal may function in neural transmission.

Deficiency Mild zinc deficiency has been described in many diseases including diabetes mellitus, AIDS, cirrhosis, alcoholism, inflammatory bowel disease, malabsorption syndromes, and sickle cell anemia. In these diseases, mild chronic zinc deficiency can cause stunted growth in children, decreased taste sensation (hypogusia), impaired immune function, and night blindness due to impaired conversion of

retinol to retinaldehyde. Severe chronic zinc deficiency has been described as a cause of hypogonadism and dwarfism in several Middle Eastern countries. In these children, hypopigmented hair is also part of the syndrome. Acrodermatitis enteropathica is a rare autosomal recessive disorder characterized by abnormalities in zinc absorption. Clinical manifestations include diarrhea, alopecia, muscle wasting, depression, irritability, and a rash involving the extremities, face, and perineum. The rash is characterized by vesicular and pustular crusting with scaling and erythema. In addition, hypopigmentation and corneal edema have been described in these patients. Occasional patients with Wilson's disease have developed zinc deficiency as a consequence of penicillamine therapy. Patients on long-term parenteral nutrition have developed deficiency when zinc has been omitted from the total parenteral nutrition (TPN) solution.

The diagnosis of zinc deficiency is usually made by a serum zinc level of <12 μmol/L (<70 μg/dL). Pregnancy and birth control pills may cause a slight depression in serum zinc levels, and hypoalbuminemia from any cause can result in hypozincemia. In acute stress situations, zinc may be redistributed from serum into tissues. Zinc deficiency may be treated with 60 mg elemental zinc, given orally twice a day. Zinc gluconate lozenges (13 mg elemental Zn every 2 h while awake) have been reported to reduce the duration and symptoms of the common cold in adults, but these studies are conflicting.

Toxicity Acute zinc toxicity after oral ingestion causes nausea and vomiting, fever, and respiratory distress. Zinc fumes from welding may also be toxic and cause fever, chills, excessive salivation, sweating, and headache. Chronic large doses of zinc may depress immune function and cause hypochromic anemia as a result of copper deficiency.

COPPER Copper is an integral part of numerous enzyme systems including amine oxidases, ferrooxidase (ceruloplasmin), cytochrome-c oxidase, superoxide dismutase, and dopamine hydroxylase. As such, copper plays a role in iron metabolism, melanin synthesis, and central nervous system function; the synthesis and cross-linking of elastin and collagen; and the scavenging of superoxide radicals.

Copper is absorbed in the proximal small intestine, and 90% of circulating copper is bound to ceruloplasmin. The body contains 50 to 120 mg of copper, and high concentrations are found in liver, brain, heart, spleen, kidney, and blood. The U.S. RDA is 1.5 to 3 mg of copper intake per day, although World Health Organization recommendations are somewhat lower. Dietary sources of copper include shellfish, liver, nuts, legumes, bran, and organ meats, whereas milk is a very poor source. Copper is primarily excreted in the feces, and small amounts are also excreted in urine.

Deficiency Dietary copper deficiency is relatively rare, although it has been described in premature infants fed milk diets and in infants with malabsorption. Signs and symptoms of copper deficiency include a hypochromic-normocytic anemia, osteopenia, depigmentation, mental retardation, and psychomotor abnormalities. Copper deficiency anemia has been reported in patients with malabsorptive diseases and nephrotic syndrome and in patients treated for Wilson's disease with chronic high doses of oral zinc, which can interfere with copper absorption. Menkes kinky hair syndrome is an X-linked metabolic disturbance of copper metabolism characterized by mental retardation, hypocupremia, and decreased circulating ceruloplasmin (Chap. 351). It is caused by mutations in a copper-transporting ATP7A gene. Children with this disease often die within 5 years due to dissecting aneurysms or cardiac rupture.

The diagnosis of copper deficiency is usually made on the basis of low serum levels of copper (<65 μg/dL) and low ceruloplasmin levels (<18 mg/dL). Serum levels of copper may be elevated in pregnancy or stress conditions since ceruloplasmin is an acute-phase reactant.

Toxicity Toxicity due to copper is usually accidental and may include nausea, vomiting, diarrhea, and hemolytic anemia. In severe cases, kidney failure, liver failure, and coma may ensue. In Wilson's disease, mutations in the copper-transporting ATP7B gene lead to accumulation of copper in the liver and brain, with low blood levels due to decreased ceruloplasmin (Chap. 348). Indian childhood cirrhosis is another hereditary disease characterized by extremely high copper levels in the liver. The World Health Organization recommends that adult females should not ingest >10 mg/d and males should not take in >12 mg/d of copper.

SELENIUM Selenium, in the form of selenocysteine, is a component of the enzyme glutathione peroxidase, which serves to protect proteins, cell membranes, lipids, and nucleic acids from oxidant molecules. Selenocysteine is also found in the deiodinase enzymes, which mediate the deiodination of thyroxine to the more active triiodothyronine (Chap. 330). Rich sources of selenium include seafood, muscle meat, and cereals, although the selenium content of cereal is determined by the soil concentration. Countries with low soil concentrations include parts of Scandinavia, China, and New Zealand. *Keshan disease* is an endemic cardiomyopathy found in children and young women residing in regions of China where dietary intake of selenium is low (<20 μg/d). Concomitant deficiencies of iodine and selenium may worsen the clinical manifestations of cretinism. The adult RDAs for selenium in the United States are 55 and 70 μg/d for females and males, respectively. Low blood levels of selenium in various populations have been correlated with an increase in coronary artery disease and certain cancers, although the data are not consistent. Selenosis occurs at intakes of ≥400 μg/d and can result in nausea, vomiting, loss of hair, nail changes, peripheral neuropathy, and fatigue.

CHROMIUM Chromium potentiates the action of insulin in patients with impaired glucose tolerance, presumably by increasing insulin receptor–mediated signaling. In addition, in some patients, improvement in blood lipid profiles has been reported. The usefulness of chromium supplements in muscle building are not substantiated. Rich food sources of chromium include yeast, meat, and grain products. Chromium deficiency has been reported to cause glucose intolerance, peripheral neuropathy, and confusion. The suggested intake of chromium for adults is 50 to 200 μg/d. Chromium in the trivalent state is found in supplements and is largely nontoxic; however, chromium-6 is a product of stainless steel welding and is a known pulmonary carcinogen, as well as causing liver, kidney, and central nervous system.

MAGNESIUM See Chap. 340

FLUORIDE, MANGANESE, AND ULTRATRACE ELEMENTS An essential function for *fluoride* in humans has not been described, although it is useful for the maintenance of structure in teeth and bone. An adequate intake for fluoride (on the basis of protection against dental caries) has been set at 3.1 and 3.8 mg/d in adult females and males, respectively. Adult fluorosis can occur at an intake of 10 mg/d for prolonged periods and results in mottled and pitted defects in tooth enamel as well as brittle bone (skeletal fluorosis). Much lower doses of fluoride (0.7 to 2 mg) can cause dental fluorosis or mottled enamel in infants and children.

Manganese and molybdenum deficiencies have been reported in patients with rare genetic abnormalities as well as in a few patients receiving prolonged TPN. Several manganese-specific enzymes have been identified (e.g., manganese superoxide dismutase). The estimated adequate daily dietary *manganese* intake for adults is 2 to 3 mg/d. Deficiencies of manganese have been reported to result in bone demineralization, poor growth, ataxia, and convulsions.

Ultratrace elements are those for which the need is <1 mg/d. Essentiality has not been established for most ultratrace elements, although *iodine* is clearly essential (Chap. 330). *Molybenum* is necessary for the activity of sulfite and xanthine oxidase, and molybdenum deficiency may result in skeletal and brain lesions. The minimum required daily molybdenum intake is estimated to be ~25 μg/d. There is circumstantial evidence to suggest that *arsenic* (impaired growth, infertility), *boron* (impaired energy metabolism, impaired brain function), *nickel* (impaired-growth and reproduction), *silicon* (impaired growth) and *vanadium* (impaired skeletal formation) might also be essential.

BIBLIOGRAPHY

THIAMINE

FLEMING JC et al: The gene mutated in thiamine-responsive anaemia with diabetes and deafness (TRMA) encodes a functional thiamine transporter. Nat Genet 22:305, 1999

SHIMON I et al: Improved left ventricular function after thiamine supplementation in patients with congestive heart failure receiving long-term furosemide therapy. Am J Med 98:485, 1995

WILKINSON TJ et al: The response to treatment of subclinical thiamine deficiency in the elderly. Am J Clin Nutr 66:925, 1997

RIBOFLAVIN

SOARES MJ et al: The effect of exercise on the riboflavin status of older men. Br J Nutr 69:541, 1993

ZEMPLENI J, GALLOWAY JR: Pharmacokinetics of orally and intravenously administered riboflavin in healthy humans. Am J Clin Nutr 63:54, 1996

NIACIN

GIBBONS LW et al: The prevalence of side effects with regular and sustained-release nicotinic acid. Am J Med 99:378, 1995

STERN RH et al: Pharmacodynamics and drug action: Tolerance to nicotinic acid flushing. Clin Pharmacol Ther 50:66, 1991

VITAMIN B₆

RIBAYA-MERCADO JD et al: Vitamin B-6 requirements of elderly men and women. J Nutr 121:1062, 1991

RIMM EB et al: Folate and vitamin B₆ from diet and supplements in relation to risk of coronary heart disease among women. JAMA 279:359, 1998

ROBINSON K et al: Hyperhomocysteinemia and low pyridoxal phosphate. Common and independent reversible risk factors for coronary artery disease. Circulation 92:2825, 1995

VITAMIN C

CARR AC, FREI B: Toward a new recommended dietary allowance for vitamin C based on antioxidant and health effect in humans. Am J Clin Nutr 69:1086, 1999

HEMILA H: Vitamin C intake and susceptibility to the common cold. Br J Nutr 77:59, 1997

WEBB PM et al: Gastric cancer, gastritis and plasma vitamin C: Results from an international correlation and cross-sectional study. Int J Cancer 73:684, 1997

VITAMIN A

OMENN GS et al: Effects of a combination of beta-carotene and vitamin A on lung cancer and cardiovascular disease. N Engl J Med 334:1150, 1996

RUSSELL RM et al: Hepatic injury from chronic hypervitaminosis A resulting in portal hypertension and ascites. N Engl J Med 291:435, 1974

TYSON JE et al: Vitamin A supplementation for extremely low birth weight infants. N Engl J Med 340:1962, 1999

VITAMIN E

HARDING AE et al: Spinocerebellar degeneration associated with a selective defect of vitamin E absorption. N Engl J Med 313:32, 1985

HEART OUTCOMES PREVENTION EVALUATION STUDY INVESTIGATORS: Vitamin E supplementation and cardiovascular events in high-risk patients. N Engl J Med 342:154, 2000

SANO M et al: A controlled trial of selegiline, alpha-tocopherol, or both as treatment for Alzheimer's disease. N Engl J Med 336:1216, 1997

VITAMIN K

DOWD P et al: The mechanism of action of vitamin K. Annu Rev Nutr 15:419, 1995

FESKANICH D et al: Vitamin K intake and hip fractures in women: A prospective study. Am J Clin Nutr 69:74, 1999

METALS

ANDERSON RA et al: Elevated intakes of supplemental chromium improve glucose and insulin variables in individuals with type 2 diabetes. Diabetes 46:1786, 1997

CLARK LC et al: Effects of selenium supplementation for cancer prevention in patients with carcinoma of the skin. A randomized controlled trial. JAMA 276:1957, 1996

MOSSAD SB, MACKNIN ML: Zinc gluconate lozenges for treating the common cold. A randomized, double-blind, placebo-controlled study. Ann Intern Med 125:81, 1996

ZINC INVESTIGATORS' COLLABORATIVE GROUP: BHJUTTA ZA et al: Prevention of diarrhea and pneumonia by zinc supplementation in children in developing countries: Pooled analysis of randomized controlled trials. J Pediatr 135:689, 1999

Lyn Howard

ENTERAL AND PARENTERAL NUTRITION THERAPY

Parenteral and enteral nutrition provide life-sustaining therapy for patients who cannot take adequate food by mouth and who consequently are at risk for malnutrition and its effects, including susceptibility to infection, weakness and immobility; these features predispose the patient to aspiration pneumonia, pulmonary embolism, and pressure sores, all of which delay recovery from illness and increase mortality.

The term *enteral* refers to feeding via the gut and hence includes normal eating, but in the present context implies the infusion of formulas via a tube into the upper gastrointestinal tract. *Parenteral* refers to the infusion of nutrient solutions into the bloodstream. While these are different approaches to nutritional support, their goals are the same. Where feasible, enteral nutrition is the preferred route because it sustains the digestive, absorptive, and immunologic barrier functions of the gastrointestinal tract. The cost of enteral tube feeding is about one-tenth the cost of parenteral feeding.

Several developments have made tube feeding easier and more acceptable to patients. Small-bore pliable tubes have largely replaced large-bore rubber tubes, and double-lumen tubes are now available for simultaneous gastric suction and jejunal feeding when there is concern about gastric retention and aspiration. Enteral tubes can be inserted into the stomach or jejunum through the nose or, for long-term use, directly through the abdominal wall, using endoscopic, radiologic, or surgical techniques. Once the enterocutaneous tract is established, the protruding tube can be replaced by a "button" entry port, flush with the abdominal wall.

Complete nutrition by vein with sufficient calories, amino acids, minerals, and vitamins to permit wound healing, restoration of normal body composition of a cachectic patient, or growth in children became feasible in the 1960s with the development of high-flow central vein catheters. Parental nutrition is now available in all large hospitals and for some patients at home. Adequate calories and other nutrients can be delivered in the form of high-energy, isotonic intravenous fat solutions via a peripheral vein. However, peripheral veins usually cannot sustain such infusions indefinitely, and long-term support requires central venous access.

THE DECISION PROCESS FOR USING PARENTERAL OR ENTERAL NUTRITION   The decision to use specialized nutrition support should be based on the likelihood that averting or redressing malnutrition will improve the quality of life or the ability to recover from a serious illness.

Approximately 15 to 20% of hospitalized patients have evidence of malnutrition. Some malnourished patients benefit from specialized nutrition support; for others, wasting is an inevitable component of a terminal disease. Selecting the appropriate form of nutritional support for the patient requires knowledge of the potential benefits and risks of nutritional support, and the physician must inform the patient and family of these issues. A flow diagram of the steps involved in deciding whether specialized nutrition support should be undertaken and, if so, how, is depicted in Fig. 76-1. Like all life-support measures, these therapies are difficult to withdraw once started.

The first step requires consideration of the nutritional implications of the disease process. Is the condition or its treatment likely to impair appetite or food ingestion and absorption for a prolonged period of time? Because prevention of malnutrition is easier than repleting a cachectic patient, this issue must be considered in the initial evaluation (Chap. 74). The second step is to determine whether the patient is already sufficiently malnourished that lean body mass is decreased and critical functions such as healing and ventilation are impaired. The presence or absence of metabolic stress should be noted, since injury

or infection can evoke the secretion of hormonal and cytokine factors that reduce the efficiency of nutrition repletion.

Weight loss without physiologic impairment is probably of no consequence. Physiologic impairment usually develops when more than 20% of body protein is lost and is more likely if key organ systems, such as the gut or liver, are directly affected by disease. Once it is recognized that the patient is malnourished or at major risk, the next question is whether specialized nutritional support will impact positively on the patient's response to the disease, improving the quality of life. While the provision of food and water is part of basic medical care, nutrition support by enteral or parenteral means is associated with risk and discomfort and should be recommended only when potential benefit exceeds risk and undertaken only with the consent of the patient.

If it is decided that preventing or treating malnutrition with specialized nutrition support would improve the prognosis and quality of life, the nutritional requirements must be determined and the route of nutrient delivery must be selected.

RISKS AND BENEFITS OF NUTRITION SUPPORT   The risks are determined primarily by the route required to deliver nutrition support. Providing nutritional requirements by special attention to oral intake of food, or by adding oral liquid supplements and monitoring food intake with frequent calorie counts, is the safest and least costly approach. It is also the most metabolically efficient since normal eating initiates the cephalic phase of digestion. Tube-fed infants grow better if the cephalic phase is stimulated by having the infant suck on a pacifier.

Anorexia, impairment of swallowing, or bowel disease may limit oral intake or the absorption of oral nutrients, in which case tube enteral nutrition is the next consideration. The bowel and its associated digestive organs derive 70% of their required nutrients directly from food in the lumen. In addition, glutamine, short-chain fatty acids, and nucleotides may have particular importance in maintaining gut integrity. Enteral feeding also supports gut function by stimulating splanchnic blood flow, neuronal activity, IgA antibody release, and secretion of gastrointestinal hormones such as epidermal growth factor that stimulate gut trophic activity. All these factors support the gut as an immunologic barrier against enteric pathogens, reducing the likelihood of bacterial overgrowth. For these reasons, some enteral nutrition should always be provided if possible, even when parenteral nutrition is required to provide most of the support. In the past, bowel rest through parenteral nutrition was thought to be the cornerstone of treatment of many severe gastrointestinal disorders, but the value of some enteral nutrition is now widely accepted, and strict bowel rest is rarely appropriate. Parenteral nutrition alone is necessary in severe hemorrhagic pancreatitis, necrotizing enterocolitis, prolonged ileus, and distal bowel obstruction.

Specialized nutrition support is expensive, accounting for >1% of all health care dollars. Consequently, hard clinical endpoints such as mortality rate, incidence of major complications, and duration of hospital stay are required of risk-benefit studies. Better nitrogen balance, increased levels of serum albumin, and improved delayed hypersensitivity are softer endpoints. Table 76-1 summarizes clinical trials that evaluate the use of specialized nutrition support in different disease states.

Perioperative Nutrition   There is a clear-cut association between preoperative malnutrition and poor surgical outcome, but it has been difficult to demonstrate the benefit of preoperative parenteral nutrition on the outcome of surgery in malnourished patients. However, a meta-analysis of several small studies and a large cooperative Veterans Administration study indicates that preoperative parenteral nutrition does improve the outcome of severely malnourished surgical patients. In treated patients, noninfectious complications (e.g., pulmonary emboli and delayed wound healing) are reduced in the postoperative period. Effective preoperative restoration of nutrition by the parenteral route requires at least 7 to 14 days. If feasible, a safer and less costly approach is preoperative enteral nutrition, especially if provided at home.

Immediate postoperative nutritional support is appropriate for patients who received preoperative support and for patients unlikely to resume oral feeding within 10 days. The parenteral route is commonly used because of postoperative ileus or concern about disrupting a new bowel anastomosis. However, cautious jejunal feeding is often tolerated. Specialized enteral formulas supplemented with conditionally essential nutrients may be particularly beneficial in debilitated and immunosuppressed postoperative patients (Table 76-2).

Critical Illness Very early nutrition support (within the first 48 h) improves survival and reduces infections and length of hospital stay in patients with severe head injuries, burns, and major abdominal trauma. Enteral therapy, where feasible, is superior to parenteral therapy in several randomized trials. Enteral nutrition equally benefits malnourished and well-nourished injured patients. Animal studies show that enteral feeding reduces translocation of gut bacteria and the systemic catabolic response; however, these phenomena have not been substantiated in humans. Early enteral feeding may prevent bacterial overgrowth and decrease aspiration pneumonia.

The practical issue is obtaining jejunal access in a critically ill patient, who is not easily transferred out of the intensive care unit for endoscopic or radiologic tube placement. Sometimes a nasal or percutaneous combined gastric suction and jejunal feeding tube can be inserted at the bedside. If a surgical laparotomy is indicated, a feeding tube can be placed simultaneously.

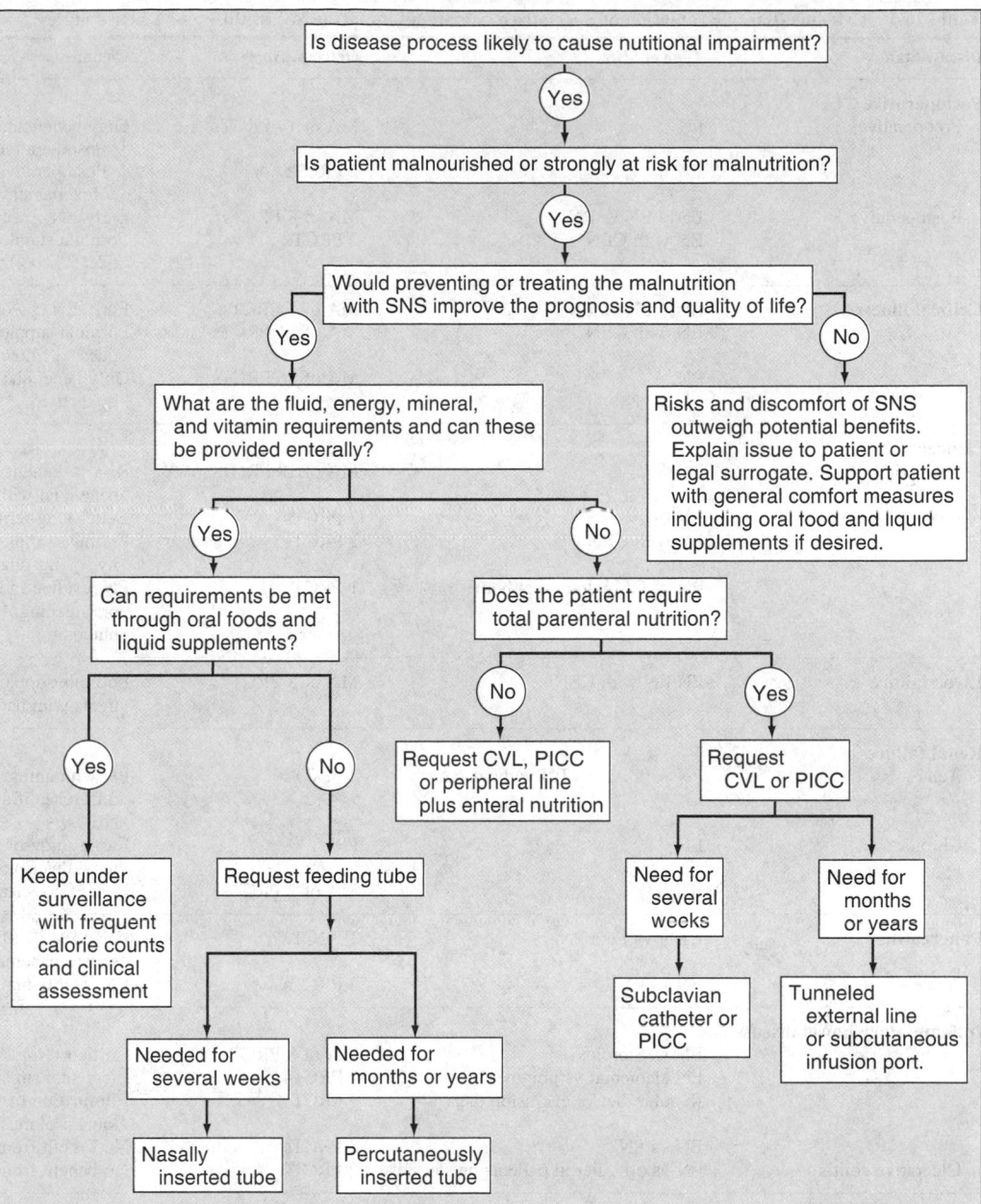

FIGURE 76-1 Should specialized nutrition support (SNS) be undertaken and if so, how? An algorithm. (PICC, peripherally inserted, central catheter; CVL, central venous line.)

Most studies of enteral feeding in critically ill patients used either a general polymeric formula or one with hydrolyzed protein. Formulas supplemented with conditionally essential nutrients reduce infections and length of hospital stay. Parenteral formulas enriched with large amounts of branched-chain amino acids (BCAA) improve nitrogen balance but do not appear to affect clinical outcome.

Cancer Cachexia Early nonrandomized studies suggested that patients with cancer cachexia benefitted from parenteral nutrition, but randomized trials demonstrated more risk than benefit for patients receiving chemotherapy or radiation. Severely malnourished cancer patients undergoing surgery benefit from preoperative parenteral nutrition, as do other malnourished patients.

In two randomized, prospective trials, patients undergoing bone marrow transplantation had better long-term survival after parenteral or enteral nutrition in the cytoreduction phase; nutrition support did not influence the initial infection rate or the frequency of graft rejection or graft-versus-host disease. Immediate morbidity is reduced if glutamine supplements are added to the parenteral nutrition solution. Parenteral nutrition continued at home delays return to oral feeding. For cancer patients with unresectable upper gastrointestinal cancer, enteral feeding is usually justified if it is desired by the patient and family. Parenteral feeding should be provided only if clinical improvement can be expected and when quality survival at home for several months is predicted.

Liver Failure Malnutrition is common in advanced liver disease. Patients with acute or chronic liver failure have decreased levels of BCAA and elevated levels of aromatic amino acids (AAA) in plasma and cerebrospinal fluid. Randomized, prospective trials with parenteral and enteral formulas high in BCAA and low in AAA have demonstrated better nitrogen balance and less risk of encephalopathy. One large multicenter study also reported improved survival. The BCAA-enriched formulas are expensive and should be used only in patients who have encephalopathy or who develop encephalopathy when fed a standard protein formula providing 0.8 g protein/kg per day.

Renal Failure Since renal failure is associated with impaired nitrogen excretion, it is rational to assume that protein restriction might

Table 76-1   Evidence-Based Evaluation of Specialized Nutrition Support (SNS) in Different Disease States[a]

Disease State	Type of SNS	Outcome Analysis	Comments
Perioperative			
Preoperative	PN	MA of 14 PRCTs	Only beneficial in severe PCM
			↓ Postoperative complications by 10%
	EN	2 PRCTs	↓ Postoperative complications by 25%;
			↓ Hospital stay
Postoperative	Early EN vs PN	MA of 8 PRCTs	Early EN ↓ septic complications
	EN with CEN	3 PRCTs	Formula supplemented with arginine, W3 FA nucleotides; ↓ postoperative complications, ↓ hospital stay
Critical illness	Early EN vs PN	MA of 8 PRCTs	Early EN ↓ septic complications
	EN with CEN	MA of 11 PRCTs	Formula supplemented with arginine, W3 FA nucleotides: ↓ infections, ↓ hospital stay
	PN	MA of 26 PRCTs	Only beneficial in severe PCM; ↓ Complications if no lipids used
Cancer			
Cachexia	PN	MA of 18 PRCTs	Risk > benefit in patients undergoing CXT or RXT, but beneficial with cancer surgery in severe PCM
BMT	PN/EN	2 PRCTs	Better long-term survival
	PN with CEN	2 PRCTs	Formula supplemented with glutamine: ↓ early mortality, ↓ hospital stay
	PN vs IV hydration at home	1 PRCT	PN resulted in less weight loss but delayed return to oral feeding. IV hydration did not result in adverse outcome
Liver failure	PN/EN with CEN	MA of 8 PRCTs	Formula supplemented with BCAA beneficial in patients with hepatic encephalopathy
Renal failure			
Acute	PN with AA vs PN without AA	2 PRCTs	PN with amino acids ↓ infectious complications. No difference if amino acids just EAA or both EAA and NEAA
Chronic	EN	PRCT	Large study of reduced protein diet did not slow rate of renal deterioration
	IDPN	MA of 2 PRCTs	Benefit not clearly established
Pancreatitis	Early vs Late PN	1 PRCT	Early PN ↓ MR and infectious complications if used in severe pancreatitis
Acute	EN vs PN	2 PRCTs	EN ↓ inflammatory response, ↓ sepsis
Inflammatory bowel disease			
Crohn's	EN vs Steroids	MA of 8 PRCTs	Corticosteroids superior to EN
	EN elemental vs polymeric	2 PRCTs	Elemental superior to polymeric
	Regular diet vs exclusion diets	1 PRCT	Elimination of foods that induce gastrointestinal symptoms prolongs remission
	EN vs PN	2 PRCTs	No benefit from bowel rest
Ulcerative colitis	PN vs oral diet in patients on steroids	2 PRCTs	No benefit from bowel rest
Short bowel syndrome	EN and CEN	PRCT, crossover design	IV HGH and oral glutamine supplements did not improve bowel function in long-term HPN patients
Pulmonary disease			
Acute, ventilated	PN and EN	2 PRCTs	↓ Glucose and ↑ fat-aided weaning process
	EN: continuous vs intermittent	1 PRCT	No difference in gastric bacterial colonization
Chronic	EN: gastric vs jejunal delivery	1 PRCT	Jejunal feeding resulted in better intake and lower incidence of pneumonia
	EN: gastric vs postpyloric delivery	1 PRCT	Equal incidence of aspiration pneumonia unless tube at Ligament of Treitz or beyond
HIV disease	PN vs EN	PRCT	PN induced greater gain of weight, fat, and H₂O, but gain in body cell mass was similar, EN led to better physical functioning
	PN vs dietary counseling	PRCT	Two months of home PN improved body composition and Karnofsky index but did not change survival
			Patients who then continued PN had longer survival: median survival on PN 199 days, with dietary counseling 57 days

[a] Only those disease states where SNS treatment has been evaluated by meta-analysis and/or prospective randomized controlled trials.

NOTE: SNS, specialized nutrition support; PN, parenteral nutrition; MA, meta-analysis; PRCT, prospective randomized control trial; PCM, protein calorie malnutrition; Early EN, tube feeding started within 48 h of onset of acute condition; EN, tube feeding; CEN, conditionally essential nutrients; W3FA, omega 3 fatty acids; CXT, chemotherapy; RXT, radiation therapy; BMT, bone marrow transplant; BCAA, branch chain amino acids; EAA, essential amino acids; NEAA, nonessential amino acids; IDPN, intradialytic parenteral nutrition; hGH, human growth hormone; HPN, home parenteral nutrition.

Table 76-2 Conditionally Essential Nutrients

Nutrient	Metabolic Function
Glutamine	Fuel for enterocyte and immunocytes; preserves hepatic glutathione
Nucleotides	Derivatives (cyclicAMP, cyclicGMP) serve as mediators for many metabolic processes
Arginine	Enhances lymphocyte cytotoxicity via nitric oxide; substrate for polyamine synthesis; promotes protein synthesis via release of human growth hormone
Branched-chain amino acids	Level in muscle regulates muscle-protein breakdown; decreased in catabolic patients, especially those with liver disease
Sulfur-containing amino acids methionine ↓ S-adenosyl methionine (SAM) ↓ Homocysteine ↓ cysteine→glutathione taurine carnitine	Glutathione, chief cytoplasmic free radical scavenger; taurine, conjugates bile salts; carnitine, transports fatty acids into mitochondria for β-oxidation; SAM donates methyl group to choline and creatine, normalizes cell wall fluidity
Short-chain fatty acids	Derived by bacterial breakdown, from soluble fibers such as pectin; fuel for enterocytes, particularly colonocytes
Omega-3 fatty acids	Promote production of prostaglandins (PG) and leukotrienes (LT) of N-3 series (PGE$_3$, LTB$_5$, etc.) and reduce production from N-6 series (PGE$_2$, LTB$_4$, etc.), which are proinflammatory

benefit patients with both acute and chronic renal failure. Patients with acute renal failure given parenteral calories and amino acids have fewer infectious complications and a better chance of leaving the hospital than similar patients given only calories. An early randomized study showed benefit when essential amino acids were the sole source of nitrogen, but in other studies, standard solutions supplying both essential and nonessential amino acids provide similar advantage. Thus, the benefit of using expensive formulas containing only essential amino acids or their keto analogues is not established. A large national study failed to show any benefit of a low-protein diet on slowing progression of renal impairment in patients on chronic dialysis. Some 15 to 20% of patients on chronic dialysis have significant nutritional impairment, usually due to profound anorexia. The anorexia may improve with stepped-up dialysis or treatment of gastritis but usually persists. The resulting growth impairment in younger patients has been treated with supplemental tube enteral nutrition. This approach has not been widely used in adult patients. Limited parenteral calories and amino acids can be provided in the last 90 min of hemodialysis treatment (intradialytic parenteral nutrition). This may improve appetite, serum protein levels, and body weight. No randomized studies have documented better survival, so the appropriateness of this regimen is not established. Standard dialysis uses glucose to provide an osmotic load, and some glucose calories are absorbed. During continuous ambulatory peritoneal dialysis, amino acids can be substituted for glucose and are also partly absorbed, offsetting the loss of endogenous amino acids into the dialysate. This approach to nutrition repletion is expensive and also awaits a randomized study.

Pancreatitis Parenteral nutrition does not improve the outcome of patients with mild or moderate pancreatitis. However, in severe pancreatitis, survival decreases as malnutrition becomes more severe. When parenteral nutrition support was delayed beyond 72 h, patients with severe pancreatitis had a threefold higher complication and mortality rate, compared to similar patients treated earlier. In the absence of severe hyperlipidemia or thrombocytopenia, intravenous lipids appear safe and are especially useful if glucose intolerance is present.

Several studies report successful enteral jejunal feeding in acute pancreatitis and, compared to parenteral nutrition, the inflammatory response and infectious complications are less.

Inflammatory Bowel Disease Evidence of nutritional deficiencies such as weight loss, growth failure, anemia, and hypoalbuminenia are common in inflammatory bowel disease (IBD), more so in Crohn's disease than in ulcerative colitis (Chap. 287). Nutrition support plays a role in correcting these nutritional deficiencies, particularly prior to elective surgery. Since IBD often improves with diversion of the fecal stream, the question is whether bowel rest and parenteral nutrition have a role as primary treatment. However, randomized, prospective studies have shown no special benefit from bowel rest. Elemental diets are not quite as effective as glucocorticoids for inducing remission in acute Crohn's disease but may be preferable in children to avoid growth impairment. Relapse is common when a regular diet is resumed. In controlled studies, remissions are prolonged if the Crohn's patient does not return to a regular diet but instead eliminates from the diet those foods that induce gastrointestinal symptoms. For the majority of Crohn's patients this leads to avoidance of cereals, yeast, green vegetables, and, early on, dairy products. Because of the possibility that diets high in omega-3 fatty acids have a beneficial effect in immune disorders by altering prostaglandin synthesis, their value in IBD is under investigation. Some studies suggest that high-fiber diets benefit IBD patients, but fiber can also cause obstruction in patients with bowel strictures.

Short Bowel Syndrome Before the advent of parenteral nutrition, patients with acute short bowel syndrome from mesenteric vascular infarction or massive small bowel surgical resection seldom survived. Parenteral nutrition has allowed many patients to survive indefinitely with only a foot or two of small intestine. In some, the remaining bowel eventually adapts and allows the absorption of adequate calories and protein. This is especially true of patients who retain their iliocecal valve and colon. However, fluid and electrolyte imbalance may persist, necessitating some parenteral fluid and electrolyte support. A gradual switch to overnight tube enteral hydration or constant sipping of an electrolyte solution may allow discontinuation of all parenteral support.

Pulmonary Disease Weight loss in patients with advanced pulmonary disease is due to increased work of breathing and poor food intake. Patients with chronic pulmonary disease who are <90% of their ideal weight have a higher 5-year mortality, independent of pulmonary status. The recommended energy intake for these patients is 1.7 times their resting energy expenditure. The use of a low-carbohydrate formula is beneficial in the weaning of patients from ventilators, but the superiority of such formulas in ambulatory patients with chronic lung disease is not established. In cystic fibrosis, malnutrition may hasten pulmonary deterioration, and enteral tube feeding enhances growth and stabilizes or improves pulmonary function, particularly in young children. Tube feeding is safest when delivered into the jejunum. Postpyloric feeding is no safer than gastric feeding.

HIV Disease Specialized nutrition support can replete body cell mass if the weight loss is due to inadequate oral intake caused by oral or esophageal disease or to inadequate intestinal absorption, which is common in HIV patients with cryptosporidosis or microsporidiosis infections (Chap. 309). The route of nutrition support has usually been parenteral, but patients respond equally well with an isocaloric semi-elemental oral diet. Patients using the oral supplement experience a better quality of life, and their medical costs are significantly lower. Wasting due to systemic infection and increased cytokine secretion is not redressed by specialized nutrition support. Survival, CD4+ counts, and intestinal function also are not improved by specialized nutrition support.

Pregnancy Severe hyperemesis gravidarum can make any oral or tube enteral nutrition impossible, and profound weight loss and ketosis may harm the developing fetus. The underlying mechanism of the disorder is not understood, but it is cured by abortion or delivery.

Table 76-3 Summary of Outcomes for Patients on Home Parenteral and Enteral Nutrition (HPEN)

Diagnosis	Number in Group	Age in Years	% Survival[a] on Therapy	Therapy Status, % at 1 year[b,c] Full Oral Nutrition	Continued on HPEN Rx	Died	Rehabilitation[c,d] Status, % in 1st year C	P	M	Complications[e] per Patient-Year HPEN[e]	NonHPEN[e]
HOME PARENTERAL NUTRITION											
Crohn's disease	562	36	96	70	25	2	60	38	2	0.9	1.1
Ischemic bowel disease	331	49	87	27	48	19	53	41	6	1.4	1.1
Motility disorder	299	45	87	31	44	21	49	39	12	1.3	1.1
Congenital bowel defect	172	5	94	42	47	9	63	27	11	2.1	1.0
Hyperemesis gravidarum	112	28	100	100	0	0	83	16	1	1.5	3.5
Chronic pancreatitis	156	42	90	82	10	5	60	38	2	1.2	2.5
Radiation enteritis	145	58	87	28	49	22	42	49	9	0.8	1.1
Chronic adhesive obstructions	120	53	83	47	34	13	23	68	10	1.7	1.4
Cystic fibrosis	51	17	50	38	13	36	24	66	16	0.8	3.7
Cancer	2122	44	20	26	8	63	29	57	14	1.1	3.3
AIDS	280	33	10	13	6	73	8	63	29	1.6	3.3
HOME ENTERAL NUTRITION											
Neurologic disorders of swallowing	1134	65	55	19	25	48	5	24	71	0.3	0.9
Cancer	1644	61	30	30	6	59	21	59	21	0.4	2.7

[a] Survival rates on therapy are values at 1 year, calculated by the life table method. This will differ from the percentage listed as died under Therapy Status, since all patients with known endpoints are considered in this latter measure. The ratio of observed versus expected deaths is equivalent to a Standard Mortality Ratio.

[b] Not shown are those patients who were back in hospital or who had changed therapy type by 12 months.

[c] Chi-square test, $p < .05$

[d] Rehabilitation is designated complete (C), partial (P), or minimal (M), relative to the patient's ability to sustain normal age-related activity.

[e] Complications refer only to those complications that resulted in rehospitalization.

SOURCE: Derived from North American HPEN Registry.

Temporary parenteral nutrition usually results in a successful outcome, but nausea and vomiting tend to persist, despite bowel rest.

Home Parenteral and Enteral Nutrition Some patients require long-term nutrition support, and for many this can be administered at home. Clinical outcomes of patients with severe intestinal disorders that used either parenteral or enteral nutrition are summarized in Table 76-3. Nutrition support is not usually appropriate in terminally ill patients but is an option if the patient is expected to survive for several months. Such therapy must make sense to the patient, and sufficient help must be available so the treatment can be given at home without undue hazard. Both home therapies are relatively safe, with <5% therapy-related mortality.

THE DESIGN OF INDIVIDUAL REGIMENS Fluid Requirements These can be estimated by adding the normal daily requirement (120 mL/kg of body weight for infants, 35 mL/kg of body weight for adults) to any abnormal loss. If the patient is on parenteral therapy, any enteral intake should be subtracted from the estimate (Table 76-4). Since abnormal loss of enteric fluid implies significant

Table 76-4 Estimation of Daily Fluid Requirements

NORMAL 70-KG MAN

Intake	Output
Normal requirement: $35 \times 70 = \sim 2500$ ml/d (derived from oral liquids of 1200 mL, or 5 glasses/cups per day and solid food providing 1300 mL, 1000 mL from water in food, 300 mL from water generated by metabolism of foods)	Urine: 1600 mL/d Insensible loss: 800 mL/d Stool: 100 mL/d [sweat loss can be up to 2 L/d; each degree of fever (C) = 200 mL/d]

TUBE ENTERAL PATIENT

58-kg woman recovering from total gastrectomy for gastric cancer and supported by jejunostomy feedings, taking nothing by mouth or intravenously but experiencing 600 mL of diarrheal losses/day:
  Normal requirement $35 \times 58 = \sim 2000$ mL/d
  Abnormal gastrointestinal loss $600 - 100 = 500$ mL/d
  Total per tube requirement = 2500 mL/d

PARENTERAL PATIENT

66-kg man with a high jejunostomy following massive bowel resection for Crohn's disease with oral intake of 2000 mL/day and jejunostomy loss of 4000 mL/day:
  Normal requirement $35 \times 66 = 2300$ mL/d
  Abnormal gastrointestinal loss $(4000 - 100)$ minus oral intake $(2000) = 1900$ mL/d
  Total parenteral requirement = 4200 mL/d

mineral losses, extra amounts of these nutrients, as well as fluid (Table 76-5), must be added to the parenteral formula.

Energy Requirements These can be determined as outlined in Chaps. 73 and 74. In the long run, energy expenditure dictates energy requirements, but in the early phase of nutrition repletion, requirements may not reflect expenditure. For example, malnourished patients are hypometabolic and may expend only 85 kJ/kg (20 kcal/kg) per day, but more calories are needed both for tissue repletion and because the metabolic rate increases with refeeding. Conversely, a highly stressed patient (sepsis, trauma) may expend 165 kJ/kg (40 kcal/kg) per day with a significant proportion of the calories coming from protein breakdown and gluconeogenesis and from catecholamine-induced lipolysis. Oxidation of exogenous glucose plateaus at 100 kJ/kg (25 kcal/kg) per day, and administering additional glucose induces hepatic steatosis. Providing such patients with additional calories as exogenous fat does not suppress endogenous lipolysis. Furthermore, lipid solutions are made from vegetable oil and egg phospholipid and lack apoproteins, which they acquire from endogenous lipoproteins. Initially, the artificial chylomicron may be taken up by the reticuloendothelial system enhancing its blockade. For all these reasons, modest hypocaloric glucose feeding with minimal parenteral fat is safer in the acutely stressed subject.

Parenteral lipid solutions are available as 10 or 20% isotonic solutions and are infused separately from amino acids and glucose or as a combined "three-in-one solution," obviating the need for an extra pump. Three-in-one solutions are less stable than the glucose and amino acid mix, and destabilized fat particles have the potential to coalesce into larger droplets, becoming fat emboli. For this reason, three-in-one solutions have a shorter storage life and must be mixed by a phar-

Table 76-5 Enteric Fluid Volumes and Their Sodium, Potassium, Chloride, and Bicarbonate Content[a]

	L/d[b]	Na, mmol/L	K,[c] mmol/L	Cl, mmol/L	HCO₃,[d] mmol/L
Oral intake	2–3				
Enteric secretions					
Saliva	1–2	10	30	10	30
Gastric juice	2	60	9	90	0
Bile	2–3	150	10	90	70
Small bowel	1	100	5	100	20
Colon	Variable	40	100	15	60

[a] Enteric secretions are also rich in divalent cations (Ca, Mg, Zn, Cu), and their loss is increased by steatorrhea, a high bowel fistula, or prolonged suction.

[b] Of the 9 L/d of oral and enteric fluid presented to the upper small bowel, normally 50% is absorbed in the jejunum, 40% in the ileum, and 10% in the colon. In short bowel patients, the colon may absorb greater amounts, up to 3 L/d.

[c] Potassium losses are small except in secretions distal to the ileocecal valve. The colon ion exchange is partly controlled by aldosterone, and therefore, Na⁺ depletion increases K⁺ loss in the stool.

[d] Bicarbonate losses must be replaced in parenteral solutions as acetate or lactate because of potential precipitation of bicarbonate with ingredients such as calcium.

macist knowledgeable about the correct mixing sequence and safe levels of electrolytes and trace elements. Iron, for example, cannot be added to this solution.

Polyunsaturated vegetable oils are used in most enteral formulas because they are absorbed better than animal fat by a diseased gastrointestinal tract. Fat must supply the essential fatty acid requirement (1 to 4% of energy from linoleic and linolenic acid) (Table 76-6). Larger amounts (30% of energy) are safe in relatively stable patients and avoid the problems of providing large amounts of glucose (e.g., hyperglycemia and hepatic steatosis). Substituting omega-3 polyunsaturated fish oils for polyunsaturated vegetable fats may reduce the catabolic response to burn injury, trauma, and radiation by reducing the synthesis of prostaglandins that enhance the inflammatory response

Table 76-6 Daily Enteral and Parenteral Requirements of Essential Fatty Acids, Minerals, and Vitamins

Nutrient	Daily Requirement, Adult Range	
	Enteral	Parenteral
Essential fatty acids, % kcal	1–2	2–4
Calcium, g	0.8–1.2	0.2–0.4
Phosphorus, g	0.8–1.2	0.4–0.8
Potassium, g	2–5	3–4
Sodium, g	1–3	1–3
Chloride, g	25–5	3–4[a]
Magnesium, g	0.3	0.3
Iron, mg	10	1–2
Zinc, mg	15	3–12
Copper, mg	2–3	0.3–0.5
Iodine, mg	0.15	0.15
Manganese, mg	2–5	2–5
Chromium, µg	50–200	15–30
Molybdenum, µg	150–300	20–120
Selenium, µg	50–200	50–100
Ascorbic acid, mg	60	100
Thiamine, mg	1.4	3.0
Riboflavin, mg	1.6	3.6
Niacin, mg	18	40
Biotin, µg	60	60
Pantothenic acid, mg	5	15
Pyridoxine, mg	2.0	4.0
Folic acid, µg	400	400
Cobalamin, µg	3.0	5
Vitamin A, µg	1000	1000
Vitamin D, µg	10	5–10
Vitamin E, mg	8–10	10–15
Vitamin K, µg	70–140	200

[a] In addition to chloride anions there is a parenteral requirement for bicarbonate equivalents to protect normal acid-base balance. These are provided as 90 mmoL or more per day of acetate or lactate because of potential precipitation of bicarbonate with ingredients such as calcium.

(Table 76-2). Such fats are available in enteral formulas and are currently being tested in parenteral formulas.

Protein or Amino Acid Requirements The recommended dietary protein allowance of 0.8 g/kg per day is adequate for nonstressed patients, such as a starved patient with a high-grade esophageal stricture. Catabolic patients, in contrast, may require up to 1.5 g/kg per day of protein to induce positive nitrogen balance and reconstitute normal body mass. Early studies showed that recombinant human growth hormone (rHGH) increases lean body mass. However, subsequent trials have shown that it is associated with increased mortality in critically ill patients, and it should not be used in this setting.

In a stable patient the adequacy of protein support can be assessed by analyzing protein balance:

$$\text{Protein balance} = \text{protein intake} - \text{protein loss}$$

where protein loss = [(24-h urine urea nitrogen (g) + 4) × 6.25]. Over a long period, protein balance is assessed by documenting wound healing, restoration of normal body composition, or resumption of longitudinal growth. In states of disturbed protein utilization (e.g., renal and hepatic failure), azotemia and abnormal plasma amino acid patterns develop. The benefit of special enteral and parenteral solutions that correct these aberrations is only established in hepatic encephalopathy (see "Risks and Benefits of Nutrition Support").

Certain nutrients that can normally be synthesized endogenously become essential in severely ill patients when endogenous production or salvage pathways are impaired. This is true of glutamine, nucleotides, and the products of methionine metabolism (Table 76-2). Glutamine, an important fuel for the enterocyte and lymphocyte, is fairly insoluble and is absent from standard parenteral formulas and present in low concentrations in most enteral formulas. Soluble glutamine-containing dipeptides are under investigation.

Nucleotides and their related metabolic products have beneficial effects on the immune system, growth of the small intestine, lipid metabolism, and hepatic function. Nucleotides can be synthesized de novo in all cells only in small amounts, and the body therefore depends on dietary nucleotides or on salvage pathways that recycle nucleotides from purine and pyrimidine turnover. Nutritionally depleted patients benefit from formulas enriched in nucleotides.

When amino acids are infused systemically, rather than via the more physiologic portal vein, methionine, the only sulfur-containing amino acid in most parenteral solutions, is transaminated in peripheral tissues rather than transulfurated in the liver. As a result, downstream sulfur products such as carnitine, taurine, and glutathione become relatively deficient (Chap. 352). Preliminary studies suggest that the addition of an intermediate compound, S-adenosyl methionine, to parenteral solutions results in less cholestasis.

Mineral and Vitamin Requirements Parenteral and enteral mineral and vitamin requirements are summarized in Table 76-6. Electrolyte modifications are necessary if the patient has significant gastrointestinal losses (Table 76-5) or renal failure. Requirements of some minerals and vitamins are higher when administered parenterally for several reasons: (1) many micronutrients delivered into the systemic rather than the portal circulation are not captured by the liver and instead pass directly into the urine; (2) patients with bowel disease may have enteric loss of sodium, potassium, chloride, and bicarbonate and malabsorption of divalent cations, fat-soluble vitamins, and vitamin B_{12}; and (3) nutrients may adhere to the tubing and delivery bags, and exposure to oxygen and light may destroy vitamins (particularly vitamin A).

PARENTERAL NUTRITION Infusion Technique and Patient Monitoring Partial and short-term total parenteral nutrition can be provided via a peripheral vein if the majority of the energy is supplied by isotonic fat solutions; long-term total parenteral nutrition using glucose as the chief energy source requires administration via a central vein catheter so the hypertonic solution can be rapidly diluted

Table 76-7 Central Venous Access for Parenteral Nutrition

Type of Catheters	Advantages	Disadvantages
Peripherally inserted central catheter Single lumen Double lumen	Insertion cost low; can be done at bedside or by vascular radiology using Doppler guidance; especially advantageous for patients with neck wounds such as tracheostomies	High incidence of skin site irritation; tendency to break at hub; patient requires assistance with weekly dressing change
Centrally inserted externalized catheter (subclavian, jugular, femoral) Single lumen Triple lumen	Can be inserted at bedside; relatively low cost; can be changed over a guidewire if clinically indicated; catheter sepsis rate within subclavian < jugular < femoral vein	10% incidence of mechanical complication with insertion, higher if physician inexperienced; need dedicated nutrition line; multiple-lumen catheters have increased sepsis rate
Centrally inserted, tunneled catheter or subcutaneous port	More stable for long-term use; when needle out, patients with ports have less disturbance of body image and can shower and swim without risk	More expensive device requiring operating room insertion; ports require needle stick.

in a high-flow system. The preferred site for central vein infusion is the superior vena cava. Access sites and catheter choices are summarized in Table 76-7. Peripherally inserted central catheters are the most economical option for short-term parenteral nutrition. In one randomized study, the number of catheter-related infections was the same with peripherally and centrally inserted catheters. Tunneled catheters and implanted subcutaneous ports require operating room insertion and are more stable for long-term use. Central catheters should be changed when clinically indicated; routine changes are costly and hazardous. Chlorhexidine solution is a more effective local antiseptic than iodophor or alcohol. Although transparent dressings are helpful in stabilizing catheters and allow easy observation of the skin site, the incidence of catheter-related sepsis is higher than with traditional dry gauze dressings; newer transparent dressings that trap less moisture are under investigation. Catheters made from Silastic material or polyurethane are associated with lower complications than polyvinylchloride catheters. Several types of needleless systems use hub valves, and contamination rates are higher with these devices when used for long-term parenteral nutrition. Appropriate clinical and laboratory monitoring for patients on parenteral nutrition are summarized in Table 76-8.

Complications (See Table 76-9) • *Mechanical* The insertion of a central venous catheter should be done only by trained personnel under aseptic techniques. Major mechanical complications include pneumothorax; hemothorax from laceration of the subclavian artery or vein; brachial plexus injury; and malpositioning of the catheter in a cerebral vein, the azygos vein, or the right ventricle. The correct catheter position must be confirmed by x-ray before hypertonic nutrient solution is infused. Catheters can subsequently dislocate, develop leaks, or become detached from the hub and embolize into the heart or pulmonary artery. Catheter thrombosis may occur, especially if the catheter is used for withdrawing blood samples, and extension of the thrombosis to the central vein is frequently coincident with infection. Thrombosed catheters can sometimes be unblocked by urokinase treatment. The addition of low-dose heparin (1000 U/L) to limit thrombosis in parenteral catheters is controversial; no randomized, controlled studies demonstrate benefit, and heparin can contribute to loss of bone mineral, which is already a problem with long-term parenteral nutrition.

Metabolic Fluid overload can cause congestive heart failure, particularly in elderly and debilitated patients. Glucose overload can cause an osmotic diuresis or stimulate insulin secretion, which in turn promotes extracellular to intracellular shifts of potassium and phosphorous. Such shifts are most dangerous in cachectic patients with depletion of potassium and phosphorus stores and can cause arrhythmias, cardiopulmonary dysfunction, and neurologic symptoms. To avoid these problems, parenteral nutrition should be started slowly and mon-

itored carefully. Glucose content is increased gradually as the patient demonstrates tolerance of the high glucose load. Late metabolic complications include cholestatic liver disease with bile sludging and gallstone formation. The exact cause of the liver disease is not understood, but lack of enteral stimulation to bile flow and defective sulfur amino acid metabolism and cholesterol solubilization appear to play a role. Cholestasis is less likely to occur if some enteral feeding is maintained. Parenteral nutrition induces hypercalciuria, which can result in negative calcium balance and osteopenia. Hypercalciuria may have several causes, including the high fixed-acid load of infused amino acids and the bisulfite preservative in parenteral solutions. Earlier, protein hydrolysates were used as an amino acid source and were contaminated with aluminum, which blocked bone mineralization. Aluminum is still a contaminant of some additives such as calcium gluconate. Once patients on long-term parenteral nutrition change from catabolic breakdown to sustained anabolism, deficiencies of micronutrients such as essential fatty acids, trace minerals, and vitamins may develop unless they are supplied in adequate amounts (Table 76-6).

Infectious Infection of the access line rarely occurs in the first 72 h, and fever during this period is usually due to infection elsewhere or some other cause. Infection of the access line is likely if the fever defervesces when the infusion of the parenteral formula is tapered.

Positive central line cultures suggest catheter sepsis, especially if no other infectious source is identified and if the organism is *Staphylococcus* or *Candida*. Although removal of the central catheter may allow fungemia to clear spontaneously, antibiotic therapy is recommended for bacterial infections and the more invasive fungi. Catheter sepsis rates are similar in single lumen central lines dedicated to parenteral nutrition whether inserted peripherally via the subclavian vein

Table 76-8 Monitoring the Patient on Total Parenteral Nutrition

CLINICAL DATA MONITORED DAILY

Sense of well-being: symptoms suggesting fluid overload, high or low blood glucose, electrolyte imbalance, etc.

Strength as judged by graded activity: getting out of bed, walking, stair climbing

Vital signs: temperature, blood pressure, pulse rate, and respiratory rate

Fluid balance: weight; fluid input (intravenous +/− enteral) versus fluid output (urine, stool, gastric suction, etc.).

Delivery equipment for parenteral nutrition: composition of nutrient solution, tubing, pump, filter, catheter, dressing (skin checked for local infection at time of dressing change)

LABORATORY DATA

Fingerstick glucose	Three times daily until patient stable
Blood glucose Na^+, K^+, CL^-, HCO_3^- Blood urea nitrogen	Daily until glucose infusion load and patient stable, then twice weekly
Liver function studies Serum creatinine, albumin PO_4^{3-}, Ca^{2+}, Mg^{2+} Hb/Hct, WBC	Baseline, then twice weekly
Clotting, INR	Baseline, then weekly
Micronutrient tests as indicated	

NOTE: Hb, hemoglobin; Hct, hematocrit; WBC, white blood cell (count); INR, international normalized ratio.

or tunneled; multiple-lumen catheters are associated with a greater incidence of sepsis. While there is no evidence to support the use of prophylactic antibiotics, recurrent catheter sepsis may be avoided if cuffs are used around the catheter exit site or small amounts of an antibiotic solution are left in the line along with a heparin lock.

ENTERAL NUTRITION

Tube Placement and Patient Monitoring The types of enteral feeding tubes, methods of insertion, their clinical uses, and potential complications are outlined in Table 76-10. The different types of enteral formulas are listed in Table 76-11. Patients on enteral feeding are at risk for many of the same metabolic complications as those receiving parenteral nutrition and should be monitored in the same way (Table 76-8). Since small-bore tubes are easily displaced, tube position should be checked at intervals by aspirating and measuring the pH of the gut fluid (<4 in stomach, >6 in jejunum).

Complications • Aspiration The debilitated patient with poor gastric emptying and impairment of swallowing and cough mechanisms is at risk for aspiration; this is particularly so for those on respirators. Tracheal suctioning induces coughing and gastric regurgitation, and cuffs on endotracheal or tracheostomy tubes seldom provide protection against aspiration. Under these circumstances, it may be safer to use a large-bore feeding tube to allow for temporary removal of gastric contents during tracheal suction or to use jejunal feeding. Constant gastric infusion of an enteral formula is better tolerated in sick patients than intermittent bolus feeding. A continuous infusion is best achieved with a pump, especially when using fine-bore tubes that

have a greater potential to clog. If long-term feeding is anticipated, endoscopic, radiologic, or surgical placement of a gastric tube is preferred by most patients. For long-term ambulatory patients, a gastrostomy tube can be converted to a gastric "button," an access device that is flush with the skin. A nasojejunal tube reduces the risk of aspiration. However, fluoroscopically guided placement of fine-bore tubes through the pylorus is time-consuming, and such tubes frequently pull back into the stomach. A percutaneous combined gastric-suction and jejunal-feeding tube is more reliable. This can be placed radiologically, endoscopically, or surgically.

Diarrhea Enteral feeding often causes diarrhea, especially if bowel function is compromised by bowel disease or drugs. The diarrhea may be controlled by the use of continuous feeding of fiber-containing formulas or by adding an anticholinergic medication to the

Table 76-9 Complications of Total Parenteral Nutrition (TPN)

First 48 h	First 2 Weeks	3 Months Onward
MECHANICAL		
Complications from catheter insertion:	Catheter coming out of vein, more common if Silastic	Detachment of line at catheter hub with blood loss or air embolism
Cephalad displacement	Detachment of line at catheter hub with blood loss or air embolism	Fractures or tears in catheter
Pneumothorax	Thrombosis	Catheter embedded in vein wall
Hemothorax		
Detachment of line at catheter hub with blood loss or air embolism		
METABOLIC		
Fluid overload	Cardiopulmonary failure	Essentially fatty acid deficiency
Hyperglycemia	Refeeding edema	Iron deficiency
Hypophosphatemia	Hyperosmolar nonketotic hyperglycemic coma	Vitamin deficiencies
Hypokalemia	Acid-base imbalance	TPN metabolic bone disease
	Electrolyte imbalance	TPN liver disease
		Zinc, copper, chromium, selenium, molybdenum, deficiency
INFECTIOUS		
	Catheter-induced sepsis	Catheter-induced sepsis
	Exit site infection	Tunnel infections
		Exit site infection

Table 76-10 Enteral Feeding Tubes

Type/Insertion Technique	Clinical Uses	Potential Complications
NASOGASTRIC TUBE		
External measurement, nostril, ear, xiphisternum; tube stiffened by ice water or stylet; position verified by injecting air and auscultating, aspirating gastric acid, or by x-ray	Short-term clinical situation (weeks) or longer periods with intermittent insertion; bolus feeding simpler, but continuous drip with pump better tolerated	Aspiration; ulceration of nasal and esophageal tissues, leading to stricture
NASOJEJUNAL TUBE		
External measurement: nostril, ear, anterior superior iliac spine (medical malleolus in infants); tube stiffened by stylet and passed through pylorus under fluoroscopy or with endoscopic loop	Short-term clinical situations where gastric emptying impaired or proximal leak suspected; requires continuous drip with pump	Spontaneous pulling back into stomach (position reverified by aspirating content pH > 6); diarrhea common, fiber-containing formula may help
GASTROSTOMY TUBE		
Percutaneous placement endoscopically, radiologically, or surgically: after tract established, can be converted to a gastric "button"	Long-term clinical situations, swallowing disorders, or impaired small-bowel absorption requiring continuous drip	Aspiration; irritation around tube exit site; peritoneal leak; balloon migration and obstruction of pylorus
JEJUNOSTOMY TUBE		
Percutaneous placement endoscopically or radiologically via pylorus or surgically into jejunum sutured to abdominal wall using fine-bore tube or larger tube	Long-term clinical situations where gastric emptying impaired; requires continuous drip with pump	Clogging or displacement of tube; jejunal fistula if large-bore tube used; diarrhea
COMBINED GASTROJEJUNOSTOMY TUBE		
Percutaneous placement endoscopically, radiologically, or surgically; intragastric arm for continuous or intermittent gastric suction; jejunal arm for enteral feeding	Used for patients with impaired gastric emptying and at high risk for aspiration or patients with acute pancreatitis or proximal leaks	Clogging; irritation around tube exit site

Table 76-11 Enteral Formulas

Composition Characteristics	Clinical Indication
STANDARD ENTERAL FORMULA	

1. Complete dietary products (+)[a]
   a. Caloric density 1 kcal/mL
   b. Protein ~14% cals, caseinates, soy, lactalbumin
   c. Fat ~30% cals, corn, soy, safflower oils
   d. CHO ~60% cals, hydrolysed corn starch, maltodextrin, sucrose
   e. Recommended daily intake of all minerals and vitamins in ≥1500 kcal/d
   f. Osmolality (mosm/kg) ~300
	Suitable for most patients requiring tube feeding; flavors available for oral use

MODIFIED ENTERAL FORMULAS	
1. Caloric density 1.5–2 kcal/mL (+)	Fluid-restricted patients
2. a. High protein ~20% cals (+)	Protein malnutrition and ↓ wound healing
b. Hydrolysed protein to small peptides (++)	↓ Protein digestion/absorption or allergy
c. ↑ Glutamine, arginine, S-containing amino acids, nucleotides (+++)	Severely immunocompromised patients
d. ↑ Branch-chain amino acids, ↓ aromatic amino acids (+++)	Liver failure patients intolerant of 0.8 g/kg per day of regular protein
e. ↓ Protein, ↓ K, Mg, and P diets (++)	Renal failure patients
f. ↓ Protein, ↑ essential amino acids, ↓ minerals and vitamins (+++)	Renal failure patients not on dialysis
3. a. Low fat, partial MCT substitution (+)	Fat malabsorption
b. ↑ Fat >40% cals (++)	Pulmonary failure with ↑ P_{CO_2} on standard formulas
c. ↑ Fat from MUFA (++)	Poorly controlled diabetes mellitus
d. Fat ↑ in ω3 (fish oil) and ↓ ω6 (+++)	Immunocompromised and autoimmune disorder
4. a. Fiber provided as soy poly saccharide (+)	Diarrhea/constipation
b. Fiber provided as blenderized fruits and vegetables (++)	↓ Binding of dilantin
5. ↑ Minerals (Zn) and vitamins (A and C) (++)	Decubitus ulcers

[a] Cost: + inexpensive; + + moderately expensive; + + + very expensive.
NOTE: CHO, carbohydrate; MCT, medium-chain triglyceride; MUFA, monunsaturated fatty acid, ω3 or ω6 polyunsatuated fat with first double bond at carbon 3 (fish oils) or carbon 6 (vegetable oils).

formula. Diarrhea associated with enteral feeding does not necessarily imply inadequate absorption of nutrients, other than water and electrolytes. Furthermore, since luminal nutrients exert trophic effects on the gut mucosa and enhance the enteric immunologic barrier, it is often appropriate to persist with tube feeding, despite the diarrhea, even when this necessitates supplemental parenteral fluid support.

THE SCOPE AND COST OF NUTRITION SUPPORT

As many as 25% of patients entering tertiary care hospitals have central catheters placed, and 20 to 30% of these catheters are used for parenteral nutrition. The incidence of catheter-related infection reflects the severity of the underlying medical condition and varies from 2 to 30 per thousand catheter days, depending on the type of patients involved. In critically ill patients, catheter sepsis is associated with a 35% mortality rate and a high cost per survivor. Most catheter-related complications derive from faulty insertion and management of the catheter rather than defects in the device. In large tertiary care hospitals, the insertion and management of these lines by specially trained teams can reduce complications by 80%, impacting significantly on outcome and costs. A growing shift from parenteral to enteral nutrition also promises significant cost savings. Home parenteral nutrition costs approximately half as much as similar treatment in the hospital, and home enteral nutrition costs much less.

BIBLIOGRAPHY

AMERICAN COLLEGE OF PHYSICIANS: Position paper: Parenteral nutrition in patients receiving cancer chemotherapy: A meta-analysis. Ann Intern Med 110:734, 1989

ANDERSON JD et al: Enteral feeding in the critically injured patient. Nutr Clin Pract 7: 117, 1992

CHARUHAS PN et al: A double-blind randomized trial comparing outpatient parenteral nutrition with intravenous hydration: Effect on resumption of oral intake after marrow transplantation. JPEN 21:157, 1997

FLYNN MB, LEIGHTTY FF: Preoperative outpatient nutritional support of patients with squamous cancer of the upper aerodigestive tract. Am J Surg 154:359, 1987

FOULKS CJ et al: An evidence-based evaluation of intradialytic parenteral nutrition. Am J Kidney Dis 33:186, 1999

GRIFFITHS AM et al: Meta-analysis of enteral nutrition as a primary treatment of active Crohn's disease. Gastroenterology 108:1056, 1995

HEYLAND DK et al: Total parenteral nutrition in the critically ill patient: A meta-analysis. JAMA 280:2013, 1998

HEYS SD et al: Enteral nutritional supplementation with key nutrients in patients with critical illness and cancer: A meta-analysis of randomized controlled clinical trials. Ann Surg 228:467, 1999

HILL GL: Body composition research: Implications for the practice of clinical nutrition. J Parenter Enter Nutr 16:197, 1992

HOWARD L et al: Current use and clinical outcome of home parenteral and enteral nutrition therapies in the United States. Gastroenterology 109:335, 1995

KALFARENTZOS F et al: Enteral nutrition is superior to parenteral nutrition in severe acute pancreatitis: Results of a randomized prospective trial. Br J Surg 84:1665, 1997

KLEIN S et al: Nutritional support in clinical practice: Review of published data and recommendations for future research directions. Am J Clin Nutr 66:683, 1997

KOTLER DP et al: Comparison of total parenteral nutrition and an oral, semielemental diet on body composition, physical function, and nutrition-related costs in patients with malabsorption due to acquired immunodeficiency syndrome. JPEN 22:120, 1998

LIPMAN TO: Clinical trials of nutrition support in cancer. Hematol Oncol Clin North Am 5:91, 1991

MELCHIOR JC et al: Improved survival by home total parenteral nutrition in AIDS patients: Follow-up of a controlled randomized prospective trial. AIDS 12:336, 1998

MOORE FA et al: Early enteral feeding, compared with parenteral, reduces postoperative septic complications. The results of a meta-analysis. Ann Surg 216:172, 1992

NAYLOR CD et al: Parenteral nutrition with branched-chain amino acids in hepatic encephalopathy: A meta-analysis. Gastroenterology 97:1033, 1989

RAAD II et al: Infectious complications of indwelling vascular catheters. Clin Infect Dis 15:197, 1992

RIORDAN AM et al: Treatment of active Crohn's disease by exclusion diet: East Anglian Multicenter Controlled Trial. Lancet 342:1131, 1993

SCOLAPIO JS et al: Effect of growth hormone, glutamine, and diet on adaption in short bowel syndrome. A randomized controlled study. Gastroenterology 113:1074, 1997

TRALLORI MA et al: Defined formula diets versus steroids in the treatment of active Crohn's disease. Scan J Gastroenterol 31:267, 1996

VETERANS ADMINISTRATION TOTAL PARENTERAL NUTRITION COOPERATIVE STUDY. Perioperative total parenteral nutrition in surgical patients. N Engl J Med 325:525, 1991

WEINSIER RL et al: Cost containment: A contribution of aggressive nutrition support in burn patients. J Burn Care Rehabil 6:436, 1985

WEISDORF S et al: Influence of prophylactic total parenteral nutrition on long-term outcome of bone marrow transplantation. Transplantation 43:833, 1987

ZIEGLER TR et al: Clinical and metabolic efficacy of glutamine-supplemented parenteral nutrition after bone marrow transplantation. Ann Intern Med 116:821, 1992

77

Jeffrey S. Flier

OBESITY

ACTH	adrenocorticotropic hormone	NIDDM	non-insulin-dependent
AgRP	Agouti-related peptide	diabetes mellitus	
BAT	brown adipose tissue	NPY	neuropeptide Y
BMI	body mass index	PPARγ	peroxisome proliferator-
CHF	congestive heart failure	activated receptor γ	
LDL	low-density lipoprotein	SHBG	sex hormone–binding globulin
MSH	melanocyte-stimulating	TNF	tumor necrosis factor
hormone		UCP	uncoupling protein

In a world where food supplies are intermittent, the ability to store energy in excess of what is required for immediate use is essential for survival. Fat cells, residing within widely distributed adipose tissue depots, are adapted to store excess energy efficiently as triglyceride and, when needed, to release stored energy as free fatty acids for use at other sites. This physiologic system, orchestrated through endocrine and neural pathways, permits humans to survive starvation for as long as several months. However, in the presence of nutritional abundance and a sedentary lifestyle, and influenced importantly by genetic endowment, this system increases adipose energy stores and produces adverse health consequences.

DEFINITION AND MEASUREMENT *Obesity* is a state of excess adipose tissue mass. Although often viewed as equivalent to increased body weight, this need not be the case—lean but very muscular individuals may be overweight by arbitrary standards without having increased adiposity. Body weights are distributed continuously in populations, so that a medically meaningful distinction between lean and obese is somewhat arbitrary. Obesity is therefore more effectively defined by assessing its linkage to morbidity or mortality.

Although not a direct measure of adiposity, the most widely used method to gauge obesity is the *body mass index* (BMI), which is equal to weight/height^2 (in kg/m^2) (Fig. 77-1). Other approaches to quantifying obesity include anthropometry (skin-fold thickness), densitometry (underwater weighing), computed tomography (CT) or magnetic resonance imaging (MRI), and electrical impedance. Using data from the Metropolitan Life Tables, BMIs for the midpoint of all heights and frames among both men and women range from 19 to 26 kg/m^2; at a similar BMI, women have more body fat than men. Based on unequivocal data of substantial morbidity, a BMI of 30 is most commonly used as a threshold for obesity in both men and women. Large-scale epidemiologic studies suggest that all-cause, metabolic, and cardiovascular morbidity begin to rise (albeit at a slow rate) when BMIs are ≥ 25, suggesting that the cut-off for obesity should be lowered. Some authorities use the term *overweight* (rather than obese) to describe individuals with BMIs between 25 or 27 and 30. A BMI between 25 and 30 should be viewed as medically significant and worthy of therapeutic intervention, especially in the presence of risk factors that are influenced by adiposity, such as hypertension and glucose intolerance.

The distribution of adipose tissue in different anatomic depots also has substantial implications for morbidity. Specifically, intraabdominal and abdominal subcutaneous fat have more significance than subcutaneous fat present in the buttocks and lower extremities. This distinction is most easily made by determining the waist-to-hip ratio, with a ratio >0.9 in women and >1.0 in men being abnormal. Many of the most important complications of obesity, such as insulin resistance, diabetes, hypertension, and hyperlipidemia, and hyperandrogenism in women, are linked more strongly to intraabdominal and/or upper body fat than to overall adiposity. The mechanism underlying this association is unknown but may relate to the fact that intraabdominal adipocytes are more lipolytically active than those from other depots. Release of free fatty acids into the portal circulation has adverse metabolic actions, especially on the liver.

PREVALENCE Recent data from the National Health and Nutrition Examination Surveys (NHANES) show that the percent of the American adult population with obesity (BMI > 30) has increased from 14.5% (between 1976 and 1980) to 22.5% (between 1998 and 1994). As many as 50% of U.S. adults ≥20 years of age were overweight (defined as BMI > 25) between the years of 1998 and 1991. Because substantial health risks exist in many individuals with BMI between 25 and 30, the increasing prevalence of medically significant obesity raises great concern. Obesity is more common among women and in the poor; the prevalence in children is also rising at a worrisome rate.

PHYSIOLOGIC REGULATION OF ENERGY BALANCE Substantial evidence suggests that body weight is regulated by both endocrine and neural components that ultimately influence the effector arms of energy intake and expenditure. This complex regulatory system is necessary because even small imbalances between energy intake and expenditure will ultimately have large effects on body weight. For example, a 0.3% positive imbalance over 30 years would result in a 9-kg (20-lb) weight gain. Alterations in stable weight by forced overfeeding or food deprivation induce physiologic changes that resist these perturbations: with weight loss, appetite increases and energy expenditure falls; with overfeeding, appetite falls and energy expenditure increases. This latter compensatory mechanism frequently fails, however, permitting obesity to develop when food is abundant and physical activity is limited. A major regulator of these adaptive responses is the adipocyte-derived hormone leptin, which acts through brain circuits (predominantly in the hypothalamus) to influence appetite, energy expenditure, and neuroendocrine function (see below).

Appetite is influenced by many factors that are integrated by the brain, most importantly within the hypothalamus (Fig. 77-2). Signals that impinge on the hypothalamic center include neural afferents, hormones, and metabolites. Vagal inputs are particularly important, bringing information from viscera, such as gut distention. Hormonal signals include leptin, insulin, cortisol, and gut peptides such as cholecystokinin, which signals to the brain through the vagus nerve. Metabolites, including glucose, can influence appetite, as seen by the effect of hypoglycemia to induce hunger; however, glucose is not normally a major regulator of appetite. These diverse hormonal, metabolic, and neural signals act by influencing the expression and release of various hypothalamic peptides [e.g., neuropeptide Y (NPY), Agouti-related peptide (AgRP), α melanocyte-stimulating hormone (MSH), and melanin concentrating hormone (MCH)] that are integrated with serotonergic, catecholaminergic, and opioid signaling pathways (see below). Psychological and cultural factors also appear to play a role in the final expression of appetite. Apart from rare syndromes involving leptin, its receptor, and the melanocortin system (see below), the defects in this complex appetite control network that account for common causes of obesity are not well understood.

Energy expenditure includes the following components: (1) resting or basal metabolic rate; (2) the energy cost of metabolizing and storing food; (3) the thermic effect of exercise; and (4) adaptive thermogenesis, which varies in response to chronic caloric intake (rising with increased intake). Basal metabolic rate accounts for about 70% of daily energy expenditure, whereas active physical activity contributes 5 to 10%. Thus, a significant component of daily energy consumption is fixed.

Adaptive thermogenesis occurs in *brown adipose tissue* (BAT), which plays an important role in energy metabolism in many mammals. In contrast to white adipose tissue, which is used to store energy in the form of lipids, BAT expends stored energy as heat. A mitochondrial *uncoupling protein* (UCP-1) in BAT dissipates the hydrogen ion gradient in the oxidative respiration chain and releases energy as heat. The metabolic activity of BAT is increased by a central action of leptin, acting through the sympathetic nervous system, which heavily innervates this tissue. In rodents, BAT deficiency causes obesity and diabetes; stimulation of BAT with a specific adrenergic agonist

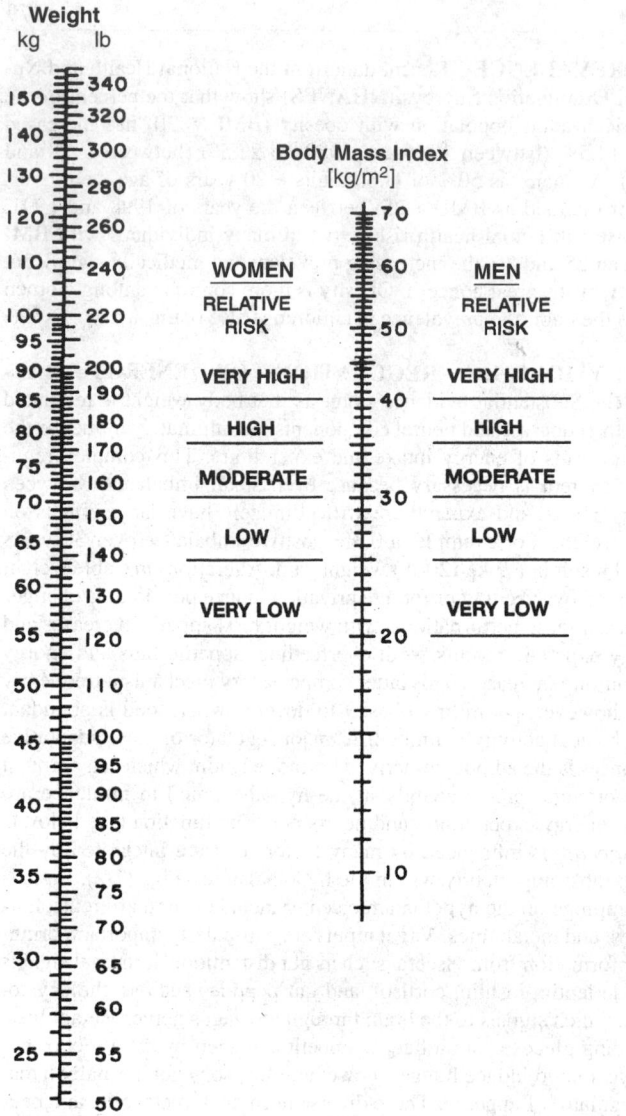

FIGURE 77-1 Nomogram for determining body mass index. To use this nomogram, place a ruler or other straight edge between the body weight (without clothes) in kilograms or pounds located on the left-hand line and the height (without shoes) in centimeters or in inches located on the right-hand line. The body mass index is read from the middle of the scale and is in metric units. (*Copyright 1978, George A. Bray, MD. Used with permission.*)

(β_3 agonist) protects against diabetes and obesity. Although BAT exists in humans (especially neonates), its physiologic role is not yet established. Homologues of UCP-1 may mediate uncoupled mitochondrial respiration in other tissues.

THE ADIPOCYTE AND ADIPOSE TISSUE Adipose tissue is composed of the lipid-storing adipose cell and a stromal/vascular compartment in which preadipocytes reside. Adipose mass increases by enlargement of adipose cells through lipid deposition, as well as by an increase in the number of adipocytes. The process by which adipose cells are derived from a mesenchymal preadipocyte involves an orchestrated series of differentiation steps mediated by a cascade of specific transcription factors. One of the key transcription factors is *peroxisome proliferator-activated receptor* γ (PPARγ), a nuclear receptor that binds the thiazoladinedione class of insulin-sensitizing drugs used in the treatment of type 2 diabetes (Chap. 333).

Although the adipocyte has generally been regarded as a storage depot for fat, it is also an endocrine cell that releases numerous molecules in a regulated fashion (Fig. 77-3). These include the energy balance-regulating hormone leptin, cytokines such as tumor necrosis factor (TNF) α, complement factors such as factor D (also known as adipsin), prothrombotic agents such as plasminogen activator inhibitor I, and a component of the blood pressure regulating system, angioten-

sinogen. These factors, and others not yet identified, play a role in the physiology of lipid homeostasis, insulin sensitivity, blood pressure control, and coagulation and are likely to contribute to obesity-related pathologies.

ETIOLOGY OF OBESITY
Though the molecular pathways regulating energy balance are beginning to be illuminated, the causes of obesity remain elusive. In part, this reflects the fact that obesity is a heterogeneous group of disorders. At one level, the pathophysiology of obesity seems simple: a chronic excess of nutrient intake relative to the level of energy expenditure. However, due to the complexity of the neuroendocrine and metabolic systems that regulate energy intake, storage, and expenditure, it has been difficult to quantitate all the relevant parameters (e.g., food intake and energy expenditure) over time in human subjects.

Role of Genes vs. Environment
Obesity is commonly seen in families. Inheritance is usually not Mendelian, however, and it is difficult to distinguish the role of genes and environmental factors. Adoptees usually resemble their biologic rather than adoptive parents with respect to obesity, providing strong support for genetic influences. Likewise, identical twins have very similar BMIs whether reared together or apart, and their BMIs are much more strongly correlated than those of dizygotic twins. These genetic effects appear to relate to both energy intake and expenditure.

Whatever the role of genes, it is clear that the environment plays a key role in obesity, as evidenced by the fact that famine prevents obesity in even the most obesity-prone individual. In addition, the recent increase in the prevalence of obesity in the United States is too rapid to be due to changes in the gene pool. Cultural factors are also important—these relate to both availability and composition of the diet and to changes in the level of physical activity.

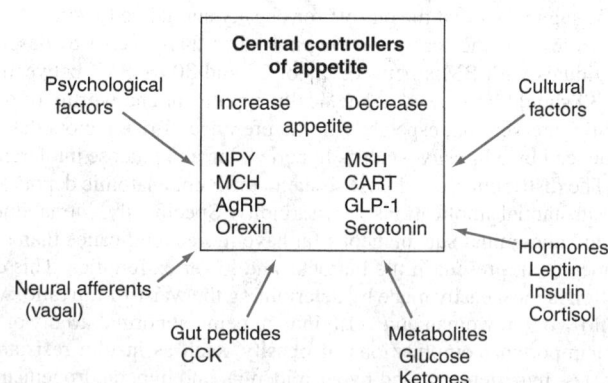

FIGURE 77-2 The factors that regulate appetite through effects on central neural circuits. Some factors that increase or decrease appetite are listed. NPY, neuropeptide Y; MCH, melanin concentrating hormone; AgRP, Agouti-related peptide; MSH, melanocyte stimulating hormone; CART, cocaine- and amphetamine-related transcript; GLP-1, glucagon-related peptide-1; CCk, cholecystokinin.

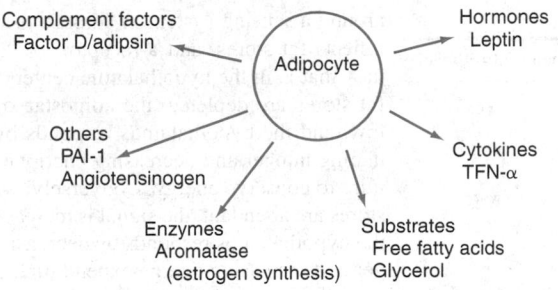

FIGURE 77-3 Factors released by the adipocyte that can affect peripheral tissues. PAI, plasminogen activator inhibitor; TNF, tumor necrosis factor.

In industrial societies, obesity is more common among poor women, whereas in underdeveloped countries, wealthier women are more often obese. In children, obesity correlates to some degree with time spent watching television. High-fat diets may promote obesity, as may diets rich in simple (as opposed to complex) carbohydrates.

Specific Genetic Syndromes Obesity in rodents has been known for many years to be caused by a number of distinct mutations distributed through the genome. Most of these single-gene mutations cause both hyperphagia and diminished energy expenditure, suggesting a link between these two parameters of energy homeostasis. Identification of the *ob* gene mutation in genetically obese (ob/ob) mice represents a major breakthrough in the field. The ob/ob mouse develops severe obesity, insulin resistance, and hyperphagia, as well as efficient metabolism (e.g., it gets fat even when given the same number of calories as lean littermates). The product of the *ob* gene is the peptide leptin, a name derived from the Greek root *leptos*, meaning thin. Leptin is secreted by adipose cells and acts through the hypothalamus. Its level of production provides an index of adipose energy stores (Fig. 77-4). High leptin levels decrease food intake and increase energy expenditure. Another mouse mutant, db/db, which is resistant to leptin, has a mutation in the leptin receptor and develops a similar syndrome. The *ob* gene is present in humans and expressed in fat. Several families with morbid, early-onset obesity due to inactivating mutations in either leptin or the leptin receptor have been described, thus demonstrating the biologic relevance of leptin in humans. The obesity in these individuals begins shortly after birth, is severe, and is accompanied by neuroendocrine abnormalities. The most prominent of these is hypogonadotropic hypogonadism, which is reversed by leptin replacement. Central hypothyroidism and growth retardation are seen in the mouse model, but their occurrence in leptin-deficient humans is less clear. To date, there is no evidence to suggest that mutations or polymorphisms in the leptin or leptin receptor genes play a prominent role in common forms of obesity.

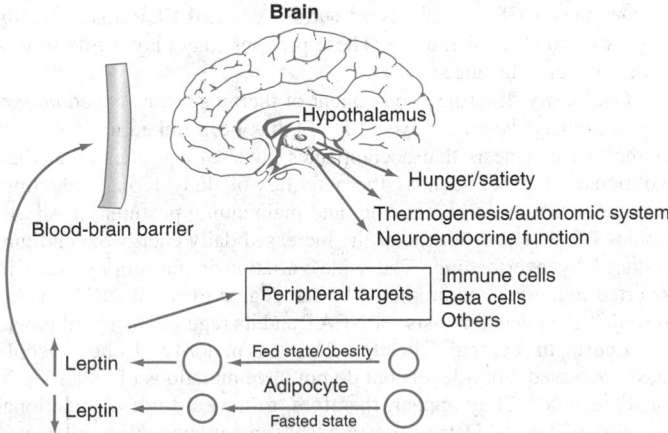

FIGURE 77-4 The physiologic system regulated by leptin. Rising or falling leptin levels act through the hypothalamus to influence appetite, energy expenditure, and neuroendocrine function and through peripheral sites to influence systems such as the immune system.

Mutations in several other genes cause severe obesity in humans (Table 77-1), each of these syndromes is rare. Mutations in the gene encoding proopiomelanocortin (POMC) cause severe obesity through failure to synthesize α-MSH, a key neuropeptide that inhibits appetite in the hypothalamus. The absence of POMC also causes secondary adrenal insufficiency due to absence of adrenocorticotropic hormone (ACTH), as well as pale skin and red hair due to absence of MSH. Proenzyme convertase 1 (PC-1) mutations are thought to cause obesity by preventing synthesis of α-MSH from its precursor peptide, POMC. α-MSH binds to the type 4 melanocortin receptor (MC4R), a key hypothalamic receptor that inhibits eating; mutations of this receptor also cause obesity. These three genetic defects, although rare, define a pathway through which leptin (by stimulating POMC and increasing MSH) restricts food intake and limits weight (Fig. 77-5).

In addition to these human obesity genes, studies in rodents reveal several other molecular candidates for hypothalamic mediators of human obesity or leanness. The *tub* gene encodes a hypothalamic peptide of unknown function; mutation of this gene causes late-onset obesity. The *fat* gene encodes carboxypeptidase E, a peptide-processing enzyme; mutation of this gene is thought to cause obesity by disrupting production of one or more neuropeptides. AgRP is coexpressed with NPY in arcuate nucleus neurons. AgRP antagonizes α-MSH action at MC4 receptors, and its overexpression induces obesity. A putative activating mutation in the gene encoding PPARγ, the adipocyte transcription factor required for adipogenesis, has been linked to obesity in a group of German subjects.

A number of complex human syndromes with defined inheritance are associated with obesity (Table 77-2). Although specific genes are undefined at present, their identification will likely enhance our understanding of more common forms of human obesity. In the Prader-Willi syndrome, obesity coexists with short stature, mental retardation, hypogonadotropic hypogonadism, hypotonia, small hands and feet, fish-shaped mouth, and hyperphagia. Most patients have a chromosome 15 deletion (Chap. 66). Laurence-Moon-Biedl syndrome involves obesity, mental retardation, retinitis pigmentosa, polydactyly, and hypogonadotropic hypogonadism.

Other Specific Syndromes Associated with Obesity • *Cushing's syndrome* Although obese patients commonly have central obesity, hypertension, and glucose intolerance, they lack other specific stigmata of Cushing's syndrome (Chap. 331). Nonetheless, a potential diagnosis of Cushing's syndrome is often entertained. Cortisol production and urinary metabolites (17OH steroids) may be increased in simple obesity. Unlike in Cushing's syndrome, however, cortisol levels in blood and urine in the basal state and in response to CRH or ACTH are normal; the overnight 1-mg dexamethasone suppression test is normal in 90%, with the remainder being normal on a standard 2-day low-dose dexamethasone suppression test.

Hypothyroidism The possibility of hypothyroidism should be considered when evaluating obesity, but it is an uncommon cause of obesity; hypothyroidism is easily ruled out by measuring thyroid stimulating hormone (TSH). Much of the weight gain that occurs in hypothyroidism is due to myxedema (Chap. 330).

Insulinoma Patients with insulinoma often gain weight as a result of overeating to avoid hypoglycemia symptoms (Chap. 334). The increased substrate plus high insulin levels promotes energy storage in fat. This can be marked in some individuals but is modest in most.

Craniopharyngioma and other disorders involving the hypothalamus Whether through tumors, trauma, or inflammation, hypothalamic dysfunction of systems controlling satiety, hunger, and energy expenditure can cause varying degrees of obesity (Chap. 328). It is uncommon to identify a discrete anatomic basis for these disorders. Subtle hypothalamic dysfunction is probably a more common cause of obesity than can be documented using currently available techniques. Growth hormone (GH), which exerts lipolytic activity, is diminished in obesity and increases with weight loss. Despite low growth hormone levels, insulin-like growth factor (IGF) I (somato-

Table 77-1 Some Obesity Genes in Humans and Mice

Gene	Gene Product	Mechanism of Obesity	In Human	In Rodent
Lep (ob)	Leptin, a fat-derived hormone	Mutation prevents leptin from delivering satiety signal; brain perceives starvation	Yes	Yes
LepR (db)	Leptin receptor	Same as above	Yes	Yes
POMC	Proopiomelanocortin, a precursor of several hormones and neuropeptides	Mutation prevents synthesis of melanocyte-stimulating hormone (MSH), a satiety signal	Yes	Yes
MC4R	Type 4 receptor for MSH	Mutation prevents reception of satiety signal from MSH	Yes	Yes
AgRP	Agouti-related peptide, a neuropeptide expressed in the hypothalamus	Overexpression inhibits signal through MC4R	No	Yes
PC-1	Prohormone convertase 1, a processing enzyme	Mutation prevents synthesis of neuropeptide, probably MSH	Yes	No
Fat	Carboxypeptidase E, a processing enzyme	Same as above	No	Yes
Tub	Tub, a hypothalamic protein of unknown function	Hypothalamic dysfunction	No	Yes
PPARγ	Peroxisome proliferator activated receptor, a transcription factor that promotes adipogenesis and modulates insulin action	Unknown	Yes	No

medin) production is normal, suggesting that GH suppression is a compensatory response to increased nutritional supply.

Pathogenesis of Common Obesity Obesity can result from increased energy intake, decreased energy expenditure, or a combination of the two. Thus, identifying the etiology of obesity should involve measurements of both parameters. However, it is nearly impossible to perform direct and accurate measurements of energy intake in free-living individuals. Obese people, in particular, appear to underreport intake. Measurements of chronic energy expenditure have only recently become available using doubly-labeled water or metabolic chamber/rooms. In subjects at stable weight and body composition, energy intake equals expenditure. Consequently, these techniques allow determination of energy intake in free-living individuals. The level of energy expenditure differs in established obesity, during periods of weight gain or loss, and in the pre- or postobese state. Studies that fail to take note of this phenomenon are not easily interpreted.

There is increased interest in the concept of a body weight "set point." This idea is supported by physiologic mechanisms centered around a sensing system in adipose tissue that reflects fat stores, and a receptor, or "adipostat," that is in the hypothalamic centers. When fat stores are depleted, the adipostat signal is low, and the hypothalamus responds by stimulating hunger and decreasing energy expenditure to conserve energy. Conversely, when fat stores are abundant, the signal is increased, and the hypothalamus responds by decreasing hunger and increasing energy expenditure. The recent discovery of the *ob* gene, and its product leptin, provides a molecular basis for this physiologic concept (see above).

What Is the Status of Food Intake in Obesity (Do the Obese Eat More Than the Lean?) This question has stimulated much debate, due in part to the methodologic difficulties inherent in determining food intake. Many obese individuals believe that they eat small quantities of food, and this claim has often been supported by the results of food intake questionnaires. However, it is now established that average energy expenditure increases as people get more obese, due primarily to the fact that metabolically active lean tissue mass increases with obesity. Given the laws of thermodynamics, the obese person must therefore eat more than the average lean person to maintain their increased weight. It may be the case, however, that a subset of individuals who are predisposed to obesity have the capacity to become obese initially without an absolute increase in caloric consumption.

What Is the State of Energy Expenditure in Obesity? The average total daily energy expenditure is higher in obese than lean individuals when measured at stable weight. However, energy expenditure falls as weight is lost, due in part to loss of lean body mass and to decreased sympathetic nerve activity. When reduced to near-normal weight and maintained there for a while, (some) obese individuals have lower energy expenditure than (some) lean individuals. There is also a tendency for those who develop obesity as infants or children to have lower resting energy expenditure rates than those who remain lean.

The physiologic basis for variable rates of energy expenditure (at a given body weight and level of energy intake) is essentially unknown. A mutation in the human β_3 adrenergic receptor may be associated with increased risk of obesity and/or insulin resistance in certain (but not all) populations. Homologues of the BAT uncoupling protein, named UCP-2 and UCP-3, have been identified in both rodents and humans. UCP-2 is expressed widely, whereas UCP-3 is primarily expressed in skeletal muscle. These proteins may play a role in disordered energy balance.

One newly described component of thermogenesis, called *nonexercise activity thermogenesis* (NEAT), has been linked to obesity. It is the thermogenesis that accompanies physical activities other than volitional exercise, such as the activities of daily living, fidgeting, spontaneous muscle contraction, and maintaining posture. NEAT accounts for about two-thirds of the increased daily energy expenditure induced by overfeeding. The wide variation in fat storage seen in overfed individuals is predicted by the degree to which NEAT is induced. The molecular basis for NEAT and its regulation are unknown.

Leptin in Typical Obesity The vast majority of obese people have increased leptin levels but do not have mutations of either leptin or its receptor. They appear, therefore, to have a form of functional "leptin resistance." Data suggesting that some individuals produce less leptin per unit fat mass than others or have a form of relative leptin deficiency that predisposes to obesity are at present contradictory and unsettled. The mechanism for leptin resistance, and whether it can be overcome by raising leptin levels, is not yet established. Some data

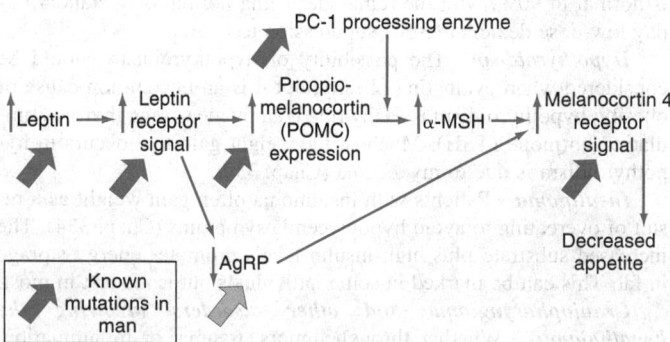

FIGURE 77-5 A central pathway through which leptin acts to regulate appetite and body weight. Leptin signals through proopiomelanocortin (POMC) neurons in the hypothalamus to induce increased production of α melanocyte stimulating hormone (α-MSH), requiring the processing enzyme PC-1 (proenzyme convertase 1). α-MSH acts as an agonist on melanocortin-4 receptors to inhibit appetite, and the neuropeptide AgRp (Agouti-related peptide) acts as an antagonist of this receptor. Mutations that cause obesity in humans are indicated by the solid blue arrows.

suggest that leptin may not effectively cross the blood-brain barrier as levels rise. It is also possible that leptin signaling inhibitors are involved in the leptin-resistant state.

PATHOLOGIC CONSEQUENCES OF OBESITY

Obesity has major adverse effects on health. Morbidly obese individuals (>200% ideal body weight) have as much as a twelvefold increase in mortality. Morality rates rise as obesity increases, particularly when obesity is associated with increased intra-abdominal fat (see above). It is also apparent that the degree to which obesity affects particular organ systems is influenced by susceptibility genes that vary in the population.

Insulin Resistance and Type 2 Diabetes Mellitus Hyperinsulinemia and insulin resistance are pervasive features of obesity, increasing with weight gain and diminishing with weight loss. Insulin resistance is more strongly linked to intraabdominal fat than to fat in other depots. The molecular link between obesity and insulin resistance has been sought for many years, with the major factors under investigation being: (1) insulin itself, by inducing receptor downregulation; (2) free fatty acids, known to be increased and capable of impairing insulin action; and (3) the cytokine TNF-α, which is produced by adipocytes, overexpressed in obese adipocytes, and capable of inhibiting insulin action. Despite insulin resistance, most obese individuals do not develop diabetes, suggesting that the onset of diabetes requires an interaction between obesity-induced insulin resistance and other factors that predispose to diabetes, such as impaired insulin secretion (Chap. 333). Obesity, however, is a major risk factor for diabetes, and as many as 80% of patients with type 2 diabetes mellitus are obese. Weight loss, even of modest degree, is associated with increased insulin sensitivity and often improves glucose control in diabetes.

Reproductive Disorders Disorders that affect the reproductive axis are associated with obesity in both men and women. Male hypogonadism is associated with increased adipose tissue, often distributed in a pattern more typical of females. In men >160% ideal body weight, plasma testosterone and sex hormone–binding globulin (SHBG) are often reduced, and estrogen levels (derived from conversion of adrenal androgens in adipose tissue) are increased (Chap. 335). Gynecomastia may be seen. However, masculinization, libido, potency, and spermatogenesis are preserved in most of these individuals. Free testosterone may be decreased in morbidly obese men whose weight exceeds 200% ideal body weight.

Obesity has long been associated with menstrual abnormalities in women, particularly in women with upper body obesity (Chaps. 52 and 336). Common findings are increased androgen production, decreased SHBG, and increased peripheral conversion of androgen to estrogen. Most obese women with oligomenorrhea have the polycystic ovarian syndrome (PCOS), with its associated anovulation and ovarian hyperandrogenism; 40% of women with PCOS are obese. Interestingly, most nonobese women with PCOS are also insulin-resistant, suggesting that insulin resistance, hyperinsulinemia, or the combination of the two are causative or contribute to the ovarian pathophysiology in PCOS in both obese and lean individuals. In obese women with PCOS, weight loss or treatment with insulin-sensitizing drugs often restores normal menses, along with a fall in estrone levels and normalized gonadotropin secretion. The increased conversion of androstenedione to estrogen, which occurs to a greater degree in women with lower body obesity, may contribute to the increased incidence of uterine cancer in postmenopausal women with obesity.

Cardiovascular Disease The Framingham Study revealed that obesity was an independent risk factor for the 26-year incidence of cardiovascular disease in men and women [including coronary disease, stroke, and congestive heart failure (CHF)]. The waist/hip ratio may be the best predictor of these risks. When the additional effects of hypertension and glucose intolerance associated with obesity are included, the adverse impact of obesity is even more evident. The effect of obesity on cardiovascular mortality in women may be seen at BMIs as low as 25. Obesity, especially abdominal obesity, is associated with an atherogenic lipid profile, with increased low-density lipoprotein (LDL) cholesterol, very low density lipoprotein and triglyceride, and decreased high-density lipoprotein cholesterol (Chap. 344). Obesity is also associated with hypertension. Measurement of blood pressure in the obese requires use of a larger cuff size to avoid artifactual increases. Obesity-induced hypertension is associated with increased peripheral resistance and cardiac output, increased sympathetic nervous system tone, increased salt sensitivity, and insulin-mediated salt retention; it is often responsive to modest weight loss.

Pulmonary Disease Obesity may be associated with a number of pulmonary abnormalities. These include reduced chest wall compliance, increased work of breathing, increased minute ventilation due to increased metabolic rate, and decreased total lung capacity and functional residual capacity (Chap. 250). Severe obesity may be associated with obstructive sleep apnea and the "obesity hypoventilation syndrome" (Chap. 263). Sleep apnea can be obstructive (most common),

Table 77-2 A Comparison of Syndromes of Obesity—Hypogonadism and Mental Retardation

Feature	Prader-Willi	Laurence-Moon-Biedl	Ahlstrom	Cohen	Carpenter
Inheritance	Sporadic; two-thirds have defect	Autosomal recessive	Autosomal recessive	Probably autosomal recessive	Autosomal recessive
Stature	Short	Normal; infrequently short	Normal; infrequently short	Short or tall	Normal
Obesity	Generalized Moderate to severe Onset 1–3 yrs	Generalized Early onset, 1–2 yrs	Truncal Early onset, 2–5 yrs	Truncal Mid-childhood, age 5	Truncal, gluteal
Craniofacies	Narrow bifrontal diameter Almond-shaped eyes Strabismus V-shaped mouth High-arched palate	Not distinctive	Not distinctive	High nasal bridge Arched palate Open mouth Short philtrum	Acrocephaly Flat nasal bridge High-arched palate
Limbs	Small hands and feet Hypotonia	Polydactyly	No abnormalities	Hypotonia Narrow hands and feet	Polydactyly Syndactyly Genu valgum
Reproductive status	1° Hypogonadism	1° Hypogonadism	Hypogonadism in males but not in females	Normal gonadal function or hypogonadotrophic hypogonadism	2° Hypogonadism
Other features	Enamel hypoplasia Hyperphagia Temper tantrums Nasal speech			Dysplastic ears Delayed puberty	
Mental retardation	Mild to moderate		Normal intelligence	Mild	Slight

central, or mixed. Weight loss (10 to 20 kg) can bring substantial improvement, as can major weight loss following gastric bypass or restrictive surgery. Continuous positive airway pressure has been used with some success.

Gallstones Obesity is associated with enhanced biliary secretion of cholesterol, supersaturation of bile, and a higher incidence of gallstones, particularly cholesterol gallstones (Chap. 302). A person 50% above ideal body weight has about a sixfold increased incidence of symptomatic gallstones. Paradoxically, fasting increases supersaturation of bile by decreasing the phospholipid component. Fasting-induced cholecystitis is a complication of extreme diets.

Cancer Obesity in males is associated with higher mortality from cancer of the colon, rectum, and prostate; obesity in females is associated with higher mortality from cancer of the gallbladder, bile ducts, breasts, endometrium, cervix, and ovaries. Some of the latter may be due to increased rates of conversion of androstenedione to estrone in adipose tissue of obese individuals.

Bone, Joint, and Cutaneous Disease Obesity is associated with an increased risk of osteoarthritis, no doubt partly due to the trauma of added weight bearing. The prevalence of gout may also be increased (Chap. 322). Among the skin problems associated with obesity is acanthosis nigricans, manifested by darkening and thickening of the skin folds on the neck, elbows, and dorsal interphalangeal spaces. Acanthosis reflects the severity of underlying insulin resistance and diminishes with weight loss. Friability of skin may be increased, especially in skin folds, enhancing the risk of fungal and yeast infections. Finally, venous stasis is increased in the obese.

℞ **TREATMENT** Obesity is a chronic medical condition. Successful treatment, defined as the sustained attainment of normal body weight without producing unacceptable treatment-induced morbidity, is rarely achieved in clinical practice. Many approaches produce short-term weight loss, and this has clear benefits for associated morbidities such as hypertension and diabetes. Despite the fact that sustained weight loss is uncommon, enormous resources are expended in pursuit of this goal.

Treatment goals should be guided by the health risks of obesity in any given individual (Fig. 77-6). The clinician should always consider the possibility that an individual has an identified cause of obesity, such as hypothyroidism, hypercortisolism, male hypogonadism, insulinoma, or central nervous system disease that affects hypothalamic function. Although they are infrequent causes of obesity, specific therapy may be available.

Behavior Modification The principles of behavior modification provide the underpinnings for many current programs of weight reduction. Typically, the patient is requested to monitor and record the circumstances related to eating, and rewards are designed to modify maladaptive behaviors. Patients may benefit from counseling offered in a stable group setting for extended periods of time, including after weight loss.

Diet Reduced caloric intake is the cornerstone of obesity treatment. The fundamental goal is the sustained reduction of energy intake below that of energy expenditure. The difficulty in achieving this goal has led to a wide array of suggested diets that vary in recommended calorie content (from total fasting to mild reductions), as well as specific food content and form (e.g., liquid vs. solid). There is no scientific evidence to validate the utility of specific "fad diets." The main diet regimens in use follow several general facts relevant to food intake and weight loss. First, a deficit of 7500 kcal will produce a weight loss of approximately 1 kg. Therefore, eating 100 kcal/d less for a year should cause a 5-kg weight loss, and a deficit of 1000 kcal/d should cause a loss of approximately 1 kg per week. The rate of weight loss on a given caloric intake is related to the rate of energy expenditure. Because obese individuals have a higher metabolic rate than lean individuals, and because men have a higher metabolic rate than women

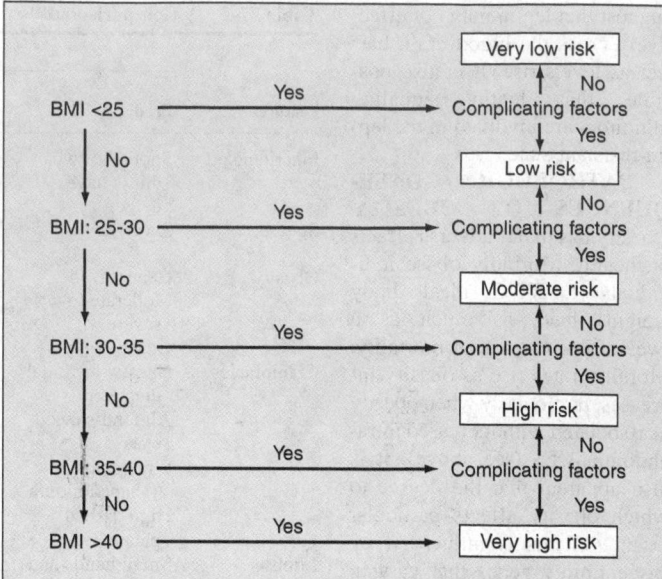

FIGURE 77-6 Risk classification algorithm. The patient is first placed into a category based on body mass index. The presence or absence of complicating factors determines the degree of health risk. Complicating factors include elevated abdominal-gluteal ratio (male: 0.95, female: 0.85), diabetes mellitus, hypertension, hyperlipidemia, male sex, and age <40. (*Copyright 1987, George A. Bray, MD. Used with permission.*)

(due to their greater lean body mass), the rate of weight loss is greater among the more obese and among men (relative to women). With chronic caloric restriction, metabolic rate diminishes, but because of reduced lean body mass (along with much greater loss in fat mass) and possibly because of other adaptations. This fall in metabolic rate with food restriction slows the rate of weight loss on a constant diet. With total starvation or diets restricted to <600 kcal/d, initial weight loss over the first week results predominantly from natriuresis and the loss of fluids.

Very low energy diets (e.g., 400 to 600 kcal/d) are widely used. The liquid protein diets popularized in the 1970s were proved to be unsafe, causing >60 deaths. Life-threatening arrhythmias were documented in the clinical research setting, a consequence of both low-quality protein and deficiencies of vitamins, minerals, and trace elements. These types of diets have now been substantially modified. A very low energy diet consisting of 45 to 70 g high-quality protein, 30 to 50 g carbohydrate, and approximately 2 g fat per day, as well as supplements of vitamins, minerals, and trace elements, appears to be safe in selected patients under medical supervision. Patients should not be started on such diets unless they are >130% of their ideal body weight. Contraindications include pregnancy, cancer, recent myocardial infarction, cerebrovascular disease, hepatic disease, or untreated psychiatric disease. When used in patients with diabetes who are receiving insulin or oral agent therapy, close supervision is required and diabetic treatment may need to be adjusted. Whenever possible, exercise regimens and behavioral modification approaches should be used in conjunction with the diet.

Advantages of very low calorie diets are the greater rate of weight loss compared to less restrictive diets, as well as the possible beneficial effect of hunger suppression brought about by the production of ketones. In patients on such diets, blood pressure, blood glucose, cholesterol, and triglyceride levels fall, and pulmonary function and exercise tolerance improve. Sleep apnea may improve within a few weeks. Complications of these very low energy diets are usually minor and include fatigue, constipation or diarrhea, dry skin, hair loss, menstrual irregularities, orthostatic dizziness, and difficulty concentrating. Cholelithiasis and pancreatitis may occur when such diets are interrupted by binge eating; gallstones have been shown to develop in as many as 25% of patients while on the diet.

Low-calorie diets, >800 kcal/d, are applicable to most patients and have fewer restrictions than the very low calorie diets. Considerable controversy has attended the question of which diet composition is most appropriate for promoting weight loss. Though commonly recommended, benefits resulting from very low fat diets are modest at best. Nonetheless, the health effects of low-fat diets—apart from curbing obesity—may be important. A diet rich in fruits, vegetables, and whole grains may promote weight loss and is preferable to low-fat diets in which large amounts of simple carbohydrates are substituted for fats. The latter may actually promote obesity. Some have advocated diets with protein replacement of simple carbohydrates in an effort to minimize insulin production. The efficacy of this strategy, aside from overall calorie reduction, is unknown.

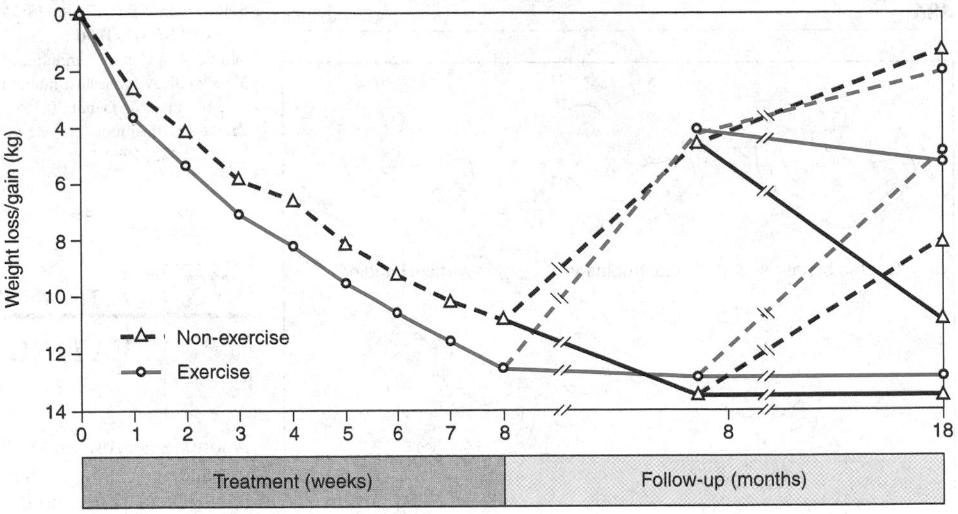

FIGURE 77-7 Weight loss and exercise. During the first 8 weeks, subjects were divided into two groups, one treated with diet and the other with diet plus exercise, with no difference in weight loss. Thereafter the subjects who exercised maintained better weight loss than those that did not. (*After KN Pavlou et al: Am J Clin Nutr 49:1115, 1989.*)

Exercise Exercise is an important component of the overall approach to treating obesity. Increased energy expenditure is the most obvious mechanism for an effect of exercise. The impact of an exercise regimen as a sole therapy of obesity has been difficult to document. On the other hand, exercise appears to be a valuable means to sustain diet therapy (Fig. 77-7). Even if exercise had no such salutary effect, it would be valuable in the obese individual for its effects on cardiovascular tone and blood pressure. Because many obese individuals have not engaged in exercise on a regular basis and may have cardiovascular risk factors, it should be introduced gradually and under medical supervision, especially in the most obese individuals.

Drugs Unfortunately, drug treatment of obesity is rarely efficacious. Despite short-term benefits, medication-induced weight loss is often associated with rebound weight gain after the cessation of drug use, side effects from the medications, and the potential for drug abuse. Given the need for effective therapies, many possible compounds have been evaluated. On the basis of placebo-controlled trials, the U.S. Food and Drug Administration (FDA) approved several amphetamine-like agents for short-term use. Phentermine is an amphetamine-like drug with low addictive potential that has shown modest efficacy (10 vs. 4.4 kg of weight loss over a 24-week period in well-controlled study). This class of drugs is thought to act centrally by reducing appetite. Effects on energy expenditure are less clear. Over-the-counter drugs, such as phenylpropanolamine HCl, have similar efficacy to prescription appetite suppressants in short-term studies. Drugs that promote serotonin release or inhibit serotonin reuptake, such as fenfluramine, also have modest efficacy. When fenfluramine was administered together with phentermine, as "fen-phen," the combination was widely used based on controlled trials that demonstrated modest but definite efficacy. However, the risk of primary pulmonary hypertension was increased up to 20-fold in association with this treatment. The FDA withdrew approval of the fen-phen combination in 1997 when reports suggested an association with right- and left-sided valvular heart disease. The histopathologic features of the valvular disease are similar to those seen in carcinoid syndrome and are thought to result from fenfluramine. Though the true incidence and long-term effects of these valvular lesions are currently unknown, the occurrence of this complication has been verified in multiple studies.

Sibutramine is a novel central reuptake inhibitor of both norepinephrine and serotonin. Using a once-daily dose over 24 weeks, it produced a 7% weight loss in a double-blind, placebo-controlled trial. It lowered cholesterol and triglyceride levels and exhibited similar clinical efficacy to fenfluramine. Sibutramine increases pulse and blood pressure in some patients, and long-term safety is not established. Orlistat is an inhibitor of intestinal lipase that causes modest weight loss due to drug-induced fat malabsorption. A randomized, double-blind trial over 2 years revealed modest weight loss (8.7 kg for 120 mg orlistat versus 5.8 kg from diet alone) during the first year and better maintenance of weight loss in a second year compared to the placebo-treated group (3.2 kg regained versus 5.6 kg regained for placebo). LDL cholesterol and insulin levels were also reduced. In patients with obesity and type 2 diabetes mellitus, the antidiabetic medication metformin tends to decrease body weight. The mechanism appears to involve inhibition of appetite. Thyroid hormone has little place in the treatment of obesity, as the vast majority of obese individuals are euthyroid. It promotes loss of lean body mass and raises the risk of complications from the hyperthyroid state.

β_3-Adrenergic receptor agonists may provide a new treatment approach for obesity. Drugs of this class are in clinical trials. In animals, β_3 agonists promote leanness by stimulating thermogenesis in BAT; they also stimulate lipolysis in white adipose tissue. These drugs also reduce insulin resistance and lower blood glucose in animal models by a mechanism that is not yet defined. Recombinant human leptin is also in clinical trials. In the rare cases of leptin deficiency caused by mutations of the leptin gene, the administration of recombinant leptin is highly effective. Preliminary reports suggest that the response to leptin is limited or absent in common causes of obesity (which are associated with hyperleptinemia and leptin resistance). New drugs are also being developed based on insights into central pathways that regulate body weight. These include antagonists for NPY receptors (subtypes Y1, Y5) and agonists for melanocortin 4 receptors.

Surgery Morbid obesity, commonly defined as either 45 kg (100 lb) or 100% above ideal body weight, is estimated to increase mortality by as much as twelvefold in men between 25 and 34 years of age and sixfold between 35 and 45 years of age. Deaths from cardiovascular disease, diabetes, and accidents have been documented. In response to ineffective treatment using diet, exercise, and available drugs, surgical approaches have been tried. The potential benefits of surgery include major weight loss and improvement in hypertension, diabetes, sleep apnea, CHF, angina, hyperlipidemia, and venous disease. Many different approaches have been used, often without adequate assessment of efficacy and complications. Jejunoileal bypass surgery has largely been abandoned because of complications, which have included electrolyte disturbances, nephrolithiasis, gallstones, gastric ulcers, arthritis, and hepatic dysfunction, with cirrhosis occurring in as many as 7% of patients. Two procedures in common use today

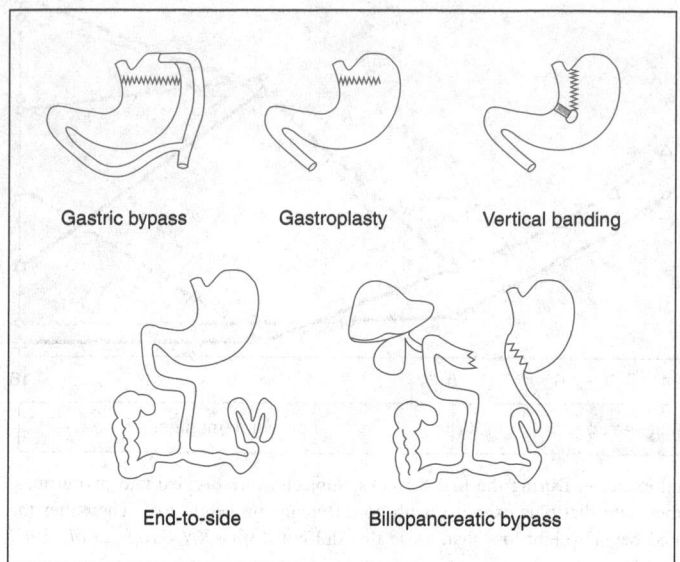

FIGURE 77-8 Examples of operative interventions used for surgical manipulation of the gastrointestinal tract.

are the vertical-banded gastroplasty and the Roux-en-Y gastric bypass (Fig. 77-8).

Following the National Institutes of Health Consensus Conference on Gastrointestinal Surgery for Severe Obesity in 1991, it was recommended that suitable patients be selected using the following criteria: (1) the presence of 45 kg (100 lb) or 100% above ideal body weight, or one or more severe medical conditions related to refractory obesity; (2) repeated failures of other therapeutic approaches; (3) at eligible weight for 3 to 5 years; (4) capability of tolerating surgery; (5) absence of alcoholism, other addictions, or major psychopathology; and (6) prior clearance by a psychiatrist. It is recommended that an appropriately experienced surgeon work together with nutritionists and other support personnel; evaluation and follow-up programs should be monitored closely.

ACKNOWLEDGMENT
The author acknowledges the contributions of Dr. George A. Bray, who wrote this chapter in the 14th edition.

BIBLIOGRAPHY

Bray GA, Greenway FL: Current and potential drugs for treatment of obesity. Endocr Rev 20:805, 1999

Burton BT et al: Report of Consensus Proceedings. Health implications of obesity: An NIH Consensus Development Conference. Int J Obesity 9:155, 1985

Connolly HM et al: Valvular heart disease associated with fenfluramine-phentermine. N Engl J Med 337:581, 1997

Flier JS: What's in a name? In search of leptin's physiologic role. J Clin Endocrinol Metab 83:1407, 1998

Gastrointestinal surgery for severe obesity: Proceedings of an NIH Consensus Development Conference, March 25–27, 1991. Am J Clin Nutr 55 (Suppl 2):615S, 1992

Heymsfield SB et al: Recombinant leptin for weight loss in obese and lean adults: A randomized, controlled, dose-escalation trial. JAMA 282:1568, 1999

Hotamisligil GS et al: Tumor necrosis factor α: A key component of the obesity-diabetes link. Diabetes 43:1271, 1994

Krude et al: Severe early onset obesity, adrenal insufficiency and red hair pigmentation caused by POMC mutations in humans. Nat Genet 19(2):155, 1998

Kuczmarski RJ et al: Increasing prevalence of overweight among US adults: JAMA 272:205, 1994

Levine JA: Role of nonexercise activity thermogenesis in resistance to fat gain in humans. Science 283:212, 1999

Montague CT: Congenital leptin deficiency is associated with severe early onset obesity in humans. Nature 387:903, 1998

Pi-Sunyer FX: Short-term medical benefits and adverse effects of weight loss. Ann Intern Med 119:722, 1993

Rosenbaum M et al: Obesity. N Engl J Med 337:396, 1997

Spiegelman BM, Flier JS: Adipogenesis and obesity: Rounding out the big picture. Cell 87:377, 1996

Willett WC et al: Guidelines for healthy weight. N Engl J Med 341:427, 1999

Yeo et al: A frameshift mutation in MC4R associated with dominantly inherited human obesity. Nat Genet 20:111, 1998

Zhang Y: Positional cloning of the mouse obese gene and its human homologue. Nature 372:425, 1994

78   *B. Timothy Walsh*

EATING DISORDERS

Anorexia nervosa and bulimia nervosa are characterized by severe disturbances of eating behavior. The salient feature of *anorexia nervosa* is a refusal to maintain a minimally normal body weight. *Bulimia nervosa* is characterized by recurrent episodes of binge eating followed by abnormal compensatory behaviors, such as self-induced vomiting. Anorexia nervosa and bulimia nervosa are closely related. Both occur primarily among previously healthy young women who become overly concerned with body shape and weight. Many patients with bulimia nervosa have past histories of anorexia nervosa, and many patients with anorexia nervosa engage in binge eating and purging behavior. In the current diagnostic system, the critical distinction between anorexia nervosa and bulimia nervosa depends on body weight: patients with anorexia nervosa are, by definition, significantly underweight, whereas the weights of patients with bulimia nervosa are in the normal range or above.

Another syndrome of disturbed eating behavior has been described recently: *Binge eating disorder* is characterized by repeated episodes of binge eating, similar to those of bulimia nervosa, in the absence of inappropriate compensatory behavior. Patients with binge eating disorder are typically middle-aged men or women with significant obesity. They have an increased frequency of anxiety and depression compared to similarly obese patients without binge eating disorder. It is not known whether patients with binge eating disorder are at increased risk for medical complications or what treatments are most useful.

EPIDEMIOLOGY

In women, the full syndrome of anorexia nervosa occurs with a lifetime prevalence of approximately 0.5%; bulimia nervosa occurs with a lifetime prevalence of 1 to 3%. Variants of these eating disorders with only some features of anorexia nervosa or bulimia nervosa are much more common and occur in 5 to 10% of young women. Both anorexia nervosa and bulimia nervosa also occur in males but at frequencies approximately one-tenth of those in females.

Anorexia nervosa and bulimia nervosa are more prevalent in cultures where food is plentiful and in which being thin is associated with attractiveness. These disorders are more frequent among young women who place a premium on thinness, such as ballet dancers and models. The incidence of anorexia nervosa appears to have increased in recent decades. The frequency of bulimia nervosa increased dramatically in the early 1970s and 1980s but may have declined somewhat in recent years.

DIAGNOSIS

The diagnosis of eating disorders is based on the presence of characteristic behavioral, psychological, and physical attributes (Tables 78-1 and 78-2). Widely accepted diagnostic criteria are provided by the American Psychiatric Association's *Diagnostic and Statistical Manual of Mental Disorders* (DSM-IV).

ANOREXIA NERVOSA For anorexia nervosa, these criteria include weight <85% of the expected weight for age and height, which

Table 78-1   Diagnostic Criteria for Anorexia Nervosa

1. Refusal to maintain body weight at or above a minimally normal weight for age and height (e.g., weight loss leading to maintenance of body weight <85% of that expected; or failure to make expected weight gain during period of growth, leading to body weight <85% of that expected).
2. Intense fear of gaining weight or becoming fat, even though underweight.
3. Disturbance in the way in which one's body weight or shape is experienced, undue influence of body weight or shape on self-evaluation, or denial of the seriousness of the current low body weight.
4. In postmenarchal females, amenorrhea, i.e., the absence of at least three consecutive menstrual cycles. (A woman is considered to have amenorrhea if her periods occur only following hormone, e.g., estrogen, administration.)

Specify type:

Restricting type: During the episode of anorexia nervosa, the person has not regularly engaged in binge-eating or purging behavior (i.e., self-induced vomiting or the misuse of laxatives, diuretics or enemas).

Binge eating/purging type: During the episode of anorexia nervosa, the person has regularly engaged in binge-eating or purging behavior (i.e., self-induced vomiting or the misuse of laxatives, diuretics, or enemas).

SOURCE: From the *Diagnostic and Statistical Manual of Mental Disorders*, 4th ed, Washington, DC, American Psychiatric Association, 1994.

is roughly equivalent to a body mass index (BMI) of 18.5 kg/m² for adult women. This weight criterion is somewhat arbitrary, so that a patient who meets all other diagnostic criteria but weighs between 85 and 90% of expected would still merit the diagnosis of anorexia nervosa. Despite being underweight, patients with anorexia nervosa are irrationally afraid of gaining weight, often out of a concern that weight gain will get "out of control." They also exhibit a distortion of body image (criterion 3, Table 78-1), which may express itself in several ways. For example, despite being emaciated, patients with anorexia nervosa may believe that their body as a whole, or some part of their body, is too fat and experience additional weight loss as a highly rewarding achievement. The current diagnostic criteria require that women with anorexia nervosa not have spontaneous menses, but occasional patients with the characteristics and complications of anorexia nervosa describe regular menses. Two mutually exclusive subtypes of anorexia nervosa are specified in DSM-IV. Patients whose weight loss is maintained primarily by caloric restriction, perhaps augmented by excessive exercise, are considered to have the "restricting" subtype of anorexia nervosa. The "binge eating/purging" subtype is characterized

Table 78-2   Diagnostic Criteria for Bulimia Nervosa

1. Recurrent episodes of binge eating. An episode of binge eating is characterized by both of the following:
   a. Eating, in a discrete period of time (e.g., within any 2-h period), an amount of food that is definitely larger than most people would eat during a similar period of time and under similar circumstances.
   b. A sense of lack of control over eating during the episode (e.g., a feeling that one cannot stop eating or control what or how much one is eating).
2. Recurrent inappropriate compensatory behavior in order to prevent weight gain, such as self-induced vomiting, misuse of laxatives or diuretics, enemas, or other medications; fasting; or excessive exercise.
3. The binge eating and inappropriate compensatory behaviors both occur, on average, at least twice a week for 3 months.
4. Self-evaluation is unduly influenced by body shape and weight.
5. The disturbance does not occur exclusively during episodes of anorexia nervosa.

Specify type:

Purging type: during the current episode of bulimia nervosa, the person has regularly engaged in self-induced vomiting or the misuse of laxatives, diuretics, or enemas.

Nonpurging type: during the current episode of bulimia nervosa, the person has used other inappropriate compensatory behaviors such as fasting or excessive exercise but has not regularly engaged in self-induced vomiting or the misuse of laxatives, diuretics, or enemas.

SOURCE: From the *Diagnostic and Statistical Manual of Mental Disorders*, 4th ed, Washington, DC, American Psychiatric Association, 1994.

by self-induced vomiting or laxative abuse. Patients with the binge/purge subtype are more prone to develop electrolyte imbalances, are more emotionally labile, and are more likely to have other problems with impulse control, such as drug abuse.

The diagnosis of anorexia nervosa can usually be made confidently on the basis of history when significant weight loss is accomplished by restrictive dieting and excessive exercise and is accompanied by a marked reluctance to gain weight. Patients with anorexia nervosa often deny that they have a serious problem and may be brought to medical attention by concerned family or friends. In atypical presentations, other causes of significant weight loss in previously healthy young people should be considered, including inflammatory bowel disease, gastric outlet obstruction, central nervous system (CNS) tumors, and neoplasm (Chap. 43).

BULIMIA NERVOSA   The critical diagnostic features of bulimia nervosa are repeated episodes of binge eating followed by inappropriate and abnormal behaviors aimed at avoiding weight gain. During binges, patients with this disorder tend to consume large amounts of sweet foods with a high fat content, such as dessert items. The most frequent compensatory behaviors are self-induced vomiting and laxative abuse, but a wide variety of techniques have been described, including the omission of insulin injections by diabetics. Typically, patients with bulimia nervosa are ashamed of their behavior and endeavor to keep their disorder hidden from family and friends. Like patients with anorexia nervosa, those with bulimia nervosa place an unusual emphasis on weight and shape as a basis for their self-esteem.

As in anorexia nervosa, there are two mutually exclusive subtypes of bulimia nervosa. Patients with the "purging" subtype utilize compensatory behaviors that directly rid the body of calories or fluids (e.g., self-induced vomiting, laxative or diuretic abuse), whereas those with the "nonpurging" subtype attempt to compensate for binges by fasting or by excessive exercise. Patients with the nonpurging subtype tend to be heavier and are less prone to fluid and electrolyte disturbances.

The diagnosis of bulimia nervosa requires a candid history from the patient detailing recurrent, large eating binges followed by the purposeful use of inappropriate mechanisms to avoid weight gain. Most patients with bulimia nervosa who present for treatment are distressed by their inability to control their eating behavior but are able to provide such details if queried in a supportive and nonjudgmental fashion.

ETIOLOGY

The fundamental etiology of the eating disorders is unknown but is believed to involve a combination of psychological, biologic, and cultural risk factors. Many of these risk factors, such as sexual or physical abuse and a family history of mood disturbance or substance abuse, are best viewed as nonspecific risk factors that increase vulnerability to a range of psychiatric disorders. Other factors appear to be more specific to the development of an eating disorder.

Patients who develop anorexia nervosa are inclined to be more obsessional and perfectionist than their peers. The disorder often begins as a diet not distinguishable at the outset from those undertaken by many adolescents and young women. As weight loss progresses, the fear of gaining weight grows; dieting becomes stricter; and psychological, behavioral, and medical aberrations increase. The fact that most cases are reported from countries where food is plentiful and where thinness, especially among women, is highly valued suggests that cultural factors play a significant role in the development of anorexia nervosa. However, it is notable that the clinical syndrome was well described over a century ago, when the cultural pressures were quite different.

Numerous physiologic disturbances, including abnormalities in a variety of neurotransmitter systems, have been described in anorexia nervosa (see below). It is difficult to distinguish neurochemical, metabolic, and hormonal changes that may have a role in the initiation or

Table 78-3 Common Characteristics of Anorexia Nervosa and Bulimia Nervosa

	Anorexia Nervosa	Bulimia Nervosa
CLINICAL CHARACTERISTICS		
Onset	Mid-adolescence	Late adolescence/early adulthood
Female:male	10:1	10:1
Prevalence in women	0.5%	1–3%
Weight	Markedly decreased	Usually normal
Menstruation	Absent	Usually normal
Binge eating	25–50%	Required for diagnosis
Mortality	~5% per decade	Low
PHYSICAL AND LABORATORY FINDINGS[a]		
Skin/extremities	Lanugo	
	Acrocyanosis	
	Edema	
Cardiovascular	Bradycardia	
	Hypotension	
Gastrointestinal	Salivary gland enlargement	Salivary gland enlargement
	Slow gastric emptying	Dental erosion
	Constipation	
	Elevated liver enzymes	
Hematopoietic	Normochromic, normocytic anemia	
	Leukopenia	
Fluid/electrolyte	Increased BUN, creatinine	Hypokalemia
	Hyponatremia	Hypochloremia
		Alkalosis
Endocrine	Hypoglycemia	
	Low estrogen or testosterone	
	Low LH and FSH	
	Low-normal thyroxine	
	Normal TSH	
	Increased cortisol	
Bone	Osteopenia	

[a] Patients with the binge-eating/purging subtype of anorexia nervosa may also exhibit the physical and laboratory findings associated with bulimia nervosa.

NOTE: BUN, blood urea nitrogen; LH, luteinizing hormone; FSH, follicle stimulating hormone; TSH, thyroid stimulating hormone.

perpetuation of the syndrome from those that are secondary to the disorder. The resolution of most of these abnormalities with weight restoration argues against their having a critical etiologic role.

Bulimia nervosa typically begins during or following an episode of dieting, often in association with depressed mood. Patients who develop bulimia nervosa describe a higher-than-expected prevalence of childhood and parental obesity, suggesting that a predisposition towards obesity may increase vulnerability to this eating disorder. The marked increase in the number of cases of bulimia nervosa during the past 25 years and the rarity of bulimia nervosa in underdeveloped countries suggest that cultural factors are important. Several biologic abnormalities in patients with bulimia nervosa may perpetuate this disorder once it has begun. These include abnormalities of CNS serotonergic function, which is involved in the regulation of eating behavior, and disruption of peripheral satiety mechanisms, including the release of cholecystokinin (CCK) from the small intestine.

Genetic factors probably contribute to the risk of development of eating disorders, as the incidence of these disorders is greater in families with one affected member and the concordance in monozygotic twins is greater than in dizygotic twins. However, specific genes have not been identified, and the range of the estimates of heritability is large.

CLINICAL FEATURES (Table 78-3)

ANOREXIA NERVOSA Anorexia nervosa typically begins in mid to late adolescence, sometimes in association with a stressful life event such as leaving home for school. The disorder occasionally develops in early puberty, before menarche, but seldom begins after age 40. Despite being underweight, patients with anorexia nervosa rarely complain of hunger or fatigue and often exercise extensively. Further weight loss is viewed by the patient as a fulfilling accomplishment,

while weight gain is seen as a personal failure. Patients tend to become socially withdrawn and increasingly committed to work or study, dieting, and exercise. As weight loss progresses, thoughts of food dominate mental life and idiosyncratic rules develop around eating. Patients with anorexia nervosa may obsessively collect cookbooks and recipes and be drawn to food-related occupations. Despite the denial of hunger, one-quarter to one-half of patients with anorexia nervosa engage in eating binges.

Physical Features Patients with anorexia nervosa typically have few physical complaints but may note cold intolerance and constipation. Some women who develop anorexia nervosa after menarche report that their menses ceased before significant weight loss occurred. Weight and height should be measured to allow calculation of BMI (kg/m^2). Vital signs may reveal bradycardia, hypotension, and hypothermia. Soft, downy hair growth (lanugo) sometimes occurs, especially on the back, and alopecia may be seen. Salivary gland enlargement, which is associated with starvation as well as with binge eating and vomiting, may make the face appear surprisingly full in contrast to the marked general wasting. Acrocyanosis of the digits is common, and peripheral edema can be seen in the absence of hypoalbuminemia, particularly when the patient begins to regain weight. Some patients who consume large amounts of vegetables containing vitamin A develop a yellow tint to the skin (*hypercarotenemia*), which is especially notable on the palms.

Laboratory Abnormalities Mild normochromic, normocytic anemia is frequent, as is mild to moderate leukopenia, with a disproportionate reduction of polymorphonuclear leukocytes. Dehydration may result in slightly increased levels of blood urea nitrogen and creatinine. Serum liver enzyme levels may increase, especially during the early phases of refeeding. The level of serum proteins is usually normal. Blood sugar is often low and serum cholesterol may be moderately elevated. Gastrointestinal motility is diminished, leading to reduced gastric emptying and constipation. A range of electrolyte disturbances may develop, reflecting the degree to which the patient restricts or overconsumes fluids and whether the patient engages in purging behavior. Hypokalemic alkalosis suggests self-induced vomiting or the use of diuretics. Hyponatremia is common and may result from excess fluid intake and disturbances in the secretion of antidiuretic hormone.

Endocrine Abnormalities The regulation of virtually every endocrine system is altered in anorexia nervosa, but the most striking changes occur in the reproductive system. Amenorrhea is hypothalamic in origin and reflects diminished production of gonadotropin-releasing hormone (GnRH). When exogenous GnRH is administered in a physiologic pulsatile manner, pituitary responses of luteinizing hormone (LH) and follicle stimulating hormone (FSH) are normalized, indicating the absence of a primary pituitary abnormality. The resulting gonadotropin deficiency causes low plasma estrogen in women and reduced testosterone in men. The hypothalamic GnRH pulse generator is exquisitely sensitive, particularly in women, to body weight, stress, and exercise, each of which may contribute to *hypothalamic amenorrhea* in anorexia nervosa (Chap. 336). Although the mechanisms underlying these effects are unknown, the decreased adipose tissue associated with weight loss leads to a marked reduction in leptin, a hormone that plays a permissive role in GnRH production (Chap. 77). In many patients, weight gain to a specific threshold triggers restoration of the GnRH pulse generator, initially recapitulating the pubertal pattern of nocturnal gonadotropin secretion before returning to the normal adult pattern.

Serum cortisol and 24-h urine free cortisol levels are generally elevated but without characteristic clinical signs of cortisol excess. Thyroid function tests resemble the pattern seen in euthyroid sick syndrome (Chap. 330). Thyroxine (T_4) and free T_4 levels are usually in the low-normal range, triiodothyronine (T_3) levels are reduced, and reverse T_3 (rT_3) is elevated. The level of thyroid stimulating hormone (TSH) is normally or partially suppressed. Growth hormone is increased, but insulin-like growth factor 1 (IGF-1), which is produced mainly by the liver, is reduced, as it is in other conditions of starvation. Diminished bone density is routinely observed in anorexia nervosa and reflects the effects of multiple nutritional deficiencies, reduced gonadal steroids, and increased cortisol. The degree of bone density reduction is proportional to the length of the illness, and patients are at risk for the development of symptomatic fractures. The occurrence of anorexia nervosa during adolescence may lead to the premature cessation of linear bone growth and a failure to achieve expected adult height.

Cardiac Abnormalities Cardiac output is reduced, and congestive heart failure occasionally occurs during rapid refeeding. The electrocardiogram usually shows sinus bradycardia, reduced QRS voltage, and nonspecific ST-T-wave abnormalities. Some patients develop a prolonged QT_c interval, which may predispose to serious arrhythmias.

BULIMIA NERVOSA The typical patient presenting for treatment of bulimia nervosa is a woman of normal weight in her mid-twenties who reports binge eating and purging 5 to 10 times a week for 5 to 10 years. The disorder usually begins in late adolescence or early adulthood during or following a diet. The self-imposed caloric restriction leads to increased hunger and to overeating. In an attempt to avoid weight gain, the patient induces vomiting, takes laxatives or diuretics, or engages in some other form of compensatory behavior. Initially, patients may experience a sense of satisfaction that appealing food can be eaten without weight gain. However, as the disorder progresses, patients perceive diminished control over eating. Binges increase in size and frequency and are provoked by a variety of stimuli, such as transient depression, anxiety, or a sense that too much food has been consumed in a normal meal. Between binges, patients attempt to restrict caloric intake, which increases hunger and sets the stage for the next binge.

Although vomiting may be triggered initially by manual stimulation of the gag reflex, most patients with bulimia nervosa develop the ability to induce vomiting at will. Rarely, patients resort to the regular use of syrup of ipecac. Laxatives and diuretics are frequently taken in impressive quantities, such as 30 or 60 laxative pills on a single occasion. The resulting fluid loss produces dehydration and a feeling of emptiness but has little impact on caloric balance.

The physical abnormalities associated with bulimia nervosa primarily result from the purging behavior. Painless bilateral salivary gland hypertrophy (sialadenosis) may be noted. A scar or callus on the dorsum of the hand may develop due to repeated trauma from the teeth among patients who manually stimulate the gag reflex. Recurrent vomiting and the exposure of the lingual surfaces of the teeth to stomach acid leads to loss of dental enamel and eventually to chipping and erosion of the front teeth. Laboratory abnormalities are surprisingly infrequent, but hypokalemia, hypochloremia, and hyponatremia are observed occasionally. Repeated vomiting may lead to alkalosis, whereas repeated laxative abuse may produce a mild metabolic acidosis. Serum amylase may be mildly elevated due to an increase in the salivary isoenzyme.

Serious physical complications resulting from bulimia nervosa are rare. Oligomenorrhea and amenorrhea are more frequent than in women without eating disorders. Arrhythmias occasionally occur secondary to electrolyte disturbances. Tearing of the esophagus and rupture of the stomach, which constitute life-threatening events, have been reported. Some patients who have chronically abused laxatives or diuretics develop transient peripheral edema when this behavior ceases, presumably due to high levels of aldosterone resulting from persistent fluid and electrolyte depletion.

PROGNOSIS

The course and outcome of anorexia nervosa are highly variable. One-quarter to one-half of patients eventually recover fully, with few psychological or physical sequelae. However, many patients have persistent difficulties with weight maintenance, depression, and eating disturbances, including bulimia nervosa. The development of obesity following anorexia nervosa is rare. The long-term mortality of anorexia nervosa is among the highest associated with any psychiatric disorder. Approximately 5% of patients die per decade of follow-up, primarily due to the physical effects of chronic starvation or by suicide.

Virtually all of the physiologic abnormalities associated with anorexia nervosa are observed in other forms of starvation and markedly improve or disappear with weight gain. A worrisome exception is the reduction in bone mass, which may not recover fully, particularly when anorexia nervosa occurs during adolescence when peak bone mass is normally achieved.

The prognosis of bulimia nervosa is much more favorable. Mortality is low, and full recovery occurs in approximately 50% of patients within 10 years. Approximately 25% of patients have persistent symptoms of bulimia nervosa over many years. Few patients progress from bulimia nervosa to anorexia nervosa.

℞ **TREATMENT   Anorexia Nervosa** Because of the profound physiological and psychological effects of starvation, there is a broad consensus that weight restoration to 90% of predicted weight is the primary goal in the treatment of anorexia nervosa. Unfortunately, because most patients resist this goal, its accomplishment is often accompanied by frustration for the patient, the family, and the physician. In attempting to engage the patient in treatment, it may be useful for the physician to elicit the patient's physical concerns (e.g., about osteoporosis, weakness, or fertility) and, if possible, educate the patient regarding the importance of normalizing nutritional status in order to address those concerns. The physician should attempt to reassure the patient that weight gain will not be permitted to get "out of control" but simultaneously emphasize that weight restoration is medically and psychologically imperative.

The intensity of the initial treatment, including the need for hospitalization, is determined by the patient's current weight, the rapidity of recent weight loss, and the severity of medical and psychological complications (Fig. 78-1). Hospitalization should be strongly considered for patients weighing <75% of expected, even if the results of routine blood studies are within normal limits. Acute medical problems, such as severe electrolyte imbalances, should be identified and addressed. Nutritional restoration can almost always be successfully accomplished by oral feeding, and parenteral methods are rarely required. For severely underweight patients, sufficient calories (approximately 1500 to 1800 kcal/d) should be provided initially in divided meals as food or liquid supplements to maintain weight and to permit stabilization of fluid and electrolyte balance. Calories can then be gradually increased to achieve a weight gain of 1 to 2 kg (2 to 4 lb) per week, typically requiring an intake of 3000 to 4000 kcal/d. Meals must be supervised, ideally by personnel who are firm regarding the necessity of food consumption, empathic regarding the challenges entailed, and reassuring regarding the patient's eventual recovery. Patients have great psychological difficulty complying with the need for increased caloric consumption, and the assistance of psychiatrists or psychologists experienced in the treatment of anorexia nervosa is usually necessary.

Psychiatric treatment focuses primarily on two issues. First, patients require much emotional support during the period of weight gain. Second, patients must learn to base their self-esteem, not on the achievement of an inappropriately low weight, but on the development of satisfying personal relationships and the attainment of reasonable academic and occupational goals. For younger patients, the active involvement of the family in treatment is crucial.

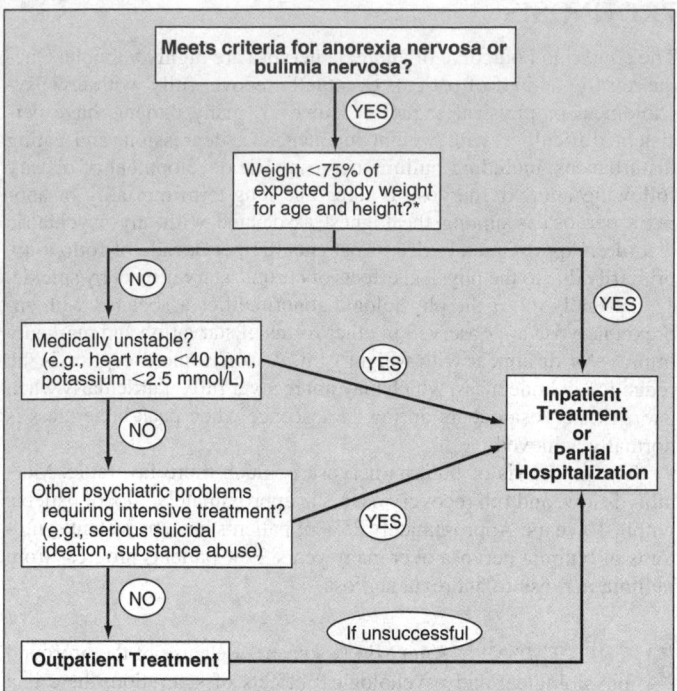

FIGURE 78-1 An algorithm for basic treatment decisions regarding patients with anorexia nervosa or bulimia nervosa. Based on the American Psychiatric Association's practice guidelines for the treatment of patients with eating disorders.* Although outpatient management may be considered for patients with anorexia nervosa weighing more than 75% of expected, there should be a low threshold for using more intensive interventions if the weight loss has been rapid or if current weight is <80% of expected.

Less severely affected patients may be treated in a partial hospitalization program where medical and psychiatric supervision is available and several meals can be monitored each day. Outpatient treatment may suffice for mildly ill patients. Weight must be monitored at frequent intervals, and explicit goals agreed on for weight gain, with the understanding that more intensive treatment will be required if the level of care initially employed is not successful.

Medical complications occasionally occur during refeeding. Most patients transiently retain excess fluid, occasionally resulting in peripheral edema. Fluid retention occurs during recovery from other forms of malnutrition and generally does not require specific treatment in the absence of cardiac, renal, or hepatic dysfunction. Congestive heart failure and acute gastric dilatation have been described when refeeding has been rapid. Transient modest elevations in serum levels of liver enzymes occasionally occur. Low levels of magnesium and phosphate should be repleted. Multivitamins should be given, and it is important to ensure adequate intake of vitamin D (400 IU/d) and calcium (1500 mg/d) to minimize bone loss.

No psychotropic medications are of established value in the treatment of anorexia nervosa; tricyclic antidepressants are contraindicated when there is prolongation of the QT_c interval. The alterations of cortisol and thyroid hormone metabolism do not require specific treatment and are corrected by weight gain. Estrogen treatment appears to have minimal impact on bone density in underweight patients but may be helpful to relieve symptoms of estrogen deficiency.

Bulimia Nervosa Bulimia nervosa can usually be treated on an outpatient basis. Cognitive behavioral therapy (CBT) is a short-term (4 to 6 months) psychological treatment that focuses on the intense concern with shape and weight, the persistent dieting, and the binge eating and purging that characterize this disorder. Patients are directed to monitor the circumstances, thoughts, and emotions associated with binge/purge episodes, to eat regularly, and to challenge their assumptions linking weight to self-esteem. CBT produces symptomatic remission in 25 to 50% of patients.

Numerous double-bind, placebo-controlled trials have documented that antidepressant medications are useful in the treatment of bulimia nervosa but are probably somewhat less effective than CBT. Although efficacy has been established for virtually all chemical classes of antidepressants, only the selective serotonin reuptake inhibitor fluoxetine (Prozac) has been approved for use in bulimia nervosa by the U.S. Food and Drug Administration. Antidepressant medications are helpful even for patients with bulimia nervosa who are not depressed, and the dose of fluoxetine recommended for bulimia nervosa (60 mg/d) is higher than that typically used to treat depression. These observations suggest that different mechanisms may underlie the utility of these medications in bulimia nervosa and in depression.

A substantial minority of patients with bulimia nervosa do not respond adequately to CBT, antidepressant medication, or their combination. More intensive forms of treatment, including hospitalization, may be required for such patients.

BIBLIOGRAPHY

AMERICAN PSYCHIATRIC ASSOCIATION: Practice guideline for the treatment of patients with eating disorders (revision). Am J Psychiatry 157(Suppl 1):1, 2000.

BECKER AE et al: Eating disorders. N Engl J Med 340:1092, 1999

DEVLIN MJ: Assessment and treatment of binge-eating disorder. Psychiatr Clin North Am 19:761, 1996

FAIRBURN CG et al: Risk factors for bulimia nervosa. A community-based case-control study. Arch Gen Psychiatry 54:509, 1997

KEEL PK et al: Long-term outcome of bulimia nervosa. Arch Gen Psychiatry 56:63, 1999

SULLIVAN PF: Mortality in anorexia nervosa. Am J Psychiatry 152:1073, 1995

WALSH BT, DEVLIN MJ: Eating disorders: Progress and problems. Science 280:1387, 1998

Section 1
NEOPLASTIC DISORDERS

79

Dan L. Longo

APPROACH TO THE PATIENT WITH CANCER

The application of current treatment techniques (surgery, radiation therapy, chemotherapy, and biological therapy) results in the cure of >50% of patients diagnosed with cancer. Nevertheless, patients experience the diagnosis of cancer as one of the most traumatic and revolutionary events that has ever happened to them. Independent of prognosis, the diagnosis brings with it a change in a person's self-image and in his or her role in the home and workplace. The prognosis of a person who has just been found to have pancreatic cancer is the same as the prognosis of the person with aortic stenosis who develops the first symptoms of congestive heart failure (median survival, about 8 months). However, the patient with heart disease may remain functional and maintain a view of him- or herself as a fully intact person with just a malfunctioning part, a diseased organ ("a bum ticker"). By contrast, the patient with pancreatic cancer has a completely altered self-image and is viewed differently by family and anyone who knows the diagnosis. He or she is being attacked and invaded by a disease that could be anywhere in the body. Every ache or pain takes on desperate significance. Cancer is an exception to the coordinated interaction among cells and organs. In general, the cells of a multicellular organism are programmed for collaboration. Many diseases occur because the specialized cells fail to perform their assigned task. Cancer takes this malfunction one step further. Not only is there a failure of the cancer cell to maintain its specialized function, but it also strikes out on its own; the cancer cell competes to survive using natural mutability and natural selection to seek advantage over normal cells in a recapitulation of evolution. One consequence of the traitorous behavior of cancer cells is that the patient feels betrayed by his or her body. The cancer patient feels that he or she, and not just a body part, is diseased.

THE MAGNITUDE OF THE PROBLEM

There is no nationwide cancer registry; therefore, the incidence of cancer is estimated on the basis of the National Cancer Institute's Surveillance, Epidemiology, and End Results (SEER) database, which tabulates cancer incidence and death figures from nine sites, accounting for about 10% of the U.S. population, and from population data from the Bureau of the Census. In 2000, 1.22 million new cases of invasive cancer (619,700 men, 600,400 women) were diagnosed and 552,200 people (284,100 men, 268,100 women) died from cancer. The percent distribution of new cancer cases and cancer deaths by site for men and women are shown in Table 79-1. Cancer incidence has been declining by about 2% each year since 1992.

The most significant risk factor for cancer overall is age; two-thirds of all cases were in people over age 65. Cancer incidence increases as the third, fourth, or fifth power of age in different sites. For the interval between birth and age 39, 1 in 62 men and 1 in 52 women will develop cancer; for the interval between ages 40 and 59, 1 in 12 men and 1 in 11 women will develop cancer; and for the interval between ages 60 and 79, 1 in 3 men and 1 in 4 women will develop cancer.

Cancer is the second leading cause of death behind heart disease.

Table 79-1 Distribution of Cancer Incidence and Deaths for 2000[a]

Male			Female		
Sites	%	Number	Sites	%	Number
CANCER INCIDENCE					
Prostate	29	180,400	Breast	30	182,800
Lung and bronchus	14	89,500	Lung and bronchus	12	74,600
Colon and rectum	10	63,600	Colon and rectum	11	66,600
Bladder	6	38,300	Endometrium	6	36,100
Lymphoma	5	31,700	Ovary	4	23,100
Melanoma	4	27,300	Lymphoma	4	23,100
Oral Cavity	3	20,200	Melanoma	3	20,400
Kidney	3	18,800	Bladder	2	14,900
Leukemia	3	16,900	Pancreas	2	14,600
Pancreas	2	13,700	Thyroid	2	13,700
All other	19	119,300	All other	22	130,500
CANCER DEATHS					
Lung and bronchus	31	89,300	Lung and bronchus	25	67,600
Prostate	11	31,900	Breast	15	40,800
Colon and rectum	10	27,800	Colon and rectum	11	28,500
Pancreas	5	13,700	Pancreas	5	14,500
Lymphoma	5	13,700	Ovary	5	14,000
Leukemia	4	12,100	Lymphoma	5	12,400
Esophagus	3	9,200	Leukemia	4	9,600
Liver and bile duct	3	8,500	Endometrium	2	6,500
			Brain	2	5,900
Bladder	3	8,100	Stomach	2	5,400
Stomach	3	7,600	Myeloma	2	5,400
All other	22	62,200	All other	21	57,500

[a] Data exclude basal and squamous cell skin cancers and carcinoma in situ except the bladder.
SOURCE: RT Greenlee et al, with permission.

Deaths from heart disease have declined 45% in the United States since 1950 and continue to decline. After a 70-year period of increases, cancer deaths began to decline in 1997 (Fig. 79-1). The five leading causes of cancer deaths are shown for various populations in Table 79-2. Along with the decrease in incidence has come an increase in survival for cancer patients. The 5-year survival for white patients was 39% in 1960–1963 and 61% in 1989–1995. Cancers are more often deadly in blacks; the 5-year survival was 48% for the 1989–1995 interval. Incidence and mortality vary among racial and ethnic groups (Table 79-3). The basis for these differences is unclear.

PATIENT MANAGEMENT

Important information is obtained from every portion of the routine history and physical examination. The duration of symptoms may reveal the chronicity of disease. The past medical history may alert the physician to the presence of underlying diseases that may affect the choice of therapy or the side effects of treatment. The social history may reveal occupational exposure to carcinogens or habits, such as smoking or alcohol consumption, that may influence the course of disease and its treatment. The family history may suggest an underlying familial cancer predisposition and point out the need to begin

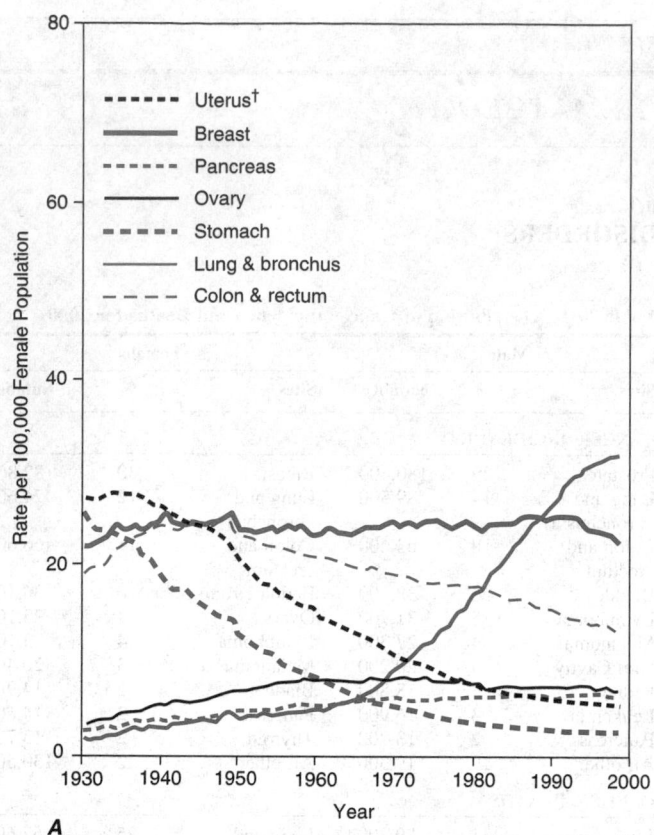

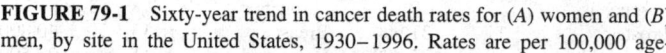

FIGURE 79-1 Sixty-year trend in cancer death rates for (*A*) women and (*B*) men, by site in the United States, 1930–1996. Rates are per 100,000 age- adjusted to the 1970 U.S. standard population. *(From Greenlee.)*

surveillance or other preventive therapy for unaffected siblings of the patient. The review of systems may suggest early symptoms of meta- static disease or a paraneoplastic syndrome.

DIAGNOSIS The diagnosis of cancer relies most heavily on invasive tissue biopsy and should never be made without obtaining tissue; no noninvasive diagnostic test is sufficient to define a disease process as cancer. Although in rare clinical settings (e.g., thyroid nod- ules) fine-needle aspiration is an acceptable diagnostic procedure, the diagnosis generally depends on obtaining adequate tissue to permit careful evaluation of the histology of the tumor, its grade, and its invasiveness and to yield further molecular diagnostic information, such as the expression of cell-surface markers or intracellular proteins that typify a particular cancer, or the presence of a molecular marker, such as the t(8;14) translocation of Burkitt's lymphoma. Increasing evidence links the expression of certain genes with the prognosis and response to therapy (Chaps. 81 and 82).

Occasionally a patient will present with a metastatic disease pro- cess that is defined as cancer on biopsy but has no apparent primary site of disease. Efforts should be made to define the primary site based on age, sex, sites of involvement, histology and tumor markers, and personal and family history. Particular attention should be focused on ruling out the most treatable causes (Chap. 99).

Once the diagnosis of cancer is made, the management of the pa- tient is best undertaken as a multidisciplinary collaboration among the primary care physician, medical oncologists, surgical oncologists, ra- diation oncologists, oncology nurse specialists, pharmacists, social workers, rehabilitation medicine specialists, and a number of other consulting professionals working closely with each other and with the patient and family.

DEFINING THE EXTENT OF DISEASE AND THE PROGNOSIS The first priority in patient management after the di- agnosis of cancer is established and shared with the patient is to de- termine the extent of disease. The curability of a tumor usually is inversely proportional to the tumor burden. Ideally, the tumor will be diagnosed before symptoms develop or as a consequence of screening efforts (Chap. 80). A very high proportion of such patients can be cured. However, most patients with cancer present with symp- toms related to the cancer, caused either by mass effects of the tu- mor or by alterations associated with the production of cytokines or hormones by the tumor.

For most cancers, the extent of disease is evaluated by a vari- ety of noninvasive and invasive diagnostic tests and procedures. This process is called *staging*. There are two types. *Clinical staging* is based on physical ex- amination, radiographs, isotopic scans, computed tomography, and other imaging procedures;

Table 79-2   The Five Leading Primary Tumor Sites for Patients Dying of Cancer Based on Age and Sex in 1997

Rank	All Ages	Under 20	20–39	40–59	60–79	>80
			Age			
1	M,F: lung	M,F: leukemia	M: lymphoma F: breast	M: lung F: breast	M,F: lung	M,F: lung
2	M: prostate F: breast	M,F: brain	M: leukemia F: cervix	M: colorectal F: lung	M: prostate F: breast	M: prostate F: colorectal
3	M,F: colorectal	M: endocrine F: soft tissue sarcoma	M: brain F: lung	M: pancreas F: colorectal	M: colorectal	M: colorectal F: breast
4	M,F: pancreas	M: bone sarcoma F: endocrine	M: lung F: leukemia	M: lymphoma F: ovary	M,F: pancreas	M: bladder F: pancreas
5	M: lymphoma F: ovary	M: lymphoma F: bone sarcoma	M: colorectal F: brain	M: esophagus F: cervix	M: lymphoma F: ovary	M: pancreas F: lymphoma

NOTE: M, male; F, female.

492

pathologic staging takes into account information obtained during a surgical procedure, which might include intraoperative palpation, resection of regional lymph nodes and/or tissue adjacent to the tumor, and inspection and biopsy of organs commonly involved in disease spread. Pathologic staging includes histologic examination of all tissues removed during the surgical procedure. Surgical procedures performed may include a simple lymph node biopsy or more extensive procedures such as thoracotomy, mediastinoscopy, or laparotomy. Surgical staging may occur in a separate procedure or may be done at the time of definitive surgical resection of the primary tumor.

Knowledge of the predilection of particular tumors for spread to adjacent or distant organs helps direct the staging evaluation.

Information obtained from staging is used to define the extent of disease either as localized, as exhibiting spread outside of the organ of origin to regional but not distant sites, or as metastatic to distant sites. The most widely used system of staging is the TNM (tumor, node, metastasis) system codified by the International Union Against Cancer and the American Joint Committee on Cancer (AJCC).[1] The TNM classification is an anatomically based system that categorizes the tumor on the basis of the size of the primary tumor lesion (T1–4, where a higher number indicates a tumor of larger size), the presence of nodal involvement (usually N0 and N1 for the absence and presence, respectively, of involved nodes, although some tumors have more elaborate systems of nodal grading), and the presence of metastatic disease (M0 and M1 for the absence and presence, respectively, of metastases). The various permutations of T, N, and M scores are then broken into stages, usually designated by the roman numerals I through IV. Tumor burden increases and curability decreases with increasing stage. Other anatomic staging systems are used for some tumors, e.g., the Dukes classification for colorectal cancers, the International Federation of Gynecologists and Obstetricians (FIGO) classification for gynecologic cancers, and the Ann Arbor classification for Hodgkin's disease.

Certain tumors cannot be grouped appropriately on the basis of anatomic considerations. For example, hematopoietic tumors such as leukemia, myeloma, and lymphoma are often disseminated at presentation and do not spread in the fashion typical of solid tumors. For these tumors, other prognostic factors have been identified (Chaps. 111, 112, and 113).

In addition to tumor burden, a second major determinant of treatment outcome is the physiologic reserve of the patient. Patients who are bedridden before developing cancer are likely to fare worse, stage for stage, than fully active patients. Physiologic reserve is a determinant of how a patient is likely to cope with the physiologic stresses imposed by the cancer and its treatment. This factor is difficult to assess directly. Instead, surrogate markers for physiologic reserve are used, such as the patient's age or Karnofsky performance status (Table 79-4). Older patients and those with a Karnofsky performance status <70 have a poor prognosis unless the poor performance is a reversible consequence of the tumor.

Increasingly, biologic features of the tumor are being related to prognosis. The expression of particular oncogenes, drug-resistance genes, apoptosis-related genes, and genes involved in metastasis are being found to influence response to therapy and prognosis. The presence of selected cytogenetic abnormalities may influence survival. Tumors with higher growth fractions, as assessed by expression of proliferation-related markers such as proliferating cell nuclear antigen (PCNA), behave more aggressively than tumors with lower growth fractions. Information obtained from studying the tumor itself will increasingly be used to influence treatment decisions.

MAKING A TREATMENT PLAN From information on the extent of disease and the prognosis and in conjunction with the patient's wishes, it is determined whether the treatment approach should be curative or palliative in intent. Cooperation among the various professionals involved in cancer treatment is of the utmost importance in treatment planning. For some cancers, chemotherapy or chemotherapy plus radiation therapy delivered before the use of definitive surgical treatment (so-called neoadjuvant therapy) may improve the outcome, as seems to be the case for locally advanced breast cancer and head and neck cancers. In certain settings in which combined modality therapy is intended, coordination among the medical oncologist, radiation oncologist, and surgeon is crucial to achieving optimal results. Sometimes the chemotherapy and radiation therapy need to be delivered sequentially, and other times concurrently. Surgical procedures may precede or follow other treatment approaches. It is best for the treat-

Table 79-3   Cancer Incidence and Mortality in Racial and Ethnic Groups 1990–1996

Site	White	Black	Asian/Pacific Islander	American Indian	Hispanic
INCIDENCE PER 100,000 POPULATION					
All	M: 480	M: 598	M: 326	M: 178	M: 327
	F: 352	F: 336	F: 245	F: 137	F: 243
Breast (F)	113	66	73	34	69
Colon	M: 53	M: 58	M: 47	M: 22	M: 36
	F: 37	F: 45	F: 23	F: 12	F: 20
Lung	M: 73	M: 112	M: 52	M: 25	M: 39
	F: 43	F: 46	F: 23	F: 14	F: 20
Prostate (M)	147	223	82	47	103
MORTALITY PER 100,000 POPULATION					
All	M: 209	M: 309	M: 129	M: 123	M: 132
	F: 140	F: 168	F: 84	F: 90	F: 86
Breast (F)	26	31	11	12	15
Colon	M: 22	M: 28	M: 13	M: 11	M: 13
	F: 15	F: 20	F: 9	F: 9	F: 8
Lung	M: 70	M: 101	M: 35	M: 41	M: 32
	F: 34	F: 33	F: 15	F: 20	F: 11
Prostate (M)	24	55	11	14	17

NOTE: M, male; F, female.

Table 79-4   Karnofsky Performance Index

Performance Status	Functional Capability of the Patient
100	Normal; no complaints; no evidence of disease
90	Able to carry on normal activity; minor signs or symptoms of disease
80	Normal activity with effort; some signs or symptoms of disease
70	Cares for self; unable to carry on normal activity or do active work
60	Requires occasional assistance but is able to care for most needs
50	Requires considerable assistance and frequent medical care
40	Disabled; requires special care and assistance
30	Severely disabled; hospitalization is indicated although death is not imminent
20	Very sick; hospitalization necessary; active supportive treatment is necessary
10	Moribund, fatal processes progressing rapidly
0	Dead

[1]The AJCC *Manual for Staging Cancer*, 5th edition, can be obtained from the AJCC at 55 East Erie Street, Chicago, Il, 60611.

Table 79-5   Tumor Markers

Tumor Markers	Cancer	Non-Neoplastic Conditions
HORMONES		
Human chorionic gonadotropin	Gestational trophoblastic disease, gonadal germ cell tumor	Pregnancy
Calcitonin	Medullary cancer of the thyroid	
Catecholamines	Pheochromocytoma	
ONCOFETAL ANTIGENS		
Alphafetoprotein	Hepatocellular carcinoma, gonadal germ cell tumor	Cirrhosis, hepatitis
Carcinoembryonic antigen	Adenocarcinomas of the colon, pancreas, lung, breast, ovary	Pancreatitis, hepatitis, inflammatory bowel disease, smoking
ENZYMES		
Prostatic acid phosphatase	Prostate cancer	Prostatitis, prostatic hypertrophy
Neuron-specific enolase	Small cell cancer of the lung, neuroblastoma	
Lactate dehydrogenase	Lymphoma, Ewing's sarcoma	Hepatitis, hemolytic anemia, many others
TUMOR-ASSOCIATED PROTEINS		
Prostate-specific antigen	Prostate cancer	Prostatitis, prostatic hypertrophy
Monoclonal immunoglobulin	Myeloma	Infection, MGUS[a]
CA-125	Ovarian cancer, some lymphomas	Menstruation, peritonitis, pregnancy
CA 19-9	Colon, pancreatic, breast cancer	Pancreatitis, ulcerative colitis
CD30	Hodgkin's disease, anaplastic large cell lymphoma	—
CD25	Hairy cell leukemia, adult T cell leukemia/lymphoma	—

[a] MGUS, monoclonal gammopathy of uncertain significance.

ment plan either to follow a standard protocol precisely or else to be part of an ongoing clinical research protocol evaluating new treatments. Ad hoc modifications of standard protocols are likely to compromise treatment results.

The choice of treatment approaches was formerly dominated by the local culture in both the university and the practice settings. However, it is now possible to gain access electronically to standard treatment protocols and to every approved clinical research study in North America through a personal computer interface with the Internet.[2]

The skilled physician also has much to offer the patient for whom curative therapy is no longer an option. Often a combination of guilt and frustration over the inability to cure the patient and the pressure of a busy schedule greatly limit the time a physician spends with a patient who is receiving only palliative care. Resist these forces. In addition to the medicines administered to alleviate symptoms (see below), it is important to remember the comfort that is provided by holding the patient's hand, continuing regular examinations, and taking time to talk.

MANAGEMENT OF DISEASE AND TREATMENT COMPLICATIONS   Because cancer therapies are toxic (Chap. 84), patient management involves addressing complications of both the disease and its treatment as well as the complex psychosocial problems

[2]The National Cancer Institute maintains a database called PDQ (Physician Data Query) that is accessible on the Internet under the name CancerNet at wwwicic.nci.nih.gov/health.htm. Information can be obtained through a facsimile machine using CancerFax by dialing 301-402-5874. Patient information is also provided by the National Cancer Institute in at least three formats: on the Internet via CancerNet at wwwicic.nci.nih.gov/patient.htm, through the CancerFax number listed above, or by calling 1-800-4-CANCER. The quality control for the information provided through these services is rigorous.

associated with cancer. In the short term during a course of curative therapy, the patient's functional status may decline. Treatment-induced toxicity is less acceptable if the goal of therapy is palliation. The most common side effects of treatment are nausea and vomiting (see below), febrile neutropenia (Chap. 85), and myelosuppression (Chap. 104). Therapeutic tools are now available to minimize the acute toxicity of cancer treatment.

New symptoms developing in the course of cancer treatment should always be assumed to be reversible until proven otherwise. The fatalistic attribution of anorexia, weight loss, and jaundice to recurrent or progressive tumor could result in a patient dying from a reversible intercurrent cholecystitis. Intestinal obstruction may be due to reversible adhesions rather than progressive tumor. Systemic infections, sometimes with unusual pathogens, may be a consequence of the immunosuppression associated with cancer therapy. Some drugs used to treat cancer or its complications (e.g., nausea) may produce central nervous system symptoms that look like metastatic disease or may mimic paraneoplastic syndromes such as the syndrome of inappropriate antidiuretic hormone. A definitive diagnosis should be pursued and may even require a repeat biopsy.

A critical component of cancer management is assessing the response to treatment. In addition to a careful physical examination in which all sites of disease are physically measured and recorded in a flow chart by date, response assessment usually requires periodic repeating of imaging tests that were abnormal at the time of staging. If imaging tests have become normal, repeat biopsy of previously involved tissue is performed to document complete response by pathologic criteria. Biopsies are not usually required if there is macroscopic residual disease. A *complete response* is defined as disappearance of all evidence of disease, and a *partial response* as >50% reduction in the sum of the products of the perpendicular diameters of all measureable lesions. *Progressive disease* is defined as the appearance of any new lesion or an increase of >25% in the sum of the products of the perpendicular diameters of all measurable lesions. Tumor shrinkage or growth that does not meet any of these criteria is considered *stable disease*. Some sites of involvement (e.g., bone) or patterns of involvement (e.g., lymphangitic lung or diffuse pulmonary infiltrates) are considered unmeasurable. No response is complete without biopsy documentation of their resolution but partial responses may exclude their assessment unless clear objective (though unmeasurable) progression has occurred.

Tumor markers may be useful in patient management in certain tumors. Response to therapy may be difficult to gauge with certainty. However, some tumors produce or elicit the production of markers that can be measured in the serum or urine and, in a particular patient, rising and falling levels of the marker are usually associated with increasing or decreasing tumor burden, respectively. Some clinically useful tumor markers are shown in Table 79-5. Tumor markers are not in themselves specific enough to permit a diagnosis of malignancy to be made, but once a malignancy has been diagnosed and shown to be associated with elevated levels of a tumor marker, the marker can be used to assess response to treatment.

The recognition and treatment of depression are important components of management. The incidence of depression in cancer patients is ~25% overall and may be greater in patients with greater debility. This diagnosis is likely in a patient with a depressed mood (dysphoria) and/or a loss of interest in pleasure (anhedonia) for at least 2 weeks.

In addition, three or more of the following symptoms are usually present: appetite change, sleep problems, psychomotor retardation or agitation, fatigue, feelings of guilt or worthlessness, inability to concentrate, and suicidal ideation. Patients with these symptoms should receive therapy. Medical therapy with a serotonin reuptake inhibitor such as fluoxetine (10 to 20 mg/d), sertraline (50 to 150 mg/d), or paroxetine (10 to 20 mg/d) or a tricyclic antidepressant such as amitriptyline (50 to 100 mg/d) or desipramine (75 to 150 mg/d) should be tried, allowing 4 to 6 weeks for response. Effective therapy should be continued at least 6 months after resolution of symptoms. If therapy is unsuccessful, other classes of antidepressants may be used. In addition to medication, psychosocial interventions such as support groups, psychotherapy, and guided imagery may be of benefit.

Many patients opt for unproven or unsound approaches to treatment when it appears that conventional medicine is unlikely to be curative. Those seeking such alternatives are often well educated and may be early in the course of their disease. Unsound approaches are usually hawked on the basis of unsubstantiated anecdotes and not only cannot help the patient but may be harmful. Physicians should strive to keep communications open and nonjudgmental, so that patients are more likely to discuss with the physician what they are actually doing. The appearance of unexpected toxicity may be an indication that a supplemental therapy is being taken.[3]

LONG-TERM FOLLOW-UP/LATE COMPLICATIONS
At the completion of treatment, sites originally involved with tumor are reassessed, usually by radiography or imaging techniques, and any persistent abnormality is biopsied. If disease persists, the multidisciplinary team discusses a new salvage treatment plan. If the patient has been rendered disease-free by the original treatment, the patient is followed regularly for disease recurrence. The optimal guidelines for follow-up care are not known. For many years, a routine practice has been to follow the patient monthly for 6 to 12 months, then every other month for a year, every 3 months for a year, every 4 months for a year, every 6 months for a year, and then annually. At each visit, a battery of laboratory and radiographic and imaging tests were obtained on the assumption that it is best to detect recurrent disease before it becomes symptomatic. However, where follow-up procedures have been examined, this assumption has been found to be untrue. Studies of breast cancer, melanoma, lung cancer, colon cancer, and lymphoma have all failed to support the notion that asymptomatic relapses are more readily cured by salvage therapy than symptomatic relapses. In view of the enormous cost of a full battery of diagnostic tests and their manifest lack of impact on survival, new guidelines are emerging for less frequent follow-up visits during which the history and physical examination are the major investigations performed.

As time passes, the likelihood of recurrence of the primary cancer diminishes. For many types of cancer, survival for 5 years without recurrence is tantamount to cure. However, important medical problems can occur in patients treated for cancer and must be examined (Chap 103). Some problems emerge as a consequence of the disease and some as a consequence of the treatment. An understanding of these disease- and treatment-related problems may help in their detection and management.

Despite these concerns, most patients who are cured of cancer return to normal lives.

SUPPORTIVE CARE
In many ways, the success of cancer therapy depends on the success of the supportive care. Failure to control the symptoms of cancer and its treatment may lead patients to abandon curative therapy. Of equal importance, supportive care is a major determinant of quality of life. Even when life cannot be prolonged, the physician must strive to preserve its quality. Quality-of-life measurements have become common end-points of clinical research studies.

Furthermore, palliative care has been shown to be cost-effective when approached in an organized fashion. A credo for oncology could be to cure sometimes, to extend life often, and to comfort always.

Pain Pain occurs with variable frequency in the cancer patient: 25 to 50% of patients present with pain at diagnosis, 33% have pain associated with treatment, and 75% have pain with progressive disease. The pain may have several causes. In about 70% of cases, pain is caused by the tumor itself—by invasion of bone, nerves, blood vessels, or mucous membranes or obstruction of a hollow viscus or duct. In about 20% of cases, pain is related to a surgical or invasive medical procedure, to radiation injury (mucositis, enteritis, or plexus or spinal cord injury), or to chemotherapy injury (mucositis, peripheral neuropathy, phlebitis, steroid-induced aseptic necrosis of the femoral head). In 10% of cases, pain is unrelated to cancer or its treatment.

Assessment of pain requires the methodical investigation of the history of the pain, its location, character, temporal features, provocative and palliative factors, and intensity (Chap. 12); a review of the oncologic history and past medical history as well as personal and social history; and a thorough physical examination. The patient should be given a 10-division visual analogue scale on which to indicate the severity of the pain. The clinical condition is often dynamic, making it necessary to reassess the patient frequently. Pain therapy should not be withheld while the cause of pain is being sought.

A variety of tools are available with which to address cancer pain. About 85% of patients will have pain relief from pharmacologic intervention. However, other modalities, including antitumor therapy (such as surgical relief of obstruction, radiation therapy, and strontium-89 or samarium-153 treatment for bone pain), neurostimulatory techniques, regional analgesia, or neuroablative procedures are effective in an additional 12% or so. Thus, very few patients will have inadequate pain relief if appropriate measures are taken.

The World Health Organization (WHO) has devised a simple and effective method for the rational titration of oral analgesia, called the *WHO ladder*. The ladder has the following three steps. (1) For mild to moderate pain, one begins with acetaminophen (650 mg every 4 h or 975 mg every 6 h), aspirin (650 mg every 4 h or 975 mg every 6 h), or a nonsteroidal anti-inflammatory agent (NSAID; e.g., ketoprofen, 25 to 60 mg every 6 h) with or without an adjuvant such as a glucocorticoid (dexamethasone) or an antidepressant (amitriptyline). (2) When pain persists or increases, an opioid such as codeine or hydrocodone (30 mg every 3 to 4 h is roughly equivalent to 10 mg of intravenous morphine) should be added (not substituted); fixed combinations such as oxycodone/acetaminophen (Percocet) or oxycodone/aspirin (Percodan) are worth testing. (3) Pain that is persistent or that is moderate to severe at the outset should be treated by increasing the potency of the opioid or using higher dosages (e.g., morphine, 15 to 30 mg every 3 to 4 h, or controlled-release morphine, 90 to 120 mg bid), and fixed opioid/NSAID combinations should be abandoned. Adjuvants may be used at all steps. The critical features of this approach are that the treatment is oral, should be given around the clock with supplemental doses as needed to control pain, and is tailored to the individual patient. Transmucosal fentanyl (in lollipop form) may aid in control of breakthrough pain. Records of pain control should be a prominent component of the medical record. When opioids are used, the patient should be placed on a prophylactic regimen to prevent constipation.

Nausea Emesis in the cancer patient is usually caused by chemotherapy (Chap. 84). Its severity can be predicted from the drugs used to treat the cancer. Three forms of emesis are recognized on the basis of their timing with regard to the noxious insult. *Acute emesis*, the most common variety, occurs within 24 h of treatment. *Delayed emesis* occurs 1 to 7 days after treatment; it is rare, but, when present, usually follows cisplatin administration. *Anticipatory emesis* occurs before administration of chemotherapy and represents a conditioned response to visual and olfactory stimuli previously associated with chemotherapy delivery.

---

[3]Information about unsound methods may be obtained from the National Council Against Health Fraud, Box 1276, Loma Linda, CA 92354, or from the Center for Medical Consumers and Health Care Information, 237 Thompson Street, New York, NY 10012.

Acute emesis is the best understood form. Stimuli that activate signals in the chemoreceptor trigger zone in the medulla, the cerebral cortex, and peripherally in the intestinal tract lead to stimulation of the vomiting center in the medulla, the motor center responsible for coordinating the secretory and muscle contraction activity that leads to emesis. Diverse receptor types participate in the process, including dopamine, serotonin, histamine, opioid, and acetylcholine receptors. The serotonin receptor antagonists ondansetron and granisetron are the most effective drugs against highly emetogenic agents, but they are expensive.

As with the analgesia ladder, emesis therapy should be tailored to the situation. For mildly and moderately emetogenic agents, prochlorperazine, 5 to 10 mg orally or 25 mg rectally, is effective. Its efficacy may be enhanced by administering the drug before the chemotherapy is delivered. Dexamethasone, 10 to 20 mg intravenously, is also effective and may enhance the efficacy of prochlorperazine. For highly emetogenic agents such as cisplatin, mechlorethamine, dacarbazine, and streptozocin, combinations of agents work best and administration should begin 6 to 24 h before treatment. Ondansetron, 8 mg orally every 6 h the day before therapy and intravenously on the day of therapy, plus dexamethasone, 20 mg intravenously before treatment, is an effective regimen. Like pain, emesis is easier to prevent than to alleviate.

Delayed emesis may be related to bowel inflammation from the therapy and can be controlled with oral dexamethasone and oral metoclopramide, a dopamine receptor antagonist that also blocks serotonin receptors at high dosages. The best strategy for preventing anticipatory emesis is to control emesis in the early cycles of therapy to prevent the conditioning from taking place. If this is unsuccessful, prophylactic antiemetics the day before treatment may help. Experimental studies are evaluating behavior modification.

Effusions   Fluid may accumulate abnormally in the pleural cavity, pericardium, or peritoneum. Asymptomatic malignant effusions may not require treatment. Symptomatic effusions occurring in tumors responsive to systemic therapy usually do not require local treatment but respond to the treatment for the underlying tumor. Symptomatic effusions occurring in tumors unresponsive to systemic therapy may require local treatment in patients with a life expectancy of at least 6 months.

Pleural effusions due to tumors may or may not contain malignant cells. Lung cancer, breast cancer, and lymphomas account for about 75% of malignant pleural effusions. Their exudative nature is usually gauged by an effusion/serum protein ratio of 0.5 or an effusion/serum lactate dehydrogenase ratio of 0.6. When the condition is symptomatic, thoracentesis is usually performed first. In most cases, symptomatic improvement occurs for <1 month. Chest tube drainage is required if symptoms recur within 2 weeks. Fluid is aspirated until the flow rate is <100 mL in 24 h. Then either 60 units of bleomycin or 1 g of doxycycline is infused into the chest tube in 50 mL of 5% dextrose in water; the tube is clamped; the patient is rotated on four sides, spending 15 min in each position; and, after 1 to 2 h, the tube is again attached to suction for another 24 h. The tube is then disconnected from suction and allowed to drain by gravity. If <100 mL drains over the next 24 h, the chest tube is pulled, and a radiograph taken 24 h later. If the chest tube continues to drain fluid at an unacceptably high rate, sclerosis can be repeated. Bleomycin may be somewhat more effective than doxycycline but is very expensive. Doxycycline is usually the drug of first choice. If neither doxycycline nor bleomycin is effective, talc can be used.

Symptomatic pericardial effusions are usually treated by creating a pericardial window or by stripping the pericardium. If the patient's condition does not permit a surgical procedure, sclerosis can be attempted with doxycycline and/or bleomycin.

Malignant ascites is usually treated with repeated paracentesis of small volumes of fluid. If the underlying malignancy is unresponsive to systemic therapy, peritoneovenous shunts may be inserted. Despite the fear of disseminating tumor cells into the circulation, widespread metastases are an unusual complication. The major complications are occlusion, leakage, and fluid overload. Patients with severe liver disease may develop disseminated intravascular coagulation.

Nutrition   Cancer and its treatment may lead to a decrease in nutrient intake of sufficient magnitude to cause weight loss and alteration of intermediary metabolism. The prevalence of this problem is difficult to estimate because of variations in the definition of cancer cachexia, but most patients with advanced cancer experience weight loss and decreased appetite. A variety of both tumor-derived factors (e.g., bombesin, adrenocorticotropic hormone) and host-derived factors (e.g., tumor necrosis factor, interleukins 1 and 6, growth hormone) contribute to the altered metabolism, and a vicious cycle is established in which protein catabolism, glucose intolerance, and lipolysis cannot be reversed by the provision of calories.

It remains controversial how to assess nutritional status and when and how to intervene. Efforts to make the assessment objective have included the use of a prognostic nutritional index based on albumin levels, triceps skin fold thickness, transferrin levels, and delayed-type hypersensitivity skin testing. However, a simpler approach has been to define the threshold for nutritional intervention as >10% unexplained body weight loss, serum transferrin level <1500 mg/L (150 mg/dL), and serum albumin <34 g/L (3.4 g/dL).

The decision is important, because it appears that cancer therapy is substantially more toxic and less effective in the face of malnutrition. Nevertheless, it remains unclear whether nutritional intervention can alter the natural history. Unless some pathology is affecting the absorptive function of the gastrointestinal tract, enteral nutrition provided orally or by tube feeding is preferred over parenteral supplementation. However, the risks associated with the tube may outweigh the benefits. Megestrol acetate, a progestational agent, has been advocated as a pharmacologic intervention to improve nutritional status. Research in this area may provide more tools in the future as cytokine-mediated mechanisms are further elucidated.

Psychosocial Support   The psychosocial needs of patients vary with their situation. Patients undergoing treatment experience fear, anxiety, and depression. Self-image is often seriously compromised by deforming surgery and loss of hair. Women who receive cosmetic advice that enables them to look better also feel better. Loss of control over how one spends time can contribute to the sense of vulnerability. Juggling the demands of work and family with the demands of treatment may create enormous stresses. Sexual dysfunction is highly prevalent and needs to be discussed openly with the patient. An empathetic health care team is sensitive to the individual patient's needs and permits negotiation where such flexibility will not adversely affect the course of treatment.

Cancer survivors have other sets of difficulties. Patients may have fears associated with the termination of a treatment they associate with their continued survival. Adjustments are required to physical losses and handicaps, real and perceived. Patients may be preoccupied with minor physical problems. They perceive a decline in their job mobility and view themselves as less desirable workers. They may be victims of job and/or insurance discrimination. Patients may experience difficulty reentering their normal past life. They may feel guilty for having survived and may carry a sense of vulnerability to colds and other illnesses. Perhaps the most pervasive and threatening concern is the ever-present fear of relapse (the Damocles syndrome).

Patients in whom therapy has been unsuccessful have other problems related to the end of life.

Death and Dying   The most common causes of death in patients with cancer are infection (leading to circulatory failure), respiratory failure, hepatic failure, and renal failure. Intestinal blockage may lead to inanition and starvation. Central nervous system disease may lead to seizures, coma, and central hypoventilation. About 70% of patients develop dyspnea preterminally. However, many months usually pass between the diagnosis of cancer and the occurrence of these complications, and during this period the patient is severely affected by the possibility of death. The path of unsuccessful cancer treatment usually occurs in three phases. First, there is optimism at the hope of cure; when the tumor recurs, there is the acknowledgment of an incurable disease, and the goal of palliative therapy is embraced in the hope of being able to live with disease; finally, at the disclosure of imminent death, another adjustment in outlook takes place. The patient imagines the worst in preparation for the end of life and may go through stages of adjustment to the diagnosis. These stages include denial, isolation, anger, bargaining, depression, acceptance, and hope. Of course, patients do not all progress through all the stages or proceed through them in the same order or at the same rate. Nevertheless, developing an understanding of how the patient has been affected by the diagnosis and is coping with it is an important goal of patient management.

It is best to speak frankly with the patient and the family regarding the likely course of disease. These discussions can be difficult for the physician as well as for the patient and family. The critical features of the interaction are to reassure the patient and family that everything that can be done to provide comfort will be done. They will not be abandoned. Many patients prefer to be cared for in their homes or in a hospice setting rather than a hospital. The American College of Physicians has published a book called *Home Care Guide for Cancer: How to Care for Family and Friends at Home* that teaches an approach to successful problem-solving in home care. With appropriate planning, it should be possible to provide the patient with the necessary medical care as well as the psychological and spiritual support that will prevent the isolation and depersonalization that can attend in-hospital death.

The care of dying patients may take a toll on the physician. A "burnout" syndrome has been described that is characterized by fatigue, disengagement from patients and colleagues, and a loss of self-fulfillment. Efforts at stress reduction, maintenance of a balanced life, and setting realistic goals may combat this disorder.

End-of-Life Decisions Unfortunately, a smooth transition in treatment goals from curative to palliative may not be possible in all cases because of the occurrence of serious treatment-related complications or rapid disease progression. Vigorous and invasive medical support for a reversible disease or treatment complication is assumed to be justified. However, if the reversibility of the condition is in doubt, the patient's wishes determine the level of medical care. These wishes should be elicited before the terminal phase of illness and reviewed periodically. This information can guide the physician should the patient be unable to speak for him- or herself. The family cannot be expected to make such decisions without guidance from the patient and support from the physician when surrogate decisions are required. Advance directives such as a living will or a durable power of attorney for health care provide guidance for the health care team and the family regarding the patient's wishes and may protect the patient's assets from depletion on expensive but unwanted care.

Only about 15% of the population has implemented an advance directive. Physicians should take the initiative to speak with patients and family members about advance directives.[4]

BIBLIOGRAPHY

Clinical Practice Guideline Number 9, Management of Cancer Pain. U.S. Department of Health and Human Services, Agency for Health Care Policy and Research publication no. 94-0592, 1994

GREENLEE RT et al: Cancer statistics, 2000. CA Cancer J Clin 50:7, 2000

GRUNBERG SM, HESKETH PJ: Control of chemotherapy-induced emesis. N Engl J Med 329:1790, 1993

LEVY MH: Pharmacologic treatment of cancer pain. N Engl J Med 335:1124, 1996

THERASSE P et al: New guidelines to evaluate response to treatment in solid tumors. J Natl Cancer Inst 92:205, 2000

WALSH D et al: The symptoms of advanced cancer: Relationship to age, gender, and performance status in 1000 patients. Support Care Cancer 8:175, 2000

---

[4]Information about advance directives can be obtained from the American Association of Retired Persons, 601 E Street, NW, Washington, DC 20049, 202-434-2277 or Choice in Dying, 250 West 57th Street, New York, NY 10107, 212-366-5540.

80   *Otis W. Brawley, Barnett S. Kramer*

PREVENTION AND EARLY DETECTION OF CANCER

The prevention and control of cancer is a burgeoning field because of advances in understanding the biology of carcinogenesis. The field has expanded beyond the identification and avoidance of carcinogens to include studies of specific interventions to lower cancer risk, as well as screening for early detection of cancer.

Central to the prevention and control of cancer is the concept that carcinogenesis is not an event but a process, a series of discrete cellular changes that result in progressively more autonomous cellular processes. *Primary prevention* concerns the identification and manipulation of the genetic, biologic, and environmental factors in the causal pathway. Smoking cessation, diet modification, and chemoprevention are primary prevention activities. *Secondary prevention* concerns the identification of asymptomatic neoplastic lesions combined with effective therapy. Screening is a form of secondary prevention. Screening may also be a form of primary prevention of invasive cancer; screening Pap smears are used to identify and treat preinvasive lesions of the cervix.

EDUCATION AND HEALTHFUL HABITS   Public education on the avoidance of identified risk factors for cancer and encouraging healthy habits were among early efforts in cancer prevention and control. Many educational messages have come to the public through commercials in the print and electronic media and through school health courses. The physician is a potentially powerful messenger in this education campaign about the hazards of smoking, the benefits of a healthful diet, and sun avoidance.

Smoking Cessation   Tobacco use through cigarettes and other means is the most avoidable risk factor for cardiovascular disease and cancer. Lung cancer mortality rates correlate with the number of cigarettes smoked per day as well as the degree of inhalation of cigarette smoke. Those who stop smoking have a lower lung cancer mortality rate than those who continue smoking, despite the persistence for years of some carcinogen-induced genetic mutations. In addition to lung cancer, cigarette smoking is a causative agent in cancers of the larynx, oropharynx, esophagus, bladder, and pancreas. Smoking cessation and avoidance have the potential to save and extend more lives than any other public health activity. About 400,000 Americans die prematurely every year because of cigarette smoking. A smoker has a one in three lifetime risk of dying prematurely of a cancer or cardiovascular or pulmonary disease caused by cigarette smoking. Indeed, more human lives are lost due to cardiovascular disease caused by smoking than from smoking-related cancer. The risk of tobacco smoke is not necessarily limited to the smoker. Epidemiologic studies suggest that environmental tobacco smoke may cause lung cancer and other pulmonary diseases in nonsmokers.

Nonsmoking persons should be encouraged not to start smoking, and persons who smoke should be encouraged to stop. Tobacco prevention is a pediatric issue. Over 80% of American smokers begin smoking before the age of 18. Nearly 20% of Americans aged 12 to 18 have smoked a cigarette in the past month. Counseling of adolescents and young adults is critical to prevent smoking. A physician's simple advice to not start smoking or to quit smoking can be of benefit. The U.S. Agency for Health Care Research and Quality recommends that physicians query patients on tobacco use on every office visit, record the answer with the vital signs, and ask smokers if they would like assistance in quitting.

Current approaches to smoking cessation recognize that smoking is an addiction (Chap. 390). The smoker who is quitting goes through a process with identifiable stages that include contemplation of quitting, an action phase in which the smoker quits, and a maintenance phase. Smokers who quit completely are more likely to be successful than those who gradually reduce the number of cigarettes smoked or change to cigarettes lower in tar or nicotine. More than 90% of the Americans who have successfully quit smoking did so on their own without participation in an organized cessation program, but cessation programs are helpful for some smokers. The Community Intervention Trial for Smoking Cessation (COMMIT) was a community-based 4-year program. One community of each of 11 matched community pairs was randomly assigned to intervention. The intervention included public education through the media and community-wide events, health care providers, worksites and other organizations, and cessation resources. COMMIT demonstrated that light smokers can benefit from simple cessation messages and cessation programs. The quit rate (fraction of the subjects followed who achieved and maintained cessation at the end of the trial) was 30.6% in the intervention communities and 27.5% in the control communities. This finding is statistically significant, but modest. The control communities enjoyed a substantial decrease in smoking through study participation. The COMMIT interventions were not successful for heavy smokers (>25 cigarettes per day). Heavy smokers need an intensive, broad-based cessation program that includes counseling, behavioral strategies, and pharmacologic adjuncts such as nicotine gum and nicotine patches.

Cigar and pipe smoking carry the same risks as tobacco smoke including lung cancer. Smokeless tobacco is the fastest growing part of the tobacco industry and represents a significant health risk. Chewing tobacco is a carcinogen linked to dental caries, gingivitis, oral leukoplakia, and oral cancer. The systemic effects of smokeless tobacco may increase risks for other cancers. Nitrosamines found in smokeless tobacco cause lung cancer in laboratory animals.

Diet Modification   Dietary modification may have significant potential for lowering cancer risk in western culture. Studies of international dietary patterns and animal studies suggest that diets high in fat increase the risk for cancers of the breast, colon, prostate, and endometrium. These cancers have their highest incidence and mortalities in western countries, where fat comprises an average of 40 to 45% of the total calories consumed. In populations at low risk for these cancers, fat accounts for <20% of dietary calories.

Nonetheless, dietary fat has not been accepted by all as important in the etiology of cancers. Case-control and cohort epidemiologic studies give conflicting results. In addition, diet is a highly complex exposure to many nutrients and chemicals. Low-fat diets may render some protection through anticarcinogens found in vegetables, fruits, legumes, nuts, and grains. Substances found in these foods that may be protective include phenols, sulfur-containing compounds, flavones, and fiber.

In observational studies, dietary fiber appears protective against colonic polyps and invasive cancer of the colon. The mechanisms involved are complex and speculative. They involve binding of oxidized bile acids, a decrease in bowel transit time, and generation of soluble fiber products, such as butyrate, that may have differentiating properties. High-fiber diets may also protect against breast and prostate cancer by absorbing and inactivating dietary estrogenic and androgenic cancer promoters. Protective effects of fiber have not been proved in a prospective clinical trial.

The U.S. National Institutes of Health (NIH) Women's Health Initiative, launched in 1994, is a long-term clinical trial enrolling more than 100,000 women aged 45 to 69. It studies the potential cancer-preventing effects of a low-fat diet and vitamin supplementation. It must be stressed that the scientific evidence does not currently establish the anticarcinogenic value of vitamin, mineral, or nutritional supplements in amounts greater than that provided by a good diet.

The Polyp Prevention Trial studied 2000 elderly persons randomly assigned to a low-fat, high-fiber diet or a routine diet followed for 4 years. No significant differences in polyp formation were noted.

A simple way to decrease dietary fat and increase fiber is to consume at least 5 to 9 servings of fruits and vegetables a day. Such a diet may lower the risk of cardiac disease as well as cancer.

Sun Avoidance   Nonmelanoma skin cancers (basal cell and squamous cell) are induced by cumulative exposure to ultraviolet radiation. Intermittent acute sun exposure and sun damage have been linked to melanoma. Sunburns, especially in childhood and adolescence, are associated with an increased risk of melanoma in adulthood. Reduction of sun exposure through use of protective clothing and changes in the pattern of outdoor activities can reduce skin cancer risk. Sunscreens decrease the risk of actinic keratoses, the precursor to squamous cell skin cancer, but melanoma risk may be increased. Sunscreens prevent burning and may encourage more prolonged exposure to the sun; yet they may not filter out wavelengths of energy that cause melanoma.

Educational interventions to help people assess their risk of developing skin cancer accurately have some impact. Self-examination for skin pigment characteristics associated with melanoma, such as freckling, may be useful in identifying people at high risk. People who recognize themselves as being at risk tend to be more compliant with sun-avoidance recommendations. Possible risk factors for melanoma include a propensity to sunburn, a large number of benign melanocytic nevi, and atypical nevi.

CANCER CHEMOPREVENTION   Chemoprevention of cancer is a relatively new concept. It involves the use of specific natural or synthetic chemical agents to reverse, suppress, or prevent carcinogenesis before the development of invasive malignancy. While the concept that pharmacologic agents can prevent a cancer is relatively new, the idea that a compound can prevent chronic disease is not. Clinicians routinely prevent heart disease, kidney disease, and stroke by treating hypertension with pharmacologic agents. Lipid-lowering drugs are used to prevent coronary artery disease.

Improved understanding of the biology of cancer makes chemoprevention a real possibility. Cancer develops through an accumulation of genetic changes that are potential points of intervention to prevent cancer. The initial genetic changes are termed *initiation*. The alteration can be inherited or acquired through the action of physical, infectious, or chemical carcinogens. Like most human diseases, cancer arises through an interaction between genetics and environmental exposures (Table 80-1). Influences that cause the initiated cell to progress through the carcinogenic process and to change phenotypically are termed *promoters*. Promoters include hormones such as androgens, linked to prostate cancer, and estrogen, linked to breast and endometrial cancer. The distinction between an initiator and a promoter is sometimes arbitrary; some components of cigarette smoke are "complete carcinogens," acting as both initiators and promoters. Cancer can be prevented or controlled through interference with the factors that cause initiation, promotion, or progression. Compounds of interest in chemoprevention often have antimutagenic, antioxidant, or antiproliferative activity.

Before a chemoprevention strategy can become standard practice, evidence of benefit must be gathered from clinical trials. These trials are usually large, long-term, randomized, placebo-controlled, and double-blinded. They often allow for the study of drugs for prevention of multiple cancers and the study of end-points beyond cancer, such as other chronic diseases. Several large clinical trials have been completed, and a number are continuing in the twenty-first century. Only tamoxifen has been approved by the U.S. Food and Drug Administration for prevention; it lowers risk of breast cancer in high-risk women.

Multiple Cancer Site Prevention Trials   The Physicians' Health Trial involves 22,071 American male physicians. Participants were randomly assigned to receive β-carotene, aspirin, and/or placebo in a 2 × 2 factorial design. All major medical events were recorded. In 1988, the aspirin arm was unblinded after the trial demonstrated that aspirin therapy causes a significant reduction in cardiovascular mortality. The β-carotene arm of the study stopped in 1998, and data analysis is proceeding.

The Women's Health Study, launched in 1992, is a 10-year trial involving 44,000 female nurses. Subjects are randomly assigned to β-carotene, α-tocopherol, aspirin, and/or placebo in a factorial design

Table 80-1   Carcinogens and Associated Cancers or Neoplasms

Carcinogens[a]	Associated Cancer or Neoplasm
Alkylating agents	Acute myelocytic leukemia, bladder cancer
Androgens	Prostate cancer
Aromatic amines (dyes)	Bladder cancer
Arsenic	Cancer of the lung, skin
Asbestos	Cancer of the lung, pleura, peritoneum
Benzene	Acute myelocytic leukemia
Chromium	Lung cancer
Diethylstilbestrol (prenatal)	Vaginal cancer (clear cell)
Epstein-Barr virus	Burkitt's lymphoma, nasal T cell lymphoma
Estrogens	Cancer of the endometrium, liver
Ethyl alcohol	Cancer of the liver, esophagus, head and neck
Helicobacter pylori	Gastric cancer
Hepatitis B or C virus	Liver cancer
Human immunodeficiency virus	Non-Hodgkin's lymphoma, Kaposi's sarcoma, squamous cell carcinomas (especially of the urogenital tract)
	Human papilloma virus
Human T cell lymphotropic virus type I (HTLV-I)	Adult T cell leukemia/lymphoma
Immunosuppressive agents (aza-thioprine, cyclosporine, gluco-corticoids)	Non-Hodgkin's lymphoma
Nitrogen mustard gas	Cancer of the lung, head and neck, nasal sinuses
Nickel dust	Cancer of the lung, nasal sinuses
Phenacetin	Cancer of the renal pelvis and bladder
Polycyclic hydrocarbons	Cancer of the lung, skin (especially squamous cell carcinoma of scrotal skin)
Schistosomiasis	Bladder cancer (squamous cell)
Sunlight (ultraviolet)	Skin cancer (squamous cell and melanoma)
Tobacco (including smokeless)	Cancer of the upper aerodigestive tract, bladder
Vinyl chloride	Liver cancer (angiosarcoma)

[a] Agents that are thought to act as cancer initiators and/or promoters.

yielding eight different treatment groups. The end-points are total epithelial cancers, breast cancer, lung cancer, colon cancer, and vascular disease.

The Women's Health Initiative uses a partial factorial design that places women in 22 intervention groups. Participants can receive calcium and vitamin D supplementation, hormone replacement therapy, and counseling to increase exercise and cease smoking. Prevention of a number of cancers, cardiovascular disease, osteoporosis, and other diseases will be assessed.

Prevention of Hormonally Driven Cancers   Hormonal manipulation is being tested in the primary prevention of breast and prostate cancer. Tamoxifen is an antiestrogen with partial estrogen agonistic activity in some tissues, such as endometrium and bone. One of its actions is to upregulate transforming growth factor β, which decreases breast cell proliferation. In randomized placebo-controlled trials to assess tamoxifen as an adjuvant in breast cancer treatment, this drug reduced the number of new breast cancers in the uninvolved breast by more than a third. In a randomized placebo-controlled trial involving >13,000 women at high risk, tamoxifen decreased the risk of developing cancer by 49% compared to placebo. Tamoxifen also reduced the risk of bone fractures; a small increase in risk of endometrial cancer, stroke, pulmonary emboli, and deep vein thrombosis was noted. A trial to compare tamoxifen with another selective estrogen receptor modulator, raloxifene, is ongoing.

Finasteride is a 5α-reductase inhibitor. It inhibits the conversion of testosterone to dihydrotestosterone, a more potent stimulator of prostate cell proliferation than testosterone. In an F344 rat model of carcinogen-induced prostate cancer, finasteride decreased the inci-

dence of cancers. Finasteride is being tested as a preventive agent for prostate cancer in a 10-year study involving 18,000 men age 55 and older.

Chemoprevention of Cancers of the Upper Aerodigestive Tract
Smoking causes diffuse epithelial injury in the head, neck, esophagus, and lung. Patients cured of squamous cell cancers of the lung, esophagus, head, and neck are at risk (as high as 5% per year) of developing a second cancer of the upper aerodigestive tract. Cessation of cigarette smoking does not markedly decrease the cured cancer patient's risk of second malignancy, even though it does lower the cancer risk in those who have never developed a malignancy. Smoking cessation may halt the early stages of the carcinogenic process (such as metaplasia), but it may have no effect on late stages of carcinogenesis. This "field carcinogenesis" hypothesis for cancer of the upper aerodigestive tract has made "cured" patients an important population for chemoprevention of second malignancies. A randomized, placebo-controlled clinical trial has demonstrated that adjuvant isoretinoin (13-*cis*-retinoic acid) can reduce the incidence of second primary tumors in patients treated with local therapy for head and neck cancer. However, overall survival was not improved due to mortality from recurrences of the primary tumor.

Oral leukoplakia, a premalignant lesion commonly found in smokers, has been used as an intermediate marker allowing the demonstration of chemopreventive activity in smaller, shorter-duration, randomized, placebo-controlled trials. Response was associated with upregulation of retinoic acid receptor β. Therapy with isoretinoin causes regression of oral leukoplakia. However, the lesions recur when the agent is withdrawn, suggesting the need for chronic administration of retinoids. Premalignant lesions in the oropharyngeal area have also responded to β-carotene, retinol, α-tocopherol (vitamin E), and selenium. Further study to improve the definition of the activity of these drugs is ongoing. The ability of isoretinoin to prevent second malignancies in patients cured of early-stage non-small cell lung cancer is also being assessed.

Several large-scale trials have assessed agents in the chemoprevention of lung cancer in patients at high risk. In the Alpha-Tocopherol/Beta-Carotene (ATBC) Lung Cancer Prevention Trial, participants were male smokers, aged 50 to 69 at entry. At entry, participants had smoked an average of one pack of cigarettes per day for 35.9 years. Participants received α-tocopherol, β-carotene, and/or placebo in a randomized, 2×2 factorial design. After a median follow-up of 6.1 years, lung cancer incidence and mortality were statistically significantly *increased* in those receiving β-carotene. α-Tocopherol had no significant impact on lung cancer mortality, and no evidence suggested interaction between the two drugs. Patients receiving α-tocopherol had a higher incidence of hemorrhagic stroke.

The Beta-Carotene and Retinol Efficacy Trial (CARET) involved 17,000 American smokers and workers with asbestos exposure. Entrants were randomly assigned to one of four arms and received β-carotene, retinol, and/or placebo in a 2×2 factorial design. This trial demonstrated harm from β-carotene: a lung cancer rate of 5 per 1000 subjects per year for those taking placebo and of 6 per 1000 subjects per year for those taking β-carotene. The difference was statistically significant.

These ATBC and CARET results demonstrate the importance of testing chemoprevention hypotheses before implementing them widely, because the results stand in contrast to a number of observational epidemiologic studies. In the ATBC trial, participants taking α-tocopherol had a one-third reduction in the incidence of prostate cancer, compared to those not taking α-tocopherol. Assessment of these findings continues. The Physicians' Health Trial showed neither an increased nor a decreased risk of lung cancer in those using β-carotene; fewer of its participants were smokers than those in the ATBC and CARET studies.

Chemoprevention of Colon Cancer   Many of the current colon cancer prevention trials are based on the premise that most colorectal cancers develop from adenomatous polyps. These trials use adenoma recurrence or disappearance as a surrogate end-point to assess colon cancer prevention. Early clinical trial results suggest that nonsteroidal anti-inflammatory drugs (NSAIDs), such as piroxicam, sulindac, and aspirin, may prevent adenoma formation or cause regression of adenomatous polyps. The mechanism of action of NSAIDs is unknown, but they are presumed to work through the cyclooxygenase pathway. In the Physicians' Health Trial, aspirin had no effect on colon cancer incidence, although the 6-year assessment period may not have been long enough to evaluate definitively this end-point.

Epidemiologic studies suggest that diets high in calcium lower colon cancer risk. Calcium binds bile and fatty acids, which cause hyperproliferation of colonic epithelium. It is hypothesized that this effect reduces intraluminal exposure to these compounds. Early data from randomized studies suggest that calcium supplementation decreases the risk of adenomatous polyp recurrence by about 20%, even though it does not decrease the proliferative rate of the colonic epithelium. Epithelial proliferative rate may not be an adequate surrogate marker in colon cancer prevention trials.

Cyclooxygenase II inhibitors may be even more effective at colon cancer prevention.

Vaccines and Cancer Prevention A number of infectious agents have been linked to the development of cancer, leading to interest in developing vaccines to protect against these agents. The hepatitis B vaccine is quite effective in preventing hepatitis and hepatomas due to chronic hepatitis B infection. Public health officials are encouraging widespread administration of this vaccine, especially in Asia, where the disease is epidemic. In the future, human papilloma virus (HPV) vaccines could be developed to prevent cervical cancer, and *Helicobacter pylori* vaccines may be developed to prevent gastric cancer.

CANCER SCREENING Screening is a means of detecting disease early in asymptomatic individuals with the goal of decreasing morbidity and mortality. Screening for cancer is intuitively appealing and has attracted great public interest as technology has generated a number of diagnostic tests and procedures that are safe, quick, and inexpensive. While screening can potentially save lives, and has been shown clearly to do so in the case of breast, cervical, and colon cancer, it is also subject to a number of biases, which can suggest a benefit when actually there is none. Bias can even mask net harm. Early detection does not in itself confer benefit. To be of value, screening must detect disease earlier, and treatment of earlier disease must yield a better outcome than treatment at the onset of symptoms. Cause-specific mortality, rather than survival after diagnosis, is the preferred end point (see below).

Because screening is done on asymptomatic, healthy persons, it should offer substantial likelihood of benefit. A critical approach to screening is necessary to ensure that benefit results. Screening tests and their appropriate use should be carefully evaluated before their use is widely encouraged in screening programs as a matter of public policy.

Screening examinations, tests, or procedures are usually not diagnostic of cancer but instead indicate that a cancer may be present. The diagnosis is then made following a workup that includes a biopsy and pathologic confirmation.

A number of genes have been identified that predispose for a disease, and many more will be identified in the near future. Testing for these genes can define a high-risk population. The ability to predict the development of a particular cancer may some day present therapeutic options as well as ethical dilemmas. It may eventually allow for early intervention to prevent a cancer or limit its severity. People at high risk will be ideal candidates for chemoprevention and screening; however, the efficacy of these interventions in the high-risk population should be investigated. Currently, persons at high risk for a particular cancer can engage in intensive screening. While this course is clinically prudent, it is not known if it saves lives in these populations.

The Accuracy of Screening A screening test's accuracy or ability to discriminate disease is described by four indices: sensitivity, specificity, positive predictive value, and negative predictive value (Table 80-2). *Sensitivity* is the proportion of persons with the disease who test positive in the screen (i.e., the ability of the test to detect disease when it is present). *Specificity* is the proportion of persons who do not have the disease and test negative in the screening test (i.e., the ability of a test to tell that the disease is not present). The *positive predictive value* is the proportion of persons who test positive who actually have the disease. Similarly, *negative predictive value* is the proportion of who test negative and do not have the disease. The sensitivity and specificity of a test are relatively independent of the underlying prevalence (or risk) of the disease in the population screened, but the predictive values depend strongly on the prevalence of the disease (Table 80-3).

Screening is most beneficial, efficient, and economical when the target disease is common in the population being screened. To be valuable, the screening test should have a high specificity; sensitivity need not be very high, as demonstrated in Table 80-3.

Potential Biases of Screening Tests The common biases of screening are lead time, length, and selection. These biases can make a screening test seem beneficial when actually it is not (or even causes net harm). Whether beneficial or not, screening can create the false impression of an epidemic by increasing the number of cancers diagnosed. It can also give the appearance of a shift in stage, thus improving survival statistics without reducing mortality (i.e., the number of deaths from a given cancer relative to the number of people at risk for

Table 80-2 Definition of Terms

Term	Definition
Sensitivity	The proportion of persons with the condition who test positive: $a/(a + c)$
Specificity	The proportion of persons without the condition who test negative: $d/(b + d)$
Positive predictive value	The proportion of persons with a positive test who have the condition: $a/(a + b)$
Negative predictive value	The proportion of persons with a negative test who do not have the condition: $d/(c + d)$

	Condition present	Condition absent
Positive test	a	b
Negative test	c	d

a = true positive
b = false positive
c = false negative
d = true negative

Table 80-3 Predictive Value Relationships[a]

Positive predictive value (PPV) is a function of sensitivity, specificity, and prevalence:

$$PPV = \frac{prevalence \times sensitivity}{(prevalence \times sensitivity) + (1 - prevalence)(1 - sensitivity)}$$

PPV for a prevalence of 5 per 1000:

	PPV for a Sensitivity of, %	
Specificity	0.8	0.95
0.95	7	9
0.999	80	83

PPV for a prevalence of 1 per 10,000:

	PPV for a Sensitivity of, %	
Specificity	0.8	0.95
0.95	0.2	0.2
0.999	7	9

[a] The positive predictive value is expressed as a percentage. It is influenced by the sensitivity and specificity of the screening test and the prevalence of the disease being screened for. As shown here, for relatively uncommon diseases, such as cancer, the positive predictive value is influenced particularly strongly by the specificity of the screening test at a given prevalence.

the cancer). In such a case, the *apparent* duration of survival increases without lives being saved or life expectancy changed.

Lead-time bias occurs when a test does not influence the natural history of the disease; the patient is merely diagnosed at an earlier date. When lead-time bias occurs, survival *appears* increased, but life is not really prolonged. The screening test only prolongs the time the subject is aware of the disease and spends as a patient.

Length bias occurs when slow-growing, less aggressive cancers are detected during screening. Cancers diagnosed owing to the onset of symptoms between scheduled screenings are on average more aggressive, and treatment outcomes are not as favorable. An extreme form of length bias is termed *overdiagnosis*, the detection of "pseudo-disease." The reservoir of some undetected slow-growing tumors is large. Many of these tumors fulfill the histologic criteria of cancer but will never become clinically significant or cause death. This problem is compounded by the fact that the most common cancers appear most frequently at ages when competing causes of death are more frequent.

Selection bias must be considered in assessing the results of any screening effort. The population most likely to seek screening may differ from the general population to which the screening test might be applied. The individuals screened may have volunteered because of a particular risk factor not found in the general population, such as a strong family history. In general, volunteers for studies may be more health conscious and thus likely to have a better prognosis or lower mortality rate, irrespective of the screening result. This is termed the *healthy volunteer effect*.

Potential Drawbacks of Screening Risks associated with screening include harm caused by the screening intervention itself, harm due to the further investigation of persons with positive test results (both true and false positives), and harm from the treatment of persons with a true-positive result, even if life is extended by treatment. The diagnosis and treatment of cancers that would never have caused medical problems can lead to the harm of unnecessary treatment and give patients the anxiety of a cancer diagnosis. The psychosocial impact of cancer screening, whether the result is positive or negative, can also be substantial when applied to the entire population.

Assessment of Screening Tests Good clinical trial design can offset some biases of screening and demonstrate the relative risks and benefits of a screening test. A randomized, controlled screening trial with cause-specific mortality as the end-point provides the strongest support for a screening intervention. In a randomized trial, two like populations are randomly established. One is given the medical standard of care (which may be no screening at all), and the other receives the screening intervention being assessed. The two populations are compared over time. Efficacy for the population studied is established when the group receiving the screening test has a better cause-specific mortality rate than the control group. Studies showing a reduction in the incidence of advanced-stage disease, an improved survival, or a stage shift are weaker evidence of benefit. These latter criteria are necessary but not sufficient to establish the value of a screening test.

Although a randomized, controlled screening trial provides the strongest evidence to support the usefulness of a screening test, it is not perfect. Unless the trial is population-based, it does not remove

Table 80-4 Screening Recommendations for Asymptomatic Normal-Risk Subjects[a]

Test or Procedure	USPSTF	ACS	CTFPHC
Sigmoidoscopy	>50, periodically <50, not recommended	≥50, every 3–5 years	Insufficient evidence
Fecal occult blood testing	≥50, every year	≥50, every year	Insufficient evidence
Digital rectal examination	No recommendation	≥40, every year	Poor evidence to include or exclude
Prostate-specific antigen	Recommendation against	M: ≥50, every year	Recommendation against
Pap test	F: 18–65, every 1–3 years	F: beginning at age 18, yearly ×3 and then at physician discretion	Fair evidence to include in examination of sexually active women
Pelvic examination	Do not recommend, advise adnexal palpation during exam for other reasons	F: 18–40, every 1–3 years with Pap test; >40, every year	Not considered
Endometrial tissue sampling	Not considered	At menopause if obese or a history of unopposed estrogen use	Not considered
Breast self-examination	No recommendation	≥20, monthly	Insufficient evidence to make a recommendation
Breast clinical examination	F: >50, every year	F: 20–40, every 3 years; >40, yearly	F: >50, every year
Mammography	F: 50–75, every 1–2 years	F: ≥40, every year	F: 50–69, every year
Complete skin examination	Not recommended	20–39, every 3 years	Poor evidence to include or exclude

[a] Summary of the screening procedures recommended for the general population by U.S. Preventive Services Task Force (USPSTF), the American Cancer Society (ACS), and the Canadian Task Force on Prevention Health Care (CTFPHC). These recommendations refer to asymptomatic persons who have no risk factors, other than age or gender, for the targeted condition. NOTE: F, female; M, male.

the issue of generalizability to the target population. Screening trials generally involve thousands of persons and last for years. Less definitive study designs are therefore often used to estimate the effectiveness of screening practices. After a randomized controlled clinical trial, in descending order of strength, evidence may be derived from:

- The findings of internally controlled trials using intervention allocation methods other than randomization (e.g., allocation determined by birth date, date of clinic visit);
- The findings of cohort or case-control analytic observational studies;
- The results of multiple time series studies with or without the intervention;
- The opinions of respected authorities based on clinical experience, descriptive studies, or consensus reports of experts (the weakest evidence because even experts can be misled by the biases described above).

Screening for Specific Cancers Widespread screening for breast, cervical, and colon cancer is beneficial for certain age groups. Special surveillance of those at high risk for a specific cancer because of a family history or a genetic risk factor may be prudent, but few studies have been carried out to assess the impact of this practice on mortality in specific high-risk populations. A number of organizations have considered whether or not to endorse routine use of certain screening tests. Because these groups have not used the same criteria to judge whether a screening test should be endorsed, they have arrived at different recommendations. The screening guidelines of the U.S. Preventive Services Task Force, the Canadian Task Force on Preventive Health Care, and the American Cancer Society are often quoted and show a range of recommendations (Table 80-4).

Breast cancer Breast self-examination, clinical breast examination by a care giver, and mammography have been advocated as useful screening tools. Only screening mammography alone and screening mammography with clinical examination have been evaluated in randomized controlled trials. A number of well-designed trials have demonstrated that annual or biennial screening with mammography or mammography plus clinical breast examination in women over the age of 50 saves lives. In these trials, the breast cancer mortality rate is decreased by about a third. Experts disagree on whether average-risk women aged 40 to 49 should receive regular screening (Table 80-4). The statistical significance of the screening effect in women aged 40 to 49 depends on the statistical test used. An analysis of eight large randomized trials showed no benefit from mammographic screening for women aged 40 to 49 when assessed 5 to 7 years after trial entry. However, a small benefit emerged 10 to 12 years after study entry. What proportion of this possible benefit is due to screening after these women turned 50 is not known. In randomized screening studies of women aged 50 to 69, the decline in mortality begins about 5 years after initiation of screening. Nearly half of women aged 40 to 49 years screened annually will have false-positive mammograms necessitating further evaluation, often including biopsy. The risk of false-positive testing should be discussed with the patient.

While no study has shown breast self-examination to decrease mortality, it is recommended as prudent by many organizations. A substantial fraction of breast cancers are first detected by the patient, even with widespread mammographic screening.

Cervical cancer   Screening with Papanicolaou smears decreases cervical cancer mortality. The cervical cancer mortality rate has fallen significantly since the widespread use of the Pap smear, although this trend actually began earlier. Most screening guidelines recommend regular Pap testing for all women who are or have been sexually active or have reached the age of 18. With the onset of sexual activity comes the risk of sexual transmission of HPV, the most common etiologic factor for cervical cancer. The recommended interval for Pap screening varies from 1 to 3 years. An upper age limit at which screening ceases to be effective is not known.

Colorectal cancer   Fecal occult blood testing, digital rectal examination, rigid and flexible sigmoidoscopy, radiographic barium contrast studies, and colonoscopy have been considered for colorectal cancer screening. Annual fecal occult blood testing using hydrated specimens could reduce colorectal cancer mortality by a third. The sensitivity for fecal occult blood is increased if specimens are rehydrated before testing, but at the cost of lower specificity. The false-positive rate for rehydrated fecal occult blood testing is high; 1 to 5% of persons tested have a positive result. About 2 to 10% of those with occult blood in the stool have cancer, and 20 to 30% have adenomas. The high false-positive rate of fecal occult blood testing dramatically increases the number of colonoscopies performed.

Two case-control studies suggest that regular screening of people over 50 with sigmoidoscopy decreases mortality. These types of studies are prone to selection biases. A quarter to a third of polyps can be discovered with the rigid sigmoidoscope; half are found with a 35-cm flexible scope, and two-thirds to three-quarters are found with a 60-cm scope. Diagnosis of polyposis by sigmoidoscopy should lead to evaluation of the entire colon with colonoscopy and/or barium enema. The most efficient interval for screening sigmoidoscopy is unknown. Case-control studies suggest that testing at intervals of up to 9 years may confer benefit. Most authorities feel that full colonoscopy is too cumbersome and invasive for widespread use as a screening tool in standard-risk populations. It may be suitable for subjects at extremely high risk, such as members of families with a genetic predisposition to colorectal cancer. Colonoscopy is accepted in screening persons with inflammatory bowel disease. Data are not available on digital rectal examination or barium enema as colon cancer screening tools, but both are insensitive.

Lung cancer   Screening chest radiographs and sputum cytology have been evaluated as methods for lung cancer screening. No reduction in lung cancer mortality has been found in these studies, although all the controlled trials performed have had low statistical power. Even screening of high-risk subjects (smokers) has not been proved to be beneficial. Spiral computed tomography (CT) can diagnose lung cancers at early stages; however, false-positive rates are high. Ongoing studies are evaluating spiral CT screening.

Ovarian cancer   Adnexal palpation, transvaginal ultrasound, and serum CA-125 determination have been considered for ovarian cancer screening. Adnexal palpation is too insensitive to detect ovarian cancer at an early enough stage to affect mortality substantially. Neither transvaginal ultrasound nor CA-125 screening has been tested in a completed randomized prospective trial. Ovarian cancer screening can lead to an invasive diagnostic workup, which may include laparotomy. In a clinical study, 0.6% of 900 adult women had a serum CA-125 level >35 U/mL. Thus, if 100,000 adult women were screened, 600 would be identified as having a high CA-125. The prevalence of ovarian cancer in the female adult population is approximately 20 per 100,000. Thus, the screening test would identify 600 women who would undergo further evaluation to identify 20 cases of ovarian cancer. Some of these 600 would only be inconvenienced by an ultrasound examination. Others would undergo an exploratory laparotomy. A large proportion of the 20 women identified as having ovarian cancer would have advanced, incurable disease and thus not benefit from screening. An NIH consensus conference in 1994 concluded that routine screening for ovarian cancer was not indicated for standard-risk women or those with a single affected family member, but that it might be worthwhile in families with genetic ovarian cancer syndromes.

Prostate cancer   The most common prostate cancer screening modalities are digital rectal examination and assays for serum prostate-specific antigen (PSA). Newer serum tests, such as measurement of the ratio of bound to free serum PSA, have yet to be fully evaluated. An emphasis on PSA screening has caused prostate cancer to become the most common non-skin cancer diagnosed in American males. Screening for this disease is very prone to lead-time bias, length bias, and overdiagnosis, and substantial debate rages among experts on whether it is effective. Some experts are concerned that prostate cancer screening, more than screening for other cancers, may cause net harm. Prostate cancer screening clearly detects many asymptomatic cancers, but the ability to distinguish tumors that are lethal but still curable from those that pose little or no threat to health is limited. Men over age 50 have a very high prevalence of indolent, clinically insignificant prostate cancers. No well-designed trial has demonstrated the true benefit of prostate cancer screening and treatment, but trials are in progress.

The effectiveness of radical prostatectomy, radiation therapy, and other treatments for low-stage prostate cancer is also under study in randomized trials. Definitive treatment of cancers detected by screening may cause morbidity for some men, such as impotence and urinary incontinence, and carries a low but finite risk of death. Pending the completion of ongoing randomized trials comparing usual care to prostate screening and comparing definitive therapy to "watchful waiting," organizations have provided conflicting recommendations on prostate cancer screening (Table 80-4). After a thorough review of the literature, the American Cancer Society and the American Urologic Association changed their guidelines from a recommendation for screening to a recommendation that men be offered screening after being informed of the potential risks and benefits. A man should have a life expectancy of at least 10 years to be eligible for screening.

Endometrial cancer   Transvaginal ultrasound and endometrial sampling have been advocated as screening tests for endometrial cancer. Benefit from routine screening has not been shown. Transvaginal ultrasound and endometrial sampling are indicated for workup of vaginal bleeding in postmenopausal women but are not considered as screening tests in symptomatic women.

Skin cancer   Visual examination of all skin surfaces by the patient or by a health care provider is used in screening for basal and squamous cell cancers and melanoma. No prospective randomized study has been performed to look for a mortality decrease. Observational epidemiologic evidence from Scotland and Australia suggests that screening programs have caused a stage shift in melanomas diagnosed. Screening may reinforce sun avoidance and other skin cancer prevention behaviors.

BLOCK G et al: Fruit, vegetables, and cancer prevention: A review of the epidemiological evidence. Nutr Cancer 18:1, 1992

BRAWLEY OW: Prostate carcinoma incidence and patient mortality: The effects of screening and early detection. Cancer 80:1857, 1997

FISHER B et al: Tamoxifen for prevention of breast cancer: Report of the National Surgical Adjuvant Breast and Bowel Project P-1 study. J Natl Cancer Inst 90:1371, 1998

GREENWALD P et al: Chemoprevention. CA Cancer J Clin 45:31, 1995

HENSCHKE CI et al: Early Lung Cancer Action Project: Overall design and findings from baseline screening. Lancet 354:99, 1999

LIPPMAN SM et al: Cancer chemoprevention. J Clin Oncol 12:851, 1994

NATIONAL INSTITUTES OF HEALTH CONSENSUS DEVELOPMENT PANEL: Breast cancer screening for women ages 40–49. J Natl Cancer Inst 89:1015, 1997

SOX HC: Preventive health services in adults. N Engl J Med 330:1589, 1995

THE ALPHA-TOCOPHEROL, BETA CAROTENE CANCER PREVENTION STUDY GROUP: The effect of vitamin E and beta carotene on the incidence of lung cancer and other cancers in male smokers. N Engl J Med 330:1029, 1994

U.S. PREVENTIVE SERVICES TASK FORCE: *Guide to Clinical Preventive Services*, 2d ed. Washington, DC, Government Printing Office, 1996

81

Francis S. Collins, Jeffrey M. Trent

CANCER GENETICS

THE CLONAL NATURE OF CANCER   Nearly all cancers originate from a single cell. While multiple cumulative events are invariably required to move a cell from normal to the transformed phenotype (see below and Chap. 82), the origin of tumors from a single clone of cells is a critical discriminating feature between neoplasia and hyperplasia.

CANCER IS A GENETIC DISEASE   Cancer arises because of alterations in DNA that result in unrestrained cellular proliferation. Most of these alterations involve actual sequence changes in the DNA (i.e., mutation). They may arise as a consequence of random replication errors, exposure to carcinogens (e.g., radiation), or faulty DNA repair processes.

While virtually all cancer is genetic, most cancer is not inherited. Certain individuals with cancer have inherited a germline mutation that predisposes them to the cancer, but even in that situation additional somatic mutations are required for a tumor to develop. In a truly sporadic cancer, *all* of the mutations responsible for the malignant phenotype arise somatically. Such a cancer is caused by genetic alterations but has no hereditary implications.

RNA AND RNA TUMOR VIRUSES   Many malignancies in animals are transmissible, and the etiologic agent is frequently a retrovirus, which possesses a single-stranded RNA genome. During the life cycle of the virus, the single-stranded RNA is converted to double-stranded DNA and is inserted at random into the host chromosome. On rare occasions the virus can be remobilized, carrying along with it an adjacent segment of host DNA. Should this host DNA contain a growth-promoting gene, then the retrovirus is potentially transforming. Although efforts to identify retroviruses in human malignancies have mostly been fruitless, retroviruses are implicated in at least one human malignancy. Human T cell lymphotropic virus (HTLV) type I causes adult T cell lymphoma/leukemia, particularly in Japan and the Caribbean (Chap. 191). Unlike animal retroviruses that induce neoplasia, HTLV-I does not contain a growth-promoting transforming oncogene. The tax protein, a 40-kDa molecule encoded in the pX region of the viral genome, induces the activation of a number of genes (including some promoting growth) through interactions with *rel* family and CREB (cyclic AMP response element binding protein) family transcription factors.

DNA tumor viruses are more commonly involved in human malignancy. Human papilloma viruses (especially types 16 and 18) cause cervical cancer (Chap. 188), and both hepatitis B and hepatitis C viruses have been implicated in hepatocellular carcinoma (Chap. 297) .

In addition, the Epstein-Barr virus, a herpesvirus that causes a mild illness in children but infectious mononucleosis in nonimmune adolescents and adults, causes Burkitt's lymphoma in Africa, nasopharyngeal carcinoma in Asia, and lymphomas in the setting of immune deficiency (Chap. 184).

GENERAL CLASSES OF CANCER GENES   In 1914 Boveri hypothesized that cells become malignant either because of overactivation of a gene that promotes cell division or because of loss of function of a gene that normally restrains growth. This hypothesis is largely correct, although defects in DNA repair genes are also involved. Genes that promote normal cell growth are referred to as *protooncogenes*, and activation of such genes by point mutation, amplification, or dysregulation converts them to *oncogenes*.

Genes that normally restrain growth are called *tumor suppressors* (use of the alternative designation of anti-oncogenes is to be discouraged), and unregulated cell growth arises if their function is lost. The diploid nature of mammalian cells allows certain predictions about the consequences of somatic mutations of tumor suppressor genes. Loss of one allele is unlikely to have significant consequences in most instances, as the remaining normal allele is usually sufficient for normal function. Thus, most cells of an individual with an inherited loss of function of one tumor suppressor allele are functionally normal. Only the rare cell that loses or develops a mutation in the remaining normal copy will exhibit uncontrolled growth. This model correctly predicts that the inheritance pattern of cancer in a family with a tumor suppressor gene mutation will be expressed as an autosomal dominant trait, though the cellular mechanism is recessive.

The third category of genes that contribute to malignancy is the DNA repair genes. Every cell division involves the copying of 6 billion base pairs (bp) of DNA. DNA polymerase has a finite error rate, and many environmental influences can damage DNA. As a consequence, repair systems are essential to protect the integrity of the genome. When the repair systems themselves are faulty, either on the basis of inherited or acquired mutation, the rate of accumulation of mutations throughout the genome rises as cell divisions occur. To the extent that these mutations involve oncogenes and tumor suppressor genes, the likelihood of developing malignancy increases.

MENDELIAN CANCER SYNDROMES   Roughly 100 syndromes of familial cancer have been reported, though many are rare. The majority are inherited as autosomal dominant traits, although some of those associated with DNA repair abnormalities (xeroderma pigmentosum, Fanconi anemia, ataxia telangiectasia) are autosomal recessives. Most of the genes responsible for the dominantly inherited cancer syndromes are tumor suppressor genes (Table 81-1). The hallmarks of a tumor suppressor gene are as follows: (1) the germline mutation that affects one allele generally causes a loss of function; (2) tumors also show loss of the second normal allele as a result of a somatic mutation; and (3) often the *normal* function of the gene is to suppress unrestrained cellular growth or to promote differentiation.

The retinoblastoma gene (*RB*) is a paradigm of such a tumor suppressor gene. In a pedigree showing dominant inheritance of susceptibility to retinoblastoma, a loss-of-function germline mutation occurs in one allele of the *RB* gene on chromosome 13. Analysis of the DNA from the tumors invariably shows that the wild-type allele has also been lost by one of several possible mechanisms (Fig. 81-1). However, not all retinoblastoma tumors arise in the context of a strong family history. Sporadic retinoblastoma, which is usually unilateral and on average occurs at a slightly older age than familial retinoblastoma, is usually a consequence of somatic mutation in both alleles of the *RB* gene without any germline predisposition.

Another tumor suppressor gene is the p53 gene on chromosome 17p, which is frequently altered in solid tumors. p53 is somewhat unusual for a tumor suppressor gene in that missense mutations that produce a dominant negative protein product may also be growth-promoting, so that not all alterations obliterate function. Mutations in p53 are found in nearly half of human tumors. Germline mutations in

Table 81-1   Selected Tumor Suppressor Genes Responsible for Familial Cancer Syndromes

Syndrome	Gene	Chromosome Location	Tumors
Basal cell nevus	PTC	9q22.3	Basal cell cancer, jaw cysts, medulloblastoma
Familial breast/ovarian cancer	BRCA1	17q21	Breast, ovarian, colon, prostate cancer
Familial breast cancer	BRCA2	13q12-13	Breast cancer, male breast cancer
Familial melanoma	p16	9p21	Melanoma, pancreatic cancer
Familial polyposis coli	APC	5q21	Intestinal polyposis, colorectal cancer
Familial retinoblastoma	RB	13q24	Retinoblastoma, osteosarcoma
Familial Wilms' tumor	WT1	11p13	Wilms' tumor, WAGR[a]
Hereditary multiple exostoses	EXT1	11p11-13	Exostoses, chondrosarcoma
Li-Fraumeni	p53	17q13	Sarcomas, breast cancer
Neurofibromatosis type 1	NF1	17q11.2	Neurofibroma, neurofibrosarcoma, brain tumor
Neurofibromatosis type 2	NF2	22q12	Acoustic neuroma, meningioma
Tuberous sclerosis	TSC2	16p13.3	Angiofibroma, renal angiomyolipoma
Von Hippel–Lindau	VHL	3p25-26	Renal cell cancer, pheochromocytoma, retinal angioma, hemangioblastoma

[a] WAGR, Wilms' tumor, aniridia, genitourinary abnormalities, and mental retardation.

p53 have dramatic consequences, resulting in a phenotype known as the *Li-Fraumeni syndrome*, where affected individuals may develop a variety of sarcomas, brain tumors, and leukemia. Figure 81-2 illustrates a typical pedigree of this devastating disorder.

In many instances the discovery of genes responsible for familial cancer syndromes has provided insight into the normal control of cell growth. For instance, in type I neurofibromatosis—one of the more common dominant disorders of humans—positional cloning efforts uncovered a previously unknown gene on chromosome 17q that, when mutated, produces a clinical phenotype of café au lait spots, neurofibromas, Lisch nodules of the iris, and a predisposition to neurofibrosarcoma and glioma. The responsible gene, which (like many of the genes in Table 81-1) has a close homologue in yeast, is neurofibromin (*NF1*), a critical participant in the regulation of the protooncogene *ras*. As shown in Fig. 81-3, the NF1 protein is a GTPase-activating protein (GAP) that normally acts to convert *ras* from its active, growth-promoting, GTP-bound form to its inactive, GDP-bound form. Loss of both copies of *NF1* (one copy by inheritance, one by somatic mutation)

thus renders a cell vulnerable to overgrowth, since *ras* is left in the "on" position.

While most autosomal dominant inherited cancer syndromes are due to mutations in tumor suppressor genes, there are a few interesting exceptions. Multiple endocrine neoplasia type II—a dominant disorder characterized by pituitary adenomas, medullary carcinoma of the thyroid, and (in some pedigrees) pheochromocytoma—is due to gain-of-function mutations in the protooncogene *ret* on chromosome 10.

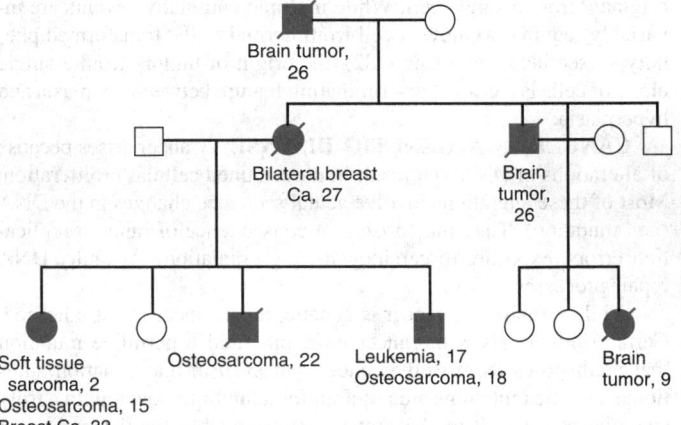

FIGURE 81-2 Pedigree of a family with the Li-Fraumeni syndrome. The affected individuals have developed sarcomas, brain tumors, leukemia, and breast cancer at an early age. All of the affected individuals were found to have a germline mutation in codon 252 of the p53 gene. (*After D Malkin et al, Science 250:1233, 1990, with permission.*)

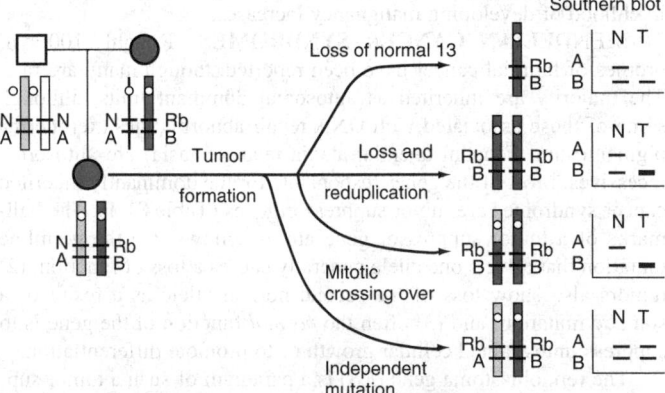

FIGURE 81-1 Diagram of possible mechanisms for tumor formation in an individual with familial retinoblastoma. On the left is shown the pedigree of an affected individual who has inherited the abnormal (Rb) allele from her affected mother. The four chromosomes of her two parents are drawn to indicate their origin. Just below the retinoblastoma locus a polymorphic marker is also analyzed in this family. The patient is AB at this locus, like her mother, whereas her father is AA. Thus the B allele must be on the chromosome carrying the retinoblastoma disease gene. Tumor formation results when the normal allele (N), which this patient inherited from her father, is inactivated. On the right are shown four possible ways in which this could occur. In each case, the resulting chromosome 13 arrangement is shown, as well as the results of a Southern blot comparing normal tissue with tumor tissue. Note that in the first three situations the normal allele (A) has been lost in the tumor tissue, which is referred to as loss of heterozygosity. (*From TD Gelehrter and FS Collins, in Principles of Medical Genetics, Baltimore, Williams & Wilkins, 1990, with permission.*)

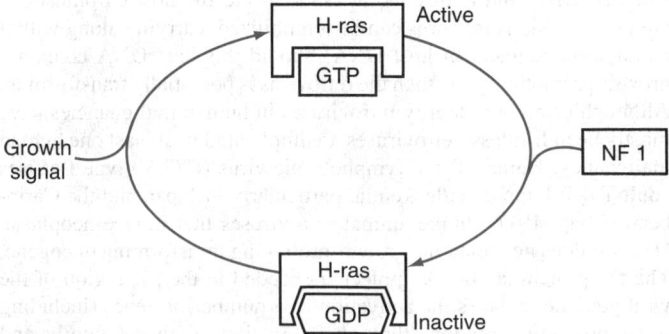

FIGURE 81-3 The *ras* pathway. The active form of the *ras* protein binds GTP and promotes cell division. The conversion to the inactive form, which binds GDP, is catalyzed by a number of proteins including the protein product of the neurofibromatosis type I (*NF1*) gene. Thus, loss of function of NF1 has the effect of leaving *ras* in the "on" position. Alternatively, mutations in the *ras* protein that block its inactivation also predispose to cancer.

Interestingly, loss-of-function mutations in *ret* cause a totally different phenotype, Hirschsprung's disease (aganglionic megacolon) (Chaps. 339 and 289).

Dominantly inherited colon cancer is sometimes associated with familial polyposis, which is usually due to mutations in the adenomatous polyposis coli (*APC*) tumor suppressor gene on chromosome 5 (Table 81-1). However, in most colon cancer families affected individuals do not have familial polyposis, but instead the cancer arises from normal-appearing epithelium. Hereditary nonpolyposis colon cancer (HNPCC, or Lynch's syndrome) is commonly defined as the occurrence of colon cancer in at least three individuals over at least two generations and with at least one individual diagnosed under the age of 50. As many as 1 in 200 individuals in the general population may have HNPCC, although this number is somewhat controversial. Most HNPCC is due to mutations in one of four DNA mismatch repair genes (Table 81-2). All four of these genes are components of a repair system that is normally responsible for correcting errors in freshly copied DNA. Tumors in patients with HNPCC are characterized by profound genomic instability, especially for short repeated sequences called *microsatellites*. Figure 81-4 shows an example of the instability in allele sizes for dinucleotide repeats in the cancers in HNPCC. The unstable phenotype [sometimes referred to as the "mutator" phenotype, or the "RER⁺" (replication error) phenotype] probably requires loss of both copies of the particular mismatch repair gene (one inherited, one somatic), so that the mechanism is similar to that typical of a tumor suppressor gene.

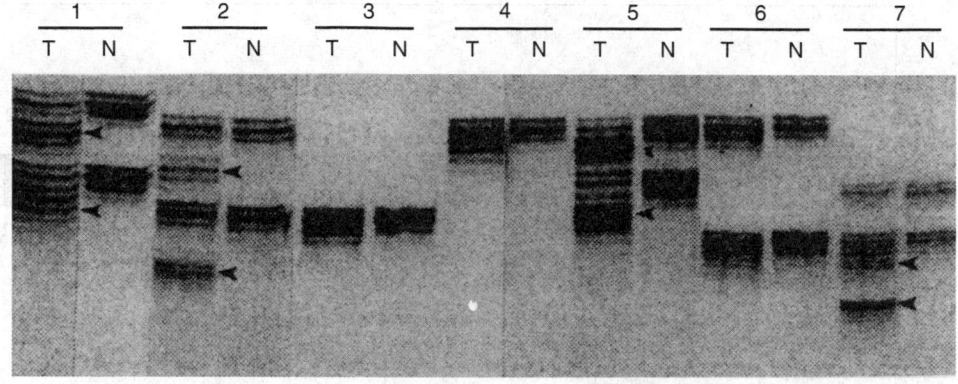

FIGURE 81-4 Demonstration of microsatellite instability in normal and tumor tissue from HNPCC (hereditary nonpolyposis colon cancer) patients. In each case the lane marked T contains DNA from a tumor, and the lane marked N contains DNA from normal tissue of the same patient. The marker (*D2S123*, located on chromosome 2) is a microsatellite composed of a tandem repeat of the dinucleotide CA, which varies in length from chromosome to chromosome. Normally, however, the length of the repeat is stable in somatic tissues. In this example, a polymerase chain reaction analysis has been applied to genomic DNA, and new alleles for the marker are apparent in tumors 1, 2, 5, and 7. Because the tumor tissue is defective in DNA mismatch repair, clonal abnormalities in copying of the CA repeat have arisen. Errors are also occurring in functional genes, eventually resulting in the malignant phenotype. (*From LA Aaltonen et al, Clues to the pathogenesis of familial colorectal cancer. Science 260:812, 1993, with permission.*)

MORE COMPLEX INHERITED FORMS OF CANCER

While the Mendelian forms of cancer described above have taught us much about mechanisms of cellular growth control, most forms of cancer do not follow such simple patterns of inheritance. In many instances (e.g., lung cancer), a strong environmental contribution is at work, but even in such circumstances some individuals may be genetically more susceptible to developing cancer given the appropriate exposure.

In the case of breast and ovarian cancer, circumstantial evidence indicates that a subset of affected individuals (5 to 10%) might be accounted for by dominantly inherited high-penetrance susceptibility genes; two of these genes have been identified by positional cloning. *BRCA1*, located on chromosome 17, is capable when mutated of producing a high risk (up to 85% lifelong) of breast cancer and also of ovarian cancer (50% lifelong risk). Roughly 1 in 500 women carries a germline *BRCA1* mutation, often giving rise to a strong family history. Men with *BRCA1* mutations may have a modestly increased risk of prostate cancer. An array of mutational heterogeneity has been described for *BRCA1* (Fig. 81-5), as is often the case for genetic disorders. An exception is the Ashkenazi Jewish population, where 1 in 100 individuals carries a particular 2-bp deletion (denoted 185delAG)

of *BRCA1*, apparently as a consequence of descent from a common ancestor.

Mutations in another gene on chromosome 13, *BRCA2*, also confer a high risk of breast cancer (and a somewhat lower risk of ovarian cancer); men with *BRCA2* mutations are prone to develop breast cancer. The frequency of *BRCA2* mutations is estimated to be about half that of *BRCA1*. About 1% of Ashkenazi Jews again have a common mutation: 6174delT.

What then of the 90 to 95% of breast cancers that arise in individuals without germline alterations in *BRCA1* or *BRCA2*? Hereditary factors may still contribute to a significant fraction of these, but those factors must be weaker and therefore more difficult to discern.

GENETIC TESTING AND COUNSELING FOR CANCER SUSCEPTIBILITY

The discovery of genes like *RB*, p53, *NF1*, *ret*, the HNPCC mismatch repair genes, *BRCA1*, and *BRCA2* raises the possibility of DNA analysis to predict risk of cancer. There are many complexities associated with such testing. First, one must know the sensitivity and specificity of the test; the mutational heterogeneity for each of these genes constitutes a considerable technical challenge, as it is often necessary to sample every nucleotide of the coding region, the splice junctions, and the promoter to identify most mutations. False-positive results—i.e., sequence alterations that turn out to be benign polymorphic variants (allelic variations) rather than disease-causing mutations—can present a thorny problem. Unless proven interventions are available and the test is sensitive, specific, and relatively inexpensive, it will be inappropriate to offer such tests to the general population; the number of false-positive tests will exceed the number of true positives and a great deal of anxiety and expense will be incurred evaluating persons who are not at an increased risk. Generally, therefore, such testing is not considered except for individuals of higher-than-normal risk, usually on the basis of their family history. In deciding whether to offer such testing, it is critical to determine whether evidence exists for effective interventions to reduce the risk of cancer in those found to be at high risk. If such interventions do not exist (as is the case for Li-Fraumeni syndrome), then the value of the information is limited, and the major negative psychological consequences of this information must be seriously considered.

For conditions such as colon and breast cancer, prophylactic measures exist (total colectomy and bilateral mastectomy, respectively), but these prophylactic measures are more radical and potentially disfiguring than the surgical procedures that would be used to treat the patient if the malignancies actually occurred (segmental bowel resection and lumpectomy, respectively). Other potential negative conse-

Table 81-2 Genetic Alterations in Kindreds with Hereditary Nonpolyposis Colon Cancer (HNPCC)

Gene	Percent of Cases
MSH2	31
MLH1	33
PMS1	2
PMS2	4

SOURCE: Liu et al, *Nature Med* 2:169, 1996, with permission.

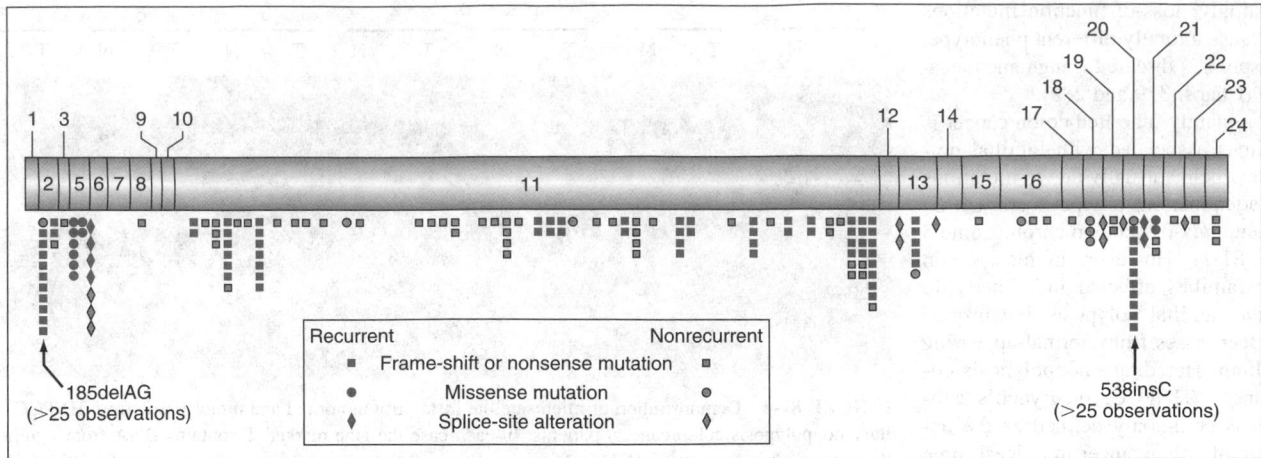

FIGURE 81-5 Germline mutations that have been reported in the *BRCA1* gene, primarily found in families with a high incidence of breast cancer, ovarian cancer, or both. The numbers refer to the exons of the gene; there is no exon 4. *(Information is provided courtesy of the Breast Cancer Information Core data base, which is accessible on the World Wide Web at www.nchgr.nih.gov/ dir/lab_transfer/bic/.)*

quences of a positive genetic test include insurance and employment discrimination. One can still argue, of course, that a close relative of an individual known to carry a mutation in a cancer-causing gene is already sensitized to his or her personal risk of cancer, and that a test establishing that an individual at risk does *not* harbor the mutation can be quite useful. Testing should never be undertaken, however, without a full consideration of how the individual will handle a positive as well as a negative result.

Despite these caveats, genetic testing for some cancer syndromes already appears to have greater benefits than risks, and in those situations it is reasonable to offer testing to individuals at high risk. This would include conditions such as multiple endocrine neoplasia type 2 (Chap. 339) and von Hippel-Lindau disease (Chap. 370). More in the gray zone, although potentially applicable to much larger numbers of individuals, are tests for *BRCA1*, *BRCA2*, and the HNPCC genes. More research is urgently needed in those situations to determine the effectiveness of various interventions (life-style, diet, surveillance, or surgery). Until those answers are available, such testing should be offered only as part of a research protocol. As more susceptibility genes are identified, better answers become available about the effectiveness of interventions, and health insurance discrimination is legislatively prohibited, genetic testing will move into the mainstream of medicine. Every physician of the future will need to have the skills of a genetic counselor.

ACQUIRED MUTATIONS IN CANCER The identification of mutations in the germline of patients with heritable cancers means that the alteration is present in every cell of the body. However, in most cancers a normal cell becomes a malignant cell by a series of mutations that arise not in the germline but in somatic cells. Usually mutations must occur in several genes to give rise to neoplasia. The underlying questions are "how many mutations cause a cancer?" and "what specific genes are affected?" rather than whether or not mutational events cause cancer.

While answers to these questions are not available for every human malignancy, advances in molecular and cellular biology and epidemiologic analyses of human and experimental cancers are providing insights in cancer causation. Table 81-3 summarizes evidence from several lines of investigation pointing to a mutational basis for cancer causation. One particularly striking feature is the fact that the overall incidence of cancer increases as the fourth to sixth power of age for most malignancies (Fig. 81-6*A*). For some tumors, the shape of the age-incidence curve suggests heterogeneity in molecular mechanisms. For example, Hodgkin's disease has a bimodal age distribution, suggesting that two etiologically (and therefore mutationally) distinct forms of this disease may exist (Fig. 81-6*B*).

MULTISTEP BASIS OF CANCER From 5 to 10 accumulated mutations are thought to be necessary for a cell to move from the normal to the fully malignant phenotype. At each step the mutated cell may gain a slight growth advantage, so that it is increased in its representation relative to its neighbors. Figure 81-7, a representation of a lineage diagram hypothesized by Peter Nowell, illustrates how a single cell, afflicted with progressive alterations in tumor suppressor genes and protooncogenes, can develop into a clonal malignancy.

We are beginning to understand the precise nature of the genetic alterations responsible for some malignancies and to get a sense of the order in which they occur. Perhaps the best studied example is colon cancer, where an analysis of DNA from tissues extending from normal epithelium through adenoma to carcinoma have identified some of the genes mutated along the way (Fig. 81-8). However, the order of mutational events is far from uniform, and the diagram in Fig. 81-8 should be considered a generalization and not a defined pathway. Similar data are being accumulated for other malignancies.

MECHANISMS OF SOMATIC MUTATION OF ONCO-GENES IN MALIGNANCY Cellular protooncogenes, their necessity and importance in normal cell growth, and their responsibility for transformation-associated change after removal of normal growth controls are discussed in Chap. 82. Mechanisms that upregulate (or activate) cellular protooncogenes can be grouped into three broad areas: point mutations, DNA amplification, and chromosome rearrangements.

Point Mutation One protooncogene that is commonly activated in solid tumors by point mutation is a member of the *ras* family of oncogenes; these were initially cloned from human bladder carcinoma cells and are critical regulators of normal and aberrant cell growth (Fig. 81-3). Mutations in one of the *ras* genes (H-*ras*, K-*ras*, or N-*ras*) are present in up to 85% of pancreatic cancers and 15% of all human cancers. In studies of K-*ras* (particularly in lung and colon cancer), the mutational spectrum of this gene has been identified. Remarkably, and in contrast to the diversity of mutations observed in the *BRCA1* gene (Fig. 81-5), most of these activated genes contain point mutations in codons 12 or 61 (which convey resistance to the inactivating action of GAP). The specificity of this pattern of mutation means that it has

Table 81-3   Evidence That Mutations Cause Cancer

Malignant tumors are clonal in nature
Some cancers show a Mendelian pattern of inheritance
DNA from malignant cells can in some instances transform normal cells to a malignant phenotype
Most tumors contain somatic mutations in oncogenes and/or tumor suppressor genes
Recurring sites of chromosome change are observed in cancers at the sites of genes involved in cellular growth control
Most carcinogens are mutagens
Defects in DNA repair systems increase the probability of cancer

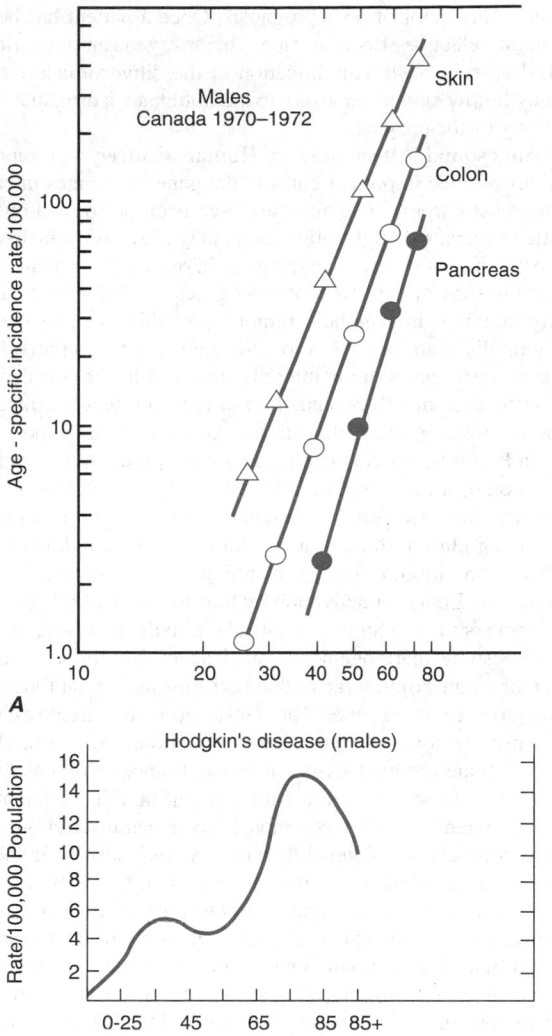

A

B

FIGURE 81-6 Relationship between age and cancer incidence. *A.* Age-specific incidence of skin, colon, and pancreas cancers in Canadian males. The curves appear as straight lines when plotted using logarithmic axes, fitting the multihit model of cancer (see text). *B.* For some tumor types (e.g., Hodgkin's disease), a bimodal age distribution is seen, perhaps indicative of a differing mutational basis (see text). *(From I Tannock and R Hall, The Basic Science of Oncology, 2d ed, New York, McGraw Hill, 1992, with permission.)*

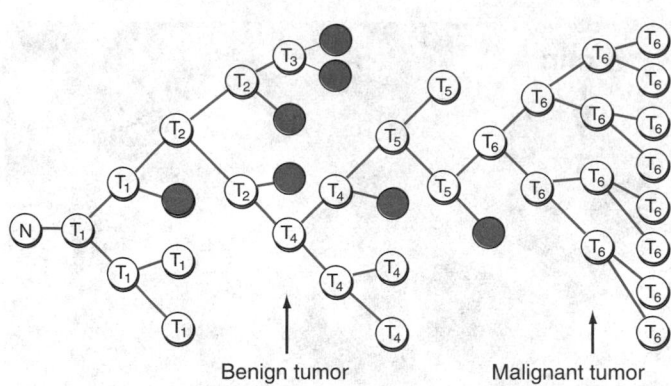

Benign tumor   Malignant tumor

FIGURE 81-7 Multistep clonal development of malignancy. In this diagram a series of five cumulative mutations (T1, T2, T4, T5, T6), each with a modest growth advantage acting alone, eventually results in a malignant tumor. Note that not all such alterations result in progression; for example, the T3 clone is a dead end. The actual number of cumulative mutations necessary to transform from the normal to the malignant state is unknown in most tumors. *(After P Nowell, Science 194:23, 1976, with permission.)*

The recognition of DNA amplification was greatly facilitated by the development of a procedure based on dual-color fluorescence in situ hybridization (FISH) called *comparative genomic hybridization* (CGH). DNA from tumor and normal cells is labeled with different fluorescent reporter molecules and then hybridized to normal metaphase chromosomes. Regions of duplications and deletions within tumor DNA are then demonstrated as quantifiable alterations in signal intensity at particular sites. With this technique the entire genome can be surveyed for gains and losses of DNA sequences, thus pinpointing chromosomal regions likely to contain genes important in the development or progression of cancer.

Numerous genes are known to be amplified in human malignancies. Several genes, including N-*myc* were identified because they were present within the amplified DNA sequences of a tumor and had homology to known oncogenes. Because the region amplified often extends to hundreds of thousands of base pairs, more than one oncogene may be amplified in some cancers (particularly sarcomas). Genes simultaneously amplified in many cases include *MDM2, GLI, CDK4, SAS,* and others implicated in cellular growth control. The clinical implications of gene amplification have been explored for some cancers [most notably *ERBB2 (HER-2/neu)* in breast cancer and N-*myc* in neuroblastoma]; demonstration of amplification of a cellular gene

potential value in diagnostic or prognostic studies of cancer. For K-*ras*, mutations may be a useful prognostic marker in lung cancer, but for most other cancers (including pancreas and colon cancer) no prognostic utility has been demonstrated. This is in part because *ras* mutations occur early in colon cancer (Fig. 81-8), being common in precancerous lesions of the bowel.

DNA Amplification The second mechanism for activation of oncogene overexpression is DNA sequence amplification. This increase in DNA sequence copy number may cause cytologically recognizable chromosome alterations referred to as *homogeneous staining regions* (HSRs), if integrated within chromosomes, or *double minutes* (dmins), if extrachromosomal in nature (Fig. 81-9).

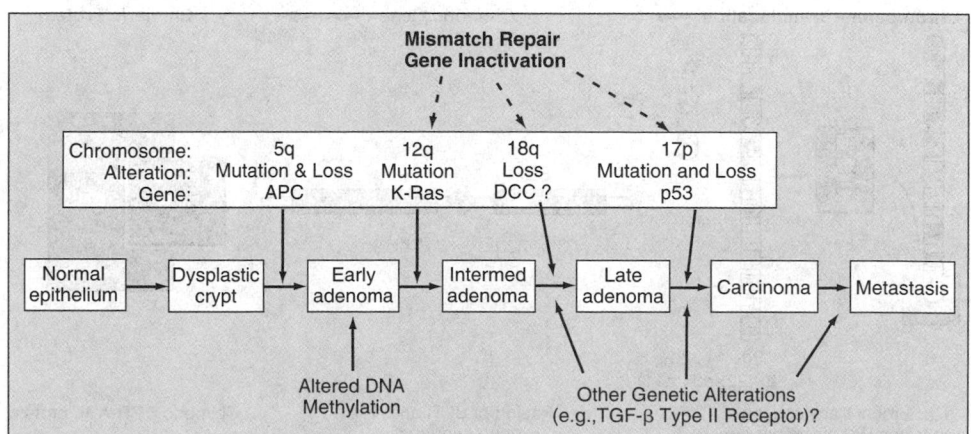

FIGURE 81-8 Progressive somatic mutational steps in the development of colon carcinoma. The accumulation of alterations in a number of different genes results in the progression from normal epithelium through early adenoma to full blown carcinoma. While the steps shown here do not always occur in this order, it is clear that an accumulation of somatic mutations is required before cancer develops. Patients with familial polyposis are already one step into this pathway, since they inherit a germline alteration of the *APC* gene.

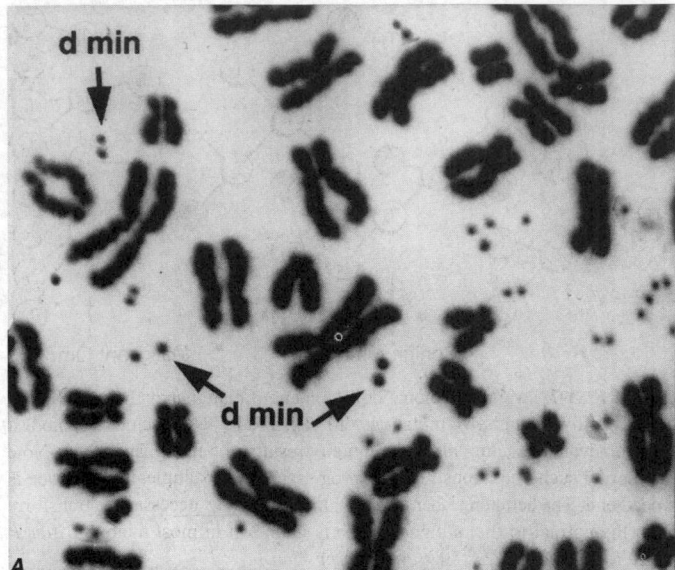

FIGURE 81-9 Representative examples of tumor cells containing cytogenetic evidence of gene amplification. *A.* Example of multiple copies of double minute (dmin) chromosomes from a patient with ovarian carcinoma. *B.* Example of a homogeneous staining region (HSR) on chromosome 7 from a patient with malignant melanoma.

is usually a predictor of poor prognosis. Once a patient has been exposed to the selective effects of chemotherapy, gene amplification may lead to drug resistance. Amplification of the dihydrofolate reductase gene may follow clinical exposure to methotrexate, a drug that inhibits the activity of the enzyme.

Chromosomal Alterations in Human Cancer Chromosomal alterations provide important clues to the genetic changes in cancers. To date, most chromosome analyses have been performed on hematopoietic cancers, although solid tumors may also have translocations. The breakpoints of several recurring chromosome abnormalities often occur at the sites of cellular protooncogenes. Translocations are particularly common in lymphoid tumors, probably because these cell types normally rearrange DNA to generate antigen receptors. Indeed, antigen receptor genes are commonly involved in the translocations, implying that an imperfect regulation of receptor gene rearrangement may be involved in the pathogenesis. An example is Burkitt's lymphoma, a B-cell tumor characterized by a reciprocal translocation between chromosomes 8 and 14. Molecular analysis of Burkitt's lymphomas demonstrated that the breakpoints occurred within or near the *myc* locus on chromosome 8 and within the immunoglobulin heavy chain locus on chromosome 14, resulting in the transcriptional activation of *myc.* Enhancer activation by translocation, although not universal, appears to play an important role in malignant progression.

Chromosome rearrangements can lead to the abnormal overexpression of a transcription factor that performs its normal function and turns on growth-related genes. The translocation may create a chimeric transcription factor that has altered function. For example, the t(15;17) of acute promyelocytic leukemia produces a retinoic acid receptor with an abnormal cell distribution that inhibits differentiation. Gene rearrangements most commonly involve transcription factors, but other components of signaling pathways may also be involved.

The first reproducible chromosome abnormality detected in human malignancy was the Philadelphia chromosome in chronic myelogenous leukemia (CML). This cytogenetic abnormality is generated by reciprocal translocation involving the *ABL* oncogene, a tyrosine kinase on chromosome 9 being placed in proximity to the *BCR* (breakpoint cluster region) on chromosome 22. Figure 81-10 illustrates the generation of the translocation and its protein product. The consequence of expression of the *BCR-ABL* gene product is the activation of signal transduction pathways, leading to cell growth independent of normal external growth factor signals.

In addition to transcription factors and signal transduction molecules, translocations may involve the overexpression of cell cycle regulatory proteins, such as cyclins, and of proteins that regulate cell death, such as bcl2. Altering control of expression of cell cycle regulatory proteins can lead to aberrant cell cycle control. The overexpression of bcl-2 can prevent the death of a cell that has endured enough genetic damage to cause its death. If such a cell survives to receive additional genetic damage, a tumor can develop. Table 81-4 lists representative examples of recurring chromosome alterations in malignancy and the associated gene(s) rearranged or dysregulated by the chromosomal change.

Technical obstacles have slowed the identification of recurring chromosome abnormalities in human solid tumors (particularly carcinomas) because of the complexity of chromosome alterations in such tumors, in contrast to the solitary, often reciprocal, nature of chromosome rearrangements in hematopoietic malignancies.

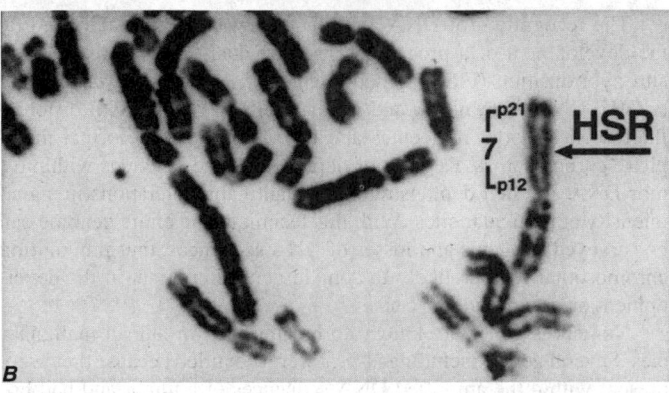

Chromosome Translocation → **Chimeric Gene** → **Chimeric Protein**

9   22   9q+   22q-
t(9;22)(q34;q11)

Reciprocal translocation generates Ph¹ chromosome

Fusion of BCR and ABL gene sequences

Chimeric BCR-ABL protein

FIGURE 81-10 Specific translocation seen in chronic myelogenous leukemia (CML). The Philadelphia chromosome (Ph) is derived from a reciprocal translocation between chromosomes 9 and 22 with the breakpoint joining the sequences of the *ABL* oncogene with the *BCR* gene. The fusion of these DNA sequences allows the generation of an entirely novel fusion protein with modified function (see text). *(Courtesy of ER Fearon and KR Cho.)*

EPIGENETIC REGULATION OF GENE EXPRESSION AND CANCER The term *epigenetic* refers

Table 81-4 Representative Oncogenes at Chromosomal Translocations

Gene (Chromosome)	Translocation	Malignancy
ABL (9q34.1)	(9;22)(q34;q11)	Chronic myelogenous leukemia
BCR (22q11)		
AML1 (21q22)	(3;21)(q26;q22)	Acute myelogenous leukemia, myelodysplasia
EAP (3q26)		
EVI1 (3q26)		
ATF1 (12q13)	(12;22)(q13;q12)	Malignant melanoma of soft parts (MMSP)
EWS (22q12)		
BCL1 (11q13.3)	(11;14)(q13;q32)	Mantle cell lymphoma
IgH (14q32)		
BCL2 (18q21.3)	(14;18)(q32;q21)	Follicular lymphoma
IgH (14q32)		
BCL3 (19q13.1)	(14;19)(q32;q13)	B cell chronic lymphocytic leukemia
IgH (14q32)		
ERG (21q22.3)	(22;21)(q12;q22)	Ewing's sarcoma
EWS (22q12)		
FLI1 (11q24)	(11;22)(q24;q12)	Ewing's sarcoma
EWS (22q12)		
LCK (1p34)	(1;7)(p34;q35)	T cell acute lymphocytic leukemia (ALL)
TCRB (7q35)		
MLL/ALL1/HRX (11q23)	(4;11)(q21;q23)	ALL
myc (8q24)	(8;14)(q24;q32)	Burkitt's lymphoma, B cell ALL
TAN1 (9q34) deletion	(7;9)(q34;q34)	T cell ALL
WT1 (11p13)	(11;22)(p13;q12)	Desmoplastic small round cell tumor (DSRCT)
EWS (22q12)		
TLS/FUS (16p11)	(12;16)(q13;p11)	Myxoid liposarcoma
CHOP (12q13)		
PAX3 (2q35)	(2;13)(q35;q14)	Alveolar rhabdomyosarcoma
FKHR/ALV(13q14)		
PAX7 (1p36)	(1;13)(p36;q14)	Alveolar rhabdomyosarcoma
KHR/ALV(13q14)		
ret (10q11.2)	(10;17)(q11.2;q23)	Papillary thyroid carcinomas

SOURCE: After Hesketh.

to mechanisms of gene regulation independent of DNA sequence. The inactivation of the second X chromosome in female cells is an example of an epigenetic mechanism that prevents gene expression from the inactivated chromosome. During embryologic development, entire regions of chromosomes from one parent are silenced and gene expression proceeds from the chromosome of the other parent. For most genes, expression occurs from both parental alleles or randomly from one parent or the other. The preferential expression of a particular gene exclusively from the allele contributed by one parent is called *parental imprinting* and is thought to be regulated by the methylation of the silenced allele.

The role of epigenetic control mechanisms in the development of human cancer is unclear. However, a general decrease in the level of DNA methylation has been noted as a common change in cancers. In addition, the loss of imprinting of the normally silent maternal allele of the insulin-like growth factor II gene at chromosome 11p15.5 has been implicated in some cases of the rare pediatric malignancy Wilms' tumor. The loss of imprinting may result in the overexpression of the growth factor and a predisposition to malignant transformation.

THE FUTURE The real challenge in oncology is to convert the growing molecular understanding of cancer into clinical advances, particularly the development of new therapies. One can anticipate that in the coming years the molecular analysis of mutations in tumors will allow stratification of malignancies into more precise subgroups than is currently possible by histologic classification, including subgroups with particularly good or bad prognoses or that have a lower or higher likelihood of responding to a particular therapy. Some of this information is already accumulating, but usually only one or two genes are assessed; the promise of the future is to obtain a detailed molecular "fingerprint" of every tumor in order to provide the maximum information about its biology and response to therapy. The application of techniques for assessing global gene expression (cDNA microarrays,

serial analysis of gene expression, or SAGE, and others) is leading to novel ways of looking at cancer that are considerably more discriminating than light microscopy, the gold standard of medical practice. The National Cancer Institute in conjunction with the National Center for Biotechnology Information have undertaken the Cancer Genome Anatomy Project (CGAP) (www.ncbi.nlm.nih.gov/ncicgap/) to collect data on the differences in gene expression between normal and malignant tissues and make it available on the Internet.

Genetics will also influence cancer prevention and early detection. The ability to identify cancer susceptibility genes presages a new era of cancer prevention, if the potential risks of such testing can be surmounted. Currently, most cancer early detection strategies (such as mammography, stool occult blood testing, or digital rectal examination) are applied to population groups. The ability to identify the individuals at highest risk and to focus preventive medicine efforts accordingly may be both better received by patients and more cost effective. Early detection strategies will be even more effective if we can develop the ability to identify very small numbers of malignant or premalignant cells at a time when the risk of metastasis is still very low.

More importantly, detailed molecular information about the regulation of the cell cycle and the interplay of tumor suppressor genes and proto-oncogenes that control it may lead to new effective therapies, based on pathophysiology rather than empiricism. Whether such strategies will rely on drugs of the traditional types or will be based on more novel strategies such as gene therapy or immunotherapy is hard to predict.

BIBLIOGRAPHY

BUNZ F et al: Disruption of p53 in human cancer cells alters the responses to therapeutic agents. J Clin Invest 104:263, 1999

BUTEL JS: Viral carcinogenesis: revelation of molecular mechanisms and etiology of human disease. Carcinogenesis 21:405, 2000

CUI H et al: Loss of imprinting in normal tissue of colorectal cancer patients with microsatellite instability. Nat Med 4:1276, 1998

EMMERT-BUCK MR et al: Molecular profiling of clinical tissue specimens: Feasibility and applications. Am J Pathol 156:1109, 2000

FEINBERG AP: DNA methylation, genomic imprinting and cancer. Curr Top Microbiol Immunol 249:87, 2000

GOLUB TR et al: Molecular classification of cancer: Class discovery and class prediction by gene expression monitoring. Science 286:531, 1999

HABER DA, FEARON ER: The promise of cancer genetics. Lancet 351(Suppl 2):S1, 1998

KORSMEYER SJ: Bcl-2 gene family and the regulation of programmed cell death. Cancer Res 59(suppl 7):1693s, 1999

LAL A et al: A public database for gene expression in human cancers. Cancer Res 59: 5403, 1999

TONIN P: Genes implicated in hereditary breast cancer syndromes. Semin Surg Oncol 18: 281, 2000

VOGELSTEIN B, KINZLER KW: The multistep nature of cancer. Trends Genet 9:138, 1993

82 *Robert G. Fenton, Dan L. Longo*

CELL BIOLOGY OF CANCER

Two characteristic features define a cancer: cell growth not regulated by external signals (i.e., autonomous) and the capacity to invade tissues and metastasize to and colonize distant sites (Chap. 83). The first of these features, the uncontrolled growth of abnormal cells, is a property of all neoplasms, or new growths. A neoplasm may be benign or malignant. If invasion, the second cardinal feature of cancer, is present, the neoplasm is malignant. Cancer is a synonym for *malignant neoplasm*. Cancers of epithelial tissues are called *carcinomas*; cancers of nonepithelial (mesenchymal) tissues are called *sarcomas*.

Cancer is a genetic disease, but the level of its expression is the single cell. Although some forms of cancer are heritable, most mutations occur in somatic cells and are caused by intrinsic errors in DNA replication or are induced by carcinogen exposure. A single genetic lesion is usually not sufficient to induce neoplastic transformation of a cell. The malignant phenotype is acquired only after several (5 to 10) mutations lead to derangements in a variety of gene products. Each genetic alteration may cause phenotypic changes typified by the progression in epithelial tissues from hyperplasia to adenoma to dysplasia to carcinoma in situ to invasive carcinoma. Cells have evolved mechanisms to resist neoplastic transformation (see below).

The >200 discrete cell types in the body are not equally susceptible to developing cancer. Some cells, such as cardiac myocytes, sensory receptor cells for light and sound, and lens fibers, persist throughout life without dividing or being replaced. Neoplasia in such tissues is exceedingly rare. Most differentiated tissues undergo constant renewal characterized by cell death and replacement.

In tissues with rapid turnover, such as skin, bone marrow, and gut, an individual cell is on one of two largely mutually exclusive paths: division or differentiation. Cells capable of dividing are undifferentiated (stem cells), whereas terminally differentiated cells are unable to divide. Stem cells produce daughter cells that can either become new stem cells (thus replenishing the stem cell compartment) or undergo terminal differentiation, depending on the circumstances and the environmental signals. Stem cells are distinguished from differentiating cells by different patterns of gene expression. Gene expression is the product of the tissue-specific programming interacting with environmental factors such as cell-to-cell contact; interactions with extracellular matrix; endocrine hormones; paracrine growth and differentiation factors; and stresses such as heat, oxidation, irradiation, and physical distortion or traction.

Cancer is most common in tissues with rapid turnover, especially those exposed to environmental carcinogens and whose proliferation is regulated by hormones. The most common genetic changes involve the activation of proto-oncogenes or the inactivation of tumor suppressor genes (Chap. 81). Although genetic damage is nearly universal in human cancer, cells with neoplastic features can be generated in vitro without genetic damage. Removal and in vitro culture of cells from the epiblast of a murine embryo lead to the uncontrolled proliferation of the cells and the generation of a teratocarcinoma cell line capable of producing tumors when inoculated into animals. The removal of these normal embryonic cells from their normal environment leads to uncontrolled growth. However, if the teratocarcinoma cells are reinjected into an early embryo, under the inductive influence of their normal neighbors they can differentiate into normal organs and tissues appropriate for the location where they are injected.

Thus, environmental factors exert potent effects on the gene expression of target cells. The panoply of signals received by a particular cell leads to the activation of particular sets of transcription factors. The pattern of gene expression determines whether a cell will divide, differentiate, or die.

PRINCIPLES OF CELL CYCLE REGULATION

The mechanism of cell division is substantially the same in all dividing cells and has been conserved throughout evolution. The process assures that the cell accurately duplicates its contents, especially its chromosomes. The cell cycle is divided into four phases. During M phase, the replicated chromosomes are separated and packaged into two new nuclei by mitosis and the cytoplasm is divided between the two daughter cells by cytokinesis. The other three phases of the cell cycle are called *interphase*: G1 (gap 1), a period of growth during which the cell determines its readiness to commit to DNA synthesis; S (DNA synthesis), during which the genetic material is replicated and no re-replication is permitted; and G2 (gap 2), during which the fidelity of DNA replication is determined and errors are corrected.

During S phase, DNA synthesis begins with the unfolding of chromatin and nucleosome complexes rendering DNA accessible for the addition of DNA helicase and single-strand binding proteins that help open the double helix. Replication origins are spaced roughly 100,000 nucleotide pairs apart throughout the genome. DNA polymerase and DNA primase attach to these sites and catalyze the polymerization of the DNA at a rate of about 50 nucleotides per second. DNA polymerase δ catalyzes leading-strand synthesis, while DNA polymerase α uses DNA primase–generated Okazaki fragments for lagging-strand synthesis. Topoisomerase I nicks DNA, relieving torsional tension of the replicating helix; topoisomerase II introduces double strand breaks to avoid DNA tangles. Topoisomerases are targets of many chemotherapeutic drugs. Once a DNA segment is replicated, chromatin is reassembled, and replication origins are relicensed by binding of specific proteins that prevent re-replication until the next S phase. Although this system for replication is efficient and accurate, occasional mistakes are made, and these are repaired by a variety of mechanisms. In some cancers, the mismatch repair mechanisms are defective and errors increase by 3 to 4 logs, greatly increasing the likelihood of mutations in growth regulatory genes in daughter cells.

DNA polymerase is unable to replicate the end of a DNA chain completely, resulting in loss of DNA with each replication. This problem has been solved by a mechanism that replicates tandem repeats of a six-nucleotide sequence (GGGTTA) to the ends of each chromosome. These repeated sequences are called *telomeres* and are replicated through an RNA-dependent DNA polymerase called *telomerase*. Normal somatic cells do not express telomerase, and the replicative lifetime of such cells is limited to approximately 30 cell divisions due to the progressive loss of telomere repeats; the limit imposed on somatic cell division is called the *Hayflick limit*, at which time replicative senescence occurs. Germ cells do express telomerase and have a long (possibly unlimited) replicative lifetime. The aberrant expression of telomerase in cancer cells is thought to be a component of the neoplastic process, assuring that the cell will be able to undergo many divisions without inducing senescence or genetic catastophe. Inhibition of telomerase activity in cancer cells could have antitumor effects.

The cell cycle transitions between G1 and S and between G2 and M are tightly regulated to ensure that cells are prepared to divide and to minimize errors in the replication process. Checkpoints in G1 and G2 determine whether a cell will enter S or M phase, respectively; these checkpoints are regulated by serine/threonine protein kinases (cyclin-dependent kinases, or cdk) and kinase-associated proteins called *cyclins*. The enzymatic activity of each cdk is determined by its association with a cyclin and its phosphorylation state. There are at least seven cdk family members, and a like number of cyclins, which generate a group of cdk/cyclin complexes with differing substrate specificities and times of action during the cell cycle. Cyclin expression varies with the cell cycle, and the synthesis of these proteins is transcriptionally regulated and their degradation is mediated by ubiquitin conjugation and destruction in proteasomes.

The cyclin B/cdc2 complex (also called *mitosis promoting factor*, or MPF) is the primary regulator of transition from G2 to M phase. It is activated by a cdk-activating kinase (CAK) and a phosphatase (cdc25c) that removes inhibitory phosphates. The cdc25C is the target of a DNA damage–induced kinase that inhibits its activity. DNA damage leads to phosphorylation of cdc25C and its transport out of the nucleus, away from cyclin B/cdc2. This prevents entry into M phase until DNA damage is repaired. The regulated movement of molecules into and out of the nucleus is a common control mechanism in signal transduction. Some of the substrates of cyclin B/cdc2 are defined; its phosphorylation of histone H1, nuclear lamins, and microtubule-associated proteins facilitates chromosome condensation, nuclear membrane breakdown, and spindle formation, respectively.

The checkpoint regulating transition from G1 to S is frequently disrupted in cancer. The product of the retinoblastoma tumor suppressor gene, the nuclear phosphoprotein Rb, governs the key transition referred to as the *reaction point*. A second pathway regulated by the p53 tumor suppressor interacts with the Rb pathway to ensure that cell proliferation can safely take place. Rb and p53 are inactivated by products encoded by DNA tumor viruses, including SV40 large T antigen, adenovirus E1A and E1B, and human papillomavirus E6 and E7. The Rb and p53 pathways each include other oncogenes and tumor suppressors that are frequently disrupted in cancer (Table 82-1).

Regulation of passage through the restriction point is complex. In early G1, Rb is hypophosphorylated and in a complex with the E2F transcription factor. This nuclear complex binds to the promoters of genes required for cell cycle progression and inhibits their expression. However, in mid and late G1, Rb becomes phosphorylated (at ~10 sites) by the sequential activity of the cyclin D/cdk4 and cyclin E/cdk2 complexes. Hyperphosphorylated Rb releases E2F, thus relieving transcriptional repression, and heterodimers of E2F and DP1 transcription factor family members activate several genes required for S phase progression, including dihydrofolate reluctase, thymidine kinase, DNA polymerase, and cdc2 (Fig. 82-1). In addition to its role in growth regulation, Rb is required for the in vitro differentiation of muscle cells and adipocytes. Cell cycle control and induction of differentiation are functions of Rb that contribute to tumor suppression.

The activity of cdk is also regulated by cdk inhibitors (cdki). These low-molecular-weight proteins are divided into two families: the Cip/Kip family encoding $p21^{Cip1/Waf1}$, $p27^{Kip1}$, $p57^{Kip2}$, which inhibit cdk activity broadly, and the Ink4 family encoding $p16^{INK4a}$, $p15^{INK4b}$, $p18^{INK4c}$, and $p19^{INK4d}$, which block cyclin D/cdk4 activity and inhibit Rb phosphorylation and G1/S transition. p21 is induced by p53 in response to DNA damage, causing G1 arrest to permit DNA repair. If DNA damage is too great, a cell suicide pathway is induced to eliminate cells that may be dysfunctional (see below).

The cdki can be induced by growth inhibitors such as transforming growth factor (TGF) β and can be inhibited by growth factors such as interleukin (IL) 2. Genetic alterations in cdki, especially p16 and p15, occur with high frequency in certain tumors. Alterations at the p16 locus on chromosome 9p21 have been detected in 75% of pancreatic cancers; 40 to 70% of glioblastomas; 50% of esophageal cancers; and about 20% of non-small cell lung cancers, soft tissue sarcomas, and bladder cancers. Mutations in p16 account for half of familial melanomas. Some tumors fail to express cdki because the genes are methylated, an epigenetic mechanism for blocking transcription. Rb pathway regulation is also circumvented by overexpression of cyclin D1 [breast cancer and the t(11;14) in mantle cell lymphoma] and by mutations in cdk4 that abrogate p16 binding.

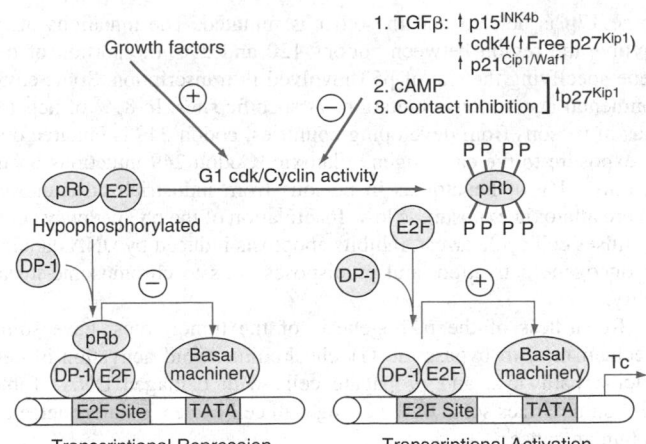

FIGURE 82-1 The retinoblastoma gene product, pRb, regulates cell cycle progression at the restriction point by sequestering the E2F transcription factor. Hypophosphorylated pRb forms an inactive complex with the E2F/DP-1 heterodimer that is bound to regulatory E2F sites of promoters of genes required for S phase. Rb recruits histone deacetylases to the promoter, rendering chromatin inaccessible to the basal transcriptional machinery. The kinase activities of *cdk*4/cyclin D and *cdk*2/cyclin E convert pRb to the hyperphosphorylated state with loss of binding pocket activity. G1 cdk activity is positively regulated by growth factors and inhibited by a variety of physiologic signals from the cell microenvironment. Hyperphosphorylated Rb dissociates from E2F/DP-1, which then associates with coactivators containing histone acetylase activity to form transcriptionally active complexes. S phase genes are expressed and cell cycle progresses.

Whereas Rb, cyclin D, cdk4, and p16 are commonly altered in cancer, E2F overexpression or p21 mutations have not yet been seen. Additional study may reveal why some components of the system are susceptible to alterations and other components are not.

p53, the "guardian of the genome," is a transcription factor that is not usually called upon to act in the course of normal replication. Levels of p53 are normally kept low by its association with mdm2, which binds p53 and shuttles it out of the nucleus for degradation. However, with DNA damage, p53 is phosphorylated by the ataxia telangiectasia gene product ATM, it dissociates from mouse double minute 2 (mdm2), and its destruction is slowed, leading to increased levels. Also, p53 influences transcription to either halt cell cycle progression (e.g., through induction of p21 expression to inhibit cdk activity) to permit repair of the DNA or, if the damage is too great, to initiate cell suicide (*apoptosis*). p53-induced genes involved in apoptosis include death receptors (DR5) and death-inducing members of the Bcl-2 family. p53 also induces expression of mdm2, thus downregulating its own activity.

Inducers of p53 include hypoxia, DNA damage, ribonucleotide depletion, and telomere shortening. Dysregulated activity of oncogenes such as *myc*, which promote aberrant G1/S transition, induces p53-mediated apoptosis. A second product of the Ink4a locus is $p14^{ARF}$, encoded by an alternative reading frame (ARF) from p16. Levels of ARF are upregulated by *myc* and E2F. ARF binds to mdm2/p53 complexes and rescues p53 from the inhibitory effects of mdm2 with subsequent activation of p53-induced genes. This oncogene checkpoint leads to the death of renegade cells that attempt to traverse the restriction point without the right signals.

Mutation in p53 is the most common genetic alteration found in human cancer (>50%) and is the causative lesion in Li-Fraumeni familial cancer sydrome. In tumors, usually one p53 allele on chromo-

Table 82-1 Cell Cycle Regulators in Human Cancer

Gene	Genetic Change	Functional Consequences
RETINOBLASTOMA PATHWAY		
Retinoblastoma	Deletion Point mutation	Loss of growth control at restriction point; loss of G1 checkpoint; TGF-β resistance
Cyclin D	Chromosome translocation Gene amplification	Aberrant increase in cyclin D/cdk4 activity with inhibition of Rb function
Cdk4	Point mutation	Loss of $p16^{INK4a}$ binding site; deregulated cyclin D/cdk4 activity
$p16^{INK4a}$	Deletion Point mutations Methylation	Failure to regulate cyclin D/cdk4 activity; leads to Rb hyperphosphorylation and aberrant entry in S phase
P53 PATHWAY		
p53	Deletion Point mutation	Loss of $p21^{Cip1/Waf1}$-mediated checkpoint control; genomic instability; resistance to apoptosis
Mdm2	Amplification	Increased p53 degradation; failure to induce p53 stess responses
$p14^{ARF}$	Homozygous deletion	Unregulated mdm2 inhibition of p53 levels and activity; loss of oncogene checkpoint
ATM	Deletion Point mutation	Decreased activation of p53 by ionizing radiation; loss of multiple checkpoints; genomic instability

NOTE: TGF, transforming growth factor.

some 17p is deleted and the other is mutated. The mutations often involve the region between codons 120 and 290, the portion of the gene specifying the site of p53 involved in transcription. Some environmental agents cause mutations at specific sites. In 81% of hepatomas in persons from developing countries, codon 249 is mutated due to exposure to the carcinogen, aflatoxin. Codon 249 mutations occur in only 11% of hepatomas in persons from industrialized countries where aflatoxin exposure is low. Inactivation of the p53 pathway compromises cell cycle arrest, inhibits apoptosis induced by DNA damage or oncogene activation, and predisposes cells to chromosome instability.

Regardless of the pathogenesis of the tumor, most have some mechanism(s) to bypass the G1 checkpoint, avoid activation of cell suicide pathways, and propagate cells with damaged DNA. Table 82-1 summarizes some of the changes in cell cycle regulators detected in human cancers.

SIGNALING FROM OUTSIDE THE CELL TO THE NUCLEUS

The behavior of cells in the body is tightly regulated by environmental signals. The ability of a cell to respond to a specific set of signals determines whether the cell will live or die, differentiate, proliferate, or remain quiescent. In normal cells and tissues, coordinated action such as wound healing or the inflammatory response is regulated by signaling pathways that convert extracellular signals into the performance of specialized action in the responding cells. In cancer cells, the process of invading and metastasizing is influenced by signal transduction pathways activated by paracrine and autocrine factors.

The coupling of extracellular signals to cell response varies for different receptor and signaling systems. The binding of a growth factor [e.g., epidermal growth factor (EGF)] to its receptor on the cell surface produces measurable changes in the cell within seconds and elicits a sequence of events that may last for days. Rapid responses are elicited by changes in ion flux, phosphorylation events, lipid metabolism, and production of second messengers. Long-term responses are mediated by the transfer of signaling information from the receptor to the nucleus, where alterations in the pattern of gene expression result in phenotypic change. Signal transduction comprises the mechanisms by which information received at the plasma membrane is imparted to the nuclear transcriptional machinery and other cell functions. Many signal transduction pathways are perturbed in cancer cells. There are three families of cell surface receptors: ion channel–linked receptors, G protein–linked receptors, and enzyme-linked receptors. Although ion channel–linked receptors are a component of growth-related activation in many cell types, they are primarily involved in neurotransmitter signal transduction and are somewhat less important in the pathogenesis of neoplasia than the other two types and will not be discussed further.

G PROTEIN–LINKED RECEPTORS The G protein–linked receptors traverse the plasma membrane seven times (serpentine receptors). They do not induce covalent modification of their substrates, as do enzyme-linked receptors, but generate second messenger molecules such as cyclic AMP, cyclic GMP, and calcium to activate downstream processes. Upon ligand binding, these receptors activate trimeric G proteins inducing the release of Gα and G$\beta\gamma$ subunits, each of which elicits downstream signals. The process is terminated by GTP hydrolysis by Gα subunits. The roles of G protein signaling pathways in human cancer include certain endocrine tumors whose cells of origin depend on cyclic AMP for growth. About half of growth hormone–secreting pituitary tumors encode mutant Gα subunits that are defective in GTPase activity and are constitutively activated even in the absence of ligand. These Gα subunits bind to and stimulate the activity of adenyl cyclase, leading to unregulated synthesis of cyclic AMP. Cyclic AMP binds to the repressor subunit of protein kinase A thus activating the kinase, which enters the nucleus and phosphorylates

CREB (cyclic AMP response element binding protein), a transcription factor that activates genes required for proliferation of the cancer cells. Growth stimulatory Gα mutations have also been described in adrenal cortical tumors and endocrine tumors of the ovary. Factors involved in normal cell and tumor cell migration also stimulate cells through G protein–coupled receptors.

ENZYME-LINKED RECEPTORS There are at least five classes of enzyme-linked receptors: receptor guanylyl cyclases, receptor tyrosine kinases, tyrosine kinase–associated receptors, receptor tyrosine phosphatases, and receptor serine/threonine kinases. The atrial natriuretic peptide receptor is a receptor guanylyl cyclase. Some disease manifestations in cancer may be related to atrial natriuretic peptide activity (such as hyponatremia), but little is known about this receptor class. Receptor phosphatases are not known to be involved in cancer. The other classes of enzyme-linked receptors are better defined and play a more important role in cancer.

Receptor Tyrosine Kinases The receptors for most growth factors are transmembrane tyrosine kinase receptors, including platelet-derived growth factor (PDGF), fibroblast growth factors (FGFs), EGF, heregulin, insulin, insulin-like growth factors (IGF) I and II, nerve growth factor (NGF), stem cell factor, vascular endothelial growth factor, macrophage colony stimulating factors (CSF), and others. Much of what we know about receptor tyrosine kinases and the events that follow their ligation emerged from the study of the proliferation-inducing altered forms of the normal cellular genes (proto-oncogenes) that are the cancer-causing genes (oncogenes) in animal retroviruses. Although downstream events vary with the receptor/ligand combinations, the activation of the receptor follows a typical pattern. Ligand binding induces dimerization or oligomerization of receptor subunits, which activates tyrosine kinase activity and causes autophosphorylation of specific tyrosine residues in the cytoplasmic domain of the receptor. Phosphorylated tyrosine residues on the receptors or on associated adaptor proteins form docking sights for other signal transduction molecules that contain one or more *src-homology region 2*, or SH2, domains, named because the sequence was first identified in the *src* nonreceptor tyrosine kinase. Phosphorylation of tyrosine residues provides a unique amplification signal because of the rapid and specific binding of SH2 domains to p-Tyr, although p-Tyr comprises only 0.05% of total cell phosphoamino acid. These associations via SH2 domains trigger subsequent events (Fig. 82-2). Signaling is terminated by the action of p-Tyr-specific phosphatases.

Protein domain interactions between evolutionarily conserved motifs play critical roles in all forms of signal transduction, ranging from tyrosine kinase pathways, death-inducing molecules, and the association of transcription complexes on gene regulatory regions. The most common docking mechanisms are based on recognition of particular protein sequences; the SH2 domains recognize p-Tyr-containing sequences with specificity conferred by surrounding amino acid residues, the SH3 domains dock with proline-rich sequences, and the pleckstrin homology domains [pleckstrin is a major protein kinase C (PKC) substrate in platelets] lead to associations with phosphatidylinositol lipids phosphorylated in the 3 position by phosphatidylinositol 3-kinase (PI3K; see below). Some molecules that do not have docking domains are brought into association with the receptors through the activity of adaptor proteins that are composed of docking domains only. Thus, the nucleotide exchange factor son of sevenless (SOS; named for its role in *Drosophila* eye development) is brought close to the membrane to activate Ras through its association with the adaptor protein grb2 (identified because it "grabbed" p-Tyr-containing proteins).

Receptor tyrosine kinases activate many signaling pathways including phospholipase C-γ, which hydrolyzes phosphoinoside 4,5-bisphosphate (PIP2) into diacylglycerol (DAG) and inositol triphosphate (IP3). DAG together with calcium ion activates PKC, a family of serine/threonine kinases with different activation requirements, subcellular locations, and substrates in different cell types. PKC is the target of tumor-promoting phorbol esters, and its activation can influence cell proliferation, differentiation, and tumorigenesis. IP3 induces the release of intracellular calcium, which binds to calmodulin, a protein

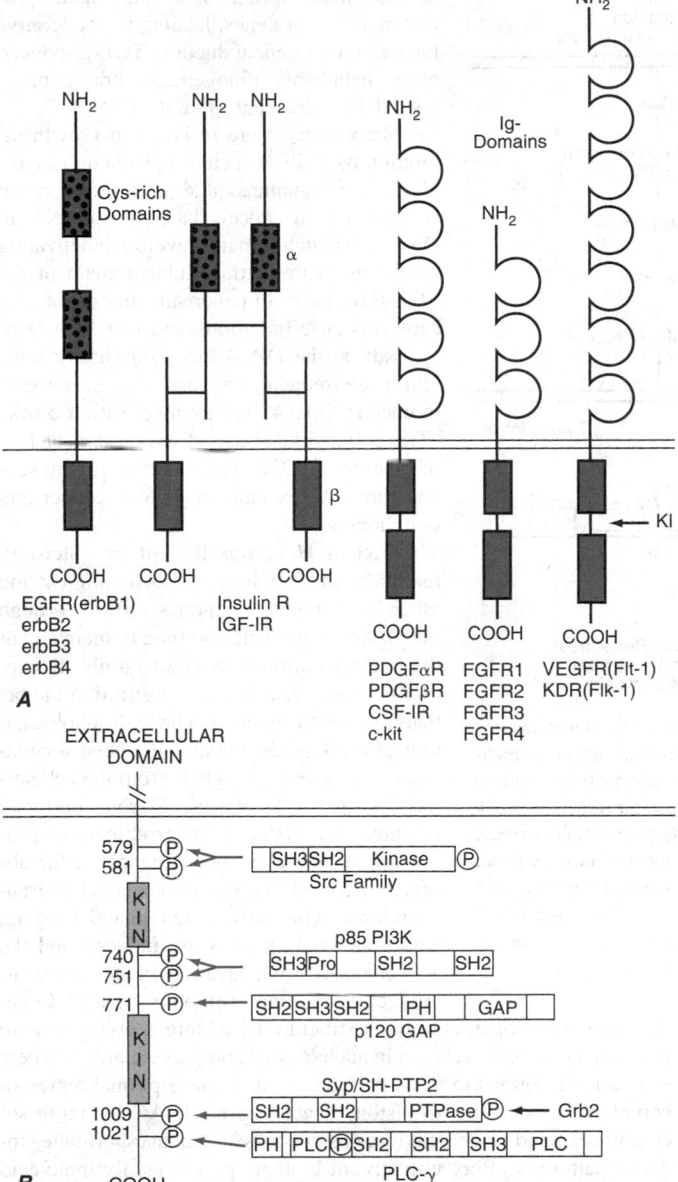

FIGURE 82-2 *A.* Structures of receptor tyrosine kinases activated by ligand-induced dimerization. Conserved extracellular domains, a single transmembrane spanning region, and a cytoplasmic domain encoding the tyrosine kinase characterize these receptors. The insulin and insulin-like growth factor (IGF) I receptors are disulfide-linked heterotetramers of α and β chains that undergo allosteric changes upon ligand binding. In the other cases shown, ligand binding induces homo- or heterodimerization within the subfamily followed by receptor autophosphorylation on tyrosine residues. Some kinase domains contain a kinase insert (KI). Flt-1 and Flk-1 are endothelial cell–specific receptors for vascular endothelial growth factor (VEGF) and are required for embryonic blood vessel differentiation and angiogenesis in the adult. Other members of the receptor tyrosine kinase family not shown share structural similarities. *B.* Multiple tyrosine autophosphorylation sites on activated platelet-derived growth factor (PDGF) receptor β chains serve as docking sites for signal transduction molecules. These include enzymes that activate downstream substrates and docking proteins to provide SH2 or p-Tyr binding sites for other proteins. These interactions lead to the formation of a signal transduction complex whose structure determines the nature of the signal transduction pathways activated by a particular ligand. SH2, SH3, pleckstrin homology (PH), proline-rich (Pro), phospholipase C (PLC), phosphoinositol 3-kinase (PI3K), GTPase activating protein (GAP), and protein tyrosine phosphatase (PTPase) domains are shown.

that regulates the activity of many enzymes, including phosphatases. Calcium fluxes within cells can be short or prolonged, and the duration has profound physiologic effects. PI3K is a lipid kinase that generates PI(3,4)P2 and PI(3,4,5)P3, membrane lipids that act as binding sites for proteins containing PH motifs. Such proteins include Akt serine/threonine kinase, which is implicated in activating survival pathways in many cells. Src family tyrosine kinases bind to p-Tyr on activated receptors and amplify signaling information by phosphorylation of distinct protein substrates within the cell. Src activity is required for G1 progression in some cells through its induction of the transcription factor c-myc. Another consequence of receptor tyrosine kinase activation is stimulation of the Ras/MAP (mitogen-activated protein) kinase pathway that leads to activation of a number of transcription factors that regulate proliferation, differentiation, and cell survival. This pathway is frequently abnormal in cancer cells.

Ras is a 21-kDa member of a large family of proteins, including rho, rac, rab, and others, that regulate cytoskeletal changes, vesicular and nuclear transport, and proliferation and that share sequence homology with the Gα subunit of G protein–linked receptors. Ras is attached to the inner cell membrane through an isoprenyl lipid group added after translation by the enzyme farnesyl transferase. If the lipid group is not added, Ras does not localize to the membrane and cannot function normally. In unstimulated cells, Ras is bound to GDP and is inactive. Following receptor tyrosine kinase activation, the guanine nucleotide exchange factor SOS is brought to the membrane by its association with grb2. SOS removes GDP from Ras and adds GTP. GTP-bound Ras then activates a cascade ending with MAP kinase, which migrates to the nucleus and phosphorylates (activates) a number of transcription factors (Fig. 82-3). The kinetics of MAP kinase activity are critical: in PC12 rat pheochromocytoma cells, stimulation with EGF results in transient stimulation of MAP kinase activity, retention of MAP kinase in the cytoplasm, and cell proliferation; stimulation of PC12 cells with NGF induces sustained activation of MAP kinase, nuclear translocation of MAP kinase, and neuronal differentiation.

Genetic defects leading to increased signaling from receptor tyrosine kinase–linked pathways are important in the etiology and progression of human cancer. About 30% of human cancers (especially pancreatic, lung, and colon adenocarcinomas) have mutated *Ras*. The mutations usually involve codons 12, 13, or 61 and result in a Ras protein that fails to hydrolyze its bound GTP and is thus constitutively active. In the hereditary disorder, neurofibromatosis, a mutation in the gene that encodes neurofibromin, a GTPase activating protein (GAP), inhibits its ability to inactivate Ras by converting the GTP to GDP. Constitutively activated Ras results in the unregulated activity of the signaling pathways downstream of Ras, including the MAP kinase pathway and activation of PI3K. Some epithelial cancers overexpress one or more members of the receptor tyrosine kinase family. EGF receptors, IGF-I receptors, and HER-2/*neu* are overexpressed in lung, bladder, breast, head and neck, and ovarian cancers. Mutations within the Ret tyrosine kinase receptor lead to constitutive receptor dimerization and kinase activation and are responsible for the dominant inherited cancer syndromes multiple endocrine neoplasia (MEN) type 2A and type 2B and familial medullary thyroid carcinoma. Autocrine and paracrine sources of the relevant growth factors have been noted in some cases.

Tyrosine Kinase–Associated Receptors The receptors for growth hormone, prolactin, erythropoietin, thrombopoietin, most interleukins, granulocyte CSF, granulocyte-macrophage CSF, interferon-α, interferon-γ, and many other cytokines are members of the tyrosine kinase–associated receptor family. These single-transmembrane receptors contain ligand-specific subunits and shared signaling subunits. Ligand binding induces the activation of receptor-associated tyrosine kinases. Three families of kinases are known to be associated with this class of receptors: *src* family (*src, yes, fgr, fyn, lck, lyn, hck, blk,* and counting), *syk* family (*syk,* ZAP-70), and Janus family (JAK1, JAK2, JAK3, Tyk2). The Janus family kinases have receptor sites that

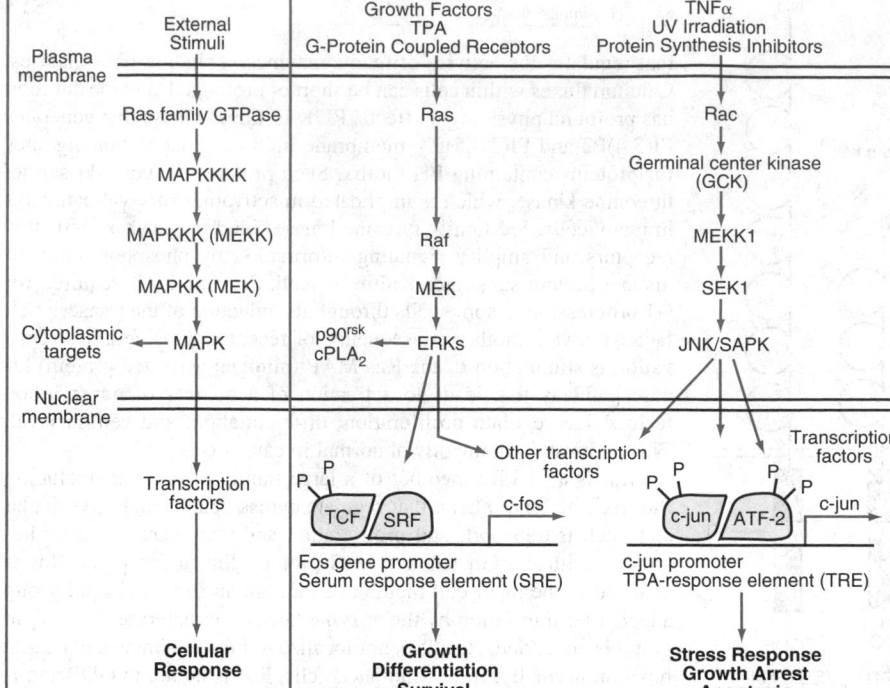

FIGURE 82-3 The mitogen-activated protein (MAP) kinase cascades. MAP kinase signal transduction cascades link *Ras* activation with the nucleus. The overall framework of the MAP kinase cascades is shown in the box at the left. A series of sequential protein kinase–mediated phosphorylations result in the activation of MAP kinase, which has cytoplasmic and nuclear targets. The nuclear targets of MAP kinase are transcription factors bound to their DNA recognition sites that require phosphorylation to induce transactivating functions. ERKs (extracellular signal response kinases) target the ternary complex factor (TCF), while JNK/SAPK targets c-*jun* and ATF-2. Transcription factors associated with other promoters also serve as targets for MAP kinases. Other MAP kinase cascades exist in the cell. Each pathway is activated by different stimuli, and the pattern of gene expression induced by each pathway is characteristic of that pathway. Interactions between pathways permit an integrated response to diverse signals.

act as docking sites for SH2-containing transcription factors called STATs (signal transducers and activators of transcription). Tyrosine phosphorylation of STATs induces their dimerization by SH2–p-Tyr association followed by translocation to target genes in the nucleus. A unique feature of JAK/STAT signaling is that the pathway from cell membrane to nucleus is traversed by a single dimeric molecule, as opposed to the cascade of kinase and adaptor molecules associated with membrane tyrosine kinases. The *src* family kinases can associate with receptor tyrosine kinases as well as tyrosine kinase–associated receptors, and, not surprisingly, signal transduction through either receptor class leads to the activation of similar signaling cascades. As a consequence of *src* family activation, *myc* is one of the transcription factors activated. The *syk* family usually activates the *src* family member in the receptor complex.

These receptors are often overexpressed on tumors of hematopoietic origin, and, similar to receptor tyrosine kinases, autocrine or paracrine stimulation may contribute to the neoplastic state of the tumor cell.

Serine/Threonine Kinase Receptors These receptors recognize TGF-β, bone morphogenetic factors, and other activins as ligands. Ligand binding leads to activation of the receptor kinase activity, but downstream events are not well defined. Bone morphogenetic factors are important in bone formation and in determining ventral vs. dorsal orientation in the developing embryo. TGF-β induces transformation of mesenchymal cells but inhibits the proliferation of most cell types through the induction of cdki, which block G1 progression in an Rb-dependent manner. Activation of TGF-β receptors leads to the phosphorylation of transcription factors Smad2 and Smad3, which then associate with their obligate partner Smad4. This complex, probably a heterotrimer, translocates into the nucleus where specific genes are activated. The direct path to the nucleus is analogous to the JAK/STAT signaling pathway. Smads bind to specific DNA sequences adjacent

to other transcription factor sites in the promoters of target genes, leading to cooperative interaction for gene induction. TGF-β induced genes include plasminogen activator inhibitor-1 (PAI-1), collagenase I, and p15^{INK4b}.

Many cancers are resistant to growth inhibition by TGF-β, including leukemias, lymphomas, melanomas, and breast and colon cancers. Colon cancers harboring defects in DNA mismatch repair develop inactivating mutations in the extracellular domain of the TGF-β receptor. In pancreatic and colon cancers, missense mutations and loss of heterozygosity at the DPC4 locus on chromosome 18q21 are frequent. This locus has been found to encode Smad4, and its inactivation blocks TGF-β signaling. Loss of expression or loss of function of TGF-β receptors occurs in several tumor types including colon cancer and lymphomas.

Nuclear Hormone Receptors Steroids, retinoids, thyroid hormone, vitamin D, and other lipid-soluble hormones diffuse through the plasma membrane and bind to members of the nuclear hormone receptor family. Receptors for these ligands are transcription factors that reside in the nucleus. The hydrophobic nature of the ligands obviates the need for machinery to transduce signals from the cell surface to the cell interior. Steroid hormone receptors are bound as heterodimers to promoter/enhancer elements of genes; in the absence of ligand, these complexes act as transcriptional repressors. Upon ligand binding, conformational changes are induced and the active transcription factor binds to coactivating factors and transcription is induced. Coactivators tend to open chromatin structure by adding acetyl groups to histones. Histone acetylation in nucleosomal complexes permits access of promoter regions to RNA polymerase II. Transcriptional repressor complexes associate with histone deacetylases (HDAC; co-repressor complexes), and chromatin remains condensed. Nuclear hormone–induced pathways affect virtually all biologic processes. Retinoic acid receptors (RAR) provide a clear link to cancer. Retinoids bind receptors composed of an RAR subunit (α, β, γ) dimerized with a retinoid-X receptor (RXR) and activate genes that influence differentiation in many cell types.

Acute promyelocytic leukemia (APL) is associated with the t(15; 17) translocation, which fuses sequences from a novel gene PML (promyelocytic leukemia) to the RARα gene, resulting in expression of a PML-RARα fusion protein. PML-RARα binds to and represses RARα-inducible genes required for myeloid differentiation. Repression is mediated by HDAC binding to PML-RARα. The developmental arrest at the promyelocyte stage of differentiation is associated with unregulated proliferation in these cells. Patients with APL can achieve complete remission with pharmacologic doses of all-trans retinoic acid (tretinoin), the ligand for RARα. Tretinoin induces the release of HDAC, permitting coactivator binding. Drugs that inhibit HDAC activity may provide a therapeutic benefit by activating genes required for the differentiation of cancer cells.

Cell-Cell and Cell–Extracellular Matrix (ECM) Communication In addition to information conveyed by soluble mediators, cell surface receptors relay important signals between cells, such as contact inhibition, and cell-ECM signals, such as anchorage-dependent growth. In cancer, these highly organized mechanisms of intercellular interaction often become disrupted or are subsumed for the purpose of metastasizing (Chap. 83). Individual cells no longer respond to signals from their neighbors, actin filaments are highly disorganized, and adherens junctions are lost. Normal patterns of growth and differentiation are disrupted, and the potential for metastasis increases.

E-cadherins are integral membrane glycoproteins that mediate calcium-dependent homophilic adhesion as the major component of adherens junctions between epithelial cells. E-cadherin cytoplasmic domains bind complexes containing α- and β-catenins, which are structurally linked to the cytoskeleton (actin cables and intermediate filaments). β-Catenin that is not sequestered in E-cadherin complexes is rapidly phosphorylated by glycogen synthesis kinase (GSK) 3β in a complex with the APC (adenomatous polyposis coli) gene product (maps to chromosome 5, mutated in familial polyposis) and is degraded by the ubiquitin/proteosome pathway. Degradation of β-catenin can be blocked by several mechanisms, including mutations that inactivate APC and mutations in serine phosphorylation sites within β-catenin that target it for degradation. Such mutations result in increased free β-catenin, which translocates into the nucleus and binds to members of the T cell factor (TCF) family of transcription factors, influencing the expression of genes such as c-*myc* and cyclin D1 that promote progression through G1. Excess free β-catenin has been implicated in hereditary and sporadic forms of colon cancer and melanoma. Decreased expression of E-cadherin has been noted in breast, colon, prostate, gastric, and other cancers and is a marker of poor prognosis.

Epithelial cell growth and survival require attachment of cells to components of the ECM that compose basement membranes, including collagen, fibronectin, vitronectin, and laminin. The integrin family of transmembrane receptors is composed of α and β subunits that adhere to the ECM and convey information to cytoplasmic membrane-associated structures called *focal adhesions*. The complexes, whose assembly is mediated by the Rho and Rac GTPases, are sites of attachment of actin cables but are also active in cell signaling through their association with focal adhesion kinase (FAK) and Src tyrosine kinases. Integrin-ECM interactions lead to activation of the Ras/MAP kinase, PI3K, and phospholipase C-γ pathways. Detachment of epithelial and endothelial cells from ECM induces their death by a form of programmed cell death called *anoikis* (Greek, "homeless"). This molecular safeguard prevents abnormal spread of cells. Invasive cancers often avoid anoikis by activating Ras or Src, which allow anchorage-independent growth of cells by activation of Akt kinase.

REGULATION OF GENE TRANSCRIPTION

One consequence of signal transduction is the activation of sequence-specific transcription factors that regulate gene expression. Whether a cell proliferates, differentiates, or undergoes apoptosis is regulated by gene products made in response to physiologic stimuli. For some transcription factors, the ligand goes directly to the nucleus where they reside (nuclear hormone receptors). For others, activated kinases enter the nucleus and phosphorylate factors already bound to DNA (MAP kinase and AP-1 transcription factor). Some transcription factors are activated in the cytoplasm and translocate to the nucleus (STATs). NF-κB is held in the cytoplasm by the negative regulator IκB, which is phosphorylated and degraded as a consequence of signal transduction. NF-κB is then released from IκB, and NF-κB translocates to the nucleus.

Transcription factors recognize short stretches of DNA of a defined nucleotide sequence 6 to 12 base pairs in length. These recognition sites may be upstream or downstream of the transcription start site [the TATA box where the first subunit of the transcription machinery, transcription factor IID (TFIID), binds]. Transcription factors may affect transcription at sites remote from the start site by looping out large intervening DNA sequences.

Transcription factors contain specific amino acid sequences capable of recognizing the DNA sequence and usually form one of several structural motifs: helix-turn-helix, homeodomain, zinc finger, leucine zipper, and helix-loop-helix are all used as DNA-binding motifs or mediate dimerization of factors required for DNA binding. Tran-

scription factors function in one or more of several ways. They can physically bend the DNA to permit the ordered addition of the components of the transcription machinery. Activated transcription factors bind to coactivator proteins in complexes that encode enzymatic activity leading to the acetylation of histones. This alters nucleosomal conformation and increases accessibility of DNA to transcription proteins. Transcription factors can inhibit transcription by blocking binding of a positive transcription factor or preventing the assembly of a transcription complex. They can form complexes with co-repressors and deacetylate histones. Promoters can also be made inaccessible by methylation of cytosine- and guanosine-rich sequences near promoters. The complex interaction between positive and negative transcription factors dictates the level of gene transcription. Individual genes may have ≥ 20 sites for transcription factor binding. The pattern of gene expression is determined by which factors are expressed in a given cell type.

Most genes are regulated at multiple levels, though transcription initiation is the dominant control point. The von Hippel–Lindau gene on chromosome 3p (a tumor suppressor gene involved in the pathogenesis of renal cell cancer) appears to act by inhibiting the elongation of an RNA chain after transcription initiation. A message may be spliced alternatively and encode different proteins in different cells. Transport of the message from the nucleus to the cytoplasm may be altered. Messenger RNA turnover may be accelerated. Some proteins, such as apoferritin and thymidylate synthase, regulate the translation of their own messages (and perhaps other messages) by binding to mRNA and preventing initiation of protein synthesis. Thus, there are many levels at which gene expression may be influenced.

Some transcription factors were identified because of their transforming effects when their genes, usually in mutated form, were incorporated into animal retroviral genomes; *myc*, *rel*, *fos*, *jun*, and others are examples of proto-oncogene transcription factors that are overexpressed in certain cancers and that contribute to the malignant phenotype of tumor cells. The mutated oncogenes are often more resistant to protein degradation and have a longer half-life than the normal cellular counterpart. Transcription factors with unusual properties may be generated by chromosome translocation that produces a chimeric protein. Novel genes may be activated that promote proliferation and inhibit apoptosis. Usually the genetic changes lead to inhibition of normal lineage-specific differentiation, resistance to apoptosis, and proliferation.

REGULATION OF CELL DEATH

The homeostasis of adult organisms requires a balance between the generation of new cells and the death of old cells. Some cells die when their telomeres no longer protect the integrity of DNA replication. Some cells die when they have sustained sufficient hypoxic, heat, oxidative, or ultraviolet irradiation damage that cannot be repaired. A cell can be killed if it becomes infected with a virus or other intracellular pathogen that destroys the cell or is recognized by the host's lymphocytes, which kill the infected cell. Multicellular organisms are models of cellular cooperation; some cells die to preserve the rest of the organism.

Genetic damage to growth-regulating genes of stem cells could be catastrophic; however, single genetic events such as activation of *myc* expression or loss of the Rb checkpoint often lead to the death of the cell by apoptosis. Apoptosis is a form of cell death initiated by extracellular or intracellular signals in which enzymes are activated to degrade nuclear DNA by making intranucleosomal cuts, causing the cell to shrink and finally break up. The core apoptosis machinery consists of a family of specialized proteases called *caspases* (they contain a cysteine at their active site and cleave substrates after *asp*artic acid residues). Like coagulation and complement systems, caspases exist as proenzymes with minimal enzymatic activity that can be rapidly induced by activators, and each enzyme acts to activate the next enzyme in the cascade. Key targets include DNA (chromatin degraded into nucleosomal multimers), nuclear lamins (nucleus shrinks and fragments), cytoskeletal regulatory proteins, DNA repair enzymes, and others. The cell shrinks, its chromatin fragments, and the cell breaks apart forming apoptotic bodies.

The latent activity of caspases is tightly regulated to prevent the death of normal cells. Assembly of initiator caspases into active complexes occurs by two main mechanisms. Members of the tumor necrosis factor (TNF) receptor superfamily, including Fas (CD95), and DR4 and DR5 death receptors encode transmembrane proteins whose cytoplasmic domains encode protein association or docking domains, called *death domains* and *death effector domains* (DED). Ligand binding induces dimerization of death domains with recruitment to the membrane of an adaptor signaling protein called *Fas-associated death domain* (FADD). FADD forms a complex with procaspase 8 mediated by DED interactions; caspase 8 is activated by self-cleavage. Caspase 8 then cleaves effector caspase 3 into active heterodimeric subunits, and death ensues (Fig. 82-4). Regulation of this pathway occurs at the level of expression of Fas receptor and ligand and the secretion of death-inducing cytokines, TNF and *t*umor necrosis factor-*r*elated *a*poptosis-*i*nducing *l*igand (TRAIL) (ligand for DR4 and -5).

The second pathway of caspase activation encompasses responses to a greater variety of noxious signals including DNA damage, growth factor deprivation, reactive oxygen damage, and heat stress. The mitochondrion plays a key role in this pathway as the storehouse of

protein cofactors required for the activation of caspases. Damage within the cell is detected by the mitochondria by unknown mechanisms. The mitochondria then lose membrane potential and release cytochrome c, which forms a complex with apoptosis-activating factor (Apaf) 1. This complex binds to procaspase 9 via a caspase recruitment domain (CARD), and caspase 9 is activated. Caspase 9 then cleaves effector caspases and induces cell death. The release of cytochrome c from the mitochondria appears to be regulated by bcl2.

The *bcl2* gene was discovered as the chromosome 18q contribution to the t(14;18) translocation in follicular lymphoma. The gene did not transform cells but prolonged the life of cells destined to die, greatly increasing a pool of cells available for subsequent genetic mutations. Members of the *bcl2* family fall into two groups: *bcl2* and *bcl*-X_L prevent cell death, whereas *bax*, *bad*, *bak*, and others promote cell death. The *bcl2* family members associate as homodimers or heterodimers; the combinatorial effects of the various dimers allow a fine level of control over cell survival. When any of the death promoters exist as homo- or heterodimers, the cell dies by apoptosis. When a death promoter heterodimerizes with either *bcl2* or *bcl*-X_L, cell death is prevented. Thus, the relative amounts of different *bcl2* family members determine whether a cell will survive potentially damaging insults. Furthermore, phosphorylation of *bcl2* family members by cellular kinases can alter the biologic activity of individual members, altering the balance in favor of death or survival.

In addition to its presumed role in the etiology of follicular lymphoma, *bcl2* is expressed in a number of cancers. It prevents the normal p53-mediated destruction of cells with damaged DNA and also appears to prevent the death of cells severely damaged by cancer chemotherapy. In addition, *bcl2* mediates drug resistance and contributes to neoplasia in a novel way, preventing the death that would normally eliminate the damaged cell, rather than promoting aberrant cell growth. Strategies to overcome *bcl2* function might well make available therapies more effective.

The apoptotic machinery is subject to regulation by multiple signal transduction pathways, and many of these are subverted in cancer cells to shift the balance toward survival of the malignant clone. In addition to *bcl2*, two other important links have been established between growth factor signaling and survival pathways. Activation of P13K by tyrosine kinases leads to activation of the serine/threonine kinase Akt. Akt directly promotes cell survival by phosphorylation of Bad and procaspase 9, inhibiting their apoptotic functions. Cancer cells can usurp the activity of Akt; in some cases, cells expressing a mutated Ras oncogene or increased levels of tyrosine kinase receptors (e.g., HER-2/*neu*) have upregulated the Akt pathway. An alternative genetic lesion leading to increased Akt kinase activity results in the loss of the PTEN tumor suppressor, a lipid phosphatase that normally downregulates the P13K pathway by dephosphorylating lipid second messengers. Another important pathway usurped by cancer cells involves NF-κB activation. NF-κB induces expression of the inhibitor of apoptosis (IAP) family of genes whose products inhibit caspase activity; one such, survivin, is expressed in lymphomas and other tumors.

Thus, cancer becomes more adaptive to its host from genetic events that alter apoptosis. Stimulation of proliferation or prevention of death can be complementary targets for cell transformation. Apoptosis pathways are important targets for treatment. Paclitaxel and other microtubule inhibitors induce the phosphorylation and inactivation of *bcl2*. One could make bone marrow cells highly resistant to chemotherapy-induced death by expressing a form of *bcl2* that lacks the loop domain in the BH1 region, as this is the site that is phosphorylated to inhibit *bcl2* function. Tumor cells and normal cells express DR4 and -5 receptors; however, tumor cells fail to express decoy receptors that protect normal cells from the DR4 and -5 ligand, TRAIL. Thus, therapies directed at DR4 or -5 may be tumor selective.

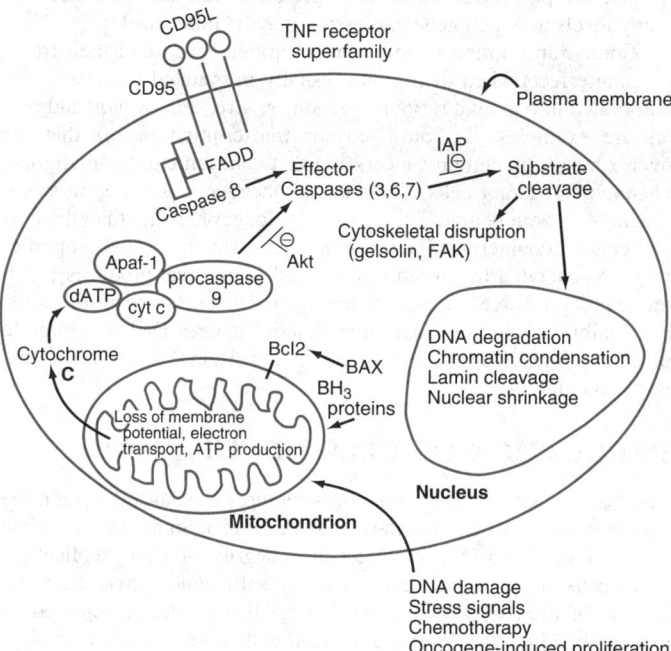

FIGURE 82-4 Mechanisms of apoptosis in eukaryotic cells. Programmed cell death is induced by two main pathways. Crosslinking of members of the tumor necrosis factor (TNF) receptor superfamily, such as CD95 (Fas) by its ligand (CD95L) lead to the binding of Fas-associated desk domain (FADD) and procaspase 8 to death domain motifs of CD95. Caspase 8 is activated by autocatalysis and subsequently cleaves and activates effector caspases such as caspase 3. Alternatively, effector caspase activation can occur when cytochrome c is released from the mitochondria in response to a variety of noxious environmental or intracellular events. The release of cytochrome c is regulated by members of the Bcl2 family, some of which form pores that traverse the mitochondrial membranes and regulate transmembrane potential. Cytochrome c, along with deoxyadenosine triphosphate (dATP), binds to Apaf-1, inducing a conformational change that permits association with procaspase 9 to form the apoptosome with subsequent activation of caspase 9. Caspase 9 activates effector caspases and the cell dies. Inhibitors of apoptosis (IAP) can inhibit caspases. One IAP member, survivin, is overexpressed in some cancer cells.

CELL BIOLOGY AND CANCER

For a cancer to arise, mutations must occur that affect a variety of pathways. Often the G1 cell cycle checkpoint is affected. Apoptosis is averted by mutations in the p53 pathway or by other mechanisms. The expression of telomerase is a common feature in cancers. Overexpression of growth factors and their receptors is frequently detected. Activation of the *Ras* proto-oncogene or other changes leading to a constitutively active MAP kinase cascade are common. Changes in cytoskeleton and responsiveness to contact-mediated growth inhibition are frequent in cancer cells. Usually when a mutation occurs in one component of a signaling pathway, other mutations are seen in other pathways rather than in another component of the same pathway. The high level of mutability of cancer cells facilitates adaptation to the environment, including the development of resistance to anticancer drugs. As tumors progress, they acquire the ability to secrete proteases that aid in the escape from local barriers so that they may metastasize (Chap. 83). Discrete steps in tumor progression lead to the production of factors by the tumor cells that permit neovascularization to supply nutrients to the growing tumor. Other mutations allow the tumor to escape immune surveillance mechanisms; for example, some tumors downregulate expression of class I major histocompatibility complex antigens so that they become invisible to T cells. The wide range of changes that must occur in a single cell to permit the behavior associated with a malignant neoplasm makes it clear why carcinogenesis is a multistep process and why human cancers may have 10 or more genetic lesions that account for the biology.

The characteristic of cancer cells that has dominated clinical thinking is their uncontrolled proliferation. However, the growth fraction of most human cancers is usually not higher than the growth fraction of normal gut epithelia or normal bone marrow, and most human tumor explants are difficult to propagate for long periods of time in culture. Cancer cell lines immortal in vitro may have additional genetic lesions that permit their growth in vitro. Naturally occurring tumors growing in vivo show a Gompertzian or exponential decline in their growth fraction because the daughter cells of a division are not uniformly capable of further division. The accumulation of genetic damage, poor oxygen or nutrient supply, and other unknown factors contribute to the senescence of some tumor cells, so that by the time a tumor becomes clinically apparent at a tumor burden of 10^8 to 10^9 cells, most of the proliferative capability of the tumor is finished. Often by this time, more malignant and highly selected clonal derivatives of the tumor have metastasized to other sites where new tumor deposits with more aggressive characteristics are formed. Thus, cancer cells can be viewed as having lost the altruism that usually characterizes cell behavior in multicellular organisms. Cancer cells operate under natural selection imposed by a hostile environment. Ironically, the more successful they are at achieving independence from environmental influences, the more assured is the destruction of their host and ultimately themselves.

Many potential therapeutic agents are in clinical development based on our concepts of tumor cell biology. They include the development of growth factor and growth factor receptor antagonists; inhibitors of phosphoryl transfer to block key kinases; selective inhibitors of PKC, P13K, phospholipase C, and other targets; farnesyl transferase inhibitors that block the insertion of *Ras* into the membrane; mutant versions of proteins such as *Ras* and p53 that may make the cell vulnerable to immunologic attack if employed as a vaccine; and inhibitors of angiogenesis or the steps in metastasis that may limit tumor growth and prevent its spread. However, it seems unlikely that a single target will be the highly sought-after point of vulnerability. More likely, combinations of inhibitors will be required to improve antitumor effects. For example, the combination of chemotherapy and antibody to EGF receptors appears to produce greater antitumor effects than the sum of the effects produced individually.

BIBLIOGRAPHY

ADAMS PD, KAELIN WG: Negative control elements of the cell cycle in human cancers. Curr Opin Cell Biol 10:791, 1998

BUNZ F et al: Disruption of p53 in human cancer cells alters the responses to therapeutic agents. J Clin Invest 104:263, 1999

DOWNWARD J: Ras signaling and apoptosis. Curr Opin Genet Dev 8:49, 1998

GIACCIA AJ, KASTAN MB: The complexity of p53 modulation: Emerging patterns from divergent signals. Genes Dev 12:2973, 1998

HUNTER T: Signaling-2000 and beyond. Cell 100:113, 2000

NUNEZ G et al: Caspases: The proteases of the apoptotic pathway. Oncogene 17:3237, 1998

PORTER AC, VAILLANCOURT RR: Tyrosine kinase receptor-activated signal transduction pathways which lead to oncogenesis. Oncogene 16:1343, 1998

SGAMBATO A et al: Multiple functions of p27 (Kip1) and its alterations in tumor cells: a review. J Cell Physiol 183:18, 2000

STRUHL K: Histone acetylation and transcriptional regulatory mechanisms. Genes Dev 12:599, 1998

TAN PB, KIM SK: Signaling specificity: The RTK/RAS/MAP kinase pathway in metazoans. Trends Genet 15:145, 1999

---

83   *Judah Folkman*

ANGIOGENESIS

aFGF	acidic FGF	PDGF	platelet-derived growth factor
bFGF	basic FGF	TIMPs	tissue inhibitors of
COX 2	cyclooxygenase 2		metalloproteinases
HIF	hypoxia-inducible factor	uPA	urokinase plasminogen activator
IFN	interferon	VEGF	vascular endothelial growth
IL	interleukin		factor
MTD	maximum tolerated dose		

Virtually every cell in the body lives adjacent to a capillary blood vessel, or at least no further than the mean oxygen diffusion distance of 100 to 200 μm. Some cell types, such as beta cells in the pancreatic islets, fat cells, and skeletal muscle cells, are surrounded by at least two capillaries (Fig. 83-1). Capillaries of 8 to 20 μm diameter are lined by a single layer of endothelial cells. These cells cover ~1000 m^2, an area the size of a tennis court. The length of capillary tubing in 1 mm^3 of human heart muscle is ~2500 mm, and 1 kg of fat contains ~3500 m of capillaries. During normal conditions vascular endothelial cell proliferation is barely detectable—<0.01% of endothelial cells are in cycle. Endothelial cell turnover is >1000 days and in retinal vasculature may be >5000 days. In contrast, in the normal adult bone marrow, ~6 billion cell divisions occur per hour and the turnover time is ~5 days, (i.e., the time during which bone marrow is completely replaced). Endothelial cells can emerge from their resting state and proliferate as rapidly as bone marrow cells during formation of new capillaries. This process is called *angiogenesis* and leads to *neovascularization*.

Physiologic angiogenesis is tightly regulated and of limited duration. It is essential to reproduction and embryonic development. During postnatal and adult life, angiogenesis in wound repair and in exercised muscle is restricted to days or weeks.

Pathologic angiogenesis, in contrast, is usually persistent and unabated. Angiogenesis that continues for months or years supports the growth and progression of solid tumors and leukemias, provides a conduit for the entry of inflammatory cells into sites of chronic inflammation (e.g., Crohn's disease and chronic cystitis), is the most common cause of blindness, destroys cartilage in rheumatoid arthritis, contributes to growth and hemorrhage of atherosclerotic plaques, leads to intraperitoneal bleeding in endometriosis, is the basis of life-threatening hemangiomas of infancy, and permits prostate growth in benign prostatic hypertrophy. These are just a few of the "angiogenic disease processes," which are found in almost all specialties of medicine. Angiogenesis inhibitors are a new *class* of drugs that suppress or reverse the pathologic neovascularization upon which these diseases are dependent.

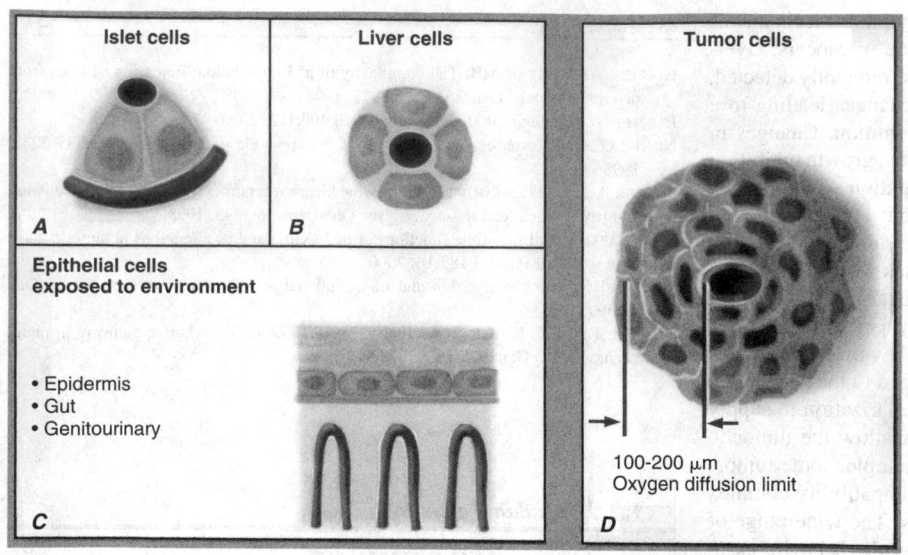

FIGURE 83-1 Diagram of three common configurations of how cells are apposed to capillary blood vessels. *A.* Islet cells are sandwiched between two capillary vessels, apical and basal. All fat cells and most skeletal cells are similar. *B.* Hepatic cells live adjacent to one capillary, and the next layer of hepatocytes are in another capillary neighborhood. Kidney, lung, and other organs are similar. *C.* Epithelial cells in the epidermis, gastrointestinal tract, and genitourinary tract are separated from vessels beneath them in dermis or submucosa but are still within the 100- to 200-μm oxygen diffusion limit. *D.* In contrast, tumor cells pile up as microcylinders around a capillary out to six or more layers. The cells at the greatest distance from the open capillary are severely hypoxic or anoxic.

NEOPLASTIC DISEASE

HISTORIC BACKGROUND Tumor hyperemia, observed during surgery since the 1870s, was for the next 100 years attributed to simple dilation of existing host vessels. Two reports, in 1939 and 1945, suggested that tumor vascularity was due to the induction of new blood vessels. This idea was dismissed by most investigators. The few who accepted it believed that new vessels were an inflammatory side effect of tumor growth.

In 1971, based on experiments carried out in the 1960s, a hypothesis was proposed that tumor growth could be angiogenesis-dependent, i.e., tumors could recruit their own private blood supply by releasing a diffusible chemical signal that stimulated angiogenesis. Tumor angiogenesis could then be a novel second target for anticancer therapy. These concepts were not accepted at the time. The conventional wisdom was that tumor neovascularization was (1) an inflammatory host response to necrotic tumor cells, (2) a host response detrimental to the tumor, or (3) "established" vasculature that could not regress. From these assumptions most scientists concluded that it was fruitless to attempt to discover an angiogenesis stimulator, to say nothing of discovering angiogenesis inhibitors. Eventual acceptance of the 1971 hypothesis was slow because it would be 2 more years before the first vascular endothelial cells were successfully cultured in vitro, 8 more years before *capillary* endothelial cells could be cultured in vitro, 11 years before the discovery of the first angiogenesis inhibitor, and 13 years before the purification of the first angiogenic protein. By the mid-1980s, after a series of reports from several laboratories demonstrating that tumor growth was angiogenesis-dependent, this hypothesis had been confirmed by genetic methods.

THE ANGIOGENIC SWITCH **The Prevascular Phase** Most human tumors arise without angiogenic activity and exist in situ as microscopic-sized lesions of 0.2 to 2 mm diameter for months to years, after which a small percentage may switch to the angiogenic phenotype. Autopsy studies of people who died of trauma but who never had cancer during their lifetime reveal that in women from 40 to 50 years of age, 39% had in situ carcinomas in their breast, but breast cancer is diagnosed in only 1% of women in this age range. In men from age 50 to 70, 46% had in situ prostate cancers at the time of death, but only 1% are diagnosed in this age range during life. In

people from age 50 to 70, >98% had small carcinomas of the thyroid (Fig. 83-2), but thyroid cancer is diagnosed in only 0.1% in this age range. In the majority of human tumors, the angiogenic phenotype appears after the malignant phenotype is recognized histologically. However, for certain human tumors (e.g., carcinoma of the cervix), the preneoplastic stage of dysplasia becomes angiogenic before the malignant phenotype is recognized histologically. When a nonangiogenic in situ carcinoma emerges in avascular epidermis or mucosa (e.g., melanoma or breast cancer), it is separated from host vessels by a basement membrane (Fig. 83-3). If a nonangiogenic tumor emerges in the midst of a vascularized tissue (e.g., an islet cell carcinoma), it may form an in situ microcylinder of tumor cells around capillary vessels (called *cooption*).

At the clinical level the angiogenic switch is recognized by expansion of tumor mass to a detectable size, local bleeding, and metastasis. For example, a positive mammogram usually represents a neovascularized tumor—a non-neovascularized in situ carcinoma is below the detectable limits of mammography. Hematuria in bladder cancer, melena in colorectal cancer, and hemoptysis in lung cancer all result from neovascularized tumors. Tumor cells are not usually shed into the circulation until after neovascularization has occurred. Furthermore, distant metastases themselves cannot be detected until they have "turned on" the angiogenic switch.

At the cellular level at least four mechanisms of the angiogenic switch have been identified in human and mouse tumors: (1) avascular in situ carcinomas can recruit their own blood supply by stimulating neovascularization in an adjacent host vascular bed—the most common process in human tumors; (2) circulating precursor endothelial cells from bone marrow may incorporate into an angiogenic focus; (3) tumors may induce host fibroblasts and/or macrophages in the tumor bed to overexpress an angiogenic factor [e.g., vascular endothelial growth factor (VEGF)]; and (4) preexisting vessels can be coopted by tumor cells. The angiogenic switch may also include combinations of these mechanisms. Once tumors have switched on angiogenesis, they rarely revert to the nonangiogenic phenotype. Neuroblastoma and retinoblastoma may be exceptions, but spontaneous loss of angiogenic activity (and tumor regression) is rare even in these two tumors. After the angiogenic switch, new microvessels converge on the tiny in situ tumor. Tumor cells grow as microcylinders, or "perivascular cuffs," around each new vessel. One endothelial cell can support from 5 to 100 tumor cells.

At the molecular level, the angiogenic switch operates as a shift in the balance of production by tumor cells of molecules that positively or negatively regulate angiogenesis. The overexpression of positive regulators of angiogenesis and the downregulation of inhibitors of angiogenesis during early tumor development are generally triggered by genetic mutations that control angiogenesis. For example, overexpression of the *ras* oncogene increases production of the angiogenic protein VEGF, while a mutation in the p53 tumor-suppressor gene or its deletion decreases production of the angiogenesis inhibitor protein, thrombospondin-1. In the normal cell wild-type p53 upregulates thrombospondin-1 and downregulates VEGF.

The angiogenic switch can be further modified by environmental conditions such as hypoxia, endogenous angiogenesis inhibitors, and genetic background of the host.

1. *Hypoxia*: After a tumor has become neovascularized, its continued expansion may lead to increased tissue pressure. This increased interstitial pressure is caused mainly by plasma that leaks from new vessels but is slow to efflux from the tumor because of a dearth of

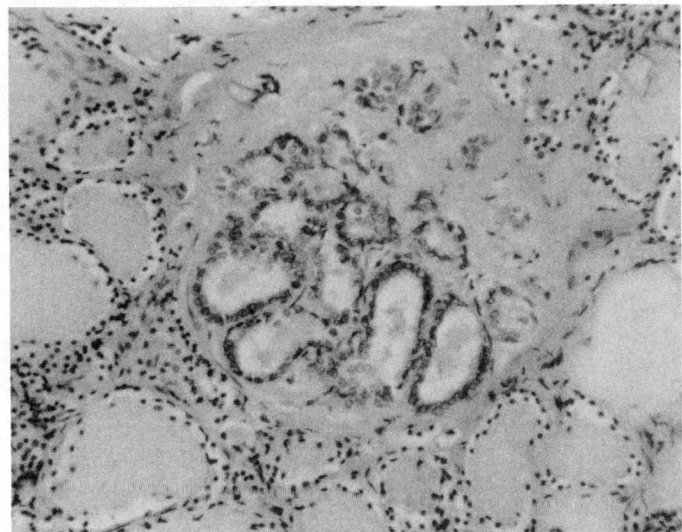

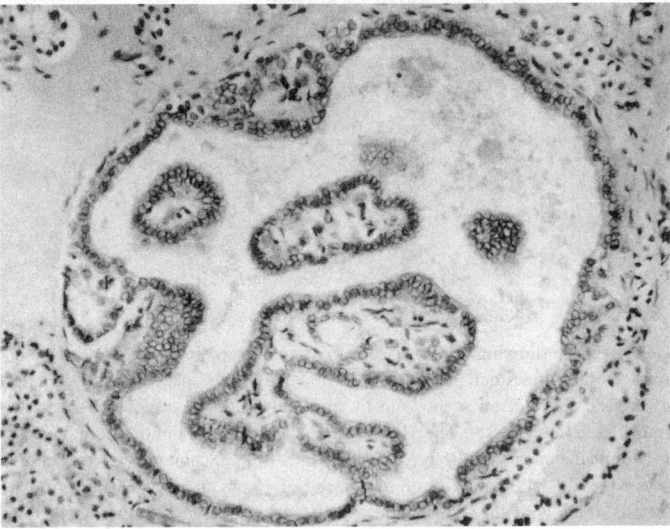

FIGURE 83-2 *A.* Papillary carcinoma of the thyroid gland at autopsy of a patient who died of trauma and who had no cancer during lifetime. The tumor is only 0.24 mm diameter and is not angiogenic. *B.* The same magnification of a similar tumor in a different patient who also died of trauma but had no cancer diagnosed during life. This lesion is 0.5 mm and is not angiogenic. *(From Harach et al.)*

intratumoral lymphatics. Microvessels in the center of the tumor are the first to be compressed, which leads to central necrosis. Hypoxia activates an hypoxia-inducible factor (HIF-1) binding sequence in the VEGF promoter. This leads to transcription of VEGF mRNA, increased stability of VEGF message, and increased production of VEGF protein beyond what may have been triggered genetically. Tumors, therefore, do not "outgrow their blood supply" but compress it. A counterintuitive lesson is that in situ tumors arising in an avascular compartment (e.g., epidermis) are *not* hypoxic, but larger neovascularized tumors become hypoxic after compressing their blood supply. Low pH and low glucose in a tumor may also upregulate production of angiogenic factors, especially VEGF.

2. *Endogenous angiogenesis inhibitors*: At the molecular level, the angiogenic switch can also be modified by endothelial inhibitors that either circulate [e.g., interferon (IFN) β, platelet factor 4, angiostatin] or are releasable from extracellular matrix [e.g., endostatin, thrombospondin-1, and tissue inhibitors of metalloproteinases (TIMPs)]. Therapeutic administration of an endogenous angiogenesis inhibitor, such as angiostatin or endostatin, can tip the balance of the angiogenic switch so that angiogenic output of a tumor is opposed or abrogated.

3. *Genetic control of host response*: Just as the angiogenic output of a given tumor is governed by oncogenes and tumor-suppressor genes, the angiogenic response of the host is genetically regulated. It is known that hemangiomas predominate in white infants and that ocular neovascularization in macular degeneration is almost never found in black patients. The genes that regulate these effects are not yet known.

Endogenous Angiogenesis Promoters The known endogenous angiogenic promoters are listed in Table 83-1. Virtually all of these proteins are produced by different types of tumors. However, acidic FGF (aFGF), basic FGF (bFGF), VEGF, and angiopoietin-1 and -2 are the most well studied and have been found in a wide variety of human tumors.

Fibroblast growth factors aFGF and bFGF stimulate endothelial cell mitosis and migration in vitro and are among the most potent angiogenic proteins in vivo. They have high affinity for heparin and heparan sulfate. They lack a signal sequence for secretion but are stored in extracellular matrix. An unsolved problem is how bFGF is exported from tumor cells in the absence of a signal sequence. Many different cells synthesize bFGF, including tumor cells of the central nervous system, sarcomas, genitourinary tumors, and even endothelial cells in the tumor vasculature. Proteinases and heparanases are thought to mobilize bFGF from the extracellular matrix. Furthermore, some tumors recruit macrophages and activate them to secrete bFGF, while others attract mast cells, which, because of their high heparin content, sequester bFGF. bFGF is not a specific endothelial mitogen but has several cell targets including fibroblasts, smooth-muscle cells, and neurons. However, experimental tumors transfected with bFGF containing an engineered signal sequence stimulate endothelial proliferation almost to the exclusion of smooth-muscle and fibroblast proliferation. This is similar to the process in human tumors. This selective attraction of vascular endothelial cells by bFGF released from a tumor may be explained by the smooth-muscle repellant activity of angiopoietin-2 elaborated from proliferating endothelial cells in a tumor bed (see below). bFGF interferes with adhesion of leukocytes to endothelium; thus, tumors that elaborate bFGF may produce a form of local immunologic tolerance.

Abnormally elevated levels of bFGF are found in the serum and urine of cancer patients and in the cerebrospinal fluid of patients with different types of brain tumors. High bFGF levels in renal carcinoma correlate with poor outcome. Also, bFGF levels in the urine of children with Wilms' tumor correlate with stage of disease and tumor grade.

Vascular endothelial growth factor/vascular permeability factor The first proposal that tumor angiogenesis is associated with increased microvascular permeability led to the identification of vascular permeability factor (VPF). VPF was subsequently sequenced and shown to be a specific inducer of angiogenesis; it was called *vascular endothelial growth factor*. VEGF is an endothelial cell mitogen and motogen that is angiogenic in vivo. Its permeability effect on capillaries is more potent than histamine and contributes to ascites in ovarian cancer and to edema in brain tumors. Its expression correlates with blood vessel growth during embryogenesis and with angiogenesis in the female reproductive tract and in tumors. VEGF is a 40- to 45-kDa homodimeric protein with a signal sequence secreted by a wide variety of cells and by the majority of human tumor cells. For example, >60% of breast cancers overexpress VEGF. VEGF exists as five different isoforms of 121, 145, 165, 189, and 206 amino acids, of which VEGF$_{165}$ is the predominant molecular species produced by a variety of normal and neoplastic cells. Two receptors for VEGF are found mainly on vascular endothelial cells, the 180-kDa fms-like tyrosine kinase (Flt-1) and the 200-kDa human kinase insert domain–containing receptor (KDR) and its mouse homologue, Flk-1. VEGF binds to both receptors, but KDR/Flk-1 transduces the signals for endothelial proliferation and chemotaxis. Other structural homologues of the VEGF family have recently been identified, including VEGF-B, -C,

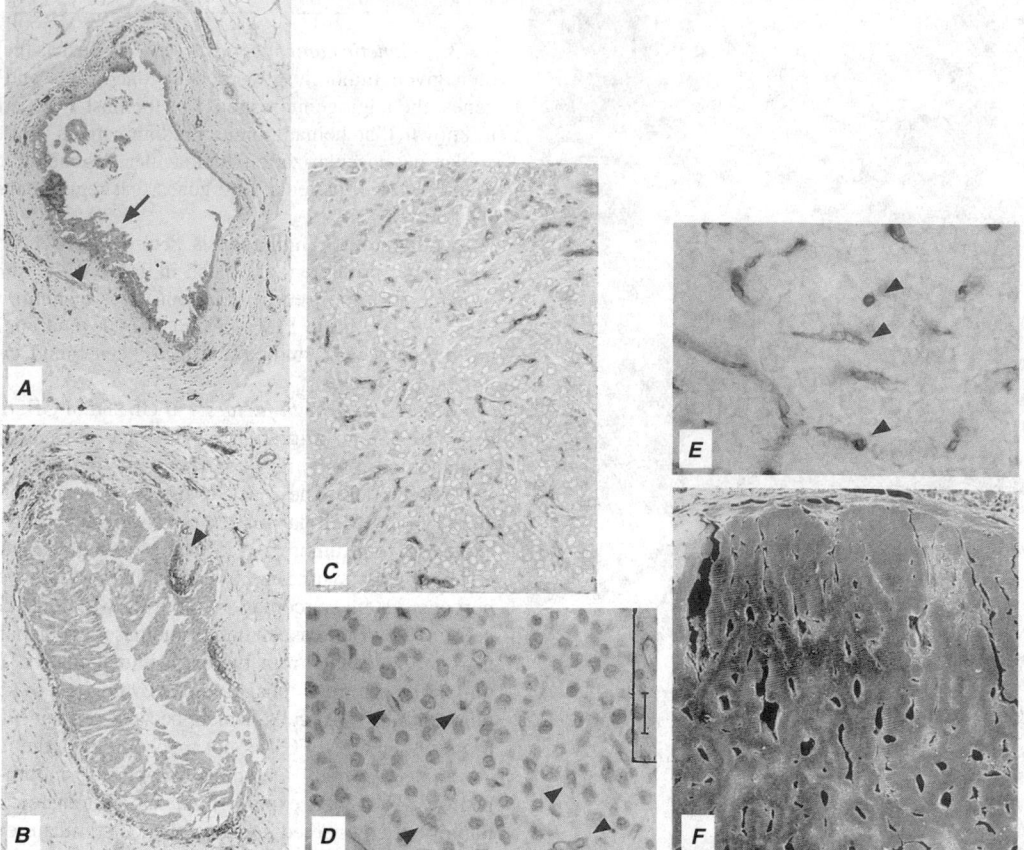

FIGURE 83-3 *A.* Human breast cancer. Large breast duct partially lined by duct carcinoma in situ (arrow) and intense angiogenesis in the immediately adjacent periductal breast stroma. Brown-staining microvessels (antibody to von Willebrand factor) are indicated by arrowhead. Note the absence of angiogenesis in the areas of breast stroma adjacent to portions of duct lined with benign duct epithelium *(From Weidner N et al, with permission of the publisher). B.* Large breast duct filled with carcinoma in situ and surrounded by new microvessels in the periductal breast stroma. Arrowhead shows invasion of microvessels through basement membrane of the duct, accompanied by invasion of tumor cells into the periductal stroma. *C.* Invasive duct carcinoma, area of highest density of microvessels. *D.* Higher power of invasive human breast carcinoma 4-μm thick section. Microvessels (brown stained with antibody to CD31) are indicated by arrowheads. *E.* 50-μm thick confocal micros-

copy section showing microvessels in three dimensions (arrowheads) surrounded by tumors cells, which fill the intercapillary space. *F.* Cross-section of breast cancer in mice showing the microcylinders of tumor cells that surround each microvessel. The 100 μm thickness of these tumor microcylinders is within the range of the oxygen diffusion limit. Scanning electron microscope view of 100-μm Vibratome section of a subcutaneous MCa-IV mouse breast tumor with the skin at the top. Blood vessels appear as black holes emptied of blood and preserved in an open state by vascular perfusion of fixative. Pale necrotic regions surround perivascular rings of tumor tissue, which are ~100 μm thick. Magnification, 25×. A 10-mm scale bar would = 400 μm. *(Courtesy of Donald M. McDonald, University of California, San Francisco. Reprinted from Folkman, with permission of the publisher.)*

-D, and -E. VEGF-C stimulates lymphatic growth and binds to Flt4, which is preferentially expressed on lymphatic endothelium. Neuropilin-1, a neuronal guidance molecule, is a recently discovered receptor for VEGF$_{165}$. Neuropilin is not a tyrosine kinase receptor and is expressed on nonendothelial cells including tumor cells. This allows VEGF that is synthesized by tumor cells to bind to their surface. Surface-bound VEGF could make endothelial cells chemotactic to tumor cells or it could act in a paracrine manner to mediate cooption of tumor cells around microvessels (Fig. 83-3).

VEGF expression is upregulated by the *ras* oncogene. The farnesyl transferase inhibitors inhibit *ras* expression. One mechanism of their antitumor effect is to inhibit angiogenesis by inhibiting VEGF expression.

VEGF expression is inhibited by the von Hippel–Lindau (VHL) protein. The VHL-tumor suppressor gene is inactivated in patients with VHL disease and in most sporadic clear-cell renal carcinomas, which leads to VEGF-mediated angiogenesis. The VHL gene normally suppresses hypoxia-inducible genes including erythropoietin. When VHL is mutated or deleted, these genes are overexpressed even under normoxic conditions. This explains why renal cell carcinomas driven by mutant VHL are associated with a high hematocrit.

Experimental evidence indicates that bFGF function may be in part dependent upon VEGF. bFGF induces the expression of VEGF. The two endothelial mitogens act synergistically to stimulate capillary tube formation in vitro. Systemic administration of a soluble receptor for VEGF (flk-1) completely blocks cornea angiogenesis induced by implanted bFGF. An important implication of these studies is that angiogenesis inhibitors that block VEGF (currently in clinical trial) may also inhibit bFGF.

Angiopoietins Tie2 is a receptor found only on vascular endothelial cells. It is a specific tyrosine kinase whose ligand is angiopoietin-1. Angiopoietin-1 induces endothelial cells to recruit pericytes and smooth-muscle cells [mainly by producing platelet-derived growth factor (PDGF) BB] to become incorporated in the vessel wall. Vessels stimulated by angiopoietin-1 are not leaky and are analogous to new vessels in a healing wound. Angiopoietin-2 blocks the Tie-2 receptor and acts to repel pericytes and smooth muscle. It is produced by vascular endothelium in a tumor bed, but it is unclear how tumor cells mediate this. Nevertheless, tumor vessels remain thin "endothelial-lined tubes" even though some of these microvessels reach the diameter of venules (Fig. 83-3). A key point is that angiopoietin-2 and VEGF together increase angiogenesis. However, if VEGF is neutral-

Table 83-1 Endogenous Stimulators of Angiogenesis

Protein	Molecular Weight, kDa	Year Reported
Basic fibroblast growth factor (FGF-2)	18	1984
Acidic fibroblast growth factor (FGF-1)	16.4	1984
Angiogenin	14.1	1985
Transforming growth factor α	5.5	1986
Transforming growth factor β	25	1986
Tumor necrosis factor α	17	1987
Vascular endothelial growth factor		
VPF	40–45	1983
VEGF		1989
Platelet-derived endothelial growth factor	45	1989
Granulocyte colony-stimulating factor	17	1989
Placental growth factor	25	1991
Interleukin 8	40	1992
Hepatocyte growth factor	92	1993
Proliferin	35	1994
Angiopoietin-1	70	1996
Leptin	16	1998

NOTE: VPF, vascular permeability factor.

Table 83-2 Endogenous Inhibitors of Angiogenesis

Name	Molecular Weight, kDa	Year	Reference
Platelet factor 4		1982	Nature 297:307
Interferon alpha		1980	Science 208:516
Prolactin fragment	16	1993	Endocrinol 133:1292
Angiostatin	38	1994	Cell 88:277
Endostatin	20	1997	Cell 79:315
Antithrombin III	53	1999	Science 285:1926
Interleukin 12		1995	J Natl Cancer Inst 87:581
Inducible protein 10		1995	J Exp Med 182:155
Vasostatin	21	1998	J Exp Med 188:2349
Canstatin	24	2000	J Biol Chem 275:1209
Restin	22	1999	Biochem Biophys Res Commun 255:735
Troponin I	22	1999	Proc Natl Acad Sci 96:2645
Pigment epithelium growth factor (PEGF)	50	1999	Science 285:1926
2-methoxyestradiol		1994	Proc Natl Acad Sci 91:3964
PEX	26	1998	Cell 92:391
Id1 and Id3		1999	Nature 401:670
VEG1		1999	FASEB J 13:181
Proliferin-related protein (PRP)		1994	Science 266:1581
Meth-1, Meth-2	110, 98	1999	J Biol Chem 274:13349
Osteopontin cleaved product		1999	Trends Bio Sci 7:182
Maspin		2000	Nat Med 6:196

SOURCE: Folkman and in part from Carmeliet and Jain.

ized or withdrawn, endothelial cells in the absence of perivascular smooth muscle and pericytes undergo apoptosis and new microvessels regress. These differences indicate that angiogenesis in tumors may be more vulnerable to certain angiogenesis inhibitors than angiogenesis in healing wounds. Endostatin inhibits tumor growth in mice without delaying wound healing.

Endogenous Angiogenesis Inhibitors   Certain endogenous inhibitors of angiogenesis are known to play a role in the angiogenic switch, including: IFN-α and platelet factor 4, and the class of angiostatic steroids typified by tetrahydrocortisol (Table 83-2).

thrombospondin-1   The production of thrombospondin-1 has been shown to be inversely related to the ability of a cell line to produce a tumor and vessels in vivo; loss of thrombospondin-1 production allowed non-tumorigenic cells to become tumorigenic. Thrombospondin-1 is regulated by wild-type p53. Loss of p53 function in tumor cells dramatically decreased the level of angiogenesis inhibitor. Restoration of p53 increased the inhibitor and suppressed the angiogenic activity of the tumor cells. The angiogenic switch was controlled by a negative regulator of angiogenesis generated by the tumor. The switch itself was viewed as a result of a shift in the "net balance" of angiogenesis stimulators and inhibitors. This led to the discovery of angiostatin, a second inhibitor found to be involved in the angiogenic switch.

Angiostatin, endostatin, and antiangiogenic antithrombin III   Several clinical and experimental observations suggested that certain tumors may produce angiogenesis inhibitors. The removal of certain tumors (e.g., breast carcinomas, colon carcinomas, and osteogenic sarcomas) can be followed by rapid growth of distant metastases. A primary tumor can suppress metastases from a different type of tumor, e.g., a breast cancer can inhibit melanoma metastases. In melanoma, partial spontaneous regression of the primary tumor may be followed by rapid growth of metastases. Regression of small cell lung cancer by ionizing radiation may be followed by rapid growth of distant metastases. If one portion of a primary tumor is removed (e.g., cytoreductive surgery for testicular cancer), the residual tumor increases its rate of expansion. A similar phenomenon is observed in animal tumors, i.e., certain primary tumors inhibit the growth, but not the number, of their own metastases. Surgical removal of a primary tumor increases growth rate of the residual tumors. Many primary tumors can suppress the growth of a second tumor inoculation. This "resistance" to a second tumor challenge is inversely proportional to the size of the tumor inoculum and directly proportional to the size of the first tumor. A threshold size is necessary for the inhibitory effect to occur.

At least three hypotheses have been advanced to explain these diverse observations and experiments: (1) "concomitant immunity"—a primary tumor induces an immunologic response against a secondary tumor or a metastasis in the same host; (2) depletion of nutrients by the primary tumor; or (3) production of antimitotic factors from the primary tumor that directly inhibit the proliferation of the secondary tumor. However, none of these ideas offers a molecular mechanism to explain all of the experiments cited above, and overall they have not been confirmed. Concomitant immunity has been ruled out as a mechanism because tumors can suppress metastasis in mice with severe combined immunodeficiency (SCID).

Once it was realized that a tumor could generate both positive and negative regulators of angiogenesis, then it also became clear that a primary tumor, while stimulating angiogenesis in its own vascular bed, could possibly inhibit angiogenesis in the vascular bed of a distant metastasis. However, at least two conditions would be necessary: (1) the primary tumor (i.e., the first tumor to grow) would need to generate an angiogenic promoter in excess of an inhibitor in its own local vascular bed, and (2) the putative inhibitor would need to have a longer half-life in the circulation than the angiogenic promoter. Research done over the past decade has identified angiostatin, endostatin, and antiangiogenic antithrombin as negative regulators of angiogenesis.

Lewis lung carcinoma generated angiostatin, a 38-kDa cleavage product of plasminogen. Systemic administration of purified angiostatin completely inhibited growth of metastases, producing dormant tumors of microscopic size ($<200\ \mu m$ in diameter) in the lung, and inhibited the growth of primary tumors. Angiostatin is not secreted by tumor cells but is generated through proteolytic cleavage of circulating plasminogen by a series of enzymes released from the tumor cells. At least one of these tumor-derived enzymes, urokinase plasminogen activator (uPA), converts plasminogen to plasmin, while a phosphoglycerate kinase from hypoxic tumor cells then reduces the plasmin so that it can be converted to angiostatin by one of several different metalloproteinases. Other types of tumors have since been reported to generate angiostatin, e.g., human prostate cancer. Prostate-specific antigen generates angiostatin-like fragments from plasminogen.

Furthermore, when murine fibrosarcoma cells were transfected with angiostatin, primary subcutaneous tumors formed. Their growth was slowed in proportion to increased levels of angiostatin production by the tumor cells. In these tumors the *total angiogenic output* of the primary tumor was decreased by transfected angiostatin, which opposed the activity of the tumor's secreted angiogenic promoter in a dose-dependent manner, but never completely counteracted it. The rate of tumor growth (expansion of tumor mass) was directly proportional to the total angiogenic output of the tumor, inversely proportional to angiostatin production and to tumor cell apoptosis, and virtually independent of tumor cell proliferation.

Murine hemangioendothelioma generated endostatin, a 20-kDa cleavage product of collagen XVIII. Human non-small cell lung carcinoma generated a 53-kDa cleavage product of antithrombin III (antiangiogenic ATIII). (This tumor does not metastasize, but the circulating angiogenesis inhibitor was detected because a subcutaneous tumor suppressed the growth of a second tumor at a remote site). All three of these proteins specifically inhibit endothelial cell proliferation and not other cell types. They have no effect on tumor cells per se. Endostatin inhibits tumor angiogenesis but not wound angiogenesis. It has no effect on pregnant mice nor on normal neonatal mice. Endostatin is present in *C. elegans* as a product of collagen XVIII and so may be at least 600 million years old on an evolutionary time scale. Other endogenous angiogenesis inhibitors are presented in Table 83-2.

Angiogenesis Inhibitors in Clinical Trial Angiogenesis inhibitors are in clinical trials in the United States for patients with cancer (Table 83-3). While a few endogenous antiangiogenic proteins have entered clinical trial [e.g., angiostatin, endostatin, and interleukin (IL) 12], these are more difficult to manufacture, and it will take some time before large quantities of these inhibitors become available for large numbers of patients. The majority of angiogenesis inhibitors currently in clinical trial for cancer are antibodies or small-molecular-weight synthetic molecules that inhibit specific targets along the angiogenic pathway.

BYSTANDER MOLECULES IN THE ANGIOGENIC PATHWAY A variety of molecules in the angiogenic pathway are not strictly endothelial cell mitogens or suppressors but operate as modifiers, markers, or receptors of the angiogenic process. They include: (1) integrins $\alpha_v\beta_3$ and $\alpha_v\beta_5$, which are upregulated on proliferating endothelial cells and act as receptors for fragments of fibronectin and other matrix components; (2) ephrins, which specify arterial or venous development of capillary vessels; (3) cyclooxygenase 2 (COX 2), the production of which is stimulated by bFGF and which converts lipid precursors to prostaglandin E_2 (PGE$_2$), an angiogenic stimulator; (4) plasminogen activator inhibitor 1 (PAI-1), which counteracts the upregulation of uPA that is produced by growing capillaries, thus restricting proteolysis to a local event at the tip of angiogenic vessels; (5) AC133, a specific marker for circulating endothelial precursor cells, which arise from bone marrow; and (6) nitric oxide synthase, which generates nitric oxide, that induces vasodilation in the vascular bed, a possible prerequisite for sprout formation.

METASTASES ARE ANGIOGENESIS-DEPENDENT Before tumors have become neovascularized in experimental animals, tumor cells rarely, if ever, shed into the circulation and metastases are essentially nonexistent. After the primary tumor becomes neovascularized, the number of tumor cells shed into the circulation increases in proportion to the increased neovascularization. Metastases that survive at a distant site must become angiogenic to be detected. Nonangiogenic metastases remain dormant at a microscopic size (<0.2 mm) indefinitely. Therefore, angiogenesis is required at both ends of the metastatic cascade.

Table 83-3   Angiogenesis Inhibitors in Clinical Trials

Drug	Sponsor	Mechanism
PHASE I		
COL-3	Collagenex, NCI	Synthetic MMP inhibitor; tetracycline derivative
BMS-275291	Bristol-Myers Squibb	Synthetic MMP inhibitor
SU6668	Sugen	Blocks VEGF, FGF, and EGF receptor signaling
Endostatin	EntreMed	Inhibits endothelial proliferation
EMD 121974	Merck KCgaA	Blocks an endothelial integrin
Angiostatin	EntreMed	Inhibits endothelial proliferation
2-methoxy-estradiol	EntreMed	Inhibits microtubule function
PHASE II		
Squalamine	Magainin	Inhibits Na/H exchanger
TNP-470	TAP Pharm.	Fumagillin analogue; inhibits endothelial proliferation
Combretastatin	Oxigene	Apoptosis in proliferating endothelium
Interleukin-12	Genetics Inst.	Induces IFN-γ and IP-10
CAI	NCI	Inhibits calcium influx
Anti-VEGF Ab	Genentech	Monoclonal antibody to VEGF
PHASE III		
Marimastat	British Biotech	Synthetic MMP inhibitor
AG3340	Agouron	Synthetic MMP inhibitor
Neovastat	Aetema	Natural MMP inhibitor
Interferon-α	Commercially available	Inhibition of bFGF production
IM862	Cytran	Endothelial inhibitor
Thalidomide	Celgene	Unknown
SU5416	Sugen	Blocks VEGF receptor signaling

NOTE: bFGF, basic fibroblast growth factor; EGF, epidermal growth factor; IFN, interferon; IP-10, inducible protein 10; MMP, a metalloproteinase inhibitor; NCI, National Cancer Institute; VEGF, vascular endothelial growth factor.
SOURCE: From National Cancer Institute Database (updated April 14, 2000).

Clinical patterns in which metastases first present may also be explained by angiogenic mechanisms. Cancer metastases are known to present in at least four different common clinical patterns and in one rare pattern. These clinical observations have previously been unrelated to each other but may be unified by angiogenic principles from tumor-bearing animals.

1. The patient whose metastases appear, sometimes explosively, a few months after surgical removal of a primary tumor (e.g., osteogenic sarcoma) may have lost a circulating angiogenesis inhibitor generated by the primary tumor. A model for this clinical presentation is the murine Lewis lung carcinoma that generates angiostatin.

2. Metastases that are not being suppressed by the primary tumor may already be present when the primary tumor is first diagnosed. The experimental model is a Lewis lung carcinoma subline that does not generate angiostatin.

3. The "unknown," or "occult," primary describes a pattern of metastases that present in the absence of a primary tumor or before it is located. In the relevant animal model lung metastases grow so rapidly that they suppress the primary tumor. However, it has not yet been

determined whether a circulating angiogenic inhibitor is generated by the metastases.

4. If metastases do not appear until years after surgical removal of the primary tumor, the patient may harbor dormant microscopic metastases that are not angiogenic. Those that eventually switch to the angiogenic phenotype can grow to detectable metastases. An example is the node-negative breast cancer patient who develops lung metastases 10 to 15 years after resection of the primary tumor. An animal model that mimics this pattern has been developed. Surgical removal of a B-16 melanoma from a syngeneic mouse leaves numerous viable lung metastases that are not angiogenic and do not expand beyond 0.1 to 0.2 mm diameter; they remain dormant for the life of the animal. They also remain viable, as evidenced by the fact that trauma to the lung or transplantation of a small piece of lung to the subcutaneous tissue of another mouse quickly generates a lethal tumor in both cases.

5. After surgical removal of a renal cell carcinoma, metastases will sometimes regress completely or partly. While this is an uncommon clinical pattern, V2 carcinoma in the rabbit most closely resembles it. Removal of a primary tumor in the leg is followed by regression of metastases. This does not appear to be an immune reaction because fresh tumor grows successfully in the same rabbit. One explanation is that the metastases were dependent upon high production of a circulating angiogenic stimulator, such as bFGF from the primary tumor. High plasma levels of bFGF have been found to correlate with high mortality in human renal cancer.

These clinical patterns are summarized in Fig. 83-4 as a unifying guide for clinicians. The hypothesis that these clinical patterns are linked by angiogenic mechanisms requires additional confirmation in the laboratory, but it provides a direction for further research.

LEUKEMIA IS ANGIOGENESIS-DEPENDENT Leukemia was assumed not to be angiogenic because it had been thought of as "liquid tumor." However, when bone marrow biopsies from children with newly diagnosed acute lymphoblastic leukemia were stained with an antibody to von Willebrand factor to highlight vascular endothelium, microvessel density was increased six- to sevenfold when compared to children with "control" bone marrow biopsies taken at the time of diagnosis of a solid tumor. Confocal microscopy further revealed that new microvessels in leukemic bone marrow were surrounded by a perivascular cuff of tumor cells like solid tumors. bFGF in the urine of the leukemic children was approximately sevenfold higher than in controls. Acute myeloid leukemia and chronic myeloid leukemia in adults are also associated with intense bone marrow neovascularization. Cellular levels of the angiogenic factor VEGF are significantly increased in acute myeloid leukemia and provide a prognostic indicator of outcome. The close physical configuration of microvessels and bone marrow cells may facilitate a two-way para-

crine pathway between vascular endothelial cells that produce mitogens for bone marrow cells [such as granulocyte colony stimulating factor (G-CSF)] and bone marrow cells that produce bFGF, a mitogen for endothelial cells.

Further work suggests that leukemia growth is dependent on angiogenesis. Murine leukemias can be suppressed or eradicated and survival of leukemia-bearing mice prolonged when they are treated with antiangiogenic therapy. The mice were treated either by systemic administration of endostatin or by chemotherapy administered on an "antiangiogenic" schedule. A conventional schedule of chemotherapy at a maximum tolerated dose was ineffective (see below).

Certain patients with multiple myeloma refractory to all conventional therapy have undergone successful remission when treated with thalidomide. This has initiated a debate about whether the beneficial effect of thalidomide is due to its antiangiogenic activity or to some other property such as its weak capacity to inhibit tumor necrosis factor (TNF-α) activity. This question arose because microvessel density did not decrease significantly in parallel with improvement of the disease. However, this result is not unexpected. In animal tumors that undergo steady regression in tumor volume as a result of antiangiogenic therapy, microvessel density (microvessels per square millimeter) may in some cases remain constant even as tumor volume is reduced by one-half, because capillary dropout and tumor cell dropout are going on at a near constant ratio. Furthermore, other effects of antiangiogenic therapy, such as the reduction of plasma leakage from tumor vessels, would not be revealed by microvessel density. Further, thalidomide is among the weakest inhibitors of TNF-α. Four other compounds that inhibit TNF-α more potently than thalidomide have no antiangiogenic effect. Pentoxifylline inhibits TNF-α at a similar potency as thalidomide, yet thalidomide inhibits cornea angiogenesis and pentoxifylline does not. Ibuprofen *increases* TNF-α in the serum of mice by twofold, yet it inhibits angiogenesis. Finally dexamethasone is a more potent inhibitor of TNF-α than thalidomide, but dexamethasone does not inhibit angiogenesis or does so only weakly.

ANTIANGIOGENIC THERAPY CIRCUMVENTS ACQUIRED DRUG RESISTANCE The emergence of drug-resistant tumor cells is a major problem accompanying almost all chemotherapy. Conventional cytotoxic chemotherapy targets the cancer cell, and it is the genetic instability and high mutation rate of these cells that are responsible in part for acquired drug resistance. However, vascular endothelial cells are genetically stable and have a low mutation rate, like bone marrow cells. Bone marrow cells do not appear to develop drug resistance against conventional chemotherapy. Thus, it is possible that tumor vessels will also maintain sensitivity to antiangiogenic therapy.

MICROVESSEL DENSITY IS A USEFUL PROGNOSTIC INDICATOR Neovascularization in human brain tumors correlates directly with tumor grade. Tumor vascularity in cutaneous melanoma also influences prognosis. Microvessel density is an independent prognostic indicator for human breast cancer. In fact, the majority of reports (52 different studies) confirm that microvessel density is a powerful and often an independent prognostic indicator for a variety of different human cancers. However, at least seven other reports fail to show the prognostic value of microvessel density. Some of these negative reports may be methodologic problems. Others may represent the co-existence of angiogenesis inhibitors and stimulators that cannot easily be measured in a tumor. Summaries of all published reports are given in (Tables 83-4 through 83-9). The best prognostic information from a histologic microsection of a tumor is obtained when the highest area of microvessel density ("hot spot") is quantified. These areas may contain the most angiogenic tumor cells, which have the highest chance of becoming an angiogenic metastasis.

Despite its usefulness as a *prognostic* marker, quantification of microvessel density is not necessarily a useful *surrogate* marker for

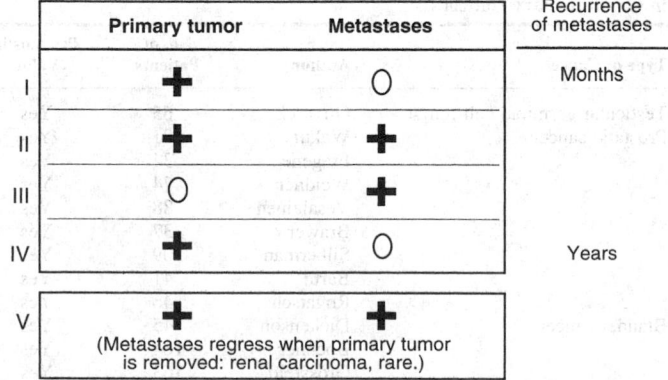

At first diagnosis:

	Primary tumor	Metastases	Recurrence of metastases
I	+	O	Months
II	+	+	
III	O	+	
IV	+	O	Years
V	+	+	

(Metastases regress when primary tumor is removed: renal carcinoma, rare.)

FIGURE 83-4 Metastatic patterns in cancer patients at the time of first diagnosis.

Table 83-4 Breast Cancer—Intratumoral Vascularization and Prognosis

Author	No. of Patients	Median Follow-up, Years	Relapse-Free Survival
Weidner	165	4.0	<.001
Bosari	180	9.0	<.03
Visscher	58	5.1	NS
Obermair	64	4.1	<.01
Ogawa	155	7.0	<.002
Fox	211	3.5	ND
Toi	125	5.1	<.01
Toi	328	4.6	<.0001
Simpson	178	6.0	0.002
Gasparini	531	6.3	<.001
Bevilacqua	211	6.6	<.0001
Obermair	230	4.6	ND
Fox	109	2.0	.04
Heimann	167	20.0	.04
Barbareschi	91	5.5	.006
Gasparini	191	5.5	<.01
Gasparini	178	5.2	<.01
Hall	87	9.5; 1.5	NS
Axelsson	220	11.5	NS
Van Hoef	93	13.0	NS

NOTE: Published positive studies. ND, not done; NS, not significant.
SOURCE: From Gasparini and Harris.

efficacy of antiangiogenic therapy. Although it is currently employed in a few early clinical trials of antiangiogenic therapy, experimental studies suggest that it will be of little value to predict efficacy of an angiogenesis inhibitor. Microvessel density is determined mainly by intercapillary distance, itself governed by the cuff thickness of tumor cells surrounding a microvessel. In experimental animals, microvessel density may remain constant as a tumor is shrinking under antiangiogenic therapy. Residual tumor cells can form cuffs around remaining vessels, so that the vessel density may not change significantly. Microvessel density also may not distinguish between benign and malignant tumors. The microvessel density in normal pituitary tissue is higher than in a pituitary adenoma, which is higher than in a pituitary carcinoma. In the normal pituitary gland, the perivascular cuff is one to two cell layers. However, in the adenoma the perivascular cuff is increased as tumor cells adapt to lower oxygen tensions. Cuff thickness is even greater in the carcinoma, thus giving the lowest microvessel density. However, for other tumors, such as breast carcinoma, microvessel density is significantly higher than in normal breast tissue. In certain animal tumors, angiogenic output exceeds the growth capacity of the tumor cells. Initial antiangiogenic therapy will lead to a reduction in microvessel density, which may then remain constant as vascular density comes into balance with tumor cell population, whether the tumor remains stable or regresses. Finally, if the first microvessel density is obtained from an open biopsy and a subsequent follow-up microvessel density is from a needle biopsy, the second density will

Table 83-5 Prognostic Value of Microvessel Density in Breast Cancer Patients Treated with Adjuvant Therapy

Author	No. of Patients	Median Follow-up, Years	Adjuvant Treatment	Relapse-Free Survival
Weidner	82	4.0	Heterogeneous	<.001
Toi	198	4.6	Heterogeneous	<.001
Gasparini	191	5.5	CD31	<.001
Macaulay	88	2.5	Tamoxifen	ND
Gasparini	178	5.2	CD31	<.001

NOTE: ND, not done.
SOURCE: From Gasparini and Harris.

Table 83-6 Prognostic Value of Microvessel Density in Non-Small Cell Lung Cancers

Author	No. of Patients	Median Follow-up, Months	Prognostic Value
Macchiarini	87	60	Yes
Yamazaki	42	71	Yes
Fontanini	253	24	Yes
Giatromanolaki	107	36	Yes
Angeletti	96	24	Yes
Apolinario	116	60	Yes
		(stage II only)	
Fontanini	470	29	Yes
Fontanini	73	47	Yes

SOURCE: From Gasparini and Harris.

be higher. This artifact is due to tissue compression by the needle biopsy.

CYTOTOXIC CHEMOTHERAPY MAY BE ANGIOGE-NESIS-DEPENDENT Certain cytotoxic chemotherapeutic agents may depend in part for their anticancer activity on their ability to inhibit proliferating endothelial cells. Proliferating and migrating microvascular endothelial cells are exposed to chemotherapeutic drugs before tumor cells. However, the endothelial cells have a chance to recover during the traditional 2-3 week off-therapy period designed to allow recovery of bone marrow. Recovering endothelium can resupply residual tumor cells with new vessels and with paracrine factors necessary for tumor cell survival. Tumor recurrence requires resumption of chemotherapy, which itself can lead to emergence of drug-resistant clones of tumor cells (but not of endothelial cells). The convention of *maximum tolerated dose* (MTD) virtually forces the prolonged off-therapy schedule.

If the schedule of the chemotherapeutic agent is altered (increased number of lower drug doses) to apply maximum cytotoxic pressure to the endothelial cells in the tumor bed (i.e., an "antiangiogenic schedule" instead of a "conventional schedule"), even large tumors in mice may be permanently cured. In contrast, all mice on the conventional schedule of MTD therapy died with drug-resistant tumors. The antiangiogenic schedule of the chemotherapeutic drug was more frequent but was administered at a threefold lower total lower dose per day so that bone marrow was not depressed. Thus, efficacy of cytotoxic chemotherapy can be improved (in mice) by applying new logic to an old drug. The new logic is that antiangiogenic properties of certain conventional cytotoxic agents are not revealed unless the drugs are administered frequently. Frequent administration requires lower doses.

These results in mice may help to explain why some patients who

Table 83-7 Prognostic Value of Microvessel Density in Genitourinary Cancers

Type of Cancer	Author	No. of Patients	Prognostic Value
Testicular germinal cell tumor	Olivarez	65	Yes
Prostatic cancer	Wakui	101	Yes
	Fregene	34	Yes
	Weidner	74	Yes
	Vesalainen	88	Yes
	Brawer	37	Yes
	Silberman	109	Yes
	Barth	41	Yes
	Rogatsch	46	Yes
Bladder cancer	Dickenson	45	Yes
	Bochner	164	Yes
	Grossfeld	163	Yes

NOTE: ND, not done.
SOURCE: From Gasparini and Harris.

Table 83-8 Prognostic Value of Microvessel Density in Esophageal and Gastrointestinal Tumors

Type of Cancer	Author	No. of Patients	Median Follow-up, Months	Prognostic Value
Esophageal	Tanigawa	43	3.1	Yes
Gastric	Maeda	124	>5	Yes
	Tanigawa	181	4.1	Yes
Colorectal	Saclarides	48	4.4	Yes
	Tomisaki	175	5.0	Yes
	Takebayashi	166	6.3	Yes
	Bossi	178	5.0	No
	Lindmark	212	4.5	Yes[a]

[a] High vascularity associated with good prognosis.
SOURCE: From Gasparini and Harris.

are receiving long-term maintenance or even palliative chemotherapy continue to have stable disease beyond the time that tumor cells would have been expected to develop drug resistance. For example, long-term stable disease has been observed in a few patients with metastatic breast cancer who have been on weekly paclitaxel for several years. Paclitaxel has been reported to have antiangiogenic activity in addition to its anticancer activity. In the future, formal clinical trials with antiangiogenic schedules of chemotherapy should be tested.

Although "fractionated" radiotherapy (i.e., increased frequency of exposures at lower doses) was found empirically to be more effective and to cause fewer side effects than higher radiation doses more widely spaced, the biologic basis of this approach may be due, in part, to the effect of ionizing radiation on endothelial cells. Conventional radiotherapy of tumor-bearing animals is greatly enhanced and with fewer side effects when the radiotherapy is administered in combination with subtherapeutic doses of angiostatin.

GUIDELINES FOR CLINICAL TRIALS OF ANGIOGENESIS INHIBITORS New guidelines are required to examine the clinical effects of angiogenesis inhibitors because this class of drugs differs so markedly from cytotoxic chemotherapy. First, end-points for efficacy require different definitions. For cytotoxic therapy, lack of tumor regression is considered a failure, and an end-point of stable disease is little valued because it has never been shown to improve patient survival. In contrast, stable disease brought about by antiangiogenic therapy may be a favorable end-point of antiangiogenic therapy if it can be shown to improve the quality or duration of life. Experience with endostatin in early phase I clinical trials shows that patients with advanced metastatic disease refractory to all conventional therapy and who have had stable disease on endostatin for up to 6 months so far have pain relief, increased appetite, normal bone marrow function, and no side effects. A similar experience has been gained from IFN-α administered daily at low dose (3 million units) for malignancies dependent upon overexpression of bFGF as their sole or main angiogenic protein (i.e., giant cell tumors of bone, angioblastoma). In fact, five of six of these patients who had failed all conven-

Table 83-9 Prognostic Value of Microvessel Density in Malignant Melanoma

Author	No. of Patients	Median Follow-up, Months	Thickness, mm	Prognostic Value
Srivastava	20	>5	0.76–4.00	Yes
Fallowfield	64	ND	0.48–18.5	Yes
Carnochan	107	>5	0.85–1.25	No
Busam	120	8.9	Invasive	No
Graham	37	>10	0.76	Yes
Vlaykova	31	>3	0.76	Yes

NOTE: ND, not done.
SOURCE: From Gasparini and Harris.

tional therapy had complete regressions of their tumors by 1 to 3 years and are now off therapy and remain tumor free. This illustrates a second difference from cytotoxic therapy: antiangiogenic therapy takes longer to achieve stable disease and tumor regression is slower. It is analogous to the use of tamoxifen or to the treatment of other chronic diseases such as tuberculosis. Nevertheless, patients enjoy a high quality of life during antiangiogenic therapy.

Third, tumor progression during a clinical trial of cytotoxic chemotherapy is considered as a failure, and patients are often discontinued from the trial. With antiangiogenic therapy, some patients with rapidly advancing metastatic disease may show some tumor progression before stable disease is achieved. In the first clinical trials of tamoxifen, some patients were discontinued early in the trials because of tumor progression. After the term *tamoxifen flare* was invented, patients stayed on long-term tamoxifen therapy for several years. Of course, very rapid tumor progression during antiangiogenic therapy requires that the inhibitor be discontinued and the patient offered a different therapy.

Fourth, unlike cytotoxic chemotherapy, antiangiogenic therapy is more effective if it is administered frequently, without gaps, for a long period of time (e.g., like tamoxifen) and at a dose that has little or no toxicity. The term *MTD* is less useful for angiogenesis inhibitors.

Fifth, angiogenesis inhibitors can be used in combination with conventional chemotherapy, radiotherapy, immunotherapy, gene therapy, or other modalities, usually without increasing side effects. Clinical trials of angiogenesis inhibitors in combination with chemotherapy or radiotherapy are already under way.

CLINICAL SIGNS IN CANCER PATIENTS BASED ON ANGIOGENESIS Certain clinical signs and symptoms from tumor neovascularization are associated with specific tumor types. For example, retinoblastomas in the posterior eye induce iris neovascularization in the anterior chamber. Some brain tumors induce angiogenesis in remote areas of the brain. Bone pain in metastatic prostate cancer may be related in part to neovascularization. A problem in the diagnosis of a primary bone tumor is that if the biopsy specimen contains only the neovascular response at the periphery of the tumor, it may be mistaken for granulation tissue or inflammation. Several cancer syndromes, such as inappropriate hormonal activity, hypercoagulation, and cachexia, are secondary to the presence of biologically active peptides released into the circulation from vascularized tumors. Therefore, an early therapeutic effect of antiangiogenic therapy could be increased appetite, weight gain, and disappearance of a cancer syndrome. The angiogenesis induced by cervical cancer may be observed by colposcopy; the appearance of telangiectasia, or "vascular spiders," in a mastectomy scar may herald local recurrence of tumor; color Doppler imaging can demonstrate neovascularization in breast cancer and other tumors; bladder carcinoma is detected by cystoscopy based, in part, on its neovascularization; and mammography may reveal the vascularized rim of a breast tumor. A wide range of radiologic signs of cancer are based on "enhancement" of lesions by radiopaque dyes sequestered transiently in the neovasculature of a tumor. Moreover, in some tumors large central areas cannot be penetrated by radiopaque dyes because of vascular compression, a situation that is unusual in prevascular tumors.

CLINICAL MISPERCEPTIONS ABOUT TUMOR ANGIOGENESIS Because angiogenesis research is such a broad and rapidly moving field (at least 30 reports each week), certain misperceptions have emerged.

One misperception is that angiogenesis is synonymous with malignancy. The presence of angiogenesis does not distinguish between a benign and a malignant tumor. Benign adrenal adenomas are highly neovascularized but appear to lack the growth potential to take advantage of the new blood vessels they have induced. Angiogenesis may not be necessary for certain tumor cells that can grow as a flat sheet between membranes, e.g., gliomatosis in the meninges. Large tumors

Table 83-10   Angiogenesis Inhibitors in U.S. Clinical Trials for Eye Disease[a]

Drug	Sponsor	Mechanism	Phase: Disease	Location
Anecortave acetate	Alcon	Angiostatic steroid	I: Macular degeneration	New York, Palo Alto, Baltimore, Cleveland
LY33531 (oral)	Lilly	Protein kinase C β inhibitor (anti-VEGF)	III: Diabetic retinopathy	U.S.
rhuFab	Genetech	Anti-VEGF	I: Macular degeneration	Boston
AG3340 (oral)	Agouron	Inhibitor of MMP-2 and -9	III: Macular degeneration	U.S.
Anti-VEGF aptamer	Gilead/EyeTECH	Anti-VEGF	I: Macular degeneration	New York, Boston, Palo Alto

[a] Updated March, 2000.

NOTE: MMP, metalloproteinase inhibitor; VEGF, vascular endothelial growth factor.

are thought to have "established" vessels that would be refractory to antiangiogenic therapy. A few feeder vessels, usually arteries, may be observed in the midst of a histologic cross-section of a tumor and could be considered as established. However, tumor cells depend on *thin-walled microvessels* for diffusion of nutrients, growth factors, and oxygen, and it is these vessels that continue to undergo high turnover rates even in a large, slowly growing or indolent tumors. These microvessels require the continuous presence of endothelial growth factors such as VEGF. Withdrawal or blockade of VEGF leads to endothelial cell apoptosis and regression of microvessels. In both animals and humans, very large tumors have regressed in response to antiangiogenic therapy, but a longer time of therapy is required. For example, a high-grade giant cell tumor (refractory to all conventional therapy) of >1 kg in the pelvis of a 17-year-old girl underwent 90% regression after 1 year of daily systemic therapy with IFN-α (3 million units). It is commonly stated that tumors "outgrow their blood supply." This is inaccurate; growing tumors can gradually *compress* their blood supply because of increasing interstitial pressure (discussed above). These areas of vascular compression become ischemic but are not avascular. Necrosis may follow. Vessel compression also interferes with the optimal delivery of therapeutic agents. Paradoxically, antiangiogenic therapy can decrease ischemia, apparently because it decreases interstitial pressure.

Another misperception is that antiangiogenic therapy will be less effective against slowly growing tumors, because this is true for cytotoxic chemotherapeutic agents. In fact the opposite has been found in experimental animals. Slowly growing mouse tumors respond more effectively to angiogenesis inhibitors (TNP-470 or angiostatin) than do rapidly growing tumors. Rapidly growing tumors require higher doses of angiogenesis inhibitors to suppress their growth to the same extent as slowly growing tumors. While cytotoxic therapy is dependent on tumor cell cycle, antiangiogenic therapy is not. It is widely assumed that only "highly vascularized" tumors are susceptible to antiangiogenic therapy. This misperception comes from attempts to estimate the angiogenic output of a tumor from an angiogram or a gross tumor specimen. A large, dark, unstained area in an angiogram is usually due to nonfilling of compressed vessels. This is often misinterpreted as "avascular" tumor. However, at the microscopic level, histologic sections reveal high microvessel density. A large tumor observed at the operating table, such as a neurofibrosarcoma, may be a hard white mass and assumed to be "poorly vascularized," when in fact the histologic microsections show intense neovascularization.

SUMMARY: TWO CELLULAR TARGETS IN A TUMOR   An important lesson from angiogenesis research is to think about a tumor as containing two cell compartments that stimulate each other: the endothelial cell compartment and the tumor cell compartment. Anticancer therapy may be more efficacious if each compartment is treated by drugs that selectively target each cell type. The mutational rate is high in the tumor cell compartment and low in the

endothelial cell compartment. This is the reason why it may be possible to employ antiangiogenic therapy for the long term, together with conventional chemotherapy or other therapies and subsequently in the postchemotherapy period.

DISEASES OF OCULAR NEOVASCULARIZATION

Pathologic angiogenesis is the most common cause of blindness worldwide. Pathologic neovascularization can occur in each compartment of the eye. For example, of >21 diseases that cause pathologic neovascularization in the cornea, contact lens wear, trauma, prior surgery, herpes simplex, and herpes zoster are the most frequently associated with pathologic neovascularization. Of ~37 diseases associated with iris neovascularization, central retinal vein occlusion, neovascular glaucoma, diabetes mellitus, and retinoblastoma are the most frequent. Of 14 diseases associated with retinal neovascularization, age-related macular degeneration, diabetes mellitus, retinopathy of prematurity, central retinal vein occlusion, branch retinal vein occlusion, and sickle cell disease are the most frequent. In western countries, age-related macular degeneration and diabetic retinopathy are the diseases of ocular neovascularization that affect the most patients. The large number of diseases listed above that are associated with ocular neovascularization and that directly or indirectly cause blindness illustrates how few effective therapies are currently available. This outline also reveals how few of these therapies can be administered systemically and how great is the opportunity to employ antiangiogenic therapy in clinical trials to reduce the incidence of blindness from pathologic neovascularization.

AGE-RELATED MACULAR DEGENERATION   In age-related macular degeneration, angiogenesis occurs in the choroid. In the severe form of the disease, microhemorrhages from these new vessels lead to blindness. Approximately 1.7 million individuals in the United States suffer from the severe form, which is the leading cause of blindness in those ≥64 years. Laser therapy is less effective than in diabetic retinopathy. The angiogenic protein VEGF is markedly elevated in macular degeneration and may be a major mediator of this disease. Of the five angiogenesis inhibitors currently in clinical trials for ocular neovascularization (Table 83-10), four are employed in the treatment of macular degeneration. One inhibitor is an antibody that neutralizes VEGF, and the other is a synthetic low-molecular-weight compound that targets a VEGF receptor.

DIABETIC RETINOPATHY   Diabetic retinopathy affects ~1.2 million of the estimated 14 million U.S. diabetic patients. It is the leading cause of blindness in persons between ages 25 and 64. Pathologic angiogenesis occurs in the retina, and new microvessels grow into the vitreous where they bleed and cause vitreous retraction. Laser therapy is more successful than in macular degeneration, but it is painful and causes gradual obliteration of the peripheral retina and loss of accompanying visual fields. Overexpression of VEGF may also mediate diabetic retinopathy but appears to be induced by upregulation of HIF-1 secondary to hypoxia in the retina. An orally available protein kinase Cβ inhibitor of VEGF is in phase III clinical trial for diabetic retinopathy. An early primary cause of the hypoxia may be adhesion of leukocytes to endothelium in retinal vessels (by upregulation of intercellular adhesion molecule 1 on retinal microvascular endothelium), leading to slow flow or periods of no flow.

RETINOPATHY OF PREMATURITY   At the time of birth, both the retina and its vascular supply are still growing. Blood vessels that supply the retina in the premature baby and in the newborn are exquisitely sensitive to changes in oxygen, a mechanism that guarantees an adequate blood supply to the growing retina. In newborn cats exposed to oxygen, VEGF levels are downregulated and vascular growth in the retina is slowed or inhibited. However, the retina continues to grow. Subsequently, when the animal is returned to room air, the mismatch between the delayed vascularization and the steadily growing retina leads to relative hypoxia, which triggers a surge of VEGF and retinal neovascularization. This may cause retinal detachment and microhemorrhage. In the United States there are currently ~180,000 cases of retinopathy of prematurity, also called *retrolental fibroplasia.*

The increased understanding of the angiogenic mechanism of retinopathy of prematurity has led to clinical trials in which infants are weaned from oxygen to room air very slowly in order to prevent the rapid rise of VEGF. A recent report showed that in newborn animals returned to room air after exposure to oxygen, pathologic neovascularization was completely prevented while normal vascular development continued if the animals were treated with angiostatin for 5 days, beginning with the first day of exposure to room air. It is not yet clear whether systemic therapy of retinopathy of prematurity will be feasible in infants.

ENDOGENOUS ANGIOGENESIS INHIBITORS IN THE EYE Normally the components of the eye that transmit light (cornea, aqueous, lens, and vitreous) are avascular. The maintenance of this avascular state is accomplished, in part, by the presence of potent inhibitors of angiogenesis. Pigment epithelium-derived factor (PEDF) is a 50-kDa serpin and is a potent angiogenesis inhibitor that is produced by retinal cells. The amount of inhibitory PEDF produced by retinal cells is directly correlated with oxygen concentrations, suggesting that its loss plays a permissive role in ischemia-driven retinal neovascularization. In other words, when oxygen is decreased PEDF is decreased and VEGF is increased. Both changes facilitate neovascularization. PEDF has the unique characteristic of inhibiting endothelial migration toward a wide variety of angiogenic inducers tested. It may be the predominant angiogenesis inhibitor in the eye. When neutralizing antibody to PEDF (but not preimmune sera) is injected into the cornea, it becomes neovascularized. PEDF has also been found in tumors.

Thrombospondin-1 has also been found in ocular tissues such as cornea and in the retina. During hypoxia-driven retinal angiogenesis in newborn mice (returned to room air after oxygen exposure), a three-fold increase in expression of thrombospondin-1 was seen corresponding to peak neovascularization and peak VEGF expression. The increased thrombospondin-1 expression during ischemia-induced angiogenesis appears to be mediated by VEGF. This suggests that thrombospondin functions in a negative-feedback system to protect the eye against surges of VEGF. It is interesting that the same balance of positive and negative regulators of angiogenesis originally found in tumors operates in normal tissues and that a shift in the net balance of these regulators mediates pathologic angiogenesis as well as its return to the normal nonangiogenic state.

ANGIOGENESIS IN SKIN DISEASE

Many dermatologic diseases are associated with angiogenesis. A caveat is that, unlike neoplastic diseases, which are virtually all angiogenesis-dependent, not all nonneoplastic diseases that are angiogenic are also angiogenesis-dependent.

ANGIOGENESIS-ASSOCIATED VS. ANGIOGENESIS-DEPENDENT SKIN DISEASE In certain diseases of the skin, angiogenesis may be an important side effect that facilitates healing or otherwise protects the host. Examples include ulcerations, delayed healing of wounds, and chronic infections, in which antiangiogenic therapy could be contraindicated. A few of the dermatologic diseases known to be angiogenesis-dependent are described.

Infantile Hemangiomas Hemangiomas consist of tumor-like clusters of proliferating capillaries. They occur in 1 out of 100 newborns and in 1 out of 4 premature infants, and by age 1 year are present in up to 10% of infants. In the first, or proliferating, stage, the lesions grow rapidly, reaching peak growth by ~4 months. By about 1 year they may enter the involuting stage, where they stop growing, following which they regress over the next 3 to 5 years (the involuted stage) and then usually disappear. During the proliferating stage the endothelial cells overexpress bFGF, VEGF, and metalloproteinases, all of which appear in the urine at abnormally high levels. In normal skin, keratinocytes express IFN-β, an angiogenesis inhibitor of similar strength as IFN-α. IFN-α or -β inhibit overexpression of aFGF and bFGF. Glucocorticoids (prednisone, 5 mg/kg) are used as first-line therapy for hemangiomas that are destroying tissue, interfering with sight, or threatening life. A dramatic slowing and subsequent regression occur in ~30% of patients, but glucocorticoids fail in the remaining 70% (i.e., either no regression, but some slowing of the disease, or continued rapid growth of the lesions). The mechanism by which glucocorticoids act as antiangiogenic agents is not clear, but they do inhibit synthesis of metalloproteinases. When glucocorticoids fail and the hemangioma is life-threatening, IFN-α is used at low dose, 3 million units/m^2 daily subcutaneously for 8 to 12 months. While ~95% of hemangiomas regress spontaneously, 5% are sight- or life-threatening. Hemangiomas in the liver, heart, airway, or brain may be associated with a 50% mortality if untreated. IFN-α is antiangiogenic on the basis of its ability to inhibit overproduction of bFGF. Urinary levels of bFGF fall toward normal as hemangiomas regress, and bFGF levels can be used as a guide to dosing of IFN-α. While IFN-α accelerates regression of hemangiomas in 85% of patients, it fails in the other 15% for unknown reasons. Many of the failures are Kaposi hemangioendotheliomas (KHE), a very aggressive form of hemangioma, often accompanied by platelet trapping and thrombocytopenia. IFN-α works well in only 50% of KHE. Regressions of hemangioma are slower with IFN-α than with glucocorticoids. In infants <1 year old, a side effect of IFN-α can be delayed walking. This occurs in ~4% of infants and can be detected early by spasticity of the lower limbs (*spastic diplegia*). It is reversible if IFN-α is discontinued; for this reason, all children on IFN-α are followed carefully by a neurologist.

A "cavernous hemangioma" is not a hemangioma but a venous malformation in which there is a dearth of smooth muscle in the wall of a large thin venous structure lined by endothelium. These never regress spontaneously, and neither glucocorticoids nor IFN-α are effective. Thus an adult with a cavernous hemangioma should not be treated with IFN-α.

Verruca Vulgaris Warts are caused by infection of keratinocytes in the skin by one of many subtypes of human papillomavirus (HPV). HPV contains two genes (E6/E7) that may increase angiogenesis. The E6 gene destabilizes the p53 tumor-suppressor gene, which upregulates VEGF and downregulates thrombospondin-1, an angiogenesis inhibitor. The HPV E7 gene inactivates the tumor suppressor gene Rb. Antiangiogenic therapy may be beneficial in these lesions, which are usually highly neovascularized.

Psoriasis Psoriasis is a proliferative disorder of epidermis accompanied by increased vascularity in the dermis in the form of elongated and widened dermal capillaries. The disease is T lymphocyte mediated. Psoriatic lesions are angiogenic. The major angiogenic mediator in psoriasis appears to be VEGF, which is upregulated, as are its receptors. In patients with psoriasis, the increased vascularity induced by VEGF may act as a conduit for delivery of T lymphocytes to the epidermal target. VEGF itself may facilitate T lymphocyte targeting. When VEGF is overexpressed in a tumor vascular bed, leukocyte rolling and adhesion are enhanced.

Up to 5 million Americans have psoriasis, but ~500,000 have a severe form that requires long-term therapy, such as with methotrexate for several years. Both glucocorticoids and retinoids are weak angiogenesis inhibitors, and they may be suppressing the angiogenic component as well as the infiltration of immune cells. More potent angiogenesis inhibitors may be useful.

Basal Cell and Squamous Cell Carcinomas Both of these skin malignancies are highly angiogenic and follow the rules for other angiogenic-dependent tumors. Inactivation of the p53 tumor-suppressor gene (in part by ultraviolet light–induced mutations) is thought to be an early event in tumorigenesis, and its inactivation downregulates the angiogenesis inhibitor thrombospondin-1 and upregulates VEGF expression. Furthermore, the normal expression of IFN-β in keratinocytes is markedly decreased, permitting upregulation of the angiogenic stimulator bFGF. These lesions comprise >90% of the ~700,000 skin cancers that are treated each year in the United States.

Cutaneous Melanoma Melanoma in the skin begins in a radial or horizontal growth phase, which usually does not exceed a thickness of 0.75 mm. This stage is not neovascularized or is poorly neovascularized. It is analogous to the avascular phase of early in situ carcinoma. In the vertical growth phase, there are increased neovascularization, increased proliferation, and increased thickness of tumor beyond 0.75 mm, and intensity of vascularization correlates directly with increased metastatic risk and mortality. Progression of melanoma often begins with inactivation of the tumor-suppressor gene p16 and is followed later by expression of $\alpha_v\beta_3$ integrin and by expression of VEGF receptors on the melanoma cells. *Ras* mutations that upregulate VEGF expression emerge later and may be followed by expression of the angiogenic proteins, IL-8, and bFGF. This sequential onset of expression of angiogenic proteins by a tumor cell is similar to progression of breast cancer. It is not clear if or how expression of $\alpha_v\beta_3$ integrin as well as VEGF receptors on the melanoma cells themselves facilitates tumor growth, unless the VEGF is acting as an autocrine growth factor for the tumor cells, while at the same time acting as a paracrine stimulator of endothelial cells. A precedent for this mechanism has been reported for human pancreatic cancer. The angiogenesis inhibitor 2-methoxyestradiol currently in a phase I trial for breast cancer also showed efficacy against melanoma in animals.

Kaposi's Sarcoma (KS) This lesion, which acts like a malignancy in patients with AIDS, may instead be a chronic inflammatory reactive process that is highly angiogenic. The angiogenesis is driven mainly by VEGF and hepatocyte growth factor. The tat protein of the HIV virus also plays a role in the angiogenic pathway for KS, but this is still being elucidated. The origin of KS cells is also not clear, but they appear to arise from the vascular system, possibly from smooth-muscle cells or pericytes. Two different angiogenesis inhibitors in phase II trials, thalidomide and TNP-470, a synthetic analogue of fumagillin, have shown efficacy against KS. However, there are currently too few cases to make any general conclusions.

Neurofibromatosis These slow-growing benign skin tumors of Schwann cell origin can grow in other organs and become very large. Neurofibromas are very neovascularized and express VEGF. This may be driven by overexpression of the *ras* oncogene. The gene for neurofibromin (NF1) is a negative regulator of *ras*, and mutation of this gene increases *ras* expression. Because of their very slow growth rate and high angiogenic activity, neurofibromas illustrate a type of tumor for which long-term antiangiogenic therapy may be more effective than cytotoxic chemotherapy. They are rich in mast cells, which may enhance tumor angiogenesis by mobilization of bFGF. If a patient with a neurofibroma had abnormally high plasma or urine levels of bFGF, daily IFN-α could be used at a low dose of 3 million units/m^2 for a prolonged period of 2 to 3 years, with slow regression as a goal.

Recessive Dystrophic Epidermolysis Bullosa This autosomal recessive disorder is characterized by subepidermal blistering, scarring, fusion of digits, and severe pruritus. Epidermis separates from dermis, in part due to a loss of collagen VII, which participates in the anchoring of these two cellular layers. Aggressive cutaneous squamous cell carcinoma, which emerges from this lesion, is the most common cause of death. Very high levels of bFGF have been found in the urine of these patients but not in patients with other blistering disorders. The source of bFGF could be its mobilization from heparan sulfate proteoglycans in the defective epidermal-dermal junction. bFGF not only stimulates angiogenesis directly but also stimulates the production of COX 2, which converts lipid precursors to prostaglandin E$_2$, another angiogenic stimulator. Keratinocyte growth is also stimulated by bFGF. Continuous keratinocyte proliferation may be a precursor to the development of squamous cell carcinoma. COX 2 inhibitors have antiangiogenic and antitumor activity in mice and may be useful in angiogenic diseases in man. Another antiangiogenic approach could be low-dose IFN-α, based on the same rationale for reducing high bFGF expression in life-threatening hemangiomas.

ANGIOGENESIS IN ARTHRITIS

The role of angiogenesis in rheumatoid arthritis and in other forms of arthritis can be most simply conceptualized as two phases: prevascular and vascular. The prevascular phase is analogous to an acute inflammatory state in which the synovium is invaded by inflammatory and immune cells, with macrophages, mast cells, and T cells predominating, among others. These cells may be the source of the angiogenic stimulators found in synovial fluid, which include VEGF, bFGF, IL-8, and hepatocyte growth factor. Activated endothelial cells can also release hepatocyte growth factor. The growth of a neovascular pannus from the synovium begins the vascular phase of arthritis. The vascular pannus can invade and destroy cartilage, a process that is enhanced by the generation of enzymatic activity, mainly metalloproteinases, at the advancing front of new proliferating endothelium. This neovascular pannus overcomes endogenous angiogenesis inhibitors in the cartilage that normally protect it from vascular invasion and maintain its avascularity. These inhibitors include, among others, TIMPs 1, 2, 3 and 4 (ranging from 21 to 29 kDa); thrombospondin-1; and troponin I. Experimental evidence that arthritis is angiogenesis-dependent is based on suppression of rat adjuvant arthritis by an angiogenesis inhibitor, TNP-470 (a synthetic analogue of fumagillin).

This somewhat simplistic model does not do justice to the complexity of the angiogenic response in arthritis, which is beyond the scope of this chapter. Nevertheless, it provides a platform to think about antiangiogenic therapy of arthritis. In principle, inhibition of neovascularization in the joint should interrupt a conduit for continuous traffic of inflammatory cells into the joint and prevent destruction of cartilage. The COX 2 inhibitors currently in wide use for arthritis have been found to be potent angiogenesis inhibitors capable of inhibiting tumor growth in mice. Other angiogenesis inhibitors currently in clinical trial for cancer may eventually also find use in antiarthritis therapy. An interesting potential candidate would be 2-methoxyestradiol.

ANGIOGENESIS IN GYNECOLOGIC DISEASE

Angiogenesis in the female reproductive tract is being actively studied because it is the principal example of physiologic angiogenesis. Angiogenesis in the ovarian follicle is driven mainly by bFGF and VEGF although other angiogenic regulatory molecules are being studied. However, while VEGF is known to be upregulated by estrogen, it is not clear whether endogenous angiogenesis inhibitors operate in combination with declining estrogen to turn off angiogenesis in the ovarian follicle. When angiogenesis is increased in any one follicle, it is suppressed in all other follicles. This is analogous to the suppression of angiogenesis in distant metastases by a primary tumor, but it is not known if the ovarian system utilizes similar endogenous inhibitors as have been discovered in various tumor systems.

A variety of diseases of the female reproductive tract are based on angiogenic processes. A few of these are mentioned here briefly to illustrate that similar molecules mediate angiogenesis in tumors and in gynecologic disease, although they may be regulated differently.

Endometriosis In this disease, endometrial glands or stroma are present outside the uterine cavity, e.g., in the ovaries, uterine ligaments, rectovaginal septum, and pelvic peritoneum. The foci of endometrium are usually under the control of the ovarian hormones and undergo cyclic menstrual changes with periodic bleeding, which is painful and may lead to fibrosis. At least one angiogenic protein, VEGF, is known to mediate the neovascularization in these lesions. VEGF is upregulated by increased estrogen and downregulated by withdrawal of estrogen. It has been suggested that endometriotic tissue may produce its own estrogen because it contains aromatase cytochrome P450, not found in normal endometrium. Approximately 780,000 women in the United States suffer from endometriosis. No clinical trials of angiogenesis inhibitors for endometriosis are currently under way, but this class of drugs holds promise as an additional treatment of endometriosis, perhaps on a monthly basis. At least three angiogenesis inhibitors are produced in the female reproductive system: 2-methoxyestradiol, proliferin-related protein, and a 16-kDa fragment of prolactin. It would be of interest to know if any of these would be therapeutic for endometriosis.

Other Pathology Angiogenesis may be increased in dysfunctional uterine bleeding such as breakthrough bleeding from contraceptives. The edema and ascites of the ovarian hyperstimulation syndrome is thought to be mediated by the ability of VEGF to increase vascular permeability. Preeclampsia during pregnancy may be related to abnormal vascular remodeling, although it is not clear how the hypertension and cerebral edema associated with this disease are mediated by an endothelial cell product.

Carcinoma of the Ovary, Endometrium, and Cervix These common gynecologic tumors are all angiogenesis-dependent. As a result, they share certain characteristics discussed under "Neoplastic Disease," above. Microvessel density in histologic sections provides independent prognostic indicators of metastatic risk and/or mortality. VEGF is a major angiogenic mediator in these tumors. The ascites in ovarian carcinoma contains concentrations of VEGF of up to 100 times higher than those in serum in the same patient. Endometrial carcinoma, which can be induced by long-term tamoxifen therapy, may operate through upregulation of IL-8 in the endometrium. The potential value of angiogenesis inhibitors in the treatment of gynecologic tumors refractory to conventional therapy is suggested by two reports: (1) experimental ovarian cancer was inhibited by administration of angiostatin and endostatin, which acted synergistically; and (2) malignant ascites and growth of human ovarian cancer were inhibited in experimental animals by inhibiting a receptor for VEGF.

ANGIOGENESIS IN CARDIOVASCULAR DISEASE

Angiogenesis in the cardiovascular system occurs under three different conditions: (1) neovascularization in atherosclerotic plaques, (2) formation of collateral vessels to an area of ischemic myocardium or ischemic muscle in a limb, and (3) neovascularization at the edges of a myocardial infarction during its repair.

Angiogenesis in Atherosclerotic Plaques Angiogenesis occurs in atherosclerotic plaques, and hypoxia is thought to be a major stimulus. The mediators of angiogenesis found in most plaques are bFGF, VEGF, transforming growth factor β (TGF-β), and PDGF-BB. Smooth-muscle cells in plaques are a source of VEGF and PDGF-BB. Macrophages, mast cells, and T cells, which are also found to infiltrate plaques, can produce bFGF and TGF-β. However, the angiogenic factor(s) directly responsible for plaque angiogenesis and the sequential order in which these factors act during the evolution of a plaque have not been worked out. The new microvessels in a plaque can be the source of intraplaque microhemorrhage. Furthermore, the production

of metalloproteinases at the advancing tips of new microvessels may contribute to plaque rupture.

The evidence that atherosclerotic plaques are angiogenesis-dependent. However, some supporting experimental evidence has been obtained in transgenic mice deficient in the gene for apolipoprotein E (ApoE-/-). When these mice are fed a western diet containing 0.15% cholesterol, they develop atherosclerotic plaques in the aorta over 6 months. Early plaques <250 μm thick are not neovascularized. Cells in the center of such a plaque would lie within the oxygen diffusion limit of oxygen arriving from the normal vasa vasorum or from the arterial lumen. However, intense neovascularization occurred as plaques enlarged to >250 μm. When mice were treated during the development of a plaque with either of the angiogenesis inhibitors TNP-470 (a synthetic fumagillin analogue in phase II clinical trial) or endostatin (in phase I clinical trial), total plaque area was reduced by 70% and 85%, respectively. This finding has important clinical implications.

If long-term antiangiogenic therapy inhibits plaque growth or reduces plaque microhemorrhage or rupture, then it will be important to document this in cancer patients who are receiving angiogenesis inhibitors over a period of $\geq$1 to 2 years. Furthermore, if antiangiogenic therapy blocks plaque angiogenesis, plaque growth, bleeding, or rupture, would this obviate the need for coronary collateral vessels? If so, then this would remove the theoretical concern that long-term antiangiogenic therapy for cancer might decrease collateral development. Another extenuating circumstance is that collateral vessels in general are thick-walled and coated with smooth muscle. They are less likely to undergo regression during exposure to an angiogenesis inhibitor than the thin-walled endothelial tubes, which are not covered or stabilized by smooth muscle in a tumor bed.

Therapeutic Angiogenesis in Ischemic Vascular Disease Experimental and clinical attempts to increase angiogenesis in ischemic tissues are very recent and have generally followed two strategies: injection into the ischemic tissue of angiogenic proteins (either VEGF or FGFs) or injection of genetic material that codes for these angiogenic stimulators. The animal data show that it is possible to increase the density of new blood vessels and flow to an ischemic area beyond what can be accomplished by hypoxia defense mechanisms in the body. It is not yet clear how durable the new vessels will be once they are induced in an ischemic tissue. We understand much more about stopping angiogenesis than starting it. However, once the techniques for therapeutic angiogenesis are further developed, the clinical need could be enormous.

FUTURE DIRECTIONS

Many other diseases are dominated by the angiogenic process. These include Crohn's disease, thyroiditis, benign prostatic hypertrophy, glomerulonephritis, ectopic bone formation, keloids, and others. However, they were not included in this chapter because the evidence that they are angiogenesis-dependent is not yet sufficiently compelling.

The diseases that were included *are* more clearly angiogenesis-dependent and serve to illustrate an important direction for the future. Oncologists, dermatologists, ophthalmologists, rheumatologists, gynecologists, and cardiologists are dealing with diseases that appear on the surface to be completely different from each other. Advances in therapy of these diseases are reported at different meetings and in different journals, and the specialists who treat them rarely go to each other's meetings or talk to each other. Nevertheless, all of these diseases are dominated by pathologic angiogenesis. The angiogenesis is driven by a small but similar set of molecules, which are regulated differently in each disease. Furthermore, a new class of drugs, the angiogenesis inhibitors, is becoming available and may permit improvements in therapy for many of these diseases. Thus, angiogenesis is a unifying process that has heuristic value across many medical specialties. The "angiogenesis-dependency" of many diseases, neoplastic and nonneoplastic, is of course not sufficiently quantitative to be called a theory, but it is similar to Stephen Wolfram's definition of a theory as "a compressed package of information, applicable to many cases."

BIBLIOGRAPHY

BROWDER T et al: Antiangiogenic scheduling of chemotherapy improves efficacy against experimental drug-resistant cancer. Cancer Res 60:1878, 2000

CARMELIET P, JAIN RK: Angiogenesis in cancer and other diseases: From genes to function to therapy. Nature, in press, 2000

FOLKMAN J: Tumor angiogenesis, in *Cancer Medicine 5*, JR Holland et al (eds). Hamilton, Ontario, BC Decker, 2000, pp 132–152

GASPARINI G, HARRIS AL: Prognostic significance of tumor vascularity, in *Antiangiogenic Agents in Cancer Therapy*, BA Teicher (ed). Totowa, NJ, Humana Press, 1999, pp 317–319

HANAHAN D, FOLKMAN J: Patterns and emerging mechanisms of the angiogenic switch during tumorigenesis. Cell 86:353, 1996.

———, WEINBERG RA: The hallmarks of cancer. Cell 100:57, 2000

HARACH HR et al: Occult papillary carcinoma of the thyroid. A normal finding in Finland. A systematic autopsy study. Cancer 56:531, 1985

MASFERRER JL et al: Antiangiogenic and antitumor activities of cyclooxygenase-2 inhibitors. Cancer Res 60:1306, 2000

ROHAN RM et al: Genetic heterogeneity of angiogenesis in mice. FASEB J 14:871, 2000

SINGHAL S et al: Antitumor activity of thalidomide in refractory multiple myeloma. N Engl J Med 341:1565, 1999

WEIDNER N et al: Tumor angiogenesis and metastasis—correlation in invasive breast carcinoma. N Engl J Med 324:1, 1991

XU L et al: Inhibition of malignant ascites and growth of human ovarian carcinoma by oral administration of a potent inhibitor of the vascular endothelial growth factor receptor tyrosine kinases. Int J Oncol 16:445, 2000

YOKOYAMA Y et al: Synergy between angiostatin and endostatin: Inhibition of ovarian cancer growth. Cancer Res 60:2190, 2000

84   *Edward A. Sausville, Dan L. Longo*

PRINCIPLES OF CANCER TREATMENT

The goal of cancer treatment is first to eradicate the cancer. If this primary goal cannot be accomplished, the goal of cancer treatment shifts to palliation, the amelioration of symptoms, and preservation of quality of life while striving to extend life. The dictum *primum non nocere* is *not* the guiding principle of cancer therapy. Every cancer treatment has the potential to cause harm, and treatment may be given that produces toxicity with no benefit. The therapeutic index of many interventions is quite narrow, and most treatments are given to the point of toxicity. The guiding principle of cancer treatment is *primum succerrere*, first hasten to help. Radical surgical procedures, large-field hyperfractionated radiation therapy, high-dose chemotherapy, and maximum tolerable doses of cytokines such as interleukin (IL) 2 are all used in certain settings where 100% of the patients will experience toxicity and side effects from the intervention, and only a fraction of the patients will experience benefit. One of the challenges of cancer treatment is to use the various treatment modalities alone and together in a fashion that maximizes the chances for patient benefit.

Cancer treatments are divided into four main groups: surgery, radiation therapy (including photodynamic therapy), chemotherapy (including hormonal therapy), and biologic therapy (including immunotherapy, differentiating agents, and agents targeting cancer cell biology). The modalities are often used in combination, and agents in one category can act by several mechanisms. For example, cancer chemotherapy agents can induce differentiation, and antibodies (a form of immunotherapy) can be used to deliver radiation therapy. Surgery and radiation therapy are considered local treatments, though their effects can influence the behavior of tumor at remote sites. Chemotherapy and biologic therapy are usually systemic treatments.

Cancer behaves in many ways as an organ that regulates its own growth. However, cancers have not set an appropriate limit on how much growth should be permitted. Normal organs and cancers share the property of having a population of cells in cycle and actively renewing and a population of cells not in cycle. In cancers, cells that are not dividing are heterogeneous; some have sustained too much genetic damage to replicate but have defects in their death pathways that permit their survival; some are starving for nutrients and oxygen; and some are reversibly out of cycle poised to be recruited back into cycle and expand if needed. Severely damaged and starving cells are unlikely to kill the patient. The problem is that the cells that are reversibly not in cycle are capable of replenishing tumor cells physically removed or damaged by radiation and chemotherapy.

Tumors follow a Gompertzian growth curve (Fig. 84-1); the growth fraction of a neoplasm starts at 100% with the first transformed cell and declines exponentially over time until by the time of diagnosis at a tumor burden of 1 to 5×10^9 tumor cells, the growth fraction is usually 1 to 4%. Cancers are actually trying to limit their own growth but are not completely successful at doing so. The peak growth rate occurs before the tumor is detectable. Folkman has suggested that tumors restrict their growth by elaborating angiogenesis inhibitors (Chap. 83). Other cellular mechanisms to withdraw cells from the cell cycle probably exist as well. Several observations support the idea of autoregulation of tumor growth. Metastases can be observed to grow more rapidly than the primary tumor, consistent with the idea that an inhibitory factor slows the growth of larger tumor masses. When a tumor recurs after surgery or chemotherapy, frequently its growth is accelerated and the growth fraction of the tumor is increased. This pattern is similar to that seen in regenerating organs. Partial resection of the liver results in the recruitment of cells into the cell cycle, and the resected liver volume is replaced. Similarly, chemotherapy-damaged bone marrow increases its growth to replace cells killed by chemotherapy. However, cancers do not recognize a limit on their expansion. Monoclonal gammopathy of uncertain significance may be an example of a clonal neoplasm with intrinsic features that stop its

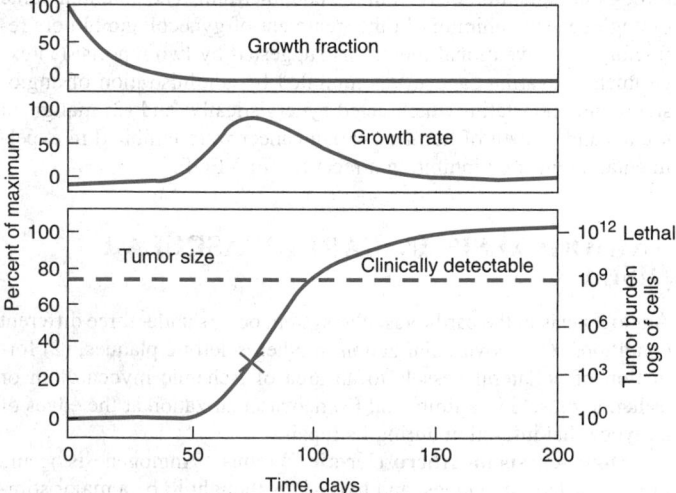

FIGURE 84-1 Gompertzian tumor growth. The growth fraction of a tumor declines exponentially over time (*top*). The growth rate of a tumor peaks before it is clinically detectable (*middle*). Tumor size increases slowly, goes through an exponential phase, and slows again as the tumor reaches the size at which it is attempting to level off. The maximum growth rate occurs at 1/e, the point at which the tumor is about 37% of its maximum size (marked with an X). Tumor becomes detectable at a burden of about 10^9 (1 cm³) and kills the patient at a tumor burden of about 10^{12} (1 kg). Efforts to treat the tumor and reduce its size can result in an increase in the growth fraction and an increase in growth rate.

growth before a lethal tumor burden is reached. A fraction of patients with this disorder go on to develop fatal multiple myeloma, but probably this occurs because of the accumulation of additional genetic lesions. Elucidation of the mechanisms that regulate this organ-like behavior may provide additional clues to cancer control and treatment.

PRINCIPLES OF CANCER SURGERY

Surgery is used in cancer prevention, diagnosis, staging, treatment (for both localized and metastatic disease), palliation, and rehabilitation.

PREVENTION Cancer can be prevented by surgery in people who have premalignant lesions resected (e.g., premalignant lesions of skin, colon, cervix) and in those who are at higher-than-normal risk of cancer from either an underlying disease (colectomy in those with pancolonic involvement with ulcerative colitis), the presence of genetic lesions (familial polyposis—colectomy; multiple endocrine neoplasia type II—thyroidectomy; familial breast or ovarian cancer—mastectomy, oophorectomy), or a developmental anomaly (orchiectomy in those with an undescended testis). In some cases, prophylactic surgery is more radical than the surgical procedures used to treat the cancer after it develops. The assessment of risk involves many factors and should be undertaken with care before advising a patient to undergo a major procedure. For breast cancer prevention, many experts use a 20% risk of developing breast cancer over the next 5 years as a threshold. However, patient fears play a major role in defining candidates for cancer prevention surgery. Counseling and education may not be enough to allay the fears of someone who has lost close family members to a malignancy.

DIAGNOSIS The ideal diagnostic procedure varies with the type of cancer, its anatomic location, and the medical condition of the patient. However, the underlying principle is to obtain as much tissue as safely possible. Tumors may be heterogeneous in appearance. Pathologists are better able to make the diagnosis when they have more tissue to examine. In addition to light-microscopic inspection of a tumor for pattern of growth, degree of cellular atypia, invasiveness, and morphologic features that aid in the differential diagnosis, sufficient tissue is of value in searching for genetic abnormalities and protein expression patterns that may aid in differential diagnosis or provide information about prognosis or likely response to treatment. Such testing requires that the tissue be handled properly (e.g., immunologic detection of proteins is more effective in fresh-frozen tissue rather than in formalin-fixed tissue); thus, coordination among the surgeon, pathologist, and primary care physician is essential to ensure that the amount of information learned from the biopsy material is maximized.

These goals are best met by an *excisional biopsy* in which the entire tumor mass is removed with a small margin of normal tissue surrounding it. If an excisional biopsy cannot be performed, *incisional biopsy* is the procedure of second choice. A wedge of tissue is removed, and an effort is made to include the majority of the cross-sectional diameter of the tumor in the biopsy to minimize sampling error. When the diagnosis is being made through an endoscope or via fluoroscopy, it may be necessary to obtain a *core-needle biopsy* of the mass; considerably less tissue is obtained and the diagnosis may be less certain. However, this procedure often provides enough information to plan a definitive surgical procedure. Least reliable in diagnosis of primary cancer is *fine-needle aspiration*. This technique generally obtains only a suspension of cells from within a mass. This approach (with stereotactic guidance of the needle) is the procedure of choice in the diagnosis of brain tumors and may be useful in diagnosing thyroid nodules and in confirming persistent or recurrent disease in a patient with known cancer, but the procedure is overutilized in primary diagnosis. It would be preferable to perform a larger open operation to obtain more tissue in most sites. The biopsy techniques that involve cutting into tumor carry with them a risk of facilitating the spread of the tumor.

STAGING As noted in Chap. 79, an important component of patient management is defining the extent of disease. Radiographic and other imaging tests can be helpful in defining the clinical stage; however, pathologic staging requires defining the extent of involvement by documenting the histologic presence of tumor in tissue biopsies obtained through a surgical procedure. Axillary lymph node sampling in breast cancer and lymph node sampling at laparotomy for lymphomas and testicular, colon, and other intraabdominal cancers provide crucial information for treatment planning and may determine the extent and nature of primary cancer treatment.

TREATMENT Surgery is perhaps the most effective means of treating cancer. About 40% of cancer patients are cured today by surgery. Unfortunately, a large fraction of patients with solid tumors (perhaps 60%) have metastatic disease that is not accessible for removal. However, even when the disease is not curable by surgery alone, the removal of tumor can obtain important benefits, including local control of tumor, preservation of organ function, debulking that permits subsequent therapy to work better, and staging information on extent of involvement. Cancer surgery aiming for cure is usually planned to excise the tumor completely with an adequate margin of normal tissue (the margin varies with the tumor and the anatomy), touching the tumor as little as possible to prevent vascular and lymphatic spread, and minimizing operative risk. Extending the procedure to resect draining lymph nodes obtains prognostic information, but such resections alone generally do not improve survival.

Increasingly, laparoscopic approaches are being taken to the primary tumor. Lymph node spread may be assessed using the *sentinel node approach*, in which the first draining lymph node a tumor would encounter is defined by injecting a dye at operation and resecting the first node to turn blue. The sentinel node evaluation is continuing to undergo clinical testing but appears to provide reliable information without the risks (lymphedema, lymphangiosarcoma) associated with resection of all the regional nodes. Advances in adjuvant chemotherapy and radiation therapy following surgery have permitted a substantial decrease in the extent of primary surgery necessary to obtain the best outcomes. Thus, lumpectomy with radiation therapy is as effective as modified radical mastectomy for breast cancer, and limb-sparing surgery followed by adjuvant radiation therapy and chemotherapy has replaced radical primary surgical procedures involving amputation and disarticulation for childhood rhabdomyosarcomas. More limited surgery is also being employed to spare organ function, as in larynx and bladder cancer. The magnitude of operations necessary to optimally control and cure cancer has also been diminished by technical advances; for example, the circular anastomotic stapler has allowed narrower (<2 cm) margins in colon cancer without compromise of local control rates, and many patients who would have had colostomies are able to maintain normal anatomy.

In some settings, e.g., bulky testicular cancer or stage III breast cancer, surgery is not the first treatment modality employed. After an initial diagnostic biopsy, chemotherapy and/or radiation therapy are delivered to reduce the size of the tumor and control clinically undetected metastatic disease, and such therapy is followed by a surgical procedure to remove residual masses. This is called *neoadjuvant therapy*. Because the sequence of treatment is critical to success and is different from the standard surgery-first approach, coordination among the surgical oncologist, radiation oncologist, and medical oncologist is crucial.

Surgery may be curative in a subset of patients with metastatic disease. Patients with lung metastases from osteosarcoma may be cured by resection of the lung lesions. In patients with colon cancer who have fewer than five liver metastases restricted to one lobe and no extrahepatic metastases, hepatic lobectomy may produce long-term disease-free survival in 25% of selected patients. Surgery can also be associated with systemic antitumor effects. In the setting of hormonally responsive tumors, oophorectomy and/or adrenalectomy may control estrogen production and orchiectomy may reduce androgen production, both with effects on metastatic tumor growth. If resection of the primary lesion takes place in the presence of metastases, any noted change in tumor behavior is most often acceleration of growth, perhaps based on the removal of a source of angiogenesis inhibitors and mass-related growth regulators in the tumor. However, on rare occasions (certain renal cancers), primary tumor resection is accompanied by regression of metastatic lesions. Similarly, splenectomy in some cases of lymphoma may be associated with regression of disease at remote sites. This phenomenon is attributed to the removal of a source of growth or angiogenic factors upon which the remote sites depend for growth.

PALLIATION Surgery is employed in a number of ways for supportive care: insertion of central venous catheters, diagnostic evaluation of pulmonary infiltrates, control of pleural and pericardial effusions and ascites, caval interruption for recurrent pulmonary emboli, stabilization of cancer-weakened weight-bearing bones, and control of hemorrhage, among others. Surgical bypass of gastrointestinal, urinary tract, or biliary tree obstruction can alleviate symptoms and prolong survival. Surgical procedures may provide relief of otherwise intractable pain or reverse neurologic dysfunction (cord decompression). Splenectomy may relieve symptoms and reverse hypersplenism. Intrathecal or intrahepatic therapy relies on surgical placement of appropriate infusion portals. Surgery may correct other treatment-related toxicities such as adhesions or strictures.

REHABILITATION Surgical procedures are also valuable in restoring a cancer patient to full health. Orthopedic procedures may be necessary to assure proper ambulation. Breast reconstruction can make an enormous impact on the patient's perception of successful therapy. Plastic and reconstructive surgery can correct the effects of disfiguring primary treatment.

PRINCIPLES OF RADIATION THERAPY

PHYSICAL PROPERTIES AND BIOLOGIC EFFECTS
Radiation therapy is a physical form of treatment that damages any tissue in its path. Tumor cells seem somewhat more sensitive to the lethal effects of radiation than normal tissues primarily because of differences in ability to repair sublethal DNA and other damage. In the target tissue, radiation damages DNA (usually single strand breaks) and generates free radicals from cell water that are capable of damaging cell membranes, proteins, and organelles. Radiation damage is dependent on oxygen; hypoxic cells are more resistant. Augmentation of oxygen is the basis for radiation sensitization. Sulfhydryl compounds interfere with free radical generation and may act as radiation protectors. The challenge for radiation treatment planning is to deliver the radiation to the tumor volume with as little normal tissue in the field as possible. →*Principles of radiation injury are discussed in Chap. 394.*

Therapeutic radiation is delivered in three ways: teletherapy with beams of radiation generated at a distance and aimed at the tumor within the patient, brachytherapy with encapsulated sources of radiation implanted directly into or adjacent to tumor tissues, and systemic therapy with radionuclides targeted in some fashion to a site of tumor. Teletherapy is the most commonly used form of radiation therapy.

Radiation from any source decreases in intensity as a function of the square of the distance from the source (inverse square law). Thus, if the radiation source is 5 cm above the skin surface and the tumor is 5 cm below the skin surface, the intensity of radiation in the tumor will be $5^2/10^2$, or 25% of the intensity at the skin. By contrast, if the radiation source is moved to 100 cm from the patient, the intensity of radiation in the tumor will be $100^2/105^2$, or 91% of the intensity at the skin. Teletherapy maintains intensity over a larger volume of target tissue by increasing the source-to-surface distance. In brachytherapy, the source-to-surface distance is small; thus, the effective treatment volume is small.

X-rays and *gamma rays* are the forms of radiation most commonly used to treat cancer. They are both electromagnetic, nonparticulate waves that cause the ejection of an orbital electron when absorbed. This orbital electron ejection is called *ionization*. X-rays are generated by linear accelerators; gamma rays are generated from decay of atomic nuclei in radioisotopes such as cobalt and radium. These waves behave biologically as packets of energy, called *photons*. Particulate forms of radiation are also used in certain circumstances. Electron beams have a very low tissue penetrance and are used to treat skin conditions such as mycosis fungoides. Neutron beams may be somewhat more effective than x-rays in treating salivary gland tumors. However, aside from these specialized uses, particulate forms of radiation such as neutrons, protons, and negative π mesons, which should do more tissue damage because of their higher linear energy transfer (LET) and be less dependent on oxygen, have not yet found wide applicability to cancer treatment.

A number of parameters influence the damage done to tissue by radiation. Hypoxic cells are relatively resistant. Nondividing cells are more resistant than dividing cells. In addition to these biologic parameters, physical parameters of the radiation are also crucial. The *energy* of the radiation determines its ability to penetrate tissue. Low-energy orthovoltage beams (150 to 400 kV) scatter when they strike the body, much like light diffuses when it strikes particles in the air. Such beams result in more damage to adjacent normal tissues and less radiation delivered to the tumor. Megavoltage radiation (≥ 1 MeV) has very low lateral scatter; this produces a skin-sparing effect, more homogeneous distribution of the radiation energy, and greater deposit of the energy in the tumor, or *target volume*. The tissues that the beam passes through to get to the tumor is called the *transit volume*. The maximum dose in the target volume is often the cause of complications to tissues in the transit volume, and the minimum dose in the target volume influences the likelihood of tumor recurrence. Dose homogeneity in the target volume is the goal.

Radiation is quantitated on the basis of the amount of radiation absorbed in the patient, not based upon the amount of radiation generated by the machine. A rad (radiation absorbed dose) is 100 ergs of energy per gram of tissue; a gray (Gy) is 100 rad. Radiation dose is measured by placing detectors at the body surface or calculating the dose based on radiating phantoms that resemble human form and substance. Radiation dose has three determinants: total absorbed dose, number of fractions, and time. A frequent error is to omit the number of fractions and the duration of treatment. This is analogous to saying that a runner completed a race in 20 s; without knowing how far he or she ran, the result is difficult to interpret. The time could be very good for a 200-m race or very poor for a 100-m race. Thus, a typical course of radiation therapy should be described as 4500 cGy delivered to a particular target (e.g., mediastinum) over 5 weeks in 180-cGy fractions. Most radiation treatment programs are delivered once a day, 5 days a week in 150- to 200-cGy fractions.

The killing of tumor cells in vivo by radiation is described in detail in Chap. 394. Although radiation can interfere with many cellular processes, many experts feel that a cell must undergo a double-stranded DNA break from radiation in order to be killed. The factors that influence tumor cell killing include the D_0 of the tumor (the dose required to deliver an average of one lethal hit to all the cells in a population), the D_q of the tumor (the threshold dose—a measure of the cell's ability to repair sublethal damage), hypoxia, tumor mass, growth fraction, and cell cycle time and phase (cells in late G_1 and S are more resistant). Rate of clinical response is not predictive; some cells do not die after radiation exposure until they attempt to replicate.

Compounds that incorporate into DNA and alter its stereochemistry (e.g., halogenated pyrimidines, cisplatin) augment radiation effects. Hydroxyurea, another DNA synthesis inhibitor, also potentiates radiation effects. Compounds that deplete thiols (e.g., buthionine sulfoximine) can also augment radiation effects. Hypoxia is the main factor that interferes with radiation effects.

APPLICATION TO PATIENTS Radiation therapy can be used alone or together with chemotherapy to produce cure of localized tumors and control of the primary site of disease in tumors that have disseminated. Therapy is planned based on the use of a simulator with the treatment field or fields designed to accommodate an individual patient's anatomic features. Individualized treatment planning employs lead shielding tailored to shape the field and limit the radiation exposure of normal tissue. Often the radiation is delivered from two or three different positions. Conformal three-dimensional treatment planning is permitting the delivery of higher doses of radiation to the target volume without increasing complications in the transit volume.

Radiation therapy is a component of curative therapy for a number of diseases including breast cancer, Hodgkin's disease, head and neck cancer, prostate cancer, and gynecologic cancers. Radiation therapy can also palliate disease symptoms in a variety of settings: relief of bone pain from metastatic disease, control of brain metastases, reversal of cord compression and superior vena caval obstruction, shrinkage of painful masses, and opening threatened airways. In high-risk settings, radiation therapy can prevent the development of leptomeningeal disease and brain metastases in acute leukemia and lung cancer.

Brachytherapy involves placing a sealed source of radiation into or adjacent to the tumor and withdrawing the radiation source after a period of time precisely calculated to deliver a chosen dose of radiation to the tumor. This approach is often used to treat brain tumors and cervical cancer. The difficulty with brachytherapy is the short range of radiation effects (the inverse square law) and the inability to shape the radiation to fit the target volume. Normal tissue may receive substantial exposure to the radiation, with attendant radiation enteritis or cystitis in cervix cancer or brain injury in brain tumors.

TOXICITY Though radiation therapy is most often administered to a local region, systemic effects, including fatigue, anorexia, nausea, and vomiting, may develop related in part to the volume of tissue irradiated, dose fractionation, radiation fields, and individual susceptibility. Bone is among the most radioresistant organs, radiation effects being manifested mainly in children through premature fusion of the epiphyseal growth plate. By contrast, the male testis, female ovary, and bone marrow are the most sensitive organs. Any bone marrow in a radiation field will be eradicated by therapeutic irradiation. Organs with less need for cell renewal, such as heart, skeletal muscle, and nerves, are more resistant to radiation effects. In radiation-resistant organs, the vascular endothelium is the most sensitive component. Organs with more self-renewal as a part of normal homeostasis, such as the hematopoietic system and mucosal lining of the intestinal tract, are more sensitive. Acute toxicities include mucositis, skin erythema (ulceration in severe cases), and bone marrow toxicity. Often these can be alleviated by interruption of treatment.

Chronic toxicities are more serious. Radiation of the head and neck region usually produces thyroid failure. Cataracts and retinal damage can lead to blindness. Salivary glands stop making saliva, which leads to dental carries and poor dentition. Taste and smell can be affected. Mediastinal irradiation leads to a threefold increased risk of *fatal* myocardial infarction. Other late vascular effects include chronic constrictive pericarditis, lung fibrosis, viscus stricture, spinal cord transection, and radiation enteritis. The most serious late toxicity is the development of second solid tumors in or adjacent to the radiation fields. Such tumors can develop in any organ or tissue and occur at a rate of about 1% per year beginning in the second decade after treatment. Some organs vary in susceptibility to radiation carcinogenesis. Women under age 30 experience a 100-fold or greater increase in the incidence of breast cancer after chest or mantle field radiation; women treated after age 30 have little or no increased risk of breast cancer. No data suggest that a threshold dose of therapeutic radiation exists below which the incidence of second cancers is decreased. High rates of second tumors have been documented in people who received as little as 1000 cGy.

RADIONUCLIDES AND RADIOIMMUNOTHERAPY Nuclear medicine physicians or radiation oncologists may administer radionuclides with therapeutic effects. Iodine-131 is used to treat thyroid cancer as iodine is naturally taken up preferentially by the thyroid. It emits gamma rays that destroy the normal thyroid as well as the tumor. Strontium-89 and samarium-153 are two radionuclides that are preferentially taken up in bone, particularly sites of new bone formation. Both are capable of controlling bone metastases and the pain associated with them, but the dose-limiting toxicity is myelosuppression.

Monoclonal antibodies and other ligands can be attached to radioisotopes by conjugation (for nonmetal isotopes) or by chelation (for metal isotopes), and the targeting moiety can result in the accumulation of the radionuclide preferentially in tumor. Iodine-131-labeled anti-CD20 and yttrium-90-labeled anti-CD20 are active in B cell lymphoma, and other labeled antibodies are being evaluated. Thyroid uptake of labeled iodine is blocked by cold iodine. Dose-limiting toxicity is myelosuppression.

PHOTODYNAMIC THERAPY Some chemical structures (porphyrins, phthalocyanines) are selectively taken up by cancer cells by mechanisms not fully defined. When light, usually delivered by laser, is shone on cells containing these compounds, free radicals are generated and the cells die. Hematoporphyrins and light are being used with increasing frequency to treat skin cancer; ovarian cancer; and cancers of the lung, colon, rectum, and esophagus. Palliation of recurrent locally advanced disease can sometimes be dramatic and last many months.

PRINCIPLES OF CHEMOTHERAPY

HISTORIC BACKGROUND The treatment of patients with cancer using chemicals in the hope of causing regressions of established tumors or to slow the rate of tumor growth arose by analogy to the proposition of Ehrlich that bacteria could be killed selectively by compounds acting as "magic bullets." Candidate compounds that might have selectivity for cancer cells were suggested by the marrow-toxic effects of sulfur and nitrogen mustards and led, in the 1940s, to the first notable regressions of hematopoietic tumors following use of these compounds by Gilman and colleagues. As these compounds caused covalent modification of DNA, the structure of DNA was thereby identified as a potential target for drug design efforts. Biochemical studies demonstrating the requirement of growing tumor cells for precursors of nucleic acids led to nearly contemporaneous studies by Farber of folate analogues. The cure of patients with advanced choriocarcinoma by methotrexate in the 1950s provided further impetus to define the value of chemotherapeutic agents in many different tumor types. This resulted in efforts to understand unique metabolic requirements for biosynthesis of nucelic acids and led to the design, rational for the time, of compounds that might selectively interdict DNA synthesis in proliferating cancer cells. The capacity of hormonal manipulations including oophorectomy and orchiectomy to cause regressions of breast and prostate cancers, respectively, provided a rationale for efforts to interdict various aspects of hormone function in hormone-dependent tumors. The serendipitous finding that certain poisons derived from bacteria or plants could affect normal DNA or mitotic spindle function allowed completion of the classic armamentatrium of "cancer chemotherapy agents" with proven safety and efficacy in the treatment of certain cancers.

END-POINTS OF DRUG ACTION Chemotherapy agents may be used for the treatment of active, clinically apparent cancer. Table 84-1A lists those tumors considered curable by conventionally available chemotherapeutic agents. Most commonly, chemotherapeutic agents are used to address metastatic cancers. If a tumor is localized to a single site, serious consideration of surgery or primary radiation therapy should be given, as these treatment modalities may be curative as local treatments. Chemotherapy may be employed after the failure of these modalities to eradicate a local tumor, or as part of multimodality approaches to offer primary treatment to a clinically localized tumor. In this event, it can allow *organ preservation* when given with radiation, as in larynx or other upper airway sites; or sensitize tumors to radiation when given, for example, to patients concurrently receiving radiation for lung or cervix cancer (Table 84-1B). Chemotherapy can be administered as an *adjuvant* to surgery (Table 84-1C) or radiation, a use that may have curative potential in breast, colon, or anorectal neoplasms. In this use, chemotherapy attempts to eliminate clinically unapparent tumor that may have already disseminated.

Table 84-1 Curability of Cancers with Chemotherapy

A. Advanced cancers with possible cure	**D. Cancers possibly cured with "high-dose" chemotherapy with stem cell support**
Acute lymphoid and acute myeloid leukemia (pediatric/adult)	Relapsed leukemias, lymphoid and myeloid
Hodgkin's disease (pediatric/adult)	Relapsed lymphomas, Hodgkin's and non-Hodgkin's
Lymphomas—certain types (pediatric/adult)	Chronic myeloid leukemia
Germ cell neoplasms	Multiple myeloma
Embryonal carcinoma	**E. Cancers responsive with useful palliation, but not cure, by chemotherapy**
Teratocarcinoma	Bladder carcinoma
Seminoma or dysgerminoma	Chronic myeloid leukemia
Choriocarcinoma	Hairy cell leukemia
Gestational trophoblastic neoplasia	Chronic lymphocytic leukemia
Pediatric neoplasms	Lymphoma—certain types
Wilm's tumor	Multiple myeloma
Embryonal rhabdomyocarcinoma	Gastric carcinoma
Ewing's sarcoma	Cervix carcinoma
Peripheral neuroepithelioma	Endometrial carcinoma
Neuroblastoma	Soft tissue sarcoma
Small cell lung carcinoma	Head and neck cancer
Ovarian carcinoma	Adrenocortical carcinoma
B. Advanced cancers possibly cured by chemotherapy and radiation	Islet-cell neoplasms
	Breast carcinoma
Squamous carcinoma (head and neck)	**F. Tumor poorly responsive in advanced stages to chemotherapy**
Squamous carcinoma (anus)	Pancreatic carcinoma
Breast carcinoma	Biliary-tract neoplasms
Carcinoma of the uterine cervix	Renal carcinoma
Non-small cell lung carcinoma (stage III)	Thyroid carcinoma
Small cell lung carcinoma	Carcinoma of the vulva
C. Cancers possibly cured with chemotherapy as adjuvant to surgery	Colorectal carcinoma
	Non-small cell lung carcinoma
Breast carcinoma	Prostate carcinoma
Colorectal carcinoma[a]	Melanoma
Osteogenic sarcoma	Hepatocellular carcinoma
Soft tissue sarcoma	

[a] Rectum also receives radiation therapy.

Chemotherapy can be used in *conventional dose* regimens. In general, these doses produce reversible acute side effects primarily consisting of transient myelosuppression with or without gastrointestinal toxicity (nausea), which are readily managed. *High-dose* chemotherapy regimens are predicated on the observation that the concentration-effect curve for many anticancer agents is rather steep, and increased dose can produce markedly increased therapeutic effect, although at the cost of potentially life-threatening complications that require intensive support, usually in the form of bone marrow or stem cell support from the patient (*autologous*) or from donors matched for histocompatibility loci (*allogeneic*). High-dose regimens nonetheless have definite curative potential in defined clinical settings (Table 84-1D).

Karnofsky was among the first to champion the evaluation of a chemotherapeutic agent's benefit by carefully quantitating its effect on tumor size and using these measurements to decide objectively the basis for further treatment of a particular patient or further clinical evaluation of a drug's potential. A partial response (PR) is defined conventionally as a decrease by at least 50% in a tumor's bi-dimensional area; a complete response (CR) connotes disappearance of all tumor; progression of disease signifies increase by >25% from baseline or best response; and "stable" disease fits into none of the above categories.

If cure is not possible, chemotherapy may be undertaken with the goal of palliating some aspect of the tumor's effect on the host. Common tumors that may be meaningfully addressed with palliative intent

are listed in Table 84-1E. Usually tumor-related symptoms may manifest as pain, weight loss, or some local symptom related to the tumor's effect on normal structures. Patients treated with palliative intent should be aware of their diagnosis and the limitations of the proposed treatment, have access to suitable palliative strategies in the event that no treatment is elected, and have a suitable "performance status" [according to assessment algorithms such as the one developed by Karnofsky or by the Eastern Cooperative Oncology Group (ECOG)]. ECOG performance status 0 (PS0) patients are without symptoms; PS1 patients have mild symptoms not requiring treatment; PS2, symptoms requiring some treatment; PS3, disabling symptoms, but allowing ambulation for >50% of the day; PS4, ambulation <50% of the day. Only PS0 to PS2 patients are generally considered suitable for palliative (noncurative) treatment. If there is curative potential, even poor performance status patients may be treated, but their prognosis is usually inferior to those of good performance patients treated with similar regimens.

PATH FOR NEW DRUG DISCOVERY AND DEVELOPMENT The usefulness of any drug is governed by the extent to which a given dose causes a useful result (therapeutic effect; in the case of anticancer agents, toxicity to tumor cells) as opposed to a toxic effect. The therapeutic index is the degree of separation between toxic and therapeutic doses. Really useful drugs have large therapeutic indices, and this usually occurs when the drug target is expressed in the disease-causing compartment as opposed to the normal compartment. Classically, selective toxicity of an agent for an organ is governed by the expression of an agent's target; or differential accumulation into or elimination from compartments where toxicity is experienced or ameliorated, respectively. Current antineoplastic agents have the unfortunate property that their targets are present in both normal and tumor tissues. In the main they therefore have relatively narrow therapeutic indices.

Agents with promise for the treatment of cancer have in the past been detected empirically through screening for antiproliferative effects in animal or human tumors in rodent hosts or through inhibition of tumor cells growing in tissue culture. An optimal schedule for demonstrating antitumor activity in animals is defined in further preclinical studies, as is the optimal drug formulation for a given route and schedule. Safety testing in two species on an analogous schedule of administration defines the starting dose for a phase I trial in humans, where escalating doses of the drug are given until reversible toxicity is observed. *Dose-limiting toxicity* (DLT) defines a dose that conveys greater toxicity than would be acceptable in routine practice, allowing definition of a *maximal tolerated dose* (MTD). The occurrence of toxicity is correlated if possible with plasma drug concentrations. The MTD or a dose just lower than the MTD is usually the dose suitable for phase II trials, where a fixed dose is administered to a relatively homogeneous set of patients in an effort to define whether the drug causes regression of tumors. An "active" agent conventionally has partial response rates of at least 20 to 25% with reversible non-life-threatening side effects, and it may then be suitable for study in phase III trials to assess efficacy in comparison to standard or no therapy. Response is but the most immediate indicator of drug effect. To be clinically valuable, responses must translate into effects on *overall survival* or at least *time to progression* as important indicators of an ultimately useful drug. More recently, active efforts to quantitate effects of anticancer agents on *quality of life* as an important outcome are being developed. Cancer drug clinical trials conventionally use a toxicity grading scale where grade I toxicities do not require treatment; grade II often require symptomatic treatment but are not life-threatening; grade III toxicities are potentially life-threatening if untreated; grade IV toxicities are actually life-threatening; and grade V toxicities ultimately lead to patient death.

The process of cancer drug development is likely to evolve in significant ways in the near future as (1) the molecular analysis of human tumors defines more precisely the molecular targets that can be the focus of drug discovery efforts, and (2) clinical trials are undertaken only after means of assessing the behavior of the drug in relation to its target have been developed. The basis for optimism and anticipated change in clinical trials methodology extends from emerging understanding of the basis for cancer incidence and progression. Cancer arises from genetic lesions that cause an excess of cell growth or division, with inadequate cell death (Chap. 82). In addition, failure of cellular differentiation results in altered cellular position and capacity to proliferate while cut off from normal cell regulatory signals. An overall schema for understanding cancer progression can be seen in Fig. 84-2. Normally, cells in a differentiated state are stimulated to enter the cell cycle from a quiescent state, or "G0," or continue after completion of a prior cell division cycle in response to environmental cues including growth factor and hormonal signals. Cells progress through G1 and enter S phase after passing through "checkpoints," which are biochemically regulated transition points, to assure that the genome is ready for replication. One important checkpoint is mediated by the p53 tumor-suppressor gene product, acting through its upregulation of the p21^{WAF1} inhibitor of cyclin-dependent kinase (CDK) function, acting on CDKs 4 or 6. These molecules can also be inhibited by the p16^{INK4A} and p27^{KIP1} CDK inhibitors and, in turn, are activated by cyclins of the D family (which appear during G1) and the proper sequence of regulatory phosphorylations. Activated CDKs 4 or 6 phosphorylate and thus inactivate the product of the retinoblastoma susceptibility gene, pRb, which in its nonphosphorylated state complexes with transcription factors of the E2F family. Phosphorylated pRb re-

leases E2Fs, which activate genes important in completing DNA replication during S phase, progression through which is promoted by CDK2 acting in concert with cylins A and E. During G2, another checkpoint occurs, in which the cell assures the completion of correct DNA synthesis. Cells then progress into M phase under the influence of CDK1 and cyclin B. Cells may then go on to a subsequent division cycle or enter into a quiescent, differentiated state.

Also shown in Fig. 84-2 are the sites of action of protooncogenes, regulators of cellular proliferation that, in an active state, promote cell growth, and whose deregulation produces oncogenes, originally discovered as the genes encoded by tumor-forming viruses in animals. Oncogenes can be divided into two families: (1) those that act in the cytoplasm to disrupt normal growth factor–related signaling, including *ras*, *raf*, and the tyrosine kinases of the *src* and *erb*B or *sis* families; and (2) nuclear oncogenes, including *jun*, *fos*, *myc*, and *myb*, that act to alter transcriptional control of cassettes of genes. In contrast, tumor-suppressor genes, including p53 and pRb, act as cellular "brakes" whose normal function is to inhibit or prevent unregulated cellular growth. The capacity to divide indefinitely is provided by activation of *telomerase*, which allows continued replication of chromosomes by addressing the unique need of chromosome ends to be continually renewed to a proper length to allow normal mitosis. The capacity to invade and metastasize is conveyed by elaboration of *matrix metalloproteases* and *plasminogen activators* and the capacity to recruit host stromal cells at the site of invasion through tumor-induced *angiogenesis*.

As will become apparent below, currently used drugs for the treatment of cancer focus principally on the proximate biochemistry of nucleic acid and mitotic spindle structure or function. Drugs of the future may seek to replace lost function of tumor-suppressor genes; counter the action of activated oncogenes; influence the capacity of cells to die; prevent normal chromosomal end replication; actually infect cells with viruses designed to replicate in the milieu of the cancer but not the normal cell; cause differentiation of cells with exit from the cell cycle by activating the appropriate genes; and utilize immunologic strategies, including antibodies and engineered cells to be directed at novel proteins expressed on the surface of cancer cells.

BIOLOGIC BASIS FOR CANCER CHEMOTHERAPY
The classic view of how cancer chemotherapeutic agents cause regressions of tumors focused on models such as the L1210 murine leukemia system, where cancer cells grow exponentially after inoculation into the peritoneal cavity of an isogenic mouse. The interaction of drug with its biochemical target in the cancer cell was proposed to result in "unbalanced growth" that was not sustainable and therefore resulted in cell death, directly as a result of interacting with the drug's proximal target. Agents could be categorized (Fig. 84-3) as cell cycle–active, phase-specific (e.g., antimetabolites, purines, and pyrimidines in S phase; vinca alkaloids in M), and phase-nonspecific agents (e.g., alkylators, and antitumor antibiotics including the anthracyclines, actinomycin, and mitomycin), which can injure DNA at any phase of the cell cycle but appear to then block in G2 before cell division at a checkpoint in the cell cycle. Cells arrested at a checkpoint may repair DNA lesions. Checkpoints have been defined at the G1 to S transition, mediated by the tumor-suppressor gene p53 (giving rise to the characterization of p53 as a "guardian of the genome"); at the G2 to M transition, mediated by the *chk1* kinase influencing the function of CDK1; and during M phase, to ensure the integrity of the mitotic spindle. The importance of the concept of checkpoints extends from the hypothesis that repair of chemotherapy-mediated damage can occur while cells are stopped at a checkpoint; therefore, manipulation of checkpoint function emerges as an important basis of affecting resistance to chemotherapeutic agents.

Resistance to drugs was postulated to arise either from cells not being in the appropriate phase of the cell cycle or from decreased uptake, increased efflux, metabolism of the drug, or alteration of the target, e.g., by mutation or overexpression. Indeed, the *p170PGP*

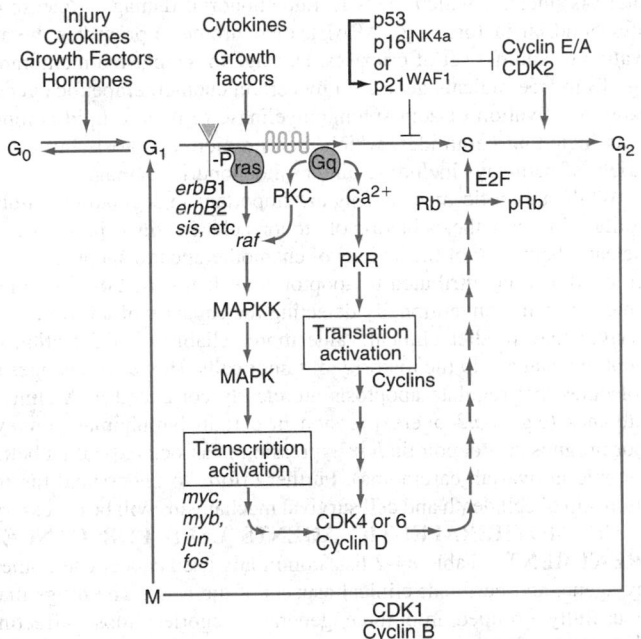

FIGURE 84-2 Basis for neoplastic growth and progression. Normally cells are stimulated to enter a proliferating state through the action of growth factors, positional signals, or cytokines. Cells enter G1 under the influence of normal signaling pathways including tyrosine kinase receptors coupled to ras protooncogenes or seven-transmembrane receptors coupled through heterotrimeric guanine nucleotide binding (G) proteins, especially G$_q$ linked to calcium- and lipid-mediated signaling pathways through protein kinase C (PKC). Cells activate transcription and translation of key regulatory molecules such as the cyclins, which activate cyclin-dependent kinases (CDKs) 4 or 6. Phosphorylation of the retinoblastoma susceptibility protein (pRb) causes release of E2F transcription factors to an active state, promoting the transcription of multiple genes allowing progression through S phase, where DNA is replicated. Tumor cells possess activated oncogenes such as *erb*B1, *erb*B2, and *sis* or mutated *ras* gene products that are tonically activated, thus driving proliferation autonomously. *Raf* and the mitogen-activated kinases, MAPKK and MAPK, amplify the growth signal in a kinase cascade. "Brakes" to cell cycle progression include the p53-mediated G1 to S phase checkpoint, mediated by the CDK inhibitors p16INK4a and p21WAF1. Progression through S phase is also promoted by CDK2 acting in concert with cyclins E and A, and initiation of cell division is governed by the action of CDK1 acting in concert with cyclin B.

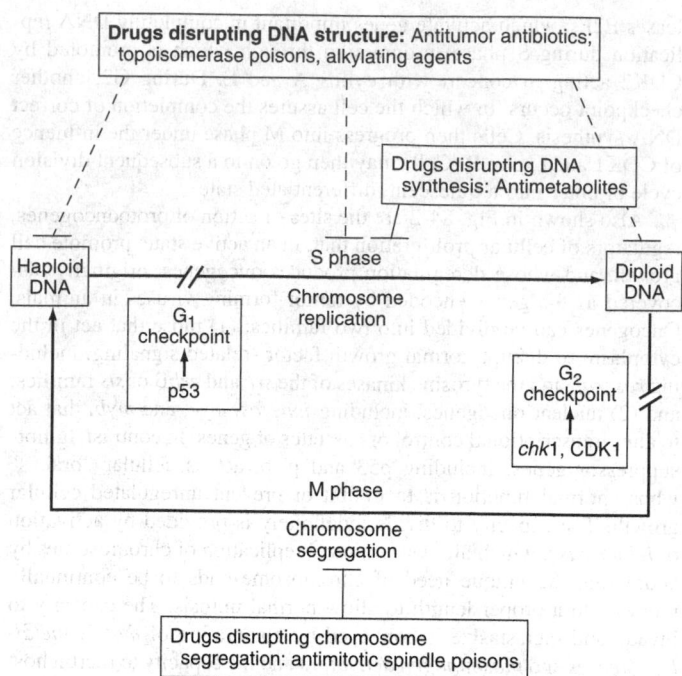

FIGURE 84-3　Location of drug action in the cell cycle. Cancer chemotherapy agents can be broadly described as phase-specific agents acting in S (antimetabolites) and M (spindle poisons) phase, respectively, and phase-nonspecific agents that injure their targets throughout the cycle but cause arrest of cell cycle progression at "checkpoints." The G1 checkpoint is mediated through p53 acting on CDKs 4,6, and 2, and the G2 checkpoint is mediated in part by the *chk1* kinase acting on CDK1.

(p170 P-glycoprotein; *mdr* gene product) was recognized from experiments with cells growing in tissue culture as mediating the efflux of chemotherapeutic agents in resistant cells. Certain neoplasms, particularly hematopoietic tumors, have an adverse prognosis if they express high levels of p170PGP, and modulation of this protein's function has been attempted by a variety of strategies.

Combinations of agents were proposed to afford the opportunity to affect many different targets or portions of the cell cycle at once, particularly if the toxic effects for the host of the different components of the combination were distinct. Combinations of agents were actually more effective in animal model systems than single agents, particularly if the tumor cell inoculum was high. This thinking led to the design of "combination chemotherapy" regimens, where drugs acting by different mechanisms (e.g., an alkylating agent plus an antimetabolite plus a mitotic spindle blocker) were combined. Particular combinations were chosen to emphasize drugs whose individual toxicities to the host were, if possible, distinct.

This view of cancer drug action is grossly oversimplified. Most tumors do not grow in an exponential pattern but rather follow Gompertzian kinetics, where the rate of tumor growth decreases as tumor mass increases (Fig. 84-1). Thus, a tumor has quiescent, differentiated compartments; proliferating compartments; and both well-vascularized and necrotic regions. Also, cell death is itself now understood to be a closely regulated process. *Necrosis* refers to cell death induced, for example, by physical damage with the hallmarks of cell swelling and membrane disruption. *Apoptosis*, or programmed cell death, refers to a highly ordered process whereby cells respond to defined stimuli by dying, and it recapitulates the necessary cell death observed during the ontogeny of the organism. *Anoikis* refers to death of epithelial cells after removal from the normal milieu of substrate, particularly from cell-to-cell contact. Cancer chemotherapeutic agents can cause both necrosis and apoptosis. Apoptosis is characterized by chromatin condensation (giving rise to "apoptotic bodies"); cell shrinkage; and, in

living animals, phagocytosis by surrounding stromal cells without evidence of inflammation. This process is regulated either by signal transduction systems that promote a cell's demise after a certain level of insult is achieved or in response to specific cell-surface receptors that mediate cell death signals. Modulation of apoptosis by manipulation of signal transduction pathways has emerged as a basis for understanding the actions of currently used drugs and designing new strategies to improve their use.

The current view envisions that the interaction of a chemotherapeutic drug with its target causes or is itself a signal that initiates a "cascade" of signaling steps to trigger an "execution phase" where proteases, nucleases, and endogenous regulators of the cell death pathway are activated. Effective cancer chemotherapeutic agents are efficient activators of apoptosis through signal transduction pathways (Fig. 84-4). For example, in the cytokine-mediated pathway, exogenous ligands such as the Fas ligand (FasL) bind to cell-surface receptors (CD95; Fas), or tumor necrosis factor (TNF) or its homologue Apo2L binds to its cognate receptors and directly recruits accessory molecules to activate a protease cascade (utilizing members of the caspase family of *cysteine asp*artyl prote*ases*), resulting in apoptosis. In a second pathway, growth factor deprivation elicits poorly defined signals that result in protease activation. Chemotherapeutic agents create molecular lesions (in DNA or cellular membranes) as a consequence of combining with their respective molecular targets. These lesions are sensed by a cellular "damage sensor," whose molecular nature is unclear, which leads to mitochondrial damage. Release of mitochondrial factors (e.g., APAF1, cytochrome c) promotes the activation of another set of caspases. Damage to the plasma membrane, e.g., from free radicals generated by certain chemotherapeutic agents, leads to activation of acid sphingomyelinase to release lipid components including ceramides, which then promote apoptosis through a variety of pathways including direct mitochondrial damage.

While apoptotic mechanisms are important in regulating cellular proliferation and the behavior of tumor cells in vitro, in vivo it is unclear whether all of the actions of chemotherapeutic agents to cause cell death can be attributed to apoptotic mechanisms. Loss of clonogenic survival (conventionally detecting the capacity of a few cells to survive) may predict clinical value more reliably than detection of apoptotic changes in the majority of tumor cells. However, changes in molecules that regulate apoptosis are clearly correlated with clinical outcomes (e.g., *bcl2* overexpression in certain lymphomas conveys poor prognosis; proapototic *bax* expression is associated with a better outcome in ovarian carcinoma). Further efforts to understand the relationship of cell death and cell survival mechanisms will be necessary.

CHEMOTHERAPEUTIC AGENTS USED FOR CANCER TREATMENT　Table 84-2 lists commonly used cancer chemotherapy agents and pertinent clinical aspects of their use. The drugs may be usefully grouped into three general categories: those affecting DNA, those affecting microtubules, and those acting at hormone-like receptors.

Direct DNA-Interactive Agents • *Formation of covalent DNA adducts*　Alkylating agents as a class break down, either spontaneously or after normal organ or tumor cell metabolism, to reactive intermediates that covalently modify bases in DNA. This leads to cross-linkage of DNA strands or the appearance of breaks in DNA as a result of repair efforts. "Broken" or cross-linked DNA is intrinsically unable to complete normal replication or cell division; in addition, it is a potent activator of cell cycle checkpoints and signaling pathways that can activate apoptosis. As a class, alkylating agents share similar toxicities, including myelosuppression, alopecia, gonadal dysfunction, mucositis, and pulmonary fibrosis. They differ greatly in a spectrum of normal organ toxicities.

Nitrogen mustard (mechlorethamine) is the prototypic agent of this class, decomposing rapidly in aqueous solution to yield potentially a bifunctional carbonium ion. It must be administered shortly after preparation into a rapidly flowing intravenous line. It is powerful vesicant, and infiltration may be symptomatically ameliorated by infiltration of the affected site with 1/6 *M* thiosulfate. Even without infiltration, aseptic thrombophlebitis is frequent. It can be used topically as a dilute solution in cutaneous lymphomas, with a notable incidence of hypersensitivity reactions. It causes moderate nausea after intravenous administration.

Cyclophosphamide is inactive unless metabolized by the liver to 4-hydroxyl-cyclophosphamide, which decomposes into alkylating species, as well as to chloroacetaldehyde and acrolein. The latter causes chemical cystitis, and therefore excellent hydration must be maintained while using cyclophosphamide. If severe, the cystitis may be effectively treated by mercaptoethanesulfonate (MESNA). Liver disease impairs drug activation. Sporadic interstitial pneumonitis leading to pulmonary fibrosis can accompany the use of cyclophosphamide, and high doses used in conditioning regimens for bone marrow transplant can cause cardiac dysfunction. Ifosfamide is a cyclophosphamide analogue also activated in the liver, but more slowly, and it requires mandatory coadministration of MESNA to prevent bladder injury. Central nervous system (CNS) effects, including somnolence, confusion, and psychosis, can follow ifosfamide use, and the incidence appears related to low body surface area or the presence of nephrectomy.

There are several less commonly used alkylating agents. Chlorambucil causes predictable myelosuppression, azospermia, nausea, and pulmonary side effects. Busulfan can cause profound myelosuppression, alopecia, and pulmonary toxicity but is relatively "lymphocyte sparing." Its routine use in treatment of chronic myeloid leukemia has been curtailed in favor of hydroxyurea or interferon (IFN), but it still is employed in marrow transplant preparation regimens. Melphalan shows variable oral bioavailability and undergoes extensive binding to albumin and α_1-acidic glycoprotein. Mucositis appears more prominently.

Nitrosoureas break down to carbamoylating species that not only cause a distinct pattern of DNA base pair–directed toxicity but also can covalently modify proteins. They share the feature of causing relatively delayed bone marrow toxicity, which can be cumulative and long-lasting. Streptozotocin is unique in that its glucose-like structure conveys specific toxicity to the islet cells of the pancreas (for whose derivative tumor types it is prominently indicated) as well as causing renal toxicity in the form of Fanconi's syndrome, including amino aciduria, glycosuria, and renal tubular acidosis. Methyl CCNU (lomustine) causes direct glomerular as well as tubular damage, cumulatively related to dose and time of exposure.

Procarbazine is metabolized in the liver and possibly in tumor cells to yield a variety of free radical and alkylating species. In addition to myelosuppression, it causes hypnotic and other CNS effects, including vivid nightmares. It can cause a disulfiram-like syndrome on ingestion of ethanol. Hexamethylmelamine and thiotepa can chemically give rise to alkylating species, although the nature of the DNA damage has not been well characterized in either case. Thiotepa can be used for intrathecal treatment of neoplastic meningitis. Dacarbazine (DTIC) is activated in the liver to yield the highly reactive methyl diazonium cation. It causes only modest myelosuppression from 21 to 25 days after a dose but causes prominent nausea on day 1.

Cisplatin was discovered fortuitously by observing that bacteria present in electrolysis solutions could not divide. Only the cis diamine configuration is active as an antitumor agent. It is hypothesized that in the intracellular environment, a chloride is lost from each position, being replaced by a water molecule. The resulting positively charged species is an efficient bifunctional interactor with DNA, forming Pt-base cross-links. Cisplatin requires administration with adequate hydration, including forced diuresis with mannitol to prevent kidney damage; even with the use of hydration, gradual decrease in kidney function is common. Hypomagnesemia frequently attends cisplatin use and can lead to hypocalcemia and symptomatic tetany. Other common toxicities include neurotoxocity with "stocking and glove" sensorimotor neuropathy. Hearing loss occurs in 50% of patients treated with

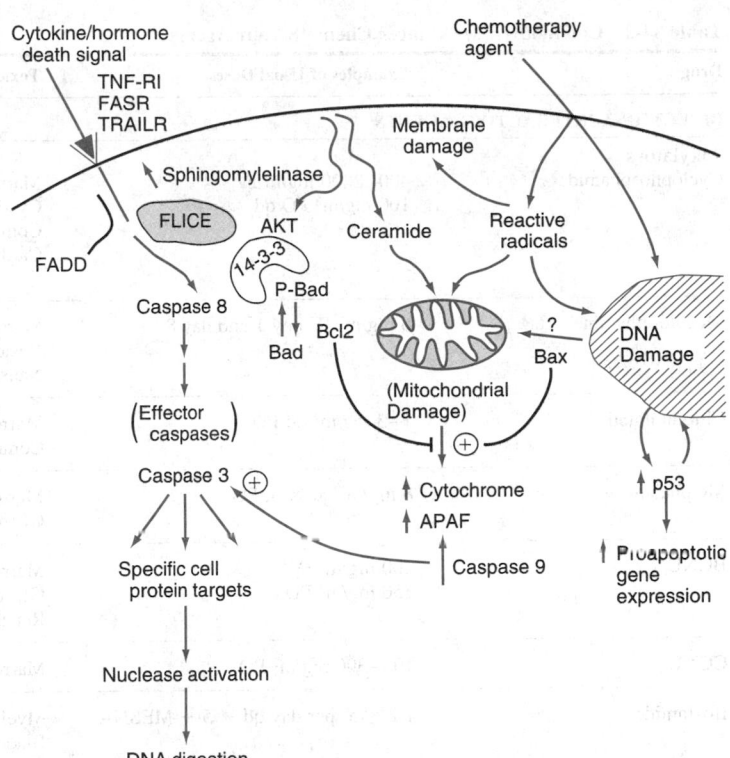

FIGURE 84-4 Integration of cell death responses. Cell death through an *apoptotic* mechanism requires active participation of the cell. In response to hormonal or cytokine death signals, receptors activate "upstream" cysteine aspartyl proteases (caspases), which then directly digest cytoplasmic and nuclear proteins, resulting in activation of "downstream" caspases; these cause activation of nucleases resulting in the characteristic DNA fragmentation that is a hallmark of apoptosis. Chemotherapy agents that create lesions in DNA seem to activate aspects of this process through a pathway that appears to result in damage to mitochondria, perhaps by activating the transcription of genes whose products can produce or modulate the toxicity of free radicals. In addition, membrane damage with activation of sphingomyelinases results in the production of ceramides that can have a direct action at mitochondria. The antiapoptotic protein *bcl2* attenuates mitochondrial toxicity, while proapoptotic gene products such as *bax* antagonize the action of *bcl2*. Damaged mitochondria release cytochrome C and "apoptosis activating factor," which can directly activate caspase 9, resulting in propagation of a direct signal to other downstream caspases through protease activation. An additional proapoptotic stimulus is the *bad* protein, which can heterodimerize with *bcl2* gene family members to antagonize apoptosis. Importantly, though, *bad* protein function can be retarded by its sequestration as phospho-*bad* through the 14-3-3 adapter proteins. The phosphorylation of *bad* is mediated by the action of the AKT kinase in a way that defines how growth factors that activate this kinase can retard apoptosis and promote cell survival.

conventional doses. Cisplatin is intensely emetogenic, requiring prophylactic antinausea agents. Myelosuppression is less evident than with other alkylating agents. Chronic vascular toxicity is a more unusual toxic phenomena, including Raynaud's syndrome and coronary artery disease. In an effort to obviate these toxicities, carboplatin was developed and clearly displays less nephro-, oto- and neurotoxicity. However, myelosuppression is more frequent, and as the drug is exclusively cleared through the kidney, adjustment of dose for creatinine clearance must be accomplished through use of various dosing nomograms.

Antitumor antibiotics and topoisomerase poisons *Antitumor antibiotics* are substances produced by bacteria that in nature appear to provide chemical defense against other hostile microorganisms. As a class they bind to DNA directly and can frequently undergo electron transfer reactions to generate free radicals in close proximity to DNA, leading to DNA damage in the form of single strand breaks or cross-links. *Topoisomerase poisons* include natural products or semi-synthetic species derived ultimately from plants, and they modify enzymes

Table 84-2 Commonly Used Cancer Chemotherapy Agents

Drug	Examples of Usual Doses	Toxicity	Interactions, Issues
DIRECT DNA-INTERACTING AGENTS			
Alkylators			
Cyclophosphamide	400–2000 mg/m²IV 100 mg/m² PO qd	Marrow (relative platelet sparing) Cystitis Common alkylator[a] Cardiac (high dose)	Liver metabolism required to activate to phosphoramide mustard + acrolein MESNA protects against "high-dose" bladder damage
Mechlorethamine	6 mg/m² IV day 1 and day 8	Marrow Vesicant Nausea	Topical use in cutaneous lymphoma
Chlorambucil	1–3 mg/m² qd PO	Marrow Common alkylator[a]	
Melphalan	8 mg/m² qd × 5, PO	Marrow (delayed nadir) GI (high dose)	Decreased renal function delays clearance
BCNU	200 mg/m² IV 150 mg/m² PO	Marrow (delayed nadir) GI, liver (high dose) Renal	
CCNU	100–300 mg/m² PO	Marrow (delayed nadir)	
Ifosfamide	1.2 g/m² per day qd × 5 + MESNA	Myelosuppressive Bladder Neurologic Metabolic acidosis Neuropathy	Isomeric analogue of cyclophosphamide More lipid soluble Greater activity vs testicular neoplasms and sarcomas Must use MESNA
Procarbazine	100 mg/m² per day qd ×14	Marrow Nausea Neurologic Common alkylator[a]	Liver and tissue metabolism required Disulfiran-like effect with ethanol Acts as MAOI HBP after tyrosinase-rich foods
DTIC	375 mg/m² IV day 1 & day 15	Marrow Nausea Flulike	Metabolic activation
Hexamethylmelamine	260 mg/m² per day qd ×14–21 as 4 divided oral doses	Nausea Neurologic (mood swing) Neuropathy Marrow (less)	Liver activation Barbiturates enchance/cimetidine diminishes
Cisplatin	20 mg/m² qd ×5 IV 1 q3–4 weeks or 100–200 mg/m²/dose IV q3–4 weeks	Nausea Neuropathy Auditory Marrow platelets > WBCs Renal Mg²⁺, Ca²⁺	Maintain high urine flow; osmotic diuresis, monitor intake/output K⁺, Mg²⁺ Emetogenic—prophylaxis needed Full dose if CrCl > 60 mL/min and tolerate fluid push
Carboplatin	365 mg/m² IV q3–4 weeks as adjusted for CrCl	Marrow platelets > WBCs Nausea Renal (high dose)	Reduce dose according to CrCl: AUC = dose/(CrCl + 25) to AUC of 5–7 mg/mL per min
Antitumor antibiotics			
Bleomycin	15–25 mg/d qd ×5 IV bolus or continuous IV	Pulmonary Skin effects Raynaud's Hypersensitivity	Inactivate by bleomycin hydrolase (decreased in lung/skin) O₂ enhances pulmonary toxicity Cisplatin-induced decrease in CrCl may increase skin/lung toxicity Reduce dose if CrCl < 60 mL/min
Actinomycin D	10–15 μg/kg per day qd ×5 IV bolus	Marrow Nausea Mucositis Vesicant Alopecia	Radiation recall

(continued)

Table 84-2—(continued)

Drug	Examples of Usual Doses	Toxicity	Interactions, Issues
Mithramycin	15–20 μg/kg qd ×4–7 (hypercal-cemia) or 50 μg/kg qod ×3–8 (antineo-plastic)	Marrow Liver Renal Mucositis Hypocalcemia Nausea Vesicant	Acute hemorrhagic syndrome
Mitomycin C	6–10 mg/m² q6 weeks	Marrow Vesicant Hemolytic-uremic syndrome Lung CV—heart failure	Treat superficial bladder cancers by intravesical infusion Delayed marrow toxicity Cumulative marrow toxicity
Etoposide (VP16-213)	100–150 mg/m² IV qd ×3–5d or 50 mg/m² PO qd ×21d or up to 1500 mg/m²/of dose (high dose with stem cell support)	Marrow (WBCs > platelet) Alopecia Hypotension Hypersensitivity (rapid IV) Nausea Mucositis (high dose)	Hepatic metabolism—renal 30% Reduce doses with renal failure Schedule-dependant (5 day better than 1 day) Late leukemogenic Accentuate antimetabolite action
Teniposide (VM-26)	150–200 mg/m² twice per week for 4 weeks	Marrow Alopecia	
Amsacrine	100–150 mg/m² IV qd ×5	Marrow Mucositis Nausea CV—arrhythmia (avoid hypokale-mia)	Decrease dose by 30% if liver or re-nal failure
Topotecan	20 mg/m² IV q3–4 weeks over 30 min or 1.5–3 mg/m² q3–4 weeks over 24 h or 0.5 mg/m² per day over 21 days	Marrow Mucositis Nausea Mild alopecia	Reduce dose with renal failure No liver toxicity
Irinotecan (CPT II)	100–150 mg/m² IV over 90 min q3–4 weeks or 30 mg/m² per day over 120 h	Diarrhea: "early onset" with cramp-ing, flushing, vomiting; "late onset" after several doses Marrow Alopecia Nausea Vomiting Pulmonary	Prodrug requires enzymatic clear-ance to active drug "SN 38" "Early diarrhea" likely due to biliary excretion Late diarrhea, use "high-dose" loper-amide (2 mg q2–4 h)
Doxorubicin and daunorubicin	45–60 mg/m² dose q3–4 weeks or 10–30 mg/m² dose q week or continuous-infusion regimen	Marrow Mucositis Alopecia Cardiovascular acute/chronic Vesicant	Heparin aggregate; coadministration increases clearance Tylenol, BCNU increase liver tox-icity Radiation recall
Idarubicin	10–15 mg/m² IV q 3 weeks or 10 mg/m² IV qd ×3	Marrow Cardiac (less than doxorubicin)	None established
Epirubicin	150 mg/m² IV q3 weeks	Marrow Cardiac	None established
Mitoxantrone	12 mg/m² qd ×3 or 12–14 mg/m² q3 weeks	Marrow Cardiac (less than doxorubicin) Vesicant (mild) Blue urine, sclerae, nails	Interacts with heparin Less alopecia, nausea than doxoru-bicin Radiation recall

INDIRECT DNA-INTERACTING AGENTS

Antimetabolites

| Deoxycoformycin | 4 mg/m² IV every other week | Nausea
 Immunosuppression
 Neurologic
 Renal | Excretes in urine
 Reduce dose for renal failure
 Inhibits adenosine deaminase |

(continued)

Table 84-2 Commonly Used Cancer Chemotherapy Agents—*(continued)*

Drug	Examples of Usual Doses	Toxicity	Interactions, Issues
6-Mercaptopurine	75 mg/m² PO *or* up 500 mg/m² PO (high dose)	Marrow Liver Nausea	Variable bioavailability Metabolize by xanthine oxidase Decrease dose with allopurinol Increased toxicity with thiopurine methyltransferase deficiency

6-Thioguanine	2–3 mg/kg per day for up to 3–4
	  weeks
		Marrow
		Liver
		Nausea
			Variable bioavailability
			Increased toxicity with thiopurine
			  methyltransferase deficiency

Azathioprine	1–5 mg/kg per day	Marrow
		Nausea
		Liver
			Metabolizes to 6-MP, therefore re-
			  duce dose with allopurinol
			Increased toxicity with thiopurine
			  methyltransferase deficiency

2-Chlorodeoxyadenosine	0.09 mg/kg per day qd ×7 as contin- uous infusion	Marrow Renal Fever	Notable use in hairy cell leukemia
Hydroxyurea	20–50 mg/kg (lean body weight) PO qd *or* 1–3 g/d	Marrow Nausea Mucositis Skin changes Rare renal, liver, lung, CNS	Decrease dose with renal failure Augments antimetabolite effect
Methotrexate	15–30 mg PO or IM qd ×3–5 *or* 30 mg IV days 1 and 8 *or* 1.5–12 g/m² per day (with leu- covorin)	Marrow Liver/lung Renal tubular Mucositis	Rescue with leucovorin Excreted in urine Decrease dose in renal failure NSAIDs increase renal toxicity
5-Fluorouracil	375 mg/m² IV qd ×5 *or* 600 mg/m² IV days 1 and 8	Marrow Mucositis Neurologic Skin changes	Toxicity enhanced by leucovorin Dihydropyrimidine dehydrogenase deficiency increases toxicity Metabolizes in tissues

Cytosine arabinoside	100 mg/m² per day qd ×7 by con-
	  tinuous infusion
	or 1–3 g/m² dose IV bolus
		Marrow
		Mucositis
		Neurologic (high dose)
		Conjunctivitis (high dose)
		Noncardiogenic pulmonary edema
			Enhances activity of alkylating
			  agents
			Metabolizes in tissues by deamina-
			  tion

Azacytidine	750 mg/m² per week
	or 150–200 mg/m² per day ×5–10
	  (bolus) or (continuous IV)
		Marrow
		Nausea
		Liver
		Neurologic
		Myalgia
			Use limited to leukemia
			Altered methylation of DNA alters
			  gene expression

Gemcitabine	1000 mg/m² IV weekly ×7	Marrow Nausea Hepatic Fever/"flu syndrome"	

Fludarabine phosphate	25 mg/m² IV qd ×5	Marrow
		Neurologic
		Lung
			Dose reduction with renal failure
			Metabolized to F-ara converted to F-
			  ara ATP in cells by deoxycytidine
			  kinase

Asparaginase	25,000 IU/m² q3–4 weeks
	or 6000 IU/m² per day qod for 3–4
	  weeks
	or 1000–2000 IU/m² for 10–20
	  days
		Protein synthesis
		Clotting factors
		Glucose
		Albumin
		Hypersensitivity
		CNS
		Pancreatitis
		Hepatic
			Blocks methotrexate action

(continued)

Table 84-2—(continued)

Drug	Examples of Usual Doses	Toxicity	Interactions, Issues
Antimitotic agents			

Vincristine	1–1.4 mg/m² per week	Vesicant
		Marrow
		Neurologic
		GI: ileus/constipation; bladder hypo-
		  toxicity; SIADH
		Cardiovascular
			Hepatic clearance
			Dose reduction for bilirubin
			  >1.5 mg/dL
			Prophylactic bowel regimen

Vinblastine	6–8 mg/m² per week	Vesicant Marrow Neurologic (less common but similar spectrum to other vincas) Hypertension Raynaud's	Hepatic clearance Dose reduction as with vincristine
Vinorelbine	15–30 mg/m² per week	Vesicant Marrow Allergic/broncospasm (immediate) Dyspnea/cough (subacute) Neurologic (less prominent but simi- lar spectrum to other vincas)	Hepatic clearance

Paclitaxel	135–175 mg/m² per 24-h infusion
	or 175 mg/m² per 3-h infusion
	or 140 mg/m² per 96-h infusion
	or 250 mg/m² per 24-h infusion plus
	  G-CSF
		Hypersensitivity
		Marrow
		Mucositis
		Alopecia
		Sensory neuropathy
		CV conduction disturbance
		Nausea—infrequent
			Premedicate with steroids, H_1 and H_2
			  blockers
			Hepatic clearance
			Dose reduction as with vincas

Docetaxel	100 mg/m² per 1-h infusion q3
	  weeks
		Hypersensitivity
		Fluid retention syndrome
		Marrow
		Dermatologic
		Sensory neuropathy
		Nausea infrequent
		Some stomatitis
			Premedicate with steroids, H_1 and H_2
			  blockers

Estramustine phosphate	14 mg/kg per day in 3–4 divided doses with water >2 h after meals Avoid Ca^{2+}-rich foods	Nausea Vomiting Diarrhea CHF Thrombosis Gynecomastia	

[a] Common alkylator: alopecia, pulmonary, infertility, plus teratogenesis.
NOTE: AUC, area under the curve; CHF, congestive heart failure; CNS, central nervous system; CrCl, creatinine clearance; CV, cardiovascular; G-CSF, granulocyte colony stimulating factor; GI, gastrointestinal; HBP, high blood pressure; MAOI, monoamine oxidase inhibitors; MESNA, mercaptoethanesulfonate; 6-MP, 6-mercaptopurine; NSAIDs, nonsteroidal anti-inflammatory drugs; SIADH, syndrome of inappropriate antidiuretic hormone; WBCs, white blood cells.

that regulate the capacity of DNA to unwind to allow normal replication or transcription.

Doxorubicin is the most widely active and frequently used antineoplastic agent. It can intercalate into DNA, thereby altering DNA structure, replication, and topoisomerase function. It can also undergo redox cycling by accepting electrons into its quinone ring system. It causes predictable myelosuppression, alopecia, nausea, and mucositis. In addition, it causes acute cardiotoxicity in the form of atrial and ventricular dysrhythmias, but these are rarely of clinical significance. In contrast, cumulative doses >550 mg/m² are associated with a 10% incidence of chronic cardiomyopathy. The incidence of cardiomyopathy appears to be related to schedule (peak serum concentration), with low dose, frequent treatment, or continuous infusions better tolerated than intermittent higher dose exposures. Radiation recall or interaction with radiation to cause local site complications is frequent. The drug is a powerful vesicant, with necrosis of tissue apparent 4 to 7 days after an extravasation; therefore it should be administered into a rapidly flowing intravenous line. The drug is metabolized by the liver, so doses must be reduced by 50 to 75% in the presence of liver dysfunction. Daunorubicin is closely related to doxorubicin and was actually introduced first into leukemia treament, where it remains part of curative regimens and has been shown preferable to doxorubicin owing

to less mucositis and colonic damage. Idarubicin is an orally acting doxorubicin analogue, whose ultimate place in therapy is uncertain.

Bleomycin refers to a mixture of glycopeptides that have the unique feature of forming complexes with Fe^{2+} while bound to DNA. Oxidation gives rise to superoxide and hydroxyl radicals. The drug is of interest clinically as it causes little, if any, myelosuppression. The drug is cleared rapidly, but augmented skin and pulmonary toxicity in the presence of renal failure has led to the recommendation that doses be reduced by 50 to 75% in the face of a creatinine clearance <25 mL/min. Bleomycin is not a vesicant, and can be administered intravenously, intramuscularly, or subcutaneously. Common side effects include fever and chills, facial flush, and Raynaud's syndrome. Hypertension can follow rapid intravenous administration, and the incidence of anaphylaxis with early preparations of the drug has led to the practice of administering a test dose of 0.5 to 1 unit before the rest of the dose. The most feared complication of bleomycin treatment is pulmonary fibrosis, which increases in incidence at >300 cumulative units administered and is at best minimally responsive to treatment (e.g., glucocorticoids). The earliest indicator of an adverse effect is a decline in the DL_{CO}, although cessation of drug immediately upon documentation of a decrease in DL_{CO} may not prevent further decline in pulmonary function. Bleomycin is inactivated by a bleomycin hydrolase, whose concentration is diminished in skin and lung. Because bleomycin-dependent electron transport is dependent on O_2, bleomycin toxicity may become apparent after exposure to transient very high inspired P_{O_2}. Thus, during surgical procedures, patients with prior exposure to bleomycin should be maintained on the lowest inspired P_{O_2} consistent with maintaining adequate tissue oxygenation.

D-Actinomycin intercalates into DNA and appears to have less, but not absent, capacity to undergo electron transfer reactions. It causes severe myelosuppression, nausea, alopecia, and mucositis. It is a notable vesicant. Mithramycin historically was used against testicular and other neoplasms; however, in addition to causing nausea, myelosuppression, and vesicant properties, it causes an "acute hemorrhagic syndrome" consisting of platelet function defects in association with indicators of disseminated intravascular coagulation. It is used in current practice to control hypercalcemia. In addition, renal and hepatic dysfunction may complicate its use.

Mitomycin C undergoes reduction of its quinone function to generate a bifunctional DNA alkylating agent. It is a broadly active antineoplastic agent with a number of unpredictable toxicities, including delayed bronchospasm 12 to 14 h after dosing and a chronic pulmonary fibrosis syndrome more frequent at doses of 50 to 60 mg/m². Cardiomyopathy has been described, particularly in the setting of prior radiation therapy. A hemolytic-uremic syndrome carries an ultimate mortality rate of 25 to 50% and is poorly treated by conventional component support and exchange transfusion. Mitomycin is a notable vesicant and causes substantial nausea and vomiting. It can be used for intravesical instillation for curative treatment of superficial transitional bladder carcinomas and, with radiation therapy, for curative treatment of anal carcinoma.

Mitoxantrone is a synthetic compound that was designed to recapitulate features of doxorubicin but with less cardiotoxicity. It is quantitatively less cardiotoxic (comparing the ratio of cardiotoxic to therapeutically effective doses), but its status in therapy is unclear as doses of 150 mg/m² have produced evidence of 10% incidence of cardiotoxicity; it also causes alopecia.

Etoposide was synthetically derived from the plant product podophyllotoxin, and it binds directly to topoisomerase II and DNA in a reversible ternary complex. In that capacity, it stabilizes the covalent intermediate in the enzyme's action where the enzyme is covalently linked to DNA. This "alkali-labile" DNA bond was historically a first hint that an activity such as topoisomerase exists. The drug therefore causes a prominent G2 arrest, reflecting the action of a DNA damage checkpoint. Prominent clinical effects include myelosuppression, nausea, and transient hypotension related to the speed of administration of the agent. Etoposide is a mild vesicant but is relatively free from other "large organ" toxicities. Teniposide is a structural relative with unique activity in childhood lymphoblastic leukemia. When given at high doses or very frequently, topoisomerase inhibitors may cause acute leukemia associated with chromosome 11q23 abnormalities in up to 1% of exposed patients.

Camptothecin was isolated from extracts of a Chinese tree and had notable antileukemia activity. Early clinical studies with the sodium salt of the hydrolyzed camptothecin lactone showed evidence of notable toxicity with little activity. Identification of topoisomerase I as the target of camptothecins and the need to preserve lactone structure allowed additional efforts to identify active members of this series. Topoisomerase I is responsible for unwinding the DNA strand by introducing single strand breaks and allowing rotation of one strand about the other. In S phase, topoisomerase I-induced breaks that are not promptly resealed lead to progress of the replication fork off the end of a DNA strand. The DNA damage is a potent signal for induction of apoptosis. Camptothecins promote the stabilization of the DNA linked to the enzyme in a so-called cleavable complex, analogous to the action of etoposide with topoisomerase II. Topotecan is a camptothecin derivative approved for use in ovarian tumors. Toxicity is limited to myelosuppression and mucositis. CPT-11, or irinotecan, is a camptothecin with evidence of activity in colon carcinoma. In addition to myelosuppression, it causes a secretory diarrhea, which can be treated effectively with loperamide or octreotide.

Indirect Effectors of DNA Function: Antimetabolites A broad definition of antimetabolites would include compounds with structural similarity to precursors of purines or pyrimidines or that interfere with purine or pyrimidine synthesis. Antimetabolites can cause DNA damage indirectly, through misincorporation into DNA, abnormal timing or progression through DNA synthesis, or altered function of pyrimidine and purine biosynthetic enzymes. They tend to convey greatest toxicity to cells in S phase, and the degree of toxicity increases with duration of exposure. Common toxic manifestations include stomatitis, diarrhea, and myelosuppression. Second malignancies are not associated with their use.

Methotrexate inhibits dihydrofolate reductase, which regenerates reduced folates from the oxidized folates produced when thymidine monophosphate is formed from deoxyuridine monophosphate. Without reduced folates, cells die a "thymineless" death. N⁵tetrahydrofolate or N⁵formyltetrahydrofolate (leucovorin) can bypass this block and rescue cells from methotrexate, which is maintained in cells by polyglutamylation. The drug and other reduced folates are transported into cells by the folate carrier, and high concentrations of drug can bypass this carrier and allow diffusion of drug directly into cells. These properties have suggested the design of "high-dose" methotrexate regimens with leucovorin rescue of normal marrow and mucosa, part of curative approaches to osteosarcoma in the adjuvant setting, and hematopoietic neoplasms of children and adults. Methotrexate is cleared by the kidney by both glomerular filtration and tubular secretion, and toxicity is augmented by renal dysfunction and drugs such as salicylates, probenecid, and nonsteroidal anti-inflammatory agents that undergo tubular secretion. With normal renal function, 15 mg/m² leucovorin will rescue 10^{-8} to 10^{-6} M methotrexate in three to four doses. However, with decreased creatinine clearance, doses of 50 to100 mg/m² are continued until methotrexate levels are $<5 \times 10^{-8}$ M. In addition to bone marrow suppression and mucosal irritation, methotrexate can cause renal failure itself at high doses owing to crystallization in renal tubules; therefore high-dose regimens require alkalinization of urine with increased flow by hydration. Methotrexate can be sequestered in third space collections and leech back into the general circulation, causing prolonged myelosuppression. Less frequent adverse effects include reversible increases in transaminases and a hypersensitivity-like pulmonary syndrome. Chronic low-dose methotrexate can cause hepatic fibrosis. When administered to the intrathecal space, methotrexate can cause chemical arachnoiditis and CNS dysfunction. Trimetrexate is a methotrexate derivative that is not polyglutamylated and does not use the reduced folate carrier.

5-Fluorouracil (5FU) represents an early example of "rational" drug design in that it originated from the observation that tumor cells incorporate uracil more efficiently into DNA than normal cells, especially gut. 5FU is metabolized in cells to 5'FdUMP, which inhibits thymidylate synthetase (TS). In addition, misincorporation can lead to single strand breaks, and RNA can aberrantly incorporate FUMP. 5FU is metabolized by dihydropyrimidine dehydrogenase, and deficiency of this enzyme can lead to excessive toxicity from 5FU. Oral bioavailability varies unreliably. Intravenous administration leads to bone marrow suppression after short infusions but to more evidence of stomatitis after prolonged infusions. Leucovorin augments the toxicity and activity of 5FU by promoting formation of the ternary covalent complex of 5FU, the reduced folate, and TS. Less frequent toxicities include CNS dysfunction, with prominent cerebellar signs, and endothelial toxicity manifested by thrombosis, including pulmonary embolus and myocardial infarction.

Cytosine arabinoside (ara-C) is incorporated into DNA after formation of ara-CTP, resulting in S phase–related toxicity. Continuous infusion schedules allow maximal efficiency of effect, with uptake maximal at 5 to 7 μM. Ara-C can be administered intrathecally. Adverse effects include nausea, diarrhea, stomatitis, chemical conjunctivitis, and cerebellar ataxia. Gemcitabine is a cytosine derivative that is similar to ara-C in that it is incorporated into DNA after anabolism to the triphosphate, rendering DNA susceptible to breakage and repair synthesis, which differs from that in ara-C in that lesions including the analogue are very inefficiently removed. In contrast to ara-C, gemcitabine appears to have useful activity in a variety of solid tumors, with limited nonmyelosuppressive toxicities. 6-Thioguanine and 6-mercaptopurine (6MP) are used in the treatment of acute lymphoid leukemia. Although administered orally, they display very variable bioavailability. 6MP is metabolized by xanthine oxidase and therefore requires dose reduction when used with allopurinol.

Fludarabine phosphate is a prodrug of F-ara-A, which in turn was designed to diminish the susceptibility of ara-A to adenosine deaminase. Ara-A is incorporated into DNA and can cause delayed cytotoxicity even in cells with low growth fraction, including chronic lymphocytic leukemia and follicular B cell lymphoma. CNS dysfunction and T cell depletion leading to opportunistic infections can occur in addition to myelosuppression. 2-Chlorodeoxyadenosine is a similar compound with activity in hairy cell leukemia. 2-Deoxycoformycin inhibits adenosine deaminase, with resulting increase in dATP levels. This causes inhibition of ribonucleotide reductase as well as augmented susceptibility to apoptosis, particularly in T cells. Renal failure and CNS dysfunction are notable toxicities in addition to immunosuppression.

Hydroxyurea inhibits ribonucleotide reductase, resulting in S phase block. It is orally bioavailable and the drug of choice for the acute management of myeloproliferative states. Asparaginase is not classically considered an antimetabolite as it causes breakdown of extracellular asparagine required for protein synthesis in certain leukemic cells. However, it effectively stops DNA synthesis by preventing the requisite concurrent protein synthesis, and therefore it has a similar functional outcome as the classic antimetabolites. As asparaginase is a foreign protein, hypersensitivity reactions are common, as are effects on organs such as pancreas and liver that require continuing protein synthesis. This results in decreased insulin secretion with hyperglycemia, with or without hyperamylasemia and clotting function abnormalities. The latter may be associated with CNS and dural vein thrombosis.

Mitotic Spindle Inhibitors Microtubules are cellular structures that form the mitotic spindle and in interphase cells are responsible for the cellular "scaffolding" along which various motile and secretory processes occur. Microtubules are composed of repeating noncovalent multimers of a hetrodimer of α and β subunits of the protein tubulin. Vincristine binds to the tubulin dimer with the result that microtubules are disaggregated. This results in the block of growing cells in M phase; however, toxic effects in G1 and S phase are also evident. The drug is bound to blood-formed elements, leading to its occasional use as vinca-loaded platelets to treat autoimmune thrombocytopenia. The drug is metabolized by the liver, and dose adjustment in the presence of hepatic dysfunction is required. It is a powerful vesicant, and infiltration can be treated by local heat and infiltration with hyaluronidase. The drug is lethal if inadvertently administered by the intrathecal route. At clinically used intravenous doses, neurotoxicity in the form of glove-and-stocking neuropathy is frequent. Children tolerate 2 mg/m², but adult doses may be capped at 2 mg total to lower the incidence of disabling chronic neuropathy; whether this compromises needed dose intensity in curative regimens is uncertain. Acute neuropathic effects include jaw pain, paralytic ileus, urinary retention, and the syndrome of inappropriate antidiuretic hormone secretion. Myelosuppression is not seen. Vinblastine is similar to vincristine, except that it tends to be more myelotoxic, with more frequent thrombocytopenia and also mucositis and stomatitis. Vinorelbine is a recently introduced vinca alkaloid that appears to have differences in resistance patterns in comparison to vincristine and vinblastine; it may be administered orally.

The taxanes include paclitaxel and docetaxel. These agents differ from the vinca alkaloids in that the taxanes stabilize microtubules against depolymerization. The "stabilized" microtubules function abnormally and are not able to undergo the normal dynamic changes of microtubule function necessary for cell cycle completion. Taxanes are

among the most broadly active antineoplastic agents for use in solid tumors, with evidence of activity in ovarian cancer, breast cancer, Kaposi's sarcoma, and lung tumors. They are administered intravenously, and paclitaxel requires use of a cremophore-containing vehicle that can cause hypersensitiviy reactions. Premedication with regimens including dexamethasone (20 mg orally or intravenously 12 and 6 h before treatment), diphenhydramine (50 mg), and cimetidine (300 mg) both 30 min before treatment decreases but does not eliminate the risk of hypersensitivity reactions to the paclitaxel vehicle. Docetaxel uses a polysorbate 80 formulation, which can cause fluid retention in addition to hypersensitivity reactions, and dexamethasone premedication with or without antihistamines is frequently used. Paclitaxel causes hypersensitivity reactions, myelosuppression, neurotoxicity in the form of glove-and-stocking numbness, and paresthesia. Cardiac rhythm disturbances were observed in phase I and II trials, most commonly asymptomatic bradycardia but, much more rarely, varying degrees of heart block. These have not emerged as clinically significant in the majority of patients. Infrequently occurring evidence of myocardial ischemia during paclitaxel administration cannot yet be clearly related to the drug. Docetaxel causes comparable degrees of myelosuppression and neuropathy. Hypersensitivity reactions, including bronchospasm, dyspnea, and hypotension, are less frequent but occur to some degree in up to 25% of patients. Fluid retention appears to result from a vascular leak syndrome that can aggravate preexisting effusions. Rash can complicate docetaxel administration, appearing prominently as a pruritic maculopapular rash affecting the forearms, but it has also been associated with fingernail ridging, breakdown, and skin discoloration. Stomatitis appears to be somewhat more frequent than with paclitaxel.

Estramustine was originally synthesized as a mustard derivative that might be useful in neoplasms that possessed estrogen receptor sites. However, no evidence of interaction with DNA was observed. Surprisingly, the drug caused metaphase arrest, and subsequent study revealed that it binds to microtubule-associated proteins, resulting in abnormal microtubule function. Estramustine binds to estramustine-binding proteins (EMBP), which have particular presence in prostate tumor tissue. The drug is approved for treatment of metastatic prostate cancer as an oral formulation. Gastrointestinal and cardiovascular adverse effects related to the estrogen moiety occur in up to 10% of patients, including worsened heart failure and thromboembolic phenomena. Gynecomastia and nipple tenderness can also occur.

Hormonal Agents The family of steroid hormone receptor–related molecules have emerged as prominent targets for "small molecules" useful in cancer treatment. When bound to their cognate ligands, these receptors can alter gene transcription and, in certain tissues, induce apoptosis. The pharmacologic effect is a mirror or parody of the normal effects of the agent acting in nontransformed tissue, although the effects on tumors are mediated by indirect effects in some cases.

Glucocorticoids are generally given in "pulsed" high-dose exposure in leukemias and lymphomas, where they induce apoptosis in tumor cells. Cushing's syndrome or inadvertent adrenal suppression on withdrawal from high-dose glucocorticoids can be significant complications, along with infections common in immunosuppressed patients, in particular *Pneumocystis* pneumonia, which classically appears a few days after completing a course of high-dose steroids. Tamoxifen is a partial estrogen receptor antagonist; it has a tenfold greater degree of antitumor activity in breast cancer patients whose tumors express estrogen receptors than in those who have low or no levels of expression. Side effects include a somewhat increased risk of estrogen-related cardiovascular complications, such as thromboembolic phenomena, and a small increased incidence of endometrial carcinoma, which appears after chronic use. Progestational agents including medroxyprogesterone acetate, androgens including halotestin, and, paradoxically, estrogens have approximately the same degeree of activity in primary hormonal treatment of breast cancers that have elevated levels of estrogen receptors. Estrogen is not used often owing to prominent cardiovascular and uterotropic activity.

Prostate cancer is classically treated by diethylstilbesterol (DES) acting as an estrogen at the level of the hypothalamus to downregulate hypothalamic luteinizing hormone (LH) production, resulting in decreased elaboration of testosterone by the testicle. For this reason, orchiectomy is equally as effective as moderate-dose DES, inducing responses in ~80% of previously untreated patients with prostate cancer but without the prominent cardiovascular side effects of DES, including thrombosis and exacerbation of coronary artery disease. In the event that orchiectomy is not accepted by the patient, testicular androgen suppression can also be effected by luteinizing hormone–releasing hormone (LHRH) agonists such as leuprolide and goserelin. These agents cause tonic stimulation of the LHRH receptor, with the loss of its normal pulsatile activation resulting in its desensitization and decreased output of LH by the anterior pituitary. Therefore, as primary hormonal manipulation in prostate cancer one can choose orchiectomy or leuprolide, not both. The addition of actual antagonists of androgens acting at the androgen receptor, including flutamide or bicalutamide, is of uncertain additional benefit in extending overall response duration, but it clearly prevents the activation of androgen receptors by adrenal androgens, and the combined use of orchiectomy or leuprolide plus flutamide is referred to as "total androgen blockade."

Interestingly, tumors that respond to a primary hormonal manipulation may frequently respond to second and third hormonal manipulations. Thus, breast tumors that had previously responded to tamoxifen have, on relapse, notable response rates to withdrawal of tamoxifen itself or to subsequent addition of a progestin. Likewise, initial treatment of prostate cancers with leuprolide plus flutamide may be followed after disease progression by response to withrawal of flutamide. These responses may result from the removal of antagonists from mutant steroid hormone receptors that have come to depend on the presence of the antagonist as a growth-promoting influence.

Additional strategies to treat refractory breast and prostate cancers that possess steroid hormone receptors may also address adrenal capacity to produce androgens and estrogens, even after orchiectomy or oophorectomy, respectively. Thus, aminoglutethimide or ketoconazole can be used to block adrenal synthesis by interfering with the enzymes of steroid hormone metabolism. Administration of these agents requires concomitant hydrocortisone replacement and additional glucocorticoid doses administered in the event of physiologic stress. Steroid hormone–inducing "aromatase" activity may be present in tumor tissue, and second- or third-line approaches to inhibition of aromatase activity may also be effected by such agents as anastrazole and letrozole.

Humoral mechanisms can also result in complications of an underlying malignancy. Adrenocortical carcinomas can cause Cushing's syndrome as well as syndromes of androgen or estrogen excess. Mitotane can counteract these by decreasing synthesis of steroid hormones. Islet cell neoplasms can cause debilitating diarrhea, treated with the somatostatin analogue octreotide. Prolactin-secreting tumors can be effectively managed by the dopaminergic agononist bromocriptine.

An additional strategy related conceptually to the use of steroid hormones is the use of retinoids, including tretinoin, the all-*trans*-isomer of retinoic acid, or isotretinoin, the 13-*cis* isomer of retinoic acid, to cause "differentiation" by acting on the retinoid receptor, which is in the steroid hormone receptor family. In particular, tretinoin is part of curative regimens for acute promyelocytic leukemia (PML) and appears to act by causing accelerated degradation of the fusion protein created by the t(15;17) translocation fusing the retinoic acid receptor α and the PML transcription factor. Acute side effects related to differentiation of promyelocytes to mature granulocytes may result in pulmonary symptoms related to granulocyte sequestration in the pulmonary vasculature; these are treated by respiratory support and glucocorticoids. Squamous neoplasms, including those of the skin and cervix, also appear to be uniquely responsive in certain cases to retinoids.

ACUTE COMPLICATIONS OF CANCER CHEMOTHERAPY Myelosuppression The common cytotoxic chemotherapeutic agents almost invariably affect bone marrow function. Titration of this effect determines in many cases the MTD of the agent on a given schedule. The normal kinetics of blood cell turnover influence the sequence and sensitivity of each of the formed elements. Polymorphonuclear leukocytes (PMNs; $T_{1/2} = 6$ to 8 h), platelets ($T_{1/2} = 5$ to 7 days), and red blood cells (RBC; $T_{1/2} \sim 120$ days) have most, less, and least susceptibility to usually administered cytotoxic agents, respectively. The *nadir count* of each cell type in response to classes of agents is characteristic. Maximal neutropenia occurs 6 to 14 days after conventional doses of anthracyclines, antifolates, and antimetabolites. Alkylating agents differ in timing of cytopenias. Nitrosoureas, DTIC, and procarbazine can display delayed marrow toxicity, first appearing 6 weeks after dosing.

Complications of myelosuppression result from the predictable sequelae of the missing cells' function. *Febrile neutropenia* refers to the clinical presentation of fever (one temperature $\geq 38.5°C$ or three readings $\geq 38°C$ but $\leq 38.5°C$ per 24 h) in a cytopenic patient with an uncontrolled neoplasm involving the bone marrow or, more usually, in a patient undergoing treatment with cytotoxic agents. Mortality from uncontrolled infection varies inversely with the PMN count. If the nadir PMN count is $>1000/\mu L$, there is little risk; if $<500/\mu L$, risk of death is markedly increased. Management of febrile neutropenia has conventionally included empirical coverage with antibiotics for the duration of neutropenia (Chap. 85). Selection of antibiotics is governed by the expected association of infections with certain underlying neoplasms; careful physical examination (with scrutiny of catheter sites, dentition, mucosal surfaces, and perirectal and genital orifices by gentle palpation); chest x-ray; and Gram stain and culture of blood, urine and sputum (if any) to define a putative site of infection. In the absence of any originating site, a broadly acting β-lactam with anti-*Pseudomonas* activity, such as ceftazidime, is begun empirically. The addition of vancomycin to cover potential cutaneous sites of origin (until these are ruled out or shown to originate from methicillin-sensitive organisms) or metronidazole or imipenem for abdominal or other sites favoring anaerobes reflects modifications tailored to individual patient presentations. The coexistence of pulmonary compromise raises a distinct set of potential pathogens, including *Legionella*, *Pneumocystis*, and fungal agents, that may require further diagnostic evaluations such as bronchoscopy with bronchoalveolar lavage. Febrile neutropenic patients can be stratified broadly into two prognostic groups. The first, with expected short duration of neutropenia and no evidence of hypotension or abdominal or other localizing symptoms, may be expected to do well even with less complex, oral regimens, e.g., ciprofloxacin plus amoxicillin/clavulinic acid. Detailed evaluation of such simple oral programs and intravenous regimens is ongoing. A less favorable prognostic group are patients with expected prolonged neutropenia, evidence of sepsis, and end-organ compromise, particularly pneumonia. These patients clearly require tailoring of their antibiotic regimen to their underlying presentation, with frequent empirical addition of antifungal agents if fever persists for 7 days without identification of an adequately treated organism or site.

Transfusion of granulocytes has no role in the management of febrile neutropenia, owing to their exceedingly short half-life, mechanical fragility, and clinical syndromes of pulmonary compromise with leukostasis after their use. Instead, *colony stimulating factors* (CSFs) are used to augment bone marrow production of PMNs. These include "early-acting" factors such as IL-1, IL-3, and stem cell factor, which act on multiple lineages, and "late-acting" lineage-specific factors such as G-CSF (granulocyte colony stimulating factor) or GM-CSF (granulocyte-macrophage colony stimulating factor), erythropoietin, thrombopoietin, IL-6, and IL-11. CSFs are overused in oncology practice. The settings in which their use has been proven effective are limited. G-CSF, GM-CSF, erythropoietin, and IL-11 are currently approved for use. The American Society of Clinical Oncology has developed practice guidelines for the use of G-CSF and GM-CSF (Table 84-3). Primary administration (i.e., shortly after completing chemo-

Preventive Uses
With the first cycle of chemotherapy (so-called primary CSF administration)
     Not needed on a routine basis
     Use if the probability of febrile neutropenia is ≤40%
     Use if patient has preexisting neutropenia or active infection
With subsequent cycles if febrile neutropenia has previously occurred (so-called secondary CSF administration)
     Not needed after short duration neutropenia without fever
     Use if patient had febrile neutropenia in previous cycle
     Use if prolonged neutropenia (even without fever) delays therapy
Therapeutic Uses
Afebrile neutropenic patients
     No evidence of benefit
Febrile neutropenic patients
     No evidence of benefit
     May feel compelled to use in the face of clinical deterioration from sepsis, pneumonia, or fungal infection, but benefit unclear
To augment dose-intensity of chemotherapy in patients with curable malignancies
     No evidence of benefit
In bone marrow or peripheral blood stem cell transplantation
     Use to mobilize stem cells from marrow
     Use to hasten myeloid recovery
In acute myeloid leukemia
     G-CSF of minor or no benefit
     GM-CSF of no benefit and may be harmful
In myelodysplastic syndromes
     Not routinely beneficial
     Use intermittently in subset with neutropenia and recurrent infection
What Dose And Schedule Should Be Used?
G-CSF: 5 μg/kg per day subcutaneously
GM-CSF: 250 μg/m^2 per day subcutaneously
When Should Therapy Begin And End?
When indicated, start 24–72 h after chemotherapy
Continue until absolute neutrophil count is 10,000/μL
Do not use concurrently with chemotherapy or radiation therapy

---

NOTE: G-CSF, granulocyte colony stimulating factor; GM-CSF, granulocyte-macrophage colony stimulating factor.
SOURCE: From the American Society of Clinical Oncology.

therapy to reduce the nadir) of G-CSF to patients receiving cytotoxic regimens associated with a 40% incidence of febrile neutropenia has reduced the incidence of febrile neutropenia in several studies by about 50%. Most patients, however, receive regimens that do not have such a high risk of expected febrile neutropenia, and therefore most patients initially should not receive G-CSF or GM-CSF. Special circumstances such as a documented history of febrile neutropenia with the regimen in a particular patient; extensive compromise of marrow by prior radiation or chemotherapy; or active, open wounds or deep-seated infection may support primary treatment with G-CSF or GM-CSF. Administration of G-CSF or GM-CSF to afebrile neutropenic patients or to patients with "low-risk" febrile neutropenia (secondary administration, use after neutropenia has developed) as defined above is not recommended, although administration to "high-risk" patients with febrile neutropenia and evidence of organ compromise is reasonable. G-CSF or GM-CSF is conventionally started 24 to 72 h after completion of chemotherapy and continued until a PMN count of 10,000/μL is achieved. Also, patients with myeloid leukemias undergoing induction therapy may have a slight reduction in the duration of neutropenia if G-CSF (not GM-CSF) is commenced after completion of therapy and may be of particular value in elderly patients, but the influence on long-term outcome has not been defined. GM-CSF probably has a more restricted utility than G-CSF, with its use currently limited to patients after autologous bone marrow transplants, although proper "head-to-head" comparisons with G-CSF have not been conducted in most instances. GM-CSF may be associated with more systemic side effects.

Dangerous degrees of thrombocytopenia do not frequently complicate the management of patients with solid tumors receiving cytotoxic chemotherapy (carboplatin-containing regimens are frequently involved), but they are frequent in patients with certain hematologic neoplasms where marrow is infiltrated with tumor. Severe bleeding related to thrombocytopenia occurs with increased frequency at platelet counts <20,000/μL and is very prevalent at counts <5000/μL. Prophylactic transfusions to keep platelets >20,000/μL are warranted in patients with leukemia (the threshold for transfusion is 10,000/μL in patients with solid tumors and no other bleeding diathesis). Careful review of medication lists to prevent exposure to nonsteroidal anti-inflammatory agents and maintenance of clotting factor levels adequate to support near-normal prothrombin and partial thromboplastin time tests are of import in minimizing the risk of bleeding in the thrombocytopenic patient. Certain cytokines in clinical investigation have shown ability to increase platelets (e.g., IL-6, IL-1, thrombopoietin), but clinical benefit and safety are not yet proven. IL-11 (oprelvekin) is approved for use in the setting of expected thrombocytopenia, but its effects on platelet counts are small and it is associated with side effects such as headache, fever, malaise, syncope, cardiac arrhythmias, and fluid retention.

Anemia associated with chemotherapy can be managed by transfusion of packed RBCs. Transfusion is not undertaken until the hemoglobin falls to <80 g/L (8 g/dL), or if compromise of end-organ function occurs or an underlying condition (e.g., coronary artery disease) calls for maintenance of hemoglobin >90 g/L (9 g/dL). Patients who are to receive therapy for >2 months on a "stable" regimen and who are likely to require continuing transfusions are also candidates for erythropoietin to maintain hemoglobin of 90 to 100 g/L (9 to 10 g/dL). In the setting of adequate iron stores and serum erythropoietin levels <100 ng/mL, erythropoietin, 150 U three times a week, can produce a slow increase in hemoglobin over about 2 months of administration. Quality of life is better at higher hemoglobin concentrations, but expense is a concern with erythropoietin use.

Nausea and Vomiting   The most common side effect of chemotherapy administration is nausea, with or without vomiting. Antineoplastic agents vary in their capacity to cause nausea and vomiting. Nitrogen mustard, nitrosoureas, streptozotocin, DTIC, cisplatin, and actinomycin are highly emetogenic and produce vomiting in virtually all patients. Doxorubicin, daunorubicin, and conventional-dose cyclophosphamide are moderately emetogenic. Antimetabolites are dose- and schedule-dependent, with single doses of methotrexate and fluorouracil producing at worst anorexia; while 5-day regimens of 5-fluorouracil and high-dose methotrexate produce nausea in ~50% of patients. Other agents such as chlorambucil, melphalan, and busulfan in conventional doses produce little tendency to emesis.

Emesis is a reflex caused by stimulation of the vomiting center in the medulla. Input to the vomiting center comes from the chemoreceptor trigger zone (CTZ) and afferents from the peripheral gastrointestinal tract, cerebral cortex, and heart. In addition, a conditioned reflex may contribute to anticipatory nausea arising after repeated cycles of chemotherapy. Accordingly, antiemesis agents differ in their locus of action. Combining agents from different classes or the sequential use of different classes of agent is the cornerstone of successful management of chemotherapy-induced nausea and vomiting. Of great importance are the prophylactic administration of agents and the use of psychological techniques including the maintenance of a supportive milieu, counseling, and relaxation to augment the action of antiemetic agents.

Antidopaminergic phenothiazines act directly at the CTZ, and include prochlorperazine (Compazine), 10 mg intramuscularly or intravenously, 10 to 25 mg orally, or 25 mg per rectum every 4 to 6 h for up to four doses; and thiethylperazine (Torecan), 10 mg by all the above routes every 6 h. Haloperidol (Haldol) is a butyrophenone dopamine antagonist given at 0.5 to 1.0 mg intramuscularly or orally every 8 h. Antihistamines such as diphenhydramine (Benadryl) have little intrinsic antiemetic capacity but are frequently given to prevent or treat dystonic reactions that can complicate use of the antidopaminergic agents. Lorazepam (Ativan) is a short-acting benzodiazepine that provides an anxiolytic effect to augment the effectiveness of a variety of agents when used at 1 to 2 mg intramuscularly, intravenously, or orally every 4 to 6 h. Dexamethasone (Decadron) likewise augments the action of a variety of agents when used at 4 to 40 mg intravenously or orally, given before treatment and repeated up to 10 mg orally every 6 h four times. Metoclopramide (Reglan) acts on peripheral dopamine receptors to augment gastric emptying and is used in high doses for highly emetogenic regimens (1 to 2 mg/kg intravenously 30 min before chemotherapy and every 2 h for up to three additional doses as needed); intravenous doses of 10 to 20 mg every 4 to 6 h as needed or 50 mg orally 4 h before and 8 and 12 h after chemotherapy are used for moderately emetogenic regimens. Serotonin antagonists are useful in moderately to severely emetogenic regimens; ondansetron (Zofran) is given as 0.15 mg/kg intravenously for three doses just before and at 4 and 8 h after chemotherapy, and granisetron (Kytril) is given as a single dose of 0.01 mg/kg just before chemotherapy. δ-9-Tetrahydrocannabinol (Marinol) is a rather weak antiemetic compared to other available agents, but it may be useful for persisting nausea and is used orally at 10 mg every 3 to 4 h as needed.

Alopecia Chemotherapeutic agents vary widely in causing alopecia, with anthracyclines, alkylating agents, and topoisomerase inhibitors reliably causing near total alopecia when given at therapeutic doses. Antimetabolites are more variably associated with alopecia. Psychologic support and the use of cosmetic resources are to be encouraged, and "chemo caps" that reduce scalp temperature to decrease the degree of alopecia should be discouraged.

Gonadal Dysfunction and Pregnancy Cessation of ovulation and azoospermia reliably result from alkylating agent– and topoisomerase poison–containing regimens. The duration of these effects varies with age and sex. Males treated for Hodgkin's disease with mechlorethamine- and procarbazine-containing regimens are effectively sterile, while fertility usually returns after regimens including cisplatin, vinblastine or etoposide, and bleomycin for testicular cancer. Sperm banking before treatment may be considered to support patients likely to be sterilized by treatment. Females experience amenorrhea with anovulation after alkylating agent therapy but are likely to recover normal menses if treatment is completed before age 30 and unlikely to recover menses after age 35. Even those who regain menses usually experience premature menopause. As the magnitude and extent of decreased fertility can be difficult to predict, patients should be counseled to maintain effective contraception, preferably by barrier means, during and after therapy. Resumption of efforts to conceive should be considered in the context of the likely prognosis of the patient. Hormone-replacement therapy should be undertaken in women who do not have a hormonally responsive tumor.

Chemotherapy agents have variable effects on the success of pregnancy (Chap. 7). All agents tend to have increased risk of adverse outcomes when administered during the first trimester, and strategies to delay chemotherapy if possible until after this milestone should be considered if the pregnancy is to continue to term. Patients in their second or third trimester can be treated with most regimens for the common neoplasms afflicting women in their child-bearing years with the exception of antimetabolites, particularly antifolates, which have notable teratogenic or fetotoxic effects throughout pregnancy. The need for anticancer chemotherapy per se is infrequently a clear basis to recommend termination of a concurrent pregnancy, although each treatment strategy in this circumstance must be tailored to the individual needs of the patient. →*Chronic effects of cancer treatment are reviewed in Chap. 103.*

BIOLOGIC THERAPY

No postulates resembling principles have emerged from efforts to develop biologic approaches to cancer treatment. The goal of biologic therapy is to manipulate the host-tumor interaction in favor of the host. Theoretically, biologic approaches should reflect a bell-shaped dose-response curve where the maximum biologic effect is less than the MTD. Empirical trial and error has led to the discovery that a number of biologic treatment approaches may produce antitumor effects, but nearly all of them are most active at their MTD.

IMMUNE MEDIATORS OF ANTITUMOR EFFECTS The very existence of a cancer in a person is testimony to the failure of the immune system to deal effectively with the cancer. Tumors have a variety of means of avoiding the immune system: (1) they are often only subtly different from their normal counterparts; (2) they are capable of downregulating their major histocompatibility complex antigens, effectively masking them from recognition by T cells; (3) they are inefficient at presenting antigens to the immune system; (4) they can cloak themselves in a protective shell of fibrin to minimize contact with surveillance mechanisms; and (5) they can produce a range of soluble molecules, including potential immune targets, that can distract the immune system from recognizing the tumor cell. Some of the cell products initially polarize the immune response away from cellular immunity (shifting from Th1 to Th2 responses, Chap. 305) and ultimately lead to defects in T cells that prevent their activation and cytotoxic activity. Cancer treatment further suppresses host immunity. A variety of strategies are being tested to overcome these barriers.

Cell-Mediated Immunity The strongest evidence that the immune system can exert clinically meaningful antitumor effects comes from allogeneic bone marrow transplantation. Adoptively transferred T cells from the donor expand in the tumor-bearing host, recognize the tumor as being foreign, and mediate impressive antitumor effects (graft-versus-tumor effects). Three types of experimental interventions are being developed to take advantage of the ability of T cells to kill tumor cells.

1. Allogeneic T cells are being transferred to cancer-bearing hosts in three major settings: in the form of allogeneic bone marrow transplantation, as pure lymphocyte transfusions following bone marrow recovery after allogeneic bone marrow transplantation, and as pure lymphocyte transfusions following immunosuppressive (but not myeloablative) therapy (so-called minitransplants). In each of these settings, the effector cells are donor T cells that recognize the tumor as being foreign, probably through minor histocompatibility differences. The main risk of such therapy is the development of graft-versus-host disease because of the minimal difference between the cancer and the normal host cells. This approach has been highly effective in hematologic cancers.

2. Autologous T cells are being removed from the tumor-bearing host, manipulated in several ways in vitro, and given back to the patient. The two major classes of autologous T cell manipulation are: (1) to develop tumor antigen–specific T cells and expand them to large numbers over many weeks ex vivo before administration, and (2) to activate the cells with polyclonal stimulators such as anti-CD3 and anti-CD28 after a short period ex vivo and try to expand them in the host after adoptive transfer with stimulation by IL-2, for example. Short periods removed from the patient permit the cells to overcome the tumor-induced T cell defects, and such cells traffic and home to sites of disease better than cells that have been in culture for many weeks. Individual centers have successful experiences with one or the other approach but not both, and whether one is superior to the other is not known.

3. Tumor vaccines are aimed at boosting T cell immunity. The finding that mutant oncogenes that are expressed only intracellularly can be recognized as targets of T cell killing greatly expanded the possibilities for tumor vaccine development. No longer is it difficult to find something different about tumor cells from normal cells. However, major difficulties remain in getting the tumor-specific peptides presented in a fashion to prime the T cells. Tumors themselves are very poor at presenting their own antigens to T cells at the first antigen exposure (*priming*). Priming is best accomplished by professional antigen-presenting cells (dendritic cells). Thus, a number of experimental strategies are aimed at priming host T cells against tumor-associated peptides. Vaccine adjuvants such as GM-CSF appear capable of attracting antigen-presenting cells to a skin site containing a tumor an-

tigen. Such an approach has been documented to eradicate microscopic residual disease in follicular lymphoma and give rise to tumor-specific T cells. Purified antigen-presenting cells can be pulsed with tumor, its membranes, or particular tumor antigens and delivered as a vaccine. Tumor cells can be transfected with genes that attract antigen-presenting cells. Other ideas are also being tested. In a variation on the theme of adoptive transfer, the tumor vaccine may be given to the normal bone marrow and lymphoid cell donor of an allogeneic transplant so that the donor immune system has more cells capable of recognizing the tumor specifically. Vaccines against viral cancers (papillomavirus in cervical cancer), lymphomas, and melanomas have had modest clinical success.

Antibodies In general, antibodies are not very effective at killing cancer cells. Because the tumor seems to influence the host toward making antibodies rather than generating cellular immunity, it is inferred that antibodies are easier to defend against. Many patients can be shown to have serum antibodies directed at their tumors, but these do not appear to influence disease progression. However, the ability to grow very large quantities of high-affinity antibody directed at a tumor by the hybridoma technique has led to the application of antibodies to the treatment of cancer. The first study of a monoclonal antibody in cancer was published in 1980 and demonstrated many hurdles that needed to be overcome to make the approach successful. It seemed best to attack a determinant that was not shed or modulated by the tumor. A target that was involved in an important function for the tumor cells might be superior to a physiologically irrelevant target. Murine antibodies were not very effective because they did not mediate human effector mechanisms well and the host nearly always made antibodies against the therapeutic antibody that prevented it from finding the target.

The lessons were learned; humanized antibodies against the CD20 molecule expressed on B cell lymphomas (rituximab) and against the HER-2/neu receptor overexpressed on epithelial cancers, especially breast cancer (herceptin), have become reliable tools in the oncologists armamentarium. Each used alone can cause tumor regression (rituximab > herceptin), and both appear to potentiate the effects of combination chemotherapy given just after antibody administration. It is likely that other antibodies against other important tumor targets will be available soon. Conjugation to drugs, toxins, isotopes, photodynamic agents, and other killing moieties may also be effective. Radioconjugates are the closest to approval. Other conjugates are associated with problems that have not yet been solved (e.g., antigenicity, instability, poor tumor penetration).

Cytokines There are >70 separate proteins and glycoproteins with biologic effects in humans: IFN-α, -β, -γ; IL-1 through -18 (so far); the tumor necrosis factor (TFN) family [including lymphotoxin, TFN-related apoptosis-inducing ligand (TRAIL), CD40 ligand, and others]; and the chemokine family. Only a fraction of these has been tested against cancer; only IFN-α and IL-2 are in routine clinical use.

About 20 different genes encode IFN-α, and their biologic effects are indistinguishable. Interferon induces the expression of many genes, inhibits protein synthesis, and exerts a number of different effects on diverse cellular processes. Its antitumor effects appear to be antagonized in vitro by thymidine, suggesting that de novo thymidylate synthesis is also affected. The two recombinant forms that are commercially available are IFN-α2a and -α2b. In general, interferon antitumor effects are dose-related, and IFN is most effective at its MTD. Interferon is not curative for any tumor but can induce partial responses in follicular lymphoma, hairy cell leukemia, chronic myeloid leukemia, melanoma, and Kaposi's sarcoma. It has been used in the adjuvant setting in stage II melanoma, multiple myeloma, and follicular lymphoma. Its effects on survival are controversial. It produces fever, fatigue, a flulike syndrome, malaise, myelosuppression, and depression and can induce clinically significant autoimmune disease.

IL-2 must exert its antitumor effects indirectly through augmentation of immune function. Its biologic activity is to promote the growth and activity of T cells and natural killer (NK) cells. High doses of IL-2 can produce tumor regressions in ~20% of patients with meta-

static melanoma and renal cell cancer. About 5% of patients may experience complete remissions that are durable, unlike any other treatment for these tumors. IL-2 is associated with myriad clinical side effects: intravascular volume depletion, capillary leak syndrome, adult respiratory distress syndrome, hypotension, fever, chills, skin rash, and impaired renal and liver function. Patients may require blood pressure support and intensive care to manage the toxicity. However, once the agent is stopped, most of the toxicities reverse completely within 3 to 6 days.

BIBLIOGRAPHY

ABELOFF MD et al (eds): *Clinical Oncology*, 2d ed. Philadelphia, Churchill Livingstone, 2000

AMERICAN SOCIETY OF CLINICAL ONCOLOGY: Update of recommendations for use of hematopoietic colony-stimulating factors: Evidence-based clinical practice guidelines. J Clin Oncol 14:1957, 1996

CHABNER BA, LONGO DL (eds): *Cancer Chemotherapy and Biotherapy: Principles and Practice*, 3d ed. Philadelphia, Lippincott Williams & Wilkins, 2001

85	*Robert Finberg*

INFECTIONS IN PATIENTS WITH CANCER

ALL	acute lymphocytic leukemia	CT	computed tomography
AML	acute myelocytic leukemia	HSV	herpes simplex virus
CLL	chronic lymphocytic leukemia	MRI	magnetic resonance imaging
CMV	cytomegalovirus	PMNs	polymorphonuclear leukocytes
CNS	central nervous system	VZV	varicella-zoster virus

Infections are a common cause of death and an even more common cause of morbidity in patients with a wide variety of neoplasms. Autopsy studies show that most deaths from acute leukemia and half of deaths from lymphoma are caused directly by infection. With more intensive chemotherapy, patients with solid tumors have become more likely to die of infection rather than their underlying disease.

A physical predisposition to infection (Table 85-1) can be a result of the neoplasm's production of a break in the skin; for example, a squamous cell carcinoma may cause local invasion of the epidermis, which allows bacteria to gain access to the subcutaneous tissue and permits the development of cellulitis. The artificial closing of a normally patent orifice can also predispose to infection: Obstruction of a ureter by a tumor can cause urinary tract infection, and obstruction of the bile duct can cause cholangitis. Part of the host's normal defense against infection depends on the continuous emptying of a viscus; without emptying, a few bacteria present as a result of bacteremia or local transit can multiply and cause disease.

A similar problem can affect patients whose lymph node integrity has been disrupted by radical surgery, particularly patients who have had radical node dissections. A common clinical problem following radical mastectomy is the development of cellulitis (usually caused by streptococci or staphylococci) because of lymphedema and/or inadequate lymph drainage. In most cases, this problem can be addressed by local measures designed to prevent fluid accumulation and breaks in the skin, but antibiotic prophylaxis has been necessary in refractory cases.

A life-threatening problem common to many cancer patients is the loss of the reticuloendothelial capacity to clear microorganisms after splenectomy. Splenectomy is common in patients with Hodgkin's disease and in the management of hairy cell leukemia, chronic lymphocytic leukemia (CLL), and refractory idiopathic thrombocytopenic purpura. Even after curative therapy for the underlying disease, the lack of a spleen predisposes such patients to rapidly fatal infections.

Table 85-1 Normal Barriers to Infections

Type of Defense	Specific Lesion	Cells Involved	Organisms	Cancer Association	Disease
Physical barrier	Breaks in skin	Skin epithelial cells	Staphylococci, streptococci	Head and neck, squamous cell carcinoma	Cellulitis, extensive skin infection
Emptying of fluid collections	Occlusion of orifices: ureters, bile duct, colon	Luminal epithelial cells	Gram-negative bacilli	Renal, ovarian, biliary tree, metastatic diseases of many cancers	Rapid, overwhelming bacteremia, urinary tract infection
Lymphatic disease	Node dissection	Lymph nodes	Staphylococci, streptococci	Breast cancer surgery	Cellulitis
Splenic clearance of microorganisms	Splenectomy	Splenic reticuloendothelial cells	*Streptococcus pneumoniae, Haemophilus influenzae, Neisseria meningitidis, Babesia, Capnocytophaga canimorsus*	Hodgkin's disease, leukemia, idiopathic thrombocytopenic purpura	Rapid, overwhelming sepsis
Phagocytosis	Lack of granulocytes	Granulocytes (neutrophils)	Staphylococci, streptococci, enteric organisms	Hairy cell, acute myelocytic, and acute lymphocytic leukemias	Bacteremia
Humoral immunity	Lack of antibody	B cells	*S. pneumoniae, H. influenzae, N. meningitidis*	Chronic lymphocytic leukemia	Infections with encapsulated organisms, sinusitis, pneumonia
Cellular immunity	Lack of T cells	T cells and macrophages	*Mycobacterium tuberculosis, Listeria,* herpesviruses, fungi, other intracellular parasites	Hodgkin's disease, leukemia, T cell lymphoma	Infections with intracellular bacteria, fungi, parasites

The loss of the spleen through trauma similarly predisposes the normal host to overwhelming infection as long as 25 years after splenectomy. The splenectomized patient should be counseled about the risks of infection with certain organisms, such as the protozoan *Babesia* (Chap. 214) and *Capnocytophaga canimorsus* (formerly dysgonic fermenter 2 or DF-2), a bacterium carried in the mouths of animals (Chap. 127). Since encapsulated bacteria (*Streptococcus pneumoniae, Haemophilus influenzae,* and *Neisseria meningitidis*) are the organisms most commonly associated with postsplenectomy sepsis, splenectomized persons should be vaccinated (and revaccinated; Table 85-2) against the capsular polysaccharides of these organisms. Many clinicians recommend giving splenectomized patients a small supply of antibiotics effective against *S. pneumoniae, N. meningitidis,* and *H. influenzae* to avert rapid, overwhelming sepsis in the event that they cannot present for medical attention immediately after the onset of fever or other symptoms of bacterial infection.

The level of suspicion of infections with certain organisms should depend on the type of cancer diagnosed (Table 85-3). Diagnosis of multiple myeloma or CLL should prompt the measurement of im-

munoglobulin levels and the consideration of either antibody replacement or antibiotic prophylaxis. (In the case of CLL, antibiotic prophylaxis for likely pathogens has proven a cost-effective preventive measure.) Similarly, patients with acute lymphocytic leukemia (ALL), patients with non-Hodgkin's lymphoma, and all cancer patients treated with high-dose glucocorticoids (or glucocorticoid-containing chemotherapy regimens) should receive antibiotic prophylaxis for *Pneumocystis carinii* infection (Table 85-3).

In addition to exhibiting susceptibility to certain infectious organisms, patients with cancer are likely to manifest their infections in characteristic ways.

SYSTEM-SPECIFIC SYNDROMES

SKIN-SPECIFIC SYNDROMES (See Plate IID-57) Skin lesions are common in cancer patients, and their appearance may permit the diagnosis of systemic bacterial or fungal infection. While cellulitis caused by skin organisms such as *Streptococcus* or *Staphylococcus* is common, neutropenic patients and those with impaired blood or lym-

Table 85-2 Vaccination of Cancer Patients Receiving Chemotherapy

	Use in Indicated Patients		
Vaccine	Intensive Chemotherapy	Hodgkin's Disease	Bone Marrow Transplantation
Diphtheria-tetanus (diphtheria, pertussis, tetanus; DPT) for children <7 years old	Primary series and boosters as necessary	No special recommendation	12 and 24 months after transplantation
Poliomyelitis[a]	Complete primary series and boosters	No special recommendation	12 and 24 months after transplantation
Haemophilus influenzae type b	Primary series and booster for children	Immunization before treatment and booster 3 months afterward	12 and 24 months after transplantation
23-Valent pneumococcal	Every 5 years	Immunization before treatment and booster 3 months afterward	12 and 24 months after transplantation
4-Valent meningococcal	Every 5 years	Immunization before treatment and booster 3 months afterward	12 and 24 months after transplantation
Influenza	Seasonal immunization	Seasonal immunization	Seasonal immunization
Measles/mumps/rubella	Contraindicated	Contraindicated	After 24 months in patients without graft-versus-host disease
Varicella-zoster virus	Contraindicated[b]	Contraindicated	Contraindicated

[a] Live-virus vaccine is contraindicated; inactivated vaccine should be used.
[b] Contact the manufacturer for more information on use in children with acute lymphocytic leukemia.

Table 85-3 Infections and Cancer

Cancer	Underlying Immune Abnormality	Organisms Causing Infection
Multiple myeloma	Hypogammaglobulinemia	*Streptococcus pneumoniae, Haemophilus influenzae, Neisseria meningitidis*
Chronic lymphocytic leukemia	Hypogammaglobulinemia	*S. pneumoniae, H. influenzae, N. meningitidis*
Acute myelocytic or lymphocytic leukemia	Granulocytopenia, skin and mucous-membrane lesions	Extracellular gram-positive and gram-negative bacteria, fungi
Hodgkin's disease	Abnormal T cell function	Intracellular pathogens (*Mycobacterium tuberculosis, Listeria, Salmonella, Cryptococcus, Mycobacterium avium*)
Non-Hodgkin's lymphoma and acute lymphocytic leukemia	Glucocorticoid chemotherapy, T and B cell dysfunction	*Pneumocystis carinii*
Colon and rectal tumors	Local abnormalities[a]	*Streptococcus bovis* (bacteremia)
Hairy cell leukemia	Abnormal T cell function	Intracellular pathogens (*M. tuberculosis, Listeria, Cryptococcus, M. avium*)

[a] The reason for this association is not well defined.

phatic drainage may develop infections with unusual organisms. Innocent-looking macules or papules may be the first sign of bacterial or fungal sepsis in immunocompromised patients. In the neutropenic host, a macule progresses rapidly to ecthyma gangrenosum, a usually painless, round, necrotic lesion consisting of a central black or gray-black eschar with surrounding erythema. Ecthyma gangrenosum is located in nonpressure areas (as distinguished from necrotic lesions associated with lack of circulation) and is often associated with *Pseudomonas aeruginosa* bacteremia (Chap. 155) but may be caused by other bacteria.

Candidemia (Chap. 205) is also associated with a variety of skin conditions and commonly presents as a maculopapular rash. Punch biopsy of the skin may be the best method for diagnosis.

Cellulitis, an acute spreading inflammation of the skin, is most often caused by infection with group A *Streptococcus* or *Staphylococcus aureus*, virulent organisms normally found on the skin (Chap. 128). Although cellulitis tends to be circumscribed in normal hosts, it may spread rapidly in neutropenic patients [those with fewer than 500 functional polymorphonuclear leukocytes (PMNs) per microliter]. A tiny break in the skin may lead to spreading cellulitis, which is characterized by pain and erythema; in such patients, signs of infection (e.g., purulence) are often lacking. What might be a furuncle in a normal host may require amputation because of uncontrolled infection in a patient presenting with leukemia. A dramatic response to an infection that might be trivial in a normal host can mark the first sign of leukemia. Fortunately, granulocytopenic patients are likely to be infected with certain types of organisms (Table 85-4); thus the selection of an antibiotic regimen is somewhat easier than it might otherwise be. (See discussion below on the selection of antibiotics for use in neutropenic patients.) It is essential to recognize cellulitis early and to treat it aggressively. Patients who are neutropenic or have previously received antibiotics for other reasons may develop cellulitis with unusual organisms (e.g., *Escherichia coli*, *Pseudomonas*, or fungi). Early treatment, even of innocent-looking lesions, is essential to prevent necrosis and loss of tissue. Debridement to prevent spread may

Table 85-4 Organisms Likely to Cause Infections in Granulocytopenic Patients

Gram-positive cocci	*Enterobacter* spp.
Staphylococcus epidermidis	*Serratia* spp.
Staphylococcus aureus	*Acinetobacter* spp.[a]
Viridans *Streptococcus*	*Citrobacter* spp.
Enterococcus faecalis	Gram-positive bacilli
Streptococcus pneumoniae	Diphtheroids
Gram-negative bacilli	JK bacillus[a]
Escherichia coli	Fungi
Klebsiella spp.	*Candida* spp.
Pseudomonas aeruginosa	*Aspergillus* spp.
Non-*aeruginosa Pseudomonas* spp.[a]	

[a] Often associated with intravenous catheters.

sometimes be necessary early in the course of disease, but it can often be performed after chemotherapy, when the PMN count increases.

Sweet's syndrome, or *febrile neutrophilic dermatosis*, was originally described in women with elevated white blood cell counts. The disease is characterized by the presence of leukocytes in the lower dermis, with edema of the papillary body. Ironically, this disease now is usually seen in neutropenic patients with cancer, most often in association with acute leukemia but also in association with a variety of other malignancies. Sweet's syndrome usually presents as red or bluish-red papules or nodules that may coalesce and form sharply bordered plaques. The edema may suggest vesicles, but on palpation the lesions are solid, and vesicles probably never arise in this disease. The lesions are most common on the face, neck, and arms. On the legs, they may be confused with erythema nodosum. The development of lesions is often accompanied by high fevers and an elevated erythrocyte sedimentation rate. Both the lesions and the temperature elevation respond dramatically to glucocorticoids. Treatment begins with high doses of glucocorticoids (60 mg of prednisone per day) followed by tapered doses over the next 2 to 3 weeks.

Data indicate that *erythema multiforme* with mucous membrane involvement is often associated with herpes simplex virus (HSV) infection and is distinct from Stevens-Johnson syndrome, which is associated with drugs and tends to have a more widespread distribution. Since cancer patients are both immunosuppressed (and therefore susceptible to herpes infections) and heavily treated with drugs (and therefore subject to Stevens-Johnson syndrome), both of these conditions are common in this population.

Cytokines, which are used as adjuvants or primary treatments for cancer, can themselves cause characteristic rashes, further complicating the differential diagnosis. This phenomenon is a particular problem in bone marrow transplant recipients (Chap. 136), who, in addition to having the usual chemotherapy-, antibiotic-, and cytokine-induced rashes, are plagued by graft-versus-host disease.

CATHETER-RELATED INFECTIONS Because intravenous catheters are commonly used in cancer chemotherapy and are prone to infection (Chap. 135), they pose a major problem in the care of patients with cancer. Reviews have emphasized that some infected catheters can be treated with antibiotics while others must be removed. If the patient has a "tunneled" catheter (which consists of an entrance site, a subcutaneous tunnel, and an exit site), a red streak over the subcutaneous part of the line (the tunnel) is grounds for immediate removal of the catheter. Failure to remove catheters under these circumstances may result in extensive cellulitis and tissue necrosis.

More common than tunnel infections are exit-site infections, often with erythema around the area where the line penetrates the skin. Most authorities (Chap. 139) recommend treatment (usually with vancomycin) for an exit-site infection caused by a coagulase-negative *Staphylococcus*. Treatment of coagulase-positive staphylococcal infection is associated with a poorer outcome, and it is advisable to remove the catheter. Similarly, many clinicians remove catheters associated with infections due to *P. aeruginosa* and *Candida* species, since such infections are difficult to treat and bloodstream infections with these organisms are likely to be deadly.

GASTROINTESTINAL TRACT–SPECIFIC SYNDROMES

Upper Gastrointestinal Tract Disease • *Infections of the mouth* The oral cavity is rich in aerobic and anaerobic bacteria (Chap. 167) that normally live in a commensal relationship with the host. The antimetabolic effects of chemotherapy cause a breakdown of host defenses, leading to ulceration of the mouth and the potential for invasion by resident bacteria. Mouth ulcerations afflict most patients receiving chemotherapy and have been associated with viridans streptococcal bacteremia. A variety of topical rinses and elixirs have been proposed to treat these ulcerations. Although some may have a local anesthetic effect, the efficacy of any of these therapies in the prevention of disease is unproven. Similarly, the efficacy of mouthwashes in the prevention of esophagitis or invasive candidiasis is doubtful. Fluconazole, on the other hand, is clearly effective in the treatment of both local infections (thrush) and systemic infections (esophagitis) due to *C. albicans*.

Noma (or *cancrum oris*), commonly seen in malnourished children, is a penetrating disease of the soft and hard tissues of the mouth and adjacent sites, with resulting necrosis and gangrene. It has a counterpart in immunocompromised patients and is thought to be due to invasion of the tissues by *Bacteroides, Fusobacterium*, and other normal inhabitants of the mouth. It is associated with debility, poor oral hygiene, and immunosuppression.

Viruses, particularly HSV, are a prominent cause of morbidity in immunocompromised patients, in whom they are associated with severe mucositis. The use of acyclovir, either prophylactically or therapeutically, is of value.

Esophageal infections The differential diagnosis of esophagitis (usually presenting as substernal chest pain upon swallowing) includes herpes simplex and candidiasis, both of which are readily treatable.

Lower Gastrointestinal Tract Disease Hepatic candidiasis (Chap. 205) results from seeding of the liver (usually from a gastrointestinal source) in neutropenic patients. It is most common in patients being treated for acute leukemia and usually develops around the time the neutropenia resolves. The characteristic picture is that of persistent fever unresponsive to antibiotics; abdominal pain and tenderness or nausea; and elevated serum levels of alkaline phosphatase in a patient with hematologic malignancy who has recently recovered from neutropenia. The diagnosis of this disease (which may present in an indolent manner and persist for several months) is based on the finding of yeasts or pseudohyphae in granulomatous lesions. Hepatic ultrasound or computed tomography (CT) may reveal bull's-eye lesions. In some cases, magnetic resonance imaging (MRI) reveals small lesions not visible by other imaging modalities. The pathology (a granulomatous response) and the timing (with resolution of neutropenia and an elevation in granulocyte count) suggest that the host response to *Candida* is an important component of the manifestations of disease. In many cases, although organisms are visible, cultures of biopsied material may be negative. The designation *hepatosplenic candidiasis* or *hepatic candidiasis* is a misnomer because the disease often involves the kidneys and other tissues; the term *chronic disseminated candidiasis* may be more appropriate. Because of the risk of bleeding with liver biopsy, diagnosis is often based on radiographic abnormalities. Amphotericin B is traditionally used for therapy (often for several months, until all manifestations of disease have disappeared), but fluconazole may be useful for outpatient therapy.

Typhlitis *Typhlitis*, sometimes referred to as necrotizing colitis, neutropenic colitis, necrotizing enteropathy, ileocecal syndrome, or cecitis, is a clinical syndrome of fever and right-lower-quadrant tenderness in an immunosuppressed host. This syndrome is almost always seen in neutropenic patients after chemotherapy with cytotoxic drugs. It may be more common among children than among adults and appears to be much more common among patients with acute myelocytic leukemia (AML) or ALL than among those with other types of cancer.

Physical examination reveals right-lower-quadrant tenderness, with or without rebound tenderness. Associated diarrhea (often bloody) is common, and the diagnosis can be confirmed by the finding of a thickened cecal wall on CT or ultrasonography. Plain films may reveal a right-lower-quadrant mass, but CT with contrast or MRI is a much more sensitive means of making the diagnosis. Although surgery is sometimes attempted to avoid perforation from ischemia, most cases resolve with medical therapy alone. The disease is sometimes associated with positive blood cultures (usually for aerobic gram-negative bacilli), and therapy is recommended for a broad spectrum of bacteria (particularly gram-negative bacilli, likely bowel flora). Recurrence is rare, and most patients recover uneventfully.

***Clostridium difficile*–Induced Diarrhea** Cancer patients seem to be predisposed to the development of *C. difficile* diarrhea (Chap. 145) as a consequence of chemotherapy alone. Thus, they may have positive toxin tests before receiving antibiotics. Obviously, such patients are also subject to *C. difficile*–induced diarrhea as a result of antibiotic pressure. It is worth noting that toxins other than *C. difficile* may be associated with diarrhea; therefore, the detection of nonspecific toxins in the stool—without a specific neutralization test—does not prove that *C. difficile* infection is present.

CENTRAL NERVOUS SYSTEM–SPECIFIC SYNDROMES

Meningitis While meningitis in immunocompetent adults is likely to be caused by *S. pneumoniae*, the same is not true in immunocompromised patients. As noted previously, splenectomized patients are susceptible to rapid overwhelming infection with encapsulated bacteria (including *S. pneumoniae, H. influenzae*, and *N. meningitidis*). Similarly, patients who are antibody-deficient (such as patients with CLL, those who have received intensive chemotherapy, or those who have undergone bone marrow transplantation) are likely to have infections with these bacteria. Other cancer patients, however, because of their defective cellular immunity, are likely to be infected with other pathogens (Table 85-3). The presentation of meningitis in patients with lymphoma, patients receiving chemotherapy (particularly with glucocorticoids) for solid tumors, and patients who have received bone marrow transplants suggests a diagnosis of cryptococcal or listerial infection.

Encephalitis The spectrum of disease resulting from viral encephalitis is expanded in immunocompromised patients. Infection with varicella-zoster virus (VZV) has been associated with encephalitis that may be caused by VZV-related vasculitis. The slow viruses (e.g., Creutzfeldt-Jakob agent) may also be associated with dementia and encephalitic presentations, and a diagnosis of progressive multifocal leukoencephalopathy should be considered when a patient who has received chemotherapy presents with dementia. Other abnormalities of the central nervous system (CNS) that may be confused with infection include normal-pressure hydrocephalus and vasculitis resulting from CNS irradiation. It may be possible to differentiate these conditions by MRI.

Brain Abscess Brain abscesses in immunocompromised patients are likely to be due to *Cryptococcus* (particularly in patients with lymphoma or those receiving glucocorticoids), *Nocardia*, or *Aspergillus*. *Aspergillus* may enter via the lungs or—like *Mucor*—may invade the hard and soft palates to cause pneumonia (see below) with or without brain abscesses.

PULMONARY INFECTIONS

Pneumonia (Chap. 255) in immunocompromised patients may be difficult to diagnose because conventional methods of diagnosis depend on the presence of neutrophils. Bacterial pneumonia in neutropenic patients may present without purulent sputum—or, in fact, without any sputum at all—and may not produce physical findings suggestive of chest consolidation (rales or egophony).

In granulocytopenic patients with persistent or recurrent fever, the chest x-ray pattern may help to localize an infection and thus to determine which investigative tests and procedures should be undertaken and which therapeutic options should be considered (Table 85-5). The difficulties encountered in the management of pulmonary infiltrates relate in part to the difficulties of performing diagnostic procedures on

Table 85-5 Differential Diagnosis of Chest Infiltrates in Immunocompromised Patients

| Infiltrate | Cause of Pneumonia | |
	Infectious	Noninfectious
Localized	Common bacterial pulmonary pathogens, *Legionella*, mycobacteria	Local hemorrhage or embolism, tumor
Nodular	Fungi (e.g., *Aspergillus* or *Mucor*), *Nocardia*	Recurrent tumor
Diffuse	Viruses (especially CMV), *Chlamydia*, *Pneumocystis carinii*, *Toxoplasma gondii*, mycobacteria	Congestive heart failure, radiation pneumonitis, drug-induced lung injury, diffuse alveolar hemorrhage (described after BMT)

ABBREVIATIONS: CMV, cytomegalovirus; BMT, bone marrow transplantation.

the patients involved. When platelet counts can be increased to adequate levels by transfusion, microscopic and microbiologic evaluation of the fluid obtained by endoscopic bronchial lavage is often diagnostic. Lavage fluid should be cultured for *Mycoplasma*, *Chlamydia*, *Legionella*, *Nocardia*, fungi, and more common bacterial pathogens. In addition, the possibility of *P. carinii* pneumonia should be considered, especially in patients with ALL or lymphoma who have not received prophylactic trimethoprim-sulfamethoxazole. The characteristics of the infiltrate may be helpful in decisions about further diagnostic and therapeutic maneuvers. Nodular infiltrates suggest fungal pneumonia (e.g., that caused by *Aspergillus* or *Mucor*). Such lesions may best be approached by visualized biopsy procedures.

Aspergillus species (Chap. 206) can colonize the skin and respiratory tract or cause fatal systemic illness. Although *Aspergillus* may cause aspergillomas in a previously existing cavity or may produce allergic bronchopulmonary aspergillosis, the major problem posed by this genus in neutropenic patients is invasive disease due to *A. fumigatus* or *A. flavus*. The organisms enter the host through colonization of the respiratory tract, with subsequent invasion of the blood vessels. The disease is likely to present as a thrombotic or embolic event because of the ability of the organisms to invade blood vessels. The risk of infection with *Aspergillus* correlates directly with the duration of neutropenia. In prolonged neutropenia, positive surveillance cultures for colonization of the nasopharynx with *Aspergillus* may predict the development of disease.

Patients with *Aspergillus* infection often present with pleuritic chest pain and fever, which are sometimes accompanied by cough. Hemoptysis may be an ominous sign. Chest x-rays may reveal new focal infiltrates or nodules. Chest CT may reveal a characteristic halo consisting of a mass-like infiltrate surrounded by an area of low attenuation. The presence of a "crescent sign" on a chest x-ray or a chest CT scan, in which the mass progresses to central cavitation, is characteristic of invasive *Aspergillus* infection but may develop only with the resolution of the lesions.

In addition to causing pulmonary presentations, *Aspergillus* may invade through the nose or palate, with deep sinus penetration. The appearance of a discolored area in the nasal passages or on the hard palate should prompt a search for invasive *Aspergillus*. This situation is likely to require surgical debridement. Treatment (Chap. 206) with high doses of amphotericin B has been successful in curing granulocytopenic patients of invasive *Aspergillus* infection after the return of granulocytes. Catheter infections with *Aspergillus* usually require both removal of the catheter and antifungal therapy.

Diffuse interstitial infiltrates suggest viral, parasitic, or *P. carinii* pneumonia. If the patient has a diffuse interstitial pattern on chest x-ray, it may be reasonable to institute empirical treatment with trimethoprim-sulfamethoxazole (for *Pneumocystis*) and an erythromycin derivative or a quinolone (for *Chlamydia*, *Mycoplasma*, and *Legionella*) while considering invasive diagnostic procedures. Noninvasive procedures, such as staining of sputum smears for *Pneumocystis* and serum cryptococcal antigen tests, may be helpful on occasion. In trans-

plant recipients who are seropositive for cytomegalovirus (CMV), culture of a nonpulmonary site for CMV may be worthwhile. Infections with viruses that cause only upper respiratory symptoms in immunocompetent hosts, such as respiratory syncytial, influenza, and parainfluenza viruses, may be associated with fatal pneumonitis in immunocompromised hosts. An attempt at early diagnosis by nasopharyngeal aspiration should be considered so that appropriate treatment can be instituted.

While bleomycin is the most common cause of chemotherapy-induced lung disease, other causes include alkylating agents (such as cyclophosphamide, chlorambucil, and melphalan), nitrosoureas [carmustine (BCNU), lomustine (CCNU), and methyl-CCNU], busulfan, procarbazine, methotrexate, and hydroxyurea. Both infectious and noninfectious (drug- and/or radiation-induced) pneumonitis can cause fever and abnormalities on chest x-ray; thus, the differential diagnosis of an infiltrate in a patient receiving chemotherapy encompasses a broad range of conditions (Table 85-5). Since the treatment of radiation pneumonitis (which may respond dramatically to glucocorticoids) or drug-induced pneumonitis is different from that of infectious pneumonia, a biopsy may be important in the diagnosis. Unfortunately, no definitive diagnosis can be made in approximately 30% of cases, even after bronchoscopy.

Open-lung biopsy is the "gold standard" of diagnostic techniques. Biopsy via a visualized thoracostomy can replace an open procedure in many cases. When a biopsy cannot be performed, empirical treatment can be undertaken with erythromycin (or an erythromycin derivative such as azithromycin) and trimethoprim-sulfamethoxazole (in the case of diffuse infiltrates) or with amphotericin B (in the case of nodular infiltrates). The risks should be weighed carefully in these cases. If inappropriate drugs are administered, empirical treatment may prove toxic or ineffective; either of these outcomes may be riskier than biopsy.

CARDIOVASCULAR INFECTIONS Patients with Hodgkin's disease are prone to persistent infections by *Salmonella*, sometimes (and particularly often in elderly patients) affecting a vascular site. The use of intravenous catheters deliberately lodged in the right atrium is associated with a high incidence of bacterial endocarditis (presumably related to valve damage followed by bacteremia). Nonbacterial thrombotic endocarditis has been described in association with a variety of malignancies (most often solid tumors) and may follow bone marrow transplantation as well. The presentation of an embolic event with a new cardiac murmur suggests this diagnosis. Blood cultures are negative in this disease of unknown pathogenesis.

ENDOCRINE SYNDROMES In addition to infections of the skin, gastrointestinal tract, and pulmonary system, infections of the endocrine system have been described in immunocompromised patients. *Candida* infection of the thyroid during neutropenia can be defined by indium-labeled white-cell scans or gallium scans after neutrophil counts increase. CMV infection can cause adrenalitis with or without resulting adrenal insufficiency. The presentation of a sudden endocrine anomaly in an immunocompromised patient may be a sign of infection in the involved end organ.

MUSCULOSKELETAL INFECTIONS Infection that is a result of vascular compromise (resulting in gangrene) can occur when a tumor compromises the blood supply to muscles, bones, or joints. The process of diagnosis and treatment of such infection is similar to that in normal hosts, with the following caveats: (1) In terms of diagnosis, a lack of physical findings resulting from a lack of granulocytes in the granulocytopenic patient should make the clinician more aggressive in obtaining tissue rather than relying on physical signs. (2) In terms of therapy, aggressive debridement of infected tissues may be required, but it is usually difficult to operate on patients who have recently received chemotherapy, both because of a lack of platelets (which results in bleeding complications) and because of a lack of white blood cells (which may lead to secondary infection). A blood culture positive for *Clostridium perfringens* (an organism commonly associated with gas gangrene) can have a number of meanings (Chap. 145). Bloodstream infections with intestinal organisms like *Streptococcus bovis* and *C. perfringens* may arise spontaneously from lower gastrointestinal lesions (tumor or polyps); alternatively, these lesions may be harbingers of invasive disease. The clinical setting must be considered in order to define the appropriate treatment for each case.

RENAL AND URETERAL INFECTIONS Infections of the urinary tract are common among patients whose ureteral excretion is compromised (Table 85-1). *Candida*, which has a predilection for the kidney, can invade either from the bloodstream or in a retrograde manner (via the ureters or bladder) in immunocompromised patients. The presence of "fungus balls" or persistent candiduria suggests invasive disease. Persistent funguria (with *Aspergillus* as well as *Candida*) should prompt a search for a nidus of infection in the kidney.

Certain viruses are typically seen only in immunosuppression. BK virus (polyomavirus hominis 1) has been documented in the urine of bone marrow transplant recipients and, like adenovirus, may be associated with hemorrhagic cystitis. BK-induced cystitis usually remits with decreasing immunosuppression. Anecdotal reports have described the treatment of adenovirus with ribavirin in cases of severe hemorrhagic cystitis in immunocompromised patients.

ABNORMALITIES THAT PREDISPOSE TO INFECTION

THE LYMPHOID SYSTEM It is beyond the scope of this chapter to detail how all the immunologic abnormalities that result from cancer or from chemotherapy for cancer lead to infections. Disorders of the immune system are discussed in other sections of this book. As has been noted, patients with antibody deficiency are predisposed to overwhelming infection with encapsulated bacteria (including *S. pneumoniae, H. influenzae*, and *N. meningitidis*). Infections that result from the lack of a functional cellular immune system are described in Chap. 309. It is worth mentioning, however, that patients undergoing intensive chemotherapy for any form of cancer will have not only defects due to granulocytopenia but also lymphocyte dysfunction, which may be profound. Thus, these patients—especially those receiving glucocorticoid-containing regimens—should be given prophylaxis for *P. carinii* pneumonia.

THE HEMATOPOIETIC SYSTEM Initial studies in the 1960s revealed a dramatic increase in the incidence of infections (fatal and nonfatal) among cancer patients with a granulocyte count of <500/μL. Recent studies have cited a figure of 48.3 infections per 100 neutropenic patients (<1000 granulocytes per microliter) with hematologic malignancies and solid tumors, or 46.3 infections per 1000 days at risk.

Neutropenic patients are unusually susceptible to infection with a wide variety of bacteria; thus, antibiotic therapy should be initiated promptly to cover likely pathogens if infection is suspected. Indeed, early initiation of antibacterial agents is mandatory to prevent deaths. These patients are susceptible to gram-positive and gram-negative organisms found commonly on the skin and in the bowel (Table 85-4). Because treatment with narrow-spectrum agents leads to infection with organisms not covered by the antibiotics used, the initial regimen should target pathogens likely to be initial causes of bacterial infection in neutropenic hosts (Fig. 85-1).

℞ **TREATMENT Antibacterial Therapy** Hundreds of antibacterial regimens have been tested for use in neutropenic patients with cancer. Many of the relevant studies involved small populations in which the outcomes were generally good, and most lacked the statistical power to detect differences among the regimens studied. Each febrile neutropenic patient should be approached as a unique problem, with particular attention given to previous infections and recent exposures to antibiotics. Several general guidelines are useful in the initial treatment of neutropenic patients with fever (Fig. 85-1):

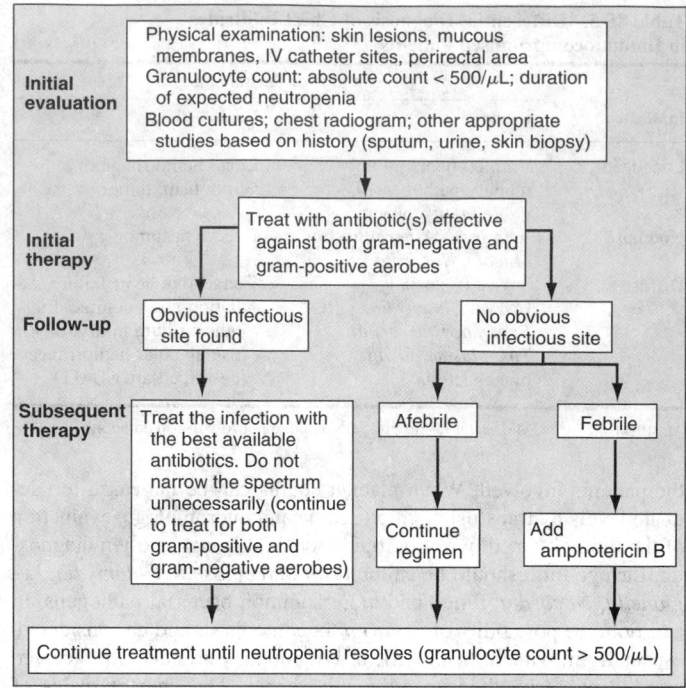

FIGURE 85-1 Diagnosis and treatment of febrile neutropenic patients: an algorithm.

1. It is necessary to use antibiotics active against both gram-negative and gram-positive bacteria (Table 85-4) in the initial regimen.
2. An aminoglycoside or an antibiotic without good activity against gram-positive organisms (e.g., ciprofloxacin) alone is not adequate in this setting.
3. The agents used should reflect both the epidemiology and the antibiotic resistance pattern of the hospital. For example, in hospitals where there is gentamicin resistance, amikacin-containing regimens should be considered; in hospitals with frequent *P. aeruginosa* infections, a regimen with the highest level of activity against this pathogen (such as tobramycin plus a semisynthetic penicillin) would be reasonable for initial therapy.
4. A single third-generation cephalosporin constitutes an appropriate initial regimen in many hospitals (if the pattern of resistance justifies its use).
5. Most standard regimens are designed for patients who have not previously received prophylactic antibiotics. The development of fever in a patient receiving antibiotics affects the choice of subsequent therapy (which should target resistant organisms and organisms known to cause infections in patients being treated with the antibiotics already administered).
6. Randomized trials have indicated that it is safe to use oral antibiotic regimens to treat "low-risk" patients with fever and neutropenia. Outpatients who are expected to remain neutropenic for <10 days and who have no concurrent medical problems (such as hypotension, pulmonary compromise, or abdominal pain) can be classified as low risk and treated with a broad-spectrum oral regimen. On the basis of large studies, it can be concluded that this therapy is safe and effective, at least when delivered in the inpatient setting. Outpatient treatment has been assessed in small studies, but data from large randomized trials demonstrating the safety of outpatient treatment of fever and neutropenia are not yet available.

The initial antibacterial regimen should be refined on the basis of culture results (Fig. 85-1). Blood cultures are the most relevant on which to base therapy; surface cultures of skin and mucous membranes may be misleading. In the case of gram-positive bacteremia or another gram-positive infection, it is important that the antibiotic be optimal for the organism isolated. If the infection is caused by certain gram-negative pathogens (such as *P. aeruginosa*), a synergistic combination of antibiotics (usually a semisynthetic penicillin, such as piperacillin, plus an aminoglycoside) may be appropriate. Although it is not desirable to leave the patient unprotected, the addition of more and more antibacterial agents to the regimen is not appropriate unless there is a clinical or microbiologic reason to do so. *Planned progressive therapy* (the serial, empirical addition of one drug after another without culture data) is not efficacious in most settings and may have unfortunate consequences. Simply adding another antibiotic for fear that a gram-negative infection is present is a dubious practice. The synergy exhibited by β-lactams and aminoglycosides against certain gram-negative organisms (especially *P. aeruginosa*) provides the rationale for using two antibiotics in this setting. Mere addition of a quinolone or another antibiotic not likely to exhibit synergy for "double coverage" has not been shown to be of benefit and may cause additional toxicities and side effects. Cephalosporins can cause bone marrow suppression, and vancomycin is associated with neutropenia in some healthy people (Chap. 137). Furthermore, the addition of multiple cephalosporins may induce β lactamase production by some organisms; cephalosporins and double β-lactam combinations should probably be avoided altogether in *Enterobacter* infections.

Antifungal Therapy Fungal infections in cancer patients are most often associated with neutropenia. Neutropenic patients are predisposed to the development of invasive fungal infections, most commonly those due to *Candida* and *Aspergillus* species and occasionally those caused by *Fusarium*, *Trichosporon*, and *Bipolaris*. Cryptococcal infection, which is common among patients taking immunosuppressive agents, is uncommon among neutropenic patients receiving chemotherapy for AML. Invasive candidal disease is usually caused by *C. albicans* or *C. tropicalis* but can be caused by *C. krusei*, *C. parapsilosis*, and *C. glabrata*.

Most clinicians add amphotericin B to antibacterial regimens if a neutropenic patient remains febrile despite 4 to 7 days of treatment with antibacterial agents. The rationale for the empirical addition of amphotericin B is that it is difficult to culture fungi before they cause disseminated disease and that mortality from disseminated fungal infections in granulocytopenic patients is high. The imidazoles (especially fluconazole) may have prophylactic efficacy in this regard, but the spectrum of activity of the currently available azoles is narrower than that of amphotericin B. Amphotericin B is the mainstay of therapy for disseminated *Candida* or *Aspergillus* infection in the neutropenic patient. The combined use of an imidazole and amphotericin B is controversial because of the theoretical antagonistic effects of these agents. The insolubility of amphotericin B has resulted in the marketing of several amphotericin B–lipid formulations. Lipid preparations have been shown to be less toxic than the amphotericin B deoxycholate complex. However, because of the high cost of the lipid preparations, at many centers their use is reserved for patients who fail to respond to standard amphotericin B. Since the side effects of the formulations differ, unnecessary switching from one to another is not recommended.

Other Therapeutic Modalities Another way to address the problems of the febrile neutropenic patient is to replenish the neutrophil population. Although granulocyte transfusions are efficacious in the treatment of refractory gram-negative bacteremia, they do not have a documented role in prophylaxis. Because of the expense, the risk of leukoagglutinin reactions (although this risk has probably been decreased by improved cell-separation procedures), and the risk of transmission of CMV from unscreened donors, granulocyte transfusion is reserved for patients unresponsive to antibiotics. This modality is efficacious for documented gram-negative bacteremia refractory to antibiotics, particularly in situations where granulocyte numbers will be depressed for only a short period.

A variety of cytokines, including granulocyte colony-stimulating factor and granulocyte-macrophage colony-stimulating factor, enhance granulocyte recovery after chemotherapy and consequently shorten the period of maximal vulnerability to fatal infections. The role of these cytokines in routine practice is still a matter of some debate. Most authorities recommend their use only when neutropenia is both severe and prolonged. The cytokines themselves may have adverse effects, including fever, hypoxemia, and pleural effusions or serositis in other areas. Since there is little evidence that their routine administration lessens the risk of death and since they are still expensive, the cytokines have not become the standard of care in all centers. The role of other cytokines (such as macrophage colony-stimulating factor for monocytes or interferon-γ) in preventing or treating infections in granulocytopenic patients is under investigation.

Once neutropenia has resolved, patients are not at high risk of infection. However, depending on what drugs they receive, patients who continue on chemotherapeutic protocols remain at high risk for certain diseases. Any patient receiving more than a maintenance dose of glucocorticoids (including many treatment regimens for diffuse lymphoma) should also receive prophylactic trimethoprim-sulfamethoxazole because of the risk of *P. carinii* infection; those with ALL should receive such prophylaxis for the duration of chemotherapy.

PREVENTION OF INFECTION IN CANCER PATIENTS

EFFECT OF THE ENVIRONMENT Outbreaks of fatal *Aspergillus* infection have been associated with construction projects and materials in several hospitals. The association between spore counts and risk of infection suggests the need for a high-efficiency air-handling system in hospitals that care for large numbers of neutropenic patients. The use of laminar-flow rooms and prophylactic antibiotics has decreased the number of infectious episodes in severely neutropenic patients. However, because of the expense of such a program and the failure to show that it dramatically affects mortality, most centers do not routinely use laminar flow to care for neutropenic patients. Some centers use "reverse isolation," in which health care providers and visitors to a patient who is neutropenic wear gowns and gloves. Since most of the infections these patients develop are due to organisms that colonize the patients' own skin and bowel, the validity of such schemes is dubious, and limited clinical data do not support their use. Hand washing by all staff caring for neutropenic patients should be required to prevent the spread of resistant organisms.

The presence of large numbers of bacteria (particularly *P. aeruginosa*) in certain foods, especially fresh vegetables, has led some authorities to recommend a special "low-bacteria" diet. A diet consisting of cooked and canned food is satisfactory to most neutropenic patients and does not involve elaborate disinfection or sterilization protocols. However, there are no studies to support even this type of dietary restriction. Counseling of patients to avoid leftovers, deli foods, and unpasteurized dairy products is recommended.

PHYSICAL MEASURES Although few studies address this issue, patients with cancer are predisposed to infections resulting from anatomic compromise (e.g., lymphedema resulting from node dissections after radical mastectomy). Surgeons who specialize in cancer surgery can provide specific guidelines for the care of such patients, and patients benefit from common-sense advice about how to prevent infections in vulnerable areas.

ANTIBIOTIC PROPHYLAXIS There is no consensus on the use of prophylactic antibiotics in neutropenic patients. The incidence of infection is lower among patients who receive broad-spectrum antibiotic prophylaxis than among those who do not. Because of the prolongation of neutropenia associated with the use of trimethoprim-sulfamethoxazole, some clinicians use broad-spectrum agents such as quinolones (e.g., ciprofloxacin). Either regimen can be given orally, and both have the advantage of inactivity against anaerobic organisms; thus, neither is likely to disrupt the bowel flora and permit colonization with new aerobes or *Candida*. However, both regimens have adverse effects and can lead to the selection of resistant organisms in a hospital. For these reasons, many clinicians reserve their use for patients with the longest periods of neutropenia (e.g., bone marrow transplant recipients). The same issues apply to the use of antifungal agents. While agents such as fluconazole may prevent infections with susceptible organisms (e.g., *C. albicans*), they can cause a concomitant increase in infections due to resistant fungi (e.g., *C. krusei*). Thus, the decision to use antifungal prophylaxis may vary with the fungi endemic in a given hospital. Prophylaxis for *P. carinii* is mandatory for patients with ALL and for all cancer patients receiving glucocorticoid-containing chemotherapy regimens.

VACCINATION OF CANCER PATIENTS   In general, patients undergoing chemotherapy respond less well to vaccines than normal hosts. Their greater need for vaccines thus leads to a dilemma in their management. Purified proteins and inactivated vaccines are almost never contraindicated and should be given to patients even during chemotherapy. For example, all adults should receive diphtheria-tetanus toxoid boosters at the indicated times as well as seasonal influenza vaccine. However, if possible, vaccination should not be undertaken concurrent with cytotoxic chemotherapy. If patients are expected to be receiving chemotherapy for several months and vaccination is indicated (for example, influenza vaccination in the fall), the vaccine should be given midcycle—as far as possible from the antimetabolic agents that will prevent an immune response. The meningococcal and pneumococcal polysaccharide vaccines should be given to patients before splenectomy, if possible. The Advisory Committee on Immunization Practices recommends reimmunization every 5 years for the pneumococcal vaccine; although no official stand has been taken, this recommendation seems reasonable for the meningococcal vaccine as well. The *H. influenzae* type b conjugate vaccine should be administered to all splenectomized patients; there is no current recommendation for reimmunization, but immunity appears to be much longer-lasting than that induced by polysaccharide vaccines.

In general, live virus (or live bacterial) vaccines should not be given to patients during intensive chemotherapy because of the risk of disseminated infection. Recommendations on vaccination are summarized in Table 85-2.

BIBLIOGRAPHY

DE PAUW BE, DOMPELING EC: Antibiotic strategy after the empiric phase in patients treated for a hematological malignancy. Ann Hematol 72:273, 1996

FREIFELD A et al: A double-blind trial of oral versus intravenous antibiotics for empirical therapy in low risk patients with fever and neutropenia from cancer chemotherapy. N Engl J Med 341:305, 1999

HUGHES WT et al: 1997 guidelines for the use of antimicrobial agents in neutropenic patients with unexplained fever. Clin Infect Dis 25:551, 1997

INTERNATIONAL ANTIMICROBIAL THERAPY COOPERATIVE GROUP OF THE EORTC: Oral versus intravenous antimicrobials as empirical therapy in cancer patients with fever and granulocytopenia. N Engl J Med 341:312, 1999

MALIK IA et al: Feasibility of outpatient management of fever in cancer patients with low-risk neutropenia: Results of a prospective randomized trial. Am J Med 98:224, 1995

RODRIGUEZ-ADRIAN LJ et al: The potential role of cytokine therapy for fungal infections in patients with cancer: Is recovery from neutropenia all that is needed? Clin Infect Dis 26:1270, 1998

WONG-BERINGER A et al: Lipid formulations of amphotericin B: Clinical efficacy and toxicities. Clin Infect Dis 27:603, 1998

86

Arthur J. Sober, Howard K. Koh, Gregory P. Wittenberg, Carl V. Washington, Jr.

MELANOMA AND OTHER SKIN CANCERS

Pigmented skin lesions are among the most common findings on physical examination. The challenge is to distinguish cutaneous melanomas, which may be lethal, from the remainder, which with rare exceptions are benign. Cutaneous neoplasms are depicted in Section IIB (**Plates IIB-20 to -27**) of the Color Atlas; benign and malignant pigmented lesions are in Section IIC (**Plates IIC-28 to -33**).

MELANOMA

Melanomas originate from melanocytes, pigment cells normally present in the epidermis and sometimes in the dermis. This tumor affects approximately 44,200 individuals per year in the United States, resulting in 7300 deaths. The tumor can affect adults of all ages, even teenagers; it has distinct clinical features that make it detectable at a time when cure by surgical excision is possible; and it is located on the skin surface, where it is visible. The incidence has increased dramatically; if the incidence continues to increase at the present rate, within a decade, lifetime risk of melanoma will exceed 1%.

The reason for the increase in melanoma incidence is thought to be increased recreational sun exposure, especially early in life. Individuals of similar ethnic background who immigrate after childhood to areas of high sun exposure (e.g., Israel and Australia) have lower melanoma rates than individuals of similar age who were either born in those countries or immigrated before age 10. The individuals most susceptible to development of melanoma are those with fair complexions, red or blond hair, blue eyes, and freckles and who tan poorly and sunburn easily. Most studies link increased melanoma risk to history of sunburn. Other factors associated with increased risk include a family history of melanoma (1 in 10 melanoma patients have an affected family member); the presence of a clinically atypical mole (dysplastic nevus), a giant congenital melanocytic nevus, or a small to medium-sized congenital melanocytic nevus (see below); the presence of a higher than average number of ordinary melanocytic nevi; and immunosuppression (Table 86-1). Individuals with 50 or more moles ≥2 mm in size have a 64-fold increased risk. About 30% of melanomas arise in a nevus. Melanoma is relatively rare in heavily pigmented peoples. Dark-skinned populations (such as those of India and Puerto Rico), blacks, and East Asians have rates 10 to 20 times lower than lighter-skinned whites. In keeping with the role of sun exposure, the incidence is inversely correlated with the latitude of residence; at any latitude, however, darker-skinned persons have a lower incidence.

CLINICAL CHARACTERISTICS   There are four types of cutaneous melanoma (Table 86-2). In three of these—superficial spreading melanoma, lentigo maligna melanoma, and acral lentiginous melanoma—the lesion has a period of superficial (so-called radial) growth during which it increases in size but does not penetrate deeply. During this period, the melanoma is most capable of being cured by surgical excision. The fourth type—nodular melanoma—does not have a recognizable radial growth phase and usually presents as a deeply invasive lesion, capable of early metastasis. When tumors begin to penetrate deeply into the skin, they are in the so-called vertical growth phase. Melanomas with a radial growth phase are characterized by irregular and sometimes notched borders, variation in pigment pattern, and variation in color. An increase in size or change in color is noted by the patient in 70% of early lesions. Bleeding, ulceration, and pain are late signs and are of little help in early recognition. Nodular melanomas are dark brown-black to blue-black nodules. Melanomas are occasionally amelanotic, in which case the diagnosis is established

Table 86-1   Risk Factors for Cutaneous Melanoma

High risk (>50-fold increase in risk)
  Persistently changing mole
  Clinically atypical moles in patient with two family members with melanoma
  Adulthood (vs. childhood)
  >50 nevi ≥2 mm in diameter
Intermediate risk (~10-fold increase in risk)
  Family history of melanoma
  Sporadic clinically atypical moles
  Congenital nevi (?)
  White ethnicity (vs black or East Asian ethnicity)
  Personal history of prior melanoma
Low risk (2- to 4-fold increase in risk)
  Immunosuppression
  Sun sensitivity or excess exposure to sun

SOURCE: Adapted from AR Rhodes et al: JAMA 258:3146, 1987.

histologically after biopsy of a new or changing skin growth. Lentigo maligna melanoma is usually confined to chronically sun-damaged sites (face, neck, back of hands) in older individuals. Acral lentiginous melanoma occurs on the palms, soles, nail beds, and mucous membranes. While this type occurs in whites, it is most frequent (along with nodular melanoma) in blacks and East Asians. Superficial spreading melanoma is most frequent in whites. Melanomas arising in dysplastic nevi (see below) are usually of this type. The back is the most common site for melanoma in men. In women, the back and the lower leg (knee to ankle) are frequent sites.

PROGNOSTIC FACTORS The most important prognostic factor is the stage at the time of presentation [see the discussion of revised American Joint Cancer Commission (AJCC) stages, below]. Five-year survival for clinical stages I and II (primary tumor; no clinical evidence of disease elsewhere) is about 85%. For clinical stage III (clinically palpable regional nodes that contain tumor), the 5-year survival is about 50% when only one node is involved and about 15 to 20% when four or more nodes are involved. The 5-year survival for clinical stage IV (disseminated disease) is <5%. Fortunately, most melanomas are diagnosed in clinical stages I and II. Within these stages, the prognosis depends on the thickness of the primary tumor (Table 86-3). This system is based on the rationale that the likelihood of metastasis should correlate with tumor volume, with thickness being the best single index of tumor volume. Melanomas <0.76 mm thick are usually cured by surgical removal (with 5-year survival rates of 96 to 99%). Approximately 40% of primary melanomas now fall in a low-risk category (thickness <1 mm). In low-risk patients who develop metastases, the primary tumors often exhibit either microscopic features of anaplasia or a vertical growth phase. More than 50% of individuals with melanomas ≥4 mm thick will develop metastatic disease and die of their melanoma (Table 86-3). These thick tumors are almost always raised above the plane of the skin. Certain anatomic sites affect the prognosis. The favorable sites appear to be the forearm and leg (excluding feet), while unfavorable sites include scalp, hands, feet, and mucous membranes. In general, women with stage I or II disease have a better survival than men, perhaps in part because of earlier diagnosis; women frequently have melanomas on the lower leg, where self-recognition is more likely and prognosis is better. Older individuals have poorer prognoses. This finding has been explained in part by a tendency toward later diagnosis (and thus thicker tumors) in men and by a higher proportion in men of acral melanomas (palmar-plantar), which have a poorer prognosis. Melanoma may recur after many years. About 10 to 15% of first-time recurrences develop more than 5 years after treatment of the original lesion. The time to recurrence varies inversely with tumor thickness. Other prognostic factors for stages I and II melanoma include the presence of an ulcer in the primary tumor, high mitotic rate, and the presence of microscopic tumor satellites (foci of tumor ≥0.05 mm in diameter in the reticular dermis or subcutaneous fat, distinct from the main body of the tumor). The presence of microscopic satellites is also predictive of microscopic metastases to the regional lymph nodes. An alternative prognostic scheme for clinical stages I and II melanoma, proposed by Clark, is based on the anatomic level of invasion in the skin. Level I is intraepidermal (in situ); level II penetrates the papillary dermis; level III spans the papillary dermis; level IV penetrates the reticular dermis; and level V penetrates into the subcutaneous fat. The 5-year survival for these stages averages 100, 95, 82, 71, and 49%, respectively.

NATURAL HISTORY Melanomas may spread by the lymphatic channels or the bloodstream. The earliest metastases are often to regional lymph nodes. Surgical lymphadenectomy usually controls regional disease. Liver, lung, bone, and brain are common sites of hematogenous spread, but unusual sites, such as the anterior chamber of the eye, may also be involved. Once metastatic disease is established, the likelihood of cure is low.

MANAGEMENT The entire cutaneous surface, including the scalp and mucous membranes, should be examined in each patient. Bright room illumination is important, and a 7× to 10× hand lens is helpful for evaluating variation in pigment pattern. A history of relevant risk factors should be elicited. Any suspicious lesions should be biopsied, evaluated by a specialist, or recorded by chart and/or photography for follow-up. Examination of the lymph nodes and palpation

Table 86-2 Clinical Features of Malignant Melanoma

Type	Site	Average Age at Diagnosis, Years	Duration of Known Existence, Years	Color
Lentigo maligna melanoma	Sun-exposed surfaces, particularly malar region of cheek and temple	70	5–20[a] or longer	In flat portions, shades of brown and tan predominant, but whitish gray occasionally present; in nodules, shades of reddish brown, bluish gray, bluish black
Superficial spreading melanoma	Any site (more common on upper back and, in women, on lower legs)	40–50	1–7	Shades of brown mixed with bluish red (violaceous), bluish black, reddish brown, and often whitish pink, and the border of lesion is at least in part visibly and/or palpably elevated
Nodular melanoma	Any site	40–50	Months to less than 5 years	Reddish blue (purple) or bluish black; either uniform in color or mixed with brown or black
Acral lentiginous melanoma	Palm, sole, nail bed, mucous membrane	60	1–10	In flat portions, dark brown predominantly; in raised lesions (plaques) brown-black or blue-black predominantly

[a] During much of this time, the precursor stage, lentigo maligna, is confined to the epidermis.
SOURCE: Adapted from AJ Sober, in *Pathophysiology of Dermatologic Diseases*, NA Soter, HP Baden (eds). New York, McGraw-Hill, 1984.

Table 86-3 Prognosis of Melanoma by Thickness (Breslow) and AJCC Stages: 5-Year Survival Rates

AJCC Stage	Thickness Range, mm	% Overall Survival
IA (localized)	≤0.75	96
IB (localized)	0.76–1.49	87
IIA (localized)	1.5–2.49	75
	2.50–3.99	66
IIB (localized)	≥4.00	47
III (metastatic to regional nodes)		45 (one node)
		<20 (two nodes)
IV (metastatic to distant sites)		8–10[a]

[a] One-year survival.

of the abdominal viscera are part of the staging examination for suspected melanoma. The patient should be advised to have other family members screened if either melanoma or clinically atypical moles (dysplastic nevi) are present. Melanoma prevention is based on protection from the sun. Routine use of a sunblock of SPF ≥15, use of protective clothing, and avoiding intense midday ultraviolet exposure should be recommended. The patient should be educated in the clinical features of melanoma and advised to report any growth or other change in a pigmented lesion. Patient education brochures are available from the American Cancer Society, the American Academy of Dermatology, the National Cancer Institute, and the Skin Cancer Foundation. Self-examination at 6- to 8-week intervals may enhance the likelihood of detecting change between follow-up visits. Routine follow-up visits for melanoma patients and patients with clinically atypical moles (dysplastic nevi) may facilitate early detection of new tumors.

Precursor Lesions Clinically atypical moles, also termed *dysplastic nevi*, occur in certain families affected by melanoma. In some families, melanomas occur nearly exclusively in the individuals with dysplastic nevi. These nevi appear to be transmitted as an autosomal dominant trait that involves chromosome 9p16. In other families, the nevi may not be present in all individuals with an increased risk of melanoma. The melanomas may arise in clinically atypical moles or in normal skin. Individuals with clinically atypical moles and two family members with melanoma have been reported to have a >50% lifetime risk for developing melanoma. Table 86-4 lists the features that are characteristic of clinically atypical moles and that differentiate them from benign acquired nevi. The number of clinically atypical moles may vary from one to several hundred. Clinically atypical moles usually differ from each other in appearance. The borders are often hazy and indistinct, and the pigment pattern is more highly varied than that in benign acquired nevi. Of the 90% of melanoma patients whose disease is regarded as sporadic (i.e., who lack a family history of melanoma), about 40% have clinically atypical moles, as compared with an estimated 5 to 10% of the population at large. The observation that at least 20% of sporadic melanomas arise in association with a clinically atypical mole makes this nevus the most important precursor for melanoma.

Less frequent precursors include the giant congenital melanocytic nevus and the small congenital melanocytic nevus (although the latter relationship is disputed by some). Congenital melanocytic nevi are present at birth or appear in the neonatal period (tardive form). The giant melanocytic nevus, also called the bathing trunk, cape, or garment nevus, is a rare malformation that affects perhaps 1 in 30,000 to 1 in 100,000 individuals. These nevi are usually >20 cm in diameter and may cover more than half the body surface. Giant nevi often occur in association with multiple small congenital nevi. The borders are sharp, and hair may be present. The lesions are usually dark brown and may have darker and lighter areas. Pigment is haphazardly displayed. The surface is smooth to rugose or cerebriform and may vary from one portion of the lesion to another. A lifetime risk of melanoma development of 6% has been estimated. The risk is greatest before age 5 and next greatest between ages 5 and 10. Early detection of melanoma is difficult in these lesions because of the deep dermal or subcutaneous origin of melanoma in these lesions and because of the large and varied surface of the nevus. Prophylactic excision early in life can be accomplished by staged removal with coverage by split-thickness skin grafts. No uniform management guidelines for giant congenital nevi have been developed.

The small- to medium-sized congenital melanocytic nevus, which affects approximately 1% of persons, usually presents as a raised dark- to medium-brown lesion with a smooth or papillomatous surface. The border is sharp, and lesions may be oriented along lines of skin cleavage. Follicular hyper- and hypopigmentation may coexist in a salt-and-pepper configuration. The lesion may have an excess of coarse hairs. Melanoma may develop in these lesions but the risk is not quantitated. Considerations of body surface area suggest that the incidence of melanomas arising in small congenital melanocytic nevi is probably higher than would be expected by chance. The remnants of a nevus with histopathologic features of a congenital nevus have been observed in 2 to 6% of melanomas. The management of small- to medium-sized congenital melanocytic nevi remains controversial; prophylactic removal under local anesthesia in the early teen years is appropriate as melanomas arise later in these lesions.

Differential Diagnosis The aim of differential diagnosis is to distinguish benign pigmented lesions from melanoma and its precursors. If melanoma is a consideration, then biopsy is appropriate. Some benign look-alikes may be removed in the process of trying to detect authentic melanoma. Table 86-5 summarizes the distinguishing features of benign lesions that may be confused with melanoma. Early detection of melanoma may be facilitated by applying the "ABCD rules": A—asymmetry, benign lesions are usually symmetric; B—border irregularity, most nevi have clear-cut borders; C—color variegation, benign lesions usually have uniform light or dark pigment; D—diameter >6 mm (the size of a pencil eraser).

Biopsy Any pigmented cutaneous lesion that has changed in size or shape or has other features suggestive of malignant melanoma should be biopsied. The recommended technique is an excisional biopsy, as that facilitates pathologic assessment of the lesion, permits accurate measurement of thickness if the lesion is melanoma, and constitutes treatment if the lesion is benign. Shave biopsy or curettage of a suspected melanoma is contraindicated. For large lesions or lesions on anatomic sites where excisional biopsy may not be feasible (such as the face, hands, or feet), an incisional biopsy through the most nodular or darkest area of the lesion is acceptable; this should include the vertical growth phase of the primary tumor, if present. Data from prospective studies do not indicate that an incisional biopsy facilitates the spread of melanoma.

Staging Once the diagnosis of malignant melanoma has been confirmed, the tumor must be staged to determine prognosis and treatment. The history should probe for evidence of metastatic disease, such as malaise, weight loss, headaches, visual difficulty, or bone pain. The physical examination should be directed especially to the skin, re-

Table 86-4 Clinical Features Distinguishing Atypical Moles from Benign Acquired Nevi

Clinical Feature	Clinically Atypical Moles	Benign Acquired Nevi
Color	Variable mixtures of tan, brown, black, or red/pink within a single nevus; nevi may look very different from each other	Uniformly tan or brown
Shape	Irregular borders; pigment may fade off into surrounding skin; macular portion at the edge of the nevus	Round; sharp, clear-cut borders between the nevus and the surrounding skin; may be flat or elevated
Size	Usually more than 6 mm in diameter; may be more than 10 mm; occasionally smaller than 6 mm	Usually less than 6 mm in diameter
Number	Often very many (more than 100), but occasionally may be only one	In a typical adult, 10 to 40 are scattered over the body; perhaps 15% of patients have no nevi
Location	Sun-exposed areas; the back is the most common site, but dysplastic nevi may also be seen on the scalp, breasts, and buttocks	Generally on the sun-exposed surfaces of the skin above the waist; the scalp, breasts, and buttocks are rarely involved

SOURCE: Modified from RJ Friedman et al (eds): *Cancer of the Skin*. Philadelphia, Saunders, 1991.

Table 86-5 Pigmented Lesions That Must Be Distinguished from Cutaneous Melanoma and Its Precursors

Lesion	Description
Blue nevus	Gunmetal or cerulean blue, blue-gray. Stable over time. One-half occur on dorsa of hands and feet. Lesions are usually single, small, 3 mm to <1 cm. Must be distinguished from nodular melanoma.
Compound nevus	Round or oval shape, well-demarcated, smooth-bordered. May be dome-shaped or papillomatous; colors range from flesh colored to very dark brown, with individual nevi being relatively homogeneous in color.
Hemangioma	Dome-shaped reddish, purple, blue nodule. Compression with a glass microscope slide may result in blanching. Must be distinguished from nodular melanoma.
Junctional nevus	Flat to barely raised brown lesion. Sharp border. Fine pigmentary stippling visible, especially upon magnification.

Lentigo
  Juvenile
  Solar
	Flat, uniformly medium or dark brown lesion with sharp border. Solar lentigines are acquired lesions on sites of chronic solar exposure (face and backs of hands). Lesions are 2 mm to ≥1 cm. Solar lentigines have reticulate pigmentation upon magnification.

Pigmented basal cell carcinoma	Papular border. May have central ulceration. Usually on a sun-exposed surface in an older patient. Patient usually has dark brown eyes and dark brown or black hair.
Pigmented dermatofibroma	Lesion is not well demarcated visually, is firm, and dimples downward when compressed laterally. Usually on extremities. Usually <6 mm.
Seborrheic keratosis	Rough, sharp-bordered lesions that feel waxy and "stuck on"; range in color from flesh to tan, to dark brown. Presence of keratin plugs in surface is helpful for discriminating especially dark lesions from melanoma.
Subungual hematoma	Maroon (red-brown) coloration. As lesion grows out from nail fold, a curving clear area is seen.
Tattoo (medical or traumatic)	In medical tattoo, lesions are small pigmentary dots, often blue or green, which make a regular pattern (rectangle). Traumatic tattoos are irregular, and pigmentation may appear black.

gional draining lymph nodes, central nervous system, liver, and spleen. In the absence of signs or symptoms of metastasis, few laboratory or radiologic tests are indicated for staging purposes. Aside from a chest radiograph, and possibly liver function tests, no other tests or scans are routinely indicated unless the history or physical examination suggests metastasis to a specific organ. Specifically, liver-spleen scans and computed tomography have a low yield and are not cost-effective. However, once signs of metastasis exist, favored sites of spread, such as the liver, lungs, bone, and brain, should be scanned. Appropriate evaluations place patients into four clinical stages (Table 86-3).

℞ **TREATMENT Surgical Management** For a newly diagnosed cutaneous melanoma, wide surgical excision of the lesion with a margin of normal skin is necessary to remove all malignant cells and minimize local recurrence. The appropriate width of the margin is a source of controversy. Based upon clinical studies, the following margins can be recommended for primary melanoma: in situ: 0.5 cm; invasive up to 1 mm thick: 1.0 cm; 1 to 4 mm thick: 2.0 cm; >4 mm thick: at least 2 cm. For lesions on the face, hands, and feet, strict adherence to these margins must give way to individual considerations about the constraints of surgery and minimization of morbidity. In all instances, however, inclusion of subcutaneous fat in the surgical specimen facilitates adequate thickness measurement and assessment of surgical margins by the pathologist.

Elective Regional Node Dissection Elective regional node dissection in AJCC stage II disease (without palpable adenopathy) has been advocated, based on the hypothesis that melanoma metastasizes in an orderly fashion from the skin to regional lymph nodes and finally to distant sites. If that is the case, surgical excision of nodal micrometastases could theoretically provide definitive treatment at a time of relatively low tumor burden and perhaps improve survival. The efficacy of this procedure remains controversial; while some retrospective series suggest a survival benefit, randomized studies examining this question showed no survival advantage for wide local excision followed by immediate elective regional node dissection compared with wide local excision followed by delayed dissection (only if nodes became palpable). Furthermore, the procedure has associated morbidity, and some lesions, especially those on the trunk, have ambiguous nodal draining sites, making it difficult to decide which area to dissect. Results of biopsy of the first drainage node—the so-called sentinel node—predicts the likelihood of metastases in higher nodes. Sentinel nodes can be identified by injecting a blue dye or radioactive isotope around the primary tumor site. A negative biopsy result appears to obviate the need for elective regional nodal dissection. Patients with lesions <1 mm thick have an excellent prognosis and need no node dissection; at the other extreme, patients with lesions >4 mm thick have such a high risk for distant metastases that elective node dissection may not alter the ultimate clinical outcome. A subset of patients with AJCC stage II lesions of intermediate thickness may benefit from elective regional node dissection, but there is no consensus about which patients should undergo this procedure.

Adjuvant Therapy For patients who are free of disease but at high risk for metastases, adjuvant therapy that complements surgery is needed to destroy occult micrometastases, prolong disease-free survival, and improve the cure rate. Many strategies have been tried unsuccessfully. However, adjuvant interferon-α may improve disease-free and overall survival, particularly in patients with nodal metastases (stage III disease). High-dose interferon, 20 million units per square meter intravenously 5 days a week for 4 weeks followed by 10 million units per square meter subcutaneously three times a week for 11 months, has been effective in some, but not all, studies. In nearly half of patients, these doses of interferon are associated with severe toxicity, including flulike illness and decline in performance status. The toxicity reverses with lower doses and when therapy is stopped. If interferon is beneficial at all, it benefits only a small fraction of treated patients.

Treatment of Metastatic Disease Melanoma can metastasize to any organ, the brain being a particularly common site. Metastatic melanoma generally is incurable, with survival in patients with visceral metastases generally <1 year. Thus, the goal of treatment is usually palliation. Patients with soft-tissue and node metastases fare better than those with liver and brain metastases. Metastases limited to regional nodes (AJCC stage III disease) warrant a therapeutic lymph node dissection. Surgical excision of a single metastasis to the lung or to a surgically accessible brain site can prolong survival. Trials of stereotactic radiosurgery will determine its future role in the treatment of brain metastases. More often, however, patients have multiple brain metastases that require radiation therapy and glucocorticoids. Radiation therapy can provide local palliation for recurrent tumors or metastases. Patients who have advanced regional disease limited to a limb may benefit from hyperthermic limb perfusion with melphalan and tumor necrosis factor. Complete response rates >90% have been reported; responses are associated with significant palliation of symptoms.

A number of drugs and biologicals have minimal antitumor activity (15 to 20% partial response rates) in metastatic melanoma, including dacarbazine (DTIC); the nitrosoureas carmustine (BCNU), lomustine (CCNU), and semustine (methyl-CCNU); platinum analogues such as cisplatin and carboplatin; vinca alkyloids such as vincristine, vinblastine, and vindesine; the taxanes paclitaxel and docetaxel; interferon; and interleukin 2 (IL-2). Single-agent dacarbazine is considered the standard treatment. This agent has been given at a number of different doses and schedules; 250 mg/m^2 intravenously every day for 5 days every 3 weeks is a standard schedule. Dacarbazine-based combination regimens are probably more effective. Interferon and IL-2 produce response rates similar to those seen with cytotoxic agents; however, at active doses, they usually cause greater toxicity than chemotherapy.

Melanomas often express cell-surface antigens that may be recognized by host immune cells. A number of melanoma-associated antigens have been discovered. Melanoma antigens (MAGEs)-1, -2, and -3 (endogenous proteins controlled by genes on the X chromosome; there are up to 12 of these genes) and tyrosinase, an enzyme involved in melanin synthesis, are antigens that are processed into peptides and presented to T cells via HLA-A antigens on the tumor, particularly the HLA-A1 and -A2 alleles, which are expressed in about 85% of patients with melanoma. In addition, a melanoma antigen called MART is recognized in the context of class II MHC antigens. These melanoma-associated antigens alone or in combination may make it possible to develop vaccination strategies against melanoma. Such strategies include the use of purified proteins as immunogens and the use of genetically altered tumor cells to elicit a T cell response. Alternative experimental approaches include efforts to expand tumor-specific T cells (obtained either from the tumor as tumor-infiltrating lymphocytes or harvested from the peripheral blood after vaccination) in vitro and transfer them into patients in large numbers. In addition, monoclonal antibodies to tumor antigens are being tested, with some early indication of efficacy in around 15% of patients. All of these experimental approaches will need considerable further development before being applicable on a wide scale. However, once an approach is found that is active in metastatic disease, it may prove most useful as adjuvant therapy.

The absence of curative therapy for patients with metastatic melanoma underscores the importance of early detection and prevention as strategies to decrease melanoma mortality.

NONMELANOMA SKIN CANCER

Nonmelanoma skin cancer is the most common cancer in the United States, with an estimated annual incidence of more than 1,000,000 cases. Basal cell carcinomas (BCCs) account for 70 to 80% of nonmelanoma skin cancers. Squamous cell carcinomas (SCCs), while representing only about 20% of nonmelanoma skin cancers, are more significant because of their ability to metastasize; they account for most of the 2300 deaths annually. Incidence rates have risen dramatically over the past decade.

ETIOLOGY　The cause of BCC and SCC is multifactorial. Cumulative exposure to sunlight, principally the ultraviolet B (UV-B) spectrum, is the most significant factor. Other factors associated with a higher incidence of skin cancer are male sex, older age, Celtic descent, a fair complexion, a tendency to sunburn easily, and an outdoor occupation. The incidence of these tumors increases with decreasing latitude. Most tumors develop on sun-exposed areas of the head and neck. Tumors are more common on the left side of the body in the United States but on the right side in England, presumably owing to asymmetric exposure during driving. As the earth's protective ozone shield continues to thin, further increases in the incidence of skin cancer can be anticipated. In certain geographic areas, exposure to arsenic in well water or from industrial sources may significantly increase the risk of BCC and SCC. Skin cancer in affected individuals may be seen with or without other cutaneous markers of chronic arsenism (e.g., arsenical keratoses). Less common is exposure to the cyclic aromatic hydrocarbons in tar, soot, or shale. The risk of lip or oral SCC is increased with cigarette smoking. Human papillomaviruses and ultraviolet radiation may act as cocarcinogens.

Host factors associated with a high risk of skin cancer include immunosuppression induced by disease or drugs. Transplant recipients receiving chronic immunosuppressive therapy are particularly prone

to SCC. The frequency of skin cancer is proportional to the duration of immunosuppression and the extent of sun exposure. Skin cancer is a not uncommon finding in patients infected with HIV, and it may be more aggressive in this setting. Other factors include ionizing radiation, thermal burns, certain scars, and chronic ulcerations. Several heritable conditions have been associated with skin cancer (e.g., albinism, xeroderma pigmentosum, and BCC nevus syndrome). Mutations in the tumor suppressor gene, *patched*, may lead to BCC.

CLINICAL PRESENTATION　Nonmelanoma skin cancers are often asymptomatic, but nonhealing ulceration, bleeding, or pain can occur.

Basal Cell Carcinoma　BCC is a malignancy arising from epidermal basal cells. The most common type is *noduloulcerative BCC*, which begins as a small, pearly nodule, often with small telangiectatic vessels on its surface. The nodule grows slowly and may undergo central ulceration. Various amounts of melanin may be present in the tumor; tumors with a heavier accumulation are referred to as *pigmented BCC*. While clinically no more aggressive than the noduloulcerative variant, the latter may be mistaken for malignant melanoma. *Superficial BCC* consists of one or several erythematous, scaling plaques that slowly enlarge. Although they are more commonly found on the trunk and extremities, the head and neck can also be affected. The lesions may be confused with benign inflammatory dermatoses, especially nummular eczema and psoriasis. *Morpheaform (fibrosing) BCC* manifests itself as a solitary, flat or slightly depressed, indurated, whitish or yellowish plaque. Borders are typically indistinct, a feature associated with a greater potential for extensive subclinical spread.

Squamous Cell Carcinoma　Primary cutaneous SCC is a malignant neoplasm of keratinizing epidermal cells. Unlike BCC, which has a very low metastatic potential, SCC can metastasize and grow rapidly. The clinical features of SCC vary widely. Commonly, SCC appears as an ulcerated nodule or a superficial erosion on the skin or lower lip, but it may present as a verrucous papule or plaque. Unlike BCC, overlying telangiectasias are uncommon. The margins of this tumor may be ill-defined, and fixation to underlying structures may occur. Cutaneous SCC may develop anywhere on the body, but it usually arises on sun-damaged skin. A related neoplasm, keratoacanthoma, typically appears as a dome-shaped papule with a central keratotic crater, expands rapidly, and commonly regresses without therapy. This lesion can be difficult to differentiate from SCC.

SCC has several premalignant forms (actinic keratosis, actinic cheilitis, and some cutaneous horns) and in situ forms (e.g., Bowen's disease) that are confined to the epidermis. Actinic keratoses and cheilitis are hyperkeratotic papules and plaques that occur on sun-exposed areas. While the potential for malignant degeneration is low in any individual lesion, the risk of SCC increases with larger numbers of lesions. Bowen's disease presents as a scaling, erythematous plaque, which may develop into invasive SCC in up to 20% of cases. Controversy exists regarding the association of Bowen's disease with internal malignancy; however, no significant relationship is noted when other predisposing factors (e.g., arsenic) are absent. Treatment of premalignant and in situ lesions reduces the subsequent risk of invasive disease.

NATURAL HISTORY　**Basal Cell Carcinoma**　The natural history of BCC is that of a slowly enlarging, locally invasive neoplasm. The degree of local destruction and risk of recurrence vary with the size, duration, and location of the tumor; the histologic subtype; the presence of recurrent disease; and various patient characteristics. Location on the central face (e.g., the nose, the nasolabial fold, or the periorbital or perioral area), the ears, or the scalp may portend a higher risk. Small nodular, pigmented, cystic, or superficial BCCs respond well to most treatments. Large nodular, noduloulcerative, and especially morpheaform BCCs may be more aggressive. The metastatic potential of BCC is about 0.0028 to 0.1%. Persons with either BCC or SCC have an increased risk of developing subsequent skin cancers.

Squamous Cell Carcinoma　The natural history of SCC depends on both tumor and host characteristics. Tumors arising on actinically damaged skin have a lower metastatic potential than those on protected surfaces. The metastatic frequency of cutaneous SCC, 0.3 to 3.7%, is lower than that of mucosal SCC. Tumors occurring on the lower lip and ear have metastatic potential approaching 13 and 11%, respectively. The metastatic potential of SCC arising in burn scars, chronic ulcerations, or the genitalia is higher. The overall metastatic rate for recurrent tumors approaches 30%. Poorly differentiated, deep tumors with perineural or lymphatic invasion often behave aggressively. Multiple tumors with rapid growth and aggressive behavior can be a therapeutic challenge in immunosuppressed patients. Regional lymph nodes are the most common site of metastasis. In patients with metastatic disease, the 5-year survival rate may be low.

℞ **TREATMENT** **Basal Cell Carcinoma** The treatment modalities used for BCC include electrodesiccation and curettage (ED&C), excision, cryosurgery, radiation therapy, Mohs micrographic surgery (MMS), and others. The mode of therapy chosen depends on tumor characteristics, age, medical status, preferences of the patient, and other factors. ED&C remains the method most commonly employed by dermatologists. This method is selected for low-risk tumors (e.g., a small primary tumor of a less aggressive subtype in a favorable location). Excision, which offers the advantage of histologic control, is usually selected for more aggressive tumors or those in high-risk locations, or, in many instances, for esthetic reasons. Cryosurgery using liquid nitrogen may be used in certain low-risk tumors, but it requires specialized equipment (cryoprobes) to be effective for advanced neoplasms. Radiation therapy, while not employed as often as surgical modalities, offers an excellent chance for cure in many cases of BCC. It is useful in patients not considered surgical candidates and as a surgical adjunct in high-risk tumors. Younger patients may not be good candidates for radiation therapy because of the risks of long-term carcinogenesis and radiodermatitis. MMS is a specialized type of surgical excision that permits the ultimate in histologic control and preservation of uninvolved tissue. It is preferred for lesions that are recurrent, in a high-risk location, or large and ill-defined, and where maximal tissue conservation is critical (e.g., the eyelids). Topical chemotherapy with 5-fluorouracil (5FU) cream has limited usefulness in the management of BCC and should be used only for treating superficial BCC. Intralesional 5FU is being investigated for BCC. Intralesional interferon is effective in certain primary tumors. Photodynamic therapy, which employs selective activation of a photoactive drug by visible light, may be useful in patients with numerous tumors. Lasers also have been used for the treatment of skin cancer.

Squamous Cell Carcinoma The therapy of cutaneous SCC should be based on an analysis of risk factors influencing the biologic behavior of the tumor. These include the size, location, and degree of histologic differentiation of the tumor and the age and physical condition of the patient. Surgical excision, MMS, and radiation are standard methods of treatment. Cryosurgery and ED&C have been used successfully for small primary tumors. Metastases are treated with lymph node dissection, irradiation, or both. 13-*Cis*-retinoic acid (1 mg orally every day) plus interferon (3 million units subcutaneously or intramuscularly every day) may produce a partial response in most patients. Systemic chemotherapy combinations that include cisplatin may also be palliative in some patients.

PREVENTION Since the vast majority of skin cancers are related to chronic UV-B exposure, they are largely preventable by blocking sun exposure. Emphasis should be placed on preventive measures beginning early in life. Patients must understand that damage from UV-B begins early, despite the fact that cancers develop years later. Regular use of sunscreens and protective clothing should be encouraged. Avoidance of tanning salons and sun exposure during midday (10 A.M. to 2 P.M.) is recommended. Precancerous and in situ lesions should be treated early. Early detection of small tumors affords simpler treatment modalities with higher cure rates and lower morbidity. In patients with a history of skin cancer, long-term follow-up for the detection of recurrence, metastasis, and new skin cancers should be emphasized. Chemoprophylaxis using synthetic retinoids is useful in controlling new lesions in some patients with multiple tumors.

OTHER TYPES OF CUTANEOUS CANCER

Neoplasms of cutaneous adnexa, and sarcomas of fibrous, mesenchymal, fatty, and vascular tissues make up 1 to 2% of nonmelanoma skin cancers. The recent rapid rise in the incidence of Kaposi's sarcoma is attributed to HIV infection and immunosuppressive therapy. Human herpesvirus 8 appears to be the cause of sporadic and HIV-associated Kaposi's sarcoma. Current therapy is palliative and depends on the symptoms and sites of involvement. Treatment modalities include cryosurgery, vinblastine, excision, radiation, interferon, and systemic combination chemotherapy (Chap. 309).

ACKNOWLEDGMENT
The authors wish to acknowledge Dr. Nhu-linh T. Tran, who was a co-author of this chapter in the 14th edition.

BIBLIOGRAPHY

AUTIER P et al: Sunscreen use and duration of sun exposure: A double-blind randomized trial. J Natl Cancer Inst 91:1304, 1999
BALCH CM et al: Efficacy of an elective regional lymph node dissection of 1 to 4 mm thick melanomas for persons 60 years of age and younger. Ann Surg 224:255, 1996
DRAKE LA et al: Guidelines of care of basal cell carcinoma. J Am Acad Dermatol 26: 117, 1992
———— et al: Guidelines of care for cutaneous squamous cell carcinoma. J Am Acad Dermatol 28:628, 1993
GAILANI MR et al: Developmental genes and cancer: Role of *patched* in basal cell carcinoma of the skin. J Natl Cancer Inst 89:1103, 1997
KIRKWOOD JM et al: Interferon-alpha-2b adjuvant therapy of high-risk resected cutaneous melanoma. The Eastern Cooperative Oncology Group trial EST1684. J Clin Oncol 14:7, 1996
RHODES AR: Benign neoplasias and hyperplasias of melanocytes, in *Fitzpatrick's Dermatology in General Medicine,* 5th ed, IM Freedberg et al (eds). New York, McGraw-Hill, 1999, pp 1018–1097
TOULOUKIAN CE, ROSENBERG SA: A survey of treatments used in patients with metastatic melanoma: Analysis of 189 patients referred to the National Cancer Institute. Cancer J Sci Am 5:269, 1999

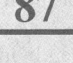 *Everett E. Vokes*

HEAD AND NECK CANCER

Epithelial carcinomas of the head and neck arise from the mucosal surfaces in the head and neck area and typically are squamous cell in origin. This category includes tumors of the paranasal sinuses, the oral cavity, and the nasopharynx, oropharynx, hypopharynx, and larynx. Tumors of the salivary glands differ from the more common carcinomas of the head and neck in etiology, histopathology, clinical presentation, and therapy. →*Thyroid malignancies are described in Chap. 330.*

INCIDENCE AND EPIDEMIOLOGY The annual number of new cases of head and neck cancers in the United States is approximately 40,000, accounting for about 5% of adult malignancies. Head and neck cancers are more common in certain other countries, and the worldwide incidence exceeds half a million cases annually. In North America and Europe, the tumors usually arise from the oral cavity, oropharynx, or larynx, whereas nasopharyngeal cancer is more common in the Mediterranean countries and in the Far East.

ETIOLOGY AND GENETICS Alcohol and tobacco use are the most common risk factors for head and neck cancer in the United States. Smokeless tobacco is an etiologic agent for oral cancers. Other potential carcinogens include marijuana and occupational exposures such as nickel refining, exposure to textile fibers, and woodworking.

Dietary factors may contribute. The incidence of head and neck cancer is highest in people with the lowest consumption of fruits and vegetables. Certain vitamins, including dietary carotenoids, may be protective; retinoids are being tested for prevention.

Some head and neck cancers may have a viral etiology. The DNA of human papilloma virus has been detected in the tissue of oral and tonsil cancers, and Epstein-Barr virus (EBV) infection is associated with nasopharyngeal cancer. Nasopharyngeal cancer occurs endemically in some countries of the Mediterranean and Far East, where EBV antibody titers can be measured to screen high-risk populations. Nasopharyngeal cancer has also been associated with other environmental factors, such as consumption of salted fish.

No specific risk factors or environmental carcinogens have been identified for salivary gland tumors.

HISTOPATHOLOGY, CARCINOGENESIS, AND MOLECULAR BIOLOGY Squamous cell head and neck carcinomas can be divided into well-differentiated, moderately well-differentiated, and poorly differentiated categories. Patients with poorly differentiated tumors have a worse prognosis than those with well-differentiated tumors. For nasopharyngeal cancers, the less common differentiated squamous cell carcinoma is distinguished from nonkeratinizing and undifferentiated carcinoma (lymphoepithelioma) that contains infiltrating (bystander) lymphocytes.

Salivary gland tumors can arise from the major (parotid, submandibular, sublingual) or minor salivary glands (located in the submucosa of the upper aerodigestive tract). Most parotid tumors are benign, but half of submandibular and sublingual gland tumors and most minor salivary gland tumors are malignant. Malignant tumors include mucoepidermoid and adenoidcystic carcinomas and adenocarcinomas.

The mucosal surface of the entire pharynx is exposed to alcohol and tobacco-related carcinogens and is at risk for the development of a premalignant or malignant lesion, such as erythroplakia or leukoplakia (hyperplasia, dysplasia), that can progress to invasive carcinoma. Alternatively, multiple synchronous or metachronous cancers can develop. In fact, patients with early-stage head and neck cancer are at greater risk of dying of a second malignancy than of dying from a recurrence of the primary disease.

Second head and neck malignancies are not therapy-induced but, instead, reflect the exposure of the upper aerodigestive mucosa to the same carcinogens that caused the first cancer. These second primaries develop in the head and neck area, the lung, or the esophagus.

Chromosomal deletions and other alterations, most frequently involving chromosomes 3p, 9p, 17p, and 13q, have been identified in both premalignant and malignant head and neck lesions, as have mutations in tumor suppressor genes, commonly the *p53* gene. Amplification of oncogenes is less common, but overexpression of PRAD-1/bcl-1 (cyclin D1), bc1-2, transforming growth factor β, and the epidermal growth factor receptor have been described. The latter finding correlates positively with tumor size and poor outcome and is a target for experimental treatments.

Resected tumor specimens with histopathologically negative margins ("complete resection") can have histopathologically undetectable residual tumor cells with persistent *p53* mutations at the margins. Thus, a tumor-specific *p53* mutation can be detected in some phenotypically "normal" surgical margins, indicating residual disease. Patients with such submicroscopic marginal involvement may have a worse prognosis than patients with negative margins.

CLINICAL PRESENTATION AND DIFFERENTIAL DIAGNOSIS Most head and neck cancers occur after age 50, although these cancers can appear in younger patients, including those without known risk factors. The manifestations vary according to the stage and primary site of the tumor. Patients with nonspecific signs and symptoms in the head and neck area should be evaluated with a thorough otolaryngologic exam, particularly if symptoms persist longer than 2 to 4 weeks.

Cancer of the nasopharynx typically does not cause early symptoms. However, on occasion it may cause unilateral serous otitis media due to obstruction of the eustachian tube, unilateral or bilateral nasal obstruction, or epistaxis. Advanced nasopharyngeal carcinoma causes neuropathies of the cranial nerves.

Carcinomas of the oral cavity present as nonhealing ulcers, changes in the fit of dentures, or painful lesions. Tumors of the tongue base or oropharynx can cause decreased tongue mobility and alterations in speech. Cancers of the oropharynx or hypopharynx rarely cause early symptoms, but they may cause sore throat and/or otalgia.

Hoarseness may be an early symptom of laryngeal cancer, and persistent hoarseness requires referral to an otorhinolaryngologist for indirect laryngoscopy and/or radiographic studies. If a head and neck lesion treated initially with antibiotics does not resolve in a short period, further workup is indicated; to simply continue the antibiotic treatment may be to lose the chance of early diagnosis of a malignancy.

Advanced head and neck cancers in any location can cause severe pain, otalgia, airway obstruction, cranial neuropathies, trismus, odynophagia, dysphagia, decreased tongue mobility, fistulas, skin involvement, and massive cervical lymphadenopathy, which may be unilateral or bilateral. Some patients have enlarged lymph nodes even though no primary lesion can be detected by endoscopy or biopsy; these patients are considered to have carcinoma of unknown primary. If the enlarged nodes are located in the upper neck and the tumor cells are of squamous cell histology, the malignancy probably arose from a mucosal surface in the head or neck. Tumor cells in supraclavicular lymph nodes may also arise from a primary site in the chest or abdomen.

The physical examination should include scrutiny of all visible mucosal surfaces and palpation of the floor of mouth and tongue and of the neck. In addition to tumors themselves, leukoplakia—a white mucosal patch—or erythroplakia—a red mucosal patch—may be observed; these "premalignant" lesions can represent hyperplasia, dysplasia, or carcinoma in situ. All visible lesions should be biopsied. Further examination should be performed by the otorhinolaryngologist. Additional staging procedures include computed tomography of the head and neck to identify the extent of the disease. Patients with lymph node involvement should have chest radiography and a bone scan to screen for distant metastases. The definitive staging procedure is an endoscopic examination under anesthesia, which may include laryngoscopy, esophagoscopy, and bronchoscopy; during this procedure, multiple biopsy samples are obtained to establish a primary diagnosis, define the extent of primary disease, and identify any additional premalignant lesions or second primaries.

Head and neck tumors are classified according to the TNM system of the American Joint Committee on Cancer. This classification varies according to the specific anatomic subsite (Tables 87-1 and 87-2). Distant metastases are found in <10% of patients at initial diagnosis, but in autopsy series, microscopic involvement of the lungs, bones, or liver is more common, particularly in patients with advanced neck lymph node disease.

In patients with lymph node involvement and no visible primary, the diagnosis should be made by lymph node excision. If the results indicate squamous cell carcinoma, a panendoscopy should be performed, with biopsy of all suspicious-appearing areas and directed biopsies of common primary sites, such as the nasopharynx, tonsil, tongue base, and pyriform sinus.

℞ **TREATMENT** Generally, patients with head and neck cancer can be categorized into three clinical groups: those with localized disease, those with locally or regionally advanced disease, and those with recurrent and/or metastatic disease. Comorbidities associated with tobacco and alcohol abuse can affect treatment outcome.

Localized Disease Approximately one-third of patients have localized disease; that is, T1 or T2 (stage I or stage II) lesions without detectable lymph node involvement or distant metastases. These lesions are treated with curative intent by surgery or radiation. The choice of modality differs according to institutional expertise. Generally, radiation therapy is preferred for laryngeal cancer to preserve voice function, and surgery is preferred for small lesions in the oral cavity to avoid the long-term complications of radiation, such as xerostomia and dental decay. Overall 5-year survival is 60 to 90%.

Table 87-1 TNM Classification for Head and Neck Cancer (except Nasopharyngeal)

T Grade	Primary Tumor Site				
	Lip	Oral Cavity	Oropharynx	Hypopharynx	Larynx
TX			Primary tumor cannot be assessed		
T0			No evidence of primary tumor		
Tis			Carcinoma in situ		
T1	0–2 cm	0–2 cm	0–2 cm	1 site	1 site or limited to vocal cords
T2	2.1–4 cm	2.1–4 cm	2.1–4 cm	>1 site, no vocal cord fixation	>1 site or impaired cord mobility
T3	>4 cm	>4 cm	>4 cm	vocal cord paralysis	Vocal cord paralysis
T4	>4 cm with massive invasion		Massive soft tissue, bone, or cartilage invasion		

REGIONAL LYMPH NODES (N)

NX	Regional lymph nodes cannot be assessed
N0	No regional lymph node metastasis
N1	Metastasis in a single ipsilateral lymph node, 3 cm or less in greatest dimension
N2	Metastasis in a single ipsilateral lymph node, more than 3 cm but not more than 6 cm in greatest dimension; or in multiple ipsilateral lymph nodes, none more than 6 cm in greatest dimension; or in bilateral or contralateral lymph nodes, none more than 6 cm in greatest dimension
N2a	Metastasis in single ipsilateral lymph node more than 3 cm but more than 6 cm in greatest dimension
N2b	Metastasis in multiple ipsilateral lymph nodes, none more than 6 cm in greatest dimension
N2c	Metastasis in bilateral or contralateral lymph nodes, none more than 6 cm in greatest dimension
N3	Metastasis in a lymph node more than 6 cm in greatest dimension

DISTANT METASTASIS (M)

MX	Presence of distant metastasis cannot be assessed
M0	No distant metastasis
M1	Distant metastasis

STAGE GROUPING

Stage 0	Tis	N0	M0	Stage IV	T4	N0	M0
Stage I	T1	N0	M0		T4	N1	M0
Stage II	T2	N0	M0		Any T	N2	M0
Stage III	T3	N0	M0		Any T	N3	M0
	T1	N1	M0		Any T	Any N	M1
	T2	N1	M0				
	T3	N1	M0				

Locally or Regionally Advanced Disease Locally or regionally advanced disease—that is, disease with a large primary tumor and/or lymph node metastases—can also be treated with curative intent, but not with surgery or radiation therapy alone. Combined modality therapy including surgery, radiation therapy and chemotherapy is most successful. Concomitant chemotherapy and radiation therapy appears to be the most effective sequencing of treatment.

Induction chemotherapy In this strategy, patients receive chemotherapy [usually cisplatin and fluorouracil (5FU)] before surgery and radiotherapy. Most patients who receive three cycles of this combination show tumor reduction, and the response is clinically "complete" in up to half of these patients. This "sequential" multimodality therapy does not cure more patients than surgery plus radiation therapy alone. Time to recurrence may be improved but survival is similar. However, induction chemotherapy allows for organ preservation in patients with laryngeal and hypopharyngeal cancer.

Concomitant chemoradiotherapy With the concomitant strategy, chemotherapy and radiation therapy are given simultaneously rather than sequentially. Because most patients with head and neck cancer develop recurrent disease in the head and neck area, this approach is aimed at killing radiation-resistant cancer cells with chemotherapy. In addi-tion, chemotherapy can enhance cell killing by radiation therapy. Toxicity (mucositis) is increased with concomitant chemoradiotherapy; however, meta-analysis of randomized trials documents an improvement in 5-year survival of 8% with concomitant 5FU and radiation therapy. Results seem even better with 5FU and cisplatin plus radiation

Table 87-2 Definition of TNM—Nasopharynx

PRIMARY TUMOR (T)

TX	Primary tumor cannot be assessed
T0	No evidence of primary tumor
Tis	carcinoma in situ
T1	Tumor confined to the nasopharynx
T2	Tumor extends to soft tissues of oropharynx and/or nasal fossa
T2a	without parapharyngeal extension
T2b	with parapharyngeal extension
T3	Tumor invades bony structures and/or paranasal sinuses
T4	Tumor with intracranial extension and/or involvement of cranial nerves, infratemporal fossa, hypopharynx, or orbit

REGIONAL LYMPH NODES (N)

The distribution and the prognostic impact of regional lymph node spread from nasopharynx cancer, particularly of the un-differentiated type, is different than that of other head and neck mucosal cancers and justifies use of a different N classi-fication scheme.

NX	Regional lymph nodes cannot be assessed
N0	No regional lymph node metastasis
N1	Unilateral metastasis in lymph nodes(s), 6 cm or less in greatest dimension, above the supraclavicular fossa
N2	Bilateral metastasis in lymph node(s), 6 cm or less in greatest dimension, above the supraclavicular fossa
N3	Metastasis in a lymph node(s)
N3a	greater than 6 cm in dimension
N3b	extension to the supraclavicular fossa

STAGE GROUPING

Stage 0	Tis	N0	M0
Stage I	T1	N0	M0
Stage IIA	T2a	N0	M0
Stage IIB	T1	N1	M0
	T2	N1	M0
	T2a	N1	M0
	T2b	N0	M0
	T2b	N1	M0
Stage III	T1	N2	M0
	T2a	N2	M0
	T2b	N2	M0
	T3	N0	M0
	T3	N1	M0
	T3	N2	M0
Stage IVA	T4	N0	M0
	T4	N1	M0
	T4	N2	M0
Stage IVB	Any T	N3	M0
Stage IVC	Any T	Any N	M1

therapy. Five-year survival is 34 to 50%. The use of radiation therapy together with cisplatin has produced markedly improved survival in patients with advanced nasopharyngeal cancer. The success of concomitant chemoradiotherapy in patients with unresectable disease has led to the testing of a similar approach in patients with resectable disease in an effort to increase organ preservation.

Recurrent and/or Metastatic Disease Patients with recurrent and/or metastatic disease are, with few exceptions, treated with palliative intent. Some patients may require local or regional radiation therapy for pain control, but most are given chemotherapy. Response rates to chemotherapy average only 30 to 50%; the duration of response averages only 3 months, and the median survival time is 6 months. Therefore, chemotherapy provides transient symptomatic benefit. Drugs with single-agent activity in this setting include methotrexate, 5FU, cisplatin, paclitaxel, and docetaxel. Combinations of cisplatin and 5FU, carboplatin and 5FU, and cisplatin and paclitaxel are also used.

CHEMOPREVENTION β-carotene and *cis*-retinoic acid can lead to the regression of leukoplakia. In addition, the use of *cis*-retinoic acid may reduce the incidence of second primaries.

TREATMENT COMPLICATIONS Complications involved in the treatment of head and neck cancer are usually related to the extent of surgery. Several attempts have been made to limit the extent of surgery or to replace it with chemotherapy and radiation therapy. Acute complications of radiation include mucositis and dysphagia. Long-term complications include xerostomia, loss of taste, decreased tongue mobility, second malignancies, and dysphagia and neck fibrosis. The complications of chemotherapy vary with the regimen used but usually include myelosuppression, mucositis, nausea and vomiting, and nephrotoxicity (with cisplatin).

SALIVARY GLAND TUMORS Most benign salivary gland tumors are treated with surgical excision, and patients with invasive salivary gland tumors are treated with surgery and radiation therapy. Neutron radiation may be particularly effective. These tumors may recur regionally; adenoidcystic carcinoma has a tendency to recur along the nerve tracks. Distant metastases may occur as late as 10 to 20 years after the initial diagnosis. For metastatic disease, therapy is given with palliative intent, usually chemotherapy with doxorubicin and/or cisplatin.

BIBLIOGRAPHY

AL-SARRAF M et al: Chemoradiotherapy versus radiotherapy in patients with advanced nasopharyngeal cancer: Phase III randomized Intergroup study 0099. J Clin Oncol 16:1310, 1998

BRIZEL DM et al: Hyperfractionated irradiation with or without concurrent chemotherapy for locally advanced head and neck cancer. N Engl J Med 338:1798, 1998

CALIFANO J et al: Genetic progression model for head and neck cancer: implications for field cancerization. Cancer Res 56:2488, 1996

RICE DH: Salivary gland disorders. Neoplastic and nonneoplastic. Med Clin North Am 83:197, 1999

SHIN DM, LIPPMAN SM: Paclitaxel-based chemotherapy for recurrent and/or metastatic head and neck squamous cell carcinoma: Current and future directions. Semin Oncol 26 (Suppl 2):100, 1999

VOKES EE, ATHANASIADIS I: Chemotherapy for squamous cell carcinoma of head and neck: The future is now. Ann Oncol 7:15, 1996

VOKES EE et al: Head and neck cancer. N Engl J Med 328:184, 1993

88 *John D. Minna*

NEOPLASMS OF THE LUNG

Each year, primary carcinoma of the lung affects 94,000 males and 78,000 females in the United States, 86% of whom die within 5 years of diagnosis, making it the leading cause of cancer death in both men and women and in all races. The incidence of lung cancer peaks between ages 55 and 65 years. Lung cancer accounts for 31% of all cancer deaths in men and 25% in women. The effects of smoking cessation efforts begun 25 years ago have been seen in a slowing of the rate of age-adjusted cancer death from lung cancer in males ($\sim$70 per 100,000 male population); but, unfortunately, the rate in females is still increasing ($\sim$35 per 100,000 female population). Only 15% of patients have local disease at diagnosis; 25% have disease spread to regional lymph nodes, and >55% have distant metastases. The 5-year survival rate of patients with local disease is 50%; it is 20% for patients with regional disease and 14% overall. The 5-year overall lung cancer survival rate has nearly doubled in the last 30 years. The improvement is due to advances in combined-modality treatment with surgery, radiotherapy, and chemotherapy. Thus, primary carcinoma of the lung is a major health problem with a generally grim prognosis. However, an orderly approach to diagnosis, staging, and treatment based on knowledge of the clinical behavior of lung cancer and involving multidisciplinary input allows choice and delivery of the best therapy for potential cure or optimal palliation of individual patients.

PATHOLOGY

The term *lung cancer* is used for tumors arising from the respiratory epithelium (bronchi, bronchioles, and alveoli). Mesotheliomas, lymphomas, and stromal tumors (sarcomas) are distinct from epithelial lung cancer. Four major cell types make up 88% of all primary lung neoplasms according to the World Health Organization classification (Table 88-1). These are *squamous* or *epidermoid carcinoma, small cell* (also called *oat cell*) *carcinoma, adenocarcinoma* (including bronchioloalveolar), and *large cell* (also called *large cell anaplastic*) *carcinoma*. The remainder include undifferentiated carcinomas, carcinoids, bronchial gland tumors (including adenoid cystic carcinomas and mucoepidermoid tumors), and rarer tumor types. The various cell types have different natural histories and responses to therapy, and thus a correct histologic diagnosis by an experienced pathologist is the first step to correct treatment. In the past 25 years, for unknown reasons, adenocarcinoma has replaced squamous cell carcinoma as the most frequent histologic subtype for all sexes and races combined (Table 88-1).

Major treatment decisions are made on the basis of whether a tumor is classified histologically as a small cell carcinoma or as one of the non-small cell varieties (epidermoid, adenocarcinoma, large cell carcinoma, bronchioloalveolar carcinoma, and mixed versions of these). Some of the distinctions are summarized in Tables 88-1 and 88-2. At presentation, small cell carcinomas usually have already spread such that surgery is unlikely to be curative, and they are managed primarily by chemotherapy with or without radiotherapy. In contrast, non-small cell cancers that are found to be localized at the time of presentation may be cured with either surgery or radiotherapy. Non-small cell cancers do not respond as well to chemotherapy as small cell cancers.

Ninety percent of patients with lung cancer of all histologic types are current or former cigarette smokers. Of the annual 171,600 new cases of lung cancer, $\sim$50% develop in former smokers. With increased success in smoking cessation efforts, the number of former smokers will grow, and these individuals will be important candidates for early detection and chemoprevention efforts. By far the most common form of lung cancer arising in lifetime nonsmokers, in women, and in young patients (<45 years) is adenocarcinoma. However, in nonsmokers with adenocarcinoma involving the lung, the possibility of other primary sites should be considered. Epidermoid and small cell cancers usually present as central masses with endobronchial growth, while adenocarcinomas and large cell cancers tend to present as peripheral nodules or masses, frequently with pleural involvement. Epidermoid and large cell cancers cavitate in $\sim$10 to 20% of cases. Bronchioloalveolar carcinoma, a form of adenocarcinoma arising from peripheral airways, can present as a single mass; as a diffuse, multinodular lesion; or as a fluffy infiltrate.

ETIOLOGY

Most lung cancers are caused by carcinogens and tumor promoters ingested via cigarette smoking. The prevalence of smoking in the United States is 28% for males and 25% for females, age 18 years or older; 38% of high school seniors smoke. The relative risk of developing lung cancer is increased about 13-fold by active smoking and about 1.5-fold by long-term passive exposure to cigarette smoke. Chronic obstructive pulmonary disease, which is also smoking-related, further increases the risk of developing lung cancer. The lung cancer death rate is related to the total amount (often expressed in "cigarette pack-years") of cigarettes smoked, such that the risk is increased 60- to 70-fold for a man smoking two packs a day for 20 years as compared with a nonsmoker.

Table 88-1 Frequency, Age-Adjusted Incidence, and Survival Rates for Different Histologic Types of Lung Cancer (All Races, Both Sexes, and All Stages)[a]

Histologic Type of Thoracic Malignancy	Frequency, %	Age-Adjusted Rate	5-year Survival Rate (All Stages)
Adenocarcinoma (and all subtypes)	32	17	17
Bronchioloalveolar carcinoma	3	1.4	42
Squamous cell (epidermoid) carcinoma	29	15	15
Small cell carcinoma	18	9	5
Large cell carcinoma	9	5	11
Carcinoid	1.0	0.5	83
Mucoepidermoid carcinoma	0.1	<0.1	39
Adenoid cystic carcinoma	<0.1	<0.1	48
Sarcoma and other soft tissue tumors	0.1	0.1	30
All others and unspecified carcinomas	11.0	6	NA
Total	100	52	14

[a] Data on histology frequency and age-adjusted incidence rates per 100,000 U.S. population are from 60,514 cases of invasive lung cancer involving all races and both sexes obtained from the data for 1983–1987 of the Surveillance, Epidemiology, and End Results (SEER) Program of the National Cancer Institute; 5-year relative survival rates for all stages, all races, and both sexes are from the SEER data on 87,128 carcinomas, 1978–1986. NA, not available.
SOURCE: Summarized from Travis et al: Cancer 75:191, 1995.

Conversely, the chance of developing lung cancer decreases with cessation of smoking but may never return to the nonsmoker level. The increase in lung cancer rate in women is also associated with a rise in cigarette smoking. Women have a higher relative risk per given exposure than men (~1.5 fold higher), and women with lung cancer are more likely to have never smoked than men. This gender difference is likely due to a higher susceptibility to tobacco carcinogens in women.

Efforts to get people to stop smoking are mandatory. However, smoking cessation is extremely difficult, because the smoking habit represents a powerful addiction to nicotine (Chap. 390). Preventing people from starting to smoke may be more effective, an effort that needs to be targeted to children.

Although human lung cancer is not thought of as a genetic disease, various molecular genetic studies have shown the acquisition by lung cancer cells of a number of genetic lesions, including activation of dominant oncogenes and inactivation of tumor suppressor or recessive oncogenes (Chaps. 81 and 82). In fact, lung cancer cells may have to accumulate a large number (perhaps ≥10) of such lesions. For the dominant oncogenes, these include point mutations in the coding regions of the *ras* family of oncogenes (particularly in the K-*ras* gene in adenocarcinoma of the lung); amplification, rearrangement, and/or loss of transcriptional control of *myc* family oncogenes (c-, N-, and L-*myc*; changes in c-*myc* are found in non-small cell cancers, while changes in all *myc* family members are found in small cell lung cancer); and overexpression of *bcl-2*, *Her-2/neu*, and the telomerase gene (Table 88-2). Tumor mutations in *ras* genes are associated with a poor prognosis in non-small cell lung cancer, while tumor amplification of c-*myc* is associated with a poor prognosis in small cell lung cancer.

For the recessive oncogenes (*tumor suppressor genes*), cytogenetic and allelotyping analyses have shown allele loss involving chromosome regions 1p, 1q, 3p12-13, 3p14 (*FHIT* gene region), 3p21, 3p24-25, 4p, 4q, 5q, 8p, 9p (*p16/CDKN2*, *p15*, *p19ARF* gene cluster), 11p13, 11p15, 13q14 (retinoblastoma, *rb*, gene), 16q, and 17p13 (*p53* gene), as well as other sites. Several candidate recessive oncogenes on chromosome 3p appear to be involved in nearly all lung cancers and may be affected early in preneoplastic lesions. The *p53* and *rb* genes are both mutated in >90% of small cell lung cancers, while *p53* is mutated in >50% and *rb* in 20% of non-small cell lung cancers. *p16/CDKN2* is abnormal in 10% of small cell and >50% of non-small cell lung cancers. Rb and *p16/CDKN2* are part of the same G1-to-S cell cycle regulatory pathway. Either one or the other of these elements appears to be mutated or to have its expression turned off (e.g., by hypermethylation of the promoter) in the large majority of lung cancers. Histologically identifiable preneoplastic lesions found in the respiratory epithelium of lung cancer patients and smokers include hyperplasia, dysplasia (progressively severe), and carcinoma in situ. 3p allele loss (hyperplasia) followed by 9p (*p16/CDKN2*) allele loss (hyperplasia) are the earliest events; 17p (*p53*) abnormalities and then *ras* mutations usually are found only in carcinoma in situ and invasive cancer. Thus, molecular changes involving allele loss and microsatellite alteration can be found in the earliest preneoplastic lesions and potentially even before any histologic changes are noted. Clinical trials of early diagnosis are needed to prove the usefulness of these molecular markers in the identification of very early lung cancer and in the monitoring of treatment and chemoprevention.

The large number of lesions shows that lung cancer, like other common epithelial malignancies, is a multistep process that is likely to involve both carcinogens and tumor promoters. Prevention can be directed at both processes. Lung cancer cells produce many peptide hormones and express receptors for these hormones, which can act to stimulate tumor cell growth in an "autocrine" fashion. Highly carcinogenic derivatives of nicotine are formed in cigarette smoke. Lung cancer cells of all histologic types express receptors for nicotine. Nicotine can prevent apoptosis in lung cancer cell lines. Thus, nicotine itself could be directly involved in lung cancer pathogenesis.

While lung cancer does not have a clear pattern of Mendelian inheritance, several features suggest a potential for familial association. Inherited mutations in *rb* (patients with retinoblastomas living to adulthood) and *p53* (Li-Fraumeni syndrome) genes may develop lung cancer. First-degree relatives of lung cancer probands have a two- to threefold excess risk of lung cancer or other cancers, many of which are not smoking-related. Genetic epidemiologic studies have proposed an association between the P450 enzyme or chromosome fragility (*mutagen sensitivity*) genotypes and the development of lung cancer. The identification of persons at very high risk of developing lung cancer would be useful in early detection and prevention efforts.

CLINICAL MANIFESTATIONS

Lung cancer gives rise to signs and symptoms caused by local tumor growth, invasion or obstruction of adjacent structures, growth in regional nodes through lymphatic spread, growth in distant metastatic sites after hematogenous dissemination, and remote effects of tumor products (paraneoplastic syndrome). Peptide hormone secretion by the tumor or immunologic cross-reaction between tumor and normal tissue antigens can produce a variety of signs and symptoms (Chap. 100).

Although 5 to 15% of patients with lung cancer are identified while they are asymptomatic, usually as a result of a routine chest radiograph, most patients present with some sign or symptom. Central or endobronchial growth of the primary tumor may cause cough, hemoptysis, wheeze and stridor, dyspnea, and postobstructive pneumonitis (fever and productive cough). Peripheral growth of the primary tumor may cause pain from pleural or chest wall involvement, cough, dyspnea on a restrictive basis, and symptoms of lung abscess resulting from

Table 88-2 Comparison of Small Cell and Non-Small Cell Lung Cancers

Feature	Small Cell	Non-Small Cell
Histology	Scant cytoplasm; small, hyperchromatic nuclei with fine chromatin pattern; nucleoli indistinct; diffuse sheets of cells	Abundant cytoplasm; pleomorphic nuclei with coarse chromatin pattern; nucleoli often prominent; glandular or squamous architecture
General neuroendocrine properties		
Dense-core granules	Present	Absent[a]
L-Dopa decarboxylase activity	High	Absent
Chromogranin	Present	Absent
Synaptophysin	Present	Absent
Neuron-specific enolase	High	Low
Creatine kinase BB isozyme	High	Low
CD56 and CD57 antigens	Present	Absent
Peptide hormone production		
Gastrin-releasing peptide gene products	Present	Absent
Other neuropeptides	ACTH, AVP, calcitonin, ANF	PTH
Autocrine loops	GRP/GRP receptor	HGF/MET
	SCF/KIT	NDF/ERBB2
Other markers		
HLA, β_2-microglobulin	Absent/low	Present
Intermediate filament pattern	"SCLC"	"Non-SCLC"
Neurofilaments	Present	Absent
Opioid receptors	Present	Present
Nicotine receptors	Present	Present
EGF receptors	Low or absent	Present
Mucin	Absent	Present in adenocarcinomas
Surfactant-associated proteins	Absent	Often present
Carcinoembryonic antigen	Present	Present
Recessive oncogene (tumor suppressor gene) and allelotype abnormalities		
3p allele loss	100%	>90%
rb mutations	~90%	~20%
p16/CDKN2 mutations/absent expression	~10%	~50%
p53 mutations/abnormal expression	>90%	>50%
4p, 4q, 5q, 8p, 11p and other allele losses	Present	Present
Microsatellite alterations	Present	Present
Dominant oncogene abnormalities		
ras mutations	<1%	~30%
myc family overexpression	>50%	10–35%
bcl-2 overexpression	>75%	>50%
Her-2/neu overexpression	<10%	~30%
Telomerase overexpression	>90%	>90%
Microsatellite alterations	35%	22%
Promoter hypermethylation (*p16*, DAP Kinase, GSTP1, MGMT, *FHIT, RARβ*)	10–40%	10–40%
Response to radiotherapy	Objective shrinkage in 80–90%; often complete response	Objective shrinkage in 30–50%; response uncommonly complete
Response to combination chemotherapy		
Overall regression rate	90%	40–60%
Rate of complete regression	30%	5%

[a] Ten percent of non-small cell lung cancers have populations of cells expressing neuroendocrine markers, and these are best demonstrated by immunohistochemical stains.

ABBREVIATIONS: ACTH, adrenocorticotropic hormone; ANF, atrial natriuretic factor; AVP, arginine vasopressin; CD56, neural cell adhesion molecule (NCAM)-1; CD57, Leu-7 or HNK-1; HLA, human leukocyte antigen; PTH, parathormone; SCLC, small cell lung cancer; GRP, gastrin-releasing peptide; SCF, stem cell factor; KIT, SCF receptor; HGF, hepatocyte growth factor; MET, met protooncogene, HGF receptor; NDF, neu differentiation factor or heregulin; ERBB2, her2/neu protooncogene receptor.

tumor cavitation. Regional spread of tumor in the thorax (by contiguous growth or by metastasis to regional lymph nodes) may cause tracheal obstruction, esophageal compression with dysphagia, recurrent laryngeal nerve paralysis with hoarseness, phrenic nerve paralysis with elevation of the hemidiaphragm and dyspnea, and sympathetic nerve paralysis with Horner's syndrome (enophthalmos, ptosis, miosis, and ipsilateral loss of sweating). *Pancoast's* (or *superior sulcus tumor) syndrome* results from local extension of a tumor (usually epidermoid) growing in the apex of the lung with involvement of the eighth cervical and first and second thoracic nerves, with shoulder pain that characteristically radiates in the ulnar distribution of the arm, often with radiologic destruction of the first and second ribs. Often Horner's syndrome and Pancoast's syndrome coexist. Other problems of regional spread include *superior vena cava syndrome* from vascular obstruction; pericardial and cardiac extension with resultant tamponade, arrhythmia, or cardiac failure; lymphatic obstruction with resultant pleural effusion; and lymphangitic spread through the lungs with hypoxemia and dyspnea. In addition, bronchioloalveolar carcinoma can spread transbronchially, producing tumor growing along multiple alveolar surfaces with impairment of gas exchange, respiratory insufficiency, dyspnea, hypoxemia, and sputum production.

Extrathoracic metastatic disease is found at autopsy in >50% of patients with epidermoid carcinoma, 80% of patients with adenocarcinoma and large cell carcinoma, and >95% of patients with small cell cancer. Lung cancer metastases may occur in virtually every organ system. Common clinical problems related to metastatic lung cancer include brain metastases with neurologic deficits; bone metastases with pain and pathologic fractures; bone marrow invasion with cytopenias or leukoerythroblastosis; liver metastases causing biochemical liver dysfunction, biliary obstruction, and pain; lymph node metastases in the supraclavicular region and occasionally in the axilla and groin; and spinal cord compression syndromes from epidural or bone metastases. Adrenal metastases are common but rarely cause adrenal insufficiency.

Paraneoplastic syndromes are common in patients with lung cancer and may be the presenting finding or first sign of recurrence. In addition, paraneoplastic syndromes may mimic metastatic disease and, unless detected, lead to inappropriate palliative rather than curative treatment. Often the paraneoplastic syndrome may be relieved with successful treatment of the tumor. In some cases, the pathophysiology of the paraneoplastic syndrome is known, particularly when a hormone with biologic activity is secreted by a tumor (Chap. 100). However, in many cases the pathophysiology is unknown. Systemic symptoms of anorexia, cachexia, weight loss (seen in 30% of patients), fever, and suppressed immunity are paraneoplastic syndromes of unknown etiology. *Endocrine syndromes* are seen in 12% of patients; hypercalcemia and hypophosphatemia resulting from the ectopic production by epidermoid tumors of parathyroid hormone (PTH) or PTH-related peptide production, hyponatremia with the syndrome of inappropriate secretion of antidiuretic hormone or possibly atrial natriuretic factor by small cell cancer, and ectopic secretion by small cell cancer of adrenocorticotropic hormone (ACTH). ACTH secretion usually results in additional electrolyte disturbances, especially hypokalemia, rather than the changes in body habitus that occur in Cushing's syndrome from a pituitary adenoma.

Skeletal–connective tissue syndromes include clubbing in 30% of cases (usually non-small cell carcinomas) and hypertrophic pulmonary osteoarthropathy in 1 to 10% of cases (usually adenocarcinomas) with periostitis and clubbing giving pain, tenderness, and swelling over the affected bones and a positive bone scan. *Neurologic-myopathic syndromes* are seen in only 1% of patients but are dramatic and include the myasthenic *Eaton-Lambert syndrome* and retinal blindness with small cell cancer, while peripheral neuropathics, subacute cerebellar degeneration, cortical degeneration, and polymyositis are seen with all lung cancer types. Many of these are caused by autoimmune responses such as the development of anti-voltage-gated calcium channel antibodies in the Eaton-Lambert syndrome (Chap. 101). Coagulation, thrombotic, or other hematologic manifestations occur in 1 to 8% of patients and include migratory venous thrombophlebitis (*Trousseau's syndrome*), nonbacterial thrombotic (marantic) endocarditis with arterial emboli, disseminated intravascular coagulation with hemorrhage, and anemia, granulocytosis, and leukoerythroblastosis. Cutaneous manifestations such as dermatomyositis and acanthosis nigricans are uncommon (≤1%), as are the renal manifestations of nephrotic syndrome or glomerulonephritis (≤1%).

DIAGNOSIS AND STAGING

EARLY DIAGNOSIS   The screening of asymptomatic persons at high risk (men older than 45 years who smoke ≥40 cigarettes per day) by means of sputum cytology and chest radiographs has not improved the survival rate. Although 90% of patients whose lung cancer is detected by screening are asymptomatic, no difference was found in the survival rates of the screened and nonscreened groups. Women have not been studied. The use of low dose spiral computed tomography (CT) lung scanning may be more sensitive, particularly for peripheral lesions. However, false positive rates are high (25% have abnormal tests, only 10% of which are cancers), and survival benefit for screening has not yet been shown (Chap. 80).

ESTABLISHING A TISSUE DIAGNOSIS OF LUNG CANCER   Once signs, symptoms, or screening studies suggest lung cancer, a tissue diagnosis must be established. Tumor tissue can be obtained by a bronchial or transbronchial biopsy during fiberoptic bronchoscopy; by node biopsy during mediastinoscopy; from the operative specimen at the time of definitive surgical resection; by percutaneous biopsy of an enlarged lymph node, soft tissue mass, lytic bone lesion, bone marrow, or pleural lesion; by fine-needle aspiration of thoracic or extrathoracic tumor masses using CT guidance; or from an adequate cell block obtained from a malignant pleural effusion. In most cases, the pathologist should be able to make a definite diagnosis of epithelial malignancy and make the crucial differentiation of small cell from non-small cell lung cancer.

STAGING PATIENTS WITH LUNG CANCER   Lung cancer staging consists of two parts: first, a determination of the location of tumor (anatomic staging) and, second, an assessment of a patient's ability to withstand various antitumor treatments (physiologic staging). In a patient with non-small cell lung cancer, *resectability* (whether the tumor can be entirely removed by a standard surgical procedure such as a lobectomy or pneumonectomy), which depends on the anatomic stage of the tumor, and *operability* (whether the patient can tolerate such a surgical procedure), which depends on the cardiopulmonary function of the patient, are determined.

Non-Small Cell Lung Cancer   The TNM International Staging System should be used for cases of non-small cell lung cancer, particularly in preparing patients for curative attempts with surgery or radiotherapy (Table 88-3). The various T (tumor size), N (regional node involvement), and M (presence or absence of distant metastasis) factors are combined to form different stage groups. At presentation, approximately one-third of patients have disease localized enough for a curative attempt with surgery or radiotherapy (patients with stage I or II disease and some with stage IIIA disease), one-third have distant

Table 88-3   TNM (Tumor, Node, Metastasis) International Staging System for Lung Cancer

Stage	TNM Descriptors	5-Year Survival Rate, %	
		Clinical Stage	Surgical-Pathologic Stage
IA	T1 N0 M0	61	67
IB	T2 N0 M0	38	57
IIA	T1 N1 M0	34	55
IIB	T2 N1 M0	24	39
IIB	T3 N0 M0	22	38
IIIA	T3 N1 M0	9	25
	T1–2–3 N2 M0	13	23
IIIB	T4 N0–1–2 M0	7	<5
	T1–2–3–4 N3 M0	3	<3
IV	Any T any N M1	1	<1

TUMOR (T) STATUS DESCRIPTOR

T0	No evidence of a primary tumor
TX	Primary tumor cannot be assessed, or tumor proven by the presence of malignant cells in sputum or bronchial washings but not visualized by imaging or bronchoscopy
TIS	Carcinoma in situ
T1	Tumor >3 cm in greatest dimension, surrounded by lung or visceral pleura, without bronchoscopic evidence of invasion more proximal than lobar bronchus (i.e., not in main bronchus)
T2	Tumor with any of following: >3 cm in greatest dimension; involves main bronchus, ≥2 cm distal to the carcina; invades visceral pleura; associated with atelectasis or obstructive pneumonitis extending to hilum but does not involve entire lung
T3	Tumor of any size that directly invades any of the following: chest wall (including superior sulcus tumors), diaphragm, mediastinal pleura, parietal pericardium; or tumor in main bronchus <2 cm distal to carina but without involvement of carina; or associated atelectasis or obstructive pneumonitis of entire lung
T4	Tumor of any size that invades any of the following: mediastinum, heart, great vessels, trachea, esophagus, vertebral body, carina; or tumor with a malignant pleural or pericardial effusion[a], or with satellite tumor nodule(s) within the ipsilateral primary-tumor lobe of the lung.

LYMPH NODE (N) INVOLVEMENT DESCRIPTOR

NX	Regional lymph nodes cannot be assessed
N0	No regional lymph node metastasis
N1	Metastasis to ipsilateral peribronchial and/or ipsilateral hilar lymph nodes, and intrapulmonary nodes involved by direct extension of the primary tumor
N2	Metastasis to ipsilateral mediastinal and/or subcarinal lymph nodes(s)
N3	Metastasis to contralateral mediastinal, contralateral hilar, ipsilateral or contralateral scalene, or supraclavicular lymph node(s)

DISTANT METASTASIS (M) DESCRIPTOR

MX	Presence of distant metastasis cannot be assessed
M0	No distant metastasis
M1	Distant metastasis present[b]

[a] Most pleural effusions associated with lung cancer are due to tumor. However, in a few patients with multiple negative cytopathologic exams of a non-bloody, non-exudative pleural or pericardial effusion that clinical judgment dictates is not related to the tumor, the effusion should be excluded as a staging element and the patient's disease staged as T1, T2, or T3.

[b] Separate metastatic pulmonary tumor nodule(s) in the ipsilateral nonprimary tumor lobe(s) of the lung are classified as M1.

SOURCE: Adapted from CF Mountain. Regional lymph node classification for lung cancer staging taken from CF Mountain and C Dresler: Chest 111:1718, 1997.

metastatic disease (stage IV disease), and one-third have local or regional disease that may or may not be amenable to a curative attempt (some patients with stage IIIA disease and others with stage IIIB disease) (see below). This staging system provides useful prognostic information.

Small Cell Lung Cancer   A simple two-stage system is used. In this system, limited-stage disease (seen in about 30% of all patients with small cell lung cancer) is defined as disease confined to one hemithorax and regional lymph nodes (including mediastinal, contralateral hilar, and usually ipsilateral supraclavicular nodes), while extensive-stage disease (seen in about 70% of patients) is defined as disease exceeding those boundaries. Clinical studies such as physical examination, x-rays, CT and bone scans, and bone marrow examination are used in staging. In part, the definition of limited-stage disease relates to whether the known tumor can be encompassed within a tolerable radiation therapy port. Thus, contralateral supraclavicular nodes, recurrent laryngeal nerve involvement, and superior vena caval obstruction can all be part of limited-stage disease. However, cardiac tamponade, malignant pleural effusion, and bilateral pulmonary parenchymal involvement generally qualify disease as extensive-stage because the organs within a curative radiation therapy port cannot safely tolerate curative radiation doses.

GENERAL STAGING PROCEDURES   (See Table 88-4) All patients with lung cancer should have a complete history and physical examination, with evaluation of all other medical problems, determination of performance status and history of weight loss, and a CT scan of the chest and abdomen with contrast. Positron emission tomography (PET) scans are sensitive in detecting metastatic disease. While not done in every patient, fiberoptic bronchoscopy provides material for pathologic examination, information on tumor size, location, degree of bronchial obstruction (i.e., assesses resectability), and recurrence.

Chest radiographs and CT scans are needed to evaluate tumor size and nodal involvement; old radiographs are useful for comparison. CT scans are of use in the preoperative staging of non-small cell lung cancer to detect mediastinal nodes and pleural extension and occult abdominal disease (e.g., of the liver and adrenal glands), as well as in the planning of curative radiation therapy to allow the design of fields to encompass all the known tumor while avoiding as much normal tissue as possible. However, mediastinal nodal involvement should be documented histologically if the findings will influence therapeutic decisions. Thus, sampling of lymph nodes via mediastinoscopy or thoracotomy to establish the presence or absence of N2 or N3 nodal involvement is crucial in considering a curative surgical approach for patients with non-small cell lung cancer with clinical stage I, II, or III disease. Likewise, unless the CT-detected abnormalities are unequivocal, histology of suspicious abdominal lesions should be confirmed by procedures such as fine-needle aspiration if the patient would otherwise be considered for curative treatment. In small cell lung cancer, CT scans are used in the planning of chest radiation treatment and in the assessment of the response to chemotherapy and radiation therapy. Surgery or radiotherapy can make interpretation of conventional chest x-rays difficult; after treatment, CT scans can provide good evidence of tumor recurrence.

If signs or symptoms suggest involvement by tumor, brain CT or bone scans are performed, as well as radiography of any suspicious bony lesions. Any accessible lesions suspicious for cancer should be biopsied if a histologic diagnosis would influence treatment.

In patients presenting with a mass lesion on chest x-ray or CT scan and no obvious contraindications to a curative approach after the initial evaluation, the mediastinum must be investigated. Approaches vary among centers and include performing chest CT scan and mediastinoscopy (for right-sided tumors) or lateral mediastinotomy (for left-sided lesions) on all patients and proceeding directly to thoracotomy for staging of the mediastinum. In patients presenting with disease that is confined to the chest but not resectable, and who thus are candidates

Table 88-4   Pretreatment Staging Procedures for Patients with Lung Cancer

All Patients
Complete history and physical examination
   Determination of performance status and weight loss
Complete blood count with platelet determination
Measurement of serum electrolytes, glucose, calcium, and phosphorus; renal and liver function tests
Electrocardiogram
Skin test for tuberculosis
Chest x-ray
CT scan of chest and abdomen
CT scan of brain and radionuclide scan of bone if any finding suggests the presence of tumor metastasis in these organs
X-rays of suspicious bony lesions detected by scan or symptom
Barium-swallow radiographic examination if esophageal symptoms exist
Pulmonary function studies and arterial blood gas measurements if signs or symptoms of respiratory insufficiency are present
Biopsy of accessible lesions suspicious for cancer if a histologic diagnosis is not yet made or if treatment or staging decisions would be based on whether or not a lesion contained cancer

Patients with non-small cell lung cancer who have no contraindication to curative surgery or radiotherapy with or without chemotherapy[a]
All the above procedures, plus the following:
   Fiberoptic bronchoscopy with washings, brushings, and biopsy of suspicious areas
   Pulmonary function tests and arterial blood gas measurements
   Coagulation tests
   CT scan of brain
   If surgical resection is planned: surgical evaluation of the mediastinum at mediastinoscopy or at thoracotomy
   If the patient is a poor surgical risk or a candidate for curative radiotherapy: transthoracic fine-needle aspiration biopsy or transbronchial forceps biopsy of peripheral lesions if material from routine fiberoptic bronchoscopy is negative

Patients presenting with small cell or advanced non-small cell lung cancer
For proven small cell lung cancer, all the procedures under ''All Patients,'' plus the following:
   Fiberoptic bronchoscopy with washings and biopsy
   CT scan of brain
   Bone marrow aspiration and biopsy (if peripheral blood counts abnormal)
For non-small cell lung cancer or cancer of unknown histology, all the procedures under ''All Patients,'' plus the following:
   Fiberoptic bronchoscopy if indicated by hemoptysis, obstruction, pneumonitis, or no histologic diagnosis of cancer
   Biopsy of accessible lesions suspicious for tumor to obtain a histologic diagnosis or if therapy would be altered by finding of tumor
   Transthoracic fine-needle aspiration biopsy or transbronchial forceps biopsy of peripheral lesions if fiberoptic bronchoscopy is negative and no other material exists for a histologic diagnosis
   Diagnostic and therapeutic thoracentesis if a pleural effusion is present

[a] Patients with non-small cell lung cancer and extrathoracic metastatic disease, malignant pleural effusion, or intrathoracic disease beyond the bounds of a tolerable radiotherapy port.

for neoadjuvant chemotherapy plus surgery or for curative radiotherapy with or without chemotherapy, other tests are done as indicated to evaluate specific symptoms. In patients presenting with non-small cell cancer that is not curable, all the general staging procedures are done, plus fiberoptic bronchoscopy as indicated to evaluate hemoptysis, obstruction, or pneumonitis, as well as thoracentesis with cytologic examination (and chest tube drainage as indicated) if fluid is present. As a rule, a radiographic finding of an isolated lesion (such as an enlarged adrenal gland) should be confirmed as cancer by fine-needle aspiration before a curative attempt is rejected.

STAGING OF SMALL CELL LUNG CANCER   Pretreatment staging for patients with small cell lung cancer includes the initial general lung cancer evaluation with chest and abdominal CT scans (because of the high frequency of hepatic and adrenal involvement) as well as fiberoptic bronchoscopy with washings and biopsies to determine the tumor extent before therapy; brain CT scan (10% of patients have metastases); bone marrow biopsy and aspiration (20 to 30% of patients have tumor in the bone marrow); and radionuclide scans (bone) if symptoms or other findings suggest disease involvement in these areas. Chest and abdominal CT scans are very useful to evaluate and follow tumor response to therapy, and chest CT scans are helpful in planning chest radiotherapy ports.

If signs or symptoms of spinal cord compression or leptomeningitis develop at any time in lung cancer patients with disease of any histologic type, a spinal CT scan or magnetic resonance imaging (MRI) scan and examination of the cerebrospinal fluid cytology are performed. If malignant cells are detected, radiation therapy to the site of compression and intrathecal chemotherapy (usually with methotrexate) are given. In addition, a brain CT or MRI scan is performed to search for brain metastases, which often are associated with spinal cord or leptomeningeal metastases.

DETERMINATION OF RESECTABILITY AND OPERABILITY In patients with non-small cell lung cancer, the following are major contraindications to curative surgery or radiotherapy alone: extrathoracic metastases; superior vena cava syndrome; vocal cord and, in most cases, phrenic nerve paralysis; malignant pleural effusion; cardiac tamponade; tumor within 2 cm of the carina (not curable by surgery but potentially curable by radiotherapy); metastasis to the contralateral lung; bilateral endobronchial tumor (potentially curable by radiotherapy); metastasis to the supraclavicular lymph nodes; contralateral mediastinal node metastases (potentially curable by radiotherapy); and involvement of the main pulmonary artery. Most patients with small cell lung cancer have unresectable disease; however, if clinical findings suggest the potential for resection (most common with peripheral lesions), that option should be considered.

PHYSIOLOGIC STAGING Patients with lung cancer often have cardiopulmonary and other problems related to chronic obstructive pulmonary disease as well as other medical problems. To improve their preoperative condition, correctable problems (e.g., anemia, electrolyte and fluid disorders, infections, and arrhythmias) should be addressed, smoking stopped, and appropriate chest therapy instituted. Since it is not always possible to predict whether a lobectomy or pneumonectomy will be required until the time of operation, a conservative approach is to restrict resectional surgery to patients who could potentially tolerate a pneumonectomy. In addition to nonambulatory performance status, a myocardial infarction within the past 3 months is a contraindication to thoracic surgery because 20% of patients will die of reinfarction, while an infarction in the past 6 months is a relative contraindication. Other major contraindications include uncontrolled major arrhythmias, a maximum breathing capacity <40% of the predicted value, an FEV_1 (forced expiratory volume in 1 s) <1 L, CO_2 retention (which is more serious than hypoxemia), and severe pulmonary hypertension. Recommending surgery when the FEV_1 is 1.1 to 2.4 L requires careful judgment, while an FEV_1 >2.5 L usually permits a pneumonectomy. In patients with borderline pulmonary status or a question of pulmonary hypertension, split pulmonary function testing by ventilation-perfusion lung scans can define physiologic operability. The activity from quantitative scans is summed for each lung in the anterior and posterior views, and the ratio of the normal to total lung activity is multiplied by the FEV_1. Pneumonectomy usually is physiologically tolerable if this predicted value is >1 L.

℞ **TREATMENT** The overall treatment approach to patients with lung cancer is shown in Table 88-5. Patients should be encouraged to stop smoking. Those who do fare better than those who continue to smoke.

Non-Small Cell Lung Cancer: Localized Disease • *Surgery* In patients with non-small cell lung cancer of stages IA, IB, IIA and IIB (Table 88-3) who can tolerate operation, the treatment of choice is pulmonary resection. In stage IIIA cases where the patient's age, cardiopulmonary function, and anatomy are favorable, resection also should be considered. If a complete resection is possible, the 5-year survival rate for N1 disease is about 50%, while it is about 20% for N2 disease. However, only 20% of cases of N2 disease are technically

Table 88-5 Summary of Treatment Approach to Patients with Lung Cancer

Non-small cell lung cancer
Stages IA, IB, IIA, IIB, and some IIIA:
  Surgical resection for stages IA, IB, IIA, and IIB
  Surgical resection with complete-mediastinal lymph node dissection and consideration of neoadjuvant CRx for stage IIIA disease with "minimal N2 involvement" (discovered at thoracotomy or mediastinoscopy)
  Postoperative RT for patients found to have N2 disease if no neoadjuvant CRx given
  Discussion of risks/benefits of adjuvant CRx with individual patients
  Curative potential RT for "nonoperable" patients
Stage IIIA with selected types of stage T3 tumors:
  Tumors with chest wall invasion (T3): en bloc resection of tumor with involved chest wall and consideration of postoperative RT
  Superior sulcus (Pancoast's) (T3) tumors: preoperative RT (30–45 Gy) followed by en bloc resection of involved lung and chest wall with consideration of postoperative RT or intraoperative brachytherapy
  Proximal airway involvement (<2 cm from carina) without mediastinal nodes: sleeve resection if possible preserving distal normal lung or pneumonectomy
Stages IIIA "advanced, bulky, clinically evident N2 disease" (discovered preoperatively) and IIIB disease that can be included in a tolerable RT port:
  Curative potential RT + CRx if performance status and general medical condition are reasonable; otherwise, RT alone
  Consider neoadjuvant CRx and surgical resection for IIIA disease with advanced N2 involvement
Stage IIIB disease with carinal invasion (T4) but without N2 involvement:
  Consider pneumonectomy with tracheal sleeve resection with direct reanastomosis to contralateral mainstem bronchus
Stage IV and more advanced IIIB disease:
  RT to symptomatic local sites
  CRx for ambulatory patients
  Chest tube drainage of large malignant pleural effusions
  Consider resection of primary tumor and metastasis for isolated brain or adrenal metastases

Small cell lung cancer
  Limited stage (good performance status): combination CRx + chest RT
  Extensive stage (good performance status): combination CRx
  Complete tumor responders (all stages): prophylactic cranial RT
  Poor-performance-status patients (all stages):
    Modified-dose combination CRx
    Palliative RT

All patients
  RT for brain metastases, spinal cord compression, weight-bearing lytic bony lesions, symptomatic local lesions (nerve paralyses, obstructed airway, hemoptysis in non-small cell lung cancer and in small cell cancer not responding to CRx)
  Appropriate diagnosis and treatment of other medical problems and supportive care during CRx
  Encouragement to stop smoking
  Entrance into clinical trial, if eligible

ABBREVIATIONS: CRx, chemotherapy; RT, radiotherapy.

resectable, and most of these are discovered to be N2 only at thoracotomy. Surgery for N2 disease is the most controversial area in the surgical management of lung cancer. Patients with N2 disease can be divided into "minimal" disease (involvement of only one node with microscopic foci, usually discovered at thoracotomy or mediastinoscopy) and the more common "advanced," bulky disease, clinically obvious on CT scans and discovered preoperatively. Patients with contralateral or bilateral positive mediastinal (N3) nodes, extracapsular nodal involvement, or fixed nodes are not considered candidates for resection. Approaches that may make resection possible include chest wall resection for direct extension of tumor, tracheal sleeve pneumonectomy, and sleeve lobectomy for lesions near the carina. Neoadjuvant (preoperative) chemotherapy has response rates of 50 to 60% and causes unresectable disease to become resectable in many patients who respond (see below). Video-assisted thoracic surgery (VATS) via thoracoscopy is not usually used for curative lung cancer resection but may be useful for peripheral lesions in patients with poor lung function.

The extent of resection is a matter of surgical judgment based on findings at exploration. Conservative resection that encompasses all known tumor gives survival equal to that obtained with more extensive procedures. However, lobectomy is superior to wedge resection in reducing the rate of local recurrence. Thus, lobectomy is preferred to pneumonectomy and wedge resection. Wedge resection and segmentectomy (potentially by VATS) are reserved for patients with poor pulmonary reserve and small peripheral lesions. About 43% of all patients with lung cancer undergo thoracotomy. Of these, 76% have a definitive resection, 12% are explored only for disease extent, and 12% have a palliative procedure with known disease left behind. About 30% of patients treated with resection for cure survive for 5 years, and 15% survive for 10 years (Table 88-3). The 30-day hospital mortality rate after pulmonary resection is 3% for lobectomy and 6% for pneumonectomy. Thus, most patients thought to have a "curative" resection ultimately die of metastatic disease (usually within 5 years of surgery).

Management of occult and stage 0 carcinomas In the uncommon situation where malignant cells are identified in a sputum or bronchial washing specimen but the chest radiograph appears normal (TX tumor stage), the lesion must be localized. More than 90% can be localized by meticulous examination of the bronchial tree with a fiberoptic bronchoscope under general anesthesia and collection of a series of differential brushings and biopsies. Often, carcinoma in situ or multicentric lesions are found in these patients. Current recommendations are for the most conservative surgical resection, allowing removal of the cancer and conservation of lung parenchyma, even if the bronchial margins are positive for carcinoma in situ. The 5-year overall survival rate for these occult cancers is ~60%. Close follow-up of these patients is indicated because of the high incidence of second primary lung cancers (5% per patient per year). One approach to in situ or multicentric lesions uses systemically administered hematoporphyrin (which localizes to tumors and sensitizes them to light) followed by bronchoscopic phototherapy.

Solitary pulmonary nodule When a patient presents with an asymptomatic, solitary pulmonary nodule (defined as an x-ray density completely surrounded by normal aerated lung, with circumscribed margins, of any shape, usually 1 to 6 cm in greatest diameter), a decision to resect or follow the nodule must be made. Approximately 35% of all such lesions in adults are malignant, most being primary lung cancer, while <1% are malignant in nonsmokers under 35 years of age. A complete history, including a smoking history, physical examination, routine laboratory tests, chest CT scan, fiberoptic bronchoscopy, and old chest x-rays are obtained. PET scans are useful in detecting lung cancers >1.5 cm in diameter. If no diagnosis is immediately apparent, the following risk factors would all argue strongly in favor of proceeding with resection to establish a histologic diagnosis: a history of cigarette smoking; age 35 years or older; a relatively large lesion; lack of calcification; chest symptoms; associated atelectasis, pneumonitis, or adenopathy; and growth of the lesion revealed by comparison with old x-rays. At present, only two radiographic criteria are reliable predictors of the benign nature of a solitary pulmonary nodule: lack of growth over a period >2 years and certain characteristic patterns of calcification. Calcification alone does not exclude malignancy. However, a dense central nidus, multiple punctate foci, and "bull's eye" (granuloma) and "popcorn ball" (hamartoma) calcifications are all highly suggestive of a benign lesion.

When old x-rays are not available and the characteristic calcification patterns are absent, the following approach is reasonable: Nonsmoking patients younger than 35 years can be followed with serial CT every 3 months for 1 year and then yearly. If any significant growth is found, a histologic diagnosis is needed. For patients older than 35 years and all patients with a smoking history, a histologic diagnosis must be made. The sample for histologic diagnosis can be obtained either at the time of nodule resection or, if the patient is a poor oper-

ative risk, via VATS or transthoracic fine-needle biopsy. Some institutions use preoperative fine-needle aspiration on all such lesions; however, all positive lesions have to be resected, and negative cytologic findings in most cases have to be confirmed by histology on a resected specimen. While much has been made of sparing patients an operation, the high probability of finding a malignancy (particularly in smokers older than 35 years) and the excellent chance for surgical cure when the tumor is small both suggest an aggressive approach to these lesions.

The application of low-dose spiral CT scanning to high-risk populations is under investigation. The test identifies a large number of asymptomatic pulmonary nodules that require evaluation. Approximately 23% of screened high-risk patients have an abnormality, and ~12% of the detected abnormalities are lung cancer. Criteria for distinguishing cancers from nonmalignant lesions short of a lobectomy are being developed. Lesions >1 cm are usually resected; those ≤1 cm are followed for change at 3-month intervals. Although a number of early lung cancers are detected in this way, it is not yet clear that survival is improved.

Radiotherapy with curative intent Patients with stage III disease, as well as patients with stage I or II disease who refuse surgery or are not candidates for pulmonary resection, should be considered for radiation therapy with curative intent. The decision to administer high-dose radiotherapy is based on the extent of disease and the volume of the chest that requires irradiation. Patients with distant metastases, malignant pleural effusion, or cardiac involvement are generally not considered for curative radiation treatment. The median survival period for patients with unresectable non-small cell lung cancer localized to the chest who undergo primary radiotherapy with curative intent is <1 year. However, 6% of these patients are alive at 5 years and are cured by radiotherapy alone. In addition to being potentially curative, radiotherapy, by controlling the primary tumor, may increase the quality and length of life of noncured patients. Treatment usually involves midplane doses of 55 to 60 Gy, and the major concern is the amount of lung parenchyma and other organs in the thorax included in the treatment plan, including the spinal cord, heart, and esophagus. In patients with a major degree of underlying pulmonary disease, the treatment plan may have to be compromised because of the deleterious effect of radiation on pulmonary function. The risk of radiation pneumonitis is proportional to the radiation dose and the volume of lung in the field. The full clinical syndrome (dyspnea, fever, and radiographic infiltrate corresponding to the treatment port) occurs in 5% of cases. Acute radiation esophagitis occurs during treatment but usually is self-limited, while spinal cord injury should be avoided by careful treatment planning. Continuous hyperfractionated accelerated radiation therapy (CHART) involves delivery of 36 treatments of 1.5 Gy given 3 times a day for 12 consecutive days to a total dose of 54 Gy. The 2-year survival rate increased from 20 to 29% with CHART, although more esophagitis occurred. Brachytherapy (local radiotherapy delivered by placing radioactive "seeds" in a catheter in the tumor bed) provides a way to give a high local dose while sparing surrounding normal tissue.

Combined-modality therapy with curative intent After apparently complete resection, adjuvant radiation therapy has not been shown to improve survival. Meta-analysis of studies with post-operative radiation therapy found it to be deleterious to survival in patients with stage I and II disease.

Carcinomas of the superior pulmonary sulcus producing *Pancoast's syndrome* are usually treated with combined radiotherapy and surgery. Patients with these carcinomas should have the usual preoperative staging procedures, including mediastinoscopy and CT scans to determine tumor extent and a neurologic examination (and sometimes nerve conduction studies) to document neurologic findings. Sometimes a histologic diagnosis is not made, but the combination of tumor location and pain distribution permit a diagnostic accuracy for cancer of >90%. If mediastinoscopy is negative, two curative approaches may be used in treating a Pancoast's syndrome tumor. Preoperative irradiation [30 Gy in 10 treatments] is given to the area, followed by an en bloc resection of the tumor and involved chest wall 3 to 6 weeks later. The 3 year survival rate is 42% for epidermoid and 21% for adeno- and large cell carcinomas. The second approach involves radiotherapy alone in curative doses and standard fractionation, which leads to survival rates similar to those from combined-modality therapy.

A meta-analysis of chemotherapy in non-small cell lung cancer used updated data on 9387 individual patients from 52 randomized trials, both published and unpublished, with the main outcome measure being survival. Regimens containing cisplatin were significantly more effective than no treatment. Trials in early-stage disease comparing surgery with surgery plus chemotherapy gave a hazard ratio of 0.87 (13% reduction in risk of death at 5 years) in favor of chemotherapy. Confidence intervals of these data are wide. However, adjuvant chemotherapy is, in general, not considered standard treatment.

The most impressive benefits were obtained when chemotherapy was added to radiotherapy for locally advanced disease (stage IIIB and some stage IIIA disease) and when chemotherapy was given preoperatively in a neoadjuvant fashion in stage IIIA disease. Preoperative neoadjuvant chemotherapy is widely used for stage IIIA disease. Preoperative combined modality therapy followed by surgical resection has given promising early results. Whether the surgery adds benefit after chemoradiotherapy has not been defined. Provided the risk/benefit ratio of using chemotherapy is discussed appropriately with patients, such therapy can be given in a noninvestigational setting. For stage IIIA disease, resection followed by postoperative radiation plus chemotherapy for N2 disease, neoadjuvant chemotherapy followed by surgical resection, or neoadjuvant chemoradiotherapy followed by resection are options. For stage IIIB and bulky IIIA disease, neoadjuvant chemotherapy (2 or 3 cycles of a cisplatin-based combination) followed by chest radiation therapy (60 Gy) has improved median survival time from 10 to 14 months and the 5-year survival rate from 7 to 17% compared to results with radiation therapy alone. Administration of radiation and chemotherapy concurrently is being tested; myelotoxicity and esophagitis are increased, but survival improvement is not yet proven. Randomized clinical trials also are needed to evaluate the usefulness of the new agents with activity against non-small cell lung cancer, including the taxanes (paclitaxel and docetaxel), vinorelbine, gemcitabine, and camptothecins (topotecan and CPT-11) in both adjuvant and neoadjuvant settings.

Disseminated Non-Small Cell Lung Cancer The 70% of patients who have unresectable non-small cell cancer have a poor prognosis. Patients with performance status scores of 0 (asymptomatic), 1 (symptomatic, fully ambulatory), 2 (in bed <50% of the time), 3 (in bed >50% of the time), and 4 (bedridden) have median survival times of 34, 25, 17, 8, and 4 weeks, respectively. Standard medical management, the judicious use of pain medications, the appropriate use of radiotherapy, and outpatient chemotherapy form the cornerstone of management. Patients whose primary tumor is causing symptoms such as bronchial obstruction with pneumonitis, hemoptysis, or upper airway or superior vena cava obstruction should have radiotherapy to the primary tumor. The case for prophylactic treatment of the asymptomatic patient is to prevent major symptoms from occurring in the thorax. However, if the patient can be followed closely, it may be appropriate to defer treatment until symptoms develop. Usually a course of 30 to 40 Gy over 2 to 4 weeks is given to the tumor. Radiation therapy provides relief of intrathoracic symptoms with the following frequencies: hemoptysis, 84%; superior vena cava syndrome, 80%; dyspnea, 60%; cough, 60%; atelectasis, 23%; and vocal cord paralysis, 6%. Cardiac tamponade (treated with pericardiocentesis and radiation therapy to the heart), painful bony metastases (with relief in 66%), brain or spinal cord compression, and brachial plexus involvement may also be palliated with radiotherapy. Usually, with brain metastases and cord compression, dexamethasone (25 to 100 mg/d in four divided doses) is also given and then rapidly tapered to the lowest dosage that relieves symptoms.

Brain metastases often are isolated instances of relapse in patients with adenocarcinoma of the lung otherwise controlled by surgery or

radiotherapy. However, there is no proven value for prophylactic cranial irradiation or for CT scans of the head in asymptomatic patients.

Pleural effusions are common and are usually treated with thoracentesis. If they recur and are symptomatic, chest tube drainage with a sclerosing agent such as intrapleural talc is used. First, the chest cavity is completely drained. Xylocaine 1% is instilled (15 mL), followed by 50 mL normal saline. Then, 10 g sterile talc is dissolved in 100 mL normal saline, and this solution is injected through the chest tube. The chest tube is clamped for 4 h if tolerated, and the patient is rotated onto different sides to distribute the sclerosing agent. The chest tube is removed 24 to 48 h later, after drainage has become slight (usually <100 mL/24 h). VATS has been used to drain and treat large malignant effusions. Symptomatic endobronchial lesions that recur after surgery or radiotherapy or that develop in patients with severely compromised pulmonary function are difficult to treat with conventional therapy. Neodynium-YAG (yttrium-aluminum-garnet) laser therapy administered through a flexible fiberoptic bronchoscope (usually under general anesthesia) can provide palliation in 80 to 90% of patients even when the tumor has relapsed after radiotherapy. Local radiotherapy delivered by brachytherapy, photodynamic therapy using a photosensitizing agent, and endobronchial stents are other measures that can relieve airway obstruction from tumor.

Chemotherapy The use of chemotherapy for non-small cell lung cancer requires careful judgment to balance potential benefits and toxicity. Modest survival benefits (of 1 to 2 months), symptom palliation, and improved quality of life may accrue from combination chemotherapy. Randomized trials in advanced disease comparing supportive care with supportive care plus chemotherapy gave a hazard ratio of 0.73 (27% reduction in risk of death at 1 year) in favor of including chemotherapy. Economic analysis has found chemotherapy to be cost-effective palliation. Combination chemotherapy produces an objective tumor response in ~30 to 40% of patients; the response is complete in <5%. Median survival for chemotherapy-treated patients is 9 to 10 months, and the 1-year survival rate is 40%. Thus, in patients with non-small cell lung cancer who desire chemotherapy, it is reasonable to give chemotherapy if the patient is ambulatory, has not received prior chemotherapy, and is able to understand and accept the risk/benefit ratio from such therapy. The chemotherapy should be one of the published standard regimens, such as paclitaxel plus carboplatin, paclitaxel plus cisplatin, or vinorelbine plus cisplatin. Improved antiemetics have made treatment tolerable on an outpatient basis. New drugs with proven activity in non-small cell lung cancer include docetaxel, irinotecan, and gemcitabine. All eligible patients should be encouraged to enter clinical studies that are designed to determine the benefits and toxicities of these new treatments.

Small Cell Lung Cancer Untreated patients with small cell lung cancer have a median survival period of 6 to 17 weeks, while patients treated with combination chemotherapy have a median survival period of 40 to 70 weeks. Thus, chemotherapy with or without radiotherapy or surgery can prolong survival in patients with small cell lung cancer. The goal of treatment is to achieve a complete clinical regression of tumor documented by repeating the initial positive staging procedures, particularly fiberoptic bronchoscopy with washings and biopsy. The initial response, determined 6 to 12 weeks after the start of therapy, predicts both the median and long-term survivals and the potential for cure. Patients who achieve a complete clinical regression survive longer than patients with only partial regression, who in turn survive longer than patients with no response. Complete response is required for long-term (>3-year) survival.

After initial staging, patients are classified as having limited or extensive disease and as being physiologically able or not able to tolerate combination chemotherapy or chemoradiotherapy. The overall mortality rate from initial combination chemotherapy even in these selected patients is 1 to 5%, comparable with the operative mortality rate for pulmonary resection. Such therapy should be reserved for ambulatory patients with no prior chemotherapy or radiotherapy; no other major medical problems; and adequate heart, liver, renal, and bone marrow function. The arterial P_{O_2} on room air should be >6.6 kPa (50 mmHg), and there should be no CO_2 retention. For patients with limitations in any of these areas, the initial combined-modality therapy or chemotherapy must be modified to prevent undue toxicity. In all patients, these treatments must be coupled with supportive care for infectious, hemorrhagic, and other medical complications.

Chemotherapy The combination most widely used is etoposide plus cisplatin or carboplatin, given every 3 weeks on an outpatient basis for 4 to 6 cycles. Another active regimen is etopside, cisplatin, and paclitaxel. Increased dose intensity of chemotherapy adds toxicity without clear survival benefit. Appropriate supportive care (antiemetic therapy, administration of fluid and saline boluses with cisplatin, monitoring of blood counts and blood chemistries, monitoring for signs of bleeding or infection, and, as required, administration of erythropoietin and granulocyte colony-stimulating factor) and adjustment of chemotherapy doses on the basis of nadir granulocyte counts are essential. The initial combination chemotherapy may result in moderate to severe granulocytopenia (e.g., granulocyte counts <500 to 1500/μL) and thrombocytopenia (platelet counts <50,000 to 100,000/μL). After the initial 4 to 6 cycles of therapy, patients should be restaged to determine if they have entered a complete clinical remission, indicated by complete disappearance of all clinically evident lesions and paraneoplastic syndromes, or a partial remission, or have no response or tumor progression (seen in 10 to 20% of patients). Chemotherapy is then stopped in responding patients. More prolonged chemotherapy has not been shown to be of value. Patients whose tumors are progressing or not responding should be switched to a new, experimental chemotherapy regimen. Oral etoposide, as a single agent, has been shown to be of clinical benefit in the initial treatment of patients who are elderly or have a very poor performance status.

Radiotherapy High-dose (40 Gy) radiotherapy to the whole brain should be given to patients with documented brain metastases. Prophylactic cranial irradiation (PCI) may be given to patients with complete responses, since it significantly decreases the development of brain metastases (which occur in 60 to 80% of patients living ≥2 years who do not receive PCI), but survival benefit is small (5%). Because some studies indicate possible deficits in cognitive ability that could be related to PCI, the long-term quality of life after PCI needs to be further studied. The patient needs to be informed of the risks and benefits. In the case of symptomatic, progressive lesions in the chest or at other critical sites, if radiotherapy has not yet been given to these areas, it may be administered in full doses (e.g., 40 Gy to the chest tumor mass).

Combined-modality therapy Most patients with limited-stage small cell lung cancer should receive combined-modality therapy with etoposide plus cisplatin (or other platinum-containing regimen) and concurrent chest radiotherapy. Acute and chronic toxicities are expected with chemoradiotherapy, particularly when the chemotherapy and radiotherapy are given concurrently. However, the addition of chest radiation therapy to chemotherapy reduces the local failure rate and improves survival. Patients should be selected (limited-stage disease, a performance status of 0 to 1, and initial good pulmonary function) such that radiotherapy can be given in full doses and in a manner that does not sacrifice too much lung function. Some studies show twice-daily radiation fractions produce less toxicity and improve survival compared to once-daily treatments, but large randomized trials are still needed.

For extensive-stage disease, initial chest radiotherapy usually is not advocated. However, for favorable patients (e.g., those with a performance status of 0 to 1, good pulmonary function, and only one site of extensive disease), the addition of chest radiotherapy to chemotherapy can be considered. For all patients, if chemotherapy is inadequate to relieve local tumor symptoms, a course of radiotherapy can be added.

About 20 to 30% of patients with limited-stage disease and 1 to

5% of patients with extensive-stage disease are cured. About 50% of patients with limited-stage and 30% of patients with extensive-stage disease enter complete remission, and 90 to 95% of all patients have complete or partial responses. These responses increase the median survival period to 10 to 12 months for patients with extensive-stage disease and to 14 to 18 months for patients with limited-stage disease, as compared with 2 to 4 months for untreated patients. In addition, most patients have relief of their tumor-related symptoms and improvement of performance status. However, the maintenance of good performance status in a patient receiving outpatient chemotherapy requires judgment and skill to avoid undue therapeutic toxicity. New treatments, such as new drug combinations, very intensive initial or "reinduction" therapy with autologous bone marrow infusion, and novel ways of combining chemotherapy, radiotherapy, and surgery, should be given only in the context of an approved clinical protocol.

Although surgical resection is not routinely recommended for small cell lung cancer, occasional patients meet the usual requirements for resectability (stage I or II disease with negative mediastinal nodes). Moreover, this histologic diagnosis is made in some patients only on review of the resected surgical specimen. Such patients have been reported to have high cure rates (>25%) if adjuvant chemotherapy is used.

LUNG CANCER PREVENTION

Deterring children from taking up smoking is likely to be the most effective lung cancer prevention. Smoking cessation programs are successful in 5 to 20% of volunteers; the poor efficacy is because of the nature of nicotine addiction. Early diagnosis strategies have the problem of high false-positive rates, which add to the expense and the failure of such strategies to result in improved survival.

Chemoprevention may be an approach to reduce lung cancer risk. Patients with head and neck cancer, who are at increased risk of developing lung cancer, experienced a decrease in second cancers when given 13-cis retinoic acid. However, the drug causes significant toxicity, and its activity is not yet confirmed. Vitamin E and β-carotene supplements actually increase the risk of lung cancer. Thus, currently no strategy for chemoprevention of lung cancer has been proven effective.

BENIGN LUNG NEOPLASMS

The benign neoplasms of the lung, representing <5% of all primary tumors, include bronchial adenomas and hamartomas (90% of such lesions) and a group of very uncommon neoplasms (chondromas, fibromas, lipomas, hemangiomas, leiomyomas, teratomas, pseudolymphomas, and endometriosis). The diagnostic and primary-treatment approach is basically the same for all these neoplasms. They can present as central masses causing airway obstruction, cough, hemoptysis, and pneumonitis. The masses may or may not be visible on radiographs but usually are accessible to fiberoptic bronchoscopy. Alternatively, they can present without symptoms as solitary pulmonary nodules and thus will be evaluated as part of a solitary pulmonary nodule workup. In all cases, the extent of surgery must be determined at operation, and a conservative procedure with appropriate reconstructions is usually performed.

BRONCHIAL ADENOMAS Bronchial adenomas (80% central) are slow-growing, endobronchial lesions; they represent 50% of all benign pulmonary neoplasms. About 80 to 90% are carcinoids, 10 to 15% are adenocystic tumors (or cylindromas), and 2 to 3% are mucoepidermoid tumors. Adenomas present in patients 15 to 60 years old (average age, 45) as endobronchial lesions and are often symptomatic for several years. Patients may have a chronic cough, recurrent hemoptysis, or obstruction with atelectasis, lobar collapse, or pneumonitis and abscess formation. Bronchial carcinoids, which usually follow a benign course, and small cell lung cancers, which are highly malignant, both express a neuroendocrine phenotype similar to the Kulchitsky cell. This cell is part of the amine precursor uptake and decarboxylation (APUD) system. Carcinoids, like small cell lung cancers, may secrete other hormones, such as ACTH or arginine vasopressin, and can cause paraneoplastic syndromes that resolve on resection. In addition, bronchial carcinoid metastases (usually to the liver) may produce the carcinoid syndrome, with cutaneous flush, bronchoconstriction, diarrhea, and cardiac valvular lesions (Chap. 93), which small cell lung cancer does not. Occasionally, pathologists may have difficulty distinguishing carcinoids from small cell lung cancers. Carcinoid tumors that have an unusually aggressive histologic appearance (referred to as *atypical carcinoids*) metastasize in 70% of cases to regional nodes, liver, or bone, compared with only a 5% rate of metastasis for carcinoids with typical histology.

Bronchial adenomas of all types, because of their endobronchial and often central location, are usually visible by fiberoptic bronchoscopy; and tissue for histologic diagnosis is obtained in this manner. Because they are hypervascular, they can bleed profusely after bronchoscopic biopsy, and this problem should be anticipated. Bronchial adenomas must be dealt with as potentially malignant and thus require removal not only for symptom relief but also because they can be locally invasive or recurrent, potentially can metastasize, and may produce paraneoplastic syndromes. Surgical excision is the primary treatment for all types of bronchial adenomas. The extent of surgery is determined at operation and should be as conservative as possible. Often bronchotomy with local excision, sleeve resection, segmental resection, or lobectomy is sufficient. Five-year survival rates after surgical resection are 95%, decreasing to 70% if regional nodes are involved. The treatment of metastatic pulmonary carcinoids is unclear because they can either be indolent or behave more like small cell lung carcinoma. Assessment of the tempo and histology of the disease in the individual patient is necessary to determine if and when chemotherapy or radiotherapy is indicated.

HAMARTOMAS Pulmonary hamartomas have a peak incidence at age 60 and are more frequent in men than in women. Histologically, they contain normal pulmonary tissue components (smooth muscle and collagen) in a disorganized fashion. They are usually peripheral, clinically silent, and benign in their behavior. Unless the radiographic findings are pathognomonic for hamartoma, with "popcorn" calcification, the lesions usually have to be resected for diagnosis, particularly if the patient is a smoker. VATS may minimize the surgical complications.

METASTATIC PULMONARY TUMORS

The lung is a frequent site of metastases from primary cancers outside the lung. Usually such metastatic disease is considered incurable. However, two special situations should be borne in mind. The first is the development of a solitary pulmonary shadow on a chest x-ray in a patient known to have an extrathoracic neoplasm. This shadow may represent a metastasis or a new primary lung cancer. Because the natural history of lung cancer is often worse than that of other primary tumors, a single pulmonary nodule in a patient with a known extrathoracic tumor is approached as though the nodule is a primary lung cancer, particularly if the patient is older than 35 years and a smoker. If a vigorous search for other sites of active cancer proves negative, the nodule is surgically resected. Second, in some cases, multiple pulmonary nodules can be resected with curative intent. This tactic is usually recommended if, after careful staging, it is found that (1) the patient can tolerate the contemplated pulmonary resection, (2) the primary tumor has been definitively and successfully treated, and (3) all known metastatic disease can be encompassed by the projected pulmonary resection. The key is selection and screening of patients to exclude those with uncontrolled primary tumors and extrapulmonary metastases. Primary tumors whose pulmonary metastases have been successfully resected for cure include osteogenic and soft tissue sarcomas; colon, rectal, uterine, cervix, and corpus tumors; head and neck, breast, testis, and salivary gland cancer; melanoma; and bladder and kidney tumors. Five-year survival rates of 20 to 30% have been found in carefully selected patients, and dramatic results have been achieved in patients with osteogenic sarcomas, where resection of pulmonary metastases (sometimes requiring several thoracotomies) is becoming a standard curative treatment approach.

BIBLIOGRAPHY

AUPERIN A et al: Prophylactic cranial irradiation for patients with small-cell lung cancer in complete remission. N Engl J Med 341:476, 1999

CHUTE J et al: Twenty years of phase III trials for patients with extensive-stage small-cell lung cancer: Perceptible progress. J Clin Oncol 17:1794, 1999

Clinical practice guidelines for the treatment of unresectable non-small-cell lung cancer. J Clin Oncol 15:2996, 1997

HECHT SS: Tobacco smoke carcinogens and lung cancer. J Natl Cancer Inst 91:1194, 1999

HENSCHKE CI et al: Early Lung Cancer Action Project: Overall design and findings from baseline screening. Lancet 354:99, 1999

MOUNTAIN CF: Revisions in the international system for staging lung cancer. Chest 111:1710, 1997

TURRISI AT III et al: Twice-daily compared with once-daily thoracic radiotherapy in limited small-cell lung cancer treated concurrently with cisplatin and etoposide. N Engl J Med 340:265, 1999

WAGNER H JR: Postoperative adjuvant therapy for patients with resected non-small cell lung cancer: Still controversial after all these years. Chest 117(Suppl 1):110S, 2000

WINGO PA et al: Annual report to the nation on the status of cancer, 1973–1996, with a special section on lung cancer and tobacco smoking. J Natl Cancer Inst 91:675, 1999

89   *Marc E. Lippman*

BREAST CANCER

Breast cancer is a malignant proliferation of epithelial cells lining the ducts or lobules of the breast. In the year 2000, about 185,000 cases of invasive breast cancer and 42,000 deaths occurred in the United States. Mortality from breast cancer has begun to decrease. Epithelial malignancies of the breast are the most common cause of cancer in women (excluding skin cancer), accounting for about one-third of all cancer in women. This chapter will not consider rare malignancies of the breast, including sarcomas and lymphomas. Human breast cancer is a clonal disease; a single transformed cell—the end result of a series of somatic (acquired) or germline mutations—is able to express full malignant potential. Thus, breast cancer may exist for a long period as either a noninvasive disease or an invasive but nonmetastatic disease.

GENETIC CONSIDERATIONS Not more than 10% of human breast cancers can be linked directly to germline mutations. Several genes have been implicated in familial cases. The Li-Fraumeni syndrome is characterized by inherited mutations in the p53 tumor suppressor gene, which lead to an increased incidence of breast cancer, osteogenic sarcomas, and other malignancies.

Another putative tumor suppressor gene, *BRCA-1*, has been identified at the chromosomal locus 17q21; this gene encodes a zinc finger protein, and the product therefore may function as a transcriptional factor. The gene appears to be involved in gene repair. Women who inherit a mutated allele of this gene from either parent have an approximately 60 to 80% lifetime chance of developing breast cancer and about a 33% chance of developing ovarian cancer. Men who carry a mutant allele of the gene have an increased incidence of prostate cancer but usually not of breast cancer. A third gene, termed *BRCA-2*, which has been localized to chromosome 11, is associated with an increased incidence of breast cancer in men and women.

BRCA-1 and *BRCA-2* can now be sequenced readily and germline mutations detected; patients with these mutations can be counseled appropriately. All women with strong family histories for breast cancer should be referred to genetic screening programs whenever possible, particularly women of Ashkenazi Jewish descent who have a high likelihood of a specific *BRCA-1* mutation (deletion of adenine and guanine at position 185).

Even more important than the role these genes play in inherited forms of breast cancer may be their role in sporadic breast cancer. The p53 mutation is present in approximately 40% of human breast cancers as an acquired defect. Evidence for *BRCA-1* mutation in primary breast cancer has not been reported. However, decreased expression of *BRCA-1* mRNA and abnormal cellular location of the *BRCA-1* protein have been found in some breast cancers. Loss of heterozygosity of some genes suggests that tumor-suppressor activity may be inactivated in sporadic cases of human breast cancer. Finally, one dominant oncogene plays a role in about a quarter of human breast cancer cases. The product of this gene, a member of the epidermal growth factor receptor superfamily, is called *erbB2* (HER-2, neu) and is overexpressed in these breast cancers due to gene amplification; this overexpression can transform human breast epithelium. ■

EPIDEMIOLOGY   Breast cancer is a hormone-dependent disease. Women without functioning ovaries who never receive estrogen replacement do not develop breast cancer. The female to male ratio is about 150 to 1. For most epithelial malignancies, a log-log plot of incidence versus age shows a straight-line increase with every year of life. A similar plot for breast cancer shows the same straight-line increase but with a decrease in slope beginning at the age of menopause. The three dates in a woman's life that have a major impact on breast cancer incidence are age at menarche, age at first full-term pregnancy, and age at menopause. Women who experience menarche at age 16 have only 50 to 60% of the breast cancer risk of a woman having menarche at age 12; the lower risk persists throughout life. Similarly, menopause occurring 10 years before the median age of menopause (52 years), whether natural or surgically induced, reduces lifetime breast cancer risk by about 35%. Women who have a first full-term pregnancy by age 18 have a reduced (30 to 40%) risk of breast cancer compared with nulliparous women. Thus, length of menstrual life— particularly the fraction occurring before first full-term pregnancy— is a substantial component of the total risk of breast cancer. This factor can account for 70 to 80% of the variation in breast cancer frequency in different countries.

International variation in incidence has provided some of the most important clues on hormonal carcinogenesis. A woman living to age 80 in North America has one chance in nine of developing invasive breast cancer. Asian women have one-fifth to one-tenth the risk of breast cancer of women in North America or Western Europe. Asian women have substantially lower concentrations of estrogens and progesterone. These differences cannot be explained on a genetic basis, because Asian women living in a western environment have sex steroid hormone concentrations and risk identical to that of their western counterparts. These women also differ markedly in height and weight from Asian women in Asia; height and weight are critical regulators of age of menarche and have substantial effects on plasma concentrations of estrogens.

The role of diet in breast cancer etiology is controversial. While there are associative links between total caloric and fat intake and breast cancer risk, the exact role of fat in the diet is unproven. However, there is a risk associated with moderate alcohol intake; the mechanism is unknown. Recommendations favoring abstinence from alcohol must be weighed against other social pressures and the possible cardioprotective effect of moderate alcohol intake.

The potential role of exogenous hormones in breast cancer is of extraordinary importance, because millions of American women regularly use oral contraceptives and postmenopausal hormone replacement therapy (HRT). The most credible meta-analyses of oral contraceptive use suggest that these agents cause little if any increased risk of breast cancer. By contrast, oral contraceptives offer a substantial protective effect against ovarian epithelial tumors and endometrial cancers. Far more controversial are the data surrounding HRT in hy-

pogonadal and/or menopausal women. First, HRT with estrogens alone, usually in the form of equine conjugated estrogens, provides less than the physiologic equivalent of premenopausal estrogens but is associated with an increased risk of endometrial cancer, a reduction in the symptoms of estrogen deprivation, a reduction in osteoporosis and resultant hip fractures, and a one-third reduction in deaths due to cardiovascular disease. Meta-analyses suggest a small increase in breast cancer incidence, particularly with high dosages and a long duration of treatment. For the average woman, the negative effect on the breast is probably outweighed by protective effects on bone and heart. Preliminary data suggest that there is a reduction in the risk of colon cancer as well.

The addition of progestogens to HRT regimens drastically reduces the risk of endometrial cancer. It is not clear whether the protective effects against cardiovascular and osteoporotic bone diseases are altered. However, progestogens are copromoters of breast cancer in model systems, and an increased risk of breast cancer is possible.

Whether a history of previous biopsy findings of atypical hyperplasia or in situ carcinoma or strong family histories of breast cancer alter the risk-to-benefit ratios for HRT is unknown. It is likely that the average woman benefits from HRT. The risks of HRT in patients with a positive family history and patients with a remote personal history of breast cancer are unknown.

In addition to the other factors, radiation may be a risk factor in younger women. Women who have been exposed before age 30 to radiation in the form of multiple fluoroscopies (200 to 300 cGy) or treatment for Hodgkin's disease (>3600 cGy) have a substantial increase in risk of breast cancer, whereas radiation exposure after age 30 appears to have a minimal carcinogenic effect on the breast.

EVALUATION OF BREAST MASSES IN MEN AND WOMEN   Because the breasts are a common site of potentially fatal malignancy in women and because they frequently provide clues to underlying systemic diseases in both men and women, examination of the breast is an essential part of the physical examination. Unfortunately, internists frequently do not examine the breast in men, and, in women, they are apt to refer this evaluation to gynecologists. Because of the association between early detection and improved outcome, it is the duty of every physician to distinguish breast abnormalities at the earliest possible stage and to institute a definite diagnostic workup. It is for this reason that all women should be trained in self-examination of the breasts. Although breast cancer in men is unusual, unilateral lesions should be evaluated in the same manner as in women, with the recognition that gynecomastia in men can sometimes begin unilaterally and is often asymmetric. Nevertheless, about as many suspicious breast lesions are now detected by screening mammography as by physical examination.

Virtually all breast cancer is diagnosed by biopsy of a nodule detected either on a mammogram or by palpation. Algorithms have been developed to enhance the likelihood of diagnosing breast cancer and reduce the frequency of unnecessary biopsy.

The Palpable Breast Mass   Women should be strongly encouraged to examine their breasts monthly. The minimum benefit of this practice is the greater likelihood of detecting a mass at a smaller size, when it can be treated with more limited surgery. Breast examination by the physician should be performed in good light so as to see retractions and other skin changes. The nipple and areolae should be inspected, and an attempt should be made to elicit nipple discharge. All regional lymph node groups should be examined, and any lesions should be measured. While lesions with certain features are more likely to be cancerous (hard, irregular, tethered or fixed, or painless lesions), physical examination alone cannot exclude malignancy. Furthermore, a negative mammogram in the presence of a persistent lump in the breast does not exclude malignancy.

In premenopausal women, lesions that are either equivocal or nonsuspicious on physical examination should be reexamined in 2 to 4 weeks, during the follicular phase of the menstrual cycle. Days 5 to 7 of the cycle are the best time for breast examination. A dominant mass in a postmenopausal woman or a dominant mass that persists through a menstrual cycle in a premenopausal woman should be aspirated by fine-needle biopsy or referred to a surgeon. If nonbloody fluid is aspirated and the lesion is thereby cured, the diagnosis (cyst) and therapy have been accomplished together. Solid lesions that are persistent, recurrent, complex or bloody cysts require mammography and biopsy, although in selected patients the so-called triple diagnostic techniques (palpation, mammography, aspiration) can be used to avoid biopsy (Figs. 89-1 to 89-3). Ultrasound can be used in place of fine-needle aspiration to distinguish cysts from solid lesions. Not all solid masses are detected by ultrasound; thus, a palpable mass that is not visualized on ultrasound must be presumed to be solid.

Several points are essential in pursuing these management decision trees. First, risk factor analysis is not part of the decision structure. Second, fine-needle aspiration should be used only in centers that have proven skill in obtaining such specimens and analyzing them. Although the likelihood of cancer is low in the setting of a "triple negative" (benign-feeling lump, negative mammogram, and negative fine-needle aspiration), it is not zero, and the patient and physician must be aware of about 1% risk of false negativity. Third, additional technologies such as magnetic resonance imaging, ultrasound, and sestamibi imaging cannot be used to exclude the need for biopsy, although in unusual circumstances they may provoke a biopsy.

The Abnormal Mammogram   Screening mammography has reduced the lethality of breast cancer by promoting detection at an earlier stage. The procedure is justified on an annual basis for women over age 40.

Screening mammography should not be confused with diagnostic mammography, which is performed after a palpable abnormality has been detected. Diagnostic mammography is aimed at evaluating the rest of the breast before biopsy is performed, or occasionally is part of the triple test strategy to exclude immediate biopsy.

Subtle abnormalities that are first detected by screening mammography should be evaluated carefully by compression or magnified views. These abnormalities include clustered microcalcifications, densities (especially if spiculated), and new or enlarging architectural distortion. For some nonpalpable lesions ultrasound may be helpful either to identify cysts or to guide biopsy. If there is no palpable lesion and detailed mammographic studies are unequivocally benign, the patient should have routine follow-up appropriate to the patient's age.

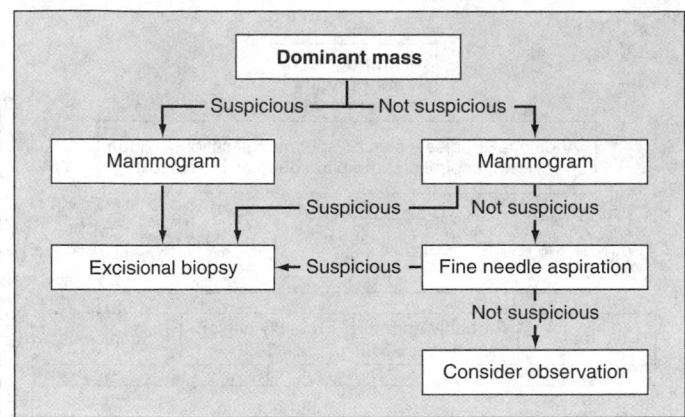

FIGURE 89-2   The "triple diagnosis" technique.

If a nonpalpable mammographic lesion has a low index of suspicion, mammographic follow-up in 3 to 6 months is reasonable. Workup of indeterminate and suspicious lesions has been rendered more complex by the advent of stereotactic biopsies. Morrow and colleagues have suggested that these procedures are indicated for lesions that require biopsy but are likely to be benign—that is, for cases in which the procedure probably will eliminate additional surgery. When a lesion is more probably malignant, open excisional biopsy should be performed with a needle localization technique. Others have proposed more widespread use of stereotactic core biopsies for nonpalpable lesions, on economic grounds and because diagnosis leads to earlier treatment planning. However, stereotactic diagnosis of a malignant lesion does not eliminate the need for definitive surgical procedures, particularly if breast conservation is attempted. For example after a breast biopsy with needle localization (i.e., local excision) of a stereotactically diagnosed malignancy, reexcision may still be necessary to achieve negative margins. To some extent, these issues are decided on the basis of referral pattern and the availability of the resources for stereotactic core biopsies. A reasonable approach is shown in Fig. 89-4.

Breast Masses in the Pregnant or Lactating Woman   During pregnancy, the breast grows under the influence of estrogen, progesterone, prolactin, and human placental lactogen. Lactation is suppressed by progesterone, which blocks the effects of prolactin. After

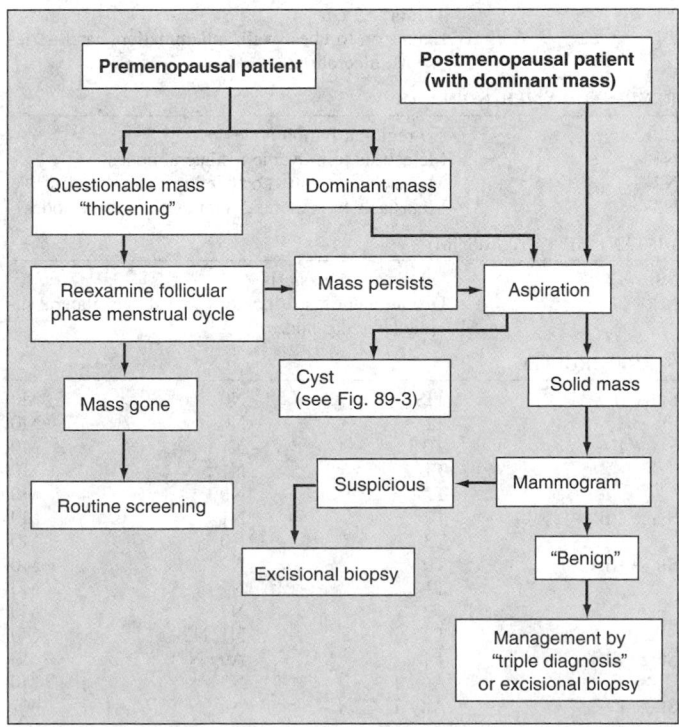

FIGURE 89-1   Approach to a palpable breast mass.

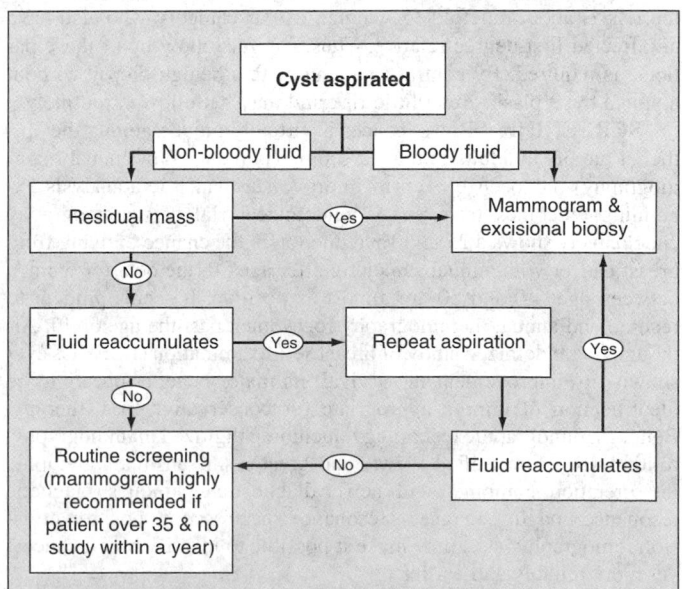

FIGURE 89-3   Management of a breast cyst.

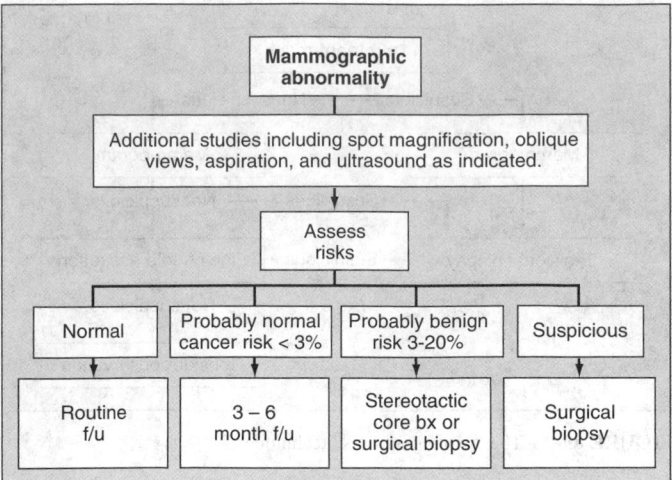

FIGURE 89-4 Approaches to abnormalities detected by mammogram. Note: f/u, follow-up.

delivery, lactation is promoted by the fall in progesterone levels, which leaves the effects of prolactin unopposed. The development of a dominant mass during pregnancy or lactation should never be attributed to hormonal changes, and biopsy should never be performed under local anesthesia. Breast cancer develops in 1 in every 3000 to 4000 pregnancies. Stage for stage, breast cancer in pregnant patients is no different from premenopausal breast cancer in nonpregnant patients. However, pregnant women often have more advanced disease because a breast mass was ignored.

Benign Breast Masses Only about 1 in every 5 to 10 breast biopsies leads to a diagnosis of cancer, although the rate of positive biopsies varies in different countries. (These differences may be related to interpretation and availability of mammograms.) The vast majority of benign breast masses are due to "fibrocystic" disease, a descriptive term for small fluid-filled cysts and modest epithelial cell and fibrous tissues hyperplasia. However, fibrocystic disease is a histologic, not a clinical, diagnosis, and women who have had a biopsy with benign findings are at greater risk of developing breast cancer than those who have not had a biopsy. The subset of women with ductal or lobular cell proliferation (about 30% of patients), particularly the small fraction (3%) with atypical hyperplasia, have a fourfold greater risk of developing breast cancer than unbiopsied women, and the increase in the risk is about ninefold for women in this category who also have an affected first-degree relative. Thus, careful follow-up of these patients is required. By contrast, patients with a benign biopsy without atypical hyperplasia are at little risk and may be followed routinely.

SCREENING Breast cancer is virtually unique among the epithelial tumors in adults in that screening (in the form of annual mammography) has been proven to improve survival. Meta-analysis examining outcomes from every randomized trial of mammography conclusively shows a 25 to 30% reduction in the chance of dying from breast cancer with annual screening after age 50; the data for women between ages 40 and 50 are almost as positive. It seems prudent to recommend annual mammography for women past the age of 40. Although no randomized study of breast self-examination (BSE) has ever shown any improvement in survival, its major benefit appears to be identification of tumors appropriate for conservative local therapy. Better mammographic technology, including digitized mammography, routine use of magnified views, and greater skill in mammographic interpretation, combined with newer diagnostic techniques (magnetic resonance imaging, magnetic resonance spectroscopy, positron emission tomography, etc.) may make it possible to identify breast cancers yet more reliably and earlier.

STAGING Correct staging of breast cancer patients is of extraordinary importance. Not only does it permit an accurate prognosis,

but in many cases therapeutic decision-making is based largely on the TNM classification (Table 89-1). Comparison with historic series should be undertaken with caution, as the staging has changed in the past 10 years.

℞ TREATMENT **Primary Breast Cancer** A series of randomized clinical trials both in the United States and abroad have shown that breast-conserving treatments, consisting of the removal of the primary tumor by some form of lumpectomy with or without irradiating the breast, results in a survival that is as good as that after extensive procedures, such as mastectomy or modified radical mastectomy, with or without further irradiation. While breast conservation is associated with a possibility of recurrence in the breast, 10-year survival is at least as good as that after more radical surgery. Postoperative radiation to regional nodes following mastectomy is also associated with an improvement in survival. Since radiation therapy can also reduce the rate of local or regional recurrence, it should be strongly considered following mastectomy for women with high-risk primary tumors (i.e., T2 in size, positive margins, positive nodes). At present, approximately one-third of women in the United States are managed by lumpectomy. Breast-conserving surgery is not suitable for all patients; it is not generally suitable for tumors >5 cm (or for smaller tumors if the breast is small), for tumors involving the nipple areola complex, for tumors with extensive intraductal disease involving multiple quadrants of the breast, for women with a history of collagen-vascular disease, and for women who either do not have the motivation for breast conservation or do not have convenient access to radiation therapy. However, these groups probably do not account for more than one-third of patients. Thus, a great many women who undergo mastectomy could safely avoid this procedure.

An extensive intraductal component is a predictor of recurrence in the breast, and so are several clinical variables. Both axillary lymph node involvement and involvement of vascular or lymphatic channels

Table 89-1 Staging of Breast Cancer

PRIMARY TUMOR (T)

T0	No evidence of primary tumor
TIS	Carcinoma in situ
T1	Tumor ≤2 cm
T2	Tumor >2 cm but ≤5 cm
T3	Tumor >5 cm
T4	Extension to chest wall, inflammation, satellite lesions, ulcerations

REGIONAL LYMPH NODES (N)

N0	No regional lymph nodes
N1	Metastasis to movable ipsilateral nodes
N2	Metastasis to matted or fixed ipsilateral nodes
N3	Metastasis to ipsilateral internal mammary nodes

DISTANT METASTASIS (M)

M0	No distant metastasis
M1	Distant metastasis (includes spread to ipsilateral supraclavicular nodes)

STAGE GROUPING

Stage 0	TIS	N0	M0
Stage I	T1	N0	M0
Stage IIA	T0	N1	M0
	T1	N1	M0
	T2	N0	M0
Stage IIB	T2	N1	M0
	T3	N0	M0
Stage IIIA	T0	N2	M0
	T1	N2	M0
	T2	N2	M0
	T3	N1, N2	M0
Stage IIIB	T4	Any N	M0
	Any T	N3	M0
Stage IV	Any T	Any N	M1

SOURCE: Modified from the American Joint Committee on Cancer, 1992.

by metastatic tumor in the breast are associated with a higher risk of relapse in the breast but are not contraindications to breast-conserving treatment. When these patients are excluded, and when lumpectomy with negative tumor margins is achieved, breast conservation is associated with a recurrence rate in the breast of less than 10%. The survival of patients who have recurrence in the breast is somewhat worse than that of women who do not. Thus, recurrence in the breast is a negative prognostic variable for long-term survival. However, recurrence in the breast is not the *cause* of distant metastasis. If recurrence in the breast caused metastatic disease, then women treated with lumpectomy, who have a higher rate of recurrence in the breast, should have poorer survival. Most patients should consult with a radiation oncologist before making a final decision concerning local therapy. However, a multimodality clinic approach in which the surgeon, radiation oncologist, medical oncologist, and other caregivers cooperate to evaluate the patient and develop a treatment is usually considered a major advantage by patients.

Adjuvant therapy One of the significant advances in the treatment of solid tumors of adults has been the improved survival resulting from the use of systemic therapy after local management of breast cancer. More than one-third of the women who would otherwise die of metastatic breast cancer remain disease-free when treated with the appropriate systemic regimen.

PROGNOSTIC VARIABLES The most important prognostic variables are provided by *tumor staging*. The size of the tumor and the status of the axillary lymph nodes provide reasonably accurate information on the likelihood of tumor relapse. The relation of pathologic stage to 5-year survival is shown in Table 89-2. For most women, the need for adjuvant therapy can be readily defined on this basis alone. In the absence of lymph node involvement, involvement of microvessels (either capillaries or lymphatic channels) in tumors is nearly equivalent to lymph node involvement. The greatest controversy concerns women with intermediate prognoses. *There is no justification for adjuvant chemotherapy in women with tumors <1 cm in size whose axillary lymph nodes are negative.*

Other prognostic variables have been sought and some appear to influence disease-free and overall survival. What is less clear is whether they add to the information from pathologic staging.

Estrogen and progesterone receptor status are of prognostic significance. Tumors that lack either or both of these receptors are more likely to recur than tumors that have them.

Several *measures of tumor growth rate* correlate with early relapse. S-phase analysis using flow cytometry is the most accurate measure, and the indirect S-phase assessments using antigens associated with the cell cycle, such as PCNA (Ki67), are also valuable. Several studies suggest that tumors with a high proportion (more than the median) of cells in the S phase pose a greater risk of relapse and that chemotherapy offers the greatest survival benefit for these tumors. For this reason, some clinicians use S-phase assessment as a deciding factor for instituting adjuvant therapy when other pathologic features are unclear. Assessment of DNA content in the form of ploidy is of modest value, with nondiploid tumors having a somewhat worse prognosis.

Histologic classification of the tumor has also been used as a prognostic factor. Tumors with a poor nuclear grade have a higher risk of recurrence than tumors with a good nuclear grade. Semiquantitative

measures such as the Elston score improve the reproducibility of this measurement.

Molecular changes in the tumor are also useful. Tumors that overexpress erbB2 (HER-2/neu) or have a mutated p53 gene have a worse prognosis. Particular interest has centered on erbB2 overexpression as measured by histochemistry. Tumors that overexpress erbB2 are more likely to respond to higher doses of doxorubicin-containing regimens. For this reason, erbB2 expression is usually worth measuring as a means of deciding on therapy.

To grow, a tumor must generate a neovasculature (Chap. 83). The presence of more microvessels in a tumor is associated with a worse prognosis.

Other variables that have also been used to evaluate prognosis include proteins associated with invasiveness, such as type IV collagenase, cathepsin D, plasminogen activator, plasminogen activator receptor, and the metastasis suppressor gene, nm23. None of these has been widely accepted as a prognostic variable for therapeutic decision-making. One problem in interpreting these prognostic variables is that most of them have not been examined in a study using a large cohort of patients.

ADJUVANT REGIMENS Selection of appropriate adjuvant chemotherapy or hormone therapy regimens is a highly controversial issue in some situations. Meta-analyses have helped to define broad limits for therapy but do not help in choosing optimal regimens or in choosing a regimen for certain subgroups of patients. A summary of recommendations is shown in Table 89-3. In general, premenopausal women for whom any form of adjuvant systemic therapy is indicated should receive chemotherapy for 6 months. The antiestrogen (tamoxifen) improves survival in premenopausal patients with positive estrogen receptor values and should be added following completion of chemotherapy. Prophylactic castration may also be associated with a substantial survival benefit (primarily in estrogen receptor–positive patients) but is not widely used in this country.

Data on postmenopausal women are also controversial. The impact of adjuvant chemotherapy is less clear-cut than in premenopausal patients, although some survival advantage has been shown. The first decision is whether chemotherapy or tamoxifen should be used. While adjuvant tamoxifen improves survival regardless of axillary lymph node status, the improvement in survival is modest for patients in whom multiple lymph nodes are involved. For this reason, it has been usual to give chemotherapy to postmenopausal patients who have no medical contraindications and who have more than one positive lymph node; tamoxifen is commonly given simultaneously or subsequently. For postmenopausal women for whom systemic therapy is warranted but who have a more favorable prognosis, tamoxifen may be used as a single agent.

Most comparisons of adjuvant chemotherapy regimens show little difference among them, although slight advantages for doxorubicin-containing regimens are usually seen.

One approach—so-called neoadjuvant chemotherapy—involves the administration of adjuvant therapy before definitive surgery and radiation therapy. Because the objective response rates of patients with breast cancer to systemic therapy in this setting exceed 75%, many patients will be "downstaged" and may become candidates for breast-conserving therapy. At least one large randomized study has failed to show any difference in survival using this approach.

Other adjuvant treatments under investigation include the use of new drugs, such as paclitaxel, and therapy based on alternative kinetic and biologic models. In such approaches, high doses of single agents are used separately in relatively dose-intensive cycling regimens. One large randomized trial for node-positive patients suggests that patients treated with doxorubicin-cyclophosphamide for four cycles followed by four cycles of paclitaxel have a substantial additional gain in survival as compared with women receiving doxorubicin-cyclophosphamide alone. Very high dose therapy with stem cell transplantation in the adjuvant setting has not proved superior.

Table 89-2 5-Year Survival Rate for Breast Cancer by Stage

Stage	5-Year Survival, %
0	99
I	92
IIA	82
IIB	65
IIIA	47
IIIB	44
IV	14

SOURCE: Modified from data of the National Cancer Institute—Surveillance, Epidemiology, and End Results (SEER).

Table 89-3 Suggested Approaches to Adjuvant Therapy

Age Group	Lymph Node Status[a]	Endocrine Receptor (ER) Status	Tumor	Recommendation
Premenopausal	Positive	Any	Any	Multidrug chemotherapy + tamoxifen if ER-positive
Premenopausal	Negative	Any	>2 cm, or 1–2 cm with other poor prognostic variables	Multidrug chemotherapy + tamoxifen if ER-positive
Postmenopausal	Positive	Negative	Any	Multidrug chemotherapy
Postmenopausal	Positive	Positive	Any	Tamoxifen with or without chemotherapy
Postmenopausal	Negative	Positive	>2 cm, or 1–2 cm with other poor prognostic variables	Tamoxifen
Postmenopausal	Negative	Negative	>2 cm, or 1–2 cm with other poor prognostic variables	Consider multidrug chemotherapy

[a] As determined by pathologic examination.

Systemic therapy of metastatic disease Nearly half of patients treated for apparently localized breast cancer develop metastatic disease. Although some of these patients can be salvaged by combinations of systemic and local therapy, most eventually succumb. Soft tissue, bony, and visceral (lung and liver) metastases each account for approximately one-third of sites of initial relapses. However, by the time of death, most patients will have bony involvement. Recurrences can appear at any time after primary therapy. Half of all initial cancer recurrences occur more than 5 years following initial therapy.

Because this diagnosis of metastatic disease alters the outlook for the patient so drastically, it should not be made without biopsy. Every oncologist has seen patients with tuberculosis, gallstones, primary hyperparathyroidism, or other nonmalignant diseases misdiagnosed and treated as though they had metastatic breast cancer. This is a catastrophic mistake and justifies biopsy for every patient at the time of initial suspicion of metastatic disease.

The choice of therapy requires consideration of local therapy needs, the overall medical condition of the patient, and the hormone receptor status of the tumor, as well as the exercise of clinical judgment. Because therapy of systemic disease is palliative, the potential toxicities of therapies should be balanced against the response rates. Several variables influence the response to systemic therapy. For example, the presence of estrogen and progesterone receptors is a strong indication for endocrine therapy, since the response rates for tumors that express both receptors may approach 70%. On the other hand, patients with short disease-free intervals, rapidly progressive visceral disease, lymphangitic pulmonary disease, or intracranial disease are unlikely to respond to endocrine therapy.

In many cases, systemic therapy can be withheld while the patient is managed with appropriate local therapy. Radiation therapy and occasionally surgery are effective at relieving the symptoms of metastatic disease, particularly when bony sites are involved. Many patients with bone-only or bone-dominant disease have a relatively indolent course. Under such circumstances, systemic chemotherapy has a modest effect, whereas radiation therapy may be effective for long periods. Other systemic treatments, such as strontium 89 and/or bisphosphonates, may provide a palliative benefit without inducing objective responses. Since the goal of therapy is to maintain well-being for as long as possible, emphasis should be placed on avoiding the most hazardous complications of metastatic disease, including pathologic fracture of the axial skeleton and spinal cord compression. New back pain in patients with cancer should be explored aggressively on an emergent basis; to wait for neurologic symptoms is a potentially catastrophic error. Metastatic involvement of endocrine organs can cause profound dysfunction, including adrenal insufficiency and hypopituitarism. Similarly, obstruction of the biliary tree or other impaired organ function

may be better managed with a local therapy than with a systemic approach.

Endocrine therapy Normal breast tissue is estrogen-dependent. Both primary and metastatic breast cancer may retain this phenotype. The best means of ascertaining whether a breast cancer is hormone-dependent is through analysis of estrogen and progesterone receptor levels on the tumor. Tumors that are positive for the estrogen receptor and negative for the progesterone receptor have a response rate of approximately 30%. Tumors that have both receptors have a response rate approaching 70%. If neither receptor is present, the objective response rates are less than 10%. Receptor analyses provide information as to the correct ordering of endocrine therapies. Because of their lack of toxicity and because some patients whose receptor analyses are reported as negative respond to endocrine therapy, an endocrine treatment should be attempted in every patient with metastatic breast cancer. Potential endocrine therapies are summarized in Table 89-4. The choice of endocrine therapy is usually determined by toxicity profile and availability. In most patients, the initial endocrine therapy is the antiestrogen tamoxifen. Newer antiestrogens that are free of agonistic effects are in clinical trial. Cases in which tumors shrink in response to tamoxifen withdrawal (as well as withdrawal of pharmacologic doses of estrogens) have been reported. Endogenous estrogen formation may be blocked by aromatase inhibitors or analogues of luteinizing hormone–releasing hormone (LHRH). Additive endocrine therapies, including treatment with progestogens, estrogens, and androgens, may also be tried in patients who respond to initial endocrine therapy; the mechanism of action of these latter therapies is unknown. However, patients who respond to one endocrine therapy have at least a 50% chance of responding to a second endocrine therapy. It is not uncommon for patients to respond to two or three sequential endocrine therapies; however, combination endocrine therapies do not appear to be superior to individual agents, and combinations of chemotherapy with endocrine therapy are not useful. The median survival of patients with metastatic disease is approximately 2 years, and many patients, particularly older persons and those with hormone-dependent disease, may respond to endocrine therapy for 3 to 5 years or longer.

Chemotherapy Unlike many other epithelial malignancies, breast cancer responds to several chemotherapeutic agents, including anthracyclines, alkylating agents, taxanes, and antimetabolites. Multiple combinations of these agents have been found to improve re-

Table 89-4 Endocrine Therapies for Breast Cancer

Therapy	Comments
Castration	For premenopausal women
Surgical	
LHRH agonists	
Antiestrogens	
Tamoxifen	Useful in pre- and postmenopausal women
"Pure" antiestrogens	Promising early clinical data
Surgical adrenalectomy	Rarely employed second-line choice
Aromatase inhibitors	Low toxicity and superiority to additive hormone therapy
High-dose progestogens	Common third line choice
Hypophysectomy	Rarely used
Additive androgens or estrogens	Plausible third-line therapies; potentially toxic

NOTE: LHRH, luteinizing hormone–releasing hormone.

sponse rates somewhat, but they have had little impact on duration of response or survival. As previously mentioned, median survival from diagnosis of metastatic disease is approximately 2 years. The choice among multidrug combinations frequently depends on whether adjuvant chemotherapy was administered and, if so, what type. While patients treated with adjuvant regimens such as cyclophosphamide, methotrexate, and fluorouracil (CMF regimens) may subsequently respond to the same combination in the metastatic disease setting, most oncologists use drugs to which the patients have not been previously exposed. Once patients have progressed after combination drug therapy, it is most common to treat them with single agents. Given the significant toxicity of most drugs, the use of a single effective agent will minimize toxicity by sparing the patient exposure to drugs that would be of little value. Unfortunately, no form of in vitro drug sensitivity testing to select the drugs most efficacious for a given patient has been demonstrated to be useful.

Most oncologists use either an anthracycline or paclitaxel following failure with the initial regimen. However, the choice has to be balanced with individual needs.

The use of a humanized antibody to *erbB2* (herceptin) combined with paclitaxel can improve response rate and survival for women whose metastatic tumors overexpress *erbB2*. The magnitude of the survival extension is modest in patients with metastatic disease. Application to adjuvant therapy may prove even more beneficial.

High-dose chemotherapy including autologous bone marrow transplantation Autologous bone marrow transplantation combined with high doses of single agents can produce improvement even in heavily pretreated patients. However, such responses are rarely, if ever, durable and are unlikely to substantially alter the clinical course for most patients with advanced metastatic disease. Randomized trials have not been encouraging, and these approaches cannot be recommended as part of clinical care outside of research settings.

Stage III Breast Cancer Between 10 and 25% of patients have so-called locally advanced or stage III breast cancer at diagnosis. Many of these cancers are technically operable, whereas others, particularly cancers with chest wall involvement, inflammatory breast cancers, or cancers with large matted axillary lymph nodes, cannot be managed with surgery initially. Although no randomized trials have proved the efficacy of induction chemotherapy, this approach has gained widespread use. More than 90% of patients with locally advanced breast cancer show a partial or better response to multidrug chemotherapy regimens that include an anthracycline. Early administration of this treatment reduces the bulk of the disease and frequently makes the patient a suitable candidate for salvage surgery and/or radiation therapy. These patients should be managed in multimodality clinics, if possible, to coordinate surgery, radiation therapy, and systemic chemotherapy. Such approaches produce long-term disease-free survival in about 30 to 50% of patients.

Breast Cancer Prevention Women who have one breast cancer are at risk of developing a contralateral breast cancer at a rate of approximately 0.5% per year. When adjuvant tamoxifen is administered to these patients, the rate of development of contralateral breast cancers is reduced. In other tissues of the body, tamoxifen has estrogen-like effects that are beneficial: preservation of bone mineral density and long-term lowering of cholesterol. However, tamoxifen has estrogen-like effects on the uterus, leading to an increased risk of uterine cancer (0.75% incidence after 5 years on tamoxifen). The Breast Cancer Prevention Trial (BCPT) revealed a >40% reduction in breast cancer amongst women with a risk of at least 1.66% taking the drug for 5 years. Raloxifene has shown similar breast cancer prevention potency but may have different effects on bone and heart. The two are being compared in a prospective randomized prevention trial (the STAR trial).

Noninvasive Breast Cancer Breast cancer develops as a series of molecular changes in the epithelial cells that lead to ever more malignant behavior. Increased use of mammography and better mammographic diagnosis have led to more frequent diagnosis of noninvasive breast cancer. These lesions fall into two groups: ductal carcinoma in situ (DCIS) and lobular carcinoma in situ (lobular neoplasia). The management of both entities is controversial.

Ductal carcinoma in situ Proliferation of cytologically malignant breast epithelial cells within the ducts is termed DCIS. Significant disagreement can occur in differentiating atypical hyperplasia from DCIS. At least one-third of the cases of untreated DCIS progress within 5 years to invasive breast cancer. For many years, the standard treatment for this disease was mastectomy. However, since treatment of this condition by lumpectomy and radiation therapy gives survival that is as good as the survival for invasive breast cancer by mastectomy, it appears paradoxical to recommend more aggressive therapy for a "less" malignant disease. In one randomized trial, the combination of wide excision plus irradiation for DCIS caused a substantial reduction in the local recurrence rate as compared with wide excision alone with negative margins, though survival is identical in the two arms. No studies have compared either of these regimens to mastectomy. Addition of tamoxifen to any DCIS surgical/radiation therapy regimen will further improve outcome.

Several prognostic features may help to identify patients at high risk for local recurrence after either lumpectomy alone or lumpectomy with radiation therapy. These include extensive disease; age less than 40; and cytologic features such as necrosis, poor nuclear grade, and comedo subtype with overexpression of erbB2. Some data suggest that adequate excision with careful determination of pathologically clear margins is associated with a low recurrence rates. When such surgery is combined with radiation therapy, recurrence (which is usually in the same quadrant) occurs with a frequency of ≤10%. Given the fact that half of these recurrences will be invasive, about 5% of the initial cohort will eventually develop invasive breast cancer. A reasonable expectation of mortality for these patients is about 1%, a figure that approximates the mortality rate for DCIS managed by mastectomy. Although this train of reasoning has not formally been proved valid, it is reasonable at present to recommend that patients who desire breast preservation, and in whom DCIS appears to be reasonably localized, be managed by adequate surgery with meticulous pathologic evaluation, followed by breast irradiation and tamoxifen. For patients with localized DCIS, there is no need for axillary lymph node dissection. More controversial is the question of what management is optimal when there is any degree of invasion. Because of a significant likelihood (10 to 15%) of axillary lymph node involvement even when the primary lesion shows only microscopic invasion, it is prudent to do at least a level 1 and 2 axillary lymph node dissection for all patients with any degree of invasion, although in centers familiar with the technique, sentinel node biopsy may be substituted. Further management is dictated by the presence of nodal spread.

Lobular neoplasia Proliferation of cytologically malignant cells within the lobules is termed *lobular neoplasia*. Approximately 30% of patients who have had adequate local excision of the lesion develop breast cancer (usually infiltrating ductal cell carcinoma) over the next 15 to 20 years. Ipsilateral and contralateral disease are equally common. Therefore, lobular neoplasia may be a premalignant lesion that suggests an elevated risk of subsequent breast cancer, rather than a form of malignancy itself, and aggressive local management seems unreasonable. Most patients should be treated with tamoxifen for 5 years and followed with careful annual mammography and semiannual physical examinations. Additional molecular analysis of these lesions may make it possible to discriminate between patients who are at risk of further progression and who require additional therapy and those in whom simple follow-up is adequate.

Male Breast Cancer Breast cancer is about 1/150th as frequent in men as in women. It usually presents as a unilateral lump in the breast and is frequently not diagnosed promptly. Given the small amount of soft tissue and the unexpected nature of the problem, locally advanced presentations are somewhat more common. When male

Table 89-5   Breast Cancer Surveillance Guidelines

Test	Frequency
RECOMMENDED	
History; eliciting symptoms; physical examination	q3–6 months × 3 years; q6–12 months × 2 years; then annually
Breast self-examination	Monthly
Mammography	Annually
Pelvic examination	Annually
Patient education about symptoms of recurrence	Ongoing
Coordination of care	Ongoing
NOT RECOMMENDED	
Complete blood count	
Serum chemistry studies	
Chest radiographs	
Bone scans	
Ultrasound examination of the liver	
Computed tomography of chest, abdomen, or pelvis	
Tumor marker CA 15-3	
Tumor marker CEA	

SOURCE: *Recommended Breast Cancer Surveillance Guidelines*, ASCO Education Book, Fall, 1997.

breast cancer is matched to female breast cancer by age and stage, its overall prognosis is identical. Although gynecomastia may initially be unilateral or asymmetric, any unilateral mass in a man over the age of 40 should receive a careful workup all the way through biopsy. On the other hand, bilateral symmetric breast development rarely represents breast cancer and is almost invariably due to endocrine disease or a drug effect. It should be kept in mind, nevertheless, that the risk of cancer is much greater in men with gynecomastia; in such men, gross asymmetry of the breasts should arouse suspicion of cancer. Male breast cancer is best managed by mastectomy and axillary lymph node dissection (modified radical mastectomy). Patients with locally advanced disease or positive nodes should also be treated with irradiation. Approximately 90% of male breast cancers contain estrogen receptors, and approximately 60% of cases with metastatic disease respond to endocrine therapy. There are no randomized studies exploring adjuvant therapy for male breast cancer. Two historic experiences suggest that the disease responds well to adjuvant systemic therapy, and, if not medically contraindicated, the same criteria for the use of adjuvant therapy in women should be applied to men.

The sites of relapse and spectrum of response to chemotherapeutic drugs are virtually identical for breast cancers in the two sexes.

FOLLOW-UP OF BREAST CANCER PATIENTS Despite the availability of sophisticated and expensive imaging techniques and a wide range of serum tumor marker tests, no studies document that survival is influenced by early diagnosis of relapse. Surveillance guidelines are given in Table 89-5.

BIBLIOGRAPHY

BENICHOU J et al: Graphs to estimate an individualized risk of breast cancer. J Clin Oncol 14:103, 1996

BERRY DA: Benefits and risks of screening mammography for women in their forties: A statistical appraisal. J Natl Cancer Inst 90:1431, 1998

BRODIE AMH, NJAR VCO: Aromatase inhibitors in advanced breast cancer: Mechanism of clinical implications. J Steroid Biochem Mol Biol 66:1, 1998

EARLY BREAST CANCER TRIALISTS' COLLABORATIVE GROUP: Polychemotherapy for early breast cancer: An overview of the randomized trials. Lancet 352:930, 1998

FISHER B et al: Effect of preoperative chemotherapy on the outcome of women with operable breast cancer. J Clin Oncol 16:2672, 1998

———— et al: Lumpectomy and radiation therapy for the treatment of intraductal breast cancer: Findings from National Surgical Adjuvant Breast and Bowel Project B-17. J Clin Oncol 16:441, 1998

HARRIS J et al (eds): *Diseases of the Breast*. 2d ed. Philadelphia, Lippincott-Raven, 1999

MORROW M et al: Local control following breast-conserving surgery for invasive cancer: Results of clinical trials. J Natl Cancer Inst 87(22):1669, 1995

RAVANDI-KASHANI F, HAYES TG: Male breast cancer: A review of the literature. Eur J Cancer 34(9):1341, 1998

STOCKLER M et al: Systematic reviews of chemotherapy and endocrine therapy for metastatic breast cancer. Cancer Treat Rev 26:151, 2000

90   *Robert J. Mayer*

GASTROINTESTINAL TRACT CANCER

The gastrointestinal tract is the second most common noncutaneous site for cancer and the second major cause of cancer-related mortality in the United States.

ESOPHAGEAL CANCER

INCIDENCE AND ETIOLOGY   Cancer of the esophagus is a relatively uncommon but extremely lethal malignancy. The diagnosis was made in 12,300 Americans in 2000 and led to 12,100 deaths. Worldwide, the incidence of esophageal cancer varies strikingly. It occurs frequently within a geographic region extending from the southern shore of the Caspian Sea on the west to northern China on the east and encompassing parts of Iran, Central Asia, Afghanistan, Siberia, and Mongolia. High-incidence "pockets" of the disease are also present in such disparate locations as Finland, Iceland, Curaçao, southeastern Africa, and northwestern France. In North America and western Europe, the disease is far more common in blacks than whites, is more common in males than females, appears most often after age 50, and seems to be associated with a lower socioeconomic status.

A variety of causative factors have been implicated in the development of the disease (Table 90-1). In the United States, esophageal cancer cases are either squamous cell carcinomas or adenocarcinomas. The etiology of squamous cell esophageal cancer is related to excess alcohol consumption and/or cigarette smoking. The relative risk increases with the amount of tobacco smoked or alcohol consumed, with these factors acting synergistically. The consumption of whiskey is linked to a higher incidence than the consumption of wine or beer. Squamous cell esophageal carcinoma has also been associated with the ingestion of nitrites, smoked opiates, and fungal toxins in pickled vegetables, as well as mucosal damage caused by such physical insults as long-term exposure to extremely hot tea, the ingestion of lye, radiation-induced strictures, and chronic achalasia. The presence of an esophageal web in association with glossitis and iron deficiency (i.e.,

Table 90-1   Some Etiologic Factors Believed to Be Associated with Esophageal Cancer

Excess alcohol consumption
Cigarette smoking
Other ingested carcinogens
   Nitrates (converted to nitrites)
   Smoked opiates
   Fungal toxins in pickled vegetables
Mucosal damage from physical agents
   Hot tea
   Lye ingestion
   Radiation-induced strictures
   Chronic achalasia
Host susceptibility
   Esophageal web with glossitis and iron deficiency (i.e., Plummer-Vinson or Paterson-Kelly syndrome)
   Congenital hyperkeratosis and pitting of the palms and soles (i.e., tylosis palmaris et plantaris)
? Dietary deficiencies molybdenum, zinc, vitamin A
? Celiac sprue
Chronic gastric reflux (i.e., Barrett's esophagus) for adenocarcinoma

Plummer-Vinson or Paterson-Kelly syndrome) and congenital hyperkeratosis and pitting of the palms and soles (i.e., tylosis palmaris et plantaris) have each been linked with squamous cell esophageal cancer, as have dietary deficiencies of molybdenum, zinc, and vitamin A.

For unclear reasons, the incidence of squamous cell esophageal cancer has decreased in both the black and white population in the United States over the past 20 years, while the rate of adenocarcinoma has risen dramatically, particularly in white males. Adenocarcinomas arise in the distal esophagus in the presence of chronic gastric reflux and gastric metaplasia of the epithelium (Barrett's esophagus), which is more common in obese persons. Adenocarcinomas arise within dysplastic columnar epithelium in the distal esophagus. Even before frank neoplasia is detectable, aneuploidy and p53 mutations are found in the dysplastic epithelium. These adenocarcinomas behave clinically like gastric adenocarcinoma and now account for >50% of esophageal cancers.

CLINICAL FEATURES About 15% of esophageal cancers occur in the upper third of the esophagus (cervical esophagus), 40% in the middle third, and 45% in the lower third. Squamous cell carcinomas and adenocarcinomas of the esophagus cannot be distinguished radiographically or endoscopically.

Progressive dysphagia and weight loss of short duration are the initial symptoms in the vast majority of patients. Dysphagia initially occurs with solid foods and gradually progresses to include semisolids and liquids. By the time these symptoms develop, the disease is usually incurable, since difficulty in swallowing does not occur until ≥60% of the esophageal circumference is infiltrated with cancer. Dysphagia may be associated with pain on swallowing (odynophagia), pain radiating to the chest and/or back, regurgitation or vomiting, and aspiration pneumonia. The disease most commonly spreads to adjacent and supraclavicular lymph nodes, liver, lungs, and pleura. Tracheoesophageal fistulas may develop as the disease advances, leading to severe suffering. As with other squamous cell carcinomas, hypercalcemia may occur in the absence of osseous metastases, probably from parathormone-related peptide secreted by tumor cells (Chap. 100).

DIAGNOSIS Attempts at endoscopic and cytologic screening for carcinoma in patients with Barrett's esophagus, while effective as a means of detecting high-grade dysplasia, have not yet been shown to improve the prognosis in individuals found to have a carcinoma. Routine contrast radiographs effectively identify esophageal lesions large enough to cause symptoms. In contrast to benign esophageal leiomyomas, which result in esophageal narrowing with preservation of a normal mucosal pattern, esophageal carcinomas characteristically cause ragged, ulcerating changes in the mucosa in association with deeper infiltration, producing a picture resembling achalasia. Smaller, potentially resectable tumors are often poorly visualized despite technically adequate esophagograms. Because of this, esophagoscopy should be performed in all patients suspected of having an esophageal abnormality, to visualize the tumor and to obtain histopathologic confirmation of the diagnosis. Because the population of persons at risk for squamous cell carcinoma of the esophagus (i.e., smokers and drinkers) also has a high rate of cancers of the lung and the head and neck region, endoscopic inspection of the larynx, trachea, and bronchi should also be done. A thorough examination of the fundus of the stomach (by retroflexing the endoscope) is imperative as well. Endoscopic biopsies of esophageal tumors fail to recover malignant tissue in one-third of cases because the biopsy forceps cannot penetrate deeply enough through normal mucosa pushed in front of the carcinoma. Cytologic examination of tumor brushings frequently complements standard biopsies and should be performed routinely. The extent of tumor spread to the mediastinum and paraaortic lymph nodes should also be assessed by computed tomography (CT) scans of the chest and abdomen and by endoscopic ultrasound.

℞ **TREATMENT** The prognosis for patients with esophageal carcinoma is poor. Fewer than 5% of patients are alive 5 years after the diagnosis; thus, management focuses on symptom control. Surgical resection of all gross tumor (i.e., total resection) is feasible in only 40% of cases, with residual tumor cells frequently present at the resection margins. Such esophagectomies have been associated with a postoperative mortality rate of ~10% due to anastomotic fistulas, subphrenic abscesses, and respiratory complications. About 20% of patients who survive a total resection live 5 years. The outcome of primary radiation therapy (5500 to 6000 cGy) for squamous cell carcinomas is similar to that of radical surgery, sparing patients perioperative morbidity but often resulting in less satisfactory palliation of obstructive symptoms. The evaluation of chemotherapeutic agents in patients with esophageal carcinoma has been hampered by ambiguity in the definition of "response" (i.e., benefit) and the debilitated physical condition of many treated individuals. Nonetheless, significant reductions in the size of measurable tumor masses have been reported in 15 to 25% of patients given single-agent treatment and in 30 to 60% of patients treated with drug combinations that include cisplatin. Combination chemotherapy and radiation therapy as the initial therapeutic approach, either alone or followed by an attempt at operative resection, may be of benefit. When administered along with radiation therapy, chemotherapy produces a better survival outcome than radiation therapy alone. The use of preoperative chemotherapy and radiation therapy followed by esophageal resection appears to prolong survival as compared with historic controls, but randomized trials have produced inconsistent results.

For the incurable, surgically unresectable patient with esophageal cancer, dysphagia, malnutrition, and the management of tracheoesophageal fistulas loom as major issues. Approaches to palliation include repeated endoscopic dilatation, the surgical placement of a gastrostomy or jejunostomy for hydration and feeding, and endoscopic placement of an expansive metal stent to bypass the tumor. Endoscopic fulguration of the obstructing tumor with lasers appears to be the most promising of these techniques.

TUMORS OF THE STOMACH

GASTRIC ADENOCARCINOMA **Incidence and Epidemiology** For unclear reasons, the incidence and mortality rates for gastric cancer have decreased markedly during the past 60 years. The mortality rate from gastric cancer in the United States has dropped in men from 28 to 5.0 per 100,000 population, while in women, the rate has decreased from 27 to 2.3 per 100,000. Nonetheless, 21,500 new cases of stomach cancer were diagnosed in the United States and 13,000 Americans died of the disease in 2000. Gastric cancer incidence has decreased worldwide but remains high in Japan, China, Chile, and Ireland.

The risk of gastric cancer is greater among lower socioeconomic classes. Migrants from high- to low-incidence nations maintain their susceptibility to gastric cancer, while the risk for their offspring approximates that of the new homeland. These findings suggest that an environmental exposure, probably beginning early in life, is related to the development of gastric cancer, with dietary carcinogens considered the most likely factor(s).

Pathology About 85% of stomach cancers are adenocarcinomas, with 15% due to lymphomas and leiomyosarcomas. Gastric adenocarcinomas may be subdivided into two categories: a *diffuse type* in which cell cohesion is absent, so that individual cells infiltrate and thicken the stomach wall without forming a discrete mass; and an *intestinal type* characterized by cohesive neoplastic cells that form glandlike tubular structures. The diffuse carcinomas occur more often in younger patients, develop throughout the stomach (including the cardia), result in a loss of distensibility of the gastric wall (so-called linitis plastica or "leather bottle" appearance), and carry a poorer prognosis. Intestinal-type lesions are frequently ulcerative, more commonly appear in the antrum and lesser curvature of the stomach, and are often preceded by a prolonged precancerous process. While the incidence of diffuse carcinomas is similar in most populations, the intestinal type tends to predominate in the high-risk geographic regions and is less likely to be found in areas where the frequency of gastric cancer is declining. Thus, different etiologic factor(s) may be involved in these two subtypes. In the United States, the distal stomach is the site of origin of ~30% of gastric cancers, ~20% arise in the midportion of the stomach, and ~37% originate in the proximal third of the stomach. The remaining 13% involve the entire stomach.

Etiology The long-term ingestion of high concentrations of nitrates in dried, smoked, and salted foods appears to be associated with a higher risk. The nitrates are thought to be converted to carcinogenic nitrites by bacteria (Table 90-2). Such bacteria may be introduced exogenously through the ingestion of partially decayed foods, which are consumed in abundance worldwide by the lower socioeconomic classes. Bacteria such as *Helicobacter pylori* may also contribute to this effect by causing chronic gastritis, loss of gastric acidity, and bacterial growth in the stomach. Loss of acidity may occur when acid-producing cells of the gastric antrum have been removed surgically to control benign peptic ulcer disease or when achlorhydria, atrophic gastritis, and even pernicious anemia develop in the elderly. Serial endoscopic examinations of the stomach in patients with atrophic gastritis have documented replacement of the usual gastric mucosa by intestinal-type cells. This process of intestinal metaplasia may lead to cellular atypia and eventual neoplasia. Since the declining incidence of gastric cancer in the United States primarily reflects a decline in distal, ulcerating, intestinal-type lesions, it is conceivable that better food preservation and the availability of refrigeration to all socioeconomic classes have decreased the dietary ingestion of exogenous bacteria.

Several additional etiologic factors have been associated with gastric carcinoma. Gastric ulcers and adenomatous polyps have occasionally been so linked, but data regarding a cause-and-effect relationship are unconvincing. The inadequate clinical distinction between benign gastric ulcers and small ulcerating carcinomas may, in part, account for this presumed association. The presence of extreme hypertrophy of gastric rugal folds (i.e., Ménétrier's disease), giving the impression of polypoid lesions, has been associated with a striking frequency of malignant transformation; such hypertrophy, however, does not represent the presence of true adenomatous polyps. Individuals with blood group A have a higher incidence of gastric cancer than persons with blood group O; this observation may be related to differences in the mucous secretion leading to altered mucosal protection from carcinogens. Duodenal ulcers are not associated with gastric cancer.

Clinical Features Gastric cancers, when superficial and surgically curable, usually produce no symptoms. As the tumor becomes more extensive, patients may complain of an insidious upper abdominal discomfort varying in intensity from a vague, postprandial fullness to a severe, steady pain. Anorexia, often with slight nausea, is very common but is not the usual presenting complaint. Weight loss may eventually be observed, and nausea and vomiting are particularly prominent with tumors of the pylorus; dysphagia may be the major symptom caused by lesions of the cardia. There are no early physical signs. A palpable abdominal mass indicates long-standing growth and predicts regional extension.

Gastric carcinomas spread by direct extension through the gastric wall to the perigastric tissues, occasionally adhering to adjacent organs such as the pancreas, colon, or liver. The disease also spreads via lymphatics or by seeding of peritoneal surfaces. Metastases to intra-abdominal and supraclavicular lymph nodes occur frequently, as do metastatic nodules to the ovary (Krukenberg's tumor), periumbilical region ("Sister Mary Joseph node") or peritoneal cul-de-sac (Blumer's shelf palpable on rectal or vaginal examination); malignant ascites may also develop. The liver is the most common site for hematogenous spread of tumor.

The presence of iron-deficiency anemia in men and of occult blood in the stool in both sexes mandate a search for an occult gastrointestinal tract lesion. A careful assessment is of particular importance in patients with atrophic gastritis or pernicious anemia. Unusual clinical features associated with gastric adenocarcinomas include migratory thrombophlebitis, microangiopathic hemolytic anemia, and acanthosis nigricans.

Diagnosis A double-contrast radiographic examination is the simplest diagnostic procedure for the evaluation of a patient with epigastric complaints. The use of double-contrast techniques helps to detect small lesions by improving mucosal detail. The stomach should be distended at some time during every radiographic examination, since decreased distensibility may be the only indication of a diffuse infiltrative carcinoma. Although gastric ulcers can be detected fairly early, distinguishing benign from malignant lesions is difficult. The anatomic location of an ulcer is not in itself an indication of the presence or absence of a cancer.

Gastric ulcers that appear benign by radiography present special problems. Some physicians believe that gastroscopy is not mandatory if the radiographic features are typically benign, if complete healing can be visualized by x-ray within 6 weeks, and if a follow-up contrast radiograph obtained several months later shows a normal appearance. However, we recommend gastroscopic biopsy and brush cytology for all patients with a gastric ulcer in order to exclude a malignancy. Malignant gastric ulcers must be recognized before they penetrate into surrounding tissues, because the rate of cure of early lesions limited to the mucosa or submucosa is >80%. Since gastric carcinomas are difficult to distinguish clinically or radiographically from gastric lymphomas, endoscopic biopsies should be made as deep as possible, due to the submucosal location of lymphoid tumors.

The staging system for gastric carcinoma is shown in Table 90-3.

℞ TREATMENT Complete surgical removal of the tumor with resection of adjacent lymph nodes offers the only chance for cure. However, this is possible in fewer than a third of patients. A subtotal gastrectomy is the treatment of choice for patients with distal carcinomas, while total or near-total gastrectomies are required for more proximal tumors. The inclusion of extended lymph node dissection to these procedures appears to confer an added risk for complications without enhancing survival. The prognosis following complete surgical resection depends on the degree of tumor penetration into the stomach wall and is adversely influenced by regional lymph node involvement, vascular invasion, and abnormal DNA content (i.e., aneuploidy), characteristics found in the vast majority of American patients. As a result, the probability of survival after 5 years for the 25 to 30% of patients able to undergo complete resection is ~20% for distal tumors and <10% for proximal tumors, with recurrences continuing to occur for at least 8 years after surgery. In the absence of ascites or extensive hepatic or peritoneal metastases, however, even patients whose disease is believed to be incurable by surgery should be offered an attempt at resection of the primary lesion, since reduction of tumor bulk is the best form of palliation and may enhance the probability of benefit from chemotherapy and/or radiation therapy.

Gastric adenocarcinoma is a relatively radioresistant tumor, and adequate control of the primary tumor requires doses of external beam irradiation that exceed the tolerance of surrounding structures, such as

---

Table 90-2 Nitrate-Converting Bacteria as a Factor in the Causation of Gastric Carcinoma[a]

Exogenous sources of nitrate-converting bacteria:
  Bacterially contaminated food (common in lower socioeconomic classes, who have a higher incidence of the disease; diminished by improved food preservation and refrigeration)
  ? *Helicobacter pylori* infection
Endogenous factors favoring growth of nitrate-converting bacteria in the stomach:
  Decreased gastric acidity
  Prior gastric surgery (antrectomy) (15 to 20 year latency period)
  Atrophic gastritis and/or pernicious anemia
  ? Prolonged exposure to histamine H_2-receptor antagonists

[a] Hypothesis: Dietary nitrates are converted to carcinogenic nitrites by bacteria.

bowel mucosa and spinal cord. As a result, the major role of radiation therapy in patients has been palliation of pain. Radiation therapy alone after a complete resection does not prolong survival. In the setting of surgically unresectable disease limited to the epigastrium, patients treated with 3500 to 4000 cGy did not live longer than similar patients not receiving radiotherapy; however, survival was prolonged slightly when 5-fluorouracil (5-FU) was given in combination with radiation therapy. In this clinical setting, the 5-FU may well be functioning as a radiosensitizer.

The administration of combinations of cytotoxic drugs to patients with advanced gastric carcinoma has been associated with partial responses in 30 to 50% of cases, providing significant benefit to individuals who respond to treatment. Such drug combinations have generally included 5-FU and doxorubicin together with mitomycin-C, cisplatin, or high doses of methotrexate. Despite this encouraging response rate, complete remissions are uncommon, the partial responses are transient, and the overall influence of multidrug therapy on survival has been a source of debate. The use of prophylactic (i.e., adjuvant) chemotherapy following the complete resection of a gastric cancer has not improved survival. However, postoperative chemotherapy combined with radiation therapy has been shown to reduce the recurrence rate and prolong survival.

Table 90-3 Staging System for Gastric Carcinoma

Stage	TNM	Features	Data from American College of Surgeons Number of Cases, %	5-Year Survival, %
0	TisN0M0	Node negative; limited to mucosa	1	90
IA	T1N0M0	Node negative; invasion of lamina propria or submucosa	7	59
IB	T2N0M0	Node negative; invasion of muscularis propria	10	44
II	T1N2M0	Node positive; invasion beyond mucosa but within wall		
	T2N1M0	*or*	17	29
	T3N0M0	Node negative; extension through wall		
IIIA	T2N2M0	Node positive; invasion of muscularis propria or through wall	21	15
	T3N1-2M0			
IIIB	T4N0-1M0	Node negative; adherence to surrounding tissue	14	9
IV	T4N2M0	Node positive; adherence to surrounding tissue		
		or	30	3
	T1-4N0-2M1	Distant metastases		

PRIMARY GASTRIC LYMPHOMA Primary lymphoma of the stomach is relatively uncommon, accounting for <15% of gastric malignancies and about 2% of all lymphomas. The stomach is, however, the most frequent extranodal site for lymphoma, and gastric lymphoma has increased in frequency during the past 25 years. The disease is difficult to distinguish clinically from gastric adenocarcinoma; both tumors are most often detected during the sixth decade of life; present with epigastric pain, early satiety, and generalized fatigue; and are usually characterized by ulcerations with a ragged, thickened mucosal pattern demonstrated by contrast radiographs. The diagnosis of lymphoma of the stomach may occasionally be made through cytologic brushings of the gastric mucosa but usually it requires a biopsy at gastroscopy or laparotomy. Failure of gastroscopic biopsies to detect lymphoma in a given case should not be interpreted as being conclusive, since superficial biopsies may miss the deeper lymphoid infiltrate. The macroscopic pathology of gastric lymphoma may also mimic adenocarcinoma, consisting of either a bulky ulcerated lesion localized in the corpus or antrum or a diffuse process spreading throughout the entire gastric submucosa and even extending into the duodenum. Microscopically, the vast majority of gastric lymphoid tumors are non-Hodgkin's lymphomas of B cell origin; Hodgkin's disease involving the stomach is extremely uncommon. Histologically, these tumors may range from well-differentiated, superficial processes [mucosa-associated lymphoid tissue (MALT)] to high-grade, large cell lymphomas. Infection with *H. pylori*, the same bacterium associated with the development of gastric adenocarcinoma, appears to increase the risk for gastric lymphoma in general and MALT lymphomas in particular. Gastric lymphomas spread initially to regional lymph nodes (often to Waldeyer's ring) and may then disseminate. Gastric lymphomas are staged like other lymphomas (Chap. 112).

℞ **TREATMENT** Primary gastric lymphoma is a far more treatable disease than adenocarcinoma of the stomach, a fact that underscores the need for making the correct diagnosis. Antibiotic treatment to eradicate *H. pylori* infection has led to regression of about 75% of gastric MALT lymphomas and should be considered before surgery, radiation therapy, or chemotherapy are undertaken in patients having such tumors. Responding patients should undergo periodic endoscopic surveillance because it remains unclear whether the neoplastic clone is eliminated or merely suppressed. Subtotal gastrectomy, usually followed by combination chemotherapy, has led to 5-year survival rates of 40 to 60% in patients with localized high-grade lymphomas. The need for a major surgical procedure is not clear, particularly in patients with preoperative radiographic evidence of nodal involvement, for whom chemotherapy alone is effective therapy. A role for radiation therapy is not defined because most recurrences develop at sites distant from the epigastrium. If widespread disease is discovered at the time of laparotomy, combination chemotherapy should be used.

GASTRIC (NONLYMPHOID) SARCOMA Leiomyosarcomas are the most common of this group of gastric malignancies and make up 1 to 3% of gastric neoplasms. They most frequently involve the anterior and posterior walls of the gastric fundus and often ulcerate and bleed. Even those lesions that appear benign on histologic examination may behave in a malignant fashion. Leiomyosarcomas rarely invade adjacent viscera and characteristically do not metastasize to lymph nodes, but they may spread to the liver and lungs. The treatment of choice is surgical resection. Combination chemotherapy should be reserved for patients with metastatic disease.

COLORECTAL CANCER

INCIDENCE Cancer of the large bowel is second only to lung cancer as a cause of cancer death in the United States. Approximately 130,200 new cases occurred in 2000, and 56,300 deaths were due to colorectal cancer. The incidence rate has declined slightly during the past 15 years and the mortality rate has decreased in recent years, particularly in females. Colorectal cancer generally occurs in individuals ≥50 years.

POLYPS AND MOLECULAR PATHOGENESIS Most colorectal cancers, regardless of etiology, arise from adenomatous polyps. A polyp is a grossly visible protrusion from the mucosal surface and may be classified pathologically as a nonneoplastic hamartoma (*juvenile polyp*), a hyperplastic mucosal proliferation (*hyperplastic polyp*), or an adenomatous polyp. Only adenomas are clearly premalignant, and only a minority of such lesions ever develop into cancer. Population-screening studies and autopsy surveys have revealed that adenomatous polyps may be found in the colons of >30% of middle-aged or elderly people; however <1% of polyps ever become malignant. Most polyps produce no symptoms and remain clinically undetected. Occult blood in the stool may be found in <5% of patients with such lesions.

A number of molecular changes have been described in DNA obtained from adenomatous polyps, dysplastic lesions, and polyps containing microscopic foci of tumor cells (carcinoma in situ), which are thought to represent a multistep process in the evolution of normal colonic mucosa to life-threatening invasive carcinoma. These developmental steps towards carcinogenesis include point mutations in the K-*ras* protooncogene; hypomethylation of DNA, leading to gene activation; loss of DNA ("allelic loss") at the site of a tumor suppressor gene [the adenomatous polyposis coli (*APC*) gene] located on the long arm of chromosome 5 (5q21); allelic loss at the site of a tumor suppressor gene located on chromosome 18q [the deleted in colorectal cancer (*DCC*) gene]; and allelic loss at chromosome 17p, associated with mutations in the *p53* tumor suppressor gene (Chap. 81). Thus, the altered proliferative pattern of the colonic mucosa, which results in progression to a polyp and then to carcinoma, may involve the mutational activation of an oncogene followed by and coupled with the loss of genes that normally suppress tumorigenesis. While the present model includes five such molecular alterations, others are likely involved in the carcinogenic process. It remains uncertain whether the genetic aberrations always occur in a defined order. Based on this model, however, it is believed that neoplasia develops only in those polyps in which all of these mutational events take place.

Clinically, the probability of an adenomatous polyp becoming a cancer depends on the gross appearance of the lesion, its histologic features, and its size. Adenomatous polyps may be pedunculated (stalked) or sessile (flat-based). Cancers develop more frequently in sessile polyps. Histologically, adenomatous polyps may be tubular, villous (i.e., papillary), or tubulovillous. Villous adenomas, most of which are sessile, become malignant more than three times as often as tubular adenomas. The likelihood that any polypoid lesion in the large bowel contains invasive cancer is related to the size of the polyp, being negligible (<2%) in lesions <1.5 cm, intermediate (2 to 10%) in lesions 1.5 to 2.5 cm in size, and substantial (10%) in lesions >2.5 cm.

Following the detection of an adenomatous polyp, the entire large bowel should be visualized endoscopically or radiographically, since synchronous lesions are present in about one-third of cases. Colonoscopy should then be repeated periodically, even in the absence of a previously documented malignancy, since such patients have a 30 to 50% probability of developing another adenoma and are at a higher-than-average risk for developing a colorectal carcinoma. Adenomatous polyps are thought to require >5 years of growth before becoming clinically significant; colonoscopy need not be carried out more frequently than every 3 years.

ETIOLOGY AND RISK FACTORS   Risk factors for the development of colorectal cancer are listed in Table 90-4.

Diet   The etiology for most cases of large-bowel cancer appears to be related to environmental factors. The disease occurs more often in upper socioeconomic populations who live in urban areas. Mortality from colorectal cancer is directly correlated with per capita consumption of calories, meat protein, and dietary fat and oil as well as elevations in the serum cholesterol concentration and mortality from coronary artery disease. Geographic variations in incidence are unrelated to genetic differences, since migrant groups tend to assume the large-bowel cancer incidence rates of their adopted countries. Furthermore, population groups such as Mormons and Seventh Day Adventists,

whose lifestyle and dietary habits differ somewhat from those of their neighbors, have significantly lower than expected incidence and mortality rates for colorectal cancer. Colorectal cancer has increased in Japan since that nation has adopted a more "western" diet. At least two hypotheses have been proposed to explain the relationship to diet, neither of which is fully satisfactory.

Animal fats   One hypothesis is that the ingestion of animal fats leads to an increased proportion of anaerobes in the gut microflora, resulting in the conversion of normal bile acids into carcinogens. This provocative hypothesis is supported by several reports of increased amounts of fecal anaerobes in the stools of patients with colorectal cancer. Diets high in animal (but not vegetable) fats are also associated with high serum cholesterol, which is also associated with enhanced risk for the development of colorectal adenomas and carcinomas.

Fiber   The observation that South African Bantus ingest a diet far higher in roughage, produce more frequent, bulkier stools, and have a lower incidence of large-bowel cancer than Americans and Europeans led to the proposal that the higher rate of colorectal cancer in western society results from low intake of dietary fiber. This theory suggests that dietary fiber accelerates intestinal transit time, thereby reducing the exposure of colonic mucosa to potential carcinogens and diluting these carcinogens because of enhanced fecal bulk. This theory has been largely discredited. Although an enhanced fiber intake increases fecal bulk, higher fiber intake has not been documented to consistently shorten stool transit time. In addition, despite the generally higher fiber intake in low-incidence countries, the environmental differences between developing and industrialized nations are myriad and include such other important dietary variables as meat and fat consumption. Furthermore, a diet low in fiber may lead to chronic constipation and diverticulosis. If a low-fiber diet were a significant risk factor in colorectal cancer, individuals with diverticulosis should be at higher risk for developing colorectal tumors; this is not the case. Finally, addition of fiber to the diet does not protect against the development of adenomatous polyps or colorectal cancer.

Thus, the weight of epidemiologic evidence implicates diet as being the major etiologic factor for colorectal cancer, particularly diets high in calories and animal fat.

HEREDITARY FACTORS AND SYNDROMES   As many as 25% of patients with colorectal cancer have a family history of the disease, suggesting a hereditary predisposition. Inherited large-bowel cancers can be divided into two main groups: the well-studied but uncommon polyposis syndromes and the more common nonpolyposis syndromes (Table 90-5).

Polyposis Coli   Polyposis coli (familial polyposis of the colon) is a rare condition characterized by the appearance of thousands of adenomatous polyps throughout the large bowel. It is transmitted as an autosomal dominant trait; the occasional patients with no family history probably developed the condition due to a spontaneous mutation. Polyposis coli is associated with a deletion in the long arm of chromosome 5 (including the *APC* gene) in both neoplastic (somatic mutation) and normal (germline mutation) cells. The loss of this genetic material (i.e., allelic loss) results in the absence of tumor suppressor genes whose protein products would normally inhibit neoplastic growth. The presence of soft tissue and bony tumors, congenital hypertrophy of the retinal pigment epithelium, mesenteric desmoid tumors, and of ampullary cancers in addition to the colonic polyps characterizes a subset of polyposis coli known as *Gardner's syndrome*. The appearance of malignant tumors of the central nervous system accompanying polyposis coli defines *Turcot's syndrome*. The colonic polyps in all these conditions are rarely present before puberty but are generally evident in affected individuals by age 25. If the polyposis is not treated surgically, colorectal cancer will develop in almost all patients before age 40. Polyposis coli results from a defect in the colonic mucosa leading to an abnormal proliferative pattern and an impaired DNA repair following exposure to radiation or ultraviolet light. Once the multiple polyps that constitute polyposis coli are detected, patients should undergo a total colectomy. The ileoanal anastomotic technique allows removal of the entire bowel while retaining the anal sphincter;

Table 90-4   Risk Factors for the Development of Colorectal Cancer

Diet
  Animal fat
Hereditary syndromes (autosomal dominant inheritance)
  Polyposis coli
  Nonpolyposis syndrome (Lynch syndrome)
Inflammatory bowel disease
Streptococcus bovis bacteremia
Ureterosigmoidostomy
? Tobacco use

this appears to be the best treatment. Medical therapy with nonsteroidal anti-inflammatory drugs such as sulindac and cyclooxygenase-2 inhibitors such as celecoxib decreases the number and size of polyps in patients with polyposis coli; however, this effect on polyps is only temporary. Colectomy remains the primary therapy. The offspring of patients with polyposis coli, who often are prepubertal when the diagnosis is made in the parent, have a 50% risk for the development of this premalignant disorder and should be carefully screened by annual flexible sigmoidoscopy until age 35. Proctosigmoidoscopy is a sufficient screening procedure because polyps tend to be evenly distributed from cecum to anus, making more invasive and expensive techniques such as colonoscopy or barium enema unnecessary. Testing for occult blood in the stool is an inadequate screening maneuver. An alternative method for identifying carriers is testing DNA from peripheral blood mononuclear cells for the presence of a mutated *APC* gene. The detection of such a germline mutation can lead to a definitive diagnosis before the development of polyps.

Hereditary Nonpolyposis Colon Cancer Hereditary nonpolyposis colon cancer (HNPCC), also known as Lynch syndrome, is another autosomal dominant trait. It is characterized by the presence of three or more relatives with histologically documented colorectal cancer, one of whom is a first-degree relative of the other two; one or more cases of colorectal cancer diagnosed before age 50 in the family; and colorectal cancer involving at least two generations. In contrast to polyposis coli, HNPCC is associated with an unusually high frequency of cancer arising in the proximal large bowel. The median age for the appearance of an adenocarcinoma is <50 years, 10 to 15 years younger than the median age for the general population. Despite having a poorly differentiated histologic appearance, the proximal colon tumors in HNPCC have a better prognosis than sporadic tumors from patients of similar age. Families with HNPCC often include individuals with multiple primary cancers; the association of colorectal cancer with either ovarian or endometrial carcinomas is especially strong in women. It has been recommended that members of such families undergo biennial colonoscopy beginning at age 25 years, with intermittent pelvic ultrasonography and endometrial biopsy offered for potentially afflicted women; such a screening strategy has not yet been validated. HNPCC is associated with germline mutations of several genes, particularly *hMSH2* on chromosome 2 and *hMLH1* on chromosome 3. These mutations lead to errors in DNA replication and are thought to result in DNA instability because of defective repair of DNA mismatches, resulting in abnormal cell growth and tumor development. Testing tumor cells for "microsatellite instability" (sequence changes reflecting defective mismatch repair) in patients under age 50 with colorectal cancer and a positive family history for colorectal or endometrial cancer may identify probands with HNPCC.

INFLAMMATORY BOWEL DISEASE (See also Chap. 287) Large-bowel cancer is increased in incidence in patients with long-standing inflammatory bowel disease. Cancers develop more commonly in patients with ulcerative colitis than in those with granulomatous colitis, but this impression may result in part from the occasional difficulty of differentiating these two conditions. The risk of colorectal cancer in a patient with inflammatory bowel disease is relatively small during the initial 10 years of the disease, but then it appears to increase at a rate of ~0.5 to 1% per year. Cancer may develop in 8 to 30% of patients after 25 years. The risk is higher in younger patients with pancolitis.

Cancer surveillance in patients with inflammatory bowel disease

is unsatisfactory. Symptoms such as bloody diarrhea, abdominal cramping, and obstruction, which may signal the appearance of a tumor, are similar to the complaints caused by a flare-up of the underlying disease. In patients with a history of inflammatory bowel disease lasting 15 years or more who continue to experience exacerbations, the surgical removal of the colon can significantly reduce the risk for cancer and also eliminate the target organ for the underlying chronic gastrointestinal disorder. The value of such surveillance techniques as colonoscopy with mucosal biopsies and brushings for less symptomatic individuals with chronic inflammatory bowel disease is uncertain. The lack of uniformity regarding the pathologic criteria that characterize dysplasia and the absence of data that such surveillance reduces the development of lethal cancers have made this costly practice an area of controversy.

OTHER HIGH-RISK CONDITIONS *Streptococcus bovis* **Bacteremia** For unknown reasons, individuals who develop endocarditis or septicemia from this fecal bacteria have a high incidence of occult colorectal tumors and, possibly, upper gastrointestinal cancers as well. Endoscopic or radiographic screening appears advisable.

Ureterosigmoidostomy There is a 5 to 10% incidence of colon cancer 15 to 30 years after ureterosigmoidostomy to correct congenital extrophy of the bladder. Neoplasms characteristically are found at a site distal to the ureteral implant where colonic mucosa is chronically exposed to both urine and feces.

Tobacco Use Cigarette smoking is linked to the development of colorectal adenomas, particularly after more than 35 years of tobacco use. No biologic explanation for this association has yet been proposed.

PRIMARY PREVENTION Several orally administered compounds have been assessed as possible inhibitors of colon cancer. The most effective class of these chemopreventive agents is aspirin and other nonsteroidal anti-inflammatory drugs, which are thought to suppress cell proliferation by inhibiting prostaglandin synthesis. Regular aspirin use reduces the risk for colonic adenomas and carcinomas as well as for death from large-bowel cancer; this inhibiting effect on colonic carcinogenesis appears to increase with the duration of drug use. Oral folic acid supplements and oral calcium supplements have been found to reduce the risk of adenomatous polyps and colorectal cancers in case-control studies. While antioxidant vitamins such as ascorbic acid, tocopherols, and β-carotene are present in diets rich in fruits and vegetables, which have been associated with lower rates of colorectal cancer, they have been found to be ineffective at reducing the incidence of subsequent adenomas in patients who had undergone the removal of a colonic adenoma. Estrogen replacement therapy has been associated with a reduction in the risk of colorectal cancer in

Table 90-5 Hereditable (Autosomal Dominant) Gastrointestinal Polyposis Syndromes

Syndrome	Distribution of Polyps	Histologic Type	Malignant Potential	Associated Lesions
Familial adenomatous polyposis	Large intestine	Adenoma	Common	None
Gardner's syndrome	Large and small intestine	Adenoma	Common	Osteomas, fibromas, lipomas, epidermoid cysts, ampullary cancers, congenital hypertrophy of retinal pigment epithelium
Turcot's syndrome	Large intestine	Adenoma	Common	Brain tumors
Nonpolyposis syndrome (Lynch syndrome)	Large intestine (often proximal)	Adenoma	Common	Endometrial and ovarian tumors
Peutz-Jeghers syndrome	Small and large intestines, stomach	Hamartoma	Rare	Mucocutaneous pigmentation; tumors of the ovary, breast, pancreas, endometrium
Juvenile polyposis	Large and small intestines, stomach	Hamartoma, rarely progressing to adenoma	Rare	Various congenital abnormalities

women, conceivably by an effect on bile acid synthesis and composition. The otherwise unexplained reduction in colorectal cancer mortality in women may be a result of the widespread use of estrogen replacement in postmenopausal individuals.

SCREENING   The rationale for colorectal cancer screening programs is that the earlier detection of localized, superficial cancers in asymptomatic individuals will increase the surgical cure rate. Such screening programs are important for individuals having a family history of the disease in first-degree relatives. The relative risk for developing colorectal cancer increases to 1.75 in such people and may be even higher if the relative was afflicted before age 60. The use of proctosigmoidoscopy as a screening tool was based on the observation that 60% of early lesions are located in the rectosigmoid. For unexplained reasons, however, the proportion of large-bowel cancers arising in the rectum has been decreasing during the past several decades, with a corresponding increase in the proportion of cancers in the more proximal descending colon. As such, the potential for rigid proctosigmoidoscopy to detect a sufficient number of occult neoplasms to make the procedure cost-effective has been questioned. Flexible, fiberoptic sigmoidoscopes permit trained operators to visualize the colon for up to 60 cm, which enhances the capability for cancer detection. However, this technique still leaves the proximal half of the large bowel unscreened.

Most programs directed at the early detection of colorectal cancers have focused on digital rectal examinations and fecal occult blood testing. The digital examination should be part of any routine physical evaluation in adults older than age 40, serving as a screening test for prostate cancer in men, a component of the pelvic examination in women, and an inexpensive maneuver for the detection of masses in the rectum. The development of the Hemoccult test has greatly facilitated the detection of occult fecal blood. Unfortunately, even when performed optimally, the Hemoccult test has major limitations as a screening technique. About 50% of patients with documented colorectal cancers have a negative fecal Hemoccult test, consistent with the intermittent bleeding pattern of these tumors. When random cohorts of asymptomatic persons have been tested, 2 to 4% have Hemoccult-positive stools. Colorectal cancers have been found in <10% of these "test-positive" cases, with benign polyps being detected in an additional 20 to 30%. Thus, a colorectal neoplasm will not be found in most asymptomatic individuals with occult blood in their stool. Nonetheless, persons found to have Hemoccult-positive stool routinely undergo further medical evaluation, including sigmoidoscopy, barium enema, and/or colonoscopy—procedures that are not only uncomfortable and expensive but also associated with a small risk for significant complications. The added cost of these studies would appear justifiable if the small number of patients found to have occult neoplasms because of Hemoccult screening could be shown to have an improved prognosis and prolonged survival. Prospectively controlled trials addressing this issue have been performed. One of these studies, conducted at the University of Minnesota and involving >46,000 participants, reported a statistically significant reduction in mortality from colorectal cancer for individuals undergoing annual screening. However, this benefit only emerged after >13 years of follow-up and was extremely expensive to achieve, since all positive tests (most of which were false-positive) were followed by colonoscopy. Moreover, these colonoscopic examinations may have represented "chance selection" for more effective endoscopic screening and may also have provided the opportunity for cancer prevention through the removal of potentially premalignant adenomatous polyps.

Screening techniques for large-bowel cancer in asymptomatic persons remain unsatisfactory. Recommendations from governmental and private agencies are conflicting. Compliance with any screening strategy within the general population is poor. At present, the American Cancer Society suggests annual digital rectal examinations beginning at age 40, annual fecal Hemoccult screening beginning at age 50, and sigmoidoscopy (preferably flexible) every 3 to 5 years beginning at age 50 for asymptomatic individuals having no colorectal cancer risk factors. The use of colonoscopy or double-contrast barium enemas for screening have not yet been systematically examined. Nonetheless, the American Cancer Society has proposed such a "total colon examination" every 10 years as an alternative to Hemoccult testing with periodic flexible sigmoidoscopy. More effective techniques for screening are needed, perhaps taking advantage of the molecular changes that have been described in these tumors. Analysis of stool for specific *ras* protooncogene mutations is being tested.

CLINICAL FEATURES   Presenting Symptoms   Symptoms vary with the anatomic location of the tumor. Since stool is relatively liquid as it passes through the ileocecal valve into the right colon, cancers arising in the cecum and ascending colon may become quite large, without resulting in any obstructive symptoms or noticeable alterations in bowel habits. Lesions of the right colon commonly ulcerate, leading to chronic, insidious blood loss without a change in the appearance of the stool. Consequently, patients with tumors of the ascending colon often present with symptoms such as fatigue, palpitations, and even angina pectoris and are found to have a hypochromic, microcytic anemia indicative of iron deficiency. Since the cancer may bleed intermittently, a random fecal occult blood test may be negative. As a result, the unexplained presence of iron-deficiency anemia in any adult (with the possible exception of a premenopausal, multiparous woman) mandates a thorough endoscopic and/or radiographic visualization of the entire large bowel (Fig. 90-1).

Since stool becomes more concentrated as it passes into the transverse and descending colon, tumors arising there tend to impede the passage of stool, resulting in the development of abdominal cramping, occasional obstruction, and even perforation. Radiographs of the abdomen often reveal characteristic annular, constricting lesions ("applecore" or "napkin-ring") (Fig. 90-2).

Cancers arising in the rectosigmoid are often associated with hematochezia, tenesmus, and narrowing of the caliber of stool; anemia is an infrequent finding. While these symptoms may lead patients and their physicians to suspect the presence of hemorrhoids, the development of rectal bleeding and/or altered bowel habits demands a prompt digital rectal examination and proctosigmoidoscopy.

Staging, Prognostic Factors, and Patterns of Spread   The prognosis for individuals having colorectal cancer is related to the depth of tumor penetration into the bowel wall and the presence of both regional lymph node involvement and distant metastases. These variables are incorporated into the staging system introduced by Dukes

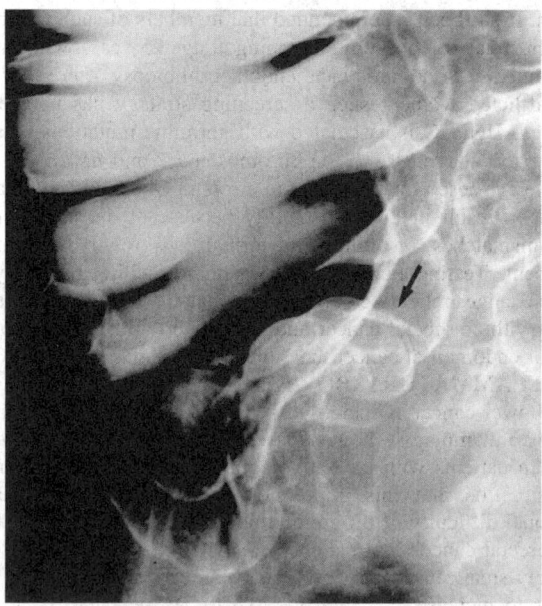

FIGURE 90-1   Double-contrast air-barium enema revealing a sessile tumor of the cecum in a patient with iron-deficiency anemia and guaiac-positive stool. The lesion at surgery was a stage B adenocarcinoma.

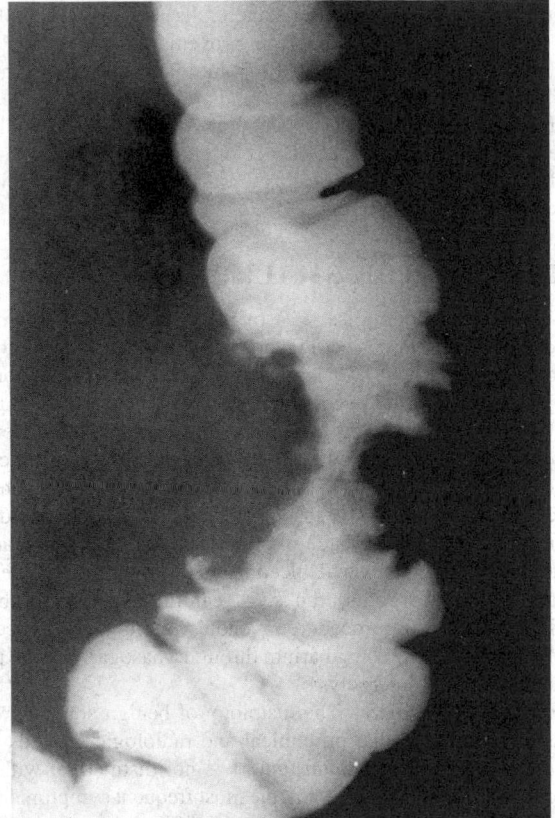

FIGURE 90-2 Annular, constricting adenocarcinoma of the descending colon. This radiographic appearance is referred to as an "apple-core" lesion and is always highly suggestive of malignancy.

and applied to a TNM classification method, in which T represents the depth of tumor penetration, N the presence of lymph node involvement, and M the presence or absence of distant metastases (Table 90-6). Superficial lesions that do not penetrate into the muscularis or involve regional lymph nodes are designated as *stage A* (T1N0M0) disease; tumors that penetrate more deeply but have not spread to lymph nodes are *stage B* disease [subclassified as *stage B₁* (T2N0M0) if lesions are restricted to the muscularis and as *stage B₂* (T3N0M0) if lesions involve or penetrate the serosa]; regional lymph node involvement defines *stage C* (TxN1M0) disease; and metastatic spread to sites such as liver, lung, or bone indicates *stage D* (TxNxM1) disease. Unless gross evidence of metastatic disease is present, disease stage cannot be determined accurately before surgical resection and pathologic analysis of the operative specimens. It is not clear whether the detection of nodal metastases by special immunohistochemical molecular techniques has the same prognostic implications as disease detected by routine light microscopy.

Table 90-6 Staging of and Prognosis for Colorectal Cancer

Stage				Approximate 5-Year Survival, %
Dukes	TNM	Numerical	Pathologic Description	
A	T1N0M0	I	Cancer limited to mucosa and submucosa	>90
B₁	T2N0M0	I	Cancer extends into muscularis	85
B₂	T3N0M0	II	Cancer extends into or through serosa	70–80
C	TxN1M0	III	Cancer involves regional lymph nodes	35–65
D	TxNxM1	IV	Distant metastases (i.e., liver, lung, etc.)	5

Most recurrences after a surgical resection of a large-bowel cancer occur within the first 4 years, making 5-year survival a fairly reliable indicator of cure. The likelihood for 5-year survival in patients with colorectal cancer is stage-related (Table 90-6). That likelihood has improved during the past several decades when similar surgical stages have been compared. The most plausible explanation for this improvement appears to be more thorough intraoperative and pathologic staging. In particular, more exacting attention to pathologic detail has revealed that the prognosis following the resection of a colorectal cancer is not related merely to the presence or absence of regional lymph node involvement but may be more precisely assessed by the number of involved lymph nodes (one to four lymph nodes versus five or more lymph nodes). Other predictors of a poor prognosis after a total surgical resection include tumor penetration through the bowel wall into pericolic fat, poorly differentiated histology, perforation and/or tumor adherence to adjacent organs (increasing the risk for an anatomically adjacent recurrence), and venous invasion by tumor (Table 90-7). Regardless of the clinicopathologic stage, a preoperative elevation of the plasma carcinoembryonic antigen (CEA) level predicts eventual tumor recurrence. The presence of aneuploidy and specific chromosomal deletions, such as allelic loss in chromosome 18q (involving the *DCC* gene) in tumor cells, appears to predict a higher risk for metastatic spread, particularly in patients with stage B₂ (T3N0M0) disease. Conversely, the detection of microsatellite instability in tumor tissue has been associated with a more favorable outcome. In contrast to most other cancers, the prognosis in colorectal cancer is not influenced by the size of the primary lesion when adjusted for nodal involvement and histologic differentiation.

Cancers of the large bowel generally spread to regional lymph nodes or to the liver via the portal venous circulation. The liver represents the most frequent visceral site of metastatic dissemination; it is the initial site of distant spread in one-third of recurring colorectal cancers and is involved in more than two-thirds of such patients at the time of death. In general, colorectal cancer rarely metastasizes to the lungs, supraclavicular lymph nodes, bone, or brain without prior spread to the liver. A major exception to this rule occurs in patients having primary tumors in the distal rectum, from which tumor cells may spread through the paravertebral venous plexus, escaping the portal venous system and thereby reaching the lungs or supraclavicular lymph nodes without hepatic involvement. The median survival after the detection of distant metastases is 6 to 9 months (hepatomegaly, abnormal liver chemistries) to 24 to 30 months (small liver nodule initially identified by elevated CEA level and subsequent CT scan).

℞ **TREATMENT** Total resection of tumor is the optimal treatment when a malignant lesion is detected endoscopically or radiographically in the large bowel. An evaluation for the presence of metastatic disease, including a thorough physical examination, chest radiograph, biochemical assessment of liver function, and measurement of the plasma CEA level, should be performed before surgery. When possible, a colonoscopy of the entire large bowel should be

Table 90-7 Predictors of Poor Outcome Following Total Surgical Resection of Colorectal Cancer

Tumor spread to regional lymph nodes
Number of regional lymph nodes involved
Tumor penetration through the bowel wall
Poorly differentiated histology
Perforation
Tumor adherence to adjacent organs
Venous invasion
Preoperative elevation of CEA titer (>5.0 ng/mL)
Aneuploidy
Specific chromosomal deletion (e.g., allelic loss on chromosome 18q)

NOTE: CEA, carcinoembryonic antigen.

performed to identify synchronous neoplasms and/or polyps. The detection of metastases should not preclude surgery in patients with tumor-related symptoms such as gastrointestinal bleeding or obstruction, but it often prompts the use of a less radical operative procedure. At the time of laparotomy, the entire peritoneal cavity should be examined, with thorough inspection of the liver, pelvis, and hemidiaphragm and careful palpation of the full length of the large bowel. Following recovery from a complete resection, patients should be observed carefully for 5 years by semiannual physical examinations and yearly blood chemistry measurements. If a complete colonoscopy was not performed preoperatively, it should be carried out within the first several postoperative months. Some authorities favor measuring plasma CEA levels at 3-month intervals because of the sensitivity of this test as a marker for otherwise undetectable tumor recurrence. Subsequent endoscopic or radiographic surveillance of the large bowel, probably at triennial intervals, is indicated, since patients who have been cured of one colorectal cancer have a 3 to 5% probability of developing an additional bowel cancer during their lifetime and a >15% risk for the development of adenomatous polyps. Anastomotic ("suture-line") recurrences are infrequent in colorectal cancer patients provided the surgical resection margins were adequate and free of tumor. Periodic CT screening, chest radiographs, or more frequent colonoscopic examinations do not affect prognosis and add unnecessary costs to postoperative surveillance.

Radiation therapy to the pelvis is recommended for patients with rectal cancer because it reduces the 30 to 40% probability of regional recurrences following complete surgical resection of stage B or C tumors, especially if they have penetrated through the serosa. This alarmingly high rate of local disease recurrence is believed to be due to the fact that the contained anatomic space within the pelvis limits the extent of the resection and because the rich lymphatic network of the pelvic side wall immediately adjacent to the rectum facilitates the early spread of malignant cells into surgically inaccessible tissue. Radiation therapy, either pre- or postoperatively, reduces the likelihood of pelvic recurrences but does not appear to prolong survival. Preoperative radiotherapy is indicated for patients with large, potentially unresectable rectal cancers; such lesions may shrink enough to permit subsequent surgical removal. Radiation therapy is not effective in the primary treatment of colon cancer.

Chemotherapy in patients with advanced colorectal cancer has proven to be of only marginal benefit. 5-FU is the most effective single agent for this disease. Partial responses are obtained in 15 to 20% of patients. The probability of tumor response appears to be somewhat greater for patients with liver metastases when chemotherapy is infused directly into the hepatic artery, but intraarterial treatment is costly and toxic and does not appear to prolong survival. The concomitant administration of folinic acid (leucovorin) improves the efficacy of 5-FU in patients with advanced colorectal cancer, presumably by enhancing the binding of 5-FU to its target enzyme, thymidylate synthase. A threefold improvement in the partial response rate is noted when folinic acid is combined with 5-FU; however, the effect on survival is marginal, and the optimal dose schedule remains to be defined.

Irinotecan (CPT-11), a topoisomerase 1 inhibitor, prolongs survival when compared to supportive care in patients whose disease has progressed on 5-FU. Furthermore, the addition of irinotecan to 5-FU and leucovorin improves response rates and survival of patients with metastatic disease. Oxaliplatin, a platinum analogue, also improves the response rate when added to 5-FU and leucovorin as initial treatment of patients with metastatic disease.

Patients with solitary hepatic metastases without clinical or radiographic evidence of additional tumor involvement should be considered for partial liver resection, because such procedures are associated with 5-year survival rates of 25 to 30% when performed on selected individuals by experienced surgeons.

The administration of 5-FU and leucovorin for 6 months after re-section of tumor in patients with stage C disease leads to a 40% decrease in recurrence rates and 30% improvement in survival. Patients with stage B_2 tumors do not benefit from adjuvant therapy. In rectal cancer, the delivery of postoperative (and probably preoperative) combined modality therapy (5-FU plus radiation therapy) reduces the risk of recurrence and increases the chance of cure for patients with stages B_2 and C tumors. The 5-FU acts as a radiosensitizer when delivered together with radiation therapy.

TUMORS OF THE SMALL INTESTINE

Small-bowel tumors comprise <5% of gastrointestinal neoplasms. Because of their rarity, a correct diagnosis is often delayed. Abdominal symptoms are usually vague and poorly defined, and conventional radiographic studies of the upper and lower intestinal tract often appear normal. Small-bowel tumors should be considered in the differential diagnosis in the following situations: (1) recurrent, unexplained episodes of crampy abdominal pain; (2) intermittent bouts of intestinal obstruction, especially in the absence of inflammatory bowel disease or prior abdominal surgery; (3) intussusception in the adult; and (4) evidence of chronic intestinal bleeding in the presence of negative conventional contrast radiographs. A careful small-bowel barium study is the diagnostic procedure of choice; the diagnostic accuracy may be improved by infusing barium through a nasogastric tube placed into the duodenum (enteroclysis).

BENIGN TUMORS The histology of benign small-bowel tumors is difficult to predict on clinical and radiologic grounds alone. The symptomatology of benign tumors is not distinctive, with pain, obstruction, and hemorrhage being the most frequent symptoms. These tumors are usually discovered during the fifth and sixth decades of life, more often in the distal rather than the proximal small intestine. The most common benign tumors are adenomas, leiomyomas, lipomas, and angiomas.

Adenomas These tumors include those of the islet cells and Brunner's glands as well as polypoid adenomas. *Islet cell adenomas* are occasionally located outside the pancreas; the associated syndromes are discussed in Chap. 93. *Brunner's gland adenomas* are not truly neoplastic but represent a hypertrophy or hyperplasia of submucosal duodenal glands. These appear as small nodules in the duodenal mucosa that secrete a highly viscous alkaline mucus. Most often, this is an incidental radiographic finding not associated with any specific clinical disorder.

Polypoid Adenomas About 25% of benign small-bowel tumors are polypoid adenomas (Table 90-5). They may present as single polypoid lesions or, less commonly, as papillary villous adenomas. As in the colon, the sessile or papillary form of the tumor is sometimes associated with a coexisting carcinoma. Occasionally, patients with Gardner's syndrome develop premalignant adenomas in the small bowel; such lesions are generally in the duodenum. Multiple polypoid tumors may occur throughout the small bowel (and occasionally the stomach and colorectum) in the Peutz-Jeghers syndrome. The polyps are usually hamartomas (juvenile polyps) having a low potential for malignant degeneration. Mucocutaneous melanin deposits as well as tumors of the ovary, breast, pancreas, and endometrium are also associated with this autosomal dominant condition.

Leiomyomas These neoplasms arise from smooth-muscle components of the intestine and are usually intramural, affecting the overlying mucosa. Ulceration of the mucosa may cause gastrointestinal hemorrhage of varying severity. Cramping, intermittent abdominal pain is frequently encountered.

Lipomas These tumors occur with greatest frequency in the distal ileum and at the ileocecal valve. They have a characteristic radiolucent appearance, are usually intramural and asymptomatic, but on occasion cause bleeding.

Angiomas While not true neoplasms, these lesions are important because they frequently cause intestinal bleeding. They may take the form of telangiectasia or hemangiomas. Multiple intestinal telangiectasias occur in a nonhereditary form confined to the gastrointestinal tract or as part of the hereditary Osler-Rendu-Weber syndrome. Vascular tumors may also take the form of isolated hemangiomas, most commonly in the jejunum. Angiography, especially during bleeding, is the best procedure for evaluating these lesions.

MALIGNANT TUMORS While rare, small-bowel malignancies occur in patients with long-standing regional enteritis and celiac sprue as well as in individuals with AIDS. Malignant tumors of the small bowel are frequently associated with fever, weight loss, anorexia, bleeding, and a palpable abdominal mass. After ampullary carcinomas (many of which arise from biliary or pancreatic ducts), the most frequently occurring small-bowel malignancies are adenocarcinomas, lymphomas, carcinoid tumors, and leiomyosarcomas.

Adenocarcinomas The most common primary cancers of the small bowel are adenocarcinomas, accounting for ~50% of malignant tumors. These cancers occur most often in the distal duodenum and proximal jejunum, where they tend to ulcerate and cause hemorrhage or obstruction. Radiologically, they may be confused with chronic duodenal ulcer disease or with Crohn's disease if the patient has long-standing regional enteritis. The diagnosis is best made by endoscopy and biopsy under direct vision. Surgical resection is the treatment of choice.

Lymphomas Lymphoma in the small bowel may be primary or secondary. A diagnosis of a primary intestinal lymphoma requires histologic confirmation in a clinical setting in which palpable adenopathy and hepatosplenomegaly are absent and no evidence of lymphoma is seen on chest radiograph, CT scan, or peripheral blood smear or on bone marrow aspiration and biopsy. Symptoms referable to the small bowel are present, usually accompanied by an anatomically discernible lesion. Secondary lymphoma of the small bowel consists of involvement of the intestine by a lymphoid malignancy extending from involved retroperitoneal or mesenteric lymph nodes (Chap. 112).

Primary intestinal lymphoma accounts for ~20% of malignancies of the small bowel. These neoplasms are non-Hodgkin's lymphomas; they usually have a diffuse, large cell histology and are of T cell origin. Intestinal lymphoma involves the ileum, jejunum, and duodenum, in decreasing frequency, a pattern that mirrors the relative amount of normal lymphoid cells in these anatomic areas. The risk of small-bowel lymphoma is increased in patients with a prior history of malabsorptive conditions (e.g., celiac sprue), regional enteritis, and depressed immune function due to congenital immunodeficiency syndromes, prior organ transplantation, autoimmune disorders, or AIDS.

The development of localized or nodular masses that narrow the lumen results in periumbilical pain (made worse by eating) as well as weight loss, vomiting, and occasional intestinal obstruction. The diagnosis of small-bowel lymphoma may be suspected from the appearance on contrast radiographs of patterns such as infiltration and thickening of mucosal folds, mucosal nodules, areas of irregular ulceration, or stasis of contrast material. The diagnosis can be confirmed by surgical exploration and resection of involved segments. Intestinal lymphoma can occasionally be diagnosed by peroral intestinal mucosal biopsy, but since the disease mainly involves the lamina propria, full-thickness surgical biopsies are usually required.

Resection of the tumor constitutes the initial treatment modality. While postoperative radiation therapy has been given to some patients following a total resection, most authorities favor short-term (three cycles) systemic treatment with combination chemotherapy. The frequent presence of widespread intraabdominal disease at the time of diagnosis and the occasional multicentricity of the tumor often make a total resection impossible. The probability of sustained remission or cure is ~75% in patients with localized disease but is ~25% in individuals with unresectable lymphoma. In patients whose tumors are not resected, chemotherapy may lead to bowel perforation.

A unique form of small-bowel lymphoma, diffusely involving the entire intestine, was first described in oriental Jews and Arabs and is referred to as *immunoproliferative small intestinal disease* (IPSID), *Mediterranean lymphoma*, or *α-heavy chain disease*. This is a B cell tumor. The typical presentation includes chronic diarrhea and steator-

rhea associated with vomiting and abdominal cramps; clubbing of the digits may be observed. A curious feature in many patients with IPSID is the presence in the blood and intestinal secretions of an abnormal IgA that contains a shortened α-heavy chain and is devoid of light chains. It is suspected that the abnormal α chains are produced by plasma cells infiltrating the small bowel. The clinical course of patients with IPSID is generally one of exacerbations and remissions, with death frequently resulting from either progressive malnutrition and wasting or the development of an aggressive lymphoma. The use of oral antibiotics such as tetracycline appears to be beneficial in the early phases of the disorder, suggesting a possible infectious etiology. Combination chemotherapy has been administered during later stages of the disease, with variable results. Results are better when antibiotics and chemotherapy are combined.

Carcinoid Tumors Carcinoid tumors arise from argentaffin cells of the crypts of Lieberkühn and are found from the distal duodenum to the ascending colon, areas embryologically derived from the midgut. More than 50% of intestinal carcinoids are found in the distal ileum, with most congregating close to the ileocecal valve. Most intestinal carcinoids are asymptomatic and of low malignant potential, but invasion and metastases may occur, leading to the carcinoid syndrome (Chap. 93).

Leiomyosarcomas Leiomyosarcomas often are >5 cm in diameter and may be palpable on abdominal examination. Bleeding, obstruction, and perforation are common.

CANCERS OF THE ANUS

Cancers of the anus account for 1 to 2% of the malignant tumors of the large bowel. Most such lesions arise in the anal canal, the anatomic area extending from the anorectal ring to a zone approximately halfway between the pectinate (or dentate) line and the anal verge. Carcinomas arising proximal to the pectinate line (i.e., in the transitional zone between the glandular mucosa of the rectum and the squamous epithelium of the distal anus) are known as basaloid, cuboidal, or cloacogenic tumors; about one-third of anal cancers have this histologic pattern. Malignancies arising distal to the pectinate line have a squamous cell histology, ulcerate more frequently, and constitute ~55% of anal cancers. The prognosis for patients with basaloid and squamous cell cancers of the anus is identical when corrected for tumor size and the presence or absence of nodal spread.

The development of anal cancer is associated with infection by human papillomavirus, the same organism etiologically linked to cervical cancer. The virus is sexually transmitted. The infection may lead to anal warts (condyloma accuminata) which may progress to anal intraepithelial neoplasia and on to squamous cell carcinoma. The risk for anal cancer is increased among homosexual males, presumably related to anal intercourse. Anal cancer risk is increased in both men and women with AIDS, possibly because their immunosuppressed state permits more severe papillomavirus infection. Anal cancers occur most commonly in middle-aged persons and are more frequent in women than men. At diagnosis, patients may experience bleeding, pain, sensation of a perianal mass, and pruritus.

Radical surgery (abdominal-perineal resection with lymph node sampling and a permanent colostomy) used to be the treatment of choice for this tumor type. The 5-year survival rate after such a procedure was 55 to 70% in the absence of spread to regional lymph nodes; <20% if nodal involvement was present. An alternative therapeutic approach combining external beam radiation therapy with concomitant chemotherapy has resulted in biopsy-proven disappearance of all tumor in >80% of patients whose initial lesion was <3 cm in size. Tumor has recurred in <10% of these patients, and ~70% of patients with anal cancers can be cured with nonoperative treatment. Surgery should be reserved for the minority of individuals who are found to have residual tumor after being managed initially with radiation therapy combined with chemotherapy.

BIBLIOGRAPHY

CRUMP W et al: Lymphoma of the gastrointestinal tract. Semin Oncol 26:324, 1999

DESCH CE et al: Recommended colorectal cancer surveillance guidelines by the American Society of Clinical Oncology. J Clin Oncol 17:1312, 1999

DEVESA SS et al: Changing patterns in the incidence of esophageal and gastric carcinomas in the United States. Cancer 83:2049, 1998

FUCHS CS, MAYER RJ: Gastric carcinoma. N Engl J Med 333:32, 1995

ISAACSON PG: Gastric MALT lymphoma: From concept to cure. Ann Oncol 10:637, 1999

JÄNNE PA, MAYER RJ: Chemoprevention of colorectal cancer. N Engl J Med 342:1960, 2000

KELSEN DP et al: Chemotherapy followed by surgery compared with surgery alone for localized esophageal cancer. N Engl J Med 339:1979, 1998

LYNCH HT et al: Hereditary colorectal cancer. Semin Oncol 26:478, 1999

RYAN DP et al: Carcinoma of the anal canal. N Engl J Med 342:792, 2000

SALTZ LB et al: Irinotecan plus fluorouracil and leucovorin for metastatic colorectal cancer. N Engl J Med 343:905, 2000

91   Jules L. Dienstag, Kurt J. Isselbacher

TUMORS OF THE LIVER AND BILIARY TRACT

BENIGN LIVER TUMORS

HEPATOCELLULAR ADENOMAS Hepatocellular adenomas are benign tumors of the liver found predominantly in women in their third and fourth decades. Their preponderance in women suggests a hormonal influence in their pathogenesis, and oral contraceptives are thought to play an etiologic role. The risk of liver adenomas is increased among those who take anabolic steroids and exogenous androgens. Multiple hepatic adenomas have been associated with glycogen storage disease type I.

Hepatic adenomas occur predominantly in the right lobe of the liver, may be multiple, and are often quite large (>10 cm). Microscopically, they consist of normal or slightly atypical hepatocytes. These cells contain increased glycogen, making them appear paler and larger than normal. Clinical features include pain and the presence of a palpable mass or features of intratumor hemorrhage (pain and circulatory collapse). The diagnosis is usually made by a combination of techniques: sonography, computed tomography (CT), magnetic resonance imaging (MRI), selective hepatic arteriography, and radionuclide scans. The angiographic appearance is typically hypervascular but often also includes hypovascular regions. Technetium 99m scans usually show a defect, because phagocytosing Kupffer cells are absent. Like hepatocellular carcinomas, adenomas have a T_1-intense MRI appearance. The risk of malignant change is small; the risk is higher for large (>10 cm) and multiple adenomas.

Management involves imaging surveillance for small tumors. If the lesion is large (8 to 10 cm), near the surface, and resectable, surgical removal is appropriate. A patient with liver adenoma should stop taking oral contraceptives. Surgical resection may be required for tumors that do not shrink after oral contraceptives are stopped. Pregnancy increases the risk of hemorrhage and should be avoided in women with large adenomas. Patients with multiple large adenomas (e.g., those with glycogen-storage disease) may benefit from liver transplantation.

FOCAL NODULAR HYPERPLASIA Focal nodular hyperplasia is a benign tumor often identified incidentally on imaging studies or at laparoscopy done for other reasons. Like hepatic adenomas, it occurs predominantly in women; however, oral contraceptives are not implicated, and hemorrhage and necrosis are rare. The risk of hemorrhage, however, appears to be higher in women taking oral contra-

ceptives. Typically, the lesion is a solid tumor, often in the right lobe, with a fibrous core and stellate projections. The fibrous projections contain atypical hepatocytes, biliary epithelium, Kupffer cells, and inflammatory cells. A technetium scan will usually show a hot spot because of the presence of Kupffer cells. The lesion appears vascular on angiography, and septations may be detectable by angiography, helical CT scan, and, most reliably, by MRI, but only rarely by ultrasound. Surgery is indicated only for symptomatic lesions.

HEMANGIOMA AND OTHER BENIGN TUMORS Hemangiomas are the most common benign liver tumors, occurring predominantly in women and usually detected incidentally. The prevalence in the general population is in the range of 0.5 to 7.0%. These asymptomatic vascular lesions can be identified by MRI, contrast-enhanced CT, labeled red blood cell nuclide scans, or hepatic angiography. They do not need to be removed unless they are large and are producing a mass effect. Hemorrhage is rare, and malignant change does not occur.

Nodular regenerative hyperplasia consists of multiple hepatic nodules resulting from periportal hepatocyte regeneration with surrounding atrophy. It may be associated with an underlying condition such as malignancy or connective tissue disease. Portal hypertension (in the absence of cirrhosis) is the most common clinical manifestation. Other less common benign hepatic lesions include *bile duct adenomas* and *cystadenomas*.

CARCINOMAS OF THE LIVER

HEPATOCELLULAR CARCINOMA Epidemiology and Etiology Primary hepatocellular carcinoma is one of the most common tumors in the world. It is especially prevalent in regions of Asia and sub-Saharan Africa, where the annual incidence is up to 500 cases per 100,000 population. In the United States and western Europe, it is much less common; however, the annual incidence in the United States has increased from 1.4/100,000 in the period 1976 to 1980 to 2.4/100,000 in 1991 to 1995. Hepatocellular carcinoma is up to four times more common in men than in women and usually arises in a cirrhotic liver. The incidence peaks in the fifth to sixth decades of life in western countries but one to two decades earlier in regions of Asia and Africa with a high prevalence of liver carcinoma.

The principal reason for the high incidence of hepatocellular carcinoma in parts of Asia and Africa is the frequency of chronic infection with *hepatitis B virus* (HBV) and *hepatitis C virus* (HCV). These chronic infections frequently lead to cirrhosis, which itself is an important risk factor for hepatocellular carcinoma (the risk of liver cancer in a cirrhotic liver is ~3% per year); 60 to 90% of these tumors occur in patients with macronodular cirrhosis. Studies in regions of Asia where hepatocellular carcinoma and HBV infection are prevalent have shown that the incidence of this cancer is about 100-fold higher in individuals with evidence of HBV infection than in noninfected controls. In China, the lifetime risk of developing hepatocellular carcinoma in patients with chronic hepatitis B approaches 40%. In patients with HBV infection and hepatocellular carcinoma, HBV DNA may be integrated into host genomic DNA, both in the tumor cells and in adjacent, uninvolved hepatocytes. In addition, modifications of cellular gene expression occur by insertional mutagenesis, chromosomal rearrangements, or the transcriptional transactivating activity of the X and the pre-S2 regions of the HBV genome.

HCV also leads to hepatocellular carcinoma. HCV genetic material does not become integrated into host genomic DNA. Therefore, the mechanism of HCV carcinogenesis is unclear. In Europe and Japan, HCV appears to be substantially more prevalent than HBV in cases of hepatocellular carcinoma. Both HBV and HCV can be demonstrated in some patients, but the clinical course of liver malignancy in these patients does not appear to differ from that when only one virus is implicated. One distinction in high-prevalence areas between hepatocellular carcinoma associated with HBV infection and with HCV infection is in the timing of onset. In Asia, HBV is acquired at birth via perinatal transmission, whereas HCV infection is acquired primarily during adulthood from transfused blood and injections. Correspondingly, the onset of liver carcinoma occurs one to two decades earlier in those with lifelong hepatitis B than in persons with adult-acquired hepatitis C. Retrospective analysis indicates that hepatocellular carcinoma occurs on average approximately 30 years after HCV infection and almost exclusively in patients with cirrhosis. The annual incidence of hepatocellular carcinoma in cirrhotic patients with chronic hepatitis C is 1.5 to 4%.

Any agent or factor that contributes to chronic, low-grade liver cell damage and mitosis makes hepatocyte DNA more susceptible to genetic alterations. Thus, as indicated above, *chronic liver disease* of any type is a risk factor and predisposes to the development of liver cell carcinoma. These conditions include alcoholic liver disease, α_1-antitrypsin deficiency, hemochromatosis, and tyrosinemia. In Africa and southern China, *aflatoxin B$_1$* is an important public health hazard. This mycotoxin appears to induce a very specific mutation at codon 249 in the tumor suppressor gene p53.

The loss, inactivation, or mutation of the p53 gene has been implicated in tumorigenesis and is the most common genetic derangement present in human cancers. Thus HBV and aflatoxin B$_1$ have been implicated in the pathogenesis of hepatocellular carcinoma in regions of Africa and southern China where both agents are prevalent.

In view of the male predominance of liver cancer, hormonal factors may also play a role. Hepatocellular tumors may occur with long-term androgenic steroid administration, with exposure to thorium dioxide or vinyl chloride (see below), and possibly with exposure to estrogens in the form of oral contraceptives.

Clinical and Laboratory Features   Cancers of the liver initially may escape clinical recognition because they occur in patients with underlying cirrhosis, and the symptoms and signs may suggest progression of the underlying disease. The most common presenting features are abdominal *pain* with detection of an abdominal mass in the right upper quadrant. There may be a *friction rub* or *bruit* over the liver. Blood-tinged ascites occurs in about 20% of cases. Jaundice is rare, unless there is significant deterioration of liver function or mechanical obstruction of the bile ducts. Serum elevations of alkaline phosphatase and α fetoprotein (AFP) are common (see below). An abnormal type of prothrombin, des-γ-carboxy prothrombin, is made and correlates with AFP elevations.

A small percentage of patients with hepatocellular carcinoma have a *paraneoplastic syndrome*; erythrocytosis may result from erythropoietin-like activity produced by the tumor; hypercalcemia may result from secretion of a parathyroid-like hormone. Other manifestations may include hypercholesterolemia, hypoglycemia, acquired porphyria, dysfibrinogenemia, and cryofibrinogenemia.

Imaging procedures to detect liver tumors include ultrasound, CT, MRI, hepatic artery angiography (Chap. 282), and technetium scans. Ultrasound is frequently used to screen high-risk populations and should be the first test if hepatocellular carcinoma is suspected; it is less costly than scans, is relatively sensitive, and can detect most tumors >3 cm. Helical CT and MRI scans are being used with increasing frequency and have higher sensitivities.

AFP levels >500 μg/L are found in about 70 to 80% of patients with hepatocellular carcinoma. Lower levels may be found in patients with large metastases from gastric or colonic tumors and in some patients with acute or chronic hepatitis. High levels of serum AFP (>500 to 1000 μg/L) in an adult with liver disease and without an obvious gastrointestinal tumor strongly suggest hepatocellular carcinoma. A rising level suggests progression of the tumor or recurrence after hepatic resection or therapeutic approaches such as chemotherapy or chemoembolization (see below).

Percutaneous *liver biopsy* can be diagnostic if the sample is taken from an area localized by ultrasound or CT. Because these tumors tend to be vascular, percutaneous biopsies should be done with caution. Cytologic examination of ascitic fluid is invariably negative for tumor cells. Occasionally, *laparoscopy* or *minilaparotomy*, to permit liver biopsy under direct vision, may be used. This approach has the additional advantage of sometimes identifying patients who have a localized resectable tumor suitable for partial hepatectomy.

℞ TREATMENT   Staging of hepatocellular carcinoma is based on tumor size (< or > 50% of the liver), ascites (absent or present), bilirubin (< or > 3), and albumin (< or >3) to establish Okuda stages I, II, and III. The Okuda system predicts clinical course better than the American Joint Cancer Commission TNM system. The natural history of each stage without treatment is: stage I, 8 months; stage II, 2 months; stage III, less than 1 month.

The course of *clinically apparent* disease is rapid; if untreated, most patients die within 3 to 6 months of diagnosis. When hepatocellular carcinoma is detected very early by serial screening of AFP and ultrasound, survival is 1 to 2 years after resection. In selected cases, therapy may prolong life. *Surgical resection* offers the only chance for cure; however, few patients have a resectable tumor at the time of presentation, because of underlying cirrhosis, involvement of both hepatic lobes, or distant metastases (common sites are lung, brain, bone, and adrenal), and the 5-year survival is low. In patients at high risk for the development of hepatocellular carcinoma, screening programs have been initiated to identify small tumors when they are still resectable. Because 20 to 30% of patients with early hepatocellular carcinoma do not have elevated levels of circulating AFP, ultrasonographic screening is recommended as well as AFP determination. In a study in the Far East, persons positive for hepatitis B surface antigen, with or without liver disease, were screened serially; a number of patients with small, subclinical tumors were identified, and surgical resection undertaken. Follow-up observation revealed a 5-year survival rate in this group of 70% and a 10-year survival rate of 50%. These Asian patients, however, were unusual in that they had minimal or no liver disease and their tumors tended to be unifocal or encapsulated. The findings are in contrast to a study in a large population of Italian patients with cirrhosis, associated in most cases with chronic HBV and/or HCV infections; screening every 3 to 12 months permitted the detection of a 3% annual incidence of cancer in this cohort but in most cases failed to achieve the goal of early detection of surgically treatable disease. No randomized study has yet shown survival benefit for screening patients at high risk of developing hepatocellular carcinoma.

Liver transplantation may be considered as a therapeutic option; tumor recurrence or metastases are the major problems. Patients who have a single lesion ≤5 cm or three or fewer lesions ≤3 cm have survival after liver transplantation that is the same as survival after transplantation for nonmalignant liver disease (Chap. 301). Other approaches include (1) hepatic artery embolization and chemotherapy (chemoembolization), (2) alcohol or radio-frequency ablation via ultrasound-guided percutaneous injection, and (3) ultrasound-guided cryoablation.

Treatment options for unresectable disease are limited. Randomized trials have not shown a survival advantage after chemoembolization. The liver cannot tolerate high doses of radiation. The disease is not responsive to chemotherapy, including newer agents such as gemcytabine. Investigative immunotherapy and gene therapy techniques have not been successful. Based on the presence of hormone receptors on the tumor, tamoxifen has been tested, but without success, and octreotide has had some modest activity. In patients with resectable tumors, polyprenoic acid (a retinoic acid formulation) and intra-arterial ^{131}I-labeled lipiodol have been reported to reduce the rate of recurrence.

Prevention is the preferred strategy. Hepatitis B vaccine can prevent infection and its sequelae, and a reduction in hepatocellular carcinoma has been seen in Taiwan with the introduction of universal vaccination of children. Interferon treatment reduces the incidence of hepatic failure, death, and liver cancer in patients infected with HBV.

Treatment with interferon may lower the risk of development of liver cancer in patients with hepatitis C–related cirrhosis (Chap. 297), but additional studies are needed.

OTHER MALIGNANT LIVER TUMORS

Fibrolamellar carcinoma differs from the typical hepatocellular carcinoma in that it tends to occur in young adults without underlying cirrhosis. This tumor is nonencapsulated but well circumscribed and contains fibrous lamellae; it grows slowly and is associated with a longer survival if treated. Surgical resection has resulted in 5-year survivals >50%; if the lesion is nonresectable, liver transplantation is an option, and the outcome far exceeds that observed in the nonfibrolamellar variety of liver cancer. *Hepatoblastoma* is a tumor of infancy that typically is associated with very high serum AFP levels. The lesions are usually solitary, may be resectable, and have a better 5-year survival than that of hepatocellular carcinoma. *Angiosarcoma* consists of vascular spaces lined by malignant endothelial cells. Etiologic factors include prior exposure to thorium dioxide (Thorotrast), polyvinyl chloride, arsenic, and androgenic anabolic steroids. *Epithelioid hemangioendothelioma* is of borderline malignancy; most cases are benign, but bone and lung metastases occur. This tumor occurs in early adulthood, presents with right upper quadrant pain, is heterogeneous on sonography, hypodense on CT, and without neovascularity on angiography. Immunohistochemical staining reveals expression of factor VIII antigen. In the absence of extrahepatic metastases, these lesions can be treated by surgical resection or liver transplantation.

METASTATIC TUMORS   Metastatic tumors of the liver are common, ranking second only to cirrhosis as a cause of fatal liver disease. In the United States, the incidence of metastatic carcinoma is at least 20 times greater than that of primary carcinoma. At autopsy, hepatic metastases occur in 30 to 50% of patients dying from malignant disease.

Pathogenesis   The liver is uniquely vulnerable to invasion by tumor cells. Its size, high rate of blood flow, double perfusion by the hepatic artery and portal vein, and its Kupffer cell filtration function combine to make it the next most common site of metastases after the lymph nodes. In addition, local tissue factors or endothelial membrane characteristics appear to enhance metastatic implants. Virtually all types of neoplasms except those primary in the brain may metastasize to the liver. The most common primary tumors are those of the gastrointestinal tract, lung, and breast, as well as melanomas. Less common are metastases from tumors of the thyroid, prostate, and skin.

Clinical Features   Most patients with metastases to the liver present with symptoms referable only to the primary tumor, and the asymptomatic hepatic involvement is discovered in the course of clinical evaluation. Sometimes hepatic involvement is reflected by nonspecific symptoms of weakness, weight loss, fever, sweating, and loss of appetite. Rarely, features indicating active hepatic disease, especially abdominal pain, hepatomegaly, or ascites, are present. Patients with widespread metastatic liver involvement usually have suggestive clinical signs of cancer and hepatic enlargement. Some have localized induration or tenderness, and, occasionally, a friction rub may be found over tender areas of the liver.

Results of liver biochemical tests are often abnormal, but the elevations in marker levels are often only mild and nonspecific. These signs reflect the effects of fever and wasting as well as those of the infiltrating neoplastic process itself. An increase in serum alkaline phosphatase is the most common and frequently the only abnormality. Hypoalbuminemia, anemia, and occasionally a mild elevation of aminotransferase levels may also be found with more widespread disease. Substantially elevated serum levels of carcinoembryonic antigen are usually found when the metastases are from primary malignancies in the gastrointestinal tract, breast, or lung.

Diagnosis   Evidence of metastatic invasion of the liver should be sought actively in any patient with a primary malignancy, especially of the lung, gastrointestinal tract, or breast, before resection of the primary lesion. An elevated level of alkaline phosphatase or a mass apparent on ultrasound, CT, or MRI examination of the liver may provide a presumptive diagnosis. Blind percutaneous needle biopsy of the liver will result in a positive diagnosis of metastatic disease in only 60 to 80% of cases with hepatomegaly and elevated alkaline phosphatase levels. Serial sectioning of specimens, two or three repeated biopsies, or cytologic examination of biopsy smears may increase the diagnostic yield by 10 to 15%. The yield is increased when biopsies are directed by ultrasound or CT or obtained during laparoscopy.

TREATMENT   Most metastatic carcinomas respond poorly to all forms of treatment, which is usually only palliative. Rarely a single, large metastasis can be removed surgically. Systemic chemotherapy may slow tumor growth and reduce symptoms, but it does not alter the prognosis. Chemoembolization, intrahepatic chemotherapy, and alcohol or radio-frequency ablation may provide palliation.

CHOLANGIOCARCINOMA   Benign tumors of the extrahepatic bile ducts are extremely rare causes of mechanical biliary obstruction. Most of these are papillomas, adenomas, or cystadenomas and present with obstructive jaundice or hemobilia. Adenocarcinoma of the extrahepatic ducts is more common. There is a slight male preponderance (60%), and the incidence peaks in the fifth to seventh decades. Apparent predisposing factors include (1) some chronic hepatobiliary parasitic infestations, (2) congenital anomalies with ectatic ducts, (3) sclerosing cholangitis and chronic ulcerative colitis, and (4) occupational exposure to possible biliary tract carcinogens (employment in rubber or automotive plants). Cholelithiasis is not clearly a predisposing factor for cholangiocarcinoma. The lesions of cholangiocarcinoma may be diffuse or nodular. Nodular lesions often arise at the bifurcation of the common bile duct (Klatskin tumors) and are usually associated with a *collapsed gallbladder*, a finding that mandates cholangiography to view proximal hepatic ducts.

Patients with cholangiocarcinoma usually present with biliary obstruction, painless jaundice, pruritus, weight loss, and acholic stools. A deep-seated, vaguely localized right upper quadrant pain may be noted. Hepatomegaly and a palpable, distended gallbladder (unless the lesion is high in the duct) are frequent accompanying signs. Fever is unusual unless associated with ascending cholangitis. Because the obstructing process is gradual, the cholangiocarcinoma is often far advanced by the time it presents clinically. The diagnosis is most frequently made by cholangiography following ultrasound demonstration of dilated intrahepatic bile ducts. Any focal strictures of the bile ducts should be considered malignant until proved otherwise. Endoscopic cholangiography permits obtaining specimens for cytology (sensitivity ~60%) and insertion of stents for biliary drainage. Survival of 1 to 2 years is possible in some cases. Perhaps 20% of patients have surgically resectable tumors, but 5-year survival is only 10 to 30%. The high recurrence rate limits the value of liver transplantation. Photodynamic therapy (intravenous hematoporphyrin with cholangioscopically delivered light) has been used with promising early results.

CARCINOMA OF THE PAPILLA OF VATER   The ampulla of Vater may be involved by extension of tumor arising elsewhere in the duodenum or may itself be the site of origin of a sarcoma, carcinoid tumor, or adenocarcinoma. Papillary adenocarcinomas are associated with slow growth and a more favorable clinical prognosis than diffuse, infiltrative cancers of the ampulla, which are more frequently widely invasive. The presenting clinical manifestation is usually obstructive jaundice. Endoscopic retrograde cannulation of the pancreatic duct is the preferred diagnostic technique when ampullary carcinoma is suspected, because it allows for direct endoscopic inspection and biopsy of the ampulla and for pancreatography to exclude a pancreatic malignancy. Cancer of the papilla is usually treated by wide surgical excision. Lymph node or other metastases are present at the time of surgery in approximately 20% of cases, and the 5-year survival rate following surgical therapy in this group is only 5 to 10%. In the absence of metastases, radical pancreaticoduodenectomy (the

Whipple procedure) is associated with 5-year survival rates as high as 40%.

CANCER OF THE GALLBLADDER Most cancers of the gallbladder develop in conjunction with stones rather than polyps. In patients with gallstones, the risk for developing gallbladder cancer, while increased, is still quite low. In one study, gallbladder cancer developed in only 5 of 2583 patients with gallstones followed for a median of 13 years. In the United States, adenocarcinomas make up the vast majority of the estimated 6500 new cases of gallbladder cancer diagnosed each year. The female/male ratio is 4:1, and the mean age at diagnosis is approximately 70 years. The clinical presentation is most often one of unremitting right upper quadrant pain associated with weight loss, jaundice, and a palpable right upper quadrant mass. Cholangitis may supervene. The preoperative diagnosis of the condition has been facilitated by ultrasound and CT. CT is also useful in guiding fine-needle aspiration and biopsy.

Once symptoms have appeared, spread of the tumor outside the gallbladder by direct extension or by lymphatic or hematogenous routes is almost invariable. Over 75% of gallbladder carcinomas are unresectable at the time of surgery, the exceptions being tumors discovered incidentally at laparotomy. If the tumor is found by the pathologist, no additional therapy is required. If the tumor is noted by the surgeon on routine cholecystectomy, a second operation is generally performed to resect the adjacent liver, bile duct, and local lymph nodes. Incidental resectable gallbladder tumors have a 50% 5-year survival. The 1-year mortality rate for unresectable disease is about 95%, and <5% of patients survive 5 years. Radical operative resection does not appear to improve survival. Trials of radiation and chemotherapy in patients with gallbladder cancer have been disappointing.

BIBLIOGRAPHY

BRUIX J et al: Transarterial embolization versus symptomatic treatment in patients with advanced hepatocellular carcinoma: Results of a randomized, controlled trial in a single institution. Hepatology 27:1578, 1998

CHANG M-H et al: Universal hepatitis B vaccination in Taiwan and the incidence of hepatocellular carcinoma in children. N Engl J Med 336:1855, 1997

DE GROEN PC et al: Biliary tract cancers. N Engl J Med 341:1368, 1999

EL-SERAG HB et al: Rising incidence of hepatocellular carcinoma in the United States. N Engl J Med 340:745, 1999

LIN S-M et al: Long-term beneficial effect of interferon therapy in patients with chronic hepatitis B virus infection. Hepatology 29:971, 1999

MOR E et al: Treatment of hepatocellular carcinoma associated with cirrhosis in the era of liver transplantation. Ann Intern Med 129:643, 1998

ORTNER MA et al: Photodynamic therapy of nonresectable cholangiocarcinoma. Gastroenterology 114:536, 1998

SCHAFER DF, SORRELL MF: Hepatocellular carcinoma. Lancet 353:1253, 1999

YOSHIDA H et al: Interferon therapy reduces the risk for hepatocellular carcinoma: National surveillance program of cirrhotic and noncirrhotic patients with chronic hepatitis C in Japan. Ann Intern Med 131:174, 1999

92 Robert J. Mayer

PANCREATIC CANCER

INCIDENCE AND ETIOLOGY The incidence of pancreatic carcinoma in the United States has increased significantly as the median life expectancy of the American population has lengthened. The tumor results in the death of >98% of afflicted patients. 28,200 individuals died of pancreatic cancer in 2000, making it the fifth most common cause of cancer-related mortality. The disease is more common in males than in females and in blacks than in whites. It rarely develops before the age of 50.

Little is known about the causes of pancreatic cancer. Cigarette smoking is the most consistent risk factor, with the disease being two to three times more common in heavy smokers than in nonsmokers. Whether this association is due to a direct carcinogenic effect of to-

bacco metabolites on the pancreas or an as yet undefined exposure that occurs more frequently in cigarette smokers is uncertain. Patients with chronic pancreatitis are at increased risk of pancreatic cancer, as are persons with long-standing diabetes mellitus. Obesity is a risk factor for pancreatic cancer; risk is directly related to increased calorie intake. Alcohol abuse or cholelithiasis are not risk factors for pancreatic cancer. Nor is pancreatic cancer associated with coffee consumption. Mutations in K-*ras* genes have been found in >85% of specimens of human pancreatic cancer. Pancreatic cancer has been associated with mutation of the $p16^{INK4}$ gene located on chromosome 9p21, a gene also implicated in the pathogenesis of malignant melanoma.

CLINICAL FEATURES More than 90% of pancreatic cancers are ductal adenocarcinomas, with islet cell tumors constituting the remaining 5 to 10%. Pancreatic cancers occur twice as frequently in the pancreatic head (70% of cases) as in the body (20%) or tail (10%) of the gland.

With the exception of jaundice, the initial symptoms associated with pancreatic cancer are often insidious and are usually present for >2 months before the cancer is diagnosed (Table 92-1). Pain and weight loss are present in >75% of patients. The pain typically has a gnawing, visceral quality, occasionally radiating from the epigastrium to the back. Pain is often a more severe problem in lesions arising in the body or tail of the gland, as such tumors may become quite large before being detected. Characteristically, the pain improves somewhat when the patient bends forward. The development of significant pain suggests retroperitoneal invasion and infiltration of the splanchnic nerves, indicating that the primary lesion is advanced and is not surgically resectable. Rarely, such pain may be transient and associated with hyperamylasemia, indicative of acute pancreatitis caused by ductal obstruction by tumor. The weight loss observed in most patients is primarily the result of anorexia, although in the initial period of the disease, subclinical malabsorption may also be a contributing factor.

Jaundice due to biliary obstruction is found in >80% of patients having tumors in the pancreatic head and is typically accompanied by dark urine, a claylike appearance of stool, and pruritus. In contrast to the "painless jaundice" sometimes observed in patients having carcinomas of the bile ducts, duodenum, or periampullary regions, most icteric individuals with ductal carcinomas of the pancreatic head will complain of significant abdominal discomfort. Although the gallbladder is usually enlarged in patients with carcinoma of the head of the pancreas, it is palpable in <50% (Courvoisier's sign). However, the presence of an enlarged gallbladder in a jaundiced patient without biliary colic should suggest malignant obstruction of the extrahepatic biliary tree.

Glucose intolerance, presumably a direct consequence of the tumor, often develops within 2 years of the clinical diagnosis. Other initial manifestations include venous thrombosis and migratory thrombophlebitis (Trousseau's syndrome), gastrointestinal hemorrhage from varices due to compression of the portal venous system by tumor, and splenomegaly caused by cancerous encasement of the splenic vein.

DIAGNOSTIC PROCEDURES (Fig. 92-1) Despite the availability of serologic tests for tumor-associated antigens, such as

Table 92-1 Presenting Signs and Symptoms of Pancreatic Carcinoma

Frequent
  Abdominal pain
  Weight loss
  Jaundice (lesions of pancreatic head only)
Infrequent
  Glucose intolerance
  Palpable gallbladder
  Migratory thrombophlebitis
  Gastrointestinal hemorrhage
  Splenomegaly

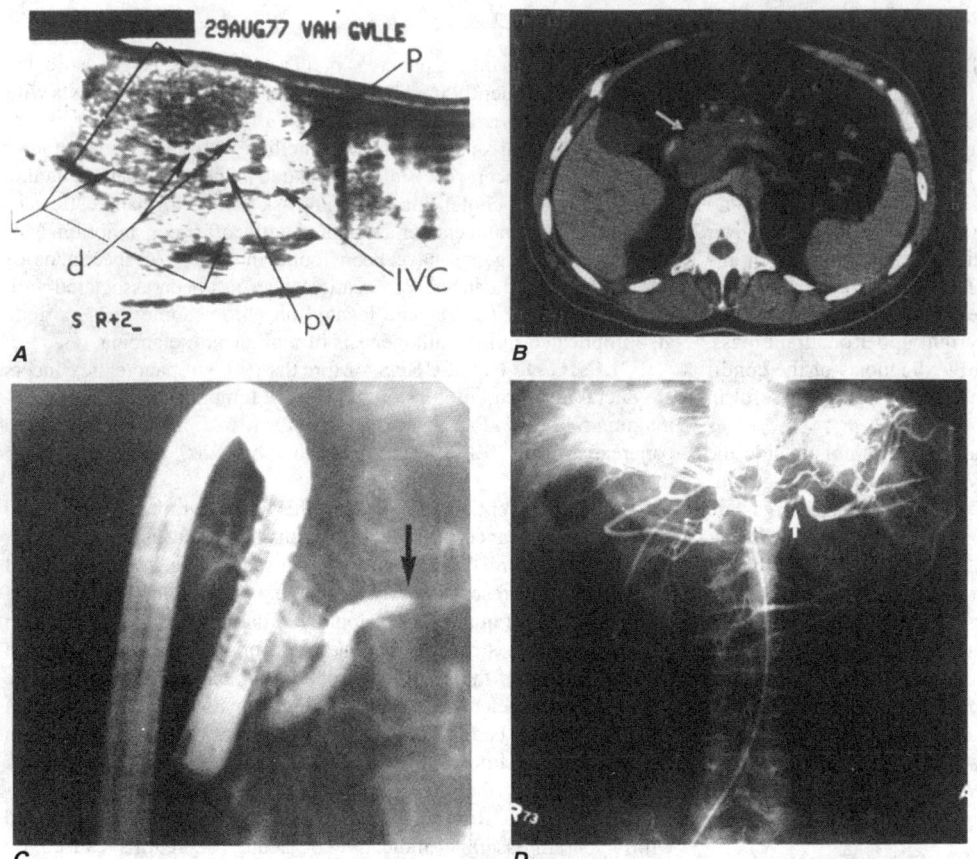

FIGURE 92-1 Carcinoma of the pancreas. *A.* Sonogram showing pancreatic carcinoma (P), dilated intrahepatic bile ducts (d), dilated portal vein (pv), and inferior vena cava (IVC). *B.* CT scan showing pancreatic carcinoma (*arrow*). *C.* Endoscopic retrograde showing abrupt cutoff of the duct of Wirsung (*arrow*). *D.* Arteriogram showing sheathing of splenic artery by tumor encasement (*arrow*).

the carcinoembryonic antigen (CEA) and CA 19-9, and noninvasive imaging techniques, such as computed tomography (CT) and ultrasonography, the early diagnosis of a potentially resectable pancreatic carcinoma remains extremely difficult. The nonspecificity of the initial symptoms and the poor sensitivity of both serologic assays and noninvasive techniques have frustrated the development of effective screening procedures. When the disease is clinically suspected in a patient having vague, persistent abdominal complaints, ultrasound should be performed to visualize the gallbladder and the pancreas, as well as upper gastrointestinal contrast radiographs to rule out a hiatal hernia or a peptic ulcer. If these studies fail to provide an explanation for the symptoms, a CT scan should be considered. It should encompass not only the pancreas but also the liver, retroperitoneal lymph nodes, and pelvis, as pancreatic cancer frequently spreads within the abdomen. While more costly than ultrasonography, CT is technically simpler, more reproducible, provides better definition of the body and tail of the pancreas, and requires less interpretive skill. CT generally detects a malignant pancreatic lesion in >80% of cases; in 5 to 15% of patients with proven pancreatic carcinoma, the CT scan shows only generalized pancreatic enlargement suggesting pancreatitis rather than malignancy. False-positive results occur in about 5 to 10% of cases where no tumor was found on laparotomy. Magnetic resonance imaging (MRI) has not been shown to be better than CT in the evaluation of pancreatic lesions. The value of positron emission tomography (PET) has not been defined. When clinical circumstances dictate additional diagnostic evaluation, endoscopic retrograde cholangiopancreatography (ERCP) with endoscopic ultrasonography (EUS) may clarify the cause of ambiguous CT or ultrasound findings. The characteristic findings are stenosis or obstruction of either the pancreatic or the common bile duct; both duct systems are abnormal in over half the cases. Carcinoma and chronic pancreatitis can be difficult to dis-

tinguish by ERCP, particularly if both diseases are present. False-negative results with ERCP are infrequent (<5%) and usually occur in the setting of islet cell, rather than ductal, carcinomas.

Selective and superselective angiography may be of value in some patients. Angiography is an effective means of detecting carcinomas in the body and tail of the pancreas by the demonstration of vascular narrowing, displacement, or occlusion by tumor. Angiography is being replaced as a diagnostic and staging procedure by spiral CT scanning with contrast imaging. This high-resolution technology predicts the resectability of the tumor if no disease is found outside the pancreas, obstruction of the superior mesenteric-portal vein confluence is absent, or tumor extension to the celiac axis and superior mesenteric arteries is not found. Radiographic staging criteria are shown in Table 92-2.

Regardless of the results of the above diagnostic studies, a histologic confirmation of pancreatic cancer is mandatory; similar findings can result from other neoplasms such as islet cell tumor or lymphoma, for which the therapeutic approach and prognosis differ from those for ductal carcinoma. In patients with unresectable disease or medical contraindications to surgical resection, tissue may be obtained through a percutaneous needle aspiration biopsy of the pancreas with CT or ultrasonographic guidance.

Unfortunately, however, even laparotomy may not provide a definitive diagnosis, because chronic pancreatitis may also produce a hard mass in the head of the pancreas indistinguishable from carcinoma by palpation. Furthermore, a superficial biopsy of such a mass may not show neoplastic tissue, revealing only evidence of pancreatitis, as the cancer is often surrounded by edematous, inflamed, and fibrotic tissue (i.e., chronic pancreatitis).

℞ **TREATMENT** Complete surgical resection of pancreatic tumors offers the only effective treatment for this disease. Unfortunately, such "curative" operations are only possible in 10 to 15% of

Table 92-2   Clinical (Radiographic) Staging of Pancreatic Cancer

Stage	Clinical/Radiographic Criteria
I	Resectable (T1–T2, selected T3,[a] NX, M0)
	No encasement of celiac axis or SMA
	Patent SMPV confluence
	No extrapancreatic disease
II	Locally advanced (T3, NX–1, M0)
	Arterial encasement (celiac axis or SMA) or venous occlusion (SMV or portal vein)
	No extrapancreatic disease
III	Metastatic (T1–3, NX–1, M1)
	Metastases typically to liver, peritoneum, and occasionally lung

[a] Resectable T3 lesions include those with isolated involvement of the SMV, portal vein, or hepatic artery without encasement of the celiac axis or SMA.
NOTE: T1, restricted to pancreas; T2, extension to duodenum, bile duct, or peripancreatic tissues; T3, extension to stomach, spleen, colon, or adjacent large vessels; NX, nodal status unknown; N0, regional nodes uninvolved; N1, regional nodes involved; M0, metastases absent; M1, metastases present; SMA, superior mesenteric artery; SMPV, superior mesenteric vein confluence with portal vein; SMV, superior mesenteric vein

patients with pancreatic cancer, usually those individuals with a tumor in the pancreatic head in whom jaundice was the initial symptom. Patients considered for such a procedure should have no evidence of metastatic spread on a chest radiograph and abdominal-pelvic CT scan and should be operated on by an experienced surgeon, as mortality rates of >15% have been associated with this procedure. Curative resection is usually preceded by laparoscopic inspection of the abdomen to confirm absence of occult disease spread to the omentum, peritoneum, or liver, which would preclude curative resection. Although the potential for cure in patients with pancreatic cancer is restricted to the few who are able to undergo a complete surgical resection, the 5-year survival rate following such operations is only 10%. Nonetheless, the procedure is worth attempting, particularly for lesions in the pancreatic head, since ductal carcinomas often cannot be distinguished preoperatively from ampullary, duodenal, and distal bile duct tumors or pancreatic cyst adenocarcinomas, all of which have far higher rates of resectability and cure. Furthermore, patients who undergo resection and eventually experience disease recurrence survive three to four times longer than those whose tumor is not excised, indicating that such operations have a palliative effect. The risk for tumor recurrence is not affected by the type of operative procedure—i.e., total pancreatectomy versus pancreaticoduodenectomy ("Whipple resection")—but it is increased by the presence of lymph node metastases or tumor invasion into adjacent viscera. As a rule, pancreaticoduodenectomy or distal pancreatectomy seems preferable to total pancreatectomy because of the retention of exocrine function and avoidance of brittle diabetes.

The median survival for patients whose pancreatic cancers are surgically unresectable is 6 months. Management is directed at palliation of symptoms. Ambulatory patients having tumors in the pancreatic head should be considered for surgical diversion of the biliary system. If jaundice has already developed, therapeutic options include either nonoperative biliary decompression by endoscopic or percutaneous, transhepatic biliary drainage or surgical biliary bypass. External beam radiation in patients with unresectable tumors that have not spread beyond the pancreas does not appear to prolong survival, although a sufficient reduction in tumor size may lead to palliation of pain. However, the addition of chemotherapy with fluorouracil (5-FU) to external beam irradiation has increased the survival time for these patients, perhaps because 5-FU acts as a radiosensitizing agent. In a small patient population, a similar combination of radiation therapy and 5-FU appears to have prolonged the survival and increased the cure rate as compared to a prospectively randomized nontreatment control group of patients who had a complete surgical resection of their pancreatic cancer. This observation needs to be confirmed before it can be accepted. The possibility of administering such chemoradiation therapy at diagnosis and before surgery ("neoadjuvant" treatment), to increase the potential for resectability, is under investigation. Intraoperative radiation therapy has the potential to deliver higher doses of radiation to the tumor while sparing neighboring tissues but does not give better results than external beam treatment.

Chemotherapy in the management of patients with widely metastatic pancreatic cancer has been disappointing. Gemcitabine, a deoxycytidine analogue, produces improvement in the quality of life for patients with advanced pancreatic cancer. However, duration of survival is only moderately improved. Newer forms of treatment, including combining gemcitabine with other cytotoxic agents or therapies directed at specific molecular targets, such as K-*ras*, or p53 are being evaluated. Experimental therapy should constitute the initial treatment for consenting, ambulatory patients. →*Pancreatic endocrine tumors are discussed in Chap. 93.*

BIBLIOGRAPHY

Burris HA et al: Improvements in survival and clinical benefit with gemcitabine as first-line therapy for patients with advanced pancreatic cancer. A randomized trial. J Clin Oncol 15:2403, 1997

Conlon KC et al: Long-term survival after curative resection for pancreatic ductal adenocarcinoma. Clinicopathologic analysis of 5-year survivors. Ann Surg 223:273, 1996

Jimenez RE et al: Impact of laparoscopic staging in the treatment of pancreatic cancer. Arch Surg 135:409, 2000

Schnall S, Macdonald JS: Chemotherapy of adenocarcinoma of the pancreas. Semin Oncol 23:220, 1996

Silverman DT et al: Dietary and nutritional factors and pancreatic cancer: A case-control study based on direct interviews. J Natl Cancer Inst 86:1510, 1994

Spitz FR et al: Preoperative and postoperative chemoradiation strategies in patients treated with pancreaticoduodenectomy for adenocarcinoma of the pancreas. J Clin Oncol 15: 928, 1997

Yeo CJ et al: Six-hundred-fifty consecutive pancreaticoduodenectomies in the 1990's. Ann Surg 226:248, 1997

93 *Robert T. Jensen*

ENDOCRINE TUMORS OF THE GASTROINTESTINAL TRACT AND PANCREAS

Gastrointestinal neuroendocrine tumors (NETs) are derived from the diffuse neuroendocrine system of the gastrointestinal (GI) tract, which is composed of amine- and acid-producing cells with different hormonal profiles, depending on the site of origin. The tumors they produce can be divided into carcinoid tumors and pancreatic endocrine tumors (PETs). These tumors were originally classified as APUDomas (for *a*mine *p*recursor *u*ptake and *d*ecarboxylation), as were pheochromocytomas, melanomas, and medullary thyroid carcinomas because they share certain cytochemical, pathologic, and biologic features (Table 93-1). APUDomas were thought to have a similar embryonic origin from neural crest cells, but the peptide-secreting cells are not of neuroectodermal origin.

CLASSIFICATION, PATHOLOGY, AND TUMOR BIOLOGY OF NETS

NETs are generally composed of monotonous sheets of small round cells with uniform nuclei; mitoses are uncommon. They can be tentatively identified on routine histology; however, these tumors are principally recognized by their histologic staining patterns due to shared cellular proteins. Historically, silver staining was used, and tumors were classified as showing an argentaffin reaction if they took

Table 93-1 General Characteristics of GI Neuroendocrine Tumors [Carcinoids, Pancreatic Endocrine Tumors (PETs)]

1. Share general neuroendocrine cell markers
   a. Chromogranins (A, B, C) are acidic monomeric soluble proteins found in the large secretory granules; chromogranin A is most widely used
   b. Neuron-specific enolase (NSE) is the γ-γ dimer of the enzyme enolase and is a cytosolic marker of neuroendocrine differentiation
   c. Synaptophysin is an integral membrane glycoprotein of molecular weight 38,000 found in small vesicles of neurons and neuroendocrine tumors
2. Pathologic similarities
   a. All PETs show amine precursor uptake and decarboxylation
   b. Ultrastructurally they have dense-core secretory granules (>80 nm)
   c. Histologically appear similar with few mitoses and uniform nuclei
   d. Frequently synthesize multiple peptides/amines, which can be detected immunocytochemically but may not be secreted
   e. Presence or absence of clinical syndrome or type can not be predicted by immunocytochemical studies
   f. Histologic classifications do not predict biologic behavior; only invasion or metastases establishes malignancy
3. Similarities of biologic behavior
   a. Generally slow growing, but a proportion are aggressive
   b. Secrete biologically active peptides/amines, which can cause clinical symptoms
   c. Generally have high densities of somatostatin receptors, which are used for both localization and treatment

up and reduced silver or as being argyrophilic if they did not reduce it. Immunocytochemical localization of chromogranins (A,B,C), neuron-specific enolase, or synaptophysin, which are all neuroendocrine cell markers, are now used (Table 93-1). Chromogranin A is the most widely used.

Ultrastructurally, these tumors possess electron-dense neurosecretory granules and frequently contain small clear vesicles that correspond to synaptic vesicles of neurons. NETs synthesize numerous peptides, growth factors, and bioactive amines that may be ectopically secreted, giving rise to a specific clinical syndrome (Table 93-2). The diagnosis of the specific syndrome, such as a VIPoma [vasoactive intestinal peptide (VIP)-secreting tumor], requires the clinical features of the disease and cannot be made from the immunocytochemistry results only (Table 93-1). Furthermore, pathologists cannot distinguish between benign and malignant NETs unless metastases or invasion are present.

Carcinoid tumors are frequently classified according to their anatomic area of origin (i.e., foregut, midgut, hindgut) because tumors with similar areas of origin share functional manifestations, histochemistry, and secretory products (Table 93-3). Foregut tumors generally have a low serotonin [5-hydroxytryptamine (5-HT)] content, are argentaffin-negative but argyrophilic, occasionally secrete adrenocorticotropic hormone (ACTH) or 5-hydroxytryptophan (5-HTP) causing an atypical carcinoid syndrome (Fig. 93-1), make several hormones, and may metastasize to bone. They uncommonly produce a clinical syndrome due to the secreted products. Midgut carcinoids are argentaffin-positive, have a high serotonin content, most frequently cause the typical carcinoid syndrome when they metastasize (Table 93-3, Fig. 93-1), release serotonin and tachykinins (substance P, neuropeptide K, substance K), rarely secrete 5-HTP or ACTH, and uncommonly metastasize to bone. Hindgut carcinoids (rectum and transverse and descending colon) are argentaffin-negative, often argyrophilic, rarely contain serotonin or cause the carcinoid syndrome, rarely secrete 5-HTP or ACTH, contain numerous peptides, and may metastasize to bone.

PETs can be classified into specific functional or nonfunctional syndromes (Table 93-2). Each of the functional syndromes is associated with symptoms due to the specific hormone released. In contrast,

Table 93-2 GI Neuroendocrine Tumor Syndromes

Name	Biologically Active Peptide(s) Secreted	Incidence (New Cases/ 10^6 Population Per Year)	Tumor Location	Malignant, %	Associated with MEN-1, %	Main Symptoms/Signs
I. ESTABLISHED SPECIFIC FUNCTIONAL SYNDROME						
Carcinoid Tumor						
Carcinoid syndrome	Serotonin, possibly tachykinins, motilin, prostaglandins	0.5–2	Midgut (75–87%) Foregut (2–33%) Hindgut (1–8%) Unknown (2–15%)	95–100	Rare	Diarrhea (32–84%) Flushing (63–75%) Pain (10–34%) Asthma (4–18%) Heart disease (11–41%)
Pancreatic endocrine tumor						
Zollinger-Ellison syndrome	Gastrin	0.5–1.5	Duodenum (70%) Pancreas (25%) Other sites (5%)	60–90	20–25	Pain (79–100%) Diarrhea (30–75%) Esophageal symptoms (31–56%)
Insulinoma	Insulin	1–2	Pancreas (>99%)	<10	4–5	Hypoglycemic symptoms (100%)
VIPoma (Verner-Morrison syndrome, pancreatic cholera, WDHA)	Vasoactive intestinal peptide	0.05–0.2	Pancreas (90%, adult) Other (10%, neural, adrenal, periganglionic)	40–70	6	Diarrhea (90–100%) Hypokalemia (80–100%) Dehydration (83%)
Glucagonoma	Glucagon	0.01–0.1	Pancreas (100%)	50–80	1–20	Rash (67–90%) Glucose intolerance (38–87%) Weight loss (66–96%)
Somatostatinoma	Somatostatin	Rare	Pancreas (55%) Duodenum-jejunum (44%)	>70	45	Diabetes mellitus (63–90%) Cholelithiases (65–90%) Diarrhea (35–90%)
GRFoma	Growth hormone–releasing hormone	Unknown	Pancreas (30%) Lung (54%) Jejunum (7%) Other (13%)	>60	16	Acromegaly (100%)
ACTHoma	ACTH	Rare	Pancreas (4–16%, all ectopic Cushing's)	>95	Rare	Cushing's syndrome (100%)
PET causing carcinoid syndrome	Serotonin, ? tachykinins	Rare (43 cases)	Pancreas (≤% all carcinoids)	60–88	Rare	Same as carcinoid syndrome above
PET causing hypercalcemia	PTHrP, others unknown	Rare	Pancreas (rare cause of hypercalcemia)	84	Rare	Abdominal pain due to hepatic metastases
II. POSSIBLE SPECIFIC FUNCTIONAL SYNDROME						
PET secreting calcitonin	Calcitonin	Rare	Pancreas (rare cause of hypercalcitonemia)	>80	16	Diarrhea (50%)
III. NO FUNCTIONAL SYNDROME						
PPoma/nonfunctional	None	1–2	Pancreas (100%)	>60	18–44	Weight loss (30–90%) Abdominal mass (10–30%) Pain (30–95%)

NOTE: MEN, multiple endocrine neoplasia; VIPoma, tumor-secreting vasoactive intestinal peptide; WDHA, watery diarrhea, hypokalemia, and achlorhydria syndrome; GRFoma, tumor-secreting growth hormone–releasing factor; ACTH, adrenocorticotrophic hormone; PET, pancreatic endocrine tumor; PTHrP, parathyroid hormone–related protein; PPoma, tumor secreting pancreatic polypeptide.

	Location (% of Total)	Incidence of Metastases	Incidence of Carcinoid Syndrome
Foregut			
Esophagus	<1	67	—
Stomach	3.8	31	9.5
Duodenum	2.1	—	3.4
Pancreas	<1	76	20
Gallbladder	<1	56	5
Ampulla	<1	—	—
Larynx	<1	0	—
Bronchus, lung	32.5	27	13
Midgut			
Jejunum	2.3	}70	9
Ileum	17.6		9
Meckel's diverticulum	0.4	—	13
Appendix	7.6	35	<1
Colon	6.3	71	5
Liver	<1	29	—
Ovary	<1	32	50
Testis	<1	—	50
Cervix	<1	67	3
Hindgut			
Rectum	10	14	—

SOURCE: Location and incidence of metastases are from 5468 cases studied from 1973–1991, reported by Modlin and Sandor. Incidence of carcinoid syndrome is from 4349 cases studied from 1950–1971, reported by JD Godwin, Cancer 36:560, 1975.

nonfunctional PETs release no products that cause a specific clinical syndrome. "Nonfunctional" is a misnomer in the strict sense because these tumors frequently ectopically secrete a number of peptides [pancreatic polypeptide (PP) chromogranin A, neurotensin]; however, they cause no specific clinical syndrome. The symptoms caused by nonfunctional PETs are entirely due to the tumor per se.

Carcinoid tumors can occur in almost any GI tissue (Table 93-3);

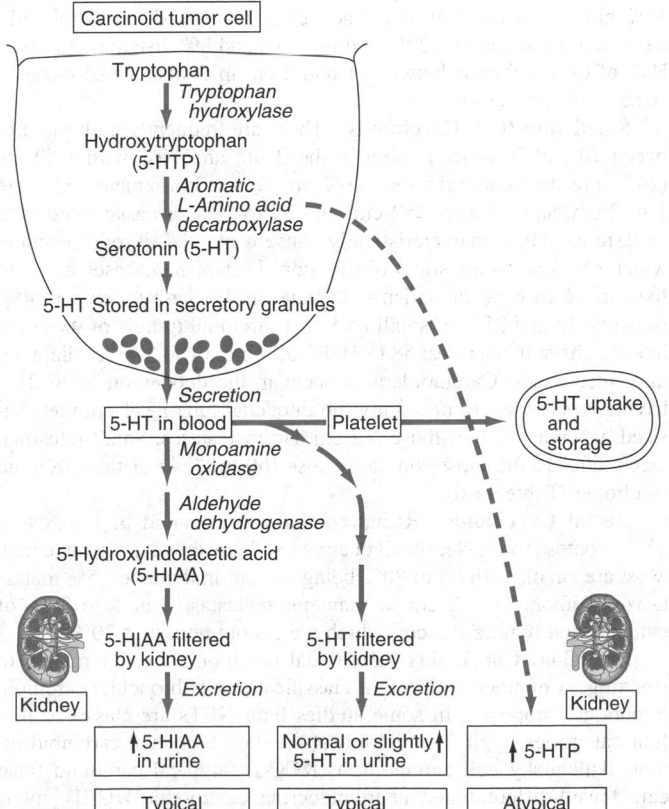

FIGURE 93-1 Synthesis, secretion, and metabolism of serotonin (5-HT) in patients with typical and atypical carcinoid syndromes.

however, most (70%) originate from one of four sites; bronchus, jejunum/ileum, rectum, or appendix. In the past, carcinoid tumors most frequently occurred in the appendix (i.e., 40%); however, the bronchus/lung is now the most common site (32%). Overall, the GI tract is the most common site for these tumors, comprising 74%, with the respiratory tract a distant second at 25%.

The term *pancreatic endocrine tumor*, although widely used, is also a misnomer, because these tumors can occur either almost exclusively in the pancreas (insulinomas, glucagonomas, nonfunctional PETs, PETs causing hypercalcemia) or at both pancreatic and extrapancreatic sites [gastrinomas, VIPomas, somatostatinomas, GRFomas (GRF, growth hormone–releasing factor)]. PETs are also called *islet cell tumors*; however, this term is discouraged because it is not established that many originate from the islets and many can occur at extrapancreatic sites.

The exact incidence of carcinoid tumors or PETs varies according to whether only symptomatic or all tumors are considered. The incidence of clinically significant carcinoids is 7 to 13 cases per million population per year, whereas malignant carcinoids are reported at autopsy in 21 to 84 cases per million population per year. Clinically significant PETs have a prevalence of 10 cases per million population, with insulinomas, gastrinomas, and nonfunctional PETs having an incidence of 0.5 to 2 cases per million population per year (Table 93-2); VIPomas are 2- to 8-fold less common, glucagonomas are 17- to 30-fold less common, and somatostatinomas the least common. In autopsy studies 0.5 to 1.5% of all cases have a PET; however, in fewer than 1 in 1000 cases was a functional tumor present.

Both carcinoid tumors and PETs commonly show malignant behavior (Tables 93-2, 93-3). With PETs, except for insulinomas in which <10% are malignant, 50 to 100% are malignant. With carcinoid tumors the percentage showing malignant behavior varies in different locations. For the four most common sites of occurrence the incidence of metastases varies greatly: jejunum/ileum (70%) > appendix (35%) > lung/bronchus (27%) > rectum (14%). A number of factors are important in determining survival and the aggressiveness of the tumor (Table 93-4). The presence of liver metastases is the single most im-

Table 93-4 Prognostic Factors in Neuroendocrine Tumors

Both carcinoid tumors and PETs
  Presence of liver metastases ($p < .001$)
  Extent of liver metastases ($p < .001$)
  Presence of lymph node metastases ($p < .001$)
  Depth of invasion ($p < .001$)
  Primary tumor site ($p < .001$)
  Primary tumor size ($p < .005$)
  Various histologic features
    Tumor differentiation ($p < .001$)
    High growth indices (high Ki-67 index, PCNA expression)
    High mitotic counts ($p < .001$)
    Vascular or perineural invasion
    Flow cytometric features (i.e., aneuploidy)
Carcinoid tumors
  Presence of carcinoid syndrome
  Laboratory results [urinary 5-HIAA level ($p < .01$), plasma neuropeptide K ($p < .05$), serum chromogranin A ($p < .01$)]
  Presence of a secondary malignancy
  Male gender ($p < .001$)
  Older age ($p < .01$)
  Mode of discovery (incidental > symptomatic)
PETs
  Ha-Ras oncogene or p53 overexpression
  Female gender
  MEN-1 syndrome absent
  Laboratory findings (increased chromogranin A in some studies; increased gastrin level in gastrinomas)

NOTE: PET, pancreatic endocrine tumor; MEN, multiple endocrine neoplasia; PCNA, proliferating cell nuclear antigen; Ki-67, proliferation-associated nuclear antigen recognized by Ki-67 monoclonal antibody.

Table 93-5 Genetic Syndromes Associated with an Increased Incidence of Neuroendocrine Tumors [NETs: Carcinoids or Pancreatic Endocrine Tumors (PETs)]

Syndrome	Location of Gene Mutation and Gene Product	NETs Seen/Frequency
Multiple endocrine neoplasia type 1 (MEN-1)	11q13 (encodes 610-amino-acid protein, menin)	80–100% develop PETs, (nonfunctional > gastrinoma > insulinoma) Carcinoids: gastric (13–30%), bronchial/thymic (8%)
von Hippel-Lindau disease	3q25 (encodes 213-amino-acid protein)	12–17% develop PETs (almost always nonfunctional)
von Recklinghausen's disease [neurofibromatosis1 (NF-1)]	17q11.2 (encodes 2485-amino-acid protein, neurofibromin)	Duodenal somatostatinomas (usually nonfunctional) Rarely insulinoma, gastrinoma
Tuberous sclerosis	9q34 (TSCI) (encodes 1164-amino-acid protein, hamartin) 16p13 (TSC2) (encodes 1807-amino-acid protein, tuberin)	Uncommonly develop PETs [nonfunctional and functional (insulinoma, gastrinoma)]

portant prognostic factor for both carcinoid tumors and PETs. The size of the primary tumor is particularly important in the development of liver metastases. For example, with small-intestinal carcinoids, which are the most frequent cause of the carcinoid syndrome due to metastatic disease in the liver (Table 93-2), metastases occur in 15 to 25% if the tumor diameter is <1 cm, in 58 to 80% if it is 1 to 2 cm and in >75% if it is >2 cm. The size of the primary tumor has also been shown to be an independent predictor of the development of liver metastases for gastrinomas and other PETs. The presence of lymph node metastases, the depth of invasion, various histologic features (differentiation, mitotic rates, growth indices), and flow cytometric results such as the presence of aneuploidy are all important prognostic factors for the development of metastatic disease. The development of the carcinoid syndrome, older age, male gender, the presence of a symptomatic tumor, or greater increases in a number of tumor markers [5-hydroxyindolacetic acid (5-HIAA), neuropeptide K, chromogranin A] also adversely affect prognosis in patients with carcinoid tumors (Table 93-4). With PETs or gastrinomas, a worse prognosis is associated with female gender, overexpression of the *Ha-Ras* oncogene or p53, the absence of multiple endocrine neoplasia (MEN) type 1, and higher levels of various tumor markers (e.g., chromogranin A, gastrin).

A number of genetic disorders are associated with an increased incidence of neuroendocrine tumors (Table 93-5). Each one is caused by a loss of a possible tumor suppressor gene. The most important is MEN-1, an autosomal dominant disorder due to a defect in a 10-exon gene on 11q13, which encodes for a 610-amino-acid nuclear protein, menin (Chap. 339). In patients with MEN-1, 95 to 100% develop hyperparathyroidism due to parathyroid hyperplasia, 80 to 100% develop nonfunctional PETs, 54 to 80% develop pituitary adenomas, and bronchial carcinoids develop in 8%, thymic carcinoids in 8%, and gastric carcinoids in 13 to 30% of patients with Zollinger-Ellison syndrome. Functional PETs occur in 80% of patients with MEN-1, with 54% developing Zollinger-Ellison syndrome, 21% insulinomas, 3% glucagonomas, and 1% VIPomas. MEN-1 is present in 20 to 25% of all patients with Zollinger-Ellison syndrome, in 4% of those with insulinomas, and in <5% of those with other PETs.

Three phakomatoses associated with NETs are von Hippel–Lindau disease, von Recklinghausen's disease, or neurofibromatosis type 1 (NF-1), and tuberous sclerosis (Bourneville's disease). Von Hippel–Lindau disease is an autosomal dominant disorder due to defects in a gene on chromosome 3p25, which encodes a 213-amino-acid protein that interacts with the elongin family of proteins as a transcriptional regulator and in abnormal protein destruction (Chap. 370). In addition to cerebellar hemangioblastomas, renal cancer, and pheochromocytomas, 10 to 17% of these patients develop a PET. Most are nonfunctional, although insulinomas and VIPomas are reported. Patients with NF-1 have defects in a gene on chromosome 17q11.2 encoding for a 2845-amino-acid protein, neurofibromin, which functions in normal cells as a suppressor of the Ras signaling cascade (Chap. 370). Up to 12% of these patients develop an upper GI carcinoid tumor, characteristically in the periampullary region (54%). Many of such tumors are classified as somatostatinomas because they contain somatostatin immunocytochemically; however, they seldom produce a clinical somatostatinoma syndrome. NF-1 has rarely been associated with insulinomas and Zollinger-Ellison syndrome. Tuberous sclerosis is caused by mutations that alter either the 1164-amino-acid protein, hamartin (TSC1), or the 1807-amino-acid protein, tuberin (TSC2) (Chap. 370). Both hamartin and tuberin interact in a pathway related to cytosolic G protein regulation. A few cases including nonfunctional and functional PETs (insulinomas and gastrinomas) have been reported (Table 93-5).

Changes in the MEN-1 gene, p16/MTS1 tumor suppressor gene, and DPC 4/Smad 4 gene; amplification of the HER-2/neu protooncogene; and deletions of unknown tumor suppressor genes on chromosomes 1 and 3p may be important in the pathogenesis of PETs. Loss of heterozygosity at the MEN-1 locus on chromosome 11q13 has been found in 93% of sporadic PETs (patients without MEN-1) and in 26 to 75% of sporadic carcinoid tumors. Mutations in the MEN-1 gene were found in 31 to 34% of sporadic gastrinomas.

CARCINOID TUMORS AND CARCINOID SYNDROME

GENERAL TUMOR CHARACTERISTICS OF THE MOST COMMON GI CARCINOID TUMORS Appendiceal Carcinoids These occur in 1 in every 200 to 300 appendectomies, usually in the appendiceal tip. More than 90% are <1 cm in diameter; 35% have metastases. In one study of 1570 appendiceal carcinoids, 62% were localized and 27% had regional and 8% distant metastases. Half of the carcinoids between 1 and 2 cm in diameter had metastasized to lymph nodes.

Small-Intestinal Carcinoids These are frequently multiple. Between 70 and 80% are present in the ileum and 70% within 60 cm (24 in.) of the ileocecal valve; 40% are <1 cm in diameter, 32% are 1 to 2 cm, and 29% are >2 cm; and 35 to 70% are associated with metastases. They characteristically cause a marked fibrotic reaction, which can lead to intestinal obstruction. Distant metastases occur to liver in 36 to 60% of patients, to bone in 3%, and to lung in 4%. Between 15 and 25% of small (<1 cm) carcinoid tumors of the small intestine have metastases; 58 to 100% of tumors 1 to 2 cm in diameter have metastases. Carcinoids also occur in the duodenum, with 21% having metastases. In one study, no duodenal tumor <1 cm metastasized, whereas 33% of those >2 cm had metastases. Small-intestinal carcinoids are the most common cause (60 to 87%) of the carcinoid syndrome (Table 93-6).

Rectal Carcinoids Rectal carcinoids are found in 1 of every 2500 proctoscopies. Nearly all occur 4 to 13 cm above the dentate line. Most are small, with 66 to 80% being <1 cm in diameter; 5% metastasize. Tumors 1 to 2 cm in diameter metastasize in 5 to 30% of patients, and tumors >2 cm, which are uncommon, in >70%.

Bronchial Carcinoids Bronchial carcinoids are not related to smoking. A number of different classifications of bronchial carcinoid tumors are proposed. In some studies lung NETs are classified into four categories: typical carcinoid (also called bronchial carcinoid tumor, Kulchitsky cell carcinoma-I, KCC-I); atypical carcinoid (also called well-differentiated neuroendocrine carcinoma, KC-II); intermediate small cell neuroendocrine carcinoma; and small cell neuroendocarcinoma (KC-III). Another proposed classification includes three categories of lung NETs: benign or low-grade malignant (typical car-

	At Presentation	During Course of Disease
Symptoms/signs		
Diarrhea	32–73%	68–84%
Flushing	23–65%	63–74%
Pain	10%	34%
Asthma/wheezing	4–8%	3–18%
Pellagra	2%	5%
None	12%	22%
Carcinoid heart disease present	11%	14–41%
Demographics		
Male	46–59%	46–61%
Age		
Mean	57 yrs	52–54 yrs
Range	25–79 yrs	9–91 yrs
Tumor location		
Foregut	5–9%	2–33%
Midgut	78–87%	60–87%
Hindgut	1–5%	1–8%
Unknown	2–11%	2–15%

cinoid); low-grade malignant (atypical carcinoid), and high-grade malignant (poorly differentiated carcinoma of the large cell or small cell type). These different categories of lung NETs have different prognoses, varying from excellent for typical carcinoid to poor for small cell neuroendocrine carcinomas.

Gastric Carcinoids   These account for 3 of every 1000 gastric neoplasms. Three different subtypes of gastric carcinoids are noted. Each originates from gastric enterochromaffin-like (ECL) cells in the gastric mucosa. Two subtypes are associated with hypergastrinemic states: (1) chronic atrophic gastritis (type I) (80% of all gastric carcinoids); and (2) Zollinger-Ellison syndrome, almost always as part of the MEN-1 syndrome (type II) (6% of all cases). These tumors generally pursue a benign course, with 9 to 30% associated with metastases. They are usually multiple and small and infiltrate only to the submucosa. The third subtype of gastric carcinoid (type III) (sporadic) occurs without hypergastrinemia (14% of all carcinoids) and pursues an aggressive course, with 54 to 66% developing metastases. Sporadic carcinoids are usually single, large tumors; 50% have atypical histology and can be a cause of the carcinoid syndrome.

CARCINOID TUMORS WITHOUT THE CARCINOID SYNDROME   The age of patients at diagnosis ranges from 10 to 93 years, with a mean age of 63 years for carcinoid tumors of the small intestine and 66 years for those of the rectum. The presentation is diverse and related to the site of origin and extent of malignant spread. In the appendix, carcinoid tumors are usually found incidentally during surgery for suspected appendicitis. Small-intestinal carcinoids in the jejunum/ileum present with periodic abdominal pain (51%), intestinal obstruction with ileus/invagination (31%), an abdominal tumor (17%), or GI bleeding (11%). Because of the vagueness of the symptoms the diagnosis is usually delayed approximately 2 years from onset of the symptoms, with a range up to 20 years. Duodenal, gastric, and rectal carcinoids are most frequently found by chance at endoscopy. The most common symptoms of rectal carcinoids are melena/bleeding (39%), constipation (17%), and diarrhea (12%). Bronchial carcinoids are frequently discovered as a lesion on a chest radiograph, and 31% of the patients are asymptomatic. Thymic carcinoids present as anterior mediastinal masses, usually on chest radiograph of computed tomography (CT) scan. Ovarian and testicular carcinoids usually present as masses discovered on physical examination or by ultrasound. Metastatic carcinoid tumor in the liver presents frequently as hepatomegaly in a patient who may have minimal symptoms and near-normal liver function test results.

CARCINOID TUMORS WITH SYSTEMIC SYMPTOMS DUE TO SECRETED PRODUCTS   Carcinoid tumors can contain numerous GI peptides: gastrin, insulin, somatostatin, motilin, neurotensin, tachykinins (substance K, substance P, neuropeptide K), glu-cagon, gastrin-releasing peptide, VIP, PP, other biologically active peptides (ACTH, calcitonin, growth hormone–releasing hormone), prostaglandins, and bioactive amines (serotonin). These substances may or may not be released in sufficient amounts to cause symptoms. In patients with carcinoid tumors, elevated serum levels of PP were found in 43%, motilin in 14%, gastrin in 15%, and VIP in 6%. Foregut carcinoids are more likely to produce various GI peptides than midgut carcinoids. Ectopic ACTH production causing Cushing's syndrome is increasingly seen with foregut carcinoids (respiratory tract primarily), and in some series foregut carcinoid was the most common cause of the ectopic ACTH syndrome, accounting for 64% of all cases. Acromegaly due to GRF release occurs with foregut carcinoids, as does the somatostatinoma syndrome with duodenal carcinoids. The most common systemic syndrome is the carcinoid syndrome.

CARCINOID SYNDROME   Clinical Features   The cardinal features at presentation as well as during the disease course are shown in Table 93-6. Flushing and diarrhea are the two most common symptoms, occurring in up to 73% initially and in up to 89% during the course of the disease. The characteristic flush is of sudden onset: it is a deep red or violaceous erythema of the upper body (especially the neck and face), often associated with a feeling of warmth, and occasionally associated with pruritus, lacrimation, diarrhea, or facial edema. Flushes may be precipitated by stress, alcohol, exercise, or certain foods such as cheese or by certain agents such as catecholamines, pentagastrin, and serotonin reuptake inhibitors. Flushing episodes may be brief, lasting 2 to 5 min, especially initially, or they may last for hours, especially later in the disease course. Flushing is usually seen with midgut carcinoids but can also occur with foregut carcinoids. With bronchial carcinoids the flushes are frequently prolonged for hours to days, reddish in color, and associated with salivation, lacrimation, diaphoresis, diarrhea, and hypotension. The flush associated with gastric carcinoids is also reddish in color but patchy in distribution over the face and neck. It may be provoked by food and have accompanying pruritus.

Diarrhea is present in 32 to 73% of patients initially and in 68 to 84% at some time in the disease course. Diarrhea usually occurs with flushing (85% of cases). The diarrhea is usually watery, with 60% having <1 L per day or diarrhea. Steatorrhea is present in 67%, and in 46% it is >15 g/day (normal <7 g). Abdominal pain may be present with the diarrhea or independently in 10 to 34% of cases.

Cardiac manifestations occur in 11% of patients initially and in 14 to 41% at some time in the disease course. The cardiac disease is due to fibrosis involving the endocardium, primarily on the right side, although left side lesions can occur also. The dense fibrous deposits are most common on the ventricular aspect of the tricuspid valve and less common on the pulmonary valve cusps. They can result in constriction of the valves and pulmonic stenosis is usually predominant, whereas the tricuspid valve is often fixed open, resulting in regurgitation. Up to 80% of patients with cardiac lesions develop heart failure. Lesions on the left side are much less extensive, are found in 30% at autopsy, and most frequently affect the mitral valve.

Other clinical manifestations include wheezing or asthma-like symptoms (8 to 18%) and pellagra-like skin lesions (2 to 25%). A variety of noncardiac problems due to increased fibrous tissue have been reported, including retroperitoneal fibrosis causing urethral obstruction, Peyronie's disease of the penis, intrabdominal fibrosis, and occlusion of the mesenteric arteries or veins.

Pathobiology   In different studies covering 8876 patients with carcinoid tumors, carcinoid syndrome occurred in 8%, with a range of 1.4 to 18.4%. It occurs only when sufficient concentrations of tumor-secreted products reach the systemic circulation. In 91% of cases this occurs after metastasis to the liver. Rarely, the carcinoid syndrome can occur without hepatic metastases, caused by primary gut carcinoids with nodal metastases with extensive retroperitoneal invasion, pancreatic carcinoids with retroperitoneal lymph nodes, or carcinoids of the lung or ovary with direct access to the systemic circulation. All carcinoid tumors do not have the same propensity to metastasize and cause the carcinoid syndrome (Table 93-3). Midgut carcinoids account for 60 to 67% of cases of carcinoid syndrome, foregut tumors for 2 to 33%, hindgut for 1 to 8%, and unknown primary sites for 2 to 15%.

One of the main secretory products of carcinoid tumors involved in the carcinoid syndrome is serotonin [5-hydroxytryptamine (5-HT)] (Fig. 93-1), which is synthesized from tryptophan. Up to 50% of dietary tryptophan can be used in this synthetic pathway by tumor cells, which can result in inadequate supplies for conversion to niacin; hence 2 to 5% of patients can develop pellagra-like lesions. Serotonin has numerous biologic effects including stimulating intestinal secretion, inhibiting absorption, stimulating increases in intestinal motility, and stimulating fibrogenesis. While 56 to 88% of carcinoid tumors are associated with serotonin overproduction, 12 to 26% of patients do not have the carcinoid syndrome. Serotonin overproduction is noted in 90 to 100% of patients with the carcinoid syndrome. Serotonin is thought to be predominantly responsible for the diarrhea by its effects on gut motility and intestinal secretion. Serotonin receptor antagonists (especially 5-HT$_3$ antagonists) relieve the diarrhea in most patients. Prostaglandin E$_2$ and tachykinins may be important mediators of the diarrhea in some patients. Flushing is not relieved by serotonin receptor antagonists. In patients with gastric carcinoids the red, patchy pruritic flush is likely due to histamine release because it can be prevented by H$_1$ and H$_2$ receptor antagonists. Numerous studies show tachykinins are stored in carcinoid tumors and released during flushing. Octreotide can relieve the flushing induced by pentagastrin in these patients without altering stimulated increase in plasma substance P, suggesting other mediators must be involved in the flushing. Both histamine and serotonin may be responsible for the wheezing as well as the fibrotic reactions involving the heart, causing Peyronie's disease and intraabdominal fibrosis. The exact mechanism of the heart disease is unclear. The valvular heart disease caused by the appetite-suppressant drug, dexfenfluramine, is histologically indistinguishable from that observed in carcinoid disease or after long exposure to 5-HT$_2$-selective ergot drugs. Metabolites of fenfluramine have high affinity for 5-HT$_2$ receptors, whose activation is known to cause fibroblast mitogenesis. Lastly, high levels of 5-HT$_{2B}$ and 5-HT$_{2C}$ receptor transcripts are known to occur in heart valves. These observations support the conclusion that serotonin overproduction is important for the valvular changes, possibly by activating 5-HT$_2$ receptors in the endocardium.

Patients may develop either a typical or atypical carcinoid syndrome (Fig. 93-1). In patients with the typical form, characteristically caused by a midgut carcinoid tumor, the conversion of tryptophan to 5-HTP is the rate-limiting step. 5-HTP is rapidly converted to 5-HT and stored in secretory granules of the tumor or in platelets. A small amount remains in plasma and is converted to 5-HIAA, which appears in large amounts in the urine. These patients have an expanded serotonin pool size, increased blood and platelet serotonin levels, and increased urinary 5-HIAA. Some carcinoid tumors cause an atypical carcinoid syndrome thought to be due to a deficiency in the enzyme dopa decarboxylase; thus, 5-HTP cannot be converted to 5-HT (serotonin) and is secreted into the bloodstream. In these patients, plasma serotonin levels are normal but urinary levels may be increased because some 5-HTP is converted to 5-HT in the kidney. Characteristically, urinary 5-HTP and 5-HT are increased, but urinary 5-HIAA levels are only slightly elevated. Foregut carcinoids are the most likely to cause an atypical carcinoid syndrome.

One of the most life-threatening complications of the carcinoid syndrome is the development of a carcinoid crisis. This is more frequent in patients who have intense symptoms from foregut tumors or have greatly increased urinary 5-HIAA levels (i.e., >200 mg/d). The crisis may occur spontaneously or be provoked by stress, anesthesia, chemotherapy, or a biopsy. Patients develop intense flushing, diarrhea, abdominal pain, and cardiac abnormalities including tachycardia, hypertension, or hypotension. If not adequately treated, it can be fatal.

Diagnosis The diagnosis of carcinoid syndrome relies on measurement of urinary or plasma serotonin or its metabolites in the urine. The measurement of 5-HIAA is most frequently used. False-positive elevations may occur if the patient is eating serotonin-rich foods (e.g., bananas, pineapple, walnuts, pecans, avocados, or hickory nuts) or taking certain medications (e.g., cough syrup containing guaifanesin, acetaminophen, salicylates, or L-dopa). The normal range in daily urinary 5-HIAA excretion is between 2 and 8 mg. The 5-HIAA level has a 73% sensitivity and 100% specificity for carcinoid syndrome.

Most physicians use only the urinary 5-HIAA excretion rate; however, plasma and platelet serotonin levels, if available, may give additional information. Platelet serotonin levels are more sensitive than urinary 5-HIAA but are not generally available. If an atypical carcinoid syndrome is suspected and the urinary 5-HIAA is minimally elevated or normal, other urinary metabolites of tryptophan such as 5-HTP or 5-HT should be measured.

Flushing occurs in a number of other conditions or diseases including systemic mastocytosis; chronic myelogenous leukemia with increased histamine release; menopause; reactions to alcohol or glutamate; and side effects of chlorpropamide, calcium channel blockers, and nicotinic acid. None of these conditions cause an increase in urinary 5-HIAA.

The diagnosis of carcinoid tumor can be suggested by the carcinoid syndrome, by recurrent abdominal symptoms in a healthy-appearing individual, or by discovering hepatomegaly or hepatic metastases associated with minimal symptoms. Ileal carcinoids, which make up 25% of all clinically detected carcinoids, should be suspected in patients with bowel obstruction, abdominal pain, flushing, or diarrhea.

Serum chromogranin A levels are elevated in 50 to 100% of patients with carcinoid tumors, and the level correlates with tumor bulk. Serum chromogranin A levels are not specific for carcinoid tumors because they are also elevated in patients with PETs and other NETs. Plasma neuron-specific enolase levels are also used as a marker of carcinoid tumors but are less sensitive than chromogranin A, being increased in only 17 to 47% of patients.

℞ **TREATMENT Carcinoid Syndrome** Treatment includes avoiding conditions that precipitate flushing, dietary supplementation with nicotinamide, treatment of heart failure with diuretics, treatment of wheezing with oral bronchodilators, and controlling the diarrhea with antidiarrheal agents such as loperamide or diphenoxylate. If patients still have symptoms, serotonin receptor antagonists or somatostatin analogues are the drugs of choice.

There are 14 subclasses of serotonin (5-HT) receptors, and antagonists for most are not available. The 5-HT$_1$ and 5-HT$_2$ receptor antagonists methysergide, cyproheptadine, and ketanserin have all been used to control the diarrhea but usually do not decrease flushing. The use of methysergide is limited because it can cause or enhance retroperitoneal fibrosis. Ketanserin diminishes diarrhea in 30 to 100% of patients. 5-HT$_3$ receptor antagonists (ondansetron, tropisetron, alosetron) can control diarrhea and nausea in up to 100% of patients and occasionally ameliorate the flushing. A combination of histamine H$_1$ and H$_2$ receptor antagonists (i.e., diphenhydramine and cimetidine or ranitidine) may control flushing in patients with foregut carcinoids.

Synthetic analogues of somatostatin (octreotide, lanreotide) are now the most widely used agents to control the symptoms of patients with carcinoid syndrome (Fig. 93-2). These drugs are effective at relieving symptoms and decreasing urinary 5-HIAA levels when self-administered every 6 to 12 h. Octreotide controls symptoms in >80% of patients, including the diarrhea and flushing, and 70% of patients show a >50% decrease in urinary 5-HIAA excretion. Patients with mild to moderate symptoms should initially be treated with 100 μg subcutaneously every 8 h. Individual responses vary, and patients have received doses as high as 3000 μg/d. About 40% of patients escape control after a median of 4 months, and the dose may need to be increased. Similar results are reported with lanreotide.

In patients with carcinoid crises, somatostatin analogues are effective at both treating the condition as well as preventing its development

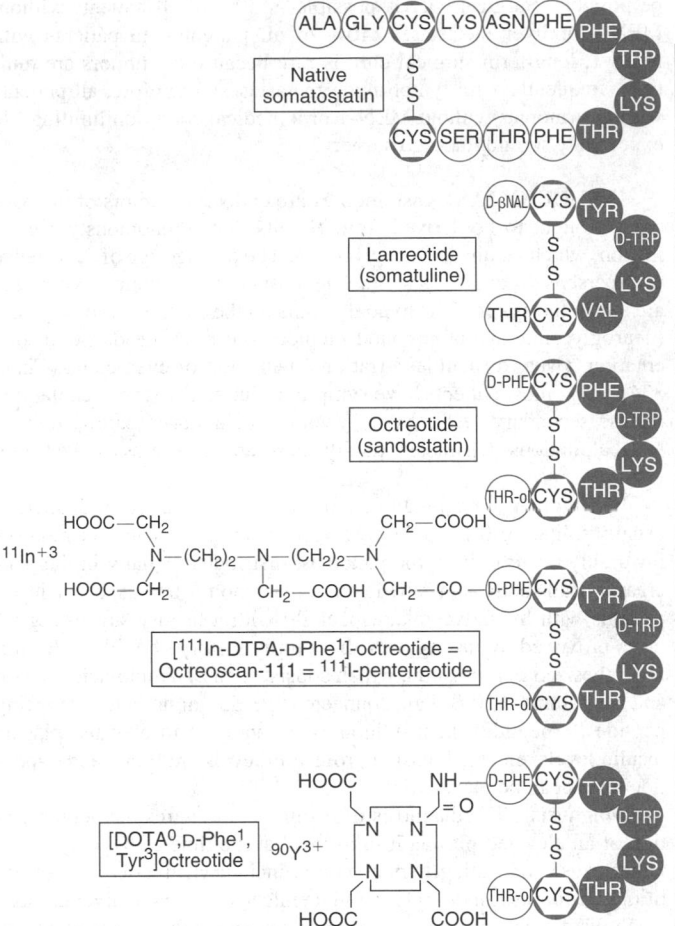

FIGURE 93-2 Structure of somatostatin and synthetic analogues used for diagnostic or therapeutic indications. DOTA, 1,4,7,10-tetra-azacylododecane-N, N', N'', N'''-tetracetic acid.

during known precipitating events such as surgery, anesthesia, chemotherapy, or stress. It is recommended that octreotide (150 to 250 μg subcutaneously every 6 to 8 h) be used 24 to 48 h before anesthesia and then continued throughout the procedure.

Sustained-release preparations of both octreotide [octreotide-LAR (long-acting release)] and lanreotide [lanreotide-PR (prolonged release)] are useful. Octreotide-LAR (30 mg/month) gives a plasma level $\geq$1 ng/mL for 25 days, whereas this level would require three to six injections per day of the non-sustained-release form. Lanreotide-PR is given intramuscularly every 10 to 14 days. Both sustained-release forms are highly effective.

Short-term side effects occur in 40 to 60% of patients receiving subcutaneous somatostatin analogues. Pain at the injection site and GI side effects (59% discomfort, 15% nausea, diarrhea) are the most common. They are usually short-lived and do not interrupt treatment. Important long-term side effects include gallstone formation, steatorrhea, and poor glucose tolerance. The overall incidence of gallstones/biliary sludge is 52%, with 7% of patients having symptomatic disease requiring surgical treatment.

Interferon α is effective in controlling symptoms of the carcinoid syndrome, either alone or combined with hepatic artery embolization. The response rate is 42% for interferon α alone; when given with hepatic artery embolization, diarrhea was controlled for 1 year in 43% and flushing in 86% of patients.

Hepatic artery embolization alone or with chemotherapy (chemoembolization) has been used to control the symptoms of carcinoid syndrome. Embolization alone controls symptoms in up to 76% of patients, and chemoembolization (5-fluorouracil, doxorubicin, cisplatin, mitomycin) in 60 to 75% of patients. Hepatic artery embolization can have major side effects including nausea, vomiting, pain, and fe-

ver. In two studies, between 5 and 7% of patients died from complications of hepatic artery occlusion.

Other drugs have been used successfully in small numbers of patients to control the symptoms of carcinoid syndrome. Parachlorophenylalanine can inhibit tryptophan hydroxylase and the conversion of tryptophan to 5-HTP (Fig. 93-1). However, its severe side effects, including psychiatric disturbances, make it intolerable for long-term use. α-Methyldopa inhibits the conversion of 5-HTP to 5-HT; however, its effects are only partial.

Carcinoid Tumors (Nonmetastatic) Surgery is the only potentially curative therapy. Because the probability of metastases increases with increasing primary tumor size, the extent of surgical resection is determined accordingly. With appendiceal carcinoids, simple appendectomy is curative. With rectal carcinoids <1 cm, local resection is curative. With small-intestinal carcinoids <1 cm there is no consensus. Because 15 to 69% of small-intestinal carcinoids this size have metastases, some recommend a wide resection with *en bloc* resection of the adjacent lymph-bearing mesentery. If the carcinoid tumor is >2 cm for rectal, appendiceal, or small intestine, a full cancer operation should be done, including a right hemicolectomy for appendiceal carcinoid, an abdominoperineal or low anterior resection for rectal carcinoids, and an *en bloc* resection of adjacent lymph nodes for small-intestinal carcinoids. For carcinoids 1 to 2 cm in diameter in the appendix, a simple appendectomy is proposed by some, whereas others favor a right hemicolectomy. For 1- to 2-cm rectal carcinoids, a wide local full-thickness excision is recommended.

With type I or II gastric carcinoids, which are usually <1 cm, endoscopic removal is recommended. In type I or II gastric carcinoids if the tumor is >2 cm or if there is local invasion, some recommend total gastrectomy, others recommend antrectomy in type 1. For types I and II gastric carcinoids 1 to 2 cm, some recommend endoscopic treatment, others surgical treatment. With type III gastric carcinoids, if >2 cm, excision and regional lymph node clearance is recommended. Most tumors <1 cm are treated endoscopically.

PANCREATIC ENDOCRINE TUMORS

Functional PETs usually present with symptoms due to hormone excess. Only late in the course of the disease does the tumor itself cause prominent symptoms such as abdominal pain. In contrast, all of the symptoms due to *nonfunctional* PETs are due to the tumor. Thus, some functional PETs may present with severe symptoms with a small or undetectable primary tumor, whereas nonfunctional tumors almost always present late in their course when they are large and often metastatic. The mean delay between onset of continuous symptoms and diagnosis of a functional PET syndrome is 4 to 7 years. Therefore, the diagnoses are frequently missed for extended periods of time.

Treatment of PETs requires two different strategies. Treatment must be directed at the hormone excess state, such as the gastric acid hypersecretion in gastrinomas or hypoglycemia in insulinomas. Ectopic hormone secretion usually causes the presenting symptoms and can cause life-threatening complications. Except for insulinomas, 50% are malignant (Table 93-2); therefore treatment must also be directed against the tumor per se. These tumors are frequently not curable by surgery due to the extent of disease. Individual PETs are discussed below.

GASTRINOMA (ZOLLINGER-ELLISON SYNDROME) (See also Chap. 285) A gastrinoma is a NET secreting gastrin, a hormone that causes gastric acid hypersecretion (Zollinger-Ellison syndrome). The chronic hypergastrinemia results in marked gastric acid hypersecretion and growth of the gastric mucosa, with increased numbers of parietal cells and proliferation of gastric ECL cells. The gastric acid hypersecretion characteristically causes peptic ulcer disease, often refractory and severe, as well as diarrhea. The most common presenting symptoms are abdominal pain (70 to 100%), diarrhea (37 to 73%), and gastroesophageal reflux disease (GERD) (30 to 35%) and 10 to 20% have diarrhea only. Although peptic ulcers may occur in unusual locations, most patients have a typical duodenal ulcer. The diagnosis of gastrinoma should be considered in patients with peptic ulcer disease with diarrhea; with peptic ulcers in an unusual or in multiple locations; and with peptic ulcer disease that is refractory to treatment or persistent, associated with prominent gastric folds, associated with findings suggestive of MEN-1 (hyperparathyroidism, family history of ulcer or endocrinopathy, pituitary tumors), or without *Helicobacter pylori* present. *H. pylori* is present in >90% of patients with idiopathic peptic ulcers but is present in <50% of patients with gastrinomas. Chronic unexplained diarrhea should also suggest gastrinoma.

About 20 to 25% of patients have MEN-1, and in most cases the hyperparathyroidism is present before the gastrinoma. These patients are treated differently from those without MEN-1; therefore, MEN-1 should be sought in all patients by family history and by measuring plasma calcium and plasma hormones (parathormone, growth hormone, prolactin).

Most gastrinomas (50 to 70%) are present in the duodenum, followed by the pancreas (20 to 40%) and other intraabdominal sites (mesentery, lymph nodes, biliary tract, liver, stomach, ovary). Gastrinomas may also occur in the left ventricular septum. In MEN-1 the gastrinomas are also usually in the duodenum (70 to 90%), followed by the pancreas (10 to 30%), and they are almost always multiple. Between 60 and 90% of gastrinomas are malignant (Table 93-2) with metastatic spread to lymph nodes and liver. Distant metastases to bone occur in 12 to 30% of patients with liver metastases.

Diagnosis   The diagnosis of gastrinoma requires the demonstration of fasting hypergastrinemia and an increased basal gastric acid output (BAO; hyperchlorhydria). More than 98% of patients with gastrinomas have fasting hypergastrinemia, although in 40 to 60% the level may be less than 10 times normal. Therefore, when the diagnosis is suspected, a fasting gastrin level should be determined first. Gastric acid–suppressant drugs such as proton pump inhibitors (omeprazole, pantoprazole, lansoprazole) can suppress acid secretion sufficiently to cause hypergastrinemia and need to be discontinued for a week before the gastrin determination. If the gastrin level is elevated, document that the gastric pH <2.5; hypergastrinemia secondary to achlorydria (atrophic gastritis, pernicious anemia) is one of the most common causes of hypergastrinemia. If the fasting gastrin is >1000 ng/L; 10 times normal) and the pH <2.5, which occurs in 40 to 60% of patients with gastrinoma, the diagnosis is established after ruling out the possibility of retained antrum syndrome by history. In patients with hypergastrinemia with fasting gastrins <1000 ng/L and gastric pH <2.5, other conditions such as *H. pylori* infections, antral G cell hyperplasia/hyperfunction, gastric outlet obstruction, or, rarely, renal failure can masquerade as a gastrinoma. To establish the diagnosis in this group, a determination of BAO and a secretin provocative test should be done. In >80% of patients with gastrinomas, BAO is elevated, i.e., 15 meq/h, and the secretin provocative test is positive, i.e., >200 ng/L increase in serum gastrin level.

℞ **TREATMENT**   The gastric acid hypersecretion in patients with gastrinomas can be controlled in almost every case by oral gastric antisecretory drugs. Because of their long duration of action and potency, the proton pump inhibitors (H^+,K^+-ATPase inhibitors) are the drugs of choice. Histamine H_2-receptor antagonists are also effective, although more frequent dosing (every 4 to 8 h) and high doses are frequently required. In patients with MEN-1 with hyperparathyroidism, correction of the hyperparathyroidism increases the sensitivity to gastric antisecretory drugs and decreases the basal acid output.

With the increased ability to control acid hypersecretion, >50% of the patients who are not cured (>60% of patients) will die from tumor-related causes. At presentation, careful imaging studies are essential to localize the extent of the tumor (see below). About one-third of patients present with hepatic metastases; in <15% of those with hepatic metastases, the disease is limited so that surgical resection may be possible. Surgical cure is possible in 30% of all patients without MEN-1 or liver metastases (40% of all patients). In patients with MEN-1, long-term surgical cure is rare because the tumors are multiple, frequently with lymph node metastases. Therefore, all patients with gastrinomas without MEN-1 or a medical condition limiting life expectancy should undergo surgery.

INSULINOMAS   Insulinomas are endocrine tumors of the pancreas thought to be derived from β cells that autonomously secrete insulin, which results in hypoglycemia. The average age of occurrence is in persons 40 to 50 years old. The most common clinical symptoms are due to the effect of the hypoglycemia on the central nervous system (neuroglycemic symptoms) and include confusion, headache, disorientation, visual difficulties, irrational behavior, or even coma (Chap. 334). Also, most patients have symptoms due to excess catecholamine release secondary to the hypoglycemia, including sweating, tremor, and palpitations. Characteristically these attacks are associated with fasting.

Insulinomas are generally small (>90% are <2 cm in diameter), usually solitary (90%), and only 5 to 15% are malignant. They almost invariably occur only in the pancreas, distributed equally in the pancreatic head, body and tail. Insulinomas should be suspected in all patients with hypoglycemia, especially with a history suggesting attacks provoked by fasting or with a family history of MEN-1. Insulin is synthesized as proinsulin, which consists of a 21-amino-acid α chain and a 30-amino-acid β chain connected by a 33-amino-acid connecting peptide (C peptide). In insulinomas, in addition to elevated plasma insulin levels, elevated plasma proinsulin levels are found and C-peptide levels can be elevated.

Diagnosis   The diagnosis of insulinoma requires the demonstration of an elevated plasma insulin level at the time of hypoglycemia. Other causes of fasting hypoglycemia include inadvertent or surreptitious use of insulin or oral hypoglycemic agents, severe liver disease, alcoholism, poor nutrition, or other extrapancreatic tumors. The most reliable test for diagnosing insulinoma is a fast up to 72 h with serum glucose, C-peptide, and insulin measurements every 4 to 8 h. If at any point the patient becomes symptomatic or glucose levels are persistently <2.2 mmol/L (40 mg/dL), the test should be terminated and repeat samples for the above studies obtained before glucose is given. Some 70 to 80% of patients will develop hypoglycemia during the first 24 h and 98% by 48 h. In nonobese normal subjects, serum insulin levels should decrease to >43 pmol/L (6 μU/mL) when blood glucose decreases to ≤2.2 mmol/L (40 mg/dL) and the ratio of insulin to glucose is <0.3 (in mg/dL). In addition to having an insulin level >6 μU/ml when blood glucose is ≤40 mg/dL, some investigators also require elevated C-peptide and serum proinsulin levels and/or insulin: glucose ratio >0.3 for the diagnosis of insulinoma. The effects of surreptitious use of insulin or hypoglycemic agents may be difficult to distinguish from the symptoms of insulinomas. The combination of proinsulin levels (normal in exogenous insulin/hypoglycemic agent users), C-peptide levels (low in exogenous insulin users), antibodies to insulin (positive in exogenous insulin users), and sulfonylurea levels in serum or plasma will allow the correct diagnosis to be made.

℞ **TREATMENT**   Only 5 to 15% of insulinomas are malignant; therefore, after appropriate imaging, surgery should be performed. Between 75 and 95% of patients are cured by surgery. Before surgery the hypoglycemia can be controlled by frequent small meals and the use of diazoxide (150 to 800 mg/d). Diazoxide is a benozthiadiazide whose hyperglycemic effect is attributed to inhibition of insulin release; 50 to 60% of patients respond to diazoxide. Its side effects are sodium retention and GI symptoms such as nausea. Other agents effective in some patients to control the hypoglycemia include verapamil and diphenylhydantoin. Long-acting somatostatin analogues such as octreotide are acutely effective in 40% of patients. However, octreotide needs to be used with care because it inhibits growth hormone secretion and can lower plasma glucagon levels and so worsen the hypoglycemia.

For the 5 to 15% of patients with malignant insulinomas, the above drugs or somatostatin analogues are used initially. If they are not effective, hepatic arterial embolization, chemoembolization, or chemotherapy have been used. These will be discussed below.

GLUCAGONOMAS Glucagonomas are endocrine tumors of the pancreas that secrete excessive amounts of glucagon that causes a distinct syndrome characterized by dermatitis, glucose intolerance or diabetes, and weight loss. Glucagonomas mainly occur in persons between 45 and 70 years old. They are heralded clinically by a characteristic dermatitis (migratory necrolytic erythema; in 67 to 90%), accompanied by glucose intolerance (40 to 90%), weight loss (66 to 96%), anemia (33 to 85%), diarrhea (15 to 29%), and thromboembolism (11 to 24%). The characteristic rash usually starts as an annular erythema at intertriginous and periorificial sites, especially in the groin or buttock. It subsequently becomes raised and bullae form; when the bullae rupture, eroded areas form. The lesions can wax and wane. A characteristic laboratory finding is hypoaminoacidemia, which occurs in 26 to 100% of patients.

Glucagonomas are generally large tumors at diagnosis, with an average size of 5 to 10 cm. Between 50 and 80% occur in the pancreatic tail and 50 to 82% have evidence of metastatic spread at presentation, usually to the liver. Glucagonomas are rarely extrapancreatic and usually occur singly.

Diagnosis The diagnosis is confirmed by demonstrating an increased plasma glucagon level [normal is <150 ng/L]. In one study plasma glucagon levels were >1000 ng/L in 90%, between 500 and 1000 ng/L in 7%, and <500 ng/L in 3%. A plasma glucagon level >1000 ng/L is considered diagnostic. Other diseases causing increased plasma glucagon levels include renal failure, acute pancreatitis, hypercortisolism, hepatic failure, prolonged fasting, or familial hyperglucagonemia. Except for cirrhosis, these disorders do not usually increase plasma glucagon to >500 ng/L.

℞ **TREATMENT** Metastases are present at presentation in 50 to 80% of patients, so curative surgical resection is not possible. Surgical debulking in patients with advanced disease or other antitumor treatments may be beneficial (see below). Long-acting somatostatin analogues (octreotide, lanreotide) improve the skin rash in 75% of patients and may improve the weight loss, pain, and diarrhea but not the glucose intolerance.

SOMATOSTATINOMA SYNDROME Somatostatinomas are endocrine tumors that secrete excessive amounts of somatostatin, which causes a syndrome characterized by diabetes melitus, gallbladder disease, diarrhea, and steatorrhea. The mean age of onset is 51 years. Somatostatinomas occur primarily in the pancreas and small intestine, and the frequency of the symptoms differs in each. The usual symptoms are more frequent in pancreatic than intestinal somatostatinomas: diabetes mellitus (95% vs. 21%), gallbladder disease (94% vs. 43%), diarrhea (92% vs. 38%), steatorrhea (83% vs. 12%), hypochlorhydria (86% vs. 12%), and weight loss (90% vs. 69%). Somatostatinomas occur in the pancreas in 56 to 74% of cases, with the primary location being in the pancreatic head. The tumors are usually solitary (90%) and large (mean diameter, 4.5 cm). Liver metastases are present in 69 to 84% of patients.

Somatostatin is a tetradecapeptide (Fig. 93-2), widely distributed in the central nervous system and gastrointestinal tract where it functions as a neurotransmitter or has paracrine and autocrine actions. It is a potent inhibitor of many processes, including release of almost all hormones, acid secretion, intestinal and pancreatic secretion, and intestinal absorption. Most of the clinical manifestations are directly related to these inhibitory actions.

Diagnosis In most cases somatostatinomas have been found incidentally either at the time of cholecystectomy or during endoscopy. The presence of psammoma bodies in a duodenal tumor should particularly raise suspicion. Duodenal somatostatin-containing tumors are increasingly associated with von Recklinghausen's disease. Most of these do not cause the somatostatinoma syndrome as patients are usually asymptomatic and have normal plasma somatostatin levels. The diagnosis of somatostatinoma requires elevated plasma somatostatin levels.

℞ **TREATMENT** Pancreatic tumors are frequently metastatic at presentation (70 to 92%), whereas 30 to 69% of small-intestinal somatostatinomas have metastases. Symptoms are improved by octreotide treatment (Fig. 93-2).

VIPOMAS VIPomas are endocrine tumors that secrete excessive amounts of VIP, which causes a distinct syndrome characterized by large-volume diarrhea, hypokalemia, and dehydration. This syndrome is also called Verner-Morrison syndrome, pancreatic cholera, or WDHA syndrome (watery *d*iarrhea, *h*ypokalemia, and *a*chlorhydria), which some patients develop. The mean age of patients is 49 years; however, the syndrome can occur in children; when it does, it is usually caused by a ganglioneuroma or ganglioneuroblastoma.

The principal symptoms are large-volume diarrhea (in 100%) severe enough to cause hypokalemia (80 to 100%), dehydration (83%), hypochlorhydria (54 to 76%), and flushing (20%). The diarrhea is secretory in nature, persists during fasting, and is almost always >1 L per day and >3 L per day in 70%. Most patients do not have accompanying steatorrhea (16%), and the increased stool volume is due to increased excretion of sodium and potassium, which, with the anions, accounts for the osmolality of the stool. Patients frequently have hyperglycemia (25 to 50%) and hypercalcemia (25 to 50%).

VIP is a 28-amino-acid peptide neurotransmitter, ubiquitously present in the central nervous system and GI tract. Its known actions include stimulation of small-intestinal chloride secretion as well as effects on smooth-muscle contractility, inhibition of acid secretion, and vasodilatory effects which explain most features of the clinical syndrome.

In adults 80 to 90% of VIPomas are pancreatic; VIP-secreting pheochromocytomas, intestinal carcinoids, and occasional ganglioneuromas account for the rest. These tumors are usually single; 50 to 75% are in the pancreatic tail and 37 to 68% have hepatic metastases at diagnosis.

Diagnosis The diagnosis requires the demonstration of an elevated plasma VIP level and the presence of large-volume diarrhea. A stool volume of <700 mL/day excludes the diagnosis of VIPoma. A number of causes of diarrhea can be excluded by fasting the patient. Other diseases that can cause secretory large-volume diarrhea include gastrinomas, chronic laxative abuse, carcinoid syndrome, systemic mastocytosis, diabetic diarrhea, AIDS, and rarely medullary thyroid cancer. Of these conditions, only VIPomas causes a marked increase in plasma VIP.

℞ **TREATMENT** The most important initial treatment in these patients is to correct their dehydration, hypokalemia, and electrolyte losses with fluid and electrolyte replacement. Patients may require 5 L/day of fluid and >350 mmol/day (350 meq/day) of potassium. Because 37 to 68% of adults with VIPomas have metastatic disease in the liver at presentation, a significant number of patients cannot be cured surgically. In these patients, long-acting somatostatin analogues such as octreotide or lanreotide (Fig. 93-2) are the drugs of choice.

Octreotide will control the diarrhea in 87% of patients. In nonresponsive patients, the combination of glucocorticoids and octreotide has proved helpful in a few. Other drugs that may be helpful include prednisone (60 to 100 mg/d), clonidine, indomethacin, phenothiazines, loperamide, lidamidine, lithium, proparanolol, and metoclopramide. Treatment of advanced disease with embolization, chemoembolization, and chemotherapy may also be helpful (see below).

NONFUNCTIONAL PANCREATIC ENDOCRINE TUMORS Nonfunctional PETs are endocrine tumors that originate in the pancreas and either secrete no products or their secreted products do not cause a specific clinical syndrome. The symptoms are due entirely to the tumor per se. Nonfunctional PETs almost always secrete chromogranin A (90 to 100%), chromogranin B (90 to 100%), PP (58%), α-human chorionic gonadotropin (hCG) (40%), and β-HCG (20%), but none cause a specific syndrome. Patients with nonfunctional PETs usually present late in their disease course with invasive tumors and hepatic metastases (in 64 to 92%), and the tumors are usually large (72% >5 cm). These tumors are usually solitary except in patients with MEN-1, where they are multiple; they occur primarily in the pancreatic head; and though they do not cause a functional syndrome, they synthesize numerous peptides and cannot be distinguished from functional tumors by immunocytomchemistry.

The most common symptoms are abdominal pain (30 to 80%), jaundice (20 to 35%), and weight loss, fatigue, or bleeding; 10 to 15% are found incidentally. The average time from the beginning of symptoms to diagnosis is 5 years.

Diagnosis The diagnosis is established by histology in a patient with a PET without either clinical symptoms or elevated plasma hormone levels of one of the established syndromes (Table 93-2). Even though chromogranin A levels are elevated in almost every patient, this can be found in functional PETs, carcinoids, and other neuroendocrine disorders. Plasma PP is increased in 22 to 71% of patients and should suggest the diagnosis in a patient with a pancreatic mass because it is usually normal in patients with pancreatic adenocarcinomas. However, elevated plasma PP is not diagnostic of this tumor because it is elevated in a number of other conditions such as chronic renal failure, old age, inflammatory conditions, and diabetes.

℞ **TREATMENT** Unfortunately, surgical curative resection can be considered in only a minority of patients because 64 to 92% present with metastatic disease. Treatment needs to be directed against the tumor itself using chemotherapy, embolization, chemoembolization, or hormonal therapy (see below).

GRFOMAS GRFomas are endocrine tumors that secrete excessive amounts of GRF that causes acromegaly. The frequency is not known. GRF (also called growth hormone–releasing hormone, GHRH) is a 44-amino-acid peptide, and 25 to 44% of PETs have GRF immunoreactivity, although excess secretion is uncommon. GRFomas are lung tumors in 47 to 54% of cases, PETs in 29 to 30%, and small-intestinal carcinoids in 8 to 10% and up to 12% occur at other sites. Patients have a mean age of 38 years, and the symptoms are usually due to either acromegaly or the tumor per se. The acromegaly caused by GRFomas is indistinguishable from classic acromegaly. The pituitary abnormality is growth hormone–secreting somatotrope cell hyperplasia rather than a pituitary adenoma. The pancreatic tumors are usually large (>6 cm), and liver metastases are present in 39%. They should be suspected in any patient with acromegaly and an abdominal tumor, in a patient with MEN-1 with acromegaly, or in a patient without a pituitary adenoma with acromegaly or associated with hyperprolactinemia, which occurs in 70% of GRFomas. GRFomas are an uncommon cause of acromegaly. The diagnosis is established by performing plasma assays for GRF and growth hormone. The normal level for GRF is <5 ng/L (5 pg/mL) in men and <10 ng/L (10 pg/mL) in women. Most GRFomas have a plasma GRF level ≥300 ng/L (300 pg/mL). Patients with GRFomas also have increased plasma insulin-like growth factor 1 levels similar to those in classic acromegaly. Surgery is the treatment of choice if diffuse metastases are not present. Long-acting somatostatin analogues such as octreotide or lanreotide (Fig. 93-2) induce responses in 75 to 100% of patients.

OTHER RARE PET SYNDROMES Cushing's syndrome (ACTHoma) due to a PET occurs in 4 to 16% of all patients with ectopic Cushing's syndrome. It occurs in 5% of cases of sporadic gastrinomas, almost invariably in patients with hepatic metastases, and is an independent, poor prognostic factor. Paraneoplastic hypercalcemia due to PETs releasing parathyroid hormone–related peptide is rare. The tumors are usually large, and liver metastases are usually present. PETs secreting calcitonin may cause a specific clinical syndrome. In one study, half the patients had diarrhea, which disappeared with resection of the tumor. In Table 93-2, this is a possible specific disorder because so few cases have been described.

TUMOR LOCALIZATION

Localization of the primary tumor and defining the extent of the disease are essential to the proper management of all carcinoids and PETs. Numerous tumor localization methods are used in both types of NETs, including conventional imaging studies [CT scanning, magnetic resonance imaging (MRI), transabdominal ultrasound, selective angiography] and somatostatin receptor scintigraphy (SRS). In PETs, endoscopic ultrasound (EUS) and functional localization by measuring venous hormonal gradients are also reported useful. Bronchial carcinoids are usually detected by a standard chest radiography and assessed by CT. Rectal, duodenal, colonic, and gastric carcinoids are usually detected by GI endoscopy.

PETs as well as carcinoid tumors possess high-affinity somatostatin receptors in both their primary tumors and their metastases. Of the five types of somatostatin receptors (sst_{1-5}), radiolabeled octreotide binds with high affinity to sst_2, lower for sst_3 and sst_5, and has very low affinity for sst_1 and sst_4. Between 90 and 100% of carcinoid tumors and PETs express sst_2, and many also have the other four sst subtypes. Interaction with these receptors can be used to localize NETs using [^{111}In-DTPA-D-Phe^1] octreotide (Fig. 93-2) and radionuclide scanning (SRS) as well as for treatment of the hormone excess state with octreotide or lanreotide. Because of its greater sensitivity than conventional imaging and its ability to localize tumor throughout the body at one time, SRS is now the imaging modality of choice for localizing both primary and metastatic NET tumors. SRS localizes tumors in 73 to 89% of patients with carcinoids and in 56 to 100% of patients with PETs, except for insulinomas. Insulinomas are usually small and have low densities of sst receptors, which results in SRS being positive in only 12 to 50% of patients with insulinomas. Figure 93-3 shows an example of the increased sensitivity of SRS in a patient with a gastrinoma. The CT scan (Fig. 93-3, *top*) did not show any disease after primary tumor resection; however, hypergastrinemia remained, and the SRS demonstrated a metastasis in the liver (Fig. 93-3, *bottom*). Occasional false-positive responses with SRS can occur (12% in one study) because numerous other normal and abnormal cells can have high densities of sst receptors including granulomas (sarcoid, tuberculosis, etc.), thyroid diseases (goiter, thyroiditis), and activated lymphocytes (lymphomas, wound infections). For PETs located in the pancreas, EUS is highly sensitive, localizing 77 to 93% of insulinomas, which occur almost exclusively within the pancreas. EUS is less sensitive for extrapancreatic tumors. If liver metastases are identified by SRS, a CT scan or MRI is then recommended to assess the size and exact location of the metastases, because SRS does not provide reliable information on tumor size. Functional localization measuring hormone gradients after intraarterial calcium injections in insulinomas (insulin) or gastrin gradients after secretin injections in gastrinoma will be positive in 80 to 100% of patients. However, this method gives only regional localization and therefore is reserved for cases where other imaging tests are negative.

℞ **TREATMENT** Advanced Disease (Diffuse Metastatic Disease) The single most important prognostic factor for survival is the presence of liver metastases (Fig. 93-4). For patients with carcinoids without hepatic metastases, the 5-year survival is 80%; with limited liver metastases, it is also 80%; but with diffuse metastases, it is 50% (Fig. 93-4, *bottom*). With gastrinomas, the 5-year survival without liver metastases is 98%; with limited metastases in one hepatic lobe it is 78%; and with diffuse metastases, 16% (Fig. 93-4, *top*). A number of different modalities are effective, including cytoreductive surgery (removal of all visible tumor), treatment with chemotherapy,

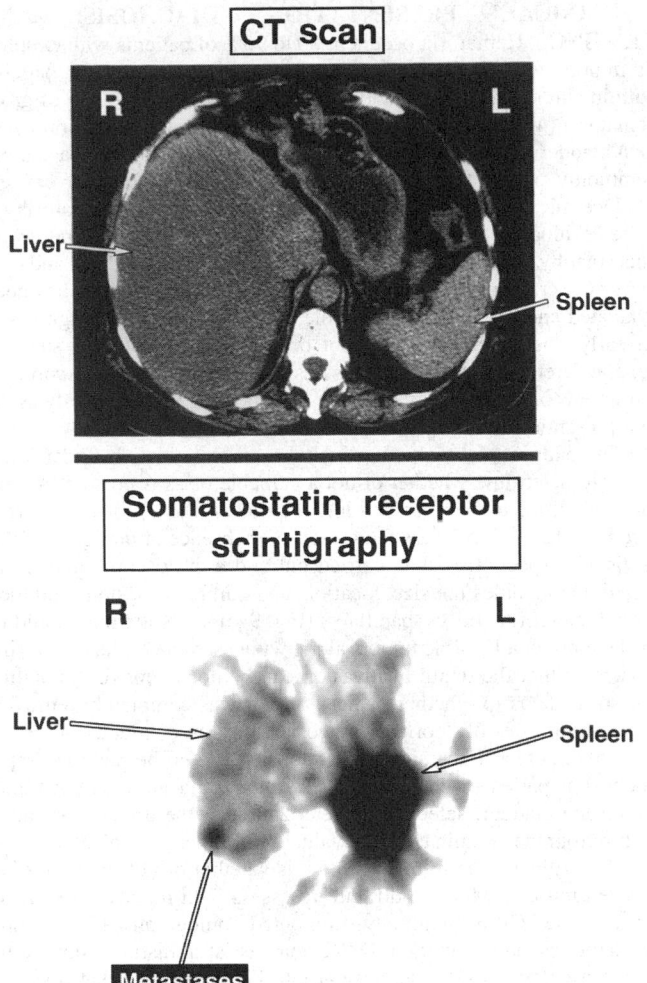

FIGURE 93-3 Ability of computed tomography (CT) (*top*) or somatostatin receptor scintigraphy (*bottom*) to localize metastatic gastrinoma in the liver in a patient with Zollinger-Ellison syndrome.

somatostatin analogues, interferon α, hepatic embolization alone or with chemotherapy (chemoembolization), radiotherapy, and liver transplantation.

Specific Antitumor Treatments Cytoreductive surgery is only possible in the 9 to 22% of patients who have limited hepatic metastases. No randomized studies have proven it extends life, but it appears to increase survival and therefore is recommended if possible.

Chemotherapy for metastatic carcinoid tumors has been disappointing, with response rates of 0 to 40% with various two- or three-drug combinations. Chemotherapy for PETs has been more successful, with tumor shrinkage reported in 30 to 70% of patients. The current regimen of choice is streptozotocin and doxorubicin.

Long-acting somatostatin analogues (octreotide, lanreotide) and interferon α rarely decrease tumor size (i.e., 0 to 17%); however, these drugs have tumoristatic effects, stopping additional growth in 50 to 95% of patients with NETs. How long tumor stabilization lasts or whether it prolongs survival has not been established.

Hepatic embolization and chemoembolization (with dacarbazine, cisplatin, doxorubicin, 5-fluorouracil, or streptozotocin) decrease tumor bulk and help control the symptoms of hormone excess. These modalities are generally reserved for patients in whom treatment with somatostatin analogues, interferon (carcinoids), or chemotherapy (PETs) fails.

Radiotherapy is being used with two different somatostatin radionuclides coupled by a DOTA-chelating group to octreotide (Fig. 93-2): [^{111}In-DTPA-D-Phe^{1}] octreotide (emits γ rays, internal conversion,

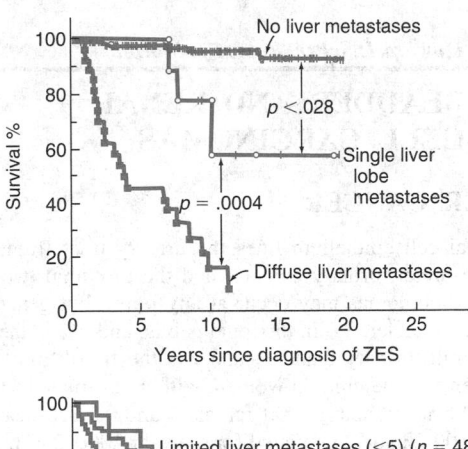

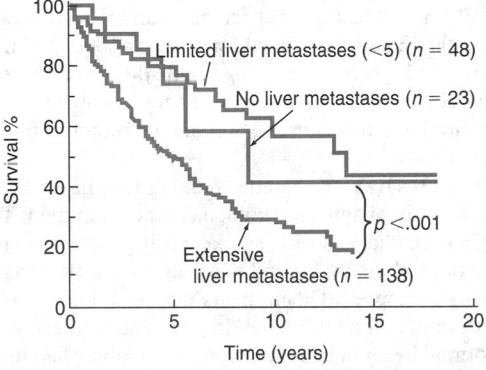

FIGURE 93-4 Effect of the presence and extent of liver metastases on survival in patients with gastrinomas (*top*) or carcinoid tumors (*bottom*). *(Top panel is drawn from data from 199 patients with gastrinomas, modified from F Yu et al: J Clin Oncol 17:615, 1999. Bottom panel is drawn from data from 209 patients with carcinoid tumors from ET Janson et al: Ann Oncol 8:685, 1997.)*

and Auger electrons) and yttrium-90 (emits high energy β particles). The ^{111}In compound showed disease stabilization in 40% and a decrease in tumor size in 30% of patients with advanced metastatic disease.

The use of liver transplantation has been abandoned for treatment of most metastatic tumors to the liver. However, for metastatic NETs it is still a consideration. Liver transplantation in 103 cases of malignant NETs (48 were PETs, 43 were carcinoids) achieved 2- and 5-year survival rates of 60% and 47%, respectively. However, recurrence-free survival was low (<24%). Liver transplantation may be justified for younger patients with metastatic NETs limited to the liver.

BIBLIOGRAPHY

CARCINOID TUMORS AND SYNDROME

CAPLIN ME et al: Carcinoid tumour. Lancet 352:799, 1998

JENSEN RT, NORTON JA: Carcinoid tumors and the carcinoid syndrome, *Cancer: Principles and Practice of Oncology*, VT DeVita Jr, S Hellman, SA Rosenberg (eds). Philadelphia, Lippincott-Raven, 1997, pp 1704–1723

KULKE MH, MAYER RJ: Carcinoid tumors. N Engl J Med 340:858, 1999

MODLIN IM, SANDOR A: An analysis of 8305 cases of carcinoid tumors. Cancer 79:813, 1997

PANCREATIC ENDOCRINE TUMORS

FRAKER DL, JENSEN RT: Pancreatic endocrine tumors, in *Cancer: Principles and Practice of Oncology*, VT DeVita Jr, S Hellman, SA Rosenberg (eds). Philadelphia, Lippincott-Raven, 1997, pp 1678–1704

JENSEN RT, NORTON JA: Endocrine neoplasma of the pancreas, in *Textbook of Gastroenterology*, 3d ed, T Yamada et al (eds). Philadelphia, Lippincott Williams & Wilkins, 1999, pp 2193–2228

MIGNON M, JENSEN RT (eds): *Endocrine Tumors of the Pancreas: Recent Advances in Research and Management.* Basel, Karger, 1995

O'SHEA D, BLOOM SR (Guest Eds): Gastrointestinal Endocrine Tumours. Bailliere's Clin Gastroenterol 10:555, 1996

Howard I. Scher, Robert J. Motzer

BLADDER AND RENAL CELL CARCINOMAS

BLADDER CANCER

A transitional cell epithelium lines the urinary tract from the renal pelvis to the ureter, urinary bladder, and the proximal two-thirds of the urethra. Carcinomas may occur at any point, but generally 90% develop in the bladder, 8% in the renal pelvis, and 2% in the ureter or urethra. Overall, urinary bladder cancer is the fourth most common cancer in men and the ninth in women, with an estimated 53,200 new cases (38,300 males and 14,900 females) and 12,200 deaths (8100 males and 4100 females) predicted for the year 2000. The median age at diagnosis is 65 years. Once diagnosed, these tumors exhibit the tendency to recur over time and in new locations in the urothelial tract. As long as urothelium is present, continuous monitoring of the urothelial tract is required.

EPIDEMIOLOGY   Cigarette smoking is believed to contribute to up to 50% of the diagnosed urothelial cancers in men. The risk of developing a urothelial cancer in smokers is increased two- to fourfold relative to nonsmoking males and may persist for 10 years or longer after smoking is stopped. Other agents that have been implicated include exposure to aniline dyes, the drugs phenacetin and chlornaphazin, and external beam radiation. Chronic cyclophosphamide exposure increases risk nine-fold. Diets rich in meat and fat predispose to bladder cancer; ingestion of vitamin A supplements appears to be protective. Exposure to *Schistosoma haematobium*, a parasite found in many developing countries, is associated with an increase in both squamous (70%) and transitional cell (30%) carcinomas of the bladder.

PATHOLOGY   In the United States, 90 to 95% of bladder tumors diagnosed are transitional cell tumors. Pure squamous tumors with keratinization comprise 3%, adenocarcinomas 2%, and small cell tumors (with paraneoplastic syndromes) <1%. Adenocarcinomas develop primarily in the urachal remnant in the dome of the bladder or in the periurethral tissues. Some assume a signet cell histology. Lymphomas or melanomas are rare. Overall, 75% of tumors present as superficial lesions, 20% with muscle invasion, and 5% with metastatic disease. Of the transitional cell tumors, low-grade papillary lesions that grow on a central stalk are most common. They are very friable, have a tendency to bleed, and are at a high risk for recurrence, yet they rarely progress to the more lethal invasive variety. In contrast, carcinoma in situ (CIS) is a high-grade tumor that is considered a precursor of the more lethal muscle-infiltrating cancers. Tumors are rated by histologic type and grade. Grade I lesions (highly differentiated tumors) rarely progress to a higher stage, while grade III tumors usually do.

PATHOGENESIS   The multicentric nature of the disease and high rate of recurrence has led to the hypothesis that a field defect develops in the urothelium. Molecular genetic analyses of bladder tumors representing defined stages and different grades have shown a series of *primary chromosomal aberrations* associated with cancer *development*, and *secondary changes* associated with *progression* to a more advanced stage. Using paired bladder tumor and normal tissues from the same patient, 9q deletions are an early event in cancer development, while 3p and 5q deletions were more prevalent in invasive vs. superficial tumors. Deletions of 17p (*TP53* locus), 18q (the *DCC* gene locus), and the *RB* gene locus on chromosome 13q24 were seen only in invasive disease, while deletions of 3p and 11p occur in both superficial and invasive tumors. p53 overexpression correlates with a higher probability of progression to a more advanced stage and bladder cancer mortality for patients with Ta, Tis, T1 and muscle-infiltrating lesions. These factors have not been routinely used for clinical decision-making.

CLINICAL PRESENTATION, DIAGNOSIS, AND STAGING   Hematuria occurs in 80 to 90% of patients with exophytic tumors, while irritative symptoms are more common for patients with in situ disease. The bladder is the most common source of gross hematuria (40%), but benign cystitis (22%) is a more common cause than bladder cancer (15%) (Chap. 48). Microscopic hematuria is more commonly of prostatic origin (25%), while 2% of bladder cancers produce microscopic hematuria. The documentation of hematuria requires evaluation with a urinary cytology, visualization of the urothelial tract by sonography or an intravenous pyelogram (IVP), and cystoscopy. Screening of asymptomatic subjects for hematuria has been evaluated and shown to increase the frequency of tumor diagnosis at an early stage. Screening has not been shown to confer a survival benefit. Ureteral obstruction may result in flank pain or discomfort. Symptoms of metastatic disease are documented less commonly as the first presenting sign of a urothelial cancer.

The endoscopic evaluation includes an examination under anesthesia to determine whether or not a palpable mass is present. A flexible endoscope is then inserted into the bladder, and a bladder barbotage is performed to assess the presence or absence of malignant cells. A visual inspection is then carried out and a cystoscopic map completed that includes the size, location, and number of lesions and their growth pattern (solid vs. papillary) (Fig. 94-1). An attempt should be made to resect all visible tumors along with a sample of the underlying muscle so that the depth of invasion can be documented. A notation is also made as to whether or not a tumor was completely removed. Random biopsies of "normal" mucosal areas are conducted to assess for a field defect. Each site that is biopsied should be recorded separately. For patients with a positive cytology and no apparent tumor within the bladder, selective catheterization of the ureter is required with retrograde examination to evaluate for upper tract disease.

The critical issue in management is whether or not the tumor has invaded muscle, which is difficult to assess with noninvasive procedures alone. Ultrasonography, computed tomography (CT) and/or magnetic resonance imaging (MRI) may assist in distinguishing a tumor that extends to the perivesical fat (T3b) from one that does not (T3a), and to document whether or not regional lymph nodes are involved (N+). They are also important in the assessment of the upper tracts. Distal metastases are assessed by CT of the abdomen, pulmonary x-rays, or radonculide imaging of the skeleton. The need for these studies is based in part on the local extent of the lesion.

The revised 1997 TNM (tumor, nodes, metastasis) staging system is illustrated in Fig. 94-2. Ta lesions grow as exophytic lesions, while CIS starts on the surface and tends to invade muscle. As the degree of muscle infiltration increases, the probability of nodal and subsequent distal spread also increases.

R_x TREATMENT   Treatments are based on the extent and depth of invasion of the tumor within the primary site and the presence or probability of metastatic spread. At a minimum, the management of a tumor that has not invaded the bladder wall is a complete endoscopic resection with or without intravesical therapy. Recurrences are seen in 50% or more of cases, of which 5 to 20% will progress to a more advanced stage. The decision to recommend additional therapy is based on the histologic subtype, the number of lesions, the depth of invasion, and whether or not CIS is present. Solitary papillary lesions are generally treated by surgery alone. Intravesical therapy is usually recommended for recurrent disease.

CIS frequently follows a more aggressive course. As such, intravesical therapy is generally recommended earlier in the clinical course. The standard treatment for a tumor that has invaded muscle, either at the time of diagnosis or following treatment for superficial disease, is radical cystectomy. Depending on the findings at surgery, systemic chemotherapy may or may not be advised.

Superficial Disease   Intravesical therapies are applied in two contexts: as an adjuvant to a complete endoscopic resection to prevent recurrence, or, less commonly, to eliminate disease that cannot be controlled by endoscopic resection alone. Intravesical treatments are advised for patients with four or more recurrences in a given year,

>40% involvement of the bladder surface by tumor, the presence of diffuse CIS, or documented T1 disease. A number of agents are available, but based on randomized comparisons, Bacillus Calmette-Guerin (BCG) is considered standard. Thiotepa, doxorubicin, mitomycin-C, and interferon have also been used. Side effects include dysuria, frequency, and, depending on the drug, myelosuppression or a contact dermatitis (from mitomycin C). Rarely, intravesical BCG may produce a systemic illness associated with granulomatous infections in multiple sites that requires anti-tuberculin therapy for control. Significant BCG toxicities occur in <6% of patients.

Following endoscopic resection, patients are reevaluated at 3-month intervals to ensure that no recurrences have developed. Those with persistent disease or new tumors are generally

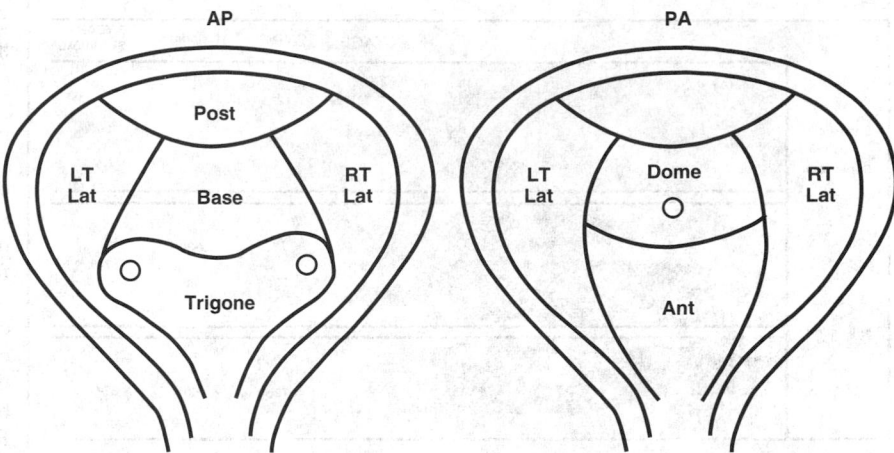

FIGURE 94-1 Bladder cancer map.

considered for a second course of BCG or intravesical chemotherapy. Those with persistent disease may be considered for cystectomy, although the specific indications vary. Obvious candidates are those with new invasive tumors or persistent CIS, and those with bladder function that has been compromised to the point where persistent pain, blood loss, frequency, or a severely limited bladder capacity is present. Recurrences may develop anywhere along the urothelial tract, including the renal pelvis, ureter, or urethra. In fact, one consequence of the "successful" treatment of tumors in the bladder is an increase in the frequency of extravesical recurrences.

Muscle-Infiltrating Disease The treatment of a tumor that has invaded muscle can be separated into control of the primary tumor and control of systemic disease. Radical cystectomy is considered the standard treatment, although in selected cases bladder-sparing approaches using an aggressive endoscopic resection, partial cystectomy, or a combined modality approach with resection, systemic chemotherapy, and external beam radiation therapy are used. The latter should not be considered outside of a research setting.

Radical cystectomy involves an evaluation of the pelvic lymph nodes, removal of the primary tumor, and creation of a conduit or reservoir for urinary flow. At the time of surgery, grossly abnormal lymph nodes are evaluated by frozen section. If metastases are confirmed, the procedure is often aborted unless a diversion is required for palliation of local symptoms. The results of treatment of node-positive disease are shown in Table 94-1. In males radical cystectomy involves the removal of the bladder, prostate, seminal vesicles, proximal vas deferens, and proximal urethra, with a margin of adipose tissue and peritoneum. Impotence is universal unless the *nervi erigentes*, responsible for erectile capacity, can be preserved. In females the procedure includes removal of the bladder, urethra, uterus, fallopian tubes, ovaries, anterior vaginal wall, and surrounding fascia.

Urine flow is directed through either an internal reservoir that drains to the urethra or the abdominal wall, or via a Bricker procedure in which urine flows through an ileal conduit from the ureters to the abdominal wall, where it is collected in an external appliance without an internal reservoir. A segment of colon, jejunum, or ileum can be used to bridge the gap between the ureters and the skin. Use of absorbable sutures may prevent formation of calculi at the sutures. A uretero-ileal conduit probably is the most widely used. A syndrome characterized by hypochloremic acidosis, hyperkalemia, hyponatremia, and uremia has been described when a segment of jejunum is utilized. Concurrent diseases in the bowel, such as ulcerative colitis or Crohn's disease, may hinder the use of resected bowel.

Alternatives to an external appliance include internal reservoirs that are created from detubularized bowel segments and are periodically self-catheterized by the patient. A number of procedures have been described that use either ileocecal or ileal reservoirs, which are anastamosed to either the abdominal wall or the urethra. When an anastomosis to the urethra is created, primarily in men with no urethral disease, the patient can then void in a manner that is similar to natural

voiding. Several indications for urethrectomy (including CIS or exophytic tumor in the urethra and diffuse CIS in the urinary bladder) preclude the creation of a urethral anastomosis. Continent reservoirs are being applied with increasing frequency, but are still not constructed for the majority of patients, for technical or disease-related reasons. Intercurrent diseases, impaired renal function, hesitancy to prolong the surgical trauma, dilated ureters, and bowel diseases all decrease the use of continent reservoirs. Patients with ureterosigmoid diversion require periodic colonoscopy because of the risk of cancer.

Cystectomy is major surgery, and appropriate medical clearance is essential. This includes optimizing cardiac medications and nutritional status. In approximately 5 to 10% of cases, depending on the location of the tumor, a partial cystectomy is possible. This procedure can be considered when a lesion develops on the dome of the bladder where a 2-cm margin can be achieved, CIS is absent in other sites of the bladder, and bladder capacity is adequate after the tumor is removed. Carcinomas in the ureter or in the renal pelvis are treated by nephroureterectomy with a bladder cuff.

Indications for cystectomy include: (1) muscle-invading tumors not suitable for segmental resection; (2) low-stage tumors unsuitable for conservative management due to, for example, multicentric and frequent recurrences resistant to intravesical instillations; (3) high grade tumors (T1G3) associated with CIS or bladder symptoms such as frequency or hemorrhage rendering the patient a "bladder cripple." Outcomes are reported on the basis of 5-year survivals. As shown in Table 94-2, survival varies inversely with depth of invasion and lymph node status. For the majority of cases, however, extension to a single lymph node predicts a poor outcome with a median time to recurrence of 22 months. In some countries external beam radiation therapy is considered standard. This is not the case in the United States, where its role is limited to those patients deemed unfit for cystectomy or those with unresectable local disease, and as part of an experimental approach that seeks to spare the bladder.

Metastatic Disease Patients with metastatic disease include those whose tumor has recurred after definitive local treatment and those who present with metastases. A number of chemotherapeutic agents have shown activity as single agents, of which cisplatin, paclitaxel, and gemcitabine are considered most active (Table 94-3). Responses to single agents are generally incomplete and not durable. Using multidrug regimens, response rates in excess of 50% have been reported with combinations such as M-VAC (methotrexate, vinblastine, doxorubicin, and cisplatin), PT (cisplatin and paclitaxel), and gemcitabine variants. Based on randomized comparisons, M-VAC is considered standard but can be associated with significant toxicities, including neutropenia and fever; mucositis in 10 to 20%; a decrease in renal and auditory function; and a peripheral neuropathy. Alopecia is universal; fatigue can be dose-limiting in some cases. More recently 2- and 3-drug combinations based on cisplatin/carboplatin, paclitaxel, and gemcitabine have been explored. In a direct comparison to M-VAC, gemcitabine/cisplatin showed similar response proportions and

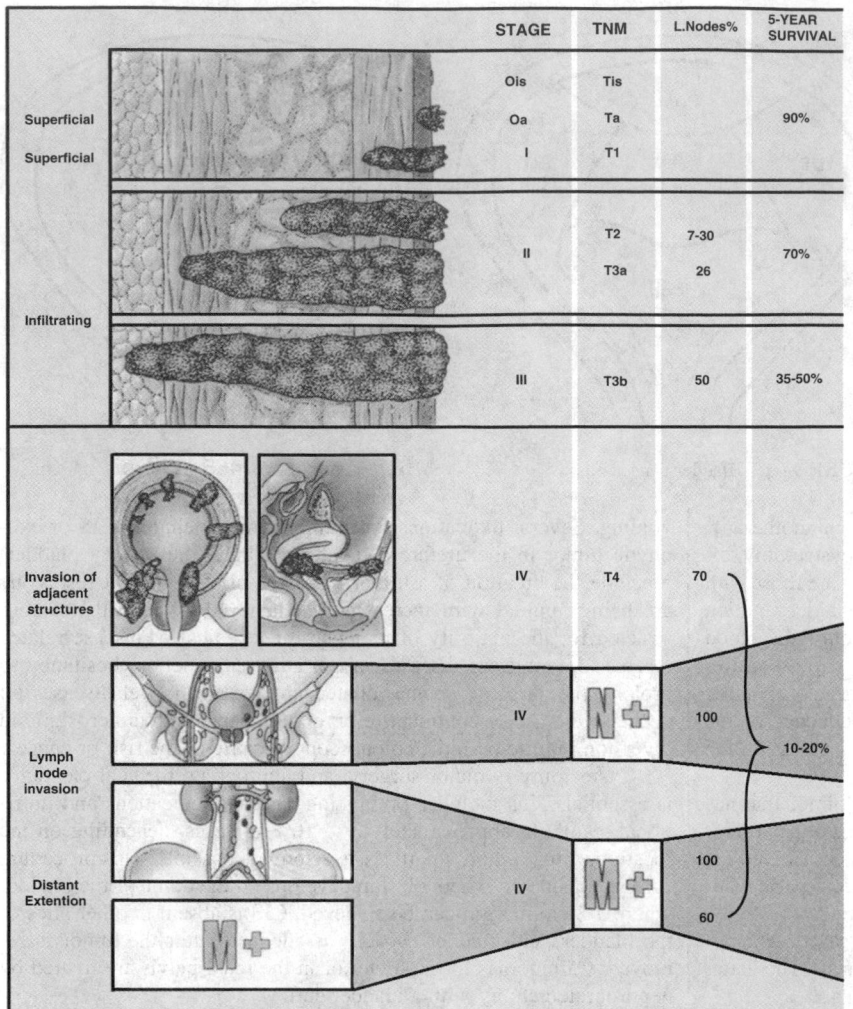

	STAGE	TNM	L.Nodes%	5-YEAR SURVIVAL
Superficial	Ois	Tis		90%
	Oa	Ta		
Superficial	I	T1		
Infiltrating	II	T2	7-30	70%
		T3a	26	
	III	T3b	50	35-50%
Invasion of adjacent structures	IV	T4	70	10-20%
Lymph node invasion	IV	N+	100	
Distant Extention	IV	M+	100	
			60	

FIGURE 94-2 Bladder staging.

survival with fewer side effects. Long-term survival may be obtained in 10 to 15% of patients with metastatic disease and 20 to 25% of patients with unresectable nodal disease at presentation. In general, the proportion of patients rendered tumor-free is higher in patients with disease limited to nodal sites as opposed to visceral or bone sites. Patients with adverse features, such as a compromised performance status, visceral disease, or bone metastases, are rarely cured with chemotherapy alone. In these cases, median survivals rarely exceed 6 months.

Chemotherapy for Invasive Disease Chemotherapy can be given before (neoadjuvant) or after (adjuvant) definitive local therapy. Cumulative results of nonrandomized phase II trials have shown that the proportion of bladders rendered free of tumor varies inversely with T stage; but only 20 to 25% of bladders are tumor-free after chemotherapy alone. To date, neoadjuvant chemotherapy has not been shown to prolong life. Several groups are investigating bladder-sparing strategies but these approaches are not considered routine practice. The need for adjuvant therapy is based on a pathologic determination of risk. In general, the finding of nodal disease at surgery, extravesical tumor extension, or vascular invasion in the resected specimen are considered indications for postoperative adjuvant therapy. When administered, a minimum of four cycles at full dose is recommended.

Overview Superficial TaG1 lesions rarely progress to an invasive lesion and can be handled with an endoscopic resection. Muscle-invasive disease may require both aggressive local therapy and systemic therapy of micrometastases for cure, while metastatic urinary bladder cancer is the most lethal for the majority of patients. Only a small proportion of patients with metastatic disease can be cured with chemotherapy. Current refinements in therapy include identifying subgroups of patients with superficial disease where the intensity of follow-up can be reduced or where intravesical therapy is needed. For muscle-invasive disease, efforts are being made to identify patients for whom organ preservation is possible without compromising overall survival, as well as those with subclinical micrometastases for whom systemic therapy is needed for cure. Efforts to improve therapy include better surgical techniques and the incorporation of newly identified chemotherapeutic agents into combination regimens. For the majority of patients, combined modality approaches are essential to optimal management.

RENAL CELL CARCINOMA

Renal cell carcinoma accounts for 90 to 95% of malignant neoplasms arising from the kidney. Notable features include refractoriness to cytotoxic agents, infrequent but reproducible responses to biologic response modifiers such as interferon α and interleukin (IL) 2, and a variable clinical course for patients with metastatic disease, including anecdotal reports of spontaneous regression.

EPIDEMIOLOGY AND ETIOLOGY In the year 2000, 31,200 new cases of renal cancer were diagnosed, and 11,900 people died of the disease. The male:female ratio is 2:1. Incidence peaks between the ages of 50 and 70, although this malignancy may be diagnosed at any age. Many environmental factors have been investigated as possible contributing causes. The strongest association is with cigarette smoking (accounting for 20 to 30% of cases) and obesity. The risk is increased for patients who have acquired cystic disease of the kidney associated with end-stage renal disease.

Most cases are sporadic, although familial forms have been reported. One is associated with von Hippel-Lindau (VHL) syndrome. Nearly 35% of patients with VHL disease develop renal cell cancer. An increased incidence has also been reported for patients with tuberous sclerosis and polycystic kidney disease.

Most of the cancers arise from the epithelial cells of the proximal tubules. A number of genetic alterations have been described, of which abnormalities on chromosome 3 are most frequent. A t(3;8) translocation was first described in a pedigree of patients with the familial form of the disease, while deletions of 3p21–26 (where *VHL* maps) have been identified in familial as well as sporadic tumors. *VHL* mutations are identified in a high proportion of sporadic, nonpapillary renal cell cancers and associated cell lines.

Table 94-1 Survival of Patients with Node Positive Bladder Cancer

Series	Year	No. of Patients	5-Year Survival, %
Whitmore	1981	134	7
Smith	1983	230	4
Skinner	1984	36	35
Bosl	1991	229	19
Pagano	1991	26	4

Table 94-2 5-Year Survival in Bladder Cancer Based on Pathologic Stage

Series	No. of Patients	Year	P2, %	P3a, %	P3b, %	Operative Mortality, %
Whitmore	137	1983	60	26	11	14
Montie	99	1983	62	74	57	9
Skinner	197	1984	83	69	29	1.0
Pagano	261	1991	63	50	15	1.8

Table 94-3 Selected Single Agents with Activity in Urothelial Tract Malignancies

Agent	No. Responding/ No. Treated	Percent	95% Confidence Interval
Cisplatin	200/706	28	26–32
Methrotrexate	8/236	45	37–50
Doxorubicin	47/274	17	13–22
Vinblastine	6/38	16	4–28
Ifosfamide	28/101	28	19–37
Gallium nitrate	9/29	29	13–45
Paclitaxel	11/26	42	23–61

PATHOLOGY Renal cell neoplasia represents a heterogeneous group of tumors with distinct histopathologic, genetic, and clinical features ranging from benign to high-grade malignant. Categories include clear cell carcinoma (60% of cases), papillary (5 to 15%), chromophobic tumors (5 to 10%), oncocytomas (5 to 10%), and collecting or Bellini duct tumors (<1%). Clear cell tumors are characterized by tumor cells with clear cytoplasm and consistently show a deletion of 3p. Papillary tumors tend to be bilateral and multifocal. Trisomy 7 and/or 17 are the most frequent genetic markers. Chromophobic tumors are characterized by multiple chromosomal losses but do not exhibit 3p deletions; they also have a more indolent clinical course. Oncocytomas have a characteristic morphology including a deeply eosinophilic cytoplasm, do not exhibit 3p deletions or trisomy 7 or 17, and are considered benign neoplasms. In contrast, Bellini duct carcinomas are very rare and are thought to arise from the collecting ducts within the renal medulla. They tend to afflict younger patients and are very aggressive tumors.

CLINICAL PRESENTATION The presenting signs and symptoms include hematuria, abdominal pain, and a flank or abdominal mass. This classic triad occurs in 10 to 20% of patients. Other symptoms are fever, weight loss, anemia, and a varicocele (Table 94-4); the tumor can be found incidentally on a radiograph.

The presentation has changed over the past two decades, due to the advent and widespread use of radiologic cross-sectional imaging procedures (CT, ultrasound, MRI). The more frequent use of sensitive abdominal imaging modalities in recent years contributes to earlier detection, including incidental low-stage renal masses detected during evaluation for other medical conditions. The increasing number of incidentally discovered low-stage tumors contributes to an improved 5-year survival for patients with renal cell carcinoma and increased use of nephron-sparing surgery (partial nephrectomy).

A spectrum of paraneoplastic syndromes has been associated with these malignancies, including erythrocytosis, hypercalcemia, nonmetastatic hepatic dysfunction (Stauffers' syndrome) and acquired dysfibrinogenemia. Erythrocytosis is present at presentation in only about 3% of patients. More frequently anemia, a sign of advanced disease, is reported.

The standard evaluation of patients with suspected renal cell tumors includes a CT scan of the abdomen and pelvis, a chest radiograph, urine analysis, and urine cytology. A CT of the chest is warranted if metastatic disease is suspected from the chest radiograph, as it will detect significantly smaller lesions, and their presence may influence the approach to the primary tumor. MRI is useful in evaluating the inferior vena cava in cases of suspected tumor involvement or invasion by thrombus, as well as for patients in whom iodinated contrast cannot be administered owing to either allergy or renal dysfunction. In clinical practice any solid renal masses should be considered malignant until proved otherwise and require a definitive diagnosis. If no metastases are demonstrated, surgery is indicated, even if there is invasion of the renal vein. The differential diagnosis of a renal mass includes cysts, benign neoplasms (adenoma, angiomyolipoma, oncocytoma), inflammatory lesions (pyelonephritis or abscesses), and other primary or metastatic malignant neoplasms. Other malignancies that may involve the kidney include transitional cell carcinomas of the renal pelvis, sarcoma, lymphoma, Wilms' tumor, and metastatic disease, especially from melanoma primaries. All of these are less common than renal cell carcinoma as kidney masses.

STAGING AND PROGNOSIS Two staging systems used commonly are the Robson classification and the American Joint Committee on Cancer (AJCC) staging system. According to the former, stage I tumors are confined to the kidney; stage II tumors extend through the renal capsule but are confined to Gerota's fascia; stage III tumors involve the renal vein or vena cava (stage III A) or the hilar lymph nodes (stage III B); and stage IV disease includes tumors that are locally invasive to adjacent organs (excluding the adrenal gland) or distant metastases. Five-year survival rate varies by stage: 66% for stage I, 64% for stage II, 42% for stage III, and 11% for stage IV. The prognosis for patients with stage IIIA lesions is similar to that of stage II disease, whereas the 5-year survival rate for patients with stage IIIB lesions is only 20%, closer to that of stage IV.

℞ TREATMENT Localized Tumors The standard management for stage I or II tumors and selected cases of stage III disease is radical nephrectomy. This procedure involves en bloc removal of Gerota's fascia; its contents including the kidney, the ipsilateral adrenal gland, and adjacent hilar lymph nodes. The role of a regional lymphadenectomy is controversial. For patients with stage IIIA disease, the tumor should be resected from the renal vein or vena cava.

In selected patients who have only one kidney, a partial nephrectomy may be performed, depending on the size and location of the lesion. Partial nephrectomy may also be performed for patients with bilateral tumors, accompanied by a radical nephrectomy on the opposite side. Partial nephrectomy techniques are being applied electively to resect small masses for patients with a normal contralateral kidney. There is no proven role for adjuvant chemotherapy, immunotherapy, or radiation therapy following successful surgical removal of the tumor, even in cases with a poor prognosis.

Advanced Disease Metastatic renal cell carcinoma, for which there is no effective therapy, is associated with dismal survival. A number of options have been explored, including hormonal therapy, chemotherapy (cytotoxic agents), and immunotherapy. Responses to hormonal therapy (progestins) are rare (1 to 2%) and of short duration. No chemotherapy agent has been shown to consistently produce tumor regressions in >20% of patients.

Two biologic therapies, interferon α and IL-2, have been studied extensively for the treatment of advanced disease. Both reproducibly produce responses in 10 to 20% of patients; the response is durable in fewer than 5% of patients. It was the observation of occasional durable complete remissions that resulted in the Food and Drug Administration's approval of IL-2 as a treatment for this disease. IL-2 is usually administered by infusion of 720,000 IU/k every 8 h per day for 5 to 7 days. Toxicities from IL-2 include a capillary leakage syndrome, fever, chills, fatigue, and hypotension.

Table 94-4 Signs and Symptoms in Patients with Renal Cell Cancer

Presenting Sign or Symptom	Incidence, %
Classic triad: hematuria, flank pain, flank mass	10–20
Hematuria	40
Flank pain	40
Palpable mass	25
Weight loss	33
Anemia	33
Fever	20
Hypertension	20
Abnormal liver function	15
Hypercalcemia	5
Erythrocytosis	3
Neuromyopathy	3
Amyloidosis	2
Increased erythrocyte sedimentation rate	55

Surgery in the Setting of Metastases Nephrectomy may be indicated in highly selected cases for the alleviation of symptoms, including pain or recurrent urinary hemorrhage, and particularly if the latter is severe or associated with obstruction. Some physicians advocate the performance of a nephrectomy in the presence of metastases in the hope either that a spontaneous regression will occur or that the sensitivity to a cytokine will be increased. The observed frequency of spontaneous regression, 0.8%, coupled with the morbidity and mortality of the procedure itself, does not justify the approach. Nephrectomy in the presence of metastatic disease followed by IFN-α is associated with a modest survival benfit over IFN-α alone.

There are reports of long-term survival at rates of 15 to 50% for patients who relapse following nephrectomy at a solitary site and undergo surgical resection of the metastasis. Because renal cell tumors are radioresistant, surgical resection is also advised for palliation of solitary central nervous system metastases, repair of actual or impending fractures in weight-bearing bones, or relief of spinal cord compression.

Observation Alone   Renal cell carcinoma is one of several malignancies in which spontaneous regressions have been reported anecdotally. A more frequent occurrence is prolonged periods of stable disease: up to 10% of patients with metastatic disease show no progression for >12 months. Because responses to systemic therapy are uncommon, and all systemic therapies are associated with treatment-related toxicity, an option for management in asymptomatic patients with metastases is close observation until evidence of disease progression or symptoms occur, at which time appropriate therapy is initiated. It is important to document the presence of progressive disease before initiating an experimental treatment; this will avoid attributing stable disease to the drug when it may be a feature of the tumor.

CARCINOMA OF THE RENAL PELVIS AND URETER

About 500 cases of renal pelvis and ureter cancer occur each year; nearly all are transitional cell carcinomas similar to bladder cancer in biology and appearance. This tumor also is associated with chronic phenacetin abuse and with Balkan nephropathy, a chronic interstitial nephritis endemic in Bulgaria, Greece, Bosnia-Herzegovina, and Romania.

The most common symptom is painless gross hematuria, and the disease usually is detected on IVP during the workup for hematuria. Patterns of spread are like those in bladder cancer. For disease localized to the renal pelvis and ureter, nephroureterectomy (including excision of the distal ureter with a portion of the bladder) is associated with a 5-year survival of 80 to 90% for low-grade lesions. More invasive or histologically poorly differentiated tumors are more likely to recur locally and metastasize. Metastatic disease is treated with M-VAC or CMV (cisplatin, methotrexate, vinblastine) chemotherapy, as used in bladder cancer, and the outcome is similar to that for metastatic transitional cell cancer of bladder origin.

BIBLIOGRAPHY

BASSELLI EC, GREENBERG RE: Intravesical therapy for superficial bladder cancer. Oncology 14:719, 2000

FIGLIN RA: Renal cell carcinoma: Management of advanced disease. J Urol 161:381, 1999

LINEHAN WM et al: Cancer of the kidney and ureter, in *Cancer: Principles and Practice of Oncology*, 5th ed, VT DeVita et al (eds). Philadelphia New York: Lippincott-Raven, 1997, pp 1271–1300

MOTZER RJ et al: Renal-cell carcinoma. N Engl J Med 335:865,1996

————: Systemic therapy for renal cell carcinoma. J Urol 163:408,2000

OZEN H, HALL MC: Bladder cancer. Curr Opin Oncol 12:255, 2000

REUTER VE et al. Contemporary approach to the classification of renal epithelial tumors. Sem Oncol 27:124, 2000

95   *Howard I. Scher*

HYPERPLASTIC AND MALIGNANT DISEASES OF THE PROSTATE

CT computed tomography	PSAD prostate-specific antigen density
DRE digital rectal examination	PIN prostatic intraepithelial neoplasia
GnRH gonadotropin-releasing hormone	3D-CRT three-dimensional conformal radiation therapy
LH luteinizing hormone	TRUS transrectal ultrasonography
MRI magnetic resonance imaging	TURP transurethral resection of the prostate
PSA prostate-specific antigen	

The process of aging is associated with an increasing frequency of both benign and malignant alterations of the prostate gland. These conditions reflect the uncontrolled growth of both the stromal and epithelial components of the gland. Autopsies of men in the eighth decade of life show hyperplastic changes in >90% and malignant changes in >70%. Most men with benign or malignant conditions of the prostate are not diagnosed during their lifetimes. The high prevalence of these diseases, coupled with comorbid conditions and competing causes of death that are frequent in this age group, mandates a careful consideration of the risk/benefit ratio of any proposed intervention. Management is centered on the continual reassessment of the disease as it unfolds in the individual. For the benign proliferative disorders, the symptoms of urinary frequency, infection, and potential for obstruction are counterbalanced by the side effects and complications of medical or surgical therapy. For malignant disease, the risk of developing symptoms or death from cancer is balanced against treatment efficacy and treatment-related morbidity for interventions proposed at different points in the natural history.

The incidence and mortality of prostate cancer have declined over the past few years. The decline is not clearly related to any meaningful decrease in the disease or its severity. Instead, the number of cases diagnosed increased dramatically in the early 1990s based on the widespread use of serum prostate-specific antigen (PSA) levels. The test led to the diagnosis of more asymptomatic cancers, some of which may never have produced symptoms—so-called lead-time bias (Chap. 80). Screening for prostate cancer has not been proven effective in prospective randomized trials. Prostate cancer is the most common cancer diagnosis and the second leading cause of cancer death in men. In 2000, 180,400 cases were diagnosed and 31,900 men died of prostate cancer, down from the peak of 352,000 new cases in 1996. The projected lifetime risk of developing prostate cancer for a 50-year-old man is 42%, of being diagnosed is 9.5%, and of dying from prostate cancer is 2.9%.

ANATOMY

The prostate is located in the pelvis and is surrounded by the rectum, bladder, dorsal and periprostatic venous complexes, musculature of the pelvic sidewall, the urethral sphincter (responsible for passive urinary control), the pelvic plexus, and cavernous nerves (which innervate the pelvic organs and corpora cavernosa). It is divided into a peripheral zone, a central zone, and a transition zone. The anterior surface is covered by the fibromuscular stroma. Most cancers develop in the peripheral zone, while nonmalignant proliferation occurs predominantly in the transition zone. The functional unit is the glandular acinus, which consists of an epithelial compartment including epithelial, basal, and neuroendocrine cells, and a stromal compartment including fibroblasts and smooth-muscle cells. These compartments are separated by a basement membrane. PSA and prostate-specific acid phosphatase are produced in the epithelial cells. Both stromal and epithelial cells express androgen receptors and depend on androgens for growth. Additional growth regulatory signals occur via paracrine signaling between the two compartments. In cancer, the relationship between stromal and epithelial elements contributes to growth both in the primary and in metastatic sites. The major circulating androgen in the blood is testosterone, which is converted to dihydrotestosterone, the active form, by 5α-reductase. Changes in prostate size occur during two distinct periods: diffuse enlargement during puberty and in focal regions in the periurethral area after the age of 55.

DIAGNOSIS AND SCREENING

Symptoms Most cancers are asymptomatic in their early stages. By contrast, benign proliferative disorders may encroach on the urethra early in the clinical course, giving rise to symptoms of outlet obstruction such as hesitancy, intermittent voiding, diminished stream, incomplete emptying, and postvoid leakage. For the patient with symptoms, the history is focused on the urinary tract to identify other causes of voiding dysfunction. For quantification of symptoms, the preferred questionnaire is the self-administered American Urological Association (AUA) *Symptom Index* in which the symptoms can be classified as mild, moderate, or severe on the basis of seven questions (Table 95-1). This index is useful in planning and in follow-up. Over time, the resistance to the flow of urine reduces the compliance of the detrusor muscle, resulting in nocturia, urgency, and bladder instability and ultimately in urinary retention. The relationship between the signs and symptoms of obstruction and prostate size is not straightforward, and a small gland does not exclude significant blockage. In severe cases the bladder may be palpable on physical examination. Infection, tranquilizing drugs, antihistamines, or alcohol can precipitate urinary retention.

Obstructive symptoms are distinct from irritative symptoms such as frequency, dysuria, or urgency, which may occur from infectious, inflammatory, or neoplastic diseases. Conditions that can mimic cancer include acute prostatitis, granulomatous prostatitis, and prostate calculus. Prostatitis usually produces induration and/or pain and is treated with antibiotics. Prostate cancer may manifest in the same manner, and the distinction can only be established histologically, but a biopsy should not be performed before a trial of antibiotics if prostatitis is a possible diagnosis. In cases where the tumor has extended beyond the confines of the gland, symptoms of hematospermia or erectile dysfunction may occur. Prostate cancer may also present with pain secondary to bone metastases, although many patients are asymptomatic despite extensive spread. Less common presentations include myelophthisic disorders, disseminated intravascular coagulation, or spinal cord compression. The proportion of men diagnosed at these late stages has also decreased significantly as a result of PSA-based detection strategies.

Physical Examination The standard evaluation for prostatic diseases includes the digital rectal examination (DRE). It should be performed with careful attention to the size and consistency of the gland, the presence of lesions within the gland, or evidence of extension beyond its confines. Its importance can not be overemphasized. The posterior surfaces of the lateral lobes, where carcinoma begins most often, are easily palpable on DRE. Carcinoma characteristically is hard, nodular, and irregular, but induration may also be due to fibrous areas in a benign hyperplastic background or to calculi. Extraprostatic extension to the seminal vesicles can often be detected by rectal examination, while scrotal and/or lower extremity lymphedema secondary to infiltration of pelvic lymph nodes indicates extensive disease. The need for establishing a histologic diagnosis is based on the finding of an abnormal DRE or an elevated serum PSA level.

Prostate-Specific Antigen PSA is a serine protease that is produced by both nonmalignant and malignant epithelial cells. In serum, it circulates as an inactive complex with two protease inhibitors—α_1-antichymotrypsin and β_2-macroglobulin. PSA is prostate specific but not prostate cancer specific and is measured most commonly by radioimmunoassay. The normal range is 0 to 4 ng/mL; ~30% of men with a PSA in the range of 4 to 10 ng/mL and 50% of those with a PSA >10 ng/mL will have cancer. Between 20 and 25% of men with an abnormal DRE have cancer at biopsy, and 20% of men have cancer detected when the PSA is in the normal range. African American men normally have higher PSA levels, even if they do not have prostate cancer. They also have a 50% higher risk of prostate cancer. The reason for the racial differences is not known.

Several refinements have been proposed to increase the sensitivity of the test for younger men more likely to die of the disease, while reducing the frequency of diagnosing cancers of low biologic potential in elderly men more likely to die of other causes. These modifications include age-specific reference ranges, using a lower "upper" limit of normal for younger males and higher "upper" limit for older individuals. Prostate-specific antigen density (PSAD) is calculated by dividing the serum PSA level by the estimated prostate weight calculated from transrectal ultrasonography (TRUS). It was proposed to correct for the influence of benign prostatic hyperplasia (BPH) on the measured level of PSA. Values <0.10 are consistent with BPH, while values >0.15 suggest the presence of cancer. PSAD levels also increase with age.

PSA velocity is derived from calculations of the rate of change in PSA before the diagnosis of cancer was established. Increases of >0.75 ng/mL per year are suggestive of cancer. For a 50-year-old male, an increase from 2.5 to 3.9 ng/mL in a 1-year period would warrant further testing, even though the level is still in the "normal" range. Free and complexed PSA measurements are used to determine which men require a biopsy when the PSA level is in the range of 4 to 10 ng/mL. In cancer, the level of free PSA is lower. Using a 25%

Table 95-1 AUA System Index

Questions to be Answered	AUA Symptom Score (Circle 1 Number on Each Line)					
	Not at All	Less than 1 Time in 5	Less than Half the Time	About Half the Time	More than Half the time	Almost Always
Over the past month, how often you have had a sensation of not emptying your bladder completely after you finished urinating?	0	1	2	3	4	5
Over the past month, how often have you had to urinate again less than 2 h after you finished urinating?	0	1	2	3	4	5
Over the past month, how often have you found you stopped and started again several times when you urinated?	0	1	2	3	4	5
Over the past month, how often have you found it difficult to postpone urination?	0	1	2	3	4	5
Over the past month, how often have you had a weak urinary stream?	0	1	2	3	4	5
Over the past month, how often have you had to push or strain to begin urination?	0	1	2	3	4	5
Over the past month, how many times did you most typically get up to urinate from the time you went to bed at night until the time you got up in the morning?	(None)	(1 time)	(2 times)	(3 times)	(4 times)	(5 times)
Sum of 7 circled numbers (AUA Symptom Score): ————						

NOTE: AUA, American Urological Association.

SOURCE: Barry MJ et al: J Urol 148:1549, 1992. Used with permission.

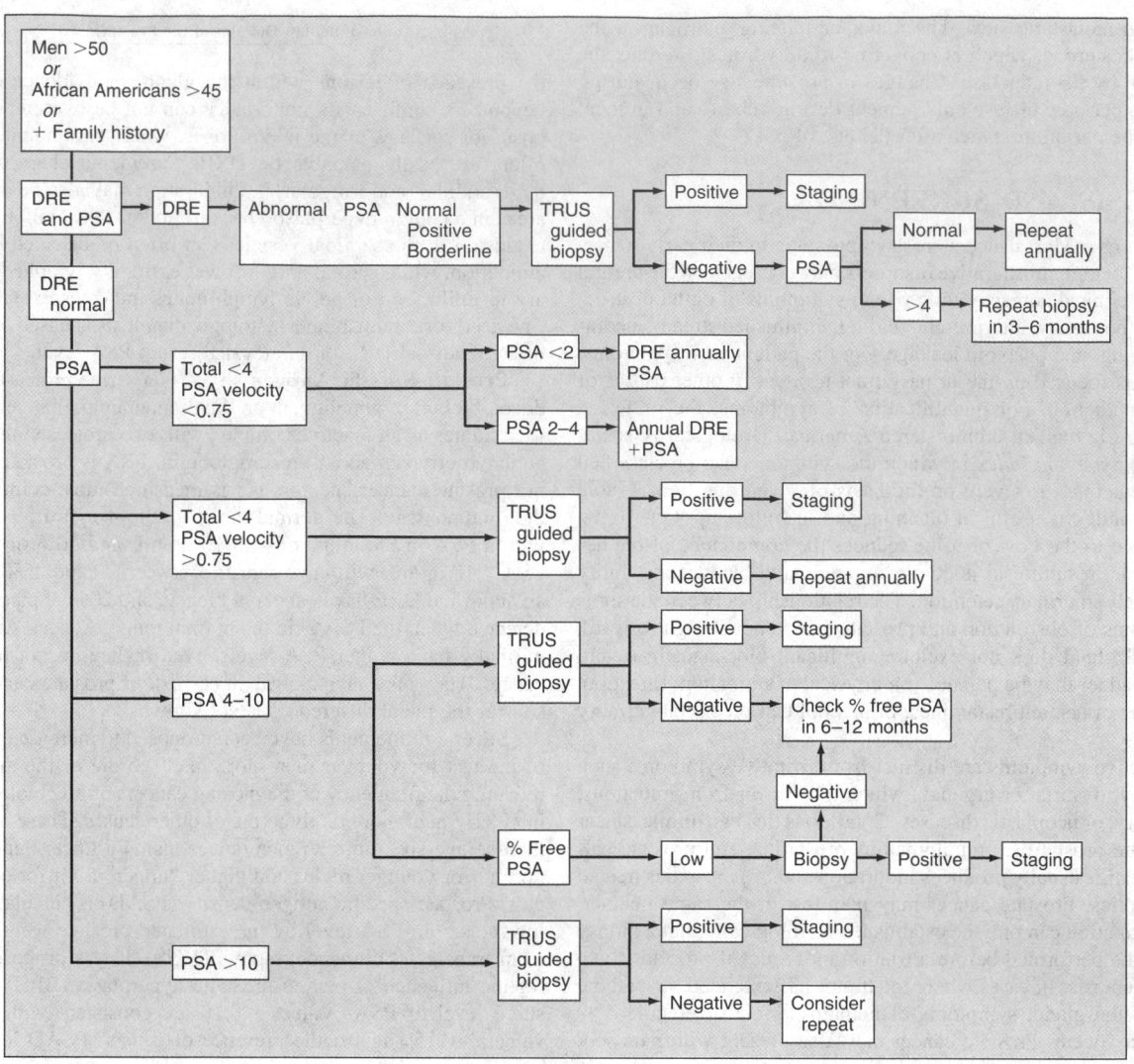

FIGURE 95-1 Men who desire early detection after discussion of pros and cons with their health care providers and who have a > 10 year life expectancy.

(Modified from NCCN Prostate Practice Guidelines)

threshold of free PSA for patients with levels in the range of 4 to 10 ng/mL, specificity was improved by 20% while maintaining a sensitivity of 95%. Further refinements to increase the specificity of distinguishing benign and malignant conditions involve the determination of the ratios of free to total, complexed to total, and free to complexed PSA. Using normal ranges for free/total PSA of >0.15, for complexed/total PSA of <0.70, and for free/complexed PSA of >0.25 improved specificity in one study by 20%. These modifications are designed to reduce the frequency of biopsies in men without cancer. Figure 95-1 illustrates a diagnostic algorithm based on the DRE and PSA findings.

Transrectal Ultrasonography Most cancers are hypoechoic by ultrasonography. Unfortunately, no single finding on ultrasound permits univeral distinction between cancer and benign conditions and identification of extracapsular disease. Cancers <5 to 7 mm, those that are well differentiated, and those located in the transition zone are difficult to distinguish from the normal prostate. The primary role of ultrasound is to ensure accurate sampling of any index lesions and of the gland during biopsy. Routine sampling includes a minimum of six cores from the peripheral zone of the gland, each of which is identified and labeled separately for histologic examination. A biopsy session, defined as one that procures four or more cores from widely separated areas of the prostate, has a sensitivity of ~80% for the detection of a cancer. TRUS has also been used in the assessment of local disease extent; accuracy is limited and is generally restricted to determining whether the tumor invades the seminal vesicles. It is also used to determine the size of the gland for the calculation of PSAD and to guide the placement of radioactive seeds during implantation.

Pathology The noninvasive proliferation of epithelial cells within ducts is termed *prostatic intraepithelial neoplasia* (PIN). It is considered the precursor of cancer, but not all PIN lesions develop into invasive cancers. Nevertheless, on a genetic level, these regions are highly unstable and typically multifocal. Of the cancers identified, >95% are adenocarcinomas; the remainder include squamous cell tumors, transitional cell tumors, and, rarely, carcinosarcomas. Metastases to the prostate are rare, but in some cases, transitional cell tumors originating in the bladder or colonic lesions may invade the gland directly. In the evaluation for adenocarcinoma, each core is examined for the presence or absence of cancer. When cancer is identified, the extent and grade are assessed and the presence or absence of perineural invasion or extracapsular extension reported. Histologic grade is based most commonly on the *Gleason system*, in which the dominant and secondary glandular histologic patterns are independently assigned numbers from 1 to 5 (best to least differentiated) and summed to give a total score of 2 to 10 for each tumor. The grading is reproducible and correlates with clinical outcomes. The most poorly differentiated area of tumor (i.e., the area with the highest histologic grade) often determines biologic behavior.

STAGING

The TNM staging system (Table 95-2) includes categories for cancers identified solely on the basis of an abnormal PSA with no palpable abnormalities on DRE (T1c), those that are palpable but clinically confined to the gland (T2), and those that have extended outside of

Table 95-2 Comparison of Clinical Stage by the TNM Classification System and the Whitmore-Jewett Staging System

TNM Stage	Description	Whitmore-Jewett Stage	Description
T1a	Nonpalpable, with 5% or less of resected tissue with cancer	A1	Well differentiated tumor on few chips from 1 lobe
T1b	Nonpalpable, with >5% of resected tissue with cancer	A2	Involvement more diffuse
T1c	Nonpalpable, detected due to elevated serum PSA		
T2a	Palpable, half of one lobe or less	BIN	Palpable, < one lobe, surrounded by normal tissue
T2b	Palpable, > half of one lobe but not both lobes	B1	Palpable, < one lobe
T2c	Palpable, involves both lobes	B2	Palpable, one entire lobe or both lobes
T3a	Palpable, unilateral extracapsular extension	C1	Palpable, outside capsule, not into seminal vesicles
T3b	Palpable, bilateral extracapsular extension		
T3c	Tumor invades seminal vesicle(s)	C2	Palpable, seminal vesicle involved
MI	Distant metastases	D	Metastatic disease

SOURCE: Adapted from FF Schroder et al: TNM classification of prostate cancer. Prostate (Suppl) 4:129, 1992; and American Joint Committee on Cancer, 1992.

the gland (T3 and T4). The presence or absence of nodal (N) and distant metastases (M) are also recorded. Clinical staging alone is inaccurate in assessing capsular invasion and the probability of spread to nodal or more distant sites. To refine this assessment, the TNM system has been modified to incorporate the results of imaging studies such as ultrasound or magnetic resonance imaging (MRI) in the assignment of T stage.

Computed tomography (CT) scans lack sensitivity and specificity to detect extraprostatic extension and in visualization of lymph nodes. MRI is an improvement, particularly with an endorectal coil and is superior to CT. T1-weighted images demonstrate the periprostatic fat, periprostatic venous plexus, perivesicular tissues, lymph nodes, and bone marrow. T2-weighted images demonstrate the internal architecture of the prostate and seminal vesicles. Most cancers have a low signal, while the normal peripheral zone has a high signal. Nevertheless, MRI lacks sensitivity and specificity. No single test accurately predicts pathologic stage at surgery.

Another limitation of the TNM system is that the majority of men are now being diagnosed with T1c or T2 disease. Thus, to refine the prediction of local disease extent, most groups are now using multiplex staging models based on a combination of the findings of the DRE, biopsy, Gleason score, and baseline PSA (Table 95-3). Others are developing models based on the number of cores and the percentage of each core involved by tumor. This information can be used to assist patients in selecting treatments, although it remains controversial how recommendations should be affected by a particular level of probability of node-positive disease.

These same parameters are also being used to assess the probability of cure (Fig. 95-2). Some tumors that have extended beyond the confines of the gland may still be curable, while others that are still organ-confined may not. Because successful surgery removes all prostatic tissues, both benign and malignant, and radiation therapy eliminates only the malignant component, different definitions of cure are needed depending on the modality used. Thus, following surgery, the PSA level should become undetectable; following radiation therapy, it should generally fall to <1.0 ng/mL. What the models do not address is what probability of cure a patient would accept to proceed with a given approach. For example, would one categorically deny a surgical procedure to a 40-year-old male if the probability of cure was only 15%? These same models can also be used to stratify patients into risk

groups to assess outcomes of specific therapies. While this form of analysis does not replace prospective trials, it does eliminate the bias associated with the tendency to refer older and more infirm patients for radiation therapy and younger, healthier individuals for surgery.

To complete the staging evaluation, patients may undergo radionuclide bone scanning. This test is highly sensitive but relatively non-specific, because areas of increased uptake are not always secondary to osteoblastic activity from metastases. Healing fractures, arthritis, Paget's disease, and numerous other conditions will also show abnormal uptake. True-positive bone scan results are rare if the PSA is <8 and uncommon when the PSA is <10 ng/mL. More common is a false-positive scan, which, in turn, leads to additional low-yield testing. CT scans yield little useful clinical information unless the probability of lymph node metastases is >30% using nomogram predictions; an MRI is more likely to detect pathologically significant nodal disease. Molecular diagnostics are being performed that seek to identify the presence of circulating prostate cancer cells using an assay for PSA based on reverse transcriptase polymerase chain reaction (RT-PCR) in the leukocyte fraction of the peripheral blood or bone marrow. A large proportion of men with tumors seemingly confined to the organ test positive; the significance is unclear. These procedures are in their infancy, and application is not advised on a routine basis.

TREATMENT SELECTION: THE MODEL OF CLINICAL STATES

The framework for evaluating the risks from an enlarging but non-malignant gland, the probability that a clinically significant cancer is present in an individual with or without urinary symptoms, and the probability that a patient with cancer will develop symptoms or die of prostate cancer are provided by the clinical states model illustrated in Fig. 95-3. It includes clinically significant milestones where interventions might be considered and allows for the assessment of the prognosis of the treated patient. In the first state are patients with no cancer diagnosis. It includes patients with benign proliferative disorders or those who warrant screening on the basis of family history or a level of PSA or symptoms. In the second state are those with a cancer that is clinically confined to the gland. For these patients the issue is to determine which tumors require treatment based on their biologic potential, which can be eradicated by local means alone, and which require a combined-modality approach that includes systemic therapy to effect cure. The third state includes those who have a rising PSA level after surgery or radiation for localized disease but who have no clinically detectable lesions on scans. Next are patients with detectable metastases who have not undergone castration, and the last level is those who have detectable disease on scan despite castration. The risk of death from cancer relative to the risk of death from comorbid conditions increases over time, being greatest for the patient who has progressed after hormonal therapy.

At any point, a patient resides in only one state and remains there until the disease progresses. Thus, a patient who presents with a localized prostate cancer who has had all cancer removed surgically remains in the state of localized disease as long as his PSA remains undetectable. In this way, both time factors and that the fact that a patient has been treated are accounted for. Overall treatment effects are assessed by measuring time within a particular state. The scheme also allows a distinction between cure, elimination of all cancer cells, with an undetectable PSA and cancer control, i.e., modulating the rate of growth so that the patient dies of other causes. In this paradigm, a patient with a detectable PSA who dies of other causes having suffered no morbidity from the disease or its treatment, PSA level, is considered a therapeutic success.

MANAGEMENT BY STATES

NO CANCER DIAGNOSIS **Screening** The American Cancer Society (ACS) and the AUA recommend an annual DRE and a

Gleason Score	PSA, 0.0–4.0 NG/ML Clinical Stage			PSA, 4.1–10.0 NG/ML Clinical Stage			PSA, 10.1–20.0 NG/ML Clinical Stage		
	T1c	T2a	T2b	T1c	T2a	T2b	T1c	T2a	T2b
ORGAN-CONFINED DISEASE									
5	81 (76–84)	68 (63–72)	57 (50–62)	71 (67–75)	55 (51–60)	43 (38–49)	60 (54–65)	43 (38–49)	32 (26–37)
6	78 (74–81)	64 (59–68)	52 (46–57)	67 (64–70)	51 (47–54)	38 (34–43)	55 (51–59)	38 (34–43)	26 (23–31)
7	63 (58–68)	47 (41–52)	34 (29–39)	49 (45–54)	33 (29–38)	22 (18–26)	35 (31–40)	22 (18–26)	13 (11–16)
8 to 10	52 (41–62)	36 (27–45)	24 (17–32)	37 (28–46)	23 (16–31)	14 (9–19)	23 (16–32)	14 (9–19)	7 (5–11)
ESTABLISHED CAPSULAR PENETRATION									
5	18 (15–22)	30 (26–35)	40 (34–46)	27 (23–30)	41 (36–46)	50 (45–55)	35 (30–40)	50 (45–56)	57 (51–63)
6	21 (18–25)	34 (30–38)	43 (38–48)	30 (27–33)	44 (41–48)	52 (48–56)	38 (34–42)	52 (48–57)	57 (51–62)
7	31 (26–36)	45 (40–50)	51 (46–57)	40 (35–44)	52 (48–57)	54 (49–59)	45 (40–50)	55 (50–60)	51 (45–57)
8 to 10	34 (27–44)	47 (38–56)	48 (40–57)	40 (33–49)	49 (42–57)	46 (39–53)	40 (33–49)	46 (38–55)	38 (30–47)
SEMINAL VESICLE INVOLVEMENT									
5	1 (1–2)	2 (1–3)	3 (2–4)	2 (1–3)	3 (2–5)	5 (3–8)	3 (2–5)	5 (3–8)	8 (5–11)
6	1 (1–2)	2 (1–3)	3 (2–4)	2 (2–3)	3 (2–4)	5 (4–7)	4 (3–5)	5 (3–7)	7 (5–10)
7	4 (2–7)	6 (4–9)	10 (6–14)	8 (5–11)	10 (8–13)	15 (11–19)	12 (8–16)	14 (10–19)	18 (13–24)
8 to 10	9 (5–16)	12 (7–19)	17 (11–25)	15 (10–22)	19 (13–26)	24 (17–31)	20 (13–28)	22 (15–31)	25 (18–34)
LYMPH NODE INVOLVEMENT									
5	0 (0–0)	0 (0–1)	1 (0–2)	0 (0–1)	1 (0–1)	2 (1–3)	1 (0–2)	2 (1–3)	4 (1–7)
6	0 (0–1)	1 (0–1)	2 (1–3)	1 (1–2)	2 (1–3)	4 (3–6)	3 (2–5)	4 (3–6)	10 (7–13)
7	1 (1–3)	2 (1–4)	5 (2–8)	3 (2–5)	4 (3–6)	9 (6–12)	8 (5–11)	9 (6–13)	17 (12–23)
8 to 10	4 (2–7)	5 (2–9)	10 (5–17)	8 (4–12)	9 (5–13)	16 (11–24)	16 (10–24)	17 (11–25)	29 (21–38)

* Modified from Partin AW, Kattan MW, Subong ENP, et al: Combination of prostate-specific antigen, clinical stage, and Gleason score to predict pathological stage of localized prostate cancer a multi-institutional update. JAMA 277:1445, 1997. Copyright 1997 American Medical Association, with permission.
† Numbers represent percent predictive probability (95% CI).
ABBREVIATION: PSA, prostate-specific antigen.

determination of PSA level for all men aged 50 to 79. Individuals with a first-degree relative with prostate cancer and African Americans, who have a higher risk of dying of the disease, are advised to begin testing at age 45. Routine screening for prostate cancer has been advised despite a lack of prospective, randomized, controlled trials proving the benefit of the approach because the disease rarely causes symptoms until it is advanced. The more widespread use of routine DREs and PSA testing has resulted in a significant increase in the proportion of men with clinically localized tumors, a reduced frequency of nodal spread, and a decreased frequency of nodal and osseous disease at presentation. Risks of screening are unnecessary morbidity or mortality from overdetection and overtreatment. Formal clinical trials are underway, but until the studies are complete and the results available, men must make an informed decision to be screened or not.

Hyperplasia A patient with an enlarged prostate who has no symptoms and normal PSA levels generally does not require treatment. Those with symptoms such as an inability to urinate, renal insufficiency, urinary tract infection, gross hematuria, or bladder stones are candidates for prostate surgery. As the natural history is not well defined, it is not always clear whether to intervene and, if so, how. The majority of men do not develop significant obstruction, and in many, minor irritative and/or obstructive symptoms change slowly or not at all. In these cases urine flow studies can identify those whose maximum flows are normal and who are unlikely to benefit from treatment. Measuring postvoid residual volume identifies patients likely to fail a "watch and wait" approach, while pressure-flow studies may identify those with primary bladder dysfunction. A cystoscopic examination is advised for all patients with hematuria and to assess the urinary outflow tract before a surgical intervention. Imaging of the upper urinary tract by ultrasonography or intravenous pyelography should be reserved for patients with indications such as hematuria, a history of stones, or prior urinary tract problems.

Most patients are monitored and/or treated medically, after a discussion with their physicians about the degree of incapacity and/or discomfort present and the likely outcome of each potential treatment strategy. A variety of decision diagrams have been proposed. Patients who opt for deferred therapy should be evaluated on an annual basis by the reassessment of symptoms and clinical manifestations. Medical therapies include finasteride, which blocks the conversion of testosterone to dihydrotestosterone, the principal androgen in the prostate, by competitively inhibiting the 5α-reductase enzyme. A dose of 5 mg/d causes an average decrease in prostate size of ~24%, an increase in urine flow rates, and, in some, improvement in symptoms. Long-term efficacy has not been documented, but symptomatic improvement

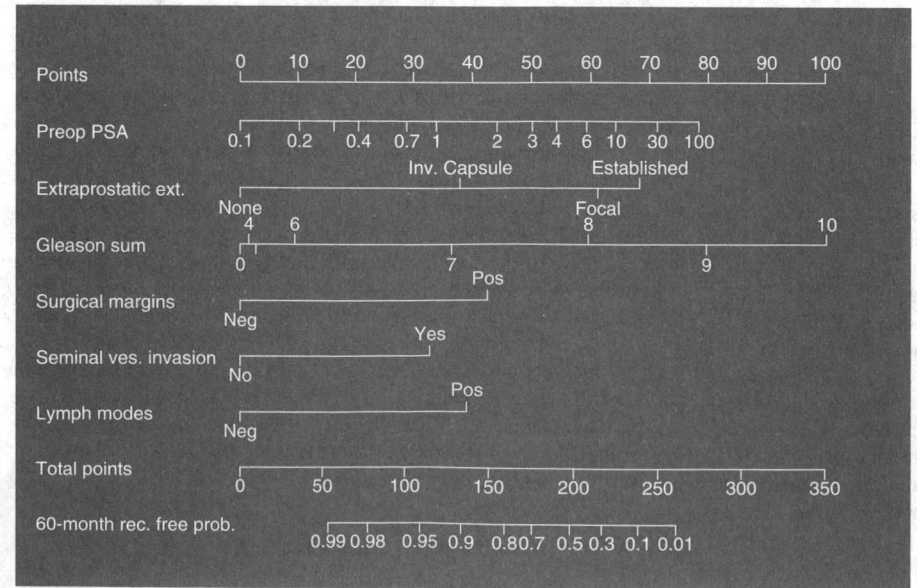

FIGURE 95-2 Kattan recurrence nomogram. *(From Kattan et al.)*

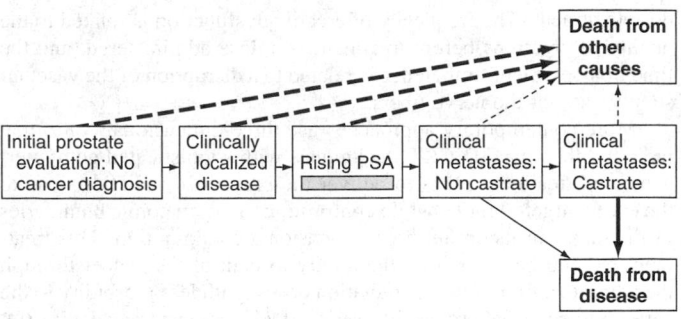

FIGURE 95-3 Clinical states. *(From Scher and Heller).*

has been documented for ≥3 years provided therapy is continued. α-Adrenergic blockers such as terazosin act by relaxing the smooth muscle of the bladder neck, increasing peak urinary flow rates and reducing symptoms. No data prove that these agents influence the progression of the disease.

Patients who do not improve or who progress on medical therapy require surgical intervention. Surgical approaches include a transurethral resection of the prostate (TURP); transurethral incision; or removal of the gland by a retropubic, suprapubic, or perineal route. Other approaches include ultrasound, coils, stents, lasers, or hyperthermia. Overall, surgery offers the best chance for improving symptoms, at the cost of the highest rate of complications. TURP is the most common surgical procedure. Transurethral incision of the prostate is of similar efficacy in men with relatively small prostates and can be performed in ambulatory settings. Open prostatectomy is usually reserved for men with massive prostates; it has the longest recovery time and the highest morbidity, particularly impotence. Transurethral incision has the least morbidity overall and is least disruptive to ejaculatory function.

Elevated PSA and No Cancer Diagnosis on Biopsy Patients who have undergone a biopsy procedure and do not have a cancer diagnosis should continue to be monitored. In some cases, a repeat biopsy session with particular attention to the transition zone is advised. The frequency of PIN is similar in men of different ethnic backgrounds around the world, while the incidence of the clinical disease varies in different ethnic groups. Prevention of progression from PIN to cancer is an area of active research. Proving the benefit of a prevention strategy is difficult because of the long-term follow-up that is necessary, the large sample sizes required to demonstrate a difference in outcome, and the absence of surrogate measures that predict for efficacy. Agents under study include the retinoids, vitamin D, selenium, soy, and modifications of dietary fat. Most are based on epidemiologic data suggesting a decreased prostate cancer risk. A large-scale, double-blind, randomized, multicenter trial of finasteride in men over age 55 has accrued 18,000 men, and follow-up is awaited.

CLINICALLY LOCALIZED DISEASE Localized prostate cancer (stages T1-2, NX or 0, M0) may require no therapy, may be curable with localized therapy, or may require combined-modality systemic and local therapy. The key is to distinguish these distinct prognostic groups. Treatment planning includes an assessment of the probability of local control, local failure, and systemic failure. The more advanced the disease, the lower the probability of local control and the higher the probability of systemic relapse. In general, these tumors are managed by watchful waiting, radical surgery, or radiation therapy. Comparisons between these approaches are limited by the lack of prospective comparative trials, referral biases, and differences in the endpoints evaluated.

Conservative Management (Watchful Waiting) The concept of watchful waiting, or deferred therapy, evolved from the recognition of the high prevalence of the disease in the population, the low probability that some cancers would affect an individual's quality-adjusted life expectancy, and the fact that morbidities associated with the local treatment options were unacceptable to many patients. Watchful waiting acknowledges the facts that the natural history of an untreated prostate cancer is to progress and that it may be difficult to monitor progression within the gland so that the "window of curability" is not

lost. That the disease is often multifocal leads to the possibility that the biopsy on which the decision to defer therapy is made may not represent accurately the malignant potential of a second unidentified cancer. Within 10 years of diagnosis, most tumors produce local symptoms such as urinary retention, incontinence, hematuria, ureteral and bowel obstruction, and pelvic pain, but these complications rarely lead to the death of the patient. Some tumors may metastasize, but few patients succumb to the disease. Case selection criteria are evolving, but in general, watchful waiting is not advised for patients with high-grade disease or for those with a >10-year life expectancy. Some physicians consider observation only for patients with low-grade tumors (Gleason score ≤6) that do not involve more than a small percentage of a single core.

Radical Prostatectomy The objective of a radical prostatectomy is the removal of all prostate tissue with a clear margin of resection, preservation of the external sphincter to maintain continence, and sparing of the autonomic nerves in the neurovascular bundle so that potency is retained. The procedure is performed through a retropubic or perineal approach. In contemporary series, hospital stays are short; mortality <0.4%; and complications such as rectal injury, deep vein thrombosis, and embolic events are rare. The procedure is recommended primarily for patients with clinically localized disease (T1c–T3a, N0 or NX, M0 or MX) who have a life expectancy of >10 years. The operation is not justified in men with a life expectancy <5 years. Properly performed, the procedure requires appropriate case selection and meticulous technique that permits the delineation of the anatomy of the gland and surrounding tissues. In one review, the overall rate of positive margins was 25%. Careful planning can reduce this rate. For example, by considering the laterality and extent of disease, it may be apparent that nerve-sparing cannot be achieved without compromising cancer control. A positive margin increases the risk of progression significantly. Through PSA-based detection, the proportion of men with positive nodes and positive margins continues to decline.

Complication rates, specifically the probability of developing a bladder neck contracture, incontinence, or impotence, vary depending on the experience of the surgeon and whether the patient or the physician is describing the outcome. Rates of incontinence based on physician reporting are 5 to 10%, compared to 19 to 31% based on independent questioning by a third party. Time is also a consideration, as full recovery of function may not occur for weeks or months following the procedure. Factors associated with incontinence include older age, functional length of the urethra, surgical technique, preservation of neurovascular bundles, and development of an anastomotic stricture. If the nerves are preserved, ~70% of men recover the ability to achieve an erection sufficient for penetration. Most men are impotent immediately after the procedure and gradually recover function over 6 to 12 months. Often the quality of the erection is decreased from preoperative levels. Nevertheless, with orally active drugs such as sildenafil, intraurethral inserts of alprostadil, and intracavernosal injections of vasodilators, many patients can achieve nearly natural erections and recover satisfactory sexual activity. Factors associated with recovery include younger age, quality of erections before the operation, and the absence of damage to the neurovascular bundles. Loss of one bundle is associated with a 75% reduction in the recovery of function.

After a successful radical prostatectomy in which all prostate tissue has been removed, serum PSA levels should become undetectable within 4 weeks, based on the half-life of 3 days. If the PSA level remains detectable or becomes detectable after having been undetectable, the patient is considered to have persistent disease or to have a recurrence. In the absence of adjuvant treatment, most patients destined to recur do so within the first 5 years after surgery. Thus, one early benchmark of "success" is the probability of freedom from PSA (or "biochemical") progression. This varies as a function of initial clinical stage, Gleason grade, and serum PSA level before surgery. In one series of 1359 men with clinical stages T1/T2 cancer followed for a mean of 44 months (range 1 to 170), the PSA relapse–free survival rates were 78% at 5 years and 73% at 10 years. In a separate series of T1c patients, 89% were free of progression at 5 years. Considered by baseline PSA levels, 95% of those with a normal level (<4 ng/mL) and 68% of those with a PSA >10 ng/mL were free of progression at 5 years. Considered by grade or Gleason sum in the biopsy specimen, 5- and 10-year PSA relapse-free survivals were 56% and 46%, respectively, for those with tumors of Gleason score of 7, and 46 to 53% at 5 years for those with tumors of Gleason score ≥8. These outcomes appear superior to those reported with watchful waiting, recognizing the limitations in comparing the results of nonrandomized selected series.

The most significant predictor of recurrence is pathologic stage. When the disease is confined to the organ and has not extended into the periprostatic soft tissue, 91 to 97% of patients remain free of progression at 5 years and 85 to 92% at 10 years. Extension to the periprostatic soft tissues (pT3a and N0) decreases PSA relapse-free probabilities to 74% and 68% at 5 and 10 years, respectively, which is decreased further to 40 to 47% and 25% if there is seminal vesicle invasion (pT3c and N0). The high frequency of extracapsular extension and positive surgical margins in patients with clinically localized prostate cancers that were presumed to be confined to the gland led to the investigation of neoadjuvant hormonal therapy. The results of several large contemporary series evaluating 3 months of hormone therapy before surgery showed that, on average, positive margins are reduced from 41% to 17%, serum PSA levels by 96%, and prostate volume by 34% with neoadjuvant hormone therapy. The surrogate of a reduction in positive margin rates was not predictive of a reduction in failure rates, as the time to PSA relapse was no different between groups receiving and not receiving hormones. As such, neoadjuvant hormonal therapy is not recommended. Several recurrence models are available that incorporate all of these factors.

Radiation Therapy Radiation therapy can be delivered externally, by implantation of radioactive sources into the gland, or a combination of both. As is the case with surgery, outcomes vary as a function of the method, the dose, the endpoints, and whether outcomes were based on clinical or pathologic staging of the lymph nodes. Some groups report local control, and others PSA relapse-free survival, time to metastases, or overall survival. Cause-specific survivals are rarely reported. Local control can be reported on the basis of a DRE alone or the more stringent criterion of a negative biopsy at 18 to 24 months following treatment. Length of follow-up can also influence the results. To standardize reporting, the American Society of Therapeutic Radiation Oncology has developed a consensus definition of PSA relapse as three consecutive rising PSA values from the nadir value.

External beam therapy Overall, outcomes with external beam therapy are similar for patients with T1 and T2a disease to those obtained with radical surgery. Outcomes for patients with locally advanced disease (T2bc and T3/T4) are less favorable, the result of both inadequate control of the primary tumor and the high rate of systemic failure associated with more advanced disease. For the latter group, 30 to 40% of patients relapse locally using standard doses.

Conventional techniques use simulators and CT scans of the pelvis to determine the location and shape of the target volume and the surrounding normal organs. Typical treatment plans use a four-field pelvic box designed to include the prostate, seminal vesicles, and the locally draining lymph nodes. Normal structures are protected by shaping the beams with cerrobend trim blocks. Therapy is delivered on a daily basis, excepting weekends, in 1.8- to 2.0-Gy fractions. Outcomes are dose-dependent; in one series of stage C patients, actuarial 7-year local recurrence rates were 36% for those receiving 60 to 64.9 Gy, 32% for those receiving 65 to 69.9 Gy, and 24% for those treated at ≥70 Gy. Complication rates also increase with increasing dose. Using standard doses, grade 2 or greater rectal and/or urinary symptoms requiring medication occur in 60% of cases, while late sequelae such as cystitis, hematuria, stricture, or bladder contracture occur in 7% of cases. The frequency of adverse events is significantly higher in patients who have undergone a TURP, while the frequency of rectal complications is directly related to the volume of the anterior rectal wall receiving full-

dose treatment. The frequency of erectile dysfunction is related to the quality of erections before treatment, the dose administered, and the time of assessment. Impotence is related to a disruption of the vascular supply and not the nerve fibers.

More contemporary approaches use three-dimensional conformal radiation therapy (3D-CRT) techniques with sophisticated computer-generated treatment plans to deliver the prescribed radiation dose to the entire target volume, while conforming to the anatomic boundaries of the tumor in its entire three-dimensional configuration. This treatment method has increased the ability to control the cancer through the administration of higher radiation doses, with less morbidity to the surrounding normal organs. In a series of 743 patients treated with 3D-CRT, 90% of patients receiving 75.6 or 81.0 Gy achieved a PSA nadir of ≤1 ng/mL compared with 76% and 56% of those treated with 70.2 Gy and 64.8 Gy, respectively ($p < .001$).

As is the case with surgically treated patients, pre-therapy nomograms can be used to stratify patient groups. In one series, the 5-year actuarial PSA relapse-free survival for patients with favorable prognostic indicators (stage T1/T2, pretreatment PSA of 10.0 ng/mL, and Gleason score of 6) was 85%; it was 65% for those with an intermediate prognosis (one of the prognostic indicators with a higher value) and 35% for those with unfavorable features (two or more indicators with higher values) ($p < .001$).

Tolerance of 3D-CRT has been excellent despite the use of higher radiation doses; grade 3 to 4 rectal or urinary toxicities were seen in 2.1% of patients. In contrast, among patients treated with conventional external-beam radiotherapy, the incidence of grade 3 to 4 toxicities for patients who received radiation doses of >70 Gy was 6.9%.

To improve outcomes for patients with unfavorable features, several groups have explored hormone therapy before radiation therapy. Prospective randomized trials showed improved local control and a delay in time to PSA relapse in patients receiving 2 to 3 years of treatment. The impact on survival has been less clear.

Interstitial therapy Interstitial brachytherapy is based on the principle that the deposition of radiation energy in tissues decreases exponentially as a function of distance from the radiation source. By infiltrating tumor tissue with radioactive sources, intensive irradiation is delivered to the prostate with minimal irradiation of the surrounding tissues. In a series of 197 patients followed for a median of three years, 5-year actuarial PSA relapse-free survival for patients with pre-therapy PSA levels of 0 to 4, 4 to 10, and >10 were 98%, 90%, and 89%, respectively. Nevertheless, many physicians feel that implantation is best reserved for patients with good or intermediate prognostic features.

Overall, the procedure is well tolerated, although most patients experience urinary frequency and urgency, which can persist for several months. Incontinence has been seen in 2 to 4% of cases. Higher complication rates are observed in patients who have undergone a prior TURP or who have obstructive symptoms at baseline. Proctitis has been reported in <2% of patients. Longer follow-up will be necessary to see whether the overall frequency of impotence is lower, higher, or the same as that observed using external radiation delivery techniques.

RISING PSA Included in the group of patients with a rising PSA and no evidence of metastatic disease on scans are those who have progressed after watchful waiting, radical prostatectomy, radiation therapy, or both surgery and radiation, with or without prior hormone exposure. For these individuals, the issue is to determine whether the rising PSA is due to local persistence or recurrence (additional therapy to the primary site might be curative) or the result of micrometastatic disease. Imaging studies such as CT, MRI, or bone scan are typically uninformative. The objective is to assess the probability of disease progressing to the point where metastases will occur or cause symptoms. This is the point in the disease where the probability of death from disease exceeds the probability of death from other causes. Difficulty in making these predictions comes from the fact that most patients with a rising PSA receive some form of therapy before the development of metastatic disease, making it virtually impossible to assess the natural history.

To estimate the probability of having a local or systemic recurrence, many investigators use the time to PSA failure or the rate of rise of PSA as predictive factors. In general, recurrences documented >1 year after primary treatment tend to be localized, while those recurring in <1 year tend to be systemic. These predictions are not hard and fast. In one series of patients with PSA recurrence after surgery who did not receive systemic therapy until metastatic disease was documented, the median time to metastatic progression was 8 years, and 63% of the patients with rising PSA values remained free of metastases at 5 years. Patients with tumors of Gleason score 8 to 10 had a probability of metastatic progression of 37%, 51%, and 71% at 3, 5, and 7 years, respectively. Combining a high-grade histology and rapid PSA doubling time, the proportion with metastases was 23%, 32%, and 53% during the same time intervals if the time to recurrence was <2 years and the PSA doubling time was >10 months and 47%, 69%, and 79% for the same recurrence interval with <10 months doubling time. For those with tumors of Gleason score 5 to 7, a PSA recurrence in the first 2 years and a doubling time of <10 months identified a group of patients with a frequency of metastases of 19%, 65%, and 85% at 3, 5, and 7 years, respectively.

Prostascint scanning uses a radioactive antibody to prostate-specific membrane antigen (PSMA), which is highly expressed on prostate epithelial cells. For a patient who has undergone a radical prostatectomy, antibody localization to the prostatic fossa is suggestive of local recurrence, in which case external beam radiation therapy might be recommended. Others recommend that a biopsy of the urethrovesical anastamosis be obtained before considering radiation. Most, however, rely on clinical criteria with the additional caveat that the probability of durable PSA control varies inversely with the level of PSA at the start of radiation therapy. Radiation therapy is usually not recommended if the PSA level exceeds 1 to 2 ng/mL or if the PSA was persistently elevated after surgery (indicating that disease-free status was not achieved). For patients with a rising PSA after radiation therapy, a salvage prostatectomy can be considered if (1) residual disease is detected in the gland based on a repeat biopsy, (2) the tumor was amenable to surgical extirpation before radiation therapy, and (3) metastatic disease is absent on imaging studies. Unfortunately, case selection is poorly defined in most series, and morbidities have been significant. As currently performed, virtually all patients are impotent, and ~45% have either incontinence or stress incontinence. Bleeding, bladder neck contractures, and rectal injury are not uncommon.

METASTATIC DISEASE Noncastrate The removal or blockade of androgens by medical or surgical means is the mainstay of treatment for patients with advanced disease. Surgical orchiectomy is the "gold standard" but is the least preferred by patients. Medical therapies can be subdivided into those that result in a lowering of serum testosterone levels, e.g., gonadotropin-releasing hormone (GnRH) agonists and antagonists and estrogens, and the antiandrogens (Fig. 95-4). Inhibitors of adrenal enzyme synthesis such as ketoconazole and aminoglutethimide are typically used as second-line treatment. The antitumor effects of agents that lower serum testosterone levels are similar, but toxicities differ. Castration is associated with gynecomastia, impotence, weakness, fatigue, hot flushes, loss of muscle mass, changes in personality, anemia, depression, and loss of skeletal mass. Loss of bone mass can be reduced by coadministration of bisphosphonates.

GnRH analogues (leuprolide acetate and goserelin acetate) initially produce a rise in luteinizing hormone (LH) and follicle-stimulating hormone (FSH), followed by a downregulation of receptors in the pituitary gland, which effects a chemical castration. The initial rise in testosterone may result in a clinical flare of the disease. As such, these agents are contraindicated in men with significant obstructive symptoms, cancer-related pain, or spinal cord compromise. The flare can be prevented by pretreatment with antiandrogens. Pure GnRH antagonists that do not produce the initial rise in testosterone will shortly be available.

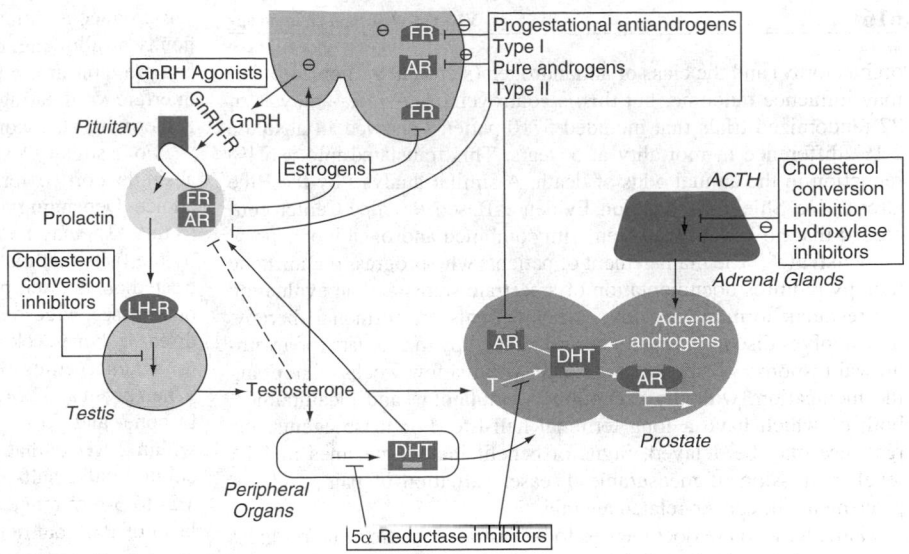

FIGURE 95-4 Sites of action of different hormone therapies.

Diethylstilbestrol (3 mg/d) produces castrate levels of testosterone in 1 to 2 weeks and is inexpensive. Its significant cardiovascular toxicities include edema, congestive heart failure, myocardial infarction, cerebrovascular accidents, phlebitis, and pulmonary embolism. Gynecomastia, a common adverse event, can be reduced by prophylactic irradiation of the breasts. Progestational agents such as medroxyprogesterone acetate (Provera) and megestrol acetate (Megace), are inferior to conventional castration and are not used as first-line treatment. The antifungal agent ketoconazole administered at a dose of 1200 mg/d (six times the antifungal dose) produces a chemical castration in 24 h. It is absorbed in an acid environment and typically prescribed with citrus juices to improve absorption; antacids or H_2 blocking agents reduce absorption and should be avoided when the pills are administered. The effects on testosterone synthesis, however, are not sustained, and long-term use is limited by hepatoxicity. It can be useful for the unusual patient who presents with a coagulopathy or spinal neurologic compromise and who requires a rapid response. Aminoglutethimide, a second adrenal synthesis inhibitor, was originally developed as an antiseizure medication. It is administered with hydrocortisone. Side effects include somnolence, fatigue, rash, and, after prolonged periods, hypothyroidism; its use is limited.

Nonsteroidal antiandrogens such as flutamide (Eulexin), bicalutamide (Casodex), or nilutamide (Anandron) block the binding of androgens to the receptor. They do not block the production of LH centrally, and as a result, serum testosterone levels increase. These drugs have been used clinically in several situations: (1) to block the flare from the initial rise in testosterone from GnRH use, (2) as monotherapy to preserve potency, and (3) as part of a combined androgen-blockade approach designed to simultaneously inhibit testicular and adrenal androgens. Toxicities differ among the agents but generally include gynecomastia (which can be significant), fatigue, elevations in serum transaminases, and diarrhea. The latter is the most common reason the drug is discontinued. Nilutamide is also associated with impaired adaptation to darkness, alcohol intolerance, and, rarely, pneumonitis.

Hormonal therapy is the treatment of choice, but the timing of treatment is not as clear. Early administration of hormones delays progression, but the survival benefit is less clear. It is controversial whether hormonal therapy should be initiated with a rising PSA level or whether treatment should be held until metastatic disease is detectable on scans. Most physicians recommend use of hormonal therapy with PSA elevation, based on evidence from clinical trials suggesting a survival advantage to such an approach.

A second controversy is whether a combined androgen-blockade that includes an antiandrogen is superior to castration without an antiandrogen. In randomized comparisons, both positive and negative trials have been reported but the majority have shown no difference. Some feel that the method of primary castration (GnRH analogue vs.

orchiectomy) and the class of antiandrogen (steroidal vs. nonsteroidal) may influence outcome, but this is controversial. A meta-analysis of 22 randomized trials that included 5710 patients showed an absolute 2.1% difference in mortality at 5 years. This translated into a 6.4% reduction in the annual odds of death. A similar analysis by the Blue Cross/Blue Shield Association Evidence-Based Practice Center concluded that no benefit was seen with combined androgen blockade.

Castrate   The management of patients who progress on hormone therapy requires documentation of a castrate status and an evaluation for residual hormone sensitivity. For patients on hormonal therapy, this involves discontinuing all hormonal therapy to evaluate for a withdrawal response. Responses are noted within a few weeks of stopping the medication, with the exception of nilutamide and bicalutamide, both of which have a long terminal half-life. For these agents, the response may be delayed. Signs of benefit include declines in PSA level, regression of measurable disease, palliation of pain, and improvements in cancer-related anemia.

Patients who are documented to be castrated, and/or who progress after a trial of withdrawal, are often given one additional hormonal manipulation. Depending on prior hormone exposure, options include inhibitors of adrenal steroid hormone synthesis such as ketoconazole and aminoglutethimide, glucocorticoids, antiandrogens, estrogens, or progestational agents. The responses are often short-lived and do not occur in the majority of patients. Nevertheless, the response can be durable in some patients and provide significant palliation in the absence of curative therapies. Glucocorticoids have been associated with clinical benefit and declines in PSA levels in 30 to 40% of cases.

Estramustine (Emcyt) is a synthetic combination of estrogen with a nitrogen mustard moiety at C17 that affects microtubule assembly and disassembly. It has no alkylating effects in vivo. About 20% of the drug is metabolized to pure estrogenic moieties, which exert an antigonadotropin effect and which account for the side effect profile. It is often used in patients who have failed hormone therapy and has additive/synergistic effects with other drugs including the vinca alkaloids (vinblastine and navelbine), taxanes (paclitaxel, docetaxel), and the podophyllotoxins (etoposide).

Patients who progress on primary hormone therapy and after hormone withdrawal and receive one additional (second-line) intervention are considered to have "hormone-independent" or "hormone-refractory" disease. At this point, chemotherapy is often considered, although some feel it has no role in the management of prostate cancer because no single agent or combination of drugs has been shown to improve survival in a prospective randomized trial. In the absence of a proven benefit in survival, it is important to consider the specific goals of therapy before it is recommended. These goals might include palliation of symptoms, delaying progression, or inducing decreases in the PSA level. Interpreting reported outcomes with individual agents is limited in part by differences in case selection and the wide range of endpoints used.

Mitoxantrone has modest activity as a single agent and is more effective at relieving pain and improving quality of life when given together with prednisone. No effect on survival has been shown. However, mitoxantrone plus prednisone and estramustine plus vinblastine are often used to palliate symptoms of disease. The most frequently utilized contemporary regimens are weekly combinations of estramustine and a taxane (paclitaxel or docetaxel). Weekly doxorubin also provides palliation.

PALLIATION OF PAIN   Pain is one of the most feared debilitating manifestations of advanced disease. Palliation of pain can be achieved with external beam radiation therapy, bone-seeking radioisotopes, cold bisphosphonates, and chemotherapy. The goals are to relieve symptoms, prevent complications, and improve quality-adjusted life expectancy. To optimize treatment selection, it is important to consider the sites and distribution of the pain and the presence or absence of neurologic compromise. Spinal cord compression is one of the most devastating complications. Once a loss of function is documented, the probability of recovery is small. Particular areas where a high index of suspicion is required are the base of the skull, which can produce a variety of symptoms including diplopia, deafness, difficulty swallowing, dysarthria, and facial weakness; and mental nerve compression in the jaw, resulting in a numb lip and chin, which can interfere with eating. In these situations, external beam radiation together with glucocorticoids are required.

For a solitary lesion that is symptomatic and can be treated through a single port, external beam radiation therapy is the treatment of choice. Depending on the clinical situation, a single high-dose fraction (6 to 9 Gy) may be all that is necessary. The overall utility is limited by the facts that metastases are rarely solitary and that additional untreated areas often become symptomatic in a relatively short time. In other cases, wide-field portals are needed. For those with more diffuse disease, bone-seeking radioisotopes are available. ^{153}Sm-EDTMP (quadramet) emits β particles and a photon; its half-life is about 22 h. When given at 37 MBq/kg (1 mCi/kg), half the administered dose goes to bone, and 70 to 95% of patients experience decreased bone pain within 2 weeks that lasts 8 to 15 weeks. ^{89}Sr (metastron) is a pure β-emitter with a half-life of 50 days that emits a 1.46-MeV electron with a 2- to 3-mm range in bone. Used alone it has modest effects on the level of PSA but does provide a degree of palliation that is similar to external beam approaches. The results of randomized comparisons suggest a systemic effect, as fewer patients treated with the isotope developed new areas of pain or required additional radiation therapy compared to patients receiving radiation therapy alone. Cold bisphosphonates have been shown to be superior to placebo in the prevention of skeletal events for patients with breast cancer, lung cancer, and multiple myeloma. They may be active in prostate cancer as well.

ACKNOWLEDGMENT

Dr. Jean Wilson and Dr. Arthur Sagalowski were the authors of this chapter in the 14th edition and parts of their chapter have been retained here.

BIBLIOGRAPHY

BENIGN PROSTATIC HYPERPLASIA

CORDON-CARDO C et al: Distinct altered patterns of p27kip1 expression in benign prostatic hyperplasia and prostatic carcinoma. J Natl Cancer Inst 90:1284, 1998

GROSSFELD GD, COAKLEY FV: Benign prostatic hyperplasia: Clinical overview and value of diagnostic imaging. Radiol Clin North Am 38:31, 2000

McCONNELL JD et al: The effect of finasteride on the risk of acute urinary retention and the need for surgical treatment among men with benign prostatic hyperplasia. N Engl J Med 338:557, 1998

PROSTATE CANCER

ALBERTSEN PC et al: Competing risk analysis of men aged 55 to 74 years at diagnosis managed conservatively for clinically localized prostate cancer. JAMA 280:975, 1998

CARTER H et al: Prostate-specific antigen testing of older men. J Natl Cancer Inst 91: 1733, 1999

KATTAN MW et al: Postoperative nomogram for disease recurrence after radical prostatectomy for prostate cancer. J Clin Oncol 17:1499, 1999

OSOBA D et al: Health-related quality of life in men with metastatic prostate cancer treated with prednisone alone or mitxantrone and prednisone. J Clin Oncol 17:1654, 1999

POUND CR et al: Natural history of progression to metastases and death from prostate cancer in men with PSA recurrence following radical prostatectomy. JAMA 281:1591, 1999

SCHER HI, HELLER G: Clinical states in prostate cancer: Towards a dynamic model of disease progression. Urology 55:323, 2000

SELTZER MA et al: Comparison of helical computerized tomography, positron emission tomography and monoclonal antibody scans for evaluation of lymph node metastases in patients with prostate specific antigen relapse after treatment for localized prostate cancer. J Urol 162:1322, 1999

96   *Robert J. Motzer, George J. Bosl*

TESTICULAR CANCER

Primary germ cell tumors (GCTs) of the testis, arising by the malignant transformation of primordial germ cells, constitute 95% of all testicular neoplasms. Infrequently, GCTs arise from an extragonadal site, including the mediastinum, retroperitoneum and, very rarely, the pineal gland. This disease is notable for the young age of the afflicted patients, the totipotent capacity for differentiation of the tumor cells, and its curability; >90% of all newly diagnosed patients will be cured. Experience in the management of GCTs leads to improved outcome.

INCIDENCE AND EPIDEMIOLOGY Nearly 6900 new cases of testicular GCT were diagnosed in the United States in 2000; the incidence of this malignancy has increased slowly over the past 40 years. The tumor occurs most frequently in men between the ages of 20 and 40. A testicular mass in a man 50 years or older should be regarded as a lymphoma until proved otherwise. GCT is at least 4 to 5 times more common in white than in African-American males, and a higher incidence has been observed in Scandinavia and New Zealand than in the United States.

ETIOLOGY AND GENETICS Cryptorchidism is associated with a severalfold higher risk of GCT. Abdominal cryptorchid testes are at a higher risk than inguinal cryptorchid testes. Orchiopexy should be performed before puberty, if possible. Early orchiopexy reduces the risk of GCT and improves the ability to save the testis. An abdominal cryptorchid testis that cannot be brought into the scrotum should be removed. About 2% of men with GCTs of one testis will develop a primary tumor in the other testis. Testicular feminization syndromes increase the risk of testicular GCT, and Klinefelter's syndrome is associated with mediastinal GCT.

An isochromosome of the short arm of chromosome 12 [i(12p)] is pathognomonic for GCT of all histologic types. Excess 12p copy number either in the form of i(12p) or as increased 12p on aberrantly banded marker chromosomes occurs in nearly all GCT, but the gene(s) on 12p involved in the pathogenesis are not yet defined.

CLINICAL PRESENTATION A painless testicular mass is pathognomonic for a testicular malignancy. More commonly, patients present with testicular discomfort or swelling suggestive of epididymitis and/or orchitis. In this circumstance, a trial of antibiotics is reasonable. However, if symptoms persist or a residual abnormality remains, then testicular ultrasound examination is indicated.

Ultrasound of the testis is indicated whenever a testicular malignancy is considered and for persistent or painful testicular swelling. If a testicular mass is detected, a radical inguinal orchiectomy should be performed. Because the testis develops from the gonadal ridge, its blood supply and lymphatic drainage originate in the abdomen and descend with the testis into the scrotum. An inguinal approach is taken to avoid breaching anatomic barriers and permitting additional pathways of spread.

Back pain from retroperitoneal metastases is common and must be distinguished from musculoskeletal pain. Dyspnea from pulmonary metastases occurs infrequently. Patients with increased serum levels of human chorionic gonadotropin (hCG) may present with gynecomastia. A delay in diagnosis is associated with a more advanced stage and possibly worse survival.

The staging evaluation for GCT includes a determination of serum levels of α fetoprotein (AFP) and hCG. After orchiectomy, a chest radiograph and a computed tomography (CT) scan of the abdomen and pelvis should be performed. A chest CT scan is required if pulmonary nodules, mediastinal or hilar disease is suspected. *Stage I disease* is limited to the testis, epididymis, or spermatic cord. *Stage II disease* is limited to retroperitoneal (regional) lymph nodes. *Stage III disease* is disease outside the retroperitoneum, involving supradiaphragmatic nodal sites or viscera. The staging may be "clinical"—defined solely by physical examination, blood marker evaluation, and radiographs—or "pathologic"—defined by an operative procedure.

The regional draining lymph nodes for the testis are in the retroperitoneum, and the vascular supply originates from the great vessels (for the right testis) or the renal vessels (for the left testis). As a result, the lymph nodes that are involved first by a right testicular tumor are the interaortocaval lymph nodes just below the renal vessels. For a left testicular tumor, the first involved lymph nodes are lateral to the aorta (para-aortic) and below the left renal vessels. In both cases, further nodal spread is inferior and contralateral and, less commonly, above the renal hilum. Lymphatic involvement can extend cephalad to the retrocrural, posterior mediastinal, and supraclavicular lymph nodes.

Treatment is determined by tumor histology (seminoma versus nonseminoma) and clinical stage (Table 96-1).

PATHOLOGY GCTs are divided into nonseminoma and seminoma subtypes. Nonseminomatous GCTs are most frequent in the third decade of life and can display the full spectrum of embryonic and adult cellular differentiation. This entity comprises four histologies: embryonal carcinoma, teratoma, choriocarcinoma, and endodermal sinus (yolk sac) tumor. Choriocarcinoma, consisting of both cytotrophoblasts and syncytiophoblasts, represents malignant trophoblastic differentiation and is invariably associated with secretion of hCG. Endodermal sinus tumor is the malignant counterpart of the fetal yolk sac and is associated with secretion of AFP. Pure embryonal carcinoma may secrete AFP or hCG, or both; this pattern is biochemical evidence of differentiation. Teratoma is composed of somatic cell types derived from two or more germ layers (ectoderm, mesoderm, or endoderm). Each of these histologies may be present alone or in combination with others. Nonseminomatous GCTs tend to metastasize early to sites such as the retroperitoneal lymph nodes and lung parenchyma. One-third of patients present with disease limited to the testis (stage I), one-third with retroperitoneal metastases (stage II), and one-third with more extensive supradiaphragmatic nodal or visceral metastases (stage III).

Seminoma represents about 50% of all GCTs, has a median age in the fourth decade, and generally follows a more indolent clinical course. Most patients (70%) present with stage I disease, about 20% with stage II disease, and 10% with stage III disease; lung or other visceral metastases are rare. Radiation therapy is the treatment of choice in patients with stage I disease and stage II disease where the nodes are <5 cm in maximum diameter. When a tumor contains both seminoma and nonseminoma components, patient management is directed by the more aggressive nonseminoma component.

TUMOR MARKERS Careful monitoring of the serum tumor markers AFP and hCG is essential in the management of patients with GCT, as these markers are important for diagnosis, as prognostic indicators, in monitoring treatment response, and in the detection of early relapse. Approximately 70% of patients presenting with disseminated nonseminomatous GCT have increased serum concentrations of AFP and/or hCG. While hCG concentrations may be increased in patients with either nonseminoma or seminoma histology, the AFP concentration is increased only in patients with nonseminoma. The presence of an increased AFP level in a patient whose tumor showed only seminoma indicates that an occult nonseminomatous component exists and that the patient should be treated accordingly for nonseminomatous GCT. The serum lactate dehydrogenase (LDH) level serves as an additional marker of all GCTs, but it is not as specific as either AFP or

Table 96-1   Germ Cell Tumor Staging and Treatment

Stage	Extent of Disease	Treatment Seminoma	Nonseminoma
I	Testis only, T1, no vascular/lymphatic invasion	Radiation therapy	RPLND or observation
II	T2–4 or vascular/lymphatic invasion present	Radiation therapy	RPLND
IIA	Nodes <2 cm	Radiation therapy	RPLND or chemotherapy often followed by RPLND
IIB	Nodes 2–5 cm	Radiation therapy	RPLND +/− adjuvant chemotherapy or chemotherapy followed by RPLND
IIC	Nodes >5 cm	Chemotherapy	Chemotherapy
III	Distant metastases	Chemotherapy	Chemotherapy, often followed by surgery (biopsy or resection)

hCG. LDH levels are increased in 50 to 60% patients with metastatic nonseminoma and in up to 80% of patients with advanced seminoma.

AFP, hCG, and LDH levels should be determined before and after orchiectomy. Increased serum AFP and hCG concentrations decay according to first-order kinetics; the half-life is 24 to 36 h for hCG and 5 to 7 days for AFP. AFP and hCG should be assayed serially during and after treatment. The reappearance of hCG and/or AFP or the failure of these markers to decline according to the predicted half-life is an indicator of persistent or recurrent tumor.

℞ **TREATMENT**   **Stage I Nonseminoma**   If, after an orchiectomy (for clinical stage I disease), radiographs and physical examination show no evidence of disease, and serum AFP and hCG concentrations either are normal or are declining to normal according to the known half-life, patients may be managed by either a nerve-sparing retroperitoneal lymph node dissection (RPLND) or surveillance. The retroperitoneal lymph nodes are pathologically involved by GCT (pathologic stage II) in 20 to 50% of these patients. The choice of surveillance or RPLND is based on the pathology of the primary tumor. If the primary tumor shows no pathologic evidence for lymphatic or vascular invasion *and* is limited to the testis (T1), then either option is reasonable. If lymphatic or vascular invasion is present *or* the tumor extends into the tunica, spermatic cord, or scrotum (T2 through T4), then surveillance should not be offered. Either approach should cure >95% of patients.

A RPLND is the standard operation for removal of the regional lymph nodes of the testis (retroperitoneal nodes). The operation removes the lymph nodes ipsilateral to the primary site and the nodal groups adjacent to the primary landing zone. The standard (modified bilateral) RPLND removes all node-bearing tissue down to the bifurcation of the great vessels, including the ipsilateral iliac nodes. The major long-term effect of this operation is retrograde ejaculation and infertility. A nerve-sparing RPLND, usually accomplished by identification and dissection of individual nerve fibers, may avoid injury to the sympathetic nerves responsible for ejaculation. Normal ejaculation is preserved in approximately 90% of patients. Patients with pathologic stage I disease are observed, and only the 10% who relapse require additional therapy. If retroperitoneal nodes are found to be involved at RPLND, then a decision regarding adjuvant chemotherapy is made on the basis of the extent of retroperitoneal disease (see below).

Surveillance is an option in the management of clinical stage I disease when no vascular/lymphatic invasion is found and the primary tumor is classified as T1. Only 20 to 30% of patients have pathologic stage II disease, implying that most RPLNDs in this situation are not therapeutic. Although surveillance has not been compared to RPLND in a randomized trial, all large studies show that surveillance and RPLND lead to equivalent long-term survival rates. Patient compliance is essential if surveillance is to be successful. Patients must be carefully followed with periodic chest radiography, physical examination, CT scan of the abdomen, and serum tumor marker determinations. The median time to relapse is about 7 months, and late relapses (later than 2 years) are rare. The 70 to 80% of patients who do not relapse require no intervention after orchiectomy; treatment is reserved for those who do relapse. When the primary tumor is classified as T2 through T4 *or* lymphatic/vascular invasion is identified, nerve-sparing RPLND is preferred. About 50% of these patients have pathologic stage II disease and are destined to relapse.

Stage II Nonseminoma   Patients with limited, ipsilateral retroperitoneal adenopathy (nodes usually ≤3 cm in largest diameter) generally undergo a modified bilateral RPLND as primary management. Nearly all patients with pathologic stage II disease whose disease is completely resected by RPLND are cured. The local recurrence rate after a properly performed RPLND is very low. Depending on the extent of disease, the postoperative management options include either surveillance or two cycles of adjuvant chemotherapy. Surveillance is

the preferred approach for patients with resected "low-volume" metastases (tumor nodes ≤2 cm in diameter, *and* <6 nodes are involved) because the probability of relapse is one-third or less. Because relapse occurs in ≥50% of patients with "high-volume" metastasis (>6 nodes involved, *or* any involved node >2 cm in largest diameter, *or* extranodal tumor extension), two cycles of adjuvant chemotherapy should be considered, as it results in cure in ≥98% of patients. Regimens consisting of etoposide (100 mg/m² daily on days 1 through 5) plus cisplatin (20 mg/m² daily on days 1 through 5) with or without bleomycin (30 units per day on days 2, 9, and 16) given at 3-week intervals are effective and well tolerated.

Stages I and II Seminoma   Inguinal orchiectomy followed by retroperitoneal radiation therapy cures about 98% of patients with stage I seminoma. The dose of radiation (2500 to 3000 cGy) is low and well tolerated, and the in-field recurrence rate is negligible. About 2% of patients relapse with supradiaphragmatic or systemic disease. Surveillance has been proposed as an option, and studies have shown that about 15% of patients relapse. The median time to relapse is 12 to 15 months, and late relapses during surveillance (>5 years) may be more frequent than with nonseminoma. The relapse is usually treated with chemotherapy. Surveillance for clinical stage I seminoma is generally not recommended.

Nonbulky retroperitoneal disease (stage IIA and IIB) is also treated with radiation therapy. Prophylactic supradiaphragmatic fields are not used. Relapses in the anterior mediastinum are unusual. Approximately 90% of patients achieve relapse-free survival with retroperitoneal masses <5 cm in diameter. Because at least one-third of patients with bulkier disease relapse, initial chemotherapy is preferred for stage IIC disease.

Chemotherapy for Advanced GCT   Regardless of histology, patients with stage IIC and stage III GCT are treated with chemotherapy. Combination chemotherapy programs based on cisplatin at doses of 100 to 120 mg/m² per cycle plus etoposide cure 70 to 80% of such patients, with or without bleomycin, depending on risk stratification (see below). A complete response (the complete disappearance of all clinical evidence of tumor on physical examination and radiography plus normal serum levels of AFP and hCG for 1 month or more) occurs after chemotherapy alone in about 60% of patients, and another 10 to 20% become disease-free with surgical resection of all sites of residual disease. Lower doses of cisplatin result in inferior survival rates.

The toxicity of the cisplatin/bleomycin/etoposide (BEP) regimen may be substantial. Nausea, vomiting, and hair loss occur in most patients, although nausea and vomiting have been markedly ameliorated by modern antiemetic regimens. Myelosuppression is frequent, and symptomatic bleomycin pulmonary toxicity occurs in about 5% of patients. Treatment-induced mortality due to neutropenia with septicemia or bleomycin-induced pulmonary failure occurs in 1 to 3% of patients. Dose reductions for myelosuppression are rarely indicated. Long-term permanent toxicities include nephrotoxicity (reduced glomerular filtration and persistent magnesium wasting), ototoxicity, and peripheral neuropathy. When bleomycin is administered by weekly bolus injection, Raynaud's phenomenon appears in 5 to 10% of patients. Less often, other evidence of small blood vessel damage has been reported, including transient ischemic attacks and myocardial infarction.

Risk-Directed Chemotherapy   Because not all patients are cured and treatment may cause significant toxicities, patients are stratified into "good-risk" and "poor-risk" groups according to pretreatment clinical features. For good-risk patients, the goal is to achieve maximum efficacy with minimal toxicity. For poor-risk patients, the goal is to identify more effective therapy with tolerable toxicity.

The International Germ Cell Cancer Consensus Group (IGCCCG) developed criteria to assign patients to three risk groups (good, intermediate, poor) (Table 96-2). Seminoma is either good or intermediate risk based on the absence or presence of nonpulmonary visceral metastases. Marker levels play no role in defining risk. No poor-risk category exists for seminoma. Nonseminomas have good-, intermediate-, and poor-risk categories based on the site of the primary tumor,

Table 96-2 IGCCCG Risk Classification for Advanced Germ Cell Tumors

Risk Group	Nonseminoma	Seminoma
Good	Gonadal or retroperitoneal primary site, no nonpulmonary visceral metastases, AFP <1000 ng/mL, beta-hCG < mIU/mL, LDH <1.5 × upper limit of normal (ULN)	Any primary site, no nonpulmonary visceral metastases, any LDH are hCG levels
Intermediate	Gonadal or retroperitoneal primary site, no nonpulmonary visceral metastases, AFP 1000–10000 ng/mL, beta-hCG 5000–50000 mIU/mL, LDH 1.5–10 × ULN	Any primary site, non-pulmonary visceral metastases present, any LDH and hCG levels
Poor	Mediastinal primary site, nonpulmonary visceral metastases present, AFP ≥10000 ng/ML, beta-hCG >50,000 mIU/mL, LDH >10 × ULN	No patients classified as poor risk

the presence or absence of nonpulmonary visceral metastases, and marker levels.

For ~90% of patients with good-risk GCTs, four cycles of etoposide plus cisplatin (EP) or three cycles of BEP produce durable, complete responses, with minimal acute and chronic toxicity. Pulmonary toxicity is absent when bleomycin is not used and is rare when therapy is limited to 9 weeks; myelosuppression with neutropenic fever is less frequent; and the treatment mortality rate is negligible. About 75% of intermediate-risk patients and 45% of poor-risk patients achieve durable complete remission with four cycles of BEP, and no regimen has proved superior. More effective therapy is needed.

Postchemotherapy Surgery Resection of residual metastases after the completion of chemotherapy is an integral part of therapy. If the initial histology is nonseminoma and the marker values have normalized, all sites of residual disease should be resected. In general, residual retroperitoneal disease requires a modified bilateral RPLND, which is associated with retrograde ejaculation. Thoracotomy (unilateral or bilateral) and neck dissection are less frequently required to remove residual mediastinal, pulmonary parenchymal, or cervical nodal disease. Viable tumor (seminoma, embryonal carcinoma, yolk sac tumor, or choriocarcinoma) will be present in 15%, mature teratoma in 40%, and necrotic debris and fibrosis in 45% of resected specimens. The frequency of teratoma or viable disease is highest in residual mediastinal tumors. If necrotic debris or mature teratoma is present, no further chemotherapy is necessary. If viable tumor is present but completely excised, two additional cycles of chemotherapy are given.

If the initial histology is seminoma, mature teratoma is rarely present, and the most frequent finding is necrotic debris. For residual retroperitoneal disease, a complete RPLND is technically difficult owing to extensive postchemotherapy fibrosis. Observation is recommended when no radiographic abnormality exists or a residual mass <3 cm is present. Controversy exists over what to do when the residual mass exceeds 3 cm in diameter. About 25% of such masses contain viable GCT. Some investigators prefer excision or biopsy, but radiation therapy and surveillance are alternatives.

Salvage Chemotherapy Of patients with advanced GCT, 20 to 30% fail to achieve a durable complete response to first-line chemotherapy. A combination of cisplatin, ifosfamide and vinblastine (VeIP) will cure about 25% of patients as a second-line therapy. Patients are more likely to achieve a durable complete response to VeIP if they had a testicular primary tumor and relapsed from a prior complete remission to first-line cisplatin-containing chemotherapy. In contrast, if the patient failed to achieve a complete response or has a primary mediastinal nonseminoma, then VeIP is rarely beneficial. Those patients are candidates for dose-intensive treatment.

Chemotherapy consisting of dose-intensive, high-dose carboplatin (≥1500 mg/m²) plus etoposide (≥1200 mg/m²), with or without cyclophosphamide or ifosfamide, with peripheral blood stem cell support induces a complete response in 25 to 40% of patients who have progressed after ifosfamide-containing salvage chemotherapy. About one-half of the complete responses will be durable. High-dose therapy is the treatment of choice and standard of care for this patient population. Paclitaxel is active in previously treated patients and is being studied as a new component in conventional-dose and dose-intensive salvage therapy. Cure is still possible in some relapsed patients.

EXTRAGONADAL GCT AND MIDLINE CARCINOMA OF UNCERTAIN HISTOGENESIS The prognosis and management of patients with extragonadal GCTs depends on the tumor histology and site of origin. All patients with a diagnosis of extragonadal GCT should have a testicular ultrasound examination. Nearly all patients with retroperitoneal or mediastinal seminoma achieve a durable complete response to BEP or EP. The clinical features of patients with primary retroperitoneal nonseminoma GCT are similar to those of patients with a primary of testis origin, and careful evaluation will find evidence of a primary testicular GCT in about two-thirds of cases. In contrast, a primary mediastinal nonseminomatous GCT is associated with a poor prognosis; one-third of patients are cured with standard therapy (four cycles of BEP). Patients with newly diagnosed mediastinal nonseminoma are considered to have poor-risk disease and should be considered for clinical trials testing regimens of possibly greater efficacy. In addition, mediastinal nonseminoma is associated with hematologic disorders, including acute myelogenous leukemia, myelodysplastic syndrome, and essential thrombocytosis unrelated to previous chemotherapy. These hematologic disorders are very refractory to treatment. Nonseminoma of any primary site may change into other malignant histologies such as embryonal rhabdomyosarcoma or adenocarcinoma. This is called malignant transformation. i(12p) has been identified in the transformed cell type, indicating GCT clonal origin.

A group of patients (most commonly men) with poorly differentiated tumors of unknown histogenesis, midline in distribution, and not associated with secretion of AFP or hCG has been described; a few (10 to 20%) are cured by standard cisplatin-containing chemotherapy. i(12p) is present in about 25% of such tumors (the fraction that are cisplatin-responsive), confirming their origin from primitive germ cells. This finding is also predictive of the response to cisplatin-based chemotherapy and resulting long-term survival. These tumors are heterogeneous; neuroepithelial tumors and lymphoma may also present in this fashion.

FERTILITY Infertility is an important consequence of the treatment of GCTs. Preexisting infertility or impaired fertility is often present. Azoospermia and/or oligospermia are present at diagnosis in at least 50% of patients with testicular GCTs. Ejaculatory dysfunction is associated with RPLND, and germ cell damage may result from cisplatin-containing chemotherapy. Nerve-sparing techniques to preserve the retroperitoneal sympathetic nerves have made retrograde ejaculation less likely in the subgroups of patients who are candidates for this operation. Spermatogenesis does recur in some patients after chemotherapy. However, because of the significant risk of impaired reproductive capacity, semen analysis and cryopreservation of sperm in a sperm bank should be recommended to all patients before radiation therapy, chemotherapy, or RPLND.

BIBLIOGRAPHY

Bosl GJ et al: Testicular germ-cell cancer. N Engl J Med 337:242, 1997

Chaganti RSK et al: Molecular biology of adult male germ cell tumors, in *Comprehensive Tetbook of Genitourinary Oncology*, NJ Vogelzang, PT Scardino, WO Shipley, DS Coffey (eds). Baltimore, Williams and Wilkins, 1999

Einhorn LH et al: Evaluation of optimal duration of chemitherapy in favorable-prognosis disseminated germ cell tumors: A Southeastern Cancer Study Group protocol. J Clin Oncol 7:387, 1989

INTERNATIONAL GERM CELL CANCER CONSENSUS GROUP: International Germ Cell Consensus Classification: A prognostic factor-based staging system for metastatic germ cell cancers. J Clin Oncol 15:594, 1997

LOEHRER PJ et al: Vinblastine plus ifosfamide plus cisplatin as initial salvage therapy in recurrent germ cell tumor. J Clin Oncol 16:2500, 1998

SIEGERT W et al: Germ cell tumors: dose-intensive therapy. Semin Oncol 25:215, 1998

97   Robert C. Young

GYNECOLOGIC MALIGNANCIES

OVARIAN CANCER

Incidence and Epidemiology Epithelial ovarian cancer is the leading cause of death from gynecologic cancer in the United States. In 2000, 23,100 new cases were diagnosed and 14,000 women died from ovarian cancer. The disease accounts for 5% of all cancer deaths in women in the United States; more women die of this disease than from cervical and endometrial cancer combined.

The age-specific incidence of the common epithelial type of ovarian cancer increases progressively and peaks in the eighth decade. Epithelial tumors, unlike germ cell and stromal tumors, are uncommon before the age of 40. Epidemiologic studies suggest higher incidences in industrialized nations and an association with disordered ovarian function, including infertility, nulliparity, frequent miscarriages, and use of ovulation-inducing drugs such as clomiphene. Each pregnancy reduces the ovarian cancer risk by about 10%, and breast feeding and tubal ligation also appear to reduce the risk. Oral contraceptives reduce the risk of ovarian cancer in patients with a familial history of cancer and in the general population. Many of these risk-reduction factors support the "incessant ovulation" hypothesis for ovarian cancer etiology, which implies that an aberrant repair process of the surface epithelium is central to ovarian cancer development. Estrogen replacement after menopause does not appear to increase the risk of ovarian cancer, although one study showed a modest increase in risk with >11 years of use.

Familial cases account for about 5% of all ovarian cancer, and a family history of ovarian cancer is a major risk factor. Compared to a lifetime risk of 1.6% in the general population, women with one affected first-degree relative have a 5% risk. In families with two or more affected first-degree relatives, the risk may exceed 50%. Three types of autosomal dominant familial cancer are recognized: (1) site-specific in which only ovarian cancer is seen, (2) families with cancer of the ovary and breast, and (3) the Lynch type II cancer family syndrome with nonpolyposis colorectal cancer, endometrial cancer, and ovarian cancer.

Etiology and Genetics In women with hereditary breast-ovarian cancer, two susceptibility loci have been identified: BRCA-1, located on chromosome 17q12-21, and BRCA-2, on 13q12-13. Both are tumor suppressor genes, and their protein products act as inhibitors of tumor growth. Both genes are large, and numerous mutations have been described; most are frameshift or nonsense mutations, and 86% produce truncated protein products. The implications of the many other mutations including many missense mutations are not known. The cumulative risk of ovarian cancer with critical mutations of BRCA-1 or -2 is 25%, compared to the lifetime risk of 50% for breast cancer for similar mutations. Men in such families have an increased risk of prostate cancer.

Cytogenetic analysis of sporadic epithelial ovarian cancers generally reveals complex karyotypic rearrangements. Structural abnormalities frequently appear on chromosomes 1 and 11, and loss of heterozygosity (LOH) is common on 3q, 6q, 11q, 13q, and 17.

Abnormalities of oncogenes are frequently found in ovarian cancer and include c-*myc*, H-*ras*, K-*ras*, and *neu*.

Ovarian tumors (usually not epithelial) are sometimes components of complex genetic syndromes. Peutz-Jeghers syndrome (mucocutaneous pigmentation and intestinal polyps) is associated with ovarian sex cord stromal tumors and Sertoli cell tumors in men. Patients with gonadal dysgenesis (46XY genotype or mosaic for Y-containing cell lines) develop gonadoblastomas, and women with nevoid basal cell carcinomas have an increased risk of ovarian fibromas.

Clinical Presentation and Differential Diagnosis Most patients with ovarian cancer are first diagnosed when the disease has already spread beyond the true pelvis. The occurrence of abdominal pain, bloating, and urinary symptoms usually indicates advanced disease. Localized ovarian cancer is generally asymptomatic. However, progressive enlargement of a localized ovarian tumor can produce urinary frequency or constipation, and rarely torsion of an ovarian mass causes acute abdominal pain or a surgical abdomen. In contrast to cervical or endometrial cancer, vaginal bleeding or discharge is rarely seen with early ovarian cancer. The diagnosis of early disease usually occurs with palpation of an asymptomatic adnexal mass during routine pelvic examination. However, most ovarian enlargements discovered this way, especially in premenopausal women, are benign functional cysts that characteristically resolve over one to three menstrual cycles. Adnexal masses in premenarchal or postmenopausal women are more likely to be pathologic. A solid, irregular, fixed pelvic mass is usually ovarian cancer. Other causes of adnexal masses include pedunculated uterine fibroids, endometriosis, benign ovarian neoplasms, and inflammatory lesions of the bowel.

Evaluation of patients with suspected ovarian cancer should include measurement of serum levels of the tumor marker CA-125. CA-125 determinants are glycoproteins with molecular masses from 220 to 1000 kDa, and a radioimmunoassay is used to determine circulating CA-125 antigen levels. Between 80 and 85% of patients with epithelial ovarian cancer have levels of CA-125 ≥35 U/mL. Other malignant tumors can also elevate CA-125 levels, including cancers of the endometrium, cervix, fallopian tubes, pancreas, breast, lung, and colon. Certain nonmalignant conditions that can elevate CA-125 levels include pregnancy, endometriosis, pelvic inflammatory disease, and uterine fibroids. About 1% of normal females have serum CA-125 levels >35 U/mL. However, in postmenopausal women with an asymptomatic pelvic mass and CA-125 levels ≥65 U/mL, the test has a sensitivity of 97% and a specificity of 78%.

Screening In contrast to patients who present with advanced disease, patients with early ovarian cancers (stages I and II) are commonly curable with conventional therapy. Thus, effective screening procedures would improve the cure rate in this disease. Although pelvic examination can occasionally detect early disease, it is a relatively insensitive screening procedure. Transvaginal sonography has replaced the slower and less sensitive abdominal sonography, but significant false-positive results are noted, particularly in premenopausal women. In one study, 67 laparotomies were required to diagnose 1 primary ovarian cancer. Doppler flow imaging coupled with transvaginal ultrasound may improve accuracy and reduce the high rate of false positives.

CA-125 has been studied as a screening tool. Unfortunately, half of women with stages I and II ovarian cancer have CA-125 levels <65 U/mL. Other nonmalignant disorders can elevate the CA-125 level, and both false-negative and -positive results have been high in most screening studies.

Attempts have been made to improve the sensitivity and specificity by combinations of procedures, commonly transvaginal ultrasound and CA-125 levels. In a screening study of 22,000 women, 42 had a positive screen and 11 had ovarian cancer (7 with advanced disease). In addition, eight women with a negative screen developed ovarian cancer. Thus, the false-positive rate would lead to a large number of unnecessary (i.e., negative) laparotomies if each positive screen resulted in a surgical exploration. The National Institutes of Health Consensus Conference recommended against screening for ovarian cancer among the general population without known risk factors for the disease. Although no evidence shows that screening saves lives, many physicians use annual pelvic examinations, transvaginal ultrasound, and CA-125 levels to screen women with a family history of ovarian cancer or breast/ovarian cancer syndromes.

Pathology Common epithelial tumors comprise most (85%) of the ovarian neoplasms. These may be benign (50%), frankly malignant (33%), or tumors of low malignant potential (16%) (tumors of borderline malignancy). Epithelial tumors of low malignant potential have the cytologic features of malignancy but do not invade the ovarian stroma. More than 75% of borderline malignancies present in early stage and generally occur in younger women. They have a much better natural history than their malignant counterpart.

There are five major subtypes of common epithelial tumors: serous (50%), mucinous (25%), endometroid (15%), clear cell (5%), and Brenner tumors (1%), the latter derived from the urothelium. Benign common epithelial tumors are almost always serous or mucinous and develop in women ages 20 to 60. They are frequently large (20 to 30 cm), bilateral, and cystic.

Malignant epithelial tumors are usually seen in women over 40. They present as solid masses, with areas of necrosis and hemorrhage. Masses >10 to 15 cm have usually already spread into the intraabdominal space. Spread eventually results in intraabdominal carcinomatosis, which leads to bowel and renal obstruction and cachexia.

Although most ovarian tumors are epithelial, two other important ovarian tumor types exist—stromal and germ cell tumors. These tumors are distinct in their cell of origin but also have different clinical presentations and natural histories and are often managed differently (see below).

Metastasis to the ovary can occur from breast, colon, gastric, and pancreatic cancers, and the Krukenberg tumor was classically described as bilateral ovarian masses from metastatic mucin-secreting gastrointestinal cancers.

Staging and Prognostic Factors Laparotomy is often the primary procedure used to establish the diagnosis. Less invasive studies useful in defining the extent of spread include chest x-rays, abdominal computed tomography scans, and abdominal and pelvic sonography. If the woman has specific gastrointestinal symptoms, a barium enema or gastrointestinal series can be performed. Symptoms of bladder or renal dysfunction can be evaluated by cystoscopy or intravenous pyelography.

A careful staging laparotomy will establish the stage and extent of disease and allow for the cytoreduction of tumor masses in patients with advanced disease. Proper laparotomy requires a vertical incision of sufficient length to ensure adequate examination of the abdominal contents. The presence, amount, and cytology of any ascites fluid should be noted. The primary tumor should be evaluated for rupture, excrescences, or dense adherence. Careful visual and manual inspection of the diaphragm and peritoneal surfaces is required. In addition to total abdominal hysterectomy and bilateral salpingo-oophorectomy, a partial omentectomy should be performed and the paracolic gutters inspected. Pelvic lymph nodes as well as para-aortic nodes in the region of the renal hilus should be biopsied. Since this surgical procedure defines stage, establishes prognosis, and determines the necessity for subsequent therapy, it should be performed by a surgeon with special expertise in ovarian cancer staging. Studies have shown that patients operated upon by gynecologic oncologists were properly staged 97% of the time, compared to 52 and 35% of cases staged by obstetricians/gynecologists and general surgeons, respectively. At the end of staging, 23% of women have stage I disease (cancer confined to the ovary or ovaries); 13% have stage II (disease confined to the true pelvis);

Table 97-1 Staging and Survival in Gynecologic Malignancies

Stage	Ovarian	5-Year Survival, %	Endometrial	5-Year Survival, %	Cervix	5-Year Survival, %
0	—		—		Carcinoma in situ	100
I	Confined to ovary	90	Confined to corpus	89	Confined to uterus	85
II	Confined to pelvis	70	Involves corpus and cervix	80	Invades beyond uterus but not to pelvic wall	60
III	Intraabdominal spread	15–20	Extends outside the uterus but not outside the true pelvis	30	Extends to pelvic wall and/or lower third of vagina, or hydronephrosis	33
IV	Spread outside abdomen	1–5	Extends outside the true pelvis or involves the bladder or rectum	9	Invades mucosa of bladder or rectum or extends beyond the true pelvis	7

47% have stage III (disease spread into but confined to the abdomen); and 16% have stage IV disease (spread outside the pelvis and abdomen). The 5-year survival correlates with stage of disease: stage I—90%, stage II—70%, stage III—15 to 20%, and stage IV—1 to 5% (Table 97-1).

Prognosis in ovarian cancer is dependent not only upon stage but on the extent of residual disease and histologic grade. Patients presenting with advanced disease but left without significant residual disease after surgery have a median survival of 39 months, compared to 17 months for those with suboptimal tumor resection.

Prognosis of epithelial tumors is also highly influenced by histologic grade but less so by histologic type. In early-stage disease, survival is better in mucinous adenocarcinoma than endometrial and serous types, and clear cell carcinomas have the worst prognosis. Although grading systems differ among pathologists, all grading systems show a better prognosis for well- or moderately differentiated tumors and a poorer prognosis for poorly differentiated histologies. Typical 5-year survivals for patients with all stages of disease are: well differentiated—88%, moderately differentiated—58%, poorly differentiated—27%.

The prognostic significance of pre- and postoperative CA-125 levels is uncertain. Serum levels generally reflect volume of disease, and high levels usually indicate unresectability and a poorer survival. Postoperative levels, if elevated, usually indicate residual disease. Nevertheless, on multivariate analysis, CA-125 is not an independent prognostic factor because of the association with volume of disease. The rate of decline of CA-125 levels during initial therapy or the absolute level after one to three cycles of chemotherapy correlates with prognosis but is not sufficiently accurate to guide individual treatment decisions. Even when the CA-125 level falls to normal after surgery or chemotherapy, "second-look" laparotomy identifies residual disease in 60% of women. Other more quantitative approaches to define prognosis include ploidy analysis and image cytometry (automated analysis of cell morphology); they remain investigational.

Genetic and biologic factors may influence prognosis. Increased tumor levels of p53 are associated with a worse prognosis in advanced disease. Epidermal growth factor receptors in ovarian cancer are associated with a high risk of progression, but the increased expression of HER-2/neu has given conflicting prognostic results, and expression of Mdr-1 has not been of prognostic value. HER-2/neu is being evaluated as a target for antibody therapy.

TREATMENT The selection of therapy for patients with epithelial ovarian cancer depends upon the stage, extent of residual tumor, and histologic grade. In general, patients are considered in three separate treatment groups: (1) those with early (stages I and II) ovarian cancer and microscopic or no residual disease; (2) patients with advanced (stage III) disease but minimal residual tumor (<1 cm) after initial surgery; and (3) patients with bulky residual tumor and advanced (stage III or IV) disease.

Patients with stage I disease, no residual tumor, and well or moderately differentiated tumors need no adjuvant therapy after definitive surgery and 5-year survival exceeds 95%. For all other patients with early disease and those stage I patients with poor prognosis histologic grade, adjuvant therapy is probably warranted, and single-agent cisplatin or platinum-containing drug combinations used in advanced disease are appropriate. Five-year survival for this group exceeds 80%.

For the patients with advanced (stage III) disease but with limited or no residual disease after definitive cytoreductive surgery (about half of all stage III patients), the primary therapy is platinum-based combination chemotherapy. Approximately 70% of women respond to initial combination chemotherapy, and 40 to 50% have a complete regression of disease. Only about half of these patients are free of disease if surgically restaged. Although a variety of combinations are active, a randomized prospective trial of paclitaxel and cisplatin compared to cyclophosphamide and cisplatin in patients with more advanced disease demonstrated better results for the paclitaxel-cisplatin combination (response rate: 77 versus 64%; complete remission rate: 54 versus 33%, median survival: 37.5 versus 24.4 months). A subsequent trial of paclitaxel, 175 mg/m^2 by 3-h infusion, and carboplatin, dosed to an AUC (area under the curve) of 7.5, showed equal antitumor activity to paclitaxel plus cisplatin but substantially less toxicity.

Patients with advanced disease (stages III and IV) and bulky residual tumor are generally treated with a paclitaxel-platinum combination regimen as well and, while the overall prognosis is poorer, 5-year survival may reach 10 to 15%. In some instances, cytoreductive surgery can be performed after initial response to chemotherapy, and a multicenter European trial demonstrated that this strategy led to a significant improvement in progression-free interval and survival.

Historically, patients who had an excellent initial response to chemotherapy and have no clinical evidence of disease have had a second-look laparotomy. For patients with stage I ovarian cancer or for germ cell tumors, the operation rarely detects residual tumor and has been largely abandoned. Even for those with stages II and III epithelial tumors, the second-look surgical procedure itself does not prolong overall survival. Its routine use cannot be recommended. Maintenance therapy does not prevent recurrences in patients in complete remission.

Patients with advanced disease whose disease recurs after initial treatment are usually not curable but may benefit significantly from limited surgery to relieve intestinal obstruction, localized radiation therapy to relieve pressure or pain from mass lesions or metastasis, or palliative chemotherapy. The selection of chemotherapy for palliation depends upon the initial regimen and evidence of drug resistance. Patients who have a complete regression of disease that lasts ≥6 months respond to reinduction with the same agents. Patients relapsing within the first 6 months of initial therapy rarely do. Chemotherapeutic agents with >15% response rates in patients relapsing after initial combination chemotherapy include gemcitabine, topotecan, ifosfamide, etoposide, and hexamethylmelamine. Intraperitoneal chemotherapy (usually cisplatin) may be used if a small residual volume (<1 cm^3) of tumor exists. Progestational agents and antiestrogens produce responses in 5 to 15% of patients and have minimal side effects.

Borderline malignancy has a 95% 5-year survival even in stage III disease when managed with surgery. Radiation and chemotherapy are not useful.

OVARIAN GERM CELL TUMORS   Fewer than 5% of all ovarian tumors are germ cell in origin. They include teratoma, dysgerminoma, endodermal sinus tumor, and embryonal carcinoma. Germ cell tumors of the ovary generally occur in younger women (75% of ovarian malignancies in women <30), display an unusually aggressive

natural history, and are commonly cured with less extensive nonsterilizing surgery and chemotherapy. Women cured of these malignancies are able to conceive and have normal children.

These neoplasms can be divided into three major groups: (1) benign tumors (usually dermoid cysts); (2) malignant tumors that arise from dermoid cysts; and (3) primitive malignant germ cell tumors including dysgerminoma, yolk sac tumors, immature teratomas, embryonal carcinomas, and choriocarcinoma.

Dermoid cysts are teratomatous cysts usually lined by epidermis and skin appendages. They often contain hair, and calcified bone or teeth can sometimes be seen on conventional pelvic x-ray. They are almost always curable by surgical resection. Approximately 1% of these tumors have malignant elements, usually squamous cell carcinoma.

Malignant germ cell tumors are usually large (median—16 cm). Bilateral disease is rare except in dysgerminoma (10 to 15% bilaterality). Abdominal or pelvic pain in young women is the usual presenting symptom. Serum human chorionic gonadoptropin (β-hCG) and α fetoprotein levels are useful in the diagnosis and management of these patients. Before the advent of chemotherapy, extensive surgery was routine but has now been replaced by careful evaluation of extent of spread followed by resection of bulky disease and preservation of one ovary, uterus, and cervix, if feasible. This allows many affected women to preserve fertility. After surgical staging, 60 to 75% of women have stage I disease and 25 to 30% have stage III disease. Stages II and IV are infrequent.

Most of the malignant germ cell tumors are managed with chemotherapy after surgery. Regimens used in testicular cancer such as PVB (cisplatin, vinblastine, bleomycin) and BEP (bleomycin 30 units IV weekly, etoposide 100 mg/m^2 days 1 to 5, and cisplatin 20 mg/m^2 days 1 to 5), with three or four courses given at 21-day intervals, have produced 95% long-term survival in patients with stages I to III disease. This regimen is the treatment of choice for all malignant germ cell tumors except grade I, stage I immature teratoma, where surgery alone is adequate, and perhaps early-stage dysgerminoma, where surgery and radiation therapy are used.

Dysgerminoma is the ovarian counterpart of testicular seminoma. The tumor is very sensitive to radiation therapy. The 5-year disease-free survival is 100% in early-stage patients and 61% in stage III disease. Unfortunately, the use of radiation therapy makes many patients infertile. BEP chemotherapy is equally or more effective and does not cause infertility. In incompletely resected patients with dysgerminoma, the 2-year disease-free survival was 95% and infertility was not observed. Combination chemotherapy (BEP) has replaced postoperative radiation therapy as the treatment of choice in women with ovarian dysgerminoma.

OVARIAN STROMAL TUMORS   Stromal tumors make up <10% of ovarian tumors. They are named for the stromal tissue involved: granulosa, theca, Sertoli, Leydig, and collagen-producing stromal cells. The granulosa and theca cell stromal cell tumors occur most frequently in the first three decades of life. Granulosa cell tumors frequently produce estrogen and cause menstrual abnormalities, bleeding, and precocious puberty. Endometrial carcinoma can be seen in 5% of these women, perhaps related to the persistent hyperestrogenism. Sertoli and Leydig cell tumors, when functional, produce androgens with resultant virilization or hirsutism. Some 75% of these stromal cell tumors present in stage I and can be cured with total abdominal hysterectomy and bilateral salpingo-oophorectomy. Stromal tumors generally grow slowly, and recurrences can occur 5 to 10 years after initial surgery. Neither radiation therapy nor chemotherapy have been documented to be consistently effective, and surgical management remains the primary treatment.

CARCINOMA OF THE FALLOPIAN TUBE

The fallopian tube is the least common site of cancer in the female genital tract although its epithelial surface far exceeds that of the ovary, where epithelial cancer is 20 times more common. Approximately 300

with the remainder being mixed mesodermal, endometroid, and transitional cell tumors. BRCA-1 and -2 mutations are found in 7% of cases. The gross and microscopic characteristics and the spread of the tumor are similar to those of ovarian cancer but can be distinguished if the tumor arises from the endosalpinx, the tubal epithelium shows a transition between benign and malignant, and the ovaries and endometrium are normal or minimally involved. The differential diagnosis includes primary or metastatic ovarian cancer, chronic salpingitis, tuberculous salpingitis, salpingitis isthmica nodosa, and cautery artifact.

Unlike patients with ovarian cancer, patients frequently present with early symptoms, usually postmenopausal vaginal bleeding, pain, and leukorrhea. Surgical staging is similar to that used for ovarian cancer, and prognosis is related to stage and extent of residual disease. Patients with stages I and II disease are generally treated with surgery alone or with surgery and pelvic radiation therapy, although radiation therapy does not clearly improve 5-year survival (5-year survival stage I: 74 versus 75%, stage II: 43 versus 48%). Patients with stages III and IV disease are treated with the same chemotherapy regimens used in advanced ovarian carcinoma, and 5-year survival is similar (stage III—20%, stage IV—5%).

UTERINE CANCER

Carcinoma of the endometrium is the most common female pelvic malignancy. Approximately 36,100 new cases are diagnosed yearly, although in most (75%) tumor is confined to the uterine corpus at diagnosis and therefore most can be cured. The 6500 deaths yearly make uterine cancer only the seventh leading cause of cancer death in females. It is primarily a disease of postmenopausal women, although 25% of cases occur in women <age 50 and 5% <age 40. The disease is common in Eastern Europe and the United States and uncommon in Asia.

Phenotypic characteristics and risk factors common in patients with endometrial cancer include obesity, altered menstruation, low fertility index, late menopause, anovulation, and postmenopausal bleeding. Exposure to unopposed estrogen from either endogenous or exogenous sources may play a central etiologic role. Women taking tamoxifen for breast cancer treatment or prevention have a twofold increased risk.

Endometrial carcinoma occurs most often in the sixth and seventh decades of life. Symptoms often include abnormal vaginal discharge (90%); abnormal bleeding (80%), which is usually postmenopausal; and leukorrhea (10%). Evaluation of such patients should include a history and physical and pelvic examinations followed by an endometrial biopsy or a fractional dilation and curettage. Outpatient procedures such as endometrial biopsy or aspiration curettage can be used but are definitive only when positive.

Between 75 and 80% of all endometrial carcinomas are adenocarcinomas, and the prognosis depends upon stage, histologic grade, and extent of myometrial invasion. Grade I tumors are highly differentiated adenocarcinomas, grade II contain some solid areas, and grade III tumors are largely solid or undifferentiated. Adenocarcinoma with squamous differentiation is seen in 10% of patients; the most differentiated form is known as *adenoacanthoma*, and the poorly differentiated form is called *adenosquamous carcinoma*. Other less common pathologies include mucinous carcinoma (5%) and papillary serous carcinoma (<10%). This latter type has a natural history similar to ovarian carcinoma and should be managed as an ovarian cancer. Rarer histologies include secretory (2%), ciliated, clear cell, and undifferentiated carcinomas.

The staging of endometrial cancer requires surgery to establish the extent of disease and the depth of myometrial invasion. Peritoneal fluid should be sampled; the abdomen and pelvis explored; and pelvic and para-aortic lymphadenectomy performed depending upon the histology, grade, and depth of invasion in the uterine specimen on frozen section. After evaluation and staging, 74% of patients are stage I, 13%

are stage II, 9% are stage III, and 3% are stage IV. Five-year survival by stage is as follows: stage I—89%, stage II—80%, stage III—30%, and stage IV—9% (Table 97-1).

Patients with uncomplicated endometrial carcinoma are effectively managed with total abdominal hysterectomy and bilateral salpingo-oophorectomy. Pre- or postoperative irradiation has been used, and although vaginal cuff recurrence is reduced, survival is not altered. In women with poor histologic grade, deep myometrial invasion, or extensive involvement of the lower uterine segment or cervix, intracavitary or external beam irradiation is warranted.

About 15% of women have endometrial carcinoma with extension to the cervix only (stage II), and management depends upon the extent of cervical invasion. Superficial cervical invasion can be managed like stage I disease, but extensive cervical invasion requires radical hysterectomy or preoperative radiotherapy followed by extrafascial hysterectomy. Once disease is outside the uterus but still confined to the true pelvis (stage III), management generally includes surgery and irradiation. Patients who have involvement only of the ovary or fallopian tubes generally do well with such therapy (5-year survivals of 80%). Other stage III patients with disease extending beyond the adnexa or those with serous carcinomas of the endometrium have a significantly poorer prognosis (5-year survival of 15%).

Patients with stage IV disease (outside the abdomen or invading the bladder or rectum) are treated palliatively with irradiation, surgery, and/or progestational agents. Progestational agents produce responses in about 25% of patients. Well-differentiated tumors respond most frequently, and response can be correlated with the level of progesterone receptor expression in the tumor. The commonly used progestational agents hydroxyprogesterone (Dilalutin), megastrol (Megace), and deoxyprogesterone (Provera) all produce similar response rates, and the antiestrogen tamoxifen (Nolvadex) produces responses in 10 to 25% of patients in a salvage setting.

Chemotherapy is not very successful in advanced endometrial carcinoma. The most active single agents with consistent response rates of ≥20% include cisplatin, carboplatin, doxorubicin, epirubicin, and paclitaxel. Combinations of drugs with or without progestational agents have generally produced response rates similar to single agents.

CERVIX CANCER

Carcinoma of the cervix was once the most common cause of cancer death in women, but over the past 30 years, the mortality rate has decreased by 50% due to widespread screening with the Pap smear. Cervix cancer trails breast, lung, colorectal, endometrium, and ovarian cancers in incidence. In 2000, ~12,800 new cases of invasive cervix cancer occurred, and >50,000 cases of carcinoma in situ were detected. There were 4600 deaths from the disease, and of those patients, ~85% had never had a Pap smear. It remains the major gynecologic cancer in underdeveloped countries. It is more common in lower socioeconomic groups, in women with early initial sexual activity and/ or multiple sexual partners, and in smokers. Venereal transmission of human papilloma virus (HPV) has an important etiologic role. Over 66 types of HPVs have been isolated, and many are associated with genital warts. Those types associated with cervical carcinoma are 16, 18, 31, 45, and 51 to 53. These, along with many other types, are also associated with cervical intraepithelial neoplasia (CIN). The protein product of HPV-16, the E7 protein, binds and inactivates the tumor suppressor gene Rb, and the E6 protein of HPV-18 has sequence homology to the SV40 large T antigen and has the capacity to bind and inactivate the tumor suppressor gene p53. E6 and E7 are both necessary and sufficient to cause cell transformation in vitro. These binding and inactivation events may explain the carcinogenic effects of the viruses (Chap. 188).

Uncomplicated HPV lower genital tract infection and condylomatous atypia of the cervix can progress to CIN. This lesion precedes invasive cervical carcinoma and is classified as low-grade squamous intraepithelial lesion (SIL), high-grade SIL, and carcinoma in situ. Carcinoma in situ demonstrates cytologic evidence of neoplasia without invasion through the basement membrane, can persist unchanged for 10 to 20 years, but eventually progresses to invasive carcinoma.

The Pap smear is 90 to 95% accurate in detecting early lesions such as CIN but is less sensitive in detecting cancer when frankly invasive cancer or fungating masses are present. Inflammation, necrosis, and hemorrhage may produce false-positive smears, and colposcopic-directed biopsy is required when any lesion is visible on the cervix, regardless of Pap smear findings. The American Cancer Society recommends that women after onset of sexual activity, or >age 20, have two consecutive yearly smears. If negative, smears should be repeated every 3 years. The American College of Obstetrics and Gynecology recommends yearly Pap smears with routine annual pelvic and breast examinations. The Pap smear can be reported as normal (includes benign, reactive or reparative changes); atypical squamous cells of undetermined significance (ASCUS); low- or high-grade CIN; or frankly malignant. Women with ASCUS or low-grade CIN should have repeat smears in 3 to 6 months and be tested for HPV. Women with high-grade CIN or frankly malignant Pap smears should have colposcopic-directed cervical biopsy. Colposcopy is a technique using a binocular microscope and 3% acetic acid applied to the cervix in which abnormal areas appear white and can be biopsied directly. Cone biopsy is still required when endocervical tumor is suspected, colposcopy is inadequate, the biopsy shows microinvasive carcinoma, or when a discrepancy is noted between the Pap smear and the colposcopic findings. Cone biopsy alone is therapeutic for CIN in many patients, although a less radical electrocautery excision may be sufficient.

Approximately 80% of invasive cervix carcinomas are squamous cell tumors, 10 to 15% are adenocarcinomas, 2 to 5% are adenosquamous with epithelial and glandular structures, and 1 to 2% are clear cell mesonephric tumors.

Patients with cervix cancer generally present with abnormal bleeding or postcoital spotting that may increase to intermenstrual or prominent menstrual bleeding. Yellowish vaginal discharge, lumbosacral back pain, and urinary symptoms can also be seen.

The staging of cervical carcinoma is clinical and generally completed with a pelvic examination under anesthesia with cystoscopy and proctoscopy. Chest x-rays, intravenous pyelograms, and computed tomography are generally required, and magnetic resonance imaging (MRI) may be used to assess extracervical extension. Stage 0 is carcinoma in situ, stage I is disease confined to the cervix, stage II disease invades beyond the cervix but not to the pelvic wall or lower third of the vagina, stage III disease extends to the pelvic wall or lower third of the vagina or causes hydronephrosis, stage IV is present when the tumor invades the mucosa of bladder or rectum or extends beyond the true pelvis. Five-year survivals are as follows: stage I—85%, stage II—60%, stage III—33%, and stage IV—7% (Table 97-1).

Carcinoma in situ (stage 0) can be managed successfully by cone biopsy or by abdominal hysterectomy. For stage I disease, results appear equivalent for either radical hysterectomy or radiation therapy. Patients with stages II to IV disease are primarily managed with radical radiation therapy or combined modality therapy. Retroperitoneal lymphadenectomy has no proven therapeutic role. Pelvic exenterations, although uncommon, are performed for centrally recurrent or persistent disease. Advances have been made in the reconstruction of the vagina, bladder, and rectum following this operation.

In women with locally advanced disease (stages IIB to IVA), platinum-based chemotherapy given concomitantly with radiation therapy improves survival compared to radiation therapy alone. Cisplatin, 75 mg/m² over 4 h, followed by 5-fluorouracil (5-FU) 4 g given by 96-h infusion on days 1 to 5 of radiation therapy, is a common regimen. Two additional cycles of chemotherapy are given at 3-week intervals. Concurrent chemoradiotherapy reduced the risk of recurrence by 30 to 50% across wide spectrum of stages and presentations and is the treatment of choice in stages IIB to IV cervix cancer.

Chemotherapy has been used in patients with unresectable advanced disease or recurrent disease. Active agents with ≥20% response rates include cisplatin, 5-FU, ifosfamide, and irinotecan. No combination of agents has proved better than single agents. Intraarterial chemotherapy has been studied, either pre-or postoperatively, but is associated with substantial local toxicity and response rates of 20%.

GESTATIONAL TROPHOBLASTIC NEOPLASIA

Gestational choriocarcinoma accounts for <1% of female gynecologic malignancies and can be cured with appropriate chemotherapy. Deaths from this disease have become rare in the United States. The spectrum of disease ranges from benign hydatidiform mole to trophoblastic malignancy (placental-site trophoblastic tumor and choriocarcinoma).

Epidemiology   In the United States, the incidence is about 1 per 1000 pregnancies; in Asia, 2 per 1000 pregnancies. Maternal age >45 years is a risk factor for hydatidiform mole. A prior history of molar pregnancy is also a risk factor. Choriocarcinoma occurs approximately once in 25,000 pregnancies or once in 20,000 live births. Prior history of hydatidiform mole is a risk factor for choriocarcinoma. A woman with a molar pregnancy is 1000 times more likely to develop choriocarcinoma than a woman with a prior normal-term pregnancy.

Pathology and Etiology   The trophoblastic neoplasms have been divided by morphology into complete or partial hydatidiform mole, invasive mole, placental-site trophoblastomas, and choriocarcinomas. Hydatidiform moles contain clusters of villi with hydropic changes, hyperplasia of the trophoblast, and the absence of fetal vessels. Invasive moles differ only by invasion into the uterine myometrium. Placental-site trophoblastic tumors are predominately made up of cytotrophoblast cells arising from the placental implantation site. Choriocarcinomas consist of anaplastic trophoblastic tissue with both cytotrophoblastic and syncytiotrophoblastic elements and no identifiable villi.

Complete moles result from uniparental disomy in which loss of the maternal genes (23 autosomes plus X) occurs by unknown mechanisms and is followed by duplication of the paternal haploid genome (23 autosomes plus X). Uncommonly (5%), moles result from dispermic fertilization of an empty egg, resulting in either 46XY or 46XX genotype. Partial moles result from dispermic fertilization of an egg with retention of the maternal haploid set of chromosomes, resulting in diandric triploidy (Chap. 65).

Clinical Presentation   Molar pregnancies are generally associated with first-trimester bleeding, ectopic pregnancies, or threatened abortions. The uterus is inappropriately large for the length of gestation, and β-hCG levels are higher than expected. Fetal parts and heart sounds are not present. The diagnosis is generally made by the passage of grapelike clusters from the uterus, but ultrasound demonstration of the hydropic mole can be diagnostic. Patients suspected of a molar pregnancy require a chest film, careful pelvic examinations, and weekly serial monitoring of β-hCG levels.

℞ TREATMENT   Patients with hydatidiform moles require surgical evacuation coupled with postevacuation monitoring of β-hCG levels. In most women (80%), the β-hCG titer progressively declines within 8 to 10 days of evacuation (serum half-life is 24 to 36 h). Patients should be monitored on a monthly basis and should not become pregnant for at least a year. Patients found to have invasive mole at curettage are generally treated with hysterectomy and chemotherapy. Approximately half of patients with choriocarcinoma develop the malignancy after a molar pregnancy, and the other half develop the malignancy after abortion, ectopic pregnancy, or occasionally after a normal full-term pregnancy.

Chemotherapy is generally used for gestational trophoblastic neoplasia and is often used in hydatidiform mole if β-hCG levels rise or plateau or if metastases develop. Patients with invasive mole or choriocarcinoma require chemotherapy. Several regimens are effective, including methotrexate at 30 mg/m² intramuscularly on a weekly basis until β-hCG titers are normal. However, methotrexate (1 mg/kg) every other day for 4 days followed by leukovorin (0.1 mg/kg) intravenously 24 h after methotrexate is associated with a cure rate of ≥90% and low toxicity. Intermittent courses are continued until the β-hCG titer becomes undetectable for 3 consecutive weeks, and then patients are monitored monthly for a year.

Patients with high-risk tumors (high β-hCG levels, disease presenting ≥4 months after antecedent pregnancy, brain or liver metastasis, or failure of single-agent methotrexate) are initially treated with combination chemotherapy. MAC chemotherapy with methotrexate, actinomycin-D, and cyclophosphamide has been the most commonly used regimen, with cycles of therapy given every 3 weeks until complete remission. Other effective regimens include EMA-CO (a cyclic non-cross-resistant combination of etoposide, methotrexate, and dactinomycin alternating with cyclophosphamide and vincristine); cisplatin, bleomycin, and vinblastine; and cisplatin, etoposide, and bleomycin. EMA-CO is now the regimen of choice for patients with high-risk disease because of excellent survival rates (>80%) and less toxicity than MAC. The use of etoposide carries a 1.5% lifetime risk of acute myeloid leukemia (16-fold relative risk). Because of this problem, etoposide-containing regimens should be reserved for patients with high risk features. Patients with brain or liver metastasis are usually treated with local irradiation to metastatic sites in conjunction with chemotherapy. Long-term studies of patients cured of trophoblastic disease have not demonstrated an increased risk of maternal complications or fetal abnormalities with subsequent pregnancies.

BIBLIOGRAPHY

BARAKAT RR et al: Corpus epithelial tumors, in *Principles and Practice of Gynecologic Oncology*, 3d ed, WJ Hoskins et al (eds). Philadelphia, Lippincott Williams & Wilkins, 2000, pp 919–959

HACKER NF: Uterine cancer, in *Practical Gynecologic Oncology*, 2d ed, JS Berek, NF Hacker (eds). Baltimore, Williams & Wilkins, 1994, pp 285–326.

MORRIS M et al: Pelvic radiation with concurrent chemotherapy compared with pelvic and para-aortic radiation for high-risk cervical cancer. N Engl J Med 340:1137, 1999

OZOLS RF et al: Epithelial ovarian cancer, in *Principles and Practice of Gynecologic Oncology*, 3d ed, WJ Hoskins et al (eds). Philadelphia, Lippincott, Williams & Wilkins, 2000, pp 981–1057

——— et al: Randomized phase III study of cisplatin/paclitaxel versus carboplatin/paclitaxel in optimal stage III epithelial ovarian cancer. Proc Am Soc Clin Oncol 18:356a, 1999

SOPER VT: Identification and management of high-risk gestational trophoblastic disease. Semin Oncol 22:172, 1995

STEHMAN FB et al: Uterine cervix, in *Principles and Practice of Gynecologic Oncology*, 3d ed, WJ Hoskins et al (eds). Philadelphia, Lippincott Williams & Wilkins, 2000, pp 841–918

VANDERBURG ME et al: Intervention debulking surgery does improve survival in advanced epithelial ovarian cancer. N Engl J Med 332:629, 1995

WILLIAMS S et al: Adjuvant therapy of ovarian germ cell tumors with cisplatin, etoposide and bleomycin: A trial of the Gynecologic Oncology Group. J Clin Oncol 12:701, 1994

YOUNG RC et al: Adjuvant therapy in stage I and stage II epithelial ovarian cancer. Results of two prospective trials. N Engl J Med 327:1021, 1990

98

Shreyaskumar R. Patel, Robert S. Benjamin

SOFT TISSUE AND BONE SARCOMAS AND BONE METASTASES

Sarcomas are rare (less than 1% of all malignancies) mesenchymal neoplasms that arise in bone and soft tissues. These tumors are usually of mesodermal origin, although a few are derived from neuroectoderm, and they are biologically distinct from the more common epithelial malignancies. Sarcomas affect all age groups; 15% are found in children younger than age 15, and 40% occur after age 55. Sarcomas are

one of the most common solid tumors of childhood and are the fifth most common cause of cancer deaths in children. Sarcomas may be divided into two groups, those derived from bone and those derived from soft tissues.

SOFT TISSUE SARCOMAS

Soft tissues include muscles, tendons, fat, fibrous tissue, synovial tissue, vessels, and nerves. Approximately 60% of soft tissue sarcomas arise in the extremities, with the lower extremities involved three times as often as the upper extremities. Thirty percent arise in the trunk, the retroperitoneum accounting for 40% of all trunk lesions. The remaining 10% arise in the head and neck.

INCIDENCE Approximately 7800 new cases of soft tissue sarcomas occurred in the United States in 1999. The annual age-adjusted incidence is approximately 2 per 100,000 population, but the incidence varies with age. Soft tissue sarcomas constitute 0.7% of all cancers in the general population and 6.5% of all cancers in children.

EPIDEMIOLOGY Malignant transformation of a benign soft tissue tumor is extremely rare, with the exception that malignant peripheral nerve sheath tumors (neurofibrosarcoma, malignant schwannoma) can arise from neurofibromas in patients with neurofibromatosis. Several etiologic factors have been implicated in soft tissue sarcomas.

Environmental Factors Trauma or previous injury is rarely involved, but sarcomas can arise in scar tissue resulting from a prior operation, burn, fracture, or foreign body implantation. Chemical carcinogens such as polycyclic hydrocarbons, asbestos, and dioxin may be involved in the pathogenesis.

Iatrogenic Factors Sarcomas in bone or soft tissues occur in patients who are treated with radiation therapy. The tumor nearly always arises in the irradiated field. The risk increases with time.

Viruses Kaposi's sarcoma (KS) in patients with HIV type 1, classic KS, and KS in HIV-negative homosexual men is caused by human herpes virus (HHV8) (Chap. 185). No other sarcomas are associated with viruses.

Immunologic Factors Congenital or acquired immunodeficiency, including therapeutic immunosuppression, increases risk of sarcoma.

Genetic Factors Li-Fraumeni syndrome is a familial cancer syndrome in which affected individuals have germ-line abnormalities of the tumor suppressor gene *p53* and an increased incidence of soft tissue sarcomas and other malignancies, including breast cancer, osteosarcoma, brain tumor, leukemia, and adrenal carcinoma (Chap. 81). Neurofibromatosis 1 (NF-1, peripheral form, von Recklinghausen's disease) is characterized by multiple neurofibromas and café au lait spots. Neurofibromas occasionally undergo malignant degeneration to become malignant peripheral nerve sheath tumors. The gene for NF-1 is located in the pericentromeric region of chromosome 17 and encodes neurofibromin, a tumor suppressor protein with GTPase-activating activity that inhibits Ras function (Chap. 370). Germ-line mutation of the *Rb-1* locus (chromosome 13q14) in patients with inherited retinoblastoma is associated with the development of osteosarcoma in those who survive the retinoblastoma and of soft tissue sarcomas unrelated to radiation therapy. Other soft tissue tumors, including desmoid tumors, lipomas, leiomyomas, neuroblastomas, and paragangliomas, occasionally show a familial predisposition.

Ninety percent of synovial sarcomas contain a characteristic chromosomal translocation t(X;18) (p11;q11) involving a nuclear transcription factor on chromosome 18 called *SYT* and two breakpoints on X. Patients with translocations to the second X breakpoint (*SSX2*) may have longer survival than those with translocations involving *SSX1*.

Insulin-like growth factor (IGF) type 2 is produced by some sarcomas and may act as an autocrine growth factor and as a motility factor that promotes metastatic spread. IGF-2 stimulates growth through IGF-1 receptors but its effects on motility are through different

Table 98-1 AJCC Staging System for Sarcomas

Histologic Grade (G)	Tumor Size (T)	Node Status (N)	Metastases (M)
Well differentiated (G1)	≤5 cm (T1)	Not involved (N0)	Absent (M0)
Moderately differentiated (G2)	>5 cm (T2)	Involved (N1)	Present (M1)
Poorly differentiated (G3)	Superficial fascial involvement (Ta)		
Undifferentiated (G4)	Deep fascial involvement (Tb)		

Disease Stage	5-year survival, %
Stage I	98.8
A: G1,2; T1a,b; N0; M0	
B: G1,2; T2a; N0; M0	
Stage II	81.8
A: G1,2; T2b; N0; M0	
B: G3,4; T1; N0; M0	
C: G3,4; T2a; N0; M0	
Stage III G3,4; T2b; N0; M0	51.7
Stage IV	<20
A: any G; any T; N1; M0	
B: any G; any T; any N; M1	

receptors. If secreted in large amounts, IGF-2 may produce hypoglycemia (Chaps. 100 and 334).

CLASSIFICATION Approximately 20 different groups of sarcomas are recognized on the basis of the pattern of differentiation toward normal tissue. For example, rhabdomyosarcoma shows evidence of skeletal muscle fibers with cross-striations; leiomyosarcomas contain interlacing fascicles of spindle cells resembling smooth muscle; and liposarcomas contain adipocytes. When precise characterization of the group is not possible, the tumors are called *unclassified sarcomas*. All of the primary bone sarcomas also can arise from soft tissues (e.g., extraskeletal osteosarcoma). The entity *malignant fibrous histiocytoma* includes many tumors previously classified as fibrosarcomas or as pleomorphic variants of other sarcomas and is characterized by a mixture of spindle (fibrous) cells and round (histiocytic) cells arranged in a storiform pattern with frequent giant cells and areas of pleomorphism.

For purposes of treatment, most soft tissue sarcomas can be considered together. However, some specific tumors have distinct features. For example, *liposarcoma* can have a spectrum of behaviors. Pleomorphic liposarcomas and dedifferentiated liposarcomas behave like other high-grade sarcomas; in contrast, well-differentiated liposarcomas (better termed *atypical lipomatous tumors*) lack metastatic potential, and myxoid liposarcomas metastasize infrequently but, when they do, have a predilection for unusual metastatic sites containing fat, such as the retroperitoneum, mediastinum, and subcutaneous tissue. Rhabdomyosarcomas, Ewing's sarcoma, and other small cell sarcomas tend to be more aggressive, and are more responsive to chemotherapy than other soft tissue sarcomas.

DIAGNOSIS The most common presentation is an asymptomatic mass. Mechanical symptoms referable to pressure, traction, or entrapment of nerves or muscles may be present. All new and persistent or growing masses should be biopsied, either by a cutting needle (core-needle biopsy) or by a small incision, placed so that it can be encompassed in the subsequent excision without compromising a definitive resection. Sarcomas tend to metastasize through the blood rather than the lymphatic system; lymph node metastases occur in 5%, except in synovial and epithelioid sarcomas, clear-cell sarcoma (melanoma of the soft parts), angiosarcoma, and rhabdomyosarcoma where nodal spread may be seen in 17%. The pulmonary parenchyma is the most common site of metastases. Exceptions are leiomyosarcomas arising in the gastrointestinal tract, which metastasize to the liver; myxoid liposarcomas, which seek fatty tissue; and clear-cell sarcomas, which may metastasize to bones. Central nervous system metastases are rare, except in alveolar soft part sarcoma.

Radiographic Evaluation Imaging of the primary tumor is best with plain radiographs and magnetic resonance imaging (MRI) for tumors of the extremities or head and neck and by computed tomography (CT) for tumors of the chest, abdomen, or retroperitoneal cavity. A radiograph and CT scan of the chest are important for the detection of lung metastases. Other imaging studies may be indicated, depending on the symptoms, signs, or histology.

STAGING AND PROGNOSIS The histologic grade, relationship to fascial planes, and size of the primary tumor are the most important prognostic factors. The newly revised American Joint Commission on Cancer (AJCC) staging system is shown in Table 98-1. Prognosis is related to the stage. Cure is common in the absence of metastatic disease, but a small number of patients with metastases can also be cured. Most patients with stage IV disease die within 6 to 12 months, but some patients may live with slowly progressive disease for many years.

TREATMENT AJCC stage I patients are adequately treated with surgery alone. Stage II patients require adjuvant radiation therapy. Stage III patients require adjuvant chemotherapy. Stage IV patients are managed primarily with chemotherapy with or without other modalities.

Surgery Soft tissue sarcomas tend to grow along fascial planes, with the surrounding soft tissues compressed to form a pseudocapsule that gives the sarcoma the appearance of a well-encapsulated lesion. This is invariably deceptive, because "shelling out" or marginal excision of such lesions results in a 50 to 90% probability of local recurrence. Wide excision with a negative margin, incorporating the biopsy site, is the standard surgical procedure for local disease. The adjuvant use of radiation therapy and/or chemotherapy improves the local control rate and permits the use of limb-sparing surgery with a local control rate (85 to 90%) comparable to that achieved by radical excisions and amputations. Limb-sparing approaches are indicated except when negative margins are not obtainable, when the risks of radiation are prohibitive, or when neurovascular structures are involved so that resection will result in serious functional consequences to the limb.

Radiation Therapy External beam radiation therapy is an adjuvant to limb-sparing surgery for improved local control. Preoperative radiation therapy allows the use of smaller fields and smaller doses but results in a higher rate of wound complications. Postoperative radiation therapy must be given to larger fields, as the entire surgical bed must be encompassed, and in higher doses to compensate for hypoxia in the operated field. Brachytherapy or interstitial therapy, in which the radiation source is inserted into the tumor bed, is comparable in efficacy (except in low grade lesions), less time consuming, and less expensive.

Adjuvant Chemotherapy Chemotherapy is the mainstay of treatment for Ewing's/peripheral neuroepithelial tumors (PNET) and rhabdomyosarcomas. Meta-analysis of 14 randomized trials revealed a highly significant improvement in local control and disease-free survival in favor of doxorubicin-based chemotherapy. Overall survival is improved only for extremity sarcomas, however. An alternative approach is to treat such patients preoperatively with chemotherapy (neoadjuvant therapy); the subset of patients who respond continue adjuvant therapy postoperatively, and the nonresponders can be spared the toxicity of systemic therapy to which they are unlikely to respond. Neither strategy has been proved superior.

Advanced Disease Metastatic soft tissue sarcomas are largely incurable, but up to 20% of patients who achieve a complete response become long-term survivors. The therapeutic intent, therefore, is to produce a complete remission with chemotherapy and/or surgery. Surgical resection of metastases, whenever possible, is an integral part of the management. Some patients benefit from repeated surgical excision of metastases. Despite their histologic heterogeneity, the sensitivity to chemotherapy of most soft tissue sarcomas is poor. The two most active chemotherapeutic agents are doxorubicin and ifosfamide. There is a steep dose-response relationship for these drugs in sarcomas. Dacarbazine (DTIC) in combination with doxorubicin may be more active than the single agents. Vincristine, etoposide, and dactinomycin are effective in Ewing's sarcoma and rhabdomyosarcoma, especially in children. Chondrosarcomas and leiomyosarcomas arising from the gastrointestinal tract are unresponsive to standard chemotherapeutic drugs.

BONE SARCOMAS

INCIDENCE AND EPIDEMIOLOGY Bone sarcomas are rarer than soft tissue sarcomas; they accounted for only 0.2% of all new malignancies and approximately 2500 new cases in the United States in 1999. Several benign bone lesions have the potential for malignant transformation. Enchondromas and osteochondromas can transform into chondrosarcoma; fibrous dysplasia, bone infarcts, and Paget's disease of bone can transform into either malignant fibrous histiocytoma or osteosarcoma.

CLASSIFICATION **Benign Tumors** The common benign bone tumors include enchondroma, osteochondroma, chondroblastoma, and chondromyxoid fibroma, of cartilage origin; osteoid osteoma and osteoblastoma, of bone origin; fibroma and desmoplastic fibroma, of fibrous tissue origin; hemangioma, of vascular origin; and giant cell tumor, of unknown origin.

Malignant Tumors The most common malignant tumors of bone are plasma cell tumors (Chap. 113). The four most common malignant nonhematopoietic bone tumors are osteosarcoma, chondrosarcoma, Ewing's sarcoma, and malignant fibrous histiocytoma. Rare malignant tumors include chordoma (of notochordal origin), malignant giant cell tumor and adamantinoma (of unknown origin), and hemangioendothelioma (of vascular origin).

Musculoskeletal Tumor Society Staging System Sarcomas of bone are staged according to the Musculoskeletal Tumor Society staging system based on grade and compartmental localization. A Roman numeral reflects the tumor grade: stage I is low-grade, stage II is high-grade, and stage III includes tumors of any grade that have lymph node or distant metastases. In addition, the tumor is given a letter reflecting its compartmental localization. Tumors designated A are intracompartmental (i.e., confined to the same soft tissue compartment as the initial tumor), and tumors designated B are extracompartmental (i.e., extending into the adjacent soft tissue compartment or into bone).

OSTEOSARCOMA Osteosarcoma, accounting for almost 45% of all bone sarcomas, is a spindle cell neoplasm that produces osteoid (unmineralized bone) or bone. About 60% of all osteosarcomas occur in children and adolescents in the second decade of life, and about 10% occur in the third decade of life. Osteosarcomas in the fifth and sixth decades of life are frequently secondary to either radiation therapy or transformation in a preexisting benign condition, such as Paget's disease. Males are affected 1.5 to 2 times as often as females. Osteosarcoma has a predilection for metaphyses of long bones; the most common sites of involvement are the distal femur, proximal tibia, and proximal humerus. The classification of osteosarcoma is complex, but 75% of osteosarcomas fall in the "classic" category, which include osteoblastic, chondroblastic, and fibroblastic osteosarcomas. The remaining 25% are classified as "variants" on the basis of (1) clinical characteristics, as in the case of osteosarcoma of the jaw, postradiation osteosarcoma, or Paget's osteosarcoma; (2) morphologic characteristics, as in the case of telangiectatic osteosarcoma, small cell osteosarcoma, or epithelioid osteosarcoma; or (3) location, as in parosteal or periosteal osteosarcoma. Diagnosis usually requires a synthesis of clinical, radiologic, and pathologic features. Patients typically present with pain and swelling of the affected area. A plain radiograph reveals a destructive lesion with a moth-eaten appearance, a spiculated periosteal reaction (sunburst appearance), and a cuff of periosteal new bone formation at the margin of the soft tissue mass (Codman's triangle). A CT scan of the primary tumor is best for defining bone destruction and the pattern of calcification, whereas MRI is better for defining intramedullary and soft tissue extension. A chest radiograph and CT scan are used to detect lung metastases. Metastases to the bony skeleton should be imaged by a bone scan. Almost all osteosarcomas are hypervascular. Angiography is not helpful for diagnosis, but it is the most sensitive test for assessing the response to preoperative chemotherapy. Pathologic diagnosis is established either with a core-needle biopsy, where feasible, or with an open biopsy with an appropriately placed incision that does not compromise future limb-sparing resection. Most osteosarcomas are high-grade. The most important prognostic factor for long-term survival is response to chemotherapy. Preoperative chemotherapy followed by limb-sparing surgery (which can be accomplished in >80% of patients) followed by postoperative chemotherapy is standard management. The effective drugs are doxorubicin, ifosfamide, cisplatin, and high-dose methotrexate with leucovorin rescue. The various combinations of these agents that have been used have all been about equally successful. Long-term survival rates in extremity osteosarcoma range from 60 to 80%. Osteosarcoma is radioresistant; radiation therapy has no role in the routine management. Malignant fibrous histiocytoma is considered a part of the spectrum of osteosarcoma and is managed similarly.

CHONDROSARCOMA Chondrosarcoma, which constitutes approximately 20 to 25% of all bone sarcomas, is a tumor of adulthood and old age with a peak incidence in the fourth to sixth decades of life. It has a predilection for the flat bones, especially the shoulder and pelvic girdles, but can also affect the diaphyseal portions of long bones. Chondrosarcomas can arise de novo or as a malignant transformation of an enchondroma or, rarely, of the cartilaginous cap of an osteochondroma. Chondrosarcomas have an indolent natural history and typically present as pain and swelling. Radiographically, the lesion may have a lobular appearance with mottled or punctate or annular calcification of the cartilaginous matrix. It is difficult to distinguish low-grade chondrosarcoma from benign lesions by x-ray or histologic examination. The diagnosis is therefore influenced by clinical history and physical examination. A new onset of pain, signs of inflammation, and progressive increase in the size of the mass suggest malignancy. The histologic classification is complex, but most tumors fall within the classic category. Like other bone sarcomas, high-grade chondrosarcomas spread to the lungs. Most chondrosarcomas are resistant to chemotherapy, and surgical resection of primary or recurrent tumors, including pulmonary metastases, is the mainstay of therapy. There are two histologic variants for which this rule does not hold, however. Dedifferentiated chondrosarcoma is a low-grade tumor that dedifferentiates into a high-grade osteosarcoma or a malignant fibrous histiocytoma, a tumor that responds to chemotherapy. Mesenchymal chondrosarcoma, a rare variant composed of a small cell element, also is responsive to systemic chemotherapy and is treated like Ewing's sarcoma.

EWING'S SARCOMA Ewing's sarcoma, which constitutes approximately 10 to 15% of all bone sarcomas, is common in adolescence and has a peak incidence in the second decade of life. It typically involves the diaphyseal region of long bones and also has an affinity for flat bones. The plain radiograph may show a characteristic "onion peel" periosteal reaction with a generous soft tissue mass, which is better demonstrated by CT or MRI. This mass is composed of sheets of monotonous, small, round, blue cells and can be confused with lymphoma, embryonal rhabdomyosarcoma, and small cell carcinoma. The presence of p30/32, the product of the *mic-2* gene (which maps to the pseudoautosomal region of the X and Y chromosomes) is a cell-surface marker for Ewing's sarcoma [and other members of a family of tumors called *peripheral primitive neuroectodermal tumors*

(*PNETs*)]. Most PNETs arise in soft tissues; they include peripheral neuroepithelioma, Askin's tumor (chest wall), and esthesioneuroblastoma. Glycogen-filled cytoplasm detected by staining with periodic acid–Schiff is also characteristic of Ewing's sarcoma cells. The classic cytogenetic abnormality associated with this disease (and other PNETs) is a reciprocal translocation of the long arms of chromosomes 11 and 22, t(11;22), which creates a chimeric gene product of unknown function with components from the *fli-1* gene on chromosome 11 and *ews* on 22. This disease is very aggressive, and it is therefore considered a systemic disease. Common sites of metastases are lung, bones, and bone marrow. Systemic chemotherapy is the mainstay of therapy, often being used before surgery. Doxorubicin, cyclophosphamide or ifosfamide, etoposide, vincristine, and dactinomycin are active drugs. Local treatment for the primary tumor includes surgical resection, usually with limb salvage or radiation therapy. Patients with lesions below the elbow and below the mid-calf have a 5-year survival rate of 80% with effective treatment. Ewing's sarcoma is a curable tumor, even in the presence of obvious metastatic disease, especially in children less than 11 years old.

TUMORS METASTATIC TO BONE

Bone is a common site of metastasis for carcinomas of the prostate, breast, lung, kidney, bladder, and thyroid and for lymphomas and sarcomas. Prostate, breast, and lung primaries account for 80% of all bone metastases. Metastatic tumors of bone are more common than primary bone tumors. Tumors usually spread to bone hematogenously, but local invasion from soft tissue masses also occurs. In descending order of frequency, the sites most often involved are the vertebrae, proximal femur, pelvis, ribs, sternum, proximal humerus, and skull. Bone metastases may be asymptomatic or may produce pain, swelling, nerve root or spinal cord compression, pathologic fracture, or myelophthisis (replacement of the marrow). Symptoms of hypercalcemia may be noted in cases of bony destruction.

Pain is the most frequent symptom. It usually develops gradually over weeks, is usually localized, and often is more severe at night. When patients with back pain develop neurologic signs or symptoms, emergency evaluation for spinal cord compression is indicated (Chap. 102). Bone metastases exert a major adverse effect on quality of life in cancer patients.

Cancer in the bone may produce osteolysis, osteogenesis, or both. Osteolytic lesions result when the tumor produces substances that can directly elicit bone resorption (vitamin D–like steroids, prostaglandins, or parathyroid hormone–related peptide) or cytokines that can induce the formation of osteoclasts (interleukin 1 and tumor necrosis factor). Osteoblastic lesions result when the tumor produces cytokines that activate osteoblasts. In general, purely osteolytic lesions are best detected by plain radiography, but they may not be apparent until they are larger than 1 cm. These lesions are more commonly associated with hypercalcemia and with the excretion of hydroxyproline-containing peptides indicative of matrix destruction. When osteoblastic activity is prominent, the lesions may be readily detected using radionuclide bone scanning (which is sensitive to new bone formation), and the radiographic appearance may show increased bone density or sclerosis. Osteoblastic lesions are associated with higher serum levels of alkaline phosphatase, and, if extensive, may produce hypocalcemia. Although some tumors may produce mainly osteolytic lesions (e.g., kidney cancer) and others mainly osteoblastic lesions (e.g., prostate cancer), most metastatic lesions produce both types of lesion and may go through stages where one or the other predominates.

In older patients, particularly women, it may be necessary to distinguish metastatic disease of the spine from osteoporosis. In osteoporosis, the cortical bone may be preserved, whereas cortical bone destruction is usually noted with metastatic cancer.

Treatment of metastatic bone disease depends on the underlying malignancy and the symptoms. Some metastatic bone tumors are cur-

able (lymphoma, Hodgkin's disease), and others are treated with palliative intent. Pain may be relieved by local radiation therapy. Hormonally responsive tumors are responsive to hormone inhibition (antiandrogens for prostate cancer, antiestrogens for breast cancer). Strontium 89 and samarium 153 are bone-seeking radionuclides that can exert antitumor effects and relieve symptoms. Bisphosphonates such as pamidronate may relieve pain and inhibit bone resorption. Monthly administration prevents bone-related clinical events and may reduce the incidence of bone metastases in women with breast cancer. When the integrity of a weight-bearing bone is threatened by an expanding metastatic lesion that is refractory to radiation therapy, prophylactic internal fixation is indicated. Overall survival is related to the prognosis of the underlying tumor. Bone pain at the end of life is particularly common; an adequate pain relief regimen including sufficient amounts of narcotic analgesics is required. →*The management of hypercalcemia is discussed in Chap. 341.*

BIBLIOGRAPHY

Evans RG et al: Multimodal therapy for the management of localized Ewing's sarcoma of pelvic and sacral bones: A report from the second intergroup study. J Clin Oncol 9:1173, 1991

Patel SR, Benjamin RS: New chemotherapeutic strategies for soft tissue sarcomas. Sem Surg Oncol 17:47, 1999

——— (eds): Sarcomas. Part I. Hematol Oncol Clin North Am 9:513, 1995

——— (eds): Sarcomas. Part II. Hematol Oncol Clin North Am 9:707, 1995

West DC: Ewing sarcoma family of tumors. Curr Opin Oncol 12:323, 2000

99   *Richard M. Stone*

METASTATIC CANCER OF UNKNOWN PRIMARY SITE

INCIDENCE AND EPIDEMIOLOGY The presenting findings in a patient with a newly discovered malignancy may not reveal its site of origin. Patients with cancer of unknown primary site (CUPS) present difficult diagnostic and therapeutic dilemmas. First, as additional studies may be many, costly, and/or uncomfortable for the patient, the strategy used in searching for the primary must assess what, if any, result the identification of the site of origin would have on the patient's treatment and survival. Second, while individuals with CUPS fare poorly overall (median survival is 4 to 11 months), certain subgroups of patients are more likely to benefit from treatment and, in some cases, to enjoy long disease-free survival. The literature is a poor guide for the care of such patients, owing to the heterogeneity of the tumors, the selection bias in small retrospective studies, and the variability in the definition of the syndrome and the thoroughness of the evaluation performed to identify a primary site.

No universally accepted definition of the CUPS syndrome exists. An occult neoplasm should fulfill all of the following criteria: (1) biopsy-proven malignancy; (2) unrevealing history, physical examination, chest film, abdominal and pelvic computed tomography (CT) scans, complete blood counts, chemistry survey, mammography (women), β human chorionic gonadotropin (βhCG) levels (men), α fetoprotein (AFP) levels (men), and prostate-specific antigen (PSA) levels (men); (3) histologic evaluation not consistent with a primary tumor at the biopsy site; and (4) failure of additional diagnostic studies (based only on findings from the laboratory and pathologic review) to identify the primary site. Such additional diagnostic tests could include, for example, colonoscopy in a patient whose rectal examination discloses guaiac-positive stool or a meticulous otolaryngologic examination in a patient who presents with squamous cell carcinoma in a cervical node. Many cases that fulfill the definition of CUPS offer clues that a given organ is the probable site of origin. Epidemiologic data suggest that the incidence of cancers for which the primary site is unknown is decreasing. CUPS accounts for about 2% of all cancer diagnoses—about 24,400 cases in the year 2000. Most patients with CUPS are over age 60.

BIOLOGIC CONSIDERATIONS The biologic behavior of CUPS is unique. In ~25% of patients, the primary site becomes apparent during the course of the illness; in about 57% of patients, the primary site can be diagnosed at autopsy; but in almost 20%, the primary site remains obscure even at autopsy. Cancers presenting as CUPS often display unusual patterns of metastatic spread (e.g., pancreatic cancer presenting with bony metastases). The fact that more tumor bulk is present at distant sites than in the tissue of origin suggests that the genetic lesions underlying cases of CUPS produce a distinctly aggressive phenotype. Microsatellite DNA analysis has shown that the same pattern of genetic alterations that appear in a cervical lymph node metastasis can be found in seemingly morphologically normal aerodigestive tissue. Such data imply that clinically evident metastases may be able to arise from microscopic primary lesions. Although physiologic and genetic data that might account for the distinctive natural history of CUPS neoplasms are scant, cell lines derived from such tumors may have abnormalities of chromosome 1, a finding generally associated with advanced malignancy. In some patients, the primary tumor spontaneously regresses (perhaps under immunologic attack) or necroses. In some, a primary lesion was resected years before presentation (e.g., melanoma).

CLINICAL PRESENTATION, DIAGNOSTIC EVALUATION, AND PATHOLOGY **History and Physical Examination** Patients present with a variety of symptoms and signs, including fatigue, weight loss, other systemic symptoms, pain, abnormal bleeding, abdominal swelling, subcutaneous masses, and lymphadenopathy. Once CUPS is considered, the physician's approach must involve reasonable efforts to identify the primary site or to determine the histology or subcategory of the metastatic tumor to decide on the optimal therapy. Though usually unrevealing, a thorough history and physical examination should be carried out to elicit easily obtainable clues regarding the primary site. The patient should be questioned concerning epigastric pain, which, if present, would mandate careful exclusion of pancreatic carcinoma as well as other gastrointestinal malignancies. Symptoms referable to a given location (e.g., new cough, hematochezia, hemoptysis, change in bowel habits, unusual vaginal bleeding, nipple discharge) should prompt an aggressive specific diagnostic approach. Occupational exposure to asbestos, for example, would raise the suspicion of mesothelioma. The absence of prior smoking reduces the likelihood of lung cancer but does not exclude it. A history of fulguration of a skin lesion, colonic polypectomy, dilatation and curettage, or prostate biopsy should prompt a review of the original histology.

Pathology Review The most important aspect of the workup of a patient with CUPS is the thorough evaluation of the tissue obtained at biopsy by light-microscopy, immunohistochemistry, ultrastructural studies, immunophenotyping, and karyotypic and molecular biologic analysis. First, if the original biopsy sample is inadequate for either confirmation of malignancy or the performance of additional specialized studies, rebiopsy is mandatory. The clinician must have a close working relationship with a pathologist skilled in the evaluation of tumor specimens, especially when the organ of origin is uncertain. Plans may be made to process the tissue for (1) routine light-microscopy, histochemical, and immunohistochemical analysis; (2) freezing for DNA and RNA isolation or for in situ genetic and immunologic evaluation; and (3) special fixation for ultrastructural analysis. Single-cell tumor suspensions in short-term culture permit cytogenetic analysis.

If routine histologic analysis fails to suggest the tissue of origin (e.g., gland formation in adenocarcinoma, psammoma bodies in ovarian or thyroid cancer, or spindle architecture in sarcomas), special histochemical studies may be helpful. For example, mucin positivity is helpful in recognizing a poorly differentiated adenocarcinoma. Light-microscopic analysis will show approximately 60% of CUPS tumors to be well or moderately differentiated adenocarcinomas, 30%

poorly differentiated carcinomas/adenocarcinomas, and 5% poorly differentiated malignant neoplasms not further classifiable. In the poorly differentiated neoplasms, immunohistochemical, cytogenetic, and molecular biologic studies can be extremely useful in identifying sarcomas, germ cell carcinomas, lymphomas, neuroendocrine neoplasms (including melanoma), and other tumors whose diagnosis would suggest a more specific therapeutic approach.

Immunohistochemical Analysis Antibodies to specific cell components make it possible to characterize tumors that are not identified by standard techniques. Table 99-1 provides a list of antigens

Table 99-1 Possible Pathologic Evaluation of Biopsy Specimens from Patients with Metastatic Cancer of Unknown Primary Site

Evaluation/Findings	Suggested Primary Site or Neoplasm
HISTOLOGY (HEMATOXYLIN AND EOSIN STAINING)	
Psammoma bodies, papillary configuration	Ovary, thyroid
Signet ring cells	Stomach
IMMUNOHISTOLOGY	
Leukocyte common antigen (LCA, CD45)	Lymphoid neoplasm
Leu-M1	Hodgkin's disease
Epithelial membrane antigen	Carcinoma
Cytokeratin	Carcinoma[a]
CEA	Carcinoma
HMB45	Melanoma
Desmin	Sarcoma
Thyroglobulin	Thyroid carcinoma
Calcitonin	Medullary carcinoma of the thyroid
Myoglobin	Rhabdomyosarcoma
PSA/prostatic acid phosphatase	Prostate
AFP	Liver, stomach, germ cell
Placental alkaline phosphatase	Germ cell
B, T cell markers	Lymphoid neoplasm
S-100 protein	Neuroendocrine tumor, melanoma
Gross cystic fluid protein	Breast, sweat gland
Factor VIII	Kaposi's sarcoma, angiosarcoma
FLOW CYTOMETRY	
B, T cell markers	Lymphoid neoplasm
ULTRASTRUCTURE	
Actin-myosin filaments	Rhabdomyosarcoma
Secretory granules	Neuroendocrine tumors
Desmosomes	Carcinoma
Premelanosomes	Melanoma
CYTOGENETICS	
Isochromosome 12p; 12q($-$)	Germ cell
t(11;22)	Ewing's sarcoma, primitive neuro-ectodermal tumor
t(8;14)[b]	Lymphoid neoplasm
3p($-$)	Small cell lung carcinoma; renal cell carcinoma, mesothelioma
t(X;18)	Synovial sarcoma
t(12;16)	Myxoid liposarcoma
t(12;22)	Clear cell sarcoma (melanoma of soft parts)
t(2;13)	Alveolar rhabdomyosarcoma
1p($-$)	Neuroblastoma
RECEPTOR ANALYSIS	
Estrogen/progesterone receptor	Breast
MOLECULAR BIOLOGIC STUDIES	
Immunoglobulin, bcl-2, T-cell receptor gene rearrangement	Lymphoid neoplasm

[a] See text for discussion of cytokeratins.
[b] Or any other rearrangement involving an antigen-receptor gene.
NOTE: CEA, carcinoembryonic antigen; PSA, prostate-specific antigen; AFP, α fetoprotein.

that may be assessed in undifferentiated or poorly differentiated specimens. A diagnosis of lymphoma should be excluded by employing antibodies reactive to the leukocyte common antigen (LCA, CD45). LCA-positive tumors are lymphomas and have the same chances of responding to therapy as if the diagnosis were unambiguous. About half of patients with aggressive-histology lymphoma can be cured with combination chemotherapy (Chap. 112). The immunohistochemical detection of specific types of filament proteins is helpful in the identification of carcinomas and sarcomas. The presence of keratin suggests carcinoma; all epithelial tumors contain this protein. Specific types of cytokeratins (CK) permit a firm diagnosis. For example, ovarian cancers are CK20−/CK7+, colorectal cancers are CK20+/CK7−, and pancreaticobiliary tumors are CK20+/CK7+. However, certain sarcomas, mesotheliomas, and germ cell tumors are also keratin-positive. Sarcomas may react with antibodies to desmin. Sarcoma subgroups may be identified by expression of myoglobin (rhabdomyosarcoma) or factor VIII (angiosarcoma or Kaposi's sarcoma). Prostate, breast, and thyroid carcinomas express, respectively, PSA, gross cystic fluid protein, or thyroglobulin. The finding of AFP, βhCG, or placental alkaline phosphatase staining is very helpful in assigning a germ cell origin. The S-100 protein is present in virtually all primary and metastatic melanomas, including the amelanotic variety. However, S-100 positivity is also found in other tumors of neuroendocrine origin (e.g., small cell lung cancer, carcinoid, neuroepithelioma); a more specific marker for melanomas is the HMB45 (human melanoma black) antigen.

Other Diagnostic Approaches Electron microscopy can identify cell junctions (i.e., desmosomes, typical of epithelial cancers), neuroendocrine granules, melanosomes, and muscle filaments. Cytogenetic analysis may identify tumors with specific chromosomal translocations or other genetic abnormalities (Table 99-1). Cytogenetic abnormalities can also be determined by fluorescence in situ hybridization with chromosome-specific probes, a technique that does not require cells to divide, as is the case with traditional karyotype analysis. Fresh tissue may be required for detection of estrogen or progesterone receptors (to assess breast cancer) or antigens that are sensitive to fixation. Lineage can be assigned by analysis of DNA for signature gene rearrangements, such as those of immunoglobulin (B cell) or T cell receptor (T cell). Technological advances promise to influence the diagnosis of cancer. Isolation of mRNA from tumor specimens may permit the molecular profiling of tumors by microarray analysis of gene expression. This could lead to novel classifications of tumors based on molecular characteristics that may predict clinical behavior and/or response to specific therapies.

Additional Studies If the pathologist does not identify the likely tissue of origin, it is unlikely that additional expensive diagnostic tests will benefit the patient. In females with metastatic adenocarcinoma or poorly differentiated carcinoma, mammography should be performed, although the diagnostic yield will be quite low except in patients with axillary metastases. Magnetic resonance imaging, positron-emission tomography, or indium-111-pentreotide scanning can identify occult primary breast lesions but are expensive. The use of abdominal/pelvic CT scans leads to the identification of the primary site (often the pancreas) in up to 35% of patients but has little effect on natural history. Whether to measure serum tumor markers such as AFP, βhCG, carcinoembryonic antigen (CEA), CA-125 (associated with ovarian cancer), and PSA is controversial; value has not been proven. Numerous studies have shown a lack of benefit of contrast studies (upper gastrointestinal series, barium enema, or intravenous pyelogram) in patients with CUPS who have no specific symptoms and no findings referable to the gastrointestinal or urinary tract. Moreover, autopsy series reveal that the most likely primary site of origin includes epithelial tissues such as lung, stomach, colon, and kidney, which give rise to tumors that respond poorly to chemotherapy, minimizing the therapeutic impact of such a diagnosis.

Additional invasive diagnostic studies are indicated if the presentation strongly suggests a particular primary site. For example, radiographic evidence of lung or mediastinal involvement would mandate fiberoptic bronchoscopy to exclude lung cancer. In the relatively unusual case of metastatic squamous cell cancer presenting in an inguinal lymph node, anoscopy and colposcopy should be performed to detect carcinoma of the vulva, cervix, vagina, penis, or anus, all of which may be cured even with lymph node spread. A summary of a reasonable diagnostic approach is found in Table 99-2.

℞ **TREATMENT** **Prognostic Subgroups** The exclusion of treatable and potentially curable neoplasms is important. Patients with squamous cell carcinoma have a somewhat longer median survival (9 months) than do those with adenocarcinoma or unclassifiable neoplasms (4 to 6 months). If laboratory studies indicate a significant likelihood that the neoplasm is a lymphoma, germ cell tumor, sarcoma, neuroendocrine tumor, or breast or prostate cancer, then disease-appropriate therapy should be administered. Patients with lymphoma or a germ cell neoplasm may be cured with combination chemotherapy. In other malignancies, effective palliative chemotherapy (for sarcoma or a breast or neuroendocrine tumor) or hormonal therapy (for breast or prostate cancer) should be strongly considered. Although often requiring electron microscopy for diagnosis, neuroendocrine tumors (especially if anaplastic) often respond to cisplatin-based chemotherapy.

Patients in whom the primary site can be identified fare somewhat better than those in whom it remains undefined. Classification and regression tree (CART) analysis has led to a prognostic index ranging from a median survival of 40 months (those with one or two organ sites involved; not adenocarcinoma in histology; and without adrenal, bone, liver, or pleural involvement) to a median survival of 5 months (liver metastases, nonneuroendocrine histology, age $\geq$62). Patients may often be categorized as having one of several clinical features or syndromes suggesting a specific form of potentially beneficial therapy (Table 99-3).

Syndrome of unrecognized extragonadal germ cell cancer A subset of patients with poorly differentiated CUPS are responsive to chemotherapy. These patients display one or more of the following features: age <50; tumor involving midline structures, lung parenchyma, or lymph nodes; an elevated serum AFP or βhCG level; evidence of rapid tumor growth; or tumor responsiveness to previously administered radiotherapy or chemotherapy. Platinum-based chemotherapy has led to long-term survival in a fraction of patients with these features, especially those who have a favorable performance status at diagnosis, suggesting that their tumors behaved like germ cell neoplasms. If all patients with poorly differentiated carcinoma (including poorly differentiated adenocarcinoma) are treated with a chemotherapy regimen designed for germ cell cancer (e.g., cisplatin plus etoposide or vinblastine, often also with bleomycin) (Chap. 96), about 25% will respond completely and 33% will have a partial response. Patients whose disease does not respond to two cycles of therapy should not continue therapy. One in six patients survives >5 years without evidence of disease. Patients with poorly differentiated carcinoma or adenocarcinoma whose tumors have abnormalities of chromosome 12 similar to those described in patients with proven germ cell cancer are more likely to respond to platinum-based chemotherapy

Table 99-2 Suggested Clinical Evaluation of Patients with Metastatic Cancer of Unknown Primary Site

History: smoking history, asbestos exposure, abdominal pain
Physical examination: lymph nodes, thyroid, skin;
  Men: prostate
  Women: breasts, pelvic examination
Laboratory evaluation: stool evaluation for occult blood; urinalysis; complete blood count; liver function tests; calcium, electrolytes, creatine; measurement of serum levels of βhCG, AFP, CEA, and CA-125 (women); chest x-ray; abdominal and pelvic CT; mammography
Pathologic evaluation: see Table 99-1

NOTE: PSA, prostate-specific antigen; βhCG, β-human chorionic gonadotropin; AFP, α fetoprotein; CEA, carcinoembryonic antigen; CT, computed tomography.

Clinicopathologic Features	Suspected Primary Site	Suggested Therapy
Squamous cell carcinoma, cervical node	Head and neck cancer	Radical neck dissection; radiotherapy ± chemotherapy
Carcinoma, axillary nodes (female)	Breast cancer	Breast radiotherapy or mastectomy, systemic adjuvant therapy
Peritoneal carcinomatosis (female)	Ovarian cancer	Debulking surgery, cisplatin-based chemotherapy
Pleural effusion, adenocarcinoma cells estrogen and/or progesterone receptor positive	Breast cancer	Systemic therapy for metastatic breast cancer
Poorly differentiated cancer, age <50, lung or retroperitoneal or mediastinal mass or lymph nodes, elevated serum βhCG or AFP levels	Germ cell tumor (extragonadal)	Cisplatin/VP-16-based chemotherapy (controversial)
Bony metastases (male)	Prostate cancer	Androgen blockade (leuprolide plus flutamide)
Adenocarcinoma, liver metastases, elevated CEA level	Gastrointestinal malignancy	Surgical resection of liver lesion feasible; colonoscopy with resection (if appropriate) of tumors; 5-fluoro-uracil/leucovorin

NOTE: βhCG, β-human chorionic gonadotropin; AFP, α fetoprotein; CEA, carcinoembryonic antigen.

than are patients with a similar presentation whose tumors lack this cytogenetic abnormality.

Peritoneal carcinomatosis in women Women who present with increased abdominal girth and a pelvic mass or pain and who are found to have adenocarcinoma throughout the peritoneal cavity without a clear site of origin also may benefit from platinum-based chemotherapy. This syndrome has been termed *primary peritoneal papillary serous carcinoma* or *multifocal extraovarian serous carcinoma*. While breast cancer or a gastrointestinal malignancy can produce these findings, peritoneal carcinomatosis is most commonly ascribed to ovarian cancer, even in patients with apparently normal ovaries at the time of laparotomy. Especially if psammoma bodies or a papillary configuration is noted in the pathology examination or if the CA-125 level is elevated, women with adenocarcinoma of the peritoneal cavity without a defined primary should receive maximum surgical cytoreduction followed by cisplatin (or carboplatin) plus paclitaxel. The stage-specific response to such therapy appears to be comparable to that for patients with proven ovarian cancer. About 10% of patients who present in this fashion may remain free of disease 2 years after diagnosis.

Carcinoma in an axillary lymph node in a female Women with adenocarcinoma or poorly differentiated carcinoma in an axillary mass should receive treatment for stage II breast cancer whether or not a careful breast examination or mammography suggests the diagnosis of primary breast cancer and whether or not estrogen or progesterone receptors are detectable in the node. Even if no lesion is found in the breast, a breast recurrence will develop in one-half of these patients if no mastectomy is performed. Modified radical mastectomy or breast irradiation reduces the risk of local recurrence. In addition, adjuvant systemic therapy (chemotherapy and/or tamoxifen, depending on menopausal and estrogen receptor status) should be given to reduce the risk of developing evident metastatic breast cancer (Chap. 89).

Adjuvant systemic therapy may be administered before definitive local radiation treatment. Women with axillary metastases without an obvious breast primary appear to have the same likelihood of prolonged disease-free survival as patients with typical stage II breast cancer.

Bone metastases in males Particularly if the lesions are osteoblastic, the serum PSA level should be measured, as the probability of prostate carcinoma is high. Empirical hormonal therapy (e.g., leuprolide and flutamide) should be strongly considered.

Cervical lymph node metastases Patients who present with a neck mass should be considered to have a primary tumor of the upper aerodigestive tract (*head and neck cancer*) until a different source is proven. Especially if the pathologist diagnoses squamous histology and the node is located in a high or midcervical area, a careful ear, nose, and throat examination including direct laryngoscopy, nasopharyngoscopy, and random blind biopsies should be undertaken. A thyroid examination and scan should be performed to rule out a primary thyroid tumor, especially if the histology is not definitely squamous. Definitive local therapy (external beam radiation or radical neck dissection) combined with platinum-based chemotherapy may lead to prolonged survival in those with head and neck primaries (Chap. 87).

Adenocarcinoma and liver metastases Liver metastases from an adenocarcinoma is not as well characterized as a syndrome as the unrecognized germ cell cancer syndrome (nor as responsive to therapy). However, such patients may have a primary stomach, biliary, or colorectal tumor. Tumors with limited hepatic involvement may be amenable to resection. A flexible sigmoidoscopy or colonoscopy may detect a potentially obstructive colonic lesion. If a tumor is found, resection may be beneficial, depending on the tumor's size; even if none is found, treatment with a combination of 5-fluorouracil plus leucovorin is palliative for some patients with presumed metastatic gastrointestinal malignancy. Given the severe diarrhea that may be a consequence of this regimen and the relative resistance of gastrointestinal tumors to chemotherapy, patients should be informed of the risks before treatment.

Patients not falling into one of the preceding categories should be treated palliatively. In some patients, observation is appropriate. For example, individuals without evidence of additional metastatic disease who have undergone resection of a solitary pulmonary nodule containing malignant cells may actually have undergone definitive therapy for a small primary lung tumor. Radiation therapy may relieve symptoms in patients with bony pain or neurologic compromise. The largest and most poorly responsive subgroup are those with moderate to well-differentiated adenocarcinomas. Combination chemotherapy is frequently employed in such patients; however, response rates to "all-purpose" regimens [e.g., FAM (5-fluorouracil, doxorubicin, mitomycin C), FACP (5-fluorouracil, doxorubicin, cyclophosphamide, cisplatin)], or to ICE (ifosfamide, carboplatin, etoposide) are generally well under 50%, especially if patients with poorly differentiated adenocarcinoma, who have a higher response rate, are excluded; complete responses are rare. Regimens containing mitomycin C are associated with the risk of hemolytic uremic syndrome. In some series, patients with a good performance status whose disease is limited to soft tissue sites or extends only above the diaphragm have shown a better rate of response to therapy. While patients whose disease responds to treatment seem to have better survival than those whose disease does not respond, the difference may be related to inherent characteristics of the tumor rather than to a beneficial effect of chemotherapy.

Before combination chemotherapy is attempted in a patient with CUPS, the potential benefits must be weighed carefully against the certainty of toxicity. While some randomized studies have reported a benefit of one form of therapy over another, these reports are generally plagued by small numbers of patients and inadequate control of potential prognostic variables. Depending on motivation, eligibility, and availability, patients with CUPS may be candidates for evaluation of new (phase I) therapies.

BIBLIOGRAPHY

ABBRUZZESE JL et al: Analysis of a diagnostic strategy for patients with suspected tumors of unknown origin. J Clin Oncol 13:2094, 1995

CALIFANO J et al: Unknown primary head and neck squamous cell carcinoma: Molecular identification of the site or origin. J Natl Cancer Inst 91:599, 1999

DE BRAUD F, AL-SERRAF M: Diagnosis and management of squamous cell carcinoma of unknown primary tumor site of the neck. Semin Oncol 20:273, 1993

ETTINGER DS et al: NCCN practice guidelines for occult primary tumors. Oncology 12:226, 1998

GOLUB TR et al: Molecular classification of cancer: Class discovery and class prediction by gene expression monitoring. Science 256:531, 1999

HESS KR et al: Classification and regression tree analysis of 1000 consecutive patients with unknown primary carcinoma. Clin Cancer Res 5:3403, 1999

HAINSWORTH JD, GRECO FA: Management of patients with cancer of an unknown primary site. Oncology 14:563, 2000

LENZI R et al: Poorly differentiated carcinoma and poorly differentiated adenocarcinoma of unknown origin: Favorable subsets of patients with unknown primary carcinoma? J Clin Oncol 15:2056, 1997

MOTZER RJ et al: Molecular and cytogenetic studies in the diagnosis of patients with poorly differentiated carcinomas of unknown primary site. J Clin Oncol 13:274, 1995

MUGGIA FM, BARANDA J: Management of peritoneal carcinomatosis of unknown primary tumor site. Semin Oncol 20:268, 1993

100   *Bruce E. Johnson*

PARANEOPLASTIC SYNDROMES

ENDOCRINE SYNDROMES

Paraneoplastic syndromes are caused by factors produced by cancer cells that often act at a distance from both the primary cancer site and its metastases. The accurate documentation of a paraneoplastic endocrine syndrome requires (1) demonstration of mRNA expression and protein production by the tumor tissue, (2) biochemical and clinical resolution of the syndrome following successful surgical resection, (3) elevated levels of the hormone in the peripheral blood, (4) a tenfold or greater concentration gradient in the blood before and after it passes through the cancer, and (5) normal or suppressed endogenous hormone production.

The three major classes of hormones are steroids, monoamines, and peptides/proteins. Production of steroid hormones by malignant tumors is rare; lymphomas may produce 1,25-dihydroxyvitamin D from circulating 1-hydroxyvitamin D, but most other steroid-producing tumors are benign tumors of the glands that normally secrete the steroid. Monoamines such as norepinephrine and epinephrine are secreted by pheochromocytomas (Chap. 332), but they are not secreted ectopically by malignant tumor cells.

Most hormonal syndromes in patients with cancer are related to the production of peptide or protein hormones. The most common of these endocrine syndromes are listed in Table 100-1, together with the protein hormones that mediate them and the tumors that most commonly produce the hormones. A peptide hormone generally is encoded by an mRNA that is translated into a larger prohormone molecule, which undergoes a number of posttranslational modifications, including cleavage, glycosylation, and/or other steps. For example, pro-opiomelanocortin can be cleaved to yield adrenocorticotropic hormone (ACTH), lipotropin, endorphin, melanocyte-stimulating hormone, and/or enkephalin, with different cell types producing different products. In addition, some cells use alternatively spliced forms of the message to produce different proteins (e.g., calcitonin vs. calcitonin gene-related peptide).

Tumor cells of nonendocrine organs often lack certain components of the pathway that leads from prohormone to biologically active hormone to secreted product. Generally, as a result of defects in protein processing or post-translational changes, tumor cells may produce pro-teins that are structurally related to but biologically less active than the normal hormones. Thus, cancer patients may have elevated levels of immunoreactive hormones in plasma in the absence of clinical syndromes of hormone excess.

The severity of paraneoplastic endocrine syndromes often parallels the clinical course of the cancer. However, with some benign or slowly growing tumors, the hormone syndrome can be the major cause of morbidity. Despite their production by tumor cells, hormones are not very good tumor markers. Human chorionic gonadotropin (hCG) is a reliable tumor marker in some forms of testicular cancer, but no other hormone is used to quantitate tumor mass.

Most endocrine cancer syndromes occur with tumors derived from neuroendocrine or neural crest tissue (small cell lung cancer, carcinoid tumors). The genetic mechanisms that account for the production of a hormone by a cell that does not usually produce it are not clear. Oncogenes may activate other cellular genes (including genes that encode hormones) that normally are silent. Alternatively, demethylation of normally methylated inactive genes may permit expression in rapidly dividing cells.

HYPERCALCEMIA OF MALIGNANCY   Hypercalcemia of malignancy, the most common paraneoplastic endocrine syndrome, is responsible for approximately 40% of all hypercalcemia (Chap. 341). Hypercalcemia with cancer is classified as humoral hypercalcemia of malignancy (HHM), which is caused by circulating hormones, or local osteolytic hypercalcemia (LOH), which is caused by local paracrine factors secreted by cancers within bone. Parathyroid hormone-related peptide (PTHrP) causes nearly all cases of HHM, while the mediators of LOH in bone are heterogeneous.

Pathogenesis   Eighty percent of patients with hypercalcemia of malignancy have HHM. PTHrP is composed of 139 to 173 amino acids; 8 of the first 13 amino acids at the amino-terminal end are identical to the amino-terminal portion of parathyroid hormone (PTH). PTHrP binds to PTH receptors in the bone and kidney and causes increased bone resorption, decreased bone formation, increased renal tubular reabsorption of calcium, increased phosphaturia, and increased urinary levels of cyclic adenosine monophosphate, leading to hypercalcemia. PTHrP is detected in the plasma in ~80% of cancer patients with hypercalcemia. Rare patients have been reported to have hypercalcemia caused by ectopically produced authentic PTH. HHM in lymphoma may be caused by the production of 1,25-dihydroxyvitamin D by the tumor.

Twenty percent of patients with hypercalcemia have LOH, in which hypercalcemia is caused by the local production of hormones or cytokines by cancers that have spread to the bone or bone marrow; such factors increase bone resorption in the area around the cancer. The ectopically produced hormones that may play a role in LOH include transforming growth factors α and β, interleukin (IL)-1, IL-6, prostaglandins, and tumor necrosis factor.

Clinical Manifestations   The initial symptoms and signs of hypercalcemia (calcium level $\geq$ 2.6 mmol/L)[1] include malaise, fatigue, confusion, anorexia, bone pain, polyuria, polydipsia, weakness, constipation, nausea, and vomiting. Neurologic symptoms and signs in profound hypercalcemia (>3.5 mmol/L) include confusion, lethargy, coma, and death. The cancers associated with HHM are non-small cell lung cancer and cancers of the breast, kidney, head and neck, and bladder. HHM is particularly common in patients with cancers of squamous cell histology. Hypercalcemia is uncommon at presentation (<1% of patients) but becomes more common as the cancer progresses and is present in 10 to 20% of patients near the time of death. LOH is responsible for hypercalcemia in patients with breast cancer, myeloma, lymphoma, and leukemia. Among hypercalcemic patients with breast cancer, approximately half have HHM and half have LOH.

---

[1]Calcium measurements given in millimoles per liter can be multiplied by 4 to convert to milligrams per deciliter or by 2 to convert to milliequivalents per liter.

Diagnosis The patient with cancer who develops hypercalcemia should be evaluated for other causes of hypercalcemia, including use of thiazide diuretics, vitamin D, or lithium, hyperthyroidism, and sarcoidosis. If the underlying cancer is controlled, elevation of serum PTH as measured by immunoassay suggests primary hyperparathyroidism, which may be responsible for as many as 10% of cases of hypercalcemia of cancer and which should be treated like other cases of hyperparathyroidism (Chap. 341). A normal PTH level and a low serum phosphorus level in the absence of bone metastases support the diagnosis of HHM, while a normal PTHrP level and normal phosphorus in a patient with bone metastases suggest LOH.

℞ **TREATMENT** The median survival of patients with hypercalcemia of malignancy is only 1 to 3 months. Intervention to reverse hypercalcemia should be undertaken when the cancer is likely to be controlled with appropriate systemic or local treatment.

The treatment of HHM and LOH is similar (Chap. 341). Patients with mild to moderate hypercalcemia (2.7 to 3.5 mmol/L) can be treated with 2 to 4 L of saline hydration per day and furosemide to prevent intravascular volume overload. The bisphosphonate pamidronate (90 mg intravenously) decreases osteoclastic bone resorption. Combined administration of diuretics and pamidronate reduces the serum calcium to normal values in 90% of patients within 7 days. Doses may be repeated as needed. In patients with LOH, glucocorticoids may inhibit the production of cytokines that promote bone resorption. Severe hypercalcemia [3.50 mmol/L (>14 mg/dL)] with alteration of mental status can be treated with all of the above plus salmon calcitonin, 4 to 8 U/kg, administered intramuscularly or subcutaneously every 12 h. Calcitonin administration will decrease the serum calcium within 24 h, and its hypocalcemic effect can be prolonged in patients with LOH by adding glucocorticoids. If these agents are not effective in reducing the serum calcium, plicamycin and gallium nitrate may be added.

HYPONATREMIA OF MALIGNANCY Hyponatremia of malignancy (Na⁺ level <130 mmol/L) is usually due to the inappropriate secretion of arginine vasopressin (AVP) and is termed the *syndrome of inappropriate antidiuretic hormone secretion* (SIADH). In rare cases, atrial natriuretic peptide produces hyponatremia.

Pathogenesis Small cell lung cancer is the malignancy chiefly responsible for producing ectopic AVP. AVP mRNA is expressed and translated, and the product is processed into the nonapeptide AVP, which is secreted into the circulation. The ectopically produced AVP binds to receptors in the kidney, causing retention of free water with resulting hypoosmolality in the plasma and hyperosmolality in urine (Chap. 329).

About 15% of cancer patients with SIADH do not have evidence of ectopic production of AVP. In some of these patients, tumors secrete atrial natriuretic peptide. This hormone inhibits sodium reabsorption in the proximal tubule and inhibits release of renin and aldosterone. How atrial natriuretic peptide leads to hyponatremia is not clear.

Clinical Manifestations SIADH is commonly recognized as asymptomatic hyponatremia on routine serum chemistry examination. It is present at the time of diagnosis in 15% of patients with small cell lung cancer, 3% of patients with head and neck cancer, and <1% of patients with non-small cell lung cancer. Hyponatremia may also occur with primary brain tumors, hematologic malignancies, melanoma, sarcoma, and gynecologic, gastrointestinal, breast, prostate, and bladder cancers. The symptoms of mild hyponatremia (>120 mmol/L) include difficulty focusing attention, fatigue, nausea, vomiting, anorexia,

Table 100-1 Common Paraneoplastic Endocrine Syndromes

Syndrome	Proteins	Tumors Typically Associated with Syndrome
Hypercalcemia of malignancy	Parathyroid hormone-related peptide (PTHrP)	Non-small cell lung cancer
		Breast cancer
	Parathyroid hormone (PTH)	Renal cell carcinoma
		Head and neck cancer
		Bladder cancer
		Myeloma
Syndrome of inappropriate antidiuretic hormone secretion (SIADH)	Arginine vasopressin (AVP)	Small cell lung cancer
	Atrial natriuretic peptide	Head and neck cancer
		Non-small cell lung cancer
Cushing's syndrome	Adrenocorticotropic hormone (ACTH)	Small cell lung cancer
		Carcinoid tumors
	Corticotropin-releasing hormone (CRH)	
Acromegaly	Growth hormone–releasing hormone (GHRH)	Carcinoid tumors
		Small cell lung cancer
	Growth hormone (GH)	Pancreatic islet cell tumors
Gynecomastia	Human chorionic gonadotropin (hCG)	Testicular cancer
		Lung cancer
		Carcinoid tumors of the lung and gastrointestinal tract
Non-islet cell tumor hypoglycemia	Insulin-like growth factor-2 (IGF-2)	Sarcomas

weakness, and headache. Profound hyponatremia (<120 mmol/L) can cause confusion, lethargy, coma, seizures, and death.

Diagnosis (See also Chap. 329) SIADH is suspected in patients with hyponatremia (serum sodium <130 mmol/L) and a concentrated urine (osmolality >300 mosm/kg). Patients are euvolemic, are not using diuretics, and have normal thyroid and adrenal function. Polydipsia is excluded by the urine osmolality. Pseudohyponatremia can be present if serum glucose, triglyceride, or protein levels are high. Conditions other than cancer that can cause SIADH include central nervous system disorders, pulmonary infections, positive-pressure breathing, pneumothorax, asthma, and a wide array of drugs, including chemotherapeutic agents (vincristine, vinblastine, cisplatin, cyclophosphamide, melphalan), thiazide diuretics, carbamazepine, antidepressants, nicotine, and narcotics.

℞ **TREATMENT** Treatment should be directed at the underlying cancer. Patients whose tumors have not been or cannot be controlled are candidates for restriction of fluid intake to 500 mL/d. Such restriction corrects hyponatremia within 7 days in most patients, but it is difficult and uncomfortable for patients to maintain fluid restriction for extended periods. Oral demeclocycline (600 to 1200 mg/d) may be useful in blocking the effects of AVP but can cause renal insufficiency. Other agents that may be used for the treatment of hyponatremia include dilantin and lithium.

Rare patients develop profound hyponatremia and altered mental status. These patients should be treated with normal saline hydration and furosemide diuresis. If that is not effective, 3% saline can be administered via a central line together with furosemide diuresis to prevent hypervolemia. Hypertonic saline is rarely required and must be given slowly; fluid balance and electrolytes should be monitored several times per day, and the increase in sodium should be limited to 0.5 mmol/L per hour to prevent pontine lysis (Chap. 329).

ECTOPIC ACTH SYNDROME Ectopic production of ACTH by cancer cells is responsible for ~15% of all cases of Cushing's syndrome and for most cases of Cushing's syndrome that occur in cancer patients (Chaps. 328, 331). In rare patients, Cushing's syndrome is caused by ectopically produced corticotropin-releasing hormone (CRH), which stimulates pituitary ACTH release.

Pathogenesis When pro-opiomelanocortin mRNA is expressed in cancer cells, the 241-amino-acid prohormone is translated and processed into a variety of molecules, including, in some cases, the 39-amino-acid hormone ACTH, which can be secreted into the circulation. The ectopically produced ACTH causes excessive secretion of glucocorticoids and mineralocorticoids by the adrenals.

Clinical Manifestations Women make up 50% of patients with ectopic ACTH syndrome and 90% of patients with pituitary Cushing's disease. Therefore, Cushing's syndrome in men is more likely to be caused by ectopic ACTH than by a pituitary tumor. Because of mineralocorticoid excess, patients with ectopic Cushing's syndrome usually have hypokalemic alkalosis at presentation, a rare finding in patients with Cushing's disease. Other common manifestations of ectopic ACTH syndrome include weakness, hypertension, and hyperglycemia. Ectopic ACTH syndrome in patients with slow-growing cancers (e.g., carcinoids) may develop typical features of central obesity, moon facies, hyperpigmentation, and hirsutism in addition to the metabolic abnormalities.

Ectopic ACTH syndrome is most commonly due to small cell lung cancer (50% of cases), bronchial carcinoid tumors (10%), thymic carcinoid tumors or thymomas (10%), pancreatic islet cell tumors (10%), pheochromocytoma or other neural crest tumors (5%), or medullary carcinoma of the thyroid (5%). About 2% of patients with small cell lung cancer and bronchial carcinoids have ectopic ACTH syndrome at the time of diagnosis. Patients with small cell lung cancer and ectopic ACTH syndrome have shorter survival rates than patients without the syndrome and are more likely to develop opportunistic infections.

Diagnosis (See also Chaps. 328, 331) Ectopic ACTH syndrome is usually characterized by elevated levels of urinary free cortisol that do not decrease after administration of high doses of dexamethasone (8 mg/d). However, in 20 to 30% of patients with ectopic ACTH syndrome, urinary cortisol levels decrease by >50% after administration of high-dose dexamethasone. The plasma levels of ACTH are markedly elevated in more than half of patients. If these tests do not provide definitive evidence of ectopic ACTH syndrome, bilateral inferior petrosal vein sampling will show an elevated ACTH level in petrosal vein blood that does not increase after administration of CRH.

TREATMENT Treatment of the ectopic ACTH syndrome should be directed at the underlying cancer: chemotherapy for small cell lung cancer; surgical resection or radiation therapy for carcinoids. Some patients with ectopic Cushing's syndrome have no evidence of tumor after extensive evaluation. These patients should be treated symptomatically and followed closely with periodic imaging studies, because they may have slow-growing tumors amenable to surgical resection.

Agents that inhibit steroidogenesis in the adrenal gland include ketoconazole (400 to 1200 mg/d), which reduces urinary cortisol excretion by more than half in two-thirds of patients, and metyrapone (1 to 4 g/d), which also reduces urinary cortisol excretion. Patients who are in good condition and whose manifestations are not controlled by drugs may be considered for adrenalectomy.

ECTOPIC ACROMEGALY Ectopic production of growth hormone-releasing hormone (GHRH) is the predominant cause of ectopic acromegaly (Chap. 328).

Pathogenesis GHRH is processed into 40- and 44-amino-acid peptides and binds to receptors in the pituitary, increasing production of growth hormone that increases insulin-like growth factor (IGF)-1 production in peripheral tissues. Rare cases of ectopic acromegaly are due to ectopic production of growth hormone itself by tumors.

Clinical Manifestations The symptoms and signs of ectopic acromegaly develop over several years and include increasing glove and shoe size, facial disfigurement, arthralgias, amenorrhea-galactorrhea or impotence, hypertension, muscle weakness, and diabetes mellitus. Ectopic acromegaly has been reported in fewer than 100 patients and accounts for 1% or less of all cases of acromegaly. The cancers associated with ectopic acromegaly include carcinoid tumors of the bron-

chus, pancreatic islet cell tumors, and cancers of the lung, breast, colon, and adrenal glands.

Diagnosis If a clinical diagnosis of acromegaly is suspected in a patient with cancer, the serum levels of GHRH and IGF-1 and the glucose-suppressed growth hormone (GH) serum level should be measured (Chap. 328). Patients with elevated GHRH levels and acromegaly have ectopic acromegaly. Patients without evidence of cancer who have elevated GHRH levels should undergo imaging of the central nervous system, chest, and abdomen to look for an occult cancer. Patients with cancer, low GHRH levels, high GH levels, and elevated IGF-1 levels should undergo magnetic resonance imaging of the pituitary and hypothalamus. If no pituitary tumor is detected, GH may be secreted directly by the known tumor. Not all GH-secreting tumors of the pituitary are demonstrable by imaging techniques, however.

TREATMENT The therapy of ectopic acromegaly should be directed at the underlying cancer and should consist of surgical resection or radiation therapy for patients with carcinoid and islet cell tumors. Medical control of ectopic acromegaly is obtained by using octreotide (100 to 250 μg every 8 h), which inhibits pituitary secretion of growth hormone. Octreotide produces symptomatic improvement in approximately two-thirds of patients.

GYNECOMASTIA Ectopic production of hCG or estrogens by tumors such as cancers of the lung and testis is responsible for approximately 3% of cases of gynecomastia detected in men (Chap. 337). Ectopic production of hCG is the most common cause of paraneoplastic gynecomastia; the hCG acts by stimulating the Leydig cells of the testis to produce increased amounts of estrogen. Alternatively, on rare occasions, a tumor (such as a hepatoma or a germ cell tumor with choriocarcinoma elements) contains aromatase enzyme activity that converts circulating androgens to estrogen. Leydig cell or Sertoli cell tumors may also secrete estradiol. In all cases, the increased ratio of estrogen to testosterone leads to the proliferation of breast tissue and gynecomastia. Other tumors rarely associated with ectopic gynecomastia include carcinoid tumors of the bronchus, intestine, and small cell lung cancer.

About 5% of men with testicular choriocarcinoma present with an enlarging breast mass. In the absence of an obvious cancer, men presenting with gynecomastia should have a careful examination of the testes and measurement of serum hCG. Patients with a testicular mass should undergo an inguinal orchiectomy for diagnosis and treatment. If no testicular mass is found by physical examination, the testes should be examined with ultrasound. Patients with an elevated hCG level and no testicular mass should undergo evaluation for an extragonadal germ cell tumor.

TREATMENT The therapy of tumor-associated gynecomastia should be directed at the underlying cancer: chemotherapy is used for testicular cancers, and surgical resection or radiation therapy for carcinoids and islet cell tumors. In patients with successfully treated testicular cancer, gynecomastia completely resolves in three-fourths of cases.

NON-ISLET CELL TUMOR HYPOGLYCEMIA Hypoglycemia that is not caused by the ectopic production of insulin (as in patients with islet cell tumors of the pancreas) can occur with large, slow-growing sarcomas, mesotheliomas, and hepatomas (Chap. 334). Ectopic production of IGF-2 is responsible for hypoglycemia in most patients with non-islet cell tumors. The ectopically produced IGF-2 inhibits glycogenolysis and gluconeogenesis in the liver, suppresses lipolysis, and increases peripheral glucose utilization, thereby causing hypoglycemia. IGF-2 may also act as an autocrine growth factor for the tumor.

Patients with large sarcomas (1 to 10 kg) may develop hypoglycemia, particularly with fasting. Headache, fatigue, confusion, or seizures may occur. Patients with a large sarcoma and hypoglycemia are likely to have non-islet cell tumor hypoglycemia. Although IGF-2 protein or mRNA is detectable in tumor tissue, the diagnosis is usually made on clinical grounds, because the plasma levels of IGF-2 are typically not elevated. Levels of IGF binding proteins may be increased.

R̲x̲ **TREATMENT** The therapy of non-islet cell hypoglycemia should be directed at the underlying cancer: surgical resection or radiation therapy. Patients whose tumors cannot be successfully resected or irradiated can be treated with frequent oral feedings or constant intravenous administration of glucose.

HEMATOLOGIC SYNDROMES

The elevation of granulocyte, platelet, and eosinophil counts in most patients with myeloproliferative disorders is caused by the proliferation of the myeloid elements due to the underlying disease rather than a paraneoplastic syndrome. The paraneoplastic hematologic syndromes in patients with solid tumors are less well characterized than the endocrine syndromes, because the ectopic hormone(s) or cytokines responsible have not been identified in most of these tumors (Table 100-2). The severity of the paraneoplastic syndromes parallels the course of the cancer.

ERYTHROCYTOSIS Ectopic production of erythropoietin by cancer cells causes most paraneoplastic erythrocytosis. The ectopically produced erythropoietin stimulates the production of red blood cells in the bone marrow and raises the hematocrit. Other lymphokines and hormones produced by cancer cells may stimulate erythropoietin release but have not been proven to cause erythrocytosis.

Most patients with erythrocytosis have an elevated hematocrit (>52% in men; 48% in women) that is detected on a routine blood count. Approximately 3% of patients with renal cell cancer, 10% of patients with hepatoma, and 15% of patients with cerebellar hemangioblastomas have erythrocytosis. In most cases the erythrocytosis is asymptomatic.

Patients with erythrocytosis due to a renal cell cancer, hepatoma, or central nervous system cancer should have measurement of red cell mass. If the red cell mass is elevated, the serum erythropoietin level should then be measured. Patients with an appropriate cancer, elevated erythropoietin levels, and no other explanation for erythrocytosis (e.g., a hemoglobinopathy that causes increased O_2 affinity, Chap. 106) have the paraneoplastic syndrome.

Table 100-2 Paraneoplastic Hematologic Syndromes

Syndrome	Proteins	Cancers Typically Associated with Syndrome
Erythrocytosis	Erythropoietin	Renal cancers
		Hepatocarcinoma
		Cerebellar hemangioblastomas
Granulocytosis	G-CSF	Lung cancer
	GM-CSF	Gastrointestinal cancer
	IL-6	Ovarian cancer
		Genitourinary cancer
Thrombocytosis	IL-6	Lung cancer
		Gastrointestinal cancer
		Breast cancer
		Ovarian cancer
		Lymphoma
Eosinophilia	IL-5	Lymphoma
		Leukemia
		Lung cancer
Thrombophlebitis	Unknown	Lung cancer
		Pancreatic cancer
		Gastrointestinal cancer
		Breast cancer
		Genitourinary cancer
		Ovarian cancer
		Prostate cancer
		Lymphoma

R̲x̲ **TREATMENT** Successful resection of the cancer usually resolves the erythrocytosis. If the tumor neither can be resected nor treated effectively with radiation therapy or chemotherapy, phlebotomy may control any symptoms related to erythrocytosis.

GRANULOCYTOSIS Approximately 30% of patients with solid tumors have granulocytosis (granulocyte count >8000/μL). In about half of patients with granulocytosis and cancer, the granulocytosis has an identifiable nonparaneoplastic etiology (infection, tumor necrosis, glucocorticoid administration, etc.). The other patients have proteins in urine and serum that stimulate the growth of bone marrow cells. Tumors and tumor cell lines from patients with lung, ovarian, and bladder cancers have been documented to produce granulocyte colony-stimulating factor (G-CSF), granulocyte-macrophage colony-stimulating factor (GM-CSF), and/or IL-6. However, the etiology of granulocytosis has not been characterized in most patients.

Patients with granulocytosis are nearly all asymptomatic, and the differential white blood cell count does not have a shift to immature forms of neutrophils. Granulocytosis occurs in 40% of patients with lung and gastrointestinal cancers, 20% of patients with breast cancer, 30% of patients with brain tumors and ovarian cancers, and 10% of patients with renal cell carcinoma. Patients with advanced-stage disease are more likely to have granulocytosis than those with early-stage disease.

Paraneoplastic granulocytosis does not require treatment. The granulocytosis resolves when the underlying cancer is successfully treated.

THROMBOCYTOSIS Thirty-five percent of patients with thrombocytosis (platelet count >400,000/μL) have an underlying diagnosis of cancer. IL-6, a candidate molecule for the etiology of paraneoplastic thrombocytosis, stimulates the production of platelets in vitro and in vivo. Some patients with cancer and thrombocytosis have elevated levels of IL-6 in plasma. Another candidate molecule is thrombopoietin, a peptide hormone that stimulates megakaryocyte proliferation and platelet production. The etiology of thrombocytosis has not been established in most cases.

Patients with thrombocytosis are nearly all asymptomatic. Thrombocytosis is not clearly linked to thrombosis in patients with cancer. Thrombocytosis is present in 40% of patients with lung and gastrointestinal cancers, 20% of patients with breast, endometrial, and ovarian cancers, and 10% of patients with lymphoma. Patients with thrombocytosis are more likely to have advanced-stage disease and have a poorer prognosis than patients without thrombocytosis. Paraneoplastic thrombocytosis does not require treatment.

EOSINOPHILIA Eosinophilia is present in ~1% of patients with cancer. Tumors and tumor cell lines from patients with lymphomas or leukemia may produce IL-5, which stimulates eosinophil growth. Activation of IL-5 transcription in lymphomas and leukemias may involve translocation of the long arm of chromosome 5, to which the genes for IL-5 and other cytokines map.

Patients with eosinophilia are typically asymptomatic. Eosinophilia is present in 10% of patients with lymphoma, 3% of patients with lung cancer, and occasional patients with cervical, gastrointestinal, renal, and breast cancer. Patients with markedly elevated eosinophil counts (>5000/μL) can develop shortness of breath and wheezing. A chest radiograph may reveal diffuse pulmonary infiltrates from eosinophil infiltration and activation in the lungs.

R̲x̲ **TREATMENT** Definitive treatment is directed at the underlying malignancy: tumors should be resected or treated with radiation or chemotherapy. In most patients who develop shortness of breath related to eosinophilia, symptoms resolve with the use of oral or inhaled glucocorticoids.

THROMBOPHLEBITIS Deep venous thrombosis and pulmonary embolism are the most common thrombotic conditions in patients with cancer. Migratory or recurrent thrombophlebitis may be the initial manifestation of cancer. Approximately 15% of patients who develop deep venous thrombosis or pulmonary embolism have a diagnosis of cancer (Chap. 117). The coexistence of peripheral venous thrombosis with visceral carcinoma, particularly pancreatic cancer, is called *Trousseau's syndrome.*

Pathogenesis Patients with cancer are predisposed to thromboembolism because they are often at bedrest or immobilized, and tumors may obstruct or slow blood flow. In addition, clotting may be promoted by release of procoagulants or cytokines from tumor cells or associated inflammatory cells, or by platelet adhesion or aggregation. The specific molecules that mediate the increased risk of thromboembolism have not been identified.

Clinical Manifestations Patients with cancer who develop deep venous thrombosis usually develop swelling or pain in the leg, and physical examination reveals tenderness, warmth, and redness. Patients who present with pulmonary embolism develop dyspnea, chest pain, and syncope, and physical examination shows tachycardia, cyanosis, and hypotension. Approximately 5% of patients with no history of cancer who have a diagnosis of deep venous thrombosis or pulmonary embolism will have a diagnosis of cancer within 1 year. The most common cancers associated with thromboembolic episodes include lung, pancreatic, gastrointestinal, breast, ovarian, and genitourinary cancers, lymphomas, and brain tumors. Patients with cancer who undergo surgical procedures requiring general anesthesia have a 20 to 30% risk of deep venous thrombosis.

Diagnosis The diagnosis of deep venous thrombosis in patients with cancer is made by impedance plethysmography or bilateral compression ultrasonography of the leg veins. Patients with a noncompressible venous segment have deep venous thrombosis. If compression ultrasonography is normal and a high clinical suspicion exists for deep venous thrombosis, venography should be done to look for a luminal filling defect. Elevation of D-dimer is not as predictive of deep venous thrombosis in patients with cancer as in patients without cancer.

Patients with symptoms and signs suggesting a pulmonary embolism should be evaluated with a chest radiograph, electrocardiogram, arterial blood gas analysis, and ventilation–perfusion scan. Patients with mismatched segmental perfusion defects have a pulmonary embolus. Patients with equivocal ventilation–perfusion findings should be evaluated as described above for deep venous thrombosis in their legs. If deep venous thrombosis is detected, they should be anticoagulated. If deep venous thrombosis is not detected, they should be considered for a pulmonary angiogram.

Patients without a diagnosis of cancer who present with an initial episode of thrombophlebitis or pulmonary embolus need no additional tests for cancer other than a careful history and physical exam. In light of the many possible primary sites, diagnostic testing in asymptomatic patients is wasteful. However, if the clot is refractory to standard treatment or is in an unusual site, or if the thrombophlebitis is migratory or recurrent, efforts to find an underlying cancer are indicated.

℞ **TREATMENT** Patients with cancer and a diagnosis of deep venous thrombosis or pulmonary embolism should be treated initially with intravenous unfractionated heparin or low molecular weight heparin for at least 5 days and coumadin started within 1 or 2 days. The coumadin dose should be adjusted so the INR is 2 to 3. Patients with proximal deep venous thrombosis and a relative contraindication to heparin anticoagulation (hemorrhagic brain metastases or pericardial effusion) should be considered for placement of a filter in the inferior vena cava (Greenfield filter) to prevent pulmonary embolism. Coumadin should be administered for 3 to 6 months. Patients with cancer who undergo a major surgical procedure should be considered for heparin prophylaxis or pneumatic boots. Breast cancer patients undergoing chemotherapy and patients with implanted catheters should be considered for prophylaxis (1 mg coumadin per day).

→*Cutaneous paraneoplastic syndromes are discussed in Chap. 57. Neurologic paraneoplastic syndromes are discussed in Chap. 101. More extensive discussion of functional endocrine tumors is given in Chap. 93.*

BIBLIOGRAPHY

BARTTER F, SCHWARTZ W: The syndrome of inappropriate secretion of antidiuretic hormone. Am J Med 42:790, 1967

BODY JJ et al: Current use of bisphosphonates in oncology. International Bone and Cancer Study Group. J Clin Oncol 16:3890, 1998

BRAUNSTEIN GD: Gynecomastia. N Engl J Med 328:490, 1993

EZZAT S: Acromegaly. Endocrinol Metab Clin North Am 26:703, 1997

JOHNSON BE et al: A prospective study of patients with lung cancer and hyponatremia of malignancy. Am J Respir Crit Care Med 156:1669, 1997

LEE AY et al: Clinical utility of a rapid whole-blood D-dimer assay in patients with cancer who present with suspected acute deep venous thrombosis. Ann Intern Med 131:417, 1999

LEVINE MN, LEE AY: Treatment of venous thromboembolism in cancer patients. Semin Thromb Hemost 25:245, 1999

NEWELL-PRICE J et al: The diagnosis and differential diagnosis of Cushing's syndrome and pseudo-Cushing's states. Endocr Rev 19:647, 1998

WINQUIST EW et al: Ketoconazole in the management of paraneoplastic Cushing's syndrome secondary to ectopic adrenocorticotropin production. J Clin Oncol 13:157, 1995

101 Muhammad T. Al-Lozi, Alan Pestronk

PARANEOPLASTIC NEUROLOGIC SYNDROMES

GENERAL PRINCIPLES

A paraneoplastic neurologic syndrome (PNNS) is a neurologic disorder that is associated with a neoplasm but lies anatomically remote from it. Paraneoplastic disorders are caused by immune or other mechanisms and are not due to direct effects of the tumor itself, metastases, opportunistic infections, complications of drug or radiation therapy, or malnutrition. Clinical features of a PNNS are often distinctive. Onset can be dramatic, arising subacutely over weeks or even days to produce neurologic symptoms that may be profoundly disabling.

PNNS associated with autoantibodies can be grouped into (1) disorders in which the neoplasm contains a surface antigen or intracellular protein that is the antigenic target, and (2) monoclonal gammopathy syndromes associated with secretion of an antibody by the neoplasm. Each subgroup has typical clinical, pathologic, and immune characteristics (Table 101-1). Some PNNS, including lymphoma-associated motor neuropathy, subacute necrotic myelopathy, dermatomyositis, and necrotizing myopathy, have no currently identified antibody or target antigen and are not yet classifiable in this scheme.

The temporal relationship of a PNNS to the associated neoplasm is variable. The PNNS may precede or follow the identification of a neoplasm by weeks, months, or occasionally years. The strength of the association between neoplasms and PNNS varies with different syndromes, different neoplasms, and the clinical context. In some PNNS, such as the sensory neuronopathy associated with anti-Hu antibodies, the association with neoplasm is very strong. By contrast, the Lambert-Eaton myasthenic syndrome (LEMS) is associated with neoplasm in approximately 50% of cases only; the relationship is probably stronger in older individuals who have a history of cigarette smoking. Disorders that are clinically identical to most PNNS also occur in the absence of cancer. Nonetheless, the development of a PNNS in a previously healthy individual should in most circumstances prompt a thorough search for its associated neoplasms.

PNNS-associated neoplasms vary considerably in terms of malignancy. Tumors associated with subacute necrotic myelopathy are often severe and unresponsive to therapy. In other syndromes, the tumor either remains small or can be effectively treated; in such cases, the

Table 101-1 General Features of Paraneoplastic Neurologic Syndromes (PNNS) Associated with Autoantibodies

Features		Intracellular Antigen	Surface Membrane Antigen	Neoplasm Produces Antibody
		Tumor Protein is Antigenic Target		
Clinical	Disease location	Central NS	Nerve or muscle	Peripheral nerve
		Occasionally peripheral NS	Rarely central NS	Occasionally muscle
	Disease course	Subacute onset → plateau	Subacute onset → plateau	Chronic progression
	Treatment	Rarely effective	Immunomodulation, many types	Immunomodulation, cytotoxic
	Disease pathology	Neural cell death	Membrane dysfunction	Damage to axons or myelin
			Focal damage to nerve or muscle cell	
	Typical disorders	Sensory neuronopathy (Hu)	Myasthenia gravis	Motor neuropathy (IgM anti-G_{M1})
		Cerebellar ataxia (Yo)	LEMS	Anti-MAG neuropathy (IgM)
		Limbic encephalitis (Hu; Ma2)	Isaac's neuromyotonia	POEMS (IgG or IgA)
				Cryoglobulinemia
				Amyloidosis
Antigen	Location	PNNS target; neoplasm	PNNS target; neoplasm	PNNS target
		Nuclear or cytoplasmic	Surface membrane	Cell surface
	Type	RNA binding proteins	Transmitter receptor	Glycolipid
		Golgi-related proteins	Ion channel	Glycoprotein
Antibody	Location	Serum	Serum	Serum
		CSF	Usually not CSF	
	Type	Polyclonal IgG	Polyclonal IgG	Monoclonal
				IgM: known target
				IgG or IgA: ? target
	Pathogenic	Rarely	Often	Probably
Neoplasm types		Small cell lung	Small cell lung	MGUS
		Gynecologic	Thymoma	Lymphoma
		Testicular	Lymphoma	
Neoplasm frequency		Nearly always: 80 to 95%	Variable: 10 to 70%	Nearly always

NOTE: NS, nervous system; LEMS, Lambert-Eaton myasthenic syndrome; G_{M1}, G_{M1} ganglioside; MAG, myelin-associated glycoprotein; CSF, cerebrospinal fluid; POEMS, polyneuropathy, organomegaly, endocrinopathy, m-protein, skin changes; MGUS, monoclonal gammopathy of unknown significance.

long-term prognosis is determined by the effectiveness of management of the paraneoplastic syndrome. Thymoma associated with myasthenia gravis is an example of a tumor in this category. In some PNNS, such as those associated with small cell lung cancer (SCLC) and anti-Hu antibodies, it has been suggested that the presence of the autoantibodies may confer a more favorable prognosis by inhibiting tumor growth.

As outlined in Table 101-2, certain syndromes are associated with particular types of tumors, and more than one syndrome may occur with a given neoplasm. For example, SCLCs are associated with a variety of PNNS, including limbic encephalitis, cerebellar ataxia, opsoclonus-myoclonus, necrotic myelopathy, sensory neuronopathy, autonomic neuropathy, and LEMS.

Prevalence estimates vary with the particular syndrome. Tumors that are most often associated with PNNS are cancers of the lung, stomach, breast, ovary, and colon. Some 30% of patients with thymoma also develop myasthenia gravis as a paraneoplastic syndrome. A poorly characterized neuromyopathy with proximal weakness and distal sensory loss is very common in patients who have lost more than 15% of their body weight. In contrast, most of the well-defined PNNS are rare, with estimated prevalence rates of <1% of the population with cancer.

The diagnosis of a PNNS depends primarily on (1) the presence of a recognized clinical paraneoplastic syndrome; (2) careful exclusion of other cancer-related disorders; and (3) appropriate confirmatory studies, including measurement of specific antibodies and neurophysiologic studies to define the anatomic distribution of the disease process.

PNNS OF THE CENTRAL NERVOUS SYSTEM

LIMBIC ENCEPHALITIS Limbic encephalitis is a feature of several paraneoplastic syndromes. It occurs in isolation or overlaps with syndromes that also involve the brainstem, cerebellum, spinal cord, and posterior root ganglia. Patients present with seizures, confusion, psychiatric symptoms (agitation, hallucinations, depression, anxiety, and changes in personality), or severe short-term memory loss. Seizures are commonly complex-partial in type, with or without secondary generalization, and may be intractable and refractory to

treatment. Other features can include vertigo, ataxia, nystagmus, numbness/paresthesias, and symmetric or asymmetric weakness. Limbic encephalitis typically progresses over a period of weeks before stabilizing. Exacerbations may occur, and remissions are rare, with or without treatment. The onset of symptoms may precede or follow the discovery of tumor. Limbic encephalitis is most commonly associated with SCLC; less frequently with testicular cancer; and occasionally with thymoma, Hodgkin's disease, non-SCLC, breast, colon, and bladder cancer. Some cases are not associated with cancer.

Magnetic resonance imaging (MRI) suggests that paraneoplastic limbic encephalitis is often a relatively widespread disease of the central nervous system. The T2 signal may be increased not only in the temporal lobes but also in the cortex or brainstem. Approximately 75% of patients show electroencephalographic abnormalities that may include focal slowing and/or paroxysmal sharp waves and spikes. Cerebrospinal fluid (CSF) often shows elevated protein, mild mononuclear pleocytosis, oligoclonal bands, or increased IgG synthesis but may be normal.

Neuropathologic features of limbic encephalitis include neuronal loss in the hippocampus, cingulate gyrus, orbital frontal lobe, brainstem, and posterior root ganglia. Additionally, there may be scattered gliosis, microglial nodules, and/or perivascular lymphocytic cuffing.

Anti-Hu antibodies (Table 101-2) are detected in the serum and CSF in the majority of patients with paraneoplastic limbic encephalitis. Most patients with anti-Hu antibodies have SCLC; however, breast and prostate cancer and neuroblastoma are also described. Approximately 20% of patients with SCLC without neurologic symptoms have low titers of anti-Hu antibodies. Anti-Hu antibodies are strongly (>90%) associated with neoplasms; patients with positive antibody titers but a negative initial malignancy workup should have a search for neoplasm repeated every 6 to 12 months. Immunotherapy [plasma exchange, intravenous immunoglobulin (IVIg), cyclophosphamide, or glucocorticoids] and/or resection of primary tumor are only rarely associated with improvement in the limbic encephalitis.

Patients with limbic and/or brainstem encephalitis and testicular cancer may have serum IgG antibodies that bind to Ma2, a 40-kD cytoplasmic and nuclear protein. Ma2 is expressed in both brain tissue

Table 101-2 Neurologic Paraneoplastic Syndromes

Syndrome	Features	Antibody Target	Neoplasm/Percentage
BRAIN			
Limbic encephalitis	Onset: subacute Confusion Memory loss Temporal lobe seizures	Hu	SCLC, testicular cancer, breast, colon, bladder, lymphoma
Brainstem encephalitis	Vertigo Cerebellar: ataxia, nystagmus Ocular: diplopia, gaze palsies	Hu	SCLC
Cerebellar degeneration	Cerebellar: ataxia, dysarthria	Yo Tr Glutamate receptors	Ovary, uterus, SCLC, Hodgkin's lymphoma
Opsoclonus/myoclonus	Involuntary eye movements: rapid, random directions Ataxia Encephalopathy	Ri (NOVA) Hu Neurofilament	Neuroblastoma, lung, breast
SPINAL CORD			
Necrotizing myelopathy	Weakness: paraplegia or quadriplegia Sensory loss: spinal level Urinary incontinence	Not known	SCLC, lymphoma
PERIPHERAL NERVE			
Neuronopathies			
Sensory neuronopathy	Onset: subacute Sensory loss; diffuse, asymmetric, numbness/paresthesias, dysesthesia/pain Sensory ataxia: pseudoathetosis ± encephalomyelitis	Hu	SCLC (90% of cases), breast, ovary, prostate
Motor neuronopathy	Onset: subacute Weakness: arms > legs Usually asymmetric	Not known	Lymphoma
Axonal neuropathies			
Sensorimotor neuropathy	Distal motor and sensory loss Most common paraneoplastic neuropathy, especially with >15% weight loss Axonal neuropathy	None	Many neoplasms
Mononeuritis multiplex	Weakness and/or sensory loss in the distribution of multiple nerves Onset: acute to subacute	Not known	Cryoglobulinemia, leukemia, lymphoma
Neuromyotonia (Isaacs)	Weakness: distal and proximal Stiffness Fasciculations	Voltage-gated potassium channels	Thymoma
Amyloid neuropathy	Distal symmetric axonal loss: small > large Autonomic symptoms prominent	Not known	Multiple myeloma
Autonomic neuropathies			
Enteric neuropathy	Gastroparesis Intestinal pseudo-obstruction Esophageal achalasia Dysphagia	Hu	Thymoma, SCLC
Demyelinating neuropathies			
Anti-MAG	Sensory > motor Distal, symmetric Gait disorder Tremor Slowly progressive NCV: Long distal latencies, Conduction block uncommon	Myelin-associated glycoprotein (MAG)	MGUS, IgM M-protein in 85%
Multifocal motor neuropathy	Slowly progressive Motor Distal > proximal Asymmetric NCV: Motor conduction block Motor axon loss (late)	G_{M1} ganglioside	MGUS, IgM M-protein in 20%
Anti-sulfatide	Slowly progressive Sensory > motor Distal, symmetric Demyelinating or axonal	Sulfatide	MGUS, IgM M-protein in 90% with demyelinating neuropathy
POEMS	Sensorimotor neuropathy Symmetric Mixed demyelinating and axonal	Not known	Multiple myeloma, IgG or IgA M-protein in 90%
CIDP	Chronic or relapsing Motor > sensory Distal and proximal weakness Usually symmetric NCV: Conduction block, slow sensory and motor conduction velocities	β-Tubulin in 20%	MGUS, IgM or IgG M-protein in 15%, lymphoma

(continued)

Table 101-2—(continued)

Syndrome	Features	Antibody Target	Neoplasm/Percentage
NEUROMUSCULAR JUNCTION			
LEMS	Weakness: proximal and distal Ocular: ptosis May improve with exercise Dry mouth Rapid repetitive stimulation: increment	Voltage-gated P/Q calcium channels	SCLC in 60% of cases, especially older and smoking history

Myasthenia gravis	Weakness
	  Cranial: ocular, face, bulbar
	  Respiratory, limbs, trunk
	Fatigue
	Slow repetitive stimulation: decrement
		Nicotinic acetylcholine receptor	Thymoma in 10%, especially >30 years

MUSCLE			
Necrotizing myopathy	Males > 40 Rapid-onset weakness Necrosis on muscle biopsy May improve with treatment of cancer	Not known	Lung, breast, alimentary tract
Dermatomyositis	Females > 40 Proximal muscle weakness Skin rash	Not known	Ovarian, nasopharyngeal
Type II atrophy	Especially with weight loss > 15% Wasting > weakness	Not known	Many neoplasms
Myopathy with anti-decorin antibodies	> 50 years of age Proximal symmetric weakness Mildly elevated creatine kinase	Decorin	Waldenström's macroglobulinemia, IgM M-protein
Rippling muscle disease	Cramps induced by touching muscle Muscle waves induced by percussion Electrically silent	Not known	Thymoma
Scleromyxedema	Skin papules Raynaud's phenomenon Proximal muscle weakness High creatine kinase Myopathic electromyography	Not known	MGUS, IgG or IgA λ M-protein

NOTE: SCLC, small cell lung cancer; NCV, nerve conduction velocity; MGUS, monoclonal gammopathy of undetermined significance; POEMS, polyneuropathy, organomegaly, endocrinopathy, m-protein, skin changes; CIDP, chronic inflammatory demyelinating polyneuropathy; LEMS, Lambert-Eaton myasthenic syndrome.

and testicular tumors. Occasional patients in this subgroup have improved after treatment of the primary neoplasm.

BRAINSTEM ENCEPHALITIS Paraneoplastic brainstem encephalitis is usually associated with disease elsewhere in the central or peripheral nervous system. Symptoms of brainstem encephalitis relate to the distribution of the disease process. The predominant symptoms are due to medullary involvement producing nausea, vomiting, nystagmus, vertigo, and ataxia. A rare syndrome of marked dysarthria and dysphagia is associated with pontine involvement. Mesencephalic inflammation and neuronal loss result in nuclear or internuclear eye movement abnormalities; diplopia and oscillopsia may be disabling. Rostral midbrain and nigral involvement may cause rigidity. Other rare disorders are deafness and hypoventilation.

PARANEOPLASTIC CEREBELLAR DEGENERATION (PCD) Approximately 90% of PCD occurs with SCLC, Hodgkin's lymphoma, or breast or ovarian cancer. Patients usually present with the subacute onset of a pancerebellar disorder consisting of nystagmus, oculomotor ataxia, dysarthric speech, and limb and gait ataxia (Chaps. 22 and 364). In many patients, especially those with the anti-Yo antibody syndrome, signs are restricted to cerebellar dysfunction. However, symptoms of more widespread central (lethargy, cognitive abnormalities) and peripheral (weakness, sensory changes, and dry mouth) nervous system involvement may be present. Symptoms usually progress over weeks and eventually stabilize, leaving the patient severely disabled.

MRI usually reveals cerebellar atrophy. The CSF may be normal or show mildly elevated protein, mononuclear pleocytosis, increased IgG index, and/or oligoclonal bands. The most consistent neuropathologic feature is a diffuse loss of Purkinje cells. Neuronal loss in the granular cell layer and deep cerebellar nuclei may also occur. Perivascular cuffing has been observed in the cerebellum and leptomeninges.

PCD may be associated with polyclonal IgG anti-Yo, anti-Tr, or anti-glutamate receptor (mGluR1) antibodies in the serum and CSF. Anti-Yo antibodies are commonly associated with breast or ovarian cancer. The Yo autoantigens are proteins that are prominently expressed in Purkinje cell cytoplasm (Golgi) and proximal dendrites but not in the nucleus. Anti-Tr and anti-mGluR1 antibodies occur with Hodgkin's lymphoma. Clinical features in the three antibody groups are similar. PCD syndromes rarely improve after treatment; however, occasional anti-Tr patients improve after treatment of Hodgkin's lymphoma. Reappearance or exacerbation of the PCD may indicate recurrence of the tumor.

PARANEOPLASTIC OPSOCLONUS-MYOCLONUS (POM) This disorder is also known as the "dancing eyes–dancing feet" syndrome. Opsoclonic eye movements are involuntary, high-amplitude, arrhythmic, multidirectional, conjugate saccades. They are often nearly continuous and persist with the eyes closed and during sleep. Opsoclonus is associated with blinking and myoclonus and increases with visual pursuit and voluntary ocular refixation. The syndrome may occur in isolation or as a component of other PNNS, including limbic or brainstem encephalitis. POM occurs in 2% of young children with neuroblastoma and may precede or follow the discovery of the neoplasm; 50% of children with POM harbor neuroblastoma. Patients may also manifest ataxia, irritability, and vomiting. Antibodies directed against neurofilaments have been described. In the pediatric population, POM may improve following treatment with adrenocorticotropic hormone (ACTH), glucocorticoids, or IVIg, but residual central nervous system signs are frequent.

In adults, opsoclonus/myoclonus syndromes may develop in association with neoplasms of the lung (anti-Hu antibodies), breast (anti-Ri antibodies), thymus, lymphoid cells, ovaries, uterus, and bladder. Anti-Ri antibodies bind to neuronal nuclear antigens, including NOVA-1, a protein that regulates RNA splicing or metabolism in a subset of developing neurons. Remissions may occur spontaneously or following treatment of the underlying tumor. Clonazepam and/or valproate may be useful for symptomatic control of opsoclonus and myoclonus.

CARCINOMA-ASSOCIATED RETINOPATHY (CAR) The chief complaint in CAR is unilateral or bilateral, symmetric or asymmetric, loss of vision. Night blindness may be the presenting symptom. The visual loss occurs either gradually or in a stepwise pattern over weeks to months. Other symptoms may include visual shimmering, sparkling, or distortions. Examination shows poor visual acuity, impaired color vision, and an afferent pupillary defect. Visual field defects most commonly consist of central and/or ring scotomas. CAR occurs mainly with SCLC (90%) but may also occur with melanoma and gynecologic neoplasms. CAR visual loss frequently precedes the discovery of SCLC. CAR associated with melanoma usually follows the discovery of cancer, with an interval of up to 10 years. Histologically, there is severe loss of the inner and outer segments of the rods and cones, with widespread degeneration of the outer nuclear layer. The electroretinogram is usually flat due to loss of the rod and cone cells. Polyclonal IgG antibodies in SCLC/CAR are directed against recoverin, a 23-kD retinal photoreceptor–specific calcium-binding protein. Other autoantigens include retinal enolase, the S-antigen, and tubby-like protein 1 (TULP1) which is a molecule expressed in synaptic terminals of photoreceptor cells. Treatment with glucocorticoids (prednisone) produces mild to moderate improvement in most patients.

PARANEOPLASTIC MYELOPATHY   Paraneoplastic myelopathy is a rare disorder that presents as acute spinal shock manifest as flaccid paraparesis with a sensory level and sphincter disturbances (Chap. 368). Spinal cord dysfunction is rapidly progressive and ascending. The prognosis is poor. The CSF is often cellular with a high protein. MRI may show T2 signal changes in the spinal cord, with cord swelling and involvement of both white and gray matter structures. The onset of the syndrome may precede or follow detection of a neoplasm, typically lymphoma, leukemia, or lung cancer.

STIFF-PERSON SYNDROME (SPS)   SPS is characterized by stiffness and painful spasms, especially in axial and proximal limb muscles, due to hyperexcitability of motor neurons (Chap. 22). The stiffness produces lumbar hyperlordosis. Muscle spasms are triggered by stretching, emotion, and sensory stimulation. A small minority of SPS occurs in association with neoplasms such as breast cancer, SCLC, thymoma, Hodgkin's disease, and colon cancer. IgG polyclonal antibodies directed against amphiphysin, a 125-kD synaptic vesicle–associated protein, have been detected in sera of some SPS patients, primarily those with breast cancer. Some patients respond to glucocorticoids or tumor resection. Treatment with diazepam, clonazepam, lioresal, or sodium valproate may produce symptomatic improvement.

PNNS OF THE NEUROMUSCULAR SYSTEM

Paraneoplastic neuromuscular syndromes may selectively involve nerve cell bodies (anterior horn or dorsal root ganglia), peripheral nerves (myelin or motor, sensory, or autonomic axons), the neuromuscular junction, or muscle. Some neuromuscular PNNS, including sensory neuronopathy with anti-Hu antibodies, are almost always associated with cancer. Other syndromes, such as myasthenia gravis, are statistically associated with neoplasms but in up to 90% of patients a neoplasm is never found. Some neuromuscular PNNS have protean clinical manifestations that are not distinctive; correct diagnosis may rely upon serologic testing for specific autoantibodies (Tables 101-2 and 101-3).

NEURONOPATHIES   Neuronopathies, indicating damage to the cell body of the neuron, are typically asymmetric and produce proximal as well as distal involvement early in their clinical course. They are generally poorly responsive to treatment.

Subacute sensory neuronopathy (SSN) presents with numbness and pain that evolves in a progressive fashion over 1 to 8 weeks. A history of smoking is found in >95% of patients. Examination shows asymmetric sensory loss that may involve the face and trunk and proximal as well as distal regions of the upper and lower extremities. All sensory modalities are affected. Patients may become disabled by severe sensory ataxia and pseudoathetosis resulting from the deafferentation. Strength is usually normal. Tendon reflexes are diffusely diminished or absent. Nerve conduction studies show diminished or absent sensory responses with normal motor studies. SSN may occur in isolation but is often associated with central nervous system signs, ranging from mild nystagmus to severe encephalopathy. CSF commonly shows a mild pleocytosis and elevated protein levels. Serum IgG antibodies that bind to the Hu family of 35- to 40-kDa nuclear proteins are characteristic of SSN and are a useful diagnostic test. Hu proteins are neuron-specific but are also found in SCLC cells. Although anti-Hu antibodies have strong specificity for SSN and other PNNS, there is no evidence that the antibodies play a pathogenic role. Morphologically there is neuronal loss with perivascular inflammatory infiltrates in the dorsal root ganglia. SSN with anti-Hu antibodies is almost always associated with a neoplasm, especially SCLC, but neoplasm is found at initial evaluation in only 50% of patients. As noted above, the presence of anti-Hu antibodies is associated with a lower degree of malignancy of the SCLC, suggesting that the antibodies may inhibit tumor growth. The differential diagnosis of SSN includes Sjögren's syndrome and drug toxicity from cisplatin or pyridoxine. Treatment consists of therapy for the associated neoplasm. There is almost never improvement in the SSN itself; however, physical therapy may allow the patient, over time, to partially compensate for the sensory loss.

Motor neuronopathy is a rare syndrome that begins subacutely and then reaches a plateau. Patients have asymmetric weakness that may involve the arms more than the legs. The bulbar muscles are spared. Sensation is normal. Motor neuronopathy often manifests after the detection of a neoplasm, typically lymphoma. CSF shows elevated protein levels and oligoclonal bands in 60% of cases.

PERIPHERAL NEUROPATHY   These disorders typically present with distal symptoms and signs in the limbs. They may be axonal, demyelinating, or a combination of the two types. The presence of circulating paraproteins or serologic markers often helps to define paraneoplastic neuropathy syndromes (Table 101-2).

Polyneuropathies associated with circulating paraproteins include: (1) chronic inflammatory demyelinating polyneuropathy (CIDP); (2) demyelinating neuropathy with serum IgM binding to antimyelin-associated glycoprotein (MAG); (3) multifocal motor neuropathy; (4) POEMS syndrome (*p*olyneuropathy, *o*rganomegaly, *e*ndocrinopathy or edema, *M* protein, and *s*kin changes); and (5) primary acquired amyloidosis. →*For further discussion of polyneuropathies associated with circulating paraproteins, see Chap. 378.*

An *axonal sensorimotor neuropathy* is frequently associated with neoplasms. This syndrome is especially common in patients with long-standing cancer and substantial weight loss (>15% of baseline weight). The neuropathy is characterized by distal, symmetric sensory loss and paresthesias, which may be painful, and by weakness and muscle wasting, which is especially prominent in the distal legs. Pathologically there is noninflammatory degeneration of axons and mild myelin loss, presumably secondary to the axonopathy. An accompanying myopathy with atrophy of type II muscle fibers may produce proximal muscle weakness. Axonal loss, with low-amplitude sensory and motor amplitudes and normal conduction velocities, is seen on electrophysiologic studies. This neuromyopathy has been described in association with a variety of solid tumors (lung, breast, stomach), lymphoma, and plasma cell dyscrasia. Successful treatment of the neoplasm may result in improvement or stabilization of the neuromyopathy.

Other axonal neuropathies may be PNNS, but their associations with neoplasms are less clearly established. *Peripheral nerve vasculitis*, producing mononeuritis multiplex or asymmetric sensorimotor polyneuropathy, has been reported with lymphomas or carcinoma of the lung, prostate, kidney, or stomach. *Polyneuropathy,* presenting

Table 101-3 Antibodies Associated with Paraneoplastic Syndromes

Antibody	Antigen Name	Antigen Location	Antigen Function/Characteristics	Neoplasm	Clinical Syndromes
ANTIBODIES AGAINST INTRACELLULAR ANTIGENS					
Anti-Hu	Hu	Neuronal nuclei, CNS, dorsal root	RNA binding protein	SCLC, neuroblastoma, non-SCLC	Encephalomyelitis Limbic encephalitis Cerebellar ataxia Sensory neuronopathy Autonomic neuropathy
Anti-Yo	CRD 1 CRD 2	Purkinje cells, cytoplasm	Possible c-*myc* binding	Ovary, breast, uterine	Cerebellar degeneration
Anti-Ri	Ri (Nova)	CNS, neuronal nuclei	RNA binding protein	Breast, SCLC	Opsoclonus/myoclonus
Anti-Ma1	Ma1	Nuclei, nucleoli, cytoplasm	Phosphoprotein? Function?	Breast, colon, parotid	Cerebellar ataxia Brainstem encephalitis
Anti-Ma2 (Ta)	Ma2	Normal brain, testicular tumor	Phosphoprotein Function?	Testicular	Limbic encephalitis Brainstem encephalitis
Anti-CV2	CV2	Oligodenodrocyte cytoplasm	?	SCLC, thymoma	Cerebellar ataxia Limbic encephalitis Polyneuropathy
Anti-Tr	Not known	Purkinje cell cytoplasm	?	Hodgkin's	Cerebellar ataxia
ANTIBODIES AGAINST CELL SURFACE ANTIGENS					
Anti-VGCC	P/Q VGCC	Peripheral cholinergic synapses	Control permeability of calcium	SCLC	Lambert-Eaton myasthenic syndrome
Anti-AChR	AChR	Neuromuscular junction	Transmitter receptor	Thymoma	Myasthenia gravis
Anti-VGKC	VGKC	Peripheral nerve	Control permeability of potassium	Thymoma	Neuromyotonia
Anti-amphiphysin	Amphiphysin	Synaptic vesicles	Synaptic vesicles	Breast	Stiff-person syndrome
Anti-mGluR1	Metabotropic glutamate receptor	Cell surface receptors	Excitatory receptor	Hodgkin's	Cerebellar ataxia
Anti-MAG	Myelin-associated glycoprotein	Non-compact myelin	Glycoprotein	MGUS	Demyelinating sensorimotor neuropathy, tremor, gait ataxia
Anti-GM1	G_{M1} ganglioside	Peripheral nerve	Glycolipid	MGUS	Multifocal motor neuropathy
Anti-Sulfatide	Sulfatide	Peripheral nerve	Glycolipid	MGUS	Demyelinating neuropathy

NOTE: CNS, central nervous system; SCLC, small cell lung cancer; VGCC, voltage-gated calcium channel; AChR, acetylcholine receptor; VGKC, voltage-gated potassium channel; MGUS, monoclonal gammopathy of undetermined significance.

with either a subacute mononeuritis multiplex or a slowly progressive distal symmetric sensorimotor polyneuropathy, occurs in approximately 20% of patients with cryoglobulinemia. *Guillain-Barré syndrome* (Chap. 378) may be associated with Hodgkin's disease; it is characterized by subacute motor weakness; sensory loss, which is often mild in comparison with the motor deficits; areflexia; and a characteristic elevation of spinal fluid protein concentration without pleocytosis. *Enteric autonomic neuropathy* with anti-Hu antibodies, commonly presenting as intestinal pseudoobstruction, has been described in association with SCLC.

NEUROMUSCULAR JUNCTION *Lambert-Eaton myasthenic syndrome* is a disorder of the presynaptic component of neuromuscular transmission. Common symptoms in LEMS are weakness, fatigue, and dryness of the mouth. Some patients complain of paresthesias, myalgia, or impotence. Weakness is symmetric, proximal, and most prominent in the lower limbs. Strength can decrease with rest and improve with exercise. Ocular (diplopia and ptosis) and bulbar (dysphagia and dysarthria) symptoms may occur in some patients. Respiratory muscle weakness is rare. Tendon reflexes are either diminished or absent at rest but may increase after exercise. About 50% of patients have an associated neoplasm, most commonly SCLC and less often a lymphoproliferative disorder. About 3% of patients with SCLC have LEMS. Almost all patients with both SCLC and LEMS have a smoking history. LEMS may precede the detection of cancer by 2 to 3 years.

The most useful diagnostic test for LEMS is repetitive nerve stimulation, specifically the finding of compound muscle action potential (CMAP) amplitudes that are small at rest but increase by at least 100% after rapid repetitive nerve stimulation (30 to 50 Hz) or maximal muscle contraction sustained for at least 10 s. LEMS is believed to be an autoimmune disorder associated with diminished quantal release of acetylcholine. IgG antibodies directed against P/Q voltage-gated calcium channels (VGCC) in the motor nerve terminal are found in the sera of ~90% of patients with LEMS and in nearly 100% when LEMS is associated with neoplasm. False-positive findings occur with hypergammaglobulinemia, chronic liver disorders, and (in <3% of normal individuals) infection. Ultrastructurally, the number of active zones, which represent the P/Q VGCC in the presynaptic nerve terminal membrane, is decreased in LEMS. This humoral immune response to P/Q VGCC may be stimulated by similar VGCC expressed by the tumor cells. Edrophonium chloride (Tensilon) generally does not improve strength. Treatment of LEMS is directed at tumor resection, enhancing the release of acetylcholine from the presynaptic terminal, and modulating the autoimmune response. Treatment modalities directed at improving neuromuscular transmission include 3,4-diaminopyridine, guanidine, and pyridostigmine. Immunomodulation may include plasmapheresis, glucocorticoids, azathioprine, and cyclosporine.

Myasthenia gravis (MG) is associated with thymoma in 10 to 15% of patients, especially those who present at ≥30 years. Fatigable weakness may involve the ocular, facial, bulbar, and/or limb muscles. Anti-acetylcholine receptor antibodies are detected in about 85% of cases. Slow repetitive nerve stimulation (5 Hz) of proximal or facial muscles produces a decrement of ≥10% in 70% of patients. Single-fiber electromyography is a sensitive but not specific confirmatory test in difficult cases. →*Myasthenia gravis is discussed in Chap. 380.*

MYOPATHY   Mild proximal muscle weakness with type II muscle fiber atrophy is commonly encountered in patients with cancer, especially when weight loss of >15% is present. Muscle wasting is more prominent than muscle weakness in this syndrome. Inflammatory myopathy, especially dermatomyositis in older females, may occur in association with a variety of neoplasms (Chap. 382).

Necrotizing myopathy presents with a subacute onset of weakness that is typically proximal and ranges from mild to severe. Some patients experience myalgia in addition to muscle weakness. The serum creatine kinase levels are very high. Muscle fiber necrosis is the predominant finding in muscle biopsy. Necrotizing myopathy is most commonly seen with adenocarcinoma and non-small cell cancer of the lung but may also be associated with a variety of other neoplasms. The overall prognosis depends on the malignancy of the associated neoplasm. Weakness may improve following tumor resection or glucocorticoid treatment.

Chronic proximal myopathies have been described with an IgM M-protein binding to decorin; scleromyxedema with IgG or IgA M-proteins; a rippling muscle disease has been reported to occur with thymoma. Hormone-secreting (ACTH or parathyroid hormone–like) tumors may also be associated with proximal myopathies.

BIBLIOGRAPHY

DALMAU J et al: Ma1, a novel neuron- and testis-specific protein, is recognized by the serum of patients with paraneoplastic syndromes. Brain 122:27, 1999

DROPCHO EJ: Neurological paraneoplastic syndromes. J Neurol Sci 153:264, 1998

GIOMETTO B et al: Autoimmunity in paraneoplastic neurological syndromes. Brain Pathol 9:261, 1999

GRISOLD W, DRLICEK M: Paraneoplastic neuropathy. Curr Opin Neurol 12:617, 1999

LEVIN M et al: Paraneoplastic necrotizing myopathy: Clinical and pathological features. Neurology 50:764, 1998

NEWSOM-DAVIS J: Paraneoplastic neurological disorders. J R Coll Physicians Lond 33: 225, 1999

PESTRONK A: Chronic immune polyneuropathies and serum autoantibodies, in *Neuroimmunology for the Clinician*, LA Polak, Y Harada (eds). Boston, Butterworth-Heinemann, 1997

———: Paraneoplastic syndromes. Neuromuscular Disease Center at Washington University in Saint Louis. www.neuro.wustl.edu/neuromuscular

REES J: Paraneoplastic syndromes. Curr Opin Neurol 11:633, 1998

SCARAVILLI F et al: The neuropathology of paraneoplastic syndromes. Brain Pathol 9: 251, 1999

SMITH PS et al: Paraneoplastic cerebellar ataxia due to autoantibodies against a glutamate receptor. N Engl J Med 342:21, 2000

102   *Rasim Gucalp, Janice Dutcher*

ONCOLOGIC EMERGENCIES

CNS central nervous system	PTH parathormone
CSF cerebrospinal fluid	SVCS superior vena cava syndrome
CT computed tomography	SVC superior vena cava
HUS hemolytic-uremic syndrome	SIADH syndrome of inappropriate
MRI magnetic resonance imaging	secretion of antidiuretic hormone
PTHrP parathormone-related	TTP thrombotic thrombocytopenic
protein	purpura

Emergencies in patients with cancer may be classified into three groups: pressure or obstruction caused by a space-occupying lesion,

metabolic or hormonal problems (paraneoplastic syndromes, Chap. 100), and complications arising from the effects of treatment.

STRUCTURAL-OBSTRUCTIVE ONCOLOGIC EMERGENCIES

SUPERIOR VENA CAVA SYNDROME   Superior vena cava syndrome (SVCS) is the clinical manifestation of superior vena cava (SVC) obstruction, with severe reduction in venous return from the head, neck, and upper extremities. Malignant tumors, such as lung cancer, lymphoma, and metastatic tumors, are responsible for more than 90% of all SVCS cases. Lung cancer, particularly of small-cell and squamous-cell histologies, accounts for approximately 85% of all cases of malignant origin. Metastatic cancers to the mediastinum, such as testicular and breast carcinomas, account for a small proportion of cases. Other causes include benign tumors, aortic aneurysm, thyroid enlargement, thrombosis, and fibrosing mediastinitis caused by prior irradiation or histoplasmosis.

Patients with SVCS usually present with neck and facial swelling (especially around the eyes), dyspnea, and cough. Other symptoms include hoarseness, tongue swelling, headaches, nasal congestion, epistaxis, hemoptysis, dysphagia, pain, dizziness, syncope, and lethargy. Bending forward or lying down may aggravate the symptoms. The characteristic physical findings are dilated neck veins, an increased number of collateral veins covering the anterior chest wall, cyanosis, and edema of the face, arms, and chest. More severe cases include proptosis, glossal and laryngeal edema, and obtundation. The clinical picture is milder if the obstruction is located above the azygos vein.

The diagnosis of SVCS is a clinical one. The most significant chest radiographic finding is widening of the superior mediastinum, most commonly on the right side. Pleural effusion occurs in only 25% of patients, often on the right side. However, a normal chest radiograph is still compatible with the diagnosis if other characteristic findings are present. Computed tomography (CT) provides the most reliable view of the mediastinal anatomy. The diagnosis of SVCS requires diminished or absent opacification of central venous structures with prominent collateral venous circulation. Magnetic resonance imaging (MRI) has no advantages over CT. Invasive procedures, including bronchoscopy, percutaneous needle biopsy, mediastinoscopy, and even thoracotomy, can be performed by a skilled clinician without any major risk of bleeding. For patients with a known cancer, a detailed workup usually is not necessary, and appropriate treatment may be started after obtaining a CT scan of the thorax. For those with no history of malignancy, a detailed evaluation is absolutely necessary to rule out benign causes and determine a specific diagnosis to direct the appropriate therapy.

℞   **TREATMENT**   The one potentially life-threatening complication of a superior mediastinal mass is tracheal obstruction. Upper airway obstruction demands emergent therapy. Diuretics with a low salt diet, head elevation, and oxygen may produce temporary symptomatic relief.

Radiation therapy is the primary treatment for SVCS caused by non-small cell lung cancer and other metastatic solid tumors. Chemotherapy is effective when the underlying cancer is small cell carcinoma of the lung or lymphoma. Recurrent SVCS occurs in 10 to 30% of patients after initial therapy; it may be palliated with the use of intravascular self-expanding stents (Fig. 102-1). Surgery may provide immediate relief for patients in whom a benign process is the cause.

Clinical improvement occurs in most patients, although this improvement may be due to the development of adequate collateral circulation. The mortality associated with SVCS does not relate to caval obstruction, but rather to the underlying cause.

SVCS and Central Venous Catheters in Adults   The use of long-term central venous catheters has become common practice in patients with cancer. Major vessel thrombosis may occur. In these cases, catheter removal should be combined with anticoagulation to

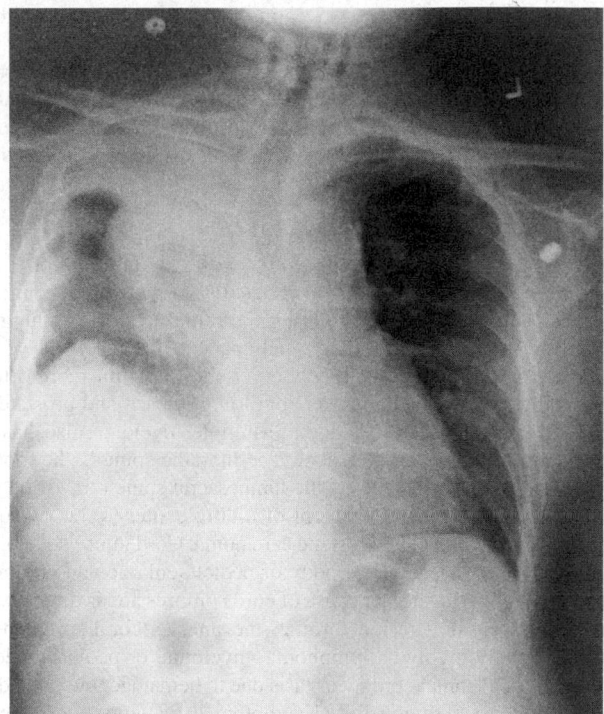

A

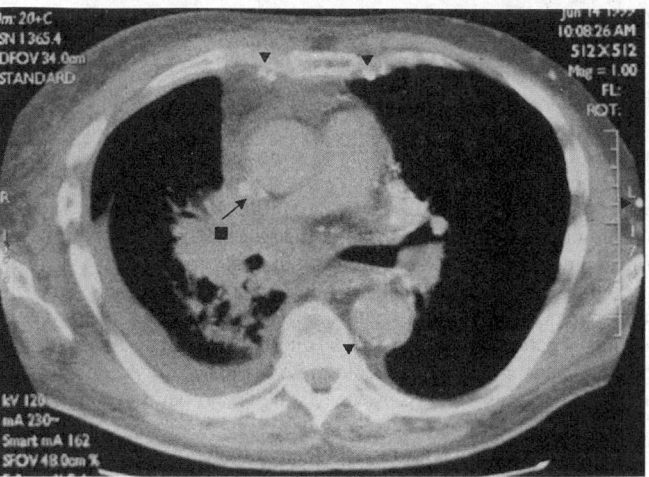

B

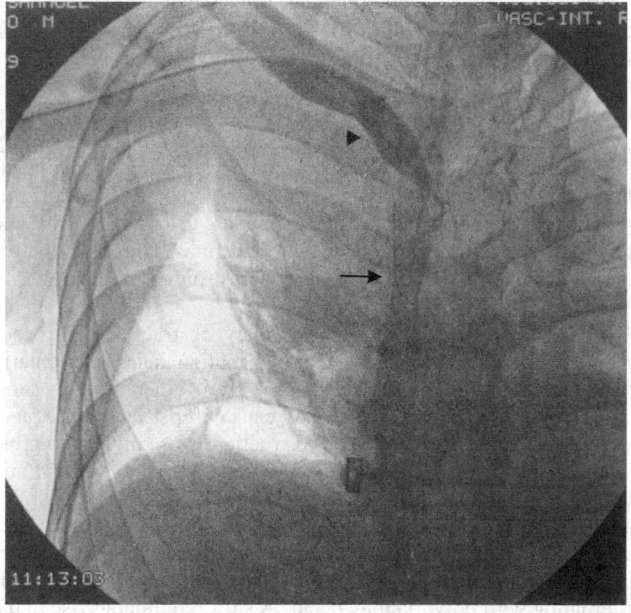

C

FIGURE 102-1 *A*. Chest radiographs of a 59-year-old man with recurrent SVCS caused by non-small cell lung cancer showing right paratracheal mass with right pleural effusion. *B*. Computed tomography of same patient demonstrating obstruction of SVC with thrombosis (arrow) by the lung cancer (square) and collaterals (arrowheads). *C*. Balloon angioplasty (arrowhead) with walstent (arrow) in same patient.

prevent embolization. SVCS in this setting, if detected early, can be treated successfully by fibrinolytic therapy without sacrificing the catheter. Warfarin (1 mg/d) reduces the incidence of thrombosis without altering coagulation tests.

PERICARDIAL EFFUSION/TAMPONADE   Malignant pericardial disease is found at autopsy in 5 to 10% of patients with cancer, most frequently with lung cancer, breast cancer, leukemias, and lymphomas. Cardiac tamponade as the initial presentation of extrathoracic malignancy is rare. The origin is not malignancy in about 50% of cancer patients with symptomatic pericardial disease, but can be related to irradiation, drug-induced pericarditis, hypothyroidism, idiopathic pericarditis, infection, or autoimmune diseases. Two types of radiation pericarditis have been described: an acute inflammatory, effusive pericarditis occurring within months of irradiation, which usually resolves spontaneously, and a chronic effusive pericarditis that may appear up to 20 years after radiotherapy and is accompanied by a thickened pericardium.

Most patients with pericardial metastasis are asymptomatic. However, the common symptoms are dyspnea, cough, chest pain, orthopnea, and weakness. Pleural effusion, sinus tachycardia, jugular venous distension, hepatomegaly, peripheral edema, and cyanosis are the most frequent physical findings. Relatively specific diagnostic findings, such as paradoxical pulse, diminished heart sounds, pulsus alternans (pulse waves alternating between those of greater and lesser amplitude with successive beats), and friction rub are less common than with nonmalignant pericardial disease. Chest radiographs and ECG reveal abnormalities in 90% of patients, but half of these abnormalities are nonspecific. Echocardiography is the most helpful diagnostic test. Pericardial fluid may be serous, serosanguineous, or hemorrhagic, and cytologic examination of pericardial fluid is diagnostic in most patients. False negative cytology may occur in patients with lymphoma and mesothelioma.

℞ TREATMENT   Pericardiocentesis with or without the introduction of sclerosing agents, the creation of a pericardial window, complete pericardial stripping, cardiac irradiation, or systemic chemotherapy are effective treatments. Acute pericardial tamponade with life-threatening hemodynamic instability requires immediate drainage of fluid. This can be quickly achieved by pericardiocentesis. Alternatively, subxyphoid pericardiotomy can be performed in 45 min under local anesthesia.

INTESTINAL OBSTRUCTION   Intestinal obstruction and reobstruction are common problems in patients with advanced cancer, particularly colorectal or ovarian carcinoma. However, other cancers, such as lung or breast cancer and melanoma, can metastasize within the abdomen, leading to intestinal obstruction. Typically, obstruction occurs at multiple sites. Intestinal pseudoobstruction is caused by infiltration of the mesentery or bowel muscle by tumor, involvement of the celiac plexus, or paraneoplastic neuropathy in patients with small cell lung cancer. Paraneoplastic neuropathy is associated with IgG antibodies reactive to neurons of the myenteric and submucosal plexuses of the jejunum and stomach. Ovarian cancer can lead either to authentic luminal obstruction or to pseudoobstruction that results when circumferential invasion of a bowel segment arrests the forward progression of peristaltic contractions.

The onset of obstruction is usually insidious. Pain is the most common symptom and is usually colicky in nature. Pain can also be due to abdominal distention, tumor masses, or hepatomegaly. Vomiting can be intermittent or continuous. Patients with complete obstruction usually have constipation. Physical examination may reveal abdominal distention with tympany, ascites, visible peristalsis, high-pitched bowel sounds, and tumor masses. Erect plain abdominal films may reveal multiple air-fluid levels and dilation of the small or large bowel. Acute cecal dilation to more than 12 to 14 cm is considered a surgical emergency because of the high likelihood of rupture. The overall prognosis for the patient with cancer who develops intestinal obstruction is poor; median survival is 3 to 4 months. About one-fourth to one-third of patients are found to have intestinal obstruction due to causes other than cancer. Adhesions from previous operations are a common benign cause. Ileus induced by vincristine is another reversible cause.

℞ TREATMENT The management of intestinal obstruction in patients with advanced malignancy depends on the extent of the underlying malignancy and the functional status of the major organs. The initial management should include surgical evaluation. Operation is not always successful and may lead to further complications with a substantial mortality rate (10 to 20%). Self-expanding metal stents placed in the gastric outlet, duodenum, proximal jejunum, colon, or rectum may palliate obstructive symptoms at those sites without major surgery. Patients known to have advanced intraabdominal malignancy should receive a prolonged course of conservative management, including nasogastric decompression. Treatment with antiemetics, antispasmodics, and analgesics may allow patients to remain outside the hospital. The somatostatin analogue octreotide may relieve obstructive symptoms through its inhibitory effect on gastrointestinal secretion.

URINARY OBSTRUCTION Urinary obstruction may occur in patients with prostatic or gynecologic malignancies, particularly cervical carcinoma, or metastatic disease from other primary sites. Radiation therapy to pelvic tumors may cause fibrosis and subsequent ureteral obstruction. Bladder outlet obstruction is usually due to prostate and cervical cancers and may lead to bilateral hydronephrosis and renal failure.

Flank pain is the most common symptom. Persistent urinary tract infection, persistent proteinuria, or hematuria in patients with a cancer should raise suspicion of ureteral obstruction. Total anuria and/or anuria alternating with polyuria may occur. A slow, continuous rise in the serum creatinine level necessitates immediate evaluation in patients with cancer. Renal ultrasound examination is the safest and cheapest way to identify hydronephrosis. The function of an obstructed kidney can be evaluated by a nuclear scan. CT can be helpful in identifying a retroperitoneal mass or retroperitoneal adenopathy.

℞ TREATMENT Obstruction associated with flank pain, sepsis, or fistula formation is an indication for immediate palliative urinary diversion. There are many newer techniques by which internal ureteral stents can be placed under local anesthesia. Percutaneous nephrostomy offers an alternative approach for drainage. In the case of bladder outlet obstruction due to malignancy, a suprapubic cystostomy can be used for urinary drainage.

MALIGNANT BILIARY OBSTRUCTION This common clinical problem can be caused by a primary carcinoma arising in the pancreas, ampulla of Vater, bile duct, or liver or by metastatic disease to the periductal lymph nodes or liver parenchyma. The most common metastatic tumors causing biliary obstruction are gastric, colon, breast, and lung cancers. Jaundice, light-colored stools, dark urine, pruritus, and weight loss due to malabsorption are usual symptoms. Pain and secondary infection are uncommon in malignant biliary obstruction. Ultrasound, CT, or percutaneous transhepatic or endoscopic retrograde cholangiography will identify the site and nature of the biliary obstruction.

℞ TREATMENT Palliative intervention is indicated only in patients with disabling pruritus resistant to medical treatment, severe malabsorption, or infection. Stenting under radiographic control, surgical bypass, or radiation therapy with or without chemotherapy may alleviate the obstruction. The choice of modality should be based on the site of obstruction (proximal versus distal), the type of tumor (sensitive to radiotherapy, chemotherapy, or neither), and the general condition of the patient. In the absence of pruritus, biliary obstruction may be a largely asymptomatic cause of death.

SPINAL CORD COMPRESSION Spinal cord compression occurs in 5 to 10% of patients with cancer. Epidural tumor is the first manifestation of malignancy in about 10% of patients. The underlying cancer is usually identified during the initial evaluation; lung cancer is most commonly the primary malignancy.

Metastatic tumor involves the vertebral column more often than any other part of the bony skeleton. Lung, breast, and prostate cancer are the most frequent offenders. Multiple myeloma also has a high incidence of spine involvement. The thoracic spine is the most common site (70%), followed by the lumbosacral spine (20%) and the cervical spine (10%). Involvement of multiple sites is most frequent in patients with breast and prostatic carcinoma. Cord injury develops when metastases to the vertebral body or pedicle enlarge and compress the underlying dura. Another cause of cord compression is direct extension of a paravertebral lesion through the intervertebral foramen. These cases usually involve a lymphoma, myeloma, or pediatric neoplasm. Parenchymal spinal cord metastasis due to hematogenous spread is rare.

The most common initial symptom in patients with spinal cord compression is localized back pain and tenderness due to involvement of vertebrae by tumor. Pain is usually present for days or months before other neurologic findings appear. It is exacerbated by movement and by coughing or sneezing. It can be differentiated from the pain of disk disease by the fact that it worsens when the patient is supine. Radicular pain is less common than localized back pain and usually develops later. Radicular pain in the cervical or lumbosacral areas may be unilateral or bilateral. Radicular pain from the thoracic roots is often bilateral and is described by patients as a feeling of tight, band-like constriction around the thorax and abdomen. Typical cervical radicular pain radiates down the arm; in the lumbar region, the radiation is down the legs. Loss of bowel or bladder control may be the presenting symptom, but usually occurs late in the course.

On physical examination, pain induced by straight leg raising, neck flexion, or vertebral percussion may help to determine the level of cord compression. Patients develop numbness and paresthesias in the extremities or trunk. Loss of sensibility to pinprick is as common as loss of sensibility to vibration or position. The upper limit of the zone of sensory loss is often one or two vertebrae below the site of compression. Motor findings include weakness, spasticity, and abnormal muscle stretching. The presence of an extensor plantar reflex reflects significant compression. Deep tendon reflexes may be brisk. Motor and sensory loss usually precede sphincter disturbance. Patients with autonomic dysfunction may present with decreased anal tonus, decreased perineal sensibility, and a distended bladder. The absence of the anal wink reflex or the bulbocavernosus reflex confirms cord (conus or cauda equina) involvement. In doubtful cases, evaluation of post-voiding urinary residual volume can be helpful. A residual volume of more than 150 mL suggests bladder dysfunction. Autonomic dysfunction is an unfavorable prognostic factor. Patients with progressive neurologic symptoms should have frequent neurologic examinations and rapid therapeutic intervention.

Patients with cancer who develop back pain should be evaluated for spinal cord compression as quickly as possible (Fig. 102-2). Treatment is more often successful in patients who are ambulatory and still have sphincter control at the time treatment is initiated. Patients should have a neurologic examination and plain films of the spine. Those whose physical examination suggests cord compression should receive dexamethasone (24 mg intravenously every 6 h), starting immediately.

Erosion of the pedicles (the "winking owl" sign) is the earliest radiologic finding of vertebral tumor. Other radiographic changes include increased intrapedicular distance, vertebral destruction, lytic or

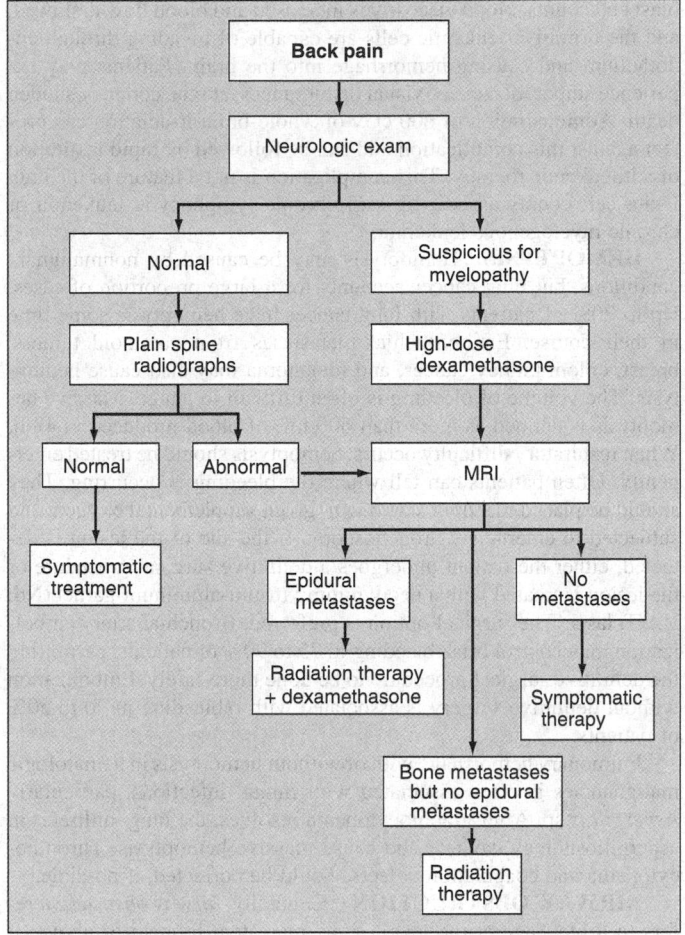

FIGURE 102-2 Management of cancer patients with back pain.

sclerotic lesions, scalloped vertebral bodies, and vertebral body collapse. Vertebral collapse is not a reliable indicator of the presence of tumor; about 20% of cases of vertebral collapse, particularly those in older patients and postmenopausal women, are due not to cancer but to osteoporosis. Also, a normal appearance on plain films of the spine does not exclude the diagnosis of cancer. The role of bone scans in the detection of cord compression is not clear; this method is sensitive but less specific than spinal radiography.

The full-length image of the cord provided by MRI is useful. On T1-weighted images, good contrast is noted between the cord, cerebrospinal fluid, and extradural lesions. Owing to their sensitivity in demonstrating the replacement of bone marrow by tumor, MRI can show which parts of a vertebra are involved by tumor (the body, pedicle, lamina, spinous process). MRI also visualizes intraspinal extradural masses compressing the cord. T2-weighted images are most useful for the demonstration of intramedullary pathology. Gadolinium-enhanced MRI can help to characterize and delineate intramedullary disease. MRI is as good as or better than myelography plus postmyelogram CT in detecting metastatic epidural disease with cord compression. Myelography should be reserved for patients who have poor MR images or who cannot undergo MRI promptly. CT in conjunction with myelography enhances the detection of small areas of spinal destruction.

In patients with spinal cord compression and an unknown primary tumor, a simple workup including chest radiography, mammography, measurement of prostate-specific antigen, and abdominal CT usually reveals the underlying malignancy.

TREATMENT The treatment of patients with spinal cord compression is aimed at relief of pain and restoration of neurologic function (Fig. 102-2).

Radiation therapy plus glucocorticoids is generally the initial treatment of choice for spinal cord compression. Up to 75% of patients treated when still ambulatory remain ambulatory, but only 10% of patients with paraplegia recover walking capacity. Indications for surgical intervention include unknown etiology, failure of radiation therapy, a radioresistant tumor type (e.g., melanoma or renal cell cancer), pathologic fracture dislocation, and rapidly evolving neurologic symptoms. Until recently, laminectomy was the standard operation for metastatic spinal cord compression, although results were poor. At present, laminectomy should be used only for tissue diagnosis and for the removal of posteriorly localized epidural deposits in the absence of vertebral disease. Because most cases of epidural spinal cord compression are due to anterior or anterolateral extradural disease, resection of the anterior vertebral body along with the tumor, followed by spinal stabilization, has achieved good results and low mortality rate. Chemotherapy may have a role in patients with chemosensitive tumors who have had prior radiation therapy to the same region and who are not candidates for surgery.

The histology of the tumor is an important determinant of both recovery and survival. Rapid onset and quick progression are poor prognostic features.

INCREASED INTRACRANIAL PRESSURE About 25% of patients with cancer die with intracranial metastases. The cancers that most often metastasize to the brain are lung and breast cancers and melanoma. Brain metastases often occur in the presence of systemic disease, and they frequently cause major symptoms, disability, and early death.

The signs and symptoms of a metastatic brain tumor are similar to those of other intracranial expanding lesions: headache, nausea, vomiting, behavioral changes, seizures, and focal, progressive neurologic changes. Occasionally the onset is abrupt, resembling a stroke, with the sudden appearance of headache, nausea, vomiting, and neurologic deficits. This picture is usually due to hemorrhage into the metastasis. Melanoma, germ cell tumors, and renal cell cancers have a particularly high incidence of intracranial bleeding. The tumor mass and surrounding edema may cause obstruction of the circulation of cerebrospinal fluid, with resulting hydrocephalus. Patients with increased intracranial pressure may have papilledema with visual disturbances and neck stiffness. As the mass enlarges, brain tissue may be displaced through the fixed cranial openings, producing various herniation syndromes.

CT and MRI are equally effective in the diagnosis of brain metastases. CT with contrast should be used as a screening procedure. The CT scan shows brain metastases as multiple enhancing lesions of various sizes with surrounding areas of low-density edema. If a single lesion or no metastases are visualized by contrast-enhanced CT, MRI of the brain should be performed. Gadolinium-enhanced MRI is more sensitive than CT at revealing small lesions, particularly in the brainstem or cerebellum.

TREATMENT If signs and symptoms of brain herniation (particularly headache, drowsiness, and papilledema) are present, the patient should be intubated and hyperventilated to maintain P_{CO_2} between 25 and 30 mmHg and should receive infusions of mannitol (1 to 1.5 g/kg) every 6 h. Dexamethasone is the best initial treatment for all symptomatic patients with brain metastases (see above). Patients with multiple lesions should receive whole-brain radiation therapy. Patients with a single brain metastasis and with controlled extracranial disease may be treated with surgical excision followed by whole-brain radiation therapy, especially if they are younger than 60 years. Radioresistant tumors should be resected if possible. Stereotactic radiosurgery is an effective treatment for inaccessible or recurrent lesions. With a gamma knife or linear accelerator, multiple small, well-colimated beams of ionizing radiation destroy lesions seen on MRI. Some patients with increased intracranial pressure associated with hydrocephalus may benefit from shunt placement.

NEOPLASTIC MENINGITIS   Tumor involving the leptomeninges is a complication of both primary tumors of the central nervous system (CNS) and tumors that metastasize to the CNS. The incidence is estimated at 3 to 8% of patients with cancer. Melanoma, breast and lung cancer, lymphoma (including AIDS-associated), and acute leukemia are the most common causes.

Patients typically present with multifocal neurologic signs and symptoms including headache, gait abnormality, mental changes, nausea, vomiting, seizures, back or radicular pain, and limb weakness. Signs include cranial nerve palsies, extremity weakness, paresthesia, and decreased deep tendon reflexes.

Diagnosis is made by demonstrating malignant cells in the cerebrospinal fluid (CSF); however, up to 40% of patients may have false negative CSF cytology. An elevated CSF protein level is nearly always present (except in HLTV-1-associated adult T cell leukemia). Patients with neurologic signs and symptoms consistent with neoplastic meningitis who have a negative CSF cytology but an elevated CSF protein level should have the spinal tap repeated at least three times for repeated cytologic examination before the diagnosis is rejected. MRI may show hydrocephalus or smooth or nodular enhancement of the meninges.

The development of neoplastic meningitis usually occurs in the setting of uncontrolled cancer outside the CNS; thus, prognosis is poor (median survival 10 to 12 weeks). However, treatment of the neoplastic meningitis may successfully alleviate symptoms and control the CNS spread.

℞ **TREATMENT**   Intrathecal chemotherapy, usually methotrexate, cytarabine, or thiotepa, is delivered by lumbar puncture or by an intraventricular reservoir (Ommaya) three times a week until the CSF is free of malignant cells. Then injections are given twice a week for a month and then weekly for a month. An extended release preparation of cytarabine (Depocyte) has a longer half-life and is more effective than regular formulations. Among solid tumors, breast cancer responds best to therapy. Patients with neoplastic meningitis from either acute leukemia or lymphoma may be cured of their CNS disease if the systemic disease can be eliminated.

SEIZURES   Seizures occurring in a patient with cancer can be caused by the tumor itself, by metabolic disturbances, by radiation injury, by cerebral infarctions, by chemotherapy-related encephalopathies, or by CNS infections. Metastatic disease to the CNS is the most common cause of seizures in patients with cancer. Seizures are a presenting symptom of CNS metastasis in 6 to 29% of cases. Approximately 10% of patients with CNS metastasis eventually develop seizures. The presence of frontal lesions correlates with early seizures, and the presence of hemispheric symptoms increases the risk for late seizures. Both early and late seizures are uncommon in patients with posterior fossa lesions. Seizures are also common in patients with CNS metastases from melanoma. Very rarely, cytotoxic drugs such as etoposide, busulfan, and chlorambucil cause seizures.

℞ **TREATMENT**   Patients in whom seizures due to CNS metastases have been demonstrated should receive anticonvulsive treatment with diphenylhydantoin. Prophylactic anticonvulsant therapy is not recommended unless the patient is at a high risk for late seizures. In those patients, serum diphenylhydantoin levels should be monitored closely and the dosage adjusted accordingly.

INTRACEREBRAL LEUKOCYTOSTASIS   Intracerebral leukocytostasis (Ball's disease) is a potentially fatal complication of acute leukemia (particularly myelogenous leukemia) that can occur when the peripheral blast cell count is greater than 100,000/μL. At such high blast cell counts, blood viscosity is increased and blood flow is slowed, and the primitive leukemic cells are capable of invading through endothelium and causing hemorrhage into the brain. Patients may experience stupor, dizziness, visual disturbances, ataxia, coma, or sudden death. Administration of 600 cGy of whole-brain irradiation can protect against this complication and can be followed by rapid institution of antileukemic therapy. This complication is not a feature of the high white cell counts associated with chronic lymphocytic leukemia or chronic myelogenous leukemia.

HEMOPTYSIS   Hemoptysis may be caused by nonmalignant conditions, but lung cancer accounts for a large proportion of cases. Up to 20% of patients with lung cancer have hemoptysis some time in their course. Endobronchial metastases from carcinoid tumors, breast, colon, kidney cancer, and melanoma may also cause hemoptysis. The volume of bleeding is often difficult to gauge. Massive hemoptysis is defined as more than 600 mL of blood produced in 48 h. When respiratory difficulty occurs, hemoptysis should be treated emergently. Often patients can tell where the bleeding is occurring. They should be placed bleeding side down, given supplemental oxygen, and subjected to emergency bronchoscopy. If the site of the lesion is detected, either the patient undergoes a definitive surgical procedure or the lesion is treated with a neodymium:yttrium-aluminum-garnet (Nd:YAG) laser. The surgical option is preferred. Bronchial artery embolization may control brisk bleeding in 75 to 90% of patients, permitting the definitive surgical procedure to be done more safely. Embolization without definitive surgery is associated with rebleeding in 20 to 50% of patients.

Pulmonary hemorrhage with or without hemoptysis in hematologic malignancies is often associated with fungal infections, particularly *Aspergillus* sp. After granulocytopenia resolves, the lung infiltrates in aspergillosis may cavitate and cause massive hemoptysis. Thrombocytopenia and coagulation defects should be corrected, if possible.

AIRWAY OBSTRUCTION   Generally, *airway obstruction* refers to a blockage at the level of the mainstem bronchi or above. It may result either from intraluminal tumor growth or from extrinsic compression of the airway. If the obstruction is proximal to the larynx, a tracheostomy may be life-saving. For more distal obstructions, particularly intrinsic lesions incompletely obstucting the airway, bronchoscopy with laser treatment, photodynamic therapy, or stenting can produce immediate relief in most patients. However, radiation therapy (either external-beam irradiation or brachytherapy) given together with glucocorticoids may also open the airway. Symptomatic extrinsic compression may be palliated by stenting.

METABOLIC EMERGENCIES

HYPERCALCEMIA   Hypercalcemia is the most common paraneoplastic syndrome (Chaps. 100 and 341), occurring in about 10% of patients with advanced cancer. It is associated most often with cancers of the lung, breast, head and neck, and kidney and with multiple myeloma and some B and T cell lymphomas.

Increased release of calcium from bone is the main factor leading to hypercalcemia. Bone resorption is increased dramatically through stimulation of the proliferation and activity of osteoclasts, and bone formation is not stimulated in parallel. The kidney may play an important role through an increase in the reabsorption of calcium in the distal tubule. Parathormone-related protein (PTHrP) produced by tumors has a central role as a mediator of hypercalcemia in cancer. PTHrP shares 80% homology with the first 13 amino acids of parathormone (PTH), which are in the region responsible for binding to the PTH receptor. PTHrP acts via the PTH hormone receptors on osteoblasts and renal tubular cells to stimulate bone resorption and renal calcium conservation, leading to hypercalcemia. Elevated plasma PTHrP levels are also found in most hypercalcemic patients with bone metastases, whose hypercalcemia has traditionally been explained by local osteolysis due to the production of osteolytic factors by tumors. Transforming growth factors, cytokines (interleukins 1 and 6), and other unknown factors could play a contributory role. True "ectopic"

PTH production by malignant tumors is rare. In lymphoma, a vitamin D–related product of the tumor may also increase calcium absorption in the gut.

The clinical features of hypercalcemia in patients with cancer are nonspecific and include fatigue, anorexia, constipation, polydipsia, muscle weakness, nausea, and vomiting. They may easily be attributed to the malignancy itself or to its treatment. Laboratory assessment should include measurement of serum electrolytes, calcium, phosphate, and albumin. Hypoalbuminemia is common in malignancy and affects the total serum concentration of calcium. If the ionized calcium level cannot be obtained, then the corrected serum calcium concentration should be calculated with the following formula:

Corrected serum calcium = measured serum calcium
+ 0.8 (4.0 − measured serum albumin)

Most patients with hypercalcemia of malignancy have obvious evidence of malignancy, and their serum PTH levels are suppressed. Measurements of PTHrP and serum 1,25 dihydroxyvitamin D are not indicated. Routine serum chemistry evaluations are not able to distinguish between malignant and nonmalignant causes of hypercalcemia.

TREATMENT Not all patients with moderate to severe hyper calcemia (corrected calcium ≥12 mg/dL) should be treated. The decision to treat will depend on the patient's quality of life, the current symptoms, and the prospect for further cancer treatment. Treatment directed at hypercalcemia only extends life in patients for whom effective cancer treatment is available. Nonetheless, therapy may be indicated to reduce symptoms and improve the quality of life. Treatment of symptomatic hypercalcemia begins with intravenous saline to restore the depleted intravascular volume, which may be 4 to 8 L below normal at presentation. Rehydration usually has little effect on calcium levels, producing a median decrease of only 1 mg/dL. Antiresorptive agents are essential to decrease osteoclastic activity and control hypercalcemia. Bisphosphonates, which are potent inhibitors of bone resorption, are easy to administer, virtually free of side effects, and rapidly effective in lowering the serum calcium level. Pamidronate is the most effective of the commercially available bisphosphonates. The recommended dose of pamidronate is 60 mg for moderate hypercalcemia (corrected calcium 12 to 13.5 mg/dL) and 90 mg for severe hypercalcemia (corrected calcium >13.5 mg/dL). The dose is given as a single infusion over 4 or 24 h.

SYNDROME OF INAPPROPRIATE SECRETION OF ANTIDIURETIC HORMONE (SIADH) SIADH is attributed to production of arginine vasopressin by the tumor cells and is characterized by hyponatremia, urine osmolarity inappropriately higher than plasma osmolarity, and high urinary sodium excretion in the absence of volume depletion. Renal, adrenal, and thyroid insufficiency must be excluded, because these disorders can also present with hyponatremia and impaired urinary dilution. Low serum levels of urea and uric acid are useful in distinguishing SIADH from conditions associated with renal hypoperfusion (Chaps. 100 and 329).

A broad spectrum of malignant tumors have been reported to cause SIADH. Ectopic vasopressin secretion may occur in some 38% of small cell carcinomas of the lung; often adrenocorticotropic hormone is also produced. The presence of hyponatremia in patients with small cell lung cancer confers a poor prognosis. SIADH may also be caused by various other conditions, such as CNS and pulmonary disorders and some surgical procedures. A variety of drugs have also been shown to produce SIADH, including antidepressants, angiotensin converting-enzyme inhibitors, and cytotoxic drugs such as vincristine, vinorelbine, ifosfamide, cyclophosphamide, cisplatin, levamisole, and melphalan.

Most patients with SIADH are asymptomatic. The severity of symptoms and signs is related to the degree of hyponatremia and the rapidity with which it develops. Early changes include anorexia, depression, lethargy, irritability, confusion, muscle weakness, and

marked personality changes. When the plasma sodium level falls below 110 mEq/L, extensor plantar responses, areflexia, and pseudobulbar palsy may be noted; and further reductions may cause coma, convulsions, and death.

TREATMENT The optimal therapy for SIADH is to treat the underlying malignancy. If that is not possible, other therapeutic approaches are available, such as water restriction or the administration of demeclocycline (900 to 1200 mg per os bid), urea, or lithium carbonate (300 mg per os tid). Demeclocycline is usually used first. Demeclocycline and lithium inhibit the effects of vasopressin on the distal renal tubule. Patients with seizure or coma from hyponatremia may require normal saline infusion plus furosemide to enhance free water clearance. The rate of sodium correction should be slow [0.5 to 1 (mEq/L)/h] to prevent rapid fluid shifts and central pontine myelinolysis. The serum calcium level should be monitored closely to avoid hypocalcemia.

LACTIC ACIDOSIS Lactic acidosis is a rare and potentially fatal metabolic complication of cancer. Lactic acidosis associated with sepsis and circulatory failure is a common preterminal event in many malignancies. Lactic acidosis in the absence of hypoxemia may occur in patients with leukemia, lymphoma, or solid tumors. Extensive involvement of the liver by tumor is present in most cases. Alteration of liver function may be responsible for the lactate accumulation. Tachypnea, tachycardia, change of mental status, and hepatomegaly may be seen. The serum level of lactic acid may reach 10 to 20 meq/L (90 to 180 mg/dL). Treatment is aimed at the underlying disease. The danger from lactic acidosis is from the acidosis, not the lactate. Sodium bicarbonate should be added if acidosis is very severe or if hydrogen ion production is very rapid and uncontrolled. The prognosis is poor.

HYPOGLYCEMIA Persistent hypoglycemia occasionally is associated with tumors other than pancreatic islet cell tumors. Usually these tumors are large, and often they are of mesenchymal origin or are hepatomas or adrenocortical tumors. Mesenchymal tumors are usually located in the retroperitoneum or thorax. In these patients, obtundation, confusion, and behavioral aberrations occur in the postabsorptive period and may precede the diagnosis of the tumor. Hypoglycemia is due to tumor overproduction of insulin-like growth factor, a peptide hormone with structural homology to proinsulin but having only about 1% of its biologic effects. Additionally, the development of hepatic dysfunction from liver metastases and increased glucose consumption by the tumor can contribute to hypoglycemia. If the tumor cannot be resected, treatment of the hypoglycemia has generally been relief of symptoms, with the administration of glucose, glucocorticoids, or glucagon.

Hypoglycemia can be artifactual; hyperleukocytosis from leukemia, myeloproliferative diseases, leukemoid reactions, or colony stimulating factor treatment can increase glucose consumption in the test tube after blood is drawn, leading to pseudohypoglycemia.

ADRENAL INSUFFICIENCY In patients with cancer, adrenal insufficiency may go unrecognized because the symptoms, such as nausea, vomiting, anorexia, and orthostatic hypotension, are nonspecific and may be mistakenly attributed to progressive cancer or to cancer therapy. Primary adrenal insufficiency may develop owing to replacement of both glands by metastases (lung, breast, colon, or kidney cancer, lymphoma), to removal of both glands, or to hemorrhagic necrosis in association with sepsis or anticoagulation. Impaired adrenal steroid synthesis occurs in patients being treated for cancer with mitotane, ketoconazole, aminoglutethimide, or the investigational agent suramin or in those undergoing rapid reduction in glucocorticoid therapy. Rarely, metastatic replacement causes primary adrenal insufficiency as the first manifestation of an occult malignancy. Metastasis to the pituitary or hypothalamus is found at autopsy in up to 5% of patients with cancer, but associated secondary adrenal insufficiency is rare. Patients abruptly discontinuing megestrol acetate therapy (for cancer cachexia) may develop Addisonian crisis from central suppression of the pituitary-adrenal axis with decreased serum levels of cortisol and adrenocorticotropic hormone.

Acute adrenal insufficiency is potentially lethal. Treatment of suspected adrenal crisis is initiated after the sampling of serum cortisol and ACTH levels (Chap. 331).

TREATMENT-RELATED EMERGENCIES

TUMOR LYSIS SYNDROME   Tumor lysis syndrome is a well-recognized clinical entity that is characterized by various combinations of hyperuricemia, hyperkalemia, hyperphosphatemia, lactic acidosis, and hypocalcemia and is caused by the destruction of a large number of rapidly proliferating neoplastic cells. Frequently, acute renal failure develops as a result of the syndrome.

Tumor lysis syndrome is most frequently associated with the treatment of Burkitt's lymphoma, acute lymphoblastic leukemia, and other high-grade lymphomas, but it also may be seen with chronic leukemias and, rarely, with solid tumors. This syndrome has been seen in patients with chronic lymphocytic leukemia after treatment with fludarabine and cladribine. Tumor lysis syndrome usually occurs during or shortly (1 to 5 days) after chemotherapy. Rarely, spontaneous necrosis of malignancies causes tumor lysis syndrome.

Hyperuricemia may be present at the time of chemotherapy. Effective treatment accelerates the destruction of malignant cells and leads to increased serum uric acid levels from the turnover of nucleic acids. Owing to the acidic local environment, uric acid can precipitate in the tubules, medulla, and collecting ducts of the kidney, leading to renal failure. Lactic acidosis and dehydration may contribute to the precipitation of uric acid in the renal tubules. The finding of uric acid crystals in the urine is strong evidence for uric acid nephropathy. The ratio of urinary uric acid to urinary creatinine is >1 in patients with acute hyperuricemic nephropathy and <1 in patients with renal failure due to other causes.

Hyperphosphatemia, which can be caused by the release of intracellular phosphate pools by tumor cell lysis, produces a reciprocal depression in serum calcium, which causes severe neuromuscular irritability and tetany. Deposition of calcium phosphate in the kidney and hyperphosphatemia may cause renal failure. Potassium is the principal intracellular cation, and massive destruction of malignant cells may lead to hyperkalemia. Hyperkalemia in patients with renal failure may rapidly become life-threatening. Hyperkalemia can cause ventricular arrhythmias and sudden death.

The likelihood that the tumor lysis syndrome will occur in patients with Burkitt's lymphoma is related to the tumor burden and renal function. Hyperuricemia and high serum levels of lactate dehydrogenase LDH (>1500 U/L), both of which correlate with total tumor burden, also correlate with the risk of tumor lysis syndrome. In patients at risk for tumor lysis, pretreatment evaluations should include a complete blood count, serum chemistry evaluation, and urine analysis. High leukocyte and platelet counts may artificially elevate potassium levels ("pseudohyperkalemia") due to lysis of these cells after the blood is drawn. In these cases, plasma potassium instead of serum potassium should be followed. In pseudohyperkalemia, no electrocardiographic abnormalities are present. In patients with abnormal baseline renal function, the kidneys and retroperitoneal area should be evaluated by sonography and/or CT. Urine output should be watched closely.

Recognition of risk and prevention are the most important steps in the management of this syndrome (Fig. 102-3). Despite aggressive prophylaxis, tumor lysis syndrome and/or oliguric or anuric renal failure may occur. Dialysis is often necessary and should be considered early in the course. Hemodialysis is preferred. The prognosis is excellent, and renal function recovers after the uric acid level is lowered to <10 to 20 mg/dL.

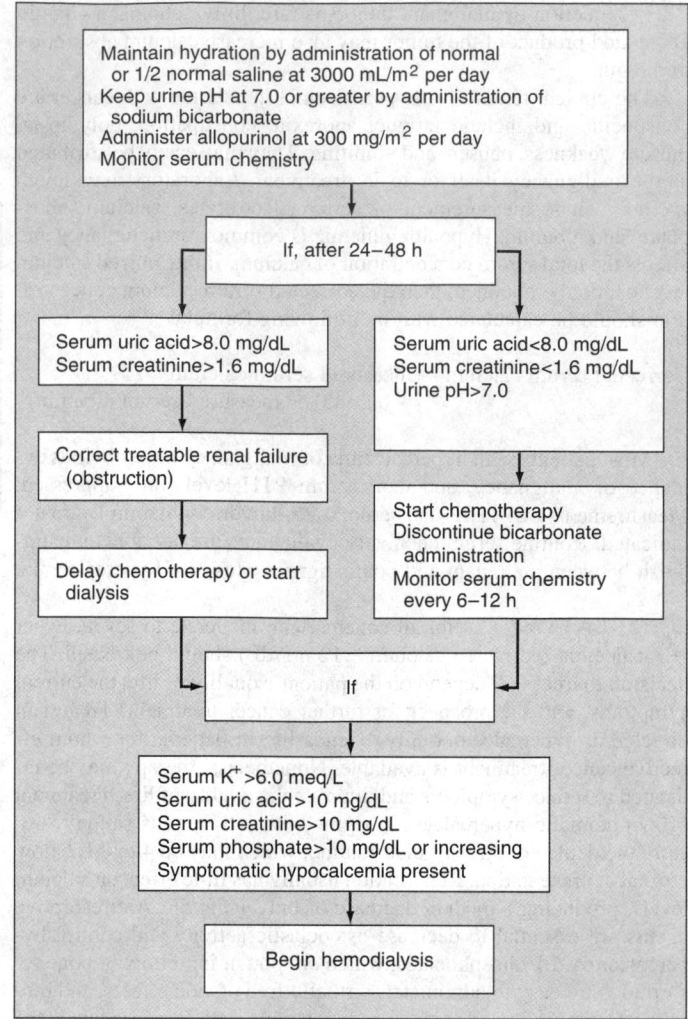

FIGURE 102-3   Management of patients at high risk for the tumor lysis syndrome.

HUMAN ANTIBODY INFUSION REACTIONS   The initial infusion of human or humanized antibodies (e.g., rituximab) is associated with fever, chills, nausea, asthenia, and headache in up to half of treated patients. Bronchospasm and hypotension occur in 1% of patients. The pathogenesis is thought to be activation of immune effector processes (cells and complement). In the presence of high levels of circulating tumor cells, thrombocytopenia, a rapid fall in circulating tumor cells, and mild tumor lysis syndrome may also occur. Diphenhydramine and acetaminophen can often prevent or suppress the symptoms. If they occur, the infusion should be stopped and restarted at half the initial infusion rate after the symptoms have abated.

HEMOLYTIC-UREMIC SYNDROME   Hemolytic-uremic syndrome (HUS) and, less commonly, thrombotic thrombocytopenic purpura (TTP) occurring after treatment with antineoplastic drugs have been described. Mitomycin is by far the most common agent causing this peculiar syndrome. Other chemotherapeutic agents, including cisplatin, bleomycin, and gemcitabine, have also been reported to be associated with this syndrome. It occurs most often in patients with gastric, colorectal, and breast carcinoma. In one series, 35% of patients were without evident cancer at the time this syndrome appeared. Secondary HUS/TTP has also been reported as a rare but sometimes fatal complication of bone marrow transplantation.

HUS usually has its onset 4 to 8 weeks after the last dose of chemotherapy, but it is not rare to detect it several months later. HUS is characterized by microangiopathic hemolytic anemia, thrombocytopenia, and renal failure. Dyspnea, weakness, fatigue, oliguria, and purpura are also common initial symptoms and findings. Systemic hypertension and pulmonary edema frequently occur. Severe hypertension, pulmonary edema, and rapid worsening of hemolysis and renal function may occur after a blood transfusion. Cardiac findings include atrial arrhythmias, pericardial friction rub, and pericardial effusion. Raynaud's phenomenon is part of the syndrome in patients treated with bleomycin.

Laboratory findings include severe to moderate anemia associated with red blood cell fragmentation and numerous schistocytes on peripheral smear. Reticulocytosis, decreased plasma haptoglobin, and an elevated lactic dehydrogenase (LDH) level document hemolysis. The serum bilirubin level is usually normal or slightly elevated. The Coombs test is negative. The white cell count is usually normal, and thrombocytopenia ($<100,000/\mu L$) is almost always present. Most patients have a normal coagulation profile, although some have mild elevations in thrombin time and in level of fibrin degradation products. The serum creatinine level is elevated at presentation and shows a pattern of subacute worsening within weeks of the initial azotemia. The urinalysis reveals hematuria, proteinuria, and granular or hyaline casts; and circulating immune complexes may be present.

The basic pathologic lesion appears to be deposition of fibrin in the walls of capillaries and arterioles, and these deposits are similar to those seen in HUS due to other causes. These microvascular abnormalities involve mainly the kidneys and rarely occur in other organs. The pathogenesis of chemotherapy-related HUS is unknown. Immune complexes have been proposed but not confirmed to be etiologic.

The case fatality rate is high; most patients die within a few months. Plasmapheresis and plasma exchange may normalize the hematologic abnormalities, but renal failure is not reversed in most patients. Immunoperfusion over a staphylococcal protein A column is the most successful treatment. About half of the patients treated with immunoperfusion respond with resolution of thrombocytopenia, improvement in anemia, and stabilization of renal failure. Treatment is well tolerated. It is not clear how the treatment works.

NEUTROPENIA AND INFECTION These remain the most common serious complications of cancer therapy. →*They are covered in detail in Chap. 85.*

PULMONARY INFILTRATES Patients with cancer may present with dyspnea associated with diffuse interstitial infiltrates on chest radiographs. Such infiltrates may be due to progression of the underlying malignancy, treatment-related toxicities, infection, and/or unrelated diseases. The cause may be multifactorial; however, most commonly they occur as a consequence of treatment. Infiltration of the lung by malignancy has been described in patients with leukemia, lymphoma, and breast and other solid cancers. Pulmonary lymphatics may be involved diffusely by neoplasm (pulmonary lymphangitic carcinomatosis), resulting in a diffuse increase in interstitial markings on chest radiographs. The patient is often mildly dyspneic at the onset, but pulmonary failure develops over a period of weeks. In some patients, dyspnea precedes changes on the chest radiographs and is accompanied by a nonproductive cough. This syndrome is characteristic of solid tumors. In patients with leukemia, diffuse microscopic neoplastic peribronchial and peribronchiolar infiltration is frequent but may be asymptomatic. However, some patients present with diffuse interstitial infiltrates, an alveolar capillary block syndrome, and respiratory distress. In these situations, glucocorticoids can provide symptomatic relief, but specific chemotherapy should always be started promptly.

In addition, accumulation of leukemic blasts in the pulmonary capillary system may cause pulmonary distress and failure in patients with acute myelogenous leukemia. This complication is strongly related to high peripheral blast counts ($>100,000/\mu L$) and a short tumor cell doubling time. Some patients with pulmonary leukostasis may have nodular and/or floccular, diffuse infiltrates on chest radiographs. In addition to dyspnea, patients may develop dizziness, confusion, tinnitus, ataxia, visual blurring, and retinal abnormalities due to leukostasis in cerebral vessels. Leukapheresis and/or chemotherapy should be started without delay. Pulmonary irradiation may reduce symptoms.

Several cytotoxic agents, such as bleomycin, methotrexate, busulfan, and the nitrosoureas, may cause pulmonary damage. The most frequent presentations are interstitial pneumonitis, alveolitis, and pulmonary fibrosis. Some cytotoxic agents, including methotrexate and procarbazine, may cause an acute hypersensitivity reaction. Cytosine arabinoside has been associated with noncardiogenic pulmonary edema. Administration of multiple cytotoxic drugs, as well as radiation therapy and preexisting lung disease, may potentiate the pulmonary toxicity. Supplemental oxygen may potentiate the effects of drugs and radiation injury. Patients should always be managed with the lowest FI_{O_2} that is sufficient to maintain hemoglobin saturation.

The onset of symptoms may be insidious, with symptoms including dyspnea, nonproductive cough, and tachycardia. Patients may have bibasilar crepitant rales, end-inspiratory crackles, fever, and cyanosis. The chest radiograph generally shows an interstitial and sometimes an intraalveolar pattern that is strongest at the lung bases and may be symmetric. A small effusion may occur. Hypoxemia with decreased carbon monoxide diffusing capacity is always present. Glucocorticoids may be helpful in patients in whom pulmonary toxicity is related to radiation therapy or to chemotherapy. Treatment is otherwise supportive.

Radiation pneumonitis and/or fibrosis is a relatively frequent side effect of thoracic radiation therapy when the dosage exceeds 40 Gy; it may be acute or chronic. It has its onset usually from 2 to 6 months after completion of radiation therapy. The clinical syndrome, which varies in severity, consists of dyspnea, cough with scanty sputum, low-grade fever, and an initial hazy infiltrate on chest radiographs. The infiltrate and tissue damage generally are confined to the radiation field. The patients subsequently may develop a patchy alveolar infiltrate and air bronchograms, which may progress to acute respiratory failure that is sometimes fatal. A lung biopsy may be necessary to make the diagnosis. Asymptomatic infiltrates found incidentally after radiation therapy need not be treated. However, prednisone should be administered to patients with fever or other symptoms. The dosage should be tapered slowly after the resolution of radiation pneumonitis, as abrupt withdrawal of glucocorticoids may cause an exacerbation of pneumonia. Delayed radiation fibrosis may occur years after radiation therapy and is signaled by dyspnea on exertion. Often it is mild, but it can progress to chronic respiratory failure. Therapy is supportive.

Classical radiation pneumonitis that leads to pulmonary fibrosis is due to radiation-induced production of local cytokines such as platelet-derived growth factor β, tumor necrosis factor, and transforming growth factor β in the radiation field. An immunologically mediated sporadic radiation pneumonitis occurs in about 10% of patients; bilateral alveolitis mediated by T cells results in infiltrates outside the radiation field. This form of radiation pneumonitis usually resolves without sequelae.

Pneumonia is a common problem in patients undergoing treatment for cancer. Bacterial pneumonia typically causes a localized infiltrate on chest radiographs. Therapy is tailored to the causative organism. When diffuse interstitial infiltrates appear in a febrile patient, the differential diagnosis is extensive and includes pneumonia due to infection with *Pneumocystis carinii*, cytomegalovirus, or intracellular pathogens such as mycoplasma and *Legionella*; effects of drugs or radiation; tumor progression; nonspecific pneumonitis; and fungal disease. Patients with cancer who are neutropenic and have fever and local infiltrates on chest radiograph should be treated with a third generation cephalosporin perhaps together with an aminoglycoside or imipenem. A new or persistent focal infiltrate not responding to broad spectrum antibiotics argues for initiation of empiric antifungal therapy. When diffuse bilateral infiltrates develop in patients with febrile neutropenia, broad spectrum antibiotics plus trimethoprim-sulfamethoxazole with or without erythromycin should be initiated. The empiric administration of trimethoprim-sulfamethoxazole plus erythromycin to patients without neutropenia and these antibiotics plus ceftazidime to patients with neutropenia covers nearly every treatable diagnosis (except tumor progression) and gives as good overall survival as a strategy based on early invasive intervention with bronchoalveolar lavage or open lung biopsy. If the patient does not improve in 4 days, open lung biopsy is the procedure of choice. Bronchoscopy with bronchoalveolar lavage may be used in patients who are poor candidates for surgery.

In patients with pulmonary infiltrates who are afebrile, heart failure and multiple pulmonary emboli form part of the differential diagnosis.

TYPHLITIS Neutropenic enterocolitis (typhlitis) is a necrosis of the cecum and adjacent colon that may complicate the treatment of acute leukemia. The patient develops right lower quadrant abdominal pain, often with rebound tenderness and a tense, distended abdomen, in a setting of fever and neutropenia. Watery diarrhea (often containing sloughed mucosa) and bacteremia are common, and bleeding may occur. Plain abdominal films are generally of little value in the diagnosis; CT scan may show marked bowel wall thickening, particularly in the cecum, with bowel wall edema. Rapid institution of broad-spectrum antibiotic coverage and nasogastric suction may reverse the disease. Surgical intervention should be considered if there is no improvement by 24 h after the start of antibiotic treatment. If the localized abdominal findings become diffuse, the prognosis is poor.

HEMORRHAGIC CYSTITIS Hemorrhagic cystitis can develop in patients receiving cyclophosphamide or ifosfamide. Both drugs are metabolized to acrolein, which is a strong chemical irritant that is excreted in the urine. Prolonged contact or high concentrations may lead to bladder irritation and hemorrhage. Symptoms include gross hematuria, frequency, dysuria, burning, urgency, incontinence, and nocturia. The best management is prevention. Maintaining a high rate of urine flow minimizes exposure. In addition, 2-mercaptoethanesulfonate (mesna) detoxifies the metabolites and can be coadministered with the instigating drugs. Mesna usually is given three times on the day of ifosfamide administration in doses that are each 20% of the total ifosfamide dose. If hemorrhagic cystitis develops, the maintenance of a high urine flow may be sufficient supportive care. If conservative management is not effective, irrigation of the bladder with an 0.37 to 0.74% formalin solution for 10 min stops the bleeding in most cases. *N*-acetylcysteine may also be an effective irrigant. Prostaglandins (carboprost tromethamine) can inhibit the progress. In extreme cases, ligation of the hypogastric arteries, urinary diversion, or cystectomy may be necessary.

In summary, the diagnosis of cancer and its treatment carry risk of a multitude of medical problems. Knowledge of both the disease process and the potential hazards of the treatment is required to anticipate and treat these emergent complications.

BIBLIOGRAPHY

ALBANELL J, BASELGA J: Systemic therapy emergencies. Semin Oncol 27:347, 2000

ALLEN KB et al: Pericardial effusion: subxiphoid pericardiostomy versus percutaneous catheter drainage. Ann Thorac Surg 67:437, 1999

BOOGERD W et al: Diagnosis and treatment of spinal cord compression in malignant disease. Cancer Treat Rev 19:129, 1993

BOYD TS et al: Radiosurgery for brain metastases. Neurosurg Clin North Am 10:337, 1999

COLLIN BA et al: Pneumonia in the compromised host including cancer patients and transplant patients. Infect Dis Clin North Am 12:781, 1998

DIAZ PL et al: Palliative treatment of malignant colorectal strictures with metallic stents. Cardiovasc Intervent Radiol 22:29, 1999

JONES DP et al: Tumor lysis syndrome: Pathogenesis and management. Pediatr Nephrol 9:206, 1995

LABLAW A et al: Emergency treatment of malignant extradural spinal cord compression. J Clin Oncol 16:1613, 1998

SEBER A et al: Risk factors for severe hemorrhagic cystitis following BMT. Bone Marrow Transplant 23:35, 1999

SNYDER HW et al: Treatment of cancer chemotherapy–associated thrombotic thrombocytopenic/hemolytic uremic syndrome by protein A immunoadsorption of plasma. Cancer 71:1882, 1993

103   *Michael C. Perry, Dan L. Longo*

LATE CONSEQUENCES OF CANCER AND ITS TREATMENT

The 5-year survival rate of all patients diagnosed with cancer is now 59%. This year alone, nearly 700,000 survivors will be added to the 7 million already considered cured. Virtually all of these survivors will bear some mark of their diagnosis and its therapy, and many will experience long-term complications, including medical problems, psychosocial disturbances, sexual dysfunction, and inability to find employment or insurance.

Problems may be related to the cancer itself (for example, patients with primary cancers of the head and neck are at increased risk for subsequent lung cancer) or to the normal aging process (surviving one cancer does not necessarily alter the risk of other common tumors that increase in frequency with age). However, many of the problems affecting cured patients are related to the treatments. Large numbers of individuals carefully followed for periods up to 30 years have taught us the spectrum of problems that can be encountered. Because of heterogeneity in treatment details and in completeness of follow-up, some treatment-related problems went undetected for many years. However, studies of long-term survivors of childhood cancers, acute leukemia, Hodgkin's disease, lymphomas, testicular cancer, and localized solid tumors have identified the features of cancer treatment that are associated with later morbidity and mortality. We have been somewhat slow to act in changing those aspects of primary treatment that contribute to these late problems. This reticence is due to the uncertainty associated with changing a treatment that is known to work before having a replacement that works as well.

The first task is always to eradicate the diagnosed malignancy. Late problems occurring in cured patients reflect the success of treatment. Such problems never develop in those who do not survive the cancer. Morbidity and mortality from iatrogenic disease should be avoided, if possible. However, the risk of late complications should not lead to the failure to apply potentially curative treatment. The challenge is to preserve or augment the cure rate while decreasing the risk of serious treatment-related illness.

The mechanisms of damage vary. Surgical procedures can create abnormal physiology (such as blind loops leading to malabsorption) or interfere with normal organ function (splenectomy leading to impaired immune response). Radiation therapy can damage organ function directly (salivary gland toxicity leading to dry mouth and dental caries), act as a carcinogen (second solid tumors in radiation ports), or promote accelerated aging-associated changes (atherosclerosis). Cancer chemotherapy can produce damage to the bone marrow and immune system and induce a spectrum of organ dysfunctions. Therapy may produce subclinical damage that may only become recognized in the presence of a second inciting factor (such as the increased incidence of melanoma in patients with dysplastic nevus syndrome treated for Hodgkin's disease with radiation therapy). Finally, although the mechanisms are not elucidated, cancer and its treatment are associated with psychosocial problems that can impair the survivor's ability to adapt to life after cancer.

Late effects by treatment modality are shown in Table 103-1. →*Toxicities associated with drugs are discussed in Chap. 84; radiation toxicity is discussed in Chap 394.*

CONSEQUENCES BY ORGAN SYSTEM   Cardiovascular Dysfunction Most anthracyclines damage the heart muscle. A dose-dependent dropout of myocardial cells is seen on endomyocardial biopsy, and eventually ventricular failure ensues. About 5% of patients who receive >550 mg/m^2 of doxorubicin will develop congestive heart failure (CHF). Coexisting cardiac disease, hypertension, advanced age, and concomitant therapy with thoracic radiation therapy or mitomycin may hasten the onset of CHF. Anthracycline-induced CHF is not readily reversible; mortality is as high as 50%, thus, prevention is the best approach. Mitoxantrone is a related drug that has less cardiac toxicity. Administration of doxorubicin by continuous infusion or encapsulated in liposomes appears to decrease the risk of heart damage. Dexrazoxane, an intracellular iron chelator, may protect the heart against anthracycline toxicity by preventing iron-dependent free-radical generation.

Mediastinal radiation therapy that includes the heart can induce acute pericarditis, chronic constrictive pericarditis, myocardial fibrosis, or accelerated premature coronary atherosclerosis. The incidence of acute pericarditis is 5 to 13%; patients may be asymptomatic or have dyspnea on exertion, fever, chest pain. Onset is insidious with a peak about 9 months after treatment. Pericardial effusion may be present. Chronic constrictive pericarditis can develop 5 to 10 years after treatment and usually presents with dyspnea on exertion. Myocardial fibrosis may present as unexplained CHF with diagnostic evaluation showing restrictive cardiomyopathy. Patients may have aortic insufficiency from valvular thickening or mitral regurgitation from papillary muscle dysfunction. Patients who receive mantle field radiation therapy have a three-fold increased risk of *fatal* myocardial infarction. Similarly, radiation of the carotids is associated with premature atherosclerosis of the carotids and can produce central nervous system (CNS) embolic disease.

At very high doses, cyclosphosphamide can produce a hemorrhagic myocarditis. Patients receiving bleomycin may develop Raynaud's phenomenon. The symptoms range from mild to debilitating; up to 40% of patients receiving bleomycin for testicular cancer report this problem.

Pulmonary Dysfunction Pulmonary fibrosis from bleomycin is dose-related, with potential exacerbation by age, preexisting lung disease, thoracic radiation, high concentrations of inhaled oxygen, and the concomitant use of other chemotherapeutic agents. Several other chemotherapy agents and radiation therapy can cause pulmonary fibrosis, and at least five can cause pulmonary venoocclusive disease, especially following high-dose therapy such as that involved in stem cell/bone marrow transplantation.

Liver Dysfunction Clinically significant long-term damage to the liver from standard dose chemotherapy is relatively infrequent, and mostly confined to patients who have received chronic methotrexate for maintenance therapy of acute lymphoblastic leukemia. Radiation doses to the liver exceeding 1500 cGy can produce liver dysfunction. Although rarely seen with standard dose chemotherapy, hepatic venoocclusive disease is more common with high-dose therapy, such as that given to prepare patients for autologous or allogeneic stem cell transplantation. Endothelial damage is probably the inciting event.

Renal/Bladder Dysfunction Reduced renal function may be produced by cisplatin and is usually asymptomatic, but may also render the patient that much more susceptible to other renal insults. Cyclophosphamide cystitis may eventually lead to the development of bladder cancer. Ifosfamide produces cystitis and a proximal tubular defect, a Fanconi-like syndrome that is usually, but not always, reversible.

Endocrine Dysfunction Long-term survivors of childhood cancer who received cranial irradiation are shorter, more likely to be obese, and have reductions in strength, exercise tolerance, and bone

Table 103-1 Late Effects of Cancer Therapy

Surgical Procedure		Effect
Amputation		Functional loss
Lymph node dissection		Risk of lymphedema
Ostomy		Psychosocial impact
Splenectomy		Risk of sepsis
Adhesions		Risk of obstruction
Bowel anastomoses		Malabsorption syndromes

Radiation Therapy		Effect
Organ		
Bone		Premature termination of growth, osteonecrosis
Soft tissues		Atrophy, fibrosis
Brain		Neuropsychiatric deficits, cognitive dysfunction
Thyroid		Hypothyroidism, Graves' disease, cancer
Salivary glands		Dry mouth, carries, dysgeusia
Eyes		Cataracts
Heart		Pericarditis, myocarditis, coronary artery disease
Lung		Pulmonary fibrosis
Kidney		Decreased function, hypertension
Liver		Decreased function
Intestine		Malabsorption, stricture
Gonads		Infertility, premature menopause
Any		Secondary neoplasia

Chemotherapy		Effect
Organ	Drug	
Bone	Glucocorticoids	Osteoporosis, avascular necrosis
Brain	Methotrexate, ara-C, others	Neuropsychiatric deficits, cognitive decline?
Peripheral nerves	Vincristine, platinum	Neuropathy, hearing loss
Eyes	Glucocorticoids	Cataracts
Heart	Anthracyclines	Cardiomyopathy
Lung	Bleomycin	Pulmonary fibrosis
	Methotrexate	Pulmonary hypersensitivity
Kidney	Platinum, others	Decreased function, hypomagnesemia
Liver	Various	Altered function
Gonads	Alkylating agents, others	Infertility, premature menopause
Bone marrow	Various	Aplasia, myelodysplasia, secondary leukemia

mineral density. The obesity may be related to alterations in leptin biology. Growth hormone deficiency is the most common hormone deficiency.

Thyroid disease is common in patients who have received radiation therapy to the neck, such as patients with Hodgkin's disease, with an incidence of up to 62% at 26 years post-therapy. Hypothyroidism is the most common abnormality, followed by Graves' disease, thyroiditis, and cancer. Such patients should have frequent thyroid-stimulating hormone (TSH) levels to detect hypothyroidism early and suppress the TSH drive, which may contribute to thyroid cancer.

Nervous System Dysfunction Although many patients experience peripheral neuropathy during chemotherapy, only a few have chronic problems, perhaps because they have other co-existing diseases such as diabetes mellitus. High doses of cisplatin can produce severe sensorimotor neuropathy. Vincristine may produce permanent numbness and tingling in the fingers and toes.

Neurocognitive sequelae from intrathecal chemotherapy, with or without radiation therapy, are recognized complications of the successful therapy of childhood acute lymphoblastic leukemia. Cognitive decline has been attributed to radiating the brain in the treatment of a variety of tumor types. In addition, cognitive decline can follow the use of adjuvant chemotherapy in women being treated for breast cancer. Because the agents are given at modest doses and are not thought to cross the blood-brain barrier, the mechanism of the cognitive decline is not defined.

Many patients suffer intrusive thoughts about cancer recurrence for many years after successful treatment. Adjustment to normal expectations can be difficult. Cancer survivors may often have more problems holding a job, staying in a stable relationship, and coping with the usual stresses of daily life.

A dose-related hearing loss can occur with the use of cisplatin, usually with doses in excess of 400 mg/m². This is irreversible and patients should be screened with audiometric exams periodically during such therapy.

Eyes   Cataracts may be caused by chronic glucocorticoid use, radiation therapy to the head, and, rarely, by tamoxifen.

Sexual and Reproductive Dysfunction   Reversible azoospermia can be caused by many chemotherapy agents. The gonads may also be permanently damaged by radiation therapy or by chemotherapeutic agents, particularly the alkylating agents. The extent of the damage depends upon the patient's age and the total dose administered. As a woman nears menopause, smaller amounts of chemotherapy will produce ovarian failure. In men, chemotherapy may produce infertility, but hormone production is not usually affected. Women, however, commonly lose both fertility and hormone production. The premature induction of menopause in a young woman can have serious medical and psychological consequences. Hormone replacement therapy is controversial, but most evidence supports its use. Paroxetine may be useful in controlling hot flashes.

Musculoskeletal Dysfunction   Late consequences of radiation therapy on the musculoskeletal system occur mostly in children and are related to the radiation dose, volume of tissue irradiated, and the age of the child at the time of therapy. Damage to the microvasculature of the epiphyseal growth zone may result in leg length discrepancy, scoliosis, and short stature.

Oral Complications   Radiation therapy can damage the salivary glands, producing dry mouth. Without saliva, dental caries develop and many patients have poor dentition. In rare patients, taste can be adversely affected and appetite can be suppressed.

SECOND MALIGNANCIES   Second malignancies are a major cause of death for those cured of cancer. Second malignancies can be grouped into three categories: those associated with the primary cancer, those caused by radiation therapy, and those caused by chemotherapy.

Primary cancers increase the risk of secondary cancers in a number of settings. Patients with head and neck cancers are at increased risk of developing a lung cancer, and vice versa, probably because of shared risk factors, especially tobacco abuse. Patients with breast cancer are at increased risk of a second breast cancer in the contralateral breast. Patients with Hodgkin's disease are at increased risk of non-Hodgkin's lymphoma. Patients with genetic syndromes, such as MEN 1 or Lynch syndrome, are at increased risk of second cancers of specific types. In none of these examples does it appear that treatment of primary cancer is the cause of the secondary cancer, but a role for treatment is difficult to exclude. These predispositions should result in heightened surveillance in persons at risk. Patients with head and neck cancer may have a reduced risk of developing lung cancer with retinoic acid treatment. Other cancer preventions have not been proved effective.

Patients treated with radiation therapy have an increasing and apparently life-long risk of developing second solid tumors, usually in or adjacent to the radiation field. The risk is modest in the first decade after treatment but reaches 1% per year in the second decade, such that populations followed for 25 years or more have a ≥25% chance of developing a second treatment-related tumor. Some organs differ in their susceptibility to radiation carcinogenesis with age; women receiving chest radiation therapy after age 30 have a small increased risk of breast cancer, but those under 30 have a 128-fold increased risk. The chances of curing the second malignancies hinge on early diagnosis. Patients who were treated with radiation therapy should be carefully examined on an annual basis and evaluated for any abnormalities in organs and tissues that were in the radiation field. Symptoms in a patient cured of cancer should not be dismissed as they may be an early sign of second cancers.

Chemotherapy produces two clinical syndromes that can be fatal: myelodysplasia and acute myeloid leukemia. Two types of acute leukemia have been described. The first occurs in patients treated with alkylating agents, especially over a protracted period. The malignant cells frequently carry genetic deletions in chromosomes 5 or 7. The lifetime risk is about 2%; the risk is increased by the addition of radiation therapy and is about 3 times higher in people treated over age 40. It peaks in incidence 4 to 6 years after treatment; the risk returns to baseline if no disease has developed within 10 years of treatment. The second type of acute leukemia occurs after exposure to topoisomerase II inhibitors such as doxorubicin or etoposide. It is morphologically indistinguishable from the first but contains a characteristic chromosome translocation involving 10q23. The incidence is <1%, and it usually occurs 1 1/2 to 3 years after treatment. Both forms of acute leukemia are highly refractory to treatment, and no preventive strategy has been developed.

Hormonal manipulations can also cause second tumors. Tamoxifen induces endometrial cancer in about 1 to 2% of women taking it 5 years or longer. Usually these tumors are found at early stage; mortality from endometrial cancer is very low compared to the benefit from tamoxifen use as adjuvant therapy in women with breast cancer.

CONSEQUENCES BY CANCER TYPE   Pediatric Cancers Quality of life is often excellent, although the majority have at least one late effect. About one-third of long-term survivors have moderate to severe problems. Cognitive function may be impaired. Late effects are worse for those with poor socioeconomic status. Functional impairments in the cardiovascular system due to radiation therapy and anthracyclines, and in the lungs due to radiation therapy, are rare. Scoliosis and/or delayed growth due to radiation of the skeleton is more common. Many have psychosocial and sexual problems. Second malignant neoplasms are a significant cause of death.

Hodgkin's Disease   The patient cured of Hodgkin's disease remains subject to long-term medical problems such as thyroid dysfunction, premature coronary artery disease, gonadal dysfunction, postsplenectomy sepsis, and second malignancies. The second malignancies encountered include myelodysplasia and acute myeloid leukemia, non-Hodgkin's lymphomas, breast cancer, lung cancer, and melanoma. The major risk factor for hematologic malignancies is treatment with alkylating agents, while solid tumors are more likely to be seen with the use of radiation therapy. Patients cured of Hodgkin's disease seem to have greater fatigue, more psychosocial and sexual problems, and report a poorer quality of life than patients cured of acute leukemia.

Non-Hodgkin's Lymphomas   The patient cured of a non-Hodgkin's lymphoma may be at increased risk of myelodysplasia and acute leukemia if high doses or prolonged alkylating agents were used. Chronic exposure to cyclophosphamide increases the risk of bladder cancer. Patients cured of lymphoma report a very good quality of life.

Acute Leukemia   The late effects of anti-leukemic therapy include second malignancies (hematologic and solid tumors), neuropsychiatric difficulties, subnormal growth, thyroid abnormalities, and infertility.

Head and Neck Cancer   Patients frequently have poor dentition, dry mouth, trismus, difficulty in eating, and poor nutrition. Those with nasopharyngeal cancer report the poorest long-term quality of life, possibly related to the volume of disease that is radiated.

Stem Cell Transplantation   Cured patients are at risk of second cancers, especially if radiation therapy was part of the treatment. They are also subject to gonadal damage and infertility. Graft-versus-host disease is the leading factor contributing to the morbidity and mortality from allogeneic bone marrow transplantation, with an immune-mediated attack against the skin, liver, and gut epithelium. About half of patients report psychosexual problems.

Breast Cancer   Patients treated with adjuvant chemotherapy and/or hormonal therapy for breast cancer are at risk for endometrial cancer from the use of tamoxifen. Those patients who have received chemotherapy may be at risk from doxorubicin or radiation-induced cardiomyopathy and acute leukemia. The development of premature ovarian failure from chemotherapy may cause hormone-deficient symptoms (hot flashes, decreased vaginal secretions, dyspareunia) and places women at risk for osteoporosis and cardiovascular deaths. Patients commonly report intrusive thoughts of cancer and psychological distress.

Testicular Cancer Depending on the modalities used for therapy, patients cured of testicular cancer can anticipate Raynaud's phenomena, renal and/or pulmonary damage from chemotherapy, and ejaculatory dysfunction from retroperitoneal lymph node dissection. Sexual dysfunction is reported by 15% of patients cured of testicular cancer.

Colon Cancer To date the major threat to patients with colorectal cancer treated with chemotherapy and or radiation therapy remains the risk of a second colorectal cancer. Quality of life is reported as high in long-term survivors.

Prostate Cancer Radical surgical treatment is often accompanied by impotence and about 10 to 15% develop some urine incontinence. Use of radiation therapy increases the risk of second cancers.

The challenge for the future is to integrate new chemotherapy and biologic agents and newer techniques of delivering radiation therapy in a fashion that increases cure rates and lowers the late effects of treatment. Additional populations at risk for late effects include those with cancers where therapy is becoming more effective, such as ovarian cancer, and cancers where chemotherapy and radiation therapy are used together in an organ-sparing approach, such as bladder cancer, anal cancer, and laryngeal cancer. Patients who have been cured of a cancer represent an important resource for cancer prevention studies.

BIBLIOGRAPHY

Bookman MA et al: Late complications of curative treatment in Hodgkin's disease. JAMA 260:680, 1988

Mackie E et al: Adult psychosocial outcomes in long-term survivors of acute lymphoblastic leukemia and Wilms' tumor: A controlled study. Lancet 355:1310, 2000

Socie G et al: New malignant disease after allogeneic marrow transplantation for childhood acute leukemia. J Clin Oncol 18:348, 2000

van Leeuwen FE et al: Long-term risk of second malignancy in survivors of Hodgkin's disease treated during adolescence or young adulthood. J Clin Oncol 18: 487, 2000

Section 2
DISORDERS OF HEMATOPOIESIS

104

Peter J. Quesenberry, Gerald A. Colvin

HEMATOPOIESIS

Hematopoiesis is the production of blood cells. It is a tightly regulated system exquisitely responsive to functional demands. The level of neutrophils, eosinophils, and basophils are maintained in discrete ranges with rapid adjustments when demands such as bacterial infection, parasitic infection, or allergic reaction are imposed. Similarly, lymphocytes, monocytes, platelets, and red cells, while maintained in normal ranges, respond rapidly to demands—lymphocytes to immune challenge, monocytes to various infections, platelets to hemorrhage or inflammation, and red cells to tissue hypoxia from many causes. Derangements in marrow function can lead to an excess of white cells, such as leukemia or leukemoid reactions, or an inadequate number of cells, such as anemia, thrombocytopenia, or leukopenia. Kinetics of cytopenia induction after marrow injury with drugs, radiation, or infections reflect the life span of these cells in peripheral blood. The first lineage to drop are the neutrophils with a blood life span of 6 to 8 h, followed by platelets with a 10-day life span. Anemia develops over a longer time in the absence of blood loss, reflecting the 120-day life span of red blood cells. All of these cell types are produced by primitive cells termed *stem cells*, which are present in the bone marrow of adult mammals.

The production of all the cell types except lymphocytes is usually very efficient, and production is controlled largely by negative feedback. When demand for production of cells of a particular lineage increases or peripheral levels of the cells fall, stimulatory cytokines are released and generate new cells with a time delay of a few days, or the time required for maturation from stem cell precursors. By contrast, production of lymphocytes is highly inefficient. Each day many more cells are generated than are required in the periphery. Most lymphocytes are destroyed during development; this is due at least in part to the destruction of cells that express antigen receptors specific for self antigens.

HEMATOPOIETIC STEM CELLS Hematopoietic stem cells are characterized by extensive proliferation and differentiation capacity, with the ability to self-renew on a population basis (Fig. 104-1). They also express a variety of cell-surface proteins and have the ability to rapidly "home" to bone marrow after intravenous injection. Human stem cells lack markers of lineage commitment (i.e., lineage-negative) and express c-Kit, c-mpl, and usually cluster of differentiation determinant-34 (CD34); a small subset of stem cells may be CD34-negative. Murine cells are also lineage-negative and express c-Kit, CD34, c-mpl, and Ly6A or Sca. The most primitive cells are characterized by low-level expression of a relatively large number of cytokine receptors and by relative exclusion (or pumping out) of the dyes rhodamine and Hoechst. These cells express a variety of adhesion proteins presumptively involved in marrow homing, including alpha$_4$, alpha$_5$, alpha$_6$, L-selectin, and platelet/endothelial cell adhesion molecule (PECAM) (Fig. 104-2). Another characteristic of the stem cell is a functional plasticity in response to cytokines as it transits the cell cycle (Fig. 104-3). Engraftment capacity is good in G$_1$ but virtually lost in late S and early G$_2$.

The stem cell is also a highly mobile cell with the capacity to evolve rapidly or involute pseudopodial extensions. The gold standard for defining the stem cell has been in vivo repopulation and long-term reconstitution of lethally irradiated mice. In vivo repopulation studies using unique radiation-induced chromosomal abnormalities or retroviral markers have shown that one or, at most, a few stem cells are capable of reconstituting the entire lymphohematopoietic system of a mouse; they also have defined classes of stem cells with short, medium, or long-term repopulating capacity. These are cell types that differ in the kinetics of hematopoietic reconstitution. Short-term cells repopulate in the first few weeks after transplantation but are not long-lasting; long-term cells account for long-lived reconstitution beginning a few months after reconstitution and lasting the entire life span; medium-term cells bridge the time between short- and long-term cells. When relatively small numbers of marked stem cells—obtained by limiting dilution of sorted marrow cells—are transplanted, lymphohematopoiesis may be clonal or oligoclonal, initially. Normal polyclonal lymphohematopoiesis derives from a relatively large number of clones. Both competitive marrow repopulation and mathematical studies support the model of polyclonal hematopoiesis. The most primitive long-term repopulating cells on activation with cytokines can rapidly alter phenotype and become short-term repopulating cells.

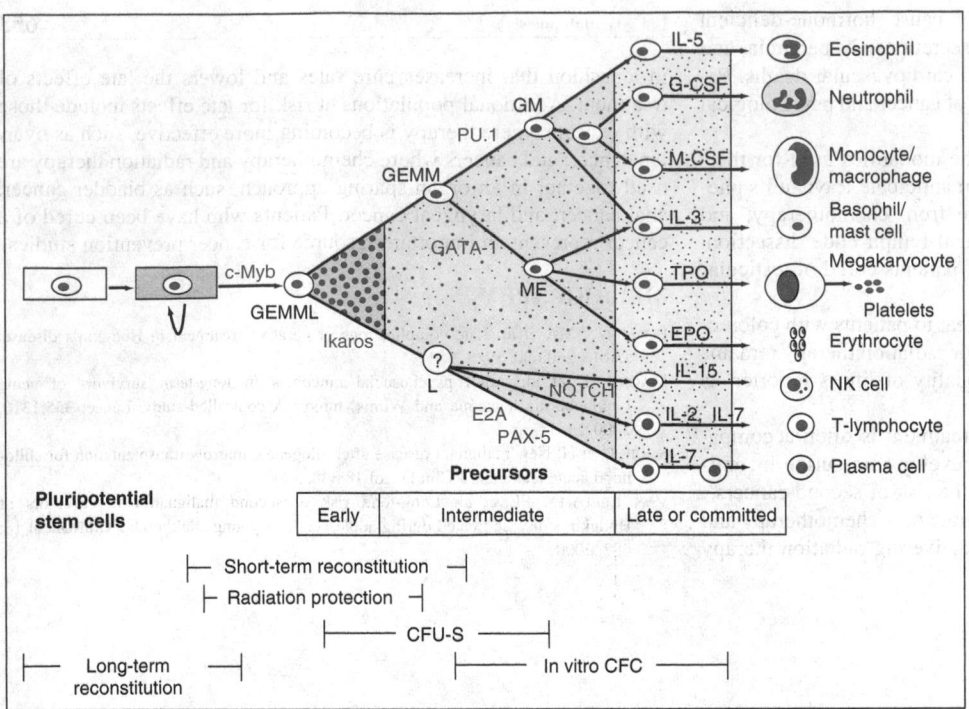

FIGURE 104-1 Cellular basis of hematopoiesis. Mature cells are derived from a common multipotent progenitor. Lineage development appears to occur as a consequence of the ordered expression of transcription factors (in blue). Thus, mice in which PU.1 expression has been blocked develop normal erythrocytes and megakaryocytes, but no other cell lineages. Once lineage commitment occurs, cytokines and colony-stimulating factors (in black) regulate development, again through the induction of transcription factors. Abbreviations: HSC, hematopoietic stem cell; GEMML, cell giving rise to granulocyte, erythroid, monocyte, megakaryocyte, and lymphoid cells: GEMM, cell giving rise to granulocyte, erythroid, monocyte, and megakaryocytic cells; GM, cell giving rise to granulocytic and monocyte cells; ME, cell giving rise to megakaryocytic and erythroid cells; L, lymphoid lineage stem cell.

While stable multilineage chimerism has been documented in humans after clinical marrow transplantation, no assay system exists for human stem cell activity. A number of surrogate assays are used for the long-term, multilineage-repopulating cell in both humans and mice. These include the multifactor-responsive, high-proliferative potential colony-forming cells (HPP-CFC) and variations of stromal-based assays including the cobblestone-forming cell, long-term culture-initiating cell (LTC-IC) or LTC-IC–extended (LTC-IC–e). The adequacy of these assays is still the subject of debate. In addition, the NOD-SCID immunodeficient mouse has become a surrogate model for assaying human hematopoietic stem cells, although lineage skewing and variability of engraftment undermine its reliability.

LINEAGE PLASTICITY OF STEM CELLS Tissue stem cells are capable of producing a wide variety of differentiated cell lineages, depending on intrinsic cell programming and the microenvironmental signals. Marrow cells may differentiate into mesenchy-

mal, myocyte, endothelial, hematopoietic, and neural cells. Neural muscle and hepatic stem cells have been reported to give rise to hematopoiesis in transplanted mice. The regulation of stem cell plasticity and life span remains incompletely understood. However, once a particular set of transcription factors has been induced, either through an intrinsic program or from extracellular signals, reversibility is limited. The sequentially ordered activation of transcription factors leads to lineage commitment.

MICROENVIRONMENT Nonhematopoietic tissues exert major influences on hematopoiesis, both short- and long-range. The nonhematopoietic tissues immediately abutting hematopoietic tissue have been termed the hematopoietic microenvironment, and the cells that comprise the environment influence hematopoiesis. For example, a surface location of adoptively transferred murine stem cells in the spleen of lethally irradiated mice favored erythropoiesis, while an intrasplenic trabecular location was biased toward granulocyte production. In both human and murine species, various cell types have been identified in stroma, including hematopoietically derived macrophages and nonhematopoietic preadipocytic fibroblasts, endothelial cells, and vascular smooth muscle. This system appears capable of supporting the most primitive stem cells and controlling their proliferation and self-renewal. Most stem cells are resting under normal physiologic conditions but can be recruited into the cell cycle by demands of increased terminally differentiated hematopoietic cells. Cell-cell contact is critical in determining the microenvironment stimulus. Stem cells and primitive cells bind tightly to the stroma, while maturing precursors and terminally differentiated cells are nonadherent. Blocking interactions between stem cells and stromal cells with antibodies to vascular cell adhesion molecule (VCAM)-1 on stromal cells

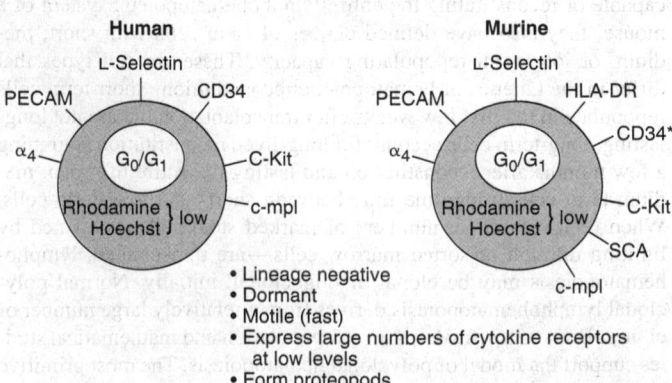

FIGURE 104-2 The phenotype of human and murine stem cells.

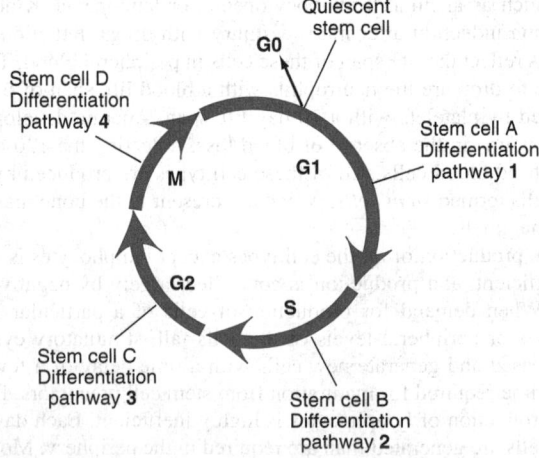

FIGURE 104-3 The functional plasticity of stem cells in response to cytokines as it transits the cell cycle. The stem cell has the capacity to differentiate into morphologically different phenotypes as it marches through the cell cycle (depicted as Stem Cell A-D). Engraftment capacity is good in G_1 but virtually lost in late S and early G_2.

or its ligand, VLA-4, on stem cells block the interaction. Cytokine receptors binding to membrane-associated cytokines like stem cell factor, or to extracellular matrix-bound ligands, contribute other adhesive interactions.

PROGENITORS Bone marrow stem cells can be induced to proliferate and differentiate into a wide variety of mature cell types in vitro in the presence of an appropriate colony-stimulating factor (CSF). Cells that give rise to mature colonies of granulocytes and macrophages are called granulocyte-macrophage colony-forming units (CFU-GM) (Fig. 104-4). The particular hematopoietic growth factor that stimulates the development of these colonies is called granulocyte-macrophage colony-stimulating factor (GM-CSF). Distinct culture conditions and supplemental growth factors, alone and in combination, are capable of producing a range of cell expansions from multilineage colonies that include lymphocytes to single-lineage clones. The different stem/progenitor clones are summarized in Table 104-1. Progenitor cells in general are found to have a higher proliferative rate and more lineage restriction than stem cells. They are also responsive to smaller numbers of cytokines. Thus, they are defined by expression of a limited variety of cytokine receptors.

The size of the colonies denotes the activity of cells at different stages of differentiation. Terminally acting cytokines produce smaller colonies called CFU (colony-forming units). When progenitors are stimulated with mixtures of early- and late-acting cytokines and are cultured for longer periods of time, the colonies are larger and multiple lineages are represented. Primitive multifactor-responsive erythroid colonies are termed burst-forming unit erythroid (BFU-E) while even more primitive colonies with great proliferative potential are termed HPP-CFC.

CYTOKINES The lymphohematopoietic stem/progenitor populations and their progeny are largely defined by their cytokine responsiveness and cytokine receptor phenotype. Major efforts to define the regulators of granulocyte, erythroid, and platelet production have culminated in the definitions of a variety of glycoproteins. Acting through cell surface receptors at very low concentrations, these glycoproteins control the production of stem cells in vivo. Most prominent have been erythropoietin for red blood cells, GM-CSF for granulocytes and macrophages, granulocyte-CSF (G-CSF) for granulocytes, and thrombopoietin for platelets. In addition, macrophage-CSF or CSF-1, was defined as a primary regulator of macrophage-monocyte production and function. These cytokines exert prominent actions on specific cell lineages, but all exert actions on different cell lineages or on cells that have the potential to differentiate along more than one lineage.

In addition to the more lineage-restricted cytokines, a large number (perhaps up to 70) act broadly on multiple lineages and at multiple stages of lymphohematopoiesis. They exert effects on renewal, proliferation, survival, and differentiation; these effects may be stimulatory or inhibitory, and the cytokines usually show additive or synergistic effects with other cytokines. The cytokines also modulate intrinsic functions of early stem cells (migration and cell adherence) and pro-

Table 104-1 Progenitor Stem Cells

In Vitro Assay	Stem/Progenitor Clones
GM-colony forming unit culture (G-CSF, GM-CSF, CSF-1)	Defined by cytokine regulators Produces colonies of granulocytes, granulocytes/macrophages, or macrophages
CFU-E	Small colonies of red cells; need only erythropoietin
CFU-MEG	Small colonies of megakaryocytes
BFU-E	Large aggregates of red cells; needs erythropoietin plus other cytokines
BFU-MEG	Large colonies of megakaryocytes; needs multiple cytokines
HPP-CFC	Stimulated by multiple factors with great proliferative and differentiative potential
	Large colonies surrogate for primitive stem cells
Colony-forming unit blast	Small colonies of undifferentiated blasts; needs multiple cytokines
Cobblestone forming or long term culture initiating cell (LTC-IC)	Forms granulocyte/macrophage colonies after culture with adherent stroma
	Relatively primitive cell
LTC-IC extended	May be a more primitive stem cell
	Long time growth on stroma produces multipotential lymphomyeloid progenitors

NOTE: CFU, colony-forming unit; BFU, burst-forming unit; HPP-CFC, high-proliferative potential colony-forming cells.

mote the effector functions of their terminally differentiated progeny. G-CSF primes neutrophils to undergo oxidative metabolism in response to formyl-methionyl-leucyl-phenylalanine (fMLF) and enhances cell migration, while interleukin (IL) 3 activates basophils, mast cells, and eosinophils. CSF-1 at low levels supports survival of murine marrow macrophages and at higher levels stimulates protein synthesis, cell division, and various macrophage functions, including antitumor activity, secretion of products of oxygen reduction, and plasminogen activator. CSF-1 also induces secretion of IL-1 from macrophages. Many of the hematopoietically active cytokines induce secretion of other cytokines, either inhibitory or stimulatory, creating multiple cytokine regulatory loops. Transforming growth factor β (TGF-β) is an inhibitory cytokine but also an autocrine factor supporting survival of pluripotent hematopoietic stem cells by blocking G1 to S phase transition. TGF-β conversely shows stimulatory effects on progenitors. Cytokines also modulate adhesion protein and integrin expression on multiple cell types. They exert their effects by interacting with surface-based receptors and initiating second-messenger cascades (see below).

The lymphohematopoietic cytokines can be broadly divided into colony-stimulating factors, erythropoietin, thrombopoietin, the interleukins, the inhibitory cytokines, chemokines that regulate cell migration and activation, and a variety of other hematopoietically active cytokines. A noninclusive overview of these cytokines emphasizing their primary, highlighted, or first-described action is presented in Tables 104-2, 104-3 and 104-4. The general characteristics of cytokines are summarized in Table 104-5.

CYTOKINE RECEPTORS, SIGNAL TRANSDUCTION, AND TRANSCRIPTION FACTORS Cytokines induce their effects through cell-surface membrane receptors. Several cytokine receptor families have been identified. The hematopoietic receptor family includes IL-2, IL-3, IL-4, IL-5, IL-6, IL-7, IL-9, G-CSF, GM-CSF, and erythropoietin. Common characteristics of this family include four conserved cysteine residues and a WSXWS motif (X is a variable, nonconserved amino acid). Some also have immunoglobulin-like structures in their extracellular domains. Receptors frequently consist of multiple chains, and dimerization on cytokine binding is a usual feature of receptor biology. These receptors have no intrinsic signaling capacity and transmit signals by attaching to intracellular signaling molecules, such as the src family and the JAK family kinases. GM-

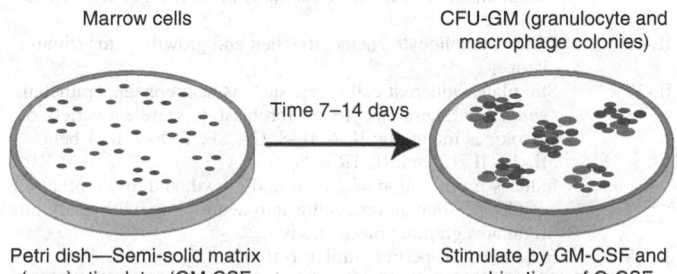

Marrow cells   CFU-GM (granulocyte and macrophage colonies)

Time 7–14 days

Petri dish—Semi-solid matrix (agar) stimulator (GM-CSF, G-CSF, CSF-1)   Stimulate by GM-CSF and combinations of G-CSF, GM-CSF and CSF-1

FIGURE 104-4 Marrow cells in semi-solid media in the presence of stimulatory factors in conditioned media or serum form colonies of granulocytes and macrophages.

Table 104-2 Lymphohematopoietic Cytokines

Growth Factor	Highlighted and/or Predominant Actions
Erythropoietin	Limited proliferative effects; modulates/stimulates survival and terminal maturation of CFU-E
	Globin synthesis and proliferation of proerythroblasts and basophilic erythroblasts
	Increases in vivo red cell production
GM-CSF	Predominant action on granulocyte/macrophage progenitors
	Action on multipotent neutrophil, macrophage megakaryocyte, eosinophil, erythroid, and dendritic progenitors
	Stimulates function of mature neutrophils and macrophages
	Inhibits neutrophil migration and stimulates cytotoxic and phagocytic activity against yeast, parasites, and antibody-coated tumor cells
	In vivo, increases granulocytes, monocytes, eosinophils, and dendritic cells
	Has a variable effect on the platelet count
G-CSF	Stimulates granulocyte and pre-B cell production in vitro and primes neutrophils for function
	Increases neutrophil levels in vivo
CSF-1	Stimulates a population of progenitors that make macrophages
	Also stimulates function and cell division of mature macrophages
IL-3 or Multi-CSF	Multilineage stimulator with direct megakaryocyte, mast cell/basophil, B cell, and eosinophil stimulatory activity
	Synergizes with EPO to stimulate primitive erythroid stem cells and with multiple factors to stimulate HPP-CFC
	In vivo, increases blood eosinophil, granulocyte, and monocyte levels as well as tissue mast cells
Thrombopoietin	Ligand for C-mpl
	Major regulator of megakaryocyte proliferation, differentiation, and platelet production
	Stimulates and supports survival of primitive stem cells
	In vivo, increases platelet production

NOTE: CFU, colony-forming unit; CSF, colony-stimulating factor; GM-CSF, granulocyte-macrophage colony-stimulating factor; G-CSF, granulocyte-CSF; EPO, erythropoietin.

CSF, IL-3, and IL-5 receptors have low-affinity alpha chains and a common high-affinity beta chain. The common beta chain may play a role in the competitive binding of these ligands.

Receptors for FLT-3 ligand, c-kit, platelet-derived growth factor (PDGF), CSF-1, and thrombopoietin constitute the tyrosine kinase receptor family. These receptors have conserved cysteines in the extracellular domain, with tyrosine kinase activity in the cytoplasmic domain, an immunoglobulin-like structure involved in ligand, and binding. Chemokine receptors are seven-transmembrane (serpin) G-protein linked receptors that signal cell activation and migration.

Cytokines typically cause receptor oligomerization on hematopoietic cells, followed by activation of intrinsic (receptor) or extrinsic tyrosine kinases, phosphorylation of the receptor and recruitment of Src-homology (SH2), and phospho-tyrosine binding (PT3) domain proteins to the receptor. Subsequent steps vary with different cytokines but essentially represent a series of phosphorylation-dephosphorylation events, with the final activation or nuclear translocation of a protein or protein complex that binds specific regions of DNA and initiates various genetic programs (i.e., acts as a transcription factor).

The complexity of these second-messenger signaling systems is illustrated by signaling through the GM-CSF, IL-3, and IL-5 receptors, which share a common beta chain. The beta chain does not have kinase activity but induces tyrosine phosphorylation of itself and a number of cytoplasmic proteins, including kinases, such as P1-3 kinase; adapters illustrated by Grb2; the insulin receptor-substrate 2 Cbl and Shc;

guanine nucleotide exchange factors such as Vav; phosphastases such as SH2-domain protein tyrosine phosphatase-2 and SH2-containing inositol phosphatase; and transcription factors such as STAT 5.

Receptor phosphorylation is mediated by receptor-associated kinases, such as JAK2 (Janus family kinase 2, named Janus for the Roman god who guards the gates and looks in two directions; original Janus kinases were felt to have both tyrosine and serine kinase activity) and Src-family kinases. These sequential protein interactions lead to the evolution of proteins or protein complexes, termed *transcription factors*, that bind to specific regions of DNA to initiate genetic pro-

Table 104-3 Interleukins

Cytokine	Action
IL-1	Regulation immune system, induction fever, acute phase protein, tissue repair and cytotoxicity
	Directly stimulates early stem cells and acts synergistically with many other cytokines to stimulate HPP-CFC
	A prominent inducer of other cytokines from many cell types
IL-2	T cell growth factor
	Increases production of gamma interferon
	Stimulates and activates B cells and natural killer cells
	Inhibits GM colony formation and erythropoiesis
IL-4	Stimulates B cell maturation, immunoglobin synthesis and generation of cytotoxic and helper T lymphocytes
	Synergizes with other cytokines to stimulate GM, mast cell, erythroid, and megakaryocyte proliferation
	Stimulates proliferation and differentiation of dendritic cells
	Inhibits monocyte cytokine production
IL-5	Stimulates B cells and supports the proliferation, maturation and function of eosinophils
IL-6	Stimulates megakaryopoiesis and synergizes with IL-1, 2, 3, 4, GM-CSF, and CSF-1 to stimulate myeloid proliferation
	Plasma cell proliferation-enhanced
	Induces hepatocyte protein synthesis
IL-7	B and T cell stimulation
	Stimulates early hematopoietic stem cells and has activity with kit-ligand in inducing pre-B cells in culture
IL-8	Chemotactic factor for granulocytes
	Mobilizes stem cells into the peripheral blood
IL-9	T cell growth factor
	Supports erythroid burst development and has mast cell growth-promoting activity
IL-10	Inhibits INF-γ production by T cells
	Increases cytotoxic T cell precursors and function
	Synergistically stimulates mast cells
IL-11	Very similar in action to IL-6
IL-12	NK cell stimulatory factor
	In synergy with IL-2 generates cytotoxic T cells
	Induces INF-γ production by NK and T cells
IL-13	Similar in action to IL-4 on B cells and monocytes
	In contrast to IL-4, induces production of IFN-γ by large granular lymphocytes and stimulates T cells
IL-14	Induces B cell proliferation and inhibits immunoglobin synthesis
IL-15	Shares biologic activity with IL-2
	Stimulates proliferation of activated CD4+, CD8+, $\gamma\delta$ subsets of T cells, NK cells, and mast cells
	Costimulator with IL-12 to facilitate production of IFN-γ and TNF-α
IL-16	CD4+ lymphocyte chemoattractant and growth factor stimulator
IL-17	Stimulates adherent cell types, such as macrophage, epithelial, endothelial, keratinocyte, or fibroblast, to secrete a variety of cytokines including: IL-6, IL-8, G-CSF, TNF-α, IL-1 beta, IL-10, IL-12, and IL-1R antagonist
	Induces proliferation of T cells and growth and differentiation of CD34+ human progenitor into neutrophils (with co-culture)
	Stimulates granulopoiesis in vivo
IL-18	Functional properties similar to IL-12
	Augments cell-mediated immunity
	Modulates T, B, and NK cell function
	Induces IFN-γ in type 1 helper T and NK cells

NOTE: GM, granulocyte-macrophage; IFN, interferon; NK, natural killer; TNF, tumor necrosis factor; IL, interleukin.

Table 104-4   Other Lymphohematopoietic Cytokines

Cytokine	Action
Kit ligand	Identical with hematolymphopoietic growth factor
	Synergizes with a large number of cytokines to stimulate HPP-CFC
	With IL-7 stimulates pre-B cell generation
	Multilineage effects in mice and primates with mast cell activation
	Acts on primitive stem/progenitor cells
FLT-3	Acts on relatively primitive progenitor/stem cells showing synergies with G-CSF, GM-CSF, M-CSF, IL-3, and kit-ligand
	Stimulates dendritic cell formation
b-FbF	Pleiotropic growth factor stimulating primitive marrow cells, megakaryocyte progenitors, and marrow stromal cells
LIF	Supports proliferation of IL-3 dependent cell line DA-1 and has multiple non-hematopoietic actions
	Sustains proliferation of embryonic stem cells
TGF-β	Inhibits early stem cells while stimulating progenitors, possibly through modulating surface cytokine receptor expression
	Probable autocrine factor for early stem cell survival
Mip-1α	Blocks stem cell entry into cell cycle and quiesces stem cells
Pentapeptide	Removes stem/progenitor cells from S phase
Tetrapeptide	Blocks entry of stem cells into S phase
Platelet-derived growth factor	Acts on erythroid and granulopoietic progenitors and, indirectly, on early multilineage stem cells
Hepatocyte growth factor	Synergizes with other growth factors at the progenitor cell level

grams determining survival, proliferation, differentiation, and function.

As with second messengers, the transcription factor field is complex and evolving, but a number of transcription factors associated with specific stem cell levels or differentiation pathways have been described. Transcription factors that act at the earliest stem cell levels include c-myb, p45-NF-E2, GATA-2, AML-1 and tal-1/SCL, while Ikaros and PU-1 may act at the earliest lymphoid level. GATA-1 influences erythroid, mast cell, and megakaryocyte lineages, while FOG (friend of GATA-1) acts in concert with GATA-1. PU-1 appears to influence granulocyte and monocyte differentiation, P45-NF-E2 affects megakaryocyte lineages, and PAX-5 B lymphoid development. These transcription factors usually act in complexes with specific conformations binding to particular DNA sequences.

MIGRATION HOMING AND ADHESION PROTEINS
The process of stem cell homing to the marrow is complex and involves a number of adhesion proteins. Very late antigen (VLA) 4, VLA-5, VLA-6, PECAM, P- and E-selectin, CD44, CXCR, and a receptor for ligand-bearing galactosyl and mannosyl residues have been shown to be expressed by hematopoietic stem/progenitor cells and

Table 104-5   General Characteristics of Cytokines

Cytokines are glycoproteins acting at very low concentrations
Almost all cytokines are pleiotropic effectors, showing multiple biologic activities
The activity of most cytokines is strictly regulated, addresses multiple target cells, is normally transient, and can be regulated at all levels of gene expression
Factors are usually produced only by activated cells in response to an induction signal
Cell surface receptor is bound to initiate second-messenger cascade
Cytokines play a pivotal role in cell-to-cell communication processes, inducing the synthesis of novel gene products once they have bound to their respective receptors
Frequently act on stem/progenitors and their differentiated progeny to stimulate *or* inhibit renewal, survival, proliferation, differentiation, and function
Usually act on multiple different lineages, activate stimulatory or inhibitory activities, and synergize or antagonize the actions of other factors
Frequently act on neoplastic counterpart of normal target cell

implicated in marrow homing. The integrins α_4 and/or α_5 are expressed on immature blasts, erythroid progenitors, monocytes, and CD34+ cells; in general, expression of α_4 appears to decrease with maturation. Hematopoietic cells also bind differentially to different extracellular matrix components: erythroid cells to fibronectin, CFU-GM and BFU-E to collagen.

Antibody to VLA-4 given in vivo causes mobilization of hematopoietic progenitors in normal or cytokine-treated primates and/or mice. Stem cell mobilization by cytokines involves down regulation of adhesion protein expression on hematopoietic stem cells. The cell-cycle related fluctuations in engraftment appear to be based on alterations on different surface adhesion proteins. The stem cells are highly motile and move in a direction of cytokine or chemokine gradients with steel factor and stromal-derived factor 1 (SDF-1) being active. Adhesion proteins act not only for motility/adhesion, but also serve a regulatory role that is similar in some cases to traditional cytokines.

PHYSIOLOGY OF HEMATOPOIESIS AND SOURCES OF CYTOKINES   Erythropoietin is produced largely by the kidney in response to tissue hypoxia. The regulation of granulocyte and monocyte production is more complex, but appears to be in response to various infectious or noxious agents, such as gram-negative bacteria, the endotoxin in the cell wall of these bacteria, and antigen stimulation. All of these interact with peripheral tissue cells to generate a variety of cytokine messages, resulting in increase production in specific cell types. Parasitic infections appear to elicit IL-5, which modulates the eosinophilia and mast cell lineages. Viral infections have specific effects on lymphocyte classes; typically bacterial infections stimulate granulocyte production. Tuberculosis or other mycobacterial infections predominantly induce increased monocyte production. All of these biologic affects appear to be mediated by the selective evolution of cytokine complexes from tissue endothelial cells, fibroblasts, macrophages, and lymphocytes. Most cells produce a large variety of cytokines, but the key is the relative levels, combinations, and timing of the production of these cytokines (Fig. 104-5).

HEMATOPOIETIC STEM CELL AND CYTOKINE DISEASES   The classic stem cell disease is *chronic myeloid leukemia*. Here a specific genetic translocation between chromosomes 9 and 22 at the stem cell level leads to excess production of granulocytes, monocytes, basophils, frequently platelets, and less frequently red cells. Other lymphohematopoietic clonal stem cell diseases include polycythemia vera, myelofibrosis with myeloid metaplasia, paroxysmal nocturnal hemoglobinuria, and acute myeloid leukemia. Out of the scope of this chapter, but relevant to these discussions, is the fact that many lymphoid neoplasms are clonal diseases at early stages of development, but probably not at the mature stage suggested by the tumor cell-surface phenotype. The vast majority of peripheral B cell and T cell malignancies have genetic lesions associated with receptor gene rearrangements, which occur early in lymphoid cell development. Aplastic anemia appears to be a disease characterized by a defective number of hematopoietic stem cells. Cyclic hematopoiesis is another disease of hematopoietic stem cells. In gray collie dogs with this disorder, levels of platelets, reticulocytes, monocytes, and granulocytes cycle. This disease can be cured or transmitted by marrow transplantation. The human disease, cyclical neutropenia—or cyclic hematopoiesis in which blood cells oscillate with a 21-day period—is caused by missense and splicing mutations in the gene encoding neutrophil elastase, thus implicating this inflammatory chymotryptic serine protease in the oscillatory timing of hematopoiesis. The stem cell diseases are summarized in Table 104-6.

A number of cytokine disorders or diseases have now been defined. The best characterized is the anemia of renal failure, an erythropoietin deficiency state that can be corrected by the administration of erythropoietin. Various tumors, particularly lung cancer, increase peripheral granulocyte counts secondary to the production of G-CSF. The IL-6 family of cytokines appears to be prominently involved in a number of inflammatory states, causes the systemic symptoms associated with

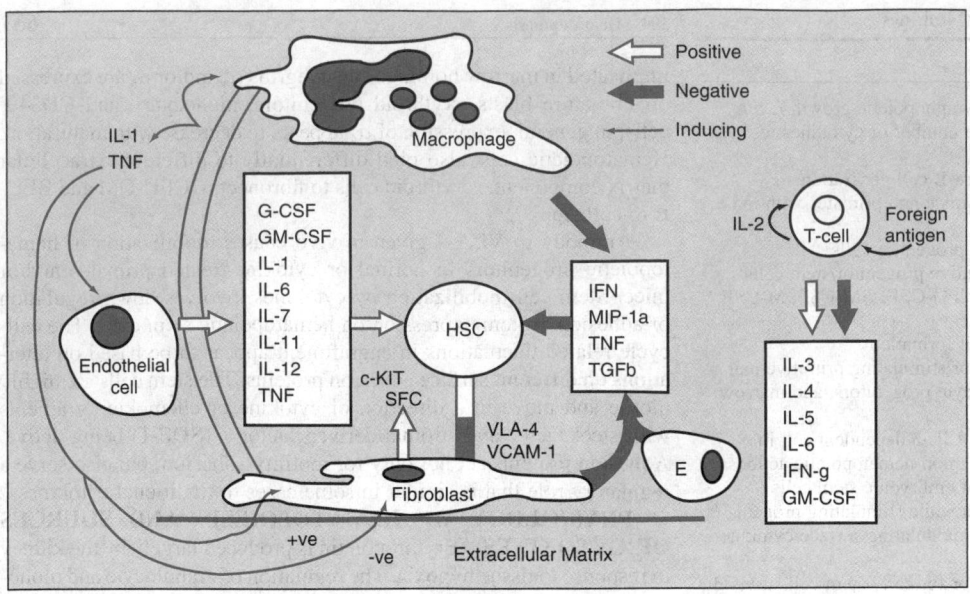

FIGURE 104-5 The cellular and humoral influence on hematopoietic stem cells.

Castleman's disease and atrial myxoma, and may be an etiologic factor in multiple myeloma. IL-6 may also be a major cause of symptoms in various lymphomas. Abnormalities of the c-Kit receptor may underlie a number of mast cell diseases in humans; IL-5 production is the proximate cause of a number of eosinophilic states. A deficiency of IL-1 is a feature of aplastic anemia. Mutations in the G-CSF receptor in chronic congenital neutropenia (Kostmann's syndrome) may be a causative factor in the evolution of acute myeloid leukemia in some of these patients.

THERAPEUTIC IMPLICATIONS OF STEM CELLS AND CYTOKINES Stem Cells Stem cell transplantation was first established as an effective therapy for relapsed acute myeloid leukemia and aplastic anemia. It is now a mainstay of therapy for virtually all leukemias and some relapsed lymphomas. Application of this treatment to a number of solid tumors has been disappointing. Major expectations with regard to its potential in breast cancer have not yet been fulfilled, although it appears to be effective in relapsed testicular cancer. The rationale is the use of very high doses of drugs or radiation designed to kill all tumor cells, but at levels where marrow toxicity would be lethal. Marrow damage is the dose-limiting toxicity for many chemotherapeutic agents. If marrow function is replaced by transplant, it might be possible to increase the dose of chemotherapy substantially before another organ toxicity becomes dose-limiting.

The strategy is somewhat different in intrinsic marrow diseases, such as aplastic anemia, where marrow function is restored without the need for killing tumor cells, or in genetic marrow diseases such as thalassemia and sickle cell anemia, where replacement of the abnormal marrow with normal marrow corrects the disease state. Aggressive autoimmune diseases are also being treated with marrow replacement. Stem cells can come from a related or unrelated allogeneic source or directly from the patient. The sources of the stem cells also vary. Initially, marrow aspirate was the predominant source, but now apheresed peripheral blood stem cells are the most utilized. In addition, umbilical vein cord blood, especially in pediatric patients, appears effective.

Table 104-6   Stem Cell Diseases

Chronic myeloid leukemia	Most lymphomas and probably multiple myeloma
Most acute leukemias	
Polycythemia vera	Many chronic neutropenias
Myelofibrosis with myeloid metaplasia	Pure red cell aplasia and Fanconi's anemia
Primary thrombocytosis	Cyclic neutropenias
Paroxysmal nocturnal hemoglobinuria	Shwachman-Diamond syndrome
	Aplastic anemia

Numbers of cells are sometimes limiting for adult recipients (Chap 115).

Cytokines Demonstration that hematopoietic cytokines could modulate red blood cell and white cell production in humans has been useful in some clinical settings. Erythropoietin treatment improves hematocrit and quality of life in patients with chronic renal failure. Erythropoietin has been tried in myelodysplastic syndromes (MDS), a group of clonal stem cell disorders. Meta-analysis shows an overall response rate of only 13%; the actual overall clinical benefit was exceedingly small. In addition, the best results were seen in patients receiving daily injections. Prohibitive costs and often poor response limits use to those patients with serum EPO levels lower than 500 mU/L, and less than 5% myeloblasts. The utilization of erythropoietin in other settings than renal failure remains controversial and its use may relate more to effective marketing than to the science.

These concerns are multiplied for the use of the myeloid growth factors, G-CSF, and GM-CSF. These agents elevate neutrophil and monocyte counts, and under very selective conditions they can result in a reduced toxicity of various chemotherapeutic regimens (Table 104-7). Unfortunately, they save about the same amount of money in hospitalizations for febrile neutropenia as they cost, and their use has not increased survival rate. Virtually all of the G-CSF and GM-CSF trials in cancer patients have been flawed by design; they involve escalation of drugs to toxic levels and reversal of toxicity without addressing the question of whether the patient's survival is affected by the treatment. GM-CSF and G-CSF are grossly overutilized; they are often used in settings where their efficacy has not been shown (e.g., patients with a low probability of neutropenia). Their use should still be considered experimental, and they should continue to be studied in a protocol setting but not used routinely. G-CSF is useful in mobilization of stem cells, and it is also effective in treatment of various chronic neutropenias, in particular cyclic neutropenia and Kostmann's syndrome. G-CSF may be involved in the evolution to acute myeloid leukemia in some patients, but overall it appears to be an effective intervention in these seriously ill patients. G-CSF may also aid in healing of diabetic skin ulcers.

IL-11 and thrombopoietin can elevate platelet counts in experimental animals, but their place in clinical practice is unclear. IL-11 has been approved for use in chemotherapy-induced thrombocytopenia, but its effects are small. Use of pegylated recombinant human megakaryocyte growth and development factor—the truncated version of thrombopoietin—has resulted in production of neutralizing antithrombopoietin antibodies and thrombocytopenia. Recombinant human thrombopoietin does not commonly elicit neutralizing antithrombopoietin antibodies. Clinical benefit (or cost effectiveness) has not yet been shown with thrombopoietin. Surrogate values of platelet counts or number of platelet transfusions are not valid criteria for clinical benefit. Thrombopoietin may eventually find a role as an expander of early stem cells in vitro. Active research in this important area continues.

Gene Therapy Hematopoietic stem cells provide an ideal vehicle for various gene therapy approaches. These cells can be easily induced into the cell cycle for retroviral integration. Long-term expression of introduced genes is currently being obtained in animal models. Initial clinical application has been disappointing, but success has been obtained in Gaucher's disease, suggesting that gene therapy will eventually become a successful approach to a number of hematopoietic diseases.

Table 104-7 Clinical Cytokine Application

Cytokine	Clinical Indications/New Directions	Clinical Toxicity
G-CSF	Clear use for G-CSF in mobilization of stem cells and perhaps in high dose chemotherapy when expected risk of febrile neutropenia is over 40%. Effective in treatment of various chronic neutropenias, in particular cyclic neutropenia, Kostmann and possible Shwachman-Diamond sydrome. *Routine use* for chemotherapy induced neutropenia is *not warranted* as a survival advantage has not been seen, and there is prohibitive cost vs. benefit ratio. Use in AIDS is FDA-approved, but actual clinical utility also in doubt.	Bone pain, splenomegaly (splenic rupture has been reported), exacerbation of psoriasis and other dermatological conditions, Sweet's syndrome (neutrophilic dermatitis), hair loss, elevation of leukocyte alkaline phosphatase and lactate dehydrogenase, and potential activation of some leukemias.
GM-CSF	FDA-approved for use in treatment of neutropenia in elderly patients undergoing induction for AML, high-dose chemotherapy and bone marrow transplant. Impressive response seen at our institution in use with low-dose ARA-c for treatment of AML arising out of a myelodysplastic syndrome (MDS). Clinical utility in solid tumors limited.	Hyperpyrexia, arthralgias, myalgias, serositis. IV administration can cause dyspnea, tachycardia, hypotension, flushing and myalgias.
Erythropoietin (EPO)	Clear use only in anemia of renal failure where the pathophysiology of that disease is pure EPO deficiency. Used in patients with cancer who are Jehovah's Witnesses (if they agree, as there is a small amount of albumin in product). Studies show improved quality of life in chemotherapy-induced anemia, but the actual benefit is probably small, with prohibitive cost versus benefit ratio. Most benefit from chemotherapy-induced anemia in platinum-treated patients. Limited use in MDS-induced anemia with a 13% overall response rate. HIV-related anemia can respond to EPO with decreased blood transfusions if the serum EPO level <500 U/L.	Hypertension, seizures, exacerbation of porphyria, potentially increased chance of thrombotic event.
IL-2	Well studied in a variety of malignancies as an immune modulator. Used alone or in conjunction with other cytokines or chemotherapy for malignant melanoma, renal cell carcinoma, lymphoma, cutaneous-T cell lymphoma. AML, and post-BMT to enhance graft-versus-tumor effect. Poor toxicity profile and very modest response rates limit clinical use. A 10 to 20% response rate was seen in melanoma and renal cell carcinoma.	Hyperpyrexia, hypotension, vascular leak syndrome, malaise, flulike symptoms, cholestasis, hepatic dysfunction, thyroiditis, vitiligo, inflammatory bowel changes, myocardial infarction, arrhythmia, ARDS, pulmonary edema, cytopenias, renal failure, and other toxicities.
Interferons (IFN-α,-β,-γ)	IFN-α: Clear use in CML, especially early stage, where up to an 80% response rate has been observed. Also quite active in treatment of hairy cell leukemia, with up to a 90% response rate. Clinical utility in treating mycosis fungoides, Sezary syndrome, HTLV-1–associated T cell leukemia/lymphoma, malignant melanoma, and multiple myeloma. IFN-β: Clinical use in relapsed, remitting multiple sclerosis. IFN-γ: May be protective in development of GVHD. May inhibit IL-6 mediated cell growth. Trials with cyclosporine to induce autologous graft-versus-host syndrome are currently being investigated. Has been used in patients with chronic granulomatous disease and idiopathic pulmonary fibrosis.	Hyperpyrexia, flulike symptoms, malaise, fatigue, chills, headache, myalgias, and hyperlipidemia. Neurologic toxicity can be seen with depression, agitation, insomnia, and seizures. Cytopenia, arrhythmia, and elevated transaminases can also be seen.
IL-11	Mild activity in chemotherapy-induced thrombocytopenia. Limited clinical application, no completed studies on use in aplastic anemia, MDS, or immune-related thrombocytopenia. Use of lower dose IL-11 is currently under investigation for use in inflammatory bowel disease and psoriasis.	Myalgias, arthralgias, fatigue, lower extremity edema, treatment-related anemia (secondary to increased plasma volume), and rarely arrhythmia. There is also increased levels of acute phase reactants such as fibrinogen, C-reactive protein, and haptoglobin.
Thrombopoietin (TPO)	Pegylated recombinant human megakaryocyte growth and development factor (truncated TPO) generated neutralizing antibodies causing thrombocytopenia in some patients. Recombinant human TPO in early trials was generally well tolerated with rare and transient antibody formation, but true clinical benefit has yet to be established. May eventually find a role as a research tool to expand early progenitor/stem cells in vitro.	Initial studies of TPO showed the development of neutralizing antibodies to endogenous regulatory proteins worsening thrombocytopenia.
Tumor necrosis factor α (TNF-α)	Remains investigational in humans with severe toxicity when given systemically. Good preliminary results when used via isolated limb perfusion in patients with sarcoma or melanoma, with up to a 51% response rate allowing limb salvage ~80% of time in these patients. Animal studies suggest direct cytotoxicity against malignant cells acting via immune mediation, and vascular changes.	Hyperpyrexia, severe hypotension limiting systemic administration.
Keratinocyte growth factor (KGF)	Exciting murine data show that administration of human recombinant KGF can decrease gut GVHD while preserving graft-versus-leukemia effect. May improve wound healing. Modulation of KGF may be used in the future as a treatment modality in prostate cancer.	Unknown.
Monocyte/Macrophage Colony Stimulating Factor (M-CSF)	Currently being investigated with phase I protocols for effectiveness in renal cell carcinoma, melanoma, other malignancies and severe fungal infections.	Malaise, iritis, periorbital inflammation, thrombocytopenia.
Stem Cell Factor (SCF)	Phase I studies in patients with metastatic lung and breast cancer showed in vitro hematopoietic progenitor stimulation but no clear clinical benefit in blood count recovery. Use of SCF with G-CSF to mobilize stem cells in phase III trials reduced the number of aphereses needed by half when compared with G-CSF alone. Modest trilineage response in phase I trials in patients with aplastic anemia.	Allergy-like reaction including respiratory difficulties and uticarial rash because of mast cell degranulation. Aggressive premedication ameliorates reaction.

(continued)

Table 104-7 Clinical Cytokine Application—(continued)

Cytokine	Clinical Indications/New Directions	Clinical Toxicity
IL-6	Preclinical data held promise as a thrombopoietic factor. Disappointing clinical results secondary to dose limitation below calculated effectiveness because of severe toxicity. No current clinical benefit when used as an antitumor agent in phase I-III trials.	Hyperpyrexia, chills, malaise, fatigue, treatment-related anemia (secondary to increased plasma volume), hepatotoxicity, and cardiac arrhythmia. There is also increased levels of acute phase reactants such as fibrinogen. C-reactive protein, and haptoglobin.
IL-12	Phase I study in patients with HIV and malignancy show increased levels of IFN-γ. Anti-tumor effect being studied currently in many types of malignancies with phase II studies.	Oral stomatitis, transient hepatic dysfunction.

NOTE: AML, acute myeloid leukemia; ARA-c, cystosine arabinoside; MDS, myelodysplastic syndrome; IL, interleukin; BMT, bone marrow transplantation; ARDS, acute respiratory distress syndrome; CML, chronic myeloid leukemia; HTLV, human T-cell leukemia; GVHD, graft-versus-host disease.

ACKNOWLEDGMENT
Dr. Francis Ruscetti and Dr. Jonathan Keller contributed this chapter in the 14th edition and portions of their chapter have been retained here.

BIBLIOGRAPHY

BJORNSON CR et al: Turning brain into blood: A hematopoietic fate adopted by adult neural stem cells in vivo. Science 283:534, 1999

ORKIN SH: Hematopoiesis: How does it happen? Curr Opin Cell Biol 7:870, 1995

QUESENBERRY PJ, BECKER PS: Stem cell homing: Rolling, crawling, and nesting. Proc Natl Acad Sci USA 95:15155, 1998

QUESENBERRY P et al: Chiaroscuro hematopoietic stem cell. Trans Am Clin Climatol Assoc 109:19, 1998

SHIVDASANI RA, ORKIN SH: The transcriptional control of hematopoiesis. Blood 87: 4025, 1996

WARD AC et al: The Jak-Stat pathway in normal and perturbed hematopoiesis. Blood 95: 19, 2000

105 *John W. Adamson*

IRON DEFICIENCY AND OTHER HYPOPROLIFERATIVE ANEMIAS

Anemias associated with normocytic and normochromic red cells and an inappropriately low reticulocyte response (reticulocyte index <2.5) are *hypoproliferative anemias*. This category includes early iron deficiency (before hypochromic microcytic red cells develop), acute and chronic inflammation (including many malignancies), renal disease, hypometabolic states such as protein malnutrition and endocrine deficiencies, and anemias from marrow damage. Marrow damage states are discussed in Chap. 109. Hypoproliferative anemias are the most common anemias and anemia associated with acute and chronic inflammation is the most common of these. The anemia of acute and chronic inflammation, like iron deficiency, is related in part to abnormal iron metabolism. The anemias associated with renal disease, inflammation, cancer, and hypometabolic states are characterized by an abnormal erythropoietin response to anemia.

IRON METABOLISM

Iron is a critical element in the function of all cells, although the amount of iron required by individual tissues varies during development. At the same time, the body must protect itself from free iron, which is highly toxic in that it participates in chemical reactions that generate free radicals such as singlet O_2 or OH^-. Consequently, elaborate mechanisms have evolved that allow iron to be made available for critical physiologic functions while at the same time conserving this element and handling it in such a way that toxicity is avoided.

The major role of iron in mammals is to carry O_2 as part of the heme protein that, in turn, is part of hemoglobin. O_2 also is bound by a heme protein in muscle, myoglobin. Iron also is a critical element in iron-containing enzymes, including the cytochrome system in mitochondria. Iron distribution in the body is shown in Table 105-1. Without iron, cells lose their capacity for electron transport and energy metabolism; in erythroid cells hemoglobin synthesis is impaired, resulting in anemia and reduced O_2 delivery to tissue.

THE IRON CYCLE IN HUMANS Figure 105-1 outlines the major pathways of internal iron exchange in humans. Iron absorbed from the diet or released from stores circulates in the plasma bound to *transferrin*, the iron transport protein. Transferrin is a bilobed glycoprotein with two iron binding sites. Transferrin that carries iron exists in two forms—*monoferric* (one iron atom) or *diferric* (two iron atoms). The turnover (half-clearance time) of transferrin-bound iron is very rapid—typically 60 to 90 min. Because the overwhelming majority of iron transported by transferrin is delivered to the erythroid marrow, the clearance time of transferrin-bound iron from the circulation is affected most by the plasma iron level and the activity of the erythroid marrow. When erythropoiesis is markedly stimulated, the pool of erythroid cells requiring iron increases and the clearance time of iron from the circulation decreases. The half-clearance time of iron in the presence of iron deficiency is as short as 10-15 min; this value reflects the limits of iron delivery as a function of the cardiac output going to the bone marrow. With suppression of the erythroid marrow, the plasma iron level typically is increased and the half-clearance time is prolonged to as much as several hours. Normally, the iron bound to transferrin turns over 10 to 20 times per day. Assuming a normal plasma iron level of 80 to 100 μg/dL, the amount of iron passing through the transferrin pool is 20 to 24 mg/d.

The iron-transferrin complex circulates in the plasma until the iron-carrying transferrin interacts with specific *transferrin receptors* on the surface of marrow erythroid cells. Diferric transferrin has the highest affinity for transferrin receptors; apotransferrin (transferrin not carrying iron) has very little affinity. While transferrin receptors are found on cells in many tissues within the body—and all cells at some time during development will display transferrin receptors—the cell having the greatest number of receptors (300,000 to 400,000/cell) is the developing erythroblast.

Once the iron-bearing transferrin interacts with its receptor, the iron-transferrin-receptor complex is internalized via clathrin-coated pits and transported to an acidic endosome, where the iron is released at the low pH. The iron is then made available for heme synthesis while the transferrin-receptor complex is recycled to the surface of the cell, where the bulk of the transferrin is released back into the circulation and the transferrin receptor reanchors into the cell membrane. At this point a certain amount of the transferrin receptor protein may be released into circulation. Within the erythroid cell, iron that is in excess of the amount needed for hemoglobin synthesis binds to a stor-

Table 105-1 Body Iron Distribution

	Iron Content, mg	
	Adult Male (80 kg)	**Adult Female (60 kg)**
Hemoglobin	2500	1700
Myoglobin/enzymes	500	300
Transferrin iron	3	3
Iron stores	600–1000	0–300

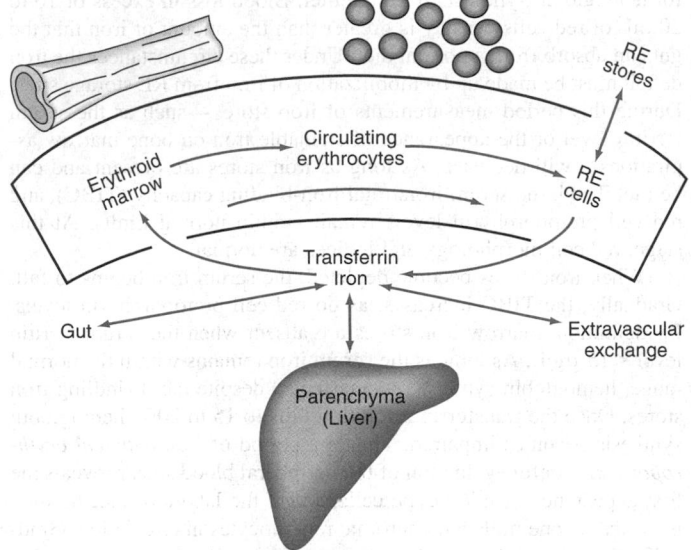

FIGURE 105-1 Internal iron exchange. Normally about 80% of iron passing through the plasma transferrin pool is recycled from broken down red cells. Absorption of about 1 mg/d is required from the diet in men, 1.4 mg/d in women to maintain homeostasis. As long as transferrin saturation is maintained between 20 to 60% and erythropoiesis is not increased, iron stores are not required. However, in the event of blood loss, dietary iron deficiency, or inadequate iron absorption, up to 40 mg/d of iron can be mobilized from stores.

age protein, *apoferritin*, forming *ferritin*. This mechanism of iron exchange also takes place in other cells of the body expressing transferrin receptors, especially liver parenchymal cells where the iron can be incorporated into heme-containing enzymes or stored. The iron incorporated into hemoglobin subsequently enters the circulation as new red cells are released from the bone marrow. The iron is then part of the red cell mass and will not become available for reutilization until the red cell dies.

In a normal individual, the average red cell life span is 120 days. Thus, 0.8 to 1.0% of red cells turn over each day. At the end of its life span, the red cell is recognized as senescent by the cells of the *reticuloendothelial (RE) system*, and the cell undergoes phagocytosis. Once within the RE cell, the hemoglobin from the ingested red cell is broken down, the globin and other proteins are returned to the amino acid pool, and the iron is shuttled back to the surface of the RE cell, where it is presented to circulating transferrin. The "harvesting" of iron from senescent red cells is both efficient and rapid, with newly recycled iron appearing in the circulation within 10 min of ingestion of the red cell. It is the efficient and highly conserved recycling of iron from senescent red cells that supports steady state (and even mildly accelerated) erythropoiesis.

Since each milliliter of red cells contains 1 mg of elemental iron, the amount of iron needed to replace those red cells lost through senescence amounts to 16 to 20 mg/day (assuming an adult with a red cell mass of 2 L). Any additional iron required for daily red cell production comes from the diet. Normally, an adult male will need to absorb at least 1 mg of elemental iron daily to meet needs, while females in the childbearing years will need to absorb an average of 1.4 mg/d. However, to achieve a maximum proliferative erythroid marrow response to anemia, additional iron must be available. With markedly stimulated erythropoiesis, demands for iron are increased by as much as six- to eightfold. With hemolytic anemias, the rate of red cell destruction is increased, but the iron recovered from the red cells is efficiently reutilized for hemoglobin synthesis. In contrast, with blood loss anemia the rate of red cell production is limited by the amount of iron that can be mobilized from ferritin and hemosiderin stores. Typically, the rate of mobilization under these circumstances will not support red cell production more than 2.5 to 3 times normal. If the delivery of iron to the stimulated marrow is suboptimal, the marrow's proliferative response is blunted and normal hemoglobin synthesis is im-

paired. The result is a hypoproliferative marrow accompanied by microcytic, hypochromic anemia.

While blood loss or hemolysis places a demand for iron to be supplied to the erythroid marrow, other conditions such as inflammation interfere with iron release from stores and can result in a rapid decrease in the serum iron (see below).

NUTRITIONAL IRON BALANCE The balance of iron metabolism in the organism is tightly controlled and designed to conserve iron for reutilization. There is no excretory pathway for iron, and the only mechanisms by which iron is lost from the body are blood loss (via gastrointestinal bleeding, menses, or other forms of bleeding) and the loss of epidermal cells from the skin and gut. Normally, the only route by which iron comes into the body is via absorption from food (dietary iron intake) or from medicinal iron taken orally. Iron may also enter the body through red cell transfusions or injection of iron complexes. The margin between the amount of iron available for absorption and the requirement for iron in growing infants and the adult female is narrow. The narrowness of this margin accounts for the great prevalence of iron deficiency worldwide—currently estimated at one-half billion people.

External iron exchange—the amount of iron required from the diet to replace losses—averages about 10% of body iron content a year in the male and 15% in women of childbearing age, equivalent to 1.0 and 1.4 mg of elemental iron daily, respectively. Dietary iron content is closely related to total caloric intake (approximately 6 mg of elemental iron per 1000 calories). Iron bioavailability is affected by the nature of the foodstuff with heme iron (e.g., red meat) being most readily absorbed. In the United States, the average iron intake in an adult male is 15 mg/d with 6% absorption; for the average female, the daily intake is 11 mg/d with 12% absorption. An individual with iron deficiency can increase iron absorption to about 20% of the iron present in a meat-containing diet but only 5 to 10% of the iron in a vegetarian diet. As a result, nearly one-third of the female population in the United States has virtually no iron stores. Vegetarians are at an additional disadvantage because certain foodstuffs that include phytates and phosphates reduce iron absorption by about 50%. When ionizable iron salts are given together with food, the amount of iron absorbed is reduced. This is particularly true with iron in the ferric state. When the percentage of iron absorbed from individual food items is compared with the percentage for an equivalent amount of ferrous salt, iron in vegetables is only about one-twentieth as available, egg iron one-eighth, liver iron one-half, and heme iron one-half to two-thirds. Therefore, liver and heme iron are absorbed nearly as well as iron salt added to food, while the iron in vegetables and eggs is much less available.

Infants, children, and adolescents may be unable to maintain normal iron balance because of the demands of body growth and lower dietary intake of iron. In pregnancy during the last two trimesters, daily iron requirements increase to 5 to 6 mg. That is the reason why iron supplements are almost universally prescribed for pregnant women in developed countries. Enthusiasm for supplementing foods such as bread and cereals with iron has waned in the face of concerns that the very prevalent hemochromatosis gene would result in an unacceptable risk of iron overload.

Iron absorption takes place largely in the proximal small intestine and is a carefully regulated process. For absorption, iron must be taken up by the luminal cell. That process is facilitated by the acidic contents of the stomach, which maintains the iron in solution. At the brush border of the absorptive cell, the ferric iron is converted to the ferrous form by a ferrireductase. Transport across the membrane is accomplished by divalent metal transporter 1 (DMT 1, also known as Nramp 2 or DCT 1). DMT 1 is a general cation transporter. Once iron is inside the gut cell, the iron may be stored as ferritin or transported through the cell to be released at the basolateral surface to plasma transferrin. It is likely another transporter acts here in concert with hephaestin, another ferroxidase. Hephaestin is similar to ceruloplasmin, the copper-carrying protein.

Iron absorption is influenced by a number of physiologic states. Erythroid hyperplasia, for example, stimulates iron absorption, even in the face of normal or increased iron stores. Patients with anemias associated with high levels of ineffective erythropoiesis absorb excess amounts of dietary iron. Over time, this may lead to iron overload and tissue damage. In iron deficiency iron is much more efficiently absorbed from a given diet while the contrary is true in the presence of iron overload. This is possibly mediated through signals that become fixed before the jejunal crypt cell migrates up the villus to become an absorptive cell. The normal individual can reduce iron absorption in situations of excessive intake or medicinal iron intake; however, while the percent of iron absorbed goes down, the absolute amount goes up. This accounts for the acute iron toxicity occasionally seen when children ingest large numbers of iron tablets. Under these circumstances, the amount of iron absorbed exceeds the transferrin binding capacity of the plasma, resulting in free iron that affects critical organs such as cardiac muscle cells.

IRON DEFICIENCY ANEMIA

STAGES OF IRON DEFICIENCY Iron deficiency anemia is the condition in which there is anemia and clear evidence of iron deficiency. However, it is worthwhile to consider the steps by which iron deficiency occurs (Fig. 105-2). These can be divided into three stages. The first stage is *negative iron balance*, in which the demands for (or losses of) iron exceed the body's ability to absorb iron from the diet. This stage can result from a number of physiologic mechanisms including blood loss, pregnancy (in which the demands for red cell production by the fetus outstrip the mother's ability to provide iron), rapid growth spurts in the adolescent, or inadequate dietary iron intake. Most commonly, the growth needs of the fetus or rapidly growing child exceed the individual's ability to absorb the iron necessary

for hemoglobin synthesis from the diet. Blood loss in excess of 10 to 20 mL of red cells per day is greater than the amount of iron that the gut can absorb from a normal diet. Under these circumstances the iron deficit must be made up by mobilization of iron from RE storage sites. During this period measurements of iron stores—such as the serum ferritin level or the appearance of stainable iron on bone marrow aspirations—will decrease. As long as iron stores are present and can be mobilized, the serum iron, total iron-binding capacity (TIBC), and red cell protoporphyrin levels remain within normal limits. At this stage, red cell morphology and indices are normal.

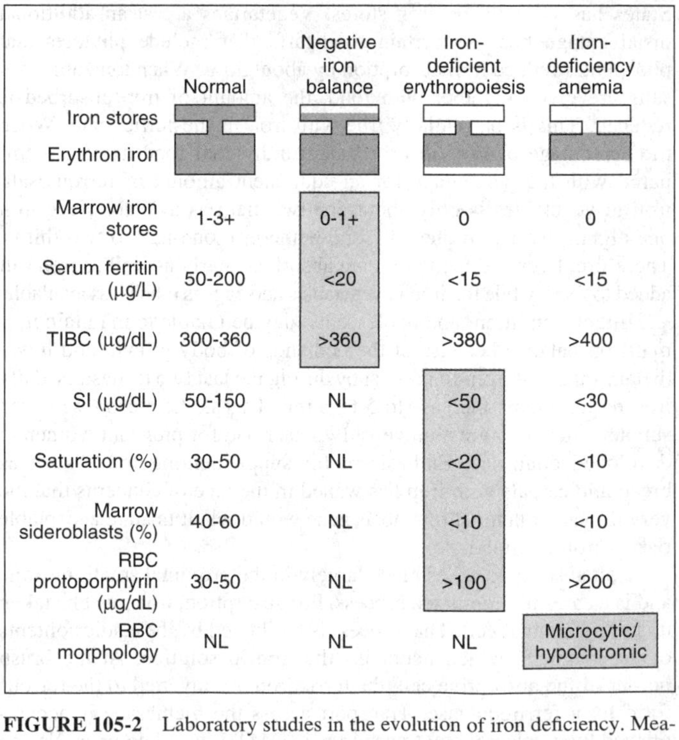

When iron stores become depleted, the serum iron begins to fall. Gradually, the TIBC increases, as do red cell protoporphyrin levels. By definition, marrow iron stores are absent when the serum ferritin level <15 μg/L. As long as the serum iron remains within the normal range, hemoglobin synthesis is unaffected despite the dwindling iron stores. Once the transferrin saturation falls to 15 to 20%, hemoglobin synthesis becomes impaired. This is a period of *iron-deficient erythropoiesis*. Careful evaluation of the peripheral blood smear reveals the first appearance of microcytic cells, and if the laboratory technology is available, one finds hypochromic reticulocytes in circulation. Gradually, the hemoglobin and hematocrit begin to fall, reflecting *iron deficiency anemia*. The transferrin saturation at this point is 10 to 15%.

When moderate anemia is present (hemoglobin 10–13 g/dL), the bone marrow remains hypoproliferative. With more severe anemia (hemoglobin 7–8 g/dL), hypochromia and microcytosis become more prominent, misshapen red cells (poikilocytes) appear on the blood smear as cigar or pencil-shaped forms and target cells, and the erythroid marrow becomes increasingly ineffective. Consequently, with severe prolonged iron deficiency anemia, erythroid hyperplasia of the marrow develops rather than hypoproliferation.

CAUSES OF IRON DEFICIENCY Conditions that increase demand for iron, increase iron loss, or decrease iron intake, absorption, or use can produce iron deficiency (Table 105-2).

CLINICAL PRESENTATION OF IRON DEFICIENCY Certain clinical conditions carry an increased likelihood of iron deficiency. Pregnancy, adolescence, periods of rapid growth, and an intermittent history of blood loss of any kind should alert the clinician to possible iron deficiency. A cardinal rule is that the appearance of iron deficiency in an adult male means gastrointestinal blood loss until proven otherwise. Signs related to iron deficiency depend upon the severity and chronicity of the anemia in addition to the usual signs of anemia—fatigue, pallor, and reduced exercise capacity. *Cheilosis* (fissures at the corners of the mouth) and *koilonychia* (spooning of the fingernails) are signs of advanced tissue iron deficiency. The diagnosis of iron deficiency is typically based on laboratory results.

LABORATORY IRON STUDIES Serum Iron and Total Iron-Binding Capacity The serum iron level represents the amount of circulating iron bound to transferrin. The TIBC is an indirect measure of the circulating transferrin. The normal range for the serum iron is 50 to 150 μg/dL; the normal range for TIBC is 300 to 360 μg/dL. Transferrin saturation, which is normally 25 to 50%, is obtained by

	Normal	Negative iron balance	Iron-deficient erythropoiesis	Iron-deficiency anemia
Iron stores				
Erythron iron				
Marrow iron stores	1-3+	0-1+	0	0
Serum ferritin (μg/L)	50-200	<20	<15	<15
TIBC (μg/dL)	300-360	>360	>380	>400
SI (μg/dL)	50-150	NL	<50	<30
Saturation (%)	30-50	NL	<20	<10
Marrow sideroblasts (%)	40-60	NL	<10	<10
RBC protoporphyrin (μg/dL)	30-50	NL	>100	>200
RBC morphology	NL	NL	NL	Microcytic/hypochromic

FIGURE 105-2 Laboratory studies in the evolution of iron deficiency. Measurements of marrow iron stores, serum ferritin, and total iron-binding capacity (TIBC) are sensitive to early iron-store depletion. Iron-deficient erythropoiesis is recognized from additional abnormalities in the serum iron (SI), percent transferrin saturation, the pattern of marrow sideroblasts, and the red cell protoporphyrin level. Patients with iron deficiency anemia demonstrate all the same abnormalities plus hypochromic microcytic anemia. *(From Hillman and Finch, with permission)*

Table 105-2 Causes of Iron Deficiency

Increased demand for iron and/or hematopoiesis
  rapid growth in infancy or adolescence
  pregnancy
  erythropoietin therapy
Increased iron loss
  chronic blood loss
  menses
  acute blood loss
  blood donation
  phlebotomy as treatment for polycythemia vera
Decreased iron intake, absorption, or use
  inadequate diet
  malabsorption from disease (sprue, Crohn's disease)
  malabsorption from surgery (post-gastrectomy)
  acute or chronic inflammation

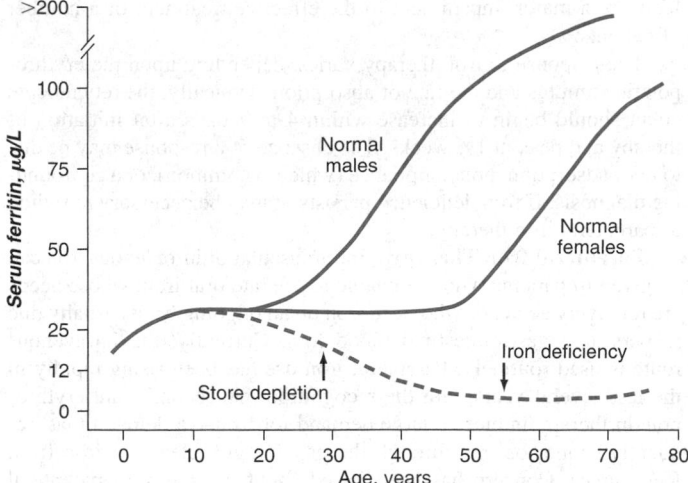

FIGURE 105-3 Serum ferritin levels as a function of sex and age. Iron store depletion and iron deficiency are accompanied by a fall in serum ferritin level below 20 μg/L. (*From Hillman and Ault*)

Table 105-3 Iron Store Measurements

Iron Stores	Marrow Iron Stain, 0–4+	Serum Ferritin, μg/L
0	0	<15
1–300 mg	Trace to 1+	15–30
300–800 mg	2+	30–60
800–1000 mg	3+	60–150
1–2 g	4+	>150
Iron overload	—	>500–1000

the following formula: serum iron × 100 ÷ TIBC. Iron deficiency states are associated with saturation levels below 18%. In evaluating the serum iron, the clinician should be aware that there is a diurnal variation in the value. A transferrin saturation rate of >50% indicates that a disproportionate amount of the iron bound to transferrin is being delivered to nonerythroid tissues. If this condition persists for an extended time, tissue iron overload may occur.

Serum Ferritin Free iron is toxic to cells, and the body has established an elaborate set of protective mechanisms to bind iron in various tissue compartments. Within cells, iron is stored complexed to protein as ferritin or hemosiderin. Apoferritin binds to free ferrous iron and stores it in the ferric state. As ferritin accumulates within cells of the RE system, protein aggregates are formed as hemosiderin. Iron in ferritin or hemosiderin can be extracted for release by the RE cells although hemosiderin is less readily available. Under steady state conditions, the serum ferritin level correlates with total body iron stores; thus, the serum ferritin level is the most convenient laboratory test to estimate iron stores. The normal value for ferritin varies according to the age and gender of the individual (Fig. 105-3). Adult males have serum ferritin values averaging about 100 μg/L, while adult females have levels averaging 30 μg/L. As iron stores are depleted, the serum ferritin falls to <15 μg/L. Such levels are virtually always diagnostic of absent body iron stores.

Evaluation of Bone Marrow Iron Stores Although RE cell iron stores can also be estimated from the iron stain of a bone marrow aspirate or biopsy, the measurement of serum ferritin has largely supplanted bone marrow aspirates for determination of storage iron (Table 105-3). The serum ferritin level is a better indicator of iron overload than the marrow iron stain. However, in addition to storage iron the marrow iron stain provides information about the effective delivery of iron to developing erythroblasts. Normally, 40 to 60% of developing erythroblasts—called *sideroblasts*—will have visible ferritin granules in their cytoplasm. This represents iron in excess of that needed for hemoglobin synthesis. In states in which release of iron from storage sites is blocked, RE iron will be detectable, and there will be few or no sideroblasts. In the myelodysplastic syndromes, mitochondrial dysfunction occurs, and accumulation of iron in mitochondria appears in a necklace fashion around the nucleus of the erythroblast. Such cells are referred to as *ringed sideroblasts*.

Red Cell Protoporphyrin Levels Protoporphyrin is an intermediate in the pathway to heme synthesis. Under conditions in which heme synthesis is impaired, protoporphyrin ac-

cumulates within the red cell. This can reflect an inadequate iron supply to erythroid precursors to support hemoglobin synthesis. Normal values are less than 30 μg/dL of red cells. In iron deficiency, values in excess of 100 μg/dL are seen. The most common causes of increased red cell protoporphyrin levels are absolute or relative iron deficiency and lead poisoning.

Serum Levels of Transferrin Receptor Protein Because erythroid cells have the highest numbers of transferrin receptors on their surface of any cell in the body, and because transferrin receptor protein (TRP) is released by cells into the circulation, serum levels of TRP reflect the total erythroid marrow mass. Another condition in which TRP levels are elevated is absolute iron deficiency. Normal values are 4 to 9 μg/L determined by immunoassay. This laboratory test is becoming increasingly available and has been proposed to measure the serial expansion of the erythroid marrow in response to recombinant erythropoietin therapy.

DIFFERENTIAL DIAGNOSIS Other than iron deficiency, only three conditions need to be considered in the differential diagnosis of a hypochromic microcytic anemia (Table 105-4). The first is inherited defects in globin chain synthesis: the thalassemias. These are differentiated from iron deficiency most readily by serum iron values, since it is characteristic to have at least normal—if not increased—serum iron levels and transferrin saturation with the thalassemias.

The second condition is chronic inflammatory disease with inadequate iron supply to the erythroid marrow. The distinction between true iron deficiency anemia and the anemia associated with chronic inflammatory states is among the most common diagnostic problems encountered by clinicians (see below). Usually the anemia of chronic disease is normocytic and normochromic. Again, the iron values usually make the differential diagnosis clear, as the ferritin level is normal or increased and the TIBC is typically below normal.

Finally, the myelodysplastic syndromes comprise the third condition. Some patients with myelodysplasia have impaired hemoglobin synthesis with mitochondrial dysfunction resulting in impaired iron incorporation into heme. The iron values again reveal normal stores and more than an adequate supply to the marrow, despite the microcytosis and hypochromia.

℞ TREATMENT The severity and cause of iron deficiency anemia will determine the appropriate approach to treatment. As an example, symptomatic elderly patients with severe iron deficiency anemia and cardiovascular instability may require red cell transfusions. Younger individuals who have compensated for their anemia can be

Table 105-4 Diagnosis of Microcytic Anemia

Tests	Iron Deficiency	Inflammation	Thalassemia	Sideroblastic Anemia
Smear	Micro/hypo	Normal micro/hypo	Micro/hypo with targeting	Variable
SI	<30	<50	Normal to high	Normal to high
TIBC	>360	<300	Normal	Normal
Percent saturation	<10	10–20	30–80	30–80
Ferritin (μg/L)	<15	30–200	50–300	50–300
Hemoglobin pattern	Normal	Normal	Abnormal	Normal

NOTE: SI, serum iron; TIBC, total iron-binding capacity

treated more conservatively with iron replacement. The foremost issue for the latter patient is the precise identification of the cause of the iron deficiency.

For the majority of cases of iron deficiency (pregnant women, growing children and adolescents, patients with infrequent episodes of bleeding, and those with inadequate dietary intake of iron), oral iron therapy will suffice. For patients with unusual blood loss or malabsorption, specific diagnostic tests and appropriate therapy take priority. Once the diagnosis of iron deficiency anemia and its cause is made, and a therapeutic approach is charted, there are three major approaches.

Red Cell Transfusion   Transfusion therapy is reserved for those individuals who have symptoms of anemia, cardiovascular instability, and continued and excessive blood loss from whatever source, and those who require immediate intervention. The management of these patients is less related to the iron deficiency than it is to the consequences of the severe anemia. Not only do transfusions correct the anemia acutely, but the transfused red cells provide a source of iron for reutilization, assuming they are not lost through continued bleeding. Transfusion therapy will stabilize the patient while other options are reviewed.

Oral Iron Therapy   In the patient with established iron deficiency anemia who is asymptomatic, treatment with oral iron is usually adequate. Multiple preparations are available ranging from simple iron salts to complex iron compounds designed for sustained release throughout the small intestine (Table 105-5). While the various preparations contain different amounts of iron, they are generally all absorbed well and are effective in treatment. Some come with other compounds designed to enhance iron absorption, such as citric acid. It is not clear whether the benefits of such compounds justify their costs. Typically, for iron replacement therapy up to 300 mg of elemental iron per day is given, usually as three or four iron tablets (each containing 50 to 65 mg elemental iron) given over the course of the day. Ideally, oral iron preparations should be taken on an empty stomach, since foods may inhibit iron absorption. Some patients with gastric disease or prior gastric surgery require special treatment with iron solutions, since the retention capacity of the stomach may be reduced. The retention capacity is necessary for dissolving the shell of the iron tablet before the release of iron. A dose of 200 to 300 mg of elemental iron per day should result in the absorption of up to 50 mg of iron per day. This supports a red cell production level of two to three times normal in an individual with a normally functioning marrow and appropriate erythropoietin stimulus. However, as the hemoglobin level rises, erythropoietin stimulation decreases, and the amount of iron absorbed is reduced. The goal of therapy in individuals with iron deficiency anemia is not only to repair the anemia, but also to provide stores of at least ½ to 1 g of iron. Sustained treatment for a period of 6 to 12 months after correction of the anemia will be necessary to achieve this.

Of the complications of oral iron therapy, gastrointestinal distress is the most prominent and is seen in 15 to 20% of patients. For these patients, abdominal pain, nausea, vomiting, or constipation often lead to noncompliance. Although small doses of iron or iron preparations with delayed release may help somewhat, the gastrointestinal side ef-

fects are a major impediment to the effective treatment of a number of patients.

The response to iron therapy varies, depending upon the erythropoietin stimulus and the rate of absorption. Typically, the reticulocyte count should begin to increase within 4 to 7 days after initiation of therapy and peak at 1½ weeks. The absence of a response may be due to poor adsorption, noncompliance (which is common), or a confounding diagnosis. If iron deficiency persists, it may be necessary to switch to parenteral iron therapy.

Parenteral Iron Therapy   Intramuscular or intravenous iron can be given to patients who are unable to tolerate oral iron, whose needs are relatively acute, or who need iron on an ongoing basis, usually due to persistent gastrointestinal blood loss. Currently, the intravenous route is used routinely. Parenteral iron use has been rising rapidly in the last several years with the recognition that recombinant erythropoietin therapy induces a large demand for iron—a demand that frequently cannot be met through the physiologic release of iron from RE sources. Concern has been raised about the safety of parenteral iron—particularly iron dextran. The serious adverse reaction rate to intravenous iron dextran is 0.7%. Fortunately, newer iron complexes are becoming available in the United States that are likely to have an even lower rate of adverse effects. The most recently approved preparation is intravenous iron gluconate (Ferrlecit).

There are two approaches to the use of parenteral iron: one is to administer the total dose of iron required to correct the hemoglobin deficit and provide the patient with at least 500 mg of iron stores; the second is to give repeated small doses of parenteral iron over a protracted period. The latter approach is common in dialysis centers, where it is not unusual for 100 mg of elemental iron to be given weekly for 10 weeks to augment the erythropoietic response to recombinant erythropoietin therapy. The amount of iron needed by an individual patient is calculated by the following formula: body weight (kg) × 2.3 × (15 − patient's hemoglobin, g/dL) + 500 or 1000 mg (for stores).

In administering intravenous iron, anaphylaxis is always a concern. Anaphylaxis is less common with the newer preparations. The factors that have correlated with a serious anaphylactic-like reaction include a history of multiple allergies or a prior allergic reaction to dextran (in the case of iron dextran). Generalized symptoms appearing several days after the infusion of a large dose of iron can include arthralgias, skin rash, and low-grade fever. This may be dose-related, but it does not preclude the further use of parenteral iron in the patient. To date, patients with sensitivity to iron dextran have been safely treated with iron gluconate. If a large dose of iron dextran is to be given (>100 mg) the iron preparation should be diluted in 5% dextrose in water or 0.9% NaCl solution. The iron solution can then be infused over a 60 to 90 min period (for larger doses) or at a rate convenient for the attending nurse or physician. While a test dose (25 mg) of parenteral iron is recommended, in reality a slow infusion of a larger dose of parenteral iron solution will afford the same kind of early warning as a separately injected test dose. Early in the infusion of iron, if chest pain, wheezing, a fall in blood pressure, or other systemic manifestations occur, the infusion of iron—whether as a large solution or a test dose—should be interrupted immediately.

OTHER HYPOPROLIFERATIVE ANEMIAS

In addition to mild to moderate iron deficiency anemia, the hypoproliferative anemias can be divided into four categories: (1) chronic inflammation/infection; (2) renal disease; (3) endocrine and nutritional deficiencies (hypometabolic states); and (4) marrow damage (Chap. 109). With chronic inflammation, renal disease, or hypometabolism, endogenous erythropoietin production is inadequate for the degree of anemia observed. For the anemia of chronic inflammation (anemia of chronic disease), the erythroid marrow also responds inadequately to stimulation in part due to defects in iron reutilization. As a result of the lack of adequate erythropoietin stimulation, an examination of the peripheral blood smear will disclose only an occasional polychromat-

Table 105-5   Oral Iron Preparations

Generic Name	Tablet (Iron Content), mg	Elixir (Iron Content), mg in 5 mL
Ferrous sulfate	325 (65)	300 (60)
	195 (39)	90 (18)
Extended release	525 (105)	
Ferrous fumarate	325 (107)	
	195 (64)	100 (33)
Ferrous gluconate	325 (39)	300 (35)
Polysaccharide iron	150 (150)	100 (100)
	50 (50)	

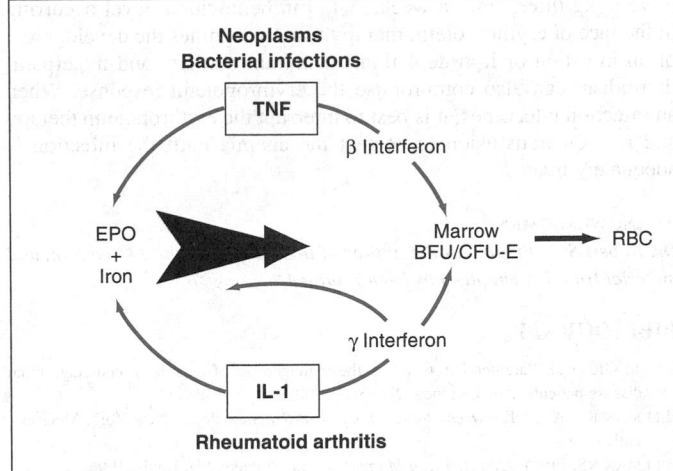

FIGURE 105-4 Suppression of erythropoiesis by inflammatory cytokines. Neoplasms and bacterial infections through the release of TNF and IFN-β suppress erythropoietin production, release of iron from reticuloendothelial stores, and the proliferation of erythroid progenitors (BFU/CFU-E). The mediators in patients with vasculitis and rheumatoid arthritis include IL-1 and IFN-γ. The blue arrows indicated sites of inflammatory cytokine inhibitory effects.

ophilic (shift) reticulocyte. In the cases of iron deficiency or marrow damage, appropriate elevations in endogenous erythropoietin levels are typically found, and "shift" reticulocytes will be present on the blood smear.

ANEMIA OF ACUTE AND CHRONIC INFLAMMATION/ INFECTION (THE ANEMIA OF CHRONIC DISEASE)
The anemia of chronic disease—which encompasses inflammation, infection, tissue injury, and conditions associated with the release of proinflammatory cytokines (such as cancer)—is one of the most common forms of anemia seen clinically and is probably the most important in the differential diagnosis of iron deficiency, since many of the features of the anemia are brought about by inadequate iron delivery to the marrow, despite the presence of normal or increased iron stores. This is reflected by a low serum iron, increased red cell protoporphyrin, a hypoproliferative marrow, transferrin saturation in the range of 15 to 20%, and a normal or increased serum ferritin. The serum ferritin values are often the most distinguishing feature between true iron deficiency anemia and the iron-deficient erythropoiesis associated with inflammation. Typically, serum ferritin values increase three-fold over basal levels in the face of inflammation. All of these changes are due to the effects of inflammatory cytokines at several levels of erythropoiesis (Fig. 105-4). IL-1 directly decreases erythropoietin production in response to anemia. IL-1, acting through accessory cell release of IFN-γ, suppresses the response of the erythroid marrow to erythropoietin—an effect that can be overcome by increased erythropoietin administration in vitro and in vivo. In addition, tumor necrosis factor (TNF), acting through the release of IFN-β by marrow stromal cells, also suppresses the response to erythropoietin; several of these same cytokines, acting in concert, block the release of iron from RE storage sites. The overall result is a chronic hypoproliferative anemia with classic changes in iron metabolism. The anemia is further compounded by a mild to moderate shortening in red cell survival.

With chronic inflammation/infection, the primary disease will determine the severity and characteristics of the anemia. For instance, many patients with cancer also have anemia that is typically normocytic and normochromic. In contrast, patients with long-standing active rheumatoid arthritis or chronic infections such as tuberculosis will have a microcytic, hypochromic anemia. In both

cases, the bone marrow is hypoproliferative, but the differences in red cell indices reflect differences in the availability of iron for hemoglobin synthesis. Occasionally, conditions associated with chronic inflammation are also associated with chronic blood loss. Under these circumstances, a bone marrow aspirate stained for iron may be necessary to rule out absolute iron deficiency. However, the administration of iron in this case will correct the iron deficiency component of the anemia and leave the inflammatory component unaffected.

The anemia associated with acute infection or inflammation is typically mild, but becomes more pronounced over time. Acute infection can produce a fall in hemoglobin levels of 2 to 3 g/dL within 1 or 2 days; this is largely related to the hemolysis of red cells near the end of their natural life span. The fever and cytokines released exert a selective pressure against cells with more limited capacity to maintain the red cell membrane. In most individuals the mild anemia is reasonably well tolerated, and symptoms, if present, are associated with the underlying disease. Occasionally, in patients with preexisting cardiac disease, moderate anemia (hemoglobin 10–11 g/dL) may be associated with angina, exercise intolerance, and shortness of breath. The red cell indices vary from normocytic, normochromic to microcytic, hypochromic. The serum iron values tend to correlate with the red cell indices. The erythropoietic profile that distinguishes the anemia of inflammation from the other causes of hypoproliferative anemias is shown in Table 105-6.

ANEMIA OF RENAL DISEASE Chronic renal failure is usually associated with a moderate to severe hypoproliferative anemia; the level of the anemia correlates with the severity of the renal failure. Red cells are typically normocytic and normochromic. Reticulocytes are decreased. The anemia is due to a failure to produce adequate amounts of erythropoietin and a reduction in red cell survival. In certain forms of acute renal failure, the correlation between the anemia and renal function is weaker. Patients with the hemolytic-uremic syndrome increase erythropoiesis in response to the hemolysis, despite renal failure requiring dialysis. Polycystic renal disease also shows a smaller degree of erythropoietin deficiency for a given level of renal failure. By contrast, patients with diabetes have more severe erythropoietin deficiency for a given level of renal failure.

Assessment of iron status provides information to distinguish the anemia of renal disease from the other forms of hypoproliferative anemia (Table 105-6) and to guide management. Patients with the anemia of renal disease usually present with normal serum iron, TIBC, and ferritin levels. However, those maintained on chronic hemodialysis may develop iron deficiency from blood loss through the dialysis procedure. Iron must be replenished in these patients to ensure an adequate response to erythropoietin therapy (see below).

ANEMIA IN HYPOMETABOLIC STATES Patients who are starving, particularly for protein, and those with a variety of endocrine disorders that produce lower metabolic rates may develop a mild to moderate hypoproliferative anemia. The release of erythropoietin from the kidney is sensitive to the need for O_2, not just O_2 levels. Thus, erythropoietin production is triggered at lower levels of O_2 tension in disease states (such as hypothyroidism and starvation) where metabolic activity and thus O_2 demand is decreased.

Table 105-6   Diagnosis of Hypoproliferative Anemias

Tests	Iron Deficiency	Inflammation	Renal Disease	Hypometabolic States
Anemia	Mild to severe	Mild	Mild to severe	Mild
MCV (fL)	70–90	80–90	90	90
Morphology	Normo-microcytic	Normocytic	Normocytic	Normocytic
SI	<30	<50	Normal	Normal
TIBC	>360	<300	Normal	Normal
Saturation (%)	<10	10–20	Normal	Normal
Serum ferritin (μg/L)	<15	30–200	115–150	Normal
Iron stores	0	2–4+	1–4+	Normal

NOTE: MCV, mean corpuscular volume; SI, serum iron; TIBC, total iron-binding capacity

Endocrine Deficiency States   The difference in the levels of hemoglobin between men and women is related to the effects of androgen and estrogen on erythropoiesis. Testosterone and anabolic steroids augment erythropoiesis; castration and estrogen administration to males decrease erythropoiesis. Patients who are hypothyroid or have deficits in pituitary hormones also may develop a mild anemia. Pathogenesis may be complicated by other nutritional deficiencies as iron and folic acid absorption can be affected by these disorders. Usually, correction of the hormone deficiency reverses the anemia.

Anemia may be more severe in Addison's disease, depending on the level of thyroid and androgen hormone dysfunction; however, anemia may be masked by decreases in plasma volume. Once such patients are given cortisol and volume replacement, the hemoglobin level may fall rapidly. Mild anemia complicating hyperparathyroidism may be due to decreased erythropoietin production as a consequence of the renal effects of hypercalcemia or to impaired proliferation of erythroid progenitors.

Protein Starvation   Decreased dietary intake of protein may lead to mild to moderate hypoproliferative anemia; this form of anemia may be prevalent in the elderly. The anemia can be more severe in patients with a greater degree of starvation. In marasmus, where patients are both protein- and calorie-deficient, the release of erythropoietin is impaired in proportion to the reduction in metabolic rate; however, the degree of anemia may be masked by volume depletion and becomes apparent after refeeding. Deficiencies in other nutrients (iron, folate) may also complicate the clinical picture but may not be apparent at diagnosis. Changes in the erythrocyte indices on refeeding should prompt evaluation of iron, folate, and B_{12} status.

Anemia in Liver Disease   A mild hypoproliferative anemia may develop in patients with chronic liver disease from nearly any cause. The peripheral blood smear may show burr cells and stomatocytes from the accumulation of excess cholesterol in the membrane from a deficiency of lecithin cholesterol acyltransferase. Red cell survival is shortened, and the production of erythropoietin is inadequate to compensate. In alcoholic liver disease, nutritional deficiencies can add complexity to the management. Folate deficiency from inadequate intake and iron deficiency from blood loss and inadequate intake can alter the red cell indices.

℞ TREATMENT   Many patients with hypoproliferative anemias experience recovery of normal hemoglobin levels when the underlying disease is appropriately treated. For those in whom such reversals are not possible—such as patients with end-stage renal failure, cancer, and chronic inflammatory diseases—symptomatic anemia requires treatment. The two major forms of treatment are transfusions and erythropoietin.

Transfusions   Thresholds for transfusion should be altered based on the patient's symptoms. In general, patients without serious underlying cardiovascular or pulmonary disease can tolerate hemoglobin levels above 8 g/dL and do not require intervention until the hemoglobin falls below that level. Patients with more physiologic compromise may need to have their hemoglobin levels kept above 11 g/dL. A typical unit of packed red cells increases the hemoglobin level by 1 g/dL. Transfusions are associated with certain infectious risks (Chap. 114) and chronic transfusions can produce iron overload.

Erythropoietin   Erythropoietin is particularly useful in anemias in which endogenous erythropoietin levels are inappropriately low, such as the hypoproliferative anemias. Iron status must be evaluated and iron repleted to obtain optimal effects from erythropoietin. In patients with chronic renal failure, the usual dose of erythropoietin is 50 to 150 U/kg three times a week subcutaneously. The dose needed to correct the anemia in patients with cancer is higher, up to 300 U/kg three times a week. Hemoglobin levels of 10 to 12 g/dL are usually reached within 4 to 6 weeks if iron levels are adequate. Once a target hemoglobin level is reached, the erythropoietin dose can be decreased

to 75 U/kg three times a week. A fall in hemoglobin level occurring in the face of erythropoietin therapy usually signifies the development of an infection or iron depletion. Aluminum toxicity and hyperparathyroidism can also compromise the erythropoietin response. When an infection intervenes, it is best to interrupt the erythropoietin therapy and rely on transfusion to correct the anemia until the infection is adequately treated.

ACKNOWLEDGMENT
Dr. Robert S. Hillman was the author of this chapter in the 14th edition, and material from his chapter has been retained.

BIBLIOGRAPHY

BAILIE GR et al: Parenteral iron use in the management of anemia in end-stage renal disease patients. Am J Kidney Dis 35:1, 2000

HILLMAN RS, AULT KA: *Hematology in Clinical Practice*, 2d ed. New York, McGraw-Hill, 1998

HILLMAN RS, FINCH CA: *Red Cell Manual*, 7th ed. Philadelphia, Davis, 1996

TSAKIRIS D: Morbidity and mortality reduction associated with the use of erythropoietin. Nephron 85 (Suppl S1):2, 2000

106   *Edward J. Benz, Jr.*

HEMOGLOBINOPATHIES

Hemoglobin is critical for normal oxygen delivery to tissues; it is also present in erythrocytes in such high concentrations that it can alter red cell shape, deformability, and viscosity. Hemoglobinopathies are disorders affecting the structure, function, or production of hemoglobin. These disorders are usually inherited and range in severity from asymptomatic laboratory abnormalities to death in utero. Different forms may present as hemolytic anemia, erythrocytosis, cyanosis, or vasoocclusive stigmata.

PROPERTIES OF THE HUMAN HEMOGLOBINS

HEMOGLOBIN STRUCTURE   Different hemoglobins are produced during embryonic, fetal, and adult life (Fig. 106-1). Each consists of a tetramer of globin polypeptide chains: a pair of α-like chains 141 amino acids long and a pair of β-like chains 146 amino acids long. The major adult hemoglobin, HbA, has the structure $\alpha_2\beta_2$. HbF ($\alpha_2\gamma_2$) predominates during most of gestation, and HbA$_2$ ($\alpha_2\delta_2$) is a minor adult hemoglobin.

Each globin chain enfolds a single heme moiety, consisting of a

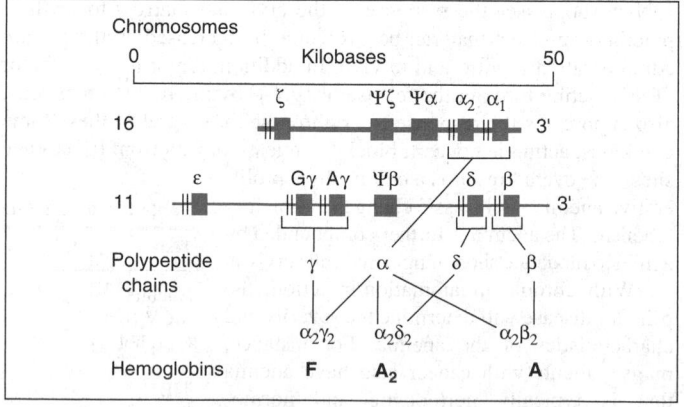

FIGURE 106-1   The globin genes. The α-like genes (α,ζ) are encoded on chromosome 16; the β-like genes ($\beta,\gamma,\delta,\epsilon$) are encoded on chromosome 11. The ζ and ϵ genes encode embryonic globins.

protoporphyrin IX ring complexed with a single iron atom in the ferrous state (Fe^{2+}), positioned in a manner optimal for reversible binding of oxygen. Each heme moiety can bind a single oxygen molecule; every molecule of hemoglobin can thus transport up to four oxygen molecules.

The amino acid sequences of the various globins are highly homologous to one another. Each has a highly helical *secondary structure*. Their globular *tertiary structures* cause the exterior surfaces to be rich in polar (hydrophilic) amino acids that enhance solubility and the interior to be lined with nonpolar groups, forming a hydrophobic "pocket" into which heme is inserted. The tetrameric *quaternary structure* of HbA contains two $\alpha\beta$ dimers. Numerous tight interactions (i.e., $\alpha_1\beta_1$ contacts) hold the α and β chains together. The complete tetramer is held together by interfaces (i.e., $\alpha_1\beta_2$ contacts) between the α-like chain of one dimer and the non-α chain of the other dimer.

The hemoglobin tetramer is highly soluble, but individual globin chains are insoluble. Unpaired globin precipitates, forming inclusions (Heinz bodies) that damage the cell. Normal globin chain synthesis is balanced so that each newly synthesized α or non-α globin chain will have an available partner with which to pair to form hemoglobin.

Solubility and reversible oxygen binding are the key properties deranged in hemoglobinopathies. Both depend most on the hydrophilic surface amino acids, the hydrophobic amino acids lining the heme pocket, a key histidine in the F helix, and the amino acids forming the $\alpha_1\beta_1$ and $\alpha_1\beta_2$ contact points. Mutations in these strategic regions tend to be the ones that alter clinical behavior.

FUNCTION OF HEMOGLOBIN To support oxygen transport, hemoglobin must bind O_2 efficiently at the partial pressure of oxygen (PO_2) of the alveolus, retain it, and release it to tissues at the PO_2 of tissue capillary beds. Oxygen acquisition and delivery over a relatively narrow range of oxygen tensions depend on a property inherent in the tetrameric arrangement of heme and globin subunits within the hemoglobin molecule called *cooperativity* or *heme-heme interaction*.

At low oxygen tensions, the hemoglobin tetramer is fully deoxygenated (Fig. 106-2). Oxygen binding begins slowly as O_2 tension rises. However, as soon as some oxygen has been bound by the tetramer, an abrupt increase occurs in the slope of the curve. Thus, hemoglobin molecules that have bound some oxygen develop a higher oxygen affinity, greatly accelerating their ability to combine with more oxygen. This S-shaped oxygen equilibrium curve, along which substantial amounts of oxygen loading *and unloading* can occur over a narrow range of oxygen tensions, is physiologically more useful than the high-affinity hyperbolic curve of individual monomers.

Oxygen affinity is modulated by several factors. The Bohr effect arises from the stabilizing action of protons on deoxyhemoglobin, which binds protons more readily than oxyhemoglobin because it is a weaker acid. Thus, hemoglobin has a lower oxygen affinity at low pH, facilitating delivery to tissues (Fig. 106-2). The major small molecule that alters oxygen affinity in humans is 2,3-bisphosphoglycerate (2,3-BPG, formerly 2,3-DPG), which lowers oxygen affinity when bound to hemoglobin. HbA has a reasonably high affinity for 2,3-BPG. HbF does not bind 2,3-BPG, so it tends to have a higher oxygen affinity in vivo. Hemoglobin may also bind nitric oxide reversibly, thereby contributing to vascular tone.

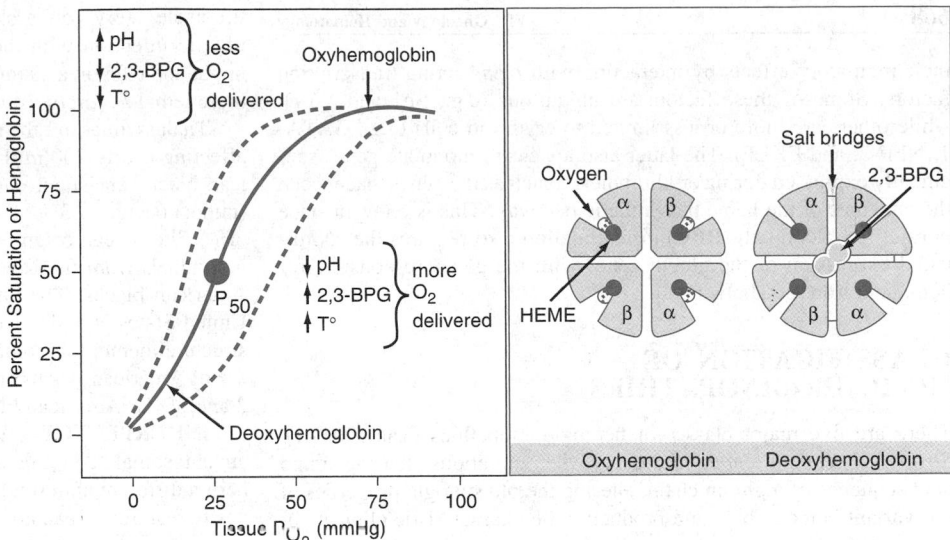

FIGURE 106-2 Hemoglobin-oxygen dissociation curve. The hemoglobin tetramer can bind up to four molecules of oxygen in the iron-containing sites of the heme molecules. As oxygen is bound, 2,3-BPG and CO_2 are expelled. Salt bridges are broken, and each of the globin molecules changes its conformation to facilitate oxygen binding. Oxygen release to the tissues is the reverse process, salt bridges being formed and 2,3-BPG and CO_2 bound. Deoxyhemoglobin does not bind oxygen efficiently until the cell returns to conditions of higher pH, the most important modulator of O_2 affinity (Bohr effect). When acid is produced in the tissues, the dissociation curve shifts to the right, facilitating oxygen release and CO_2 binding. Alkalosis has the opposite effect, reducing oxygen delivery.

To understand hemoglobinopathies, it is sufficient to understand that proper oxygen transport depends on the tetrameric structure of the proteins, the proper arrangement of the charged amino acids, and interaction with low-molecular-weight substances such as protons or 2,3-BPG.

DEVELOPMENTAL BIOLOGY Red cells first appearing at about 6 weeks after conception contain the embryonic hemoglobins Hb Portland ($\zeta_2\gamma_2$), Hb Gower I ($\zeta_2\varepsilon_2$), and Hb Gower II ($\alpha_2\varepsilon_2$). At 10 to 11 weeks, fetal hemoglobin (HbF; $\alpha_2\gamma_2$) becomes predominant. The switch to nearly exclusive synthesis of adult hemoglobin (HbA; $\alpha_2\beta_2$) occurs at about 38 weeks (Fig. 106-1). Fetuses and newborns therefore require α-globin but not β-globin for normal gestation. Small amounts of HbF are produced during postnatal life. A few red cell clones called *F cells* are progeny of a small pool of immature committed erythroid precursors (BFU-e) that retain the ability to produce HbF. Profound erythroid stress, such as that seen in severe hemolytic anemias, after bone marrow transplant, or during chemotherapy, cause more of the "F potent" BFU-e to be recruited. HbF levels thus tend to rise in some patients with sickle cell anemia or thalassemia. This phenomenon is also important because it probably explains the ability of hydroxyurea to increase levels of HbF in adults. Fetal globin genes can also be partially activated after birth by agents such as butyrate, which inhibit histone deacetylase and modify the structure of chromatin.

GENETICS AND BIOSYNTHESIS OF HUMAN HEMOGLOBIN The human hemoglobins are encoded in two tightly linked gene clusters; the α-like globin genes are clustered on chromosome 16, and the β-like genes on chromosome 11 (Fig. 106-1). The α-like cluster consists of two α-globin genes and a single copy of the ζ gene. The non-α gene cluster consists of a single ε gene, the $G\gamma$ and $A\gamma$ fetal globin genes, and the adult δ and β genes.

Important regulatory sequences flank each gene. Immediately upstream are typical promoter elements needed for the assembly of the transcription initiation complex. Sequences in the 5' flanking region of the γ and the β genes appear to be crucial for the correct developmental regulation of these genes, while elements that function like classic enhancers and silencers are in the 3' flanking regions. The locus control region (LCR) elements located far upstream appear to control the overall level of expression of each cluster. These elements achieve their regulatory effects by interacting with *trans*-acting transcription factors. Some of these factors are ubiquitous (e.g., Sp1 and YY1), while others are more or less limited to erythroid cells (e.g., GATA-1, NFE-2, and EKLF). The latter also appear to modulate genes specifically expressed during erythropoiesis, such as the genes that encode the enzymes of the heme biosynthetic pathway. This is relevant since normal red blood cell (RBC) differentiation also requires the coordinated expression of the globin genes with the genes responsible for heme and iron metabolism.

CLASSIFICATION OF HEMOGLOBINOPATHIES

There are five major classes of hemoglobinopathies (Table 106-1). *Structural hemoglobinopathies* occur when mutations alter the amino acid sequence of a globin chain, altering the physiologic properties of the variant hemoglobins and producing the characteristic clinical abnormalities. The variant hemoglobins relevant to this chapter polymerize abnormally, as in sickle cell anemia, or exhibit altered solubility or oxygen-binding affinity. *Thalassemia syndromes* arise from mutations that impair production or translation of globin mRNA, leading to deficient globin chain biosynthesis. Clinical abnormalities are attributable to the inadequate supply of hemoglobin and the imbalances in the production of individual globin chains, leading to premature destruction of erythroblasts and red cells. *Thalassemic hemoglobin variants* combine features of thalassemia (e.g., abnormal globin biosynthesis) and of structural hemoglobinopathies (e.g., an abnormal amino acid sequence). Hereditary persistence of fetal hemoglobin (HPFH) is characterized by synthesis of high levels of fetal hemoglobin in adult life. *Acquired hemoglobinopathies* include modifications of the hemoglobin molecule by toxins (e.g., acquired methemoglobinemia) and abnormal hemoglobin synthesis (e.g., high levels of HbF production in preleukemia and α-thalassemia in myeloproliferative disorders).

EPIDEMIOLOGY Hemoglobinopathies are especially common in areas where malaria is endemic. This clustering of hemoglobinopathies is assumed to reflect a selective survival advantage for the abnormal red cells, which presumably provide a less hospitable environment during the obligate intraerythrocytic stages of the parasitic

Table 106-1   Classification of Hemoglobinopathies

I. Structural hemoglobinopathies—hemoglobins with altered amino acid sequences that result in deranged function or altered physical or chemical properties
   A. Abnormal hemoglobin polymerization—HbS, hemoglobin sickling
   B. Altered O_2 affinity
      1. High affinity—polycythemia
      2. Low affinity—cyanosis, pseudoanemia
   C. Hemoglobins that oxidize readily
      1. Unstable hemoglobins—hemolytic anemia, jaundice
      2. M hemoglobins—methemoglobinemia, cyanosis
II. Thalassemias—defective biosynthesis of globin chains
   A. α Thalassemias
   B. β Thalassemias
   C. $\delta\beta$, $\gamma\delta\beta$, $\alpha\beta$ Thalassemias
III. Thalassemic hemoglobin variants—structurally abnormal Hb associated with coinherited thalassemic phenotype
   A. HbE
   B. Hb Constant Spring
   C. Hb Lepore
IV. Hereditary persistence of fetal hemoglobin—persistence of high levels of HbF in adults
V. Acquired hemoglobinopathies
   A. Methemoglobin due to toxic exposures
   B. Sulfhemoglobin due to toxic exposures
   C. Carboxyhemoglobin
   D. HbH in erythroleukemia
   E. Elevated HbF in states of erythroid stress and bone marrow dysplasia

life cycle. Very young children with α-thalassemia are *more* susceptible to infection with the nonlethal *Plasmodium vivax*. Thalassemia might then favor a natural "vaccination" against infection with the more lethal *P. falciparum*.

Thalassemias are the most common genetic disorders in the world, affecting nearly 200 million people worldwide. About 15% of American blacks are silent carriers for α thalassemia; α-thalassemia trait (minor) occurs in 3% of American blacks and in 1 to 15% of persons of Mediterranean origin. β Thalassemia has a 10 to 15% incidence in individuals from the Mediterranean and Southeast Asia and 0.8% in American blacks. The number of severe cases of thalassemia in the United States is about 1000. Sickle cell disease is the most common structural hemoglobinopathy occurring in heterozygous form in about 8% of American blacks and in homozygous form in 1 in 400. Between 2 and 3% of American blacks carry a hemoglobin C allele.

INHERITANCE AND ONTOGENY Hemoglobinopathies are autosomal "codominant" traits—compound heterozygotes that inherit a different abnormal mutant allele from each parent exhibit composite features of each. For example, patients inheriting sickle β thalassemia exhibit features of β thalassemia and sickle cell anemia. The α-chain is present in HbA, HBA$_2$, and HbF; α-chain mutations thus cause abnormalities in all three. The α-globin hemoglobinopathies are symptomatic in utero and after birth because normal function of the α-globin gene is required throughout gestation and adult life. In contrast, infants with β-globin hemoglobinopathies tend to be asymptomatic until 3 to 9 months of age, when HbA has largely replaced HbF.

DETECTION AND CHARACTERIZATION OF HEMOGLOBINOPATHIES— GENERAL METHODS

Electrophoretic techniques are used for routine hemoglobin analysis. Electrophoresis at pH-8.6 on cellulose acetate membranes is simple, inexpensive, and reliable for initial screening. Hemoglobins S, G, and D have the same mobility at pH-8.6. Agar gel electrophoresis at pH-6.1 in citrate buffer is often used as a complementary method because it detects different variants (S migration differs from G and D). Comparison of results obtained in each system usually allows unambiguous diagnosis, but some important variants are electrophoretically silent. These mutant hemoglobins can usually be characterized by more specialized techniques such as isoelectric focusing and/or high-pressure liquid chromatography (HPLC).

Quantitation of the hemoglobin profile is often desirable. HbA$_2$ is frequently elevated in β-thalassemia trait and depressed in iron deficiency. HbF is elevated in HPFH, some β thalassemia syndromes, and occasional periods of erythroid stress or marrow dysplasia. For characterization of sickle cell trait, sickle thalassemia syndromes, or hemoglobin SC disease, and for monitoring the progress of exchange transfusion therapy to lower the percentage of circulating HbS, quantitation of individual hemoglobins is also required. In most laboratories, quantitation is performed only if the test is specifically ordered.

Because some variants can comigrate with HbA or HbS (sickle hemoglobin), electrophoretic assessment should always be regarded as incomplete unless functional assays for hemoglobin sickling, solubility, or oxygen affinity are also performed, as dictated by the clinical presentation. The best sickling assays involve measurement of the degree to which the hemoglobin becomes insoluble, or gelated, as it is deoxygenated (i.e., sickle solubility test). Unstable hemoglobins are detected by their precipitation in isopropanol or after heating to 50°C. High-O_2 affinity and low-O_2 affinity variants are detected by quantitating the partial pressure of oxygen at which the hemoglobin sample becomes 50% saturated with oxygen (P$_{50}$ test). Direct tests for the percentages of carboxyhemoglobin and methemoglobin, employing spectrophotometric techniques, can readily be obtained from most clinical laboratories on an urgent basis.

Complete characterization, including amino acid sequencing or gene cloning and sequencing, is available from several investigational

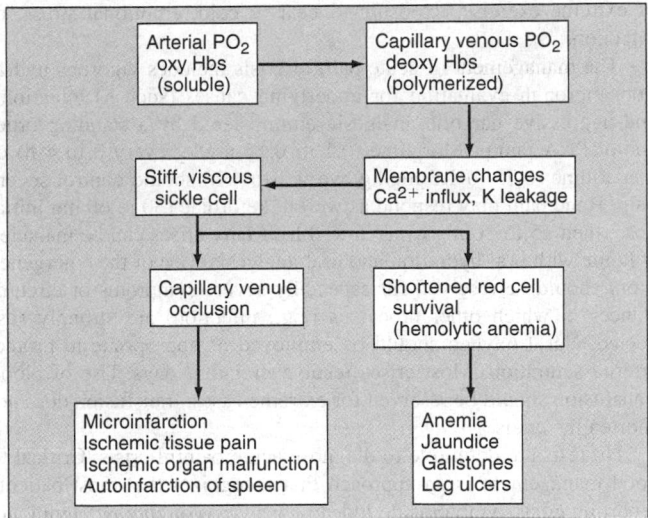

FIGURE 106-3 Pathophysiology of sickle cell crisis.

laboratories around the world. The advent of the polymerase chain reaction (PCR), allele-specific oligonucleotide hybridization, and automated DNA sequencing has made it possible to identify globin gene mutations in a few days.

Diagnosis is best established by recognition of a characteristic history, physical findings, peripheral blood smear morphology, and abnormalities of the complete blood cell count (e.g., profound microcytosis with minimal anemia in thalassemia trait). Laboratory evaluation identifies the specific hemoglobinopathy suspected clinically.

STRUCTURALLY ABNORMAL HEMOGLOBINS

SICKLE CELL SYNDROMES The sickle cell syndromes are caused by a mutation in the β-globin gene that changes the sixth amino acid from glutamic acid to valine. HbS ($\alpha_2\beta_2^{6Glu \rightarrow Val}$) polymerizes reversibly when deoxygenated to form a gelatinous network of fibrous polymers that stiffen the erythrocyte membrane, increase viscosity, and cause dehydration due to potassium leakage and calcium influx (Fig. 106-3). These changes also produce the characteristic sickle shape. Sickled cells lose the pliability needed to traverse small capillaries. They possess altered "sticky" membranes (especially reticulocytes) that are abnormally adherent to the endothelium of small venules. These abnormalities provoke unpredictable episodes of microvascular vasoocclusion and premature red cell destruction (hemolytic anemia). Hemolysis occurs because the abnormal erythrocytes are destroyed by the spleen. The rigid adherent cells also clog small capillaries and venules, causing tissue ischemia, acute pain, and gradual end-organ damage. This venoocclusive component usually dominates the clinical course. Prominent manifestations include episodes of ischemic pain (i.e., painful crises) and ischemic malfunction or frank infarction in the spleen, central nervous system, bones, liver, kidneys, and lungs.

The prototype disease, sickle cell anemia, is the homozygous state for HbS (Table 106-2). Several sickle syndromes occur as the result of inheritance of HbS from one parent and another hemoglobinopathy, such as β thalassemia or HbC ($\alpha_2\beta_2^{6Glu \rightarrow Lys}$) from the other parent.

Clinical Manifestations • *Sickle cell anemia* Most patients with sickling syndromes suffer from hemolytic anemia, with hematocrits of 15 to 30%, and significant reticulocytosis. Anemia was once thought to exert protective effects against vasoocclusion by reducing blood viscosity. Natural history and drug therapy trials suggest that an *increase* in the hematocrit with feedback inhibition of reticulocytosis might be beneficial, even at the expense of increased blood viscosity. The role of adhesive reticulocytes in vasoocclusion might account for these paradoxical effects.

Granulocytosis is common. The white cell count can fluctuate substantially and unpredictably during and between painful crises, infectious episodes, and other intercurrent illnesses.

Vasoocclusion causes protean manifestations; intermittent episodes in connective and musculoskeletal structures produce painful ischemia manifested by acute pain and tenderness, fever, tachycardia, and anxiety. These recurrent episodes, called *painful crises*, are the most common clinical manifestation. Their frequency and severity vary greatly. Pain can develop almost anywhere in the body and may last from a few hours to 2 weeks. Repeated crises requiring hospitalization (more than three per year) correlate with reduced survival in adult life, suggesting that these episodes are associated with accumulation of chronic end-organ damage. Provocative factors include infection, fever, excessive exercise, anxiety, abrupt changes in temperature, hypoxia, or hypertonic dyes.

Repeated microinfarction can destroy tissues having microvascular beds that promote sickling. Thus, the spleen is frequently infarcted within the first 18 to 36 months of life, causing susceptibility to infection, particularly from pneumococci. Acute venous obstruction of the spleen (*splenic sequestration crisis*), a rare occurrence in early childhood, may require emergency transfusion and/or splenectomy to prevent trapping of the entire arterial output in the obstructed spleen. Occlusion of retinal vessels can produce hemorrhage, neovascularization, and eventual detachments. Renal papillary necrosis invariably produces isosthenuria. More widespread renal necrosis leads to renal failure in adults, a common late cause of death. Bone and joint ischemia can lead to aseptic necrosis (especially of the femoral or humeral heads), chronic arthropathy, and unusual susceptibility to osteomyelitis, which may be caused by organisms such as *Salmonella*, rarely encountered in other settings. The *hand-foot syndrome* is caused by painful infarcts of the digits and dactylitis. Stroke is especially common in children, a small subset of whom tend to suffer repeated episodes; stroke is less common in adults and is often hemorrhagic. A particularly painful complication in males is priapism, due to infarction of the penile venous outflow tracts; permanent impotence is a frequent consequence. Chronic lower leg ulcers probably arise from ischemia and superinfection in the distal circulation.

Acute chest syndrome is a distinctive manifestation characterized

Table 106-2   Clinical Features of Sickle Hemoglobinopathies

Condition	Clinical Abnormalities	Hemoglobin Level g/L (g/dL)	Mean Corpuscular Volume, fL	Hemoglobin Electrophoresis
Sickle cell trait	None; rare painless hematuria	Normal	Normal	Hb S/A:40/60
Sickle cell anemia	Vasoocclusive crises with infarction of spleen, brain, marrow, kidney, lung; aseptic necrosis of bone; gallstones; priapism; ankle ulcers	70–100 (7–10)	80–100	Hb S/A:100/0 Hb F:2–25%
S/β^0 thalassemia	Vasoocclusive crises; aseptic necrosis of bone	70–100 (7–10)	60–80	Hb S/A:100/0 Hb F:1–10%
S/β^+ thalassemia	Rare crises and aseptic necrosis	100–140 (10–14)	70–80	Hb S/A:60/40
Hemoglobin SC	Rare crises and aseptic necrosis; painless hematuria	100–140 (10–14)	80–100	Hb S/A:50/0 Hb C:50%

by chest pain, tachypnea, fever, cough, and arterial oxygen desaturation. It can mimic pneumonia, pulmonary emboli, bone marrow infarction and embolism, myocardial ischemia, or in situ lung infarction. Acute chest syndrome is thought to reflect in situ sickling within the lung, producing pain and temporary pulmonary dysfunction. Acute chest syndrome may be difficult or impossible to distinguish from other entities. Pulmonary infarction and pneumonia are the most frequent underlying or concomitant conditions in patients with this syndrome. Repeated episodes of acute chest pain correlate with reduced survival. Acutely, reduction in arterial oxygen saturation is especially ominous because it promotes sickling on a massive scale. Repeated acute or subacute pulmonary crises lead to pulmonary hypertension and cor pulmonale, an increasingly common cause of death as patients survive further into adult life.

Sickle cell syndromes are remarkable for their clinical heterogeneity. Some patients remain virtually asymptomatic into or even through adult life, while others suffer repeated crises requiring hospitalization from early childhood. At least five haplotypes of sickle cell disease are recognized based upon their origin: Senegal, Cameroon, Benin, Central African Republic, and India. Among these, patients of the Central African Republic have the worst disease and those of Senegal the least severe. Patients with sickle thalassemia and sickle-HbE tend to have similar, slightly milder, symptoms, perhaps because of the ameliorating effects of production of other hemoglobins within the red cell. Hemoglobin SC disease, one of the more common variants of sickle cell anemia, is frequently marked by lesser degrees of hemolytic anemia and a greater propensity for the development of retinopathy and aseptic necrosis of bones. In most respects, however, the clinical manifestations resemble sickle cell anemia. Some rare hemoglobin variants actually aggravate the sickling phenomenon.

Sickle cell trait　Sickle cell trait is usually asymptomatic. Anemia and painful crises are exceedingly rare. An uncommon, but highly distinctive, symptom is painless hematuria, often occurring in adolescent males, probably due to papillary necrosis. Sloughing of papillae with ureteral obstruction has been reported, as have isolated cases of massive sickling or sudden death due to exposure to high altitudes or extraordinary extremes of exercise and dehydration.

Diagnosis　Sickle cell syndromes are readily suspected on the basis of characteristic hemolytic anemia, red cell morphology (**Plate V-39**), and intermittent episodes of ischemic pain. Diagnosis is confirmed by hemoglobin electrophoresis and sickling tests. Thorough characterization of the exact hemoglobin profile of the patient is important, because sickle thalassemia and hemoglobin SC disease are correlated with alterations in prognosis or clinical features. The diagnosis is usually established in childhood, but occasional patients, often with compound heterozygous states, do not develop symptoms until the onset of puberty, pregnancy, or early adult life. Genotyping of family members and potential parental partners is critical for genetic counseling. Details of the childhood history help to establish prognosis and eligibility for aggressive or experimental therapies. Factors associated with increased morbidity and mortality are more than three crises requiring hospitalization per year, chronic neutrophilia, a history of splenic sequestration or hand-foot syndrome, and second episodes of acute chest syndrome. Patients with a history of cerebrovascular accidents are at higher risk for repeated episodes and require especially close monitoring.

℞ **TREATMENT**　Patients with sickle cell syndromes require ongoing continuity of care. Familiarity with the pattern of symptoms provides the best safeguard against excessive use of the emergency room, hospitalization, and habituation to addictive narcotics. Additional preventive measures include regular slit-lamp examinations to monitor development of retinopathy; antibiotic prophylaxis appropriate for splenectomized patients during dental or other invasive procedures; vaccination against pneumococci and *Haemophilus influenzae*; and vigorous oral hydration before or during periods of extreme exercise, exposure to heat or cold, emotional stress, or infection.

The management of acute painful crisis includes vigorous hydration, thorough evaluation for underlying causes (such as infection), and aggressive narcotic analgesia administered by a standing order and/or PCA pump. Morphine (0.1 to 0.15 mg/kg every 3 to 4 h) or meperidine (0.75 to 1.5 mg/kg every 2 to 4 h) should control severe pain. Bone pain may respond as well to ketorolac (30 to 60 mg initial dose, then 15 to 30 mg every 6 to 8 h). Many crises can be managed at home with oral hydration and oral analgesia. Use of the emergency room should be reserved for especially severe symptoms or circumstances in which other processes (e.g., infection) are strongly suspected. Nasal oxygen should be employed as appropriate to protect arterial saturation. Most crises resolve in 1 to 7 days. Use of blood transfusion should be reserved for extreme cases; transfusion does not shorten the crisis.

No tests are definitive to diagnose acute painful crisis. Critical to good management is an approach that recognizes that most patients reporting crisis symptoms do indeed have crisis or another significant medical problem. Diligent diagnostic evaluation for underlying causes is imperative, even though these are found infrequently. In adults, the possibility of aseptic necrosis or sickle arthropathy must be considered, especially if pain and immobility become repeated or chronic at a single site. Nonsteroidal anti-inflammatory agents are often effective for sickle cell arthropathy.

Acute chest syndrome is a medical emergency that may require management in an intensive care unit. Hydration should be monitored carefully to avoid the development of pulmonary edema, and oxygen therapy should be especially vigorous for protection of arterial saturation. Diagnostic evaluation for pneumonia and pulmonary embolism should be thorough, since these may occur with atypical symptoms. Critical interventions are transfusion to maintain a hematocrit >30 and emergency exchange transfusion if arterial saturation drops below 90%.

As patients with sickle cell syndromes increasingly survive into their fifth and sixth decades (median age at death is 42 years for men, 48 years for women), end-stage renal failure and pulmonary hypertension are becoming increasingly prominent causes of end-stage morbidity; anecdotal evidence suggests that a sickle cell cardiomyopathy and/or premature coronary artery disease may compromise cardiac function in later years. Sickle cell patients have received kidney transplants, but they often experience an increase in the frequency and severity of crises, possibly due to increased infection as a consequence of immunosuppression.

The most significant advance in the therapy of sickle cell anemia has been the introduction of hydroxyurea as a mainstay of therapy for patients with severe symptoms. Hydroxyurea (10 to 30 mg/kg/per day) increases fetal hemoglobin and may also exert beneficial affects on red cell hydration, vascular wall adherence, and suppression of the granulocyte and reticulocyte counts; indeed, dosage is titrated to maintain a white cell count between 5,000 and 8,000. White cells and reticulocytes may play a major role in the pathogenesis of sickle cell crisis, and their suppression may be an important benefit of hydroxyurea therapy.

Hydroxyurea should be considered in patients experiencing repeated episodes of acute chest syndrome or more than three crises per year requiring hospitalization. The utility of this agent for reducing the incidence of other complications (e.g., priapism, retinopathy) is under evaluation, as are the long-term side effects. Therefore, when possible, treatment should be instituted as part of a clinical trial. Most patients respond within a few months with elevations of fetal hemoglobin.

Bone marrow transplantation can provide definitive cures but is known to be effective and safe only in children. Prognostic features justifying bone marrow transplant are the presence of repeated crises early in life, a high neutrophil count, or the development of hand-foot syndrome. Children at risk for stroke can be identified through the use of Doppler ultrasound techniques. Prophylactic exchange transfusion appears to reduce the risk of stroke substantially in this population. Children who do suffer a cerebrovascular accident should be maintained for at least 3 to 5 years on a program of vigorous exchange transfusion, since the risk of second strokes is extremely high in this population.

Gene therapy for sickle cell anemia is under investigation, but no safe therapy is currently available. Agents blocking red cell hydration or vascular adhesion, such as clotrimazole, may have value as an adjunct to hydroxyurea therapy; trials are ongoing.

UNSTABLE HEMOGLOBINS Amino acid substitutions that reduce solubility or increase susceptibility to oxidation produce "unstable" hemoglobins that precipitate, forming inclusion bodies injurious to the red cell membrane. Representative mutations are those that interfere with contact points between the α and β subunits [e.g., Hb Philly ($\beta^{35Tyr \to Phe}$)], alter the helical segments [e.g., Hb Genova ($\beta^{28Leu \to Pro}$)], or disrupt interactions of the hydrophobic pockets of the globin subunits with heme [e.g., Hb Koln ($\beta^{98Val \to Met}$)] (Table 106-3). The inclusions, called *Heinz bodies*, are clinically detectable by staining with supravital dyes such as crystal violet (Heinz body test). Removal of these inclusions by the spleen generates pitted, rigid cells that have shortened life spans, producing hemolytic anemia of variable severity, sometimes requiring chronic transfusion support. Splenectomy may be needed to correct the anemia. Leg ulcers and premature gallbladder disease due to bilirubin turnover are frequent stigmata.

Unstable hemoglobins occur sporadically, often by spontaneous new mutations. Heterozygotes are often symptomatic because a significant Heinz body burden can develop even when the unstable variant accounts for a portion of the total hemoglobin. Symptomatic unstable hemoglobins tend to be β-globin variants, because sporadic mutations affecting only one of the four α globins would generate only 20 to 30% abnormal hemoglobin.

HEMOGLOBINS WITH ALTERED OXYGEN AFFINITY High-affinity hemoglobins [e.g., Hb Yakima ($\beta^{99Asp \to His}$)] bind oxygen more readily but deliver less O_2 to tissues at normal capillary P_{O_2} levels (Fig. 106-2). Mild tissue hypoxia ensues, stimulating RBC production and erythrocytosis (Table 106-3). In extreme cases, the hematocrit can rise to 60 to 65%, increasing blood viscosity and producing typical symptoms (headache, somnolence, or dizziness). Phlebotomy may be required. Typical mutations alter interactions within the heme pocket or disrupt the Bohr effect or salt-bond site. Mutations that impair the interaction of HbA with 2,3-BPG can increase O_2 affinity, because 2,3-BPG binding lowers O_2 affinity.

Low-affinity hemoglobins [e.g., Hb Kansas ($\beta^{102Asn \to Thr}$)] bind sufficient oxygen in the lungs, despite their lower oxygen affinity, to achieve nearly full saturation. At capillary oxygen tensions, they lose sufficient amounts of oxygen to maintain homeostasis at a low hematocrit (Fig. 106-2) (pseudoanemia). Capillary hemoglobin desaturation can also be sufficient to produce clinically apparent cyanosis. Despite these findings, patients usually require no specific treatment.

METHEMOGLOBINEMIAS Methemoglobin is generated by oxidation of the heme iron moieties to the ferric state, causing a char-

acteristic bluish-brown, muddy color resembling cyanosis. Methemoglobin has such high oxygen affinity that virtually no oxygen is delivered to tissues. Levels >50 to 60% are often fatal.

Congenital methemoglobinemia arises from globin mutations that stabilize iron in the ferric state [e.g., HbM Iwata ($\alpha^{87His \to Tyr}$), Table 106-3] or from mutations that impair the enzymes that reduce methemoglobin to hemoglobin (e.g., methemoglobin reductase, NADP diaphorase). Acquired methemoglobinemia is caused by toxins that oxidize heme iron, notably nitrate and nitrite-containing compounds.

DIAGNOSIS AND MANAGEMENT OF PATIENTS WITH UNSTABLE HEMOGLOBINS, HIGH-AFFINITY HEMOGLOBINS, AND METHEMOGLOBINEMIA *Unstable hemoglobin variants* should be suspected in patients with nonimmune hemolytic anemia, jaundice, splenomegaly, or premature biliary tract disease. Severe hemolysis usually presents during infancy as neonatal jaundice or anemia. Milder cases may present in adult life with anemia or only as unexplained reticulocytosis, hepatosplenomegaly, premature biliary tract disease, or leg ulcers. Because spontaneous mutation is common, family history of anemia may be absent. The peripheral blood smear often shows anisocytosis, abundant cells with punctate inclusions, and irregular shapes (i.e., poikilocytosis).

The two best tests for diagnosing unstable hemoglobins are the Heinz body preparation and the isopropanol or heat stability test. Many unstable Hb variants are electrophoretically silent. A normal electrophoresis does not rule out the diagnosis.

Severely affected patients may require transfusion support for the first 3 years of life, because splenectomy before age 3 is associated with a significantly greater immune deficit. Splenectomy is usually effective thereafter, but occasional patients may require lifelong transfusion support. Even after splenectomy, patients can develop cholelithiasis and leg ulcers. Splenectomy can also be considered in patients exhibiting severe secondary complications of chronic hemolysis, even if anemia is absent. Precipitation of unstable hemoglobins is aggravated by oxidative stress, e.g., infection, antimalarial drugs.

High-O_2-affinity hemoglobin variants should be suspected in patients with erythrocytosis. The best test for confirmation is measurement of the P_{50}. A high-O_2-affinity Hb causes a significant left shift (i.e., lower numeric value of the P_{50}); confounding conditions, e.g., tobacco smoking or carbon monoxide exposure, can also lower the P_{50}.

Patients with high-affinity hemoglobin are often asymptomatic; rubor or plethora may be telltale signs. When the hematocrit reaches 55 to 60%, symptoms of high blood viscosity and sluggish flow (headache, lethargy, dizziness, etc.) may be present. These symptoms respond to judicious phlebotomy. Erythrocytosis represents an appropriate attempt to compensate for the impaired oxygen delivery by the abnormal variant. Overzealous phlebotomy may stimulate increased erythropoiesis or aggravate symptoms by thwarting this compensatory mechanism. The guiding principle of phlebotomy should be to improve oxygen delivery by reducing blood viscosity and increasing blood flow rather than restoration of a normal hematocrit. Modest iron deficiency may aid in control.

Low-affinity hemoglobins should be considered in patients with cyanosis or a low hematocrit with no other cause apparent after thorough evaluation. The P_{50} test confirms the diagnosis. Counseling and reassurance are the interventions of choice.

Methemoglobin should be suspected in patients with hypoxic symptoms who appear cyanotic but have a Pa_{O_2} sufficiently high that hemoglobin should be fully saturated with oxygen. A history of nitrite or other oxidant ingestions may not always be available; some exposures may be unapparent to the patient, and others may result from suicide attempts. The characteristic muddy appearance of freshly drawn blood can be a critical clue. The diagnostic test of choice is measurement of the methemoglobin content, which is usually available on an emergency basis.

Methemoglobinemia often causes symptoms of cerebral ischemia

Table 106-3 Representative Abnormal Hemoglobins with Altered Synthesis or Function

Designation	Mutation	Population	Main Clinical Effects[a]
Sickle or S	$\beta^{6Glu \to Val}$	African	Anemia, ischemic infarcts
C	$\beta^{6Glu \to Lys}$	African	Mild anemia; interacts with HbS
E	$\beta^{26Glu \to Lys}$	Southeast Asian	Microcytic anemia, splenomegaly, thalassemic phenotype
Köln	$\beta^{98Val \to Met}$	Sporadic	Hemolytic anemia, Heinz bodies when splenectomized
Yakima	$\beta^{99Asp \to His}$	Sporadic	Polycythemia
Kansas	$\beta^{102Asn \to Lys}$	Sporadic	Mild anemia
M. Iwata	$\alpha^{87His \to Tyr}$	Sporadic	Methemoglobinemia

[a] See text for details.

Table 106-4 The α Thalassemias

Condition	Hemoglobin A, %	Hemoglobin H (β^4), %	Hemoglobin level, g/L (g/dL)	MCV, fL
Normal	97	0	150 (15)	90
Silent thalassemia: $-\alpha/\alpha\alpha$	98–100	0	150 (15)	90
Thalassemia trait: $-\alpha/-\alpha$ homozygous α-thal-2[a] or $--/\alpha\alpha$ heterozygous α-thal-1[a]	85–95	Rare red blood cell inclusions	120–130 (12–13)	70–80
Hemoglobin H disease: $--/-\alpha$ heterozygous α-thal-1/α-thal-2	70–95	5–30	60–100 (6–10)	60–70
Hydrops fetalis: $--/--$ homozygous α-thal-1	0	5–10[b]	Fatal in utero or at birth	

[a] When both α alleles on one chromosome are deleted, the locus is called α-thal-1; when only a single α allele on one chromosome is deleted, the locus is called α-thal-2.
[b] 90–95% of the hemoglobin is hemoglobin Barts (tetramers of γ chains).

at levels >15%; levels >60% are usually lethal. Intravenous injection of 1 mg/kg of methylene blue is effective emergency therapy. Milder cases and follow-up of severe cases can be treated orally with methylene blue (60 mg three to four times each day) or ascorbic acid (300 to 600 mg/d).

THALASSEMIA SYNDROMES

The thalassemia syndromes are inherited disorders of α- or β-globin biosynthesis. The reduced supply of globin diminishes production of hemoglobin tetramers, causing hypochromia and microcytosis. Unbalanced accumulation of α and β subunits occurs because the synthesis of the unaffected globins proceeds at normal rate. Unbalanced chain accumulation dominates the clinical phenotype. Clinical severity varies widely, depending on the degree to which the synthesis of the affected globin is impaired, altered synthesis of other globin chains, and coinheritance of other abnormal globin alleles.

β-THALASSEMIA SYNDROMES Mutations causing thalassemia can affect any step in the pathway of globin gene expression: transcription, processing of the mRNA precursor, translation, and post-translational metabolism of the β-globin polypeptide chain. The most common forms arise from mutations that derange splicing of the mRNA precursor or prematurely terminate translation of the mRNA.

Hypochromia and microcytosis due to reduced amounts of hemoglobin tetramers characterize all forms of β thalassemia. In heterozygotes (β-thalassemia trait), this is the only abnormality seen; anemia is minimal. In homozygous states, unbalanced α- and β-globin accumulation causes accumulation of highly insoluble unpaired α chains, which form toxic inclusion bodies that kill developing erythroblasts in the marrow. Few of the proerythroblasts beginning erythroid maturation survive. The few surviving red cells bear a burden of inclusion bodies, detected in the spleen, shortening the red cell life span and producing severe hemolytic anemia. The resulting profound anemia stimulates erythropoietin release and compensatory erythroid hyperplasia, but the marrow response is sabotaged by ineffective erythropoiesis. Anemia persists. Erythroid hyperplasia can become exuberant and produce extramedullary erythropoietic tissue in the liver and spleen.

Massive bone marrow expansion deranges growth and development. Children develop characteristic "chipmunk" facies due to maxillary marrow hyperplasia and frontal bossing, thinning and pathologic fracture of long bones and vertebrae due to cortical invasion by erythroid elements, and profound growth retardation. Hemolytic anemia causes hepatosplenomegaly, leg ulcers, gallstones, and high-output congestive heart failure. The conscription of caloric resources to support erythropoiesis leads to inanition, susceptibility to infection, endocrine dysfunction, and, in the most severe cases, death during the first decade of life. Chronic transfusions with red cells improves oxygen delivery, suppresses the excessive ineffective erythropoiesis, and prolongs life, but the inevitable side effects, notably iron overload, usually prove fatal by age 30. Bone marrow transplantation in childhood is the only curative therapy.

Severity is highly variable. Known modulating factors are those that ameliorate the burden of unpaired α-globin inclusions. Alleles associated with milder synthetic defects and coinheritance of α-thalassemia trait reduce clinical severity by reducing accumulation of excess α globin. HbF persists to various degrees in β thalassemias. γ-Globin gene chains can substitute for β chains, simultaneously generating more hemoglobin and reducing the burden of α-globin inclusions. The terms *β-thalassemia major* and *β-thalassemia intermedia* are used to reflect the clinical heterogeneity. Patients with β-thalassemia major require intensive transfusion support to survive. Patients with β-thalassemia intermedia have a somewhat milder phenotype and can survive without transfusion. The terms *β-thalassemia minor* and *β-thalassemia trait* describe asymptomatic heterozygotes for β thalassemia.

α-THALASSEMIA SYNDROMES The four classic α thalassemias, most common in Asians, are α-thalassemia-2 trait, in which one of the four α-globin loci is deleted; α-thalassemia-1 trait, with two deleted loci; HbH disease, with three loci deleted; and hydrops fetalis with Hb Bart's, with all four loci deleted (Table 106-4). Nondeletion forms of α thalassemia also exist.

α-Thalassemia-2 trait is an asymptomatic, silent carrier state. *α-Thalassemia-1 trait* resembles β-thalassemia minor. Offspring doubly heterozygous for α-thalassemia-2 and α-thalassemia-1 exhibit a more severe phenotype, called HbH disease. Heterozygosity for a deletion that removes both genes from the same chromosome (*cis* deletion) is common in Asians and Mediterranean individuals, as is homozygosity for α-thalassemia-2 (*trans* deletion). Both produce asymptomatic hypochromia and microcytosis.

In *HbH disease*, HbA production is only 25 to 30% of normal. Fetuses accumulate some unpaired β chains. In adults, unpaired β chains accumulate and are soluble enough to form β_4 tetramers called *HbH*. HbH forms few inclusions in erythroblasts but does precipitate in circulating red cells. Patients with HbH disease have thalassemia intermedia characterized by moderately severe hemolytic anemia but milder ineffective erythropoiesis. Survival into midadult life without transfusions is common.

The homozygous state for the α-thalassemia-1 *cis* deletion (hydrops fetalis) causes total absence of α-globin synthesis. No physiologically useful hemoglobin is produced beyond the embryonic stage. Excess γ globin forms tetramers called *Hb Bart's* (γ_4), which has an extraordinarily high oxygen affinity. It delivers almost no O_2 to fetal tissues, causing tissue asphyxia, edema (hydrops fetalis), congestive heart failure, and death in utero. α-Thalassemia-2 trait is common (15 to 20%) among people of African descent. The *cis* α-thalassemia-1 deletion is almost never seen, however. Thus, α-thalassemia-2 and the *trans* form of α-thalassemia-1 are very common, but HbH disease and hydrops fetalis are almost never encountered.

DIAGNOSIS AND MANAGEMENT The diagnosis of β-thalassemia major is readily made during childhood on the basis of severe anemia accompanied by hepatosplenomegaly; profound microcytosis; a characteristic blood smear (**Plate V-2**); and elevated levels of HbF, HbA$_2$, or both. Many patients require chronic hypertransfusion therapy designed to maintain a hematocrit of at least 27 to 30% so that erythropoiesis is suppressed. Splenectomy is required if the annual transfusion requirement (volume of RBCs per kilogram body weight per year) increases by >50%. Folic acid supplements may be useful. Vaccination with pneumococcal vaccine in anticipation of eventual splenectomy is advised, as is close monitoring for infection, leg ulcers, and biliary tract disease. Early endocrine evaluation is required for glucose intolerance, thyroid dysfunction, and delayed onset of puberty or secondary sexual characteristics. Many patients develop endocrine deficiencies as a result of iron overload.

Patients with β-thalassemia intermedia exhibit similar stigmata but can survive without chronic hypertransfusion. Management is particularly challenging because a number of factors can aggravate the anemia, including infection, onset of puberty, and development of splenomegaly and hypersplenism. Some patients may eventually benefit from splenectomy. The expanded erythron can cause excess absorption of dietary iron and hemosiderosis, even without transfusion.

β-Thalassemia minor (i.e., thalassemia trait) usually presents as profound microcytosis and hypochromia with target cells but only minimal or mild anemia. The mean corpuscular volume is rarely >75 fL; the hematocrit is rarely <30 to 33%. Hemoglobin electrophoresis classically reveals an elevated HbA$_2$ (3.5 to 7.5%), but some forms are associated with normal HbA$_2$ and/or elevated HbF. Genetic counseling and patient education are essential. Patients with β-thalassemia trait should be warned that their blood picture resembles iron deficiency and can be misdiagnosed. They should eschew routine use of iron but know that iron deficiency requiring supplementation can develop, as in other persons, during pregnancy or from chronic bleeding.

Persons with α-thalassemia trait may exhibit mild hypochromia and microcytosis, usually without anemia. HbA$_2$ and HbF levels are normal. Affected individuals usually require only genetic counseling. HbH disease resembles β-thalassemia intermedia, with the added complication that the HbH molecule behaves like a moderately unstable hemoglobin. Patients with HbH disease should undergo splenectomy if excessive anemia or a transfusion requirement develops. Oxidative drugs should be avoided. Iron overload leading to death can occur in more severely affected patients.

PREVENTION Antenatal diagnosis of thalassemia syndromes is now widely available. DNA diagnosis is based on PCR amplification of fetal DNA, obtained by amniocentesis or chorionic villus biopsy followed by hybridization to allele-specific oligonucleotides probes. The probes can be designed to detect simultaneously the subset of mutations that account for 95 to 99% of the α or β thalassemias that occur in a particular ethnic group.

THALASSEMIC STRUCTURAL VARIANTS

Thalassemic structural variants are characterized by both defective synthesis and abnormal structure.

HEMOGLOBIN LEPORE Hb Lepore [$\alpha_2(\delta\beta)_2$] arises by an unequal crossover and recombination event that fuses the proximal end of the δ gene with the distal end of the closely linked β gene. The resulting chromosome contains only the fused $\delta\beta$ gene. The Lepore ($\delta\beta$) globin is synthesized poorly because the fused gene is under the control of the weak δ-globin promoter. Hb Lepore alleles have a phenotype like β-thalassemia, except for the added presence of 2 to 20% Hb Lepore. Compound heterozygotes for Hb Lepore and a classic β-thalassemia allele may also have severe thalassemia.

HEMOGLOBIN E HbE (i.e., $\alpha_2\beta_2^{26Glu\rightarrow Lys}$) is extremely common in Cambodia, Thailand, and Vietnam. The gene has become far more prevalent in the United States as a result of immigration of Asian persons, especially in California, where HbE is the most common variant detected. HbE is mildly unstable but not enough to affect RBC life span significantly. The high frequency of the HbE gene may be a result of the thalassemia phenotype associated with its inheritance. Heterozygotes resemble individuals with mild β-thalassemia trait. Homozygotes have somewhat more marked abnormalities but are asymptomatic. Compound heterozygotes for HbE and a β-thalassemia gene can have β-thalassemia intermedia or β-thalassemia major, depending on the severity of the coinherited thalassemic gene.

The β^E allele contains only a single base change, in codon 26, that causes the amino acid substitution. However, this mutation activates a cryptic RNA splice site generating a structurally abnormal globin mRNA that cannot be translated from about 50% of the initial pre-mRNA molecules. The remaining 40 to 50%, which are normally spliced, generate functional mRNA that is translated into β^E globin because the mature mRNA carries the base change that alters codon 26.

Genetic counseling of the persons at risk for HbE should focus on the interaction of HbE with β-thalassemia rather than HbE homozygosity, a condition associated with microcytosis and hypchromia that is usually asymptomatic, with hemoglobin levels rarely <10 gm/dL.

OTHER UNCOMMON HEMOGLOBINOPATHIES

HEREDITARY PERSISTENCE OF FETAL HEMOGLOBIN HPFH is characterized by continued synthesis of high levels of HbF in adult life. No deleterious effects are apparent, even when all of the hemoglobin produced is HbF. These rare patients demonstrate convincingly that prevention or reversal of the fetal to adult hemoglobin switch would provide efficacious therapy for sickle cell anemia and β thalassemia.

ACQUIRED HEMOGLOBINOPATHIES The two most important acquired hemoglobinopathies are carbon monoxide poisoning and methemoglobinemia (see above). Carbon monoxide has a higher affinity for hemoglobin than does oxygen; it can replace oxygen and diminish O$_2$ delivery. Chronic elevation of carboxyhemoglobin levels to 10 or 15%, as occurs in smokers, can lead to secondary polycythemia. Carboxyhemoglobin is cherry red in color and masks the development of cyanosis usually associated with poor O$_2$ delivery to tissues.

Abnormalities of hemoglobin biosynthesis have also been described in blood dyscrasias. In some patients with myelodysplastic, erythroleukemic, or myeloproliferative disorders, a mild form of HbH disease may also be seen. The abnormalities are not severe enough to alter the course of the underlying disease.

MANAGEMENT OF TRANSFUSIONAL HEMOSIDEROSIS

Chronic blood transfusion can lead to blood-borne infection, alloimmunization, febrile reactions, and lethal iron overload. A unit of packed RBCs contains 250 to 300 mg iron (1 mg/mL). The iron assimilated by a single transfusion of two units of packed RBCs is thus equal to a 1- to 2-year intake of iron. Iron accumulates in chronically transfused patients because no mechanisms exist for increasing iron excretion; an expanded erythron causes especially rapid development of iron overload because accelerated erythropoiesis promotes excessive absorption of dietary iron. Vitamin C should not be supplemented because it generates free radicals in iron excess states.

Patients who receive >100 units of packed RBCs usually develop hemosiderosis. The ferritin level rises, followed by early endocrine dysfunction (glucose intolerance and delayed puberty), cirrhosis, and cardiomyopathy. Liver biopsy shows both parenchymal and reticuloendothelial iron. Newer methods for assessing hepatic iron such as the superconducting quantum-interference device (SQUID) are accurate but not widely available. Cardiac toxicity is often insidious. Early development of pericarditis is followed by dysrhythmia and pump failure. The onset of heart failure is ominous, often presaging death within a year (Chap. 345).

The decision to start long-term transfusion support should be accompanied by therapy with iron-chelating agents. The only approved and available iron chelator, desferoxamine (Desferal), is expensive and poorly absorbed from the gastrointestinal tract. Its iron-binding kinetics require chronic slow infusion via a metering pump. The constant presence of the drug improves the efficiency of chelation and protects tissues from occasional releases of the most toxic fraction of iron—low-molecular-weight iron—which may not be sequestered by protective proteins. Oral iron-chelating agents such as deferiprone showed initial promise, but long-term trials have raised serious doubts about their efficacy and safety.

Desferoxamine is relatively nontoxic. Occasional cataracts, deafness, and local skin reactions, including urticaria, occur. Skin reactions can usually be managed with antihistamines. Negative iron balance can be achieved, even in the face of a high transfusion requirement, but this alone does not prevent long-term morbidity and mortality in chronically transfused patients. Irreversible end-organ deterioration develops at relatively modest levels of iron overload, even if symptoms do not appear for many years thereafter. To obtain a significant survival advantage, chelation must begin before 5 to 8 years of age.

EXPERIMENTAL THERAPIES

Bone marrow transplantation provides stem cells able to express normal hemoglobin; it has been used in a large number of patients with β thalassemia and a smaller number of patients with sickle cell anemia. Early in the course of disease, before end-organ damage occurs, transplantation is curative in 80 to 90% of patients. In highly experienced centers, the treatment-related mortality is <10%. Since survival into adult life is possible with conventional therapy, the decision to transplant is best made in consultation with specialized centers.

Gene therapy of thalassemia and sickle cell disease has proved to be an elusive goal. Uptake of gene vectors into the nondividing hematopoietic stem cells has been disappointingly inefficient.

Reestablishing high levels of fetal hemoglobin synthesis should ameliorate the symptoms of β thalassemia. Cytotoxic agents such as hydroxyurea and cytarabine promote high levels of HbF synthesis, probably by stimulating proliferation of the primitive HbF-producing progenitor cell population (i.e., F cell progenitors). Unfortunately, no regimen has yet been identified that ameliorates the clinical manifestations of β thalassemia. Butyrates stimulate HbF production, but only transiently. Pulsed or intermittent administration has been found to sustain HbF induction in the majority of patients with sickle cell disease. It is unclear whether butyrate will have similar activity in patients with β thalassemia.

APLASTIC AND HYPOPLASTIC CRISIS IN PATIENTS WITH HEMOGLOBINOPATHIES

Patients with hemolytic anemia sometimes exhibit an alarming decline in hematocrit during and immediately after acute illnesses. Bone marrow suppression occurs in almost everyone during acute inflammatory illnesses. In patients with shortened red cell life spans, suppression can cause anemia. These hypoplastic crises are usually transient and do not require transfusion.

Aplastic crisis refers to a profound cessation of erythroid activity in patients with chronic hemolytic anemia. It is associated with a rapidly falling hematocrit. Episodes are usually self-limited. Aplastic crises are caused by infection with a particular strain of parvovirus (B19A). Children infected with this virus usually develop permanent immunity. Aplastic crises do not often recur and are rarely seen in adults. Management requires close monitoring of the hematocrit and reticulocyte count. If anemia becomes symptomatic, transfusion support is indicated. Most crises resolve spontaneously within 1 to 2 weeks.

ACKNOWLEDGMENT
Some material from Chap. 107 by Dr. Ernest Beutler in the last edition has been retained in this edition. In addition, portions of this chapter describe well-established aspects of this topic and are revised and updated from earlier chapters on this topic by the author.

BIBLIOGRAPHY

BENZ EJ: Hemoglobin variants associated with hemolytic anemia, altered oxygen affinity, and methemoglobinemias, in *Hematology: Basic Principles and Practice*, 3d ed, R Hoffman et al (eds). New York, Churchill Livingstone, 2000, pp 554–561

EMBURY SH, VICHINSKY EP: Sickle cell disease, in *Hematology: Basic Principles and Practice*. 3d ed, R Hoffman et al (eds). New York, Churchill Livingstone, 2000, pp 510–554

FORGET BG: Thalassemia syndromes, in *Hematology: Basic Principles and Practice*, 3d ed, R Hoffman et al (eds). New York, Churchill Livingstone, 2000, pp 485–510

OLIVIERI NF: The beta-thalassemias. N Engl J Med 341:99, 1999

STEINBERG MH: Drug therapy: Management of sickle cell disease. N Engl J Med 340: 1021, 1999

———, BENZ EJ JR: Pathobiology of the human erythrocyte and its hemoglobins, in *Hematology: Basic Principles and Practice*, 3d ed, R Hoffman et al (eds). New York. Churchill Livingstone, 2000, pp 356–367

107 *Bernard M. Babior, H. Franklin Bunn*

MEGALOBLASTIC ANEMIAS

The megaloblastic anemias are disorders caused by impaired DNA synthesis. Cells primarily affected are those having relatively rapid turnover, especially hematopoietic precursors and gastrointestinal epithelial cells. Cell division is sluggish, but cytoplasmic development progresses normally, so megaloblastic cells tend to be large, with an increased ratio of RNA to DNA. Megaloblastic erythroid progenitors tend to be destroyed in the marrow. Thus, marrow cellularity is often increased but production of red blood cells (RBC) is decreased, an abnormality termed *ineffective erythropoiesis* (Chap. 61).

Most megaloblastic anemias are due to a deficiency of cobalamin (vitamin B_{12}) and/or folic acid. The various clinical entities associated with megaloblastic anemia are listed in Table 107-1.

PHYSIOLOGIC AND BIOCHEMICAL CONSIDERATIONS

FOLIC ACID Folic acid is the common name for pteroylmonoglutamic acid. It is synthesized by many different plants and bacteria. Fruits and vegetables constitute the primary dietary source of the vitamin. Some forms of dietary folic acid are labile and may be destroyed by cooking. The minimum daily requirement is normally about 50 μg, but this may be increased severalfold during periods of enhanced metabolic demand such as pregnancy.

The assimilation of adequate amounts of folic acid depends on the nature of the diet and its means of preparation. Folates in various foodstuffs are largely conjugated to a chain of glutamic acid residues. This highly polar side chain impairs the intestinal absorption of the vitamin. However, conjugases (γ-glutamyl carboxypeptidases) in the lumen of the gut convert polyglutamates to mono- and diglutamates, which are readily absorbed in the proximal jejunum.

Plasma folate is primarily in the form of N^5-methyltetrahydrofolate, a monoglutamate, which is transported into cells by a carrier that is specific for the tetrahydro forms of the vitamin. Once in the cell, the N^5-methyl group is removed in a cobalamin-requiring reaction (see below), and the folate is then reconverted to the polyglutamate form. The polyglutamate form may be useful for retention of folate by the cell.

A folate-binding protein occurs in plasma, milk, and other body fluids. The function of this folate binder and its membrane-bound precursor is unknown. Neither the binder nor its precursor is related to the tetrahydrofolate carrier.

Normal individuals have about 5 to 20 mg folic acid in various body stores, half in the liver. In light of the minimum daily requirement, it is not surprising that a deficiency will occur within months if dietary intake or intestinal absorption is curtailed.

The prime function of folate compounds is to transfer 1-carbon moieties such as methyl and formyl groups to various organic compounds (Fig. 107-1). The sources of these 1-carbon moieties is usually serine, which reacts with tetrahydrofolate to produce glycine and $N^{5,10}$-methylenetetrahydrofolate. An alternative source is forminoglutamic acid, an intermediate in histidine catabolism, which gives up its formimino group to tetrahydrofolate to yield N^5-formiminotetrahydrofol-

COBALAMIN DEFICIENCY

I. Inadequate intake: vegetarians (rare)
II. Malabsorption
  A. Defective release of cobalamin from food
    1. Gastric achlorhydria
    2. Partial gastrectomy
    3. Drugs that block acid secretion
  B. Inadequate production of intrinsic factor (IF)
    1. Pernicious anemia
    2. Total gastrectomy
    3. Congenital absence or functional abnormality of IF (rare)
  C. Disorders of terminal ileum
    1. Tropical sprue
    2. Nontropical sprue
    3. Regional enteritis
    4. Intestinal resection
    5. Neoplasms and granulomatous disorders (rare)
    6. Selective cobalamin malabsorption (Imerslund's syndrome) (rare)
  D. Competition for cobalamin
    1. Fish tapeworm (Diphyllobothrium latum)
    2. Bacteria: "blind loop" syndrome
  E. Drugs: p-aminosalicylic acid, colchicine, neomycin
III. Other
  A. Nitrous oxide
  B. Transcobalamin II deficiency (rare)
  C. Congenital enzyme defects (rare)

FOLIC ACID DEFICIENCY

I. Inadequate intake: unbalanced diet (common in alcoholics, teenagers, some infants)
II. Increased requirements
  A. Pregnancy
  B. Infancy
  C. Malignancy
  D. Increased hematopoiesis (chronic hemolytic anemias)
  E. Chronic exfoliative skin disorders
  F. Hemodialysis
III. Malabsorption
  A. Tropical sprue
  B. Nontropical sprue
  C. Drugs: Phenytoin, barbiturates, (?) ethanol
IV. Impaired metabolism
  A. Inhibitors of dihydrofolate reductase: methotrexate, pyrimethamine, triamterene, pentamidine, trimethoprim
  B. Alcohol
  C. Rare enzyme deficiencies: dihydrofolate reductase, others

OTHER CAUSES

I. Drugs that impair DNA metabolism
  A. Purine antagonists: 6-mercaptopurine, azathioprine, etc.
  B. Pyrimidine antagonists: 5-fluorouracil, cytosine arabinoside, etc.
  C. Others: procarbazine, hydroxyurea, acyclovir, zidovudine
II. Metabolic disorders (rare)
  A. Hereditary orotic aciduria
  B. Lesch-Nyhan syndrome
  C. Others
III. Megaloblastic anemia of unknown etiology
  A. Refractory megaloblastic anemia
  B. Di Guglielmo's syndrome[a]
  C. Congenital dyserythropoietic anemia

---

[a] A form of acute myeloid leukemia with atypical, dysplastic changes in erythroid series.

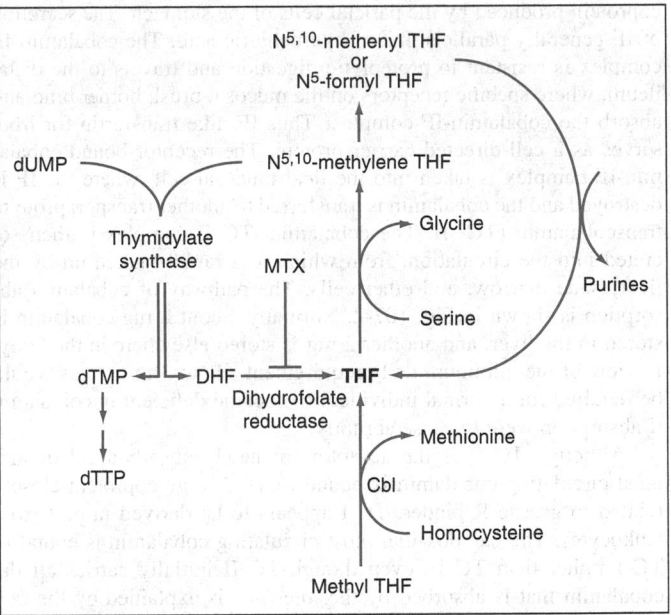

FIGURE 107-1   Folate metabolism. Folate is essential for the de novo synthesis of purines, deoxythymidylate monophosphate (dTMP) and methionine, serving as an intermediate carrier of 1-carbon fragments used in the biosynthesis of these compounds. Its active form is tetrahydrofolate (THF). THF acquires the 1-carbon fragment principally from serine, which is converted to glycine in the course of the reaction. For purine synthesis, the 1-carbon fragment is first oxidized to the level of formic acid, then transferred to substrate. For methionine synthesis, a cobalamin-requiring reaction, the 1-carbon fragment is first reduced to the level of a methyl group, then transferred to homocysteine. In these reactions the cofactor is released as THF, which can immediately participate in another 1-carbon transfer cycle. During the production of dTMP from dUMP, however, the 1-carbon fragment is reduced from formaldehyde to a methyl group in the course of the transfer reaction. The hydrogen atoms used for this reduction come from the cofactor, which is therefore released, not as THF, but as dihydrofolate (DHF). To participate further in the 1-carbon transfer cycle, the DHF has to be re-reduced to THF, a reaction catalyzed by dihydrofolate reductase.

ate and glutamic acid. These derivatives provide entry into an interconvertible donor pool consisting of tetrahydrofolate derivatives carrying various 1-carbon moieties. The constituents of this pool can donate their 1-carbon moieties to appropriate acceptor compounds to form metabolic intermediates, which are ultimately converted to building blocks used in the synthesis of macromolecules. The most important building blocks are (1) purines, in which the C-2 and C-8 atoms are introduced in folate-dependent reactions; (2) deoxythymidylate monophosphate (dTMP), synthesized from $N^{5,10}$-methylenetetrahydrofolate and deoxyuridylate monophosphate (dUMP); and (3) methio-

nine, formed by the transfer of a methyl group from N^5-methyltetrahydrofolate to homocysteine (two of these three reactions are shown in Fig. 107-1).

In all but one of the 1-carbon transfer reactions, tetrahydrofolate is produced. It can immediately accept a 1-carbon moiety and reenter the donor pool. The single exception is the thymidylate synthase reaction (dUMP → dTMP), in which dihydrofolate is the product (Fig. 107-1). This must be reduced to tetrahydrofolate by the enzyme dihydrofolate reductase before it can reenter the donor pool. A number of drugs are able to inhibit dihydrofolate reductase (Table 107-1), thereby diverting folate from the donor pool and producing what amounts to a state of folate deficiency in the face of normal tissue folate concentrations.

COBALAMIN   This vitamin is a complex organometallic compound in which a cobalt atom is situated within a corrin ring, a structure similar to the porphyrin from which heme is formed. Unlike heme, however, cobalamin cannot be synthesized in the human body and must be supplied in the diet. The only dietary source of cobalamin is animal products: meat and dairy foods. The minimum daily requirement for cobalamin is about 2.5 μg.

During gastric digestion, cobalamin in food is released and forms a stable complex with gastric R binder, one of a closely related group of glycoproteins of unknown function that are found in secretions (e.g., saliva, milk, gastric juice, bile), phagocytes, and plasma. On entering the duodenum, the cobalamin–R binder complex is digested, releasing the cobalamin, which then binds to intrinsic factor (IF), a 50-kDa glycoprotein produced by the parietal cells of the stomach. The secretion of IF generally parallels that of hydrochloric acid. The cobalamin-IF complex is resistant to proteolytic digestion and travels to the distal ileum, where specific receptors on the mucosal brush border bind and absorb the cobalamin-IF complex. Thus IF, like transferrin for iron, serves as a cell-directed carrier protein. The receptor-bound cobalamin-IF complex is taken into the ileal mucosal cell, where the IF is destroyed and the cobalamin is transferred to another transport protein, transcobalamin (TC) II. The cobalamin–TC II complex is then secreted into the circulation, from which it is rapidly taken up by the liver, bone marrow, and other cells. The pathway of cobalamin absorption is shown in Fig. 107-2. Normally, about 2 mg cobalamin is stored in the liver, and another 2 mg is stored elsewhere in the body. In view of the minimum daily requirement, about 3 to 6 years would be required for a normal individual to become deficient in cobalamin if absorption were to cease abruptly.

Although TC II is the acceptor for newly absorbed cobalamin, most circulating cobalamin is bound to TC I, a glycoprotein closely related to gastric R binder. TC I appears to be derived in part from leukocytes. The paradox that most circulating cobalamin is bound to TC I rather than TC II, even though TC II initially carries all the cobalamin that is absorbed by the intestine, is explained by the fact that cobalamin bound to TC II is rapidly cleared from the blood ($t_{1/2}$ about 1 h), while clearance of cobalamin bound to TC I requires many days. The function of TC I is unknown.

Cobalamin is an essential cofactor for two enzymes in human cells:

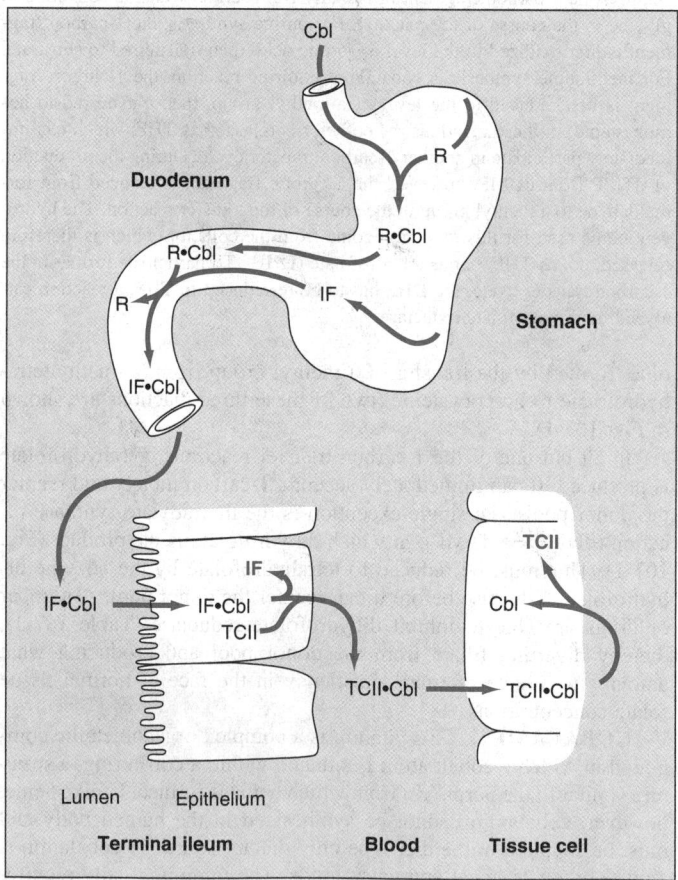

FIGURE 107-2 The assimilation of cobalamin. On entering the stomach, dietary cobalamin (Cbl) forms a complex with R binding protein. As this protein is digested in the small intestine, cobalamin is transferred to intrinsic factor (IF). This complex passes through the intestine until it reaches specific receptors on the mucosa of the distal ileum. The internalized Cbl is then transferred to transcobalamin II (TC II), which circulates in the plasma until it binds to receptors on cells throughout the body and is internalized.

methionine synthase and methylmalonyl-CoA synthase. Cobalamin exists in two metabolically active forms, identified by the alkyl group attached to the sixth coordination position of the cobalt atom: methylcobalamin and adenosylcobalamin. The vitamin preparation that is used therapeutically is cyanocobalamin (also called vitamin B_{12}). Cyanocobalamin has no known physiologic role and must be converted to a biologically active form before it can be used by tissues.

Methylcobalamin is the form required for methionine synthase, which catalyzes the conversion of homocysteine to methionine (Fig. 107-1). When this reaction is impaired, folate metabolism is deranged, and it is this derangement that underlies the defect in DNA synthesis and the megaloblastic maturation pattern in patients who are deficient in cobalamin. In cobalamin deficiency, the unconjugated N^5-methyltetrahydrofolate newly taken from the bloodstream cannot be converted to other forms of tetrahydrofolate by methyl transfer. This is the so-called folate trap hypothesis. Because N^5-methyltetrahydrofolate is a poor substrate for the conjugating enzyme, it largely remains in the unconjugated form and slowly leaks from the cell. Tissue folate deficiency therefore develops, and this results in megaloblastic hematopoiesis. This hypothesis explains why tissue folate stores in cobalamin deficiency are substantially reduced, with a disproportionate reduction in conjugated, as compared with unconjugated, folates, despite normal or supranormal serum folate levels. It also explains why large doses of folate can produce a partial hematologic remission in patients with cobalamin deficiency.

Megaloblastic changes in both cobalamin and folate deficiency as well as in methotrexate treatment are related to a deficiency in production of dTMP. In addition, the excess deoxyuridylate that accumulates can be phosphorylated and mistakenly incorporated into DNA in place of thymidylate; base pairing can be affected by this U-for-T substitution.

Plasma homocysteine levels are elevated in both folate and cobalamin deficiency, and high levels of plasma homocysteine appear to be a risk factor for thrombosis in both veins and arteries. It is not yet known, however, if hyperhomocysteinemia due to folate or cobalamin deficiency predisposes to thrombosis or alters its response to treatment.

Impairment in the conversion of homocysteine to methionine may also be partly responsible for the neurologic complications of cobalamin deficiency (see below). The methionine formed in this reaction is needed for the production of choline and choline-containing phospholipids. Nervous system damage is postulated to result at least in part from interference with these processes due to decreased methionine production in cobalamin deficiency.

Adenosylcobalamin is required for the conversion of methylmalonyl CoA to succinyl CoA. Lack of this cofactor leads to large increases in the tissue levels of methylmalonyl CoA and its precursor, propionyl CoA. As a consequence, nonphysiologic fatty acids containing an odd number of carbon atoms are synthesized and incorporated into neuronal lipids. This biochemical abnormality may also contribute to the neurologic complications of cobalamin deficiency (see below).

CLINICAL DISORDERS

CLASSIFICATION OF MEGALOBLASTIC ANEMIAS
(Table 107-1) The cause of megaloblastic anemia varies in different parts of the world. In temperate zones, folate deficiency in alcoholics and pernicious anemia are the common types of megaloblastic anemias. In certain areas close to the equator, tropical sprue is endemic and an important cause of megaloblastic anemia, while in Scandinavia, infestations by the fish tapeworm, *Diphyllobothrium latum*, may be a cause.

The dietary intake of cobalamin is more than adequate for the body's requirements, except in true vegetarians and their breast-fed infants. Thus deficiency of cobalamin is almost always due to malabsorption. Malabsorption can occur at several levels. In contrast, the dietary intake of folic acid is marginal in many parts of the world. Furthermore, because the body's stores of folate are relatively low, folic acid deficiency can arise rather suddenly during periods of decreased dietary intake or increased metabolic demand. Finally, folic acid deficiency may be due to malabsorption. Often two or more of these factors coexist in a given patient.

Combined deficiencies of cobalamin and folic acid are not uncommon. Patients with tropical sprue are often deficient in both vitamins. The biochemical lesion that results in megaloblastic maturation of bone marrow cells also causes structural and functional abnormalities of the rapidly proliferating epithelial cells of the intestinal mucosa. Thus severe deficiency of one vitamin can lead to malabsorption of the other. Furthermore, as discussed above, a deficiency of cobalamin causes a secondary reduction in cellular folic acid.

Finally, megaloblastic anemias may occasionally be induced by factors unrelated to a vitamin deficiency. Most such cases are caused by one or more of the many drugs that interfere with DNA synthesis. Less commonly, megaloblastic maturation is encountered in certain acquired defects of hematopoietic stem cells. Rarest of all are specific congenital enzyme deficiencies.

COBALAMIN DEFICIENCY The clinical features of cobalamin deficiency involve the blood, the gastrointestinal tract, and the nervous system.

The hematologic manifestations are almost entirely the result of anemia, although very rarely purpura may appear, due to thrombocytopenia. Symptoms of anemia may include weakness, light-headedness, vertigo, and tinnitus, as well as palpitations, angina, and the symptoms of congestive failure. On physical examination, the patient with florid cobalamin deficiency is pale, with slightly icteric skin and eyes. Elevated bilirubin levels are related to high erythroid cell turnover in the marrow. The pulse is rapid, and the heart may be enlarged; auscultation will usually reveal a systolic flow murmur.

The gastrointestinal manifestations reflect the effect of cobalamin deficiency on the rapidly proliferating gastrointestinal epithelium. The patient sometimes complains of a sore tongue, which on inspection will be smooth and beefy red. Anorexia with moderate weight loss may also be evident, possibly accompanied by diarrhea and other gastrointestinal symptoms. These latter manifestations may be caused in part by megaloblastosis of the small intestinal epithelium, which results in malabsorption.

The neurologic manifestations often fail to remit fully on treatment. They begin pathologically with demyelination, followed by axonal degeneration and eventual neuronal death; the final stage, of course, is irreversible. Sites of involvement include peripheral nerves; the spinal cord, where the posterior and lateral columns undergo demyelination; and the cerebrum itself. Signs and symptoms include numbness and paresthesia in the extremities (the earliest neurologic manifestations), weakness, and ataxia. There may be sphincter disturbances. Reflexes may be diminished or increased. The Romberg and Babinski signs may be positive, and position and vibration senses are usually diminished. Disturbances of mentation will vary from mild irritability and forgetfulness to severe dementia or frank psychosis. It should be emphasized that *neurologic disease may occur in a patient with a normal hematocrit* and normal RBC indexes. Although it has many benefits, folate supplementation of food may increase the likelihood of neurologic presentations of cobalamin deficiency.

In the classic patient, in whom hematologic problems predominate, the blood and bone marrow show characteristic megaloblastic changes (described under "Diagnosis," below). The anemia may be very severe—hematocrits of 15 to 20 are not infrequent—but is surprisingly well tolerated by the patient because it develops so slowly.

Defective Release of Cobalamin from Food Cobalamin in food is tightly bound to enzymes in meat and is split from these enzymes by hydrochloric acid and pepsin in the stomach. People older than 70 years are commonly unable to release cobalamin from food sources but retain the ability to absorb crystalline B_{12}, the form most commonly found in multivitamins. The exact incidence of the defect in cobalamin release from food has not been well defined; estimates vary from 10 to greater than 50% of those over age 70 years. Only a minority of these persons go on to develop frank cobalamin deficiency, but many have biochemical changes, including low levels of cobala-

min bound to TC II and elevated homocysteine levels, that augur cobalamin deficiency (see below).

Similarly, patients on drugs that suppress gastric acid production, such as omeprazole, may also fail to release cobalamin from food.

Pernicious Anemia Pernicious anemia, considered the most common cause of cobalamin deficiency, is caused by the absence of IF, from either atrophy of the gastric mucosa or autoimmune destruction of parietal cells. It is most frequently seen in individuals of northern European descent and African Americans and is much less common in southern Europeans and Asians. Men and women are equally affected. It is a disease of the elderly, the average patient presenting near age 60; it is rare under age 30, although typical pernicious anemia can be seen in children under age 10 (juvenile pernicious anemia). Inherited conditions in which a histologically normal stomach secretes either an abnormal IF or none at all will induce cobalamin deficiency in infancy or early childhood.

The incidence of pernicious anemia is substantially increased in patients with other diseases thought to be of immunologic origin, including Graves' disease, myxedema, thyroiditis, idiopathic adrenocortical insufficiency, vitiligo, and hypoparathyroidism. Patients with pernicious anemia also have abnormal circulating antibodies related to their disease: 90% have antiparietal cell antibody, which is directed against the H^+,K^+-ATPase, while 60% have anti-IF antibody. Antiparietal cell antibody is also found in 50% of patients with gastric atrophy without pernicious anemia, as well as in 10 to 15% of an unselected patient population, but anti-IF antibody is usually absent from these patients. Relatives of patients with pernicious anemia have an increased incidence of the disease, and even clinically unaffected relatives may have anti-IF antibody in their serum. Finally, treatment with glucocorticoids may reverse the disease.

The destruction of parietal cells in pernicious anemia is thought to be mediated by cytotoxic T cells. Pernicious anemia is unusually common in patients with agammaglobulinemia, suggesting that the cellular immune system plays a role in its pathogenesis. In contrast, *Helicobacter pylori* does not cause parietal cell destruction in pernicious anemia.

The most characteristic finding in pernicious anemia is gastric atrophy affecting the acid- and pepsin-secreting portion of the stomach; the antrum is spared. Other pathologic changes are secondary to the deficiency of cobalamin; these include megaloblastic alterations in the gastric and intestinal epithelium and the neurologic changes described above. The abnormalities in the gastric epithelium appear as cellular atypia in gastric cytology specimens, a finding that must be carefully distinguished from the cytologic abnormalities seen in gastric malignancy.

The *clinical manifestations* are primarily those of cobalamin deficiency, as described above. The disease is of insidious onset and progresses slowly. Laboratory examination will reveal hypergastrinemia and pentagastrin-fast achlorhydria as well as the hematologic and other laboratory abnormalities discussed under "Diagnosis."

Through appropriate replacement therapy, patients with pernicious anemia should experience complete and lifelong correction of all abnormalities that are due to cobalamin deficiency, except to the extent that irreversible changes in the nervous system may have occurred before treatment. These patients, however, are unusually subject to gastric polyps and have about twice the normal incidence of cancer of the stomach. Thus, patients should be followed with frequent stool guaiac examinations and endoscopy when indicated.

Postgastrectomy Following total gastrectomy or extensive damage to gastric mucosa as, for example, by ingestion of corrosive agents, megaloblastic anemia will develop because the source of IF has been removed. In all such patients, the absorption of orally administered cobalamin is impaired. Megaloblastic anemia may also follow partial gastrectomy, but the incidence is lower than after total gastrectomy. The cause of cobalamin deficiency after partial gastrectomy is not clear; defective release of cobalamin from food and intestinal overgrowth of bacteria have been suggested, but response to antibiotics is not common.

Intestinal Organisms Megaloblastic anemia may occur with intestinal stasis due to anatomic lesions (strictures, diverticula, anastomoses, "blind loops") or pseudoobstruction (diabetes mellitus, scleroderma, amyloid). This anemia is caused by colonization of the small intestine by large masses of bacteria that consume intestinal cobalamin before absorption. Steatorrhea may also be seen under these circumstances because bile salt metabolism is disturbed when the intestine is heavily colonized with bacteria. Hematologic responses have been observed after administration of oral antibiotics such as tetracycline and ampicillin. Megaloblastic anemia is seen in persons harboring the fish tapeworm, *D. latum*, due to competition by the worm for cobalamin. Destruction of the worm eliminates the problem.

Ileal Abnormalities Cobalamin deficiency is common in tropical sprue, while it is an unusual complication of nontropical sprue (gluten-sensitive enteropathy; Chap. 286). Virtually any disorder that compromises the absorptive capacity of the distal ileum can result in cobalamin deficiency. Specific entities include regional enteritis, Whipple's disease, and tuberculosis. Segmental involvement of the distal ileum by disease can cause megaloblastic anemia without any other manifestations of intestinal malabsorption such as steatorrhea. Cobalamin malabsorption is also seen after ileal resection. The Zollinger-Ellison syndrome (intense gastric hyperacidity due to a gastrin-secreting tumor) may cause cobalamin malabsorption by acidifying the small intestine, retarding the transfer of the vitamin from R binder to IF and impairing the binding of the cobalamin-IF complex to the ileal receptors. Chronic pancreatitis may also cause cobalamin malabsorption by impairing the transfer of the vitamin from R binder to IF. This abnormality can be detected by tests of cobalamin absorption (see below, Schilling test), but it is invariably mild and never causes clinical cobalamin deficiency. Finally, there is a rare congenital disorder, Imerslund-Gräsbeck disease, in which a selective defect in cobalamin absorption is accompanied by proteinuria. Affected individuals have a mutation in cubulin, a receptor that mediates intestinal absorption of the cobalamin-IF complex.

Nitrous Oxide Inhalation of nitrous oxide as an anesthetic destroys endogenous cobalamin. As ordinarily used, the magnitude of the effects are not sufficient to cause clinical cobalamin deficiency, but repeated or protracted exposure (>6 h), particularly in older patients with borderline cobalamin stores, can lead to severe megaloblastic anemia and/or acute neurologic deficits.

FOLIC ACID DEFICIENCY Since January, 1998, folic acid has been added to all enriched grain products by order of the U.S. Food and Drug Administration; accordingly, the incidence of folic acid deficiency has fallen markedly. Patients with folic acid deficiency are more often malnourished than those with cobalamin deficiency. The gastrointestinal manifestations are similar to but may be more widespread and more severe than those of pernicious anemia. Diarrhea is often present, and cheilosis and glossitis are also encountered. However, in contrast to cobalamin deficiency, neurologic abnormalities do not occur.

The hematologic manifestations of folic acid deficiency are the same as those of cobalamin deficiency. Folic acid deficiency can generally be attributed to one or more of the following factors: inadequate intake, increased demand, or malabsorption.

Inadequate Intake Alcoholics may become folate deficient because their main source of caloric intake is alcoholic beverages. Distilled spirits are virtually devoid of folic acid, while beer and wine do not contain enough of the vitamin to satisfy the daily requirement. In addition, alcohol may interfere with folate metabolism. Narcotic addicts are also prone to become folate deficient because of malnutrition. Many indigent and elderly individuals who subsist primarily on canned foods or "tea and toast" and occasional teenagers whose diet consists of "junk food" develop folate deficiency. Food folate supplementation has made folate deficiency very rare.

Increased Demand Tissues with a relatively high rate of cell division such as the bone marrow or gut mucosa have a large requirement for folate. Therefore, patients with chronic hemolytic anemias or other causes of very active erythropoiesis may become deficient. Pregnant women formerly were at risk to become deficient in folic acid because of the high demand of the developing fetus. Deficiency in the first weeks of pregnancy can cause neural tube defects in newborns. Often the pregnancy was not detected until the defect had developed; thus, provision of folate supplementation to women after they learned they were pregnant was ineffective. However, folate food supplementation has decreased neural tube defects by more than 50%. Folate deficiency may also occur during the growth spurts of infancy and adolescence. Patients on chronic hemodialysis may require supplementary folate to replace that lost in the dialysate.

Malabsorption Folic acid deficiency is a common accompaniment of tropical sprue. Both the gastrointestinal symptoms and malabsorption are improved by the administration of either folic acid or antibiotics by mouth. Patients with nontropical sprue (gluten-sensitive enteropathy) may also develop significant folic acid deficiency that parallels other parameters of malabsorption. Similarly, folate deficiency in alcoholics may be due in part to malabsorption. In addition, other primary small-bowel disorders are sometimes associated with folate deficiency (Chap. 286).

DRUGS Next to deficiency of folate or cobalamin, the most common cause of megaloblastic anemia is drugs. Agents that cause megaloblastic anemia do so by interfering with DNA synthesis, either directly or by antagonizing the action of folate. They can be classified as follows:

1. *Direct inhibitors of DNA synthesis*. They include purine analogues (6-thioguanine, azathioprine, 6-mercaptopurine), pyrimidine analogues (5-fluorouracil, cytosine arabinoside), and other drugs that interfere with DNA synthesis by a variety of mechanisms (hydroxyurea, procarbazine). The antiviral agent zidovudine (AZT), used for treating HIV, often causes severe megaloblastic anemia.

2. *Folate antagonists*. The most toxic of these is methotrexate, a powerful inhibitor of dihydrofolate reductase which is used in the treatment of certain malignancies. Much less toxic but still capable of inducing a megaloblastic anemia are several weak dihydrofolate reductase inhibitors used to treat a variety of nonmalignant conditions including pentamidine, trimethoprim, triamterene, and pyrimethamine.

3. *Others*. A number of drugs antagonize folate by mechanisms that are poorly understood but are thought to involve an effect on absorption of the vitamin by the intestine. In this category are the anticonvulsants phenytoin, primidone, and phenobarbital. Megaloblastic anemia induced by these agents is mild.

OTHER MECHANISMS Hereditary Megaloblastic anemia may be seen in several hereditary disorders. Orotic aciduria is a deficiency of orotidylic decarboxylase and phosphorylase, leading to a defect in pyrimidine metabolism and characterized by retarded growth and development as well as by the excretion of large amounts of orotic acid. Megaloblastic anemia has been reported in a single case of the Lesch-Nyhan syndrome, a condition resulting from a deficiency of hypoxanthine-guanine phosphoribosyltransferase whose clinical manifestations include gout, mental retardation, and self-mutilation. It has also been described in methylmalonic aciduria due to a combined defect in the biosynthesis of methyl and adenosyl cobalamins, although it is not seen in methylmalonic aciduria due to methylmalonyl CoA mutase deficiency. Congenital folate malabsorption causes megaloblastic anemia, accompanied by ataxia and mental retardation. Megaloblastic anemia has been reported to accompany the congenital deficiency of two other folate-metabolizing enzymes: dihydrofolate reductase and N^5-methyltetrahydrofolate:homocysteine methyltransferase. These deficiencies are less well documented than is congenital folate malabsorption. A thiamine-responsive megaloblastic anemia accompanied by nerve deafness and diabetes mellitus has been reported in several children. Megaloblastic changes as well as multinuclearity of red blood cell precursors are seen in the marrow of certain patients with congenital dyserythropoietic anemia, a group of inherited disorders characterized by mild to moderate anemia and a benign course.

107 Megaloblastic Anemias
679

TC II deficiency, like the congenital abnormalities in cobalamin absorption described previously, causes pronounced deficiency in cobalamin in infancy or early childhood, with all the accompanying manifestations. Megaloblastic anemia is not seen in hereditary TC I deficiency.

Refractory Megaloblastic Anemia This is a form of myelodysplasia in which megaloblastic erythropoiesis may sometimes be seen. Megaloblastic changes are restricted to the RBC series (see below). As with other forms of myelodysplasia, refractory megaloblastic anemia is associated with an increased incidence of acute leukemia.

Megaloblastic changes are seen in erythremic myelosis and acute erythroleukemia (di Guglielmo), where RBC precursors are prominently involved. Here, the marrow is characterized by bizarre erythroid maturation, with multinuclearity and multipolar mitotic figures in the RBC precursors (Chap. 111).

MEGALOBLASTIC DISEASE WITHOUT ANEMIA

Megaloblastic disease is easily overlooked in nonanemic patients. It can present in one of two ways.

Acute Megaloblastic Anemia Occasionally, a full-blown megaloblastic state can develop over the course of just a few days. This is usually seen following nitrous oxide anesthesia but may occur in any patient with a serious illness requiring intensive care, especially a patient receiving multiple transfusions, dialysis, or total parenteral nutrition. An acute megaloblastic state can also be precipitated by the administration of a weak antifolate (e.g., trimethoprim) to a patient with marginal tissue folate stores.

The condition resembles an immune cytopenia, with a rapidly developing thrombocytopenia and/or leukopenia in the absence of anemia. The blood smear may be completely normal, but the marrow is floridly megaloblastic. Acute megaloblastic anemia responds rapidly to treatment with folate plus cobalamin in the usual therapeutic doses.

Cobalamin Deficiency without Anemia Cobalamin deficiency without hematologic abnormalities is surprisingly common, especially in the elderly. The risk of a nonhematologic presentation for cobalamin deficiency is increased by the folate food fortification because folate can mask the hematologic effects of cobalamin deficiency. Between 10 and 30% of persons over age 70 years have metabolic evidence of cobalamin deficiency, either elevated homocysteine levels, low cobalamin-TCII levels, or both. Only 10% of these patients have defective production of IF, and the remainder often cannot release cobalamin from their food (see above). These patients may present with neuropsychiatric abnormalities, including peripheral neuropathies, gait disturbance, memory loss, and psychiatric symptoms, sometimes with abnormal evoked potentials. Serum cobalamin levels may be normal or low, but serum levels of methylmalonic acid are almost invariably increased due to a deficiency of cobalamin at the tissue level. The neuropsychiatric abnormalities tend to improve and serum methylmalonic acid levels generally return to normal after treatment with cobalamin. Neurologic defects do not always reverse with cobalamin supplementation.

DIAGNOSIS The finding of significant macrocytosis [mean corpuscular volume (MCV) > 100 fL] suggests the presence of a megaloblastic anemia. Other causes of macrocytosis include hemolysis, liver disease, alcoholism, hypothyroidism, and aplastic anemia. If the macrocytosis is marked (MCV > 110 fL), the patient is much more likely to have a megaloblastic anemia. Macrocytosis is less marked with concurrent iron deficiency or thalassemia. The reticulocyte count is low, and the leukocyte and platelet count may also be decreased, particularly in severely anemic patients. The blood smear (**see Plate V-24**) demonstrates marked anisocytosis and poikilocytosis, together with macroovalocytes, which are large, oval, fully hemoglobinized erythrocytes typical of megaloblastic anemias. There is some basophilic stippling, and an occasional nucleated RBC may be seen. In the white blood cell series, the neutrophils show hypersegmentation of the nucleus (**see Plate V-38**). This is such a characteristic finding that a single cell with a nucleus of six lobes or more should raise the im-

mediate suspicion of a megaloblastic anemia. A rare myelocyte may also be seen. Bizarre, misshapen platelets are also observed. The reticulocyte index is low. The bone marrow is hypercellular with a decreased myeloid/erythroid ratio and abundant stainable iron. RBC precursors are abnormally large and have nuclei that appear much less mature than would be expected from the development of the cytoplasm (nuclear-cytoplasmic asynchrony). The nuclear chromatin is more dispersed than expected, and it condenses in a peculiar fenestrated pattern that is very characteristic of megaloblastic erythropoiesis. Abnormal mitoses may be seen. Granulocyte precursors are also affected, many being larger than normal, including giant bands and metamyelocytes. Megakaryocytes are decreased and show abnormal morphology.

Megaloblastic anemias are characterized by ineffective erythropoiesis (Chap. 61). In a severely megaloblastic patient, as many as 90% of the RBC precursors may be destroyed before they are released into the bloodstream, compared with 10 to 15% in normal individuals. Enhanced intramedullary destruction of erythroblasts results in an increase in unconjugated bilirubin and lactic acid dehydrogenase (isoenzyme 1) in plasma. Abnormalities in iron kinetics also attest to the presence of ineffective erythropoiesis, with increased iron turnover but low incorporation of labeled iron into circulating RBCs.

In evaluating a patient with megaloblastic anemia, it is important to determine whether there is a specific vitamin deficiency by measuring serum cobalamin and folate levels. The normal range of cobalamin in serum is 200 to 900 pg/mL; values <100 pg/mL indicate clinically significant deficiency. Measurements of cobalamin bound to TC II would be a more physiologic measure of cobalamin status, but such assays are not yet routinely available. The normal serum concentration of folic acid ranges from 6 to 20 ng/mL; values ≤4 ng/mL are generally considered to be diagnostic of folate deficiency. Unlike serum cobalamin, serum folate levels may reflect recent alterations in dietary intake. Measurement of RBC folate level provides useful information because it is not subject to short-term fluctuations in folate intake and is better than serum folate as an index of folate stores.

Once cobalamin deficiency has been established, its pathogenesis can be delineated by means of a Schilling test. A patient is given radioactive cobalamin by mouth, followed shortly thereafter by an intramuscular injection of unlabeled cobalamin. The proportion of the administered radioactivity excreted in the urine during the next 24 h provides an accurate measure of absorption of cobalamin, assuming that a complete urine sample has been collected. Because cobalamin deficiency is almost always due to malabsorption (Table 107-1), this first stage of the Schilling test should be abnormal (i.e., small amounts of radioactivity in the urine). The patient is then given labeled cobalamin bound to IF. Absorption of the vitamin will now approach normal if the patient has pernicious anemia or some other type of IF deficiency. If cobalamin absorption is still decreased, the patient may have bacterial overgrowth (blind loop syndrome) or ileal disease (including an ileal absorptive defect secondary to the cobalamin deficiency itself). Cobalamin malabsorption due to bacterial overgrowth can frequently be corrected by the administration of antibiotics. The Schilling test can provide equally reliable information after the patient has had adequate therapy with parenteral cobalamin.

A normal Schilling test in a patient with documented cobalamin deficiency may indicate poor absorption of the vitamin when mixed with food. This can be established by repeating the Schilling test with radioactive cobalamin scrambled with an egg.

Serum methylmalonic acid and homocysteine levels are also useful in the diagnosis of megaloblastic anemias. Both are elevated in cobalamin deficiency, while elevated levels of homocysteine but not methylmalonic acid are seen in folate deficiency. These tests measure tissue vitamin stores and may demonstrate a deficiency even when the more traditional but less reliable folate and cobalamin levels are borderline or even normal. Patients (particularly older patients) without anemia and with normal serum cobalamin levels but elevated levels of serum methylmalonic acid may develop neuropsychiatric abnormalities. Treatment of patients with this "subtle" cobalamin deficiency will usually prevent further deterioration and may result in improvement.

℞ **TREATMENT   Cobalamin Deficiency**   Apart from specific therapy related to the underlying disorder (e.g., antibiotics for intestinal overgrowth with bacteria), the mainstay of treatment for cobalamin deficiency is replacement therapy. Because the defect is nearly always malabsorption, patients are generally given parenteral treatment, specifically in the form of intramuscular cyanocobalamin. Parenteral treatment begins with 1000 μg cobalamin per week for 8 weeks, followed by 1000 μg cyanocobalamin intramuscularly every month for the rest of the patient's life. However, cobalamin deficiency can also be managed very effectively by oral replacement therapy with 2 mg crystalline B_{12} per day.

The response to treatment is gratifying. Shortly after treatment is begun, and several days before a hematologic response is evident in the peripheral blood, the patient will experience an increase in strength and an improved sense of well-being. Marrow morphology begins to revert toward normal within a few hours after treatment is initiated. Reticulocytosis begins 4 to 5 days after therapy is started and peaks at about day 7 (Fig. 107-3), with subsequent remission of the anemia over the next several weeks. If a reticulocytosis does not occur, or if it is less brisk than expected from the level of the hematocrit, a search should be made for other factors contributing to the anemia (e.g., infection, coexisting iron and/or folate deficiency, or hypothyroidism). Hypokalemia and salt retention may occur early in the course of therapy. Thrombocytosis may also be seen.

In most cases, replacement therapy is all that is needed for the treatment of cobalamin deficiency. Occasionally, however, a patient with a severe anemia will have such a precarious cardiovascular status that emergency transfusion is necessary. This must be done with great care, because such patients may develop heart failure from fluid overload. Blood must be administered slowly in the form of packed RBCs, with very close observation. A small volume of packed RBCs will frequently be enough to ameliorate the acute cardiovascular problems. If necessary, blood may be administered by exchanging patient blood (mostly plasma) for packed cells.

With lifelong treatment, patients should experience no further manifestations of cobalamin deficiency, although neurologic symptoms may not be fully corrected even by optimal therapy. The potential for late development of gastric carcinoma in pernicious anemia necessitates careful follow-up of the patient.

Folate, particularly in large doses, can correct the megaloblastic anemia of cobalamin deficiency without altering the neurologic abnormalities. The neurologic manifestations may even be aggravated by folate therapy. Cobalamin deficiency can thus be masked in patients who are taking large doses of folate. For this reason, a hematologic response to folate must never be used to rule out cobalamin deficiency in a given patient; cobalamin deficiency can be excluded only by appropriate laboratory evaluation.

In light of the high frequency of defective cobalamin absorption in older people and the possible increased risk that overt cobalamin deficiency will present with neurologic rather than hematologic symptoms (because of folate food fortification), some experts have recommended the use of 0.1 mg oral crystalline cobalamin prophylaxis daily in people over age 65 years.

Folate Deficiency   As for cobalamin deficiency, folate deficiency is treated by replacement therapy. The usual dose of folate is 1 mg/d, by mouth, but higher doses (up to 5 mg/d) may be required for folate deficiency due to malabsorption. Parenteral folate is rarely necessary. The hematologic response is similar to that seen after replacement therapy for cobalamin deficiency, i.e., a brisk reticulocytosis after about 4 days, followed by correction of the anemia over the next 1 to 2 months. The duration of therapy depends on the basis of the deficiency state. Patients with a continuously increased requirement (such as patients with hemolytic anemia) or those with malabsorption or chronic malnutrition should continue to receive oral folic acid indefinitely. In addition, the patient should be encouraged to maintain an optimal diet containing adequate amounts of folate.

Other Causes of Megaloblastic Anemia   Megaloblastic anemia due to drugs can be treated, if necessary, by reducing the dose of the drug or eliminating it altogether. The effects of folate antagonists that inhibit dihydrofolate reductase can be counteracted by folinic acid [5-formyl tetrahydrofolate (THF)] in a dose of 100 to 200 mg/d (Fig. 107-1), which circumvents the block in folate metabolism by providing a form of folate that can be converted to 5,10-methylene THF. For the megaloblastic forms of sideroblastic anemia, pyridoxine in pharmacologic doses (as high as 300 mg/d) should be tried. If this fails, pyridoxal phosphate may work, presumably in part by promoting the conversion of THF to 5,10-methylene THF. Simple supportive measures are all that appear to be in order for treatment of refractory megaloblastic anemia. Acute erythroleukemia (di Guglielmo's disease) is usually treated like other types of acute myeloid leukemia (Chap. 111).

BIBLIOGRAPHY

ALLEN RH et al: Metabolic abnormalities in cobalamin [vitamin B_{12}] and folate deficiencies. FASEB J 7:1344, 1993

BABIOR BM: The megaloblastic anemias, in *Williams' Hematology*, 6th ed, E Beutler et al (eds). New York, McGraw-Hill, 2000

CARMEL R : Prevalence of undiagnosed pernicious anemia in the elderly. Arch Intern Med 156:1097, 1996

——: Cobalamin, the stomach and aging. Am J Clin Nutr 66:750, 1997.

—— et al: The frequently low cobalamin levels in dementia usually signify treatable metabolic, neurologic and electrophysiologic abnormalities. Eur J Haematol 54:245, 1995

COOPER TR, ROSENBLATT DS: Inherited defects of vitamin B_{12} metabolism. Annu Rev Nutr 7:291, 1987

D'ANGELO A, SELHUB J: Homocysteine and thrombotic disease. Blood 90:1, 1997

HSING AW et al: Pernicious anemia and subsequent cancer. Cancer 71:745, 1993

JACQUES PF et al: The effect of folic acid fortification on plasma folate and total homocysteine concentrations. N Engl J Med 340:1449, 1999

JOSTEN E et al: Metabolic evidence that deficiencies of vitamin B_{12}, folate, and vitamin B_6 occur commonly in the elderly. Am J Clin Nutr 58:468, 1993

KUZMINSKI AM et al: Effective treatment of cobalamin deficiency with oral cobalamin. Blood 92:1191, 1998

LINDENBAUM J et al: Neuropsychiatric disorders caused by cobalamin deficiency in the absence of anemia or macrocytosis. N Engl J Med 318:1720, 1988

METZ J et al: The significance of subnormal vitamin B_{12} concentration in older people: A case-control study. J Am Geriatr Soc 44:1355, 1996

SAVAGE DG et al: Sensitivity of serum methylmalonic acid and total homocysteine determinations for diagnosing cobalamin and folate deficiencies. Am J Med 96:239, 1994

SCHILLING RF, WILLIAMS WJ: Vitamin B_{12} deficiency: Underdiagnosed, overtreated? Hosp Pract (Off Ed) 30:47, 1995

TOH BH et al: Pernicious anemia. N Engl J Med 337:1441, 1997

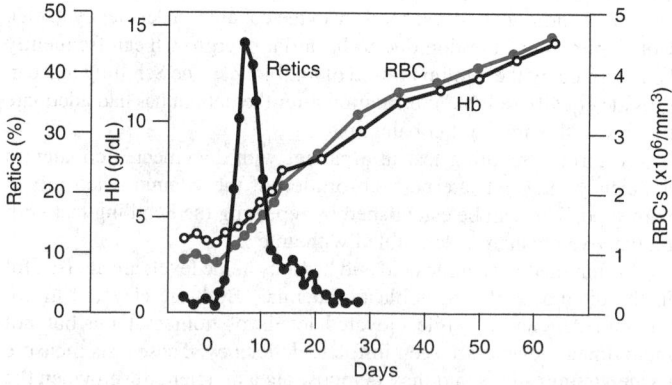

FIGURE 107-3   Hematologic response of a patient with pernicious anemia to an intramuscular injection of 100 μg cobalamin on day 0. (From A Erslev, TG Gabuzda, *Pathophysiology of Blood,* Philadelphia, Saunders, 1975, with permission.)

108

H. Franklin Bunn, Wendell Rosse

HEMOLYTIC ANEMIAS AND ACUTE BLOOD LOSS

DIC disseminated intravascular coagulation	PCH paroxysmal cold hemoglobinuria
G6PD glucose-6-phosphate dehydrogenase	PNH paroxysmal nocturnal hemoglobinuria
LDH lactate dehydrogenase	PK pyruvate kinase
MCHC mean corpuscular hemoglobin concentration	RBC red blood cells
MCV mean corpuscular volume	TTP thrombotic thrombocytopenia purpura

The loss of red cells either through hemorrhage or, less commonly, through premature destruction of the red cells (hemolysis) may cause anemia. Hemolysis or blood loss normally leads to an increase in red cell production, which is clinically manifested by an increase in reticulocytes.

HEMOLYTIC ANEMIAS

Red blood cells (RBC) normally survive 90 to 120 days in the circulation. The life span of RBC may be shortened in a number of disorders, often resulting in anemia if the bone marrow is not able to replenish adequately the prematurely destroyed RBC. The disorders associated with hemolytic anemias are generally identified by the abnormality that brings about the premature destruction of the RBC.

In all patients with hemolytic anemia, a careful history and physical examination provide important clues to the diagnosis. The patient may complain of fatigue and other symptoms of anemia (Chap. 61). Less commonly, jaundice and even red-brown urine (hemoglobinuria) are reported. A complete drug and toxin exposure history and the family history often provide crucial information. The physical examination may show jaundice of skin and mucosae. Splenomegaly is encountered in a variety of hemolytic anemias. A wide array of other historic and physical findings is associated with specific hemolytic anemias (see below).

Laboratory tests may be used initially to demonstrate the presence of hemolysis (Table 108-1) and define its cause. An elevated reticulocyte count in the patient with anemia is the most useful indicator of hemolysis, reflecting erythroid hyperplasia of the bone marrow; biopsy of the bone marrow is often unnecessary. Reticulocytes are also elevated in patients with active blood loss, those with myelophthisis, and those who are recovering from suppression of erythropoiesis (Chap. 61). The morphology of the RBC may provide evidence both of hemolysis and of its cause; the characteristic abnormalities and their

associated causes and syndromes are listed in Table 108-2. While the findings on the peripheral blood smear alone are rarely pathognomonic, they may provide important clues to the presence of hemolysis and to diagnosis.

RBC may be prematurely removed from the circulation by macrophages, particularly those of the spleen and liver (extravascular lysis), or, less commonly, by disruption of their membranes during their circulation (intravascular hemolysis). Both mechanisms result in increased heme catabolism and enhanced formation of unconjugated bilirubin, which is normally conjugated by the liver and excreted. The plasma level of unconjugated bilirubin may be high enough to produce readily apparent jaundice (detectable usually when serum bilirubin is >34 μmol/L or 2 mg/dL). The unconjugated (indirect) bilirubin level can be further elevated by a commonly encountered defect in conjugation of bilirubin (Gilbert's syndrome) (Chap. 294). In patients with hemolysis, the level of unconjugated bilirubin never exceeds 70 to 85 μmol/L (4 to 5 mg/dL), unless liver function is impaired.

In the absence of tissue damage in other organs, serum enzyme levels can be useful in the diagnosis and monitoring of patients with hemolysis. Lactate dehydrogenase (LDH), particularly LDH-2, is elevated by accelerated RBC destruction. Serum AST (SGOT) may be somewhat elevated, whereas ALT (SGPT) is not.

Haptoglobin is an α globulin that is present in high concentration (~1.0 g/L) in the plasma (and serum). It binds specifically and tightly to the globin in hemoglobin. The hemoglobin-haptoglobin complex is cleared within minutes by the mononuclear phagocyte system. Thus patients with significant hemolysis, either intravascular or extravascular, have low or absent levels of serum haptoglobin. The fact that haptoglobin synthesis is decreased in patients with hepatocellular disease and increased in inflammatory states must be considered in the interpretation of serum haptoglobin.

Intravascular hemolysis (which is uncommon) results in the release of hemoglobin into the plasma. In these cases, plasma hemoglobin is increased in proportion to the degree of hemolysis. Plasma hemoglobin may be falsely elevated due to lysis of RBC in vitro. If the haptoglobin-binding capacity of the plasma is exceeded, free hemoglobin passes through renal glomeruli. This filtered hemoglobin is reabsorbed by the proximal tubule, where it is catabolized in situ, and the heme iron is incorporated into storage proteins (ferritin and hemosiderin). The presence of hemosiderin in the urine, detected by staining the sediment with Prussian blue, indicates that a significant amount of circulating free hemoglobin has been filtered by the kidneys. Hemosiderin appears 3 to 4 days after the onset of hemoglobinuria and may persist for weeks after its cessation. When the absorptive capacity of the tubular cells is exceeded, hemoglobinuria ensues. Hemoglobinuria indicates severe intravascular hemolysis. Hemoglobinuria must be distinguished from

Table 108-1 Laboratory Evaluation of Hemolysis

	Extravascular	Intravascular
HEMATOLOGIC		
Routine blood film	Polychromatophilia	Polychromatophilia
Reticulocyte count	↑	↑
Bone marrow examination	Erythroid hyperplasia	Erythroid hyperplasia
PLASMA OR SERUM		
Bilirubin	↑ Unconjugated	↑ Unconjugated
Haptoglobin	↓, Absent	Absent
Plasma hemoglobin	N– ↑	↑ ↑
Lactate dehydrogenase	↑ (Variable)	↑ ↑ (Variable)
URINE		
Bilirubin	0	0
Hemosiderin	0	+
Hemoglobin	0	+ in severe cases

NOTE: N, normal.

Table 108-2 Red Blood Cell Morphology in the Diagnosis of Hemolytic Anemia

Morphology	Cause	Syndromes
Spherocytes	Loss of membrane	Hereditary spherocytosis, autoimmune hemolytic anemia
Target cells	Increased ratio of RBC surface area to volume	Hemoglobin disorders: thalassemias, hemoglobin S, C, etc.; liver disease
Schistocytes	Traumatic disruption of membrane	Microangiopathy, intravascular prostheses
Sickled cells	Polymerization of hemoglobin S	Sickle cell syndromes
Acanthocytes	?Abnormal membrane lipids	Severe liver disease (spur cell anemia)
Agglutinated cells	Presence of IgM antibody	Cold agglutinin disease
Heinz bodies	Precipitated hemoglobin	Unstable hemoglobin, oxidant stress

hematuria (in which case RBC are seen on urine examination) and from myoglobin due to rhabdomyolysis; in all three cases, the urine is positive with the benzidine reaction, commonly used in analysis of urine. The distinction between hemoglobinuria and myoglobinuria can best be made by specific tests that exploit immunologic differences or differences in solubility. After centrifugation of an anticoagulated blood specimen, the plasma of patients with hemoglobinuria has a reddish-brown color, whereas that of patients with myoglobinuria is normal in color. Because of its higher molecular weight, hemoglobin has lower glomerular permeability than myoglobin and is less rapidly cleared by the kidneys.

CLASSIFICATION The hemolytic anemias can be grouped in three different ways, shown in Table 108-3. The cause of accelerated RBC destruction can be regarded as (1) a molecular defect (hemoglobinopathy or enzymopathy) inside the red cell, (2) an abnormality in membrane structure and function, or (3) an environmental factor such as mechanical trauma or an autoantibody. In *intracorpuscular types* of hemolysis, the patient's RBC have an abnormally short life span in a normal recipient (with a compatible blood type), while compatible normal RBC survive normally in the patient. The opposite is true in *extracorpuscular types* of hemolysis. Finally, hemolytic disorders can be classified as either inherited or acquired.

INHERITED HEMOLYTIC ANEMIAS The inherited hemolytic anemias are due to inborn defects in one of three main components of red cells: the membrane, the enzymes, or hemoglobin. These defects are often known at the genomic level, but their identification still largely depends on their clinical and laboratory manifestations.

Red Cell Membrane Disorders These are usually readily detected by morphologic abnormalities of the RBC on the blood film. There are three types of inherited RBC membrane abnormalities: hereditary spherocytosis, hereditary elliptocytosis (including hereditary pyropoikilocytosis), and hereditary stomatocytosis.

Hereditary spherocytosis This condition is characterized by spherical RBC due to a molecular defect in one of the proteins in the cytoskeleton of the RBC membrane, leading to a loss of membrane and hence decreased ratio of surface area to volume and consequently spherocytosis. This disorder usually has an autosomal dominant inheritance pattern and an incidence of approximately 1:1000 to 1:4500. In ~20% of patients, the absence of hematologic abnormalities in family members suggests either autosomal recessive inheritance or a spontaneous mutation. The disorder is sometimes clinically apparent in early infancy but often escapes detection until adult life.

CLINICAL MANIFESTATIONS The major clinical features of hereditary spherocytosis are anemia, splenomegaly, and jaundice. The prominence of jaundice accounts for the disorder's prior designation as "congenital hemolytic jaundice" and is due to an increased concentration of unconjugated (indirect-reacting) bilirubin in plasma. Jaundice may be intermittent and tends to be less pronounced in early childhood. Because of the increased bile pigment production, pig-

mented gallstones are common, even in childhood. Compensatory erythroid hyperplasia of the bone marrow occurs, with the extension of red marrow into the midshafts of long bones and occasionally with extramedullary erythropoiesis, at times leading to the formation of paravertebral masses visible on chest x-ray. Because the bone marrow's capacity to increase erythropoiesis by six- to eightfold exceeds the usual rate of hemolysis, anemia is usually mild or moderate and may even be absent in an otherwise healthy individual. Compensation may be temporarily interrupted by episodes of relative erythroid hypoplasia precipitated by infections, particularly parvovirus, trauma, surgery, and pregnancy. Splenomegaly is very common. The hemolytic rate may increase transiently during systemic infections, which induce further splenic enlargement. Chronic leg ulcers, similar to those observed in sickle cell anemia, occur occasionally.

The characteristic erythrocyte abnormality is the spherocyte (**Plate V-26**). The mean corpuscular volume (MCV) is usually normal or slightly decreased, and the mean corpuscular hemoglobin concentration (MCHC) is increased to 350 to 400 g/L. Spheroidicity may be quantitatively assessed by measurement of the osmotic fragility of the RBC on exposure to hypoosmotic solutions causing a net influx of water (Fig. 108-1). Because spherocytes have a decreased surface area per unit volume, they are able to take in less water and hence lyse at a higher concentration of saline than normal cells. On microscopic examination, spherocytes are usually detected as small cells without central pallor. They will ordinarily not influence the osmotic fragility test unless they constitute more than 1 or 2% of the total cell population. The autohemolysis test, which measures the amount of spontaneous hemolysis occurring after 48 h of sterile incubation, is also useful.

PATHOGENESIS The molecular abnormality in hereditary spherocytosis primarily involves the proteins responsible for tethering the lipid bilayer to the underlying cytoskeletal network. Nearly all patients have a significant deficiency of spectrin, which is sometimes secondary to an inherited molecular defect in that protein. About 50% of patients have a defect in ankyrin, the protein that forms a bridge between protein 3 and spectrin (Fig. 108-2). Homozygotes who have a recessive inheritance pattern for ankyrin deficiency have more severe anemia than heterozygotes with the more common dominant form. About 25% of patients have a mutation of protein 3, resulting in a deficiency of that protein and mild anemia with dominant inheritance. Most of the remaining 25% have mutations of spectrin, leading to impaired synthesis or self-association; β-spectrin deficiency is generally mild, with dominant inheritance, while α-spectrin deficiency is severe, with a recessive inheritance pattern. Because the lipid bilayer is not well anchored when these proteins are defective, part of it is lost by vesiculation, resulting in a more spherical and less deformable cell. Because of their shape and rigidity, spherocytes cannot traverse the interstices of the spleen where their increased metabolic rate cannot be sustained, causing a further loss of surface membrane. This "conditioning" produces a subpopulation of hyperspheroidal RBC in the peripheral blood.

Table 108-3 Classification of Hemolytic Anemias

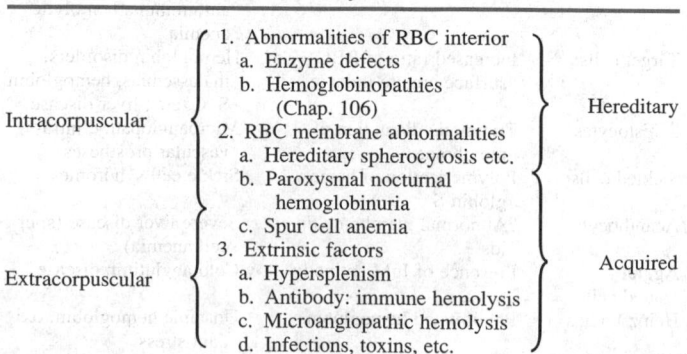

Intracorpuscular	1. Abnormalities of RBC interior a. Enzyme defects b. Hemoglobinopathies 　 (Chap. 106) 2. RBC membrane abnormalities a. Hereditary spherocytosis etc. b. Paroxysmal nocturnal 　 hemoglobinuria c. Spur cell anemia	Hereditary
Extracorpuscular	3. Extrinsic factors a. Hypersplenism b. Antibody: immune hemolysis c. Microangiopathic hemolysis d. Infections, toxins, etc.	Acquired

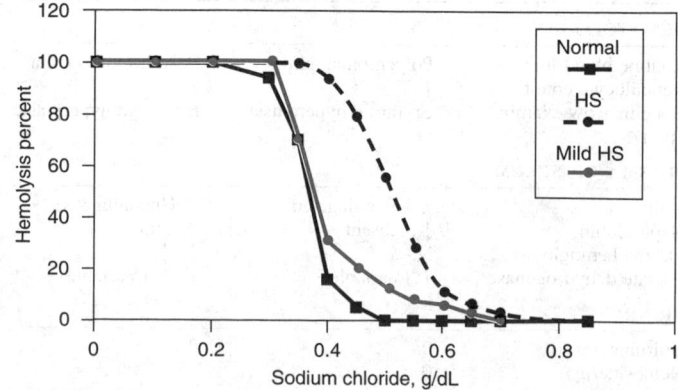

FIGURE 108-1 Osmotic fragility of RBC in hereditary spherocytosis (HS). The results from two patients are compared to that from a normal individual.

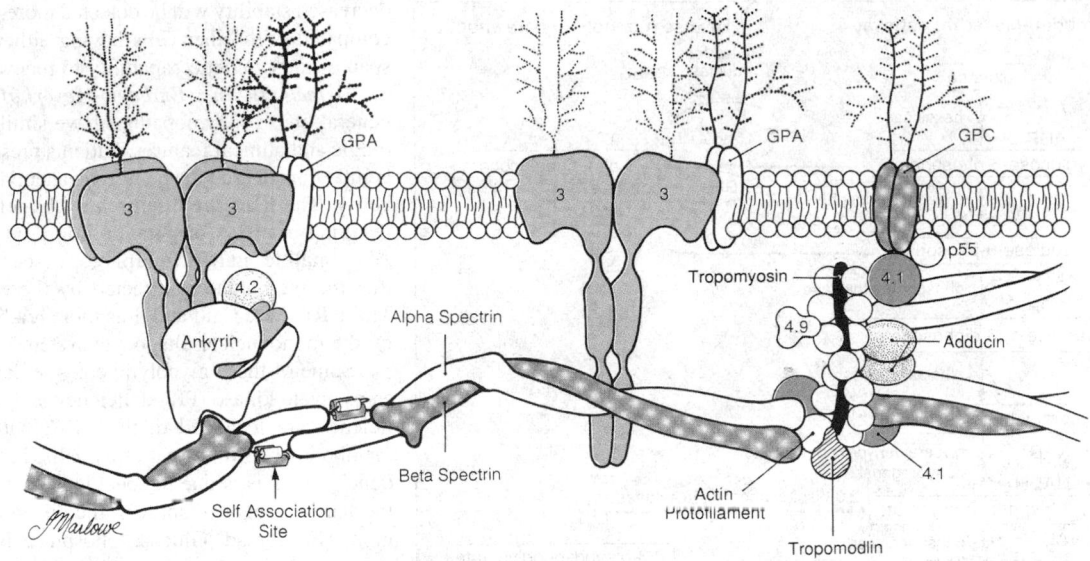

FIGURE 108-2 Diagram of a cross section of the RBC membrane. Spectrin, actin, tropomyosin, adducin, and protein 4.1 form a meshwork that laminates the inner surface of the membrane. In contrast, other proteins such as the glycophorins (GPA and GPC) and protein 3 (anion transport channel) traverse the lipid bilayer. Long polysaccharide chains are covalently attached to these proteins on the outer surface of the cell and also to glycolipid. Ankyrin and protein 4.2 form a bridge between spectrin and a fraction of the anion transport proteins. Protein 4.1 binds to GPC. *(Lux SE, Palek, J, with permission.)*

DIAGNOSIS   Hereditary spherocytosis must be distinguished primarily from the spherocytic hemolytic anemias associated with RBC antibodies. The family history of anemia and/or splenectomy is helpful, when present. The diagnosis of immune spherocytosis is usually readily established by a positive direct Coombs test (see below). Spherocytes are also seen in association with hemolysis induced by splenomegaly in patients with cirrhosis, in clostridial infections, and in certain snake envenomations (due to the action of phospholipases on the membrane). A few spherocytes are seen in the course of a wide variety of hemolytic disorders, particularly glucose-6-phosphate dehydrogenase (G6PD) deficiency.

℞   TREATMENT   Splenectomy reliably corrects the anemia, although the RBC defect and its consequent morphology persist. The operative risk is low. RBC survival after splenectomy is normal or nearly so; if it is not, an accessory spleen or another diagnosis should be sought. Because of the potential for gallstones and for episodes of bone marrow hypoplasia or hemolytic crises, splenectomy should be performed in symptomatic individuals; cholecystectomy should not be performed without splenectomy, as intrahepatic gallstones may result. Splenectomy in children should be postponed until age 4, if possible, to minimize the risk of severe infections with grampositive encapsulated organisms. Polyvalent pneumococcal vaccine should be administered at least 2 weeks before splenectomy. In patients with severe hemolysis, folic acid (1 mg/d) should be administered prophylactically.

Hereditary elliptocytosis and hereditary pyropoikilocytosis
Oval or elliptic RBC are normally found in birds, reptiles, camels, and llamas; however, they occur in appreciable numbers in humans only in *hereditary elliptocytosis,* a disorder that is transmitted as an autosomal dominant trait and affects 1 per 4000 to 5000 people, a frequency similar to that of hereditary spherocytosis (rarely, patients with myelodysplastic disorders of the bone marrow may have acquired elliptocytosis). The elliptic shape is acquired as the cell deforms to traverse the microcirculation but does not spring back to its initial biconcave shape. In most affected individuals, a structural abnormality of erythrocyte spectrin that leads to impaired assembly of the cytoskeleton. In some families, affected individuals have a deficiency of erythrocyte membrane protein 4.1, which stabilizes the interaction of spectrin and actin in the cytoskeleton (Fig. 108-2); homozygotes with absence of this protein have more marked hemolysis. In Southeast

Asia, there is a high incidence of hereditary ovalocytosis, in which a small internal deletion of protein 3 makes the membrane rigid and confers resistance against malaria.

The great majority of patients manifest only mild hemolysis, with hemoglobin levels >120 g/L, reticulocytes <4% (0.2×10^{12}/L), depressed haptoglobin levels, and RBC survival times just under the normal range. In 10 to 15% of patients with more severe abnormalities, the rate of hemolysis is substantially increased, with median survival times of RBC as short as 5 days and reticulocytes ranging up to 20%. Hemoglobin levels rarely fall below 90 to 100 g/L. RBC destruction occurs predominantly in the spleen, which is enlarged in patients with overt hemolysis. Hemolysis is corrected by splenectomy.

In both the anemic and nonanemic varieties of this disorder, at least 25% and, more commonly, >75% of RBC are elliptic, with an axial ratio (width/length) of <0.78. Patients with hemolysis frequently have microovalocytes, bizarre-shaped RBC, and RBC fragments, all of which increase in number after splenectomy. The degree of hemolysis does not correlate with the percentage of elliptocytes. Osmotic fragility is usually normal but may be increased in patients with overt hemolysis.

Hereditary pyropoikilocytosis is a rare disorder related to hereditary elliptocytosis and is characterized by bizarre-shaped, microcytic RBC that undergo disruption at temperatures of 44 to 45°C (in contrast, normal RBC are stable up to 49°C). This condition results from a deficiency of spectrin and an abnormality of spectrin self-assembly. Hemolysis is usually severe, is recognized in childhood, and is partially responsive to splenectomy.

Hereditary stomatocytosis   Stomatocytes are cup-shaped RBC (concave on one face and convex on the other). This formation results in a slitlike central zone of pallor on dried smears. The syndrome of hereditary hemolytic anemia and stomatocytic RBC is inherited in an autosomal dominant pattern. RBC have an increased permeability to sodium and potassium, which is compensated for by an increased active transport of these cations. In some patients, the RBC are swollen with an excess of ions and water and a decreased mean corpuscular hemoglobin concentration (overhydrated stomatocytes, "hydrocytosis"); many of these patients lack the RBC membrane protein 7.2 (stomatin). In other patients, the RBC are shrunken, with a decreased ion and water content and an increased mean corpuscular hemoglobin concentration (dehydrated stomatocytes, "desiccytosis" or "xerocytosis"). Those patients in whom the RBC are overhydrated have true stomatocytes on dried smears. Dehydrated stomatocytes assume the mor-

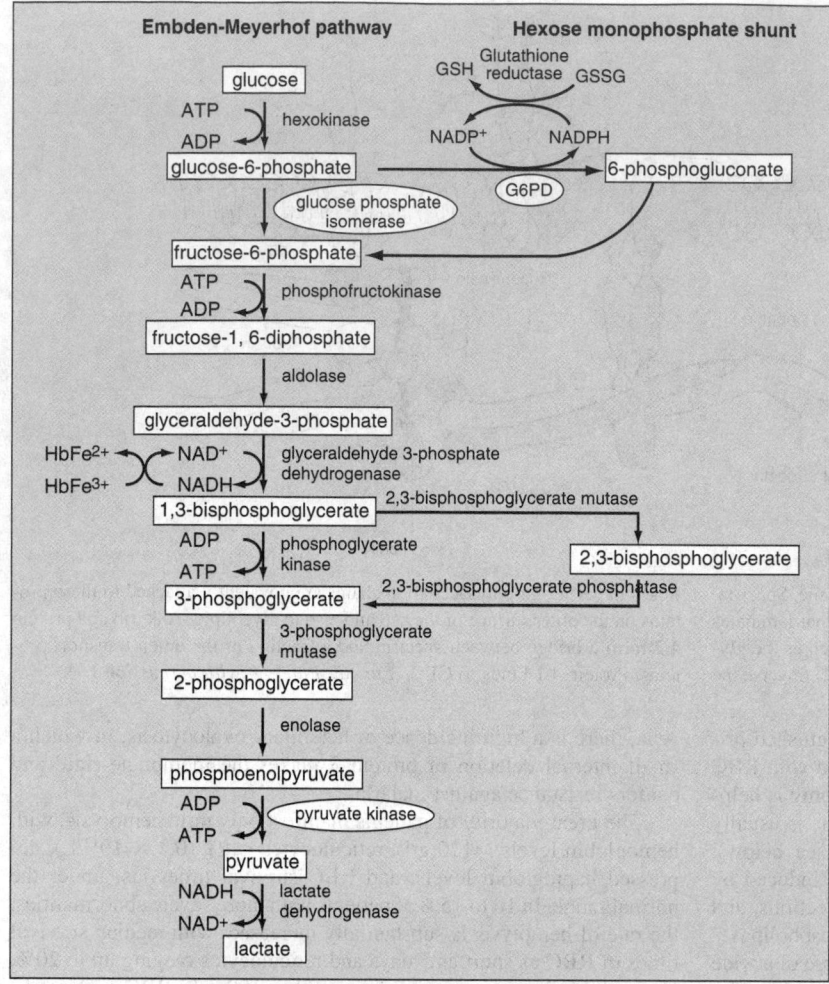

Embden-Meyerhof pathway   **Hexose monophosphate shunt**

FIGURE 108-3 RBC metabolism. The Embden-Meyerhof pathway (glycolysis) generates ATP for energy and membrane maintenance. The generation of NADPH maintains hemoglobin in a reduced state. The hexose monophosphate shunt generates NADPH that is used to reduce glutathione, which protects the red cell against oxidant stress. The Rapaport-Luebering shunt regulates 2,3-bisphosphoglycerate levels, a critical determinant of oxygen affinity of hemoglobin. Enzyme deficiency states in order of prevalence: glucose-6-phosphate dehydrogenase (G6PD) $\gg$ pyruvate kinase > glucose-6-phosphate isomerase > rare deficiencies of other enzymes in the pathway. The more common enzyme deficiencies are encircled.

phology of target cells on dried smears. Osmotic fragility is increased in overhydrated stomatocytes and decreased in underhydrated stomatocytes. RBC lacking Rh proteins (Rh_{null} cells) are stomatocytic and have a shortened life span.

Most patients have splenomegaly and mild anemia. Splenectomy decreases but does not totally correct the hemolytic process.

Red Cell Enzyme Defects During its maturation, the RBC loses its nucleus, ribosomes, and mitochondria and thus its capability for protein synthesis and oxidative phosphorylation. The mature circulating RBC has a relatively simple pattern of intermediary metabolism (Fig. 108-3) in keeping with its modest metabolic obligations. ATP must be generated from the Embden-Meyerhof pathway to drive the cation pump that maintains the ionic milieu in the RBC. Smaller amounts of energy are needed for the preservation of hemoglobin iron in the ferrous (Fe^{2+}) state and perhaps for the renewal of the lipids in the RBC membrane. About 10% of the glucose consumed by the RBC is metabolized via the hexose-monophosphate shunt (Fig. 108-3), which protects both hemoglobin and the membrane from exogenous oxidants, including certain drugs.

Deficiency states have been reported for most of the enzymes shown in Fig. 108-3. Many of these enzyme abnormalities appear to be restricted to RBC. Mutations can result in no protein product, a dysfunctional product, or an unstable product. Mutations resulting in

decreased stability will be detected more readily in RBC compared with other cells having either a shorter life span or the synthetic capability to renew the enzyme.

Defects in the Embden-Meyerhof pathway In general, these enzymopathies have similar pathophysiologic and clinical features. Patients present with a congenital nonspherocytic hemolytic anemia of variable severity. The RBC are often relatively deficient in ATP, resulting in a leak of potassium ion out of these cells. Abnormalities in RBC morphology (see below) indicate that the membrane is affected by the enzyme defect. These RBC are rigid and thus more readily sequestered by the mononuclear phagocyte system.

Some of these glycolytic enzyme deficiencies such as pyruvate kinase (PK) deficiency and hexokinase deficiency are localized to the RBC, with no apparent metabolic abnormality in other cells; in the case of PK deficiency, this is due to specific isozymes confined to the RBC. In other disorders, the enzyme deficiency is more widespread. Glucose phosphate isomerase deficiency and phosphoglycerate kinase deficiency also involve leukocytes, although affected individuals have no apparent abnormalities of leukocyte function. Individuals with deficiency of triose phosphate isomerase have decreased levels of enzyme in leukocytes, muscle cells, and cerebrospinal fluid, and they have a progressive neurologic disorder. Some patients with phosphofructokinase deficiency have a myopathy.

About 95% of the clinically significant defects in the glycolytic pathway are due to PK deficiency, and about 4% are due to glucose phosphate isomerase deficiency. The remainder, shown in Fig. 108-3, are extremely rare. Most have been encountered in isolated families; clinical manifestations are variable. A number of different mutations result in PK deficiency. Some missense mutations in decreased reaction with substrate (phosphoenolpyruvate), an enhancing molecule (fructose 1,6 diphosphate), or ADP. Thus, there is considerable variability in the clinical manifestations and laboratory findings among individuals reported as having PK deficiency. Most of these patients are compound heterozygotes who have inherited a different defective enzyme from each parent.

Most of the glycolytic enzyme defects are inherited in an autosomal recessive pattern. The parents of affected patients are heterozygotes and express half-normal levels of enzyme activity, which are more than adequate for normal metabolic function. Thus, the parents are entirely asymptomatic. Since the gene frequency for this group of enzymopathies is low, true homozygotes are often the offspring of a consanguineous mating. More often, affected individuals are compound heterozygotes. Phosphoglycerate kinase deficiency is inherited as a sex-linked disorder. Affected males have a severe hemolytic anemia, while female carriers may have a mild hemolytic process.

CLINICAL MANIFESTATIONS Patients with severe hemolysis usually present during early childhood with anemia, jaundice, and splenomegaly.

LABORATORY FINDINGS Patients have a normocytic (or slightly macrocytic), normochromic anemia with reticulocytosis. In those with PK deficiency, bizarre erythrocytes, including spiculated cells, are noted on the peripheral smear, especially after splenectomy. Spherocytes are usually absent; hence the term *congenital nonspherocytic hemolytic anemia* has been applied to these disorders. Unlike hereditary spherocytosis, the osmotic fragility of freshly drawn blood is usually normal. Incubation brings out an osmotically fragile population of RBC, an abnormality not corrected by the addition of glucose.

The diagnosis of this group of anemias depends on specific enzymatic assays; care must be taken to provide an appropriate concentration of substrate to detect those variants with a low affinity for substrate or enhancing molecule. An abnormality in enzyme kinetics, differences in electrophoretic mobility, pH optimum, or heat stability may be useful in documenting heterogeneity among enzyme variants.

℞ **TREATMENT** Most patients do not require therapy. Those with severe hemolysis should be given folic acid (1 mg/d). Blood transfusions may be necessary during a hypoplastic crisis. Women with PK deficiency may become very anemic during pregnancy, sometimes leading to the diagnosis for the first time.

Because of their enzymatic defect, the younger cells (reticulocytes) depend on mitochondrial respiration rather than glycolysis for maintenance of ATP. However, in the hypoxic environment of the spleen, aerobic metabolism is curtailed and the ATP-depleted cells are destroyed in situ. Reticulocytes are normally retained in the spleen for 24 to 48 h. Patients with PK deficiency may benefit from splenectomy, which usually leads to a marked increase in circulating reticulocytes. Patients with deficiency of glucose phosphate isomerase also may improve after splenectomy. Splenectomy has not been proven effective in individuals with other glycolytic enzymopathies.

Defects in the hexose-monophosphate shunt The normal RBC is well protected against oxidant stress. When the cell is exposed to a drug or toxin that generates oxygen radicals, glucose metabolism via the hexose-monophosphate shunt is normally increased severalfold. Reduced glutathione is regenerated, protecting the sulfhydryl groups of hemoglobin and the RBC membrane from oxidation. Individuals with an inherited defect in the hexose-monophosphate shunt are unable to maintain an adequate level of reduced glutathione in their RBC, hemoglobin sulfhydryl groups become oxidized, and the hemoglobin precipitates within the RBC, forming Heinz bodies.

G6PD DEFICIENCY This is by far the most common congenital shunt defect, affecting more than 200 million people throughout the world; like hemoglobin S, it partially protects the patient from malaria by providing a defective home for the merozoite. Considerable genetic heterogeneity exists among affected individuals, and over 400 variants of G6PD have been described. In most cases, the alteration is a base substitution, leading to an amino acid replacement rather than a deletion or truncation of the protein. The mutations generate enzymes with differences in electrophoretic mobility, enzyme kinetics, pH optimum, and heat stability. These differences result in great variation of clinical severity, ranging from nonspherocytic hemolytic anemia without demonstrable oxidant stress (particularly shortly after birth), through hemolytic anemia only when stimulated by marked to mild oxidant stress, to no clinically detectable abnormality. The normal G6PD is designated as type B. About 20% of individuals of African descent have a G6PD (designated A+) that differs by a single amino acid and is electrophoretically distinguishable but functionally normal. Among the clinically significant G6PD variants, the most common, the so-called A— type, is due to two base substitutions and is encountered primarily in individuals of central African descent. The A— G6PD has the same electrophoretic mobility as the A+ type, but it is unstable and has abnormal kinetic properties. This variant is found in about 11% of African American males. A second relatively common G6PD variant is encountered among peoples of Mediterranean origin, particularly Sardinians and Sephardic Jews; this variant is more severe than the A— variant and may result in nonspherocytic hemolytic anemia in the absence of known oxidative stress. A third relatively common and slightly less severe variant occurs in southern Chinese populations.

The G6PD gene is located on the X chromosome; thus the deficiency state is a sex-linked trait. Affected males (hemizygotes) inherit the abnormal gene from their mothers who are usually carriers (heterozygotes). Because of inactivation of one of the two X chromosomes (Lyon hypothesis: Chap. 65), the heterozygote has two populations of RBC: normal and deficient in G6PD. Most female carriers are asymptomatic. Those who happen to have a high proportion of deficient cells

resemble the male hemizygotes. G6PD activity normally declines ~50% during the 120-day life span of the RBC. This decay is moderately accelerated in A— RBC and markedly so in RBC containing the Mediterranean variant. Individuals with the A— variant normally have a slightly shortened RBC survival time, but they are not anemic. Clinical problems arise only when the affected individual is subjected to some type of environmental stress. Most often, hemolytic episodes are triggered by viral and bacterial infections. The mechanism is unknown. In addition, drugs or toxins that pose an oxidant threat to the RBC (most commonly sulfa drugs, antimalarials, and nitrofurantoin) cause hemolysis in individuals deficient in G6PD (Table 108-4). Although aspirin is frequently mentioned as a likely offender, it has no deleterious effect in A— individuals. Accidental ingestion of toxic compounds such as naphthalene (moth balls) may cause severe hemolysis. Metabolic acidosis can precipitate an episode of hemolysis in individuals deficient in G6PD.

CLINICAL AND LABORATORY FEATURES The patient may experience an acute hemolytic crisis within hours of exposure to the oxidant stress, leading to hemoglobinuria and peripheral vascular collapse in severe cases. Since only the older population of RBC is rapidly destroyed, the hemolytic crisis is usually self-limited, even if the exposure to the oxidant continues. Among black males with the A— variant, the RBC mass decreases by a maximum of 25 to 30%. During acute hemolysis, a rapid drop in hematocrit is accompanied by a rise in plasma hemoglobin and unconjugated bilirubin and a decrease in plasma haptoglobin. The oxidation of hemoglobin leads to the formation of Heinz bodies, visualized by means of a supravital stain such as crystal violet. However, Heinz bodies are usually not seen after the first day or so, since these inclusions are readily removed by the spleen. Their removal leads to the formation of "bite cells" (RBC that have lost a peripheral portion of the cell). Multiple bites cause the formation of fragments. A few spherocytes also may be present. Individuals with the Mediterranean type G6PD have a more unstable enzyme and, therefore, a much lower overall enzyme activity than individuals with the A— variant. As a result, they have more severe clinical manifestations. A minority of patients are exquisitely sensitive to fava beans and develop a fulminant hemolytic crisis after exposure. The oxidants in *Vicia fava* are two β-glycosides whose aglycones, when autooxidized, produce oxygen free radicals. The incidence of favism is highly variable due to variations in concentration, in absorption, or in metabolism of the aglycones. Favism is not encountered in individuals with the A— variant.

The *diagnosis* of G6PD deficiency should be considered in any individual, particularly a male of African or Mediterranean descent, who experiences an acute hemolytic episode. The patient should be questioned about possible exposure to oxidant agents. The diagnosis can be established by a number of tests that assess either the enzyme activity or the effects of its deficiency. However, the test may yield a false-negative result during a hemolytic episode when the old RBC containing the defective enzyme have already lysed.

℞ **TREATMENT** Since hemolysis in patients deficient in A— G6PD is usually self-limited, no specific treatment is necessary. Splenectomy does not benefit Mediterranean patients with chronic hemolysis. Blood transfusions are rarely indicated. Adequate urine flow should be maintained if hemoglobinuria develops during an acute hemolytic episode.

Table 108-4 Drugs Causing Hemolysis in Subjects Deficient in G6PD

Antimalarials: Primaquine, pamaquine, dapsone
Sulfonamides: Sulfamethoxazole
Nitrofurantoin
Analgesics: Acetanilid
Miscellaneous: Vitamin K (water-soluble form), doxorubicin, methylene blue, nalidixic acid, furazolidone, niridazole, phenazopyridine

Prevention of hemolytic episodes is best. Infections ought to be treated promptly. Patients should be warned about risks posed by oxidant drugs and fava beans. Any patient of African or Mediterranean ancestry about to be given an oxidant drug should be screened for G6PD deficiency.

OTHER DEFECTS OF THE HEXOSE-MONOPHOSPHATE SHUNT   A few kindreds have been found to have congenital deficiency in RBC glutathione due to a defect in either of the two enzymes responsible for the synthesis of this tripeptide. Affected individuals have a hemolytic anemia with Heinz bodies that is aggravated by oxidant drugs. Deficiency of glutathione reductase has been reported, but its relationship to clinically significant hemolysis is not well established. Sometimes the deficiency state can be corrected by the administration of riboflavin (5 mg/d). Deficiencies of glutathione peroxidase and 6-phosphogluconate dehydrogenase have been observed, but their association with hemolysis is uncertain.

Other enzyme defects   Hemolytic anemia may sometimes be caused by abnormalities in enzymes of nucleotide metabolism. Individuals with pyrimidine 5′-nucleotidase deficiency have marked coarse basophilic stippling in their RBC because the mRNA of the cell is not properly metabolized. Hemolytic anemia also has been noted in individuals whose RBC have supranormal levels of adenosine deaminase and relatively low levels of ATP.

Hemoglobinopathies   The sickling disorders constitute an important form of congenital hemolytic anemia. Less commonly, hemolysis may be due to the inheritance of an unstable hemoglobin variant. →*For further discussion, see Chap. 106.*

ACQUIRED HEMOLYTIC ANEMIAS   In most patients with acquired hemolytic anemia, RBC are made normally but are prematurely destroyed because of damage acquired in the circulation. (The exceptions are rare disorders characterized by acquired dysplasia of the cells of the bone marrow and the production of structurally and functionally abnormal RBC.) The damage that occurs may be mediated by antibodies or toxins or may be due to abnormalities in the circulation, including an overactive mononuclear phagocyte system or traumatic lysis by natural or artificial impediments to circulation. The acquired hemolytic anemias can be classified into five categories (Table 108-5).

Hypersplenism   The spleen is particularly efficient in trapping and destroying RBC that have minimal defects. This unique ability of the spleen to filter mildly damaged RBC results from its unusual vascular anatomy (Chap. 63). Almost all the blood circulating through the spleen flows rapidly from arterioles in the white pulp to sinuses in the spleen's red pulp and then into the venous system. In contrast, a small portion of splenic blood flow (normally 1 to 2%) passes into the "marginal zone" of the lymphatic white pulp. Although the cells that occupy this zone are not phagocytic, they serve as a mechanical filter that hinders the progress of severely damaged blood cells. As RBC leave this zone and enter the red pulp, they flow into narrow cords, rich in macrophages, that end blindly but communicate with sinuses through small openings between the lining cells of the sinuses. These openings, averaging 3 μm in diameter, test the ability of RBC (4.5 μm in diameter) to undergo a deformation. RBC that cannot re-enter the vascular sinuses are engulfed by phagocytic cells and destroyed (see Fig. 63-1).

The normal spleen retains reticulocytes for 1 to 2 days but otherwise poses no threat to normal RBC until they become senescent. However, in the face of splenomegaly, increased destruction of the cells of the blood, including the RBC, may take place due to pooling of the blood in a relatively nutrient-poor environment full of phagocytic cells. When splenic sequestration causes cytopenia, hypersplenism is diagnosed. In infiltrative diseases of the spleen, substantial splenomegaly may exist with no apparent hemolysis; inflammatory and congestive splenomegaly is commonly associated with modest shortening of RBC survival time, along with more marked granulocytopenia and thrombocytopenia. Patients with cytopenia(s) sufficient to produce symptoms generally benefit from splenectomy.

Immunologic Causes of Hemolysis   Immune hemolysis in the adult is usually induced by IgG or IgM antibodies with specificity for antigens associated with the patient's RBC (often called "autoantibodies") (Table 108-6); rarely, transfused RBC may be hemolyzed by alloantibodies directed against foreign antigens on those cells (Chap. 114).

The Coombs antiglobulin test is the major tool for diagnosing autoimmune hemolysis. This test relies on the ability of antibodies specific for immunoglobulins (especially IgG) or complement components (especially C3) to agglutinate RBC when these proteins are present on the RBC. The *direct Coombs test* measures the ability of anti-IgG or anti-C3 antisera to agglutinate the patient's RBC. The presence or absence of IgG and/or C3 may help define the origin of the immune hemolytic anemia (Table 108-6). Rarely, neither IgG nor complement may be found on the RBC of the patient (Coombs-negative immune hemolytic anemia).

Antibodies to particular RBC antigens in the serum of the patient can be detected by reacting the serum with normal RBC bearing the antigen. IgM antibodies (usually cold-reacting) may be detected by agglutination of normal or fetal RBC. IgG antibodies may be detected by the *indirect Coombs test*, in which the serum of the patient is incubated with normal RBC and antibody is detected with anti-IgG, as in the direct Coombs test.

"Warm" antibodies   Antibodies that react with protein antigens are nearly always IgG and react at body temperature; occasionally, they are IgA and rarely IgM. Hemolysis due to autologous antibodies is called *autoimmune hemolytic (or immunohemolytic) anemia, warm antibody type.*

Table 108-5   Causes of Acquired Hemolytic Anemia

I. Entrapment
II. Immune
   A. Warm-reactive (IgG) antibody
   B. Cold-reactive IgM antibody (cold agglutinin disease)
   C. Cold-reactive IgG antibody (paroxysmal cold hemoglobinuria)
   D. Drug-dependent antibody
      1. Autoimmune
      2. Haptene
III. Traumatic hemolytic anemia
   A. Impact hemolysis
   B. Macrovascular defects—prostheses
   C. Microvascular causes
      1. Thrombotic thrombocytopenic purpura/hemolytic-uremic syndrome
      2. Other causes of microvascular abnormalities
      3. Disseminated intravascular hemolysis
IV. Hemolytic anemia due to toxic effects on the membrane
   A. Spur cell anemia
   B. External toxins
      1. Animal or spider bites
      2. Metals (e.g., copper)
      3. Organic compounds
V. Paroxysmal nocturnal hemoglobinuria

Table 108-6   Use of the Direct Coombs Test in Diagnosing the Cause of Autoimmune Hemolytic Anemia

Reaction with		Causes
Anti-IgG	**Anti-C3**	
Yes	No	Antibodies to Rh proteins, hemolysis caused by α-methyldopa or penicillin
Yes	Yes	Antibodies to glycoprotein antigens, SLE
No	Yes	Cold-reacting antibodies (agglutinins or Donath-Landsteiner antibody), most drug-related antibodies, IgM antibodies, IgG antibodies of low affinity, activation of complement by immune complexes

CLINICAL MANIFESTATIONS Immunohemolytic anemia of the warm antibody type is induced by IgG antibody and occurs at all ages, but it is more common in adults, particularly women. In approximately one-fourth of patients this disorder occurs as a complication of an underlying disease affecting the immune system, especially lymphoid neoplasms (Chap. 112); collagen vascular diseases, especially systemic lupus erythematosus (SLE); and congenital immunodeficiency diseases (Table 108-7). In the initial evaluation of the patient, drugs that are known to cause immunohemolytic anemia must be ruled out (see below). The presentation and course of IgG immunohemolytic anemia are quite variable. In its mildest form, the only manifestation is a positive direct Coombs test. In this instance, insufficient antibody is present on the RBC surface to permit the reticuloendothelial system to recognize the cell as abnormal.

Most symptomatic patients have a moderate to severe anemia [hemoglobin levels 60 to 100 g/L and reticulocyte counts 10 to 30% (200 to 600 $\times$ 10^3/μL)], spherocytosis (**Plate V-8**), and splenomegaly.

Severe immunohemolytic anemia presents with fulminant hemolysis associated with hemoglobinemia, hemoglobinuria, and shock; this syndrome may be rapidly fatal unless aggressively treated.

The direct Coombs test is positive in 98% of patients; usually IgG is detected with or without C3. Rarely, the cells may be agglutinated by the antibody, causing difficulty in analysis by flow cytometry.

Immune thrombocytopenia also may be present (*Evans's syndrome*), a disorder in which separate antibodies are directed against platelets and RBC. Occasionally, venous thrombosis occurs.

PATHOGENESIS IgG antibodies lyse RBC by two mechanisms: (1) immune adherence of RBC to phagocytes mediated by the antibody and by complement components that become fixed to the membrane (by far the more important mechanism of destruction), and (2) complement activation. Upon binding to Fc receptors on macrophages, the antibody-coated red cell is engulfed and destroyed. If internalization is only partial, the RBC membrane is removed, resulting in the formation of spherocytes, which are destroyed in the spleen. Complement-mediated immune adherence involves the interaction of C3b and C4b with receptors on the macrophage; while much less likely to lead to RBC lysis, this mechanism markedly increases the immune adherence due to IgG. Immune adherence, particularly that due to the IgG antibody, is also enhanced by the transit of RBC into the cords and sinuses of the spleen, which brings cells into intimate contact with phagocytic cells.

℞ **TREATMENT** Patients having a mild degree of hemolysis usually do not require therapy. In those with clinically significant hemolysis, initial therapy consists of glucocorticoids (e.g., prednisone, 1.0 mg/kg per day). A rise in hemoglobin is frequently noted within 3 or 4 days and occurs in most patients within 1 to 2 weeks. Prednisone is continued until the hemoglobin level has risen to normal values, and thereafter it is tapered rapidly to about 20 mg/d, then slowly over the course of several months. An algorithm for this tapering process is given in Fig. 108-4. For chronic therapy with prednisone, alternate-day administration is preferred. More than 75% of patients achieve an initial significant and sustained reduction in hemolysis; however, in half these patients the disease recurs, either during glucocorticoid tapering or after its cessation. Glucocorticoids have two modes of action: an immediate effect due to inhibition of the clearance of IgG-coated RBC by the mononuclear phagocyte system and a later effect due to inhibition of antibody synthesis. Splenectomy is recommended for patients who cannot tolerate or fail to respond to glucocorticoid therapy.

Patients who have been refractory to glucocorticoid therapy and to splenectomy are treated with immunosuppressive drugs such as azathioprine and cyclophosphamide. A success rate of ~50% has been reported with each. Intravenous gamma globulin may cause rapid cessation of hemolysis; however, it is not nearly as effective in this disorder as in immune thrombocytopenia.

Patients with severe anemia may require blood transfusions. Because the antibody in this disease is usually a "panagglutinin," reacting with nearly all normal donor cells, cross-matching is impossible. The goal in selecting blood for transfusion is to avoid administering RBC with antigens to which the patient may have alloantibodies. A common procedure is to adsorb the panagglutinin present in the patient's serum with the patient's own RBC from which antibody has been previously eluted. Serum cleared of autoantibody can then be tested for the presence of alloantibody to donor blood groups. ABO-compatible RBC matched in this fashion are administered slowly, with watchfulness for signs of an immediate-type hemolytic transfusion reaction.

PROGNOSIS In most patients, hemolysis is controlled by glucocorticoid therapy alone, by splenectomy, or by a combination. Fatalities occur among three rare subsets of patients: (1) those with overwhelming hemolysis who die from anemia; (2) those whose host defenses are impaired by glucocorticoids, splenectomy, and/or immunosuppressive agents; and (3) those with major thrombotic events coincident with active hemolysis.

When immunohemolysis develops as a complication of an under-

Table 108-7 Hemolysis due to Antibodies

WARM-ANTIBODY IMMUNOHEMOLYTIC ANEMIA

1. Idiopathic
2. Lymphomas: Chronic lymphocytic leukemia, non-Hodgkin's lymphomas, Hodgkin's disease (infrequent)
3. SLE and other collagen-vascular diseases
4. Drugs
   a. α-Methyldopa type (autoantibody to Rh antigens)
   b. Penicillin type (stable hapten)
   c. Quinidine type (unstable hapten)
5. Postviral infections
6. Other tumors (rare)

COLD-ANTIBODY IMMUNOHEMOLYTIC ANEMIA

1. Cold agglutinin disease
   a. Acute: *Mycoplasma* infection, infectious mononucleosis
   b. Chronic: Idiopathic, lymphoma
2. Paroxysmal cold hemoglobinuria

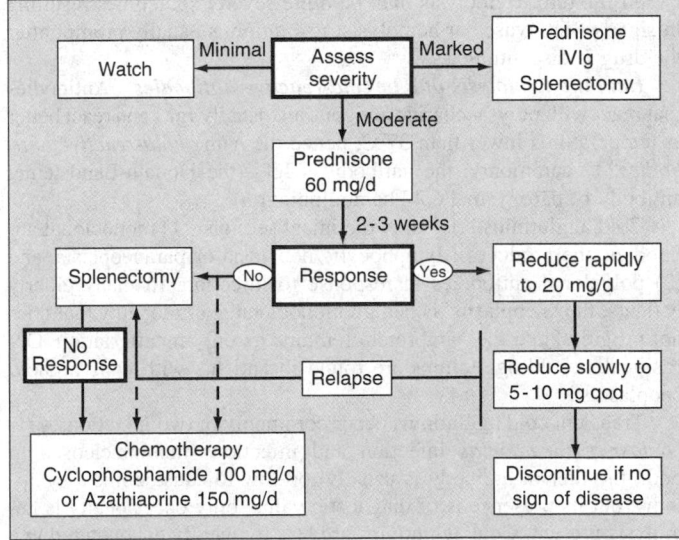

FIGURE 108-4 Algorithm for the treatment of patients with IgG-mediated immune hemolytic anemia. The patient with minimal disease may be watched carefully. The patient with very severe disease may need all modalities of treatment applied at once. The more common patient with moderate disease may be treated with prednisone at a high dose; if no response is seen, then either splenectomy or chemotherapy is given. If a response is seen, the dose of prednisone is reduced over time. If relapse occurs during this process, splenectomy or chemotherapy may be needed.

lying disorder, the prognosis is often dominated by that of the primary disease.

Immunohemolytic anemia secondary to drugs   Drugs cause immunohemolytic anemia by two mechanisms of action: (1) they induce a disorder identical in almost every respect to warm-antibody immunohemolytic anemia (e.g., α-methyldopa (an antihypertensive; Chap. 246), and (2) they become associated as haptenes with the RBC surface and induce the formation of an antibody directed against the RBC-drug complex (e.g., penicillin, quinidine).

A positive direct Coombs test is observed in up to 10% of patients receiving α-methyldopa therapy in doses of 2 g/d or higher. A small minority of these patients develop spherocytosis and hemolysis, which may be severe. α-Methyldopa alters and makes immunogenic the protein(s) of the Rh complex; the resulting antibodies cross-react with the normal Rh protein. Thus the antibody does not react with the drug, and the indirect Coombs test is positive in almost all patients even when the drug is not added to the test. The RBC are coated with IgG but not C3. Hemolysis decreases over the course of several weeks after cessation of drug therapy, although the direct Coombs test may remain positive for more than 1 year.

In most other cases of drug-induced hemolysis, the antibody is directed against the combination of the drug and the membrane glycoprotein to which it is attached. The hemolytic reaction in vivo is dependent on the presence of the drug and usually ceases shortly after the drug has been discontinued. Penicillin and its congeners may cause this type of reaction if the drug is given in very high doses (10 million units per day or more). The drug adheres relatively firmly to the protein of the RBC membrane. Complement is not usually fixed, and the hemolysis in vivo is usually not severe. Since the antibody is usually IgG, spherocytosis and splenic destruction may occur. Most other drugs (such as quinine, quinidine, sulfonamides, sulfonureas, phenacetin, stibophen, and dipyrone) do not adhere as tightly to their glycoproteins, and the drug-antibody complexes are removed during the washing steps of the direct and indirect Coombs reactions. These antibodies (particularly IgM) are usually able to fix complement, and these components remain on the RBC surface; thus the direct Coombs test is positive with anti-C3 but not anti-IgG. The antibody is detected in the *indirect* Coombs test only when the drug is added to the incubation mixture. Hemolysis may be quite severe, sometimes resulting in signs of intravascular hemolysis; resolution is usually prompt after the drug is discontinued.

Immune hemolysis due to cold-reactive antibodies   Antibodies that react with polysaccharide antigens are usually IgM and react better at temperatures lower than 37°C, hence the name *cold-reactive antibodies*. Uncommonly, the antibody is IgG (the Donath-Landsteiner antibody of paroxysmal cold hemoglobinuria).

Cold agglutinins arise in two clinical settings: (1) monoclonal antibodies, the product of lymphocytic neoplasia or paraneoplasia, and (2) polyclonal antibodies in response to infection. In many elderly patients, the "neoplasm" is benign monoclonal gammopathy that does not progress, and the paraprotein remains its only manifestation. Occasionally, cold agglutinins are found in patients with nonlymphoid neoplasms.

Transient cold agglutinins occur commonly in two infections: *Mycoplasma pneumoniae* infection and infectious mononucleosis. In both, the titer of antibody is usually too low to cause clinical symptoms, but its presence is of diagnostic value; only occasionally is hemolysis present. Cold agglutinins are less frequently encountered in a number of other viral infections. Their manifestations are usually benign.

The specificity of the antibody may be of diagnostic value. Cold agglutinins reacting more strongly with adult RBC than fetal (cord) RBC are called *anti-I*; these antibodies are seen in benign lymphoproliferation (chronic cold agglutinin monoclonal gammopathy) and in *Mycoplasma* infections. Those reacting more strongly with cord RBC cells are called *anti-i*; these antibodies are seen in aggressive

lymphomas and in infectious mononucleosis. Rarely, the antibody may react with other antigens that are equally expressed on adult and cord RBC. The clinical manifestations elicited by the antibody on exposure to cold are of two sorts: intravascular agglutination (acrocyanosis) and hemolysis. Acrocyanosis is the marked purpling of the extremities, ears, and nose when the blood becomes cold enough to agglutinate in the veins; it clears on warming and does not have the vasospastic characteristics of Raynaud's phenomenon (Chap. 248). Patients may also have symptoms when swallowing cold food or drinks.

The hemolysis is usually not severe and is manifested by a mild reticulocytosis, agglutination on the blood film, and agglutination during analysis of the blood by particle analysis (giving rise to a falsely high mean corpuscular volume). The degree of hemolysis depends on several variables.

1. *Antibody titer.* In general, the titer in symptomatic patients is above 1:2000 dilution of serum and may range to as high as 1:50,000. When collecting samples, great care must be taken that the serum is separated from the cells while the sample is maintained at 37°C so that the antibody will not adsorb onto the patient's own cells.

2. *Thermal amplitude of the antibody* (the highest temperature at which the antibody will react with the RBC). For most antibodies, this is 23 to 30°C. Those with a higher thermal amplitude (up to 37°C) are more hemolytic, since it is more likely that these temperatures will be encountered during RBC circulation.

3. *Environmental temperature.* Since the reaction can occur only at temperatures below body temperature, frequency and degree of exposure to cold are major determinants of the rate of hemolysis.

The hemolysis that occurs is due primarily to the hemolytic action of complement, since there are no functional Fc receptors for the IgM antibody. Complement is readily fixed; a single molecule of IgM is enough to effect binding of C1 and initiate the cascade. However, the normal human RBC is remarkably resistant to the hemolytic action of complement because of several defense mechanisms. Therefore, severe hemolysis with hemoglobinuria occurs only with massive activation of the antibody, such as by sudden cooling. The activation of complement is always marked by the accumulation of a degradation product of C3, C3dg, on the surface; this product is what is detected with appropriate antisera in the direct Coombs test in all patients with significant cold agglutinin disease. The cutaneous manifestations and hemolysis are best treated by maintaining the patient in a warm environment.

Splenectomy is usually not of value in this disorder. Glucocorticoids are of limited value, although patients with the panthermal variety of cold agglutinin disease may respond. Chlorambucil and cyclophosphamide are commonly used to treat patients who have hemolysis associated with monoclonal gammopathy, but their efficacy is usually marginal. Successful treatment of the malignant neoplasm responsible for the cold agglutinin often reduces the titer of antibody and the severity of the hemolysis.

Chronic cold agglutinin disease tends to be unremitting. The overall prognosis is dominated by the underlying lymphoproliferative disease, if present. In those patients in whom cold agglutinin disease appears to arise spontaneously, malignant lymphoma may develop after several years.

Paroxysmal cold hemoglobinuria (PCH)   Now a rare disorder, PCH was more frequent when tertiary syphilis was prevalent; now, most cases are either secondary to a viral infection or are autoimmune. PCH results from the formation of the Donath-Landsteiner antibody, an IgG antibody that is directed against the P antigen (Chap. 114) and that can induce complement-mediated lysis. Attacks are precipitated by exposure to cold and are associated with hemoglobinemia and hemoglobinuria; chills and fever; back, leg, and abdominal pain; headache; and malaise. Recovery from the acute episode is prompt, and between episodes patients are usually asymptomatic. When this syndrome accompanies acute viral infections (e.g., measles and mumps in children), it is self-limited but may be severe. Although the direct Coombs test may show complement to be present (seldom IgG), this test may be negative. The diagnosis is made by demonstrating cold-reacting IgG antibodies either by lytic tests (when the titer is very high) or by special antiglobulin tests. When PCH is secondary to syphilis, it responds to therapy for syphilis. Chronic autoimmune PCH may respond to prednisone or cytotoxic therapy (azathioprine or cyclophosphamide) but does not respond to splenectomy. The natural history of this disease often extends over many years.

Hemolysis due to Trauma in the Circulation RBC may be fragmented by mechanical trauma as they circulate; this circumstance leads to intravascular hemolysis and in most cases to RBC fragments called *schistocytes*. Schistocytes are identified by the sharp points that result from the faulty resealing of the fractured membrane (**Plate V-28**). Mechanical trauma leading to hemolysis occurs in three clinical settings: (1) when RBC flow through small vessels over the surface of bony prominences and are subject to external impact during various physical activities, (2) when RBC flow across a pressure gradient created by an abnormal heart valve or valve prosthesis (macrovascular), and (3) when the deposition of fibrin or small platelet thrombi in the microvasculature exposes RBC to a physical impediment that fragments them (microvascular) (Table 108-8).

External impact Hemoglobinemia and hemoglobinuria have been observed in a small proportion of individuals who have undergone a prolonged march or a prolonged run, most typically on a hard surface and while wearing thin-soled shoes. The role of direct external trauma in this process has been demonstrated by the fact that hemolysis can be prevented by the insertion of a soft inner sole in the runner's shoes. Similar types of hemolysis have been described following karate and the playing of bongo drums. No abnormality of RBC has been demonstrated, even during the acute episode. Susceptible individuals will develop hemoglobinemia and hemoglobinuria when exposed to the conditions described above. Muscle damage during some of these activities may produce myoglobinuria, but renal function is preserved. No specific therapy is required except to obtain better running shoes.

Macrovascular traumatic hemolysis Hemolysis associated with fragmented RBC (**Plate V-28**) occurs in approximately 10% of patients with artificial aortic valve prostheses. This incidence is somewhat greater with valves having stellite rather than Silastic occluders, greater with small valves as compared with larger valves, and greater when valves are cloth-covered or when there is a paravalvular leak. Traumatic hemolysis is rare in recipients of porcine valves. Severe hemolysis may occur after repair of ostium primum or endocardial cushion defects with a prosthetic patch. Mitral valve prostheses may produce hemolysis, but since the pressure gradient across these valves is lower than across aortic prostheses, the incidence is lower. A moderately shortened RBC survival time with little or no anemia occurs in some patients with severe calcific aortic stenosis. Indeed, almost any intracardiac lesion that alters hemodynamics may lead to some shortening of RBC survival. Traumatic hemolysis has been observed in patients who have undergone aortofemoral bypass.

Table 108-8   Changes in RBC and Platelets Induced by Intravascular Trauma

Etiology	Fragments	Hemolysis	Thrombocytopenia
Impact: march hemoglobinuria, etc.	0	+	0
Cardiac (turbulence):			
Aortic valve prosthesis	++++	++++	0
Mitral valve prosthesis	++	++	0
Calcific aortic stenoses	+	±	0
Vessel disease[a]	+++	+	+
Thrombotic thrombocytopenic purpura	++++	++++	++++
Hemolytic-uremic syndrome	++++	++++	++++
Adenocarcinoma	++++	++++	++++
Disseminated intravascular coagulation	++	±	++++

[a] Malignant hypertension, eclampsia, renal graft rejection, hemangiomas, immune disease (scleroderma).

CLINICAL MANIFESTATIONS In severe cases, hemoglobin levels fall to 50 to 70 g/L with reticulocytosis, fragmented RBC in the peripheral blood, depressed haptoglobin, elevated serum LDH, and hemoglobinemia and hemoglobinuria. Iron loss (as hemoglobin or hemosiderin) in the urine may lead to iron deficiency. The direct Coombs test may rarely become positive.

PATHOGENESIS A number of factors combine to cause the fragmentation of RBC by prostheses: (1) the shear stress resulting from turbulent blood flow, particularly when blood is forced through a small aperture by high pressure (e.g., a paravalvular leak around an aortic valve); (2) direct mechanical trauma of RBC at the time of seating of the occluder of the prosthetic valve; and (3) the deposition of fibrin across disrupted attachment points.

℞ **TREATMENT** Iron deficiency should be corrected by the administration of oral iron. The elevated hemoglobin that results may permit a decrease in the cardiac output and a slowing of the hemolytic rate. Limitation in physical activity also lessens the hemolytic rate. When these measures fail, any paravalvular leak must be repaired or the prosthetic valve replaced.

Microvascular traumatic hemolysis If fibrin or platelet microthrombi are deposited in arteriolar sites, RBC may be trapped on the meshwork and fragmented by high shear forces.

ABNORMALITIES OF THE VESSEL WALL Disorders such as malignant hypertension, eclampsia, renal allograft rejection, disseminated cancer, hemangiomas, or disseminated intravascular coagulation (DIC) may cause traumatic hemolysis. The degree of hemolysis induced by this family of disorders is usually quite mild, but a large number of fragments may be seen in the peripheral blood. In some patients, thrombocytopenia may be severe. Therapy is best directed at the primary disease. Thus, reversal of renal graft rejection, treatment of malignant hypertension and eclampsia, control of cancer, and the like, lead to a cessation of hemolysis. The relative importance of the primary vascular abnormality versus fibrin deposition is unclear.

Thrombotic thrombocytopenia purpura (TTP) This disorder is characterized by arteriolar lesions in various organs that contain platelet thrombi and produce thrombocytopenia and hemolytic anemia due to fragmentation of RBC. Tissue hypoxia resulting from vessel occlusion may cause organ dysfunction, most frequently manifest in the nervous system or the kidney. The disease affects individuals of all ages, but primarily young adults and more often women.

CLINICAL MANIFESTATIONS The classic pentad of TTP includes hemolytic anemia with fragmentation of erythrocytes and signs of intravascular hemolysis, thrombocytopenia, diffuse and nonfocal neurologic findings, decreased renal function, and fever. These signs and symptoms occur variably, depending on the number and sites of the arteriolar lesions. The anemia may be very mild to very severe, and the thrombocytopenia often parallels it. The neurologic and renal symptoms are usually seen only when the platelet count is markedly diminished (<20 to $30 \times 10^3/\mu L$). Fever is not reliably present. TTP may be acute in onset, but its course spans days to weeks in most patients and occasionally continues for months. Proteinuria and a moderate elevation of blood urea nitrogen may be found on initial presentation; the latter continues to rise while urine output falls if the patient develops renal failure. Neurologic symptoms develop in $>90\%$ of patients whose disease terminates in death. Initially, changes in mental status such as confusion, delirium, or altered states of consciousness may occur. Focal findings include seizures, hemiparesis, aphasia, and visual field defects. These neurologic symptoms may fluctuate and terminate in coma. Involvement of myocardial blood vessels may be a cause of sudden death. The severity of the disorder can be estimated from the degree of anemia and thrombocytopenia and the serum LDH level. Prothrombin time, partial thromboplastin time, fibrinogen concentration, and the level of fibrin split products are usually normal or only mildly abnormal. If the coagulation tests indicate a major consumption of clotting factors, the diagnosis of TTP is doubtful. A positive antinuclear antibody (ANA) determination is obtained in approximately 20% of patients.

PATHOGENESIS The manifestations of TTP can be explained by *localized* platelet thrombi. The agglutination of platelets is mediated by unusually large multimers of von Willebrand factor. Patients with TTP have acquired an antibody that inhibits a protease that normally cleaves von Willebrand factor. Arterioles are filled with hyalin material, presumably fibrin and platelets, and similar material may be seen beneath the endothelium of otherwise uninvolved vessels. Immunofluorescence studies have shown the presence of immunoglobulin and complement in arterioles. Microaneurysms of arterioles are often present. An association with pregnancy, AIDS, systemic lupus erythematosus (SLE), scleroderma, and Sjögren's syndrome suggests an immunologic origin.

DIAGNOSIS The combination of hemolytic anemia with fragmented RBC, thrombocytopenia, normal coagulation tests, fever, neurologic disorders, and renal dysfunction is virtually pathognomonic of TTP. Although they are not usually required for diagnosis, biopsies of skin and muscle, gingiva, lymph node, or bone marrow may show the typical arteriolar abnormalities. TTP must be distinguished from idiopathic thrombocytopenic purpura or Evans's syndrome (the former plus immunohemolytic anemia) by the finding of fragmented but not spherocytic RBC in the peripheral blood and a negative direct Coombs test.

R̲x̲ **TREATMENT** Plasma exhange permits >90% of patients to survive if therapy is promptly instituted. Many patients require daily or even twice daily plasmapheresis with plasma replacement. If a response is obtained (as indicated by increasing platelet count and decreasing plasma LDH and fragmented RBC), plasmapheresis may be done less frequently but sometimes must be continued for several weeks to months. Most patients also receive high doses of glucocorticoids and some receive platelet-active agents (dipyridamole, sulfinpyrazone, dextran, aspirin), but their efficacy is not proven. Vincristine, cyclophosphamide, or splenectomy has been used to treat patients who do not respond to plasma exchange. Even coma is not a contraindication to therapy, since full neurologic recovery is the rule in patients responding to therapy. Relapses have been noted in ~10% of patients but are usually responsive to retreatment. Platelet transfusions should not be given because they can precipitate thrombotic events.

Hemolytic-uremic syndrome This disorder is similar to TTP and is characterized by the same arteriolar lesions, which may be confined to the kidney, and by similar laboratory findings. It is usually encountered in young children. Often the patient has a prodrome of a gastroenteritic bloody diarrhea caused by *Escherichia coli* 0157:H7, and the lesions are thought to be due to the elaboration of Shiga-like verotoxins that damage renal vascular endothelial cells. This disorder has been associated with eating undercooked meat. Very rarely, the disorder appears to be familial. Patients present with acute hemolytic anemia, thrombocytopenic purpura, and acute oliguric renal failure. Most patients have either hemoglobinuria or anuria. Unlike TTP, neurologic manifestations are uncommon. The peripheral blood and coagulation tests are usually indistinguishable from those of TTP.

Patients are treated with plasmapheresis, dialysis, and transfusions. The efficacy of glucocorticoids, dextran, and heparin is uncertain. The mortality rate in children ranges from 5 to 20% but is considerably higher in adults. A disorder resembling the hemolytic-uremic syndrome has been described in adults treated with the antineoplastic drug mitomycin C, usually in combination with other drugs. It may also occur in patients receiving high-dose chemotherapy with autologous stem cell transplantation.

Disseminated intravascular coagulation Inappropriate activation of the clotting system with deposition of fibrin in small vessels may lead to RBC fragmentation in the microvasculature. RBC

fragmentation occurs in about one-fourth of patients with DIC (Chap. 117). The degree of hemolysis is much less in DIC than in either TTP or the hemolytic-uremic syndrome, and anemia with reticulocytosis is rare.

Environmental Alteration of the Red Cell Membrane by "Toxic" Effects A variety of infections may be associated with severe hemolysis. The microbes that cause bartonellosis (Chap. 163), as well as malaria and babesiosis (Chap. 214) directly parasitize RBC. *Clostridium welchii* (Chap. 145) produces a phospholipase that can cleave the phosphoryl bond of lecithin, thereby lysing human RBC. A mild, transient hemolysis frequently accompanies bacteremia with diverse organisms such as pneumococci, staphylococci, and *E. coli*.

Hemolysis may result from the direct action of snake and spider venoms on the RBC. Although cobra venom is directly lytic in vitro, the clinical disease induced by the bite of the cobra is one of moderate hemolysis associated with spherocytosis. Spider bites, particularly the bite of the brown recluse spider, induce acute intravascular hemolysis associated with spherocytosis and fragments of complement components on the RBC. The hemolysis continues for several days up to 1 week.

Copper has a direct hemolytic effect on RBC. Hemolysis has been observed after exposure of individuals to copper salts (such as during hemodialysis). Transient episodes of hemolysis occur in patients with Wilson's disease (Chap. 348).

The RBC membrane is unstable at temperatures above 49°C due to denaturation of the cytoskeletal protein spectrin. The RBC undergoes a process of budding, cleavage, and resealing above this temperature. Patients with extensive burns have prominent spherocytosis, hemoglobinemia, and sometimes hemoglobinuria.

Spur Cell Anemia Hemolytic anemia with bizarre-shaped RBC occurs in about 5% of patients with severe hepatocellular disease, particularly advanced Laennec's cirrhosis.

Clinical manifestations Anemia is more severe than is observed in otherwise uncomplicated cirrhosis. Hematocrit levels range between 15 and 25%. Splenomegaly is always present and is greater than in patients who have cirrhosis without spur cell anemia. Jaundice may be severe because of the hemolysis and liver dysfunction, and hepatic encephalopathy is common. The RBC are irregularly shaped with multiple spicules, and a small number of bizarre-shaped fragments are commonly seen on peripheral blood smears (**Plate V-27**). Reticulocytosis and other signs of hemolysis are present. The tests of liver function are typical of patients with severe cirrhosis.

RBC half-life is decreased to as short as 6 days (normal being 26 to 32 days); RBC destruction is localized to the spleen. Normal transfused RBC acquire the defect and have a survival time similar to that of the patient's own RBC.

Pathogenesis The surface membrane of a spur cell contains 50 to 70% excess cholesterol, but its total phospholipid content is normal. By contrast, the target-shaped RBC is more common in liver disease and has an excess of both cholesterol and phospholipid. The selective cholesterol excess in the spur cell is due to abnormal low-density lipoprotein with an increased mole ratio of free (unesterified) cholesterol to phospholipid. Cholesterol out of proportion to phospholipid decreases the fluidity of the spur cell membrane, and cell deformability is decreased. These rigid, cholesterol-laden RBC cannot pass through the filtering system of the spleen, further impeded by congestive splenomegaly in cirrhosis.

Diagnosis Patients with spur cell anemia have severe hemolysis and characteristic RBC morphology. Increasing anemia in a patient with chronic cirrhosis most commonly results from blood loss, folic acid deficiency, or iron deficiency.

RBC of similar morphology are seen in patients with abetalipoproteinemia. However, hemolysis is minimal.

Spur cells or acanthocytes have irregular spikes (irregular in length of projections and their spacing) and must be distinguished from regularly spaced, crenated RBC (echinocytes). Echinocytes are a frequent artifact on portions of some blood smears, and they are uniformly present in some patients with uremia ("burr cells") (**Plate V-3**). Small, dense crenated spheres (spheroechinocytes) are sometimes seen in congenital nonspherocytic hemolytic anemia due to enzyme deficiencies in the Embden-Meyerhof pathway (see above).

R̲x̲ **TREATMENT** Transfusion therapy is of limited benefit. Attempts to influence RBC cholesterol with various lipid-lowering agents have been unsuccessful. Splenectomy has been reported to prevent both the conditioning of RBC in the spleen and their premature destruction. However, splenectomy carries a high risk in patients with severe liver disease complicated by portal hypertension and coagulation defects. It must be reserved for patients in whom hemolysis is a major problem and who are relatively good surgical risks.

Prognosis Spur cell anemia occurs during the late stages of cirrhosis, and >90% of patients succumb to their underlying liver disease within 1 year of the diagnosis of spur cell anemia.

Paroxysmal Nocturnal Hemoglobinuria (PNH) This hemolytic disorder is distinctive because it is an intracorpuscular defect acquired at the stem cell level.

Clinical manifestations The three common manifestations of PNH are: hemolytic anemia, venous thrombosis, and deficient hematopoiesis. Anemia is highly variable with hematocrit values ranging from ≤20% to normal. RBC are normochromic and normocytic unless iron deficiency has occurred from chronic iron loss in the urine.

Granulocytopenia and thrombocytopenia are common and reflect deficient hematopoiesis. Clinical hemoglobinuria is intermittent in most patients and never occurs in some, but hemosiderinuria is usually present. The lack of two proteins, decay-accelerating factor (DAF, CD55) and a membrane inhibitor of reactive lysis (MIRL, CD59) (see below) make the RBC more sensitive to the lytic effect of complement.

DAF normally disrupts the enzyme complexes from either the classical (antibody-driven) pathway or the alternative pathway that activate C3 and C5; CD59 inhibits the conversion of C9 by the membrane attack complex C5b-8 to a polymeric complex capable of penetrating the membrane.

The platelets also lack these proteins, but the life span of the platelet is normal. However, the activation of complement indirectly stimulates platelet aggregation and hypercoagulability; this probably accounts for the tendency to thrombosis seen in PNH.

Venous thrombosis is a common complication of patients of European origin, affecting ~40% at one time or another; it is less common in Asian patients. It occurs primarily in intraabdominal veins (hepatic, portal, mesenteric) and results in the Budd-Chiari syndrome, congestive splenomegaly, and abdominal pain. It may occur in cerebral venous sinuses and is a common cause of death in patients with PNH. The bone marrow may appear normocellular, but in vitro marrow progenitor assays are abnormal. In about 15 to 30% of long-term survivors of aplastic anemia, PNH cells appear in the circulation; in some patients, the manifestations of PNH become dominant. Patients with PNH may have aplastic periods lasting from weeks to years. PNH may be seen in association with other stem cell disorders, including myelofibrosis, and (rarely) other myelodysplastic or myeloproliferative disorders.

Pathogenesis PNH is an acquired clonal disease, arising from an inactivating somatic mutation in a single abnormal stem cell of a gene on the X-chromosome (*pig-A*) important for the biosynthesis of the glycosylphosphatidylinositol (GPI) anchor. This anchor is necessary for the attachment of a number of proteins to the external membrane surface, and its partial or complete absence results in the absence of those proteins; to date, about 20 proteins have been found to be missing on the blood cells of patients with PNH. The normal clone of stem cells does not completely disappear, and the proportion of cells that are abnormal varies among patients and over time in a single patient.

Diagnosis PNH should be suspected in anyone with otherwise unexplained hemolytic anemia, especially with leukopenia and/or thrombocytopenia and with evidence of intravascular hemolysis (hemoglobinemia, hemoglobinuria, hemosiderinuria, elevated LDH). Any-

one recovering from aplastic anemia should be examined at intervals for the appearance of the diagnostic cells. The diagnosis is often delayed because (1) it is not considered, (2) hemoglobinuria is confused with hematuria, (3) elevation of the LDH is attributed to liver disease, and (4) the diagnostic tests (Ham's test and the sucrose lysis test) are not reliable.

For many years, the diagnosis of PNH depended on the demonstration of the lysis of RBC after complement activation either by acid (Ham or acidified serum lysis test) or by reduction in ionic strength (sucrose lysis test). These tests are inferior to the analysis of GPI-linked proteins (e.g., CD59, DAF) on RBC and granulocytes by flow cytometry.

R̲x̲ **TREATMENT** Transfusion therapy is useful in PNH not only for raising the hemoglobin level but also for suppressing the marrow production of RBC during episodes of sustained hemoglobinuria. Washed RBC are the preferred source to prevent exacerbation of hemolysis. Therapy with androgens sometimes results in a rise in hemoglobin level. Glucocorticoids reduce the rate of hemolysis in moderate doses (15 to 30 mg prednisone) on alternate days.

Iron deficiency is common. Iron replacement may exacerbate hemolysis because of the formation of many new RBC, which may be sensitive to complement. This occurrence may be minimized by giving prednisone (60 mg/d) or by suppressing the bone marrow with transfusions.

Acute thrombosis in PNH, particularly the Budd-Chiari syndrome and cerebral thrombosis, should be treated with thrombolytic agents. Heparin therapy should be instituted rapidly and maintained for several days before changing to coumadin therapy. Antithymoctye globulin (total dose of 150 mg/kg over 4 to 10 days) is often of use in treating marrow hypoplasia; prednisone counteracts the immune-complex disease that results from the administration of this foreign protein.

In patients with either hypoplasia or thrombosis who have an appropriate sibling donor, marrow transplantation should be considered early in the course of the disease. The usual conditioning programs are sufficient to eradicate the aberrant clone.

ANEMIA OF ACUTE BLOOD LOSS

The normal capacity to compensate for acute blood loss involves cardiovascular mechanisms, an adjustment in the oxygen affinity of hemoglobin, and an increase in erythropoiesis in the marrow. The signs and symptoms of blood loss relate to the volume of the blood loss and the time frame over which the hemorrhage occurs (Table 108-9). Losses of up to 20% of the blood volume are normally tolerated by redistribution of blood flow mediated by reflex venospasm, but the presence of fever or pain may interfere with this compensation. With larger losses, blood volume redistribution is not adequate to maintain normal blood pressure: initially, hypotension is only seen on standing, but with greater losses progressively greater problems are encountered

Table 108-9 Signs and Symptoms of Acute Blood Loss

Blood Loss		Symptoms	Signs
%,[a]	Volume, mL		
<20	<1000	Restlessness	+/- Vasovagal reaction
20–30	1000–1500	Anxiety, DOE	Orthostatic hypotension, tachycardia on exertion
30–40	1500–2000	Syncope on sitting or standing	Orthostatic hypotension, tachycardia at rest
>40	>2000	Confusion, shortness of breath	Shock, poor perfusion

[a] Based on an estimated total blood volume of 5000 mL (70-kg adult).

in maintaining blood pressure in sitting or supine positions. If the blood loss is more gradual, plasma volume increases, but albumin production usually lags behind the fluid shifts. It may take 2 to 3 days for the liver to generate the albumin lost in a 1500-mL bleed.

The most rapid hematologic adjustment to acute blood loss is an increase in oxygen delivery to the tissues. This is first mediated by the Bohr effect, where the more acidic milieu of the hypoperfused hypoxic tissues shifts the hemoglobin oxygen dissociation curve to the right. Over several hours the RBC increase their production of 2,3-bisphosphoglycerate, which also enhances the unloading of oxygen to tissues. These two mechanisms can substantially increase the capacity of RBC to deliver oxygen to the tissues.

The marrow response to hemorrhage is related to the generation of erythropoietin in the kidney in response to decreased oxygen tensions. A normal response depends on the production of erythropoietin, the presence of normal erythroid progenitors in the marrow, and an adequate supply of iron. If these three elements are normal, reticulocytes begin to increase in number in the first 2 days based on early release of reticulocytes from the marrow. However, it takes 3 to 6 days for erythroid hyperplasia to appear and 7 to 10 days before the erythropoietic response is maximal, producing reticulocyte counts up to 20 to 30%, a reticulocyte index of ≥ 3, and a marked increase in the marrow erythoid/granulocytic ratio.

DIAGNOSIS   Usually it is clear that a patient is bleeding; however, in some cases, large volumes of blood loss can occur internally from the gastrointestinal tract (esophageal varicies, cancer in the stomach or colon), a ruptured spleen, fractures and other trauma, or other lesions that can cause massive hemorrhage into the peritoneal cavity, pleural cavity, or the retroperitoneal space. Patients who have bled sufficiently to develop hypotension generally develop anemia, which is apparent only after volume replacement. The granulocyte count may increase to $\geq 20,000$ cells/μL and include immature cell types such as metamyelocytes and myelocytes. Epinephrine-induced demargination of peripheral granulocytes and release of cells from the marrow may account for this change. Nucleated RBC may appear in the circulation, and platelet counts may exceed $1 \times 10^6/\mu$L. The basis for the increased platelet count is unclear. Hemorrhage in an internal cavity is accompanied by a rise in unconjugated bilirubin and a fall in serum haptoglobin.

℞ TREATMENT   Treatment of the underlying cause of the hemorrhage is of paramount importance. If the patient is severely anemic or sufficiently hypovolemic, packed RBC should be transfused. In less severe cases, if the patient has normal kidneys (and presumably a normal erythropoietin response to anemia), normal bone marrow function, and an adequate supply of iron, no specific therapy for the anemia is required.

BIBLIOGRAPHY

AMIDON TM et al: Mitral and aortic paravalvular leaks with hemolytic anemia. Am Heart J 125:266, 1993

BEUTLER E: Study of glucose-6-phosphate dehydrogenase: History and molecular biology. Am J Hematol 42:53, 1993

FURLAN M et al: Von Willebrand factor-cleaving protease in thrombotic thrombocytopenic purpura and the hemolytic-uremic syndrome. N Engl J Med 339:1578, 1998

HIRONO A et al: Enzymatic diagnosis in non-spherocytic hemolytic anemia. Medicine 67:110, 1988

LUX SE, PALEK J: Disorders of the red cell membrane, in Blood: Principles and Practice of Hematology, RI Handin et al (eds). Philadelphia, Lippincott, 1995

MIWA S, FUJII H: Molecular basis of erythroenzymopathies associated with hemolytic anemia: Tabulation of mutant enzymes. Am J Hematol 51:122, 1996

ROSE M et al: The changing course of thrombotic thrombocytopenic purpura and modern therapy. Blood Rev 7:94, 1993

ROSSE WF: Paroxysmal nocturnal hemoglobinuria as a molecular disease. Medicine 76:63, 1997

TSAI H-M, LIAN E C-Y: Antibodies to von Willebrand factor-cleaving protease in acute thrombotic thrombocytopenic purpura. N Engl J Med 339:1585, 1998

109   Neal S. Young

APLASTIC ANEMIA, MYELODYSPLASIA, AND RELATED BONE MARROW FAILURE SYNDROMES

The hypoproliferative anemias associated with marrow damage include aplastic anemia, myelodysplasia (MDS), pure red cell aplasia (PRCA), and myelopthisis. Anemia in these disorders, which is normochromic, normocytic, or macrocytic and characterized by low reticulocyte count, is not a solitary or even the major finding in these diseases, which are better described as marrow failure states. In bone marrow failure, pancytopenia—anemia, leukopenia, and thrombocytopenia (sometimes in various combinations)—results from deficient hematopoiesis, as distinguished from blood count depression due to peripheral destruction of red cells (hemolytic anemias), platelets (idiopathic thrombocytopenic purpura or due to splenomegaly), and granulocytes (as in the immune leukopenias).

Hematopoietic failure syndromes are classified by dominant morphologic features of the bone marrow (Table 109-1). While practical distinction among these syndromes is clear in stereotypical cases, they can, of course, occur secondary to other diseases, and are so closely related that the differential diagnosis may be arbitrary, patients may seem to suffer from two or three related diseases simultaneously, or one diagnosis may appear to evolve into another. Finally, there is an important pathophysiologic relationship among these syndromes in their sharing of immune-mediated mechanisms of marrow destruction and some element of genomic instability resulting in a higher rate of malignant transformation.

APLASTIC ANEMIA

DEFINITION   Aplastic anemia is pancytopenia with bone marrow hypocellularity. Acquired aplastic anemia is distinguished from iatrogenic marrow aplasia, the common occurrence of marrow hypo-

Table 109-1   Differential Diagnosis of Pancytopenia

Pancytopenia with hypocellular bone marrow
  Acquired aplastic anemia
  Inherited aplastic anemia (Fanconi's anemia)
  Some myelodysplasia syndromes
  Rare aleukemic leukemia (AML)
  Some acute lymphoid leukemia
  Some lymphomas of bone marrow
Pancytopenia with cellular bone marrow
  Primary bone marrow diseases
    Myelodysplasia syndromes
    Paroxysmal nocturnal hemoglobinuria
    Myelofibrosis
    Some aleukemic leukemia
    Myelophthisis
    Bone marrow lymphoma
    Hairy cell leukemia
  Secondary to systemic diseases
    Systemic lupus erythematosus
    Hypersplenism
    B_{12}, folate deficiency
    Overwhelming infection
    Alcohol
    Brucellosis
    Sarcoidosis
    Tuberculosis
    Leishmaniasis
Hypocellular bone marrow ± cytopenia
  Q fever
  Legionnaires' disease
  Anorexia nervosa, starvation
  Mycobacteria

cellularity after intensive cytotoxic chemotherapy for cancer. Aplastic anemia can also be constitutional: the genetic disease Fanconi's anemia, while frequently associated with typical physical anomalies and the development of pancytopenia early in life, can also present as marrow failure in normal-appearing adults. Acquired aplastic anemia is often stereotypical in its manifestations, with the abrupt onset of low blood counts in a previously well young adult; seronegative hepatitis or a course of an incriminated medical drug may precede the onset. The diagnosis in these instances is uncomplicated. Sometimes blood count depression is moderate or incomplete, resulting in anemia, leukopenia, and thrombocytopenia in some combination. Aplastic anemia is related to both paroxysmal nocturnal hemoglobinuria (PNH; Chap. 108) and to MDS, and in some cases a clear distinction among these disorders may not be possible.

EPIDEMIOLOGY The incidence of acquired aplastic anemia in Europe and Israel is 2 cases per million persons annually. In Thailand and China, rates of 5 to 7 per million have been established. In general, men and women are affected with equal frequency, but there is a biphasic age distribution, with the major peak among older children and young adults and a second rise in the elderly.

ETIOLOGY The origins of aplastic anemia have been inferred from several recurring clinical associations (Table 109-2); unfortunately, these relationships are neither a reliable guide in an individual patient nor necessarily etiologic. In addition, while most cases of aplastic anemia are idiopathic, little other than history separates these cases from those with a presumed etiology such as a drug exposure.

Radiation Marrow aplasia is a major acute sequela of radiation. Radiation damages DNA; tissues dependent on active mitosis are par-

ticularly susceptible. Nuclear accidents can involve not only power plant workers but also employees of hospitals, laboratories, and industry (food sterilization, metal radiography, etc.), as well as innocents exposed to stolen, misplaced, or misused sources. While the radiation dose can be approximated from the rate and degree of decline in blood counts, dosimetry by reconstruction of the exposure can help to estimate the patient's prognosis and also to protect medical personnel from contact with radioactive tissue and excreta. MDS and leukemia, but probably not aplastic anemia, are late effects of irradiation.

Chemicals Benzene is a notorious cause of bone marrow failure. Vast quantities of epidemiologic, clinical, and laboratory data link benzene to aplastic anemia, acute leukemia, and blood and marrow abnormalities. The occurrence of leukemia is roughly correlated with cumulative exposure, but susceptibility must also be important, as only a minority of even heavily exposed workers develop benzene myelotoxicity. The employment history is important, especially in industries where benzene is used for a secondary purpose, usually as a solvent. Benzene-related blood diseases have declined with regulation of industrial exposure. Although benzene is no longer generally available as a household solvent, exposure to its metabolites occurs in the normal diet and in the use of lead-free gasoline. The association between marrow failure and other chemicals that contain a benzene ring is much less well substantiated; these chemicals may have been contaminated with benzene in manufacture, or petroleum distillates may have been used to dissolve the product.

Drugs (See Table 109-3) Many chemotherapeutic drugs have marrow suppression as a major toxicity; effects are dose-dependent and will occur in all recipients. In contrast, idiosyncratic reactions to

Table 109-2   Classification of Aplastic Anemia and Single Cytopenias

Acquired	Inherited
APLASTIC ANEMIA	
Secondary	Fanconi's anemia
Radiation	Dyskeratosis congenita
Drugs and chemicals	Shwachman-Diamond syndrome
Regular effects	Reticular dysgenesis
Idiosyncratic reactions	Amegakaryocytic thrombocytopenia
Viruses	Familial aplastic anemias
Epstein-Barr virus (infectious	Preleukemia (monosomy 7, etc.)
mononucleosis)	Nonhematologic syndrome
Hepatitis (non-A, non-B, non-	(Down's, Dubowitz, Seckel)
C hepatitis)	
Parvovirus B19 (transient	
aplastic crisis, PRCA)	
HIV-1 (AIDS)	
Immune diseases	
Eosinophilic fasciitis	
Hypoimmunoglobulinemia	
Thymoma/thymic carcinoma	
Graft-versus-host disease in	
immunodeficiency	
Paroxysmal nocturnal hemoglobi-	
nuria	
Pregnancy	
Idiopathic	
CYTOPENIAS	
PRCA (see Table 109-4)	Congenital PRCA (Diamond-Black-
	fan anemia)
	Transient erythroblastopenia of
	childhood
Neutropenia/Agranulocytosis	
Idiopathic	Kostmann's Syndrome
Drugs, toxins	Shwachman-Diamond syndrome
Pure white cell aplasia	Reticular dysgenesis
Thrombocytopenia	
Drugs, toxins	Amegakaryocytic thrombocytopenia
Idiopathic amegakaryocytic	Thrombocytopenia with absent radii

NOTE: PRCA, pure red cell aplasia.

Table 109-3   Some Drugs and Chemicals Associated with Aplastic Anemia

Agents that regularly produce marrow depression as major toxicity in commonly employed doses or normal exposures:
  Cytotoxic drugs used in cancer chemotherapy: *alkylating agents*, antimetabolites, antimitotics, some antibiotics

Agents that frequently but not inevitably produce marrow aplasia:
  Benzene (and benzene-containing chemicals such as kerosene, carbon tetrachloride, Stoddard's solvent, chlorophenols)

Agents associated with aplastic anemia but with a relatively low probability:
  Chloramphenicol
  Insecticides
  Antiprotozoals: *quinacrine* and chloroquine, mepacrine
  Nonsteroidal anti-inflammatory drugs (including *phenylbutazone*, indomethacin, ibuprofen, sulindac, aspirin)
  Anticonvulsants (*hydantoins*, *carbamazepine*, phenacemide, felbamate)
  Heavy metals (*gold*, arsenic, bismuth, mercury)
  Sulfonamides: some antibiotics, antithyroid drugs (methimazole, methylthiouracil, propylthiouracil), antidiabetes drugs (tolbutamide, chlorpropamide), carbonic anhydrase inhibitors (acetazolamide and methazolamide)
  Antihistamines (*cimetidine*, chlorpheniramine)
  D-Penicillamine
  Estrogens (in pregnancy and in high doses in animals)

Agents whose association with aplastic anemia is more tenuous:
  Other antibiotics (streptomycin, tetracycline, methicillin, mebendazole, trimethoprim/sulfamethoxazole, flucytosine)
  Sedatives and tranquilizers (chlorpromazine, prochlorperazine, piperacetazine, chlordiazepoxide, meprobamate, methyprylon)
  Allopurinol
  Methyldopa
  Quinidine
  Lithium
  Guanidine
  Potassium perchlorate
  Thiocyanate
  Carbimazole

NOTE: Terms set in italic show the most consistent association with aplastic anemia.

a large and diverse group of drugs may lead to aplastic anemia without a clear dose-response relationship. These associations rest largely on accumulated case reports, but a massive international study in Europe in the 1980s quantitated drug relationships, especially for nonsteroidal analgesics, sulfonamides, thyrostatic drugs, some psychotropics, penicillamine, allopurinol, and gold. Not all associations necessarily reflect causation: a drug may have been used to treat the first symptoms of bone marrow failure (antibiotics for fever or the preceding viral illness) or provoked the first symptom of a preexisting disease (petechiae by nonsteroidal anti-inflammatory agents administered to the thrombocytopenic patient). In the context of total drug use, idiosyncratic reactions, while individually devastating, are exceedingly rare events. Chloramphenicol, the most infamous culprit, reportedly produced aplasia in only about 1/60,000 therapy courses, and even this number is almost certainly an overestimate (risks are almost invariably exaggerated when based on collections of cases; although the introduction of chloramphenicol was perceived to have created an epidemic of aplastic anemia, its diminished use was not followed by a changed frequency of marrow failure). Risk estimates are usually lower when determined in population-based studies; furthermore, the low absolute risk is also made more obvious: even a 10- or 20-fold increase in risk translates, in a rare disease, to but a handful of drug-induced aplastic anemia cases among hundreds of thousands of exposed patients.

Infections   Hepatitis is the most common preceding infection, and posthepatitis marrow failure accounts for about 5% of etiologic associations in most series. Patients are usually young men who have recovered from a mild bout of liver inflammation 1 to 2 months earlier; the subsequent pancytopenia is very severe. The hepatitis is almost invariably seronegative (non-A, non-B, non-C, non-G) and presumably due to a novel, as yet undiscovered, virus. Fulminant liver failure in childhood can follow seronegative hepatitis, and marrow failure occurs at a high rate in these patients as well. Aplastic anemia can rarely follow infectious mononucleosis, and Epstein-Barr virus has been found in the marrow of a few aplastic anemia patients, some without a suggestive preceding history. Parvovirus B19, the cause of transient aplastic crisis in hemolytic anemias and of some pure red cell aplasia (see below), does not usually cause generalized bone marrow failure. Blood count depression is frequent in the course of many viral and bacterial infections but is comparatively moderate and resolves with the infection.

Immunologic Diseases   Aplasia is a major consequence and the cause of death in *transfusion-associated graft-versus-host disease*, which can occur after infusion of unirradiated blood products to an immunodeficient recipient. Aplastic anemia is strongly associated with the rare collagen vascular syndrome called *eosinophilic fasciitis*, which is characterized by painful induration of subcutaneous tissues (Chap. 313). Pancytopenia with marrow hypoplasia can also occur in systemic lupus erythematosus.

Pregnancy   Aplastic anemia very rarely may occur and recur during pregnancy and resolve with delivery or with spontaneous or induced abortion.

Paroxysmal Nocturnal Hemoglobinuria   An acquired mutation in the *PIG-A* gene in a hematopoietic stem cell is required for the development of PNH, but *PIG-A* mutations probably occur commonly in normal individuals. If the PIG-A mutant stem cell proliferates, the result is a clone of progeny deficient in glycosylphosphatidylinositol-linked cell surface membrane proteins (Chap. 108). Such PNH cells are now most accurately enumerated using fluorescence-activated flow cytometry of CD55 or CD59 expression on granulocytes rather than Ham or sucrose lysis tests on red cells. Deficient cells can be detected in about a quarter of patients with aplastic anemia at the time of presentation [and PNH cells are also seen in cases of hypocellular MDS (see below)]. In addition, functional studies of bone marrow from PNH patients, even those with mainly hemolytic manifestations, show evidence of defective hematopoiesis. Patients with an initial clinical di-

agnosis of PNH, especially younger individuals, may later develop frank marrow aplasia and pancytopenia; patients with an initial diagnosis of aplastic anemia may suffer from hemolytic PNH years after recovery of blood counts. One explanation for the aplastic anemia/PNH syndrome is selection of the deficient clones, perhaps because they are favored for proliferation in the peculiar environment of immune-mediated marrow destruction.

Congenital Disorders   Fanconi's anemia, an autosomal recessive disorder, manifests as progressive pancytopenia, increased chromosome fragility, congenital developmental anomalies, and an increased risk of malignancy. Patients with Fanconi's anemia typically have short stature; café au lait spots; and anomalies involving the thumb, radius, and genitourinary tract. At least seven different genetic defects have been defined by complementation analysis. The most common, type A Fanconi's anemia, is due to a mutation in *FANCA*. The function of the four cloned genes so far identified in Fanconi's anemia remains unknown.

Patients with Shwachman-Diamond syndrome may develop pancreatic insufficiency, malabsorption, and neutropenia and are at risk of aplastic anemia. Dyskeratosis congenita is an X-linked disorder characterized by mucous membrane leukoplasia, dystrophic nails, reticular hyperpigmentation, and the later development of aplastic anemia in about half of patients. Mutation in the *DKC1 (dyskerin)* gene has been found in some cases.

PATHOPHYSIOLOGY   Bone marrow failure results from severe damage to the hematopoietic cell compartment. In aplastic anemia, replacement of the bone marrow by fat is apparent in the morphology of the biopsy specimen (Fig. 109-1; **Plate V-13**) and magnetic resonance imaging of the spine; cells bearing the CD34 antigen, a marker of early hematopoietic cells, are greatly diminished; and in functional studies, committed and primitive progenitor cells are virtually absent—in vitro assays have suggested that the stem cell pool is reduced to ≤1% of normal in severe disease at the time of presentation. Qualitative abnormalities, such as limited number of operating stem cell clones or shortened telomere length, may follow from the quantitative deficiency, reflecting the shrunken and stressed state of hematopoiesis. An intrinsic stem cell defect exists for constitutional aplastic anemia, as cells from patients with Fanconi's anemia exhibit chromosome damage and death on exposure to certain chemical agents, but there is no convenient mechanism for the propagation of an *acquired* genetic abnormality that would produce a hypoproliferative (as opposed to neoplastic) disease. Aplastic anemia does not appear to result from defective stroma or growth factor production.

Drug Injury   Extrinsic damage to the marrow follows massive physical or chemical insults such as high doses of radiation and toxic chemicals. For the more common idiosyncratic reaction to modest doses of medical drugs, altered drug metabolism has been invoked as a likely mechanism. The metabolic pathways of many drugs and chemicals, especially if they are polar and have limited water solubility, involve enzymatic degradation to highly reactive electrophilic compounds; these intermediates are toxic because of their propensity to bind to cellular macromolecules. For example, derivative hydroquinones and quinolones are responsible for benzene-induced tissue injury. Excessive generation of toxic intermediates or failure to detoxify the intermediates may be genetically determined and apparent only on specific drug challenge; the complexity and specificity of the pathways imply multiple susceptible loci and would provide an explanation for the rarity of idiosyncratic drug reactions.

Immune-Mediated Injury   The recovery of marrow function in some patients prepared for bone marrow transplantation with antilymphocyte globulin (ALG) first suggested that aplastic anemia might be immune-mediated. Consistent with this hypothesis was the frequent failure of simple bone marrow transplantation from a syngeneic twin, without conditioning cytotoxic chemotherapy, which also argued both *against* simple stem cell absence as the cause and *for* the presence of a host factor producing marrow failure. Laboratory data support an important role for the immune system in aplastic anemia. Blood and bone marrow cells of patients can suppress normal hematopoietic pro-

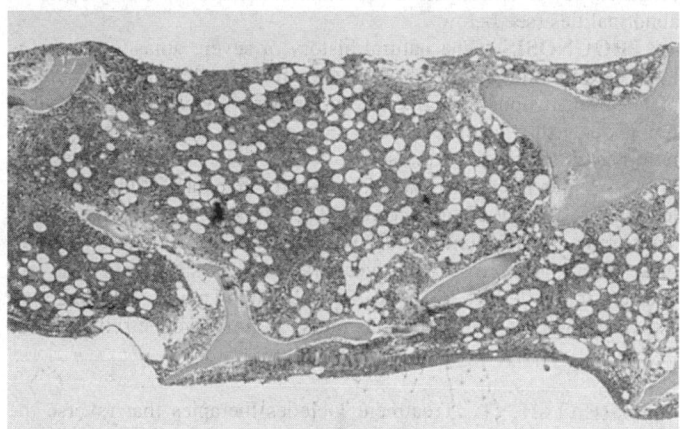
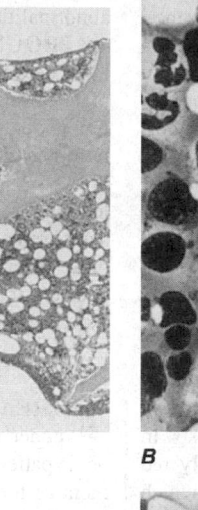

A

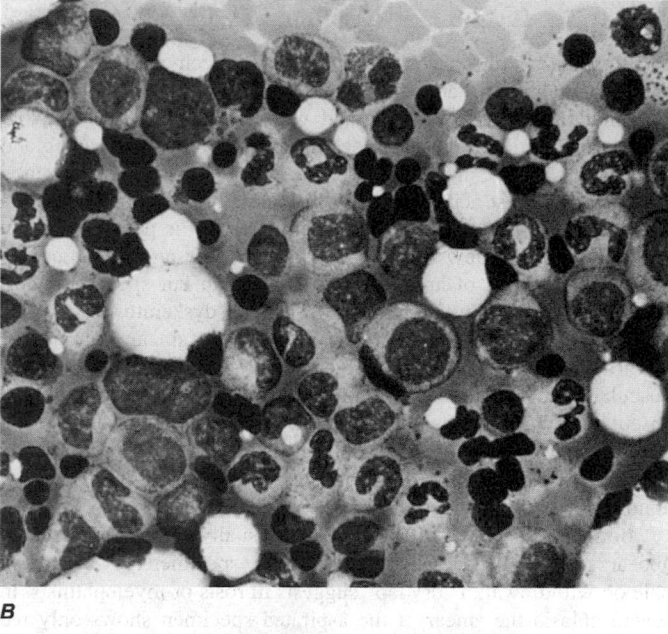

B

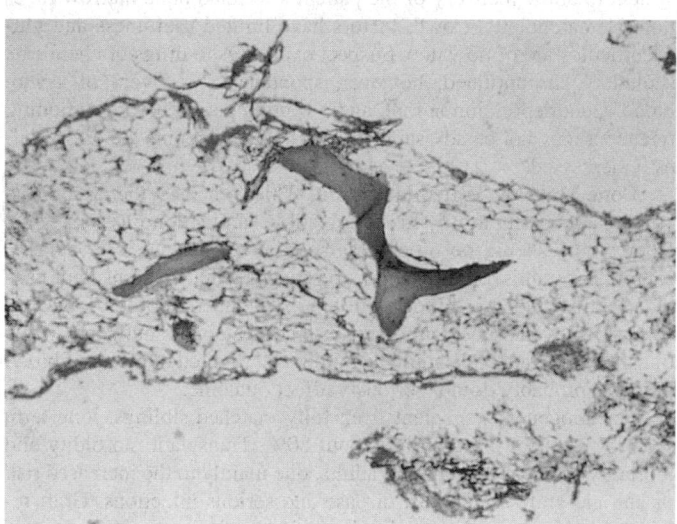

C

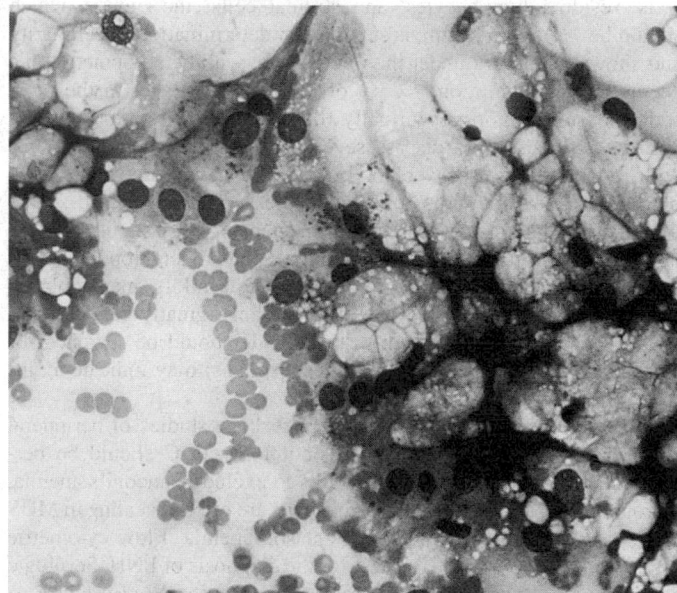

D

FIGURE 109-1 *A.* Normal bone marrow biopsy. *B.* Normal bone marrow aspirate smear. The marrow is normally 30 to 70% cellular, and there is a heterogeneous mix of myeloid, erythroid, and lymphoid cells. *C.* Aplastic ane-mia biopsy. *D.* Smear in aplastic anemia, showing replacement of hematopoietic tissue by fat and only residual stromal and lymphoid cells.

genitor cell growth, and removal of T cells from aplastic anemia bone marrow improves colony formation in vitro. Increased numbers of activated cytotoxic T cells are observed in aplastic anemia patients and usually decline with successful immunosuppressive therapy; cytokine measurements suggest a predominant T_H1 immune response (interferon γ, interleukin 2, and tumor necrosis factor). Interferon and tumor necrosis factor induce Fas expression on CD34 cells, leading to apoptotic cell death; localization of activated T cells to bone marrow and local production of their soluble factors are probably important in stem cell destruction.

Early immune system events in aplastic anemia are not well understood. Many different exogenous antigens appear capable of initiating a pathologic immune response, but at least some of the active T cells recognize true self-antigens. The rarity of occurrence of aplastic anemia despite common exposures (medical drugs, hepatitis virus) suggests that genetically determined features of the immune response can convert a normal physiologic response into a sustained abnormal autoimmune process.

CLINICAL FEATURES **History** Aplastic anemia can appear with seeming abruptness or have a more insidious onset. Bleeding is the most common early symptom; a complaint of days to weeks of easy bruising, oozing from the gums, nose bleeds, heavy menstrual flow, and sometimes petechiae will have been noticed. With thrombocytopenia, massive hemorrhage is unusual, but small amounts of bleeding in the central nervous system can result in catastrophic intracranial or retinal hemorrhage. Symptoms of anemia are also frequent, including lassitude, weakness, shortness of breath, and a pounding sensation in the ears. Infection is an unusual first symptom in aplastic anemia (unlike in agranulocytosis, where pharyngitis, anorectal infection, or frank sepsis occur early). A striking feature of aplastic anemia is the restriction of symptoms to the hematologic system, and patients often feel and look remarkably well despite drastically reduced blood counts. Systemic complaints and weight loss should point to other etiologies of pancytopenia. History of drug use, chemical exposure, and preceding viral illnesses must often be elicited with repeated questioning.

Physical Examination Petechiae and ecchymoses are often present, and retinal hemorrhages may be present. Pelvic and rectal examinations should be performed with great gentleness to avoid trauma; these will often show bleeding from the cervical os and blood in the stool. Pallor of the skin and mucous membranes is common except in the most acute cases or those already transfused. Infection on presentation is unusual but may be present if the patient has been symptomatic for a few weeks. Lymphadenopathy and splenomegaly are highly atypical of aplastic anemia. Café au lait spots and short stature suggest Fanconi's anemia; peculiar nails, dyskeratosis congenita.

LABORATORY STUDIES Blood The smear shows large erythrocytes and a paucity of platelets and granulocytes. Mean corpuscular volume (MCV) is commonly increased. Reticulocytes are absent or few, and lymphocyte numbers may be normal or reduced. The presence of immature myeloid forms suggests leukemia or MDS; nucleated red blood cells suggest marrow fibrosis or tumor invasion; abnormal platelets suggest either peripheral destruction or MDS.

Bone Marrow The bone marrow is usually readily aspirated but appears dilute on smear, and the fatty biopsy specimen may be grossly pale on withdrawal; a "dry tap" suggests fibrosis or myelophthisis. In severe aplasia the smear of the aspirated specimen shows only red cells, residual lymphocytes, and stromal cells; the biopsy, which should be >1 cm in length, is superior for determination of cellularity and shows mainly fat under the microscope, with hematopoietic cells occupying, by definition, <25% of the marrow space. In the most serious cases the biopsy is virtually 100% fat. The correlation between marrow cellularity and disease severity is imperfect. Some patients with moderate disease by blood counts will have empty iliac crest biopsies, while "hot spots" of hematopoiesis may be seen in severe cases. If an iliac crest specimen is inadequate, cells should also be obtained by aspiration from the sternum. Residual hematopoietic cells should have normal morphology, except for mildly megaloblastic erythropoiesis; megakaryocytes are invariably greatly reduced and usually absent. Areas adjacent to the spicule should be searched for myeloblasts. Granulomas (in cellular specimens) may indicate an infectious etiology of the marrow failure.

Ancillary Studies Chromosome breakage studies of peripheral blood using diepoxybutane (DEB) or mitomycin C should be performed on children and younger adults to exclude Fanconi's anemia. Chromosome studies of bone marrow cells are often revealing in MDS and should be negative in typical aplastic anemia. Flow cytometric assays have replaced the Ham test for the diagnosis of PNH. Serologic studies may show evidence of viral infection, especially Epstein-Barr virus and HIV. Posthepatitis aplastic anemia is typically seronegative. The spleen size should be determined by scanning if the physical examination of the abdomen is unsatisfactory. Magnetic resonance imaging may be helpful to assess the fat content on a few vertebrae in order to distinguish aplasia from MDS.

DIAGNOSIS The diagnosis of aplastic anemia is usually straightforward, based on the combination of pancytopenia with a fatty, empty bone marrow. Aplastic anemia is a disease of the young and should be a leading diagnosis in the pancytopenic adolescent or young adult. When pancytopenia is secondary, the primary diagnosis is usually obvious from either history or physical examination: the massive spleen of alcoholic cirrhosis, the history or metastatic cancer or systemic lupus erythematosus, or obvious miliary tuberculosis on chest radiograph (Table 109-1).

Diagnostic problems can occur with atypical presentations and among related hematologic diseases. While pancytopenia is most common, some patients with bone marrow hypocellularity have depression of only one or two of three blood lines, sometimes showing later progression to more recognizable aplastic anemia. The bone marrow in constitutional or Fanconi's anemia is indistinguishable morphologically from the aspirate in acquired disease. The diagnosis can be suggested by family history, abnormal blood counts since childhood, or the presence of associated anomalies of the skeletal and urogenital

systems. Patients with Fanconi's anemia may have no peculiar physical findings and can present with aplastic anemia as adults, in the third and fourth decades and, rarely, even later. Aplastic anemia may be difficult to distinguish from the hypocellular variety of MDS: MDS is favored by finding morphologic abnormalities, particularly of megakaryocytes and myeloid precursor cells, and typical cytogenetic abnormalities (see below).

PROGNOSIS The natural history of severe aplastic anemia is rapid deterioration and death. Provision first of red blood cell and later platelet transfusions and effective antibiotics were of some benefit, but few patients showed spontaneous recovery. The major prognostic determinant is the blood count; severe disease is defined by the presence of two of three parameters: absolute neutrophil count <500/μL, platelet count <20,000/μL, and corrected reticulocyte count <1% (or absolute reticulocyte count <50,000/μL). Survival of patients who fulfill these criteria is about 20% at 1 year after diagnosis; patients with very severe disease, defined by an absolute neutrophil count <200/μL, fare even more poorly. Treatment has markedly improved survival in this disease.

TREATMENT Treatment includes therapies that reverse the underlying marrow failure and supportive care of the pancytopenic patient. Severe acquired aplastic anemia can be cured by replacement of the absent hematopoietic cells (and the immune system) by stem cell transplant, or ameliorated by suppression of the immune system to allow recovery of the patient's residual bone marrow function. Hematopoietic growth factors have limited usefulness and glucocorticoids are of no value. Suspect exposures to drugs or chemicals should be discontinued; however, spontaneous recovery of severe blood count depression is rare, and a waiting period before beginning treatment may not be advisable unless the blood counts are only modestly depressed.

Bone Marrow Transplantation This is the best therapy for the young patient with a fully histocompatible sibling donor (Chap. 115). HLA typing should be ordered as soon as the diagnosis of aplastic anemia is established in a child or younger adult. In transplant candidates, transfusion of blood from family members should be avoided so as to prevent sensitization to histocompatability antigens; while transfusions in general should be minimized, limited numbers of blood products probably do not seriously affect outcome.

For allogeneic transplant from fully matched siblings, long-term survival rates for children are about 80%. Transplant morbidity and mortality are increased among adults, due mainly to the increased risk of chronic graft-versus-host disease and serious infections. Graft rejection was historically a major determinant of outcome in bone marrow transplant for aplastic anemia; high rates of primary or secondary graft failure may be related to the pathophysiology of marrow failure as well as to alloimmunization from transfusions.

Most patients do not have a suitable sibling donor. Occasionally, a full phenotypic match can be found within the family and serve as well. Far more available are other alternative donors, either unrelated but histocompatible volunteers, or closely but not perfectly matched family members. Survival using alternative donors is about half that of conventional sibling transplants. These patients will be at risk for late complications, especially a higher rate of cancer, if radiation is used as a component of conditioning. The majority of adults who undergo alternative donor transplants succumb to transplant-related complications.

Immunosuppression Used alone, ALG or antithymocyte globulin (ATG) induces hematologic recovery (independence from transfusion and a leukocyte count adequate to prevent infection) in about 50% of patients. The addition of cyclosporine to either ALG or ATG has further increased response rates to about 70 to 80% and especially improved outcomes for children and for severely neutropenic patients. Combined treatment is now standard for patients with severe disease. Hematologic response strongly correlates with survival. Improvement in granulocyte number is generally apparent within 2 months of treatment. Most recovered patients continue to have some degree of blood count depression, the MCV remains elevated, and the bone marrow cellularity returns towards normal only very slowly, if at all. Relapse (recurrent pancytopenia) is frequent, often occurring as cyclosporine is discontinued; most, but not all, patients respond to reinstitution of immunosuppression, and some responders become dependent on continued cyclosporine administration. Development of MDS, with typical marrow morphologic or cytogenetic abnormalities, occurs in about 15% of treated patients, usually but not invariably associated with a return of pancytopenia, and some patients develop leukemia. Although the laboratory diagnosis of PNH can generally be made at the time of presentation of aplastic anemia by flow cytometry, recovered patients showing frank hemolysis or, less commonly, thrombosis should be retested for PNH. Bone marrow examinations should be performed annually or if there is an unfavorable change in blood counts.

Horse ATG (ATGAM; Upjohn) is given at 40 mg/kg per day for 4 days; rabbit ALG (Thymoglobulin; SangStat), is administered at 3.5 mg/kg per day for 5 days. For ATG, anaphylaxis is a rare but occasionally fatal complication; allergy should be tested by a prick skin test with an undiluted solution and immediate observation, desensitization is feasible. ATG binds to peripheral blood cells, and therefore, platelet and granulocyte numbers may fall further during active treatment. Serum sickness, a flulike illness with a characteristic cutaneous eruption and arthralgia, often develops about 10 days after initiating treatment. Most patients are given methylprednisolone, 1 mg/kg per day for 2 weeks, to ameliorate the immune consequences of heterologous protein infusion. Excessive or extended glucocorticoid therapy is associated with avascular joint necrosis. Cyclosporine is administered orally at an initial dose of 12 mg/kg per day in adults (15 mg/kg per day in children), with subsequent adjustment according to blood levels obtained every 2 weeks. Trough levels should be between 150 and 200 ng/mL. The most important side effects of chronic cyclosporine treatment are nephrotoxicity, hypertension, seizures, and opportunistic infections, especially *Pneumocystis carinii* (prophylactic treatment with monthly inhaled pentamidine is recommended).

Most patients with aplastic anemia lack a suitable marrow donor and immunosuppression is the treatment of choice. Long-term survival is equivalent with transplantation and immunosuppression. However, successful transplant cures marrow failure, while patients who recover adequate blood counts after immunosuppression remain at risk of relapse and malignant evolution. Because of the excellent results in children, allogeneic transplant should always be performed in the pediatric population if a suitable sibling donor is available. Increasing age and the severity of neutropenia are the most important factors weighing in the decision between transplant and immunosuppression in adults who have a matched family donor: older patients do better with ATG and cyclosporine, while transplant is preferred if granulocytopenia is profound. Some reluctant patients may be treated by immunosuppression followed by transplant for failure to recover blood counts or occurrence of late complications.

Outcomes following both transplant and immunosuppression have improved with time. High doses of cyclophosphamide, without stem cell rescue, have been reported to produce durable hematologic recovery, without relapse or evolution to MDS, but this treatment can produce sustained severe neutropenia and response is often delayed. Novel immunosuppressive drugs such as mycophenolate mofetil may further improve outcome.

Other Therapies The effectiveness of androgen therapy has not been verified in controlled trials, but occasional patients will respond or even demonstrate blood count dependence on continued therapy. For patients with moderate disease or those with severe pancytopenia who have failed immunosuppression, a 3- to 4-month trial is appropriate. Hematopoietic growth factors, granulocyte colony stimulating factor (G-CSF), granulocyte-macrophage CSF (GM-CSF), and interleukin 3, are not recommended as initial therapy for severe aplastic anemia, and even their role as adjuncts to immunosuppression is not well defined. Some patients may respond to chronic administration of growth factors in combination after failing immunosuppression. Sple-

nectomy may occasionally increase blood counts in relapsed or refractory cases.

Supportive Care Meticulous medical attention is required so that the patient may survive to benefit from definitive therapy or, having failed treatment, to maintain a reasonable existence in the face of pancytopenia. First and most important, infection in the presence of severe neutropenia must be aggressively treated by prompt institution of parenteral, broad-spectrum antibiotics, usually ceftazadime or a combination of an aminoglycoside, cephalosporin, and semisynthetic penicillin. Therapy is empirical and must not await results of culture, although specific foci of infection such as oropharyngeal or anorectal abscesses, pneumonia, sinusitis, and typhlitis (necrotizing colitis) should be sought on physical examination and with radiographic studies. When indwelling plastic catheters become contaminated, vancomycin should be added. Persistent or recrudescent fever implies fungal disease: *Candida* or *Aspergillus* are common, especially after several courses of antibacterial antibiotics, and a progressive course may be averted by timely initiation of amphotericin. Granulocyte transfusions using G-CSF–mobilized peripheral blood have been effective in the treatment of overwhelming infections in a few patients. Hand washing, the single most effective method of preventing the spread of infection, remains a neglected practice. Nonabsorbed antibiotics for gut decontamination are poorly tolerated and not of proven value. Total reverse isolation is not clearly beneficial in reducing mortality from infections.

Both platelet and erythrocyte numbers can be maintained by transfusion. Alloimmunization limits the usefulness of platelet transfusions and can be avoided or minimized by several strategies, including use of single donors to reduce exposure and physical or chemical methods to diminish leukocytes in the product; HLA-matched platelets are often effective in patients refractory to random donor products. Inhibitors of fibrinolysis such as aminocaproic acid have not been shown to relieve mucosal oozing; the use of low-dose glucocorticoids to induce "vascular stability" is unproven. Whether platelet transfusions are better used prophylactically or only as needed remains unclear. Any rational regimen of prophylaxis requires transfusions once or twice weekly in order to maintain the platelet count $>10,000/\mu L$ (oozing from the gut, and presumably also from other vascular beds, increases precipitously at counts $<5000/\mu L$). Menstruation should be suppressed either by oral estrogens or nasal follicle-stimulating hormone/luteinizing hormone (FSH/LH) antagonists. Aspirin and other nonsteroidal anti-inflammatory agents inhibit platelet function and must be avoided.

Red blood cells should be transfused to maintain a normal level of activity, usually at a hemoglobin value of 70 g/L (90 g/L if there is underlying cardiac or pulmonary disease); a regimen of 2 units every 2 weeks will replace normal losses in a patient without a functioning bone marrow. In chronic anemia, the iron chelator deferoxamine should be added at the time of the fiftieth transfusion in order to avoid secondary hemochromatosis.

PURE RED CELL APLASIA

More restricted forms of marrow failure occur, in which only a single circulating cell type is affected and the aregenerative marrow shows corresponding absence or decreased numbers of specific precursor cells: aregenerative anemia as in PRCA (see below), thrombocytopenia with amegakaryocytosis (Chap. 116), and neutropenia without marrow myeloid cells in agranulocytosis (Chap. 64). In general, and in contrast to aplastic anemia and MDS, the unaffected lineages appear quantitatively and qualitatively normal. Agranulocytosis, the most frequent of these syndromes, is usually a complication of medical drug use (with agents similar to those related to aplastic anemia), either by a mechanism of direct chemical toxicity or by immunologic mediation. Agranulocytosis has an incidence similar to aplastic anemia but is especially frequent among the elderly and in women. The syndrome should resolve with discontinuation of exposure, but significant mortality is attached to neutropenia in the older and often previously unwell patient. Both pure white cell aplasia (agranulocytosis without incriminating drug exposure) and amegakaryocytic thrombocytopenia are exceedingly rare and, like PRCA, appear to be due to destructive antibodies or lymphocytes and can respond to immunosuppressive therapies. In all the single lineage failure syndromes, progression to pancytopenia or leukemia is unusual.

DEFINITION AND DIFFERENTIAL DIAGNOSIS   PRCA is characterized by anemia, reticulocytopenia, and absent or rare erythroid precursor cells in the bone marrow. The classification of PRCA is shown in Table 109-4. In adults, PRCA is acquired. An identical syndrome can occur constitutionally: Diamond-Blackfan anemia, or congenital PRCA, is diagnosed at birth or in early childhood and often responds to glucocorticoid treatment. Temporary red cell failure occurs in transient aplastic crisis of hemolytic anemias, due to acute parvovirus infection (Chap. 187), and in transient erythroblastopenia of childhood, which affects normal children.

CLINICAL ASSOCIATIONS AND ETIOLOGY   PRCA has important associations with immune system diseases. A small minority of cases occur with a thymoma. More frequently, red cell aplasia can be the major manifestation of large granular lymphocytosis or may occur in chronic lymphocytic leukemia. Some patients may be hypogammaglobulinemic. As with agranulocytosis, PRCA can be due to an idiosyncratic reaction to a drug.

Like aplastic anemia, PRCA results from diverse mechanisms. Antibodies to red blood cell precursors are frequently present in the blood, but T cell inhibition is probably the more common immune mechanism. Cytotoxic lymphocyte activity restricted by histocompatibility locus or specific for human T cell leukemia/lymphoma virus I–infected cells, as well as natural killer cell activity inhibitory of erythropoiesis, have been demonstrated in particularly well-studied individual cases.

Persistent Parvovirus B19 Infection   Chronic parvovirus infection is an important, treatable cause of PRCA. This common virus causes a benign exanthem of childhood (fifth disease) and a polyarthralgia syndrome in adults. In patients with underlying hemolysis (or any condition that increases demand for red blood cell production), parvovirus infection can cause a transient aplastic crisis and an abrupt but temporary worsening of the anemia due to failed erythropoiesis. In normal individuals, acute infection is resolved by production of neutralizing antibodies to the virus, but in the setting of congenital, acquired, or iatrogenic immunodeficiency, persistent viral infection

may occur. The bone marrow shows red cell aplasia and the presence of giant pronormoblasts (Fig. 109-2), the cytopathic sign of B19 parvovirus infection and highly suggestive of the diagnosis. Viral tropism for human erythroid progenitor cells is due to its use of erythrocyte P antigen as a cellular receptor for entry. Direct cytotoxicity of virus causes anemia if demands on erythrocyte production are high; in normal individuals, the temporary cessation of red cell production is not clinically apparent, and skin and joint symptoms are mediated by immune complex deposition.

TREATMENT   History, physical examination, and routine laboratory studies may disclose an underlying disease or a suspect drug exposure. Thymoma should be sought by radiographic procedures. Tumor excision is indicated, but anemia does not necessarily improve with surgery. The diagnosis of parvovirus infection requires detection of viral DNA sequences in the blood (IgG and IgM antibodies are commonly absent). The presence of erythroid colonies has been considered predictive of response to immunosuppressive therapy in idiopathic PRCA.

Red cell aplasia is compatible with long survival with supportive care alone, a combination of erythrocyte transfusions and iron chelation. For persistent B19 parvovirus infection, almost all patients respond to intravenous immunoglobulin therapy (for example, 0.4 g/kg daily for 5 days), although relapse and retreatment may be expected, especially in patients with AIDS. The majority of patients with idiopathic PRCA respond favorably to immunosuppression. Most first receive a course of glucocorticoids, followed in the absence of a response by cyclosporine, ATG, azathioprine, or cyclophosphamide.

MYELODYSPLASIA

DEFINITION   The myelodysplastic syndromes are a heterogeneous group of hematologic disorders broadly characterized by cytopenias associated with a dysmorphic (or abnormal appearing) and usually cellular bone marrow, and consequent ineffective blood cell production (Table 109-5). The current nomenclature was developed by the French-American-British (FAB) Cooperative Group and, while increasing recognition of the syndromes, is not entirely satisfactory: chronic myelomonocytic leukemia, while associated with dysplastic morphology, behaves as a myeloproliferative disease; sideroblastic anemias likely have a distinctive etiology; and the borderline between refractory anemia with excess blasts in transformation and acute myeloid leukemia is so arbitrary as to have been abandoned in the most recent World Health Organization classification. The FAB scheme has been recently supplemented by the International Prognostic Scoring System (IPSS; Table 109-6).

EPIDEMIOLOGY   Idiopathic MDS is a disease of the elderly; the mean age at onset is 68 years. There is a slight male preponderance. MDS is a relatively common form of bone marrow failure, with incidence rates reported of 35 to >100 per million persons in the general population and 120 to >500 per million in the aged. MDS is rare in children, but monocytic leukemia can be seen. Therapy-related MDS is not age-related and may occur in as many as 15% of patients within a decade following intensive combined modality treatment for cancer. Rates of MDS have increased over time, due to the recognition of the syndrome by physicians and the aging of the population.

ETIOLOGY AND PATHOPHYSIOLOGY   The myelodysplastic syndromes have been convincingly linked to environmental exposures such as radiation and benzene; other risk factors have been reported inconsistently. Secondary MDS occurs as a stereotypical late toxicity of cancer treatment, usually with a combination of radiation and the radiomimetic alkylating agents such as busulfan, nitrosourea, or procarbazine (with a latent period of 5 to 7 years) or the DNA topoisomerase inhibitors (2 years). Both acquired aplastic anemia following immunosuppressive treatment and Fanconi's anemia can evolve into MDS.

MDS is a clonal hematopoietic stem cell disorder leading to impaired cell proliferation and differentiation. Cytogenetic abnormalities

---

Table 109-4   Classification of Pure Red Cell Aplasia

Self-limited
  Transient erythroblastopenia of childhood
  Transient aplastic crisis of hemolysis (B19 parvovirus infection)
Fetal red blood cell aplasia
  Nonimmune hydrops fetalis (in utero B19 parvovirus infection)
Hereditary pure red cell aplasia
  Congenital pure red cell aplasia (Diamond-Blackfan syndrome)
Acquired pure red cell aplasia
  Thymoma and malignancy
    Thymoma
    Lymphoid malignancies (and more rarely other hematologic diseases)
    Paraneoplastic to solid tumors
  Connective tissue disorders with immunologic abnormalities
    Systemic lupus erythematosus, juvenile rheumatoid arthritis, rheumatoid arthritis
    Multiple endocrine gland insufficiency
  Virus
    B19 parvovirus, hepatitis, adult T cell leukemia virus, Epstein-Barr virus
  Pregnancy
  Drugs
    Especially phenytoin, azathioprine, chloramphenicol, procaineamide, isoniazid
  Idiopathic

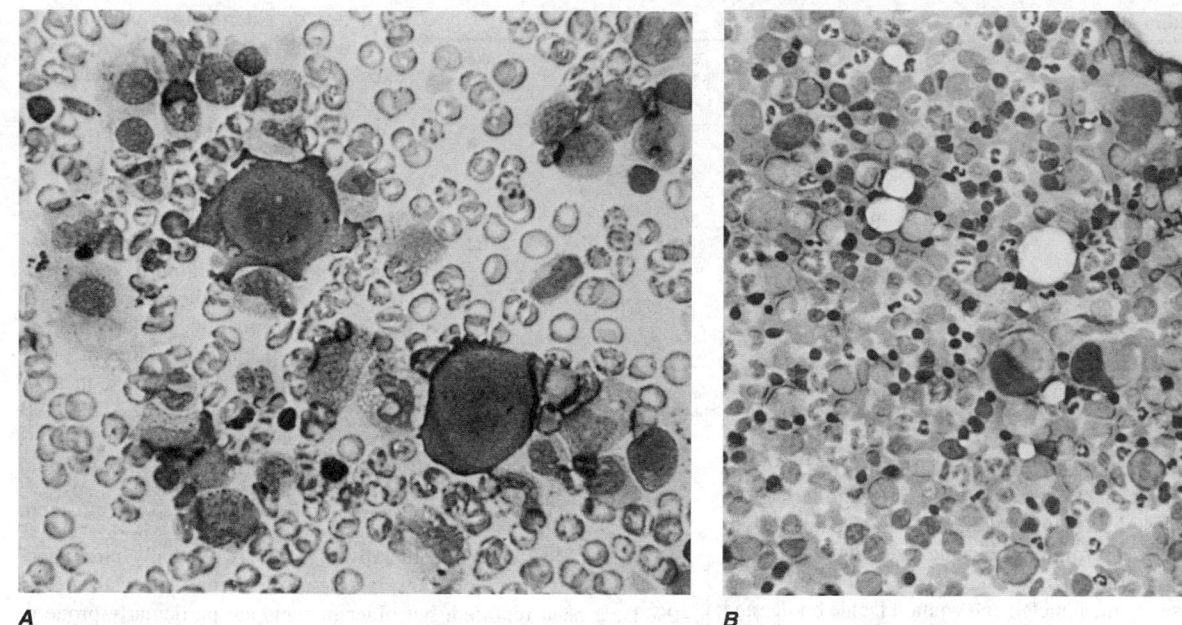

A

B

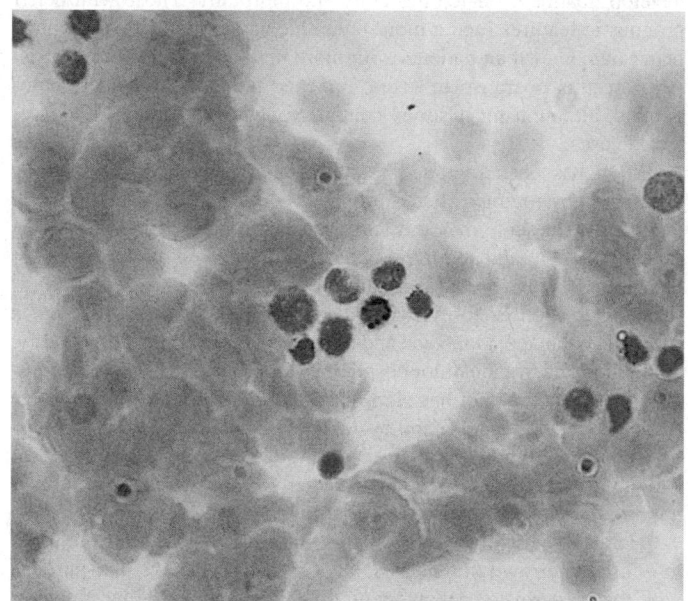

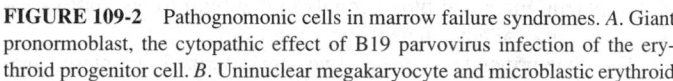

C

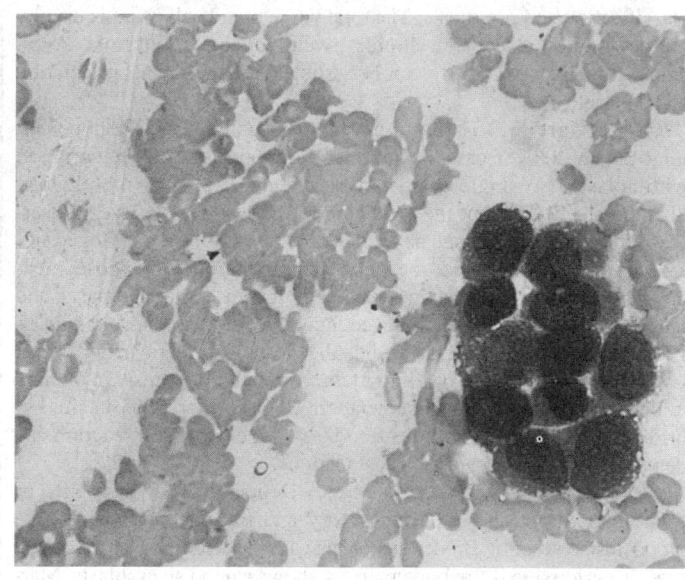

D

FIGURE 109-2 Pathognomonic cells in marrow failure syndromes. *A*. Giant pronormoblast, the cytopathic effect of B19 parvovirus infection of the erythroid progenitor cell. *B*. Uninuclear megakaryocyte and microblastic erythroid precursors typical of the 5q- myelodysplasia syndrome. *C*. Ringed sideroblast showing perinuclear iron granules. *D*. Tumor cells present on a touch preparation made from the marrow biopsy of a patient with metastatic carcinoma.

are found in about half of patients, and some of the same specific lesions are also seen in frank leukemia; deletions are more frequent than translocations. Both presenting and evolving hematologic manifestations result from the accumulation of multiple genetic lesions, loss of tumor suppressor genes, activating oncogene mutations, or other harmful alterations. Cytogenetic abnormalities are not random (loss of all or part of 5, 7, and 20, trisomy of 8) and may be related to etiology (11q23 following topoisomerase II inhibitors); chronic myelomonocytic leukemia is often associated with t(5;12) that creates a chimeric *tel-PDGFβ* gene. The type and number of cytogenetic abnormalities strongly correlate with the probability of leukemic transformation and survival. Mutations of N-*ras* (an oncogene), *p53* and *IRF-1* (tumor suppressor genes), *Bcl-2* (an antiapoptotic gene), and others have been reported in some patients but may occur relatively late in the sequence leading to leukemic transformation. Apoptosis of marrow cells is increased in MDS, presumably due to these acquired genetic alterations or possibly to an overlaid immune response. Sideroblastic anemia may be related to mutations in mitochondrial genes. Ineffective erythropoiesis and disordered iron metabolism are the functional consequences of the genetic alterations.

CLINICAL FEATURES Anemia dominates the early course. Most symptomatic patients complain of the gradual onset of fatigue and weakness, dyspnea, and pallor, but at least half the patients are asymptomatic and MDS is discovered only incidentally on routine blood counts. Previous chemotherapy or radiation exposure is an important historic fact. Fever and weight loss should point to a myeloproliferative rather than myelodysplastic process. Children with Down's syndrome are susceptible to MDS, and a family history may indicate a hereditary form of sideroblastic anemia or Fanconi's anemia.

The physical examination is remarkable for signs of anemia; about 20% of patients have splenomegaly. Some unusual skin lesions, including Sweet's syndrome (febrile neutrophilic dermatosis), have been associated with MDS.

LABORATORY STUDIES **Blood** Anemia is present in the majority of cases, either alone or as part of bi- or pancytopenia; isolated neutropenia or thrombocytopenia is more unusual. Macrocytosis

Table 109-5 Classification of Myelodysplasia (MDS)

Subtype	Blood	Marrow[a]	% of MDS Cases	Median Survival, Months	Leukemic Evolution, %[b]
Refractory anemia	Blasts <1%	Blasts <5%	27	50	16
Refractory anemia with ringed sidero-blasts	Blasts <1%	Blasts <5%	20	65	15
Refractory anemia with excess blasts	Blasts ≤5%	Blasts 5–20%	26	15	48
Refractory anemia with excess blasts in transformation	Blasts >5%	Blasts 20–30% or Auer rods	13	9	62
Chronic myelomonocytic leukemia	≥1 × 10⁹/L monocytes	Any number	14	23	29

[a] By definition, the bone marrow of acute myeloid leukemia contains >30% blasts.
[b] Leukemic evolution refers to the percentage of cases that transform into acute myeloid leukemia.

is common, and the smear may be dimorphic with a distinctive population of large red blood cells. Platelets are also large and lack granules. In functional studies, they may show marked abnormalities, and patients may have bleeding symptoms despite seemingly adequate numbers. Neutrophils are hypogranulated; have hyposegmented, ringed, or abnormally segmented nuclei; and contain Dohle bodies and may be functionally deficient. Circulating myeloblasts usually correlate with marrow blast numbers, and their quantitation is important for classification and prognosis. The total white blood cell count is usually normal or low, except in chronic myelomonocytic leukemia. As in aplastic anemia, MDS also can be associated with a clonal population of PNH cells.

Bone Marrow The bone marrow is usually normal or hypercellular but in 20% of cases is sufficiently hypocellular to be confused with aplasia. No single characteristic feature of marrow morphology distinguishes MDS, but the following are commonly observed: dyserythropoietic changes (especially nuclear abnormalities) and ringed sideroblasts in the erythroid lineage; hypogranulation and hyposegmentation in granulocytic precursors, with an increase in myeloblasts; and megakaryocytes showing reduced numbers of disorganized nuclei. Prognosis strongly correlates with the proportion of marrow blasts. Cytogenetic analysis also is important. A much more sensitive method to detect infrequent chromosome aberrations is fluorescent in situ hybridization, and gene amplification by polymerase chain reaction can detect known chromosomal translocations.

DIFFERENTIAL DIAGNOSIS Deficiencies of vitamin B₁₂ or folate should be suggested by history and excluded by appropriate blood tests; vitamin B₆ deficiency can be assessed by a therapeutic trial of pyridoxine if the bone marrow shows ringed sideroblasts. Marrow dysplasia can be observed in acute viral infections, drug reactions, or chemical toxicity but should be transient. More difficult (arbitrary) are the distinctions between hypocellular MDS and aplasia or between refractory anemia with excess blasts in transformation and early acute leukemia.

PROGNOSIS The median survival varies greatly with FAB type and, according to IPSS calculations, ranges from years for patients with 5q- or sideroblastic anemia to a few months in refractory anemia with excess blasts or severe pancytopenia associated with monosomy 7. Most patients die as a result of complications of pancytopenia and not due to leukemic transformation; perhaps one-third will succumb to other diseases unrelated to their MDS. Precipitous worsening of pancytopenia, acquisition of new chromosomal abnormalities on serial cytogenetic determination, and increase in the number of blasts are all poor prognostic indicators. The outlook in therapy-related MDS, regardless of FAB type, is very poor, and most patients will progress within a few months to refractory acute myeloid leukemia.

TREATMENT The therapy of MDS is generally unsatisfactory. Only stem cell transplantation offers cure: survival rates of 40% have been reported, but older patients are particularly prone to develop treatment-related mortality and morbidity. Those with better prognostic features (and a more favorable natural history) have much better outcomes than patients with more malignant subtypes. Surprisingly, results of transplant using matched unrelated donor are comparable, although most series contain younger and more highly selected cases.

MDS has been regarded as particularly refractory to cytotoxic chemotherapy regimens but is probably no more resistant to effective treatment than acute myeloid leukemia in the elderly, in whom drug toxicity is often fatal and remissions, if achieved, are brief. Low doses of cytotoxic drugs have been administered for their "differentiating" potential: responses to cytosine arabinoside did not translate into a survival advantage; etoposide and 5-azacytidine are under active study. Amifostine, an organic thiophosphonate that blocks apoptosis, can improve blood counts but has significant toxicities. Immunosuppressive therapies, including ATG and cyclosporine, that are effective in aplastic anemia may induce sustained remissions in a high proportion of patients with refractory anemia, especially in those with hypocellular marrows or without cytogenetic abnormalities.

Hematopoietic growth factors can improve blood counts but, as in most other marrow failure states, have been most beneficial in patients with the least severe pancytopenia. G-CSF treatment alone failed to improve survival in a controlled trial. The combination of G-CSF and erythropoietin increased blood counts in one-third to one-half of patients, but survival advantage is not yet proven.

The same principles of supportive care described for aplastic anemia apply to MDS. Because many patients will be anemic for years, erythrocyte transfusion support should be accompanied by iron chelation in order to prevent secondary hemochromatosis.

Table 109-6 International Prognostic Scoring System

Prognostic Variable	Score Value				
	0	0.5	1.0	1.5	2.0
Bone marrow blasts (%)	<5%	5–10%		11–20%	21–30%
Karyotype[a]	Good	Intermediate	Poor		
Cytopenia[b] (lineages affected)	0 or 1	2 or 3			
Risk Group Scores	**Score**				
Low	0				
Intermediate-1	0.5–1.0				
Intermediate-2	1.5–2.0				
High	≥2.5				

[a] Good = normal, -Y, del(5q), del (20q); intermediate = all other abnormalities; poor = complex (≥3 abnormalities) or chromosome 7 abnormalities.
[b] Cytopenias defined as Hb <100 g/L, platelet count < 100,000/μL, absolute neutrophil count <1500/μL.

MYELOPHTHISIC ANEMIAS

Fibrosis of the bone marrow (see **Plate V-19**), usually accompanied by a characteristic blood smear picture called *leukoerythroblastosis*, can occur as a primary hematologic disease, called *myelofibrosis* or *myeloid metaplasia* (Chap. 110), and as a secondary process, called *myelophthisis*. Myelophthisis, or secondary myelofibrosis, is reactive. Fibrosis can be a response to invading tumor cells, usually of an epithelial cancer of breast, lung, and prostate or neuroblastoma. Marrow fibrosis may occur with infection of mycobacteria (both *Mycobacterium tuberculosis* and *M. avium*) fungi, or

HIV, and in sarcoidosis. Intracellular lipid deposition in Gaucher's disease and obliteration of the marrow space related to absence of osteoclast remodeling in congenital osteopetrosis also can produce fibrosis. Secondary myelofibrosis is a late consequence of radiation therapy or treatment with radiomimetic drugs. Usually, the infectious or malignant underlying processes are obvious. Marrow fibrosis can also be a feature of a variety of hematologic syndromes, especially chronic myeloid leukemia, multiple myeloma, lymphomas, myeloma, and hairy cell leukemia.

The pathophysiology has three distinct features: proliferation of fibroblasts in the marrow space (myelofibrosis); the extension of hematopoiesis into the long bones and most particularly into extramedullary sites, usually the spleen, liver, and lymph nodes (myeloid metaplasia); and ineffective erythropoiesis. The etiology of fibrosis is unknown but most likely involves dysregulated production of growth factors: platelet-derived growth factor and transforming growth factor β have been implicated. Abnormal regulation of other hematopoietins would lead to localization of blood-producing cells in nonhematopoietic tissues and uncoupling of the usually balanced processes of stem cell proliferation and differentiation. Myelofibrosis is remarkable for pancytopenia despite extraordinarily large numbers of circulating hematopoietic progenitor cells.

Anemia is dominant in secondary myelofibrosis, usually normocytic and normochromic. The diagnosis is suggested by the characteristic leukoerythroblastic smear (see Plate V-9). Erythrocyte morphology is very abnormal, with circulating nucleated red blood cells, teardrops, and shape distortions. White blood cell numbers are often elevated, sometimes mimicking a leukemoid reaction, with circulating myelocytes, promyelocytes, and myeloblasts. Platelets may be abundant and are often giant size. Inability to aspirate the bone marrow, the characteristic "dry tap," can allow a presumptive diagnosis before the biopsy is decalcified.

The course of secondary myelofibrosis is determined by its cause, usually a metastatic tumor or an advanced hematologic malignancy. Treatable causes must be excluded, especially tuberculosis and fungus. Transfusion support can relieve symptoms.

BIBLIOGRAPHY

BROWN KE, YOUNG NS: Parvovirus B19 in human disease. Annu Rev Med 48:59, 1997

ERSLEV AJ, SOLTAN A: Pure red cell aplasia: A review. Blood Rev 10:20, 1996

GREENBERG P et al: International scoring system for evaluating prognosis in myelodysplastic syndromes. Blood 89:2079, 1997

HEANEY ML, GOLDE DW: Myelodysplasia. N Engl J Med 340:1649, 1999

YOUNG NS: *The Bone Marrow Failure Syndromes.* Philadelphia, Saunders, 2000

———, ALTER BP: *Aplastic Anemia, Acquired and Inherited.* Philadelphia, Saunders, 1994

———, BARRETT AJ: The treatment of severe acquired aplastic anemia. Blood 85:3367, 1995

| 110 | *Jerry L. Spivak* |

POLYCYTHEMIA VERA AND OTHER MYELOPROLIFERATIVE DISEASES

Polycythemia vera, idiopathic myelofibrosis, essential thrombocytosis, and chronic myeloid leukemia (CML) are commonly classified together under the rubric *the chronic myeloproliferative disorders*, because their pathophysiology involves the clonal expansion of a multipotent hematopoietic progenitor cell with the overproduction of one or more of the formed elements of the blood. These entities may transform into acute leukemia naturally or as a consequence of mutagenic treatment. However, while polycythemia vera, idiopathic myelofibrosis, essential thrombocytosis, and CML share similar phenotypic characteristics, CML is genotypically distinct from the other three disorders because it alone is associated with translocation of genetic material between the long arms of chromosomes 9 and 22, resulting in the production of the unique fusion protein, bcr-abl. Furthermore, based on its natural history, CML is more appropriately considered as a form of leukemia. →*CML is discussed with the acute myeloid leukemias in Chap. 111.*

POLYCYTHEMIA VERA

Polycythemia vera is a clonal disorder involving a multipotent hematopoietic progenitor cell in which there is accumulation of phenotypically normal red cells, granulocytes, and platelets in the absence of a recognizable physiologic stimulus. Polycythemia vera, the most common of the chronic myeloproliferative disorders, occurs in about 2 per 100,000 people. It spares no adult age group. Vertical transmission has been documented, establishing a genetic basis for the disorder. A slight overall male predominance has been observed, but females predominate within the reproductive age range.

ETIOLOGY The etiology of polycythemia vera is unknown. Although nonrandom chromosome abnormalities such as 20q-, trisomy 8 or 9 have been documented in a small percentage of untreated polycythemia vera patients, no consistent cytogenetic abnormality has been associated with the disorder and no specific genetic defect has yet been identified. Impaired posttranslational processing of the thrombopoietin receptor, Mpl, has been noted in polycythemia vera patients; the extent of the defect correlated with disease duration and splenomegaly. While this defect is specific for polycythemia vera and is not found in secondary polycythemias, its role in the pathophysiology of the disorder is still undefined. In contrast to normal erythroid progenitor cells, polycythemia vera erythroid progenitor cells can grow in vitro in the absence of erythropoietin due to hypersensitivity to insulin-like growth factor I. However, this phenotypic abnormality is not specific for polycythemia vera and has been documented in essential thrombocytosis and secondary polycythemias. Polycythemia vera erythroid progenitor cells are more resistant to apoptosis induced by erythropoietin deprivation, due to upregulation of bcl-X_L, an antiapoptotic protein. The polycythemia vera erythroid progenitors do not divide more rapidly than their normal counterparts, but they accumulate because they do not die normally. Additionally, the transformed hematopoietic progenitor cells in polycythemia vera, as in other neoplastic disorders, exhibit clonal dominance and suppress the proliferation of normal hematopoietic progenitor cells by an unknown mechanism. Consequently, the circulating formed elements of the blood represent only progeny of the transformed clone.

CLINICAL FEATURES Although massive splenomegaly may be the initial presenting sign in polycythemia vera, most often the disorder is first recognized by the discovery of a high hemoglobin or hematocrit, and with the exception of aquagenic pruritus, no symptoms distinguish polycythemia vera from other causes of erythrocytosis.

Uncontrolled erythrocytosis can lead to neurologic symptoms such as vertigo, tinnitus, headache, and visual disturbances. Systolic hypertension also accompanies an elevated red cell mass. In some patients, venous or arterial thrombosis may be the presenting manifestation of polycythemia vera. Intraabdominal venous thrombosis is particularly common and may be catastrophic when there is sudden compromise of the hepatic vein. Polycythemia vera should be suspected in any patient who develops the Budd-Chiari syndrome. Digital ischemia may also occur. Easy bruising, epistaxis, or gastrointestinal hemorrhage may be observed, and polycythemia vera patients are frequently hypermetabolic. Hypercuricemia with secondary gout and uric acid stones and acid-peptic disease also complicate the disorder. Because isolated erythrocytosis is a common initial presentation for polycythemia vera but no clonal marker is available for the disease, the first task of the physician is to distinguish this autonomous clonal form of erythrocytosis from the many other types of erythrocytosis, most of which are correctable (Table 110-1).

Erythropoiesis is normally regulated by the glycoprotein hormone erythropoietin. Erythropoietin, which in adults is produced primarily in the kidneys and to a small extent in the liver, promotes the proliferation of erythroid progenitor cells, maintains their survival, and facilitates their differentiation. Because erythropoietin acts as a survival factor, it is constitutively produced and, like the red cell mass, its level is constant as long as tissue oxygenation is adequate. The plasma erythropoietin level, like the red cell mass, differs among individuals but in adults is not affected by either age or gender. Erythropoietin production is regulated at the level of gene transcription. Hypoxia is the only physiologic stimulus that increases the number of cells producing erythropoietin, and thus the production and metabolism of erythropoietin are independent of its plasma level. In the absence of renal or hepatic disease, plasma erythropoietin levels reflect erythropoietin production, and therefore the assay for plasma erythropoietin is a surrogate assay for tissue hypoxia. Erythropoietin is active at the picomolar level, and its production is tightly regulated. Thus, the plasma erythropoietin level does not rise outside the normal range until the hemoglobin level falls below 105 g/L. This is not meant to imply that an increase in erythropoietin production does not occur as the hemoglobin level falls below normal, but because the normal range for plasma erythropoietin is wide (4 to 26 mU/mL), unless the patient's baseline level is known, any increase will not be recognized until the hemoglobin falls below 105 g/L. Thereafter, there is a log-linear inverse correlation between the levels of plasma erythropoietin and hemoglobin. With erythrocytosis, erythropoietin production is suppressed; this suppression reflects not only the increase in tissue oxygen transport associated with the increase in red cell number but also additional negative-feedback mechanism unrelated to oxygen transport but related to the increase in blood viscosity and an increase in red cell precursors capable of taking up erythropoietin. The summation of these mechanisms accounts for the paradoxical observation that many patients with hypoxic erythrocytosis due to cyanotic congenital heart disease or obstructive lung disease have a "normal" plasma erythropoietin level. The plasma erythropoietin level is a useful diagnostic test in patients with isolated erythrocytosis, because an elevated level essentially excludes polycythemia vera as the cause for the erythrocytosis.

DIAGNOSIS When confronted with an elevated hemoglobin or hematocrit level, it is important to obtain previous values to determine the duration of this laboratory abnormality. Because the hemoglobin or hematocrit level is affected by the plasma volume, and hematocrit and red cell mass are not linearly related, a red cell mass determination must also be performed to distinguish absolute erythrocytosis from relative erythrocytosis due to a reduction in plasma volume alone (also known as *stress* or *spurious erythrocytosis* or *Geisböck's syndrome*). Red cell mass determination is important because in polycythemia vera, in contrast to erythropoietin-driven erythrocytosis, the plasma volume is frequently elevated, not only masking the true extent of red cell mass expansion but often its presence. Indeed, a significant proportion of patients with polycythemia vera have a hematocrit within the normal range, particularly in patients with a substantial splenomegaly. Failure to recognize this phenomenon is undoubtedly the basis for many of the reported instances of hepatic or portal vein thrombosis in patients with a so-called undefined myeloproliferative disorder.

Red cell mass is reliably determined by isotope dilution using the patient's ^{51}Cr-tagged red cells; extrapolations made by determining directly only the plasma volume are unacceptable. Furthermore, to allow ample time for equilibration of the labeled red cells, measurements should be made over a period of ≥90 min.

Once the presence of absolute erythrocytosis has been established, its cause must be determined. An elevated plasma erythropoietin level suggests either an hypoxic cause for erythrocytosis or autonomous erythropoietin production, in which case assessment of pulmonary function and an abdominal computed tomography scan to evaluate renal and hepatic anatomy are appropriate. A normal erythropoietin level does not exclude an hypoxic cause for erythrocytosis. In polycythemia vera, in contrast to hypoxic erythrocytosis, the arterial oxygen saturation is normal. However, a normal oxygen saturation does not exclude a high-affinity hemoglobin as a cause for erythrocytosis, and it is here that documentation of previous hemoglobin levels and a family study become important. Because there is no clonal marker for polycythemia vera, clinical guidelines have been proposed to define the disease. A modified version is provided in Table 110-2. However, these guidelines do not establish clonality, and in some patients only with time will the underlying disorder become apparent. Diagnostic ambiguity does not preclude the initiation of therapy.

Other laboratory studies that may aid in diagnosis include the red cell count, mean corpuscular volume, and red cell distribution width (RDW). Only three situations cause microcytic erythrocytosis: β-thalassemia trait, hypoxic erythrocytosis, and polycythemia vera. However, with β-thalassemia trait the RDW is normal, whereas with hypoxic erythrocytosis and polycythemia vera, the RDW is usually elevated. A properly made blood smear from a patient with erythrocytosis will be virtually unreadable due to the marked elevation in red cell count, but no specific morphologic abnormalities are seen in the leukocytes or platelets in polycythemia vera. However, when these are also elevated the diagnosis is assured. In many patients, the leukocyte alkaline phosphatase level is also increased, as is the uric acid level. Elevated serum vitamin B_{12} or B_{12}-binding capacity may be present. In patients with associated acid-peptic disease, occult gastrointestinal bleeding may lead to presentation with hypochromic, microcytic anemia.

A bone marrow aspirate and biopsy will provide no specific diagnostic information, and unless there is a need to establish the presence of myelofibrosis or exclude some other disorder, these procedures need not be done. Although the presence of a cytogenetic abnormality such as trisomy 8 or 9 or 20q- in the setting of an expansion of the red cell mass supports the clonal etiology, no specific cytogenetic abnormality is associated with polycythemia vera, and the absence of a cytogenetic marker does not exclude the diagnosis.

COMPLICATIONS The major clinical complications of polycythemia vera relate directly to the increase in blood viscosity asso-

Table 110-1 Causes of Absolute Erythrocytosis

Hypoxia	Tumors
Carbon monoxide intoxication	Hypernephroma
High altitude	Hepatoma
Pulmonary disease	Cerebellar hemangioblastoma
High-affinity hemoglobin	Adrenal adenoma
Sleep-apnea syndrome	Pheochromocytoma
Respiratory center	Meningioma
dysfunction	Uterine fibromyoma
Supine hypoventilation	Familial (with normal hemoglobin
Right-to-left cardiac shunts	function)
Renal disease	Erythropoietin receptor mutations
Renal cysts	DPG mutase deficiency
Hydronephrosis	Bartter's syndrome
Renal artery stenosis	Androgen therapy
Focal glomerulonephritis	Recombinant erythropoietin therapy
Renal transplantation	Polycythemia vera

NOTE: DPG, diphosphoglycerate

Table 110-2 Suggested Criteria for the Clinical Diagnosis of Polycythemia Vera[a]

Elevated red cell mass
Normal arterial oxygen saturation
Splenomegaly
In the absence of splenomegaly:
  Leukocytosis and thrombocytosis

[a] It must be emphasized that these criteria do not establish clonality.

ciated with elevation of the red cell mass and indirectly to the increased turnover of red cells, leukocytes, and platelets and the attendant increase in uric acid and histamine production. The latter appears to be responsible for the increase in peptic ulcer disease and for the pruritus associated with this disorder, although little formal proof for this has been obtained. A sudden massive increase in spleen size is another problem and can be associated with splenic infarction or progressive cachexia. Myelofibrosis and myeloid metaplasia can also develop with transfusion-dependent anemia, but the frequency is low in those not receiving chemotherapy or irradiation. Although acute nonlymphocytic leukemia is reported to be increased in polycythemia vera, the incidence of acute leukemia in patients not exposed to chemotherapy or radiation is low and the development of leukemia is not related to disease duration, suggesting that the treatment exposure may be a more important risk factor than the disease itself.

Erythromelalgia is a curious syndrome of unknown etiology involving primarily the lower extremities and manifested usually by erythema, warmth, and pain of the affected appendage and occasionally digital infarction. It occurs with a variable frequency in patients with a myeloproliferative disorder and is usually responsive to salicylates. Some of the central nervous system symptoms observed in patients with polycythemia vera may represent a variant of erythromelalgia.

If left uncontrolled, erythrocytosis can lead to intravascular thrombosis involving vital organs such as the liver, heart, brain, or lungs. Patients with massive splenomegaly are particularly prone to thrombotic events because the associated increase in plasma volume masks the true extent of the red cell mass elevation as measured by the hematocrit or hemoglobin level. A "normal" hematocrit or hemoglobin level in a polycythemia vera patient with massive splenomegaly should be considered as indicative of an elevated red cell mass until proven otherwise.

℞ TREATMENT Polycythemia vera is generally an indolent disorder whose clinical course can run many decades, and its medical management should reflect the tempo of the disorder. Maintenance of the hemoglobin level at ≤ 140 g/L in men and ≤ 120 g/L in women is mandatory to avoid the thrombotic complications. Thrombosis due to erythrocytosis is the most significant complication of this disorder. Phlebotomy serves initially to reduce hyperviscosity by bringing the red cell mass into the normal range. Periodic phlebotomies thereafter serve to maintain the red cell mass within the range of normal and to induce a state of iron deficiency, which prevents an accelerated reexpansion of the red cell mass. In most polycythemia vera patients, once an iron-deficient state is achieved, phlebotomy is usually required only at 3-month intervals. Although both phlebotomy and iron deficiency, in addition to the disease itself, tend to increase the platelet count, thrombocytosis is not correlated with thrombosis in polycythemia vera, in contrast to the strong correlation between erythrocytosis and thrombosis in this disease. The use of salicylates as a tonic against thrombosis in polycythemia vera patients is potentially harmful, and salicylates should be employed only to treat erythromelalgia. Oral anticoagulants are not routinely indicated and are difficult to assess owing to the artifactual imbalance between the test tube anticoagulant and plasma that occurs when blood from these patients is assayed for prothrombin or partial thromboplastin activity. Asymptomatic hyperuricemia requires no therapy, but allopurinol should be administered to avoid further elevation of the uric acid when chemotherapy is employed to reduce splenomegaly or leukocytosis-associated pruritus. Generalized pruritus intractable to antihistamines can be a major problem in polycythemia vera, and hydroxyurea, interferon (IFN)-α, and psoralens with ultraviolet light in the A range (PUVA) therapy may have some palliative effects. Asymptomatic thrombocytosis requires no therapy. Symptomatic thrombocytosis or splenomegaly can be treated with hydroxyurea or IFN-α, although each can be associated with significant side effects. Anagrelide, a quinazolin derivative and platelet antiaggregant that also lowers the platelet count, can control thrombocytosis. A reduction in platelet number may be necessary in the treatment of erythromelalgia if salicylates are not effective or if

the thrombocytosis is associated with migraine-like symptoms. However, the highest priority for treatment is reduction of the red cell mass to normal. Alkylating agents and ^{32}P are leukemogenic in polycythemia vera, and their use should be avoided. If a cytotoxic agent must be used, hydroxyurea is preferred, but it also may be leukemogenic with chronic use. Chemotherapy should be used for as short a time as possible. In some patients, massive splenomegaly unresponsive to reduction by hydroxyurea or IFN-α therapy and associated with intractable weight loss will require splenectomy. Allogeneic bone marrow transplantation may be effective in young patients.

Patients with polycythemia vera can be expected to live long and useful lives when their red cell mass is effectively managed with phlebotomy. Chemotherapy is never indicated to control the red cell mass unless venous access is impossible.

IDIOPATHIC MYELOFIBROSIS

Idiopathic myelofibrosis (other designations include *agnogenic myeloid metaplasia* or *myelofibrosis with myeloid metaplasia*) is a clonal disorder of a multipotent hematopoietic progenitor cell of unknown etiology characterized by marrow fibrosis, myeloid metaplasia with extramedullary hematopoiesis, and splenomegaly. Idiopathic myelofibrosis is uncommon; in the absence of a specific clonal marker, establishing this diagnosis is difficult because myelofibrosis and myeloid metaplasia with splenomegaly are also features of both polycythemia vera and CML. Furthermore, myelofibrosis and splenomegaly occur in a variety of benign and malignant disorders (Table 110-3), many of which are amenable to specific therapies not effective in idiopathic myelofibrosis. In contrast to the other chronic myeloproliferative disorders and so-called acute or malignant myelofibrosis, which can occur at any age, idiopathic myelofibrosis primarily afflicts individuals in their sixth decade or later.

ETIOLOGY The etiology of idiopathic myelofibrosis is unknown. Although nonrandom chromosome abnormalities such as 20q-, 13q-, and trisomy 1q are not uncommon, no specific cytogenetic abnormality has been identified. The degree of myelofibrosis and the extent of extramedullary hematopoiesis are not related. This disorder is associated with overproduction of type III collagen, a finding that has been attributed to platelet-derived growth factor or transforming growth factor β, but no proof has been forthcoming. Importantly, fibroblasts in idiopathic myelofibrosis are not part of the neoplastic clone.

CLINICAL FEATURES No specific signs or symptoms are associated with idiopathic myelofibrosis. Most patients are asymptomatic at presentation and are usually detected by the discovery of splenic enlargement and/or abnormal blood counts during a routine examination. A blood smear reveals the characteristic features of extramedullary hematopoiesis: teardrop-shaped red cells, nucleated red cells, myelocytes, and promyelocytes; myeloblasts may also be present but have no prognostic significance. Anemia, usually mild initially, is the rule, while the leukocyte and platelet counts are either normal or increased but either can be depressed. Mild hepatomegaly may accompany the splenomegaly, and both the lactate dehydrogenase and serum alkaline phosphatase levels can be elevated. The level of leukocyte

Table 110-3 Causes of Myelofibrosis

Carcinoma metastatic to the marrow	Chronic myeloid leukemia
Infection	Polycythemia vera
Lymphoma	Idiopathic myelofibrosis
Hodgkin's disease	Systemic mastocytosis
Acute leukemia (lymphoid or myeloid)	Thorium dioxide (Thorotrast) exposure
Hairy cell leukemia	Systemic lupus erythematosus
Multiple myeloma	Renal osteodystrophy

alkaline phosphatase can be low, normal, or elevated. Marrow may be unaspirable due to the myelofibrosis, and bone x-rays may reveal osteosclerosis. Exuberant extramedullary hematopoiesis can cause ascites, pulmonary hypertension, intestinal or ureteral obstruction, intracranial hypertension, pericardial tamponade, spinal cord compression, or skin nodules. Splenic enlargement can be sufficiently rapid to cause splenic infarctions with fever and pleuritic chest pain. Hyperuricemia and secondary gout may ensue.

DIAGNOSIS While the clinical picture described above is characteristic of idiopathic myelofibrosis, all of the clinical features described can be observed in polycythemia vera or CML. Massive splenomegaly commonly masks erythrocytosis in polycythemia vera, and reports of intraabdominal thromboses in idiopathic myelofibrosis likely represent instances of unrecognized polycythemia vera. Furthermore, many other disorders have features that overlap with idiopathic myelofibrosis but respond to distinctly different therapies. Therefore, the diagnosis of idiopathic myelofibrosis is one of exclusion, which requires that the disorders listed in Table 110-3 be ruled out.

The presence of teardrop-shaped red cells, nucleated red cells, myelocytes, and promyelocytes establishes the presence of extramedullary hematopoiesis; the presence of leukocytosis, thrombocytosis with large and bizarre platelets, as well as circulating myeloblasts suggests the presence of a myeloproliferative disorder as opposed to a secondary form of myelofibrosis (Table 110-3). Marrow is usually not aspirable due to increased marrow reticulin, but marrow biopsy will reveal a hypercellular marrow with trilineage hyperplasia and, in particular, increased megakaryocytes, but there are no characteristic morphologic abnormalities that distinguish idiopathic myelofibrosis from the other chronic myeloproliferative disorders. Splenomegaly due to extramedullary hematopoiesis may be sufficiently massive to cause portal hypertension and variceal formation. In some patients, exuberant extramedullary hematopoiesis can dominate the clinical picture. An intriguing feature of idiopathic myelofibrosis is the occurrence of autoimmune abnormalities such as immune complexes, antinuclear antibodies, rheumatoid factor, or a positive Coombs' test. Whether these represent a host reaction to the disorder or are involved in its pathogenesis is unknown. Cytogenetic analysis of blood or marrow is useful both to exclude CML and for prognostic purposes, because complex karyotype abnormalities portend a poor prognosis in idiopathic myelofibrosis.

COMPLICATIONS Idiopathic myelofibrosis is a chronic disorder but with a median survival of only 5 years (range 1 to 15 years), a duration much shorter than for polycythemia vera or essential thrombocytosis. The natural history of idiopathic myelofibrosis is one of inexorable marrow failure with transfusion-dependent anemia and increasing organomegaly. Patients are prone to deep-seated tissue infections, particularly of the lungs. As with CML, idiopathic myelofibrosis can evolve from a chronic phase to an accelerated phase with constitutional symptoms and increasing marrow failure. About 10% of patients develop an aggressive form of acute leukemia for which therapy is usually ineffective. Important prognostic factors for disease acceleration include anemia; thrombocytopenia; age; the presence of complex cytogenetic abnormalities; and constitutional symptoms such as unexplained fever, night sweats, or weight loss. Any nonrandom cytogenetic abnormality is associated with a shortened life span, and the presence or development of multiple cytogenetic abnormalities is highly indicative of disease acceleration.

℞ **TREATMENT** There is no specific therapy for idiopathic myelofibrosis. Anemia may be exacerbated by deficiency of folic acid or iron, and in rare instances, pyridoxine therapy has been effective. However, anemia is more often due to ineffective erythropoiesis not compensated for by the extramedullary hematopoiesis in the spleen and liver; neither androgens nor erythropoietin has been consistently effective therapy. Erythropoietin may worsen splenomegaly. A red cell

splenic sequestration study can establish the presence of hypersplenism, for which splenectomy is indicated. Splenectomy may also be necessary if splenomegaly impairs alimentation and should be performed before cachexia sets in. In this situation, splenectomy should not be avoided because of concern over rebound thrombocytosis, loss of hematopoietic capacity, or compensatory hepatomegaly. However, for unexplained reasons, splenectomy increases the risk of blastic transformation. Allopurinol can control significant hyperuricemia and hydroxyurea has proved useful for controlling organomegaly. The role of interferon-α is undefined, and its side effects are more pronounced in the older individuals who are affected with this disorder, but reversal of myelofibrosis has been observed. Glucocorticoids are used to control autoimmune complications. Allogeneic bone marrow transplantation should be considered in younger patients.

ESSENTIAL THROMBOCYTOSIS

Essential thrombocytosis (other designations include *essential thrombocythemia, idiopathic thrombocytosis, primary thrombocytosis, hemorrhagic thrombocythemia*) is a clonal disorder of unknown etiology involving a multipotent hematopoietic progenitor cell and is manifested clinically by the overproduction of platelets without a definable cause. Essential thrombocytosis is an uncommon disorder, but its exact frequency is unknown. No clonal marker distinguishes it from the more common nonclonal, reactive forms of thrombocytosis (Table 110-4). Clinical recognition of thrombocytosis is unlikely in the largely asymptomatic persons affected by this disorder. As a consequence, essential thrombocytosis was formerly considered to be a disease of the elderly and to be responsible for significant morbidity due to hemorrhage or thrombosis. However, with the widespread application of platelet counting, it is now clear that essential thrombocytosis can occur at any age in adults and often occurs without symptoms or disturbances of hemostasis. There is an unexplained female predominance, in contrast to the reactive forms of thrombocytosis where no sex bias exists. Because no clonal marker is available for the disorder, clinical criteria have been proposed to distinguish it from the other chronic myeloproliferative disorders, which may also present with thrombocytosis but have distinct prognosis and treatment (Table 110-5). These criteria do not establish clonality; therefore, they are truly useful only in identifying disorders such as CML, polycythemia vera, or myelodysplasia, which can masquerade as essential thrombocytosis, as opposed to establishing the presence of essential thrombocytosis. Furthermore, as with "primary" erythrocytosis, nonclonal, benign forms of thrombocytosis exist (such as hereditary overproduction of thrombopoietin) that are not widely recognized because we currently lack the diagnostic tools to do so.

ETIOLOGY Megakaryocytopoiesis and platelet production depend upon thrombopoietin and its receptor, Mpl. As in the case of early erythroid and myeloid progenitor cells, early megakaryocytic progenitors require the presence of interleukin (IL) 3 and stem cell factor for optimal proliferation, and their subsequent development is enhanced by IL-6 and -11. However, megakaryocyte maturation and differentiation require thrombopoietin.

Megakaryocytes are unique amongst hematopoietic progenitor

Table 110-4 Causes of Thrombocytosis

Iron-deficiency anemia	Idiopathic myelofibrosis
Hyposplenism	Essential thrombocytosis
Postsplenectomy[a]	Chronic myeloid leukemia
Malignancy	Idiopathic sideroblastic anemia
Collagen vascular disease	Myelodysplasia (5q- syndrome)
Inflammatory bowel disease	Postsurgery
Infection	Rebound (cessation of ethanol intake,
Hemolysis	correction of vitamin B_{12} or folate
Hemorrhage	deficiency)
Polycythemia vera	

[a] If the platelet count is greater than $2 \times 10^6/\mu L$, the etiology is most likely a myeloproliferative disorder.

Table 110-5 Suggested Criteria for the Clinical Diagnosis of Essential Thrombocytosis[a]

Platelet count ≥ 500,000/μL
Absence of a known cause of reactive thrombocytosis (see Table 110-4)
Absence of the Ph chromosome and the bcr-abl gene rearrangement
Normal red cell mass
Presence of marrow iron
Absence of myelofibrosis
Absence of myelodysplasia clinically and by cytogenetic analysis
Splenomegaly

[a] The concept that a platelet count greater than $1 \times 10^6/\mu L$ distinguishes essential thrombocytosis from other causes of thrombocytosis has no clinical validity.

cells because they undergo endomitotic as opposed to mitotic reduplication of their genome. In the absence of thrombopoietin, endomitotic megakaryocytic reduplication and, by extension, the cytoplasmic development necessary for platelet production are impaired. Like erythropoietin, thrombopoietin is produced in both the liver and the kidneys, and an inverse correlation between the platelet count and plasma thrombopoietic activity exists. Like erythropoietin, plasma levels of thrombopoietin are controlled in part by the size of its progenitor cell pool. In contrast to erythropoietin, but like its myeloid counterparts granulocyte and granulocyte-macrophage colony stimulating factors, thrombopoietin not only enhances the proliferation of its target cells but also enhances the reactivity of their end-stage product, the platelet. In addition to its role in thrombopoiesis, thrombopoietin enhances the survival of multipotent hematopoietic stem cells.

The clonality of essential thrombocytosis has been established by the use of the isoenzymes of glucose-6-phosphate dehydrogenase in patients who are hemizygous for this gene, by the use of X-linked DNA polymorphisms, and by the identification of nonrandom, although variable cytogenetic abnormalities. The multipotent hematopoietic progenitor cell involved in this disorder can vary; in some patients lymphocytes contained the same clonal marker as the megakaryocytes, erythrocytes, and myeloid cells, whereas in others the lymphocytes were not involved. Similar observations have been made in polycythemia vera. Furthermore, a number of families have been described in which essential thrombocytosis was inherited, in one instance as an autosomal dominant trait. In one kindred, in addition to essential thrombocytosis, idiopathic myelofibrosis and polycythemia vera were also individually documented.

CLINICAL FEATURES Clinically, essential thrombocytosis is most often identified incidentally when a platelet count is obtained during the course of a routine evaluation. Occasionally, review of previous platelet counts will reveal that an elevation was present but overlooked. No symptoms or signs are specific for essential thrombocytosis, but patients do have hemorrhagic and thrombotic tendencies expressed as easy bruising for the former or microvascular occlusions for the latter, which may be manifested by erythromelalgia, migraine, or transient ischemic attacks. Physical examination is generally unremarkable except for the presence of mild splenomegaly. Massive splenomegaly is more characteristic of the other myeloproliferative disorders, particularly polycythemia vera or idiopathic myelofibrosis.

Anemia is unusual, but a mild neutrophilic leukocytosis is not. The blood smear, however, is most remarkable for the number of platelets present, some of which may be very large. The leukocyte alkaline phosphatase score is either normal or elevated. The large mass of circulating platelets may prevent the accurate measurement of serum potassium due to the release of platelet potassium upon blood clotting. This hyperkalemia is a laboratory artifact and is not associated with any electrocardiographic abnormalities. Similarly, arterial oxygen measurements can be inaccurate unless the blood is collected on ice. The prothrombin and partial thromboplastin times are normal, while abnormalities of platelet function such as a prolonged bleeding time and impaired platelet aggregation can be present. However, in spite of much study, characteristic platelet function abnormalities associated are not defined, and no platelet function test predicts the presence of clinically significant bleeding or thrombosis.

The elevated platelet count may hinder the collection of a marrow aspirate, but marrow biopsy usually reveals both megakaryocyte hyperplasia and hypertrophy, as well as an overall increase in marrow cellularity. An increase in marrow reticulin may be present, but if extensive, another diagnosis should be considered. The absence of stainable iron demands an explanation, because iron deficiency alone can cause thrombocytosis and absent marrow iron is a feature of polycythemia vera.

While nonrandom cytogenetic abnormalities have been identified in essential thrombocytosis, no consistently identifiable abnormality is noted, even involving chromosomes 3 and 1 where the genes for thrombopoietin and its receptor Mpl, respectively, are located.

DIAGNOSIS Thrombocytosis is encountered in a variety of clinical disorders (Table 110-4) in which production of cytokines is increased. Thus, the first obligation when confronted with a high platelet count is to determine if it is a consequence of another disorder. Cytogenetic evaluation is mandatory to determine if the thrombocytosis is due to CML or a myelodysplastic disorder such as the 5q-syndrome. Because the bcr-abl translocation can be present in the absence of the Ph chromosome, polymerase chain reaction analysis for bcr-abl expression should be performed in all patients with thrombocytosis in whom a cytogenetic study is normal. Anemia and ringed sideroblasts are not features of essential thrombocytosis, but they are features of idiopathic refractory sideroblastic anemia, in which thrombocytosis can also occur. The presence of massive splenomegaly should suggest the possibility of another myeloproliferative disorder, and in this setting a red cell mass determination is mandatory because substantial splenomegaly can mask the presence of erythrocytosis. What appears to be essential thrombocytosis can evolve into polycythemia vera, revealing the true nature of the underlying myeloproliferative disorder.

COMPLICATIONS Perhaps no other condition in clinical medicine has caused otherwise astute physicians to intervene inappropriately more often than thrombocytosis, particularly if the platelet count is greater than $1 \times 10^6/\mu L$. It is commonly believed that a high platelet count must cause intravascular stasis and thrombosis; however, no controlled clinical study has ever established either association.

To the contrary, very high platelet counts are associated primarily with hemorrhage, while platelet counts of $<1 \times 10^6/\mu L$ are more often associated with thrombosis. This is not meant to imply that an elevated platelet count cannot cause symptoms in a patient with essential thrombocytosis, but rather that the focus should be on the patient, not the platelet count. For example, some of the most dramatic neurologic problems in essential thrombocytosis are migraine-related but may respond only to lowering of the platelet count; other symptoms may be a manifestation of erythromelalgia and respond simply to platelet cyclooxygenase inhibitors such as aspirin, without a reduction in platelet number. Still others may represent an interaction between an atherosclerotic vascular system and a high platelet count, and others may have no relationship to the platelet count whatsoever. Progress in distinguishing essential thrombocytosis from polycythemia vera and in defining new causes of hypercoagulability (like factor V Leiden) make the older literature on thrombocytosis less reliable.

℞ **TREATMENT** An elevated platelet count in an asymptomatic patient requires no therapy, and before any therapy is initiated in a patient with thrombocytosis, the cause of symptoms must be clearly identified to be a consequence of the elevated platelet count. Plasmapheresis and cytotoxic therapy have never been proven efficacious and cannot be recommended. Furthermore, patients with essential thrombocytosis treated with ^{32}P, hydroxyurea, or alkylating agents are placed at risk of developed acute leukemia without any proof of benefit from such therapy. If platelet reduction is deemed necessary on the basis of neurologic symptoms refractory to salicylates, IFN-α or anagrelide, a quinazolin derivative, can reduce the platelet count, but neither is uniformly effective nor without significant side effects. Bleeding associated with thrombocytosis usually responds to ϵ-aminocaproic acid, which can be given prophylactically before and after elective surgery. As more clinical experience is acquired, it appears that essential thrombocytosis is more benign than previously thought, and that evolution to acute leukemia is more likely to be a consequence of prior therapy than of the disease itself. In managing patients with thrombocytosis, the physician's first obligation is to do no harm.

BIBLIOGRAPHY

ADAMSON JW et al: Polycythemia vera: Stem cell and probable clonal origin of the disease. N Engl J Med 295:913, 1976

BAROSI G: Myelofibrosis with myeloid metaplasia: Diagnostic definition and prognostic classification for clinical studies and treatment guidelines. J Clin Oncol 17:2954, 1999

BUSS DH et al: The incidence of thrombotic and hemorrhagic disorders in association with extreme thrombocytosis: An analysis of 129 cases. Am J Hematol 20:365, 1985

MOLITERNO AR et al: Posttranslational processing of the thrombopoietin receptor is impaired in polycythemia vera platelets. Blood 94:2555, 1999

REILLY JT et al: Cytogenetic abnormalities and their prognostic significance in idiopathic myelofibrosis: A study of 106 cases. Br J Haematol 98:96, 1997

SCHAFER AI: Bleeding and thrombosis in the myeloproliferative disorders. Blood 64:1, 1984

STERKERS Y et al: Acute myeloid leukemia and myelodysplastic syndromes following essential thrombocythemia treated with hydroxyurea: High proportion of cases with 17p deletion. Blood 91:616, 1998

TARTAGLIA AP et al: Adverse effects of antiaggregating platelet therapy in the treatment of polycythemia vera. Semin Hematol 23:172, 1986

111   *Meir Wetzler, John C. Byrd, Clara D. Bloomfield*

ACUTE AND CHRONIC MYELOID LEUKEMIA

The myeloid leukemias are a heterogeneous group of diseases characterized by infiltration of the blood, bone marrow, and other tissues by neoplastic cells of the hematopoietic system. In 2000, the estimated number of new myeloid leukemia cases in the United States was 10,100. These leukemias comprise a spectrum of malignancies that, untreated, range from rapidly fatal to slowly growing. Based on their untreated course, the myeloid leukemias have traditionally been designated *acute* or *chronic*.

ACUTE MYELOID LEUKEMIA

INCIDENCE The incidence of acute myeloid leukemia (AML) is approximately 2.3 per 100,000 people per year, and the age-adjusted incidence is higher in men than in women (2.9 versus 1.9). AML incidence increases with age; it is 1.3 in individuals younger than 65 years and 12.2 in those older than 65. No significant change in AML incidence has occurred over the past 20 years.

ETIOLOGY Heredity, radiation, chemical and other occupational exposures, and drugs have been implicated in the development of AML. No direct evidence suggests a viral etiology.

Heredity Certain syndromes with somatic cell chromosome aneuploidy, e.g., Down (chromosome 21 trisomy), Klinefelter (XXY and variants), and Patau (chromosome 13 trisomy), are associated with an increased incidence of AML. Inherited diseases with excessive chromatin fragility, e.g., Fanconi anemia, Bloom syndrome, ataxia telangiectasia, and Kostmann syndrome, are also associated with AML.

Radiation Survivors of the atomic bomb explosions in Japan had an increased incidence of myeloid leukemias that peaked 5 to 7 years after exposure. Therapeutic radiation alone seems to add little risk of AML but can increase the risk in people exposed to alkylating agents (see below).

Chemical and Other Exposures Exposure to benzene, which is used as a solvent in the chemical, plastic, rubber, and pharmaceutical industries, is associated with an increased incidence of AML. Smoking and exposure to petroleum products, paint, embalming fluids, ethylene oxide, herbicides, and pesticides, have also been associated with an increased risk of AML.

Drugs Anticancer drugs are the leading cause of treatment-associated AML. Alkylating agent–associated leukemias occur on average 4 to 6 years after exposure, and affected individuals have aberrations in chromosomes 5 and 7. Topoisomerase II inhibitor–associated leukemias occur 1 to 3 years after exposure, and affected individuals usually have aberrations involving chromosome 11q23. Chloramphenicol, phenylbutazone, and, less commonly, chloroquine and methoxypsoralen can result in bone marrow failure that may evolve into AML.

CLASSIFICATION The categorization of acute leukemia into biologically distinct groups is based on morphology, cytochemistry, and immunophenotype as well as cytogenetic and molecular techniques.

Morphologic and Cytochemical Classification The diagnosis of AML is established by the presence of >20% myeloblasts in blood and/or bone marrow. Myeloblasts have nuclear chromatin that is uniformly fine or lacelike in appearance and large nucleoli (two to five per cell). If specific cytoplasmic granules, Auer rods, or the nuclear folding and clefting characteristic of monocytoid cells are not present, the morphologic features observed under light microscopy may not be sufficient to clarify the diagnosis. A positive myeloperoxidase reaction in >3% of the blasts may be the only feature distinguishing AML from acute lymphoblastic leukemia (ALL).

AML is classified based on morphology and cytochemistry according to the French, American, and British (FAB) schema, which includes eight major subtypes, M0 to M7 (Table 111-1). The World Health Organization classification incorporates molecular (including cytogenetic), morphologic, and clinical features (such as prior hematologic disorder) in defining disease entities (Table 111-1).

Immunophenotypic Classification The phenotype of human myeloid leukemia cells can be studied by multiparameter flow cytometry after the cells are labeled with monoclonal antibodies to cell-surface antigens. For example, M0, which is characterized by immature morphology and no lineage-specific cytochemical reactions, is diagnosed by flow cytometric demonstration of the myeloid-specific antigens cluster designation (CD) 13 or 33. Similarly, M7 can often be diagnosed only by expression of the platelet-specific antigen CD41 or by electron-microscopic demonstration of myeloperoxidase.

Chromosomal Classification Chromosomal analysis of the leukemic cell provides the most important pretreatment prognostic information in AML. Only two cytogenetic abnormalities have been invariably associated with a specific FAB group: t(15;17)(q22;q12) with M3 and inv(16)(p13q22) with M4Eo. However, many chromosomal abnormalities have been associated primarily with one FAB group, including t(8;21)(q22;q22) with M2, and t(9;11)(p22;q23), and other translocations involving 11q23, with M5. Many of the recurring chromosomal abnormalities in AML have been associated with specific clinical characteristics. More commonly associated with younger age are t(8;21) and t(15;17), and with older age, del(5q) and del(7q). Granulocytic sarcomas are associated with t(8;21); disseminated intravascular coagulation (DIC) with t(15;17); and diabetes insipidus, fever, and infection all with monosomy 7. The reasons for most associations of chromosomal abnormalities with specific clinical features are unknown.

Molecular Classification The many recurring cytogenetic abnormalities led to molecular studies, which have revealed genes that may be involved in leukemogenesis. The 15;17 translocation, characteristic of M3, encodes a chimeric protein, Pml/Rarα, which is formed by the fusion of the retinoic acid receptor-α (*RARα*) gene from chromosome 17 and the promyelocytic leukemia (*PML*) gene from chromosome 15. The *RARα* gene encodes a member of the nuclear

Table 111-1   Acute Myeloid Leukemia (AML) Classification Systems

French-American-British (FAB) Classification[a]
M0: Minimally differentiated leukemia
M1: Myeloblastic leukemia without maturation
M2: Myeloblastic leukemia with maturation
M3: Hypergranular promyelocytic leukemia
M4Eo: Variant: Increase in abnormal marrow eosinophils
M4: Myelomonocytic leukemia
M5: Moncytic leukemia
M6: Erythroleukemia (DiGuglielmo's disease)
M7: Megakaryoblastic leukemia

World Health Organization Classification[b]
I. AML with recurrent cytogenetic translocations
   AML with t(8;21)(q22;q22);*AML1(CBFα)/ETO*
   Acute promyelocytic leukemia [AML with t(15;17)(q22;q12) and variants; *PML/RARα*]
   AML with abnormal bone marrow eosinophils [inv(16)(p13q22) or t(16;16)(p13;q22) *CBFβ/MYH11*]
   AML with 11q23 (*MLL*) abnormalities
II. AML with multilineage dysplasia
   With prior myelodysplastic syndrome
   Without prior myelodysplastic syndrome
III. AML and myelodysplastic syndrome, therapy-related
   Alkylating agent-related
   Epipodophyllotoxin-related
   Other types
IV. AML not otherwise categorized
   AML minimally differentiated
   AML without maturation
   AML with maturation
   Acute myelomonocytic leukemia
   Acute monocytic leukemia
   Acute erythroid leukemia
   Acute megakaryocytic leukemia
   Acute basophilic leukemia
   Acute panmyelosis with myelofibrosis

[a] JM Bennett et al: Ann Intern Med 103:620, 1985
[b] NL Harris et al: J Clin Oncol 17:3835, 1999

hormone receptor family of transcription factors. After binding retinoic acid, *RARα* can promote expression of a variety of genes. The 15;17 translocation juxtaposes *PML* with *RARα* in a head-to-tail configuration that is under the transcriptional control of *PML*. Three different breakpoints in the *PML* gene lead to various fusion proteins. The Pml-Rarα fusion protein tends to suppress gene transcription and blocks differentiation of the cells. Pharmacologic doses of the Rarα ligand, all-trans-retinoic acid (tretinoin or ATRA), relieve the block and promote differentiation (see below).

The inv(16), characteristic of M4Eo or AML with abnormal bone marrow eosinophils, and the t(8;21) characteristic of M2 both involve subunits of the transcription factor complex core-binding factor (Cbf), also known as polyomavirus enhancer binding protein 2. This transcription factor contains two subunits, an α subunit, the Am11 protein, and a β subunit, the Pebp2 protein, and is involved in the expression of a number of differentiation-dependent genes in myeloid cells. The inv(16) results in a fusion of the core-binding factor β (*CBFB*) gene on the q arm (encodes Pebp2 protein) and the myosin heavy chain (*MYH11*) gene on the p arm. The 8;21 translocation involves the core-binding factor α (*CBFA*) gene on chromosome 21, called the *AML1* gene, joining the *ETO* gene on chromosome 8. Similar to the t(15;17) gene product, the Am11/Eto protein acts to block transcription of *CBFA-CBFB*-controlled genes.

Most translocations that involve 11q23 rearrange the *MLL* (myeloid-lymphoid or mixed-lineage leukemia) gene. The *MLL* gene has two regions that encompass multiple zinc fingers and has at least two additional potential DNA-binding motifs. Abnormalities in the *MLL* gene are relatively common in patients with AML who do not have 11q23 rearrangements cytogenetically.

These molecular aberrations are increasingly being used for diagnosis and detection of residual disease after treatment.

CLINICAL PRESENTATION   Symptoms   Patients with AML most often present with nonspecific symptoms that begin gradually or abruptly and are the consequence of anemia, leukocytosis, leukopenia or leukocyte dysfunction, or thrombocytopenia. Nearly half have had symptoms for 3 months or more before the leukemia is diagnosed.

Half mention fatigue as the first symptom, but most complain of fatigue or weakness at the time of diagnosis. Anorexia and weight loss are common. Fever with or without an identifiable infection is the initial symptom in ~10% of patients. Signs of abnormal hemostasis (bleeding, easy bruising) are noted first in 5% of patients. On occasion, bone pain, lymphadenopathy, nonspecific cough, headache, or diaphoresis is the presenting symptom.

Rarely patients may present with symptoms from a mass lesion located in the soft tissues, breast, uterus, ovary, cranial or spinal dura, gastrointestinal tract, lung, mediastinum, prostate, bone, or other organs. The mass lesion represents a tumor of leukemic cells and is called a *granulocytic sarcoma*, or *chloroma*. Typical AML may occur simultaneously, later, or not at all in these patients. This rare presentation is more common in patients with 8;21 translocations.

Physical Findings   Fever, splenomegaly, hepatomegaly, lymphadenopathy, sternal tenderness, and evidence of infection and hemorrhage are often found at diagnosis. Significant gastrointestinal bleeding, intrapulmonary hemorrhage, or intracranial hemorrhage occur most often in M3 AML. Bleeding associated with coagulopathies may also occur in M5 AML and with extreme degrees of leukocytosis or thrombocytopenia in other FAB subtypes. Retinal hemorrhages are detected in 15% of patients. Infiltration of the gingivae, skin, soft tissues, or the meninges with leukemic blasts at diagnosis is characteristic of the monocytic subtypes (M4 and M5).

Hematologic Findings   Anemia is usually present at diagnosis and can be severe. The degree varies considerably irrespective of other hematologic findings, splenomegaly, or the duration of symptoms. The anemia is usually normochromic normocytic. Decreased erythropoiesis often results in a reduced reticulocyte count, and erythrocyte survival is decreased by accelerated destruction. Active blood loss also contributes to the anemia.

The median presenting leukocyte count is about 15,000/μL. Twenty-five to 40% of patients have counts <5000/μL, and 20% have counts >100,000/μL. Fewer than 5% have no detectable leukemic cells in the blood. Poor neutrophil function may be noted functionally by impaired phagocytosis and migration and morphologically by abnormal lobulation and deficient granulation.

Platelet counts <100,000/μL are found at diagnosis in ~75% of patients, and about 25% have counts <25,000/μL. Both morphologic and functional platelet abnormalities can be observed, including large and bizarre shapes with abnormal granulation and inability of platelets to aggregate or adhere normally to one another.

Pretreatment Evaluation   Once the diagnosis of AML is suspected, a rapid evaluation and initiation of appropriate therapy should follow (Table 111-2). In addition to clarifying the subtype of leukemia, initial studies should evaluate the overall functional integrity of the major organ systems, including the cardiovascular, pulmonary, hepatic, and renal systems. Factors that have prognostic significance, either for achieving complete remission (CR) or for predicting the duration of CR, should also be assessed before initiating treatment. Leukemic cells should be obtained from all patients and cryopreserved for future use as new tests become available. All patients should be evaluated for infection.

Most patients are anemic and thrombocytopenic at presentation. Replacement of the appropriate blood components, if necessary, should begin promptly. Because qualitative platelet dysfunction or the presence of an infection may increase the likelihood of bleeding, evidence of hemorrhage justifies the immediate use of platelet transfusion, even if the platelet count is only moderately decreased.

About 50% of patients have a mild to moderate elevation of serum

Table 111-2 Initial Diagnostic Evaluation and Management of Adult Patients with AML

History
  Increasing fatigue or decreased exercise tolerance (anemia)
  Excess bleeding or bleeding from unusual sites (DIC, thrombocytopenia)
  Fevers or recurrent infections (granulocytopenia)
  Headache, vision changes, nonfocal neurologic abnormalities (CNS leukemia or bleed)
  Early satiety (splenomegaly)
  Family history of AML (Fanconi, Bloom or Kostmann syndromes or ataxia telangiectasia)
  History of cancer (exposure to alkylating agents, radiation, topoisomerase II inhibitors)
  Occupational exposures (radiation, benzene, petroleum products, paint, smoking, pesticides
Physical Examination
  Performance status (prognostic factor)
  Ecchymosis and oozing from IV sites (DIC, possible acute promyelocytic leukemia)
  Fever and tachycardia (signs of infection)
  Papilledema, retinal infiltrates, cranial nerve abnormalities (CNS leukemia)
  Poor dentition, dental abscesses
  Gum hypertrophy (leukemic infiltration, most common in monocytic leukemia)
  Skin infiltration or nodules (leukemia infiltration, most common in monocytic leukemia)
  Lymphadenopathy, splenomegaly, hepatosplenomegaly
  Back pain, lower extremity weakness [spinal granulocytic sarcoma, most likely in t(8;21) patients]
Laboratory and Radiologic Studies
  CBC with manual differential cell count
  Chemistry tests (electrolytes, creatinine, hepatic enzymes, BUN, calcium, phosphorus, LDH, uric acid, bilirubin, amylase, lipase)
  Clotting studies (prothrombin time, partial thromboplastin time, fibrinogen, D-dimer)
  Viral serologies (CMV, HSV-1, Varicella zoster)
  RBC type and screen
  HLA-typing of patient, siblings, and parents for potential allogeneic SCT
  Bone marrow aspirate and biopsy (morphology, cytochemistry, cytogenetics, flow cytometry, molecular studies)
  Cryopreservation of viable leukemia cells (for later study)
  Echocardiogram
  PA and lateral chest radiograph
  Placement of central venous access device
Interventions for Specific Patients
  Dental evaluation (for those with poor dentition)
  Lumbar puncture (for those with symptoms of CNS involvement)
  Screening spine MRI (for patients with back pain, lower extremity weakness, paresthesias)
  Social work referral for patient and family psychosocial support
Counseling for All Patients
  Provide patient with disease information, financial information, support group information

uric acid at presentation. Only 10% have marked elevations, but renal precipitation of uric acid and the nephropathy that may result is a serious but uncommon complication. The initiation of chemotherapy may aggravate hyperuricemia, and patients are usually immediately started on allopurinol and hydration at diagnosis. Finally, the presence in high concentrations of lysozyme, a marker for monocytic differentiation, may be etiologic in renal tubular dysfunction, which could worsen other renal problems that arise during the initial phases of therapy.

PROGNOSTIC FACTORS The single most important prognostic factor is attainment of CR. CR is defined after examination of both blood and bone marrow and should last ≥4 weeks. The blood neutrophil count must be ≥1500/μL and the platelet count ≥100,000/μL. Hemoglobin concentration or hematocrit are not considered in determining CR. Circulating blasts should be absent. While rare blasts may be detected in the blood during marrow regeneration, they should disappear on successive studies. Bone marrow cellularity should be

>20% with trilineage maturation. The bone marrow should contain <5% blasts, and Auer rods should be absent. Extramedullary leukemia should not be present. For patients in CR, reverse transcriptase polymerase chain reaction (RT-PCR) to detect AML-associated molecular abnormalities, and fluorescence in situ hybridization (FISH) to detect AML-associated cytogenetic aberrations are currently used to detect residual disease. Such detection of minimal residual disease may become a reliable discriminator between patients in CR who do or do not require additional and/or alternative therapies.

Many factors influence the likelihood of entering CR, the length of CR, and the curability of AML. Prognostic factors are influenced by the treatment used. Age at diagnosis remains among the most important pretreatment risk factors, with >60 years being associated with a poorer prognosis primarily because of its influence on the patient's ability to survive induction therapy and thus achieve CR. Chronic and intercurrent diseases impair tolerance to rigorous therapy; acute medical problems at diagnosis reduce the likelihood of survival. Performance status, independent of age, also influences ability to survive induction therapy and thus respond to treatment. Age may also influence outcome because AML in older patients differs biologically. The leukemic cells in elderly patients more commonly express CD34 and the mdr1 efflux pump that conveys resistance to natural product-derived agents such as the anthracyclines (see below). With each successive decade of age, a greater proportion of patients have more resistant disease.

Chromosome findings at diagnosis are an independent prognostic factor. Patients with t(8;21), inv(16), or t(15;17) have extremely good prognoses, while those with no cytogenetic abnormality have a moderately favorable outcome when treated with high-dose cytarabine. Patients with del(5q), -7, and abnormalities involving 12p have a very poor prognosis. Patients with certain abnormalities, such as inv(3), rarely achieve CR with standard induction chemotherapy.

A prolonged symptomatic interval with cytopenias preceding diagnosis or a history of an antecedent hematologic disorder are other pretreatment clinical features that are associated with a lower CR rate and shorter survival time. The CR rate is lower in patients who have had anemia, leukopenia, and/or thrombocytopenia for >1 month before the diagnosis of AML when compared to those without such a history. Responsiveness to chemotherapy declines as the duration of the antecedent disorder(s) increases. Secondary AML developing after treatment with cytotoxic agents and/or irradiation for other malignancies is extremely difficult to treat successfully.

A high presenting leukocyte count is an independent prognostic factor; duration of CR is inversely related to the presenting leukocyte count or absolute circulating myeloblast count. Among patients with hyperleukocytosis (>100,000/μL), early central nervous system bleeding and pulmonary leukostasis and late relapse contribute to poor outcome.

The FAB classification diagnosis has been found to be an independent prognostic factor in some series. Other characteristics of the leukemic cell have been reported to have prognostic significance, including Auer rods, ultrastructural features, in vitro and in vivo growth characteristics and chemotherapeutic sensitivity, and immunophenotype. Expression of the *MDR1* gene adversely influences outcome. This gene encodes a protein that actively pumps out a variety of lipophilic compounds (e.g., anthracyclines) from the cell.

In addition to pretreatment variables, several treatment factors have been reported to correlate with prognosis in AML, in particular with CR duration. One is the rapidity with which the blast cells disappear from the blood after the institution of therapy. In addition, patients who achieve CR after one induction cycle have longer CR than those requiring multiple cycles.

℞ **TREATMENT** Treatment of the newly diagnosed patient with AML is usually divided into two phases, induction and postremission management (Fig. 111-1). The initial goal is to quickly induce CR. Once CR is obtained, further therapy must be used to prolong survival.

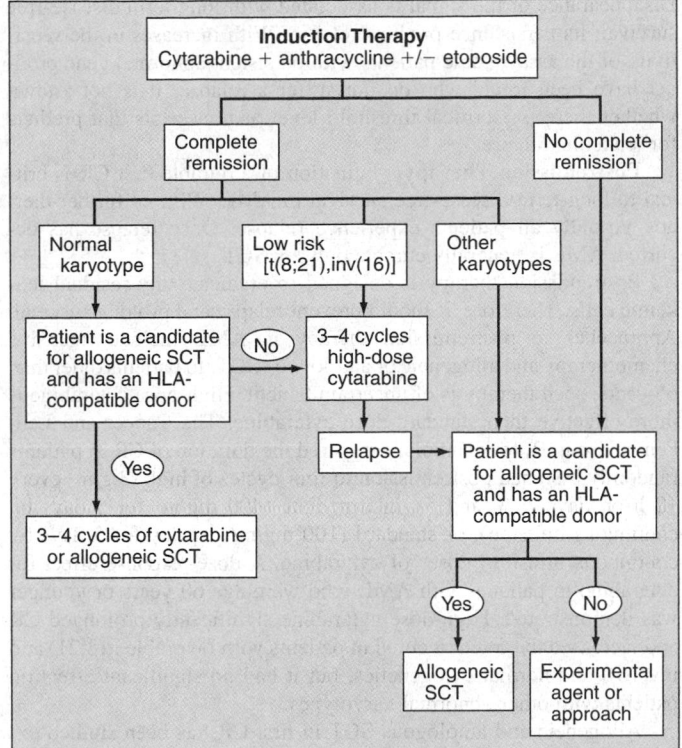

Induction Therapy
Cytarabine + anthracycline +/− etoposide

FIGURE 111-1 Flow chart for the therapy of newly diagnosed AML. For all forms of AML except acute promyelocytic leukemia, standard therapy includes a 7-day continuous infusion of cytarabine (100–200 mg/m² per day) and a 3-day course of daunorubicin (45 mg/m² per day) or idarubicin (12–13 mg/m² per day) with or without 3 days of etoposide. Patients who achieve CR undergo some form of consolidation therapy, including sequential courses of high-dose cytarabine, high-dose combination chemotherapy with allogeneic SCT or novel therapies, based on their predicted risk of relapse (i.e., risk-stratified therapy). Patients with acute promyelocytic leukemia usually receive tretinoin together with combination chemotherapy for remission induction and then receive consolidation chemotherapy (daunorubicin and cytarabine) followed by maintenance tretinoin.

Induction Chemotherapy The most commonly used CR induction regimens (for patients with all FAB subtypes except M3) consist of combination chemotherapy with cytarabine (cytosine arabinoside) and an anthracycline. Cytarabine is a cell cycle S-phase-specific antimetabolite that becomes phosphorylated to an active triphosphate form that interferes with DNA synthesis. Anthracyclines are DNA intercalaters. Their primary mode of action is thought to be inhibition of topoisomerase II, leading to DNA breaks. Cytarabine is usually administered as a continuous intravenous infusion at 100 to 200 mg/m² per day for 7 days. Anthracycline therapy generally consists of daunorubicin, 45 mg/m² intravenously on days 1, 2, and 3 (*the 7 and 3 regimen*). Treatment with idarubicin at 12 or 13 mg/m² per day for 3 days in conjunction with cytarabine by 7-day continuous infusion is at least as effective and may be superior to daunorubicin in younger patients. The addition of etoposide or other agents does not increase the CR rate but may improve the CR duration.

After induction chemotherapy, the bone marrow is examined to determine if the leukemia has been eliminated. If >5% blasts exist with ≥20% cellularity, the patient has traditionally been retreated with cytarabine and an anthracycline in doses similar to those given initially, but for 5 and 2 days, respectively. Our recommendation, however, is to consider changing therapy in this setting. Patients who fail to attain CR after two induction courses should immediately proceed to an allogeneic stem cell transplant (SCT) if an appropriate donor exists.

With the 7 and 3 cytarabine/daunorubicin regimen outlined above, 65 to 75% of adults with de novo AML achieve CR. Two-thirds

achieve CR after a single course of therapy, and one-third require two courses. About 50% of patients who do not achieve CR have a drug-resistant leukemia, and 50% do not achieve CR because of fatal complications of bone marrow aplasia or impaired recovery of normal stem cells.

High-dose cytarabine-based regimens have very high CR rates after a single cycle of therapy. When given in high doses, more cytarabine may enter the cells, saturate the cytarabine-inactivating enzymes, and increase the intracellular levels of 1-β-D-arabinofuranylcytosine-triphosphate, the active metabolite incorporated into DNA. Thus, higher doses of cytarabine may increase the inhibition of DNA synthesis and thereby overcome resistance to standard-dose cytarabine. In two randomized studies, one by the Southwest Oncology Group (SWOG) and one by the Australian Leukemia Study Group (ALSG), high-dose cytarabine with an anthracycline produced CR rates similar to those achieved with standard 7 and 3 regimens. However, the ALSG demonstrated that the CR duration was much longer after high dose cytarabine than after standard-dose cytarabine.

The hematologic toxicity of high-dose cytarabine-based induction regimens has typically been greater than that associated with 7 and 3 regimens. Toxicity with high-dose cytarabine includes myelosuppression, pulmonary toxicity, and significant and occasionally irreversible cerebellar toxicity. All patients treated with high-dose cytarabine must be closely monitored for cerebellar toxicity. Full cerebellar testing should be performed before each dose, and further high-dose cytarabine should be withheld if evidence of cerebellar toxicity develops.

Supportive Care Measures geared to supporting patients through several weeks of granulocytopenia and thrombocytopenia are critical to the success of AML therapy. Patients with AML should be treated in centers expert in providing supportive measures for their management.

Recombinant hematopoietic growth factors have been incorporated into clinical trials in AML. These trials have been designed to lower the infection rate after chemotherapy or to sensitize (prime) the leukemic blasts to chemotherapy, or both. Both granulocyte colony stimulating factor (G-CSF) and granulocyte-macrophage colony stimulating factor (GM-CSF) have reduced the median time to neutrophil recovery by an average of 5 to 7 days. This accelerated rate of neutrophil recovery, however, has not always translated into significant reductions in infection rates. In most randomized studies, both G-CSF and GM-CSF have failed to improve the CR rate, disease-free survival, or overall survival. Although receptors for both G-CSF and GM-CSF are present on AML blasts, therapeutic efficacy is neither enhanced nor inhibited by these agents. The use of growth factors as supportive care for AML patients is controversial. We favor their use in elderly patients, those receiving intensive regimens, patients with uncontrolled infections, or those participating in clinical trials.

Multilumen right atrial catheters should be inserted through a subcutaneous tunnel as soon as patients with newly diagnosed AML have been stabilized. They should be used thereafter for administration of intravenous medications and transfusions, as well as for blood drawing. The separation between the vascular access site and the exit site and the presence of a Dacron cuff in the subcutaneous channel reduce the risk of infection. With meticulous attention to sterile technique in catheter placement and maintenance, catheters may often be left in place for months.

Adequate and prompt blood bank support is critical to therapy of AML. Platelet transfusions should be given as needed to maintain a platelet count >10,000 to 20,000/μL. We believe that the platelet count should be kept at higher levels in febrile patients and during episodes of active bleeding or DIC. Patients with poor posttransfusion platelet count increments may benefit from administration of platelets from human leukocyte antigen (HLA)-matched donors. Red blood cell transfusions should be administered to keep the hemoglobin level >80 g/L (8 g/dL) in the absence of active bleeding or DIC. Blood products leukodepleted by filtration should be used to avert or delay alloimmunization as well as febrile reactions. Blood products should also be irradiated to prevent graft-versus-host disease (GVHD). Cytomegalovirus (CMV)-negative blood products should be used for CMV-seronegative patients who are potential candidates for allogeneic SCT. Leukodepleted products are also effective for these patients if CMV-negative products are not available.

Infectious complications remain the major cause of morbidity and death during induction and postremission chemotherapy for AML. Prophylactic administration of antibiotics in the absence of fever is controversial. Oral nystatin or clotrimazole are recommended to prevent localized candidiasis. For patients who are herpes simplex virus antibody titer–positive, acyclovir prophylaxis is effective in preventing reactivation of latent oral herpes infections.

Fever develops in most patients with AML, but infections are documented in only half of febrile patients. Early initiation of empiric broad-spectrum antibacterial and antifungal antibiotics has significantly reduced the number of patients dying of infectious complications (Chap. 85). An antibiotic regimen adequate to treat gram-negative and gram-positive organisms should be instituted at the onset of fever in a granulocytopenic patient after clinical evaluation, including a detailed physical examination with inspection of the indwelling catheter exit site and a perirectal examination, as well as procurement of cultures and radiographs aimed at documenting the source of fever. Specific antibiotic regimens should be based on antibiotic sensitivity data obtained from the institution at which the patient is being treated. Acceptable regimens include imipenem-cilastin, an antipseudomonal semisynthetic penicillin (e.g., piperacillin) combined with an aminoglycoside, a third-generation cephalosporin with antipseudomonal activity (i.e., ceftazidine or cefapime) or double β-lactam combinations (ceftazidine and piperacillin). Empiric vancomycin is not given initially in the absence of suspected gram-positive infection or mucositis. Aminoglycosides should be avoided if possible in patients with renal insufficiency. For patients with known immediate-type hypersensitivity reactions to penicillin, aztreonam may be substituted for β-lactams. Aztreonam should be combined with an aminoglycoside or a quinolone antibiotic rather than used alone. Empiric vancomycin should be initiated in neutropenic patients who remain febrile for 3 days, and amphotericin B is added at 7 days if fever persists. Liposomal amphotericin is at least equivalent to regular amphotericin for empiric antifungal treatment and has less renal toxicity. Antibacterial and antifungal antibiotics should be continued until patients are no longer neutropenic, regardless of whether a specific source has been found for the fever.

Treatment of Promyelocytic Leukemia   ATRA is an oral drug that induces the differentiation of leukemic cells bearing the t(15;17); it is not effective in other forms of AML. Acute promyelocytic leukemia is responsive to cytarabine and daunarubicin, but about 10% of patients treated with these drugs die from DIC induced by the release of granule components by dying tumor cells. ATRA does not produce DIC but produces another complication called the retinoic acid syndrome. Occurring within the first 3 weeks of treatment, it is characterized by fever, dyspnea, chest pain, pulmonary infiltrates, pleural and pericardial effusions, and hypoxia. The syndrome is related to the adhesion of differentiated neoplastic cells in the pulmonary vasculature. Glucocorticoids, chemotherapy, and/or supportive measures can be effective. About 10% of patients die from this syndrome.

ATRA (45 mg/m^2 per day orally until remission is documented) plus concurrent chemotherapy (7 and 3) appears to be the safest and most effective treatment for acute promyelocytic leukemia. Unlike patients with other types of AML, patients with this subtype may benefit from maintenance therapy with either ATRA or chemotherapy. The optimal regimen is being sought in clinical studies.

Arsenic trioxide produces meaningful responses in patients refractory to ATRA.

The detection of minimal residual disease by RT-PCR amplification of the t(15;17) chimeric gene product appears to predict relapse.

Disappearance of the signal is associated with long-term disease-free survival; its persistence predicts relapse. With increases in the sensitivity of the assay, some patients with persistent abnormal gene product have been found who do not suffer a relapse. It is not known whether there is a critical threshold level of transcripts that predicts for leukemia relapse.

Postremission Therapy   Induction of a durable first CR is critical to long-term disease-free survival in AML. Without further therapy virtually all patients experience relapse. Once relapse has occurred, AML is generally curable only by SCT.

Postremission therapy is designed to eradicate any residual leukemic cells. Therefore, it should prevent relapse and prolong survival. Approaches to postremission therapy in AML include intensive chemotherapy and allogeneic or autologous SCT. In patients older than 65 years, such therapy is of uncertain benefit. High-dose cytarabine is more effective than standard-dose cytarabine. The Cancer and Leukemia Group B, for example, compared the duration of CR in patients randomly assigned postremission to four cycles of high (3 g/m^2 every 12 h on days 1, 3, and 5), intermediate (400 mg/m^2 for 5 days by continuous infusion), or standard (100 mg/m^2 per day for 5 days by continuous infusion) doses of cytarabine. A dose-response effect for cytarabine in patients with AML who were age 60 years or younger was demonstrated. High-dose cytarabine significantly prolonged CR and increased the fraction cured in patients with favorable [t(8;21) and inv(16)] and normal cytogenetics, but it had no significant effect on patients with other abnormal karyotypes.

Allogeneic and autologous SCT in first CR has been studied extensively in younger patients with no major organ dysfunction. Allogeneic SCT is used in patients <55 years with an HLA-compatible donor. Relapse with this therapy occurs in only a small fraction of patients, but toxicity is relatively high from treatment; complications include veno-occlusive disease, GVHD, and infections. Autologous transplantation can be used in young and older patients and uses the same type of high-dose therapy. Patients subsequently receive their own stem cells collected while in remission. The toxicity is lower with autologous SCT (5% mortality rate), but the relapse rate is higher than with allogeneic SCT. The increased relapse rate is due to the absence of the graft-vs-leukemia effect seen with allogeneic SCT and possible contamination of the autologous stem cells with tumor cells. Purging the autologous stem cells does not lower the relapse rate with autologous SCT.

Randomized trials comparing intensive therapy and autologous and allogeneic SCT have shown improved duration of remission with allogeneic SCT compared to autologous SCT or chemotherapy alone. However, overall survival is generally not different; the improved disease control with allogeneic SCT is erased by the increase in fatal toxicity. Prognostic factors may help select patients in first CR for whom transplant is most effective.

Our approach includes strong consideration for allogeneic SCT in first CR for patients with high risk karyotypes. Patients with normal karyotypes who have other poor risk factors (antecedent hematologic disorder, failure to attain remission with a single induction course, hyperleukocytosis, *MLL* gene abnormalities) are also potential candidates. If a suitable HLA donor does not exist, autologous SCT or novel therapeutic approaches are considered. Patients with t(8;21) and inv(16) are treated with repetitive doses of high-dose cytarabine, which offers a high frequency of cure without the morbidity of transplant.

Relapse   Once relapse occurs after the standard induction and postremission chemotherapy approach described above and outlined in Fig. 111-1, patients are rarely cured with further standard-dose chemotherapy. Patients eligible for allogeneic SCT should receive transplants expeditiously at the first sign of relapse. Long-term disease-free survival is approximately the same (30 to 50%) with allogeneic SCT in first relapse or in second remission. Autologous SCT rescues about 20% of relapsed patients with AML who have chemosensitive disease. The most important factors predicting response at relapse are the length of the previous CR, whether initial CR was achieved with one or two courses of chemotherapy, and the type of postremission

Table 111-3 Selected New Agents Under Study for the Treatment of Adults with AML

Class of Drugs	Example Agent(s)
MDR1 modulator	Cyclosporine analogues, PSC-833
Demethylating agent	Decitabine, 5-azacytidine
Histone deacetylase inhibitor	Phenylbutyrate, depsipeptide
Heavy metals	Arsenic trioxide, antimony
Protein kinase C inhibitor	Bryostatin, UCN-01
Cell cycle inhibitor	Flavopiridol
Humanized antibodies	Anti-CD33 (HuM195)
Toxin-conjugated antibodies	CMA-676 (anti-CD33 linked to calicheamicin)
Radiolabeled antibodies	Yttrium-90-labeled human M195
Cytokines	Recombinant human IL-2 and IL-12

therapy. Because of the poor outcome of patients in early (<12 months) first relapse, it is justified (for patients without HLA-compatible donors) to explore innovative approaches, such as new drugs or immunotherapies (Table 111-3). Patients with longer (>12 months) first CR generally relapse with drug-sensitive disease and may achieve a second remission with the original induction regimen. However, cure for these patients is uncommon, and treatment with novel approaches should be considered if SCT is not possible. It is not yet clear whether careful monitoring for residual disease by RT-PCR, FISH and quantitative PCR identifies patients destined to relapse who are more readily cured by salvage therapy given before overt clinical relapse.

CHRONIC MYELOID LEUKEMIA

INCIDENCE The incidence of chronic myeloid leukemia (CML) is 1.3 per 100,000 people per year, and the age-adjusted incidence is higher in men than in women (1.7 versus 1.0). CML incidence decreased slightly between 1973 and 1991 (1.5 versus 1.3). The incidence of CML increases slowly with age until the middle forties, when it starts to rise rapidly.

DEFINITION The diagnosis of CML is established by identifying a clonal expansion of a hematopoietic stem cell possessing a reciprocal translocation between chromosomes 9 and 22. This translocation results in the head-to-tail fusion of the breakpoint cluster region (*BCR*) gene on chromosome 22q11 with the *ABL* (named after the abelson murine leukemia virus) gene located on chromosome 9q34. Untreated, the disease is characterized by the inevitable transition from a chronic phase to an accelerated phase and on to blast crisis.

ETIOLOGY No clear correlation with exposure to cytotoxic drugs, such as alkylating agents, has been found, and there is no direct evidence of a viral etiology. Cigarette smoking has been shown to accelerate the progression to blast crisis and therefore has an adverse effect on survival in CML. The effect of radiation was demonstrated in the study of the atomic bomb survivors, where it has been estimated that the development of a CML cell mass of 10,000/μL takes 6.3 years. No increase in CML incidence was found in the survivors of the Chernobyl accident, suggesting that only large doses of radiation can induce CML.

PATHOPHYSIOLOGY The product of the fusion gene resulting from the t(9;22) plays a central role in the development of CML. This chimeric gene is transcribed into a hybrid *BCR/ABL* mRNA in which exon 1 of ABL is replaced by variable numbers of 5' BCR exons. Bcr/Abl fusion proteins, p210$^{BCR-ABL}$, are produced that contain NH$_2$-terminal domains of Bcr and the COOH-terminal domains of Abl. Bcr/Abl fusion proteins can transform hematopoietic progenitor cells in vitro. Furthermore, reconstituting lethally irradiated mice with bone marrow cells infected with retrovirus carrying the gene encoding the p210$^{BCR-ABL}$ leads to the development of a myeloproliferative syndrome resembling CML in 50% of the mice. Specific antisense oligomers to the *BCR/ABL* junctions inhibit the growth of t(9;22)-positive leukemic cells without affecting normal colony formation.

The mechanism(s) by which p210$^{BCR-ABL}$ promotes the transition from the benign state to the fully malignant one is still unclear. Messenger RNA for *BCR/ABL* can occasionally be detected in normal individuals. However, attachment of the *BCR* sequences to *ABL* results in three critical functional changes: (1) the Abl protein becomes constitutively active as a tyrosine kinase enzyme, (2) the DNA protein–binding activity of Abl is attenuated, and (3) the binding of Abl to cytoskeletal actin microfilaments is enhanced.

Disease Progression The events associated with transition to the acute phase are poorly understood. Chromosomal instability of the malignant clone, resulting, for example, in the acquisition of an additional t(9;22), trisomy 8, or 17p- (p53 loss), is a fundamental characteristic of CML. Acquisition of these additional genetic and/or molecular abnormalities is critical to the phenotypic transformation. The site of the breakpoint within the *BCR* gene may predict the time to development of blast crisis, but this claim has been refuted by others. Heterogeneous structural alterations of the p53 gene, as well as structural alterations and lack of protein production of the retinoblastoma gene, have been associated with disease progression in a subset of patients. Rare patients show alterations in *RAS*. Sporadic reports also document the presence of an altered *MYC* (named after the myelocytomatosis virus) gene or the appearance of p190$^{BCR-ABL}$, the protein commonly found in adult ALL and occasionally in AML, during the clinical evolution of small numbers of patients with CML. Progressive de novo DNA methylation at the *BCR/ABL* locus has also been shown to herald blastic transformation. Finally, interleukin (IL)-1β may be involved in the progression of CML to the blastic phase. Multiple pathways to disease transformation exist, but the exact timing and relevance of each of these remains unclear.

CLINICAL PRESENTATION Symptoms The clinical onset of the chronic phase is generally insidious. Accordingly, some patients are diagnosed while still asymptomatic, during health screening tests; other patients present with fatigue, malaise, and weight loss or have symptoms resulting from splenic enlargement, such as early satiety and left upper quadrant pain or mass. Less common are features related to granulocyte or platelet dysfunction, such as infections, thrombosis, or bleeding. Occasionally, patients present with leukostatic manifestations due to severe leukocytosis or thrombosis such as vasoocclusive disease, cerebrovascular accidents, myocardial infarction, venous thrombosis, priapism, visual disturbances, and pulmonary insufficiency.

Progression of CML is associated with worsening symptoms. Unexplained fever, significant weight loss, increasing dose requirement of the drugs controlling the disease, bone and joint pain, bleeding, thrombosis, and infections suggest transformation into accelerated or blastic phases. Fewer than 10 to 15% of newly diagnosed patients present with accelerated disease or with de novo blastic phase CML.

Physical Findings In most patients the abnormal finding on physical examination at diagnosis is minimal to moderate splenomegaly; mild hepatomegaly is found occasionally. Persistent splenomegaly despite continued therapy is a sign of disease acceleration. Lymphadenopathy and extramedullary myeloid tumors (granulocytic sarcomas) are unusual except late in the course of the disease; when they are present, the prognosis is poor.

Hematologic Findings Elevated white blood cell counts, with various degrees of immaturity of the granulocytic series, are present at diagnosis. Usually <5% circulating blasts and <10% blasts and promyelocytes are noted. Cycling of the counts may be observed in patients followed without treatment. Platelet counts are almost always elevated at diagnosis, and a mild degree of normochromic normocytic anemia is present. Leukocyte alkaline phosphatase is characteristically low in CML cells. Serum levels of vitamin B$_{12}$ and vitamin B$_{12}$–binding proteins are generally elevated. Phagocytic functions are usually normal at diagnosis and remain normal during the chronic phase. Histamine production secondary to basophilia is increased in later stages, causing pruritus, diarrhea, and flushing.

At diagnosis, bone marrow cellularity, primarily of the myeloid and megakaryocytic lineages, with a greatly altered myeloid to erythroid ratio, is increased in almost all patients with CML. The marrow blast percentage is generally normal or slightly elevated. Marrow or blood basophilia, eosinophilia, and monocytosis may be present. While collagen fibrosis in the marrow is unusual at presentation, significant degrees of reticulin stain–measured fibrosis are noted in about half of the patients.

Disease acceleration is defined by the development of increasing degrees of anemia unaccounted for by bleeding or chemotherapy, cytogenetic clonal evolution, or blood or marrow blasts between 10 and 20%, blood or marrow basophils ≥20%, or platelet count <100,000/μL. *Blast crisis* is defined as acute leukemia, with blood or marrow blasts ≥20%. Hyposegmented neutrophils may appear (Pelger-Huët anomaly). Blast cells can be classified as myeloid, lymphoid, erythroid, or undifferentiated, based on morphologic, cytochemical, and immunologic features. About half the cases are myeloid, one-third lymphoid, 10% erythroid, and the rest are undifferentiated.

Chromosomal Findings The cytogenetic hallmark of CML, found in 90 to 95% of patients, is the t(9;22)(q34;q11). Originally, this was recognized by the presence of a shortened chromosome 22 (22q-), designated as the *Philadelphia chromosome*, that arises from the reciprocal 9;22 translocation. Some patients may have complex translocations (designated as *variant translocations*) involving three, four, or five chromosomes (usually including chromosomes 9 and 22). However, the molecular consequences of these changes appear similar to those resulting from the typical t(9;22).

PROGNOSTIC FACTORS The clinical outcome of patients with CML is variable. Death is expected in 10% of patients within 2 years and in about 20% yearly thereafter. The median survival time is ~4 years. Therefore, several prognostic models that identify different risk groups in CML have been developed. The most commonly used staging systems have been derived from multivariate analyses of prognostic factors. The Sokal index identified percentage of circulating blasts, spleen size, platelet count, cytogenetic clonal evolution, and age as the most important prognostic indicators. Two models, that of Tura and the combined model of Kantarjian, divide patients according to the number of negative prognostic factors. Age ≥60 years, spleen ≥10 cm below the costal margin, blasts ≥3% in blood or ≥5% in marrow, basophils ≥7% in blood or ≥3% in marrow, platelets ≥700,000/μL, or any of the characteristics of accelerated disease are associated with a very poor short-term prognosis and a threefold higher hazard rate, or risk of death per unit of time, in the first year. A prognostic scoring system to estimate the survival of CML patients treated with interferon (IFN) α has been developed.

℞ **TREATMENT** The goal of therapy in CML is to achieve prolonged, durable, nonneoplastic, nonclonal hematopoiesis, which entails the eradication of any residual cells containing the BCR/ABL transcript. Hence the goal is complete molecular remission and cure (Table 111-4). A proposed treatment plan for the newly diagnosed patient with CML is presented in Fig. 111-2.

Allogeneic SCT Allogeneic SCT is the only curative therapy for CML and, when feasible, is the treatment of choice. However, it is complicated by a high early mortality rate owing to the transplant procedure. When the outcome of all patients undergoing allogeneic SCT reported to the International Bone Marrow Transplant Registry was compared with the outcome of all patients treated with hydroxyurea or interferon (IFN) α by the German CML Study Group, the survival for the former group was statistically better, but only starting 5 years after transplant. When only low-risk patients (by Sokal's criteria) were evaluated, the benefit in survival for allogeneic SCT was seen after 6 years. Outcome of SCT depends on multiple factors including: (1) the patient (i.e., age and phase of disease); (2) the type of donor [i.e., syngeneic (monozygotic twins) or HLA-compatible allogeneic, related or unrelated]; (3) the preparative regimen; (4) GVHD; and (5) posttransplantation treatment.

Table 111-4   Response Criteria in CML

Hematologic	
Complete response[a]	White blood cell count <10,000/μL, normal morphology
	Normal hemoglobin and platelet counts
Incomplete response	White blood cell count ≥10,000/μL
Cytogenetic	Percentage of bone marrow metaphases with t(9;22)
Complete response	0
Partial response	≤35
Minor response	36–85[b]
No response	85–100
Molecular	Presence of BCR/ABL transcript by RT-PCR
Complete response	None
Incomplete response	Any

[a] Complete hematologic response requires the disappearance of splenomegaly.
[b] Up to 15% normal metaphases are occasionally seen at diagnosis (when 30 metaphases are analyzed).

The patient As experience has been gained and safety and efficacy have been established, it has become clear that patients should be younger than 65 years and have a healthy and histocompatible donor. Furthermore, survival after SCT in the accelerated and blastic phases of the disease is significantly diminished and is associated with a very high rate of relapse. The Seattle data demonstrate that SCT early in the chronic phase (1 to 2 years from diagnosis) is superior to later SCT. While overall survival, disease-free survival, and relapse rates are not influenced by prior IFN-α treatment, incidence and severity of acute and chronic GVHD correlate with prior IFN-α treatment in the unrelated donor and possibly also in the related donor setting. Therefore, because early SCT is more effective than late SCT, the decision to perform allogeneic SCT should probably be made within a year of diagnosis when IFN-α is the initial therapy; a 3-month hiatus is recommended between discontinuing IFN-α and initiating SCT.

The donor Transplantation from a family donor, who is either fully matched or mismatched at only one HLA locus, should be considered standard therapy for any patient with CML who is a candidate for an HLA-related sibling transplant. Syngeneic SCT in patients with chronic phase CML has been reported from the Seattle group to result in 7-year disease-free survival in 55%, with a 30% relapse rate. With HLA-identical sibling SCT in the chronic phase, many groups have reported 5-year disease-free survival in 40 to 70% of patients, with a 25% relapse rate. SCT from an HLA-matched unrelated donor has

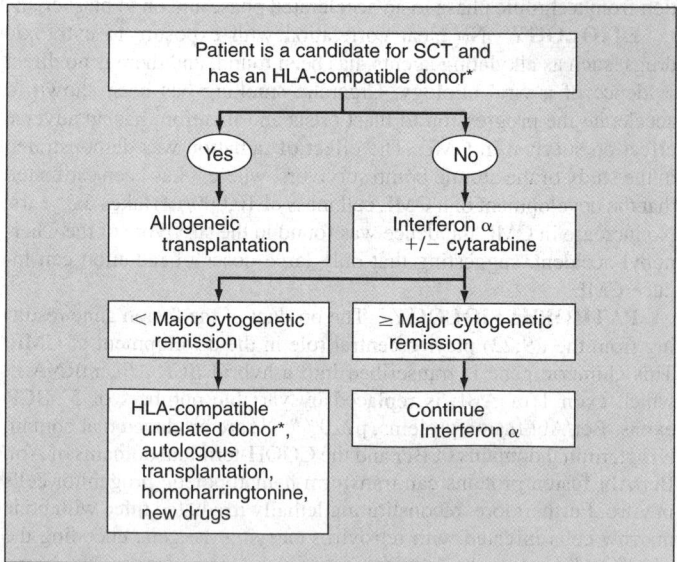

FIGURE 111-2 Flow chart for the therapy of newly diagnosed CML. Please refer to text for details. The asterisk denotes that some centers use an HLA-compatible unrelated donor for SCT at this time and some only use unrelated donors if interferon α fails.

been reported by the Seattle group to result in a 74% probability of surviving 3 years for patients transplanted in chronic phase less than 1 year from diagnosis and younger than 50 years. A 2-year disease-free (based on hematologic analyses) survival of 45% ($\pm$21%) for patients receiving SCT from unrelated individuals, matched or mismatched at only one locus, transplanted less than 1 year from diagnosis was reported by the National Marrow Donor Program. Patients age 40 to 50 years fared poorly (15 of 55 survived). The probability of 2-year disease-free (based on cytogenetic analyses) survival in a report on unrelated transplants from the Medical College of Wisconsin, using a standardized conditioning regimen and T cell depletion, was 52% for patients transplanted in chronic phase (regardless of the time from diagnosis). Patients receiving transplants from unrelated individuals have higher rates of graft failure and acute and chronic GVHD and prolonged convalescence after treatment, compared to those who receive allogeneic transplants from related individuals. Peripheral blood is now being studied as a source of hematopoietic progenitor cells; it may offer rapid engraftment and less risk for the donor. Umbilical-cord blood may permit mismatched SCT with notably less GVHD; graft-versus-leukemia (GVL) effects do not appear to be impaired. A problem with cord blood is obtaining an appropriate number of progenitor cells to reconstitute hematopoiesis in an adult.

Preparative regimens These regimens have been studied by several groups. A randomized study by the Seattle group compared cyclophosphamide and total-body irradiation with busulphan and cyclophosphamide. They found no significant differences in the 3-year probabilities of survival, relapse, event-free survival, speed of engraftment, or incidence of venoocclusive disease of the liver. Significantly more patients in the total-body irradiation arm experienced major elevations of creatinine, acute GVHD, longer periods of fever, positive blood cultures, hospital admissions, and longer inpatient hospital stays. However, increased chronic GVHD, obstructive bronchiolitis and alopecia were noted with busulphan. Intravenous busulphan may permit better control of serum levels. Minitransplants in which the preparative regimen is aimed at eliminating host lymphocytes rather than bone marrow are being tested. Reduced toxicity with preserved antitumor efficacy is the goal.

Development and type of GVHD Development of grade I GVHD, as compared to no GVHD, decreases the risk of relapse. A lower relapse rate was observed also in patients with grade II GVHD but was accompanied by a substantially higher transplant-related mortality rate. The decreased relapse rate may be caused by a GVL effect. Depletion of T lymphocytes from donor marrow can prevent GVHD but results in an increased risk of relapse, which exceeds the relapse rate after syngeneic SCT. Thus, T lymphocytes from the donor marrow mediate a significant antileukemic, or GVL, effect, and even syngeneic marrow may exhibit limited GVL activity in CML.

Posttransplantation treatment Further support for the existence of an immunologically mediated GVL effect comes from the observation that donor leukocyte infusions (without prior conditioning or GVHD prophylaxis) can induce hematologic and cytogenetic remissions in patients with CML who have relapsed after allogeneic SCT.

The activity of IFN-α in patients with early chronic-phase CML was the basis for the use of IFN-α after SCT, either to induce cytogenetic remissions in relapsed patients or to prevent relapse after SCT for high-risk patients. The main concern about IFN-α use after allogeneic SCT has been the development or worsening of GVHD, because IFN-α acts as an immunomodulator. However, in published reports encompassing 52 allogeneic recipients who were free of GVHD and were either at high risk for relapse or had already relapsed, only 6 subsequently developed GVHD after IFN-α therapy was initiated. IFN-α has also been combined with mononuclear cells obtained from donor blood to induce cytogenetic remissions in relapsed patients. Cytogenetic remissions have been achieved, but the exact role of IFN-α as opposed to the mononuclear cells is unclear. IL-2, with or without IFN-α, is also being evaluated for its ability to restore complete cytogenetic remission in patients who suffer relapses after SCT.

IFN-α has been used after SCT to prevent relapse in patients with advanced disease at time of transplant (patients at high risk for relapse). Cytogenetic CR has been maintained for as long as 2 years posttransplantation in small numbers of patients with blast crisis or second chronic phase. Similarly, IL-2 (2.5×10^6 to 6×10^6 units/m^2 per day) has been given to patients after T cell–depleted allogeneic SCT in an effort to induce GVL without GVHD, and thus prevent relapse. Compared with historical control subjects, patients treated with IL-2 have a lower risk of disease relapse. A randomized trial is warranted.

Interferons When allogeneic SCT is not feasible, IFN-α therapy is the treatment of choice. The interferons are a complex group of naturally occurring proteins produced by eukaryotic cells in response to viruses, antigens, and mitogens. Three distinct groups of IFN species have been identified: IFN-α, -β, and -γ. Although various interferons have become available for clinical investigation, most data have been generated with IFN-α preparations.

Interferons have potent, pleiotropic biologic effects, spanning a spectrum of antiviral, microbicidal, immunomodulatory, and antiproliferative properties. While interferons downregulate the expression of several oncogenes and cytokines, they also upregulate the expression of IFN regulatory factor-1 (a transcriptional activator with antioncogenic activity), adhesion molecules, and the histocompatibility genes. Interferons also inhibit angiogenesis and induce a cellular immune response. However, their mode(s) of action are still unknown.

In seven randomized studies comparing IFN-α and chemotherapy, both modalities have been found to be effective in achieving hematologic remissions. However, patients treated with IFN-α survived longer than patients treated with hydroxyurea or busulphan. The 5-year survival rate was 51% with IFN-α and 42% with chemotherapy.

Patients develop both acute and chronic side effects from IFN-α therapy. Acute side effects (flulike symptoms) appear early in the course of the treatment. Most flulike symptoms respond to acetaminophen, and tachyphylaxis develops within 1 to 2 weeks. Chronic reactions, such as fatigue and lethargy, depression, weight loss, myalgias, and arthralgias, occur in about half of the patients and may require dose reduction. Patients also report cough, postnasal drip, and dryness of the skin. Infrequently, immune-mediated thrombocytopenia and anemia develop. In addition, long-term therapy has been associated with late autoimmune side effects, such as hypothyroidism and occasionally generalized autoimmune phenomena.

The most important persistent side effects in patients with CML who are treated with IFN-α are neurologic. All patients treated with IFN-α are subject to some neurologic toxicity, the most common symptom being lethargy. Up to 20% of patients have neurologic side effects that are associated with compromised quality of life and reduced ability to carry out their regular activity, such as full-time work. In addition, at the required doses, impotence in men is not infrequent.

Hematologic remissions are generally achieved within 1 to 2 months of starting IFN-α. However, some patients have a cyclic response pattern with progressively lower peak and nadir counts over a period of months. The increase in counts during the cycling that occurs in the first few months of therapy should not be confused with resistance. Cytogenetic responses generally start at 3 to 12 months, and complete cytogenetic responses may require 6 months to 4 years of therapy. However, most complete cytogenetic responses are achieved within 12 to 18 months; and in single-agent, single-arm studies they have been identified in up to 26% of patients.

The combination of IFN-α with cytarabine has produced better results than those with IFN-α alone; cytogenetic responses occurred earlier, but the influence on survival is not yet known.

Chemotherapy Initial management of patients with chemotherapy is currently reserved for rapid lowering of white blood cell counts, reduction of symptoms, and reversal of symptomatic splenomegaly. Hydroxyurea, a ribonucleotide reductase inhibitor, induces rapid disease control. The initial dose is 1 to 4 g/d, and the dose should be reduced by half with each 50% reduction of the leukocyte count. Unfortunately, cytogenetic remissions with hydroxyurea are uncommon. Busulphan, an alkylating agent that acts on early progenitor cells, has a more prolonged effect. However, we do not recommend its use because of its serious side effects, which include unexpected, and occasionally fatal, myelosuppression in 5 to 10% of patients; pulmonary, endocardial, and marrow fibrosis; and an Addison-like wasting syndrome.

Homoharringtonine (HHT) is a plant alkaloid derived from a tree, *Cephalotaxus fortuneii* sp. *harringtonii*. HHT blocks peptide bond formation after binding of the aminoacyl-transfer RNA to the ribosome. In patients whose disease progressed during treatment with IFN-α or who were in later chronic phase ($>$1 year from diagnosis), HHT induced 72% complete hematologic responses and 22% complete or major cytogenetic responses. The use of HHT before IFN-α in early chronic phase resulted in a 92% complete hematologic response rate and a 27% major cytogenetic response rate. Toxicity is mainly related to myelosuppression.

Intensive combination chemotherapy has also been used in chronic phase CML, with 30 to 50% of patients achieving complete cytogenetic responses. However these cytogenetic remissions have been short lived. Consequently, intensive combination chemotherapy regimens are being used today only to mobilize normal progenitors in the blood in order to collect circulating stem cells for autologous transplantation.

Autologous SCT   Autologous SCT could potentially cure CML if a means to select the residual normal progenitors, which coexist with their malignant counterparts, could be developed. As a source of autologous hematopoietic stem cells for transplantation, blood offers certain advantages over marrow (e.g., faster engraftment and no general anesthesia). Normal hematopoietic stem cells appear with increased frequency in the blood of patients with CML during the recovery phase after chemotherapy and G-CSF.

A retrospective analysis of $>$200 autologous SCT performed for CML at eight centers worldwide suggests that autologous SCT prolongs survival in chronic- or accelerated-phase patients when compared with conventional therapy. At transplant 93 patients were in chronic phase, 25 were in accelerated phase, and 114 were in blast crisis or second chronic phase. Patients received autologous bone marrow and/or blood hematopoietic stem cells. In 42 cases the hematopoietic progenitors were subjected to ex vivo manipulation by long-term bone marrow culture, by incubation with recombinant IFN-γ, or by chemotherapy. In 49 cases the hematopoietic progenitors were harvested during the recovery phase after various chemotherapy regimens. After autologous SCT, 29 of 93 (31%) patients in first chronic phase achieved complete cytogenetic remissions. The median duration of cytogenetic remission was 14 months, with a range of 2 to 68 months. Approaches to treat minimal residual disease after autologous transplantation, such as immune modulation, are currently being investigated.

Leukapheresis and Splenectomy   Intensive leukapheresis may control the blood counts in chronic phase CML; however, it is expensive and cumbersome. It is useful in emergencies where leukostasis-related complications such as pulmonary failure or cerebrovascular accidents are likely. It may also have a role in the treatment of pregnant women in whom it is important to avoid potentially teratogenic drugs.

Splenectomy was used in CML in the past because of the suggestion that evolution to the acute phase might occur in the spleen. However, this does not appear to be the case, and splenectomy is now reserved for symptomatic relief of painful splenomegaly unresponsive to chemotherapy or for significant anemia or thrombocytopenia associated with hypersplenism. Splenic radiation is used rarely to reduce the size of the spleen.

Minimal Residual Disease   The correlation between residual cells with the t(9;22) and disease recurrence is not completely understood. In initial studies with RT-PCR used to predict disease recurrence after IFN-α therapy, residual disease was found in all samples tested from patients with complete cytogenetic remissions. Later stud-

ies demonstrated the elimination of the BCR/ABL mRNA transcript after more prolonged IFN-α treatment in some cases. It is now possible to quantitate transcripts, and longer follow-up may indicate whether quantitation of the BCR/ABL transcript is useful for predicting cytogenetic and clinical relapse.

After allogeneic SCT, RT-PCR analysis may be positive for residual disease during the first 6 months in patients who subsequently achieve a long-lasting remission. However, late persistence of RT-PCR positivity appears to indicate a reduced probability of cure. RT-PCR positivity at any single time point is not predictive of imminent relapse. After allogeneic SCT, patients are often divided according to RT-PCR results into one of three groups: (1) persistently positive, (2) intermittently negative, and (3) persistently negative. These three groups have low, intermediate, and high probability of maintaining remission and disease free-survival, respectively. Although these data suggest that patients who are persistently RT-PCR positive more than 6 months after allogeneic SCT need additional therapeutic interventions, this conclusion has not been rigorously established. The studies have used an assortment of techniques for measuring minimal residual disease, the level of sensitivity has been variable, and the follow-up durations of patients are short. Real-time RT-PCR may provide a more sensitive tool to predict relapse in CML and in other cancers. In patients who do not have any evidence for GVHD and are intermittently RT-PCR negative, GVL may be induced by alloreactive donor cells (without the side effects of GVHD) to suppress the proliferation of the leukemic cells.

Future Directions   The synthetic inhibitor of the BCR/ABL kinase, STI571, induces selective inhibition in the growth of t(9;22)-bearing tumor cells in vitro and some responses in patients. Inhibition of *RAS* with a farnesyl transferase inhibitor that blocks its insertion into the membrane may have antitumor activity in CML on the basis of early clinical trials. Preclinical efforts to use BCR/ABL peptides as a tumor vaccine appear promising. The use of BCR/ABL antisense oligonucleotides to purge residual leukemic cells from autologous hematopoietic progenitors before reinfusion, as well as approaches to induce GVL in the setting of minimal residual disease without inducing GVHD, are underway.

Treatment of Blast Crisis   The treatment for all forms of blast crisis is generally ineffective. Treatment is tailored to the phenotype of the blast cell. Myeloid crises and erythroid crisis are treated as for AML, but remissions occur in only a minority of cases and are generally short lived. Patients may present without having had a chronic phase. AML with a t(9;22) is probably blast crisis of CML and carries a poor prognosis.

Lymphoid blast crisis is treated like ALL (Chap. 112) with vincristine (1.4 mg/m^2 weekly) plus prednisone (60 mg/m^2 orally qd) induction therapy with or without an anthracycline. About one-third of patients will reenter chronic phase after 2 to 3 weeks of treatment, but the remissions last only a median of ~4 months. Even SCT is minimally effective during blast crises. Novel treatment approaches are needed.

BIBLIOGRAPHY

BLOOMFIELD CD et al: Frequency of prolonged remission duration following high-dose cytarabine intensification in acute myeloid leukemia varies by cytogenetic subtype. Cancer Res 58:4173, 1998

DRUKER BJ, LYDON NB: Lessons learned from the development of an abl tyrosine kinase inhibitor. Clin Invest 105:3, 2000

FADERL S et al: The biology of chronic myeloid leukemia. N Engl J Med 341:164, 1999

HIDDEMANN W et al: Management of acute myeloid leukemia in elderly patients. J Clin Oncol 17:3569, 1999

LOWENBERG B et al: Acute myeloid leukemia. N Engl J Med 341:1051, 1999

SAWYERS CL: Chronic myeloid leukemia. N Engl J Med 340:1330, 1999

SILVER RT et al: An evidence-based analysis of the effect of busulfan, hydroxyurea, interferon, and allogeneic bone marrow transplantation in treating the chronic phase of chronic myeloid leukemia: Developed for the American Society of Hematology. Blood 94:1517, 1999

SLACK JL: The biology and treatment of acute progranulocytic leukemia. Curr Opin Oncol 11:93, 1999

MALIGNANCIES OF LYMPHOID CELLS

ABVD doxorubicin, bleomycin, vinblastine, and dacarbazine	EBV Epstein-Barr virus
ALLs acute lymphoid leukemias	HTLV human T cell lymphotropic virus
ATL adult T cell lymphoma	IPI International Prognostic Index
CHOP cyclophosphamide, doxorubicin, vincristine, and prednisone	LDH lactate dehydrogenase
	MALT mucosa-associated lymphoid tissue
CLL chronic lymphoid leukemia	MOPP mechlorethamine, vincristine, procarbazine, and prednisone
CNS central nervous system	
CT computed tomography	NK natural killer
CVP cyclophosphamide, vincristine, and prednisone	

Malignancies of lymphoid cells range from the most indolent to the most aggressive human malignancies. These cancers arise from cells of the immune system at different stages of differentiation, resulting in a wide range of morphologic, immunologic, and clinical findings. Advances in our understanding of the normal immune system have allowed a better understanding of these sometimes confusing disorders.

Some malignancies of lymphoid cells almost always present as leukemia (i.e., primary involvement of bone marrow and blood), while others almost always present as lymphomas (i.e., solid tumors of the immune system). However, other malignancies of lymphoid cells can present as either leukemia or lymphoma. In addition, the clinical pattern can change over the course of the illness. This change is more often seen in a patient who seems to have a lymphoma and then develops the manifestations of leukemia over the course of the illness.

BIOLOGY OF LYMPHOID MALIGNANCIES: CONCEPTS OF THE WHO CLASSIFICATION OF LYMPHOID MALIGNANCIES

The classification of lymphoid malignancy evolved steadily throughout the twentieth century. The distinction between leukemia and lymphoma was made early, and separate classification systems were developed for each. Leukemias were first divided into acute and chronic subtypes based on average survival. Chronic leukemias were easily subdivided into those of lymphoid or myeloid origin based on morphologic characteristics. However, in recent years, a spectrum of diseases that were formerly all called chronic lymphoid leukemia has become apparent (Table 112-1). The acute leukemias were usually malignancies of blast cells with few identifying characteristics. When cytochemical stains became available, it was possible to divide these objectively into myeloid malignancies and acute leukemias of lymphoid cells. Acute leukemias of lymphoid cells have been subdivided based on morphologic characteristics by the French-American-British (FAB) group (Table 112-2). Using this system, lymphoid malignancies of small uniform blasts (e.g., typical childhood acute lymphoblastic

Table 112-1 Lymphoid Disorders that Can Present as "Chronic Leukemia" and Be Confused with Typical B Cell Chronic Lymphoid Leukemia.

Follicular lymphoma
Splenic marginal zone lymphoma
Nodal marginal zone lymphoma
Mantle cell lymphoma
Hairy cell leukemia
Prolymphocytic leukemia (B cell or T cell)
Lymphoplasmacytic lymphoma
Sézary syndrome
Smoldering adult T cell leukemia/lymphoma

Table 112-2 Classification of Acute Lymphoid Leukemia (ALL)

Immunologic Subtype	% of Cases	FAB Subtype	Cytogenetic Abnormalities
Pre-B ALL	75	L1, L2	t(9;22), t(4;11), t(1;19)
T cell ALL	20	L1, L2	14q11 or 7q34
B cell ALL	5	L3	t(8;14), t(8;22), t(2;8)

NOTE: FAB, French-American-British classification.

leukemia) were called L1, lymphoid malignancies with larger and more variable size cells were called L2, and lymphoid malignancies of uniform cells with basophilic and sometimes vacuolated cytoplasm were called L3 (e.g., typical Burkitt's lymphoma cells). Acute leukemias of lymphoid cells have also been subdivided based on immunologic (i.e., T vs. B) and cytogenetic abnormalities (Table 112-2). Major cytogenetic subgroups include the t(9;22) (e.g., Philadelphia chromosome–positive acute lymphoblastic leukemia) and the t(8;14) found in the L3 or Burkitt's leukemia.

Non-Hodgkin's lymphomas were separated from Hodgkin's disease by recognition of the Sternberg-Reed cells early in the twentieth century. The first systematic classification for non-Hodgkin's lymphomas was proposed by Gall and Mallory in the first half of the twentieth century and divided non-Hodgkin's lymphomas into giant follicular lymphoma, lymphosarcoma, and reticulum cell sarcoma. Unfortunately, this fairly simple system proved to be imprecise in its definitions and only marginally clinically useful. In the 1950s, Henry Rappaport and colleagues recognized the importance of growth pattern in subdividing non-Hodgkin's lymphomas and used pattern in addition to cell size and shape as the basis for a new classification that proved more clinically relevant. In the 1970s, it was recognized that non-Hodgkin's lymphomas were all tumors of lymphocytes and were derived from either T or B cells. This led to immunologically based classifications of lymphomas such as the Lukes-Collins classification in the United States and the Kiel classification proposed by Lennert and associates in Europe. In an attempt to unify terminology and improve the effectiveness of communication between pathologists and clinicians, the Working Formulation was proposed in 1982. Over the next two decades the Kiel classification dominated clinical practice in Europe, whereas the Working Formulation became the main classification system used in North America.

In the past two decades, increased understanding of the immune system and the genetic abnormalities associated with non-Hodgkin's lymphoma have led to the identification of several previously unrecognized types of lymphoma. The recognition of these new and clinically relevant lymphomas led to proposals for changing existing classifications. A new proposal that is part of the basis of the new World Health Organization classification of lymphoid malignancies takes into account morphologic, clinical, immunologic, and genetic information and attempts to divide non-Hodgkin's lymphomas and other lymphoid malignancies into clinical/pathological entities that have clinical and therapeutic relevance. This system is presented in Table 112-3. Clinical studies have shown that this new system is clinically relevant and has a higher degree of diagnostic accuracy than those used previously. The possibilities for subdividing lymphoid malignancies are extensive. However, Table 112-3 presents in bold those malignancies that occur in at least 1% of patients. Specific lymphoma subtypes will be dealt with in more detail below.

GENERAL ASPECTS OF LYMPHOID MALIGNANCIES

ETIOLOGY AND EPIDEMIOLOGY Chronic lymphoid leukemia (CLL) is the most prevalent form of leukemia in western countries. It occurs most frequently in older adults and is exceedingly rare in children. Approximately 13,000 new cases are diagnosed in the

Table 112-3 WHO Classification of Lymphoid Malignancies

B Cell	T Cell	Hodgkin's Disease
Precursor B cell neoplasm	Precursor T cell neoplasm	Nodular lymphocyte-predominant Hodgkin's disease
Precursor B lymphoblastic leukemia/lymphoma (precursor B cell acute lymphoblastic leukemia)	**Precursor T lymphoblastic lymphoma/leukemia (precursor T cell acute lymphoblastic leukemia)**	
Mature (peripheral) B cell neoplasms	Mature (peripheral) T cell neoplasms	Classical Hodgkin's disease
B cell chronic lymphocytic leukemia/small lymphocytic lymphoma	T cell prolymphocytic leukemia	Nodular sclerosis Hodgkin's disease
B cell prolymphocytic leukemia	T cell granular lymphocytic leukemia	Lymphocyte-rich classical Hodgkin's disease
Lymphoplasmacytic lymphoma	Aggressive NK cell leukemia	Mixed-cellularity Hodgkin's disease
Splenic marginal zone B cell lymphoma (± villous lymphocytes)	Adult T cell lymphoma/leukemia (HTLV-I+)	Lymphocyte-depletion Hodgkin's disease
Hairy cell leukemia	Extranodal NK/T cell lymphoma, nasal type	
Plasma cell myeloma/plasmacytoma	Enteropathy-type T cell lymphoma	
Extranodal marginal zone B cell lymphoma of MALT type	Hepatosplenic γδ T cell lymphoma	
Mantle cell lymphoma	Subcutaneous panniculitis-like T cell lymphoma	
Follicular lymphoma	**Mycosis fungoides/Sézary syndrome**	
Nodal marginal zone B cell lymphoma (± monocytoid B cells)	Anaplastic large cell lymphoma, primary cutaneous type	
Diffuse large B cell lymphoma	**Peripheral T cell lymphoma, not otherwise specified (NOS)**	
Burkitt's lymphoma/Burkitt cell leukemia	**Angioimmunoblastic T cell lymphoma**	
	Anaplastic large cell lymphoma, primary systemic type	

NOTE: HTLV, human T cell lymphotropic virus; MALT, mucosa-associated lymphoid tissue; NK, natural killer; WHO, World Health Organization.
SOURCE: Adapted from Harris et al.

United States each year, but because of the prolonged survival associated with this disorder, the total prevalence is many times higher. CLL is more common in men than in women and more common in whites than in blacks. This is an uncommon malignancy in Asia. The etiologic factors for typical CLL are unknown.

In contrast to CLL, acute lymphoid leukemias (ALLs) are predominantly cancers of children and young adults. The L3 or Burkitt's leukemia occurring in children in developing countries seems to be associated with infection by the Epstein-Barr virus (EBV) in infancy. However, the explanation for the etiology of more common subtypes of ALL is much less certain. Childhood ALL occurs more often in higher socioeconomic subgroups. Children with trisomy 21 (Down's syndrome) have an increased risk for childhood acute lymphoblastic leukemia as well as acute myeloid leukemia. Exposure to high-energy radiation in early childhood increases the risk of developing T cell acute lymphoblastic leukemia.

The etiology of ALL in adults is also uncertain. ALL is unusual in middle-aged adults but increases in incidence in the elderly. However, acute myeloid leukemia is still much more common in these patients. Environmental exposures including certain industrial exposures, exposure to agricultural chemicals, and smoking might increase the risk of developing ALL as an adult.

The cell of origin of Hodgkin's disease has not been determined definitively, but molecular evidence suggests that most are of B cell origin. The incidence of Hodgkin's disease appears fairly stable, with approximately 8000 new cases diagnosed each year in the United States. Hodgkin's disease is more common in whites than in blacks

and more common in males than in females. A bimodal distribution of age at diagnosis has been observed, with one peak incidence occurring in patients in their 20s and the other in those in their 80s. Patients in the younger age groups diagnosed in the United States largely have the nodular sclerosing subtype of Hodgkin's disease. Elderly patients, patients infected with HIV, and patients in third world countries more commonly have mixed-cellularity Hodgkin's disease or lymphocyte-depleted Hodgkin's disease. Infection by HIV is a risk factor for developing Hodgkin's disease. In addition, an association between infection by EBV and Hodgkin's disease has been demonstrated. A monoclonal or oligoclonal proliferation of EBV-infected cells in 20 to 40% of the patients with Hodgkin's disease has led to proposals for this virus having an etiologic role in Hodgkin's disease. However, the matter is not settled definitively.

For unknown reasons, non-Hodgkin's lymphomas have increased in frequency in the United States at the rate of 4% per year since 1950. Almost 60,000 new cases of non-Hodgkin's lymphoma were diagnosed in the United States in the year 2000. Non-Hodgkin's lymphomas are more frequent in the elderly and more frequent in men. Patients with both primary and secondary immunodeficiency states are predisposed to developing non-Hodgkin's lymphomas. These include patients with HIV infection; patients who have undergone organ transplantation; and patients with inherited immune deficiencies, the sicca syndrome, and rheumatoid arthritis.

The incidence of non-Hodgkin's lymphomas and the patterns of expression of the various subtypes differ geographically. T cell lymphomas are more common in Asia than in western countries, while certain subtypes of B cell lymphomas such as follicular lymphoma are more common in western countries. A specific subtype of non-Hodgkin's lymphoma known as the angiocentric nasal T/natural killer (NK) cell lymphoma has a striking geographic occurrence, being most frequent in Southern Asia and parts of Latin America. Another subtype of non-Hodgkin's lymphoma associated with infection by human T cell lymphotropic virus (HTLV) I is seen particularly in southern Japan and the Caribbean.

A number of environmental factors have been implicated in the occurrence of non-Hodgkin's lymphoma, including infectious agents, chemical exposures, and medical treatments. Several studies have demonstrated an association between exposure to agricultural chemicals and an increased incidence in non-Hodgkin's lymphoma. Patients treated for Hodgkin's disease can develop non-Hodgkin's lymphoma; it is unclear whether this is a consequence of the Hodgkin's disease or its treatment. However, the infectious etiology of non-Hodgkin's lymphoma is the area where evidence has been expanding most rapidly in recent years. Table 112-4 illustrates those infectious agents associated with the development of non-Hodgkin's lymphoma. HTLV-I infects T cells and leads directly to the development of adult T cell lymphoma (ATL) in a small percentage of infected patients. The cumulative lifetime risk of developing lymphoma in an infected patient is 2.5%. The virus is transmitted by infected lymphocytes ingested by nursing babies of infected mothers, blood-borne transmission, or sexually. The median age of patients with ATL is about 56 years, emphasizing the long latency.

EBV is associated with the development of Burkitt's lymphoma

Table 112-4 Infectious Agents Associated with the Development of Lymphoid Malignancies

Infectious Agent	Lymphoid Malignancy
Epstein-Barr virus	Burkitt's lymphoma
	Post–organ transplant lymphoma
	Primary CNS diffuse large B cell lymphoma
	Hodgkin's disease
	Extranodal NK/T cell lymphoma, nasal type
HTLV-I	Adult T cell leukemia/lymphoma
HIV	Diffuse large B cell lymphoma
	Burkitt's lymphoma
Hepatitis C virus	Lymphoplasmacytic lymphoma
Helicobacter pylori	Gastric MALT lymphoma
Human herpesvirus 8	Primary effusion lymphoma
	Multicentric Castleman's disease

NOTE: CNS, central nervous system; HTLV, human T cell lymphotropic virus; MALT, mucosa-associated lymphoid tissue; NK, natural killer.

in Central Africa and the occurrence of aggressive non-Hodgkin's lymphomas in immunosuppressed patients in western countries. EBV infection is strongly associated with the occurrence of extranodal nasal T/NK cell lymphomas in Asia and South America. Infection with HIV predisposes to the development of aggressive, B cell non-Hodgkin's lymphoma. This may be through overexpression of interleukin 6 by infected macrophages. Infection of the stomach by the bacterium *Helicobacter pylori* induces the development of gastric MALT (mucosa-associated lymphoid tissue) lymphomas. This association is supported by evidence that patients treated with antibiotics to eradicate *H. pylori* have regression of their MALT lymphoma. The bacterium does not transform lymphocytes to produce the lymphoma; instead, a vigorous immune response is made to the bacterium and the chronic antigenic stimulation leads to the neoplasia.

Chronic hepatitis C virus infection has been associated with the development of lymphoplasmacytic lymphoma. Human herpesvirus 8 is associated with primary effusion lymphoma in HIV-infected persons and multicentric Castleman's disease, a diffuse lymphadenopathy associated with systemic symptoms of fever, malaise, and weight loss.

In addition to infectious agents, a number of other diseases or exposures may predispose to developing lymphoma (Table 112-5).

IMMUNOLOGY All lymphoid cells are derived from a common hematopoietic progenitor that gives rise to lymphoid, myeloid, erythroid, monocyte, and megakaryocyte lineages. Through the ordered and sequential activation of a series of transcription factors, the cell first becomes committed to the lymphoid lineage and then gives rise to B and T cells. About 75% of all lymphoid leukemias and 90% of all lymphomas are of B cell origin. A cell becomes committed to B cell development when it begins to rearrange its immunoglobulin genes. The sequence of cellular changes, including changes in cell-surface phenotype, that characterize normal B cell development are shown in Fig. 112-1. A cell becomes committed to T cell differentiation upon migration to the thymus and rearrangement of T cell antigen

Table 112-5 Diseases or Exposures Associated with Increased Risk of Development of Malignant Lymphoma

Inherited immunodeficiency disease	Autoimmune disease
Klinefelter's syndrome	Sjögren's syndrome
Chédiak-Higashi syndrome	Celiac sprue
Ataxia telangiectasia syndrome	Rheumatoid arthritis and sys-
Wiscott-Aldrich syndrome	temic lupus erythematosus
Common variable immunodefi-	Chemical or drug exposures
ciency disease	Phenytoin
Acquired immunodeficiency dis-	Dioxin, phenoxyherbicides
eases	Radiation
Iatrogenic immunosuppression	Prior chemotherapy and radiation
HIV-1 infection	therapy
Acquired hypogammaglobulin-	
emia	

receptor genes. The sequence of the events that characterize T cell development are depicted in Fig. 112-2.

Although lymphoid malignancies often retain the cell-surface phenotype of lymphoid cells at particular stages of differentiation, this information is of little consequence. The so-called stage of differentiation of a malignant lymphoma does not predict its natural history. For example, the clinically most aggressive lymphoid leukemia is Burkitt's leukemia, which has the phenotype of a mature follicle center IgM-bearing B cell. Leukemias bearing the immunologic cell-surface phenotype of more primitive cells (e.g., pre-B ALL, CD10+) are less aggressive and more amenable to curative therapy than the "more mature" appearing Burkitt's leukemia cells. Furthermore, the apparent stage of differentiation of the malignant cell does not reflect the stage at which the genetic lesions that gave rise to the malignancy developed. For example, follicular lymphoma has the cell-surface phenotype of a follicle center cell, but its characteristic chromosomal translocation, the t(14;18), which involves juxtaposition of the anti-apoptotic *bcl-2* gene next to the immunoglobulin heavy chain gene (see below), had to develop early in ontogeny as an error in the process of immunoglobulin gene rearrangement. Why the subsequent steps that led to transformation became manifest in a cell of follicle center differentiation is not clear.

The major value of cell-surface phenotyping is to aid in the differential diagnosis of lymphoid tumors that appear similar by light microscopy. For example, benign follicular hyperplasia may resemble follicular lymphoma; however, the demonstration that all the cells bear the same immunoglobulin light chain isotype strongly suggests the mass is a clonal proliferation rather than a polyclonal response to an exogenous stimulus.

GENETIC CONSIDERATIONS Malignancies of lymphoid cells are associated with recurring genetic abnormalities. While specific genetic abnormalities have not been identified for all subtypes of lymphoid malignancies, it is presumed that they exist. Genetic abnormalities can be identified at a variety of levels including gross chromosomal changes (i.e., translocations, additions, or deletions); rearrangement of specific genes that may or may not be apparent from cytogenetic studies; and overexpression, underexpression, or mutation of specific oncogenes. Altered expression or mutation of specific proteins is particularly important. Many lymphomas contain balanced chromosomal translocations involving the antigen receptor genes; immunoglobulin genes on chromosomes 2, 14, and 22 in B cells; and T cell antigen receptor genes on chromosomes 7 and 14 in T cells. The rearrangement of chromosome segments to generate mature antigen receptors must create a site of vulnerability to aberrant recombination. B cells are even more susceptible to acquiring mutations during their maturation in germinal centers; the generation of antibody of higher affinity requires the introduction of mutations into the variable region genes in the germinal centers. Other nonimmunoglobulin genes, for example *bcl-6*, may acquire mutations as well.

In the case of diffuse large B cell lymphoma, the translocation t(14;18) occurs in approximately 30% of patients and leads to overexpression of the *bcl-2* gene found on chromosome 18. Some other patients without the translocation also overexpress the BCL-2 protein. This protein is involved in suppressing apoptosis—i.e., the mechanism of cell death most often induced by cytotoxic chemotherapeutic agents. A higher relapse rate has been observed in patients whose tumors overexpress the BCL-2 protein, but not in those patients whose lymphoma cells show only the translocation. Thus, particular genetic mechanisms have clinical ramifications.

Table 112-6 presents the best documented translocations and associated oncogenes for various subtypes of lymphoid malignancies. In some cases, such as the association of the t(14;18) in follicular lymphoma, the t(2;5) in anaplastic large T/null-cell lymphoma, the t(8;14) in Burkitt's lymphoma, and the t(11;14) in mantle cell lymphoma, the great majority of tumors in patients with these diagnoses display these

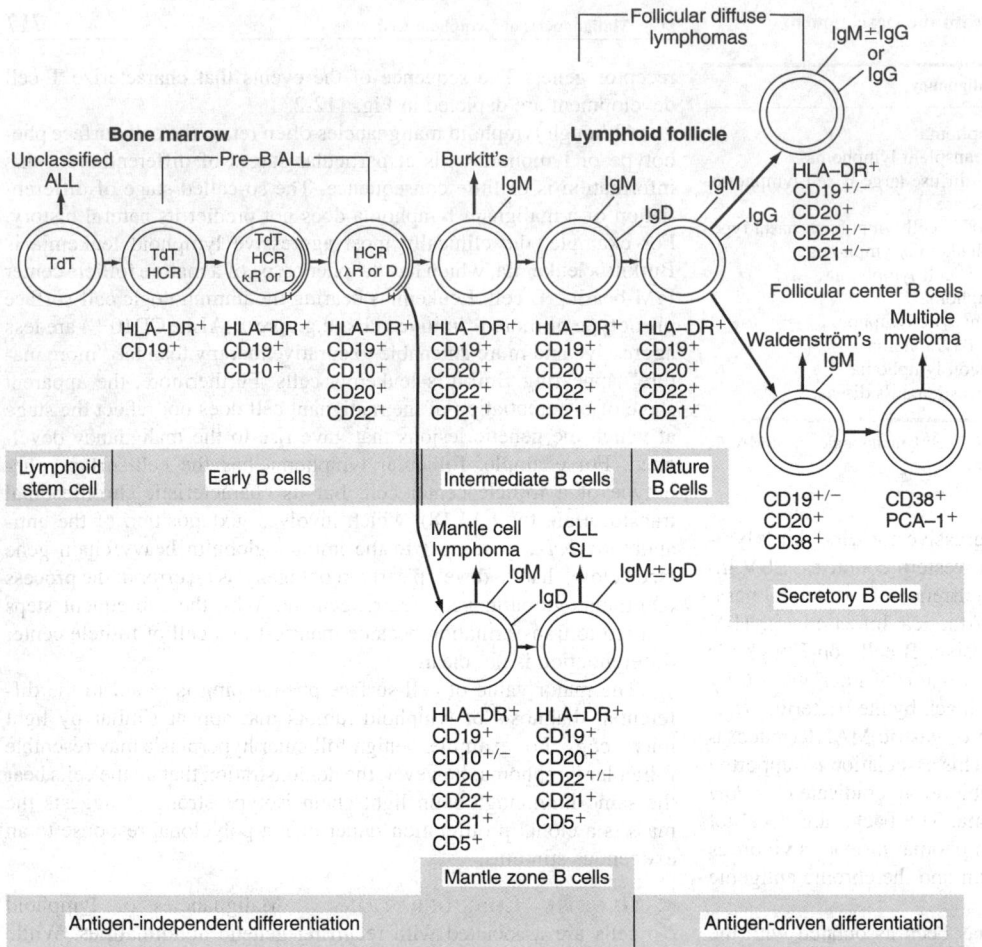

FIGURE 112-1 Pathway of normal B cell differentiation and relationship to B cell lymphomas. HLA-DR, CD10, CD19, CD20, CD21, CD22, CD5, and CD38 are cell markers used to distinguish stages of development. Terminal transferase (TdT) is a cellular enzyme. Immunoglobulin heavy chain gene rearrangement (HCR) and light chain gene rearrangement or deletion (κ R or D, λ R or D) occur early in B cell development. The approximate normal stage of differentiation associated with particular lymphomas is shown. ALL, acute lymphoid leukemia; CLL, chronic lymphoid leukemia; SL, small lymphocytic lymphoma.

abnormalities. In other types of lymphoma where a minority of the patients have tumors expressing specific genetic abnormalities, the defects may have prognostic significance. No specific genetic abnormalities have been identified in Hodgkin's disease.

In typical B cell CLL, trisomy 12 conveys a poorer prognosis. In ALL in both adults and children, genetic abnormalities have important prognostic significance. Patients whose tumor cells display the t(9;22) have a much poorer outlook than patients who do not have this translocation. Other genetic abnormalities that occur frequently in adults with ALL include the t(4;11) and the t(8;14). The t(4;11) is associated with younger age, female predominance, high white cell counts, and L1 morphology. The t(8;14) is associated with older age, male predominance, frequent central nervous system (CNS) involvement, and L3 morphology. Both are associated with a poor prognosis. In childhood ALL, hyperdiploidy has been shown to have a favorable prognosis. ∎

Approach to the Patient

Regardless of the type of lymphoid malignancy, the initial evaluation of the patient should include performance of a careful history and physical examination. These will help confirm the diagnosis, identify those manifestations of the disease that might require prompt attention, and aid in the selection of further studies to optimally characterize the patient's status to allow the best choice of therapy. It is difficult to overemphasize the importance of a carefully done history and physical examination. They might provide observations that lead to reconsid-

ering the diagnosis, provide hints at etiology, clarify the stage, and allow the physician to establish rapport with the patient that will make it possible to develop and carry out a therapeutic plan.

For patients with ALL, evaluation is usually completed after a complete blood count, chemistry studies reflecting major organ function, a bone marrow biopsy with genetic and immunologic studies, and a lumbar puncture. The latter is necessary to rule out occult CNS involvement. At this point, most patients would be ready to begin therapy. In ALL, prognosis is dependent upon the genetic characteristics of the tumor, the patient's age, the white cell count, and the patient's overall clinical status and major organ function.

In CLL, the patient evaluation should include a complete blood count, chemistry tests to measure major organ function, serum protein electrophoresis, and a bone marrow biopsy. However, some physicians believe that the diagnosis would not always require a bone marrow biopsy. Patients often have imaging studies of the chest and abdomen looking for pathologic lymphadenopathy. Patients with typical B cell CLL can be subdivided into three major prognostic groups. Those patients with only blood and bone marrow involvement by leukemia but no lymphadenopathy, organomegaly, or signs of bone marrow failure have the best prognosis. Those with lymphadenopathy and organomegaly have an intermediate prognosis, and patients with bone marrow failure, defined as hemoglobin <100 g/L (10 g/dL) or platelet count <100,000/μL, have the worst prognosis. The

pathogenesis of the anemia or thrombocytopenia is important to discern. The prognosis is adversely affected when either or both of these abnormalities are due to progressive marrow infiltration and loss of productive marrow. However, either or both may be due to autoimmune phenomena or to hypersplenism that can develop during the course of the disease. These destructive mechanisms are usually completely reversible (glucocorticoids for autoimmune disease; splenectomy for hypersplenism) and do not influence disease prognosis.

Two popular staging systems have been developed to reflect these prognostic groupings (Table 112-7). Patients with typical B cell CLL can have their course complicated by immunologic abnormalities including autoimmune hemolytic anemia, autoimmune thrombocytopenia, and hypogammaglobulinemia. Patients with hypogammaglobulinemia benefit from regular (monthly) γ globulin administration. Because of expense, γ globulin is often withheld until the patient experiences a significant infection. These abnormalities do not have a clear prognostic significance and should not be used to assign a higher stage.

The initial evaluation of a patient with Hodgkin's disease or non-Hodgkin's lymphoma is similar. In both situations, the determination of an accurate anatomic stage is an important part of the evaluation. The staging system that is utilized is the Ann Arbor staging system originally developed for Hodgkin's disease (Table 112-8).

Evaluation of patients with Hodgkin's disease will typically include a complete blood count; erythrocyte sedimentation rate; chemistry studies reflecting major organ function; computed tomography

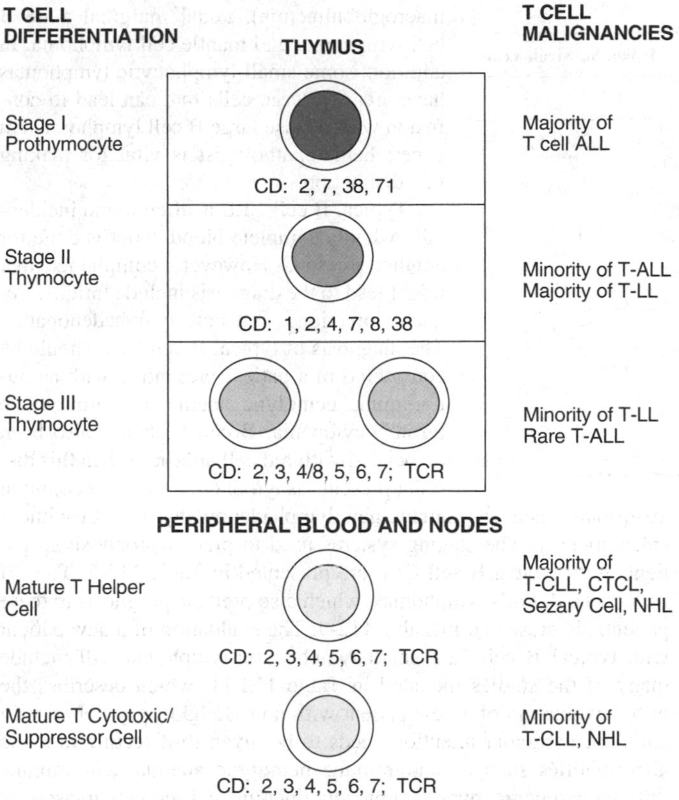

T CELL DIFFERENTIATION

THYMUS

T CELL MALIGNANCIES

Stage I
Prothymocyte

CD: 2, 7, 38, 71

Majority of
T cell ALL

Stage II
Thymocyte

CD: 1, 2, 4, 7, 8, 38

Minority of T-ALL
Majority of T-LL

Stage III
Thymocyte

CD: 2, 3, 4/8, 5, 6, 7; TCR

Minority of T-LL
Rare T-ALL

PERIPHERAL BLOOD AND NODES

Mature T Helper
Cell

CD: 2, 3, 4, 5, 6, 7; TCR

Majority of
T-CLL, CTCL,
Sezary Cell, NHL

Mature T Cytotoxic/
Suppressor Cell

CD: 2, 3, 4, 5, 6, 7; TCR

Minority of
T-CLL, NHL

FIGURE 112-2 Pathway of normal T cell differentiation and relationship to T cell lymphomas. CD1, CD2, CD3, CD4, CD5, CD6, CD7, CD8, CD38, and CD71 are cell markers used to distinguish stages of development. T cell antigen receptors (TCR) rearrange in the thymus, and mature T cells emigrate to nodes and peripheral blood. ALL, acute lymphoid leukemia; T-ALL, T cell ALL; T-LL, T cell lymphoblastic lymphoma; T-CLL, T cell chronic lymphoid leukemia; CTCL, cutaneous T cell lymphoma; NHL, non-Hodgkin's lymphoma.

(CT) scans of the chest, abdomen, and pelvis; and a bone marrow biopsy. A gallium scan is not necessary for primary staging, but when it is performed at the completion of therapy it allows evaluation of persistent radiographic abnormalities, particularly the mediastinum. In most cases, these studies will allow assignment of anatomic stage and the development of a therapeutic plan.

In patients with non-Hodgkin's lymphoma, the same evaluation

Table 112-6 Cytogenetic Translocation and Associated Oncogenes Often Seen in Lymphoid Malignancies

Disease	Cytogenetic Abnormality	Oncogene
CLL/small lymphocytic lymphoma	t(14;15)(q32;q13)	—
MALT lymphoma	t(11;18)(q21;q21)	—
Precursor B cell acute lymphoid leukemia	t(9;22)(q34;q11) or variant t(4;11)(q21;q23)	BCR/ABL AF4, ALLI
Precursor acute lymphoid leukemia	t(9;22) t(1;19) t(17;19) t(5;14)	BCR, ABL E2A, PBX HLF, E2A IL3, IGμ
Mantle cell lymphoma	t(11;14)(q13;q32)	BCL-1
Follicular lymphoma	t(14;18)(q32;q21)	BCL-2
Diffuse large-cell lymphoma	t(3;-)(q27;-)^a t(17;-)(p13-)	BCL-6 p53
Burkitt's lymphoma, Burkitt's leukemia	t(8;-)(q24;-)^a	C-MYC
CD30+ Anaplastic large cell lymphoma	t(2;5)(p23;q35)	ALK
Lymphoplasmacytoid lymphoma	t(9;14)(p13;q32)	—

^{a} Numerous sites of translocation may be involved with these genes.
NOTE: CLL, chronic lymphoid leukemia; MALT, mucosa-associated lymphoid tissue.

described for patients with Hodgkin's disease is usually carried out. In addition, serum levels of lactate dehydrogenase (LDH) and β_2-microglobulin and serum protein electrophoresis are often included in the evaluation. Anatomic stage is assigned in the same manner as used for Hodgkin's disease. However, the prognosis of patients with non-Hodgkin's lymphoma is best assigned using the International Prognostic Index (IPI) (Table 112-9). This is a powerful predictor of outcome in all subtypes of non-Hodgkin's lymphoma. Patients are assigned an IPI score based on the presence or absence of five adverse prognostic factors and may have none or all five of these adverse prognostic factors. Figure 112-3 shows the prognostic significance of this score in 1300 patients with all types of non-Hodgkin's lymphoma.

CLINICAL FEATURES, TREATMENT, AND PROGNOSIS OF SPECIFIC LYMPHOID MALIGNANCIES

PRECURSOR CELL B CELL NEOPLASMS Precursor B Cell Lymphoblastic Leukemia/Lymphoma The most common cancer in childhood is B cell acute lymphoblastic leukemia (ALL). Although this disorder can also present as a lymphoma in either adults or children, presentation as lymphoma is quite rare.

The malignant cells in patients with precursor B cell lymphoblastic leukemia are most commonly of pre-B cell origin. Patients typically present with signs of bone marrow failure such as pallor, fatigue, bleeding, fever, and infection related to peripheral blood cytopenias. Peripheral blood counts regularly show anemia and thrombocytopenia but might show leukopenia, a normal leukocyte count, or leukocytosis based largely on the number of circulating malignant cells (**see Plate V-24**). Extranodal sites of disease are frequently involved in patients who present with leukemia, which might be manifested by lymphadenopathy, hepato- or splenomegaly, CNS disease, testicular enlargement, and/or cutaneous infiltration.

The diagnosis is usually made by bone marrow biopsy, which shows infiltration by malignant lymphoblasts. Demonstration of a pre-B cell immunophenotype (Fig. 112-1) and, often, characteristic cytogenetic abnormalities (Table 112-6) confirm the diagnosis. An adverse prognosis in patients with precursor B cell ALL is predicted by a very high white cell count, the presence of symptomatic CNS disease, and unfavorable cytogenetic abnormalities. For example, t(9;22) is frequently found in adults with B cell lymphoblastic leukemia and is associated with a very poor outlook.

℞ **TREATMENT** The treatment of patients with precursor B cell lymphoblastic leukemia involves remission induction with combination chemotherapy, a consolidation phase that includes administration of high-dose systemic therapy and treatment to eliminate disease in the CNS, and a period of continuing therapy to prevent relapse and effect cure. The overall cure rate in children is 85%, while about 50% of adults are long-term disease-free survivors. This reflects the high proportion of adverse cytogenetic abnormalities seen in adults with precursor B cell lymphoblastic leukemia.

Precursor B cell lymphoblastic lymphoma is a rare presentation of precursor B cell lymphoblastic malignancy. These patients often have a rapid transformation to leukemia, and similar treatment approaches as are used in patients presenting with leukemia are appropriate. In the few patients who present with the disease confined to lymph nodes, a high cure rate has been reported.

MATURE (PERIPHERAL) B CELL NEOPLASMS
B Cell Chronic Lymphoid Leukemia/Small Lymphocytic Lymphoma B cell CLL/small lymphocytic lymphoma represents by far the most common lymphoid leukemia, and when presenting as a lymphoma, it accounts for ~7% of non-Hodgkin's lymphomas. As the name implies, presentation can be as either leukemia or lymphoma.

Table 112-7   Staging of Typical B Cell Lymphoid Leukemia

Stage	Clinical Features	Median Survival, Years
RAI SYSTEM		
0: Low risk	Lymphocytosis only in blood and marrow	>10
I: Intermediate risk	Lymphocytosis + lymphadenopathy + splenomegaly ± hepatomegaly	7
II		
III: High risk	Lymphocytosis + anemia + thrombocytopenia	1.5
IV		
BINET SYSTEM		
A	Fewer than three areas of clinical lymphadenopathy; no anemia or thrombocytopenia	>10
B	Three or more involved node areas; no anemia or thrombocytopenia	7
C	Hemoglobin ≤10 g/dL and/or platelets <100,000/μl	2

The major clinical characteristics of B cell CLL/small lymphocytic lymphoma are presented in Table 112-10.

The diagnosis of typical B cell CLL is made when an increased number of circulating lymphocytes (i.e., $>4 \times 10^9$/L and usually $>10 \times 10^9$/L) is found (**see Plate V-17**) that are monoclonal B cells and display the CD5 antigen. Confirmation of bone marrow infiltration by the same cells confirms the diagnosis. The peripheral blood smear in such patients typically shows many "smudge" or "basket" cells, nuclear remnants of cells damaged by the physical shear stress of making the blood smear. If cytogenetic studies are performed, trisomy 12 is found in ~25 to 30% of patients. Abnormalities in chromosome 13 are also seen.

If the primary presentation is lymphadenopathy and a lymph node biopsy is performed, pathologists usually have little difficulty in making the diagnosis of small lymphocytic lymphoma based on morphologic findings and immunophenotype. However, even in these patients ~70 to 75% will be found to have bone marrow involvement and the search for circulating monoclonal B lymphocytes is often positive.

The differential diagnosis of typical B cell CLL is extensive and presented in Table 112-1. Immunophenotyping will eliminate the T cell disorders and can often help sort out other B cell malignancies. For example, only mantle cell lymphoma and typical B cell CLL are usually CD5 positive. Typical B cell small lymphocytic lymphoma can be confused with other B cell disorders including lymphoplasmacytic lymphoma (i.e., the tissue manifestation of Waldenström's

Table 112-8   The Ann Arbor Staging System for Hodgkin's Disease

Stage	Definition
I	Involvement of a single lymph node region or lymphoid structure (e.g., spleen, thymus, Waldeyer's ring)
II	Involvement of two or more lymph node regions on the same side of the diaphragm (the mediastinum is a single site; hilar lymph nodes should be considered "lateralized" and, when involved on both sides, constitute stage II disease)
III	Involvement of lymph node regions or lymphoid structures on both sides of the diaphragm
III₁	Subdiaphragmatic involvement limited to spleen, splenic hilar nodes, celiac nodes, or portal nodes
III₂	Subdiaphragmatic involvement includes paraaortic, iliac, or mesenteric nodes plus structures in III₁
IV	Involvement of extranodal site(s) beyond that designated as "E" More than one extranodal deposit at any location Any involvement of liver or bone marrow
A	No symptoms
B	Unexplained weight loss of >10% of the body weight during the 6 months before staging investigation Unexplained, persistent, or recurrent fever with temperatures >38°C during the previous month Recurrent drenching night sweats during the previous month
E	Localized, solitary involvement of extralymphatic tissue, excluding liver and bone marrow

macroglobulinemia), nodal marginal zone B cell lymphoma, and mantle cell lymphoma. In addition, some small lymphocytic lymphomas have areas of large cells that can lead to confusion with diffuse large B cell lymphoma. An expert hematopathologist is vital for making this distinction.

Typical B cell CLL is often found incidentally when a complete blood count is done for another reason. However, complaints that might lead to the diagnosis include fatigue, frequent infections, and new lymphadenopathy. The diagnosis of typical B cell CLL should be considered in a patient presenting with an autoimmune hemolytic anemia or autoimmune thrombocytopenia. B cell CLL has also been associated with red cell aplasia. When this disorder presents as lymphoma, the most common abnormality is asymptomatic new lymphadenopathy, with or without splenomegaly. The staging systems used to predict prognosis in patients with typical B cell CLL are presented in Table 112-7. The IPI for non-Hodgkin's lymphomas, which also predicts prognosis in these patients, is presented in Table 112-9. The evaluation of a new patient with typical B cell CLL/small lymphocytic lymphoma will include many of the studies included in Table 112-11, which describes the initial evaluation of a new patient with non-Hodgkin's lymphoma. In addition, particular attention needs to be given to detecting immune abnormalities such as autoimmune hemolytic anemia, autoimmune thrombocytopenia, hypogammaglobulinemia, and red cell aplasia.

TREATMENT   Patients whose presentation is typical B cell CLL with no manifestations of the disease other than bone marrow involvement and lymphocytosis (i.e., Rai stage O and Binet stage A; Table 112-7) can be followed without specific therapy for their malignancy. These patients have a median survival >10 years, and some will never require therapy for this disorder. If the patient has an adequate number of circulating normal blood cells and is asymptomatic, many physicians would not initiate therapy for patients in the intermediate stage of the disease manifested by lymphadenopathy and/or hepatosplenomegaly. However, the median survival for these patients is ~7 years, and most will require treatment in the first few years of follow-up. Patients who present with bone marrow failure (i.e., Rai stage III or IV or Binet stage C) will require initial therapy in almost all cases. These patients have a serious disorder with a median survival of only 1.5 years. It must be remembered that immune manifestations of typical B cell CLL should be managed independently of specific antileukemia therapy. For example, glucocorticoid therapy for autoimmune cytopenias and γ globulin replacement for patients with hypogammaglobulinanemia should be used whether or not antileukemia therapy is given.

Patients who present primarily with lymphoma and have a low IPI score have a 5-year survival of ~75%, but those with a high IPI score

Table 112-9   International Prognostic Index for Non-Hodgkin's Lymphoma

Five clinical risk factors
  age ≥ 60 years
  serum lactate dehydrogenase levels elevated
  performance status ≥ 2 (ECOG) or ≤ 70 (Karnofsky)
  Ann Arbor stage III or IV
  >1 site of extranodal involvement
Patients are assigned a number for each risk factor they have
Patients are grouped differently based upon the type of lymphoma
For diffuse large B cell lymphoma:

0,1 factor = low risk	35% of cases; 5-year survival, 73%
2 factors = low-intermediate risk	27% of cases; 5-year survival, 51%
3 factors = high-intermediate risk	22% of cases; 5-year survival, 43%
4,5 factors = high risk	16% of cases; 5-year survival, 26%

have a 5-year survival of <40% and are more likely to require early therapy.

The most common treatments for patients with typical B cell CLL/small lymphocytic lymphoma have been the use of single-agent chlorambucil or single-agent fludarabine. Chlorambucil can be administered orally with few immediate side effects, while fludarabine is administered intravenously and is associated with significant immune suppression. However, fludarabine is by far the more active agent and is the only drug associated with a significant incidence of complete remission. For young patients presenting with leukemia requiring therapy, fludarabine is today the treatment of choice. Because fludarabine is an effective second-line agent in patients with tumors unresponsive to chlorambucil, the latter agent is often chosen in elderly patients who require therapy. Many patients who present with lymphoma will receive a combination chemotherapy regimen used in other lymphomas such as CVP (cyclophosphamide, vincristine, and prednisone), or CHOP (cyclophosphamide, doxorubicin, vincristine, and prednisone). Young patients with this disease can be candidates for bone marrow transplantation. Allogeneic bone marrow transplantation can be curative but is associated with a significant treatment-related mortality. The place of autologous transplantation in patients with this disorder remains uncertain.

Molecular analysis of immunoglobulin gene sequences in CLL has demonstrated that about half the patients have tumors expressing mutated immunoglobulin genes and half have tumors expressing unmutated or germ-line immunoglobulin sequences. Patients with unmutated immunoglobulins tend to have a more aggressive clinical course and are less responsive to therapy. Unfortunately, immunoglobulin gene sequencing is not routinely available. CD38 expression is said to be low in the better-prognosis patients expressing mutated immunoglobulin and high in poorer-prognosis patients expressing unmutated immunoglobulin, but this test has not been confirmed as a reliable means of distinguishing the two groups.

Extranodal Marginal Zone B Cell Lymphoma of MALT Type
Extranodal marginal zone B cell lymphoma of MALT type makes up approximately 8% of non-Hodgkin's lymphomas. This small-cell lymphoma presents in extranodal sites. It was previously considered a

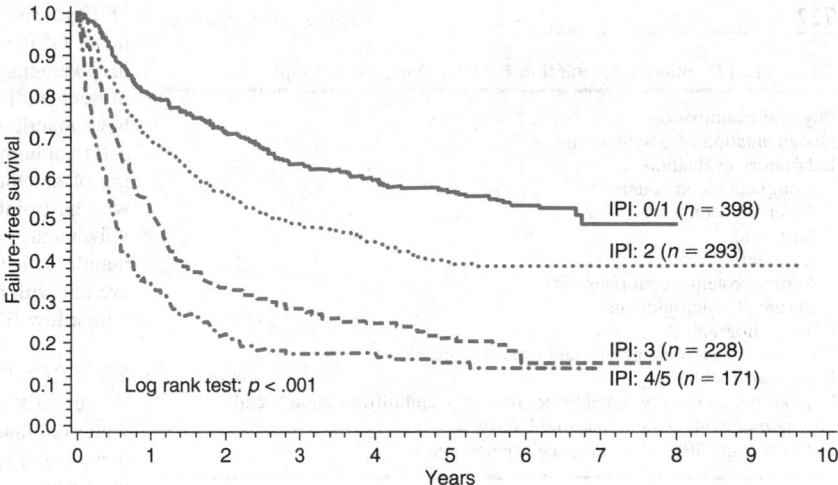

FIGURE 112-3 Relationship of International Prognostic Index (IPI) to survival. Kaplan-Meier survival curves for 1300 patients with various kinds of lymphoma stratified according to the IPI.

small lymphocytic lymphoma or sometimes a pseudolymphoma. The recognition that the gastric presentation of this lymphoma was associated with *H. pylori* infection was an important step in recognizing it as a separate entity. The clinical characteristics of extranodal marginal zone B cell lymphoma of MALT type are presented in Table 112-10.

The diagnosis of extranodal marginal zone B cell lymphoma of MALT type can be made accurately by an expert hematopathologist based on a characteristic pattern of infiltration of small lymphocytes that are monoclonal B cells and CD5 negative. In some cases, transformation to diffuse large B cell lymphoma occurs, and both diagnoses may be made in the same biopsy. The differential diagnosis includes benign lymphocytic infiltration of extranodal organs and other small-cell B cell lymphomas.

Extranodal marginal zone B cell lymphoma of MALT type may occur in the stomach, orbit, intestine, lung, thyroid, salivary gland, skin, soft tissues, bladder, kidney, and CNS. It may present as a new mass, be found on routine imaging studies, or be associated with local symptoms such as upper abdominal discomfort in gastric lymphoma. These lymphomas are localized to the organ in question in ~40% of cases and to the organ and regional lymph nodes in ~30% of patients. However, distant metastasis can occur—particularly with transformation to diffuse large B cell lymphoma. Many patients who develop

Table 112-10 Clinical Characteristics of Patients with Common Types of Non-Hodgkin's Lymphomas (NHL)

Disease	Median Age, years	Frequency in Children	% Male	Stage I/II vs III/IV, %	B Symptoms, %	Bone Marrow Involvement, %	Gastrointestinal Tract Involvement, %	% Surviving 5 years
B cell chronic lymphocytic leukemia/small lymphocytic lymphoma	65	Rare	53	9 vs 91	33	72	3	51
Mantle cell lymphoma	63	Rare	74	20 vs 80	28	64	9	27
Extranodal marginal zone B cell lymphoma of MALT type	60	Rare	48	67 vs 33	19	14	50	74
Follicular lymphoma	59	Rare	42	33 vs 67	28	42	4	72
Diffuse large B cell lymphoma	64	~25% of childhood NHL	55	54 vs 46	33	16	18	46
Burkitt's lymphoma	31	~30% of childhood NHL	89	62 vs 38	22	33	11	45
Precursor T cell lymphoblastic lymphoma	28	~40% of childhood NHL	64	11 vs 89	21	50	4	26
Anaplastic large T/null cell lymphoma	34	Common	69	51 vs 49	53	13	9	77
Peripheral T cell non-Hodgkin's lymphoma	61	~5% of childhood NHL	55	20 vs 80	50	36	15	25

NOTE: MALT, mucosa-associated lymphoid tissue.

Table 112-11 Staging Evaluation for Non-Hodgkin's Lymphoma

Physical examination
Documentation of B symptoms
Laboratory evaluation
   Complete blood counts
   Liver function tests
   Uric acid
   Calcium
   Serum protein electrophoresis
   Serum β_2-microglobulin
Chest radiograph
CT scan of abdomen, pelvis, and usually chest
Bone marrow biopsy
Lumbar puncture in lymphoblastic, Burkitt's, and diffuse large B cell
 lymphoma with positive marrow biopsy
Gallium scan (SPECT) in large-cell lymphoma

NOTE: CT, computed tomography; SPECT, single photon emission CT.

this lymphoma will have an autoimmune or inflammatory process such as Sjögren's syndrome (salivary gland MALT), Hashimoto's thyroiditis (thyroid MALT), or *Helicobacter* gastritis (gastric MALT).

Evaluation of patients with extranodal marginal zone B cell lymphoma of MALT type follows the pattern set forth in Table 112-11 for staging a patient with non-Hodgkin's lymphoma. In particular, patients with gastric lymphoma need to have studies performed to document the presence or absence of *H. pylori* infection. Endoscopic studies including ultrasound can help define the extent of gastric involvement. Most patients with extranodal marginal zone B cell lymphoma of MALT type have a good prognosis, with a 5-year survival of ~75%. In patients with a low IPI score, the 5-year survival is ~90%, while it drops to ~40% in patients with a high IPI score.

℞ **TREATMENT** Extranodal marginal zone B cell lymphoma of MALT type is curable when localized. Local therapy such as radiation or surgery can effect cure, and this is one of the few times where surgery might be a reasonable primary therapy for a patient with non-Hodgkin's lymphoma. Patients with gastric MALT lymphomas who are infected with *H. pylori* can achieve remission in the majority of cases with eradication of the infection. These remissions can be durable. Patients who present with more extensive disease are most often treated with single-agent chemotherapy such as chlorambucil. Coexistent diffuse large B cell lymphoma must be treated with combination chemotherapy. The additional acquired mutations that mediate the histologic progression also convey *Helicobacter* independence to the growth.

Mantle Cell Lymphoma Mantle cell lymphoma makes up ~6% of all non-Hodgkin's lymphomas. Recognized as a separate entity only in the past decade, this lymphoma was previously placed in a number of other subtypes. Its existence was confirmed by the recognition that these lymphomas have a characteristic chromosomal translocation, t(11;14) between the immunoglobulin heavy chain gene on chromosome 14 and the *bcl-1* gene on chromosome 11, and regularly overexpress the BCL-1 protein. The clinical characteristics of mantle cell lymphoma are presented in Table 112-10.

The diagnosis of mantle cell lymphoma can be made accurately by an expert hematopathologist based on morphologic findings and proof that the tumor is a B cell lymphoma. As with all subtypes of lymphoma, an adequate biopsy is important. The differential diagnosis of mantle cell lymphoma includes other small-cell B cell lymphomas. In particular, mantle cell lymphoma and small lymphocytic lymphoma share a characteristic expression of CD5. Mantle cell lymphoma usually has a slightly indented nucleus.

The most common presentation of mantle cell lymphoma is with palpable lymphadenopathy, frequently accompanied by systemic symptoms. Approximately 70% of patients will be stage IV at the time

of diagnosis, with frequent bone marrow and peripheral blood involvement. Of the extranodal organs that can be involved, gastrointestinal involvement is particularly important to recognize. Patients who present with lymphomatosis polyposis in the large intestine usually have mantle cell lymphoma. The evaluation of patients with mantle cell lymphoma involves the studies presented in Table 112-11 for staging of patients with non-Hodgkin's lymphoma. Patients who present with gastrointestinal tract involvement often have Waldeyer's ring involvement, and vice versa. The 5-year survival for all patients with mantle cell lymphoma is ~25%, with only occasional patients who present with a high IPI score surviving 5 years and ~50% of patients with a low IPI score surviving 5 years.

℞ **TREATMENT** Current therapies for mantle cell lymphoma are unsatisfactory. Patients with localized disease might be treated with combination chemotherapy followed by radiotherapy; however, these patients are exceedingly rare. For the usual presentation with disseminated disease, treatments are unsatisfactory, with the minority of patients achieving complete remission. Aggressive combination chemotherapy regimens followed by autologous or allogeneic bone marrow transplantation are frequently offered to younger patients. For the occasional elderly, asymptomatic patient, observation followed by single-agent chemotherapy might be the most practical approach. Combined used of rituximab (anti-CD20 antibody) and chemotherapy may be associated with better response rates.

Follicular Lymphoma Follicular lymphomas make up 22% of non-Hodgkin's lymphomas worldwide and at least 30% of non-Hodgkin's lymphomas diagnosed in the United States. This type of lymphoma can be diagnosed accurately on morphologic findings alone and has been the diagnosis in the majority of patients in therapeutic trials for "low-grade" lymphoma in the past. The clinical characteristics of follicular lymphoma are presented in Table 112-10.

Evaluation of an adequate biopsy by an expert hematopathologist is sufficient to make a diagnosis of follicular lymphoma. The tumor is composed of small cleaved and large cells in varying proportions organized in a follicular pattern of growth (**see Plate V-30**). Confirmation of B cell immunophenotype and the existence of the t(14;18) and abnormal expression of BCL-2 protein are confirmatory. The major differential diagnosis is between lymphoma and reactive follicular hyperplasia. The coexistence of diffuse large B cell lymphoma must be considered. Patients with follicular lymphoma are often subclassified into those with predominantly small cells, those with a mixture of small and large cells, and those with predominantly large cells. While this distinction cannot be made simply or very accurately, these subdivisions do have prognostic significance. Patients with follicular lymphoma with predominantly large cells have a higher proliferative fraction, progress more rapidly, and have a shorter overall survival with simple chemotherapy regimens.

The most common presentation for follicular lymphoma is with new, painless lymphadenopathy. Multiple sites of lymphoid involvement are typical, and unusual sites such as epitrochlear nodes are sometimes seen. However, essentially any organ can be involved, and extranodal presentations do occur. Most patients do not have fevers, sweats, or weight loss, and an IPI score of 0 or 1 is found in ~50% of patients. Fewer than 10% of patients have a high (i.e., 4 or 5) IPI score. The staging evaluation for patients with follicular lymphoma should include the studies included in Table 112-11 for the staging of patients with non-Hodgkin's lymphoma.

℞ **TREATMENT** Follicular lymphoma is one of the malignancies most responsive to chemotherapy and radiotherapy. In addition, as many as 25% of the patients undergo spontaneous regression—usually transient—when followed without therapy. In an asymptomatic patient, no initial treatment and watchful waiting can be an appropriate management strategy and is particularly likely to be adopted for older patients. For patients who do require treatment, single-agent chlorambucil or cyclophosphamide or combination chemotherapy with CVP or CHOP are most frequently used. With adequate treatment, between 50 and 75% of patients will achieve a complete remission. While most patients relapse (median response duration is about 2 years), at least 20% of complete responders will remain in remission for >10 years. For the rare patient with localized follicular lymphoma, involved field radiotherapy produces an excellent treatment result.

A number of new therapies have been shown to be active in the treatment of patients with follicular lymphoma. These include new cytotoxic agents such as fludarabine, interferon α, monoclonal antibodies with or without radionuclides, and lymphoma vaccines. In patients treated with a doxorubicin-containing combination chemotherapy regimen, interferon α given to patients in complete remission seems to prolong survival. The monoclonal antibody rituximab can cause objective responses in 35 to 50% of patients with relapsed follicular lymphoma, and radiolabeled antibodies appear to have response rates well in excess of 50%. Trials with tumor vaccines have been encouraging. Both autologous and allogeneic hematopoietic stem cell transplantation yield high complete response rates in patients with relapsed follicular lymphoma, and long-term remissions can occur.

Patients with follicular lymphoma with a predominance of large cells have a shorter survival when treated with single-agent chemotherapy but seem to benefit from receiving an anthracycline-containing combination chemotherapy regimen. When their disease is treated aggressively, the overall survival for such patients is no lower than for patients with other follicular lymphomas, and the failure-free survival is superior.

Patients with follicular lymphoma have a high rate of histologic transformation to diffuse large B cell lymphoma ($\sim$7% per year). This is recognized $\sim$40% of the time during the course of the illness by repeat biopsy and is present in almost all patients at autopsy. This transformation is usually heralded by rapid growths of lymph nodes—often localized—and the development of systemic symptoms such as fevers, sweats, and weight loss. Although these patients have a poor prognosis, aggressive combination chemotherapy regimens can sometimes cause a complete remission in the diffuse large B cell lymphoma, usually leaving the patient with persisting follicular lymphoma.

Diffuse Large B Cell Lymphoma Diffuse large B cell lymphoma is the most common type of non-Hodgkin's lymphoma, representing approximately one-third of all cases. This lymphoma makes up the majority of cases in previous clinical trials of "aggressive" or "intermediate-grade" lymphoma. The clinical characteristics of diffuse large B cell lymphoma are presented in Table 112-10.

The diagnosis of diffuse large B cell lymphoma can be made accurately by an expert hematopathologist when review of an adequate biopsy and proof of B cell immunophenotype are available (see Plate V-22). Cytogenetic and molecular genetic studies are not necessary for diagnosis, but some evidence has accumulated that patients who overexpress the BCL-2 protein might be more likely to relapse than others. Patients with prominent mediastinal involvement are sometimes diagnosed as a separate subgroup having primary mediastinal diffuse large B cell lymphoma. This latter group of patients has a younger median age (i.e., 37 years) and a female predominance (66%). Subtypes of diffuse large B cell lymphoma, including those with an immunoblastic subtype and tumors with extensive fibrosis, are recognized by pathologists but do not appear to have important, independent prognostic significance.

Diffuse large B cell lymphoma can present as either primary lymph node disease or at extranodal sites. More than 50% of patients will have some site of extranodal involvement at diagnosis, with the most common sites being the gastrointestinal tract and bone marrow, each being involved in 15 to 20% of patients. Essentially any organ can be involved, making a diagnostic biopsy imperative. For example, diffuse large B cell lymphoma of the pancreas has a much better prognosis than pancreatic carcinoma but would be missed without biopsy. Primary diffuse large B cell lymphoma of the brain is being diagnosed with increasing frequency.

The initial evaluation of patients with diffuse large B cell lymphoma involves the studies presented in Table 112-11 for staging of patients with non-Hodgkin's lymphoma. After a careful staging evaluation, $\sim$50% of patients will be found to have stage I or II disease and $\sim$50% will have widely disseminated lymphoma. Bone marrow biopsy shows involvement by lymphoma in about 15% of cases, with marrow involvement by small cells more frequent than with large cells.

TREATMENT The initial treatment of all patients with diffuse large B cell lymphoma should be with a combination chemotherapy regimen. The most popular regimen in the United States is CHOP, although a variety of other anthracycline-containing combination chemotherapy regimens appear to be equally efficacious. Patients with stage I or nonbulky stage II can be effectively treated with three to four cycles of combination chemotherapy followed by involved field radiotherapy. The results are at least equal and probably superior to six to eight cycles of combination therapy, and cure rates of 60 to 70% in stage II disease and 80 to 90% in stage I disease can be expected.

For patients with bulky stage II, stage III, or stage IV, six to eight cycles of combination chemotherapy regimen such as CHOP are usually administered. A frequent approach would be to administer four cycles of therapy and then reevaluate. If the patient has achieved a complete remission after four cycles, two more cycles of treatment might be given and then therapy discontinued. Using this approach, $\sim$60 to 70% of patients can be expected to achieve a complete remission, and 50 to 70% of complete responders will be cured. The chances for a favorable response to treatment are predicted by the IPI. In fact, the IPI was developed specifically to predict outcome in patients with diffuse large-cell lymphoma. For the 35% of patients with a low IPI score of 0 to 1, the 5-year survival is >70%, while for the 20% of patients with a high IPI score of 4 to 5, the 5-year survival is $\sim$20%. A number of other factors, including molecular features of the tumor, levels of circulating cytokines and soluble receptors, and other surrogate markers, have been shown to influence prognosis. However, they have not been validated as rigorously as the IPI and have not been uniformly applied clinically.

Because a large number of patients with diffuse large B cell lymphoma are either initially refractory to therapy or relapse after apparently effective chemotherapy, >50% of patients will be candidates for salvage treatment at some point. Alternative combination chemotherapy regimens can induce complete remission in as many as 50% of these patients, but long-term disease-free survival is seen in $\leq$10%. Autologous bone marrow transplantation has been shown to be superior to salvage chemotherapy at usual doses and leads to long-term disease-free survival in $\sim$40% of patients whose lymphomas remain chemotherapy-sensitive after relapse.

Burkitt's Lymphoma/Leukemia Burkitt's lymphoma/leukemia is a rare disease in adults in the United States, making up <1% of non-Hodgkin's lymphomas, but it makes up $\sim$30% of childhood non-Hodgkin's lymphoma. Burkitt's leukemia, or L3 ALL, makes up a small proportion of childhood and adult acute leukemias. The clinical features of Burkitt's lymphoma occurring in adults are presented in Table 112-10.

Burkitt's lymphoma can be diagnosed morphologically by an expert hematopathologist with a high degree of accuracy. The cells are homogeneous in size and shape (see Plate V-4). Demonstration of a very high proliferative fraction and the presence of the t(8;14) or one of its variants, t(2;8) (c-myc and the λ light chain gene) or t(8;22) (c-myc and the κ light chain gene), can be confirmatory. Burkitt's cell leukemia is recognized by the typical medium-sized cells with round nuclei, multiple nucleoli, and basophilic cytoplasm with cytoplasmic vacuoles. Demonstration of a B cell immunophenotype and one of the above-noted cytogenetic abnormalities is confirmatory.

The three distinct clinical forms of Burkitt's lymphoma that are recognized are endemic, sporadic, and immunodeficiency-associated.

Endemic and sporadic Burkitt's lymphomas occur frequently in children in Africa, and the sporadic form in western countries. Immuno-deficiency-associated Burkitt's lymphoma is seen in patients with HIV infection.

Pathologists sometimes have difficulty distinguishing between Burkitt's lymphoma and diffuse large B cell lymphoma. In the past, a separate subgroup of non-Hodgkin's lymphoma intermediate between the two was recognized. When tested, this subgroup could not be diagnosed accurately. Distinction between the two major types of B cell aggressive non-Hodgkin's lymphoma can sometimes be made based on the extremely high proliferative fraction seen in patients with Burkitt's lymphoma (i.e., essentially 100% of tumor cells are in cycle) caused by *c-myc* deregulation.

Most patients in the United States with Burkitt's lymphoma present with peripheral lymphadenopathy or an intraabdominal mass. The disease is typically rapidly progressive and has a propensity to metastasize to the CNS. Initial evaluation should always include an examination of cerebral spinal fluid to rule out metastasis in addition to the other staging evaluations noted in Table 112-11. Once the diagnosis of Burkitt's lymphoma is suspected, a diagnosis must be made promptly and staging evaluation must be accomplished expeditiously. This is the most rapidly progressive human tumor, and any delay in initiating therapy can adversely affect the patient's prognosis.

℞ **TREATMENT**   Treatment of Burkitt's lymphoma in both children and adults involves the use of intensive combination chemotherapy regimens incorporating administered high doses of cyclophosphamide. Prophylactic therapy to the CNS is mandatory and incorporated in all modern regimens. Burkitt's lymphoma was one of the first cancers shown to be curable by chemotherapy. Today, cure can be expected in 70% of both children and young adults when effective therapy is administered precisely. Salvage therapy has been generally ineffective in patients failing the initial treatment, emphasizing the importance of the initial treatment approach.

Other B Cell Lymphoid Malignancies   *B-cell prolymphocytic leukemia* involves blood and marrow infiltration by large lymphocytes with prominent nucleoli. Patients typically have a high white cell count, splenomegaly, and minimal lymphadenopathy. The chances for a complete response to therapy are poor.

Hairy cell leukemia is a rare disease that presents predominantly in older males. Typical presentation involves pancytopenia, although occasional patients will have a leukemic presentation. Splenomegaly is usual. The malignant cells appear to have "hairy" projections on light and electron microscopy and show a characteristic staining pattern with tartrate-resistant acid phosphatase. Bone marrow is typically not able to be aspirated, and biopsy shows a pattern of fibrosis with diffuse infiltration by the malignant cells. Patients with this disorder are prone to unusual infections including infection by *Mycobacterium avium intracellulare*, and vasculitic syndromes have been described. Hairy cell leukemia is responsive to chemotherapy with interferon α, pentostatin, or cladribine, with the latter being the usually preferred treatment. Clinical complete remissions with cladribine occur in the majority of patients, and long-term disease-free survival is frequent.

Splenic marginal zone lymphoma involves infiltration of the splenic white pulp by small, monoclonal B lymphocytes. This is a rare disorder that can present as leukemia as well as lymphoma. Definitive diagnosis is often made at splenectomy, which is also an effective therapy. This is an extremely indolent disorder, but when chemotherapy is required, the most usual treatment has been chlorambucil.

Lymphoplasmacytic lymphoma is the tissue manifestation of Waldenström's macroglobulinemia (Chap. 113). This type of lymphoma has been associated with chronic hepatitis C virus infection, and an etiologic association has been proposed. Patients typically present with lymphadenopathy, splenomegaly, bone marrow onvolvement, and occasionally peripheral blood involvement. The tumor cells do not ex-

press CD5. Patients often have a monoclonal IgM protein, high levels of which can dominate the clinical picture with the symptoms of hyperviscosity. Treatment of lymphoplasmacytic lymphoma can be aimed primarily at reducing the abnormal protein, if present, but will usually also involve chemotherapy. Chlorambucil, fludarabine, and cladribine have been utilized. The median 5-year survival for patients with this disorder is ~60%.

Nodal marginal zone lymphoma, also known as *monocytoid B cell lymphoma*, represents ~1% of non-Hodgkin's lymphomas. This lymphoma has a slight female predominance and presents with disseminated disease (i.e., stage III or IV) in 75% of patients. Approximately one-third of patients have bone marrow involvement, and a leukemic presentation occasionally occurs. The staging evaluation and therapy should use the same approach as used for patients with follicular lymphoma. Approximately 60% of the patients with nodal marginal zone lymphoma will survive 5 years after diagnosis.

PRECURSOR CELL T CELL MALIGNANCIES   Precursor T Cell Lymphoblastic Leukemia/Lymphoma   Precursor T cell malignancies can present either as ALL or as an aggressive lymphoma. These malignancies are more common in children and young adults, with males more frequently affected than females.

Precursor T cell ALL can present with bone marrow failure, although the severity of anemia, neutropenia, and thrombocytopenia is often less than in precursor B cell ALL. These patients sometimes have very high white cell counts, a mediastinal mass, lymphadenopathy, and hepatosplenomegaly. Precursor T cell lymphoblastic lymphoma is most often found in young men presenting with a large mediastinal mass and pleural effusions. Both presentations have a propensity to metastasize to the CNS, and CNS involvement is often present at diagnosis.

℞ **TREATMENT**   Children with precursor T cell ALL seem to benefit from very intensive remission induction and consolidation regimens. The majority of patients treated in this manner can be cured. Older children and young adults with precursor T cell lymphoblastic lymphoma are also often treated with "leukemia-like" regimens. Patients who present with localized disease have an excellent prognosis. However, advanced age is an adverse prognostic factor. Adults with precursor T cell lymphoblastic lymphoma who present with high LDH levels or bone marrow or CNS involvement are often offered bone marrow transplantation as part of their primary therapy.

MATURE (PERIPHERAL) T CELL DISORDERS   Mycosis Fungoides   Mycosis fungoides is also known as *cutaneous T cell lymphoma*. This lymphoma is more often seen by dermatologists than internists. The median age of onset is in the mid-fifties, and the disease is more common in males and in blacks.

Mycosis fungoides is an indolent lymphoma with patients often having several years of eczematous or dermatitic skin lesions before the diagnosis is finally established. The skin lesions progress from patch stage to plaque stage to cutaneous tumors. Early in the disease, biopsies are often difficult to interpret, and the diagnosis may only become apparent by observing the patient over time. In advanced stages, the lymphoma can metastasize to lymph nodes and visceral organs. A particular syndrome in patients with this lymphoma involves erythroderma and circulating tumor cells. This is known as Sézary's syndrome.

Rare patients with localized early stage mycosis fungoides can be cured with radiotherapy, often total-skin electron beam irradiation. More advanced disease has been treated with topical glucocorticoids, topical nitrogen mustard, phototherapy, psoralen with ultraviolet A (PUVA), electron beam radiation, interferon, and systemic cytotoxic therapy. Unfortunately, these treatments are palliative.

Adult T Cell Lymphoma/Leukemia   Adult T cell lymphoma/leukemia is one manifestation of infection by the HTLV-I retrovirus. Patients can be infected through transplacental transmission, blood transfusion, and by sexual transmission of the virus. Patients who acquire the virus from their mother through breast milk are most likely to develop lymphoma, but the risk is still only 2.5% and the latency averages 55 years. Tropical spastic paraparesis, another manifestation of HTLV-I infection (Chap. 191), occurs after a shorter latency (1 to 3 years) and is most common in people who acquire the virus during adulthood from transfusion or sex.

The diagnosis of adult T cell lymphoma/leukemia is made when an expert hematopathologist recognizes the typical morphologic picture, a T cell immunophenotype (i.e., CD4 positive) of malignant cells has been demonstrated, and the existence of antibodies to HTLV-I is proven. Examination of the peripheral blood will usually reveal characteristic, pleomorphic abnormal CD4-positive cells with indented nuclei, which have been called "flower" cells (see Plate V-40).

A subset of patients have a smoldering clinical course and long survival, but most patients present with an aggressive disease manifested by lymphadenopathy, hepatosplenomegaly, skin infiltration, hypercalcemia, lytic bone lesions, and elevated LDH levels. The skin lesions can be papules, plaques, tumors, and ulcerations. Bone marrow involvement is not usually extensive, and anemia and thrombocytopenia are not usually prominent. Although treatment by combination chemotherapy regimens can result in objective responses, true complete remissions are unusual, and the median survival of patients is about 7 months.

Anaplastic Large T/Null Cell Lymphoma Anaplastic large T/null cell lymphoma was previously usually diagnosed as undifferentiated carcinoma or malignant histiocytosis. Discovery of the CD30, or Ki-1, antigen and the recognition that some patients with previously unclassified malignancies displayed this antigen led to the identification of a new type of lymphoma. Subsequently, discovery of the t(2;5) and the resultant frequent overexpression of the anaplastic lymphoma kinase (alk) protein confirmed the existence of this entity. This lymphoma accounts for ~2% of all non-Hodgkin's lymphomas. The clinical characteristics of patients with anaplastic large T/null cell lymphoma are presented in Table 112-10.

The diagnosis of anaplastic large T/null cell lymphoma is made when an expert hematopathologist recognizes the typical morphologic picture and a T cell or null cell immunophenotype is demonstrated along with CD30 positivity. Documentation of the t(2;5) and/or overexpression of alk protein confirm the diagnosis. Some diffuse large B cell lymphomas can also have an anaplastic appearance but have the same clinical course or response to therapy as other diffuse large B cell lymphomas.

Patients with anaplastic large T/cell null cell lymphoma are typically young (median age, 33 years) and male (~70%). Some 50% of patients present in stage I/II, and the remainder with more extensive disease. Systemic symptoms and elevated LDH levels are seen in about one-half of patients. Bone marrow and the gastrointestinal tract are rarely involved, but skin involvement is frequent. Some patients with disease confined to the skin have a different and more indolent disorder that has been termed *cutaneous anaplastic large T/null cell lymphoma* and might be related to lymphomatoid papulosis.

Rx TREATMENT Treatment regimens appropriate for other aggressive lymphomas, such as diffuse large B cell lymphoma, should be utilized in patients with anaplastic large T/null cell lymphoma. Surprisingly, given the anaplastic appearance, this disorder has the best survival rate of any aggressive lymphoma. The 5-year survival is >75%. While traditional prognostic factors such as the IPI predict treatment outcome, overexpression of the alk protein is an important prognostic factor, with patients overexpressing this protein having a superior treatment outcome.

Peripheral T Cell Lymphoma The peripheral T cell lymphomas make up a heterogenous morphologic group of aggressive neoplasms that share a mature T cell immunophenotype. They represent ~7% of all cases of non-Hodgkin's lymphoma. A number of distinct clinical syndromes are included in this group of disorders. The clinical characteristics of patients with peripheral T cell lymphoma are presented in Table 112-10.

The diagnosis of peripheral T cell lymphoma, or any of its specific subtypes, requires an expert hematopathologist, an adequate biopsy, and immunophenotyping. Most peripheral T cell lymphomas are CD4-positive, but a few will be CD8-positive, both CD4- and CD8-positive, or have an NK-cell immunophenotype. No characteristic genetic abnormalities have yet been identified, but translocations involving the T cell antigen receptor genes on chromosomes 7 or 14 may be detected. The differential diagnosis of patients suspected of having peripheral T cell lymphoma includes reactive T cell infiltrative processes. In some cases, demonstration of a monoclonal T cell population using T cell receptor gene rearrangement studies will be required to make a diagnosis.

The initial evaluation of a patient with a peripheral T cell lymphoma should include the studies in Table 112-11 for staging patients with non-Hodgkin's lymphoma. Unfortunately, patients with peripheral T cell lymphoma usually present with adverse prognostic factors, with >80% of patients having an IPI score ≥2 and >30% having an IPI score ≥4. As this would predict, peripheral T cell lymphomas are associated with a poor outcome, and only 25% of the patients survive 5 years after diagnosis. Treatment regimens are the same as those used for diffuse large B cell lymphoma, but patients with peripheral T cell lymphoma have a poorer response to treatment. Because of this poor treatment outcome, hematopoietic stem cell transplantation is often considered early in the care of young patients.

A number of specific clinical syndromes are seen in the peripheral T cell lymphomas. *Angioimmunoblastic T cell lymphoma* is one of the more common subtypes, making up ~20% of T cell lymphomas. These patients typically present with generalized lymphadenopathy, fever, weight loss, skin rash, and polyclonal hypergammaglobunenemia. In some cases, it is difficult to separate patients with a reactive disorder from those with true lymphoma.

Extranodal T/NK cell lymphoma of nasal type has also been called *angiocentric lymphoma* and was previously termed *lethal midline granuloma*. This disorder is more frequent in Asia and South America than in the United States and Europe. Although most frequent in the upper airway, it can involve other organs. The course is aggressive, and patients frequently have the hemophagocytic syndrome. When marrow and blood involvement occur, distinction between this disease and leukemia might be difficult. Some patients will respond to aggressive combination chemotherapy regimens, but the overall outlook is poor.

Enteropathy-type intestinal T cell lymphoma is a rare disorder that occurs in patients with untreated gluten-sensitive enteropathy. Patients are frequently wasted and sometimes present with intestinal perforation. The prognosis is poor. *Hepatosplenic γδ T cell lymphoma* is a systemic illness that presents with sinusoidal infiltration of the liver, spleen, and bone marrow by malignant T cells. Tumor masses generally do not occur. The disease is associated with systemic symptoms and is often difficult to diagnosis. Treatment outcome is poor. *Subcutaneous panniculitis-like T cell lymphoma* is a rare disorder that is often confused with panniculitis. Patients present with multiple subcutaneous nodules, which progress and can ulcerate. Hemophagocytic syndrome is common. Response to therapy is poor. The development of the hemophagocytic syndrome (profound anemia, ingestion of erythrocytes by monocytes and macrophages) in the course of any peripheral T cell lymphoma is generally associated with a fatal outcome.

HODGKIN'S DISEASE Nodular Lymphocyte-Predominant Hodgkin's Disease Nodular lymphocyte predominant Hodgkin's disease is now recognized as an entity distinct from classic Hodgkin's disease. Previous classification systems recognized that biopsies from a subset of patients diagnosed as having Hodgkin's disease contained a predominance of small lymphocytes and rare Sternberg-Reed cells. In recent years, it was recognized that a subset of these patients had a nodular growth pattern and a clinical course that varied from that of patients with classic Hodgkin's disease. This is an unusual clinical entity and represents <5% of cases of Hodgkin's disease.

Nodular lymphocyte-predominant Hodgkin's disease has a number of characteristics that suggest its relationship to non-Hodgkin's lymphoma. These include a clonal proliferation of B cells and a distinctive immunophenotype; tumor cells express J chain and display CD45 and epithelial membrane antigen (ema) and do not express two markers normally found on Sternberg-Reed cells, CD30 and CD15. This lymphoma tends to have a chronic, relapsing course and sometimes transforms to diffuse large B cell lymphoma.

The treatment of patients with nodular lymphocyte-predominant Hodgkin's disease is controversial. Some clinicians favor no treatment and merely close follow-up. In the United States, most physicians will treat localized disease with radiotherapy and disseminated disease with regimens utilized for patients with classic Hodgkin's disease. Regardless of the therapy utilized, most series report a long-term survival of >80%.

Classical Hodgkin's Disease   Hodgkin's disease occurs in ~8000 patients in the United States each year, and the disease does not appear to be increasing in frequency. Most patients present with palpable lymphadenopathy that is nontender; in most patients, these lymph nodes are in the neck, supraclavicular area, and axilla. More than half the patients will have mediastinal adenopathy at diagnosis, and this is sometimes the initial manifestation. Subdiaphragmatic presentation of Hodgkin's disease is unusual and more common in older males. Approximately one-third of patients present with fevers, night sweats, and/or weight loss—B symptoms in the Ann Arbor staging classification (Table 112-8). Occasionally, Hodgkin's disease can present as a fever of unknown origin. This is more common in older patients who are found to have mixed-cellularity Hodgkin's disease in an abdominal site. Rarely, the fevers persist for days to weeks, followed by afebrile intervals and then recurrence of the fever. This pattern is known as *Pel-Epstein fever*. Hodgkin's disease can occasionally present with unusual manifestations. These include severe and unexplained itching, cutaneous disorders such as erythema nodosum and ichthyosiform atrophy, paraneoplastic cerebellar degeneration and other distant effects on the CNS, nephrotic syndrome, immune hemolytic anemia and thrombocytopenia, hypercalcemia, and pain in lymph nodes on alcohol ingestion.

The diagnosis of Hodgkin's disease is established by review of an adequate biopsy specimen by an expert hematopathologist. In the United States, most patients would be classified as having nodular sclerosing Hodgkin's disease, with a minority of patients having mixed-cellularity Hodgkin's disease. Lymphocyte-predominant and lymphocyte-depleted Hodgkin's disease are rare. Mixed-cellularity Hodgkin's disease or lymphocyte-depletion Hodgkin's disease are seen more frequently in patients infected by HIV (see Plate V-18). The differential diagnosis of a lymph node biopsy suspicious for Hodgkin's disease includes inflammatory processes, mononucleosis, non-Hodgkin's lymphoma, diphenylhydantoin-induced lymphadenopathy, and nonlymphomatous malignancies.

The staging evaluation for a patient with Hodgkin's disease would typically include a careful history and physical examination; complete blood count; erythrocyte sedimentation rate; serum chemistry studies including LDH; chest radiograph; CT scan of the chest, abdomen, and pelvis; and bone marrow biopsy. Many patients would also have a gallium scan. If radiologic expertise is available, a bipedal lymphangiogram can be helpful. Gallium scans are most useful at the completion of therapy to document remission. Staging laparotomies were once popular for most patients with Hodgkin's disease but are now done rarely because of an increased reliance on systemic rather than local therapy.

℞ TREATMENT   Patients with localized Hodgkin's disease are cured >90% of the time. In patients with good prognostic factors, extended field radiotherapy has a high cure rate. Increasingly, patients with all stages of Hodgkin's disease are treated initially with chemotherapy. Patients with localized or good-prognosis disease receive a brief course of chemotherapy followed by radiotherapy to sites of node involvement. Patients with more extensive disease or those with B symptoms receive a complete course of chemotherapy. The most popular chemotherapy regimens used in the treatment of Hodgkin's disease include doxorubicin, bleomycin, vinblastine, and dacarbazine (ABVD) and mechlorethamine, vincristine, procarbazine, and prednisone (MOPP), or combinations of the drugs in these two regimens. Today, most patients in the United States receive ABVD. Long-term disease-free survival in patients with advanced disease can be achieved in >75% of patients who lack systemic symptoms and in 50 to 70% of patients with systemic symptoms.

Patients who relapse after primary therapy of Hodgkin's disease can frequently still be cured. Patients who relapse after initial treatment only with radiotherapy have an excellent outcome when treated with chemotherapy. Patients who relapse after an effective chemotherapy regimen are usually not curable with subsequent chemotherapy administered at standard doses. However, patients with a long initial remission can be an exception to this rule. Autologous bone marrow transplantation can cure half of patients who fail effective chemotherapy regimens.

Because of the very high cure rate in patients with Hodgkin's disease, long-term complications have become a major focus for clinical research. In fact, in some series of patients with early-stage disease, more patients died from late complications of therapy than from Hodgkin's disease itself. This is particularly true in patients with localized disease. The most serious late side effects include second malignancies and cardiac injury. Patients are at risk for the development of acute leukemia in the first 10 years after treatment with combination chemotherapy regimens that contain alkylating agents. The risk for development of acute leukemia appears to be greater after MOPP-like regimens than with ABVD. The development of carcinomas as a complication of treatment for Hodgkin's disease has become a major problem. These tumors usually occur ≥10 years after treatment and are associated more with radiotherapy than with chemotherapy. For this reason, young women treated with thoracic radiotherapy for Hodgkin's disease should institute screening mammograms 5 to 10 years after treatment, and all patients who receive thoracic radiotherapy for Hodgkin's disease should be discouraged from smoking. Thoracic radiation also accelerates coronary artery disease, and patients should be encouraged to minimize risk factors for coronary artery disease such as smoking and elevated cholesterol levels.

A number of other late side effects from the treatment of Hodgkin's disease are well known. Patients who receive thoracic radiotherapy are at very high risk for the eventual development of hypothyroidism and should be observed for this complication; intermittent measurement of thyrotropin should be made to identify the condition before it becomes symptomatic. Lhermitte's syndrome occurs in ~15% of patients who receive thoracic radiotherapy. This syndrome is manifested by an "electric shock" sensation into the lower extremities on flexion of the neck. Infertility is a concern for all patients undergoing treatment for Hodgkin's disease. In both women and men, the risk of permanent infertility is age-related, with younger patients more likely to recover fertility. In addition, treatment with ABVD rather than MOPP increases the chances to retain fertility.

LYMPHOMA-LIKE DISORDERS

The most common condition that pathologists and clinicians might confuse with lymphoma is reactive, atypical lymphoid hyperplasia. Patients might have localized or disseminated lymphadenopathy and might have the systemic symptoms characteristic of lymphoma. Underlying causes include a drug reaction to diphenylhydantoin or carbamezepine. Immune disorders such as rheumatoid arthritis and lupus erythematosus, viral infections such as cytomegalovirus and EBV, and bacterial infections such as cat-scratch disease may cause adenopathy (Chap. 63). In the absence of a definitive diagnosis after initial biopsy, continued follow-up, further testing, and repeated biopsies, if necessary, are the appropriate approach rather than instituting therapy.

Specific conditions that can be confused with lymphoma include *Castleman's disease*, which can present with localized or disseminated lymphadenopathy; some patients have systemic symptoms. The disseminated form is often accompanied by anemia and polyclonal hypergammaglobulinemia, and the condition seems to be related to an overproduction of interleukin 6, possibly produced by human herpesvirus 8. Patients with localized disease can be treated effectively with local therapy, while the initial treatment for patients with disseminated disease is usually with systemic glucocorticoids.

Sinus histiocytosis with massive lymphadenopathy (Rosai-Dorfman's disease) usually presents with bulky lymphadenopathy in children or young adults. The disease is usually nonprogressive and self-limited, but patients can manifest autoimmune hemolytic anemia.

Lymphomatoid papulosis is a cutaneous lymphoproliferative disorder that is often confused with anaplastic large-cell lymphoma involving the skin. The cells of lymphomatoid papulosis are similar to those seen in lymphoma and stain for CD30, and T cell receptor gene rearrangements are sometimes seen. However, the condition is characterized by waxing and waning skin lesions that usually heal, leaving small scars. In the absence of effective communication between the clinician and the pathologist regarding the clinical course in the patient, this disease will be misdiagnosed. Since the clinical picture is usually benign, misdiagnosis is a serious mistake.

ACKNOWLEDGMENT

Dr. Arnold Freedman and Dr. Lee Nadler contributed this chapter to the 14th edition, and some elements of that chapter were retained here.

BIBLIOGRAPHY

ARMITAGE JO et al: *Text Atlas of Lymphomas.* London, Martin Dunitz, 1999

HARRIS NL et al: World Health Organization classification of neoplastic diseases of the hematopoietic and lymphoid tissues: Report of the Clinical Advisory Committee Meeting, Airlie House, Virginia, November, 1997. J Clin Oncol 17:3835, 1999

HAUKE RJ, ARMITAGE JO: A new approach to non-Hodgkin's lymphoma. Intern Med 39:197, 2000

URBA WJ, LONGO DL: Hodgkin's disease. N Engl J Med 326:678, 1992

---

113   *Dan L. Longo*

PLASMA CELL DISORDERS

GENERAL PRINCIPLES The *plasma cell disorders* are monoclonal neoplasms related to each other by virtue of their development from common progenitors in the B lymphocyte lineage. Multiple myeloma, Waldenström's macroglobulinemia, primary amyloidosis (Chap. 319), and the heavy chain diseases comprise this group and may be designated by a variety of synonyms such as *monoclonal gammopathies, paraproteinemias, plasma cell dyscrasias,* and *dysproteinemias.* Mature B lymphocytes destined to produce IgG bear surface immunoglobulin molecules of both M and G heavy chain isotypes with both isotypes having identical idiotypes (variable regions). Under normal circumstances, maturation to antibody-secreting plasma cells is stimulated by exposure to the antigen for which the surface immunoglobulin is specific; however, in the plasma cell disorders the control over this process is lost. The clinical manifestations of all the plasma cell disorders relate to the expansion of the neoplastic cells, to the secretion of cell products (immunoglobulin molecules or subunits, lymphokines), and to some extent to the host's response to the tumor. →*Normal development of B lymphocytes is discussed in Chap. 305.*

There are three categories of structural variation among immunoglobulin molecules that form antigenic determinants, and these are used to classify immunoglobulins (Chap. 305). *Isotypes* are those determinants that distinguish among the main classes of antibodies of a given species and are the same in all normal individuals of that species.

Therefore, isotypic determinants are, by definition, recognized by antibodies from a distinct species (heterologous sera) but not by antibodies from the same species (homologous sera). There are five heavy chain isotypes (M, G, A, D, E) and two light chain isotypes (κ, λ). *Allotypes* are distinct determinants that reflect regular small differences between individuals of the same species in the amino acid sequences of otherwise similar immunoglobulins. These differences are determined by allelic genes; by definition, they are detected by antibodies made in the same species. *Idiotypes* are the third category of antigenic determinants. They are unique to the molecules produced by a given clone of antibody-producing cells. Idiotypes are formed by the unique structure of the antigen-binding portion of the molecule.

Antibody molecules (Fig. 305-8) are composed of two heavy chains (mol wt ~50,000) and two light chains (mol wt ~25,000). Each chain has a constant portion (limited amino acid sequence variability) and a variable region (extensive sequence variability). The light and heavy chains are linked by disulfide bonds and are aligned so that their variable regions are adjacent to one another. This variable region forms the antigen recognition site of the antibody molecule; its unique structural features form a particular set of determinants, or idiotypes, that are reliable markers for a particular clone of cells because each antibody is formed and secreted by a single clone. Each chain is specified by distinct genes, synthesized separately, and assembled into an intact antibody molecule after translation (Fig. 113-1). Because of the mechanics of the gene rearrangements necessary to specify the immunoglobulin variable regions (VDJ joining for the heavy chain, VJ joining for the light chain), a particular clone rearranges only one of the two chromosomes to produce an immunoglobulin molecule of only one light chain isotype and only one allotype (allelic exclusion). After exposure to antigen, the variable region may become associated with a new heavy chain isotype (class switch). Each clone of cells performs these sequential gene arrangements in a unique way. This results in each clone producing a unique immunoglobulin molecule. In most cells, light chains are synthesized in slight excess, are secreted as free light chains by plasma cells, and are cleared by the kidney, but <10 mg of such light chains is excreted per day.

Electrophoretic analysis of components of the serum proteins permits determination of the amount of immunoglobulin in the serum (Fig. 113-2). The variety of immunoglobulins move heterogeneously in an electric field and form a broad peak in the gamma region. The gamma globulin region of the electrophoretic pattern is usually increased in the sera of patients and animals with plasma cell tumors. There is a sharp spike in this region called an *M component* (M for monoclonal). Less commonly, the M component may appear in the beta$_2$ or alpha$_2$ globulin region. The antibody must be present at a concentration of at least 5 g/L (0.5 g/dL) to be detectable by this method. This corresponds to approximately 10^9 cells producing the antibody. Confirmation that such an M component is truly monoclonal relies on the use of immunoelectrophoresis that shows a single light and heavy chain type. Hence immunoelectrophoresis and electrophoresis provide qualitative and quantitative assessment of the M component, respectively. Once the presence of an M component has been confirmed, electrophoresis provides the more practical information for managing patients with monoclonal gammopathies. In a given patient, the amount of M component in the serum is a reliable measure of the tumor burden. This makes the M component an excellent tumor marker, yet it is not specific enough to be used to screen asymptomatic patients. In addition to the plasma cell disorders, M components may be detected in other lymphoid neoplasms such as chronic lymphocytic leukemia and lymphomas of B or T cell origin; nonlymphoid neoplasms such as chronic myeloid leukemia, breast cancer, and colon cancer; a variety of nonneoplastic conditions such as cirrhosis, sarcoidosis, parasitic diseases, Gaucher's disease, and pyoderma gangrenosum; and a number of autoimmune conditions, including rheumatoid arthritis, myasthenia gravis, and cold agglutinin disease. A very rare skin disease known as lichen myxedematosus or papular muci-

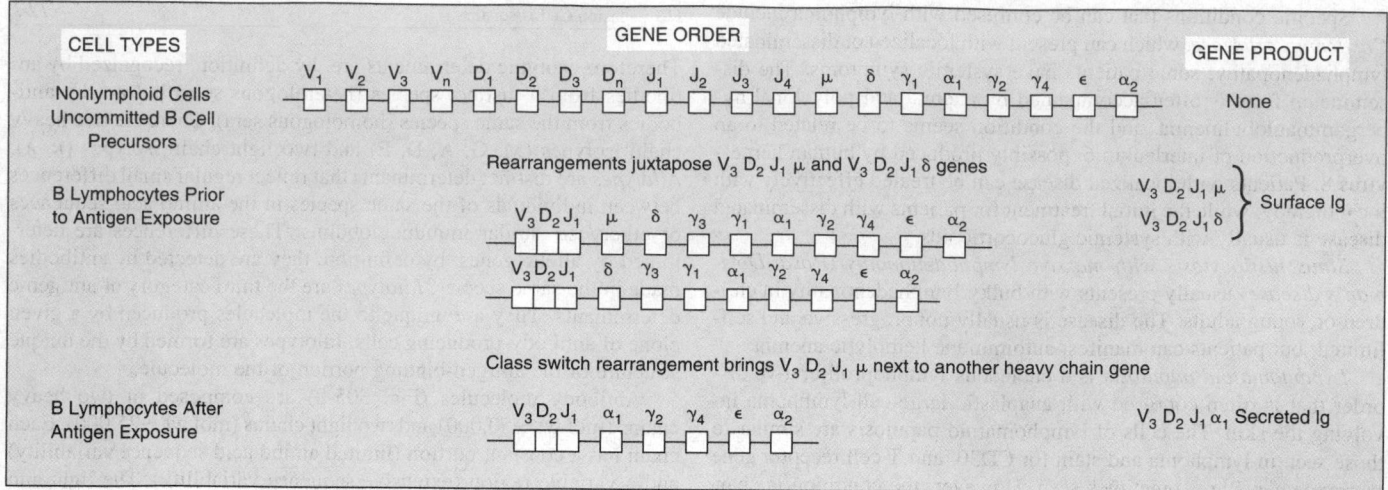

FIGURE 113-1 Immunoglobulin heavy chains are encoded by four distinct genetic elements: variable (Igh-V), diversity (Igh-D), joining (Igh-J), and constant (Igh-C) genes. The variable region of the immunoglobulin heavy chain is encoded by the V, D, and J genes. The same variable region may be associated with any of the 10 heavy chain constant region genes. In the germ-line genome (all cells except B cells) the V, D, and J genes are widely separated and exist in numerous forms. Once a cell becomes committed to B cell differ-entiation, a single V gene and a single D gene translocate to a single J gene, and the intervening genetic material is excised (VDJ joining). The newly formed VDJ gene is transcribed into a single message along with either an M or D isotype C gene. Upon exposure to antigen, another rearrangement may occur so that the VDJ gene may be associated with a G, A, or E isotype C gene. In light chain genes there appear to be no D genes, and thus light chain variable regions are formed by VJ joining.

nosis is associated with a monoclonal gammopathy. Highly cationic IgG is deposited in the dermis of patients with this disease. This organ specificity may reflect the specificity of the antibody for some antigenic component of the dermis.

The nature of the M component is variable in plasma cell disorders. It may be an intact antibody molecule of any heavy chain subclass, or it may be an altered antibody or fragment. Isolated light or heavy chains may be produced. In some plasma cell tumors such as extramedullary or solitary bone plasmacytomas, less than a third of patients will have an M component. In about 20% of myelomas, only light chains are produced and in most cases are secreted in the urine as Bence Jones proteins. The frequency of myelomas of a particular heavy chain class is roughly proportional to the serum concentration, and therefore IgG myelomas are more common than IgA and IgD myelomas.

MULTIPLE MYELOMA **Definition** Multiple myeloma represents a malignant proliferation of plasma cells derived from a single clone. The terms *multiple myeloma* and *myeloma* may be used interchangeably. The tumor, its products, and the host response to it result in a number of organ dysfunctions and symptoms of bone pain or fracture, renal failure, susceptibility to infection, anemia, hypercalcemia, and occasionally clotting abnormalities, neurologic symptoms, and vascular manifestations of hyperviscosity.

Etiology The cause of myeloma is not known. Myeloma occurred with increased frequency in those exposed to the radiation of nuclear warheads in World War II after a 20-year latency. A variety of chromosomal alterations have been found in patients with myeloma; 13q14 deletions, 17p13 deletions, and 11q abnormalities predominate. The most common translocation is t(11;14)(q13;q32), and evidence is strong that errors in switch recombination—the genetic mechanism to change antibody heavy chain isotype—participate in the transformation pathway. Overexpression of *myc* or *ras* genes has been noted in some cases. Mutations in p53 and Rb-1 have also been described, but no common molecular pathogenesis has yet emerged.

Myeloma has been seen more commonly than expected among farmers, wood workers, leather workers, and those exposed to petroleum products. The neoplastic event in myeloma may involve cells earlier in B cell differentiation than the plasma cell. Circulating B cells bearing surface immunoglobulin that share the idiotype of the M component are present in myeloma patients. Interleukin (IL) 6 may play a role in driving myeloma cell proliferation; a large fraction of myeloma cells exposed to IL-6 in vitro respond by proliferating. The IL-6 de-pendency of myeloma is controversial. Infection of marrow macrophages with human herpesvirus 8 has been noted in some cases leading to the hypothesis that viral IL-6 may contribute to the pathogenesis. This notion is also debated. It remains difficult to distinguish benign from malignant plasma cells on the basis of morphologic criteria in all but a few cases (**see Plate V-27**).

Incidence and Prevalence About 13,200 cases of myeloma were diagnosed in 2000, and 11,200 people died from the disease. Myeloma increases in incidence with age. The median age at diagnosis is 68 years; it is rare under age 40. The yearly incidence is around 4 per 100,000 and remarkably similar throughout the world. Males are slightly more commonly affected than females, and blacks have nearly twice the incidence of whites. In the age group over 25 the incidence is 30 per 100,000. Myeloma accounts for about 1% of all malignancies in whites and 2% in blacks; 13% of all hematologic cancers in whites and 33% in blacks.

Pathogenesis and Clinical Manifestations (Table 113-1) Bone pain is the most common symptom in myeloma, affecting nearly 70% of patients. The pain usually involves the back and ribs, and unlike the pain of metastatic carcinoma, which often is worse at night, the pain of myeloma is precipitated by movement. Persistent localized pain in a patient with myeloma usually signifies a pathologic fracture. The bone lesions of myeloma are caused by the proliferation of tumor cells and the activation of osteoclasts that destroy the bone. The osteoclasts respond to osteoclast activating factors (OAF) made by the myeloma cells [OAF activity can be mediated by several cytokines, including IL-1, lymphotoxin, and tumor necrosis factor (TNF)]. However, production of these factors stops following administration of glucocorticoids or interferon (IFN)-α. The bone lesions are lytic in nature and are rarely associated with osteoblastic new bone formation. Therefore, radioisotopic bone scanning is less useful in diagnosis than is plain radiography. The bony lysis results in substantial mobilization of calcium from bone, and serious acute and chronic complications of hypercalcemia may dominate the clinical picture (see below). Localized bone lesions may expand to the point that mass lesions may be palpated, especially on the skull (Fig. 113-3), clavicles, and sternum, and the collapse of vertebrae may lead to spinal cord compression.

The next most common clinical problem in patients with myeloma is susceptibility to bacterial infections. The most common infections are pneumonias and pyelonephritis, and the most frequent pathogens are *Streptococcus pneumoniae*, *Staphylococcus aureus*, and *Klebsiella pneumoniae* in the lungs and *Escherichia coli* and other gram-negative

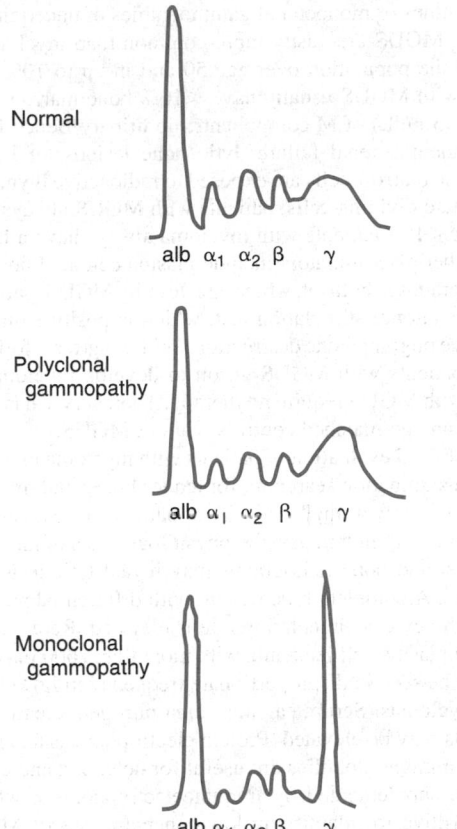

FIGURE 113-2 Representative patterns of serum electrophoresis. The upper panel illustrates the normal pattern of serum protein on electrophoresis. Since there are many different immunoglobulins in the serum, their differing mobilities in an electric field produce a broad peak. In conditions associated with increases in polyclonal immunoglobulin, the broad peak is more prominent (middle panel). In monoclonal gammopathies, the predominance of a product of a single cell produces a "church spire" sharp peak, usually in the gamma globulin region (bottom panel).

Table 113-1 Pathogenesis and Clinical Manifestations of Multiple Myeloma

Clinical Finding	Underlying Cause	Pathogenic Mechanism
Hypercalcemia, pathologic fractures, cord compression, lytic bone lesions, osteoporosis, bone pain	Skeletal destruction	Tumor expansion; production of osteoclast activating factors (OAF) by tumor cells
Renal failure	Light chain proteinuria, hypercalcemia, urate nephropathy, amyloid glomerulopathy (rare) Pyelonephritis	Toxic effects of tumor products, light chains, OAF, DNA breakdown products Hypogammaglobulinemia
Anemia	Myelophthisis, decreased production, increased destruction	Tumor expansion; production of inhibitory factors and autoantibodies by tumor cells
Infection	Hypogammaglobulinemia, decreased neutrophil migration	Decreased production due to tumor-induced suppression; increased IgG catabolism
Neurologic symptoms	Hyperviscosity, cryoglobulins, amyloid deposits Hypercalcemia, cord compression	Products of tumor; properties of M component; light chains OAF
Bleeding	Interference with clotting factors, amyloid damage of endothelium, platelet dysfunction	Products of tumor; antibodies to clotting factors; light chains; antibody coating of platelets
Mass lesions		Tumor expansion

organisms in the urinary tract. In about 25% of patients, recurrent infections are the presenting features, and over 75% of patients will have a serious infection at some time in their course. The susceptibility to infection has several contributing causes. First, patients with myeloma have diffuse hypogammaglobulinemia if the M component is excluded. The hypogammaglobulinemia is related to both decreased production and increased destruction of normal antibodies. Moreover, some patients generate a population of circulating regulatory cells in response to their myeloma that can suppress normal antibody synthesis. In the case of IgG myeloma, normal IgG antibodies are broken down more rapidly than normal because the catabolic rate for IgG antibodies varies directly with the serum concentration. The large M component results in fractional catabolic rates of 8 to 16% instead of the normal 2%. These patients have very poor antibody responses, especially to polysaccharide antigens such as those on bacterial cell walls. Most measures of T cell function in myeloma are normal, but a subset of CD4+ cells may be decreased. Granulocyte lysozyme content is low, and granulocyte migration is not as rapid as normal in patients with myeloma, probably the result of a tumor product. There are also a variety of abnormalities in complement functions in myeloma patients. All these factors contribute to the immune deficiency of these patients.

Renal failure occurs in nearly 25% of myeloma patients, and some renal pathology is noted in over half. Many factors contribute to this. Hypercalcemia is the most common cause of renal failure. Glomerular deposits of amyloid, hyperuricemia, recurrent infections, and occasional infiltration of the kidney by myeloma cells all may contribute to renal dysfunction. However, tubular damage associated with the

excretion of light chains is almost always present. Normally, light chains are filtered, reabsorbed in the tubules, and catabolized. With the increase in the amount of light chains presented to the tubule, the tubular cells become overloaded with these proteins, and tubular damage results either directly from light chain toxic effects or indirectly from the release of intracellular lysosomal enzymes. The earliest manifestation of this tubular damage is the adult Fanconi syndrome (a type

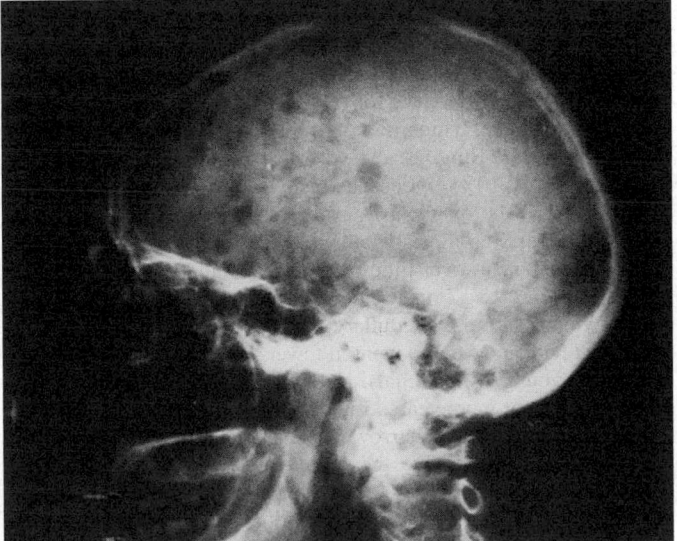

FIGURE 113-3 Bony lesions in multiple myeloma. The skull demonstrates the typical "punched out" lesions characteristic of multiple myeloma. The lesion represents a purely osteolytic lesion with little or no osteoblastic activity. (*Courtesy of Dr. Geraldine Schechter.*)

2 proximal renal tubular acidosis), with increased loss of glucose, amino acids, and defects in the ability of the kidney to acidify and concentrate the urine. The proteinuria is not accompanied by hypertension, and the protein is nearly all light chains. Generally, very little albumin is in the urine because glomerular function is usually normal. When the glomeruli are involved, the proteinuria is nonselective. Patients with myeloma also have a decreased anion gap [i.e., $Na^+ - (Cl^- + HCO_3^-)$] because the M component is cationic, resulting in retention of chloride. This is often accompanied by hyponatremia that is felt to be artificial (pseudohyponatremia) because each volume of serum has less water as a result of the increased protein. Myeloma patients are susceptible to developing acute renal failure if they become dehydrated.

Anemia occurs in about 80% of myeloma patients. It is usually normocytic and normochromic and related both to the replacement of normal marrow by expanding tumor cells and to the inhibition of hematopoiesis by factors made by the tumor. In addition, mild hemolysis may contribute to the anemia. A larger than expected fraction of patients may have megaloblastic anemia due to either folate or vitamin B_{12} deficiency. Granulocytopenia and thrombocytopenia are very rare. Clotting abnormalities may be seen due to the failure of antibody-coated platelets to function properly or to the interaction of the M component with clotting factors I, II, V, VII, or VIII. Raynaud's phenomenon and impaired circulation may result if the M component forms cryoglobulins, and hyperviscosity syndromes may develop depending on the physical properties of the M component (most common with IgM, IgG3, and IgA paraproteins). Hyperviscosity is defined on the basis of the relative viscosity of serum as compared with water. Normal relative serum viscosity is 1.8 (i.e., serum is normally almost twice as viscous as water). Symptoms of hyperviscosity occur at a level of 5 to 6, a level usually reached at paraprotein concentrations of around 40 g/L (4 g/dL) for IgM, 50 g/L (5 g/dL) for IgG3, and 70 g/L (7 g/dL) for IgA.

Although neurologic symptoms occur in a minority of patients, they may have many causes. Hypercalcemia may produce lethargy, weakness, depression, and confusion. Hyperviscosity may lead to headache, fatigue, visual disturbances, and retinopathy. Bony damage and collapse may lead to cord compression, radicular pain, and loss of bowel and bladder control. Infiltration of peripheral nerves by amyloid can be a cause of carpal tunnel syndrome and other sensorimotor mono- and polyneuropathies.

Many of the clinical features of myeloma, e.g., cord compression, pathologic fractures, hyperviscosity, sepsis, and hypercalcemia, can present as medical emergencies. Despite the widespread distribution of plasma cells in the body, tumor expansion is dominantly within bone and bone marrow and, for reasons unknown, rarely causes enlargement of spleen, lymph nodes, or gut-associated lymphatic tissue.

Diagnosis and Staging   The classic triad of myeloma is marrow plasmacytosis (>10%), lytic bone lesions, and a serum and/or urine M component. The diagnosis may be made in the absence of bone lesions if the plasmacytosis is associated with a progressive increase in the M component over time or if extramedullary mass lesions develop. There are two important variants of myeloma, solitary bone plasmacytoma and extramedullary plasmacytoma. These lesions are associated with an M component in fewer than 30% of the cases, they may affect younger individuals, and both are associated with median survivals of 10 or more years. Solitary bone plasmacytoma is a single lytic bone lesion without marrow plasmacytosis. Extramedullary plasmacytomas usually involve the submucosal lymphoid tissue of the nasopharynx or paranasal sinuses without marrow plasmacytosis. Both tumors are highly responsive to local radiation therapy. If an M component is present, it should disappear after treatment. Solitary bone plasmacytomas may recur in other bony sites or evolve into myeloma. Extramedullary plasmacytomas rarely recur or progress.

The most difficult differential diagnosis in patients with myeloma involves their separation from individuals with benign monoclonal gammopathies or monoclonal gammopathies of uncertain significance (MGUS). MGUS are vastly more common than myeloma, occurring in 1% of the population over age 50 and in up to 10% over age 75. Patients with MGUS usually have <10% bone marrow plasma cells; <30 g/L (3 g/dL) of M components; no urinary Bence Jones protein; and no anemia, renal failure, lytic bone lesions, or hypercalcemia. When bone marrow cells are exposed to radioactive thymidine in order to quantitate dividing cells, patients with MGUS always have a labeling index <1%; patients with myeloma always have a labeling index >1%. Other discriminators include plasma cell acid phosphatase and β-glucuronidase, both of which are low in MGUS patients, and the salmon calcitonin stimulation test, which is positive only in patients with active ongoing bone destruction. With long-term follow-up, about 25% of patients with MGUS go on to develop myeloma. Typically, patients with MGUS require no therapy. Their survival is about 2 years shorter than age-matched controls without MGUS.

The clinical evaluation of patients with myeloma includes a careful physical examination searching for tender bones and masses. It is paradoxical that only a small minority of patients have an enlargement of the spleen and lymph nodes, the physiologic sites of antibody production. Chest and bone radiographs may reveal lytic lesions or diffuse osteopenia. A complete blood count with differential may reveal anemia. Erythrocyte sedimentation rate is elevated. Rare patients (~2%) may have plasma cell leukemia with more than 2000 plasma cells/μL. This may be seen in disproportionate frequency in IgD (12%) and IgE (25%) myelomas. Serum calcium, urea nitrogen, creatinine, and uric acid levels may be elevated. Protein electrophoresis and measurement of serum immunoglobulins are useful for detecting and characterizing M spikes, supplemented by immunoelectrophoresis, which is especially sensitive for identifying low concentrations of M components not detectable by protein electrophoresis. A 24-h urine specimen is necessary to quantitate protein excretion, and a concentrated aliquot is used for electrophoresis and immunologic typing of any M component. Serum alkaline phosphatase is usually normal even with extensive bone involvement because of the absence of osteoblastic activity. It is also important to quantitate serum β_2-microglobulin (see below). Serum soluble IL-6 receptor levels and C-reactive protein may reflect physiologic IL-6 levels in the patient.

The serum M component will be IgG in 53% of patients, IgA in 25%, and IgD in 1%; 20% of patients will have only light chains in serum and urine. Dipsticks for detecting proteinuria are not reliable at identifying light chains, and the heat test for detecting Bence Jones protein is falsely negative in about 50% of patients with light chain myeloma. Fewer than 1% of patients have no identifiable M component; these patients usually have light chain myelomas in which renal catabolism has made the light chains undetectable in the urine. IgD myeloma may also present as light chain myeloma. About two-thirds of patients with serum M components also have urinary light chains. The light chain isotype may have an impact on survival. Patients secreting lambda light chains have a significantly shorter overall survival than those secreting kappa light chains. It is not clear whether this is due to some genetically important determinant of cell proliferation or because lambda light chains are more likely to cause renal damage and form amyloid than are kappa light chains. The heavy chain isotype may have an impact on patient management as well. About half of patients with IgM paraproteins develop hyperviscosity compared with only 2 to 4% of patients with IgA and IgG M components. Among IgG myelomas, it is the IgG3 subclass that has the highest tendency to form both concentration- and temperature-dependent aggregates, leading to hyperviscosity and cold agglutination at lower serum concentrations.

The staging system for patients with myeloma is a functional system for predicting survival and is based on a variety of clinical and laboratory tests, unlike the anatomic staging systems for solid tumors. Details of the staging system are given in Table 113-2. Based on the hemoglobin, calcium, M component, and degree of skeletal involvement, the total-body tumor burden is estimated to be low (stage I, $<0.6 \times 10^{12}$ cells/m²), intermediate (stage II, 0.6 to 1.2×10^{12} cells/

Table 113-2 Myeloma Staging System

Stage	Criteria	Estimated Tumor Burden, $\times 10^{12}$ cells/m^2

I	All of the following:
	1. Hemoglobin >100 g/L (>10 g/dL)
	2. Serum calcium <3 mmol/L (<12 mg/dL)
	3. Normal bone x-ray or solitary lesion
	4. Low M-component production
	   a. IgG level <50 g/L (<5 g/dL)
	   b. IgA level <30 g/L (<3 g/dL)
	   c. Urine light chain <4 g/24 h
		<0.6 (low)

II	Fitting neither I nor III	0.6–1.20 (intermediate)

III	One or more of the following:
	1. Hemoglobin <85 g/L (<8.5 g/dL)
	2. Serum calcium >3 mmol/L (>12 mg/dL)
	3. Advanced lytic bone lesions
	4. High M-component production
	   a. IgG level >70 g/L (>7 g/dL)
	   b. IgA level >50 g/L (>5 g/dL)
	   c. Urine light chains >12 g/24 h
		>1.20 (high)

SUBCLASSIFICATION BASED ON SERUM CREATININE LEVELS

Level	Stage	Median Survival, Months
A < 177 μmol/L (<2 mg/dL)	IA	61
B > 177 μmol/L (>2 mg/dL)	IIA,B	55
	IIIA	30
	IIIB	15

STAGING BASED ON SERUM β_2-MICROGLOBULIN LEVELS

Level	Stage	Median Survival, Months
<0.004 g/L (<4 μg/mL)	I	43
>0.004 g/L (>4 μg/mL)	II	12

m^2), or high (stage III, >1.2 × 10^{12} cells/m^2), and the stages are further subdivided on the basis of renal function [A if serum creatinine <177 mol/L (<2 mg/dL), B if >177 (>2)]. Patients in stage IA have a median survival of more than 5 years and those in stage IIIB about 15 months. β_2-Microglobulin is a protein of 11,000 mol wt with homologies with the constant region of immunoglobulins that is the light chain of the class I major histocompatibility antigens (HLA-A, -B, -C) on the surface of every cell. Serum β_2-microglobulin is the single most powerful predictor of survival and can substitute for staging. Patients with β_2-microglobulin levels <0.004 g/L have a median survival of 43 months and those with levels >0.004 g/L only 12 months. It is also felt that once the diagnosis of myeloma is firm, histologic features of atypia may also exert an influence on prognosis. IL-6 may be an autocrine and/or paracrine growth factor for myeloma cells; elevated levels are associated with more aggressive disease. High labeling index and high levels of lactate dehydrogenase and thymidine kinase are also associated with poor prognosis.

Other factors that may influence prognosis are the number of cytogenetic abnormalities, % plasma cells in the marrow, performance status, and serum levels of IL-6, soluble IL-6 receptors, C-reactive protein, hepatocyte growth factor, C-terminal cross-linked telopeptide of collagen I, TGF-β, and syndecan-1.

℞ **TREATMENT** About 10% of patients with myeloma will have an indolent course demonstrating only very slow progression of disease over many years. Such patients only require antitumor therapy when the serum myeloma protein level rises above 50 g/L (5 g/dL) or progressive bone lesions develop. Patients with solitary bone plasmacytomas and extramedullary plasmacytomas may be expected to enjoy prolonged disease-free survival after local radiation therapy to a dose of around 40 Gy. There is a low incidence of occult marrow involvement in patients with solitary bone plasmacytoma. Such pa-

tients are usually detected because their serum M component falls slowly or disappears initially only to return after a few months. These patients respond well to systemic chemotherapy.

The vast majority of patients with myeloma require therapeutic intervention. In general such therapy is of two sorts: systemic chemotherapy to control the progression of myeloma, and symptomatic supportive care to prevent serious morbidity from the complications of the disease. All patients with stage II or III disease and stage I patients exhibiting Bence Jones proteinuria, progressive lytic bone lesions, vertebral compression fractures, recurrent infections, or rising serum M component should be treated with systemic combination chemotherapy. Therapy can prolong and improve the quality of life for myeloma patients.

The standard treatment has consisted of intermittent pulses of an alkylating agent [L-phenylalanine mustard (L-PAM, melphalan), cyclophosphamide, or chlorambucil] and prednisone administered for 4 to 7 days every 4 to 6 weeks. The alkylating agents appear to be roughly equally active, but resistance to one agent is often accompanied by resistance to the others. The usual doses are as follows: melphalan, 8 mg/m^2 per day; cyclophosphamide, 200 mg/m^2 per day; chlorambucil, 8 mg/m^2 per day; prednisone, 25 to 60 mg/m^2 per day. Melphalan is used most commonly, but because of their near equivalence in antitumor efficacy, we favor cyclophosphamide as the alkylating agent because it is less toxic to the marrow stem cell compartment and results in a lower incidence of acute myelodysplastic syndromes than do the other alkylating agents. Doses may need adjustment based on marrow tolerance. However, there are few constraints on the dose of the steroid pulse, and it appears that more is better. Patients responding to therapy generally have a prompt and gratifying reduction in bone pain, hypercalcemia, and anemia, and often have fewer infections. The serum M component lags substantially behind the symptomatic improvement, often taking 4 to 6 weeks to fall. This fall depends on the rate of tumor kill and the fractional catabolic rate of immunoglobulin, which in turn depends on the serum concentration (for IgG). Light chain excretion, with a functional half-life of approximately 6 h, may fall within the first week of treatment. However, since urine light chain levels may relate to renal tubular function, they are not a reliable measure of tumor cell kill. Calculations of tumor cell kill are made by extrapolation of the serum M component level and rely heavily on the assumption that every tumor cell produces immunoglobulin at a constant rate. About 60% of patients will achieve at least a 75% reduction in serum M component level and tumor cell mass in response to an alkylating agent and prednisone. Although this is a tumor reduction of less than one log, clinical responses may last many months. The important feature of the level of the M protein is not how far or how fast it falls, but the rate of its increase after therapy. Efforts to improve the fraction of patients responding and the degree of response have involved adding other active chemotherapeutic agents to the treatment program. Patients with more advanced disease may benefit most from such an approach. High-dose therapy with hematopoietic support is also being tested in younger patients. Sequential treatment with combination chemotherapy regimens followed by two successive high-dose melphalan treatments, each supported with peripheral blood stem cell transplants, have achieved complete responses in 50% of patients treated within a year of diagnosis. Complete responses are rare (<10%) with standard therapy. Long-term follow-up is not yet available. Allogeneic transplants may also produce high response rates, but treatment-related mortality may be as high as 40%.

The ideal duration of therapy has not been determined. Most physicians treat every 4 to 6 weeks for 1 or 2 years. Cessation of therapy is followed by relapse, usually within a year. Retreatment may be associated with a second response in up to 80% of patients. Maintenance therapy (e.g., with IFN-α) may prolong the duration of response, but this therapy is toxic and has generally not prolonged survival. The regrowth rate of the tumor during relapse accelerates with each relapse. This observation suggests that kinetic resistance to therapy (i.e., increase in cycling cells) is perhaps more important than drug resistance controlled by mdr-1 expression. Patients often respond to treatment, but the length of the response progressively shortens. Patients primarily resistant to initial therapy have a median survival of less than a year. High-dose pulsed steroids used alone (200 mg prednisone every other day or 1 g/m^2 per day methylprednisolone for 5 days) or VAD combination chemotherapy (vincristine, 0.4 mg/d in a 4-day continuous infusion; doxorubicin, 9 mg/m^2 per day in a 4-day continuous infusion; dexamethasone, 40 mg/d for 4 days per week for 3 weeks) may offer useful palliation in patients resistant to primary therapy. High-dose melphalan has activity in patients with refractory disease. Thalidomide, which inhibits angiogenesis, also produces responses in refractory cases, but at doses that may cause somnolence.

About 15% of patients die within the first 3 months after diagnosis; subsequently, the death rate is about 15% per year. The disease usually follows a chronic course for 2 to 5 years before developing an acute terminal phase, usually marked by the development of pancytopenia with a cellular marrow that is refractory to treatment. Widespread organ infiltration by myeloma cells occurs, and survival is less than 6 months. About 46% of patients die in the chronic phase of disease from progressive myeloma (16%) and renal failure (10%), sepsis (14%), or both (6%). Death in the acute terminal phase (26%) is chiefly from progressive myeloma (13%) and sepsis (9%). Five percent of patients die of acute leukemia, myeloblastic or monocytic. Although it has been debated that this is related to the primary disease, it appears more likely to be the result of chronic therapy with alkylating agents. Nearly 23% of patients die of myocardial infarction, chronic lung disease, diabetes, or stroke, all intercurrent illnesses related more to the age of the patient group than to the tumor.

Supportive care directed at the anticipated complications of the disease may be as important as primary antitumor therapy. The hypercalcemia generally responds well to glucocorticoid therapy, hydration, and natriuresis. Calcitonin may add to the inhibitory effects of steroids on bone resorption. Bisphosphonates (e.g., pamidronate 90 mg once a month) reduce osteoclastic bone resorption and preserve performance status and quality of life; antitumor effects are also possible. Treatments aimed at strengthening the skeleton, such as fluorides, calcium, and vitamin D, with or without androgens, have been suggested but are not of proven efficacy. Iatrogenic worsening of renal function may be prevented by the use of allopurinol during chemotherapy to avoid urate nephropathy and by maintaining a high fluid intake to prevent dehydration and to help excrete light chains and calcium. In the event of acute renal failure, plasmapheresis is approximately 10 times more effective at clearing light chains than peritoneal dialysis, and acutely reducing the protein load may result in functional improvement. Urinary tract infections should be watched for and treated early. Chronic dialysis probably should not be initiated in patients who have failed to respond to antitumor therapy. Plasmapheresis may be the treatment of choice for hyperviscosity syndromes. Although the pneumococcus is a dreaded pathogen in myeloma patients, pneumococcal polysaccharide vaccines may not elicit an antibody response. The advent of intravenous gamma globulin preparations raises some hope that prophylactic administration may prevent some serious infections, but this has not been tested. Chronic oral antibiotic prophylaxis is probably not warranted. Patients developing neurologic symptoms in the lower extremities, severe localized back pain, or problems with bowel and bladder control may need emergency myelography and radiation therapy for palliation. Most bone lesions respond to analgesics and chemotherapy, but certain painful lesions may respond most promptly to localized radiation. The chronic anemia may respond to hematinics (iron, folate, cobalamin), and some have responded to androgens. The pathogenesis of the anemia should be established and specific therapy instituted, where possible.

WALDENSTRÖM'S MACROGLOBULINEMIA   In 1948, Waldenström described a malignancy of lymphoplasmacytoid cells

that secreted IgM. In contrast to myeloma, the disease was associated with lymphadenopathy and hepatosplenomegaly, but the major clinical manifestation was the hyperviscosity syndrome. The disease resembles the related diseases chronic lymphocytic leukemia, myeloma, and lymphocytic lymphoma. Waldenström's macroglobulinemia and IgM myeloma both follow a similar clinical course. The diagnosis of IgM myeloma is usually reserved for patients with lytic bone lesions and is important only because of the hazard of pathologic fractures.

The cause of macroglobulinemia is unknown. The disease is similar to myeloma in being slightly more common in men and occurring with increased incidence with age (median 64 years). There have been reports that the IgM in some patients with macroglobulinemia may have specificity for myelin-associated glycoprotein (MAG), a protein that has been associated with demyelinating disease of the peripheral nervous system and may be lost earlier and to a greater extent than the better known myelin basic protein in patients with multiple sclerosis. Sometimes patients with macroglobulinemia develop a peripheral neuropathy before the appearance of the neoplasm. There is speculation that the whole process begins with a viral infection that may elicit an antibody response that cross-reacts with a normal tissue component.

Like myeloma, the disease involves the bone marrow, but unlike myeloma, it does not cause bone lesions or hypercalcemia. Like myeloma, a serum M component is present in the serum in excess of 30 g/L (3 g/dL), but unlike myeloma, the size of the IgM paraprotein results in little renal excretion and only around 20% of patients excrete light chains. Therefore, renal disease is not common. The light chain isotype is kappa in 80% of the cases. Patients present with weakness, fatigue, and recurrent infections, similar to myeloma patients, but epistaxis, visual disturbances, and neurologic symptoms such as peripheral neuropathy, dizziness, headache, and transient paresis are much more common in macroglobulinemia. Physical examination reveals adenopathy and hepatosplenomegaly, and ophthalmoscopic examination may reveal vascular segmentation and dilatation of the retinal veins characteristic of hyperviscosity states. Patients may have a normocytic, normochromic anemia, but rouleaux formation and a positive Coombs' test are much more common than in myeloma. Malignant lymphocytes are usually present in the peripheral blood. About 10% of macroglobulins are cryoglobulins. These are pure M components and are not the mixed cryoglobulins seen in rheumatoid arthritis and other autoimmune diseases. Mixed cryoglobulins are composed of IgM or IgA complexed with IgG, for which they are specific. In both cases, Raynaud's phenomenon and serious vascular symptoms precipitated by the cold may occur, but mixed cryoglobulins are not commonly associated with malignancy. Patients suspected of having a cryoglobulin based on history and physical examination should have their blood drawn into a warm syringe and delivered to the laboratory in a container of warm water to avoid errors in quantitating the cryoglobulin.

TREATMENT   Control of serious hyperviscosity symptoms such as an altered state of consciousness or paresis can be achieved acutely by plasmapheresis because 80% of the IgM paraprotein is intravascular. Fludarabine (25 mg/m^2 per day for 5 days every 4 weeks) or cladribine (0.1 mg/kg per day for 7 days every 4 weeks) are highly effective single agents. About 80% of patients respond to chemotherapy, and their median survival is over 3 years. The absence of other serious organ toxicities results in a longer life span of patients with macroglobulinemia compared with those with myeloma.

POEMS SYNDROME   The features of this syndrome are *poly*neuropathy, *o*rganomegaly, *e*ndocrinopathy, *m*ultiple myeloma, and *s*kin changes (POEMS). Patients usually have a severe, progressive sensorimotor polyneuropathy associated with sclerotic bone lesions from myeloma. Polyneuropathy occurs in about 1.4% of myelomas, but the POEMS syndrome is only a rare subset of that group. Unlike typical myeloma, hepatomegaly and lymphadenopathy occur in about two-thirds of patients, and splenomegaly is seen in one-third. The lymphadenopathy frequently resembles Castleman's disease histologically, a condition that has been linked to IL-6 overproduction. The endocrine manifestations include amenorrhea in women and impotence and gynecomastia in men. Hyperprolactinemia due to loss of normal inhibitory control by the hypothalamus may be associated with other central nervous system manifestations such as papilledema and elevated cerebrospinal fluid pressure and protein. Type 2 diabetes mellitus occurs in about one-third of patients. Hypothyroidism and adrenal insufficiency are occasionally noted. Skin changes are diverse: hyperpigmentation, hypertrichosis, skin thickening, and digital clubbing. Other manifestations include peripheral edema, ascites, pleural effusions, fever, and thrombocytosis.

The pathogenesis of the disease is unclear, but high circulating levels of the proinflammatory cytokines IL-1, IL-6, and TNF have been documented and levels of the inhibitory cytokine transforming growth factor β (TGF-β) are lower than expected. Treatment of the myeloma may result in an improvement in the other disease manifestations.

HEAVY CHAIN DISEASES The heavy chain diseases are rare lymphoplasmacytic malignancies. Their clinical manifestations vary with the heavy chain isotype. Patients secrete a defective heavy chain that usually has an intact Fc fragment and a deletion in the Fd region. Gamma, alpha, and mu heavy chain diseases have been described, but no reports of delta or epsilon heavy chain diseases have appeared. Molecular biologic analysis of these tumors has revealed structural genetic defects that may account for the aberrant chain secreted.

Gamma Heavy Chain Disease (Franklin's Disease) This disease affects people of widely different age groups and countries of origin. It is characterized by lymphadenopathy, fever, anemia, malaise, hepatosplenomegaly, and weakness. Its most distinctive symptom is palatal edema, resulting from node involvement of Waldeyer's ring, and this may progress to produce respiratory compromise. The diagnosis depends on the demonstration of an anomalous serum M component [often <20 g/L (<2 g/dL)] that reacts with anti-IgG but not anti-light chain reagents. *The M component is typically present in both serum and urine.* Most of the paraproteins have been of the gamma$_1$ subclass, but other subclasses have been seen. The patients may have thrombocytopenia, eosinophilia, and nondiagnostic bone marrow. Patients usually have a rapid downhill course and die of infection; however, some patients have survived 5 years with chemotherapy.

Alpha Heavy Chain Disease (Seligmann's Disease) This is the most common of the heavy chain diseases. It is closely related to a malignancy known as *Mediterranean lymphoma*, a disease that affects young people in parts of the world where intestinal parasites are common, such as the Mediterranean, Asia, and South America. The disease is characterized by an infiltration of the lamina propria of the small intestine with lymphoplasmacytoid cells that secrete truncated alpha chains. Demonstrating alpha heavy chains is difficult because the alpha chains tend to polymerize and appear as a smear instead of a sharp peak on electrophoretic profiles. Despite the polymerization, hyperviscosity is not a common problem in alpha heavy chain disease. Without J chain–facilitated dimerization, viscosity does not increase dramatically. Light chains are absent from serum and urine. The patients present with chronic diarrhea, weight loss, and malabsorption and have extensive mesenteric and para-aortic adenopathy. Respiratory tract involvement occurs rarely. Patients may vary widely in their clinical course. Some may develop diffuse aggressive histologies of malignant lymphoma. Chemotherapy may produce long-term remissions. Rare patients appear to have responded to antibiotic therapy, raising the question of the etiologic role of antigenic stimulation, perhaps by some chronic intestinal infection. Chemotherapy plus antibiotics may be more effective than chemotherapy alone.

Mu Heavy Chain Disease The secretion of isolated mu heavy chains into the serum appears to occur in a very rare subset of patients with chronic lymphocytic leukemia. The only features that may distinguish patients with mu heavy chain disease are the presence of vacuoles in the malignant lymphocytes and the excretion of kappa light chains in the urine. The diagnosis requires ultracentrifugation or gel filtration to confirm the nonreactivity of the paraprotein with the light chain reagents, because some intact macroglobulins fail to interact with these serums. The tumor cells seem to have a defect in the assembly of light and heavy chains, because they appear to contain both in their cytoplasm. There is no evidence that such patients should be treated differently from other patients with chronic lymphocytic leukemia (Chap. 112).

BIBLIOGRAPHY

BATAILLE R, HAROUSSEAU J-L: Multiple myeloma. N Engl J Med 336:1657, 1997

DIMOPOULOS MA, ALEXANIAN R: Waldenström's macroglobulinemia. Blood 83:1452, 1994

GARCIA-SANZ R et al: Primary plasma cell leukemia: Clinical, immunophenotypic, DNA ploidy, and cytogenetic characteristics. Blood 93:1032, 1999

GHERARDI RK et al: Overproduction of proinflammatory cytokines imbalanced by their antagonists in POEMS syndrome. Blood 87:1458, 1996

HU K, YAHALOM J: Radiotherapy in the management of plasma cell tumors. Oncology 14:101, 2000

KONINGSBERG R et al: Predictive role of interphase cytogenetics for survival of patients with multiple myeloma. J Clin Oncol 18:804, 2000

KYLE RA: "Benign" monoclonal gammopathy—after 20–35 years of follow-up. Mayo Clin Proc 68:26, 1993

———: Plasma cell disorders. Hematol/Oncol Clin North Am 13:1117, 1999

LENHOFF S et al: Impact on survival of high-dose therpy with autologous stem cell support in patients younger than 60 years with newly diagnosed multiple myeloma: A population-based study. Blood 95:7, 2000

SINGHAL S et al: Antitumor activity of thalidomide in refractory myeloma. N Engl J Med 341:1565, 1999

VESOLE DH et al: High-dose melphalan with autotransplanation for refractory multiple myeloma: Results of a Southwest Oncology Group phase II trial. J Clin Oncol 17:2173, 1999

114 *Jeffery S. Dzieczkowski, Kenneth C. Anderson*

TRANSFUSION BIOLOGY AND THERAPY

ACE	angiotensin-converting enzyme	HBV	hepatitis B virus
CCI	corrected count increment	HCV	hepatitis C virus
CMV	cytomegalovirus	HGV	hepatitis G virus
DAT	direct antiglobulin test	HTLV	human T lymphotropic virus
DHTRs	delayed hemolytic transfusion reactions	PRBC	packed RBC
		RBC	red blood cell
DIC	disseminated intravascular coagulation	RD	random donor
		SDAP	single-donor apheresis platelets
FFP	fresh frozen plasma		
FNHTR	febrile nonhemolytic transfusion reaction	TA-GVHD	transfusion-associated
		vWF	von Willebrand factor
GVHD	graft-versus-host disease		

BLOOD GROUP ANTIGENS AND ANTIBODIES

The study of red blood cell (RBC) antigens and antibodies forms the foundation of transfusion medicine. Serologic studies initially characterized these antigens, but now the molecular composition and structure of many are known. Antigens, either carbohydrate or protein, are assigned to a blood group system based upon the structure and the similarity of the determinant epitopes. Other cellular blood elements and plasma proteins are also antigenic and can result in *alloimmunization*, the production of antibodies directed against the blood group antigens of another individual. These antibodies are called *alloantibodies*.

Antibodies directed against RBC antigens may result from "natural" exposure, particularly to carbohydrates that mimic some blood group antigens. Those antibodies that occur via natural stimuli are usually produced by a T cell–independent response (thus, generating no memory) and are IgM isotype. *Autoantibodies* (antibodies against autologous blood group antigens) arise spontaneously or as the result of infectious sequelae (e.g., from *Mycoplasma pneumoniae*) and are also often IgM. These antibodies are often clinically insignificant due to their low affinity for antigen at body temperature. However, IgM antibodies can activate the complement cascade and result in hemolysis. Antibodies that result from allogeneic exposure, such as transfusion or pregnancy, are usually IgG. IgG antibodies commonly bind to antigen at warmer temperatures and may hemolyze RBCs. Unlike IgM antibodies, IgG antibodies can cross the placenta and bind fetal erythrocytes bearing the corresponding antigen, resulting in hemolytic disease of the newborn, or *hydrops fetalis*.

Alloimmunization to leukocytes, platelets, and plasma proteins may also result in transfusion complications such as fevers and urticaria but generally does not cause hemolysis. Assay for these other alloantibodies is not routinely performed; however, they may be detected using special assays.

ABO ANTIGENS AND ANTIBODIES   The first blood group antigen system, recognized in 1900, was ABO, the most important in transfusion medicine. The major blood groups of this system are A, B, AB, and O. O type RBCs lack A or B antigens. These antigens are carbohydrates attached to a precursor backbone, may be found on the cellular membrane either as glycosphingolipids or glycoproteins, and are secreted into plasma and body fluids as glycoproteins. H substance is the immediate precursor upon which the A and B antigens are added. This H substance is formed by the addition of fucose to the glycolipid or glycoprotein backbone. The subsequent addition of *N*-acetylgalactosamine creates the A antigen, while the addition of galactose produces the B antigen.

The genes that determine the A and B phenotypes are found on chromosome 9p and are expressed in a Mendelian codominant manner. The gene products are glycosyl transferases, which confer the enzymatic capability of attaching the specific antigenic carbohydrate. Individuals who lack the "A" and "B" transferases are phenotypically type "O," while those who inherit both transferases are type "AB." Rare individuals lack the H gene, which codes for fucose transferase, and cannot form H substance. These individuals are homozygous for the silent h allele (hh) and have Bombay phenotype (O_h).

The ABO blood group system is important because essentially all individuals produce antibodies to the ABH carbohydrate antigen that they lack. The naturally occurring anti-A and anti-B antibodies are termed *isoagglutinins*. Thus, type A individuals produce anti-B, while type B individuals make anti-A. Neither isoagglutinin is found in type AB individuals, while type O individuals produce both anti-A and anti-B. Thus, persons with type AB are "universal recipients" because they do not have antibodies against any ABO phenotype, while persons with type O blood can donate to essentially all recipients because their cells are not recognized by any ABO isoagglutinins. The rare individuals with Bombay phenotype produce antibodies to H substance (which is present on all red cells except those of hh phenotype) as well as to both A and B antigens and are therefore compatible only with other hh donors.

In most people, A and B antigens are secreted by the cells and are present in the circulation. Nonsecretors are susceptible to a variety of infections (e.g., *Candida albicans*, *Neisseria meningitidis*, *Streptococcus pneumoniae*, *Haemophilus influenzae*) as many organisms may bind to polysaccharides on cells. Soluble blood group antigens may block this binding.

Rh SYSTEM   The Rh system is the second most important blood group system in pretransfusion testing. The Rh antigens are found on a 30- to 32-kDa RBC membrane protein, which has no defined function. Although more than 40 different antigens in the Rh system have been described, five determinants account for the vast majority of phenotypes. The presence of the D antigen confers Rh "positivity," while people who lack the D antigen are Rh negative. Two allelic antigen pairs, E/e and C/c, are also found on the Rh protein.

The three Rh genes, E/e, D, and C/c, are arranged in tandem on chromosome 1 and inherited as a haplotype, i.e., cDE or Cde. Two haplotypes can result in the phenotypic expression of two to five Rh antigens.

The D antigen is a potent alloantigen. About 15% of people lack this antigen. Exposure of these Rh-negative people to even small amounts of Rh-positive cells, by either transfusion or pregnancy, can result in the production of anti-D alloantibody.

OTHER BLOOD GROUP SYSTEMS AND ALLOANTIBODIES   More than 100 blood group systems are recognized, composed of more than 500 antigens. The presence or absence of certain antigens has been associated with various diseases and anomalies; antigens also act as receptors for infectious agents. Alloantibodies of importance in routine clinical practice are listed in Table 114-1.

Antibodies to *Lewis system* carbohydrate antigens are the most common cause of incompatibility during pretransfusion screening. The Lewis gene product is a fucosyl transferase and maps to chromosome 19. The antigen is not an integral membrane structure but is adsorbed to the RBC membrane from the plasma. Antibodies to Lewis antigens are usually IgM and cannot cross the placenta. Lewis antigens may be adsorbed onto tumor cells and may be targets of therapy.

I system antigens are also oligosaccharides related to H, A, B, and Le. I and i are not allelic pairs but are carbohydrate antigens that differ only in the extent of branching. The i antigen is an unbranched chain that is converted by the I gene product, a glycosyltransferase, into a branched chain. The branching process affects all the ABH antigens, which become progressively more branched in the first 2 years of life. Some patients with cold agglutinin disease or lymphomas can produce anti-I autoantibodies that cause RBC destruction. Occasional patients with mononucleosis or *Mycoplasma* pneumonia may develop cold agglutinins of either anti-I or anti-i specificity. Most adults lack i expression; thus, finding a donor for patients with anti-i is not difficult. Even though most adults express I antigen, binding is generally low at body temperature. Thus, administration of warm blood prevents isoagglutination.

The *P system* is another group of carbohydrate antigens controlled by specific glycosyltransferases. Its clinical significance is in rare cases of syphilis and viral infection that lead to paroxysmal cold hemoglobinuria. In these cases, an unusual autoantibody to P is produced that binds to RBCs in the cold and fixes complement upon warming. Antibodies with these biphasic properties are called *Donath-Landsteiner antibodies*. The P antigen is also expressed on urothelial cells and may be a receptor for *Escherichia coli* binding.

The *MNSsU system* is regulated by genes on chromosome 4. M and N are determinants on glycophorin A, an RBC membrane protein, and S and s are determinants on glycophorin B. Anti-S and anti-s IgG antibodies may develop after pregnancy or transfusion and lead to hemolysis. Anti-U antibodies are rare but problematic; virtually every donor is incompatible because nearly all persons express U.

The *Kell* protein is very large (720 amino acids) and its secondary structure contains many different antigenic epitopes. The immunoge-

Table 114-1   RBC Blood Group Systems and Alloantigens

Blood Group System	Antigen	Alloantibody	Clinical Significance
Rh (D, C/c, E/e)	RBC protein	IgG	HTR, HDN
Lewis (Le^a, Le^b)	Oligosaccharide	IgM/IgG	Rare HTR
Kell (K/k)	RBC protein	IgG	HTR, HDN
Duffy (Fy^a/Fy^b)	RBC protein	IgG	HTR, HDN
Kidd (Jk^a/Jk^b)	RBC protein	IgG	HTR (often delayed), HDN (mild)
I/i	Carbohydrate	IgM	None
MNSsU	RBC protein	IgM/IgG	Anti-M rare HDN, anti-S, -s, and -U HDN, HTR

NOTE: RBC, red blood cell; HDN, hemolytic disease of the newborn; HTR, hemolytic transfusion reaction.

nicity of Kell is third behind the ABO and Rh systems. The absence of the Kell precursor protein (controlled by a gene on X) is associated with acanthocytosis, shortened RBC survival, and a progressive form of muscular dystrophy that includes cardiac defects. This rare condition is called the *McLeod phenotype*. The K_x gene is linked to the 91-kDa component of the NADPH-oxidase on the X chromosome, deletion or mutation of which accounts for about 60% of cases of chronic granulomatous disease.

The *Duffy* antigens are codominant alleles, Fy^a and Fy^b, that also serve as receptors for *Plasmodium vivax*. More than 70% of persons in malaria-endemic areas lack these antigens, probably from selective influences of the infection on the population.

The *Kidd* antigens, Jk^a and Jk^b, may elicit antibodies transiently. A delayed hemolytic transfusion reaction that occurs with blood tested as compatible is often related to delayed appearance of anti-Jk^a.

PRETRANSFUSION TESTING

Pretransfusion testing of a potential recipient consists of the "type and screen." The "forward type" determines the ABO and Rh phenotype of the recipient's RBC by using antisera directed against the A, B, and D antigens. The "reverse type" detects isoagglutinins in the patient's serum and should correlate with the ABO phenotype, or forward type.

The alloantibody screen identifies antibodies directed against other RBC antigens. The alloantibody screen is performed by mixing patient serum with type O RBCs that contain the major antigens of most blood group systems and whose extended phenotype is known. The specificity of the alloantibody is identified by correlating the presence or absence of antigen with the results of the agglutination.

Cross matching is ordered when there is a high probability that the patient will require a packed RBC (PRBC) transfusion. Blood selected for cross matching must be ABO compatible and lack antigens for which the patient has alloantibodies. Nonreactive cross matching confirms the absence of any major incompatibility and reserves that unit for the patient.

In the case of Rh-negative patients, every attempt must be made to provide Rh-negative blood components to prevent alloimmunization to the D antigen. In an emergency, Rh-positive blood can be safely transfused to a Rh-negative patient who lacks anti-D; however, the recipient is likely to become alloimmunized and produce anti-D. Rh-negative women of child-bearing age who are transfused with products containing Rh-positive RBCs should receive passive immunization with anti-D (RhoGam or WinRho) to reduce or prevent sensitization.

BLOOD COMPONENTS

Blood products intended for transfusion are routinely collected as whole blood (450 mL) in various anticoagulants. Most donated blood is processed into components: PRBCs, platelets, and fresh frozen plasma (FFP) or cryoprecipitate (Table 114-2). Whole blood is first separated into PRBCs and platelet-rich plasma by slow centrifugation. The platelet-rich plasma is then centrifuged at high speed to yield one unit of random donor (RD) platelets and one unit of FFP. Cryoprecipitate is produced by thawing FFP to precipitate the plasma proteins, which are then separated by centrifugation.

Apheresis technology is used for the collection of multiple units of platelets from a single donor. These single-donor apheresis platelets (SDAP) contain the equivalent of at least six units of RD platelets and have fewer contaminating leukocytes than pooled RD platelets.

Table 114-2 Characteristics of Selected Blood Components

Component	Volume, mL	Content	Clinical Response
PRBC	180–200	RBCs with variable leukocyte content and small amount of plasma	Increase hemoglobin 10 g/L and hematocrit 3%
Platelets	50–70	5.5×10^{10}/RD unit	Increase platelet count 5000–10,000/μL
	200–400	$\geq 3.0 \times 10^{11}$/SDAP product	CCI $\geq 10 \times 10^9$/L within 1 h and $\geq 7.5 \times 10^9$/L within 24 h post-transfusion
FFP	200–250	Plasma proteins—coagulation factors, proteins C and S, antithrombin	Increases coagulation factors about 2%
Cryoprecipitate	10–15	Cold-insoluble plasma proteins, fibrinogen, factor VIII, vWF	Topical fibrin glue, also 80 IU factor VIII

NOTE: PRBC , packed red blood cells; RBC, red blood cell; RD, random donor; SDAP, single-donor apheresis platelets; CCI, corrected count increment; FFP, fresh frozen plasma; vWF, von Willebrand factor.

Plasma may also be collected by apheresis. Plasma derivatives such as albumin, intravenous immunoglobulin, antithrombin, and coagulation factor concentrates are prepared from pooled plasma from many donors and are treated to eliminate infectious agents.

WHOLE BLOOD Whole blood provides both oxygen-carrying capacity and volume expansion. It is the ideal component for patients who have sustained acute hemorrhage of 25% or greater total blood volume loss. Whole blood is stored at 4°C to maintain erythrocyte viability, but platelet dysfunction and degradation of some coagulation factors occurs. In addition, 2,3-BPG levels fall over time, leading to an increase in the oxygen affinity of the hemoglobin and a decreased capacity to deliver oxygen to the tissues, a problem with all red cell storage. Whole blood is not readily available since it is routinely processed into components.

PACKED RED BLOOD CELLS This product increases oxygen-carrying capacity in the anemic patient. Adequate oxygenation can be maintained with a hemoglobin content of 70 g/L in the normovolemic patient without cardiac disease; however, comorbid factors often necessitate transfusion at a higher threshold. The decision to transfuse should be guided by the clinical situation and not by an arbitrary laboratory value. In the critical care setting, liberal use of transfusions to maintain near normal levels of hemoglobin may have unexpected negative effects on survival. In most patients requiring transfusion, levels of hemoglobin of 100 g/L are sufficient to keep oxygen supply from being critically low.

PRBCs may be modified to prevent certain adverse reactions. Contaminating leukocytes are responsible for inducing fevers and causing alloimmunization to HLA antigens. Leukocytes can be removed by several methods. Bedside filtration is the most popular method and removes 99.9% of donor leukocytes. Leukoreduction may be done in the blood bank before storage of cellular components; this practice results in less cytokine release from the cells. Plasma, which may cause allergic reactions, can be removed from cellular blood components by washing.

PLATELETS Thrombocytopenia is a risk factor for hemorrhage, and platelet transfusion reduces the incidence of bleeding. The threshold for prophylactic platelet transfusion is 10,000/μL. In patients without fever or infections, a threshold of 5000/μL may be sufficient to prevent spontaneous hemorrhage. For invasive procedures, 50,000/μL platelets is the usual target level.

Platelets are given either as pools prepared from five to eight RDs or as SDAPs from a single donor. In an unsensitized patient without increased platelet consumption [splenomegaly, fever, disseminated intravascular coagulation (DIC)], six to eight units of RD platelets (about 1 unit per 10 kg body weight) are transfused, and each unit is anticipated to increase the platelet count 5000 to 10,000/μL. Patients who have received multiple transfusions may be alloimmunized to many HLA- and platelet-specific antigens and have little or no increase in their posttransfusion platelet counts. Patients who may require multiple transfusions are best served by receiving SDAP and leukocyte-reduced components to lower the risk of alloimmunization.

Refractoriness to platelet transfusion may be evaluated using the corrected count increment (CCI):

$$CCI = \frac{posttransfusion\ count - pretransfusion\ count}{number\ of\ platelets\ transfused \times 10^{11}} \times BSA$$

where BSA is body surface area measured in square meters. The platelet count performed 1 h after the transfusion is acceptable if the CCI is 10×10^9/mL, and after 18 to 24 h an increment of 7.5×10^9/mL is expected. Patients who have suboptimal responses are likely to have received multiple transfusions and have antibodies directed against class I HLA antigens. Refractoriness can be investigated by detecting anti-HLA antibodies in the recipient's serum. Patients who are sensitized will often react with 100% of the lymphocytes used for the HLA-antibody screen, and HLA-matched SDAPs should be considered for those patients who require transfusion. Although ABO-identical HLA-matched SDAPs provide the best chance for increasing the platelet count, locating these products is difficult. Platelet cross matching is available in some centers. Additional clinical causes for a low platelet CCI include fever, bleeding, splenomegaly, DIC, or medications in the recipient.

FRESH FROZEN PLASMA   FFP contains stable coagulation factors and plasma proteins: fibrinogen, antithrombin, albumin, as well as proteins C and S. Indications for FFP include correction of coagulopathies, including the rapid reversal of coumadin; supplying deficient plasma proteins; and treatment of thrombotic thrombocytopenic purpura. FFP should not be routinely used to expand blood volume. FFP is an acellular component and does not transmit intracellular infections, e.g., cytomegalovirus (CMV). Patients who are IgA-deficient and require plasma support should receive FFP from IgA-deficient donors to prevent anaphylaxis (see below).

CRYOPRECIPITATE   Cryoprecipitate is a source of fibrinogen, factor VIII, and von Willebrand factor (vWF). It is ideal for supplying fibrinogen to the volume-sensitive patient. When factor VIII concentrates are not available, cyroprecipitate may be used since each unit contains approximately 80 units of factor VIII. Cryoprecipitate may also be used as a source of vWF for patients with dysfunctional (type II) or absent (type III) von Willebrand disease.

PLASMA DERIVATIVES   Plasma from thousands of donors may be pooled to derive specific protein concentrates, including albumin, intravenous immunoglobulin, antithrombin, and coagulation factors. In addition, donors who have high-titer antibodies to specific agents or antigens provide hyperimmune globulins, such as anti-D (RhoGam, WinRho), and antisera to hepatitis B virus (HBV), varicella-zoster virus, CMV, and other infectious agents.

ADVERSE REACTIONS TO BLOOD TRANSFUSION

Adverse reactions to transfused blood components occur despite multiple tests, inspections, and checks. Fortunately, the most common reactions are not life-threatening, although serious reactions can present with mild symptoms and signs. Some reactions can be reduced or prevented by modified (filtered, washed, or irradiated) blood components. When an adverse reaction is suspected, the transfusion should be stopped and reported to the blood bank for investigation.

Transfusion reactions may result from immune and nonimmune mechanisms. Immune-mediated reactions are often due to preformed donor or recipient antibody; however, cellular elements may also cause adverse effects. Nonimmune causes of reactions are due to the chemical and physical properties of the stored blood component and its additives.

Infectious complications of transfusion have become less frequent, although fear of these complications remains a primary concern. The incidence of transfusion-related infections has been reduced substan-

tially due to improved donor screening and testing of collected blood. Infections, like any adverse transfusion reaction, must be brought to the attention of the blood bank for appropriate studies (Table 114-3).

IMMUNE-MEDIATED REACTIONS Acute Hemolytic Transfusion Reactions   Immune-mediated hemolysis occurs when the recipient has preformed antibodies that lyse donor erythrocytes. The ABO isoagglutinins are responsible for the majority of these reactions, although alloantibodies directed against other RBC antigens, i.e., Rh, Kell, and Duffy, may result in hemolysis.

Acute hemolytic reactions may present with hypotension, tachypnea, tachycardia, fever, chills, hemoglobinemia, hemoglobinuria, chest and/or flank pain, and discomfort at the infusion site. Monitoring the patient's vital signs before and during the transfusion is important to identify reactions promptly. When acute hemolysis is suspected, the transfusion must be stopped immediately, intravenous access maintained, and the reaction reported to the blood bank. A correctly labeled posttransfusion blood sample and any untransfused blood should be sent to the blood bank for analysis. The laboratory evaluation for hemolysis includes the measurement of serum haptoglobin, lactate dehydrogenase (LDH), and indirect bilirubin levels.

The immune complexes that result in RBC lysis can cause renal dysfunction and failure. Diuresis should be induced with intravenous fluids and furosemide or mannitol. Tissue factor released from the lysed erythrocytes may initiate DIC. Coagulation studies including prothrombin time (PT), activated partial thromboplastin time (aPTT), fibrinogen, and platelet count should be monitored in patients with hemolytic reactions.

Errors at the patient's bedside, such as mislabeling the sample or transfusing the wrong patient, are responsible for the majority of these reactions. The blood bank investigation of these reactions includes examination of the pre- and posttransfusion samples for hemolysis and repeat typing of the patient samples; direct antiglobulin test (DAT), sometimes called the direct Coombs test, of the posttransfusion sample; repeating the cross matching of the blood component; and checking all clerical records for errors. DAT detects the presence of antibody or complement bound to RBCs in vivo.

Delayed Hemolytic and Serologic Transfusion Reactions   Delayed hemolytic transfusion reactions (DHTRs) are not completely preventable. These reactions occur in patients previously sensitized to RBC alloantigens who have a negative alloantibody screen due to low antibody levels. When the patient is transfused with antigen-positive blood, an anamnestic response results in the early production of al-

Table 114-3   Risks of Transfusion Complications

	Frequency, Episodes:Unit
Reactions	
Febrile (FNHTR)	1–4:100
Allergic	1–4:100
Delayed hemolytic	1:1,000
TRALI	1:5,000
Acute hemolytic	1:12,000
Fatal hemolytic	1:100,000
Anaphylactic	1:150,000
Infections[a]	
Hepatitis B	1:66,000
Hepatitis C	1:103,000
HIV-1	1:676,000
HIV-2	None reported
HTLV-I and -II	1:641,000
Malaria	1:4,000,000
Other complications	
RBC allosensitization	1:100
HLA allosensitization	1:10
Graft-versus-host disease	Rare

[a] Infectious agents rarely associated with transfusion, theoretically possible or of unknown risk include: Hepatitis A virus, parvovirus B-19, *Babesia microti* (babesiosis), *Borrelia burgdorferi* (Lyme disease), *Trypanosoma cruzi* (Chagas' disease), and *Treponema pallidum*, human herpesvirus-8 and hepatitis G virus.

NOTE: FNHTR, febrile nonhemolytic transfusion reaction; TRALI, transfusion-related acute lung injury; HTLV, human T lymphotropic virus; RBC, red blood cell

loantibody that binds donor RBCs. The alloantibody is detectable 1 to 2 weeks following the transfusion, and the posttransfusion DAT may become positive due to circulating donor RBCs coated with antibody or complement. The transfused, alloantibody-coated erythrocytes are cleared by the extravascular reticuloendothelial system. These reactions are detected most commonly in the blood bank when a subsequent patient sample reveals a positive alloantibody screen or a new alloantibody in a recently transfused recipient.

No specific therapy is usually required, although additional RBC transfusions may be necessary. Delayed serologic transfusion reactions (DSTR) are similar to DHTR, as the DAT is positive and alloantibody is detected; however, RBC clearance is not increased.

Febrile Nonhemolytic Transfusion Reaction The most frequent reaction associated with the transfusion of cellular blood components is a febrile nonhemolytic transfusion reaction (FNHTR). These reactions are characterized by chills and rigors and a 1°C or greater rise in temperature. FNHTR is diagnosed when other causes of fever in the transfused patient are ruled out. Antibodies directed against donor leukocyte and HLA antigens may mediate these reactions; thus, multiply transfused patients and multiparous women are felt to be at increased risk. Although antibodies may be demonstrated in the recipient's serum, investigation is not routinely done because of the mild nature of most FNHTR. The use of leukocyte-reduced blood products may prevent or delay sensitization to leukocyte antigens and thereby reduce the incidence of these febrile episodes. Cytokines released from cells within stored blood components may mediate FNHTR; thus, leukoreduction before storage may prevent these reactions. The incidence and severity of these reactions can be decreased in patients with recurrent reactions by premedicating with acetaminophen or other antipyretic agents.

Allergic Reactions Urticarial reactions are related to plasma proteins found in transfused components. Mild reactions may be treated symptomatically by temporarily stopping the transfusion and administering antihistamines (diphenhydramine, 50 mg orally or intramuscularly). The transfusion may be completed after the signs and/or symptoms resolve. Patients with a history of allergic transfusion reaction should be premedicated with an antihistamine. Cellular components can be washed to remove residual plasma for the extremely sensitized patient.

Anaphylactic Reaction This severe reaction presents after transfusion of only a few milliliters of the blood component. Symptoms and signs include difficulty breathing, coughing, nausea and vomiting, hypotension, bronchospasm, loss of consciousness, respiratory arrest, and shock. Treatment includes stopping the transfusion, maintaining vascular access, and administering epinephrine (0.5 to 1.0 mL of 1:1000 dilution SQ). Glucocorticoids may be required in severe cases.

Patients who are IgA-deficient may be sensitized to this Ig class and are at risk for anaphylactic reactions associated with plasma transfusion. Individuals with severe IgA deficiency should therefore receive only IgA-deficient plasma and washed cellular blood components. Patients who have anaphylactic or repeated allergic reactions to blood components should be tested for IgA deficiency.

Graft-Versus-Host Disease Graft-versus-host disease (GVHD) is a frequent complication of allogeneic bone marrow transplantation, in which viable lymphocytes from donor marrow attack and cannot be eliminated by an immunodeficient host. Transfusion-related GVHD is mediated by donor T lymphocytes that recognize host HLA antigens as foreign and mount an immune response, which is manifested clinically by the development of fever, a characteristic cutaneous eruption, diarrhea, and liver function abnormalities. GVHD can also occur when blood components that contain viable T lymphocytes are transfused to immunodeficient recipients or to immunocompetent recipients who share HLA antigens with the donor (e.g., a family donor). In addition to the aforementioned clinical features of GVHD, transfusion-associated GVHD (TA-GVHD) is characterized by marrow aplasia and pancytopenia. TA-GVHD is highly resistant to treatment with immunosuppressive therapies, including glucocorticoids, cyclosporine, antithymocyte globulin, and ablative therapy followed by allogeneic

bone marrow transplantation. Clinical manifestations appear at 8 to 10 days, and death occurs at 3 to 4 weeks posttransfusion.

TA-GVHD can be prevented by irradiation of cellular components (minimum of 2500 cGy) before transfusion to patients at risk. Patients at risk for TA-GVHD include fetuses receiving intrauterine transfusions, selected immunocompetent (e.g., lymphoma patients) or immunocompromised recipients, recipients of donor units known to be from a blood relative, and recipients who have undergone marrow transplantation. Directed donations by family members should be discouraged (they are not less likely to transmit infection); lacking other options, the blood products from family members should always be irradiated.

Transfusion-Related Acute Lung Injury This uncommon reaction results from the transfusion of donor plasma that contains high titer anti-HLA antibodies that bind recipient leukocytes. The leukocytes aggregate in the pulmonary vasculature and release mediators that increase capillary permeability. The recipient develops symptoms of respiratory compromise and signs of noncardiogenic pulmonary edema, including bilateral interstitial infiltrates on chest x-ray. Treatment is supportive, and patients usually recover without sequelae. Testing the donor's plasma for anti-HLA antibodies can support this diagnosis. The implicated donors are frequently multiparous women, and transfusion of their plasma component should be avoided.

Posttransfusion Purpura This reaction presents as thrombocytopenia 7 to 10 days after platelet transfusion and occurs predominantly in women. Platelet-specific antibodies are found in the recipient's serum, and the most frequently recognized antigen is HPA-1a found on the platelet glycoprotein IIIa receptor. The delayed thrombocytopenia is due to the production of antibodies that react to both donor and recipient platelets. Additional platelet transfusions can worsen the thrombocytopenia and should be avoided. Treatment with intravenous immunoglobulin may neutralize the effector antibodies, or plasmapheresis can be used to remove the antibodies.

Alloimmunization A recipient may become alloimmunized to a number of antigens on cellular blood elements and plasma proteins. Alloantibodies to RBC antigens are detected during pretransfusion testing, and their presence may delay finding antigen-negative crossmatch-compatible products for transfusion. Women of child-bearing age who are sensitized to certain RBC antigens (i.e., D, c, E, Kell, or Duffy) are at risk for bearing a fetus with hemolytic disease of the newborn. Matching for D antigen is the only pretransfusion selection test to prevent RBC alloimmunization.

Alloimmunization to antigens on leukocytes and platelets can result in refractoriness to platelet transfusions. Once alloimmunization has developed, HLA-compatible platelets from donors who share similar antigens with the recipient may be difficult to find. Hence, prudent transfusion practice is directed at preventing sensitization through the use of leukocyte-reduced cellular components, as well as limiting antigenic exposure by the judicious use of transfusions and use of SDAPs.

NONIMMUNOLOGIC REACTIONS **Fluid Overload** Blood components are excellent volume expanders, and transfusion may quickly lead to volume overload. Monitoring the rate and volume of the transfusion, along with the use of a diuretic, can minimize this problem.

Hypothermia Refrigerated (4°C) or frozen (−18°C or below) blood components can result in hypothermia when rapidly infused. Cardiac dysrhythmias can result from exposing the sinoatrial node to cold fluid. Use of an in-line warmer will prevent this complication.

Electrolyte Toxicity RBC leakage during storage increases the concentration of potassium in the unit. Neonates and patients in renal failure are at risk for hyperkalemia. Preventive measures, such as using fresh or washed RBCs, are warranted for neonatal transfusions because this complication can be fatal.

Citrate, commonly used to anticoagulate blood components, chelates calcium and thereby inhibits the coagulation cascade. Hypocalcemia, manifested by circumoral numbness and/or tingling sensation of the fingers and toes, may result from multiple rapid transfusions. Because citrate is quickly metabolized to bicarbonate, calcium infusion is seldom required in this setting. If calcium or any other intravenous infusion is necessary, it must be given through a separate intravenous line.

Iron Overload Each unit of RBCs contains 200 to 250 mg of iron. Symptoms and signs of iron overload affecting endocrine, hepatic, and cardiac function are common after 100 units of RBCs have been transfused (total body iron load of 20 g). Preventing this complication by using alternative therapies (e.g., erythropoietin) and judicious transfusion is preferable and cost effective. Deferoxamine and other chelating agents are available, but the response is often suboptimal.

Hypotensive Reactions Transient hypotension may be noted among transfused patients who take angiotensin-converting enzyme (ACE) inhibitors. Since blood products contain bradykinin that is normally degraded by ACE, patients on ACE inhibitors may have increased bradykinin levels that cause hypotension. The blood pressure typically returns to normal without intervention.

Immunomodulation Transfusion of allogeneic blood is immunosuppressive. Multiply transfused renal transplant recipients are less likely to reject the graft. However, in postoperative settings and in cancer patients, immune suppression is dangerous. The use of leukocyte-depleted cellular products may reduce the immunosuppression, though controlled data have not been obtained.

INFECTIOUS COMPLICATIONS Viral Infections • Hepatitis C virus (HCV) The use of an improved screening test for HCV antibodies has reduced the incidence of posttransfusion HCV infection to 1 in 103,000 transfusions. Infection with HCV may be asymptomatic or lead to chronic active hepatitis, cirrhosis, and liver failure.

Hepatitis B virus Transfusion-associated HBV infection has been reduced with improved donor selection and screening, along with increased vaccination of the donor and recipient population. However, some data suggest that HBV is more commonly transmitted by transfusion than HCV. Vaccination of individuals who require long-term transfusion therapy can prevent this complication.

Hepatitis G virus (HGV) This hepatotropic virus is transmitted by transfusion. Infection with HGV results in no apparent adverse effects. Routine testing is not available and does not appear to be warranted.

Human immunodeficiency virus type 1 Intensive donor screening and testing has dramatically reduced the risk of HIV-1 infection by blood transfusion. Donated blood is tested for HIV-1 p24 antigen. Two antigen-positive seronegative donors have been identified. The risk of HIV-1 infection per transfusion episode is 1 in 676,000. A specific assay to detect antibodies to HIV-2 is also performed on donated blood. No cases of HIV-2 infection have been reported in the United States since 1992, and only three donors have been found to have HIV-2 antibodies.

Cytomegalovirus This ubiquitous virus infects 50% or more of the general population and is transmitted by the infected "passenger" white blood cells found in transfused PRBCs or platelet components. Donated blood is not routinely tested for serologic evidence of donor exposure, but assays can be performed to identify CMV-seronegative donors, if needed. Alternatively, cellular components that are leukocyte-reduced have a decreased risk of transmitting CMV, regardless of the serologic status of the donor. Groups at risk for CMV infections include immunosuppressed patients, CMV-seronegative transplant recipients, and neonates; these patients should receive seronegative or leukocyte-depleted components.

Human T lymphotropic virus (HTLV) type I Assays to detect HTLV-I and -II are used to screen all donated blood. HTLV-1 is associated with adult T cell leukemia/lymphoma and tropical spastic paraparesis in a small percentage of infected persons (Chap. 191). The reported risk of HTLV-I infection via transfusion is 1 in 641,000 transfusion episodes. HTLV-II is not clearly associated with any disease.

Parvovirus B-19 Blood components and products derived from pooled plasma can transmit this virus, the etiologic agent of erythema infectiosum, or fifth disease, in children. Parvovirus B-19 shows tropism for erythroid precursors and inhibits both erythrocyte production and maturation. Pure red cell aplasia, presenting either as acute aplastic crisis or chronic anemia with shortened RBC survival, may occur in individuals with an underlying hematologic disease, such as sickle cell disease or thalassemia. The fetus of a seronegative woman is at risk for developing hydrops if infected with this virus.

Bacterial Contamination Most bacteria do not grow well at cold temperatures; thus, PRBCs and FFP are not common sources of bacterial contamination. However, some gram-negative bacteria, notably *Yersinia* and *Pseudomonas* species, can grow at 1° to 6°C. Platelet concentrates, which are stored at room temperature, are more likely to be contaminated with skin contaminants such as gram-positive organisms, including coagulase-negative staphylococci.

Recipients of transfusions contaminated with bacteria may develop fever and chills, which can progress to septic shock and DIC. These reactions may occur abruptly, within minutes of initiating the transfusion, or after several hours. The onset of symptoms and signs is often sudden and fulminant, which aids in differentiating bacterial contamination from a FNHTR. The reactions, particularly those related to gram-negative contaminants, are the result of infused endotoxins formed within the contaminated stored component.

When contaminated transfusions are suspected (i.e., when there is sudden development of shock), the transfusion must be stopped immediately. Therapy is directed at supporting the recipient's blood pressure, cardiac output, oxygenation, and renal function. The laboratory investigation should include cultures of any untransfused component, along with the routine blood bank clerical checks and serologic studies. Broad-spectrum antibiotic coverage should be started immediately and may be adjusted based on culture and sensitivity.

Parasites Various parasites including those causing malaria, babesiosis, and Chagas' disease can be transmitted by blood transfusion rarely. Geographical migration and travel of donors can shift the incidence of these rare infections. Because these infections can prove fatal, they should be considered in the transfused patient in the appropriate clinical setting.

ALTERNATIVES TO TRANSFUSION

Alternatives to allogeneic blood transfusions that avoid homologous donor exposures with attendant immunologic and infectious risks remain attractive. Autologous blood is the best option when transfusion is anticipated. However, the cost:benefit ratio of autologous transfusion remains high. No transfusion is a zero-risk event; clerical errors and bacterial contamination remain potential complications even with autologous transfusions. Additional methods of autologous transfusion in the surgical patient include preoperative hemodilution, recovery of shed blood from sterile surgical sites, and postoperative drainage collection. Directed or designated donation from friends and family of the potential recipient has not been safer than volunteer donor component transfusions. Such directed donations may in fact place the recipient at higher risk for complications such as GVHD and alloimmunization.

Oxygen-carrying blood substitutes, such as perfluorocarbons and aggregated hemoglobin solution, are presently in various stages of clinical trials. Granulocyte- and granulocyte-macrophage colony stimulating factor (G- or GM-CSF) are clinically useful to hasten leukocyte recovery in patients with leukopenia related to high-dose chemotherapy. Erythropoietin stimulates erythrocyte production in patients with anemia of chronic renal failure and other conditions, thus avoiding or reducing the need for transfusion. This hormone can also stimulate erythropoiesis in the autologous donor to enable additional donation. Thrombopoietin, a cytokine that promotes megakaryocyte proliferation and maturation, is being tested for its ability to reduce the need for platelet transfusion.

BIBLIOGRAPHY

ANDERSON KC, NESS PM (eds): *Scientific Basis of Transfusion Medicine, Implications for Clinical Practice.* Philadelphia, Saunders, 1999

CARSON JL et al: Perioperative blood transfusion and postoperative mortality. JAMA 279: 199, 1998

ETCHSON J et al: The cost effectiveness of preoperative autologous blood donations. N Engl J Med 332:719, 1995

GOODNOUGH LT et al: Transfusion medicine (2 parts). N Engl J Med 340:438, 525, 1999

HEBERT PC et al: A multicenter, randomized, controlled clinical trial of transfusion requirements in critical care. N Engl J Med 340:409, 1999

KUTER DJ et al: Platelet growth factors: Potential impact on transfusion medicine. Transfusion 39:321, 1999

MENITOVE JE et al: *The Technical Manual,* 18th ed. Arlington VA, American Association of Blood Banks, 1997

RUBELLA P et al: A multicenter randomized study of the threshold for prophylactic platelet transfusions in adults with acute myeloid leukemia. N Engl J Med 337:1870, 1997

SAGMEISTER M et al: A restrictive platelet transfusion policy allowing long-term support of outpatients with severe aplastic anemia. Blood 93:3124, 1999

SCHREIBER GB et al: The risk of transfusion-transmitted viral infections. N Engl J Med 334:1685, 1996

115 *Frederick R. Appelbaum*

BONE MARROW AND STEM CELL TRANSPLANTATION

Bone marrow transplantation is the generic term used to describe the collection and transplantation of hematopoietic stem cells. The procedure is usually carried out for one of two purposes: (1) to replace an abnormal but nonmalignant lymphohematopoietic system with one from a normal donor, or (2) to treat malignancy by allowing the administration of higher doses of myelosuppressive therapy than would otherwise be possible. The use of bone marrow transplantation has been steadily increasing, both because of the its demonstrated effectiveness in selected diseases and because of increasing availability of donors. The International Bone Marrow Transplant Registry estimates that about 50,000 transplants were performed during 1999.

THE HEMATOPOIETIC STEM CELL

Several features of the hematopoietic stem cell make bone marrow transplantation clinically feasible, including its remarkable regenerative capacity, its ability to home to the marrow space following intravenous injection, and the ability of the stem cell to be cryopreserved. Transplantation of a single stem cell can replace the entire lymphohematopoietic system of an adult mouse. In humans, transplantation of a few percent of a donor's bone marrow volume regularly results in complete and sustained replacement of the recipient's entire lymphohematopoietic system, including all red cells, granulocytes, B and T lymphocytes, and platelets, as well as cells comprising the fixed macrophage population, including Kupffer cells of the liver, pulmonary alveolar macrophages, osteoclasts, Langerhans cells of the skin, and brain microglial cells. The ability of the hematopoietic stem cell to home to the marrow following intravenous injection is mediated, at least in part, by the interaction of specific cell molecules, termed *selectins*, on bone marrow endothelial cells with their unique ligands, termed *integrins*, on early hematopoietic cells. Human hematopoietic stem cells can survive freezing and thawing with little, if any, damage, making it possible to remove and store a portion of the patient's own bone marrow for later reinfusion following treatment of the patient with high-dose myelotoxic therapy.

CATEGORIES OF BONE MARROW TRANSPLANTATION

Bone marrow transplantation can be described according to the relationship between the patient and the donor and by the anatomic source of stem cells. In approximately 1% of cases, patients have identical twins who can serve as donors. Syngeneic donors represent the best source of stem cells; unlike allogeneic donors, there is no risk of graft-versus-host disease (GVHD) and, unlike use of autologous marrow, there is no risk that the stem cells are contaminated with tumor cells.

Allogeneic transplantation involves a donor and recipient who are not immunologically identical. Following allogeneic transplantation immune cells transplanted with the marrow or developing from it can react against the patient, causing GVHD. Alternatively, if the immunosuppressive preparative regimen used to treat the patient before transplant is inadequate, immunocompetent cells of the patient can cause graft rejection. The risks of these complications are greatly influenced by the degree of matching between donor and recipient for antigens encoded by genes of the major histocompatibility complex.

The human leukocyte antigen (HLA) molecules are responsible for binding antigenic proteins and presenting them to T cells. The antigens presented by HLA molecules may derive from exogenous sources (e.g., during active infections) or may be endogenous proteins produced by the cell. If individuals are not matched for HLA, T cells from one individual will react strongly to the mismatched HLA, or "major antigens," of the second. Even if the individuals are HLA-matched, the T cells of the donor may react to differing endogenous, or "minor antigens," presented by the HLA of the recipient. Reactions to minor antigens tend to be less vigorous. The genes of major relevance to transplantation include HLA-A, -B, -C, and -D; they are closely linked and therefore tend to be inherited as haplotypes, with only rare crossovers between them. Thus, the odds that any one full sibling will match a patient are one in four, and the probability that the patient has an HLA-identical sibling is $1 - (0.75)^n$ where n equals the number of siblings.

With current techniques, the risk of graft rejection is 1 to 3%, and the risk of severe, life-threatening acute GVHD is approximately 15% following transplantation between HLA-identical siblings. The incidence of graft rejection and GVHD increases progressively with the use of family member donors mismatched for one, two, or three antigens. While survival following a one-antigen mismatched transplant is not markedly altered, survival following two- or three-antigen mismatched transplants is significantly impaired, and such transplants should only be performed as part of clinical trials.

The formation of the National Marrow Donor Program has allowed for the identification of HLA-matched unrelated donors for many patients. The genes encoding HLA antigens are highly polymorphic, and thus the odds of any two unrelated individuals being HLA-identical are extremely low, somewhat less than 1 in 10,000. However, by identifying and typing >3 million volunteer donors, HLA-matched donors now can found for approximately 50% of patients for whom a search is initiated. It takes, on average, 3 to 4 months to complete a search and schedule and initiate an unrelated donor transplant. Results so far suggest that GVHD is somewhat increased and survival somewhat poorer with such donors than with HLA-matched siblings.

Autologous transplantation involves the removal and storage of the patient's own stem cells with subsequent reinfusion after the patient receives high-dose myeloablative therapy. Unlike allogeneic transplantation, there is no risk of GVHD or graft rejection with autologous transplantation. On the other hand, autologous transplantation lacks a graft-versus-tumor effect, and the autologous stem cell product can be contaminated with tumor cells that could lead to relapse. A variety of techniques have been developed to "purge" autologous products of tumor cells. Some use antibodies directed at tumor-associated antigens plus complement, antibodies linked to toxins, or antibodies conjugated to immunomagnetic beads. In vitro incubation with certain chemotherapeutic agents such as 4-hydroperoxycylophosphamide and long-term culture of bone marrow has also been shown to diminish tumor cell numbers in stem cell products. Another technique is positive selection of stem cells using antibodies to CD34, with subsequent column adherence or flow techniques to select normal stem cells while leaving tumor cells behind. All these approaches can reduce the number of tumor cells from 1000- to 10,000-fold and are clinically feasible; however, no prospective randomized trials have yet shown that any of these approaches results in a decrease in relapse rates or improvements in disease-free or overall survival.

Bone marrow aspirated from the posterior and anterior iliac crests has traditionally been the source of hematopoietic stem cells for transplantation. Typically, anywhere from 1.5 to 5 × 10^8 nucleated marrow cells per kilogram are collected for allogeneic transplantation. Several recent studies have found improved survival in the settings of both matched sibling and unrelated transplantation by transplanting higher numbers of bone marrow cells.

Hematopoietic stem cells circulate in the peripheral blood but in very low concentrations. Following the administration of certain hematopoietic growth factors, including granulocyte colony stimulating factor (G-CSF) or granulocyte-macrophage colony stimulating factor (GM-CSF), and during recovery from intensive chemotherapy, the concentration of hematopoietic progenitor cells in blood, as measured either by colony forming units or expression of the CD34 antigen, increases markedly. This has made it possible to harvest adequate numbers of stem cells from the peripheral blood for transplantation. Donors are typically treated with 4 or 5 days of hematopoietic growth factor, following which stem cells are collected in one or two 4-h pheresis sessions. In the autologous setting, transplantation of >2.5 × 10^6 CD34 cells per kilogram, a number easily collected in most circumstances, leads to rapid and sustained engraftment in virtually all cases. Compared to the use of autologous marrow, use of peripheral blood stem cells results in more rapid hematopoietic recovery, with granulocytes recovering to 500/μL by day 12 and platelets recovering to 20,000/μL by day 14. While this more rapid recovery diminishes the morbidity of transplantation, no studies show an improvement in survival.

Hesitation in studying the use of peripheral blood stem cells for allogeneic transplantation was because peripheral blood stem cell products contain as much as one log more T cells than are contained in the typical marrow harvest; in animal models, the incidence of GVHD is related to the number of T cells transplanted. Nonetheless, phase II and now randomized phase III trials have shown that the use of growth factor–mobilized peripheral blood stem cells from HLA-matched family members leads to faster engraftment without an increase in acute GVHD. Chronic GVHD may be increased with peripheral blood stem cells, but in trials conducted so far, this has been more than balanced by reductions in relapse rates and nonrelapse mortality, with the use of peripheral blood stem cells resulting in improved overall survival.

Umbilical cord blood contains a high concentration of hematopoietic progenitor cells, allowing for its use as a source of stem cells for transplantation. Cord blood transplantation from family members has been explored in the setting where the immediate need for transplantation precludes waiting the 9 or so months generally required for the baby to mature to the point of donating marrow. Use of cord blood in such settings results in somewhat slower engraftment than seen with marrow but a low incidence of GVHD, perhaps reflecting the low number of T cells in cord blood. More recently, several banks have been developed to harvest and store cord blood for possible transplantation to unrelated patients from material that would otherwise be discarded. A summary of the first 272 unrelated cord blood transplants, facilitated by the New York Blood Center, reported engraftment in approximately 90% of patients but at a slower pace than seen with a marrow. Significant GVHD was seen in 40% of patients. The risk of graft failure was related to the dose of cord blood cells per kilogram infused. The low cell content of most cord blood collections has limited the use of this approach as a source of stem cells for adult patients.

THE TRANSPLANT PREPARATIVE REGIMEN

The treatment regimen administered to patients immediately preceding transplantation is designed to eradicate the patient's underlying disease and, in the setting of allogeneic transplantation, immunosuppress the patient adequately to prevent rejection of the transplanted marrow. The appropriate regimen, therefore, depends on the disease setting and source of marrow. For example, when transplantation is performed to treat severe combined immunodeficiency and the donor is a histocompatible sibling, no treatment is required because no host cells require eradication and the patient is already too immunoincompetent to reject the transplanted marrow. For aplastic anemia, there is no large population of cells to eradicate and high-dose cyclophosphamide plus antithymocyte globulin is sufficient to immunosuppress the patient adequately to accept the marrow graft. In the setting of thalassemia and sickle cell anemia, high-dose busulfan is frequently added to cyclophosphamide in order to eradicate the hyperplastic host hematopoiesis. A variety of different regimens have been developed to treat malignant diseases. Most of these regimens included agents that have high activity against the tumor in question at conventional doses and have myelosuppression as their predominant dose-limiting toxicity. Therefore, these regimens commonly include busulfan, cyclophosphamide, melphalan, thiotepa, carmustine, etoposide, and total-body irradiation in various combinations.

THE TRANSPLANT PROCEDURE

Marrow is usually collected from the donor's posterior and sometimes anterior iliac crests with the donor under general or spinal anesthesia. Typically, 10 to 15 mL/kg of marrow is aspirated, placed in heparinized media, and filtered through 0.3- and 0.2-mm screens to remove fat and bony spicules. The collected marrow may undergo further processing depending on the clinical situation, such as the removal of red cells to prevent hemolysis in ABO-incompatible transplants, the removal of donor T cells to prevent GVHD, or attempts to remove possible contaminating tumor cells in autologous transplantation. Marrow donation is a safe procedure, with only very rare complications reported.

Peripheral blood stem cells are collected by leukopheresis after the donor has been treated with hematopoietic growth factors or, in the setting of autologous transplantation, sometimes after treatment with a combination of chemotherapy and growth factors. Stem cells for transplantation are generally infused through a large-bore central venous catheter. Such infusions are usually well tolerated, although occasionally patients develop fever, cough, or shortness of breath. These symptoms usually resolve with slowing of the infusion. When the stem cell product has been cryopreserved using dimethyl sulfoxide, patients more often experience short-lived nausea or vomiting due to the odor and taste of the cryoprotectant.

ENGRAFTMENT

Peripheral blood counts usually reach their nadir several days to a week posttransplant as a consequence of the preparative regimen, then cells produced by the transplanted stem cells begin to appear in the peripheral blood. The rate of recovery depends on the source of stem cells, the use of posttransplant growth factors, and the form of GVHD prophylaxis employed. If marrow is the source of stem cells, recovery to 100 granulocytes per microliter occurs by day 16 and 500/μL by day 22. Use of G-CSF-mobilized peripheral blood stem cells speeds the rate of recovery by approximately 1 week when compared to marrow. Use of myeloid growth factor (G-CSF or GM-CSF) posttransplant can further accelerate recovery by 3 to 5 days, while use of methotrexate to prevent GVHD delays engraftment by a similar period. Following allogeneic transplantation, engraftment can be documented using fluorescence in situ hybridization of sex chromosomes if donor and recipient are sex-mismatched, HLA-typing if HLA-mismatched, or restriction fragment length polymorphism analysis if sex- and HLA-matched.

COMPLICATIONS FOLLOWING BONE MARROW TRANSPLANT

EARLY DIRECT CHEMORADIO-TOXICITIES The transplant preparative regimens commonly used cause a spectrum of acute toxicities that vary according to the specific regimen but frequently result in nausea, vomiting, and mild skin erythema (Fig. 115-1). Regimens that include high-dose cyclophosphamide can result in hemorrhagic cystitis, which can usually be prevented by bladder irrigation or therapy with the sulfhydryl compound, mercaptoethanesulfonate (MESNA); rarely, acute hemorrhagic carditis is seen. Most preparative regimens will result in oral mucositis, which typically develops approximately 5 to 7 days posttransplant and often requires narcotic analgesia. Use of a patient-controlled analgesic pump provides the greatest patient satisfaction and results in a lower cumulative dose of narcotic. Patients begin losing their hair 5 to 6 days posttransplant and by 1 week are usually profoundly pancytopenic.

Approximately 10% of patients will develop venoocclusive disease of the liver, a syndrome resulting from direct cytotoxic injury to hepatic-venular and sinusoidal endothelium, with subsequent deposition of fibrin and the development of a local hypercoagulable state. This chain of events results in the clinical symptoms of tender hepatomegaly, ascites, jaundice, and fluid retention. These symptoms can develop any time during the first month posttransplant, with the peak incidence at day 16. The mortality of venoocclusive disease is approximately 30%, with progressive hepatic failure culminating in a terminal hepatorenal syndrome. Both thrombolytic and antithrombotic agents, such as tissue plasminogen activator, heparin, and prostaglandin E, have been studied as therapy, but none has proven of consistent major benefit in controlled trials and all have significant toxicity. Early studies with defibrotide, a polydeoxyribonucleotide, seem encouraging.

Although most pneumonias developing posttransplant are caused by infectious agents, in approximately 5% of patients a diffuse interstitial pneumonia will develop that is thought to be the result of direct toxicity of the preparative regimen. Bronchoalveolar lavage typically shows alveolar hemorrhage, and biopsies are typically characterized by diffuse alveolar damage, although some cases may have a more clearly interstitial pattern. High-dose glucocorticoids are often used as treatment, although randomized trials testing their utility have not been reported.

LATE DIRECT CHEMORADIOTOXICITIES Late complications of the preparative regimen include decreased growth velocity in children and delayed development of secondary sex characteristics. These complications can be partly ameliorated with the use of appropriate growth and sex hormone replacement. Most men become azoospermic, and most postpubertal women will develop ovarian failure, which should be treated. Thyroid dysfunction, usually well compensated, is sometimes seen. Cataracts develop in 10 to 20% of patients and are most common in patients treated with total-body irradiation and those who receive glucocorticoid therapy posttransplant for treatment of GVHD. Aseptic necrosis of the femoral head is seen in 10% of patients and is particularly frequent in those receiving chronic glucocorticoid therapy.

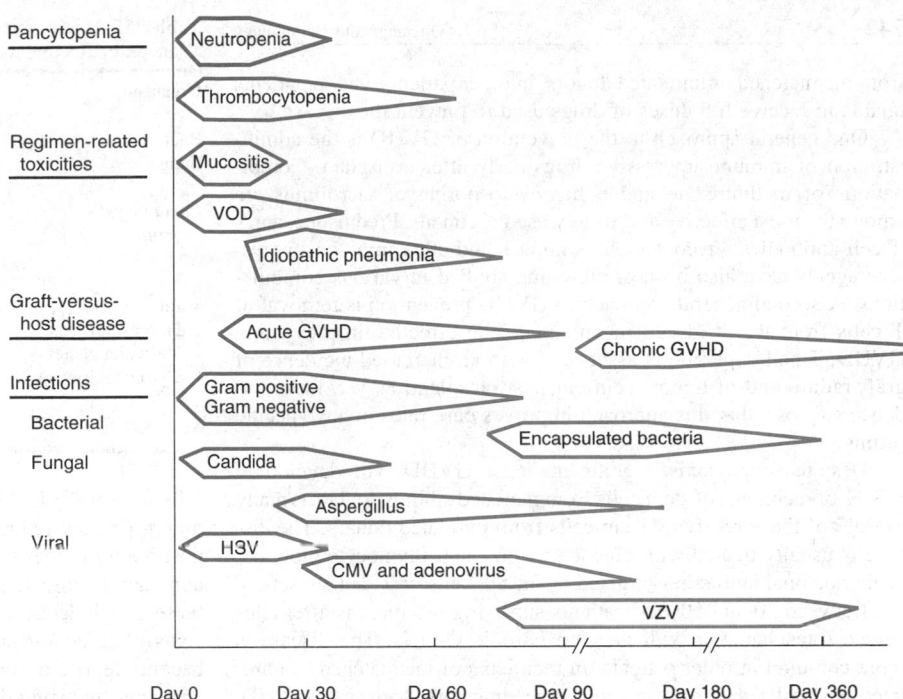

FIGURE 115-1 Major syndromes complicating marrow transplantation. VOD, venocclusive disease; GVHD, graft-versus-host disease; HSV, herpes simplex virus; CMV, cytomegalovirus; VZV, varicella-zoster virus. The size of the box roughly reflects the risk of the complication.

GRAFT-VERSUS-HOST DISEASE GVHD is the result of allogeneic T cells that were either transferred with the donor's stem cell inoculum or develop from it, reacting with antigenic targets on host cells. GVHD developing within the first 3 months posttransplant is termed *acute GVHD*, while GVHD developing or persisting beyond 3 months posttransplant is termed *chronic GVHD*. Acute GVHD most often first becomes apparent between 2 and 4 weeks posttransplant and is characterized by an erythematous maculopapular rash; persistent anorexia or diarrhea, or both; and by liver disease with increased serum levels of bilirubin, alanine and aspartate aminotransferase, and alkaline phosphatase. Since many conditions can mimic acute GVHD, diagnosis usually requires skin, liver, or endoscopic biopsy for confirmation. In all these organs, endothelial damage and lymphocytic infiltrates are seen. In skin, the epidermis and hair follicles are damaged; in liver, the small bile ducts show segmental disruption; and in intestines, destruction of the crypts and mucosal ulceration may be noted. A commonly used rating system for acute GVHD is shown in Table 115-1. Grade I acute GVHD is of little clinical significance, does not affect the likelihood of survival, and does not require treatment. In contrast, grades II to IV GVHD are associated with significant symptoms and a poorer probability of survival and require aggressive therapy. The incidence of acute GVHD is higher in recipients of stem cells

Table 115-1 Clinical Staging and Grading of Acute Graft-Versus-Host Disease

Clinical Stage	Skin	Liver—Bilirubin, μmol/L (mg/dL)	Gut
1	Rash <25% body surface	34–51 (2–3)	Diarrhea 500–1000 mL/d
2	Rash <25–50% body surface	51–103 (3–6)	Diarrhea 1000–1500 mL/d
3	Generalized erythroderma	103–257 (6–15)	Diarrhea > 1500 mL/d
4	Desquamation and bullae	>257 (> 15)	Ileus

OVERALL CLINICAL GRADE	SKIN STAGE	LIVER STAGE	GUT STAGE
I	1–2	0	0
II	1–3	1	1
III	1–3	2–3	2–3
IV	2–4	2–4	2–4

from mismatched or unrelated donors, in older patients, and in patients unable to receive full doses of drugs used to prevent the disease.

One general approach to the prevention of GVHD is the administration of immunosuppressive drugs early after transplant. Combinations of methotrexate and either cyclosporine or tacrolimus are among the most effective and widely used regimens. Prednisone, anti-T cell antibodies, mycophenolate mofetil, and other immunosuppressive agents have also been or are being studied in various combinations. A second general approach to GVHD prevention is removal of T cells from the stem cell inoculum. While effective in preventing GVHD, T cell depletion is associated with an increased incidence of graft failure and of tumor recurrent posttransplant; as yet, little evidence suggests that this approach improves cure rates in any specific setting.

Despite prophylaxis, significant acute GVHD will develop in ~30% of recipients of stem cells from matched siblings and in as many as 60% of those receiving stem cells from unrelated donors. The disease is usually treated with glucocorticoids, anti-thymocyte globulin, or monoclonal antibodies targeted against T cells or T cell subsets.

Between 20 and 50% of patients surviving >6 months after allogeneic transplantation will develop chronic GVHD. The disease is more common in older patients, in recipients of mismatched or unrelated stem cells, and in those with a preceding episode of acute GVHD. The disease resembles an autoimmune disorder with malar rash, sicca syndrome, arthritis, obliterative bronchiolitis, and bile duct degeneration and cholestasis. Single-agent prednisone or cyclosporine is standard treatment at present, although trials of other agents, including thalidomide, are under way. In most patients, chronic GVHD resolves, but it may require 1 to 3 years of immunosuppressive treatment before these agents can be withdrawn without the disease recurring. Because patients with chronic GVHD are susceptible to significant infection, they should receive prophylactic trimethoprim-sulfamethoxazole, and all suspected infections should be investigated and treated aggressively.

GRAFT FAILURE While complete and sustained engraftment are usually seen posttransplant, occasionally marrow function either does not return or, after a brief period of engraftment, is lost. Graft failure after autologous transplantation can be the result of inadequate numbers of stem cells being transplanted, damage during ex vivo treatment or storage, or exposure of the patient to myelotoxic agents posttransplant. Infections with cytomegalovirus (CMV) or human herpes virus type 6 have also been associated with loss of marrow function. Graft failure after allogeneic transplantation can also be due to immunologic rejection of the graft by immunocompetent host cells. Immunologically based graft rejection is more common following use of less immunosuppressive preparative regimens, in recipients of T cell–depleted stem cell products, and in patients receiving grafts from HLA-mismatched donors.

Treatment of graft failure usually involves removing all potentially myelotoxic agents from the patient's regimen and attempting a short trial of myeloid growth factor. Persistence of lymphocytes of host origin in allogeneic transplant recipients with graft failure indicates immunologic rejection. Reinfusion of donor stem cells in such patients is usually unsuccessful unless preceded by a second immunosuppressive preparative regimen. Standard preparative regimens are generally tolerated poorly if administered within 100 days of a first transplant because of cumulative toxicities. However, use of regimens combining, for example, anti-CD3 antibodies with high-dose glucocorticoids have been successful in achieving engraftment in >50% of patients.

INFECTION The general problem of infection in the immunocompromised host is discussed in Chap. 136. Posttransplant patients, particularly recipients of allogeneic transplantation, require unique approaches. Early after transplantation, patients are profoundly neutropenic, and because the risk of bacterial infection is so great, most centers initiate antibiotic treatment once the granulocyte count

Table 115-2 An Approach to Infection Prophylaxis in Allogeneic Transplant Recipients

Organism		Approach
Bacterial	Ceftazidime	2 g IV q8h while neutropenic
Fungal	Fluconazole	400 mg PO qd to day 75 posttransplant
Pneumocystis carinii	Trimethoprim-sulfamethoxazole	1 double-strength tablet PO bid 2 days/week until day 180 or off immunosuppression
Viral		
Herpes simplex	Acyclovir	800 mg PO bid to day 30
Varicella zoster	Acyclovir	800 mg PO bid to day 365
Cytomegalovirus	Ganciclovir	5 mg/kg IV bid for 7 days, then 5 (mg/kg)/d 5 days/week to day 100

falls to <500/μL. Fluconazole prophylaxis at a dose of 200 to 400 mg/kg per day reduces the risk of candidal infections. Patients seropositive for herpes simplex should receive acyclovir prophylaxis. One approach to infection prophylaxis is shown in Table 115-2. Despite these prophylactic measures, most patients will develop fever and signs of infection posttransplant. The management of patients who become febrile despite bacterial and fungal prophylaxis is a difficult challenge and is guided by individual aspects of the patient and by the institution's experience.

Once patients engraft, the incidence of bacterial infection diminishes; however, patients, particularly allogeneic transplant recipients, remain at significant risk of infection. During the period from engraftment until about 3 months posttransplant, the most common causes of infection are gram-positive bacteria, fungi (particularly *Aspergillus*) and viruses including CMV. CMV infection, which in the past was frequently seen and often fatal, can be prevented in seronegative patients by the use of seronegative blood products. The use of ganciclovir, either as prophylaxis beginning at the time of engraftment or initiated when CMV first reactivates as evidenced by development of antigenemia, can significantly reduce the risk of CMV disease in seropositive patients. Foscarnet is effective for some patients who develop CMV antigenemia or infection despite the use of ganciclovir or who cannot tolerate the drug.

Pneumocystis carinii pneumonia, once seen in 5 to 10% of patients, can be prevented by treating patients with oral trimethoprim-sulfamethoxazole for 1 week pretransplant and resuming the treatment once patients have engrafted.

The risk of infection diminishes considerably beyond 3 months after transplant unless chronic GVHD develops, requiring continuous immunosuppression. Most transplant centers recommend continuing trimethoprim-sulfamethoxazole prophylaxis while patients are receiving any immunosuppressive drugs and also recommend careful monitoring for late CMV reactivation. In addition, most centers recommend prophylaxis against varicella zoster, using acyclovir for 1 year posttransplant.

TREATMENT OF SPECIFIC DISEASES USING BONE MARROW TRANSPLANTATION

NONMALIGNANT DISEASES   **Immunodeficiency Disorders** By replacing abnormal stem cells with cells from a normal donor, marrow transplantation can cure patients of a variety of immunodeficiency disorders including severe combined immunodeficiency, Wiskott-Aldrich syndrome, and Chédiak-Higashi syndrome. The widest experience has been with severe combined immunodeficiency disease, where cure rates of 90% can be expected with HLA-identical donors and success rates of 50 to 70% have been reported using haplotype-mismatched parents as donors (Table 115-3).

Aplastic Anemia Transplantation from matched siblings after a preparative regimen of high-dose cyclophosphamide and antithymo-

Disease	Allogeneic, %	Autologous, %
Severe combined immunodeficiency	90	N/A
Aplastic anemia	90	N/A
Thalassemia	90	N/A
Acute myeloid leukemia		
First remission	55–60	50
Second remission	40	30
Acute lymphoblastic leukemia		
First remission	50	40
Second remission	40	30
Chronic myeloid leukemia		
Chronic phase	70	ID
Accelerated phase	40	ID
Blast crisis	15	ID
Chronic lymphoblastic leukemia	50	ID
Myelodysplasia	45	ID
Multiple myeloma	30	35
Non-Hodgkin's lymphoma		
First relapse/second remission	40	40
Hodgkin's disease		
First relapse/second remission	40	50
Breast cancer		
High-risk stage II	N/A	70
Stage IV	N/A	15

[a] These estimates are generally based on data reported by the International Bone Marrow Transplant Registry. The analysis has not been reviewed by their Advisory Committee.
NOTE: N/A, not applicable; ID, insufficient data.

cyte globulin can cure up to 90% of patients younger than age 40 with severe aplastic anemia. Results in older patients and in recipients of mismatched family member or unrelated marrow are less favorable; therefore, a trial of immunosuppressive therapy is generally recommended for such patients before considering transplantation. Transplantation is effective in all forms of aplastic anemia including, for example, the syndromes associated with paroxysmal nocturnal hemoglobinuria and Fanconi's anemia. Patients with Fanconi's anemia are abnormally sensitive to the toxic effects of alkylating agents and so less intensive preparative regimens must be used in their treatment (Chap. 109).

Hemoglobinopathies Marrow transplantation from an HLA-identical sibling following a preparative regimen of busulfan and cyclophosphamide can cure 70 to 90% of patients with thalassemia major. The best outcomes can be expected if patients are transplanted before they develop hepatomegaly or portal fibrosis and if they have been given adequate iron chelation therapy. Among such patients, the probabilities of 5-year survival and disease-free survival are 95 and 90%, respectively. Although prolonged survival can be achieved with aggressive chelation therapy, transplantation is the only curative treatment for thalassemia. Transplantation is being studied as a curative approach to patients with sickle cell anemia. Two-year survival and disease-free survival rates of 90 and 80%, respectively, have been reported following matched sibling transplantation. Decisions about patient selection and the timing of transplantation remain difficult, but transplantation seems to represent a reasonable option for younger patients who suffer repeated crises or other significant complications and who have not responded to other interventions (Chap 106).

Other Nonmalignant Diseases Theoretically, marrow transplantation should be able to cure any disease that results from an inborn error of the lymphohematopoietic system. Transplantation has been used successfully to treat congenital disorders of white blood cells such as Kostmann's syndrome, chronic granulomatous disease, and leukocyte adhesion deficiency. Congenital anemias such as Blackfan-Diamond anemia can also be cured with transplantation. Infantile malignant osteopetrosis is due to an inability of the osteoclast to resorb bone, and since osteoclasts derive from the marrow, transplantation can cure this rare inherited disorder.

Marrow transplantation has been used as treatment for a number

of storage diseases caused by enzymatic deficiencies, such as Gaucher's disease, Hurler's syndrome, Hunter's syndrome, and infantile metachromatic leukodystrophy. Transplantation for these diseases has not been uniformly successful, but treatment early in the course of these diseases, before irreversible damage to extramedullary organs has occurred, increases the chance for success.

Transplantation is being explored as a treatment for severe acquired autoimmune disorders. These trials are based on studies demonstrating that transplantation can reverse autoimmune disorders in animal models and on the observation that occasional patients with coexisting autoimmune disorders and hematologic malignancies have been cured of both with transplantation.

MALIGNANT DISEASES Acute Leukemia Allogeneic marrow transplantation cures 15 to 20% of patients who do not achieve complete response from induction chemotherapy for acute myeloid leukemia (AML) and is the only form of therapy that can cure such patients. Cure rates of 30 to 35% are seen when patients are transplanted in second remission or in first relapse. The best results with allogeneic transplantation are achieved when applied during first remission, with disease-free survival rates averaging between 55 and 60%. Chemotherapy alone can cure a portion of AML patients, and so the relative merits of transplanting all patients during first remission versus only transplanting very high risk patients and those who relapse continue to be discussed. Autologous transplantation is also able to cure a portion of patients with AML. The rates of disease recurrence with autologous transplantation are higher than seen after allogeneic transplantation, and cure rates are generally somewhat less.

Similar to patients with AML, adults with acute lymphoblastic leukemia who do not achieve a complete response to induction chemotherapy can be cured in 15 to 20% of cases with immediate marrow transplantation. Cure rates improve to 30 to 50% in second remission, and therefore transplantation can be recommended for adults who have persistent disease after induction chemotherapy or who have subsequently relapsed. Transplantation in first remission results in cure rates around 55%. While transplantation appears to offer a clear advantage over chemotherapy for patients with high-risk disease, such as those with Philadelphia chromosome–positive disease, debate continues about whether adults with standard-risk disease would be transplanted in first remission or whether transplantation should be reserved until relapse. Autologous transplantation is associated with a higher relapse rate but a somewhat lower risk of nonrelapse mortality when compared to allogeneic transplantation. On balance, most experts recommend use of allogeneic stem cells if an appropriate donor is available.

Chronic Leukemia Allogeneic marrow transplantation is the only therapy shown to cure a substantial portion of patients with chronic myeloid leukemia. Five-year disease-free survival rates are 60 to 70% for patients transplanted during chronic phase, 30 to 40% for patients transplanted during accelerated phase, and 15 to 20% for patients transplanted in blast crisis. Time from diagnosis to transplantation influences outcome, with best results obtained among patients transplanted within 1 year of diagnosis. Use of unrelated donors results in more GVHD and slightly worse survival than seen with matched siblings, although, at some large centers, 3-year disease-free survival rates of 70% have been reported. Autologous transplantation is being studied; however, few data suggest that this approach has curative potential in this disease. Given the excellent results obtained with matched sibling transplantation, most experts recommend early transplantation for younger patients with matched siblings. For older patients or those without matched siblings, it is not unreasonable to consider a trial of an interferon α–containing regimen to see if a major cytogenetic response can be achieved before making a decision about transplantation (Chap. 111).

Allogeneic transplantation has been used to only a limited extent for chronic lymphocytic leukemia, in large part because of the chronic nature of the disease and because of the age profile of patients. With allogeneic transplantation, complete remissions have been achieved in the majority of patients so far reported, with disease-free survival rates of approximately 50% at 3 years. However, treatment-related mortality has been substantial, and further follow-up is needed. There is even less experience with autologous transplantation in this disorder.

Myelodysplasia Between 40 and 50% of patients with myelo-dysplasia appear to be cured with allogeneic marrow transplantation. Results are better among younger patients and those with less advanced disease. However, some patients with myelodysplasia can live for extended periods without intervention, and so transplantation is generally recommended only for patients with disease categorized as intermediate risk I or greater according to the International Prognostic Scoring System (Chap. 109).

Lymphoma Patients with disseminated intermediate- or high-grade non-Hodgkin's lymphoma who have not been cured by first-line chemotherapy and are transplanted in first relapse or second remission can still be cured in 40 to 50% of cases. This represents a clear advantage over results obtained with salvage chemotherapy. It is unsettled whether patients with high-risk disease benefit from transplantation in first remission. Most experts favor the use of autologous rather than allogeneic transplantation for patients with non-Hodgkin's lymphoma, because fewer complications occur with this approach and survival appears equivalent. The role of transplantation in patients with indolent non-Hodgkin's lymphoma is less well defined. Long-term remissions can be obtained in many patients with acceptable toxicity and results with transplantation in patients with recurrent disease generally appear better than one would expect with conventional-dose chemotherapy. However, late relapses are seen after transplantation, and no randomized study has confirmed its superiority.

The role of transplantation in Hodgkin's disease is similar to that in non-Hodgkin's lymphoma. With transplantation, 5-year disease-free survival ranges from 20 to 30% in patients who never achieve a first remission with standard chemotherapy and up to 60% for those transplanted in second remission. Transplantation has no defined role in first remission in Hodgkin's disease.

Myeloma Patients with myeloma who have progressed on first-line therapy can sometimes benefit from allogeneic or autologous transplantation. Autologous transplantation has been studied as part of the initial therapy of patients, and in randomized trials, both disease-free survival as well as overall survival were improved with this approach.

Solid Tumors Among women with metastatic breast cancer, between 15 and 20% disease-free survival rates at 3 years have been reported, with better results seen in younger patients who have responded completely to standard-dose therapy before undergoing transplantation. Randomized trials have not shown superior survival for patients treated for metastatic disease with high-dose chemotherapy plus stem cell support. Randomized trials evaluating transplantation as treatment for primary breast cancer are being conducted, but final results are not yet available.

Patients with testicular cancer who have failed first-line chemotherapy have been treated with autologous transplantation. Approximately 10 to 20% of such patients apparently have been cured with this approach.

The use of high-dose chemotherapy with autologous stem cell support is being studied for several other solid tumors, including ovarian cancer, small-cell lung cancer, neuroblastoma, and pediatric sarcomas. As in most other settings, the best results have been obtained in patients with limited amounts of disease and where the remaining tumor retains sensitivity to conventional-dose chemotherapy. Few randomized trials of transplantation in these diseases have been completed.

Posttransplant Relapse Patients who relapse following autologous transplantation sometimes respond to further chemotherapy, particularly if the remission following transplantation was long. More options are available for patients who relapse following allogeneic transplantation. Of particular interest are the response rates seen with infusion of unirradiated donor lymphocytes. Complete responses in as many as 75% of patients with chronic myeloid leukemia, 40% in myelodysplasia, 25% in AML, and 15% in myeloma have been reported. Major complications of donor lymphocyte infusions include transient myelosuppression and the development of GVHD. These complications appear to be dependent on the number of donor lymphocytes infused. The impressive responses seen with donor lymphocyte infusions in some patients has encouraged investigation into the use of "nonablative" transplant regimens as treatment for various malignancies. In this approach, preparative regimens and posttransplant immunosuppression are selected that allow for engraftment without regard to their direct antitumor activities. The antitumor effects are the result of a graft-versus-tumor effect arising from the transplanted stem cells or subsequent infusion of donor lymphocytes. While engraftment can be reliably achieved with this approach, with little toxicity, and complete responses are seen, neither the rate of complete responses nor their duration have yet been entirely determined for any specific disease category.

BIBLIOGRAPHY

CURTIS RE et al: Solid cancers after bone marrow transplantation. N Engl J Med 336: 897, 1997

FISCHER A: Thirty years of bone marrow transplantation for severe combined immunodeficiency (Editorial). N Engl J Med 340:559, 1999

GOODMAN JL et al: A controlled trial of fluconazole to prevent fungal infections in patients undergoing bone marrow transplantation. N Engl J Med 326:845, 1992

GOODRICH JM et al: Ganciclovir prophylaxis to prevent cytomegalovirus disease after allogeneic marrow transplant. Ann Intern Med 118:173, 1993

HANSEN JA et al: Bone marrow transplants from unrelated donors for patients with chronic myeloid leukemia. N Engl J Med 338:962, 1998

PHILIP T et al: Autologous bone marrow transplantation as compared with salvage chemotherapy in relapses of chemotherapy-sensitive non-Hodgkin's lymphoma. N Engl J Med 333:1540, 1995

ROWLINGS PA et al: Factors correlated with progression-free survival after high-dose chemotherapy and hematopoietic stem cell transplantation for metastatic breast cancer. JAMA 282:1335, 1999

RUBINSTEIN P et al: Outcomes among 562 recipients of placental-blood transplants from unrelated donors. N Engl J Med 339:1565, 1998

WALTERS MC et al: Bone marrow transplantation for sickle cell disease. N Engl J Med 335:369, 1996

ZITTOUN RA et al: Autologous or allogeneic bone marrow transplantation compared with intensive chemotherapy in acute myelogenous leukemia. N Engl J Med 332:217, 1995

Robert I. Handin

116

DISORDERS OF THE PLATELET AND VESSEL WALL

Patients with platelet or vessel wall disorders usually bleed into superficial sites such as the skin, mucous membranes, or genitourinary or gastrointestinal tract. Bleeding begins immediately after trauma and either responds to simple measures such as pressure and packing or requires systemic therapy with glucocorticoids, desmopressin [1-desamino-8-D-arginine vasopressin (DDAVP)], plasma fractions, or platelet concentrates. The most common platelet/vessel wall disorders are (1) various forms of thrombocytopenia, (2) von Willebrand's disease (vWD), and (3) drug-induced platelet dysfunction. This chapter reviews the diagnosis and treatment of quantitative and qualitative platelet disorders as well as vessel wall defects that cause bleeding. →*For further discussion of the physiology of normal hemostasis and the cardinal manifestations of bleeding arising from hemostatic disorders, see Chap. 62.*

PLATELET DISORDERS

Platelets arise from the fragmentation of megakaryocytes, which are very large, polyploid bone marrow cells produced by the process of endomitosis. They undergo from three to five cycles of chromosomal duplication without cytoplasmic division. After leaving the marrow space, about one-third of the platelets are sequestered in the spleen, while the other two-thirds circulate for 7 to 10 days. Normally, only a small fraction of the platelet mass is consumed in the process of hemostasis, so most platelets circulate until they become senescent and are removed by phagocytic cells. The normal blood platelet count is 150,000 to 450,000/μl. A decrease in platelet count stimulates an increase in the number, size, and ploidy of megakaryocytes, releasing additional platelets into the circulation. This process is regulated by thrombopoietin (TPO) binding to its megakaryocyte receptor, a proto-oncogene c-mpl. TPO (c-mpl ligand) is secreted continuously at a low level and binds tightly to circulating platelets. A reduction in platelet count increases the level of free TPO and thereby stimulates megakaryocyte and platelet production.

The platelet count varies during the menstrual cycle, rising following ovulation and falling at the onset of menses. It is also influenced by the patient's nutritional state and can be decreased in severe iron, folic acid, or vitamin B_{12} deficiency. Platelets are *acute-phase reactants*, and patients with systemic inflammation, tumors, bleeding, and mild iron deficiency may have an increased platelet count, a benign condition called *secondary* or *reactive thrombocytosis*. The cytokines interleukin (IL)-3, IL-6, and IL-11 may stimulate platelet production in acute inflammation. In contrast, the increase in platelet count that is characteristic of the myeloproliferative disorders such as polycythemia vera, chronic myelogenous leukemia, myeloid metaplasia, and essential thrombocytosis can cause either severe bleeding or thrombosis. In these patients, unregulated platelet production is secondary to a clonal stem cell abnormality affecting all the bone marrow progenitors.

THROMBOCYTOPENIA Thrombocytopenia is caused by one of three mechanisms—decreased bone marrow production, increased splenic sequestration, or accelerated destruction of platelets. In order to determine the etiology of thrombocytopenia, each patient should have a careful examination of the peripheral blood film, an assessment of marrow morphology by examination of an aspirate or biopsy, and an estimate of splenic size by bedside palpation supplemented, if necessary, by ultrasonography or computed tomographic

(CT) scan. Occasional patients have "pseudothrombocytopenia," a benign condition in which platelets agglutinate or adhere to leukocytes when blood is collected with EDTA as anticoagulant. This is a laboratory artifact, and the actual platelet count in vivo is normal. A scheme for classifying patients with thrombocytopenia based on these clinical observations and laboratory tests is outlined in Fig. 116-1.

Impaired Production Disorders that injure stem cells or prevent their proliferation frequently cause thrombocytopenia. They usually affect multiple hematopoietic cell lines so that thrombocytopenia is accompanied by varying degrees of anemia and leukopenia. Diagnosis of a platelet production defect is readily established by examination of a bone marrow aspirate or biopsy, which should show a reduced number of megakaryocytes. The most common causes of decreased platelet production are marrow aplasia, fibrosis, or infiltration with malignant cells, all of which produce highly characteristic marrow abnormalities. Occasionally, thrombocytopenia is the presenting laboratory abnormality in these disorders. Cytotoxic drugs impair megakaryocyte proliferation and maturation and frequently cause thrombocytopenia. Rare marrow disorders such as congenital amegakaryocytic hypoplasia and *t*hrombocytopenia with *a*bsent *r*adii (TAR syndrome), produce a selective decrease in megakaryocyte production.

Splenic Sequestration Since one-third of the platelet mass is normally sequestered in the spleen, splenectomy will increase the platelet count by 30%. Postsplenectomy thrombocytosis is a benign self-limited condition that does not require specific therapy. In contrast, when the spleen enlarges, the fraction of sequestered platelets increases, lowering the platelet count. The most common causes of splenomegaly are portal hypertension secondary to liver disease and splenic infiltration with tumor cells in myeloproliferative or lymphoproliferative disorders (Chap. 63). Isolated splenomegaly is rare, and in most patients it is accompanied by other clinical manifestations of an underlying disease. Many patients with leukemia, lymphoma, or a myeloproliferative syndrome have both marrow infiltration and splenomegaly and develop thrombocytopenia from a combination of impaired marrow production and splenic sequestration of platelets.

Accelerated Destruction Abnormal vessels, fibrin thrombi, and intravascular prostheses can all shorten platelet survival and cause *nonimmunologic thrombocytopenia*. Thrombocytopenia is common in patients with vasculitis, the hemolytic uremic syndrome (HUS), thrombotic thrombocytopenic purpura (TTP), or as a manifestation of disseminated intravascular coagulation (DIC). In addition, platelets coated with antibody, immune complexes, or complement are rapidly cleared by mononuclear phagocytes in the spleen or other tissues, inducing *immunologic thrombocytopenia*. The most common causes of immunologic thrombocytopenia are viral or bacterial infections, drugs, and a chronic autoimmune disorder referred to as *idiopathic thrombocytopenic purpura* (ITP). Patients with immunologic thrombocytopenia do not usually have splenomegaly and have an increased number of bone marrow megakaryocytes.

DRUG-INDUCED THROMBOCYTOPENIA Many common drugs can cause thrombocytopenia (Table 116-1). Cancer chemotherapeutic agents may depress megakaryocyte production. Ingestion of large quantities of alcohol has a marrow-depressing effect leading to transient thrombocytopenia, particularly in binge drinkers. Thiazide diuretics, used to treat hypertension or congestive heart failure, impair megakaryocyte production and can produce mild thrombocytopenia (50,000 to 100,000/μL), which may persist for several months after the drug is discontinued.

Most drugs induce thrombocytopenia by eliciting an immune response in which the platelet is an innocent bystander. The platelet is damaged by complement activation following the formation of drug-antibody complexes. Current laboratory tests can identify the causative agent in 10% of patients with clinical evidence of drug-induced thrombocytopenia. The best proof of a drug-induced etiology is a prompt

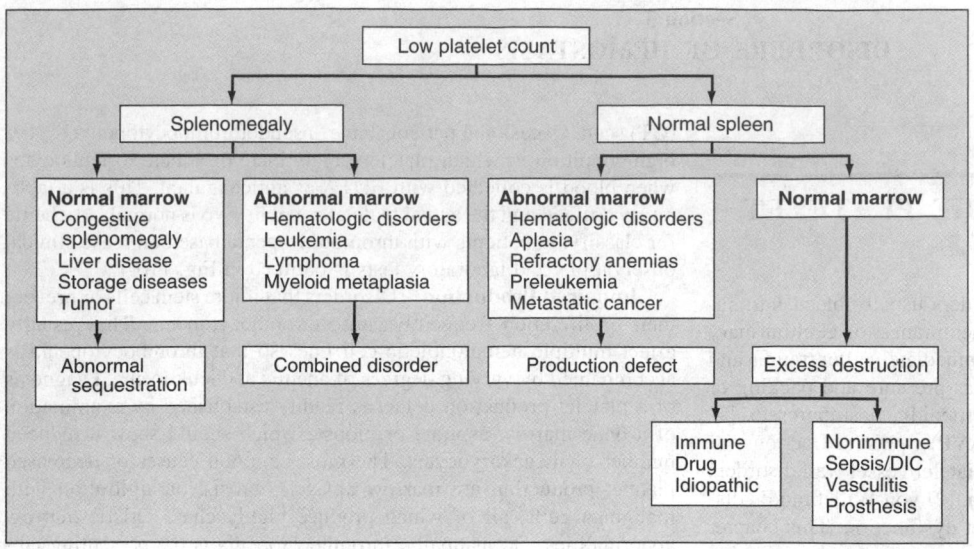

FIGURE 116-1 Clinical evaluation of patients with thrombocytopenia. [*Modified from RI Handin, in W Beck (ed), Hematology, 4th ed. Cambridge, MA, MIT Press, 1985.*]

rise in the platelet count when the suspected drug is discontinued. Patients with drug-induced platelet destruction may also have a secondary increase in megakaryocyte number without other marrow abnormalities.

Although most patients recover within 7 to 10 days and do not require therapy, occasional patients with platelet counts <10,000 to 20,000/μL have severe hemorrhage and may require temporary support with glucocorticoids, plasmapheresis, or platelet transfusions while waiting for the platelet count to rise. A patient who has recovered from drug-induced immunologic thrombocytopenia should be instructed to avoid the offending drug in the future, since only minute amounts of drug are needed to set up subsequent immune reactions. Certain drugs that are cleared from body storage depots quite slowly, such as phenytoin, may induce prolonged thrombocytopenia.

Heparin is a common cause of thrombocytopenia in hospitalized patients. Between 10 and 15% of patients receiving therapeutic doses of heparin develop thrombocytopenia and, occasionally, may have severe bleeding or intravascular platelet aggregation and paradoxical thrombosis. Heparin-induced thrombosis, sometimes called the "white clot syndrome," can be fatal unless recognized promptly. Most cases of heparin thrombocytopenia are due to drug-antibody binding to platelets; some are secondary to direct platelet agglutination by heparin. The offending antigen is a complex formed between heparin and the platelet-derived heparin neutralizing protein, platelet factor 4. Prompt cessation of heparin will reverse both thrombocytopenia and heparin-induced thrombosis. Low-molecular-weight heparin products have reduced the incidence of heparin-induced thrombocytopenia. They are effective antithrombotic agents (Chap. 118) and are less immunogenic. Unfortunately, 80 to 90% of the antibodies generated against conventional heparins cross-react with low-molecular-weight heparins, so only a minority of patients with preformed antibody can be treated with this product.

IDIOPATHIC THROMBOCYTOPENIC PURPURA The immunologic thrombocytopenias can be classified on the basis of the pathologic mechanism, the inciting agent, or the duration of the illness. The explosive onset of severe thrombocytopenia following recovery

from a viral exanthem or upper respiratory illness (*acute ITP*) is common in children and accounts for 90% of the pediatric cases of immunologic thrombocytopenia. Of these patients, 60% recover in 4 to 6 weeks and >90% recover within 3 to 6 months. Transient immunologic thrombocytopenia also complicates some cases of infectious mononucleosis, acute toxoplasmosis, or cytomegalovirus infection and can be part of the prodromal phase of viral hepatitis and initial infection with HIV. Acute ITP is rare in adults and accounts for <10% of postpubertal patients with immune thrombocytopenia. Acute ITP is caused by immune complexes containing viral antigens that bind to platelet Fc receptors or by antibodies produced against viral antigens that cross-react with the platelet. In addition to these viral disorders, the differential diagnosis includes atypical presentations of aplastic anemia, acute leukemias, or metastatic tumor. A bone marrow examination is essential to exclude these disorders, which can occasionally mimic acute ITP.

Most adults present with a more indolent form of thrombocytopenia that may persist for many years and is referred to as *chronic ITP*. Women age 20 to 40 are afflicted most commonly and outnumber men by a ratio of 3:1. They may present with an abrupt fall in platelet count and bleeding similar to patients with acute ITP. More often they have a prior history of easy bruising or menometrorrhagia. These patients have an autoimmune disorder with antibodies directed against target antigens on the glycoprotein IIb-IIIa or glycoprotein Ib-IX complex (Fig. 62-2). Although most antibodies function as opsonins and accelerate platelet clearance by phagocytic cells, occasional antibodies bind to epitopes on critical regions of these glycoproteins and impair platelet function. Platelet-associated IgG can be measured but specificity is a problem. High "background" level of IgG on normal platelets and elevations in plasma immunoglobulin levels or in circulating immune complexes will nonspecifically increase platelet-associated IgG. Few clinical situations require platelet-associated IgG testing.

A low platelet count may be the initial manifestation of systemic lupus erythematosus (SLE) or the first sign of a primary hematologic disorder. Thus, patients with chronic ITP should have a bone marrow examination and an antinuclear antibody determination. In addition, patients with hepatic or splenic enlargement, lymphadenopathy, or atypical lymphocytes should have serologic studies for hepatitis viruses, cytomegalovirus, Epstein-Barr virus, toxoplasma, and HIV. HIV infection is a common cause of immunologic thrombocytopenia. Thrombocytopenia can be the initial symptom of HIV infection or a complication of fully developed clinical AIDS.

TREATMENT Treatment of patients with ITP must take into account the age of the patient, the severity of the illness, and the anticipated natural history. Although adults have a higher incidence of intracranial bleeding than children, specific therapy may not be necessary unless the platelet count is <20,000/μL or there is extensive bleeding. Hemorrhage in patients with either acute or chronic ITP can usually be controlled with glucocorticoids but, in rare cases, may require temporary phagocytic blockade with intravenous immunoglobulin (IVIG) or anti-RhD (WinRho). Although antibody preparations are effective, they are expensive and should be reserved for patients with severe thrombocytopenia and clinical bleeding who are refractory to other measures. Emergency splenectomy is usually reserved for patients with acute or chronic ITP who are desperately ill and have not responded to any medical measures. The treatment of symptomatic thrombocytopenia in patients with HIV infection is more complex be-

Table 116-1 Drugs that May Cause Thrombocytopenia

1. Chemotherapeutic agents—especially carboplatin, alkylating agents, anthracyclines, antimetabolites
2. Antibiotics—sulfonamides, penicillins, cephalosporins
3. Heparins—highest incidence is with unfractionated products
4. Cardiovascular agents—thiazide diuretics, rarely angiotensin converting enzyme inhibitors

cause the administration of glucocorticoids or splenectomy may increase susceptibility to opportunistic infections. Splenectomy has been effective in the course of HIV before the onset of symptomatic AIDS. Treatment with zidovudine (AZT) and other antiviral agents that reduce viral load can improve the platelet count in patients with HIV-induced thrombocytopenia.

Symptomatic patients with chronic ITP are usually placed on prednisone, 60 mg/d for 4 to 6 weeks. The drug is then decreased slowly over another few weeks. About 50% of patients with chronic ITP will normalize their platelet count on high doses of prednisone. However, the majority will have a fall in platelet count following steroid withdrawal. Patients with chronic ITP who fail to maintain a normal platelet count after a course of prednisone are eligible for elective splenectomy. These steroid-responsive but steroid-dependent patients are very likely to respond to splenectomy, and 70% will have a normal platelet count within 1 week after surgery. Some patients who do not respond to glucocorticoids may still respond to splenectomy. Occasionally, patients may fail to respond to splenectomy because of the failure to remove an accessory spleen. In other patients, a small, inactive accessory spleen may grow or new splenic foci may develop from splenic cells shed at the time of surgery and cause the late onset of thrombocytopenia. In either case, the presence of splenic tissue can be diagnosed by examination of the blood smear for Howell-Jolly bodies that appear in the red cells of asplenic individuals. Persistent splenic tissue can be confirmed by a radionuclide scan.

Patients still thrombocytopenic after splenectomy or who relapse months to years after initial therapy have received a variety of immunosuppressive drugs including azathioprine, cyclophosphamide, vincristine, vinblastine, and cyclosporine. Danazol has also been used with some success. Although each of these drugs may be beneficial, they have serious side effects and should be used judiciously. IVIG and anti-RhD are only transiently effective and expensive. IVIG can cause meningismus and headache, and some lots have carried hepatitis C virus. Anti-RhD can cause hemolysis. These drugs should be used to raise the platelet count temporarily and to support patients before surgery or labor and delivery; they are not substitutes for splenectomy. If a patient is not bleeding and maintains a platelet count >20,000/μL, consideration should be given to withholding therapy. Patients with severe chronic thrombocytopenia may live with their disease for two or three decades.

FUNCTIONAL PLATELET DISORDERS

As described in Chap. 62, normal hemostasis requires three critical platelet reactions—adhesion, aggregation, and granule release. Clinical bleeding can result from a failure of any of these important functions. Table 116-2 lists the major functional platelet disorders. Table 116-3 lists methods to assess platelet function.

Von Willebrand's Disease vWD is the most common inherited bleeding disorder, occurring in 1 in 800 to 1000 individuals. The von Willebrand factor (vWF) is a heterogeneous multimeric plasma glycoprotein with two major functions: (1) It facilitates platelet adhesion under conditions of high shear stress by linking platelet membrane receptors to vascular subendothelium; and (2) it serves as the plasma carrier for factor VIII, the antihemophilic factor, a critical blood coagulation protein. Discrete domains in each vWF subunit mediate each of these important functions. The normal plasma vWF level is 10 mg/L. The vWF activity is distributed among a series of plasma multimers with estimated molecular weights ranging from 400,000 to >20 million. A single large vWF precursor subunit is synthesized in endothelial cells and megakaryocytes, where it is cleaved and assembled into the disulfide-linked multimers present in plasma, platelets, and vascular subendothelium. A modest reduction in plasma vWF concentration or a selective loss in the high-molecular-weight multimers decreases platelet adhesion and causes clinical bleeding.

Although vWD is heterogeneous, certain clinical features are common to all the syndromes. With one exception (type III disease), all forms are inherited as autosomal dominant traits, and affected patients are heterozygous with one normal and one abnormal vWF allele. In

Table 116-2 Classification of Functional Platelet Disorders

I. Disorders of adhesion
   A. Inherited
      1. Bernard-Soulier syndrome
      2. von Willebrand's disease (vWD)
   B. Acquired
      1. Uremia
      2. Acquired vWD
II. Disorders of aggregation
   A. Inherited
      1. Glanzmann's thrombasthenia
      2. Afibrinogenemia
   B. Acquired
      1. Fibrin degradation product inhibition
      2. Dysproteinemias
      3. Drugs—e.g., ticlopidine, Gp IIb/IIIa inhibitors
III. Disorders of granule release
   A. Inherited
      1. Oculocutaneous albinism (Hermansky-Pudlak syndrome)
      2. Chédiak-Higashi syndrome
      3. Isolated dense (δ) granule deficiency
      4. Gray-platelet syndrome—combined α and β granule deficiency
   B. Acquired
      1. Cardiopulmonary bypass
      2. Myeloproliferative disorders
      3. Drugs—aspirin and other nonsteroidal anti-inflammatory agents

mild cases, bleeding occurs only after surgery or trauma. More severely affected patients have spontaneous epistaxis or oral mucosal, gastrointestinal, or genitourinary bleeding. The laboratory findings are variable. The most diagnostic pattern is the combination of (1) a prolonged bleeding time, (2) a reduction in plasma vWF concentration, (3) a parallel reduction in biologic activity as measured with the ristocetin cofactor assay, and (4) reduced factor VIII activity. The variability in laboratory tests is related to both the heterogeneous nature of the defects in vWD and the fact that plasma levels are influenced by ABO blood group type, central nervous system disorders, systemic inflammation, and pregnancy. Since vWD is an autosomal dominant disorder, some vWF is produced by the remaining normal allele. Thus patients with mild defects may have laboratory values that fluctuate over time and may occasionally be within the normal range.

There are three major types of vWD. Their mode of inheritance and laboratory findings are shown in Fig. 116-2. Patients with *type I disease*, the most common abnormality, have a mild to moderate de-

Table 116-3 Evaluation of Platelet Function

Bleeding time
  Modified Ivy method
  Skin incision—time to stop bleeding
  Global screen of platelet role in hemostasis
von Willebrand factor assays
  vWF Ag—immunoassay of total vWF protein
  vWF R:Cof—bioassay of vWF that measures ability of patient plasma to support agglutination of normal platelets in the presence of ristocetin
  Factor VIII—coagulation assay of factor VIII bound and carried by plasma vWF
Platelet aggregometry
  Measures platelet aggregation in response to a panel of agonists, usually ADP, collagen, arachidonic acid, and epinephrine
Membrane glycoproteins
  Presence of glycoproteins Ib-IX and IIb-IIIa can be measured using monoclonal antibodies and flow cytometry
Platelet granule content
  Dense granules—electron microscopy or uptake and retention of radiolabeled serotonin
  Alpha granules—electron microscopy and/or immunoassays for platelet-associated proteins—vWF, fibrinogen, platelet factor four

NOTE: vWF, von Willebrand factor; ADP, adenosine diphosphate; Ag, antigen, R:Cof, ristocetin cofactor.

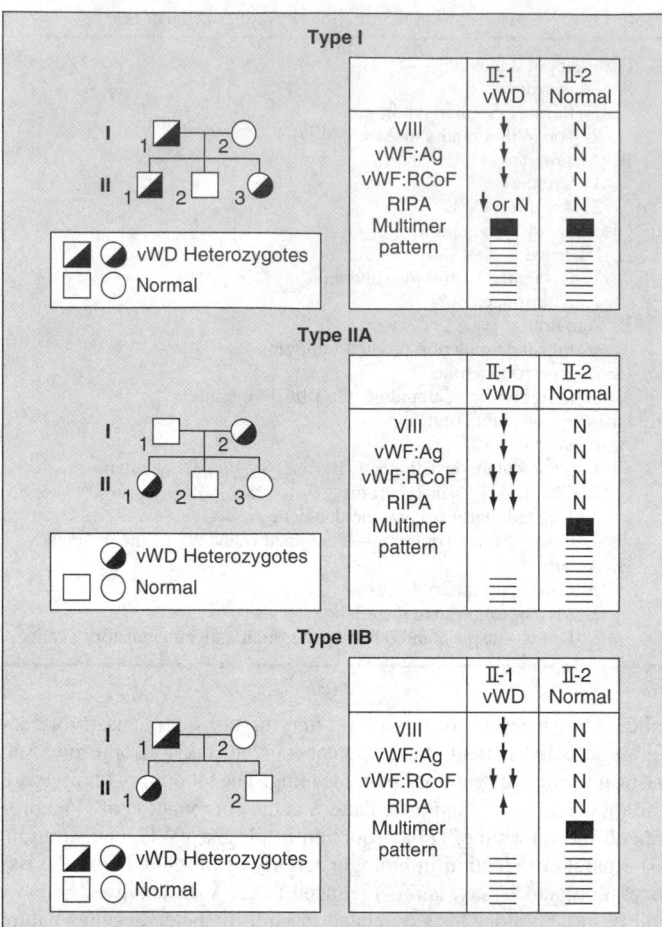

FIGURE 116-2 Pattern of inheritance and laboratory findings in von Willebrand's disease. The assays of platelet function include a coagulation assay of factor VIII bound and carried by von Willebrand factor (vWF), abbreviated as VIII; immunoassay of total vWF protein, abbreviated vWF:Ag; bioassay of the ability of patient plasma to support ristocetin-induced agglutination of normal platelets, abbreviated vWF:RCoF; and ristocetin-induced aggregation of patient platelets, abbreviated RIPA. The multimer pattern illustrates the protein bonds present when plasma is electrophoresed in a polyacrylamide gel. The II-1 and II-2 columns refer to the phenotypes of the second-generation offspring.

crease in plasma vWF. In the milder cases, although hemostasis is impaired, the vWF level is just below normal (50% activity, or 5 mg/L). In type I disease, vWF antigen, factor VIII activity, and ristocetin cofactor activity are decreased with a normal spectrum of multimers detected by sodium dodecyl sulfate (SDS)–agarose gel electrophoresis.

The variant forms of vWD (*type II disease*) are much less common and characterized by normal or near-normal levels of a dysfunctional protein. Patients with the *type IIa variant* of vWD have a deficiency in the high- and medium-molecular-weight forms of vWF multimer detected by SDS-agarose electrophoresis. This is due either to an inability to secrete the high-molecular-weight vWF multimers or to proteolysis of the multimers soon after they leave the endothelial cell and enter the circulation. Mutations in a localized region of the vWF A-2 domain have been identified in families with type IIa vWD (Fig. 116-3). The quantity of vWF antigen and the amount of associated factor VIII are usually normal. In the *type IIb variant*, high-molecular-weight multimers are also decreased; however, the decrease is due to the inappropriate binding of vWF to platelets. Intravascular platelet aggregates form that are rapidly cleared from the circulation, causing mild, variable thrombocytopenia. Mutations in a disulfide-bonded loop in the A-1 domain that binds to glycoprotein Ib-IX are the cause of the type IIb defect (Fig. 116-3). A few patients have a platelet mem-

brane disorder that mimics type IIb vWD—*platelet-type vWD*. It is due to mutations in the portion of glycoprotein Ib-IX that interacts with vWF. Levels of total vWF antigen and factor VIII are normal.

Approximately 1 in 1 million individuals has a very severe form of vWD that is phenotypically recessive (*type III disease*). Type III patients are usually the offspring of two parents (usually asymptomatic) with mild type I disease. Type III patients may inherit a different abnormality from each parent (a doubly heterozygous or compound heterozygous state) or be homozygous for a single defect. Type III patients have severe mucosal bleeding and no detectable vWF antigen or activity and, like patients with mild hemophilia, may have sufficiently low factor VIII that they have occasional hemarthroses. Major deletions in the vWF gene have been found in some type III families. Families with nonsense mutations and the combination of a deleted and nonsense mutant allele have also been described.

Type IIN disease is due to a defect in the factor VIII binding site of vWF. Patients resemble those with mild hemophilia and have low levels of factor VIII. The presence of disease in both males and females in a family is a clue to the role of vWF in this disease.

℞ TREATMENT There are two therapeutic options. Factor VIII concentrates retain high-molecular-weight vWF multimers (Humate-P, Alfanate), are highly purified and heat-treated to destroy HIV, and are appropriate treatments for all the inherited forms of vWD. During surgery or after major trauma, patients should receive factor VIII concentrates twice daily for 2 or 3 days to assure optimal hemostasis. Minor bleeding episodes such as prolonged epistaxis or severe menorrhagia may respond to a single infusion. Recurrent menorrhagia, a major problem for women with severe vWD, can be treated effectively with oral contraceptive agents that suppress menses.

A second therapeutic option, which avoids the use of plasma, is the use of DDAVP or desmopressin, a vasopressin analogue that has minimal blood pressure–elevating and fluid-retaining properties and raises the plasma vWF level in both normal individuals and patients with mild vWD. Patients with type I disease are the best candidates for DDAVP therapy. However, they must be tested for an adequate response before anticipated surgery, and vWF levels must be monitored closely during therapy, since the patient may develop tachyphylaxis when therapy is continued for more than 48 h. DDAVP should not be given to patients with variant forms of vWD without prior testing, since it may not improve multimer pattern or hemostasis in type IIa patients and may actually worsen the defect by depleting high-molecular-weight multimers, inducing intravascular platelet aggregation, and lowering the platelet count in type IIb patients. It is ineffective therapy for the severe (type III) form of vWD.

Acquired vWD Although most cases of vWD are inherited, acquired vWD may be caused by antibodies that inhibit vWF function or by lymphoid or other tumors that selectively adsorb vWF multimers onto their surfaces. Anti-vWF antibodies have developed in patients with severe vWD following multiple transfusions, as well as in patients with autoimmune and lymphoproliferative disorders. Adsorption of vWF to tumor surfaces has been documented in patients with Waldenström's macroglobulinemia and Wilms' tumor and inferred in other patients with lymphoma. Treatment of acquired vWD should focus on the underlying disease, since plasma derivatives and DDAVP are often not effective and the disorder can be fatal.

Platelet Membrane Defects Receptors that modulate platelet adhesion and aggregation are located on the two major platelet surface glycoproteins. vWF facilitates platelet adhesion by binding to glycoprotein Ib-IX, while fibrinogen links platelets into aggregates via sites on the glycoprotein IIb-IIIa complex. Two rare platelet defects are characterized by a loss of or a defect in these glycoprotein receptors. Patients with the *Bernard-Soulier syndrome* have markedly reduced platelet adhesion and cannot bind vWF to their platelets due to deficiency or dysfunction of the glycoprotein Ib-IX complex. They also have reduced levels of several other membrane proteins, mild thrombocytopenia, and extremely large, lymphocytoid platelets. Platelets from patients with *Glanzmann's disease* or *thrombasthenia* are deficient or defective in the glycoprotein IIb-IIIa complex. Their platelets do not bind fibrinogen and cannot form aggregates, although the platelets undergo shape change and secretion and are of normal size.

Both these disorders are autosomal recessive traits and are characterized by markedly impaired hemostasis and recurrent episodes of severe mucosal hemorrhage. Bernard-Soulier platelets react normally to all stimuli except ristocetin. In contrast, thrombasthenic platelets adhere normally and will agglutinate with ristocetin but will not aggregate with any of the agonists that require fibrinogen binding, such as adenosine diphosphate (ADP), thrombin, or epinephrine.

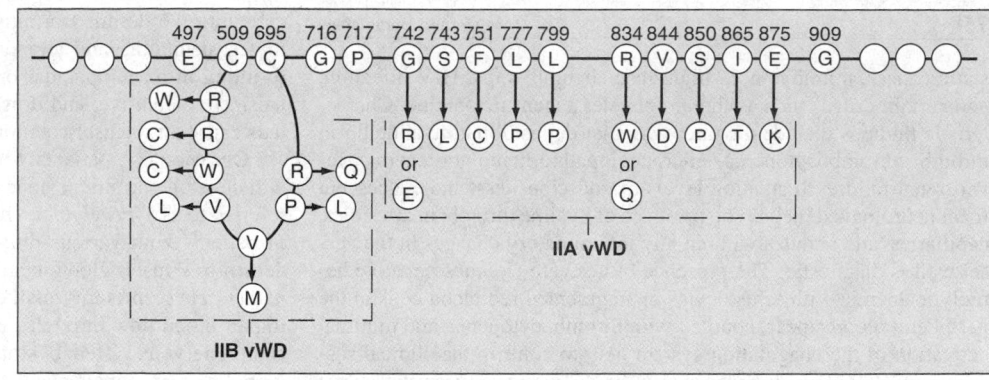

FIGURE 116-3 Location of mutations in types IIa and IIb von Willebrand's disease. Mutations in the region of the protein between amino acids 742 and 875 have been identified in patients with type IIa disease. These result in a deficiency in high- and medium-molecular-weight multimers due either to failure to secrete high-molecular-weight forms of vWF or to their proteolytic degradation in the circulation. In type IIb disease, there is also a decrease in high-molecular-weight vWF, but the defect is due to the failure of vWF with mutations in the A-1 domain of the protein (amino acids 509–695) to bind properly to platelet glycoprotein Ib-IX.

The only effective therapy for hemorrhagic episodes in these two disorders is transfusion with normal platelets. Alloimmunization will eventually limit the life span of infused platelets. In addition, a few patients have developed inhibitor antibodies with specificity for the missing protein. These antibodies bind to the protein that is expressed on the transfused normal platelets and impair their function.

Platelet Release Defects The most common mild bleeding disorders arise from the ingestion of aspirin and other nonsteroidal antiinflammatory drugs (NSAIDs) that inhibit platelet production of thromboxane A_2, an important mediator of platelet secretion and aggregation (Figs. 62-3 and 62-4). These drugs inhibit cyclooxygenase, which converts arachidonic acid to a labile endoperoxide intermediate that is critical for thromboxane formation. Aspirin is the most potent agent, since it irreversibly acetylates the platelet enzyme so that a single dose impairs hemostasis for 5 to 7 days. The other agents are competitive and reversible inhibitors with more transient effects. Blocking thromboxane A_2 synthesis partially inhibits platelet release and aggregation with weak agonists, such as ADP and epinephrine, and produces a mild hemostatic defect. The administration of high doses of certain antibiotics, particularly penicillin, can coat the platelet surface, block platelet release, and impair hemostasis.

Patients generally have minimal symptoms such as easy bruising, and bleeding is usually confined to the skin. Occasional patients will have prolonged oozing after surgery, particularly with procedures involving mucous membranes such as periodontal, oral, or reconstructive plastic surgery. The antiplatelet effect of drugs such as aspirin is more dramatic when they are administered to patients with underlying defects such as vWD or hemophilia. Patients with drug-induced cyclooxygenase deficiency often have a mildly prolonged bleeding time, and their platelets fail to aggregate when incubated with arachidonic acid, epinephrine, or low doses of ADP. Patients who have taken aspirin should be treated as if they have a mild hemostatic defect for the next 5 to 7 days. Platelet responses to collagen and thrombin are impaired at low doses but normal at higher doses. Symptomatic patients should be encouraged to use drugs such as acetaminophen that do not impair platelet function. Although most cases of cyclooxygenase deficiency are drug-induced, occasional patients have inherited disorders in platelet cyclooxygenase activity that impair thromboxane production or receptor level defects that prevent platelets from responding to thromboxane A_2.

Of the metabolic disorders that can perturb hemostasis, uremic platelet dysfunction is clinically the most important. The mechanism by which uremia impairs platelet function is not well understood, and retention of phenolic and guanidinosuccinic acids, excess prostacyclin production, or impaired vWF-platelet interactions have all been implicated. The degree of uremia correlates with bleeding symptoms and anemia. Bleeding can usually be reversed by dialysis and often improves after red cell transfusion or treatment with erythropoietin. In addition, factor VIII concentrate or DDAVP, both of which raise plasma vWF levels, can also improve hemostasis. Conjugated estrogens improve hemostasis and can be used as long-term therapy.

Storage Pool Defects Platelet granules have considerable amounts of adenine nucleotides, calcium, and adhesive glycoproteins such as thrombospondin, fibronectin, and vWF, all of which promote platelet adhesion and aggregation. Patients with defective platelet granules have a mild bleeding disorder. Platelet storage pool defects may be inherited as an isolated disorder or be part of systemic granule packaging defects such as oculocutaneous albinism or the Hermansky-Pudlak or Chédiak-Higashi syndromes. Clinically, these patients cannot be distinguished from those with other functional platelet disorders, since they all have easy bruising, mucosal bleeding, and a prolonged bleeding time. They can be differentiated from patients with the cyclooxygenase defects because their platelets will usually aggregate in response to arachidonic acid. In addition, their platelets have decreased levels of specific granule constituents such as ADP and serotonin and abnormalities in granule morphology that are best visualized by electron microscopy.

Occasionally, patients with acute or chronic leukemia or one of the myeloproliferative disorders develop an acquired storage pool disorder due to dysplastic megakaryocyte development. In addition, patients with liver disease and some patients with SLE or other immune complex–mediated disorders may have circulating platelets that have degranulated prematurely. Platelet degranulation and a transient storage pool disorder may occur after prolonged cardiopulmonary bypass. Fortunately, most patients with storage pool defects have only mildly impaired hemostasis. They can be treated with platelet transfusions. Occasional patients have responded to DDAVP.

VESSEL WALL DISORDERS

Bleeding from vascular disorders (nonthrombocytopenic purpura) is usually mild and confined to the skin and mucous membranes. The pathogenesis of bleeding is poorly defined in many of the syndromes, and classic tests of hemostasis, including the bleeding time and tests of platelet function, are usually normal. Vascular purpura arises from damage to capillary endothelium, abnormalities in the vascular subendothelial matrix or extravascular connective tissues that support blood vessels, or from the formation of abnormal blood vessels. Several idiopathic disorders involve the vessel wall and can cause more severe bleeding and organ dysfunction.

THROMBOTIC THROMBOCYTOPENIC PURPURA TTP is a fulminant, often lethal disorder that may be initiated by endothelial injury and subsequent release of vWF and other procoagulant materials from the endothelial cell. Causes include pregnancy, metastatic cancer, mitomycin C, high-dose chemotherapy, HIV infection, and certain drugs, such as the antiplatelet angent ticlopidine. Characteristic findings include the microvascular deposition of hyaline fibrin thrombi, thrombocytopenia, microangiopathic hemolytic anemia, fever, renal failure, fluctuating levels of consciousness, and evanescent focal neurologic deficits. The presence of hyaline thrombi in arterioles, capillaries, and venules without any inflammatory changes in the vessel wall is diagnostic. The presence of a severe Coombs-negative hemolytic anemia with schistocytes or fragmented red blood cells in the peripheral blood smear, coupled with thrombocytopenia, and minimal activation of the coagulation system help to confirm the clinical suspicion of TTP. This disorder should be distinguished from vasculitis and SLE, which can predispose patients to TTP. Platelet-associated IgG and complement levels are usually normal in TTP.

The treatment of acute TTP has focused on the use of exchange transfusion or intensive plasmapheresis coupled with infusion of fresh frozen plasma. Patients with TTP become transiently deficient in a plasma enzyme that depolymerizes ultra-high-molecular-weight vWF released from endothelial cells. Therapy may remove abnormal forms of vWF and replenish the deficient enzyme. Overall mortality has been markedly reduced, and the majority of patients with TTP recover from this formerly fatal disorder. Most patients surviving the acute illness recover completely, with no residual renal or neurologic disease. Occasional patients with a chronic, relapsing form of TTP require maintenance plasmapheresis and plasma infusion, and a few patients are controlled only with glucocorticoids.

HEMOLYTIC-UREMIC SYNDROME HUS is a disease of infancy and early childhood that closely resembles TTP. Patients present with fever, thrombocytopenia, microangiopathic hemolytic anemia, hypertension, and varying degrees of acute renal failure. In many cases, onset is preceded by a minor febrile or viral illness, and an infectious or immune complex–mediated cause has been proposed. Epidemics related to infection with a specific strain of *Escherichia coli* (O157:H7) have been documented. As in TTP, disseminated intravascular coagulation is not found. In contrast to TTP, the disorder remains localized to the kidney, where hyaline thrombi are seen in the afferent arterioles and glomerular capillaries. Such thrombi are not present in other vessels, and neurologic symptoms, other than those associated with uremia, are uncommon. No therapy is proven effective; however, with dialysis for acute renal failure, the initial mortality is only 5%. Between 10 and 50% of patients have some chronic renal impairment.

HENOCH-SCHÖNLEIN PURPURA Henoch-Schönlein, or anaphylactoid, purpura is a distinct, self-limited type of vasculitis that occurs in children and young adults. Patients have an acute inflammatory reaction in capillaries, mesangial tissues, and small arterioles that leads to increased vascular permeability, exudation, and hemorrhage. Vessel lesions contain IgA and complement components. The syndrome may be preceded by an upper respiratory infection or streptococcal pharyngitis or be associated with food or drug allergies. Patients develop a purpuric or urticarial rash on the extensor surfaces of the arms and legs and on the buttocks as well as polyarthralgias or arthritis, colicky abdominal pain, and hematuria from focal glomerulonephritis. Despite the hemorrhagic features, all coagulation tests are normal. A small number of patients may develop fatal acute renal failure, and 5 to 10% develop chronic nephritis. Glucocorticoids provide symptomatic relief of the joint and abdominal pains but do not alter the course of the illness.

METABOLIC AND INFLAMMATORY DISORDERS Acute febrile illnesses may cause capillary fragility and skin bleeding. Immune complexes containing viral antigens or the viruses themselves may damage endothelial cells. In addition, certain pathogens such as the rickettsiae that cause Rocky Mountain spotted fever replicate in endothelial cells and damage them. Thrombocytopenia is also a frequent finding in acute infectious disorders and may contribute to skin bleeding. In addition, whenever the platelet count is $<10,000/\mu L$, gaps develop between endothelial cells, which allow the diapedesis of red cells into the dermis, forming petechiae. Drugs such as the sulfonamides, penicillin, and allopurinol may cause vascular inflammation, resulting in maculopapular or urticarial rashes. Some of these mechanisms are additive, and drug reactions in thrombocytopenic individuals cause an intensely hemorrhagic rash.

Occasionally, patients with diffuse polyclonal hyperglobulinemia will develop purpuric lesions on the lower limbs—a benign condition referred to as *hyperglobulinemic purpura*. Vascular purpura may occur in patients with various monoclonal gammopathies, including Waldenström's macroglobulinemia, multiple myeloma, and cryoglobulinemia. These proteins markedly increase serum viscosity and may impair blood flow through capillaries and lead to retinal hemorrhage, central nervous system dysfunction, and skin necrosis. In addition, the globulins may impair platelet aggregation and adhesion and interfere with fibrin polymerization. Patients with mixed cryoglobulinemia develop a more extensive maculopapular lesion due to immune complex–mediated damage to the vessel wall. The mixed cryoglobulinemia (usually IgG and anti-IgG) may be associated with arthralgias, diffuse weakness, and unexplained nephritis. Plasmapheresis will temporarily lower the level of globulins, remove immune complexes, and improve symptoms in these patients. However, long-term management must include control of the underlying disease that produces the abnormal globulins or immune complexes.

Patients with *scurvy* (vitamin C deficiency) develop painful episodes of perifollicular skin bleeding as well as bleeding into muscles and, occasionally, into the gastrointestinal and genitourinary tracts. The diagnosis is confirmed by the presence of hyperkeratosis of skin, gum swelling, and low levels of the vitamin in leukocytes. Vitamin C is needed to synthesize hydroxyproline, an essential constituent of collagen. Thus, collagen synthesis is impaired by scurvy. Patients with *Cushing's syndrome*, an excess production of glucocorticoids, or patients on large doses of glucocorticoids develop generalized protein wasting and may show skin bleeding or easy bruising due to atrophy of the supporting connective tissue around blood vessels. Aging causes a similar atrophy of perivascular connective tissue on the extensor surfaces of the hands and arms, leading to *senile purpura*—dark purple, irregularly shaped hemorrhagic areas due to abnormal skin mobility that tears small blood vessels.

Patients with inherited disorders of the connective tissue matrix such as *Marfan's syndrome*, *Ehlers-Danlos syndrome*, and *pseudoxanthoma elasticum* also have easy bruising. In addition to having fragile skin vessels and easy bruising, patients with Ehlers-Danlos syndrome may develop aneurysms in intraabdominal vessels and apoplectic rupture and hemorrhage due to defects in the vascular collagen network. Primary vascular abnormalities can also lead to bleeding. Patients with *Osler-Weber-Rendu disease* (hereditary hemorrhagic telangiectasia), an inherited autosomal dominant disorder, have frequent episodes of nasal and gastrointestinal bleeding from abnormal telangiectatic capillaries. They may develop pulmonary arteriovenous fistulas. Two genetic defects have been identified in these patients both involving proteins that bind to transforming growth factor β (TGF-β); HHT-1 has mutations in endoglin, and HHT-2 has mutations in ALK-1. Patients with *angiodysplasia* of the colon have increased incidence of gastrointestinal bleeding. In the *Kasabach-Merritt syndrome*, patients may have very extensive and progressively enlarging vascular malformation that may involve large portions of their extremities. Bleeding is secondary to disseminated intravascular coagulation triggered by stagnant blood flow through the tortuous vessels.

BIBLIOGRAPHY

AMERICAN SOCIETY OF HEMATOLOGY PRACTICE GUIDELINE PANEL: Diagnosis and treatment of idiopathic thrombocytopenic purpura. Ann Intern Med 126:316, 1997

EWENSTEIN BM, HANDIN RI: von Willebrand's disease, in *Blood: Principles and Practice of Hematology*, RI Handin et al (eds). Philadelphia, Lippincott, 1994, pp 1069–1094

KELTON JG: The clinical management of heparin-induced thrombocytopenia. Semin Hematol 36:17, 1999

WARKENTON TE, KELTON J: The platelet life cycle: Quantitative disorders in blood, in *Blood: Principles and Practice of Hematology*, RI Handin et al (eds). Philadelphia, Lippincott, 1994, pp 973–1049

DISORDERS OF COAGULATION AND THROMBOSIS

Patients with congenital plasma coagulation defects characteristically bleed into muscles, joints, and body cavities hours or days after an injury. Most of the *inherited* plasma coagulation disorders are due to defects in single coagulation proteins, with the two X-linked disorders, factors VIII and IX deficiency, accounting for the majority. These patients may have severe bleeding and chronic disability and require specialized medical therapy. With rare exceptions, the known disorders prolong either the prothrombin time (PT), partial thromboplastin time (PTT), or both. If they are abnormal, quantitative assays of specific coagulation proteins are then carried out using the PT or PTT tests with plasma from congenitally deficient individuals as substrate. The corrective effect of varying concentrations of patient plasma is measured and expressed as a percentage of a normal pooled plasma standard. The interval range for most coagulation factors is from 50 to 150% of this average value, and the minimal level of most individual factors needed for adequate hemostasis is 25%.

Acquired coagulation disorders are both more frequent and more complex, arising from deficiencies of multiple coagulation proteins and simultaneously affecting both primary and secondary hemostasis. The most common acquired hemorrhagic disorders are (1) disseminated intravascular coagulation (DIC), (2) the hemorrhagic diathesis of liver disease, and (3) vitamin K deficiency and complications of anticoagulant therapy.

Although congenital and acquired bleeding disorders are relatively rare, venous and arterial thrombosis and embolism are common medical disorders that have been recognized for >100 years. Although risk factors such as atherosclerotic vascular disease, congestive heart failure, malignancy, and immobility predispose patients to thrombosis, specific coagulation defects have not yet been identified in most patients with thromboembolism. Several inherited coagulation abnormalities induce a hypercoagulable or prethrombotic state and predispose patients to thrombosis. These disorders affect young people, cause recurrent episodes of thromboembolism, and may involve multiple members of a single family. An understanding of the biochemical basis of thromboembolism is also important because anticoagulant and antithrombotic regimens are based on the premise that modifying critical coagulation reactions will reduce the incidence of thrombosis. →*For further discussion of the physiology of normal hemostasis and the cardinal manifestations of the hemorrhagic and thrombotic disorders, see Chap. 62.*

FACTOR VIII DEFICIENCY—HEMOPHILIA A Pathogenesis and Clinical Manifestations The antihemophilic factor (AHF), or factor VIII coagulant protein, is a large (265-kDa), single-chain protein that regulates the activation of factor X by proteases generated in the intrinsic coagulation pathway (Figs. 62-5 and 62-6). It is synthesized in liver and circulates complexed to the von Willebrand factor (vWF) protein. Factor VIII molecule is present in low concentration (10 μg/L) and is susceptible to proteolysis. The gene for factor VIII is on the X chromosome, and carrier detection and prenatal diagnosis are well established.

One in 10,000 males is born with deficiency or dysfunction of the factor VIII molecule. The resulting disorder, *hemophilia A*, is characterized by bleeding into soft tissues, muscles, and weight-bearing joints. Symptomatic patients usually have factor VIII levels <5%, with a close correlation between the clinical severity of hemophilia and plasma AHF level. Patients with <1% factor VIII activity have *severe* disease; they bleed frequently even without discernible trauma. Patients with levels of 1 to 5% have *moderate* disease with less frequent bleeding episodes. Those with levels >5% have *mild* disease with infrequent bleeding that is usually secondary to trauma. Occasional patients with factor VIII levels as high as 25% are discovered when they bleed after major trauma or surgery. The majority of patients with hemophilia A have factor VIII levels below <5%.

Hemophilic bleeding occurs hours or days after injury, can involve any organ, and, if untreated, may continue for days or weeks. This can result in large collections of partially clotted blood putting pressure on adjacent normal tissues and can cause necrosis of muscle (compartment syndromes), venous congestion (pseudophlebitis), or ischemic damage to nerves. Patients with hemophilia often develop femoral neuropathy due to pressure from an unsuspected retroperitoneal hematoma. They can also develop large calcified masses of blood and inflammatory tissue that are mistaken for cancers (pseudotumor syndrome).

Patients with severe hemophilia are usually diagnosed shortly after birth because of an extensive cephalhematoma or profuse bleeding at circumcision. However, young children with moderate disease may not bleed until they begin to walk or crawl, and individuals with mild hemophilia may not be diagnosed until they are adolescents or young adults. Typically, a hemophilia patient presents with pain followed by swelling in a weight-bearing joint, such as the hip, knee, or ankle. The presence of blood in the joint (*hemarthrosis*) causes synovial inflammation, and repetitive bleeding erodes articular cartilage and causes osteoarthritis, articular fibrosis, joint ankylosis, and eventually muscle atrophy. Bleeding may occur into any joint, but after a joint has been damaged, it may become a site for subsequent bleeding episodes.

Hematuria, without any genitourinary pathology, is also common. It is usually self-limited and may not require specific therapy. The most feared complications of hemophilia are oropharyngeal and central nervous system bleeding. Patients with oropharyngeal bleeding may require emergency intubation to maintain an adequate airway. Central nervous system bleeding can occur without antecedent trauma or without evidence of a specific lesion.

Patients suspected of having hemophilia should have a platelet count, bleeding time, PT, and PTT. Typically, the patient will have a prolonged PTT with all other tests normal. Because of the clinical similarity of factor VIII deficiency and factor IX deficiency, any male with an appropriate bleeding history and a prolonged PTT should have specific assays for factor VIII and factor IX.

℞ TREATMENT Tenets regarding the treatment of bleeding in hemophilia patients include the following: (1) Symptoms often precede objective evidence of bleeding. (2) Signs of bleeding may not appear until several days after well-documented trauma. The patients can generally be relied upon to identify early symptoms, usually pain. Early treatment is more effective, less costly, and can be lifesaving. (3) Avoid the use of aspirin or aspirin-containing drugs, which impair platelet function and may cause severe hemorrhage. COX-2 inhibitors can be used, as they do not impair platelet function.

Plasma products enriched in factor VIII have revolutionized the care of hemophilia patients, reduced the degree of orthopedic deformity, and permitted virtually any form of elective and emergency surgery. The widespread use of factor VIII concentrates has also produced serious complications, including viral hepatitis, chronic liver disease, and AIDS. *Cryoprecipitate*, which contains about half the factor VIII activity of fresh-frozen plasma in one-tenth the original volume, is simple to prepare and is produced in hospital or regional blood banks.

Three developments have increased the safety of factor VIII therapy and have changed medical practice. First, heating of lyophilized factor VIII concentrates under carefully controlled conditions can inactivate HIV without destroying factor VIII activity. Second, highly purified factor VIII can be produced by adsorbing and eluting factor VIII from monoclonal antibody columns. Third, recombinant factor VIII is now available. Patients with hemophilia should receive either monoclonal purified or recombinant factor VIII to minimize viral infections and exposure to irrelevant proteins.

Each unit of factor VIII infused, defined as the amount present in 1 mL normal plasma, will raise the plasma level of the recipient by

2%/kg of body weight. Factor VIII has a half-life of 8 to 12 h, making it necessary to infuse it continuously or at least twice daily to sustain a chosen factor VIII level. In patients with mild hemophilia, an alternative treatment is desmopressin (DDAVP), which transiently increases the factor VIII level. DDAVP will increase the factor level two- to threefold. Although generally safe, it occasionally causes hyponatremia or may precipitate thrombosis in elderly patients.

An uncomplicated episode of soft tissue bleeding or an early hemarthrosis can be treated with one infusion of sufficient factor VIII concentrate to raise the factor VIII level to 15 or 20%. A more extensive hemarthrosis or retroperitoneal bleeding requires twice-daily or continuous infusions in order to keep the factor VIII level at 25 to 50% for at least 72 h. Life-threatening bleeding into the central nervous system or major surgery may require therapy for 2 weeks with levels kept at a minimum of 50% normal. Patients also need skilled orthopedic care, with immobilization of inflamed joints to promote healing and to prevent contractures, and physical therapy to strengthen muscles and maintain joint mobility.

Before surgery, every hemophilia patient should be screened for the presence of an inhibitor to factor VIII. Patients with hemophilia who do not have an inhibitor should receive factor VIII infusions just before surgery and will require daily monitoring so that the factor VIII level is maintained >50% for 10 to 14 days after surgery. When patients undergo joint replacement or other major orthopedic surgery, therapy should be continued for 3 weeks to permit wound healing and the institution of physical therapy.

Hemophilia patients also require treatment before dental procedures. Filling of a carious tooth can be managed by a single infusion of factor VIII concentrate coupled with the administration of 4 to 6 g of ε-aminocaproic acid (EACA) four times daily for 3 to 4 days after the dental procedure. EACA is a potent antifibrinolytic agent that inhibits plasminogen activators present in oral secretions and stabilizes clot formation in oral tissue. Alternatives include tranexamic acid, a longer-acting antifibrinolytic. EACA is also effective when used as a mouthwash. For major oral and periodontal surgery and extractions of permanent teeth, patients should probably be hospitalized briefly and also treated with factor VIII concentrates. Therapy should begin just before surgery and continue for at least 2 to 3 days.

Many centers have organized home-care programs so that patients can administer their own factor VIII infusions with the onset of symptoms. Occasional patients with very frequent bleeding receive regularly scheduled infusions. Despite the expense and inconvenience of "prophylactic" infusions, their use in early childhood has reduced or eliminated hemarthroses. Concern about transmission of AIDS has made some patients reluctant to treat themselves, despite the fact that current blood products carry a very low or no risk of transmitting HIV.

The prospects for correcting factor VIII deficiency by gene therapy are promising; some success has been achieved in dogs. Clinical studies in humans are underway.

Complications   Most hemophilia patients have had multiple episodes of hepatitis, and a majority have elevated hepatocellular enzyme levels and abnormalities on liver biopsy. Ten to 20% of patients also have hepatosplenomegaly, and a small number develop chronic active or persistent hepatitis or cirrhosis. A few patients with hemophilia and end-stage liver disease have received liver transplants with cure of both diseases. Along with homosexuals and intravenous drug abusers, hemophilia patients are at high risk for AIDS because they frequently receive blood products; they can also present with the full range of AIDS-related syndromes, including diffuse lymphadenopathy and immune thrombocytopenia. Although up to 50% of multiply transfused hemophiliacs are HIV-positive and many have clinical AIDS, the advances in factor VIII concentrate production should prevent future HIV infection.

Despite frequent bleeding, severe iron-deficiency anemia is uncommon because most of the bleeding is internal and iron is effectively recycled. Mild iron deficiency from chronic epistaxis or gastrointestinal bleeding occurs in some patients. In addition, some patients have developed a mild Coombs-positive hemolytic anemia due to small amounts of anti-A and anti-B antibody that are present in intermediate purity factor VIII concentrates.

Following multiple transfusions, 10 to 20% of patients with severe hemophilia develop inhibitors to factor VIII. Inhibitors are usually IgG antibodies that rapidly neutralize factor VIII activity. Two types of inhibitors are found with different biologic characteristics and different clinical presentations. Patients with type I inhibitors have a typical anamnestic response and raise their antibody titer following exposure to factor VIII. Patients with a type II inhibitor have a low antibody titer that is not stimulated by factor VIII infusion. Patients with the type I inhibitor should not receive factor VIII. Control of bleeding may require the infusion of either porcine factor VIII concentrates, which may not be affected by inhibitors, or prothrombin complex concentrates, which contain trace quantities of activated coagulation factors and can bypass the block in coagulation produced by the inhibitor. Patients with low-titer type II antibodies may respond to higher doses of factor VIII.

Protocols to induce tolerance to human factor VIII use massive doses of the factor coupled with immunosuppression. Tolerance induction is expensive and not always effective; it should be reserved for severely affected patients.

Genetic Counseling and Carrier Detection   It is possible to trace the defective allele in some families by examining the inheritance of restriction fragment length polymorphisms (RFLP) linked to the factor VIII gene. In addition, in families in which a specific mutation has been defined in the factor VIII gene, it can be readily detected by gene amplification and allele-specific oligonucleotide hybridization. For example, 45% of patients with severe hemophilia A have a chromosomal inversion arising from homologous recombination between sequences in intron 22 and an upstream gene. The inversion is readily detected by polymerase chain reaction (PCR) or Southern blotting. Precise diagnosis is possible early in pregnancy from either chorionic villus biopsy or amniocentesis.

Female carriers of hemophilia, who are heterozygotes, usually produce sufficient factor VIII from the factor VIII allele on their normal X chromosome for normal hemostasis. However, occasional hemophilia carriers will have factor VIII levels far below 50% due to random inactivation of normal X chromosomes in tissue producing factor VIII. These symptomatic carriers may bleed with major surgery or bleed occasionally with menses. Rarely, true female hemophiliacs arise from consanguinity within families with hemophilia or from concomitant Turner's syndrome or XO mosaicism in a carrier female.

FACTOR IX DEFICIENCY—HEMOPHILIA B   Factor IX is a single-chain, 55-kDa proenzyme that is converted to an active protease (IXa) by factor XIa or by the tissue factor–VIIa complex. Factor IXa then activates factor X in conjunction with activated factor VIII. Factor IX is one of six proteins synthesized in the liver that require vitamin K for biologic activity. Vitamin K is a cofactor for a unique posttranslational modification that inserts a second carboxyl group onto certain glutamic acid residues on factor IX (Chap. 62). This modification permits calcium binding and adsorption onto phospholipid surfaces. Factor IX gene is on the X chromosome.

Factor IX deficiency or dysfunction (hemophilia B, Christmas disease) occurs in 1 in 100,000 male births. Accurate laboratory diagnosis is critical, since it is indistinguishable clinically from factor VIII deficiency (hemophilia A) but requires different treatment. Either fresh-frozen plasma or a plasma fraction enriched in the prothrombin complex proteins is used. Monoclonally purified or recombinant factor IX preparations are now available. In addition to the expected complications of hepatitis, chronic liver disease, and AIDS, the therapy of factor IX deficiency has a special hazard. Trace quantities of activated coagulation factors in prothrombin complex concentrates may activate the coagulation system and cause thrombosis and embolism. This is particularly common in immobilized surgical patients and patients with liver disease. As a result, some centers have returned to fresh-frozen plasma for factor IX–deficient surgical patients, while others have recommended the addition of small doses of heparin to the concentrate to activate antithrombin III during the infusion and reduce hypercoagulability. The recombinant or monoclonally purified products are less likely to be thrombogenic.

FACTOR XI DEFICIENCY Factor XI is a 160-kDa dimeric protein activated to an active protease (XIa) by factor XIIa, in conjunction with high-molecular-weight kininogen and kallikrein (Figs. 62-5 and 62-6). Factor XI deficiency is inherited as an autosomal recessive trait and is especially common in Ashkenazi Jews. In contrast to deficiency in factors VIII and IX, the correlation between factor level and propensity to bleed is not as precise, spontaneous bleeding is less, and hemarthroses are rare. Many patients with factor XI deficiency present with posttraumatic bleeding or with bleeding in the perioperative period, and occasional factor XI–deficient women have menorrhagia. Daily infusions of fresh-frozen plasma are sufficient, since the half-life of factor XI is approximately 24 h. The majority of defective factor XI alleles were accounted for by a limited number of mutations.

OTHER FACTOR DEFICIENCIES Deficiencies in factors V, VII, X, and prothrombin (factor II) are exceedingly rare autosomal recessive disorders. Spontaneous or posttraumatic musculoskeletal bleeding or menorrhagia can occur with these deficiencies, but hemarthroses are uncommon. Fresh-frozen plasma is the appropriate therapy, although prothrombin concentrates may be employed for patients with severe prothrombin deficiency or decreases in factors VII and X as long as the risks of hepatitis and thrombosis are recognized.

Defects in the contact activation pathway involving Hageman factor (factor XII), high-molecular-weight kininogen, and prekallikrein cause laboratory abnormalities but no clinical bleeding. Despite dramatic prolongation of the PTT, often to greater than 100 s, deficient individuals have normal hemostasis and can undergo major surgery without plasma replacement therapy. Direct activation of factor IX by the tissue factor–VIIa complex may bypass this defective step in coagulation (Fig. 62-7). Recognition of these disorders is important because such patients should neither be treated inappropriately with plasma nor denied indicated surgery on the basis of these laboratory abnormalities.

AFIBRINOGENEMIA AND DYSFIBRINOGENEMIA Fibrinogen is a 340-kDa dimeric molecule made up of two sets of three covalently linked polypeptide chains. Thrombin sequentially cleaves fibrinopeptides A and B from the Aα and Bβ chains of fibrinogen to produce fibrin monomer, which then polymerizes to form a fibrin clot. Although fibrinogen is needed for platelet aggregation and fibrin formation, severe fibrinogen deficiency does not usually cause serious bleeding except after surgery. Patients with afibrinogenemia, who have no detectable fibrinogen in plasma or platelets, may have infrequent, mild bleeding episodes. Preliminary genetic analyses do not show any gross deletion or structural changes in the genes encoding the α, β, and γ chains of fibrinogen despite the total absence of plasma fibrinogen.

Fibrinogen is an abundant plasma protein (2.5 g/L). Mutations have been identified that alter the release of fibrinopeptides from the Aα and Bβ chains of fibrinogen, the rate of polymerization of fibrin monomers, and the sites for fibrin cross-linking. These dysfibrinogenemias are almost always inherited as autosomal dominant traits, so patients have nearly equal concentrations of normal and mutant fibrinogen in their plasma. Patients with dysfibrinogenemia have a slightly prolonged PT and PTT, a prolonged thrombin time, and a disparity in levels of fibrinogen measured with functional and immunologic assays. Despite these abnormalities, most patients have no symptoms or only moderate bleeding. A few dysfibrinogenemias induce a hypercoagulable state and increase the risk of thrombosis, and others have been associated with an increased incidence of abortion (Chap. 118). Some patients with liver disease, hepatomas, AIDS, and lymphoproliferative disorders develop an acquired form of dysfibrinogenemia.

FACTOR XIII DEFICIENCY AND DEFECTIVE FIBRIN CROSS-LINKING Factor XIII is a transglutaminase that stabilizes fibrin clots by forming ε-amino–γ-glutamyl cross-links between ad-

jacent α and γ chains of fibrin. Factor XIII deficiency is an extremely rare inherited syndrome. Patients usually bleed in the neonatal period from their umbilical stump or circumcision. In addition to hemorrhage, these patients may have poor wound healing, a high incidence of infertility among males and abortion among affected females, and a high incidence of intracerebral hemorrhage. These observations suggest that the enzyme may be important in other physiologic and pathologic processes beyond hemostasis, including placental implantation, spermatogenesis, and wound healing. Several drugs, including isoniazid, may bind to cross-linking sites on fibrinogen and mimic factor XIII deficiency by blocking enzyme activity. Normal hemostasis requires only 1% of normal enzyme activity, which can be achieved with a single infusion of fresh-frozen plasma or a purified factor XIII–rich product derived from human placenta called Fibrogammin. Factor XIII has a 14-day half-life.

VITAMIN K DEFICIENCY Vitamin K is a fat-soluble vitamin that plays a critical role in hemostasis. Dietary vitamin K is absorbed in the small intestine and stored in the liver. The vitamin is also synthesized by endogenous bacterial flora in the small intestine and colon; however, the quantity of endogenous vitamin K absorbed from the large intestine is debated. Following absorption and transport, vitamin K is converted to an active epoxide in liver microsomes and serves as a cofactor in the enzymatic carboxylation of glutamic acid residues on prothrombin complex proteins (Fig. 117-1).

The three major causes of vitamin K deficiency are inadequate dietary intake, intestinal malabsorption, and loss of storage sites due to hepatocellular disease. Neonatal vitamin K deficiency, which causes hemorrhagic disease of the newborn, has disappeared from western countries with the routine administration of vitamin K to all newborn infants. Although a 30-day supply of vitamin K is stored in the normal liver, acutely ill patients can become deficient within 7 to 10 days. Acute vitamin K deficiency is particularly common in patients recovering from biliary tract surgery who have no dietary intake of vitamin K, have T-tube drainage of bile, and are on broad-spectrum antibiotics. Vitamin K deficiency is also seen in chronic liver disease, particularly primary biliary cirrhosis, and in some malabsorption states (Chaps. 286 and 298). The cephalosporins inhibit the reduction and recycling of vitamin K, much like coumarin.

With vitamin K deficiency, plasma levels of all the prothrombin complex proteins (factors II, VII, IX, X; proteins C and S) decrease. Factor VII and protein C, which have the shortest half-lives, decrease first. Because of the rapid fall in factor VII, patients with mild vitamin K deficiency may have a prolonged PT and a normal PTT. Later, as the levels of the other factors fall, the PTT will also become prolonged. Parenteral administration of 10 mg vitamin K rapidly restores vitamin K levels in the liver and permits normal production of prothrombin complex proteins within 8 to 10 h. Severe hemorrhage can be treated with fresh-frozen plasma, which immediately corrects the hemostatic

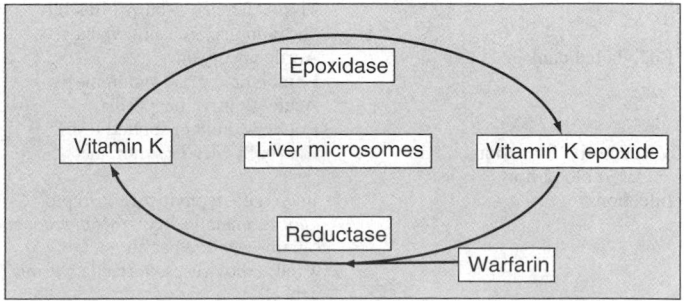

FIGURE 117-1 The mechanism of action of vitamin K, a cofactor in the formation of di-γ-carboxyglutamic acid residues on coagulation proteins, is depicted. Vitamin K is converted to an epoxide in liver microsomes. The epoxide is the active form and is reduced back to vitamin K by a liver membrane reductase. Warfarin blocks the action of the reductase and competitively inhibits the effects of vitamin K.

defect. If the cause of vitamin K deficiency cannot be eliminated, patients may need monthly injections. Purified prothrombin complex concentrates should be avoided because they contain trace quantities of activated forms of the prothrombin complex proteins and can cause thrombosis in patients with liver disease. They also carry an increased risk of hepatitis.

DISSEMINATED INTRAVASCULAR COAGULATION

DIC can be either an explosive and life-threatening bleeding disorder or a relatively mild or subclinical disorder. Although a long list of diseases can be complicated by DIC, it is most frequently associated with obstetric catastrophes, metastatic malignancy, massive trauma, and bacterial sepsis (Table 117-1). In each case, a tentative triggering mechanism has been identified. For example, tumors and traumatized or necrotic tissue release tissue factor into the circulation, while endotoxin from gram-negative bacteria activates several steps in the coagulation cascade. In addition to a direct effect on the activation of Hageman factor (factor XII), endotoxin induces the expression of tissue factor on the surface of monocytes and endothelial cells. These activated cell surfaces then accelerate coagulation reactions. These potent thrombogenic stimuli cause the deposition of small thrombi and emboli throughout the microvasculature. This early thrombotic phase of DIC is then followed by a phase of procoagulant consumption and secondary fibrinolysis. Continued fibrin formation and fibrinolysis lead to hemorrhage from the coagulation factor and platelet depletion and the antihemostatic effects of fibrin degradation products (Fig. 117-2).

The clinical presentation varies with the stage and severity of the syndrome. Most patients have extensive skin and mucous membrane bleeding and hemorrhage from surgical incisions or venipuncture or catheter sites. Less often, patients present with peripheral acrocyanosis, thrombosis, and pregangrenous changes in digits, genitalia, and nose—areas where blood flow is markedly reduced by vasospasm or microthrombi. Some patients, particularly those with chronic DIC secondary to malignancy, have laboratory abnormalities without any evidence of thrombosis or hemorrhage.

The laboratory manifestations include thrombocytopenia and the

Table 117-1   Etiologic Factors and Disorders Causing Disseminated Intravascular Coagulation

Liberation of tissue factors	Obstetric syndromes—abruptio placentae, amniotic fluid embolism, retained dead fetus, second trimester abortion
	Hemolysis
	Neoplasms, particularly mucinous adenocarcinomas, acute promyelocytic leukemia
	Intravascular hemolysis
	Fat embolism
	Tissue damage—burns, frostbite, head injury, gunshot wounds
Endothelial damage	Aortic aneurysm
	Hemolytic uremic syndrome
	Acute glomerulonephritis
	Rocky Mountain spotted fever
Vascular malformation and decreased blood flow	Kasabach-Merritt syndrome
Infections	Bacterial: staphylococci, streptococci, pneumococci, meningococci, gram-negative bacilli
	Viral: arboviruses, varicella, variola, rubella
	Parasitic: malaria, kala-azar
	Rickettsial: Rocky Mountain spotted fever
	Mycotic: acute histoplasmosis

SOURCE: Modified from RI Handin, RD Rosenberg, in *Hematology*, 4th ed, WS Beck (ed), Cambridge, MA, MIT Press, 1985.

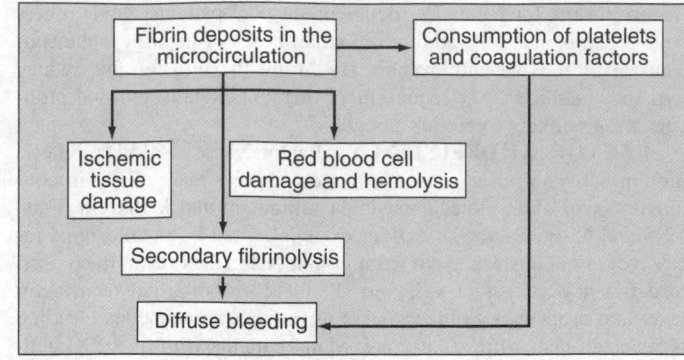

FIGURE 117-2   The pathophysiology of disseminated intravascular coagulation (DIC). Shown are the interactions between coagulation and fibrinolytic pathways that result in bleeding in patients with DIC.

presence of schistocytes or fragmented red blood cells that arise from cell trapping and damage within fibrin thrombi; prolonged PT and PTT and thrombin time and a reduced fibrinogen level from depletion of coagulation proteins; and elevated fibrin degradation products (FDP) from intense secondary fibrinolysis. The D dimer immunoassay, which specifically measures cross-linked fibrin derivatives, is a more specific FDP assay. The abnormality in DIC that predicts bleeding is the plasma fibrinogen level; low fibrinogen levels are associated with more bleeding.

℞ TREATMENT   DIC, although sometimes indolent, can cause life-threatening hemorrhage and may require emergency treatment. This should include (1) an attempt to correct any reversible cause of DIC; (2) measures to control the major symptom, either bleeding or thrombosis; and (3) a prophylactic regimen to prevent recurrence in cases of chronic DIC. Treatment will vary with the clinical presentation. In patients with an obstetric complication such as abruptio placentae or acute bacterial sepsis, the underlying disorder is easy to correct, and prompt delivery of the fetus and placenta or treatment with appropriate antibiotics will reverse the DIC syndrome. In patients with metastatic tumor causing DIC, control of the primary disease may not be possible, and long-term prophylaxis may be necessary.

Patients with bleeding as a major symptom should receive fresh-frozen plasma to replace depleted clotting factors and platelet concentrates to correct thrombocytopenia. Those with acrocyanosis and incipient gangrene or other thrombotic problems need immediate anticoagulation with intravenous heparin. The use of heparin in the treatment of bleeding is still controversial. Although it is a logical way to reduce thrombin generation and prevent further consumption of clotting proteins, it should be reserved for patients with thrombosis or who continue to bleed despite vigorous treatment with plasma and platelets.

Patients who initially have mild DIC and may not be symptomatic may begin to bleed following surgery or chemotherapy. For example, mild DIC, without clinical bleeding, has been documented during saline- or prostaglandin-induced midtrimester abortions. Prophylactic treatment of patients with heparin may prevent progression of a mild DIC syndrome and has been used in the treatment of patients with acute promyelocytic leukemia and in some patients with a retained dead fetus who require surgical extraction. However, most patients with low-grade DIC can be managed with plasma and platelet replacement and do not require heparin. Chronic DIC does not respond to oral warfarin anticoagulants, but it can be controlled with long-term heparin infusion. Occasional patients with indolent tumors and severe DIC have been maintained on heparin administered by intermittent subcutaneous injection or continuous infusion with portable pumps.

Despite our detailed understanding of the pathophysiology of DIC and a vigorous approach to therapy, treatment does not change the natural history of the underlying disorder. Therapy will only stabilize the patient, prevent exsanguination or massive thrombosis, and permit institution of definitive therapy.

Liver dysfunction is frequently accompanied by a hemostatic defect. The major causes of hemorrhage in patients with liver disease are shown in Table 117-2. Bleeding is usually due to an anatomic lesion that is exacerbated by a hemostatic defect. Most patients bleed from complications of portal hypertension, esophageal varices, or gastritis and peptic ulcer disease. Portal hypertension also causes splenomegaly, with splenic sequestration of platelets and thrombocytopenia, which contributes to the hemostatic defect (Chap. 298).

Patients with hepatocellular liver disease cannot store vitamin K optimally and may have some degree of vitamin K deficiency. Cholestasis, a frequent feature of liver disease, impairs vitamin K absorption and further decreases liver vitamin K stores. Abnormalities in the γ-carboxylation of prothrombin complex proteins independent of vitamin K and the production of abnormal proteins have also been described. Patients may also have decreased production of other coagulation proteins, including fibrinogen and factor V. The liver also produces inhibitors of coagulation such as antithrombin III and proteins C and S and is the clearance site for activated coagulation factors and fibrinolytic enzymes. Thus patients with liver disease are also "hypercoagulable" and predisposed to developing DIC or systemic fibrinolysis. Coagulation defects in advanced liver failure are often difficult to distinguish from those of DIC.

Each patient with hemorrhage and liver disease should have a PT, PTT, platelet count, and fibrinogen determination, although it is not always possible to determine the major hemostatic abnormality from a single set of laboratory values. It is helpful to have previous laboratory data available for patients with chronic liver disease who develop an acute complication. The degree of prolongation of the PT predicts the risk of bleeding. Most patients present with moderate prolongation of the PT and PTT, mild thrombocytopenia, and a normal fibrinogen level. However, they may also present with a more complex defect combining defective synthesis, abnormal clearance, and active consumption of coagulation proteins. Since vitamin K deficiency is so common, a single parenteral dose of vitamin K is given after initial laboratory studies have been obtained, even though this may only partially correct the laboratory abnormalities. The presence of severe thrombocytopenia or a low fibrinogen level suggests the additional complication of DIC and may require further studies and therapy.

The safest replacement therapy for a patient with liver disease is fresh-frozen plasma, since it supplies all known coagulation factors. However, even this form of therapy has drawbacks, since large quantities of plasma may precipitate hepatic encephalopathy and cause fluid and sodium overload. Prothrombin complex concentrates should be avoided because they replace only the vitamin K–dependent factors, may be contaminated with hepatitis and AIDS virus, and contain trace quantities of activated coagulation proteins. Similarly, fibrinogen concentrates (or cryoprecipitate), rich in factor VIII and fibrinogen, should not be used without additional fresh-frozen plasma. Anticoagulation with heparin has been advocated to control DIC, but this is particularly hazardous and not recommended in cirrhosis because heparin is metabolized erratically and may lead to severe bleeding.

FIBRINOLYTIC DEFECTS Bleeding can also occur from defects in the fibrinolytic system. Patients with α_2 plasmin inhibitor deficiency or plasminogen activator inhibitor (PAI) 1 have rapid fibrinolysis following fibrin deposition after trauma or surgery and may experience recurrent hemorrhage. Similarly, patients with cirrhosis have an impaired clearance of tissue plasminogen activator (tPA) and systemic fibrinolysis that may contribute to their hemorrhagic defect. Rarely, patients with tumors such as metastatic prostatic cancer may develop diffuse bleeding from primary fibrinolysis rather than DIC. Clues to the diagnosis include a disproportionately low fibrinogen level with a relatively normal PT and PTT and the presence of a normal or nearly normal platelet count. With rare exceptions, patients with primary fibrinolysis should have an elevated titer of FDP but a normal D dimer level. However, it is sometimes difficult or impossible to differentiate primary fibrinolysis from the secondary fibrinolysis accompanying DIC. Patients with clearly established primary fibrinolysis should not receive heparin; they require plasma therapy and, occasionally, fibrinolytic inhibitors such as EACA. However, EACA should not be given to patients suspected of having DIC unless they are also receiving heparin, since EACA can cause massive, often fatal, thrombosis in a patient with DIC.

CIRCULATING ANTICOAGULANTS Circulating anticoagulants, or inhibitors, are usually IgG antibodies that interfere with coagulation reactions. Specific inhibitors inactivate individual coagulation proteins and may cause severe hemorrhage. They arise in 15 to 20% of patients with factor VIII or factor IX deficiency who have received plasma infusions. *Specific* inhibitors also occur in previously normal individuals. Although the most common target protein is factor VIII, inhibitors with specificity for each of the coagulation proteins occur. In addition to hemophiliacs, anti-factor VIII antibodies are seen in postpartum females, in patients on various drugs, as part of the spectrum of autoantibodies in systemic lupus erythematosus (SLE) patients, and in normal elderly individuals. Circulating anticoagulants also occur in patients with AIDS.

Nonspecific (lupus-like) inhibitors prolong coagulation tests by binding to phospholipids. They are assayed by their anticoagulant effect [lupus anticoagulant (LA) activity] or their ability to bind to the complex phospholipid cardiolipin [anticardiolipin antibody (ACLA) activity]. While most often encountered in patients with SLE, these nonspecific inhibitors may develop in patients with many other disorders and also in otherwise normal individuals.

The critical laboratory feature that identifies the presence of either type of inhibitor is the failure of normal plasma to correct a prolonged PT, PTT, or both. Plasma from patients with a specific inhibitor will progressively inactivate a coagulation protein and thus prolong whichever of these screening tests requires the participation of that clotting factor. This effect persists after dilution. Nonspecific inhibitors immediately prolong the PT and PTT and, at low dilution, block multiple coagulation reactions. However, these effects can be overcome by altering the quantity or type of phospholipid or by diluting the plasma.

Hemorrhage in patients with specific inhibitors may require treatment with massive plasma or concentrate infusion, the use of activated prothrombin complex concentrates to bypass the antibodies against factors VIII or IX, and plasmapheresis or exchange transfusion to lower antibody titer. Chronic immunosuppressive regimens have been particularly useful in otherwise normal individuals with an acquired factor VIII antibody. Many patients lose their antibody and recover within 6 to 12 months, although the acute mortality rate from uncontrollable bleeding may approach 10%.

Patients with LA activity have normal hemostasis and will not bleed unless they have concomitant thrombocytopenia or prothrombin

---

Table 117-2   Causes of Bleeding in Liver Disease

Anatomic Factors
  Portal hypertension
    Varices
    Splenomegaly and secondary thrombocytopenia
  Peptic ulceration
  Gastritis
Hepatic Function Abnormalities
  Decreased synthesis of procoagulant proteins: fibrinogen, prothrombin, factors V, VII, IX, X, XI
  Decreased synthesis of coagulation inhibitors: protein C, protein S, antithrombin III
  Impaired absorption and metabolism of vitamin K
  Failure to clear activated coagulation proteins leading to:
    Disseminated intravascular coagulation
    Systemic fibrinolysis
Complications of Therapy
  Dilution of platelets and coagulation proteins from massive transfusions
  Infusion of activated coagulation proteins in prothrombin complex concentrates
  Bleeding from heparin; thrombosis from ε-aminocaproic acid (EACA)

deficiency. Both thrombocytopenia and hypoprothrombinemia are secondary to autoantibodies that bind either to platelets or the prothrombin molecule. While these antibodies have no effect on function, they accelerate clearance of the coated platelets or the antibody-prothrombin complexes.

The presence of LA activity may predispose patients to venous and arterial thromboembolism and may cause midtrimester abortions. However, the risk of thrombosis is difficult to estimate and the appropriate therapy for individual patients difficult to choose. Tests for either LA or ACLA activity are not well standardized, and results vary among and within patients. The best predictor is a consistent prolongation of more than one coagulation test coupled with a high titer of ACLA activity. Second, the risk of thrombosis is increased in patients who have SLE compared with those with idiopathic LA or ACLA activity. Prophylactic therapy is not clearly beneficial, and treatments aimed at reducing the titer of antibody are not superior to conventional antithrombotic therapy.

Therapy should be individualized. Patients with SLE and either LA or ACLA activity who have had a thrombotic episode are at high risk for a recurrence and should receive long-term anticoagulant therapy. Women who have had more than one midtrimester abortion, especially those with SLE, should have a trial of anticoagulant therapy. Patients with a single thrombotic episode (stroke or pulmonary embolus) and no other risk factor except LA or ACLA activity should be treated. No consensus has been reached about treatment after an initial minor event [deep venous thrombosis (DVT)]. Asymptomatic patients with only laboratory abnormalities should not be treated. Glucocorticoids should be administered only in conjunction with antithrombotic agents and are not of proven efficacy.

INHERITED PRETHROMBOTIC DISORDERS Coagulation is carefully regulated by a series of inhibitors that limit thrombin generation and fibrin formation and by the fibrinolytic system, which effectively removes fibrin thrombi (Figs. 62-5 and 62-6). Inherited defects in the natural coagulation inhibitors (i.e., antithrombin, proteins C and S), abnormalities in the fibrinolytic system, and certain dysfibrinogenemias predispose patients to thrombosis (Table 62-5). A single point mutation in the factor V gene (factor V Leiden), which converts arginine 506 to glutamine and makes the molecule resistant to degradation by activated protein C, may account for 25% of inherited prethrombotic states. Antithrombin, protein C, and protein S defects are all autosomal dominant traits, so heterozygous individuals, who have a 50% reduction in protein concentration or a mixture of mutant and normal molecules, will have an increased risk of thrombosis. The patients have similar clinical presentations with a strong family history of thrombosis, episodes of recurrent venous thromboembolism, and symptoms by their early twenties. Any patient with this distinctive history should be tested for specific abnormalities.

ANTITHROMBIN DEFICIENCY Antithrombin complexes with activated coagulation proteins and blocks their biologic activity (Fig. 62-5). The rate of this reaction is enhanced by heparin-like molecules within the vessel wall or on endothelial cells. Plasma antithrombin III content is 5 to 15 mg/L (50 to 150%), with values only slightly below normal increasing the risk of thrombosis. For optimal screening, the antithrombin III concentration is measured by immunoassay and the plasma antithrombin and heparin cofactor activity assessed with functional assays. The most common defect (1 in 2000 indidivuals) is mild (heterozygous) antithrombin deficiency. Dysfunctional antithrombin molecules with mutations affecting either the serine protease or heparin-binding site or activation of inhibitor by heparin have also been described.

Patients with antithrombin deficiency who develop acute thrombosis or embolism can be treated with intravenous heparin, since there is usually sufficient normal antithrombin to act as a heparin cofactor. Following their first episode of thromboembolism, patients should be placed on oral anticoagulants for life to prevent recurrent thrombosis. Family studies should be conducted when an antithrombin-deficient

individual is discovered, since up to half the members of a kindred may be affected. Asymptomatic individuals with antithrombin deficiency should receive prophylactic anticoagulation with heparin or plasma infusions to raise their antithrombin level before medical or surgical procedures that may increase their risk of thrombosis. Chronic oral anticoagulation is not recommended until individuals at risk have a thrombotic episode.

DEFICIENCIES OF PROTEINS C AND S Protein C is a vitamin K–dependent hepatic protein that binds to the endothelial cell surface protein thrombomodulin and is converted to an active protease by thrombin (Fig. 62-5). Activated protein C, in conjunction with protein S, proteolyzes factors Va and VIIIa, which shuts off fibrin formation. Activated protein C may also stimulate fibrinolysis and accelerate clot lysis. Deficiencies of proteins C and S are usually autosomal dominant disorders, and deficiencies in the two proteins cause an identical syndrome of recurrent venous thrombosis and pulmonary embolism. Dysfunctional molecules have also been identified in some patients with thrombosis. Rare patients with homozygous protein C deficiency have fulminant neonatal intravascular coagulation and require prompt diagnosis and treatment.

The correlation between protein C and S levels and the risk of thrombosis is not as precise as for antithrombin III deficiency. In fact, some asymptomatic individuals with protein C "deficiency" have been discovered. In some well-studied protein C–deficient kindreds, asymptomatic individuals may have protein C levels as low as or lower than relatives with recurrent thrombosis. It is possible that an undiscovered cofactor is present in symptomatic patients. Finally, since a fraction of the available protein S is bound to C4b-binding protein and is unavailable for coagulation reactions, both free and total protein S levels or C4b-binding protein levels should be assessed for maximum accuracy.

Heterozygous patients with protein C or S deficiencies who develop acute thrombosis should be heparinized and then placed on oral anticoagulants. There are, however, two potential problems with the use of coumarin anticoagulants in these patients. First, these vitamin K antagonists (Fig. 117-1; Fig. 62-5), which lower the level of the procoagulant factors II, VII, IX, and X, may also reduce the concentration of proteins C and S sufficiently to nullify the desired antithrombotic effect. In addition, patients who are protein C–deficient may develop coumarin-induced skin necrosis; this defect may predispose patients to a rare but serious complication. Patients with homozygous protein C deficiency require periodic plasma infusions rather than oral anticoagulants to prevent recurrent intravascular coagulation and thrombosis.

RESISTANCE TO ACTIVATED PROTEIN C AND THE FACTOR V LEIDEN MUTATION Some patients with familial or recurrent venous thromboembolism were found not to prolong their PTT when activated protein C was added to their plasma. These patients were found to have an identical mutation in which arginine 506 in factor V is converted to glutamine. This amino acid substitution abolishes a protein C cleavage site in factor V and thus prolongs the thrombogenic effect of factor V activation. About 3% of the population worldwide is heterozygous for this mutation. The mutation is absent in certain populations, e.g., Asians, African Americans, and Native Americans. It may account for 25% of patients with recurrent deep venous thrombosis or pulmonary embolism.

Heterozygosity at this allele increases an individual's lifetime risk of venous thromboembolism sevenfold. The risk rises steadily with age. A homozygote has a twentyfold increased risk of thrombosis. Heterozygosity coupled with ingestion of oral contraceptives or pregnancy increases the risk at least fifteenfold. Coinheritance of factor V Leiden and another low-penetrance defect such as protein C or S deficiency is also additive. Many previous studies of risk factors predisposing patients to venous thromboembolism are being reevaluated to take into account this common mutation.

PROTHROMBIN GENE MUTATION A specific point mutation in the prothrombin gene [conversion of G to A at position 20210 (G20210A)] also predisposes to venous thrombosis and embolism.

This mutation is in the 3'-untranslated region of the gene and results in a 30% increase in plasma prothrombin levels, either through more efficient translation or greater stability of the message. Heterozygotes account for ~18% of cases with family histories of venous thrombosis and 6% of patients with first episodes of DVT.

The inheritance of multiple mutations increases the risk of thrombosis. The relationship between known mutations and the type of thrombosis is shown in Table 117-3. The fraction of patients with DVT with known mutations is shown in Table 117-4.

℞ TREATMENT Patients who develop venous thromboembolism without a clear predisposing factor, have a strong family history, present under the age 30, or have more than one episode should have assays for antithrombin III, proteins C and S, and factor V Leiden. Patients who present with DVT or pulmonary embolism during pregnancy or while using oral contraceptives have a 30% chance of having factor V Leiden.

Treatment recommendations for patients with the inherited prethrombotic disorders are still evolving. All patients should receive standard initial therapy with heparin, either conventional or low dose (Chap. 118), followed by 3 months of oral warfarin. This regimen should allow for maximal healing and reendothelialization of the thrombosed vessels and minimize recurrence in the damaged vascular beds. It is not clear which patients should go on to receive long-term (perhaps lifelong) anticoagulation, a judgment that depends on assessing the risk/benefit ratio.

Patients with antithrombin III deficiency who become symptomatic have a high likelihood of recurrent events and should be placed on lifelong anticoagulation. Patients with protein C or S deficiency or heterozygous factor V Leiden and prothrombin G20210A patients have a lower likelihood of recurrent disease. Long-term anticoagulation should be reserved until their second or subsequent episode of thromboembolism. Homozygous factor V Leiden patients should be placed on long-term anticoagulation after their initial episode, and all patients should receive replacement therapy or receive heparin prophylaxis during surgery or after trauma; women with these defects should avoid the use of oral contraceptives. The asymptomatic relatives of patients shown to have these disorders should be screened to determine if they have inherited the defective gene. If so, they should receive appropriate prophylaxis but not start anticoagulation until they are symptomatic. In the absence of a congenital defect predisposing a patient to thrombosis, recurring or migratory thrombophlebitis may indicate an underlying malignancy.

DYSFIBRINOGENEMIAS AND FIBRINOLYTIC DEFECTS Recurrent venous thrombosis and embolism may be due to familial defects in fibrinogen or plasminogen or decreased synthesis or release of tPA. While most dysfibrinogenemias cause bleeding, several variants have excessively rapid release of fibrinopeptides and recurrent thromboembolism. Patients with this disorder and those with an abnormal plasminogen that resists activation by streptokinase and urokinase have been treated successfully with heparin and oral anticoagulants. Defects in tPA content or release have not been completely characterized. One group of patients with recurrent venous thrombosis and embolism failed to increase venous blood fibrinolytic activity when challenged with local ischemia or physical exercise. The other group had impaired fibrinolytic activity in extracts prepared from biopsied veins. Young patients with acute myocardial infarction may have impaired fibrinolysis due to increased plasma levels of PAI, a serine protease inhibitor that binds to tPA and is derived from endothelial cells.

Many common illnesses are associated with an increased risk of thrombosis (Table 62-5). These patients are said to have a "hypercoagulable" or "prethrombotic" state. This increased risk is seen in patients with chronic congestive heart failure and metastatic cancer and in patients undergoing major surgery. The generation of tissue factor activity in damaged or ischemic tissue or metastatic tumor, coupled with venous stasis and endothelial injury, induces the formation of venous and, more rarely, arterial thrombi. Several hematologic disorders, paroxysmal nocturnal hemoglobinuria, essential thrombocythemia, and polycythemia vera predispose patients to venous and arterial thrombosis through diverse mechanisms related to increased blood viscosity and abnormal blood cells. Diseases that affect the endothelial cell, such as Behçet's syndrome, Kawasaki's disease, and homocystinuria, or the administration of drugs such as the oral contraceptives, which lower antithrombin III levels, or L-asparaginase, which inhibits production of multiple coagulation factors, may also predispose patients to thrombosis. Infusion of granulocyte-macrophage colony stimulating factor (GM-CSF) has been associated with thrombosis. Tamoxifen, an estrogen receptor antagonist, can cause venous thrombosis. The mechanism is unclear.

Plasma homocysteine levels influence the risk of both venous and arterial thromboembolism. Individuals with the congenital homocystinuria syndrome have, in addition to their Marfanoid habitus, an increased incidence of strokes and coronary artery disease. These patients have well-recognized enzyme defects (Chap. 352), excrete homocysteine in their urine, and have very high plasma levels of the amino acid. Some patients with early-onset cerebral vascular events have mild homocystinuria that can be brought out by a methionine loading test. Epidemiologic studies show a relationship between homocysteine levels that are nearer to the normal range and coronary artery disease. Although this correlation is not yet definitive, the relationship remains intriguing and of potential clinical relevance. Vitamin B_{12} deficiency occurs in about 30% of people over age 70, produces elevated homocysteine levels, and may be a reversible cause of thrombotic disease.

Table 117-4 Prevalence of Coagulation Defects in Patients with Venous Thrombosis

Defect	Prevalence, %
Factor V Leiden (Arg506Gln) R506 Q	12–40
Hyperhomocysteinemia	10–20
Prothrombin G20210A	6–18
Deficiencies of antithrombin III, proteins C and S	5–15
Antiphospholipid antibody syndrome	10–20

Table 117-3 Relationship Between Coagulation Defect and Site of Thrombosis

Abnormality	Arterial	Venous
Factor V Leiden R506 Q	–	+
Prothrombin G20210A	–	+
Antithrombin III	–	+
Protein C	–	+
Protein S	–	+
Homocysteinemia	+	+
Antiphospholipid antibody[a]	+	+

[a] Anticardiolipin antibody—lupus anticoagulant.

BIBLIOGRAPHY

ANTONARAKIS SE: Molecular genetics of factor VIII gene and haemophilia A. Haemophilia 4:1, 1998

FEINSTEIN DI: Lupus anticoagulant, anticardiolipin antibodies, fetal loss and systemic lupus erythematosus. Blood 80:859, 1992

GREAVES M: Antiphospholipid antibodies and thrombosis. Lancet 353:1348, 1999

KAY MA, HIGH K: Gene therapy for the hemophilias. Proc Natl Acad Sci USA 96:10379, 1999

LEE C: Recombinant clotting factors in the treatment of hemophilia. Thromb Haemost 82:516, 1999

LEVI M, TEN CATE H: Current concepts: Disseminated intravascular coagulation. N Engl J Med 341:586, 1999

MANUCC PM, TUDDENHAM EG: The hemophilias: Progress and problems. Semin Hematol 36:104, 1999

118   *Robert I. Handin*

ANTICOAGULANT, FIBRINOLYTIC, AND ANTIPLATELET THERAPY

ANTICOAGULANT AND FIBRINOLYTIC THERAPY

Anticoagulation with heparin, followed by treatment with oral vitamin K antagonists, is the standard treatment for acute venous thrombosis and pulmonary embolism. In addition, chronic oral anticoagulation is used to prevent cerebral arterial embolism from cardiac sources such as ventricular mural thrombi or atrial thrombi or from an atherosclerotic, partially stenosed carotid or vertebral artery. Anticoagulants are also used, less successfully, to treat peripheral or mesenteric arterial thrombosis. These agents retard fibrin deposition on established thrombi and prevent the formation of new thrombi. The induction of a fibrinolytic state by the infusion of plasminogen activators such as recombinant tissue plasminogen activator (rtPA), streptokinase (SK), or urokinase (UK) has become an accepted mode of therapy for some thromboembolic disorders. Fibrinolytic therapy has been proposed for patients with massive pulmonary embolism and systemic hypotension and to restore the patency of acutely occluded peripheral and coronary arteries. Prompt fibrinolytic therapy can reduce both myocardial damage and mortality following acute coronary occlusion (Chap. 243), though mechanical interventions such as angioplasty and stent placement are also effective ways to restore vessel patency. Fibrinolytic therapy may also be effective in acute thrombotic strokes and in venoocclusive disease of the liver.

ACUTE ANTICOAGULATION WITH HEPARIN   Heparin is a naturally occurring mucopolysaccharide polymer with tetrasaccharide sequences that bind to and activate antithrombin III. It can dramatically reduce thrombin generation and fibrin formation in patients with acute venous and arterial thrombosis or embolism (Table

118-1). Heparin is administered to patients with acute thrombosis or embolism by giving an initial loading dose of 5000 to 10,000 units followed by a continuous intravenous infusion at a rate sufficient to keep the activated partial thromboplastin time (APTT) at 1.5 to 2 times the patient's preheparin APTT. This requires infusion of 800 to 1000 U.S.P. units per hour and is continued while patients are begun on oral anticoagulants and achieve appropriate prolongation of the prothrombin time. The usual duration of combined heparin-warfarin therapy is 5 to 7 days. Heparin is then discontinued, and the patient is maintained on warfarin. Alternatives to a continuous infusion include the administration of 5000 U.S.P. units of heparin four times a day either subcutaneously or intravenously. Unfractionated conventional heparin preparations are heterogeneous, with only 20% of the product biologically active. In addition, active heparin fractions may vary considerably in molecular weight. Biologically active, low-molecular-weight heparin (LMWH) preparations, while more expensive than unfractionated heparin, have several advantages: (1) they can be administered subcutaneously once or twice daily, (2) their pharmacokinetics are so predictable that APTT monitoring is not necessary, and (3) they are less immunogenic and less likely to cause thrombocytopenia. Many patients with deep venous thrombosis, a frequent cause for hospitalization, can be given LMWH as outpatients. Given their other advantages and equivalent efficacy, LMWH preparations have largely replaced unfractionated heparin (Table 118-1).

Patients with recurrent thromboembolism refractory to oral anticoagulants, pregnant women with thromboembolism, and patients with chronic disseminated intravascular coagulation (DIC) may be treated with daily injections of LMWH preparations such as enoxoparin or dalteparin. These agents are also effective in prevention of venous thrombosis in high-risk surgical and medical patients, including those with congestive heart failure, myocardial infarction, or cardiomyopathy.

The major complication of unfractionated heparin therapy is bleeding—especially from surgical sites and into the retroperitoneum. Aspirin or aspirin-containing drugs impair platelet function. Thus, intramuscular injections in patients on both heparin and an antiplatelet drug may cause significant bleeding. Heparin's anticoagulant effect can be rapidly reversed by the administration of protamine sulfate. However, this is usually not necessary, since reduction or omission of a heparin-dose usually improves hemostasis and stops bleeding. Thrombocytopenia occurs in ~10% of recipients and is usually mild, with the platelet count falling to 50,000 to 100,000/μL. Thrombocytopenia is more common in patients receiving heparin derived from beef lung as opposed to porcine intestinal mucosa. LMWH is less likely to cause either thrombocytopenia or bleeding. However, antibodies arising from exposure to unfractionated heparin often cross-react with LMWH. Thus, LMWH cannot usually be used to treat patients with established thrombocytopenia.

Heparin-induced thrombocytopenia (HIT) results from generation of an autoantibody to a complex of unfractionated heparin with the anti-heparin protein platelet factor 4 (PF-4). Heparin-PF-4-antibody complexes can bind to the platelet Fc receptor and cause platelet activation, agglutination, and arterial thrombosis. Recognition of the rare complication of thrombocytopenia and paradoxical thrombosis is critical, since discontinuing heparin can promptly reverse the syndrome and may be lifesaving. Heparin administration for >5 months also carries a risk of osteoporosis, perhaps through its activation of osteoclasts. LMWH causes less osteoporosis on chronic administration.

Table 118-1   Anticoagulant Therapy with Low-Molecular-Weight and Unfractionated Heparin

Clinical Indication	Heparin Dose and Schedule	Target PTT[a]	LMWH Dose and Schedule[b]
Venous thrombosis pulmonary embolism			
Treatment	5000 U IV bolus; 1000–1500 U/h	2–2.5	100 U/kg SC bid
Prophylaxis	5000 U SC q8–12h	<1.5	100 U/kg SC bid
Acute myocardial infarction			
With thrombolytic therapy	5000 U IV bolus; 1000 U/h	1.5–2.5	100 U/kg SC bid
With mural thrombus	8000 U SC q8h + warfarin	1.5–2.0	100 U /kg SC bid
Unstable angina	5000 U IV bolus; 1000 U/h	1.5–2.5	100 U/kg SC bid
Prophylaxis			
General surgery	5000 U SC bid	<1.5	100 U/kg SC before and bid
Orthopedic surgery	10000 U SC bid	1.5	100 U/kg SC before and bid
Medical patients with CHF, MI	10000 U SC bid	1.5	100 U/kg SC bid

[a] Times normal control; assumes PTT has been standardized to heparin levels so that 1.5–2.5× normal equals 0.2–0.4 U/mL; if PTT is normal (27–35 S), start with 5000 U bolus 1300 U/h infusion monitoring PTT; if PTT at recheck is <50 S, rebolus with 5000 U and increase infusion by 100 U/h; if PTT at recheck is 50–60 s, increase infusion rate by 100 U/h; if PTT at recheck is 60–85 s, no change; if PTT at recheck is 85–100 s, decrease infusion rate 100 U/h; if PTT at recheck is 100–120 s, stop infusion for 30 min and decrease rate 100 U/h at restart; if PTT at recheck is >120 s, stop infusion for 60 min and decrease rate 200 U/h at restart.
[b] LMWH does not affect PTT and PTT is not used to adjust dosage.
NOTE: PTT, partial thromboplastin time; LMWH, low-molecular-weight heparin; CHF, congestive heart failure; MI, myocardial infarction.

CHRONIC ORAL ANTICOAGULATION

The coumarin anticoagulants, which include warfarin and dicumarol (dicoumarol), prevent the reduction of vitamin K epoxides in liver microsomes and induce a state of vitamin K deficiency (see Fig. 117-1). They slow thrombin generation and clot formation by impairing the biologic activity of the prothrombin complex proteins and are used to prevent the recurrence of venous thrombosis and pulmonary embolism. Although regimens employing loading doses of drug have been advocated, the simplest way to induce anticoagulation is to administer a single dose of a coumarin compound and monitor the prothrombin time (PT) until the desired prolongation is achieved. For example, treatment can be initiated with 5 mg/d of warfarin or equivalent, with the goal of prolonging the PT to 1.5 to 2 times the control value. Although the PT may reach this value after a few days of therapy, effective anticoagulation, with stable reduction of all the prothrombin complex proteins, requires at least 1 week of warfarin administration. Most patients require a daily maintenance dose of 2.5 to 7.5 mg of warfarin to remain anticoagulated.

Because commercial thromboplastins have different potencies, the PT can vary widely. In an effort to standardize oral anticoagulation, the International Normalized Ratio (INR) method has been adopted by most hospital laboratories and clinicians. In this reporting method, the ratio of the patient's PT is compared to the mean PT for a group of normal individuals. The ratio is adjusted for the sensitivity of the laboratory's thromboplastin determined by the International Sensitivity Index (ISI). Thus, $INR = (PT_{patient}/PT_{normal})^{ISI}$. Use of the INR permits physicians to obtain the appropriate level of anticoagulation independent of laboratory reagents and to follow published recommendations for intensity of anticoagulation. The intensity of anticoagulation may be varied somewhat depending on the clinical indication (Table 118-2). Patients with chronic indwelling venous catheters have been maintained on 1 mg/d of warfarin to prevent clot formation at the catheter tip; such a dose has no effect on the PT.

Although warfarin anticoagulants reduce the recurrence of deep venous thrombosis and pulmonary or cerebral embolism, they may also cause bleeding. Any patient who takes oral anticoagulants requires frequent monitoring of the PT. Despite the most careful management, fluctuations in PT can occur. Various drugs that alter liver microsomal metabolism of coumarins or compete for albumin-binding sites can increase or decrease the potency of these drugs (Table 118-3).

The risk of bleeding increases and, up to a point, the risk of recurrent thrombosis declines with the duration of anticoagulation. Patients with a single uncomplicated thromboembolic event achieve maximal benefit after 3 to 6 months of anticoagulation. About 10% of patients on an oral anticoagulant for 1 year have a bleeding complication requiring medical supervision, and 0.5 to 1% have a fatal hemorrhage. The anticoagulant effects of coumarins can be reversed by infusion of fresh-frozen plasma or by the administration of vitamin K. Fresh-frozen plasma works immediately, but the effects last only a few hours. Vitamin K takes 8 to 12 h to become effective; after vitamin K administration, vitamin K antagonists are more difficult to use for reinduction of anticoagulation. In many cases, reduction or omission of several doses of warfarin improves hemostasis and stops hemorrhage.

Table 118-2 INR Target Ranges for Oral Anticoagulation

Condition	INR	Duration
Venous thrombosis		
Treatment	2–3	3–6 months
Prevention	1.5–1.5	Chronic
Atrial fibrillation	1.5–2	Chronic
Myocardial infarction	2–3	2–3 months
Lupus-like anticoagulants	3–4	Chronic
Mechanical heart valves		
Tissue valves	2–2.5	Chronic
Mechanical valves	3–4	Chronic
Cardiomyopathy	2–3	Chronic

NOTE: INR, International Normalized Ratio.

Table 118-3 Effect of Drugs and Metabolic Changes on Oral Anticoagulant Potency

I. Factors leading to enhanced potency and increased prothrombin time
  A. Reduced coumarin clearance
    1. Disulfiram
    2. Metronidazole
    3. Trimethoprim-sulfamethoxazole
  B. Reduced albumin binding
    Phenylbutazone
  C. Additive hemostatic effect of certain drugs or disorders
    1. Aspirin
    2. Heparin
    3. Liver disease
    4. Thrombocytopenia
    5. Vitamin K deficiency
  D. Increased turnover of vitamin K
    1. Clofibrate
    2. Hypermetabolism (e.g., hyperthyroidism)
II. Factors leading to diminished potency and decreased prothrombin time
  A. Accelerated coumarin clearance—induction of hepatic metabolizing enzymes
    1. Barbiturates
    2. Rifampin
  B. Reduced absorption
    Cholestyramine
  C. Impaired metabolism
    Genetic coumarin resistance

Despite the risk of bleeding, some patients may require lifelong anticoagulation.

Hemorrhagic skin necrosis is a rare complication. Some patients with this complication are deficient in protein C, an anticoagulant protein whose activity is reduced by vitamin K antagonists. Patients suspected of protein C deficiency should only begin oral anticoagulant therapy when combined with heparin or plasma infusions to restore protein C levels to normal. Patients with an inherited coumarin resistance may require extremely high doses to get an anticoagulant effect. Psychologically disturbed patients may surreptitiously ingest coumarin and present with unexplained bleeding and a prolonged PT. Plasma coumarin levels can be measured to confirm such ingestion.

FIBRINOLYTIC THERAPY

Fibrinolysis, an important part of the normal hemostatic process, is initiated by the release of either tissue plasminogen activator (tPA) or pro-urokinase (proUK) from endothelial cells. These agents preferentially activate plasminogen adsorbed onto fibrin clots, a mechanism that localizes the lytic process to sites that contain fibrin thrombi. Although fibrinolysis begins immediately after vascular injury, clot lysis and vessel recanalization may not be complete for 7 to 10 days. The fibrinolytic pathway is important in normal hemostasis; defects can predispose patients to either hemorrhage or recurrent thrombosis (Chap. 117). Activators of the fibrinolytic system are frequently used to accelerate clot lysis in patients with thromboembolism (Fig. 118-1; Table 118-4).

The pharmacologic agents being used to accelerate clot lysis are either derived from natural products or are chemically modified derivatives. They differ with respect to fibrin specificity and some types of complications (Table 118-4). For example, many individuals have antistreptococcal antibodies that react with SK and reduce its potency and cause febrile reactions. All fibrinolytic agents cause hemorrhage. In addition to tPA and proUK, several other agents are relatively "fibrin-specific" and preferentially activate plasminogen in the presence of fibrin. Although this makes it theoretically possible to achieve selective clot lysis, in practice the efficacy and toxicity of the "specific" and "nonspecific" fibrinolytic agents are similar. However, equivalent doses of rtPA cost 10 times more than SK.

Some systemic fibrinolysis always occurs after the infusion of clinically effective doses of fibrin-specific agents. Fibrinogen level falls ~25% after infusion of lytic doses of rtPA. In addition, both the fibrin-specific and -nonspecific agents can cause hemorrhage as they cannot

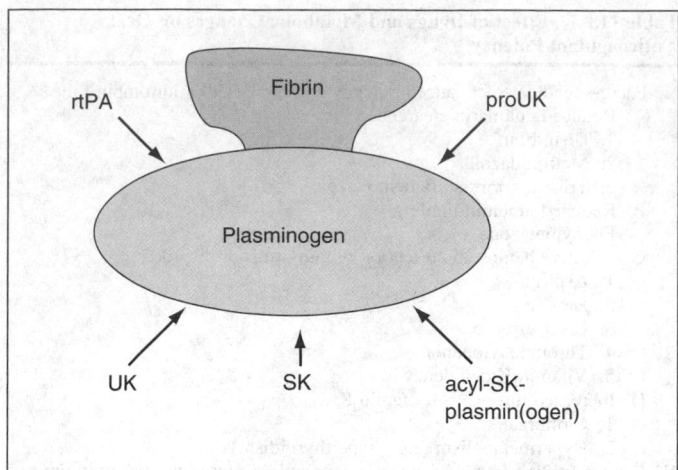

FIGURE 118-1 The mechanism of action of various plasminogen activators used for thrombolytic therapy. Recombinant tissue plasminogen activator (rtPA) and pro-urokinase (proUK) preferentially activate plasminogen bound to fibrin and are called "fibrin-specific" activators. Urokinase (UK), streptokinase (SK), and acylated streptokinase-plasminogen conjugates activate both free and fibrin-bound plasminogen.

differentiate between vital hemostatic plugs and pathologic thrombi. To minimize the risk of bleeding, systemic lytic therapy is not recommended for patients with recent surgery or a history of neurologic lesions, gastrointestinal bleeding, or hypertension.

The current indications for fibrinolytic therapy are listed in Table 118-5. Fibrinolytic therapy is currently recommended for patients with massive pulmonary embolism that is complicated by hypotension, hypoxemia, and right heart strain. It is also used for selected patients with peripheral arterial embolism or occlusion and for patients with extensive iliofemoral thrombophlebitis. While lytic therapy may hasten the resolution of venous thrombi, the long-term benefit still remains unproven, and no firm evidence proves that lytic therapy reduces postphlebitic complications. In contrast, fibrinolytic therapy may be of distinct benefit in patients with axillary vein thrombosis, a condition that does not usually respond to conventional anticoagulation. Fibrinolytic agents are also used to restore the patency of occluded venous catheters and dialysis shunts. For this indication the agents are instilled locally. The extensive literature on the use of fibrinolytic agents to treat patients with coronary artery disease and myocardial infarction is reviewed in Chap. 243. When given within a few hours of infarction, fibrinolytic therapy reduces mortality and myocardial damage.

Although the doses and mode of administration may differ slightly, the general principles and complications are the same for all the fibrinolytic agents. SK and UK are the oldest and most extensively studied

Table 118-5   Possible Indications for Fibrinolytic Therapy

Acute coronary occlusion
Acute peripheral arterial occlusion
Massive pulmonary embolism with severe hypoxemia and hypotension
Axillary vein thrombosis
Massive iliofemoral vein thrombosis—efficacy as yet unproven
Occluded arterial or venous cannulae—low dose, direct infusion into cannula
Venoocclusive disease of the liver

fibrinolytic agents. SK is a bacterial enzyme, and UK is a product of renal tubular epithelial cells. SK is an indirect plasminogen activator that interacts with circulating plasminogen to form an equimolar complex with proteolytic activity. The SK-plasminogen complex then activates additional plasminogen molecules that initiate fibrinolysis. In contrast, UK has intrinsic proteolytic activity and can activate plasminogen directly.

In the case of SK, a loading dose of 250,000 units is usually given irrespective of body weight. Since patients may have antistreptococcal antibodies, the loading dose may need to be repeated. In addition, patients may develop acute allergic symptoms including urticaria and, occasionally, serum sickness reactions. With UK, a loading dose of 4400 units per kilogram body weight is administered over 10 to 30 min. Both regimens induce an intense lytic state as evidenced by a drop in fibrinogen, prolongation of the thrombin time, and a prolongation of the euglobulin lysis time—an in vitro measure of fibrinolytic activity. After the initial loading dose, 100,000 units of SK or 4400 units of UK per kilogram body weight are administered hourly for 24 to 72 h. At the desired time, the lytic state is reversed by discontinuing UK or SK and by administering heparin for 7 to 10 days. Heparin can be started at the same time as the fibrinolytic agent. Fibrinolytic therapy should be initiated as soon as possible after the onset of thrombosis or embolism.

Fibrin-specific agents such as rtPA or proUK are also administered intravenously. Systemic infusion of 100 mg rtPA over 6 h restores coronary artery patency in ~75% of patients. Patients are then maintained on heparin for several days. ProUK given in a similar manner has almost identical effects, but large clinical trials suggest that rtPA is superior to other fibrinolytic agents in maintaining patency of acutely occluded coronary arteries.

ANTIPLATELET DRUG THERAPY

Antiplatelet drugs play a critical role in the management of patients with arterial vascular disease and thromboembolism. Aspirin is the most widely studied of these drugs because of its unique pharmacology. A single dose of aspirin irreversibly acetylates and inactivates the enzyme cyclooxygenase and thereby inhibits platelet production of thromboxane A_2. Although aspirin may also inactivate cyclooxygenase in other tissues, including endothelial cells, such cells recover rapidly by synthesizing new enzyme. Platelets, which are anucleate, cannot synthesize new enzyme and remain inactive for the rest of their life span. As little as one 160-mg tablet of aspirin daily or a 325-mg tablet every other day inhibits platelet thromboxane production and aggregation.

Patients with coronary artery disease who have unstable angina are at high risk for myocardial infarction (Chap. 243). The prompt administration of aspirin dramatically reduces progression to myocardial infarction in this group, although aspirin has no effect on the frequency, intensity, or duration of chronic angina. Aspirin also reduces the incidence of second infarction by 25% when administered to patients who have had a myocardial infarct.

Table 118-4   Fibrinolytic Activators

Product	Source	Molecular Weight	Fibrin-Specific	Complications
Recombinant tissue plasminogen activator (rtPA)	Recombinant	70,000	+	Bleeding
Pro-urokinase (proUK)	Melanoma cell cultures	55,000	+	Bleeding
Urokinase (UK)	Renal tubular cell cultures	33,000	−	Bleeding
Streptokinase (SK)	β-Hemolytic streptococci	47,000	−	Immune reactions—hypotension, fever Bleeding
Acyl-SK-plasmin(ogen)	Chemical synthesis	139,000	+/−	Immune reactions—hypotension, fever Bleeding

Daily aspirin therapy also reduces the incidence of first infarcts. The combination of aspirin and dipyridamole, when begun before surgery, may also increase the patency of coronary bypass grafts; the same combination reduces the incidence of cerebral emboli in patients on warfarin who have prosthetic intracardiac valves. Although dipyridamole has been a popular antithrombotic agent, it has little efficacy when given alone. Aspirin may be the active agent in the combination aspirin-dipyridamole trials.

Aspirin also reduces the frequency of transient ischemic attacks in patients with occlusive cerebrovascular disease. It has largely supplanted anticoagulation with the coumarin compounds in patients with transient ischemia. Aspirin also reduces the incidence of a second stroke by 25% when administered to men following a first stroke. Aspirin is also effective in maintaining the patency of arteriovenous cannulas inserted into patients with renal failure who require hemodialysis. Aspirin plus dipyridamole may also slow the progression of some forms of glomerulonephritis, although these drugs are not widely used in the treatment of renal disease. Aspirin is not effective in maintaining the patency of vessels following percutaneous angioplasty or stent placement.

Although aspirin is clearly the most efficacious antiplatelet agent in clinical use today, a large number of new drugs are being tested that may supplement aspirin therapy. Ticlopidine, a potent inhibitor of platelet function, is effective as an alternative to aspirin in patients with cerebrovascular disease and is superior to aspirin or warfarin in maintaining coronary stent patency. Ticlopidine is more expensive than aspirin and causes some serious side effects, including neutropenia and occasional rare episodes of thrombotic thrombocytopenic purpura (TTP). A related drug, clopidogrel (Plavix), has been proposed as a substitute, but rare cases of TTP have also been noted with its use.

Monoclonal antibodies and both recombinant and chemically synthesized peptides that block either platelet adhesion or aggregation are being tested in clinical trials. A monoclonal antibody Fab fragment that blocks fibrinogen binding to platelet GpIIb/IIIa, thus inhibiting platelet aggregation (abciximab, RheoPro), is used in patients with coronary artery disease who undergo angioplasty. RheoPro is also being evaluated in other settings, e.g., as an adjunct to fibrinolytic therapy in patients with an acute myocardial infarction. A cyclic peptide based on the consensus fibronectin adhesion sequence RGD (arginine, glycine, aspartic acid) called eptifibatide (Integrilin) is as effective as RheoPro for maintaining patency after angioplasty and stent placement as is a small molecule inhibitor (Aggrestat). Orally active GpIIb/IIIa inhibitors have not been proven safe or effective.

The uses of antithrombotic therapy are evolving rapidly. However, aspirin is the current mainstay for chronic therapy and should be used (325 qd or qod) indefinitely in any patient who has had a coronary or cerebral thrombosis. It will reduce ischemic events by 25% or more. Patients undergoing angioplasty or stent placement should receive RheoPro/Integrilin or Aggrestat acutely, followed by 3 weeks of ticlopidine or clopidogrel.

BIBLIOGRAPHY

ANANTHASUBRAMANIAM K et al: Heparin-induced thrombocytopenia and thrombosis. Prog Cardiovasc Dis 42:247, 2000

AWTRY EH, LOSCALZO J: Aspirin. Circulation 101:1206, 2000

BHATT DL, TOPOL EJ: Antiplatelet and anticoagulant therapy in the secondary prevention of ischemic heart disease. Med Clin North Am 84:163, 2000

TCHENG JE: Clinical challenges of platelet glycoprotein IIb/IIIa receptor inhibitor therapy: Bleeding, reversal, thrombocytopenia, and retreatment. Am Heart J 139:538, 2000

NOBEL PRIZE IN PHYSIOLOGY OR MEDICINE, 1930

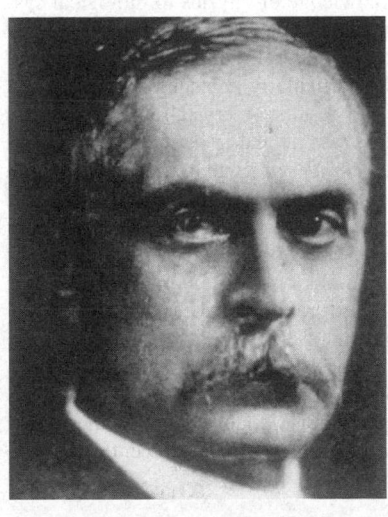

Karl Landsteiner was born in Vienna, Austria, on June 14, 1868, the only child of Leopold and Fanny Landsteiner. He was only 6 years old when his father died. After *Gymnasium* (German high school), he entered the University of Vienna Medical School at age 17. On graduation from medical school in 1891, he decided on a career in laboratory research rather than the practice of medicine. Landsteiner undertook research with Emil Fischer (a Nobel laureate in 1902) at the University of Würzburg. In 1899 at the age of 31, while working as an assistant in Anton Weichselbaum's laboratory in the Department of Pathology at the University of Vienna, he discovered the blood groups A, B, and O using agglutination techniques. The fourth group, AB, was added a year later by Landsteiner. The original publication of the identification of groups was only three pages, and Landsteiner was the sole author. In the next 8 years little attention was paid to this highly significant discovery. However, in 1910 it was demonstrated that these blood groups were transmitted by Gregor Mendel's laws of inheritance—A, B, and AB were autosomal dominant, and O was recessive. Until Landsteiner's discovery, blood transfusions had been abandoned because of serious complications. Subsequently, blood typing allowed the use of blood transfusions to save millions of lives.

With the devastation of Vienna during World War I, Landsteiner was forced to move to a small hospital in Leiden, Holland, where he worked as a pathologist until he was invited to become a member of the Rockefeller Institute in New York in 1922. In 1930 Landsteiner received the Nobel Prize, some 30 years after his discovery of blood groups. His family only learned that Landsteiner (a modest man) had received the Nobel Prize when a friend arrived at his home to congratulate him. In 1940 at the age of 72, Landsteiner and his co-workers made another important discovery—a new factor in the blood named the rhesus (Rh) factor. This discovery explained the deaths of newborn babies from erythroblastosis fetalis when there was incompatibility between an Rh-negative mother and an Rh-positive baby. This discovery also allowed incompatibilities in blood transfusion due to Rh factor incompatibility to be avoided. At the age of 75 Landsteiner had a fatal heart attack while at his laboratory workbench, with a pipette in his hand, at the Rockefeller Institute. It was written, "Landsteiner belonged to those scholars for whom the aim of science is first of all the honour of the human spirit."

REFERENCES

1. Magill FN (ed): *Nobel Prize Winners: Physiology or Medicine*, vol 1. Pasadena, Salem Press, 1993
2. Schrier RW: *A Salute to Nobel Laureates in Physiology and Medicine*, Proceedings of the Association of American Physicians 108(1): Jan 1996
3. Sourkes TL: *Nobel Prize Winners in Medicine and Physiology 1910–1965*. London, Abelard-Schuman, 1967

Robert W. Schrier, MD

NOBEL PRIZE IN PHYSIOLOGY OR MEDICINE, 1962

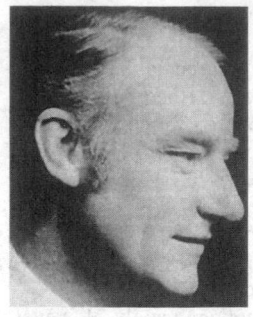

Francis Harry Compton Crick was born in Northampton, England, on June 8, 1916. He had his early education in Northampton and then received his B.Sc. degree in physics from University College London. The German bombing in World War II destroyed the physics laboratory at UCL, forcing Crick to abandon his Ph.D. research. Instead, he became a research scientist for the British Admiralty, studying magnetic and acoustic mines. In 1949 Crick decided to change his interests to biology and entered a doctorate program at the Medical Research Council's Cavendish Laboratory at Cambridge. He worked with Nobel Laureates Laurence Bragg and Max Perutz, using x-ray diffraction studies of biological molecules, particularly proteins. At Cambridge he met 23-year-old James D. Watson and began a scientific collaboration that would change the world of science.

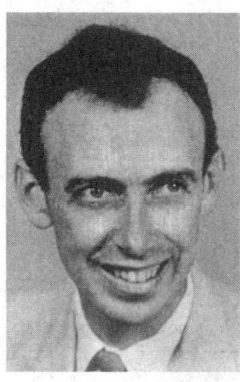

James Dewey Watson was born in Chicago, Illinois, on April 6, 1928. He was a brilliant student and received a scholarship to enter the University of Chicago at the age of 15. He received his B.S. degree there in zoology in 1947 and then entered Indiana University to obtain a Ph.D. degree in the same field, writing his thesis on bacteriophage proliferation and the effects of x-rays on the process, under the supervision of Nobel Laureates Salvador Edward Luria and Hermann Joseph Muller. After receiving his Ph.D. he moved to Copenhagen, Denmark, to study phage infection of bacteria. At a meeting in Italy, he met Maurice Wilkins, who presented a paper on x-ray diffraction through crystalline DNA, which indicated that DNA might be helical in nature. This work enhanced Watson's interest in DNA, and he decided in 1952 to move to the Cavendish Laboratory in Cambridge where he met Francis Crick, who was also interested in the structure of DNA. At that time DNA was felt to be the genetic material of heredity; thus an understanding of its structure could lead to the genetic code whereby proteins, cells, and organisms are created.

The challenge of understanding the structure of DNA excited Crick and Watson more than their primary work at the Cavendish—the study of the hemoglobin structure and the genetics of viruses, respectively. With their knowledge of the chemistry of nucleotides and the x-ray diffraction results from Rosalind Franklin and Maurice Wilkins, in 1951 Crick and Watson initially proposed a single structure chain helical model of DNA. Franklin, however, found this proposal incompatible with her x-ray diffraction studies. After this failure, Crick and Watson were ordered by their supervisors at the Cavendish to return to their primary tasks; they assumed that Watson and Crick could not compete with the senior and established Wilkins-Franklin group at King's College in London. Even Wilkins told them: "DNA, you know, is Midas' gold. Everyone who touches it goes mad."

A great coincidence then occurred. Although Linus Pauling, who had described the helix in protein structure, was not allowed to travel outside the United States because of his antinuclear views, his son, Peter Pauling, was working at the Cavendish at the same time as Watson and Crick. Peter Pauling shared with Crick and Watson a paper that had been submitted to the *Proceedings of the National Academy of Science*, purporting to have described the structure of DNA as a triple helix. Crick and Watson immediately recognized the flaws in this proposal and thus were allowed to return to their real passion, the study of the structure of DNA. On this second attempt, however, they were equipped with more knowledge about the molecule. They had seen Franklin's excellent DNA diffraction photographs that suggested that there were two helically arranged polynucleotide chains. Moreover, Erwin Chargaff had shown that in various species, including humans, the amount of thymine equalled the amount of adenine and the amount of guanine equalled the amount of cytosine. Crick and Watson then began to build a cardboard and metal model of DNA. Their structure this time consisted of two polynucleotide chains running in opposite directions in a double helical shape like a right-handed spiral staircase.

This time, the Crick and Watson double-helix structure of DNA was supported by the x-ray diffraction results of Rosalind Franklin. Thus, Crick and Watson quickly published three brief papers in the spring of 1953 that drastically changed genetic research.

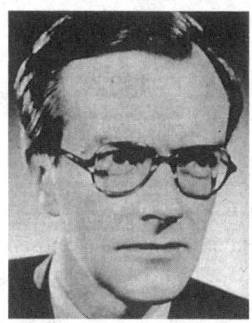

Maurice Hugh Frederick Wilkins was born on December 15, 1916, in Pongaroa, New Zealand, to Edgar Henry and Eveline Constance Jane Wilkins, both of Dublin, Ireland. Edgar Wilkins was a school physician who had been interested in research but had little time to pursue it because of his practice. Maurice was sent to England at an early age to pursue his education, first at King Edward's School in Birmingham, and at St. John's College at the University of Cambridge for his B.A. He earned his Ph.D. from Birmingham University with a thesis on the luminescence of solids and the electron trap theory of phosphorescence. During World War II he joined the Manhattan Project team in Berkeley, California, where he was involved in the mass spectrography studies of the separation of uranium isotopes. After the war and the devastating explosion of atomic bombs at Hiroshima and Nagasaki, Wilkins decided to apply his knowledge of physics to biological systems to try to obtain a better understanding of heredity and disease.

Wilkins became quite interested in the structure of DNA. He found that the DNA fibers in gel were particularly amenable to analysis by x-ray diffraction techniques. The results of crystallography studies suggested that the DNA structure was helical in nature. The width of the helix suggested that it was composed of two strands, that is, a double helix. He and Rosalind Franklin shared this information with Crick and Watson, who ultimately published the double-helix structure of DNA. In 1962 Wilkins shared the Nobel Prize in Physiology or Medicine with Crick and Watson. His only disappointment was that Franklin could not share in this deserved honor because in 1957 she had died of cancer at the young age of 37.

The discovery of the structure of DNA has been compared to finding the Rosetta Stone or to splitting the atom, or to the greatest step in understanding genetics since Gregor Mendel illustrated the fundamentals of inheritance in the middle of the nineteenth century.

REFERENCES

1. Aaseng N: *The Disease Fighters.* Minneapolis, Lerner Publications, 1987
2. Magill FN (ed): *Nobel Prize Winners: Physiology and Medicine,* vol 2. Pasadena, Salem Press, 1993
3. Schrier RW: *A Salute to Nobel Laureates in Physiology and Medicine,* Proceedings of the Association of American Physicians 108(1): Jan 1996
4. Sourkes TL: *Nobel Prize Winners in Medicine and Physiology 1901–1965.* London, Abelard-Schuman, 1967
5. Watson JD: *The Double Helix.* New York, Penguin Books, 1968

Robert W. Schrier, MD

119

Lawrence C. Madoff, Dennis L. Kasper

INTRODUCTION TO INFECTIOUS DISEASES: HOST–PARASITE INTERACTIONS

Despite decades of dramatic progress in their treatment and prevention, infectious diseases remain a major cause of death and debility and are responsible for worsening the living conditions of many millions of people around the world. Infections frequently challenge the physician's diagnostic skill and must be considered in the differential diagnoses of syndromes affecting every organ system.

CHANGING EPIDEMIOLOGY OF INFECTIOUS DISEASES With the advent of antimicrobial agents, some medical leaders believed that infectious diseases would soon be eliminated and become of historic interest only. Indeed, the hundreds of chemotherapeutic agents developed since World War II, most of which are potent and safe, include drugs effective not only against bacteria but also against viruses, fungi, and parasites. Nevertheless, we now realize that as we developed antimicrobial agents, microbes developed the ability to elude our best weapons and to counterattack with new survival strategies. Antibiotic resistance occurs at an alarming rate among all classes of mammalian pathogens. Pneumococci resistant to penicillin and enterococci resistant to vancomycin have become commonplace. Even *Staphylococcus aureus* with reduced susceptibility to vancomycin has appeared. Such pathogens present real clinical problems in managing infections that were easily treatable just a few years ago. Diseases once thought to have been nearly eradicated from the developed world—tuberculosis, cholera, and rheumatic fever, for example—have rebounded with renewed ferocity. Newly discovered and emerging infectious agents appear to have been brought into contact with humans by changes in the environment and by movements of human and animal populations. An example of the propensity for pathogens to escape from their usual niche is the alarming 1999 outbreak in New York of encephalitis due to a flavivirus similar or identical to West Nile virus, which had never previously been isolated in the Americas.

Many infectious agents have been discovered only in recent decades. Ebola virus, hantavirus, the agent of human granulocytotropic ehrlichiosis, and retroviruses such as HIV humble us despite our deepening understanding of pathogenesis at the most basic molecular level. Even in developed countries, infectious diseases have made a resurgence. Between 1980 and 1996, mortality from infectious diseases in the United States increased by 64% to levels not seen since the 1940s.

The role of infectious agents in the etiology of diseases once believed to be noninfectious is being increasingly recognized. For example, it is now widely accepted that *Helicobacter pylori* is the causative agent of peptic ulcer disease and perhaps of gastric malignancy. Human papillomavirus is likely to be the most important cause of invasive cervical cancer. A new human herpesvirus (HHV-8) is believed to be the cause of most cases of Kaposi's sarcoma. Epstein-Barr virus is a cause of certain lymphomas and may play a role in the genesis of Hodgkin's disease. The possibility certainly exists that other diseases of unknown cause, such as rheumatoid arthritis, sarcoidosis, or inflammatory bowel disease, have infectious etiologies. There is even evidence that atherosclerosis may have an infectious component.

Medical advances over infectious diseases have been hindered by changes in the patient population. Immunocompromised hosts now constitute a significant proportion of the seriously infected population. Physicians immunosuppress their patients to prevent the rejection of transplants and to treat neoplastic and inflammatory diseases. Some infections, most notably that caused by HIV, immunocompromise the host in and of themselves. Lesser degrees of immunosuppression are associated with other infections, such as influenza and syphilis. Infectious agents that coexist peacefully with immunocompetent hosts wreak havoc in those who lack a complete immune system. AIDS has brought to prominence once-obscure organisms such as *Pneumocystis carinii*, *Cryptosporidium parvum*, and *Mycobacterium avium*.

BIOTERRORISM In recent years, the efforts of some governments and terrorist organizations to use biological weaponry have refocused public concern on the topic. To date, there is little evidence that biological weapons have ever been effectively used; indeed, their ease of use may be overstated. However, the ability of infectious agents to inflict widespread illness and thus to cause societal disruption and panic, together with the relatively low cost of these agents, has led to their being called a "poor man's nuclear arsenal."

Several pathogens have been considered likely candidates for biological warfare. *Bacillus anthracis*, which causes the zoonosis anthrax, is widely viewed as the leading contender. The hardy spores of the bacillus can be distributed by bombardment or other dispersal mechanisms. Inhalation of this pathogen results in severe pneumonia with a mortality rate of 95% in untreated persons. A World Health Organization report estimated that 50 kg of *B. anthracis* released upwind of a city with a population of 500,000 would result in up to 95,000 fatalities, with an additional 125,000 persons incapacitated. Moreover, the attack might go undetected until large numbers of seriously ill individuals presented with overt disease. In 1979, an accidental release from a military microbiology facility near Sverdlovsk in the former Soviet Union caused at least 66 deaths from inhalational anthrax along a 4-km-wide path downwind of the facility. The vast scope of the Soviet Union's biological warfare program, employing 60,000 people at its height, has only recently come to light. This endeavor is thought to be echoed by efforts in many other countries in the world today. In response to the perceived threat of anthrax as a biological weapon, the U.S. military recently decided to vaccinate more than 2 million of its members against this infection.

Smallpox, an ancient scourge caused by variola virus, has also been considered as a bioweapon owing to its contagiousness and high mortality rate and to the declining population of immunized persons. Indeed, one of the earliest accounts of biological warfare involved the distribution of smallpox-infected blankets to Native American tribes by British troops. Debate continues about whether to eradicate the two known existing stocks of the virus in U.S. and Russian government laboratories. Many investigators believe that additional undocumented stockpiles of the virus exist around the world.

Other infectious organisms that combine the virulence and stability necessary for biological weapons include *Yersinia pestis*, the agent of plague, and *Francisella tularensis*, the agent of tularemia. Viral hemorrhagic fever agents such as the Ebola and Marburg viruses as well as toxins such as that from *Clostridium botulinum* have also been considered as biological weapons. While some of the diseases caused by these agents can be effectively treated or prevented if sufficient resources exist to do so, it may also be possible for an aggressor to render organisms resistant to antibiotics or even to vaccines through genetic manipulation or other means.

HOST FACTORS IN INFECTION For any infectious process to occur, the parasite and the host must first encounter each other. Factors such as geography, environment, and behavior thus influence the likelihood of infection. Though the initial encounter between a susceptible host and a virulent organism frequently results in disease, some organisms can be harbored in the host for years before disease becomes clinically evident. For a complete view, individual patients must be considered in the context of the population to which they belong. Infectious diseases do not often occur in isolation; rather, they spread through a group exposed from a point source (e.g., a contaminated water supply) or from individual to individual (e.g., via respiratory droplets). Thus, the clinician must be alert to infections prevalent in the community as a whole. A detailed history, including information on travel, behavioral factors, exposures to animals or potentially contaminated environments, and living and occupational conditions, must be elicited. For example, the likelihood of infection by *Plasmodium falciparum* can be significantly affected by altitude, climate, terrain, season, and even time of day. Antibiotic-resistant strains are localized to specific geographic regions, and a seemingly minor alteration in a travel itinerary can dramatically influence the likelihood of acquiring chloroquine-resistant malaria. If such important details in the history are overlooked, inappropriate treatment may result in the death of the patient. Likewise, the chance of acquiring a sexually transmitted disease can be greatly affected by a relatively minor variation in sexual practices, such as the method used for birth control. Knowledge of the relationship between specific risk factors and disease allows the physician to influence a patient's health even before the development of infection by modification of these risk factors and—when a vaccine is available—by immunization.

Many specific host factors influence the likelihood of acquiring an infectious disease. Age, immunization history, prior illnesses, level of nutrition, pregnancy, coexisting illness, and perhaps emotional state all have some impact on the risk of infection after exposure to a potential pathogen. The importance of individual host defense mechanisms, either specific or nonspecific, becomes apparent in their absence, and our understanding of these immune mechanisms is enhanced by studies of clinical syndromes developing in immunodeficient patients (Table 119-1). For example, the frequent occurrence of meningococcal disease in people with deficiencies in specific complement proteins of the "membrane attack complex" underscores the importance of an intact complement system in the prevention of meningococcal infection.

Medical care itself increases the patient's risk of acquiring an infection in several ways: (1) through contact with pathogens during hospitalization, (2) through breaching of the skin (with intravenous devices or surgical incisions) or mucosal surfaces (with endotracheal tubes or bladder catheters), (3) through introduction of foreign bodies, (4) through alteration of the natural flora with antibiotics, and (5) through treatment with immunosuppressive drugs.

THE IMMUNE RESPONSE Infection involves complicated interactions of parasite and host and inevitably affects both. In most cases, a pathogenic process consisting of several steps is required for the development of infections. Since the competent host has a complex series of barricades in place to prevent infection, the successful parasite must utilize specific strategies at each of these steps. The specific strategies used by bacteria, viruses, and parasites (Chaps. 120 and 180) have some remarkable conceptual similarities, but the strategic details are unique not only for each class of organism but also for individual species within a class.

Once in the bloodstream or a normally sterile body site, the microorganism faces the host's tightly integrated cellular and humoral immune systems. Cellular immunity (Chap. 305), comprising T lymphocytes, macrophages, and natural killer cells, primarily recognizes and combats pathogens that proliferate intracellularly. Cellular immune mechanisms are important in immunity to all classes of infectious agents, including most viruses and many bacteria (e.g., *Mycoplasma*, *Chlamydia*, *Listeria*, *Salmonella*, and *Mycobacterium*), parasites (e.g., *Trypanosoma*, *Toxoplasma*, and *Leishmania*), and fungi (e.g., *Histoplasma*, *Cryptococcus*, and *Coccidioides*). Usually, T lymphocytes are activated by macrophages and B lymphocytes, which present foreign antigens along with the host's own major histocompatibility complex antigen. Activated T cells may then act in several ways to fight infection. Cytotoxic T cells may directly attack and lyse host cells that express foreign antigens. Helper T cells stimulate the proliferation of B cells and the production of immunoglobulins. B cells and T cells communicate with each other via a variety of signals, and often more than one signal is employed simultaneously. For example, costimulation through the CD40-CD40 ligand increases B cell responses, and costimulation via the B7-CD28 axis is required for activation of the CD4+ helper T cell. T cells elaborate cytokines (e.g., interferon), which directly inhibit the growth of pathogens or stimulate killing by host macrophages and cytotoxic cells. Cytokines also augment the host's immunity by stimulating the inflammatory response (fever, the production of acute-phase serum components, and the proliferation of leukocytes). Cytokine stimulation does not always result in a favorable response in the host; septic shock (Chap. 124) and toxic shock syndrome (Chaps. 139 and 140) are among the conditions that are mediated by these inflammatory substances.

The reticuloendothelial system comprises monocyte-derived phagocytic cells that are located in the liver (Kupffer cells), lung (alveolar macrophages), spleen, kidney (mesangial cells), brain (microglia), and lymph nodes and that clear circulating microorganisms. Although these tissue macrophages and polymorphonuclear leukocytes (PMNs) are capable of killing microorganisms without help, they function much more efficiently when pathogens are first *opsonized* (Greek, "to prepare for eating") by components of the complement system such as C3b and/or by antibodies.

Extracellular pathogens, including most encapsulated bacteria, are attacked by the humoral immune system, which includes antibodies, the complement cascade, and phagocytic cells. Antibodies are complex glycoproteins (also called immunoglobulins) that are produced by mature B lymphocytes, circulate in body fluids, and are secreted on mucosal surfaces. Antibodies specifically recognize and bind to foreign antigens. One of the most impressive features of the immune system is the ability to generate an incredible diversity of antibodies capable of recognizing virtually every foreign antigen yet not reacting with self. In addition to being exquisitely specific for antigens, antibodies come in different structural and functional classes: IgG predominates in the circulation and persists for many years after exposure; IgM is the earliest specific antibody to appear in response to infection; secretory IgA is important in immunity at mucosal surfaces, while monomeric IgA appears in the serum; and IgE is important in allergic and parasitic diseases. Antibodies may directly impede the function of an invading organism, neutralize secreted toxins and enzymes, or facilitate the removal of the antigen (invading organism) by phagocytic cells. Immunoglobulins participate in cell-mediated immunity by promoting the antibody-dependent cellular cytotoxicity functions of certain T lymphocytes. Antibodies also promote the deposition of complement components on the surface of the invader.

The complement system (Chap. 305) consists of a group of serum proteins functioning as a cooperative, self-regulating cascade of enzymes that adhere to—and in some cases disrupt—the surface of invading organisms. Some of these surface-adherent proteins (e.g., C3b) can then act as opsonins for destruction of microbes by phagocytes. The later, "terminal" components (C7, C8, and C9) can directly kill some bacterial invaders (notably, many of the neisseriae) by forming a "membrane attack complex" and disrupting the integrity of the bacterial membrane, thus causing bacteriolysis. Other complement components, such as C5a, act as chemoattractants for PMNs. Complement activation and deposition occur by either or both of two pathways: the

Table 119-1 Infections Associated with Selected Defects in Immunity

Host Defect	Disease or Therapy Associated with Defect	Common Etiologic Agent of Infection
NONSPECIFIC IMMUNITY		
Impaired cough	Rib fracture, neuromuscular dysfunction	Bacteria causing pneumonia, aerobic and anaerobic oral flora
Loss of gastric acidity	Achlorhydria, histamine blockade	*Salmonella* spp., enteric pathogens
Loss of cutaneous integrity	Penetrating trauma, athlete's foot	*Staphylococcus* spp., *Streptococcus* spp.
	Burn	*Pseudomonas aeruginosa*
	Intravenous catheter	*Staphylococcus* spp., *Streptococcus* spp., gram-negative rods, coagulase-negative staphylococci
Implantable device	Heart valve	*Streptococcus* spp., coagulase-negative staphylococci, *Staphylococcus aureus*
	Artificial joint	*Staphylococcus* spp., *Streptococcus* spp., gram-negative rods
Loss of normal bacterial flora	Antibiotic use	*Clostridium difficile*, *Candida* spp.
Impaired clearance		
Poor drainage	Urinary tract infection	*Escherichia coli*
Abnormal secretions	Cystic fibrosis	Chronic pulmonary infection with *P. aeruginosa*
INFLAMMATORY RESPONSE		
Neutropenia	Hematologic malignancy, cytotoxic chemotherapy, aplastic anemia, HIV infection	Gram-negative enteric bacilli, *Pseudomonas* spp., *Staphylococcus* spp., *Candida* spp.
Chemotaxis	Chédiak-Higashi syndrome, Job's syndrome, protein-calorie malnutrition	*S. aureus*, *Streptococcus pyogenes*, *Haemophilus influenzae*, gram-negative bacilli
	Leukocyte adhesion defects 1 and 2	Bacteria causing skin and systemic infections, gingivitis
Phagocytosis (cellular)	Systemic lupus erythematosus, chronic myelogenous leukemia, megaloblastic anemia	*Streptococcus pneumoniae*, *H. influenzae*
Splenectomy	—	*H. influenzae*, *S. pneumoniae*, other streptococci, *Capnocytophaga* spp., *Babesia microti*, *Salmonella* spp.
Microbicidal defect	Chronic granulomatous disease	Catalase-positive bacteria and fungi: staphylococci, *E. coli*, *Klebsiella* spp., *P. aeruginosa*, *Aspergillus* spp., *Nocardia* spp.
	Chédiak-Higashi syndrome	*S. aureus*, *S. pyogenes*
	Interferon γ receptor defect, interleukin 12 deficiency, interleukin 12 receptor defect	*Mycobacterium* spp., *Salmonella* spp.
COMPLEMENT SYSTEM		
C3	Congenital liver disease, systemic lupus erythematosus, nephrotic syndrome	*S. aureus*, *S. pneumoniae*, *Pseudomonas* spp., *Proteus* spp.
C5	Congenital	*Neisseria* spp., gram-negative rods
C6, C7, C8	Congenital, systemic lupus erythematosus	*Neisseria meningitidis*, *N. gonorrhoeae*
Alternative pathway	Sickle cell disease	*S. pneumoniae*, *Salmonella* spp.
IMMUNE RESPONSE		
T lymphocyte deficiency/dysfunction	Thymic aplasia, thymic hypoplasia, Hodgkin's disease, sarcoidosis, lepromatous leprosy	*Listeria monocytogenes*, *Mycobacterium* spp., *Candida* spp., *Aspergillus* spp., *Cryptococcus neoformans*, herpes simplex virus, varicella-zoster virus
	AIDS	*Pneumocystis carinii*, cytomegalovirus, herpes simplex virus, *Mycobacterium avium-intracellulare*, *C. neoformans*, *Candida* spp.
	Mucocutaneous candidiasis	*Candida* spp.
	Purine nucleoside phosphorylase deficiency	Fungi, viruses
B cell deficiency/dysfunction	Bruton's X-linked agammaglobulinemia	*S. pneumoniae*, other streptococci
	Agammaglobulinemia, chronic lymphocytic leukemia, multiple myeloma, dysglobulinemia	*H. influenzae*, *N. meningitidis*, *S. aureus*, *Klebsiella pneumoniae*, *E. coli*, *Giardia lamblia*, *P. carinii*, enteroviruses
	Selective IgM deficiency	*S. pneumoniae*, *H. influenzae*, *E. coli*
	Selective IgA deficiency	*G. lamblia*, hepatitis virus, *S. pneumoniae*, *H. influenzae*
Mixed T and B cell deficiency/dysfunction	Common variable hypogammaglobulinemia	*P. carinii*, cytomegalovirus, *S. pneumoniae*, *H. influenzae*, various other bacteria
	Ataxia-telangiectasia	*S. pneumoniae*, *H. influenzae*, *S. aureus*, rubella virus, *G. lamblia*
	Severe combined immunodeficiency	*S. aureus*, *S. pneumoniae*, *H. influenzae*, *Candida albicans*, *P. carinii*, varicella-zoster virus, rubella virus, cytomegalovirus
	Wiskott-Aldrich syndrome	Agents of infections associated with T and B cell abnormalities
	X-linked hyper-IgM syndrome	*P. carinii*, cytomegalovirus, *Cryptosporidium parvum*

SOURCE: Adapted from H Masur and A Fauci, in *Harrison's Principles of Internal Medicine*, 13th ed, KJ Isselbacher et al (eds), New York, McGraw-Hill, 1994.

classic pathway is activated primarily by immune complexes (i.e., antibody bound to antigen), and the alternative pathway is activated by microbial components, frequently in the absence of antibody. PMNs have receptors for both antibody and C3b, and antibody and complement function together to aid in the clearance of infectious agents.

PMNs, short-lived white blood cells that engulf and kill invading microbes, are first attracted to inflammatory sites by chemoattractants such as C5a, which is a product of complement activation at the site of infection. PMNs localize to the site of infection by adhering to cellular adhesion molecules expressed by endothelial cells. Endothelial cells express these receptors, called *selectins* (CD-62, ELAM-1), in response to inflammatory cytokines such as tumor necrosis factor

(TNF) α and interleukin 1. The binding of these selectin molecules to specific receptors on PMNs results in the adherence of the PMNs to the endothelium. Cytokine-mediated upregulation and expression of intercellular adhesion molecule 1 (ICAM 1) on endothelial cells then take place, and this latter receptor binds to β_2 integrins on PMNs, thereby facilitating diapedesis into the extravascular compartment. Once the PMNs are in the extravascular compartment, various molecules such as arachidonic acids further enhance the inflammatory process.

Approach to the Patient

The clinical manifestations of infectious diseases at presentation are myriad, varying from fulminant life-threatening processes to brief and self-limited conditions to indolent chronic maladies. The clinician must use all the skills of medicine to diagnose the infection and prescribe appropriate treatment. First, a careful history is essential and must include details on underlying chronic diseases; medications; occupation; travel; and risk factors for exposure to certain types of pathogens, such as those associated with sexual contacts, family illnesses, illicit drug use, particular animals, blood transfusions, ingestion of contaminated liquids or foods, or bites of insect vectors. Since infectious diseases may involve many organ systems, a careful review of systems may elicit important clues as to the disease process. The physical examination must be thorough, and attention must be paid to seemingly minor details: a soft heart murmur that might indicate bacterial endocarditis; an evanescent skin rash that suggests rheumatic fever; or a retinal lesion that suggests disseminated candidiasis or cytomegalovirus (CMV) infection.

LABORATORY INVESTIGATIONS   Laboratory studies must be carefully considered and directed toward establishing an etiologic diagnosis in the shortest possible time, at the lowest possible cost, and with the least possible discomfort to the patient. Cultures must be performed in a manner that minimizes the likelihood of contamination with normal flora while maximizing the yield. A sputum sample is far more likely to be valuable when elicited with careful coaching by the clinician than when collected in a container simply left at the bedside with cursory instructions. Gram's stains of specimens should be interpreted carefully and the quality of the specimen assessed. The findings on Gram's staining should correspond to the results of culture; a discrepancy may suggest diagnostic possibilities such as infection due to fastidious or anaerobic bacteria.

The microbiology laboratory must be an ally in the diagnostic endeavor (Chap. 121). Astute laboratory personnel will suggest optimal culture and transport conditions or alternative tests to facilitate diagnosis. If informed about specific potential pathogens, an alert laboratory staff will allow sufficient time for these organisms to become evident in culture, even when present in small numbers or when slow-growing. The parasitology technician who is attuned to the specific diagnostic considerations relevant to a particular case may be able to detect the rare, otherwise-elusive egg or cyst in a stool specimen. In cases where a diagnosis appears difficult, serum should be stored during the early acute phase of the illness so that a diagnostic rise in titer of antibody to a specific pathogen can be detected later. Bacterial and fungal antigens can sometimes be detected in body fluids, even when cultures are negative or are rendered sterile by antibiotic therapy. Techniques such as the polymerase chain reaction allow the amplification of specific DNA sequences so that minute quantities of foreign nucleic acids can be recognized in host specimens.

℞   **TREATMENT**   Optimal therapy for infectious diseases requires a broad knowledge of medicine and careful clinical judgment. Life-threatening infections such as bacterial meningitis or sepsis, viral encephalitis, or falciparum malaria must be treated immediately, often before a specific causative organism is identified. Antimicrobial

agents must be chosen empirically and must be active against the range of potential infectious agents consistent with the clinical scenario. In contrast, good clinical judgment sometimes dictates withholding of antimicrobials in a self-limited process or until a specific diagnosis is made. The dictum *primum non nocere* should be adhered to, and it should be remembered that all antimicrobials carry a risk (and a cost) to the patient. Direct toxicity may be encountered—e.g., ototoxicity due to aminoglycosides, lipodystrophy due to HIV protease inhibitors, and hepatotoxicity due to antituberculous agents such as isoniazid and rifampin. Allergic reactions are common and can be serious. Since superinfection sometimes follows the eradication of the normal flora and colonization by a resistant organism, one invariable principle is that infectious disease therapy should be directed toward as narrow a spectrum of infectious agents as possible. Treatment specific for the pathogen should result in as little perturbation as possible of the host's microflora. With few exceptions, abscesses require surgical or percutaneous drainage for cure. Foreign bodies, including medical devices, must generally be removed in order to eliminate an infection of the device or of the adjacent tissue. Other infections, such as necrotizing fasciitis, peritonitis due to a perforated organ, gas gangrene, and chronic osteomyelitis, require surgery as the primary means of cure; in these conditions, antibiotics play only an adjunctive role.

The role of immunomodulators in the management of infectious diseases has received increasing attention. Glucocorticoids have been shown to be of benefit in the treatment of *Haemophilus influenzae* meningitis in children and in therapy for *P. carinii* pneumonia in patients with AIDS. The use of these agents in other infectious processes remains less clear and in some cases (in cerebral malaria and septic shock, for example) is detrimental. Other agents that modulate the immune response include prostaglandin inhibitors, specific lymphokines, and TNF inhibitors. Specific antibody therapy plays a role in the treatment and prevention of many diseases. Specific immunoglobulins have long been known to prevent the development of symptomatic rabies and tetanus. More recently, CMV immune globulin has been recognized as important not only in preventing the transmission of the virus during organ transplantation but also in treating CMV pneumonia in bone marrow transplant recipients. There is a strong need for well-designed clinical trials to evaluate each new interventional modality.

PERSPECTIVE   The genetic simplicity of many infectious agents allows them to undergo rapid evolution and to develop selective advantages that result in constant variation in the clinical manifestations of infection. Moreover, changes in the environment and the host can predispose new populations to a particular infection. An epidemic of lethal respiratory failure—later identified as hantavirus pulmonary syndrome—on a Navajo reservation in the southwestern United States in 1993 caused nationwide alarm, exemplifying the fear that new plagues induce in the human psyche.

The potential for infectious agents to emerge in novel and unexpected ways requires that physicians and public health officials be knowledgeable, vigilant, and open-minded in their approach to unexplained illness. The emergence of antimicrobial-resistant pathogens (e.g., enterococci that are resistant to all known antimicrobial agents and cause infections that are essentially untreatable) has led some to conclude that we are entering the "postantibiotic era." Others have held to the perception that infectious diseases no longer represent as serious a concern to world health as they once did. The progress that science, medicine, and society as a whole have made in combating these maladies is impressive, and it is ironic that, as we stand on the threshold of an understanding of the most basic biology of the microbe, infectious diseases are posing renewed problems. We are threatened by the appearance of new diseases such as AIDS, hepatitis C, and Ebola virus infection and by the reemergence of old foes such as tuberculosis, cholera, plague, and *Streptococcus pyogenes* infection. True students of infectious diseases were perhaps less surprised than anyone else by these developments. Those who know pathogens are aware of their incredible adaptability and diversity. As ingenious and successful as therapeutic approaches may be, our ability to develop methods to counter infectious agents so far has not matched the myriad strategies employed by the sea of microbes that surrounds us. Their sheer numbers and the rate at which they can evolve are daunting. Moreover, environmental changes, rapid global travel, population movements, and medicine itself—through its use of antibiotics and immunosuppressive agents—all increase the impact of infectious diseases. Although new vaccines, new antibiotics, improved global communication, and new modalities for treating and preventing infection will be developed, pathogenic microbes will continue to develop new strategies of their own, presenting us with an unending and dynamic challenge.

BIBLIOGRAPHY

ARMSTRONG G et al: Trends in infectious disease mortality in the United States during the 20th century. JAMA 281:61, 1999

BERKELMAN RI, HUGHES JM: The conquest of infectious diseases: Who are we kidding? Ann Intern Med 119:426, 1993

BUCKLEY RH: Immunodeficiency diseases. JAMA 268:2797, 1992

DE JONG R et al: Severe mycobacterial and *Salmonella* infections in interleukin-12 receptor-deficient patients. Science 280:1435, 1998

FIELDS BN: Pathogenesis of viral infections, in *Virology*, BN Fields (ed). New York, Raven, 1996, pp 191–239

GOLD HS, EISENSTEIN BI: Introduction to bacterial diseases, in *Principles and Practice of Infectious Diseases*, 5th ed, GL Mandell et al (eds). New York, Churchill Livingstone, 2000, p 2065

GRAYSTON JT, CAMPBELL LA: Editorial response: The role of *Chlamydia pneumoniae* in atherosclerosis. Clin Infect Dis 28:993, 1999

HENDERSON DA: Bioterrorism as a public health threat. Emerg Infect Dis 4:488, 1998

NEWPORT MJ et al: A mutation in the interferon-γ-receptor gene and susceptibility to mycobacterial infection. N Engl J Med 335:1941, 1996

PILE JC et al: Anthrax as a potential biological warfare agent. Arch Intern Med 158:429, 1998

PUCK JM: Primary immunodeficiency diseases. JAMA 278:1835, 1997

QUAGLIARELLO V, SCHELD MW: Bacterial meningitis: Pathogenesis, pathophysiology, and progress. N Engl J Med 327:864, 1992

120 *Gerald B. Pier*

MOLECULAR MECHANISMS OF MICROBIAL PATHOGENESIS

Over the past two decades, molecular studies of microbial pathogenesis have yielded an explosion of information about the various microbial and host molecules that contribute to the processes of infection and disease. These processes can be classified into several stages: microbial encounter with and entry into the host; microbial growth after entry; avoidance of innate host defenses; tissue invasion and tropism; tissue damage; and transmission to new hosts. Virulence is the measure of an organism's capacity to cause disease and is a function of the pathogenic factors elaborated by microbes. These factors promote colonization (the simple presence of potentially pathogenic microbes in or on a host), infection (attachment and growth of pathogens and avoidance of host defenses), and disease (often, but not always, the activities of secreted toxins or toxic metabolites). In addition, the host's inflammatory response to infection greatly contributes to disease and its attendant clinical signs and symptoms. Knowledge of the molecular structures of the microbial surface, their interactions with the host, and the host response is critical to an understanding of the basic processes of infection and disease.

MICROBIAL ENTRY AND ADHERENCE

ENTRY SITES A microbial pathogen can potentially enter any part of a host organism. In general, the type of disease produced by a particular microbe is often a direct consequence of its route of entry into the body. The most common sites of entry are body parts in contact with the external environment, including mucosal surfaces (particularly those of the respiratory, alimentary, and urogenital tracts) and the skin. Ingestion, inhalation, and sexual contact are typical routes of microbial entry. Other portals of entry include injuries to the skin (cuts, bites, burns, trauma) along with injection via natural (i.e., vector-borne) or artificial (i.e., needle-stick injury) routes. A few pathogens, such as *Schistosoma* spp., can penetrate unbroken skin. The conjunctiva can serve as an entry point for pathogens of the eye.

Microbial entry usually relies on the organism's biologic characteristics and reflects the presence of specific microbial factors needed for persistence and growth in a tissue. Fecal-oral spread via the alimentary tract requires a biology consistent with survival in the varied environments of the gastrointestinal tract (including the low pH of the stomach and the high bile content of the intestine) as well as in contaminated food or water outside the host. Organisms that gain entry via the respiratory tract are most often those that survive well in small moist droplets produced during sneezing and coughing; most such pathogens do not survive well once they dry out. Pathogens that enter by venereal routes often survive best on the warm moist environment of the urogenital mucosa. Many sexually transmitted human pathogens have restricted host ranges and do not infect other animals (e.g., *Neisseria gonorrhoeae*, *Treponema pallidum*, and HIV).

The biology of microbes entering through the skin is highly varied. Some of these organisms can survive in a broad range of environments, such as the salivary glands or alimentary tracts of arthropod vectors, the mouths of larger animals, soil, and water. A complex biology allows protozoan parasites such as *Plasmodium*, *Leishmania*, and *Trypanosoma* spp. to undergo morphogenic changes that allow the organism to be transmitted to mammalian hosts during insect feeding for blood meals. Plasmodia are injected as infective sporozoites from the salivary glands during mosquito feeding. *Leishmania* parasites are regurgitated as promastigotes from the alimentary tract of sandflies and injected by bite into a susceptible host. Trypanosomes are first ingested from infected hosts by reduviid bugs; the pathogens then multiply in the gastrointestinal tract of the insects and are released in feces onto the host's skin during subsequent feedings. Most microbes that land directly on intact skin are destined to die, as survival on the skin or in hair follicles requires resistance to fatty acids, low pH, and other antimicrobial factors on skin. Once it is damaged (and particularly if it becomes necrotic), the skin can be a major portal of growth and entry for pathogens or their toxic products. Tetanus and burn wound infections are clear examples. After animal bites, pathogens resident in the animal's saliva gain access through the skin to the victim's tissues. Rabies is the paradigm for this pathogenic process; rabies virus grows in striated muscle cells at the site of inoculation.

MICROBIAL ADHERENCE Once in or on a host, most microbes must anchor themselves to a tissue or tissue factor; the possible exceptions are organisms that directly enter the bloodstream and multiply there. Specific microbial ligands or adhesins for host receptors constitute a major area of study in the field of microbial pathogenesis. Adhesins comprise a wide range of surface structures, not only anchoring the microbe to a tissue and promoting cellular entry where appropriate but also eliciting host responses critical to the pathogenic process (Table 120-1). Most microbes produce multiple adhesins specific for multiple host receptors. These adhesins are often redundant, are serologically variable, and act additively or synergistically with other microbial factors to promote microbial sticking to host tissues. In addition, some microbes (such as *Mycobacterium tuberculosis* and *Legionella pneumophila*) adsorb host proteins (such as complement components) onto their surface and utilize the natural host protein receptor for microbial binding and entry into target cells.

All viral pathogens must bind to host cells, enter them, and replicate within them. Viral coat proteins serve as the ligands for cellular entry, and more than one ligand-receptor interaction may be needed; for example, HIV utilizes its envelope glycoprotein (gp) 120 to enter host cells by binding to both CD4 and one of several receptors for

Table 120-1 Examples of Microbial Ligand-Receptor Interactions

Microorganism	Type of Microbial Ligand	Host Receptor
VIRAL PATHOGENS		
Influenza virus	Hemagglutinin	Sialic acid
Measles virus	H glycoprotein	CD46/moesin
Herpes simplex virus	gC protein	Heparin sulfate
Human herpesvirus type 6	?	CD46
HIV	Surface glycoprotein	CD4 and chemokine
Epstein-Barr virus	Envelope protein	CD21 (=CR2)
Adenovirus and coxsackie-virus	Fiber protein	Coxsackie-adenovirus receptor (CAR) and major histocompatibility class I antigens
BACTERIAL PATHOGENS		
Neisseria spp.	Pili	Membrane cofactor protein (CD46)
Pseudomonas aeruginosa	Pili and flagella	Asialo-GM1
	Lipopolysaccharide	Cystic fibrosis transmembrane conductance regulator
Escherichia coli	Pili	Ceramides/mannose and digalactosyl residues
Streptococcus pyogenes	Hyaluronic acid capsule	CD44
Yersinia spp.	Invasin/accessory invasin locus	β_1 Integrins
Bordetella pertussis	Filamentous hemagglutinin	CR3
Legionella pneumophila	Adsorbed C3bi	CR3
Mycobacterium tuberculosis	Adsorbed C3bi	CR3
FUNGAL PATHOGENS		
Blastomyces dermatitidis	WI-1	Possibly matrix proteins and integrins
Candida albicans	int1p	Extracellular matrix proteins
PROTOZOAL PATHOGENS		
Plasmodium vivax	Merozoite form	Duffy Fy antigen
Plasmodium falciparum	EBA-175	Glycophorin A
Entamoeba histolytica	Surface lectin	*N*-Acetylglucosamine

meningitidis, the pili are critical for attachment to mucosal epithelial cells. For others, such as *P. aeruginosa*, the pili only partially mediate the cells' adherence to host tissues. *V. cholerae* cells appear to use two different types of pili for intestinal colonization. Whereas interference with this stage of colonization would appear to be an effective antibacterial strategy, attempts to develop pilus-based vaccines for human diseases have not been highly successful to date.

Flagella are long appendages attached at either one or both ends of the bacterial cell (polar flagella) or distributed over the entire cell surface (peritrichous flagella). Flagella, like pili, are composed of a polymerized or aggregated basic protein. In flagella, the protein subunits form a tight helical structure and vary serologically with the species. Spirochetes such as *T. pallidum* and *Borrelia burgdorferi* have axial filaments similar to flagella running down the long axis of the center of the cell, and they "swim" by rotation around these filaments. Some bacteria can glide over a surface in the absence of obvious motility structures.

Other bacterial structures involved in adherence to host tissues include specific staphylococcal and streptococcal proteins that bind to human extracellular matrix proteins such as fibrin, fibronectin, laminin, and collagen. Fibronectin appears to be a commonly used receptor for various pathogens; a particular sequence, Arg-Gly-Asp or RGD, is critical for bacterial binding. Surface lipoteichoic acids may also promote streptococcal adherence to mucosal surfaces. The surface lipopolysaccharide (LPS) of *P. aeruginosa* mediates binding to the cystic fibrosis transmembrane conductance regulator (CFTR) on airway epithelial cells. Coagulase-negative staphylococci readily colonize prosthetic devices and catheters commonly used in medical care; the surface capsular polysaccharide of these organisms promotes binding to the prosthetic material. It has been reported that *Staphylococcus aureus* produces the same capsular polysaccharide and may also use this material to colonize prosthetic devices.

FUNGAL ADHESINS Several fungal adhesins have been described that mediate colonization of epithelial surfaces, particularly adherence to structures like fibronectin, laminin, and collagen. The product of the *Candida albicans INT1* gene, int1p, bears similarity to mammalian integrins that bind to extracellular matrix proteins. Transformation of normally nonadherent *Saccharomyces cerevisiae* with this gene allows these yeast cells to adhere to human epithelial cells. Disruption of *INT1* in *C. albicans* diminishes but does not eliminate epithelial cell adhesion; this result indicates that both int1p and other adhesins mediate binding of *C. albicans* to epithelial cells. Moreover, int1p is needed for filamentous growth of *C. albicans*—a phenotype linked to virulence, and particularly to the ability to penetrate keratinized epithelium. *INT1*-deficient *C. albicans* exhibits markedly reduced virulence in a mouse model of infection.

For several fungal pathogens that initiate infections after inhalation of infectious material, the inoculum is ingested by alveolar macrophages, in which the cells transform to pathogenic phenotypes. Like *C. albicans*, *Blastomyces dermatitidis* binds to CD11b/CD18 integrins as well as to CD14 on macrophages. *B. dermatitidis* produces a 120-kDa surface protein, designated WI-1, that mediates this adherence. The binding domain of WI-1 is homologous to the invasin protein of *Yersinia* that binds to the same type of host cell receptor. An unidentified factor on *Histoplasma capsulatum* also mediates binding of this fungal pathogen to the integrin surface proteins.

chemokines. Similarly, the measles virus H glycoprotein binds to both CD46 and the membrane-organizing protein moesin. The gC protein on herpes simplex virus binds to heparin sulfate; this step is followed by attachment to cells mediated by the viral gD (and possibly gH) protein. CD46 has now been shown to be the cellular receptor for human herpesvirus type 6. Eukaryotic parasites use complicated surface glycoproteins as adhesins, some of which are lectins with specificity for carbohydrates on host cells.

Among the microbial adhesins studied in greatest detail are bacterial pili and flagella. *Pili* or *fimbriae* are commonly used by gram-negative bacteria for attachment to host cells and tissues. In electron micrographs, these hairlike projections (up to several hundred per cell) may be confined to one end of the organism (polar pili) or distributed more evenly over the surface. An individual cell may have pili with a variety of functions. Most pili are made up of a major pilin protein subunit (molecular weight, 17,000 to 30,000) that polymerizes to form the pilus. Many strains of *Escherichia coli* express mucus-binding type 1 pili, whose binding to host tissues is inhibited by D-mannose. Other strains produce the Pap (pyelonephritis-associated) or P pilus adhesin that mediates binding to digalactose (gal-gal) residues on globosides of the human P blood groups. These pili have proteins located at the tips of the main pilus unit that are critical to the binding specificity of the whole pilus unit. Immunization with the mannose-binding FimH tip protein of type 1 pili prevents experimental *E. coli* bladder infections in mice and monkeys. *E. coli* cells causing diarrheal disease express pilus-like receptors for enterocytes on the small bowel, along with other receptors termed *colonization factors*.

A common type of pilus found in *Neisseria* spp., *Moraxella* spp., *Vibrio cholerae*, and *Pseudomonas aeruginosa* mediates adherence of these organisms to target surfaces. These pili tend to have a relatively conserved amino-terminal region and a more variable carboxyl-terminal region. For some species such as *N. gonorrhoeae* and *Neisseria*

HOST RECEPTORS Host receptors are found both on target cells (such as epithelial cells lining mucosal surfaces) and within the mucus layer covering these cells. Microbial pathogens bind to a wide range of host receptors to establish infection (Table 120-1). Selective loss of host receptors for a pathogen may confer natural resistance to an otherwise susceptible population. For example, *Plasmodium vivax*, one of four *Plasmodium* species causing malaria, binds to the Duffy blood group antigen, Fy, on erythrocytes. In West Africa, 70% of individuals lack Fy antigens and are resistant to *P. vivax* infection. *Salmonella typhi*, the etiologic agent of typhoid fever, uses CFTR to enter the gastrointestinal submucosa after being ingested. As homozygous mutations in *CFTR* are the cause of the life-shortening disease cystic fibrosis, heterozygote carriers (e.g., 4 to 5% of individuals of European ancestry) may have had a selective advantage due to decreased susceptibility to *S. typhi* infection.

Numerous virus–target cell interactions have been described, and it is now clear that different viruses can use similar host cell receptors for entry. The list of certain and likely host receptors for viral pathogens is long. Among the host membrane components that can serve as receptors for viruses are sialic acids, gangliosides, glycosaminoglycans, integrins and other members of the immunoglobulin superfamily, histocompatibility antigens, and regulators and receptors for complement components.

MICROBIAL GROWTH AFTER ENTRY

Once established on a mucosal or skin site, pathogenic microbes must replicate before causing full-blown infection and disease. Within cells, viral particles release their nucleic acids, which may be directly translated into viral proteins (positive-strand RNA viruses), transcribed from a negative strand of RNA into a complementary mRNA (negative-strand RNA viruses), or transcribed into a complementary strand of DNA (retroviruses); for DNA viruses, mRNA may be transcribed directly from viral DNA, either in the cell nucleus or in the cytoplasm. To grow, bacteria must acquire specific nutrients or synthesize them from precursors in host tissues. For example, since aromatic amino acids are not available as nutrients in host tissues, pathogenic bacteria must synthesize them from precursors. Many infectious processes are usually confined to specific epithelial surfaces—influenza to the respiratory mucosa, gonorrhea to the urogenital epithelium, shigellosis to the gastrointestinal epithelium. While there are multiple reasons for this specificity, one important consideration is probably the ability of these pathogens to obtain from these specific environments the nutrients needed for growth and survival.

Temperature restrictions also play a role in limiting certain pathogens to specific tissues. Rhinoviruses, a cause of the common cold, grow best at 33°C and replicate in cooler nasal tissues but not in the lung. Leprosy lesions due to *Mycobacterium leprae* are found in and on relatively cool body sites. Fungal pathogens that infect the skin, hair follicles, and nails (dermatophyte infections) remain confined to the cooler, exterior, keratinous layer of the epithelium.

A topic of major interest is the ability of many bacterial, fungal, and protozoal species to grow in multicellular masses referred to as *biofilms*. These masses are biochemically and morphologically quite distinct from the free-living individual cells referred to as *planktonic cells*. Growth in biofilms leads to altered microbial metabolism, production of extracellular virulence factors, and decreased susceptibility to biocides, antimicrobial agents, and host defense molecules and cells. Regulation of biofilm morphogenesis is controlled by bacterial quorum-sensing systems. Quorum sensing for some organisms involves the production of homoserine lactone molecules such as *N*-(3-oxodo-decanoyl)homoserine lactone and *N*-butyrylhomoserine lactone, which combine with transcriptional activators to control gene expression. *P. aeruginosa* growing on the bronchial mucosa during chronic infection, staphylococci and other pathogens growing on implanted medical devices, and dental pathogens growing on tooth surfaces to form plaques represent several examples of microbial biofilm growth associated with human disease. Many other pathogens can form biofilms during

in vitro growth, including *Helicobacter pylori*, the cause of stomach ulcers; *E. coli* O157, one cause of the hemolytic-uremic syndrome; and *Gardnerella vaginalis*, an organism associated with bacterial vaginosis.

AVOIDANCE OF INNATE HOST DEFENSES

As microbes have probably interacted with mucosal/epithelial surfaces since the emergence of multicellular organisms, it is not surprising that multicellular hosts have a variety of innate surface defense mechanisms that can sense when pathogens are present and contribute to their elimination. The skin, a formidable physical barrier to microbial entry, is both acidic and bathed with fatty acids toxic to many microbes. Successful skin pathogens such as staphylococci must tolerate these adverse conditions. Mucosal surfaces themselves present a barrier composed of a thick mucus layer that entraps microbes and facilitates their transport out of the body by such processes as mucociliary clearance, coughing, and urination. Mucous secretions, saliva, and tears contain antibacterial factors such as lysozyme and antiviral factors such as interferons. Gastric acidity is inimical to the survival of many ingested pathogens, and many mucosal surfaces—particularly the nasopharynx, the vaginal tract, and the gastrointestinal tract—contain a resident flora of commensal microbes that interfere with the ability of pathogens to colonize and infect a host.

Pathogens that survive these factors must still contend with host endocytic, phagocytic, and inflammatory responses as well as with host genetic factors that determine the degree to which a pathogen can survive and grow. The growth of viral pathogens entering skin or mucosal epithelial cells can be limited by a variety of host genetic factors, including production of interferons, modulation of receptors for viral entry, and age- and hormone-related susceptibility factors; by nutritional status; and even by personal habits such as smoking and exercise.

ENCOUNTERS WITH EPITHELIAL CELLS Over the past decade, many bacterial pathogens have been shown to enter epithelial cells (Fig. 120-1), often using specialized surface structures that bind to receptors for internalization. However, the exact role and the importance of this process in infection and disease are not well defined for most of these pathogens. Bacterial entry into host epithelial cells is seen as a means for dissemination to adjacent or deeper tissues or as a route to sanctuary to avoid ingestion and killing by professional phagocytes. Epithelial cell entry appears, for instance, to be a critical aspect of dysentery induction by *Shigella*.

Curiously, the less virulent strains of many bacterial pathogens are more adept at entering epithelial cells than are more virulent strains; examples include pathogens that lack the surface polysaccharide capsule needed to cause serious disease. Thus, for *Haemophilus influenzae*, *Streptococcus pneumoniae*, *S. agalactiae* (group B *Streptococcus*), and *S. pyogenes*, isogenic mutants or variants lacking capsules enter epithelial cells better than the wild-type, encapsulated parental forms that cause disseminated disease. These observations have led to the proposal that epithelial cell entry may be a manifestation of host defense, resulting in bacterial clearance by both shedding of epithelial cells containing internalized bacteria and initiation of a subclinical inflammatory response. However, a consequence of this process would be the opening of a hole in the epithelium, potentially allowing un-ingested organisms to enter the submucosa. This scenario has been documented in murine *Salmonella typhimurium* infections and in experimental bladder infections with uropathogenic *E. coli*. In the latter system, bacterial pili mediate cell attachment to integral membrane glycoproteins called uroplakins that coat the host cells, resulting in exfoliation of the cells with attached bacteria. Subsequently, infection is produced by residual bacterial cells that invade the denuded epithelium. Perhaps at low bacterial inocula epithelial cell ingestion and subclinical inflammation are efficient means to eliminate pathogens, while at higher inocula a proportion of surviving bacterial cells enter the host tissue through the damaged mucosal surface and multiply,

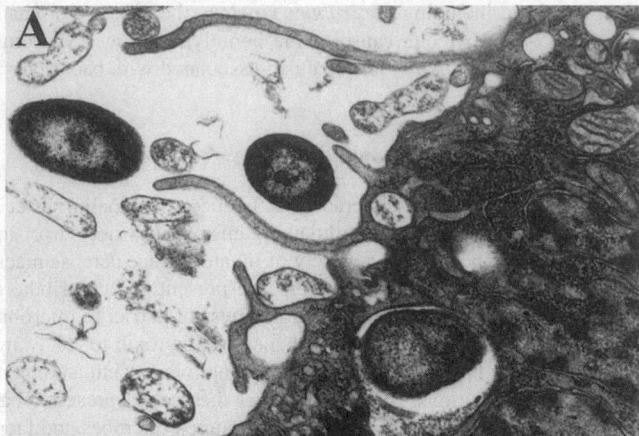

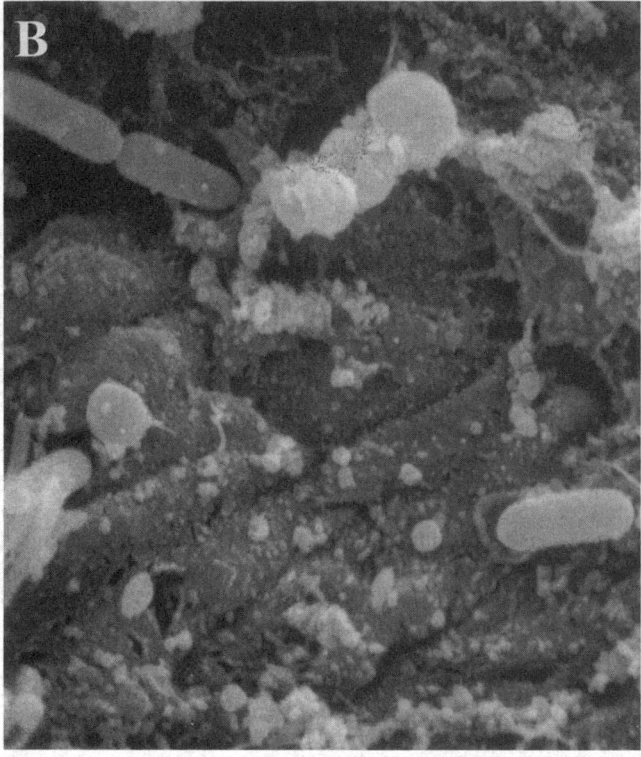

FIGURE 120-1   Entry of bacteria into epithelial cells. *A.* Internalization of *P. aeruginosa* by cultured airway epithelial cells expressing wild-type cystic fibrosis transmembrane conductance regulator (CFTR), the cell receptor for bacterial ingestion. *B.* Entry of *P. aeruginosa* into murine tracheal epithelial cells after murine infection by the intranasal route.

producing disease. Alternatively, failure of the appropriate epithelial cell response to a pathogen may allow the organism to survive on a mucosal surface where, if it avoids other host defenses, it can grow and cause a local infection. Along these lines, as noted above, *P. aeruginosa* is taken into epithelial cells by CFTR, a protein missing or nonfunctional in most severe cases of cystic fibrosis. The major clinical consequence of this disease is chronic airway-surface infection with *P. aeruginosa* in 80 to 90% of patients with cystic fibrosis. The failure of airway epithelial cells to ingest and promote the removal of *P. aeruginosa* has been proposed as a key component of the hypersusceptibility of these patients to chronic airway infection.

ENCOUNTERS WITH PHAGOCYTES   Phagocytosis of microbes is a major innate host defense that limits the growth and spread of pathogens. Phagocytes appear rapidly at sites of infection in conjunction with the initiation of inflammation. Ingestion of microbes

by both tissue-fixed macrophages and migrating phagocytes probably accounts for the limited ability of most microbial agents to cause disease. A family of related molecules called *collectins*, *soluble defense collagens*, or *pattern recognition molecules* are found in blood (mannose-binding lectin), in lung (surfactant proteins A and D), and most likely in other tissues as well and bind to carbohydrates on microbial surfaces to promote phagocyte clearance. Bacterial pathogens seem to be ingested principally by polymorphonuclear neutrophils (PMNs), while eosinophils are frequently found at sites of infection by protozoan or multicellular parasites. Successful pathogens, by definition, must avoid being cleared by professional phagocytes. One of several antiphagocytic strategies employed by bacteria and by the fungal pathogen *Cryptococcus neoformans* is to elaborate large-molecular-weight surface polysaccharide antigens, often in the form of a capsule that coats the cell surface. Most pathogenic bacteria produce such antiphagocytic capsules.

As activation of local phagocytes in tissues is a key step in initiating inflammation and migration of additional phagocytes into infected sites, much attention has been paid to microbial factors that initiate inflammation. Encounters with phagocytes are governed largely by the structure of the microbial constituents that elicit inflammation, and detailed knowledge of these structures for bacterial pathogens has contributed greatly to our understanding of molecular mechanisms of microbial pathogenesis (Fig. 120-2). The best-studied system involves the interaction of LPS from gram-negative bacteria and the glycosylphosphatidylinositol (GPI)-anchored membrane protein CD14 found on the surface of professional phagocytes, including migrating and tissue-fixed macrophages and PMNs. A soluble form of CD14 is also found in plasma and on mucosal surfaces. A plasma protein, LPS-binding protein (LBP), transfers LPS to membrane-bound CD14 on myeloid cells and promotes binding of LPS to soluble CD14. Soluble CD14/LPS/LBP complexes bind to many cell types and may be internalized to initiate cellular responses to microbial pathogens. It has been shown that peptidoglycan and lipoteichoic acid from gram-positive bacteria and cell-surface products of mycobacteria and spirochetes can interact with CD14 (Fig. 120-2).

GPI-anchored receptors do not have intracellular signaling domains, and mammalian Toll-like receptors (TLRs) transduce signals for cellular activation due to LPS binding. TLRs initiate cellular activation through a series of signal-transducing molecules (Fig. 120-2) that lead to nuclear translocation of the transcription factor NF-κB, a master-switch for production of important inflammatory cytokines such as tumor necrosis factor α (TNF-α) and interleukin (IL) 1.

The initiation of inflammation can occur not only with LPS and peptidoglycan but also with viral particles and other microbial products such as polysaccharides, enzymes, and toxins.

Bacterial Cell Wall Structure   Gram-positive bacteria have a rigid cell wall that gives the organisms their characteristic shape, differentiates them from eukaryotic cells, and allows them to survive in osmotically unfavorable environments. The cell wall is composed mainly of peptidoglycan (Fig. 120-3, panel *C*; a polymer of *N*-acetylglucosamine and its lactyl ether, *N*-acetylmuramic acid), with peptide side chains covalently bound to the lactyl group (Fig. 120-3, panel *A*). The peptide chains consist of alternating D and L amino acids and are usually linked to each other by a pentaglycine bridge binding a terminal D-alanine on one peptide substituent to the penultimate L-lysine on a neighboring peptide. Variations in this basic structure have been described for a number of bacterial genera. In addition, the cell walls of gram-positive bacteria contain teichoic acids (Fig. 120-3, panel *D*), phosphate-linked polymers of ribitol or glycerol that can have additional compounds linked to available side groups. Lipid tails anchor these acids to the cytoplasmic membrane, giving rise to lipoteichoic acids.

Gram-negative bacteria possess a cytoplasmic membrane and a peptidoglycan layer similar to but reduced from that found in gram-positive organisms, but these organisms also produce an outer membrane that is covalently linked to the tetrapeptides of the peptidoglycan layer by a lipoprotein (Fig. 120-3, panel *B*). Embedded in the outer membrane are special proteins with important functions, including maintaining the outer membrane's integrity, acting as a selective barrier for diffusion of molecules into the cell, serving as receptors for bacteriophages, and binding siderophores that scavenge iron for transport into the bacterial cell. The exterior layer of the outer membrane contains the major surface glycolipid, which can be either a classical bacterial LPS or a lipooligosaccharide (LOS); pathogens such as *Neisseria* and *Haemophilus* spp. express LOS, which contains smaller polysaccharide constituents. Although LPS/LOS was thought to be essential to the viability of gram-negative bacteria, a viable strain of *N. meningitidis* lacking LOS has now been made.

Exterior to the LPS for many, but not all, gram-negative pathogens is a capsular polysaccharide, which (along with LPS for some pathogenic species) confers resistance to phagocytosis by preventing innate host opsonins, such as the complement proteins C3 and C4, from coating the organisms—a process that promotes their uptake by phagocytes. Capsular polysaccharides are also important extracellular components of gram-positive bacteria, serving as critical factors in bacterial resistance to opsonophagocytosis and phagocytic killing. Variation in the expression of the capsule in *S. pneumoniae* accounts for the different morphologies of colonies of this pathogen on agar plates (smooth and rough phenotypes); this property was exploited in studies proving that DNA carries genetic information in a cell.

Lipopolysaccharide Most of the important biologic properties associated with LPS (endotoxin) are due to the lipid A portion (Fig. 120-3, panel *E*), a relatively conserved, highly acylated di-*N*-acetylglucosamine backbone linked β 1→6 and containing phosphate groups on the reducing 1 and nonreducing 4′ carbons. Attached to carbon 6′ is the inner polysaccharide core, which

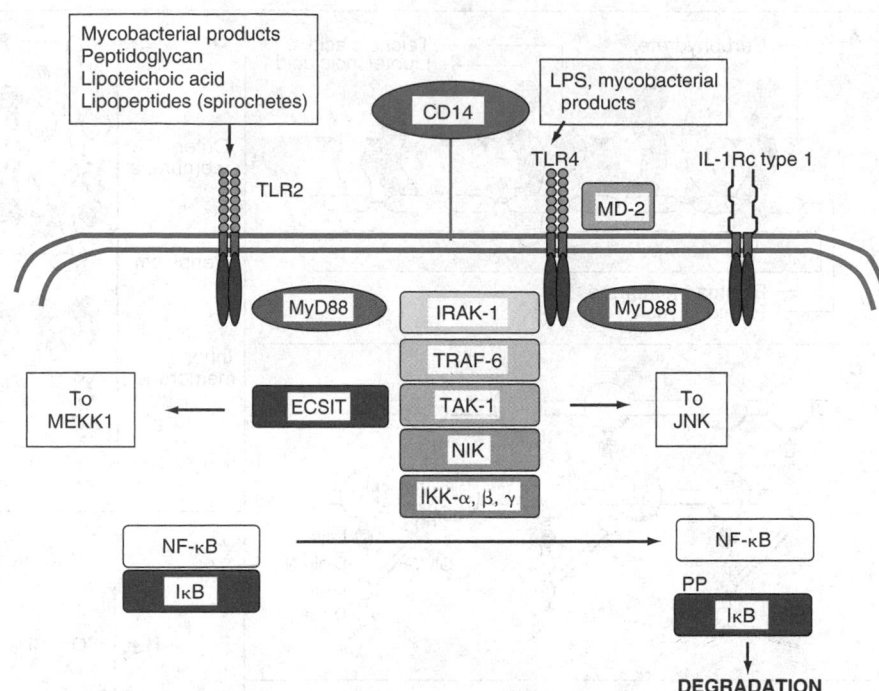

FIGURE 120-2 Cellular signaling pathways for production of inflammatory cytokines in response to microbial products. Various microbial cell-surface constituents interact with CD14, which in turn interacts in a currently unknown fashion with toll-like receptors (TLR). Both CD14 and TLRs contain extracellular leucine-rich domains. The cytoplasmic domains of TLRs are oligomerized for binding to the general adaptor protein MyD88, which also binds to members of the interleukin-1 receptor (IL-1Rc) transmembrane proteins due to homology in the intracellular domain. Oligomerization is followed by activation of signal-transducing molecules such as IRAK-1 (IL-1Rc-associated kinase 1), TRAF-6 (tumor necrosis factor receptor–associated factor 6), TAK-1 (transforming growth factor β–activating kinase 1), and NIK (Nck-interacting kinase). In addition to activating other signaling pathways leading to cytokine production and stress responses, such as the c-Jun *N*-terminal kinase (JNK) pathway and MAP kinase kinase kinase (MEKK1) pathway [via evolutionarily conserved signaling intermediate in Toll pathways (ECSIT)], TLR-mediated signaling leads to activation of the inducible kinase complex, IKK-α, -β, and -γ. These are part of a larger complex that phosphorylates the inhibitory portion (I) of nuclear factor κB (NF-κB), resulting in release of IκB from NF-κB. Phosphorylated (PP) IκB is then degraded and NF-κB translocates to the nucleus, where it binds to transcriptional sites on target genes, many of which encode inflammatory proteins. *(Figure courtesy of Dr. Terry Means and Dr. Douglas Golenbock.)*

is usually, but not always, composed of a di- or trisaccharide of 2-keto-3-deoxyoctonate (KDO). Additional sugar substituents are linked to the inner core, forming a complete core. Attached to the complete core are either short polysaccharide side chains (forming LOS) or longer O polysaccharide side chains (forming complete LPS) composed of a variety of monosaccharides, substituted with a variety of components, such as formyl, acetyl, and hydroxybutyryl side chains; amino acids or peptides; and phosphate groups. Further biologic functions of LOS/LPS that are important to the survival of microbes after entry into a host include resistance to the bacteriolytic effects of complement and protection against antimicrobial factors such as defensins and bactericidal permeability-increasing protein, a molecule closely related to LBP in structure and function. Defensins are found in high concentrations in granules of myeloid cells, including platelets, and are usually highly cationic peptides capable of insertion into bacterial cells and killing of these cells.

Additional Interactions of Microbial Pathogens and Phagocytes Other ways that microbial pathogens avoid destruction by phagocytes include production of factors that are toxic to the phagocytes or that interfere with the chemotactic and ingestion function of phagocytes. Hemolysins, leukocidins, and the like are microbial proteins that can kill phagocytes that are attempting to ingest organisms elaborating these substances. For example, staphylococcal hemolysins

inhibit macrophage chemotaxis and kill these phagocytes. Streptolysin O made by *S. pyogenes* binds to cholesterol in phagocyte membranes and initiates a process of internal degranulation, with the release of normally granule-sequestered toxic components into the phagocyte's cytoplasm. *Entamoeba histolytica*, an intestinal protozoan that causes amebic dysentery, can disrupt phagocyte membranes after direct contact via the release of protozoal phospholipase A and pore-forming peptides.

Microbial Survival Inside Phagocytes Many important microbial pathogens use a variety of strategies to survive inside phagocytes (particularly macrophages) after ingestion. Inhibition of fusion of the phagocytic vacuole (the phagosome) containing the ingested microbe with the lysosomal granules containing antimicrobial substances (the lysosome) allows *M. tuberculosis*, *S. typhi*, and *Toxoplasma gondii* to survive inside macrophages. Some organisms, such as *Listeria monocytogenes*, escape into the phagocyte's cytoplasm to grow and eventually spread to other cells. Resistance to killing within the macrophage and subsequent growth are critical to successful infection by herpes-type viruses, measles virus, poxviruses, *Salmonella*, *Yersinia*, *Legionella*, *Mycobacterium*, *Trypanosoma*, *Nocardia*, *Histoplasma*, *Toxoplasma*, and *Rickettsia*. *Salmonella* spp. use a master regulatory system, in which the *PhoP/PhoQ* genes control other genes, to enter and survive within cells, with intracellular survival entailing structural changes in the cell envelope LPS.

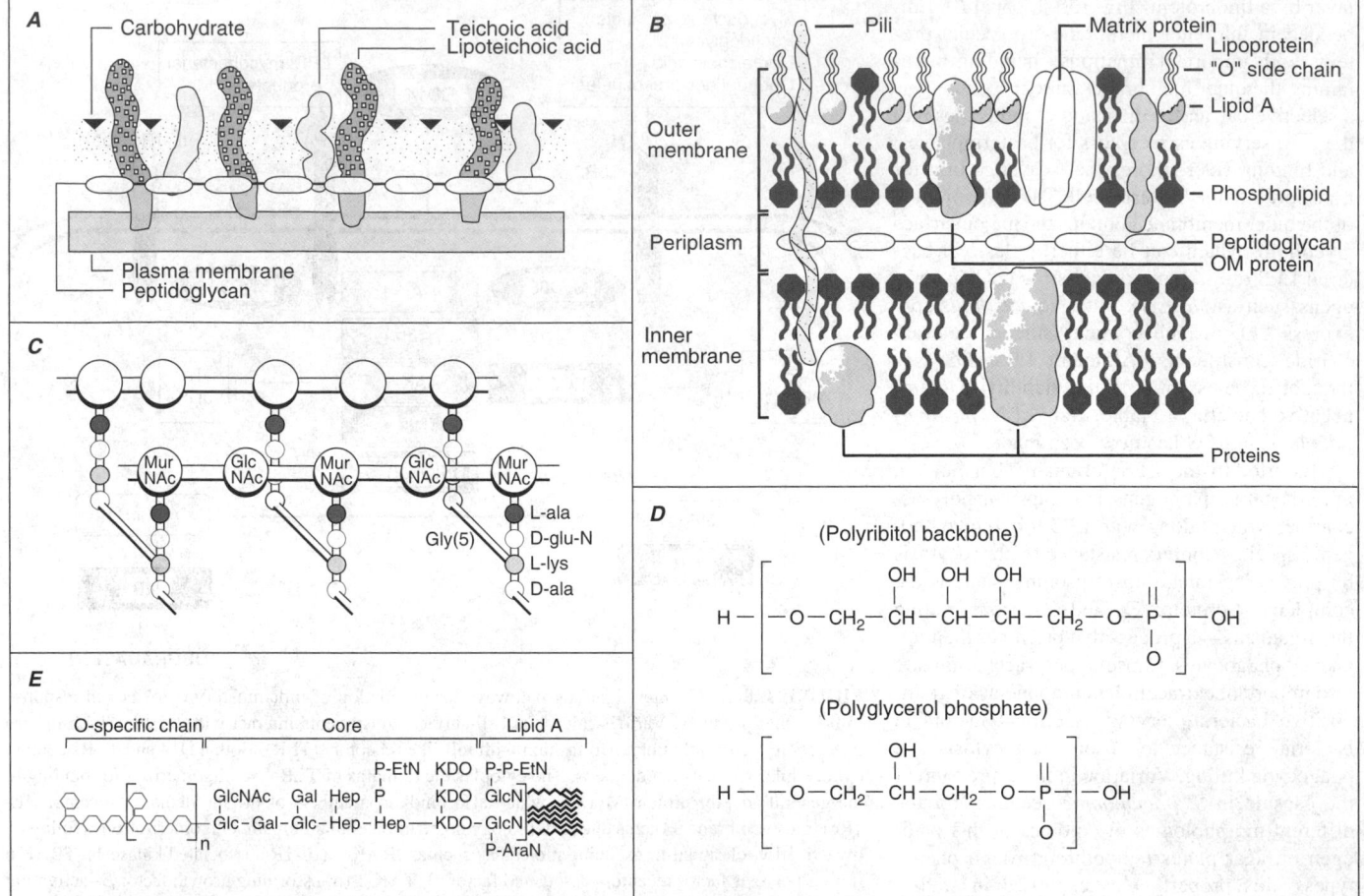

FIGURE 120-3 Schematic representations of bacterial surface structures. *A.* Cytoplasmic membrane and cell wall typical of gram-positive bacteria. *B.* Outer structure of a gram-negative organism (OM = outer membrane). *C.* Detailed structure of peptidoglycan showing backbone of *N*-acetylmuramic acid (MurNAc) and *N*-acetylglucosamine (GlcNAc); tetrapeptide bridges composed of L-alanine (L-ala), D-glutamate (D-glu-N), L-lysine (L-lys), and D-alanine (D-ala); and pentaglycine [Gly(5)] cross-bridges. *D.* Teichoic acid backbone. *E.* Detailed structure of lipopolysaccharide typical of *Salmonella* spp., including the lipid A sugars glucosamine (GlcN) and 4-amino arabinose (AraN) and the core sugars 2-keto-3-deoxyoctonate (KDO), heptose (Hep), glucose (Glc), galactose (Gal), and *N*-acetylglucosamine (GlcNAc). Hexagons depicting the O-specific chain represent variable monosaccharide residues that comprise this structure. *(Drawing courtesy of TJ DiCesare.)*

TISSUE INVASION AND TISSUE TROPISM

TISSUE INVASION Most viral pathogens cause disease by growth at skin or mucosal entry sites, but some pathogens spread from the initial site to deeper tissues. Virus can spread via the nerves (rabies virus) or plasma (picornaviruses) or within migratory blood cells (poliovirus, Epstein-Barr virus, and many others). Specific viral genes determine where and how individual viral strains can spread.

Bacteria may invade deeper layers of mucosal tissue via intracellular uptake by epithelial cells, traversal of epithelial cell junctions, or penetration through denuded epithelial surfaces. Among virulent *Shigella* strains and invasive *E. coli*, outer-membrane proteins are critical to epithelial cell invasion and bacterial multiplication. *Neisseria* and *Haemophilus* spp. penetrate mucosal cells by poorly understood mechanisms before dissemination into the bloodstream. Staphylococci and streptococci elaborate a variety of extracellular enzymes, such as hyaluronidase, lipases, nucleases, and hemolysins, that are probably important in breaking down cellular and matrix structures and allowing the bacteria access to deeper tissues and blood. Organisms that colonize the gastrointestinal tract can often translocate through the mucosa into the blood and, under circumstances in which host defenses are inadequate, cause bacteremia. *Yersinia enterocolitica* can invade the mucosa through the activity of the invasin protein. Some bacteria (e.g., *Brucella*) can be carried from a mucosal site to a distant site by phagocytic cells (e.g., PMNs) that ingest but fail to kill the bacteria.

Fungal pathogens almost always take advantage of host immunocompromise to spread hematogenously to deeper tissues. The AIDS epidemic has resoundingly illustrated this principle: the immunodeficiency of many HIV-infected patients permits the development of life-threatening fungal infections of the lung, blood, and brain. Other than the capsule of *C. neoformans*, specific fungal antigens involved in tissue invasion are not well characterized. Both fungal pathogens and protozoal pathogens (e.g., *Plasmodium* spp. and *E. histolytica*) undergo morphologic changes to spread within a host. Malarial parasites grow in liver cells as merozoites and are released into the blood to invade erythrocytes and become trophozoites. *E. histolytica* is found as both a cyst and a trophozoite in the intestinal lumen, through which this pathogen enters the host, but only the trophozoite form can spread systemically to cause amebic liver abscesses. Other protozoal pathogens, such as *T. gondii*, *Giardia lamblia*, and *Cryptosporidium*, also undergo extensive morphologic changes after initial infection to spread to other tissues.

TISSUE TROPISM The propensity of certain microbes to cause disease by infecting specific tissues has been known since the early days of bacteriology, yet the molecular basis for this propensity is understood somewhat better for viral pathogens than for other agents of infectious disease. Specific receptor-ligand interactions clearly underlie the ability of certain viruses to enter cells within tissues and disrupt normal tissue function, but the mere presence of a receptor for a virus on a target tissue is not sufficient for tissue tropism. Factors in the cell, route of viral entry, viral capacity to penetrate into cells, viral genetic elements that regulate gene expression, and pathways of viral spread in a tissue all affect tissue tropism. Some viral genes are best transcribed in specific target cells, such as hepatitis B genes in liver cells and Epstein-Barr virus genes in B lymphocytes. The route of inoculation of poliovirus determines its neurotropism, although the molecular basis for this circumstance is not understood.

The lesser understanding of the tissue tropism of bacterial and parasitic infections is exemplified by *Neisseria* spp. There is no well-accepted explanation of why *N. gonorrhoeae* colonizes and infects the human genital tract while the closely related species *N. meningitidis* principally colonizes the human oropharynx. *N. meningitidis* expresses a capsular polysaccharide, while *N. gonorrhoeae* does not; however, there is no indication that this property plays a role in the different tissue tropisms displayed by these two bacterial species. *N. gonorrhoeae* can use cytidine monophosphate *N*-acetylneuraminic acid from host tissues to add *N*-acetylneuraminic acid (sialic acid) to its LOS O side chain, and this alteration appears to make the organism resistant to host defenses. Lactate, present at high levels on genital mucosal surfaces, stimulates sialylation of gonococcal LOS. Bacteria with sialic acid sugars in their capsules, such as *N. meningitidis*, *E. coli* K-1, and group B streptococci, have a propensity to cause meningitis, but this generalization has many exceptions. For example, all recognized serotypes of group B streptococci contain sialic acid in their capsules, but only one serotype (III) is responsible for most cases of group B streptococcal meningitis. Moreover, both *H. influenzae* and *S. pneumoniae* can readily cause meningitis, but these organisms do not have sialic acid in their capsules.

TISSUE DAMAGE AND DISEASE

Disease is a complex phenomenon resulting from tissue invasion and destruction, toxin elaboration, and host response. Viruses cause much of their damage by exerting a cytopathic effect on host cells and inhibiting host defenses. The growth of bacterial, fungal, and protozoal parasites in tissue, which may or may not be accompanied by toxin elaboration, can also compromise tissue function and lead to disease. For some bacterial and possibly some fungal pathogens, toxin production is one of the best-characterized molecular mechanisms of pathogenesis, while host factors such as IL-1, TNF-α, kinins, inflammatory proteins, products of complement activation, and mediators derived from arachidonic acid metabolites (leukotrienes) and cellular degranulation (histamines) readily contribute to the severity of disease.

VIRAL DISEASE Viral pathogens are well known to inhibit host immune responses by a variety of mechanisms. Immune responses can be affected by down-regulating production of most major histocompatibility complex (MHC) molecules (adenovirus E3 protein), by diminishing cytotoxic T cell recognition of virus-infected cells (Epstein-Barr virus EBNA1 antigen and cytomegalovirus IE protein), by producing virus-encoded complement receptor proteins (herpesvirus and vaccinia virus) that protect infected cells from complement-mediated lysis, by making proteins that interfere with the action of interferon (influenza virus and poxvirus), and by elaborating superantigen-like proteins (mouse mammary tumor virus and related retroviruses, rabies nucleocapsid, and possibly the Nef protein of HIV). Superantigens activate large populations of T cells that express particular subsets of the T cell receptor β protein, causing massive cytokine release and subsequent host reactions. Another molecular mechanism of viral virulence involves the production of peptide growth factors for host cells, which disrupt normal cellular growth, proliferation, and differentiation. In addition, viral factors can bind to and interfere with the function of host receptors for signaling molecules. Modulation of cytokine production during viral infection can stimulate viral growth inside cells with receptors for the cytokine, and virus-encoded cytokine homologues (e.g., the Epstein-Barr virus BCRF1 protein, which is highly homologous to the immunoinhibitory IL-10 molecule) can potentially prevent immune-mediated clearance

of viral particles. Viruses can cause disease in neural cells by interfering with levels of neurotransmitters without necessarily destroying the cells, or they may induce either programmed cell death (apoptosis) to destroy tissues or inhibitors of apoptosis to allow for prolonged viral infection of cells. Overall, any disruption of normal cellular and tissue function due to viral infection can underlie the resultant clinical disease.

BACTERIAL TOXINS Among the first infectious diseases to be understood were those due to toxin-elaborating bacteria. Diphtheria, botulism, and tetanus toxins are responsible for the diseases associated with local infections due to *Corynebacterium diphtheriae*, *Clostridium botulinum*, and *Clostridium tetani*, respectively. Enterotoxins produced by *E. coli*, *Salmonella*, *Shigella*, *Staphylococcus*, and *V. cholerae* contribute to diarrheal disease caused by these organisms. Staphylococci, streptococci, *P. aeruginosa*, and *Bordetella* elaborate various toxins that cause or contribute to disease, including toxic shock syndrome toxin 1 (TSST-1); erythrogenic toxin; exotoxins A, S, and U; and pertussis toxin. A number of these toxins (e.g., cholera toxin, diphtheria toxin, pertussis toxin, *E. coli* heat-labile toxin, and *P. aeruginosa* exotoxin) have adenosine diphosphate (ADP)-ribosyltransferase activity; i.e., the toxins enzymatically catalyze the transfer of the ADP-ribosyl portion of nicotinamide adenine diphosphate to target proteins and inactivate them. The staphylococcal enterotoxins, TSST-1, and the streptococcal pyogenic exotoxins behave as superantigens, stimulating certain T cells to proliferate without processing of the protein toxin by antigen-presenting cells. Part of this process involves stimulation of the antigen-presenting cells to produce IL-1 and TNF-α, which have been implicated in many of the clinical features of diseases like toxic shock syndrome and scarlet fever. A number of gram-negative pathogens (*Salmonella*, *Yersinia*, and *P. aeruginosa*) possess the ability to inject toxins directly into host target cells by means of a complex set of proteins referred to as the type III secretion system.

ENDOTOXIN The lipid A portion of gram-negative LPS has potent biologic activities that cause many of the clinical manifestations of gram-negative bacterial sepsis, including fever, muscle proteolysis, uncontrolled intravascular coagulation, and shock. The effects of lipid A appear to be mediated by the production of potent cytokines due to LPS binding to CD14 and signal transduction via TLRs, particularly TLR4. Cytokines exhibit potent hypothermic activity through effects on the hypothalamus; they also increase vascular permeability, alter the activity of endothelial cells, and induce endothelial-cell procoagulant activity. Numerous therapeutic strategies aimed at neutralizing the effects of endotoxin are under investigation, but so far the results have been disappointing.

INVASION Many diseases are caused primarily by pathogens growing in tissue sites that are normally sterile. Pneumococcal pneumonia is mostly attributable to the growth of *S. pneumoniae* in the lung and the attendant host inflammatory response, although specific factors that enhance this process (e.g., pneumolysin) may be responsible for some of the pathogenic potential of the pneumococcus. Disease that follows bacteremia and invasion of the meninges by meningitis-producing bacteria such as *N. meningitidis*, *H. influenzae*, *E. coli* K1, and group B streptococci appears to be due solely to the ability of these organisms to gain access to these tissues, multiply in them, and provoke cytokine production leading to tissue-damaging host inflammation.

Specific molecular mechanisms accounting for tissue invasion by fungal and protozoal pathogens are less well described. Except for studies pointing to factors like capsule and melanin production by *C. neoformans* and possibly levels of cell wall glucans in some pathogenic fungi, the molecular basis for fungal invasiveness is not well defined. Melanism has been shown to protect the fungal cell against death caused by phagocyte factors such as nitric oxide, superoxide, and hypochlorite. Morphogenic variation and production of proteases (e.g., the *Candida* aspartyl proteinase) have been implicated in fungal invasion of host tissues.

If pathogens are effectively to invade host tissues (particularly the blood), they must avoid the major host defenses represented by complement and phagocytic cells. Bacteria most often avoid these defenses through their cell surface polysaccharides—either capsular polysaccharides or long O-side-chain antigens characteristic of the smooth LPS of gram-negative bacteria. These molecules can prevent the activation and/or deposition of complement opsonins or limit the access of phagocytic cells with receptors for complement opsonins to these molecules when they are deposited on the bacterial surface below the capsular layer. Another potential mechanism of microbial virulence is the ability of some organisms to present the capsule as an apparent self antigen through molecular mimicry. For example, the polysialic acid capsule of group B *N. meningitidis* is chemically identical to an oligosaccharide found on human brain cells.

Immunochemical studies of capsular polysaccharides have led to an appreciation of the tremendous chemical diversity that can result from the linking of a few monosaccharides. For example, three hexoses can link up in more than 300 different, potentially serologically distinct ways, while three amino acids have only six possible peptide combinations. Capsular polysaccharides have been used as effective vaccines against meningococcal meningitis as well as against pneumococcal and *H. influenzae* infections and may prove to be of value as vaccines against any organisms that express a nontoxic, immunogenic capsular polysaccharide. In addition, most encapsulated pathogens become virtually avirulent when capsule production is interrupted by genetic manipulation; this observation emphasizes the importance of this structure in pathogenesis.

HOST RESPONSE   The inflammatory response of the host is critical for interruption and resolution of the infectious process but also is often responsible for the signs and symptoms of disease. Infection promotes a complex series of host responses involving the complement, kinin, and coagulation pathways. The production of cytokines such as IL-1, TNF-α, and other factors regulated in part by the NF-κB transcription factor leads to fever, muscle proteolysis, and other effects, as noted above. An inability to kill or contain the microbe usually results in further damage due to the progression of inflammation and infection. For example, in many chronic infections, degranulation of host inflammatory cells can lead to release of host proteases, elastases, histamines, and other toxic substances that can degrade host tissues. Chronic inflammation in any tissue can lead to the destruction of that tissue and to clinical disease associated with loss of organ function, such as sterility from pelvic inflammatory disease caused by chronic infection with *N. gonorrhoeae*.

The nature of the host response elicited by the pathogen often determines the pathology of a particular infection. Local inflammation produces local tissue damage, while systemic inflammation, such as that seen during sepsis, can result in the signs and symptoms of septic shock. The severity of septic shock is associated with the degree of production of host effectors. Disease due to intracellular parasitism results from the formation of granulomas, wherein the host attempts to wall off the parasite inside a fibrotic lesion surrounded by fused epithelial cells that make up so-called multinucleated giant cells. A number of pathogens, particularly anaerobic bacteria, staphylococci, and streptococci, provoke the formation of an abscess, probably because of the presence of zwitterionic surface polysaccharides such as the capsular polysaccharide of *Bacteroides fragilis*. The outcome of an infection depends on the balance between an effective host response that eliminates a pathogen and an excessive inflammatory response that is associated with an inability to eliminate a pathogen and with the resultant tissue damage that leads to disease.

TRANSMISSION TO NEW HOSTS

As part of the pathogenic process, most microbes are shed from the host, often in a form infectious for susceptible individuals. However, the rate of transmissibility may not necessarily be high, even if the disease is severe in the infected individual, as these traits are not linked. Most pathogens exit via the same route by which they entered: respiratory pathogens by aerosols from sneezing or coughing or through salivary spread, gastrointestinal pathogens by fecal-oral spread, sexually transmitted diseases by venereal spread, and vector-borne organisms by either direct contact with the vector through a blood meal or indirect contact with organisms shed into environmental sources such as water. Microbial factors that specifically promote transmission are not well characterized. Respiratory shedding is facilitated by overproduction of mucous secretions, with consequently enhanced sneezing and coughing. Diarrheal toxins such as cholera toxin, *E. coli* heat-labile toxins, and *Shigella* toxins probably facilitate fecal-oral spread of microbial cells in the high volumes of diarrheal fluid produced during infection. The ability to produce phenotypic variants that resist hostile environmental factors (e.g., the highly resistant cysts of *E. histolytica* shed in feces) represents another mechanism of pathogenesis relevant to transmission. Blood parasites such as *Plasmodium* spp. change phenotype after ingestion by a mosquito—a prerequisite for the continued transmission of this pathogen. Venereally transmitted pathogens may undergo phenotypic variation due to the production of specific factors to facilitate transmission, but shedding of these pathogens into the environment does not result in the formation of infectious foci.

In summary, the molecular mechanisms used by pathogens to colonize, invade, infect, and disrupt the host are numerous and diverse. Each phase of the infectious process involves a variety of microbial and host factors interacting in a manner that can result in disease. Recognition of the coordinated genetic regulation of virulence factor elaboration when organisms move from their natural environment into the mammalian host emphasizes the complex nature of the host-parasite interaction. Fortunately, the need for diverse factors in successful infection and disease implies that a variety of therapeutic strategies may be developed to interrupt this process and thereby prevent and treat microbial infections.

BIBLIOGRAPHY

ANDERSON DM, SCHNEEWIND O: Type III machines of gram-negative pathogens: Injecting virulence factors into host cells and more. Curr Opin Microbiol 2:18, 1999

BERGER EA et al: Chemokine receptors as HIV-1 coreceptors: Roles in viral entry, tropism, and disease. Annu Rev Immunol 17:657, 1999

BRANDHORST TT: Targeted gene disruption reveals an adhesin indispensable for pathogenicity of *Blastomyces dermatitidis*. J Exp Med 189:1207, 1999

CHOW JC et al: Toll-like receptor-4 mediates lipopolysaccharide-induced signal transduction. J Biol Chem 274:10689, 1999

DAVIES DG et al: The involvement of cell-to-cell signals in the development of a bacterial biofilm. Science 280:295, 1998

ERNST RK et al: How intracellular bacteria survive: Surface modifications that promote resistance to host innate immune responses. J Infect Dis 179(Suppl 2):S326, 1999

GALE CA et al: Linkage of adhesion, filamentous growth, and virulence in *Candida albicans* to a single gene, *INT1*. Science 279:1355, 1998

GARTEN W, KLENK H-D: Understanding influenza virus pathogenicity. Trends Microbiol 7:99, 1999

MULVEY MA et al: Induction and evasion of host defenses by type 1–piliated uropathogenic *Escherichia coli*. Science 282:1494, 1998

PIER GB et al: *Salmonella typhi* uses CFTR to enter intestinal epithelial cells. Nature 392:79, 1998

SCHNEIDER-SCHAULIES S, TER MEULEN V: Pathogenic aspects of measles virus infections. Arch Virol Suppl 15:139, 1999

SOTO GE, HULTGREN SJ: Bacterial adhesins: Common themes and variations in architecture and assembly. J Bacteriol 181:1059, 1999

SVANBORG C et al: Cytokine responses during mucosal infections: Role in disease pathogenesis and host defence. Curr Opin Microbiol 2:99, 1999

121 *Andrew B. Onderdonk*

LABORATORY DIAGNOSIS OF INFECTIOUS DISEASES

The laboratory diagnosis of infection requires the demonstration, either direct or indirect, of viral, bacterial, fungal, or parasitic agents in tissues, fluids, or excreta of the host. Clinical microbiology laboratories are responsible for processing these specimens and also for determining the antibiotic susceptibility of bacterial pathogens. Traditionally, detection of pathogenic agents has relied largely on either the microscopic visualization of pathogens in clinical material or the growth of microorganisms in the laboratory. Identification is generally based on phenotypic characteristics, such as fermentation profiles for bacteria, cytopathic effects in tissue culture for viral agents, and microscopic morphology for fungi and parasites. These techniques are reliable but are often time-consuming. Increasingly, the use of nucleic acid probes is becoming a standard detection and/or identification method in the clinical microbiology laboratory, gradually replacing phenotypic characterization and microscopic visualization methods.

DETECTION METHODS

Reappraisal of the methods employed in the clinical microbiology laboratory has led to the development of strategies for detection of pathogenic agents through nonvisual biologic signal detection systems. Much of this methodology is based on either computerization of detection systems with relatively inexpensive but sophisticated computers or the use of nucleic acid probes directed at specific DNA or RNA targets. This chapter discusses both the methods that are currently available and those that are being developed.

BIOLOGIC SIGNALS A *biologic signal* is a material that can be reproducibly differentiated from other substances present in the same physical environment. Key issues in the use of a biologic (or electronic) signal are distinguishing it from background noise and translating it into meaningful information. Examples of biologic signals applicable to clinical microbiology include structural components of bacteria, fungi, and viruses; specific antigens; metabolic end products; unique DNA or RNA base sequences; enzymes; toxins or other proteins; and surface polysaccharides.

DETECTION SYSTEMS A detector is used to sense a signal and to discriminate between the signal and background noise. Detection systems range from the trained eyes of a technologist assessing morphologic variations to sensitive electronic instruments, such as gas-liquid chromatographs coupled to computer systems for signal analysis. The sensitivity with which signals can be detected varies widely. It is essential to use a detection system that discerns small amounts of signal even when biologic background noise is present—i.e., that is both sensitive and specific. Common detection systems include immunofluorescence; chemiluminescence for DNA/RNA probes; flame ionization detection of short- or long-chain fatty acids; and detection of substrate utilization or end-product formation as color changes, of enzyme activity as a change in light absorbance, of turbidity changes, of cytopathic effects in cell lines, and of particle agglutination.

AMPLIFICATION Amplification enhances the sensitivity with which weak signals can be detected. The most common microbiologic amplification technique is growth of a single bacterium into a discrete colony on an agar plate or into a suspension containing many identical organisms. The advantage of growth as an amplification method is that it requires only an appropriate growth medium; the disadvantage is the amount of time required for amplification. More rapid specific amplification of biologic signals can be achieved with techniques such as polymerase (ligase) chain reactions (PCRs, for DNA/RNA), enzyme immunoassays (EIAs, for antigens and antibodies), electronic amplification (for gas-liquid chromatography assays), antibody capture methods (for concentration and/or separation), and selective filtration or centrifugation. Although a variety of methods are available for the amplification and detection of biologic signals in research, thorough testing is required before they are validated as diagnostic assays.

DIRECT DETECTION

MICROSCOPY The field of microbiology has been defined largely by the development and use of the microscope. The examination of specimens by microscopic methods rapidly provides useful diagnostic information. Staining techniques permit organisms to be seen more clearly.

The simplest method for microscopic evaluation is the wet mount, which is used, for example, to examine cerebrospinal fluid (CSF) for the presence of *Cryptococcus neoformans*, with India ink as a background against which to visualize large-capsuled yeast cells. Wet mounts with dark-field illumination are also used to detect spirochetes from genital lesions and to reveal *Borrelia* or *Leptospira* in blood. Skin scrapings and hair samples can be examined with use of either 10% KOH wet-mount preparations or the calcofluor white method and ultraviolet illumination to detect fungal elements as fluorescing structures. Staining of wet mounts—for example, with lactophenol cotton blue stain for fungal elements—is often used for morphologic identification. These techniques enhance signal detection and decrease the background, making it easier to identify specific fungal structures.

STAINING Gram's Stain Without staining, bacteria are difficult to see at the magnifications (400 to 1000×) used for their detection. Although simple one-step stains can be used, differential stains are more common. Gram's stain differentiates between organisms with thick peptidoglycan cell walls (gram-positive) and those with outer membranes that can be dissolved with alcohol or acetone (gram-negative).

Gram's stain is particularly useful for examining sputum for polymorphonuclear leukocytes (PMNs) and bacteria. Sputum specimens with 25 or more PMNs and fewer than 10 epithelial cells per low-power field often provide clinically useful information. However, the presence in "sputum" samples of more than 10 epithelial cells per low-power field and of multiple bacterial types suggests contamination with oral microflora. Despite the difficulty of discriminating between normal microflora and pathogens, Gram's stain may prove useful for specimens from areas with a large resident microflora if a useful biologic marker (signal) is available. Gram's staining of vaginal swab specimens can be used to detect epithelial cells covered with gram-positive bacteria in the absence of lactobacilli and the presence of gram-negative rods—a scenario regarded as a sign of bacterial vaginosis. Similarly, examination of stained stool specimens for leukocytes is useful as a screening procedure before testing for *Clostridium difficile* toxin or other enteric pathogens.

The examination of CSF and joint, pleural, or peritoneal fluid with Gram's stain is useful for determining whether bacteria and/or PMNs are present. The sensitivity is such that $>10^4$ bacteria per milliliter should be detected. Centrifugation is often performed before staining to concentrate specimens thought to contain low numbers of organisms. The pellet is examined after staining. This simple method is particularly useful for examination of CSF for bacteria and white blood cells or of sputum for acid-fast bacilli (AFB).

Acid-Fast Stain The acid-fast stain identifies organisms that retain carbol fuchsin dye after acid/organic solvent disruption (e.g., *Mycobacterium* spp.). Modifications of this procedure allow the differentiation of *Actinomyces* from *Nocardia* or other weakly acid-fast organisms. The acid-fast stain is applied to sputum, other fluids, and tissue samples when AFB (e.g., *Mycobacterium* spp.) are suspected. The identification of the pink/red AFB against the blue background of the counterstain requires a trained eye, since few AFB may be detected in an entire smear, even when the specimen has been concentrated by centrifugation. An alternative method is the auramine-rhodamine combination fluorescent dye technique.

Fluorochrome Stains Fluorochrome stains, such as acridine orange, are used to identify white blood cells, yeasts, and bacteria in body fluids. Other specialized stains, such as Dappe's stain, may be used for the detection of *Mycoplasma* in cell cultures. Capsular, flagellar, and spore stains are used for identification or demonstration of characteristic structures.

Immunofluorescent Stains The direct immunofluorescent antibody technique uses antibody coupled to a fluorescing compound, such as fluorescein, and directed at a specific antigenic target to visualize organisms or subcellular structures. When samples are examined under appropriate conditions, the fluorescing compound absorbs ultraviolet light and reemits light at a higher (visible) wavelength detectable by the human eye. In the indirect immunofluorescent antibody technique, an unlabeled (target) antibody binds a specific antigen. The specimen is then stained with fluorescein-labeled polyclonal antibody directed at the target antibody. Because each unlabeled target antibody attached to the appropriate antigen has multiple sites for attachment of the second antibody, the visual signal can be intensified (i.e., amplified). This form of staining is called *indirect* because a two-antibody system is used to generate the signal for detection of the antigen. Both direct and indirect methods detect viral inclusions (e.g., cytomegalovirus and herpes simplex virus) within cultured cells as well as many difficult-to-grow bacterial agents (e.g., *Legionella pneumophila*) directly in clinical specimens.

MACROSCOPIC ANTIGEN DETECTION Latex agglutination assays and EIAs are rapid and inexpensive methods for identifying organisms, extracellular toxins, and viral agents by means of protein and polysaccharide antigens. Such assays may be performed directly on clinical samples or after growth of organisms on agar plates or in viral cell cultures. The biologic signal in each case is the antigen to be detected. Monoclonal or polyclonal antibodies coupled to a reporter (such as latex particles or an enzyme) are used for detection of antibody-antigen binding reactions.

Techniques such as direct agglutination of bacterial cells with specific antibody are simple but relatively insensitive, while latex agglutination and EIAs are more sensitive. Some cell-associated antigens, such as capsular polysaccharides and lipopolysaccharides, can be detected by agglutination of a suspension of bacterial cells when antibody is added; this method is useful for typing of the somatic antigens of *Shigella* and *Salmonella*. In systems such as EIAs, which employ antibodies coupled to an enzyme, an antigen-antibody reaction results in the conversion of a colorless substrate to a colored product. Because the coupling of an enzyme to the antibody can amplify a weak biologic signal, the sensitivity of such assays is often high. In each instance, the basis for antigen detection is antigen-antibody binding, with the detection system changed to accommodate the biologic signal. Most such assays provide information as to whether antigen is present but do not quantify the antigen. EIAs are also useful for detecting bacterial toxins—e.g., *C. difficile* toxins A and B in stool.

DETECTION OF PATHOGENIC AGENTS BY CULTURE

SPECIMEN COLLECTION AND TRANSPORT To culture bacterial, mycotic, or viral pathogens, an appropriate sample must be placed into the proper medium for growth (amplification). The success of efforts to identify a specific pathogen often depends on the collection and transport process coupled to a laboratory-processing algorithm suitable for the specific sample/agent. In some instances, it is better for specimens to be plated at the time of collection rather than first being transported to the laboratory (e.g., urethral swabs being cultured for *Neisseria gonorrhoeae* or sputum specimens for pneumococci). In general, the more rapidly a specimen is plated onto appropriate media, the better the chance for isolating bacterial pathogens. Appendix B lists procedures for collection and transport of common

specimens. Because there are many pathogen-specific paradigms for these procedures, it is important to seek advice from the microbiology laboratory when in doubt about a particular situation.

ISOLATION OF BACTERIAL PATHOGENS Isolation of suspect pathogen(s) from clinical material relies on the use of artificial media that support bacterial growth in vitro. Such media are composed of agar, which is not metabolized by bacteria; nutrients to support the growth of the species of interest; and sometimes substances to inhibit the growth of other bacteria. Broth is employed for growth (amplification) of organisms from specimens with few bacteria, such as peritoneal dialysis fluid, CSF, or samples in which anaerobes or other fastidious organisms may be present. The general use of liquid medium for all specimens is not worthwhile.

Two basic strategies are used to isolate pathogenic bacteria. The first is to employ enriched media that support the growth of any bacteria that may be present in a sample such as blood or CSF, which contain no bacteria under normal conditions. Broths that allow the growth of small numbers of organisms may be subcultured to solid media when growth is detected. The second strategy is to isolate (amplify) specific bacterial species from stool, genital tract secretions, or sputum—sites that contain many bacteria under normal conditions. Antimicrobial agents or other inhibitory substances are incorporated into the agar medium to inhibit growth of all but the bacteria of interest. After incubation, organisms that grow on such media are further characterized to determine whether they are pathogens. Selection for organisms that may be pathogens from the normal microflora shortens the time required for diagnosis (Fig. 121-1).

ISOLATION OF VIRAL AGENTS (See also Chap. 180) Pathogenic viral agents often are cultured when the presence of serum antibody is not a criterion for active infection or when an increase in serum antibody may not be detected during infection. The biologic signal—virus—is amplified to a detectable level. Although a number of techniques are available, an essential element is a monolayer of cultured mammalian cells sensitive to infection with the suspected virus. These cells serve as the amplification system by allowing the proliferation of viral particles. Virus may be detected by direct observation of the cultured cells for cytopathic effects or by immunofluorescent detection of viral antigens following incubation. Culture methods are particularly useful for detection of rapidly propagated agents, such as cytomegalovirus or herpes simplex virus.

AUTOMATION OF MICROBIAL DETECTION IN BLOOD

The detection of microbial pathogens in blood is difficult because the number of organisms present in the sample is often low and the organisms' integrity and ability to replicate may be damaged by humoral defense mechanisms or antimicrobial agents. Over the years, systems that rely on the detection of CO_2 produced by bacteria and yeasts in blood culture medium have allowed the automation of the detection procedure. The most common systems involve either the insertion of a sampling device into each culture bottle at periodic intervals, with drawing off of the head-space gas for analysis by an infrared monitor, or the use of reflectance optics, with a light-emitting diode and photodiode employed to detect a color change in a CO_2-sensitive indicator built into the bottom of the culture bottle. These systems measure CO_2 concentration as indicative of microbial growth. Sophisticated algorithms are used to evaluate the rate at which CO_2 is being produced and then to determine whether the rate of change is consistent with microbial growth. Such methods are no more sensitive than the human eye in detecting a positive culture; however, because the bottles in an automated system are monitored more frequently, a positive culture is often detected more rapidly than by manual techniques, and important information, including the result of Gram's stain and preliminary susceptibility assays, can be obtained sooner. One advantage of reflectance optic systems is that the bottles are scanned continuously in a

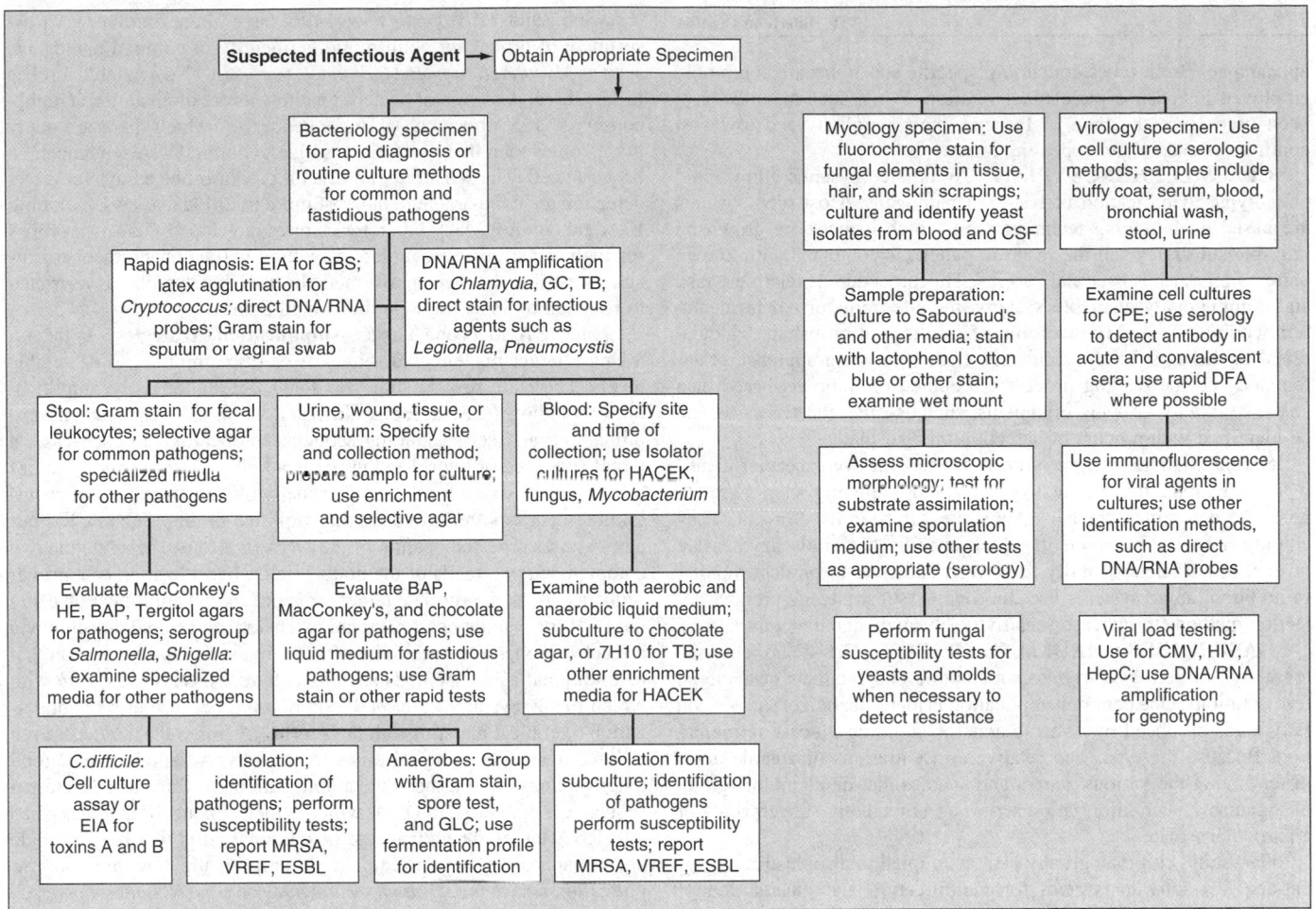

FIGURE 121-1 Common specimen-processing algorithms used in clinical microbiology laboratories. Abbreviations: BAP, blood agar plate; CMV, cytomegalovirus; CPE, cytopathic effects; CSF, cerebrospinal fluid; DFA, direct fluorescent antibody; EIA, enzyme immunoassay; ESBL, extended-spectrum β-lactamase; GBS, group B *Streptococcus*; GC, *Neisseria gonorrhoeae*; GLC, gas-liquid chromatography; HACEK, *Haemophilus aphrophilus/* *parainfluenzae/paraphrophilus*, *Actinobacillus actinomycetemcomitans*, *Cardiobacterium hominis*, *Eikenella corrodens*, and *Kingella kingae*; HE, Hektoen enteric medium; HcpC, hepatitis C virus; HIV, human immunodeficiency virus; MRSA, methicillin-resistant *Staphylococcus aureus*; TB, *Mycobacterium tuberculosis*; VREF, vancomycin-resistant *Enterococcus faecium*.

noninvasive monitoring procedure, and thus the likelihood of laboratory contamination is decreased.

Automated systems also have been applied to the detection of microbial growth from specimens other than blood, such as peritoneal and other normally sterile fluids. *Mycobacterium* spp. can be detected in certain automated systems if appropriate liquid media are used for culture.

DETECTION OF PATHOGENIC AGENTS BY SEROLOGIC METHODS

Measurement of serum antibody provides an indirect marker for past or current infection with a specific viral agent or other pathogens, including *Brucella*, *Legionella*, *Rickettsia*, and *Helicobacter pylori*. The biologic signal is usually either IgM or IgG antibody directed at surface-expressed antigen(s). The detection systems include those used for bacterial antigens (agglutination reactions, immunofluorescence, and EIA) and unique systems such as hemolysis inhibition and complement fixation. Serologic methods generally fall into two categories: those that determine protective antibody levels and those that measure changing antibody titers during infection. Determination of an antibody response as a measure of current immunity is important in the case of viral agents for which there are vaccines, such as rubella virus or varicella-zoster virus; assays for this purpose normally use one or two dilutions of serum for a qualitative determination of protective antibody levels. Quantitative serologic assays to detect increases in antibody titers most often employ paired serum samples obtained 10 to 14 days apart (i.e., acute- and convalescent-phase samples). Since the incubation period before symptoms are noted may be long enough for an antibody response to occur, the demonstration of acute-phase antibody alone is often insufficient to establish the diagnosis of active infection as opposed to past exposure. In such circumstances, IgM may be useful as a measure of an early, acute-phase antibody response. A fourfold increase in total antibody titer or in EIA activity between the acute- and convalescent-phase samples is also regarded as evidence for active infection.

For certain viral agents, such as Epstein-Barr virus, the antibodies produced may be directed at different antigens during different phases of the infection. For this reason, most laboratories test for antibody directed at both viral capsid antigens and antigens associated with recently infected host cells to determine the stage of infection.

IDENTIFICATION METHODS

Once bacteria are isolated, traditional methods of phenotypic characterization are often used to identify specific isolates. An organism's phenotypic characteristics include traits that are readily detectable after growth on agar media (colony size, color, hemolytic reactions, odor), use of specific substrates and carbon sources (such as carbohydrates), formation of specific end products during growth, and microscopic appearance. Broth tubes containing specific substrates are commonly employed for phenotypic characterization. While such methods have been used since the time of Pasteur, their simplicity and low cost continue to make them appealing today.

CLASSIC PHENOTYPING Automated systems allow rapid phenotypic identification of bacterial pathogens. Most such systems are based on biotyping techniques, in which isolates are grown on multiple substrates and the reaction pattern is compared with known patterns for various bacterial species. This procedure is relatively fast, and commercially available systems include miniaturized fermentation, coding to simplify recording of results, and probability calculations for the most likely pathogens. If the biotyping approach is automated and the reading process is coupled to computer-based data analysis, rapidly growing organisms, such as Enterobacteriaceae, can be identified within hours of detection on agar plates.

Several systems use preformed enzymes for even speedier identification (within 2 to 3 h). Such systems do not rely on bacterial growth per se to determine whether a substrate has been used or not. They employ a heavy inoculum in which specific bacterial enzymes are present in sufficient quantity to convert substrate to product rapidly. In addition, some systems use fluorogenic substrate/end-product detection methods to increase sensitivity (through signal amplification).

GAS-LIQUID CHROMATOGRAPHY Gas-liquid chromatography is often used to detect metabolic end products of bacterial fermentations. One common application is identification of short-chain fatty acids produced by obligate anaerobes during glucose fermentation. Because the types and relative concentrations of volatile acids differ among the various genera and species that make up this group of organisms, such information serves as a metabolic "fingerprint" for a particular isolate.

Gas-liquid chromatography can be coupled to a sophisticated signal-analysis software system for identification and quantitation of long-chain fatty acids (LCFAs) in the outer membranes and cell walls of bacteria and fungi. For any given species, the types and relative concentrations of LCFAs are distinctive enough to allow identification of even closely related species. An organism may be identified definitively within a few hours after detection of growth on appropriate media. LCFA analysis is one of the most advanced procedures currently available for phenotypic characterization.

NUCLEIC ACID PROBES Techniques for the detection and quantitation of specific DNA and RNA base sequences in clinical specimens have become powerful tools for the diagnosis of bacterial, viral, parasitic, and fungal infections. The basic strategy is to detect a relatively short sequence of bases specific for a particular pathogen on single-stranded DNA or RNA by hybridization of a complementary sequence of bases (probe) coupled to a "reporter" system that serves as the signal for detection. Detection of an organism by nucleic acid probes offers a decided advantage over culture methods for difficult-to-grow organisms. Current technology encompasses a wide array of methods for amplification and signal detection, some of which have been approved by the U.S. Food and Drug Administration (FDA) for clinical diagnosis.

Use of nucleic acid probes generally involves lysis of intact cells and denaturation of the DNA or RNA to render it single-stranded. The probe may be hybridized to the target sequence in a solution or on a solid support, depending on the system employed. In situ hybridization of a probe to a target is also possible and allows the use of probes with agents present in tissue specimens. Once the probe has been hybridized to the target (biologic signal), a variety of strategies may be employed to amplify and/or quantify the target-probe complex (Fig. 121-2).

Probes for Direct Detection of Pathogens in Clinical Specimens Nucleic acid probes are available commercially for direct detection of various bacterial and parasitic pathogens, including *L. pneumophila*, *Chlamydia trachomatis*, *N. gonorrhoeae*, group A *Streptococcus*, *Gardnerella vaginalis*, *Mycoplasma hominis*, and *Giardia lamblia*. In addition, probes for direct detection of human papillomavirus, *Can-*

dida spp., and *Trichomonas vaginalis* have been approved. An assortment of probes for confirming the identity of cultured pathogens, such as *Mycobacterium* and *Salmonella* spp., are also available. Probes for the direct detection of bacterial pathogens are often aimed at highly conserved 16S ribosomal RNA sequences, of which there are many more copies than there are of any single genomic DNA sequence in a bacterial cell. The sensitivity and specificity of probe assays for direct detection are comparable to those of more traditional assays, including EIA and culture. Many laboratories have developed their own probes for pathogens; however, unless a method-validation protocol for diagnostic testing has been performed, the use of such probes is restricted to research by federal law in the United States.

Nucleic Acid Probe Target-Amplification Strategies In theory, a single target nucleic acid sequence can be amplified to detectable levels. There are several strategies for target and/or probe amplification, including PCR, ligase chain reaction, strand displacement amplification, and self-sustaining sequence replication. In each case, a target sequence or hybridized probe is amplified exponentially to obtain sufficient signal for detection, usually by the attachment of chemiluminescent reporter groups to the amplified product. The PCR strategy requires repeated heating of the DNA or RNA to separate the two complementary strands of the double helix, hybridization of a primer sequence to the appropriate target sequence, target amplification using the PCR for complementary strand extension, and signal detection via a labeled probe. The sensitivity of such assays is far greater than that of traditional assay methods such as culture. However, the care with which the assays are performed is important, because cross-contamination of clinical material with DNA or RNA from other sources (even at low levels) can cause false-positive results. An alternative method employs transcription-mediated amplification, in which an RNA target sequence is converted to DNA, which is then exponentially transcribed into RNA target. The advantage of this method is that only a single heating/annealing step is required for amplification. At present, amplification assays for *Mycobacterium tuberculosis*, *N. gonorrhoeae*, *C. trachomatis*, and *M. hominis* are on the market. Again, many laboratories have used commercially available *taq* polymerase, probe sequences, and reagents to develop "in-house" assays for diagnostic use. Issues related to quality control, interpretation of results, sample processing, and regulatory requirements have slowed the commercial development of diagnostic assay kits.

Signal Amplification Strategies Alternative systems for signal amplification have great appeal, particularly for quantitative determination of the amount of target present in a given specimen. With the advent of newer therapeutic regimens for HIV-associated disease, cytomegalovirus infection, and hepatitis C virus infection, the response to therapy has been monitored by determining both genotype and "viral load" at various times after treatment initiation. Target amplification (PCR, transcription-mediated amplification) is difficult to control in a manner that allows accurate determination of the original target (genome) concentration. In other systems, probes attached to complementary target sequences are amplified by the attachment of a second probe and an amplification multimer to the original probe. In one such system, branched-chain DNA (bDNA)-based amplification, bDNA is attached to a site different from the target-binding sequence of the original probe. Chemiluminescent-labeled oligonucleotides can then bind to multiple repeating sequences on the bDNA. The amplified bDNA signal is detected by chemiluminescence. Alternatively, a DNA probe may be attached to an RNA target and the resulting DNA/RNA hybrid captured on a solid support by antibody specific for DNA/RNA hybrids (concentration/amplification) and detected by chemiluminescent-labeled antibody specific for DNA/RNA hybrids. Both methods can be used to determine the approximate number of target copies (virus) in the starting material. The advantage of these systems over PCR is that only a single heating/annealing step is required to hybridize the target-binding probe to the target sequence for amplification.

Application of Nucleic Acid Probe Technology Nucleic acid probe technology is being used to identify difficult-to-grow or noncultivable bacterial pathogens, such as *Mycobacterium*, *Legionella*,

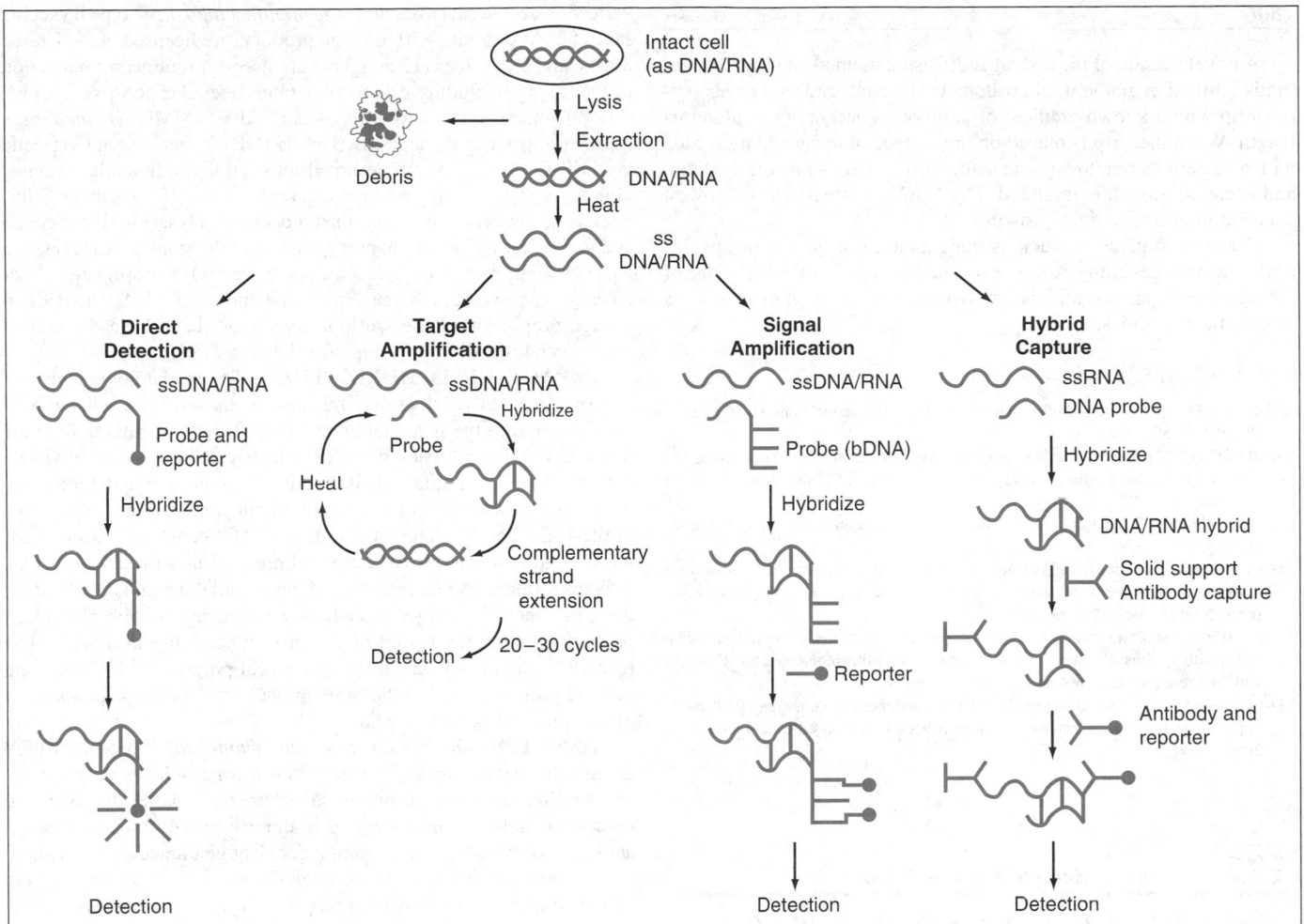

FIGURE 121-2 Strategies for amplification and/or detection of a target-probe complex. DNA or RNA extracted from microorganisms is heated to create single-stranded (ss) DNA/RNA containing appropriate target sequences. These target sequences may be hybridized directly (direct detection) with probes attached to reporter molecules; they may be amplified by repetitive cycles of complementary strand extension (polymerase chain reaction) before attachment of a reporter probe; or the original target-probe signal may be amplified via hybridization with an additional probe containing multiple copies of a secondary reporter target sequence (branched-chain DNA, or bDNA). DNA/RNA hybrids can also be "captured" on a solid support (hybrid capture), with antibody directed at the DNA/RNA hybrids used to concentrate them and a second antibody coupled to a reporter molecule attached to the captured hybrid.

Ehrlichia, *Rickettsia*, *Babesia*, *Borrelia*, and *Tropheryma whippelii*. Amplification methods are also being used to detect chronic viral infections, such as herpes simplex encephalitis, cytomegalovirus infection, and hepatitis C. The monitoring of therapy with quantitative viral-load testing is a significant new application of nucleic acid technology. Further applications will likely include the replacement of culture for identification of many pathogens with solid-state DNA/RNA chip technology, in which thousands of unique nucleic acid sequences can be detected on a single computer chip. Probe technology also has the potential to detect viral pathogens faster than is possible with current culture techniques. However, if laboratories are to take full advantage of probe technology, the cost of reagents and assay automation must be competitive with the cost of existing methodology. At present, the detection of agents such as *C. trachomatis* or *N. gonorrhoeae* by probe technology is more expensive for most laboratories than detection by traditional culture or EIA. Moreover, because automated processing equipment is just beginning to find its way into the laboratory for these assays, nucleic acid amplification methods are both more labor-intensive and more expensive than other detection systems. In the absence of clear documentation of clinical utility, many laboratories continue to wait for FDA approval of commercially available DNA/RNA probe assays rather than validating in-house assays.

SUSCEPTIBILITY TESTING A principal responsibility of the clinical microbiology laboratory is to determine which antimicrobial agents inhibit a specific bacterial isolate. Such testing is used to screen for infection control problems, such as methicillin-resistant *Staphylococcus aureus*, vancomycin-resistant *Enterococcus faecium*, or extended-spectrum β-lactamase-producing organisms. Two approaches are useful. The first is a qualitative assessment of susceptibility, with responses categorized as susceptible, resistant, or intermediate. This approach can involve either the placement of paper disks containing antibiotics on an agar surface inoculated with the bacterial strain to be tested (Kirby-Bauer or disk/agar diffusion method), with measurement of the zones of growth inhibition following incubation, or the use of broth tubes containing a set concentration of antibiotic (breakpoint method). These methods have been carefully calibrated against quantitative methods and clinical experience with each antibiotic, and zones of inhibition and breakpoints have been calculated on a species-by-species basis.

The second approach is to inoculate the test strain of bacteria into a series of broth tubes (or agar plates) with increasing concentrations of antibiotic. The lowest concentration of antibiotic that inhibits microbial growth in this test system is known as the *minimum inhibitory concentration* (MIC). If tubes in which no growth occurs are subcultured, the minimum concentration of antibiotic required to kill the starting inoculum can also be determined (*minimum bactericidal concentration*, or MBC). Quantitative susceptibility testing by the microbroth dilution technique, a miniaturized version of the broth dilution technique using microwell plates, lends itself to automation and is commonly used in larger clinical laboratories.

A novel version of the disk/agar diffusion method employs a quantitative diffusion gradient, or epsilometer (E-test), and uses an absorbent strip with a known gradient of antibiotic concentrations along its length. When the strip is placed on the surface of an agar plate seeded with a bacterial strain to be tested, antibiotic diffuses into the medium, and bacterial growth is inhibited. The MIC is estimated as the lowest concentration that inhibits growth.

For some organisms, such as obligate anaerobes, routine susceptibility testing generally is not performed because of the difficulty of growing the organisms and the predictable sensitivity of most isolates to specific antibiotics.

BIBLIOGRAPHY

McNicol AM et al: In situ hybridization and its diagnostic applications in pathology. J Pathol 182:250, 1997

Miller JM et al: Specimen collection, transport and storage, in *Manual of Clinical Microbiology*, 6th ed, P Murray et al (eds). Washington, DC, American Society for Microbiology, 1995

Salfinger M et al: Diagnostic tools in tuberculosis. Present and future. Respiration 65:163, 1998

Sarasini A et al: Diagnostic significance and clinical impact of quantitative assays for diagnosis of human cytomegalovirus infection/disease in immunocompromised patients. New Microbiol 21:293, 1998

Trabaud MA et al: Comparison of HCV RNA assays for the detection and quantification of hepatitis C virus RNA levels in serum of patients with chronic hepatitis C treated with interferon. J Med Virol 52:105, 1997

Yeghiazarian T et al: Quantitation of human immunodeficiency virus type 1 RNA levels in plasma by using small-volume-format branched-DNA assays. J Clin Microbiol 36:2096, 1998

122　*Gerald T. Keusch, Kenneth J. Bart*

IMMUNIZATION PRINCIPLES AND VACCINE USE

CDC Centers for Disease Control and Prevention	HBV hepatitis B virus
DTaP diphtheria/tetanus/acellular pertussis vaccine	Hib *H. influenzae* type b
	IPV inactivated poliovirus vaccine
DTP diphtheria/tetanus/pertussis	MMR measles/mumps/rubella
FDA Food and Drug Administration	NCVIA National Childhood Vaccine Injury Act
GMPs good manufacturing practices	OPV oral poliovirus vaccine
HBsAg hepatitis B surface antigen	Td tetanus/diphtheria

Most humans live their lives ignoring the certainty of their own mortality. Perhaps this fact explains why the adage "an ounce of prevention is worth a pound of cure" has so little effect on their everyday behavior. Even when it comes to acting to protect their young, parents are capable of ignoring the potential for mortality among their children (in the developed world) and of accepting the certainty of childhood deaths (in the developing world). In both settings, parents all too often fail to seek out and demand the best preventive measures available. Unless mandated by the law in the former setting or provided by benevolent organizations or governments in the latter, universal immunization has invariably remained an unattained goal. Compulsion and benevolence, it seems, are two essential components of immunization.

However, the integration of immunization practices (a major component of primary disease prevention) into routine health care services has provided caregivers with control over a substantial proportion of the disease and mortality that plagued the United States during the first half of the twentieth century (Table 122-1). For society today, immunization represents one of the most cost-effective means of preventing infectious disease. For every dollar spent, diphtheria/tetanus/pertussis (DTP) vaccine saves $29, measles/mumps/rubella (MMR) vaccine saves $21, trivalent oral poliovirus vaccine (OPV) saves $6, varicella vaccine saves $5, and *Haemophilus influenzae* type b vaccine saves $2. At present, >50 biologic products are licensed in the United States, and 6 vaccines (12 antigens) are used for routine immunization in the young, including diphtheria/tetanus/acellular pertussis vaccine (DTaP), inactivated poliovirus vaccine (IPV), MMR, *H. influenzae* type b (Hib) vaccine, hepatitis B virus (HBV) vaccine, and varicella vaccine. Five vaccines are designed for routine use in adults: tetanus/diphtheria (Td) toxoids, adsorbed, for adult use; HBV vaccine; influenza virus vaccine; polyvalent pneumococcal polysaccharide vaccine; and varicella vaccine. Some preparations are designated as special-use vaccines (e.g., hepatitis A vaccine for travelers). Unfortunately, vaccines for eukaryotic pathogens (protozoa and helminths), which affect a large proportion of the world's population, have been difficult to develop and remain only a hope for the future.

IMPACT OF IMMUNIZATION The epidemiologically appropriate use of vaccines has resulted in the global eradication of smallpox and in the potential eradication of poliomyelitis in the next few years and of measles by 2020. Already achieved are the virtual elimination of congenital rubella syndrome, tetanus, and diphtheria as well as a dramatic reduction in pertussis, rubella, measles, and mumps in the United States. The introduction of Hib conjugate vaccines for immunization of infants has all but eliminated invasive *Haemophilus* infections (including meningitis and pneumonia), presumably because these vaccines also reduce nasopharyngeal carriage of Hib and induce protection before the period of greatest vulnerability in infancy. The recently licensed polyvalent pneumococcal polysaccharide conjugate vaccine promises to have the same impact on invasive pneumococcal disease, including otitis media.

DEFINITIONS *Vaccination* and *immunization* are often used as interchangeable terms. However, the former denotes only the administration of a vaccine or toxoid, whereas the latter describes the process of inducing or providing immunity by any means, whether active or passive. Thus, vaccination does not guarantee immunization. *Active immunization* refers to the induction of immune defenses by the administration of antigens in appropriate forms, whereas *passive immunization* involves the provision of temporary protection by the administration of exogenously produced immune substances. Immunizing agents thus include vaccines, toxoids, and antibody-containing immunoglobulin preparations from human or animal donors (Table 122-2).

PRINCIPLES OF IMMUNIZATION Artificial induction of immunity closely follows two well-tested principles of nature. The first, active immunization, can be traced at least as far back as Thucydides, who noted that people surviving epidemics of plague in Athens were spared during later outbreaks of the same disease. The second, passive immunization, is a natural process as well and is exemplified by the transplacental transmission of maternal antibodies to the fetus to provide protection against several diseases during the first months of life. Use of the two measures together may produce a complementary effect (as with HBV vaccine plus hepatitis B immune globulin) or may actually interfere with the development of immunity (as when measles vaccine is administered within 6 weeks of immunoglobulin). Depending on whether there are multiple species or serotypes of an organism and—if so—whether there are common, cross-reactive, protective antigens, a specific vaccine may induce protection against all representative forms of an infectious agent or against the immunizing strain only. One of the intrinsic virtues of whole-organism vaccines is that they potentially contain all protective antigens of the organism. However, this virtue is counterbalanced by an inherent problem with such vaccines: the possibility of adverse responses to reactive but nonprotective antigens present in the mix. Because the immune response to specific antigens is controlled genetically, all individuals cannot be expected to respond identically to the same vaccine.

APPROACHES TO ACTIVE IMMUNIZATION The two standard approaches to active immunization are (1) the use of live, generally attenuated, infectious agents (e.g., measles virus); and (2) the use of inactivated agents or their constituents or products obtained by genetic recombination (e.g., acellular pertussis vaccines). For many diseases (e.g., poliomyelitis, influenza), both approaches have been employed. Live attenuated vaccines are believed to induce an immunologic response more nearly like that resulting from natural infection than the response induced by killed vaccines. Currently available inactivated or killed vaccines consist of inactivated whole organisms (e.g., plague vaccine); detoxified protein exotoxins (e.g., tetanus toxoid); recombinant protein antigens (e.g., HBV vaccine); or carbohydrate antigens, either present as soluble purified capsular material (e.g., *Streptococcus pneumoniae* polysaccharides) or conjugated to a protein carrier (e.g., Hib polysaccharide conjugated to diphtheria or tetanus toxoids).

Table 122-1 Changes in Morbidity due to Vaccine-Preventable Diseases in the United States

Disease	Baseline 20th-Century Annual Morbidity	Year Vaccine Introduced	1998 Provisional Morbidity	Decrease, %
Diphtheria	175,885	1923	1	>99.99
Pertussis	147,271	1926	6279	95.7
Tetanus	1314	1927	34	97.4
Poliomyelitis, paralytic	16,316	1955	0	100
Measles	503,282	1963	89	>99.99
Mumps	152,209	1967	606	99.6
Rubella (congenital)	47,745 (823)	1969	345 (5)	99.3 (99.4)
Haemophilus influenzae type b	20,000	1985	54	99.7

SOURCE: National Vaccine Program Office, Centers for Disease Control and Prevention [MMWR 48(12):243, 1999].

APPROACHES TO PASSIVE IMMUNIZATION Passive immunization is generally used to provide temporary immunity in an unimmunized subject exposed to an infectious disease when active immunization either is unavailable (e.g., for cytomegalovirus infection) or has not been implemented before exposure (e.g., for rabies). Passive immunization is used in the treatment of certain disorders associated with toxins (e.g., diphtheria), in certain bites (those of snakes and spiders), and as a specific or nonspecific immunosuppressant [Rho(D) immune globulin and antilymphocyte globulin, respectively].

Three types of preparations are used in passive immunization: (1) standard human immune serum globulin for general use (e.g., gamma globulin), administered intramuscularly or intravenously; (2) special immune serum globulins with a known content of antibody for specific agents (e.g., HBV or varicella-zoster immune globulin); and (3) animal sera and antitoxins.

ROUTE OF ADMINISTRATION The route of administration in part determines the rapidity and nature of the immune responses to vaccines. Vaccines can be administered orally, intranasally, intradermally, subcutaneously, or intramuscularly. Parenterally administered vaccine may not induce mucosal secretory IgA, and mucosal immunization may not induce good systemic responses. Vaccines must be administered by the licensed route to ensure immunogenicity and safety. For example, administration of HBV vaccine into the gluteal rather than the deltoid muscle often fails to induce an adequate immune response, while subcutaneous rather than intramuscular administration of DTP increases the risk of reactions.

AGE Because age influences the response to vaccines, schedules for immunization are based on age-dependent responses determined empirically from clinical trials. The presence of high levels of maternal antibody and/or the immaturity of the immune system in the early months of life impairs the initial immune response to some vaccines (e.g., measles or Hib polysaccharide but not HBV). In the elderly, vaccine responses may be diminished because of natural waning of the immune system. Hence, larger amounts of an antigen may be required to produce the desired response (e.g., in vaccination against influenza).

ADJUVANT POTENTIATION The immune response to some antigens is potentiated by the addition of adjuvants such as aluminum salts or, in the case of polysaccharides (e.g., the polyribose phosphate oligosaccharide of Hib), by conjugation to a carrier protein. Adjuvants, nonspecific boosters of immune responses, are used with inactivated products such as diphtheria and tetanus toxoids, acellular pertussis (aP) vaccine, and HBV vaccine. The mechanism for adjuvant enhancement of immunogenicity is not well defined but relates in part to the rendering of soluble antigens into a particulate form, the mobilization of phagocytes to the site of antigen deposition, and the slowing down of the release of antigens, which prolongs stimulation of the immune response.

THE IMMUNE RESPONSE While many constituents of infectious microorganisms and their products, such as exotoxins, are or can be made to be immunogenic, only a limited number stimulate a protective immune response. The immune system is complex, and antigen composition and presentation are critical for stimulation of the desired immune responses.

The Primary Response In the primary response to a vaccine antigen, an apparent latent period of several days precedes the detection of humoral and cell-mediated immunity. Although the immune response is turned on by contact with the antigen and the immune system, measurable circulating antibodies do not appear for 7 to 10 days. The immunoglobulin class of the response also changes over time. Early-appearing IgM antibodies generally exhibit only low affinity for the antigen, whereas later-appearing IgG antibodies display high affinity. For "thymus-dependent" antigens, CD4+ T helper lymphocytes control the switch from IgM to IgG. Some individuals do not respond, even when presented repeatedly with a vaccine antigen, often because they lack the major histocompatibility complex determinants required to recognize the antigen. This situation is known as *primary vaccine failure*.

The Secondary Response Heightened humoral or cell-mediated responses are elicited by a second exposure to the same antigen. These secondary responses occur rapidly, usually within 4 or 5 days, and result, for example, in increased titers of IgG antibody. The secondary response depends on immunologic memory after the first exposure and is characterized by a marked proliferation of antibody-producing B lymphocytes and/or effector T cells. Polysaccharide vaccines, such as that for *S. pneumoniae*, evoke immune responses that are independent of T cells and are not enhanced by repeated administration. Covalent linking of polysaccharides to proteins converts the former to T cell–dependent antigens that induce immunologic memory and secondary responses to revaccination. Although levels of vaccine-induced antibodies may decline over time (*secondary vaccine failure*), revaccination or exposure to the organism may elicit a rapid protective secondary response consisting of IgG antibodies with little or no detectable IgM. This *anamnestic response* indicates that immunity has persisted. The lack of measurable antibody does not necessarily mean that the

Table 122-2 Definitions of Immunizing Agents

Term	Definition
Vaccine	A suspension of attenuated live or killed microorganisms or antigenic portions of these agents presented to a potential host to induce immunity and prevent disease
Toxoid	A modified bacterial toxin that has been made nontoxic but retains the capacity to stimulate the formation of antitoxin
Immune globulin	An antibody-containing solution derived from human blood by cold ethanol fractionation of large pools of plasma and used primarily for maintenance of the immunity of immunodeficient persons or for passive immunization; intramuscular and intravenous preparations available
Antitoxin	An antibody derived from the serum of animals after stimulation with specific antigens and used to provide passive immunity

individual is unprotected. Furthermore, the mere presence of detectable antibodies after the administration of some vaccines and toxoids does not ensure clinical protection. A minimal circulating level of antibody is known to be required for protection from some diseases (e.g., 0.01 IU/mL for tetanus antitoxin).

Hypersensitivity Reactions Independent of antibody production, the stimulation of the immune system by vaccination may elicit unanticipated responses, especially hypersensitivity reactions. In the past, killed measles vaccine induced incomplete humoral immunity and cell-mediated hypersensitivity, resulting in the development of a syndrome of atypical measles in some children after subsequent exposure; thus this type of vaccine is no longer in use.

Mucosal Immunity Some pathogens are confined to and replicate only at mucosal surfaces (e.g., *Vibrio cholerae*), while others are able to penetrate the mucosa and replicate (e.g., poliovirus, rubella virus, and influenza virus). At the mucosal site, these organisms induce secretory IgA. The induction of secretory IgA by vaccines may be an efficient way to block the essential first steps in pathogenesis, whether the organism is restricted to mucosal surfaces or systemically invades the host across mucosal surfaces.

Measurement of the Immune Response Immune responses to vaccines are often gauged by the concentration of specific antibody in serum. While seroconversion serves as a dependable indicator of an immune response, it measures only one immunologic parameter and does not necessarily indicate protection. The development of circulating antibodies after immunization often correlates directly with clinical protection (e.g., against measles or rubella). Some responses may not in themselves confer immunity but may be sufficiently associated with protection that they remain useful proxy measures of protective immunity (e.g., vibriocidal serum antibodies in cholera).

HERD IMMUNITY It is not necessary to immunize every person in order to stop transmission of an infectious agent through a population. For those organisms dependent on person-to-person transmission, there may be a definable prevalence of immunity in the population above which it becomes difficult for the organism to circulate and reach new susceptibles. This prevalence is called *herd immunity*. When herd immunity is operative, the goals of immunization are converted from the immunization of every person in the community to the immunization of a specified minimum percentage of persons at risk. Herd immunity may wane if immunization capacity fails (as in diphtheria in the new independent states of the former Soviet Union) or if a sufficient percentage of individuals refuse to be immunized (as in pertussis in the United Kingdom and Japan in the 1970s because concern about infrequent—albeit severe—vaccine reactions came to exceed the fear of the disease itself). In both situations, loss of herd immunity led to renewed circulation of the organism and increased susceptibility to infection, with subsequent large outbreaks.

TARGET POPULATIONS AND TIMING OF IMMUNIZATION For common and highly communicable childhood diseases like measles, the target population is the universe of susceptible individuals, and the time to immunize is as early in life as is feasible. Epidemiologic differences in measles in different settings, however, dictate different strategies of immunization. In the industrialized world, immunization with live-virus vaccine at 12 to 15 months of age has been the norm because the vaccine protects >95% of those immunized at this age and there is little measles morbidity/mortality among very young infants. In contrast, in the developing world, measles accounts for a significant proportion of deaths of young infants. Thus it is desirable to immunize children during the first few months of life in order to narrow the window of vulnerability between the rapid decline of maternal antibody after 4 to 6 months and the development of vaccine-induced active immunity.

Hib causes meningitis, epiglottitis, and pneumonia in early childhood, with rates rising sharply after the disappearance of maternally derived antibody. The first Hib vaccines often failed when administered during infancy; this failure was due mainly to an age-related inability to respond to polysaccharide antigens. To overcome this problem, the protective polysaccharide was coupled to protein and converted to a T cell–dependent antigen to which young infants could respond.

In contrast to measles and Hib infection, rubella is primarily a threat to the fetus; young infants and children are not at risk of serious illness. Given the susceptibility of the fetus, immunization of all women of reproductive age before pregnancy would be an ideal strategy. However, it is difficult to systematically vaccinate adolescent and young-adult females. Thus, to assure the protection of as many women as possible, the rubella component is included in a combination vaccine with mumps and measles (MMR) that is administered during infancy.

Some vaccines are now used primarily for adults. For example, influenza virus and polyvalent pneumococcal polysaccharide vaccines are used to prevent pneumonia deaths in the elderly. Unfortunately, these vaccines are underutilized, in part because physicians and otherwise healthy individuals in the target group ignore the indications and in part because there is still a tendency to think about disease prevention with vaccines as a strategy for children. Pneumococcal polysaccharide vaccine is also recommended for children >2 years old who are at risk of severe or even life-threatening pneumococcal infection, such as those with sickle cell disease, asplenia (whether functional or anatomic), renal failure with nephrotic syndrome, cerebrospinal fluid leak, and HIV infection or other immunosuppressive disease states.

THE DEVELOPMENT OF VACCINES

BIOLOGIC IMPEDIMENTS There are often major technical problems to overcome in vaccine development. Although just one major antigenic type of influenza virus is typically in circulation at any one time, the virus is characterized biologically by its antigenic drift. Thus, a new antigenic version capable of causing a global pandemic emerges periodically, and a new vaccine must be rapidly devised, produced, and distributed. In contrast, many prevalent pneumococcal polysaccharide serotypes circulate at all times. Because immunity to the pneumococcus is serotype specific, an individual is susceptible to all serotypes against which he or she lacks antibody. Serotype-specific protection has made it more difficult to develop an effective pneumococcal vaccine than it was to develop a vaccine against *H. influenzae*, of which one capsular serotype (type b) is associated with nearly all cases of severe disease. To overcome this problem, pneumococcal vaccine currently includes 23 polysaccharides that represent ~80% of the virulent serotypes commonly encountered in the United States. Unfortunately, some serotypes are poorly immunogenic, and immunized individuals remain susceptible to the serotypes not included in the vaccine.

STRATEGY FOR VACCINE DEVELOPMENT Vaccine development depends on the systematic application of a four-phase strategy: (1) studies in animals to identify protective antigen, (2) determination of how to present this antigen effectively to the immune system, (3) assessment of the safety and immunogenicity of the preparation in small and then in large human populations at various ages, and (4) evaluation of safety and efficacy in the target population. Each of these steps is simple in concept but difficult in execution, not least because of the clinical trials necessary to assess safety and efficacy; failure at any level stops the process. Thus, in 1995, >190 candidate vaccines were under investigation, but just 5 new products were licensed in the United States. Progress in immunology has taught us much about the organization and function of the immune system (Chap. 305); it has also taught us that the immune system is complicated and that details of antigen composition and presentation are critical for stimulating desired immune responses.

Ultimately, vaccines for humans must be tested in humans. After initial animal studies and small phase 1 and 2 human studies to assess immune responses, optimal dosage, and safety, clinical trials of vaccine efficacy are performed, sometimes with informed volunteers who are challenged with a virulent strain. Larger clinical effectiveness trials in the community, typically involving 1000 to 10,000 vaccinees, may lead to application for licensure. Because of their limited size, however, these trials cannot be expected to detect rare adverse effects. Thus, licensing does not guarantee that a new vaccine is completely safe, and postlicensing monitoring is needed to ensure effectiveness and to document the occurrence of adverse events of low frequency. In 1999, the recently licensed rhesus rotavirus vaccine was withdrawn because postmarketing surveillance uncovered an association with a rare event in infants, intussusception of the bowel.

The development of vaccines goes beyond technology and proof of principle to issues such as development costs, manufacturers' liability and indemnity, perceived public health needs, and the likelihood that a product will be used or sold. Given the complex science required, the costs of vaccine development are high and success is uncertain, adding risk to the development decision. It is unfortunate that the one sure implication of uncertainty in vaccine development is increased cost. In addition, a rational assignment of costs for development between the public and private sectors in the United States has never been achieved.

VACCINE FORMULATIONS Studies of clinical immunology have shown that living and dead antigens do not necessarily induce the same immune responses and that the requirements for the development of protective immunity differ with the organism. These insights, together with the refinement of epidemiologic concepts surrounding immunization, have changed the strategy of vaccine development. The goal is not only to select the correct antigens but also to ensure that the vaccines will result in the type of immune response needed for protection, whether the T cell–mediated activation of macrophages or the generation of cytotoxic T cells, B cell–mediated secretory IgA, or a particular IgG subtype response to a specific polysaccharide epitope.

Live vaccines consist of selected or genetically altered organisms that are avirulent or dramatically attenuated yet remain immunogenic. These agents are expected to cause a subclinical illness that mimics natural infection except for the lack of clinically significant disease. They offer the advantage of replication in vivo, which increases the antigenic load presented to the host's immune system; they may confer lifelong protection with one dose; they present all expressed antigens, thus overcoming immunogenetic restrictions in some hosts; they may reach the local sites most relevant to the induction of protective immunity; and they may produce important protective antigens in vivo that are not efficiently expressed in vitro.

Nonviable vaccines may fail to elicit mucosal IgA-mediated immunity, as they lack a delivery system that will effectively transport them to local antigen-processing cells. Moreover, except for pure polysaccharide antigens, these preparations must almost always be given in multiple doses to induce effective responses. However, killed vaccines can be extremely effective. For example, the nonviable hepatitis A vaccine formulation appears to be close to 100% effective in inducing protective immunity. Methods are under development to incorporate vaccine antigens into degradable polymers that may release antigen at predictable times after a single inoculation and simulate multiple injections over time of the same vaccine.

In spite of their advantages, live vaccines are not always to be preferred. For example, live OPV is contraindicated for use in children with immune-deficiency diseases and in their adult contacts. In addition, even though killed poliovirus vaccine does not completely immunize the gut and can neither reduce the circulation of wild-type poliovirus nor immunize contacts of vaccine recipients, the United States has now switched to a four-dose schedule of this vaccine because of the risk of vaccine-associated polio posed by live OPV.

To create a deliverable vaccine, constituents other than the antigens are required (Table 122-3). These constituents can affect the immunogenicity, efficacy, and safety of a vaccine and can render one formulation superior to another.

NEW VACCINE APPROACHES The first generation of vaccines included whole killed—or, more recently, live—attenuated microorganisms or partially purified microbial products, such as teta-

Table 122-3   Constituents of Vaccines

Constituent(s)	Examples/Purpose
Preservatives, stabilizers, antibiotics	These components are used to prevent the vaccine's deterioration before use, to inhibit or prevent bacterial growth, or to stabilize the antigen. Any of these additives may elicit allergic reactions.
Adjuvants	An aluminum salt is used in some vaccines (e.g., toxoids, hepatitis B vaccine) to enhance the immune response.
Suspending fluid	The suspending fluid can be sterile water, saline, buffer, or more complex fluids derived from the growth medium or biologic system in which the agent is produced (e.g., egg antigens, cell culture ingredients, serum proteins).

nus toxoid, that induced protective antibodies. The second generation of vaccines has taken advantage of molecular genetics and protein chemistry to isolate and manipulate purified proteins or components or subunits of organisms or to generate genetically engineered and attenuated live native organisms or cloned antigens expressed by harmless vector organisms. One conceptual leap is the production of transgenic plants expressing protective vaccine antigens (cloned, for example, in potatoes or bananas) that, when ingested orally, induce mucosal and systemic immune responses to homologous infectious challenges. While the practical use of this technique awaits further refinement, the concept that protective immunity can be induced in this manner has been proven in both animals and humans. Ease of production, stability, ease of administration without equipment, and low cost are the obvious advantages.

Another conceptual leap has led to a third generation of vaccines, in which nucleic acids (either DNA or RNA) are used to induce immunity. Development of DNA vaccines is at a more advanced stage. The principle is simple. First, a DNA plasmid containing the gene sequence for the immunogenic protein or fragment of interest is assembled, and the gene is placed under the control of a strong promoter and an appropriate transcription termination sequence. A single immunization with the plasmid (via intramuscular or intradermal injection, helium-accelerated gene gun injection of DNA-coated gold particles, compressed-air pneumatic jet injection of soluble DNA, direct skin application after suitable preparation, or even insertion of biodegradable stents loaded with the DNA of interest) results in DNA uptake into cells where the gene is expressed and processed normally; thus the product stimulates an immune response. Alteration of the DNA construct or of the mode of administration or the coadministration of cytokine genes can determine whether the immune response is humoral or cellular or whether it involves primarily Th1, Th2, or cytotoxic T cells. Such decisions can be used to optimize the protective immunity induced.

This form of immunization offers real advantages and only theoretical and remote disadvantages (Table 122-4). Moreover, DNA vaccines may be useful in inducing tumor immunity, treating allergy (by suppressing IgE production), or even administering genes for gene therapy. RNA vaccines would avoid some of the potential concerns raised by DNA vaccines because RNA is less stable and does not persist or integrate into the chromosome or cause insertional mutagenesis. However, this lack of stability and the likely need for multiple doses, along with the increased cost of producing, storing, and transporting RNA, are significant disadvantages that remain to be overcome. The concept of nucleic acid vaccines—whether based on DNA or RNA—has been validated experimentally, and early human trials have begun. There is great optimism for the future but much to be learned if we are to apply this powerful new immunization technique successfully.

PRODUCTION OF VACCINES As products to be given to healthy individuals to prevent disease, vaccines must not only be ef-

Table 122-4 Advantages and Disadvantages of DNA Vaccines

Advantages	Disadvantages
Safe; cannot cause infection; stable and heat resistant	Potential risk of integration of viral oncogenes from the vector
No need to express or purify antigens in vitro; no need for adjuvants; can be genetically engineered	Tumor promotion from integration near proto-oncogene or tumor suppressor genes
Normal processing of gene product closely resembling native conformation	Possible induction of tolerance or autoimmunity by vaccine persistence causing a persistent immune response
Persistence for prolonged periods; induction of durable immune response	Possible influence of strong promoter on expression of host genes, with adverse consequences
Induction of both humoral and cell-mediated immunity, including cytotoxic T cells	
Likely to be safe in pregnant women, immunosuppressed patients, or infants in the presence of maternal antibodies	

ficacious but also cause no harm. In the United States, quality assurance is the responsibility of vaccine manufacturers. Standards of manufacture of biologics [known as good manufacturing practices (GMPs)] are regulated and supervised by the U.S. Food and Drug Administration (FDA). Proof of the safety, efficacy, sterility, and purity of products is required before licensure, and sterility and purity are continually monitored for all lots of vaccine after licensure. Post-marketing studies of safety (phase IV studies) are part of routine regulatory control. On rare occasions, either GMP or quality assurance is inadequate; for example, the release of incompletely killed Salk polio vaccine in 1955 caused an outbreak of poliomyelitis in nearly 200 vaccine recipients and their contacts. Unregulated and uncontrolled manufacture of vaccines in developing countries has sometimes led to immunization with inactive products that fail to provide the expected protective immunity.

Another problem in the production of vaccines has unexpectedly cropped up in the past decade. For various reasons, including the high costs of vaccine development and the prospect of much higher profitability from investments in other products, the number of vaccine manufacturers in the United States has declined and the cost of some basic childhood vaccines has increased. Concern therefore exists about the future availability of these essential biologics for national use. Furthermore, pricing decisions made within the private-sector pharmaceutical industry can have a major impact on vaccine use. This situation has stimulated an initiative toward increased public involvement in supplying vaccine to individuals for whom price is an issue as well as in oversight of the vaccine supply and of price negotiations with the industry.

ADMINISTRATION OF VACCINES   Health care workers administering vaccines must take the precautions necessary to minimize the risk of spreading disease—for example, hand washing between immunizations. They should be immunized against hepatitis B, measles, rubella, influenza, and varicella. Different vaccines should not be mixed in the same syringe unless such a practice is specifically endorsed by licensure. Disposable needles and syringes should be discarded in labeled, puncture-proof containers to prevent inadvertent needlestick injury or reuse.

The addition of new, individually injectable vaccines to the immunization schedule has heightened parental concerns about the administration of up to four injections at a single clinic visit. The development and use of combinations of vaccines are intended to mitigate these concerns. Even when multiple injections are required, providers must make every effort to administer all indicated vaccines at each visit.

Wherever effective primary health care systems ensure access to medical services for the majority and the population is educated about the need for and efficacy of vaccines, coverage rates for basic immunization are usually high, regardless of the route of vaccine administration or the number of doses necessary. However, without systematic attention to the completion of multiple-dose vaccine schedules, coverage rates for second, third, and booster doses may drop off significantly.

USE OF VACCINES

Recommendations for vaccine use in the United States are developed by several different groups. These recommendations are the result of a collaborative process among the recommending groups, the pharmaceutical industry, and the FDA.

Vaccines recommended in 1999 for routine administration to infants, children, and adults are shown in Table 122-5; vaccines recommended for special use are shown in Table 122-6; and schedules for immunization of children and adults are shown in Fig. 122-1 and Table 122-7, respectively. The recommendations on route, site, and dosages for vaccination are derived from theoretical considerations, experimental trials, and clinical experience; deviation from these recommendations can result in inadequate protection. The administration of doses at intervals longer than those recommended does not diminish the ultimate protective response but merely delays it. It is not necessary to restart an interrupted series from the beginning or to add an extra dose. In contrast, giving vaccines at shorter-than-recommended intervals may result in poor responses.

RECORDING AND REPORTING REQUIREMENTS   Certain aspects of vaccine use are regulated by the National Childhood Vaccine Injury Act (NCVIA) of 1986 (modified in 1995). The act requires that all mandated childhood vaccinations be recorded by health care providers in the child's permanent medical record, including date of administration, manufacturer and lot number, and name of the provider administering the vaccine. State-based immunization information systems and registries are being developed to help public and private providers manage their immunization activities and particularly to address the problem of assessing immunization coverage when an individual's records are divided among multiple medical facilities.

Parents must be informed about the benefits and risks of immunization and should maintain an up-to-date immunization record on their children. Educational materials providing the required information (Vaccine Information Statements, VISs) are available from the American Academy of Pediatrics (AAP) or the Centers for Disease Control and Prevention (CDC).

VACCINES FOR ROUTINE USE Infants and Children   Recommended routine-use vaccines and schedules for their administration to infants and children are shown in Table 122-5 and Fig. 122-1, respectively. It is current practice for all children in the United States to receive DTaP, poliovirus, MMR, Hib, HBV, and varicella vaccines unless there are specific contraindications. Hepatitis A vaccine is currently recommended when there is a special risk of exposure to infection due to residence in communities with elevated rates of hepatitis A or travel to highly endemic countries.

Adults (See Table 122-7)   All adults should be immune to diphtheria and tetanus. If not previously immunized, adults require a primary immunizing course of Td. Many individuals remain immune to tetanus into adulthood because they have received tetanus toxoid rather than Td after injuries, but they are commonly at risk of diphtheria because of the decline in titer of diphtheria antitoxin and the lack of boosting against diphtheria. The development of acellular pertussis vaccines that appear to be safe in adults may lead to a recommendation for booster immunization of adults if clinical trials confirm safety and efficacy. Routine immunization against polio is not recommended for adults unless they are at particular risk of exposure (e.g., through travel to endemic regions, as discussed below) or are the parents or guardians of a child with an immunodeficiency disorder. Adults should be pro-

Table 122-5 Routinely Recommended Vaccines for Infants, Children, and Adults

Vaccine	Year Licensed	Type of Immunizing Agent	Protective Antibody	Route of Administration	Efficacy, %	Adverse Events
DT	1949	Toxoid	Diphtheria and tetanus neu-	IM	D: 95	Local reactions
Td	1955		tralizing antitoxins, ≥ 0.1 IU/mL each		T: 95	Hypersensitivity to tetanus toxoid
aP	1993	Inactivated bacterial anti- gen	Not known	IM	80–90	Reduced local reactions compared with whole-cell
	1996	Acellular (DTaP)				vaccines; no serious reac- tions reported
Hib	1987	Bacterial polysaccharide- protein conjugate	Antibody to capsular poly- saccharide, 0.15 μg/mL	IM	90	Few local, no serious reac- tions
HBV	1981	Inactivated serum-derived viral antigen	Antibody to surface anti- gen, 10 mIU/mL	IM	80–95	Few (? Guillain-Barré syn- drome)
	1987	Recombinant antigen				
Influenza	1945	Inactivated virus or viral components[a]	Neutralizing antibody	IM	40–60	? Guillain-Barré syndrome with swine influenza vac- cine
MMR	1971	Live viruses	Neutralizing measles anti- body, ≥ 200 mIU/mL, not known for mumps or rubella	SC	M: 95	Acute encephalopathy (measles)
					Mu: 90	Rare parotitis or orchitis (mumps)
					R: 95	Arthralgia and rare arthrop- athy (rubella)
Pneumococcus	1983	Bacterial polysaccharide of 23 types	Antibody to capsular poly- saccharide	IM or SC	60–80	Local reactions; rare ana- phylaxis
Poliomyelitis	1963	OPV, live virus of 3 sero- types	Neutralizing antibody at any detectable titer	Oral	95[b]	Rare vaccine-associated polio
	1967	IPV, inactivated virus of 3 serotypes		SC	95	No significant reactions

[a] Only "split-virus" influenza vaccine should be given to children <13 years old since whole-virus influenza vaccines are associated with higher rates of adverse reactions in young children.

[b] In developing countries, OPV efficacy is only 70 to 90%, presumably because of inter- fering enteroviruses in the intestinal tract.

NOTE: DT, diphtheria and tetanus toxoids, adsorbed; Td, tetanus and diphtheria toxoids,

adsorbed, for adult use; aP, acellular pertussis; Hib, *Haemophilus influenzae* type b; HBV, hepatitis B virus; MMR, measles-mumps-rubella; OPV, trivalent oral poliovirus vaccine; IPV, inactivated poliovirus vaccine; IM, intramuscular; SC, subcutaneous.

SOURCE: Recommendations of the Advisory Committee on Immunization Practices, the American Academy of Pediatrics, and the American College of Physicans.

tected from measles, mumps, and rubella; they should be vaccinated unless they are known to have received vaccine on or after their first birthday or to have had physician-diagnosed disease. Rubella vaccine should be given to all women of childbearing age unless they have documentary proof of immunization after their first birthday or labo- ratory evidence of immunity. An unsupported history of rubella dis- ease is unreliable and should not be accepted. Adults without a clear history of chickenpox should receive varicella vaccine. College stu- dents, particularly freshmen living in a dormitory, are at increased risk of meningococcal meningitis. They should be made aware of the poly- saccharide vaccine for serogroups A, C, Y, and W-135 and should be offered the option of immunization.

Current recommendations also include influenza vaccine for rou- tine annual administration to adults ≥ 65 years of age and to individ- uals with chronic illness at any age. Polyvalent pneumococcal poly- saccharide vaccine is similarly recommended for the elderly or chronically ill. HBV vaccine is recommended for individuals at high risk of exposure, including health care workers exposed to potentially infected blood or blood products, homosexuals, injection drug users, individuals living and working in institutions for the mentally retarded, and household contacts of known carriers of hepatitis B surface antigen (HBsAg). A new recombinant outer-surface protein A (rOspA) is li- censed for persons 15 to 70 years of age for Lyme disease (LYMErix, SmithKline Beecham Pharmaceuticals), with use based on individual risk (geography and risk of exposure to ticks).

Adverse Events Modern vaccines, while safe and effective, are associated with adverse effects that range from infrequent and very mild to rare and life-threatening. The decision to use a vaccine involves an assessment of the risks of disease, the benefits of vaccination, and the risks associated with vaccination. Because these factors may change over time, continued assessment is essential. Table 122-8 lists valid and invalid contraindications to immunization and describes ap- propriate precautions in the use of specific vaccines. Antivaccine ad- vocacy groups actively encourage avoidance of immunization because

of their unproven belief that vaccines may cause certain disorders (for example, autism). This situation presents a challenge to the physician in educating parents about vaccine benefits and risks.

Vaccine components, including protective antigens, animal pro- teins introduced during vaccine production, and antibiotics or other preservatives or stabilizers, can cause allergic reactions in some recip- ients. These reactions may be local or systemic and may include ur- ticaria and serious anaphylaxis. The most common extraneous allergen is egg protein introduced when vaccines such as those for measles, mumps, influenza, and yellow fever are prepared in embryonated eggs. Local or systemic reactions can result from too-frequent administration of vaccines such as Td, diphtheria/tetanus (DT), or rabies; these re- actions are probably due to antigen-antibody complexes. In addition, live-virus vaccines can interfere with tuberculin test responses. When a tuberculin skin test is indicated, it should be done either on the day of immunization or 6 weeks later. When influenza vaccine is given to children <13 years old, only "split-virus" preparations should be used since whole-virus vaccines are associated with higher rates of adverse reactions in young children. Cumulative exposure to mercury in thi- merosal-preserved vaccines is a concern, and plans are under way to replace current vaccines with thimerosal-free products. In the interim, infants born to HBsAg-negative mothers should not receive the initial dose of HBV vaccine at birth.

All detected adverse events temporally related to vaccination are expected to be reported to both the local health department and the vaccine manufacturer. The NCVIA requires health care providers to report certain suspected adverse events following the receipt of a man- dated vaccine to the FDA's Vaccine Adverse Events Reporting System (Table 122-9). Although a temporal relationship does not establish cause and effect, this surveillance system remains the only mechanism for collecting the data needed to form conclusions and make decisions.

USE OF VACCINES IN SPECIAL CIRCUMSTANCES
Pregnancy Because of theoretical risk to the fetus and real risk of litigation to the practitioner, routine immunization of pregnant women

Table 122-6   Special-Use Vaccines

Vaccine	Year Licensed in United States	Type of Immunizing Agent	Route of Administration	Indications	Efficacy	Adverse Events
Anthrax	1970	Inactivated avirulent bacteria	SC (6 doses primary; annual booster)	For high risk of exposure (i.e., persons in contact with or involved in manufacture of animal hides, furs, bone meal, wool, goat hair)	90% antibody response but efficacy uncertain	No serious adverse effects known
Tuberculosis (BCG)	1950	Living bacteria (attenuated *Mycobacterium bovis*)	ID	PPD-negative individuals in prolonged contact with active TB patient	Controversial; reduces disseminated disease in children (0–80% protection against pulmonary TB; 75–86% protection against miliary and meningitic TB)	Regional adenitis, disseminated BCG infection, osteitis
Hepatitis A	1995	Killed virus antigen	IM	Travelers or persons living in high-risk areas	94%	Local reactions
Cholera	1914	Inactivated bacteria	SC or IM	Not recommended for public health use	50% (short-lived)	Frequent fever, local pain, swelling
Meningococcus A, C, Y, W-135	1981	Bacterial polysaccharide of 4 serotypes	SC	Military personnel; principally travelers to epidemic areas	90% for 2- to 3-year-olds	Rare
Plague	1911	Inactivated bacteria	IM	Laboratory workers; foresters in endemic areas; travelers	90% antibody response but efficacy uncertain	10% local reactions; rare sterile abscesses and hypersensitivity
Rabies (human diploid)	1980	Inactivated virus	IM or ID	Travelers; laboratory workers; veterinarians	Virtually 100%	25% local reactions; 6% arthropathy, arthritis, angioedema
Yellow fever	1953	Live virus	SC	Laboratory workers; travelers	High	Encephalitis; encephalopathy
Japanese encephalitis	1993	Inactivated virus	SC	Travelers	80–90%	Anaphylactic/severe delayed allergic reactions common; recipient should be observed for 10 days
Typhoid						
Phenol and heat-killed	1952	Killed whole bacteria	IM	Not routinely recommended in U.S.; used for travelers, contacts of carriers	50–70% (short-lived)	Frequent fever, local swelling, pain
Ty$_{21a}$	1992	Live mutant bacteria	Oral	Travelers, contacts of carriers	50–70%	None
Vi	1995	Vi capsular polysaccharide	IM	Travelers	70–75%	Local reactions
Lyme disease	1999	Recombinant outer-surface protein	IM	For high risk of exposure to infected ticks	76% (3 doses)	Local reactions

NOTE: SC, subcutaneous; BCG, bacille Calmette-Guérin; ID, intradermal; PPD, purified protein derivative; TB, tuberculosis; IM, intramuscular.

SOURCE: Recommendations of the Advisory Committee on Immunization Practices, the American Academy of Pediatrics, and the American College of Physicians.

is best avoided. However, wherever hygienic conditions during delivery cannot be guaranteed, it is essential to ensure that pregnant women are immune to tetanus: the transfer of maternal antitoxin is an important means of preventing neonatal tetanus, and pregnant women can safely receive tetanus as well as diphtheria toxoids. Although live-virus vaccines in general should be withheld during pregnancy, polio and yellow fever vaccines are exceptions and may be administered if the risk of exposure to disease is great. If indicated, some inactivated vaccines (e.g., HBV, influenza, and pneumococcal vaccines) are safe for pregnant women. Known pregnancy is considered a contraindication to the receipt of rubella, measles, mumps, and varicella vaccines. Although of theoretical concern, no cases of congenital rubella syndrome or abnormalities attributable to rubella vaccine virus have been observed in infants born to susceptible mothers who received rubella vaccine during pregnancy.

Breast Feeding   Neither killed nor live vaccine affects the safety of breast feeding for either mother or infant. Breast-fed infants can be immunized on a normal schedule.

Occupational Exposure   Immunization recommendations for most occupational groups remain to be developed. Specific practices are now mandated by the Occupational Safety and Health Administration for the immunization of health care workers against hepatitis B in the United States. Rubella is transmitted to and from health care workers in medical facilities, particularly in pediatric practice. Health care workers who might transmit rubella to pregnant patients should be immune to rubella; it is prudent to screen these employees for antibodies to rubella virus and to immunize susceptible individuals. Persons providing health care are also at greater risk from measles and varicella than the general public, and those who are likely to come into contact with measles- and varicella-infected patients should be immune. Persons employed in caring for patients with chronic diseases can transmit influenza; such workers should be vaccinated annually. Unfortunately, these recommendations often are not fully implemented, even in academic institutions.

HIV Infection and Other Immunocompromised States   Limited studies in HIV-infected individuals have found no increase in the risk of adverse events from live or inactivated vaccines. However, immune responses may not be as vigorous in immunocompromised individuals as in those with a normal immune system. Persons known to be infected with HIV should be immunized with recommended vaccines in the same manner as individuals with a normal immune system and as early in the course of their disease as possible, before immune function becomes significantly impaired. Live attenuated MMR vaccine can be administered to this group, but OPV cannot (Table 122-10). IPV should be used when vaccination against polio is indicated. Household contacts of immunocompromised individuals should be immune to polio; when vaccinated, they should receive IPV. In practice, it is not necessary to test for HIV before making decisions about the immunization of asymptomatic individuals from known HIV risk groups.

Live attenuated vaccines are normally contraindicated in immunocompromised patients, including those with congenital immunodeficiency syndromes and those receiving immunosuppressive therapy. Passive immunization with immunoglobulin preparations or antitoxins can be considered in individual cases, either as postexposure prophylaxis or as part of the treatment of established infection.

Postexposure Immunization

For certain infections, active or passive immunization soon after exposure prevents or attenuates disease expression. Recommended postexposure immunization regimens are compiled in Table 122-11. Measles immune globulin given within 6 days of exposure may prevent or modify infection, and measles vaccine given within the first few days after exposure may prevent symptomatic infection. Although clinical manifestations of rubella in pregnant women are minimized by postexposure passive immunization, this approach may not prevent maternal viremia, fetal infection, and congenital rubella syndrome. Therefore, the administration of immune globulin is recommended only for women developing rubella during pregnancy who will not consider abortion under any circumstances. Tetanus immune globulin can be used in patients with tetanus. Survivors with no history of tetanus immunization should receive a primary series of toxoid injections since disease does not result in the

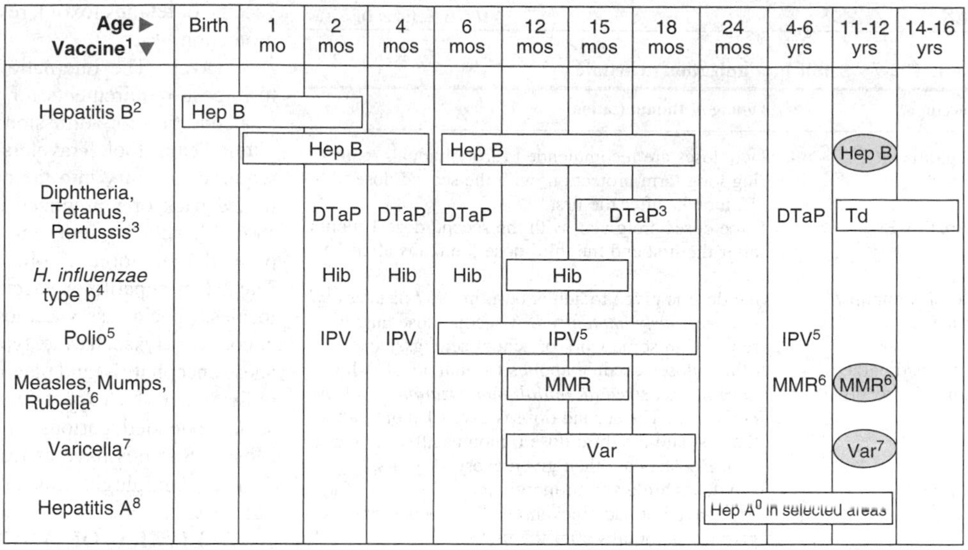

Age ▶ Vaccine[1] ▼	Birth	1 mo	2 mos	4 mos	6 mos	12 mos	15 mos	18 mos	24 mos	4-6 yrs	11-12 yrs	14-16 yrs
Hepatitis B[2]	Hep B											
			Hep B		Hep B						Hep B	
Diphtheria, Tetanus, Pertussis[3]			DTaP	DTaP	DTaP		DTaP[3]			DTaP	Td	
H. influenzae type b[4]			Hib	Hib	Hib	Hib						
Polio[5]			IPV	IPV		IPV[5]				IPV[5]		
Measles, Mumps, Rubella[6]						MMR				MMR[6]	MMR[6]	
Varicella[7]						Var					Var[7]	
Hepatitis A[8]										Hep A[8] in selected areas		

FIGURE 122-1 Recommended childhood immunization schedule in the United States for January through December 2000. Vaccines are listed under the routinely recommended ages. Clear bars indicate a range of acceptable ages for vaccination; shaded ovals indicate timing of catch-up vaccination: at 11 or 12 years of age, hepatitis B vaccine and measles/mumps/rubella vaccine should be administered to children not previously vaccinated, and varicella vaccine should be administered to children not previously vaccinated who lack a reliable history of chickenpox. Vaccine abbreviations: Hep B, hepatitis B; DTaP, diphtheria/tetanus/acellular pertussis; Hib, *Haemophilus influenzae* type b; Td, tetanus/diphtheria toxoids, adsorbed; IPV, inactivated poliovirus vaccine; MMR, measles/ mumps/rubella; Var, varicella-zoster; Hep A, hepatitis A. **Key to footnotes:** [1]*This schedule indicates the recommended ages* for routine administration of licensed childhood vaccines as of November 1, 1999. Additional vaccines may subsequently be licensed and recommended. A licensed combination vaccine may be used whenever any of its components is indicated and its other components are not contraindicated. Because clinical studies of infants have demonstrated that some combination products may induce a weaker immune response to the Hib vaccine component, DTaP/Hib combination products should not be used for primary immunization of infants at 2, 4, or 6 months of age unless approved by the FDA for these ages. Providers should consult the manufacturers' package inserts for detailed recommendations. [2]*The hepatitis B surface antigen (HBsAg) status of pregnant women,* if not known, should be determined as soon as possible during pregnancy. *Infants born to HBsAg-negative mothers* should receive the first dose of Hep B vaccine by age 2 months. The second dose should be given at least 1 month after the first dose. The third dose should be administered at least 4 months after the first dose and at least 2 months after the second dose, but not before 6 months of age. In this setting, a licensed combination Hep B/Hib vaccine may be used (e.g., ComVax; Merck) at 2, 4, and 12 to 15 months of age in place of the usual immunization schedule for each vaccine given independently. *Infants born to HBsAg-positive mothers* should receive Hep B vaccine and immunoprophylaxis with 0.5 mL of hepatitis B immune globulin (HBIG)—at separate sites—within 12 h of birth. The second dose is recommended at 1 month of age and the third dose at 6 months of age. *Infants born to mothers whose HBsAg status is unknown* should receive Hep B vaccine within 12 h of birth. Maternal blood should be drawn at delivery and HBsAg status determined; if the mother's HBsAg test is positive, the infant should receive HBIG no later than 1 week of age. All children and adolescents through 18 years of age who have not been immunized against hepatitis B may begin the series during any visit. Special efforts should be made to immunize children who were born in, or whose parents were born in, areas of the world with moderate or high endemicity of hepatitis B virus infection. [3]*DTaP is the preferred vaccine for all doses.* The fourth dose of DTaP may be administered as early as 12 months of age, provided 6 months have elapsed since the third dose and the child is unlikely to return at age 15 to 18 months. Td is recommended at 11 to 12 years of age if at least 5 years have elapsed since the last dose of DTaP, diphtheria/ tetanus/pertussis (DTP) vaccine, or diphtheria/tetanus (DT) vaccine. Subsequent routine Td boosters are recommended every 10 years. [4]*Three Hib conjugate vaccines* are licensed for infant use. If PRP-OMP [PedvaxHIB or ComVax (Merck)] is administered at 2 and 4 months of age, a dose at 6 months is not required. [5]*To eliminate the risk of vaccine-associated paralytic polio* (VAPP), an all-IPV schedule is now recommended for routine childhood polio vaccination in the United States. All children should receive four doses of IPV at 2, 4, and 6 to 18 months and 4 to 6 years. If available, trivalent oral poliovirus vaccine (OPV) may be used *only* for mass vaccination campaigns to control outbreaks of paralytic polio, for unvaccinated children who will be traveling in <4 weeks to areas where polio is endemic or epidemic, and for children of parents who do not accept the recommended number of vaccine injections. The latter children may receive OPV only for the third and/or fourth dose; in this situation, health care professionals should administer OPV only after discussing the risk for VAPP with parents or caregivers. [6]The second dose of MMR vaccine is recommended routinely at 4 to 6 years but may be administered during any visit, provided that at least 4 weeks have elapsed since receipt of the first dose and that both doses are administered beginning at or after 12 months of age. Children who have not previously received the second dose should complete the schedule by the 11- to 12-year-old visit. [7]Var vaccine is recommended at any visit on or after the first birthday for susceptible children, i.e., those who lack a reliable history of chickenpox (as judged by a health care professional) and who have not been immunized. Susceptible persons ≥13 years of age should receive two doses at least 4 weeks apart. [8]Hep A vaccine is recommended for use in selected states and/or regions with higher-than-average infection rates. Information may be obtained from local public health departments. *(From the Advisory Committee on Immunization Practices, the American Academy of Pediatrics, and the American Academy of Family Physicians.)*

Table 122-7 Adult Immunization Schedule

Vaccine	Timing of Immunization
Hepatitis A[a]	Two doses are recommended for individuals requiring long-term protection, with the second dose 6–12 months after the first.
Hepatitis B[a]	Three doses are given, with the second dose 1 month after the first and the third dose 5 months after the second.
Measles/mumps/ rubella	One dose is given to adults born in 1957 or later *and not previously immunized*. A second dose may be required in some work or school settings.
Tetanus/diphtheria toxoids, adsorbed	A three-dose schedule applies for individuals who *have not received an initial immunization series in childhood*. The second dose is given 1 month after the first and the third dose 6 months after the second. Boosters are then given every 10 years.
Varicella	Two doses are given to individuals ≥13 years of age who have not had chickenpox. The second dose is given 1–2 months after the first.
Influenza	Vaccine is administered yearly to individuals ≥65 years of age; to younger people with chronic medical problems, such as heart disease and diabetes; and to those who work or live with high-risk persons.
Streptococcus pneumoniae (polysaccharide)	Vaccine is usually given once to individuals ≥65 years of age. A repeat dose may be given 5 years later for those at highest risk. Immunization is also recommended for younger people with chronic medical problems, such as heart disease, diabetes, renal failure, and sickle cell anemia, and for those who work or live with high-risk persons.

[a] For individuals at risk.
SOURCE: National Coalition for Adult Immunization.

development of protective levels of antitoxin. Administration of rabies immune globulin plus rabies vaccine in the immediate postexposure period is highly effective in preventing disease. Similarly, for persons who have not been actively immunized, the use of immune globulin within 2 weeks of exposure to hepatitis A is likely to prevent clinical illness. Good data indicate the efficacy of human hepatitis B immune globulin in preventing disease after exposure. While no high-titer preparation is available for postexposure protection against non-A, non-B hepatitis, standard human immune serum globulin is efficacious.

Simultaneous Administration of Multiple Vaccines The simultaneous administration of the most widely used live and inactivated vaccines has not resulted in impaired antibody responses or in increased rates of adverse reactions. Simultaneous administration of vaccines is advantageous in that it increases the probability that a child will ultimately be fully immunized; it is also useful in any age group when the potential exists for exposure to multiple infectious diseases during travel to endemic countries. However, combination DTaP/Hib vaccines should not be used for primary immunization of infants because the response to Hib is blunted and suboptimal. Live-virus vaccines not given together on the same day should generally be administered at least 30 days apart.

High doses of immune globulin may inhibit the efficacy of measles and rubella vaccines, and an interval of at least 3 months is recommended between the administration of immune globulin and that of MMR vaccine or its components. Postpartum vaccination of rubella-susceptible women should not be delayed because of the administration of anti-Rho(D) immune globulin or any other blood product during the last trimester or at delivery. Should administration of an immune globulin preparation become necessary after vaccination, it should be postponed, if possible, for at least 14 days to allow time for vaccine-virus replication and development of immunity. In general, there is little interaction of immune globulin with inactivated vaccines, and postexposure passive prophylaxis can be given together with HBV

vaccine or tetanus toxoid, resulting in both immediate and long-lasting protection.

Travel The International Sanitary Regulations allow countries to impose requirements for yellow fever and killed cholera vaccines as a condition for admission, even though the latter is not an effective public health tool. Travelers should know whether these vaccines are required for entry into the countries on their itinerary to avoid being turned back or immunized on the spot. Infants, children, and adults should have all routine immunizations updated before traveling, with particular attention to polio, measles, and DTP/DTaP or Td vaccines. The use of hepatitis A vaccine may be advisable for travelers to some locales. Special-use vaccines (Table 122-6), including rabies, meningococcal polysaccharide, typhoid (oral live or Vi polysaccharide), Japanese encephalitis, and plague vaccines, should be considered for those individuals who expect to go beyond the usual tourist routes or to spend extended periods in rural areas in disease-endemic regions. Most U.S. cities have at least one travel clinic that maintains up-to-date epidemiologic information and can provide the appropriate vaccines.

DELIVERY OF VACCINES Over the past 25 years, considerable progress has been made to ensure that every child in the United States is fully immunized by the time of school entry. All 50 states now require immunization for school entry, and most have laws addressing attendance at preschools and day-care centers. The impact of immunization and of other improvements in the health care provided to the American population on the incidence of vaccine-preventable illness is shown in Table 122-1. Nonetheless, many children are not fully immunized, especially in poor and underserved communities. The failure to vaccinate preschool children was largely responsible for the resurgence of measles between 1989 and 1991, with >55,000 cases and >130 measles-related deaths. Outbreaks of pertussis, mumps, and congenital rubella syndrome have occurred for the same reason: low immunization rates among preschool children.

ACCESS TO IMMUNIZATION Four major barriers to infant and childhood immunization have been identified within the health care system: (1) low public awareness and lack of public demand for immunization, (2) inadequate access to immunization services, (3) missed opportunities to administer vaccines, and (4) inadequate resources for public health and preventive programs. These problems are sources of public concern, and their solution is a priority for national health policy in the United States. In response, the Children's Immunization Initiative was begun in 1990. At the national level, this program includes outreach and educational campaigns to promote parental awareness of the value of vaccination and to encourage health care providers to use every opportunity to vaccinate the children in their care. At the state and local levels, community and business groups, religious and service groups, schools, and the media have joined together in community-based networks. A National Immunization Week each April has been established to focus attention on the vaccination needs of infants and children. To improve the quality and quantity of vaccination services, expanded immunization-clinic hours and computerization of immunization records are being implemented as well.

There has been only modest progress towards the goals for adult immunization in the United States. Adult-immunization goals are important: As many as 60,000 adults die each year of vaccine-preventable diseases for which effective vaccines are not being optimally used. Most persons ≥65 years of age do not receive influenza vaccine each year, and even fewer have ever received pneumococcal vaccine. Health care providers more often miss vaccination opportunities with adults than with infants and children. From 60 to 90% of adults hospitalized for or dying of influenza-associated respiratory disease have received medical care during the previous year and could have been immunized at that time. Medicare reimbursement for excess hospitalization during influenza epidemics ranges from $750 million to $1 billion. Additional efforts are required to ensure that adults receive pneumococcal, Td, and HBV vaccines as well.

A special setting for adult immunization is the administration of

Table 122-8 Immunization Contraindications and Precautions

Vaccine	Contraindication or Precaution[a] Valid	Contraindication or Precaution[a] Invalid
General[b]	Anaphylactic reaction to vaccine (contraindication to further doses of that vaccine) Anaphylactic reaction to vaccine constituent (contraindication to use of vaccines containing that substance) Moderate or severe illnesses, with or without fever	Mild to moderate local reaction (soreness, redness, swelling) following dose of injectable antigen Mild acute illness, with or without low-grade fever Current antimicrobial therapy Convalescent phase of illness Prematurity (same dosage and indications as for normal, full-term infants) Recent exposure to an infectious disease History of penicillin or other nonspecific allergies or family history of such allergies
DTaP/DTP	Encephalopathy within 72 h after dose Fever of ≥40.5°C (105°F) within 48 h after dose (P) Collapse or shocklike state (hypotonic-hyporesponsive episode) within 48 h after dose (P) Seizures within 3 days after dose (P) Persistent, inconsolable crying lasting ≥3 h within 48 h after dose (P)	Temperature of <40.5°C (105°F) after dose Family history of convulsions[c] Family history of an adverse event following vaccination Family history of sudden infant death syndrome
OPV[d]	Infection with HIV or a household contact infected with HIV Known immunodeficiency (hematologic and solid tumors, congenital immunodeficiency, and long-term immunosuppressive therapy) Immunodeficient household contact Pregnancy[e] (P)	Breast feeding Current antimicrobial therapy Diarrhea
IPV	Anaphylactic reactions to neomycin or streptomycin Pregnancy[e]	—
MMR	Anaphylactic reactions to eggs or to neomycin[f] Pregnancy Known immunodeficiency (hematologic and solid tumors, congenital immunodeficiency syndrome, and long-term immunosuppressive therapy) Recent IG administration (P)	Tuberculosis or positive PPD test Simultaneous TB skin testing[g] Breast feeding Pregnancy of mother of recipient Immunodeficient family member or household contact Infection with HIV Nonanaphylactic reactions to eggs or neomycin
Hib	None identified	History of Hib disease
HBV	None identified	Pregnancy
Influenza	First trimester of pregnancy (vaccination avoided on theoretical grounds) Anaphylactic reactions to eggs	—
Pneumococcus	Has not been evaluated in pregnancy	
Varicella	Primary acquired immunodeficiency History of anaphylactic reaction to neomycin Pregnancy	Contact dermatitis in response to neomycin

[a] Precautions are followed by "(P)." The events or conditions listed as precautions, although not contraindications, should be carefully reviewed. The benefits and risks of administering a specific vaccine to an individual under the circumstances should be considered. If the risks are believed to outweigh the benefits, the vaccine should be withheld; if the benefits are believed to outweigh the risks (for example, during an outbreak or foreign travel), the vaccine should be administered. Whether and when to administer DTaP to children with proven or suspected underlying neurologic disorders should be decided on an individual basis.

[b] For DTP/DTaP, OPV, IPV, MMR, Hib, HBV, influenza, pneumococcus, and varicella.

[c] If a child has a precaution to the receipt of a subsequent dose of whole-cell DTP, the child should not routinely receive DTP. If a child has a contraindication to the receipt of a subsequent dose of whole-cell DTP, the child should not receive DTaP. Acetaminophen given before DTaP and thereafter every 4 h for 24 h should be considered for children with a personal or family (sibling or parent) history of convulsions.

[d] No data exist to substantiate the theoretical risk of a suboptimal immune response when OPV and MMR are given within 30 days of each other.

[e] It is prudent on theoretical grounds to avoid vaccinating pregnant women. However, if immediate protection against poliomyelitis is needed, OPV is preferred, although IPV may be considered if vaccination can be completed before the anticipated imminent exposure.

[f] Persons with a history of anaphylactic reactions following egg ingestion should be vaccinated only with caution. Protocols have been developed for vaccinating such persons and should be consulted (J Pediatr 102:196, 1983; J Pediatr 113:504, 1988).

[g] Measles vaccination may temporarily suppress tuberculin reactivity. If skin testing cannot be done on the day of MMR vaccination, the test should be postponed for 4 to 6 weeks.

NOTE: IPV, inactivated polio vaccine; PPD, purified protein derivative; TB, tuberculosis; IG, immunoglobulin.

SOURCES: This information is based on the recommendations of the Advisory Committee on Immunization Practices (ACIP) and those of the Committee on Infectious Diseases (Red Book Committee) of the American Academy of Pediatrics (AAP). Sometimes these recommendations vary from those contained in the manufacturers' package inserts. For more detailed information, providers should consult the published recommendations of the ACIP (Vaccine side effects, adverse reactions, contraindications, and precautions. MMWR 45:1, 1996) and the AAP as well as the manufacturers' package inserts.

certain vaccines to pregnant women to enhance passive immunity in their offspring (e.g., tetanus toxoid). In most cases the mother herself derives important benefits as well. Immunization of the mother should be undertaken at least 6 weeks before delivery to allow for efficient transplacental transfer of antibody to the fetus.

STANDARDS FOR IMMUNIZATION PRACTICES National standards of immunization for adult and pediatric practice have been established to define common policies and practices for public health clinics and in physicians' private offices (Table 122-12). These guidelines highlight the need to distinguish between valid contraindications and conditions that are often considered but are not in fact contraindications (Table 122-8). Among the valid contraindications applicable to all vaccines are a history of anaphylaxis or other serious allergic reactions to a vaccine or vaccine component and the presence of a moderate or severe illness, with or without fever. Infants who develop encephalopathy within 72 h of a dose of DTP or DTaP should not receive further doses; those who develop a "precaution" (Table 122-8) should not normally receive further doses. Because of theoretical risks to the fetus, pregnant women should not receive MMR or varicella vaccine. Diarrhea, minor respiratory illness with or without fever, mild to moderate local reactions to a previous dose of vaccine, the concurrent or recent use of antimicrobial agents, mild to moderate malnutrition, or the convalescent phase of an acute illness are not valid contraindications to routine immunization. Failure to vaccinate chil-

Table 122-9   Reportable Events Following Vaccination, as Required by the National Childhood Vaccine Injury Act of 1986 (Modified in 1995)[a]

Vaccine/Toxoid	Event	Interval from Vaccination
DTaP; P; DTP-Hib; DT; Td or TT	Anaphylaxis	4 h
	Encephalopathy (or encephalitis)	72 h
MMR, MR, or M	Anaphylaxis	4 h
	Encephalopathy (or encephalitis)	5–15 days
	Residual seizure disorder	5–15 days
Rubella-containing vaccines (MMR, MR, R)	Chronic arthritis	42 days
	Anaphylaxis	4 h
	Encephalopathy (or encephalitis)	5–15 days
	Residual seizure disorder	5–15 days
OPV	Paralytic poliomyelitis	
	In an immunocompetent recipient	30 days
	In an immunocompromised recipient	6 months
	In a vaccine-associated community case	No limits
IPV	Anaphylaxis	4 h

[a] Compensation (under the NCVIA) is effective for claims filed on or after March 10, 1995. Any acute complications or sequelae of an illness, disability, injury, or condition that arose within the prescribed period (including deaths) are also covered.

NOTE: P, pertussis; TT, tetanus toxoid; MR, measles/rubella; M, measles; R, rubella.

dren because of these conditions is increasingly viewed as a missed opportunity for immunization.

BIOTERRORISM The end of the twentieth century witnessed a rise in the risk of bioterrorism. While smallpox has been eradicated, known stocks of smallpox virus still exist in the United States and Russia, and unknown stocks probably exist in other countries considered likely to engage in terrorism. Global supplies of smallpox vaccine for use in case of deliberate release of smallpox virus are inadequate, and millions of people are likely to become infected and die in the event of such a release. Steps are only now being taken to ensure sufficient stockpiles of vaccine for this eventuality, and it will be several more years before these reach a critical size.

THE NATIONAL VACCINE INJURY COMPENSATION PROGRAM The use of mandated vaccines benefits society as a whole by reducing morbidity and the cost of care for preventable diseases and by reducing childhood mortality. Thus, in the United States, society has assumed the obligation to care for those injured by the administration of mandated vaccines. The NCVIA of 1986 (modified in 1995) is the instrument in use to ensure fairness to injured persons as well as protection for federal, state, and local immunization programs; private immunization providers; and vaccine manufacturers. The act was designed to implement two vital public policies: (1) to provide prompt and fair compensation to the families of children who have died or have been injured as a result of routine mandated immunization; and (2) to reduce the adverse impact of the tort system on vaccine supply, cost, and innovation/development. The success of immunization programs in the United States depends upon the continued viability of the National Vaccine Injury Compensation Program.

CONTROL OF VACCINE-PREVENTABLE DISEASE

A continuing task of public health practice is to maintain individual and herd immunity. The job is not over once a population is fully vaccinated; rather, it is imperative to immunize each subsequent generation as long as the threat of the disease persists. Ongoing surveillance and prompt reporting of disease to local or state health departments are essential to this goal, ensuring a continuing awareness of the possibility of vaccine-preventable illness. Nearly all vaccine-preventable diseases are now notifiable, and individual case data are routinely forwarded to the CDC. These data are used to detect outbreaks or other unusual events that require investigation and to evaluate prevention and control policies, practices, and strategies.

As a direct consequence of successes in immunization, vaccine-preventable diseases have become less visible; ironically, this situation may foster complacency among parents and health care providers about routine immunization of children. Even among the affluent and educated, immunization levels may be low, reflecting a misunderstanding of the continuing threat of disease with which parents and health care providers have limited experience or perhaps an unjustifiably greater fear of adverse reactions to vaccination than of the potential for illness and death due to vaccine-preventable diseases. Health care workers play an essential role in influencing the attitudes of patients regarding appropriate immunization; therefore, it is essential that these professionals continually update their own knowledge about vaccines and about the epidemiology of vaccine-preventable illnesses.

RESEARCH ON VACCINES AND IMMUNIZATION

The potential to eradicate selected diseases and to build sustainable immunization programs that reach every child is not being fulfilled with existing vaccines and delivery technology. New vaccines or new formulations that will not only improve protective responses but also simplify the immunization schedule are needed. The ideal would be vaccines that can be administered orally early in life, that provide lifelong protection against multiple infections, that can be given as one or only a few doses, and that are less reactive and more heat stable than current vaccines. To attain these ambitious goals may take decades, but progress is already being made in the development of new combinations of current vaccines to facilitate complete immunization. The results will be applicable to immunization programs in both developed and developing countries.

REEMERGENCE OF CONTROLLED DISEASE AND EMERGENCE OF NEW DISEASE The emergence of new pathogens is fostered

Table 122-10   Recommendations for Routine Immunization of HIV-Infected Persons in the United States

Vaccine	HIV Clinical Status		Comments
	Asymptomatic	Symptomatic	
DTaP/Td	Yes	Yes	No change in usual immunization schedule
OPV	No	No	Increased risk of vaccine virus proliferation and paralytic polio; IPV used for household contacts of HIV-infected persons
IPV	Yes	Yes	Antibody response potentially impaired in symptomatic patients
MMR	Yes	Yes	No change in usual immunization schedule; with high risk of exposure to measles, first dose given at 6–11 months of age, second dose at >12 months of age; with documented infection, measles immune globulin potentially administered (see Table 122-11)
Hib conjugate	Yes	Yes	No change in usual immunization schedule
HBV	Yes	Yes	Antibody response potentially impaired; higher-dose vaccine available, but no data address optimal dose; possibly wise to check antibody titer after immunization and give additional doses if titer is inadequate
Pneumococcus	Yes	Yes	Should be given to all ≥2 years old
Influenza	Yes	Yes	Antibody response potentially impaired in symptomatic patients
Varicella	No	No	Use in asymptomatic HIV-infected persons not studied

SOURCE: Centers for Disease Control and Prevention.

by the genetic potential of microbes to evolve as well as by rapid changes in human demographics and behavior and in a global ecology that creates new or more favorable hosts. Proof of the need for continuing vaccine research is found in the emergence of new infectious diseases such as HIV infection, Lyme borreliosis, hantavirus pulmonary syndrome, and hepatitis C; the appearance of a new epidemic cholera strain (serotype O139 Bengal) that exhibits no cross-immunity with the traditional O1 serotype; and the increase in global incidence and in drug resistance of familiar diseases that were once considered under control, such as tuberculosis and malaria. In addition, some common illnesses without a previously known etiology, such as peptic ulcer disease and cervical and nasopharyngeal cancer, have now been epidemiologically linked to specific infectious agents and have thus become potentially vaccine-preventable conditions.

DEVELOPMENT OF NEW VACCINES For many serious or even life-threatening infectious diseases, no effective vaccines are available. Although many new vaccines are undergoing human trials, the task of developing vaccines is proving very complex. Priorities for the United States currently include research on the following vaccines: HIV, pneumococcus (conjugate), group B *Streptococcus*, respiratory syncytial virus, rotavirus, *Mycobacterium tuberculosis*, herpes simplex virus, influenza A and B viruses, and hepatitis C virus. Also of high priority are vaccines for two virus-associated tumors: cervical cancer (human papillomavirus) and nasopharyngeal cancer (Epstein-Barr virus).

INTERNATIONAL CONSIDERATIONS

Since the establishment of the World Health Organization's Expanded Programme on Immunization in 1981, levels of coverage for the recommended basic children's vaccines (bacille Calmette-Guérin, polio, DTP/DTaP, measles, and HBV) have risen from 5% to ~80% worldwide. Each year, at least 2.7 million deaths from measles, neonatal tetanus, and pertussis and 200,000 cases of paralysis due to polio are prevented by immunization. Despite the successes of this program, many vaccine-preventable diseases remain prevalent in the developing world. Measles, for example, continues to kill an estimated 1.5 million children each year, and cases of diphtheria, whooping cough, polio, and neonatal tetanus still occur at unacceptably high rates. It is estimated that between 20 and 35% of all deaths of children under the age of 5 years are still associated with vaccine-preventable diseases.

In addition to the antigens included in the Expanded Programme for routine use in the developing world, others (Hib, Japanese B encephalitis, yellow fever, group A meningococcus, mumps, and rubella) are used regionally, depending on disease epidemiology and resources. Polio has been targeted for eradication; this disease has already been eliminated in the Americas and Europe and is close to elimination in the Western Pacific.

Table 122-11 Recommended Postexposure Immunization with Immunoglobulin Preparations in the United States

Disease	Indicated	Comments
Measles	Yes	Standard human immune globulin is recommended for exposed infants and adults with normal immunocompetence (but with a contraindication to measles vaccine) and for immunocompromised patients exposed to measles (regardless of immunization status). Patients should be immunized 3–6 months after immunoglobulin administration. Recommended dose: 0.25–0.5 mL/kg (40–80 mg of IgG/kg) IM; 80 mg of IgG/kg for immunocompromised contact; maximum, 15 mL.
Rubella	No	Efficacy is unreliable; therefore, standard human immune globulin is recommended for administration only to antibody-negative pregnant women in the first trimester who have a documented rubella exposure and who will not consider terminating the pregnancy. Recommended dose: 0.55 mL/kg (90 mg of IgG/kg) IM.
Tetanus	Yes	Human tetanus immune globulin (TIG) has replaced equine tetanus antitoxin because of the risk of serum sickness with equine serum. Recommended dose for postexposure prophylaxis: 250–500 units of TIG (10–20 mg of IgG/kg) IM. Recommended dose for treatment of tetanus: 3000–6000 units of TIG IM.
Rabies	Yes	Human rabies immune globulin (RIG) is preferred over equine rabies antiserum because of the risk of serum sickness. RIG or antiserum is recommended for nonimmunized individuals with animal bites in which rabies cannot be ruled out and with other exposures to known rabid animals. Recommended dose of RIG: 20 IU/kg (22 mg of IgG/kg). Recommended dose of antiserum: 40 IU/kg. Rabies vaccine is given as well at 0, 3, 7, 14, and 28 days.
Hepatitis A	Yes	Standard immune serum globulin is given in a single dose of 0.02–0.04 mL/kg or (for continuous exposure) in a dose of up to 0.06 mL/kg every 5 months. Postexposure treatment with hepatitis A immune globulin has not been studied.
Hepatitis B	Yes	Standard immune serum globulin is not reliably effective. Special human hepatitis B immune globulin is useful and is recommended for neonates born to an infected mother and after mucous-membrane or parenteral contact with infected persons or infected blood or serum. Recommended dose for neonates: 0.5 mL IM within 12 h of birth. Recommended dose for percutaneous or mucosal exposure: 0.06 mL/kg (10 mg of IgG/kg) IM.
Non-A, non-B hepatitis	Yes	Standard immune serum globulin may be valuable. Recommended dose: 0.12 mL/kg (10 mg of IgG/kg) IM, up to 10 mL.

Because infectious diseases know no geographic or political boundaries, uncontrolled disease anywhere in the world poses a threat to the United States. Vaccines offer the opportunity to control and even eradicate some diseases, and eradication means that vaccines are no longer needed. Vaccines represent the best hope for stopping the pandemic of HIV infection throughout the world. The experience with smallpox has shown that the eradication of disease is a remarkably good economic investment. The entire sum that the United States spent for the global smallpox eradication campaign has been recouped, in 1968 dollars, every 2.5 months since 1971. The global eradication of polio will save the United States over $300 million a year in vaccine and associated delivery costs and will save over $1.5 billion a year worldwide.

Issues of cost, liability, risk, and profitability limit the interest of the pharmaceutical industry in the development of vaccines (e.g., for malaria) that will be used primarily in poor developing countries. Efforts have been made to create partnerships in public research and privately funded development. Activities of established international organizations (such as the World Health Organization) and some new organizations (such as the Global Alliance for Vaccines and Immunization, the International AIDS Vaccine Initiative, and the Bill and Melinda Gates Foundation) have helped to move the process forward with strategy development and implementation or new funding. New international schemes are being considered by wealthy industrial nations; for example, advance-purchase schemes are being proposed in which the purchase of effective vaccines is guaranteed, ensuring the profitability that the marketplace has provided for industry in the wealthy countries. The effectiveness of such approaches remains to be seen, but they offer much-needed hope for at-risk populations around the world.

Table 122-12   Standards for Immunization Practices

Standard Number	Standard
Pediatric Practice	
1.	Immunization services are readily available.
2.	There are no barriers to or unnecessary prerequisites for the receipt of vaccines.
3.	Immunization services are available free or for a minimal fee.
4.	Providers use all clinical encounters to screen and, when indicated, immunize children.
5.	Providers educate parents and guardians about immunization in general terms.
6.	Providers question parents or guardians about contraindications and, before immunizing a child, inform them in specific terms about the risks and benefits of the immunizations their child is to receive.
7.	Providers follow only true contraindications.
8.	Providers administer simultaneously all vaccine doses for which a child is eligible at the time of each visit.
9.	Providers use accurate and complete recording procedures.
10.	Providers coschedule immunization appointments in conjunction with appointments for other child health services.
11.	Providers report adverse events following immunization promptly, accurately, and completely.
12.	Providers operate a tracking system.
13.	Providers adhere to appropriate procedures for vaccine management.
14.	Providers conduct semiannual audits to assess immunization coverage levels and to review immunization records for the patient populations they serve.
15.	Providers maintain up-to-date, easily retrievable medical protocols at all locations where vaccines are administered.
16.	Providers operate with patient-oriented and community-based approaches.
17.	Vaccines are administered by properly trained individuals.
18.	Providers receive ongoing education and training on current immunization recommendations.
Adult Practice	
1.	Appropriate vaccine use is promoted through information campaigns for health care practitioners and trainees, employers, and the public about the benefits of immunizations.
2.	Providers are completely immunized to protect themselves and prevent transmission to patients.
3.	Providers routinely determine the immunization status of their adult patients, offer vaccines to those for whom they are indicated, and maintain complete immunization records.
4.	Providers identify high-risk patients in need of influenza vaccine and develop a system to recall them for annual immunization.
5.	Providers and institutions identify high-risk adult patients in hospitals and other treatment centers and ensure that appropriate vaccination is considered either before discharge or as part of discharge planning.
6.	Licensing/accreditation agencies support the development by health care institutions of comprehensive immunization programs for staff, trainees, volunteer workers, inpatients, and outpatients.
7.	States establish preenrollment immunization requirements for colleges and other institutions of higher education.
8.	Institutions that train health care professionals, deliver health care, or provide laboratory or other medical support services require appropriate immunizations for persons at risk of contracting or transmitting vaccine-preventable illnesses.
9.	Health care benefit programs, third-party payers, and government health care programs provide coverage for adult immunization services.
10.	A standard personal and institutional immunization record is adopted as a means of verifying the immunization status of patients and staff.

SOURCE: For pediatric standards: Ad Hoc Working Group for the Development of Standards for Pediatric Immunization Practices. JAMA 269:1817, 1993; for adult standards: The National Coalition for Adult Immunization.

SOURCES OF INFORMATION ON IMMUNIZATION

- Official vaccine package circulars and Vaccine Administration Statements from the Centers for Disease Control and Prevention
- Report of the Committee on Infectious Diseases of the American Academy of Pediatrics ("Red Book")
- Recommendations of the Advisory Committee on Immunization Practices, Centers for Disease Control and Prevention
- Guide for Adult Immunization, American College of Physicians
- Health Information for International Travel (published yearly) and Advisory Memoranda on Travel (published periodically), Centers for Disease Control and Prevention
- Control of Communicable Diseases in Man, American Public Health Association
- Technical Bulletin of the College of Obstetrics and Gynecology
- National Network for Immunization Information, Infectious Diseases Society of America/Pediatric Infectious Diseases Society/American Academy of Pediatrics/American Nurses Association

BIBLIOGRAPHY

ADVISORY COMMITTEE ON IMMUNIZATION PRACTICES: Recommended childhood immunization schedule—United States. MMWR 48:12, 1999

ALARCON JB et al: DNA vaccines: Technology and application as anti-parasite and antimicrobial agents. Adv Parasitol 42:343, 1999

CASADEVALL A: Passive antibody therapies: Progress and continuing challenges. Clin Immunol 93:5, 1999

CHAPEL HM: Safety and availability of immunoglobulin replacement therapy in relation to potentially transmissible agents. IUIS Committee on Primary Immunodeficiency Disease. International Union of Immunological Societies. Clin Exp Immunol 118(Suppl 1):29, 1999

CLELAND JL: Single-administration vaccines: Controlled-release technology to mimic repeated immunizations. Trends Biotechnol 17:25, 1999

CUTTS FT et al: Measles elimination: Progress and challenges. Vaccine 17(Suppl 2):S47, 1999

CZERKINSKY C et al: Mucosal immunity and tolerance: Relevance to vaccine development. Immunol Rev 170:197, 1999

GARDNER P: Indications for acellular pertussis vaccines in adults: The case for selective, rather than universal, recommendations. Clin Infect Dis 28(Suppl 2):S131, 1999

GELLIN BG et al: Adult immunization: Principles and practice. Adv Intern Med 44:327, 1999

GLEZEN WP, ALPERS M: Maternal immunization. Clin Infect Dis 28:219, 1999

JONG EC: Travel immunization. Med Clin North Am 83:903, 1999

KEITEL WA: Cellular and acellular pertussis vaccines in adults. Clin Infect Dis 28(Suppl 2):S118, 1999

KILLEEN K et al: Bacterial mucosal vaccines: *Vibrio cholerae* as a live attenuated vaccine/vector paradigm. Curr Top Microbiol Immunol 236:237, 1999

LINDBERG AA: Glycoprotein conjugate vaccines. Vaccine 17(Suppl 2):S28, 1999

MAHONEY RT, MAYNARD JE: The introduction of new vaccines into developing countries. Vaccine 17:646, 1999

MOLRINE DC et al: Normal IgG and impaired IgM responses to polysaccharide vaccines in asplenic patients. J Infect Dis 179:513, 1999

RICHTER L, KIPP B: Transgenic plants as edible vaccines. Curr Top Microbiol Immunol 240:159, 1999

SINGHAL S, MEHTA J: Reimmunization after blood or marrow stem cell transplantation. Bone Marrow Transplant 23:637, 1999

Vaccine-preventable diseases: Improving vaccination coverage in children, adolescents, and adults. A report on recommendations from the Task Force on Community Preventive Services. MMWR 48(RR-8):1, 1999

WEBSITES OF INTEREST

www.cdc.gov/nip
www.idsociety.org/vaccine/resources.html
www.nfid.org/factsheets
www.genweb.com/Dnavax/dnavax.html

HEALTH ADVICE FOR INTERNATIONAL TRAVEL

In 1991, the World Health Organization estimated that more than 30 million persons traveled from industrialized countries to the developing world. Studies show that between 50 and 75% of short-term travelers to the tropics or subtropics report some health impairment. Most of these health problems are minor, with only 5% requiring medical attention and fewer than 1% requiring hospitalization.

Although infectious agents contribute substantially to morbidity in travelers, these pathogens account for only about 1% of deaths among this population. Cardiovascular disease and injuries are the most frequent causes of death among travelers from the United States, accounting for 49 and 22% of deaths, respectively. Age-specific rates of mortality due to cardiovascular disease are similar to those among nontravelers. In contrast, rates of death due to injury—the majority from motor vehicle, drowning, or aircraft accidents—are several times higher among travelers. Figure 123-1 summarizes the monthly incidence of health problems during travel in developing countries.

GENERAL ADVICE

Staying healthy during travel requires familiarity with the health risks that may be encountered at a given destination. However, health maintenance recommendations are based not only on the traveler's destination but also on risk assessment, which is determined by health status, specific itinerary, and lifestyle during travel. Detailed information regarding country-specific risks and recommendations may be obtained from many sources, including those listed under "Sources of Information on Travel Medicine."

IMMUNIZATIONS FOR TRAVEL Immunizations for travel are generally divided into three categories: routine (childhood/adult boosters that are necessary regardless of travel), required (immunizations that are mandated by international regulations for entry into certain areas or for border crossings), and recommended (immunizations that are desirable because they confer protection against a variety of

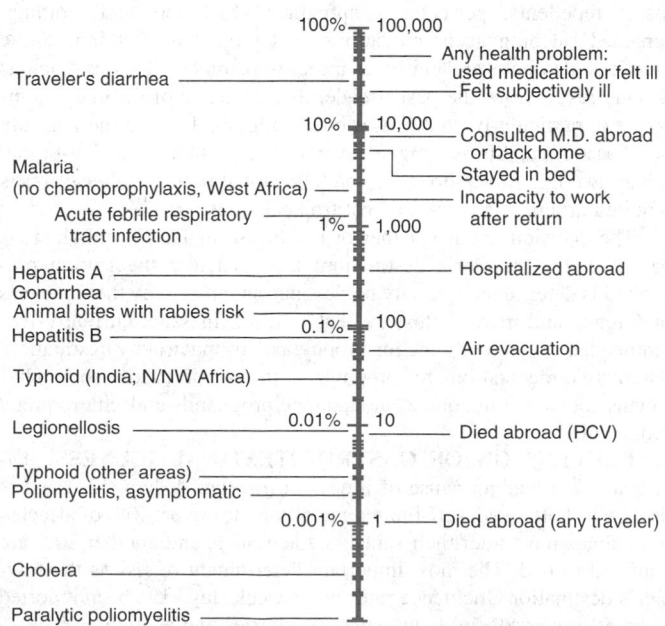

FIGURE 123-1 Incidence rate, per month, of health problems during a stay in developing countries. PCV, Peace Corps volunteer. *(From Steffen and Lobel, with permission from Chapman and Hall, New York.)*

illnesses for which travel increases the risk). Vaccines commonly given to travelers are listed in Table 123-1.

Routine Immunizations • *Diphtheria, tetanus, and polio* Diphtheria continues to be a problem worldwide, with large outbreaks in the independent states formerly encompassed by the Soviet Union. Serosurveys show that tetanus antitoxin is lacking in many North Americans, especially those over the age of 50. Although the risk of polio to the international traveler is extremely low and although polio has been eradicated from the western hemisphere, studies in the United States have found varying levels of immunity in the general population; data indicate that 12% of adult American travelers are unprotected against at least one poliovirus serogroup. Foreign travel offers an ideal opportunity to have these immunizations updated.

Measles Measles (rubeola) continues to be a major cause of morbidity and mortality in the developing world (Chap. 194). Several outbreaks of measles in the United States have been linked to imported cases. The group at highest risk consists of persons born after 1956 and vaccinated before 1980, in many of whom primary vaccination failed. Travelers in this group should be reimmunized.

Influenza Influenza occurs year-round in the tropics and during the summer months in the southern hemisphere (which coincide with the winter months in the northern hemisphere). Vaccination should be considered for all travelers to these regions, particularly those who are elderly or chronically ill. The largest outbreak of travel-related influenza occurred in the summer of 1998 in Alaska and the Northwest Territories of Canada among cruise ship passengers and staff (Chap. 190).

Pneumococcal infection Pneumococcal vaccine should be administered routinely to persons at high risk of serious pneumococcal infection, such as individuals with chronic heart, lung, or renal disease and those who have been splenectomized or have sickle cell disease.

Required Immunizations • *Yellow fever* Documentation of yellow fever vaccination may be required for entry into countries of sub-Saharan Africa and equatorial South America, where the disease is endemic or epidemic, or into countries that are at risk of having the infection introduced. This vaccine is given only by state-authorized yellow fever centers, and its administration must be documented on an official International Certificate of Vaccination. The incidence of yellow fever among travelers is extremely low, probably because the vaccine is highly efficacious.

Cholera According to the World Health Organization, cholera vaccine should no longer be required for entry into any country. (However, see *recommended* use below.)

Meningococcal meningitis Meningococcal vaccination is required for entry into Saudi Arabia during the Hajj. (For information on *recommended* use, see below.)

Recommended Immunizations • *Hepatitis A and B* Hepatitis A is the most frequent vaccine-preventable infection of travelers; the incidence of symptomatic infection during a 1-month stay in a developing country ranges from 3 to 6 cases per 1000. The risk is six times greater for those who stray from the usual tourist routes. The mortality rate for hepatitis A increases with age, reaching almost 3% among symptomatic individuals over age 50. Several vaccines are available in North America, each of which has an efficacy rate of >95%. The monthly incidence of hepatitis B infection, both symptomatic and asymptomatic, is 80 to 240 cases per 100,000. For reasons that are not entirely clear, long-stay overseas workers are at considerable risk for hepatitis B infection. In the near future, a combined hepatitis A and B vaccine should become available in the United States.

Typhoid fever The attack rate for typhoid fever is 1 case per 30,000 per month of travel to the developing world (Chap. 156). However, the rates in India, Senegal, and North Africa are tenfold higher, and, within these areas, rates are especially high among travelers to relatively remote destinations and among persons who are returning to their homelands to stay with relatives or friends. Each of the three

Table 123-1 Vaccines Commonly Used for Travel

Vaccine	Primary Series	Booster Interval
Cholera, parenteral	2 doses, ≥1 week apart, SC or IM	6 months
Cholera, live oral (CVD 103 - HgR)	1 dose	6 months
Hepatitis A (Havrix), 1440 enzyme immunoassay units/mL	2 doses, 6–12 months apart, IM	>10 years
Hepatitis A (VAQTA)[a]	2 doses, 6–12 months apart, IM	>10 years
Hepatitis A/B combined (Twinrix)	3 doses at 0, 1, and 6–12 months, IM	>10 years
Hepatitis B (Engerix B): accelerated schedule	3 doses at 0, 1, and 2 months *or* 0, 7, and 21 days, IM	12 months, once only
Hepatitis B (Engerix B or Recombivax): standard schedule	3 doses at 0, 1, and 6 months, IM	None required
Immune globulin (hepatitis A prevention)	1 dose IM	Intervals of 3–5 months, depending on initial dose
Japanese encephalitis (JEV, Biken)	3 doses, 1 week apart, SC	12–18 months (first booster), then 4 years
Lyme disease (PMC)	3 doses at 0, 1, and 12 months, IM	Optimum booster schedule not yet determined
Meningococcus, quadrivalent	1 dose SC	>3 years (optimum booster schedule not yet determined)
Rabies, human diploid cell vaccine (HDCV)	3 doses at 0, 7, and 21 or 28 days, ID	None required except with exposure
Rabies (HDCV), rabies vaccine absorbed (RVA), or purified chick embryo cell vaccine (PCEC)	3 doses at 0, 7, and 21 or 28 days, IM	None required except with exposure
Typhoid, heat-phenol-inactivated	2 doses, ≥4 weeks apart, SC	3 years
Typhoid Ty21a, oral live attenuated (Vivotif)	1 capsule every other day × 4 doses	5 years
Typhoid Vi capsular polysaccharide, injectable (Typhim Vi)	1 dose IM	2 years
Yellow fever	1 dose SC	10 years

[a] Two new vaccines have been marketed (AVAXIM and EPAXAL).

available vaccines—one oral and two injectable—has an efficacy rate of approximately 70%.

Meningococcal meningitis Although the risk of meningococcal disease among travelers has not been quantified, it is likely to be higher among those who live with poor indigenous populations in overcrowded conditions. The vaccine is recommended for persons traveling to sub-Saharan Africa during the dry season or to areas of the world where there are epidemics. Meningococcal vaccine, which protects against serogroups A/C/Y/W-135, has an efficacy rate of >90%.

Japanese encephalitis The risk of Japanese encephalitis, an infection transmitted by mosquitoes in rural Asia and Southeast Asia, is approximately 1 case per 5000 per month of stay in an endemic area. Most symptomatic infections in U.S. residents have involved military personnel or their families. The vaccine efficacy rate is >80%. Serious allergic reactions sometimes occur; these reactions may be delayed in onset, developing up to 10 days after immunization. The vaccine is recommended for persons staying >1 month in endemic areas.

Cholera The risk of cholera is extremely low, with approximately 1 case per 500,000 journeys to endemic areas. Cholera vaccine is rarely recommended but should be considered for aid workers in refugee camps or in disaster/war-torn areas. The injectable vaccine available in the United States is only 30 to 50% effective, and its protective effect persists for only a short period. A more effective oral cholera vaccine is available in other countries.

Rabies Many cases of rabies have been reported in travelers, but there are no data on the risk of infection. Domestic animals are the major transmitters of rabies in developing countries (Chap. 197). Countries where canine rabies is highly endemic include Mexico, the Philippines, Sri Lanka, India, Thailand, and Vietnam. Each of the three vaccines available in the United States provides >90% protection. Rabies vaccine is recommended for long-stay travelers, particularly children, and persons who may be occupationally exposed in endemic areas.

PREVENTION OF MALARIA AND OTHER INSECT-BORNE DISEASES It is estimated that more than 30,000 Ameri-

can and European travelers develop malaria each year (Chap. 214). Nevertheless, several studies indicate that fewer than 50% of U.S. travelers to malaria-endemic regions adhere to basic recommendations for malaria prevention.

The risk of malaria is highest in sub-Saharan Africa and Oceania (1:50 to 1:1000) and during the past decade has increased by more than fivefold for travelers to Kenya. The risk is intermediate (1:1000 to 1:12,000) for travelers to Haiti and the Indian subcontinent and is low (<1:50,000) for travelers to Asia and to Central and South America. Of the 1000 cases of malaria reported annually in the United States, 90% of those due to *Plasmodium falciparum* occur in travelers returning or immigrating from Africa and Oceania. With the worldwide increase in chloroquine- and multidrug-resistant falciparum malaria, decisions about chemoprophylaxis have become more difficult. Moreover, the spread of malaria due to primaquine- and chloroquine-resistant strains of *P. vivax* has added to the complexity of treatment. The case-fatality rate of falciparum malaria in the United States is 4%; however, in only one-third of patients who die is the diagnosis of malaria considered before death.

Compliance with chemoprophylaxis regimens and use of personal protection measures are keys to the prevention of malaria. Personal protection measures are aimed at preventing mosquito bites, especially between dusk and dawn, and include the use of DEET-containing insect repellents, permethrin-impregnated bed nets and clothing, screened sleeping accommodations, and protective clothing. These practices also help prevent other insect-transmitted illnesses, such as dengue fever. Over the past decade, the incidence of dengue has increased, particularly in the Caribbean region, Latin America, and Southeast Asia. Since dengue fever is transmitted by a day-biting, urban-dwelling mosquito, attention to personal protection measures is required around the clock in most tropical areas.

The decision about whether or not to use malaria prophylaxis is based on the traveler's destination; the particular medication prescribed is determined not only by destination but also by the traveler's preference and medical history. Table 123-2 lists the currently recommended drugs of choice for prophylaxis of malaria by destination. Alternative medications for prophylaxis that are in use by some physicians include primaquine, atovaquone/proguanil, and chloroquine/proguanil.

PREVENTION OF GASTROINTESTINAL ILLNESS Diarrhea is the leading cause of illness in travelers (Chap. 131) and is usually a short-lived, self-limited condition; however, 40% of affected individuals must alter their scheduled activities, and another 20% are confined to bed. The most important determinant of risk is the traveler's destination. Incidence rates per 2-week stay have been reported to be as low as 8% in industrialized countries and as high as 55% in parts of Africa, Central and South America, and Southeast Asia. Infants and young adults are at particularly high risk. The incidence of diarrhea is proportional to the number of dietary indiscretions. Studies of U.S. students in Mexico showed that eating meals in restaurants and cafe-

Geographic Area	Drug of Choice	Alternatives
Central America (north of Panama), Haiti, Dominican Republic, Iraq, Egypt, Turkey, northern Argentina, and Paraguay	Chloroquine	Mefloquine Doxycycline Atovaquone/proguanil
South America including Panama (except northern Argentina and Paraguay); Asia (including Southeast Asia); Africa; and Oceania	Mefloquine	Doxycycline Atovaquone/proguanil
Thai, Myanmar, and Cambodian borders	Doxycycline	Atovaquone/proguanil Primaquine?

[a] See CDC's *Health Information for International Travel 1999–2000.*
NOTE: See also Chap. 214.

terias or consuming food from street vendors was associated with increased risk.

The most frequently identified pathogen causing traveler's diarrhea is toxigenic *Escherichia coli*, although in some parts of the world (notably northern Africa and Southeast Asia) *Campylobacter* infections appear to predominate. Other common causative organisms include *Salmonella*, *Shigella*, rotavirus, and the Norwalk agent. Except for giardiasis, parasitic infections are uncommon causes of traveler's diarrhea. A growing problem for travelers is the development of antibiotic resistance in many bacterial pathogens, including strains of *Campylobacter* and *Salmonella* resistant to quinolones and strains of *E. coli*, *Shigella*, and *Salmonella* resistant to trimethoprim-sulfamethoxazole.

Although the mainstay of prevention of traveler's diarrhea involves food and water precautions, the literature has repeatedly documented dietary indiscretions in 98% of travelers within the first 48 h after arrival at their destination. The old maxim "Boil it, cook it, peel it, or forget it!" is easy to remember but appears to be difficult to adhere to. General food and water precautions include eating foods piping hot; avoiding foods that are raw, poorly cooked, or sold by street vendors; and drinking boiled or commercially bottled beverages, particularly those that are carbonated. Heating kills diarrhea-causing organisms, whereas freezing does not; therefore, ice cubes made from unpurified water should be avoided.

As traveler's diarrhea can occur despite rigorous food and water precautions, travelers should carry medications for self-treatment. For mild to moderate diarrhea, loperamide and fluid replacement may be sufficient. An antibiotic is useful in reducing the frequency of bowel movements and duration of illness in moderate to severe diarrhea. The standard regimen is a 3-day course of a quinolone taken twice daily or (in the case of some of the newer agents) once daily. However, studies have shown that a single large dose of a quinolone may be as effective as the 3-day regimen, particularly if infection with a multidrug-resistant organism is not suspected. For diarrhea acquired in areas such as Thailand, where >70% of *Campylobacter* infections are quinolone resistant, azithromycin may be a better choice.

Prophylaxis of traveler's diarrhea with bismuth subsalicylate is widely used but only about 60% effective. For certain individuals (e.g., athletes who must be in peak physical condition to perform, persons with a repeated history of traveler's diarrhea, and some persons with chronic diseases), a single daily dose of a quinolone antibiotic during travel of <1 month's duration is highly effective.

PREVENTION OF OTHER TRAVEL-RELATED PROBLEMS Travelers are at high risk for *sexually transmitted diseases.* Surveys have shown that large numbers engage in casual sex, and there is a reluctance to use condoms consistently. An increasing number of travelers are being diagnosed with *schistosomiasis.* Travelers should be cautioned to avoid bathing, swimming, or wading in freshwater lakes, streams, or rivers in the parts of tropical South America, the Caribbean, Africa, and Southeast Asia where this infection can be

acquired. Travelers are cautioned to avoid walking barefoot because of the risk of *hookworm* and *strongyloidiasis* and, at night, *snakebites.* Prevention of *travel-associated injury* depends mostly on commonsense precautions. Riding on motorcycles and overcrowded public vehicles is not recommended; in particular, individuals should not travel by road after dark in rural areas. In addition to its association with motor vehicle accidents, excessive alcohol use has been a significant factor in drownings, assaults, and injuries.

THE TRAVELER'S MEDICAL KIT A traveler's medical kit is strongly advisable, particularly for long-stay travelers. The contents may vary widely, depending on the itinerary, duration of stay, style of travel, and local medical facilities. While many medications are available abroad, often over the counter, directions for their use may be nonexistent or in a foreign language, and, more important, a product may be outdated or counterfeit. Therefore, if possible, a complete supply of medications should accompany the traveler. In the kit, the short-term traveler should consider carrying an analgesic, an antidiarrheal agent, antihistamines, a laxative, oral rehydration salts, sunscreen with a skin protection factor of at least 30, insect repellents (DEET) for the skin, an insecticide for clothing (permethrin), and (if necessary) an antimalarial. To these medications the long-stay traveler might add a broad-spectrum general-purpose antibiotic, an antibacterial eye and skin ointment, and a topical antifungal cream. Regardless of the duration of travel, a first-aid kit containing items such as scissors, tweezers, and bandages should be considered.

TRAVEL AND SPECIAL HOSTS

PREGNANCY AND TRAVEL A woman's medical history and itinerary, the quality of medical care at her destinations, and her degree of flexibility determine whether travel is wise during pregnancy. According to the American College of Obstetrics and Gynecology, the safest part of pregnancy in which to travel is the second trimester (between 18 and 24 weeks), when there is the least danger of spontaneous abortion or premature labor. Some obstetricians prefer that women stay within a few hundred miles of home after the 28th week of pregnancy in case problems arise; in general, however, healthy women may be advised that it is acceptable to travel.

Despite this general recommendation, there are some relative contraindications to international travel during pregnancy, including certain obstetric risk factors: a history of miscarriage, premature labor, incompetent cervix, or toxemia. General medical problems such as diabetes, heart failure, severe anemia, or a history of thromboembolic disease should also prompt the pregnant woman to postpone her travels. Finally, regions in which the pregnant woman and her fetus may be at excessive risk (e.g., those at high altitudes and those where livevirus vaccines are required or where multidrug-resistant malaria is endemic) are not ideal destinations during any trimester.

Malaria Malaria during pregnancy carries a significant risk of morbidity and death. Levels of parasitemia are highest and failure to clear the parasites after chloroquine treatment are most frequent among primigravidae. Severe disease, with complications such as cerebral malaria, massive hemolysis, and renal failure, is especially likely in pregnancy. Fetal sequelae include spontaneous abortion, stillbirth, preterm delivery, and congenital infection.

Traveler's Diarrhea Because dehydration due to traveler's diarrhea can lead to inadequate placental blood flow, pregnant travelers must be extremely cautious regarding their food and beverage intake. The exclusive consumption of bottled (carbonated) or boiled drinks without ice, the eating of well-cooked meats and pasteurized dairy products, and the avoidance of pre-prepared salad items should help protect against traveler's diarrhea due to the usual causes as well as against infections such as toxoplasmosis, hepatitis E, and listeriosis, which can have serious sequelae in pregnancy.

The mainstay of therapy for traveler's diarrhea is rehydration. Kaolin-pectin combinations and loperamide may be used if necessary, but many of the usual antibiotics (e.g., quinolones) are contraindicated during pregnancy. Ampicillin alone or with clavulanic acid may be used, but many strains of *E. coli* and other organisms implicated in traveler's diarrhea are resistant. Azithromycin or an oral third-generation cephalosporin may be the best option.

Because of the major problems encountered when infants are given local foods and beverages, women are strongly encouraged to breast-feed when traveling with a neonate. A nursing mother with traveler's diarrhea should not stop breast-feeding but should increase her fluid intake.

Air Travel and High-Altitude Destinations   Commercial air travel is not a risk to the healthy pregnant woman or to the fetus. Fetal oxygenation is not adversely affected by the decreased cabin pressures because of the fetal hemoglobin dissociation curve; the higher radiation levels reported at altitudes >10,500 m (35,000 ft) should pose no problem to the healthy pregnant traveler. Since each airline has a policy regarding pregnancy and flying, it is best to check with the specific carrier when booking reservations. Domestic air travel is usually permitted until the 36th week, whereas international air travel is generally curtailed after the 32nd week.

There are no known risks for pregnant women who travel to high-altitude destinations and stay for short periods. However, there are likewise no data on the safety of pregnant women at altitudes >4500 m (15,000 ft). Because of the harsh conditions usually associated with such trips, they are generally contraindicated for other reasons.

THE HIV-INFECTED TRAVELER   The traveler infected with HIV is at special risk of serious infections due to a number of pathogens that may be more prevalent at travel destinations than at home. However, the degree of risk depends primarily on the state of the immune system at the time of travel. For persons whose CD4+ cell counts are normal or >500/μL, no data suggest a greater risk during travel than for persons without HIV infection. Individuals with AIDS (CD4+ counts <200/μL) and others who are symptomatic need special counseling and should visit a travel medicine practitioner before departure, especially when traveling to the developing world.

Several countries now routinely deny entry to HIV-positive individuals, even though no data show that these restrictions decrease rates of transmission of the virus. In general, HIV testing is required of those individuals who wish to stay abroad longer than 3 months or who intend to work or study abroad. Some countries will accept an HIV serologic test done within 6 months of departure, whereas others will not accept a blood test done at any time in the traveler's home country. In addition, border officials often have the authority to make inquiries of individuals entering a country and to check the medications they are carrying. If a drug such as zidovudine (AZT) is identified, the person may be barred from entering the country. Information on testing requirements for specific countries is available from consular offices but is subject to frequent change.

Health insurance policies should be checked to make sure they are valid for care in other countries. The HIV-positive traveler should strongly consider obtaining trip cancellation insurance and evacuation insurance in case of illness. It is ideal to have the name of a physician at the travel destination who is familiar with the treatment of patients with AIDS, as the clinical findings associated with infection may be atypical in a patient with AIDS, and several infections may exist simultaneously. The traveler should be encouraged to visit the physician promptly if problems arise.

Immunizations   All of the HIV-infected traveler's routine immunizations should be up to date (Chap. 122). The response to immunization may be impaired at CD4+ cell counts of <200/μL (and in some cases at even higher counts). However, when the risk of illness is high or the sequelae of illness are serious, immunization is recommended. In certain circumstances, it may be prudent to check the adequacy of the serum antibody response before departure (e.g., yellow fever neutralization inhibition if exposure is unavoidable).

Because of the increased risk of infections due to *Streptococcus pneumoniae* and other bacterial pathogens that cause pneumonia following influenza, pneumococcal polysaccharide and influenza vaccines should be administered. The estimated rates of response to influenza vaccine are >80% among persons with asymptomatic HIV infection and <50% among those with AIDS.

In general, live attenuated vaccines are contraindicated for persons with immune dysfunction. Live oral polio vaccine should not be given to HIV-infected patients or to members of their households. Instead, inactivated polio vaccine (eIPV) should be used; most HIV-infected individuals without AIDS will develop protective antibody levels in response to this vaccine.

Because measles (rubeola) can be a severe and lethal infection in HIV-positive patients, the measles vaccine (or the combination measles-mumps-rubella vaccine) should be given to these individuals. Although this is a live vaccine, there have been no reports of serious complications in this population. Between 18 and 58% of symptomatic HIV-infected vaccinees develop adequate antibody titers, and between 50 and 100% of those who are infected but asymptomatic seroconvert.

The decision of whether or not to administer any of the special vaccines to an HIV-infected traveler should be based on the individual's risk. Inactivated vaccines can be administered without concern for safety but with concern about adequate protection. For example, data suggest that HIV-infected persons do not have as strong an antibody response to the meningococcal meningitis vaccine as do uninfected persons. Moreover, few data are available on the efficacy of many of the other vaccines (e.g., those for hepatitis A, typhoid, and cholera).

It is recommended that the live yellow fever vaccine not be given to HIV-infected travelers. Nevertheless, when inadvertently administered to HIV-positive military personnel, this vaccine elicited no adverse reactions. Therefore, if the traveler's CD4+ count is >200/μL and travel in an endemic area is absolutely necessary, the vaccine can probably be administered safely. HIV-infected persons whose CD4+ count is <200/μL should be discouraged from traveling to endemic regions. If the traveler is passing through or traveling to an area where the vaccine is required but the disease risk is low, a physician's waiver should be issued. Bacille Calmette-Guérin vaccine should not be given because of reports of disseminated infection in HIV-infected persons.

A transient (days to weeks) burst of viremia has been demonstrated in HIV-infected individuals following immunization with vaccines for such diseases as influenza, pneumococcal infection, and tetanus (Chap. 309). However, at this point, there is no evidence that this transient increase in viremia is detrimental over time. Furthermore, it is likely that immune activation associated with infection with the live organisms in question would result in increases in viremia of greater magnitude and duration than those associated with vaccination. Therefore, the vaccination recommendations discussed above need not be modified at this time.

Gastrointestinal Illness   Decreased levels of gastric acid, abnormal gastrointestinal mucosal immunity, other complications of HIV infection, and medications taken by HIV-infected patients make traveler's diarrhea especially problematic in these individuals. Traveler's diarrhea is likely to occur more frequently, be more severe, and be more difficult to treat in association with HIV infection. *Salmonella*, *Shigella*, and *Campylobacter* infections are also more protracted and more often accompanied by bacteremia in HIV-infected persons.

Cryptosporidium (Chap. 218), a common cause of diarrhea in tropical countries, produces severe chronic diarrhea and cholecystitis with increased mortality among patients with AIDS. *Isospora belli* causes infections at high rates among AIDS patients in the developing world; this infection is associated with malabsorption, weight loss, and relapses after treatment. Persistent diarrhea due to microsporidiosis has been reported.

Because of these potential problems, the HIV-infected traveler must be careful to consume only appropriately prepared foods and beverages. In addition, this group of individuals may benefit from prophylaxis for traveler's diarrhea, using bismuth subsalicylate or a daily antibiotic (ideally a quinolone derivative) for short-term travel to the developing world. If the traveler is already taking a sulfonamide preparation for prophylaxis of *Pneumocystis* pneumonia, a regimen of self-treatment with a quinolone would be appropriate.

Other Travel-Related Infections   Data are lacking on the severity of vector-borne diseases in HIV-infected individuals. Malaria is especially severe in asplenic and certain immunocompromised hosts, although increased severity has not been demonstrated in AIDS. *Babesia* infection is known to cause serious illness and to recur in HIV-infected patients; this tick-transmitted illness occurs in parts of the United States but is not known to be a widespread problem.

Visceral leishmaniasis (Chap. 215) has been reported in numerous HIV-infected travelers. Because the usual signs—splenomegaly and hyperglobulinemia—are nonspecific and may even be lacking, the diagnosis is difficult to make. In addition, serologic results are often negative. This infection is difficult to treat, and its associated mortality is high. Even short-term travelers to southern Europe have developed the illness; thus, the avoidance of sandfly bites is critical.

Certain respiratory illnesses, such as histoplasmosis and coccidioidomycosis, cause greater morbidity and mortality among patients with AIDS than in the general population. Though tuberculosis is common among HIV-infected persons (especially in developing countries), the acquisition of this infection by the short-term traveler is not a major concern. The possibility of acquiring *Legionella* infections from spas should be considered, although no data confirm an increase in the severity of such infections in AIDS.

Finally, the HIV-infected traveler should always be cautioned about safe sexual practices, which may help prevent both the transmission of HIV to others and the acquisition by the traveler of other sexually transmitted diseases that may be drug resistant or may result in serious sequelae (e.g., syphilis).

Medications   Adverse events due to medications and drug interactions are common and raise complex issues for HIV-infected persons. In addition, rates of cutaneous reaction are unusually high among patients with AIDS. Physicians advising these travelers need to consider the problems that may arise from the use of agents such as antimalarial drugs, medications for altitude acclimatization, or antidiarrheal compounds; one example is increased cutaneous sensitivity to sulfonamides. Since zidovudine is metabolized by hepatic glucuronidation, inhibitors of this process may elevate serum levels of the drug. Though quinine does not affect levels of zidovudine, there are no relevant data on chloroquine, primaquine, or mefloquine. Furthermore, it is not known whether the antagonistic effect of zidovudine on pyrimethamine has clinical relevance in the treatment or prevention of plasmodial infections.

CHRONIC ILLNESS, DISABILITY, AND TRAVEL

Evaluating fitness for travel is a growing issue in view of the increased number of elderly and chronically ill individuals journeying to exotic destinations. Conditions encountered during flight are of particular concern in these cases. Since most commercial aircraft are pressurized to 2500 m (8000 ft) above sea level, corresponding to a Pa_{O_2} of about 55 mmHg, individuals with serious cardiopulmonary problems should be evaluated before travel. In addition, those who have recently had surgery, a myocardial infarction, a cerebrovascular accident, or another medical crisis may be at high risk for adverse events in flight. A summary of current recommendations regarding fitness to fly has been published by the Aerospace Medical Association Air Transport Medical Committee. Chronic health problems should not prevent travel, but special measures can make the journey safer and more comfortable.

Heart Disease   Cardiovascular events are the main cause of deaths among travelers and of in-flight emergencies on commercial aircraft. Persons with underlying heart disease should review their itineraries with a physician prior to departure; travel in harsh environments or to remote destinations is not wise. Extra supplies of all medications should be kept in carry-on luggage, along with a recent copy of an electrocardiogram and the name and telephone number of the traveler's physician at home. Pacemakers are not affected by airport security devices, but electronic telephone checks of pacemaker function cannot be transmitted by international satellites. The traveler may benefit from supplemental oxygen, which should be ordered by a physician (since oxygen delivery systems are not standard) 48 to 72 h before flight time. Personal oxygen tanks are not permitted on aircraft. Travelers should request aisle seating and should walk, perform stretching and flexing exercises, and remain hydrated during the flight to prevent venous thrombosis and pulmonary embolism.

Chronic Lung Disease   Chronic obstructive pulmonary disease (COPD) is one of the most common diagnoses in patients who require emergency-room evaluation for symptoms occurring during airline flights. Patients with COPD experience dyspnea, edema, wheezing, cyanosis, and chest pain. The best predictor of the development of these symptoms is the sea level Pa_{O_2}. A Pa_{O_2} of at least 72 mmHg corresponds to an in-flight Pa_{O_2} of 55 mmHg when the cabin is pressurized to 2500 m (8000 ft). Therefore, if the traveler's baseline Pa_{O_2} is <72 mmHg, the provision of supplemental oxygen during the flight should be considered. Pulmonary function is also maximized by continuing bronchodilator treatment and the use of glucocorticoids as prescribed. Contraindications to flight include active bronchospasm, lower respiratory infection, phlebitis, pulmonary hypertension, and recent thoracic surgery (within the preceding 3 weeks) or pneumothorax. Consideration should be given to decreasing the amount of outdoor activity at the destination if there is excessive air pollution.

Diabetes Mellitus   Alterations in glucose control and changes in insulin requirements are common problems when diabetic patients travel. Changes in time zone, in the amount and timing of food intake, and in physical activity demand more vigilant assessment of metabolic control. The diabetic traveler should pack medication (including a bottle of regular insulin for emergencies), insulin syringes and needles, equipment and supplies for glucose monitoring, and snacks in carry-on luggage. Insulin is stable for about 3 months at room temperature but should be kept as cool as possible. The name and telephone number of the home physician and a card and necklace listing the medical problems and the type and dose of insulin used should accompany the traveler. When six or more time zones are crossed, insulin requirements may be temporarily altered, depending on food intake and physical activity. In traveling eastward (e.g., from the United States to Europe), the morning insulin dose on arrival may need to be decreased. The blood glucose can then be checked during the day to determine whether additional insulin is required. For flights westward, with lengthening of the day, an additional dose of regular insulin may be required. Comfortable footwear is essential for the diabetic traveler.

Other Special Groups   Other groups for whom special travel measures are now being encouraged include patients undergoing dialysis, those with transplants, and those with other disabilities. Up to 13% of travelers have some disability, but few advocacy groups and tour companies dedicate themselves to this growing population. The key to safe travel in each case is adequate research ahead of time. Patients undergoing chronic ambulatory peritoneal dialysis may ship their dialysis solutions to their destinations before traveling. They should carry essential medical records as well as antibiotics for self-treatment of presumed peritonitis. Hemodialysis patients need to reserve appointments at dialysis centers prior to their departure from home. Travel by transplant recipients to distant destinations should ideally be scheduled at least 1 year after surgery, as most rejection episodes occur early. Medication interactions are a source of serious concern for these travelers, and appropriate medical information should be carried, along with the home physician's name and telephone number. Some travelers taking glucocorticoids carry stress doses in case they become ill. Immunization of these immunocompromised travelers may result in less than adequate protection against certain diseases. Thus, the traveler and physician must carefully consider which destinations are appropriate.

PROBLEMS AFTER RETURN

The most frequent medical problems encountered by travelers after their return home are diarrhea, fever, respiratory illnesses, and skin diseases. Frequently ignored problems are fatigue and emotional stress, especially in long-stay travelers. The approach to diagnosis requires some knowledge of geographic medicine, in particular the epidemiology and clinical presentation of infectious disorders. A geographic history should focus on the traveler's exact itinerary, including dates of arrival and departure; exposure history (food indiscretions, drinking-water sources, freshwater contact, sexual activity, animal contact, insect bites); location and style of travel (urban vs. rural, first-class hotel accommodation vs. camping); immunization history; and use of antimalarial chemosuppression.

DIARRHEA   Although extremely common, acute traveler's diarrhea is usually self-limited or amenable to antibiotic therapy. Bowel symptoms that persist after the traveler's return home have a less well-defined etiology and may require medical attention from a specialist. Infectious agents appear to be responsible for only a small proportion of cases with persistent bowel symptoms. Of the pathogens detected in these instances, *Giardia lamblia* (Chap. 218) is by far the most common; *Cyclospora cayetanensis*, *Cryptosporidium* spp., and *Entamoeba histolytica* are rare isolates. The most frequent causes of persistent diarrhea after travel are postinfectious sequelae, such as lactose intolerance or an irritable bowel syndrome. When no infectious etiology can be identified, a trial of metronidazole therapy for presumed giardiasis, a strict lactose-free diet for 1 week, or a several-week trial of high-dose hydrophilic mucilloid relieves the symptoms of many patients.

FEVER   Fever in a traveler who has returned from a malarious area should be considered a medical emergency because death from *P. falciparum* malaria can follow an illness of only several days' duration. Although "fever from the tropics" does not always have a tropical cause, malaria should be the first diagnosis considered. The risk of *P. falciparum* malaria is highest among travelers returning from Africa or Oceania and among those who become symptomatic within the first 2 months after return. Other important causes of fever after travel include viral hepatitis (hepatitis A and E), typhoid fever, bacterial enteritis, arbovirus infections (e.g., dengue fever), rickettsial infections (including tick and scrub typhus or Q fever) and—in rare instances—leptospirosis, acute HIV infection, and amebic liver abscess. In at least 25% of cases, no etiology can be found, and the illness resolves spontaneously. Clinicians should keep in mind that no present-day antimalarial agent guarantees protection from malaria and that some immunizations—notably, those against typhoid and cholera—are only partially protective.

As noted above, the approach to the febrile returned traveler begins with a detailed medical and geographic history. Knowing exact dates of arrival and departure from tropical areas enables the physician to ascertain the shortest and longest possible incubation periods for illnesses in the differential diagnosis. For example, a traveler who develops fever <1 week after arrival in a malarious area cannot have malaria because the incubation period is too short, whereas a fever whose onset comes >2 weeks after departure from an endemic area cannot be dengue fever because the incubation period is too long. In the physical examination, particular attention should be given to the skin so as not to miss a subtle rash or eschar.

When no specific diagnosis is forthcoming, the following investigations may be helpful: complete blood count, liver function tests, thick/thin blood films for malaria (repeated twice if necessary), urinalysis, blood cultures (repeated once if necessary), and collection of an acute-phase serum sample to be held for later examination along with a paired convalescent-phase serum sample.

SKIN DISEASES   Pyodermas, sunburn, insect bites, skin ulcers, and cutaneous larva migrans are the most common skin conditions encountered in travelers after their return home. In those with persistent skin ulcers, the diagnoses of cutaneous leishmaniasis, mycobacterial infection, or fungal infection should be considered. Careful, complete inspection of the skin is important in detecting the rickettsial eschar in a febrile patient or the central breathing hole in a "boil" due to myiasis.

EMERGING INFECTIOUS DISEASES   In recent years, travel and commerce have fostered the worldwide spread of HIV infection, led to the reemergence of cholera as a global health threat, and created considerable fear about the possible spread of Ebola virus infection and plague. For travelers, there are more realistic concerns. One of the largest outbreaks of dengue fever ever documented is now raging in Latin America; schistosomiasis is being described in previously unaffected lakes in Africa; and antibiotic-resistant strains of sexually transmitted and enteric pathogens are emerging at an alarming rate in the developing world. As Nobel Laureate Dr. Joshua Lederberg pointed out, "The microbe that felled one child in a distant continent yesterday can reach yours today and seed a global pandemic tomorrow." The vigilant clinician understands that the importance of a thorough travel history cannot be overemphasized.

SOURCES OF INFORMATION ON TRAVEL MEDICINE

- CDC publication *Health Information for International Travel*
- CDC home page: www.cdc.gov
- CDC travel information: www.cdc.gov/travel/travel.html
- Health Canada: www.hwc.ca/hpb/lcdc
- International Society of Travel Medicine: www.istm.org

BIBLIOGRAPHY

AEROSPACE MEDICAL ASSOCIATION, AIR TRANSPORT MEDICINE COMMITTEE: Medical guidelines for air travel. Aviat Space Environ Med 67(Suppl 10):b1, 1996

CAUMES E et al: Dermatoses associated with travel to tropical countries: A prospective study of the diagnosis and management of 269 patients presenting to a tropical disease unit. Clin Infect Dis 20:542, 1995

CENTERS FOR DISEASE CONTROL AND PREVENTION: *Health Information for International Travel 1999–2000*, publication no. (CDC) 92-8280. Washington, DC, Government Printing Office, 1999

ERICSSON CD: Travelers' diarrhea: Epidemiology, prevention and self-treatment. Infect Dis Clin North Am 12:285, 1998

FRADIN MS: Mosquitoes and mosquito repellents: A clinician's guide. Ann Intern Med 128:931, 1998

KEMMERER TP et al: Health problems of corporate travelers: Risk factors and management. J Trav Med 5:184, 1998

MAGILL AJ: Fever in the returned traveler. Infect Dis Clin North Am 12:455, 1998

MILENO MD, BIA FS: The compromised traveler. Infect Dis Clin North Am 12:369, 1998

SAMUEL B, BARRY M: The pregnant traveler. Infect Dis Clin North Am 12:323, 1998

STEFFEN R, LOBEL HO: Epidemiologic basis for the practice of travel medicine. J Wilderness Med 5:56, 1994

WILSON ME: *A World Guide to Infectious Diseases, Distribution, Diagnosis*. New York, Oxford University Press, 1991

124 *Robert S. Munford*

SEPSIS AND SEPTIC SHOCK

ARDS acute respiratory distress syndrome	LPS lipopolysaccharide
DIC disseminated intravascular coagulation	PAF platelet-activating factor
	SIRS systemic inflammatory response syndrome
IL interleukin	TGF-β transforming growth factor β
IL-1Ra IL-1 receptor antagonist	
iNOS inducible nitric oxide synthase	TNF tumor necrosis factor
LBP LPS-binding protein	

DEFINITIONS (See Table 124-1) The host's reaction to invading microbes involves a rapidly amplifying polyphony of signals and responses that may spread beyond the invaded tissue. Fever or hypothermia, tachypnea, and tachycardia often herald the onset of *sepsis*, the systemic response to microbial invasion. When counterregulatory control mechanisms are overwhelmed, homeostasis may fail, and dysfunction of major organs may supervene (*severe sepsis*). Further regulatory imbalance leads to *septic shock*, which is characterized by hypotension as well as organ dysfunction. As sepsis progresses to septic shock, the risk of dying increases substantially. Sepsis is usually reversible, whereas patients with septic shock often succumb despite aggressive therapy.

The *systemic inflammatory response syndrome* (SIRS), as defined in the early 1990s by critical care specialists, may have an infectious or a noninfectious etiology. If infection is suspected or proven, a patient with SIRS is said to have sepsis.

ETIOLOGY Sepsis can be a response to any class of microorganism. Microbial invasion of the bloodstream is not essential for the development of sepsis, since local or systemic spread of microbial

signal molecules or toxins can also elicit the response. Blood cultures yield bacteria or fungi in ~20 to 40% of cases of severe sepsis and 40 to 70% of cases of septic shock. Individual gram-negative or gram-positive bacteria account for ~70% of these isolates; the remainder are fungi or a mixture of microorganisms (Table 124-2). In patients whose blood cultures are negative, the etiologic agent is often established by culture or microscopic examination of infected material from a local site. In some case series, a majority of patients with a clinical picture of severe sepsis or septic shock have had negative microbiologic data.

Factors that predispose to gram-negative bacillary bacteremia include diabetes mellitus, lymphoproliferative diseases, cirrhosis of the liver, burns, invasive procedures or devices, and treatment with drugs that cause neutropenia. Major risk factors for gram-positive bacteremia include vascular catheterization, the presence of indwelling mechanical devices, burns, and intravenous drug use. Fungemia occurs most often in immunosuppressed patients with neutropenia, often after broad-spectrum antimicrobial therapy. In patients who experience bacteremia, factors that increase the risk of developing severe sepsis include age (>50 years) and a primary pulmonary, abdominal, or neuromeningeal site of infection. Bacteremia that arises from an intravascular catheter or the urinary tract is less likely to induce severe sepsis.

EPIDEMIOLOGY The septic response is now a contributing factor in >100,000 deaths per year in the United States. The incidence of severe sepsis and septic shock has increased over the last 15 years and is now probably between 300,000 and 500,000 cases per year. Approximately two-thirds of cases occur in patients hospitalized for other illnesses. The increasing incidence of severe sepsis in the United States is attributable to the aging of the population, the increasing longevity of patients with chronic diseases, and the relatively high frequency with which sepsis develops in patients with AIDS. The widespread use of antimicrobial agents, glucocorticoids, indwelling catheters and mechanical devices, and mechanical ventilation also plays a role.

PATHOPHYSIOLOGY The septic response is often triggered when microorganisms spread from the gastrointestinal tract or skin into contiguous tissues. Localized tissue infection may then lead to bacteremia or fungemia. Alternatively, microorganisms may be introduced directly into the bloodstream (for example, via intravenous catheters). In general, the septic response occurs when immune defenses fail to contain an invading microbe. Since most cases are triggered by microbes that do not ordinarily cause systemic disease in normal hosts (Table 124-2), deficiencies in nonadaptive host factors may be most important. The septic response may also be induced by microbial ex-

Table 124-1 Definitions Used to Describe the Condition of Patients with Sepsis

Bacteremia	Presence of bacteria in the blood, as evidenced by positive blood cultures
Septicemia	Presence of microbes or their toxins in blood
Systemic inflammatory response syndrome (SIRS)	Two or more of the following conditions: (1) fever (oral temperature >38°C) or hypothermia (<36°C); (2) tachypnea (>24 breaths/min); (3) tachycardia (heart rate >90 beats/min); (4) leukocytosis (>12,000/μL), leukopenia (<4,000/μL), or >10% bands. May have an infectious or a noninfectious etiology
Sepsis	SIRS that has a proven or suspected microbial etiology
Severe sepsis (similar to "sepsis syndrome")	Sepsis with one or more signs of organ dysfunction (such as metabolic acidosis, acute encephalopathy, oliguria, hypoxemia, or disseminated intravascular coagulation) or hypotension
Septic shock	Sepsis with hypotension (arterial blood pressure of <90 mmHg systolic or 40 mmHg less than patient's normal blood pressure) that is unresponsive to fluid resuscitation, along with organ dysfunction (see severe sepsis)
Refractory septic shock	Septic shock that lasts for >1 h and does not respond to fluid or pressor administration
Multiple-organ dysfunction syndrome (MODS)	Dysfunction of more than one organ, requiring intervention to maintain homeostasis

SOURCE: Adapted from American College of Chest Physicians/Society of Critical Care Medicine Consensus Conference Committee.

Table 124-2 Microorganisms Involved in Episodes of Severe Sepsis at Eight Academic Medical Centers

Microorganisms	Episodes with Bloodstream Infection, % (n = 436)	Episodes with Documented Infection but No Bloodstream Infection, % (n = 430)	Total Episodes, % (n = 866)
Gram-negative bacteria[a]	35	44	40
Gram-positive bacteria[b]	40	24	31
Fungi	7	5	6
Polymicrobial	11	21	16
Classic pathogens[c]	<5	<5	<5

[a] Enterobacteriaceae, pseudomonads, *Haemophilus* spp., other gram-negative bacteria.
[b] *Staphylococcus aureus*, coagulase-negative staphylococci, enterococci, *Streptococcus pneumoniae*, other streptococci, other gram-positive bacteria.
[c] Such as *Neisseria meningitidis*, *S. pneumoniae*, *H. influenzae*, and *Streptococcus pyogenes*.
SOURCE: Adapted from Sands et al.

otoxins that act as superantigens (e.g., toxic shock syndrome toxin 1; Chap. 139).

Microbial Signals Animals recognize certain microbial molecules as signals that microorganisms have invaded. Lipopolysaccharide (LPS, also called *endotoxin*) is the most potent and best-studied gram-negative bacterial signal molecule. A plasma protein (LPS-binding protein, or LBP) transfers LPS to CD14 on the surfaces of monocytes, macrophages, and neutrophils. This interaction rapidly triggers the production and release of mediators, such as tumor necrosis factor (TNF) α (see below), that amplify the LPS signal and transmit it to other cells and tissues. Soluble CD14 may also bind LPS in plasma and transfer it to cells that lack cell-surface CD14. The peptidoglycan and lipoteichoic acids of gram-positive bacteria, certain polysaccharides, extracellular enzymes, and toxins elicit responses in animals that are similar to those induced by LPS; some of these molecules may also bind CD14. CD14 thus attracts numerous non-self molecules to the surfaces of myeloid cells, greatly increasing the sensitivity with which these molecules can be recognized by the host. Evidence suggests that signal specificity occurs in or on the plasma membrane and is conferred, at least in part, by members of the toll-like receptor family of transmembrane proteins. Other innate immune mechanisms for recognizing microbial molecules include complement (principally the alternative pathway), mannose-binding protein, and C-reactive protein.

Host Responses The septic response involves complex interactions among microbial signal molecules, leukocytes, humoral mediators, and the vascular endothelium.

Cytokines Inflammatory cytokines amplify and diversify the response. These proteins can exert endocrine, paracrine, and autocrine effects (Chap. 305). TNF-α stimulates leukocytes and vascular endothelial cells to release other cytokines (as well as additional TNF-α), to express cell-surface adhesion molecules, and to increase arachidonic acid turnover. Blood levels of TNF-α are high in most patients with severe sepsis or septic shock. Moreover, intravenous infusion of TNF-α can elicit many of the characteristic abnormalities of sepsis, including fever, tachycardia, tachypnea, leukocytosis, myalgias, and somnolence. In animals, larger doses of TNF-α induce shock, disseminated intravascular coagulation (DIC), and death. Specific TNF-α antagonists can abrogate the septic response and prevent the deaths of experimental animals challenged with endotoxin.

Although TNF-α is a central mediator, it is only one of many cytokines that contribute to the septic process. Interleukin (IL) 1β, for example, which exhibits many of the same activities as TNF-α, seems to play an increasingly significant role as sepsis intensifies. TNF-α, IL-1β, interferon-γ, IL-8, and other cytokines probably interact synergistically with each other and with additional mediators. Moreover, some mediators (such as IL-1β and TNF-α) may enhance their own rates of synthesis by positive feedback. As sepsis progresses, the mixture of cytokines and other molecules becomes very complex: elevated blood levels of >50 molecules have been found in patients with septic shock. In animal models, the septic response can be interrupted by early interventions that neutralize one or another of its many components; this observation testifies to the importance of mediator interactions for the overall outcome. It has been much more difficult to rescue animals from severe sepsis and septic shock.

Phospholipid-derived mediators Arachidonic acid, released from membrane phospholipids by phospholipase A$_2$, is converted by the cyclooxygenase pathway into prostaglandins and thromboxanes. Prostaglandin E$_2$ and prostacyclin cause peripheral vasodilatation, whereas thromboxane is a vasoconstrictor and promotes platelet aggregation. Administration of the cyclooxygenase inhibitor ibuprofen for 48 h to patients with severe sepsis suppressed production of these metabolites and decreased body temperature, heart rate, and metabolic acidosis without reducing mortality. Leukotrienes are also potent mediators of ischemia and shock; the fact that the reaction to endotoxin challenge is normal in mice that lack the 5-lipoxygenase gene, however, casts doubt on the role of leukotrienes in the septic response.

Another important phospholipid-derived mediator is platelet-activating factor (PAF; 1-*O*-alkyl-2-acetyl-*sn*-glycero-3-phosphorylcholine). PAF potently stimulates neutrophil aggregation and degranulation, promotes platelet aggregation, and may contribute to tissue injury.

Coagulation factors Intravascular fibrin deposition, thrombosis, and DIC are important features of the septic response. IL-6 and other mediators promote intravascular coagulation initially by inducing blood monocytes to express tissue factor (Chap. 62). When tissue factor is expressed on monocytes, it binds to factor VIIa to form an active complex that can convert factors X and IX to enzymatically active forms. The result is activation of both extrinsic and intrinsic clotting pathways, culminating in the generation of fibrin. Clotting is also favored by impaired function of the protein C–protein S inhibitory pathway and depletion of antithrombin, while fibrinolysis is prevented by increased plasma levels of plasminogen activator inhibitor 1. Thus, there may be a striking propensity to intravascular fibrin deposition, thrombosis, and bleeding (Chap. 146). Contact-system activation occurs during sepsis but contributes more to the development of hypotension than to DIC.

Complement C5a and other products of complement activation may promote neutrophil reactions such as chemotaxis, aggregation, degranulation, and oxygen-radical production. When administered to animals, C5a induces hypotension, pulmonary vasoconstriction, neutropenia, and vascular leakiness due in part to endothelial damage.

Activation of the vascular endothelium Many tissues may be damaged by the septic response. The probable underlying mechanism is widespread vascular endothelial injury, with fluid extravasation and microthrombosis that decrease oxygen and substrate utilization by the affected tissues. Leukocyte-derived mediators and platelet-leukocyte-fibrin thrombi contribute to this injury, but the vascular endothelium itself seems to play an active role. Stimuli such as TNF-α induce vascular endothelial cells to produce and release cytokines, procoagulant molecules, PAF, endothelium-derived relaxing factor (nitric oxide), and other mediators. In addition, regulated cell-adhesion molecules promote the adherence of neutrophils to endothelial cells. While these responses may attract phagocytes to infected sites and activate their antimicrobial arsenals, endothelial cell activation can also promote increased vascular permeability, microvascular thrombosis, DIC, and hypotension. Moreover, vascular integrity may be damaged by neutrophil enzymes (such as elastase) and toxic oxygen metabolites so that local hemorrhage ensues. Blocking the adhesion of leukocytes to endothelial cell surfaces, as with monoclonal antibodies to intercellular adhesion molecule 1, can prevent tissue necrosis in response to endotoxin administration in animals.

Septic shock Much evidence now implicates nitric oxide, produced by inducible nitric oxide synthase (iNOS), as a mediator of septic shock in experimental animals and probably in humans. Mice that lack the *iNOS* gene may not be resistant to endotoxic shock, however. Other prominent hypotensive molecules are β-endorphin, bradykinin, PAF, and prostacyclin. Agents that inhibit the synthesis or action of each of these mediators can prevent or reverse endotoxic shock in animals. However, in clinical trials, neither a PAF receptor antagonist nor a bradykinin antagonist improved the survival rate of patients with septic shock, and a NOS inhibitor, L-N^G-methylarginine HCl, actually increased the mortality rate.

Control mechanisms Elaborate host mechanisms regulate both microbial signals and the inflammatory response. While plasma LBP promotes the inflammatory response by facilitating the interaction of LPS with monocyte cell-surface CD14, LBP and other plasma proteins (such as phospholipid transfer protein) also can prevent LPS signaling by transferring LPS molecules into plasma lipoprotein particles. The relative plasma concentrations of LPS, LBP, CD14, and lipoproteins may therefore govern the intensity with which LPS—and probably other microbial molecules—can trigger host responses. The mechanisms that control the inflammatory response are also complex, overlapping, and poorly understood. Glucocorticoids inhibit cytokine synthesis by monocytes in vitro and, when administered with or shortly after an inflammatory stimulus, may protect animals from septic shock. The increase in blood cortisol levels early in the septic response presumably plays a similar inhibitory role. In addition, certain cytokine antagonists may contribute. Blood levels of IL-1 receptor antagonist (IL-1Ra) often greatly exceed those of circulating IL-1β, and this excess may result in inhibition of the binding of IL-1β to its receptors. Transforming growth factor β (TGF-β) and IL-10 can also inhibit LPS-induced responses by human monocytes in vitro and prevent endotoxic death in animals. Blood and tissue levels of prostaglandin E$_2$, TGF-β, α-melanocyte-stimulating hormone, cortisol, IL-1Ra, soluble TNF receptors, and IL-10 increase during the septic response, and these molecules probably act in concert to diminish its intensity. In fact, very high concentrations of many anti-inflammatory molecules are found in the blood of patients with severe sepsis or septic shock, so that the net mediator balance in the blood of these extremely sick patients may actually be anti-inflammatory. In addition, blood leukocytes from patients with severe sepsis are often hyporesponsive to agonists such as LPS. In patients with severe sepsis, persistence of leukocyte hyporesponsiveness has been associated with an increased risk of dying. Research is needed to clarify the role of the anti-inflammatory response in the septic process.

CLINICAL MANIFESTATIONS   The manifestations of the septic response are usually superimposed on the symptoms and signs of the patient's underlying illness and primary infection. The systemic response to infection often intensifies over time from mild (sepsis) to extremely severe (septic shock). The rate at which the response increases may differ from patient to patient, and there are striking individual variations in its manifestations. For example, some patients with sepsis are normo- or hypothermic; the absence of fever is most common in neonates, in elderly patients, and in persons with uremia or alcoholism.

Hyperventilation is often an early sign. Disorientation, confusion, and other manifestations of encephalopathy may also develop early in the septic response, particularly in the elderly and in individuals with preexisting neurologic impairment. Focal neurologic signs are uncommon, although preexisting focal deficits may become more prominent.

Hypotension and DIC predispose to acrocyanosis and ischemic necrosis of peripheral tissues, most commonly the digits. Cellulitis, pustules, bullae, or hemorrhagic lesions may develop when hematogenous bacteria or fungi seed the skin or underlying soft tissue. Bacterial toxins may also be distributed hematogenously to elicit diffuse cutaneous reactions. On occasion, skin lesions may suggest specific pathogens. When sepsis is accompanied by cutaneous petechiae or purpura, infection with *Neisseria meningitidis* (or, less commonly, *Haemophilus influenzae*) should be suspected **(Plate IID-44)**; in a patient who has been bitten by a tick while in an endemic area, petechial lesions also suggest Rocky Mountain spotted fever **(Plate IID-45)**. A cutaneous lesion seen almost exclusively in neutropenic patients is ecthyma gangrenosum, usually caused by *Pseudomonas aeruginosa*. It is a bullous lesion, surrounded by edema, that undergoes central hemorrhage and necrosis **(Plate IID-57C)**. Histopathologic examination shows bacteria in and around the wall of a small vessel, with little or no neutrophilic response. Hemorrhagic or bullous lesions in a septic patient who has recently eaten raw oysters suggest *Vibrio vulnificus* bacteremia, while such lesions in a patient who has recently suffered a dog bite may indicate bloodstream infection due to *Capnocytophaga canimorsus* or *C. cynodegmi*. Generalized erythroderma in a septic patient suggests the toxic shock syndrome due to *Staphylococcus aureus* or *Streptococcus pyogenes*.

Gastrointestinal manifestations such as nausea, vomiting, diarrhea, and ileus may suggest acute gastroenteritis. Stress ulceration can lead to upper gastrointestinal bleeding. Cholestatic jaundice, with elevated levels of serum bilirubin (mostly conjugated) and alkaline phosphatase, may precede other signs of sepsis. Hepatocellular or canalicular dysfunction appears to underlie most cases, and the results of hepatic function tests return to normal with resolution of the infection. Prolonged or severe hypotension may induce acute hepatic injury or ischemic bowel necrosis.

Many tissues may be unable to extract oxygen normally from the blood, so that anaerobic metabolism occurs despite near-normal mixed venous oxygen saturation. Blood lactate levels rise early, in part because of increased glycolysis with impaired clearance of the resulting lactate and pyruvate by the liver and kidneys. As hypoperfusion develops, tissue hypoxia generates more lactic acid, contributing to metabolic acidosis. The blood glucose concentration often increases, particularly in patients with diabetes, although impaired gluconeogenesis and excessive insulin release on occasion produce hypoglycemia. The cytokine-driven acute-phase response inhibits the synthesis of albumin and transthyretin while enhancing the production of C-reactive protein, LBP, fibrinogen, and complement components. Protein catabolism is often markedly accelerated.

MAJOR COMPLICATIONS   Cardiopulmonary Complications   Ventilation-perfusion mismatching produces a fall in arterial P$_{O_2}$ early in the course. Increasing alveolar capillary permeability results in an increased pulmonary water content, which decreases pulmonary compliance and interferes with oxygen exchange. Progressive diffuse pulmonary infiltrates and arterial hypoxemia (Pa$_{O_2}$/FI$_{O_2}$, <200 mmHg) indicate the development of the acute respiratory distress syndrome (ARDS). ARDS develops in ~50% of patients with severe sepsis or septic shock. The failure of the respiratory muscles can exacerbate hypoxemia and hypercapnia. An elevated pulmonary capillary wedge pressure (>18 mmHg) suggests fluid volume overload or cardiac failure rather than ARDS. Pneumonia caused by viruses or by *Pneumocystis carinii* may be clinically indistinguishable from ARDS.

Sepsis-induced hypotension usually results from a generalized maldistribution of blood flow and blood volume and from hypovolemia that is due, at least in part, to diffuse capillary leakage of intravascular fluid. Other factors that may decrease effective intravascular volume include dehydration from antecedent disease or insensible fluid losses, vomiting or diarrhea, and polyuria. During early septic shock, systemic vascular resistance is usually elevated and cardiac output may be low. After fluid repletion, in contrast, cardiac output typically increases and systemic vascular resistance falls. Indeed, normal or increased cardiac output and decreased systemic vascular resistance distinguish septic shock from cardiogenic, extracardiac obstructive, and hypovolemic shock; other processes that can produce this combination include anaphylaxis, beriberi, cirrhosis, and overdoses of nitroprusside or narcotics (Chap. 38).

Depression of myocardial function, manifested as increased end-diastolic and systolic ventricular volumes with a decreased ejection fraction, develops within 24 h in most patients with severe sepsis. Cardiac output is maintained despite the low ejection fraction because ventricular dilatation permits a normal stroke volume. In survivors, myocardial function returns to normal over several days. Although myocardial dysfunction may contribute to hypotension, refractory hypotension is usually due to a low systemic vascular resistance, and death results from refractory shock or the failure of multiple organs rather than from cardiac dysfunction per se.

Renal Complications   Oliguria, azotemia, proteinuria, and nonspecific urinary casts are frequently found. Many patients are inappropriately polyuric; hyperglycemia may exacerbate this tendency. Most renal failure is due to acute tubular necrosis induced by hypotension or capillary injury, although some patients also have glomerulonephritis, renal cortical necrosis, or interstitial nephritis. Drug-induced renal damage may complicate therapy, particularly when hypotensive patients are given aminoglycoside antibiotics.

Coagulation   Although thrombocytopenia occurs in 10 to 30% of patients, the underlying mechanism(s) are not understood. Platelet counts are usually very low (<50,000/μL) in patients with DIC; these low counts typically reflect diffuse endothelial injury or microvascular thrombosis.

Neurologic Complications   When the septic illness lasts for weeks to months, "critical-illness" polyneuropathy may prevent weaning from ventilatory support and produce distal motor weakness. Electrophysiologic studies are diagnostic. Guillain-Barré syndrome, metabolic disturbances, and toxin activity must be ruled out.

LABORATORY FINDINGS Abnormalities that occur early in the septic response may include leukocytosis with a left shift, thrombocytopenia, hyperbilirubinemia, and proteinuria. Leukopenia may develop. The neutrophils may contain toxic granulations, Döhle bodies, or cytoplasmic vacuoles. As the septic response becomes more severe, thrombocytopenia worsens (often with prolongation of the thrombin time, decreased fibrinogen, and the presence of D-dimers, suggesting DIC), azotemia and hyperbilirubinemia become more prominent, and levels of aminotransferases rise. Active hemolysis suggests clostridial bacteremia, malaria, a drug reaction, or DIC; in the case of DIC, microangiopathic changes may be seen on a blood smear.

During early sepsis, hyperventilation induces respiratory alkalosis. With respiratory muscle fatigue and the accumulation of lactate, metabolic acidosis (with increased anion gap) typically supervenes. Evaluation of arterial blood gases reveals hypoxemia, which is initially correctable with supplemental oxygen but whose later refractoriness to 100% oxygen inhalation indicates right-to-left shunting. The chest radiograph may be normal or may show evidence of underlying pneumonia, volume overload, or the diffuse infiltrates of ARDS. The electrocardiogram may show only sinus tachycardia or nonspecific ST-T wave abnormalities.

Most diabetic patients with sepsis develop hyperglycemia. Severe infection may precipitate diabetic ketoacidosis, which may exacerbate hypotension (Chap. 333). Hypoglycemia occurs rarely. The serum albumin level, initially within the normal range, declines as sepsis continues. Serum lipid concentrations are often elevated. Hypocalcemia is rare.

DIAGNOSIS There is no specific test. Diagnostically sensitive findings in a patient with suspected or proven infection include fever or hypothermia, tachypnea, tachycardia, and leukocytosis or leukopenia (Table 124-1); acutely altered mental status, thrombocytopenia, or hypotension also suggests the diagnosis. The septic response can be quite variable, however. In one study, 36% of patients with severe sepsis had a normal temperature, 40% had a normal respiratory rate, 10% had a normal pulse rate, and 33% had normal white blood cell counts. Moreover, the systemic responses of uninfected patients with other conditions may be similar to those characteristic of sepsis. Noninfectious etiologies of SIRS (Table 124-1) include pancreatitis, burns, trauma, adrenal insufficiency, pulmonary embolism, dissecting or ruptured aortic aneurysm, myocardial infarction, occult hemorrhage, cardiac tamponade, post-cardiopulmonary bypass syndrome, anaphylaxis, and drug overdose.

Definitive etiologic diagnosis requires isolation of the microorganism from blood or a local site of infection. At least two blood samples (10 mL each) should be obtained (from different venipuncture sites) for culture. Because gram-negative bacteremia is typically low-grade (<10 organisms per milliliter of blood), multiple blood cultures or prolonged incubation of cultures may be necessary; *S. aureus* grows more readily and is detectable in blood cultures within 48 h in most instances. In many cases, blood cultures are negative; this result can reflect prior antibiotic administration, the presence of slow-growing or fastidious organisms, or the absence of microbial invasion of the bloodstream. In these cases, Gram's staining and culture of material from the primary site of infection or of infected cutaneous lesions may help establish the microbial etiology. The skin and mucosae should be examined carefully and repeatedly for lesions that might yield diagnostic information. With overwhelming bacteremia (e.g., pneumococcal sepsis in splenectomized individuals or fulminant meningococcemia), microorganisms are sometimes visible on buffy coat smears of peripheral blood.

Detection of endotoxin in blood by the limulus lysate test may portend a poor outcome, but this assay is not useful for diagnosing gram-negative bacterial infections, including gram-negative bacteremia. Although blood levels of IL-6 also may correlate with prognosis,

cytokine assays are poorly standardized and currently have limited clinical value.

℞ TREATMENT Patients in whom sepsis is suspected must be managed expeditiously. This task is best accomplished in an intensive care unit by personnel who are experienced in the care of the critically ill. Successful management requires urgent measures to treat the local site of infection, to provide hemodynamic and respiratory support, and to eliminate the offending microorganism. The outcome is also influenced by the patient's underlying disease, which should be managed aggressively.

Antimicrobial Agents Antimicrobial chemotherapy should be initiated as soon as samples of blood and other relevant sites have been cultured. The choice of initial therapy is based on knowledge of the likely pathogens at specific sites of local infection. Available information about patterns of antimicrobial susceptibility among bacterial isolates from the community, the hospital, and the patient also should be taken into account. It is important, pending culture results, to initiate empirical antimicrobial therapy that is effective against both gram-positive and gram-negative bacteria (Table 124-3). Maximal recommended doses of antimicrobial drugs should be given intravenously, with adjustment for impaired renal function when necessary. When

Table 124-3 Initial Antimicrobial Therapy for Severe Sepsis with No Obvious Source in Adults with Normal Renal Function

Clinical Condition	Antimicrobial Regimens (Intravenous Therapy)
Immunocompetent adult	The many acceptable regimens include (1) ceftriaxone (1 g q12h) *or* ticarcillin-clavulanate (3.1 g q4-6h) *or* piperacillin-tazobactam (3.75 g q4–6h); (2) imipenem-cilastatin (0.5 g q6h) *or* meropenem (1 g q8h). Gentamicin or tobramycin (5 mg/kg q24h) may be *added* to either regimen. If the patient is allergic to β-lactam agents, use ciprofloxacin (400 mg q12h) *plus* clindamycin (600 mg q8h). If the institution has a high incidence of MRSA infections, *add* vancomycin (15 mg/kg q12h) to each of the above regimens.
Neutropenia[a] (<500 neutrophils/μL)	Regimens include (1) ceftazidime (2 g q8h) *or* ticarcillin-clavulanate (3.1 g q4h) *or* piperacillin-tazobactam (3.75 g q4h) *plus* tobramycin (5 mg/kg q24h); (2) imipenem-cilastatin (0.5 g q6h) *or* meropenem (1 g q8h) *or* ceftazidime *or* cefepime (2 g q12h). Vancomycin (15 mg/kg q12h) and ceftazidime should be used if the patient has an infected vascular catheter, if staphylococci are suspected, if the patient has received quinolone prophylaxis, if the patient has received intensive chemotherapy that produces mucosal damage, or if the institution has a high incidence of MRSA infections.
Splenectomy	Cefotaxime (2 g q6–8h) *or* ceftriaxone (2 g q12h) should be used. If the local prevalence of cephalosporin-resistant pneumococci is high, *add* vancomycin. If the patient is allergic to β-lactam drugs, vancomycin (15 mg/kg q12h) *plus* ciprofloxacin (400 mg q12h) *or* aztreonam (2 g q8h) should be used.
IV drug user	Nafcillin *or* oxacillin (2 g q4h) *plus* gentamicin (5 mg/kg q24h). If the local prevalence of MRSA is high or if the patient is allergic to β-lactam drugs, vancomycin (15 mg/kg q12h) with gentamicin should be used.
AIDS	Ceftazidime (2 g q8h), ticarcillin-clavulanate (3.1 g q4h), *or* piperacillin-tazobactam (3.75 g q4h) *plus* tobramycin (5 mg/kg q24h) should be used. If the patient is allergic to β-lactam drugs, ciprofloxacin (400 mg q12h) *plus* vancomycin (15 mg/kg q12h) *plus* tobramycin should be used.

[a] Adapted in part from WT Hughes et al: Clin Infect Dis 25:551, 1997.
NOTE: MRSA, methicillin-resistant *Staphylococcus aureus*.

culture results become available, the regimen can often be simplified, as a single antimicrobial agent is frequently adequate for the treatment of a known pathogen. Most patients require antimicrobial therapy for at least 1 week; the duration of treatment is typically influenced by factors such as the site of tissue infection, the adequacy of surgical drainage, the patient's underlying disease, and the antimicrobial susceptibility of the bacterial isolate(s).

Removal of the Source of Infection Removal or drainage of a focal source of infection is essential. Sites of occult infection should be sought carefully. Indwelling intravenous catheters should be removed, the tip rolled over a blood agar plate for quantitative culture, and a new catheter inserted at a different site. Foley and drainage catheters should be replaced. The possibility of paranasal sinusitis (often caused by gram-negative bacteria) should be considered if the patient has undergone nasal intubation. In the neutropenic patient, cutaneous sites of tenderness and erythema, particularly in the perianal region, must be carefully sought. In patients with sacral or ischial decubitus ulcers, it is important to exclude pelvic or other soft-tissue pus collections (by computed tomography or magnetic resonance imaging, if necessary). In patients with severe sepsis arising from the urinary tract, sonography or computed tomography should be used to rule out ureteral obstruction, perinephric abscess, and renal abscess. These studies are not so urgent in patients with less severe urosepsis, provided that a clinical response is evident within 48 to 72 h.

Hemodynamic, Respiratory, and Metabolic Support (See also Chap. 38) The primary goal is to restore adequate oxygen and substrate delivery to the tissues. Adequate organ perfusion is essential. Effective intravascular volume depletion is common in patients with sepsis, and initial management of hypotension should include the administration of intravenous fluids, typically 1 to 2 L of normal saline over 1 to 2 h. The pulmonary capillary wedge pressure or the central venous pressure must be monitored in patients with refractory shock or underlying cardiac or renal disease. To avoid pulmonary edema, the pulmonary capillary wedge pressure should be maintained between 12 and 16 mmHg or the central venous pressure between 10 and 12 cmH$_2$O. The urine output rate should be kept above 30 mL/h by continuing fluid administration; a diuretic such as furosemide may be used if needed. In about one-third of patients, hypotension and organ hypoperfusion respond to fluid resuscitation; a reasonable goal is to maintain a mean arterial blood pressure of >60 mmHg (systolic pressure, >90 mmHg) and a cardiac index of ≥4 (L/min)/m^2. If these guidelines cannot be met by volume infusion, inotropic and vasopressor therapy is indicated (Chap. 38). Circulatory adequacy is also assessed by clinical parameters (mentation, urine output, skin perfusion) and, when possible, by measurements of oxygen delivery and consumption.

Adrenal insufficiency should be considered in septic patients with refractory hypotension, fulminant *N. meningitidis* bacteremia, prior glucocorticoid use, disseminated tuberculosis, or AIDS. The cosyntropin (α^{1-24}-ACTH) stimulation test (Chap. 331) may suggest absolute or partial adrenal insufficiency. Supplemental hydrocortisone (50 mg intravenously every 6 h) may be given while the results of the cosyntropin test are awaited.

Ventilator therapy is indicated for progressive hypoxemia, hypercapnia, neurologic deterioration, or respiratory muscle failure. Sustained tachypnea (respiratory rate, >30 breaths/min) is frequently a harbinger of impending respiratory collapse; mechanical ventilation is often initiated to ensure adequate oxygenation, divert blood from the muscles of respiration, prevent aspiration of oropharyngeal contents, and reduce the cardiac afterload. Blood or erythrocyte transfusion is indicated if oxygen delivery is compromised by a low hemoglobin concentration (<8 to 10 g/dL).

Bicarbonate is sometimes administered for severe metabolic acidosis (arterial pH < 7.2). DIC, if complicated by major bleeding, should be treated with transfusion of fresh-frozen plasma and platelets. Successful treatment of the underlying infection is essential to reverse both acidosis and DIC.

These are consensus recommendations; none of these generally accepted components of resuscitative care has been validated in randomized clinical trials.

General Support In patients with prolonged severe sepsis (i.e., that lasting more than 2 or 3 days), nutritional supplementation may reduce the impact of protein hypercatabolism; available evidence favors the enteral delivery route. Recovery is also assisted by preventing skin breakdown, deep venous thrombosis, nosocomial infections, and stress ulcers.

Other Measures Despite aggressive management, many patients with severe sepsis or septic shock die. Two kinds of agents that may help prevent these deaths are being investigated: (1) drugs that neutralize bacterial endotoxin, thereby potentially benefiting the fraction (approximately half) of septic patients who have gram-negative bacterial infection, and (2) drugs that interfere with one or more mediators of the inflammatory response and may benefit all patients with sepsis.

Antiendotoxin agents Lipid A, the toxic moiety of endotoxin, is conserved in the LPS of gram-negative bacteria. Despite much effort to develop drugs that bind lipid A and neutralize endotoxin in vivo, the potential of endotoxin as a target for therapeutic intervention remains controversial. In placebo-controlled clinical trials, two monoclonal antibodies to endotoxin did not prevent the death of patients with severe gram-negative bacterial sepsis. In retrospective studies, these antibodies did not bind to LPS with high affinity, and one was reported to be a polyreactive autoantibody. A theoretically more promising agent is bactericidal permeability-increasing protein, a human neutrophil protein that neutralizes the toxicity of lipid A and may be bactericidal to many gram-negative bacteria. In one clinical trial, this protein decreased morbidity and mortality among children with fulminant meningococcemia. Other investigational drugs include nontoxic lipid A analogs that reduce host responses to endotoxins and lipoproteins (such as high-density lipoprotein) that bind and neutralize endotoxin in the circulation and can remove it from the surfaces of myeloid cells.

Antimediator agents Other adjunctive therapies are intended to control the inflammatory response, regardless of the microbial stimulus. However, numerous agents that directly or indirectly interfere with the actions of inflammatory mediators have not prevented the death of patients with severe sepsis or septic shock. Many factors have probably contributed to the unsuccessful outcomes of these trials, including problems with study design (inappropriate end points, inadequate sample size, population heterogeneity, multiple covariates) and drug administration (wrong dose, time, or duration of administration). Anti-inflammatory drugs tested in clinical trials include methylprednisolone, ibuprofen, recombinant IL-1Ra, genetically engineered soluble receptors for TNF-α, and monoclonal antibodies to TNF-α. Because TNF-α and IL-1β doubtless play key roles in antimicrobial host defense, neutralizing these cytokines could be detrimental in some cases. In addition, studies suggest that many anti-inflammatory molecules, including soluble TNF receptors and IL-1Ra, may already be present at high concentrations in the plasma of patients with septic shock. Identifying beneficial regimens of treatment with drugs that neutralize TNF-α and IL-1β may therefore be very difficult. Clinical trials are testing drugs (antithrombin, activated protein C, tissue factor pathway inhibitor) intended to prevent or reverse microthombosis and evaluating regimens in which low doses of glucocorticoids are administered for prolonged periods.

All of the more recent clinical trials have enrolled patients with severe sepsis or septic shock. Neither the ability of adjunctive agents to prevent severe sepsis or septic shock in high-risk patients nor the value of combination therapy with two or more adjunctive drugs has been tested.

PROGNOSIS Approximately 20 to 35% of patients with severe sepsis and 40 to 60% of patients with septic shock die within 30 days. Others die within the ensuing 6 months. Late deaths often result from poorly controlled infection, complications of intensive care, failure of multiple organs, or the patient's underlying disease.

Several prognostic stratification systems indicate that factoring in the patient's age, underlying condition, and various physiologic variables can yield estimates of the risk of dying of severe sepsis. Of the individual covariates, the severity of underlying disease most strongly influences the risk of dying. Septic shock is also a strong predictor of short- and long-term mortality. Case-fatality rates are similar for culture-positive and culture-negative severe sepsis.

PREVENTION   Prevention offers the best opportunity to reduce morbidity and mortality. Most episodes of severe sepsis and septic shock are nosocomial. These cases might be prevented by reducing the number of invasive procedures undertaken, by limiting the use (and duration of use) of indwelling vascular and bladder catheters, by reducing the incidence and duration of profound neutropenia (<500 neutrophils/μL), and by more aggressively treating localized nosocomial infections. Indiscriminate use of antimicrobial agents and glucocorticoids should be avoided, and optimal infection-control measures (Chap. 134) should be used. In addition, prompt and aggressive management of patients with sepsis is imperative. Studies indicate that 50 to 70% of patients who develop nosocomial severe sepsis or septic shock have experienced a less severe stage of the septic response (e.g., SIRS, sepsis) on at least one previous day in the hospital. Research is needed to identify patients at high risk for severe sepsis and to develop adjunctive agents that can damp the septic response before organ dysfunction or hypotension occurs.

BIBLIOGRAPHY

AMERICAN COLLEGE OF CHEST PHYSICIANS/SOCIETY OF CRITICAL CARE MEDICINE CONSENSUS CONFERENCE COMMITTEE: Definitions for sepsis and organ failure and guidelines for the use of innovative therapies in sepsis. Crit Care Med 20:864, 1992

ASTIZ ME, RACKOW EC: Septic shock. Lancet 351:1501, 1998

BRUN-BUISSON C et al: Bacteremia and severe sepsis in adults: A multicenter prospective survey in ICUs and wards of 24 hospitals. Am J Respir Crit Care Med 154:617, 1996

CAIN BS et al: The physiologic basis for anticytokine clinical trials in the treatment of sepsis. J Am Coll Surg 186:337, 1998

EIDELMAN LA et al: The spectrum of septic encephalopathy. Definitions, etiologies, and mortalities. JAMA 275:470, 1996

JAMES JH et al: Lactate is an unreliable indicator of tissue hypoxia in injury or sepsis. Lancet 354:505, 1999

LEVI M et al: The cytokine-mediated imbalance between coagulant and anticoagulant mechanisms in sepsis and endotoxaemia. Eur J Clin Invest 27:3, 1997

QUARTIN AA et al: Magnitude and duration of the effect of sepsis on survival. JAMA 277:1058, 1997

RANGEL-FRAUSTO MS et al: The natural history of the systemic inflammatory response syndrome (SIRS). A prospective study. JAMA 273:117, 1995

SANDS KE et al: Epidemiology of sepsis syndrome in 8 academic medical centers. JAMA 278:234, 1997

WHEELER AP, BERNARD GR: Treating patients with severe sepsis. N Engl J Med 340:207, 1999

| **125** | *Jeffrey A. Gelfand* |

FEVER OF UNKNOWN ORIGIN

CMV cytomegalovirus	MRI magnetic resonance imaging
CSF cerebrospinal fluid	NSAIDs nonsteroidal anti-
CT computed tomography	inflammatory agents
ESR erythrocyte sedimentation rate	PCR polymerase chain reaction
FUO fever of unknown origin	PPD purified protein derivative
IDSA Infectious Diseases Society of	
America	

DEFINITION AND CLASSIFICATION   *Fever of unknown origin* (FUO) was defined by Petersdorf and Beeson in 1961 as (1)

temperatures >38.3°C (101°F) on several occasions; (2) a duration of fever of >3 weeks; and (3) failure to reach a diagnosis despite 1 week of inpatient investigation. While this classification has stood for more than 30 years, Durack and Street have proposed a new system for classification of FUO: (1) classic FUO; (2) nosocomial FUO; (3) neutropenic FUO; and (4) FUO associated with HIV infection (Table 125-1).

Classic FUO   Classic FUO corresponds closely to the earlier definition of FUO, differing only with regard to the prior requirement for 1 week's study in the hospital. The new definition is broader, stipulating three outpatient visits or 3 days in the hospital without elucidation of a cause or 1 week of "intelligent and invasive" ambulatory investigation.

Nosocomial FUO   In nosocomial FUO, a temperature of ≥38.3°C (101°F) develops on several occasions in a hospitalized patient who is receiving acute care and in whom infection was not manifest or incubating on admission. Three days of investigation, including at least 2 days' incubation of cultures, is the minimum requirement for this diagnosis.

Neutropenic FUO   Neutropenic FUO is defined as a temperature of ≥38.3°C (101°F) on several occasions in a patient whose neutrophil count is <500/μL or is expected to fall to that level in 1 to 2 days. The diagnosis of neutropenic FUO is invoked if a specific cause is not identified after 3 days of investigation, including at least 2 days' incubation of cultures.

HIV-Associated FUO   FUO associated with HIV infection is defined by a temperature of ≥38.3°C (101°F) on several occasions over a period of >4 weeks for outpatients or >3 days for hospitalized patients with HIV infection. This diagnosis is invoked if appropriate investigation over 3 days, including 2 days' incubation of cultures, reveals no source.

Adoption of these categories of FUO on a wide scale in the literature would allow a more rational compilation of data regarding these disparate groups. In the remainder of this chapter, the discussion will focus on classic FUO unless otherwise specified.

CAUSES OF CLASSIC FUO   Table 125-2 summarizes the findings of several large studies of FUO carried out since the advent of the antibiotic era, including a prospective study of 167 adult patients with FUO encompassing all 8 university hospitals in the Netherlands and using a standardized protocol in which the first author reviewed every patient. Coincident with the widespread use of antibiotics, increasingly useful diagnostic technologies—both noninvasive and invasive—have been developed. Newer studies reflect not only changing patterns of disease but also the impact of diagnostic techniques that make it possible to eliminate many patients with specific illness from the FUO category. The ubiquitous use of microbiologic cultures and the widespread use of potent broad-spectrum antibiotics may have decreased the number of infections causing FUO. The wide availability of ultrasonography, computed tomography (CT), and magnetic resonance imaging (MRI) has enhanced the detection of occult neoplasms and lymphomas in patients previously thought to have FUO. Likewise, the widespread availability of highly specific and sensitive immunologic testing has reduced the number of undetected cases of systemic lupus erythematosus and other autoimmune diseases.

Several generalizations can be made. Infections, especially extrapulmonary tuberculosis, remain the leading diagnosable cause of FUO. Prolonged mononucleosis syndromes caused by Epstein-Barr virus, cytomegalovirus (CMV), or HIV are conditions whose consideration as a cause of FUO is sometimes confounded by delayed antibody responses. Intraabdominal abscesses (sometimes poorly localized) and renal, retroperitoneal, and paraspinal abscesses continue to be difficult to diagnose. Renal malacoplakia, with submucosal plaques or nodules involving the urinary tract, may cause FUO and is often fatal if untreated. It is associated with coliform infection, is seen most often in patients with defects of intracellular bacterial killing, and is treated with fluoroquinolones or trimethoprim-sulfamethoxazole. Occasionally, other organs may be involved. Osteomyelitis, especially where prosthetic devices have been implanted, and infective endocarditis

Table 125-1   Categories of FUO[a]

	Category of FUO			
Feature	**Nosocomial**	**Neutropenic**	**HIV-Associated**	**Classic**
Patient's situation	Hospitalized, acute care, no infection when admitted	Neutrophil count either <500/μL or expected to reach that level in 1–2 days	Confirmed HIV-positive	All others with fevers for $\geq$3 weeks
Duration of illness while under investigation	3 days[b]	3 days[b]	3 days[b] (or 4 weeks as outpatient)	3 days[b] or three outpatient visits
Examples of cause	Septic thrombophlebitis, sinusitis, *Clostridium difficile* colitis, drug fever	Perianal infection, aspergillosis, candidemia	MAI[c] infection, tuberculosis, non-Hodgkin's lymphoma, drug fever	Infections, malignancy, inflammatory diseases, drug fever

[a] All require temperatures of $\geq$38.3°C (101°F) on several occasions.
[b] Includes at least 2 days' incubation of microbiology cultures.
[c] *M. avium/M. intracellulare.*

SOURCE: Modified from DT Durack, AC Street, in JS Remington, MN Swartz (eds): *Current Clinical Topics in Infectious Diseases.* Cambridge, MA, Blackwell, 1991.

Table 125-2   Classic FUO in Adults

Authors (Year of Publication)	Years of Study	No. of Cases	Infections (%)	Neoplasms (%)	Noninfectious Inflammatory Diseases (%)	Miscellaneous Causes (%)	Undiagnosed Causes (%)
Petersdorf and Beeson (1961)	1952–1957	100	36	19	19[a]	19[a]	7
Larson and Featherstone (1982)	1970–1980	105	32	20	16[a]	11[a]	7
Knockaert and Vanneste (1992)	1980–1989	199	22.5	7	23[a]	21.5[a]	25.5
DeKleijn et al. (1997, Part I)	1992–1994	167	26	12.5	24	8	30

[a] Authors' raw data retabulated to conform to altered diagnostic categories.

SOURCE: Modified from DeKleijn et al., 1997 (Part I).

must be considered. Although true culture-negative infective endocarditis is rare, one may be misled by slow-growing organisms of the HACEK group (*Haemophilus aphrophilus, Actinobacillus actinomycetemcomitans, Cardiobacterium hominis, Eikenella corrodens,* and *Kingella kingae*; Chap. 150), *Bartonella* spp. (previously *Rochalimaea*), *Legionella* spp., *Coxiella burnetii, Chlamydia psittaci,* and fungi. Prostatitis, dental abscesses, sinusitis, and cholangitis continue to be sources of occult fever.

Fungal disease, most notably histoplasmosis involving the reticuloendothelial system, may cause FUO. FUO with headache should prompt examination of spinal fluid for *Cryptococcus neoformans.* Malaria (which may result from transfusion, the failure to take a prescribed prophylactic agent, or infection with a drug-resistant strain) continues to be a cause, particularly of nonsynchronized FUO. A related protozoan species, *Babesia,* may cause FUO and is increasing in incidence.

In most earlier series, neoplasms were the next most common cause of FUO after infections (Table 125-3). In the two most recent series, a decrease in the percentage of FUO cases due to malignancy was attributed to improvement in diagnostic technologies. This observation does not diminish the importance of considering neoplasia in the initial diagnostic evaluation of a patient with fever. A number of patients in these series had temporal arteritis, adult Still's disease, drug-related fever, and factitious fever. In recent series, approximately 25 to 30% of cases of FUO have remained undiagnosed. The general term *noninfectious inflammatory diseases* applies to systemic rheumatologic or vasculitic diseases such as polymyalgia rheumatica, lupus, and adult Still's disease as well as to granulomatous diseases such as sarcoidosis and Crohn's and granulomatous hepatitis.

Table 125-3   Malignancies Commonly Associated with FUO

Hodgkin's disease
Non-Hodgkin's lymphoma
Leukemia (including preleukemic and aleukemic phases)
Renal cell carcinoma
Hepatoma
Colon carcinoma

In the elderly, multisystem disease is the most frequent cause of FUO, giant cell arteritis being the leading etiologic entity in this category. Tuberculosis is the most common infection causing FUO in the elderly, and colon cancer is an important cause of FUO with malignancy.

Many diseases have been grouped in the various studies as "miscellaneous." On this list are drug fever, pulmonary embolism, factitious fever, familial Mediterranean fever, and Fabry's disease.

A drug-related etiology must be considered in any case of prolonged fever. Any febrile pattern may be elicited by a drug, and both relative bradycardia and hypotension are uncommon. Eosinophilia and/or rash is found in only one-fifth of patients with drug fever, which usually begins 1 to 3 weeks after the start of therapy and remits 2 to 3 days after therapy is stopped. Virtually all classes of drugs cause fever, but antimicrobials (especially β-lactam antibiotics), cardiovascular drugs (e.g., quinidine), antineoplastic drugs, and drugs acting on the central nervous system (e.g., phenytoin) are particularly common causes.

It is axiomatic that, as the duration of fever increases, the likelihood of an infectious cause decreases (Table 125-4). In a series of 347

Table 125-4   Causes of FUO Lasting >6 Months

Cause	Cases (%)
None identified	19
Miscellaneous causes	13
Factitious causes	9
Granulomatous hepatitis	8
Neoplasm	7
Still's disease	6
Infection	6
Collagen vascular disease	4
Familial Mediterranean fever	3
No fever[a]	27

[a] No actual fever observed during 2 to 3 weeks of inpatient observation. Includes patients with exaggerated circadian rhythm.
SOURCE: From a study of 347 patients referred to the National Institutes of Health from 1961 to 1977 with a presumptive diagnosis of FUO of >6 months' duration (Aduan et al.)

patients referred to the National Institutes of Health from 1961 to 1977, only 6% had an infection. A significant proportion (9%) had factitious fevers—i.e., fevers due either to false elevations of temperature or to self-induced disease. A substantial number of these factitious cases were in young women in the health professions. It is worth noting that 8% of the patients with prolonged fevers (some of whom had completely normal liver function studies) had granulomatous hepatitis, and 6% had adult Still's disease. After prolonged investigation, 19% of cases still had no specific diagnosis. A total of 27% of patients either

had no actual fever during the weeks of inpatient observation or had an exaggerated circadian temperature rhythm without chills, elevated pulse, or other abnormalities.

The conditions that may be considered in a differential diagnosis of classic FUO in adults are listed in Table 125-5. This list applies strictly to the United States; the frequency of global travel underscores the need for a detailed travel history, and the continuing emergence of new infectious diseases makes this listing potentially incomplete.

SPECIALIZED DIAGNOSTIC STUDIES   Classic FUO Certain specific diagnostic maneuvers become critical in dealing with prolonged fevers. If factitious fever is suspected, electronic thermom-

Table 125-5   Causes of FUO in Adults in the United States

Infections
  Localized pyogenic infections
    Appendicitis
    Cat-scratch disease
    Cholangitis
    Cholecystitis
    Dental abscess
    Diverticulitis/abscess
    Lesser sac abscess
    Liver abscess
    Mesenteric lymphadenitis
    Osteomyelitis
    Pancreatic abscess
    Pelvic inflammatory disease
    Perinephric/intrarenal abscess
    Prostatic abscess
    Renal malacoplakia
    Sinusitis
    Subphrenic abscess
    Suppurative thrombophlebitis
    Tuboovarian abscess
  Intravascular infections
    Bacterial aortitis
    Bacterial endocarditis
    Vascular catheter infection
  Systemic bacterial infections
    Bartonellosis
    Brucellosis
    Campylobacter infection
    Cat-scratch disease/bacillary angiomatosis
      (*B. henselae*)
    Gonococcemia
    Legionnaires' disease
    Leptospirosis
    Listeriosis
    Lyme disease
    Melioidosis
    Meningococcemia
    Rat-bite fever
    Relapsing fever
    Salmonellosis
    Syphilis
    Tularemia
    Typhoid fever
    Vibriosis
    Yersinia infection
  Mycobacterial infections
    M. avium/M. intracellulare infections
    Other atypical mycobacterial infections
    Tuberculosis
  Fungal infections
    Aspergillosis
    Blastomycosis
    Candidiasis
    Coccidioidomycosis
    Cryptococcosis
    Histoplasmosis
    Mucormycosis
    Paracoccidioidomycosis
    Sporotrichosis

  Other bacterial infections
    Actinomycosis
    Nocardiosis
    Whipple's disease
  Rickettsial infections
    Ehrlichiosis
    Murine typhus
    Q fever
    Rickettsialpox
    Rocky Mountain spotted fever
  Mycoplasmal infections
  Chlamydial infections
    Lymphogranuloma venereum
    Psittacosis
    TWAR (*C. pneumoniae*) infection
  Viral infections
    Colorado tick fever
    Coxsackievirus group B infection
    Cytomegalovirus infection
    Dengue
    Epstein-Barr virus infection
    Hepatitis A, B, C, D, and E
    Human herpesvirus 6 infection
    Human immunodeficiency virus infection
    Lymphocytic choriomeningitis
    Parvovirus B19 infection
  Parasitic infections
    Amebiasis
    Babesiosis
    Chagas' disease
    Leishmaniasis
    Malaria
    P. carinii infection
    Strongyloidiasis
    Toxocariasis
    Toxoplasmosis
    Trichinosis
  Presumed infections, agent undetermined
    Kawasaki's disease (mucocutaneous lymph
      node syndrome)
    Kikuchi's disease (necrotizing lymphadeni-
      tis)
Neoplasms
  Malignant
    Colon cancer
    Hepatoma
    Hodgkin's lymphoma
    Immunoblastic lymphadenopathy
    Leukemia
    Lymphomatoid granulomatosis
    Malignant histiocytosis
    Nephroma
    Non-Hodgkin's lymphoma
    Pancreatic cancer
    Sarcoma
  Benign
    Atrial myxoma
    Castleman's disease
    Renal angiomyolipoma

Collagen vascular/hypersensitivity diseases
  Adult Still's disease
  Behçet's disease
  Erythema multiforme
  Erythema nodosum
  Giant-cell arteritis/polymyalgia rheumatica
  Hypersensitivity pneumonitis (e.g., "metal fume
    fever," "farmer's lung," "air-conditioner lung")
  Hypersensitivity vasculitis
  Mixed connective-tissue disease
  Polyarteritis nodosa
  Relapsing polychondritis
  Rheumatic fever
  Rheumatoid arthritis
  Schnitzler's syndrome
  Systemic lupus erythematosus
  Takayasu's aortitis
  Weber-Christian disease
  Wegener's granulomatosis
Granulomatous diseases
  Crohn's disease
  Idiopathic granulomatous hepatitis
  Midline granuloma
  Sarcoidosis
Miscellaneous conditions
  Aortic dissection
  Drug fever
  Gout
  Hematomas
  Hemolytic diseases/hemoglobinopathies
  Laennec's cirrhosis
  PFPA syndrome: periodic fever, adenitis, phar-
    yngitis, aphthae
  Postmyocardial infarction syndrome
  Recurrent pulmonary emboli
  Subacute thyroiditis (de Quervain's)
  Tissue infarction/necrosis
Inherited and metabolic diseases
  Adrenal insufficiency
  Cyclic neutropenia
  Deafness, urticaria, and amyloidosis
  Fabry's disease
  Familial Mediterranean fever
  Hyperimmunoglobulinemia D and periodic fever
  Type V hypertriglyceridemia
Thermoregulatory disorders
  Central
    Brain tumor
    Cerebrovascular accident
    Encephalitis
    Hypothalamic dysfunction
  Peripheral
    Hyperthyroidism
    Pheochromocytoma
Factitious fevers
"Afebrile" FUO (<38.3°C)
Habitual hyperthermia (exaggerated circadian
  rhythm)

SOURCE: Modified from RK Root, RG Petersdorf, in JD Wilson et al (eds): *Harrison's Principles of Internal Medicine*, 12th ed. New York, McGraw-Hill, 1991.

eters should be used, temperature-taking should be supervised, and simultaneous urine and body temperatures should be measured. Any tissue removed during prior relevant surgery should be reexamined; slides should be requested, and, if need be, paraffin blocks of fixed pathologic material should be reexamined and additional special studies performed. Relevant x-rays should be reexamined; reviewing of prior radiologic reports may be insufficient. Serum should be set aside in the laboratory as soon as possible and retained for future examination for rising antibody titers. *Febrile agglutinins* is a vague term that in most laboratories refers to serologic studies for salmonellosis, brucellosis, and rickettsial diseases. These studies are seldom useful, having low sensitivity and variable specificity. Rising titers of antibody to *Brucella* (Chap. 160) are usually diagnostic, but false-positive results may be obtained in typhoid fever, tularemia, and yersinial infections. Infection with *Brucella canis* may be missed with standard antibody tests for *Brucella. Salmonella* infection (Chap. 156) elevates antibody titers to the H and O antigens. High titers of antibody to the H antigen persist for years and may reflect previous infection or immunization. Serology for *Yersinia enterocolitica* may be useful. The measurement of specific antirickettsial titers should be requested for the diagnosis of Rocky Mountain spotted fever and Q fever. Multiple blood samples (no fewer than three, rarely more than six), including samples for anaerobic culture, should be cultured in the laboratory for at least 2 weeks to ensure that any HACEK-group organisms that may be present have ample time to grow (Chap. 150). Lysis-centrifugation blood culture techniques should be employed in cases where prior antimicrobial therapy or fungal or atypical mycobacterial infection is suspected. Blood culture media should be supplemented with L-cysteine or pyridoxal to assist in the isolation of nutritionally variant streptococci. It should be noted that sequential cultures positive for multiple organisms may reflect self-injection of contaminated substances. Urine cultures, including cultures for mycobacteria, fungi, and CMV, are indicated. Blood, urine, or cerebrospinal fluid (CSF) can now be tested for a variety of pathogens such as CMV or hepatitis C virus by using the polymerase chain reaction (PCR) to amplify and hence detect viral nucleic acid (Chap. 121). Liver biopsy, even when the results of liver function studies are normal, should be considered and pursued if the diagnosis remains elusive. Specimens should be cultured for mycobacteria and fungi. Likewise, bone marrow biopsy (not simple aspiration) should be used to obtain specimens for histology and culture. The blood smear should be examined for *Plasmodium, Babesia, Trypanosoma, Leishmania,* and *Borrelia.*

In an FUO workup, the erythrocyte sedimentation rate (ESR) should be determined. Striking elevation of the ESR and anemia of chronic disease are frequently seen in association with giant cell arteritis or polymyalgia rheumatica, common causes of FUO in patients over 50 years of age. Still's disease is also suggested by elevations of ESR, leukocytosis, and anemia and is often accompanied by arthralgias, polyserositis (pleuritis, pericarditis), lymphadenopathy, splenomegaly, and rash. Antinuclear antibody, antineutrophil cytoplasmic antibody, rheumatoid factor, and serum cryoglobulins should be measured to rule out other collagen vascular diseases and vasculitis. Another cause of an extremely high ESR may be a false-positive value attributable to a cold agglutinin with a broad thermal amplitude. The ESR test is nonspecific, yielding values that depend on certain serum proteins (most notably fibrinogen) known to interfere with the zeta-potential that keeps erythrocytes from clumping. When fibrinogen levels go up, the zeta-potential is inhibited, erythrocytes clump, and the ESR is high. A cold agglutinin, by binding to erythrocytes, can produce a false-positive agglutinin that mimics an acute-phase response; cold agglutinins may be seen in *Mycoplasma* and Epstein-Barr virus infections and in lymphomas.

With rare exceptions, the intermediate-strength purified protein derivative (PPD) skin test should be used to screen for tuberculosis in patients with classic FUO. Concurrent control tests, such as the CMI test (Connaught Labs, Swiftwater, PA), which is especially effective, should be employed. It should be kept in mind that both the PPD skin test and control tests may yield negative results in miliary tuberculosis,

sarcoidosis, Hodgkin's disease, malnutrition, or AIDS. Noninvasive procedures should include an upper gastrointestinal contrast study with small-bowel follow-through and barium enema to include the terminal ileum and cecum. Chest x-rays should be repeated if new symptoms arise. In some cases, pulmonary function studies may be necessary. A diminished carbon monoxide diffusing capacity may indicate a restrictive lung disease such as sarcoidosis, even with a normal chest x-ray. In such cases, transbronchial biopsy may prove diagnostic. Flexible colonoscopy may be advisable, since colon carcinoma is a cause of FUO and easily escapes detection by ultrasound and CT.

CT of the chest and abdomen should be performed. If a spinal or paraspinal lesion is suspected, however, MRI is preferred. MRI may be superior to CT in demonstrating intraabdominal abscesses and aortic dissection, but the relative utility of MRI and CT in the diagnosis of FUO is unknown. At present, it appears that abdominal CT, with oral and intravenous contrast, should be used unless MRI is specifically indicated. Arteriography may be useful for patients in whom systemic necrotizing vasculitis is suspected. Saccular aneurysms may be seen, most commonly in renal or hepatic vessels, and may permit diagnosis of arteritis when biopsy is difficult. Figure 125-1 shows a renal angiogram of a patient with polyarteritis nodosa. Ultrasonography of the abdomen is useful for the investigation of the hepatobiliary tract, kidneys, spleen, and pelvis. Echocardiography may be helpful in an evaluation for bacterial endocarditis, pericarditis, nonbacterial thrombotic endocarditis, and atrial myxomas. Transesophageal echocardiography is especially sensitive for these lesions.

Radionuclide scanning procedures using technetium (Tc) 99m sulfur colloid, gallium (Ga) 67 citrate, or indium (In) 111–labeled leukocytes or immunoglobulin may be useful in identifying and/or localizing inflammatory processes. In a recent study, Ga scintigraphy yielded useful diagnostic information in almost one-third of cases, and it was suggested that this procedure might actually be used before other

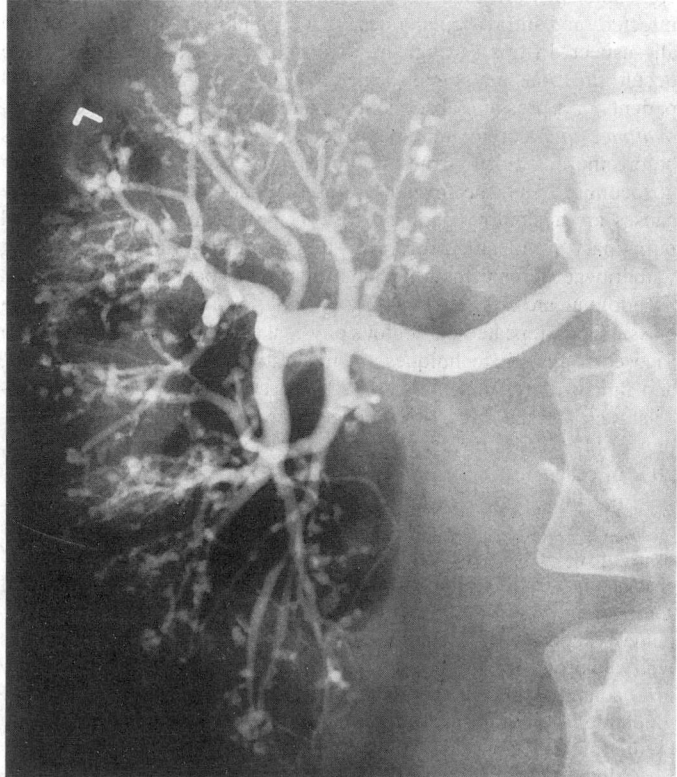

FIGURE 125-1 Renal arteriogram from a patient with fever. Arteriography showed a remarkable number of sacculated aneurysms, associated with narrowing and tapering of the arteries, consistent with systemic vasculitis—in this case, polyarteritis nodosa. (Photo courtesy of Dr. Neil Haline.)

imaging techniques if no specific organ is suspected of being abnormal. Tc bone scan should be undertaken to look for osteomyelitis or bony metastases; ^{67}Ga scan may be used to identify sarcoidosis (Chap. 318) or *Pneumocystis carinii* (Chap. 209) in the lungs or Crohn's disease (Chap. 287) in the abdomen. ^{111}In-labeled white blood cell (WBC) scan may be used to locate abscesses; ^{111}In-labeled immunoglobulin scan also shows promise in this regard. With ^{67}Ga, ^{111}In-WBC, and ^{111}In-immunoglobulin scans, false-positive and false-negative findings are common.

Biopsy of the liver and bone marrow should be considered routine in the workup of FUO if the studies mentioned above are unrevealing or if fever is prolonged. It goes without saying that areas of suspected abnormality should be sampled for pathologic examination whenever practical. When possible, a section of the tissue block should be retained for further sections or stains. PCR technology makes it possible to identify and speciate mycobacterial DNA in paraffin-embedded, fixed tissues. Thus, in some cases, it is possible to make a retrospective diagnosis based on studies of long-fixed pathologic tissues. In a patient over age 50 (or occasionally in a younger patient) with the appropriate symptoms and laboratory findings, "blind biopsy" of one or both temporal arteries may yield a diagnosis of arteritis. If noted, tenderness or decreased pulsation should guide the selection of a site for biopsy. Lymph node biopsy may be helpful if nodes are enlarged, but inguinal nodes are often palpable and are seldom diagnostically useful.

Exploratory laparotomy has been performed when all other diagnostic procedures fail but has largely been replaced by modern imaging and guided-biopsy techniques. Laparoscopic biopsy may provide more adequate guided sampling of lymph nodes or liver.

Nosocomial FUO The primary considerations in diagnosing nosocomial FUO are the underlying susceptibility of the patient coupled with the potential complications of hospitalization. The original surgical or procedural field is the place to begin a directed physical and laboratory examination for abscesses, hematomas, or infected foreign bodies. More than 50% of patients with nosocomial FUO are infected, and intravascular lines, septic phlebitis, and prostheses are all suspect. In this setting, the approach is to focus on sites where occult infections may be sequestered, such as the sinuses of intubated patients or a prostatic abscess in a man with a urinary catheter. *Clostridium difficile* colitis may be associated with fever and leukocytosis before the onset of diarrhea. In approximately 25% of patients with nosocomial FUO, the fever has a noninfectious cause. Among these causes are acalculous cholecystitis, deep vein thrombophlebitis, and pulmonary embolism. Drug fever, transfusion reactions, alcohol/drug withdrawal, adrenal insufficiency, thyroiditis, pancreatitis, gout, and pseudogout are among the many possible causes to consider. As in classic FUO, repeated meticulous physical examinations, coupled with focused diagnostic techniques, are imperative. Multiple blood, wound, and fluid cultures are mandatory. The pace of diagnostic tests is accelerated, and the threshold for procedures—CT scans, ultrasonography, ^{111}In-WBC scans, noninvasive venous studies—is low. Even so, 20% of cases of nosocomial FUO may go undiagnosed.

Like diagnostic measures, therapeutic maneuvers must be swift and decisive, as many patients are already critically ill. Intravenous lines must be changed (and cultured), drugs stopped for 72 h, and empirical therapy started if bacteremia is a threat. In many hospital settings, empirical antibiotic coverage for nosocomial FUO now includes vancomycin for methicillin-resistant *Staphylococcus aureus* as well as broad-spectrum gram-negative coverage with piperacillin/tazobactam, ticarcillin/clavulanate, imipenem, or meropenem. Practice guidelines covering many of these issues have been published jointly by the Infectious Diseases Society of America (IDSA) and the Society for Critical Care Medicine and can be accessed on the IDSA website (www.idsociety.org/practice/index.html).

Neutropenic FUO (See also Chap. 85) Neutropenic patients are susceptible to focal bacterial and fungal infections, to bacteremic infections, to infections involving catheters (including septic thrombo-phlebitis), and to perianal infections. *Candida* and *Aspergillus* infections are common. Infections due to herpes simplex virus or CMV are sometimes causes of FUO in this group. While the duration of illness may be short in these patients, the consequences of untreated infection may be catastrophic, with 50 to 60% infected, and 20% bacteremic. The IDSA has published extensive practice guidelines covering these critically ill neutropenic patients; these guidelines appear on the website cited in the previous section. In these patients, severe mucositis, quinolone prophylaxis, colonization with methicillin-resistant *S. aureus*, obvious catheter-related infection, or hypotension would dictate the use of vancomycin plus ceftazidime or imipenem to provide empirical coverage for bacterial sepsis.

HIV-Associated FUO HIV infection alone may be a cause of fever. Infection due to *Mycobacterium avium* or *Mycobacterium intracellulare*, tuberculosis, toxoplasmosis, CMV infection, *P. carinii* infection, salmonellosis, cryptococcosis, histoplasmosis, non-Hodgkin's lymphoma, and (of particular importance) drug fever are all possible causes of FUO. Mycobacterial infection can be diagnosed by blood cultures and by liver, bone marrow, and lymph node biopsies. Chest CT should be performed to identify enlarged mediastinal nodes. Serologic studies may reveal cryptococcal antigen, and ^{67}Ga scan may help identify *P. carinii* pulmonary infection. More than 80% of HIV patients with FUO are infected, but drug fever and lymphoma remain important considerations. →*Treatment of HIV-associated FUO depends on many factors and is discussed in Chap. 309.*

℞ **TREATMENT** The emphasis in patients with classic FUO is on continued observation and examination, with the avoidance of "shotgun" empirical therapy. Empirical treatment for endocarditis, for example, should be avoided unless there are specific reasons beyond fever to invoke this diagnosis. Every patient with FUO should undergo an exhaustive examination for tuberculosis. If the PPD skin test is positive or if granulomatous hepatitis or other granulomatous disease is present with anergy (and sarcoid seems unlikely), then a therapeutic trial with isoniazid and rifampin (and possibly a third drug) should be undertaken, with treatment usually continued for up to 6 weeks. A failure of the fever to respond over this period suggests an alternative diagnosis.

The response of rheumatic fever and Still's disease to aspirin and nonsteroidal anti-inflammatory agents (NSAIDs) may be dramatic. The effects of glucocorticoids on temporal arteritis, polymyalgia rheumatica, and granulomatous hepatitis are equally dramatic. Colchicine is highly effective in preventing attacks of familial Mediterranean fever but is of little use once an attack is well under way. The ability of glucocorticoids and NSAIDs to mask fever while permitting the spread of infection dictates that their use be avoided unless infection has been largely ruled out and unless inflammatory disease is both probable and debilitating or threatening.

When no underlying source of FUO is identified after prolonged observation (>6 months), the prognosis is generally good, however vexing the fever may be to the patient. Under such circumstances, debilitating symptoms are treated with NSAIDs, and glucocorticoids are the last resort. The initiation of empirical therapy does not mark the end of the diagnostic workup; rather, it commits the physician to continued thoughtful reexamination and evaluation. Patience, compassion, equanimity, and intellectual flexibility are indispensable attributes for the clinician in dealing successfully with FUO.

ACKNOWLEDGMENT
Sheldon M. Wolff, MD, now deceased, was an author of a previous version of this chapter. It is to his memory that the chapter is dedicated.

BIBLIOGRAPHY

ADUAN R et al: Prolonged fever of unknown origin. Clin Res 26:558A, 1978
DEKLEIJN EMHA et al: Fever of unknown origin (FUO): I. A prospective multicenter study of 167 patients with FUO, using fixed epidemiologic entry criteria. Medicine 76:392, 1997

—— et al: Fever of unknown origin (FUO): II. Diagnostic procedures in a prospective multicenter study of 167 patients. Medicine 76:401, 1997

HIRSCHMANN JV: Fever of unknown origin in adults. Clin Infect Dis 24:291, 1997

HOEN B et al: The Duke criteria for diagnosing infective endocarditis are specific: Analysis of 100 patients with acute fever or fever of unknown origin. Clin Infect Dis 23:298, 1996

HUGHES WT et al: 1997 guidelines for the use of antimicrobial agents in neutropenic patients with unexplained fever. Clin Infect Dis 25:551, 1997

KAZANJIAN PH: Fever of unknown origin: Review of 86 patients treated in community hospitals. Clin Infect Dis 15:968, 1992

KNOCKAERT DC et al: Long-term follow-up of patients with undiagnosed fever of unknown origin. Arch Intern Med 156:618, 1996

——, VANNESTE LJ: Fever of unknown origin in the 1980s. Arch Intern Med 152:51, 1992

——, VANNESTE LJ: Fever of unknown origin in elderly patients. J Am Geriatr Soc 41:1187, 1993

LARSON EB, FEATHERSTONE HJ: Fever of undetermined origin: Diagnosis and follow-up of 105 cases, 1970–80. Medicine 61:269, 1982

MITCHELL MA et al: Bilateral renal parenchymal malacoplakia presenting as fever of unknown origin: Case report and review. Clin Infect Dis 18:704, 1994

O'GRADY NP et al: Practice guidelines for evaluating new fever in critically ill adult patients. Clin Infect Dis 26:1042, 1998

PETERS AM: The use of nuclear medicine in infections. Br J Radiol 71:252, 1998

PETERSDORF RC, BEESON PB: Fever of unexplained origin. Medicine 40:1, 1961

VOLK EE et al: The diagnostic usefulness of bone marrow cultures in patients with fever of unknown origin. Am J Clin Pathol 110:150, 1998

126

Adolf W. Karchmer

INFECTIVE ENDOCARDITIS

The proliferation of microorganisms on the endothelium of the heart results in infective endocarditis. The prototypic lesion at the site of infection, the *vegetation* (see Plate IID-59), is a mass of platelets, fibrin, microcolonies of microorganisms, and scant inflammatory cells. Infection most commonly involves heart valves (either native or prosthetic) but may also occur on the low-pressure side of the ventricular septum at the site of a defect, on the mural endocardium where it is damaged by aberrant jets of blood or foreign bodies, or on intracardiac devices themselves. The analogous process involving arteriovenous shunts, arterioarterial shunts (patent ductus arteriosus), or a coarctation of the aorta is called *infective endarteritis.*

Endocarditis may be classified according to the temporal evolution of disease, the site of infection, the cause of infection, or a predisposing risk factor such as injection drug use. While each classification criterion provides therapeutic and prognostic insight, the methods overlap and none is sufficient alone. The classification of endocarditis as acute and subacute was initially used to describe the illness and the time elapsed until death; presently it is applied to the features and progression of infection until diagnosis. *Acute endocarditis* is a hectically febrile illness, rapidly damages cardiac structures, hematogenously seeds extracardiac sites, and, if untreated, progresses to death within weeks. *Subacute endocarditis* follows an indolent course; causes structural cardiac damage only slowly, if at all; rarely causes metastatic infection; and is gradually progressive unless complicated by a major embolic event or ruptured mycotic aneurysm.

In developed countries, the incidence of endocarditis ranges from 1.5 to 6.2 cases per 100,000 population per year. In the late 1980s in a metropolitan area of the United States (Philadelphia), endocarditis occurred in 9.3 persons per 100,000 population per year. However, half of these cases arose as a consequence of injection drug use. The incidence of endocarditis is notably increased among the elderly. The cumulative rate of prosthetic valve endocarditis is 1.5 to 3.0% at 1 year after valve replacement and 3 to 6% at 5 years; the risk is greatest during the first 6 months after valve replacement.

ETIOLOGY A vast array of microorganisms, including many species of bacteria and fungi, have been reported to cause sporadic episodes of endocarditis. Nevertheless, a small number of bacterial species cause the majority of cases (Table 126-1). The causative microorganisms vary somewhat among the major clinical types of endocarditis, in part because of the different portals of entry. The oral cavity, skin, and upper respiratory tract are the respective primary portals for the viridans streptococci, staphylococci, and HACEK organisms (*Haemophilus, Actinobacillus, Cardiobacterium, Eikenella,* and *Kingella*) causing community-acquired native valve endocarditis. *Streptococcus bovis* originates from the gastrointestinal tract, where it is associated with polyps and colonic tumors, and enterococci enter the bloodstream from the genitourinary tract. Nosocomial native valve endocarditis is largely the consequence of bacteremia arising from intravascular catheters and less commonly from nosocomial wound and urinary tract infection. Endocarditis complicates 6 to 25% of episodes of catheter-associated *Staphylococcus aureus* bacteremia; higher rates are detected by careful transesophageal echocardiography (TEE) screening (see "Echocardiography," below).

Prosthetic valve endocarditis arising within 2 months of valve surgery is generally the result of intraoperative contamination of the prosthesis or a bacteremic postoperative complication. The nosocomial nature of these infections is reflected in their primary microbial causes: coagulase-negative staphylococci, *S. aureus,* facultative gram-negative bacilli, diphtheroids, and fungi. The portals of entry and organisms causing cases beginning >12 months after surgery are similar to those in community-acquired native valve endocarditis. Epidemiologic evidence suggests that prosthetic valve endocarditis due to coagulase-negative staphylococci that presents between 2 and 12 months after surgery is often nosocomial in origin but with a delayed onset. At least 85% of coagulase-negative staphylococci that cause prosthetic valve endocarditis within 12 months of surgery are methicillin-resistant; the rate of methicillin resistance decreases to 25% among coagulase-negative staphylococci causing prosthetic endocarditis that presents >1 year after valve surgery.

Transvenous pacemaker lead and/or implanted defibrillator–associated endocarditis is usually a nosocomial infection. The majority of episodes occur within weeks of implantation or generator change and are caused by *S. aureus* or coagulase-negative staphylococci.

Endocarditis occurring among injection drug users, especially when infection involves the tricuspid valve, is commonly caused by *S. aureus* strains, many of which are methicillin-resistant. The causes of left-sided valve infection in addicts are more varied, and the involved valves have often been damaged by prior episodes of endocarditis. A number of these cases are caused by *Pseudomonas aeruginosa* and *Candida* species, and sporadic cases are due to unusual organisms such as *Bacillus, Lactobacillus,* and *Corynebacterium* species. Polymicrobial endocarditis occurs more frequently in injection drug users than in patients who do not inject drugs. The presence of HIV in this population does not significantly impact the causes of endocarditis.

From 5 to 15% of patients with endocarditis have negative blood cultures; in one-third to one-half of these cases, cultures are negative because of prior antibiotic exposure. The remainder of these patients are infected by fastidious organisms, such as pyridoxal-requiring streptococci (now designated *Abiotrophia* species), the gram-negative coccobacillary HACEK organisms, *Bartonella henselae,* or *Bartonella quintana.* Some fastidious organisms that cause endocarditis have characteristic epidemiologic settings (e.g., *Coxiella burnetii* in Europe, *Brucella* species in the Middle East). *Tropheryma whippelii* causes an indolent, culture-negative, afebrile form of endocarditis.

PATHOGENESIS Unless it is injured, the normal endothelium is resistant to infection by most bacteria and to thrombus formation. Endothelial injury (e.g., at the site of impact of high-velocity jets or on the low-pressure side of a cardiac structural lesion) causes aberrant flow and allows either direct infection by virulent organisms or the development of an uninfected platelet-fibrin thrombus—a condition called *nonbacterial thrombotic endocarditis* (NBTE). The thrombus subsequently serves as a site of bacterial attachment during transient

Table 126-1 Organisms Causing Major Clinical Forms of Endocarditis

	Native Valve Endocarditis		Prosthetic Valve Endocarditis at Indicated Time of Onset (Months) After Valve Surgery			Endocarditis in Injection Drug Users		
Organism	Community-Acquired (n = 683)	Nosocomial (n = 82)	< 2 (n = 144)	2–12 (n = 31)	> 12 (n = 194)	Right-Sided (n = 346)	Left-Sided (n = 204)	Total (n = 675)
Streptococci[a]	32	7	1	9	31	5	15	12
Pneumococci	1	—	—	—	—	—	—	—
Enterococci	8	16	8	12	11	2	24	9
Staphylococcus aureus	35	55	22	12	18	77	23	57
Coagulase-negative staphylococci	4	10	33	32	11	—	—	—
Fastidious gram-negative coccobacilli (HACEK group)[b]	3	—	—	—	6	—	—	—
Gram-negative bacilli	3	5	13	3	6	5	13	7
Candida spp.	1	4	8	12	1	—	12	4
Polymicrobial/miscellaneous	6	1	3	6	5	8	10	7
Diphtheroids	—	—	6	—	3	—	—	0.1
Culture-negative	5	2	5	6	8	3	3	3

[a] Includes viridans streptococci; *Streptococcus bovis*; other non–group A, groupable streptococci; and *Abiotrophia* spp. (nutritionally variant, pyridoxal-requiring streptococci).
[b] Includes *Haemophilus* spp., *Actinobacillus actinomycetemcomitans*, *Cardiobacterium hominis*, *Eikenella* spp., and *Kingella kingae*.
NOTE: Data are compiled from multiple studies.

bacteremia. The cardiac lesions most commonly resulting in NBTE are mitral regurgitation, aortic stenosis, aortic regurgitation, ventricular septal defects, and complex congenital heart disease. These lesions result from rheumatic heart disease (particularly in the developing world, where rheumatic fever remains prevalent), mitral valve prolapse, degenerative heart disease, and congenital malformations. NBTE also arises as a result of a hypercoagulable state; this phenomenon gives rise to the clinical entity of *marantic endocarditis* (seen in patients with malignancy) and to bland vegetations complicating systemic lupus erythematosus and the antiphospholipid antibody syndrome.

Organisms that cause endocarditis generally enter the bloodstream from mucosal surfaces, the skin, or sites of focal infection. Except for more virulent bacteria (e.g., *S. aureus*) that can adhere directly to intact endothelium or exposed subendothelial tissue, microorganisms in the blood adhere to thrombi. If resistant to the bactericidal activity of serum and the microbicidal peptides released by platelets, the organisms proliferate and either stimulate tissues to produce a procoagulant or themselves exert procoagulant activity leading to further platelet-fibrin deposition and vegetation formation. Although an enormous variety of microorganisms circulate transiently in the bloodstream, only a limited number commonly cause endocarditis. The etiologic organisms of endocarditis bear surface components that facilitate adherence to injured endothelium and host proteins or to thrombi. Experiments suggest that fibronectin receptors present on many gram-positive bacteria, clumping factor (a fibrinogen-binding surface protein) on *S. aureus*, and dextrans on streptococci facilitate adherence. Organisms become enmeshed in the growing platelet-fibrin vegetation and, in the absence of host defenses, proliferate to form dense microcolonies. More than 90% of the organisms in vegetations are metabolically inactive (nongrowing) and thus are relatively resistant to killing by antimicrobial agents. Proliferating surface organisms are shed into the bloodstream continuously, whereupon some are cleared by the reticuloendothelial system and others are redeposited on the vegetation and stimulate further vegetation growth.

The pathophysiologic consequences and clinical manifestations of endocarditis—other than constitutional symptoms, which are probably a result of cytokine production—arise from damage to intracardiac structures; embolization of vegetation fragments, leading to infection or infarction of remote tissues; hematogenous infection of sites during bacteremia; and tissue injury due to the deposition of circulating immune complexes or immune responses to deposited bacterial antigens.

CLINICAL MANIFESTATIONS The clinical syndrome of infective endocarditis is highly variable, may involve multiple organs, and spans a continuum between acute and subacute presentations. Na-

tive valve endocarditis (whether acquired in the community or nosocomially), prosthetic valve endocarditis, and endocarditis due to injection drug use share clinical and laboratory manifestations (Table 126-2). Although the relationship is not absolute, the causative microorganism is primarily responsible for the temporal course of endocarditis. β-Hemolytic streptococci, *S. aureus*, and pneumococci typically result in an acute course, although *S. aureus* occasionally causes subacute disease. Endocarditis caused by *Staphylococcus lugdunensis* (a coagulase-negative species) or by enterococci may present acutely. Subacute endocarditis is typically caused by viridans streptococci, enterococci, coagulase-negative staphylococci, and the HACEK group. Endocarditis caused by *Bartonella* species and the agent of Q fever, *C. burnetii*, is exceptionally indolent.

The clinical features of endocarditis are nonspecific. However, these symptoms in a febrile patient with valvular abnormalities or a behavior pattern (injection drug use) that predisposes to endocarditis suggest the diagnosis, as do bacteremia with organisms that frequently cause endocarditis, otherwise unexplained arterial emboli, and progressive cardiac valvular incompetence. In patients with subacute presentations, fever is typically low-grade and rarely exceeds 39.4°C (103°F); in contrast, temperatures between 39.4 and 40°C (103 and

Table 126-2 Clinical and Laboratory Features of Infective Endocarditis

Feature	Frequency, %
Fever	80–90
Chills and sweats	40–75
Anorexia, weight loss, malaise	25–50
Myalgias, arthralgias	15–30
Back pain	7–15
Heart murmur	80–85
New/worsened regurgitant murmur	10–40
Arterial emboli	20–50
Splenomegaly	15–50
Clubbing	10–20
Neurologic manifestations	20–40
Peripheral manifestations (Osler's nodes, subungual hemorrhages, Janeway lesions, Roth's spots)	2–15
Petechiae	10–40
Laboratory manifestations	
Anemia	70–90
Leukocytosis	20–30
Microscopic hematuria	30–50
Elevated erythrocyte sedimentation rate	>90
Rheumatoid factor	50
Circulating immune complexes	65–100
Decreased serum complement	5–40

104°F) are often noted in acute endocarditis. Fever may be blunted or absent in patients who are elderly or severely debilitated or who have marked cardiac or renal failure.

Cardiac Manifestations Although heart murmurs are usually indicative of the predisposing cardiac pathology rather than of endocarditis, valvular damage and ruptured chordae may result in new regurgitant murmurs. In acute endocarditis involving a normal valve, murmurs are heard on presentation in only 30 to 45% of patients but ultimately are detected in 85%. Congestive heart failure develops in 30 to 40% of patients; it is usually a consequence of valvular dysfunction but occasionally is due to endocarditis-associated myocarditis or an intracardiac fistula. The temporal progression of heart failure is variable and depends upon the severity of valvular dysfunction; failure due to aortic valve dysfunction progresses more rapidly than that due to mitral valve dysfunction. Extension of infection beyond valve leaflets into adjacent annular or myocardial tissue results in perivalvular abscesses, which in turn may cause fistulae (from the root of the aorta into cardiac chambers or between cardiac chambers) with new murmurs. Abscesses may burrow from the aortic valve annulus through the epicardium, causing pericarditis. Extension of infection into paravalvular tissue adjacent to either the right or the noncoronary cusp of the aortic valve may interrupt the conduction system in the upper interventricular septum, leading to varying degrees of heart block. Although perivalvular abscesses arising from the mitral valve may potentially interrupt conduction pathways near the atrioventricular node or in the proximal bundle of His, such interruption occurs infrequently. Emboli to a coronary artery may result in myocardial infarction; nevertheless, embolic transmural infarcts are rare.

Noncardiac Manifestations The classic nonsuppurative peripheral manifestations of subacute endocarditis are related to the duration of infection and, with early diagnosis and treatment, have become infrequent. In contrast, septic embolization mimicking some of these lesions (subungual hemorrhage, Osler's nodes) is common in patients with acute *S. aureus* endocarditis (**see Plate IID-58**). Musculoskeletal symptoms, including nonspecific inflammatory arthritis and back pain, usually remit promptly with treatment but must be distinguished from the symptoms of focal metastatic infection. Hematogenously seeded focal infection may involve any organ but most often is clinically evident in the skin, spleen, kidneys, skeletal system, and meninges. Arterial emboli, which may be asymptomatic and discovered only at autopsy, are clinically apparent in up to 50% of patients. Vegetations >10 mm in diameter (as measured by echocardiography) and those located on the mitral valve are more likely to embolize than are smaller or nonmitral vegetations. Embolic events—often with infarction—involving the extremities, spleen, kidneys (Fig. 126-1), bowel, or brain

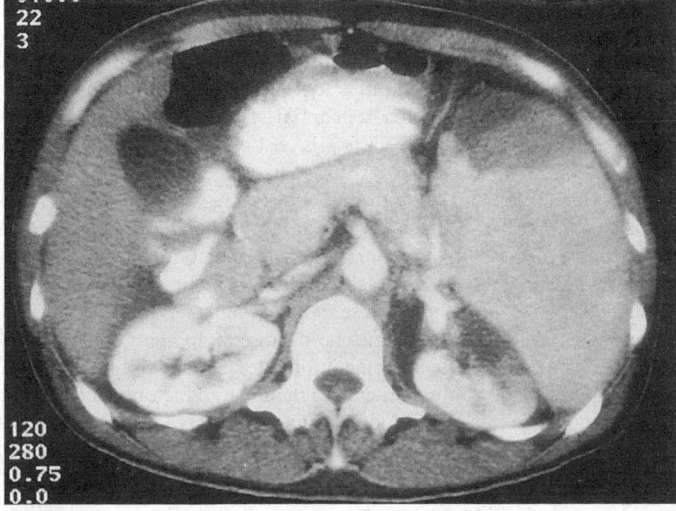

FIGURE 126-1 Computed tomography of the abdomen showing large embolic infarcts in the spleen and left kidney of a patient with *Bartonella* endocarditis.

are often noted at presentation. With antibiotic treatment, the frequency of embolic events decreases from 13 per 1000 patient-days during the initial week to 1.2 per 1000 patient-days after the third week. Emboli occurring late during or after effective therapy do not in themselves constitute evidence of failed antimicrobial treatment. Neurologic symptoms, most often resulting from embolic strokes, occur in up to 40% of patients. Other neurologic complications include aseptic or purulent meningitis, intracranial hemorrhage due to hemorrhagic infarcts or ruptured mycotic aneurysms, seizures, and encephalopathy. Microabscesses in brain and meninges occur commonly in *S. aureus* endocarditis; surgically drainable abscesses are infrequent.

Immune complex deposition on the glomerular basement membrane causes diffuse hypocomplementemic glomerulonephritis and renal dysfunction, which typically improve with effective antimicrobial therapy. Embolic renal infarcts cause flank pain and hematuria but rarely cause renal dysfunction.

Manifestations of Specific Predisposing Conditions Among injection drug users, infection involving valves on the left side of the heart presents with the typical clinical features of endocarditis. In almost 50% of patients with endocarditis associated with injection drug use, infection is limited to the tricuspid valve. These patients present with fever, faint or no murmur, and (in 75% of cases) prominent pulmonary findings, including cough, pleuritic chest pain, nodular pulmonary infiltrates, and occasionally pyopneumothorax.

Nosocomial endocarditis (defined as that which results from hospital care within the prior month and most commonly presenting as intravascular catheter–associated bacteremia), if not associated with a retained intracardiac device, has typical manifestations. Endocarditis associated with flow-directed pulmonary artery catheters is often cryptic, with symptoms masked by comorbid critical illness, and is commonly diagnosed at autopsy. Transvenous pacemaker lead and/or implanted defibrillator–associated endocarditis commonly follows initial implantation or a generator unit change; may be associated with obvious or cryptic generator pocket infection; and results in fever, minimal murmur, and pulmonary symptoms similar to those encountered in addicts with tricuspid endocarditis.

Prosthetic valve endocarditis presents with typical clinical features. Cases arising within 60 days of valve surgery (early onset) lack peripheral vascular manifestations and may be obscured by comorbidity associated with recent surgery. In both early-onset and more delayed presentations, paravalvular infection is common and often results in partial valve dehiscence, regurgitant murmurs, congestive heart failure, or disruption of the conduction system.

DIAGNOSIS The Duke Criteria The diagnosis of infective endocarditis is established with certainty only when vegetations obtained at cardiac surgery, at autopsy, or from an artery (an embolus) are examined histologically and microbiologically. Nevertheless, a highly sensitive and specific diagnostic schema—known as the *Duke criteria*—has been developed on the basis of clinical, laboratory, and echocardiographic findings (Table 126-3). Documentation of two major criteria, of one major and three minor criteria, or of five minor criteria allows a clinical diagnosis of definite endocarditis. The diagnosis of endocarditis is rejected if an alternative diagnosis is established, if symptoms resolve and do not recur with ≤4 days of antibiotic therapy, or if surgery or autopsy after ≤4 days of antimicrobial therapy yields no histologic evidence of endocarditis. Illnesses not classified as definite endocarditis or rejected are considered cases of possible infective endocarditis. When pathologically confirmed cases have been scored retrospectively by these criteria, 90% fulfill the definition of definite or possible endocarditis; 10% are rejected (primarily because of an incomplete echocardiographic evaluation). In comparison with expert opinion, the Duke criteria identify cases considered to be endocarditis but also accept a small percentage of cases rejected by the experts. This potential for a false-positive diagnosis is the major deficiency in this schema when used clinically. If all patients with a diagnosis of definite or possible endocarditis are fully treated for en-

Table 126-3 The Duke Criteria for the Clinical Diagnosis of Infective Endocarditis

MAJOR CRITERIA

Positive blood culture
  Typical microorganism for infective endocarditis from two separate blood
    cultures
      Viridans streptococci, *Streptococcus bovis*, HACEK group, *or*
      Community-acquired *Staphylococcus aureus* or enterococci in the ab-
        sence of a primary focus, *or*
  Persistently positive blood culture, defined as recovery of a microorganism
    consistent with infective endocarditis from:
      Blood cultures drawn >12 h apart; *or*
      All of three or a majority of four or more separate blood cultures, with
        first and last drawn at least 1 h apart
Evidence of endocardial involvement
  Positive echocardiogram
      Oscillating intracardiac mass on valve or supporting structures or in the
        path of regurgitant jets or in implanted material, in the absence of an
        alternative anatomic explanation, *or*
      Abscess, *or*
      New partial dehiscence of prosthetic valve, *or*
  New valvular regurgitation (increase or change in preexisting murmur not
    sufficient)

MINOR CRITERIA

Predisposition: predisposing heart condition or injection drug use
Fever ≥38.0°C (≥100.4°F)
Vascular phenomena: major arterial emboli, septic pulmonary infarcts, mycotic aneurysm, intracranial hemorrhage, conjunctival hemorrhages, Janeway lesions
Immunologic phenomena: glomerulonephritis, Osler's nodes, Roth's spots,
  rheumatoid factor
Microbiologic evidence: positive blood culture but not meeting major criterion as noted previously[a] or serologic evidence of active infection with organism consistent with infective endocarditis
Echocardiogram: consistent with infective endocarditis but not meeting major
  criterion

---

[a] Excluding single positive cultures for coagulase-negative staphylococci and diphtheroids, which are common culture contaminants, and organisms that do not cause endocarditis frequently, such as gram-negative bacilli.
NOTE: HACEK, *Haemophilus* spp., *Actinobacillus actinomycetemcomitans*, *Cardiobacterium hominis*, *Eikenella corrodens*, *Kingella kingae*.
SOURCE: Adapted from Durack et al., with permission from Excerpta Medica, Inc.

---

docarditis, this reduced specificity results in excess treatment for some
patients. A modification of the schema has been proposed in order to
increase its specificity without significantly reducing its sensitivity.
This modification would require documentation of at least one major
or three minor criteria for cases to be categorized as possible endocarditis.

The roles of bacteremia and echocardiographic findings in the diagnosis of endocarditis are appropriately emphasized in the Duke criteria. That multiple blood cultures obtained over time are positive is
consistent with the known continuous low-density nature of bacteremia in patients with endocarditis (≤100 organisms per milliliter).
Among untreated endocarditis patients who ultimately have a positive
blood culture, 95% of all blood cultures are positive, and in 98% of
cases one of the initial two sets of cultures yields the microorganism.
The diagnostic criteria attach significance to the species of organism
isolated from blood cultures. To fulfill a major criterion, the isolation
of an organism that causes both endocarditis and bacteremia in the
absence of endocarditis (e.g., *S. aureus*, enterococci) must take place
repeatedly (i.e., persistent bacteremia) and in the absence of a primary
focus of infection. Organisms that rarely cause endocarditis but commonly contaminate blood cultures (e.g., diphtheroids, coagulase-negative species) must be isolated repeatedly if their isolation is to serve
as a major criterion.

Blood Cultures   Isolation of the causative microorganism from
blood cultures is critical not only for diagnosis but also for determination of antimicrobial susceptibility and planning of treatment. In the

absence of prior antibiotic therapy, a total of three blood culture sets,
ideally with the first separated from the last by at least 1 h, should be
obtained from different venipuncture sites over 24 h. If the cultures
remain negative after 48 to 72 h, two or three additional blood cultures,
including a lysis-centrifugation culture, should be obtained, and the
laboratory should be asked to pursue fastidious microorganisms by
prolonging incubation time and performing special subcultures. Empirical antimicrobial therapy should not be administered initially to
hemodynamically stable patients with subacute endocarditis, especially those who have received antibiotics within the preceding 2
weeks; thus, if necessary, additional blood cultures can be obtained
without the confounding effect of empirical treatment. Patients with
acute endocarditis or with deteriorating hemodynamics that may require urgent surgery should be treated empirically immediately after
obtaining the initial three sets of blood cultures.

Non-Blood-Culture Tests for the Etiologic Agent   Serologic
tests can be used to identify some organisms causing endocarditis that
are difficult to recover by blood culture: *Brucella*, *Bartonella*, *Legionella*, and *C. burnetii*. Pathogens can also be identified in vegetations by culture, by microscopic examination with special stains, and
by use of polymerase chain reaction to recover unique microbial DNA
or 16S rRNA.

Echocardiography   Cardiac imaging with echocardiography allows anatomic confirmation of infective endocarditis, sizing of vegetations, detection of intracardiac complications, and assessment of cardiac function. A two-dimensional study with color flow and
continuous as well as pulsed Doppler is optimal. Transthoracic echocardiography (TTE) is noninvasive and exceptionally specific; however, it cannot image vegetations <2 mm in diameter, and in 20% of
patients it is technically inadequate because of emphysema or body
habitus. Thus, TTE detects vegetations in only 65% of patients with
definite clinical endocarditis (i.e., it has a sensitivity of 65%). Moreover, TTE is not adequate for evaluating prosthetic valves or detecting
intracardiac complications. Transesophageal echocardiography (TEE)
is safe and significantly more sensitive than TTE. It detects vegetations
in >90% of patients with definite endocarditis; nevertheless, false-
negative studies are noted in 6 to 18% of endocarditis patients. TEE
is the optimal method for the diagnosis of prosthetic endocarditis or
the detection of myocardial abscess, valve perforation, or intracardiac
fistulae.

Experts favor echocardiographic evaluation of all patients with a
clinical diagnosis of endocarditis; however, the test should not be used
to screen patients with otherwise explained positive blood cultures or
patients with unexplained fever. In patients with a low pretest likelihood of endocarditis (<5%), a high-quality TTE that is negative is
sufficient to exclude endocarditis. For patients whose habitus makes
them difficult to study with TTE and for those who may have prosthetic valve endocarditis or who are at high risk of intracardiac complications, TEE is the preferred imaging modality. For patients with a
pretest probability of endocarditis ranging from 5 to 50%, initial evaluation by TEE—in lieu of a sequential strategy of TTE, which, if
negative, will be followed by TEE—is cost-effective. A negative TEE
when endocarditis is likely does not exclude the diagnosis but rather
warrants repetition of the study in 7 to 10 days with optimal multi-
planar technique.

Other Studies   Many laboratory studies that do not aid in diagnostic evaluation are nevertheless important in the management of
patients with endocarditis; these studies include complete blood
counts, creatinine measurement, chest radiography, and electrocardiography. The erythrocyte sedimentation rate, C-reactive protein level,
circulating immune complex titer, and rheumatoid factor concentration
are commonly increased in endocarditis (Table 126-2). Cardiac catheterization is useful only to assess coronary artery patency in older
individuals who are to undergo surgery for endocarditis.

TREATMENT Antimicrobial Therapy   It is difficult to
eradicate bacteria from the avascular vegetation in infective endocarditis because this site is relatively inaccessible to host defenses

and because the bacteria are nongrowing and metabolically inactive. Since all bacteria in the vegetation must be killed, therapy for endocarditis must be bactericidal and must be given for prolonged periods. Antibiotics are generally given parenterally and must reach high serum concentrations that will, through passive diffusion, lead to effective concentrations in the depths of the vegetation. The choice of effective therapy requires precise knowledge of the susceptibility of the causative microorganisms. The initiation of treatment before a cause is defined must balance the need to establish a microbiologic diagnosis against the potential progression of disease or the need for urgent surgery (see "Blood Cultures" above). The individual vulnerabilities of the patient should be weighed in the selection of therapy—e.g., allergies, end-organ dysfunction, interactions with concomitant medications, and risks of adverse events.

Although given for several weeks longer, the regimens recommended for the treatment of endocarditis involving prosthetic valves (except for staphylococcal infections) are similar to those used to treat native valve infection (Table 126-4). Recommended doses and duration of therapy should be adhered to unless alterations are required by adverse events.

Organism-specific therapies* • *STREPTOCOCCI Although most strains of viridans streptococci and *S. bovis* that cause endocarditis are susceptible to penicillin [minimum inhibitory concentration (MIC) ≤ 0.1 μg/mL], recent reports indicate increasing penicillin resistance among viridans streptococci recovered from blood cultures. In the selection of optimal therapy, the penicillin MIC must be determined

Table 126-4 Antibiotic Treatment for Infective Endocarditis Caused by Common Organisms[a]

Organism	Drug, Dose, Duration	Comments
Streptococci		
Penicillin-susceptible[b] streptococci, S. bovis	Penicillin G 2–3 million units IV q4h for 4 weeks	—
	Penicillin G 2–3 million units IV q4h *plus* gentamicin[c] 1 mg/kg IM or IV q8h, both for 2 weeks	Avoid penicillin plus gentamicin if risks of aminoglycoside toxicity are increased or case is complicated
	Ceftriaxone 2 g/d IV as single dose for 4 weeks	Can use ceftriaxone in patients with nonimmediate penicillin allergy
	Vancomycin[d] 15 mg/kg IV q12h for 4 weeks	Use vancomycin in patients with severe or immediate β-lactam allergy
Relatively penicillin-resistant[e] streptococci	Penicillin G 3 million units IV q4h for 4–6 weeks *plus* gentamicin[c] 1 mg/kg IV q8h for 2 weeks	Preferred for treatment of prosthetic valve endocarditis caused by penicillin-susceptible streptococci; continue penicillin for 6 weeks in this setting
Penicillin-resistant[f] streptococci, pyridoxal-requiring streptococci (*Abiotrophia* spp.)	Penicillin G 3–4 million units IV q4h *plus* gentamicin[c] 1 mg/kg IV q8h, both for 4–6 weeks	—
Enterococci[g]	Penicillin G 3–4 million units IV q4h *plus* gentamicin[c] 1 mg/kg IV q8h, both for 4–6 weeks	Can use streptomycin 7.5 mg/kg q12h in lieu of gentamicin if there is not high-level resistance to streptomycin
	Ampicillin 2 g IV q4h *plus* gentamicin[c] 1 mg/kg IV q8h, both for 4–6 weeks	Do not use cephalosporins or carbapenems for treatment of enterococcal endocarditis
	Vancomycin[d] 15 mg/kg IV q12h *plus* gentamicin[c] 1 mg/kg IV q8h, both for 4–6 weeks	Use vancomycin plus gentamicin for penicillin-allergic patients or desensitize to penicillin
Staphylococci		
Methicillin-susceptible, infecting native valves (no foreign devices)	Nafcillin or oxacillin 2 g IV q4h for 4–6 weeks *plus* (optional) gentamicin[c] 1 mg/kg IM or IV q8h for 3–5 days	May use penicillin 3–4 million units q6h if isolate is penicillin-susceptible (does not produce β-lactamase)
	Cefazolin 2 g IV q8h for 4–6 weeks *plus* (optional) gentamicin[c] 1 mg/kg IM or IV q8h for 3–5 days	Can use cefazolin regimen for patients with nonimmediate penicillin allergy
	Vancomycin[d] 15 mg/kg IV q12h for 4–6 weeks	Use vancomycin for patients with immediate (urticarial) or severe penicillin allergy
Methicillin-resistant, infecting native valves (no foreign devices)	Vancomycin[d] 15 mg/kg IV q12h for 4–6 weeks	No role for routine use of rifampin
Methicillin-susceptible, infecting prosthetic valves	Nafcillin or oxacillin 2 g IV q4h for 6–8 weeks *plus* gentamicin[c] 1 mg/kg IM or IV q8h for 2 weeks *plus* rifampin[h] 300 mg PO q8h for 6–8 weeks	Use gentamicin during initial 2 weeks; determine susceptibility to gentamicin before initiating rifampin (see text); if patient is highly allergic to penicillin, use regimen for methicillin-resistant staphylococci; if β-lactam allergy is of the minor, nonimmediate type, can substitute cefazolin for oxacillin/nafcillin
Methicillin-resistant, infecting prosthetic valves	Vancomycin[d] 15 mg/kg IV q12h for 6–8 weeks *plus* gentamicin[c] 1 mg/kg IM or IV q8h for 2 weeks *plus* rifampin[h] 300 mg PO q8h for 6–8 weeks	Use gentamicin during initial 2 weeks; determine gentamicin susceptibility before initiating rifampin (see text)
HACEK organisms	Ceftriaxone 2 g/d IV as single dose for 4 weeks	May use another third-generation cephalosporin at comparable dosage
	Ampicillin 2 g IV q4h *plus* gentamicin[c] 1 mg/kg IM or IV q8h, both for 4 weeks	Determine ampicillin susceptibility; do not use ampicillin if β-lactamase is produced

[a] Doses are for adults with normal renal function. Doses of gentamicin, streptomycin, and vancomycin must be adjusted for reduced renal function. Ideal body weight is used to calculate doses per kilogram (men = 50 kg + 2.3 kg per inch over 5 feet; women = 45.5 kg + 2.3 kg per inch over 5 feet).
[b] MIC ≤ 0.1 μg/mL.
[c] Aminoglycosides should not be administered as single daily doses and should be introduced as part of the initial treatment. Target peak and trough serum concentrations of gentamicin 1 h after a 20- to 30-min infusion or IM injection are 3–5 μg/mL and ≤ 1 μg/mL, respectively; the target peak serum concentration of streptomycin (timing as with gentamicin) is 20–25 μg/mL.
[d] Desirable peak vancomycin level 1 h after completion of a 1-h infusion is 30–45 μg/mL.
[e] MIC > 0.1 μg/mL and <0.5 μg/mL.
[f] MIC ≥ 0.5 μg/mL.
[g] Antimicrobial susceptibility must be evaluated; see text.
[h] Rifampin increases warfarin and dicumarol requirements for anticoagulation.

(Table 126-4). The 2-week penicillin/gentamicin regimen should not be used to treat complicated native valve infection or prosthetic valve endocarditis. Although small studies have suggested that a 2-week regimen of single daily doses of ceftriaxone (2 g IV) plus gentamicin (3 mg/kg) or netilmicin (4 mg/kg) is effective for penicillin-susceptible streptococcal endocarditis, the data are not sufficient to support routine use of this regimen. Penicillin/gentamicin is recommended for the treatment of endocarditis caused by group B strepto-cocci.

ENTEROCOCCI Enterococci are resistant to oxacillin, nafcillin, and the cephalosporins and are inhibited only by penicillin, ampicillin, teicoplanin (not available in the United States), and vancomycin. To kill enterococci requires the synergistic interaction of a cell wall–active antibiotic (penicillin, ampicillin, vancomycin, or teicoplanin) that is effective at achievable serum concentrations and an aminogly-coside (gentamicin or streptomycin) to which the isolate does not ex-hibit high-level resistance. An isolate's resistance to cell wall–active agents or ability to replicate in the presence of gentamicin at $\geq$500 μg/mL or streptomycin at 2000 μg/mL—a phenomenon called *high-level aminoglycoside resistance*—indicates that the ineffective anti-microbial cannot participate in the interaction to produce killing. High-level resistance to gentamicin predicts that tobramycin, netilmicin, amikacin, and kanamycin will also be ineffective. In fact, even when enterococci are not highly resistant to gentamicin, it is difficult to predict the ability of these other aminoglycosides to participate in syn-ergistic killing; consequently, they should not in general be used to treat enterococcal endocarditis.

Clearly, enterococci causing endocarditis must be tested for high-level resistance to streptomycin and gentamicin, β-lactamase produc-tion, and susceptibility to penicillin and ampicillin (MIC, $\leq$16 μg/ mL) and to vancomycin (MIC, $\leq$8 μg/mL). If the isolate produces β-lactamase, ampicillin/sulbactam or vancomycin can be used as the cell wall–active component; if the penicillin/ampicillin MIC is >16 μg/mL, vancomycin can be considered; and if the vancomycin MIC is >8 μg/mL, penicillin or ampicillin may be considered. Based on the absence of high-level resistance, gentamicin or streptomycin should be used as the aminoglycoside. If there is high-level resistance to both these drugs, no aminoglycoside should be given; instead, an 8- to 12-week course of a single cell wall–active agent is suggested. If single-drug therapy fails or the isolate is resistant to all of the com-monly used agents, surgical treatment is advised. The role of newer agents potentially active against multidrug-resistant enterococci (quin-upristin/dalfopristin, linezolid, and daptomycin) in the treatment of endocarditis has not been established.

STAPHYLOCOCCI The regimens used to treat staphylococcal en-docarditis are not based upon coagulase production but rather upon the presence or absence of a prosthetic valve or foreign device, the native valve(s) involved, and the resistance of the isolate to penicillin and methicillin. Penicillinase is produced by 95% of staphylococci; thus, all isolates should be considered penicillin-resistant until shown not to produce this enzyme. The addition of gentamicin (if the isolate is susceptible) to a β-lactam antibiotic to enhance therapy for native mitral or aortic valve endocarditis is optional. Its addition hastens erad-ication of bacteremia but does not improve survival rates. If added, gentamicin should be limited to the initial 3 to 5 days of therapy to avoid nephrotoxicity. Gentamicin generally is not added to the van-comycin regimen in this setting.

Methicillin-susceptible *S. aureus* endocarditis that is uncompli-cated and limited to the tricuspid or pulmonic valve—a condition occurring almost exclusively in injection drug users—can often be treated with a 2-week course that combines oxacillin or nafcillin (but not vancomycin) with gentamicin. Prolonged fevers ($\geq$ 5 days) during therapy suggest that these patients should receive standard therapy.

Staphylococcal prosthetic valve endocarditis is treated for 6 to 8 weeks with a multidrug regimen. Rifampin is an essential component because it kills staphylococci that are adherent to foreign material. Two other agents (selected on the basis of susceptibility testing) are com-bined with rifampin to prevent in vivo emergence of resistance. Be-cause many staphylococci, particularly methicillin-resistant *S. aureus* and *S. epidermidis*, are resistant to gentamicin, the utility of gentamicin should be established before rifampin treatment is begun. If the isolate is resistant to gentamicin, another aminoglycoside or a fluoroquinolone (chosen in light of susceptibility results) should be substituted.

OTHER ORGANISMS Although penicillin is the therapy of choice for endocarditis caused by *S. pneumoniae*, therapy should be initiated with ceftriaxone and vancomycin until susceptibility to penicillin is established. *P. aeruginosa* endocarditis is treated with an antipseu-domonal penicillin (ticarcillin or piperacillin) and high doses of tobra-mycin (8 mg/kg per day in three divided doses). Endocarditis caused by Enterobacteriaceae is treated with a potent β-lactam antibiotic plus an aminoglycoside. Corynebacterial endocarditis is treated with pen-icillin plus an aminoglycoside (if the organism is susceptible to the aminoglycoside) or with vancomycin, which is highly bactericidal for most strains. Therapy for *Candida* endocarditis consists of amphoter-icin B plus flucytosine and early surgery; long-term (if not indefinite) suppression with fluconazole is used increasingly.

Empirical therapy In designing and executing therapy without culture data (i.e., before culture results are known or when cultures are negative), clinical and epidemiologic clues to etiology must be weighed, and both the pathogens associated with the specific endo-carditis syndrome and the hazards of suboptimal therapy must be con-sidered. Thus, empirical therapy for acute endocarditis in an injection drug user should cover methicillin-resistant *S. aureus* and gram-neg-ative bacilli. The initiation of treatment with vancomycin plus genta-micin immediately after blood is obtained for cultures covers these as well as many other potential causes. In treating culture-negative epi-sodes, marantic endocarditis must be excluded and fastidious organ-isms sought serologically. In the absence of confounding prior anti-biotic therapy, it is unlikely that *S. aureus* or enterococcal infection will present with negative blood cultures. Thus, in this situation, these organisms are not the determinants of therapy for subacute endocar-ditis. Blood culture–negative native valve endocarditis is treated with ceftriaxone (or ampicillin) plus gentamicin; these two anti-microbials plus vancomycin should be used if prosthetic valves are involved.

Outpatient antimicrobial therapy Fully compliant patients who have sterile blood cultures, are afebrile during therapy, and have no clinical or echocardiographic findings that suggest an impending com-plication may complete therapy as outpatients. Careful follow-up and a stable home setting are necessary, as are predictable intravenous access and selection of antimicrobials that are stable in solution.

Monitoring antimicrobial therapy The serum bactericidal ti-ter—the highest dilution of the patient's serum during therapy that kills 99.9% of the standard inoculum of the infecting organism—is no longer recommended for assessment of patients receiving standard regimens. However, in the treatment of endocarditis caused by unusual organisms, this measurement, although not standardized and difficult to interpret, may provide a patient-specific assessment of in vivo an-tibiotic effect. Serum concentrations of aminoglycosides and vanco-mycin should be monitored.

Antibiotic toxicities, including allergic reactions, occur in 25 to 40% of patients and commonly arise during the third week of therapy. Blood tests to detect antibiotic-specific potential end-organ toxicity should be performed periodically.

In most patients effective antibiotic therapy results in subjective improvement and resolution of fever within 5 to 7 days. Blood cultures should be repeated daily until sterile, rechecked if there is recrudescent fever, and performed again 4 to 6 weeks after therapy to document cure. Blood cultures become sterile within 2 days after the start of appropriate therapy when infection is caused by viridans streptococci, enterococci, or HACEK organisms. In *S. aureus* endocarditis, β-lac-tam therapy results in sterile cultures in 3 to 5 days, whereas positive cultures may persist for 7 to 9 days with vancomycin treatment. When fever persists for 7 days in spite of appropriate antibiotic therapy, patients should be evaluated for paravalvular abscess and for extra-cardiac abscesses (spleen, kidney) or complications (embolic events). Recrudescent fever raises the question of these complications but also of drug reactions or complications of hospitalization. Serologic abnormalities (e.g., erythrocyte sedimentation rate, rheumatoid factor) resolve slowly and do not reflect response to treatment. Vegetations become smaller with effective therapy, but at 3 months after cure half are unchanged and 25% are slightly larger.

Surgical Treatment Intracardiac and central nervous system complications of endocarditis are important causes of the morbidity and mortality associated with this infection. In some cases, effective treatment for these complications requires surgery. Most of the clinical indications for surgical treatment of endocarditis are not absolute (Table 126-5). The risks and benefits as well as the timing of surgical treatment must therefore be individualized.

Intracardiac surgical indications Most surgical interventions are clearly warranted by intracardiac findings, often detected by echocardiography. Because of the highly invasive nature of prosthetic valve endocarditis, as many as 40% of affected patients merit surgical treatment. In many patients, coincident rather than single intracardiac events necessitate surgery.

CONGESTIVE HEART FAILURE Moderate to severe refractory congestive heart failure caused by new or worsening valve dysfunction is the major indication for cardiac surgical treatment of endocarditis. Of patients with moderate to severe heart failure due to valve dysfunction who are treated medically, 60 to 90% die within 6 months. In the setting of similar hemodynamic dysfunction, surgical treatment is associated with mortality rates of 20 to 40% with native valve endocarditis and 35 to 55% with prosthetic valve infection. Surgery may be required to relieve functional stenosis due to large vegetations or to restore competence to damaged regurgitant valves.

PERIVALVULAR INFECTION This complication, which occurs in 10 to 15% of native valve and 45 to 60% of prosthetic valve infections, is suggested by persistent unexplained fever during appropriate therapy, new electrocardiographic conduction disturbances, and pericarditis. Extension can occur from any valve but is most common with aortic valve infection. TEE with color Doppler is the test of choice to detect perivalvular abscesses (sensitivity, ≥85%). Although occasional perivalvular infections are cured medically, surgery is warranted when fever persists, fistulae develop, prostheses are dehisced and unstable, and infection relapses after appropriate treatment. Cardiac rhythm must be monitored since high-grade heart block may require insertion of a pacemaker.

Table 126-5 Indications for Cardiac Surgical Intervention in Patients with Endocarditis

Surgery required for optimal outcome
  Moderate to severe congestive heart failure due to valve dysfunction
  Partially dehisced unstable prosthetic valve
  Persistent bacteremia despite optimal antimicrobial therapy
  Lack of effective microbicidal therapy (e.g., fungal or *Brucella* endocarditis)
  S. aureus prosthetic valve endocarditis with an intracardiac complication
  Relapse of prosthetic valve endocarditis after optimal antimicrobial therapy
  Persistent unexplained fever (≥10 days) in culture-negative prosthetic valve endocarditis
Surgery to be strongly considered for improved outcome[a]
  Perivalvular extension of infection
  Poorly responsive *S. aureus* endocarditis involving the aortic or mitral valve
  Large (>10-mm diameter) hypermobile vegetations with increased risk of embolism
  Persistent unexplained fever (≥10 days) in culture-negative native valve endocarditis
  Poorly responsive or relapsed endocarditis due to highly antibiotic-resistant enterococci or gram-negative bacilli

[a] Surgery must be carefully considered; findings are often combined with other indications to prompt surgery.

UNCONTROLLED INFECTION Continued positive blood cultures or otherwise unexplained persistent fevers (in patients with either blood culture–positive or –negative endocarditis) despite optimal antibiotic therapy may reflect uncontrolled infection and warrant surgery. Surgical treatment is also advised for endocarditis caused by those organisms against which clinical experience indicates that effective antimicrobial therapy is lacking. This category includes infections caused by yeasts, fungi, *P. aeruginosa*, other highly resistant gram-negative bacilli, *Brucella* species, and probably *C. burnetii*.

S. AUREUS ENDOCARDITIS Mortality rates for *S. aureus* prosthetic valve endocarditis exceed 70% with medical treatment but are reduced to 25% with surgical treatment. In patients with intracardiac complications associated with *S. aureus* prosthetic valve infection, surgical treatment reduces mortality by twentyfold. Surgical treatment should be considered for patients with *S. aureus* native aortic or mitral valve infection who have TTE-demonstrable vegetations and remain septic during the initial week of therapy. Isolated tricuspid valve endocarditis, even with persistent fever, rarely requires surgery.

PREVENTION OF SYSTEMIC EMBOLI Mortality and persisting morbidity due to emboli are largely limited to patients suffering occlusion of cerebral or coronary arteries. Echocardiographic determination of vegetation size and anatomy, although predictive of patients at high risk of systemic emboli, does not identify those patients in whom the benefits of surgery to prevent emboli clearly exceed the risks of the surgical procedure. Net benefits favoring surgery are most likely when the risk of embolism is high and other surgical benefits can be achieved simultaneously—e.g., repair of a moderately dysfunctional valve or debridement of a paravalvular abscess.

Timing of cardiac surgery Surgery to correct valvular dysfunction and progressive congestive heart failure should not be delayed simply to permit additional antibiotic therapy, since this course of action increases the risk of mortality. Similarly, surgery should not be delayed when the indication is uncontrolled or perivalvular infection. Delay is justified only when infection is controlled and congestive heart failure is fully compensated with medical therapy. Recrudescent endocarditis involving a prosthetic valve follows surgery in 2% of patients with culture-positive native valve endocarditis and 15% of patients with active prosthetic valve endocarditis. These risks are more acceptable than the high mortality rates that result when surgery is inappropriately delayed or not performed.

Among patients who have experienced a neurologic complication of endocarditis, further neurologic deterioration can occur as a consequence of cardiac surgery. The risk of significant neurologic exacerbation is related to the interval between the complication and surgery. Where feasible, cardiac surgery should be delayed for 2 to 3 weeks after a nonhemorrhagic embolic stroke and for 4 weeks after a hemorrhagic embolic stroke. A ruptured mycotic aneurysm should be clipped and cerebral edema allowed to resolve prior to cardiac surgery.

Extracardiac complications Splenic abscess develops in 3 to 5% of patients with endocarditis. Effective therapy requires either computed tomography–guided percutaneous drainage or splenectomy. Mycotic aneurysms occur in 2 to 15% of endocarditis patients; half of these cases involve the cerebral arteries and present as headaches, focal neurologic symptoms, or hemorrhage. Cerebral aneurysms should be monitored by angiography. Some will resolve, but those that persist, enlarge, or leak should be treated surgically if possible. Extracerebral aneurysms present as local pain, a mass, local ischemia, or bleeding; generally these aneurysms are treated by resection.

OUTCOME The outcome of infective endocarditis is affected by a variety of factors, some of which are interrelated. Factors with an adverse impact include older age, severe comorbid conditions, delayed diagnosis, involvement of prosthetic valves or the aortic valve, an invasive (*S. aureus*) or antibiotic-resistant (*P. aeruginosa*, yeast) pathogen, intracardiac complications, and major neurologic complications. Death and poor outcome often are related not to failure of

Table 126-6 Procedures for Which Endocarditis Prophylaxis Is Advised in Patients at High or Moderate Risk for Endocarditis[a]

Dental procedures
   Extractions
   Periodontal procedures, cleaning causing gingival bleeding
   Implant placement, reimplantation of avulsed teeth
   Endodontic instrumentation (root canal) or surgery beyond the apex
   Subgingival placement of antibiotic fibers or strips
   Placement of orthodontic bands but not brackets
   Intraligamentary injections (anesthetic)
Respiratory procedures
   Operations involving the mucosa
   Bronchoscopy with rigid bronchoscope
Gastrointestinal procedures[b]
   Esophageal: Sclerotherapy of varices, stricture dilation
   Biliary tract: Endoscopic retrograde cholangiography with biliary obstruction, biliary tract surgery
   Intestinal tract: Surgery involving the mucosa
Genitourinary procedures
   Urethral dilation, prostate or urethral surgery
   Cystoscopy

[a] Prophylaxis is optional for high-risk patients undergoing bronchoscopy or gastrointestinal endoscopy with/without biopsy, vaginal delivery, vaginal hysterectomy, or transesophageal echocardiography.
[b] Prophylaxis is recommended for high-risk patients and optional for moderate-risk group (see Table 126-7).
SOURCE: Adapted from Dajani et al.

antibiotic therapy but rather to the interactions of comorbidities and endocarditis-related end-organ complications. The overall survival rate for patients with native valve endocarditis caused by viridans streptococci, HACEK organisms, or enterococci (susceptible to synergistic therapy) ranges from 85 to 90%. For *S. aureus* native valve endocarditis in patients who do not inject drugs, survival rates are 55 to 70%, whereas 85 to 90% of injection drug users survive this infection. Prosthetic valve endocarditis beginning within 2 months of valve replacement results in mortality rates of 40 to 50%, whereas rates are only 10 to 20% in later-onset cases.

PREVENTION   Antibiotics have been administered in conjunction with selected procedures considered to entail a risk for bacteremia and endocarditis. The benefits of antibiotic prophylaxis are not established and in fact may be modest: only 50% of patients with native valve endocarditis knew that they had a valve lesion predisposing to infection, most endocarditis cases do not follow a procedure, and 35% of cases are caused by organisms not targeted by prophylaxis. Dental treatments, the procedures most widely accepted as predisposing to endocarditis, are no more frequent during the 3 months preceding this diagnosis than in uninfected matched controls. Nevertheless, an expert committee of the American Heart Association, along with similar advisory groups in other developed countries, has identified procedures that may precipitate bacteremia with organisms that cause endocarditis (Table 126-6), patients who should receive prophylaxis based on the relative risk for developing endocarditis and the severity of subsequent

Table 126-7 Cardiac Lesions for Which Endocarditis Prophylaxis Is Advised

High Risk	Moderate Risk
Prosthetic heart valves	Congenital cardiac malformations (other than high-/low-risk lesions), ventricular septal defect, bicuspid aortic valve
Prior bacterial endocarditis	
Complex cyanotic congenital heart disease; other complex congenital lesions after correction (see text)	
Patent ductus arteriosus	Acquired aortic and mitral valve dysfunction
Coarctation of the aorta	Hypertrophic cardiomyopathy (asymmetric septal hypertrophy)
Surgically constructed systemic-pulmonary shunts	Mitral valve prolapse with valvular regurgitation and/or thickened leaflets

Table 126-8 Antibiotic Regimens for Prophylaxis of Endocarditis in Adults at Moderate or High Risk[a]

I. Oral cavity, respiratory tract, or esophageal procedures[b]
   A. Standard regimen
      1. Amoxicillin 2.0 g PO 1 h before procedure
   B. Inability to take oral medication
      1. Ampicillin 2.0 g IV or IM within 30 min of procedure
   C. Penicillin allergy
      1. Clarithromycin 500 mg PO 1 h before procedure
      2. Cephalexin[c] or cefadroxil[c] 2.0 g PO 1 h before procedure
      3. Clindamycin 600 mg PO 1 h before procedure or IV 30 min before procedure
   D. Inability to take oral medication
      1. Cefazolin[c] 1.0 g IV or IM 30 min before procedure
II. Genitourinary and gastrointestinal tract[d] procedures
   A. High-risk patients
      1. Ampicillin 2.0 g IV or IM *plus* gentamicin 1.5 mg/kg (not to exceed 120 mg) IV or IM within 30 min of procedure; repeat ampicillin 1.0 g IV or IM or amoxicillin 1.0 g PO 6 h later
   B. High-risk, penicillin-allergic patients
      1. Vancomycin 1.0 g IV over 1-2 h *plus* gentamicin 1.5 mg/kg (not to exceed 120 mg) IV or IM within 30 min before procedure; no second dose recommended
   C. Moderate-risk patients
      1. Amoxicillin 2.0 g PO 1 h before procedure or ampicillin 2.0 g IV or IM within 30 min before procedure
   D. Moderate-risk, penicillin-allergic patients
      1. Vancomycin 1.0 g IV infused over 1-2 h and completed within 30 min of procedure

[a] Dosing for children: for amoxicillin, ampicillin, cephalexin, or cefadroxil, use 50 mg/kg PO; cefazolin, 25 mg/kg IV; clindamycin, 20 mg/kg PO, 25 mg/kg IV; clarithromycin, 15 mg/kg PO; gentamicin, 1.5 mg/kg IV or IM; and vancomycin, 20 mg/kg IV.
[b] For patients at high risk (Table 126-7), administer a half-dose 6 h after the initial dose.
[c] Do not use cephalosporins in patients with immediate hypersensitivity (urticaria, angioedema, anaphylaxis) to penicillin.
[d] Excludes esophageal procedures.
SOURCE: Adapted from Dajani et al.

infection (Table 126-7), and regimens that may be used for prophylaxis (Table 126-8). Except for an isolated secundum atrial septal defect and a totally corrected patent ductus arteriosus, ventricular septal defect, or pulmonary stenosis, patients with congenital heart defects continue to experience high rates of endocarditis despite total surgical correction of the defect. In vulnerable patients, maintaining good dental hygiene and aggressively treating local infections may reduce the risk of endocarditis.

BIBLIOGRAPHY

BAYER AS et al: Diagnosis and management of infective endocarditis and its complications. Circulation 98:2936, 1998

DAJANI AS et al: Prevention of bacterial endocarditis: Recommendations by the American Heart Association, from the Committee on Rheumatic Fever, Endocarditis, and Kawasaki Disease, Council on Cardiovascular Diseases in the Young. JAMA 277:1794, 1997

D'UDEKEM Y et al: Long-term results of operation for paravalvular abscess. Ann Thorac Surg 62:48, 1996

DURACK D et al: New criteria for diagnosis of infective endocarditis: Utilization of specific echocardiographic findings. Am J Med 96:200, 1994

HEIDENREICH PA et al: Echocardiography in patients with suspected endocarditis: A cost-effective analysis. Am J Med 107:198, 1999

KARCHMER AW: Infections of prosthetic valves and intravascular devices, in *Mandell, Douglas, and Bennett's Principles and Practice of Infectious Diseases*, 5th ed, GL Mandell et al (eds). New York, Churchill Livingstone, 2000, pp 903–917

————: Infective endocarditis, in *Heart Disease*, 6th ed, E Braunwald et al (eds). Philadelphia, Saunders, 2000

KAYE D (ed): *Infective Endocarditis*, 2d ed. New York, Raven, 1992

MORRIS CD et al: Thirty-year incidence of infective endocarditis after surgery for congenital heart defect. JAMA 279:599, 1998

RAOULT D et al: Cultivation of the bacillus of Whipple's disease. N Engl J Med 342:620, 2000

STROM BL et al: Dental and cardiac risk factors for infective endocarditis: A population-based, case-control study. Ann Intern Med 129:761, 1998

WILSON WR et al: Antibiotic treatment of adults with infective endocarditis due to viridans streptococci, enterococci, other streptococci, staphylococci, and HACEK microorganisms. JAMA 274:1706, 1995

INFECTIOUS COMPLICATIONS OF BITES AND BURNS

The skin is an essential component of the nonspecific immune system, protecting the host from potential pathogens in the environment. Breaches in this protective barrier thus represent a form of immunocompromise that predisposes the patient to infection. Bites and scratches from animals and humans allow the inoculation of microorganisms past the skin's protective barrier into deeper, susceptible host tissues. Thermal burns may cause massive destruction of the integument as well as derangements in humoral and cellular immunity, enabling environmental opportunists and components of the host's own skin flora to cause infection.

ANIMAL BITES AND SCRATCHES   Each year in the United States, between 1 and 2 million animal-bite wounds are sustained; the vast majority are inflicted by pet dogs and cats, which number more than 100 million. Other bite wounds are a consequence of encounters with animals in the wild or in occupational settings. While many of these wounds require minimal or no therapy, a significant number result in infection, which may be life-threatening. The microbiology of bite-wound infections in general reflects the oropharyngeal flora of the biting animal, although organisms from the soil, the skin of the animal and victim, and the animal's feces may also be involved.

Dog Bites   Dogs are responsible for approximately 80% of bite wounds, an estimated 15 to 20% of which become infected. A study for the period 1992 through 1994 found that dog bites resulted in more than 900 emergency department visits each day in the United States. Most dog bites are provoked and are inflicted by the victim's pet or by a dog known to the victim. These bites frequently occur during efforts to break up a dogfight. Victims tend to be male, and bites most often involve a lower extremity. Infection typically manifests 8 to 24 h after the bite as pain at the site of injury with cellulitis accompanied by purulent, sometimes foul-smelling discharge. Septic arthritis and osteomyelitis may develop if the canine tooth penetrates synovium or bone. Systemic manifestations such as fever, lymphadenopathy, and lymphangitis may also occur. The microbiology of dog-bite wound infections is usually mixed and includes α-hemolytic streptococci, *Pasteurella* spp., *Staphylococcus* spp., *Eikenella corrodens*, and *Capnocytophaga canimorsus* (formerly designated DF-2). Many wounds also include anaerobic bacteria such as *Actinomyces*, *Fusobacterium*, *Prevotella*, and *Porphyromonas* spp.

While most infections resulting from dog-bite injuries are localized to the area of injury, many of the microorganisms involved are capable of causing systemic infection, including bacteremia, meningitis, brain abscess, endocarditis, and chorioamnionitis. These infections are particularly likely in hosts with edema or compromised lymphatic drainage in the involved extremity (e.g., following a bite on the arm after radical or modified radical mastectomy) and in patients who are immunocompromised by medication or disease (e.g., glucocorticoid use, systemic lupus erythematosus, acute leukemia, or hepatic cirrhosis). In addition, dog bites and scratches may result in systemic illnesses such as rabies (Chap. 197) and tetanus (Chap. 143).

Infection with *C. canimorsus* following dog-bite wounds may result in fulminant sepsis, disseminated intravascular coagulation, and renal failure, particularly in hosts who have impaired hepatic function, who have undergone splenectomy, or who are immunosuppressed. This organism is a thin gram-negative rod that is difficult to culture on most solid media but grows in a variety of liquid media. The bacteria are occasionally seen within polymorphonuclear leukocytes on Wright-stained smears of peripheral blood from septic patients.

Cat Bites   Although less common than dog bites, cat bites and scratches result in infection in more than half of all cases. Because the narrow, sharp feline incisors penetrate deeply into tissue, cat bites are more likely than dog bites to cause septic arthritis and osteomyelitis; the development of these conditions is particularly likely when punctures are located over or near a joint, especially in the hand. Women sustain cat bites more frequently than do men. These bites most often involve the hands and arms. Both bites and scratches from cats are prone to infection from organisms in the cat's oropharynx. *Pasteurella multocida*, a normal component of the feline oral flora, is a small gram-negative coccobacillus implicated in the majority of cat-bite wound infections. Like that of dog-bite wound infections, however, the microflora of cat-bite wound infections is usually mixed. Other microorganisms causing infection after cat bites are similar to those causing dog-bite wound infections.

The same risk factors for systemic infection following dog-bite wounds apply to cat-bite wounds. *Pasteurella* infections tend to advance rapidly, often within hours, causing severe inflammation accompanied by purulent drainage; *Pasteurella* may also be spread by respiratory droplets from animals, resulting in pneumonia or bacteremia. Like dog-bite wounds, cat-bite wounds may result in the transmission of rabies or in the development of tetanus. Infection with *Bartonella henselae* causes cat-scratch disease (Chap. 163) and is an important late consequence of cat bites and scratches. Tularemia (Chap. 161) has also been reported to follow cat bites.

Other Animal Bites   Infections have been attributed to bites from many animal species, often as a consequence of occupational exposure (farmers, laboratory workers, veterinarians) or recreational exposure (hunters and trappers, wilderness campers, owners of exotic pets). Generally, the microflora of bite wounds reflects the oral flora of the biting animal. Most members of the cat family, including feral cats, harbor *P. multocida*. Bite wounds from aquatic animals such as alligators or piranhas may contain *Aeromonas hydrophila*. Venomous snakebites (Chap. 397) result in severe inflammatory responses and tissue necrosis—conditions that render these injuries prone to infection. The snake's oral flora includes many species of aerobes and anaerobes, such as *Pseudomonas aeruginosa*, *Proteus* spp., *Staphylococcus epidermidis*, *Bacteroides fragilis*, and *Clostridium* spp. Bites from nonhuman primates are highly susceptible to infection with pathogens similar to those isolated from human bites (which are discussed later in this chapter). Bites from Old World monkeys (*Macaca*) may also result in the transmission of B virus (*Herpesvirus simiae*, cercopithecine herpesvirus), a cause of serious infection of the human central nervous system. Bites of seals, walruses, and polar bears may cause a chronic suppurative infection known as *seal finger*, which is probably due to one or more species of *Mycoplasma* colonizing these animals.

Small rodents, including rats, mice, and gerbils, as well as animals that prey on rodents may transmit *Streptobacillus moniliformis* (a microaerophilic, pleomorphic gram-negative rod) or *Spirillum minor* (a spirochete), which cause a clinical illness known as *rat-bite fever*. The vast majority of cases in the United States are streptobacillary, whereas *Spirillum* infection occurs mainly in Asia.

In the United States, the risk of rodent bite mainly affects laboratory workers or inhabitants of rodent-infested dwellings (particularly children). Rat-bite fever is distinguished from acute bite-wound infection by its typical manifestation after the initial wound has healed. Streptobacillary disease follows an incubation period of 3 to 10 days. Fever, chills, myalgias, headache, and severe migratory arthralgias are usually followed by a maculopapular rash, which characteristically involves the palms and soles and may become confluent or purpuric. Complications include endocarditis, myocarditis, meningitis, pneumonia, and abscesses in many organs. *Haverhill fever* is an *S. moniliformis* infection acquired from contaminated milk or drinking water and has similar manifestations. Streptobacillary rat-bite fever was frequently fatal in the preantibiotic era. The differential diagnosis includes Rocky Mountain spotted fever, Lyme disease, leptospirosis, and secondary syphilis. The diagnosis is made by direct observation of the causative organisms in tissue or blood, by culture on enriched media, or by serologic testing with specific agglutinins.

Spirillum infection (referred to in Japan as *sodoku*) causes pain and purple swelling at the site of the initial bite, with associated lymphangitis and regional lymphadenopathy, after an incubation period of 1 to 4 weeks. The systemic illness includes fever, chills, and headache. The original lesion may eventually progress to an eschar. The infection is diagnosed by direct visualization of the spirochetes in blood or tissue or by animal inoculation.

Human Bites Human bites may be self-inflicted; may be sustained by medical personnel caring for patients; or may take place during fights, domestic abuse, or sexual activity. Human bites more frequently become infected than do bites inflicted by other animals. These infections reflect the diverse oral microflora of humans, which includes multiple species of aerobic and anaerobic bacteria. Common aerobic isolates include viridans streptococci, *Staphylococcus aureus*, *E. corrodens* (which is particularly common in clenched-fist injury; see below), and *Haemophilus influenzae*. Anaerobic species, including *Fusobacterium nucleatum* and *Prevotella*, *Porphyromonas*, and *Peptostreptococcus* spp., are isolated from 50% of human-bite wound infections; many of these isolates produce β-lactamases. The oral flora of hospitalized and debilitated patients often includes Enterobacteriaceae in addition to the usual organisms. Both HIV and hepatitis B virus have been reported to be transmitted by human bite, but these instances appear to be quite rare.

Human bites are categorized as "occlusional" injuries, which are inflicted by actual biting, and "clenched-fist" injuries, which are sustained when the fist of one individual strikes the teeth of another, causing traumatic laceration of the hand. For several reasons, clenched-fist injuries result in particularly serious infections. The deep spaces of the hand, including the bone, joint, and tendons, are frequently inoculated with organisms in the course of such injuries. The clenched position of the fist during injury, followed by extension of the hand, may further promote the introduction of bacteria as contaminated tendons retract beneath the skin's surface. Moreover, medical attention is often sought only after frank infection develops.

℞ **TREATMENT** **Initial Assessment** A careful history should be elicited, including the type of biting animal, the type of attack (provoked or unprovoked), and the amount of time elapsed since injury. Local and regional authorities should be contacted to determine whether an individual species could be rabid and/or to locate and observe the biting animal when rabies prophylaxis may be indicated (Chap. 197). Suspicious human-bite wounds should provoke careful questioning regarding domestic or child abuse. Details on antibiotic allergies, immunosuppression, splenectomy, liver disease, mastectomy, and immunization history should be obtained. The wound should be inspected carefully for evidence of infection, including redness, exudate, and foul odor. The type of wound (puncture, laceration, or scratch); the depth of penetration; and the possible involvement of joints, tendons, nerves, and bone should be assessed. It is often useful to include a diagram or photograph of the wound in the medical record. In addition, a general physical examination should be conducted and should include an assessment of vital signs as well as an evaluation for evidence of lymphangitis, lymphadenopathy, dermatologic lesions, and functional limitations. Injuries to the hand warrant consultation with a hand surgeon for the assessment of tendon, nerve, and muscular damage. Radiographs should be obtained when the bone may have been penetrated or a tooth fragment may be present. Culture and Gram's staining of all infected wounds are essential; anaerobic cultures should be undertaken if abscesses, devitalized tissue, or foul-smelling exudate is present. A small-tipped swab may be used to culture deep punctures or small lacerations. It is also reasonable to culture samples from uninfected wounds due to bites inflicted by animals other than dogs and cats, since the microorganisms causing disease are less predictable in these cases. A white blood cell count should be determined and blood cultured if systemic infection is suspected.

Wound Management Wound closure is controversial in bite injuries. Many authorities prefer not to attempt primary closure of wounds that are or may become infected, preferring to irrigate these wounds copiously, debride devitalized tissue, remove foreign bodies, and approximate the wound edges. Delayed primary closure may be undertaken after the risk of infection is over. Small uninfected wounds may be allowed to close by secondary intention. Puncture wounds due to cat bites should be left unsutured because of the high rate at which they become infected. Facial wounds are usually sutured after thorough cleaning and irrigation because of the importance of a good cosmetic result in this area and because anatomic factors such as an excellent blood supply and the absence of dependent edema lessen the risk of infection.

Antibiotic Therapy • *Established infection* Antibiotics should be administered in all established bite-wound infections and should be chosen in light of the most likely potential pathogens, as indicated by the biting species and by Gram's stain and culture results (Table 127-1). For dog and cat bites, antibiotics should be effective against *S. aureus*, *Pasteurella* spp., *C. canimorsus*, streptococci, and oral anaerobes. For human bites, agents with activity against *S. aureus*, *H. influenzae*, and β-lactamase-positive oral anaerobes should be used. The combination of an extended-spectrum penicillin with a β-lactamase inhibitor (amoxicillin/clavulanic acid, ticarcillin/clavulanic acid, ampicillin/sulbactam) appears to offer the most reliable coverage for these pathogens. Second-generation cephalosporins (cefuroxime, cefoxitin) also offer substantial coverage. The choice of antibiotics in penicillin-allergic patients (particularly those in whom immediate-type hypersensitivity makes the use of cephalosporins hazardous) is more difficult and is based primarily on in vitro sensitivity since data on clinical efficacy are inadequate. The combination of an antibiotic active against gram-positive cocci and anaerobes (such as clindamycin) with trimethoprim-sulfamethoxazole or a fluoroquinolone, which is active against many of the other potential pathogens, would appear reasonable. In vitro data suggest that either trovafloxacin or azithromycin alone provides coverage against most commonly isolated bite-wound pathogens.

Antibiotics are normally given for 10 to 14 days, but the response to therapy must be carefully monitored. Failure to respond should prompt a consideration of diagnostic alternatives and surgical evaluation for possible drainage or debridement. Complications such as osteomyelitis or septic arthritis mandate a longer duration of therapy.

Management of *C. canimorsus* sepsis requires a 2-week course of intravenous penicillin G (2 million units intravenously every 4 h) and supportive measures. Alternative agents for the treatment of *C. canimorsus* infection include cephalosporins and fluoroquinolones. Serious infection with *P. multocida* (e.g., pneumonia, sepsis, or meningitis) should also be treated with intravenous penicillin G. Alternative agents include second- or third-generation cephalosporins or ciprofloxacin.

Bites by venomous snakes may not require antibiotic treatment, but it is often difficult to distinguish signs of infection from tissue damage caused by the envenomation. Thus many authorities continue to recommend treatment directed against the snake's oral flora—i.e., the administration of broadly active agents such as ceftriaxone (1 to 2 g intravenously every 12 to 24 h) or ampicillin/sulbactam (1.5 to 3.0 g intravenously every 6 h).

Seal finger appears to respond to doxycycline (100 mg twice daily for an interval guided by the response to therapy).

Presumptive or prophylactic therapy The use of antibiotics in patients presenting early after bite injury (within 8 h) is controversial. Although symptomatic infection will not yet be manifest in many of these wounds at this point, many early wounds will harbor pathogens, and many will become infected. Studies of the use of prophylactic antibiotics in wound infections are limited and have often included small numbers of cases in which various types of wounds have been managed according to various protocols. A recent meta-analysis of eight randomized trials of prophylactic antibiotics in patients with dog-bite wounds demonstrated a reduction of the rate of infection by approximately 50% with prophylaxis. However, in the absence of sound

Table 127-1 Management of Wound Infections Following Animal Bites

Biting Species	Commonly Isolated Pathogens	Preferred Antibiotic(s)[a]	Alternative Agent(s) for Penicillin-Allergic Patients	Recommendation for Prophylaxis in Patients with Recent Uninfected Wounds[b]	Other Considerations
Dog	*Staphylococcus aureus, Streptococcus* spp., *Pasteurella* spp., anaerobes, *Capnocytophaga canimorsus*	Amoxicillin/clavulanic acid (250–500 mg PO tid); or ampicillin/sulbactam (1.5–3.0 g IV q6h)	Clindamycin (150–300 mg PO qid) plus either TMP-SMZ (1 double-strength tablet bid) or ciprofloxacin (500 mg PO bid)	Sometimes[c]	Consider rabies prophylaxis.
Cat	*Pasteurella multocida, S. aureus, Streptococcus* spp., anaerobes	Amoxicillin/clavulanic acid or ampicillin/sulbactam, as for dog bite	Clindamycin plus either TMP-SMZ or a fluoroquinolone	Usually	Consider rabies prophylaxis; carefully evaluate for joint/bone penetration.
Human; occlusional bite	Viridans streptococci, *S. aureus, Haemophilus influenzae*, anaerobes	Amoxicillin/clavulanic acid or ampicillin/sulbactam, as for dog bite	Erythromycin, fluoroquinolone	Always	—
Human; clenched-fist injury	As for occlusional bite plus *Eikenella corrodens*	Ampicillin/sulbactam, as for dog bite, or imipenem	Cefoxitin[d] (1.5 g IV q6h)	Always	Examine for tendon/nerve/joint involvement.
Monkey	As for human bite	As for human bite	As for human bite	Always	For macaque monkeys, consider B virus prophylaxis with acyclovir.
Snake	*Pseudomonas aeruginosa, Proteus* spp., *Bacteroides fragilis, Clostridium* spp.	Ceftriaxone (1–2 g IV q12–24h); or ampicillin/sulbactam, as for dog bite	Clindamycin plus either TMP-SMZ or a fluoroquinolone	Sometimes, especially for venomous snakebite	Use antivenin for venomous snakebite.
Rodent	*Streptobacillus moniliformis, Leptospira* spp., *P. multocida*	Penicillin VK (500 mg PO bid)	Doxycycline (100 mg PO qd)	Sometimes[c]	—

[a] Antibiotic choices should be based on culture data, when available. Duration of therapy must be guided by response, but normally a minimum course of 10 to 14 days is required for established soft tissue infection. Osteomyelitis and septic arthritis require longer treatment. These suggestions for empirical therapy need to be tailored to individual circumstances and local conditions. Intravenous regimens should be used for hospitalized patients. When the patient is to be discharged after initial management, a single intravenous dose of antibiotic may be given and followed by oral therapy.

[b] Prophylactic antibiotics are usually given for 3 to 5 days.

[c] Prophylactic antibiotics are suggested for severe or extensive wounds, facial wounds, or crush injuries; when bone or joint may be involved; or when comorbidity exists (see text).

[d] Cefoxitin may be hazardous to patients with immediate-type hypersensitivity to penicillin.

NOTE: TMP-SMZ, trimethoprim-sulfamethoxazole.

clinical trials, many clinicians base the decision to treat bite wounds with empirical antibiotics on the species of the biting animal; the location, severity, and extent of the bite wound; and the existence of comorbid conditions in the host. All human- and monkey-bite wounds should be treated presumptively because of the high rate of infection. Most cat-bite wounds, particularly those involving the hand, should be treated. Other factors favoring treatment for bite wounds include severe injury, as in crush wounds; potential bone or joint involvement; involvement of the hands or genital region; host immunocompromise, including that due to liver disease or splenectomy; and prior mastectomy on the side of an involved upper extremity. When prophylactic antibiotics are administered, they are usually given for 3 to 5 days.

Rabies and Tetanus Prophylaxis Rabies prophylaxis, consisting of both passive administration of rabies immune globulin (with as much of the dose as possible infiltrated in and around the wound) and active immunization with rabies vaccine, should be given in consultation with local and regional public health authorities for many wild-animal (and some domestic-animal) bites and scratches as well as for certain nonbite exposures (Chap. 197). Rabies is endemic in a variety of animals, including dogs and cats in many areas of the world. Many local health authorities require the reporting of all animal bites. A tetanus booster immunization should be given if the patient has undergone primary immunization but has not received a booster dose in the past 5 years. Patients who have not previously completed primary immunization should be immunized and should also receive tetanus immune globulin. Elevation of the site of injury is an important adjunct to antimicrobial therapy. Immobilization of the infected area, especially the hand, is also beneficial.

BURNS Epidemiology More than 2 million burn injuries are brought to medical attention in the United States each year. While many burn injuries are minor and require little or no intervention, approximately 70,000 persons are hospitalized for these injuries, and 20,000 of this number are burned severely enough to require admission to a specialized burn unit. Scalds, structural fires, and flammable liquids and gases are the major causes of burns, but electrical, chemical, and smoking-related sources are also important. Burns predispose to infection by damaging the protective barrier function of the skin, thus facilitating the entry of pathogenic microorganisms, and by inducing systemic immunosuppression. It is therefore not surprising that infectious complications are the major cause of morbidity and mortality in serious burn injury and that as many as 10,000 patients in the United States die of burn-related infections each year.

Pathophysiology Loss of the cutaneous barrier facilitates entry of the patient's own flora and of organisms from the hospital environment into the burn wound. The wound often contains devitalized or frankly necrotic tissue that quickly becomes contaminated with bacteria. Invasive infection—localized and/or systemic—occurs when bacteria penetrate viable tissue, usually below the eschar. Streptococci and staphylococci were the predominant causes of burn-wound infection in the preantibiotic era and remain important pathogens at present. With the advent of antimicrobial agents, *P. aeruginosa* became a major problem in burn-wound management. As antibiotics more effective against *Pseudomonas* have become available, fungi (particularly *Candida albicans, Aspergillus* spp., and the agents of mucormycosis) have emerged as increasingly important pathogens in burn-wound patients. Herpes simplex virus infection has also been found in burn wounds, especially on the face.

The frequency of infection parallels the extent and severity of burn injury. Severe burns cause defects in both cellular and humoral immunity that have a major impact on infection. For example, decreases in the number and activity of circulating helper T cells, increases in suppressor T cells, and diminution in levels of immunoglobulin follow major burns. Neutrophil function has also been shown to be impaired after burns. The increased levels of multiple cytokines detected in burn patients are compatible with the widely held belief that the inflammatory response becomes dysregulated in these individuals. Increased permeability of the gut wall to bacteria and their components, such as endotoxin, also contributes to immune dysregulation and sepsis. Thus, the burn patient is predisposed to infection at remote sites (see below) as well as at the sites of burn injury.

Clinical Manifestations Since clinical indications of wound infection are difficult to interpret, wounds must be monitored carefully for changes that may reflect infection. A margin of erythema frequently surrounds the sites of burns and by itself is not usually indicative of infection. Signs of infection include the conversion of a partial-thickness to a full-thickness burn, color changes (e.g., the appearance of a dark brown or black discoloration of the wound), the new appearance of erythema or violaceous edema in normal tissue at the wound margins, the sudden separation of the eschar from subcutaneous tissues, and the degeneration of the wound with the appearance of a new eschar. The appearance of a green discoloration of the wound or subcutaneous fat or the development of ecthyma gangrenosum at a remote site points to a diagnosis of invasive *P. aeruginosa* infection. Changes in body temperature, hypotension, tachycardia, altered mentation, neutropenia or neutrophilia, thrombocytopenia, and renal failure may result from invasive burn wounds and sepsis. However, because profound alterations in homeostasis occur as a consequence of burns per se and because inflammation without infection is a normal component of these injuries, the assessment of these changes is complicated. Alterations in body temperature, for example, are attributable to thermoregulatory dysfunction; tachycardia and hyperventilation accompany the metabolic changes induced by extensive burn injury and are not necessarily indicative of bacterial sepsis.

Given the difficulty of evaluating burn wounds solely on the basis of clinical observation and laboratory data, wound biopsies are necessary for definitive diagnosis of infection. The timing of these biopsies can be guided by clinical changes, but in some centers burn wounds are routinely biopsied at regular intervals. The biopsy specimen is examined for histologic evidence of bacterial invasion, and quantitative microbiologic cultures are performed. The presence of $>10^5$ viable bacteria per gram of tissue is highly suggestive of invasive infection and of a dramatically increased risk of sepsis. Histopathologic evidence of invasion of viable tissue by microorganisms is a more definitive indicator of infection. A blood culture positive for the same organism seen in large quantities in biopsied tissue is a reliable indicator of burn sepsis. Surface cultures may provide some indication of the microorganisms present in the hospital environment but are not indicative of the etiology of infection.

In addition to infection of the burn wound itself, a number of other infections due to the immunosuppression caused by extensive burns and the manipulations necessary for clinical care put burn patients at risk. Pneumonia, now the most common infectious complication among hospitalized burn patients, is most often nosocomially acquired via the respiratory route; septic pulmonary emboli may also occur. Suppurative thrombophlebitis may complicate the vascular catheterization necessary for fluid and nutritional support in burns. Endocarditis, urinary tract infection, bacterial chondritis (particularly in patients with burned ears), and intraabdominal infection also complicate serious burn injury.

℞ **TREATMENT** The ultimate goal of burn-wound management is closure and healing of the wound. Early surgical excision of burned tissue, with extensive debridement of necrotic tissue and grafting of skin or skin substitutes, greatly decreases the mortality associated with severe burns. In addition, the three widely used topical antimicrobial agents—silver sulfadiazine cream, mafenide acetate cream, and silver nitrate—dramatically decrease the bacterial burden of burn wounds and reduce the incidence of burn-wound infection; they are routinely applied to partial- and full-thickness burns. All three agents are broadly active against many bacteria and against some fungi and are useful before bacterial colonization is established. Silver sulfadiazine is often used initially, but its value can be limited by bacterial resistance. Mafenide acetate has broader activity; the cream penetrates eschars and thus can prevent or treat infection beneath the eschars. The foremost disadvantages of this agent are that it can inhibit carbonic anhydrase, resulting in metabolic acidosis, and that it elicits hypersensitivity reactions in up to 7% of patients. This agent is most often used when gram-negative bacteria invade the burn wound and when treatment with silver sulfadiazine fails.

When invasive wound infection is diagnosed, topical therapy should be changed to mafenide acetate. Subeschar clysis (the direct instillation of an antibiotic, often piperacillin, under the eschar into wound tissues) is a useful adjunct to surgical and systemic antimicrobial therapy. Systemic treatment with antibiotics active against the pathogens present in the wound should be instituted. In the absence of culture data, treatment is broad and should cover organisms commonly encountered in the particular burn unit. Usually such coverage is achieved with an antibiotic active against gram-positive pathogens, such as oxacillin (2 g intravenously every 4 h), and with antibiotics active against *P. aeruginosa* and other gram-negative rods, such as mezlocillin (3 g intravenously every 4 h) and gentamicin (5 mg/kg intravenously per day). In the penicillin-allergic patient, vancomycin (1 g intravenously every 12 h) may be substituted for oxacillin (and is efficacious when methicillin-resistant *S. aureus* is present), and ciprofloxacin (400 mg intravenously every 12 h) may be substituted for mezlocillin. Patients with burn wounds frequently have alterations in metabolism and renal clearance mechanisms that mandate the monitoring of serum antibiotic levels; the levels achieved with standard doses are often subtherapeutic.

In general, prophylactic systemic antibiotics have no role in the management of burn wounds (except for minor burns in outpatients) and can in fact lead to colonization with resistant microorganisms. An exception involves cases requiring burn-wound manipulation. Since procedures such as debridement, excision, or grafting frequently result in bacteremia, prophylactic systemic antibiotics are administered at the time of burn-wound manipulation; the particular agents used should be chosen on the basis of data obtained by wound culture or data on the hospital's resident flora. All burn-injury patients should undergo tetanus booster immunization if they have completed primary immunization but have not received a booster dose in the past 5 years. Patients without prior immunization should receive tetanus immune globulin and undergo primary immunization. Infection control measures play a major role in preventing burn-wound infection and limiting the spread of antibiotic-resistant nosocomial pathogens.

BIBLIOGRAPHY

BAKER AS et al: Isolation of *Mycoplasma* species from a patient with seal finger. Clin Infect Dis 27:1168, 1998

CUMMINGS P: Antibiotics to prevent infection in patients with dog bite wounds: A meta-analysis of randomized trials. Ann Emerg Med 23:535, 1994

FLEISHER GR: The management of bite wounds. N Engl J Med 340:138, 1999

GOLDSTEIN EJ: Bite wounds and infection. Clin Infect Dis 14:633, 1992

KULLBERG BJ et al: Purpura fulminans and symmetrical peripheral gangrene caused by *Capnocytophaga canimorsus* (formerly DF-2) septicemia—a complication of dog bite. Medicine (Baltimore) 70:287, 1991

PRUITT BJ et al: The changing epidemiology of infection in burn patients. World J Surg 16:57, 1992

TALAN DA et al: Bacteriological analysis of infected dog and cat bites. N Engl J Med 340:85, 1999

WEBER DJ et al: Infections resulting from animal bites. Infect Dis Clin North Am 5:663, 1991

WEISS HB et al: Incidence of dog bite injuries treated in emergency departments. JAMA 279:51, 1998

YURT R: Burns, in *Mandell, Douglas and Bennett's Principles and Practice of Infectious Diseases*, 4th ed, G Mandell et al (eds). New York, Churchill Livingstone, 1995, pp 2761–2765

INFESTIONS OF THE SKIN, MUSCLE, AND SOFT TISSUES

ANATOMIC RELATIONSHIPS: CLUES TO THE DIAGNOSIS OF SOFT TISSUE INFECTIONS Protection against infection of the epidermis is dependent on the mechanical barrier afforded by the stratum corneum, since the epidermis itself is devoid of blood vessels (Fig. 128-1). Disruption of this layer by burns or bites (Chap. 127), abrasions, foreign bodies, primary dermatologic disorders (e.g., herpes simplex, varicella, and ecthyma gangrenosum), surgery, or vascular or pressure ulcer allows penetration of bacteria to the deeper structures. Similarly, the hair follicle can serve as a portal either for components of the normal flora (e.g., *Staphylococcus*) or for extrinsic bacteria (e.g., *Pseudomonas* in hot-tub folliculitis). Intracellular infection of the squamous epithelium with vesicle formation may arise from cutaneous inoculation, as in infection with herpes simplex virus (HSV) type 1; from the dermal capillary plexus, as in varicella and infections due to other viruses associated with viremia; or from cutaneous nerve roots, as in herpes zoster. Bacteria infecting the epidermis, such as *Streptococcus pyogenes*, may be translocated laterally to deeper structures via lymphatics, an event that results in the rapid superficial spread of erysipelas. Later, engorgement or obstruction of lymphatics causes flaccid edema of the epidermis, another characteristic of erysipelas.

The rich plexus of capillaries beneath the dermal papillae provides nutrition to the stratum germinativum, and physiologic responses of this plexus produce important clinical signs and symptoms. For example, infective vasculitis of the plexus results in petechiae, Osler's nodes, Janeway lesions, and palpable purpura, which are important clues to the existence of endocarditis (Chap. 126). In addition, metastatic infection within this plexus can result in cutaneous manifestations of disseminated fungal infection (Chap. 205), gonococcal infection (Chap. 147), *Salmonella* infection (Chap. 156), *Pseudomonas* infection (i.e., ecthyma gangrenosum; Chap. 155), meningococcemia (Chap. 146), and staphylococcal infection (Chap. 139). The plexus also provides access for bacteria to the circulation, thereby facilitating local spread or bacteremia. The postcapillary venules of this plexus are a major site of polymorphonuclear leukocyte sequestration, diapedesis, and chemotaxis to the site of cutaneous infection.

Exaggeration of these physiologic mechanisms by excessive levels of cytokines or bacterial toxins causes leukostasis, venous occlusion, and pitting edema. Edema with purple bullae, ecchymosis, and cutaneous anesthesia suggests loss of vascular integrity and necessitates exploration of the deeper structures for evidence of necrotizing fasciitis or myonecrosis. An early diagnosis requires a high level of suspicion in instances of unexplained fever and of pain and tenderness in the soft tissue, even in the absence of acute cutaneous inflammation.

INFECTIONS ASSOCIATED WITH VESICLES (Table 128-1) Vesicle formation due to infection is caused by viral proliferation within the epidermis. In varicella and variola, viremia precedes the onset of a diffuse centripetal rash that progresses from macules to vesicles, then to pustules, and finally to scabs over the course of 1 to 2 weeks. Vesicles of varicella have a "dewdrop" appearance and develop in crops randomly about the trunk, extremities, and face over 3 to 4 days. Herpes zoster occurs in a single dermatome; the appearance of vesicles is preceded by pain for several days. Zoster may occur in persons of any age but is most common among immunosuppressed individuals and elderly patients, whereas most cases of varicella occur in young children. Vesicles due to HSV are found on or around the lips (HSV-1) or genitals (HSV-2) but may appear on the head and neck of young wrestlers (herpes gladiatorum) or on the digits of health care workers (herpetic whitlow). Coxsackievirus A16 characteristically causes vesicles on the hands, feet, and mouth of children. Orf is caused by a DNA virus related to smallpox virus and infects the fingers of individuals who work around goats and sheep. Molluscum contagiosum virus induces flaccid vesicles on the skin of healthy and immunocompromised individuals.

Rickettsialpox begins following mite-bite inoculation of *Rickettsia akari* into the skin. A papule with a central vesicle evolves to form a 1- to 2.5-cm painless crusted black eschar with an erythematous halo and proximal adenopathy. While more common in the northeastern United States and the Ukraine in 1940–1950, rickettsialpox has recently been described in Ohio, Arizona, and Utah. Blistering dactylitis is a painful, vesicular, localized *Staphylococcus aureus* or group A streptococcal infection of the pulps of the distal digits of the hands.

INFECTIONS ASSOCIATED WITH BULLAE (Table 128-1) Staphylococcal scalded-skin syndrome (SSSS) in neonates is caused by a toxin (exfoliatin) from phage group II *S. aureus*. SSSS must be distinguished from toxic epidermal necrolysis (TEN), which occurs primarily in adults, is drug-induced, and has a higher mortality. Punch biopsy with frozen section is useful in making this distinction since the cleavage plane is the stratum corneum in SSSS (Fig. 128-1) and the stratum germinativum in TEN. Intravenous γ-globulin is a promising treatment for TEN. Necrotizing fasciitis and gas gangrene also induce bulla formation (see "Necrotizing Fasciitis," below). Halophilic vibrio infection can be as aggressive and fulminant as necrotizing fasciitis; a helpful clue in its diagnosis is a history of exposure to waters of the Gulf of Mexico or the Atlantic seaboard or (in a patient with cirrhosis) the ingestion of raw seafood. The etiologic organism (*Vibrio vulnificus*) is highly susceptible to tetracycline.

INFECTIONS ASSOCIATED WITH CRUSTED LESIONS (Table 128-1) Impetigo contagiosa is caused by *S. pyogenes*, and bullous impetigo is due to *S. aureus*. Both skin lesions may have an early bullous stage but then appear as thick crusts with a golden-brown color. Streptococcal lesions are most common among children 2 to 5 years of age, and epidemics may occur in settings of poor hygiene, particularly among children of lower socioeconomic status in tropical climates. It is important to recognize impetigo contagiosa because of its relationship to poststreptococcal glomerulonephritis. Superficial dermatophyte infection (ringworm) can occur on any skin surface, and skin scrapings with KOH staining are diagnostic. Primary infections with dimorphic fungi such as *Blastomyces dermatitidis* and *Sporothrix schenckii* can initially present as crusted skin lesions resembling ringworm. Disseminated infection with *Coccidioides immitis* can also involve the skin, and biopsy and culture should be performed on crusted lesions in patients from endemic areas.

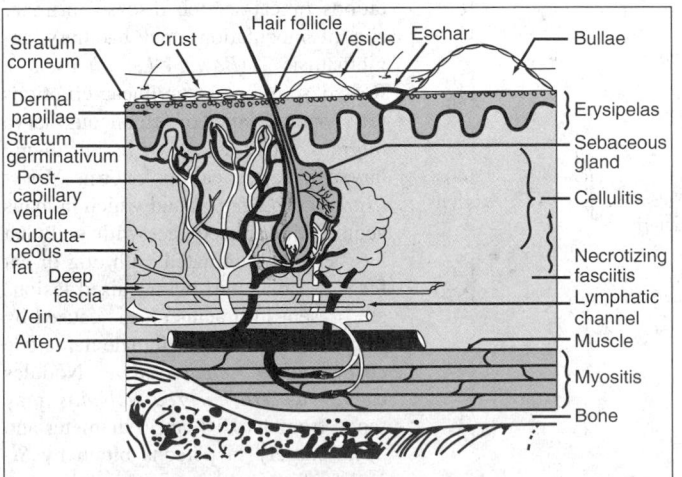

FIGURE 128-1 Structural components of the skin and soft tissue, superficial infections, and infections of the deeper structures. The rich capillary network beneath the dermal papillae plays a key role in the localization of infection and in the development of the acute inflammatory reaction.

Table 128-1 Skin and Soft Tissue Infections

Lesion, Clinical Syndrome	Infectious Agent	Chapter(s)
Vesicles		
Smallpox	Variola virus	186
Chickenpox	Varicella-zoster virus	183
Shingles (herpes zoster)	Varicella-zoster virus	183
Cold sores, herpetic whitlow, herpes gladiatorum	Herpes simplex virus	182
Hand-foot-and-mouth disease	Coxsackievirus A16	193
Orf	Parapoxvirus	186
Molluscum contagiosum	Pox-like virus	186
Rickettsialpox	*Rickettsia akari*	177
Bullae		
Staphylococcal scalded-skin syndrome	*Staphylococcus aureus*	139
Blistering distal dactylitis	*S. aureus* or *Streptococcus pyogenes*	139, 140
Necrotizing fasciitis	*S. pyogenes, Clostridium* spp., mixed aerobes and anaerobes	167
Gas gangrene	*Clostridium* spp.	145
Halophilic vibrio	*Vibrio vulnificus*	159
Crusted lesions		
Bullous impetigo/ecthyma	*S. aureus*	139
Impetigo contagiosa	*S. pyogenes*	140
Ringworm	Superficial dermatophyte fungi	208
Sporotrichosis	*Sporothrix schenckii*	208
Histoplasmosis	*Histoplasma capsulatum*	201
Coccidioidomycosis	*Coccidioides immitis*	202
Blastomycosis	*Blastomyces dermatitidis*	203
Cutaneous leishmaniasis	*Leishmania* spp.	215
Cutaneous tuberculosis	*Mycobacterium tuberculosis*	169
Nocardiosis	*Nocardia asteroides*	165
Folliculitis		
Furunculosis	*S. aureus*	139
Hot-tub folliculitis	*Pseudomonas aeruginosa*	155
Swimmer's itch	*Schistosoma* spp.	222
Acne vulgaris	*Propionibacterium acnes*	56
Papular and nodular lesions		
Fish-tank or swimming-pool granuloma	*Mycobacterium marinum*	171
Creeping eruption (cutaneous larva migrans)	*Ancylostoma braziliense*	219
Dracunculiasis	*Dracunculus medinensis*	221
Cercarial dermatitis	*Schistosoma mansoni*	222
Verruca vulgaris	Human papillomaviruses 1, 2, 4	188
Condylomata acuminata (anogenital warts)	Human papillomaviruses 6, 11, 16, 18	188
Onchocerciasis nodule	*Onchocerca volvulus*	221
Cutaneous myiasis	*Dermatobia hominis*	398
Verruca peruana	*Bartonella bacilliformis*	163
Cat-scratch disease	*Bartonella henselae*	163
Lepromatous leprosy	*Mycobacterium leprae*	170
Secondary syphilis (papulosquamous, nodular, and condylomata lata lesions)	*Treponema pallidum*	172
Tertiary syphilis (nodular gummatous lesions)	*T. pallidum*	172
Ulcers with or without eschars		
Anthrax	*Bacillus anthracis*	141
Ulceroglandular tularemia	*Francisella tularensis*	161
Bubonic plague	*Yersinia pestis*	162
Buruli ulcer	*Mycobacterium ulcerans*	171
Leprosy	*M. leprae*	170
Cutaneous tuberculosis	*M. tuberculosis*	169
Chancroid	*Haemophilus ducreyi*	149
Primary syphilis	*T. pallidum*	172
Erysipelas	*S. pyogenes*	140
Cellulitis	*Staphylococcus* spp., *Streptococcus* spp., various other bacteria	Various
Necrotizing fasciitis		
Streptococcal gangrene	*S. pyogenes*	140
Fournier's gangrene	Mixed aerobic and anaerobic bacteria	167
Myositis and myonecrosis		
Pyomyositis	*S. aureus*	139
Streptococcal necrotizing myositis	*S. pyogenes*	140
Gas gangrene	*Clostridium* spp.	145
Nonclostridial (crepitant) myositis	Mixed aerobic and anaerobic bacteria	167
Synergistic nonclostridial anaerobic myonecrosis	Mixed aerobic and anaerobic bacteria	167

Crusted nodular lesions caused by *Mycobacterium chelonei* have been described in HIV-seropositive patients. Treatment with clarithromycin looks promising.

FOLLICULITIS (Table 128-1) Hair follicles serve as a portal for a number of bacteria, though *S. aureus* is the most common cause of localized folliculitis. Sebaceous glands empty into hair follicles and ducts and, if blocked, form sebaceous cysts, which may resemble staphylococcal abscesses or may become secondarily infected. Infection of sweat glands (hidradenitis suppurativa) can also mimic infection of hair follicles, particularly in the axillae. Chronic folliculitis is uncommon except in acne vulgaris, where constituents of the normal flora (e.g., *Propionibacterium acnes*) may play a role.

Diffuse folliculitis occurs in two settings. "Hot-tub folliculitis" is caused by *Pseudomonas aeruginosa* in waters that are insufficiently chlorinated and maintained at temperatures between 37 and 40°C. Infection is usually self-limited, though bacteremia and shock have been reported. Swimmer's itch occurs when a skin surface is exposed to water infested with freshwater avian schistosomes. Warm water temperatures and alkaline pH are suitable for mollusks that serve as intermediate hosts between birds and humans. Free-swimming schistosomal cercariae readily penetrate human hair follicles or pores but quickly die and elicit a brisk allergic reaction causing intense itching and erythema.

PAPULAR AND NODULAR LESIONS (Table 128-1) Raised lesions of the skin occur in many different forms. *Mycobacterium marinum* infections of the skin may present as cellulitis or as raised erythematous nodules. Erythematous papules are early manifestations of cat-scratch disease (primary site of inoculation) and bacillary angiomatosis (*Bartonella henselae*). Raised serpiginous or linear eruptions are characteristic of cutaneous larva migrans, which is caused by burrowing larvae of dog or cat hookworms (*Ancylostoma braziliense*) and which humans acquire through contact with soil that has been contaminated with dog or cat feces. Similar burrowing raised lesions are present in dracunculiasis caused by migration of the adult female nematode *Dracunculus medinensis*. Nodules caused by *Onchocerca volvulus* may range from 1 to 10 cm in diameter and occur largely in persons bitten by *Simulium* flies in Africa. The nodules contain the adult worm encased in fibrous tissue. Migration of microfilariae into the eyes may result in blindness. Verruca peruana is caused by *Bartonella* *bacilliformis*, which is transmitted to humans by the sandfly *Phlebotomus*. This condition can take the form of single gigantic lesions (several centimeters in diameter) or multiple small lesions (several millimeters in diameter). Numerous subcutaneous nodules may also be present in cysticercosis caused by larvae of *Taenia solium*. Multiple erythematous papules develop in schistosomiasis; each represents a cercarial invasion site. Skin nodules as well as thickened subcutaneous tissue are prominent features of lepromatous leprosy. Large nodules or gummas are features of tertiary syphilis, whereas flat papulosquamous lesions are characteristic of secondary syphilis. Human papillomavirus may cause singular warts (verruca vulgaris) or multiple warts in the anogenital area (condylomata acuminata).

ULCERS WITH OR WITHOUT ESCHARS (Table 128-1) Cutaneous anthrax begins as a pruritic papule, which develops within days into an ulcer with surrounding vesicles and edema and then into an enlarging ulcer with a black eschar. Cutaneous anthrax may cause chronic nonhealing ulcers with an overlying dirty-gray membrane, though lesions may also mimic psoriasis, eczema, or impetigo. Ulceroglandular tularemia may have associated ulcerated skin lesions with painful regional adenopathy. Although buboes are the major cutaneous manifestation of plague, in 25% of cases ulcers with eschars, papules, or pustules are also present.

Mycobacterium ulcerans typically causes chronic skin ulcers on the extremities of individuals living in the tropics. *Mycobacterium leprae* may be associated with cutaneous ulcerations in patients with lepromatous leprosy related to Lucio's phenomenon or during reversal reactions. *Mycobacterium tuberculosis* may also cause ulcerations, papules, or erythematous macular lesions of the skin in both normal and immunocompromised patients.

Decubitus ulcers are due to tissue hypoxia secondary to pressure-induced vascular insufficiency and may become secondarily infected with components of the skin and gastrointestinal flora, including anaerobes. Ulcerative lesions on the anterior shins may be due to pyoderma gangrenosum, which must be distinguished from similar lesions of infectious etiology by histologic evaluation of biopsy sites. Ulcerated lesions on the genitals may be either painful (chancroid) or painless (primary syphilis).

ERYSIPELAS (Table 128-1) Erysipelas is due to *S. pyogenes* and is characterized by an abrupt onset of fiery-red swelling of the face or extremities. The distinctive features of erysipelas are well-defined indurated margins, particularly along the nasolabial fold; rapid progression; and intense pain. Flaccid bullae may develop during the second or third day of illness, but extension to deeper soft tissues is rare. Treatment with penicillin is effective; swelling may progress despite appropriate treatment, though fever, pain, and the intense red color diminish. Desquamation of the involved skin occurs 5 to 10 days into the illness. Infants and elderly adults are most commonly afflicted, and the severity of systemic toxicity varies.

CELLULITIS (Table 128-1) Cellulitis is an acute inflammatory condition of the skin that is characterized by localized pain, erythema, swelling, and heat. Cellulitis may be caused by indigenous flora colonizing the skin and appendages (e.g., *S. aureus* and *S. pyogenes*) or by a wide variety of exogenous bacteria. Because the exogenous bacteria involved in cellulitis occupy unique niches in nature, a thorough history including epidemiologic data provides important clues to etiology. When there is drainage, an open wound, or an obvious portal of entry, Gram's stain and culture provide a definitive diagnosis. In the absence of these findings, the bacterial etiology of cellulitis is difficult to establish, and in some cases staphylococcal and streptococcal cellulitis may have similar features. Even with needle aspiration of the leading edge or a punch biopsy of the cellulitis tissue itself, cultures are positive in only 20% of cases. This observation suggests that relatively low numbers of bacteria may cause cellulitis and that the expanding area of erythema within the skin may be a direct effect of extracellular toxins or of the soluble mediators of inflammation elicited by the host.

Bacteria may gain access to the epidermis through cracks in the skin, abrasions, cuts, burns, insect bites, surgical incisions, and intra-

venous catheters. Cellulitis caused by *S. aureus* spreads from a central localized infection, such as an abscess, folliculitis, or an infected foreign body (e.g., a splinter, a prosthetic device, or an intravenous catheter). In contrast, cellulitis due to *Staphylococcus pyogenes* is a more rapidly spreading, diffuse process frequently associated with lymphangitis and fever. Recurrent streptococcal cellulitis of the lower extremities may be caused by organisms of group A, C, or G in association with chronic venous stasis or with saphenous venectomy for coronary artery bypass surgery. Streptococci also cause recurrent cellulitis among patients with chronic lymphedema resulting from elephantiasis, lymph node dissection, or Milroy's disease. Recurrent staphylococcal cutaneous infections are more common among individuals who have eosinophilia and elevated serum levels of IgE (Job's syndrome) and among nasal carriers of staphylococci. Cellulitis caused by *S. agalactiae* (group B streptococci) occurs primarily in elderly patients and those with diabetes mellitus or peripheral vascular disease. *Haemophilus influenzae* typically causes periorbital cellulitis in children in association with sinusitis, otitis media, or epiglottitis. It is unclear whether this form of cellulitis will (like meningitis) become less common as a result of the impressive efficacy of the *H. influenzae* type b vaccine.

Many other bacteria also cause cellulitis. Fortunately, these organisms occur in such characteristic settings that a good history provides useful clues to the diagnosis. Cellulitis associated with cat bites and, to a lesser degree, with dog bites is commonly caused by *Pasteurella multocida*, though in the latter case *Staphylococcus intermedius* and *Capnocytophaga canimorsus* (formerly DF-2) must also be considered. Sites of cellulitis and abscesses associated with dog bites and human bites also contain a variety of anaerobic organisms, including *Fusobacterium*, *Bacteroides*, aerobic and anaerobic streptococci, and *Eikenella corrodens*. *Pasteurella* is notoriously resistant to dicloxacillin and nafcillin but is sensitive to all other β-lactam antimicrobials as well as to quinolones, tetracycline, and erythromycin. Ampicillin/clavulanate, ampicillin/sulbactam, and cefoxitin are good choices for the treatment of animal or human bite infections. *Aeromonas hydrophila* causes aggressive cellulitis in tissues surrounding lacerations sustained in fresh water (lakes, rivers, and streams). This organism remains sensitive to aminoglycosides, fluoroquinolones, chloramphenicol, trimethoprim-sulfamethoxazole, and third-generation cephalosporins; it is resistant to ampicillin, however.

P. aeruginosa causes three types of soft tissue infection: ecthyma gangrenosum in neutropenic patients, hot-tub folliculitis, and cellulitis following penetrating injury. Most commonly, *P. aeruginosa* is introduced into the deep tissues when a person steps on a nail. Treatment includes surgical inspection and drainage, particularly if the injury also involves bone or joint capsule. Choices for empirical treatment while antimicrobial susceptibility data are awaited include an aminoglycoside, a third-generation cephalosporin (ceftazidime, cefoperazone, or cefotaxime), a semisynthetic penicillin (ticarcillin, mezlocillin, or piperacillin), or a fluoroquinolone (though drugs of the last class are not indicated for the treatment of children <13 years old).

Gram-negative bacillary cellulitis, including that due to *P. aeruginosa*, is most common among hospitalized, immunocompromised hosts. Cultures and sensitivity tests are critically important in this setting because of multidrug resistance (Chap. 155).

The gram-positive aerobic rod *Erysipelothrix rhusiopathiae* is most often associated with fish and domestic swine and causes cellulitis primarily in bone renderers and fishmongers. *E. rhusiopathiae* remains susceptible to most β-lactam antibiotics (including penicillin), erythromycin, clindamycin, tetracycline, and cephalosporins but is resistant to sulfonamides, chloramphenicol, and vancomycin. Its resistance to vancomycin, which is unusual among gram-positive bacteria, is of potential clinical significance since this agent is sometimes used in empirical therapy for skin infection. Fish food containing the water flea *Daphnia* is sometimes contaminated with *M. marinum*, which can cause cellulitis or granulomas on skin surfaces exposed to the water in aquariums or injured in swimming pools. Rifampin plus ethambutol has been an effective therapeutic combination in some cases, though no comprehensive studies have been undertaken. In addition, some strains of *M. marinum* are susceptible to tetracycline or to trimethoprim-sulfamethoxazole.

NECROTIZING FASCIITIS (Table 128-1) Necrotizing fasciitis, formerly called streptococcal gangrene, may be associated with group A *Streptococcus* or mixed aerobic-anaerobic bacteria or may occur as part of gas gangrene caused by *Clostridium perfringens*. Early diagnosis may be difficult when pain or unexplained fever is the only presenting manifestation. Swelling then develops and is followed by brawny edema and tenderness. With progression, dark red induration of the epidermis appears along with bullae filled with blue or purple fluid. Later the skin becomes friable and takes on a bluish, maroon, or black color. By this stage, thrombosis of blood vessels in the dermal papillae (Fig. 128-1) is extensive. Extension of infection to the level of the deep fascia causes this tissue to take on a brownish-gray appearance. Rapid spread occurs along fascial planes, through venous channels and lymphatics. Patients in the later stages are toxic and frequently manifest shock and multiorgan failure.

Necrotizing fasciitis caused by mixed aerobic-anaerobic bacteria begins with a breach in the integrity of a mucous membrane barrier, such as the mucosa of the gastrointestinal or genitourinary tract. The portal can be a malignancy, diverticulum, hemorrhoid, anal fissure, or urethral tear. Other predisposing factors include peripheral vascular disease, diabetes mellitus, surgery, and penetrating injury to the abdomen. Leakage into the perineal area results in a syndrome called *Fournier's gangrene*, characterized by massive swelling of the scrotum and penis with extension into the perineum or the abdominal wall and legs.

Necrotizing fasciitis caused by *S. pyogenes* has increased in frequency and severity since 1985. It frequently begins deep at the site of a nonpenetrating minor trauma such as a bruise or a muscle strain. Seeding of the site via transient bacteremia is likely, though most patients deny antecedent streptococcal infection. Alternatively, *S. pyogenes* may reach the deep fascia from a site of cutaneous infection or penetrating trauma. Toxicity is severe, and renal impairment may precede the development of shock. In 20 to 40% of cases, myositis occurs concomitantly, and, as in gas gangrene (see below), serum creatinine phosphokinase values may be markedly elevated. Necrotizing fasciitis due to mixed aerobic-anaerobic bacteria may be associated with gas in the deep tissue, but gas is not usually present when the cause is *S. pyogenes*. Prompt surgical exploration down to the deep fascia and muscle is essential. Necrotic tissue must be surgically removed, and Gram's staining and culture of excised tissue are useful in establishing whether group A streptococci, mixed aerobic-anaerobic bacteria, or *Clostridium* spp. are present (see "Treatment" below).

MYOSITIS/MYONECROSIS (Table 128-1) Muscle involvement can occur with virus infection (e.g., influenza virus, dengue virus, or coxsackievirus B) or parasitic invasion (e.g., trichinosis, cysticercosis, or toxoplasmosis). Although myalgia can occur in most of these infections, severe muscle pain is the hallmark of pleurodynia (cox-

Table 128-2   Treatment of Common Infections of the Skin

Diagnosis/Condition	Primary Treatment	Alternative Treatment	See Also Chap(s).
Animal bite (prophylaxis or early infection)[a]	Amoxicillin/clavulanate, 875/125 mg PO bid	Doxycycline, 100 mg PO bid	127
Animal bite[a] (established infection)	Ampicillin/sulbactam, 1.5 g IV q6h	Clindamycin, 600–900 mg IV q8h, *plus* Ciprofloxacin, 400 mg IV q12H *or* Cefoxitin, 2 g IV q6h	127
Bacillary angiomatosis	Erythromycin, 500 mg PO qid	Doxycycline, 100 mg PO bid	163
Herpes simplex (primary genital)	Acyclovir, 400 mg PO tid for 10 days	Famciclovir, 250 mg PO tid for 5–10 days *or* Valacyclovir, 1000 mg PO bid for 10 days	182
Herpes zoster (immunocompetent host >50 years of age)	Acyclovir, 800 mg PO 5 times daily for 7–10 days	Famciclovir, 500 mg PO tid for 7–10 days *or* Valacyclovir, 1000 mg PO tid for 7 days	183
Cellulitis (staphylococcal or streptococcal[b,c])	Nafcillin or oxacillin, 2 g IV q4–6h	Cefazolin, 1–2 g q8h, *plus* Ampicillin/sulbactam, 1.5–3.0 g IV q6h *or* Erythromycin, 0.5–1.0 g IV q6h *or* Clindamycin, 600–900 mg IV q8h	139, 140
Necrotizing fasciitis (group A streptococcal[b])	Clindamycin, 600–900 mg IV q6–8h, *plus* Penicillin G, 4 million units IV q4h	Clindamycin, 600–900 mg IV q6–8h, *plus* Cephalosporin (first- or second-generation)	140
Necrotizing fasciitis (mixed aerobes and anaerobes)	Ampicillin, 2 g IV q4h, *plus* Clindamycin, 600–900 mg IV q6–8h, *plus* Ciprofloxacin, 400 mg IV q6–8h	Vancomycin, 1 g IV q6h, *plus* Metronidazole, 500 mg IV q6h, *plus* Ciprofloxacin, 400 mg IV q6–8h	167
Gas gangrene	Clindamycin, 600–900 mg IV q6–8h, *plus* Penicillin G, 4 million units IV q4–6h	Clindamycin, 600–900 mg IV q6–8h, *plus* Cefoxitin, 2 g IV q6h	145

[a] *Pasteurella multocida*, a species commonly associated with both dog and cat bites, is resistant to cephalexin, dicloxacillin, clindamycin, and erythromycin. *Eikenella corrodens*, a bacterium commonly associated with human bites, is resistant to clindamycin, penicillinase-resistant penicillins, and metronidazole but is sensitive to trimethoprim-sulfamethoxazole and fluoroquinolones.
[b] The frequency of erythromycin resistance in group A *Streptococcus* is currently about 5% in the United States but has reached 70 to 100% in some other countries. Most, but not all, erythromycin-resistant group A streptococci are susceptible to clindamycin. Approximately 90 to 95% of *Staphylococcus aureus* strains are sensitive to clindamycin.
[c] Severe hospital-acquired *S. aureus* infections or community-acquired *S. aureus* infections that are not responding to the β-lactam antibiotics recommended in this table may be caused by methicillin-resistant strains, requiring a switch to vancomycin.

sackie virus B), trichinosis, and bacterial infection. Acute rhabdomyolysis predictably occurs with clostridial and streptococcal myositis but may also be associated with influenza virus, echovirus, coxsackievirus, Epstein-Barr virus, and *Legionella* infection.

Pyomyositis is usually due to *S. aureus*, is common in tropical areas, and generally has no known portal of entry. Infection remains localized, and shock does not develop unless organisms produce toxic shock syndrome toxin 1 or certain enterotoxins and the patient lacks antibodies to the toxin produced by the infecting organisms. In contrast, *S. pyogenes* may induce primary myositis referred to as *streptococcal necrotizing myositis*, which is associated with severe systemic toxicity. Myonecrosis occurs concomitantly with necrotizing fasciitis in about 50% of cases. Both are part of the streptococcal toxic shock syndrome.

Gas gangrene usually follows severe penetrating injuries that result in interruption of the blood supply and introduction of soil into wounds. Such cases of traumatic gangrene are usually caused by *C. perfringens*, *C. septicum*, or *C. histolyticum*. Rarely, latent or recurrent gangrene can occur years after penetrating trauma, most likely owing to dormant spores that reside at the site of previous injury. Spontaneous nontraumatic gangrene among patients with neutropenia, gastrointestinal malignancy, diverticulosis, or recent radiation therapy to the abdomen is caused by several clostridial species, although *C. septicum* is most common. The tolerance of this anaerobe to oxygen probably explains why it can initiate infection spontaneously in normal tissue anywhere in the body.

Synergistic nonclostridial anaerobic myonecrosis, also known as necrotizing cutaneous myositis and synergistic necrotizing cellulitis, is a variant of necrotizing fasciitis caused by mixed aerobic and anaerobic bacteria with the exclusion of clostridial organisms (see "Necrotizing Fasciitis," above).

DIAGNOSIS This chapter has emphasized the physical appearance and location of lesions within the soft tissues as important diagnostic clues. The temporal progression of the lesions as well as the patient's travel history, animal exposure or bite history, age, underlying disease status, and lifestyle are also crucial considerations in the formulation of a narrowed differential diagnosis. However, even the astute clinician may find it challenging to diagnose all infections of the soft tissues by history and inspection alone. Soft tissue radiography, computed tomography, and magnetic resonance imaging may be useful in determining the depth of infection and should be performed in patients with rapidly progressing lesions or in those with evidence of systemic inflammatory response syndrome. These tests are particularly valuable for defining a localized abscess or detecting gas in tissue. Unfortunately, they may reveal only soft tissue swelling and thus are not specific for fulminant infections such as necrotizing fasciitis or myonecrosis caused by group A *Streptococcus*, where gas is not found in lesions.

Aspiration of the leading edge or punch biopsy with frozen section may be helpful if the results are positive, but false-negative results occur in approximately 80% of cases. There is some evidence that aspiration alone may be superior to injection and aspiration using normal saline. Frozen sections are especially useful in distinguishing SSSS from TEN and are quite valuable in cases of necrotizing fasciitis. Open surgical inspection with debridement as indicated is clearly the best way to determine the extent and severity of infection and to obtain material for Gram's staining and culture. Such an aggressive approach is important and may be lifesaving if undertaken early in the course of fulminant infections where there is evidence of systemic toxicity.

℞ **TREATMENT** A full description of the treatment of all the clinical entities described herein is beyond the scope of this chapter. As a guide to the clinician in selecting appropriate treatment, the antimicrobial agents useful in the most common and the most fulminant cutaneous infections are listed in Table 128-2.

Early and aggressive surgical exploration is essential in patients with suspected necrotizing fasciitis, myositis, or gangrene in order to (1) visualize the deep structures, (2) remove necrotic tissue, (3) reduce compartment pressure, and (4) obtain suitable material for Gram's staining and for aerobic and anaerobic cultures. Appropriate empirical antibiotic treatment for mixed aerobic-anaerobic infections could consist of ampicillin/sulbactam, cefoxitin, or the following combination: (1) clindamycin (600 to 900 mg intravenously every 8 h) or metronidazole (750 mg every 6 h) plus (2) ampicillin or ampicillin/sulbactam (2 to 3 g intravenously every 6 h) plus (3) gentamicin (1.0 to 1.5 mg/kg every 8 h). Group A streptococcal and clostridial infection of the fascia and/or muscle carries a mortality rate of 20 to 50% with penicillin treatment. In experimental models of streptococcal and clostridial necrotizing fasciitis/myositis, clindamycin has exhibited markedly superior efficacy, but no comparative trials have been performed in humans. Hyperbaric oxygen treatment may also be useful in gas gangrene due to clostridial species. Antibiotic treatment should be continued until all signs of systemic toxicity have resolved, all devitalized tissue has been removed, and granulation tissue has developed (Chaps. 140, 145, and 167).

In summary, infections of the skin and soft tissues are diverse in presentation and severity and offer a great challenge to the clinician. This chapter provides an approach to diagnosis and understanding of the pathophysiologic mechanisms involved in these infections. More in-depth information is found in chapters on specific infections.

BIBLIOGRAPHY

BISNO AI, STEVENS DL: Streptococcal infections in skin and soft tissues. N Engl J Med 334:240, 1996

FRANCIS JS, NEFF J: Viral infections of the skin and soft tissues, in *Atlas of Infectious Diseases*, DL Stevens (ed). Philadelphia, Churchill Livingstone, 1994

GARDAM MA et al: Group B streptococcal necrotizing fasciitis and streptococcal toxic shock–like syndrome in adults. Arch Intern Med 158:1704, 1998

GOLDSTEIN EJC: Bite wounds and infection. Clin Infect Dis 14:633, 1992

HOOK EW et al: Microbiologic evaluation of cutaneous cellulitis in adults. Arch Intern Med 146:295, 1986

NORRBY-TEGLUND A, STEVENS DL: Novel therapies in streptococcal toxic shock syndrome: Attenuation of virulence factor expression and modulation of host response. Curr Opin Infect Dis 11:285, 1998

SIMMONS RL, AHRENHOLZ DH: Infections of the skin and soft tissue, in *Surgical Infectious Diseases*, 2d ed, RJ Howard, RL Simmons (eds). Norwalk, CT, Appleton & Lange, 1988, p 377

STEVENS DL: Invasive group A streptococcus infections. Clin Infect Dis 14:2, 1992

———: Necrotizing infections of the skin and soft tissues, in *Atlas of Infectious Diseases*, DL Stevens (ed). Philadelphia, Churchill Livingstone, 1994

———: Streptococcal toxic shock syndrome: Spectrum of disease, pathogenesis and new concepts in treatment. Emerging Infect Dis 1:69, 1995

———: The flesh-eating bacterium: What's next? J Infect Dis 179:S366, 1999

——— et al: Effect of antibiotics on toxin production and viability of *Clostridium perfringens*. Antimicrob Agents Chemother 31:213, 1987

——— et al: Spontaneous, nontraumatic gangrene due to *Clostridium septicum*. Rev Infect Dis 12:286, 1990

——— et al: Penicillin binding protein expression at different growth stages determines penicillin efficacy in vitro and in vivo: An explanation for the inoculum effect. J Infect Dis 167:1401, 1993

TRAYLOR KK, TODD JK: Needle aspirate culture method in soft tissue infections: Injection of saline vs. direct aspiration. Pediatr Infect Dis J 17:840, 1998

WALLACE RJ et al: Clinical trial of clarithromycin for cutaneous (disseminated) infection due to *Mycobacterium chelonae*. Ann Intern Med 119:482, 1993

129 *James H. Maguire*

OSTEOMYELITIS

Osteomyelitis, an infection of bone, is caused most commonly by pyogenic bacteria and mycobacteria. Classification of cases on the basis of the causative agent; the route, duration, and anatomic location of infection; and local and systemic host factors provides a useful framework for evaluating the patient and planning treatment.

PATHOGENESIS AND PATHOLOGY Microorganisms enter bone by the hematogenous route, by direct introduction from a contiguous focus of infection, or by a penetrating wound. Trauma, ischemia, and foreign bodies enhance the susceptibility of bone to microbial invasion by exposing sites to which bacteria can bind. Phagocytes attempt to contain the infections and, in the process, release enzymes that lyse bone. Pus spreads into vascular channels, raising intraosseous pressure and impairing the flow of blood; as the untreated infection becomes chronic, ischemic necrosis of bone results in the separation of large devascularized fragments (*sequestra*). When pus breaks through the cortex, subperiosteal or soft tissue abscesses form, and the elevated periosteum deposits new bone (the *involucrum*) around the sequestrum. Bacteria escape host defenses by adhering tightly to damaged bone, by entering and persisting within osteoblasts, and by coating themselves and underlying surfaces with a protective polysaccharide-rich biofilm.

Microorganisms, infiltrates of neutrophils, and congested or thrombosed blood vessels are the principal histologic findings of acute osteomyelitis. The distinguishing feature of chronic osteomyelitis is necrotic bone, which is characterized by the absence of living osteocytes. Mononuclear cells predominate in chronic infections, and granulation and fibrous tissues replace bone that has been resorbed by osteoclasts. In the chronic stage, organisms may be too few to be seen.

HEMATOGENOUS OSTEOMYELITIS Hematogenous infection accounts for ~20% of cases of osteomyelitis and primarily affects children, in whom the long bones are infected, and older adults and intravenous drug users, in whom the spine is the usual site of infection.

Acute Hematogenous Osteomyelitis Infection usually involves a single bone, most commonly the tibia, femur, or humerus. Bacteria settle in the well-perfused metaphysis, where functioning phagocytes are scarce, a network of venous sinusoids slows the flow of blood, and fenestrations in capillaries allow organisms to escape into the extravascular space. Because vascular anatomy changes with age, hematogenous infection of long bones is uncommon during adulthood and, when it occurs, usually involves the diaphysis.

In children, the source of bacteremia is often inapparent, although there may have been recent blunt trauma to the extremity leading to a small intraosseous hematoma or vascular obstruction. On presentation, the child usually appears acutely ill, with high fever, chills, localized pain and tenderness, and leukocytosis. Cutaneous erythema and swelling indicate extension of pus through the cortex. During infancy and after puberty, infection may spread through the epiphysis into the joint space. In children of other ages (i.e., between infancy and puberty), extension of infection through the cortex results in involvement of joints if the metaphysis is intracapsular. Thus, septic arthritis of the elbow, shoulder, and hip may complicate osteomyelitis of the proximal radius, humerus, and femur, respectively.

Plain radiographs initially show soft tissue swelling, but the first change in bone—a periosteal reaction—is not evident until at least 10 days after the onset of infection. Lytic changes can be detected after 2 to 6 weeks, when 50 to 75% of bone density has been lost. Rarely, a well-circumscribed lytic lesion, or *Brodie's abscess*, is seen in a child who has been in pain for several months but has had no fever.

Chronic Hematogenous Osteomyelitis With prompt treatment, <5% of cases of acute hematogenous osteomyelitis progress to chronic osteomyelitis. On average, 10 days are required for the formation of necrotic bone, but plain radiographs are unable to detect sequestra or sclerotic new bone for many weeks.

A protracted clinical course, long periods of quiescence, and recurrent exacerbations are characteristic of chronic osteomyelitis. Sinus tracts between bone and skin may drain purulent material and occasionally pieces of necrotic bone. An increase in drainage, pain, or the erythrocyte sedimentation rate (ESR) signals an exacerbation. Fever is unusual except when obstruction of a sinus tract leads to soft tissue

infection. Rare late complications include pathologic fractures, squamous cell carcinoma of the sinus tract, and amyloidosis.

Vertebral Osteomyelitis Organisms reach the well-perfused vertebral body of adults via spinal arteries and quickly spread from the end plate into the disk space and then to the adjacent vertebral body. The infection may originate in the urinary tract, and it does so particularly often among elderly men. Other sources of bacteremia include endocarditis, soft tissue infection, and a contaminated intravenous line; these sources are usually obvious. Diabetes mellitus, hemodialysis, and intravenous drug use carry an increased risk of spinal infection. Penetrating injuries and surgical procedures to the spine may cause nonhematogenous vertebral osteomyelitis or infection localized to the disk.

Most patients with vertebral osteomyelitis report neck or back pain; 15% describe atypical pain in the chest, the abdomen, or an extremity that is due to irritation of nerve roots. Symptoms are localized to the lumbar spine more often than to the thoracic spine (>50% vs. 35% of cases) or the cervical spine in pyogenic infections, but the thoracic spine is involved most commonly in tuberculous spondylitis (Pott's disease). Percussion over the involved vertebra elicits tenderness, and physical examination may reveal spasm of the paraspinal muscles and a limitation of motion. More than 50% of patients experience a subacute illness in which a vague, dull pain gradually intensifies over 2 to 3 months; fever is low grade or absent, and the white blood cell count is normal. An acute presentation with high fever and toxicity is less common and suggests ongoing bacteremia.

Usually, by the time the patient seeks medical attention, the ESR is elevated, and plain radiographs show irregular erosions in the end plates of adjacent vertebral bodies and narrowing of the intervening disk space. This radiographic pattern is virtually diagnostic of bacterial infection because tumors and other diseases of the spine rarely cross the disk space. Computed tomography (CT) or magnetic resonance imaging (MRI) may demonstrate epidural, paraspinal, retropharyngeal, mediastinal, retroperitoneal, or psoas abscesses that originate in the spine. An epidural abscess may evolve suddenly or over several weeks; irreversible paralysis may result from failure to recognize the classic clinical presentation of a spinal epidural abscess: spinal pain progressing to radicular pain and weakness.

Microbiology More than 95% of cases of hematogenous osteomyelitis are caused by a single organism. *Staphylococcus aureus* accounts for 50% of isolates. Other common pathogens include group B streptococci and *Escherichia coli* during the newborn period and group A streptococci and *Haemophilus influenzae* in early childhood. Vertebral osteomyelitis is due to *E. coli* and other enteric bacilli in ~25% of cases. *S. aureus*, *Pseudomonas aeruginosa*, and *Serratia* infections are associated with intravenous drug use in some parts of the United States and may involve the sacroiliac, sternoclavicular, or pubic joints as well as the spine. *Salmonella* spp. and *S. aureus* are the major causes of long-bone osteomyelitis complicating sickle cell anemia and other hemoglobinopathies. Tuberculosis and brucellosis affect the spine more often than other bones. Other common sites of tuberculous osteomyelitis include the small bones of the hands and feet, the metaphyses of long bones, the ribs, and the sternum.

Unusual causes of hematogenous osteomyelitis include disseminated histoplasmosis, coccidioidomycosis, and blastomycosis in endemic areas. Immunocompromised persons on rare occasions develop osteomyelitis due to atypical mycobacteria, *Bartonella henselae*, or *Pneumocystis carinii* or to species of *Candida*, *Cryptococcus*, or *Aspergillus*. Syphilis, yaws, varicella, and vaccinia may involve bone. The etiology of chronic relapsing multifocal osteomyelitis, an inflammatory condition of children that is characterized by recurrent episodes of painful lytic lesions in multiple bones, has not yet been identified.

OSTEOMYELITIS SECONDARY TO A CONTIGUOUS FOCUS OF INFECTION **Clinical Features** This broad category of osteomyelitis includes infections introduced by penetrating injuries and surgical procedures and by direct extension of infection from adjacent soft tissues. It accounts for the greatest number of cases of osteomyelitis and occurs most commonly in adults.

Frequently, the diagnosis is not made until the infection has already become chronic. The pain, fever, and inflammatory signs due to acute osteomyelitis may be attributed to the original injury or soft tissue infection. An indolent infection may become apparent only weeks or months later, when a sinus tract develops, a surgical wound breaks down, or a fracture fails to heal. It may be impossible to distinguish radiographic abnormalities due to osteomyelitis from those due to the precipitating condition.

A special type of contiguous-focus osteomyelitis occurs in the setting of peripheral vascular disease and nearly always involves the small bones of the feet of adult diabetic patients. Diabetic neuropathy exposes the foot to frequent trauma and pressure sores, and the patient may be unaware of infection as it spreads into bone. Poor tissue perfusion impairs normal inflammatory responses and wound healing and creates a milieu that is conducive to anaerobic infections. It is often during the evaluation of a nonhealing ulcer, a swollen toe, or acute cellulitis that a radiograph provides the first evidence of osteomyelitis. If bone is palpable during examination of the base of an ulcer with a blunt surgical probe, osteomyelitis is likely.

Microbiology *S. aureus* is a pathogen in more than half of cases of contiguous-focus osteomyelitis. However, in contrast to hematogenous osteomyelitis, these infections are often polymicrobial and are more likely to involve gram-negative and anaerobic bacteria. Hence a mixture of staphylococci, streptococci, enteric organisms, and anaerobic bacteria may be isolated from a diabetic foot infection or pelvic osteomyelitis underlying a decubitus ulcer. Aerobic and anaerobic bacteria cause osteomyelitis following surgery or soft tissue infection of the oropharynx, paranasal sinuses, gastrointestinal tract, or female genital tract. *S. aureus* is the principal cause of postoperative infections; coagulase-negative staphylococci are common pathogens after implantation of orthopedic appliances; and these organisms as well as gram-negative enteric bacilli, atypical mycobacteria, and *Mycoplasma* may cause sternal osteomyelitis after cardiac surgery. Infection with *P. aeruginosa* is frequently associated with puncture wounds of the foot or with thermal burns, and *Pasteurella multocida* infection commonly follows cat bites (Chap. 127).

DIAGNOSIS Early diagnosis of acute osteomyelitis is critical because prompt antibiotic therapy may prevent the necrosis of bone. The evaluation usually begins with plain radiographs because of their ready availability, although they frequently show no abnormalities during early infection. The ESR and C-reactive protein levels are elevated in most cases of active osteomyelitis, including those in which constitutional symptoms and leukocytosis are lacking. These findings are not specific to osteomyelitis, however, and the ESR is occasionally normal in early infections. In 95% of cases, the technetium radionuclide scan using ^{99m}Tc diphosphonate is positive within 24 h of the onset of symptoms. Falsely negative scans usually indicate obstruction of blood flow to the bone. Because the uptake of technetium reflects osteoblastic activity and skeletal vascularity, the bone scan cannot differentiate osteomyelitis from fractures, tumors, infarction, or neuropathic osteopathy. ^{67}Ga citrate– and ^{111}In-labeled leukocyte or immunoglobulin scans, which have greater specificity for inflammation, may help distinguish infectious from noninfectious processes and indicate inflammatory changes within bones that for other reasons are already abnormal on radiography and technetium scanning. Ultrasound can be used to diagnose osteomyelitis by the detection of subperiosteal fluid collections, soft tissue abscesses adjacent to bone, and periosteal thickening and elevation.

MRI is as sensitive as the bone scan for the diagnosis of acute osteomyelitis because it is able to detect changes in the water content of marrow. MRI yields better anatomic resolution of epidural abscesses and other soft tissue processes than CT and is currently the imaging technique of choice for vertebral osteomyelitis (Fig. 129-1).

The role of diagnostic imaging in chronic osteomyelitis is to determine the presence of active infection and delineate the extent of debridement necessary to remove necrotic bone and abnormal soft tissues. Although plain films accurately reflect chronic changes, the

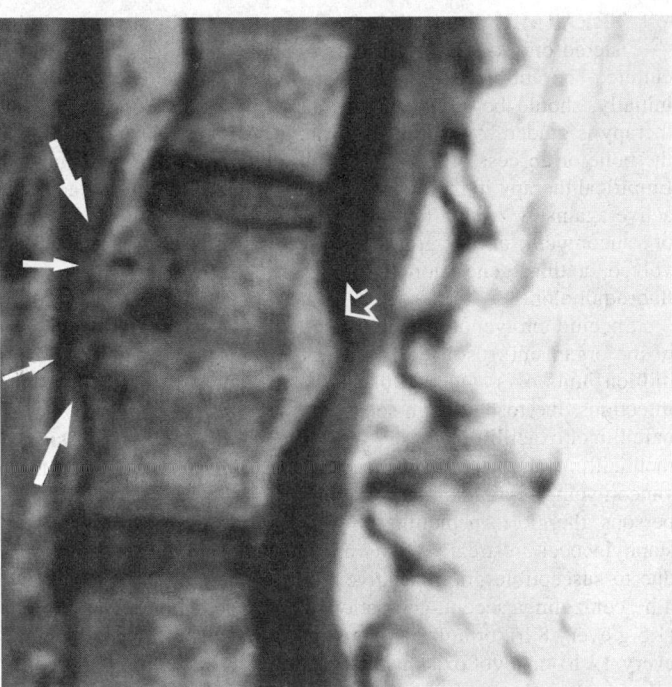

FIGURE 129-1 Osteomyelitis of the lumbar spine demonstrated on a sagittal T1-weighted magnetic resonance image after the administration of intravenous gadolinium. At L2–L3 there is involvement of the adjacent vertebral bodies and intervening disk. An epidural abscess compresses the thecal sac (open arrow), and the inflammatory process extends into the anterior prevertebral space (closed arrows).

CT scan is more sensitive for the detection of sequestra, sinus tracts, and soft tissue abscesses. Both CT and ultrasound are useful for guiding percutaneous aspiration of subperiosteal and soft tissue fluid collections. Sequential technetium and gallium or indium scans may help determine whether infection is active and may distinguish infection from noninflammatory bone changes; these methods do not, however, provide good anatomic detail. MRI provides detailed information about the activity and the anatomic extent of infection but does not always distinguish osteomyelitis from healing fractures and tumors. MRI is particularly useful in distinguishing cellulitis from osteomyelitis in the diabetic foot; however, no imaging modality consistently distinguishes infection from neuropathic osteopathy.

Appropriate samples for microbiologic studies should be obtained in all cases of suspected osteomyelitis before the initiation of antimicrobial therapy. Blood cultures are indicated in acute cases and are positive in more than one-third of cases of hematogenous osteomyelitis in children and in 25% of cases of vertebral osteomyelitis in adults. If the clinical picture demands immediate antibiotic therapy or if blood cultures are negative, samples from needle aspiration of pus in bone or soft tissues or from a bone biopsy should be obtained for culture.

The results of culture of specimens obtained by swabbing of a sinus tract or the base of an ulcer correlate poorly with the organisms infecting the bone. For this reason, in cases of chronic osteomyelitis and contiguous-focus osteomyelitis, samples for aerobic and anaerobic culture should be obtained from several sites by percutaneous needle aspiration, percutaneous biopsy, or intraoperative biopsy at the time of debridement. Isolates of coagulase-negative staphylococci and other organisms of low virulence should not automatically be disregarded as contaminants, especially in the presence of prosthetic materials. Special culture media may be necessary for the isolation of mycobacteria, fungi, and less common pathogens. In some cases, histopathologic examination of biopsy specimens may be the only way to make a diagnosis.

℞ **TREATMENT Antibiotic Therapy** Antibiotics are administered only after appropriate specimens have been obtained for culture. The antibiotics selected should be bactericidal and, at least initially, should be given intravenously. When necessary, empirical therapy is guided by findings on Gram's staining of a specimen from the bone or abscess or is chosen to cover the most likely pathogens. Empirical therapy in most cases should include high doses of an agent active against *S. aureus* (such as oxacillin, nafcillin, a cephalosporin, or vancomycin) and, if gram-negative organisms are likely to be involved, a third-generation cephalosporin, an aminoglycoside, or a fluoroquinolone.

Specific intravenous therapy is based on the in vitro susceptibility of the organism(s) isolated from bone or blood. Penicillin G (3 to 4 million units every 4 h) is the drug of choice for the treatment of infections due to penicillin-sensitive staphylococci and streptococci; nafcillin or oxacillin (2 g every 4 h) is preferred for penicillin-resistant, methicillin-sensitive staphylococci. Cefazolin (1 to 2 g every 8 h) or vancomycin [15 mg/kg (up to 1 g) every 12 h] is an alternative for persons allergic to penicillins. Infections due to methicillin-resistant staphylococci are treated with vancomycin. Regimens for infections due to susceptible gram-negative rods include ampicillin (2 g every 4 h), cefazolin, a second-generation cephalosporin such as cefuroxime (1.5 g every 8 h), or a fluoroquinolone such as ciprofloxacin (400 mg every 12 h) or levofloxacin (500 mg every 24 h). Initial therapy for osteomyelitis due to *P. aeruginosa* or *Enterobacter* spp. should not consist of a β-lactam antibiotic alone because of the potential for these organisms to develop resistance during therapy. Appropriate intravenous therapies for *P. aeruginosa* infections include tobramycin (1.7 mg/kg every 8 h, or 5 to 7 mg/kg every 24 h) and a broad-spectrum β-lactam compound such as ticarcillin (3 g every 4 h), ceftazidime (1 to 2 g every 8 h), or aztreonam (1 to 2 g every 8 h); a fluoroquinolone may be substituted for one of the latter. *Enterobacter* infections can be treated with a fluoroquinolone alone or with combinations of a broad-spectrum β-lactam antibiotic and gentamicin in the same doses as tobramycin. Serum levels of aminoglycosides should be monitored closely to avoid toxicity.

The duration of therapy is typically 4 to 6 weeks; at-home intravenous administration of antibiotics or oral therapy is appropriate for motivated and medically stable patients. Antibiotics that require infrequent dosing, such as ceftriaxone and vancomycin, facilitate home therapy. Children with acute hematogenous osteomyelitis routinely receive oral antibiotics after 5 to 10 days of parenteral therapy if signs of active infection have resolved; such treatment has been as successful as standard parenteral therapy. The doses of oral penicillins or cephalosporins required for the treatment of osteomyelitis are several times higher than the doses of these drugs given for common infections. Adults may not tolerate these high doses as well as children, and, except in the case of the fluoroquinolones, few data support the use of oral antibiotics by adults. For treatment of osteomyelitis due to Enterobacteriaceae, oral administration of an agent such as ciprofloxacin (750 mg every 12 h) or levofloxacin (500 mg every 24 h) has been as successful as intravenous administration of β-lactam antibiotics. Caution should be exercised in the use of fluoroquinolones as the sole agents for treatment of infection due to *S. aureus* or *P. aeruginosa* because resistance may develop during therapy. Addition of rifampin to a quinolone has yielded encouraging results in infections due to *S. aureus*, but further studies are necessary to confirm these findings. Oral administration of clindamycin (300 to 450 mg every 6 h) or metronidazole (500 mg every 8 h) results in high drug levels in serum and can take the place of intravenous regimens for the treatment of *Bacteroides* infections. Oral clindamycin has produced good results in therapy for osteomyelitis due to *S. aureus*, especially in children. There are few data to support the routine use of the serum minimal bactericidal concentration (MBC) other than to document adherence to treatment.

Acute Osteomyelitis Early treatment of acute hematogenous osteomyelitis of childhood with 4 to 6 weeks of an appropriate antibiotic is usually successful; treatment for <3 weeks has resulted in a 10-fold greater rate of failure. Surgical intervention in childhood cases is indicated for intraosseous or subperiosteal abscesses, concomitant septic arthritis, and failure of the acute signs of infection to improve in 24 to 48 h. Acute hematogenous osteomyelitis of bones other than the spine in adults often requires surgical debridement.

Vertebral Osteomyelitis A 4- to 6-week course of treatment with an appropriate antibiotic is usually sufficient to cure vertebral osteomyelitis. Failure of the ESR to drop by two-thirds or more of its pretreatment level is an indication for longer treatment. Surgery is seldom necessary, even in cases of many months' duration, except in instances of spinal instability, new or progressive neurologic deficits, large soft tissue abscesses that cannot be drained percutaneously, or a failure of medical treatment. Patients should maintain bed rest until back pain has declined to the point at which ambulation is possible. Body casts are no longer used. Spontaneous fusion of involved vertebrae occurs in the majority of cases after successful treatment.

Contiguous-Focus Osteomyelitis Even when diagnosed early, contiguous-focus osteomyelitis usually requires surgery in addition to 4 to 6 weeks of appropriate antibiotic therapy because of underlying soft tissue infection or damage to bone from an injury or surgery. A 2-week course of antibiotics following thorough debridement and soft tissue coverage has yielded excellent results in treatment of superficial osteomyelitis involving only the outer cortex of bone.

Chronic Osteomyelitis The risks and benefits of aggressive therapy for chronic osteomyelitis should be weighed before any attempt is made to eradicate the infection. Some patients with extensive disease prefer to live with their infections rather than undergo multiple surgical procedures, take prolonged courses of antimicrobial therapy, and face the risk of loss of an extremity. Such persons often benefit from intermittent courses of oral antibiotics to suppress acute exacerbations.

Once the decision has been made to treat chronic osteomyelitis aggressively, the patient's nutritional and metabolic status should be optimized to expedite healing of soft tissues and bone. Antibiotic administration should be started several days before surgery to reduce inflammation if the etiology of the infection is known preoperatively. If not, antibiotic therapy should be withheld until surgical debridement. An empirical antibiotic regimen is started intraoperatively after culture specimens are obtained. A 4- to 6-week course of appropriate antibiotic therapy is given postoperatively on the basis of the susceptibility pattern of organisms isolated from the bone. The benefit of prolonged oral antibiotic therapy after 4 to 6 weeks of parenteral therapy remains unproven. There is insufficient information to recommend the routine use of hyperbaric oxygen to enhance the killing of microorganisms by phagocytes or of instillation pumps and antibiotic-impregnated methacrylate beads to deliver high levels of antibiotics to the bone.

The success of therapy for chronic osteomyelitis rests largely on the complete surgical removal of necrotic bone and abnormal soft tissues. Modern imaging techniques allow accurate preoperative delineation of tissues to be debrided, but it remains difficult for the surgeon to determine intraoperatively whether all necrotic and infected tissue has been removed. In the past, the inability to repair large defects in bone and soft tissue limited the extent of debridement. Muscle flaps and skin grafts are now used routinely to cover large soft tissue defects and fill dead space, and bone grafts and vascularized bone transfer may restore a seriously compromised bone to a functional state.

In infections of recent fractures, internal fixators are often left in place, and the infection is controlled by limited debridement and suppressive antibiotic therapy. Definitive surgical/antimicrobial therapy is delayed until after bony union of the fracture is achieved. If there is nonunion of the fracture or loosening of the fixator, the appliance should be removed, the bone debrided, and an external fixator or a new internal fixator applied.

Osteomyelitis of the small bones of the feet in persons with vascular disease also requires surgical treatment. The effectiveness of the surgery is limited by the blood supply to the site and the body's ability to heal the wound. Revascularization of the extremity is indicated if the vascular disease involves large arteries. In cases of decreased perfusion due to small-vessel disease, foot-sparing surgery may fail, and the best option is suppressive therapy or amputation. The duration of antibiotic therapy depends on the surgical procedure performed. When the infected bone is removed entirely but residual infection of soft tissues remains, antibiotic therapy should be given for 2 weeks; if amputation eliminates infected bone and soft tissue, standard surgical prophylaxis is given; otherwise, postoperative antibiotics must be given for 4 to 6 weeks.

BIBLIOGRAPHY

LEW DP, WALDVOGEL FA: Osteomyelitis. N Engl J Med 336:999, 1997

——, ——: Use of quinolones in osteomyelitis and infected orthopaedic prosthesis. Drugs 58(Suppl 2):85, 1999

LIPSKY BA: Osteomyelitis of the foot in diabetic patients. Clin Infect Dis 25:1318, 1997

MADER JT et al: Staging and staging application in osteomyelitis. Clin Infect Dis 25:1303, 1997

NORDEN C et al: *Infections in Bones and Joints*. Boston, Blackwell Scientific, 1994

REZAI AR et al: Contemporary management of spinal osteomyelitis. Neurosurgery 44:1018, 1999

SAMMAK B et al: Osteomyelitis: A review of currently used imaging techniques. Eur Radiol 9:894, 1999

SWIONTKOWSKI MF et al: A comparison of short- and long-term intravenous antibiotic therapy in the postoperative management of adult osteomyelitis. J Bone Joint Surg (Br) 81:1046, 1999

TICE AD: Outpatient parenteral antimicrobial therapy for osteomyelitis. Infect Dis Clin North Am 12:903, 1998

TSUKAYAMA DT: Pathophysiology of posttraumatic osteomyelitis. Clin Orthop 360:22, 1999

130

Dori F. Zaleznik, Dennis L. Kasper

INTRAABDOMINAL INFECTIONS AND ABSCESSES

CAPD continuous ambulatory peritoneal dialysis	SBP spontaneous bacterial peritonitis
CPC capsular polysaccharide complex	TNF-α tumor necrosis factor α
CT computed tomography	VISA vancomycin-intermediate
FUO fever of unknown origin	*S. aureus*
ICAM-1 intercellular adhesion molecule 1	VRE vancomycin-resistant enterococci
PMNs polymorphonuclear leukocytes	WBCs white blood cells
PS A surface polysaccharide A	

Intraperitoneal infections generally arise because a normal anatomic barrier is disrupted. This disruption may occur when the appendix, a diverticulum, or an ulcer ruptures; when the bowel wall is weakened by ischemia, tumor, or inflammation (e.g., in inflammatory bowel disease); or with adjacent inflammatory processes, such as pancreatitis or pelvic inflammatory disease, in which enzymes (in the former case) or organisms (in the latter) may leak into the peritoneal cavity. Whatever the inciting event, once inflammation develops and organisms usually contained within the bowel or another organ enter the normally sterile peritoneal space, a predictable series of events takes place. Intraabdominal infections occur in two stages: peritonitis and—if it goes untreated—abscess formation. The types of microorganisms predominating in each stage of infection are responsible for the pathogenesis of disease.

PERITONITIS

The peritoneal cavity is large but is divided into compartments. The upper and lower peritoneal cavities are divided by the transverse mesocolon; the greater omentum extends from the transverse mesocolon and from the lower pole of the stomach to line the lower peritoneal cavity. The pancreas, duodenum, and ascending and descending colon are located in the anterior retroperitoneal space; the kidneys, ureters, and adrenals are found in the posterior retroperitoneal space. The other organs, including liver, stomach, gallbladder, spleen, jejunum, ileum, transverse and sigmoid colon, cecum, and appendix, are found within the peritoneal cavity itself. Normally the cavity is lined with a serous membrane that can serve as a conduit for fluids—a property utilized in peritoneal dialysis. A small amount of fluid, sufficient to allow movement of organs, is normally present in the peritoneal space. This fluid is serous, with a protein content (consisting mainly of albumin) of <30 g/L and fewer than 300 white blood cells (WBCs, generally mononuclear cells) per microliter. In the presence of infection, some of these compartments collect fluid or pus more often than others. These compartments include the pelvis (the lowest portion), the subphrenic spaces on the right and left sides, and Morrison's pouch, which is a posterosuperior extension of the subhepatic spaces and is the lowest part of the paravertebral groove when a patient is recumbent. The falciform ligament separating the right and left subphrenic spaces appears to act as a barrier to the spread of infection; consequently, it is unusual to find bilateral subphrenic collections.

SPONTANEOUS BACTERIAL PERITONITIS Peritonitis is either primary (without an apparent source of contamination) or secondary. The types of organisms found and the clinical presentation of these two processes are different. In adults, primary or spontaneous bacterial peritonitis (SBP) occurs most commonly in conjunction with cirrhosis of the liver (frequently the result of alcoholism). It virtually always develops in patients with ascites. Nevertheless, it is not a common event, occurring in ≤10% of cirrhotic patients. The cause of SBP has not been established definitively but is believed to involve hematogenous spread of organisms in a patient in whom a diseased liver and altered portal circulation result in a defect in the usual filtration function. Organisms are able to multiply in ascites, a good medium for growth. The proteins of the complement cascade have been found in peritoneal fluid, with lower levels in cirrhotic patients than in patients with ascites of other etiologies. The opsonic and phagocytic properties of neutrophils are decreased in patients with advanced liver disease.

The presentation of SBP differs from that of secondary peritonitis. The most common manifestation is fever, which is reported in as many as 80% of patients. Ascites is found but virtually always predates infection. Abdominal pain, an acute onset of symptoms, and peritoneal irritation detected during physical examination can be helpful diagnostically, but the absence of any of these findings does not exclude this often-subtle diagnosis. It is vital to sample the peritoneal fluid of any cirrhotic patient with ascites and fever. The finding of >300 polymorphonuclear leukocytes (PMNs) per microliter is diagnostic for SBP, according to Conn. The microbiology of SBP is also distinctive. While enteric gram-negative bacilli such as *Escherichia coli* are most commonly encountered, gram-positive organisms such as streptococci, enterococci, or even pneumococci are sometimes found. In SBP, a single organism is typically isolated; anaerobes are found less frequently in SBP than in secondary peritonitis, in which a mixed flora including anaerobes is the rule. In fact, if SBP is suspected and multiple organisms including anaerobes are recovered from the peritoneal fluid, the diagnosis must be reconsidered and a source of secondary peritonitis sought.

The diagnosis of SBP is not easy. It depends on the exclusion of a primary intraabdominal source of infection. Contrast-enhanced computed tomography (CT) is very useful in identifying an intraabdominal source for infection. It may be difficult to recover organisms from cultures of peritoneal fluid, presumably because the burden of organisms is low. However, the yield can be improved if 10 mL of peritoneal fluid is placed directly into a blood culture bottle. Bacteremia frequently accompanies SBP; therefore, blood should be cultured simultaneously. No specific radiographic studies are helpful in the diagnosis of SBP. A plain film of the abdomen would be expected to show ascites. Chest and abdominal radiography should be performed in patients with abdominal pain to exclude free air, which signals a perforation.

℞ **TREATMENT**   Treatment for SBP is directed at the isolate from blood or peritoneal fluid. Gram's staining of peritoneal fluid often gives negative results in primary peritonitis; therefore, until culture results become available, empirical therapy should cover gram-negative aerobic bacilli and gram-positive cocci. Ampicillin plus gentamicin is a reasonable initial regimen. Third-generation cephalosporins, carbapenems, or broad-spectrum penicillin/β-lactamase inhibitor combinations are also options. Empirical coverage for anaerobes is not necessary. After the infecting organism is identified, therapy should be narrowed to target that specific pathogen. Patients with SBP usually respond within 72 h to appropriate antibiotic therapy.

SECONDARY PERITONITIS   Secondary peritonitis develops when bacteria contaminate the peritoneum as a result of spillage from an intraabdominal viscus. The organisms found almost always constitute a mixed flora in which facultative gram-negative bacilli and anaerobes predominate, especially when the contaminating source is colonic. Early in the course of infection, when the host response is directed toward containment of the infection, exudate containing fibrin and PMNs is found. Early death in this setting is attributable to gram-negative bacillary sepsis and to potent endotoxins circulating in the bloodstream (Chap. 124). Gram-negative bacilli, particularly *E. coli*, are common bloodstream isolates, but *Bacteroides fragilis* bacteremia occurs as well. The severity of abdominal pain and the clinical course depend on the inciting process. The species of organisms isolated from the peritoneum also vary with the source of the initial process and the normal flora present at that site. Peritonitis can result primarily from chemical irritation or bacterial contamination. For example, as long as the patient is not achlorhydric, a ruptured gastric ulcer will release low-pH gastric contents that will serve as a chemical irritant. The normal flora of the stomach comprises the same organisms found in the oropharynx (Chap. 167) but in lower numbers. The surfaces of teeth contain ~10^7 aerobic and 10^7 anaerobic organisms per milliliter of saliva; the normally acidic stomach contains an equal ratio of aerobic and anaerobic species, but in concentrations more in the range of 10^5/mL. After meals, when gastric acidity is highest, this number may fall to 10^3/mL. Thus, the bacterial burden in a ruptured gastric ulcer—or even a duodenal ulcer—is negligible compared with that in a ruptured appendix. The normal flora of the colon below the ligament of Treitz contains ~10^{11} anaerobic organisms per gram of feces but only 10^8 aerobes per gram; therefore, anaerobic species account for 99% of the bacteria. Leakage of colonic contents (pH 7 to 8) does not cause significant chemical peritonitis, but infection is intense because of the heavy bacterial load.

Depending on the inciting event, local symptoms may initially be found in secondary peritonitis—for example, epigastric pain from a ruptured gastric ulcer. In appendicitis (Chap. 291), the initial presenting symptoms are often vague, with periumbilical discomfort and nausea followed in a number of hours by pain more localized to the right lower quadrant. Unusual locations of the appendix (including a retrocecal position) can complicate this presentation further. Once infection has spread to the peritoneal cavity, however, pain increases, particularly with infection involving the parietal peritoneum, which is innervated extensively. Patients usually lie motionless, often with knees drawn up to avoid stretching the nerve fibers of the peritoneal cavity.

Coughing and sneezing, which increase pressure within the peritoneal cavity, are associated with sharp pain. There may or may not be pain localized to the infected or diseased organ from which secondary peritonitis has arisen. Patients with secondary peritonitis generally have abnormal findings on abdominal examination, with marked voluntary and involuntary guarding of the anterior abdominal musculature. Later findings include tenderness, especially rebound tenderness. In addition, there may be localized findings in the area of the inciting event. In general, patients are febrile, with marked leukocytosis and a left shift of the WBCs to earlier granulocyte forms.

While recovery of organisms from peritoneal fluid is easier in secondary than in primary peritonitis, a tap of the abdomen is rarely the procedure of choice in secondary peritonitis. An exception is in cases involving trauma, where the possibility of a hemoperitoneum may need to be excluded early.

℞ **TREATMENT**   Treatment for secondary peritonitis includes early administration of antibiotics aimed particularly at aerobic gram-negative bacilli and anaerobes (see below) as well as etiologic studies. Secondary peritonitis usually requires both surgical intervention to address the inciting process and antibiotic administration to treat early bacteremia, to decrease the incidence of abscess formation and wound infection, and to prevent more distant spread of infection. In SBP in adults, surgery is rarely indicated. In secondary peritonitis, surgery may be life-saving.

PERITONITIS IN PATIENTS UNDERGOING CAPD   A third type of peritonitis arises in patients who are undergoing continuous ambulatory peritoneal dialysis (CAPD). Unlike primary and secondary peritonitis, which are caused by endogenous bacteria, peritonitis in CAPD patients usually involves skin organisms. The pathogenesis of infection is similar to that of intravascular-device infection, in which skin organisms migrate along the catheter, which both serves as an entry point and exerts the effects of a foreign body. Exit-site or tunnel infection may or may not accompany CAPD peritonitis. Like primary peritonitis, CAPD peritonitis is usually caused by a single organism. Peritonitis is, in fact, the most common reason for discontinuation of CAPD. Improvements in equipment design, especially that of the Y-set connector, have resulted in a decrease from one case of peritonitis per 9 months of CAPD to one case per 15 months.

The clinical presentation of CAPD peritonitis resembles that of secondary peritonitis in that diffuse pain and peritoneal signs are common. The dialysate is usually cloudy and contains >100 WBCs per microliter, >50% of which are neutrophils. The most common etiologic organism is coagulase-negative *Staphylococcus*, which accounts for ~30% of cases. *S. aureus* causes ~10% of cases, is more commonly identified among patients who are nasal carriers of the organism, and is the most frequent pathogen in those with an overt exit-site infection. Gram-negative bacilli and fungi such as *Candida* species are also found. Vancomycin-resistant enterococci (VRE) and vancomycin-intermediate *S. aureus* (VISA) have been reported to produce peritonitis in CAPD patients. The finding of more than one organism in dialysate culture should prompt a search for a cause of secondary peritonitis. As with primary peritonitis, culture of dialysate fluid in blood culture bottles improves the yield.

℞ **TREATMENT**   Empirical therapy for CAPD peritonitis should be directed at coagulase-negative *Staphylococcus*, *S. aureus*, and gram-negative bacilli until the results of cultures are available. Since the advent of VRE and VISA, recommended treatment has changed from vancomycin and an aminoglycoside to a first-generation cephalosporin such as cefazolin and an aminoglycoside, which can be administered together in the same bag. A loading dose of cefazolin (500 mg/L) is administered intraperitoneally, with a maintenance dose of 125 mg/L in each bag. Ototoxicity is a significant concern in patients receiving aminoglycosides; some data suggest that administration of a single daily dose lessens this risk. Thus, gentamicin is usually administered at a dose of 20 mg/L once a day. If methicillin-resistant *S.*

aureus is a relatively common isolate in a community, vancomycin may still be a reasonable first choice for empirical therapy, especially in a toxic-appearing patient or a patient with an overt exit-site infection. The dose (2 g) is allowed to remain in the peritoneal cavity for 6 h. The clinical response to an empirical treatment regimen should be rapid; if the patient has not responded after 48 h of treatment, catheter removal should be considered.

INTRAPERITONEAL ABSCESSES

Abscess formation is common in untreated peritonitis if overt gram-negative sepsis either does not develop or develops but is not fatal. In experimental models of abscess formation, mixed aerobic and anaerobic organisms have been implanted intraperitoneally. Without therapy directed at anaerobes, animals develop intraabdominal abscesses. As in humans, these experimental abscesses may stud the peritoneal cavity, lie within the omentum or mesentery, or even develop on the surface of or within viscera such as the liver.

PATHOGENESIS AND IMMUNITY There is often disagreement about whether an abscess represents a disease state or a host response. In a sense, it represents both: While an abscess is an infection in which viable infecting organisms and PMNs are contained in a fibrous capsule, it is also a process by which the host confines microbes to a limited space, thereby preventing further spread of infection. Experimental work has helped to define both the host cells and the bacterial virulence factors responsible—most notably, in the case of *B. fragilis*. This organism, although accounting for only 0.5% of the normal colonic flora, is the anaerobe most frequently isolated from intraabdominal infections and is the most common anaerobic bloodstream isolate. On clinical grounds, therefore, *B. fragilis* appears to be uniquely virulent. Moreover, *B. fragilis* causes abscesses in animal models of intraabdominal infection, whereas most other *Bacteroides* species must act synergistically with a facultative organism to induce abscess formation.

Of the several virulence factors identified in *B. fragilis*, one is critical—the capsular polysaccharide complex (CPC) found on the bacterial surface. The CPC comprises several distinct surface polysaccharides. Structural analysis of the polysaccharides in the CPC has shown an unusual motif of oppositely charged sugars. Polysaccharides having these *zwitterionic* characteristics evoke a host response in the peritoneal cavity that localizes bacteria into abscesses. *B. fragilis* and the CPC have been found to adhere to primary mesothelial cells in vitro; this adherence, in turn, stimulates the production of tumor necrosis factor α (TNF-α) and intercellular adhesion molecule 1 (ICAM-1) by peritoneal macrophages. Mice treated with antibodies to TNF-α or ICAM-1 did not develop abscesses in the mouse peritonitis model. Although abscesses characteristically contain PMNs, the process of abscess induction depends on the stimulation of T lymphocytes by these unique polysaccharides. Experimentally, the essential role of T cells in initiating abscess formation has been proven following blockage of the CD28-B7 costimulatory pathway. The alternative pathways of complement and fibrinogen also participate in abscess formation.

While antibodies to the CPC are not critical in immunity to abscesses, they enhance bloodstream clearance of *B. fragilis*. When administered subcutaneously, *B. fragilis* surface polysaccharide A (PS A) has immunomodulatory characteristics and stimulates T cells via an interleukin-2-dependent mechanism to inhibit the host response of abscess formation to intraperitoneal challenge with *B. fragilis*. Treatment of experimental animals with PS A or other zwitterionic molecules reduces abscess development and can be administered after bacterial contamination of the peritoneal cavity.

CLINICAL PRESENTATION Most intraperitoneal abscesses result from fecal spillage from a colonic source, such as an inflamed appendix. Of all intraabdominal abscesses, 74% are intraperitoneal or retroperitoneal and are not visceral. Abscesses can also arise from a number of other processes. They usually form within weeks of the development of peritonitis and may be found in a variety of locations, from omentum to mesentery, pelvis to psoas muscles, and subphrenic

space to a visceral organ such as the liver, where they may develop either on the surface of the organ or within it. Periappendiceal and diverticular abscesses have traditionally been frequent. Diverticular abscesses are least likely to rupture. Infections of the female genital tract and pancreatitis are also among the more common causative events. When abscesses occur in the female genital tract—either as a primary infection (e.g., tuboovarian abscess) or as an infection extending into the pelvic cavity or peritoneum—*B. fragilis* figures prominently among the organisms isolated. *B. fragilis* is not found in large numbers in the normal vaginal flora. It is encountered less commonly in pelvic inflammatory disease and endometritis, for example, without an associated abscess. In pancreatitis with leakage of damaging pancreatic enzymes, inflammation is prominent. Therefore, clinical findings such as fever, leukocytosis, and even abdominal pain do not distinguish pancreatitis itself from complications such as pancreatic pseudocyst, pancreatic abscess (Chap. 304), or intraabdominal collections of pus. Especially in cases of necrotizing pancreatitis, in which the incidence of local pancreatic infection may be as high as 30%, needle aspiration under CT guidance is performed as often as once a week to sample fluid for culture. Many centers prescribe prophylactic antibiotics to prevent infection in patients with necrotizing pancreatitis. Imipenem is the most frequently used drug for this purpose since it achieves high tissue levels in the pancreas, although it is not unique in this regard. If infected fluid is removed during needle aspiration, most experts agree that surgery is superior to percutaneous drainage.

The psoas muscle of the anterior back is another location in which abscesses are encountered. These abscesses may arise from a presumed hematogenous source, by contiguous spread from an intraabdominal or pelvic process, or by contiguous spread from nearby bony structures such as vertebral bodies. Associated osteomyelitis due to spread from bone to muscle or from muscle to bone is common in psoas abscesses. When Pott's disease was common, *Mycobacterium tuberculosis* was a frequent cause of psoas abscess. Currently in the United States, the usual isolates from psoas abscesses are either *S. aureus* or a mixture of enteric organisms including aerobic gram-negative bacilli. *S. aureus* is most likely to be isolated when a psoas abscess arises from hematogenous spread or a contiguous focus of osteomyelitis; a mixed enteric flora is most likely when the abscess has an intraabdominal or pelvic source.

DIAGNOSIS A variety of scanning procedures have considerably facilitated the diagnosis of intraabdominal abscesses. Abdominal CT probably has the highest yield, although ultrasonography is particularly useful for the right upper quadrant, kidneys, and pelvis. Both indium-labeled WBCs and gallium tend to localize in abscesses and may be useful in finding a collection. Since gallium is taken up in the bowel, indium-labeled WBCs may have a slightly greater yield for abscesses near the bowel. Neither indium-labeled WBC nor gallium scans serve as a basis for a definitive diagnosis, however; both need to be followed by other, more specific studies, such as CT, if an area of possible abnormality is identified. Abscesses contiguous with or contained within outpouchings of bowel are particularly difficult to diagnose with scanning procedures. Occasionally, a barium enema may detect a diverticular abscess not diagnosed by other procedures, although barium should not be injected if a free perforation is suspected. If one study is negative, a second study sometimes reveals a collection. On occasion, exploratory laparotomy still must be undertaken if an abscess is strongly suspected on clinical grounds, although this procedure has been less commonly used since the advent of CT.

TREATMENT An algorithm for the management of patients with intraabdominal abcesses is presented in Fig. 130-1. The treatment of intraabdominal infections involves the determination of the initial focus of infection, the administration of broad-spectrum antibiotics targeted at organisms involved in the associated infection, and the performance of a drainage procedure if one or more definitive abscesses have formed already. It cannot be overemphasized that an-

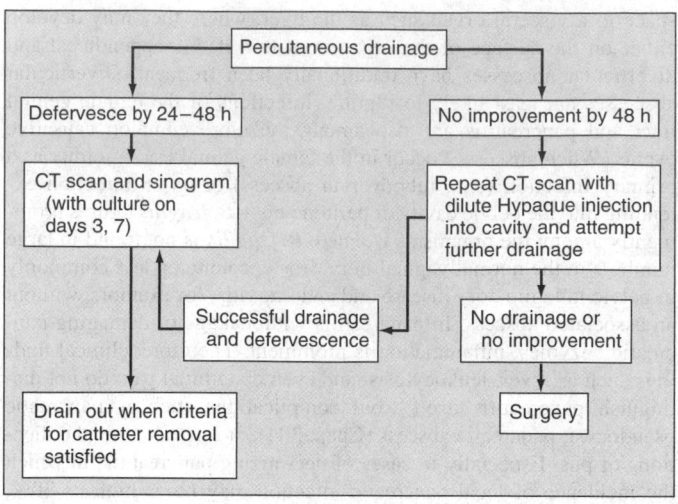

FIGURE 130-1 Algorithm for the management of patients with intraabdominal abscesses using percutaneous drainage. Antimicrobial therapy should be administered concomitantly. CT, computed tomography. *[Reprinted with permission from Lorber B (ed): Atlas of Infectious Diseases, vol VII: Intra-abdominal Infections, Hepatitis, and Gastroenteritis. Philadelphia, Current Medicine, 1995, pp 1–101, as adapted from OD Rotstein, RL Simmons, Intraabdominal abscesses, in SL Gorbach et al (eds): Infectious Diseases, Philadelphia, Saunders, 1992, p. 668.]*

timicrobial therapy, in general, is adjunctive to drainage and/or surgical correction of an underlying lesion or process in intraabdominal abscesses. Unlike the intraabdominal abscesses precipitated by most infections, for which drainage of some kind is generally required, abscesses associated with diverticulitis usually wall off locally after rupture of a diverticulum, so that surgical intervention is not routinely required.

A number of antimicrobial agents exhibit excellent activity against aerobic gram-negative bacilli. Since mortality in intraabdominal sepsis is linked to gram-negative bacteremia, empirical therapy for intraabdominal infection always needs to include adequate coverage of gram-negative aerobic and facultative organisms. Aminoglycosides and second- and third-generation cephalosporins are the agents most widely tested and used in intraabdominal processes. Newer antibiotics, such as aztreonam, imipenem, ticarcillin/clavulanic acid, piperacillin/tazobactam, and quinolones (e.g., ciprofloxacin), cover these organisms as well, although at a higher cost. Second-generation cephalosporins, such as cefoxitin or cefotetan, are not as uniformly active as the other agents against all of the aerobic gram-negative species. Aztreonam, ciprofloxacin, aminoglycosides, and most of the third-generation cephalosporins are not active against anaerobes; for the treatment of intraabdominal infections, these drugs need to be used in combination with another antibiotic. Since a number of antibiotics highly effective against anaerobes are available, third-generation cephalosporins generally should not be considered for use against the anaerobic bacteria involved in intraabdominal sepsis.

The most active and cost-effective antibiotic for anaerobic coverage currently is metronidazole (Chap. 167). Only rare isolates of *B. fragilis* have been reported to be resistant to this drug. In a study of 3177 anaerobic isolates from eight centers in the United States over a 5-year period, no strains resistant to metronidazole were documented among *B. fragilis* isolates, and resistance to imipenem, ampicillin/sulbactam, and piperacillin/tazobactam was exceedingly rare. In contrast, resistance to cefotetan, ceftizoxime, and clindamycin increased during this interval, and resistance to cefoxitin was measurable but unchanged during the study. Despite increasing reports of in vitro resistance of *B. fragilis* to a number of agents, clinical failures are still limited to case reports; therefore, the clinical significance of antimicrobial resistance in anaerobes is uncertain. One report describes a bloodstream isolate of *B. fragilis* with resistance to metronidazole and with reduced susceptibility to imipenem and amoxicillin/clavulanic acid that became resistant to both of the latter two drugs after treatment of the patient with imipenem. Among newer agents, imipenem, ticarcillin/clavulanic acid, piperacillin/tazobactam, meropenem, and ampicillin/sulbactam are highly active against anaerobes. Chloramphenicol, which exhibits strong activity against *B. fragilis* in vitro, nevertheless should probably not be considered a first-line drug for use against anaerobes, since failures of treatment have been documented in both experimental and clinical intraabdominal infections. Neither metronidazole nor clindamycin covers aerobic gram-negative bacilli; thus, these drugs must be combined with other agents for use in this setting. Metronidazole is also less active against gram-positive than against gram-negative anaerobic species.

VISCERAL ABSCESSES   Liver Abscesses   The liver is the organ most subject to the development of abscesses. Altemeier and associates studied 540 intraabdominal abscesses over a 12-year period. Of these abscesses 26% were visceral. Liver abscesses made up 13% of the total number of abscesses, or 48% of all visceral abscesses. Liver abscesses may be solitary or multiple; they may arise from hematogenous spread of bacteria or from local spread from contiguous sites of infection within the peritoneal cavity. In the past, appendicitis with rupture and subsequent spread of infection was the most common route for the development of a liver abscess. Currently, associated disease of the biliary tract is most often the etiology. Suppurative pylephlebitis (suppurative thrombosis of the portal vein), usually arising from infection in the pelvis but sometimes from infection elsewhere in the peritoneal cavity, is another common source for bacterial seeding of the liver.

Fever is the most common presenting sign of liver abscess. Some patients, particularly those with active associated disease of the biliary tract, have symptoms and signs localized to the right upper quadrant, including pain, guarding, punch tenderness, and even rebound tenderness. Nonspecific symptoms, such as chills, anorexia, weight loss, nausea, and vomiting, may also develop. Only 50% of patients with liver abscesses, however, have hepatomegaly, right-upper-quadrant tenderness, or jaundice; thus, half of patients have no symptoms or signs that would direct attention to the liver. Fever of unknown origin (FUO) may be the only presenting manifestation of liver abscess, especially in the elderly. Diagnostic studies of the abdomen, especially the right upper quadrant, should be a part of any FUO workup. The single most reliable laboratory finding is an elevated serum concentration of alkaline phosphatase, which is documented in 70% of patients with liver abscesses. Other tests of liver function may yield normal results, but 50% of patients have elevated serum levels of bilirubin, and 48% have elevated concentrations of aspartate aminotransferase. Other associated laboratory findings include leukocytosis in 77% of patients, anemia (usually normochromic, normocytic) in 50%, and hypoalbuminemia in 33%. Concomitant bacteremia is found in one-third of patients. A liver abscess is sometimes suggested by chest radiography, especially if a new elevation of the right hemidiaphragm is seen; other suggestive findings include a right basilar infiltrate and a right pleural effusion.

Imaging studies are the most reliable methods for diagnosing liver abscesses. These studies include ultrasonography, CT, indium-labeled WBC or gallium scans, and even magnetic resonance imaging. In an occasional case, more than one such study may be required. Organisms recovered from liver abscesses vary with the etiology. In liver infection arising from the biliary tree, enteric gram-negative aerobic bacilli and enterococci are common isolates. Unless previous surgery has been performed, anaerobes are not generally involved in liver abscesses arising from biliary infections. In contrast, in liver abscesses arising from pelvic and other intraperitoneal sources, a mixed flora including aerobic and anaerobic species (especially *B. fragilis*) is common. With hematogenous spread of infection, usually only a single organism is encountered; this species may be *S. aureus* or a streptococcal species such as *S. milleri*.

Liver abscesses may also be caused by *Candida* species; such abscesses usually follow fungemia in patients receiving chemotherapy for cancer and often present when neutrophils return after a period of neutropenia. Amebic liver abscesses are not an uncommon problem (Chap. 213). Amebic serologic testing gives positive results in >95% of cases; thus, a negative result helps to exclude this diagnosis.

TREATMENT While drainage—either percutaneous (with a pigtail catheter kept in place) or surgical—remains the mainstay of therapy for intraabdominal abscesses (including liver abscesses), there is growing interest in medical management alone for pyogenic liver abscesses. The drugs used in empirical broad-spectrum antibiotic therapy include the same ones used in intraabdominal sepsis. Usually, a diagnostic aspirate of abscess contents should be obtained before the initiation of empirical therapy, with antibiotic choices adjusted when the results of Gram's staining and culture become available. Cases treated without definitive drainage generally require longer courses of antibiotic therapy. When percutaneous drainage was compared with open surgical drainage, the average length of hospital stay for the former was almost twice that for the latter, although both the time required for fever to resolve and mortality were the same for the two procedures. Mortality was appreciable despite treatment, averaging 15%. Several factors may predict the failure of percutaneous drainage and therefore may favor primary surgical intervention. These factors include the presence of multiple, sizable abscesses; viscous abscess contents that tend to plug the catheter; associated disease (e.g., disease of the biliary tract) that requires surgery; or the lack of a clinical response to percutaneous drainage in 4 to 7 days.

Treatment of candidal liver abscesses usually entails lengthy administration of amphotericin B, although reports have described successful maintenance therapy with fluconazole after an initial course of amphotericin (Chap. 205).

Splenic Abscesses Splenic abscesses are much less common than liver abscesses. In fact, no splenic abscesses were observed in Altemeier's series of 540 intraabdominal abscesses. The incidence of splenic abscesses has ranged from 0.14 to 0.7% in various autopsy series. The clinical setting and the organisms isolated usually differ from those for liver abscesses. The degree of clinical suspicion for splenic abscess needs to be high, as this condition is frequently fatal if left untreated. Even in the most recently published series, diagnosis was made only at autopsy in 37% of cases. While splenic abscesses may arise occasionally from contiguous spread of infection or from direct trauma to the spleen, hematogenous spread of infection is the usual mode of development. Bacterial endocarditis is the most common associated infection. Splenic abscesses can develop in patients who have received extensive immunosuppressive therapy (particularly those with malignancy involving the spleen) and in patients with hemoglobinopathies or other hematologic disorders (especially sickle cell anemia).

While ~50% of patients with splenic abscesses have abdominal pain, the pain is localized to the left upper quadrant in only half of these cases. Splenomegaly is found in ~50% of cases. Fever and leukocytosis are generally present; the development of fever preceded diagnosis by an average of 20 days in one series. Left-sided chest findings may include abnormalities to auscultation, and chest radiographic findings may include an infiltrate or a left-sided pleural effusion. When splenic abscesses are being considered in a differential diagnosis, CT scan of the abdomen has been the most sensitive diagnostic tool. Ultrasonography can yield the diagnosis, but cases have been missed with this modality. Liver-spleen scan or gallium scan may also be useful. Streptococcal species are the most common bacterial isolates from splenic abscesses, and *S. aureus* is the next most common; presumably these prevalences reflect the bacterial cause of the associated endocarditis. An increase in the frequency of isolation of gram-negative aerobic organisms from splenic abscesses has been reported; these organisms often derive from a urinary tract focus, with associated bacteremia, or from another intraabdominal source. *Sal-*

monella species are seen fairly commonly, especially in patients with sickle cell hemoglobinopathy. Anaerobic species accounted for only 5% of isolates in the largest collected series, but the reporting of a number of "sterile abscesses" may indicate that optimal techniques for the isolation of anaerobes were not employed.

TREATMENT Because of the high mortality figures reported for splenic abscesses, the treatment of choice is splenectomy with adjunctive antibiotics. However, percutaneous drainage has been successful. The most important factor in successful treatment of splenic abscesses is early consideration of the diagnosis.

Perinephric and Renal Abscesses Perinephric and renal abscesses are not common: The former accounted for only ~0.02% of hospital admissions and the latter for ~0.2% in Altemeier's series of 540 intraabdominal abscesses. While liver abscesses generally arise from contiguous foci of infection or track from other intraabdominal sources and splenic abscesses usually arise from hematogenous spread (e.g., spread from bacterial endocarditis), perinephric and renal abscesses have a different pathogenesis. Before antibiotics became available, most renal and perinephric abscesses were hematogenous in origin, with *S. aureus* most commonly recovered. Now, in contrast, >75% of perinephric and renal abscesses arise from an initial urinary tract infection. Infection ascends from the bladder to the kidney, with pyelonephritis occurring first. Bacteria may directly invade the renal parenchyma from medulla to cortex. Local vascular channels within the kidney may also facilitate the transport of organisms. Areas of abscess developing within the parenchyma may rupture into the perinephric space. The kidneys and adrenal glands are surrounded by a layer of perirenal fat that, in turn, is surrounded by Gerota's fascia, which extends superiorly to the diaphragm and inferiorly to the pelvic fat. When abscesses extend into the perinephric space, tracking may occur through Gerota's fascia into the psoas or transversalis muscles, into the anterior peritoneal cavity, superiorly to the subdiaphragmatic space, or inferiorly to the pelvis. Of the several risk factors that have been associated with the development of perinephric abscesses, the most important is the presence of concomitant nephrolithiasis producing local obstruction to urinary flow. Of patients with perinephric abscess, 20 to 60% have renal stones. In addition, other structural abnormalities of the urinary tract, a history of urologic surgery, trauma, and diabetes mellitus have all been identified as risk factors.

The organisms most frequently encountered in perinephric and renal abscesses are *E. coli*, *Proteus* species, and *Klebsiella* species. *E. coli*, the aerobic species most commonly found in colonic flora, seems to have unique virulence properties in the urinary tract, including factors promoting adherence to uroepithelial cells. The urease of *Proteus* species splits urea, thereby creating a more alkaline and hospitable environment for bacterial proliferation. *Proteus* species are frequently found in association with large struvite stones caused by the precipitation of magnesium ammonium sulfate in an alkaline environment. These stones serve as a nidus for recurrent urinary tract infection. While a single bacterial species is usually recovered from a perinephric or renal abscess, multiple species may also be found. If a urine culture is not contaminated with periurethral flora and is found to contain more than one organism, a perinephric abscess or renal abscess should be considered in the differential diagnosis. Urine cultures may also be polymicrobial in cases of bladder diverticulum.

Candida species should be considered in the etiology of renal abscesses. This fungus may spread to the kidney via the hematogenous route or by ascension from the bladder. The hallmark of the latter route of infection is ureteral obstruction with large fungal balls.

The presentation of perinephric and renal abscesses is quite nonspecific. Flank pain and abdominal pain are common. At least 50% of patients are febrile. Pain may be referred to the groin or leg, particularly with extension of infection. The diagnosis of perinephric abscess, like that of splenic abscess, is frequently delayed, and mortality in some series is appreciable, although lower than in the past. Perinephric or renal abscess should be most seriously considered when a patient presents with symptoms and signs of pyelonephritis and remains febrile after 4 or 5 days, by which time the fever should have resolved. Moreover, when a urine culture yields a polymicrobial flora, when a patient is known to have renal stone disease, or when fever and pyuria coexist with a sterile urine culture, the diagnosis of perinephric or renal abscess should be entertained.

Renal ultrasonography and abdominal CT are the most useful diagnostic modalities. If a renal abscess or perinephric abscess is diagnosed, nephrolithiasis should be excluded, especially when a high urinary pH suggests the presence of a urea-splitting organism.

℞ TREATMENT   Treatment for perinephric or renal abscesses, like that for other intraabdominal abscesses, includes drainage of pus and antibiotic therapy directed at the organism(s) recovered. For perinephric abscesses, percutaneous drainage is usually successful.

Pancreatic Abscesses   →*See Chap. 304.*

BIBLIOGRAPHY

ALTEMEIER WA et al: Intra-abdominal abscesses. Am J Surg 125:70, 1973

BASSI C et al: Controlled clinical trial of pefloxacin versus imipenem in severe acute pancreatitis. Gastroenterology 115:1513, 1998

CHOU YH et al: Ultrasound-guided interventional procedures in splenic abscesses. Eur J Radiol 28:167, 1998

FINEGOLD SM: Anaerobic bacteria: General concepts, in *Principles and Practice of Infectious Diseases*, 5th ed, GL Mandell et al (eds). New York, Churchill Livingstone, 2000, pp 2519–2537

GIBSON FC III et al: Cellular mechanism of intraabdominal abscess formation by *Bacteroides fragilis*. J Immunol 160:5000, 1998

HUTCHISON FN, KAYSEN GA: Perinephric abscess: The missed diagnosis. Med Clin North Am 72:993, 1988

LEVISON ME, BUSH LM: Peritonitis and other intra-abdominal infections, in *Principles and Practice of Infectious Diseases*, 5th ed, GL Mandell et al (eds). New York, Churchill Livingstone, 2000, pp 821–856

SNYDMAN DR et al: Analysis of trends in antimicrobial resistance patterns among clinical isolates of *Bacteroides fragilis* group species from 1990 to 1994. Clin Infect Dis 23: S54, 1996

SOLOMKIN JS et al: Results of a randomized trial comparing sequential intravenous/oral treatment with ciprofloxacin plus metronidazole to imipenem/cilastatin for intra-abdominal infections. Ann Surg 223:303, 1996

TZIANABOS AO et al: Polysaccharide-mediated protection against abscess formation in experimental intra-abdominal sepsis. J Clin Invest 96:2727, 1995

———— et al: T cells activated by zwitterionic molecules prevent abscesses induced by pathogenic bacteria. J Biol Chem 275:6733, 2000

131   *Joan R. Butterton, Stephen B. Calderwood*

ACUTE INFECTIOUS DIARRHEAL DISEASES AND BACTERIAL FOOD POISONING

Ranging from mild annoyances during vacations to devastating dehydrating illnesses that can kill within hours, acute gastrointestinal illnesses rank second only to acute upper respiratory illnesses as the most common diseases worldwide. In children <5 years old, attack rates range from 2 to 3 illnesses per child per year in developed countries to as high as 10 to 18 illnesses per child per year in developing countries. In Asia, Africa, and Latin America, acute diarrheal illnesses are not only a leading cause of morbidity in children—with an estimated 1 billion cases per year—but also the major cause of mortality, being responsible for 4 to 6 million deaths per year, or a sobering total of 12,600 deaths per day. In some areas, more than 50% of childhood deaths are directly attributable to acute diarrheal illnesses. In addition, by contributing to malnutrition and thereby reducing resistance to other infectious agents, gastrointestinal illnesses may be indirect factors in a far greater burden of disease.

The wide range of clinical manifestations of acute gastrointestinal illnesses is matched by the wide variety of infectious agents involved, including viruses, bacteria, and parasitic pathogens (Table 131-1). This chapter will discuss factors that enable gastrointestinal pathogens to cause disease, will review host defense mechanisms, and will delineate an approach to the evaluation and treatment of patients presenting with acute diarrhea. Individual organisms causing acute gastrointestinal illnesses are discussed in detail in subsequent chapters.

PATHOGENIC MECHANISMS   Enteric pathogens have developed a variety of tactics to overcome host defenses. Understanding the virulence factors employed by these organisms is important in the diagnosis and treatment of clinical disease.

Inoculum Size   The number of microorganisms that must be ingested to cause disease varies considerably from species to species. For *Shigella*, enterohemorrhagic *Escherichia coli*, *Giardia lamblia*, or *Entamoeba*, as few as 10 to 100 bacteria or cysts can produce infection, while 10^5 to 10^8 *Vibrio cholerae* organisms must be ingested orally to cause disease. The infective dose of *Salmonella* varies widely, depending on the species, host, and food vehicle. The ability of organisms to overcome host defenses has important implications for transmission; *Shigella*, enterohemorrhagic *E. coli*, *Entamoeba*, and *Giardia* can spread by person-to-person contact, whereas under some circumstances *Salmonella* may have to grow in food for several hours before reaching an effective infectious dose.

Adherence   Many organisms must adhere to the gastrointestinal mucosa as an initial step in the pathogenic process; thus, organisms that can compete with the normal bowel flora and colonize the mucosa have an important advantage in causing disease. Specific cell-surface proteins involved in attachment of bacteria to intestinal cells are important virulence determinants. *V. cholerae*, for example, adheres to the brush border of small-intestinal enterocytes via specific surface adhesins, including the toxin-coregulated pilus and other accessory colonization factors. Enterotoxigenic *E. coli* produces an adherence protein called *colonization factor antigen* that is necessary for colonization of the upper small intestine by the organism prior to the production of enterotoxin. Enteropathogenic and enterohemorrhagic strains of *E. coli* produce virulence determinants that allow these organisms to attach to and efface the brush border of the intestinal epithelium.

Toxin Production   The production of one or more exotoxins is important in the pathogenesis of numerous enteric organisms. Such toxins include *enterotoxins*, which cause watery diarrhea by acting directly on secretory mechanisms in the intestinal mucosa; *cytotoxins*, which cause destruction of mucosal cells and associated inflammatory diarrhea; and *neurotoxins*, which act directly on the central or peripheral nervous system. Some exotoxins act by more than one mechanism; *Shigella dysenteriae* type 1, for example, produces an exotoxin that has both enterotoxic and cytotoxic activities.

The prototypical enterotoxin is cholera toxin, a heterodimeric protein composed of one A and five B subunits. The A subunit contains the enzymatic activity of the toxin, while the B subunit pentamer binds holotoxin to the enterocyte surface receptor, the ganglioside G_{M1}. After the binding of holotoxin, a fragment of the A subunit is translocated across the eukaryotic cell membrane into the cytoplasm, where it catalyzes the ADP-ribosylation of a GTP-binding protein and causes persistent activation of adenylate cyclase. The end result is an increase of cyclic AMP in the intestinal mucosa, which increases Cl^- secretion and decreases Na^+ absorption, leading to loss of fluid and the production of diarrhea.

Enterotoxigenic strains of *E. coli* may produce a protein called *heat-labile enterotoxin* (LT) that is similar to cholera toxin and causes secretory diarrhea by the same mechanism. Alternatively, enterotoxigenic strains of *E. coli* may produce *heat-stable enterotoxin* (ST), one form of which causes diarrhea by activation of guanylate cyclase and elevation of intracellular cyclic GMP. Some enterotoxigenic strains produce both LT and ST.

Bacterial cytotoxins, in contrast, destroy intestinal mucosal cells and produce the syndrome of dysentery, with bloody stools containing inflammatory cells. Enteric pathogens that produce such cytotoxins include *S. dysenteriae* type 1, *Vibrio parahaemolyticus*, and *Clostridium difficile*. Shiga toxin–producing strains of *E. coli*, most commonly serotype O157:H7 in the United States, produce potent cytotoxins that are highly related to the Shiga toxin of *S. dysenteriae* type 1. Such strains of *E. coli* have been associated with outbreaks of hemorrhagic colitis and hemolytic-uremic syndrome.

Neurotoxins usually are produced by the responsible organism outside the host and therefore cause symptoms soon after ingestion. Included are the staphylococcal and *Bacillus cereus* toxins, which act on the central nervous system to produce vomiting.

Invasion Dysentery may result not only from the production of cytotoxins but also from bacterial invasion and destruction of intestinal mucosal cells. Infections due to *Shigella* and enteroinvasive *E. coli*, for example, are characterized by the organisms' invasion of mucosal epithelial cells, intraepithelial multiplication, and subsequent spread to adjacent cells. *Salmonella*, on the other hand, causes inflammatory diarrhea by invasion of the bowel mucosa but generally is not associated with the destruction of enterocytes or the full clinical syndrome of dysentery. *Salmonella typhi* and *Yersinia enterocolitica* can penetrate intact intestinal mucosa, multiply intracellularly in Peyer's patches and intestinal lymph nodes, and then disseminate through the bloodstream to cause enteric fever, a syndrome characterized by fever, headache, relative bradycardia, abdominal pain, splenomegaly, and leukopenia.

HOST DEFENSES Given the enormous number of microorganisms ingested with every meal, the normal host must possess effective defense mechanisms to combat a constant influx of potential enteric pathogens. Studies of infections in patients with alterations in these defenses have led to a greater understanding of the variety of ways in which the normal host can protect itself against disease.

Normal Flora The large numbers of bacteria that normally inhabit the intestine act as an important host defense by preventing colonization by potential enteric pathogens. Persons with fewer intestinal bacteria, such as infants who have not yet developed normal enteric colonization or patients receiving antibiotics, are at significantly greater risk of developing infections with enteric pathogens. The composition of the intestinal flora is as important as the number of organisms present. More than 99% of the normal colonic flora is made up of anaerobic bacteria, and the acidic pH and volatile fatty acids produced by these organisms appear to be critical elements in resistance to colonization.

Gastric Acid The acidic pH of the stomach is an important barrier to enteric pathogens, and an increased frequency of infections due to *Salmonella*, *G. lamblia*, and a variety of helminths has been reported among patients who have undergone gastric surgery or are achlorhydric for some other reason. Neutralization of gastric acid with antacids or H_2 blockers—common among hospitalized patients—similarly increases the risk of enteric colonization. Some microorganisms, however, can survive the extreme acidity of the gastric environment; rotavirus, for example, is highly stable to acidity.

Table 131-1 Gastrointestinal Pathogens Causing Acute Diarrhea

Mechanism	Location	Illness	Stool Findings	Examples of Pathogens Involved
Noninflammatory (enterotoxin)	Proximal small bowel	Watery diarrhea	No fecal leukocytes	*Vibrio cholerae*, enterotoxigenic *Escherichia coli* (LT and/or ST), *Clostridium perfringens*, *Bacillus cereus*, *Staphylococcus aureus*, *Aeromonas hydrophila*, *Plesiomonas shigelloides*, rotavirus, Norwalk-like viruses, enteric adenoviruses, *Giardia lamblia*, *Cryptosporidium* spp., *Cyclospora* spp.
Inflammatory (invasion or cytotoxin)	Colon or distal small bowel	Dysentery or inflammatory diarrhea	Fecal polymorphonuclear leukocytes	*Shigella* spp., *Salmonella* spp., *Campylobacter jejuni*, enterohemorrhagic *E. coli*, enteroinvasive *E. coli*, *Yersinia enterocolitica*, *Vibrio parahaemolyticus*, *Clostridium difficile*, ? *A. hydrophila*, ? *P. shigelloides*, *Entamoeba histolytica*
Penetrating	Distal small bowel	Enteric fever	Fecal mononuclear leukocytes	*Salmonella typhi*, *Y. enterocolitica*

SOURCE: After Guerrant.

Intestinal Motility Normal peristalsis is the major mechanism for clearance of bacteria from the proximal small intestine, although gastric acidity and secreted immunoglobulins also play a role in limiting the number of organisms present. When intestinal motility is impaired—for example, by treatment with opiates or other antimotility drugs, anatomic abnormalities (diverticula, fistulas, or afferent-loop stasis following surgery), or hypomotility states (as in diabetes mellitus or scleroderma)—the frequency of bacterial overgrowth and infection of the small bowel with enteric pathogens is much increased. Some patients in whom *Shigella* infection is treated with diphenoxylate hydrochloride with atropine (Lomotil) experience prolonged fever and shedding of organisms, while patients treated with opiates for mild *Salmonella* gastroenteritis have a higher frequency of bacteremia than those not treated with opiates.

Immunity Both cellular immune responses and antibody production play important roles in protecting susceptible hosts from enteric infections. The wide spectrum of viral, bacterial, parasitic, and fungal gastrointestinal infections in patients with AIDS highlights the significance of cell-mediated immunity in protecting the normal host from these pathogens. Humoral immunity is also important and consists of systemic IgG and IgM as well as secretory IgA. Growing evidence supports the concept of a mucosal immune system for secretory IgA in which binding of bacterial antigens to the luminal surface of M cells in the distal small bowel and subsequent presentation of the antigens to subepithelial lymphoid tissue lead to the proliferation of sensitized lymphocytes. These lymphocytes circulate and populate all of the mucosal tissues of the body as IgA-secreting plasma cells.

Approach to the Patient

The approach to the patient with possible infectious diarrhea or bacterial food poisoning is shown in Fig. 131-1.

History The answers to questions with high discriminating value can quickly narrow the range of potential causes of diarrhea and help determine whether treatment is needed. Important elements of the narrative history are detailed in Fig. 131-1.

Physical Examination The examination of patients for signs of dehydration provides essential information about the severity of the diarrheal illness and the need for rapid therapy. Mild dehydration is indicated by thirst, dry mouth, decreased axillary sweat, decreased urine output, and slight weight loss. Signs of moderate dehydration include an orthostatic fall in blood pressure, skin tenting, and sunken eyes (or, in infants, a sunken fontanelle). Signs of severe dehydration range from hypotension and tachycardia to confusion and frank shock.

Diagnostic Approach   After the severity of illness is assessed, the most important distinction that the clinician must make is between *inflammatory* and *noninflammatory* disease. Using the history and epidemiologic features of the case as guides in making this distinction, the clinician can rapidly evaluate the need for further efforts to define a specific etiology and for therapeutic intervention. Examination of a stool sample is an important supplement to the narrative history. Grossly bloody or mucoid stool suggests an inflammatory process, but all stools should be examined for fecal leukocytes; the latter task is accomplished by the preparation of a thin smear of the stool on a glass slide, the addition of a drop of methylene blue, and examination of the wet mount. Causes of acute infectious diarrhea, categorized as inflammatory and noninflammatory, are listed in Table 131-1.

EPIDEMIOLOGY   Travel History   Of the 12 to 20 million people who travel from temperate industrialized countries to tropical regions of Asia, Africa, and Central and South America each year, 20 to 50% experience a sudden onset of abdominal cramps, anorexia, and watery diarrhea; thus *traveler's diarrhea* is the most common travel-related illness (Chap. 123). The time of onset is usually 3 days to 2 weeks after the traveler's arrival in a tropical area; most cases begin within the first 3 to 5 days. The illness is generally self-limited, lasting 1 to 5 days. The high rate of diarrhea among travelers to underdeveloped areas is related to the ingestion of contaminated food or water.

The organisms that cause traveler's diarrhea vary considerably with location. In all areas, enterotoxigenic *E. coli* is the most common isolate from persons with the classic secretory traveler's diarrhea syndrome; the proportion of cases accounted for by this organism ranges from a high of approximately 50% in Latin America to a low of 15% in Asia. *Shigella, Salmonella,* and *Campylobacter* spp. are classically considered to cause more invasive dysenteric disease than enterotoxigenic *E. coli*, but clinical differentiation of infections attributable to these organisms can be difficult. *Shigella, Salmonella,* and *Campylobacter* are isolated in 1 to 15% of cases, with different organisms being more common in different locations. *Vibrio* spp. are most common in Asia, although *V. cholerae* O1 reached epidemic proportions in parts of Central and South America in 1991 and remains a significant source of concern to travelers to these regions. Epidemic *V. cholerae* O139 Bengal has spread throughout India and Southeast Asia since 1992. Less frequently isolated bacteria are *Aeromonas hydrophila* and *Plesiomonas shigelloides*, which are more common among travelers to Thailand. Parasitic causes of traveler's diarrhea include *Entamoeba histolytica*, which is responsible for up to 5% of cases in Mexico and Thailand, and *G. lamblia*, which has been associated with contaminated freshwater supplies in many areas of the world. *Giardia* is found in association with zoonotic reservoirs in the northern United States and poses a risk to hikers and campers who drink from freshwater streams. A striking association of *Giardia* with contaminated water supplies has likewise been noted in Russia. *Cryptosporidium* has been recognized as a problem in travelers to the former Soviet Republics, Mexico, and Africa and has caused large-scale urban outbreaks of infection in the United States. Disease due to *Cyclospora* and microsporidia has recently been recognized. Viruses such as rotavirus and Norwalk-like viruses have been isolated from as many as 10 to 40% of visitors to areas of Latin America, Asia, and Africa who develop traveler's diarrhea.

Location   Day-care centers are sites of particularly high attack rates of enteric infections. Rotavirus is most common among children <2 years old, with attack rates of 75 to 100% among those exposed.

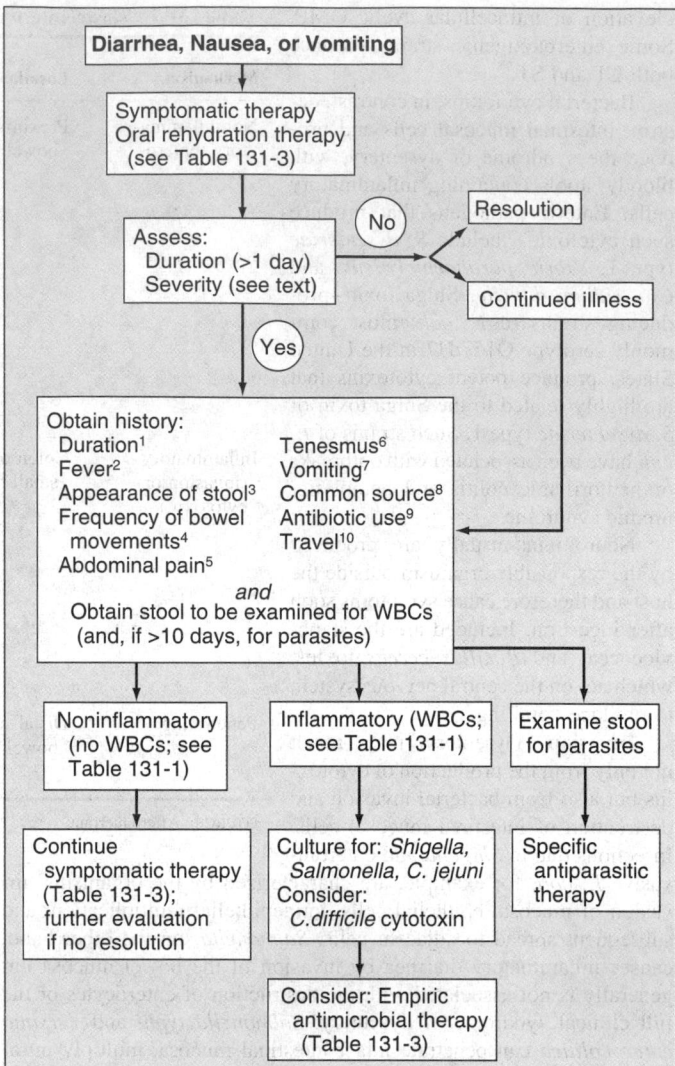

FIGURE 131-1   Clinical algorithm for the approach to patients with community-acquired infectious diarrhea or bacterial food poisoning. Key to superscripts: 1. Diarrhea lasting more than 2 weeks generally is defined as chronic; in such cases, many of the causes of acute diarrhea are much less likely, and a new spectrum of causes needs to be considered. 2. Fever often implies invasive disease, although fever and diarrhea also may result from infection outside the gastrointestinal tract, as in malaria. 3. Stools that contain blood or mucus indicate ulceration of the large bowel. Bloody stools without fecal leukocytes should alert the laboratory to the possibility of infection with Shiga toxin–producing enterohemorrhagic *Escherichia coli*. Bulky white stools suggest a small-intestinal process that is causing malabsorption. Profuse "rice-water" stools suggest cholera or a similar toxigenic process. 4. Frequent stools over a given period can provide the first warning of impending dehydration. 5. Abdominal pain may be most severe in inflammatory processes like those due to *Shigella, Campylobacter,* and necrotizing toxins. Painful abdominal muscle cramps, caused by electrolyte loss, can develop in severe cases of cholera. Bloating is common in giardiasis. An appendicitis-like syndrome should prompt a culture for *Yersinia enterocolitica* with cold enrichment. 6. Tenesmus (cramps in the rectum felt after a bowel movement) may be a feature of cases with inflammation of the rectum, as in shigellosis. 7. Vomiting implies an acute infection (e.g., a toxin-mediated illness or food poisoning) but can also be prominent in a variety of systemic illnesses (e.g., malaria) and in intestinal obstruction. 8. Asking patients whether anyone else they know is sick is a more efficient means of identifying a common source than is constructing a list of recently eaten foods. If a common source seems likely, specific foods can be investigated. See text for a discussion of bacterial food poisoning. 9. Stop antibiotic treatment if possible and consider culture for cytotoxigenic *Clostridium difficile*. Antibiotic use may increase the risk of other infections, such as salmonellosis. 10. See text for a discussion of traveler's diarrhea. (*After Guerrant and Guerrant and Bobak.*)

G. lamblia is more common among older children, with somewhat lower attack rates. Other common organisms, often spread by fecal-oral contact, are *Shigella, Campylobacter jejuni,* and *Cryptosporidium.* A characteristic feature of infection in day-care centers is the high rate of secondary cases among family members.

Similarly, hospitals are sites for concentrations of enteric infections. In medical intensive-care units and pediatric wards, diarrhea is among the most common nosocomial infections. *C. difficile* is the predominant cause of nosocomial diarrhea among adults in the United States; viral pathogens, especially rotavirus, can spread rapidly in pediatric wards. Enteropathogenic *E. coli* has been associated with outbreaks of diarrhea in nurseries for newborns. One-third of elderly patients in chronic-care institutions develop a significant diarrheal illness each year. Surveillance stool cultures suggest that 25% of the residents of these institutions harbor cytotoxin-producing *C. difficile,* which causes more than half of all cases of diarrhea in this population. Antimicrobial therapy can predispose to pseudomembranous colitis by altering the normal colonic flora and allowing the multiplication of *C. difficile.*

Age   Most of the morbidity and mortality from enteric pathogens involves children <5 years of age. Breast-fed infants are protected from contaminated food and water and derive some protection from maternal antibodies, but their risk of infection rises dramatically when they begin to eat solid foods. Infants and younger children are more likely than adults to develop rotaviral disease, while older children and adults are more commonly infected with Norwalk-like viruses. Other organisms with higher attack rates among children than among adults include enterotoxigenic, enteropathogenic, and enterohemorrhagic *E. coli; C. jejuni;* and *G. lamblia.* In children, the incidence of *Salmonella* infections is highest among infants <1 year of age, while the attack rate for *Shigella* infections is greatest among children aged 6 months to 4 years.

Bacterial Food Poisoning   If the history and the stool examination indicate a noninflammatory etiology of diarrhea and there is evidence of a common-source outbreak, questions concerning the ingestion of specific foods and the time of onset of the diarrhea after a meal can provide clues to the bacterial cause of the illness. Potential causes of bacterial food poisoning are shown in Table 131-2.

Bacterial disease caused by an enterotoxin elaborated outside the host, such as that due to *Staphylococcus aureus* or *B. cereus,* has the shortest incubation period (1 to 6 h) and generally lasts <12 h. Most cases of staphylococcal food poisoning are caused by contamination from infected human carriers. Staphylococci can multiply at a wide range of temperatures; thus, if food is left to cool slowly and remains at room temperature after cooking, the organisms will have the opportunity to form enterotoxin. Outbreaks following picnics where potato salad, mayonnaise, and cream pastries have been served offer classic examples of staphylococcal food poisoning. Diarrhea, nausea, vomiting, and abdominal cramping are common, while fever is less so.

B. cereus can produce either a syndrome with a short incubation period—the *emetic* form, mediated by a staphylococcal type of enterotoxin—or one with a longer incubation period (8 to 16 h)—the *diarrheal* form, caused by an enterotoxin resembling *E. coli* LT, in which diarrhea and abdominal cramps are characteristic but vomiting is uncommon. The emetic form of *B. cereus* food poisoning is associated with contaminated fried rice; the organism is common in uncooked rice, and its heat-resistant spores survive boiling. If cooked rice is not refrigerated, the spores can germinate and produce toxin. Frying before serving may not destroy the preformed, heat-stable toxin.

Food poisoning due to *C. perfringens* also has a slightly longer incubation period (8 to 14 h) and results from the survival of heat-resistant spores in inadequately cooked meat, poultry, or legumes. After ingestion, toxin is produced in the intestinal tract, causing moderately severe abdominal cramps and diarrhea; vomiting is rare, as is fever. The illness is self-limited, rarely lasting for more than 24 h.

Not all food poisoning has a bacterial cause. Diagnostic confusion

Table 131-2   Bacterial Food Poisoning

Incubation Period, Organisms	Symptoms	Common Food Sources
1 TO 6 H		
Staphylococcus aureus	Nausea, vomiting, diarrhea	Ham, poultry, potato or egg salad, mayonnaise, cream pastries
Bacillus cereus	Nausea, vomiting, diarrhea	Fried rice
8 TO 16 H		
Clostridium perfringens	Abdominal cramps, diarrhea (vomiting rare)	Beef, poultry, legumes, gravies
B. cereus	Abdominal cramps, diarrhea (vomiting rare)	Meats, vegetables, dried beans, cereals
>16 H		
Vibrio cholerae	Watery diarrhea	Shellfish
Enterotoxigenic *Escherichia coli*	Watery diarrhea	Salads, cheese, meats, water
Enterohemorrhagic *E. coli*	Bloody diarrhea	Ground beef, roast beef, salami, raw milk, raw vegetables, apple juice
Salmonella spp.	Inflammatory diarrhea	Beef, poultry, eggs, dairy products
Shigella spp.	Dysentery	Potato or egg salad, lettuce, raw vegetables
Vibrio parahaemolyticus	Dysentery	Mollusks, crustaceans

can result from diarrhea caused by nonbacterial agents of short-incubation food poisoning, including capsaicin, which is found in hot peppers, and a variety of toxins found in fish and shellfish (Chap. 397).

LABORATORY EVALUATION   Many cases of noninflammatory diarrhea are self-limited or can be treated empirically, and in these instances the clinician may not need to determine a specific etiology. Potentially pathogenic *E. coli* cannot be distinguished from normal fecal flora by routine culture. Special tests to detect LT and ST are not available in most clinical laboratories. In situations in which cholera is a concern, stool should be cultured on thiosulfate-citrate-bile salts-sucrose (TCBS) agar. A latex agglutination test has made the rapid detection of rotavirus in stool practical for many laboratories, while reverse transcriptase polymerase chain reaction and specific antigen enzyme immunoassays have been developed for the identification of Norwalk-like viruses. At least three stool specimens should be examined for *Giardia* cysts or stained for *Cryptosporidium* if the level of clinical suspicion regarding the involvement of these organisms is high.

All patients with fever and evidence of inflammatory disease acquired outside the hospital should have stool cultured for *Salmonella, Shigella,* and *Campylobacter. Salmonella* and *Shigella* can be selected on MacConkey's agar as non-lactose-fermenting (colorless) colonies or can be grown on *Salmonella-Shigella* agar or in selenite enrichment broth, both of which inhibit most organisms except these pathogens. Evaluation of nosocomial diarrhea should initially focus on *C. difficile;* stool culture for other pathogens in this setting has an extremely low yield and is not cost-effective. Pathogenic strains of *C. difficile* generally produce two toxins, A and B. Toxin B can be detected with a cytotoxin assay; if the toxin is present, a monolayer culture of fibroblasts will show cytopathic effects within 6 to 24 h. Rapid enzyme immunoassays and latex agglutination tests for both toxin A and toxin B have recently been developed (Chap. 145). Isolation of *C. jejuni* requires inoculation of fresh stool onto selective growth medium and incubation at 42°C in a microaerophilic atmosphere. In many laboratories in the United States, *E. coli* O157:H7 is among the most common pathogens isolated from visible bloody stools. Strains of this enterohemorrhagic serotype can be identified in specialized laboratories by serotyping but also can be identified presumptively as lactose-fermenting, indole-positive colonies of sorbitol nonfermenters (white colonies) on sorbitol MacConkey plates. Fresh stools should be examined for amebic cysts and trophozoites.

℞ **TREATMENT** In many cases, a specific diagnosis is not necessary or not available to guide treatment. The clinician can proceed with the information obtained from the history, stool examination, and evaluation of the severity of dehydration. Empirical regimens for the treatment of traveler's diarrhea are listed in Table 131-3.

The mainstay of treatment is adequate rehydration. The treatment of cholera and other dehydrating diarrheal diseases was revolutionized by the promotion of oral rehydration solutions, the efficacy of which depends on the fact that glucose-facilitated absorption of sodium and water in the small intestine remains intact in the presence of cholera toxin. The use of oral rehydration solutions has reduced mortality due to cholera from >50% (in untreated cases) to <1%. The World Health Organization recommends a solution containing 3.5 g sodium chloride, 2.5 g sodium bicarbonate, 1.5 g potassium chloride, and 20 g glucose (or 40 g sucrose) per liter of water. Patients who are severely dehydrated or in whom vomiting precludes the use of oral therapy should receive intravenous solutions such as Ringer's lactate.

Although most secretory forms of traveler's diarrhea—usually due to enterotoxigenic *E. coli*—can be treated effectively with rehydration, bismuth subsalicylate, or antiperistaltic agents, antimicrobial agents can shorten the duration of illness from between 3 and 4 days to between 24 and 36 h.

PROPHYLAXIS Improvements in hygiene to limit fecal-oral spread of enteric pathogens will be necessary if the prevalence of diarrheal diseases is to be significantly reduced in developing countries. Travelers can reduce their risk of diarrhea by eating only hot, freshly cooked food; by avoiding raw vegetables, salads, and unpeeled fruit; and by drinking only boiled or treated water and avoiding ice. In one cross-sectional epidemiologic survey, fewer than 3% of all European and North American travelers to Jamaica adhered to prescribed dietary restrictions, and travel health advice had no impact on the incidence of traveler's diarrhea; overall, the diarrhea attack rate among these travelers was 23.6%, with classic traveler's diarrhea in 11.7%.

Bismuth subsalicylate is an inexpensive agent for the prophylaxis of traveler's diarrhea; it is taken at a dosage of 2 tablets (525 mg) four times a day. Treatment appears to be effective and safe for up to 3 weeks. Prophylactic antimicrobial agents, although effective, are not generally recommended for the prevention of traveler's diarrhea, except when travelers are immunosuppressed or have other underlying illnesses that place them at high risk for morbidity from gastrointestinal infection. The risk of side effects and the possibility of developing an infection with a drug-resistant organism or with more harmful, invasive bacteria make it more reasonable to institute a short course of treatment once symptoms have developed.

The possibility of exerting a major impact on the worldwide morbidity and mortality associated with diarrheal diseases has led to intense efforts to develop effective vaccines against the common bacterial and viral enteric pathogens. Recent research has shown promising advances in the development of vaccines against rotavirus, *Shigella*, *V. cholerae*, *S. typhi*, and enterotoxigenic *E. coli*.

Table 131-3 Treatment of Traveler's Diarrhea on the Basis of Clinical Features

Clinical Syndrome	Suggested Therapy
Watery diarrhea (no blood in stool, no fever), 1 or 2 unformed stools per day without distressing enteric symptoms	Oral fluids (Pedialyte, Lytren, or flavored mineral water) and saltine crackers
Watery diarrhea (no blood in stool, no fever), 1 or 2 unformed stools per day with distressing enteric symptoms	Bismuth subsalicylate (for adults): 30 mL or 2 tablets (262 mg/tablet) every 30 min for 8 doses; or loperamide[a]: 4 mg initially followed by 2 mg after passage of each unformed stool, not to exceed 8 tablets (16 mg) per day (prescription dose) or 4 caplets (8 mg) per day (over-the-counter dose); drugs can be taken for 2 days
Watery diarrhea (no blood in stool, no distressing abdominal pain, no fever), >2 unformed stools per day	Antibacterial drug[b] plus (for adults) loperamide[a] (see dose above)
Dysentery (passage of bloody stools) or fever (>37.8°C)	Antibacterial drug[b]
Vomiting, minimal diarrhea	Bismuth subsalicylate (for adults; see dose above)
Diarrhea in infants (<2 y old)	Fluids and electrolytes (Pedialyte, Lytren); continue feeding, especially with breast milk; seek medical attention for moderate dehydration, fever lasting >24 h, bloody stools, or diarrhea lasting more than several days
Diarrhea in pregnant women	Fluids and electrolytes; can consider attapulgite, 3 g initially, with dose repeated after passage of each unformed stool or every 2 h (whichever is earlier), for a total dosage of 9 g/d; seek medical attention for persistent or severe symptoms
Diarrhea despite trimethoprim-sulfamethoxazole prophylaxis	Fluoroquinolone—with loperamide[a] (see dose above) if no fever and no blood in stool, alone in cases of fever/dysentery
Diarrhea despite fluoroquinolone prophylaxis	Bismuth subsalicylate (see dose above) for mild to moderate disease; consult physician for moderate to severe disease or if disease persists

[a] Loperamide should not be used by patients with fever or dysentery; its use may prolong diarrhea in patients with infection due to *Shigella* or other invasive organisms.
[b] The recommended antibacterial drugs are as follows:
Travel to Mexican interior, summer: *Adults:* Trimethoprim-sulfamethoxazole (TMP-SMZ), 160 mg/800 mg bid for 3 days
Children: TMP-SMZ, 4/20 mg/kg per day, given bid for 3 days
Travel to other areas in other seasons: *Adults:* A quinolone, such as norfloxacin, 400 mg bid; ciprofloxacin, 500 mg bid; ofloxacin, 400 mg bid; or levofloxacin, 500 mg/d, for 3 days

Children: TMP-SMZ (above dose) plus erythromycin at dose based on weight (<11 kg, 250 mg/d; 11–18 kg, 375 mg/d; 18.5–25 kg, 500 mg/d; 25.5–36 kg, 750 mg/d; and >36 kg, 1000 mg/d) in four divided doses for 5 days. Alternative single agents: azithromycin, 10 mg/kg per day for 3 days; or furazolidone, 7.5 mg/kg per day in four divided doses for 5 days
All patients should take oral fluids (Pedialyte, Lytren, or flavored mineral water) plus saltine crackers. If diarrhea becomes moderate or severe, if fever persists, or if bloody stools or dehydration develops, the patient should seek medical attention.
SOURCE: After Dupont.

BIBLIOGRAPHY

BLASER MJ: Epidemiologic and clinical features of *Campylobacter jejuni* infections. J Infect Dis 176(Suppl 2):S103, 1997

DUPONT HL: Travelers' diarrhea, in *Infections of the Gastrointestinal Tract*, MJ Blaser et al (eds). New York, Raven, 1995, chap 22

GLYNN KM et al: Emergence of multidrug-resistant *Salmonella enterica* serotype typhimurium DT104 infections in the United States. N Engl J Med 338:1333, 1998

GUERRANT RL: Principles and syndromes of enteric infection, in *Mandell, Douglas and Bennett's Principles and Practice of Infectious Diseases*, 4th ed, GL Mandell et al (eds). New York, Churchill Livingstone, 1995, chap 75

———, BOBAK DA: Bacterial and protozoal gastroenteritis. N Engl J Med 325:327, 1991

MEAD PS, GRIFFIN PM: *Escherichia coli* O157:H7. Lancet 352:1207, 1998

PASSARO DJ, PARSONNET J: Advances in the prevention and management of traveler's diarrhea. Curr Clin Top Infect Dis 18:217, 1998

SLUTSKER L et al: A nationwide case-control study of *Escherichia coli* O157:H7 infection in the United States. J Infect Dis 177:962, 1998

STEFFEN R et al: Epidemiology, etiology, and impact of traveler's diarrhea in Jamaica. JAMA 281:811, 1999

TAUXE RV, HUGHES JM: Food-borne disease, in *Mandell, Douglas and Bennett's Principles and Practice of Infectious Diseases*, 4th ed, GL Mandell et al (eds). New York, Churchill Livingstone, 1995, chap 81

132 King K. Holmes

SEXUALLY TRANSMITTED DISEASES: OVERVIEW AND CLINICAL APPROACH

HBV	hepatitis B virus	PCR	polymerase chain reaction
HPV	human papillomavirus	PID	pelvic inflammatory disease
HSV	herpes simplex virus	STDs	sexually transmitted diseases
LGV	lymphogranuloma venereum	STI	sexually transmitted infection
MPC	mucopurulent cervicitis	UTI	urinary tract infection
NGU	nongonococcal urethritis		

In all societies, sexually transmitted diseases (STDs) rank among the most common of all infectious diseases, with over 30 infections now classified as predominantly sexually transmitted or as frequently sexually transmissible (Table 132-1). The many new sexually transmitted pathogens recognized and characterized since 1980 include HIV types 1 and 2, human T cell lymphotropic virus (HTLV) types I and II, many genital types of human papillomavirus (HPV), *Mycoplasma genitalium*, two species of *Mobiluncus* (associated with bacterial vaginosis), two species of *Helicobacter* (initially associated with proctocolitis in homosexual men and later, during the AIDS era, with bacteremia, dermatitis, and fever among immunosuppressed individuals), and the Kaposi's sarcoma–associated herpesvirus (human herpesvirus type 8, or HHV-8).

In developing countries, with three-quarters of the world's population and 90% of the world's STDs, such factors as population growth (especially in adolescent and young-adult age groups), rural-to-urban migration, wars, and poverty create exceptional vulnerability to disease resulting from risky sexual behaviors. This situation leads to the spread of STD, with the emergence of new pathogens and new variants of old pathogens. During the 1990s, in China, Russia, the states of the former Soviet Union, and South Africa, internal social structures changed rapidly as borders opened to the West, unleashing enormous new epidemics of HIV infection and other STDs. HIV has become the leading cause of death in some developing countries, and HPV and hepatitis B virus (HBV) remain important causes of cervical and hepatocellular carcinoma, respectively—two of the commonest malignancies in the developing world. Sexually transmitted herpes simplex virus (HSV) infections now cause most genital ulcer disease throughout the world and an increasing proportion of cases of genital herpes in developing countries with generalized HIV epidemics, where the positive feedback loop between HSV and HIV transmission is a growing, intractable problem. Globally, the agents of curable STDs—gonorrhea, chlamydial infections, syphilis, chancroid, and trichomoniasis—caused ~350 million new infections annually in the mid-1990s. Bacterial vaginosis (arguably acquired sexually) occurs in up to 50% of women of reproductive age in developing countries. Thus, there are probably close to 1 billion cases of these curable infections annually, all six of which are associated with increased risk of HIV transmission or acquisition.

In the industrialized countries, fear of HIV infection since the mid-1980s, coupled with widespread behavioral interventions and better-organized systems of care for the curable STDs, have helped curb the transmission of the latter diseases. Nonetheless, viral STDs, such as genital herpes and HPV infection, had not obviously decreased in incidence at the turn of the millennium, and infection with HIV remains a leading cause of death in persons 25 to 44 years of age in the United States, as in developing countries, despite the advent of potent antiretroviral therapy.

Although rates of the bacterial STDs have fallen in all industrialized countries over the past 20 years, foci of hyperendemic transmission persist in the southeastern United States and in most large U.S. cities. Rates of gonorrhea and syphilis remain higher in the United States than in any other Western industrialized country. The reemergence of syphilis and gonorrhea epidemics in Russia and the former Soviet states has created similar foci for reintroduction of these STDs into western Europe. The remarkable return of high rates of gonorrhea and syphilis among homosexual and bisexual men in many parts of the United States reflects increased risk-taking since the advent of potent antiretroviral therapy and may portend resurgent transmission of HIV in this group.

CLASSIFICATION AND EPIDEMIOLOGY

Sexually transmitted infection (STI) may or may not result in disease (STD). Some prefer the term *reproductive tract infection* to destigmatize the diagnosis and treatment of STIs and to encompass conditions such as bacterial vaginosis, whose designation as an STD is debated.

Certain STDs (such as syphilis, gonorrhea, HIV infection, hepatitis B, and chancroid) are most concentrated within "core populations" having high rates of partner change, concurrent partners, or "dense" sexual networks—for example, prostitutes and their clients and persons involved in the use of illicit drugs, particularly crack cocaine. Poor access to or low motivation for obtaining early treatment also fosters spread of the curable STIs. In most of the United States, groups most vulnerable to STDs, including HIV infection, consist predominantly of young unmarried individuals of low socioeconomic status who often reside within crowded urban neighborhoods, although some rural areas (e.g., in the southeastern United States) also have high rates of STIs. Other STDs are distributed more evenly in society. For example, chlamydial infections can persist for many months, often asymptomatically, and can propagate widely in populations that do not share all of the characteristics of core groups described above. Similarly, genital HPV infections and genital herpes persist and spread efficiently in relatively low-risk populations.

In general, the product of three factors determines the initial rate of spread of any STI within a population: rate of exposure, efficiency of transmission per exposure, and duration of infectivity of those infected. Efforts to prevent and control STIs attempt to decrease the duration of infectivity (through early diagnosis and curative or suppressive treatment), to decrease the efficiency of transmission (e.g., through promotion of condom use and safer sexual practices), and to decrease the rate of exposure of susceptibles to infected persons (e.g., through provision of information, health education, and counseling and efforts to change the norms of sexual behavior).

Table 132-1   Sexually Transmitted and Sexually Transmissible Microorganisms

Bacteria	Viruses	Other[a]
TRANSMITTED IN ADULTS PREDOMINANTLY BY SEXUAL INTERCOURSE		
Neisseria gonorrhoeae	HIV (types 1 and 2)	Trichomonas vaginalis
Chlamydia trachomatis	Human T cell lymphotropic virus	Phthirus pubis
Treponema pallidum	type I	
Haemophilus ducreyi	Herpes simplex virus type 2	
Calymmatobacterium granulomatis	Human papillomavirus (multiple	
Ureaplasma urealyticum	genotypes)	
	Hepatitis B virus[b]	
	Molluscum contagiosum virus	
SEXUAL TRANSMISSION REPEATEDLY DESCRIBED BUT NOT WELL DEFINED OR NOT THE PREDOMINANT MODE		
Mycoplasma hominis	Cytomegalovirus	Candida albicans
Mycoplasma genitalium	Human T cell lymphotropic virus	Sarcoptes scabiei
Gardnerella vaginalis and other	type II	
vaginal bacteria	(?) Hepatitis C, D viruses	
Group B Streptococcus	Herpes simplex virus type 1	
Mobiluncus spp.	(?) Epstein-Barr virus	
Helicobacter cinaedi	Kaposi's sarcoma–associated	
Helicobacter fennelliae	herpesvirus[c]	
	Transfusion-transmitted virus	
TRANSMITTED BY SEXUAL CONTACT INVOLVING ORAL-FECAL EXPOSURE; OF DECLINING IMPORTANCE IN HOMOSEXUAL MEN		
Shigella spp.	Hepatitis A virus	Giardia lamblia
Campylobacter spp.		Entamoeba histolytica

[a] Includes protozoa, ectoparasites, and fungi.
[b] Among U.S. patients for whom a risk factor can be ascertained, most hepatitis B virus infections are transmitted sexually or by injection drug use.
[c] Human herpesvirus type 8.

MANAGEMENT OF COMMON STD SYNDROMES

Although other chapters discuss management of specific STIs, delineating treatment based on diagnosis of a specific infection, most patients are actually managed (at least initially) on the basis of presenting symptoms and signs and associated risk factors, even in industrialized countries. Table 132-2 lists some of the most common clinical STD syndromes and their microbial etiologies. Strategies for their management are outlined below. Chaps. 191 and 309 address the management of infections with human retroviruses.

RISK ASSESSMENT   Routine patient care begins with risk assessment (e.g., for heart disease, cancer). An overall risk assessment interview should include STD/HIV in primary care, urgent care, and emergency care settings as well as in specialty clinics providing adolescent, prenatal, and family planning services. STD/HIV risk assessment guides interpretation of symptoms that could reflect an STD; decisions on screening or prophylactic/preventive treatment; risk reduction counseling and intervention (e.g., hepatitis B vaccination); and notification of partners of patients with known infections. Consideration of routine demographic data (e.g., gender, age, marital status, area of residence) is a simple first step in STD/HIV risk assessment. For example, national guidelines recommend routine screening of sexually active females ≤25 years of age for C. trachomatis infection. Table 132-3 provides a set of 10 STD/HIV risk assessment questions that clinicians can pose verbally or that health care systems can adapt (with yes/no responses) into a routine self-administered questionnaire for use in clinics. The initial framing statement gives permission to discuss taboo topics.

Risk assessment is followed by clinical assessment (elicitation of information on specific current symptoms and signs of STDs). Confirmatory diagnostic tests (for those with symptoms or signs) or screening tests (for those without symptoms or signs) may involve microscopic examination, culture, antigen detection tests, genetic probe or amplification tests, or serology. Initial syndrome-based treatment should cover the most likely causes. For certain syndromes, results of rapid tests can narrow the spectrum of this initial therapy (e.g., wet mount of vaginal fluid for women with vaginal discharge, Gram's stain of urethral discharge for men with urethral discharge, rapid plasma reagin test for genital ulcer). After the institution of treatment, STD management proceeds to the "4 C's" of prevention and control: contact tracing (see "Prevention and Control of STDs," below), ensuring compliance with therapy, and counseling on risk reduction, including condom promotion and provision.

URETHRITIS IN MEN   The incidence of reported gonococcal urethritis in the United States has fallen to the lowest level since reporting began, while that of nongonococcal urethritis (NGU) remains high—a pattern typical of all industrialized countries. Until recently, Chlamydia trachomatis caused ~30 to 40% of NGU cases, but the proportion of cases due to this organism may have declined in some populations served by effective chlamydial control programs. HSV and Trichomonas vaginalis each cause a small proportion of NGU cases in the United States. Case-control studies have also implicated Ureaplasma urealyticum and M. genitalium as probable causes of many Chlamydia-negative cases, and coliform bacteria can cause urethritis in men who practice insertive anal intercourse. The initial diagnosis of urethritis in men currently includes specific tests only for Neisseria gonorrhoeae and C. trachomatis. Table 132-4 summarizes the steps in management of sexually active men with symptoms of urethral discharge and/or dysuria.

1. *Establish the presence of urethritis.* If proximal-to-distal "milking" of the urethra does not express a purulent or mucopurulent discharge, even after the patient has not voided for several hours or preferably overnight, the centrifuged sediment of the first 20 to 30 mL of voided urine can be examined for inflammatory cells, either by microscopy or by the leukocyte esterase test. In urethral gonococcal or chlamydial infection, a Gram's-stained smear of overt discharge or of an anterior urethral specimen obtained by passage of a small urethrogenital swab 2 to 3 cm into the urethra usually reveals ≥5 neutrophils per 1000× field in areas containing cells; in gonococcal infection, such a smear also usually reveals gram-negative intracellular diplococci. Patients with symptoms who lack objective evidence of urethritis may have functional rather than organic problems and generally do not benefit from repeated courses of antibiotics.

2. *Evaluate for complications or alternative diagnoses.* A brief history and examination will exclude epididymitis and systemic complications, such as disseminated gonococcal infection and Reiter's syndrome. Although digital examination of the prostate gland seldom contributes to the evaluation of sexually active young men with urethritis, men with dysuria who lack evidence of urethritis as well as sexually inactive men with urethritis should undergo prostate palpation, urinalysis, and urine culture to exclude bacterial prostatitis and cystitis.

3. *Evaluate for gonococcal and chlamydial infection.* An absence of typical gram-negative diplococci on Gram's-stained smear of urethral exudate containing inflammatory cells warrants a preliminary diagnosis of NGU and should lead to testing of the urethral specimen for C. trachomatis. Culture or DNA detection tests for N. gonorrhoeae may be positive when Gram's staining is negative; certain strains of N. gonorrhoeae reportedly can result in negative urethral Gram's stains in up to 30% of cases of urethritis. Results of tests for gonococcal and chlamydial infection predict the patient's prognosis (with greater risk for recurrent NGU if neither

Table 132-2   Major STD Syndromes and Sexually Transmitted (ST) Microbial Etiologies

Syndrome	ST Microbial Etiologies
AIDS	HIV types 1 and 2
Urethritis: males	*Neisseria gonorrhoeae, Chlamydia trachomatis, Ureaplasma urealyticum, Trichomonas vaginalis,* HSV
Epididymitis	*C. trachomatis, N. gonorrhoeae*
Lower genital tract infections: females	
Cystitis/urethritis	*C. trachomatis, N. gonorrhoeae,* HSV
Mucopurulent cervicitis	*C. trachomatis, N. gonorrhoeae*
Vulvitis	*Candida albicans,* HSV
Vulvovaginitis	*C. albicans, T. vaginalis*
Bacterial vaginosis (BV)	BV-associated bacteria (see text)
Acute pelvic inflammatory disease	*N. gonorrhoeae, C. trachomatis,* BV-associated bacteria, group B streptococci
Infertility	*N. gonorrhoeae, C. trachomatis,* BV-associated bacteria
Ulcerative lesions of the genitalia	HSV-1, HSV-2, *Treponema pallidum, Haemophilus ducreyi, C. trachomatis* (LGV strains), *Calymmatobacterium granulomatis*
Complications of pregnancy/puerperium	Several agents implicated
Intestinal infections	
Proctitis	*C. trachomatis, N. gonorrhoeae,* HSV, *T. pallidum*
Proctocolitis or enterocolitis	*Campylobacter* spp., *Shigella* spp., *Entamoeba histolytica,* other enteric pathogens
Enteritis	*Giardia lamblia*
Acute arthritis with urogenital infection or viremia	*N. gonorrhoeae* (e.g., DGI), *C. trachomatis* (e.g., Reiter's syndrome), HBV
Genital and anal warts	HPV (30 genital types)
Mononucleosis syndrome	CMV, HIV, EBV
Hepatitis	Hepatitis viruses, *T. pallidum* , CMV, EBV
Neoplasias	
Squamous cell dysplasias and cancers of the cervix, anus, vulva, vagina, or penis	HPV (especially types 16, 18, 31, 45)
Kaposi's sarcoma, body-cavity lymphomas	HHV-8
T cell leukemia	HTLV-I
Hepatocellular carcinoma	HBV
Tropical spastic paraparesis	HTLV-I
Scabies	*Sarcoptes scabiei*
Pubic lice	*Phthirus pubis*

NOTE: HSV, herpes simplex virus; LGV, lymphogranuloma venereum; DGI, disseminated gonococcal infection; HPV, human papillomavirus; CMV, cytomegalovirus; EBV, Epstein-Barr virus; HBV, hepatitis B virus; HTLV, human T cell lymphotropic virus; HHV-8, human herpesvirus type 8.

chlamydiae nor gonococci are found than if either is detected) and can guide both the counseling given to the patient and the management of the patient's sexual partner(s).

4. *Treat urethritis.*

℞ **TREATMENT**   In practice, if Gram's stain does not reveal gonococci, urethritis is treated with a regimen effective for NGU, such as azithromycin (1.0 g orally in a single dose). If gonococci are demonstrated by Gram's stain or if no diagnostic tests are performed to definitively exclude gonorrhea, treatment should also include a single-dose regimen for gonorrhea (Chap. 147). Sexual partners should be tested for gonorrhea and chlamydial infection and should receive the same regimen given to the male index case.

EPIDIDYMITIS   Acute epididymitis, almost always unilateral, must be differentiated from testicular torsion, tumor, and trauma. Torsion, a surgical emergency, usually occurs in the second or third decade of life and produces a sudden onset of pain, elevation of the testicle

Table 132-3   Ten-Question STD/HIV Risk Assessment

Framing Statement:
In order to provide the best care for you today and to understand your risk for certain infections, it is necessary for us to talk about your sexual behavior.
Screening Questions:
1) Do you have any reason to think you might have an STD? If so, what reason?
2) For all adolescents <18 years old: Have you begun having any kind of sex yet?
STD History:
3) Have you ever had any sexually transmitted diseases or any genital infections? If so, which ones?
Sexual Preference:
4) Have you had sex with men, women, or both?
Injection Drug Use:
5) Have you ever injected yourself ("shot up") with drugs? (If yes, have you ever shared needles or injection equipment?)
6) Have you ever had sex with a gay or bisexual man or with anyone who had ever injected drugs?
Characteristics of Partner(s):
7) Has your sex partner(s) had any sexually transmitted infections? If so, which ones?
STD Symptoms Checklist:
8) Have you recently developed any of these symptoms?

For Men	For Women
a) Discharge of pus (drip) from the penis	a) Abnormal vaginal discharge (increased amount, abnormal odor, abnormal yellow color)
b) Genital sores (ulcers) or rash	b) Genital sores (ulcers), rash, or itching

Sexual Practices, Past 2 Months (for patients answering yes to any of the above questions, to guide examination and testing):
9) Now I'd like to ask what parts of your body may have been sexually exposed to an STD (e.g., your penis, mouth, vagina, anus)?
Query about Interest in STD Screening Tests (for patients answering no to all of the above questions):
10) Would you like to be tested for HIV or any other STDs today? (If yes, clinician can explore which STD and why.)

SOURCE: Adapted from JR Curtis and KK Holmes. Individual-level risk assessment for STD/HIV infections. In KK Holmes et al (eds): *Sexually Transmitted Diseases,* 3rd ed. New York, McGraw-Hill, 1999, pp 669–683.

within the scrotal sac, rotation of the epididymis from a posterior to an anterior position, and absence of blood flow on Doppler examination or ^{99m}Tc scan. Persistence of symptoms after a course of therapy for epididymitis suggests the possibility of testicular tumor. In sexually active men under age 35, acute epididymitis is caused most frequently by *C. trachomatis* and less commonly by *N. gonorrhoeae* and is usually associated with overt or subclinical urethritis. Acute epididymitis in older men or following urinary tract instrumentation is usually caused by urinary pathogens. Similarly, epididymitis in men who have practiced insertive rectal intercourse is often caused by Enterobacteriaceae. These men usually have no urethritis but do have bacteriuria.

℞ **TREATMENT**   Ofloxacin (300 mg orally bid for 10 days) is an optimal agent for syndrome-based treatment of epididymitis because of its effectiveness against *N. gonorrhoeae, C. trachomatis,* and Enterobacteriaceae. Alternatively, ceftriaxone (250 mg intramuscularly) followed by doxycycline (100 mg orally bid for 10 days) is effective for epididymitis caused by *N. gonorrhoeae* or *C. trachomatis.*

URETHRITIS AND THE URETHRAL SYNDROME IN WOMEN   *C. trachomatis, N. gonorrhoeae,* and occasionally HSV cause symptomatic urethritis—known as the urethral syndrome in women—characterized by "internal" dysuria (usually without urinary urgency or frequency) and pyuria, with *Escherichia coli* or other uropathogens not present in urine at counts of $\geq 10^2$/mL. In contrast, the

Table 132-4   Management of Urethral Discharge in Men

Usual causes	Usual initial evaluation
Chlamydia trachomatis	Demonstration of urethral discharge or
Neisseria gonorrhoeae	pyuria
Ureaplasma urealyticum	Exclusion of local or systemic complications
Trichomonas vaginalis	Urethral Gram's stain to confirm urethritis,
Herpes simplex virus	detect gram-negative diplococci
Mycoplasma genitalium	Test for *N. gonorrhoeae*, *C. trachomatis*

INITIAL TREATMENT FOR PATIENT AND PARTNERS

Treat gonorrhea (unless excluded):	plus	Treat chlamydial infection:
Cefixime, 400 mg PO; *or* Ceftriaxone, 125 mg IM; *or* Fluoroquinolone (e.g., cipro-floxacin, 500 mg PO)		Azithromycin, 1 g PO; *or* Doxycycline, 100 mg bid for 7 days

MANAGEMENT OF RECURRENCE

Confirm objective evidence of urethritis. If patient was reexposed to untreated or new partner, repeat treatment of patient and partner.

If patient was not reexposed, consider infection with *T. vaginalis*[a] or doxycycline-resistant *Ureaplasma*, and consider treatment with metronidazole or azithromycin.

[a] In men, the diagnosis of *T. vaginalis* infection requires culture of early-morning first-voided urine sediment or of a urethral swab specimen obtained before voiding.

dysuria associated with vulvar herpes or vulvovaginal candidiasis (and perhaps with trichomoniasis) is often described as "external," being caused by painful contact of urine with the inflamed or ulcerated labia or introitus. Acute onset, association with urinary urgency or frequency, hematuria, or suprapubic bladder tenderness suggests bacterial cystitis. Among women with symptoms of acute bacterial cystitis, costovertebral pain and tenderness or fever suggests acute pyelonephritis. The management of bacterial urinary tract infection (UTI) is discussed in Chap. 280.

Signs of vulvovaginitis, coupled with symptoms of external dysuria, suggest vulvar infection (e.g., with HSV or *Candida albicans*). Among dysuric women without signs of vulvovaginitis, bacterial UTI must be differentiated from the urethral syndrome by assessment of risk, evaluation of the pattern of symptoms and signs, and specific microbiologic testing. An STD etiology of the urethral syndrome is suggested by young age, more than one current sexual partner or a new partner within the past month, or coexisting mucopurulent cervicitis (MPC; see below). The finding of a single urinary pathogen, such as *E. coli* or *Staphylococcus saprophyticus*, at a concentration of $\geq 10^2$/mL in a properly collected specimen of midstream urine from a dysuric woman with pyuria indicates probable bacterial UTI, whereas pyuria with $< 10^2$ conventional uropathogens per milliliter of urine ("sterile" pyuria) suggests acute urethral syndrome due to *C. trachomatis* or *N. gonorrhoeae*. Gonorrhea and chlamydial infection should be sought by specific tests. Among women with sterile pyuria caused by chlamydial infection, treatment with doxycycline (100 mg bid for 7 days) alleviates dysuria.

VULVOVAGINAL INFECTIONS   Abnormal Vaginal Discharge   If directly questioned during routine health checkups, many women acknowledge having nonspecific symptoms of vaginal discharge that do not correlate with objective signs of inflammation or with actual infection. However, unsolicited reporting of abnormal vaginal discharge does suggest bacterial vaginosis or trichomoniasis. Specifically, an abnormally increased amount, an abnormal odor, and an abnormal yellow color of the discharge are associated with one or both of these conditions. Cervical infection with *N. gonorrhoeae* or *C. trachomatis* does not appear to cause an increased amount or abnormal odor of discharge, but cervicitis, like trichomoniasis, can include the production of an increased number of neutrophils in vaginal fluid, resulting in a yellow color. Vulvar conditions such as genital herpes or vulvovaginal candidiasis can cause vulvar pruritus, burning,

irritation, or lesions as well as external dysuria (as urine passes over the inflamed vulva) or vulvar dyspareunia.

Certain vulvovaginal infections may have serious sequelae. Trichomoniasis, bacterial vaginosis, and vulvovaginal candidiasis have all been associated with increased risk of acquisition of HIV infection. Vaginal trichomoniasis and bacterial vaginosis early in pregnancy independently predict premature onset of labor. Bacterial vaginosis can also lead to anaerobic bacterial infection of the endometrium and salpinges. Vaginitis may be an early and prominent feature of toxic shock syndrome, and recurrent or chronic vulvovaginal candidiasis develops with increased frequency among women with systemic illnesses, such as diabetes mellitus or HIV-related immunosuppression (although only a very small proportion of women with recurrent vulvovaginal candidiasis in the United States actually have a serious predisposing illness).

Thus vulvovaginal symptoms or signs warrant careful evaluation, including pelvic examination, simple rapid diagnostic tests, and appropriate therapy specific for the anatomic site and type of infection. Unfortunately, a recent survey in the United States indicated that clinicians seldom perform the tests required to establish the cause of such symptoms. The diagnosis and treatment of the three most common types of vaginal infection are summarized in Table 132-5.

Inspection of the vulva and perineum may reveal tender genital ulcerations (typically due to HSV infection, occasionally to chancroid) or fissures (typically due to vulvovaginal candidiasis) or discharge visible at the introitus before insertion of a speculum (suggestive of bacterial vaginosis or trichomoniasis). Speculum examination permits the clinician to discern whether the discharge in fact looks abnormal and whether any abnormal discharge in the vagina emanates from the cervical os (mucoid and, if abnormal, yellow) or from the vagina (not mucoid, since the vaginal epithelium does not produce mucus). Symptoms or signs of abnormal vaginal discharge should prompt testing of vaginal fluid for pH, odor when mixed with 10% KOH, and microscopic features when mixed with saline and with 10% KOH. Additional objective laboratory tests useful for establishing the cause of abnormal vaginal discharge include Gram's staining to detect alterations in the vaginal flora; new card and dipstick tests for bacterial vaginosis, as described below; and a new DNA probe test purported to detect *T. vaginalis* and *C. albicans* as well as the increased concentrations of *Gardnerella vaginalis* associated with bacterial vaginosis.

℞ **TREATMENT**   Patterns of treatment for vaginal discharge vary widely. In developing countries, where clinics or pharmacies often dispense treatment based on symptoms alone without examination or testing, oral treatment with metronidazole, either as a 2-g single dose or as a 7-day regimen, provides reasonable coverage against both trichomoniasis and bacterial vaginosis, the usual causes of symptoms of vaginal discharge; metronidazole treatment of sex partners would prevent reinfection of women with trichomoniasis even if it does not help prevent the recurrence of bacterial vaginosis. Guidelines promulgated during the 1990s by the World Health Organization suggested treatment for cervical infection and for vulvovaginal candidiasis in women with symptoms of abnormal vaginal discharge; in retrospect, these recommendations were faulty, since these conditions seldom produce such symptoms.

In industrialized countries, clinicians treating symptoms and signs of abnormal vaginal discharge should at least differentiate between bacterial vaginosis and trichomoniasis, because optimal management of patients and partners differs for these two conditions, as discussed briefly below.

Vaginal Trichomoniasis (See also Chap. 218)   Symptomatic trichomoniasis characteristically produces a profuse, yellow, purulent, homogeneous vaginal discharge and vulvar irritation, often with visible inflammation of the vaginal and vulvar epithelium and petechial lesions on the cervix (the so-called strawberry cervix, usually evident only by colposcopy). The pH of vaginal fluid usually rises to ≥ 5.0. In women with typical symptoms and signs of trichomoniasis, micro-

Table 132-5 Diagnostic Features and Management of Vaginal Infection

Feature	Normal Vaginal Examination	Vulvovaginal Candidiasis	Trichomonal Vaginitis	Bacterial Vaginosis
Etiology	Uninfected; lactobacilli predominant	*Candida albicans*	*Trichomonas vaginalis*	Associated with *Gardnerella vaginalis*, various anaerobic bacteria, and mycoplasmas
Typical symptoms	None	Vulvar itching and/or irritation	Profuse purulent discharge; vulvar itching	Malodorous, slightly increased discharge
Discharge				
Amount	Variable; usually scant	Scant	Profuse	Moderate
Color[a]	Clear or white	White	Yellow	White or gray
Consistency	Nonhomogeneous, floccular	Clumped; adherent plaques	Homogeneous	Homogeneous, low viscosity; uniformly coats vaginal walls
Inflammation of vulvar or vaginal epithelium	None	Erythema of vaginal epithelium, introitus; vulvar dermatitis common	Erythema of vaginal and vulvar epithelium; colpitis macularis	None
pH of vaginal fluid[b]	Usually ≤4.5	Usually ≤4.5	Usually ≥5.0	Usually >4.5
Amine ("fishy") odor with 10% KOH	None	None	May be present	Present
Microscopy[c]	Normal epithelial cells; lactobacilli predominant	Leukocytes, epithelial cells; mycelia or pseudomycelia in up to 80% of *C. albicans* culture-positive persons with typical symptoms	Leukocytes; motile trichomonads seen in 80 to 90% of symptomatic patients, less often in the absence of symptoms	Clue cells; few leukocytes; no lactobacilli or only a few outnumbered by profuse mixed flora, nearly always including *G. vaginalis* plus anaerobic species on Gram's stain
Usual treatment	None	Azole cream, tablet, or suppository—e.g., miconazole 100-mg vaginal suppository or clotrimazole 100-mg vaginal tablet, once daily for 7 days. Fluconazole, 150 mg orally (single dose)	Metronidazole, 2 g orally (single dose) Metronidazole, 500 mg PO bid for 7 days	Metronidazole, 500 mg PO bid for 7 days Clindamycin, 2% cream, one full applicator vaginally each night for 7 days Metronidazole gel, 0.75%, one full applicator vaginally twice daily for 5 days Metronidazole, 2 g PO (single dose)[d]
Usual management of sexual partner	None	None; topical treatment if candidal dermatitis of penis is detected	Examination for STD; treatment with metronidazole, 2 g PO (single dose)	Examination for STD; no treatment if normal

[a] Color of discharge is best determined by examination against the white background of a swab.

[b] pH determination is not useful if blood is present.

[c] To detect fungal elements, vaginal fluid is digested with 10% KOH prior to microscopic examination; to examine for other features, fluid is mixed (1:1) with physiologic saline.

Gram's stain is also excellent for detecting yeasts and pseudomycelia and for distinguishing normal flora from the mixed flora seen in bacterial vaginosis, but it is less sensitive than the saline preparation for detection of *T. vaginalis*.

[d] Single-dose regimen is less effective than 7-day metronidazole regimen.

scopic examination of vaginal discharge mixed with saline reveals motile trichomonads in at least 80% of culture-positive cases. However, in the absence of symptoms or signs, culture is often required for detection of the organism. Treatment of asymptomatic as well as symptomatic cases reduces rates of transmission and prevents later development of symptoms.

R꜀ TREATMENT Only nitroimidazoles consistently cure trichomoniasis. Tinidazole and ornidazole have longer half-lives than metronidazole but do not give better results than a single 2-g oral dose of metronidazole, the treatment of choice. Treatment of male sexual partners—often facilitated by dispensing metronidazole to the female patient to give to her partner(s), with a warning about avoiding the concurrent use of alcohol—reduces both the risk of reinfection and the reservoir of infection. Treatment with 0.75% metronidazole gel intravaginally, although effective for bacterial vaginosis, is not reliable for vaginal trichomoniasis. Systemic use of metronidazole is not recommended during the first trimester of pregnancy but is considered safe thereafter.

Bacterial Vaginosis This syndrome (formerly termed *nonspecific vaginitis, Haemophilus vaginitis, anaerobic vaginitis,* or *Gardnerella-associated vaginal discharge*) is characterized by symptoms of vaginal malodor and a slightly to moderately increased white discharge, which appears homogeneous, is low in viscosity, and smoothly coats the vaginal mucosa. Risk factors include multiple sexual partners and recent intercourse with a new partner, but antibiotic treatment of male partners has not reduced the rate of recurrence among affected women.

The vaginal fluid of women with bacterial vaginosis is characterized by markedly increased prevalences and concentrations of *G. vaginalis, Mycoplasma hominis,* and several anaerobic bacteria [e.g., *Mobiluncus* spp., *Prevotella* spp. (formerly *Bacteroides* spp.), and some *Peptostreptococcus* spp.]. The vaginal fluid usually lacks hydrogen peroxide–producing *Lactobacillus* spp., which constitute most of the normal vaginal flora and perhaps help protect against certain cervical and vaginal infections. Vaginal douching, use of intravaginal nonoxynol-9 spermicide, and new sexual partners can all result in loss of vaginal colonization by hydrogen peroxide–producing lactobacilli.

Bacterial vaginosis is conventionally diagnosed clinically with the *Amsel criteria,* which include any three of the following four clinical abnormalities: (1) objective signs of increased white homogeneous vaginal discharge; (2) a vaginal discharge pH of >4.5; (3) liberation of a distinct fishy odor (attributable to volatile amines such as trimethylamine) immediately after vaginal secretions are mixed with a 10% solution of KOH; and (4) microscopic demonstration of "clue cells" (vaginal epithelial cells coated with coccobacillary organisms giving them a granular appearance and indistinct borders; Fig. 132-1) on a wet mount prepared by mixing vaginal secretions with normal

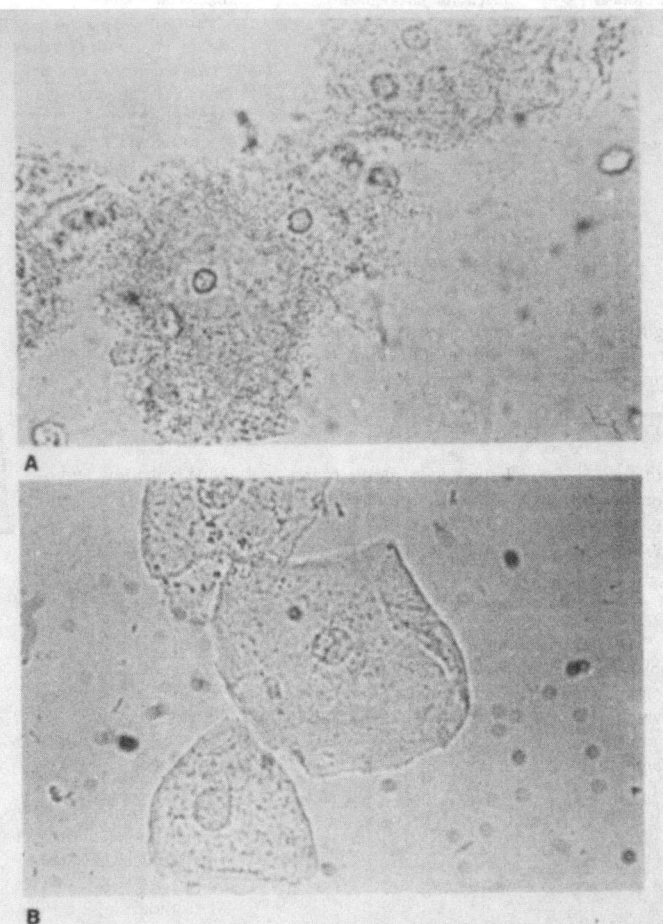

FIGURE 132-1 *A*. Vaginal epithelial "clue cells." Note granular appearance due to adherent *G. vaginalis* and indistinct cell margins (400×). *B*. Normal vaginal epithelial cells. The cell margins are distinct and lack granularity.

saline in a ratio of ~1:1. A new card test now facilitates screening of vaginal fluid for pH >4.5 and trimethylamine, and a new dipstick test detects proline aminopeptidase, an enzyme associated with this syndrome.

Alternatively, the microbiology laboratory can determine the *Nugent score* by examining a Gram-stained smear of vaginal discharge. A score of 7 to 10, based on reduced numbers or the absence of large gram-positive rods (lactobacilli) and the presence of small gram-negative or variable rods (*Gardnerella* and anaerobic rods) and of curved gram-negative or variable rods (*Mobiluncus*), has high sensitivity and specificity for the diagnosis of bacterial vaginosis. Attempts to isolate *G. vaginalis*, genital mycoplasmas, or anaerobic bacteria do not aid in the diagnosis of bacterial vaginosis because these organisms occur (albeit in much lower concentrations) in the vaginal flora of many women without the syndrome.

℞ **TREATMENT** The standard dosage of metronidazole for the treatment of bacterial vaginosis is 500 mg orally bid for 7 days. Alternatively, the single 2-g oral dose of metronidazole recommended for trichomoniasis produces short-term rates of recurrence of bacterial vaginosis somewhat higher than those obtained with the 7-day regimen. Intravaginal treatment with 2% clindamycin cream [one full applicator (5 g containing 100 mg of clindamycin phosphate) each night for 7 nights] or with 0.75% metronidazole gel [one full applicator (5 g containing 37.5 mg of metronidazole) twice daily for 5 days] is also effective and does not elicit systemic adverse reactions. Nonetheless, long-term recurrence (i.e., after several months) is distressingly common after either oral or intravaginal treatment. Treatment of male partners with metronidazole does not prevent recurrence of bacterial vaginosis, even though new sexual partners have been implicated as a risk factor for recurrence.

No controlled data support the use of currently available vaginal or oral preparations of lactobacilli for the treatment or prevention of recurrence of bacterial vaginosis. Clinical trials are evaluating prevention of recurrence by repeated intravaginal inoculation of a vaginal *Lactobacillus* species that produces hydrogen peroxide and adheres to vaginal epithelium.

Vulvovaginal Pruritus, Burning, or Irritation Vulvovaginal candidiasis produces vulvar pruritus, burning, or irritation, generally without symptoms of increased vaginal discharge or malodor. Genital herpes can produce similar symptoms, with lesions sometimes difficult to distinguish from the fissures caused by candidiasis. Signs of vulvovaginal candidiasis include vulvar erythema, edema, fissures, and tenderness. With candidiasis, a white scanty vaginal discharge sometimes takes the form of white thrushlike plaques or cottage cheese–like curds adhering loosely to the vaginal mucosa. *C. albicans* accounts for nearly all cases of symptomatic vulvovaginal candidiasis, which probably arise from endogenous strains of *C. albicans* that have colonized the vagina or the intestinal tract.

The diagnosis of vulvovaginal candidiasis usually involves the demonstration of pseudohyphae or hyphae by microscopic examination of vaginal fluid mixed with saline or 10% KOH or subjected to Gram's staining. Microscopic examination is less sensitive than culture but correlates better with symptoms.

℞ **TREATMENT** Symptoms and signs of vulvovaginal candidiasis warrant treatment, usually intravaginal administration of any of several imidazole antibiotics (e.g., miconazole or clotrimazole) for 3 to 7 days. Over-the-counter marketing of such preparations has reduced the cost of care and made treatment more convenient for many women with recurrent yeast vulvovaginitis. However, most women who purchase these preparations do not have vulvovaginal candidiasis, while many do have other vaginal infections that require different treatment. Therefore, only women with classic symptoms of vulvar pruritus and a history of previous episodes of yeast vulvovaginitis documented by an experienced clinician should self-treat. Single-dose oral treatment with fluconazole (150 mg) is also effective and is preferred by many patients. Prolonged or periodic oral therapy may benefit women with severe or frequently recurrent vulvovaginal candidiasis and those who do not respond to intravaginal or single-dose oral therapy. Such patients probably should be evaluated for diabetes and HIV infection, although such systemic illnesses seldom explain recurrent vulvovaginal candidiasis. Treatment of sexual partners is not routinely indicated.

Other Causes of Vaginal Discharge or Vaginitis In the ulcerative vaginitis associated with staphylococcal toxic shock syndrome, *Staphylococcus aureus* should be promptly identified in vaginal fluid by Gram's stain and by culture. In desquamative inflammatory vaginitis, smears of vaginal fluid reveal neutrophils, massive vaginal epithelial cell exfoliation with increased numbers of parabasal cells, and gram-positive cocci; this syndrome responds to treatment with 2% clindamycin cream. Additional causes of vaginitis and vulvovaginal symptoms in women include retained foreign bodies (e.g., tampons), cervical caps, vaginal spermicides, vaginal antiseptic preparations or douches, vaginal epithelial atrophy in postmenopausal women or in the postpartum period during prolonged breast-feeding, allergic reactions to latex condoms, vaginal aphthae associated with HIV infection or Behçet's syndrome, and vestibulitis (a poorly understood syndrome).

MUCOPURULENT CERVICITIS MPC refers to inflammation of the columnar epithelium and subepithelium of the endocervix and of any contiguous columnar epithelium that lies exposed in an ectopic position on the exocervix. MPC in women represents the "silent partner" of urethritis in men, being equally common and often caused by the same agents (*N. gonorrhoeae* or *C. trachomatis*) but more difficult to recognize. As the most common manifestation of these serious bacterial infections in women, MPC can be a harbinger or sign of pelvic inflammatory disease (PID) and—in pregnant women—can lead to obstetric complications. More than half of all cases of this syndrome in the United States today remain idiopathic.

The diagnosis of MPC rests on the detection of yellow mucopurulent discharge from the cervical os or of increased numbers of polymorphonuclear leukocytes in Gram-stained or Papanicolaou-stained smears of endocervical mucus. MPC due to *C. trachomatis* can also produce edematous cervical ectopy (see below) and endocervical bleeding upon gentle swabbing. Unlike the endocervicitis produced by gonococcal or chlamydial infection, cervicitis caused by HSV produces ulcerative lesions on the stratified squamous epithelium of the exocervix as well as on the columnar epithelium. Yellow cervical mucus on a white swab removed from the endocervix indicates the presence of polymorphonuclear leukocytes. The mucus should be rolled thinly on a slide for Gram's staining. The presence of ≥ 20 polymorphonuclear cells per $1000\times$ microscopic field within strands of cervical mucus not contaminated by vaginal squamous epithelial cells or vaginal bacteria indicates endocervicitis (Fig. 132-2). Detection of intracellular gram-negative diplococci in carefully collected endocervical mucus is quite specific but $\leq 50\%$ sensitive for gonorrhea. Therefore, specific and sensitive tests for *N. gonorrhoeae* as well as *C. trachomatis* are also indicated in evaluation of MPC.

℞ **TREATMENT** Although the above criteria for MPC are neither highly specific nor highly predictive of gonococcal or chlamydial infection in many settings, current guidelines of the Centers for Disease Control and Prevention call for consideration of empirical treatment for MPC, pending test results, "for a patient who has suspected gonorrhea or chlamydial infection, if the prevalences of these infections are high in the patient population, and the patient might be difficult to locate after treatment." In this situation, therapy should

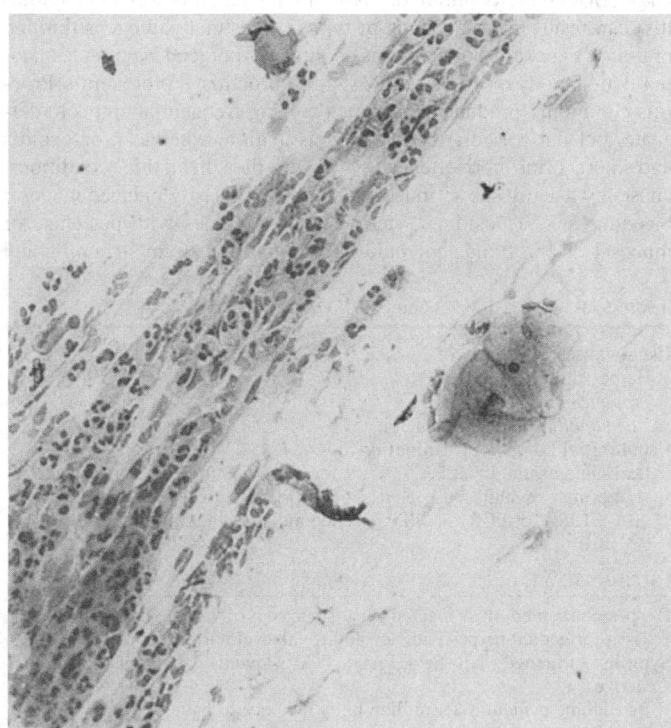

FIGURE 132-2 Gram's stain of cervical mucus, showing a strand of cervical mucus containing many polymorphonuclear leukocytes. This picture is typical of mucopurulent cervicitis. Note that leukocytes are not seen in areas of the slide containing vaginal epithelial cells, adjacent to the mucus strands. *[(From KK Holmes and WE Stamm: Lower genital tract infection in women, in KK Holmes et al (eds). Sexually Transmitted Diseases, 3d ed. New York, McGraw-Hill, 1999, pp 761–781.)]*

include a single-dose regimen effective for gonorrhea plus treatment for chlamydial infection, as outlined in Table 132-4 for treatment of urethritis. In settings where gonorrhea is much less common than chlamydial infection, initial therapy for chlamydial infection alone suffices. The etiology and potential benefit of treatment of endocervicitis not associated with gonorrhea or chlamydial infection remain undefined. Sexual partner(s) of a woman with MPC should be examined and given a regimen similar to that chosen for the woman unless results of tests for gonorrhea or chlamydial infection in either partner warrant different therapy or no therapy.

CERVICAL ECTOPY Cervical ectopy, often mislabeled "cervical erosion," is easily confused with infectious endocervicitis. Ectopy represents the presence of the one-cell-thick columnar epithelium extending from the endocervix out onto the visible ectocervix. In ectopy, the cervical os may contain clear or slightly cloudy mucus but usually not yellow mucopus. Colposcopy shows intact epithelium. Normally found during adolescence and early adulthood, ectopy gradually recedes through the second and third decades of life, as squamous metaplasia replaces the ectopic columnar epithelium. Oral contraceptive use favors the persistence or reappearance of ectopy, while smoking apparently accelerates squamous metaplasia. Cauterization for the elimination of ectopy is not warranted. Ectopy may render the cervix more susceptible to infection with *N. gonorrhoeae*, *C. trachomatis*, or HIV by exposing a larger area of susceptible columnar epithelium on the exocervix.

PELVIC INFLAMMATORY DISEASE See Chap. 133.

ULCERATIVE GENITAL LESIONS Genital ulceration reflects a set of important STIs, most of which also sharply increase the risk of sexual acquisition and shedding of HIV. Accurate diagnosis, treatment, and prevention of these infections are high priorities. In a study of genital ulcers carried out in 1996 in 10 of the U.S. cities with the highest rates of primary syphilis, polymerase chain reaction (PCR) testing of ulcer specimens demonstrated HSV in 62% of patients, *Treponema pallidum* in 13%, and *Haemophilus ducreyi* in 12 to 20%.

In Asia and Africa, chancroid was once considered the most common type of genital ulcer, followed by primary syphilis and then genital herpes. With increased efforts to control chancroid and syphilis, together with more frequent recurrences or persistence of genital herpes attributable to the growing numbers of immunosuppressed persons with HIV infection, PCR testing of genital ulcers now clearly implicates genital herpes as the most common cause of genital ulceration in some developing countries. Lymphogranuloma venereum (LGV) and donovanosis (granuloma inguinale) continue to cause genital ulceration in developing countries but rarely occur today in North America or Europe. Other causes of genital ulcer include (1) candidiasis and traumatized genital warts—both readily recognized; (2) lesions due to genital involvement of more widespread dermatoses; and (3) cutaneous manifestations of systemic diseases, such as genital mucosal ulceration in Stevens-Johnson syndrome.

Although most genital ulcerations cannot be diagnosed confidently on clinical grounds alone, clinical findings plus epidemiologic considerations (Table 132-6) can usually guide initial management (Table 132-7) pending results of further tests. Clinicians should order a rapid serologic test for syphilis in all cases of genital ulcer and a dark-field, direct immunofluorescence, or PCR test for *T. pallidum* from all lesions except those highly characteristic of infection with HSV (i.e., those with herpetic vesicles).

Typical vesicles or pustules or a cluster of painful ulcers preceded by vesiculopustular lesions suggests genital herpes. These typical clinical presentations make detection of the virus optional; however, many patients want confirmation of the diagnosis, and differentiation of HSV-1 from HSV-2 has prognostic implications, since the latter causes more frequent recurrences.

Painless, nontender, indurated ulcers with firm, nontender inguinal adenopathy suggest primary syphilis. If the results of dark-field ex-

Table 132-6 Clinical Features of Genital Ulcers

Feature	Syphilis	Herpes	Chancroid	Lymphogranuloma Venereum	Donovanosis
Incubation period	9–90 days	2–7 days	1–14 days	3 days–6 weeks	1–4 weeks (up to 6 months)
Early primary lesions	Papule	Vesicle	Pustule	Papule, pustule, or vesicle	Papule
No. of lesions	Usually one	Multiple, may coalesce	Usually multiple, may coalesce	Usually one	Variable
Diameter	5–15 mm	1–2 mm	Variable	2–10 mm	Variable
Edges	Sharply demarcated, elevated, round, or oval	Erythematous	Undermined, ragged, irregular	Elevated, round, or oval	Elevated, irregular
Depth	Superficial or deep	Superficial	Excavated	Superficial or deep	Elevated
Base	Smooth, nonpurulent, relatively nonvascular	Serous, erythematous, nonvascular	Purulent, bleeds easily	Variable, nonvascular	Red and velvety, bleeds readily
Induration	Firm	None	Soft	Occasionally firm	Firm
Pain	Uncommon	Frequently tender	Usually very tender	Variable	Uncommon
Lymphadenopathy	Firm, nontender, bilateral	Firm, tender, often bilateral with initial episode	Tender, may suppurate, loculated, usually unilateral	Tender, may suppurate, loculated, usually unilateral	None; pseudobuboes

SOURCE: From RM Ballard, KK Holmes et al (eds): *Sexually Transmitted Diseases*, 3rd ed. New York, McGraw-Hill, 1999.

amination and a rapid serologic test for syphilis are initially negative and the patient will comply with follow-up and sexual abstinence, the performance of two more dark-field examinations on successive days before treatment is begun will improve the sensitivity of diagnosis of syphilis, as will repeated serologic testing for syphilis 1 or 2 weeks later.

"Atypical" or clinically trivial ulcers may be more common manifestations of genital herpes than classic vesiculopustular lesions. Specific tests for HSV in the lesions are therefore indicated (Chap. 182). Type-specific serologic tests for serum antibody to HSV-2, now commercially available, may give negative results, especially when patients present early with the initial episode of genital herpes or when HSV-1 is the cause of genital herpes (as in 15 to 30% of cases today). Furthermore, a positive test for HSV-2 antibody does not prove that the current lesions are herpetic, since nearly one-fourth of the general population of the United States becomes seropositive for HSV-2 during early adulthood. Nonetheless, a positive HSV-2 serology does enable the clinician to tell the patient that he or she has had genital herpes, should learn to recognize symptoms, should avoid sex during recurrences, and should consider use of condoms at other times.

Demonstration of *H. ducreyi* by culture (or by PCR test, when available) is most useful when ulcers are painful and purulent, especially when inguinal lymphadenopathy with fluctance or overlying erythema is noted; if chancroid is prevalent in the community; or if the patient has recently had a sexual exposure in a chancroid-endemic area (e.g., a developing country or certain North American cities). Enlarged, fluctuant lymph nodes should be aspirated for culture or PCR tests to detect *H. ducreyi* as well as for Gram's staining and culture to rule out the presence of other pyogenic bacteria.

When genital ulcers persist beyond the natural history of initial episodes of herpes (2 to 3 weeks) or of chancroid or syphilis (up to 6 weeks) and do not resolve with syndrome-based antimicrobial therapy, then—in addition to the usual tests for herpes, syphilis, and chancroid—biopsy is indicated to exclude donovanosis, carcinoma, and other nonvenereal dermatoses. HIV serology should also be undertaken, since chronic, persistent genital herpes is common in AIDS.

Immediate syndrome-based treatment for acute genital ulcerations (after collection of all necessary diagnostic specimens) is often appropriate. Patients with typical initial or recurrent episodes of genital or anorectal herpes can benefit from prompt oral antiviral therapy (Chap. 182). The patient with nonvesicular ulcerative lesions who may not return for follow-up or may continue sexual activity should receive initial treatment for syphilis, together with empirical therapy for chancroid if exposed in an area where chancroid occurs or if regional lymph node suppuration is evident. In resource-poor settings lacking ready access to diagnostic tests, this approach to syndromic treatment for syphilis and chancroid has helped bring these two diseases under better control. Finally, empirical antimicrobial therapy may be indicated if ulcers persist and the diagnosis remains unclear after a week of observation despite attempts to diagnose herpes, syphilis, and chancroid.

PROCTITIS, PROCTOCOLITIS, ENTEROCOLITIS, AND ENTERITIS Sexually acquired proctitis, with inflammation limited to the rectal mucosa, results from direct rectal inoculation of typical STD pathogens. In contrast, inflammation extending from the rectum to the colon (proctocolitis), involving both the small and the large bowel (enterocolitis), or involving the small bowel alone (enteritis) can result from ingestion of typical intestinal pathogens through oral-anal exposure during sexual contact. Anorectal pain and mucopurulent, bloody rectal discharge suggest proctitis or protocolitis. Proctitis commonly produces tenesmus (causing frequent attempts to defecate, but not true diarrhea) and constipation, whereas proctocolitis and enterocolitis more often cause true diarrhea. In all three conditions, anoscopy usually shows mucosal exudate and easily induced mucosal bleeding (i.e., a positive "wipe test"), sometimes with petechiae or mucosal ulcers. Exudate should be sampled for Gram's staining and

Table 132-7 Initial Management of Genital Ulcer

Usual causes
Herpes simplex virus (HSV)
Treponema pallidum (primary syphilis)
Haemophilus ducreyi (chancroid)
Usual initial laboratory evaluation
Dark-field exam, direct FA, or PCR for *T. pallidum*; RPR test (if negative but primary syphilis suspected, repeat RPR in 1 week); culture, direct FA, ELISA, or PCR for HSV. In endemic area: PCR or culture for *H. ducreyi*

INITIAL TREATMENT

Herpes confirmed or suspected (history or sign of vesicles):
Treat for genital herpes with acyclovir, valacyclovir, or famciclovir
Syphilis confirmed (dark-field, FA, or PCR showing *T. pallidum*, or RPR reactive):
Benzathine penicillin 2.4 million units IM once to patient, recent (e.g., within 3 months) seronegative partner(s), and all seropositive partner(s)
Chancroid confirmed or suspected (diagnostic test positive, or HSV and syphilis excluded, and lesion persists):
Ciprofloxacin 500 mg PO as single dose
or
Ceftriaxone 250 mg IM as single dose

NOTE: FA, fluorescent antibody; PCR, polymerase chain reaction; RPR, rapid plasma reagin; ELISA, enzyme-linked immunosorbent assay; HSV, herpes simplex virus.

other microbiologic studies. Sigmoidoscopy or colonoscopy shows inflammation limited to the rectum in proctitis or disease extending at least into the sigmoid colon in proctocolitis.

The AIDS era has brought an extraordinary shift in the clinical and etiologic spectrum of intestinal infections among homosexual men. The number of cases of the acute intestinal STIs described above has fallen as high-risk sexual behaviors have become less common in this group. At the same time, the number of AIDS-related opportunistic intestinal infections has risen rapidly, many associated with chronic or recurrent symptoms. Acquisition of *N. gonorrhoeae*, HSV, or *C. trachomatis* during receptive anorectal intercourse causes most cases of infectious proctitis. Primary and secondary syphilis can also produce anal or anorectal lesions, with or without symptoms. Gonococcal or chlamydial proctitis typically involves the most distal rectal mucosa and the anal crypts and is clinically mild, without systemic manifestations. In contrast, primary proctitis due to HSV and proctocolitis due to the strains of *C. trachomatis* that cause LGV usually produce severe anorectal pain and often cause fever. Perianal ulcers and inguinal lymphadenopathy, most commonly due to HSV, can also occur in LGV or syphilis. Sacral nerve root radiculopathies, usually presenting as urinary retention, laxity of the anal sphincter, or constipation, may complicate primary herpetic proctitis. In LGV, rectal biopsy typically shows crypt abscesses, granulomas, and giant cells—findings resembling those in Crohn's disease; such findings should always prompt rectal culture and serology for LGV, which is a curable infection. Syphilis can also produce rectal granulomas, usually in association with infiltration by plasma cells or other mononuclear cells.

Diarrhea and abdominal bloating or cramping pain without anorectal symptoms and with normal findings on anoscopy and sigmoidoscopy occur with inflammation of the small intestine (enteritis) or with proximal colitis. In homosexual men without HIV infection, enteritis is often attributable to *Giardia lamblia*. Sexually acquired proctocolitis is most often due to *Campylobacter* or *Shigella* spp.

PREVENTION AND CONTROL OF STDS

Although rates of all curable STDs fell in the United States throughout the 1990s, all other industrialized countries of comparable economic development have made greater progress. For example, Sweden has virtually eliminated the transmission of gonorrhea, syphilis, and chancroid and has achieved very low rates of HIV transmission. Elimination of syphilis as an endemic disease is now a national goal in the United States, but stronger efforts toward prevention and control of all STDs are necessary.

Prevention and control of STDs require (1) reduction of the average rate of sexual exposure through alteration of behaviors and behavioral norms among both susceptible and infected persons in all population groups; (2) reduction of the efficiency of transmission through the promotion of safer sexual practices, the use of condoms during casual or commercial sex, hepatitis B immunization, and many other approaches (e.g., early detection and treatment of other STIs to reduce the efficiency of sexual transmission of HIV); and (3) shortening of the duration of infectivity of STDs through early detection and curative or suppressive treatment of patients and their sexual partners.

Primary care physicians usually do not screen for illicit drug use or sexual risk behaviors, even when typical patients have classic presentations for HIV infection or another STD. In fact, clinicians often focus only on detection and treatment of curable STDs to reduce the duration of infectivity. They generally have relatively little training or experience in risk assessment, counseling on risk reduction, tracing and treatment of sexual contacts, or condom promotion. Financial and time constraints imposed by managed-care practice patterns may further curtail screening and prevention services. As outlined in Fig. 132-3, the efforts of clinicians simply to detect and treat STDs depend in part on societal efforts to teach young people how to recognize symptoms of STDs; to motivate those with symptoms to seek care promptly; and to make such care accessible, affordable, and acceptable, especially to the young indigent patients most likely to acquire an STD.

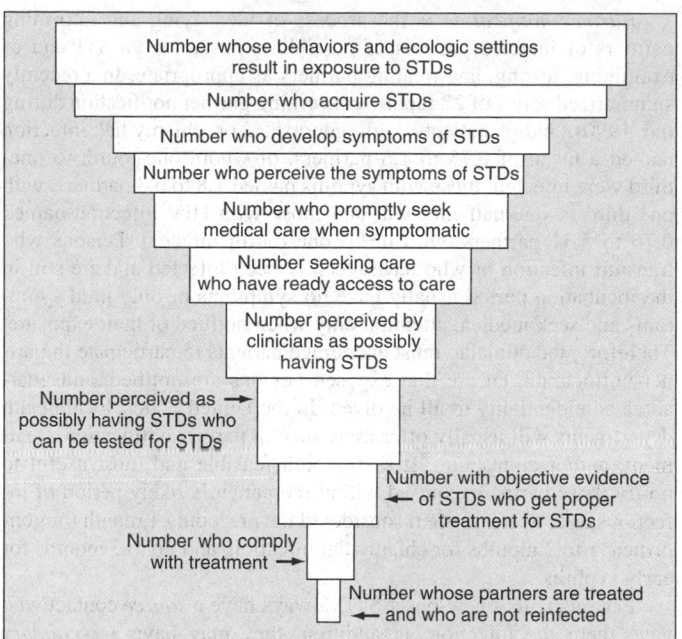

FIGURE 132-3 Critical control points for preventive and clinical interventions against sexually transmitted diseases (STDs). *(Adapted from HT Waller and MA Piot: Bull World Health Organ 41:75, 1969 and 43:1, 1970; and from "Resource allocation model for public health planning—a case study of tuberculosis control," Bull World Health Organ 84(Suppl) 1973.)*

Since many infected individuals develop no symptoms or fail to recognize and report symptoms, clinicians should routinely perform an STI risk assessment for teenagers and young adults as a selective screen. U.S. Preventive Services Task Force Guidelines recommend screening sexually active females ≤25 years of age for *C. trachomatis* whenever they present for health care (at least once a year); older women should be tested if they have more than one sexual partner, have begun a new sexual relationship since the previous test, or have another STD diagnosed. In the United States, widespread selective screening of young women for cervical *C. trachomatis* infection in some regions has been associated with a 50 to 60% drop in prevalence, and such screening also protects the individual woman from PID. Sensitive urine-based genetic amplification tests permit expansion of screening to men and teenage boys and to women in settings where a pelvic examination is not planned or is impractical.

Although gonorrhea is now substantially less common than chlamydial infection in industrialized countries, screening tests for *N. gonorrhoeae* are still appropriate for women and teenage girls attending STD clinics and for sexually active teens and young women from areas of high gonorrhea prevalence. Routine screening of asymptomatic men for urethral gonorrhea has a very low yield in the primary care setting. However, genetic amplification tests that combine screening for *N. gonorrhoeae* and *C. trachomatis* in a single low-cost assay may facilitate the prevention and control of both infections in populations at high risk.

All patients with newly detected STIs or at high risk for STIs according to routine risk assessment as well as all pregnant women should be encouraged to undergo serologic testing for syphilis and HIV infection, with appropriate HIV counseling before and after testing. Several randomized trials have shown that *risk reduction counseling* of patients with STDs significantly lowers subsequent risk of acquiring an STD. Preimmunization serologic testing for antibody to HBV is indicated for unvaccinated persons who are known to be at high risk, such as homosexually active men and injection drug users. In most young persons, however, it is more cost-effective to vaccinate against HBV without serologic screening.

Partner notification is the process of identifying and informing partners of infected patients of possible exposure to an STI and of examining, testing, and treating partners as appropriate. In a recently summarized series of 22 reports concerning partner notification during the 1990s, index patients with gonorrhea or chlamydial infection named a mean of 0.75 to 1.6 partners, of whom one-fourth to one-third were infected; those with syphilis named 1.8 to 6.3 partners, with one-third to one-half infected; and those with HIV infection named 0.76 to 5.31 partners, with up to one-fourth infected. Persons who transmit infection or who have recently been infected and are still in the incubation period usually have no symptoms or only mild symptoms and seek medical attention only when notified of their exposure. Therefore, the clinician must encourage patients to participate in partner notification, ensure that exposed persons are notified, and guarantee confidentiality to all involved. In the United States, local health departments will usually offer assistance in partner notification, treatment, and/or counseling. It seems both feasible and most useful to notify those partners exposed within the patient's likely period of infectiousness, which is often considered the preceding 1 month for gonorrhea, 1 to 2 months for chlamydial infection, and up to 3 months for early syphilis.

Persons with a new-onset STD always have a *source* contact who gave them the infection; in addition, they may have a *secondary* (*spread* or *exposed*) contact with whom they had sex after becoming infected. The identification and treatment of these two types of contacts have different objectives. Treatment of the source contact (often a casual contact) benefits the community by preventing further transmission; treatment of the recently exposed secondary contact (typically a spouse or another steady sexual partner) prevents both the development of serious complications (such as PID) in the partner and reinfection of the index patient.

In summary, clinicians and public health agencies share responsibility for the prevention and control of STDs. In the managed-care era, the role of primary care clinicians has become increasingly important in prevention as well as in diagnosis and treatment.

BIBLIOGRAPHY

CENTERS FOR DISEASE CONTROL AND PREVENTION: 1998 Guidelines for treatment of sexually transmitted diseases. MMWR 47(RR-1):1, 1998

CHERNESKY MA: Nucleic acid tests for the diagnosis of sexually transmitted diseases. FEMS Immunol Med Microbiol 24:437, 1999

CURTIS R, HOLMES KK: Individual-level risk assessment for STD/HIV, in *Sexually Transmitted Diseases*, 3d ed, KK Holmes et al (eds). New York, McGraw-Hill, 1999, pp 669–683

DALABETTA G et al (eds): Syndromic management of sexually transmitted diseases. Sex Transm Dis 74(Suppl 1):S1, 1998

DIVISION OF STD PREVENTION: *Sexually Transmitted Disease Surveillance, 1998*. Atlanta, Centers for Disease Control and Prevention, 1999

ECKERT LO et al: Vulvovaginal candidiasis: Clinical manifestations, risk factors, and algorithm for case management. Obstet Gynecol 92:757, 1998

HOLMES KK et al (eds): *Sexually Transmitted Diseases*, 3d ed. New York, McGraw-Hill, 1999

INSTITUTE OF MEDICINE: *The Hidden Epidemic: Confronting Sexually Transmitted Diseases*, TR Eng, WT Butler (eds). Washington, DC, National Academy Press, 1997

JOINT UNITED NATIONS PROGRAMME ON HIV/AIDS (UNAIDS) AND WORLD HEALTH ORGANIZATION (WHO): *Sexually Transmitted Diseases: Policies and Principles for Prevention and Care*. UNAIDS/97.6, Geneva, 1999

KAMB ML et al: Efficacy of risk-reduction counseling to prevent human immunodeficiency virus and sexually transmitted diseases: A randomized controlled trial. Project RESPECT Study Group. JAMA 280:1161, 1998

MERTZ KJ et al: Etiology of genital ulcers and prevalence of human immunodeficiency virus coinfection in 10 US cities. The Genital Ulcer Disease Surveillance Group. J Infect Dis 178:1795, 1998

ROTHENBERG R, POTTERAT J: Partner notification for sexually transmitted diseases and HIV infection, in *Sexually Transmitted Diseases*, 3d ed, KK Holmes et al (eds). New York, McGraw-Hill, 1999

TAO G et al: Missed opportunities to assess sexually transmitted diseases in U.S. adults during routine medical checkups. Am J Prev Med 18:109, 2000

VAN DYCK E et al (eds): *Laboratory Diagnosis of Sexually Transmitted Diseases*. Albany, NY, World Health Organization, 1999

133

King K. Holmes, Robert C. Brunham

PELVIC INFLAMMATORY DISEASE

DEFINITION The term *pelvic inflammatory disease* (PID) usually refers to infection that ascends from the cervix or vagina to involve the endometrium and/or fallopian tubes. Infection can extend beyond the reproductive tract to cause pelvic peritonitis, generalized peritonitis, perihepatitis, or pelvic abscess. In rare instances, infection extends secondarily to the pelvic organs from adjacent foci of inflammation (e.g., sites of appendicitis, regional ileitis, or diverticulitis), as a result of hematogenous dissemination (e.g., of tuberculosis), or as a rare complication of certain tropical diseases (e.g., schistosomiasis). Intrauterine infection can be primary (spontaneously occurring and usually sexually transmitted) or secondary to invasive intrauterine surgical procedures (e.g., dilatation and curettage, termination of pregnancy, insertion of an intrauterine device, or hysterosalpingography) or to parturition. Endometritis or endomyometritis is particularly common following delivery by emergency cesarean section when antibiotic prophylaxis is not used.

PID is uncommon during pregnancy itself. The uterotubal junction is closed as early as the seventh week of pregnancy, and the chorioamnion becomes approximated to the endocervical os, sealing off the intrauterine cavity, at the twelfth to fifteenth week of gestation. As a consequence, ascending intrauterine infection prior to the twelfth week of gestation may be associated (as either cause or effect) with endometritis and spontaneous abortion, while ascending infection after the twelfth week may be associated with chorioamnionitis.

Spontaneously occurring PID can be of the chronic or the acute type. Chronic PID due to *Mycobacterium tuberculosis* has become uncommon in industrialized countries. However, subacute or chronic PID caused by persistent or repeated infection with *Chlamydia trachomatis* is thought to be common.

Although the clinical diagnosis of PID is imprecise, the use of endometrial biopsy together with laparoscopy provides objective evidence of a continuum progressing from cervicitis alone to endometritis, to salpingitis, and to peritonitis. In this chapter, *PID* is used to refer to the clinical syndrome that includes these conditions, while the term *salpingitis* is restricted to cases of visually or histopathologically confirmed inflammation of the fallopian tubes. The distinction between endometritis and salpingitis may be important, because long-term sequelae are much more common after salpingitis. These sequelae include infertility due to bilateral tubal occlusion, peritubal adhesions, ectopic pregnancy due to tubal damage without occlusion, chronic pelvic pain, and recurrent PID.

ETIOLOGY The etiology of PID has varied greatly among studies for reasons related to the selection of patients, the prevalence of sexually transmitted disease (STD) pathogens at the time and place of the study, and methodology. As is summarized in Table 133-1, the agents most often implicated in acute PID include those that are primary causes of cervicitis (*Neisseria gonorrhoeae* and *C. trachomatis*) and those that can be regarded as components of an altered vaginal flora.

Table 133-1   Cervical and Vaginal Organisms Most Often Implicated in Acute PID

Cervical Pathogens	Vaginal Flora Components
Neisseria gonorrhoeae *Chlamydia trachomatis*	Anaerobic bacteria *Prevotella, Peptostreptococcus, Mobiluncus,* and *Actinomyces* Facultative bacteria Enterobacteriaceae, *Haemophilus influenzae, Gardnerella vaginalis,* group B *Streptococcus* Mycoplasmas *Mycoplasma hominis, Ureaplasma urealyticum,* ?*Mycoplasma genitalium*

During the 1980s, *N. gonorrhoeae* and/or *C. trachomatis* was found in 65% of women with a clinical diagnosis of PID at San Francisco General Hospital and in 85% of patients with proven salpingitis and endometritis in Seattle; in both studies, gonorrhea was nearly twice as common as chlamydial infection and dual infection was common. However, in Western Europe and parts of the United States, as gonococcal infection has come under much better control, endocervical gonococcal infection has been found in a declining proportion of women with PID, and the microbial etiology cannot be defined in a substantial proportion of cases. In general, PID is most often associated with gonorrhea where there is a high incidence of gonorrhea—e.g., in developing countries and in indigent, inner-city populations in the United States. In several studies of women with PID, up to two-thirds of women with endocervical cultures positive for *N. gonorrhoeae* have also had endometrial, peritoneal, or tubal cultures positive for this organism. Similarly, studies of women with proven PID have shown that *C. trachomatis* can be demonstrated by culture or immunofluorescent staining in the endometrium or tubes of the majority of those who have endocervical chlamydial infection.

Anaerobic and facultative anaerobic organisms (especially *Prevotella* species, peptostreptococci, *Escherichia coli*, and group B streptococci) and genital mycoplasmas have been isolated from specimens obtained at laparoscopy from the peritoneal fluid or fallopian tubes in a varying proportion—typically one-fourth to one-third—of women with PID studied in the United States. These vaginal organisms can be found in association with chlamydial or gonococcal infection as well as in the absence of such infection. The importance of vaginal organisms in salpingitis has probably been overestimated in some studies in which specimens were obtained for cultures by culdocentesis or endometrial aspiration, procedures in which contamination of the aspirated specimen by vaginal flora is possible. However, specimens obtained by laparoscopy from some patients with PID have also contained anaerobic and facultative species. A compilation of seven studies of the microbial etiology of PID showed that 5 to 78% of patients had anaerobes and facultative bacteria isolated from the upper genital tract. It is extremely difficult to determine the exact microbial etiology of an individual case of PID because of the frequency of mixed infection, the difficulty in sampling the fallopian tube itself, and the complexity of the microbiologic techniques required to detect the various fastidious pathogens involved. This situation has implications for the approach to empirical antimicrobial treatment of PID.

In general, first episodes of acute PID are particularly likely to be caused by *N. gonorrhoeae* and/or *C. trachomatis*. These sexually transmitted pathogens are implicated somewhat less often in recurrent bouts of acute PID, in episodes occurring in women with intrauterine devices (IUDs), in episodes precipitated by invasive intrauterine diagnostic or therapeutic procedures (which are often associated with ascending infection caused by endogenous vaginal flora), and perhaps in HIV-associated PID.

EPIDEMIOLOGY It has been estimated that about 850,000 cases of PID occurred in the United States each year during the mid-1970s. PID is not a reportable disease in the United States; surveillance of physicians in private practice and of hospital discharges suggests that the incidence of PID increased from the mid-1960s through the mid-1970s and may then have decreased. Hospitalization for acute PID declined steadily from 1982 through 1997, and initial visits to physicians' offices for PID have been declining since the mid-1980s. Furthermore, the number of hospitalizations for ectopic pregnancy in the United States fell by about two-thirds from 1989 to 1997.

Acute PID is almost exclusively a disease of sexually active women. Important risk factors include a history of salpingitis or of recent vaginal douching; the use of an IUD, particularly the Dalkon shield, has also been a risk factor. In most studies, the relative risk of PID among IUD users is higher in nulliparous than in parous women and is greatest during the first few months after IUD insertion. The increased risk of PID among IUD users is evident mainly among those with multiple sex partners. In contrast, women using oral contraceptives appear to be at decreased risk of PID. Barrier methods of contraception also make PID less likely by reducing the risk of chlamydial and gonococcal infection. Tubal sterilization reduces (but does not completely eliminate) the risk of salpingitis by preventing intraluminal spread of infection into the tubes.

PATHOGENESIS Factors cited as possibly contributing to the upward spread of gonococci and chlamydiae from the endocervix to the endometrium and endosalpinx include estrogen-dominated (thin) cervical mucus, attachment to sperm that migrate upward into the tubes, use of an IUD, vaginal douching, menstruation, and subendometrial myometrial contractions, which move particulate matter from the cervix to the fundus of the uterus between days 5 and 14 of the menstrual cycle. It is important that the onset of symptoms of *N. gonorrhoeae*–associated and *C. trachomatis*–associated PID often occurs during or soon after the menstrual period. In fallopian tube organ cultures in vitro, gonococci attach to the surface of the secretory columnar cells (but not the ciliated cells) of the endosalpinx. Gonococcal pili and perhaps other surface proteins are important in this attachment. Gonococci are then taken into the secretory cells by endocytosis. They pass through the cells—and perhaps between cells—and are extruded through the base of the cell into the submucosal connective tissue. Ciliary motion ceases, and then ciliated cells, although not directly invaded by gonococci, are sloughed from the mucosa—a factor that may render the tubes more susceptible to superinfection by other organisms. It is uncertain whether this loss of ciliated cells is irreversible in vivo. Gonococcal endotoxin and peptidoglycan as well as certain cytokines (such as tumor necrosis factor α) appear to be responsible for these cytotoxic effects.

C. trachomatis also infects the columnar cells of the fallopian tube but produces little damage in tubal organ cultures, perhaps because the host response is more important than directly toxic effects of bacterial products in the pathogenesis of chlamydial salpingitis. *Chlamydia*-infected epithelial cells secrete a number of proinflammatory cytokines, which are chemotactic for neutrophils and mononuclear cells. Routine endometrial biopsies from women with chlamydial mucopurulent cervicitis (MPC) show endometritis in approximately one-half of cases. Endometritis detected in this way is sometimes but not always associated with symptoms of severe abdominal pain, presentation during days 1 through 7 of the menstrual cycle, signs of uterine tenderness, and an erythrocyte sedimentation rate (ESR) of ≥ 20 mm/h. Adnexal tenderness, cervical motion tenderness, and rebound tenderness as well as leukocytosis and elevated C-reactive protein levels are all more common in women with laparoscopic evidence of salpingitis than in those with endometritis alone. Chlamydial inclusions are demonstrable by direct immunofluorescence in columnar epithelial cells of the endometrium and endosalpinx. The endometrial biopsies usually show neutrophils infiltrating the epithelium and plasma cells infiltrating the stroma, findings also seen in gonococcal endometritis but not in the uninfected endometrium. Experimental inoculation of the fallopian tubes of lower primates with *C. trachomatis* has shown that repeated exposure to *C. trachomatis* leads to the greatest degree of tissue inflammation and damage; this finding suggests that immunopathology also underlies the pathogenesis of chlamydial disease.

The pathogenesis of PID attributable to mycoplasmas or other vaginal anaerobic or facultative organisms is less well studied. It is possible that other vaginal organisms implicated in PID often cause tubal infection in women whose tubes have already been damaged by a primary sexually transmitted pathogen (i.e., *N. gonorrhoeae* or *C. trachomatis*). The vaginal organisms implicated in PID are found in the vagina most often and in greatest concentration in bacterial vaginosis, and there is epidemiologic evidence that bacterial vaginosis itself is a predisposing factor for PID (just as poor oral hygiene is a risk factor for aspiration pneumonia).

Certain other iatrogenic factors, such as dilatation and curettage or cesarean section, can increase the risk of PID in women with endocervical gonococcal or chlamydial infection. Evidence indicates that among women undergoing cesarean section, the presence of bacterial vaginosis increases the risk of postpartum endometritis.

CLINICAL MANIFESTATIONS   Tuberculous Salpingitis Unlike nontuberculous salpingitis, genital tuberculosis often occurs in older women, many of whom are postmenopausal. Presenting symptoms include abnormal vaginal bleeding, pain (including dysmenorrhea), and infertility. Bimanual pelvic examination may be normal, though about one-quarter of these women have had adnexal masses. Endometrial biopsy shows tuberculous granulomas and provides optimal specimens for culture.

Nontuberculous Salpingitis   Symptoms of nontuberculous salpingitis classically evolve from a yellow or malodorous vaginal discharge caused by MPC and/or bacterial vaginosis to midline abdominal pain and abnormal vaginal bleeding caused by endometritis and then to bilateral lower abdominal and pelvic pain caused by salpingitis, with nausea and vomiting and increased abdominal tenderness caused by peritonitis. Some patients have diffuse abdominal pain caused by generalized peritonitis or pleuritic right upper quadrant pain caused by perihepatitis. The pattern in which symptoms evolve varies from patient to patient and is also related to the etiology of the PID.

The onset of IUD-associated PID is typically gradual and may be preceded by the malodorous vaginal discharge characteristic of bacterial vaginosis. The onset of gonococcal PID may be more acute than that of chlamydial PID, and PID of either etiology usually presents during the first half of the menstrual cycle.

The abdominal pain in nontuberculous salpingitis is usually described as dull or aching. In some cases, pain is lacking or is atypical, and active inflammatory changes are found in the course of an unrelated evaluation or procedure, such as a tubal ligation or a laparoscopic evaluation for infertility. Abnormal uterine bleeding precedes or coincides with the onset of pain in ~40% of women with PID, symptoms of urethritis (dysuria) occur in 20%, and symptoms of proctitis (anorectal pain, tenesmus, and rectal discharge or bleeding) are occasionally seen in women with gonococcal or chlamydial infection.

Speculum examination shows evidence of MPC (yellow endocervical discharge, easily induced endocervical bleeding) in the majority of women with gonococcal or chlamydial PID. Cervical motion tenderness is produced by stretching of the adnexal attachments on the side toward which the cervix is pushed. Bimanual examination reveals uterine fundal tenderness due to endometritis and abnormal adnexal tenderness due to salpingitis that is usually, but not necessarily, bilateral. Adnexal swelling is palpable in about one-half of women with acute salpingitis, but evaluation of the adnexae in a patient with marked tenderness—even by an experienced examiner—is not reliable. The initial temperature is >38°C in only about one-third of patients with acute salpingitis; thus fever is not required for the diagnosis. Laboratory findings include elevation of the ESR in 75% of patients with acute salpingitis and elevation of the peripheral white blood cell count in up to 60%.

Certain clinical manifestations of acute PID have been correlated with microbial etiology. For example, the onset of salpingitis is related to menses in women with gonococcal or chlamydial infection. Women with *N. gonorrhoeae*- or *C. trachomatis*-associated salpingitis are significantly younger than women with salpingitis of other etiologies. In a Swedish study, women with *Chlamydia*-associated salpingitis had more indolent disease, with mild symptoms of significantly longer duration and less fever, than women with gonorrhea-associated salpingitis. Women with polymicrobial PID more often have tubal or pelvic abscess formation. It is suspected that, for all recognized cases of symptomatic acute chlamydial salpingitis, there is a comparable number of unrecognized cases of indolent or mildly symptomatic chlamydial salpingitis. Furthermore, it is thought that subclinical chronic or recurrent chlamydial salpingitis may be a major cause of female infertility.

Perihepatitis and Periappendicitis   Symptoms of perihepatitis, including pleuritic upper abdominal pain and tenderness (usually localized to the right upper quadrant), develop in 3 to 10% of women with acute PID. The onset of symptoms of perihepatitis takes place during or after the onset of symptoms of PID and may overshadow lower abdominal symptoms, thereby leading to a mistaken diagnosis of cholecystitis. In perhaps 5% of cases of acute salpingitis, early laparoscopy reveals inflammation ranging from edema and erythema of the liver capsule to exudate with fibrinous adhesions between the visceral and parietal peritoneum. When treatment is delayed and laparoscopy is performed late, dense "violin-string" adhesions are seen over the liver; chronic exertional or positional right upper quadrant pain ensues when traction is placed on the adhesions. Although perihepatitis, also known as the *Fitz-Hugh–Curtis syndrome*, was for many years specifically attributed to gonococcal PID, most cases are now attributed to chlamydial salpingitis. In patients with chlamydial salpingitis, serum titers of microimmunofluorescent antibody to *C. trachomatis* are typically much higher when perihepatitis is present than when it is absent, and it has been suggested that repeated chlamydial infections are responsible for perihepatitis.

Physical findings include right upper quadrant tenderness and usually include adnexal tenderness and cervicitis, even in patients whose symptoms are not suggestive of salpingitis. Liver function tests are nearly always normal, since inflammation is largely limited to the liver capsule and usually spares the parenchyma. Ultrasonography of the right upper quadrant is normal. The presence of MPC and pelvic tenderness in a young woman with subacute pleuritic right upper quadrant pain and normal ultrasonography of the gallbladder points to a diagnosis of perihepatitis.

Periappendicitis (appendiceal serositis without involvement of the intestinal mucosa) has been found in ~5% of patients undergoing appendectomy for suspected appendicitis and can occur as a complication of gonococcal or chlamydial salpingitis.

Influence of HIV Infection   HIV infection with immunosuppression increases the risk of repeated gonococcal and chlamydial infections among repeatedly exposed female sex workers, presumably by attenuating the immune response to repeated infection. Further, among women who acquire gonococcal or chlamydial infection of the cervix, HIV infection with immunosuppression increases the likelihood of developing clinical manifestations of salpingitis. Finally, among women with salpingitis, HIV infection is associated with increased severity of salpingitis and with tuboovarian abscess requiring hospitalization and surgical drainage. However, among African women with confirmed PID, those with HIV infection appear less likely to have gonorrhea or chlamydial infection than those without HIV infection, a difference suggesting that other etiologies are especially important in the immunosuppressed patient. Nonetheless, among women with HIV infection and salpingitis, the clinical reponse to conventional antimicrobial therapy (coupled with drainage of tuboovarian abscess, when found) has been satisfactory.

DIAGNOSIS   Early diagnosis and initiation of therapy are essential to minimize tubal scarring. A reanalysis of Weström's cohort of Swedish women with proven salpingitis showed that those who delayed seeking care were three times more likely than those who sought care promptly to experience subsequent infertility or ectopic pregnancy. Appropriate treatment must not be withheld from patients who have an equivocal diagnosis; it is better to err on the side of overdiagnosis and overtreatment. On the other hand, it is essential to differentiate between salpingitis and other pelvic pathology, particularly surgical emergencies such as appendicitis and ectopic pregnancy.

No readily available clinical finding or laboratory test, short of laparoscopy, definitively identifies salpingitis, and routine laparoscopy to confirm suspected salpingitis is generally impractical. Most patients with acute PID have lower abdominal pain of <3 weeks' duration, pelvic tenderness on bimanual pelvic examination, and evidence of lower genital tract infection (e.g., MPC). Approximately 60% of such patients have salpingitis at laparoscopy. Among the patients with these findings, a rectal temperature >38°C, a palpable adnexal mass, and elevation of the ESR over 15 mm/h also raise the probability of salpingitis, which has been found at laparoscopy in 68% of patients with one of these additional findings, 90% of patients with two, and 96% of patients with three. However, only 17% of all patients with laparoscopy-confirmed salpingitis have had all three additional findings.

MPC is probably responsible for the presence of neutrophils in vaginal fluid in PID. In a woman with pelvic pain and tenderness, demonstration of an increased number of neutrophils (30 per 1000× microscopic field in strands of cervical mucus) increases the predictive value of a clinical diagnosis of acute PID.

Several clinical features other than the presence of cervicitis also favor the diagnosis of acute PID. These include onset with menses, history of recent abnormal menstrual bleeding, presence of an IUD, history of salpingitis, and sexual exposure to a male with urethritis. Detection of polymorphonuclear leukocytes in pelvic peritoneal fluid aspirated by culdocentesis supports a diagnosis of suspected salpingitis. Urethritis or proctitis may occur in chlamydial or gonococcal infection but may also represent a urinary tract source or an intestinal source, respectively. Appendicitis or another disorder of the gut is favored by the early onset of anorexia, nausea, or vomiting; the onset of pain later than day 14 of the menstrual cycle; or unilateral pain limited to the right or left lower quadrant. All women in whom the diagnosis of PID is being considered should be evaluated for ectopic pregnancy. The more sensitive serum assays for human β-chorionic gonadotropin are usually positive when ectopic pregnancy is the diagnosis. Ultrasonography and magnetic resonance imaging (MRI) can be useful for the identification of tuboovarian or pelvic abscess. MRI or intravaginal ultrasound assessment of the tubes has been reported to show increased tubal diameter, intratubal fluid, or tubal wall thickening in cases of salpingitis.

Laparoscopy is the most specific method for diagnosis of acute salpingitis. Although laparoscopic findings may be normal if inflammation is limited to the endosalpinx or the endometrium, patients with suspected PID who have a normal laparoscopy have a better prognosis (with no sequelae at all or fewer sequelae) than patients who have abnormal laparoscopic findings. The primary and uncontested value of laparoscopy in women with lower abdominal pain is for the exclusion of other surgical problems. Some of the most common or serious problems that may be confused with salpingitis (e.g., acute appendicitis, ectopic pregnancy, corpus luteum bleeding, ovarian tumor) are unilateral. Unilateral pain or pelvic mass, though not incompatible with PID, is a strong indication for laparoscopy unless the clinical picture warrants laparotomy instead. Atypical clinical findings, such as the absence of lower genital tract infection, a missed menstrual period, a positive pregnancy test, or failure to respond to appropriate therapy, are other frequent indications for laparoscopy.

Laparoscopic criteria used for the diagnosis of salpingitis include (1) erythema of the fallopian tube, (2) edema of the fallopian tube, and (3) seropurulent exudate or fresh, easily lysed adhesions at the fimbriated end or on the serosal surface of a fallopian tube.

Endometrial biopsy is relatively sensitive and specific for the diagnosis of endometritis when the endometrial changes described above are found, and the presence of endometritis correlates well with the presence of salpingitis. Endometritis is found in at least three-fourths of women with laparoscopically confirmed salpingitis and is not found in women without PID.

The etiologic diagnosis of PID can be further studied by culture or other testing of specimens obtained by endocervical swab, endometrial aspiration, or culdocentesis or by laparoscopy or laparotomy. Endocervical swab specimens should be examined by Gram's staining for neutrophils and gram-negative diplococci and by culture or DNA amplification test for *N. gonorrhoeae*. Compared with culture, the sensitivity of Gram's staining is ~60% and the specificity is >95%. The endocervical swab specimen should also be tested for *C. trachomatis* by culture or amplification assays for chlamydial DNA or RNA. Although detection of either *N. gonorrhoeae* or *C. trachomatis* in the endocervix does not prove that either agent is also present in the upper genital tract, this finding strongly supports the diagnosis of PID. The clinical diagnosis of PID made by expert gynecologists is confirmed by laparoscopy or endometrial biopsy in only ~60% of patients but

in ~90% of those who also have cultures positive for *N. gonorrhoeae* or *C. trachomatis*. There is no evidence that the isolation of anaerobes or facultative aerobes from the cervix or vagina correlates with the presence of these organisms in the upper genital tract in acute PID, but this point has not been well studied. In one study, the isolation of *Haemophilus influenzae* from the endocervix was highly correlated with this organism's recovery from the fallopian tube in cases of salpingitis. Despite the risk of contamination of endometrial specimens with components of the vaginal flora, one study showed a 2.6-fold increase in the rate of recovery of anaerobic gram-negative rods (especially *Prevotella*, black-pigmented rods, and *Fusobacterium*) by endometrial biopsy in women with endometritis compared with control women. When laparoscopy is performed, material can be obtained directly from the cul-de-sac or the fimbriated opening of the tube or by tubal aspiration if pyosalpinx is present. Such specimens should be cultured for anaerobic and facultative pathogens as well as for *N. gonorrhoeae* and *C. trachomatis*.

TREATMENT Women with PID can be treated as either outpatients or inpatients. Over the past decade, the costs of PID treatment have declined considerably because of the increased management of patients in the ambulatory setting, with use of highly active, well-absorbed antimicrobial agents. Nonetheless, hospitalization may be necessary and should be considered when (1) the diagnosis is uncertain and surgical emergencies such as appendicitis and ectopic pregnancy cannot be excluded, (2) pelvic abscess is suspected, (3) severe illness or nausea and vomiting preclude outpatient management, (4) the patient has HIV infection, (5) the patient is assessed as unable to follow or tolerate an outpatient regimen, or (6) the patient has failed to respond to outpatient therapy. If outpatient treatment is embarked on, clinical follow-up after 48 to 72 h of antibiotic treatment should be arranged. Treatment should cover *N. gonorrhoeae*, *C. trachomatis*, gram-negative facultative bacteria (especially *E. coli* and *H. influenzae*), vaginal anaerobes, and group B streptococci. Several antimicrobial combinations do provide a broad spectrum of activity against the major pathogens in vitro, but many have not been adequately evaluated for clinical efficacy in PID (Table 133-2).

Examples of Combination Regimens with Broad Activity Against Major Pathogens in PID Recommended combination regimens for ambulatory or parenteral management of PID are presented in Table 133-3.

Women managed as outpatients should receive a combined regimen with broad activity, such as ceftriaxone [250 mg intramuscularly (IM)] followed by doxycycline (100 mg by mouth, twice a day for 14 days). Metronidazole (500 mg by mouth twice daily) can be added, if tolerated, to enhance activity against anaerobes. Alternatively, ofloxacin (400 mg twice daily) plus metronidazole (500 mg twice daily), both continued for 14 days, provide good coverage of the major pathogens.

The following two parenteral regimens have given nearly identical results in a multicenter randomized trial:

1. Doxycycline [100 mg twice a day, given intravenously (IV) or orally] plus cefotetan (2.0 g IV every 12 h) or cefoxitin (2.0 g IV every 6 h). These drugs should be continued by the IV route for at least 48 h after the patient's condition improves, then followed with doxycycline (100 mg by mouth, twice a day) to complete 14 days of therapy.

2. Clindamycin (900 mg IV every 8 h) plus gentamicin (2.0 mg/kg IV or IM followed by 1.5 mg/kg every 8 h) in patients with normal renal function. Once-daily dosing of gentamicin (with combination of the total daily dose into a single daily dose) has not been evaluated in PID but has been efficacious in other serious infections and could be substituted. Treatment with these drugs should be continued for at least 48 h after the patient's condition improves, then followed with doxycycline (100 mg orally twice a day) or with clindamycin (450 mg orally four times a day) to complete 14 days of therapy. In cases with

Table 133-2 Relative Activities of the Antimicrobial Agents Most Commonly Used to Treat PID

Agent	N. gonorrhoeae	C. trachomatis	Vaginal Anaerobes		PID-Associated Facultative GNR	M. hominis
			GPC[b]	GNR[c]		
Ampicillin/ amoxicillin	2+	2+	4+	2+	2+	0
Doxycycline	2+	4+	2+	1+	1+	2+
Cefoxitin, cefotetan	3+	0	4+	3+	3+	0
Ceftriaxone	4+	0	3+	2+	4+	0
Gentamicin/ tobramycin	2+	0	1+	0	4+	2+?
Ciprofloxacin	4+	0	1+	0	3+	2+
Ofloxacin	4+	3+	1+	1+	4+	1+
Levofloxacin	4+	3+	2+	1+	4+	3+
Azithromycin	2+	4+	2+	?+	2+	?
Clindamycin	1+	3+	4+	4+	0	3+
Metronidazole	0	0	4+	4+	0	0

Relative Activity Against Indicated Pathogen[a]

[a] No single antimicrobial agent offers optimal activity against all of these pathogens, but certain combinations (e.g., cefoxitin plus doxycycline, gentamicin plus clindamycin, and ofloxacin plus metronidazole) have complementary activity. Relative activity is indicated on a scale of 0 to 4+.

[b] GPC, gram-positive cocci (peptostreptococci).

[c] GNR, gram-negative rods. Anaerobic GNR include *Prevotella*; facultative GNR include Enterobacteriaceae and *Haemophilus influenzae*.

SOURCE: Adapted from Kato N et al: Clin Infect Dis 23(Suppl 1):S31, 1996; and Waites KB et al: Antimicrob Agents Chemother 43:2571, 1999.

tuboovarian abscess, many experts use oral clindamycin rather than doxycycline for continued therapy to provide better coverage for anaerobic infection.

Management of Sexual Partners Sexual partners of patients with acute PID—particularly those who have been partners within the 1 to 2 months before the onset of symptoms of PID—should be examined for STDs and promptly treated with a regimen effective against uncomplicated gonococcal and chlamydial infection. An important point is that ≥50% of the sexual partners of women with gonococcal and/or chlamydial PID have subclinical urethral infection and may be unaware of their infection status. Treatment of PID should be considered inadequate until sexual partners have been properly evaluated and treated.

Follow-Up Hospitalized patients should show substantial clinical improvement within 3 to 5 days. Women treated as outpatients should be clinically reevaluated within 72 h. A follow-up telephone survey of women seen in an emergency room and given a prescription

Table 133-3 Combination Antimicrobial Regimens Recommended for Outpatient Treatment or for Parenteral Treatment of PID

Outpatient Regimens	Parenteral Regimens
Regimen A Ofloxacin 400 mg PO bid for 14 days *plus* Metronidazole 500 mg PO bid for 14 days	**Regimen A** Initiate parenteral therapy with either of the following regimens; continue parenteral therapy until 48 h after clinical improvement; then change to outpatient therapy, as described in text.
Regimen B Ceftriaxone 250 mg IM once *plus* Doxycycline 100 mg PO bid for 14 days *plus*[a] Metronidazole 500 mg PO bid for 14 days	Cefotetan 2 g IV q12h *or* Cefoxitin 2 g IV q6h *plus* Doxycycline 100 mg IV or PO q12h **Regimen B** Clindamycin 900 mg IV q8h *plus* Gentamicin, loading dose of 2 mg/kg IV or IM, then maintenance dose of 1.5 mg/kg q8h

[a] The addition of metronidazole is recommended by some experts.

SOURCE: Adapted from Centers for Disease Control and Prevention: MMWR 47:1, 1998.

for 10 days of oral doxycycline for PID found that 28% never filled the prescription and 41% stopped taking medication early (after an average of 4.1 days), often because of persistent symptoms, lack of symptoms, or side effects. Women not responding favorably to ambulatory therapy should be hospitalized. After completion of treatment, tests for persistent or recurrent infection with *N. gonorrhoeae* or *C. trachomatis* should be performed if symptoms persist or recur or if the patient has not complied with therapy or has been reexposed to an untreated sex partner.

Removal of an IUD Although a beneficial impact of IUD removal on the response of acute salpingitis to antimicrobial therapy and on the risk of recurrent salpingitis has not been proven, removal of the IUD 2 or 3 days after the initiation of antimicrobial therapy seems reasonable. When an IUD is removed, contraceptive counseling is essential.

Surgery Surgery is necessary for the treatment of salpingitis only in the face of life-threatening infection (such as rupture or threatened rupture of a tuboovarian abscess) or for drainage of an abscess. Ultrasonography and MRI are useful for diagnosing and monitoring pelvic abscesses. Conservative surgical procedures are usually sufficient. Pelvic abscesses can often be drained by posterior colpotomy, and peritoneal lavage can be used if there is generalized peritonitis.

PROGNOSIS Among 900 women who underwent long-term follow-up for a mean period of 8 years after successful treatment of an acute episode of PID with various regimens in Sweden, late sequelae included infertility due to bilateral tubal occlusion, ectopic pregnancy due to tubal scarring without occlusion, chronic pelvic pain, and recurrent salpingitis. Chronic pain lasting >6 months was seen in 18% of patients, and infertility due to tubal occlusion in 17%; 4% of the pregnancies that did occur were ectopic, representing approximately a sixfold increase over the expected rate of ectopic pregnancies. The rate of infertility after salpingitis was found to be related to the age of the patient, the duration of symptoms when treatment was started, the severity of salpingitis (as determined by laparoscopy) at the time of diagnosis, and the number of episodes of salpingitis. The postsalpingitis risk of infertility due to tubal occlusion among sexually active women not using contraceptives was 14% at 15 to 24 years of age and 26% at 25 to 34 years of age; the risk for women of all ages combined was 11% after one episode of salpingitis, 23% after two episodes, and 54% after three or more episodes. Women with chlamydial salpingitis who developed more severe inflammatory damage to the reproductive tract had significantly increased titers of antibody to the chlamydial heat-shock protein HSP60, as did women with infertility or ectopic pregnancy following chlamydial salpingitis. The risk of infertility after treated gonococcal salpingitis appeared lower than that after chlamydial salpingitis or polymicrobial PID. A study of outcomes of PID at the University of Washington found a sevenfold increase in the risk of ectopic pregnancy and an eightfold increase in the rate of hysterectomy after PID.

In several countries, a striking relationship has also been found between infertility due to tubal occlusion and the prevalence and titer of antibody to *C. trachomatis*. Recurrent salpingitis has been seen in ~15 to 25% of women treated for salpingitis in various studies.

PREVENTION Prevention of PID depends first on the effective control of gonococcal and chlamydial infection in the general population. Effective methods include the promotion of changes in sexual behavior and the use of barrier contraceptives together with ensuring ready access to modern methods of diagnosis of these infections and effective treatment of sex partners to control further spread. The decline in popularity of the IUD, particularly among nulliparous women, has undoubtedly helped to reduce the incidence of PID. It is also possible, but not proven, that the use of oral contraceptives and the declining proportion of women who have practiced vaginal douching since the link between douching and PID became known have contributed to lower rates of PID. A randomized controlled trial designed to determine whether selective screening for chlamydial infection reduced the risk of subsequent PID showed that women randomized to undergo screening had a 56% lower rate of PID over the following year than did women receiving the usual care without screening. This report strongly supports risk-based screening for *Chlamydia* as a highly effective way to reduce the incidence of PID and the prevalence of post-PID sequelae.

The complications and sequelae of salpingitis are minimized by early diagnosis and prompt effective treatment. It seems logical, but is unproven, that broad-spectrum therapy effective against all of the common causes of PID offers the best outcome. Although few methodologically sound clinical trials (especially with prolonged follow-up) have been conducted, one meta-analysis showed a benefit of providing good coverage against anaerobes. One placebo-controlled study showed that concurrent anti-inflammatory therapy with prednisolone hastened the reduction of acute inflammatory changes but did not improve the end results, as measured by fertility, hysterosalpingographic findings, or chronic pain. The potential value of anti-inflammatory therapy remains to be evaluated adequately.

BIBLIOGRAPHY

CENTERS FOR DISEASE CONTROL AND PREVENTION: 1998 Guidelines for treatment of sexually transmitted diseases. MMWR 47(RR-1):1, 1998

COHEN CR et al: Effect of human immunodeficiency virus type 1 infection upon acute salpingitis: A laparoscopic study. J Infect Dis 178:1352, 1998

HILLIER SL et al: Role of bacterial vaginosis–associated microorganisms in endometritis. Am J Obstet Gynecol 175:435, 1996

KIVIAT N et al: Endometrial histopathology in patients with culture-proven upper genital tract infection and laparoscopically diagnosed acute salpingitis. Am J Surg Pathol 14: 167, 1990

RASMUSSEN SJ et al: Secretion of proinflammatory cytokines by epithelial cells in response to chlamydial infection suggests a central role for chlamydial pathogenesis. J Clin Invest 99:77, 1997

SCHOLES D et al: Prevention of pelvic inflammatory disease by screening for cervical chlamydial infection. N Engl J Med 334:1362, 1996

WALKER CK et al: Pelvic inflammatory disease: Meta-analysis of antimicrobial regimen efficacy. J Infect Dis 168:969, 1993

——— et al: Anaerobes in pelvic inflammatory disease: Implications for the Centers for Disease Control and Prevention's guidelines for the treatment of sexually transmitted diseases. Clin Infect Dis 28(Suppl 1):S29, 1999

WASSERHEIT JN et al: Microbial causes of proven pelvic inflammatory disease and efficacy of clindamycin with tobramycin. Ann Intern Med 104:187, 1986

WØLNER-HANSSEN P: Silent pelvic inflammatory disease: Is it overstated? Obstet Gynecol 86:321, 1995

Section 3
CLINICAL SYNDROMES: NOSOCOMIAL INFECTIONS

134   *Robert A. Weinstein*

INFECTION CONTROL IN THE HOSPITAL

The costs of nosocomial (hospital-acquired) infections are great. It is estimated that nosocomial infections cost $4.5 billion and contribute to 88,000 deaths annually. Although infection-control and hospital epidemiology activities have been the subjects of increasing scientific study over the past 30 years, efforts to lower infection risks have been continually challenged by the growing numbers of immunocompromised patients, antibiotic-resistant bacteria, fungal and viral superinfections, and invasive devices and procedures. Four international decennial conferences on infection control, organized by the Centers for Disease Control and Prevention (CDC), have clearly documented these formidable trends. This chapter reviews the basic surveillance and prevention activities that have been developed to deal with these problems and that form the foundation for current hospital epidemiology programs.

ORGANIZATION AND RESPONSIBILITIES OF INFECTION-CONTROL PROGRAMS   The standards of the Joint Commission on Accreditation of Healthcare Organizations require all accredited hospitals to have an active program for surveillance, prevention, and control of nosocomial infections; a multidisciplinary infection-control committee usually oversees the program. The agents of the committee are the chairperson, who is preferably an infectious disease physician, and the infection-control practitioners, who are usually trained in nursing or medical technology and in epidemiology and public health. Education of physicians in infection control and hospital epidemiology is required in infectious disease fellowship programs and is available in courses provided by professional societies, primarily the Society for Healthcare Epidemiology of America.

In the 1970s, the CDC's extensive Study on the Efficacy of Nosocomial Infection Control found that nosocomial infection rates fell by 32% in hospitals that established programs with organized surveillance and control activities; a trained, effectual infection-control physician; and one infection-control practitioner per 250 beds. In contrast, rates in hospitals without effective programs increased by 18%. Since that study, the responsibilities and roles of hospital epidemiology programs have expanded in several directions. Diagnosis-related reimbursement has led hospital administrators to place increased emphasis on cost containment and on documentation of the cost-effectiveness of infection control. The quality-improvement movements and the Joint Commission have redirected infection-control attention, in part, beyond the mere writing of policies and procedures to improvement of the actual processes and optimization of outcomes. In a few hospitals, epidemiology programs have taken on additional pharmaco-epidemiologic and antibiotic-use review responsibilities. Finally, all programs must now respond to increasing governmental regulation of hospital waste and to standards mandated by the Occupational Safety and Health Administration for protecting health care workers from occupational exposure to bloodborne pathogens and tuberculosis.

SURVEILLANCE   Traditionally, infection-control practitioners survey inpatients for nosocomial infections (defined as those neither present nor incubating at the time of admission). Surveillance involves a review of microbiology laboratory results, "shoe-leather" epidemiology on the nursing wards, application of standardized definitions of infection, ongoing dialogue with hospital workers, and common sense. Some innovative infection-control programs have taken advantage of the increased use of computerized pharmacy, microbiology, and other databases in hospitals to create algorithm-driven surveillance activities.

Most hospitals aim surveillance at infections that (1) are associated with a high level of morbidity, e.g., intensive care unit (ICU)–related infections and nosocomial pneumonia; (2) are costly, e.g., cardiac surgical wound infections; (3) are difficult to treat, e.g., infections due to antibiotic-resistant bacteria; (4) pose recurring epidemic problems, e.g., *Clostridium difficile*–related diarrhea; and (5) are potentially preventable, e.g., vascular access–related infections. Quality-assurance activities in infection control have led to increased surveillance of the compliance of personnel with infection-control policies (e.g., monitoring of actual adherence to hand-washing recommendations).

The results of surveillance are expressed as rates; for example, 5 to 10% of patients develop nosocomial infections. Although such overall statistics are often requested of hospitals by administrators or surveyors, they have little value unless qualified by site of infection, by patient population, and by exposure to risk factors. Meaningful denominators for infection rates include the number of patients exposed to a specific risk (e.g., rates of pneumonia among patients using mechanical ventilators) and the number of intervention days (e.g., rates of pneumonia per 1000 patient-days on a ventilator).

Temporal trends in rates should be reviewed, and rates should be compared with regional and national norms. However, even comparison rates generated by the CDC's ongoing National Nosocomial Infections Surveillance System, which collects data from more than 270 hospitals that use standardized definitions of nosocomial infections, have not been validated independently and represent a nonrandom sample of hospitals. Interhospital comparisons are easily confounded by the wide range in risk factors and in severity of underlying illnesses; unless rates are adjusted for these factors, comparisons may be misleading. Unfortunately, systems for making such adjustments either are rudimentary or have not been well validated.

The ongoing analysis of an individual hospital's infection rates helps to determine whether control efforts are succeeding and where increased education and control measures should be focused. Knowledge of infection rates is also useful in discussions with the hospital administration regarding areas to which additional resources should be directed.

PREVENTION AND CONTROL MEASURES Epidemiologic Basis and General Measures Nosocomial infections follow basic epidemiologic patterns that can help to direct prevention and control measures. Nosocomial pathogens have reservoirs, are transmitted by predictable routes, and require susceptible hosts. Reservoirs and sources exist in the inanimate environment (e.g., tap water contaminated with *Legionella*) and in the animate environment (e.g., infected or colonized health care workers, patients, and hospital visitors). The mode of transmission most often is either cross-infection (e.g., indirect spread of pathogens from one patient to another on the inadequately washed hands of hospital personnel) or autoinoculation (e.g., aspiration of oropharyngeal flora into the lung along an endotracheal tube). Occasionally, pathogens (e.g., group A streptococci and many respiratory viruses) are spread indirectly from person to person via infectious droplets released by coughing or sneezing. Much less common—but often devastating in terms of epidemic risk—is true airborne spread of droplet nuclei (as in nosocomial chickenpox) or common-source spread by contaminated materials (e.g., iodophors contaminated with *Pseudomonas*). Factors that increase host susceptibility include underlying conditions and the many medical-surgical interventions and procedures that bypass or compromise normal host defenses.

Through its program, the hospital's infection-control committee must determine the general and specific measures used to control infections and must review and recommend specific antiseptics and disinfectants for hospital use. Given the prominence of cross-infection, hand washing is the single most important preventive measure in hospitals. Many studies have examined the antimicrobial activity of a wide variety of antiseptic-containing hand-washing agents. The use of such medicated agents is important before invasive procedures and possibly in ICU settings. In light of the poor general compliance with hand-washing recommendations, the importance of using any hand cleanser between patient contacts cannot be overemphasized (Table 134-1).

Table 134-1 Examples of Ways in Which Physicians Can Contribute to Infection-Control Efforts

- Act as role models for other personnel by paying careful attention to hand-washing recommendations and barrier precautions during contact with patients and by observing posted isolation precautions.
- Give corrective feedback to caregivers who do not adhere to hand-washing recommendations or isolation precautions.
- Place invasive devices based on clinical need (not just on convenience).
- Remove invasive devices promptly when they are no longer needed clinically.
- Limit surgical antimicrobial prophylaxis to the perioperative period.
- Exercise care in initial empirical antibiotic selection (avoid "shotgun" approaches).
- Narrow the spectrum of antibiotic therapy once a pathogen is recovered.
- Discontinue antibiotic therapy in a timely fashion.
- Become familiar with the hospital's bloodborne pathogen and tuberculosis control plans.
- Order appropriate isolation precautions promptly for infected patients.
- During patient rounds, alert nursing staff to lapses in asepsis (e.g., soiled dressings at sites of intravascular catheters) and to infection-predisposing situations (e.g., aspiration-prone positioning of patients).
- Notify infection-control practitioners of potential infection-control problems (e.g., surgical wound infections that manifest after a patient's discharge).

The fact that 25 to 50% of nosocomial infections are due to the combined effect of the patient's own flora and invasive devices highlights the importance of improvements in the use and design of such devices (Chap. 135). Intensive educational programs can be associated with at least a temporary reduction in infection rates through improved asepsis in handling and earlier removal of invasive devices, but the maintenance of such gains is often difficult. Epidemiologic studies are used increasingly to assess the value of newer devices and site-specific control measures and to debunk some traditional yet ineffective and costly measures, such as routine culturing of the environment and personnel for "pathogens."

Urinary Tract Infections Approaches to the prevention of urinary tract infections have included the use of topical meatal antimicrobials, drainage bag disinfectants, antimicrobial-coated catheters, and sealed catheter–drainage tube junctions to eliminate inadvertent breaks in the system. Because of conflicting study results, none of these measures is considered routine. Systemic antimicrobials given for other purposes decrease the risk of urinary tract infection during the first 4 days of catheterization, after which resistant bacteria or yeasts emerge as pathogens. Selective decontamination of the gut is also associated with a reduced risk. Again, however, neither approach is routine. Irrigation of catheters, with or without antimicrobials, may actually increase the risk of infection.

Pneumonia Control measures for pneumonia are aimed at the remediation of risk factors in general patient care (e.g., minimizing aspiration-prone supine positioning) and at meticulous aseptic care of respirator equipment (e.g., disinfecting or sterilizing all in-line reusable components such as nebulizers, replacing tubing circuits at intervals of >48 h—rather than more frequently—to lessen the number of breaks in the system, and teaching aseptic technique for suctioning). In a large multicenter trial, sucralfate, which provides stress-ulcer prophylaxis without altering gastric pH, did not reduce the risk of ventilator-associated pneumonia, despite the theoretical advantage of lessened risk for gastric colonization by gram-negative bacilli. The benefit of selective decontamination of the oropharynx and gut with nonabsorbable antimicrobials has been controversial.

Surgical Wound Infections The most important control measures for surgical wound infections include the use of antimicrobial prophylaxis at the start of high-risk procedures, attention to technical surgical issues and operating-room asepsis (e.g., not shaving the operative site until surgery and avoiding open or prophylactic drains), and preoperative therapy for active infection. In one study, rates of postoperative infection were lower among patients who had normothermia maintained during colorectal surgery. Reporting of surveil-

The increasingly extensive review of infection rates by regulatory agencies and third-party payers emphasizes the importance of stratifying rates by patient-related risk factors and of developing meaningful systems for interhospital comparisons and for wound surveillance after the patient's discharge from the hospital or clinic (when more than 50% of infections first become apparent).

Infections Related to Vascular Access and Monitoring (See also Chap. 135)   Control measures for infections associated with vascular access and monitoring include the moving of peripheral or arterial catheters to a new site at specified intervals (e.g., every 72 h for peripheral intravenous catheters), which may be facilitated by use of an intravenous team; application of disposable transducers and aseptic technique for the accessing of transducers or other vascular ports; removal of "idle" catheters; and consideration of use of central venous catheters impregnated with anti-infective agents. Unresolved issues include the best frequency for the rotation of central venous catheter sites (guidewire-assisted catheter changes at the same site do not lessen infection risk); the best antiseptics for site preparation and for catheter dressing; the appropriate role for mupirocin ointment, a topical antibiotic with excellent antistaphylococcal activity, in site care; and the relative degrees of risk posed by percutaneous central catheters and by newer designs—tunneled, totally implanted, or peripherally inserted central catheters (PICC lines). Improvements in composition of semitransparent access-site dressings and potential nursing benefits (ease of bathing and site inspection and protection of the site from secretions) favor use of such coverings.

Isolation Techniques   Written policies for the isolation of infectious patients are a standard component of infection-control programs. In 1996, the CDC revised its isolation guidelines to be simpler; to recognize the importance of all body fluids, secretions, and excretions in the transmission of nosocomial pathogens; and to focus precautions on the major routes of infection transmission.

The revised guidelines contain two tiers of precautions. *Standard precautions* are designed for the care of all patients in hospitals to reduce the risk of transmission of microorganisms from both recognized and unrecognized sources of infection. These precautions include gloving, as well as hand washing, for potential contact with blood; with all other body fluids, secretions, and excretions, regardless of whether they contain visible blood; with nonintact skin; and with mucous membranes. Depending on exposure risks, standard precautions also include use of masks, eye protection, and gowns.

In the second tier are precautions for the care of patients with suspected or diagnosed colonization or infection with transmissible pathogens. These transmission-based guidelines collapse the older category- and disease-specific isolation guidelines into three sets of precautions based on probable routes of transmission: *airborne precautions*, *droplet precautions*, and *contact precautions*. Sets of precautions may be combined for diseases that have more than one route of transmission (e.g., varicella). Potentially contagious clinical syndromes, such as acute diarrhea, are included in the revised guidelines.

Because some prevalent antibiotic-resistant pathogens, particularly vancomycin-resistant enterococci (VRE), may be present on *intact* skin of patients in hospitals, some experts recommend gloving for all contact with patients who are acutely ill and/or from high-risk units, such as ICUs. In recent trials, wearing gloves did not replace the need for hand washing because hands occasionally became contaminated during wearing or removal of gloves. Some studies have suggested that use of gowns and gloves compared with routine care of patients (i.e., using neither of these barriers) decreases the risk of nosocomial infection; however, more recent evaluation suggests that gowning by personnel does not add benefit beyond that conferred by gloving and hand washing. Nevertheless, requiring increased precaution levels can improve the compliance of health care workers with isolation recommendations by 30%.

EPIDEMIC PROBLEMS   Outbreaks are always big news but probably account for fewer than 5% of nosocomial infections. The investigation and control of epidemics in hospitals require that infection-control personnel develop a case definition, confirm that an outbreak really exists (since many apparent epidemics are actually pseudo-outbreaks due to surveillance or laboratory artifacts), review aseptic practices and disinfectant use, determine the extent of the outbreak, perform an epidemiologic investigation to determine modes of transmission, work closely with microbiology personnel to culture for common sources or personnel carriers as appropriate and to type epidemiologically important isolates, and heighten surveillance to judge the effect of control measures. Control measures generally include the early reinforcement of routine aseptic practices during a search for compliance problems that may have fostered the outbreak, the ensuring of the appropriate isolation of cases (and the institution of cohort isolation and nursing if needed), and the implementation of further controls on the basis of the findings of the investigation. Examples of some potential epidemic problems follow.

Chickenpox   When health care workers are exposed to chickenpox in the community or through patients with initially unrecognized infections, or when these employees work during the 24 h before developing chickenpox, infection-control practitioners institute a varicella exposure investigation and control plan. The names of exposed workers and patients are obtained; medical histories are reviewed, and (if necessary) serologic tests for immunity are conducted; physicians are notified of susceptible exposed patients; postexposure prophylaxis with varicella-zoster immune globulin (VZIG) is considered for immunocompromised or pregnant contacts (see Table 183-1); preemptive use of acyclovir is considered as an alternative strategy in some susceptible persons; and susceptible exposed employees are furloughed during the at-risk period for disease (8 to 21 days, or 28 days if VZIG has been administered). Preexposure varicella vaccination can markedly decrease risk for susceptible employees.

Tuberculosis   The resurgence of pulmonary tuberculosis in the United States since 1987 and a series of nosocomial outbreaks of infection with multidrug-resistant strains—primarily involving patients with AIDS and their caregivers—have led to a reevaluation of tuberculosis control. Important control measures include prompt recognition, isolation, and treatment of cases; recognition of atypical presentations (e.g., lower-lobe infiltrates without cavitation); use of negative pressure, 100% exhaust, private isolation rooms with closed doors, and six air changes per hour; use of face masks (approved by the National Institute for Occupational Safety and Health) by caregivers entering isolation rooms; possible use of high-efficiency particulate air filter units and/or ultraviolet lights for disinfecting air when other engineering controls are not feasible or reliable; and follow-up skin-testing of susceptible personnel who have been exposed to infectious patients before isolation.

Group A Streptococci   The potential for a group A streptococcal outbreak should be considered when even a single nosocomial case occurs. Most outbreaks involve surgical wounds and are due to the presence of an asymptomatic carrier in the operating room. Investigation can be confounded by carriage at extrapharyngeal sites such as the rectum and vagina. Health care workers in whom carriage has been linked to nosocomial transmission of group A streptococci are removed from the patient-care setting and are not permitted to return until carriage has been eliminated by antimicrobial therapy.

Aspergillus   *Aspergillus* spores are common in the environment, particularly on dusty surfaces. When hospital ceiling tiles are removed to provide access for electrical wiring or plumbing or when dusty areas are disturbed during hospital renovation, the spores become airborne. Inhalation of spores by immunosuppressed (particularly neutropenic) patients creates a risk of pulmonary and/or paranasal sinus infection and disseminated aspergillosis. Routine surveillance among neutropenic patients for infections with filamentous fungi, such as *Aspergillus* and *Fusarium*, helps hospitals to determine whether they have unduly large environmental loads of these organisms. To lower the risk, hospitals should inspect and clean air-handling equipment on a routine schedule, review all planned hospital renovations with infection-control personnel and subsequently construct appropriate barriers, remove immunosuppressed patients from renovation sites, and consider the use of high-efficiency particulate air filters for rooms housing immunosuppressed patients.

Legionella Sporadic and epidemic cases of nosocomial *Legionella* pneumonia are most often due to the contamination of potable water and predominantly affect immunosuppressed patients, particularly those receiving glucocorticoid medication. The risk varies greatly within and among geographic regions, depending on the extent of hospital hot-water contamination, on the presence or absence of high-risk patient populations, and on specific hospital practices (e.g., inappropriate use of nonsterile water in respiratory therapy equipment). Laboratory-based surveillance for nosocomial *Legionella* should be performed, and a diagnosis of legionellosis should probably be considered more often than it is. If cases are detected, environmental samples (e.g., tap water) should be cultured. If cultures yield *Legionella* and if typing of clinical and environmental isolates reveals a correlation, eradication measures should be pursued (Chap. 151). An alternative approach is to periodically culture tap water on wards housing high-risk patients. If *Legionella* is found, a concerted effort should be made to culture samples from all patients with nosocomial pneumonia for *Legionella*.

Antibiotic-Resistant Bacteria Outbreaks of antibiotic resistance can depend on any of the following events: Darwinian selection of bacterial chromosomal mutations, spread of plasmid- and/or transposon-borne resistance among bacterial species, and (re)admission to the hospital of patients chronically infected with resistant bacteria. After the introduction of resistant strains, dissemination occurs by cross-infection on unwashed hands of caregivers or, occasionally, via personnel carriage and/or environmental contamination. Outbreak control depends on close laboratory surveillance, with early detection of problems; on the reinforcement of routine asepsis (e.g., hand washing); on the implementation of barrier precautions for all colonized and/or infected patients; on the use of patient-surveillance cultures to more fully ascertain the extent of patient colonization; and on the timely initiation of an epidemiologic investigation when rates increase. Colonized personnel who are implicated in nosocomial transmission and patients who pose a threat may be decontaminated; for example, colonization with methicillin-resistant *Staphylococcus aureus* may be controlled with oral antibiotics, including trimethoprim-sulfamethoxazole and rifampin, and with topical agents, including hexachlorophene or chlorhexidine and mupirocin. In a few ICUs, selective decontamination has been used successfully as a temporary emergency control measure for outbreaks of infection due to gram-negative bacilli.

The most recent bacterial-resistance problem to plague hospitals is the emergence of VRE. Initially an ICU problem, VRE have now spread onto general wards in many hospitals. VRE are particularly problematic because of a substantial "iceberg" effect (i.e., the fact that, for each individual with a clinical infection, many other patients are colonized); the occurrence of both gastrointestinal and skin colonization (reflecting fecal contamination on the skin of ill, hospitalized patients); and the propensity for these organisms to contaminate the patient's environment, which may increase the risk of cross-infection. Control of VRE requires strict attention to hand washing by personnel, concerted use of barrier precautions or cohort nursing for patients known to be colonized or infected, and emphasis on thorough cleaning of the rooms of these patients.

Spread of vancomycin resistance to *S. aureus* is a major concern. Clinical infections with methicillin-resistant *S. aureus* strains that exhibit reduced susceptibility to vancomycin have been reported in a few patients, usually in the setting of prolonged or repeated treatment with vancomycin. The detection of these strains requires augmented laboratory activities, and their identification should trigger an aggressive epidemiologic investigation and aggressive infection-control measures.

Because the excessive use of broad-spectrum antibiotics underlies many resistance problems, antibiotic-control policies (Table 134-2)

Table 134-2 Elements of an Antibiotic-Control Program

- Review antimicrobial agents and select a basic formulary.
- Establish prophylactic, empirical, and therapeutic guidelines.
- Restrict the use of agents that have special limited indications, cause excessive toxicity, or are costly.
- Release restricted agents for use in predetermined circumstances or after prospective approval.
- Ensure that the antibiotics on the formulary are the same as those being used for susceptibility testing by the microbiology laboratory.
- Monitor patterns of antibiotic susceptibility and trends in antibiotic use, providing regular feedback to the medical staff.
- Audit the use of specific antibiotics.
- Conduct ongoing educational programs.
- Regulate in-hospital promotional efforts of pharmaceutical companies.

SOURCE: After JP Flaherty, RA Weinstein, Infect Control Hosp Epidemiol 17:236, 1996.

must be considered a cornerstone of resistance-control efforts. Although the efficacy of antibiotic-control measures in reducing rates of antimicrobial resistance has not been proved in prospective controlled trials, it seems worthwhile to restrict the use of particular agents to narrowly defined indications or possibly to cycle the use of antibiotic classes to limit selective pressure on the nosocomial flora.

EMPLOYEE HEALTH SERVICE ISSUES An institution's employee health service is a critical component of its infection-control efforts. New employees should be processed through the service, where a contagious-disease history can be taken; evidence of immunity to a variety of diseases, such as hepatitis B, chickenpox, measles, and rubella, can be sought; immunizations for hepatitis B, measles, rubella, and varicella can be given as needed and a reminder about the need for yearly influenza immunization can be imparted; baseline and "booster" purified protein derivative of tuberculin skin-testing can be performed; and education about personal responsibility for infection control can be initiated. Evaluations of employees should be codified to meet the requirements of accrediting and regulatory agencies.

The employee health service must have protocols for dealing with workers who have been exposed to contagious diseases, such as those percutaneously or mucosally exposed to the blood of patients infected with HIV. Postexposure HIV prophylaxis with a combination of antiretroviral agents (e.g., zidovudine and lamivudine, with or without indinavir or nelfinavir) is recommended. Protocols are also needed for dealing with caregivers who have common contagious diseases, such as chickenpox, group A streptococcal infections, respiratory infections, and infectious diarrhea, and for those who have less common but high-visibility public health problems, such as chronic hepatitis B or C or HIV infection, for which exposure-control guidelines have been published by the CDC and by the Society for Healthcare Epidemiology of America.

BIBLIOGRAPHY

BENNETT JV, BRACHMAN PS (eds): *Hospital Infections*, 5th ed. Philadelphia, Lippincott-Raven, 1998

BOLYARD EA et al: Guideline for infection control in healthcare personnel, 1998. Infect Control Hosp Epidemiol 19:411, 1998

CENTERS FOR DISEASE CONTROL: Report of the National Nosocomial Infections Surveillance (NNIS) System: Nosocomial infection rates for interhospital comparison: Limitations and possible solutions. Infect Control Hosp Epidemiol 12:609, 1991

GARNER JS, INFECTION CONTROL PRACTICES ADVISORY COMMITTEE: Guideline for isolation precautions in hospitals. Infect Control Hosp Epidemiol 17:53, 1996

GOLDMANN DA et al: Strategies to prevent and control the emergence and spread of antimicrobial-resistant microorganisms in hospitals—a challenge to hospital leadership. JAMA 275:234, 1996

KLEMPNER MS (ed): Hospital infections and health-care epidemiology, in *Infectious Diseases Medical Knowledge Self-Assessment Program*, 2d ed. Philadelphia, American College of Physicians, 1998

MAYHALL CG (ed): *Hospital Epidemiology and Infection Control*, 2d ed. New York, Lippincott Williams & Wilkins, 1999

SCHECKLER WE et al: Requirements for infrastructure and essential activities of infection control and epidemiology in hospitals: A consensus panel report. Infect Control Hosp Epidemiol 19:114, 1998

WEINSTEIN RA: Nosocomial infection update. Emerg Infect Dis 4:416, 1998

135

Dori F. Zaleznik

HOSPITAL-ACQUIRED
AND INTRAVASCULAR
DEVICE–RELATED INFECTIONS

Nosocomial infections are defined as infections acquired during or as a result of hospitalization. Generally, a patient who has been in the hospital for <48 h and develops an infection is considered to have been incubating the infection before hospital admission. Most infections that become manifest after 48 h are considered to be nosocomial. A patient may develop a nosocomial infection after being discharged from the hospital if the organism apparently was acquired in the hospital. Surgical wound infection developing in the weeks after hospital discharge is an example of such nosocomial infection.

INCIDENCE AND COSTS Nosocomial infections contribute significantly to morbidity and mortality as well as to excess costs for hospitalized patients. It is estimated that 5% of patients admitted to an acute care hospital in the United States acquire a new infection, with >2 million nosocomial infections per year and an annual cost of >$2 billion. Some authorities estimate that the odds of death are doubled for patients who develop a nosocomial infection, although clearly such factors as underlying disease and severity of illness also play an important role in outcome.

Although immunosuppressed hosts are especially vulnerable to infections acquired in a hospital, common nosocomial infections occur even in immunocompetent hosts. The National Nosocomial Infections Surveillance (NNIS) Registry has been monitoring nosocomial infection rates since 1970. Its most recent report covers the period from October 1996 through April 1998 and includes both teaching and non-teaching hospitals and both small and large facilities. The most common nosocomial infections have remained the same. Urinary tract infections (UTIs), pneumonia, and surgical-site infections (SSIs, formerly termed wound infections) are most frequent. However, primary bloodstream infections, especially those associated with intravascular devices, have increased in frequency, as have infections in medical and surgical intensive care units (ICUs) and infections caused by antimicrobial-resistant pathogens.

The potential impact of nosocomial infections is considerable when assessed in terms of incidence, morbidity, mortality, and financial burden. Analyses of these factors examine nosocomial infections as both medical and economic issues. The clinical problem facing the physician is the development of a new fever in a patient in the hospital. In the evaluation of such a patient, information about the most common categories of infection may not be sufficient. Rather, the clinician must also use clinical clues from the patient's presentation and hospitalization to diagnose a nosocomial infection.

Approach to the Patient

The evaluation of a hospitalized patient with new fever should include a careful history (Chap. 17). Particular attention should be paid to symptoms of headache, cough, abdominal pain, diarrhea, flank pain, dysuria, urinary frequency, and leg pain. Other features related to the patient's hospitalization are also important, such as the presence and type of intravenous devices, the past or current use of a urinary catheter, the surgical procedure conducted (if any), and the new medications administered, including those for surgical prophylaxis. The physical examination should be directed at possible sources of infection and should focus particularly on the skin (with a search for rash or embolic lesions); the lungs; the abdomen (especially the right upper quadrant); the costovertebral angles; surgical wounds; the calves; and current and old intravenous access sites (for signs of phlebitis). The laboratory evaluation of all hospitalized patients with new fever should include a complete blood count with differential, a chest radiograph, and blood and urine cultures. Other diagnostic tests to consider include liver function tests, plain-film or other studies of the abdomen, routine aerobic cultures of sputum or other relevant body fluids, and (in cases of diarrhea) testing of stool for *Clostridium difficile* toxin.

CATEGORIES OF INFECTION **Pneumonia** Certainly the astute clinician will question the patient thoroughly and perform a rapid comprehensive physical examination. One way to continue the approach to the hospitalized patient with a new fever is to consider potential infections that may be life-threatening, such as pneumonia. Most at risk for developing nosocomial pneumonia are patients in an ICU, especially those who are intubated; patients with an altered level of consciousness, especially those with nasogastric tubes; elderly patients; patients with chronic lung disease; postoperative patients; and any of the above patients taking H_2 blockers or antacids. Nosocomial pneumonia in the NNIS Registry is diagnosed 4 to 7 times per 1000 hospitalizations. Among patients on ventilators, the occurrence of pneumonia is estimated at 15 cases per 1000 ventilator days in medical and surgical ICUs. Mortality figures for nosocomial pneumonia are as high as 50%.

Oropharyngeal and gastric colonization plays a critical role in the pathogenesis of pneumonia in hospitalized patients. The oropharynx can become colonized by many species of aerobic gram-negative organisms within 48 h of the patient's hospitalization; aspiration occurs commonly during sleep and is increased by such factors as a nasogastric tube, altered consciousness, decreased gag reflex, or delayed gastric emptying. As for gastric colonization, bacterial counts in the stomach rise in the presence of medications that raise gastric pH, such as H_2 blockers and antacids, as well as in malnourished, achlorhydric, and some elderly patients. The prevalence of pneumonia is reportedly two to three times higher among intubated patients receiving H_2 blockers or antacids for stress-ulcer prophylaxis than among intubated patients receiving sucralfate, a medication that heals ulcers without altering gastric pH. Gastric colonization is believed to influence the development of pneumonia by retrograde colonization of the oropharynx. Ventilated patients are also at risk of developing pneumonia by exposure to bacteria leaking around the cuff of the endotracheal tube or to bacteria from nebulizers, condensate within ventilator circuits, or humidifiers.

Outside the ICU, pneumonia should be suspected when a patient develops a new cough, fever, leukocytosis, sputum production, and a new infiltrate on chest x-ray. Diagnosis can be complicated in patients with congestive heart failure who have concomitant chest x-ray abnormalities or in patients with chronic sputum production. Some organisms, such as *Legionella* spp., may not be associated with peripheral leukocytosis.

In ICU patients, especially those who are intubated, the signs of pneumonia are relatively subtle, and thus the diagnosis is often relatively complex. In particular, the chest x-rays are difficult to interpret, because fluid overload, congestive heart failure, and acute respiratory distress syndrome (ARDS) are all common findings in intubated patients. Polymorphonuclear leukocytes (PMNs) are often present on Gram-stained preparations of purulent secretions from these patients. An important clue to pneumonia is a change in the output or character of these secretions. If their volume or thickness increases or their color changes, a sputum Gram's stain should be performed and pneumonia seriously considered in the differential diagnosis. Serial Gram's stains are useful, as the number of PMNs may increase substantially and the type(s) of organisms may shift with the development of pneumonia. For example, the baseline sputum sample from an intubated patient may contain about 25 PMNs per high-power field and have mixed gram-positive and gram-negative organisms of several morphologic types in moderate numbers. On the day of a new fever, the same patient may have copious amounts of more tenacious sputum with more PMNs and a predominance of enteric-appearing gram-negative rods. Even without distinct changes in the chest x-ray, this patient would be considered to have developed pneumonia. Another subtle sign of pneumonia in the intubated patient is a requirement for change in ventilator settings in the absence of fluid overload, a mechanical alteration (e.g., a shift in endotracheal tube placement), or a pneumothorax.

The major organisms of concern in nosocomial pneumonia are gram-negative aerobic bacteria. *Pseudomonas aeruginosa* was the most common isolate in the NNIS survey of ICUs, with a frequency of 21%; *Staphylococcus aureus* was next most common at 20%. *Acinetobacter* has become a more common pathogen in ventilator-associated pneumonia. While surveys of organisms are useful, it is essential to know which pathogens are common in a given institution, as hospitals and especially ICUs differ in their resident flora. In some institutions, methicillin-resistant *S. aureus, Stenotrophomonas* (formerly *Xanthomonas*) *maltophilia, Flavobacterium* spp., and even *Legionella* spp. may be of particular concern. Viruses such as respiratory syncytial virus and adenovirus are receiving increased attention as etiologic agents of nosocomial pneumonia in both adults and children. In the past, viruses have been underrepresented in statistics on the agents of nosocomial pneumonia because the diagnosis of viral infection is more difficult and because many microbiology laboratories do not have the capability to isolate viruses.

Antibiotic resistance is another important issue to address in the management of a hospitalized patient. An outgrowth of the NNIS surveys is Project ICARE, which tracks antibiotic usage patterns and resistance rates in a subset of NNIS institutions. Rates of resistance are generally higher in ICUs and track with increased use of antibiotics. *P. aeruginosa, Enterobacter* spp., and enterococci are the pathogens of greatest concern in the development of antibiotic resistance. In addition to knowing the sensitivity patterns of the hospital flora, one must consider whether a patient has received continuous or multiple courses of antibiotic therapy. To reduce the likelihood of altering the sensitivity patterns of the patient's flora, antibiotic courses for pneumonia should be kept as short as possible, with coverage as narrow as possible for the organism(s) involved.

Bacteremia　Another potentially life-threatening nosocomial infection to consider in the evaluation of the patient with a new fever is bacteremia, which is usually related to the presence of an intravascular device (Chap. 134). While many common nosocomial infections such as pneumonia or UTI can be accompanied by bacteremia, primary bacteremia is defined by isolation of a recognized pathogen from the blood without an infection at another site. One carefully controlled study reported bloodstream infection in 2.7% of admissions to a surgical ICU, with 50% mortality and a prolongation of hospitalization by 24 days in survivors.

One difficulty in assessing the significance of bacteremia is to distinguish true pathogens from contaminating skin flora. This distinction is especially important in establishing an infection of an indwelling intravascular catheter because organisms that inhabit the skin, such as coagulase-negative staphylococci, also frequently cause infection. The most common point of entry for infection related to intravascular devices is the insertion site, with spread of the infection along the outside of the device initially. Other means of entry for infecting organisms include introduction via contaminated infusates or tubing, ports, or leaking connections and hematogenous seeding of a catheter during bacteremia. While gram-negative aerobic bacilli are probably the most feared nosocomial bloodstream pathogens, the NNIS data for 1980 through 1989 showed that the isolation of these organisms had not increased in frequency over the decade. The frequency of bloodstream isolation increased the most for coagulase-negative staphylococci, with the next highest increase for *Candida* spp. Other leading causes of line-related bacteremia were *S. aureus* and enterococci. Subsequent studies confirmed these findings. Nosocomial endocarditis is an important, newly recognized entity that develops largely as a complication of invasive procedures or intravascular devices and may account for as many as 10% of cases of infective endocarditis.

Establishing an infection of an intravascular device or primary bacteremia as the cause of fever in a hospitalized patient is a diagnosis of exclusion. If a patient has a fever and signs of cutaneous involvement (erythema, induration, tenderness, or purulent drainage) at the insertion site of a catheter, full cultures should be performed, the vascular-access line removed, and the catheter tip sent for quantitative culture. Studies have correlated the growth of ≥15 colonies from a catheter tip with infection of the line. More commonly, the exit site does not show signs of infection, and there is considerable debate about the necessity of removing a line from a febrile patient at that point. Although line changes over a guidewire have been shown to be safe, unless another site of infection is obvious, it is generally advisable to remove the line and to change the site when a patient develops a new fever. The traditional teaching is that an infected intravenous device should be removed. In current practice, however, especially with surgically implanted intravenous catheters, a decision may be made to attempt treatment with antibiotics while leaving the catheter in place. This practice is often successful when the infecting organism is a coagulase-negative *Staphylococcus* species but is less often effective with other organisms, particularly *Candida* spp. and gram-negative bacilli. Salvage of catheters used for hemodialysis is especially important and has been successfully accomplished with infections caused by a variety of organisms.

Another controversial management issue is whether to draw blood for culture through a line. While some studies report a correlation in the 90% range between culture results for blood drawn through vascular-access lines and those for peripheral blood, the former cultures can be either false-positive or false-negative. If the line culture is positive and no peripheral blood has been drawn, it is impossible to determine whether the patient has true bacteremia or the culture merely reflects bacteria associated with the line. Whether bacteremia is high- or low-grade and whether it is sustained or transient may influence the duration of antibiotic therapy and cannot be determined from cultures of blood specimens obtained through a line.

An area of considerable interest and controversy is the prevention of catheter-related infections through the use of intravenous devices impregnated with chlorhexidine/silver sulfadiazine or minocycline/rifampin. A meta-analysis of 11 studies found a decrease in both catheter colonization and catheter-related bacteremia with chlorhexidine/silver sulfadiazine–impregnated catheters, with associated cost savings. One multicenter prospective randomized trial directly compared the two types of catheters and found the minocycline/rifampin-impregnated catheter to be superior. Antibiotic-resistant strains were not recovered in this trial, although concern has been raised that antibiotic impregnation may increase the development of resistance. The several other studies that do not support these findings include one in which the incidence of bacteremia did not decrease with the use of chlorhexidine/silver sulfadiazine–impregnated catheters.

Surgical-Site Infection　Evaluation of fever in the postoperative patient must include careful evaluation of the surgical wound. Although SSI reportedly accounts for 19% of nosocomial infections, the true incidence of postoperative wound infection is difficult to assess, particularly at a time when many patients are hospitalized for relatively short periods. In a number of studies, careful follow-up for the development of SSI after discharge—especially observation of the wound by a trained observer, such as a nurse—has shown the actual rates of SSI in all categories of surgery to be greater than the reported rates. SSI rates vary from 4.6 to 8.2% for nonteaching and large teaching hospitals, respectively. Rates also vary by procedure, with abdominal surgery resulting in the highest rates.

Risk factors for the development of postoperative wound infection include the presence of a drain; a long preoperative length of stay, with the rates doubling for each week of preoperative hospitalization; preoperative shaving of the field, especially if performed ≥24 h beforehand; a long duration of surgery; and the presence of an untreated remote infection. Infection rates also vary with the surgeon. Perioperative antibiotic prophylaxis has been shown to decrease rates of wound infection in a number of careful studies, including those of clean surgical procedures. Antibiotic coverage after the surgical wound is closed has not been shown to provide additional benefit.

A surgical wound should be examined for localized tenderness and induration, fluctuance, drainage of purulent material, and dehiscence of sutures. Mechanical factors, as well as infection, can cause wound dehiscence. Sternal wounds following cardiac surgery are of special concern because the consequences of infection can be severe. The surface of the wound may not present an obvious cause for concern, but ongoing fevers, serous drainage, and especially the development of rocking or instability of the sternum may be sufficient cause for surgical exploration of the wound in some cases. Mediastinitis or sternal osteomyelitis is a severe complication of cardiac surgery. Wounds associated with the placement of prosthetic devices, such as mechanical joints, are also of special concern. Infection of these wounds can lead to infection of the prosthesis, and clearance of prosthetic joint infections generally requires surgical removal of the device.

The most common pathogens causing SSI are coagulase-negative *Staphylococcus* and *S. aureus*, but antibiotic-resistant bacteria and fungi are also becoming more frequent etiologies. Early infections may be associated with organisms that produce rapid, progressive skin infection, such as group A *Streptococcus* and *Clostridium* spp. Group A *Streptococcus* has been identified in some cases of recurrent infection of saphenous-vein graft harvest sites.

Urinary Tract Infection UTI, the most common type of nosocomial infection, is generally the easiest to treat and has the least severe sequelae. Four principal risk factors have been associated repeatedly with the development of UTI in hospitalized patients: female sex, prolonged urinary catheterization, lack of systemic antibiotic therapy, and breach of appropriate catheter care. The administration of systemic antibiotics to patients with urinary catheters in place for 1 to 5 days has been associated with a decrease in rates of bacteriuria. For patients with catheters in place for ≥6 days, however, this benefit is not observed.

The pathogenesis of catheter-associated UTI appears to differ in men and women. In women, the typical mechanism involves periurethral colonization with fecal flora and tracking of organisms up the catheter to the bladder; thus the pathogenesis resembles that of UTI in noncatheterized female patients, in whom bacteria track up the short female urethra. In contrast, periurethral colonization often cannot be demonstrated in men; most infections seem to arise from intraluminal spread of organisms to the bladder. Some organisms, such as *Proteus* and *Pseudomonas* spp., appear to facilitate the growth along the inside of the urinary catheter of a biofilm that encrusts and obstructs the flow of urine.

UTI is certainly an extremely common nosocomial infection; however, it is important to define this type of infection precisely. Especially in the evaluation of a febrile hospitalized patient, it is crucial to think carefully about all possible sources of infection and not to assume that UTI is the probable cause. In patients who have had urinary catheters in place for a number of days, fever, dysuria, frequency, leukocytosis, and especially flank pain or costovertebral angle tenderness are highly suggestive of bladder infection or pyelonephritis. In patients with fever but no other symptoms or signs referable to the urinary tract, one should look for ancillary findings suggestive of urinary tract involvement, such as white blood cells without epithelial cells in the urine sediment or leukocyte esterase or nitrite on urinalysis. A urine culture positive for a single organism should not be accepted as definitive evidence of UTI in an asymptomatic patient. While one might treat the febrile patient who has a positive urine culture with antibiotics, it is prudent to repeat the culture before the institution of therapy. Inability to recover any organism or the same organism on repeat culture, particularly if the patient does not respond to antibiotics, should raise questions about the validity of the diagnosis of UTI. In addition, isolation of two or more bacteria from a single specimen is most likely due to contamination unless there is reason to suspect a bladder diverticulum or a perinephric abscess.

Other Infectious Sources of Fever Several other types of infection may cause fever in the hospitalized patient and should be considered in the differential diagnosis of new fever. In patients who have received antibiotics (even a single dose as surgical prophylaxis), antibiotic-associated diarrhea may develop. This condition is usually caused by the spore-forming organism *C. difficile*, which produces toxins that cause diarrhea. Some patients may appear quite toxic with this infection, with high fevers, leukocytosis, and profuse diarrhea. The organism is quite hardy and is difficult to eradicate from the hospital environment. The hands of hospital personnel have been implicated as a mode of transmission of this organism, as have electronic rectal thermometers. The colon may become colonized with *C. difficile* while the patient is in the hospital, but—particularly if the patient is still taking antibiotics when sent home—diarrhea may not develop until after discharge.

Unless patients are consuming foods from outside the hospital, food-borne diarrheal illness is uncommon among hospitalized patients. Thus, an extensive stool evaluation is generally not cost-effective in the management of these patients.

Other infections to consider in the hospitalized patient include decubitus ulcers, particularly in patients in chronic-care wards or confined to bed rest for prolonged periods, and sinusitis, especially in intubated patients.

NONINFECTIOUS SOURCES OF FEVER A consideration of several common noninfectious causes of fever in hospitalized patients is part of a thorough evaluation of new fever. Drug treatment is the foremost noninfectious cause of fever. Drug fever may occur with or without an accompanying rash or eosinophilia and can be caused by a new medication or by medications the patient has been receiving for some time. Particular agents associated with drug fever include phenytoin, H_2 blockers, procainamide, and antibiotics, most notably sulfonamides. Even drug-associated fevers can be quite high in some patients and may take up to 5 days to resolve after discontinuation of treatment with the offending agent. Other noninfectious causes of fever include phlebitis, often at the site of an old intravenous line and sometimes followed by suppurative thrombophlebitis with clots or septic emboli, and pulmonary emboli, especially in patients undergoing prolonged bed rest; prophylactic heparin or mechanical boots are often used to reduce the risk of pulmonary embolism in the latter patients. Other entities to consider include tissue necrosis following surgery, trauma, or burns; hematomas; pancreatitis; atelectasis; and acalculous cholecystitis.

CONCLUSION The range of possibilities for the etiology of a new fever in a hospitalized patient is quite broad. An attention to detail, a careful history and physical examination, and a knowledge of the infections and organisms likely to cause nosocomial problems usually lead to an accurate diagnosis.

BIBLIOGRAPHY

DAROUICHE RO et al: A comparison of two antimicrobial-impregnated central venous catheters. N Engl J Med 340:1, 1999

FRIDKIN SK et al: Surveillance of antimicrobial use and antimicrobial resistance in United States hospitals: Project ICARE phase 2. Project Intensive Care Antimicrobial Resistance Epidemiology (ICARE) hospitals. Clin Infect Dis 29:245, 1999

GARROUSTE-OREGEAS M et al: Oropharyngeal or gastric colonization and nosocomial pneumonia in adult intensive care unit patients. Am J Respir Crit Care Med 156:1647, 1997

GOLUB R et al: Laparoscopic versus open appendectomy: A meta-analysis. J Am Coll Surg 186:545, 1998

MARR KA et al: Catheter-related bacteremia and outcome of attempted catheter salvage in patients undergoing hemodialysis. Ann Intern Med 127:275, 1997

NATIONAL NOSOCOMIAL INFECTIONS SURVEILLANCE (NNIS) SYSTEM: Report, data summary from October 1986–April 1998, issued June 1998. Am J Infect Control 26:522, 1998

RICHARDS MJ et al: Nosocomial infections in medical intensive care units in the United States. National Nosocomial Infections Surveillance System. Crit Care Med 27:887, 1999

VEENSTRA D et al: Efficacy of antiseptic-impregnated central venous catheters in preventing catheter-related bloodstream infection. A meta-analysis. JAMA 281:261, 1999

136   *Robert Finberg, Joyce Fingeroth*

INFECTIONS IN TRANSPLANT RECIPIENTS

BMT	bone marrow transplant	HSCT	hematopoietic stem cell
CMV	cytomegalovirus		transplant
CNS	central nervous system	HSV	herpes simplex virus
CSF	cerebrospinal fluid	IVIG	intravenous immune globulin
EBV	Epstein-Barr virus	LPD	lymphoproliferative disease
GVHD	graft-versus-host disease	MMR	measles/mumps/rubella
HHV	human herpesvirus	RSV	respiratory syncytial virus
HPVs	human papillomaviruses	VZV	varicella-zoster virus

The evaluation of infections in transplant recipients involves consideration of both the donor and the recipient of the transplanted organ. Infections following transplantation are complicated by the use of drugs that are necessary to enhance the likelihood of survival of the transplanted organ but that also cause the host to be immunocompromised. Thus what might have been a latent or asymptomatic infection in an immunocompetent donor or in the recipient prior to therapy becomes a life-threatening problem when the recipient becomes immunosuppressed.

A variety of organisms have been transmitted by organ transplantation (Table 136-1). Careful attention to the sterility of the medium used to process the organ combined with meticulous microbiologic evaluation reduces rates of transmission of bacteria that may be present or grow in the organ culture medium. From 2% to >20% of donor kidneys are estimated to be contaminated with bacteria—in most cases, with the organisms that colonize the skin or grow in the tissue culture medium used to bathe the donor kidney while it awaits implantation. The reported rate of bacterial contamination of transplanted

Table 136-1   Organisms Transmitted by Organ Transplantation and Common Sites of Reactivation Disease

	Site					
Organism	Blood	Lungs	Heart	Brain	Liver	Skin
Viruses						
Cytomegalovirus[a]	+	+	+/−	+	+	+
Epstein-Barr virus[b]	+	+	+	+	+	+
Herpes simplex virus		+			+	+
Human herpesvirus 6	+	+		+		+
Human herpesvirus 8	+					+
Hepatitis B and C viruses					+	
Fungi						
Candida albicans	+	+			+	+
Histoplasma capsulatum	+	+			+	
Cryptococcus	+	+		+		+
Parasites						
Toxoplasma gondii[c]		+	+	+		
Strongyloides stercoralis[d,e]	+					
Trypanosoma cruzi[e]			+			
Plasmodium falciparum[e]	+					

[a] Cytomegalovirus reactivation is prone to occur in the transplanted organ.
[b] Epstein-Barr virus reactivation usually presents as a proliferation of transformed B cells and can either be a diffuse disease or produce a mass lesion in a single organ.
[c] *T. gondii* usually causes disease in the brain. In bone marrow transplant recipients, acute pulmonary disease may also occur.
[d] *Strongyloides* "hyperinfection" may present with pulmonary disease—often associated with bacterial pneumonia.
[e] While transmission with organs has been described, it is unusual.

bone marrow is as high as 17% but is most commonly ~1%. The use of enrichment columns and monoclonal-antibody depletion procedures results in a higher incidence of contamination. Approximately 2% of cryopreserved marrow and peripheral blood stem cells transfused as part of treatment for cancer are contaminated. In one series of patients receiving contaminated products, 14% had fever or bacteremia, but none died. Results of cultures performed at the time of cryopreservation and at the time of thawing were helpful in guiding therapy for the recipient.

In many transplantation centers, transmission of infections that may be latent or clinically inapparent in the donor organ has resulted in the development of specific donor-screening protocols. In addition to ordering serologic studies focusing on viruses such as herpes-group viruses [herpes simplex virus (HSV) 1, HSV-2], varicella-zoster virus (VZV), cytomegalovirus (CMV), human herpesvirus (HHV) 6, Epstein-Barr virus (EBV), HHV-8, hepatitis B and C viruses, and HIV and on parasites such as *Toxoplasma gondii*, clinicians caring for organ donors should consider assessing stool (for parasites) and skin testing for *Mycobacterium tuberculosis*. It is expected that the recipient will have been likewise assessed. This chapter considers aspects of infection unique to various transplantation settings.

INFECTIONS IN BONE MARROW AND HEMATOPOIETIC STEM CELL TRANSPLANT RECIPIENTS

Bone marrow or hematopoietic stem cell transplantation for either immunodeficiency or cancer results in a transient state of complete immune incompetence. Immediately after transplantation, both phagocytes and immune cells (T and B cells) are absent, and the host is extremely susceptible to infection. The reconstitution that follows transplantation has been likened to maturation of the immune system in neonates. The analogy does not entirely predict infections seen in bone marrow transplant (BMT) and hematopoietic stem cell transplant (HSCT) recipients, however, because the new marrow matures in an old host who has several latent infections already.

TIMING OF INFECTIONS   In the first month after bone marrow or hematopoietic stem cell transplantation, infectious complications are similar to those in granulocytopenic patients receiving chemotherapy for acute leukemia (Chap. 85). Because of the anticipated 1- to 4-week duration of neutropenia in this population, many centers give prophylactic antibiotics to patients upon initiation of chemotherapy. Prophylactic trimethoprim-sulfamethoxazole or ciprofloxacin decreases the incidence of gram-negative bacteremia among these patients.

In the second month after transplantation, a major concern (particularly in allogeneic BMT/HSCT recipients) is CMV disease (Chap. 185), which rarely has its onset earlier than 14 days after transplantation and may become evident up to 4 months after the procedure (most commonly at 1 to 3 months). In cases in which the donor marrow is depleted of T cells [to prevent graft-versus-host disease (GVHD) or eliminate a T cell tumor], the disease may be manifested earlier. Patients who receive ganciclovir (for prophylaxis, preemptive treatment, or treatment; see below) may develop CMV infection even later than 4 months after transplantation; treatment appears to delay the development of the normal immune response to CMV infection. Although CMV disease may present as isolated fever, cytopenia, or gastrointestinal disease, the foremost cause of death from CMV infection in this setting is pneumonia.

The diagnosis of pneumonia in BMT/HSCT recipients poses some special problems (Table 85-5). Because patients have undergone treatment with multiple chemotherapeutic agents and sometimes radiation, their differential diagnosis should include—in addition to bacterial pneumonia—CMV pneumonitis, pneumonia of other viral or fungal etiology, parasitic pneumonia, diffuse alveolar hemorrhage, and chemical- or radiation-associated pneumonitis. Since fungal disease and viruses such as respiratory syncytial virus (RSV), parainfluenza virus (types 1, 2, and 3), influenza A and B viruses, and adenovirus are also causes of pneumonia in this setting, it is important to diagnose CMV specifically (see below). *M. tuberculosis* has been an uncommon cause of pneumonia among BMT/HSCT recipients in western countries (<0.1 to 0.2%) but is common in Hong Kong (5.5%) and in countries where the prevalence of tuberculosis is high. The exposure history of the recipient is clearly critical in an assessment of posttransplantation infections.

Episodes of bacteremia due to encapsulated organisms and reactivation of VZV mark the late posttransplantation period (6 months after bone marrow reconstitution). Because of the high and prolonged risk of *Pneumocystis carinii* pneumonia (especially among patients being treated for hematologic malignancies), most patients should be maintained on prophylactic doses of trimethoprim-sulfamethoxazole starting 1 month after engraftment and continuing for at least 1 year. Such prophylaxis may also protect patients seropositive for *T. gondii*, which may cause pneumonia as well as central nervous system (CNS) lesions. The advantages of maintaining patients on daily trimethoprim-sulfamethoxazole for 1 year after transplantation include protection against *Listeria monocytogenes* and nocardial disease as well as late bacterial infections with pneumococci and *Haemophilus influenzae*, which are a consequence of the inability of the immature bone marrow to respond to polysaccharide antigens. In patients with GVHD who require prolonged or indefinite courses of steroids and other immunosuppressive agents (e.g., cyclosporine, tacrolimus), there is a high risk of fungal infections (usually with *Candida* or *Aspergillus*), even after engraftment and resolution of neutropenia.

VIRAL INFECTIONS BMT/HSCT recipients are susceptible to infection with a variety of viruses, including reactivation syndromes caused by most HHVs (Table 136-2) and infections caused by viruses that circulate in the community.

Herpes Simplex Virus Within the first 2 weeks after transplantation, most patients who are seropositive for HSV-1 excrete the virus in the oropharynx. The ability to isolate HSV declines with time. Administration of prophylactic acyclovir to seropositive BMT/HSCT recipients has been shown to reduce mucositis and prevent HSV pneumonia (a rare condition reported almost exclusively in BMT recipients). Both esophagitis (usually due to HSV-1) and anogenital disease (commonly induced by HSV-2) may be prevented with acyclovir prophylaxis. →*For further discussion, see Chap. 182.*

Varicella-Zoster Virus Reactivation of herpes zoster may occur within the first month but more commonly occurs several months after transplantation (see Plate IID-37). Reactivation rates are ~40% for allogeneic recipients and 25% for autologous recipients. Localized zoster can spread in an immunosuppressed patient. Fortunately, disseminated disease can usually be controlled with high doses of acyclovir. Because of the high incidence of dissemination of herpes zoster among patients with skin lesions, acyclovir is given prophylactically in some centers to prevent severe disease. Low doses of acyclovir (400 mg orally, three times daily) appear to be effective in preventing reactivation of VZV. However, acyclovir also inhibits the development of VZV-specific immunity. Thus, its administration for only 6 months after transplantation does not prevent zoster from occurring when treatment is stopped. Some data suggest that administration of low doses of acyclovir for an entire year after transplantation is effective and may eliminate most cases of posttransplantation zoster. →*For further discussion, see Chap. 183.*

Cytomegalovirus The onset of CMV disease usually comes between 30 and 90 days after transplantation, when the granulocyte count is adequate but immunologic reconstitution has not occurred. CMV may cause interstitial pneumonia, bone marrow suppression, or graft failure. With the standard use of CMV-negative or filtered blood products, primary CMV infection should be a risk in allogeneic transplantation only when the donor is CMV-seropositive and the recipient is CMV-seronegative. Reactivation disease or superinfection with another strain from the donor is also common in CMV-positive recipients, and most seropositive patients who undergo bone marrow transplantation excrete CMV, with or without clinical findings. Serious CMV disease is much more common among allogeneic recipients and is often associated with GVHD. In addition to pneumonia and marrow suppression (and, less often, graft failure), manifestations of CMV disease in BMT/HSCT recipients include fever with or without arthralgias, myalgias, and esophagitis. CMV ulcerations occur in both the lower and upper gastrointestinal tract, and it may be difficult to distinguish diarrhea due to GVHD from that due to CMV infection. The finding of CMV in the liver of a patient with GVHD does not necessarily mean that CMV is responsible for hepatic enzyme abnormalities.

Management of CMV disease in BMT/HSCT recipients includes strategies directed at prophylaxis, suppression, preemptive therapy, or treatment. Prophylaxis results in a lower incidence of disease at the cost of treating many patients who otherwise would not require therapy. Because of the high fatality rate associated with CMV pneumonia in these patients and the difficulty of early diagnosis of CMV infection, prophylactic ganciclovir has been used in some centers and has been shown to abort CMV disease during the period of maximal vulnerability (from engraftment to day 120 after transplantation). The foremost problem with the administration of this drug relates to adverse effects, which include dose-related bone marrow suppression (thrombocytopenia, leukopenia, anemia, and pancytopenia). Because the frequency of CMV pneumonia is lower among autologous BMT recipients (2 to 7%) than among allogeneic BMT recipients (10 to 40%), prophylaxis in the former group will not become the rule until a less toxic antiviral agent becomes available.

Like prophylaxis, suppressive treatment, which targets patients with polymerase chain reaction evidence of CMV or CMV-positive urine cultures, entails the unnecessary treatment of many individuals (on the basis of a laboratory test that is not highly predictive of disease) with drugs that have adverse effects. Currently, because of the neutropenia associated with ganciclovir in BMT/HSCT recipients, a preemptive approach—treatment of those patients in whose blood CMV is detected by an antigen or DNA test—is used at most centers. This approach is almost as effective as prophylaxis or suppression and causes less toxicity. The use of the leukocyte antigen test for CMV disease (fluorescent staining of leukocytes for CMV antigens) allows earlier diagnosis but leads to treatment of more patients than would be treated on the basis of blood cultures, with a consequent increase in very late disease (>120 days after transplantation). The use of quantitative viral load assays, which are not dependent on circulating polymorphonuclear leukocytes, should permit early accurate diagnosis in the future.

Table 136-2 Herpes-Group Virus Syndromes in Transplant Recipients

Virus	Reactivation Disease
Herpes simplex virus type 1	Oral lesions, sometimes with spread
	Pneumonia, described only in BMT patients
	Hepatitis
Herpes simplex virus type 2	Severe and/or persistent anogenital lesions
	Hepatitis
Varicella-zoster virus	Zoster (dissemination may occur)
Cytomegalovirus	Associated with graft rejection, fever, bone marrow failure, pneumonitis, gastrointestinal disease
Epstein-Barr virus	B cell lymphoproliferative disease (EBV-LPD)
	Oral hairy leukoplakia (rare)
Human herpesvirus 6	Fever, rash,[a] pneumonitis, bone marrow suppression, encephalitis (manifestations are controversial)
Human herpesvirus 7	Undefined
Kaposi's sarcoma–associated virus/human herpesvirus 8	Kaposi's sarcoma
	Primary effusion lymphoma (rare)
	Multicentric Castleman's disease (rare)

[a] A rash may be seen with primary infections, but it is difficult to distinguish from other rashes seen in these patients.

NOTE: BMT, bone marrow transplant.

Treatment of CMV pneumonia in BMT/HSCT recipients requires both intravenous immune globulin (IVIG) and ganciclovir. In patients who cannot tolerate ganciclovir, foscarnet is a useful alternative, although it may produce nephrotoxicity and electrolyte imbalance. Transfusion of CMV-specific T cells from the donor decreased viral load in a small series of patients; this result suggests that immunotherapy may play a role in the treatment of this disease in the future. →*For further discussion, see Chap. 185.*

Human Herpesviruses 6 and 7   HHV-6, the cause of exanthem subitum in children (Chap. 185), is a ubiquitous herpesvirus that reactivates (as determined by culture of the virus from the blood) in ~50% of transplant recipients between 2 and 4 weeks after surgery. In some cases, reactivation of HHV-6 appears to be associated with neutropenia; since, like CMV, this virus can be found in marrow cells, it is possible that HHV-6 reactivation is responsible for some of the neutropenia that follows bone marrow transplantation. Although encephalitis developing after transplantation has been associated with HHV-6 in cerebrospinal fluid (CSF), the causality of the association is not well defined. HHV-6 DNA is sometimes found in lung samples after transplantation. However, its role in pneumonitis is unclear. While HHV-6 has been shown to be sensitive to foscarnet (and in some instances to ganciclovir) in vitro, the efficacy of antiviral treatment has not been well studied. Little is known about the related herpesvirus HHV-7 or its role in posttransplantation infection. →*For further discussion, see Chap. 185.*

Epstein-Barr Virus   Primary EBV infection can be fatal to transplant recipients; EBV reactivation can cause EBV–B cell lymphoproliferative disease (LPD), which may also be fatal to patients taking immunosuppressive drugs. The localization of EBV to B cells leads to several interesting phenomena in BMT/HSCT recipients. The marrow ablation that occurs as part of the BMT/HSCT procedure may eliminate latent EBV from the host. Infection can then be reacquired immediately after transplantation by transfer of infected donor B cells. Alternatively, transplantation from a seronegative donor may result in cure. The recipient is then at risk for a second primary infection.

EBV-LPD can develop in the recipient's B cells (if any should survive marrow ablation) but is more likely to be a consequence of outgrowth of infected donor cells. Both lytic and latent EBV replication are more likely during immunosuppression (e.g., they are associated with GVHD and the use of antibodies to T cells). Although less likely in autologous transplantation, reactivation can occur in T cell–depleted autologous recipients (e.g., patients being treated for a T cell lymphoma with marrow depletion using antibodies to T cells). EBV-LPD, which usually becomes apparent 1 to 3 months after engraftment, can cause high fevers and cervical adenopathy resembling the symptoms of infectious mononucleosis but more commonly presents as an extranodal mass. The incidence of 0.6% among allogeneic BMT/HSCT recipients contrasts with figures of ~5% for renal transplant recipients and up to 20% for cardiac transplant patients. In all cases, EBV-LPD is more likely to occur with continued immunosuppression (especially that caused by the use of antibodies to T cells and cyclosporine or tacrolimus).

EBV-specific T cells generated from the donor have been used experimentally to prevent and to treat EBV-LPD in the allogeneic recipient. Some studies indicate that EBV-LPD can be treated with antibodies to B cell surface antigens. Use of an anti-CD20 monoclonal antibody (Rituximab) to treat B cell lymphomas that express this surface protein has elicited some dramatic responses. Studies are in progress to assess efficacy in EBV-LPD, in which the involved B cells commonly bear CD20. The role of antivirals is uncertain because no available agents have been documented to have activity against latent EBV infection. Ganciclovir has been postulated to have activity on the basis of its ability to inhibit proliferation of B cells, but this activity is associated with toxicity. Both interferon α and retinoic acid have been used in the treatment of EBV-LPD, as has IVIG, but no large studies have assessed the efficacy of these agents. Chemotherapeutic regimens have been used as a last resort, even though patients' tolerance and long-term results have been disappointing in this setting. →*For further discussion, see Chap. 184.*

Human Herpesvirus 8   The EBV-related gamma herpesvirus HHV-8, which is causally associated with Kaposi's sarcoma, with primary effusion lymphoma, and sometimes with multicentric Castleman's disease, has rarely resulted in disease in BMT/HSCT recipients. The reasons may be a relatively low seroprevalence in the population and the limited duration of profound T cell suppression after bone marrow/hematopoietic stem cell transplantation. →*For further discussion, see Chap. 185.*

Other (Nonherpes) Viruses   Both RSV and parainfluenza viruses, particularly type 3, can cause severe or even fatal pneumonia in BMT recipients. Infections with both of these agents sometimes occur as disastrous nosocomial epidemics. Therapy with aerosolized ribavirin as well as RSV immunoglobulin or monoclonal antibody to RSV (Palivizumab) has been reported to lessen the severity of RSV disease, but there are no large studies to prove efficacy. Influenza is also seen in BMT recipients and generally mirrors the presence of infection in the community. Several drugs are available for the treatment of influenza (amantadine/rimantadine, ribavirin?) but have limited effects, primarily reducing symptoms and shortening the duration of illness. The newly approved neuraminidase inhibitors are active against both influenza A virus and influenza B virus. Their role in ameliorating disease in this patient population is unknown. Adenovirus can be isolated from BMT recipients at rates varying from 5 to 18%. Although hemorrhagic cystitis, pneumonia, and fatal disseminated infection have been reported, adenovirus infection, which (like CMV infection) usually occurs in the first or second month after transplantation, is often asymptomatic. Therapy with intravenous ribavirin is questionably effective. Cidofovir has proved effective in animal models and in case reports. Infections with parvovirus B19 (presenting as anemia or occasionally pancytopenia) and enteroviruses (sometimes fatal) can occur. Pleconaril, a newly developed capsid-binding agent, is being studied for treatment of enterovirus infection. Rotaviruses are a common cause of gastroenteritis in BMT/HSCT recipients. BK and, to a lesser extent, JC virus (polyomavirus hominis 1 and 2, respectively) are found in the urine of some transplant recipients. BK viruria may be associated with hemorrhagic cystitis. Progressive multifocal leukoencephalopathy caused by JC virus is rare among BMT/HSCT recipients compared with the rate among patients with impaired T cell function due to HIV infection. There is no known treatment for this disease; however, cidofovir and other agents are under study.

INFECTIONS IN SOLID ORGAN TRANSPLANT RECIPIENTS

Morbidity and mortality among solid organ transplant recipients have been reduced by the use of more effective antibiotics. The organisms that cause infections in recipients of solid organ transplants are different from those that infect BMT/HSCT recipients because solid organ recipients do not go through a period of neutropenia. As the transplantation procedure involves surgery, however, solid organ recipients are subject to infections at anastomotic sites and to wound infections. Compared with BMT/HSCT recipients, organ transplant patients are immunosuppressed for more prolonged periods (often permanently). Thus they are susceptible to the same organisms as patients with chronically impaired T cell immunity (Chap. 85, especially Table 85-1).

During the early period (<1 month after transplantation), infections are most often caused by extracellular bacteria (staphylococci, streptococci, *Escherichia coli*, other gram-negative organisms), which often originate in surgical wound or anastomotic sites. The spectrum of infection is largely determined by the type of transplant.

In subsequent weeks, the consequences of the administration of agents that suppress cell-mediated immunity and of the acquisition or reactivation (from the transplanted organ) of viruses and parasites become apparent. CMV infection is often a problem in the first 6 months after transplantation and may present as severe systemic disease or as an infection of the transplanted organ. HHV-6 reactivation (assessed by blood culture) occurs within the first 2 to 4 weeks after transplantation and may be associated with fever and granulocytopenia.

CMV is associated not only with generalized immunosuppression but also with organ-specific, rejection-related syndromes: glomerulopathy in kidney transplant recipients, bronchiolitis obliterans in lung transplant recipients, vasculopathy in heart transplant recipients, and the vanishing bile duct syndrome in liver transplant recipients. A complex interplay between increased CMV replication and enhanced graft rejection is well established: Increasing immunosuppression leads to increased CMV replication, which is associated with graft rejection. For this reason, considerable attention has been focused on the diagnosis, treatment, and prophylaxis of CMV infection in organ transplant recipients.

Beyond 6 months after transplantation, infections characteristic of patients with defects in cell-mediated immunity—e.g., infections with *Listeria*, *Nocardia*, various fungi, and other intracellular pathogens—may be a problem. Elimination of these late infections will not be possible until specific tolerance to the transplanted organ can be achieved without the administration of drugs that lead to generalized immunosuppression. Meanwhile, vigilance, prophylaxis/preemptive therapy (when indicated), and rapid diagnosis and treatment of infections can be lifesaving in solid organ transplant recipients, who, unlike most BMT recipients, continue to be immunosuppressed.

Solid organ transplant recipients are susceptible to EBV-LPD from as early as 2 months to many years after transplantation. The prevalence of this complication is increased by potent and prolonged use of T cell–suppressive drugs. The condition may be reversed (in some cases) by decreasing the degree of immunosuppression. Among organ transplant patients, those with heart and lung transplants—who receive the most intensive immunosuppressive regimens—are most likely to develop EBV-LPD, particularly in the lungs. Although disease usually originates in recipient B cells, several cases of donor origin have been reported. There is a notable tendency for EBV-LPD to develop in the transplanted organ. High organ-specific content of B lymphoid tissues (i.e., bronchial-associated lymphoid tissue in the lung), anatomic factors (i.e., lack of access of host T cells to the transplanted organ because of disturbed lymphatics), and differences in major histocompatibility loci between the host T cells and the organ (i.e., lack of cell migration or lack of effective T cell/macrophage cooperation) may result in defective elimination of EBV-infected B cells.

INFECTIOUS COMPLICATIONS OF KIDNEY TRANSPLANTATION (See Table 136-3)
Early Infections Infections developing soon after kidney transplantation are often caused by bacteria associated with skin or wound infections. Some data indicate a role for perioperative antibiotic prophylaxis, and many centers give cephalosporins or a penicillin with an aminoglycoside to decrease the risk of postoperative complications. Urinary tract infections developing soon after transplantation are usually related to anatomic alterations resulting from surgery. Such early infections may require prolonged treatment (e.g., 6 weeks of antibiotic administration for pyelonephritis). Urinary tract infections that occur >6 months after transplantation do not seem to be associated with the high rate of pyelo-

nephritis or relapse seen with infections that occur in the first 3 months and may be treated for shorter periods.

Prophylaxis with trimethoprim-sulfamethoxazole [1 double-strength tablet (800 mg sulfamethoxazole, 160 mg trimethoprim) per day] for the first 4 months after transplantation decreases the incidence of early and middle-period infections (see below and Table 136-4).

Middle-Period Infections Because of continuing immunosuppression, kidney transplant recipients are predisposed to lung infections characteristic of those in patients with T cell deficiency (i.e., infections with intracellular bacteria, mycobacteria, nocardiae, fungi, viruses, and parasites). The high mortality associated with *Legionella pneumophila* infection (Chap. 151) led to the closing of renal transplant units in hospitals with endemic legionellosis.

About 50% of all renal transplant recipients presenting with fever 1 to 4 months after transplantation have evidence of CMV disease; CMV itself accounts for the fever in over two-thirds of cases and thus is the predominant pathogen during this period. CMV infection (Chap. 185) may also present as arthralgias or myalgias. During this period, this infection may represent primary disease (in the case of a seronegative recipient of a kidney from a seropositive donor) or may present as reactivation disease or superinfection. Patients may have atypical lymphocytosis. Unlike immunocompetent patients, however, they often do not have lymphadenopathy or splenomegaly. Therefore, clinical suspicion and laboratory confirmation are necessary for diagnosis. The clinical syndrome may be accompanied by bone marrow suppression

Table 136-3   Infections After Kidney Transplantation

Site	Period After Transplantation		
	Early (<1 month)	Middle (1–4 months)	Late (>6 months)
Urinary tract	Bacteria (*Escherichia coli*, *Klebsiella*, Enterobacteriaceae, *Pseudomonas*, *Enterococcus*) associated with bacteremia and pyelonephritis, *Candida*	CMV (fever alone is common)	Bacteria; late UTIs usually not associated with bacteremia
Lungs	Bacteria (*Legionella* in endemic settings)	CMV diffuse interstitial pneumonitis, *Pneumocystis carinii*, *Aspergillus*, *Legionella*	*Nocardia*, *Aspergillus*, *Mucor*
Central nervous system	—	*Listeria* meningitis, CMV encephalitis, toxoplasmosis	CMV retinitis, *Listeria* meningitis, cryptococcal meningitis, *Aspergillus*, *Nocardia*

NOTE: CMV, cytomegalovirus; UTIs, urinary tract infections.

Table 136-4   Prophylaxis of Infections in Transplant Recipients

Risk Factor	Infection or Organism	Prophylactic Antibiotics	Examinations
Travel or residence in area with known risk of fungal infection	Coccidioidomycosis, histoplasmosis, blastomycosis	Imidazoles[a] or amphotericin B	Chest radiography
Latent viruses	HSV, VZV, EBV, CMV	Acyclovir after BMT for HSV and VZV; ganciclovir in some settings	Serologic testing for HSV, VZV, CMV, HHV-6, EBV, HHV-8
Latent fungi/parasites	*Pneumocystis carinii*, *Toxoplasma gondii*	Trimethoprim-sulfamethoxazole or dapsone plus pyrimethamine	Serologic testing for *Toxoplasma*
History of exposure to tuberculosis	*Mycobacterium tuberculosis*	Isoniazid in cases with recent conversion of PPD to positive and no previous treatment	PPD skin testing and chest radiography

[a] The use of imidazoles in this setting is under study.
NOTE: HSV, herpes simplex virus; VZV, varicella-zoster virus; EBV, Epstein-Barr virus; CMV, cytomegalovirus; BMT, bone marrow transplantation; HHV, human herpesvirus; PPD, purified protein derivative.

(particularly leukopenia). CMV also causes glomerulopathy and is associated with an increased incidence of other opportunistic infections. Because of the frequency and severity of CMV disease, a considerable effort has been made to prevent and treat it in renal transplant recipients. Administration of an immune globulin preparation enriched with antibodies to CMV (CMV-Ig) decreases the incidence in the group at highest risk for severe infections (seronegative recipients of seropositive kidneys). Ganciclovir is useful for the treatment of serious CMV disease. One study showed a significant (50%) reduction in CMV disease and rejection at 6 months in patients who received prophylactic valacyclovir (an acyclovir congener) for the first 90 days after renal transplantation. If confirmed, these results will likely change practice.

Infection with the other herpes-group viruses may become evident within 6 months after transplantation or later. Early after transplantation, HSV may cause either oral or anogenital lesions that are usually responsive to acyclovir. Large ulcerating lesions in the anogenital area may lead to bladder and rectal dysfunction as well as predisposing to bacterial infection. VZV may cause fatal disseminated infection in nonimmune kidney transplant recipients, but in immune patients reactivation zoster usually does not disseminate outside the dermatome; thus disseminated VZV infection is a less fearsome complication in kidney transplantation than in bone marrow transplantation. HHV-6 may reactivate and (although usually asymptomatic) may be associated with fever, rash, marrow suppression, or encephalitis.

EBV reactivation disease is more serious; it may present as an extranodal proliferation of B cells that invade the CNS, nasopharynx, liver, small bowel, heart, and transplanted kidney. The disease is diagnosed by the finding of a proliferation of EBV-positive B cells. The incidence of EBV-LPD is higher among patients given high doses of cyclosporine, tacrolimus, or other immunosuppressive agents (including anti-T cell antibodies). Fortunately, disease often regresses once immunocompetence is restored. HHV-8 infection can be transmitted with the donor kidney and is associated with the development of Kaposi's sarcoma in the recipient. Kaposi's sarcoma (primary vs. reactivation of HHV-8) often appears within 1 year after transplantation, although the range of onset times is wide (1 month to ~20 years).

The papovaviruses BK and JC (polyomaviruses hominis 1 and 2) have been cultured from the urine of kidney transplant recipients (as they have from that of BMT recipients). The excretion of BK virus is associated with ureteral strictures and that of JC virus with progressive multifocal leukoencephalopathy (rare). Adenoviruses may persist with continued immunosuppression in these patients.

Kidney transplant recipients are also subject to infections with other intracellular organisms. These patients may develop pulmonary infections with *Nocardia*, *Aspergillus*, and *Mucor* as well as infections with other pathogens in which the T cell/macrophage axis plays an important role. In patients without intravenous catheters, *L. monocytogenes* is the most common cause of bacteremia ≥1 month after renal transplantation. Kidney transplant recipients may develop *Salmonella* bacteremia, which can lead to endovascular infections and require prolonged therapy. Pulmonary infections with *P. carinii* are common unless the patient is maintained on trimethoprim-sulfamethoxazole prophylaxis. *Nocardia* infection (Chap. 165) may present in the skin, bones, lungs, or CNS (where it usually takes the form of single or multiple brain abscesses). *Nocardia* infection generally occurs ≥1 month after transplantation and may follow immunosuppressive treatment for an episode of rejection. Pulmonary findings are nonspecific: localized disease with or without cavities is most common, but the disease may disseminate. The diagnosis is made by culture of the organism from sputum or from the involved nodule. As with *P. carinii*, prophylaxis with trimethoprim-sulfamethoxazole appears to be efficacious in the prevention of disease. The occurrence of *Nocardia* infections >2 years after transplantation suggests that a long-term prophylactic regimen may be justified.

Toxoplasmosis can occur in seropositive patients, usually developing in the first few months after kidney transplantation. Again, trimethoprim-sulfamethoxazole is helpful in prevention. In endemic areas, histoplasmosis, coccidioidomycosis, and blastomycosis may cause pulmonary infiltrates or disseminated disease.

Late Infections Late infections (>6 months after kidney transplantation) include CMV retinitis and a variety of CNS complications. Patients (particularly those whose immunosuppression has been increased) are at risk for subacute meningitis due to *Cryptococcus neoformans*. Cryptococcal disease may present in an insidious manner (sometimes as a skin infection before the development of clear CNS findings). *Listeria* meningitis may have an acute presentation and requires prompt therapy to avoid a fatal outcome.

Patients who continue to take glucocorticoids are predisposed to infection. "Transplant elbow" is a recurrent bacterial infection in and around the elbow that is thought to result from a combination of poor tensile strength of the skin of steroid-treated patients and steroid-induced proximal myopathy that requires patients to push themselves up with their elbows to get out of chairs. Bouts of cellulitis (usually caused by *Staphylococcus aureus*) recur until patients are provided with elbow protection.

Kidney transplant recipients are susceptible to invasive fungal infections—such as those due to *Aspergillus* and *Rhizopus*, which may present as superficial lesions before dissemination. Mycobacterial infection (particularly that with *M. marinum*) can be diagnosed by skin examination. Infection with *Prototheca wickerhamii* (an achlorophyllic alga) has been diagnosed by skin biopsy. Warts caused by human papillomaviruses (HPVs) are a late consequence of persistent immunosuppression; local therapy is usually satisfactory.

HEART TRANSPLANTATION **Early Infections** Sternal wound infection and mediastinitis are early complications of heart transplantation. An indolent course is common, with fever or a mildly elevated white blood cell count preceding the development of site tenderness or drainage. Clinical suspicion based on evidence of sternal instability and failure to heal may lead to the diagnosis. Although common residents of the skin (e.g., *S. aureus* and *S. epidermidis*) as well as gram-negative organisms (e.g., *Pseudomonas aeruginosa*) and fungi (e.g., *Candida*) are often involved, mediastinitis in these patients (in rare cases) can also be due to *Mycoplasma hominis* (Chap. 178). Since this organism requires an anaerobic environment for growth and may be difficult to see on conventional medium, the laboratory should be alerted that *M. hominis* infection is suspected. *M. hominis* mediastinitis has been cured with a combination of surgical debridement (sometimes requiring muscle-flap placement) plus clindamycin and tetracycline. Organisms associated with mediastinitis may be cultured from accompanying pericardial fluid.

Middle-Period Infections *T. gondii* (Chap. 217) resident in the heart of a seropositive donor may be transmitted to a seronegative recipient. Thus serologic screening for *T. gondii* infection is important before and in the months after cardiac transplantation. Rarely, active disease can be introduced at the time of transplantation. The overall incidence of toxoplasmosis is so high in this setting that some prophylaxis is warranted. Although alternatives are available, the most frequently used agent is trimethoprim-sulfamethoxazole, which prevents infection with *Pneumocystis*, *Nocardia*, and other bacterial pathogens. CMV has also been transmitted by heart transplantation. CNS infections can be caused by *Toxoplasma*, *Nocardia*, and *Aspergillus*. *L. monocytogenes* meningitis should be considered in heart transplant recipients with fever and headache.

CMV infection is associated with poor outcomes after heart transplantation. The virus is usually cultivable 1 to 2 months after transplantation, causes manifestations (usually fever and atypical lymphocytosis, often associated with leukopenia and thrombocytopenia) at 2 to 3 months, and produces severe disease (e.g., pneumonia) at 3 to 4 months. Seropositive recipients usually develop cultivable virus faster than patients whose primary CMV infection is a consequence of transplantation. Between 40 and 70% of patients develop symptomatic CMV disease in the form of (1) CMV pneumonia, the most likely form of CMV disease to be fatal; (2) CMV esophagitis and gastritis, sometimes accompanied by abdominal pain with or without ulcerations and bleeding; and (3) the CMV syndrome consisting of CMV in the blood with fever, leukopenia, thrombocytopenia, and hepatic enzyme abnormalities. Ganciclovir is efficacious in the treatment of CMV infection; prophylaxis with ganciclovir or possibly with other antivirals, as described for renal transplantation, may reduce the incidence of CMV-related disease.

Late Infections EBV infection usually presents as a lymphoma-like proliferation of B cells late after heart transplantation, particularly in patients maintained on heavy immunosuppression. A subset of heart and heart-lung transplant recipients may develop early (within 2 months) fulminant EBV-LPD. Treatment includes the reduction of immunosuppression if possible and the consideration of B cell antibodies (Rituximab), immunomodulatory agents, or chemotherapy, as discussed earlier under bone marrow/hematopoietic stem cell transplantation. HHV-8-associated disease, including primary effusion lymphoma, has been reported in heart transplant recipients. Prophylaxis for *P. carinii* infection is required for these patients (see below).

LUNG TRANSPLANTATION **Early Infections** It is not surprising that lung transplants are predisposed to the development of pneumonia. The combination of ischemia and the resulting mucosal damage together with accompanying denervation and lack of lymph drainage probably contributes to the high rate of pneumonia (66% in one series). The prophylactic use of high doses of broad-spectrum antibiotics for the first 3 or 4 days after surgery decreases the incidence of pneumonia. Gram-negative pathogens (Enterobacteriaceae and *Pseudomonas* species) are troublesome in the first 2 weeks after surgery (the period of maximal vulnerability). Pneumonia can also be caused by *Candida* (possibly as a result of colonization of the donor lung), *Aspergillus*, and *Cryptococcus*.

Mediastinitis may occur at an even higher rate among lung transplant recipients than among heart transplant recipients and most commonly develops within 2 weeks of surgery. Pneumonitis due to CMV (which may be transmitted as a consequence of transplantation) usually presents between 2 weeks and 3 months after surgery, with primary disease occurring later than reactivation disease.

Middle-Period Infections The incidence of CMV infection, either reactivated or primary, is between 75 and 100% if either the donor or the recipient is seropositive for CMV. CMV-induced disease appears to be most severe in recipients of lung and heart-lung transplants. Whether this severity relates to the mismatch in lung antigen-presenting and host immune cells or is attributable to other (nonimmune) factors is not known. More than half of lung transplant recipients with symptomatic CMV disease have pneumonia. Difficulty in distinguishing the radiographic picture of CMV infection from organ rejection further complicates therapy. CMV can also cause bronchiolitis obliterans in lung transplants. The development of pneumonitis related to HSV has led to the prophylactic use of acyclovir. Such prophylaxis may also decrease rates of CMV disease, but ganciclovir is more active against CMV and is also active against HSV. Ganciclovir prophylaxis for CMV disease in lung transplant recipients is recommended.

Late Infections The incidence of *P. carinii* infection (which may present with a paucity of findings) is high among lung and heart-lung transplant recipients. Some form of prophylaxis for *P. carinii* pneumonia is indicated in all organ transplant situations (Tables 136-4 and 136-5). Trimethoprim-sulfamethoxazole prophylaxis for 12 months after transplantation may be sufficient to prevent *P. carinii* disease in patients whose degree of immunosuppression is not increased.

As in other transplant recipients, infection with EBV may cause either a mononucleosis-like syndrome or LPD. The tendency of the B cell blasts to present in the lung appears to be greater after lung transplantation than after the transplantation of other organs. Reduction of immunosuppression causes remission in some cases, but airway compression can be fatal and more rapid intervention may therefore become necessary. The approach to EBV-LPD is similar to that described in other sections.

LIVER TRANSPLANTATION **Early Infections** As in other types of transplantation, early bacterial infections are a major problem after liver transplantation. Many centers administer systemic

Table 136-5 Prophylactic Antibiotics or Vaccination for Immunocompromised Patients

Underlying Problem	Therapy
Splenectomy	Vaccination against pneumococci, *Haemophilus influenzae*, meningococci[a]
T cell defects (e.g., solid organ transplantation)	Prophylaxis for *P. carinii* while patient is immunosuppressed
Antibody defects (bone marrow/hematopoietic stem cell transplantation)	Vaccination for pneumococcus, *H. influenzae*, meningococci; intravenous immune globulin in some settings

[a] Patients should be advised of the importance of seeking immediate medical attention for suspected infections; it may be advisable for patients to have antibiotics (e.g., amoxicillin or amoxicillin/clavulanate) at home.

broad-spectrum antibiotics for the first 5 days after surgery, even in the absence of documented infection. However, despite prophylaxis, infectious complications are common and are correlated with the duration of the surgical procedure and the type of biliary drainage. An operation lasting >12 h is associated with an increased likelihood of infection. Patients who have a choledochojejunostomy with drainage of the biliary duct to a Roux-en-Y jejunal bowel loop have more fungal infections than those whose bile is drained via a choledochocholedochostomy with anastomosis of the donor common bile duct to the recipient common bile duct.

Peritonitis and intraabdominal abscesses are common complications of liver transplantation. Bacterial peritonitis may result from biliary leaks and primary or secondary infection after leakage of bile. Peritonitis in liver transplant recipients is often polymicrobial, commonly involving enterococci, aerobic gram-negative bacteria, staphylococci, anaerobes, or *Candida*. Only one-third of patients with intraabdominal abscesses have bacteremia. Abscesses within the first month after surgery may occur not only over the liver but also in the spleen, pericolic area, and pelvis. Treatment includes antibiotic administration and drainage as necessary.

Liver transplant patients have a high incidence of fungal infections, and the occurrence of fungal infection (often candidiasis) correlates with preoperative use of glucocorticoids, a long duration of treatment with antibacterial agents, and posttransplantation use of immunosuppressive agents.

Middle-Period Infections The development of postsurgical biliary stricture predisposes patients to cholangitis. These patients may lack the characteristic signs and symptoms of cholangitis: fever, abdominal pain, and jaundice. Alternatively, these findings may be present but may suggest graft rejection. The diagnosis of cholangitis in liver transplant recipients therefore requires documentation of bacteremia or demonstration of aggregated neutrophils in bile duct biopsy specimens. Unfortunately, invasive studies of the biliary tract (either T-tube cholangiography or endoscopic retrograde cholangiopancreatography) may themselves lead to cholangitis. For this reason, many clinicians recommend prophylaxis with antibiotics covering gram-negative organisms and anaerobes when these procedures are performed in liver transplant recipients.

Viral hepatitis is a common complication of liver transplantation (Chap. 295). Reactivation of hepatitis B and C infections, for which transplantation may be performed, is problematic. To prevent hepatitis B infection, high-dose intravenous hepatitis B immune globulin is often administered. The long-term efficacy of lamivudine (3TC) in inhibiting hepatitis B viral replication after transplantation is being studied. A combination of interferon α and ribavirin is being tested for treatment/prophylaxis of hepatitis C infection.

As in other transplantation settings, reactivation disease with herpes-group viruses is common (Table 136-2). Herpesviruses can be transmitted in donor organs. Although CMV hepatitis occurs in ~4% of liver transplant recipients, it is usually not so severe as to require retransplantation. CMV disease develops in the majority of seronegative recipients of organs from CMV-positive donors, but fatality rates are lower in liver transplant recipients than in lung or heart-lung transplant recipients. Disease due to CMV is associated with the vanishing bile duct syndrome after liver transplantation. Patients respond to treatment with ganciclovir; prophylaxis with CMV immune globulin and acyclovir or oral ganciclovir may modify disease. A role for HHV-6 in posttransplantation fever and leukopenia has been proposed. EBV-LPD after liver transplantation shows a propensity for involvement of the liver, and such disease may be of donor origin.

PANCREAS TRANSPLANTATION Transplantation of the pancreas is complicated by early abdominal infection in ~20 to 40% of cases. To prevent contamination of the allograft with enteric bacteria and yeasts, some surgeons, instead of draining the pancreas through the bowel, drain secretions into the urinary tract or bladder. A cuff of duodenum is often used in the anastomosis between the pancreatic graft and the bladder. In addition to bicarbonate loss, this technique causes a high rate of urinary tract infection (30 to 40%) and sterile cystitis. Over the long term, bowel drainage is better tolerated. An alternative method—the transplantation of islet cells only—may eliminate the problems characteristically posed by wound and urinary tract sepsis in pancreas transplant recipients.

Issues related to the development of CMV infection, EBV-LPD, and infections with opportunistic pathogens in patients receiving a pancreas are similar to those in other solid organ transplant recipients.

MISCELLANEOUS INFECTIONS IN SOLID ORGAN TRANSPLANTATION **Indwelling Intravenous Catheter Infections** The prolonged use of indwelling intravenous catheters for administration of medication, blood products, and nutrition is common in diverse transplantation settings and poses a risk of local and bloodstream infection. Significant insertion-site infection is most commonly caused by *S. aureus*. Bloodstream infection most frequently develops within a week of catheter placement or in patients who become neutropenic. Coagulase-negative staphylococci are the most common isolates from the blood. →*For further discussion of differential diagnosis and therapeutic options, see Chap. 85.*

Tuberculosis The incidence of tuberculosis occurring within 12 months after solid organ transplantation ranges broadly worldwide (0.35 to 15%), reflecting prevalences in local populations. Nonrenal transplantation, GVHD within 6 months, and intensity of immunosuppression are predictive of tuberculosis reactivation and development of disseminated disease in a host with latent disease. Tuberculosis has rarely been transmitted from the donor organ. In contrast to the low mortality in BMT/HSCT recipients, mortality in solid organ transplant patients is reported to be 29%. Isoniazid toxicity has not been a significant problem except in the liver transplantation setting.

Virus-Associated Malignancies In addition to malignancy associated with gammaherpesvirus infection (EBV, HHV-8) and simple warts (HPV), transplant recipients, particularly those who require long-term immunosuppression, are more likely than the general population to develop tumors that are virus-associated or suspected of being virus-associated. The interval to tumor development is usually >1 year. Transplant recipients develop nonmelanoma skin or lip cancers that, in contrast to de novo skin cancers, have a high squamous cell-to-basal cell ratio. Whether HPV plays a major role in these lesions is being investigated. Cervical and vulvar carcinomas, quite clearly associated with HPV, develop with increased frequency in female transplant recipients. In renal transplant recipients, rates of melanoma are modestly increased and rates of cancers of the kidney and bladder are increased.

VACCINATION OF TRANSPLANT RECIPIENTS

In addition to receiving antibiotic prophylaxis, transplant recipients should be vaccinated against likely pathogens (Table 136-6). In the

Table 136-6 Vaccination for Bone Marrow or Solid Organ Transplant Recipients

Vaccine	Use with Indicated Type of Transplantation	
	Bone Marrow	Solid Organ
Pneumococcal, *Haemophilus influenzae*, meningococcal infections	Immunize after transplantation (optimal timing not established); preimmunize[a]	Immunize before transplantation and every 5 years for Pneumovax (others not established)
Seasonal influenza	Vaccinate in the fall Vaccinate close contacts	Vaccinate before transplantation if possible
Poliomyelitis	Administer inactivated vaccine	Administer inactivated vaccine
Measles/mumps/rubella	Immunize 24 months after transplantation if graft-versus-host disease does not develop	Immunize before transplantation
Tetanus, diphtheria	Reimmunize after transplantation	Immunize before transplantation; give boosters at 10 years or as required; new primary series not required

[a] Studies indicate that it is possible to "immunize the graft" before transplantation.

case of BMT recipients, optimal responses cannot be achieved until after reconstitution, despite previous immunization of both donor and recipient. Recipients of allogeneic BMTs must be reimmunized if they are to be protected against pathogens. The situation is less clear-cut in the case of autologous transplantation. T and B cells in the peripheral blood may reconstitute the response if they are transferred in adequate numbers. However, cancer patients (particularly those with Hodgkin's disease, in whom vaccination has been extensively studied) who are undergoing chemotherapy do not respond normally to immunization, and titers of antibodies to infectious agents fall more rapidly than in healthy individuals. Therefore, even immunosuppressed patients who have not had marrow transplants may need booster vaccine injections. If memory cells are specifically eliminated as part of a marrow "cleanup" procedure, it will be necessary to reimmunize the recipient with a new primary series. Optimal times for immunizations of different transplant populations are being evaluated. Immunization of household and other contacts (including health care personnel) against influenza every season is likely to benefit the patient by preventing local spread.

In the absence of compelling data as to optimal timing, it is reasonable to administer the pneumococcal and *H. influenzae* type b conjugate vaccines to both autologous and allogeneic BMT recipients 12 months after transplantation and again 12 months later (since the response to the initial vaccine dose is weak in the early posttransplantation period). These two vaccines are particularly important for patients who have undergone splenectomy. In addition, *Neisseria meningitidis* polysaccharide vaccine, diphtheria vaccine, tetanus vaccine, and inactivated polio vaccine can all be given at these same intervals (12 and 24 months after transplantation). Some authorities recommend a new primary series for tetanus/diphtheria and inactivated polio vaccine (vaccination 12, 14, and 16 months after transplantation). Because of the risk of spread, household contacts of BMT recipients (or of patients immunosuppressed as a result of chemotherapy) should receive only inactivated polio vaccine. Live-virus measles/mumps/rubella (MMR) vaccine can be given to autologous BMT recipients 24 months after transplantation and to most allogeneic BMT recipients at the same point if they are not receiving maintenance therapy with immunosuppressive drugs and do not have ongoing GVHD. The risk of spread from a household contact is lower for MMR than for polio vaccine. In patients who have active GVHD and/or are taking high maintenance doses of glucocorticoids, it may be prudent to avoid all live-virus vaccines. In the absence of detectable antibody titers, vaccination to prevent hepatitis B and hepatitis A also seems advisable.

In the case of solid organ transplant recipients, administration of all the usual vaccines and of the indicated booster doses should be completed before immunosuppression, if possible, to maximize responses. For patients taking immunosuppressive agents, the administration of pneumococcal vaccine should be repeated every 5 years. No data are available for meningococcal polysaccharide vaccine, but it is probably reasonable to administer it along with the pneumococcal vaccine or more frequently (every 3 years for persons with significant exposure risk). *H. influenzae* conjugate vaccine is safe and should be efficacious in this population; therefore, its administration before transplantation is recommended. Booster doses of this vaccine are not recommended for adults. Solid organ transplant recipients who continue to receive immunosuppressive drugs (glucocorticoids, cyclosporine) should not receive live-virus vaccines. A person in this group exposed to measles should be given immune globulin. Similarly, an immunocompromised patient who is seronegative for varicella and who comes into contact with a person who has chickenpox should be given varicella-zoster immune globulin as soon as possible (and certainly within 96 h) or, if this is not possible, started immediately on a 10- to 14-day course of acyclovir therapy. Susceptible household contacts of transplant recipients should receive live attenuated VZV vaccine, but vaccinees should avoid direct contact with the patient if a rash develops.

Immunocompromised patients who travel may benefit from some but not all vaccines. In general, they should receive any killed or inactivated vaccine preparation appropriate to the area they are visiting; this recommendation includes the vaccines for Japanese encephalitis, hepatitis A and B, poliomyelitis, meningococcal infection, and typhoid. The live typhoid vaccines are not recommended for use in most immunocompromised patients, but inactivated typhoid or the purified polysaccharide vaccine can be used. Live yellow fever vaccine should not be administered. Phenol-inactivated cholera vaccine is probably of little use in this setting. On the other hand, immunization with the purified-protein hepatitis B vaccine is indicated if patients are likely to be exposed. Patients who will reside for >6 months in areas where hepatitis B is common (Africa, Southeast Asia, the Middle East, Eastern Europe, parts of South America, and the Caribbean) should receive hepatitis B vaccine. Inactivated hepatitis A vaccine should be used in the appropriate setting (Chap. 122). If hepatitis A vaccine is not administered, travelers should consider receiving passive protection with immune globulin (the dose depending on the duration of travel in the high-risk area).

BIBLIOGRAPHY

CHANG FY et al: Fever in liver transplant recipients: Changing spectrum of etiologic agents. Clin Infect Dis 26:59, 1998

CONE RW et al: Human herpesvirus 6 infections after bone marrow transplantation: Clinical and virologic manifestations. J Infect Dis 179:311, 1999

DE OTERO J et al: Cytomegalovirus disease as a risk factor for graft loss and death after orthotopic liver transplantation. Clin Infect Dis 26:865, 1998

ENGELS EA et al: Early infection in bone marrow transplantation: Quantitative study of clinical factors that affect risk. Clin Infect Dis 28:256, 1999

FISHMAN JA, RUBIN RH: Infection in organ-transplant recipients. N Engl J Med 338: 1741, 1998

MUELLER N: Overview of the epidemiology of malignancy in immune-deficiency. J AIDS 21 (Suppl 1):S5, 1999

PRENTICE HG, KHO P: Clinical strategies for the management of cytomegalovirus infection and disease in allogeneic bone marrow transplant. Bone Marrow Transplant 19: 135, 1997

REGAMEY N et al: Transmission of human herpesvirus 8 infections from renal-transplant donors to recipients. N Engl J Med 339:1358, 1998

ROONEY CM et al: Use of gene-modified virus-specific T lymphocytes to control Epstein-Barr-virus related lymphoproliferation. Lancet 345:9, 1995

SOMANI J, LARSON RA: Reimmunization after allogeneic bone marrow transplantation. Am J Med 98:389, 1995

WEBB IJ et al: Sources and sequelae of bacterial contamination of hematopoietic stem cell products: Implications for safety and hematotherapy and graft engineering. Transfusion 36:782, 1996

Section 4
APPROACH TO THERAPY FOR BACTERIAL DISEASES

137

Gordon L. Archer, Ronald E. Polk

TREATMENT AND PROPHYLAXIS OF BACTERIAL INFECTIONS

The development of drugs that prevent and cure bacterial infections is one of the twentieth century's major contributions to human longevity and quality of life. Antibacterial agents are among the most commonly prescribed drugs of any kind worldwide. Used appropriately, these drugs are lifesaving. However, their indiscriminate use drives up the cost of health care, leads to a plethora of side effects and drug interactions, and fosters the emergence of bacterial resistance, rendering previously valuable drugs useless. The rational use of antibacterial agents depends on an understanding of their mechanisms of action, pharmacokinetics, toxicities, and interactions; bacterial strategies for resistance; and bacterial susceptibility in vitro. In addition, patient-associated parameters, such as the site of infection and the immune and excretory status of the host, are critically important to appropriate therapeutic decisions. This chapter provides specific data required for making an informed choice of antibacterial agent.

MECHANISMS OF ACTION

Antibacterial agents, like all antimicrobial drugs, are directed against unique targets not present in mammalian cells. The goal is to limit toxicity to the host and maximize chemotherapeutic activity affecting invading microbes only. The mechanisms of action of the antibacterial agents to be discussed in this section are summarized in Table 137-1 and are depicted in Fig. 137-1.

INHIBITION OF CELL-WALL SYNTHESIS One major difference between bacterial and mammalian cells is the presence in bacteria of a rigid wall external to the cell membrane. The wall protects bacterial cells from osmotic rupture, which would result from the cell's usual marked hyperosmolarity (by up to 20 atm) relative to the host environment. The structure conferring cell-wall rigidity and resistance to osmotic lysis in both gram-positive and -negative bacteria is peptidoglycan, a large, covalently linked sacculus that surrounds the bacterium. In gram-positive bacteria, peptidoglycan is the only layered structure external to the cell membrane and is thick (20 to 80 nm); in gram-negative bacteria, there is an outer membrane external to a very thin (1-nm) peptidoglycan layer.

Chemotherapeutic agents directed at any stage of the synthesis, export, assembly, or cross-linking of peptidoglycan lead to inhibition

Table 137-1 Mechanisms of Action of and Resistance to Major Classes of Antibacterial Agents

Letter for Fig. 137-1	Antibacterial Agent[a]	Major Cellular Target	Mechanism of Action	Major Mechanisms of Resistance
A	β-Lactams (penicillins and cephalosporins)	Cell wall	Inhibit cell-wall cross-linking	1. Drug inactivation (β-lactamase) 2. Insensitivity of target (altered penicillin-binding proteins) 3. Decreased permeability (altered gram-negative outer-membrane porins) 4. Active efflux
B	Vancomycin	Cell wall	Interferes with addition of new cell-wall subunits (muramyl pentapeptides)	Alteration of target (substitution of terminal amino acid of peptidoglycan subunit)
	Bacitracin	Cell wall	Prevents addition of cell-wall subunits by inhibiting recycling of membrane lipid carrier	Not defined
C	Macrolides (erythromycin)	Protein synthesis	Bind to 50S ribosomal subunit	1. Alteration of target (ribosomal methylation) 2. Active efflux
	Lincosamides (clindamycin)	Protein synthesis	Bind to 50S ribosomal subunit	Alteration of target (ribosomal methylation)
D	Chloramphenicol	Protein synthesis	Binds to 50S ribosomal subunit	1. Drug inactivation (chloramphenicol acetyltransferase) 2. Active efflux
E	Tetracycline	Protein synthesis	Binds to 30S ribosomal subunit	1. Decreased intracellular drug accumulation (active efflux) 2. Insensitivity of target
F	Aminoglycosides (gentamicin)	Protein synthesis	Bind to 30S ribosomal subunit	1. Drug inactivation (aminoglycoside-modifying enzyme) 2. Decreased permeability through gram-negative outer membrane 3. Active efflux
G	Mupirocin	Protein synthesis	Inhibits isoleucine tRNA synthetase	Mutation of gene for target protein or acquisition of new gene for drug-insensitive target
H	Sulfonamides and trimethoprim	Cell metabolism	Competitively inhibit enzymes involved in two steps of folic acid biosynthesis	Production of insensitive targets [dihydropteroate synthetase (sulfonamides) and dihydrofolate reductase (trimethoprim)] that bypass metabolic block
I	Rifampin	Nucleic acid synthesis	Inhibits DNA-dependent RNA polymerase	Insensitivity of target (mutation of polymerase gene)
J	Metronidazole	Nucleic acid synthesis	Intracellularly generates short-lived reactive intermediates by electron transfer system	Not defined
K	Quinolones (ciprofloxacin)	DNA synthesis	Inhibit DNA gyrase (A subunit) and topoisomerase IV	1. Insensitivity of target (mutation of gyrase genes) 2. Decreased intracellular drug accumulation (active efflux)
	Novobiocin	DNA synthesis	Inhibits DNA gyrase (B subunit)	Not defined
L	Polymyxins (polymyxin B)	Cell membrane	Disrupt membrane permeability by charge alteration	Not defined
	Gramicidin	Cell membrane	Forms pores	Not defined

[a] Compounds in parentheses are major representatives for the class.

of bacterial cell growth and, in most cases, to cell death. Peptidoglycan is composed of (1) a backbone of two alternating sugars, *N*-acetylglucosamine and *N*-acetylmuramic acid; (2) a chain of four amino acids that extends down from the backbone (stem peptides); and (3) a peptide bridge that cross-links the peptide chains. Peptidoglycan is formed by the addition of subunits (a sugar with its five attached amino acids) that are assembled in the cytoplasm and transported through the cytoplasmic membrane to the cell surface. Subsequent cross-linking is driven by cleavage of the terminal stem-peptide amino acid. Antibacterial agents act to inhibit cell-wall synthesis in several ways, as described below.

Bacitracin, a cyclic peptide antibiotic, inhibits the conversion to its active form of the lipid carrier that moves the water-soluble cytoplasmic peptidoglycan subunits through the cell membrane to the cell exterior. Cell-wall subunits accumulate in the cytoplasm and cannot be added to the growing peptidoglycan chain.

Glycopeptides (vancomycin and teicoplanin) are high-molecular-weight antibiotics that bind to the terminal D-alanine–D-alanine component of the stem peptide while the subunits are external to the cell membrane but still linked to the lipid carrier. This binding sterically inhibits the addition of subunits to the peptidoglycan backbone.

β-Lactam antibiotics (penicillins, cephalosporins, carbapenems, and monobactams; Table 137-2), characterized by a four-membered β-lactam ring, prevent the cross-linking reaction called *transpeptidation*. The energy for attaching a peptide cross-bridge from the stem peptide of one peptidoglycan subunit to another is derived from the cleavage of a terminal D-alanine residue from the subunit stem peptide. The cross-bridge amino acid is then attached to the penultimate D-alanine by transpeptidase enzymes. The β-lactam ring of the antibiotic forms an irreversible covalent acyl bond with the transpeptidase enzyme (probably because of the antibiotic's steric similarity to the enzyme's D-alanine–D-alanine target), preventing the cross-linking reaction. Transpeptidases and similar enzymes involved in cross-linking are called *penicillin-binding proteins* (PBPs) because they all have active sites that bind β-lactam antibiotics.

Virtually all the antibiotics that inhibit bacterial cell-wall synthesis are bactericidal. That is, they eventually result in the cell's death due to osmotic lysis. However, much of the loss of cell-wall integrity following treatment with cell wall–active agents is due to the bacteria's own cell-wall remodeling enzymes (autolysins) that cleave peptidoglycan bonds in the normal course of cell growth. In the presence of antibacterial agents that inhibit cell-wall growth, autolysis proceeds without normal cell-wall repair; weakness and eventual cellular lysis occur.

Mechanisms of Action

| GRAM NEGATIVE | GRAM POSITIVE |

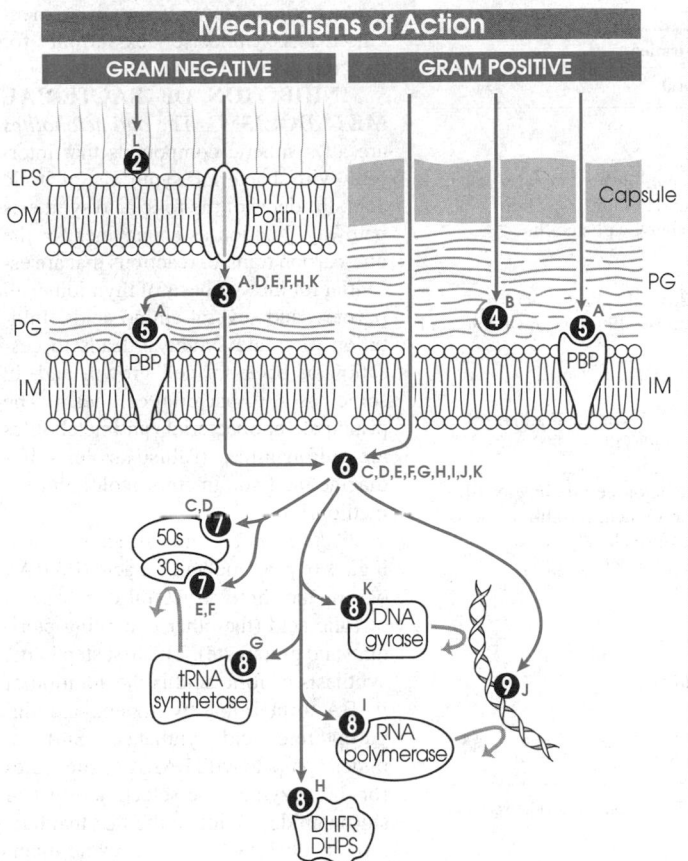

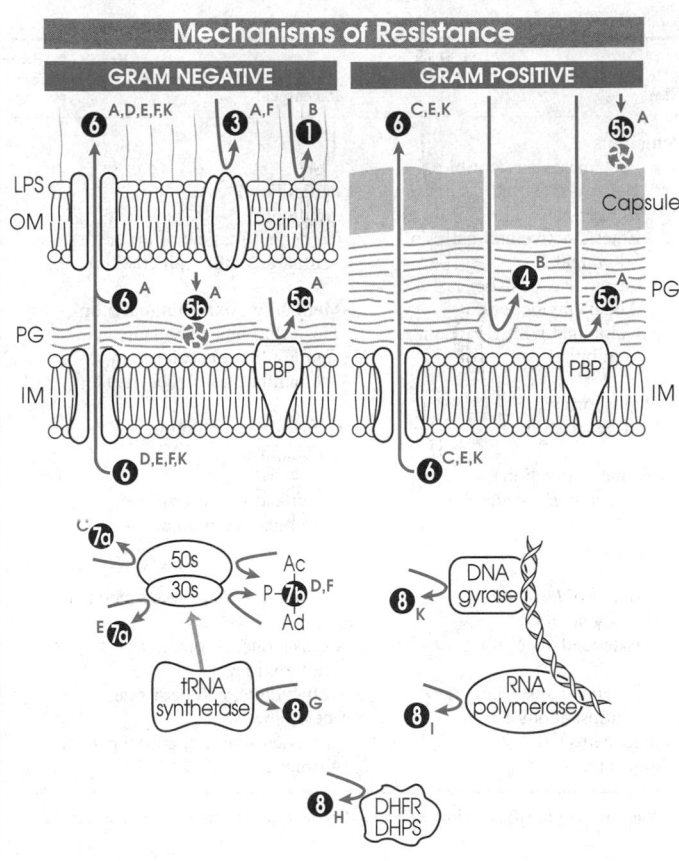

❷ Detergent action on lipid gram-negative OM.

❸ Penetration of hydrophilic drugs through porin channels in gram-negative OM.

❹ Free diffusion through gram-positive cell envelope with binding to cell-wall PG *or*

❺ Binding to cell-membrane PBP. Drug confined to space external to IM.

❻ Diffusion or transport of drugs with intracellular target through IM.

❼ Binding to ribosomal target for protein synthesis inhibition.

❽ Antibiotic interaction with target protein leading to metabolic (DHFR, DHPS), protein synthetic (tRNA synthetase), or nucleic acid (DNA gyrase, RNA polymerase) abnormalities.

❾ Direct interaction of reactive intermediates with nucleic acid.

❶ *Intrinsic resistance*: Inability of antibiotic to penetrate gram-negative envelope (e.g., vancomycin).

❸ Mutant porin channels *decrease* antimicrobial *penetration*.

❹ *Production of insensitive target* by acquired gene mediating production of altered PG.

❺ₐ *Production of β-lactam-insensitive PBP target* by mutation of gene or acquisition of new gene.

❺ᵦ *Inactivation of β-lactam antibiotic by β-lactamases in periplasm (gram-negative) or surrounding medium (gram-positive).*

❻ *Active efflux* of drugs from cytoplasm or from gram-negative periplasm.

❼ₐ Decreased ribosomal binding due to *target site alteration*.

❼ᵦ *Inactivation* of drug by chemical modification leading to decreased ribosomal interaction.

❽ Mutation of target gene or acquisition of new gene producing a *drug-insensitive target* protein.

FIGURE 137-1 Mechanisms of action of and resistance to antibacterial agents. Blue lines trace the routes of drug interaction with bacterial cells, from entry to target site. The letters in each figure indicate specific antibacterial agents or classes of agents, as shown in Table 137-1. The numbers correspond to mechanisms listed beneath each panel. Abbreviations: LPS, lipopolysaccha-ride; OM, outer membrane; PG, peptidoglycan; PBP, penicillin-binding protein; IM, inner (cytoplasmic) membrane; 50s and 30s, large and small ribosome subunits; DHFR, dihydrofolate reductase; DHPS, dihydropteroate synthetase; Ac, acetylation; Ad, adenylation; P, phosphorylation.

INHIBITION OF PROTEIN SYNTHESIS Most of the antibacterial agents that inhibit protein synthesis interact with the bacterial ribosome. The difference between the composition of bacterial and mammalian ribosomes gives these compounds their selectivity.

Aminoglycosides (gentamicin, kanamycin, tobramycin, streptomycin, netilmicin, neomycin, and amikacin) are a group of structurally related compounds containing three linked hexose sugars. They exert a bactericidal effect by binding irreversibly to the 30S subunit of the bacterial ribosome and blocking initiation of protein synthesis. The reason for the lethal effect of aminoglycosides (as opposed to the largely bacteriostatic effect of other protein synthesis–inhibiting antibacterial drugs, including the macrolides, the lincosamides, chloramphenicol, and tetracycline) is not completely understood. Uptake of aminoglycosides and their penetration through the cell membrane constitute an aerobic, energy-dependent process. Thus, aminoglycoside activity is markedly reduced in an anaerobic environment. *Spectinomycin*, an aminocyclitol antibiotic, also acts on the 30S ribosomal

Table 137-2 Classification of β-Lactam Antibiotics

Class	Route of Administration	
	Parenteral	Oral
Penicillins		
β-Lactamase–susceptible		
Narrow-spectrum	Penicillin G	Penicillin V
Enteric-active	Ampicillin	Amoxicillin, ampicillin
Enteric-active and antipseudomonal	Carbenicillin, ticarcillin, mezlocillin, azlocillin, piperacillin	Indanyl carbenicillin
β-Lactamase–resistant		
Antistaphylococcal	Methicillin, oxacillin, nafcillin	Cloxacillin, dicloxacillin
Combined with β-lactamase inhibitors	Ticarcillin plus clavulanic acid, ampicillin plus sulbactam, piperacillin plus tazobactam	Amoxicillin plus clavulanic acid
Cephalosporins		
First-generation	Cefazolin, cephalothin, cephapirin	Cephalexin, cephradine, cefadroxil
Second-generation		
Haemophilus-active	Cefamandole, cefuroxime, cefonicid, ceforanide	Cefaclor, cefuroxime axetil, ceftibuten, cefdinir, cefixime,[a] cefprozil, cefpodoxime,[a] loracarbef
Bacteroides-active	Cefoxitin, cefotetan, cefmetazole	None
Third-generation		
Extended-spectrum	Ceftriaxone, cefotaxime, ceftizoxime	None
Extended-spectrum and antipseudomonal	Ceftazidime, cefoperazone, cefepime	None
Carbapenems	Imipenem-cilastatin, meropenem	None
Monobactams	Aztreonam	None

[a] Some sources classify cefixime and cefpodoxime as third-generation oral agents because of a marginally broader spectrum.

subunit but has a different mechanism of action from the aminoglycosides and is bacteriostatic rather than bactericidal.

Macrolides (erythromycin, clarithromycin, and azithromycin) consist of a large lactone ring to which sugars are attached. They bind specifically to the 50S portion of the bacterial ribosome. After attachment of mRNA to the initiation site of the 30S ribosomal subunit (the process blocked by aminoglycosides), the 50S subunit becomes bound to the 30S component to form the 70S ribosomal complex, and protein chain elongation proceeds. Binding of macrolides to the 50S ribosomal subunit inhibits protein chain elongation.

Lincosamides (clindamycin and lincomycin), although structurally unrelated to macrolides, bind to a site on the 50S ribosome nearly identical to the binding site for macrolides. Although the mechanism and site of action of macrolides and lincosamides are similar, the number and types of bacteria against which these two groups of agents are active differ.

Chloramphenicol consists of a single aromatic ring and a short side chain. This antibiotic binds reversibly to the 50S portion of the bacterial ribosome at a site close to but not identical with the binding sites of the macrolides and lincosamides. The ribosomal binding of chloramphenicol inhibits peptide bond formation.

Tetracyclines (tetracycline, doxycycline, and minocycline) consist of four aromatic rings with various substituent groups. They interact reversibly with the bacterial 30S ribosomal subunit, blocking the binding of aminoacyl tRNA to the mRNA-ribosome complex. This mechanism is markedly different from that of the aminoglycosides, which also bind to the 30S subunit. The specificity of tetracyclines for bacteria depends both on their selectivity for bacterial ribosomes and on their requirement for active, energy-dependent transport into the bacterial cell by a system not found in mammalian cell membranes.

Mupirocin (pseudomonic acid) is produced by the bacterium *Pseudomonas fluorescens*. Its mechanism of action is unique in that it inhibits the enzyme isoleucine tRNA synthetase by competing with bacterial isoleucine for its binding site on the enzyme. Inhibition of this enzyme depletes cellular stores of isoleucine-charged tRNA and therefore leads to a cessation of protein synthesis. The antibiotic is selective for bacteria because mammalian isoleucine tRNA synthetase lacks affinity for the compound.

INHIBITION OF BACTERIAL METABOLISM The *antimetabolites* are all synthetic compounds that interfere with bacterial synthesis of folic acid. Products of the folic acid synthesis pathway function as coenzymes for the one-carbon transfer reactions that are essential for the synthesis of thymidine, all purines, and several amino acids. Inhibition of folate synthesis leads to cessation of bacterial cell growth and, in some cases, to bacterial cell death. The principal antibacterial antimetabolites are sulfonamides (sulfisoxazole, sulfadiazine, and sulfamethoxazole) and trimethoprim.

Sulfonamides are structural analogues of p-aminobenzoic acid (PABA), one of the three structural components of folic acid (the other two being pteridine and glutamate). The first step in the synthesis of folic acid is the addition of PABA to pteridine by the enzyme dihydropteroic acid synthetase. Sulfonamides compete with PABA as substrates for the enzyme. The selective effect of sulfonamides is due to the fact that bacteria synthesize folic acid, while mammalian cells cannot synthesize the cofactor and must have exogenous supplies. However, the activity of sulfonamides can be greatly reduced by the presence of excess PABA or by the exogenous addition of end products of one-carbon transfer reactions (e.g., thymidine and purines). High concentrations of the latter substances may be present in some infections as a result of tissue and white cell breakdown, compromising sulfonamide activity.

Trimethoprim is a diaminopyrimidine, a structural analogue of the pteridine moiety of folic acid. It is a competitive inhibitor of dihydrofolate reductase; this enzyme is responsible for reduction of dihydrofolic acid to tetrahydrofolic acid, the essential final component in the folic acid synthesis pathway that is necessary for all one-carbon transfer reactions. Like the sulfonamides, trimethoprim is bactericidal in the absence of thymine but is only bacteriostatic when this pyrimidine is present in high concentration. The selective antibacterial activity of trimethoprim is based on the extreme sensitivity of bacterial dihydrofolate reductase to inhibition by this drug in comparison with the mammalian enzyme. The bacterial enzyme is approximately 50,000 times more sensitive to such inhibition.

INHIBITION OF NUCLEIC ACID SYNTHESIS OR ACTIVITY Numerous antibacterial compounds have disparate effects on nucleic acids. The *quinolones*, including nalidixic acid and its fluorinated derivatives (norfloxacin, ciprofloxacin, ofloxacin, levofloxacin, sparfloxacin, grepafloxacin, and trovafloxacin), are synthetic compounds that inhibit the activity of the A subunit of the bacterial enzyme DNA gyrase as well as topoisomerase IV. DNA gyrase and topoisomerases are responsible for negative supercoiling of DNA, an essential conformation for DNA replication in the intact cell. Inhibition of the activity of DNA gyrase and topoisomerase IV is lethal to bacterial cells. The antibiotic *novobiocin* also interferes with the activity of DNA gyrase, but it interferes with the B subunit.

Rifampin, used primarily against *Mycobacterium tuberculosis*, is also active against a variety of other bacteria. Rifampin binds tightly to the B subunit of bacterial DNA-dependent RNA polymerase, thus inhibiting transcription of DNA into RNA. Mammalian-cell RNA polymerase is not sensitive to the compound.

Nitrofurantoin, a synthetic compound, causes DNA damage. The nitrofurans, compounds containing a single five-membered ring, are reduced by a bacterial enzyme to highly reactive, short-lived intermediates that are thought to cause DNA strand breakage, either directly or indirectly.

Metronidazole, a synthetic imidazole, is active against a wide range of anaerobic bacteria and protozoa. This activity is totally dependent on the organism's anaerobic electron-transport system for energy production. In the presence of this system, the nitro group of metronidazole is reduced to a series of transiently produced, reactive intermediates that are thought to cause DNA damage. The unique redox system of anaerobes accounts for the selective antibacterial activity of metronidazole. This compound is also a mutagen and a radiosensitizer of hypoxic mammalian cells.

ALTERATION OF CELL-MEMBRANE PERMEABILITY
The *polymyxins* (polymyxin B and colistin, or polymyxin E) are cyclic, basic polypeptides. They behave as cationic, surface-active compounds that disrupt the permeability of both the outer and the cytoplasmic membranes of gram-negative bacteria.

Gramicidin A is a polypeptide of 15 amino acids that acts as an ionophore, forming pores or channels in lipid bilayers.

MECHANISMS OF RESISTANCE

Some bacteria have *intrinsic resistance* to certain classes of antibacterial agents (e.g., obligate anaerobic bacteria to aminoglycosides and gram-negative bacteria to vancomycin). Clearly these agents can never be used alone in the treatment of infections caused by resistant bacteria. In addition, bacteria that are ordinarily susceptible to antibacterial agents can acquire resistance. *Acquired resistance* is one of the major limitations to effective antibacterial chemotherapy. Resistance can develop by mutation of resident genes or by acquisition of new genes. New genes mediating resistance are usually spread from cell to cell by way of mobile genetic elements such as plasmids, transposons, and bacteriophages. The resistant bacterial populations flourish in areas of high antimicrobial use, where they enjoy a selective advantage over susceptible populations.

The major mechanisms used by bacteria to resist the action of antimicrobial agents are inactivation of the compound, alteration or overproduction of the antibacterial target through mutation of the target protein's gene, acquisition of a new gene that encodes a drug-insensitive target, decreased permeability of the cell envelope to the agent, and active elimination of the compound from the periplasm or interior of the cell. Specific mechanisms of bacterial resistance to the major antibacterial agents are outlined below, summarized in Table 137-1, and depicted in Fig. 137-1.

β-LACTAMS Bacteria develop resistance to β-lactam antibiotics by a variety of mechanisms. Most common is the destruction of the drug by β-lactamases. The β-lactamases of gram-negative bacteria are confined to the periplasm, between the inner and outer membranes, while gram-positive bacteria secrete their β-lactamases into the surrounding medium. These enzymes have a higher affinity for the antibiotic than the antibiotic has for its target. Binding results in hydrolysis of the β-lactam ring. Genes encoding β-lactamases have been found in both chromosomal and extrachromosomal locations and in both gram-positive and -negative bacteria; these genes are often on mobile genetic elements. One strategy that has been devised for circumventing resistance mediated by β-lactamases is to combine the susceptible β-lactam with an inhibitor that avidly binds the inactivating enzyme, preventing its attack on the antibiotic. Unfortunately, the inhibitors (e.g., clavulanic acid, sulbactam, and tazobactam) do not bind all classes of β-lactamase and thus cannot be depended on to prevent the inactivation of β-lactam antibiotics by such enzymes. No β-lactam antibiotic or inhibitor has been produced that can resist all of the many β-lactamases that have been identified.

A second mechanism of bacterial resistance to β-lactam antibiotics is an alteration in PBP targets so that the PBPs have a markedly reduced affinity for the drug. While this alteration may occur by mutation of existing genes, the acquisition of new PBP genes (as in staphylococcal resistance to methicillin) or of new pieces of PBP genes (as in streptococcal, gonococcal, and meningococcal resistance to penicillin) is more important.

A final resistance mechanism is the coupling, in gram-negative bacteria, of a decrease in outer-membrane permeability with rapid efflux of the antibiotic from the periplasm to the cell exterior. Mutations of genes encoding outer-membrane proteins called *porins* decrease the entry of β-lactam antibiotics into the cell, while additional proteins form channels that actively pump β-lactams out of the cell. Resistance of Enterobacteriaceae to some cephalosporins and resistance of *Pseudomonas* spp. to cephalosporins and ureidopenicillins are the best examples of this mechanism.

VANCOMYCIN Clinically important resistance to vancomycin was first described among enterococci in France in 1988. Vancomycin-resistant enterococci have subsequently become disseminated worldwide. The genes encoding resistance are carried on plasmids that can transfer themselves from cell to cell. Resistance is mediated by enzymes that substitute D-lactate for D-alanine on the peptidoglycan stem peptide so that there is no longer an appropriate target for vancomycin binding. This alteration does not appear to affect cell-wall integrity, however. This type of acquired vancomycin resistance is so far confined to enterococci and is seen in *Enterococcus faecium* rather than in the more common pathogen *E. faecalis*. Most clinically important staphylococci (i.e., *Staphylococcus aureus* and *S. epidermidis*) remain susceptible. However, in 1996, an isolate of *S. aureus* recovered from an infected patient in Japan was shown to be eight times less susceptible to vancomycin than were usual isolates. Since that report, an additional three *S. aureus* isolates with intermediate susceptibility to vancomycin have been recovered from infected patients in the United States, as have numerous coagulase-negative staphylococci with reduced vancomycin susceptibility. These isolates have not acquired the genes that mediate vancomycin resistance in enterococci but are mutant bacteria with markedly thickened cell walls. These mutants were apparently selected in patients who were undergoing prolonged vancomycin therapy.

AMINOGLYCOSIDES The most common aminoglycoside resistance mechanism is inactivation of the antibiotic. Aminoglycoside-modifying enzymes, usually encoded on plasmids, transfer phosphate, adenyl, or acetyl residues from intracellular molecules to hydroxyl or amino side groups on the antibiotic. The modified antibiotic is less active because of diminished binding to its ribosomal target. Modifying enzymes that can inactivate any of the available aminoglycosides have been found in both gram-positive and -negative bacteria.

A second aminoglycoside resistance mechanism that has been identified predominantly in clinical isolates of *Pseudomonas aeruginosa* is decreased antibiotic uptake, presumably due to alterations in the bacterial outer membrane.

MACROLIDES AND LINCOSAMIDES Resistance in gram-positive bacteria, the usual target organisms for macrolides and lincosamides, is due to the production of an enzyme—most commonly plasmid-encoded—that methylates ribosomal RNA, interfering with binding of the antibiotics to their target. Methylation mediates resistance to erythromycin, clarithromycin, azithromycin, and clindamycin. Streptococci can also actively efflux these compounds.

CHLORAMPHENICOL Most bacteria resistant to chloramphenicol produce a plasmid-encoded enzyme, chloramphenicol acetyltransferase, that inactivates the compound by acetylation.

TETRACYCLINES The most common mechanism of tetracycline resistance in gram-negative bacteria is a plasmid-encoded active-efflux pump that is inserted into the cytoplasmic membrane and extrudes antibiotic from the cell. Resistance in gram-positive bacteria is due either to active efflux or to ribosomal alterations that diminish binding of the antibiotic to its target. Genes involved in ribosomal protection are found on mobile genetic elements.

MUPIROCIN Although the topical compound mupirocin was relatively recently introduced into clinical use, resistance is already becoming widespread in some areas. The mechanism appears to be either mutation of the target isoleucine tRNA synthetase so that it is no longer inhibited by the antibiotic or plasmid-encoded production of a form of the target enzyme that binds mupirocin poorly.

TRIMETHOPRIM AND SULFONAMIDES The most prevalent mechanism of resistance to trimethoprim and the sulfonamides in both gram-positive and -negative bacteria is the acquisition of plasmid-encoded genes that produce a new, drug-insensitive target—specifically, an insensitive dihydrofolate reductase for trimethoprim and an altered dihydropteroate synthetase for sulfonamides.

QUINOLONES Resistance to the newer fluoroquinolones emerged rapidly among *Staphylococcus* and *Pseudomonas* spp. after the introduction of these agents. The most common mechanism is the development of one or more mutations in target DNA gyrases and topoisomerase IV that prevent the antibacterial agent from interfering with the activity of the enzyme. Some gram-negative bacteria develop mutations that both decrease outer-membrane porin permeability and cause active drug efflux from the cytoplasm. Mutations that result in active quinolone efflux are also found in gram-positive bacteria.

RIFAMPIN Bacteria rapidly become resistant to rifampin by developing mutations in the B subunit of RNA polymerase that render the enzyme unable to bind the antibiotic. The rapid selection of resistant mutants is the major limitation to the use of this antibiotic against otherwise-susceptible staphylococci and requires that it be used in combination with another antistaphylococcal agent.

MULTIPLE ANTIBIOTIC RESISTANCE The acquisition by one bacterium of resistance to multiple antibacterial agents is becoming increasingly common. The two major mechanisms are the acquisition of multiple unrelated resistance genes and the development of mutations in a single gene or gene complex that mediate resistance to a series of unrelated compounds. The construction of multiresistant strains by acquisition of multiple genes occurs by sequential steps of gene transfer and environmental selection in areas of high-level antimicrobial use. In contrast, mutations in a single gene can conceivably be selected in a single step. Bacteria that are multiresistant by virtue of the acquisition of new genes include hospital-associated gram-negative bacteria, enterococci, and staphylococci and community-acquired strains of salmonellae, gonococci, and pneumococci. Mutations that confer resistance to multiple unrelated antimicrobial agents occur in the genes encoding outer-membrane porins and efflux proteins of gram-negative bacteria. These mutations decrease bacterial intracellular and periplasmic accumulation of β-lactams, quinolones, tetracycline, chloramphenicol, and trimethoprim. Multiresistant bacterial isolates pose increasing problems in U.S. hospitals; strains resistant to all available antibacterial chemotherapy have already been identified.

PHARMACOKINETICS

The *pharmacokinetic profile* of an antibacterial agent refers to concentrations in serum and tissue versus time and reflects the processes of absorption, distribution, metabolism, and excretion. Important characteristics include peak and trough serum concentrations and mathematically derived parameters such as half-life, clearance, and distribution volume. Pharmacokinetic information is useful for estimating the appropriate antibacterial dose and frequency of administration, for adjusting dosages in patients with impaired excretory capacity, and for comparing one drug with another. →*For further discussion of basic pharmacokinetic principles, see Chap. 70.*

ABSORPTION Data on absorption can refer to oral, intramuscular, or intravenous administration.

Oral Administration Most patients with infection are treated with oral antibacterial agents in the outpatient setting. Advantages of oral therapy over parenteral therapy include lower cost, generally fewer adverse effects (including complications of indwelling lines), and greater acceptance by patients. The percentage of an orally administered antibacterial agent that is absorbed (i.e., the agent's *bioavailability*) ranges from as little as 10 to 20% (erythromycin and penicillin G) to nearly 100% (clindamycin, metronidazole, doxycycline, and trimethoprim-sulfamethoxazole). These differences in bioavailability are not clinically important as long as concentrations at the site of infection are sufficient to inhibit or kill the pathogen. However, therapeutic efficacy may be compromised when absorption is reduced as a result of physiologic or pathologic conditions (such as the presence of food for some drugs or the shunting of blood away from the gastrointestinal tract in patients with hypotension), drug interactions (such as that of quinolones and metal cations), or noncompliance. The oral route is usually used for patients with relatively mild infections in whom absorption is not thought to be compromised by the preceding conditions. In addition, the oral route can be used in more severely ill patients after they have responded to parenteral therapy.

Intramuscular Administration Although the intramuscular route of administration usually results in 100% bioavailability, it is not as widely used in the United States as the oral and intravenous routes, in part because of the pain often associated with intramuscular injections and the relative ease of intravenous access in the hospitalized patient. Intramuscular injection may be suitable for specific indications requiring an "immediate" and reliable effect (e.g., with long-acting forms of penicillin, including benzathine and procaine, and with single doses of ceftriaxone for uncomplicated gonococcal infection).

Intravenous Administration The intravenous route is appropriate when oral antibacterial agents are not effective against a particular pathogen, when bioavailability is uncertain, or when larger doses are required than are feasible with the oral route. After intravenous administration, bioavailability is 100%; serum concentrations are maximal at the end of the infusion. For many patients requiring long-term antimicrobial therapy, outpatient intravenous administration with the use of convenient portable pumps may be cost-effective and safe when oral therapy is not feasible. Alternatively, some oral antibacterial drugs such as fluoroquinolones are sufficiently active against Enterobacteriaceae to rival parenteral therapy; their use may allow the patient to return home from the hospital earlier or to avoid hospitalization entirely.

DISTRIBUTION To be effective, an antibacterial agent must exceed the minimal concentration required to inhibit bacterial growth (MIC; Chap. 121). Serum concentrations usually exceed the MIC for susceptible bacteria, but since most infections are extravascular, the antibiotic must also distribute to the site of the infection. Concentrations of most antibacterials in interstitial fluid are similar to free drug concentrations in serum. However, when the infection is located in a "protected" site where penetration is poor, such as cerebrospinal fluid (CSF), the eye, the prostate, or infected cardiac vegetations, high parenteral doses or local administration for prolonged periods may be required for cure. In addition, even though an antibacterial agent may penetrate to the site of infection, its activity may be antagonized by factors in the local environment, such as an unfavorable pH or inactivation by cellular degradation products. For example, since the activity of aminoglycosides is reduced at acidic pH, the acidic environment in many infected tissues may be partly responsible for the relatively poor efficacy of aminoglycoside monotherapy. In addition, the abscess milieu reduces the activity of many antibacterial compounds, so that surgical drainage may be required for cure.

Most bacteria that cause human infections are located extracellularly. Intracellular pathogens such as *Legionella*, *Chlamydia*, *Brucella*, and *Salmonella* may persist or cause relapse if the antibacterial agent does not enter the cell. In general, β-lactams, vancomycin, and aminoglycosides penetrate cells poorly, whereas macrolides, tetracyclines, metronidazole, chloramphenicol, rifampin, trimethoprim-sulfamethoxazole, and quinolones penetrate cells well.

METABOLISM AND ELIMINATION Like other drugs, antibacterial agents are disposed of by hepatic elimination (metabolism or biliary elimination), by renal excretion in unchanged or metabolized form, or by a combination of the two processes. For most antibacterial drugs, metabolism leads to loss of in vitro activity, although some agents, such as cefotaxime, rifampin, and clarithromycin, have bioactive metabolites that may contribute to their overall efficacy.

The most practical application of knowing the mode of excretion of an antibacterial agent is adjustment of the dosage when elimination capability is impaired. Direct, nonidiosyncratic toxicity from antibacterial drugs most often results from failure to reduce the dosage appropriately in a patient with impaired elimination. For agents that are primarily cleared intact by glomerular filtration, drug clearance is linearly correlated with creatinine clearance. Unfortunately, for drugs whose elimination is primarily hepatic, no simple marker (such as serum creatinine) is useful for dosage adjustment in subjects with liver disease. Even in patients with severe hepatic disease, residual metabolic capability is usually sufficient to preclude accumulation and toxic effects. However, for drugs that undergo hepatic metabolism and have a narrow therapeutic index (such as chloramphenicol), alternative therapy may be warranted in patients with liver disease, since the technology for the monitoring of serum levels is not widely available.

PRINCIPLES OF ANTIBACTERIAL CHEMOTHERAPY

The choice of an antibacterial compound for a particular patient and a specific infection involves more than just a knowledge of the agent's mechanism of action and pharmacokinetic profile. The basic tenets of chemotherapy, to be elaborated below, include the following: First, material containing the infecting organism(s) should be obtained before the start of treatment so that presumptive identification can be made by microscopic examination of stained specimens and the organism can be grown for definitive identification and susceptibility testing. Second, once the organism is identified and its susceptibility to antibacterial agents is determined, the regimen with the narrowest effective spectrum should be chosen. Third, the choice of antibacterial agent is guided by the pharmacokinetic and adverse-reaction profile of active compounds, the site of infection, the immune status of the host, and evidence of efficacy from well-performed clinical trials. Finally, if all other factors are equal, the least expensive antibacterial regimen should be chosen.

SUSCEPTIBILITY OF BACTERIA TO ANTIBACTERIAL DRUGS IN VITRO The determination of the susceptibility of the patient's infecting organism to a panel of appropriate antibacterial agents is an essential first step in devising a chemotherapeutic regimen. The details of susceptibility testing are discussed elsewhere (Chap. 121). Such testing is designed to estimate the susceptibility of a bacterial isolate to an antibacterial drug under standardized conditions that favor rapidly growing aerobic or facultative organisms and to assess bacteriostasis only. Specialized testing is required for the assessment of bactericidal antimicrobial activity; for the detection of resistance among such fastidious organisms as obligate anaerobes, *Haemophilus* spp., and pneumococci; and for the determination of resistance phenotypes with variable expression, such as resistance to methicillin or oxacillin among staphylococci.

RELATIONSHIP OF PHARMACOKINETICS AND IN VITRO SUSCEPTIBILITY TO CLINICAL RESPONSE The relationship between the report of susceptibility in vitro and the clinical pharmacokinetics of the antibacterial agent helps predict clinical response. Bacteria are usually considered to be *susceptible* to a drug if the achievable peak serum concentration exceeds the MIC by at least fourfold. The *breakpoint* is the concentration of the antibiotic that separates susceptible from resistant bacteria (Fig. 137-2). When a majority of the isolates of a given bacterial species are inhibited at concentrations below the breakpoint, the species is considered to be within the spectrum of the antibiotic (see "Choice of Antibacterial Therapy," below).

The pharmacodynamic profile of an antibiotic is the quantitative relationship among the time course of antibiotic concentrations in se-

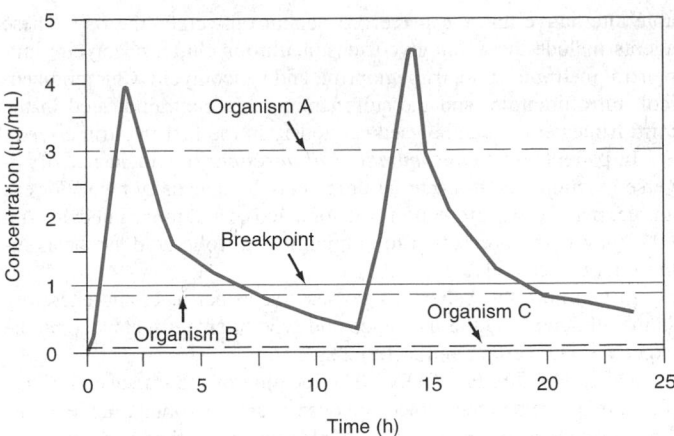

FIGURE 137-2 Relationship between pharmacokinetics of an antibiotic and susceptibility. Organism A is resistant, organism B is moderately susceptible, and organism C is very susceptible.

rum and tissue, in vitro susceptibility, and microbial response. Three pharmacodynamic parameters quantify these relationships: the ratio of the area under the curve (AUC) for the plasma concentration vs. time curve to MIC (AUC/MIC), the ratio of the maximal serum concentration to the MIC (C_{max}/MIC), and the time during a dosing interval that plasma concentrations exceed the MIC ($t > $ MIC). The pharmacodynamic profile of an antibiotic class is characterized as either concentration dependent (fluoroquinolones, aminoglycosides), such that the increase in antibiotic concentration leads to a more rapid rate of bacterial death, or time dependent (β-lactams, vancomycin), such that the reduction in bacterial density is proportional to the time that concentrations exceed the MIC. For concentration-dependent antibiotics, the C_{max}/MIC or AUC/MIC ratio correlates best with the reduction in microbial density in vitro and in animal investigations. Dosing strategies attempt to maximize these ratios by the administration of a "large" dose relative to the MIC for anticipated pathogens, often at "long" intervals (relative to the serum half-life). Once-daily dosing of aminoglycoside antibiotics is the practical consequence of these relationships. In contrast, dosage strategies for time-dependent antibiotics emphasize the administration of sufficient doses at appropriate intervals to maintain serum concentrations above the MIC, typically for at least 40 to 50% of the dosing interval. The clinical implications of these relationships are in the early stages of investigation, but their elucidation should eventually result in more rational antibacterial regimens.

STATUS OF THE HOST Various host factors must be considered in the devising of antibacterial chemotherapy. The host's antibacterial *immune function* is of importance, particularly as it relates to opsonophagocytic function. Since the major host defense against acute, overwhelming bacterial infection is the polymorphonuclear leukocyte, patients with neutropenia must be treated aggressively and empirically with bactericidal drugs for suspected infection (Chap. 85). Likewise, patients who have deficient humoral immunity (e.g., those with chronic lymphocytic leukemia and multiple myeloma) and individuals with surgical or functional asplenia (e.g., those with sickle cell disease) should be treated empirically for infections with encapsulated organisms, especially the pneumococcus.

Pregnancy increases the risk of toxicity of certain antibacterial drugs for the mother (e.g., the hepatic toxicity of tetracycline), affects drug disposition and pharmacokinetics, and—because of the risk of fetal toxicity—severely limits the choice of agents for treating infections. Certain antibacterials are contraindicated in pregnancy either because their safety has not been established or because they are known to be toxic. These agents include all fluoroquinolones, clarithromycin, erythromycin estolate (but not erythromycin base), and tetracyclines. Data on the safety of many other antibacterial drugs are limited, but these drugs may be used cautiously when there is no suitable alternative and the perceived benefit outweighs the risk. These agents include the aminoglycosides, azithromycin, clindamycin, imipenem, metronidazole, trimethoprim, and vancomycin. Chloramphenicol, nitrofurantoin, and the sulfonamides are contraindicated in the third trimester but can be used cautiously in the first two trimesters.

In patients with *concomitant viral infections*, the incidence of adverse reactions to antibacterial drugs may be unusually high. For example, persons with infectious mononucleosis and those infected with HIV may react more often to ampicillin and folic acid synthesis inhibitors, respectively.

In addition, the patient's age, sex, racial heritage, and excretory status all determine the incidence and type of side effects that can be expected with certain antibacterial agents.

SITE OF INFECTION   The location of the infected site may play a major role in the choice and dose of antimicrobial drug. Patients with suspected *meningitis* should receive drugs that can cross the blood-CSF barrier; in addition, because of the relative paucity of phagocytes and opsonins at the site of infection, the agents should be bactericidal. Chloramphenicol, one of the standard drugs used in the treatment of meningitis, is bactericidal for common organisms causing meningitis (i.e., meningococci, pneumococci, and *Haemophilus influenzae*, but *not* enteric gram-negative bacilli), is highly lipid-soluble, and enters the CSF well. However, β-lactams, the mainstay of therapy for most of these infections, do not normally reach high levels in CSF. Their efficacy is based on the increased permeability of the blood-brain and blood-CSF barriers to hydrophilic molecules during inflammation and the extreme susceptibility of most infectious organisms to even small amounts of β-lactam drug.

The vegetation, which is the major site of infection in *bacterial endocarditis*, is also a focus that is protected from normal host-defense mechanisms. Antibacterial therapy needs to be bactericidal, with the selected agent administered parenterally over a long period and at a dose that produces serum levels at least eight times higher than the minimal bactericidal concentration (MBC) for the infecting organism. Likewise, *osteomyelitis* involves a site that is somewhat resistant to opsonophagocytic removal of infecting bacteria; furthermore, avascular bone (sequestrum) represents a foreign body that thwarts normal host-defense mechanisms. *Chronic prostatitis* is exceedingly difficult to cure because most antibiotics do not penetrate the nonfenestrated capillaries serving the prostate, especially when acute inflammation is absent. Drugs that are "ion trapped" after entering prostatic tissue, such as trimethoprim and fluoroquinolones, may be uniquely effective because of this mechanism. *Intraocular infections*, especially endophthalmitis, are difficult to treat because drug penetration into the vitreous from blood is hindered by retinal capillaries lacking fenestration. Inflammation does little to disrupt this barrier. Thus, direct injection into the vitreous is necessary in many cases. Antibiotic penetration into *abscesses* is usually poor. Even when an antibiotic does penetrate into the abscess, local conditions, such as low pH or the presence of enzymes that hydrolyze the drug, may antagonize its activity.

In contrast, *urinary tract infections*, when confined to the bladder, are relatively easy to cure, in part because of the higher concentration of most antibiotics in urine than in blood. Since blood is the usual reference fluid in defining susceptibility, even organisms found to be "resistant" to achievable serum concentrations may be susceptible to achievable urine concentrations. For drugs that are used only for the treatment of urinary tract infections, such as nitrofurantoin and methenamine salts, achievable urine concentrations are used to determine susceptibility.

COMBINATION CHEMOTHERAPY   One of the tenets of antibacterial chemotherapy is that if the infecting bacterium has been identified, the most specific chemotherapy possible should be used. The use of a single agent with a narrow spectrum of activity against the pathogen diminishes the alteration of normal flora and thus limits the overgrowth of resistant nosocomial organisms (e.g., *Candida albicans*, enterococci, *Clostridium difficile*, or methicillin-resistant

staphylococci), avoids the potential toxicity of multiple-drug regimens, and reduces cost. However, certain circumstances call for the use of more than one antibacterial agent. These are summarized below.

1. *Prevention of the emergence of resistant mutants.* Spontaneous mutations occur at a detectable frequency in certain genes encoding the target proteins for some antibacterial agents. The use of these agents can eliminate the susceptible population, select out resistant mutants at the site of infection, and result in the failure of chemotherapy. Resistant mutants are usually selected when the MIC of the antibacterial agent for the infecting bacterium is close to achievable levels in serum or tissues and/or when the site of infection limits the access or activity of the agent. Among the most common examples are rifampin for staphylococci, imipenem for *Pseudomonas*, and ciprofloxacin for staphylococci and *Pseudomonas*. Small-colony variants of staphylococci resistant to aminoglycosides also emerge during monotherapy with these antibiotics. A second antibacterial agent with a mechanism of action different from that of the first is added to prevent the emergence of these resistant mutants (e.g., imipenem plus an aminoglycoside for systemic *Pseudomonas* infections). However, since resistant mutants have emerged following combination chemotherapy, this approach is not uniformly successful.

2. *Synergistic or additive activity.* Against some bacteria, two or more agents are clearly more active than one; whether or not this is the case is usually judged on the basis of testing in vitro. Synergistic or additive activity involves a lowering of the MIC or MBC of each or all of the drugs tested in combination against a specific bacterium. In *synergy*, *each* agent is more active when combined with a second drug than it would be alone, and the drugs' combined activity is therefore greater than the sum of the individual activities of each drug. In an *additive relationship*, the combined activity of the drugs is equal to the sum of their individual activities. Among the best examples of a synergistic or additive effect, confirmed both in vitro and by animal studies, are the enhanced bactericidal activities of certain β-lactam/aminoglycoside combinations against enterococci, viridans streptococci, and *P. aeruginosa*. The synergistic or additive activity of these combinations has also been demonstrated for selected isolates of enteric gram-negative bacteria and staphylococci. The combination of trimethoprim and sulfamethoxazole has synergistic or additive activity against many enteric gram-negative bacteria. Most other antimicrobial combinations display indifferent activity (i.e., the combination is *no better* than the more active of the two agents alone), and some combinations (e.g., penicillin plus tetracycline against pneumococci) may be antagonistic (i.e., the combination is *worse* than either drug alone).

3. *Therapy directed against multiple potential pathogens.* For certain infections, either a mixture of pathogens is suspected or the patient is desperately ill with an as-yet-unidentified infection (see "Empirical Therapy," below). In these situations, the most important of the likely infecting bacteria must be covered by therapy until culture and susceptibility results become available. Examples of the former infections are intraabdominal or brain abscesses and infections of limbs in diabetic patients with microvascular disease. The latter situations include fevers in neutropenic patients, acute pneumonia from aspiration of oral flora by hospitalized patients, and septic shock or sepsis syndrome.

EMPIRICAL THERAPY   In certain situations, antibacterial therapy is begun before a specific bacterial pathogen has been identified. The choice of agent is guided by the results of studies identifying the usual pathogens at that site or in that clinical setting, by pharmacodynamic considerations, and by the resistance profile of the expected pathogens in a particular hospital or geographic area. Situations in which empirical therapy is appropriate include the following:

1. *Life-threatening infection.* Any suspected bacterial infection in a patient with a life-threatening illness should be treated presumptively. Therapy is usually begun with more than one agent and is later tailored to a specific pathogen if one is eventually identified.

2. *Treatment of infections in unhospitalized patients with no cultures performed.* In many situations, it is appropriate to treat non-life-threatening infections without obtaining cultures. These situations in-

CHOICE OF ANTIBACTERIAL THERAPY

The antibacterial spectrum of specific agents and the infections for which they represent the treatment of choice are detailed below. No attempt has been made to include all the potential situations in which antibacterial agents may be used. A more detailed discussion of specific bacteria and infections that they cause can be found elsewhere in this volume.

β-LACTAMS (Table 137-2) All *penicillins* (except for the semisynthetic, penicillinase-resistant antistaphylococcal agents) are hydrolyzed by *β*-lactamases and are ineffective against isolates that produce these enzymes. Penicillin G has a spectrum that includes spirochetes (*Treponema pallidum*, *Borrelia*, and *Leptospira*), streptococci (groups A and B, viridans, and *Streptococcus pneumoniae*), enterococci, most *Neisseria* spp., a few staphylococci, many fastidious oral bacteria (including many *Porphyromonas* and *Prevotella* spp., streptococci, *Actinomyces*, and *Fusobacterium*), *Clostridium* spp. (except *C. difficile*), *Pasteurella multocida*, *Erysipelothrix rhusiopathiae*, and *Streptobacillus moniliformis*. However, penicillin G resistance is widespread among staphylococci; is increasing rapidly among gonococci, enterococci, and pneumococci; and is emerging among meningococci, viridans streptococci, and oral anaerobes such as *Porphyromonas* and *Prevotella*. Penicillin G is the *drug of choice* for syphilis, yaws, leptospirosis, group A and B streptococcal infections, actinomycosis, oral and periodontal infections, meningococcal meningitis and meningococcemia, viridans streptococcal endocarditis, clostridial myonecrosis, tetanus, anthrax, rat-bite fever, *P. multocida* infections, and erysipeloid (*E. rhusiopathiae*).

Ampicillin extends the spectrum of penicillin G to some gram-negative rods. It is active against some isolates of *Escherichia coli*, *Proteus mirabilis*, *Salmonella*, *Shigella*, and *H. influenzae* and is one of the *drugs of choice* for susceptible organisms causing urinary tract infections, salmonellosis, *H. influenzae* meningitis and epiglottitis, and *Listeria monocytogenes* meningitis. High rates of resistance have lessened its value as empirical therapy in some situations. For example, more than 80% of isolates of *E. coli* and *P. mirabilis* are resistant in some hospitals, as are 10 to 30% of isolates of *H. influenzae*; moreover, in some outbreaks of infection due to salmonellae, all isolates are ampicillin-resistant.

The *penicillinase-resistant penicillins* are used solely for the treatment of staphylococcal infections and are the *drugs of choice* for systemic or deep staphylococcal infections caused by susceptible organisms. Unfortunately, on average, approximately 30% of *S. aureus* isolates and more than 60% of coagulase-negative staphylococcal isolates acquired in U.S. hospitals are resistant to these agents (i.e., methicillin-resistant). The spectrum of these agents also includes most of the same gram-positive bacteria that are susceptible to penicillin G.

The spectrum of the *antipseudomonal penicillins* includes the bacteria covered by ampicillin as well as some additional nonpseudomonal enteric gram-negative bacilli. For example, piperacillin is active against many indole-positive *Proteus*, *Enterobacter*, *Klebsiella*, *Providencia*, and *Serratia* spp. However, the susceptibility of these penicillins to *β*-lactamase markedly limits their utility as empirical therapy when infections caused by gram-negative enteric organisms are suspected. The major use of these compounds is in the treatment of proven or suspected infections with *P. aeruginosa* and *Acinetobacter*, for which they are among the *drugs of choice*. Their relative antipseudomonal activities can be ranked as follows: piperacillin > mezlocillin/ticarcillin > carbenicillin.

The addition of *β*-lactamase inhibitors (clavulanic acid, sulbactam, or tazobactam) to ampicillin, amoxicillin, ticarcillin, or piperacillin extends the spectrum of these agents to include many organisms that are resistant by virtue of *β*-lactamase production. These organisms include *E. coli*, *Klebsiella* spp., all *Proteus* spp., *H. influenzae*, *Moraxella catarrhalis*, *Providencia* spp., and *Bacteroides* spp. Such combinations are also active against staphylococci that produce *β*-lactamase but are not methicillin-resistant. However, the efficacy of these combinations in serious staphylococcal infections has not been adequately proven. Furthermore, *Enterobacter*, *Pseudomonas*, *Acinetobacter*, and various enteric gram-negative isolates either produce *β*-lactamases not inhibited by these compounds or develop resistance attributable to non-*β*-lactamase-mediated mechanisms.

The *first-generation cephalosporins* have a spectrum that includes penicillinase-producing, methicillin-susceptible staphylococci and streptococci. While these drugs may be used when infections with gram-positive bacteria are suspected, they are *not* the drugs of choice for such infections. They have excellent activity against many isolates of *E. coli*, *Klebsiella pneumoniae*, and *P. mirabilis* and are among the drugs of choice in presumptive therapy for community-acquired urinary tract infections. They have no activity against *Bacteroides fragilis*, enterococci, methicillin-resistant staphylococci, *Pseudomonas*, *Acinetobacter*, *Enterobacter*, indole-positive *Proteus*, and *Serratia* and poor activity against *H. influenzae*.

The *parenteral second-generation cephalosporins* extend the gram-negative spectrum of first-generation compounds. The various second-generation agents have differing activities. Cefuroxime and cefamandole retain activity against gram-positive cocci and are also active against *H. influenzae*, *Neisseria*, some *Enterobacter* isolates, and indole-positive *Proteus* but exhibit poor activity against *B. fragilis*. Cefoxitin and cefotetan have reasonably good activity against *B. fragilis*, but cefotetan is less effective against some other *Bacteroides* spp. (Chaps. 130 and 167). Both of the latter drugs display poor activity against gram-positive cocci and *Enterobacter*. No second-generation cephalosporin is active against *Pseudomonas* or *Acinetobacter*.

Oral second-generation cephalosporins have fair activity against gram-positive cocci and *H. influenzae* and are widely used in outpatient therapy for otitis media, sinusitis, and lower respiratory tract infections, although cheaper agents that are equally effective are preferable. Cefixime, cefuroxime axetil, and cefpodoxime are among the *drugs of choice* for single-dose treatment of gonococcal urethritis.

Third-generation cephalosporins all have a broad spectrum of activity against enteric gram-negative rods and are especially useful for treating hospital-acquired infections caused by multiresistant organisms. In addition, ceftazidime and cefepime have excellent antipseudomonal activity. The other third-generation cephalosporins have poor antipseudomonal activity. Since resistance to third-generation cephalosporins is increasing among all nosocomial gram-negative rods, the use of these agents should be guided by susceptibility testing. The gram-positive spectrum of the third-generation cephalosporins is variable. All are less active than first-generation cephalosporins against methicillin-susceptible staphylococci; ceftazidime has the least antistaphylococcal activity of this group. However, ceftriaxone, ceftizoxime, and cefotaxime have excellent activity against streptococci, especially *S. pneumoniae*. Ceftazidime is not recommended for treatment of streptococcal infections.

Because of its excellent gram-negative spectrum; its activity against *Haemophilus*, many *S. pneumoniae* strains, and penicillin-resistant *Neisseria*; its long serum half-life; and its high serum and CSF levels, ceftriaxone has become one of the *drugs of choice* for empirical therapy for bacterial meningitis (except that caused by *Listeria* and by highly penicillin-resistant pneumococcal strains), all gonococcal infections, salmonellosis, and typhoid fever. The third-generation cephalosporins are among the *drugs of choice* for nonpseudomonal hospital-acquired pneumonia. Cefepime is more resistant to chromosomal *β*-lactamase produced by *Enterobacter* spp. than are other third-generation cephalosporins. Third-generation cephalosporins have poor activity against *Bacteroides* and no activity against methicillin-resistant staphylococci, *Enterococcus*, *Acinetobacter*, or *Stenotrophomonas*.

The *carbapenems* currently available in the United States are imipenem and meropenem. Imipenem is marketed in combination with the renal dipeptidase inhibitor cilastatin, which enables imipenem to escape renal inactivation and thus to reach higher urinary levels. Imipenem and meropenem have excellent activity in vitro against virtually all bacterial pathogens except *Stenotrophomonas*, methicillin-resistant staphylococci, and *E. faecium*. Limitations to their use are their relatively low blood levels, short serum half-life, and high cost. Imipenem has dose-related central nervous system side effects that appear to be less frequent with meropenem. Resistance to imipenem and meropenem is a problem only among nosocomial isolates of *P. aeruginosa*, approximately 20% of which are resistant. Because of their broad spectrum, carbapenems can be used as empirical therapy for serious nosocomial infections thought to be caused by multiple bacterial species or multiresistant organisms. Imipenem and meropenem are often used to treat hospital-acquired infections caused by *Enterobacter* spp. because these organisms produce inducible β-lactamases that inactivate third-generation cephalosporins but not the carbapenems. The latter antibiotics are often held in reserve as therapy for nosocomial infections due to gram-negative pathogens resistant to third-generation cephalosporins.

The only *monobactam* currently available is aztreonam. This antibiotic has a spectrum limited to facultative gram-negative enteric bacilli. It has no activity against any gram-positive or anaerobic bacterium. Its gram-negative spectrum is similar to that of ceftazidime, with equally good activity against *Pseudomonas*. Its primary advantages are its theoretical ability to preserve the normal gram-positive and anaerobic flora and the lack of cross-reactive immediate hypersensitivity in patients who have had this type of reaction to other β-lactam antibiotics.

VANCOMYCIN The spectrum of vancomycin is limited to gram-positive cocci, especially enterococci, streptococci, and staphylococci. Vancomycin serves as second-line therapy for most gram-positive bacterial infections but is the *drug of choice* for infections caused by methicillin-resistant staphylococci or *Corynebacterium jeikeium* and for serious infections in penicillin-allergic patients. Given orally (a route by which it is not absorbed), vancomycin can be used to treat antibiotic-associated pseudomembranous colitis caused by *C. difficile* in patients who have failed to respond to metronidazole, the *drug of choice*. Vancomycin has also been recommended as initial empirical therapy for presumed pneumococcal meningitis because of increasing pneumococcal resistance to penicillins and cephalosporins. Resistance to vancomycin is increasing rapidly among isolates of *E. faecium* in large hospitals, particularly in areas of high vancomycin use. In addition, *S. aureus* isolates with reduced susceptibility to vancomycin have now been detected. Because of the growing threat of vancomycin-resistant enterococci and the potential for increasing resistance among staphylococci, a national advisory committee has established guidelines for appropriate and limited use of this antibiotic.

AMINOGLYCOSIDES The aminoglycosides are rapidly bactericidal in vitro at low concentrations, with activity limited to facultative gram-negative bacteria and staphylococci. They have no activity against anaerobic bacteria and are not effective in environments that are acidic or have a low oxygen tension. However, their spectrum includes virtually all gram-negative bacteria that are not strict anaerobes, and they are among the *drugs of choice* for any suspected gram-negative bacteremic infection, particularly in neutropenic patients. Aminoglycosides are synergistically bactericidal in combination with a penicillin for the treatment of staphylococcal, enterococcal, or viridans streptococcal endocarditis and are usually combined with a β-lactam antibiotic for the treatment of gram-negative bacteremia. Aminoglycosides are also among the *drugs of choice* for severe infections of the upper urinary tract. The major limitations to use of aminoglycosides are their renal and otic toxicity, their diminished activity at certain sites of infection (e.g., abscesses and the central nervous system), and the resistance of target bacteria. Among the available agents, gentamicin is generally preferred because of its low cost; however, tobramycin has slightly greater activity against *P. aeruginosa*, and amikacin retains activity against many tobramycin- and gentamicin-resistant gram-negative bacteria because it is inactivated by fewer aminoglycoside-modifying enzymes. Streptomycin is still one of the *drugs of choice* in initial therapy for tularemia, plague, glanders, and brucellosis and is a second-line agent for the treatment of tuberculosis.

MACROLIDES Erythromycin has broad-spectrum activity against gram-positive bacteria, with additional activity against *Legionella*, *Mycoplasma*, *Campylobacter*, and some *Chlamydia* isolates. It is the *drug of choice* for infections due to *Legionella*, *Campylobacter*, and *Mycoplasma* and is among the *drugs of choice* for community-acquired pneumococcal pneumonia and group A streptococcal pharyngitis in penicillin-allergic patients. However, resistance to erythromycin among group A streptococci and pneumococci is increasing dramatically in some areas. Erythromycin also appears to be one of the *drugs of choice* for infections caused by the agent of bacillary angiomatosis (*Bartonella henselae*) in immunocompromised patients. The newer macrolides clarithromycin and azithromycin have an antibacterial spectrum similar to that of erythromycin in vitro. However, azithromycin has greater activity against *Chlamydia*. Clarithromycin, in combination with a proton pump inhibitor, has been designated a *drug of choice* for the treatment of gastric infections due to *Helicobacter pylori* (gastritis, gastric and duodenal ulcers). Both azithromycin and clarithromycin are active against nontuberculous mycobacteria, and both appear to have fewer gastrointestinal side effects than does erythromycin.

LINCOSAMIDES The only lincosamide used in the United States is clindamycin. It shares the gram-positive coccal spectrum of erythromycin but is more active, in some cases showing bactericidal activity, against susceptible staphylococci. However, resistance among staphylococci and some streptococci, mediated by the same genes responsible for macrolide resistance, limits clindamycin's usefulness against gram-positive cocci. In general, all staphylococci resistant to erythromycin should be considered resistant to clindamycin regardless of the results of in vitro susceptibility testing. However, at least half of the streptococci resistant to erythromycin are truly susceptible to clindamycin. In these bacteria, resistance is mediated by a drug-efflux pump that removes macrolides but not lincosamides. Despite increasing resistance, clindamycin remains useful for most anaerobic infections because of its broad spectrum of activity against both gram-positive and -negative strict anaerobes. It is also a *drug of choice* for the treatment of severe, invasive group A streptococcal infections. In contrast, clindamycin, like erythromycin, has no clinically significant activity against facultative gram-negative enteric bacilli. Appropriate use is limited only by resistance or the development of pseudomembranous colitis, the major serious side effect of this drug.

CHLORAMPHENICOL Chloramphenicol has a broad spectrum of activity against gram-positive and -negative bacteria, although plasmid-mediated resistance has diminished its effective spectrum. This antibiotic is rarely used in adult infections because of the rare idiosyncratic side effect of irreversible bone-marrow aplasia and the availability of other agents with similar activity. It remains one of the *drugs of choice* for the treatment of typhoid fever and plague and is still useful for the treatment of brucellosis and both pneumococcal and meningococcal meningitis in penicillin-allergic patients.

TETRACYCLINES Tetracyclines have a broad spectrum of bacteriostatic activity against gram-positive and -negative bacteria and are widely used in a variety of community-acquired infections. These agents are among the *drugs of choice* for chronic bronchitis, granuloma inguinale, brucellosis (with streptomycin), tularemia, glanders, melioidosis, spirochetal infections caused by *Borrelia* (Lyme disease and relapsing fever; doxycycline), infections caused by *Vibrio vulnificus*, some *Aeromonas* infections, infections due to *Stenotrophomonas* (minocycline), plague, and ehrlichiosis (doxycycline). The tetracyclines are also used in penicillin-allergic patients for the treatment of leptospirosis, syphilis, actinomycosis, and skin and soft-tissue infections caused by gram-positive cocci. They are among the *drugs of*

ehrlichiae and for granulomatous skin infection due to *Mycobacterium marinum* (minocycline). Doxycycline is also among the drugs recommended for the treatment of community-acquired pneumonia.

SULFONAMIDES AND TRIMETHOPRIM The folic acid synthesis inhibitors have a broad spectrum of bacteriostatic activity individually; in combination, they can be bactericidal against facultative gram-negative bacteria and staphylococci. The fixed combination of sulfamethoxazole and trimethoprim, the major folic acid synthesis inhibitors used in therapy for bacterial infections, has modest activity against some streptococci and no activity against strict anaerobes. However, resistance to the combination of sulfamethoxazole and trimethoprim is common among methicillin-resistant staphylococci and penicillin-resistant pneumococci and is increasing among *E. coli* strains that cause urinary tract infections. The individual sulfonamides are rarely used in the treatment of bacterial infections but are among the *drugs of choice* for the treatment of nocardial infections, leprosy (dapsone, a sulfone), and toxoplasmosis (sulfadiazine). Although increasing resistance has been reported among gram-negative organisms, trimethoprim-sulfamethoxazole remains one of the *drugs of choice* for the treatment of uncomplicated urinary tract infections (except for those caused by enterococci) and is widely used in the treatment of otitis media. It can be used in therapy for upper respiratory tract infections in which *S. pneumoniae*, *H. influenzae*, or *M. catarrhalis* is suspected; for gonococcal and meningococcal infections; for chancroid; and for infections thought to be caused by *Aeromonas*, *Stenotrophomonas*, *Burkholderia cepacia*, *Acinetobacter*, and *Yersinia enterocolitica*. For nosocomial infections due to *Stenotrophomonas*, trimethoprim-sulfamethoxazole is the *drug of choice*.

FLUOROQUINOLONES The fluoroquinolones have excellent activity against most facultative gram-negative rods and variable activity against gram-positive cocci; only trovafloxacin is active against obligate anaerobes. The quinolones are the oral agents with greatest activity against *P. aeruginosa*; ciprofloxacin is the most active against this species. All the quinolones except norfloxacin are well absorbed orally; ciprofloxacin, levofloxacin, trovafloxacin, and ofloxacin are also administered as intravenous formulations. The quinolones are among the *drugs of choice* for urinary tract infections, bacterial gastroenteritis, community-acquired pneumonia, and enteric fever and may be useful in therapy for serious hospital-acquired infections caused by gram-negative organisms. While older quinolones (ciprofloxacin, ofloxacin, and norfloxacin) have limited activity against gram-positive bacteria, the newer quinolones have an expanded spectrum of activity against gram-positive cocci, including staphylococci (both methicillin-susceptible and methicillin-resistant) and streptococci (especially *S. pneumoniae*). However, because of the potential for development of severe liver toxicity, it has been recommended that trovafloxacin use be limited to hospitalized patients with serious or life-threatening infections. Quinolones can also be used as prophylaxis for persons at risk for meningococcal meningitis. However, rapid expansion in the use of quinolones should be coupled with a consideration of the potential for development of resistance among all bacteria targeted by these drugs.

RIFAMPIN Rifampin has been used in combinations for the treatment of serious infections due to methicillin-resistant staphylococci (e.g., coagulase-negative staphylococcal foreign-body infections). Because the spontaneous selection of rifampin-resistant mutants occurs rapidly, rifampin should never be used alone in the treatment of staphylococcal infections. Rifampin is also used for chemoprophylaxis in persons at risk of meningococcal meningitis and for the treatment of *Legionella* pneumonia.

METRONIDAZOLE Metronidazole has a spectrum limited to anaerobic bacteria. It is one of the *drugs of choice* for the treatment of any abscess in which the involvement of obligate anaerobes is suspected (e.g., lung, brain, or intraabdominal abscesses) because of its spectrum and its ability to penetrate into the area of infection. Other antibacterial agents should be used in combination with metronidazole if facultative and aerobic pathogens are also thought to be involved.

Metronidazole is the *drug of choice* for the treatment of bacterial vaginosis and antibiotic-associated pseudomembranous colitis.

URINARY TRACT ANTISEPTICS Urinary tract antiseptics are active only in the lower urinary tract and cannot be used for the treatment of upper urinary tract or systemic infections. Their activity is limited to susceptible gram-negative enteric bacteria. The available agents in this category include nitrofurantoin and methenamine salts.

TOPICAL ANTIBACTERIAL AGENTS Mupirocin is available only as a topical preparation for use against staphylococci and streptococci. Its major applications are for impetigo and eradication of the staphylococcal carrier state. It is the *drug of choice* for the elimination of nasal carriage of both methicillin-susceptible and methicillin-resistant staphylococci. Unfortunately, the emergence of resistance is limiting its usefulness in some hospitals.

Although their efficacy has never been well documented, topical preparations that include sulfonamides, polymyxin B, neomycin, bacitracin, gramicidin, and novobiocin in a variety of combinations are widely used as eye drops, irrigation solutions, and ointments for superficial skin infections.

ADVERSE REACTIONS

Adverse drug reactions are frequently classified by mechanism as either dose-related ("toxic") effects or unpredictable reactions. Unpredictable reactions are further categorized as either idiosyncratic or allergic. Dose-related reactions include aminoglycoside-induced nephrotoxicity, penicillin-induced seizures, and vancomycin-induced anaphylactoid reactions. Many of these reactions can be avoided by reducing dosage, limiting the duration of therapy, or reducing the frequency or rate of administration. Adverse reactions to antibacterial agents are a common cause of morbidity, requiring alteration in therapy and additional expense, and they occasionally result in death. The elderly, often those with the more severe infections, may be especially prone to certain adverse reactions. →*For further discussion of adverse drug reactions, see Chap. 71.*

β-LACTAMS The therapeutic index for β-lactam antibiotics is broad, and dose-related adverse reactions are uncommon and largely preventable. The greatest concern is allergic reactions. All types can occur, including anaphylaxis (type 1, hypersensitivity reactions), nephritis and Coombs-positive hemolytic anemia (type 2, cytotoxic reactions), drug fever and serum sickness (type 3, immune-complex formation), contact dermatitis (type 4, cell-mediated effects), and maculopapular eruption (type 5, idiopathic reactions). Approximately 1 to 4% of treatment courses result in an allergic reaction, and approximately 0.004 to 0.015% of treatment courses result in anaphylaxis. Fewer than half the patients who claim an allergy to penicillin react to skin testing with the major and minor determinants (penicilloyl-polylysine and benzylpenicillin degradation products, respectively); those with negative skin tests only rarely react adversely to subsequent therapeutic doses. Generally, a suitable alternative to β-lactams is available for patients who have a severe allergy, and penicillin desensitization can be carefully undertaken if there is no suitable alternative. A small proportion (<2%) of persons who are allergic to penicillin react similarly when a cephalosporin is administered; thus, cephalosporins are contraindicated in patients with a history of an immediate reaction to penicillin, although they are often used in patients with a history of mild reactions. The same precaution applies to imipenem, but aztreonam is antigenically distinct and can be administered safely to the penicillin-allergic patient.

Other reactions thought to have an allergic basis include nephritis (associated with methicillin and occasionally nafcillin), hepatitis (related to oxacillin), leukopenia (following high doses of most β-lactams administered for prolonged periods), and severe skin rashes (toxic epidermal necrolysis and Stevens-Johnson syndrome). These reactions are not IgE-mediated, and skin testing is not predictive of their occurrence. For unclear reasons, most patients who have infectious mononucleosis develop a rash when given ampicillin or amoxicillin.

Miscellaneous reactions to β-lactams include gastrointestinal side effects ranging in severity from mild diarrhea (5 to 10%) to pseudomembranous colitis (<1%). Although the probability of antibiotic-associated colitis is low, a large number of cases occur because β-lactams are so commonly prescribed. Drugs excreted to a large extent through the bile, such as ampicillin and ceftriaxone, may be especially prone to cause diarrhea. The addition of clavulanic acid to amoxicillin further increases the frequency of diarrhea. Ceftriaxone, because of extremely high concentrations in bile, can cause "sludging" in the gallbladder and occasionally produces symptoms compatible with acute cholecystitis.

In high doses—and most often in patients with renal impairment who receive an excessive dose—penicillins (especially ticarcillin and penicillin G) can cause bleeding from impaired platelet aggregation. Ticarcillin is a disodium salt and in high doses can cause hypokalemia and fluid overload.

Seizures are occasionally observed with β-lactams, especially penicillin G and imipenem. This reaction is most common when excessive doses relative to renal function are administered or when the patient has a history of seizures.

VANCOMYCIN   When vancomycin was first used clinically in 1956, local intolerance at the infusion site was common, as were systemic reactions, including ototoxicity and nephrotoxicity. Current formulations are of higher purity and, when proper dosage guidelines are followed, are very safe, although phlebitis can still be troublesome. The most common adverse reaction is called *red man syndrome* and is characterized by pruritus, flushing, and erythema of the head and upper torso. This anaphylactoid reaction usually follows the first dose, is dependent on dose size and infusion time, and results from vancomycin-induced release of histamine. The reaction is usually mild in adult patients who receive 1 g over 60 min and diminishes with repeated doses. If vancomycin is mistakenly given as a bolus, severe hypotension may result. In unusually sensitive patients, extending the infusion time or administering H_1 receptor antagonists is usually effective in preventing this reaction or reducing its severity. Patients with this reaction must not be mislabeled as having an allergy to vancomycin, since vancomycin may be the only effective treatment for certain infections, such as those due to methicillin-resistant staphylococci.

Nephrotoxicity from vancomycin is mild and occurs in fewer than 5% of patients. Although some data suggest that aminoglycosides and vancomycin are synergistically nephrotoxic, this point is difficult to prove, and the simultaneous use of these agents should not be avoided if clinically indicated, as in the treatment of enterococcal endocarditis in penicillin-allergic patients.

Ototoxicity from vancomycin is rare as long as doses are appropriately reduced in patients with renal insufficiency. Other uncommon adverse reactions include leukopenia, skin rashes, and true allergy. Serum concentrations of vancomycin are of little use in predicting toxicity but may be of value in selecting dosages for patients with unstable renal function.

AMINOGLYCOSIDES   Aminoglycoside antibiotics have a narrow therapeutic index. The two most common adverse reactions are nephrotoxicity and ototoxicity. Rarely, respiratory depression is observed. Nephrotoxicity results from accumulation of the aminoglycoside in the peritubular space, with damage to the proximal tubule and a corresponding reduction in the glomerular filtration rate. The incidence of nephrotoxicity, defined as a >0.5% increase over baseline in the serum creatinine level, is approximately 5 to 10% among adult patients who receive therapy for 10 to 14 days. However, many cofactors also influence the frequency of toxicity, such as extremes of age (toxicity is uncommon among children, more common among the elderly), concomitant drug therapy, and hydration status. Nephrotoxicity is manifested clinically by a gradual rise in serum creatinine levels after a few days of therapy and is reversible if the dosage is reduced

or treatment is discontinued. Serum creatinine levels should be monitored every 3 to 5 days or more often if changes are seen. There is not an important difference among the most useful agents (gentamicin, tobramycin, and amikacin) in terms of the frequency of nephrotoxicity; streptomycin is a rare cause of nephrotoxicity. Some data suggest that once-daily administration may cause less nephrotoxicity.

Ototoxicity from aminoglycoside therapy presents as either auditory or vestibular damage. Since the aminoglycosides can destroy hair cells in the inner ear, ototoxicity may be permanent. The risk of ototoxicity increases with prolonged therapy, higher serum concentrations (especially in patients with renal impairment), hypovolemia, and concurrent treatment with other ototoxins, especially ethacrynic acid. Clinically apparent ototoxicity, manifested by diminished acuity or vestibular imbalance, is uncommon (probably occurring in <1% of cases) when the duration of therapy is kept to a minimum. With more sensitive monitoring (e.g., audiograms), asymptomatic high-tone hearing loss is more commonly noted. There are no clinically important differences among the aminoglycosides in the overall frequency of ototoxicity.

Neuromuscular depression from aminoglycosides is caused by reduced acetylcholine activity at postsynaptic membranes and can result in rare but severe respiratory depression. Risk factors include hypocalcemia, peritoneal administration, use of neuromuscular blockers, and preexisting respiratory depression. This complication can be largely avoided if the aminoglycoside is administered intravenously over 30 min or by intramuscular injection; if respiratory depression occurs, it is reversed by the administration of calcium.

Fear of toxicity should not prevent the use of aminoglycosides for a legitimate indication, since toxicity is usually mild and reversible. The value of measuring serum concentrations is controversial; these measurements are usually unnecessary when the patient is receiving once-daily therapy.

MACROLIDES   Serious adverse reactions to the macrolide antibiotics are very rare. Gastrointestinal effects, such as burning, nausea, and vomiting, are the most common adverse reactions to the macrolides; depending on dosage, these reactions may occur in up to 50% of patients, occasionally requiring early discontinuation of therapy. The mechanism is thought to be the binding of erythromycin to motilin receptors, with a consequent increase in gastrointestinal motility. Gastrointestinal side effects appear equally common for all the oral formulations and also occur with intravenous administration. Clarithromycin and azithromycin are better tolerated than erythromycin, although gastrointestinal distress is still their most common adverse effect.

Less common reactions include hepatotoxicity and ototoxicity. Hepatotoxicity is a rare, nonfatal complication that is usually associated with erythromycin estolate and presents as an allergic cholestatic jaundice. Ototoxicity is rare after oral administration but may occur in a dose-dependent pattern in up to 20% of adults who receive intravenous erythromycin (4 g/d) and have audiograms performed. Ototoxicity is usually reversible and mild. Allergic cutaneous reactions are observed in rare cases.

LINCOSAMIDES   The most common adverse effect of clindamycin is gastrointestinal distress. Diarrhea has been reported in up to 20% of patients and pseudomembranous colitis in 0.01 to 10%. The mechanism of pseudomembranous colitis is production of a toxin by *C. difficile* (Chap. 145). *C. difficile* colonizes the gastrointestinal tract and may produce a toxin when the normal flora is suppressed by clindamycin and other antibiotics, especially β-lactams. This toxin causes mucosal damage that results in cramps, pain, and diarrhea that may be bloody. Pseudomembranous colitis may follow both intravenous and oral administration and may not become manifest until after completion of therapy. Oral metronidazole or oral vancomycin is effective in treating symptomatic patients with toxin-positive stools, but some spores may survive, and relapse is frequent. Metronidazole is the *drug of choice* since oral treatment with vancomycin can select for vancomycin-resistant enterococci. Although diarrhea and pseudomembranous colitis can be caused by most antibacterial agents, the incidence in relation to the amount used appears to be highest for clindamycin. Allergic reactions (such as rashes and fever), hepatotoxicity, and neutropenia are observed only rarely.

CHLORAMPHENICOL Chloramphenicol causes two types of bone marrow suppression: a dose-related, reversible suppression of all elements, which occurs commonly during therapy at the maximal recommended doses (4 g/d in adults), and an idiosyncratic, irreversible aplastic anemia, which occurs in approximately 1 in every 25,000 to 40,000 exposures. The irreversible form has been reported to follow all types of chloramphenicol treatment, including ocular administration, and often develops months after therapy is discontinued.

In premature neonates and infants, chloramphenicol can cause a dose-related "gray syndrome" that is characterized by cyanosis, hypotension, and death and that results from an inability of the newborn to metabolize the drug. These potentially serious toxicities and the availability of newer drugs have substantially reduced the indications for chloramphenicol.

TETRACYCLINES Gastrointestinal effects are the most common adverse reactions to the tetracyclines. These problems may be related to a direct irritant effect, since tetracyclines can also cause esophageal ulceration when they dissolve before reaching the stomach. It is important that nighttime doses be taken with sufficient fluid. Concurrent food intake may improve tolerance, but absorption of tetracycline HCl is impaired when the drug is taken with food.

Hepatotoxicity has been reported after administration of >2 g of tetracycline intravenously and at lower doses during pregnancy. There are currently no indications for intravenous tetracycline treatment in pregnancy. All tetracyclines can cause phototoxic skin reactions; these reactions are most common with doxycycline. Other dermal reactions, including rash, are uncommon. Tetracyclines are contraindicated in children <8 years of age because of mottling of the permanent teeth; doxycycline may be less likely than the other tetracyclines to cause this problem. Worsening of renal function in patients with preexisting renal dysfunction has been reported with use of tetracycline, although some of the increased azotemia may be due to amino acid catabolism. Doxycycline and perhaps minocycline appear to be free from these renal side effects. Alternative effective agents are nearly always available for use in patients with renal dysfunction. Minocycline can cause vertigo in up to 70% of women receiving therapeutic doses and in a lower percentage of men.

SULFONAMIDES AND TRIMETHOPRIM The sulfonamides are generally safe, but the list of possible adverse reactions is very long. These compounds occasionally cause a number of allergic reactions, from relatively minor skin rashes (including maculopapular rashes and urticarial reactions typically appearing after a week of therapy) to severe or even life-threatening reactions such as erythema multiforme, Stevens-Johnson syndrome, and toxic epidermal necrolysis. The severe hypersensitivity reactions have occurred most commonly after treatment with the long-acting sulfonamides, such as sulfamethoxypyridazine, which are no longer used. Pyrimethamine plus sulfadoxine (Fansidar), used for malaria prophylaxis, may cause severe allergic reactions, including hepatic and hematologic toxicities, in addition to dermatologic toxicity. Photosensitivity reactions are also relatively common with sulfonamides.

Many patients infected with HIV who receive trimethoprim-sulfamethoxazole have adverse dermatologic reactions. These reactions are usually not life-threatening and appear to regress in many cases despite continuation of therapy. In high doses, trimethoprim interferes with the renal secretion of potassium. Hyperkalemia is relatively common among HIV-positive patients and is most often found after 7 days of trimethoprim-sulfamethoxazole therapy for pneumonia caused by *Pneumocystis carinii*.

Sulfonamides and trimethoprim may also cause severe hematologic complications, including agranulocytosis, hemolytic and megaloblastic anemia, and thrombocytopenia. These dose-related side effects may be greater in patients with renal insufficiency. Hemolytic anemia is most common in patients with glucose-6-phosphate dehydrogenase deficiency who take long-acting compounds; trimethoprim-

sulfamethoxazole rarely causes hemolysis in such subjects. Granulocytopenia from trimethoprim-sulfamethoxazole is especially common in HIV-infected patients, occurring in 10 to 50% of this group.

Renal insufficiency, caused by crystals of the relatively insoluble acetyl metabolite, is observed primarily with the long-acting sulfonamides. Many cases of crystalluria in HIV-infected patients taking sulfadiazine for toxoplasmosis have been reported. A high level of fluid intake may prevent this complication.

It is recommended that sulfonamides not be administered to the newborn because of concerns that bilirubin may be displaced from protein-binding sites, with subsequent jaundice and kernicterus.

In addition to the preceding problems, sulfonamides may occasionally cause drug fever with serum sickness, hepatic toxicity (including necrosis), and systemic lupus erythematosus.

FLUOROQUINOLONES Fluoroquinolones are relatively safe; adverse reactions rarely require discontinuation of therapy. The most common reactions include gastrointestinal distress, such as nausea or diarrhea (<5%), and central nervous system effects, including insomnia and dizziness (<5%). Trovafloxacin is prone to causing dizziness, especially among women. However, of more serious concern is the report of more than 100 cases of symptomatic liver toxicity in patients receiving trovafloxacin, including 14 cases of acute liver failure strongly associated with trovafloxacin exposure. As a result, the Food and Drug Administration has recommended that this quinolone be used only in hospitalized patients with serious or life-threatening conditions in which the benefits offered by the drug outweigh its potential risks. Phototoxicity can be severe, especially with sparfloxacin. Rarely, hepatic and renal dysfunction and anaphylactoid and allergic reactions are observed. Tendon rupture has also been associated with quinolone use in rare instances. The use of these drugs is contraindicated in patients <18 years of age because of evidence in animals of cartilage damage in developing joints. In carefully selected situations in which the perceived benefits outweigh the risks (e.g., in adolescent patients with cystic fibrosis who have pulmonary exacerbations), fluoroquinolones may be useful for short-term therapy. They are contraindicated in pregnancy because of concern for the developing fetus.

RIFAMPIN Rifampin is generally well tolerated but has several important side effects. Some patients have transient rises in hepatic aminotransferases, but these levels usually return to normal without discontinuation of the drug. Although hepatitis from rifampin itself develops only rarely, the drug is thought by some investigators to potentiate the hepatic toxicity of concomitantly administered isoniazid. Intermittent administration of rifampin (usually fewer than three times per week) has been associated with symptoms that seem to have an immunologic basis. These include flulike symptoms and (rarely) hemolysis, thrombocytopenia, shock, and renal failure. Minor gastrointestinal side effects, skin rashes, and interstitial nephritis have also been reported. Patients should be warned that rifampin and its metabolites cause secretions such as urine, tears, sweat, and saliva to turn orange and that contact lenses may be stained.

METRONIDAZOLE Serious adverse reactions to metronidazole are uncommon. Gastrointestinal side effects such as nausea are most frequent but rarely necessitate discontinuation of therapy. Pseudomembranous colitis in association with metronidazole has been reported but is very rare. A metallic taste is relatively common, and stomatitis and glossitis are occasionally reported. Disulfiram-like reactions can occur if ethanol is ingested concurrently. Peripheral neuropathy develops in some patients, and seizures and encephalopathy have been reported after high doses and in patients with hepatic failure.

Concerns about mutagenicity and carcinogenicity from metronidazole have led to recommendations that it not be used in pregnancy (especially during the first trimester) when alternative agents are available. Although retrospective studies have found no association between metronidazole and carcinogenesis, long-term administration of high doses should be avoided when therapeutic alternatives exist.

Table 137-3 Interactions of Antibacterial Agents with Other Drugs

Antibiotic	Interacts with	Potential Consequence (Clinical Significance[a])
Erythromycin/ clarithromycin	Theophylline	Theophylline toxicity—e.g., seizures (1)
	Carbamazepine	Central nervous system depression (1)
	Digoxin	Digoxin toxicity (3)
	Triazolam/midazolam	Central nervous system depression (2)
	Ergotamine	Ergotism (1)
	Warfarin	Bleeding (2)
	Cyclosporine/tacrolimus	Nephrotoxicity (1)
	Astemizole, terfenadine, cisapride, pimozide	Cardiac arrhythmias (1)
	"Statins"	Rhabdomyolysis (2)
	Valproate	Valproate toxicity (2)
Fluoroquinolones[b]	Theophylline	Theophylline toxicity (2)
	Antacids/sucralfate	Subtherapeutic antibiotic levels (1)
Tetracycline	Antacids/sucralfate	Subtherapeutic antibiotic levels (1)
Trimethoprim- sulfamethoxazole	Phenytoin	Phenytoin toxicity (2)
	Oral hypoglycemics	Hypoglycemia (2)
	Digoxin	Digoxin toxicity (3)
	Warfarin	Bleeding (2)
Metronidazole	Ethanol	Disulfiram-like reactions (2)
	Fluorouracil	Bone marrow suppression (1)
	Warfarin	Bleeding (2)
Rifampin	Warfarin	Clot formation (1)
	Oral contraceptives	Pregnancy (1)
	Cyclosporine/tacrolimus	Rejection (1)
	HIV-1 protease inhibitors	Increased viral load, resistance (1)
	Nonnucleoside reverse transcriptase inhibitors	Increased viral load, resistance (1)
	Glucocorticoids	Loss of steroid effect (1)
	Methadone	Withdrawal (1)
	Digoxin	Subtherapeutic digoxin levels (1)
	Itraconazole	Subtherapeutic itraconazole levels (1)
	Phenytoin	Loss of seizure control (1)
	"Statins"	Hypercholesterolemia (1)
	Diltiazem	Subtherapeutic diltiazem levels (1)
	Verapamil	Subtherapeutic verapamil levels (1)

[a] 1, a well-documented interaction with clinically important consequences; 2, an interaction of uncertain frequency but of potential clinical importance; 3, an unusual interaction of possible clinical importance.

[b] Ciprofloxacin, grepafloxacin > levofloxacin, trovafloxacin.

DRUG INTERACTIONS

Historically, clinically important interactions involving antibacterial drugs were generally of little concern, since β-lactams were the most widely used agents and rarely interacted with other drugs in a manner that affected the patient adversely. However, fluoroquinolones, macrolides, and rifampin are now more widely used, and interactions are of increasing concern. Table 137-3 lists the most common and best-documented interactions of antibacterial agents with other drugs and characterizes the clinical relevance of these interactions. Coadministration of drugs paired in Table 137-3 does not necessarily have clinically important adverse consequences. The result depends on the timing of administration, the dose and duration of therapy, the baseline serum concentration of the non-antibacterial drug administered, the patient's susceptibility to the pharmacologic effect of the non-antibacterial drug, and other, less-well-described cofactors. Recognition of the potential for an interaction before the administration of an antibacterial agent is crucial to the rational use of these drugs, since adverse consequences can often be prevented if the interaction is anticipated. Table 137-3 is intended only to heighten awareness of the potential for an interaction. Additional sources should be consulted to identify appropriate options. →*For further discussion of drug interactions, see Chap. 70.*

MACROLIDES Erythromycin and clarithromycin can inhibit the P450 enzyme CYP3A and thus the metabolism of many concurrently administered drugs, such as cisapride, theophylline, carbamazepine, terfenadine, astemizole, warfarin, and ergot alkaloids. The magnitude of the theophylline interaction is highly variable and is proportional to the dose and duration of erythromycin treatment. In contrast, cyclosporine levels predictably increase when erythromycin is administered, since CYP3A is responsible for cyclosporine metabolism. Decreased metabolism of terfenadine, astemizole, cisapride, and pimozide has been reported to cause severe cardiac dysfunction. Azithromycin has little effect on the metabolism of other drugs. In approximately 10% of patients receiving digoxin, concentrations increase when erythromycin is also given.

TETRACYCLINES The most important interaction involving tetracyclines is the reduction in absorption when these drugs are coadministered with di- and trivalent cations, such as antacids, iron compounds, or dairy products. A similar interaction is seen with quinolones (see below). Food also adversely affects absorption of most tetracyclines. Inducers of hepatic isoenzymes, such as phenytoin and barbiturates, increase the clearance of doxycycline; although the clinical significance of this effect is unknown, use of an alternative antibiotic may be appropriate.

SULFONAMIDES Sulfonamides may increase the hypoprothrombinemic effect of warfarin by inhibition of its metabolism and possibly by protein-binding displacement. Sulfonamides may also potentiate the effects of oral hypoglycemic agents and phenytoin through reduction in metabolism or displacement from serum protein.

FLUOROQUINOLONES There are two clinically important drug interactions involving fluoroquinolones. First, like tetracyclines, all fluoroquinolones are chelated by divalent and trivalent cations, which prevent most of the dose from being absorbed. Second, certain fluoroquinolones (grepafloxacin, ciprofloxacin, and—to a much lesser extent—levofloxacin and trovafloxacin) can inhibit hepatic enzymes that metabolize theophylline, with resultant theophylline toxicity. The same mechanism accounts for increases in serum caffeine concentrations, but the clinical significance of this interaction is unknown. Scattered reports indicate that quinolones can also potentiate the nephrotoxicity of cyclosporine, exaggerate the effects of warfarin, and increase neurotoxicity when coadministered with nonsteroidal anti-inflammatory agents. However, these interactions have not been confirmed by controlled trials.

RIFAMPIN Rifampin is an excellent inducer of many cytochrome P450 enzymes and increases the hepatic clearance of a number of drugs, including the following (with the indicated predictable outcomes): HIV-1 protease inhibitors (loss of viral suppression), oral contraceptives (pregnancy), warfarin (decreased prothrombin times), cyclosporine and prednisone (organ rejection or exacerbations of any underlying inflammatory condition), and verapamil and diltiazem (increased dosage requirements). Before rifampin is prescribed for any patient, a review of concomitant drug therapy is essential.

METRONIDAZOLE Metronidazole can cause a disulfiram-like syndrome when alcohol is ingested; thus, patients taking metronidazole should be instructed to avoid alcohol. Inhibition of the metabolism of warfarin by metronidazole leads to significant rises in prothrombin times.

PROPHYLAXIS OF BACTERIAL INFECTIONS

Antibacterial agents are occasionally indicated for use in patients who have no evidence of infection but who have been or are expected to be exposed to bacterial pathogens under circumstances that constitute a major risk of infection. The basic tenets of antimicrobial prophylaxis are as follows: First, the risk or potential severity of infection should be greater than the risk of side effects from the antibacterial agent. Second, the antibacterial agent should be given for the shortest period necessary to prevent target infections. Third, the antibacterial agent should be given before the expected period of risk (e.g., surgical prophylaxis) or as soon as possible after contact with an infected individual (e.g., prophylaxis for meningococcal meningitis).

Table 137-4 lists the major indications for antibacterial prophylaxis in adults. (The use of antibacterial agents in children to prevent rheumatic fever and otitis media under certain circumstances is also common practice.) The table includes only those indications that are widely accepted, supported by well-designed studies, or recommended by expert panels. Prophylaxis is also used but is less widely accepted for recurrent cellulitis in conjunction with lymphedema, recurrent pneumococcal meningitis in conjunction with deficiencies in humoral immunity or CSF leaks, traveler's diarrhea, gram-negative sepsis in conjunction with neutropenia, and spontaneous bacterial peritonitis in conjunction with ascites.

The major use of antibacterial prophylaxis in the United States is for infections following surgical procedures. Antibacterial agents are administered just before the surgical procedure—and, for long operations, during the procedure as well—to ensure high levels in serum and tissues during surgery. The objective is to eradicate bacteria originating from the air of the operating suite, the skin of the surgical team, or the patient's own flora that may contaminate the wound. In all but colorectal surgical procedures, prophylaxis is predominantly directed against staphylococci. Prophylaxis is intended to prevent wound infection or infection of implanted devices, not all infections that may occur during the postoperative period (e.g., urinary tract infections or pneumonia). Prolonged prophylaxis merely alters the normal flora and favors infections with organisms resistant to the antibacterial agents used.

ANTIBACTERIAL COSTS AND INAPPROPRIATE USE

Use of antibacterial agents in hospitals in the United States accounts for an important percentage of all drug costs and may represent the largest expenditure for any pharmacologic class. In the outpatient setting, the costs of antibacterial drugs are second only to those of cardiovascular agents. A survey of office-based physicians found that between 1980 and 1992 there was a marked increase in the use of expensive broad-spectrum antimicrobials. It is not unusual for the purchase cost (in 2000 dollars) of a newer parenteral antibiotic to be $1000 to $2000 for a 10- to 14-day course of treatment. Therapy with a new oral antibiotic can easily cost $50 to $75. Administration costs, monitoring costs, and pharmacy charges must be added to these figures. While some newer antibacterial agents undeniably represent important

Table 137-4 Prophylaxis of Bacterial Infections in Adults

Condition	Antibacterial Agent	Timing or Duration of Prophylaxis
Nonsurgical		
Cardiac lesions susceptible to bacterial endocarditis	Amoxicillin[a]	Before and after procedures causing bacteremia
Recurrent S. aureus infections	Mupirocin	5 days (intranasal)
Contact with patient with meningococcal meningitis	Rifampin Ciprofloxacin or ofloxacin	2 days Single dose
Bite wounds[b]	Penicillin V or amoxicillin/clavulanic acid	3–5 days
Recurrent cystitis	Trimethoprim-sulfamethoxazole or a quinolone or nitrofurantoin	3 times per week for up to 1 year or after sexual intercourse
Surgical		
Clean (cardiac, vascular, neurologic, or orthopedic surgery)	Cefazolin (vancomycin)[c]	Before and during procedure
Ocular	Topical combinations and sub-conjunctival cefazolin	During and at end of procedure
Clean-contaminated (head and neck, high-risk gastroduodenal or biliary tract surgery; high-risk cesarean section; hysterectomy)	Cefazolin (or clindamycin for head and neck)	Before and during procedure
Clean-contaminated (vaginal or abdominal hysterectomy)	Cefazolin or cefoxitin or cefotetan	Before and during procedure
Clean-contaminated (high-risk genitourinary surgery)	Ciprofloxacin	Before and during procedure
Clean-contaminated (colorectal surgery or appendectomy)	Cefoxitin or cefotetan (add oral neomycin + erythromycin for colorectal)	Before and during procedure
Dirty[b] (ruptured viscus)	Cefoxitin or cefotetan ± gentamicin (clindamycin + gentamicin) or another appropriate regimen directed at anaerobes and gram-negative aerobes	Before and for 3–5 days after procedure
Dirty[b] (traumatic wound)	Cefazolin	Before and for 3–5 days after trauma

[a] Gentamicin should be added to the amoxicillin regimen for high-risk gastrointestinal and genitourinary procedures; vancomycin should be used in penicillin-allergic patients.
[b] In these cases, use of antibacterial agents actually constitutes treatment of infection rather than prophylaxis.
[c] Vancomycin is recommended only in institutions that have a high incidence of infection with methicillin-resistant staphylococci.

advances in therapy, many newer drugs offer no advantage over older, less expensive agents.

Clinicians are understandably confused by the bewildering array of available drugs. Numerous surveys have reported that approximately 50% of antibiotic use is in some way "inappropriate." Aside from the monetary cost of unnecessary antibiotics, there are the costs of excess morbidity from adverse effects and drug interactions and the eventual costs of treating more resistant organisms. The following suggestions are intended to provide guidance through the antibiotic maze.

First, objective evidence regarding the merits of newer drugs is available through publications such as *The Medical Letter*, including the annual update of *Drugs of Choice*. Second, clinicians should become comfortable using a few drugs recommended by independent experts and should resist the temptation to use a new drug unless the merits are clear. A new antibacterial agent with a "broader spectrum and greater potency" or a "longer half-life and higher tissue levels" does not necessarily mean greater clinical efficacy. Third, the clinician must become familiar with local bacterial susceptibility profiles. It may not be necessary to use a new drug with "improved activity against *P. aeruginosa*" if that pathogen is rarely encountered or if it retains full susceptibility to older drugs. Finally, with regard to inpatient use of antibacterial drugs, appropriate empirical treatment with one or more broad-spectrum agents may often be simplified, with use of a narrower-spectrum agent or even an oral drug, once the results of cultures and susceptibility tests become available. While there is an understandable temptation not to alter effective therapy, switching to a more specific agent, once the patient has improved clinically, does not compromise eventual outcome. If these guidelines are followed, the care of patients will not be undermined, many unnecessary complications and expenses will be avoided, and the useful life of valuable drugs will be extended.

BIBLIOGRAPHY

ANNÉ S, REISMAN RE: Risk of administering cephalosporin antibiotics to patients with histories of penicillin allergy. Ann Allergy Asthma Immunol 74:167, 1995

Antimicrobial prophylaxis in surgery. Med Lett Drugs Ther 39:97, 1997

BARTLETT JG et al: Community-acquired pneumonia in adults: Guidelines for management. Clin Infect Dis 26:811, 1998

CRAIG WA: Pharmacokinetic/pharmacodynamic parameters: Rationale for antibacterial dosing of mice and men. Clin Infect Dis 26:1, 1998

GONZALES R et al: Antibiotic prescribing for adults with colds, upper respiratory tract infections, and bronchitis by ambulatory care physicians. JAMA 278:901, 1997

HOSPITAL INFECTION CONTROL PRACTICES ADVISORY COMMITTEE: Recommendations for preventing the spread of vancomycin resistance. Infect Control Hosp Epidemiol 16:105, 1995

POLK R: Optimal use of modern antibiotics: Emerging trends. Clin Infect Dis 29:264, 1999

SEPPALA H et al: The effects of changes in the consumption of macrolide antibiotics on erythromycin resistance in group A streptococci in Finland. N Engl J Med 337:441, 1997

SHLAES DM et al: Guidelines for the prevention of antimicrobial resistance in hospitals. Clin Infect Dis 25:584, 1997

SMITH T et al: Emergence of vancomycin resistance in Staphylococcus aureus. N Engl J Med 340:493, 1999

The choice of antibacterial drugs. Med Lett Drugs Ther 40:33, 1998

Section 5
DISEASES CAUSED BY GRAM-POSITIVE BACTERIA

138   *Daniel M. Musher*

PNEUMOCOCCAL INFECTIONS

Streptococcus pneumoniae (the pneumococcus) was recognized as a major cause of pneumonia in the 1880s and has been a central focus of study leading to the modern understanding of humoral immunity. The name *Diplococcus pneumoniae* was assigned to the organism in 1926 on the basis of its appearance in Gram-stained sputum. In 1974, the organism was renamed *Streptococcus pneumoniae* because of its growth in chains in liquid medium. Around 1900, pneumococcal serotypes were recognized when the injection of killed organisms into a rabbit stimulated the production of serum antibody that agglutinated and caused increased capsular density of the immunizing strain as well as of some but not all other pneumococcal isolates. Ninety serotypes have now been identified, each possessing a unique polysaccharide capsule.

MICROBIOLOGY   Pneumococci are identified in the clinical laboratory as gram-positive cocci that grow in chains and are catalase-negative. They produce pneumolysin, a toxin that breaks down hemoglobin into a greenish degeneration product, thereby causing α hemolysis on blood agar. More than 98% of pneumococcal isolates are susceptible to ethylhydrocupreine (optochin), and virtually all pneumococcal colonies are dissolved by bile salts.

Peptidoglycan and teichoic acid are the principal constituents of the pneumococcal cell wall. The cell wall's integrity depends on the presence of numerous peptide side chains cross-linked by the activity of enzymes such as trans- and carboxypeptidases. β-Lactam antibiotics inactivate these enzymes by covalently binding their active site. Unique to *S. pneumoniae* and present in all strains is C (for "cell-wall") substance, a polysaccharide consisting of teichoic acid with a phosphorylcholine residue. Surface-exposed choline-binding proteins serve as a site of attachment for potential virulence factors, such as PspA, which may prevent phagocytosis. Nearly every clinical isolate of *S. pneumoniae* has a polysaccharide capsule.

There are two systems for numbering the 90 known distinct capsules of *S. pneumoniae*. In the American system, serotypes are numbered in the order in which they were identified. The strains that most frequently cause human disease were generally the earliest to be identified and thus tend to have lower numbers. The more widely accepted Danish system places serotypes into groups based on antigenic similarities; for example, Danish group 19 includes types 19F ("first rec-

ognized"), 19A, 19B, and 19C, which in the American system would be types 19, 57, 58, and 59, respectively. Serotyping was clinically relevant in the 1930s, when type-specific antisera were administered as therapy, and (although genetic typing is more specific) it has again become important for epidemiologic studies of the spread of antibiotic-resistant isolates in communities and among countries. Capsule switching has been documented and to some extent limits the epidemiologic reliability of serotyping.

EPIDEMIOLOGY   *S. pneumoniae* colonizes the nasopharynx and can be isolated from 5 to 10% of healthy adults and from 20 to 40% of healthy children. Once the organisms have colonized an adult, they are likely to persist for 2 to 4 weeks but may persist for as long as 6 months. Pneumococci spread from one individual to another as a result of extensive close contact; transmission may be enhanced by poor ventilation. Day-care centers have been a site of spread, especially of penicillin-resistant strains of serotypes 6B, 14, 19F, and 23F. Outbreaks occur among adults in crowded living conditions—e.g., in military barracks, prisons, and shelters for the homeless—as well as among susceptible populations in settings such as nursing homes. The risk of pneumococcal pneumonia is not increased by contact in schools or workplaces (including hospitals).

The incidence of pneumococcal bacteremia is relatively high among infants up to 2 years of age and low among teenagers and young adults; rates increase beginning at around age 55. A surveillance study in South Carolina showed the incidences of pneumococcal bacteremia among infants, young adults, and persons ≥70 years of age to be 160, 5, and 70 cases per 100,000 population, respectively. Most cases of pneumococcal bacteremia in adults are due to pneumonia, and there are three to four cases of nonbacteremic pneumonia for every bacteremic case. Thus, it is estimated that there are 20 cases of pneumococcal pneumonia annually per 100,000 young adults and 280 cases annually per 100,000 persons over the age of 70. The incidence of pneumococcal bacteremia among adults exhibits a distinct midwinter peak and a striking dip in summer. In children, the incidence of bacteremia is relatively constant throughout the year except for a marked dip in midsummer. For reasons that are unclear, certain populations, including Native Americans, Native Alaskans, and African Americans, appear to be unusually susceptible to invasive pneumococcal disease. This enhanced susceptibility, not unlike that to infection with *Haemophilus influenzae*, is thought to have a genetic basic that thus far remains unelucidated.

PATHOGENETIC MECHANISMS   *S. pneumoniae* attaches to human nasopharyngeal cells through the specific interaction of bacterial surface adhesins, such as pneumococcal surface antigen A or choline-binding proteins, with epithelial cell receptors. Epithelial cell glycoconjugates containing the disaccharide GlcNAcβ1-4Gal or asialo-GM1 glycolipid are possible binding sites. Pneumococcal phase variation, in which organisms switch between transparent and opaque, may also play a role in adherence. Upon culture, a mixed population of transparent and opaque pneumococcal colonies can be identified. Organisms from opaque colonies have relatively little peptidoglycan and relatively large capsules; those from transparent colonies have much more phosphorylcholine (which contributes to their capacity to adhere to mammalian cells) and less capsular polysaccharide. When an opaque colony is inoculated intranasally into an experimental animal, only those organisms that form transparent colonies persist. In contrast, after intraperitoneal inoculation, organisms that yield transparent colonies are rapidly cleared from the blood, while those that make opaque colonies resist clearance.

Once the nasopharynx has been colonized, infection results if the organisms are carried into anatomically contiguous areas such as the eustachian tubes or the nasal sinuses and if their clearance is hindered, for example, by mucosal edema due to allergy or viral infection. Similarly, pneumonia ensues if organisms are inhaled or aspirated into the bronchioles or alveoli and then are not cleared—in many cases, because viral infection or cigarette smoke or other toxic substances have increased mucus production and/or damaged ciliary action. A mechanism by which pneumococci may bind to pneumocytes after viral infection has been suggested. Pneumocytes activated by cytokines have been shown to express the receptor for platelet-activating factor. This receptor binds the phosphorylcholine residue on pneumococcal C substance, facilitating the adherence of pneumococci. Studies suggest that pneumococci may invade tissues by penetrating mucosal layers; the clinical significance of this finding remains to be determined.

Once pneumococci reach an area where they do not naturally belong, they activate complement by classic and alternative pathways and stimulate cytokine production, which leads to the attraction of polymorphonuclear neutrophils (PMNs). The polysaccharide capsule, however, renders the organisms resistant to phagocytosis. In the absence of anticapsular antibody, phagocytic cells such as alveolar macrophages have a limited capacity to ingest and kill pneumococci; a large bacterial inoculum and/or the compromise of phagocytic function allows the initiation of lung infection. Infection of the meninges, joint spaces, bones, and peritoneal cavity results from the spread of pneumococci through the bloodstream, usually but not always from a recognized focus of infection in the respiratory tract.

The capacity to cause disease reflects the ability of pneumococci to escape ingestion and killing by host phagocytic cells, on the one hand, and to stimulate an inflammatory response and damage tissues, on the other. Encapsulated pneumococci are poorly ingested and killed in vivo in the immunologically naive host or in vitro by mammalian phagocytic cells in the absence of anticapsular antibody and complement. Unencapsulated pneumococci virtually never cause invasive disease (although they can cause conjunctivitis), and mutants lacking a capsule are essentially avirulent in experimental animals. Symptoms of disease are largely attributable to the generation of an inflammatory response that may cause pain by increasing pressure (as in otitis media) or may interfere with vital bodily functions, such as oxygenation of blood (as in pneumonia) or cerebral function (as in meningitis). Cell-wall constituents of *S. pneumoniae*, including teichoic acid, C substance, and (in particular) peptidoglycan, activate complement by the alternative pathway; the reaction between cell-wall structures and antibody also activates the classic complement pathway. The result is the release of C5a, a potent attractant for PMNs, into the surrounding medium. Inflammation is also facilitated by the ability of peptidoglycan to stimulate cytokine production, which activates endothelial cells to express selectin and integrin receptors for inflammatory cells. Inflammation in the central nervous system (CNS) during meningitis is a major contributor to neuronal cell injury. Pneumolysin, a thiol-activated toxin, exerts a variety of effects on ciliary cells and PMNs and also activates the classic complement pathway by direct binding to Clq. Injection of pneumolysin into the lungs of experimental animals

produces the histologic features of pneumonia; in mice, immunization with this substance or challenge with genetically engineered mutants that do not produce pneumolysin is associated with a significant reduction in virulence. Autolysin may contribute to the pathogenesis of pneumococcal disease by lysing bacteria, thereby releasing their constituents and heightening the reaction with human tissues. The release of excitatory amino acids in neuronal tissue may contribute to damage caused by meningitis.

HOST DEFENSE MECHANISMS Mechanisms of host defense may be immunologically nonspecific or specific. Nonspecific mechanisms include laminar airflow across mucous layers that filter inspired air, the glottal reflex, laryngeal closure, the cough reflex, the clearance of organisms from the lower airways by ciliated cells, and the ingestion by pulmonary macrophages and PMNs of small bacterial inocula that manage to reach alveolar spaces. Respiratory virus infection, chronic pulmonary disease, or heart failure compromises these mechanisms, predisposing to the development of pneumococcal pneumonia. Antibody to PspA and other pneumococcal constituents such as pneumolysin may be prevalent in the population and may contribute to immunity that is immunologically specific but not type specific.

Anticapsular antibody provides serotype-specific protection against pneumococcal infection. However, most healthy adults lack IgG antibody to most pneumococcal capsular polysaccharides. Antibody appears after colonization, infection, or vaccination. In the first few weeks after colonization, nonspecific mechanisms probably protect the host from infection. Thereafter, newly developed anticapsular antibody provides a high degree of specific protection. In contrast to this normal situation, adults who are at risk of aspirating pharyngeal contents and/or who have diminished mechanisms of lower airway clearance are at risk of developing pneumonia before antibody is produced. Similarly, children whose nasal mucosal membranes become acutely congested around the time of colonization are at risk of developing otitis media. Persons with a diminished capacity to form antibody remain susceptible for as long as they are colonized.

The risk of serious pneumococcal infection is greatly increased in persons with conditions that compromise IgG synthesis and/or the phagocytic function of PMNs and macrophages; this risk is also elevated in the presence of conditions associated with debilitation or malnutrition. Nearly all adults who are hospitalized for pneumococcal pneumonia have at least one of the conditions listed in Table 138-1 and/or fall into one of the groups known to be at high risk on epidemiologic grounds. Prior hospitalization either predisposes to or serves as a strong marker for pneumococcal infection. The susceptibility of elderly individuals to pneumococcal pneumonia may reflect diminished clearance mechanisms as well as debilitation, malnutrition, and comorbid diseases. Although IgG responses to capsular polysaccharides, as measured by enzyme-linked immunosorbent assay (ELISA), are more or less normal in elderly persons, the functional capacity of the antibody appears to be decreased. The remarkably high incidence of pneumococcal infection—perhaps 100-fold above baseline—among persons with AIDS is noteworthy.

Once a pneumococcal infection has been initiated, the absence of a spleen predisposes to fulminant disease. The liver is able to remove opsonized (antibody-coated) pneumococci from the circulation; in the absence of antibody, however, only the slow passage of blood through the splenic sinuses and prolonged contact with reticuloendothelial cells in the cords of Billroth allow time for bacterial clearance. Patients without spleens may die of pneumococcal pneumonia and sepsis at such an early stage of the illness that pulmonary consolidation is not evident on x-ray before death but rather is found only at autopsy.

SPECIFIC INFECTIONS CAUSED BY *S. PNEUMONIAE* *S. pneumoniae* causes infections of the middle ear, sinuses, trachea, bronchi, and lungs (Table 138-2) by direct spread from the nasopharyngeal site of colonization. Infections of the CNS, heart valves, bones, joints, and peritoneal cavity usually arise by hematogenous spread; in rare cases peritoneal infection develops via ascent through the fallo-

Table 138-1   Conditions That Commonly Predispose to Pneumococcal Infection

Defective antibody formation
    Common variable hypogammaglobulinemia
    Selective IgG-subclass deficiency
    Multiple myeloma
    Chronic lymphocytic leukemia
    Lymphoma
Defective complement function
Defective clearance of pneumococcal bacteremia[a]
    Congenital asplenia, hyposplenia
    Splenectomy
    Sickle cell disease
Multifactorial conditions
    Infancy and aging
    Chronic disease, hospitalization
    Glucocorticoid treatment
    Malnutrition
    Infection with HIV
    Alcoholism
    Cirrhosis of the liver
    Renal insufficiency
    Diabetes mellitus
    Fatigue, stress, and/or exposure to cold
Increased risk of exposure
    Day-care centers
    Military training camps
    Prisons
    Shelters for the homeless
Respiratory infection, inflammation[b]
    Influenza, other viral respiratory infections
    Air pollution
    Allergies
    Cigarette smoking
    Chronic obstructive pulmonary disease
    Other causes of chronic pulmonary inflammation or obstruction
Anatomic disruption of meninges (dural tear)[c]

[a] The absence of a spleen predisposes to more fulminant infection (see text).
[b] Predisposes specifically to infections of the upper or lower respiratory tract.
[c] Predisposes to recurrent bacterial meningitis.

pian tubes. The CNS may also be infected by contiguous spread of organisms, as in patients who have a tear in the dura. Primary bacteremia—i.e., the presence of pneumococci in the blood with no apparent source—occurs commonly in children under 2 years of age and as a small percentage of all pneumococcal bacteremias in adults; if no therapy is given, a source may become apparent. Pleural infection results either from direct extension of pneumonia to the visceral pleura or from hematogenous spread of bacteria from a pulmonary or extrapulmonary focus; the route cannot be determined in any individual case.

Otitis Media and Sinusitis   When fluid from the middle ear is cultured during acute otitis media or fluid from a paranasal sinus is cultured during acute sinusitis, *S. pneumoniae* is the most common isolate or is second only to nontypable *H. influenzae*. Whether in adults or in children, pneumococci are identified in about 40 to 50% of cases of otitis in which an etiologic agent is isolated. Prior infection by a

Table 138-2   Most Common Infections Caused by *Streptococcus pneumoniae*

Acute sinusitis	Osteomyelitis
Pneumonia	Septic arthritis
Acute purulent tracheobronchitis	Peritonitis
Otitis media	Endocarditis
Empyema	Pericarditis
Meningitis	Endometritis
Primary bacteremia	Cellulitis
	Brain abscess

NOTE: The order of the list very roughly approximates the order of frequency among adults, from most to least common.

respiratory virus or allergy is thought to contribute significantly to these pneumococcal infections by causing congestion of the openings to the eustachian tubes or the paranasal sinuses. Prospective studies of young children have shown that colonization precedes infection in most cases. For reasons that are unclear, serotypes 6B, 14, 19F, and 23F predominate both as colonizing and as infecting organisms of children; therefore, these serotypes are currently being studied most intensively for use in vaccines to be administered to young children.

Meningitis   Except during outbreaks of meningococcal infection, *S. pneumoniae* is the most common etiologic agent of bacterial meningitis in adults. Because of the remarkable success of *H. influenzae* type b vaccine, *S. pneumoniae* now predominates among cases in infants and toddlers as well (but not among those in newborns). Meningitis develops either by the direct extension of infection from the sinuses or the middle ear or as a result of bacteremia with seeding of the choroid plexus. Favoring the former possibility are the association between acute otitis media and meningitis as well as the documented role of *S. pneumoniae* as the most common cause of recurrent bacterial meningitis associated with head trauma, cerebrospinal fluid (CSF) leak, and/or dural tear. Favoring the latter are the association between pneumococcal bacteremia from any source and meningitis as well as an autopsy study of temporal bone from children who died of bacterial meningitis, which yielded no evidence of extension from the middle ear.

In the meninges and subarachnoid space, pneumococcal peptidoglycan stimulates an intense inflammatory response mediated by the release of interleukin (IL)1, IL-6, C5a, tumor necrosis factor (TNF), and other proinflammatory cytokines. This inflammatory response results in raised intracranial pressure, brain edema, and decreased blood flow leading to meningismus, drowsiness, or coma. Focal neurologic signs may result from vasculitis with venous or arterial thrombosis, from cranial neuropathy due to entrapment or infarction, from local cerebritis, from subdural effusion, or from brain herniation (Chap. 372).

No distinctive clinical or laboratory feature differentiates meningitis due to *S. pneumoniae* from that due to other bacteria. Patients note the sudden onset of fever, headache, and stiffness or pain in the neck. Without treatment, there is a progression over 24 to 48 h to confusion and then obtundation. On physical examination, the patient looks acutely ill and has a rigid neck. In such cases lumbar puncture should not be delayed for computed tomography (CT) of the head unless papilledema or focal neurologic signs are evident. Typical CSF findings consist of pleocytosis (500 to 10,000 cells/μL) with a predominance of PMNs, an elevated protein level (100 to 500 mg/dL), and a decrease in glucose content. If antibiotics have not been given, large numbers of pneumococci can be seen in a Gram-stained specimen of CSF in nearly all cases, and specific therapy can be administered, although *Listeria* may be misidentified as the pneumococcus. If an effective antibiotic has already been given, the number of bacteria may be greatly decreased and microscopic examination of a Gram-stained specimen may yield negative results. In this situation, immunologic methods for the detection of pneumococcal capsule in the CSF may identify an etiologic agent in up to two-thirds of cases, although these methods have fallen out of favor. Most physicians prefer to use empirical broad-spectrum antibiotic therapy until the etiologic agent has been definitively identified and its susceptibility has been reported.

Pneumonia   The distinctive symptoms and signs of pneumococcal pneumonia are (1) cough and sputum production, which reflect the proliferation of bacteria and the resulting inflammatory response in the alveoli; (2) fever; and (3) radiographic detection of an infiltrate.

Predisposing conditions   Pneumococcal pneumonia is most common at the extremes of age. Despite the undisputed role of *S. pneumoniae* as a major pathogenic bacterium for humans, the great majority of adults with pneumococcal pneumonia have underlying diseases that predispose them to infection. Otherwise-healthy military recruits involved in outbreaks of infection may be an exception to this rule; however, many of those affected have an antecedent viral-type illness that may reduce normal host resistance. In addition to prior alcoholism, malnutrition, chronic pulmonary disease of any kind, cigarette smoking, infection with HIV, diabetes mellitus, cirrhosis of the liver, anemia, prior hospitalization for any reason, renal insufficiency, and coronary artery disease (with or without recognized congestive heart failure). HIV infection is such an important predisposing factor that some authorities recommend that any young adult with pneumococcal pneumonia be tested for antibody to HIV.

Presenting symptoms Patients often present with a preexisting respiratory condition that has distinctly deteriorated. If a viral upper respiratory illness is the predisposing factor, the patient may have felt unwell for several days, with coryza or a nonproductive cough and low-grade fever; at the time of onset of pneumonia, the temperature may rise to 38.9 to 39.4°C (102 to 103°F), and sputum production becomes prominent. In a patient who has chronic bronchitis, the sputum may increase in volume, become yellow or green and thicker than usual, and be associated with a fever that becomes progressively higher over 48 to 72 h. In a small proportion of cases, the onset of disease follows a hyperacute pattern in which the patient suddenly has a single episode of shaking chills followed by sustained fever and a cough productive of blood-tinged sputum. This clinical picture is unfortunately called "classic," a vague term that is best avoided because many physicians believe that it means "most common," which is clearly not the case. In elderly subjects, the onset of disease may be especially insidious and may not suggest pneumonia at all. Persons in their eighties may have minimal cough, no sputum production, and no fever, instead appearing tired or confused. For the reasons noted above, the most abrupt progression of pneumococcal disease is seen in patients who have previously undergone splenectomy; these individuals may go from apparent good health to death in as little as 24 h. In pneumonia, pleuritic chest pain may result from extension of the inflammatory process to the visceral pleura; persistence of this pain, especially after the first day or two of treatment, raises concern about empyema (see "Complications," below). Nausea and vomiting or diarrhea, sometimes quite prominent, occur in up to 20% of cases. Clearly, the range of symptoms is sufficiently broad that there is no characteristic presentation to distinguish pneumococcal from other types of bacterial pneumonia (or from some types of nonbacterial pneumonia).

Physical findings Patients with pneumococcal pneumonia usually appear ill and have a grayish, anxious appearance that differs from that of persons with viral or mycoplasmal pneumonia. Typically, the temperature is 38.9 to 39.4°C (102 to 103°F), the pulse 90 to 110 beats per minute, and the respiratory rate >20 breaths per minute. Elderly patients may have only a slight temperature elevation or be afebrile. Hypothermia is associated with increased morbidity and mortality. Herpes labialis appears in a small percentage of cases. Pain may cause diminished respiratory excursion (splinting) on the affected side. Dullness to percussion is noted in about half of cases, and vocal fremitus is increased. Breath sounds may be bronchial or tubular, and crackles are heard in most cases if enough air is being moved to generate them. Flatness to percussion at the lung base and inability to detect the expected degree of diaphragmatic motion suggest the presence of pleural fluid, which raises the possibility of empyema; the failure to assess fremitus, to distinguish dullness from flatness by percussion, or to examine for diaphragmatic excursion may leave the physician at the mercy of often ambiguous radiologic interpretations. The finding of a heart murmur, certainly if new, raises concern about endocarditis, a rare but serious complication. Hypoxia or the generalized response to pneumonia may cause the patient to be confused, but the appearance of confusion should raise concern about meningitis. Obtundation or neck stiffness should lead to an immediate consideration of this complication.

Radiographic findings Pneumococcal pneumonia involves only one lung segment or a portion thereof in one-fourth of cases; it involves more than one segment but only one lobe or a portion thereof in another one-fourth of instances. Thus multilobar disease is seen in half of cases. Air-space consolidation is the predominant finding and

is detected in 80% of cases. Air bronchogram (visualization of the air-filled bronchus against a background of consolidation in the alveoli) is evident in fewer than half of cases and is more common in bacteremic than in nonbacteremic disease. In rare instances, pneumococcal pneumonia leads to a lung abscess; a malignancy or a mixture of anaerobic and microaerophilic organisms is likely to be implicated as well. Although some pleural fluid may actually be present in half of cases, no more than 20% of patients have a sufficient volume of fluid to allow aspiration, and in only a minority of these patients is empyema documented.

General laboratory findings The peripheral-blood white blood cell (WBC) count exceeds 12,000/μL in the great majority of patients with pneumococcal pneumonia. However, the count is <6000/μL in 5 to 10% of persons hospitalized for pneumococcal pneumonia. Such a low count is strongly associated with lethal disease and is often but not always associated with bone marrow suppression due to alcohol ingestion. The serum bilirubin level may be modestly elevated; hypoxia, inflammatory changes in the liver, and breakdown of red blood cells in the lung are all thought to contribute to this increase. Levels of lactate dehydrogenase may be elevated. A variety of other abnormalities may be present, reflecting the contributory role of underlying diseases. →*Abnormalities of pleural fluid in empyema are reviewed in Chap. 255.*

Differential diagnosis Patients who present with community-acquired pneumonia may actually have infection of the lungs due to one of many organisms. The extensive list includes the following: *H. influenzae* or *Moraxella catarrhalis* in persons with little to predispose them other than chronic or acute inflammation of the airways; *Staphylococcus aureus* in persons who take glucocorticoids or who have major anatomic disruption of the airways; *Streptococcus pyogenes*; *Neisseria meningitidis*; anaerobic species in persons who have seizures or may have aspirated oropharyngeal or gastric secretions for some other reason; *Legionella*; *Pasteurella multocida* in dog or cat owners; gram-negative bacilli, especially in persons with severely damaged lungs who are taking glucocorticoids; viruses, especially influenza virus (in season), adenovirus, or respiratory syncytial virus; *Mycobacterium tuberculosis*; fungi, including *Pneumocystis carinii* (depending upon epidemiologic factors and the possible presence of HIV infection); *Mycoplasma*; *Chlamydia pneumoniae*, especially in older adults; and *Chlamydia psittaci* in bird owners. Many older men with lung cancer present with pneumonia, as do persons who have acute-onset inflammatory pulmonary conditions of uncertain etiology or those with pulmonary embolus and infarction. The breadth of this list vividly illustrates the difficulty of using empirical therapy for community-acquired pneumonia. Many of these diseases require evaluation, and specific therapy is available for an increasing number. Moreover, pneumococci—perhaps the most common cause of community-acquired pneumonia—are increasingly resistant to available antibiotics. Taken together, these factors favor precise determination of the etiology of a pneumonia syndrome whenever possible.

Diagnostic microbiology An etiologic role for the pneumococcus in pneumonia is strongly suggested by the microscopic demonstration of large numbers of PMNs and slightly elongated gram-positive cocci in pairs and chains in the sputum (**Plate VI-2**). Capsules may be seen surrounding the bacterial forms. Examined areas of the slide must be free of buccal epithelial cells, which indicate the admixture of saliva with sputum; saliva may contain 10^7 viridans streptococci per milliliter. When characteristic microscopic findings are noted, the identification of *S. pneumoniae* in sputum culture strongly indicates pneumococcal infection of the lower respiratory tract. In the absence of such microscopic findings, the identification of pneumococci by culture may be nonspecific, reflecting colonization of the upper airways. Culture is also less sensitive than microscopic examination for identifying pneumococci. Since most pneumococci do not produce distinctly mucoid colonies, their identification in the laboratory depends on the ability to select putative pneumococcal colonies for further study from among α-hemolytic streptococci of the mouth. In short, laboratory diagnosis by sputum culture relies on the quality of the specimen provided, the care with which the relevant purulent component is separated for culture, and the assiduity with which α-hemolytic colonies are studied. These factors need to be considered when sputum cultures from patients who appear to have pneumococcal pneumonia are said to yield only "normal mouth flora" and when the medical literature describes what appear to be poor results of sputum culture. Because of the central role of microscopic examination in diagnosis, physicians may wish to view the slides with the microbiologist. Blood cultures yield *S. pneumoniae* in about 25% of cases of pneumococcal pneumonia. Modern, automated systems often yield positive blood cultures within 12 h after the sample is obtained.

Complications Empyema is the most common complication of pneumococcal pneumonia, occurring in about 2% of cases. As noted above, some fluid appears in the pleural space in a substantial proportion of cases of pneumococcal pneumonia, but this parapneumonic effusion usually reflects an inflammatory response to infection that has been contained within the lung, and its presence is self-limited. When bacteria reach the pleural space—either hematogenously or as a result of contiguous spread, possibly across lymphatics of the visceral pleura—empyema results. The finding of frank pus, a positive result on Gram's staining, or the presence of fluid with a pH of ≤7.1 indicates the need for aggressive and complete drainage, preferably by prompt insertion of a chest tube, with verification by CT that fluid has been removed. If there is no response, thoracotomy is indicated. Persistence of fever (even if low-grade) and leukocytosis after 4 or 5 days of appropriate antibiotic treatment for pneumococcal pneumonia suggests empyema. In this setting, the diagnosis is exceedingly likely if the x-ray shows the persistence of pleural fluid. At this stage, thoracotomy is often needed for cure. Aggressive drainage is likely to reduce morbidity and mortality from empyema (Chap. 262).

Other Syndromes The appearance of pneumococcal infection at other, usually sterile body sites indicates hematogenous spread, either during frank pneumonia or, in a smaller proportion of cases, from an inapparent focus of infection. A case of pneumococcal endocarditis is seen every few years at large tertiary-care hospitals. Purulent pericarditis due to this organism, occurring as a separate entity or together with endocarditis, is even rarer. Most cases of spontaneous bacterial peritonitis in children and some cases in adults are caused by *S. pneumoniae*. Peritonitis in women may be related to the use of an intrauterine contraceptive device, and pneumococcal infections of the female reproductive organs continue to be described. Septic arthritis can arise spontaneously in a natural or prosthetic joint or as a complication of rheumatoid arthritis. Osteomyelitis in adults tends to involve vertebral bones. Epidural and brain abscesses are rarely described. Cellulitis can develop and does so most often in persons who have connective tissue diseases or HIV infection. The appearance of any of these unusual pneumococcal infections in a young adult may suggest that tests for HIV infection should be undertaken.

℞ TREATMENT **Antibiotic Susceptibility** β-Lactam antibiotics, the cornerstone of therapy for serious pneumococcal infection, bind covalently to the active site and thereby block the action of the cell-membrane enzymes (endo-, trans-, and carboxypeptidases) that are responsible for cell-wall synthesis. These enzymes were identified by their reaction with radiolabeled penicillin and thus are called *penicillin-binding proteins*. In the 1960s, virtually all clinical isolates of *S. pneumoniae* were susceptible to penicillin (i.e., were inhibited in vitro by concentrations of <0.06 μg/mL). During the past 20 years in Europe and the past 10 years or so in the United States, a steadily increasing number of pneumococcal isolates have shown some degree of resistance to penicillin. Resistance results when spontaneous mutation or acquisition of new genetic material alters penicillin-binding proteins in a manner that reduces their affinity for penicillin, thereby necessitating a higher concentration of penicillin for their saturation. The genetic information acquired also conveys resistance to other antibiotics. Mutation and selection of strains in communities in the United States—especially in areas of high antibiotic use, such as day-care centers—and spread of identifiable strains from other countries where antibiotics are available without prescription have contributed to the prevalence of resistance.

For most of the antibiotic era, pneumococcal susceptibility was not studied in vitro because of the organism's high degree of susceptibility to virtually all recommended antibiotics. Clearly, the situation has changed, and it seems important to study pneumococcal isolates, especially those causing invasive disease, for antibiotic susceptibility. In 1997, about 20% of pneumococcal isolates in the United States were intermediately susceptible to penicillin [minimal inhibitory concentration (MIC), 0.1 to 1.0 μg/mL] and 15% were resistant (MIC, ≥ 2.0 μg/mL; Table 138-3). The clinical significance of the MIC varies with the infection being treated. An intermediately resistant strain (e.g., MIC = 0.5 μg/mL) behaves as a susceptible organism when it causes pneumonia, but probably not when it causes otitis and certainly not when it causes meningitis. As a result, susceptibility may eventually be redefined on the basis of the site infected—a concept supported by pharmacokinetic considerations and validated by outcome studies. Amoxicillin, with two- and fourfold lower MICs, appears to be more active against *S. pneumoniae* than penicillin—thus the emerging preference for amoxicillin. Penicillin-susceptible pneumococci are susceptible to all commonly used cephalosporins. Penicillin-intermediate strains are resistant to all first- and many second-generation cephalosporins (of which cefuroxime retains the best efficacy) but are susceptible to some third-generation cephalosporins, including cefotaxime, ceftriaxone, cefepime, and cefpodoxime. One-half of highly penicillin-resistant pneumococci are also resistant to cefotaxime and ceftriaxone, a higher proportion are resistant to cefepime, and nearly all are resistant to cefpodoxime. Pneumonia caused by intermediately penicillin-resistant strains responds well to β-lactam antibiotics. Pneumonia due to fully resistant strains also responds, but probably not as reliably; data that address this issue are currently being examined. Sinusitis and otitis media caused by intermediately resistant *S. pneumoniae* do not reliably respond to therapy, and failure of therapy may be common when these conditions are caused by highly resistant pneumococcal strains.

Resistance to erythromycin extends to the new macrolides, including azithromycin and clarithromycin. This resistance will certainly affect empirical therapy for bronchitis, sinusitis, and pneumonia. In the United States, the majority of macrolide-resistant pneumococci bear the so-called M phenotype (erythromycin MIC = 1 to 8 μg/mL) and

Table 138-3 Antibiotic Susceptibility of Pneumococci Stratified According to Penicillin Susceptibility

Status of Strain	Percentage of Isolates Susceptible to Indicated Agent									
	Tet	Em	TMP-SMZ	Cfur	Ctax or Ctri	Clin	Newer Mac	Quin	Imi	Vm
Pen-S	90	95	90	100	100	100	95	98	100	100
Pen-I	80	80	70	75	95	90	80	98	90	100
Pen-R	60	50	23	25	50	85	50	98	80	100

Abbreviations: Pen-S, sensitive to penicillin; Pen-I, intermediately resistant to penicillin; Pen-R, resistant to penicillin; Tet, tetracycline; Em, erythromycin; TMP-SMZ, trimethoprim-sulfamethoxazole; Cfur, cefuroxime; Ctax, cefotaxime; Ctri, ceftriaxone; Clin, clin-damycin; Mac, macrolides; Quin, quinolones; Imi, imipenem; Vm, vancomycin.
NOTE: These percentages reflect a composite of the data available in March 1999; actual results vary with the time and locale.

are susceptible to clindamycin. In this case, resistance is mediated by an efflux pump mechanism; it is not yet known whether M-type resistance can be overcome by clinically achievable levels of macrolides. In Europe, most macrolide resistance is due to a mutation in *ermB*, which confers high-level resistance not only to macrolides but also to clindamycin. Rates of resistance to doxycycline among pneumococci of varying susceptibility to penicillin are similar to those observed for macrolides, whereas the overall rate of pneumococcal resistance to trimethoprim-sulfamethoxazole (25%) is sufficiently high to discourage therapy with this agent unless an isolate is known to be susceptible.

The newer fluoroquinolones remain highly effective against pneumococci, with equal efficacy against penicillin-susceptible and -resistant strains. All pneumococci are susceptible to vancomycin, although it is feared that the acquisition of vancomycin resistance by enterococci and other gram-positive bacteria may eventually lead to pneumococcal transformation to resistance. Of drugs under study, the oxazolidinones and glycopeptides appear to be most promising, with MICs for drug-resistant *S. pneumoniae* strains no higher than for penicillin-susceptible strains. Resistance to streptogramins parallels that to macrolides and limits the usefulness of these drugs for the treatment of pneumonia.

Pneumococcal susceptibility patterns vary greatly between and even within individual communities and the data are in a state of flux. It does appear, however, that the constant trend is toward more widespread resistance.

General Therapy   There has been increased emphasis on outpatient therapy in patients who are at low risk (as determined by PORT score according to criteria described by the Pneumonia Outcomes Research Team; Chap. 255). This approach appears to be safe. However, if the physician is in doubt about the severity of illness, the social circumstances, or the likelihood of compliance with the prescribed antibiotic regimen, it may be best to hospitalize the patient, at least briefly.

Specific Antibiotic Therapy • *Pneumonia*   This section will deal primarily with the treatment of pneumonia that is known to be due to *S. pneumoniae*. The broader issue of empirical therapy for community-acquired pneumonia is covered in detail elsewhere (Chap. 255). However, a few general comments on empirical therapy apply. An important problem in treating pneumonia is that, without a good sputum sample that can be Gram-stained and examined microscopically, the etiologic agent is not known at the time when treatment needs to be initiated and is not likely to become known later. Empirical therapy in such cases must be effective against *S. pneumoniae*, which remains the most likely causative agent of community-acquired pneumonia, unless epidemiologic, clinical, and radiologic findings strongly favor another etiologic entity. If a good sputum sample is obtained and only *S. pneumoniae* is visible, therapy can be focused on this organism, although additional treatment may be added for organisms that are not visualized microscopically—e.g., influenza virus in a patient hospitalized during an influenza outbreak. Even if the pneumococcus is suspected, a certain degree of empiricism is required, because the antibiotic susceptibility of the strain involved will not be known for 1 or 2 days.

OUTPATIENT THERAPY   Amoxicillin (500 mg four times daily) effectively treats all cases of pneumococcal pneumonia except those caused by the most highly penicillin-resistant isolates. Neither cefuroxime nor cefpodoxime offers any advantages over amoxicillin since these drugs are less likely, even at high dosages, to be active against highly resistant pneumococcal strains. One of the newer fluoroquinolones in an accepted dosage for pneumonia is highly likely to be effective. Doxycycline, azithromycin, or clarithromycin will be effective in 85 to 90% of cases and clindamycin in a higher proportion. The trend toward increasing resistance to all these drugs is worrisome. Because one-fourth of all isolates are now resistant to trimethoprim-sulfamethoxazole, this agent can no longer be recommended. Since none of these therapies ensures the kind of antibiotic coverage that it would have had in the past, patients should be instructed to remain in close contact with the prescribing physician, especially if there is any de-

terioration in their condition. It is worth noting that an outcomes study using data from the mid-1990s, when the rate of resistance was lower, showed that treatment with any of the above-mentioned antibiotics was associated with a good outcome; the majority of cases in which an etiologic agent was identified were due to *S. pneumoniae*.

INPATIENT THERAPY   Pneumonia caused by penicillin-susceptible or intermediately penicillin-resistant pneumococcal isolates is readily treatable with penicillin. The dosages that follow are acceptable against intermediately resistant strains and against many or most fully resistant isolates, although they are excessive for use against susceptible isolates. Lower doses, however, cannot be recommended initially because susceptibility is not known until 24 to 72 h after treatment is begun. Patients who are sick enough to be hospitalized should be treated promptly. Most physicians favor parenteral antibiotics, although oral administration of well-absorbed drugs may be acceptable if the patient is not vomiting or hypotensive. Recommended regimens include ceftriaxone (1 to 2 g/d) or cefotaxime (1 to 2 g every 6 to 8 h). Ampicillin (1 to 2 g every 6 h) is also widely used. A quinolone or azithromycin can be given parenterally or orally. About 10 to 15% of all pneumococci are resistant to macrolides, and 1 to 2% are resistant to quinolones. Much of the resistance to macrolides among pneumococcal isolates may be overcome by the administration of azithromycin at a dosage of 500 mg on the first day and 250 mg/d thereafter. Clindamycin is effective against a higher proportion of resistant pneumococci than are the macrolides. Vancomycin is uniformly effective against pneumococci and should be used for initial therapy if there is reason to believe that a patient is infected with a strain that is resistant to the drugs listed above. As antimicrobial resistance among pneumococci evolves, updated recommendations will be issued by the Infectious Diseases Society of America, the American Thoracic Society, and the Centers for Disease Control and Prevention (CDC).

Patients with severe allergic reactions to β-lactam antibiotics should receive vancomycin (500 mg intravenously every 6 h) or a quinolone. As noted above, there have always been treatment failures unrelated to the antimicrobial susceptibility of the organism; nevertheless, the failure of a patient to respond promptly should raise the question of resistance, and vancomycin should be given until the susceptibility of the infecting strain to other drugs has been documented. Of course, evidence for loculated infections (such as empyema) and/or other causes of fever should be sought.

DURATION OF THERAPY   The optimal duration of treatment for pneumococcal pneumonia is uncertain. Penicillin-susceptible strains disappear from the sputum within several hours of the first dose of penicillin, and a single dose of procaine penicillin, which results in the maintenance of an effective antimicrobial level for 24 h, was said to cure pneumococcal pneumonia in otherwise-healthy young adults at the time when all isolates were susceptible. Most older physicians treat pneumococcal pneumonia for 5 to 10 days. In the absence of reports of therapy failure, younger physicians have tended to treat the infection for 10 to 14 days. Prolongation of therapy is a two-edged sword, especially in debilitated patients, because the risk of complications increases with each day of antibiotic treatment, particularly in the hospital setting. A few days of close observation and parenteral therapy followed by an oral antibiotic—with the entire course of treatment continuing for no more than 5 days after the patient becomes afebrile—may be the best approach.

Otitis media and acute sinusitis   Current treatment recommendations for otitis media and acute sinusitis—conditions whose pathogenesis and microbial etiology are similar—are based on the following points: (1) Acute otitis media is the most common infection for which antibiotics are prescribed in the United States. (2) As noted above, *S. pneumoniae* is the most likely treatable cause; taken together, *H. influenzae* and *M. catarrhalis*, many strains of which produce β-lactamases, are implicated nearly as frequently as pneumococci. (3) In the absence of diagnostic tympanocentesis, the etiologic diagnosis is nearly always presumptive. (4) Because penetration into a closed space is required, high serum levels of an effective antibiotic are required to treat otitis caused by intermediately or fully resistant pneumococci. (5) Otitis due to *S. pneumoniae* is more likely to fail to respond and to produce complications without specific therapy. (6) Antibiotics that are effective against pneumococci and yet resist β-lactamases tend to be very expensive compared with amoxicillin.

As a result of these considerations, the CDC's Otitis Media Working Group recommends that initial therapy be amoxicillin in a high dosage—e.g., 80 mg/kg for infants and toddlers or 500 mg four times daily for adults. If this regimen fails, highly penicillin-resistant pneumococci or β-lactamase-producing bacteria may be responsible, and a course of cefpodoxime, perhaps preceded by a single parenteral dose of ceftriaxone, is recommended. Once therapy has begun, patients must be monitored closely for a response. Despite the detection (by molecular analysis) of pneumococcal DNA in middle-ear fluid, chronic serous otitis ("glue ear") is probably not due to active infection and does not require antibiotic therapy.

Meningitis A reasonable recommendation is that pneumococcal meningitis be treated initially with cefotaxime (2 g every 6 h) or ceftriaxone (1 to 2 g every 12 h) plus vancomycin (500 mg every 6 h or 1 g every 12 h). Two drugs are given initially because the cephalosporin is likely to be effective against most isolates and readily penetrates the blood-brain barrier, whereas vancomycin is uniformly effective but has a somewhat unpredictable capacity to cross the blood-brain barrier. If the isolate is shown to be penicillin-susceptible, treatment can be continued with 24 million units of penicillin every 24 h, given every 4 h in divided doses or continuously. If the isolate exhibits reduced susceptibility to penicillin but is susceptible to cefotaxime or ceftriaxone, the administration of vancomycin may be discontinued. Rifampin inhibits the bactericidal activity of β-lactam antibiotics and probably should not be added to the regimen. The total duration of therapy for pneumococcal meningitis is 10 to 14 days. Despite the central pathogenic role of inflammation in meningitis, the use of glucocorticoids or other anti-inflammatory agents is controversial, even in children, in whom most of the relevant studies have been done. Data simply do not exist on which to base an informed decision regarding the administration of glucocorticoids or cyclooxygenase inhibitors to adults with pneumococcal meningitis (Chap. 372). Meningitis should be treated in an intensive care unit and with the participation of appropriate consultants, generally including a neurologist and a specialist in infectious diseases.

Endocarditis Pneumococcal endocarditis is associated with rapid destruction of heart valves. Vancomycin should be given pending assays for the minimal bactericidal concentrations of β-lactam antibiotics. There is no clear evidence that the addition of another antibiotic to the regimen is beneficial; aminoglycosides are somewhat synergistic and rifampin or quinolones are antagonistic with β-lactams. Endocarditis and meningitis should be treated initially in an intensive care unit, with the participation of appropriate consultants. Patients with endocarditis should probably be treated in collaboration with an infectious disease consultant, a cardiologist, and a cardiovascular surgeon.

Other Therapeutic Modalities A variety of agents that block the action of TNF-α, IL-1, or platelet-activating factor have conferred no benefit in and may have had a detrimental effect on pneumococcal sepsis. Similar results have been obtained with glucocorticoids.

PREVENTION Pneumococcal vaccine contains 25 μg of capsular polysaccharide from the 23 most prevalent serotypes of *S. pneumoniae*; vaccination stimulates antibody to most serotypes in most recipients. In adults under 55 years old, protection rates are at least 85%, even 5 years or longer after vaccination. The level and duration of protection decrease with advancing age, perhaps because of a diminished avidity of the antibody for the capsular polysaccharide. As a result, persons in their eighties have 50% protection for 3 years and very little or no protection thereafter. In subgroups of the population at high risk (e.g., debilitated elderly persons and individuals with severe chronic lung disease), vaccine has not been shown conclusively to be effective. Persons who most need the vaccine because of poor IgG responses are not likely to respond to immunization with significant increases in antibody level. Nevertheless, the poor average rate of response should not deter the physician from administering vaccine to individual patients who are at increased risk of pneumococcal infection. In light of the safety, low cost, and efficacy of vaccine and the emergence of antibiotic-resistant strains, the failure to vaccinate elderly persons and individuals who have conditions predisposing to pneumococcal disease is viewed by some authorities as a missed opportunity in public health policy.

The CDC's Immunization Practices Advisory Committee has broadened its recommendations for pneumococcal vaccination to include all persons over the age of 2 years who are at substantially increased risk of developing pneumococcal infection and/or a serious complication of such an infection. General categories included within these recommendations are as follows: (1) persons over the age of 65; (2) persons with anatomic or functional asplenia, CSF leak, diabetes mellitus, alcoholism, cirrhosis, chronic renal insufficiency, chronic pulmonary disease, or advanced cardiovascular disease; (3) persons who have an immunocompromising condition associated with increased risk of pneumococcal disease, such as multiple myeloma, lymphoma, Hodgkin's disease, HIV infection, organ transplantation, or chronic use of glucocorticoids; (4) persons who are genetically at increased risk, such as Native Americans and Alaskans; and (5) persons who live in special environments where outbreaks are particularly likely to occur, such as nursing homes. This list should not be regarded as all-inclusive.

Recommendations regarding revaccination seem to be somewhat inconsistent. A single revaccination is advocated for persons over the age of 65. Since antibody levels decline and there is no anamnestic response, it seems more reasonable simply to recommend revaccination at 5-year intervals, especially in persons over the age of 65, who tend to have almost no local reaction, and in splenectomized patients, who are most in need. If penicillin-resistant pneumococci continue to increase in prevalence, routine immunization of children over the age of 2 years should be considered. Pneumococcal vaccine has not been useful in children <2 years of age, who do not respond well to polysaccharide antigens. In a recent field trial, a heptavalent protein-conjugate pneumococcal polysaccharide vaccine protected infants and children against pneumococcal pneumonia, bacteremia, and meningitis; this vaccine is likely to be released for administration to young children in the next few years.

BIBLIOGRAPHY

AFESSA B et al: Pneumococcal bacteremia in adults: A 14-year experience in an inner-city university hospital. Clin Infect Dis 21:345, 1995

BARTLETT JG et al: Community-acquired pneumonia in adults: Guidelines for management. Clin Infect Dis 26:811, 1998

DAGAN R et al: Bacteriologic response to oral cephalosporins: Are established susceptibility breakpoints appropriate in the case of acute otitis media? J Infect Dis 176:1253, 1997

DOERN GV et al: Prevalence of antimicrobial resistance among respiratory tract isolates of *Streptococcus pneumoniae* in North America: 1997 results from the SENTRY antimicrobial surveillance program. Clin Infect Dis 27:111, 1998

——— et al: Antimicrobial resistance with *Streptococcus pneumoniae* in the United States, 1997–98. Emerg Infect Dis 5:757, 1999

DOWELL SF et al: Otitis media—management and surveillance in the era of pneumococcal resistance: A report from the Drug-Resistant *Streptococcus pneumoniae* Therapeutic Working Group. Pediatr Infect Dis J 18:1, 1999

FEDSON DS, MUSHER DM: Pneumococcal vaccine, in *Vaccines*, 3d ed, SA Plotkin, EA Mortimer Jr (eds). Philadelphia, Saunders, 1998

HAUSDORFF WP et al: The contribution of specific pneumococcal serogroups to different disease manifestations: Implications for conjugate vaccine formulation and use, part II. Clin Infect Dis 30:122, 2000

HEFFRON R: *Pneumonia: With Special Reference to Pneumococcus Lobar Pneumonia*. A Commonwealth Fund Book, © 1939. Reprinted by Harvard University Press, Cambridge, MA, 1979

MUSHER DM: *Streptococcus pneumoniae*, in *Principles and Practice of Infectious Diseases*, 5th ed, GL Mandell et al (eds). New York, Churchill Livingstone, 1999

———— et al: Antibody to capsular polysaccharides of *Streptococcus pneumoniae* in adults: Prevalence, persistence, relation to carriage, and resistance to infection. Clin Infect Dis 17:66, 1993

PASTOR P et al: Invasive pneumococcal disease in Dallas County, Texas: Results from population-based surveillance in 1995. Clin Infect Dis 26:590, 1998

PATON JC et al: Molecular analysis of putative pneumococcal virulence proteins. Microb Drug Resist 3:1, 1997

PLOUFFE JF et al: Bacteremia with *Streptococcus pneumoniae*: Implications for therapy and prevention. Franklin County Pneumonia Study Group. JAMA 275:194, 1996

RAHAV G et al: Invasive pneumococcal infections: A comparison between adults and children. Medicine 76:295, 1997

RODRIGUEZ MC et al: Unusual manifestations of pneumococcal infection in HIV-infected individuals: The past revisited. Clin Infect Dis 14:192, 1992

SHAPIRO ED et al: The protective efficacy of polyvalent pneumococcal polysaccharide vaccine. N Engl J Med 325:1453, 1991

TUOMANEN EI et al: Pathogenesis of pneumococcal infection. N Engl J Med 332:1280, 1995

WATANAKUNAKORN C et al: Adult bacteremic pneumococcal pneumonia in a community teaching hospital, 1992–1996. A detailed analyis of 108 cases. Arch Intern Med 157: 1965, 1997

staphylococcal species, the only important human pathogen is *S. aureus*, whose colonies are larger than those of *S. epidermidis*, are often pigmented (golden yellow), and are usually β-hemolytic on sheep blood agar. Twenty-eight species of CoNS are recognized. Of these, *S. epidermidis* is by far the most common nonurinary human isolate. Strains of *S. epidermidis* are typically white and nonhemolytic and may be tenaciously adherent as a result of their production of polysaccharide adhesin. *S. epidermidis* is followed in frequency by *S. hominis*, *S. haemolyticus*, and *S. warneri*. *S. lugdunensis* is increasingly recognized as a cause of serious human infection. *S. saprophyticus* is the most common staphylococcal urinary isolate.

STAPHYLOCOCCUS AUREUS

EPIDEMIOLOGY Humans constitute the major reservoir of *S. aureus* in nature. The mucous membranes of the anterior nasopharynx are the principal site of carriage, with roughly 30% of healthy adults being so colonized at any point in time. Other common sites of colonization include the axillae, the vagina, damaged skin, and the perineum. Among postmenarcheal U.S. women, the rate of vaginal colonization by *S. aureus* ranges from 5 to 15% but rises to 30% during menses—a change that is relevant to the pathogenesis of the toxic shock syndrome (TSS). Most adults are colonized by *S. aureus* intermittently, whereas 10 to 20% have persistent colonization and about the same percentage are never found to harbor the organism. Colonization is influenced by both microbial and host factors as well as by the nature of the competing nonstaphylococcal flora. Carriage is more common among persons with frequent staphylococcal exposure and those with habitual or chronic disruption of cutaneous epithelial integrity. Thus, colonization rates are higher among health care workers, dialysis patients, patients with type 1 diabetes, injection drug users, persons infected with HIV, and individuals with chronic dermatologic conditions. After 2 weeks in a hospital, colonization rates rise to 30 to 50%, and colonizing strains are more likely to be resistant to antibiotics.

Colonization of mucocutaneous sites is an important risk factor for staphylococcal infection. For example, surgical wound infection following cardiothoracic surgery is up to 10 times more likely among patients who harbor *S. aureus* in the nares preoperatively than among those who do not. The vast majority of postoperative wound infections of all types are caused by a strain of *S. aureus* that was present in the nares before surgery. Furthermore, presurgical clearance of carriage with topical and systemic antibiotics decreases the incidence of postoperative staphylococcal infection, but it is not yet standard practice to screen and treat patients before surgery.

PATHOGENESIS AND HOST DEFENSE *S. aureus* causes two types of syndrome: *intoxications* and *infections*. The clinical manifestations of intoxications are attributable to the action of one or a few secreted products of the microorganism (toxins), and these clinical features can be reproduced by administration of the toxin(s) in the absence of the microorganism. The toxin can be produced either in vivo (as in TSS or staphylococcal scalded skin syndrome) or in a suitable vector that subsequently delivers it to the host (as in staphylococcal food poisoning). Infections, in contrast, involve bacterial proliferation, invasion or destruction of host tissues, and—in most cases—local and systemic inflammatory responses by the host to these events. The ability of a microorganism to infect is predicated on its ability to produce certain products that enable it to survive and prosper in the host (*virulence factors*), and *S. aureus* is particularly well-armed in this regard.

Steps in Pathogenesis The pathogenesis of staphylococcal intoxications is straightforward and involves four steps: colonization by a toxigenic strain of the bacterium, toxin production, toxin absorption, and intoxication. The pathogenesis of invasive infections is more complex and the steps are less discrete. They include colonization, invasion of the bacterium across epithelial or mucosal barriers, adherence to

139

Jeffrey Parsonnet, Robert L. Deresiewicz

STAPHYLOCOCCAL INFECTIONS

CoNS coagulase-negative staphylococci	TEE transesophageal echocardiography
CSF cerebrospinal fluid	TEN toxic epidermal necrolysis
CT computed tomography	TSS toxic shock syndrome
ETs exfoliative toxins	TSST-1 toxic shock syndrome toxin 1
MICs minimum inhibitory concentrations	TTE transthoracic echocardiography
MRI magnetic resonance imaging	VISA vancomycin-intermediate *S. aureus*
MRSA methicillin-resistant *S. aureus*	VRE vancomycin-resistant enterococci
PBPs penicillin-binding proteins	
SCVs small-colony variants	
SEs staphylococcal enterotoxins	

The staphylococci are hardy and ubiquitous colonizers of human skin and mucous membranes and were among the first human pathogens identified. They cause a variety of syndromes, including superficial and deep pyogenic infections, systemic intoxications, and urinary tract infections. Staphylococci are the leading cause of bacteremia, surgical wound infections, and infections of bioprosthetic materials in the United States; in addition, they are the second leading cause of nosocomial infections. Organisms of this genus are also a significant cause of bacterial food poisoning.

Staphylococcus aureus is the most important human pathogen in the genus. It remains a major public health concern due to its tenacity, potential destructiveness, and increasing resistance to antimicrobial agents. Although less virulent, the coagulase-negative staphylococci (CoNS), especially *S. epidermidis*, adhere avidly to prosthetic materials and are important nosocomial pathogens, especially of compromised hosts. Another CoNS species, *S. saprophyticus*, is a common cause of urinary tract infections.

TAXONOMY AND MICROBIOLOGY Members of the genus *Staphylococcus* are nonmotile, nonsporulating gram-positive cocci, 0.5 to 1.5 μm in diameter, that occur singly and in pairs, short chains, and the irregular three-dimensional clusters from which their name is derived (Greek *staphulé*, "grape-like"). Staphylococci can grow over a wide range of environmental conditions, but they grow best at temperatures between 30°C and 37°C and at a pH around neutrality. They are resistant to desiccation and to chemical disinfectants, and they tolerate NaCl concentrations up to 12%. With rare exceptions, the staphylococci are facultatively anaerobic. The more virulent staphylococci can clot plasma (coagulase-positive), while the less virulent cannot (coagulase-negative). Of the six recognized coagulase-positive

materials in the extracellular matrix, evasion or neutralization of host defenses, and destruction of host tissues. For both intoxications and infections, the entire process is carefully orchestrated by the bacterium in response to specific environmental conditions.

Physical preservation of cellular integrity Staphylococci are robust and adaptable organisms that can survive under relatively harsh environmental conditions. A rigid cell wall confers shape and strength to the organisms. The major component of the cell wall, *peptidoglycan*, is responsible for its physical properties. Disruption of peptidoglycan cross-linking by cell wall–active antibiotics (β-lactams or glycopeptides) renders staphylococci susceptible to lysis mediated by endogenous peptidoglycan hydrolases (*autolysins*). The osmotolerance exhibited by *S. aureus* enables the organism to grow without microbial competition in foods of low water activity and so sets the stage for contamination of food by staphylococcal enterotoxins (SEs), which cause food poisoning.

Colonization Staphylococcal colonization of the nasal mucosa is mediated by adherence of cell-surface components to host molecules (e.g., mucin carbohydrate). Factors contributing to colonization of other surfaces, such as the vaginal mucosa, are poorly understood. After colonization, the production of certain staphylococcal toxins [toxic shock syndrome toxin 1 (TSST-1), exfoliative toxins, or SEs] can ensue under the appropriate environmental conditions. Colonization may be transient or persistent; the latter condition increases the likelihood that organisms will gain access to deeper tissues, beginning the process of infection.

Invasion and adherence to the extracellular matrix Staphylococci generally cannot invade through intact epithelial surfaces, which represent the primary line of antistaphylococcal defense. Invasion is facilitated by a mechanical break in the epithelium or by plugging of a gland or hair follicle. Once the epithelial barrier is breached, colonization of host tissues is facilitated by adherence of *S. aureus* to molecules present either on host cell surfaces or in the extracellular matrix. Several staphylococcal surface proteins, including protein A, function as adhesins by binding extracellular matrix molecules. These proteins have been designated "microbial-surface components recognizing adhesive matrix molecules" and may adhere to fibrinogen, fibronectin, collagen, elastin, and other serum constituents.

Destruction of host cells and alteration of the host microenvironment A number of products of *S. aureus* alter the host environment in a way that benefits the bacterium. *Coagulase* is a secreted enzyme that binds prothrombin and thereby causes the conversion of fibrinogen to fibrin; it may aid in the establishment of an environment within host tissues that is protected from cells of the immune system or from antibiotics. *S. aureus* produces a number of *lipases*, which may enhance the organism's survival in sebaceous areas of the human body. *Hyaluronidase* hydrolyzes hyaluronic acid, a mucopolysaccharide present in extracellular ground substance; its action may facilitate the spread of the organism through the extracellular matrix to adjoining tissues. *Staphylokinase, thermonuclease,* and *serine protease* are other extracellular enzymatic products that may play roles in pathogenesis.

S. aureus produces a number of membrane-active toxins that probably contribute to pathogenesis by damaging host cells, although their exact role in pathogenesis remains uncertain. These toxins include α-, β-, and δ-hemolysins and the synergohymenotropic toxins (γ-hemolysin and Panton-Valentine leukocidin). α-Hemolysin (α-toxin) is the prototypic pore-forming toxin; it inserts into the cell membrane, creating ion-conductive channels that destroy membrane integrity. The toxin is dermonecrotic on subcutaneous injection, induces proinflammatory changes in mammalian cells, and—in animal models—induces many findings seen in sepsis, including hypotension and thrombocytopenia. The *synergohymenotropic toxins* are a family of bicomponent toxins. Their name derives from the fact that their two components are tropic for cell membranes and are synergistically active against them. Like α-toxin, the synergohymenotropic toxins are

pore-forming toxins. *Panton-Valentine leukocidin* is most active against polymorphonuclear cells, monocytes, and macrophages. It is dermonecrotic to rabbit skin, and strains producing it are strongly associated with human furunculosis.

Evasion of host defense Once staphylococci have breached mucosal or epithelial barriers, the host's immune response is directed at containing and eliminating them, principally by polymorphonuclear recruitment and phagocytic killing. The bacteria fight back by cloaking antigenic determinants on their surface, by interfering with the function of opsonins, by directly killing the phagocytes, and by developing strategies to survive within them. The pyogenic abscess, the histologic hallmark of staphylococcal infection, represents the battlefield for this encounter, in which the microorganism survives in an environment in which leukocyte function is impaired and into which antibiotics penetrate poorly. Although the abscess may contain the spread of the bacteria, patients with abscesses are symptomatic and usually require surgical drainage for relief.

Some staphylococcal components and products are direct chemoattractants for polymorphonuclear leukocytes; others provoke the release of chemoattractant cytokines that recruit phagocytic cells to the infected area. Histologic sections of early lesions typically reveal a central focus of organisms surrounded by a zone of necrotic debris, which in turn is surrounded by a zone of viable inflammatory cells. The toxic action of staphylococcal leukocidin may in part explain the zone of necrosis. After several days, fibroblasts populate the margin of the abscess and there elaborate collagen, which creates a true capsule around the abscess.

Staphylococcal cell-wall peptidoglycan activates complement, which is an important opsonin in persons lacking antibody to staphylococcal surface components. Peptidoglycan also acts as a general stimulator of inflammatory cytokine release and may thereby contribute to sepsis, but it is weaker in this regard than gram-negative lipopolysaccharide. Opsonic antibodies specific for peptidoglycan or capsule mediate phagocytosis by polymorphonuclear leukocytes and macrophages in vitro, although the role of antibody in vivo is less certain. There is considerable interstrain variation in susceptibility to opsonization, and acquired protective immunity to staphylococcal infection is generally thought *not* to develop. (In contrast, acquired antibody-mediated immunity to systemic staphylococcal intoxications does occur; e.g., >90% of healthy adults have protective antibody to the most common TSS toxin, TSST-1.) Mitigating against opsonization is *protein A*, an important cell-surface component; protein A binds the Fc portion of IgG subclasses 1, 2, and 4 and thereby interferes with antibody-mediated opsonization. Polysaccharide capsule, which is produced by most clinical isolates, may also interfere with opsonization.

S. aureus has numerous defenses against killing after phagocytosis. Intracellular bacteria are usually killed rapidly by the oxidative burst within the phagosome, but staphylococcal catalase, which converts hydrogen peroxide to oxygen and water, detoxifies oxygen radicals and potentiates intracellular survival. Staphylococci are also taken up by nondedicated phagocytes, such as endothelial cells and osteoblasts, and may survive within them. One strategy for intracellular survival is the genesis of small-colony variants (SCVs). These slow-growing cells exhibit alterations in electron transport and generally produce reduced amounts of virulence determinants such as α-toxin and coagulase. They are relatively resistant to cell wall–active antibiotics and aminoglycosides and are capable of persisting intracellularly for extended periods, thereby evading host defenses. Their slow growth also makes them less likely to be recovered in the clinical laboratory and then targeted for treatment. Their existence may in part explain the startling capacity of certain *S. aureus* infections (e.g., chronic osteomyelitis) to recrudesce after years of dormancy and the difficulty of curing infections in intravascular sites and bone. Prolonged exposure to aminoglycosides or to trimethoprim-sulfamethoxazole appears to be a risk factor for the development of SCVs.

Hosts at particular risk for staphylococcal infection include those with frequent or chronic disruptions in epithelial or mucosal integrity;

those with disordered leukocyte chemotaxis, such as patients with the Chédiak-Higashi or Wiskott-Aldrich syndrome; those whose phagocytes are defective in oxidative killing, as in chronic granulomatous disease; those with neutropenia or acquired functional deficiencies (e.g., deficiencies induced by exogenous glucocorticoids); and those with indwelling foreign bodies, which provide a matrix for staphylococcal adherence and biofilm formation and seriously impair phagocytic function. Patients with disorders of immunoglobulin or complement (especially C1–C4 deficiencies) are also at increased risk for *S. aureus* infection.

Superantigens The superantigens are V_β-restricted T cell mitogens: they bind directly and without prior processing to major histocompatibility class II molecules on the surface of antigen-presenting cells, thereby stimulating T cells on the basis of the sequence of the variable region of the β chain of the T cell

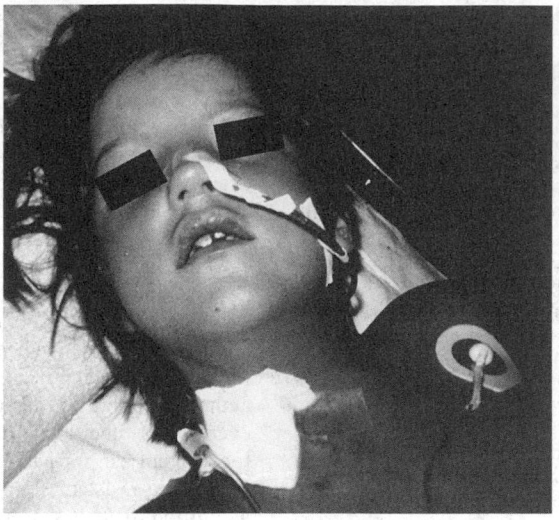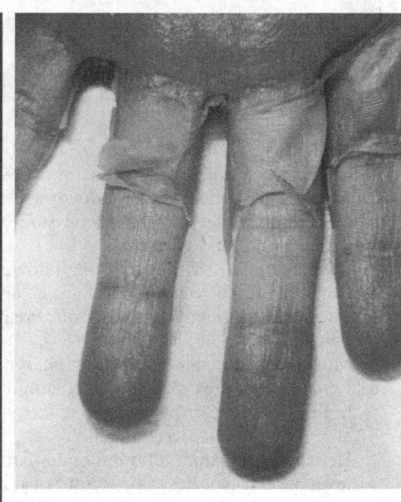

FIGURE 139-1 Cutaneous manifestations of toxic shock syndrome. The patient was a 7-year-old child with osteomyelitis and nonmenstrual TSS. *Left:* Diffuse erythroderma. The rubor was intense on the chest wall of this patient and is accurately represented in this photograph. Circumoral pallor is evident. *Right:* Desquamation of the fingers during convalescence. *(From Deresiewicz, with permission.)*

receptor rather than on the basis of the epitope specified by this receptor. Accordingly, a superantigen may be able to stimulate >10% of the T cells in a given individual—a percentage much higher than the ~1 in 10^6 cells stimulated by conventional antigens. This massive T cell stimulation provokes an exuberant and dysregulated immune response characterized by the release of the cytokines interleukins 1 and 2, tumor necrosis factor, and interferon γ. TSS is a manifestation of this process, as some aspects of septic shock may be as well. *S. aureus* produces a number of superantigens, including the SEs, TSST-1, and possibly the exfoliative toxins (ETs). Ten SEs have been identified to date, several of which are common causative agents of staphylococcal food poisoning. The mechanism by which the SEs cause vomiting is uncertain but may involve direct neural stimulation of the autonomic nervous system rather than a local effect on the gastrointestinal mucosa. The superantigenic properties of TSST-1 and the SEs are thought to explain their ability to cause TSS, although the exact mechanism by which they craft the various clinical manifestations of TSS is uncertain. There is conflicting evidence as to whether the ETs, which cause scalded skin syndrome, are superantigens; structural data suggest that they may instead be related to the serine proteases.

Genetic Regulation of Virulence Genes The production of virulence factors by bacteria is typically tightly and coordinately regulated by genetic apparatuses that sense and respond to environmental cues. Such coordinate regulation enables an organism to rapidly tailor its repertoire of proteins to suit its changing needs, either as it passes between microenvironments or as the environment evolves around it. Many of the staphylococcal exoproteins are typical virulence factors in this regard. For example, α-, β-, and δ-hemolysins, TSST-1, staphylococcal enterotoxin B, serine protease, and thermonuclease are all produced during the late logarithmic phase of growth in batch culture, at a time when nutrients become scarce and cell density reaches saturation. Their production is coordinately regulated and occurs reciprocally to that of the cell wall–associated staphylococcal proteins protein A and coagulase. Several genetic regulatory loci modulate these events, as do specific environmental conditions that presumably operate through those genetic loci. Foreign materials that increase the risk of TSS and conditions in food that predispose to staphylococcal food poisoning probably do so by presenting microenvironments that stimulate production of the relevant toxins. Similar events are undoubtedly operative within the environment of host tissues during infection, even in the absence of a foreign body.

Several distinct genetic loci regulate exoprotein production in *S. aureus*, the best-studied of which are *agr* (accessory gene regulator) and *sar* (staphylococcal accessory regulator). Both affect gene expression primarily at the level of transcription, and both activate the expression of secreted proteins and diminish the expression of cell wall–associated proteins during the late logarithmic phase of bacterial growth. Data suggest that *agr* may function primarily as a "quorum sensor," an apparatus that informs the bacterium of the density of staphylococci in its environment. Exoprotein regulation in *S. aureus* apparently results from a complex interplay of environmental factors and gene products.

STAPHYLOCOCCAL INTOXICATIONS   Toxic Shock Syndrome TSS is an acute, life-threatening intoxication characterized by fever, hypotension, rash, multiorgan dysfunction, and desquamation during the early convalescent period (Fig. 139-1). The disease was first characterized in 1978 but gained notoriety in 1980 upon the recognition of many cases among menstruating women. It is a relatively uncommon illness, with a reported annual incidence (among menstruating women) of 1 case per 100,000; it is likely, however, that the disease is substantially underreported, especially nonmenstrual cases. About half of all cases occur in settings other than menstruation and are distributed among individuals of both sexes and all ages. Menstrual and nonmenstrual cases are clinically indistinguishable. Among cases reported to the Centers for Disease Control and Prevention between 1985 and 1994, the minimum case-fatality rate was 2.5% for menstrual cases and 6.4% for nonmenstrual cases.

TSS is caused by any of several related exoproteins produced by *S. aureus*. TSST-1 is the toxin most frequently implicated (causing virtually all menstrual cases), and staphylococcal enterotoxin B is the second most frequent. For illness to develop, an individual must be colonized or infected with a toxigenic strain of *S. aureus* and must lack a protective level of antibody to the toxin made by that strain. That TSS is primarily a disease of the young reflects the fact that >90% of adults have antibodies to TSS toxins.

Menstruation remains the most common setting for TSS, but the disease can also complicate the use of barrier contraceptives and childbirth. Moreover, nonmenstrual TSS can ensue after superinfection of skin lesions of many types, including burns, insect bites, varicella lesions, and surgical wounds. Postoperative disease can develop from hours to weeks after any surgical procedure. Staphylococcal superinfection after influenza is a common setting for TSS, as is acute sinusitis. Overt infection with *S. aureus* is not required for the development of TSS; mere colonization with a toxigenic strain may suffice. Accordingly, the primary site of toxin production in TSS may appear entirely benign.

TSS remains a clinically defined syndrome (Table 139-1). Patients

Table 139-1　Staphylococcal Toxic Shock Syndrome: Case Definition

1. Fever: temperature of ≥38.9°C (≥102°F)
2. Rash: diffuse macular erythroderma ("sunburn" rash)
3. Hypotension: systolic blood pressure of ≤90 mmHg (adults) or <5th percentile for age (children <16 years of age); or orthostatic hypotension (orthostatic drop in diastolic blood pressure by ≥15 mmHg, orthostatic dizziness, or orthostatic syncope)
4. Involvement of at least three of the following organ systems:
   a. Gastrointestinal: vomiting or diarrhea at onset of illness
   b. Muscular: severe myalgias or serum creatine phosphokinase level at least twice the upper limit of normal
   c. Mucous membranes: vaginal, oropharyngeal, or conjunctival hyperemia
   d. Renal: blood urea nitrogen or creatinine level at least twice the upper limit of normal; or pyuria (≥5 leukocytes per high-power field) in the absence of urinary tract infection
   e. Hepatic: total serum bilirubin or aminotransferase (alanine or aspartate) level at least twice the upper limit of normal
   f. Hematologic: thrombocytopenia (platelet count ≤100,000/μL)
   g. Central nervous: disorientation or alteration in consciousness but no focal neurologic signs at a time when fever and hypotension are absent
5. Desquamation: 1 to 2 weeks after the onset of illness (typically palms and soles)
6. Evidence against an alternative diagnosis: negative results of cultures of blood, throat, or CSF (if performed);[a] no rise in titers of antibody to the agents of Rocky Mountain spotted fever, leptospirosis, and rubeola (if obtained)

---

[a] Blood culture may be positive for *S. aureus*. CSF, cerebrospinal fluid.
SOURCE: AL Reingold et al, Ann Intern Med 96(part 2):875, 1982.

meeting the case definition are severely ill, although milder forms of "staphylococcal toxin-mediated disease" do occur. The illness usually begins precipitously, with high fever and a complex of symptoms that may include nausea, vomiting, abdominal pain, diarrhea, muscular pain, sore throat, and headache. Dizziness is common as a manifestation of orthostatic or frank hypotension. The characteristic macular erythroderma develops over the first 2 days of illness. It is usually generalized but is sometimes locally confined; it can be evanescent or persistent. The patient's mental status is often abnormal to a degree that is out of proportion to the degree of hypotension. Conjunctival suffusion, pharyngeal injection, and peripheral edema are evident in many cases; a so-called strawberry tongue develops in up to half of patients. In menstrual disease, the vaginal mucosa may be erythematous and a purulent vaginal discharge may be present, but these findings are not universal. Common laboratory abnormalities include azotemia, hypoalbuminemia, hypocalcemia, hypophosphatemia, creatine phosphokinase elevation, leukocytosis or leukopenia with a left shift, thrombocytopenia, and pyuria.

The early signs and symptoms of TSS resolve within the first few days of illness, after which complications of organ hypoperfusion, such as renal and myocardial dysfunction, fluid overload, and adult respiratory distress syndrome, dominate the picture. After about a week of illness, desquamation begins with superficial flaking of the skin of the torso, face, and extremities, which may be followed by full-thickness desquamation of the palms, soles, and digits. Common late sequelae include peripheral gangrene, reversible nail and hair loss, muscle weakness, and lingering asthenia and neuropsychiatric dysfunction.

The differential diagnosis of TSS is that of a severe febrile exanthem with hypotension. In the setting of menstruation accompanied by purulent vaginal discharge, the diagnosis may be obvious. The challenge is to recognize the less obvious cases, in which the exanthem may be fleeting, multiorgan dysfunction may be subtle, or (in nonmenstrual cases) a primary site of infection may be inapparent. Recovery of *S. aureus* supports the diagnosis, as does demonstration of toxin production by the strain and serologic susceptibility to the toxin. Other diagnoses to consider include streptococcal TSS, staphylococcal scalded skin syndrome, Kawasaki syndrome, Rocky Mountain spotted fever, leptospirosis, meningococcemia, gram-negative sepsis, exan-

thematous viral syndromes, and severe drug reactions. Staphylococcal TSS and streptococcal TSS (Chap. 140) can be clinically indistinguishable.

Treatment of TSS involves drainage of the site of toxin production, aggressive fluid resuscitation, and administration of antistaphylococcal antibiotics. Recent surgical wounds should be explored and irrigated, even when signs of inflammation are lacking; foreign bodies should be removed. Pressors should be used for sustained hypotension that is unresponsive to fluids. Electrolyte abnormalities, particularly hypocalcemia and hypomagnesemia, must be corrected. Penicillinase-resistant penicillins (nafcillin, oxacillin) and first-generation cephalosporins have been widely used in TSS. A growing body of clinical and laboratory evidence indicates, however, that a protein synthesis inhibitor, such as clindamycin, might be superior to β-lactam agents. The authors recommend therapy with clindamycin (900 mg intravenously every 8 h), either alone or in combination with a β-lactam antibiotic [or vancomycin for patients perceived to be at risk for infection with methicillin-resistant *S. aureus* (MRSA)]. For a seriously ill patient in whom the diagnosis of TSS is uncertain, broad-spectrum antibiotics may be appropriate until the diagnosis is confirmed. A 14-day course of therapy—some of which may be administered perorally—is reasonable. Patients whose illness is severe enough to warrant vasopressors, who require mechanical ventilation, who have worsening renal function, or who have an undrainable focus of infection should be treated with intravenous immunoglobulin, which contains high levels of neutralizing antibody to TSS toxins. A single infusion of 400 mg/kg generates a protective level of antibody to TSST-1 that persists for weeks. Glucocorticoids have not been shown to be of significant benefit.

Because vaginal staphylococcal carriage can be persistent or recurrent and because in more than half of all cases TSS does not elicit immunity, recurrent menstrual TSS is a concern; recurrent nonmenstrual TSS has also been reported. The risk of recurrent illness can be assessed by tests for seroconversion to TSST-1. Women who do not seroconvert after acute illness (or who are not tested for antibody) should refrain indefinitely from using tampons or barrier contraceptives.

Staphylococcal Scalded Skin Syndrome　This syndrome encompasses a range of cutaneous diseases of varying severity caused by ET-producing strains of *S. aureus*. The most severe form of staphylococcal scalded skin syndrome is termed *Ritter's disease* in newborns and *toxic epidermal necrolysis* (TEN) in older individuals. Milder and more common forms include *pemphigus neonatorum* and (in children and adults) *bullous impetigo* (see "Skin and Soft Tissue Infections," below). Persons >5 years old rarely develop staphylococcal TEN; those who do almost invariably have underlying disease (renal insufficiency, systemic immunosuppression). The rarity of the syndrome in adults has been ascribed to acquired immunity to the inciting toxins, to enhanced renal clearance of the toxins, and perhaps to diminished sensitivity to the action of the toxins.

Staphylococcal TEN, or Ritter's disease, often begins with a nonspecific prodrome. The acute phase starts with the onset of an erythematous rash. The erythema begins in the periorbital and perioral areas and spreads to the trunk and centrifugally to the limbs. Pastia's lines may be apparent. The skin has a sandpaper texture and is often tender. Periorbital edema is common. In infants and children, fever and irritability or lethargy are common, but systemic toxicity is not. Within hours or days, wrinkling and sloughing of the epidermis begin; sloughing can be provoked by gentle stroking of the skin (Nikolsky's sign), even in areas that appear uninvolved. The denuded areas are red and glistening but not purulent, and staphylococci are not present. Exfoliation may continue in large sheets or in ragged snippets of tissue. Large, flaccid bullae may develop. As in thermal burns, significant fluid and electrolyte loss can occur at this stage, as can secondary infection. Within about 48 h, the exfoliated areas dry and secondary desquamation begins. The entire illness resolves within about 10 days. Mortality (from hypovolemia or sepsis) is ~3% among children but approaches 50% among adults. Treatment includes the administration of antistaphylococcal agents, fluid and electrolyte management, and local care to the denuded skin.

Staphylococcal Food Poisoning Between 2 and 6 h after ingestion of contaminated food, staphylococcal food poisoning begins abruptly with nausea, vomiting, crampy abdominal pain, and diarrhea. The diarrhea is usually noninflammatory and is of lower volume than that in cholera or toxigenic *Escherichia coli* infection. Fever and rash are absent, and the patient is neurologically normal. The majority of cases are self-limited and resolve between 8 and 24 h after onset. In severe cases, hypovolemia and hypotension can develop. Although most cases probably do not come to medical attention and are not diagnosed, staphylococcal intoxication is the second or third leading cause of diagnosed food poisoning in the United States.

Food poisoning is caused by the ingestion of any of the SEs, which are produced by *S. aureus* in contaminated food before it is eaten. The presence of SEs in the food vector before its consumption accounts for the short incubation period of this illness. The SEs are heat stable, thus tolerating cooking conditions that kill the organisms that produced them. The disease has a high attack rate and is somewhat more common during the summer than at other times of the year. Processed meats and custard-filled baked goods are common food vectors, perhaps because staphylococci can tolerate conditions of high protein, salt, or sugar and so grow without competition in these environments. The most important epidemiologic risk factor in outbreaks of this disease is the ingestion of food that has been left at warm temperatures for prolonged periods, thereby allowing toxin production to occur before consumption. Contaminated preparation equipment and poor personal hygiene of food handlers are frequently implicated as well.

STAPHYLOCOCCAL INFECTIONS *S. aureus* causes invasive disease by breaching host defense barriers, often after disruption or dysfunction of such barriers. The most common portals of entry leading to staphylococcal invasion are the skin and associated structures. A nidus for staphylococcal colonization and subsequent invasion is provided by chronic skin conditions, such as eczema and psoriasis; acute breaks in the skin, such as puncture wounds, abrasions, and lacerations; and abnormalities of skin appendages, such as hair follicles and nails. Colonization of the nasopharynx predisposes to respiratory tract infection after aspiration, obstruction (e.g., of a bronchus by carcinoma or of sinus ostia by trauma, edema, or polyps), or impaired ciliary function (e.g., in chronic bronchitis or acute viral infection). Intubation of the trachea provides a conduit by which upper respiratory flora, including pathogens such as *S. aureus*, can reach the lower respiratory tract.

Skin and Soft Tissue Infections *S. aureus* is the most common etiologic agent of skin and soft tissue infections (Chap. 128). Such infections are usually caused by endogenous flora—i.e., strains of *S. aureus* that are harbored in the nares or other sites of colonization. Infection may represent a primary pathologic process, with direct invasion of skin and adjacent tissues, or a secondary process complicating preexisting lesions.

Staphylococcal infections originating in hair follicles range in severity from trivial to life-threatening. *Folliculitis* is an infection of follicular ostia; the appearance is that of a domed yellow pustule with a narrow red margin. Infection is often self-limited, although healing may be hastened by topical antiseptics and more severe cases may benefit from topical or systemic antibiotics. A *furuncle* (often called a *boil*) is a deep-seated necrotic infection of a hair follicle, most often located on the buttocks, face, or neck. Furuncles are painful and tender, and their appearance is often accompanied by fever and constitutional symptoms. Surgical drainage and systemic antibiotic treatment may hasten recovery and limit scar formation. Deep infection of a group of contiguous follicles is called a *carbuncle*. This type of painful necrotic lesion occurs most commonly on the back of the neck, shoulders, hips, and thighs, typically in middle-aged or elderly men. There is intense inflammation of surrounding and underlying connective tissue, and the infection may be complicated by bacteremia. Surgical drainage and systemic antibiotic administration are indicated. *S. aureus* is also the most common cause of acute *paronychia*, infection of the lateral nail folds.

S. aureus causes *bullous impetigo*, a superficial cutaneous disorder occurring predominantly in children. An epidermal split caused by ET results in the formation of 1- to 2-cm bullae containing neutrophils and organisms. *Nonbullous impetigo* is most often caused by β-hemolytic streptococci, but *S. aureus* can secondarily infect impetiginous lesions. Treatment of impetigo with a topical antibiotic, such as mupirocin, may suffice for mild and localized infection, whereas systemic therapy is indicated for widespread or severe disease or for infection accompanied by lymphadenopathy.

Cellulitis, a spreading infection of subcutaneous tissue, is occasionally caused by *S. aureus*, but β-hemolytic streptococci are more common agents of this disease (Chap. 140). Secondary infection of surgical and traumatic wounds is more likely to be staphylococcal in etiology than is cellulitis arising from minor or inapparent breaks in the skin, and empiric treatment directed against both *S. aureus* and streptococci is reasonable in these settings. *Erysipelas*, the hallmark of which is a well-demarcated raised border, is a more superficial infection of the dermis and subcutaneous tissue; it is usually caused by group A streptococci and only rarely, if ever, by *S. aureus*.

Respiratory Tract Infections *S. aureus* can gain access to the lung parenchyma by two routes: aspiration of upper respiratory flora and hematogenous spread. Staphylococcal pneumonia is a relatively uncommon but severe infection, characterized clinically by chest pain, systemic toxicity, and dyspnea and pathologically by intense neutrophilic infiltration, necrosis, and abscess formation. *Pleural empyema* is a common complication and increases the already-considerable morbidity associated with this infection. Only rarely does *S. aureus* cause pneumonia without predisposing epidemiologic or host factors that favor colonization of the respiratory tract and/or that impair defense mechanisms. Residence in a chronic care facility, recent use of antibiotics, and hospitalization favor colonization—and hence respiratory tract infection—with *S. aureus*. Staphylococcal pneumonia most commonly follows tracheal intubation of a hospitalized patient or viral infection of the respiratory tract. Influenza virus is known both to increase respiratory colonization by *S. aureus* and to impair ciliary function (and therefore clearance of staphylococci). In a classic scenario, a patient (often elderly and/or institutionalized) develops a flu-like respiratory illness and then, after several days, deteriorates rapidly, with high fever, dyspnea, productive cough, and obtundation. The diagnosis of staphylococcal pneumonia is readily established by Gram's staining of expectorated sputum, which reveals abundant clusters of gram-positive cocci.

Hematogenous seeding of the lungs with *S. aureus* follows embolization from an intravascular nidus of infection. Common settings for septic pulmonary embolization are right-sided endocarditis (especially common among injection drug users) and septic thrombophlebitis, which is most often a complication of an indwelling venous catheter. Pneumonia is heralded by the acute onset of pleuritic chest pain and dyspnea; although diagnostic sputum may be lacking, a chest radiograph typically shows multiple nodular infiltrates, providing an important clue to both the diagnosis and the pathogenesis of disease.

Although not typically considered in the differential diagnosis of sore throat, *S. aureus* is occasionally isolated as the dominant organism from patients (especially children) with exudative *pharyngitis*. The illness may be accompanied by a scarlatiniform rash and may result in systemic toxicity (like that seen in TSS). Staphylococcal *tracheitis* may be diagnosed in children who have systemic toxicity and positive respiratory cultures but who lack pulmonary infiltrates. *S. aureus* is a prominent cause of *chronic sinusitis*, typically following the selection pressure of antimicrobial regimens that lack activity against this organism. Finally, *S. aureus* is a major etiologic agent of *sphenoid sinusitis*.

Infections of the Central Nervous System *S. aureus* gains access to structures of the central nervous system by hematogenous spread or by direct extension from contiguous structures. This organism is a prominent cause of *brain abscess*, especially as a result of embolization during mitral or aortic valve endocarditis. Such abscesses are often multiple, small, and scattered diffusely throughout the brain. Brain abscess can also develop by direct extension from frontoethmoid or sphenoid sinuses or from infected soft tissue after surgery or penetrating trauma. Patients with staphylococcal brain abscesses are more likely to have fever, meningismus, and other signs of infection than are patients with anaerobic bacterial or mixed-etiology brain abscesses. Purulent *meningitis* may accompany staphylococcal brain abscess or may develop during bacteremia in the absence of demonstrable abscesses.

S. aureus is the organism most likely to cause a variety of other space-occupying, suppurative intracranial infections. *Subdural empyema* usually develops by direct extension of osteomyelitis of the skull, after surgery or trauma, or in the setting of sinusitis. This condition may be accompanied by meningitis, epidural abscess, or intracranial phlebitis. The cardinal features of subdural empyema are fever, headache, vomiting, and signs of meningeal irritation. As the infection progresses, cerebral edema, often with infarction, may ensue and may be accompanied by alteration in mental status, seizures, and focal neurologic signs, which sometimes progress rapidly. The diagnosis should be suspected in any patient with meningeal signs and focal neurologic findings. Magnetic resonance imaging (MRI) is the diagnostic procedure of choice; lumbar puncture is contraindicated because of the danger of brainstem herniation. Early surgical drainage and treatment with an antibiotic that penetrates well into the central nervous system may be curative, although neurologic sequelae are not uncommon.

S. aureus is the most common cause of *spinal epidural abscess*, which develops most often in association with vertebral osteomyelitis or diskitis. The diagnosis is suggested by some combination of fever, back pain, radicular pain, lower-extremity weakness, and bowel or bladder dysfunction, but the presentation is often subtle, resulting in delayed diagnosis. Patients may report only difficulty in walking or weakness, and objective findings may initially be lacking. The principal danger is the potential for necrosis of the spinal cord by compression and/or venous involvement. Early recognition of this condition is critical if long-term sequelae, such as paraplegia, are to be averted. An MRI scan of the spine establishes whether or not an epidural collection is present. Fluoroscopy- or computed tomography (CT)-guided needle aspiration may confirm the diagnosis, but an open procedure offers a higher yield. Prompt surgical decompression by laminectomy is often required for preservation of neurologic function, although a trial of antibiotic therapy alone may be considered if no focal neurologic deficits are detected at the time of diagnosis. Any deterioration in neurologic status should prompt urgent surgical intervention. The pathogenesis of *intracerebral epidural abscess* is similar to that of subdural empyema, with staphylococcal infection usually following sinusitis, craniotomy, or trauma. Clinical manifestations reflect the anatomy of the underlying osteomyelitis plus the mass effect of the abscess, cerebral edema, and (often) secondary involvement of the subdural space. Emergent surgical drainage is usually required for cure.

Finally, *S. aureus* is the most common cause of *septic intracranial thrombophlebitis*, typically following sinusitis, mastoiditis, or soft tissue infection of the face. Clinical manifestations reflect the underlying condition and the anatomic structures in contiguity with the infected vein or sinus. Focal neurologic deficits, particularly of cranial nerve function, are characteristic of cavernous sinus thrombosis. Sagittal sinus thrombosis may be manifested by leg and arm weakness and by altered mental status; infections of the lateral and petrosal sinuses also produce characteristic clinical syndromes. Intracranial phlebitis may accompany epidural abscess, subdural empyema, and meningitis and is sometimes clinically indistinguishable from other types of intracranial infection. MRI is the diagnostic procedure of choice.

Urinary Tract Infections *S. aureus* is an uncommon cause of urinary tract infection. Ascending infection almost exclusively follows instrumentation of the bladder (e.g., cystoscopy or placement of an indwelling catheter). Under other circumstances, the presence of *S. aureus* in the urine, even in low numbers, suggests staphylococcal bacteremia and hematogenous seeding of the kidneys, with or without abscess formation; staphylococcal endocarditis should be considered in this setting.

Endovascular Infections *S. aureus* is the most common cause of acute bacterial *endocarditis* of both native and prosthetic valves (Chap. 126). The organism may infect previously normal valves. Staphylococcal endocarditis presents as an acute febrile illness, rarely of more than a few weeks' duration; complications such as meningitis, brain or visceral abscess, peripheral vascular embolization, valvular incompetence with heart failure, myocardial abscess, and purulent pericarditis have often developed by the time a patient seeks medical attention. The valves most commonly involved are the mitral and/or the aortic except among injection drug users, in whom infection of the tricuspid valve is most common.

The diagnosis of endocarditis is suggested by a heart murmur and the presence of conjunctival hemorrhages, subungual petechiae, or purpuric lesions on the distal extremities; it is readily confirmed by demonstration of high-grade bacteremia and echocardiography showing valvular vegetations. Echocardiography also helps establish which valve(s) are infected, the degree of valvular dysfunction or destruction, the quality of left ventricular function, and the presence or absence of annular or myocardial abscess. Transesophageal echocardiography (TEE) is more sensitive than transthoracic echocardiography (TTE) in detecting vegetations and abscesses, but it is also more invasive. TEE need not be performed in all cases of proven or suspected endocarditis. This approach is useful, however, in the setting of persistent bacteremia or fever (to evaluate for abscess) and in anticipation of surgery if TTE has not been sufficiently informative.

Native valve staphylococcal endocarditis carries a high mortality rate (on the order of 40%) and mandates prompt initiation of antimicrobial therapy. In addition to blood cultures and echocardiography, evaluation may include CT of the head and lumbar puncture if brain abscess or meningitis is suspected; a radionucleotide study if osteomyelitis is suspected; and abdominal CT if visceral abscess is suggested by abdominal pain or persistent fever or bacteremia. Indications for valve replacement are the same as those in endocarditis caused by other organisms: persistent bacteremia (beyond 5 to 7 days of therapy), valvular dysfunction resulting in heart failure, perivalvular or myocardial abscess, or recurrent embolization. Early consultation with a cardiothoracic surgeon is advisable in all cases because of the high proportion of patients with *S. aureus* endocarditis (around half) who develop one of these complications and therefore require valve replacement, often urgently. Once there is an indication for removal of an infected valve, nothing is gained and much can be lost by delaying surgery. *S. aureus* infection of a prosthetic valve (as an early or a late complication of valve replacement) almost always requires surgery for one of the above indications.

Right-sided endocarditis, which most often develops in association with injection drug use or venous catheterization, is frequently complicated by septic pulmonary emboli but otherwise carries a lower rate of serious complications than left-sided disease. Surgery is rarely required for right-sided infection. A relatively short course of parenteral combination therapy (2 weeks) may be curative, and the prognosis is relatively good.

The propensity of *S. aureus* to adhere to and infect damaged tissues makes it the foremost cause of endovascular infections other than endocarditis. Vascular infection is a consequence of hematogenous seeding of damaged vessels, especially large arteries with atheromatous plaques, resulting in the development of a mycotic aneurysm. It may also develop by spread from a contiguous focus of infection (e.g., after vascular surgery), often resulting in an infected pseudoaneurysm, or by contamination of an intravascular device, resulting in septic phlebitis. Staphylococcal infection of an atherosclerotic artery (most commonly the abdominal aorta or iliac arteries), which may be aneurysmal to begin with, is a potentially catastrophic event. Such infections are associated with high-grade bacteremia, may result in rupture and massive hemorrhage, and require surgical resection and bypass of the infected vessel. Septic phlebitis is also associated with high-grade bacteremia and systemic toxicity but is less likely than arteritis to result in rupture. Persistent bacteremia suggests the need for surgical removal of infected thrombus or vein, but the technical difficulty of such surgery may warrant an attempt at cure with antibiotics and anticoagulants alone.

Bacteremia A classic clinical scenario is that of a patient presenting with *S. aureus* bacteremia but without a demonstrable primary site of infection. Even in the absence of a changing murmur, peripheral embolic lesions, or a diagnostic echocardiogram, the possibility of endocarditis must be considered carefully in this situation. It is often hard to differentiate between endocarditis and bacteremia arising from another primary site; in addition, *S. aureus* may secondarily seed endovascular sites, such as heart valves or atheromatous plaques. Several criteria increase the likelihood that a patient has endocarditis as opposed to simple bacteremia: community (vs. nosocomial) acquisition of infection, absence of an apparent primary site of infection, and evidence of metastatic infection. The evaluation of a bacteremic patient should be tailored to the individual but may include an abdominal CT scan and a bone scan or gallium scan to detect an occult visceral abscess or osteomyelitis. TEE has demonstrated valvular abnormalities suggestive of endocarditis in up to one-fourth of bacteremic patients who lack clinical or TTE evidence of endocarditis. This finding has prompted some authorities to recommend TEE for all patients with staphylococcal bacteremia. The authors favor performance of this test for patients with persistent fever or bacteremia.

Complications of *S. aureus* bacteremia include abscesses of abdominal viscera, brain abscess, meningitis, septic arthritis, osteomyelitis, epidural abscess, and mycotic aneurysm. High-grade or persistent bacteremia mandates a thorough evaluation for these complications, even if a primary site of infection has been identified. The reported mortality rate for staphylococcal bacteremia ranges from 11 to 43%, with catheter-related infections carrying lower rates of complications and mortality than noncatheter infections.

Musculoskeletal Infections *S. aureus* is the most common cause of *acute osteomyelitis* (Chap. 129) in adults and one of the leading causes in children. Acute osteomyelitis develops as a result of either hematogenous seeding of bone (especially damaged bone) or direct extension from a contiguous focus of infection. The most common sites of hematogenous staphylococcal osteomyelitis in adults are the vertebral bodies; in children, the highly vascular metaphyses of long bones are most often affected. Acute osteomyelitis in adults usually presents with constitutional symptoms and pain over the affected area, often developing over several weeks or months. Leukocytosis and an elevated erythrocyte sedimentation rate or C-reactive protein level are laboratory clues to the diagnosis. Bacteremia may or may not be demonstrable. Four weeks of parenteral antibiotic therapy is usually curative.

S. aureus is also a prominent cause of *chronic osteomyelitis*, which develops at sites of previous surgery, trauma, or devascularization. In light of the hectic pace of many infections caused by *S. aureus*, chronic staphylococcal osteomyelitis can be impressively indolent; the infection may be asymptomatic for years or even decades, only to reawaken spontaneously and cause pain, sinus tract formation, and purulent drainage. A plain film of the affected area reveals bony destruction. The staphylococcal etiology of infection is best established by biopsy and culture of bone, as cultures of superficial or sinus tract drainage may yield misleading results. Cure requires surgical debridement of necrotic bone followed by a prolonged course of antibiotics. →*For consensus definitions of acute and chronic osteomyelitis, see Chap. 129.*

A special form of osteomyelitis is that associated with prosthetic joints or with internal or external fixation devices. Pain, fever, swelling, and decreased range of motion are cardinal features of an infected prosthesis. A plain film may suggest loosening of the prosthesis, often as radiolucency at the interface between bone and cement. *S. aureus* osteomyelitis associated with a prosthesis is infrequently cured by antibiotics alone. Persistent sepsis, persistent bacteremia, and clinical or radiologic evidence of loosening are absolute indications for removal of the prosthesis. *S. aureus* infection of fixation devices requires their removal, although this procedure may occasionally be delayed long enough to allow healing of the underlying fracture. Late relapses after apparent medical cure are not uncommon. A strategy of microbial suppression with oral antibiotics after a course of high-dose parenteral therapy is occasionally employed when removal of hardware is deemed too aggressive a measure for a particular patient.

S. aureus is a major cause of *septic arthritis* in adults (Chap. 323). Predisposing factors include injection drug use, rheumatoid arthritis, use of systemic or intraarticular steroids, penetrating trauma, and joints previously damaged by trauma or disease. Knees, hips, and sacroiliac joints are most frequently infected. In addition to parenteral antibiotics, cure requires either repeated joint aspirations—the end points being sterilization of the joint space, a decrease in the number of leukocytes in the joint aspirate, and no reaccumulation of fluid—or open or arthroscopic debridement and drainage. Failure to adequately drain joints infected with *S. aureus* poses a risk of permanent loss of function. *S. aureus* is also the most common cause of *septic bursitis* (Chap. 325), which most often involves bursae of the elbows, knees, and shoulders. As in arthritis, adequate drainage (via repeat aspiration, placement of a drain, or open debridement) hastens recovery and minimizes loss of function.

S. aureus infection of muscle (*pyomyositis*; Chap. 128) is relatively uncommon in temperate climates; *psoas abscess* is the most common such infection. The psoas muscle is seeded either hematogenously or by direct extension from the site of vertebral osteomyelitis; the results are pain upon extension of the hip and fever. Although formerly a cause of fever of unknown origin, psoas abscess is now relatively easy to diagnose by abdominal CT or MRI. Psoas abscesses are occasionally amenable to drainage via a percutaneous catheter; if not, then surgical drainage is indicated. For reasons that are not well understood, most other cases of staphylococcal pyomyositis occur in the tropics (tropical pyomyositis); in the United States, pyomyositis is seen most often in patients with underlying conditions such as diabetes mellitus, alcoholism, immunosuppressive therapy, and hematologic malignancy.

DIAGNOSIS The diagnosis of *S. aureus* infection is generally straightforward and is based on the isolation of the organism either from purulent material or from a normally sterile body fluid. Rarely should *S. aureus* growing from even a single blood culture be considered a contaminant. Clinical samples require no special transport media to preserve the viability of the organisms. Gram's staining of purulent material from a staphylococcal abscess invariably reveals abundant neutrophils and intra- and extracellular gram-positive cocci, which may be found singly or in pairs, tetrads, or clusters. *S. aureus* grows readily on standard laboratory media. Colonies that are catalase-positive and coagulase- or thermonuclease-positive are identified presumptively as *S. aureus*. Commercial kits are also available for the identification of gram-positive cocci and are generally reliable for identification of *S. aureus*.

The diagnosis of staphylococcal intoxications (such as TSS) may be more difficult and may in fact rely entirely on clinical data. The contribution of the laboratory may be confirmatory—for example, the demonstration of seroconversion to TSST-1 following a compatible illness, the demonstration of toxin production in vitro by a strain isolated from a patient, or the detection of SE in a food sample.

℞ **TREATMENT** The essential elements of therapy for staphylococcal infections are drainage of purulent collections of pus, debridement of necrotic tissue, removal of foreign bodies, and administration of antimicrobial agents. The importance of adequate drainage cannot be overemphasized; all but the smallest of staphylococcal abscesses require drainage for cure. In skin and soft tissue infections, surgical drainage is occasionally all that is required for cure. It is very difficult to eradicate *S. aureus* infection in the presence of a foreign body, such as a piece of orthopedic hardware, an intravascular catheter or other device, or a pacemaker. For example, patients with catheter-associated bacteremia who are treated with antibiotics but do not have their catheters removed have been found to be six times more likely to experience a relapse or to die of their infection than are patients whose catheters are removed. Only under extraordinary circumstances should an attempt be made to cure such infections without removal of foreign material or debridement of necrotic tissue.

Antimicrobial resistance   The relentless spread of antibiotic resistance among strains of *S. aureus* is one of the great challenges facing clinicians today. Within 4 years of the introduction of penicillin G into clinical practice in 1941, β-lactamase-mediated resistance to penicillin was reported. As additional antibiotics became available in the 1950s, resistance rapidly emerged to them as well. Bacterial killing by β-lactam antibiotics depends on binding of the drugs to penicillin-binding proteins (PBPs), a group of transpeptidases that catalyze the terminal steps in peptidoglycan assembly. *S. aureus* normally produces four PBPs, all of which are inhibited by β-lactam antibiotics and several of which are essential for bacterial integrity and multiplication. Penicillin resistance in *S. aureus* is largely due to bacterial production of β-lactamase, a serine peptidase that enzymatically degrades the β-lactam ring of penicillin, thereby inactivating the drug before it can interact with the PBPs. In most communities, >90% of *S. aureus* strains produce β-lactamase and hence are resistant to penicillin.

Methicillin, the first β-lactamase-stable semisynthetic penicillin, was introduced in 1960; it took only 1 year, however, for an MRSA strain to be isolated. Classic methicillin resistance is encoded by the methicillin resistance determinant (*mec*), a 30- to 50-kb transposon-like segment of DNA that is present in MRSA strains and absent from sensitive strains. The *mecA* gene encodes a variant PBP called *PBP2′* or *PBP2a*. PBP2′ has reduced affinity for β-lactam antibiotics and can substitute for the essential PBPs if they have been inactivated by β-lactams. MRSA strains are resistant to the action of all β-lactam antibiotics, including penicillins, cephalosporins, and carbapenems. Since the early 1980s, these strains have tended to be resistant to most other antibiotics as well, including chloramphenicol, tetracyclines, and macrolides, through other resistance mechanisms. Nosocomial (as opposed to community-acquired) isolates of MRSA are especially likely to be multidrug-resistant. Classic methicillin resistance can be detected readily in the clinical microbiology laboratory by a variety of techniques. An additional mechanism of relative resistance to methicillin—hyperproduction of β-lactamase—has been described, but the clinical significance of this form of resistance is uncertain.

Until recently, all strains of MRSA remained susceptible to vancomycin (if nothing else), making this the drug of choice for the treatment of infections caused by suspected or proven MRSA. Unfortunately, the efficacy of vancomycin for serious *S. aureus* infections, regardless of susceptibility to other agents, is suboptimal (see "Selection of Antibiotics," below). Furthermore, resistance of *S. aureus* to vancomycin has now emerged as well (see below), making the search for new antistaphylococcal agents all the more urgent. If isolates are shown to be susceptible to clindamycin or trimethoprim-sulfamethoxazole, these agents can be effective for treatment of MRSA infection—but again, many strains are resistant. Two newly licensed antibiotics, representing the vanguard of two new classes of drugs, may prove to be useful for treatment of infections caused by MRSA. A new antibiotic that combines two streptogramins, quinupristin and dalfopristin, blocks protein synthesis at two ribosomal sites, resulting in a synergistic bactericidal effect on *S. aureus* and other gram-positive cocci. Linezolid, the first representative of the new oxazolidinone class of antibiotics, also demonstrates excellent activity against *S. aureus*, including multidrug-resistant strains of MRSA. Oxazolidinones are

bacteriostatic, but resistance to them is unusual and there is no cross-resistance with other classes of compounds. Until data reveal the relative efficacies and toxicities of vancomycin and these new compounds, however, vancomycin remains the drug of choice for treatment of MRSA infections.

In 1996, a long-predicted monster—*S. aureus* with decreased susceptibility to vancomycin—finally emerged from the theoretical nightmares of microbiologists into the clinical realm. The term *vancomycin-intermediate S. aureus* (VISA) has been widely used to describe these strains, whose minimum inhibitory concentrations (MICs) of vancomycin (8 to 16 μg/mL) should theoretically confer only intermediate resistance to this agent. The clinical experience has been one of treatment failure, however. In 1997, four patients with VISA infection were reported from Japan and the United States; all died, although only one death was a direct result of the VISA infection. As of this writing, about a dozen additional cases have been reported from Asia, North America, and Europe, and the VISA genotype is already widespread in Japan. The risk factors for infection with VISA are uncertain because of the small number of reported cases, but they appear to include a history of dialysis, multiple prior courses of antibiotics (including vancomycin), admission to an intensive care unit, and prior infection with MRSA.

The mechanism for decreased susceptibility to vancomycin in *S. aureus* appears to be novel and unrelated to the mechanism of resistance of vancomycin-resistant enterococci (VRE). VISA strains have unusually thick extracellular matrices that make it more difficult for vancomycin to reach its binding site at the level of the murein monomer of the cell wall. In addition, peptidoglycan from VISA appears to bind more vancomycin than does peptidoglycan from susceptible strains of *S. aureus*. These two factors create a "vancomycin sink," resulting in an increase in the MIC of vancomycin. VISA strains may also be characterized by increased expression of PBPs, slower growth, and decreased autolysis, all potentially contributing to antimicrobial resistance. Vancomycin resistance within a population of organisms is expressed in a heterogeneous manner, which may lead to difficulty in detection of the phenotype by usual susceptibility testing and may explain the failure of antimicrobial therapy in some cases. Therefore, infection with VISA should be suspected in any patient for whom seemingly appropriate therapy with vancomycin is ineffective. Removal of prosthetic material associated with infection is even more critical than usual in treating a patient infected with MRSA or VISA. Antimicrobial therapy for infections caused by VISA is discussed below (see "Selection of antibiotics").

In recent years, the percentage of staphylococcal isolates that are methicillin-resistant has risen substantially in U.S. hospitals; this trend has been driven by widespread (and often indiscriminate) antibiotic use. In some tertiary care institutions, up to 40% of *S. aureus* isolates are now resistant to methicillin, although rates of 5 to 15% are more typical. This situation is problematic for several reasons. Hospitalized patients colonized with MRSA are at increased risk (up to fourfold higher) of developing staphylococcal bacteremia than are patients colonized with methicillin-sensitive strains. The extent to which this difference reflects differences in bacterial virulence (as opposed to host factors or appropriateness of therapy) remains unclear; MRSA strains have not been shown consistently to be more virulent than sensitive strains, but the breadth of their resistance renders colonization more persistent, which in turn increases the rate of infection. In addition, higher rates of MRSA infection within an institution cause increased use of vancomycin, which contributes to the emergence of VRE and apparently puts additional pressure on MRSA to develop resistance to vancomycin as well.

A second development over the past decade has been an apparent increase in the incidence in some communities of MRSA infection among individuals without apparent risk factors for MRSA. Previously identified risk factors for MRSA include residence in a long-term-care facility; hospitalization; chronic liver, lung, or vascular disease; dialysis; malignancy; and prolonged exposure to antibiotics. An increase in community-acquired cases of MRSA infection has been reported in several locations in the United States and suggests a change in the epidemiology of infection with this organism. It is hypothesized that strains of MRSA spread from the hospital to the community, where continued exposure to antibiotics (both appropriate and unnecessary) leads to their survival advantage and persistence. These reports have been based on retrospective observations, however, and have not yet been confirmed by prospective studies. The obvious question is whether β-lactam antibiotics should continue to be used as the empirical agents of choice for community-acquired staphylococcal infections. For the time being, the incidence of MRSA infection in the community seems too low to justify more widespread use of vancomycin in this setting. There are situations, however, in which empirical use of vancomycin for community-acquired infections is justifiable and even advisable, as discussed below.

Selection of antibiotics (Table 139-2)   Although most pathogenic strains of *S. aureus* are resistant to penicillin, the development of penicillins and cephalosporins that are resistant to β-lactamase has allowed these classes of antibiotics to remain useful for treatment of most *S. aureus* infections. Nafcillin and oxacillin, both of which are β-lactamase-resistant penicillins, are the drugs of choice for parenteral treatment of serious staphylococcal infections. Penicillin remains the drug of choice for infections caused by susceptible organisms. Drug combinations consisting of a penicillin plus a β-lactamase inhibitor are also effective but are best reserved for treatment of polymicrobial infections. Penicillin-allergic patients can usually be given a cephalosporin, although caution should be exercised if the prior adverse reaction to penicillin was anaphylaxis. Of the cephalosporins, the first-generation agents (e.g., cefazolin) are preferred for reasons related to cost and breadth of spectrum. For patients who are intolerant of all β-lactam agents, the best alternatives for parenteral administration are vancomycin and clindamycin. Dicloxacillin and cephalexin are recommended for oral treatment of minor infections or for continuation therapy; clindamycin is an alternative oral agent for most strains. Routine use of quinolones is not recommended because of the possibility of emergent resistance during therapy.

Use of vancomycin has increased dramatically over the past 20 years in response to the emergence of MRSA, for which it has often been the sole therapeutic option, and the increasing number of infections caused by CoNS and other gram-positive cocci. Vancomycin's favorable pharmacokinetic properties and relatively low toxicity profile have also contributed to its widespread use. Unfortunately, increased use of vancomycin has resulted in the emergence of both VRE and VISA, which are now poised to be the microbial scourges of the next decade. Equally important, however, is the fact—often not recognized by practitioners—that vancomycin is *less effective* than numerous other agents at our disposal. Vancomycin is generally only weakly bactericidal or even bacteriostatic for many strains of *S. aureus*. Studies of animal models have repeatedly shown vancomycin to be inferior to β-lactam agents for treatment of serious staphylococcal infections. Bacteremia is cleared more slowly in patients treated with vancomycin than in those treated with β-lactams, and clinical cure rates with vancomycin are significantly lower than with β-lactams as well. For all of these reasons, use of vancomycin should be reserved for situations in which there are no suitable alternative agents. It should not be used routinely for prophylaxis of staphylococcal infections, for empirical therapy in patients with fever and neutropenia (unless staphylococcal infection is especially likely), for decontamination of the digestive tract, for clearance of MRSA colonization, or for treatment of established gram-positive infections not due to resistant organisms. It is hoped that judicious use of vancomycin will help limit the spread of VRE and VISA and ensure that patients receive the most potent therapeutic agents.

Vancomycin remains the drug of choice for treatment of infections caused by MRSA, although sensitive strains may be amenable to therapy with clindamycin or trimethoprim-sulfamethoxazole. As discussed above, two new agents, quinupristin/dalfopristin and linezolid, offer promise for treatment of MRSA, but further studies are needed before they can be recommended for routine or preferential use. Optimal ther-

apy for infections caused by VISA is unknown. To date, all isolates of VISA have been susceptible to alternative agents. Therapeutic options include the combination of vancomycin plus a β-lactam (based largely on in vitro data), quinupristin/dalfopristin, linezolid, or one of the new quinolone antibiotics, although the potential for development of resistance to the quinolones during therapy makes their use a questionable approach for infections requiring a prolonged course of antibiotic.

In most clinical settings, no significant benefit is attained by treating *S. aureus* infections with more than one drug to which the organism is known to be susceptible. Synergy has been demonstrated in vitro for β-lactam/aminoglycoside combinations, which hasten sterilization of the blood in endocarditis. Accordingly, therapy for *S. aureus* bacteremia is often initiated with such a combination for a brief period (e.g., 5 to 7 days)—a strategy that seems reasonable when rapid clearance of bacteremia is deemed to be critical, as in prosthetic valve endocarditis. Thereafter, the toxicity of an aminoglycoside cannot be justified. Use of rifampin in conjunction with a β-lactam antibiotic (or vancomycin) occasionally results in microbial eradication and clinical cure of otherwise refractory infections, particularly those involving foreign bodies that are judged to be unremovable or those involving avascular tissue. These successes may relate to the high level of activity of rifampin against intracellular organisms, including SCVs. Chronic osteomyelitis, parameningeal infections, and septic phlebitis have all been successfully treated with rifampin plus a cell wall–active agent. Nevertheless, routine use of rifampin for serious *S. aureus* infections is not recommended because of potential added toxicity, drug interactions, and theoretical antimicrobial antagonism. Rifampin should be reserved for refractory, relapsing, or inoperable infections and should never be administered as monotherapy, which rapidly leads to resistance.

Route and duration of therapy   Because of poor bioavailability of most oral antistaphylococcal agents, parenteral therapy should be used for infections that require high concentrations of antibiotic, such as endovascular infections, infections of poorly vascularized tissue (including abscesses), and infections of the central nervous system. Given the propensity of *S. aureus* to adhere to endovascular and devitalized or damaged tissues, high doses of antibiotics (e.g., 12 g/d of nafcillin) should be used for bacteremic infections. When high serum levels of antibiotic are required to produce adequate tissue levels (e.g., in endocarditis or osteomyelitis), the parenteral route should be used for the duration of therapy. Oral agents may suffice for the treatment of nonbacteremic infections in which high serum levels of antibiotic are not requisite (e.g., skin, soft tissue, and upper respiratory tract infections).

With the notable exceptions of bacteremia (including endocarditis) and osteomyelitis, the duration of therapy for *S. aureus* infections can be tailored to the severity of illness, the immunologic status of the host, and the response to treatment. Because antibiotics penetrate bone poorly, treatment of acute osteomyelitis in adults requires at least 4 weeks of parenteral therapy. Chronic osteomyelitis is often treated with 6 to 8 weeks of parenterally administered antibiotics followed by several months of oral therapy, especially if the adequacy of debridement is uncertain.

Acute endocarditis and other endovascular infections caused by *S. aureus* should be treated with parenteral antibiotics for 4 weeks (6 weeks in the case of prosthetic valves). Simple bacteremia, as might occur with a removable or drainable focus of infection, is curable with a shorter duration of therapy, but a 2-week course of *parenteral* therapy has traditionally been recommended *for all patients* with *S. aureus* bacteremia, even under these circumstances. The costs and effort implicit in this recommendation are apparent, but shorter courses of therapy are associated with an unacceptable rate of secondary complications. Data suggest that a 7-day course of parenteral therapy may be adequate for simple bacteremia if the clinical response to therapy is prompt, if cultures of blood obtained after 2 days of therapy are neg-

Table 139-2 Antimicrobial Therapy for Infections Caused by *Staphylococcus aureus*

Infection	Antibiotic of Choice and Dose	Alternative Agents	Duration of Therapy
INTOXICATIONS			
Toxic shock syndrome	Clindamycin 900 mg IV q8h[a] or nafcillin 2 g IV q4h[a] *plus* IVIG 400 mg/kg once for severe illness (see text)	Cefazolin 1 g IV q8h for penicillin-allergic patients (instead of nafcillin);[a] vancomycin 1 g IV q12h for suspected MRSA	Total of 14 days; conversion from IV to PO therapy after resolution of fever, hypotension, and gastrointestinal symptoms; oral agents: dicloxacillin 500 mg qid, cephalexin 500 mg qid, clindamycin 300 mg qid
Scalded skin syndrome	Nafcillin or clindamycin IV at high doses, adjusted for age in children	Cefazolin	Total of 10–14 days, parenteral followed by oral therapy
Food poisoning	None	—	—
INVASIVE INFECTIONS			
Skin and soft tissue			
Folliculitis	Topical agent (e.g., mupirocin) or oral antibiotic: dicloxacillin or cephalexin 250 mg qid	Clindamycin 150–300 mg PO tid, TMP-SMZ DS 1 tablet bid, tetracycline 250 mg qid	Until resolution of infection, often 5–7 days
Furuncle/carbuncle	For severe infections (e.g., with systemic toxicity): nafcillin 1–2 g IV q4h; for mild infections: dicloxacillin or cephalexin 250–500 mg PO qid	Cefazolin 1 g IV q8h, clindamycin 600 mg IV q8h or 300 mg PO tid, vancomycin 1 g IV q12h (for severe penicillin allergy or suspected MRSA)	Until resolution of infection, often 7–10 days
Paronychia	Dicloxacillin or cephalexin 250 mg PO qid	Clindamycin 150–300 mg PO tid, TMP-SMZ DS 1 tablet bid, tetracycline 250 mg qid	Until resolution of infection, often 5–7 days
Cellulitis	Nafcillin 2 g IV q4–6h	Cefazolin 1 g IV q8h, clindamycin 600 mg IV q8h; vancomycin 1 g IV q12h for suspected infection with MRSA	Total of 10–14 days; conversion from IV to PO agent (as for TSS) after erythema and systemic symptoms have resolved
Respiratory tract			
Sinusitis	Dicloxacillin or cephalexin 500 mg PO qid or amoxicillin/clavulanate 875 mg PO bid	TMP-SMZ DS 1 tablet bid, clindamycin 300 mg PO tid, clarithromycin 500 mg PO bid	Generally 14–21 days, in accordance with severity of illness and response to therapy
Pneumonia	Nafcillin 2 g IV q4h[b]	Cefazolin 1 g IV q8h[b] or cefuroxime 1.5 g IV q8h or clindamycin 900 mg IV q8h;[b] vancomycin 1 g IV q12h for suspected MRSA	Prolonged course of parenteral therapy, often 14–21 days, as dictated by severity of illness and response to therapy; longer course of therapy in pneumonia caused by hematogenous seeding of lung parenchyma
Empyema	Nafcillin 2 g IV q4h;[b] possible addition of rifampin 300 mg PO bid for loculated empyema or persistent systemic toxicity	Cefazolin 1 g IV q8h[b] or clindamycin 900 mg IV q8h;[b] vancomycin 1 g IV q12h for suspected MRSA	Prolonged course of parenteral therapy, as dictated by clinical and radiographic response to therapy
Central nervous system			
Meningitis	Nafcillin 2 g IV q4h[a]	Vancomycin 1 g IV q12h (for severe penicillin allergy or MRSA)	Prolonged course of parenteral therapy, at least 14–21 days, depending on pathogenesis of infection and clinical response to therapy
Subdural empyema, septic phlebitis, brain abscess	Nafcillin 2 g IV q4h;[a] possible addition of rifampin 300 mg PO bid for infections not amenable to drainage	Vancomycin 1 g IV q12h (for severe penicillin allergy or MRSA)	Prolonged course of parenteral therapy, at least 4 weeks, as dictated by clinical and radiographic response to therapy
Epidural abscess (without meningitis)	Nafcillin 2 g IV q4h[b]	Cefazolin 1 g IV q8h[b] or clindamycin 900 mg IV q8h;[b] vancomycin 1 g IV q12h for MRSA	Prolonged course of parenteral therapy, at least 4 weeks
Endovascular			
Native valve endocarditis, left-sided	Nafcillin 2 g IV q4h,[b] ± gentamicin 1 mg/kg q8h for first 5–7 days	Cephalothin 2 g IV q4h or cefazolin 1 g IV q8h[b] (penicillin allergy) or vancomycin 1 g IV q12h (for MRSA or severe penicillin allergy), ± gentamicin	4 weeks of parenteral therapy
Native valve endocarditis, right-sided	Nafcillin 2 g IV q4h; or nafcillin plus gentamicin 1 mg/kg q8h for short-course therapy	Cefazolin 1 g IV q8h or vancomycin 1 g IV q12h, plus gentamicin; ciprofloxacin 750 mg PO bid plus rifampin 300 mg PO bid	4 weeks of parenteral monotherapy or oral combination therapy; 2 weeks of combination parenteral therapy

(continued)

Table 139-2—(continued)

Infection	Antibiotic of Choice and Dose	Alternative Agents	Duration of Therapy
Prosthetic valve endocarditis	Nafcillin 2 g IV q4h[b] plus rifampin 300 mg PO tid plus gentamicin 1 mg/kg q8h for first 2 weeks	Cephalothin 2 g IV q4h or cefazolin 1 g IV q8h,[b] or vancomycin 1 g IV q12h (as above) plus gentamicin, ± rifampin	6 weeks
Simple bacteremia	Nafcillin 2 g IV q4h[b]	Cefazolin 1 g IV q8h or vancomycin 1 g IV q12h (as above)	14 days of parenteral therapy; 7 days probably adequate under some circumstances (see text)
Complicated bacteremia	Nafcillin 2 g IV q4h[b]	Cefazolin 1 g IV q8h or vancomycin 1 g IV q12h (as above)	4 weeks of parenteral therapy
Mycotic aneurysm, pseudoaneurysm	Nafcillin 2 g IV q4h[b]	Cefazolin 1 g IV q8h[b] or vancomycin 1 g IV q12h (as above)	4 weeks of parenteral therapy
Musculoskeletal			
Acute osteomyelitis	Nafcillin 2 g IV q4h	Cefazolin 1 g IV q8h, clindamycin 900 mg IV q8h, or vancomycin 1 g IV q12h (for MRSA)	4 weeks of parenteral therapy
Chronic osteomyelitis	Nafcillin 2 g IV q4h, ± rifampin 300 mg PO bid	Cefazolin 1 g IV q8h, clindamycin 900 mg IV q8h, or vancomycin 1 g IV q12h (for MRSA), ± rifampin	6 to 8 weeks of parenteral therapy, often followed by several months of oral therapy (dicloxacillin or cephalexin 500 mg qid, clindamycin 300 mg qid, TMP-SMZ DS 1 tablet bid)
Septic arthritis, native joint	Nafcillin 2 g IV q4h	Cefazolin 1 g IV q8h or vancomycin 1 g IV q12h (for severe penicillin allergy or MRSA)	At least 3 weeks of parenteral therapy, as indicated by cultures and clinical course
Septic arthritis, prosthetic joint	Nafcillin 2 g IV q4h; add rifampin 300 mg PO bid if retention of prosthesis is to be attempted	Cefazolin 1 g IV q8h or vancomycin 1 g IV q12h (for severe penicillin allergy or MRSA)	4 weeks
Septic bursitis	Nafcillin 2 g IV q4h	Cefazolin 1 g IV q8h (penicillin allergy), vancomycin 1 g IV q12h (MRSA)	Parenteral therapy until resolution of systemic and local signs and symptoms, followed by several weeks of oral therapy (dicloxacillin, cephalexin, or clindamycin, as above)
Pyomyositis	Nafcillin 2 g IV q4h	Cefazolin 1 g IV q8h (penicillin allergy), vancomycin 1 g IV q12h (MRSA)	Usually 4 weeks of parenteral therapy, assuming hematogenous route of infection

[a] Vancomycin 1 g IV q12h should be given in addition to the antibiotic listed as part of initial therapy when the risk of infection with MRSA is thought to be significant (see text) or in life-threatening illness; vancomycin should be discontinued when susceptibilities are known, as appropriate.

[b] Vancomycin may be substituted for the antibiotic shown when the risk of infection with MRSA is thought to be significant (see text) or in life-threatening illness; switch to alternative agent if possible when susceptibilities are known.

ABBREVIATIONS: IVIG, intravenous immunoglobulin; MRSA, methicillin-resistant *S. aureus*; TMP-SMZ, trimethoprim-sulfamethoxazole; DS, double-strength.

COMMENTS: A. Penicillin is the β-lactam antibiotic of choice for strains of *S. aureus* that are shown to be susceptible. Penicillin should not be used before results of sensitivity testing are known, however, because of the high prevalence of resistance.

B. Patients with a history of hypersensitivity reactions to penicillin *other than anaphylaxis* may generally be treated with cephalosporins. Patients with a history of anaphylaxis to penicillin should be treated with non-β-lactam agents until hypersensitivity testing can be performed.

C. Oxacillin may be substituted for nafcillin, at the same dosages, for all indications.

D. Additional agents with excellent antistaphylococcal activity in vitro are linezolid (available in peroral and parenteral formulations), quinupristin/dalfopristin (parenteral only), and new quinolones. Until additional experience is gained with these agents, however, they should be reserved for situations in which antibiotics with established efficacies cannot be used for reasons of tolerability or antimicrobial resistance.

ative, and if TEE is negative for vegetations. These data require confirmation, however. One of the more challenging aspects of treating staphylococcal bacteremia is deciding whether to administer parenteral therapy for 2 or 4 weeks. A conservative approach (one that is supported by numerous studies) dictates that *4 weeks* should be standard unless specific criteria are met (Fig. 139-2).

PREVENTION AND CONTROL Nosocomial staphylococcal outbreaks and the spread of resistant strains of *S. aureus* are serious global problems. Within an institution, the most important vector of transmission of *S. aureus* is the hands of health care workers. Patients with exposed wounds or with nasal colonization are important reservoirs of the organisms. Transmission of *S. aureus*—and hence the incidence of staphylococcal infection within an institution—can be reduced most effectively by meticulous hand washing before and after contact with patients. The incidence of postoperative staphylococcal infection can be reduced by perioperative administration of an antibiotic with a favorable spectrum of activity and favorable pharmacokinetic properties, such as cefazolin, cefuroxime, or vancomycin. Elimination of nasal carriage before surgery (see below) may also prove to be effective in this regard.

More stringent infection-control measures must be taken to prevent the nosocomial spread of MRSA. Such measures include assigning patients colonized or infected with MRSA to private rooms, wearing gloves for contact with contaminated wounds and mucous membranes as well as a gown if contamination of clothing is likely, and hand washing with an antiseptic soap after patient contact. Patients who are colonized but not infected with MRSA should not be treated with vancomycin merely for the sake of eliminating carriage of this organism.

Staphylococcal skin and soft tissue infections may recur once a person has been colonized with a virulent strain. In this context, therapy directed at the elimination of staphylococcal colonization may be warranted, especially for patients at particular risk for complications of infection. Use of an oral β-lactam antibiotic alone is ineffective, but combination therapy for 10 to 14 days with dicloxacillin or cephalexin (500 mg four times a day) plus rifampin (300 mg twice a day) plus mupirocin (2% ointment applied topically to both nares twice a day) is usually effective at clearing the carrier state, at least for a period of months.

COAGULASE-NEGATIVE STAPHYLOCOCCI

CoNS are a major cause of nosocomial infection and are the organisms most frequently isolated from the blood of hospitalized patients. The

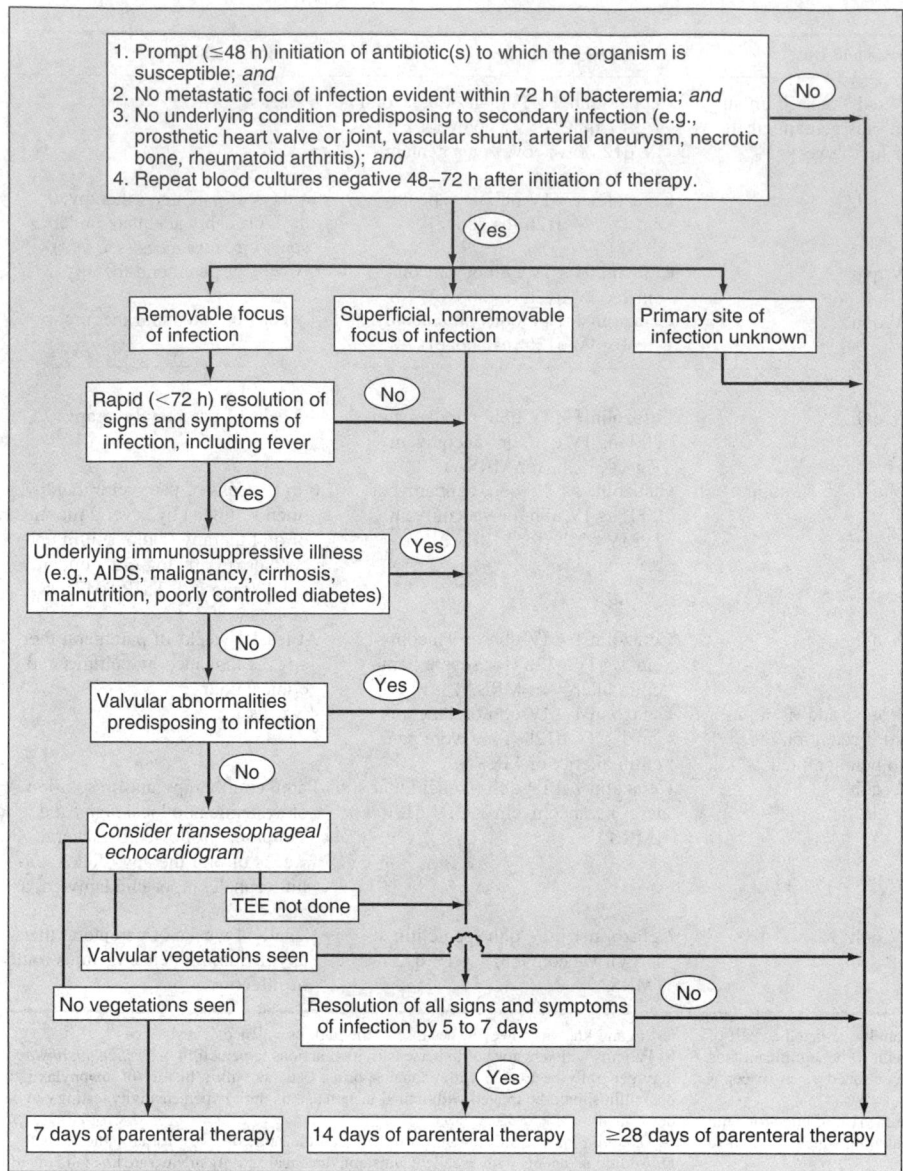

1. Prompt (≤48 h) initiation of antibiotic(s) to which the organism is susceptible; *and*
2. No metastatic foci of infection evident within 72 h of bacteremia; *and*
3. No underlying condition predisposing to secondary infection (e.g., prosthetic heart valve or joint, vascular shunt, arterial aneurysm, necrotic bone, rheumatoid arthritis); *and*
4. Repeat blood cultures negative 48–72 h after initiation of therapy.

No

Yes

Removable focus of infection

Superficial, nonremovable focus of infection

Primary site of infection unknown

Rapid (<72 h) resolution of signs and symptoms of infection, including fever

No

Yes

Underlying immunosuppressive illness (e.g., AIDS, malignancy, cirrhosis, malnutrition, poorly controlled diabetes)

Yes

No

Valvular abnormalities predisposing to infection

Yes

No

Consider transesophageal echocardiogram

TEE not done

Valvular vegetations seen

No vegetations seen

Resolution of all signs and symptoms of infection by 5 to 7 days

No

Yes

7 days of parenteral therapy

14 days of parenteral therapy

≥28 days of parenteral therapy

FIGURE 139-2 Factors to be considered in determining the duration of therapy for *S. aureus* bacteremia. *(Modified from Fowler VG Jr et al: Outcome of Staphylococcus aureus bacteremia according to compliance with recommendations of infectious disease specialists: Experience with 244 patients. Clin Infect Dis 27:478, 1998.)*

frequency with which they cause opportunistic infection in immuno-compromised hosts attests more to the increased vulnerability of such hosts in modern medical practice than to the intrinsic virulence of the organisms. Despite the weak pathogenicity of these bacteria, the global impact of CoNS infection is considerable, including increased length and cost of hospital stay; increased use of antibiotics in general; and increased use of vancomycin in particular, which has contributed to the recent emergence of vancomycin-resistant gram-positive bacteria.

Although the variety of clinical syndromes caused by CoNS is impressive, several characteristics apply to most such infections. First, they tend to be *indolent*. There is often a long latent period between the time of contamination (e.g., of a medical device) and the onset of clinical illness; bacteremia in neutropenic patients can be an exception to this rule. Second, most CoNS infections are nosocomial in origin; important exceptions are prosthetic valve endocarditis and *S. saprophyticus* infections of the urinary tract. Third, most clinically significant infections are caused by strains of CoNS that are resistant to multiple antibiotics, including penicillins and cephalosporins. Finally, most CoNS infections are associated with a medical device of some kind, and removal of such devices is often required for cure.

EPIDEMIOLOGY AND PATHOGENESIS CoNS, particularly *S. epidermidis*, are invariable and prominent constituents of the normal human skin flora. Infection most often results from direct inoculation of a foreign body at the time it is inserted, although hematogenous seeding can also occur.

CoNS are the quintessential pathogens of medical devices. The array of virulence factors produced by CoNS is meager compared with that of the virulence factors produced by *S. aureus*, but among these few factors are substances that promote bacterial adherence to and persistence on foreign bodies. A variety of surface antigens that promote colonization of medical devices by CoNS (particularly *S. epidermidis*) have been proposed; the best-studied of these is capsular polysaccharide adhesin, which serves as the organism's capsule and promotes the initial interaction of the bacteria and a foreign body. This polysaccharide is a major component of the *S. epidermidis* biofilm, which is important in the persistence of infection; the biofilm thwarts host defenses by coating staphylococcal cells onto foreign materials and impairing phagocytic killing. CoNS appear not to make toxic exoproteins or toxins; rather, they cause disease by tenaciously persisting on foreign materials, resulting in a local and occasionally a systemic inflammatory response.

The most important risk factor for infection with CoNS is the presence of a foreign body, especially an indwelling catheter. A second major risk factor for infection is deficient phagocyte function—especially neutropenia, which is most often an iatrogenic complication of chemotherapy for cancer but may also reflect an underlying disease process (such as leukemia). The likelihood of catheter-related infection depends upon a number of variables, including the experience and skill of the person who inserts the catheter, the length of time that a catheter is left in place, and the quality of postinsertion care of the catheter site. CoNS only rarely cause infections (other than urinary tract infections) in immunologically normal hosts and typically do so only under extenuating circumstances.

CLINICAL SYNDROMES Because CoNS can adhere to a variety of materials, virtually all *foreign bodies* are susceptible to colonization by these organisms. CoNS are the most common pathogens complicating the use of intravenous catheters, hemodialysis shunts and grafts, cerebrospinal fluid (CSF) shunts, peritoneal dialysis catheters, pacemaker wires and electrodes, prosthetic joints, vascular grafts, and prosthetic valves. CoNS infection of intravenous catheters may or may not be accompanied by signs of inflammation at the site of catheter insertion, and the degree of systemic toxicity (including fever) ranges from minimal to moderately severe. The diagnosis can be established by the culturing of blood drawn from the catheter and by venipuncture. Infection of CSF shunts is usually evident within several weeks of implantation. Signs of meningitis are sometimes readily apparent but more often are subtle or absent; malfunction of the shunt may be the only manifestation of shunt infection. CoNS infection of a prosthetic joint often does not become evident until long after implantation, although the inciting contamination usually occurs at the time of implantation. Infection of vascular grafts may result in the development of an aneurysm or a pseudoaneurysm, with catastrophic consequences.

CoNS are a prominent cause of *bacteremia* in immunosuppressed patients. While such infections in immunocompetent hosts are relatively benign, patients with neutropenia may have high-grade bacteremia that results in significant systemic toxicity. A serious consequence of bacteremia is the seeding of a secondary foreign body, such as a prosthetic heart valve or joint or a pacemaker.

CoNS are the organisms most commonly responsible for *prosthetic valve endocarditis*, causing the majority of infections that develop within several months of implantation as well as a substantial percentage of late infections. The syndrome is one of subacute endocarditis (thus contrasting with the syndrome produced by *S. aureus*), with an illness that is clinically indistinguishable from that caused by viridans streptococci. Infection of prosthetic valves is often complicated by valvular dysfunction secondary either to dehiscence of the sewing ring or obstruction of the valve's orifice by bulky vegetations. CoNS are a less frequent but important cause of *native valve endocarditis*, accounting for <5% of such infections and usually affecting abnormal valves.

S. saprophyticus is a common cause of *urinary tract infection* among sexually active young women, in whom it is second only to *E. coli* in frequency. Exposure to spermicide-coated condoms may increase the incidence of infection. *S. saprophyticus* produces a syndrome indistinguishable from that caused by other etiologic agents, with pyuria and symptoms of dysuria, frequency, and abdominal pain. Infection with *S. saprophyticus* is readily amenable to therapy with most agents commonly used to treat urinary tract infections. CoNS can also cause urinary tract infection in hospitalized patients who have undergone invasive procedures; such infections are especially likely to be asymptomatic and may be difficult to treat because of antimicrobial resistance.

DIAGNOSIS Although CoNS are the most common cause of nosocomial bacteremia, they are also the most common contaminants of blood cultures; differentiation between infection and contamination often poses a challenge, with major therapeutic implications. Positive blood cultures are more likely to be "true positives" when there is a clinical illness suggestive of infection, when there is an indwelling catheter or some other risk factor for CoNS infection, and when cultures of blood drawn from multiple sites are positive for phenotypically identical organisms with the same antimicrobial susceptibility patterns. Except in the setting of neutropenia, physicians often have the luxury of awaiting the results of repeat cultures when the significance of CoNS growing from a blood culture is questionable.

℞ **TREATMENT** Removal of the foreign body (especially when it is an intravenous catheter) often constitutes adequate therapy for CoNS infection related to that device. Most infections involving a foreign body require the removal of the device—whether a prosthetic valve, prosthetic joint, CSF shunt, vascular graft, pacemaker or defibrillator and associated hardware, or hemodialysis shunt. Cures of all such infections with antibiotics alone have been reported, however, and a patient's poor medical condition or the hazards of surgery occasionally warrant an attempt at medical cure without extirpation of the device (see below). Infections of peritoneal dialysis catheters can be cured with antibiotics alone often enough that an attempt should be made to do so. CoNS infections of central venous catheters are also amenable to medical therapy, although relapses are common. Persistent bacteremia during therapy is an absolute indication for removal of a catheter, and bacteremia after a catheter's removal suggests seeding of a secondary site.

It is difficult to make generalizations about the optimal duration of therapy for CoNS infections. In general, the duration of treatment is the same as for infection syndromes caused by other bacteria. For example, native valve endocarditis should be treated for 4 weeks, prosthetic valve endocarditis for 6. Transient bacteremia in an immunocompetent host may require no antimicrobial therapy after removal of an offending catheter. The efficacy of therapy can occasionally be enhanced by the delivery of antibiotics directly to the site of infection—e.g., by intraventricular administration of vancomycin for central nervous system infections or by intraperitoneal administration of antibiotic for infections of peritoneal dialysis catheters.

Despite the low degree of pathogenicity of CoNS, treatment of serious infections due to these organisms is often problematic because of the high percentage of strains that are resistant to commonly used antibiotics, including most oral agents. Most strains of CoNS isolated from patients in U.S. hospitals are resistant not only to penicillin but also to the penicillinase-resistant penicillins and cephalosporins. Nosocomial isolates are usually resistant to other classes of antibiotics as well. Vancomycin, to which the vast majority of CoNS remain susceptible, is of necessity the drug of choice for *empirical* therapy for serious CoNS infections. Strains proved to be susceptible to nafcillin (oxacillin) or penicillin should be treated with one of these agents or with a first-generation cephalosporin.

Synergistic combinations of antibiotics are often useful in the treatment of CoNS infections. Rifampin plays a unique role in this endeavor by virtue of its potency against most staphylococci, its excellent penetration into tissues (including those that are poorly vascularized), and the high levels it reaches within human cells and biofilm. Rifampin must be used in combination with other antibiotics because of the frequent and rapid emergence of microbial resistance to the drug when it is used alone. If an effort must be made to eradicate infection of a medical device without its removal, the concomitant use of a β-lactam antibiotic to which the organism is susceptible plus rifampin (300 mg twice daily by mouth) plus gentamicin affords the best chance for success. Vancomycin can be substituted for the β-lactam agent if so dictated by an organism's susceptibility pattern or by a patient's drug allergy.

BIBLIOGRAPHY

CHAMBERS HF: Methicillin resistance in staphylococci: Molecular and biochemical basis and clinical implications. Clin Microbiol Rev 10:781, 1997

DERESIEWICZ RL: Staphylococcal toxic shock syndrome, in *Superantigens: Molecular Biology, Immunology, and Relevance to Human Disease*, DYM Leung et al (eds). New York, Marcel Dekker, 1997, pp 435–479

FOWLER VG JR et al: Role of echocardiography in evaluation of patients with *Staphylococcus aureus* bacteremia: Experience in 103 patients. J Am Coll Cardiol 30:1072, 1997

HEROLD BC et al: Community-acquired methicillin-resistant *Staphylococcus aureus* in children with no identified predisposing risk. JAMA 279:593, 1998

JERNIGAN JA, FARR BM: Short-course therapy of catheter-related *Staphylococcus aureus* bacteremia: A meta-analysis. Ann Intern Med 119:304, 1993

MARRACK P, KAPPLER J: The staphylococcal enterotoxins and their relatives. Science 248:705, 1990

MUSHER DM et al: The current spectrum of *Staphylococcus aureus* infection in a tertiary care hospital. Medicine 73:186, 1994

PROCTOR RA, PETERS G: Small colony variants in staphylococcal infections: Diagnostic and therapeutic implications. Clin Infect Dis 27:419, 1998

RUPP ME, ARCHER GL: Coagulase-negative staphylococci: Pathogens associated with medical progress. Clin Infect Dis 19:231, 1994

SMITH TL et al: Emergence of vancomycin resistance in *Staphylococcus aureus*. N Engl J Med 340:493, 1999

140 *Michael R. Wessels*

STREPTOCOCCAL AND ENTEROCOCCAL INFECTIONS

Many varieties of streptococci are found as part of the normal human flora colonizing the respiratory, gastrointestinal, and genitourinary tracts. Several species are important causes of human disease. Group A *Streptococcus*, or *S. pyogenes*, is responsible for streptococcal pharyngitis, one of the most common bacterial infections of school-age-

Table 140-1 Classification of Streptococci Responsible for Human Infections

Lancefield Group	Representative Species	Hemolysis	Typical Infections
A	S. pyogenes	β	Pharyngitis, impetigo, cellulitis, scarlet fever
B	S. agalactiae	β	Neonatal sepsis and meningitis, puerperal infection, UTI, diabetic ulcer infection, endocarditis
C	S. equisimilis	β	Cellulitis, bacteremia, endocarditis
D	Enterococci: E. faecalis; E. faecium	Usually nonhemolytic	UTI, nosocomial bacteremia, endocarditis
	Nonenterococci: S. bovis	Usually nonhemolytic	Bacteremia, endocarditis
G	S. canis	β	Cellulitis, bacteremia, endocarditis, septic arthritis
Variable or nongroupable	Viridans streptococci: S. sanguis; S. mitis	α	Endocarditis, dental abscess, brain abscess
	Intermedius, milleri or anginosus group S. intermedius; S. anginosus; S. constellatus	Variable	Brain abscess, visceral abscess
	Anaerobic streptococci: Peptostreptococcus magnus	Usually nonhemolytic	Sinusitis, pneumonia, empyema, brain abscess, liver abscess

children, and for the postinfectious syndromes of acute rheumatic fever and poststreptococcal glomerulonephritis. Group B *Streptococcus*, or *S. agalactiae*, is the leading cause of bacterial sepsis and meningitis in newborns and a major cause of endometritis and fever in parturient women. Enterococci are important causes of urinary tract infection, nosocomial bacteremia, and endocarditis. Viridans streptococci are the most common cause of bacterial endocarditis.

Streptococci are gram-positive bacteria of spherical to ovoid shape that characteristically form chains when grown in liquid media. Most streptococci that cause human infections are facultative anaerobes, although some are strict anaerobes. Streptococci are relatively fastidious organisms, requiring enriched media for growth in the laboratory. No single scheme for classification of streptococci is entirely satisfactory. Consequently, clinicians and clinical microbiologists often identify streptococci by any of several classification systems, including hemolytic pattern, Lancefield group, species name, and common or trivial name. Many of the streptococci associated with human infection produce a zone of complete hemolysis around the bacterial colony when cultured on blood agar, a pattern known as β *hemolysis*. The β-hemolytic streptococci can be classified by the Lancefield system, a serologic grouping based on the reaction of specific antisera with cell-wall carbohydrate antigens of the bacteria. With rare exceptions, organisms belonging to Lancefield groups A, B, C, and G are all β-hemolytic streptococci, and each is associated with characteristic patterns of human infection. Other streptococci produce a zone of partial (α) hemolysis, often imparting a greenish appearance to the agar. These α-hemolytic streptococci are further identified by biochemical testing and include *S. pneumoniae*, an important cause of pneumonia, meningitis, and other infections, and several species of streptococci referred to collectively as the *viridans streptococci*, which are part of the normal oral flora and are important as agents of subacute bacterial endocarditis. Finally, some streptococci are nonhemolytic, a pattern sometimes called γ *hemolysis*. The classification of the major groups of streptococci responsible for human infections is outlined in Table 140-1. Among the organisms classified serologically as group D streptococci, the enterococci are now considered to constitute a separate genus on the basis of DNA homology studies. Thus, species previously designated as *S. faecalis* and *S. faecium* have been renamed *Enterococcus faecalis* and *E. faecium*, respectively. →*For further discussion of pneumococcal infections, see Chap. 138.*

GROUP A STREPTOCOCCI

Lancefield's group A consists of a single species, *S. pyogenes*. As its species name implies, this organism is associated with a variety of suppurative infections. In addition, group A streptococci can trigger the postinfectious syndromes of acute rheumatic fever (which is uniquely associated with *S. pyogenes* infection; Chap. 235) and poststreptococcal glomerulonephritis (Chap. 274).

PATHOGENESIS Group A streptococci elaborate a number of cell-surface components and extracellular products important both in the pathogenesis of infection and in the immune response of the human host. The cell wall contains a carbohydrate antigen that may be released by treatment with acid. The reaction of such acid extracts with group A–specific antiserum is the basis for the definitive identification of a streptococcal strain as *S. pyogenes*. The major surface protein of group A streptococci is M protein, which occurs in more than 100 antigenically distinct types and is the basis for the serotyping of strains with specific antisera. The M protein molecules are fibrillar structures anchored in the cell wall of the organism and extending as hairlike projections away from the cell surface. The amino acid sequence of the distal or amino-terminal portion of the M protein molecule is quite variable, accounting for the antigenic variation of the different M types, while more proximal regions of the protein are relatively conserved. A newer technique for assignment of M type to group A streptococcal isolates uses the polymerase chain reaction to amplify the variable region of the M protein gene. DNA sequence analysis of the amplified gene segment can be compared with an extensive data base [developed at the Centers for Disease Control and Prevention (CDC)] for assignment of M type. This method eliminates the need for typing sera, which are available in only a few reference laboratories. The presence of M protein on a group A streptococcal isolate correlates with its capacity to resist phagocytic killing in fresh human blood; this phenomenon appears to be due, at least in part, to the binding of plasma fibrinogen to M protein molecules on the streptococcal surface, which interferes with complement activation and deposition of opsonic complement fragments on the bacterial cell. This resistance to phagocytosis may be overcome by M protein–specific antibodies, and thus individuals with antibodies to a given M type acquired as a result of prior infection are protected against subsequent infection with organisms of the same M type but not against that with different M types.

Group A streptococci also elaborate, to varying degrees, a polysaccharide capsule composed of hyaluronic acid. The production of large amounts of hyaluronic acid capsule by certain strains lends a characteristic mucoid appearance to the bacterial colonies. The capsular polysaccharide also plays an important role in protecting the organisms from ingestion and killing by phagocytes. In contrast to M protein, the hyaluronic acid capsule is a weak immunogen, and antibodies to hyaluronate have not been shown to be important in protective immunity; the presumed explanation is the apparent structural identity between streptococcal hyaluronic acid and the hyaluronic acid of mammalian connective tissues. The capsular polysaccharide may also play a role in group A streptococcal colonization of the pharynx by binding to CD44, a hyaluronic acid–binding protein expressed on human pharyngeal epithelial cells.

Group A streptococci produce a large number of extracellular products that may be important in local and systemic toxicity and in the spread of infection through tissues. These products include streptolysins S and O, toxins that damage cell membranes and account for the hemolysis produced by the organisms; streptokinase; DNases; protease; and pyrogenic exotoxins A, B, and C. The pyrogenic exotoxins, previously known as erythrogenic toxins, cause the rash of scarlet fever. Since the mid-1980s, pyrogenic exotoxin-producing strains of group A *Streptococcus* have been linked to unusually severe invasive infections, including necrotizing fasciitis and a systemic syndrome termed the *streptococcal toxic shock syndrome*. Several extracellular products stimulate specific antibody responses useful in the serodiagnosis of recent streptococcal infection. Tests for these antibodies are used primarily for the detection of preceding streptococcal infection in cases of suspected acute rheumatic fever or poststreptococcal glomerulonephritis.

CLINICAL MANIFESTATIONS **Pharyngitis** Although seen in patients of all ages, group A streptococcal pharyngitis is one of the most common bacterial infections of childhood, accounting for 20 to 40% of all cases of exudative pharyngitis in children. It is rare among those under the age of 3. Younger children may manifest streptococcal infection with a syndrome of fever, malaise, and lymphadenopathy without exudative pharyngitis. Infection is acquired through contact with another individual carrying the organism. Respiratory droplets are the usual mechanism of spread, although other routes, including food-borne outbreaks, have been well described.

The incubation period is 1 to 4 days. Symptoms include sore throat, fever and chills, malaise, and sometimes abdominal complaints and vomiting, particularly in children. Both symptoms and signs are quite variable, ranging from mild throat discomfort with minimal physical findings to high fever and severe sore throat associated with intense erythema and swelling of the pharyngeal mucosa and the presence of purulent exudate over the posterior pharyngeal wall and tonsillar pillars. Enlarged, tender anterior cervical lymph nodes commonly accompany exudative pharyngitis.

The differential diagnosis of streptococcal pharyngitis includes the many other bacterial and viral causes of pharyngitis. Streptococcal infection is unlikely to be the cause of pharyngitis when symptoms and signs suggestive of viral infection are prominent (conjunctivitis, coryza, cough, hoarseness, or discrete ulcerative lesions of the buccal or pharyngeal mucosa). Other infections commonly producing exudative pharyngitis include infectious mononucleosis and adenovirus infection. Now rare in the United States, the pseudomembrane of diphtheria may give a similar appearance. The coryneform organism *Arcanobacterium haemolyticum* may cause pharyngitis, often in association with a scarlet fever–like rash (Chap. 141). Other causes of pharyngitis, usually without a purulent exudate, include coxsackievirus, influenza virus, mycoplasmas, and *Neisseria gonorrhoeae* and acute infection with HIV. Because of the range of clinical presentations of streptococcal pharyngitis and the large number of other agents that can produce the same clinical picture, diagnosis of streptococcal pharyngitis on clinical grounds alone is not reliable.

The throat culture remains the diagnostic "gold standard." Culture of a throat specimen that is properly collected (i.e., by vigorous rubbing of a sterile swab over both tonsillar pillars) and properly processed is the most sensitive and specific means available to make a definitive diagnosis. A rapid diagnostic kit using latex agglutination or enzyme immunoassay of swab specimens can serve as a useful adjunct to the throat culture. While precise figures on sensitivity and specificity vary among studies, the rapid diagnostic kits generally are >95% specific. Thus a positive result can be relied upon for definitive diagnosis and eliminates the need for a throat culture. However, because the rapid diagnostic tests are less sensitive than throat culture (with a relative sensitivity ranging from 55 to 90% in comparative studies), a negative result should be confirmed with a throat culture.

℞ **TREATMENT** In the usual course of uncomplicated streptococcal pharyngitis, symptoms resolve after 3 to 5 days. The course is shortened little by treatment, which is given primarily to prevent suppurative complications and rheumatic fever. Prevention of rheumatic fever depends on eradication of the organism from the pharynx,

not simply on resolution of symptoms, and requires 10 days of penicillin treatment—either a single intramuscular dose of benzathine penicillin G or a 10-day course of oral penicillin (Table 140-2). Erythromycin may be substituted for penicillin in the treatment of individuals allergic to penicillin. Follow-up culture after treatment is no longer routinely recommended but may be warranted in selected cases, such as those involving patients or families with frequent streptococcal infections or those occurring in situations in which the risk of rheumatic fever is thought to be high (e.g., when cases of rheumatic fever have recently been reported in the community).

Complications Suppurative complications of streptococcal pharyngitis have become uncommon with the widespread use of antibiotics for most cases of symptomatic streptococcal infection. The complications result from the spread of infection from the pharyngeal mucosa to deeper tissues by direct extension or by the hematogenous or lymphatic route and may include cervical lymphadenitis, peritonsillar or retropharyngeal abscess, sinusitis, otitis media, meningitis, bacteremia, endocarditis, and pneumonia. Local complications, such as abscess formation in the peritonsillar or parapharyngeal space, should be considered in a patient with unusually severe or prolonged symptoms or localized pain associated with high fever and a toxic appearance.

Asymptomatic Carrier State Surveillance cultures have shown that up to 20% of individuals in certain populations may have asymptomatic pharyngeal colonization with group A streptococci. There are no definitive guidelines for management of these asymptomatic carriers or of asymptomatic individuals who still have a positive throat culture after a full course of treatment for symptomatic pharyngitis. A reasonable course of action is to give a single 10-day course of penicillin for symptomatic pharyngitis and, if positive cultures persist, not to re-treat unless symptoms recur. Studies of the natural history of streptococcal carriage and infection have shown that the risk both of developing rheumatic fever and of transmitting infection to others is substantially lower among asymptomatic carriers than among individuals with symptomatic pharyngitis. Therefore, overly aggressive attempts to eradicate carriage are probably not justified under most circumstances. An exception is the situation in which an asymptomatic carrier is a potential source of infection to others. Outbreaks of food-borne infection and nosocomial puerperal infection have been traced to asymptomatic carriers who may harbor the organisms in the throat, on the skin, or in the vagina or anus.

℞ **TREATMENT** In cases in which a carrier is transmitting infection to others, attempts to eradicate carriage are warranted, although data are limited on the best regimen to use to clear the organism after penicillin alone has failed. The combination of penicillin

Table 140-2 Treatment of Group A Streptococcal Infections

Infection	Treatment[a]
Pharyngitis	Benzathine penicillin G, 1.2 mU IM; or penicillin V, 250 mg PO qid × 10 days (Children <27 kg: Benzathine penicillin G, 600,000 units IM; or penicillin V, 125 mg PO qid × 10 days)
Impetigo	Same as pharyngitis
Erysipelas/cellulitis	Severe: Penicillin G, 1–2 mU IV q4h Mild to moderate: Procaine penicillin, 1.2 mU IM bid
Necrotizing fasciitis/myositis	Surgical debridement plus penicillin G, 2–4 mU IV q4h
Pneumonia/empyema	Penicillin G, 2–4 mU IV q4h plus drainage of empyema

[a] Penicillin allergy: Erythromycin (10 mg/kg PO qid up to maximum of 250 mg per dose) may be substituted for oral penicillin. Alternative agents for parenteral therapy include first-generation cephalosporins—if the allergy does not manifest as immediate hypersensitivity (anaphylaxis or urticaria) or as another potentially life-threatening reaction (e.g., severe rash and fever)—or vancomycin.

V (500 mg four times daily for 10 days) and rifampin (600 mg twice daily for the last 4 days) has been used to eliminate pharyngeal carriage. A 10-day course of oral vancomycin (250 mg four times daily) and rifampin (600 mg twice daily) has eradicated rectal colonization. However, experience is not extensive with any regimen.

Scarlet Fever Scarlet fever consists of streptococcal infection, usually pharyngitis, accompanied by a characteristic rash. The rash arises from the effects of one of three toxins, currently designated streptococcal pyrogenic exotoxins A, B, and C and previously known as erythrogenic or scarlet fever toxins. In the past, scarlet fever was thought to reflect infection of an individual lacking toxin-specific immunity with a toxin-producing strain of group A *Streptococcus*. Susceptibility to scarlet fever was correlated with results of the Dick test. A small amount of erythrogenic toxin injected intradermally produced local erythema in susceptible individuals but elicited no reaction in those with specific immunity. Subsequent studies have suggested that development of the scarlet fever rash may reflect a hypersensitivity reaction requiring prior exposure to the toxin. For reasons that are not clear, scarlet fever has become less common in recent years, although strains of group A streptococci that produce pyrogenic exotoxins continue to be prevalent in the population.

The symptoms of scarlet fever are the same as those of pharyngitis alone. The rash typically begins on the first or second day of illness over the upper trunk, spreading to involve the extremities but sparing the palms and soles. The rash is made up of minute papules, giving a characteristic "sandpaper" feel to the skin. Associated findings include circumoral pallor, "strawberry tongue" (enlarged papillae on a coated tongue, which later may become denuded), and accentuation of the rash in the skin folds (Pastia's lines). Subsidence of the rash in 6 to 9 days is followed after several days by desquamation of the palms and soles. The differential diagnosis of scarlet fever includes other causes of fever and generalized rash, such as measles and other viral exanthems, Kawasaki disease, toxic shock syndrome, and systemic allergic reactions (e.g., drug eruptions).

Skin and Soft Tissue Infections Group A streptococci—and occasionally other streptococcal species—cause a variety of infections involving the skin, subcutaneous tissues, muscles, and fascia. While several clinical syndromes, recognized according to the tissues involved, offer a useful means for classification of skin and soft tissue infections, not all cases fit exactly into a single category. The classic syndromes should be considered as general guides to predicting the level of tissue involvement in a particular patient, the probable clinical course, and the likelihood that surgical intervention or aggressive life-support will be required.

Impetigo (pyoderma) Impetigo is a superficial infection of the skin caused primarily by group A streptococci and occasionally by other streptococci or by *Staphylococcus aureus*. Impetigo is seen most often in young children, tends to occur during the warmer months, and is more common in semitropical or tropical climates than in cooler regions. Infection is more common among children living under conditions of poor hygiene. Prospective studies have shown that colonization of unbroken skin with group A streptococci precedes the development of clinical infection. Minor trauma, such as a scratch or an insect bite, may then serve to inoculate organisms into the skin. Impetigo is best prevented, therefore, by attention to adequate hygiene. The usual sites of involvement are the face (particularly around the nose and mouth) and the legs, although lesions may occur at other locations. Individual lesions begin as red papules, which evolve quickly into vesicular and then pustular lesions that break down and coalesce to form characteristic honeycomb-like crusts (**Plate IID-38**). Lesions are generally not painful, and patients do not appear ill. Fever is not a feature of impetigo and, if present, suggests either infection extending to deeper tissues or another diagnosis.

The classic presentation of impetigo usually poses little diagnostic difficulty. Cultures of impetiginous lesions often yield *S. aureus* as

well as group A streptococci, but longitudinal studies have shown that, in almost all cases, streptococci can be isolated initially, with staphylococci appearing later, presumably as secondary colonizing flora. In the past, penicillin was nearly always effective against these infections; in recent years, however, penicillin treatment failures have become more common, an observation suggesting that *S. aureus* infection may have become more prominent as a cause of impetigo. *Bullous impetigo* due to *S. aureus* is distinguished from typical streptococcal infection by the presence of more extensive, bullous lesions that break down and leave thin paper-like crusts instead of the thick amber crusts of streptococcal impetigo. Other skin lesions that may be confused with impetigo include herpetic lesions—either those of orolabial herpes simplex or those of chickenpox or zoster. Herpetic lesions can generally be distinguished by their appearance as more discrete, grouped vesicles and by a positive Tzanck test. In difficult cases, cultures of vesicular fluid should yield group A streptococci in impetigo and the responsible virus in *Herpesvirus* infections.

℞ TREATMENT Treatment of streptococcal impetigo is the same as that for streptococcal pharyngitis. In view of evidence that *S. aureus* has become a relatively frequent cause of impetigo, empirical regimens should cover both streptococci and *S. aureus*. For example, either dicloxacillin or cephalexin can be given at a dose of 250 mg four times daily for 10 days. Topical mupirocin ointment is also effective. Rheumatic fever (unlike pharyngitis) is not a sequela to streptococcal skin infections, although poststreptococcal glomerulonephritis may follow either skin or throat infection. The reason for this difference is not known. One hypothesis is that the immune response necessary for development of rheumatic fever occurs only after infection of the pharyngeal mucosa. In addition, the strains of group A streptococci that cause pharyngitis are generally of different M protein types than those associated with skin infections; thus the strains that cause pharyngitis may have rheumatogenic potential, while the skin-infecting strains may not.

Cellulitis Inoculation of organisms into the skin may lead to infection involving the skin and subcutaneous tissues, or *cellulitis*. The portal of entry may be a traumatic or surgical wound, an insect bite, or any other break in skin integrity. Often, no entry site is apparent.

One form of streptococcal cellulitis, *erysipelas*, is characterized by a bright red appearance of the involved skin, which forms a plateau sharply demarcated from surrounding normal skin (**Plate IID-34**). The lesion is warm to the touch, may be tender, and appears shiny and swollen. The skin often has a *peau d'orange* texture, which is thought to reflect involvement of superficial lymphatics; superficial blebs or bullae may form, usually 2 or 3 days after onset. The lesion typically develops over a few hours and is associated with fever and chills. Erysipelas tends to occur in certain characteristic locations: the malar area of the face (often with extension over the bridge of the nose to the contralateral malar region) and the lower extremities. After one episode, recurrence at the same site—sometimes years later—is not uncommon.

Classic cases of erysipelas, with the typical features described above, are almost always due to β-hemolytic streptococci, usually those of group A and occasionally those of group C or G. Often, however, the appearance of streptococcal cellulitis is not sufficiently distinctive to permit a specific diagnosis on clinical grounds. The area of involvement may not be one of the typical sites for erysipelas, the lesion may be less intensely red than usual and may fade into surrounding skin, and/or the patient may appear only mildly ill. In such cases, it is prudent to broaden the spectrum of empiric antimicrobial therapy to include other pathogens, particularly *S. aureus*, that can produce cellulitis with the same appearance. Staphylococcal infection should be suspected if cellulitis develops around a wound or ulcer.

Streptococcal cellulitis tends to develop at anatomic sites in which normal lymphatic drainage has been disrupted, such as sites of prior episodes of cellulitis, the arm ipsilateral to a mastectomy and axillary lymph node dissection, a lower extremity previously involved in deep venous thrombosis or chronic lymphedema, and the leg from which a saphenous vein has been harvested for coronary artery bypass grafting. The organism may enter via a breach in the dermal barrier at a location some distance from the eventual site of clinical cellulitis. For example, some patients with recurrent episodes of leg cellulitis following saphenous vein removal stop having recurrent episodes only after treatment of tinea pedis on the affected extremity, fissures in the skin presumably having served as a portal of entry for streptococci, which then produced infection more proximally in the leg at the site of previous injury. Streptococcal cellulitis may also involve recent surgical wounds. Group A streptococci are among the few bacterial pathogens that typically produce signs of wound infection and surrounding cellulitis within the first 24 h after surgery. These wound infections are usually associated with a thin exudate and may spread rapidly, either as cellulitis in the skin and subcutaneous tissue or as a deeper tissue infection (see below). Streptococcal wound infection or localized cellulitis may also be associated with *lymphangitis*, manifested by red streaks extending proximally along superficial lymphatics from the site of infection.

 TREATMENT   See Table 140-2 and Chap. 128.

Deep soft tissue infections   *Necrotizing fasciitis*, also referred to as *hemolytic streptococcal gangrene*, is an infection involving the superficial and/or deep fascia investing the muscles of an extremity or the trunk. The source of the infection is either the skin, with organisms introduced into the tissue as a result of trauma (sometimes trivial), or the bowel flora, with organisms released during abdominal surgery or from an occult enteric source, such as a diverticular or appendiceal abscess. The site of inoculation in both forms of necrotizing fasciitis may be inapparent and is often some distance from the site of clinical involvement; e.g., the introduction of organisms via minor trauma to the hand may be associated with clinical infection of the tissues overlying the shoulder or chest. In cases associated with the bowel flora, the infection is usually polymicrobial, involving a mixture of anaerobic bacteria (such as *Bacteroides fragilis* or anaerobic streptococci) and facultative organisms (usually gram-negative bacilli). Cases unrelated to contamination from bowel organisms are most commonly caused by group A streptococci, either alone or in combination with other organisms (most often *S. aureus*). Overall, group A streptococci are implicated in about 60% of cases of necrotizing fasciitis. The onset of symptoms is usually quite acute and is marked by severe pain at the site of involvement, malaise, fever, chills, and a toxic appearance. The physical findings, particularly early in the illness, may not be striking, with only minimal erythema of the overlying skin. Pain and tenderness are usually severe; in contrast, in more superficial cellulitis, the skin appearance is more abnormal, but pain and tenderness are only mild or moderate. As the infection progresses (often in a matter of several hours), the severity and extent of symptoms worsen, and skin changes become more evident, with the appearance of dusky or mottled erythema and edema. The marked tenderness of the involved area may evolve into anesthesia as the spreading inflammatory process produces infarction of cutaneous nerves.

Although myositis is more commonly due to *S. aureus* infection, group A streptococci occasionally produce abscesses in skeletal muscles (*streptococcal myositis*), with little or no involvement of the surrounding fascia or overlying skin. The presentation is usually subacute, but a fulminant form has been described in association with severe systemic toxicity, bacteremia, and a high mortality rate. The fulminant form may reflect the same basic disease process as that seen in necrotizing fasciitis, but with the necrotizing inflammatory process extending into the muscles themselves rather than remaining limited to the fascial layers.

 TREATMENT   Once necrotizing fasciitis is suspected, early surgical exploration is both diagnostically and therapeutically indicated. Surgery reveals necrosis and inflammatory fluid tracking along the fascial planes above and between muscle groups, without involvement of the muscles themselves. The process usually extends beyond the area of clinical involvement, and extensive debridement is required. Drainage and debridement are central to the management of necrotizing fasciitis; antibiotic treatment is a useful adjunct (Table 140-2), but surgery is life-saving.

Treatment for streptococcal myositis consists of surgical drainage—usually by an open procedure that permits evaluation of the extent of the infection and ensures adequate debridement of involved tissues—and high-dose penicillin (Table 140-2).

Pneumonia and Empyema   Group A streptococci are an occasional cause of pneumonia, generally in previously healthy individuals. The onset of symptoms may be abrupt or gradual. Pleuritic chest pain, fever, chills, and dyspnea are the characteristic symptoms. Cough is usually present but may not be prominent. Approximately one-half of patients with group A streptococcal pneumonia have an accompanying pleural effusion. In contrast to the sterile parapneumonic effusions typical of pneumococcal pneumonia, those complicating streptococcal pneumonia are almost always infected. The empyema fluid is usually visible by chest radiography on initial presentation and may enlarge rapidly. These pleural collections should be drained early, as they tend to become loculated rapidly, resulting in a chronic fibrotic reaction that may require thoracotomy for removal.

Bacteremia, Puerperal Sepsis, and Streptococcal Toxic Shock Syndrome   Group A streptococcal bacteremia is usually associated with an identifiable local infection. Bacteremia occurs rarely with otherwise uncomplicated pharyngitis, occasionally with cellulitis or pneumonia, and relatively frequently with necrotizing fasciitis. Bacteremia without an identified source raises the possibility of endocarditis, an occult abscess, or osteomyelitis. A variety of focal infections may arise secondarily from streptococcal bacteremia, including endocarditis, meningitis, septic arthritis, osteomyelitis, peritonitis, and visceral abscesses.

Group A streptococci are occasionally implicated in infectious complications of childbirth, usually endometritis and associated bacteremia. In the preantibiotic era, puerperal sepsis was commonly caused by group A streptococci, but currently it is more often caused by group B streptococci. Several nosocomial outbreaks of puerperal infection due to group A streptococci have been traced to an asymptomatic carrier, usually an individual present at the delivery of the infant. The site of carriage may be the skin, throat, anus, or vagina.

Beginning in the late 1980s, several reports described patients who had group A streptococcal infections associated with shock and multisystem organ failure. This syndrome has been called the streptococcal toxic shock syndrome because it shares certain features with staphylococcal toxic shock syndrome. In 1993, a case definition for group A streptococcal toxic shock syndrome was formulated by a group of clinicians, microbiologists, and epidemiologists in conjunction with the CDC (Table 140-3). The general features of the illness include fever, hypotension, renal impairment, and respiratory distress syndrome. Various types of rash have been described, but rash usually does not develop. Laboratory abnormalities include a marked shift to the left in the white blood cell differential, with many immature granulocytes; hypocalcemia; hypoalbuminemia; and thrombocytopenia, which usually becomes more pronounced on the second or third day of illness. In contrast to those with staphylococcal toxic shock, the majority of patients with the streptococcal syndrome are bacteremic. The most common associated infection is a soft tissue infection—necrotizing fasciitis, myositis, or cellulitis—although a variety of other associated local infections have been described, including pneumonia, peritonitis, osteomyelitis, and myometritis. Streptococcal toxic shock syndrome is associated with a mortality rate of 30%, with most deaths secondary to shock and respiratory failure. Because of its rapidly progressive and lethal course, early recognition of the syndrome is essential. Patients should be given aggressive supportive care in the

Table 140-3 Proposed Case Definition for the Streptococcal Toxic Shock Syndrome[a]

I. Isolation of group A streptococci (*S. pyogenes*)
  A. From a normally sterile site (e.g., blood, cerebrospinal fluid, pleural or peritoneal fluid, tissue biopsy, surgical wound)
  B. From a nonsterile site (e.g., throat, sputum, vagina, superficial skin lesion)
II. Clinical signs of severity
  A. Hypotension: Systolic blood pressure of ≤90 mmHg in adults or in the 5th percentile for age in children **and**
  B. Two or more of the following signs:
    1. Renal impairment: Serum creatinine level of ≥177 μmol/L (≥2 mg/dL) for adults or at least twice the upper limit of normal for age; in patients with preexisting renal disease, an elevation over the baseline level by a factor of 2 or more
    2. Coagulopathy: Platelet count of ≤100 × 10⁹/L (100,000/μL) or disseminated intravascular coagulation, defined by prolonged clotting times, low fibrinogen level, and the presence of fibrin degradation products
    3. Liver involvement: Alanine aminotransferase (SGOT), aspartate aminotransferase (SGPT), or total bilirubin level at least twice the upper limit of normal for age; in patients with preexisting liver disease, an elevation over the baseline level by a factor of 2 or more
    4. Adult respiratory distress syndrome, defined by acute onset of diffuse pulmonary infiltrates and hypoxemia in the absence of cardiac failure; or evidence of diffuse capillary leakage manifested by acute onset of generalized edema; or pleural or peritoneal effusions with hypoalbuminemia
    5. Generalized erythematous macular rash that may desquamate
    6. Soft tissue necrosis, including necrotizing fasciitis or myositis, or gangrene

[a] An illness fulfilling criteria IA, IIA, and IIB is defined as a *definite* case. An illness fulfilling criteria IB, IIA, and IIB is defined as a *probable* case if no other etiology is identified.
SOURCE: Working Group.

form of fluid resuscitation, pressors, and mechanical ventilation in addition to antimicrobial therapy and, in cases associated with necrotizing fasciitis, surgical debridement. Exactly why certain patients develop this fulminant syndrome is not known; however, early studies of the streptococcal strains isolated from these patients demonstrated a strong association with the production of pyrogenic exotoxin A. In subsequent case series, particularly from Europe, the syndrome was also associated with strains producing exotoxin B or C.

℞ **TREATMENT** In light of the possible role of exotoxins or other streptococcal toxins in streptococcal toxic shock syndrome, treatment of the affected patients with clindamycin has been advocated by some authorities, who argue that, through its direct action on protein synthesis, clindamycin is more effective in rapidly terminating toxin production than penicillin—a cell-wall agent. Support for this view comes from studies of an experimental model of streptococcal myositis, in which mice treated with clindamycin had a higher rate of survival than those given penicillin. Comparable data on the treatment of human infections are not available. Although clindamycin resistance in group A streptococci is uncommon (<2% among U.S. isolates), it has been documented. Thus, if clindamycin is used for initial treatment of a critically ill patient, penicillin should be given as well until the antibiotic susceptibility of the streptococcal isolate is known.

Intravenous immunoglobulin has been suggested as adjunctive therapy for streptococcal toxic shock; pooled immunoglobulin preparations are likely to contain antibodies capable of neutralizing the effects of streptococcal toxins. Anecdotal reports have suggested favorable clinical responses to intravenous immunoglobulin, but no controlled trials of this modality of therapy have yet been reported.

STREPTOCOCCI OF GROUPS C AND G

Group C and group G streptococci are β-hemolytic bacteria that occasionally cause human infections similar to those caused by group A streptococci, including pharyngitis, cellulitis and soft-tissue infections, pneumonia, bacteremia, endocarditis, and septic arthritis. Puerperal sepsis, meningitis, epidural abscess, intraabdominal abscess, urinary tract infection, and neonatal sepsis have also been reported. Group C streptococci are a common cause of infection in domesticated animals, especially horses and cattle, and some human infections have been acquired through contact with animals or through consumption of unpasteurized milk. Bacteremia and septic arthritis more frequently involve group G than group C streptococci. Group C or G streptococcal bacteremia occurs most often in patients who are elderly or chronically ill and, in the absence of an obvious local infection, is likely to reflect endocarditis. Septic arthritis, sometimes involving multiple joints, may complicate endocarditis or develop in its absence.

℞ **TREATMENT** Penicillin is the drug of choice for therapy of infections due to group C or G streptococci. Antibiotic treatment is the same as for patients with similar syndromes due to group A *Streptococcus* (Table 140-2). Patients with bacteremia or septic arthritis should receive intravenous penicillin (2 to 4 mU every 4 h). All group C and G streptococci are sensitive to penicillin; nearly all are inhibited in vitro by concentrations of ≤0.03 μg/mL. Occasional isolates exhibit tolerance: although inhibited by low concentrations of penicillin, they are killed only by significantly higher concentrations. The clinical significance of tolerance is unknown. Because of the poor clinical response of some patients to penicillin alone, the addition of gentamicin (1 mg/kg every 8 h for patients with normal renal function) is recommended by some authors for treatment of endocarditis or septic arthritis due to group C or G streptococci; however, combination therapy has not been shown to be superior to treatment with penicillin alone.

Patients with joint infections often require repeated aspiration or open drainage and debridement for cure; the response to treatment may be slow, particularly in debilitated patients and those with involvement of more than one joint. Infection of prosthetic joints almost always requires removal of the prosthesis in addition to antibiotic therapy.

GROUP B STREPTOCOCCI

Identified first as a cause of mastitis in cows, streptococci belonging to Lancefield's group B have since been recognized as a major cause of sepsis and meningitis in human neonates. Group B streptococci are also a frequent cause of peripartum fever in women and an occasional cause of serious infection in nonpregnant adults. Lancefield group B consists of a single species, *S. agalactiae*, which is definitively identified with specific antiserum to the group B cell wall–associated carbohydrate antigen. A streptococcal isolate can be classified presumptively as belonging to group B on the basis of biochemical tests, including hydrolysis of sodium hippurate (in which 99% of isolates are positive), hydrolysis of bile esculin agar (in which 99 to 100% are negative), bacitracin susceptibility (in which 92% are resistant), and production of CAMP factor (in which 98 to 100% are positive). CAMP factor is a phospholipase produced by group B streptococci that results in synergistic hemolysis with β lysin produced by certain strains of *S. aureus*. Its presence can be demonstrated by cross-streaking of the test isolate and an appropriate staphylococcal strain on a blood agar plate. Group B streptococci causing human infections are encapsulated by one of nine antigenically distinct polysaccharides. The capsular polysaccharide has been shown experimentally to be important in the virulence of the organism. Antibodies to the capsular polysaccharide afford protection against group B streptococci of the same (but not of a different) capsular type.

INFECTION IN NEONATES Two general types of group B streptococcal infection in infants are defined by the age of the patient at presentation. *Early-onset infections* occur within the first week of life, with a median age of 20 h at the onset of illness. Approximately half of these infants have signs of group B streptococcal disease at birth. The infection is acquired during or shortly before birth from organisms colonizing the maternal genital tract. Surveillance studies have shown that 5 to 40% of women are vaginal or rectal carriers of group B streptococci. Approximately 50% of infants delivered vaginally by carrier mothers become colonized, although only 1 to 2% of those colonized develop clinically evident infection. Prematurity and maternal risk factors (prolonged labor, obstetric complications, and maternal fever) are often involved. The presentation of early-onset infection is the same as that of other forms of neonatal sepsis. Typical findings include respiratory distress, lethargy, and hypotension. Essentially all infants with early-onset disease are bacteremic, one-third to one-half have pneumonia and/or respiratory distress syndrome, and one-third have meningitis.

Late-onset infections occur in infants between 1 week and 3 months of age, with a mean age at onset of 3 to 4 weeks. The infecting organism may be acquired during delivery (as in early-onset cases) or during later contact with a colonized mother, nursery personnel, or another source. Meningitis is the most common manifestation of late-onset infection and in most cases is associated with a strain of capsular type III. Infants present with fever, lethargy or irritability, poor feeding, and seizures. The various other types of late-onset infection include bacteremia without an identified source, osteomyelitis, septic arthritis, and facial cellulitis associated with submandibular or preauricular adenitis.

TREATMENT Penicillin is the treatment of choice for all group B streptococcal infections. Empirical broad-spectrum therapy for suspected bacterial sepsis, consisting of ampicillin and gentamicin, is generally administered until culture results become available. If cultures yield group B streptococci, many pediatricians continue to administer gentamicin, along with ampicillin or penicillin, for a few days until clinical improvement becomes evident. Infants with bacteremia or soft-tissue infection should receive penicillin at a dosage of 200,000 units/kg per day in divided doses; those with meningitis should receive 400,000 units/kg per day. Meningitis should be treated for at least 14 days because of the risk of relapse with shorter courses.

Prevention The incidence of group B streptococcal infection is unusually high among infants of women with risk factors: preterm delivery, early rupture of membranes (>24 h before delivery), prolonged labor, fever, or chorioamnionitis. Because the usual source of the organisms infecting a neonate is the mother's birth canal, efforts have been made to prevent group B streptococcal infections by the identification of high-risk carrier mothers and their treatment with various forms of antibiotic or immunoprophylaxis. Prophylactic administration of ampicillin or penicillin to such patients during delivery has been shown to reduce the risk of infection in the newborn. This approach has been hampered by the logistical difficulties of identifying colonized women before delivery, since the results of vaginal cultures early in pregnancy are poor predictors of carrier status at delivery. The CDC has suggested two alternative approaches to the prevention of neonatal group B streptococcal infection: In the first approach, women are screened for anogenital colonization at 35 to 37 weeks of pregnancy by means of a swab culture of the lower vagina and anorectum; intrapartum chemoprophylaxis is offered to carriers and is *recommended* for those carriers with any of the risk factors noted above, those anticipating multiple births, and those who have previously given birth to an infant with group B streptococcal infection. In the second approach, screening cultures need not be performed, but intrapartum chemoprophylaxis is recommended for *all* women with one or more of the risk factors noted above. The recommended regimen for chemoprophylaxis is 5 million units of penicillin G followed by 2.5 million units every 4 h until delivery. Clindamycin or erythromycin may be substituted in women allergic to penicillin.

Treatment of all pregnant women who are colonized or who have risk factors for neonatal infection will result in exposure of 15 to 25% of pregnant women and newborns to antibiotics, with the attendant risks of allergic reactions and selection for resistant organisms. Al-

though still in the developmental stages, a group B streptococcal vaccine may ultimately offer a better solution to prevention. Because transplacental passage of maternal antibodies produces protective antibody levels in the newborn, efforts are under way to develop a vaccine against group B streptococci that can be given to childbearing women before or during pregnancy. Results of phase 1 clinical trials of group B streptococcal capsular polysaccharide–protein conjugate vaccines suggest that a multivalent conjugate vaccine would be safe and highly immunogenic.

INFECTION IN ADULTS The majority of group B streptococcal infections in adults are related to pregnancy and parturition. Peripartum fever, the most common manifestation, is sometimes accompanied by symptoms and signs of endometritis or chorioamnionitis (abdominal distention and uterine or adnexal tenderness). Blood cultures are often positive, as are cultures of vaginal swabs. Bacteremia is usually transitory but occasionally results in meningitis or endocarditis. Infections in adults that are not associated with the peripartum period generally involve individuals who are elderly or have some underlying chronic illness, such as diabetes mellitus or a malignancy. Among the infections that develop with some frequency in adults are cellulitis and soft tissue infection (including infected diabetic skin ulcers), urinary tract infection, pneumonia, endocarditis, and septic arthritis. Other reported infections include meningitis, osteomyelitis, and intraabdominal or pelvic abscesses.

TREATMENT Group B streptococci are less sensitive to penicillin than group A organisms, requiring somewhat higher doses. Adults with serious localized infections (pneumonia, pyelonephritis, abscess) should receive doses in the range of 12 million units of penicillin G daily, while patients with endocarditis or meningitis should receive 18 to 24 million units per day in divided doses. Vancomycin is an acceptable alternative for patients allergic to penicillin.

ENTEROCOCCI, GROUP D STREPTOCOCCI

ENTEROCOCCI Lancefield group D includes the enterococci, organisms now classified in a separate genus from other streptococci, and nonenterococcal group D streptococci. Enterococci are distinguished from nonenterococcal group D streptococci by their ability to grow in the presence of 6.5% sodium chloride and by the results of other biochemical tests. The enterococcal species that are significant pathogens for humans are *E. faecalis* and *E. faecium*. These organisms tend to produce infection in patients who are elderly or debilitated or in whom mucosal or epithelial barriers have been disrupted or the balance of the normal flora altered by antibiotic treatment. Urinary tract infections due to enterococci are quite common, particularly among patients who have received antibiotic treatment or undergone instrumentation of the urinary tract. Enterococci are a frequent cause of nosocomial bacteremia in patients with intravascular catheters. These organisms account for 10 to 20% of cases of bacterial endocarditis on both native and prosthetic valves. The presentation of enterococcal endocarditis is usually subacute but may be acute, with rapidly progressive valve destruction. Enterococci are frequently cultured from bile and are involved in infectious complications of biliary surgery and in liver abscesses. Moreover, enterococci are often isolated from polymicrobial infections arising from the bowel flora (e.g., intraabdominal abscesses), from abdominal surgical wounds, and from diabetic foot ulcers. While such mixed infections are frequently cured by antimicrobials not active against enterococci, specific therapy directed against enterococci is warranted when these organisms are the predominant species or are isolated from blood cultures.

TREATMENT Unlike other streptococci, enterococci are not reliably killed by penicillin or ampicillin alone at concentrations achieved clinically in the blood or tissues. Ampicillin reaches sufficiently high urinary concentrations to constitute adequate monotherapy for uncomplicated urinary tract infections. Because in vitro testing has shown evidence of synergistic killing of most enterococcal strains by the combination of penicillin or ampicillin with an aminoglycoside, combined therapy is recommended for enterococcal endocarditis and meningitis; the regimen is penicillin (3 to 4 million units every 4 h) or ampicillin (2 g every 4 h) plus moderate-dose gentamicin (1 mg/kg every 8 h for patients with normal renal function). Enterococcal endocarditis should be treated for a minimum of 4 weeks and for 6 weeks if symptoms have been present for ≥3 months or if the infection involves a prosthetic heart valve. For nonendocarditis bacteremia and other serious enterococcal infections, it is not known whether the efficacy of single-agent β-lactam therapy is improved by the addition of gentamicin, but many infectious disease specialists use combination therapy for such infections, especially in critically ill patients. Vancomycin, in combination with gentamicin, may be substituted for penicillin in allergic patients. Enterococci are resistant to all cephalosporins; therefore, this class of antibiotics should not be used for treatment of enterococcal infections.

Antimicrobial susceptibility testing should be performed routinely on enterococcal isolates from patients with serious infections, and therapy should be adjusted according to the results (Table 140-4). Most enterococci are resistant to streptomycin, and this drug should not be used for treatment of enterococcal infection unless in vitro testing of the strain indicates susceptibility. Though less widespread than streptomycin resistance, high-level resistance to gentamicin—with a minimum inhibitory concentration (MIC) of >2000 μg/mL—has become common. Gentamicin-resistant enterococci should be tested for susceptibility to streptomycin; occasional gentamicin-resistant enterococci are sensitive to streptomycin. If the isolate is resistant to all aminoglycosides, treatment with penicillin or ampicillin alone may be successful. The prolonged administration (i.e., for at least 6 weeks) of high-dose ampicillin (e.g., 12 g/d) is recommended for endocarditis due to these highly resistant enterococci.

Enterococci may be resistant to penicillins via two distinct mechanisms. The first is the production of β-lactamase (mediating resistance to penicillin and ampicillin), which has been reported for E. faecalis isolates from several locations in the United States and other countries. Because the amount of β-lactamase produced by enterococci may be insufficient for detection by routine antibiotic susceptibility testing, isolates from serious infections should be screened specifically for β-lactamase production with use of a chromogenic cephalosporin or by another method. For the treatment of β-lactamase-producing strains, vancomycin, ampicillin/sulbactam, amoxicillin/clavulanate, or imipenem may be used in combination with gentamicin.

The second mechanism of penicillin resistance is not mediated by β-lactamase and may be due to altered penicillin-binding proteins. This intrinsic penicillin resistance is common among E. faecium isolates, which routinely are more resistant to β-lactam antibiotics than

are isolates of E. faecalis. Moderately resistant enterococci (MICs of penicillin and ampicillin, 16 to 64 μg/mL) may be susceptible to high-dose penicillin or ampicillin plus gentamicin, but strains with MICs of ≥200 μg/mL must be considered resistant to clinically achievable levels of β-lactam antibiotics, including imipenem. Vancomycin plus gentamicin is the recommended regimen for infections due to enterococci with high-level intrinsic resistance to β-lactams.

Vancomycin-resistant enterococci, first reported from clinical sources in the late 1980s, have become common in many hospitals. Three major vancomycin resistance phenotypes have been described: VanA, VanB, and VanC. The VanA phenotype is associated with high-level resistance to vancomycin and to teicoplanin, a related glycopeptide antibiotic not currently available in the United States. VanB and VanC strains are resistant to vancomycin but susceptible to teicoplanin, although teicoplanin resistance may develop during treatment in VanB strains. For enterococci resistant to both vancomycin and β-lactams, there are no established therapies. Regimens that have been tried with some success in individual cases or experimentally include ciprofloxacin plus rifampin plus gentamicin; ampicillin plus vancomycin (particularly if in vitro testing shows synergistic bacteriostatic activity); and chloramphenicol or tetracycline (if the strain is susceptible in vitro). Quinupristin/dalfopristin (Synercid) is a streptogramin combination with in vitro activity against E. faecium, including vancomycin-resistant isolates, but not against E. faecalis or other enterococcal species. The evidence for clinical efficacy of this agent in serious enterococcal infections is limited, and, as of this writing, quinupristin/dalfopristin is not yet licensed for use in the United States.

OTHER GROUP D STREPTOCOCCI   The main nonenterococcal group D streptococcal species that causes human infections is S. bovis. S. bovis endocarditis is often associated with neoplasms of the gastrointestinal tract—most frequently a colon carcinoma or polyp—but is also reported in association with other bowel lesions. When occult gastrointestinal lesions are carefully sought, abnormalities are found in ≥60% of patients with S. bovis endocarditis. In contrast to the enterococci, nonenterococcal group D streptococci like S. bovis are reliably killed by penicillin as a single agent, and penicillin is the treatment of choice for S. bovis infections.

VIRIDANS AND OTHER STREPTOCOCCI

VIRIDANS STREPTOCOCCI   Consisting of multiple species of α-hemolytic streptococci, the viridans streptococci are a heterogeneous group of organisms that are important as agents of bacterial endocarditis (Chap. 126). Several species of viridans streptococci, including S. salivarius, S. mitis, S. sanguis, and S. mutans, are part of the normal flora of the mouth, where they live in close association with the teeth and gingiva. Some species contribute to the development of dental caries. The transient viridans streptococcal bacteremia induced by eating, tooth-brushing, flossing, and other sources of minor trauma, together with adherence to biologic surfaces, is thought to account for the predilection of these organisms to cause endocarditis. Viridans streptococci are also isolated, often as part of a mixed flora, from sites of sinusitis, brain abscess, and liver abscess.

Viridans streptococcal bacteremia occurs relatively frequently in neutropenic patients, particularly after bone marrow transplantation or high-dose chemotherapy for cancer. Some of these patients develop a sepsis syndrome with high fever and shock. Risk factors for viridans streptococcal bacteremia include chemotherapy with high-dose cytosine arabinoside, prior treatment with trimethoprim-sulfamethoxazole or a fluoroquinolone, treatment with antacids or histamine antagonists, mucositis, and profound neutropenia.

The S. milleri group (also referred to as the S. intermedius or S. anginosus group) includes three species that cause human disease: S. intermedius, S. anginosus, and S. constellatus. These organisms are often considered viridans streptococci, although they differ somewhat from other viridans streptococci in both their hemolytic pattern (they may be α-, β-, or nonhemolytic) and the disease syndromes they

Table 140-4   Treatment Options for Antibiotic-Resistant Enterococcal Infections

Resistance Pattern	Recommended Therapy
β-Lactamase production	Gentamicin plus ampicillin/sulbactam, amoxicillin/clavulanate, imipenem, or vancomycin
β-Lactam resistance, but no β-lactamase production	Gentamicin plus vancomycin
High-level gentamicin resistance	Streptomycin-sensitive isolate: Streptomycin plus ampicillin or vancomycin Streptomycin-resistant isolate: No proven therapy (continuous-infusion ampicillin, prolonged treatment)
Vancomycin resistance	Ampicillin plus gentamicin
Vancomycin and β-lactam resistance	Unknown; teicoplanin active against strains with low-level vancomycin resistance (VanB or VanC phenotype, but not VanA)

cause. This group commonly produces suppurative infections, particularly abscesses of brain and abdominal viscera, and infections related to the oral cavity or respiratory tract, such as peritonsillar abscess, lung abscess, and empyema.

℞ TREATMENT Isolates from neutropenic patients with bacteremia often are resistant to penicillin; thus these patients should be treated presumptively with vancomycin until the results of susceptibility testing become available. Viridans streptococci isolated in other clinical settings usually are sensitive to penicillin.

NUTRITIONALLY VARIANT STREPTOCOCCI Occasional isolates cultured from the blood of patients with endocarditis fail to grow when subcultured on solid media. These *nutritionally variant streptococci* require supplemental thiol compounds or active forms of vitamin B$_6$ (pyridoxal or pyridoxamine) for growth in the laboratory. The nutritionally variant streptococci are generally grouped with the viridans streptococci because they cause similar types of infections. However, they have been reclassified on the basis of 16S RNA sequence comparisons into a separate genus, *Abiotrophia*, with two species: *A. defectivus* and *A. adjacens*.

℞ TREATMENT Because treatment failure and relapse appear to be more common for cases of endocarditis due to nutritionally variant streptococci than for usual viridans streptococci, the addition of gentamicin (1 mg/kg every 8 h for patients with normal renal function) to the penicillin regimen is recommended in therapy for endocarditis due to these organisms.

OTHER STREPTOCOCCI *S. suis* is an important pathogen in swine and has been reported to cause meningitis in humans, usually in individuals with occupational exposure to pigs. Strains of *S. suis* associated with human infections have generally reacted with Lancefield group R typing serum and sometimes with group D typing serum as well. Isolates may be α- or β-hemolytic and are sensitive to penicillin. *S. iniae*, a pathogen of fish, has been associated with infections in humans who have handled live or freshly killed fish. Cellulitis of the hand is the most common form of human infection, although bacteremia and endocarditis have been reported. *Anaerobic streptococci*, or *peptostreptococci*, are part of the normal flora of the oral cavity, bowel, and vagina. Infections caused by the anaerobic streptococci are discussed in Chap. 167.

BIBLIOGRAPHY

BISNO AL, STEVENS DL: Streptococcal infections of skin and soft tissues. N Engl J Med 334:240, 1996
———— et al: Diagnosis and management of group A streptococcal pharyngitis: A practice guideline. Clin Infect Dis 25:574, 1997
BRADLEY SF et al: Group C streptococcal bacteremia: Analysis of 88 cases. Rev Infect Dis 13:270, 1991
CENTERS FOR DISEASE CONTROL AND PREVENTION: Prevention of perinatal group B streptococcal disease: A public health perspective. MMWR 45(RR-7):1, 1996
EDWARDS MS, BAKER CJ: *Streptococcus agalactiae* (group B *Streptococcus*), in *Principles and Practice of Infectious Diseases*, 4th ed, GL Mandell et al (eds). New York, Churchill Livingstone, 1995
ELIOPOULOS GM: Vancomycin-resistant enterococci. Mechanism and clinical relevance. Infect Dis Clin North Am 11:851, 1997
JACKSON LA et al: Risk factors for group B streptococcal disease in adults. Ann Intern Med 123:415, 1995
MOELLERING RC JR: Emergence of *Enterococcus* as a significant pathogen. Clin Infect Dis 14:1173, 1992
RICHARD P et al: Viridans streptococcal bacteraemia in patients with neutropenia. Lancet 345:1607, 1995
VARTIAN C et al: Infections due to Lancefield group G streptococci. Medicine 6:75, 1985
WEINSTEIN MR et al: Invasive infections due to a fish pathogen, *Streptococcus iniae*. S. iniae Study Group. N Engl J Med 337:589, 1997
WORKING GROUP ON SEVERE STREPTOCOCCAL INFECTIONS: Defining the group A streptococcal toxic shock syndrome: Rationale and consensus definitions. JAMA 269:390, 1993
ZURAWSKI CA et al: Invasive group A streptococcal disease in metropolitan Atlanta: A population-based assessment. Clin Infect Dis 27:150, 1998

141 Randall K. Holmes

DIPHTHERIA, OTHER CORYNEBACTERIAL INFECTIONS, AND ANTHRAX

DIPHTHERIA

DEFINITION Diphtheria is a localized infection of mucous membranes or skin caused by *Corynebacterium diphtheriae*. A characteristic pseudomembrane may be present at the site of infection. Some strains of *C. diphtheriae* produce diphtheria toxin, a protein that can cause myocarditis, polyneuritis, and other systemic toxic effects. Respiratory diphtheria is usually caused by toxinogenic (*tox*$^+$) *C. diphtheriae*, but cutaneous diphtheria is frequently caused by nontoxinogenic (*tox*$^-$) strains.

ETIOLOGY *C. diphtheriae* is an aerobic, nonmotile, nonsporulating, irregularly staining, gram-positive rod. The bacteria are club-shaped and are often arranged in clusters (*Chinese letters*) or parallel arrays (*palisades*). *C. diphtheriae* forms gray to black colonies on selective media containing tellurite. The gravis, mitis, and intermedius biotypes are distinguished by colonial morphology and laboratory tests. Both *tox*$^+$ and *tox*$^-$ strains cause infections, and *tox*$^+$ strains of all three biotypes can cause severe disease. The gene for diphtheria toxin is present in specific corynephages, and *tox*$^-$ *C. diphtheriae* can acquire the ability to produce diphtheria toxin by infection with *tox*$^+$ phages (*phage conversion*). Growth of *C. diphtheriae* under low-iron conditions that mimic the environment of host tissues induces production of diphtheria toxin and expression of systems for siderophore-dependent iron uptake and utilization of iron from heme.

IMMUNOLOGY Treatment of diphtheria toxin with formaldehyde converts it to a nontoxic but immunogenic product (*diphtheria toxoid*). Immunization with toxoid elicits antibody (*antitoxin*) that neutralizes the toxin and prevents diphtheria. The attack rate and mortality rate for diphtheria are low in immune individuals with antitoxin titers of >0.01 unit per milliliter. Antitoxin neither prevents colonization by *C. diphtheriae* nor eradicates the *carrier state*. When most individuals in a population have protective levels of antitoxin (*herd immunity*), the carrier rate for *tox*$^+$ strains of *C. diphtheriae* falls to a low level, and the risk that susceptible individuals will be exposed to *tox*$^+$ *C. diphtheriae* decreases dramatically. Susceptible individuals may contract diphtheria if they travel to regions where the disease is present or if *tox*$^+$ strains of *C. diphtheriae* are introduced into their community.

EPIDEMIOLOGY AND IMMUNITY Humans are the principal reservoir for *C. diphtheriae*. Transmission occurs primarily by close personal contact. The risk is greater that *C. diphtheriae* will be transmitted to susceptible individuals from patients with diphtheria than from carriers. The incubation period for respiratory diphtheria is typically 2 to 5 days and rarely up to 8 days. Cutaneous diphtheria is usually a secondary infection whose signs develop an average of 7 days (range, 1 to >21 days) after the appearance of primary dermatologic lesions of other etiologies.

In temperate climates, diphtheria primarily involves the respiratory tract; occurs throughout the year, with a peak incidence in colder months; and is usually caused by *tox*$^+$ *C. diphtheriae*. Before immunization was introduced, diphtheria was primarily a disease of children; it affected up to 10% of individuals in this group and sometimes caused devastating epidemics. Most young infants were immune because of transplacental transfer of maternal IgG antitoxin, but children became susceptible by 6 to 12 months of age. Approximately 75% of individuals became immune by age 10 as a result of contact with *C. diphtheriae*. Mortality rates of 30 to 40% were common in untreated disease and were sometimes >50% in epidemics. Treatment with antitoxin reduced the case-fatality rate to 5 to 10%.

Routine immunization of children in the United States resulted in a progressive decrease of diphtheria from the peak of 206,939 cases (incidence rate, 191 cases per 100,000 population) in 1921 to <5 cases per year since 1980. Concomitantly, circulation of tox⁺ strains of C. diphtheriae among the population decreased dramatically, although an endemic focus for transmission of tox⁺ and tox⁻ strains without clinical disease was recently identified in North Dakota. As the incidence rate of diphtheria decreased, a higher proportion of cases occurred in older persons (who were never immunized or whose immunity waned because it was not boosted by either booster doses of vaccine or contact with C. diphtheriae), but the case-fatality ratio remained unchanged at 5 to 10%. High rates of immunization are currently achieved by school entry (>96%), but immunization rates for younger children are substantially lower. Among adults >20 years of age, 19 to 77% are susceptible as a consequence of failure to receive periodic booster immunizations and lack of contact with C. diphtheriae. The most recent large diphtheria outbreak in the United States (about 1100 cases) occurred in Seattle, Washington, between 1972 and 1982. Alcoholism, low socioeconomic status, crowded living conditions, and Native-American ethnic background were significant risk factors in this outbreak.

A massive diphtheria epidemic (>157,000 cases and 5000 deaths) occurred recently in the states of the former Soviet Union and accounted for >80% of diphtheria cases reported worldwide during that interval. The epidemic began in 1990 with 1436 cases (0.49 per 100,000 population), peaked in 1995 with 50,425 cases (17.29 per 100,000 population), and waned by 1998 with 2720 cases (0.93 per 100,000 population) as the result of a mass immunization program. The progression of the epidemic was associated with emergence of a previously uncommon clonal group of tox⁺ C. diphtheriae strains that accounted for >80% of isolates by 1994; molecular analysis of the tox gene from these strains demonstrated that the existing diphtheria toxoid vaccine remained appropriate for control of the epidemic by vaccination.

A majority of cases throughout this epidemic occurred in persons ≥15 years old, and adults from 40 to 49 years old had very high incidence and death rates. In 1994, case-fatality rates varied from 2.8% in the Russian Federation to 23% in Lithuania and Turkmenistan. Factors that facilitated the spread of this epidemic included large-scale population movements, socioeconomic instability, deteriorating health infrastructure, delayed implementation of aggressive control measures in response to the epidemic, inadequate information for physicians and the public, and frequent shortages of supplies for prevention and treatment of the disease. The most important risk factor for diphtheria in the Republic of Georgia was lack of vaccination (matched odds ratio, 19.2), but household diphtheria exposure, exposure to skin lesions, the presence of tonsils, a history of eczema, preceding fever with myalgia, sharing a bed, sharing glasses and cups, and taking a bath less often than weekly were also significant risk factors. Although small numbers of imported cases from this epidemic occurred in western European countries, none resulted in secondary transmission of diphtheria, notwithstanding a high proportion of susceptible adults in countries with imported cases. Inadequate primary immunization of children in the states of the former Soviet Union in the years preceding the epidemic, along with failure to maintain adequate immunity in adults by booster immunization, may have synergistically facilitated transmission of diphtheria and emergence of the massive epidemic in this region.

In the tropics, cutaneous diphtheria is more common than respiratory diphtheria, occurs throughout the year, and often develops as a secondary infection complicating other dermatoses. Isolates of C. diphtheriae from skin lesions are more often tox⁻ than tox⁺. Cutaneous diphtheria is increasingly recognized in temperate climates and accounted for 86% of the 1100 cases in the Seattle epidemic of 1972 to 1982. Since 1980, cutaneous diphtheria has not been a reportable disease in the United States, and recent health statistics include only respiratory diphtheria.

During the 1990s, tox⁻ strains of C. diphtheriae were associated with new types of infections. In the United Kingdom, these strains caused symptomatic pharyngitis, predominantly among homosexual men, that was sometimes accompanied by tonsillar exudate. In Switzerland, strains with a high potential for invasiveness were isolated from 38 intravenous drug users and shown by ribotyping to be clonally related. The latter strains caused infections of the skin (15 cases), respiratory tract (10 cases), and blood (13 cases). Among the patients with bloodstream infections, 9 had endocarditis, and 4 of these 9 patients died.

PATHOLOGY AND PATHOGENESIS C. diphtheriae infects mucous membranes, most commonly in the respiratory tract, and also invades open skin lesions resulting from insect bites or trauma. In infections caused by tox⁺ C. diphtheriae, initial edema and hyperemia are often followed by epithelial necrosis and acute inflammation. Coagulation of the dense fibrinopurulent exudate produces a pseudomembrane, and the inflammatory reaction accompanied by vascular congestion extends into the underlying tissues. The pseudomembrane contains large numbers of C. diphtheriae organisms, but the bacteria are rarely isolated from the blood or internal organs.

Diphtheria toxin acts both locally and systemically, and the lethal dose for humans is ~0.1 μg/kg. Toxin contributes locally to pseudomembrane formation; systemically, it can cause myocarditis, neuritis, and focal necrosis in various organs, including the kidneys, liver, and adrenal glands. Changes in the myocardium include cloudy swelling of muscle fibers and interstitial edema. These changes are followed within weeks by hyaline and granular degeneration (sometimes with fatty degeneration), progressing to myolysis and finally to the replacement of lost muscle by fibrosis. Thus, diphtheria can cause permanent cardiac damage. In diphtheritic polyneuritis, pathologic changes include patchy breakdown of myelin sheaths in peripheral and autonomic nerves, but recovery of nerve damage is the rule if the patient survives.

Diphtheria toxin is produced by C. diphtheriae as an extracellular polypeptide. Proteolytic cleavage forms nicked toxin consisting of fragments A and B. Fragment B binds to a plasma-membrane receptor (a precursor of a heparin-binding growth factor resembling epidermal growth factor), and the bound toxin is internalized by receptor-mediated endocytosis. Fragment A is translocated across the endosomal membrane and released into the cytoplasm, where it catalyzes the transfer of the adenosine diphosphate ribose moiety from nicotinamide adenine dinucleotide (NAD) to a modified histidine residue (diphthamide) on elongation factor 2 (EF-2), thereby inactivating EF-2 and inhibiting protein synthesis. One molecule of fragment A in the cytoplasm can kill a cell. Other metabolic alterations are secondary to inhibition of protein synthesis.

CLINICAL MANIFESTATIONS Patients with C. diphtheriae in the respiratory tract are classified as diphtheria cases if pseudomembranes are present and as diphtheria carriers if pseudomembranes are absent. The disease is graded as *tonsillar* if pseudomembranes are localized to the tonsils, as *combined types* or *delayed diagnosis* if more extensive pseudomembranes are present, and as *severe* if cervical adenopathy or cervical edema is also present. Onset is often gradual, but most patients seek medical care within a few days of becoming ill. Fever of 37.8° to 38.9°C (100° to 102°F), sore throat, and weakness are the most common symptoms, while dysphagia, headache, and change of voice occur in fewer than half of patients. Neck edema and difficulty breathing are noted in ≤10% of patients and are associated with an increased risk of death. Systemic manifestations are due primarily to toxic effects of diphtheria toxin. Patients without toxicity exhibit discomfort and malaise associated with local infection, whereas severely toxic patients may develop listlessness, pallor, and tachycardia that can progress rapidly to vascular collapse.

Primary infection in the respiratory tract is most often tonsillopharyngeal but may also be (in decreasing order) laryngeal, nasal, and tracheobronchial. Multiple sites are frequently involved, and secondary spread of pharyngeal infection upward to the nasal mucosa or downward to the larynx and tracheobronchial tree is much more common than primary infection at those sites. Systemic toxicity is usually most severe when extensive pseudomembrane extends from the tonsils and pharynx into contiguous regions. A small percentage of patients present with malignant or "bull-neck" diphtheria, with extensive pseudomembrane formation, foul breath, massive swelling of the tonsils and uvula, thick speech, cervical lymphadenopathy, striking edematous swelling of the submandibular region and anterior neck, and severe toxicity.

In tonsillopharyngeal diphtheria, isolated spots of gray or white exudate may appear first. These spots often extend and coalesce within a day to form a confluent, sharply demarcated pseudomembrane that becomes progressively thicker, more tightly adherent to the underlying tissue, and darker gray in color. Unlike the exudate in streptococcal pharyngitis, the diphtheritic pseudomembrane often extends beyond the margin of the tonsils onto the tonsillar pillars, palate, or uvula. Dislodging the membrane is likely to cause bleeding. Laryngeal diphtheria often presents as hoarseness and cough. Demonstration of laryngeal pseudomembrane by laryngoscopy helps distinguish diphtheria from other infectious forms of laryngitis. Patients with nasal diphtheria may present with unilateral or bilateral serosanguineous nasal discharge associated with irritation of the nares or lip. Primary or secondary diphtheritic infection occasionally involves other mucous membranes, including the conjunctiva and the membranes of the genitourinary and gastrointestinal tracts.

Cutaneous diphtheria usually presents as an infection by *C. diphtheriae* of preexisting dermatoses involving the lower extremities, upper extremities, head, or trunk. The clinical features are similar to those of other secondary cutaneous bacterial infections. In the tropics, cutaneous diphtheria may present as a primary cutaneous lesion, typically with morphologically distinct "punched-out" ulcers that are covered by necrotic slough or membrane and have well-demarcated edges.

C. diphtheriae is an occasional cause of invasive infections, including endocarditis and septic arthritis. Risk factors for such infections include preexisting cardiac abnormalities, abuse of intravenous drugs, and alcoholic cirrhosis.

COMPLICATIONS Obstruction of the respiratory tract can be caused by extensive pseudomembrane formation and swelling early in the disease or by sloughed pseudomembrane that becomes lodged in the airways later in the disease. The risk is greater when infection involves the larynx or the tracheobronchial tree and in children because of the small size of the airways.

Myocarditis and polyneuritis are the most prominent toxic manifestations of diphtheria. The risk of each is proportional to the severity of local disease. Myocarditis occurred in 22% and neuritis in 5% of 656 hospitalized patients (54% female, 70% ≥15 years old) with diphtheria in the Kyrgyz Republic in 1995; 7% of patients with myocarditis and 2% of patients without myocarditis died. The median interval from hospitalization to death was 4.5 days (range, 0 to 13 days).

Bulbar dysfunction in diphtheritic neuritis typically develops during the first 2 weeks. Palatal and pharyngeal paralysis usually develops first. Swallowing is difficult, the voice is nasal, and ingested fluids may be regurgitated through the nose. Additional bulbar signs may develop over several weeks, with oculomotor and ciliary paralysis more common than facial or laryngeal paralysis. Peripheral polyneuritis typically begins from 1 to 3 months after the onset of diphtheria with proximal weakness of the extremities, which spreads distally. Paresthesia may occur, most often in a glove-and-stocking distribution. Polyneuritis usually resolves completely, with the time needed for improvement approximately equal to that elapsing from exposure to the development of symptoms.

Pneumonia occurs in more than one-half of fatal cases of diphtheria. Less common complications include renal failure, encephalitis, cerebral infarction, pulmonary embolism, and bacteremia or endocarditis due to invasive infection by *C. diphtheriae*. Serum sickness may result from antitoxin therapy.

COURSE AND PROGNOSIS Most cases of diphtheria develop in nonimmunized patients. The attack rate, severity of disease, and risk of complications are much lower in immunized patients. The pseudomembrane may continue to increase in size during the first day after administration of antitoxin. During the next several days to a week, it becomes softer, less adherent, and nonconfluent and eventually disappears. In the preantibiotic era, *C. diphtheriae* persisted in the throat for ~2 weeks in one-half of patients and for ≥1 month in about one-fifth. Mortality increases with the severity of local disease, the extent of pseudomembrane formation, and the delay between onset of local disease and administration of antitoxin. The death rate is highest during the first week of illness; among patients with bull-neck diphtheria; among patients with myocarditis who develop ventricular tachycardia, atrial fibrillation, or complete heart block; among patients with laryngeal or tracheobronchial involvement; among infants and patients >60 years of age; and among alcoholics. Both the mortality rate and the risk of myocarditis or peripheral neuropathy are significantly lower in cutaneous diphtheria than in respiratory diphtheria.

DIAGNOSIS A characteristic pseudomembrane on the mucosa of the tonsils, palate, oropharynx, nasopharynx, nose, or larynx suggests diphtheria but is not uniformly present. Diphtheritic pseudomembrane must be distinguished from other pharyngeal exudates, including those of group A β-hemolytic streptococcal infections, infectious mononucleosis, viral pharyngitis, fusospirochetal infection, and candidiasis. Diphtheria should be considered in patients with sore throat, cervical adenopathy or swelling, and low-grade fever, especially when these manifestations are accompanied by systemic toxicity, hoarseness, stridor, palatal paralysis, or serosanguineous nasal discharge with or without demonstrable pseudomembrane. Treatment with diphtheria antitoxin should begin as soon as the clinical diagnosis of diphtheria is made.

Definitive diagnosis of diphtheria depends on the isolation of *C. diphtheriae* from local lesions. The laboratory should be notified that diphtheria is suspected to ensure the use of selective tellurite medium appropriate for the isolation of *C. diphtheriae*. All isolates of *C. diphtheriae* should be subjected to toxicity testing. Primary isolates can be screened rapidly for the presence of the *tox* gene by the polymerase chain reaction, although occasional strains of *C. diphtheriae* that carry an inactive toxin gene give false-positive results. Biochemical tests needed to differentiate *C. diphtheriae* from corynebacteria of the normal flora (diphtheroids) require several days. Group A β-hemolytic streptococci and *Staphylococcus aureus* are also isolated frequently from patients with diphtheria.

Cutaneous diphtheria may present as a characteristic "punched-out" ulcer with a membrane, but it is more often indistinguishable from other inflammatory dermatoses. Diagnosis depends on a high degree of suspicion and on culture of cutaneous lesions on laboratory media appropriate for isolation of *C. diphtheriae*. Throat samples from all patients with cutaneous diphtheria should be cultured for *C. diphtheriae*.

℞ TREATMENT The decision to administer diphtheria antitoxin must be based on the clinical diagnosis of diphtheria without definitive laboratory confirmation, since each day of delay in treatment is associated with increased mortality. Because diphtheria antitoxin is produced in horses, it is necessary to inquire about possible allergy to horse serum and to perform a conjunctival or intracutaneous test with diluted antitoxin for immediate hypersensitivity. Epinephrine must be available for immediate administration to patients with severe allergic reactions. Patients with immediate hypersensitivity should be desensitized before a full therapeutic dose of antitoxin is given. The dose of diphtheria antitoxin currently recommended by the Committee on Infectious Diseases of the American Academy of Pediatrics is based on the site of the primary infection and the duration and severity of disease: 20,000 to 40,000 units for disease that has been present for ≤48 h and involves the pharynx or larynx; 40,000 to 60,000 units for nasopharyngeal infections; and 80,000 to 100,000 units for disease that is extensive, has been present for ≥3 days, or is accompanied by diffuse swelling of the neck. Antitoxin is administered intravenously by infusion in saline over 60 min to neutralize unbound toxin rapidly. The ~10% risk of serum sickness is acceptable because of the established therapeutic value of antitoxin in decreasing mortality from respiratory diphtheria. The risk of systemic toxicity is lower in cutaneous diphtheria than in respiratory diphtheria and must be weighed against the potential adverse effects of antitoxin treatment; authorities are not unanimous in recommending antitoxin therapy for cutaneous diphtheria.

Antibiotics have little demonstrated effect on the healing of local infection in diphtheria patients treated with antitoxin. The primary goal of antibiotic therapy for patients or carriers is therefore to eradicate *C. diphtheriae* and prevent its transmission from the patient to susceptible contacts. Erythromycin, penicillin G, rifampin, or clindamycin is recommended by most authorities. Commonly recommended regimens for the treatment of adults with respiratory diphtheria are erythromycin (500 mg four times daily, given parenterally or orally) or intramuscular procaine penicillin G (600,000 units at 12-h intervals) for 14 days. Patients with cutaneous diphtheria and carriers can be treated orally with erythromycin (500 mg four times daily) or rifampin (600 mg once daily) for 7 days. If compliance is in question, a single dose of benzathine penicillin G (1.2 to 2.4 million units intramuscularly) can be substituted. Eradication of *C. diphtheriae* should be documented by negative cultures of samples taken on two or three successive days, beginning at least 24 h after the completion of antibiotic therapy. Some authorities also recommend a repeat throat culture 2 weeks later. The small percentage of patients who continue to be infected with *C. diphtheriae* after treatment should receive an additional 10-day course of oral erythromycin or rifampin. Plasmid-mediated resistance to erythromycin of the MLS type emerged transiently in *C. diphtheriae* during the Seattle epidemic, but its frequency declined dramatically after the routine use of erythromycin was discontinued.

Patients with respiratory or cutaneous diphtheria caused by tox[+] *C. diphtheriae* or by strains of unknown toxinogenicity should be hospitalized, kept in bed initially, handled with isolation procedures appropriate for the site of infection, and given supportive care as needed. Respiratory and cardiac function must be monitored closely. Early intubation or tracheostomy is recommended when the larynx is involved or signs of impending airway obstruction are detected. Tracheobronchial membrane can sometimes be removed mechanically via the endotracheal tube or tracheostomy. Primary or secondary pneumonia should be diagnosed and treated promptly. Sedative or hypnotic drugs that may mask respiratory symptoms are contraindicated. Close electrocardiographic monitoring, treatment of arrhythmias, and electrical pacing for heart block are essential. Congestive heart failure should be treated as described in Chap. 232. Glucocorticoids do not reduce the risk of diphtheritic myocarditis or polyneuritis. Ulcerative or ecthymatous cutaneous lesions should be treated with Burow's solution applied on wet compresses after debridement of necrotic areas, and treatment for associated conditions such as pediculosis, scabies, or underlying dermatoses should be instituted. Recovery from diphtheria does not always confer active immunity, and initiation of an immunization regimen for diphtheria that is appropriate for the patient's age should be an integral part of the treatment plan.

PREVENTION Vaccines available in the United States for immunization against diphtheria include diphtheria and tetanus toxoids and pertussis vaccine adsorbed (DTP), diphtheria and tetanus toxoids and acellular pertussis vaccine adsorbed (DTaP), diphtheria and tetanus toxoids adsorbed (DT; for pediatric use), and tetanus and diphtheria toxoids adsorbed (Td; for adult use). DTaP is preferred over DTP for primary immunization of children without contraindications, and use of DTP is no longer recommended. Td contains less diphtheria toxoid than DTP, DTaP, or DT and causes fewer adverse reactions in adults. Current guidelines for primary immunization of children and

adults against diphtheria and for maintaining immunity by periodic booster doses of appropriate vaccines throughout life are summarized in Chap. 122.

Close contacts of diphtheria patients should be cultured for *C. diphtheriae*, kept under surveillance for 1 week, and treated with appropriate antibiotics if cultures are positive. Previously immunized close contacts should receive an appropriate booster containing diphtheria toxoid if their last booster was given >5 years previously. If immunization status is uncertain, close contacts should receive an antibiotic regimen appropriate for carriers and a primary immunization series appropriate for their age.

OTHER CORYNEBACTERIAL INFECTIONS

DEFINITION Medically important coryneform bacteria (formerly called *diphtheroids*) include members of the normal flora that cause opportunistic infections, human pathogens of relatively low virulence, and animal pathogens that cause occasional zoonotic infections. Reported infections caused by coryneform bacteria have increased substantially in number over the past two decades. Isolates of *C. jeikeium* and *C. urealyticum* are often resistant to multiple antibiotics.

ETIOLOGY AND LABORATORY DIAGNOSIS Because coryneform bacteria are potential pathogens, it is important not to dismiss them as constituents of the normal flora or as contaminants when they are found in clinical specimens. Laboratory differentiation of coryneform bacteria is important when they are isolated repeatedly, when they are recovered in pure culture or in large numbers, or when they form pigmented or hemolytic colonies.

The coryneform bacteria are a large, heterogeneous group of gram-positive, pleomorphic, irregularly staining bacilli or coccobacilli that superficially resemble *C. diphtheriae* and are difficult to identify and classify. The genus *Corynebacterium* is currently divided into three groups of species: the nonlipophilic, fermentative corynebacteria (including *C. diphtheriae*, *C. xerosis*, *C. striatum*, *C. minutissimum*, and others); the nonlipophilic, nonfermentative corynebacteria (including *C. pseudodiphtheriticum* and others); and the lipophilic corynebacteria (including *C. jeikeium*, *C. urealyticum*, and others). Coryneform bacteria also belong to many other genera (including *Actinomyces*, *Arcanobacterium*, and *Rhodococcus*) as well as to several groups that have not yet been assigned to genera and species by the U.S. Centers for Disease Control and Prevention (CDC).

ECOLOGY AND EPIDEMIOLOGY Humans are the probable natural reservoir for *C. xerosis*, *C. pseudodiphtheriticum* (formerly *C. hofmannii*), *C. striatum*, *C. minutissimum*, *C. jeikeium* (formerly CDC group JK), *C. urealyticum* (formerly CDC group D2), and *Arcanobacterium haemolyticum* (formerly *C. haemolyticum*). Animals are the probable natural reservoir for *Actinomyces pyogenes* (formerly *C. pyogenes*; cows, sheep, pigs), *C. ulcerans* (cows, horses), and *C. pseudotuberculosis* (sheep, horses, goats, cattle). The natural reservoir for *Rhodococcus equi* (formerly *C. equi*) is soil. The ecologic niches for many other coryneform bacteria of medical importance are not well defined.

The coryneform bacteria found most frequently as components of the normal flora include *C. pseudodiphtheriticum* (pharynx, skin), *C. xerosis* (conjunctival sac, nasopharynx, skin), and *C. striatum* (anterior nares, skin). Coryneform bacteria that commonly colonize the skin of hospitalized patients include *C. jeikeium* (axilla, groin, perineum) and *C. urealyticum*. *C. jeikeium* most often colonizes patients with malignancies or severe immunodeficiency; it is also isolated from environmental sources (surfaces, air) in hospitals and from the hands of ward staff. *C. ulcerans* infections are acquired by consumption of raw milk. *C. pseudotuberculosis* infections are acquired by contact with animals or animal products or by consumption of raw milk.

PATHOGENESIS AND CLINICAL MANIFESTATIONS *C. jeikeium* was recognized in 1976 as a cause of infections in immunocompromised hosts. This organism also causes infections in immunocompetent hosts, but severe infections continue to be most frequent in patients with hematologic malignancies and neutropenia. Skin colonization precedes clinical infection. Additional risk factors for nosocomial *C. jeikeium* sepsis include prolonged hospitalization, breaks in the integument, chronic intravascular catheterization, and prior treatment with broad-spectrum antibiotics. Other presentations of *C. jeikeium* infection include endocarditis, device-related infections, pulmonary infiltrates, cutaneous septic emboli, soft tissue infections, and rashes. Endocarditis due to *C. jeikeium* occurs primarily in patients with prosthetic heart valves. *C. jeikeium* is a rare cause of central nervous system infections in patients with ventricular shunts.

C. urealyticum (formerly CDC group D2) was identified in 1985 as a significant cause of nosocomial urinary tract infections, including acute and chronic cystitis and pyelonephritis. The organism closely resembles *C. jeikeium* but differs from the latter by producing urease and failing to convert glucose to acidic metabolites. Hydrolysis of urea by urease causes alkalinization of the urine and formation of ammonium magnesium phosphate (struvite) stones. *C. urealyticum* is a cause of alkaline-encrusted cystitis in patients with preexisting bladder lesions that serve as foci for precipitation of struvite crystals. Risk factors associated with symptomatic urinary tract infections include preexisting immunosuppression, recent urologic procedures (including renal transplantation), underlying disorders of the genitourinary tract, and a history of urinary tract infections.

A. haemolyticum causes pharyngitis and chronic skin ulcers; less frequently, it causes a variety of deep tissue infections, septicemia, and endocarditis. Some 90% of *A. haemolyticum* infections occur in patients between 10 and 30 years old. *A. haemolyticum* pharyngitis in this age group is 5 to 13% as frequent as *Streptococcus pyogenes* pharyngitis. An erythematous rash is present in 30 to 67% of cases. The rash is usually scarlatiniform and most pronounced on the trunk and proximal extremities, but it sometimes resembles urticaria or erythema multiforme. Because rash is more frequent in *A. haemolyticum* infections than in *S. pyogenes* infections, *A. haemolyticum* should be considered as a possible etiology in older children and adults who present with the scarlet fever syndrome. Infection due to *A. haemolyticum* can also present as extensive pharyngeal exudate and can mimic diphtheria. *A. haemolyticum* occasionally causes peritonsillar abscess, sepsis, endocarditis, or meningitis.

C. minutissimum is frequently isolated from the lesions of erythrasma, a common superficial skin infection characterized by the presence in intertriginous areas of reddish-brown, scaly, pruritic, macular patches that exhibit coral-red fluorescence under a Wood's light. The etiology of erythrasma appears to be polymicrobial; infection of the skin by *C. minutissimum* has been shown to follow the onset of maceration and scaling. Deep infections caused by *C. minutissimum* are rare and include abscesses, bacteremia, endocarditis, peritonitis, pyelonephritis, and infection of central venous catheters.

Among coryneform bacteria that cause disease in animals and occasionally in humans, *R. equi* has emerged as an important intracellular opportunistic pathogen in immunocompromised patients. Most reported cases are necrotizing pulmonary infections that resemble tuberculosis or nocardiosis in patients with severely defective cell-mediated immunity. Cases of *R. equi* infection are being diagnosed with increasing frequency in patients with AIDS.

A. pyogenes causes bovine mastitis, a disease transmitted by flies. Yearly epidemics of leg ulcers infected with *A. pyogenes* occurred among schoolchildren in Thailand between 1979 and 1984 and were postulated to have resulted from introduction of the organism into traumatic skin lesions by flies. Reported *A. pyogenes* infections in adults in Denmark have included abscesses, cystitis, intraabdominal infections, and mastoiditis with bacteremia.

C. ulcerans infections in humans usually present as pharyngitis and can mimic respiratory diphtheria, whereas infections caused by *C. pseudotuberculosis* typically present as suppurative granulomatous lymphadenitis. Some strains of *C. ulcerans* and *C. pseudotuberculosis* produce diphtheria toxin. Human infections by *tox+* strains of *C. ul-*

cerans—but not by *tox+* strains of *C. pseudotuberculosis*—have been reported, and administration of diphtheria antitoxin is therefore warranted in infections by *C. ulcerans* that are presumed on clinical grounds to be caused by toxinogenic strains.

C. pseudodiphtheriticum, a commensal of low virulence, is an uncommon cause of pneumonia in men with AIDS and of endocarditis, necrotizing tracheitis, tracheobronchitis, and urinary tract infection in patients without known immune deficiencies. Likewise, *C. xerosis* and *C. striatum* only occasionally cause human infections.

DIAGNOSIS The clinical features of *C. jeikeium* infections are not pathognomonic. The diagnosis of these infections is based on a high index of suspicion, identification of the organism by culture in appropriate clinical specimens, and exclusion of other likely causes of infection.

C. urealyticum often goes undetected by routine urine cultures; rather, it is necessary to incubate the cultures for 24 to 48 h on blood agar or on special media. Cultivation should be prolonged in selected cases—i.e., those involving patients (especially elderly men with preexisting genitourinary abnormalities) with alkaline urine, ammonium magnesium phosphate stones, gram-positive bacilli in the urine, or negative standard urine cultures despite clinical evidence of bacteriuria. Other microbes that can cause urinary tract infections with alkaline urine include *Proteus*, *Ureaplasma*, and some staphylococci and streptococci. Alkaline-encrusted cystitis is an anatomic diagnosis made by cystoscopy.

The differential diagnosis of *A. haemolyticum* pharyngitis with rash includes scarlet fever; rubella; staphylococcal and streptococcal toxic shock syndromes; infections caused by Epstein-Barr virus, cytomegalovirus, and enteroviruses (especially coxsackieviruses); disseminated gonococcal infection; secondary syphilis; and drug allergy. Routine diagnostic methods for throat cultures are not ideal for the detection of *A. haemolyticum*, nor is this organism detected by the rapid tests for *S. pyogenes* that are sometimes substituted for throat cultures. Pharyngitis caused by *A. haemolyticum* in adolescents and adults is likely to be underdiagnosed until improved tests for the organism are used by diagnostic laboratories.

Erythrasma is diagnosed clinically. Because of uncertainty about the etiologic role of *C. minutissimum*, culture of erythrasma lesions is not currently recommended. Pharyngitis caused by *tox+* strains of *C. ulcerans* may be clinically indistinguishable from diphtheria. The presentations of infections caused by other coryneform bacteria are not usually diagnostic; cultures are required for identification of the causal organisms.

℞ **TREATMENT** Strains of *C. jeikeium* are typically resistant to most antibiotics. Vancomycin is the drug of choice for empirical treatment of infections caused by this organism, although antimicrobial susceptibility testing may reveal other antibiotic options for some isolates. For device-related *C. jeikeium* infections, removal of the infected device is usually required in addition to appropriate antibiotic therapy.

C. urealyticum is often resistant to the antibiotics used commonly for the treatment of urinary tract infections. Empirical treatment with vancomycin is appropriate pending the results of antimicrobial susceptibility testing. Several courses of antibiotic therapy may be necessary for bacteriologic cure. Patients with alkaline-encrusted cystitis require resection of the encrusted lesions in addition to antibiotic therapy.

No controlled trials of treatment for *A. haemolyticum* infections have been performed. In vitro tests usually demonstrate susceptibility to penicillins, erythromycin, azithromycin, clindamycin, doxycycline, ciprofloxacin, and vancomycin, but treatment failures have been reported with appropriate doses of penicillins. Limited data suggest that the clinical course of *A. haemolyticum* pharyngitis may be shortened by treatment with erythromycin.

Infections with *C. ulcerans* that present like diphtheria or are known to be caused by *tox⁺* strains should be treated like diphtheria. Oral erythromycin is usually effective for treatment of erythrasma. For infections caused by *R. equi*, vancomycin is the drug of choice. Possible alternatives include erythromycin, rifampin, aminoglycosides, and chloramphenicol; the combination of erythromycin and rifampin is attractive because of possible synergy. Penicillins should not be used, because *R. equi* rapidly develops resistance. Many weeks of antibiotic treatment, sometimes supplemented by surgical intervention, are often needed for infections caused by *R. equi*. Suppressive therapy with antibiotics should be continued indefinitely in patients with AIDS after initial treatment of infections caused by *R. equi*. Initial treatment of infections caused by other coryneform bacteria should be based on the identity of the organism and published data regarding antibiotic susceptibility. Therapy should be modified, when necessary, in light of the results of antibiotic susceptibility tests.

ANTHRAX

DEFINITION Anthrax is an infection caused by *Bacillus anthracis* that occurs primarily in herbivores. Humans become infected when *B. anthracis* spores are introduced into the body by contact with infected animals or contaminated animal products, insect bites, ingestion, or inhalation. Aerosolized spores of *B. anthracis* have the potential for use in biological warfare or bioterrorism. Cutaneous anthrax is most common and is characterized by the development of a localized skin lesion with a central eschar surrounded by marked nonpitting edema. Inhalation anthrax (woolsorters' disease) typically involves hemorrhagic mediastinitis, rapidly progressive systemic infection, and a very high mortality rate. Gastrointestinal anthrax is rare and is associated with a high mortality rate.

ETIOLOGIC AGENT AND EPIDEMIOLOGY *B. anthracis* is a large, aerobic, spore-forming, gram-positive rod that is encapsulated and nonmotile and grows in chains. Sporulation does not take place in living animals. The rectangular shape of the individual bacteria gives chains of *B. anthracis* a boxcar-like appearance. Virulent strains of *B. anthracis* are pathogenic for animals, including mice and guinea pigs. Spores of *B. anthracis* can survive for years in dry earth but are destroyed by boiling for 10 min, by treatment with oxidizing agents such as potassium permanganate or hydrogen peroxide, or by dilute formaldehyde. Most strains of *B. anthracis* are susceptible to penicillin.

Anthrax occurs worldwide and is most prevalent among domestic herbivores (including cattle, sheep, horses, and goats) and wild herbivores. Grazing animals become infected when they forage for food in areas contaminated with spores of *B. anthracis*. Anthrax in herbivores tends to be severe, with high mortality. Terminally ill animals with overwhelming bacteremic infections often bleed from the nose, mouth, and bowel, thereby contaminating soil or water with vegetative *B. anthracis* that can sporulate and persist in the environment. The carcasses of infected animals provide additional potential foci of contamination.

Humans are more resistant to anthrax than are herbivorous animals. The estimated number of human cases worldwide is 20,000 to 100,000 per year. Human cases are classified as agricultural or industrial. Agricultural cases result most often from contact with animals that have anthrax (e.g., during skinning, butchering, or dissecting), from bites of contaminated or infected flies, and (in rare instances) from consumption of contaminated meat. Industrial cases are associated with exposure to contaminated hides, goat hair, wool, or bones. Only three cases of cutaneous anthrax were reported to the CDC from 1984 through 1993, and gastrointestinal anthrax has never been documented in the United States. In an epidemic in the former Soviet Union at Sverdlovsk in 1979, cases were initially reported as cutaneous and gastrointestinal anthrax associated with contaminated meat; however, subsequent analysis of epidemiologic data and autopsy findings for most of the fatal cases established that the disease was inhalational anthrax associated with accidental airborne release of *B. anthracis* from a nearby military biological weapons facility. A massive outbreak in Zimbabwe between 1978 and the early 1980s involved more than 9700 cases of agricultural anthrax in humans. This outbreak occurred during wartime and was associated with disruption of the veterinary and medical infrastructure and cessation of veterinary anthrax vaccination programs.

PATHOGENESIS *B. anthracis* can evade phagocytosis, invade the bloodstream, multiply rapidly to a high population density in vivo, and kill quickly. The poly-D-glutamic acid capsule of *B. anthracis* confers resistance to phagocytosis. Anthrax toxin consists of three different proteins called *protective antigen* (PA), *edema factor* (EF), and *lethal factor* (LF). The toxin was discovered in studies demonstrating that transfer of sterile blood from guinea pigs dying of anthrax to uninfected guinea pigs killed the recipients. PA binds to plasma membranes of target cells and is cleaved by a cellular protease into two fragments. The larger fragment remains on the cell surface, displays a binding site for a domain that is present in both EF and LF, and serves as a specific receptor that mediates endocytic entry of EF or LF into the target cells. The catalytic activity of EF, a calmodulin-dependent adenylate cyclase, is expressed in the cytoplasm of human or animal cells that contain both calmodulin and ATP. The biologic effects of EF, which include formation of edema in anthrax lesions and inhibition of polymorphonuclear leukocyte functions, are mediated by the intracellular cyclic AMP that is produced by the enzymatic action of EF. In contrast, LF is a highly specific endopeptidase that cleaves several members of the MAP-kinase-kinase protein family and inactivates their functions in signal transduction pathways. Macrophages appear to be the principal targets of LF in animals, and intoxication of macrophages by LF is associated with production of reactive oxygen species, release of cytokines (including tumor necrosis factor α and interleukin 1β), shock, and death.

Cutaneous anthrax is initiated when spores of *B. anthracis* are introduced into the skin through cuts or abrasions or by biting flies. The spores germinate within hours, and the vegetative cells multiply and produce anthrax toxin. The cutaneous anthrax lesion is characterized by necrosis, vascular congestion, hemorrhage, and gelatinous edema, but few leukocytes are present.

In inhalational anthrax, *B. anthracis* spores in airborne particles <5 μm in diameter are deposited directly into the alveoli or alveolar ducts. The spores are phagocytized by alveolar macrophages, and some are carried to and germinate in mediastinal nodes. Hemorrhagic necrosis of the nodes, associated with hemorrhagic mediastinitis and overwhelming *B. anthracis* bacteremia, may develop rapidly. Secondary pneumonia sometimes occurs.

Gastrointestinal anthrax usually results from ingestion of inadequately cooked meat from animals with anthrax. Primary infection can be initiated in the intestine by organisms that survive passage through the stomach. An oropharyngeal form of the disease has also been described. Lesions in the throat or intestine are usually accompanied by hemorrhagic lymphadenitis.

B. anthracis bacteremia occurs in almost all cases of anthrax that progress to a fatal outcome.

CLINICAL MANIFESTATIONS Approximately 95% of human cases of anthrax are the cutaneous form, and ~5% are the inhalational form. Gastrointestinal anthrax is very rare. Anthrax meningitis can occur as a complication of overwhelming *B. anthracis* bacteremia.

Cutaneous Anthrax The cutaneous lesion in anthrax is most often found on exposed areas of skin. A small red macule develops within days after inoculation of *B. anthracis* spores into skin. During the next week, the lesion typically progresses through papular and vesicular or pustular stages to the formation of an ulcer with a blackened necrotic eschar surrounded by a highly characteristic expanding zone of brawny edema. The early lesion may be pruritic, and the fully developed lesion is painless. Small satellite vesicles may surround the original lesion, and painful nonspecific regional lymphadenitis is common. Most patients are afebrile, with mild or no constitutional symptoms; in severe cases, edema may be extensive and associated with shock. Spontaneous healing occurs in 80 to 90% of untreated cases, but edema may persist for weeks. In the 10 to 20% of untreated patients who have progressive infection, bacteremia develops and is often associated with high fever and rapid death. The differential diagnosis includes staphylococcal skin infections, tularemia, plague, and orf. Cutaneous anthrax should be considered when patients have painless ulcers associated with vesicles and edema and have had contact with animals or animal products.

Inhalational Anthrax The presenting symptoms of inhalational anthrax (woolsorters' disease) resemble those of severe viral respiratory diseases. Early diagnosis of inhalational anthrax that occurs naturally or as a consequence of biological warfare or bioterrorism is difficult. After 1 to 3 days, an acute phase supervenes, with increasing fever, dyspnea, stridor, hypoxia, and hypotension usually leading to death within 24 h. Occasionally, patients present with fulminant disease. A characteristic radiologic finding associated with hemorrhagic mediastinitis is symmetric mediastinal widening, which may provide an early clue to the diagnosis of inhalational anthrax

Gastrointestinal Anthrax Symptoms of gastrointestinal anthrax are variable and include fever, nausea and vomiting, abdominal pain, bloody diarrhea, and sometimes rapidly developing ascites. Diarrhea is occasionally massive in volume. The major features of oropharyngeal anthrax are fever, sore throat, dysphagia, painful regional lymphadenopathy, and toxemia; respiratory distress may be evident. The primary lesion is most often located on the tonsils.

LABORATORY DIAGNOSIS *B. anthracis* is present in large numbers in cutaneous lesions of anthrax and can be demonstrated by Gram's staining, direct fluorescent antibody staining, or culture unless the patient has been treated with antibiotics. A small proportion of patients with anthrax have bacteremia. Patients with anthrax meningitis have bloody spinal fluid containing large numbers of *B. anthracis* demonstrable by staining or culture. Patients with mild disease usually have normal leukocyte counts, but those with disseminated disease typically have polymorphonuclear leukocytosis. Tests for antibody to *B. anthracis* are useful in confirming the diagnosis of anthrax.

℞ **TREATMENT** Viable *B. anthracis* disappears from the lesions of cutaneous anthrax within 5 h of the initiation of treatment with parenteral penicillin G. The recommended regimen for adults is 2 million units of penicillin G at intervals of 6 h until edema subsides, with the subsequent administration of oral penicillin to complete a 7- to 10-day course. For penicillin-sensitive adults, treatment with ciprofloxacin, erythromycin, tetracycline, or chloramphenicol can be substituted. Antibiotics decrease local edema and systemic toxicity in cutaneous anthrax but do not prevent eschar formation. Cutaneous lesions should be cleaned and covered, and used dressings should be decontaminated. For inhalational or gastrointestinal anthrax, high-dose penicillin (8 to 12 million units per day in divided doses at intervals of 4 to 6 h) is recommended. A rational case can be made for passive immunization with anthrax antitoxin in addition to antibiotic therapy in severely ill patients with anthrax, but no appropriate antitoxin is commercially available.

PREVENTION Inhalational anthrax was essentially eliminated in England before 1940 through the development of methods to decontaminate wool and goat hair and the improvement of working conditions for handlers of animal products.

Nonliving vaccines consisting of alum-precipitated or aluminum hydroxide–adsorbed extracellular components of unencapsulated *B. anthracis* are used in the United States for military personnel, agricultural workers, veterinary personnel, and others at risk of exposure to anthrax. The major active component of these vaccines is protective antigen. Live attenuated vaccines containing spores of *B. anthracis* are used in both developed and developing countries to immunize domestic herbivores; these preparations are also used to immunize humans in Russia but not in the United States. The probable basis for attenuation of the original Pasteur spore vaccine is partial loss of a plasmid that encodes anthrax toxin. The basis for attenuation of the current Sterne spore vaccine is loss of a plasmid that encodes capsular polypeptide.

Improved anthrax vaccines for humans are needed because the current vaccines are impure and chemically complex, elicit only slow onset of protective immunity, provide incomplete protection, and cause significant adverse reactions. In addition to agricultural and industrial anthrax, the possible use of *B. anthracis* as an agent of biological warfare or bioterrorism is a stimulus for the development of an improved vaccine. Current strategies for vaccine development include purification of candidate protective antigens, expression of protective antigens in recombinant microbial vaccines, and construction of improved live attenuated strains of *B. anthracis*.

Carcasses of animals that succumb to anthrax should be buried intact or cremated. Necropsy or butchering of infected animals should be avoided because sporulation of *B. anthracis* occurs only in the presence of oxygen.

PROGNOSIS The mortality rate is 10 to 20% for untreated cutaneous anthrax but is very low with appropriate antibiotic therapy. In contrast, the mortality rate for inhalational anthrax approaches 100%, and therapy is usually unsuccessful. The mortality rate in treated gastrointestinal anthrax is ~50%. Anthrax meningitis is usually fatal.

BIBLIOGRAPHY

BROWN AE: Other corynebacteria and *Rhodococcus*, in *Mandell, Douglas, and Bennett's Principles and Practice of Infectious Diseases*, vol 2, 5th ed, GL Mandell et al (eds). Philadelphia, Churchill Livingstone, 2000, pp 2198–2208

DITTMAN S et al: Successful control of epidemic diphtheria in the states of the former Union of Soviet Socialist Republics: Lessons learned. J Infect Dis 181(Suppl 1):S10, 2000

DIXON TC et al: Anthrax. N Engl J Med 341:815, 1999

DUESBERY NS, VANDE WOUDE GF: Anthrax toxins. Cell Mol Life Sci 55:1599, 1999

FRIEDLANDER AM et al: Anthrax vaccine: Evidence for safety and efficacy against inhalational anthrax. JAMA 282:2104, 1999

FUNKE G et al: Clinical microbiology of coryneform bacteria. Clin Microbiol Rev 10:125, 1997

GUBLER J et al: An outbreak of nontoxigenic *Corynebacterium diphtheriae* infection: Single bacterial clone causing invasive infection among Swiss drug users. Clin Infect Dis 27:1295, 1998

HADFIELD TL: The pathology of diphtheria. J Infect Dis 181(Suppl 1):S116, 2000

HOLMES RK: Biology and molecular epidemiology of diphtheria toxin and the *tox* gene. J Infect Dis 181(Suppl 1):S156, 2000

KADIROVA R et al: Clinical characteristics and management of 676 hospitalized diphtheria cases, Kyrgyz Republic, 1995. J Infect Dis 181(Suppl 1):S110, 2000

LITTLE SF, IVINS BE: Molecular pathogenesis of *Bacillus anthracis* infection. Microbes and Infection 2:131, 1999

PILE JC et al: Anthrax as a potential biological warfare agent. Arch Intern Med 158:429, 1998

POPOVIC T et al: Use of molecular subtyping to document long-term persistence of *Corynebacterium diphtheriae* in South Dakota. J Clin Microbiol 37:1092, 1999

QUICK ML et al: Risk factors for diphtheria: A prospective case-control study in the Republic of Georgia, 1995–1996. J Infect Dis 181(Suppl 1):S121, 2000

142 *Anne Schuchat, Claire V. Broome*

INFECTIONS CAUSED BY *LISTERIA MONOCYTOGENES*

Listeria monocytogenes is a gram-positive rod that can be isolated from soil, vegetation, and many animal reservoirs. Human disease due to *L. monocytogenes* generally occurs in the setting of pregnancy or of immunosuppression caused by illness or medication. Increasing evidence suggests that a substantial portion of cases of human listeriosis are attributable to the food-borne transmission of *L. monocytogenes*. Unlike most food-borne pathogens, which cause primarily gastrointestinal illness, *L. monocytogenes* causes invasive syndromes, such as meningitis, sepsis, chorioamnionitis, and stillbirth.

ETIOLOGY Listeriae are aerobic or facultatively anaerobic nonsporulating bacilli that grow at 1 to 45°C and typically have tumbling motility when cultured at 20 to 25°C. Characteristics that help distinguish *L. monocytogenes* from other *Listeria* spp. include the formation of a narrow zone of β hemolysis on sheep blood agar and the production of acid from glucose, maltose, L-rhamnose, and α-methyl-D-mannoside but not from D-xylose. Determination of the serotype of *L. monocytogenes* is based on somatic (O) and flagellar (H) antigens. Most cases of human disease are caused by serotypes 1/2a, 1/2b, and 4b. Molecular subtyping techniques have made it easier to discriminate among strains of *Listeria* and thus to link environmental or food isolates with clinical infections.

PATHOGENESIS *L. monocytogenes* is an intracellular pathogen—a characteristic consistent with its predilection for causing illness in persons with deficient cell-mediated immunity. The organism can be found as part of the gastrointestinal flora in healthy individuals. Lack of gastric acidity and abnormal gastrointestinal functioning may increase the risk of invasive disease following exposure to the organism in the gastrointestinal tract. The increased risk of *L. monocytogenes* infection in pregnant women may be due to both systemic and local immunologic changes associated with pregnancy. For example, local immunosuppression at the maternal-fetal interface of the placenta may facilitate intrauterine infection following transient maternal bacteremia.

The molecular pathogenesis of *L. monocytogenes* has recently been elucidated. The cell-surface protein internalin interacts with specific receptors to induce phagocytosis. Both listeriolysin O and phospholipases permit the organism to escape from the phagosome into the cytosol while avoiding intracellular killing. Through the surface protein Act A, *L. monocytogenes* uses actin-based motility to move to the cell membrane. Efficient cell-to-cell spread is accomplished by both actin filament formation and phospholipase production. Genetic determinants of these proteins have been characterized. Because the organism is adapted for both intracellular survival and direct cell-to-cell spread, it is not eliminated by antibodies.

EPIDEMIOLOGY Long recognized as a veterinary pathogen, *L. monocytogenes* causes basilar meningitis ("circling disease") and stillbirth in sheep and cattle. The occurrence of listeriosis among humans has received increasing attention as the role of contaminated foods in the pathogenesis of epidemic listeriosis has been recognized and reports of disease associated with the expanding immunosuppressed population have accumulated.

Invasive listeriosis—confirmed by culture of blood or cerebrospinal fluid (CSF)—occurs in approximately 5 individuals per million population annually in the United States, for an estimated 1400 cases per year. Perinatal listeriosis complicates 9 births per 100,000. A 40% decline in incidence since the period from 1986 through 1990 may be attributable to aggressive food regulation and industrial clean-up efforts. Multistate surveillance for sporadic listeriosis suggests that 20% of infections are fatal or result in stillbirth, although higher case-fatality rates have been reported during listeriosis epidemics and were described in early series. Most cases of disease due to *L. monocytogenes* are sporadic; however, investigation of several outbreaks of listeriosis during the 1980s and 1990s demonstrated common-source food-borne transmission as a cause of human illness and showed that the incubation period for disease following consumption of contaminated food can be 2 to 6 weeks. The largest North American outbreak, which took place in Los Angeles in 1985, involved more than 100 cases and 48 deaths or stillbirths. A nationwide outbreak in France in 1992 involved 279 cases and 63 deaths. Foods implicated in outbreaks

of listeriosis include contaminated coleslaw, pasteurized milk, soft cheeses, pâté, ready-to-eat pork products, and hot dogs, while epidemiologic studies have implicated undercooked chicken, uncooked hot dogs, soft cheeses, and food from store delicatessen counters in sporadic disease. Listerial contamination of foods is relatively common. Among foods contaminated with the organism, those that are purchased ready to eat, are contaminated with serotype 4b, and are contaminated at a relatively high level may be the most likely to cause illness. The long incubation period associated with listeriosis contributes to the difficulty of implicating specific foods as the cause of either common-source outbreaks or sporadic cases.

Although food-borne transmission appears to be the foremost cause of epidemic and sporadic disease, several clusters of late-onset neonatal infection suggest nosocomial transmission of *L. monocytogenes*. Contaminated multiuse materials and equipment have been suggested as causes of some nosocomial clusters. Listeriosis has been reported in veterinarians and other persons in close contact with infected animals.

CLINICAL PRESENTATION *Pregnancy-associated listeriosis* may occur during any stage of pregnancy, although most infections are detected during the third trimester, possibly because of failure to obtain specimens for bacterial culture earlier during gestation in instances of abortion and stillbirth. One-half to two-thirds of pregnant women with perinatal listeriosis experience a mild illness characterized by fever, myalgias, malaise, and backache, which sometimes are accompanied by diarrhea, abdominal pain, nausea, and/or vomiting during the bacteremic phase. Blood cultures should be used for diagnosis. Transplacental spread of the organism results in intrauterine infection, which can lead to chorioamnionitis, premature labor, intrauterine fetal demise, or early-onset disease of the newborn. Women with listeriosis diagnosed during pregnancy have a favorable clinical outcome after antibiotic therapy or delivery. Although often included in the differential diagnosis of recurrent spontaneous abortion, infection with *L. monocytogenes* appears to cause fewer than 2% of stillbirths.

Neonatal listeriosis can be classified under the same categories used for group B streptococcal infection (Chap. 140), with early-onset disease evident during the first week of life and late-onset disease developing thereafter. Infants may be symptomatic at birth; most infants with early-onset disease are symptomatic by the second day of life. Aspiration of infected amniotic fluid contributes to pathogenesis. Early-onset disease may include sepsis, respiratory distress, skin lesions, and the syndrome called *granulomatosis infantisepticum*, which is characterized by disseminated abscesses involving the liver, spleen, adrenal glands, lungs, and other sites. Infants with late-onset neonatal disease are more likely than those with early-onset disease to develop meningitis. While early-onset disease is often associated with obstetric complications such as premature delivery and chorioamnionitis, late-onset disease typically affects infants born at term by uncomplicated deliveries. Infants may acquire *L. monocytogenes* during passage through the birth canal; except in several clusters of late-onset neonatal infections linked to nosocomial transmission, the pathogenesis of late-onset disease is not well understood.

Listeriosis not associated with pregnancy usually affects persons with immunosuppressive conditions, although invasive disease can also affect immunocompetent adults, particularly elderly persons. The most common underlying conditions in nonpregnant adults with listeriosis are chronic glucocorticoid therapy, solid or hematologic malignancies, diabetes mellitus, renal disease, liver disease, and AIDS. Although the prevalence of listeriosis among persons infected with HIV is much higher than that in the general population, listeriosis is a relatively uncommon opportunistic infection in AIDS.

Sepsis Clinical studies have shown that bacteremic infection without an evident focus is the most common clinical manifestation of listeriosis among immunocompromised hosts, while infection of the central nervous system (CNS) ranks second in frequency. Listerial sepsis cannot be distinguished clinically from bacteremia involving other organisms. Patients are usually febrile, often appear extremely ill, and may have prodromal symptoms including myalgia, nausea, vomiting, and diarrhea. Immunocompromised patients with listeriosis are less likely than other adults to present with CNS infection, possibly because they are more likely to have blood cultured during febrile episodes and thus to have transient listerial bacteremia recognized.

CNS Infection The most common presentation of CNS infection due to *L. monocytogenes* is meningitis, which can present as either an acute or (less often) a subacute illness. Presenting symptoms include fever, headache, and an altered level of consciousness. Examination of CSF usually reveals pleocytosis, increased protein concentrations, and normal glucose levels, although other patterns are sometimes found. Gram's stain is often unrevealing. The diagnosis is made when *L. monocytogenes* is identified on culture. Despite its name, *L. monocytogenes* is rarely associated with monocytosis of either CSF or blood. Other syndromes seen in CNS infection include meningoencephalitis; cerebritis; and brainstem, spinal cord, or intracranial abscesses. The unusual syndrome of rhombencephalitis includes asymmetric cranial-nerve palsies, altered consciousness, cerebellar signs, and motor or sensory loss. Symptoms of other nonmeningitic CNS infections include fever, ataxia, seizures, personality changes, and coma. Nuchal rigidity is rare in nonmeningitic infections. CSF cultures may be sterile; blood cultures are usually diagnostic.

Endocarditis Like most forms of bacterial endocarditis, listerial endocarditis typically occurs in patients with prosthetic or previously damaged valves. The organism has a predilection for the left side of the heart. Endocarditis due to *L. monocytogenes* is often associated with systemic embolization.

Focal Infections Other focal infections that can follow unrecognized bacteremia include endophthalmitis, peritonitis, osteomyelitis, visceral abscess, pleuropulmonary infection, and cholecystitis. Cutaneous lesions may develop without systemic involvement and have been reported in veterinarians and poultry workers.

Recurrences Recurrent infection with *L. monocytogenes* has been reported but is rare. Many recurrences are due to the subtype responsible for the initial infection. The implication is that such recurrences result either from insufficient treatment of a focus of primary infection or from repeated exposure to a persistently contaminated source.

Gastrointestinal Illness Several common-source outbreaks of acute gastroenteritis suggest that *L. monocytogenes* can cause an acute diarrheal syndrome in persons without immunocompromising conditions. The importance of *L. monocytogenes* in sporadic diarrheal illness is unclear. Although the organism is not identified by the culture methods routinely used for stool specimens, studies using selective enrichment media for evaluation of consecutive specimens from patients hospitalized with acute diarrhea have suggested that *L. monocytogenes* is not a major cause of sporadic diarrhea.

DIAGNOSIS Invasive listeriosis is diagnosed when the organism is cultured from a site that is usually sterile, such as blood, CSF, or amniotic fluid. The organism grows readily within 36 h on routine culture media, but morphologic similarities between *Listeria* and both diphtheroids and streptococci make it necessary to use biochemical tests to identify the species. Serologic assays with whole-cell antigens have not been useful for the diagnosis of listeriosis, both because exposure to the organism (and thus the presence of antibody) may be common and because infected individuals may not produce antibody. Assays for antibody to listeriolysin O have been applied in epidemiologic investigations and, retrospectively, in the diagnosis of culture-negative CNS infection. Culture of the organism from nonsterile sites such as the vagina and rectum is not useful for clinical diagnosis, as the organism may be carried at these sites by approximately 5% of healthy individuals.

Differential diagnosis of prematurity, spontaneous abortion, or stillbirth includes infectious diseases such as group B streptococcal infection, congenital syphilis, and toxoplasmosis; pathogens such as group B streptococci and *Escherichia coli* are more common than *L. monocytogenes* as causes of meningitis and sepsis in the newborn pe-

riod. Listerial infection should always be considered in the differential diagnosis of meningitis in immunosuppressed persons, particularly transplant recipients and others undergoing glucocorticoid treatment, patients with hematologic malignancy, and HIV-infected patients. Among healthy adults, meningitis is much more likely to be caused by *Neisseria meningitidis*, *Streptococcus pneumoniae*, or viral pathogens than by *L. monocytogenes*.

TREATMENT The treatment of choice for listeriosis is intravenous administration of either ampicillin or penicillin, often in combination with an aminoglycoside for synergy. Trimethoprim-sulfamethoxazole is bactericidal against *L. monocytogenes* and has been used successfully in the treatment of patients with penicillin allergy. *L. monocytogenes* is susceptible in vitro to penicillin G, ampicillin, erythromycin, trimethoprim-sulfamethoxazole, chloramphenicol, rifampin, tetracyclines, aminoglycosides, and imipenem. However, chloramphenicol and rifampin may antagonize the bactericidal effect of penicillins. Because *L. monocytogenes* is not sensitive to cephalosporins, these agents should not be used for single-agent empirical treatment of neonatal sepsis or of meningitis in newborns or immunocompromised hosts.

Dosages and durations of therapy have not been subjected to controlled trials. For nonpregnant adults with listeriosis, the regimen of choice is either ampicillin (12 g intravenously per day in six divided doses) or penicillin G (15 to 20 million units intravenously per day in six divided doses); for immunosuppressed patients with meningitis, some experts add gentamicin (1.3 mg/kg intravenously every 8 h) for synergy. Penicillin-allergic patients may be treated with trimethoprim-sulfamethoxazole (15/75 mg/kg intravenously per day in three equal portions every 8 h). Meningitis in an immunocompetent patient may require 2 to 3 weeks of antibiotic therapy after defervescence. Meningitis, bacteremia, endocarditis, and nonmeningitic listeriosis in immunosuppressed patients should be treated longer, probably for 4 to 6 weeks. Neonatal listeriosis can be treated with a 2-week course of ampicillin. Infants weighing <2000 g should receive 100 mg/kg per day in two equal doses during the first week of life and 150 mg/kg per day during the second week. Infants weighing ≥2000 g should receive 150 mg/kg per day in three equal doses during the first week of life and 200 mg/kg per day during the second week. The addition of an aminoglycoside should be considered for neonatal infection (gentamicin, 5 mg/kg per day in two divided doses during the first week of life; 7.5 mg/kg per day in three equal doses during the second week). For listeriosis in pregnant women, a 2-week course of ampicillin (4 to 6 g per day in four equal doses) is recommended. During the last month of pregnancy, infected women with serious penicillin allergies may be treated with erythromycin.

PROGNOSIS Treatment of maternal bacteremia during pregnancy can prevent neonatal infection. Antibiotic therapy for the newborn can limit sequelae, although the widely disseminated disease characteristic of granulomatosis infantisepticum is frequently fatal regardless of treatment. Early-onset disease carries a higher mortality risk than late-onset infection, and immunocompromised hosts have a worse prognosis than do otherwise healthy adults with listeriosis.

PREVENTION *L. monocytogenes* is frequently isolated from food; the Food and Drug Administration, the U.S. Department of Agriculture, and manufacturers are pursuing further measures to reduce *L. monocytogenes* contamination of foods that have been subjected to listericidal processing. Prevention of listeriosis requires dietary counseling of persons at increased risk of disease (Table 142-1). There is no role for the administration of prophylaxis to contacts of patients with listeriosis. Clinicians are encouraged to report cases of listeriosis to local or state health departments. Case reporting and subtyping of clinical isolates can facilitate early recognition of outbreaks and prevention of subsequent cases.

Table 142-1   Dietary Recommendations for the Prevention of Food-Borne Listeriosis

Recommendations to all individuals
1. Thoroughly cook raw food from animal sources, such as beef, pork, and poultry.
2. Wash raw vegetables thoroughly before eating them.
3. Keep uncooked meats separate from vegetables and from cooked and ready-to-eat foods.
4. Avoid raw (unpasteurized) milk or foods made from raw milk.
5. Wash hands, knives, and cutting boards after handling uncooked foods.

Additional recommendations to high-risk individuals[a]
- Avoid soft cheeses such as Mexican-style, feta, Brie, Camembert, and blue-veined cheese. There is no need to avoid hard cheeses, cream cheese, cottage cheese, or yogurt.
- Leftover foods or ready-to-eat foods, such as hot dogs, should be reheated until steaming hot before being eaten.
- Although the risk of listeriosis associated with foods from delicatessen counters is relatively low and poorly characterized, pregnant women and immunosuppressed persons may choose to avoid these foods or to thoroughly reheat cold cuts before eating them.

[a] Persons immunocompromised by illness or medications; pregnant women.

BIBLIOGRAPHY

DALTON CB et al: Listeriosis from chocolate milk: Linking of an outbreak of febrile gastroenteritis and "sporadic" invasive disease. N Engl J Med 336:100, 1997

LORBER B: Listeriosis. Clin Infect Dis 24:1, 1997

PINNER RW et al: Role of foods in sporadic listeriosis: II. Microbiologic and epidemiologic investigation. JAMA 267:2046, 1992

RYSER ET, MARTH EH (eds): *Listeria, Listeriosis, and Food Safety*, 2d ed. New York, Marcel Dekker, 1999

SCHLECH WF et al: Epidemic listeriosis—evidence for transmission by food. N Engl J Med 308:203, 1983

SCHUCHAT A et al: Role of foods in sporadic listeriosis: I. Case-control study of dietary risk factors. JAMA 267:2041, 1992

——— et al: Epidemiology of human listeriosis. Clin Microbiol Rev 4:169, 1991

SOUTHWICK FS, PURICH DL: Intracellular pathogenesis of listeriosis. N Engl J Med 334:770, 1996

SWAMINATHAN B et al: *Listeria*, in *Manual of Clinical Microbiology*, PR Murray et al (eds). Washington, DC, ASM Press, 1995, p 341

TAPPERO JW et al: Reduction in the incidence of human listeriosis in the United States—effectiveness of prevention efforts? JAMA 273:1118, 1995

143   *Elias Abrutyn*

TETANUS

DEFINITION   Tetanus is a neurologic disorder, characterized by increased muscle tone and spasms, that is caused by tetanospasmin, a powerful protein toxin elaborated by *Clostridium tetani*. Tetanus occurs in several clinical forms, including generalized, neonatal, and localized disease.

ETIOLOGIC AGENT   *C. tetani* is an anaerobic, motile gram-positive rod that forms an oval, colorless, terminal spore and thus assumes a shape resembling a tennis racket or drumstick. The organism is found worldwide in soil, in the inanimate environment, in animal feces, and occasionally in human feces. Spores may survive for years in some environments and are resistant to various disinfectants and to boiling for 20 min. Vegetative cells, however, are easily inactivated and are susceptible to several antibiotics (metronidazole, penicillin, and others).

Tetanospasmin is formed in vegetative cells under plasmid control. It is a single-polypeptide chain. With autolysis, the single-chain toxin is released and cleaved to form a heterodimer consisting of a heavy chain (100 kDa), which mediates binding to nerve-cell receptors and entry into these cells, and a light chain (50 kDa), which acts to block

neurotransmitter release. The amino acid structures of the two most powerful toxins known, botulinum toxin and tetanus toxin, are partially homologous.

EPIDEMIOLOGY   Tetanus occurs sporadically and almost always affects nonimmunized persons, partially immunized persons, or fully immunized individuals who fail to maintain adequate immunity with booster doses of vaccine. Although tetanus is entirely preventable by immunization, the burden of disease is large worldwide. The disease is common in areas where soil is cultivated, in rural areas, in warm climates, during summer months, and among males. In countries without a comprehensive immunization program, tetanus occurs predominantly in neonates and other young children; an estimated 490,000 neonates died of tetanus worldwide in 1994—a reduction from 550,000 in 1993. In the United States and other nations with successful immunization programs, neonatal tetanus is rare and the disease affects other age groups and groups inadequately covered by immunization (such as nonwhites). The risk for the development of tetanus and for the most severe illness is highest among the elderly. Only 27% of persons aged 70 or older—as opposed to 88% of 6- to 11-year-olds—have protective antibody levels. During the years 1995 through 1997, a total of 124 cases were reported to the Centers for Disease Control and Prevention; both the overall incidence (0.15 cases per 100,000 population) and the annual average (41 cases) were the lowest ever reported in the United States. The actual burden of illness, however, was greater, because reporting is incomplete. Although the elderly customarily account for the highest proportion of cases, in 1995 through 1997 individuals ≥ 60 years of age accounted for only 35% of cases, whereas those 20 to 59 years of age accounted for 60% and those under 20 for 5% (with one case of neonatal tetanus). The change is attributed to a decrease in incidence in both the ≥ 60 and the < 20 age groups, along with an increase among persons 20 to 59 years of age, particularly injection drug users.

In the United States, most cases of tetanus follow an acute injury, such as a puncture wound, laceration, or abrasion. Tetanus is acquired indoors or during farming, gardening, and other outdoor activities. The injury may be major but often is trivial, so that medical attention is not sought; in some instances no injury can be identified. The disease may complicate chronic conditions such as skin ulcers, abscesses, and gangrene. Tetanus is also associated with burns, frostbite, middle-ear infection, surgery, abortion, childbirth, and drug abuse, notably "skin popping." In some patients no portal of entry for the organism can be identified.

PATHOGENESIS   Contamination of wounds with spores of *C. tetani* is probably frequent. Germination and toxin production, however, take place only in wounds with low oxidation-reduction potential, such as those with devitalized tissue, foreign bodies, or active infection. *C. tetani* does not itself evoke inflammation, and the portal of entry retains a benign appearance unless infection with other organisms is present.

Toxin released in the wound binds to peripheral motor neuron terminals, enters the axon, and is transported to the nerve-cell body in the brainstem and spinal cord by retrograde intraneuronal transport. The toxin then migrates across the synapse to presynaptic terminals, where it blocks release of the inhibitory neurotransmitters glycine and γ-aminobutyric acid (GABA). The blocking of neurotransmitter release by tetanospasmin, a zinc metalloprotease, involves the cleavage of protein(s) critical to proper function of the synaptic vesicle release apparatus. With diminished inhibition, the resting firing rate of the α motor neuron increases, producing rigidity. With lessened activity of reflexes that limit polysynaptic spread of impulses (a glycinergic activity), agonists and antagonists may be recruited rather than inhibited, with the consequent production of spasms. Loss of inhibition may also affect preganglionic sympathetic neurons in the lateral gray matter of the spinal cord and produce sympathetic hyperactivity and high circulating catecholamine levels. Tetanospasmin, like botulinum toxin, may block neurotransmitter release at the neuromuscular junction and produce weakness or paralysis; recovery requires sprouting of new nerve terminals.

In local tetanus, only the nerves supplying the affected muscles are involved. Generalized tetanus occurs when toxin released in the wound enters the lymphatics and bloodstream and is spread widely to distant nerve terminals; the blood-brain barrier blocks direct entry into the central nervous system. If it is assumed that intraneuronal transport times are equal for all nerves, short nerves are affected before long nerves: this fact explains the sequential involvement of nerves of the head, trunk, and extremities in generalized tetanus.

CLINICAL MANIFESTATIONS *Generalized tetanus*, the most common form of the disease, is characterized by increased muscle tone and generalized spasms. The median time of onset after injury is 7 days; 15% of cases occur within 3 days and 10% after 14 days.

Typically, the patient first notices increased tone in the masseter muscles (trismus, or lockjaw). Dysphagia or stiffness or pain in the neck, shoulder, and back muscles appears concurrently or soon thereafter. The subsequent involvement of other muscles produces a rigid abdomen and stiff proximal limb muscles; the hands and feet are relatively spared. Sustained contraction of the facial muscles results in a grimace or sneer (risus sardonicus), and contraction of the back muscles produces an arched back (opisthotonos). Some patients develop paroxysmal, violent, painful, generalized muscle spasms that may cause cyanosis and threaten ventilation. These spasms occur repetitively and may be spontaneous or provoked by even the slightest stimulation. A constant threat during generalized spasms is reduced ventilation or apnea or laryngospasm. The severity of illness may be mild (muscle rigidity and few or no spasms), moderate (trismus, dysphagia, rigidity, and spasms), or severe (frequent explosive paroxysms). The patient may be febrile, although many have no fever; mentation is unimpaired. Deep tendon reflexes may be increased. Dysphagia or ileus may preclude oral feeding.

Autonomic dysfunction commonly complicates severe cases and is characterized by labile or sustained hypertension, tachycardia, dysrhythmia, hyperpyrexia, profuse sweating, peripheral vasoconstriction, and increased plasma and urinary catecholamine levels. Periods of bradycardia and hypotension may also be documented. Sudden cardiac arrest sometimes occurs, but its basis is unknown. Other complications include aspiration pneumonia, fractures, muscle rupture, deep vein thrombophlebitis, pulmonary emboli, decubitus ulcer, and rhabdomyolysis.

Neonatal tetanus usually occurs as the generalized form and is usually fatal if left untreated. It develops in children born to inadequately immunized mothers, frequently after unsterile treatment of the umbilical cord stump. Its onset generally comes during the first 2 weeks of life. Poor feeding, rigidity, and spasms are typical features of neonatal tetanus.

Local tetanus is an uncommon form in which manifestations are restricted to muscles near the wound. The prognosis is excellent.

Cephalic tetanus, a rare form of local tetanus, follows head injury or ear infection. Trismus and dysfunction of one or more cranial nerves, often the seventh nerve, are found. The incubation period is a few days and the mortality is high.

DIAGNOSIS The diagnosis of tetanus is based entirely on clinical findings. Tetanus is unlikely if a reliable history indicates the completion of a primary vaccination series and the receipt of appropriate booster doses. Wounds should be cultured in suspected cases. However, *C. tetani* can be isolated from wounds of patients without tetanus and frequently cannot be recovered from wounds of those with tetanus. The leukocyte count may be elevated. Cerebrospinal fluid examination yields normal results. Electromyograms may show continuous discharge of motor units and shortening or absence of the silent interval normally seen after an action potential. Nonspecific changes may be evident on the electrocardiogram. Muscle enzyme levels may be raised. Serum antitoxin levels of ≥ 0.01 U/mL are considered protective and make tetanus unlikely, although cases developing despite protective antitoxin levels have been reported.

The differential diagnosis includes local conditions also producing trismus, such as alveolar abscess, strychnine poisoning, dystonic drug reactions (e.g., to phenothiazines and metoclopramide), and hypocalcemic tetany. Other conditions sometimes confused with tetanus include meningitis/encephalitis, rabies, and an acute intraabdominal process (because of the rigid abdomen). Markedly increased tone in central muscles (face, neck, chest, back, and abdomen) with superimposed generalized spasms and relative sparing of the hands and feet strongly suggests tetanus.

℞ TREATMENT **General Measures** The goals of therapy are to eliminate the source of toxin, neutralize unbound toxin, and prevent muscle spasms, monitoring the patient's condition and providing support—especially respiratory support—until recovery. Patients should be admitted to a quiet room in an intensive care unit, where observation and cardiopulmonary monitoring can be maintained continuously but stimulation can be minimized. Protection of the airway is vital. Wounds should be explored, carefully cleansed, and thoroughly debrided.

Antibiotic Therapy Although of unproven value, antibiotic therapy is administered to eradicate vegetative cells—the source of toxin. The use of penicillin (10 to 12 million units intravenously, given daily for 10 days) has been recommended, but metronidazole (500 mg every 6 h or 1 g every 12 h) is preferred by some experts on the basis of this drug's excellent antimicrobial activity, a survival rate higher than that obtained with penicillin in one nonrandomized trial, and the absence of the GABA antagonistic activity seen with penicillin. Clindamycin and erythromycin are also alternatives for the treatment of penicillin-allergic patients. Additional specific antimicrobial therapy should be given for active infection with other organisms.

Antitoxin Given to neutralize circulating toxin and unbound toxin in the wound, antitoxin effectively lowers mortality; toxin already bound to neural tissue is unaffected. Human tetanus immune globulin (TIG) is the preparation of choice and should be given promptly. The dose is 3000 to 6000 units intramuscularly, usually in divided doses because the volume is large. The optimal dose is not known, however, and results from one study indicated that a 500-unit dose was as effective as higher doses. Pooled intravenous immunoglobulin may be an alternative to TIG, but the specific antitoxin concentration in this formulation is not standardized. It may be best to administer antitoxin before manipulating the wound; the value of injecting a dose proximal to the wound or infiltrating the wound is unclear. Additional doses are unnecessary because the half-life of antitoxin is long. Antibody does not penetrate the blood-brain barrier. Intrathecal administration should be considered experimental. Equine tetanus antitoxin (TAT) is not available in the United States but is used elsewhere. It is cheaper than human antitoxin, but its half-life is shorter and its administration commonly elicits hypersensitivity and serum sickness.

Control of Muscle Spasms Many agents, alone and in combination, have been used to treat the muscle spasms of tetanus, which are painful and can threaten ventilation by causing laryngospasm or sustained contraction of ventilatory muscles. The ideal therapeutic regimen would abolish spasmodic activity without causing oversedation and hypoventilation. Diazepam, a benzodiazepine and GABA agonist, is in wide use. The dose is titrated, and large doses (≥ 250 mg/d) may be required. Lorazepam, with a longer duration of action, and midazolam, with a short half-life, are other options. Barbiturates and chlorpromazine are considered second-line agents. Therapeutic paralysis with a nondepolarizing neuromuscular blocking agent and mechanical ventilation may be required for the treatment of spasms unresponsive to medication or spasms that threaten ventilation. However, prolonged paralysis after the discontinuation of therapy with such agents has been described, and both the need for continued paralysis and the occurrence of complications should be assessed daily. Alternative agents include propofol, which is expensive, and dantrolene and baclofen, which are being investigated in the hope of shortening the period of therapeutic paralysis.

Respiratory Care   Intubation or tracheostomy, with or without mechanical ventilation, may be required for hypoventilation due to oversedation or laryngospasm or for the avoidance of aspiration by patients with trismus, disordered swallowing, or dysphagia. The need for these procedures should be anticipated, and they should be undertaken electively and early.

Autonomic Dysfunction   The optimal therapy for sympathetic overactivity has not been defined. Agents that have been considered include labetalol (an α- and β-adrenergic blocking agent that is recommended by some experts but that reportedly has caused sudden death), esmolol administered by continuous infusion (a beta blocker whose short half-life may be advantageous in the event of severe hypertension from unopposed α-adrenergic activity), clonidine (a central-acting antiadrenergic drug), and morphine sulfate. Parenteral magnesium sulfate and continuous spinal or epidural anesthesia have been used but may be more difficult to administer and monitor. The relative efficacy of these modalities has yet to be determined. Hypotension or bradycardia may require volume expansion, use of vasopressors or chronotropic agents, or pacemaker insertion.

Vaccine   Patients recovering from tetanus should be actively immunized (see below) because immunity is not induced by the small amount of toxin that produces disease.

Additional Measures   Additional therapeutic measures include hydration to control insensible and other fluid losses, which may be significant; the meeting of the patient's increased nutritional requirements by enteral or parenteral means; physiotherapy to prevent contractures; and administration of heparin or another anticoagulant to prevent pulmonary emboli. Bowel, bladder, and renal function must be monitored. Gastrointestinal bleeding and decubitus ulcers must be prevented, and intercurrent infection should be treated.

PREVENTION   Active Immunization   All partially immunized and unimmunized adults should receive vaccine, as should those recovering from tetanus. The primary series for adults consists of three doses: the first and second doses are given 4 to 8 weeks apart, and the third dose is given 6 to 12 months after the second. A booster dose is required every 10 years and may be given at mid-decade ages—35, 45, and so on. Combined tetanus and diphtheria toxoid (Td) adsorbed (for adult use), rather than single-antigen tetanus toxoid, is preferred for persons >7 years of age.

Wound Management   Proper wound management requires consideration of the need for (1) passive immunization with TIG and (2) active immunization with vaccine, preferably Td in persons over age 7. For clean minor wounds, Td is administered to persons who (1) have unknown tetanus immunization histories; (2) have received fewer than three doses of adsorbed tetanus toxoid; (3) have received three or more doses of adsorbed vaccine, with the last dose given >10 years previously; and (4) have received three doses of *fluid* (nonadsorbed) vaccine. The recommendations for contaminated or severe wounds are identical, except that vaccine should be given to those who have received three or more doses of adsorbed tetanus toxoid if >5 years have elapsed since the last dose. Passive immunization with TIG is not recommended for clean minor wounds but is given for all other wounds if the patient's vaccination history indicates unknown or partial immunization. The dose of TIG for passive immunization of persons with wounds of average severity is 250 units intramuscularly, which produces a protective antibody level in the serum for at least 4 to 6 weeks; the appropriate dose of TAT is 3000 to 6000 units. Vaccine and tetanus antitoxin should be administered at separate sites in separate syringes.

Neonatal Tetanus   Measures aimed at preventing neonatal tetanus include maternal vaccination, even during pregnancy; efforts to increase the proportion of births that take place in the hospital; and the provision of training for nonmedical birth attendants.

PROGNOSIS   The application of methods to monitor and support oxygenation has markedly improved the prognosis in tetanus;

mortality rates as low as 10% have been reported from units accustomed to handling such cases. In the United States during the period 1995 through 1997, the case-fatality rate was 11%; 11 deaths from tetanus were reported in 1990, 11 in 1991, and 9 in 1992. The outcome is poor in neonates and the elderly and in patients with a short incubation period, a short interval from the onset of symptoms to admission, or a short period from onset of symptoms to the first spasm (period of onset). Outcome is also related to the extent of prior vaccination.

The course of tetanus extends over 4 to 6 weeks, and patients may require ventilatory support for 3 weeks during this period. Increased tone and minor spasms can last for months, but recovery is usually complete.

BIBLIOGRAPHY

ABRUTYN E, BERLIN JA: Intrathecal therapy of tetanus: A meta-analysis. JAMA 266: 2262, 1991

AHMADSYAH I, SALIM A: Treatment of tetanus: An open study to compare the efficacy of procaine penicillin and metronidazole. BMJ 291:648, 1985

BARDENHEIER B et al: Tetanus surveillance—United States, 1995–1997. MMWR 47:1, 1998

BLECK TP: *Clostridium tetani* (tetanus), in *Principles and Practice of Infectious Diseases*, 5th ed, GL Mandell et al (eds). New York, Churchill Livingstone, 2000, pp 2537–2543

CENTERS FOR DISEASE CONTROL AND PREVENTION: Tetanus among injecting-drug users—California, 1997. MMWR 47:149, 1998

TOBIAS JD: Anesthetic implications of tetanus. South Med J 91:384, 1998

144   *Elias Abrutyn*

BOTULISM

DEFINITION   Botulism is a paralytic disease that begins with cranial nerve involvement and progresses caudally to involve the extremities. It is caused by potent protein neurotoxins elaborated by *Clostridium botulinum*. The toxins' high potency has led to consideration of their use in bioterrorism or biological warfare. Cases may be classified as (1) *food-borne botulism*, from ingestion of preformed toxin in food contaminated with *C. botulinum*; (2) *wound botulism*, from toxin produced in wounds contaminated with the organism; (3) *infant botulism*, from ingestion of spores and production of toxin in the intestine of infants; or (4) *adult infectious botulism*, a group that includes some cases in older children and adults in which disease is produced by a mechanism similar to that described for infant botulism.

ETIOLOGIC AGENT   *C. botulinum*, a species encompassing a heterogeneous group of anaerobic gram-positive organisms that form subterminal spores, is found in soil and marine environments throughout the world and elaborates the most potent bacterial toxin known. Organisms of types A through G have been distinguished by the antigenic specificities of their toxins; a classification system based on physiologic characteristics has also been described. Rare strains of other clostridial species—*C. butyricum* and *C. baratii*—have also been found to produce toxin. *C. botulinum* strains with proteolytic activity can digest food and produce a spoiled appearance; nonproteolytic types leave the appearance of food unchanged.

Of the eight distinct toxin types described (A, B, C_1, C_2, D, E, F, and G), all except C_2 are neurotoxins; C_2 is a cytotoxin of unknown clinical significance. Botulinum neurotoxin, whether ingested or produced in the intestine or a wound, enters the vascular system and is transported to peripheral cholinergic nerve terminals, including neuromuscular junctions, postganglionic parasympathetic nerve endings, and peripheral ganglia. The central nervous system is not involved. Active neurotoxin (150 kDa) is composed of a heavy chain (a 100-kDa fragment responsible for neurospecific binding and translocation into the nerve cell) and a light chain (a 50-kDa fragment responsible for intracellular catalytic activity). The steps involved in neurotoxin activity include (1) specific binding to presynaptic nerve cells at the myoneural junction, (2) internalization of the toxin inside the nerve cell in endocytic vesicles, (3) translocation of the toxin into the cytosol, and (4) proteolysis by toxin (a zinc endopeptidase) of components of the neuroexocytosis apparatus curtailing release of the neurotransmitter acetylcholine. Cure follows sprouting of new nerve terminals.

Toxin is heat-labile, but spores are highly heat-resistant; both can be inactivated under appropriate conditions (see "Prevention," below). In the gastrointestinal tract, toxin is complexed with nontoxin proteins and resists degradation.

Toxin types A, B, E, and (in rare instances) F cause human disease; type G (now called *C. argentinense*) has been associated with sudden death, but not with neuroparalytic illness, in a few patients in Switzerland; and types C and D cause animal disease.

EPIDEMIOLOGY Human botulism occurs worldwide. In the United States, the geographic distribution of cases by toxin type parallels the distribution of organism types found in the environment. Type A predominates west of the Rocky Mountains; type B is generally distributed but is more common in the East; and type E is found in the Pacific Northwest, Alaska, and the Great Lakes area. In the United States, food-borne botulism has been associated primarily with home-canned food, particularly vegetables, fruit, and condiments, and less commonly with meat and fish. Type E outbreaks are frequently associated with fish products. Commercial products occasionally cause outbreaks, but some of these outbreaks have resulted from improper handling after purchase. Outbreaks in restaurants, schools, and private homes have been traced to uncommon sources (commercial potpies, beef stew, turkey loaf, sauteed onions, baked potatoes, and chopped garlic in oil). Food-borne botulism can occur when (1) a food to be preserved is contaminated with spores, (2) preservation does not inactivate the spores but kills other putrefactive bacteria that might inhibit the growth of *C. botulinum* and provides anaerobic conditions at a pH and temperature that allow germination and toxin production, and (3) food is not heated to a temperature that destroys toxin before being eaten.

CLINICAL MANIFESTATIONS **Food-Borne Botulism** Following ingestion of food containing toxin, illness varies from a mild condition for which no medical advice is sought to very severe disease that can result in death within 24 h. The incubation period is usually 18 to 36 h but, depending on toxin dose, can extend from a few hours to several days. Symmetric descending paralysis is characteristic and can lead to respiratory failure and death. Cranial nerve involvement, which almost always marks the onset of symptoms, usually produces diplopia, dysarthria, and/or dysphagia. Weakness progresses, often rapidly, from the head to involve the neck, arms, thorax, and legs; the weakness is occasionally asymmetric. Nausea, vomiting, and abdominal pain may precede or follow the onset of paralysis. Dizziness, blurred vision, dry mouth, and very dry, occasionally sore throat are common. Patients are generally alert and oriented, but they may be drowsy, agitated, and anxious. Typically, they have no fever. Ptosis is frequent; the pupillary reflexes may be depressed, and fixed or dilated pupils are noted in half of patients. The gag reflex may be suppressed, and deep tendon reflexes may be normal or decreased. Paralytic ileus, severe constipation, and urinary retention are common.

Wound Botulism When wounds are contaminated with *C. botulinum* spores, the spores may germinate into vegetative organisms that produce toxin. This rare condition resembles food-borne illness except that the incubation period is longer, averaging about 10 days, and gastrointestinal symptoms are lacking. Wound botulism has been documented after traumatic injury involving contamination with soil; in injection drug users, for whom black-tar heroin use has been identified as a risk factor; and after cesarean delivery. The illness has occurred even after antibiotics have been given to prevent wound infection. When present, fever is probably attributable to concurrent infection with other bacteria. The wound may appear benign.

Infant Botulism In infant botulism, the most common form of the disease, toxin is produced in and absorbed from the intestine after the germination of ingested spores. The severity ranges from mild illness with failure to thrive to fulminant severe paralysis with respiratory failure and may be one cause of sudden infant death. The identification of contaminated honey as one source of spores has led to the recommendation that honey not be fed to children <12 months of age. Most cases cannot be attributed to a particular food source. The factors permitting intestinal colonization with *C. botulinum* are not fully defined, but cases usually involve infants <6 months of age; susceptibility may decrease as the normal intestinal flora develops.

Adult Infectious Botulism Rarely, botulism in adults is produced by a mechanism similar to that operative in infant botulism: intestinal colonization and toxin production. The patient may have a history of gastrointestinal disease, surgery, or recent antibiotic therapy. Toxin and organisms may be identified in the stool.

DIAGNOSIS A diagnosis of botulism must be considered in afebrile, mentally intact patients who have symmetric descending paralysis without sensory findings. The diagnosis must be suspected on clinical grounds in the context of an appropriate history. Conditions often confused with botulism include myasthenia gravis, which may be ruled out by electromyography and antibody studies, and Guillain-Barré syndrome, which is characterized by ascending paralysis, sensory abnormalities, and elevation of the protein concentration in cerebrospinal fluid. The Fisher variant of Guillain-Barré—a descending paralysis—can indeed be difficult to differentiate from botulism. Other conditions that may resemble botulism include Lambert-Eaton syndrome, poliomyelitis, tick paralysis, diphtheria, and intoxications from mushrooms, medications, or chemicals. Hypermagnesemia should be considered.

The demonstration of toxin in serum by bioassay in mice is definitive, but this test may be negative, particularly in wound and infant botulism. It is performed only by specific laboratories, which can be identified through regional public health authorities. Other assays are being developed and remain experimental. The demonstration of the organism or its toxin in vomitus, gastric fluid, or stool is strongly suggestive of the diagnosis, because intestinal carriage is rare. Isolation of the organism from food without toxin is insufficient grounds for the diagnosis. Wound cultures yielding the organism are suggestive of botulism. The edrophonium chloride (Tensilon) test for myasthenia gravis may be falsely positive in botulism but is usually less dramatically positive than in the former condition. Nerve conduction velocity is normal, but compound muscle action potentials on routine nerve stimulation studies are decreased with a supramaximal stimulus, and facilitation is evident after repetitive stimulation at high frequency. Single-fiber electromyography may be helpful. The white blood cell count and erythrocyte sedimentation rate are normal.

TREATMENT Patients should be hospitalized and monitored closely, both clinically and by spirometry, pulse oximetry, and measurement of arterial blood gases for incipient respiratory failure. Intubation and mechanical ventilation should be strongly considered when the vital capacity is <30% of predicted, especially when paralysis is progressing rapidly and hypoxemia with absolute or relative hypercarbia is documented (Chap. 266). Serial measurements of the maximal static inspiratory pressure may be useful in predicting respiratory failure.

In food-borne illness, trivalent (types A, B, and E) equine antitoxin should be administered as soon as possible after specimens are obtained for laboratory analysis. The initiation of treatment should not await laboratory confirmation, which may take days. After testing for hypersensitivity to horse serum, a vial of antitoxin is given; repeated doses are not considered necessary. Anaphylaxis and serum sickness are risks inherent in use of the equine product, and desensitization of allergic patients may be required. If there is no ileus, cathartics and enemas may be given to purge the gut of toxin; emetics or gastric lavage can also be used if the time since ingestion is brief (only a few hours). Use of antibiotics to eliminate an intestinal source for possible continued toxin production and of guanidine hydrochloride and other drugs to reverse paralysis is of unproven value. In the United States, antitoxin as well as help in clinical management and laboratory confirmation are available at *any* time from state health departments or from the Centers for Disease Control and Prevention [at (404)639-2206; emergency number: (404)639-2888].

Treatment of infant botulism requires supportive care. Neither equine antitoxin nor antibiotics have been shown to be beneficial, and the value of human botulism immune globulin, an experimental preparation, is still being evaluated. In wound botulism, equine antitoxin is administered. The wound should be thoroughly explored and debrided, and an antibiotic such as penicillin should be given to eradicate *C. botulinum* from the site, even though the benefit of this therapy is unproven. Results of wound cultures should guide the use of other antibiotics.

Botulinum toxin is being used as therapy for strabismus, blepharospasm, and other dystonias and appears safe and effective. Generalized botulism-like weakness complicating therapy has been reported.

PROGNOSIS Type A disease is generally more severe than type B, and mortality from botulism is higher among patients above age 60 than among younger patients. With improved respiratory and intensive care, the case-fatality rate in food-borne illness has been reduced to ~7.5% and is low in infant botulism as well. Artificial respiratory support may be required for months in severe cases. Some patients experience residual weakness and autonomic dysfunction for as long as a year after disease onset.

PREVENTION A pentavalent vaccine (A–E) is available for use in highly exposed individuals. Spores can be inactivated by exposure to a temperature of 116° to 121°C (e.g., in steam sterilizers or pressure cookers). Toxin can be inactivated by exposure to a temperature of 100°C for 10 min. Newly identified cases should be reported immediately to public health authorities.

BIBLIOGRAPHY

ANGULO FJ et al: Large outbreak of botulism: The hazardous baked potato. Clin Infect Dis 178:172, 1998

BHATIA KP et al: Generalised muscular weakness after botulinum toxin injection for dystonia: A report of three cases. J Neurol Neurosurg Psychiatry 67:90, 1999

CHERINGTON M: Clinical spectrum of botulism. Muscle Nerve 21:701, 1998

HATHEWAY CL: Botulism: The present status of disease. Curr Top Microbiol Immunol 195:55, 1995

MONTECUCCO C et al: Botulinum neurotoxins: Mechanism of action and therapeutic implications. Mol Med Today 2:418, 1996

PASSARO DJ et al: Wound botulism associated with black tar heroin among injecting drug users. JAMA 279:859, 1998

SHAPIRO RL et al: Botulism in the United States: A clinical and epidemiologic review. Ann Intern Med 129:221, 1998

145   *Dennis L. Kasper, Dori F. Zaleznik*

GAS GANGRENE, ANTIBIOTIC-ASSOCIATED COLITIS, AND OTHER CLOSTRIDIAL INFECTIONS

DEFINITION Bacteria of the genus *Clostridium* are gram-positive, spore-forming, obligate anaerobes that are ubiquitous in nature. There are more than 60 recognized species of clostridia, many of which are generally considered saprophytic. Some of these species are pathogenic for humans and animals, particularly under conditions of lowered oxidation-reduction potential. Infections associated with these organisms range from localized wound contamination to overwhelming systemic disease. The four major disease categories for which clostridia are responsible are intestinal disorders, deep tissue suppurative infections, skin and soft tissue infections, and bacteremia (Table 145-1). Toxins play a major role in some of these syndromes.

ETIOLOGY In humans, clostridia normally reside in the gastrointestinal tract and in the female genital tract, although they occasionally are isolated from the skin or the mouth. Of the known species of the genus *Clostridium*, at least 30 have been isolated from human infections. Like several other pathogenic anaerobic bacterial species, clostridia are quite aerotolerant, but they do not grow on artificial media in the presence of oxygen. Clostridia characteristically produce abundant gas in artificial media and form subterminal endospores. *C. perfringens*, one of the most important species, is encapsulated and nonmotile and rarely sporulates in artificial media; the spores can usually be destroyed by boiling. *C. tetani* and *C. botulinum* are discussed in detail in Chaps. 143 and 144, respectively.

Clostridia are present in the normal colonic flora at concentrations of 10^9 to 10^{10} per gram. Of the 30 or more species that normally colonize humans, *C. ramosum* is the most common and is followed in frequency by *C. perfringens*. These organisms are universally present in soil at concentrations of up to 10^4 per gram. Although clostridia are gram-positive organisms, many species may appear to be gram-negative in clinical specimens or stationary-phase cultures. Therefore, the results of Gram's staining of cultures or clinical material should be interpreted with great care.

C. perfringens is the most common of the clostridial species isolated from tissue infections and bacteremias; next in frequency are *C. novyi* and *C. septicum*. In the category of enteric infections, *C. difficile* is an important cause of antibiotic-associated colitis, and *C. perfringens* is associated with food poisoning (type A) and enteritis necroticans (type C).

PATHOGENESIS Despite the isolation of clostridial species from many serious traumatic wounds, the prevalence of severe infections due to these organisms is low. Two factors that appear to be essential to the development of severe disease are tissue necrosis and a low oxidation-reduction potential. *C. perfringens* requires about 14 amino acids and at least 6 additional growth factors for optimal growth. These nutrients are not found in appreciable concentrations in normal body fluids but are present in necrotic tissue. When *C. perfringens* grows in necrotic tissue, a zone of tissue damage due to the toxins elaborated by the organism allows progressive growth. In contrast, when only a few bacteria leak into the bloodstream from a small defect in the intestinal wall, the organisms do not have the opportunity to multiply rapidly because blood as a medium for growth is relatively deficient in certain amino acids and growth factors. Therefore, in a patient without tissue necrosis, bacteremia is usually benign.

C. perfringens possesses at least 17 possible virulence factors, including 12 active tissue toxins and enterotoxins. This species has been divided into five types (A through E) on the basis of four major lethal toxins: α, β, ϵ, and ι. The α toxin is a phospholipase C (lecithinase) that splits lecithin into phosphorylcholine and diglyceride. This α toxin has been associated with gas gangrene and is known to be hemolytic, to destroy platelets and polymorphonuclear leukocytes (PMNs), and to cause widespread capillary damage. When injected intravenously, it causes massive intravascular hemolysis and damages liver mitochondria. The α toxin may be important in the initiation of muscle

Table 145-1   Classification of Diseases Caused by Clostridia

1. Intestinal disorders
   a. Food poisoning
   b. Enteritis necroticans
   c. Antibiotic-associated colitis
2. Suppurative deep tissue infections
   a. Mixed bacterial infections
   b. Monobacterial infections
3. Skin and soft tissue infections
   a. Simple contamination
   b. Local infection without systemic signs
   c. Spreading cellulitis and fasciitis
   d. Myonecrosis (gas gangrene)
4. Bacteremia
   a. Transient bacteremia
   b. Sepsis

infections that may progress to gas gangrene. Experimentally, the higher the concentration of α toxin in the culture fluid, the smaller the dose of *C. perfringens* required to produce infection. The protective effect of antiserum is directly proportional to its content of α antitoxin. Studies suggest that θ toxin may also play an important role in pathogenesis by promoting vascular leukostasis, endothelial cell injury, and regional tissue hypoxia. The resulting perfusion defects extend the anaerobic environment and contribute to rapidly advancing tissue destruction. A characteristic pathologic finding in gas gangrene is the near absence of PMNs despite extensive tissue destruction. Experimental data indicate that both α and θ toxins are essential in the leukocyte aggregation that occurs at the margins of tissue injury instead of the expected infiltration of these cells into the area of damage. Genetically altered strains induce less leukocyte aggregation when α toxin is absent and none when θ toxin is missing. The other major toxins, β, ϵ, and ι, are known to increase capillary permeability.

C. difficile produces two major toxins, designated A and B. Both toxins appear to act by the same mechanism, but toxin B is 1000 times more potent. These toxins exert their effect by binding to small guanosine triphosphate–binding proteins in the Rho family within target cells. The toxins are uridine diphosphoglucose hydrolases and glucosyltransferases that glycosylate the guanosine triphosphatases, inactivating these proteins and resulting in disruption of actin. Once the actin filaments are destroyed, the cell is unable to function. Toxin B has 100-fold greater enzymatic activity than toxin A.

Diarrheal disease due to *C. difficile* is toxin-mediated. Earlier teaching about the pathogenesis of this disease centered on the overgrowth of *C. difficile* when antibiotics suppress the normal bowel flora. Actually, the mechanism is probably more complex, since many of the antibiotics that cause this disease are active against *C. difficile* as well as other members of the bowel flora and since many patients who become colonized with *C. difficile* do not develop diarrhea. Critical features in the pathogenesis of this disease include mechanisms of toxin production and the interaction of *C. difficile* with other components of the bowel flora. Some antibiotics may actually trigger toxin production by the organism. In turn, other constituents of the bowel flora may suppress or inhibit toxin production. *C. sordellii*, for example, neutralizes cytotoxin B in vitro. In addition, when antibiotics eliminate more sensitive members of the bowel flora, more resistant organisms may produce enzymes such as β-lactamases that can inactivate antibiotics and thereby facilitate the growth of *C. difficile*.

CLINICAL MANIFESTATIONS   Intestinal Disorders •
Food poisoning   *C. perfringens*, primarily type A, is the second or third most common cause of food poisoning in the United States (Chap. 131). The responsible toxin is thought to be a cytotoxin produced by more than 75% of strains isolated from cases of foodborne disease. The cytotoxin binds to a receptor on the small-bowel brush border and induces a calcium ion–dependent alteration in permeability. The associated loss of ions alters intracellular metabolism, resulting in cell death. Outbreaks generally have resulted from problems in the cooling and storage of food cooked in bulk. The food sources primarily involved are meat, meat products, and poultry. Generally, the implicated meats have been cooked, allowed to cool, and then recooked the following day, often in a stew or hash. Strains of *C. perfringens* that contaminate meat manage to survive initial cooking. During reheating, the organisms sporulate and germinate. The disease is associated with an attack rate that is often as high as 70%. Symptoms of food poisoning from type A strains develop 8 to 24 h after ingestion of foods heavily contaminated with the organism. The primary symptoms include epigastric pain, nausea, and watery diarrhea usually lasting 12 to 24 h. Fever and vomiting are uncommon. Molecular methods including ribotyping and pulsed-field gel electrophoresis have been used to detect fecal cytotoxin in outbreaks of food poisoning caused by *C. perfringens*.

C. perfringens has also been implicated in a more severe form of diarrhea than that of classic food poisoning. This more severe disease tends to occur in the elderly and has been associated with antibiotic use in hospitalized populations. In this form of disease, diarrhea is generally more profuse, of longer duration, and accompanied by abdominal pain. Blood and mucus have been detected in the feces of the affected patients. In one hospital-based study of a cluster of cases, widespread environmental contamination with *C. perfringens* spores was documented.

Enteritis necroticans   Necrotizing enteritis (enteritis necroticans, or *pigbel*) is caused by β toxin produced by type C strains of *C. perfringens* following ingestion of a high-protein meal in conjunction with trypsin inhibitors (e.g., in sweet potatoes) by a susceptible host who has limited intestinal proteolytic activity. This disease has been reported among children and adults in New Guinea. A similar disease, *darmbrand*, was epidemic in Germany after World War II. Clinical features of pigbel include acute abdominal pain, bloody diarrhea, vomiting, shock, and peritonitis; 40% of patients die. Pathologic studies reveal an acute ulcerative process of the bowel restricted to the small intestine. The mucosa is lifted off the submucosa, with the formation of large denuded areas. Pseudomembranes composed of sloughed epithelium are common, and gas may dissect into the submucosa. The source of the organisms may be the patient's own intestinal flora; cultures of ingested pork have failed to yield the organism. Antibodies to the β toxin of *C. perfringens* have been of considerable benefit in changing the course of established disease. In a large-scale trial, children immunized with *C. perfringens* β toxoid were protected.

Neutropenic enterocolitis (typhlitis)   See Chaps. 85 and 167.

Antibiotic-associated colitis   Strains of *C. difficile* that produce toxins detectable in the stool are the only identified cause of colitis induced by antibiotic use. The diagnosis of this type of colitis requires that there be no other identifiable cause of diarrhea and that the onset of symptoms occur either during antimicrobial administration or within 4 weeks after treatment with the implicated agent has been discontinued. Essentially any antibiotic can cause this syndrome; even metronidazole and vancomycin, which are used to treat the disease, have been implicated as etiologic agents in some cases. On a per-use basis, clindamycin, which was the first antibiotic described to cause this entity, is the most commonly implicated antibiotic. However, since other antibiotics are prescribed more often than clindamycin in the United States, cephalosporins are currently the antibiotics that most commonly cause *C. difficile* enterocolitis, and penicillins rank next in frequency. Diarrhea due to *C. difficile* has been reported in patients with some forms of malignancy or renal transplantation who have received tacrolimus without concomitant or previous antibiotic administration.

Antimicrobial-associated diarrhea can be divided into four categories based on the appearance of the colon: (1) normal colonic mucosa; (2) mild erythema with some edema; (3) granular, friable, or hemorrhagic mucosa; and (4) pseudomembrane formation. Most patients with antibiotic-associated diarrhea have a normal, minimally erythematous colonic mucosa with some edema. Occasionally, colitis is more severe and is characterized by a granular, friable, or hemorrhagic mucosa. Examination of stool from the affected patients may reveal large numbers of red blood cells and some leukocytes. Biopsy shows subepithelial edema with round cell infiltration of the lamina propria and focal extravasation of erythrocytes. *C. difficile* cytotoxin B has been found in 15 to 75% of stools from patients in the first three categories, which suggests that other factors are involved in the pathogenesis of antibiotic-associated diarrhea.

The most characteristic form of antibiotic-associated colitis caused by *C. difficile* is pseudomembranous colitis (PMC). More than 95% of patients with documented PMC have positive stool toxin assays. Close inspection of pseudomembranes reveals exudative, punctate, raised plaques with skip areas or edematous hyperemic mucosa. These plaques can enlarge and coalesce over large segments of intestine in the later stages of disease. The clinical spectrum of antibiotic-associated PMC is diverse. Diarrhea is the key feature; stools are usually watery, voluminous, and without gross blood or mucus. Most patients have abdominal cramps and tenderness, fever, and leukocytosis. However, the symptoms vary considerably. At one end of the spectrum are many patients with annoying diarrhea but no systemic signs or symptoms, while at the other end are those with severe systemic toxicity, fever (40° to 40.6°C, or 104° to 105°F), and peripheral white blood cell counts of up to 50,000/μL with a marked left shift. Fecal examination frequently reveals leukocytes. Without specific therapy, the course is highly variable. Some patients, particularly those with clinically mild disease, experience prompt resolution of symptoms with discontinuation of drug treatment, while others have protracted diarrhea with large stool volumes for up to 8 weeks, with resultant hypoalbuminemia and electrolyte imbalance. Severely ill patients with toxic megacolon and colonic perforation have been reported. Among patients who are severely ill mortality rates may be as high as 30%, while in most of those with minimal symptoms disease may resolve with the discontinuation of antibiotic treatment alone. In the majority of patients, symptoms begin 4 to 10 days after antibiotic therapy is initiated. However, ~25% of patients do not develop symptoms until use of the implicated antimicrobial has been discontinued, in some instances as long as 4 weeks afterward. Some cases have been reported within hours after initiation of antibiotic therapy or after a single dose of antibiotic administered for surgical prophylaxis.

Suppurative Deep Tissue Infections   Clostridia are frequently recovered from various suppurative conditions in conjunction with other anaerobic and aerobic bacteria but can also be the only organisms isolated. These suppurative conditions, which exist with severe local inflammation but usually without the characteristic systemic signs induced by clostridial toxins, include intraabdominal sepsis, empyema, pelvic abscess, subcutaneous abscess, frostbite with gas gangrene, infection of a stump in an amputee, brain abscess, prostatic abscess, perianal abscess, conjunctivitis, infection of a renal cell carcinoma, and infection of an aortic graft.

Clostridia are isolated from approximately two-thirds of patients with intraabdominal infections resulting from intestinal perforation. *C. ramosum*, *C. perfringens*, and *C. bifermentans* are the most commonly isolated species. The presence of clostridial species does not affect the clinical presentation or outcome of these infections (Chap. 167).

An association has been made between malignancy and the isolation of *C. septicum* in the absence of grossly contaminated deep traumatic wounds. A major site for such a malignancy is the gastrointestinal tract, particularly the colon. An association with leukemia or with other solid tumors has also been noted, and one case of fatal myonecrosis has been reported in a patient with ovarian cancer. Some of these patients present with *C. septicum* bacteremia; these cases have a fulminant clinical course (discussed below). Others develop localized suppurative infection in the abdomen or the abdominal wall without bacteremia. Presumably, this infection arises from a silent perforation that leads to intraabdominal abscess formation.

Clostridia have been isolated from suppurative infections of the female genital tract, particularly tuboovarian and pelvic abscesses. The major species involved has been *C. perfringens*. Most of these are mild suppurative infections without evidence of uterine gangrene. *C. perfringens* has been isolated from as many as 20% of diseased gallbladders at surgery. One clinical syndrome, emphysematous cholecystitis, is caused by clostridial species at least 50% of the time. In this syndrome, gas forms in the biliary radicles and the wall of the gallbladder. It is seen most often in diabetic patients. Although the mortality rate in this entity is higher than in more common forms of cholecystitis, there is no evidence of myonecrosis.

Clostridia are among the many organisms found in empyema fluid or isolated by transtracheal aspiration from patients with lung abscesses. There is no unique clinical clue to the presence of clostridia (as opposed to other organisms) in these infections. *C. perfringens* has been reported as a cause of empyema arising from aspiration pneumonia, pulmonary emboli, and infarction. However, the majority of cases of clostridial empyema are secondary to trauma.

Skin and Soft Tissue Infections   Various categories of traumatic wound infections due to clostridia have been described: simple contamination, anaerobic cellulitis, fasciitis with or without systemic manifestations, and anaerobic myonecrosis.

Simple contamination   Clostridia are cultured most often from wounds in the absence of clinical signs of sepsis. As many as 30% of battle wounds are contaminated by clostridia without signs of suppuration, and 16% of penetrating abdominal wounds yield clostridia on culture despite treatment with cephalothin and kanamycin. In cases of trauma, clostridia are isolated with equal frequency from suppurative and well-healing wounds. Thus the diagnosis of clostridial infection should be based on clinical rather than bacteriologic criteria.

Localized infection of the skin and soft tissue without systemic signs   This condition, originally referred to as *anaerobic cellulitis*, is a localized infection involving the skin and soft tissue and is due to clostridia alone or with other bacteria. There are no systemic signs of toxicity, although the infection may invade locally, producing necrosis. These infections tend to be relatively indolent, spreading slowly to contiguous areas. Localized infections are relatively free of pain and edema. Perhaps because of the lack of edema, gas that is limited to the wound and the immediately surrounding tissue may be more evident than in gas gangrene. In these localized infections, gas is never found intramuscularly. Cellulitis, perirectal abscesses, and diabetic foot ulcers are typical infections from which clostridial species can be isolated. If inadequately treated, these localized infections advance by extension through subcutaneous tissue and fascial planes into muscle and may produce severe systemic disease with signs of toxemia.

A localized form of suppurative myositis has been described in heroin addicts. These patients develop local pain and tenderness in discrete areas (particularly the thigh and forearm), with the subsequent appearance of fluctuance and crepitance that require surgical drainage. The unusual aspect of these infections is that they remain localized without systemic signs of toxicity. Moreover, the affected local areas are not necessarily sites of trauma or heroin injection. Pathologic examination reveals subcutaneous abscesses, purulent myositis, and fasciitis from which clostridia are recovered in pure culture; on occasion, mixed infections involving aerobes and anaerobes are found. Wound botulism has been reported in association with the injection of black tar heroin.

Spreading cellulitis and fasciitis with systemic toxicity   This condition involves diffuse spreading cellulitis and fasciitis, without myonecrosis and with only mild inflammation in muscle. Patients present with the abrupt onset of a syndrome that progresses rapidly (within hours) through the fascial planes. In cases with suppuration and gas in soft tissues as well as overwhelming toxemia, the infection is rapidly fatal. On physical examination there is subcutaneous crepitation but little localized pain. Surgery is of no proven value because there are no discretely involved tissues amenable to resection, as may be the case in myonecrosis. However, in rapidly advancing fasciitis, incision of the affected area is still the cornerstone of therapy. The initial local lesion may be quite innocuous and arises from an area involved by tumor or other infection and not by injury. The systemic toxic effects include hemolysis and injury of capillary membranes. Usually, this infection is uniformly fatal within 48 h, despite intensive therapy involving antitoxin and exchange transfusion. This syndrome is seen most commonly in patients with carcinoma, especially of the sigmoid or the cecum. Presumably, the tumor invades the fascia, and colonic contents leak into the abdominal wall. Patients present with extreme toxicity and occasionally with total-body crepitation. The syndrome differs from necrotizing fasciitis caused by other organisms in three respects: (1) rapid mortality, (2) rapid tissue invasion, and (3) the systemic effects of the toxin, typified by massive hemolysis.

Clostridial myonecrosis (gas gangrene)   Clostridial myonecrosis occurs when bacteria invade healthy muscle from adjacent traumatized muscle or soft tissue. The infection originates in a wound contaminated with clostridia. Although >30% of deep wounds are infected with clostridia, the incidence of clostridial myonecrosis is quite low. These infections occur in both military and civilian settings. An essential factor in the genesis of gas gangrene appears to be trauma, particularly involving deep muscle laceration. The entity of clostridial myonecrosis is relatively uncommon after simple, through-and-through bullet wounds without shattering of bone and is relatively common following shrapnel fragmentation wounds, particularly when deep muscle is involved. In civilian cases, gas gangrene can follow trauma, surgery, or intramuscular injection. The trauma need not be severe; however, the wound must be deep, necrotic, and without communication to the surface.

The incubation period of gas gangrene is usually short: almost always <3 days and frequently <24 h. Some 80% of cases are caused by *C. perfringens*, while *C. novyi*, *C. septicum*, and *C. histolyticum* cause most of the other cases. Typically, gas gangrene begins with the sudden onset of pain in the region of the wound, which helps to differentiate it from spreading cellulitis. Once established, the pain increases steadily in severity but remains localized to the infected area and spreads only if the infection spreads. Soon after pain develops, local swelling and edema—ac-

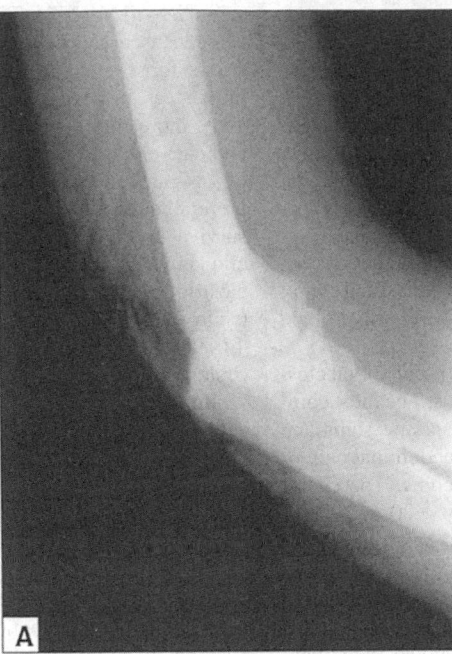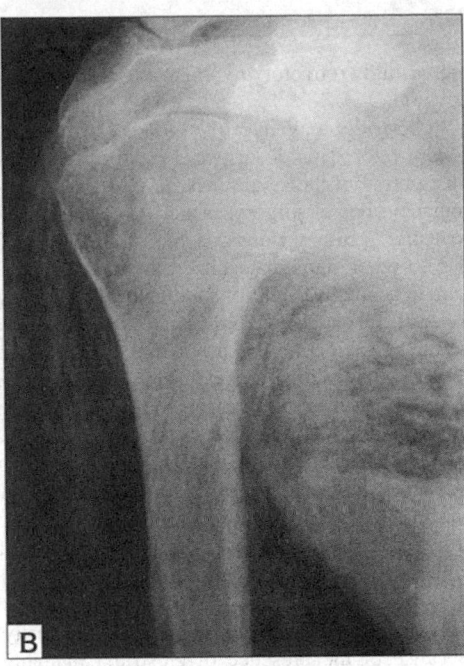

FIGURE 145-1 Spontaneous gas gangrene. Radiographs of the elbow (*A*) and shoulder (*B*) show gas in tissue. The patient developed spontaneous gas gangrene of the hand, which spread rapidly up the arm and onto the thorax. *C. septicum* was grown from blood and necrotic tissue of the arm. *[Reprinted with permission from DL Stevens (ed): Atlas of Infectious Diseases, vol II: Skin, Soft Tissue, Bone and Joint Infections. Philadelphia, Current Medicine, 1995.]*

companied by a thin, often hemorrhagic exudate—appear. Patients frequently develop marked tachycardia, but elevation in temperature may be only minimal. Gas is usually not obvious at this early stage and may be completely absent. Frothiness of the wound exudate may be noted. The skin is tense, white, often marbled with blue, and cooler than normal. The symptoms progress rapidly; swelling, edema, and toxemia increase, and a profuse serous discharge, which may have a peculiar sweetish smell, appears. Gram's staining of the wound exudate shows many gram-positive rods with relatively few inflammatory cells.

At surgery, muscle may appear pale because of the intensity of edema, but it does not contract when probed with a scalpel. When dissected, the muscle is beefy red and nonviable and can progress to become black, friable, and gangrenous. It is important to establish a diagnosis early, preferably by frozen-section biopsy of muscle.

Despite hypotension, renal failure, and (often) body crepitation, patients with myonecrosis frequently have a heightened awareness of their surroundings until just before death, when they lapse into toxic delirium and coma. In untreated cases, as the local wounds progress, the skin becomes bronzed; bullae appear, become filled with dark red fluid, and are accompanied by dark patches of cutaneous gangrene. Gas appears in later phases (Fig. 145-1) but may not be as obvious as in anaerobic cellulitis. Jaundice is rare in wound gas gangrene (in contrast to uterine infections) and, when it does appear, is almost invariably associated with hemoglobinuria, hemoglobinemia, and septicemia. Cases of clostridial myonecrosis without a history of trauma have been reported. These patients have bullous lesions and crepitation of the skin; they present with a rapidly worsening course that includes myonecrosis, especially of the extremities.

Bacteremia and Clostridial Sepsis The relatively common entity of transient clostridial bacteremia can arise in any hospitalized patient but is most common with a predisposing focus in the gastrointestinal tract, biliary tract, or uterus. Fever frequently resolves within 24 to 48 h without therapy. Despite the finding of clostridial bacteremia following septic abortions and the frequent isolation of clostridia from the lochia, most of the patients involved do not have evidence of sepsis. In one series of 60 patients with clostridial bacteremia, half had an infected site that could be associated with the bacteremia, while

the other half had a totally unrelated illness, such as tuberculous pneumonia, meningitis, or benign gastroenteritis. By the time blood culture reports are returned, patients frequently are completely well and sometimes have been discharged. Therefore, when a blood culture is positive for clostridia, the patient must be assessed clinically rather than simply treated on the basis of the culture result.

Clostridial sepsis is an uncommon but almost invariably fatal illness following clostridial infection—primarily that of the uterus, colon, or biliary tract. This entity must be differentiated from transient clostridial bacteremia, which is much more common. *C. perfringens* causes the majority of cases of sepsis as well as the majority of cases of transient bacteremia. *C. septicum*, *C. sordellii*, and *C. novyi* account for most of the remainder of cases. Clostridia account for 1 to 2.5% of all positive blood cultures in major hospital centers.

The majority of cases of clostridial sepsis originate from the female genital tract and follow septic abortion. Introduction of a foreign body is a common antecedent event. In the uterus, residual necrotic fetal and placental tissues and traumatized endometrium may allow the growth of clostridia. Only a small fraction of cases of septic abortion (1%) are followed by serious sepsis. In these patients, sepsis, fever, and chills begin from 1 to 3 days after the attempted abortion. The initial signs are malaise, headache, severe myalgias, abdominal pain, nausea, vomiting, and occasionally diarrhea. Frequently, a bloody or brown vaginal discharge is noted. Patients may rapidly develop oliguria, hypotension, jaundice, and hemoglobinuria. The hemolysis, which is secondary to *C. perfringens* α toxin, causes a characteristic bronzing of the skin. As in myonecrosis, the mental status of severely ill patients is characterized by increased alertness and apprehension. Local examination of the pelvis reveals foul cervical discharge, occasionally with gas. Frequently, laceration marks around the cervix or perforation of the cervical segment is evident. If the infection involves the myometrium or has spread to the adnexa, extreme tenderness, guarding, and an adnexal mass may be found.

Laboratory studies in patients with sepsis reveal an elevated white blood cell count and may show pink, hemoglobin-tinged plasma. Anemia is proportional to the degree of hemolysis, and the hematocrit may be extremely low. Platelet counts may be reduced, and there is often evidence of disseminated intravascular coagulation. Oliguria or anuria, increasingly refractory hypotension, and hemorrhage and bruising may develop.

Clostridia may enter the bloodstream from the gastrointestinal or biliary tract. This occurrence is associated with ulcerative lesions or obstruction of the small or large intestine, necrotic or infiltrating malignancy, bowel surgery, or various abdominal catastrophes. The patient may present with an acute febrile illness, with chills and fever but no other signs of localized infection. Intravascular hemolysis occurs in as many as half of such cases. Biliary or gastrointestinal symptoms, if present, may be the only clue to the etiology. Positive blood cultures provide the definitive clue to the diagnosis.

Patients with malignant disease can also develop rapidly fatal clostridial sepsis, particularly from a gastrointestinal focus. The most common species in this setting is *C. septicum*. Characteristic signs and symptoms include fever, tachycardia, hypotension, abdominal pain or tenderness, nausea, vomiting, and (preterminally) coma. The tachycardia may be out of proportion to the fever. Only ~20 to 30% of patients develop hemolysis. A striking feature of this syndrome is the rapidity of death, which frequently occurs in <12 h.

DIAGNOSIS The diagnosis of clostridial disease, in association with positive cultures, must be based primarily on clinical findings. Because of the presence of clostridia in many wounds, their mere isolation from any site, including the blood, does not necessarily indicate severe disease. Smears of wound exudates, uterine scrapings, or cervical discharge may show abundant large gram-positive rods as well as other organisms. Cultures should be placed in selective media and incubated anaerobically for identification of clostridia. The diagnosis of clostridial myonecrosis can be established by frozen-section biopsy of muscle.

The urine of patients with severe clostridial sepsis may contain protein and casts, and some patients may develop severe uremia. Profound alterations of circulating erythrocytes are seen in severely toxemic patients. Patients have hemolytic anemia, which develops extremely rapidly, along with hemoglobinemia, hemoglobinuria, and elevated levels of serum bilirubin. Spherocytosis, increased osmotic and mechanical red blood cell fragility, erythrophagocytosis, and methemoglobinemia have been described. Disseminated intravascular coagulation may develop in patients with severe infection. In patients with severe sepsis, Wright's or Gram's staining of a smear of peripheral blood or buffy coat may demonstrate clostridia.

X-ray examination sometimes provides an important clue to the diagnosis by revealing gas in muscles, subcutaneous tissue, or the uterus. However, the finding of gas is not pathognomonic for clostridial infection. Other anaerobic bacteria, frequently mixed with aerobic organisms, may produce gas.

The diagnosis of *C. difficile*–associated colitis is most often made by an enzyme-linked immunosorbent assay (ELISA) for toxin A. Compared with the "gold standard" tissue culture assay used primarily for the detection of toxin B, the ELISA exhibits comparable specificity and only slightly lower sensitivity (70 to 90%). The cytotoxicity assay requires a tissue culture facility, skilled laboratory technicians, and time (usually 48 h), since neutralization of the cytopathic effect with *C. sordellii* or *C. difficile* antitoxin is required before the test can be labeled positive. ELISA is more rapid and easier to perform. However, in difficult situations where the clinical diagnosis remains a possibility and ELISA results are negative, consideration should be given to requesting the cytotoxicity assay since it may detect 5 to 10% more cases. Repeat stool testing with the same assay generally does not increase the diagnostic yield for this entity. Endoscopy, although useful in establishing the presence of PMC, does not establish the etiology and should be reserved for cases with more serious disease manifestations, in which it can be used to exclude alternative diagnoses. Isolation of *C. difficile* from stool cultures is difficult. This approach should be reserved for epidemiologic studies of outbreaks since asymptomatic persons may harbor the pathogen, but production of toxin is the hallmark of disease.

℞ **TREATMENT** Traumatic wounds should be thoroughly cleansed and debrided. Traditionally, the antibiotic treatment of choice for severe clostridial infection has been penicillin G (20 million units a day in adults). Penicillin G treatment of gas gangrene has become more controversial because of increasing resistance to this drug and data obtained from animal models of infection. In a mouse model of gas gangrene, antibiotics inhibiting toxin synthesis appeared to be preferable to cell wall–active drugs; clindamycin treatment enhanced survival more than therapy with penicillin; and the combination of clindamycin and penicillin was superior to penicillin alone. For severe clostridial sepsis, clindamycin may be used at a dose of 600 mg every 6 h in combination with high-dose penicillin (3 to 4 million units every 4 h). Although no clinical trials validate this choice, it is gaining acceptance in the infectious disease community.

In cases of penicillin sensitivity or allergy, other antibiotics should be considered, but all should be tested for in vitro activity because of the occasional isolation of resistant strains. Clostridia are frequently, but not universally, susceptible in vitro to cefoxitin, carbenicillin, chloramphenicol, clindamycin, metronidazole, doxycycline, imipenem, minocycline, tetracycline, third-generation cephalosporins, and vancomycin. For severe clostridial infections, sensitivity testing should be done before an antimicrobial with unpredictable activity is used. Simple contamination of a wound with clostridia should not be treated with antibiotics. Localized skin and soft tissue infection can be managed by debridement rather than with systemic antibiotics. Drugs are required when the process extends into adjacent tissue or when fever and systemic signs of sepsis are present. Surgery is a mainstay of therapy for clostridial myonecrosis or gas gangrene. Amputation may be required for rapidly spreading infection involving a limb. Hysterectomy is required for uterine myonecrosis. Abdominal wall myonecrosis usually continues despite initial aggressive surgery and antibiotic therapy and requires repeated surgical debridement of all involved muscle.

Suppurative infections should be treated with antibiotics. Frequently, broad-spectrum antibiotics must be used because of the mixed flora involved in these infections. Aminoglycosides can be used for the aerobic gram-negative bacteria involved in mixed infections.

The use of a polyvalent gas gangrene antitoxin is still recommended by some authorities. At present, no such antitoxin is produced in the United States, and most centers have discontinued its use in the management of patients with suspected gas gangrene or clostridial postabortion sepsis because of questionable efficacy and the substantial risk of hypersensitivity to horse serum, from which the antitoxin is derived.

The use of hyperbaric oxygen in the treatment of gas gangrene is also controversial. Studies in humans are not well designed to answer questions on efficacy, but several knowledgeable authors believe that hyperbaric oxygen therapy has contributed to dramatic clinical improvement. Such therapy may, however, be associated with untoward effects due to oxygen toxicity and high atmospheric pressure. Some centers without hyperbaric chambers have reported acceptable mortality rates; thus expert surgical and medical management and control of complications are probably the most important factors in the treatment of gas gangrene. Fasciotomy should not be delayed for hyperbaric oxygen therapy.

The treatment of *C. difficile*–associated colitis requires discontinuation of therapy with the offending antimicrobial agent. In some patients, symptoms will resolve over a period of 2 weeks if the infection is left untreated. However, specific therapy shortens the duration of symptoms.

Diarrhea due to *C. difficile* should be treated with metronidazole (500 mg orally tid for 10 to 14 days). A randomized trial comparing metronidazole (250 mg qid) with oral vancomycin showed equal efficacy and relapse rates of ~9% for both regimens. Since both treatment regimens are effective, metronidazole is preferred because it is far less costly and has not been linked to the development of vancomycin-resistant enterococci. When a patient relapses, antibiotic resistance should not be inferred since it is rare; a repeat course of metronidazole is appropriate. When a patient with *C. difficile*–associated diarrhea requires continued antibiotic treatment for a serious infection such as infective endocarditis, it is often reasonable to continue therapy against *C. difficile* for the duration of the offending antibiotic treatment course and for a full 10 to 14 days following its completion. When vancomycin is used for the treatment of *C. difficile*–associated diarrhea, the starting dose should be 125 mg orally qid, although doses as high as 500 mg qid can be used if needed. When a patient requires parenteral therapy for antibiotic-associated diarrhea, intravenous metronidazole can be administered. Vancomycin is effective only if used orally; the drug is poorly absorbed after oral administration. If patients continue to have diarrhea and have signs of systemic toxicity (e.g., fever and/or leukocytosis) after 48 h of treatment with metronidazole, it is reasonable to switch to vancomycin. For especially severe disease, some experts advocate treatment with both oral vancomycin and metronidazole, although there are no trials to support this regimen.

A number of patients who respond to initial therapy present with a relapse of symptoms and a repeat positive toxin assay. Relapses following therapy are much more frequent than failures to respond to initial therapy. Most relapses occur 3 to 10 days after discontinuation of treatment. Most relapsing patients respond to a second course of antibiotics, but some go on to suffer multiple relapses. A number of options are available in this situation. Some authors report success with tapering regimens of vancomycin given daily or every other day for 1 to 2 months to avoid relapse. The resin cholestyramine binds the cytotoxin of *C. difficile* and has been used with some success to treat severe cases. Since cholestyramine also binds vancomycin, the two agents should not be used in combination. Repopulation of the normal colonic flora has also been tried in relapsing disease. Ingestion of capsules of the yeast *Saccharomyces boulardii* showed some promise in one trial; oral lactobacilli have also been used in uncontrolled studies. The administration of intravenous immunoglobulin has been tried with success in a few children and adults with relapsing infection, although this approach is not yet considered to be recommended therapy.

BIBLIOGRAPHY

BORRIELLO SP: Clostridial disease of the gut. Clin Infect Dis 20:S242, 1995

CASTAGLIUOLO I et al: *Clostridium difficile* toxin A stimulates macrophage-inflammatory protein-2 production in rat intestinal epithelial cells. J Immunol 160:6039, 1998

CHAVES-OLARTE E et al: Toxins A and B from *Clostridium difficile* differ with respect to enzymatic potencies, cellular substrate specificities, and surface binding to cultured cells. J Clin Invest 100:1734, 1997

CLEARY RK: *Clostridium difficile*–associated diarrhea and colitis: Clinical manifestations, diagnosis, and treatment. Dis Colon Rectum 41:1435, 1998

ELLEMOR DM et al: Use of genetically manipulated strains of *Clostridium perfringens* reveals that both alpha-toxin and theta-toxin are required for vascular leukostasis to occur in experimental gas gangrene. Infect Immun 67:4902, 1999

GERDING DN et al: *Clostridium difficile*–associated diarrhea and colitis. Infect Control Hosp Epidemiol 16:459, 1995

JOHNSON S et al: Epidemics of diarrhea caused by a clindamycin-resistant strain of *Clostridium difficile* in four hospitals. N Engl J Med 341:1645, 1999

JUST I et al: Glucosylation of Rho proteins by *Clostridium difficile* toxin B. Nature 375:500, 1995

KYNE L et al: Asymptomatic carriage of *Clostridium difficile* and serum levels of IgG antibody against toxin A. N Engl J Med 342:390, 2000

LORBER B: Gas gangrene and other *Clostridium*-associated diseases, in *Principles and Practice of Infectious Diseases*, 5th ed, GL Mandell et al (eds). New York, Churchill Livingstone, 2000, pp 2549–2560

PRINSSEN HM et al: *Clostridium septicum* myonecrosis and ovarian cancer: A case report and review of literature. Gynecol Oncol 72:116, 1999

ROOD JI: Virulence genes of *Clostridium perfringens*. Annu Rev Microbiol 52:333, 1998

SCHALCH B et al: Molecular methods for the analysis of *Clostridium perfringens* relevant to food hygiene. FEMS Immunol Med Microbiol 24:281, 1999

SHARMA AK, HOLDER FE: *Clostridium difficile* diarrhea after use of tacrolimus following renal transplantation. Clin Infect Dis 27:1540, 1998

TIBBLES PM, EDELSBERG JS: Medical progress: Hyperbaric-oxygen therapy. N Engl J Med 334:1642, 1996

Section 6
DISEASES CAUSED BY GRAM-NEGATIVE BACTERIA

146 *Robert S. Munford*

MENINGOCOCCAL INFECTIONS

DEFINITION *Neisseria meningitidis* is the etiologic agent of two life-threatening diseases: meningococcal meningitis and fulminant meningococcemia. Meningococci also cause pneumonia, septic arthritis, pericarditis, urethritis, and conjunctivitis. Most cases are potentially preventable by vaccination.

ETIOLOGIC AGENT *N. meningitidis* bacteria are gram-negative aerobic diplococci. Unlike the other neisseriae, they have a polysaccharide capsule. They are transmitted among humans, their only known habitat, via respiratory secretions. Colonization of the nasopharynx or pharynx is much more common than invasive disease.

EPIDEMIOLOGY Meningococcal disease occurs worldwide as isolated (sporadic) cases, institution- or community-based outbreaks, and large epidemics.

Meningococci are classified into serogroups based on the antigenicity of their capsular polysaccharides. Antigenicity reflects structural differences in these polysaccharides. Five serogroups (A, B, C, Y, and W-135) are responsible for >90% of cases of meningococcal disease worldwide. Serogroup A strains, which caused most of the large epidemics of meningococcal disease during the first half of the twentieth century, are now associated with recurring epidemics in sub-Saharan Africa and other locales in the developing world. Serogroups B, C, and Y cause most cases of sporadic and epidemic meningococcal disease in industrialized countries. In the United States and Canada during the 1990s, serogroup B was the most common cause of sporadic disease, while serogroup C was a more frequent cause of outbreaks. Serogroup Y has recently been isolated from almost one-third of cases of meningococcal disease in the United States. In general, patients with serogroup Y disease are older and more likely to have a chronic underlying illness than are patients with disease caused by other serogroups. Serogroups Y and W-135 are isolated more often than the other serogroups from patients with pneumonia.

One limitation of the serogroup classification is that the genes for capsule biosynthesis can be transferred from one strain to another, with consequent changes in the capsule structure of the recipient strain and therefore in its serogroup. Other methods for tracking meningococcal strains have thus become increasingly useful. Meningococcal serotypes and subtypes are defined by antigenic differences in specific outer-membrane proteins (OMPs), whereas multilocus enzyme electrophoresis classifies bacteria into electrophoretic types (ETs). Other techniques for establishing strain identity or nonidentity are pulsed-field gel electrophoresis and amplification of bacterial genomic sequences by polymerase chain reaction. The virulent III-1 clonal complex of serogroup A was first recognized in Nepal in 1983 to 1984; it spread to Mecca, then to sub-Saharan Africa, and subsequently to temperate Africa. Increased virulence and epidemic potential have also been ascribed to the serogroup B ET-5 complex, which was first identified in Norway in the 1970s and later caused outbreaks in Europe, Cuba, and South and North America (most recently, in the Pacific Northwest). Serogroup C ET-24 (the ET-37 complex) has caused sporadic cases and outbreaks in Canada and the United States and in some analyses has been associated with high mortality and morbidity.

Meningococcal colonization of the nasopharynx (asymptomatic carriage) can persist for months. In nonepidemic periods, ~10% of healthy individuals are colonized. Factors that predispose individuals to colonization with *N. meningitidis* include residence in the same household with a person who has meningococcal disease or is a carrier, household or institutional crowding, active or passive exposure to tobacco smoke, and a recent history of a viral upper respiratory infection. These factors have also been associated with an increased risk of meningococcal disease.

In countries with temperate climates, the attack rate for sporadic meningococcal disease is ~1 case per 100,000 persons per year. Peak disease incidence coincides with the winter peak of respiratory viral illnesses. Disease attack rates are highest among infants 3 to 9 months of age (10 to 15 cases per 100,000 infants per year). Children also have higher attack rates than adults, and there is a second peak of incidence among teenagers, in whom outbreaks have often been tied to residence in barracks, dormitories, or other crowded conditions. Although the age-specific incidence is much lower among adults (<1 case per 100,000 persons per year), approximately one-third of all cases of sporadic meningococcal disease occur in individuals ≥18 years of age. During epidemics, disease incidence increases disproportionately among teenagers and young adults and during the summer and autumn.

Meningococcal disease occurs more commonly in the household contacts of primary cases. The secondary attack rate is 400 to 1000 per 100,000 household members. School-based clusters of cases have also been described; the attack rate among school contacts of cases has been estimated at 2 to 4 cases per 100,000 exposed individuals. In outbreaks on college campuses, attack rates have been highest among students living in dormitories. Most secondary cases occur within 2 weeks of the primary case, although some may develop as long as several months later. Secondary cases account for <2% of all cases reported each year in the United States.

In an outbreak, the case isolates of *N. meningitidis* are identical when they are assessed by molecular typing methods. Recent outbreaks of meningococcal disease have occurred among persons whose common exposure took place in military barracks, schools, a university campus tavern, a jail, a school bus, a disco bar, a sports club, and a hotel.

PATHOGENESIS Meningococci that colonize the upper respiratory tract are internalized by nonciliated mucosal cells and may traverse them to enter the submucosa, from which they can make their way into the bloodstream. While meningococcal colonization occurs often in healthy humans, bloodstream infection is an infrequent event that is not essential for the organisms' survival and spread; as is often the case, the production of human disease has no obvious evolutionary advantage for either pathogen or host. Although some strains of *N. meningitidis* are thought to cause more severe disease in humans than do other strains, the basis for this difference is not understood. Meningococci may undergo important phenotypic changes when they adapt to growth in vivo; presumed virulence traits include the antiphagocytic capsular polysaccharide, an ability to sialylate the cell wall lipooligosaccharide (LOS) so that it mimics host cell carbohydrate moieties, the secretion of IgA protease, and mechanisms for iron acquisition. The ET-5 strain of serogroup B *N. meningitidis* has been associated with high case-fatality rates in some populations but not in others, however, suggesting that host factors also contribute importantly to disease pathogenesis.

A meningococcus that enters the blood from the nasopharynx and survives host defenses generally has one of two fates. If multiplication occurs slowly, the bacteria eventually seed local sites, such as the meninges, joints, or pericardium. More rapid multiplication in the blood is associated with disseminated intravascular coagulation (DIC) and shock, which usually cause symptoms before local sites become infected. There is thus a remarkable compartmentalization of bacterial growth and host inflammation in either the blood or a local site, usually the meninges.

Fulminant Meningococcemia (Purpura Fulminans) Fulminant meningococcemia is perhaps the most rapidly lethal form of septic shock experienced by humans. It differs from most other forms of septic shock by the prominence of hemorrhagic skin lesions (petechiae, purpura) and the consistent development of DIC.

The dominant proinflammatory molecule in the meningococcal cell wall is the endotoxin or LOS, and the outer membrane that contains it is poorly tethered to the underlying peptidoglycan. This structural peculiarity seems to account for the fact that meningococci shed LOS-containing membrane blebs as they grow. The bacteria can multiply to very high concentrations in the blood. The concentrations of endotoxin detected in the blood of patients with fulminant meningococcemia are 10- to 1000-fold greater than those found in the blood of patients with bacteremia due to other gram-negative bacteria. The bacteria and endotoxin-containing blebs stimulate monocytes, neutrophils, and endothelial cells, which then release cytokines and other mediators that can activate many distant targets, including other leukocytes and endothelial cells. In addition, meningococci can invade the vascular endothelium. When activated, the endothelium produces molecules that can be procoagulant as well as adhesive for leukocytes.

Patients with fulminant meningococcemia usually have extremely high blood levels of both proinflammatory mediators—i.e., tumor necrosis factor (TNF) α, interleukin (IL) 1, interferon γ, and IL-8—and anti-inflammatory mediators—i.e., IL-1 receptor antagonist (IL-1Ra), soluble IL-1 receptors, soluble TNF receptors, and IL-10. The plasma of patients with meningococcal shock can decrease the responses of normal leukocytes to stimuli such as LOS; the implication is that anti-inflammatory mediators predominate in the blood.

Procoagulant, antifibrinolytic forces are predominant in the blood of patients with fulminant meningococcemia (Fig. 146-1). Monocytes express large amounts of tissue factor. Fibrinopeptide A and thrombin-antithrombin levels are high, reflecting active clotting, while antithrombin and fibrinogen levels are low. Although the tissue factor–regulated ("extrinsic") arm of coagulation predominates, the contact system (factors XII and XI, prekallikrein, high-molecular-weight kininogen) is also activated. Striking deficiencies of antithrombin and proteins C and S can occur; studies have found a strong negative correlation between protein C activity and both the size of purpuric skin lesions and mortality. Plasminogen levels are decreased, while plas-

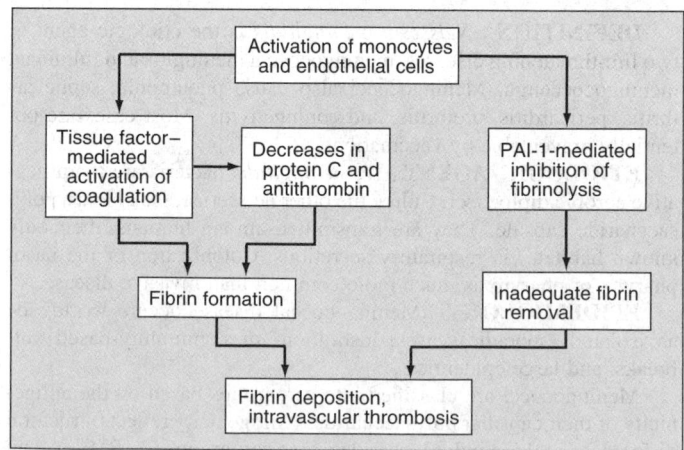

FIGURE 146-1 The pathogenesis of fibrin deposition in patients with fulminant meningococcemia. PAI-1, plasminogen activator inhibitor 1. *(Adapted from M Levi et al: Eur J Clin Invest 27:3, 1997.)*

min-antiplasmin complexes and plasminogen activator inhibitor 1 (PAI-1) levels in the blood are very high. PAI-1 levels have been correlated with mortality risk, as has a function-related polymorphism in the promoter of the PAI-1 gene.

Fibrin deposition is therefore favored both by the *procoagulant* tendency, promoted through activation of tissue factor and deficiencies of proteins C and S and antithrombin, and by an *antifibrinolytic* tendency, favored by excessive PAI-1. Both platelets and leukocytes doubtless contribute to the formation of microthrombi and to the vascular injury that ensues. Thrombosis of larger vessels leads to peripheral necrosis and gangrene that may require limb or digit amputation.

None of the candidate mediators of septic shock has proven primacy (Chaps. 38 and 124). Numerous studies have suggested that shock and DIC are not intimately linked and that the contact arm of clotting, which is of secondary importance in the pathogenesis of DIC, plays at least a contributory role in the pathogenesis of shock. The independence of DIC and shock suggests that therapies that prevent or reverse DIC may not be helpful for patients with septic shock.

Meningitis *N. meningitidis* has a striking tropism for the meninges. Infection of the central nervous system begins in the choroid plexus or in the ependyma that lines the cerebral ventricles. Meningococci adhere to cerebral capillary endothelial cells and then enter the subarachnoid space. A vigorous local inflammatory response ensues, probably triggered by endotoxin-containing meningococcal membranes. Both bacterial growth and the inflammatory response occur within the cerebrospinal fluid (CSF), where levels of endotoxin, IL-6, TNF-α, IL-1β, IL-1Ra, and IL-10 exceed the concentrations found in plasma by 100- to 1000-fold. The inflammatory response is largely confined to the subarachnoid space and contiguous structures.

Patients who develop meningitis may be individuals in whom meningococci do not grow rapidly in the blood; they may have a more vigorous initial inflammatory response to invading meningococci, may have antibodies or phagocytes that slow meningococcal growth, or may lack the (unknown) factors that allow *N. meningitidis* to multiply rapidly in vivo. The prognosis of patients with meningococcal meningitis is substantially better than that of patients with fulminant meningococcemia (Table 146-1).

HOST DEFENSE MECHANISMS Preventing meningococcal growth in blood requires bactericidal and opsonic antibodies, complement, and phagocytes (Fig. 146-2). The major bactericidal antibodies are IgM and IgG, which bind to the capsular polysaccharide. Immunity to meningococci is therefore serogroup specific. Antibodies to other surface (subcapsular) antigens may confer cross-serogroup protection. Infants are protected from meningococcal disease during the first months of life by passively transferred maternal IgG antibodies. As maternal antibody levels wane, the attack rate increases, peaking

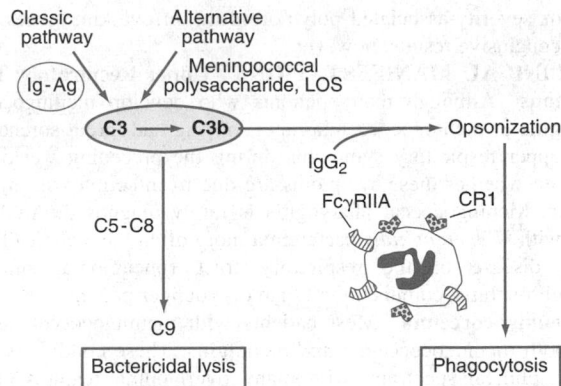

FIGURE 146-2 Protection from meningococcal disease involves both antimeningococcal immunoglobulins and complement. Activation of complement by antimeningococcal IgM or IgG promotes bacterial lysis via the membrane attack complex (C5–C9), while C3b (produced by either alternative or classic pathway activation) and antimeningococcal IgG$_2$ cooperate to produce effective opsonophagocytosis. A neutrophil defect in binding IgG$_2$ (the FcγRIIA R131 allele) has been associated with more severe meningococcal disease. CR1, complement receptor 1; LOS, lipooligosaccharide.

from 3 to 9 months of age. Disease incidence declines as protective antibodies are induced by colonization with nonpathogenic bacteria that have cross-reactive antigens. In addition to *N. lactamica*, which frequently colonizes young children, some enteric bacteria have antigens that cross-react with those of meningococci. One theory relates the occurrence of meningococcal disease to the presence of high levels of IgA antibodies to meningococci, since these antibodies can block the bactericidal activity of IgM.

Complement is required for bactericidal activity and for efficient opsonophagocytosis. Individuals deficient in any of the late complement components (C5 to C9) cannot assemble the membrane attack complex needed to kill *Neisseria*. These persons typically develop less severe meningococcal disease than complement-sufficient individuals, do so at an older age, and tend to have disease due to uncommon serogroups (W-135, X, Y, Z, and 29E). Although only one-half of individuals with known late-complement-component deficiency ever experience meningococcal disease, some affected persons have several episodes. Deficiency of each of the terminal complement components is inherited in an autosomal recessive fashion. Properdin deficiency, in contrast, is X-linked; some affected males develop overwhelming meningococcal disease, an observation indicating that the alternative complement pathway is also needed for antimeningococcal host defense. The age of disease onset in properdin-deficient individuals is typically in the teens or twenties.

Activation of the classic pathway of complement by antigen-antibody complexes or of the alternative pathway by LOS or capsular polysaccharide is important for producing and maintaining C3b (Fig. 146-2). Without C3b, neither bactericidal lysis nor phagocytosis can proceed effectively. When C3b is generated, meningococcal growth is probably checked by the membrane attack complex, which produces bacterial lysis, and by robust phagocytosis. Most IgG antibodies to the meningococcal polysaccharide are of the IgG$_2$ isotype; a phagocytic cell defect (the FcγRIIA R131 allele) that impairs the phagocytosis of IgG$_2$-coated particles has been associated with more severe meningococcal disease. This allele has also been associated with a more severe clinical course in patients with late-complement-component deficiency; thus effective phagocytosis may contribute to the relatively mild meningococcal disease usually observed in these individuals.

Indirect evidence indicates that persons who mount a vigorous inflammatory response to meningococcal LOS may experience less severe disease than those whose initial response is anti-inflammatory. This observation suggests that the inflammatory response may be critical for restraining meningococcal growth. Attempts to identify dis-

Table 146-1 Clinical Spectrum of Meningococcal Meningitis and Fulminant Meningococcemia

Feature	Fulminant Meningococcemia	Meningococcal Meningitis
Interval from onset of symptoms to presentation for medical care	Short (median, 12 h)	Longer ($\geq$1 day)
Symptoms, signs	Prostration, petechiae/purpura, fever	Fever, headache, meningismus, altered mental status, seizures
CSF culture	Often negative	Usually positive
CSF endotoxin, cytokine levels	Low	High
Blood endotoxin, cytokine levels	High	Low
Case-fatality rate	20–40%	3–10%
Fraction of total cases	~10–30%	~30–40%

NOTE: CSF, cerebrospinal fluid.

ease- or severity-associated polymorphisms in cytokine genes have had inconclusive results, however.

CLINICAL MANIFESTATIONS   Upper Respiratory Tract Infections   Although many patients who develop meningococcal meningitis or meningococcemia report having had throat soreness or other upper respiratory symptoms during the preceding week, it is uncertain whether these symptoms are due to infection with meningococci. Meningococcal pharyngitis is rarely diagnosed. Adult patients with *N. meningitidis* bacteremia more often have clinically apparent disease of the respiratory tract (pneumonia, sinusitis, tracheobronchitis, conjunctivitis) than do younger patients.

Meningococcemia   Most patients with meningococcal disease have both meningococcemia *and* meningitis. These conditions have a wide clinical spectrum, with many overlapping features (Table 146-1).

Approximately 10 to 30% of patients with meningococcal disease have meningococcemia without clinically apparent meningitis. Although meningococcemia is occasionally transient and asymptomatic, in most individuals it is associated with fever, chills, nausea, vomiting, and myalgias. Prostration is common. The most distinctive feature is rash. Erythematous macules rapidly become petechial and, in severe cases, purpuric. Although the lesions are typically found on the trunk and lower extremities, they may also occur on the face, arms, and mucous membranes. The petechiae may coalesce into hemorrhagic bullae or may undergo necrosis and ulcerate. Patients with severe coagulopathy may develop ischemic extremities or digits, often with a sharp line of demarcation between normal and ischemic tissue.

In many patients with fulminant meningococcemia, the CSF is normal and the CSF culture is negative. Indeed, the absence of meningitis in a patient with meningococcemia is a poor prognostic sign; it suggests that the bacteria have multiplied so rapidly in the blood that meningeal seeding has not yet had time to elicit inflammation in the CSF. Most of these patients also lack evidence of an acute-phase response; i.e., the erythrocyte sedimentation rate is normal, and the C-reactive protein concentration in blood is low.

The Waterhouse-Friderichsen syndrome is a dramatic example of DIC-induced microthrombosis, hemorrhage, and tissue injury. Although overt adrenal failure is infrequently documented in patients with fulminant meningococcemia, patients may have partial adrenal insufficiency and be unable to mount the normal hypercortisolemic response to severe stress or cosyntropin stimulation. Almost all patients who die from fulminant meningococcemia have adrenal hemorrhages at autopsy.

Chronic meningococcemia is a rare syndrome of episodic fever, rash, and arthralgias that can last for weeks to months. The rash may be maculopapular; it is occasionally petechial. Splenomegaly may develop. If untreated or if treated with glucocorticoids, chronic meningococcemia may evolve into meningitis, fulminant meningococcemia, or (rarely) endocarditis.

Meningitis (See also Chap. 372)   Patients with meningococcal meningitis have usually been sick for ≥24 h before they seek medical attention. Common presenting symptoms include nausea and vomiting, headache, neck stiffness, lethargy, and confusion. The symptoms and signs of meningococcal meningitis cannot be distinguished from those elicited by other meningeal pathogens. Many patients with meningococcal meningitis have concurrent meningococcemia, however, and petechial or purpuric skin lesions may suggest the correct diagnosis. CSF findings are consistent with those of purulent meningitis: hypoglycorrhachia, an elevated protein concentration, and a neutrophilic leukocytosis. A Gram's stain of CSF is usually positive (see "Diagnosis," below); when this finding is unaccompanied by CSF leukocytosis, the prognosis for normal recovery is often poor.

Other Manifestations   Arthritis occurs in ~10% of patients with meningococcal disease. When arthritis develops during the first few days of the patient's illness, it usually reflects direct meningococcal invasion of the joint. Arthritis that begins later in the course is thought to be due to immune complex deposition. Primary meningococcal pneumonia occurs principally in adults, often in military populations, and is most often due to serogroup Y. While meningococcal pericarditis is occasionally seen, endocarditis due to *N. meningitidis* is now exceedingly rare. Primary meningococcal conjunctivitis can be complicated by meningococcemia; systemic therapy is therefore warranted when this condition is diagnosed. Meningococcal urethritis has been reported in individuals who practice oral sex.

Complications   Patients with meningococcal meningitis may develop cranial nerve palsies, cortical venous thrombophlebitis, and cerebral edema. In children subdural effusions may occur. Permanent sequelae can include mental retardation, deafness, and hemiparesis. The major long-term morbidity of fulminant meningococcemia is the loss of skin, limbs, or digits that results from ischemic necrosis and infarction.

DIAGNOSIS   Few clinical clues help the physician distinguish the patient with early meningococcal disease from patients with other acute systemic infections. The most useful clinical finding is the petechial or purpuric rash **(see Plate IID-44)**, but it must be differentiated from the petechial lesions seen with gonococcemia **(see Plate IID-60)**, Rocky Mountain spotted fever **(see Plate IID-45)**, hypersensitivity vasculitis **(see Plate IIE-71)**, endemic typhus, and some viruses. In one case series, one-half of the adults with meningococcal bacteremia had neither meningitis nor a rash.

The definitive diagnosis is established by recovering *N. meningitidis*, its antigens, or its DNA from normally sterile body fluids, such as blood, CSF, or synovial fluid, or from skin lesions. Meningococci grow best on Mueller-Hinton or chocolate blood agar at 35°C in an atmosphere that contains 5 to 10% CO_2. Specimens should be plated without delay. *N. meningitidis* bacteria are oxidase-positive, gram-negative diplococci that typically utilize maltose and glucose.

A Gram's stain of CSF reveals intra- or extracellular organisms in ~85% of patients with meningococcal meningitis. The latex agglutination test for meningococcal polysaccharides is somewhat less sensitive. Reports suggest that polymerase chain reaction amplification of DNA in buffy coat or CSF samples may be more sensitive than either of these tests, and, like the latex agglutination test, this method is not affected by prior antibiotic therapy.

Throat or nasopharyngeal specimens should be cultured on Thayer-Martin medium, which suppresses the competing oral flora. Throat or nasopharyngeal cultures are recommended only for research or epidemiologic purposes, since a positive result merely confirms the carrier state and does not establish the existence of systemic disease.

℞ TREATMENT   A second-generation cephalosporin, such as cefotaxime (2 g intravenously every 8 h) or ceftriaxone (1 g intravenously every 12 h), is preferred for initial therapy, as it may cover other bacteria (such as *Streptococcus pneumoniae* and *Haemophilus influenzae*) that can cause the same syndromes (Chap. 372). Penicillin G (4 million units intravenously every 4 h) remains an acceptable alternative in most countries; high-level penicillin resistance has been reported from Spain. In the patient who is allergic to β-lactam drugs, chloramphenicol (75 to 100 mg/kg every 6 h) is a suitable alternative; chloramphenicol-resistant meningococci have been reported from Vietnam and France, however. Although some cases of mild disease may be cured with only 2 days of treatment, most patients with meningococcal meningitis should be given antimicrobial therapy for at least 5 days. While glucocorticoid therapy for meningitis in adults is controversial, many experts administer dexamethasone, beginning if possible before antibiotic therapy is initiated (Chap. 372).

Patients with fulminant meningococcemia often experience diffuse leakage of fluid into extravascular spaces, shock, and multiple-organ dysfunction (Chaps. 38 and 124). Myocardial depression may be prominent. Supportive therapy has never been studied in randomized, placebo-controlled trials. Standard measures include vigorous fluid resuscitation (often requiring several liters over the first 24 h), elective ventilation, and pressors (epinephrine or dopamine). Some authorities recommend early hemodialysis or hemofiltration. Fresh frozen plasma is often given to patients who are bleeding extensively or who have severely deranged clotting parameters. Many European experts prefer to administer antithrombin to such patients. Patients with fulminant meningococcemia in whom shock persists despite vigorous fluid resuscitation should receive supplemental glucocorticoid treatment (hydrocortisone, 1 mg/kg every 6 h) pending tests of adrenal reserve. Investigational drugs for fulminant meningococcemia include bactericidal permeability-increasing (BPI) protein—a bactericidal neutrophil protein that binds and neutralizes meningococcal LOS—as well as several anticoagulants (activated protein C, antithrombin, and tissue factor pathway inhibitor). In a recent clinical trial, recombinant BPI protein reduced long-term complications in children with fulminant meningococcemia without definitely reducing mortality.

PROGNOSIS When patients are first evaluated, the clinical features most strongly associated with a fatal outcome are shock, a purpuric or ecchymotic rash, a low or normal blood leukocyte count, an age ≥60 years, and coma. The absence of meningitis, the presence of thrombocytopenia, low blood concentrations of antithrombin or proteins S and C, high blood levels of PAI-1, and a low erythrocyte sedimentation rate (or C-reactive protein level) have also been associated with increased mortality from meningococcal disease. In contrast, having received antibiotics prior to hospital admission has been associated with lower mortality in some studies.

PREVENTION Meningococcal Polysaccharide Vaccines A single injection of quadrivalent meningococcal polysaccharide vaccine (serogroups A, C, W-135, and Y) immunizes ~80 to 95% of immunocompetent adults. Children ≥3 months of age can be vaccinated to prevent serogroup A disease, but multiple doses are required; the vaccine is otherwise ineffective in children <2 years old. The duration of vaccine-induced immunity in adults is probably <5 years. There is currently no vaccine for serogroup B; its polysaccharide is a sialic acid homopolymer that is poorly immunogenic in humans. In addition to individuals with late-complement-component or properdin deficiency, persons with sickle cell anemia, asplenia, or splenectomy should receive the quadrivalent vaccine. Vaccination is also recommended for military recruits and for individuals traveling to sub-Saharan Africa during the dry months (June to December) or to other areas with epidemic meningococcal disease. Some authorities recommend vaccination of incoming college freshmen who will live in dormitories. In general, the vaccine should be given only to persons ≥2 years of age. Investigational polysaccharide-protein conjugate meningococcal vaccines appear promising; a serogroup C conjugate vaccine was licensed for use in the United Kingdom in 1999.

Screening tests for late-complement-component deficiency should be done in family members of patients who have a family history of meningococcal disease, in patients who have a recurrence, in those whose first case occurs at ≥15 years of age, and in those with cases caused by serogroups other than A, B, or C.

Antimicrobial Chemoprophylaxis The attack rate for meningococcal disease among household contacts of cases is ~500-fold greater than that in the population as a whole. Close contacts of cases should receive chemoprophylaxis with rifampin (adult dosage, 600 mg orally every 12 h for four doses), ciprofloxacin (a single oral dose of 500 mg), or ofloxacin (a single oral dose of 400 mg). A single intramuscular injection of ceftriaxone (250 mg) is also effective. Close contacts include persons who live in the same household, day-care center contacts, and anyone directly exposed to the patient's oral secretions. Casual contacts are not at increased risk. Chemoprophylaxis should be administered as soon as possible after the case is identified.

Isolation Precautions The Centers for Disease Control and Prevention recommend that patients with meningococcal disease who are hospitalized be placed in respiratory isolation for the first 24 h.

Outbreak Control An organization- or community-based outbreak of meningococcal disease is defined as the occurrence of three or more cases within ≤3 months in persons who have a common affiliation or reside in the same area but who are not close contacts of one another; in addition, the primary disease attack rate must exceed

10 cases per 100,000 persons, and the case strains of *N. meningitidis* must be of the same molecular type. Mass vaccination should be considered when such outbreaks occur, and mass chemoprophylaxis may be used to control school- or other institution-based outbreaks. Consultation with public health authorities is recommended when such campaigns are contemplated.

BIBLIOGRAPHY

BRANDTZAEG P et al: Net inflammatory capacity of human septic shock plasma evaluated by a monocyte-based target cell assay: Identification of interleukin-10 as a major functional deactivator of human monocytes. J Exp Med 184:51, 1996

CENTERS FOR DISEASE CONTROL AND PREVENTION: Control and prevention of meningococcal disease. MMWR 46 (RR-5), 1997

FIJEN CA et al: Assessment of complement deficiency in patients with meningococcal disease in the Netherlands. Clin Infect Dis 28:98, 1999

KIRSCH EA et al: Pathophysiology, treatment and outcome of meningococcemia: A review and recent experience. Pediatr Infect Dis J 15:967, 1996

LEVIN P et al: Recombinant bactericidal/permeability-increasing protein (rBPI21) as adjunctive treatment for children with severe meningococcal sepsis: A randomised trial. Lancet 356:961, 2000

MACDONALD NE et al: Induction of immunologic memory by conjugated vs plain meningococcal C polysaccharide vaccine in toddlers—a randomized controlled trial. JAMA 280:1685, 1998

PLATONOV AE et al: Meningococcal disease and polymorphism of FcγRIIA (CD32) in late complement component–deficient individuals. Clin Exp Immunol 111:97, 1998

ROSENSTEIN N et al: Efficacy of meningococcal vaccine and barriers to vaccination. JAMA 279:435, 1998

———— et al: The changing epidemiology of meningococcal disease in the United States, 1992–1996. J Infect Dis 180:1894, 1999

STEPHENS DS et al: Sporadic meningococcal disease in adults: Results of a 5-year population-based study. Ann Intern Med 123:937, 1995

WESTENDORP RGJ et al: Genetic influence on cytokine production and fatal meningococcal disease. Lancet 349:170, 1997

147 Sanjay Ram, Peter A. Rice

GONOCOCCAL INFECTIONS

DEFINITION Gonorrhea is a sexually transmitted infection of epithelium and commonly manifests as cervicitis, urethritis, proctitis, and conjunctivitis. If untreated, infections at these sites can lead to local complications such as endometritis, salpingitis, tuboovarian abscess, bartholinitis, peritonitis, and perihepatitis in the female; periurethritis and epididymitis in the male; and ophthalmia neonatorum in the newborn. Disseminated gonococcemia is an uncommon event whose manifestations include skin lesions, tenosynovitis, arthritis, and (in rare cases) endocarditis or meningitis.

Neisseria gonorrhoeae is a gram-negative, nonmotile, non-spore-forming organism that grows in pairs (diplococci). Each individual organism is shaped like a coffee bean, with adjacent concave sides seen on Gram's stain. Gonococci, like all other *Neisseria* spp., are oxidase positive. They are distinguished from other *Neisseria* by their ability to grow on selective media and to utilize glucose but not maltose, sucrose, or lactose.

EPIDEMIOLOGY The incidence of gonorrhea has declined significantly in the United States, but there are still ~315,000 newly reported cases each year. Gonorrhea remains a major public health problem worldwide, is a significant cause of morbidity in developing countries, and may play a role in enhancing transmission of HIV.

Gonorrhea predominantly affects young, nonwhite, unmarried, less educated members of urban populations. The number of reported cases probably represents half of the true number of cases—a discrepancy resulting from underreporting, self-treatment, and nonspecific treatment without a culture-proven diagnosis. The number of reported cases of gonorrhea in the United States rose from ~250,000 in the early 1960s to a high of 1.01 million in 1978. The peak recorded incidence of gonorrhea in modern times was noted in 1975, with 468 cases per 100,000 population in the United States. This peak was attributable to the interaction of several variables, including improved accuracy of diagnosis, changes in patterns of contraceptive use, and changes in sexual behavior. The incidence of the disease has since gradually declined and is currently estimated at 120 cases per 100,000, a figure that is still the highest among industrialized countries. A further decline in the overall incidence of gonorrhea in the United States over the past decade may reflect increased condom use resulting from public health efforts to curtail HIV transmission. Presently, the attack rate in the United States is highest in the 20- to 24-year age group, in which 75% of all cases occur. With adjustment for sexual experience, the risk is highest among sexually active 15- to 19-year-old women. In terms of ethnicity, rates are highest among African-Americans and lowest among persons of Asian or Pacific Island descent.

The highest incidence of gonorrhea occurs in developing countries. The exact incidence of any of the sexually transmitted diseases (STDs) is difficult to ascertain in developing countries because of limited surveillance and variable diagnostic criteria. For example, in Kenya, it was estimated in 1987 that 10% of all live births were adversely affected by STDs, and gonococcal ophthalmia neonatorum reportedly affected 4% of all live-born infants. The median prevalence of gonorrhea in unselected populations of pregnant women has been estimated at 10% in Africa, 5% in Latin America, and 4% in Asia. Studies in Africa have clearly demonstrated that nonulcerative STDs such as gonorrhea are an independent risk factor for the transmission of HIV (Chap. 309).

Gonorrhea is transmitted from males to females more efficiently than in the opposite direction. The rate of transmission to a woman following a single unprotected sexual encounter with an infected man is on the order of 40 to 60%. Oropharyngeal gonorrhea occurs in ~20% of women who practice fellatio with infected partners. Transmission in either direction by cunnilingus is rare.

There exists in any population a small minority of individuals who have high rates of new partner acquisition. These "core-group members" or "high-frequency transmitters" are vital in sustaining STD transmission at the population level. Another instrumental factor in sustaining gonorrhea in the population is the large number of infected individuals who are asymptomatic or have minor symptoms that are ignored. These persons, unlike symptomatic individuals, do not cease sexual activity and therefore continue to transmit the disease. This situation underscores the importance of contact tracing and empirical treatment of sex partners of index cases.

PATHOGENESIS AND IMMUNOLOGY   Outer-Membrane Proteins • Pili   Fresh clinical isolates of *N. gonorrhoeae* initially form piliated (fimbriated) colonies distinguishable on translucent agar. Pilus expression is rapidly switched off with unselected subculture because of rearrangements in pilus genes. This change is a basis for phase variation of gonococci. Piliated strains adhere better to cells derived from human mucosal surfaces and are more virulent in organ culture models and human inoculation experiments than nonpiliated variants. In a fallopian tube explant model, pili mediate gonococcal attachment to nonciliated columnar epithelial cells. This event initiates gonococcal phagocytosis and transport through these cells to intercellular spaces near the basement membrane or directly into the subepithelial tissue. Damage to nearby ciliated columnar epithelial cells, which is caused by the release of cytokines, results in loss of cilia and sloughing of ciliated cells and diminishes the integrity of the fallopian tube. Nonpiliated gonococci cause epithelial damage at a much slower rate. CD46 (membrane cofactor protein) is present on urogenital epithelial cells in both men and women and has been determined to be a receptor for PilC; this subunit is located at the tip of the pilus molecule and is critical in mediating adherence. Pili are also essential for genetic competence and transformation of *N. gonorrhoeae*, which permits horizontal transfer of genetic material between different gonococcal lineages in vivo.

Opacity-associated protein   Another gonococcal surface protein that is important in adherence to epithelial cells is opacity-associated protein (Opa, formerly called protein II). Opa contributes to intergonococcal adhesion, which is responsible for the opaque nature of gonococcal colonies on translucent agar and the organism's adherence to a variety of eukaryotic cells, including polymorphonuclear leukocytes (PMNs). Certain Opa variants promote invasion of epithelial cells, and this effect has been linked with the ability of Opa to bind vitronectin, glycosaminoglycans, and several members of the carcinoembryonic antigen family (CD66). Each strain of *N. gonorrhoeae* possesses as many as 11 different *opa* genes, but usually only up to 3 types are expressed at any given time. Isolates from normally sterile sites such as the fallopian tube and synovial fluid usually fail to express Opa, while isolates from mucosal sites usually form opaque colonies. Female commercial sex workers with antibodies to Opa may be less likely to develop pelvic inflammatory disease (PID) than women without such antibodies.

Porin   Porin (previously designated protein I) is the most abundant gonococcal surface protein, accounting for >50% of the organism's total outer-membrane protein. Porin molecules exist as trimers that provide anion aqueous channels through the otherwise hydrophobic outer membrane. Porin shows stable interstrain antigenic variation and forms the basis for gonococcal serotyping. Two main serotypes have been identified: Por1A strains are often associated with disseminated gonococcal infection (DGI), while Por1B strains usually cause local genital infections only. DGI strains are generally resistant to the killing action of normal human serum, do not incite a significant local inflammatory response, and therefore may not cause symptoms at genital sites. These characteristics may be related to the ability of Por1A strains to bind complement-downregulatory molecules, resulting in a diminished inflammatory response. Porin can translocate to the cytoplasmic membrane of host cells—a process that could initiate gonococcal endocytosis and invasion. In addition, porin is an immunologic target of bactericidal and opsonophagocytic antibodies that may arise in response to immune stimulation resulting from infection or immunization with porin-containing vaccine candidates.

Other outer-membrane proteins   Other notable outer-membrane proteins include H.8, a lipoprotein that is present on the surface of all gonococcal strains in high concentration and is an excellent target for antibody-based diagnostic testing, as well as transferrin-binding proteins (Tbp1 and Tbp2) and lactoferrin-binding protein, which are required for scavenging iron from transferrin and lactoferrin in vivo. Transferrin and iron have been shown to increase attachment of iron-deprived *N. gonorrhoeae* to human endometrial cells. Gonococci deficient in transferrin- and lactoferrin-binding proteins cannot establish infection in male volunteers. IgA1 protease is produced by *N. gonorrhoeae* and may protect the organism from the action of mucosal IgA.

Lipooligosaccharide   Gonococcal lipooligosaccharide (LOS) consists of a lipid A and a core oligosaccharide that lacks the repeating O-carbohydrate antigenic side chain seen in other gram-negative bacteria (Chap. 120). Gonococcal LOS possesses marked endotoxic activity and contributes to the local cytotoxic effect in the fallopian tube model. LOS core sugars undergo a high degree of antigenic variation under different conditions of growth; this variation reflects genetic regulation and expression of glycotransferase genes that dictate the carbohydrate structure of LOS. These phenotypic changes may affect interactions of *N. gonorrhoeae* with elements of the humoral immune system (antibodies and complement) and may also influence direct binding of organisms to both professional and nonprofessional phagocytes (epithelial cells). For example, gonococci that are sialylated at their LOS sites bind complement factor H and downregulate the alternative pathway of complement. LOS sialylation may also mask bactericidal antibody–binding epitopes on LOS and porin and may decrease opsonophagocytosis and inhibit the oxidative burst in PMNs. While sialylation of LOS confers on the bacteria the ability to attenuate the inflammatory response and evade the innate immune system, experiments in male volunteers suggest that sialylated gonococci may be less capable of establishing infection than their unsialylated counterparts. This difference could be explained by the observation that the unsialylated terminal lactosamine residue of LOS binds to an asialoglycoprotein receptor on epithelial cells that would otherwise facilitate binding and subsequent gonococcal invasion of these cells.

Host Factors In addition to gonococcal structures that interact with epithelial cells, host factors seem to be important in mediating entry of gonococci into nonphagocytic cells. Activation of phosphatidylcholine-specific phospholipase C and acidic sphingomyelinase by *N. gonorrhoeae*, which results in the release of diacylglycerol and ceramide, is an essential requirement for the entry of *N. gonorrhoeae* into epithelial cells. Ceramide accumulation within cells leads to apoptosis, which may disrupt epithelial integrity and facilitate entry of gonococci into subepithelial tissue. Release of chemotactic factors as a result of complement activation contributes to inflammation, as does the toxic effect of LOS in provoking the release of inflammatory cytokines.

The importance of humoral immunity in host defenses against neisserial infections is best illustrated by the predisposition of persons deficient in terminal complement components (C5 through C9) to recurrent bacteremic gonococcal infections and to recurrent meningococcal meningitis or meningococcemia. Gonococcal porin induces T cell proliferative responses in persons with urogenital gonococcal disease. A significant increase in porin-specific interleukin (IL) 4−producing CD4+ as well as CD8+ lymphocytes is seen in individuals with mucosal gonococcal disease. A portion of these lymphocytes that show a porin-specific T_H2-type response could traffic to mucosal surfaces and play a role in immune protection against the disease. Few data clearly indicate that protective immunity is acquired from a previous gonococcal infection, although bactericidal and opsonophagocytic antibodies to porin and LOS may offer partial protection. On the other hand, women who are infected and acquire high levels of antibody to another outer-membrane protein, Rmp (reduction modifiable protein, formerly called protein III), may be especially likely to become reinfected with *N. gonorrhoeae* because Rmp antibodies block the effect of bactericidal antibodies to porin and LOS. Rmp shows little, if any, interstrain antigenic variation; therefore, Rmp antibodies potentially may block antibody-mediated killing of all gonococci. The mechanism of blocking has not been fully characterized, but Rmp antibodies noncompetitively inhibit binding of porin and LOS antibodies because of the proximity of these structures in the gonococcal outer membrane. Less well understood is how blocking antibody may divert complement binding to the gonococcal surface or otherwise hasten inactivation of complement. In male volunteers who have no history of gonorrhea, the net effect of these events may influence the outcome of experimental challenge with *N. gonorrhoeae*. Because Rmp bears extensive homology to enterobacterial OmpA and meningococcal class 4 proteins, it is possible that these blocking antibodies result from prior exposure to cross-reacting proteins from these species and also play a role in first-time infection with *N. gonorrhoeae*.

CLINICAL MANIFESTATIONS **Gonococcal Infection in Males** Acute urethritis is the most common clinical manifestation of gonorrhea in males. The usual incubation period following exposure is 2 to 7 days, although the interval can be longer and some men remain asymptomatic. Strains of the Por1A serotype, with nutritional requirements for arginine, hypoxanthine, and uracil (i.e., the AHU auxotype), tend to cause a greater proportion of cases of mild and asymptomatic urethritis than Por1B strains. Urethral discharge and dysuria, usually without urinary frequency or urgency, are the major symptoms. The discharge initially is scant and mucoid but becomes profuse and purulent within a day or two. The clinical manifestations of gonococcal urethritis are usually more severe and overt than those of nongonococcal urethritis, including urethritis caused by *Chlamydia trachomatis* (Chap. 179); however, exceptions are common, and it is often impossible to differentiate the causes of urethritis on clinical grounds alone. Most symptomatic males seek treatment and cease to be infectious. The remaining men, who are largely asymptomatic, accumulate in number over time and constitute about two-thirds of all infected men

at any point in time. Together with men incubating the organism (who shed the organism but are asymptomatic), they serve as the source of spread of infection. Prior to the antibiotic era, symptoms of urethritis persisted for about 8 weeks. Epididymitis is now an uncommon complication, and gonococcal prostatitis occurs rarely, if at all. Other unusual local complications of gonococcal urethritis include edema of the penis due to dorsal lymphangitis or thrombophlebitis, submucous inflammatory "soft" infiltration of the urethral wall, periurethral abscess or fistulae, inflammation or abscess of Cowper's gland, and seminal vesiculitis. Balanitis may develop in uncircumcised men. After a decline in gonococcal infections among homosexual men early in the era of AIDS, a disturbing increase in gonorrhea was observed among young homosexual men in the 1990s, probably related to decreased condom use. The clinical features of anorectal and pharyngeal gonorrhea are discussed below.

Gonococcal Infections in Females • *Gonococcal cervicitis* Mucopurulent cervicitis is the most common STD diagnosis in American women and may be caused by *N. gonorrhoeae*, *C. trachomatis*, and other organisms. Cervicitis may coexist with candidal or trichomonal vaginitis. *N. gonorrhoeae* primarily infects the cervical os but can also infect more peripheral areas of the cervix where columnar epithelium meets stratified squamous epithelium. Except in rare instances, the vaginal mucosa, which is lined by stratified squamous epithelium, does not become infected. Bartholin's glands occasionally become infected.

Women infected with *N. gonorrhoeae* usually develop symptoms. However, the women who either remain asymptomatic or have only minor symptoms may delay in seeking medical attention. Increased vaginal discharge and dysuria (often without urgency or frequency) are the most common symptoms. Although the incubation period of gonorrhea is less well defined in women than in men, symptoms usually develop within 10 days of infection and are more acute and intense than those of chlamydial cervicitis.

The physical examination may reveal a mucopurulent discharge (mucopus) issuing from the cervical os. The examiner may check for mucopurulent discharge by swabbing a sample of mucus from the endocervix and observing its color against the white background of the swab; yellow or green mucus suggests mucopus. However, only 35% of women with gonococcal cervicitis actually have a mucopurulent discharge defined by these criteria. Since Gram's stain is not sensitive for the diagnosis of gonorrhea in women, specimens should be submitted for culture or a nonculture assay (see below). Edematous and friable cervical ectopy as well as endocervical bleeding induced by gentle swabbing are more often seen in chlamydial infection.

N. gonorrhoeae may be recovered from the urethra and rectum of women with cervicitis, but these are rarely the sole infected sites. Urethritis in women may produce symptoms of internal dysuria, which is often attributed to "cystitis." Pyuria in the absence of bacteriuria seen on Gram's stain of unspun urine, accompanied by urine cultures that fail to yield $>10^5$ colonies of bacteria usually associated with urinary tract infection, signifies the possibility of urethritis due to *C. trachomatis*. Urethral infection with *N. gonorrhoeae* may also occur in this context, but in this instance urethral cultures will usually be positive. Compression of the urethra through the anterior vaginal wall against the symphysis pubis may express urethral exudate.

Complications of gonococcal cervicitis Gonococcal infection may extend deep enough to produce dyspareunia and lower abdominal or back pain. In such cases, it is imperative to consider a diagnosis of PID and to administer treatment for that disease (Chap. 133). Ascending infection of the genital tract follows ~20% of cases of gonococcal cervicitis and may result in acute endometritis accompanied by abnormal menstrual bleeding, midline lower abdominal pain and tenderness, and dyspareunia. Spread to the fallopian tubes results in acute salpingitis, whose symptoms may be accompanied by signs of cervical motion tenderness and abnormal adnexal mass on pelvic examination. Patients may be febrile, and leukocytosis and an elevated erythrocyte sedimentation rate or C-reactive protein level may be detected. Co-infection with *C. trachomatis* may increase the risk of PID, which is the clinical counterpart of endometritis and salpingitis. Tubal scarring leading to infertility is the most devastating sequela of salpingitis; the increased risk of ectopic pregnancy is also significant. Prompt and appropriate antibiotic therapy for gonococcal salpingitis (prior to the development of an adnexal mass) can prevent tubal infertility in nearly all cases. Bilateral tubal damage occurs in ~20% of women with an adnexal mass. More than half of women with tubal infertility give no history of PID. These women with "silent salpingitis" may report abdominal or pelvic discomfort (such as dysmenorrhea or dyspareunia) that may be attributed to other diagnoses (such as endometriosis). Spread of infection to the pelvis may result in pelvic peritonitis characterized by nausea and vomiting. Spread of gonococci—or, more commonly, of chlamydiae—via the peritoneal cavity to the upper abdomen may cause perihepatitis (Fitz-Hugh–Curtis syndrome; Chap. 133).

Gonococcal vaginitis The vaginal mucosa of healthy women is lined by stratified squamous epithelium and is usually not infected by *N. gonorrhoeae*. However, gonococcal vaginitis can occur in anestrogenic women (e.g., prepubertal girls and postmenopausal women), in whom the vaginal stratified squamous epithelial layers are often thinned down to the basilar layer, which can be infected by *N. gonorrhoeae*. The intense inflammation of the vagina makes the physical (speculum and bimanual) examination extremely painful. The vaginal mucosa is red and edematous, and an abundant purulent discharge is present. Infection in the urethra and in Skene's and Bartholin's glands often accompanies gonococcal vaginitis. Inflamed cervical erosion or abscesses in nabothian cysts may also occur. Coexisting cervicitis may result in pus in the cervical os.

Anorectal Gonorrhea Because the female anatomy permits the spread of cervical exudate to the rectum, *N. gonorrhoeae* is sometimes recovered from the rectum of women with uncomplicated gonococcal cervicitis. The rectum is the sole site of infection in only 5% of women with gonorrhea. Such women are usually asymptomatic but occasionally have acute proctitis manifested by anorectal pain or pruritus, tenesmus, purulent rectal discharge, and rectal bleeding. Among homosexual men, the frequency of gonococcal infection, including rectal infection, fell by ≥90% throughout the United States in the early 1980s, but a resurgence of gonorrhea among homosexual men was documented in several cities during the 1990s. Gonococcal isolates from the rectum of homosexual men tend to be more resistant than other gonococcal isolates to antimicrobials. Gonococci with multidrug resistance (*mtr*) are more resistant to bile salts and fatty acids in feces and thus are found with increased frequency in homosexual men. The *mtr* mutation involves a DNA-binding protein and results in the derepression of genes encoding an efflux mechanism of resistance. This situation may have been responsible for higher rates of treatment failure for rectal gonorrhea with older regimens consisting of penicillin or tetracyclines.

Pharyngeal Gonorrhea Pharyngeal gonorrhea is usually mild or asymptomatic, although symptomatic pharyngitis does occasionally occur with cervical lymphadenitis. The mode of acquisition is oral-genital sexual exposure, with fellatio being a more efficient means of transmission than cunnilingus. Most cases resolve spontaneously, and transmission from the pharynx to sexual contacts is rare. Pharyngeal infection almost always coexists with genital infection. Swabs from the pharynx should be plated directly onto gonococcal selective media. Because pharyngeal colonization with *N. meningitidis* needs to be differentiated from that with other *Neisseria* species, the diagnosis of pharyngeal gonorrhea is more expensive and difficult than that of anogenital gonorrhea.

Ocular Gonorrhea in Adults Ocular gonorrhea in an adult usually results from autoinoculation from an infected genital site. As in genital infection, the manifestations range from severe to occasionally mild or asymptomatic disease. The variability in clinical manifesta-tions may result from differences in the ability of the infecting strain to elicit an inflammatory response.

Infection may result in a markedly swollen eyelid, severe hyperemia and chemosis, and a profuse purulent discharge. The massively inflamed conjunctiva may be draped over the cornea and limbus. Lytic enzymes from the infiltrating PMNs occasionally cause corneal ulceration and rarely cause perforation.

Prompt recognition and treatment of this condition are of paramount importance. Gram's stain and culture of the purulent discharge establish the diagnosis. Genital cultures should also be performed.

Gonorrhea in Pregnant Women, Neonates, and Children Gonorrhea in pregnancy can have serious consequences for both the mother and the infant. Therefore, early detection and eradication of the disease in the mother are extremely important. Recognition of gonorrhea early in pregnancy also identifies a population at risk for other STDs, particularly *Chlamydia* infection and syphilis. These women should be monitored closely for these infections throughout pregnancy. The incidence of gonorrhea in pregnancy ranges from rare to ~10%, depending upon the population surveyed. Salpingitis and PID can occur during the first trimester and are associated with a high rate of fetal loss. In the second and third trimesters, the relative impermeability of the cervical mucus (under the influence of progesterone) and the obliteration of the intrauterine cavity (resulting from the attachment of the chorion to the endometrial decidua by around the twelfth week of gestation) pose physical barriers that usually prevent ascending infection. Pharyngeal infection, most often asymptomatic, may be more common during pregnancy because of altered sexual practices. Acquisition of gonococcal infection late in pregnancy can adversely affect labor and delivery as well as the well-being of the fetus. Prolonged rupture of the membranes, premature delivery, chorioamnionitis, funisitis (infection of the umbilical cord stump), and sepsis in the infant (with *N. gonorrhoeae* detected in the gastric aspirate of the newborn during delivery) are common complications of maternal gonococcal infection at term. Hazards to the fetus include spontaneous abortion, perinatal death, premature delivery, perinatal distress, and premature rupture of membranes. Other microorganisms and conditions, including *Mycoplasma hominis*, *Ureaplasma urealyticum*, *C. trachomatis*, and bacterial vaginosis, have been associated with similar complications.

The most common form of gonorrhea in neonates is *ophthalmia neonatorum*, which results from exposure to infected cervical secretions during parturition. Ocular neonatal instillation of a prophylactic agent (e.g., 1% silver nitrate eyedrops or ophthalmic preparations containing erythromycin or tetracycline) is a cost-effective measure for the prevention of ophthalmia neonatorum but is not effective for its treatment, which requires systemic antibiotics. The clinical manifestations are acute and begin 2 to 5 days after birth. A small inoculum of organisms, low virulence of the infecting strain, or partial suppression by ophthalmic prophylaxis can result in a more indolent course. Therefore, gonococcal infection must be ruled out by culture in every case of conjunctivitis in infants. An initial nonspecific conjunctivitis with a serosanguineous discharge is followed by tense edema of both eyelids, chemosis, and a profuse, thick, purulent discharge. Corneal ulcerations that result in nebulae or perforation may lead to anterior synechiae, anterior staphyloma, panophthalmitis, and blindness. Infections described at other mucosal sites in infants, including vaginitis, rhinitis, and anorectal infection, are likely to be asymptomatic. Pharyngeal colonization has been demonstrated in 35% of infants with gonococcal ophthalmia, and coughing is the most prominent symptom in these cases. Septic arthritis is the most common manifestation of systemic gonococcal infection in the newborn. The primary focus of DGI in most of these cases is uncertain. The onset usually comes at 3 to 21 days of age, and polyarticular involvement is common. Sepsis, meningitis, and pneumonia are seen in rare instances.

Any STD in children beyond the neonatal period raises the possibility of sexual abuse. In most cases of abuse, the perpetrator is a male assailant known to the child. Gonococcal vulvovaginitis is the most common manifestation of gonococcal infection in children beyond infancy. Anorectal and pharyngeal infections are common in these children and are frequently asymptomatic. The urethra, Bartholin's and Skene's glands, and the upper genital tract are rarely involved. All children with gonococcal infection should also be evaluated for *Chlamydia* infection, syphilis, and possibly HIV infection. All cases of suspected and confirmed child abuse should be reported to the appropriate social service agency in the county where the child resides.

Disseminated Gonococcal Infection DGI results from gonococcal bacteremia. In the 1970s, DGI occurred in ~0.5% to 3% of persons with untreated gonococcal mucosal infection. The lower incidence at present is probably attributable to a decline in the prevalence of particular strains that are likely to disseminate. DGI strains resist the bactericidal action of human serum and generally do not incite inflammation at genital sites, probably because of limited generation of chemotactic factors. These strains are often of the Por1A serotype, are highly susceptible to penicillin, and have special nutritional requirements (i.e., the AHU auxotype). Menstruation is a risk factor for dissemination, and approximately two-thirds of cases of DGI are in women. In about half of affected women, symptoms of DGI begin within 7 days of onset of menses. Complement deficiencies, especially of the components involved in the assembly of the membrane attack complex (C5 through C9), predispose to neisserial bacteremia. Up to 13% of patients with DGI have complement deficiencies, and persons with more than one episode of DGI should be screened with an assay for total hemolytic complement activity.

The clinical manifestations of DGI have sometimes been classified into two stages: a bacteremic stage and a joint-localized stage with suppurative arthritis. A clear-cut progression usually is not evident. Patients in the bacteremic stage have higher temperatures, and their fever is more frequently accompanied by chills. Painful joints are common and often occur in conjunction with tenosynovitis and skin lesions.

Polyarthralgias usually include the knees, elbows, and more distal joints; the axial skeleton is generally spared. Skin lesions are seen in ~75% of patients and include papules and pustules, often with a hemorrhagic component (**see Plate IID-60**). These lesions are usually on the extremities and number between 5 and 40. Frank arthritis, when it develops, involves one or two joints, most often (in decreasing order of frequency) the knees, wrists, ankles, and elbows. The occurrence of arthritis in the absence of signs and symptoms of the bacteremic stage has led to the suggestion that these are separate syndromes. Other joints, such as the small joints of the hands and feet and the sternoclavicular and temporomandibular joints, are occasionally involved. Most patients who develop gonococcal septic arthritis do so without prior polyarthralgias or skin lesions; in the absence of symptomatic genital infection, this disease cannot be distinguished from septic arthritis caused by other pathogens. Rarely, osteomyelitis complicates septic arthritis involving small joints.

Although it has been postulated that the initial arthritis and skin lesions are due to direct tissue invasion by *N. gonorrhoeae*, the organism has been recovered from fewer than 5% of skin lesions cultured. This low isolation rate has been attributed to either a small inoculum of infecting organisms or the fastidious growth requirements of *N. gonorrhoeae* strains that disseminate. Gonococcal antigens have been identified in "sterile" skin lesions by immunofluorescent staining techniques. There is also evidence that immune-mediated or hypersensitivity phenomena caused by gonococcal antigens account for skin lesions. Other manifestations of noninfectious dermatitis, such as nodular lesions, urticaria, and erythema multiforme, have been described. Gonococcal endocarditis, although rare today, was relatively common in the preantibiotic era, causing about one-quarter of reported cases of endocarditis. Another unusual complication of DGI is meningitis.

Gonococcal Infection in HIV-Infected Persons The association between gonorrhea and the acquisition of HIV has been demonstrated in several well-controlled studies, mainly in Kenya and Zaire. The nonulcerative STDs enhance the transmission of HIV by three- to fivefold, possibly because of increased viral shedding in persons with urethritis or cervicitis (Chap. 309). HIV has been detected by polymerase chain reaction (PCR) more commonly in ejaculates from HIV-positive men with gonococcal urethritis than in those from HIV-positive men with nongonococcal urethritis. PCR positivity diminishes by twofold following appropriate therapy for urethritis. Not only does gonorrhea enhance the transmission of HIV; it may also increase the individual's risk for acquisition of HIV. A proposed mechanism is the significantly greater number of CD4+ lymphocytes and dendritic cells that can be infected by HIV in endocervical secretions of women with nonulcerative STDs than in those of women with ulcerative STDs.

DIFFERENTIAL DIAGNOSIS The clinical features of uncomplicated gonococcal infections closely resemble those of genital infections caused by *C. trachomatis*. Although the symptoms produced by chlamydial infections tend to be milder, the two infections are often indistinguishable on clinical grounds alone. Co-infection with *N. gonorrhoeae* and *C. trachomatis* is seen in up to 40% of cases. The differential diagnosis of urethritis, epididymitis, and proctitis in men, of cervicitis in women, and of vaginitis in prepubertal girls is discussed in Chap. 132; that of PID in Chap. 133; and that of acute arthritis in young adults in Chap. 323. The differential diagnosis of the bacteremic stage of DGI includes acute rheumatoid arthritis, sarcoidosis, erythema nodosum, drug-induced arthritis, and viral infections (e.g., hepatitis B and acute HIV infection).

LABORATORY DIAGNOSIS A rapid diagnosis of gonococcal infection in men may be obtained by Gram's staining of urethral exudates. The detection of gram-negative intracellular diplococci (GNID) is usually highly specific and sensitive in diagnosing gonococcal urethritis in symptomatic males but is only ~50% sensitive in diagnosing gonococcal cervicitis. Samples should be collected with Dacron or rayon swabs. Part of the sample should be inoculated onto a plate of modified Thayer-Martin or other gonococcal selective medium for culture. It is important to process all samples immediately because gonococci do not tolerate drying. If plates cannot be incubated immediately, they can be held safely for several hours at room temperature in candle extinction jars prior to incubation. If processing is to occur within 6 h, transport of specimens may be facilitated by the use of nonnutritive swab transport systems such as Stuart or Amies medium. For longer holding periods (e.g., when specimens for culture are to be mailed), culture media with self-contained CO_2-generating systems (such as the JEMBEC or Gono-Pak systems) may be used. Specimens should also be obtained for the diagnosis of chlamydial infection.

PMNs are often seen in the endocervix on a Gram's stain, and an abnormally increased number ($\geq$30 PMNs per field in five 1000$\times$ oil-immersion fields) establishes the presence of an inflammatory discharge (mucopurulent cervicitis). Unfortunately, the presence or absence of GNID in cervical smears does not accurately predict which patients have gonorrhea, and the diagnosis in this setting should be made by culture. The sensitivity of a single endocervical culture is ~80 to 90%, with the precise figure depending on the quality of the medium and the adequacy of the clinical specimen. The yield can be enhanced by culture of a second cervical specimen. If a history of rectal sex is elicited, a rectal wall swab (uncontaminated with feces) should be cultured. A presumptive diagnosis of gonorrhea cannot be made on the basis of gram-negative diplococci in smears from the pharynx, where other *Neisseria* species are components of the normal flora.

Nucleic acid probe tests are now widely used for the direct detection of *N. gonorrhoeae* in urogenital specimens. A common assay employs a nonisotopic chemiluminescent DNA probe that hybridizes specifically with gonococcal 16S ribosomal RNA. Studies assessing the utility of the nucleic acid probe system in high-risk outpatients undergoing screening for STDs have revealed that it is at least as sensitive as conventional culture techniques and may be a cost-effective alternative to culture, especially in high-risk males. A disadvantage of non-culture-based assays in general is that specimens submitted in probe-transport systems cannot be cultured subsequently. Therefore, a culture-confirmatory test is not possible, and formal antimicrobial susceptibility testing, if needed, cannot be performed. Low-cost point-of-care tests are under development for use in resource-poor settings, where specific diagnosis often gives way to syndromic management. DNA amplification techniques such as PCR may eventually prove to be equivalent to or more sensitive than culture methods.

Because of the legal implications, gonococcal infection in children must be diagnosed only with standard culture systems. Nonculture tests for gonococcal infection should not be used alone and have not been approved by the U.S. Food and Drug Administration for use with specimens obtained from the genital tract, pharynx, and rectum of infected children. Cultures should be obtained from the pharynx and anus of both girls and boys, the vagina of girls, and the urethra of boys. Cervical specimens are not recommended for prepubertal girls. For boys with a urethral discharge, a meatal specimen of the discharge is adequate for culture. Presumptive colonies of *N. gonorrhoeae* should be identified definitively by at least two independent methods (e.g., biochemical, enzyme substrate, or serologic).

Blood should be cultured in suspected cases of DGI. The use of Isolator blood culture tubes may enhance the yield. The probability of positive blood cultures decreases after 48 h of illness. Synovial fluid should be inoculated into blood culture broth medium and plated onto chocolate agar rather than selective medium because this fluid is not likely to be contaminated with commensal bacteria. Gonococci are infrequently recovered from early joint effusions containing <20,000 leukocytes/μL but may be recovered from effusions containing >80,000 leukocytes/μL. The organisms are seldom recovered from blood and synovial fluid of the same patient.

℞ TREATMENT It is no surprise that *N. gonorrhoeae*, with its remarkable capacity to alter its antigenic structure and adapt to changes in the microenvironment, has become resistant to numerous antibiotics. The first effective agents against gonorrhea were the sulfonamides, which were introduced in the 1930s. Within a decade, antibiotic resistance emerged, resulting in treatment failures in one-third of patients. Penicillin was then employed as the drug of choice for the treatment of gonorrhea. By 1965, 42% of gonococcal isolates had developed low-level resistance to penicillin G. To prevent treatment failures, the Centers for Disease Control and Prevention (CDC) at that time recommended doubling the dose of penicillin for the treatment of gonorrhea. Resistance due to the production of penicillinase arose later.

Gonococci become fully resistant to antibiotics either by chromosomal mutations or by acquisition of R factors (plasmids). Two types of chromosomal mutations have been described. The first type, which is drug specific, is a single-step mutation leading to high-level resistance. The second type involves mutations at several chromosomal loci that combine to determine the level as well as the pattern of resistance. Strains with mutations in chromosomal genes were first observed in the late 1950s. As recently as 1997, strains with chromosomal resistance (CMRNG) accounted for resistance to penicillin, tetracycline, or both in ~20% of strains surveyed in the United States.

β-Lactamase (penicillinase)–producing strains of *N. gonorrhoeae* (PPNG) carrying plasmids with the Pc^r determinant were seen almost simultaneously in the United States, England, western Africa, and the Philippines in the late 1970s. PPNG strains have since spread worldwide and by the early 1980s accounted for >50% of all gonococcal isolates in some parts of the developing world. The average prevalence of PPNG in the United States dropped by two-thirds after most penicillin use was discontinued and is now on the order of 4%, with higher rates reported from certain areas. *N. gonorrhoeae* strains with plasmid-borne tetracycline resistance (TRNG) can mobilize some β-lactamase plasmids, and PPNG and TRNG occur together, sometimes along with CMRNG. Penicillin, ampicillin, and tetracycline are no longer reliable agents for the treatment of gonorrhea and should not be used. Third-generation cephalosporins have remained highly effective as single-dose therapy for gonorrhea. Even though the minimal inhibitory concentrations (MICs) of ceftriaxone for certain strains may reach 0.015 to 0.125 mg/L [higher than MICs for fully susceptible strains (0.0001 to 0.008 mg/L)], these levels are greatly exceeded in blood, the urethra, and the cervix when the routinely recommended ceftriaxone and cefixime regimens are administered (see below). These regimens almost always result in an effective cure.

Quinolone-containing regimens are also recommended for treatment of gonococcal infections; the fluoroquinolones offer the advantage of antichlamydial activity when administered for 7 days. Serum concentrations following therapeutic dosages of the quinolones exceed the MIC for *N. gonorrhoeae* by ~100-fold. However, quinolone-resistant *N. gonorrhoeae* (QRNG) appeared soon after these agents were first used to treat gonorrhea, particularly in Southeast Asia. QRNG strains have been reported recently in the United States, mostly in the far western states. Alterations in DNA gyrase and topoisomerase IV have been implicated as mechanisms of fluoroquinolone resistance.

Resistance to spectinomycin, which is used as an alternative agent, has been reported, but resistance to this agent is usually not associated with resistance to other antibiotics. Therefore, spectinomycin can be reserved for use against multiresistant strains of *N. gonorrhoeae*. Nevertheless, outbreaks caused by strains resistant to spectinomycin have been documented in Korea and England when the drug was used as a primary agent to treat gonorrhea.

Although clinical isolates of *N. gonorrhoeae* vary in their antimicrobial susceptibility patterns in different parts of the world, they remain susceptible to a wide variety of agents. Because failure of treatment can lead to continued transmission and the emergence of antibiotic resistance, the importance of adequate treatment with a regimen that the patient will adhere to cannot be overemphasized. Thus highly effective single-dose regimens have been developed for the treatment of uncomplicated gonococcal infections. The 1998 CDC treatment guidelines for gonococcal infections are summarized in Table 147-1; the recommendations for uncomplicated gonorrhea apply to HIV-infected as well as HIV-uninfected patients. The third-generation cephalosporins cefixime and ceftriaxone are the mainstay of therapy for uncomplicated gonococcal infection of the urethra, cervix, rectum, or pharynx. Single doses of ciprofloxacin or ofloxacin are also effective first-line regimens. Because of resistance to fluoroquinolones in several parts of Southeast Asia, these agents can no longer be considered effective in that region. Because co-infection with *C. trachomatis* occurs frequently, initial treatment regimens must incorporate an agent (e.g., azithromycin or doxycycline) effective against chlamydial infection. Pregnant women with gonorrhea should receive concurrent treatment with a macrolide antibiotic for possible *Chlamydia* infection; doxycycline should not be used during pregnancy. A single 1-g dose of azithromycin, which is effective therapy for uncomplicated chlamydial infections, results in an unacceptably low cure rate (93%) for gonococcal infections and should not be used alone. Uncomplicated gonococcal infections in penicillin-allergic persons who cannot tolerate quinolones may be treated with a single dose of spectinomycin. Persons with uncomplicated infections who receive a recommended regimen need not return for a test of cure. Cultures for *N. gonorrhoeae* should be performed if symptoms persist after therapy with an established regimen, and any gonococci isolated should be tested for antimicrobial susceptibility.

Symptomatic gonococcal pharyngitis is more difficult to eradicate than genital infection. Few regimens result in cure rates of >90%. Persons who cannot tolerate cephalosporins or quinolones can be treated with spectinomycin, but this agent results in a cure rate of ≤52%. Therefore, persons given spectinomycin should have a pharyngeal culture performed 3 to 5 days after treatment as a test of cure.

Treatments for gonococcal epididymitis and PID are discussed in Chaps. 132 and 133, respectively. Ocular gonococcal infections in older children and adults should be managed with a single dose of ceftriaxone combined with saline irrigation of the conjunctivae (both undertaken expeditiously), and patients should undergo a careful ophthalmologic evaluation that includes a slit-lamp examination.

Table 147-1 Recommended Treatment for Gonococcal Infections: 1998 Guidelines of the Centers for Disease Control and Prevention

Diagnosis	Treatment of Choice
Uncomplicated gonococcal infection of the cervix, urethra, pharynx, or rectum[a]	
First-line regimens	Cefixime (400 mg PO, single dose) *or* Ceftriaxone (125 mg IM, single dose) *or* Ciprofloxacin (500 mg PO, single dose) *or* Ofloxacin (400 mg PO, single dose) *plus* A regimen effective against possible *Chlamydia* co-infection, such as: Azithromycin (1 g PO, single dose) *or* Doxycycline (100 mg PO bid for 7 days)
Alternative regimens	Spectinomycin (2 g IM, single dose) *or* Ceftizoxime (500 mg IM, single dose) *or* Cefotaxime (500 mg IM, single dose) *or* Cefotetan (1 g IM, single dose) *or* Cefoxitin (2 g IM, single dose) *plus* probenecid (1 g PO, single dose)
Epididymitis	See Chap. 132
Pelvic inflammatory disease	See Chap. 133
Gonococcal conjunctivitis in an adult	Ceftriaxone (1 g IM, single dose)[b]
Ophthalmia neonatorum[c]	Ceftriaxone (25–50 mg/kg IV or IM, single dose, not to exceed 125 mg)
Disseminated gonococcal infection[d]	
Initial therapy[e]	
Patients tolerant of β-lactam drugs	Ceftriaxone (1 g IM or IV q24h; *recommended*) *or* Cefotaxime (1 g IV q8h) *or* Ceftizoxime (1 g IV q8h)
Patients allergic to β-lactam drugs	Ciprofloxacin (500 mg IV q12h) *or* Ofloxacin (400 mg IV q12h) *or* Spectinomycin (2 g IM q12h)
Continuation therapy	Cefixime (400 mg PO bid) *or* Ciprofloxacin (500 mg PO bid) *or* Ofloxacin (400 mg PO bid)
Meningitis or endocarditis	See text[f]

[a] True failure of treatment with a recommended regimen is rare and should prompt an evaluation for reinfection or consideration of an alternative diagnosis. In cases of quinolone failure, the isolate should be tested for drug resistance if possible.
[b] Plus lavage of the infected eye with saline solution (once).
[c] Prophylactic regimens are discussed in the text.
[d] Hospitalization is indicated if the diagnosis is uncertain, if the patient has frank arthritis with an effusion, or if the patient cannot be relied on to comply with treatment.
[e] All initial regimens should be continued for 24–48 h after clinical improvement begins, at which time therapy may be switched to one of the continuation regimens to complete a full week of antimicrobial treatment.
[f] Hospitalization is recommended to exclude suspected meningitis or endocarditis.

DGI may require higher dosages and longer durations of therapy (Table 147-1). Hospitalization is indicated if the diagnosis is uncertain, if the patient has localized joint disease that requires aspiration, or if the patient cannot be relied on to comply with treatment. Open drainage is necessary only occasionally, e.g., for management of hip infections that may be difficult to drain percutaneously. Nonsteroidal anti-inflammatory agents may be indicated to alleviate pain and hasten improvement of affected joints. Gonococcal meningitis and endocarditis should be treated in the hospital with high-dose intravenous ceftriaxone (1 to 2 g every 12 h); therapy should continue for 10 to 14 days for meningitis and for at least 4 weeks for endocarditis. All persons who experience more than one episode of DGI should be evaluated for complement deficiency.

PREVENTION AND CONTROL Condoms, if properly used, provide effective protection against the transmission and acquisition of gonorrhea as well as other infections that are transmitted to and from genital mucosal surfaces. Spermicidal preparations used with a diaphragm or cervical sponges impregnated with nonoxynol 9 offer some protection against gonorrhea and chlamydial infection. However, the frequent use of preparations that contain nonoxynol 9 is associated with mucosal disruption that paradoxically may enhance the risk of HIV infection in the event of exposure. All patients should be instructed to refer sex partners for evaluation and treatment. All sex partners of persons with gonorrhea should be evaluated and treated for *N. gonorrhoeae* and *C. trachomatis* infections if their last contact with the patient took place within 60 days before the onset of symptoms or the diagnosis of infection in the patient. If the patient's last sexual encounter was >60 days before onset of symptoms or diagnosis, the patient's most recent sex partner should be treated. Patients should be instructed to abstain from sexual intercourse until therapy is completed and until they and their sex partners no longer have symptoms. Greater emphasis must be placed on prevention by public health education, individual patient counseling, and behavior modification. Preventing the spread of gonorrhea may help reduce the transmission of HIV. No effective vaccine for gonorrhea is yet available, but efforts to test a porin vaccine candidate are under way.

ACKNOWLEDGMENT
The authors acknowledge the contributions of Dr. King K. Holmes and Dr. Stephen A. Morse to the chapter on this subject in the earlier editions.

BIBLIOGRAPHY
BLAKE MS, WETZLER LM: Vaccines for gonorrhea: Where are we on the curve? Trends Microbiol 3:469, 1995

CENTERS FOR DISEASE CONTROL AND PREVENTION: Annual Report; Gonococcal Isolate Surveillance Project (GISP); www.cdc.gov/ncidod/dastlr/gcdir/Resist/gisp.html

———: 1998 Guidelines for treatment of sexually transmitted diseases. MMWR 47 (RR-1):1, 1998

COHEN MS, CANNON JG: Human experimentation with *Neisseria gonorrhoeae*: Progress and goals. J Infect Dis 179:S375, 1999

HOOK EW III, HOLMES KK: Gonococcal infections. Ann Intern Med 102:229, 1985

JERSE AE, REST RF: Adhesion and invasion by the pathogenic *Neisseria*. Trends Microbiol 5:217, 1997

LAGA M et al: Non-ulcerative sexually transmitted diseases as risk factors for HIV-1 transmission in women: Results from a cohort study. AIDS 7:95, 1993

MCQUILLEN DP et al: Complement processing and immunoglobulin binding to *Neisseria gonorrhoeae* determined in vitro simulates in vivo effects. J Infect Dis 179:124, 1999

O'BRIEN JP et al: Disseminated gonococcal infection: A prospective analysis of 49 patients and a review of pathophysiology and immune mechanisms. Medicine (Baltimore) 62:395, 1983

US DEPARTMENT OF HEALTH AND HUMAN SERVICES: Sexually transmitted disease surveillance 1997:1, 1998

148 *Daniel M. Musher*

MORAXELLA CATARRHALIS AND OTHER MORAXELLA SPECIES

MORAXELLA CATARRHALIS

The gram-negative coccus now known as *Moraxella catarrhalis* has undergone three changes of name in as many decades. Originally called *Micrococcus catarrhalis*, it was renamed *Neisseria catarrhalis* in the 1960s because of its morphologic similarity to *Neisseria* spp. Then, in 1970, it was elevated to the status of a distinct genus, *Branhamella*, on the basis of DNA homology. In 1979 this organism was placed into the genus *Moraxella*, of which *Branhamella* may be a subgenus. A component of the normal bacterial flora of the upper airways, *M. catarrhalis* has been increasingly recognized as a cause of otitis media, sinusitis, and bronchopulmonary infection.

BACTERIOLOGY AND IMMUNITY On Gram's staining, *M. catarrhalis* organisms appear as gram-negative cocci, sometimes occurring in pairs and retaining the side-by-side kidney-bean configuration of *Neisseria* (**Plate VI-1**). These cocci tend to retain crystal violet during the decolorizing step and may be confused with *Staphylococcus aureus*. *Moraxella* colonies grow well on blood or chocolate agar but may be overlooked because of their resemblance to *Neisseria* spp. (a major component of the normal pharyngeal flora). *Moraxella* is readily distinguishable from *Neisseria* spp. by biochemical tests.

Strains of *M. catarrhalis* show a surprising degree of homogeneity in terms of their outer-membrane proteins. Antibody to some of these proteins is generally present in serum of children over the age of 4 years; however, colonizing or disease-causing isolates may survive in serum despite this naturally present antibody and complement. Bactericidal antibody emerges following natural infection and may be directed against one or more conserved outer-membrane proteins—a property of potential value in vaccine development. The presence of certain outer-membrane proteins is associated with virulence in mice, and antibody may be protective. These proteins are under investigation for use as vaccines.

EPIDEMIOLOGY With repeated cultures and the use of selective media, *M. catarrhalis* can be isolated from the upper respiratory tract or saliva of 50% of healthy schoolchildren and of up to 7% of healthy adults. When conventional microbiologic techniques are used, *Moraxella* can be isolated from sputum of about 10% of persons who have chronic bronchitis and 25% of those who have bronchiectasis in the absence of acute infection. Investigators in both the northern and southern hemispheres have reported a striking seasonal variation in the isolation of this organism from clinical specimens, with a peak in late winter/early spring and a nadir in late summer/early fall. Direct contact has not been shown to contribute to community-acquired infection, but nosocomial spread of infection has been documented occasionally.

OTITIS MEDIA AND SINUSITIS *M. catarrhalis* has repeatedly been shown to be the third most common bacterial isolate from middle-ear fluid of children who have otitis media, being surpassed only by *Streptococcus pneumoniae* and nontypable *Haemophilus influenzae*. Recent studies have shown that this organism is also a prominent isolate from sinus cavities in acute and chronic sinusitis.

PURULENT TRACHEOBRONCHITIS AND PNEUMONIA *M. catarrhalis* causes acute exacerbations of chronic bronchitis (increased production and/or purulence of sputum), purulent tracheobronchitis (the latter also involving fever and leukocytosis), and pneumonia. The great majority of infected persons are >50 years old and have a long history of cigarette smoking and underlying chronic obstructive pulmonary disease (COPD); many have lung cancer as well. In one study, 76% of affected persons had COPD (severe in many cases), and one-third of those with COPD had lung cancer; most patients also had clinical evidence of malnutrition. In one extensive series of cases, *M. catarrhalis* pneumonia did not occur in otherwise-healthy hosts.

Symptoms of *M. catarrhalis* infection have been regarded as modest in severity. Both cough and the amount and purulence of sputum are usually increased above baseline. Chills are reported in one-quarter of patients, pleuritic pain in one-third, and malaise in 40%. Most patients have peak temperatures of <38.3°C (<101°F), and peripheral white blood cell counts are <10,000/μL in nearly one-quarter of cases. Microscopic examination of a good sputum specimen following Gram's staining regularly reveals profuse organisms, and quantitative culture yields ~ 2 × 10^8 colony-forming units per milliliter (**Plate VI-1**). The radiologic appearance is variable; in one study, 43% of subjects had segmental or lobar infiltrates, and the remainder had a mixed pattern of subsegmental, segmental, interstitial, and diffuse involvement. These clinical, laboratory, and radiographic findings do not differ from those of pneumococcal or *Haemophilus* pneumonia in an older patient population. However, a far lesser degree of bloodstream invasion occurs in *M. catarrhalis* infection; in one series, none of 25 patients with *M. catarrhalis* pneumonia had bacteremia. Nevertheless, pneumonia due to *M. catarrhalis* is a marker for severe underlying disease: nearly half of patients die within 3 months of onset.

OTHER SYNDROMES Local extension causing empyema is very uncommon, and, as might be inferred from the low rate of bacteremia, metastatic complications of *M. catarrhalis* pneumonia, such as septic arthritis, are exceedingly rare. As of 1995, 58 cases of bacteremic infection due to *M. catarrhalis* had been reported, mainly in children <10 years old or adults >60 years old; most of these patients were immunocompromised. The syndromes reported have included bacteremia with no apparent focus, pneumonia, endocarditis, and meningitis. A petechial or purpuric rash, reminiscent of that observed in meningococcal sepsis and associated with disseminated intravascular coagulation, has been described in a few cases.

TREATMENT Treatment of *M. catarrhalis* infection with a penicillin/clavulanic acid combination seems highly appropriate. Penicillin resistance first appeared in *Branhamella* isolates in the mid-1970s and is now found in 85% of clinical isolates. Resistance is mediated by two closely related β-lactamases, BRO-1 and BRO-2, which are present in 90% and 10% of resistant isolates, respectively. These enzymes are active against penicillin, ampicillin, and amoxicillin but less so against cephalosporins, especially third-generation cephalosporins, and they bind avidly to clavulanic acid and sulbactam.

Cephalosporins, especially those of the second and third generations, are effective alternatives. Isolates in the United States are also nearly uniformly susceptible to tetracycline, erythromycin, trimethoprim-sulfamethoxazole, quinolones, and chloramphenicol, although tetracycline resistance—perhaps due to TetB determinants—is increasing in Europe and Asia and has been documented in the United States. A 5-day course of therapy has been shown to cure respiratory infection, although a slightly longer course may be required in sinusitis.

During the period between the identification of gram-negative cocci in a Gram-stained specimen and the final identification of the organisms by culture, the severity of the condition and the potential presence of other infecting organisms should guide antibiotic selection. For example, an exacerbation of bronchitis caused by *M. catarrhalis* might be treated with tetracycline or trimethoprim-sulfamethoxazole; however, in a patient with pneumonia, the possibility that pneumococci resistant to these agents also might be present dictates the choice of ampicillin/sulbactam or a third-generation cephalosporin, at least until culture results become available.

OTHER MORAXELLA SPECIES

Other *Moraxella* species cause a wide range of infections, including bronchitis, pneumonia, empyema, endocarditis, meningitis, conjunctivitis, urinary tract infection, septic arthritis, and wound infection. In a report on all *Moraxella* isolates submitted to the Centers for Disease

Table 148-1 *Moraxella* Species

Moraxella Species	Number of Isolates	Common Sites/ Clinical Association	Number (Percent) for Each Site
M. osloensis[a]	199	Blood	44 (22)
		CSF	18 (9)
		Urine	17 (9)
		Respiratory tract	24 (12)
M. nonliquefaciens	356	Blood	27 (8)
		CSF	6 (2)
		Respiratory tract	196 (55)
M. canis	74	Dog-bite wound	53 (72)
M-6	47	Blood, bone	15 (32)
M. lacunata	33	Conjunctivitis, keratitis	23 (70)
M. urethralis	28	Urine	16 (57)
		Genital tract	3 (11)
M. phenylpyruvica	73	Blood	19 (26)
		CSF	8 (11)
		Urine	12 (16)
M. atlantae	44	Blood	20 (45)
		CSF	5 (11)

[a] Some of these isolates would now be distinguished as a new species, *Moraxella lincolnii*.
NOTE: CSF, cerebrospinal fluid.
SOURCE: Adapted from a summary of CDC experience (Graham et al).

Control and Prevention between 1953 and 1980, certain clinical associations were apparent (Table 148-1). *M. osloensis* and *M. nonliquefaciens*, the most commonly isolated species, were cultured from a wide range of normally sterile body sites, including blood, cerebrospinal fluid, and joints. *M. osloensis* was the *Moraxella* species most frequently isolated from blood; *M. nonliquefaciens* tended to be isolated from the ears, nose, or throat (47%) or the sputum (8%) and has since been implicated as a cause of conjunctivitis and keratitis. *M. urethralis* was isolated most often from urine and the genital tract and probably represents the *Moraxella* species implicated previously in urethritis. More than half of isolates of *M. phenylpyruvica* and *M. atlantae* were obtained from normally sterile sites. A recent study found *Moraxella* spp., including *M. catarrhalis*, in 35% of infected wounds following cat bites and in 10% of those following dog bites. The clinical features of infections due to *Moraxella* spp. other than *M. catarrhalis* and the nature of the hosts in which they occur have not been fully characterized.

BIBLIOGRAPHY

GRAHAM D et al: Infections caused by *Moraxella*, *Moraxella urethralis*, *Moraxella*-like groups M-5 and M-6, and *Kingella kingae* in the United States, 1953–1980. Rev Infect Dis 12:423, 1990

IOANNIDIS JPA et al: Spectrum and significance of bacteremia due to *Moraxella catarrhalis*. Clin Infect Dis 21:390, 1995

MURPHY TF: *Branhamella catarrhalis*: Epidemiology, surface antigenic structure and immune response. Microbiol Rev 60:267, 1996

TALAN DA et al: Bacteriologic analysis of infected dog and cat bites. N Engl J Med 340:85, 1999

WRIGHT PW et al: A descriptive study of 42 cases of *Branhamella catarrhalis* pneumonia. Am J Med 88(Suppl 5A):2S, 1990

149 *Timothy F. Murphy*

HAEMOPHILUS INFECTIONS

HAEMOPHILUS INFLUENZAE

MICROBIOLOGY *Haemophilus influenzae* was first recognized in 1892 by Pfeiffer, who erroneously concluded that the bacterium was the cause of influenza. The bacterium is a small (1- by 0.3-μm) gram-negative organism of variable shape; hence, it is often described as a pleomorphic coccobacillus. In clinical specimens such as cerebrospinal fluid (CSF) and sputum, it frequently stains only faintly with phenosafranin and therefore can easily be overlooked.

H. influenzae grows both aerobically and anaerobically. Its aerobic growth requires two factors: hemin (X factor) and nicotinamide adenine dinucleotide (V factor). These requirements are used in the clinical laboratory to identify the bacterium. Six major serotypes of *H. influenzae* have been identified; designated *a* through *f*, they are based on antigenically distinct polysaccharide capsules. In addition, some strains lack a polysaccharide capsule and are referred to as *nontypable* strains. Type b and nontypable strains are the most relevant strains clinically, although encapsulated strains other than type b can cause disease. *H. influenzae* was the first free-living organism to have its entire genome sequenced.

The antigenically distinct type b capsule is a linear polymer composed of ribosyl-ribitol phosphate. Strains of *H. influenzae* type b (Hib) cause disease primarily in infants and children under the age of 6 years. Nontypable strains are primarily mucosal pathogens, although the incidence of invasive disease caused by these strains is increasing.

EPIDEMIOLOGY AND TRANSMISSION *H. influenzae* is an exclusively human pathogen. The organism is spread by airborne droplets or by direct contact with secretions or fomites. Nontypable strains colonize the upper respiratory tract of up to three-fourths of healthy adults. Colonization with nontypable *H. influenzae* is a dynamic process; new strains are acquired and other strains are replaced periodically.

Hib strains colonize the nasopharynx of children at a rate of 3 to 5%; before the introduction of type b vaccine, higher rates were seen in day-care centers. The widespread use of conjugate vaccines has resulted in a striking decrease not only in the rate of nasopharyngeal colonization by Hib but also in the incidence of meningitis due to Hib. Studies in selected populations suggest the reemergence of invasive Hib infections and higher than expected rates of nasopharyngeal colonization by Hib in vaccinated children. Continued surveillance of Hib disease and colonization rates will be important in evaluating the success of current vaccination strategies.

Certain population groups have a higher incidence of invasive Hib disease than the general population. The incidence of meningitis due to Hib has been three to four times higher among black children than among white children in several studies. In some Native American groups, the incidence of invasive Hib disease is 10 times higher than that in the general population. Although this increased incidence has not yet been accounted for, several factors may be relevant, including age at exposure to the bacterium, socioeconomic conditions, and genetic differences in the ability to mount an immune response.

PATHOGENESIS Hib strains cause systemic disease by invasion and hematogenous spread to distant sites such as the meninges, bones, and joints. The type b polysaccharide capsule is an important virulence factor affecting the bacterium's ability to avoid opsonization and cause systemic disease.

Nontypable strains cause disease by local invasion of mucosal surfaces. Otitis media results when bacteria reach the middle ear by way of the eustachian tube. Adults with chronic bronchitis experience recurrent lower respiratory tract infection due to nontypable strains. The incidence of invasive disease caused by nontypable strains is low but increasing.

IMMUNE RESPONSE Antibody to capsule is important in protection from infection by Hib strains. The level of (maternally acquired) serum antibody to the capsular polysaccharide, which is a polymer of polyribitol ribose phosphate (PRP), declines from birth to 6 months of age and, in the absence of vaccination, remains low until around 2 or 3 years of age. The age at the antibody nadir correlates with that of the peak incidence of type b disease. Antibody to PRP then appears partly as a result of exposure to Hib or cross-reacting antigens. Systemic Hib disease is unusual after the age of 6 years because of the presence of protective antibody. Vaccines in which PRP is conjugated to protein carrier molecules have been developed and are now used widely. These vaccines generate an antibody response to PRP in infants and are effective in preventing invasive infections in infants and children.

Since nontypable strains lack a capsule, the immune response to infection is directed at noncapsular antigens. These noncapsular antigens of *H. influenzae* have generated considerable interest as targets of the human immune response and as potential vaccine components.

CLINICAL MANIFESTATIONS Hib The most serious manifestation of infection with Hib is meningitis. The age of peak incidence varies somewhat among populations, depending in part on the use of vaccine, but this infection primarily affects infants under 2 years of age. The clinical manifestations of meningitis caused by Hib are similar to those of meningitis caused by other bacterial pathogens. Fever and altered central nervous system function are the most common features at presentation. Nuchal rigidity may or may not be evident. Subdural effusion, the most common complication, is suspected when, despite 2 or 3 days of appropriate antibiotic therapy, the infant has seizures, hemiparesis, or continued obtundation. The overall mortality from meningitis caused by Hib is approximately 5%, and the rate of morbidity is high. Of survivors, 6% have permanent sensorineural hearing loss, and about one-fourth have a significant handicap of some type. If more subtle handicaps are sought, up to half of survivors are found to have some neurologic sequelae, such as partial hearing loss and delay in language development.

Epiglottitis is a life-threatening infection involving cellulitis of the epiglottis and supraglottic tissues. It can lead to acute upper airway obstruction. Its unique epidemiologic features are its occurrence in an older age group (2 to 7 years old) than other Hib infections and its absence among Navajo Indians and Alaskan Eskimos. Sore throat and fever rapidly progress to dysphagia, drooling, and airway obstruction.

Cellulitis due to Hib occurs in young children. The most common location is on the head or neck, and the involved area sometimes takes on a characteristic bluish-red color. Most patients have bacteremia, and 10% have an additional focus of infection.

Hib causes *pneumonia* in infants. The infection is clinically indistinguishable from other types of bacterial pneumonia (e.g., pneumococcal pneumonia) except that Hib is more likely to involve the pleura.

Several less common invasive conditions can be important clinical manifestations of Hib infection in children. These include osteomyelitis, septic arthritis, pericarditis, orbital cellulitis, endophthalmitis, urinary tract infection, abscesses, and bacteremia without an identifiable focus. As has already been mentioned, infections due to Hib are unusual among patients older than 6 years.

Nontypable *H. influenzae* Nontypable *H. influenzae* is the second most common cause (after *Streptococcus pneumoniae*) of community-acquired bacterial pneumonia in adults. Nontypable *H. influenzae* pneumonia is especially common among patients with chronic obstructive pulmonary disease (COPD) or AIDS. The clinical features of pneumonia due to *H. influenzae* are similar to those of other types of bacterial pneumonia (including pneumococcal pneumonia). Patients present with fever, cough, and purulent sputum, usually of several days' duration. Chest radiography reveals alveolar infiltrates in a patchy or lobar distribution. Gram-stained sputum contains a predominance of small, pleomorphic, coccobacillary gram-negative bacteria.

Exacerbations of COPD caused by nontypable *H. influenzae* are characterized by increased cough, sputum production, and shortness of breath. Fever is low-grade, and no infiltrates are evident on chest x-ray.

Nontypable *H. influenzae* is one of the three most common causes of childhood otitis media (the other two being *S. pneumoniae* and *Moraxella catarrhalis*). Infants are febrile and irritable, while older children report ear pain. Symptoms of viral upper respiratory infection often precede otitis media. The diagnosis is made by pneumatic otoscopy. An etiologic diagnosis, although not routinely sought, can be established by tympanocentesis and culture of middle-ear fluid.

Nontypable *H. influenzae* also causes puerperal sepsis and is an important cause of neonatal bacteremia. These nontypable strains tend to be of biotype IV and cause invasive disease after colonizing the female genital tract.

Nontypable *H. influenzae* causes sinusitis in adults and children. In addition, the bacterium is a less common cause of various invasive infections that are reported primarily as small-series descriptions and case reports. These infections include empyema, adult epiglottitis, pericarditis, cellulitis, septic arthritis, osteomyelitis, endocarditis, cholecystitis, intraabdominal infections, urinary tract infections, mastoiditis, aortic graft infection, and bacteremia without a detectable focus.

DIAGNOSIS The most reliable method for establishing a diagnosis of Hib infection is recovery of the organism in culture. The CSF of a patient in whom meningitis is suspected should be subjected to Gram's staining and culture. The presence of gram-negative coccobacilli in Gram-stained CSF is strong evidence for Hib meningitis. Recovery of the organism from CSF confirms the diagnosis. Cultures of other normally sterile body fluids, such as blood, joint fluid, pleural fluid, pericardial fluid, and subdural effusion, are confirmatory in other infections.

Detection of PRP is an important adjunct to culture in rapid diagnosis. Immunoelectrophoresis, latex agglutination, coagglutination, and enzyme-linked immunosorbent assay are effective in detecting PRP. These assays are particularly helpful when patients have received prior antimicrobial therapy and thus are especially likely to have negative cultures.

Before the early 1980s, nontypable strains of *H. influenzae* were frequently misidentified as Hib because of their autoagglutination when serotypes were determined in agglutination assays. Since nontypable *H. influenzae* is primarily a mucosal pathogen, it is a component of a mixed flora; this situation makes etiologic diagnosis challenging. Nontypable *H. influenzae* infection is strongly suggested by the predominance of gram-negative coccobacilli among abundant polymorphonuclear leukocytes in a Gram-stained sputum specimen from a patient in whom pneumonia or tracheobronchitis is suspected. A sputum culture is helpful when interpreted along with the results of Gram's staining. Although bacteremia is detectable in a small proportion of patients with pneumonia due to nontypable *H. influenzae*, most such patients have negative blood cultures.

A diagnosis of otitis media is based on the detection by pneumatic otoscopy of fluid in the middle ear. An etiologic diagnosis requires tympanocentesis but is not routinely sought. An invasive procedure is also required to determine the etiology of sinusitis; thus, treatment is often empirical once the diagnosis is suspected in light of clinical symptoms and sinus radiographs.

TREATMENT Initial therapy for meningitis due to Hib should consist of a cephalosporin such as ceftriaxone or cefotaxime. For children, the dose of ceftriaxone is 75 to 100 mg/kg daily given in two doses 12 h apart. The pediatric dose of cefotaxime is 200 mg/kg daily given in four doses 6 h apart. Adult doses are 2 g every 12 h for ceftriaxone and 2 g every 4 to 6 h for cefotaxime. An alternative regimen for initial therapy is ampicillin (200 to 300 mg/kg daily in four divided doses) plus chloramphenicol (75 to 100 mg/kg daily in four divided doses). Therapy should continue for a total of 1 to 2 weeks.

Administration of glucocorticoids to patients with Hib meningitis reduces the incidence of neurologic sequelae. The presumed mechanism is reduction of the inflammation induced by bacterial cell-wall mediators of inflammation when cells are killed by antimicrobial agents. Dexamethasone (0.6 mg/kg per day intravenously in four divided doses for 2 days) is recommended for the treatment of Hib meningitis in children over 2 months of age.

Invasive infections other than meningitis are treated with the same antimicrobial agents. For epiglottitis, the dose of ceftriaxone is 50 mg/kg daily, and the dose of cefotaxime is 150 mg/kg daily, given in three divided doses 8 h apart. Epiglottitis constitutes a medical emergency, and maintenance of an airway is critical. The duration of therapy is determined by the clinical response. A course of 1 to 2 weeks is usually appropriate.

149 *Haemophilus* Infections **941**

Many infections caused by nontypable strains of *H. influenzae*, such as otitis media, sinusitis, and exacerbations of COPD, can be treated with oral antimicrobial agents. Approximately 25% of nontypable strains produce β-lactamase and are resistant to ampicillin. Infections caused by ampicillin-resistant strains can be treated with a variety of agents, including trimethoprim-sulfamethoxazole, amoxicillin/clavulanic acid, various extended-spectrum cephalosporins, and newer macrolides (azithromycin and clarithromycin). Fluoroquinolones are highly active against *H. influenzae* but are not currently recommended for the treatment of children or pregnant women because of possible effects on articular cartilage.

PREVENTION **Vaccination** The development of conjugate vaccines that prevent invasive infections with Hib in infants and children has been a dramatic success. Four such vaccines are licensed in the United States. In addition to eliciting protective antibody, these vaccines prevent disease by reducing pharyngeal colonization with Hib.

All children should be immunized with an Hib conjugate vaccine, receiving the first dose at approximately 2 months of age, the rest of the primary series between 2 and 6 months of age, and a booster dose at 12 to 15 months of age. Specific recommendations vary for the different conjugate vaccines. The reader is referred to the recommendations of the American Academy of Pediatrics. Currently, no vaccines are available for the prevention of disease caused by nontypable *H. influenzae*.

Chemoprophylaxis The risk of secondary disease is greater than normal among household contacts of patients with Hib disease. The attack rate is as high as 4% among susceptible infants. Therefore, all children and adults in households where there are contacts <4 years old should receive prophylaxis with oral rifampin. (This rule does not apply when all household contacts under the age of 4 years have been completely immunized with conjugate vaccine.) Children <12 years old should receive rifampin at a dose of 20 mg/kg once daily for 4 days, and adults should receive 600 mg daily for 4 days. The index case should receive rifampin before or at the time of discharge from the hospital because antimicrobial agents used for the treatment of meningitis do not reliably eradicate Hib from the nasopharynx.

When two or more cases of invasive Hib disease have occurred within 60 days at a child-care facility attended by incompletely vaccinated children, administration of rifampin to all attendees and personnel is indicated, as is recommended for household contacts. The data on secondary cases among contacts in child-care facilities following a single case are less clear. The administration of rifampin prophylaxis to contacts should be considered, but each decision should be individualized and in part based on the contacts' immunization history, the size of the center, and the extent of contact.

HAEMOPHILUS INFLUENZAE BIOGROUP AEGYPTIUS

H. influenzae biogroup aegyptius was formerly called *Haemophilus aegyptius* because of phenotypic characteristics distinct from those of *H. influenzae*. However, later studies involving DNA hybridization and DNA transformation demonstrated that *H. aegyptius* and *H. influenzae* are members of the same species.

H. influenzae biogroup aegyptius has long been associated with conjunctivitis. Moreover, this strain is now known to be the cause of Brazilian purpuric fever (BPF), which was first recognized in 1984 in the rural Brazilian town of Promissao. The sharing of many phenotypic and genotypic characteristics by the various strains of *H. influenzae* biogroup aegyptius that cause BPF indicates that these strains represent a clone of *H. influenzae*. The age of peak incidence of BPF is 1 to 4 years, with a range of 3 months to 8 years. The illness can occur sporadically or in outbreaks. Typically, after an episode of purulent conjunctivitis, high fever occurs in association with vomiting and abdominal pain. Within 12 to 48 h after onset, the patient develops petechiae, purpura, and peripheral necrosis and experiences vascular collapse. The characteristic laboratory features are thrombocytopenia, prolonged prothrombin time, uniformly unrevealing CSF findings, and blood cultures positive for *H. influenzae* biogroup aegyptius. Initial reports cited high mortality (70%), but subsequent studies have indicated that milder forms of the illness exist. Most patients have resolved or resolving purulent conjunctivitis, and culture of the conjunctiva is positive in approximately one-third of cases. BPF has been seen in several towns in Brazil and on two occasions in Australia.

HAEMOPHILUS DUCREYI

Haemophilus ducreyi is the etiologic agent of chancroid, a sexually transmitted disease characterized by genital ulceration and inguinal adenitis. *H. ducreyi* poses a significant health problem in developing countries. Although this infection is less common in the United States, its incidence has increased dramatically in the past several years. In addition to being a cause of morbidity in itself, chancroid is associated with infection with HIV because of the role of genital ulceration in the transmission of HIV.

MICROBIOLOGY *H. ducreyi* is a highly fastidious coccobacillary gram-negative bacterium whose growth requires X factor (hemin). Although, in light of this requirement, the bacterium has been classified in the genus *Haemophilus*, DNA homology and chemotaxonomic studies have established substantial differences between *H. ducreyi* and other *Haemophilus* species. Taxonomic reclassification of the organism is likely in the future but awaits further study.

The histology of the genital ulcer of chancroid is characterized by perivascular and interstitial infiltrates of macrophages and of CD4+ and CD8+ lymphocytes. The appearance is consistent with a delayed-type hypersensitivity, cell-mediated immune response. The presence of CD4+ cells and macrophages in the ulcer may explain, in part, the facilitation of transmission of HIV in patients with chancroid.

EPIDEMIOLOGY AND PREVALENCE (See also Chap. 132) Chancroid is a common cause of genital ulcers in developing countries. In the United States, chancroid is now endemic in some regions, and several large outbreaks have occurred since 1981. Recurring epidemiologic themes have been apparent in these outbreaks: (1) transmission has been predominantly heterosexual; (2) males have outnumbered females by ratios of 3:1 to 25:1; (3) prostitutes have been important in transmission of the infection; and (4) chancroid has been strongly associated with illicit drug use. The incidence of chancroid in the United States will undoubtedly increase in the coming years, and the genital ulcers associated with this infection will continue to play a role in the transmission of HIV.

CLINICAL MANIFESTATIONS Infection is acquired as the result of a break in the epithelium during sexual contact with an infected individual. After an incubation period of 4 to 7 days, the initial lesion—a papule with surrounding erythema—appears (**Plate IID-54**). In 2 to 3 days, the papule evolves into a pustule, which spontaneously ruptures and forms a sharply circumscribed ulcer that is generally not indurated. The ulcers are painful and bleed easily; little or no inflammation of the surrounding skin is evident. Approximately half of patients develop enlarged, tender inguinal lymph nodes, which frequently become fluctuant and spontaneously rupture.

The presentation of chancroid does not usually include all of the typical clinical features and is sometimes atypical. Multiple ulcers can coalesce to form giant ulcers. Ulcers can appear and then resolve, with inguinal adenitis and suppuration following 1 to 3 weeks later; this clinical picture can be confused with that of lymphogranuloma venereum. Multiple small ulcers can resemble folliculitis. Other differential diagnostic considerations include the various infections causing genital ulceration, such as primary syphilis, condyloma latum of secondary syphilis, genital herpes, and donovanosis. In rare cases chancroid lesions become secondarily infected with bacteria; the result is extensive inflammation.

DIAGNOSIS Clinical diagnosis of chancroid is often inaccurate, and laboratory confirmation should be attempted in suspected cases. Gram's staining of a swab of the lesion may reveal a predominance of characteristic gram-negative coccobacilli, but the presence of other bacteria often makes it difficult to interpret this result. An accurate diagnosis of chancroid relies on cultures of *H. ducreyi* from the lesion. In addition, aspiration and culture of suppurative lymph nodes should be considered. Since the organism can be difficult to grow, the use of selective and supplemented media is necessary.

℞ **TREATMENT** Clinical isolates of *H. ducreyi* often exhibit plasmid-mediated resistance to ampicillin, chloramphenicol, tetracyclines, and sulfonamides. Nevertheless, chancroid can be treated effectively with several regimens, including (1) ceftriaxone, 250 mg intramuscularly as a single dose; (2) azithromycin, 1 g orally as a single dose; (3) erythromycin, 500 mg orally four times daily for 7 days; and (4) ciprofloxacin, 500 mg orally twice daily for 3 days. Ciprofloxacin should not be administered to pregnant or lactating women or to persons <18 years old. Any therapeutic regimen may fail; single-dose ceftriaxone has a high failure rate in HIV-positive individuals. Isolates from patients who do not respond promptly to treatment should be tested for antimicrobial susceptibility. In patients with HIV infection, healing may be slow and longer courses of treatment may be necessary. Contacts of patients with chancroid should be identified and treated whenever possible.

OTHER *HAEMOPHILUS* SPECIES

Haemophilus species are often recovered as components of the flora of the normal human upper respiratory tract. However, these bacteria are infrequent causes of infection because of their low pathogenic potential. *Haemophilus* species have fastidious growth requirements and are generally rather slow-growing. The species implicated in human infections include *H. parainfluenzae*, *H. aphrophilus*, and *H. paraphrophilus* (Chap. 150); *H. parahaemolyticus*; *H. haemolyticus*; and *H. segnis*. *Haemophilus* species are differentiated from one another by several characteristics, primarily their requirements for X and V factors. Species designated *para-* require V factor but not X factor for growth, whereas the others require either X and V or X only.

A variety of infections involving almost all organ systems can be caused by *Haemophilus* species. Most of these unusual manifestations have been reported as single cases and small series.

The antimicrobial susceptibility characteristics of other *Haemophilus* species are similar to those of *H. influenzae*. Some strains produce β-lactamase and are thereby resistant to ampicillin. Other strains are sensitive to ampicillin, and this agent has been used successfully to treat many infections. Alternative agents with good activity against most *Haemophilus* species include trimethoprim-sulfamethoxazole, third-generation cephalosporins, tetracycline, chloramphenicol, and aminoglycosides. Endocarditis caused by ampicillin-sensitive strains should be treated with ampicillin plus an aminoglycoside.

BIBLIOGRAPHY

COMMITTEE ON INFECTIOUS DISEASES: *Haemophilus influenzae* infections, in *1997 Red Book, Report of the Committee on Infectious Diseases*, G Peter et al (eds). Elk Grove Village, IL, American Academy of Pediatrics, 1997

DOERN GV et al: *Haemophilus influenzae* and *Moraxella catarrhalis* from patients with community-acquired respiratory tract infections: Antimicrobial susceptibility patterns from the SENTRY Antimicrobial Surveillance Program (United States and Canada, 1997). Antimicrob Agents Chemother 43:385, 1999

FADEN H et al: Relationship between nasopharyngeal colonization and the development of otitis media in children. J Infect Dis 175:1440, 1997

FOXWELL AR et al: Nontypeable *Haemophilus influenzae*: Pathogenesis and prevention. Microbiol Mol Biol Rev 62:294, 1998

GALIL K et al: Reemergence of invasive *Haemophilus influenzae* type b disease in a well-vaccinated population in remote Alaska. J Infect Dis 179:101, 1999

KING R et al: An immunohistochemical analysis of naturally occurring chancroid. J Infect Dis 174:427, 1996

KLEIN JO: Clinical implications of antibiotic resistance for management of acute otitis media. Pediatr Infect Dis J 17:1084, 1998

MERTZ KJ et al: An investigation of genital ulcers in Jackson, Mississippi, with use of a multiplex polymerase chain reaction assay: High prevalence of chancroid and human immunodeficiency virus infection. J Infect Dis 178:1060, 1998

PELTOLA H et al: Perspective: A five-country analysis of the impact of four different *Haemophilus influenzae* type b conjugates and vaccination strategies in Scandinavia. J Infect Dis 179:223, 1999

QUAGLIARELLO VJ, SCHELD WM: Treatment of bacterial meningitis. N Engl J Med 336:708, 1997

SCHMID GP: Treatment of chancroid, 1997. Clin Infect Dis 28(Suppl 1):S14, 1999

YI K et al: Human immune response to nontypeable *Haemophilus influenzae* in chronic bronchitis. J Infect Dis 176:1247, 1997

---

150 *Dennis L. Kasper, Tamar F. Barlam*

INFECTIONS DUE TO THE HACEK GROUP AND MISCELLANEOUS GRAM-NEGATIVE BACTERIA

HACEK GROUP ORGANISMS

HACEK organisms are a group of fastidious, slow-growing, gram-negative bacteria whose growth requires an atmosphere of carbon dioxide. Species belonging to this group include several *Haemophilus* species, *Actinobacillus actinomycetemcomitans*, *Cardiobacterium hominis*, *Eikenella corrodens*, and *Kingella kingae*. HACEK bacteria normally reside in the oral cavity and have been associated with local infections in the mouth. They are also known to cause severe systemic infections, most often bacterial endocarditis (Chap. 126).

Of the HACEK group, the *Haemophilus* species, *A. actinomycetemcomitans*, and *C. hominis* are most frequently associated with endocarditis, which can develop on either native or prosthetic valves. In large series, up to 3% of cases of infective endocarditis are attributable to HACEK organisms. The clinical course of HACEK endocarditis tends to be subacute; however, embolization is common. The overall prevalence of major emboli associated with HACEK endocarditis ranges from 28 to 60% in different series. Cultures of blood from patients with suspected HACEK endocarditis may require up to 30 days to become positive, although most are positive within the first week. Because of this slow growth, antimicrobial testing may be difficult, and strains producing β-lactamase may not be identified accurately. This factor should be considered when choosing a therapeutic regimen.

The cure rates for HACEK prosthetic valve endocarditis appear to be high. Unlike prosthetic valve endocarditis caused by other gram-negative organisms, HACEK endocarditis is often cured with antibiotic treatment alone—i.e., without surgical intervention.

***Haemophilus* Species** *Haemophilus* species cause over half of all cases of HACEK endocarditis. *H. parainfluenzae* is most common, with *H. aphrophilus* and *H. paraphrophilus* less common. Up to 50% of patients with native valve endocarditis due to *Haemophilus* species report a history of cardiac valvular disease, 60% have been ill for <2 months before presentation, and 50% are anemic at presentation. Some 19% of these patients develop congestive heart failure. Mortality rates of up to 30% have been reported, with most deaths attributed to cerebral embolism; however, recent studies have documented mortality rates of <5%. In rare cases, *H. parainfluenzae* has been isolated from other infections, such as meningitis; brain, dental, and liver abscess; pneumonia; and septicemia.

TREATMENT   Therapy for endocarditis due to *Haemophilus* species should be based on antibiotic sensitivity testing. Empirical combination therapy with ampicillin and gentamicin, successful in prior studies, is no longer recommended because of increasing β-lactamase production by these strains. Treatment with ceftriaxone (2 g/d) is a reasonable initial approach.

Actinobacillus actinomycetemcomitans   *A. actinomycetemcomitans*, another slow-growing inhabitant of the oral cavity, can be isolated from soft tissue infections and abscesses in association with *Actinomyces israelii*. About 30% of actinomycotic lesions also yield *A. actinomycetemcomitans* on culture. *A. actinomycetemcomitans* has been associated with severe destructive periodontal disease, characterized by loss of alveolar bone of the molars and incisors, in both children and adults. Patients who develop endocarditis with this organism typically have severe periodontal disease and underlying cardiac valvular damage as well as high rates of embolic phenomena. *A. actinomycetemcomitans* has been isolated from patients with brain abscess, meningitis, parotitis, osteomyelitis, urinary tract infection, pneumonia, and empyema, among other infections.

TREATMENT   Most isolates are susceptible to third-generation cephalosporins such as ceftriaxone (2 g/d), semisynthetic penicillins such as mezlocillin, trimethoprim-sulfamethoxazole, quinolones, and azithromycin. However, because of the variability among strains, susceptibility testing should be undertaken. Endocarditis should normally be treated for 4 weeks; however, prosthetic valve infections or infections in patients with complications such as embolization justify 6 weeks of therapy.

Cardiobacterium hominis   *C. hominis* primarily causes endocarditis in patients with underlying valvular heart disease or with prosthetic valves. Many patients have signs and symptoms of long-standing infection before diagnosis and have evidence of arterial embolization, vasculitis, cerebrovascular accidents, immune complex glomerulonephritis, or arthritis at presentation. As in endocarditis due to other HACEK organisms, embolization, mycotic aneurysms, and congestive heart failure are frequent.

TREATMENT   Antibiotic sensitivity testing of *C. hominis* is difficult. Most cases of infection due to *C. hominis* are treated with penicillin (16 to 18 million units per day in 6 divided doses), either alone or in combination with an aminoglycoside (e.g., gentamicin, 5 to 6 mg/kg per day in 3 divided doses). The value of the aminoglycoside in this situation has not been established.

Eikenella corrodens   *E. corrodens*, a fastidious, facultative gram-negative organism, is part of the endogenous flora of the mouth and nasopharynx. It is most frequently recovered from sites of infection in conjunction with other bacterial species. Clinical sources of *E. corrodens* include sites of human bite wounds (clenched-fist injuries), endocarditis, soft tissue infections of the head and neck, soft tissue infections in injection drug users, osteomyelitis, respiratory infections, chorioamnionitis, gynecologic infections associated with intrauterine devices, meningitis and brain abscesses, and visceral abscesses.

TREATMENT   *E. corrodens*–associated infections can be treated with ampicillin (2 g every 4 h) or with second- or third-generation cephalosporins. The organism is susceptible to the fluoroquinolones in vitro but is resistant to metronidazole and clindamycin.

Kingella kingae   *K. kingae* is a β-hemolytic, fastidious, non-motile gram-negative rod. Because of improved microbiologic methodology, isolation of this organism is increasingly common. In young children, *K. kingae* causes septic arthritis and osteomyelitis. In several series, *K. kingae* has been the third most common cause of septic arthritis in children <24 months of age; staphylococcal and strepto-

coccal species remain most prevalent. In children <4 years of age, there is evidence for prolonged nasopharyngeal colonization, with carriage rates of 10%. Invasive *K. kingae* infections with bacteremia are associated with stomatitis. Both *K. kingae* colonization and primary herpes—a major cause of stomatitis—peak in children 6 to 48 months of age. *K. kingae* bacteremia can present with a petechial rash similar to that seen with *Neisseria meningitidis* sepsis.

Infective endocarditis, unlike other infections with *K. kingae*, occurs in older children and adults. The majority of patients have pre-existing valvular disease. As in endocarditis caused by the other HACEK organisms, there is a high incidence of complications, including arterial emboli, cerebrovascular accidents, tricuspid insufficiency, and congestive heart failure with cardiovascular collapse.

TREATMENT   *K. kingae* can be susceptible to ampicillin, second- and third-generation cephalosporins, fluoroquinolones, vancomycin, clindamycin, macrolides, and trimethoprim-sulfamethoxazole. Because of increasing β-lactamase production in *K. kingae* strains, susceptibility testing should be performed to guide therapy. Ceftriaxone (2 g/d) or ampicillin-sulbactam (3 g of ampicillin every 6 h) are both appropriate choices for initial therapy.

OTHER GRAM-NEGATIVE BACTERIA

***Acinetobacter* Species**   See Chap. 153.

Achromobacter xylosoxidans   Previously known as *Alcaligenes xylosoxidans*, the gram-negative bacillus *Achromobacter xylosoxidans* is probably part of the endogenous intestinal flora and has been isolated from water sources. Immunocompromised hosts appear to be at increased risk for infection with this organism. Nosocomial sources to which outbreaks of infection with *A. xylosoxidans* have been attributed include contaminated intravenous fluids, pressure transducers, and disinfectants. Clinical illness has been associated with isolates from many sites, including blood (often in the setting of infected intravascular devices), urine, respiratory secretions, cerebrospinal fluid, peritoneal and pleural fluids, and endocarditic prosthetic valves. Community-acquired bacteremia with *A. xylosoxidans* usually occurs in the setting of pneumonia. Metastatic skin lesions are present in one-fifth of cases. The reported mortality rate is 67%, similar to rates for other bacteremic gram-negative pneumonias.

TREATMENT   In vitro susceptibility testing of all clinically relevant isolates is essential to the selection of appropriate therapy.

Agrobacterium radiobacter (tumefaciens)   This organism has been associated with intravascular catheter–related infections in immunocompromised hosts, especially individuals infected with HIV. Clinically important infections associated with *A. radiobacter* include prosthetic joint and prosthetic valve infections, bacteremia, peritonitis, and urinary tract infections.

TREATMENT   Antibiotic sensitivity testing is essential in the choice of therapy.

***Capnocytophaga* Species**   This genus of fusiform, long, thin, gram-negative coccobacilli is facultatively anaerobic and requires an atmosphere enriched in carbon dioxide for optimal growth. *C. ochracea, C. gingivalis,* and *C. sputigena* are inhabitants of the healthy human oral cavity and have been isolated from the female genital tract. Their isolation has also been reported from blood, cerebrospinal fluid, and respiratory fluids (including pleural collections). These organisms have been associated with sepsis in immunocompromised hosts; particularly at risk are patients with acute myelogenous leukemia or acute lymphocytic leukemia. In the immunocompetent host, these three species probably play a role in localized juvenile periodontitis; however, they have been isolated from many other sites as well, usually as part of a polymicrobial infection. In vitro sensitivity testing of these organisms is difficult because they are slow-growing and fastidious.

C. canimorsus and *C. cynodegmi* are endogenous to the canine mouth. Patients infected with these species frequently have a history of dog bites or of exposure to dogs without scratches or bites. Asplenia, glucocorticoid therapy, and alcohol abuse are predisposing conditions and are associated with relatively fulminant infections. The interval from dog bite to presentation averages 5 days but ranges from 1 day to 1 month. *C. canimorsus* causes a wide range of infections, including severe sepsis with shock and disseminated intravascular coagulation, meningitis, endocarditis, cellulitis, and septic arthritis. In the asplenic individual who has recently sustained a dog bite, infection with this organism must be considered early because of a potentially rapid progression to death.

℞ TREATMENT Although penicillin has been considered first-line therapy for infections due to *C. ochracea*, *C. gingivalis*, and *C. sputigena*, an increasing number of isolates reportedly produce β-lactamase. Clindamycin (600 to 900 mg every 6 to 8 h) or drug combinations including a penicillin derivative plus a β-lactamase inhibitor—such as ampicillin/sulbactam (1.5 to 3.0 g of ampicillin every 6 h)—are currently recommended for empirical therapy. Penicillin (12 to 18 million units daily in 6 divided doses) is the drug of choice for infections with *C. canimorsus*. This regimen should also be given prophylactically to asplenic patients sustaining dog-bite injuries. Patients with suspected infection due to *C. canimorsus* should be treated empirically, because identification of this organism and determination of its antibiotic sensitivity can take many days. Other drugs to which *C. canimorsus* is reportedly susceptible include clindamycin, imipenem, quinolones, and third-generation cephalosporins.

Chromobacterium violaceum This organism is rarely a human pathogen but reportedly has been responsible for life-threatening infections with severe sepsis and metastatic abscesses. A slender, slightly curved, gram-negative rod that is facultatively anaerobic, *C. violaceum* inhabits tropical water and soil and causes infection after contamination of skin wounds. Patients with defective neutrophil function (e.g., those with chronic granulomatous disease) are infected by this organism with unusual frequency. The mortality rate in the United States from infection with *C. violaceum* has been reported at >60%.

℞ TREATMENT *C. violaceum* is generally susceptible to ciprofloxacin (500 mg every 12 h orally or 400 mg every 12 h intravenously), trimethoprim-sulfamethoxazole, gentamicin, and chloramphenicol.

***Chryseobacterium* Species** *C. meningosepticum* and *C. indologenes* were previously classified as *Flavobacterium* species. *C. meningosepticum* is a ubiquitous organism and an important cause of nosocomial infections. It has been associated with outbreaks due to contaminated fluids, such as disinfectants, arterial catheter flush solutions, and aerosolized antibiotics, and with sporadic infections due to indwelling devices, vials, sink traps, feeding tubes, and other fluid-associated apparatus. Patients with nosocomial *C. meningosepticum* infection usually have underlying immunosuppression (e.g., related to malignancy). *C. meningosepticum* has been reported to cause meningitis (primarily in neonates), sepsis, endocarditis, bacteremia, soft tissue infections, and pneumonia. *C. indologenes* has caused bacteremia, sepsis, and pneumonia, typically in immunocompromised patients with indwelling devices.

℞ TREATMENT Antibiotic treatment should be based on susceptibility results because of the high likelihood that *C. meningosepticum* will produce β-lactamase. Early reports suggested that vancomycin might be efficacious, but more recent data refute this conclusion.

Plesiomonas shigelloides This freshwater organism is a cause of acute diarrhea (Chap. 131) and occasionally of serious extraintestinal disease. *P. shigelloides* is transmitted to humans via contaminated water or food. This motile, facultatively anaerobic gram-negative rod most often produces mild diarrhea with mucoid, bloody feces containing leukocytes. Severe extraintestinal infections have been reported, most commonly in immunocompromised hosts, and include bacteremia, cellulitis, neonatal sepsis and meningitis, and septic arthritis.

℞ TREATMENT There is great variability among strains in terms of antibiotic sensitivity patterns, and isolates must be tested before appropriate therapy can be selected.

***Aeromonas* Species** Five species of *Aeromonas* are known to be associated with disease in humans, but >85% of these infections are caused by *A. hydrophila*, *A. caviae*, and *A. veronii* biovar. *sobria*. *Aeromonas* proliferates in potable and fresh water and in soil. It remains controversial whether *Aeromonas* is a cause of bacterial gastroenteritis. Although many case reports have associated *Aeromonas* with gastroenteritis, no clear outbreaks with a single isolate have been documented, no conclusive animal model exists, and asymptomatic colonization of the intestinal tract with *Aeromonas* occurs frequently. However, rare cases of hemolytic-uremic syndrome occurring after bloody diarrhea have been shown to be secondary to the presence of *Aeromonas*. In addition, identification of an enterotoxin (different from the Shiga-like toxin produced by *Escherichia coli* O157:H7) in these cases supports the hypothesis that *Aeromonas* causes gastroenteritis.

Aeromonas causes sepsis and bacteremia in infants with multiple medical problems and in immunocompromised hosts, particularly those with cancer or hepatobiliary disease. *Aeromonas* infection and sepsis can occur in trauma patients with myonecrosis or in burn patients exposed to *Aeromonas* by environmental contamination of their wounds from fresh water or soil sources. Mortality ranges from 25% for sepsis in immunocompromised adults to >90% in patients with myonecrosis. *Aeromonas* can produce skin lesions resembling the ecthyma gangrenosum lesions seen in *Pseudomonas aeruginosa* infection. These lesions are hemorrhagic vesicles surrounded by a rim of erythema with central necrosis and ulceration.

Aeromonas wound infections can occur in healthy adults who sustain minor trauma with environmental contamination, usually water-related; after severe trauma and crush injuries with sepsis and environmental exposure, usually to soil; and in nosocomial infections related to catheters, surgical incisions, or use of leeches. Other clinical manifestations include meningitis, peritonitis, pneumonia, and ocular infections.

℞ TREATMENT Treatment should be guided by antimicrobial susceptibility testing. *Aeromonas* species are generally susceptible to fluoroquinolones (e.g., ciprofloxacin at a dosage of 500 mg every 12 h orally or 400 mg every 12 h intravenously), trimethoprim-sulfamethoxazole at a trimethoprim dosage of 10 mg/kg per day in 3 or 4 divided doses, third-generation cephalosporins, and aminoglycosides. However, resistance is increasing.

Miscellaneous Organisms Many other gram-negative rods have been reported to cause occasional infections in hosts who are immunologically unprepared to deal with relatively avirulent organisms or who are unfortunate enough to encounter an exceptionally large inoculum. Such organisms include *Weeksella* species; various CDC groups, such as EF-4, Ve-2 (*Flavimonas* species), IVc-2, NO-1, WO-1, and Gilardi Group WO-1; *Sphingobacterium* species; *Protomonas* species; *Ochrobactrum anthropi*; *Oligella urethralis*; and *Shewanella putrefaciens*. The reader is advised to consult subspecialty texts and references for further guidance on these organisms.

BILGRAMI S et al: *Capnocytophaga* bacteremia in a patient with Hodgkin's disease following bone marrow transplantation: Case report and review. Clin Infect Dis 14:1045, 1992

BLOCK KC et al: *Chryseobacterium meningosepticum*: An emerging pathogen among immunocompromised adults. Medicine 76:30, 1997

DARRAS-JOLY C et al: *Haemophilus* endocarditis: Report of 42 cases in adults and review. Clin Infect Dis 24:1087, 1997

DAS M et al: Infective endocarditis caused by HACEK microorganisms. Annu Rev Med 48:25, 1997

HULSE M et al: *Agrobacterium* infection in humans: Experience at one hospital and review. Clin Infect Dis 16:112, 1993

JANDA JM et al: Evolving concepts regarding the genus *Aeromonas*: An expanding panorama of species, disease presentations, and unanswered questions. Clin Infect Dis 27:332, 1998

KUGLER KC et al: Determination of the antimicrobial activity of 29 clinically important compounds tested against fastidious HACEK group organisms. Diagn Microbiol Infect Dis 34:73, 1999

KULLBERG JB et al: Purpura fulminans and symmetrical peripheral gangrene caused by *Capnocytophaga canimorsus* (formerly DF-2) septicemia—a complication of dog bite. Medicine 70:287, 1991

MAURY S et al: Bacteremia due to *Capnocytophaga* species in patients with neutropenia: High frequency of beta-lactamase producing strains. Clin Infect Dis 28:1172, 1999

PAJU S et al: Heterogeneity of *Actinobacillus actinomycetemcomitans* strains in various human infections and relationships between serotype, genotype and antimicrobial susceptibility. J Clin Microbiol 38:79, 2000

PATRICK WD et al: Infective endocarditis due to *Eikenella corrodens*: Case report and review of the literature. Can J Infect Dis 1:139, 1990

TI T-Y et al: Nonfatal and fatal infections caused by *Chromobacterium violaceum*. Clin Infect Dis 17:505, 1993

WALSH RD et al: *Achromobacter xylosoxidans* osteomyelitis. Clin Infect Dis 16:176, 1993

WILSON ME: Prosthetic valve endocarditis and paravalvular abscess caused by *Actinobacillus actinomycetemcomitans*. Rev Infect Dis 11:665, 1989

YAGUPSKY P et al: *Kingella kingae*: An emerging cause of invasive infections in young children. Clin Infect Dis 24:86, 1997

151 *Feng-Yee Chang, Victor L. Yu*

LEGIONELLA INFECTION

DEFINITION *Legionellosis* refers to the two clinical syndromes caused by bacteria of the genus *Legionella*. *Pontiac fever* is an acute, febrile, self-limited illness that has been serologically linked to *Legionella* species, whereas *Legionnaires' disease* is the designation for pneumonia caused by these species.

HISTORY Legionnaires' disease was first recognized in 1976, when an outbreak of pneumonia took place at a hotel in Philadelphia during the American Legion Convention. Investigators from the Centers for Disease Control and Prevention (CDC) identified the causative aerobic gram-negative bacterium in lung specimens obtained from the victims at autopsy and named this organism *L. pneumophila*. Retrospective studies of stored serum samples revealed that an epidemic of Legionnaires' disease had occurred in 1957 in Austin, Minnesota. In this epidemic 78 persons were hospitalized with acute respiratory infection. Antibody determinations showed seroconversion to *L. pneumophila* in most cases.

MICROBIOLOGY At present, the family Legionellaceae comprises 41 species with 64 serogroups. The species *L. pneumophila* causes 80 to 90% of human infections and includes at least 14 serogroups; serogroups 1, 4, and 6 are most commonly implicated in human infections. To date, 17 species other than *L. pneumophila* have been associated with human infections, among which *L. micdadei*

(Pittsburgh pneumonia agent), *L. bozemanii*, *L. dumoffii*, and *L. longbeachae* are the most common.

Members of the Legionellaceae are aerobic, thin, gram-negative bacilli that do not grow on routine microbiologic media. Buffered charcoal yeast extract (BCYE) agar is the medium used to grow *Legionella*. This highly enhanced medium contains the amino acid L-cysteine, which is an absolute growth requirement for *Legionella*. Growth of the organism on BCYE medium is usually visible in 3 to 5 days at 35 to 37°C. *L. micdadei* and *L. maceachernii* produce blue colonies on BCYE medium containing bromocresol purple and bromothymol blue dyes, while the other species produce green colonies.

Antimicrobial agents, including polymyxin B, cefamandole, and vancomycin, are used in *Legionella*-selective media to suppress competing components of the microflora. Although *L. pneumophila* is relatively tolerant to these antibiotics, the drugs may inhibit the growth of other legionellae; for example, cefamandole-containing media suppress the growth of *L. micdadei*.

Traditional biochemical tests are not particularly helpful in distinguishing one *Legionella* species from another. Fatty-acid profile determination by gas-liquid chromatography and ubiquinone analysis allow identification to the genus level. The direct fluorescent antibody (DFA) test can definitively identify a number of individual species. In *L. pneumophila*, lipopolysaccharide is a prominent constituent of the outer membrane, and the serogroup-specific antigen and antibodies detected by immunofluorescence are directed primarily at the lipopolysaccharide. Both polyclonal and monoclonal DFA reagents are commercially available. The monoclonal antibody reagent is less cross-reactive but is specific for *L. pneumophila*. Genetic analysis has been considered the definitive arbiter for the identification of individual species, with the degree of DNA sequence homology the most common criterion employed. A nucleic-acid hybridization probe reactive to *Legionella* ribosomal RNA, used with a single reagent, can identify a member of the genus within hours.

ECOLOGY AND TRANSMISSION The natural habitats for *L. pneumophila* are aquatic bodies, including lakes and streams; *L. longbeachae* has been isolated from soil. Legionellae can survive under a wide range of environmental conditions; for example, the organisms can live for years in refrigerated water samples. Natural bodies of water contain only small numbers of legionellae. However, once the organisms enter human-constructed aquatic reservoirs (such as cooling towers or water-distribution systems), they can grow and proliferate. Factors known to enhance colonization by and amplification of legionellae include warm temperatures (25° to 42°C), stagnation, and scale and sediment. The presence of symbiotic microorganisms, including algae, amebas, ciliated protozoa, and other water-dwelling bacteria, likewise promotes growth of *L. pneumophila*.

Hot-water tanks colonized with *L. pneumophila* are significantly more likely than uncolonized tanks to be cooler (<60°C), to have a vertical configuration, to be older, and to have higher concentrations of calcium and magnesium. Vertical tanks, especially those that are electric coil-heated rather than gas-heated, have a pronounced temperature stratification and thick sediment accumulation at the bottom. Studies have shown that neither a high degree of outward cleanliness nor routine application of maintenance measures decreases the frequency or intensity of *Legionella* colonization. Thus, engineering guidelines and building codes, although often advocated as preventive measures, have relatively little impact on *Legionella* colonization.

The source of *Legionella* is water, but the mode of transmission from the environmental reservoir to the patient remains controversial. Early investigations that implicated cooling towers antedated the discovery that the organism could also exist in potable water distribution systems. It is now known that, in many outbreaks, cases of Legionnaires' disease continued to occur despite disinfection of cooling towers and the potable water supply was the actual source. Koch's postulates have been fulfilled in epidemiologic studies using molecular fingerprinting methods to link potable water sources (rather than cooling towers) to *Legionella* infection in humans. Community-acquired Legionnaires' disease has been linked to colonization of residential and industrial water supplies.

Multiple modes of transmission of *Legionella* to humans exist, including aerosolization, aspiration, and direct instillation into the lung during respiratory tract manipulations. Aspiration may be the predominant mode of transmission, but it is unclear whether *Legionella* enters the lung via oropharyngeal colonization or directly via the drinking of contaminated water. Nasogastric tubes have been linked to nosocomial Legionnaires' disease in several reports; microaspiration of contaminated water was the hypothesized mode of transmission. Surgery with general anesthesia is a known risk factor that is consistent with aspiration. Especially compelling is the reported 30% incidence of postoperative *Legionella* pneumonia among patients undergoing head and neck surgery in a hospital with a contaminated water supply; aspiration is a recognized sequela in such cases. Studies of patients with hospital-acquired Legionnaires' disease showed that these individuals underwent endotracheal intubation significantly more often and for a significantly longer duration than patients with nosocomial pneumonia of other etiologies.

Aerosolization of legionellae by devices filled with tap water, including nebulizers and humidifiers, has caused cases of Legionnaires' disease. An ultrasonic mist machine in the produce section of a grocery store was implicated in a community outbreak. Pontiac fever has been linked to *Legionella*-containing aerosols from water-using machinery, a cooling tower, air-conditioners, and whirlpools.

EPIDEMIOLOGY   The incidence of Legionnaires' disease depends on the degree of contamination of the aquatic reservoir, the susceptibility and immune status of the persons exposed to the water from that reservoir, the intensity of exposure, and the availability of specialized laboratory tests on which the correct diagnosis can be based.

Numerous prospective studies have found *Legionella* to rank among the top four microbial causes of community-acquired pneumonia (*Streptococcus pneumoniae*, *Haemophilus influenzae*, and *Chlamydia pneumoniae* usually ranking first, second, and third), accounting for 3 to 15% of cases. On the basis of a multihospital study of community-acquired pneumonia in Ohio, the CDC has estimated that only 3% of sporadic cases of Legionnaires' disease are correctly diagnosed. Legionellae are responsible for 10 to 50% of nosocomial pneumonias when a hospital's water system is colonized with the organisms. One situation in which the diagnosis of Legionnaires' disease should be considered is that in which the presenting patient has been hospitalized within 10 days before the onset of symptoms. In one study, a number of patients had been discharged from the hospital and readmitted with Legionnaires' disease; molecular fingerprinting showed that the isolates obtained from patients and the isolate from the hospital's water supply were similar.

The most common risk factors for Legionnaires' disease are cigarette smoking, chronic lung disease, advanced age, and immunosuppression. The disease most often develops in elderly men; this predilection is probably related to cigarette smoking. Surgery is a prominent predisposing factor in nosocomial infection, with transplant recipients at highest risk. Nosocomial cases are now being recognized among neonates and among children with immunosuppression or underlying pulmonary disease.

Pontiac fever occurs in epidemics. The high attack rate (>90%) reflects airborne transmission.

PATHOGENESIS   Legionellae enter the lungs through aspiration or direct inhalation. The organisms possess pili that may mediate adherence to respiratory tract epithelial cells. Thus, conditions that impair mucociliary clearance, including cigarette smoking, lung disease, or alcoholism, predispose to Legionnaires' disease.

Cell-mediated immunity is the primary mechanism of host defense against *Legionella*, as it is against other intracellular pathogens, including *Mycobacterium tuberculosis*, *Listeria*, and *Toxoplasma*. Al-

veolar macrophages readily phagocytose legionellae. The attachment of the bacteria to phagocytes is mediated via complement receptors, which attach to the bacterial major outer-membrane protein. Binding to these receptors promotes phagocytosis but fails to trigger an oxidative burst. Although many legionellae are killed, some proliferate intracellularly until the cells rupture; the bacteria are then phagocytosed again by newly recruited phagocytes, and the cycle begins anew. Legionnaires' disease is more common and the disease manifestations are more severe in patients with depressed cell-mediated immunity, including transplant recipients, patients infected with HIV, and patients receiving glucocorticoids. The disease also occurs with unusual frequency among patients with hairy cell leukemia (which is characterized by monocyte deficiency and dysfunction) but not among patients with other types of leukemia.

The role of neutrophils in immunity appears to be minimal: neutropenic patients are not predisposed to Legionnaires' disease. Although *L. pneumophila* is susceptible to oxygen-dependent microbiologic systems in vitro, it resists killing by neutrophils.

The humoral immune system is active against *Legionella*. Type-specific IgM and IgG antibodies are measurable within weeks of infection. In vitro, antibodies promote killing of legionellae by phagocytes (neutrophils, monocytes, and alveolar macrophages). However, antibodies neither enhance lysis by complement nor inhibit intracellular multiplication within phagocytes. Immunized animals develop a specific antibody response, with subsequent resistance to *Legionella* challenge.

Some *L. pneumophila* strains are clearly more virulent than others, although the precise factors mediating virulence remain uncertain. For example, although multiple strains may colonize water-distribution systems, only a few cause disease in patients exposed to that water. At least one surface epitope of *L. pneumophila* serogroup 1 is associated with virulence. *L. pneumophila* serogroup 6 is more commonly involved in nosocomial Legionnaires' disease and is more likely to be associated with a poor outcome.

PATHOLOGY   The consistent pathologic features of Legionnaires' disease are confined to the lungs. Findings in infected lung tissue range from multifocal pneumonia with patchy lobular inflammation to extensive multilobar consolidation. Visible abscesses with central necrosis were seen in 20% of autopsied cases in one study. On histologic examination, fibrinopurulent pneumonia with intensive alveolitis and bronchiolitis is evident. Lesions of longer standing can have a nodular appearance with a central area of necrosis surrounded by macrophages and other cells. The alveoli are filled with fibrin, neutrophils, and alveolar macrophages.

Usual tissue stains, including Gram's, hematoxylin and eosin, Brown-Brenn, and methenamine silver, do not reveal the organism. Giminez stain can be used for imprints on fresh or fixed tissue. Dieterle's silver stain or modified Giminez stain, although nonspecific and relatively insensitive, can be used for paraffin-fixed specimens. The DFA stain is not only specific but also the most sensitive option for visualization of the organism in tissues. Polyvalent DFA stains but not monoclonal DFA stain can be used for formalinized specimens. Because the DFA stains are species and serogroup specific, false-negative results can be obtained if the incorrect reagent is used. Thus, culture is the preferred method for diagnosis based on clinical specimens.

CLINICAL AND LABORATORY FEATURES   **Pontiac Fever**   Pontiac fever is an acute, self-limiting, flulike illness with a 24- to 48-h incubation period. Pneumonia does not develop in Pontiac fever. Malaise, fatigue, and myalgias are the most frequent symptoms, occurring in 97% of cases. Fever (usually with chills) develops in 80 to 90% of cases and headache in 80%. Other symptoms (seen in fewer than 50% of cases) include arthralgias, nausea, cough, abdominal pain, and diarrhea. Modest leukocytosis with a neutrophilic predominance is sometimes detected. Complete recovery takes place within only a few days without antibiotic therapy; a few patients may experience lassitude for many weeks thereafter. The diagnosis is established by antibody seroconversion.

Legionnaires' Disease (Pneumonia) Clinical findings that raise the possibility of Legionnaires' disease are summarized in Table 151-1. Although these manifestations may provide clues to the diagnosis, prospective comparative studies have shown that they are generally nonspecific and do not serve to distinguish Legionnaires' disease from pneumonia of other etiologies. Legionnaires' disease is often included in the differential diagnosis of "atypical pneumonia," along with infection due to *Chlamydia pneumoniae*, *C. psittaci*, *Mycoplasma pneumoniae*, *Coxiella burnetii*, and some viruses. The clinical similarities among these types of pneumonia include a relatively nonproductive cough and a low incidence of grossly purulent sputum. However, the clinical manifestations of Legionnaires' disease are usually more severe than those of most "atypical" pneumonias, and the course and prognosis of *Legionella* pneumonia more resemble those of bacteremic pneumococcal pneumonia than those of pneumonia due to other "atypical" pathogens. Patients with community-acquired Legionnaires' disease are significantly more likely than patients with pneumonia of other etiologies to be admitted to an intensive care unit on presentation.

The incubation period for Legionnaires' disease is 2 to 10 days. The symptoms and signs may range from a mild cough and a slight fever to stupor with widespread pulmonary infiltrates and multisystem failure. Nonspecific symptoms—malaise, fatigue, anorexia, and headache—are seen early in the illness. Myalgias and arthralgias are uncommon but are unusually marked in a few patients. Upper respiratory symptoms, including coryza, are rare.

The mild cough of Legionnaires' disease is only slightly productive. Sometimes the sputum is streaked with blood. Chest pain—either pleuritic or nonpleuritic—can be a prominent feature and, when coupled with hemoptysis, can lead to an incorrect diagnosis of pulmonary embolism. Shortness of breath is reported by one-third to one-half of patients.

Gastrointestinal difficulties are often pronounced; abdominal pain, nausea, and vomiting affect 10 to 20% of patients. Diarrhea (watery rather than bloody) is reported in 25 to 50% of cases. The most common neurologic abnormalities are confusion or changes in mental status; however, the multitudinous neurologic symptoms reported range from headache and lethargy to encephalopathy.

Patients with Legionnaires' disease virtually always have fever. Temperatures in excess of 40.5°C (104.9°F) were recorded in 20% of the cases in one series. Relative bradycardia has been overemphasized as a useful diagnostic finding; it occurs infrequently, primarily affecting older patients with severe pneumonia. Chest examination reveals rales early in the course and evidence of consolidations as the disease progresses. Abdominal examination may reveal generalized or local tenderness.

Diarrhea and hyponatremia occur significantly more often in Legionnaires' disease than in other forms of pneumonia. Hyponatremia is most common in severe cases. The mechanism of hyponatremia does not appear to be related to inappropriate secretion of antidiuretic hormone but instead to salt and water loss. Besides hyponatremia, other laboratory abnormalities include abnormal liver function tests, hypophosphatemia, hematuria, hematologic abnormalities, and thrombocytopenia; although common, these abnormalities are not found significantly more frequently in Legionnaires' disease than in pneumonias of other etiologies.

Table 151-1 Clinical Clues Suggestive of Legionnaires' Disease

Diarrhea
High fever (>40°C or >104°F))
Numerous neutrophils but no organisms revealed by Gram's staining of respiratory secretions
Hyponatremia (serum sodium level of <131 meq/L)
Failure to respond to β-lactam drugs (penicillins or cephalosporins) and aminoglycoside antibiotics
Occurrence of illness in an environment in which the potable water supply is known to be contaminated with *Legionella*
Onset of symptoms within 10 days after discharge from the hospital

Extrapulmonary Legionellosis Since the portal of entry for legionellae is the lung in virtually all cases, extrapulmonary manifestations usually result from bloodborne dissemination from the lung. In a prospective survey of patients with Legionnaires' disease diagnosed by isolation of the organism from sputum, legionellae were isolated from the blood by a special culture method in 38% of cases.

Legionella has been identified in the spleen, liver, or kidneys in 50% of autopsied cases of Legionnaires' disease. The organism has also been isolated from intrathoracic and inguinal lymph nodes—a finding suggesting dissemination by lymphatic pathways. Extrapulmonary involvement, including sinusitis, peritonitis, pyelonephritis, cellulitis, and pancreatitis, has been documented predominantly in immunosuppressed patients.

The most common extrapulmonary site of legionellosis is the heart; numerous reports have described myocarditis, pericarditis, postcardiotomy syndrome, and prosthetic-valve endocarditis. Most cases have been hospital-acquired. Since many of the patients involved have not had overt pneumonia, the lung may not have been the portal of entry. Rather, in these cardiac infections, the organisms may have gained entry through a postoperative sternal wound exposed to contaminated tap water or through a mediastinal-tube insertion site.

Various other sources of or factors promoting *Legionella* infection at various extrapulmonary sites have been postulated, including the presence of foreign bodies, such as sutures and draining tubes (wound infection after cardiothoracic surgery); immersion in a Hubbard tank (superinfection of a hip wound); bloodborne dissemination from a pulmonary infection site (perirectal abscess); and ingestion of contaminated water (peritonitis).

Chest Radiographic Abnormalities Virtually all patients with Legionnaires' disease have abnormal chest radiographs showing pulmonary infiltrates at the time of clinical presentation. In a few cases of nosocomial disease, fever and respiratory tract symptoms have preceded the appearance of the infiltrate on chest radiography. Findings on chest radiography are nonspecific and do not serve to distinguish Legionnaires' disease from pneumonias of other etiologies. Pleural effusion is evident in one-third of cases, and the diagnosis is often based on culture and antigen testing (by the method designed for use with urine) of pleural fluid obtained by thoracentesis.

In immunosuppressed patients, especially those receiving glucocorticoids, distinctive rounded nodular opacities may be seen; these lesions may expand and cavitate (Fig. 151-1). Likewise, pulmonary abscesses can occur in immunosuppressed hosts. The progression of infiltrates on chest radiography despite appropriate antibiotic therapy is common, and radiographic improvement lags behind clinical improvement by several days. Complete clearing of infiltrates requires 1 to 4 months.

DIAGNOSIS The diagnosis of Legionnaires' disease requires special microbiologic tests (Table 151-2). The sensitivity of bronchoscopy specimens is approximately the same as that of sputum samples; if sputum is not available, bronchoscopy specimens may yield the organism. Bronchoalveolar lavage fluid gives higher yields than bronchial wash specimens. Thoracentesis should be performed if pleural effusion is found, and the fluid should be evaluated by DFA staining, culture, and the antigen test designed for use with urine.

Staining Gram's staining of material from normally sterile sites, such as pleural fluid or lung tissue, occasionally suggests the diagnosis; efforts to detect legionellae in sputum by Gram's staining typically reveal numerous leukocytes, but no organisms. When they are visualized, the organisms appear as small, pleomorphic, faint, gram-negative bacilli. *L. micdadei* organisms can be detected as weakly or partially acid-fast bacilli in clinical specimens. Modified acid-fast staining substitutes 1% sulfuric acid for the traditional 3% hydrochloric acid; the less aggressive decolorizer increases the yield of *L. micdadei*. *Legionella*-infected patients have often been treated empirically with antituberculosis medications because of false-positive acid-fast smears.

The DFA test is rapid and highly specific but is less sensitive than

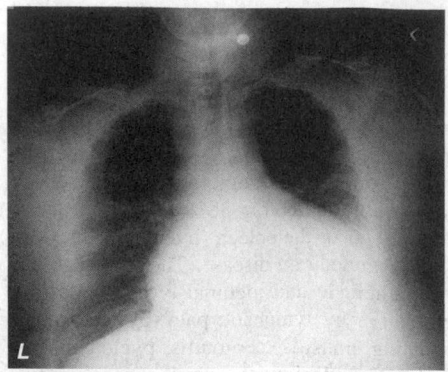
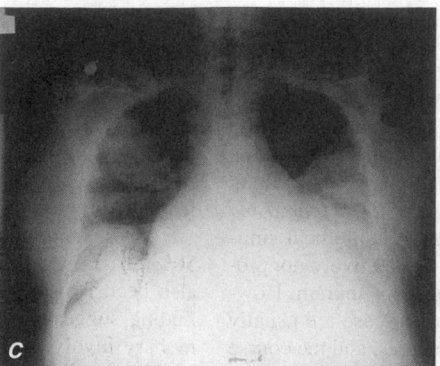
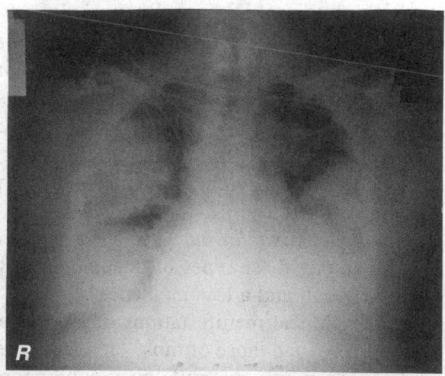

FIGURE 151-1 Chest radiographic findings in a 52-year-old man who presented with pneumonia subsequently diagnosed as Legionnaires' disease. The patient was a cigarette smoker with chronic obstructive pulmonary disease and alcoholic cardiomyopathy; he had received glucocorticoids. *L. pneumophila* was identified by DFA staining and culture of sputum. *Left:* Baseline chest radiograph showing long-standing cardiomegaly. *Center:* Admission chest radiograph showing new rounded opacities. *Right:* Chest radiograph taken 3 days after admission, during treatment with erythromycin.

culture because large numbers of organisms are required for microscopic visualization. This test is more likely to be positive in advanced than in early disease.

Culture The definitive method for diagnosis of *Legionella* infection is isolation of the organism from respiratory secretions or other specimens. As has been mentioned, BCYE agar supplemented with antibiotics and dyes is the most sensitive medium, and colonies grow slowly, requiring 3 to 5 days to become grossly visible. When culture plates are overgrown with other microflora, pretreatment of the specimen with acid or heat can markedly improve the yield. *L. pneumophila* is often isolated from sputum that is not grossly or microscopically purulent; sputum containing more than 25 epithelial cells per high-power field (a finding that classically suggests contamination) may still yield *L. pneumophila*.

Antibody Detection Antibody testing of both acute- and convalescent-phase sera may be necessary. A fourfold rise in titer is diagnostic; 4 to 12 weeks are often required for the detection of an antibody response, and some patients never seroconvert. A single titer of 1:128 in a patient with pneumonia constitutes presumptive (but not definitive) evidence for Legionnaires' disease. Serology is of use primarily in epidemiologic studies. The specificity of serology for the non–*L. pneumophila* species is uncertain; there is cross-reactivity with *L. pneumophila* and some gram-negative bacilli.

Urinary Antigen The assay for *Legionella* soluble antigen in urine (Binax, Portland, ME) is rapid, relative inexpensive, easy to perform, second only to culture in terms of sensitivity, and highly specific. Its use in every clinical laboratory is recommended. The test is available only for *L. pneumophila* serogroup 1, which, as has been mentioned, causes about 80% of *Legionella* infections. Antigen in urine is detectable 3 days after the onset of clinical disease, even if specific therapy has been started; furthermore, urinary antigen persists for several weeks.

Molecular Methods Polymerase chain reaction (PCR) with DNA probes is theoretically more sensitive and specific than other methods, but results have been disappointing to date. PCR has proved useful in the identification of legionellae from environmental water specimens.

TREATMENT Controlled evaluations of antibiotic therapy for Legionnaires' disease have never been conducted. In the 1976 American Legion outbreak, patients treated with erythromycin and tetracycline appeared to have a better outcome than those treated with other agents. These two antibiotics also exhibited intracellular activity against legionellae and were effective in animal models. The fact that *Legionella* is an intracellular pathogen provided the biologic basis for the success of erythromycin and tetracycline, given that relatively high intracellular penetration. Antibiotics capable of achieving intracellular concentrations higher than the minimal inhibitory concentration are the most likely to be efficacious in the clinical setting. The dosages for various drugs used in the treatment of *Legionella* infection are listed in Table 151-3.

The newer macrolides (especially azithromycin) and quinolones are now the antibiotics of choice, displacing erythromycin. Compared with erythromycin, the newer agents azithromycin, clarithromycin, and roxithromycin have superior in vitro activity, display greater intracellular activity, and reach higher concentrations in respiratory secretions and in lung tissue. The pharmacokinetics of the newer macrolides and quinolones also allow once- or twice-daily dosing, in

Table 151-2 Utility of Special Laboratory Tests for the Diagnosis of Legionnaires' Disease

Test	Sensitivity, %	Specificity, %
Culture		
Sputum[a]	80	100
Transtracheal aspirate	90	100
DFA staining of sputum	50–70	96–99
Urinary antigen testing[b]	70	100
Antibody serology[c]	40–60	96–99

[a] Use of multiple selective media with dyes.
[b] Serogroup 1 only.
[c] IgG and IgM testing of both acute- and convalescent-phase sera. A single titer of ≥1:128 is considered presumptive, while a single titer of ≥1:256 or fourfold seroconversion is considered definitive.

Table 151-3 Antibiotic Therapy for *Legionella* Infection[a]

Antimicrobial Agent	Dose, mg[b]	Route[c]	Frequency
Azithromycin	500[d]	PO, IV	q24h
Clarithromycin	500	PO, IV[e]	q12h
Roxithromycin	300[e]	PO	q12h
Erythromycin[f]	1000 (1 g)	IV	q6h
	500	PO	q6h
Ciprofloxacin	400	IV	q8h
	750	PO	q12h
Levofloxacin	500[d]	PO, IV	q24h
Ofloxacin	400	PO, IV	q12h
Doxycycline	100[d]	PO, IV	q12h
Minocycline	100[d]	PO, IV	q12h
Tetracycline	500	PO, IV	q6h
Trimethoprim-sulfamethoxazole	160/800	IV	q8h
	160/800	PO	q12h
Rifampin	300–600	PO, IV	q12h

[a] Total duration of therapy should be 10 to 14 days in immunocompetent hosts and 3 weeks in immunosuppressed patients and in those with advanced disease.
[b] Except as indicated.
[c] Intravenous therapy should be used until the patient's clinical condition improves, after which oral therapy can be substituted.
[d] Doubling of the first dose is recommended.
[e] Investigational in the United States.
[f] Now replaced by newer macrolides (see text).

contrast to the four-times-daily dosing required for erythromycin. Finally, the large fluid volume required for intravenous administration, symptomatic ototoxicity, and gastrointestinal side effects have rendered erythromycin obsolete for the treatment of *Legionella* infection.

The quinolones (levofloxacin, ciprofloxacin, pefloxacin, gemifloxacin, and moxifloxacin) are more active than any of the macrolides against *Legionella* in in vitro dilution susceptibility tests, intracellular models, and animal models. Furthermore, in open noncomparative studies of pneumonia, numerous cases of Legionnaires' disease have been successfully treated with quinolones. Quinolones are the preferred antibiotics for transplant recipients because both macrolides (except azithromycin) and rifampin interact pharmacologically with cyclosporine and tacrolimus.

Alternative agents include tetracycline and its analogues doxycycline and minocycline. Anecdotal reports have described both successes and failures with trimethoprim-sulfamethoxazole, imipenem, and clindamycin. For severely ill patients with Legionnaires' disease, the combination of rifampin plus a macrolide or a quinolone can be used for initial treatment.

Initial therapy should be given by the intravenous route. Usually, a clinical response occurs within 3 to 5 days, after which oral therapy can be substituted. The total duration of therapy in the immunocompetent host is 10 to 14 days; a longer course (3 weeks) may be appropriate for immunosuppressed patients and those with advanced disease. In the oral phase, 5 to 10 days of azithromycin is therapy sufficient.

Mortality rates for Legionnaires' disease vary, depending on the patient's underlying disease and its severity, the patient's immune status, the severity of pneumonia, and the timing of administration of appropriate antimicrobial therapy. Mortality rates are highest (80%) among immunosuppressed patients who do not receive appropriate antimicrobial therapy. With appropriate and timely antibiotic treatment, mortality from community-acquired Legionnaires' disease among immunocompetent patients ranges from 0 to 11%; without treatment, the figure may be as high as 31%. Pontiac fever requires only symptom-based treatment, not antimicrobial therapy.

PREVENTION Routine environmental culture of the hospital water supply is recommended as an approach to the prevention of hospital-acquired Legionnaires' disease. Positive cultures from the water supply mandate the use of specialized laboratory tests (especially culture on selective media and urinary antigen assay) for patients with hospital-acquired pneumonia.

Disinfection of the water supply is now feasible. Two methods have proven reliable and cost-effective. The superheat and flush method requires heating of the water so that the distal-outlet temperature is 70 to 80°C and flushing of the distal outlets with hot water for at least 30 min. This method is ideal for emergency situations. A commercial copper and silver ionization method has proved effective in numerous hospitals. Hyperchlorination is no longer recommended because of its expense, carcinogenicity, corrosive effects on piping, and unreliable efficacy.

BIBLIOGRAPHY

BARBAREE JM et al (eds): *Legionella—Current Status and Emerging Perspectives.* Washington, DC, American Society for Microbiology, 1993

CUNHA B et al: Legionnaires' disease: A symposium. Semin Resp Infect 13:83, 1998

FANG GD et al: Disease due to Legionellaceae (other than *Legionella pneumophila*): Historical, microbiological, clinical and epidemiologic review. Medicine 68:116, 1989

FIORE AE et al: A survey of methods used to detect nosocomial legionellosis among participants in the NNIS system. Infect Control Hosp Epidemiol 20:412, 1999

LIEBERMAN D et al: *Legionella* species community-acquired pneumonia: A review of 56 hospitalized adult patients. Chest 109:1243, 1996

LOWRY PW, TOMPKINS LS: Nosocomial legionellosis: A review of pulmonary and extrapulmonary syndromes. Am J Infect Control 21:21, 1993

SHUMAN HA et al: Intracellular multiplication of *Legionella pneumophila*: Human pathogen or accidental tourist? Curr Top Microbiol Immunol 225:99, 1998

STOUT JE, YU VL: Current concepts: Legionellosis. N Engl J Med 337:682, 1997

YU VL: Could aspiration be the major mode of transmission for *Legionella*? Am J Med 95:13, 1993

———: Resolving the controversy on environmental cultures for *Legionella*. Infect Control Hosp Epidemiol 19:893, 1998

152 Scott A. Halperin

PERTUSSIS AND OTHER *BORDETELLA* INFECTIONS

Pertussis is an acute infection of the respiratory tract caused by *Bordetella pertussis*. The name *pertussis* means "violent cough," which aptly describes the most consistent and prominent feature of the illness. The inspiratory sound made at the end of an episode of paroxysmal coughing gives rise to the common name for the illness, "whooping cough"; however, this feature is variable, being uncommon in infants ≤6 months of age and frequently absent in older children and adults. The Chinese name for pertussis is "the 100-day cough," which accurately describes the clinical course of the illness. The identification of *B. pertussis* was first reported by Bordet and Gengou in 1906, and vaccines were produced over the following two decades.

MICROBIOLOGY Six species have been identified in the genus *Bordetella*: *B. pertussis*. *B. parapertussis*, *B. bronchiseptica*, *B. avium*, *B. holmesii*, and *B. hinzii*. *B. pertussis* infects only humans and is the most important *Bordetella* species causing human disease. *B. parapertussis* causes an illness in humans that is similar to pertussis but is typically milder; co-infections with *B. parapertussis* and *B. pertussis* have been documented. *B. bronchiseptica* is an important pathogen of domestic animals that causes kennel cough in dogs, atrophic rhinitis and pneumonia in pigs, and pneumonia in cats. Both respiratory infection and opportunistic infection are occasionally reported in humans. *B. avium* is an important cause of respiratory illness in turkeys. The remaining two species, *B. hinzii* and *B. holmesii*, have been recognized as unusual causes of bacteremia. Both of these species have been isolated from patients with sepsis, most often from those who are immunocompromised.

Bordetella species are gram-negative pleomorphic aerobic bacilli that share common genotypic characteristics. *B. pertussis* and *B. parapertussis* are the most similar of the species but differ in that *B. parapertussis* does not express the gene coding for pertussis toxin. *B. pertussis* is a slow-growing fastidious organism that requires selective medium and forms small glistening bifurcated colonies. Suspicious colonies are presumptively identified as *B. pertussis* by direct fluorescent antibody testing or by agglutination with species-specific antiserum. *B. pertussis* is further differentiated from other *Bordetella* species by biochemical and motility characteristics.

B. pertussis produces a wide array of toxins and biologically active products that are important in its pathogenesis and in immunity. Most of these virulence factors are under the control of a single genetic locus that regulates their production, resulting in antigenic modulation and phase variation. Although these processes occur both in vitro and in vivo, their importance in the pathobiology of the organism is unknown; they may play a role in intracellular persistence and person-to-person spread. The organism's most important virulence factor is *pertussis toxin*, which is composed of a B oligomer-binding subunit and an enzymatically active A protomer that ADP-ribosylates a guanine nucleotide-binding regulatory protein (G protein) in target cells, producing a variety of biologic effects. Pertussis toxin has important mitogenic activity, affects the circulation of lymphocytes, and serves as an adhesin for bacterial binding to respiratory ciliated cells. In animal models, the toxin's effects include histamine sensitization, lymphocytosis promotion, and insulin secretion. Another virulence factor is *filamentous hemagglutinin*, a component of the cell wall and a bacterial adhesin. *Pertactin* is an outer-membrane protein and another important adhesin. *Fimbriae* are bacterial appendages that also play a role in bacterial attachment; they are the major antigens against which agglutinating antibodies are directed. These agglutinating antibodies have historically been the primary means of serotyping *B. pertussis* strains. Other virulence factors include tracheal cytotoxin, which causes respiratory epithelial damage; adenylate cyclase toxin, which impairs host immune cell function; dermonecrotic toxin, which may contribute to respiratory mucosal damage; and lipo-oligosaccharide, which has properties similar to those of other gram-negative bacterial endotoxins.

PATHOGENESIS Infection with *B. pertussis* is initiated by attachment of the organism to the ciliated epithelial cells of the nasopharynx. Attachment is mediated by surface adhesins (e.g., pertactin and filamentous hemagglutinin), which bind to the integrin family of cell-surface proteins, probably in conjunction with pertussis toxin. The role of fimbriae in adhesion or maintenance of infection has not been fully delineated. At the site of attachment, the organism multiplies, producing a variety of other toxins that cause local mucosal damage (tracheal cytotoxin, dermatonecrotic toxin). Impairment of host defense by *B. pertussis* is mediated by pertussis toxin and adenylate cyclase toxin. There is local cellular invasion, with intracellular bacterial persistence; however, systemic dissemination does not occur. Systemic manifestations (lymphocytosis) result from the effects of the toxins.

The pathogenesis of the clinical manifestations of pertussis is poorly understood. It is not known what causes the paroxysmal cough that is the hallmark of pertussis. A pivotal role for pertussis toxin has been proposed. Proponents of this position point to the efficacy of preventing clinical symptoms with a vaccine containing only pertussis toxoid. Detractors counter that pertussis toxin is not the critical factor because paroxysmal cough also occurs in patients infected with *B. parapertussis*, which does not produce pertussis toxin. It is thought that the neurologic events observed in pertussis, such as seizures or encephalopathy, are due to hypoxia from coughing paroxysms or apnea rather than to the effects of specific bacterial products. *B. pertussis* pneumonia, which occurs in up to 10% of infants with pertussis, is usually a diffuse bilateral primary infection. In older children and adults with pertussis, pneumonia is often due to secondary bacterial infection with streptococci or staphylococci.

IMMUNITY Both humoral and cell-mediated immunity are thought to be important in pertussis. Antibodies to pertussis toxin, filamentous hemagglutinin, pertactin, and fimbriae are all protective in animal models. Pertussis agglutinins were correlated with protection in early studies of whole-cell pertussis vaccines. Serologic correlates of protection conferred by acellular pertussis vaccines have not been established, although antibody to pertactin, fimbriae, and (to a lesser degree) pertussis toxin correlated best with protection in two acellular pertussis vaccine efficacy trials. The duration of immunity after whole-cell pertussis vaccination is short-lived, with little protection remaining after 10 to 12 years. Data on the duration of protection after acellular pertussis vaccination are still being collected. Although immunity after natural infection has been said to be lifelong, seroepidemiologic evidence suggests that it may not be and that subsequent episodes of clinical pertussis are prevented by intermittent subclinical infection.

EPIDEMIOLOGY Pertussis is a highly communicable disease, with attack rates of 80 to 100% among unimmunized household contacts and 20% within households in well-immunized populations. The infection has a worldwide distribution, with cyclical outbreaks every 3 to 5 years (a pattern that has persisted despite widespread immunization). Pertussis occurs in all months; however, in North America, pertussis activity peaks in the summer and autumn.

Before the institution of widespread immunization programs, pertussis was one of the most common infectious causes of morbidity and death. In the United States prior to the 1940s, between 115,000 and 270,000 cases of pertussis were reported annually, with an average yearly rate of 150 cases per 100,000 population. With universal childhood immunization, the number of reported cases fell by >95%, with even more dramatic decreases in mortality. Only 1010 cases of pertussis were reported in 1976. Since that time, however, rates have slowly increased. In 1994, over 15,000 cases of pertussis were reported in the United States.

Although thought of as a disease of childhood, pertussis can affect people of all ages and is increasingly being identified as a cause of prolonged coughing illness in adolescents and adults. In unimmunized populations, pertussis incidence peaks in the preschool years, and well over half of children have the disease before reaching adulthood. In highly immunized populations such as those in North America, the peak incidence is in infants <1 year of age who have not completed the three-dose primary immunization series. Recent trends, however, show an increasing incidence of pertussis in adolescents and adults. In the United States in 1997, ~30% of patients were ≤6 months of age, 25% were adolescents, and 20% were adults. The figures for adolescents and adults are probably underestimates because of a greater degree of underrecognition and underreporting in these age groups. A number of studies of prolonged coughing illness suggest that pertussis may be the etiologic agent in 12 to 30% of adults with cough that does not improve within 2 weeks. A seroprevalence study in the United States estimated an annual incidence of pertussis of 176 cases per 100,000 healthy adults. This high incidence undoubtedly includes subclinical and mild cases that would not be readily identified as pertussis; this fact accounts for infection rates similar to those reported before the introduction of routine immunization.

Severe morbidity and mortality, however, are virtually restricted to infants. In Canada, there were 10 deaths from pertussis between 1991 and 1998; all those who died were infants ≤6 months of age. Although school-age children are the source of infection for most households, adults are the likely source for high-risk infants and may serve as the reservoir of infection between epidemic years. In developing countries, pertussis remains an important cause of infant morbidity and mortality. The World Health Organization estimated that in 1995 over 40 million people worldwide were infected by *B. pertussis* and that 355,000 children died of pertussis.

CLINICAL MANIFESTATIONS Pertussis is a prolonged coughing illness with clinical manifestations that vary by age (Table 152-1). Classic pertussis is most often seen in preschool and school-age children, although it is not uncommon among adolescents and adults. After an incubation period averaging 7 to 10 days, an illness develops that is indistinguishable from the common cold and is characterized by coryza, lacrimation, mild cough, low-grade fever, and malaise. After 1 to 2 weeks, this *catarrhal phase* evolves into the *paroxysmal phase*: the cough becomes more frequent and spasmodic with repetitive bursts of 5 to 10 coughs, often within a single expiration. Posttussive vomiting is frequent, with a mucous plug occasionally expelled at the end of an episode. The episode may be terminated by an audible whoop, which occurs upon rapid inspiration against a closed glottis at the end of a paroxysm. During a spasm, there may be

Table 152-1 Clinical Features of Pertussis, by Age Group and Diagnostic Status

Feature	Percentage of Patients		
	Adolescents and Adults		
	Laboratory Confirmation	No Laboratory Confirmation	Children
Cough	95–100	95–100	95–100
Prolonged	60–80	60–80	60–95
Paroxysmal	60–90	50–90	80–95
Sleep-disturbing	50–80	50–80	90–100
Whoop	10–40	5–30	40–80
Posttussive vomiting	20–50	5–30	80–90

impressive neck-vein distension, bulging eyes, tongue protrusion, and cyanosis. Paroxysms may be precipitated by noise, eating, or physical contact. Between attacks, the patient's appearance is normal but increasing fatigue is evident. The frequency of paroxysmal episodes varies widely, from several per hour to 5 to 10 per day. Episodes are often worse at night and interfere with sleep. Weight loss is not uncommon as a result of interference with eating. Most complications occur during the paroxysmal stage. Fever is uncommon and suggests bacterial superinfection.

After 2 to 4 weeks, the coughing episodes become less frequent and less severe—changes heralding the onset of the *convalescent phase*. This phase can last from 1 to 3 months and is characterized by a gradual resolution of the coughing episodes. For 6 months to a year, intercurrent viral infections may be associated with a recrudescence of paroxysmal cough.

Not all children who develop pertussis have classic disease. Although cough (typically paroxysmal) is nearly always present, whoop may occur in only half of cases. In infants, the illness may be atypical; often apnea and cyanosis are the only symptoms at presentation. Seizures, encephalopathy, and pneumonia are all more common in infants ≤6 months old. Pertussis-associated infant deaths due to apnea may be confused with sudden infant death syndrome. The clinical manifestations in adolescents and adults may be classic but are more often atypical. In a German study of pertussis in adults, over two-thirds had paroxysmal cough and over one-third had whoop. Adult illness in North America differs from this experience: the cough may be severe and prolonged but is less frequently paroxysmal, and a whoop is uncommon. Vomiting with cough is the best predictor of pertussis as the cause of a prolonged cough in adults. Other features predictive of the disease are a cough at night and exposure to other individuals with a prolonged coughing illness.

COMPLICATIONS Complications are frequently associated with pertussis and are more common among infants than among older children or adults. Subconjunctival hemorrhages, abdominal and inguinal hernias, pneumothoraces, and facial and truncal petechiae can result from increased intrathoracic pressure generated by severe fits of coughing. Weight loss can follow decreased caloric intake. In a series of over 1100 children <2 years of age who were hospitalized with pertussis, 27.1% had apnea, 9.4% had pneumonia, 2.6% had seizures, and 0.4% had encephalopathy; 10 children (0.9%) died. Pneumonia is reported in fewer than 5% of adolescents and adults and is usually caused by encapsulated organisms such as *Streptococcus pneumoniae* or *Haemophilus influenzae*; in contrast, infants develop primary *B. pertussis* pneumonia. Pneumothorax, severe weight loss, inguinal hernia, rib fracture, and cough syncope have all been reported in adolescents and adults with pertussis.

DIAGNOSIS If the classic symptoms of pertussis are present, clinical diagnosis is not difficult. However, particularly in older children and adults, it is difficult to differentiate infections caused by *B. pertussis* and *B. parapertussis* from other respiratory tract infections on clinical grounds. Therefore, laboratory confirmation should be attempted in all cases. Lymphocytosis (absolute neutrophil count, $>10 \times 10^9$/L) is common among young children (in whom it is unusual with other infections) but not among adolescents and adults. Culture of nasopharyngeal secretions remains the "gold standard" of diagnosis; the best specimen is collected by nasopharyngeal aspiration, in which a fine flexible plastic catheter attached to a 10-mL syringe is passed into the nasopharynx and withdrawn while gentle suction is applied. Since *B. pertussis* is highly sensitive to drying, secretions should be inoculated without delay onto appropriate media (Bordet-Gengou or Regan-Lowe) or the catheter should be flushed with a phosphate-buffered saline solution. An alternative is a nasopharyngeal culture with a calcium alginate swab; again, inoculation of culture plates should be immediate or an appropriate transport medium (such as Regan-Lowe charcoal medium) should be used. Cultures become positive by day 5 of incubation, and *B. pertussis* and *B. parapertussis* can be differentiated by agglutination with specific antisera or by direct immunofluorescence.

Nasopharyngeal cultures in untreated pertussis remain positive for a mean of 3 weeks after the onset of illness; these cultures become negative within 5 days of the institution of appropriate antimicrobial therapy. Since much of the period during which the organism can be recovered from the naropharynx falls in the catarrhal phase, when the etiology of the infection is not suspected, there is only a small window of opportunity for culture-proven diagnosis. Cultures from infants and young children are more frequently positive than those from older children and adults; this difference may reflect earlier presentation of the former age group for medical care. The increasing availability of the polymerase chain reaction for pertussis in diagnostic laboratories is enhancing the sensitivity of the organism's detection. This method may further laboratory confirmation but does not solve problems related to the long delays in specimen procurement that often are encountered in pertussis cases. Direct fluorescent antibody tests of nasopharyngeal secretions for direct diagnosis may still be available in some laboratories but should not be used because of poor sensitivity and specificity.

As a result of the difficulties with laboratory diagnosis of pertussis in adolescents, adults, and any patient who has been symptomatic for >4 weeks, increasing attention is being given to serologic diagnosis. Enzyme immunoassays detecting IgA and IgG antibodies to pertussis toxin, filamentous hemagglutinin, pertactin, and fimbriae have been developed and assessed for their reproducibility. Two- or fourfold increases in antibody are suggestive of pertussis, although cross-reactivity of some antigens (such as filamentous hemagglutinin) among *Bordetella* species makes it difficult to depend diagnostically on seroconversion involving a single type of antibody. Late presentation for medical care and prior immunization also complicate serologic diagnosis because the first sample obtained may in fact be a convalescent-phase specimen. Proposed criteria for serologic diagnosis based on a single serum specimen call for comparison of the patient's antibody levels with established population values; for example, a patient with serologically confirmed pertussis might be required to have a titer greater than two or three standard deviations above the mean titer for a normal population. However, at present, no antibody test is widely or commercially available, and no specific serologic criteria are universally accepted.

DIFFERENTIAL DIAGNOSIS A child presenting with paroxysmal cough, posttussive vomiting, and whoop is likely to have an infection caused by *B. pertussis* or *B. parapertussis*; lymphocytosis increases the likelihood of a *B. pertussis* etiology. Viruses such as respiratory syncytial virus and adenovirus have been isolated from patients with clinical pertussis but probably represent co-infection. In adolescents and adults, among whom paroxysmal cough and whoop are frequently absent, the differential diagnosis of a prolonged coughing illness is more extensive. Pertussis should be suspected in anyone with a cough that does not improve within 14 days, a paroxysmal cough of any duration, or any respiratory symptoms after contact with a laboratory-confirmed case of pertussis. Other etiologies to consider include infections caused by *Mycoplasma pneumoniae*, *Chlamydia pneumoniae*, adenovirus, influenza virus, and other respiratory viruses. Use of angiotensin-converting enzyme (ACE) inhibitors, reactive airway disease, and gastroesophageal reflux disease are well-described noninfectious causes of prolonged cough in adults.

TREATMENT **Antibiotics** The purpose of antibiotic therapy for pertussis is to eradicate the infecting bacteria from the nasopharynx; therapy does not substantially alter the clinical course unless given early in the catarrhal phase. Erythromycin (preferably the estolate form) is recommended at a dose of 50 mg/kg (maximum, 2 g/d) in three divided doses and reliably clears *B. pertussis* from the nasopharynx after 5 days. A dose of 1 g/d has also been shown to be effective and may be better tolerated. Although a 14-day course of therapy has been recommended to prevent relapse, one study showed that a 7-day course was equally effective. Erythromycin is also effective against other pathogens implicated in cough illness, such as *Mycoplasma* and *Chlamydia*.

Other macrolide antibiotics, such as azithromycin and clarithromycin, are active against *B. pertussis* in vitro, but data on their clinical efficacy are limited; clinical trials are under way. Trimethoprim-sulfamethoxazole (8/40 mg/kg per day in two divided doses) is recommended as an alternative for individuals who cannot use erythromycin, although good clinical data to support this recommendation are lacking. A macrolide-resistant *B. pertussis* strain has been reported from a single case in an outbreak in Arizona.

Immune Globulin   Although immune globulin was used widely to treat pertussis in the preantibiotic era, evidence for its effectiveness was lacking and the commercially available product was removed from the market. There is renewed interest in the therapeutic use of immune globulin, particularly for infants who develop pertussis while still too young to have completed their primary immunization series. A high-titer pertussis toxin immune globulin for intravenous use is undergoing clinical trials.

Supportive Care   Infants have the highest rates of complication and death from pertussis; therefore, most infants and older children with severe disease should be hospitalized. Monitoring for apnea and cyanosis, administration of supplemental oxygen, management of secretions, hydration, and nutritional support are the mainstays of care. A quiet environment may decrease the stimulation that can trigger paroxysmal episodes. Assisted ventilation may be required for management of apnea or pneumonia. Use of β-adrenergic agonists and/or glucocorticoids has been advocated by some but has not been proved to be effective. Cough suppressants are not effective and play no role in the management of pertussis.

Infection Control Measures   Hospitalized patients with pertussis should be placed in respiratory isolation, with the use of precautions appropriate for pathogens spread by large respiratory droplets. Isolation should continue for 5 days after initiation of erythromycin therapy or for 3 weeks (i.e., until nasopharyngeal cultures are consistently negative) in those individuals unable to tolerate antimicrobial therapy.

PREVENTION   Chemoprophylaxis   Because the risk of transmission of *B. pertussis* within households is high, chemoprophylaxis is widely recommended for household contacts of pertussis cases. The effectiveness of chemoprophylaxis, although unproven, is supported by several epidemiologic studies of institutional and community outbreaks of pertussis. In the only randomized placebo-controlled study, erythromycin estolate (50 mg/kg per day in three divided doses; maximum dose, 1 g/d) was effective in reducing bacteriologically confirmed pertussis by 67%; however, there was no decrease in the incidence of clinical disease. Despite these disappointing results, many authorities continue to recommend chemoprophylaxis, particularly in households with members at high risk of severe disease (children <1 year of age). Data are not yet available on use of the newer macrolides for chemoprophylaxis.

Immunization (See also Chap. 122)   The mainstay of pertussis prevention is active immunization. Pertussis vaccine has been available for over 70 years and became widely used in North America after 1940; reported cases of pertussis have since fallen by >90%. Whole-cell pertussis vaccines are prepared through the heating, chemical inactivation, and purification of whole *B. pertussis* organisms. Although effective (average efficacy estimate, 85%, with results in various studies of different products ranging from 30 to 100%), whole-cell pertussis vaccines are associated with adverse events—both common (fever; injection site pain, erythema, and swelling; irritability) and uncommon (febrile seizures, hypotonic hyporesponsive episodes). Alleged associations of whole-cell pertussis vaccine with encephalopathy, sudden infant death syndrome, and autism, although not substantiated, have spawned an active anti-immunization lobby. The development of acellular pertussis vaccines, which are effective but less reactogenic, has greatly alleviated concerns about the inclusion of pertussis vaccine in the combined infant immunization series. In some countries (Canada, Sweden, Germany), acellular pertussis vaccines are used exclusively for childhood immunization; in the United States, acellular pertussis vaccines are now the preferred product but whole-cell vaccine is still considered acceptable. In North America, both whole-cell and acellular pertussis vaccines are given as a three-dose primary series at 2, 4, and 6 months of age, with a reinforcing dose between 15 and 18 months of age and a booster dose at 4 to 6 years of age.

A wide variety of acellular pertussis vaccines have been developed, although not all are available in every country. All acellular pertussis vaccines currently available contain pertussis toxoid. Only one monovalent pertussis toxoid vaccine has been licensed in the United States; the remainder of the fully developed vaccines contain filamentous hemagglutinin as well as toxoid. At least four acellular pertussis vaccines also contain pertactin, and two products also contain one or more types of fimbriae. All of the licensed acellular pertussis vaccines have undergone phase 3 efficacy testing. Although differences in study design make direct comparisons difficult, an effort to standardize case definitions and the similarity of some of the studies, which used common vaccine arms to allow "bridging" of the data between studies, have permitted some general conclusions. Even though some would still disagree, most experts have concluded that two-component acellular pertussis vaccines are more effective than monocomponent vaccines and that the addition of pertactin further increases efficacy. The further addition of fimbriae appears to provide some additional protective efficacy against milder disease. In two studies, protection against pertussis by vaccines correlated best with the production of antibody to pertactin, fimbriae, and pertussis toxin.

The development of acellular pertussis vaccines has sparked interest in the potential for control of pertussis in adolescents and adults and in the possibility that pertussis control in those groups will enhance the protection of infants too young to be immunized. Whole-cell pertussis vaccine is contraindicated in individuals ≥7 years of age because of their poor toleration of possible adverse events. However, adult formulations of acellular pertussis vaccines, both alone and in combination with adult-formulation diphtheria-tetanus toxoid, have been demonstrated to be safe and immunogenic in clinical trials in adolescents and adults. Further epidemiologic studies and an efficacy study are under way to better delineate the scope of pertussis illness in adolescents and adults as well as the efficacy of a single dose of acellular pertussis vaccine. These data, along with the results of other studies characterizing the spectrum of pertussis disease in adolescents and adults, will help public health authorities and advisory committees to determine the role of adolescent and adult pertussis immunization.

BIBLIOGRAPHY

CHERRY JD et al: A search for serologic correlates of immunity to *Bordetella pertussis* cough illnesses. Vaccine 16:1901, 1998

GRECO D et al: A controlled trial of two acellular vaccines and one whole-cell vaccine against pertussis. Progetto Pertosse Working Group. N Engl J Med 334:341, 1996

GUSTAFSSON L et al: A controlled trial of a two-component acellular, a five-component acellular, and a whole-cell pertussis vaccine. N Engl J Med 334:349, 1996 (published erratum appears in N Engl J Med 334:1207, 1996)

HALPERIN SA et al: Seven days of erythromycin estolate is as effective as fourteen days for the treatment of *Bordetella pertussis* infections. Pediatrics 100:65, 1997

——— et al: A randomized, placebo-controlled trial of erythromycin estolate chemoprophylaxis for household contacts of children with culture-positive *Bordetella pertussis* infection. Pediatrics 104:4, 1999

——— et al: Epidemiological features of hospitalized pertussis cases in Canada, 1991–1997: A report of the immunization monitoring program, Active (IMPACT). Clin Infect Dis 28:1238, 1999

SCHMITT-GROHÉ S et al: Pertussis in German adults. Clin Infect Dis 21:860, 1995

TROLLFORS B et al: A placebo-controlled trial of a pertussis-toxoid vaccine. N Engl J Med 333:1045, 1995

WIRSING VON KÖNIG CH et al: Pertussis in adults: Frequency of transmission after household exposure. Lancet 346:1326, 1995

WRIGHT SW et al: Pertussis infection in adults with persistent cough. JAMA 273:1044, 1995

DISEASES CAUSED BY GRAM-NEGATIVE ENTERIC BACILLI

DAEC	diffusely adherent *E. coli*	GNB	gram-negative bacilli
EAEC	enteroaggregative *E. coli*	HUS	hemolytic-uremic syndrome
EHEC	enterohemorrhagic *E. coli*	ICUs	intensive care units
EIEC	enteroinvasive *E. coli*	LPS	lipopolysaccharide
EPEC	enteropathogenic *E. coli*	NNIS	National Nosocomial
ESBLs	extended-spectrum *β*-lactamases		Infections Study
		STEC	Shiga toxin–producing *E. coli*
ETEC	enterotoxigenic *E. coli*	TMP-SMZ	trimethoprim-sulfamethoxazole
ExPEC	extraintestinal pathogenic strains of *E. coli*	UTI	urinary tract infection

GENERAL FEATURES AND PRINCIPLES

EPIDEMIOLOGY This chapter discusses gram-negative bacilli (GNB) belonging to the medically important genera of the family Enterobacteriaceae (*Escherichia*, *Klebsiella*, *Proteus*, *Enterobacter*, *Serratia*, *Citrobacter*, *Morganella*, *Providencia*, and *Edwardsiella*) as well as the genus *Actinetobacter* from the family Neisseriaceae. These bacteria are members of normal animal and human colonic flora and/or residents of a variety of environmental habitats, including long-term-care facilities and hospitals. In healthy humans, *Escherichia coli* is the predominant species of GNB in the colonic flora. GNB (primarily *E. coli*, *Klebsiella*, and *Proteus*) only transiently colonize the oropharynx and skin. In contrast, in the long-term-care and hospital settings, a variety of GNB emerge as the dominant components of the colonizing flora of both mucosal and skin surfaces, particularly with antimicrobial use and increasing severity of disease. Acquisition of these GNB from a variety of reservoirs leads to infection.

STRUCTURE AND FUNCTION Structurally, these organisms possess an extracytoplasmic outer membrane, a feature shared among gram-negative bacteria. The outer membrane consists of a lipid bilayer and associated proteins, lipoproteins, and polysaccharides [capsule, lipopolysaccharide (LPS)]. This structure interfaces with the environment, including the human host. A variety of components of the outer membrane are critical determinants in mediating the pathogenesis of infection and antimicrobial resistance.

INFECTIOUS SYNDROMES Depending on both the host and the pathogen, nearly every organ and body cavity can be infected with GNB. *Escherichia* and, to a lesser degree, *Klebsiella* and *Proteus* account for the majority of infections and are the most virulent pathogens of this group. However, the other genera are becoming increasingly important, particularly in long-term-care or hospitalized patients, in large part because of the organisms' innate or acquired resistance to antimicrobial agents and the increasing number of immunocompromised hosts. The mortality rate is significant in many GNB infections and correlates with the severity of illness. Especially problematic are pneumonitis and bacteremia from any source complicated by shock, which have associated mortality rates of 20 to 50%.

DIAGNOSIS Isolation of GNB from sterile sites almost always implies infection. Their isolation from nonsterile sites, particularly from soft tissue and respiratory cultures, requires clinical correlation to differentiate colonization from infection.

TREATMENT AND PREVENTION The antimicrobial resistance of GNB is variable and is influenced by both location and regional antibiotic use. Empirical antimicrobial choices should be based on local susceptibility patterns, but it is critical to be cognizant of emerging resistance. The acquisition of transferable plasmids that possess genes for extended-spectrum *β*-lactamases (ESBLs) is increasing. To date, these plasmids are most prevalent in *Klebsiella* and *E. coli*, but they have also been described (albeit less frequently) in most of the enteric GNB. The plasmids confer resistance to third-generation cephalosporins and aztreonam and frequently contain linked resistance determinants for aminoglycosides, tetracyclines, and trimethoprim-sulfamethoxazole (TMP-SMZ). In some outbreaks, strains with ESBLs also exhibit associated fluoroquinolone resistance. Derepression of inducible chromosomal *β*-lactamases, another important resistance mechanism, may be preexisting or may develop during therapy. This determinant confers resistance to second- and third-generation cephalosporins, to aztreonam, and often to *β*-lactam/*β*-lactamase inhibitor combinations. Of the enteric GNB, *Enterobacter*, *Serratia*, *Citrobacter*, *Proteus vulgaris*, *Proteus penneri*, *Providencia*, and *Morganella* possess this determinant. Although relevant data are suboptimal or conflicting, combination therapy may increase antimicrobial efficacy (particularly in serious infections, such as pneumonitis) and diminish the emergence of resistance. Further, drainage of abscesses and removal of infected foreign bodies are often needed for cure. GNB are commonly part of a polymicrobial infection in which it is difficult to determine the role of each specific pathogen. Although some species are more pathogenic than others, it is usually prudent, if possible, to design an antimicrobial regimen that includes activity against all of the GNB identified, since each is capable of pathogenicity in its own right. Diligent hand washing by health care personnel and avoidance of inappropriate antimicrobial use are the two most important measures for the prevention of infection.

PATHOGENESIS Multiple bacterial traits are required for various aspects of the pathogenesis of GNB. The possession of specialized virulence genes is what defines pathogens and enables them to infect the host efficiently. As more is learned about these genes, it is becoming clear that hosts and their cognate pathogens have been coadapting throughout evolutionary history. In fact, it has been speculated that infection is just a point on the spectrum of evolutionary development between microbes and the host. At one end of this spectrum is a commensal/symbiotic interaction (e.g., mitochondria—formerly bacteria—within eukaryotic cells); at the other is a lethal outcome that results in a "dead-end relationship" (e.g., Ebola virus). During this host-pathogen "chess match" over time, a variety and redundancy of solutions have emerged in both pathogens and hosts that enable the partners to maintain their coexistence (Table 153-1).

Intestinal Infection Intestinal pathogenic strains of *E. coli* cause gastroenteritis by a variety of unique pathogenic mechanisms. Their virulence traits are for the most part distinct from those of *E. coli* strains that cause disease outside the bowel. This difference is not

Table 153-1 Interactions of Extraintestinal Pathogenic *E. coli* and Humans: A Paradigm for Extracellular, Extraintestinal Gram-Negative Bacterial Pathogens

Bacterial Goal	Host Obstacle	Bacterial Solution
Extraintestinal attachment	Flow of urine Mucociliary blanket	Multiple adhesins (e.g., type I, Sfa/Foc, P pili)
Nutrient acquisition for growth	Nutrient sequestration (e.g., iron via intracellular storage and extracellular scavenging via lactoferrin and transferrin)	Cellular lysis (e.g., hemolysin); multiple mechanisms for competing for extracellular iron (e.g., siderophores) and other nutrients
Initial avoidance of host bactericidal activity	Complement Phagocytic cells Defensins	Capsular polysaccharide, lipopolysaccharide
Transmission	Hygiene Infection control Public health measures	Irritant tissue damage resulting in increased excretion (e.g., toxins such as hemolysin)
Late avoidance of host bactericidal activity	Acquired immunity (e.g., specific antibodies) Treatment with antibiotics	? Cell entry Acquisition of antimicrobial resistance

surprising in light of site-dependent differences in host environments and defense mechanisms.

Extraintestinal Infection Extraintestinal pathogenic strains of *E. coli* (ExPEC) and the other genera discussed in this chapter cause infection outside the bowel. All are extracellular pathogens and therefore share certain pathogenic features. Innate defense systems (complement, phagocytes) and humoral immunity are the most critical host defense components. As a result, both susceptibility to and severity of infection are increased with dysfunction or deficiencies of these components (e.g., neutrophils). A given pathogen usually possesses multiple adhesins for binding to a variety of host cells (e.g., in *E. coli*: type I, Sfa/Foc, P pili). Nutrient acquisition (e.g., iron via siderophores) requires many genes that are necessary but not sufficient for pathogenesis. The ability to resist the bactericidal activity of complement and professional phagocytes in the absence of antibody (e.g., conferred by capsule or O antigen of LPS) is one of the defining traits of an extracellular pathogen. Tissue damage (e.g., hemolysis in the case of *E. coli*) may facilitate spread. However, many important virulence genes await identification, and our understanding of many aspects of the pathogenesis of GNB is in its infancy (Chap. 120). The ability to induce septic shock is another defining feature of these genera. GNB are the most common cause of this dangerous complication. The lipid A moiety of LPS and probably other bacterial factors as well (e.g., capsule) stimulate a proinflammatory host response, which, if overexuberant, results in shock (Chap. 124). Lastly, a large number of serotypes (e.g., in *E. coli*, >100 O-specific and >80 capsular antigens) exist within most genera of GNB. This antigenic variability enables immune evasion and successful recurrent infection by strains of the same species and has also impeded vaccine development (Chap. 122).

ESCHERICHIA COLI INFECTIONS

From a clinical perspective, *E. coli* can be divided into three categories: commensal strains, intestinal pathogenic (enteric or diarrheagenic) strains, and ExPEC.

ETIOLOGY, EPIDEMIOLOGY, AND MANIFESTATIONS **Commensal Strains** Commensal strains of *E. coli* constitute the bulk of the facultative fecal flora in most healthy humans. Such strains appear to be adapted for peaceful coexistence with the host and appear not to cause disease within the intestinal tract. Further, in humans, these microorganisms do not usually cause disease outside the intestinal tract except in the presence of precipitating factors, such as an indwelling foreign body or an impairment of host defenses. Commensal *E. coli* strains typically lack the specialized virulence traits of intestinal and ExPEC strains.

Intestinal Pathogenic Strains In contrast to commensal *E. coli*, intestinal pathogenic strains of *E. coli* are rarely encountered in the fecal flora of healthy hosts and instead appear to be essentially obligate pathogens, causing gastroenteritis or colitis whenever ingested in sufficient quantities by a naive host. At least six distinct "pathotypes" of intestinal pathogenic *E. coli* exist: (1) enterotoxigenic *E. coli* (ETEC); (2) Shiga toxin–producing *E. coli* (STEC)/enterohemorrhagic *E. coli* (EHEC); (3) enteropathogenic *E. coli* (EPEC); (4) enteroinvasive *E. coli* (EIEC); (5) enteroaggregative *E. coli* (EAEC); and (6) diffusely adherent *E. coli* (DAEC). Organisms of these pathotypes are acquired via the fecal-oral route. Transmission occurs predominantly via contaminated food and water for ETEC, STEC, EIEC, EAEC, and DAEC and by person-to-person spread for EPEC (and occasionally STEC). Humans appear to be the major reservoir (except for STEC), since the host range appears to be dictated by species-specific attachment factors. Although there is some overlap, each pathotype possesses a unique combination of virulence traits that results in a distinctive intestinal pathogenic mechanism; however, these strains are largely incapable of causing disease outside the intestinal tract.

ETEC In tropical or developing countries, several separate episodes of ETEC infection occur in children over the first 3 years of life.

The incidence of disease diminishes with age, a pattern suggesting the development of immunity. In industrialized countries, infection usually follows travel to endemic areas. ETEC is the most common cause of traveler's diarrhea (Chap. 123), being responsible for 25 to 75% of cases. Cases usually develop within the first few weeks of travel. The incidence of infection is decreased by the prudent avoidance of potentially contaminated fluids and foods. ETEC infection is uncommon in the United States, but outbreaks have taken place secondary to contamination of domestic food products. A high inoculum (10^6 to 10^{10} CFU) is needed to cause disease. After ingestion of contaminated water or food (particularly items poorly cooked, unpeeled, or unrefrigerated), the small bowel is colonized during a 1- to 7-day incubation period. Disease is mediated in part by heat-labile (LT) and/or heat-stable (STa) toxin encoded by genes present on transferable plasmids. These toxins stimulate fluid secretion via activation of adenylate cyclase (LT) and/or guanylate cyclase (STa); the result is watery diarrhea accompanied by cramps. Characteristically absent are histopathologic changes of the small bowel; mucus, blood, and inflammatory cells in stool; and fever. The disease spectrum ranges from mild illness to a life-threatening cholera-like illness. Although symptoms are usually self-limited (2 to 6 days), infection may result in significant morbidity and mortality when health care is poor and small and/or undernourished children are affected.

STEC/EHEC STEC strains constitute an emerging group of pathogens that have received substantial media attention as a result of several large outbreaks attributable to the consumption of undercooked ground beef and other foods. Serotype O157:H7 is the most prominent of the more than 30 serotypes associated with the STEC syndrome (see below). Other common serogroups include O26, O39, O103, O104, and O111. The ability to produce Shiga-like toxin (Stx2 and/or Stx1) or related toxins is the critical factor dictating whether a bacterium can cause the clinical syndrome associated with STEC. *Citrobacter* isolates that produce Stx2 and *Shigella* strains that produce related toxins can cause the same syndrome.

A combination of factors are responsible for the emergence of STEC disease. A number of animals, including cattle and young calves, serve as a major reservoir for these strains. Ground beef, the most common food source, is frequently contaminated during processing. Further, cattle or other animal manure used as fertilizer can contaminate produce (potatoes, lettuce, sprouts, fallen apples) and water (fecal runoff). It is estimated that <10^3 CFU of STEC can cause disease. Therefore, not only can low levels of food or environmental contamination (e.g., water swallowed when swimming) result in disease, but person-to-person transmission becomes an important vehicle for secondary spread (e.g., at day-care centers and in institutions). Because of the low infective dose (which is similar to that of *Shigella*), laboratory-associated infections also take place. Both outbreaks and sporadic disease occur with this group of pathogens, with a seasonal peak in the summer.

In contrast to infection with the other five pathotypes, infection with STEC occurs more frequently in developed countries, where consumption of processed foods is more common than in developing regions. FoodNet data indicate that O157 strains are the fourth most common reported cause of bacterial diarrhea in the United States (behind *Campylobacter*, *Salmonella*, and *Shigella*). Colonization of the colon and perhaps of the ileum results in symptoms after an incubation period of 3 or 4 days. Maximal disease expression requires Stx2 (produced by most O157 isolates) and/or Stx1 (more commonly produced by non-O157 isolates) as well as other virulence genes (e.g., *eaeA*). Colonic edema and an initial secretory diarrhea may develop into the syndrome's hallmark trait of grossly bloody diarrhea (detected by history or examination) in >90% of cases. Significant abdominal pain and fecal leukocytes are commonly present (70% of cases), but fever is usually absent. Occasionally, *Clostridium difficile*, *Campylobacter*, and *Salmonella* infection present in a similar fashion, as do noninfectious diseases (e.g., appendicitis, inflammatory bowel disease). STEC disease is usually self-limited, lasting 5 to 10 days. This infection can be complicated by the hemolytic-uremic syndrome (HUS), which occurs 2 to 14 days after diarrhea in 2 to 8% of cases, most often in the very young and the elderly. An estimated 50% of all cases of HUS in the United States are caused by STEC infection. This complication is probably mediated by the systemic translocation of Shiga-like toxins and subsequent cellular damage, particularly to endothelial cells in the renal and cerebral microvasculature. HUS is characterized by microangiopathic hemolytic anemia, thrombocytopenia, and renal failure. Neurologic symptoms, with or without fever, can also occur. Although mortality with dialysis support is <10%, residual renal dysfunction and neurologic sequelae may persist.

EPEC EPEC causes disease primarily in young children, including neonates. This *E. coli* group was recognized as a cause of diarrheal disease when it was found in outbreaks of infantile diarrhea (some in hospital nurseries) in industrialized countries in the 1940s and 1950s. Presently, however, infection due to EPEC is uncommon in developed countries. In contrast, EPEC is an important cause of infant diarrhea (both sporadic and epidemic) in developing countries. Breast-feeding diminishes the incidence of infection. Rapid person-to-person spread may occur. Upon colonization of the small bowel, symptoms develop after an incubation period of 1 or 2 days. Disease is not toxin-mediated. Studies have identified a variety of virulence traits responsible for adherence and a characteristic effacement of microvilli with formation of cuplike, actin-rich pedestals to which the bacteria attach. Diarrheal stool often contains mucus but not blood. Although usually self-limiting, EPEC diarrhea may persist for weeks.

EIEC EIEC is a relatively uncommon cause of diarrhea and is rarely identified in the United States, although a few food-related outbreaks have been described. In less developed countries, sporadic disease is infrequently recognized in children and travelers. EIEC shares many features with *Shigella* infection; however, unlike *Shigella*, EIEC causes disease only at a high inoculum (10^8 to 10^{10} CFU). Invasion of and replication within the colonic mucosa result in the development of symptoms after an incubation period of 1 to 3 days. Secretory diarrhea may evolve into inflammatory colitis characterized by fever, abdominal pain, tenesmus, and scant stool containing mucus, blood, and inflammatory cells. Symptoms are usually self-limited, lasting 7 to 10 days.

EAEC and DAEC These pathotypes have been described primarily in developing countries and mostly affect young children. These strains may also cause some cases of traveler's diarrhea. A high inoculum is required for infection. In vitro, the organisms exhibit a diffuse or "stacked-brick" adherence pattern. Clinical disease has been associated with persistent diarrhea.

DIAGNOSIS A practical approach in evaluating diarrhea is to distinguish noninflammatory from inflammatory cases (Chap. 131). ETEC, EPEC, EAEC, and DAEC are uncommon causes of noninflammatory diarrhea in the United States. Their diagnosis requires specialized assays that are not routinely available and whose use is rarely indicated since these diseases are self-limiting. ETEC causes the majority of cases of noninflammatory traveler's diarrhea; EAEC and DAEC cause a minority of these cases. Definitive diagnosis generally is not necessary, and empirical antimicrobial treatment is a reasonable approach. If diarrhea persists with treatment, *Giardia* or *Cryptosporidium* should be sought. The diagnosis of infection with EIEC, a rare cause of inflammatory diarrhea in the United States, also requires specialized assays. However, evaluation for STEC, particularly when bloody diarrhea is reported or observed, is appropriate. Although screening for *E. coli* strains that do not ferment sorbitol and subsequent serotyping for O157 constitute the most common method presently used to detect STEC, testing for Shiga-like toxins or toxin genes is more sensitive, specific, and rapid. The latter approach offers another advantage: it detects both non-O157 strains and sorbitol-fermenting strains of O157, which otherwise are difficult to identify. DNA-based, enzyme-linked immunosorbent, and cytotoxicity assays are in various stages of development and will probably become the diagnostic standards in time.

Extraintestinal Pathogenic Strains From both pathogenic and clinical viewpoints, ExPEC strains are distinct from commensal and

intestinal pathogenic strains of *E. coli*. ExPEC strains also make up part of the normal human fecal flora, but, in contrast to commensal strains, possess specialized genes that encode virulence factors enabling the organisms to cause extraintestinal infections (Table 153-1). ExPEC (as opposed to commensal *E. coli*) causes the majority of cases of urinary tract infection (UTI), bacteremia, and neonatal meningitis. It is likely that ExPEC also causes the majority of other extraintestinal infections due to *E. coli*. Entry into an extraintestinal site (e.g., the urinary tract or the peritoneum)—not acquisition—is the limiting factor for infection. All age groups, all types of hosts, and nearly every organ and site are susceptible to infection by ExPEC. Normal, previously healthy hosts infected with ExPEC can become severely ill and die. However, adverse outcomes are more prevalent in the presence of coincidental disease and abnormalities in host defenses. Typical extraintestinal infections include UTI, diverse intraabdominal infections, pneumonia (particularly in hospitalized and institutionalized patients), meningitis (mainly in neonates and patients who have undergone neurosurgery), intravascular device infection, osteomyelitis, and soft tissue infection (which usually occurs in the setting of tissue compromise). Bacteremia can accompany infection at any of these sites. Although *E. coli* is considered to be primarily a community-acquired pathogen, it is the most frequently isolated of the GNB in the ambulatory, long-term-care, and hospital settings. The scope and magnitude of infection caused by ExPEC are as great as for any other invasive bacterial pathogen. Although these isolates do not make headlines, billions of health care dollars, millions of workdays, and thousands of lives are lost to this group of pathogens each year.

Infectious syndromes • URINARY TRACT INFECTION (UTI) The urinary tract is the site most frequently infected by ExPEC. About 90% of ambulatory UTIs and 25 to 35% of long-term-care and hospital UTIs are due to *E. coli*. The majority of UTIs occur in seven epidemiologically defined groups: children <1 year of age, school-age girls, premenopausal women, men with prostatic or other causes of urinary tract obstruction, postmenopausal women, individuals with neurogenic bladders, and patients with indwelling urinary catheters. In premenopausal women, diaphragm-spermicide use, sexual activity, and a history of UTI are risk factors for infection; 20% of women with an initial infection have frequent recurrences (0.3 to >20 per year). In postmenopausal women, estrogen replacement decreases the incidence of UTI. Acceptance of the diagnosis of UTI in males (beyond the first year of life) requires clear documentation since this infection is unusual in the absence of a history of instrumentation or anal intercourse. UTI in premenopausal women alone accounts for an estimated 7 million office visits and >$1 billion in direct medical costs annually. UTI is the second most common infection (behind lower respiratory tract infection) responsible for hospitalization.

Uncomplicated urethritis or cystitis occurs most commonly and is characterized by symptoms of dysuria, frequency, and suprapubic pain. Fever and/or back pain suggests progression to pyelonephritis. Pregnant women are at unusually high risk for this complication, which can adversely affect the outcome of pregnancy. As a result, prenatal screening for bacteriuria, with treatment when the results are positive, is the standard of care. Fever may take 5 to 7 days to resolve completely in appropriately treated patients with pyelonephritis but should fall over time. Persistently elevated or increasing fever and neutrophil counts should prompt evaluation for intrarenal or perinephric abscess and/or obstruction. Renal parenchymal damage and loss of renal function occur primarily in the setting of obstruction. Prostatic infection is generally a complication of UTI in men with a history of instrumentation and/or prostatic hypertrophy. The diagnosis and treatment of UTI are detailed in Chap. 280 and are tailored according to the host, the nature and site of infection, and the local pattern of antimicrobial susceptibility.

ABDOMINAL INFECTION The abdomen is the second most frequent site of extraintestinal infection due to *E. coli*. The majority of abdominal *E. coli* infections develop outside the hospital. Any inciting event that results in disruption of the bowel mucosa (particularly the colonic mucosa) often leads to acute peritonitis (secondary peritonitis; Chap. 130). This process is usually polymicrobial, but *E. coli* is isolated in most cases. Bacteremia often complicates this acute stage of infection. Abscess formation within the peritoneum may follow the acute stage or may develop as a consequence of subclinical fecal spillage (e.g., diverticulitis, chronic appendicitis). Intraperitoneal abscesses are almost always polymicrobial, with *E. coli* as the most common GNB isolated. *E. coli* is also the GNB most often responsible for primary hepatic abscesses, hepatic abscesses in the setting of biliary disease and obstruction, septic cholangitis/cholecystitis, pancreatic abscesses, and infected pancreatic pseudocysts. This organism is the leading cause of spontaneous bacterial peritonitis, usually seen in patients who have ascites associated with cirrhosis or occasionally with malignancy. *E. coli* occasionally causes splenic abscesses and peritoneal dialysis–associated peritonitis (Chap. 130).

PNEUMONIA   *E. coli* is not usually considered a cause of pneumonia (Chap. 255). Enteric GNB are responsible for only 2 to 5% of cases of community-acquired pneumonia, in part because these organisms only transiently colonize the oropharynx in a minority of healthy individuals. In contrast, oral colonization with *E. coli* and other GNB increases with the severity of illness and with antibiotic use. Thus, GNB are a common cause of pneumonia acquired by residents of long-term-care institutions and are the most frequent cause of hospital-acquired pneumonia (Chap. 135), particularly in postoperative and intensive care patients. Despite significant institutional variation, *E. coli* is generally the third or fourth most commonly isolated GNB in these settings, behind *Pseudomonas* and *Klebsiella*. Regardless of the host, severe disease and high mortality rates (20 to 60%) are usually seen when GNB cause pneumonia. Tissue necrosis, probably due to cytotoxins produced by GNB, is common. Infection is usually acquired by small-volume aspiration but occasionally occurs via hematogenous spread, in which case multifocal nodular infiltrates can be seen.

MENINGITIS (See Chap. 372)   ExPEC are a leading cause of meningitis in the first month of life. The majority of responsible strains possess the K1 capsular serotype. Outside this setting, meningitis due to *E. coli* is uncommon, occurring predominantly with cirrhosis (Chap. 299) or disruption of the meninges due to surgery or trauma.

CELLULITIS/MUSCULOSKELETAL INFECTION   Infections of decubitus ulcers and the lower extremities in diabetic patients (or other hosts with neurovascular compromise) are usually polymicrobial. *E. coli* frequently contributes to infection of decubiti and occasionally to lower-extremity infections in these patients. It may occasionally cause cellulitis or burn site or surgical wound infection, particularly when the infection originates close to the perineum. Osteomyelitis secondary to contiguous spread can occur in these settings. Hematogenously acquired osteomyelitis, particularly of vertebral bodies, is more common than is appreciated, accounting for 10% of cases in some series (Chap. 129). *E. coli* occasionally causes orthopedic device–associated infection and is a rare cause of hematogenously acquired myositis. Myositis or fasciitis of the upper leg should prompt an evaluation for an abdominal source with contiguous spread.

ENDOVASCULAR INFECTION   Extraintestinal isolates of *E. coli* cause a significant minority of intravascular device–associated infections (Chap. 135). Despite being one of the most common causes of bacteremia, however, *E. coli* rarely seeds native heart valves and is an uncommon cause of prosthetic valve endocarditis. Likewise, *E. coli* infections of aneurysms and vascular grafts are uncommon.

MISCELLANEOUS INFECTIONS   *E. coli* can cause infection in nearly every organ and site. This organism causes a minority—but still a significant number—of surgical site infections (e.g., mediastinitis), and cases of complicated sinusitis. It uncommonly causes endophthalmitis.

BACTEREMIA   *E. coli* bacteremia can result from extraintestinal infection of any site. The incidences of community-acquired and long-term-care/hospital-acquired bacteremia are roughly equal. Overall, it has been amply documented that *E. coli* and *Staphylococcus aureus* are the most common blood isolates (range for *E. coli*, 16 to 37%). *E. coli* is the GNB most frequently isolated from blood in the ambulatory setting and in most long-term-care and hospital settings. When *E. coli* is isolated from the blood, it is almost always clinically significant. Approximately 15% of bacteremias are complicated by septic shock. Two-thirds of bacteremias arise from the urinary tract; these infections are particularly common in the setting of pyelonephritis or obstruction (including kinked urinary catheters) or instrumentation of the urinary tract in the presence of *E. coli*. However, one should be cautious in identifying the urinary tract as the source of *E. coli* bacteremia in the absence of appropriate symptoms, despite a positive urine culture. Asymptomatic bacteriuria is common, particularly in women, even in the absence of an indwelling bladder catheter, with a prevalence of 15 to 25% after the age of 60. Therefore, occult abdominal or other sources should be considered. The abdomen is the second most common source, accounting for 25% of episodes. Although obstructive biliary tract disease (stones, tumor) and overt disruption of the bowel are responsible for many cases of *E. coli* bacteremia, some abdominal sources, such as abscesses, are remarkably silent clinically and require identification via imaging studies (e.g., computed tomography). Soft tissue, bone, and pulmonary infection are the next most frequent sources for bacteremia. As stated above, endocarditis is uncommon, occurring in only 2 of 861 bacteremias in a recent series. In the setting of chemotherapy-induced fever and neutropenia, *E. coli* is a common cause of bacteremia, usually secondary to intestinal mucositis. It is prudent in this situation, however, to exclude perirectal infection or typhlitis (Chap. 89). ExPEC strains are among the most common causes of sepsis in neonates.

Diagnosis   Strains of *E. coli* that cause extraintestinal infections usually grow both aerobically and anaerobically within 24 h on standard diagnostic media and are easily identified by the clinical microbiology laboratory using standard biochemical criteria (Chap. 121). More than 90% of these strains are rapid lactose fermenters.

℞ TREATMENT   Although *E. coli* is generally perceived as an "antibiotic-friendly" pathogen, resistance has increased over the past decade. In general, the frequency of ampicillin resistance precludes its empirical use, even in community-acquired infections. Rates of resistance to first-generation cephalosporins and TMP-SMZ in community-acquired strains are increasing in the United States (5 to 25%) and are even higher in Europe and developing countries. Not surprisingly, long-term-care and hospital isolates are more resistant than community isolates. Significant resistance (30 to 40%) to amoxicillin/clavulanic acid and piperacillin has been increasingly reported. Fortunately, resistance to second- and third-generation cephalosporins [mean rate, 3.2% according to 1998 National Nosocomial Infections Study (NNIS) data], fourth-generation cephalosporins, quinolones, monobactams (e.g., aztreonam), carbapenems (e.g., imipenem), and aminoglycosides is generally found in <10% of strains. An exception is in settings where quinolone prophylaxis is used extensively (patients with leukemia, transplant recipients); in these settings, significant quinolone resistance has emerged. Acquisition of plasmids containing ESBLs and other resistance determinants is likely to increase.

The mainstay of treatment for all diarrheal syndromes is the appropriate replacement of water and electrolytes (Chap. 159). The use of prophylactic antibiotics to prevent traveler's diarrhea should be discouraged, especially in light of high rates of antibiotic resistance. When diarrhea is free of mucus and blood, early patient-initiated treatment with a quinolone significantly decreases the duration of illness, and the use of loperamide may halt symptoms in a few hours (Chap. 123). Treatment of STEC is controversial since antibiotics may increase the incidence of HUS, perhaps via increased release of Shiga-like toxin.

KLEBSIELLA INFECTIONS *K. pneumoniae* is the most important *Klebsiella* species medically, causing community-acquired, long-term-care, and hospital infections. *K. oxytoca* is primarily a pathogen in long-term-care and hospital settings. *K. rhinoscleromatis* and *K. ozaenae* are usually isolated from patients in tropical climates. *Klebsiella* species are broadly prevalent in the environment and colonize mucosal surfaces of mammals. In healthy humans, *K. pneumoniae* colonization rates range from 5 to 35% in the colon and from 1 to 5% in the oropharynx; the skin is usually colonized only transiently. In long-term-care facilities and hospitals, colonization occurs with *K. oxytoxa* as well, and carriage rates are significant among both workers and patients. Person-to-person spread is thought to be the predominant mode of acquisition. Classically, *Klebsiella* is associated with community-acquired pneumonia, primarily in alcoholics. However, the majority of *Klebsiella* infections now occur in long-term-care facilities and hospitals. *Klebsiella* causes a spectrum of extraintestinal infections similar to that caused by *E. coli.* However, extraintestinal infections due to *Klebsiella* occur at a lower incidence in all sites except the respiratory tract. These variances in infection rates are probably due to differences in colonization and site-specific virulence traits. Antibiotic-resistant strains have been responsible for a number of nosocomial outbreaks of infection in intensive care units (ICUs) and neonatal nurseries. The most common clinical syndromes are pneumonia, UTI, abdominal infection, surgical site infection, soft tissue infection, and subsequent bacteremia. *K. rhinoscleromatis* is the causative agent of rhinoscleroma, a slowly progressive (months to years) mucosal upper respiratory infection that causes necrosis and occasional obstruction of the nasal passages. *K. ozaenae* has been implicated as a cause of chronic atrophic rhinitis.

Infectious Syndromes • *Pneumonia* *K. pneumoniae* causes only a small proportion of cases of community-acquired pneumonia (Chap. 255). This infection occurs primarily in hosts with underlying disease, such as alcoholics, diabetics, and individuals with chronic lung disease. As in all pneumonias due to enteric GNB, purulent sputum production and "airspace" disease on x-ray are typical. Presentation with earlier, less extensive infection is more common than that with the classic lobar infiltrate with a bulging fissure. Pulmonary necrosis, pleural effusion, and empyema occur with progression. Pulmonary infection in residents of long-term-care facilities and in hospitalized patients is especially frequent because of increased oropharyngeal colonization rates. Mechanical ventilation is an important risk factor.

UTI The incidence of *K. pneumoniae* UTI among healthy adults is only 1 to 2%. However, in complicated UTIs (including those associated with indwelling bladder catheters), the incidence of *Klebsiella* infection increases to 5 to 17%.

Abdominal infection *Klebsiella* causes a spectrum of abdominal infections similar to that caused by *E. coli* but is less frequently isolated from these infections.

Other infections *Klebsiella* cellulitis or soft tissue infection occurs most frequently in devitalized tissue (e.g., decubitus ulcers, diabetes, burn sites) or in immunocompromised hosts. *Klebsiella* causes a significant minority of surgical site infections and nosocomial sinusitis cases as well as occasional cases of osteomyelitis contiguous to soft tissue infection, temperate myositis, and neonatal meningitis or meningitis associated with neurosurgery.

Bacteremia *Klebsiella* infection at any site can result in bacteremia. Infections of the urinary tract, respiratory tract, and abdomen each account for 15 to 30% of *Klebsiella* bacteremias. Intravascular device–related infection is another important source (5 to 15%). Surgical site infection and other miscellaneous infections account for the rest. *Klebsiella* is one of the agents that causes sepsis neonatorum and bacteremia with fever and neutropenia. Like enteric GNB in general, *Klebsiella* rarely causes endocarditis or endovascular infection.

Diagnosis Except for *K. rhinoscleromatis* and *K. ozaenae*, klebsiellae are readily isolated and identified by the laboratory and usually ferment lactose.

℞ TREATMENT *K. pneumoniae* and *K. oxytoca* have similar antibiotic resistance profiles. They are intrinsically resistant to ampicillin and ticarcillin. NNIS data from 1998 indicated that 10.7% of ICU patients were infected with strains resistant to third-generation cephalosporins. This increasing degree of resistance is primarily mediated by transferable plasmids containing genes that encode ESBLs. In addition, these plasmids usually possess linked resistance determinants for aminoglycosides, tetracyclines, and TMP-SMZ. Resistance to β-lactam/β-lactamase inhibitor combinations and second-generation cephalosporins independent of ESBL-containing plasmids has also been increasingly described. In some outbreaks, ESBL-containing strains have displayed associated fluoroquinolone resistance. At this time, resistance to quinolones, cephamycins (e.g., cefoxitin), fourth-generation cephalosporins (e.g., cefepime), and amikacin is generally <10% but will probably increase. Carbapenems (e.g., imipenem) remain the most active antibiotic class against *Klebsiella.*

PROTEUS INFECTIONS *P. mirabilis* causes 90% of *Proteus* infections. These infections occur in the community, in long-term-care facilities, and in hospitals. *P. vulgaris* and *P. penneri* are isolated primarily from infections contracted in long-term-care facilities or hospitals. *Proteus* species are part of the colonic flora of a wide variety of mammals, birds, fish, and reptiles. Their ability to generate histamine from contaminated fish has implicated these GNB in the pathogenesis of scombroid (fish) poisoning (Chap. 131). *P. mirabilis* colonizes healthy humans (prevalence, 50%), but *P. vulgaris* and *P. penneri* are isolated primarily from individuals with underlying disease. The urinary tract is overwhelmingly the favored site of *Proteus* infection, in part because of unique pathogenic properties of the organisms. However, *Proteus* less commonly causes infection in a variety of extraintestinal sites.

Infectious Syndromes • *UTI* *P. mirabilis* causes only 1 to 2% of cases of UTI in healthy women, and *Proteus* species cause only 5% of cases of hospital-acquired UTI. However, *Proteus* is responsible for 10 to 15% of cases of complicated UTI, primarily those associated with catheterization; in the setting of long-term catheterization, their prevalence rate ranges from 20 to 45%. This high prevalence is due to the ability of *Proteus* to produce high levels of urease, which hydrolyzes urea to ammonia and results in alkalization of the urine. This situation, in turn, leads to precipitation of organic and inorganic compounds, with the formation of struvite and carbonate-apatite crystals, biofilm formation on catheters, and/or the development of calculi. *Proteus* becomes associated with the stones and usually can be eradicated only by complete stone removal. Over time, staghorn calculi may form and lead to obstruction and renal failure. Therefore, an unexplained alkaline urine should be cultured for *Proteus*, and identification of a *Proteus* species should prompt an evaluation for calculi.

Other infections Although the majority of *Proteus* infections arise from the urinary tract, these bacteria occasionally cause pneumonia (primarily in long-term-care or hospitalized patients), nosocomial sinusitis, intraabdominal abscesses, biliary tract infection, surgical site infection, soft tissue infection (especially decubitus and diabetic ulcers), and osteomyelitis (primarily contiguous); they rarely cause temperate myositis. In addition, *Proteus* occasionally causes neonatal meningitis (with the umbilicus often implicated as the source), and cerebral abscess is a common complication.

Bacteremia The majority of *Proteus* bacteremias originate from the urinary tract; however, any of the less common sites of infection are also potential sources. Infection of intravascular devices should also be considered. Endovascular infection is rare. *Proteus* species are occasional agents of sepsis neonatorum and bacteremia with fever and neutropenia.

Diagnosis　*Proteus* is readily isolated and identified by the laboratory. The majority of strains are lactose negative, and most demonstrate characteristic "swarming" motility on agar plates.

> ℞　**TREATMENT**　*P. mirabilis* remains susceptible to most antimicrobial agents except tetracycline. Resistance to ampicillin and first-generation cephalosporins has been acquired by 10 to 20% of strains. Acquisition of ESBLs remains uncommon. *P. vulgaris* and *P. penneri* are more resistant. Resistance to ampicillin and first-generation cephalosporins is the rule for these species. Derepression of an inducible chromosomal β-lactamase (not present in *P. mirabilis*) occurs in up to 30% of strains. Imipenem, fourth-generation cephalosporins (e.g., cefepime), aminoglycosides, TMP-SMZ, and quinolones have excellent activity (90 to 100%).

ENTEROBACTER **INFECTIONS**　*E. cloacae* and *E. aerogenes* are responsible for most *Enterobacter* infections (65 to 75% and 15 to 25%, respectively); *E. agglomerans*, *E. sakazakii*, and *E. gergoviae* are less commonly isolated (5%, 1%, and <1%, respectively). These organisms cause primarily health care– or hospital-related infections. They are prevalent in foods, environmental sources (including health care facility equipment), and a wide variety of animals. Only a minority of healthy humans are colonized, but the percentage increases significantly in the setting of long-term care or hospitalization. Although colonization is an important prelude to infection, direct introduction via intravenous lines (e.g., contaminated intravenous fluids, pressure monitors) also occurs. Significant antibiotic resistance has developed in *Enterobacter* species and has contributed to their emergence as prominent nosocomial pathogens. Individuals who have received prior antibiotic treatment, who have comorbid disease, and who are patients in ICUs are at greatest risk for infection. *Enterobacter* causes a spectrum of extraintestinal infections similar to that described for other GNB in this chapter.

Infectious Syndromes　Pneumonitis, UTI (particularly catheter-related), intravascular device–related infection, surgical wound/site infection, and abdominal infection (primarily postoperative or device-related—e.g., biliary stents) are the most common syndromes encountered. Nosocomial sinusitis, meningitis related to neurosurgical procedures (including use of pressure monitors), osteomyelitis, and endophthalmitis after eye surgery are less frequent. *E. sakazakii* is commonly responsible for neonatal meningitis/sepsis (particularly in premature infants), and contaminated formula has been implicated as a source of this infection. Neonatal meningitis is frequently associated with brain abscesses. Bacteremia can result from infection at any of these sites. In the setting of *Enterobacter* bacteremia, contamination of intravenous fluids, blood products, catheter-flushing fluids, pressure monitors, and dialysis equipment should always be considered, particularly with epidemic infection. *Enterobacter* can also cause bacteremia in patients with fever and neutropenia. *Enterobacter* endocarditis is rare, primarily affecting abnormal native or prosthetic valves.

Diagnosis　*Enterobacter* is readily isolated and identified by the laboratory. Most strains are lactose positive.

> ℞　**TREATMENT**　Significant antimicrobial resistance exists among *Enterobacter* strains. Ampicillin and the first- and second-generation cephalosporins have little or no activity. The extensive use of third-generation cephalosporins has resulted in the selection of strains that produce high levels of β-lactamase (i.e., derepression of β-lactamase), which confers resistance to second- and third-generation cephalosporins, monobactams (e.g., aztreonam), and (frequently) β-lactam/β-lactamase inhibitor combinations. Resistant isolates may emerge during therapy; their presence should be considered a possibility when clinical deterioration follows several days of improvement. A 34% resistance rate to third-generation cephalosporins was reported

in ICU isolates in 1998 (NNIS data). Imipenem, fourth-generation cephalosporins (e.g., cefepime), aminoglycosides (amikacin > gentamicin), TMP-SMZ, and quinolones have retained excellent activity (90 to 99%). However, increasing resistance to quinolones, in conjunction with the increased use of these agents, is a concern.

ACINETOBACTER **INFECTIONS**　*A. baumannii* is responsible for the majority of *Acinetobacter* infections; a minority are due to *A. calcoaceticus* and *Acinetobacter* genospecies 3 and 13TU. *Acinetobacter* is highly prevalent in the environment. It is found in most water and soil samples and has a wide habitat. *Acinetobacter* has been cultured from the moist skin of healthy humans; increased colonization of the skin and the respiratory and gastrointestinal tracts occurs in individuals in long-term-care facilities and hospitals. Reservoirs for acquisition in these settings include health care personnel, medical equipment, food, and the surrounding environment. Infections in healthy people in the community are unusual, but a few reports of pneumonia have been published. The overwhelming majority of infections are acquired in the hospital and long-term-care facilities. The spectrum of extraintestinal infections caused by *Acinetobacter* is similar to that caused by other GNB. *Acinetobacter* species account for 1 to 3% of hospital-acquired infections and affect primarily immunocompromised hosts and patients with comorbid disease. ICUs are a prominent site of *Acinetobacter* infection. In some centers, the incidence of *Acinetobacter* infections, particularly those due to antibiotic-resistant strains, is increasing. Both sporadic and epidemic infection occurs, usually after the first week of hospitalization.

Infectious Syndromes　The respiratory tract (particularly in ventilated patients) and intravascular devices (particularly for non–*A. baumannii* species) are the favored sites of infection. A catheterized urinary tract, postoperative sites, burn sites, biliary stents, sinuses (with tube-related ostial obstruction), and neurosurgical infections (site- or device-associated—e.g., pressure monitors) are less common. Uncommon infections include contiguous osteomyelitis, peritonitis associated with continuous ambulatory peritoneal dialysis, and ophthalmic infection. The respiratory tract and intravascular devices are the most common sources for bacteremia.

Diagnosis　On Gram's stain, *Acinetobacter* organisms usually appear as short GNB or coccobacilli. They are strictly aerobic, nonfermenting, and readily isolated and identified.

> ℞　**TREATMENT**　Many strains of *Acinetobacter* are highly resistant to antimicrobial agents. Empirical combination therapy is prudent pending susceptibility studies. Ampicillin, aztreonam, and the first- and second-generation cephalosporins possess little or no activity against these species. The activity of mezlocillin, piperacillin, quinolones, third- and fourth-generation cephalosporins, aminoglycosides, and β-lactam/β-lactamase inhibitor combinations is variable. Imipenem is presently the most active antimicrobial (>95% sensitivity), and β-lactam/sulbactam combinations are often active. Amikacin, third- and fourth-generation cephalosporins, quinolones, and combinations consisting of a β-lactam other than sulbactam plus a β-lactamase inhibitor retain significant activity in some centers, while highly resistant strains are more common in other centers.

SERRATIA **INFECTIONS**　*S. marcescens* causes the majority of *Serratia* infections (>90%), and *S. liquefaciens* is occasionally isolated. Serratiae are found primarily in the environment, including health care institutions and particularly in moist foci. Although strains have been isolated from a variety of animals, healthy humans are rarely colonized. In long-term-care facilities or hospitals, diverse reservoirs for the organisms include the hands of health care personnel, food, sinks, respiratory and other hospital equipment, intravenous solutions, blood products (e.g., platelets), lotions, irrigation solutions, and even disinfectants. Infection results from either direct inoculation (e.g., via intravenous fluid) or colonization (primarily of the respiratory tract) and subsequent infection. Sporadic infection is most common, but occasional epidemics and common-source outbreaks occur. The spectrum of extraintestinal infections caused by *Serratia* is similar to that for other GNB. *Serratia* species account for 1 to 3% of hospital-acquired infections.

Infectious Syndromes The respiratory tract, the genitourinary tract, intravascular devices, and surgical wounds and sites are the most common sites of *Serratia* infection and sources of *Serratia* bacteremia. Soft tissue infections, including myositis, osteomyelitis, abdominal and biliary tract infection (postprocedural), contact lens–associated infection, endophthalmitis, septic arthritis (primarily with intraarticular injections), and infusion-related bacteremias occur less commonly. Serratiae are uncommon causes of neonatal or postsurgical meningitis and bacteremia associated with fever and neutropenia. Endocarditis is rare.

Diagnosis Serratiae are readily cultured and identified by the laboratory and are usually lactose negative. A minority of *S. marcescens* strains are red-pigmented.

℞ TREATMENT A high proportion of *Serratia* strains (>80%) are resistant to ampicillin and the first-generation cephalosporins. Significant resistance to ticarcillin, piperacillin, gentamicin, second- and third-generation cephalosporins, β-lactam/β-lactamase inhibitor combinations, and aztreonam has developed and may evolve during therapy. Imipenem, amikacin, cefepime, and quinolones are the most active agents, with >90% of strains susceptible.

CITROBACTER INFECTIONS *C. freundii* and *C. koseri* (formerly *C. diversus*) cause the majority of human *Citrobacter* infections, which are similar epidemiologically and clinically to *Enterobacter* and *Acinetobacter* infections. *Citrobacter* organisms are commonly present in water, food, soil, and the intestinal tracts of animals. *Citrobacter* is part of the normal fecal flora in a minority of healthy humans, but colonization rates increase in long-term care facilities and hospitals—the settings in which nearly all infections occur. *Citrobacter* species account for 1 to 2% of nosocomial infections. The affected hosts are usually immunocompromised or have comorbid disease. *Citrobacter* causes extraintestinal infections whose spectrum is similar to that described for other GNB.

Infectious Syndromes The urinary tract is the site of 40 to 50% of infections due to *Citrobacter*. Less commonly infected sites include the biliary tree (particularly with stones or obstruction), the respiratory tract, surgical sites, soft tissue (e.g., decubitus ulcers), the peritoneum, and intravascular devices. Osteomyelitis (usually contiguous), neurosurgery-related infection, and myositis occur rarely. *Citrobacter* is also an uncommon cause of neonatal meningitis; *C. koseri* accounts for 90% of cases due to this genus. A frequent and devastating complication of this infection (occurring in 50 to 80% of cases) is the development of brain abscesses. Bacteremia is most commonly due to UTI, biliary or abdominal infection, or intravascular devices. *Citrobacter* is an uncommon cause of bacteremia in the setting of fever and neutropenia. Endocarditis or endovascular infection is rare.

Diagnosis *Citrobacter* species are readily isolated and identified, often as part of a polymicrobial culture; 35 to 50% of isolates are lactose positive.

℞ TREATMENT *C. freundii* is generally more resistant to antibiotics than *C. koseri*. Ampicillin and the first- and second-generation cephalosporins display poor activity against *Citrobacter*. Resistance is variable but increasing to ticarcillin, mezlocillin, piperacillin, aztreonam, quinolones, gentamicin, and third-generation cephalosporins; such resistance may evolve during therapy. The β-lactamase inhibitors usually do not improve susceptibility to β-lactam agents. Imipenem, amikacin, and the fourth-generation cephalosporins are most active, with >90% of strains sensitive.

MORGANELLA AND PROVIDENCIA INFECTIONS *M. morganii* (formerly *Proteus morganii*), *P. stuartii*, and (to a lesser degree) *P. rettgeri* (formerly *Proteus rettgeri*) are the members of these genera that are responsible for human infections. The epidemiologic,

pathogenic, and clinical manifestations of these organisms are similar to those of *Proteus* species; however, *Morganella* and *Providencia* are almost exclusively pathogens of persons in long-term-care facilities and, to a lesser degree, hospitalized patients.

Infectious Syndromes These species are primarily urinary tract pathogens, most often associated with long-term (>30-day) catheterization. UTI in uncatheterized or short-term-catheterized individuals is uncommon. Biofilm formation or encrustation of the catheter usually develops and may lead to catheter obstruction. Likewise, infection may result in the development of struvite bladder or renal stones, which, in turn, may lead to renal obstruction and serve as foci for relapse. Other infectious syndromes occur less commonly but include surgical wound/site infections, soft tissue infection (primarily decubitus and diabetic ulcers), burn site infection, pneumonia (particularly ventilator-associated), intravascular device infection, and intraabdominal infection. Rarely, the other extraintestinal infections described for GNB also occur. Bacteremia is uncommon; although any infected site can serve as the source, the urinary tract accounts for the majority of cases, with surgical wound/site and soft tissue infections less frequently responsible.

Diagnosis *M. morganii* and *Providencia* are readily isolated and identified. Nearly all isolates are unable to ferment lactose.

℞ TREATMENT *Morganella* and *Providencia* may be highly resistant to antimicrobial agents. Ampicillin and the first-generation cephalosporins exhibit poor activity against these organisms. Variable resistance is emerging (and may evolve during therapy) against ticarcillin, mezlocillin, piperacillin, aztreonam, gentamicin, TMP-SMZ, and the second- and third-generation cephalosporins and quinolones. The β-lactamase inhibitor tazobactam (but not sulbactam or clavulanic acid) improves susceptibility to β-lactam agents somewhat. Imipenem, amikacin, and the fourth-generation cephalosporins are most active, with >90% of strains susceptible. Removal of an infected catheter or stones is critical for eradication of the organisms from the urinary tract.

EDWARDSIELLA INFECTION *E. tarda* is the only member of this genus associated with human disease. This organism is found predominantly in both freshwater and marine environments and in the animals that live in these environments. Human acquisition occurs primarily during interaction with these reservoirs. *E. tarda* infection is rare in the United States; most recently reported cases are from Southeast Asia. This pathogen shares some of the clinical features of both *Salmonella* species and *Vibrio vulnificus*.

Infectious Syndromes Gastroenteritis is the predominant infectious syndrome reported (50 to 80% of infections). Self-limiting watery diarrhea is most frequent; however, cases of severe colitis responding to therapy have also been described. The most common extraintestinal infection is wound infection due to direct inoculation, which is often associated with freshwater, marine, or snake-related injuries. Other infectious syndromes appear to be due to invasion of the gastrointestinal tract and subsequent bacteremia. The majority of afflicted hosts have either liver disease or an iron-overload state (e.g., sickle cell disease). A primary bacteremic syndrome, sometimes complicated by meningitis, has been described and has a 40% case-fatality rate. Visceral (primarily hepatic) or intraperitoneal abscesses have also been reported.

Diagnosis Although *E. tarda* can readily be isolated and identified, most laboratories do not routinely identify it from stool.

℞ TREATMENT *E. tarda* is sensitive to most GNB-appropriate antimicrobial agents. Gastroenteritis is generally self-limiting, but treatment with TMP-SMZ or a quinolone may expedite its resolution. In the setting of overwhelming sepsis, quinolones, third- or fourth-generation cephalosporins, imipenem, and aminoglycosides—alone or in combination—are the safest choices pending susceptibility information.

INFECTIONS CAUSED BY MISCELLANEOUS GENERA Species from genera of GNB such as *Hafnia, Kluyvera, Cedecea, Pantoea,* and *Ewingella* are occasionally isolated from a variety of clinical specimens, including blood, sputum, cerebrospinal fluid, joint fluid, biliary drainage, wounds, and sputum. Although their role in disease has not always been defined, these strains appear to be rare and usually opportunistic human pathogens. The primary medical literature should be consulted for details on their potential role as infectious agents.

BIBLIOGRAPHY

BERGOGNE-BEREZIN E, TOWNER KJ: *Acinetobacter* spp. as nosocomial pathogens: Microbiological, clinical, and epidemiological features. Clin Microbiol Rev 9:148, 1996

GRANSDEN WR et al: Bacteremia due to *Escherichia coli*: A study of 861 episodes. Rev Infect Dis 12:1008, 1990

HEJAZI A, FALKINER FR: *Serratia marcescens.* J Med Microbiol 46:903, 1997

HUSNI RN et al: Risk factors for an outbreak of multi-drug-resistant *Acinetobacter* nosocomial pneumonia among intubated patients. Chest 115:1378, 1999

JANDA JM, ABBOTT SL: Infections associated with the genus *Edwardsiella*: The role of *Edwardsiella tarda* in human disease. Clin Infect Dis 17:742, 1993

NATARO JP, KAPER JB: Diarrheagenic *Escherichia coli.* Clin Microbiol Rev 11:142, 1998 [erratum appears in Clin Microbiol Rev 11:403, 1998]

PODSCHUN R, ULLMANN U: *Klebsiella* spp. as nosocomial pathogens: Epidemiology, taxonomy, typing methods, and pathogenicity factors. Clin Microbiol Rev 11:589, 1998

SANDERS WE JR, SANDERS CC: *Enterobacter* spp.: Pathogens poised to flourish at the turn of the century. Clin Microbiol Rev 10:220, 1997

SHIH CC et al: Bacteremia due to *Citrobacter* species: Significance of primary intraabdominal infection. Clin Infect Dis 23:543, 1996

STAMM WE: Catheter-associated urinary tract infections: Epidemiology, pathogenesis, and prevention. Am J Med 91:65S, 1991

VILLERS D et al: Nosocomial *Acinetobacter baumannii* infections: Microbiological and clinical epidemiology. Ann Intern Med 129:182, 1998

WATANAKUNAKORN C, PERNI SC: *Proteus mirabilis* bacteremia: A review of 176 cases during 1980–1992. Scand J Infect Dis 26:361, 1994

WOODS TD, WATANAKUNAKORN C: Bacteremia due to *Providencia stuartii*: Review of 49 episodes. South Med J 89:221, 1996

154   *John C. Atherton, Martin J. Blaser*

HELICOBACTER PYLORI INFECTIONS

DEFINITION *Helicobacter pylori* colonizes the human stomach and is of etiologic importance in peptic ulcer disease and gastric malignancy. Other gastric *Helicobacter* species colonize animals, some with a narrow range and others with a broad range of host species specificity. Those with broad specificity are occasionally found in humans, possibly as zoonoses. It is unclear whether *Helicobacter heilmanii* (formerly known as *Gastrospirillum hominis*), the most common of these species among isolates from humans, is associated with human disease. Numerous species of nongastric helicobacters are found in animals, and some have been isolated from human stool and gall bladder; whether these species cause disease is unknown.

ETIOLOGIC AGENT *H. pylori* is a gram-negative, spiral, flagellate bacillus that naturally colonizes humans and monkeys. It is noninvasive, living in gastric mucus; a small proportion of the bacterial cells are adherent to the mucosa. Its spiral shape and flagellae render *H. pylori* motile in the mucous environment, and its efficient urease protects it against acid by catalyzing urea hydrolysis to produce buffering ammonia. In vitro, *H. pylori* is microaerophilic and slow-growing and requires complex growth media. In 1997, the complete genomic sequence of *H. pylori* was published, and this information has greatly advanced the understanding of metabolic pathways and other aspects of the organism's biology. *H. heilmanii* is a longer, more

tightly coiled spiral than *H. pylori* and cannot easily be cultured in vitro at present.

EPIDEMIOLOGY The prevalence of *H. pylori* colonization is about 30% in the United States and other developed countries as opposed to >80% in most developing countries. In the United States, prevalence varies with age; around 50% of 60-year-old persons as opposed to 25% of 30-year-old persons are colonized. Spontaneous acquisition or loss of the bacterium in adulthood is uncommon. *H. pylori* is usually acquired in childhood. (The age association is mostly due to a birth-cohort effect.) Other than age, the main risk factor for colonization is low socioeconomic status; crowding and low family income in childhood are especially strong correlates of colonization.

Humans are the only important reservoir of *H. pylori*. Members of a family may carry the same strain, and colonization is particularly common in childhood institutions. These findings imply direct person-to-person spread, but whether transmission takes place by the fecal-oral or oral-oral route is unknown. *H. pylori* DNA has been found in water sources, and indirect epidemiological evidence indicates that contaminated water may lead to human colonization in developing countries. Much research is focused on determining which of these possible routes of acquisition is most important.

CLINICAL MANIFESTATIONS Essentially all *H. pylori*–colonized persons have gastric inflammation, but this condition in itself is asymptomatic (Fig. 154-1). Symptoms are due to illnesses such as peptic ulceration or gastric malignancy, which develop in fewer than 10% of individuals colonized with *H. pylori*. More than 80% of peptic ulcers are related to *H. pylori* colonization, most of the remainder being due to damage caused by aspirin or nonsteroidal anti-inflammatory drugs (NSAIDs). The main lines of evidence for an ulcer-promoting role of *H. pylori* are (1) that the presence of the organism is a risk factor for the development of ulcers, (2) that (non-NSAID-induced) ulcers rarely develop in the absence of *H. pylori*, (3) that eradication of *H. pylori* results in a dramatic drop in the rate of ulcer relapse (from about 80% to 15% in the first year), and (4) that experimental infection of gerbils and mice causes gastroduodenal injury.

Prospective case-control studies have shown that *H. pylori* colonization is a risk factor for adenocarcinomas of the stomach (other than those arising in the gastric cardia). However, persons who have had documented duodenal ulcers are less likely than other persons to develop gastric adenocarcinoma later in life; the implication is that, whereas *H. pylori* colonization increases risk for both duodenal ulcerogenesis and gastric carcinogenesis, other factors determine which disease path is taken. The presence of *H. pylori* is strongly associated with gastric lymphoma. Low-grade B-cell mucosa-associated lymphoid tissue (MALT) lymphomas, which are antigen driven, often regress following *H. pylori* eradication. Whether all such diagnosed cases represent true malignancies remains to be determined.

Most *H. pylori* colonization is asymptomatic. Whether colonization occasionally causes symptoms (nonulcer dyspepsia) in the absence of ulcers or malignancy is controversial. Some but not all trials of *H. pylori* eradication in nonulcer dyspepsia have shown a reduction of symptoms in a small proportion of patients. As there is no prospective method for identifying this small group, eradication of *H. pylori* in patients with nonulcer dyspepsia is not currently indicated.

Much interest has focused on a possible protective role for *H. pylori* in gastroesophageal reflux disease (GERD) and adenocarcinoma of the esophagus and gastric cardia. The main lines of evidence for this role are that (1) there is a temporal relationship between a falling prevalence of *H. pylori* colonization and a rising incidence of these conditions; (2) in most studies, the prevalence of *H. pylori* colonization, especially with *cagA⁺* strains, is lower among patients with these esophageal diseases than among control subjects; and (3) eradication of *H. pylori* often leads to the development or worsening of GERD or its symptoms. Although there are plausible mechanisms for a protective effect of *H. pylori* against these diseases, none has yet been definitively identified. Thus a causal link remains probable but unproven.

Several extra-gastrointestinal pathologies have been linked epidemiologically with *H. pylori* colonization. The most notable are ischemic heart disease and cerebrovascular disease. The associations have been found more commonly in small than in large studies, and most authorities consider them to be noncausal and due to confounding factors.

PATHOLOGY AND PATHOGENESIS   *H. pylori* colonization induces chronic superficial gastritis, which includes both mononuclear and polymorphonuclear cell infiltration of the mucosa. (The term *gastritis* should be used specifically to describe histologic features; it also has been used to describe endoscopic appearances and even symptoms, neither of which have been linked to microscopic findings or to the presence of *H. pylori*.) The immune response to *H. pylori* includes both the production of antibody (local and systemic) and a cell-mediated response but is ineffective in clearing the bacterium. *H. pylori* and associated inflammation are most evident in the stomach but are also found in areas of gastric metaplasia and heterotopia (e.g., the duodenal bulb).The pattern of gastric inflammation is associated with disease risk: antral-predominant gastritis is most closely linked with duodenal ulceration and is common in the United States and other developed countries, whereas the predominant form in developing countries is pangastritis, which is epidemiologically linked with gastric ulceration and adenocarcinoma. Longitudinal analyses of gastric biopsy specimens taken years apart from the same patient show that inflammation may progress to atrophy, intestinal metaplasia, and dysplasia and then (by implication) to carcinoma. Patients with atrophic gastritis are at risk for vitamin B_{12} deficiency and its associated hematologic and neurologic sequelae. Continuous omeprazole therapy (for example, for GERD) may speed progression to atrophy when *H. pylori* is present.

Most *H. pylori*–colonized persons do not develop clinical sequelae. That some persons develop overt disease whereas others do not is probably due to a combination of bacterial strain differences, host susceptibility to disease, and environmental factors; of these, bacterial factors are best studied.

The two major disease-associated *H. pylori* virulence factors described so far are a vacuolating cytotoxin, VacA, and a group of genes termed the *cag* pathogenicity island (*cag* PaI). VacA occurs in several forms, and its level of production varies between strains; thus, although all strains have the gene (*vacA*) encoding the protein, not all exhibit vacuolating activity in vitro. Cytotoxic strains are more commonly isolated from patients with peptic ulcer disease than from persons without ulcers. The *cag* PaI includes genes that confer enhanced virulence on *H. pylori* strains, at least partly by inducing epithelial cells to produce proinflammatory cytokines. The gene *cagA*, an imperfect marker for the *cag* PaI, is useful for epidemiologic studies because it encodes a highly immunogenic protein, CagA. Patients with peptic ulcers or gastric adenocarcinoma are more likely to have CagA antibodies than persons without these conditions. However, patients with esophageal dysplasia or adenocarcinoma or with the premalignant condition Barrett's esophagus are less likely to harbor *cagA*+ strains than are *H. pylori*–positive controls. Thus, eradication of *cagA*+ strains from asymptomatic persons to prevent disease is not recommended.

How does gastric *H. pylori* colonization increase risk for duodenal ulceration? One explanation is that antral *H. pylori* colonization diminishes the number of somatostatin-producing cells; somatostatin-mediated inhibition of gastrin release leads to hypergastrinemia. Individuals with antral-predominant gastritis (and thus a normally functioning acid-producing gastric corpus) develop increased acid secretion, which may increase the risk of duodenal ulceration per se or may induce gastric metaplasia in the duodenum, which becomes col-

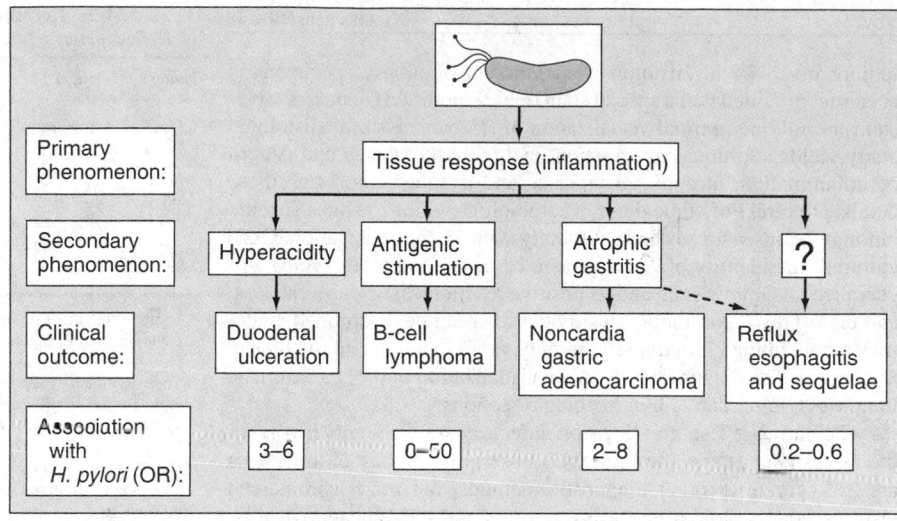

FIGURE 154-1   Schematic of the relationships between colonization with *Helicobacter pylori* and diseases of the upper gastrointestinal tract among persons in developed countries. Essentially all persons colonized with *H. pylori* develop a host response, which is generally termed *chronic gastritis*. The nature of the interaction of the host with the particular bacterial population determines the clinical outcome. *H. pylori* colonization increases the lifetime risk of peptic ulcer disease, noncardia gastric cancer, and B-cell non-Hodgkin's gastric lymphoma [odds ratios (ORs) for all, >1]. In contrast, a growing body of evidence indicates that *H. pylori* colonization protects against adenocarcinoma of the esophagus (and the related gastric cardia) and premalignant lesions such as Barrett's esophagus (OR, <1). While the incidences of peptic ulcer disease (cases not due to nonsteroidal anti-inflammatory drugs) and noncardia gastric cancer are declining in developed countries, the incidence of adenocarcinoma of the esophagus is rapidly increasing. (*Adapted from Blaser 1999, with permission.*)

onized by *H. pylori*, then inflamed, and finally ulcerated. After eradication of *H. pylori* from patients with duodenal ulcer disease, the level of acid secretion often falls.

DIAGNOSIS   Tests for *H. pylori* can be divided into two groups: invasive tests, which require upper gastrointestinal endoscopy and are based on the analysis of gastric biopsy specimens, and noninvasive tests (Table 154-1). Invasive tests are preferred for (1) the initial management of dyspeptic patients, because the decision of whether or not to eradicate *H. pylori* depends on ulcer disease status, and (2) follow-up after treatment of patients with gastric ulceration to be certain that the ulcer was not malignant. Follow-up endoscopy should be performed at least 4 weeks after cessation of all anti-*Helicobacter* drugs, since at earlier points the *H. pylori* load may be low and tests may be falsely negative. The most convenient endoscopy-based test is the biopsy urease test, in which two antral biopsy specimens are put into a gel containing urea and an indicator. The presence of *H. pylori* urease elicits a color change, which often takes place within minutes but can

Table 154-1   Commonly Used Tests to Detect *Helicobacter pylori* Infection

Test	Advantages	Disadvantages
INVASIVE (ENDOSCOPIC BIOPSY–BASED)		
Biopsy urease test	Quick, simple	Rapid test not fully sensitive, 24-h test not fully specific
Histology	Widely available; may give additional histologic information	Sensitivity dependent on experience
Culture	Permits determination of antibiotic susceptibilities	Sensitivity dependent on experience
NONINVASIVE		
Serology	Cheap and convenient	Cannot be used for early follow-up
^{13}C or ^{14}C urea breath test	Safer and cheaper than endoscopy	Low-dose irradiation in ^{14}C test

require up to 24 h. Histologic examination of biopsy specimens is accurate, provided that a special stain (e.g., a modified Giemsa or silver stain) permitting optimal visualization of *H. pylori* is used. Histologic study yields additional information, including the degree and pattern of inflammation, atrophy, metaplasia, and dysplasia, although these details are rarely of clinical use. Microbiologic culture is most specific but may be insensitive due to difficulty with *H. pylori* isolation. Once cultured, the identity of *H. pylori* can be confirmed by its typical appearance on Gram's stain and its positive reactions in oxidase, catalase, and urease tests. Antibiotic sensitivities also can be determined. Specimens containing *H. heilmanii* are only weakly positive in the biopsy urease test. The diagnosis is based on visualization of the characteristic long, tight spiral bacteria in histologic sections.

The simplest tests for *H. pylori* infection are serologic, involving the assessment of specific IgG levels in serum. The best of these tests are as accurate as other diagnostic methods, but many commercial tests, especially rapid office tests, perform poorly. In quantitative tests, a defined drop in antibody titer between matched serum samples taken before and 6 months after treatment (no sooner because of the slow decline in antibody titer) accurately indicates that *H. pylori* infection has been eradicated. The other major noninvasive tests are the ^{13}C and ^{14}C urea breath tests. In these simple tests, the patient drinks a labeled urea solution and then blows into a tube. The urea is labeled with either the nonradioactive isotope ^{13}C or a minute dose of the radioactive isotope ^{14}C (which exposes the patient to less radiation than a standard chest x-ray). If *H. pylori* urease is present, the urea is hydrolyzed and labeled carbon dioxide is detected in breath samples. Unlike serologic tests, urea breath tests can be used to assess the outcome of treatment 1 month after its completion and thus may replace endoscopy for this purpose in the follow-up of duodenal ulcer patients. As for endoscopic tests, all anti-*Helicobacter* drugs should be avoided in this period or the test may be falsely negative.

℞ **TREATMENT** At present, the only clear indications for treatment are *H. pylori*–related duodenal and gastric ulceration and the rare low-grade B-cell MALT lymphoma. *H. pylori* should be eradicated in patients with documented ulcer disease, whether or not the ulcers are currently active, to reduce the likelihood of relapse. At present, treatment is not recommended for nonulcer dyspepsia or for prophylaxis against ulcers or gastric adenocarcinoma (although it may be reasonable to eradicate *H. pylori* in persons with a strong family history of gastric cancer). Reasons for avoiding treatment for these other potential indications include the expense, the induction of morbidity in otherwise healthy people, the risk of inducing widespread antibiotic resistance in *H. pylori* and in other colonizing bacteria, and the risk of inducing or worsening GERD.

H. pylori is susceptible to a wide range of antibiotics in vitro, but monotherapy has been disappointing in vivo, probably because of inadequate antibiotic delivery to the full locus of colonization. Failure of monotherapy has led to the development of multidrug regimens, the most successful of which are triple and quadruple combinations that achieve *H. pylori* eradication rates of >90% in many trials and >75% in clinical practice. Current 7- to 14-day drug regimens consisting of a proton pump inhibitor and two or three antimicrobial agents often require only twice-daily dosing (Table 154-2).

The two most important goals in *H. pylori* eradication are to obtain the patient's compliance with the dosing regimen and to use drugs to which *H. pylori* has not acquired resistance. Treatment failure following minor lapses in compliance is common and often leads to acquired resistance to metronidazole or clarithromycin. To stress the importance of compliance, written instructions should be given to the patient, and minor side effects of the regimen should be explained. Resistance to metronidazole and clarithromycin is of growing concern; however, in multidrug regimens, the clinical significance of single-drug resistance is diminished. Assessment of antibiotic susceptibilities before treatment would be optimal but is not usually undertaken. In the absence

Table 154-2 Recommended 7- to 14-Day Regimens for the Eradication of *Helicobacter pylori*

Name	Drug 1[a]	Drug 2	Drug 3	Drug 4
OCA[b]	Omeprazole (20 mg bid)	Clarithromycin (500 mg bid)	Amoxicillin (1 g bid)	—
OCM[b]	Omeprazole (20 mg bid)	Clarithromycin (250 mg bid)	Metronidazole[c] (500 mg bid)	—
OBTM[d]	Omeprazole (20 mg bid)	Bismuth subsalicylate (2 tabs qid)	Tetracycline HCl (500 mg qid)	Metronidazole[c] (500 mg tid)

[a] In any of the three regimens, omeprazole may be replaced by lansoprazole (30 mg bid), pantoprazole (40 mg bid), ranitidine bismuth citrate (400 mg bid), or possibly ranitidine (150 mg bid). Most available data are for omeprazole.
[b] These regimens may be given for 7 to 14 days; meta-analysis suggests that 14-day regimens are slightly more effective.
[c] The optimal dose of metronidazole is not known. Tinidazole (500 mg bid) can be used in place of metronidazole.
[d] Data for this regimen are mainly from Europe and are based on bismuth subcitrate. Omeprazole is given for 10 days, and the other three agents are given on days 4 through 10.

of susceptibility information, a history of antibiotic use should be obtained, and, if resistance is likely, metronidazole-containing regimens should be avoided. Metronidazole resistance is common among persons who have taken the agent previously, even years earlier, for other conditions such as giardiasis or trichomoniasis. If initial *H. pylori* treatment fails, compliance should be checked and re-treatment should be based on known antibiotic susceptibilities. When this information cannot be obtained, the recommended course is quadruple therapy without clarithromycin (if a clarithromycin-containing regimen was given first) or triple therapy with omeprazole/clarithromycin/amoxicillin (if clarithromycin has not been used) (Table 154-2).

Given the high efficacy of treatment regimens, it is unclear whether the success of attempted *H. pylori* eradication should be checked. For gastric ulceration, the opportunity to retest for *H. pylori* is present at the repeat endoscopy, which is performed to evaluate healing. For duodenal ulceration, although many clinicians prefer to retest only if symptoms recur, a urea breath test or endoscopy should be performed no sooner than 1 month after treatment. This test will provide reassurance if treatment has been successful and will prompt re-treatment in cases of persistence.

Clearance of *H. heilmanii* has been described following the use of bismuth compounds alone or triple-therapy regimens. However, in the absence of trials, it is unclear whether this result represents successful treatment or natural clearance of the bacterium.

PREVENTION Carriage of *H. pylori* has public health significance in developing countries, where gastric adenocarcinoma is a common cause of cancer death. However, *H. pylori* has co-evolved with its human host over millennia, and there may be disadvantages in preventing or eliminating colonization. For example, as has been mentioned, the absence of *H. pylori* appears to increase the risk of developing GERD and esophageal adenocarcinoma. If mass prevention were contemplated, vaccination would be preferred, and experimental immunization of animals has given promising results. However, in the United States and other developed countries, the incidences of *H. pylori* carriage, peptic ulceration, and gastric adenocarcinoma are dropping. Thus, prevention of colonization in these countries may be unnecessary or even unwise.

BIBLIOGRAPHY

ATHERTON JC: *H. pylori* virulence factors. Br Med Bull 54:105, 1998

BLASER MJ: The changing relationships of *Helicobacter pylori* and humans: Implications for health and disease. J Infect Dis 179:1523, 1999

HANSSON L-E et al: The risk of stomach cancer in patients with gastric or duodenal ulcer disease. N Engl J Med 335:242, 1996

KUIPERS E et al: Atrophic gastritis and *Helicobacter pylori* infection in patients with reflux esophagitis treated with omeprazole or fundoplication. N Engl J Med 334:1018, 1996

MARSHALL BJ, WARREN JR: Unidentified curved bacilli in the stomach of patients with gastritis and peptic ulceration. Lancet 1:1311, 1984

NIH CONSENSUS DEVELOPMENT PANEL: *Helicobacter pylori* and peptic ulcer disease. JAMA 272:65, 1994

NOMURA A et al: *Helicobacter pylori* infection and gastric carcinoma in a population of Japanese-Americans in Hawaii. N Engl J Med 325:1132, 1991

PARSONNET J et al: *Helicobacter pylori* infection and gastric lymphoma. N Engl J Med 330:1267, 1994

TOMB JF et al: The complete genome sequence of the gastric pathogen *Helicobacter pylori*. Nature 338:539, 1997

ZUCCA E et al:Molecular analysis of the progression from *Helicobacter pylori*–associated chronic gastritis to mucosa-associated lymphoid-tissue lymphoma of the stomach. N Engl J Med 328:804, 1998

155 Christopher A. Ohl, Matthew Pollack

INFECTIONS DUE TO *PSEUDOMONAS* SPECIES AND RELATED ORGANISMS

Pseudomonas species and phylogenetically related bacteria are ubiquitous, free-living, opportunistic gram-negative pathogens. *P. aeruginosa*, the most common human pathogen in this group, is the primary subject of this chapter. Also discussed are two pathogens of increasing importance: *Burkholderia cepacia* (formerly *P. cepacia*), primarily an opportunistic pathogen, and *Stenotrophomonas maltophilia* (formerly *Xanthomonas maltophilia*), which principally infects hospitalized patients. In addition, melioidosis, a tropical systemic disease with acute and chronic manifestations caused by *B. pseudomallei* (formerly *P. pseudomallei*), will be considered.

INFECTIONS DUE TO *P. AERUGINOSA*

P. aeruginosa is a small, nonsporulating, aerobic gram-negative rod belonging to the family Pseudomonadaceae. It is motile by virtue of its single polar flagellum. More than half of all clinical isolates produce the blue-green pigment pyocyanin; this pigment is helpful in the identification of the organism and accounts for the species name *aeruginosa*, which refers to the distinctive color of copper oxide.

EPIDEMIOLOGY *P. aeruginosa* is widespread in nature, inhabiting soil, water, plants, and animals (including humans). It has a predilection for moist environments. This organism occasionally colonizes the skin, external ear, upper respiratory tract, or large bowel of healthy humans. Rates of carriage are relatively low, however, except among patients who have serious underlying disease, whose host defenses have been naturally or iatrogenically compromised, who have previously received antibiotic therapy, and/or who have been exposed to the hospital environment. Under these circumstances, colonization with *P. aeruginosa* frequently precedes infection, and factors that predispose to the former also increase the likelihood of the latter.

Most *P. aeruginosa* infections are acquired in the hospital, where intensive care units account for the highest rates of infection. According to the National Nosocomial Infections Surveillance (NNIS) system, between 1992 and 1999, *P. aeruginosa* was the second most common cause of pneumonia, the fourth most common cause of urinary tract infection, and the sixth most frequent bloodstream isolate in intensive care units. Many potential reservoirs of infection have been identified in the hospital environment, including respiratory equipment, cleaning solutions, disinfectants, sinks, vegetables, flowers, endoscopes, and physiotherapy pools. Most reservoirs are associated with moisture. It is assumed that the organism is transmitted to patients via the hands of hospital personnel or via fomites. While some infecting strains of *P. aeruginosa* appear to be endemic within the hospital, others are traced to a common source associated with a specific outbreak or epidemic. Epidemiologic investigation is facilitated by serotyping (immunotyping) of strains on the basis of differences in lipopolysaccharide (LPS) structure and by the use of molecular techniques such as pulsed-field gel electrophoresis.

PATHOGENESIS That the pathogenesis of infections due to *P. aeruginosa* is complex is evidenced by the clinical diversity of the diseases related to this organism and by the multiplicity of virulence factors it produces. *P. aeruginosa* rarely causes disease in the healthy host. Relative risk for infection is greatly increased, however, when normal cutaneous or mucosal barriers have been breached or bypassed, when immunologic defense mechanisms have been compromised, or when the protective function of the normal bacterial flora has been disrupted (Table 155-1). The ubiquity of the organism, its flexible nutritional and metabolic requirements, its environmental resiliency, and its relative resistance to antibiotics help account for the frequency and success with which it acts as an opportunistic pathogen.

Infections caused by *P. aeruginosa* usually begin with bacterial attachment and superficial colonization of cutaneous or mucosal surfaces and progress to localized bacterial invasion and damage to underlying tissues. The infection may remain anatomically localized or may spread by direct extension to contiguous structures. This process may continue with bloodstream invasion, dissemination, the systemic inflammatory-response syndrome (SIRS), multiple-organ dysfunction, and ultimately death. Not only is local infection more likely to occur in immunocompromised hosts, such as those with profound neutropenia, but it is more likely to culminate in bloodstream invasion and dissemination. LPS (endotoxin), which is a structural component of the bacterial outer membrane, is thought to play a pivotal role in the pathogenesis of the sepsis syndrome or SIRS.

The initial attachment of *P. aeruginosa* to the respiratory epithelium and other epithelial surfaces appears to be mediated by bacterial organelles called *pili* or *fimbriae* and facilitated by *alginate*, a mucoid exopolysaccharide produced by most strains of the bacterium under appropriate environmental conditions. Alginate plays an important role in colonization and infection of the respiratory tract in patients with cystic fibrosis and in the formation of biofilms within which sessile colonies of *P. aeruginosa* enjoy relative protection from host defenses and antimicrobial agents.

P. aeruginosa produces a number of extracellular virulence factors, including alkaline protease, elastase, phospholipase, cytotoxin, and exoenzymes (or exotoxins) A and S. The breakdown of host tissues by these bacterial products creates conditions conducive to enhanced bacterial proliferation, invasion, and tissue injury. Production and secretion of many of these extracellular virulence factors are under the regulatory control of a cell-to-cell signaling system that has been termed *quorum sensing*. Through lactones and other signal molecules secreted by individual *P. aeruginosa* bacteria, the entire bacterial population is able to sense its environment, communicate, and discern its own cell density. This regulatory system conceivably allows *P. aeruginosa* to produce extracellular virulence factors in a coordinated

Table 155-1 Factors Associated with *Pseudomonas aeruginosa* Infections

Disruption of cutaneous or mucosal barriers	Immunosuppression
Burn injury	Neutropenia
Dermatitis	Qualitative white blood cell defects
Penetrating trauma	Hypogammaglobulinemia
Surgery	Defective cell-mediated immunity
Endotracheal intubation	Extremes of age
Indwelling central venous catheterization	Diabetes mellitus
	Steroid therapy
Urinary bladder catheterization	Cystic fibrosis
	Cancer
Injection drug use	AIDS
Disruption of normal bacterial flora	
Broad-spectrum antibiotic therapy	
Exposure to the hospital environment	

manner dependent on cell density and may give the pathogen an appreciable advantage over host defense mechanisms.

The extracellular enzyme exotoxin A—a diphtheria-like toxin—is produced by most clinical isolates of *P. aeruginosa*. Exotoxin A inhibits mammalian protein synthesis by transferring the adenosine diphosphate (ADP) ribose moiety of the nicotinamide adenine dinucleotide into covalent linkage with elongation factor 2, inactivating this factor's ability to catalyze the elongation step in polypeptide assembly. Another extracellular cytotoxin, exoenzyme S, is also an adenosine diphosphate ribosyltransferase but, unlike exotoxin A, preferentially ribosylates guanosine triphosphate–binding proteins, resulting in disruption of host cell actin cytoskeletons. Exoenzyme S is one of several extracellular virulence factors of *P. aeruginosa* that is directly introduced from the bacterial cytosol into the host cell cytoplasm via a complex array of transmembrane proteins termed the *type III secretion apparatus*. This process requires direct cell contact and allows the injection of virulence factors from the bacterium into host cells without interference from humoral immune defenses.

CLINICAL MANIFESTATIONS AND DIAGNOSIS Respiratory Tract Infections

Primary pneumonia, or *nonbacteremic pneumonia*, results from aspiration of upper respiratory tract secretions; often develops in patients with chronic lung disease, congestive heart failure, or AIDS; and is most common in an intensive care setting in association with mechanical ventilator use. Fever, chills, severe dyspnea, cyanosis, productive cough, apprehension, confusion, and other signs of severe systemic toxicity characterize this acute, often life-threatening infection. Chest roentgenograms typically show bilateral bronchopneumonia with nodular infiltrates and small areas of radiolucency; pleural effusions are common; empyema is relatively uncommon; and lobar consolidation is occasionally seen. Cavitary lesions are particularly common in AIDS patients with *P. aeruginosa* pneumonia. Pathologic lesions include alveolar necrosis, focal hemorrhages, and microabscesses.

Bacteremic pneumonia due to *P. aeruginosa* begins as a respiratory infection but, in contrast to primary pneumonia, is typically associated with neutropenia, subsequent bloodstream invasion, and metastatic spread that produces characteristic lesions in the lungs and other viscera. Alveolar hemorrhage and necrosis are common. The signs and symptoms of this fulminant disease include those described for nonbacteremic pneumonia caused by this organism as well as those associated with gram-negative sepsis. Chest roentgenograms characteristically demonstrate a rapid progression from pulmonary vascular congestion to interstitial edema, then to pulmonary edema, and finally to diffuse necrotizing bronchopneumonia with cavity formation. The patient typically dies 3 or 4 days after initial presentation.

Chronic infection of the lower respiratory tract with *P. aeruginosa* is caused almost exclusively by mucoid strains, which produce alginate. Such infection is prevalent among older children and young adults with cystic fibrosis and also develops in some patients with AIDS. In patients with cystic fibrosis, mucoid strains invariably colonize and infect patients with increasing prevalence over time, contributing to the acute exacerbations and chronic progression that characterize pulmonary disease in these individuals. Airway obstruction appears to begin with bronchiolitis, which causes mucus plugging and predisposes to *P. aeruginosa* infection. The infection produces more mucus plugging, chronic suppuration, bronchiectasis, atelectasis, and ultimately fibrosis. This process progresses to pulmonary insufficiency, hypoxemia, and alterations in cardiopulmonary dynamics resulting in pulmonary hypertension and cor pulmonale.

Clinical manifestations of lower respiratory tract infections due to *P. aeruginosa* in patients with cystic fibrosis vary with the severity and duration of underlying lung disease, the frequency and intensity of acute episodes, and the presence of coinfecting pathogens such as *B. cepacia* (Chap. 257). Soon after colonization, patients may experience recurrent upper respiratory symptoms followed by a lingering cough. Episodes of pneumonia develop later, with persistent cough

between acute episodes. Eventually, patients exhibit a chronic productive cough, wheezing, diminished appetite, weight loss, growth retardation, and decreased activity. Acute exacerbations are typically accompanied by low-grade fever and heightened respiratory symptoms. Physical signs include evidence of malnutrition, an increase in anteroposterior diameter, intercostal retractions, cyanosis, inspiratory and expiratory wheezing, rhonchi, moist rales, abdominal distention, and clubbing of the fingers and toes. Laboratory abnormalities include leukocytosis with a left shift and hypoxemia with or without hypercarbia. Tests of pulmonary function demonstrate obstructive and restrictive defects. Chest roentgenograms reveal overaeration, patchy atelectasis, peribronchial fibrosis, and patchy infiltrates associated with pneumonia. In more advanced disease, there may be evidence of severe overaeration, depressed diaphragm, further increased anteroposterior diameter, extensive peribronchial infiltration, generalized bronchiectasis, and cyst formation.

Bacteremia *P. aeruginosa* remains an important cause of life-threatening bloodstream infection in immunocompromised patients. Bacteremia is frequently iatrogenic and is usually seen in hospitalized patients with various comorbid conditions (Table 155-1). Bloodstream infection can be either primary (with no identifiable source) or secondary to a discrete focus of infection.

The clinical features of *P. aeruginosa* bacteremia are similar to those of other forms of bacteremia. Common primary sites of infection include the urinary tract, gastrointestinal tract, lungs, skin and soft tissues, and intravascular foci, including indwelling central venous catheters. Fever, tachypnea, tachycardia, and prostration are common. Disorientation, confusion, or obtundation may be evident. Hypotension can progress to refractory shock. Renal failure, adult respiratory distress syndrome, and disseminated intravascular coagulation occur as complications.

Pathognomonic skin lesions termed *ecthyma gangrenosum* develop in a relatively small minority of patients with *P. aeruginosa* bacteremia. The lesions begin as small hemorrhagic vesicles surrounded by a rim of erythema and undergo central necrosis with subsequent ulceration (**see Plate IID-57C**). They occur singly or in small numbers on the perineum, buttocks, and extremities; in the axillae; or elsewhere. Histologically, these lesions contain numerous bacteria invading blood vessels but few inflammatory cells. Bacteria are readily visible on Gram's staining and may be cultured from aspirated material.

Endocarditis *P. aeruginosa* infects native heart valves in injection drug users as well as prosthetic heart valves. The source of *P. aeruginosa* strains infecting drug users appears to be standing water contaminating drug paraphernalia. Foreign materials mixed with heroin may cause injury to valve leaflets or mural endocardium, with resulting fibrosis and an increased risk for valve infection. Exposure of the tricuspid valve to both trauma and bacteria apparently accounts for the high incidence of tricuspid involvement in association with injection drug use.

The pulmonic, mitral, or aortic valve and the mural endocardium of either atrium may be affected in *P. aeruginosa* endocarditis. Multiple-valve infections are common. Tricuspid or right-sided involvement is often associated with septic pulmonary emboli. Right-sided *P. aeruginosa* endocarditis usually presents subacutely, while the appearance of left-sided disease is likely to be more acute or even fulminant. Fever is virtually invariable, and murmurs are usually detectable at initial presentation or shortly thereafter. Septic pulmonary emboli associated with right-sided disease result in cough, pleuritic chest pain, sputum production, pulmonary infiltration (with or without abscess formation), and pleural effusion. Left-sided infections may present as intractable heart failure or large systemic emboli. Mycotic aneurysms, cerebritis, or brain abscess may occur; septic infarcts are occasionally found in the spleen. Skin and soft tissue manifestations, including Janeway lesions, Osler's nodes, and ecthyma gangrenosum, are relatively uncommon.

The diagnosis of *P. aeruginosa* endocarditis is based on positive blood culture in the absence of an extracardiac source; an indication of valvular dysfunction or vegetation on an echocardiogram; evidence of septic pulmonary lesions on a chest roentgenogram (in right-sided disease); and the actual demonstration of infected heart valves at the time of surgery.

Central Nervous System Infections *P. aeruginosa* infections of the central nervous system include meningitis and brain abscess. These infections follow extension from a contiguous parameningeal structure such as the ear, mastoid, or paranasal sinus; direct inoculation into the subarachnoid space or brain through head trauma, surgery, or diagnostic procedures; or bacteremic spread from infection at a distant site. Like *P. aeruginosa* infections at other anatomic sites, central nervous system infections are documented almost exclusively in patients with compromised local or systemic immune-defense mechanisms.

The clinical signs of *P. aeruginosa* meningitis, like those of other forms of acute bacterial meningitis, include fever, headache, stiff neck, confusion, and obtundation. The onset of illness may be acute or even fulminant, particularly in bacteremic patients, with a precipitous downhill course, shock, coma, and early death. In nonbacteremic patients, *P. aeruginosa* meningitis or brain abscess may present more insidiously, with a paucity of systemic symptoms. This presentation is especially common in infections resulting from recent neurosurgery, cancer of the head and neck, or direct extension from a parameningeal focus of chronic infection. Occasionally, *P. aeruginosa* meningitis runs a subacute or relapsing course that is thought to be related to the intermittent release of bacteria from a loculated site of infection.

Ear Infections *P. aeruginosa* is often found in the external auditory canal, particularly under moist conditions and in the presence of inflammation or maceration (as in "swimmer's ear"). Moreover, this organism is the predominant pathogen associated with external otitis, a usually benign inflammatory process affecting the external auditory canal. The ear is painful or merely itchy, there is a purulent discharge, and pain is elicited by pulling on the pinna. The external canal appears edematous and is filled with detritus that often prevents visualization of the tympanic membrane.

P. aeruginosa occasionally penetrates the epithelium overlying the floor of the external auditory canal at the junction between bone and cartilage and invades underlying soft tissue. The ensuing invasive process, which involves soft tissue, cartilage, and cortical bone, is typically slow but destructive. Termed *malignant external otitis*, this condition occurs predominantly in elderly diabetic patients but is reported occasionally in infants with other underlying diseases and rarely in elderly nondiabetic patients. Virtually all cases of malignant external otitis are caused by *P. aeruginosa*. From the external ear, the infection advances to the retromandibular area or parotid space and enters the mastoid air cells and temporal bone. Advancing osteomyelitis at the base of the skull often involves the seventh, ninth, tenth, and eleventh cranial nerves. The cavernous sinus can become involved, as can the contralateral petrous apex. The middle ear is commonly spared; meningitis and brain abscess are relatively rare complications.

Otorrhea and severe otalgia are common presenting symptoms of malignant external otitis. Facial-nerve paralysis tends to occur early, while other cranial-nerve palsies appear later. There may be a loss of hearing. Constitutional symptoms such as fever and weight loss are relatively uncommon. Physical examination almost always reveals remarkable tenderness of the pinna of the ear and abnormalities of the external auditory canal, including swelling, erythema, purulent discharge, debris, and granulation tissue in the canal wall. The tympanic membrane is often hidden from view and is sometimes perforated. Inflammation may involve the pinna as well as the periauricular, retromandibular, and mastoid areas.

Peripheral leukocytosis is relatively infrequent in malignant external otitis, while the erythrocyte sedimentation rate is usually markedly elevated. Cerebrospinal fluid occasionally exhibits pleocytosis and an elevation in the protein level. Computed tomography (CT) or magnetic resonance imaging (MRI) of the mastoid or temporal bone typically reveals bony erosions and new bone formation, while the floor of the skull may have soft tissue densities associated with areas of cellulitis. In addition, technetium 99m bone scans and gallium 67 scans fre-

quently give positive results. Cultures of samples from the external auditory canal and of surgical specimens are almost always positive for *P. aeruginosa*.

Eye Infections (See also Chap. 28) *P. aeruginosa* causes bacterial keratitis or corneal ulcer and endophthalmitis in the human eye. Keratitis due to *P. aeruginosa* may result from even minor corneal injury, which interrupts the integrity of the superficial epithelial surface and permits bacterial access to the underlying stroma. Corneal ulcer may complicate contact lens use, particularly when extended-wear soft contact lenses are involved. Contact lens solutions or the lenses themselves may be the source of the organism, which is probably inoculated into the eye at sites of minor lens-induced corneal damage. Patients who have sustained serious burns, have undergone ocular irradiation or tracheostomy, have been exposed to the intensive care environment, and/or are in a coma are also susceptible to *P. aeruginosa*–associated corneal ulcers. *P. aeruginosa* keratitis usually starts as a small central ulcer; spreads concentrically to involve a large portion of the cornea, sclera, and underlying stroma; and in some cases progresses to posterior corneal perforation.

The clinical manifestations of *P. aeruginosa* keratitis include a rapidly expanding, necrotic stromal infiltrate in the bed of an epithelial injury; surrounding epithelial edema; an anterior chamber reaction; and mucopurulent discharge adherent to the ulcer's surface. Corneal ulcer due to *P. aeruginosa* may advance rapidly to involve the entire cornea in ≤2 days or may evolve subacutely over several days. Systemic symptoms are uncommon. Complications include corneal perforation, anterior chamber involvement, and endophthalmitis.

P. aeruginosa endophthalmitis is typically a rapidly progressive, sight-threatening condition that demands immediate therapeutic intervention. It may complicate penetrating injuries of the eye, intraocular surgery, hematogenous spread from other sites of *Pseudomonas* infection, or posterior perforation of corneal ulcers. Clinical manifestations may include eye pain, conjunctival hyperemia, chemosis, lid edema, decreased visual acuity, hypopyon, severe anterior uveitis, and signs of possible vitreous involvement. Panophthalmitis may result from this intraocular infection.

Bone and Joint Infections Vertebral osteomyelitis due to *P. aeruginosa* is associated with complicated urinary tract infection, genitourinary instrumentation or surgery, and injection drug use. Vertebral infections that are associated with a urinary tract source most often develop in the elderly and usually affect the lumbosacral spine. Presumably the route of infection in these patients is a shared venous plexus between the pelvis and spine. Injection drug use–related infections typically occur in younger patients and may affect the cervical or lumbosacral spine. *P. aeruginosa* vertebral osteomyelitis is usually an indolent disease. Accordingly, symptoms may develop weeks or even months before diagnosis. Back or neck pain is generally reported, while fever and systemic symptoms are relatively uncommon. Local tenderness and decreased range of motion of the affected spine are typical. Leukocytosis may be noted, the erythrocyte sedimentation rate is almost always markedly elevated, and blood cultures are sometimes positive. Roentgenograms reveal loss of bone density, narrowed intervertebral space, destruction of vertebral end plates, lytic lesions of vertebral bodies, sclerosis, and occasionally osteophyte formation. CT and MRI are the most sensitive and specific means of defining lesions. Technetium bone scans and gallium scans usually yield positive results. An etiologic diagnosis requires the culture of material obtained by needle aspiration or biopsy of the affected spine under fluoroscopic guidance; open biopsy is sometimes needed.

Sternoclavicular pyarthrosis caused by *P. aeruginosa* is another complication of injection drug use; in some cases it is associated with *P. aeruginosa* endocarditis, but more often it is not. Joint involvement is usually monoarticular, with the sternoclavicular joint more often affected than sternochondral joints. Patients present with acute or chronic pain in the anterior chest wall, often associated with fever and restricted movement of the homolateral shoulder. Physical examination reveals tenderness, erythema, and swelling over the affected joint. Leukocytosis is common, and the erythrocyte sedimentation rate is almost invariably elevated. Roentgenograms show soft tissue edema; bone demineralization; lytic lesions; and periosteal elevation of the clavicular head, rib, or sternum. Material obtained by arthrocentesis or synovial biopsy yields *P. aeruginosa* in culture.

P. aeruginosa infections of the symphysis pubis are associated with pelvic surgery and injection drug use. The symphysis pubis, like other fibrocartilaginous joints, exhibits a peculiar susceptibility to bloodborne infection with *P. aeruginosa*. Affected patients report pain in the groin, hip, thigh, and/or lower abdomen that is made worse by walking. Fever is variable, and the duration of symptoms before diagnosis ranges from days to months. The erythrocyte sedimentation rate is markedly elevated. Roentgenography or CT shows irregularities of the pubic margins, separation of the symphysis pubis, and osteomyelitic abnormalities of the pubic rami that may be extensive. Bone scans are usually positive. Needle aspiration or biopsy is necessary to obtain material for culture. A positive culture is particularly important for the discrimination of *P. aeruginosa* infections and other pyogenic infections from osteitis pubis, which is thought to be a noninfectious condition complicating pelvic surgery, childbirth, or trauma.

P. aeruginosa osteochondritis of the foot follows puncture wounds of the foot, primarily in children. The organism infects the small joints and bones, including the proximal phalanges, metatarsals, metatarsophalangeal joints, tarsal bones, and calcaneus. On average, local pain and swelling last for several weeks, and systemic symptoms are usually lacking. There may be plantar cellulitis over the involved area or tenderness upon deep palpation. Results of roentgenograms and bone scans are generally positive. Aspiration of the affected joint frequently yields purulent material in which *P. aeruginosa* can be demonstrated by Gram's staining and by culture.

P. aeruginosa is one of the most common causative agents in a variety of other, less specific syndromes involving nonhematogenous infections of bones and joints and collectively referred to as *chronic contiguous osteomyelitis*. These infections may result, for example, from compound fractures, contamination associated with open reduction and fixation of closed fractures, sternotomy performed in conjunction with cardiac surgery, contiguous spread from infected ischemic ulcers related to peripheral vascular disease or diabetes mellitus, and cellulitis in general. The chronicity, indolence, and heterogeneity of these infections explain their varied clinical manifestations and the frequent need for complicated long-term management.

Urinary Tract Infections *P. aeruginosa* is one of the most common causes of complicated and nosocomial infections of the urinary tract. These infections may result from urinary tract catheterization, instrumentation, surgery, or obstruction; they may arise from persistent foci (e.g., the prostate or stones) and may be chronic or recurrent. The urinary tract may be a target for bloodborne infection in patients with *P. aeruginosa* bacteremia but more often is the source of bacteremia. Chronic *P. aeruginosa* infections of the urinary tract are relatively common among patients with indwelling urinary catheters, altered urinary tract anatomy secondary to diversionary procedures, and paraplegia.

The clinical features of urinary tract infections due to *P. aeruginosa* are usually indistinguishable from those of other bacterial infections. However, *P. aeruginosa* infections exhibit a propensity for persistence, chronicity, resistance to antibiotic therapy, and recurrence. More unusual forms of urinary tract involvement peculiar to *P. aeruginosa* include (1) ulcerative lesions of the renal pelvis, ureters, and bladder that cause sloughing of vesical membranes in the urine; and (2) ecthyma-like lesions of the renal cortex that are seen in association with *Pseudomonas* sepsis.

Skin and Soft Tissue Infections As indicated above, *P. aeruginosa* bacteremia may be associated with the disseminated skin lesions of ecthyma gangrenosum (**see Plate IID-57C**). Less common skin manifestations of *P. aeruginosa* sepsis include vesicular or pus-

tular lesions, bullae, subcutaneous nodules, deep abscesses, and cellulitis. Metastatic lesions of the skin or mucous membranes complicate *Pseudomonas* sepsis and occasionally produce massive necrosis or gangrene of the extremities, perineum, face, or oropharynx.

Primary *P. aeruginosa* pyoderma occurs when the skin breaks down secondary to trauma, burn injury, dermatitis, or ulcers related to peripheral vascular disease or pressure sores. Moist conditions and neutropenia may predispose to this condition. The clinical appearance of primary *P. aeruginosa* pyoderma, which frequently includes hemorrhage and necrosis, resembles that of metastatic *P. aeruginosa* skin lesions. Histologic studies document vascular invasion by bacteria in both diseases. A rare distinguishing feature of *P. aeruginosa* pyoderma is its association with a blue-green exudate and a characteristic fruity odor.

P. aeruginosa wound sepsis complicating extensive third-degree burn injuries is associated with an extremely high mortality rate. This infection results from colonization of the burn site or burn eschar, invasion of the subeschar space and underlying dermis, vascular invasion, and systemic spread. The development and progression of *P. aeruginosa* burn wound sepsis are facilitated by the injury-associated breakdown of normal skin, selection of empirical antibiotics with inadequate coverage for this pathogen, and burn-related immune defects. Local manifestations include black, dark brown, or violaceous discoloration of the burn eschar; degeneration of underlying granulation tissue, hemorrhage, and premature eschar separation; edema, hemorrhage, and necrosis of skin adjacent to the burn site; and erythematous nodular lesions in unburned skin. Systemic manifestations include fever or hypothermia and other signs of sepsis, SIRS, or multiple-organ system failure. The diagnosis of *P. aeruginosa* burn sepsis is based on these local and systemic clinical manifestations and on a burn wound biopsy that reveals both $>10^5$ colony-forming units of *P. aeruginosa* per gram of tissue and histologic evidence of bacterial invasion of unburned tissue, vasculitis, or intense inflammation at the burn margin.

P. aeruginosa causes diffuse pruritic maculopapular and vesiculopustular rashes associated with exposure to contaminated hot tubs, spas, whirlpools, and swimming pools. Many cases of *P. aeruginosa* dermatitis have occurred in conjunction with a common-source outbreak. At least two nosocomial common-source outbreaks—one related to a physiotherapy pool—have been reported. Skin rashes may be limited to areas covered by swimsuits or may be more diffuse, sparing only the head and neck. Low-grade fever or other associated symptoms are uncommon. The illness is usually self-limited, and the rash resolves without specific therapy after cessation of exposure.

***P. aeruginosa* Infections in Patients with AIDS** During the 1980s and 1990s, *P. aeruginosa* infections were increasingly associated with AIDS. The vast majority of these infections are currently seen in patients with advanced AIDS, previous opportunistic infections, and CD4+ lymphocyte counts $<100/\mu L$ (often $<50/\mu L$). The specific immunologic factors that lead to *P. aeruginosa* infections in patients with AIDS are not well understood but are speculated to be a loss of mucosal integrity, defects in cellular and humoral immunity, and qualitative leukocyte abnormalities. Of note is that the majority of *P. aeruginosa* infections in this population are community-acquired, in contrast to the nosocomial transmission documented for most *P. aeruginosa* infections in non-AIDS patients.

Pneumonia accounts for a substantial proportion of the *P. aeruginosa* infections in patients with AIDS. In most instances, pneumonia presents as a necrotizing infection of the pulmonary parenchyma, frequently with cavitary lesions, or as a chronic relapsing bronchopulmonary infection reminiscent of the bronchopulmonary disease seen in patients with cystic fibrosis. Also frequent are bloodstream infections, including those associated with indwelling central venous catheters, and infections of the paranasal sinuses, skin and soft tissue, and urinary tract. Bacteremia, either primary or secondary to infection at a remote site, is often recurrent, associated with high mortality, and occasionally accompanied by skin manifestations similar to those seen in non-AIDS patients.

Because *P. aeruginosa* infections occur in patients with advanced

AIDS, survival after recovery from the initial infection may be limited to a few months. However, with the widespread use of highly active antiretroviral therapy and the consequent increase in CD4+ cell counts, the incidence of *P. aeruginosa* infection in patients with AIDS is likely to decline and the natural history of infection to change. For example, a few patients with recalcitrant, relapsing *P. aeruginosa* bronchopulmonary infections have reportedly experienced the resolution of infection soon after initiation of intensive antiretroviral therapy.

℞ **TREATMENT** Table 155-2 lists antimicrobial agents available in the United States that are generally active against *P. aeruginosa*. Table 155-3 outlines suggested antibiotic choices and an approach to therapy for selected sites of infection. The initial antibiotic selection should take into account the local patterns of antimicrobial susceptibility, while the susceptibilities of the isolate from a particular case should guide definitive antibiotic therapy.

In most severe or life-threatening infections due to *P. aeruginosa*, two antipseudomonal antibiotics to which the infecting strain is (or is likely to be) sensitive should be administered together. The benefits of this combined therapy, as determined by in vitro studies, are to increase efficacy, to achieve additive or synergistic killing, and to prevent the emergence of antibiotic resistance. Despite widespread acceptance of combination therapy for *P. aeruginosa* infections, there are few clinical data since the advent of newer β-lactam antibiotics documenting that combination therapy is more efficacious than monotherapy or that it actually forestalls the acquisition of antimicrobial resistance. Nevertheless, combination therapy continues to be recommended for most acute or fulminant infections, as outlined in Table 155-3.

The appropriate duration of antibiotic therapy for disease caused by *P. aeruginosa* depends on the type, location, and severity of infection. In general, chronic infections associated with extensive tissue injury, disruption of normal anatomy, foreign or prosthetic material, or suboptimal antibiotic accessibility require therapy for weeks or even months rather than days. More acute infections may be treated aggressively but for shorter periods.

P. aeruginosa infections of the lower respiratory tract in cystic fibrosis pose a special challenge because of their long-standing nature. In general, antibiotic therapy for acute exacerbations results in short-term clinical improvement, while periodic expectant courses of antimicrobial therapy may limit disease progression. A more novel approach utilizing intermittent, cyclical administration of inhaled tobramycin has been shown to improve pulmonary function, decrease the risk of hospitalization, and reduce the density of *P. aeruginosa* in sputum of older patients with cystic fibrosis. Lung transplantation has also been employed with good results in selected cystic fibrosis patients with severe, progressive lower respiratory tract infections due to *P. aeruginosa*.

Table 155-2 Antimicrobials Available in the United States with Activity Against *Pseudomonas aeruginosa*

Antimicrobial	Dose[a], Route	Comments
Antipseudomonal penicillins Piperacillin Piperacillin/tazobactam Mezlocillin Ticarcillin Ticarcillin/clavulanate	 3–4 g q4–6h IV 3.375 g q4h IV 3 g q4h IV 3 g q3–4h IV 3.1 g q4h IV	Class is listed in order of decreasing in vitro activity. Piperacillin/tazobactam or ticarcillin/clavulanate has no more activity against *P. aeruginosa* than piperacillin or ticarcillin alone. Monotherapy should not be used for serious infections.
Antipseudomonal cephalosporins Ceftazidime[b] Cefoperazone[b] Cefepime	 2 g q8–12h IV 2 g q6h IV 2 g q8–12h IV	Use higher indicated doses for neutropenic or severely immunocompromised patients. Ceftazidime reaches the highest CSF levels of the antipseudomonals (use higher indicated dose). Cefepime has less potential for β-lactamase induction than ceftazidime.
Carbapenems[b] Imipenem/cilastatin Meropenem	 0.5 g q6h IV 1 g q8h IV	Class is active against strains producing β-lactamases. Imipenem may cause seizures in patients with renal failure (avoid by reducing dose) or with CNS infections or lesions. Meropenem is slightly more active in vitro against *P. aeruginosa* than imipenem.
Monobactams Aztreonam	 2 g q6–8h IV	Drug can usually be administered to patients with β-lactam hypersensitivity.
Aminoglycosides[b] Tobramycin Gentamicin Amikacin	 MD: 2 mg/kg load, then 1.7 mg/kg q8h IV ODD: 5–7 mg/kg q24h IV Aerosolized for CF: 300 mg TOBI q12h via jet nebulizer MD: Same as tobramycin ODD: Same as tobramycin MD: 7.5 mg/kg load, then 7.5 mg/kg q12h IV ODD: 15 mg/kg q24h IV	Tobramycin has greater in vitro activity against *P. aeruginosa* than gentamicin, but the drugs' clinical efficacies are probably equivalent. Some *P. aeruginosa* isolates that are resistant to tobramycin or gentamicin may be susceptible to amikacin. Except for UTI, this class should not be used for monotherapy. ODD may reduce adverse effects. Serum levels must be monitored for MD and ODD.
Fluoroquinolones[b,c] Ciprofloxacin Levofloxacin	 0.4 g q12h IV 0.5–0.75 g bid PO 0.5 g q24h IV or PO	Of the available fluoroquinolones, ciprofloxacin is the most active against *P. aeruginosa*. Serum levels achieved with oral therapy approximate those obtained with IV therapy; thus oral dosing is useful for long-term therapy in selected patients.

[a] Indicated dosages are for the treatment of *P. aeruginosa* infections in adults. Doses should be adjusted for renal insufficiency. Higher doses may be required in patients with cystic fibrosis, and lower doses may be adequate for the treatment of uncomplicated urinary tract infections.
[b] Some strains of *P. aeruginosa* may develop resistance to these agents during therapy.
[c] Trovafloxacin, an additional fluoroquinolone with antipseudomonal activity, has been associated with hepatotoxicity. Although gatifloxacin and moxifloxacin have in vitro activity against *P. aeruginosa*, there are no clinical studies to support their use in *Pseudomonas* or nosocomial infections.
NOTE: CSF, cerebrospinal fluid; CF, cystic fibrosis; MD, multidose; ODD, once-daily dosing; CNS, central nervous system; TOBI, tobramycin inhalation solution; UTI, urinary tract infection.

ANTIMICROBIAL RESISTANCE Antibiotic resistance in *P. aeruginosa* is both intrinsic, as reflected by the relative paucity of antibiotics with inherent antimicrobial activity against wild-type strains, and acquired, as defined by high-level resistance to agents that would be expected to exhibit antimicrobial activity. Acquired resistance is rapidly increasing among *P. aeruginosa* isolates, particularly those associated with cystic fibrosis and with intensive care units. Escalating resistance among intensive care unit isolates is especially

Table 155-3 Recommended Antimicrobial Therapy for Selected Infections due to *Pseudomonas aeruginosa*

Anatomic Site or Diagnosis	Preferred Therapy[a,b]	Alternative Therapy[a,b]	Comments
Bacteremia, endocarditis, wound infections, or pneumonia	Antipseudomonal penicillin *plus* aminoglycoside	Antipseudomonal penicillin *plus* ciprofloxacin (IV) *or* Antipseudomonal cephalosporin *or* aztreonam *or* carbapenem *plus* aminoglycoside *or* ciprofloxacin (IV)	*Bacteremia*: Bacteremia due to infection of an indwelling central venous catheter usually necessitates catheter removal. Monotherapy is often acceptable if the catheter is removed. *Endocarditis*: Use highest indicated doses from Table 155-2. MD is preferable to ODD for aminoglycosides. Serum aminoglycoside levels should be 10X the MBC for the isolate. Valve replacement is often required. *Wounds*: Debridement is required. *Pneumonia*: Combination therapy should be employed initially for severe pneumonia if *P. aeruginosa* is highly suspected or confirmed by culture. Repeated or prolonged therapy may be required in patients with AIDS.
Central nervous system	Ceftazidime *plus or minus* aminoglycoside	Ciprofloxacin (IV)[c] *or* aztreonam[c] *or* meropenem[c]	Aminoglycosides should be administered intrathecally for CNS infections not responding to initial IV therapy. Brain abscesses >2 cm in diameter require drainage.
Bones and joints	Antipseudomonal penicillin *plus* aminoglycoside	Antipseudomonal cephalosporin *or* aztreonam *or* fluoroquinolone *or* carbapenem[c]	A 4- to 6-week course of therapy is often suggested. Limited data suggest that prolonged therapy with an oral fluoroquinolone may be as effective as IV administration. Surgical debridement is often required for osteomyelitis that is chronic or associated with trauma, direct inoculation of bone, or extension from adjacent tissues.
Malignant external otitis	Antipseudomonal cephalosporin *or* carbapenem *or* ciprofloxacin (IV or PO)	Antipseudomonal penicillin or cephalosporin *plus* aminoglycoside	Surgical debridement is usually required. At least 4–6 weeks of therapy is suggested. Oral ciprofloxacin can be used with close follow-up for limited disease or after initial IV therapy.
Eye			
Keratitis and corneal ulcer	Tobramycin 14 mg/mL topical solution[d] *plus or minus* piperacillin *or* ticarcillin 6–12 mg/mL topical solution[d]	Ciprofloxacin *or* ofloxacin 0.3% topical solution[d]	Fortified aminoglycoside eye drops require pharmacy preparation. Systemic antibiotics are reserved for severe infections with impending perforation or extension beyond the cornea (see endophthalmitis). If combination therapy is used, the second agent should be administered at least 5 minutes after the first.
Endophthalmitis	Same as for corneal ulcer above *plus* intravitreal amikacin 0.4 mg in 0.1 mL *or* ceftazidime 2.25 mg in 0.1 mL	Same as for corneal ulcer above *plus* intravitreal amikacin 0.4 mg in 0.1 mL *or* ceftazidime 2.25 mg in 0.1 mL	Surgical vitrectomy is usually indicated. Addition of systemic therapy with ceftazidime or an antipseudomonal penicillin plus ciprofloxacin or an aminoglycoside and subconjunctival injection of an intravitreal agent may be beneficial.
Urinary tract	Ciprofloxacin (PO or IV)	Aminoglycoside *or* antipseudomonal penicillin *or* cephalosporin *or* carbapenem	Obstructions (e.g., stones) should be relieved and foreign bodies (e.g., chronic urinary catheters) removed. Monotherapy is usually sufficient.
Dermatitis or folliculitis	None	None	Diffuse folliculitis related to spas, whirlpools, or hot tubs does not require therapy in immunocompetent hosts.

[a] Susceptibility testing should be performed on all significant *Pseudomonas* isolates in order to direct definitive therapy. Empirical antibiotic therapy for suspected *Pseudomonas* infections should take into account the institution's antimicrobial susceptibility patterns.
[b] Dosages for individual agents from each antimicrobial class are listed in Table 155-2.
[c] Clinical experience is limited for treatment of this infection with this agent. Addition of a second antipseudomonal agent is advised.
[d] 1 qqts q5min for 1 h, then q15–30min for 24–48 h; frequency can then be gradually decreased.
NOTE: MD, multidose; ODD, once-daily dosing; CNS, central nervous system; MBC, minimal bactericidal concentration.

alarming. Data from the NNIS system show an increase in rates of resistance to imipenem and fluoroquinolones from 12% during previous years to 18.5% and 23.0%, respectively, during 1999. Factors responsible for this increase may include expanding use of immunosuppressive therapies, increased severity of illness in hospitalized patients, inadequate infection control procedures, and growing antibiotic use. Resistant organisms can be transmitted directly to patients from the hospital staff, other patients, or the environment, or they may arise de novo during therapy with any given agent. Emergence of multidrug-resistant strains has been associated with increases in secondary bacteremia and mortality and has led in some cases to longer hospital stays and increased hospitalization costs. Therapy for patients with resistant *P. aeruginosa* infections should consist of antimicrobial agents selected on the basis of extended susceptibility testing. Increased treatment duration and surgical drainage or removal of infected tissues may be necessary.

INFECTIONS CAUSED BY OTHER *PSEUDOMONAS* SPECIES OR RELATED BACTERIA

Burkholderia cepacia *B. cepacia*, like *P. aeruginosa*, is primarily an opportunistic pathogen that is implicated in both sporadic endemic infections and occasional nosocomial outbreaks. Hospital epidemics are most frequently associated with a liquid reservoir or a moist environmental surface. Colonization by *B. cepacia* precedes infection, and distinction between the two is often difficult. *B. cepacia* has been reported to cause pneumonia, urinary tract infections, meningitis, peritonitis, surgical and burn wound infections, bacteremia, and endocarditis related to injection drug use. In addition, *B. cepacia* has been implicated as a cause of chronic lower respiratory tract infections in patients with chronic granulomatous disease, in patients with sickle cell hemoglobinopathies, and—together with *P. aeruginosa*—in patients with cystic fibrosis. In some patients with cystic fibrosis, the appearance of *B. cepacia* has been associated with fulminant necrotizing pneumonia, bacteremia, and a rapid downhill course.

℞ **TREATMENT**   The treatment of *B. cepacia* infections is complicated by intrinsic resistance of the organism to aminoglycosides and many β-lactam agents. Although trimethoprim-sulfamethoxazole and chloramphenicol have been used successfully in the treatment of *B. cepacia* infections, resistance to these two antimicrobial agents has been reported. Carbapenems, third-generation cephalosporins, and fluoroquinolones may offer activity against sensitive strains, but relevant clinical experience is limited. Some but not all cystic fibrosis centers segregate patients infected with *B. cepacia* in an attempt to reduce horizontal transmission to uninfected patients. In addition, many centers consider lung transplantation contraindicated in these patients because of an unacceptably high mortality rate after surgery.

Stenotrophomonas maltophilia   *S. maltophilia* is a ubiquitous, free-living opportunistic bacterium that has emerged as an important pathogen in hospitalized patients, particularly in cancer centers and intensive care units. Factors that lead to colonization and infection include prolonged hospitalization, malignancy, instrumentation (including urinary, peritoneal, and central venous catheterization), and prior administration of broad-spectrum antibiotics. This organism has most commonly been associated with pneumonia but also causes bacteremia, urinary tract infection, wound infection, peritonitis, cholangitis, meningitis, and (rarely) endocarditis. Acute *S. maltophilia* pneumonia—an often devastating disease associated with bacteremia—is being seen with increasing frequency in debilitated patients on intensive care units. Antibiotic resistance in *S. maltophilia*, based on both low outer-membrane permeability and inducible β-lactamases, is at least partly responsible for the emergence of this organism as a nosocomial pathogen under the selective pressure of antibiotic treatment.

℞ **TREATMENT**   Trimethoprim-sulfamethoxazole (at a trimethoprim dose of 15 to 20 mg/kg per day for patients with normal renal function) is the drug of choice for treatment of most *S. maltophilia* infections. Alternative agents include ticarcillin/clavulanate, minocycline, and doxycycline. The third-generation cephalosporins cefoperazone and ceftazidime are occasionally active against *S. maltophilia*, but in vitro susceptibilities may not reflect clinical efficacy. The aminoglycosides and imipenem are almost always inactive. Indwelling catheters or appliances that are associated with infection should be removed.

Melioidosis   Infections caused by *B. pseudomallei* constitute a broad spectrum of acute and chronic, local and systemic, clinical and subclinical disease processes collectively called *melioidosis*. *B. pseudomallei* and the infections it causes are found mainly in the tropics and are endemic in Southeast Asia and surrounding areas. *B. pseudomallei* is a free-living, small, motile, aerobic, gram-negative bacillary saprophyte normally found in soil, ponds, and rice paddies and on produce from endemic areas. It is occasionally a pathogen for animals. Humans contract the disease through soil contamination of abrasions, ingestion, or inhalation. In contrast to *B. cepacia*, *B. pseudomallei* does not establish colonization without causing infection and is rarely transmitted from person to person.

Melioidosis presents in different forms. High rates of seropositivity in endemic areas such as Vietnam, Thailand, and Malaysia suggest that many infections are clinically inapparent. The occasional diagnosis based solely on abnormal routine chest roentgenograms represents asymptomatic pneumonitis. Acute pulmonary infections may originate in the respiratory tract or result from hematogenous spread, their severity varying from mild bronchitis to extensive necrotizing pneumonia. Onset may be sudden or gradual. Fever, productive cough, and marked tachypnea are frequent. Chest roentgenograms typically reveal upper-lobe infiltrates or thin-walled cavities that may mimic

tuberculosis. Acute, localized, suppurative skin infections associated with nodular lymphangitis and regional lymphadenitis result from direct inoculation at sites of minor skin trauma. Recrudescent disease arising from inactive sites of infection and perhaps triggered by intercurrent illness or other events may present in an acute or chronic form.

Either acute suppurative infections or pulmonary disease may give rise to hematogenous dissemination and the acute septicemic form of melioidosis. This progression is more likely in chronically debilitated patients, such as those with diabetes mellitus or alcoholism. Septicemic patients may present with severe tachypnea, confusion, headache, pharyngitis, diarrhea, and pustular lesions of the head, trunk, and extremities. The skin may be flushed or cyanotic, signs of meningitis or arthritis may be apparent, the liver and spleen may be enlarged, and muscle tenderness may be striking. Chest roentgenograms show diffuse nodular densities that may expand, coalesce, and finally cavitate. The acute septicemic form of melioidosis usually follows a rapid downhill course, ending in early death. Mortality remains high despite optimal therapy.

The diagnosis of melioidosis should be entertained when a febrile patient who has been in an endemic area presents with an acute lower respiratory tract illness associated with tachypnea, exhibits unusual skin or subcutaneous lesions, or has a chest roentgenogram suggesting tuberculosis in the absence of sputum-associated tubercle bacilli. An etiologic diagnosis may be made by microscopic demonstration of small, irregularly staining, gram-negative rods in exudate material; by characteristic bipolar ("safety-pin") staining of organisms with methylene blue; and by a culture positive for *B. pseudomallei* and/or a fourfold or greater rise in the titer of serum antibody to the organism.

℞ **TREATMENT**   The mainstay of treatment for melioidosis is antibiotic administration combined with appropriate surgical drainage of abscesses and aggressive support for patients with septicemic forms of the disease. The guidelines for antibiotic therapy are somewhat imprecise. Subclinical infection or mere seropositivity does not usually require specific therapy. Ceftazidime or imipenem appears to be the agent of choice for clinical disease, including severe infections, while trimethoprim-sulfamethoxazole, cefotaxime, and amoxicillin/clavulanate are possible alternatives. Combination therapy with ceftazidime or imipenem plus trimethoprim-sulfamethoxazole may be indicated in severe forms of melioidosis, including septicemia. Unfortunately, increasing resistance of many strains of *B. pseudomallei* to trimethoprim-sulfamethoxazole, particularly in Southeast Asia, is of concern. Patients with acute pulmonary infections who are treated with either ceftazidime or imipenem should receive antibiotics until they show definite evidence of clinical improvement (often after 10 to 30 days), at which time therapy can be switched to an oral maintenance regimen—a combination of chloramphenicol, trimethoprim-sulfamethoxazole, and doxycycline or the single agent amoxicillin/clavulanate—and continued for 12 to 20 weeks. Chronic disease associated with persistently positive sputum cultures and extrapulmonary suppurative disease may require treatment for up to 1 year.

Other Species   *Pseudomonas fluorescens* occasionally causes human disease; it is implicated particularly often in infections related to the administration of contaminated (stored) blood products and in pseudoinfections. Additional species that are associated only rarely with human infections include *P. putida*, *P. stutzeri*, *P. pseudoalcaligenes*, and (all formerly *Pseudomonas* species) *Burkholderia gladioli*, *B. pickettii*, *Comamonas acidovorans*, *C. testosteroni*, *Brevundimonas diminuta*, and *B. vesicularis*.

BIBLIOGRAPHY

P. AERUGINOSA INFECTIONS

BALTCH AL, SMITH RP (eds): *Pseudomonas aeruginosa Infections and Treatment*. New York, Marcel Dekker, 1994

CARMELLI Y et al: Health and economic outcomes of antibiotic resistance in *Pseudomonas aeruginosa*. Arch Intern Med 159:1127, 1999

KORVICK JA, YU VL: Antimicrobial agent therapy for *Pseudomonas aeruginosa*. Antimicrob Agents Chemother 35:2167, 1991

MORRISON AF, WENZEL RP: Epidemiology of infections due to *Pseudomonas aeruginosa*. Rev Infect Dis 6(Suppl):S267, 1984

POLLACK M: The virulence of *Pseudomonas aeruginosa*. Rev Infect Dis 6(Suppl):S617, 1984

————: *Pseudomonas aeruginosa*, in *Mandell, Douglas, and Bennett's Principles and Practice of Infectious Diseases*, 5th ed, GL Mandell et al (eds). New York, Churchill Livingstone, 2000, pp 2310–2335

SHEPP DH et al: Serious *Pseudomonas aeruginosa* infection in AIDS. J Acquir Immun Defic Syndr 7:823, 1994

VAN DELDEN C, IGLEWSKI BH: Cell-to-cell signaling and *Pseudomonas aeruginosa* infections. Emerg Infect Dis 4:551, 1998

INFECTIONS DUE TO RELATED ORGANISMS

SIMPSON AJ et al: Comparison of imipenem and ceftazidime as therapy for severe melioidosis. Clin Infect Dis 29:381, 1999

VARTIVARIAN S, ANAISSIE E: *Stenotrophomonas maltophilia* and *Burkholderia cepacia*, in *Mandell, Douglas, and Bennett's Principles and Practice of Infectious Diseases*, 5th ed, GL Mandell et al (eds). New York, Churchill Livingstone, 2000, pp 2335–2339

WHITE NJ: Melioidosis, in *Hunter's Tropical Medicine and Emerging Infectious Diseases*, 8th ed, GT Strickland et al (eds). Philadelphia, Saunders, 2000, pp 313–316

156   *Cammie F. Lesser, Samuel I. Miller*

SALMONELLOSIS

The salmonellae constitute a genus of over 2300 serotypes that are highly adapted for growth in both human and animal hosts and cause a wide spectrum of disease. A subset of *Salmonella* serotypes that includes *S. typhi* and *S. paratyphi* causes enteric (typhoid) fever and is restricted to growth in human hosts. The remainder of *Salmonella* serotypes, referred to as nontyphoidal *Salmonella*, are prevalent in the gastrointestinal tracts of a broad range of animals, including mammals, reptiles, birds, and insects. Over 200 of these serotypes are pathogenic to humans; these pathogenic serotypes cause gastroenteritis and can be associated with localized infections and/or bacteremia.

ETIOLOGY   *Salmonella* is a large genus of gram-negative bacilli within the family Enterobacteriaceae. The nomenclature and classification of these bacteria have undergone numerous revisions, most recently in 1983 when—on the basis of a high degree of DNA similarity between the bacterial genomes—over 2000 bacterial strains were grouped into one species, *S. choleraesuis*. This species was further divided into seven subgroups based on host range specificity and additional DNA similarity. Almost all the strains pathogenic for humans are in subgroup 1 (*enterica* or *choleraesuis*) except for those causing rare infections (subgroups 3a and 3b). The nomenclature of this large species is quite complex. For example, the correct taxonomic name for the organism that causes enteric fever is *Salmonella choleraesuis* ssp. *choleraesuis* (or subgroup 1), serovar *typhi*. Given the cumbersome nature of this nomenclature system, a simplified system is in widespread use, in which the common species name that existed before the reclassification of the species is accepted. For example, *S. choleraesuis* ssp. *choleraesuis*, serovar *typhi*, is referred to by its common name, *S. typhi*.

The initial identification of this genus in the clinical laboratory relies on growth characteristics. Like other Enterobacteriaceae, salmonellae produce acid on glucose fermentation, reduce nitrates, and do not produce cytochrome oxidase. They are non-spore-forming and facultatively anaerobic. With few exceptions, salmonellae are motile by means of peritrichous flagella (exception: *S. gallinarum-pullorum*) and produce gas (H_2S) on sugar fermentation (exception: *S. typhi*).

Since 99% of clinical isolates are lactose nonfermenters, rare clinical isolates may not be detected if a high level of suspicion is not maintained.

Salmonella can be further divided into serovars based on the detection of three major antigenic determinants: the somatic O antigen [lipopolysaccharide (LPS) cell-wall components], the surface Vi antigen (restricted to *S. typhi* and *S. paratyphi* C), and the flagellar H antigen. In general, clinical laboratories initially divide *Salmonella* into serogroups (A, B, C_1, C_2, D, and E) based on reactivity to somatic O-antigen antisera. These initial groupings provide only limited clinical information, given their high degree of cross-reactivity. Thus, additional biochemical and serologic tests are needed to determine serotype. For the epidemiologic evaluation of *Salmonella* outbreaks, specific *Salmonella* strains within serovars can be distinguished by bacteriophage typing, plasmid profile determination, and restriction length polymorphism analysis.

PATHOGENESIS   Salmonellae are transmitted to humans orally by contaminated food or water. The bacteria traverse the gastrointestinal tract, including the acidic environment of the stomach, to colonize the small intestines. In the case of enteric fever (a systemic illness), salmonellae cross the intestinal barrier, where phagocytosis by macrophages results in their dissemination throughout the reticuloendothelial system. In nontyphoidal salmonellosis, the bacteria generally cause a localized infection resulting in an influx of neutrophils to the intestines and self-limited gastroenteritis.

Numerous attempts have been made to determine the infectious dose (ID_{50}) of *Salmonella*, both in the laboratory and in the field. Controlled experiments, in which healthy volunteers were exposed to laboratory-grown strains of *S. typhi*, concluded that the ID_{50} was 10^6 colony-forming units (CFU); increases in the ID_{50} corresponded to decreases in incubation time. However, analyses of salmonellosis outbreaks with a known source indicate that the ID_{50} can be as low as 10^3 CFU. Host defenses, the most important of which appears to be the acidity of the stomach, most likely account for variations in the ID_{50}. Conditions that decrease stomach acidity (an age of <1 year, antacid ingestion, or achlorhydric disease) increase susceptibility to *Salmonella* infection, as do conditions that decrease intestinal integrity (inflammatory bowel disease, history of gastrointestinal surgery, or alteration of the intestinal flora by antibiotic administration).

Once salmonellae reach the small intestine, the bacteria resist a variety of innate immune factors (including bile salts, lysozyme, complement, and cationic antimicrobial peptides) before penetrating the mucus layer. The organisms enter the intestines through phagocytic microfold or M cells overlying the Peyer's patches. Salmonellae also enter normally nonphagocytic epithelial cells by a process known as *bacteria-mediated endocytosis*, whose mechanism is not entirely clear but depends on the direct translocation of *Salmonella* proteins into the host cell cytoplasm by a specialized secretion apparatus (type III secretion).

In enteric (typhoid) fever, salmonellae (*S. typhi* or *S. paratyphi*) undergo phagocytosis by macrophages after crossing the epithelial layer of the small intestine. Once phagocytosed, the bacteria are protected from polymorphonuclear leukocytes (PMNs), the complement system, and the acquired immune response (antibodies). Salmonellae have evolved mechanisms to avoid or delay killing by macrophages. Upon phagocytosis, the bacteria form a "spacious phagosome" and alter the regulation of ~200 bacterial proteins. The best-characterized regulatory system is PhoP/PhoQ, a two-component regulon that senses changes in bacterial location and alters bacterial protein expression. The alterations mediated by PhoP/PhoQ include modifications in LPS and in the synthesis of outer-membrane proteins; these changes presumably remodel the bacteria's outer surface such that the organisms can resist microbicidal activities and possibly alter host cell signaling. PhoP/PhoQ also mediates the synthesis of divalent cationic transporters that scavenge magnesium. By a second type III secretion mechanism, salmonellae can directly translocate bacterial proteins into the macrophage, a phenomenon that is believed to promote survival within phagocytes.

After phagocytosis, salmonellae disseminate throughout the body in macrophages via the lymphatics and colonize reticuloendothelial tissues (liver, spleen, lymph nodes, and bone marrow). During this initial incubation stage, patients are relatively asymptomatic. Signs and symptoms, including fever and abdominal pain, probably result from secretion of cytokines by macrophages when a critical number of organisms have replicated. For example, the observed hepatosplenomegaly is likely to be related to the recruitment of mononuclear cells and the development of a cell-mediated immune response to *S. typhi* colonization. The recruitment of additional mononuclear cells and lymphocytes to Peyer's patches during the several weeks after initial colonization/infection can result in marked enlargement and necrosis of the Peyer's patches, with right-lower-quadrant abdominal pain.

It is not known why *S. typhi* and *S. paratyphi* cause systemic disease while the vast majority of pathogenic *Salmonella* strains cause gastroenteritis. In contrast to enteric fever, which is characterized by an infiltration of mononuclear cells into the small-bowel mucosa, nontyphoidal *Salmonella* gastroenteritis is characterized by massive PMN infiltration into both the large- and the small-bowel mucosa. This response appears to depend on the induction of interleukin (IL) 8, a strong neutrophil chemotactic factor, which is secreted by intestinal cells. The degranulation and release of toxic substances by neutrophils may result in damage to the intestinal mucosa, causing inflammatory diarrhea.

ENTERIC (TYPHOID) FEVER

Typhoid fever is a systemic disease characterized by fever and abdominal pain caused by dissemination of *S. typhi* or *S. paratyphi*. The disease was initially called *typhoid fever* because of its clinical similarity to typhus. However, in the early 1800s, typhoid fever was clearly defined pathologically as a unique illness on the basis of its association with enlarged Peyer's patches and mesenteric lymph nodes. In 1869, given the anatomic site of infection, the term *enteric fever* was proposed as an alternative designation to distinguish typhoid fever from typhus. However, to this day, the two designations are used interchangeably.

EPIDEMIOLOGY In contrast to other *Salmonella* serotypes, the etiologic agents of enteric fever—*S. typhi* and *S. paratyphi*—have no known hosts other than humans. Thus, enteric fever is transmitted only through close contact with acutely infected individuals or chronic carriers. While direct person-to-person transmission through the fecal-oral route has been documented, it is quite rare. Rather, most cases of disease result from ingestion of contaminated food or water. Health care workers occasionally acquire enteric fever after exposure to infected patients, while laboratory workers can acquire the disease after laboratory accidents.

Over the past four decades, with the advent of improvements in food handling and water/sewage treatment, enteric fever has become a rare occurrence in developed nations. Over the past 10 years, ~400 cases of typhoid fever and even fewer cases of paratyphoid fever have been reported annually in the United States. In contrast, enteric fever continues to be a global health problem, with an estimated 13 to 17 million cases worldwide resulting in ~600,000 deaths per year. Children <1 year of age appear to be most susceptible to initial infection and to the development of severe disease.

Enteric fever is endemic in most developing regions, especially the Indian subcontinent, South and Central America, and Asia, and is related to rapid population growth, increased urbanization, inadequate human waste treatment, limited water supply, and overburdened health care systems. These conditions most likely account for the recent epidemics of typhoid fever in eastern Europe. Antibiotic resistance among salmonellae is also a rising concern and has recently been linked to antibiotic use in livestock. Many *S. typhi* strains contain plasmids encoding resistance to chloramphenicol, ampicillin, and trimethoprim—the antibiotics that have long been used to treat enteric fever. In addition, resistance to ciprofloxacin, either chromosomally or plasmid encoded, has been observed in Asia. Morbidity and mortality are increased in outbreaks associated with antibiotic-resistant strains, presumably because of inadequate or delayed appropriate treatment.

The high worldwide prevalence of enteric fever serves as a reservoir for cases in the United States. Over 70% of U.S. cases are related to international travel within 30 days before onset. Only 3% of travelers diagnosed with enteric fever give a history of vaccination against *S. typhi* within the previous 2 years. Of U.S. cases of internationally acquired enteric fever, 80% can be linked to travel in six countries: Mexico (28%), India (25%), the Philippines (10%), Pakistan (8%), El Salvador (5%), and Haiti (4%). While the percentage of cases associated with travel to Mexico is declining, travel to the Indian subcontinent is becoming much riskier, with an incidence 18 times higher than for any other area. The recent trend toward an increased incidence of multidrug-resistant (MDR) *Salmonella* (see "Treatment," below) in developing countries is reflected by the increase in the proportion of U.S. cases caused by MDR strains from 0.6% in 1985–1989 to 12% in 1990–1994.

Almost 30% of the reported cases of enteric fever in the United States are domestically acquired. Although the majority of these cases (80%) are sporadic, large outbreaks do occur. In the most notable outbreak in the past 15 years, 47 culture-proven and 24 potential cases were linked to contaminated orange juice at a resort in New York. Evaluation of this outbreak led to the identification of a previously unknown chronic carrier. Similarly, evaluation of 25% of the 571 cases of domestically acquired enteric fever reported between 1985 and 1994 led to the identification of previously unknown chronic carriers.

CLINICAL COURSE Enteric fever is a misnomer, in that the hallmark features of this disease—fever and abdominal pain—are variable. While fever is documented at presentation in >75% of cases, abdominal pain is reported in only 20 to 40%. Thus, a high index of suspicion for this potentially lethal systemic illness is necessary when a person presents with fever and a history of recent travel to a developing country.

The incubation period for *S. typhi* ranges from 3 to 21 days. This variability is most likely related to the size of the initial inoculum and the health and immune status of the host. The most prominent symptom of this systemic infection is prolonged fever (38.8° to 40.5°C, or 101.8° to 104.9°F). A prodrome of nonspecific symptoms often precedes fever and includes chills, headache, anorexia, cough, weakness, sore throat, dizziness, and muscle pains. Gastrointestinal symptoms are quite variable. Patients can present with either diarrhea or constipation; diarrhea is more common among patients with AIDS and among children <1 year of age. As stated above, only 20 to 40% of patients present with abdominal pain, although the majority have abdominal tenderness over the course of the disease. In general, the symptoms associated with *S. typhi* are more severe than those associated with *S. paratyphi*.

Early physical findings of enteric fever include rash ("rose spots"), hepatosplenomegaly, epistaxis, and relative bradycardia. Rose spots make up a faint, salmon-colored, blanching, maculopapular rash located primarily on the trunk and chest. The rash is evident in ~30% of patients at the end of the first week and resolves after 2 to 5 days without leaving a trace. Patients can have two or three crops of lesions, and *Salmonella* can be cultured from punch biopsies of these lesions. The faintness of the rash makes it difficult to detect in dark-skinned patients. On occasion, patients who remain toxic manifest neuropsychiatric symptoms described as a "muttering delirium" or "coma vigil," with picking at bedclothes or imaginary objects.

Late complications, occurring in the third and fourth weeks of infection, are most common in untreated adults and include intestinal perforation and/or gastrointestinal hemorrhage. These complications can develop despite clinical improvement and presumably result from necrosis at the initial site of *Salmonella* infiltration in the Peyer's patches of the small intestine. Both complications are life-threatening and require immediate medical and surgical interventions, with broadened antibiotic coverage for polymicrobial peritonitis (Chap. 130) and treatment of gastrointestinal hemorrhages, including bowel resection.

Rare complications whose incidences are reduced by prompt antibiotic treatment include pancreatitis, hepatic and splenic abscesses, endocarditis, pericarditis, orchitis, hepatitis, meningitis, nephritis, myocarditis, pneumonia, arthritis, osteomyelitis, and parotitis. Despite prompt antibiotic treatment, relapse rates remain at ~10% in immunocompetent hosts.

Approximately 1 to 5% of patients with enteric fever become long-term, asymptomatic, chronic carriers who shed *S. typhi* in either urine or stool for >1 year. The incidence of chronic carriage is higher among women and among persons with biliary abnormalities (e.g., gallstones, carcinoma of the gallbladder) and gastrointestinal malignancies. The anatomic abnormalities associated with these conditions presumably allow prolonged colonization.

DIAGNOSIS Other than a positive culture, no specific laboratory test is diagnostic for enteric fever. In 15 to 25% of cases, leukopenia and neutropenia are detectable. In the majority of cases, the white blood cell count is normal despite high fever. However, leukocytosis can develop in typhoid fever (especially in children) during the first 10 days of the illness, or later if the disease course is complicated by intestinal perforation or secondary infection. Other nonspecific laboratory results include moderately elevated values in liver function tests (aminotransferases, alkaline phosphatase, and lactate dehydrogenase). In addition, nonspecific ST and T wave abnormalities can be seen on electrocardiograms.

The diagnostic "gold standard" is a culture positive for *S. typhi* or *S. paratyphi*. The yield of blood cultures is quite variable: it can be as high as 90% during the first week of infection and decrease to 50% by the third week. A low yield is related to low numbers of *Salmonella* (<15 organisms per milliliter) in infected patients and/or to recent antibiotic treatment. Centrifugation to isolate and culture the buffy coat, which contains abundant blood mononuclear cells associated with the bacteria, decreases time to isolation but does not affect culture sensitivity.

A diagnosis can also be based on positive cultures of stool, urine, rose spots, bone marrow, and gastric or intestinal secretions. Unlike blood cultures, bone marrow cultures remain highly (90%) sensitive despite ≤5 days of antibiotic therapy. Culture of intestinal secretions (best obtained by a noninvasive duodenal string test) can be positive despite a negative bone marrow culture. If blood, bone marrow, and intestinal secretions are all cultured, the yield of a positive culture is >90%. Stool cultures, while negative in 60 to 70% of cases during the first week, can become positive during the third week of infection in untreated patients. Although the majority of patients (90%) clear bacteria from the stool by the eighth week, a small percentage become chronic carriers and continue to have positive stool cultures for at least 1 year.

Several serologic tests, including the classic Widal test for "febrile agglutinins," are available; however, given high rates of false-positivity and false-negativity, these tests are not clinically useful. Polymerase chain reaction and DNA probe assays are being developed.

℞ **TREATMENT** In the preantibiotic era, the mortality rate from typhoid fever was as high as 15%. The introduction of treatment with chloramphenicol in 1948 greatly altered the disease course, decreasing mortality to <1% and the duration of fever from 14–28 days to 3–5 days. Chloramphenicol remained the standard treatment for enteric fever until the emergence of plasmid-mediated resistance to this drug in the 1970s. Given the increased mortality associated with resistance to chloramphenicol and the rare chloramphenicol-induced bone marrow toxicity, ampicillin (1 g orally every 6 h) and trimethoprim-sulfamethoxazole (TMP-SMZ; one double-strength tablet twice daily) became the mainstays of treatment.

In 1989, MDR *S. typhi* emerged. These bacteria are resistant to chloramphenicol, ampicillin, trimethoprim, streptomycin, sulfonamides, and tetracycline. Like chloramphenicol resistance, resistance to ampicillin and trimethoprim is plasmid-encoded. In 1994, 12% of *S. typhi* isolates in the United States were MDR. Thus either quinolones or third-generation cephalosporins are currently recommended for empirical antibiotic treatment. Despite efficient in vitro killing of *Salmonella*, first- and second-generation cephalosporins as well as aminoglycosides are ineffective in treating clinical infections.

Ceftriaxone (1 to 2 g intravenously or intramuscularly) for 10 to 14 days is equivalent to oral or intravenous chloramphenicol in the treatment of susceptible strains. Preliminary studies indicate that a 5- to 7-day course of ceftriaxone is likely to be sufficient for treatment of uncomplicated cases. However, one recent report describes a ceftriaxone-resistant *Salmonella* strain isolated from a child with diarrhea and apparently acquired from antibiotic-treated cattle.

Quinolones are the only available oral antibiotics for the treatment of MDR *S. typhi* infections. The greatest experience has been gained for ciprofloxacin (500 mg orally twice a day for 10 days). Shorter courses of ofloxacin (10 to 15 mg/kg in divided doses twice daily for 2 to 3 days) have also been successful. However, quinolone resistance is emerging. In 1993, an outbreak of nalidixic acid–resistant *S. typhi* (NARST) infections in Vietnam was linked to chromosomal mutations in the gene encoding DNA gyrase (the target of the quinolones). NARST strains have also been isolated in India. Thus, all strains of *S. typhi* must be screened for resistance to nalidixic acid and tested for sensitivity to a clinically appropriate quinolone. Patients infected with NARST strains need to be treated with higher doses of ciprofloxacin (10 mg/kg twice a day for 10 days) or longer courses of ofloxacin (10 to 15 mg/kg in divided doses twice daily for 7 to 10 days) or with other antibiotics to which the strains are sensitive.

In cases of severe typhoid fever (fever; an abnormal state of consciousness—i.e., delirium, obtundation, stupor, or coma—or septic shock; and a positive culture for *S. typhi* or *S. paratyphi* A), dexamethasone treatment should be considered. In a single trial in Jakarta in the early 1980s in chloramphenicol-treated patients, treatment with dexamethasone (a single dose of 3 mg/kg followed by eight doses of 1 mg/kg, given every 6 h) decreased mortality from 56% to 10%.

The 1 to 4% of patients who develop chronic carriage of *Salmonella* can be treated for 6 weeks with an appropriate antibiotic. Treatment with oral amoxicillin, TMP-SMZ, ciprofloxacin, or norfloxacin has been shown to be ~80% effective in eradicating chronic carriage of susceptible organisms. However, in cases of anatomic abnormality (e.g., biliary or kidney stones), eradication of the infection often cannot be achieved by antibiotic therapy alone but also requires surgical correction of the abnormalities.

PREVENTION AND CONTROL Theoretically, it is possible to eliminate salmonellae that cause enteric fever since the bacteria survive only in human hosts and are spread by contaminated food and water. However, given the high prevalence of the disease in developing countries that lack good facilities for sewage disposal and water treatment, this goal is currently unrealistic. Thus, travelers to developing countries should be advised to monitor their food and water intake carefully and to consider vaccination.

Three vaccine alternatives are available: (1) a heat-killed, phenol-extracted, whole-cell vaccine (two parenteral doses); (2) Ty21a, an attenuated *S. typhi* vaccine (four oral doses); and (3) ViCPS, consisting of purified Vi polysaccharide from the bacterial capsule (one parenteral dose). In addition, an acetone-killed whole-cell vaccine is available only for use by the U.S. military. The minimal ages for vaccination with the whole-cell, Ty21a, and ViCPS vaccines are 6 years, 2 years, and 6 months, respectively. A large-scale meta-analysis of vaccine trials in populations of endemic areas indicates that, while all three vaccines have similar efficacy for the first year, the 3-year cumulative efficacy of the whole-cell vaccine (73%) exceeds that of both Ty21a (51%) and purified Vi (55%). In addition, the heat-killed whole-cell vaccine maintains its efficacy for 5 years, while Ty21a and ViCPS most likely maintain their efficacy for 4 and 2 years, respectively. However, the whole-cell vaccine is associated with a much higher incidence of side effects than the other two vaccines: 16% of whole-cell vaccine recipients develop fever and 10% miss a day of work or school, while only 1 to 2% of persons receiving the alternative vaccines have any fever.

Although data on typhoid vaccines in travelers are limited, some evidence suggests that efficacy may be substantially lower than those for populations in endemic areas. The Centers for Disease Control and Prevention (CDC) currently recommends vaccination for persons traveling to developing countries who will have prolonged exposure to contaminated food and water or close contact with indigenous populations in rural areas. The only recommendations for domestic vaccination include people who have intimate or household contact with a chronic carrier or laboratory workers who frequently work with *S. typhi*. Given the decreased incidence of side effects and the similar short-term efficacy, the current bias is toward vaccination of travelers with either Ty21a or ViCPS.

Enteric fever is a reportable disease in the United States. This reporting system enables public health departments to track down potential source patients and thus to identify and treat chronic carriers in order to prevent further outbreaks. In addition, since 1 to 4% of patients with *S. typhi* infection become chronic carriers, it is important to monitor patients (especially those employed in child care or food handling) for chronic carriage and to treat this condition if indicated.

NONTYPHOIDAL SALMONELLOSIS

EPIDEMIOLOGY The incidence of nontyphoidal salmonellosis has doubled in the United States over the past two decades. Currently, the CDC estimates that there are 2 million cases annually, with 500 to 2000 deaths. Although over 200 serovars of *Salmonella* are considered to be human pathogens, the majority of the reported cases in the United States is caused by *S. typhimurium* or *S. enteritidis*. The incidence of salmonellosis is highest during the rainy season in tropical climates and during the warmer months in temperate climates, coinciding with the peak in food-borne outbreaks. Morbidity and mortality associated with salmonellosis are highest among the elderly, infants, and immunocompromised individuals, including those with hemoglobinopathies and those infected with HIV or with pathogens that cause blockade of the reticuloendothelial system (e.g., patients with bartonellosis, malaria, schistosomiasis, or histoplasmosis).

Unlike *S. typhi* and *S. paratyphi*, whose only reservoir is humans, nontyphoidal salmonellosis is acquired from multiple animal reservoirs. The main mode of transmission is from food products contaminated with animal products or waste—most commonly eggs and poultry but also undercooked meat, unpasteurized dairy products, seafood, and fresh produce.

S. enteritidis associated with chicken eggs is emerging as a major cause of food-borne disease. *S. enteritidis* causes infection of the ovaries and upper oviduct tissue of hens, resulting in contamination of the contents of eggs prior to shell deposition. Approximately 1 in 20,000 eggs is thought to be infected with *S. enteritidis*. Between 1974 and 1994, there was a fivefold increase (from 5% to 25%) in the isolation of *S. enteritidis* from eggs in the United States; in 1998, the U.S. Department of Agriculture estimated that 80% of all salmonellosis cases were caused by infected eggs. Eradication of *S. enteritidis* from hens has proven difficult, given that infection is spread to egg-laying hens both vertically from breeding flocks and horizontally through contact with rodents and manure. Transmission via contaminated eggs can be prevented by cooking of eggs such that the liquid yolk is solidified or through pasteurization of egg products.

Another factor in the increasing incidence of nontyphoidal salmonellosis in developed countries, including the United States, is related to the centralization of food processing and widespread distribution. For example, a 1994 outbreak of ~250,000 cases was linked to a pasteurized ice-cream premix most likely contaminated in tanker trucks that had previously carried unpasteurized eggs. Similar outbreaks have been traced to manufactured foods including pasteurized milk, infant formula, powdered-milk products, paprika-powdered potato chips, and a ready-to-eat savory snack. In addition, large outbreaks have been linked to fresh produce, including alfalfa sprouts, cantaloupe, fresh-squeezed orange juice, and sliced tomatoes, contaminated by manure or water at a single site and then broadly distributed.

A less common source of nontyphoidal *Salmonella* infections is exposure to exotic pets, especially reptiles. Fecal carriage rates in reptiles can be >90%. In the 1970s, 14% of cases of salmonellosis were attributed to small turtles; the distribution of these pets was subsequently prohibited by the U.S. Food and Drug Administration, with a resultant decline in rates of reptile-associated salmonellosis. However, since 1986, an increase in the popularity of nonbanned reptiles, including iguanas, has been followed by increases in rates of *Salmonella* infections. Other pets, including African hedgehogs, snakes, birds, rodents, baby chicks, ducklings, dogs, and cats, can also serve as potential vectors.

Antibiotic resistance is an increasing phenomenon among nontyphoidal *Salmonella* serovars. In particular, *S. typhimurium* of definitive phage type 104 (DT104)—a serotype resistant to ampicillin, chloramphenicol, streptomycin, sulfonamides, and tetracyclines—has become prominent in the United Kingdom. This serotype is associated with greater mortality and morbidity than other nontyphoidal *Salmonella* serotypes. Its acquisition is associated with exposure to ill farm animals and to a variety of meat products. The prevalence of *S. typhimurium* DT104 in the United States increased from 0.6% in 1979–1980 to 34% in 1996. Of concern is the isolation in the United Kingdom in 1996 of *S. typhimurium* DT104 strains resistant to ciprofloxacin (14%) or trimethoprim (24%).

CLINICAL MANIFESTATIONS **Gastroenteritis** Infection with nontyphoidal *Salmonella* most often results in gastroenteritis indistinguishable from that caused by other bacterial and viral pathogens. Nausea, vomiting, and diarrhea occur 6 to 48 h after the ingestion of contaminated food or water. Patients often experience abdominal cramping and fever (38 to 39°C, or 100.5 to 102.2°F). The diarrhea is usually characterized as loose, nonbloody stools of moderate volume. However, large-volume watery stools, bloody stools, or symptoms of dysentery do not rule out the diagnosis. Rarely, *Salmonella* causes a syndrome of pseudoappendicitis or an illness that mimics inflammatory bowel disease.

Gastroenteritis caused by nontyphoidal *Salmonella* is usually self-limited. Diarrhea resolves within 3 to 7 days and fever within 72 h. Stool cultures remain positive for 4 to 5 weeks after infection and—in rare cases of chronic carriage (<1%)—remain positive for >1 year. Antibiotic treatment is usually not recommended and in some studies has prolonged carriage of *Salmonella*. Neonates, the elderly, and the immunosuppressed (e.g., HIV-infected patients) with nontyphoidal *Salmonella* gastroenteritis are especially susceptible to dehydration and dissemination and may require hospitalization and antibiotic therapy.

Bacteremia and Endovascular Infections Up to 5% of patients with nontyphoidal *Salmonella* gastroenteritis have positive blood cultures, and 5 to 10% of these bacteremic persons develop localized infections. Bacteremia is particularly common and persistent among infants, the elderly, and patients with severe underlying infection or immunosuppression (e.g., transplant recipients, HIV-infected patients). Salmonellae have a propensity for infection of vascular sites; if >50% of three or more blood cultures are positive, an endovascular infection should be suspected. Preexisting valvular heart disease is a strong risk factor for the development of endocarditis, while atherosclerotic plaque, prosthetic grafts, and aortic aneurysms are associated with arteritis. Arteritis should be suspected in elderly patients who have a history of prolonged fever with associated back, chest, or abdominal pain preceded by gastroenteritis. Endocarditis and arteritis are rare (<1% of cases) but are associated with potentially morbid complications. Endocarditis can be complicated by cardiac valve perforation or by ring or septal abscesses, while arteritis can be associated with mycotic aneurysms, ruptured aneurysms, or vertebral osteomyelitis.

Unlike most nontyphoidal *Salmonella* serotypes, *S. choleraesuis* and *S. dublin* are frequently associated with sustained bacteremia and fever, often in the absence of a history of gastroenteritis. Similarly, these serotypes appear to be especially invasive and are often associated with metastatic infection.

Localized Infections · *Intraabdominal infections* Intraabdominal infections due to nontyphoidal *Salmonella* are rare and usually manifest as hepatic or splenic abscesses or as cholecystitis. Involvement of the pancreas and adrenals and even an infected pheochromocytoma have been reported. Risk factors include anatomic abnormalities of the hepatobiliary system, including gallstones; abdominal malignancy; and sickle cell disease (especially with splenic abscesses). Eradication of the infection often requires surgical correction of anatomic abnormalities and drainage of abscesses.

Central nervous system infections *Salmonella* infections of the central nervous system usually manifest as meningitis, although cerebral abscesses have been found. Meningitis is usually seen in neonates (<4 months old) and is associated with severe sequelae, including residual seizures, hydrocephalus, ventriculitis, abscess formation, subdural empyema, and permanent disability (e.g., mental retardation and paralysis).

Pulmonary infections Nontyphoidal *Salmonella* pulmonary infections usually present as lobar pneumonia, sometimes complicated by lung abscesses, empyemas, pleural effusions, and bronchopleural fistulas. The majority of cases occur in patients with a preexisting abnormality of lung or pleura, including malignancy. Additional risk factors include sickle cell disease and glucocorticoid use. It is important to determine whether the pulmonary infection is in fact due to *Salmonella* or whether it is a secondary infection.

Urinary and genital tract infections Urinary tract infections caused by nontyphoidal salmonellae present as either cystitis or pyelonephritis, usually in association with malignancy, urolithiasis, structural abnormalities, or immunosuppression (HIV infection, renal transplantation). Genital infections due to these bacteria are rare and present as ovarian and testicular abscesses, prostatitis, or epididymitis. Like other focal infections, both genital and urinary tract infections can be complicated by abscess formation.

Bone, joint, and soft tissue infections *Salmonella* osteomyelitis most commonly affects the femur, tibia, humerus, or lumbar vertebrae and is most often seen in association with sickle cell disease, hemoglobinopathies, or preexisting bone disease (e.g., fractures). Prolonged antibiotic treatment is recommended to decrease the incidence of relapse and chronic osteomyelitis. Septic arthritis occurs in the same patient population as osteomyelitis and usually presents in the knee, hip, or shoulder joints. Reactive arthritis (Reiter's syndrome) can follow *Salmonella* gastroenteritis and is seen most frequently in persons with the HLA-B27 histocompatibility antigen. *Salmonella* can cause rare soft tissue infections, usually at sites of local trauma in immunosuppressed patients.

DIAGNOSIS Nontyphoidal *Salmonella* gastroenteritis is diagnosed when *Salmonella* is cultured from stool. All salmonellae isolated in clinical laboratories should be sent to local public health departments. In cases where there is concern about bacteremia (i.e., those including prolonged or recurrent fever), blood cultures are indicated. Once bacteremia is documented, it is important to determine whether it is high-grade (>50% of three or more blood cultures positive); if so, endovascular infection is possible and further evaluation to identify the source is indicated. In addition, depending on clinical symptoms and on whether metastatic disease is suspected, other body fluids, such as joint fluid or cerebrospinal fluid, should be cultured.

℞ **TREATMENT** Antibiotic treatment is not generally recommended for *Salmonella* gastroenteritis. The symptoms are usually self-limited and have not been demonstrated to be altered by short courses of antibiotics. In addition, in case-control and double-blind placebo-controlled trials, antibiotic treatment has been associated with increased rates of relapse and prolonged gastrointestinal carriage. Dehydration secondary to diarrhea should be treated with fluid and electrolyte replacement.

However, preemptive antibiotic treatment should be considered in patients at increased risk for metastatic infection. These patients include neonates (probably up to 3 months of age); persons >50 years old (because of the high risk of atherosclerotic plaque or aneurysm); transplant recipients; and patients with lymphoproliferative disease, HIV infection, prosthetic joints, vascular grafts, significant joint disease, or underlying sickle cell disease. This group should receive a course of oral or intravenous antibiotics lasting for 2 or 3 days or until defervescence. Longer courses of antibiotics are not recommended because they have been associated with higher rates of chronic carriage and relapse. Rare cases of chronic nontyphoidal *Salmonella* carriage should be treated with a prolonged antibiotic course, as described above for chronic carriage of *S. typhi*.

Focal infections or life-threatening bacteremia with nontyphoidal *Salmonella* should be treated with antibiotics (at the same doses used for enteric fever). Given the increasing prevalence of antibiotic resistance, empirical therapy should include a third-generation cephalosporin and/or a quinolone. If the bacteremia is low-grade (<50% of blood cultures positive), the patient should be treated for 7 to 14 days. Patients with AIDS and *Salmonella* bacteremia should receive 1 to 2 weeks of intravenous antibiotic therapy followed by 4 weeks of oral therapy with quinolones. Patients who relapse after this regimen should receive long-term suppressive therapy with a quinolone or TMP-SMZ, as indicated by bacterial sensitivities.

If the patient has an endovascular infection or endocarditis, treatment for 6 weeks with intravenous β-lactam antibiotics is indicated. Chloramphenicol treatment has been associated with high failure rates and is not recommended. Limited case reports have described the successful treatment of *Salmonella* endovascular infections with quinolones, which may prove an alternative approach in cases caused by sensitive strains. However, concern remains about the development of quinolone resistance during prolonged therapy. Surgical resection of infected aneurysms or other infected endovascular sites is often required. If surgical resection is not possible, lifelong suppressive antibiotic therapy may be indicated. For extraintestinal nonvascular infections, 2 to 4 weeks of antibiotic therapy (depending on the site) are usually recommended. In cases of chronic osteomyelitis, abscesses, and urinary or biliary tract abnormality, surgical interventions may be required in addition to prolonged antibiotic therapy to eradicate infection.

PREVENTION AND CONTROL The incidence of nontyphoidal salmonellosis continues to rise along with rates of emergence of antibiotic-resistant strains. The increased centralization of food production plays a prominent role in the growing incidence, as one oversight can result in rapid, widespread distribution of contaminated food. Thus, it is important to monitor every step of food production, from handling of raw products to preparation of finished foods. In particular, with the increasing prevalence of *S. enteritidis* in egg-laying hens, it is recommended that pasteurized eggs be substituted for bulk-pooled eggs at all nursing homes, hospitals, and commercial food-service establishments. All cases of nontyphoidal salmonellosis should be reported to public health departments, since tracking and monitoring of these cases result in the identification of the sources of local outbreaks and help authorities anticipate large-scale international outbreaks. Lastly, the prudent use of antimicrobial agents in both humans and animals is necessary to minimize the further emergence of antibiotic-resistant strains.

BIBLIOGRAPHY

COHEN JI et al: Extra-manifestations of *Salmonella* infections. Medicine 66:349, 1987

ENGELS EA et al: Typhoid fever vaccines: A meta-analysis of studies on efficacy and toxicity. BMJ 316:110, 1998

FEY PD et al: Ceftriaxone-resistant *Salmonella* infection acquired by a child from cattle. N Engl J Med 342:1242, 2000

GLYNN MK et al: Emergence of multidrug-resistant *Salmonella enterica* serotype typhimurium DT104 infections in the United States. N Engl J Med 338:1333, 1998

HOFFMAN SL et al: Reduction in mortality in chloramphenicol-treated severe typhoid fever by high-dose dexamethasone. N Engl J Med 310:82, 1984

HOFFMAN TA et al: Waterborne typhoid fever in Dade County, Florida: Clinical and therapeutic evaluation of 105 bacteremic patients. Am J Med 59:481, 1975

MERMIN JH et al: Typhoid fever in the United States, 1985–1994: Changing risks of international travel and increasing antimicrobial resistance. Arch Intern Med 158:633, 1998

SCHERER CA, MILLER SI: Molecular pathogenesis of salmonellae, in *Molecular Pathogenesis of Salmonellae*, EA Groisman (ed). San Diego, Academic Press, 2000, in press

STUART BM, PULLEN RL: Typhoid: Clinical analysis of three hundred and sixty cases. Arch Intern Med 78:629, 1946

TAUXE RV: Emerging foodborne diseases: An evolving public health challenge. Emerg Infect Dis 3:425, 1997

157 Gerald T. Keusch

SHIGELLOSIS

DEFINITION *Shigellosis* is an acute infectious inflammatory colitis due to one of the members of the genus *Shigella*. Although the disease is often referred to as "bacillary dysentery," many patients have only mild watery diarrhea and never develop dysenteric symptoms. Less severe illness predominates in industrialized countries such as the United States, whereas more severe, often fatal dysentery occurs in patients in developing countries.

ETIOLOGIC AGENT Shigellae are slender, gram-negative, nonmotile bacilli and are members of the family Enterobacteriaceae and the tribe Escherichieae. They are so closely related to *Escherichia coli* that the two genera cannot be distinguished by DNA hybridization methods. In fact, *Shigella* can be thought of as a differentiated pathogenic *E. coli*. The four *Shigella* species (*S. dysenteriae, S. flexneri, S. boydii*, and *S. sonnei*) are defined on the basis of surface somatic O antigens and carbohydrate fermentation patterns. Most are lactose-negative (*S. sonnei* is a late lactose fermenter) and produce acid but not gas from glucose, resulting in a typical acid butt and alkaline slant in triple sugar iron agar without H_2S production. The genus is characterized by its ability to invade intestinal epithelial cells and to cause infection and illness in humans, even when the inoculum is small (a few hundred to a few thousand organisms).

EPIDEMIOLOGY Worldwide, it is estimated that at least 140 million cases of shigellosis and almost 600,000 deaths due to shigellosis occur annually among children under the age of 5 years, primarily in developing countries. The organism is found everywhere in the world but is most common where poor environmental sanitation and crowding facilitate transmission from person to person. A major outbreak took place in the makeshift camps for refugees fleeing the Rwandan civil war in 1994, with thousands of cases and high mortality.

Data collected by the Centers for Disease Control and Prevention in the United States from 1967 through 1988 suggest an average annual incidence of 6 *Shigella* infections per 100,000 population, with periodic hyperendemic increases (primarily due to large outbreaks of *S. sonnei* infection) raising the rate to between 9 and 10 per 100,000. On the basis of these data, the annual number of episodes of shigellosis in the United States is estimated at 25,000 to 30,000. Incidence rates approximate 27 per 100,000 among children 1 to 4 years of age but are only 2.6 per 100,000 among persons 20 years of age or older. Cases are detected most commonly in counties with a relatively high proportion of low-income minority-group residents, including African Americans, Hispanics, and Native Americans; rates are especially high in poor urban communities, in day-care centers, and among retarded children in custodial care.

A comparison with rates among rural Guatemalan Indian children during the same period puts this disease burden into perspective. A prospective surveillance study among 321 such children revealed an annual incidence of nearly 10,000 per 100,000.

Since the description of the genus *Shigella*, major global shifts in the prevalence of its four species have been noted. Until World War I, *S. dysenteriae* type 1 was the predominant isolate, frequently causing devastating epidemics with high mortality until it was replaced by *S. flexneri*. Since World War II, however, *S. flexneri* has been steadily replaced by *S. sonnei* in the industrialized countries. The reasons for these shifts are not clear. *S. boydii*, the fourth species, has remained largely confined to the Indian subcontinent.

Shigella is highly host-adapted and is a natural pathogen only of humans and a few other primates. Transmission from person to person takes place by the fecal-oral route, generally via direct contact but sometimes through contaminated vectors such as food, water, flies, and fomites. Contaminated imported parsley from Mexico was responsible for one multistate outbreak of *S. sonnei* diarrhea. The organism can even be transmitted during participation in recreational water sports in fecally contaminated pools or lakes and can spread rapidly among confined populations in close contact—for example, in day-care centers, in institutions for the mentally retarded, on cruise ships, or among military personnel. *Shigella* can be transmitted by anal-oral sexual practices among gay men; these cases are almost always due to *S. flexneri*. Rates of *Shigella* infection among HIV-infected individuals greatly exceed those in the non-HIV-infected population (Chap. 309).

Shigellosis is associated with a high rate of secondary household transmission. As many as 40% of children and 20% of adults who are household contacts of a case (generally a preschool child) will develop *Shigella* infection; the infection is often symptomatic in children but asymptomatic in adults, who seem to have an acquired immunity. In contrast, epidemic disease affects all ages, with clusters of severe and fatal cases in the very young and the very old. Since 1969, epidemic *S. dysenteriae* type 1 has reappeared in Latin America, in the Indian subcontinent and elsewhere in Asia, and in central and southern Africa and has been associated with relatively high mortality rates due to antimicrobial resistance and inadequate diagnosis and case management. Prolonged asymptomatic carriage is uncommon; unless there is underlying malnutrition, the organisms are generally cleared in a few weeks.

PATHOGENESIS AND PATHOLOGY Shigellae are orally ingested and, because they survive low pH more easily than other enteric pathogens (a genetically regulated property), seem to have little difficulty in passing the gastric acid barrier. An essential step in pathogenesis is invasion of colonic epithelial cells and cell-to-cell spread of infection. This step involves initial attachment of the organism to colonic cells, entry by an endocytic mechanism in which organisms are initially encased in and then escape from plasma membrane–enclosed vesicles, and a jet propulsion–like movement to the cell membrane, from which the organism can invade the adjacent cell. This sequence of events not only provides the organism with a means to evade host defenses but also allows its effective local spread. Although invasion is initially innocuous, subsequent intracellular multiplication causes cell damage and death, ultimately resulting in characteristic mucosal ulcerations.

These events are extremely complicated and require the functions of multiple genes and regulatory elements encoded on both the chromosome and a large 120- to 140-MDa plasmid present in all virulent shigellae as well as enteroinvasive *E. coli* (EIEC), which can cause a *Shigella*-like disease. The number of structural and regulatory genes known to be involved in pathogenesis continues to increase as the process continues to be dissected. Some of these gene products induce the phagocytosis-like uptake of the organism by causing rearrangements of the host cell's cytoskeleton. Once a single *Shigella* organism has invaded a single host cell, the entire process of bacterial escape from the phagocytic vesicle into the host cell's cytoplasm, multiplication, and cell-to-cell spread can take place without exposure of the bacterium to the extracellular milieu and to the host's defenses.

It was originally thought that shigellae invade the host across the intestinal epithelial cells; however, studies using cell culture or a rabbit-ileum in vivo model have suggested that the initial invasion may occur via the antigen-sampling M cell. The resulting limited penetration by organisms initiates an inflammatory response with neutrophil infiltration of the lamina propria, which alters the functional integrity of tight junctions between epithelial cells. These changes allow more organisms to breach the mucosal barrier at intercellular junctions and are essential for the development of illness. If neutrophil migration is directly inhibited by the treatment of animals with antibody to CD18, the escalating invasion by microorganisms does not take place.

Escape from the phagocytic vesicle is necessary for the virulence of shigellae and permits multiplication of the organisms in the cytoplasm. The multiplying organisms spread within the cytoplasm to the plasma membrane of the host cell and then from cell to cell. This spread is achieved by the polymerization of actin at the back end of the dividing bacteria (defined relative to the subsequent direction of motion). Binding and cross-linking by the host protein plastin result in a sphincter-like contraction that provides a forward propulsive force. This so-called actin motor is energized by ATP generated by a microbial-encoded ATPase called *IcsA*, which is, at the same time, phosphorylated and regulated by cyclic nucleotide-dependent protein kinases of the host. Phosphorylation may serve as a molecular host-defense mechanism to modulate virulence, limiting microbial spread.

Another important host protein involved in pathogenesis of shigellosis is the cadherin L-CAM, which is essential in the cell-to-cell spread of infection. Mutations in L-CAM alter the long finger-like protrusions induced by shigellae when they reach the plasma membrane and impair their subsequent fusion with the plasma membrane of the adjacent cell, thus inhibiting the transfer of the bacterium from one cell to another. Ultimately, the invaded host cell dies, possibly as a result of apoptosis induced by or during the process of microbial invasion.

Another property of apparent importance in virulence for *S. dysenteriae* type 1 is the ability to produce Shiga toxin, which is encoded by the iron-regulated chromosomal gene *stx*. Shiga toxin is composed of two distinct peptide subunits, each with highly conserved active regions. The first, located on the larger A subunit, is an *N*-glycosidase that hydrolyzes adenine from specific sites of ribosomal RNA of the mammalian 60S ribosomal subunit, irreversibly inhibiting protein synthesis. The second common region is a binding site on the B subunit that recognizes glycolipids of target cell membranes that terminate in a galactose $\alpha 1 \rightarrow$ 4-galactose disaccharide. The glycolipid Gb3, containing a gal-gal-glu trisaccharide, is a specific receptor present on toxin-sensitive rabbit intestinal villus cells but not crypt cells, and toxin action is specific for the former.

Wild-type toxigenic *S. dysenteriae* causes more severe illness in primates than does an isogenic toxin-negative mutant. The toxin of this organism, the prototype of a family of related toxin proteins produced by enterohemorrhagic *E. coli* (EHEC), appears to play a role in the pathogenesis of microangiopathic complications, hemolytic-uremic syndrome (HUS), and thrombotic thrombocytopenic purpura: only toxin-producing shigellae and *E. coli* are associated with these systemic illnesses. Two new *Shigella* enterotoxins, ShET-1 and -2, have been described; the former is restricted almost exclusively to *S. flexneri* 2a, whereas the latter is distributed more widely (e.g., in the physiologically similar EIEC). The two enterotoxins are encoded by chromosomal and plasmid genes, respectively. Both toxins alter electrolyte transport by segments of gut in vitro and cause net fluid secretion in vivo in ligated rabbit ileal loops. Moreover, both toxins induce antibody in infected humans. However, their role (if any) in the pathogenesis of the watery diarrhea phase of shigellosis remains uncertain.

In shigellosis, the epithelial surface of the human colon shows extensive ulcerations, with an exudate consisting of desquamated colonic cells, polymorphonuclear leukocytes, and erythrocytes; the ulcerations may resemble a pseudomembrane in severely affected areas. Marked mucus depletion and increased mitotic activity are evident in the crypt regions and presumably reflect a response to the loss of surface colonic cells. The lamina propria is edematous and hemorrhagic and is infiltrated by neutrophils and plasma cells. There is also swelling of capillary and venular endothelial cells, with margination of neutrophils. At the ultrastructural level, bacteria can be seen within vesicles as well as free in the cytoplasm. Histologic examination of colon from dysenteric humans shows an alteration of mucosal endothelial cells similar to that induced by endotoxin [lipopolysaccharide (LPS)]. Shiga toxin (protein) targets endothelial cells as well, especially when toxin receptor expression is upregulated by exposure to LPS or proinflammatory cytokines. Levels of circulating LPS are high in *S. dysenteriae* type 1 infection and somewhat lower in *S. flexneri* infection, even without bacteremia. The frequency of endotoxemia in shigellosis suggests a broader role for LPS in the pathogenesis of the disease. One likely mechanism is related to the ability of LPS to induce cytokine gene transcription and the strong association of cytokine secretion and inflammation. However, bacterial invasion of the mucosa itself activates the transcription factor NF-κB, which is involved in regulation of cytokine synthesis. Cytokine-producing cells are present in the mucosa of patients infected with *S. dysenteriae* or *S. flexneri* and in their stools as well. In fact, the number of cells producing interleukin 1, interleukin 6, interferon α, and transforming growth factor β is directly related to the severity of the inflammation. Inflammatory changes in *Shigella* infection thus appear to be components of the pathogenesis of dysentery as much as they are a consequence of the bacterial invasive process.

Epidemiologic evidence indicates that immunity develops and is serotype-specific. The precise nature of this immunity is not known. Common surface outer-membrane proteins involved in invasion elicit serum antibodies; although these are cross-reactive among *Shigella* species and serotypes, they do not seem to be protective. The serotype-specific determinants are likely to be somatic antigens, as serum antibody to LPS predicts resistance to infection, and there is evidence of IgA-mediated mucosal responses to LPS during convalescence from shigellosis.

CLINICAL MANIFESTATIONS Shigellosis in the United States, due primarily to *S. sonnei*, is typically an ambulatory disease, presenting as a self-limited nonbloody watery diarrhea chock full of neutrophils. The spectrum of clinical shigellosis was shown in a study in which adult volunteers ingested 10,000 organisms of *S. flexneri* type 2a. While approximately one-quarter of the volunteers never became ill, over the first 24 to 48 h ~25% developed transient fever, another 25% had fever and self-limited watery diarrhea, and the remaining 25% had fever and watery diarrhea that progressed to bloody diarrhea and dysentery. In young children in particular, the temperature can rise rapidly to 40° to 41°C and sometimes results in generalized seizures. These seizures rarely recur or result in serious sequelae. Dysentery is characterized by frequent passage (usually 10 to 30 times per day) of small-volume stools consisting of blood, mucus, and pus; this diarrhea is accompanied by abdominal cramps and tenesmus—the painful straining with stooling that may lead to rectal prolapse, especially in young children. Severe dysentery is most likely in infection due to *S. dysenteriae* type 1, occurs less commonly with *S. flexneri*, and is least likely in *S. sonnei* infection. Patients with mild disease generally recover without specific therapy in a few days to a week. Severe shigellosis can progress to toxic dilatation and colonic perforation, which may be fatal.

Endoscopy shows the mucosa to be hemorrhagic, with mucous discharge and focal ulcerations and sometimes with overlying exudate. The majority of lesions are in the distal colon and progressively diminish in the more proximal segments of large bowel. Mild dehydration is common among patients with watery diarrhea; severe dehydration is very rare. With extensive colonic involvement, protein-losing enteropathy can occur and can have important adverse nutritional consequences, especially for already poorly nourished children.

A variety of *extraintestinal complications* of shigellosis have been described. The majority arise in patients in developing countries and are related both to the prevalence of infections due to *S. dysenteriae* type 1 and *S. flexneri* and to the poor nutritional state of the host. For example, bacteremia, thought to be relatively infrequent in the United States, develops in up to 8% of patients hospitalized for shigellosis in Dacca, Bangladesh. The causative *Shigella* species is isolated from half the patients; other Enterobacteriaceae are found in the remainder. Bacteremia is associated with higher-than-usual mortality and is more common among infants <1 year of age and among persons with protein-energy malnutrition. Persistent and clinically severe *Shigella* bacteremia has been encountered in the United States in patients with AIDS (Chap. 309).

HUS may occur with *S. dysenteriae* type 1 infection. In the United States, the more likely cause of HUS is one of the hemorrhagic colitis–causing strains of *E. coli* (such as *E. coli* O157:H7) that produce high levels of Shiga-family toxins. HUS usually develops toward the end of the first week of shigellosis, when dysentery is already resolving. Oliguria and a marked drop in hematocrit (by as much as 10% within 24 h) are the first signs and may progress to anuria with renal failure and to severe anemia with congestive heart failure, respectively. Even with advanced therapy, 5 to 10% of patients with HUS die of the acute illness. In addition, renal damage progresses slowly over several decades in survivors, an estimated 50% of whom develop significant renal failure and most of whom require long-term dialysis or renal transplantation. Leukemoid reactions, with leukocyte counts of >50,000/μL, may occur along with HUS; thrombocytopenia (with 30,000 to 100,000 platelets/μL) is common. Profound hyponatremia and severe hypoglycemia may be documented. Central nervous system abnormalities include encephalopathic symptoms, seizures, altered consciousness, and bizarre posturing.

Less common extraintestinal manifestations include seizures in some patients and reactive arthritis in others; both of these manifestations are usually due to infection with *S. flexneri* strains. In patients expressing histocompatibility antigen HLA-B27, the full triad of Reiter's syndrome sometimes develops (Chap. 315). Pneumonia, meningitis, vaginitis (in prepubertal girls), keratoconjunctivitis, and "rose spot" rashes are rare events.

DIAGNOSIS AND LABORATORY FINDINGS Shigellosis is the principal bacterial cause of dysentery and should be considered whenever a patient presents with bloody diarrhea. However, in the United States, because *S. sonnei* is the most common species, most patients present with fever and nonbloody watery diarrhea indistinguishable from signs caused by other bacterial or viral agents of mild to moderate diarrhea, while many patients with bloody diarrhea have EHEC as the cause. The specific diagnosis is based on culture of *Shigella* from the stool; however, diagnosis by the polymerase chain reaction is possible, and a commercial enzyme immunoassay to detect Shiga-family toxins in stool can identify most patients infected with *S. dysenteriae* type 1 or EHEC within 3 h. The yield of *Shigella* is increased if the organism is sought by stool culture when the patient has fecal leukocytes or bloody diarrhea. The organism is very labile and must be transferred quickly to plates or holding media (such as buffered glycerol saline) if it is to survive. Stool samples are preferable to swabs; when the latter are used, a rectal sample should be obtained. More than one selective medium should be used for culture—i.e., MacConkey and one other, such as Hektoen enteric or xylose-lysine-deoxycholate. Stool cultures to diagnose nonbloody watery diarrhea have a very low yield of positives and are not cost-effective.

Serologic tests can be performed, since antibodies to somatic antigens develop early in the acute phase of disease. However, the resources for such tests are not generally available, and serologic assessments usually are used only for epidemiologic studies.

The differential diagnosis includes inflammatory colitis due to other microbial agents: EHEC, EIEC, *Campylobacter jejuni*, *Salmonella enteritidis*, *Yersinia enterocolitica*, *Clostridium difficile*, and the protozoan *Entamoeba histolytica*. Ulcerative colitis and Crohn's colitis are among the "noninfectious" conditions that should be considered (Chap. 287). All these infections except that due to *E. histolytica* are associated with the presence of large numbers of fecal leukocytes. Amebiasis can be diagnosed by the detection of erythrophagocytic trophozoites in the stool (Chap. 213).

Other laboratory studies are nonspecific and may disclose neutrophilic leukocytosis, anemia due to blood loss with hemorrhagic diarrhea, prerenal azotemia, or (if watery diarrhea has been pronounced) hyperchloremic acidosis. Laboratory findings in shigellosis complicated by HUS are discussed above.

℞ **TREATMENT** The mild to moderate dehydration in shigellosis is readily corrected with oral rehydration solutions (Chap. 159). The role of antibiotic therapy is variable and depends on the organism and the severity of disease. Since *S. sonnei* infection is usually self-limited, culture results generally do not become available until the patient is better and there is little clinical need for further therapy. The use of antibiotics in severe cases with bloody diarrhea or dysentery reduces the duration of illness and can shorten the carriage state. Resistance to sulfonamides, streptomycin, chloramphenicol, and tetracyclines is almost universal, and many shigellae are now resistant to ampicillin and trimethoprim-sulfamethoxazole as well. Knowledge of the pattern of resistance in a given population, which can change with time, is useful. In the United States, multiresistant strains are most likely to be acquired during travel abroad; either ampicillin (50 to 100 mg/kg per day in children or 2 g/d in adults, in divided doses) or trimethoprim-sulfamethoxazole (8/40 mg/kg per day in children or 2 regular-strength tablets twice a day in adults, given for 5 days) is generally recommended for domestically acquired infection. Short courses of treatment (1 or 3 days) or even single doses of drugs like tetracycline and ciprofloxacin have been employed with success and may soon become the standard. Amoxicillin should *not* be substituted for ampicillin because it is not effective against shigellosis. In developing countries, where resistance to both of these drugs is commonplace, the drug of choice for the treatment of multiresistant *S. dysenteriae* type 1 infections has been nalidixic acid (55 mg/kg per day for 5 days); however, resistance to the latter agent is increasing in prevalence. The 4-fluoroquinolones (e.g., ciprofloxacin) are highly effective against all strains (Chap. 137) but are currently too costly in the developing world and are not yet approved for use in children under 17 in the United States; these drugs have caused cartilage damage in young rodents during toxicity tests, although there is no evidence for a similar effect of therapeutic doses in humans. Alternative drugs shown to be effective include oral pivamdinocillin (amdinocillin, pivoxil, pivmecillinam; still not available in the United States), azithromycin, and intravenous ceftriaxone (50 mg/kg per day for 5 days). In small-scale clinical trials, cephalexin has had no effect in limiting symptoms; single doses of ceftriaxone may be effective, but more information is needed. No antibiotic treatment is recommended for the convalescent carrier state, which usually lasts no more than several weeks. Patients with AIDS may develop chronic carriage of *Shigella* and may be subject to relapsing infection with bacteremia (Chap. 309). This cycle may be interrupted by prolonged (several weeks') treatment with a quinolone.

The role of antimotility agents such as atropine sulfate and diphenoxylate (Lomotil) and loperamide (Imodium) in the early phases of shigellosis is controversial. Loperamide, in particular, may reduce diarrhea and in one study was highly effective in combination with antimicrobials. However, these antimotility drugs are suspected of enhancing the severity of disease by delaying excretion of organisms and thus facilitating further invasion of the mucosa and complicating toxic megacolon. Therefore, they are contraindicated in infants and young children. In adults, these agents are contraindicated for use in the dysenteric phase of disease.

Treatment of complications of shigellosis often differs in developed and developing countries. For example, antibiotic-unresponsive toxic megacolon, with or without perforation, is often managed by colectomy in the United States. Surgery is less often employed in developing countries because of a lack of availability or difficulties in ileostomy management. HUS often requires dialysis. In developing countries, dialysis may be needed relatively infrequently because azotemia is slow to develop and the risk of significant hyperkalemia is often diminished by a preexisting deficiency in total-body potassium, with malnutrition and wasting of lean body mass. The management of hyponatremia, usually caused by inappropriate secretion of antidiuretic hormone (vasopressin), is governed by the severity of the condition and the symptomatic state of the patient, as outlined in Chap. 49. Infusion of glucose can reverse clinical manifestations caused by hypoglycemia, and responses can be monitored by finger-stick blood glucose tests if no biochemistry laboratory is available. Optimal nutritional management is needed to correct deficiencies due to underlying malnutrition as well as the superimposed catabolic stress and protein-losing enteropathy of shigellosis. Nutritional support should begin during the acute illness and may be required for months thereafter (Chap. 76).

PREVENTION   Direct-contact transmission of shigellosis can be prevented by appropriate environmental and personal hygiene. Hand washing with soap and water, decontamination of water supplies, use of sanitary latrines or toilets, and precautions in the preparation and storage of food can all reduce the primary and secondary transmission of *Shigella* infection. In highly endemic developing countries, infants are protected during the period of exclusive breast feeding, which should be encouraged. Any measures that reduce the burden of malnutrition will also reduce the burden of shigellosis in the population. Stool precautions should be instituted for hospitalized infected patients to ensure safe disposal of infected excreta and linens, and hospital personnel must wash their hands and medical instruments (such as stethoscopes) after each contact with an infected patient. Cohorting of asymptomatic infected children, use of antibiotics to reduce infectiousness, and scrupulous attention to hygiene are usually successful in nosocomial outbreaks. Children in day care must be kept at home while clinically ill and ideally should have a negative stool culture before returning to the day-care facility. Likewise, food handlers who develop shigellosis should be culture-negative before returning to work. Antibiotic treatment is not indicated for the asymptomatic carrier state. No effective vaccine is available, although promising initial results have been reported with an *S. sonnei* LPS-protein conjugate vaccine.

BIBLIOGRAPHY

BAER JT et al: HIV infection as a risk factor for shigellosis. Emerg Infect Dis 5:820, 1999

FARUQUE AS et al: Shigellosis in children: A clinico-epidemiological comparison between *Shigella dysenteriae* type I and *Shigella flexneri*. Ann Trop Paediatr 18:197, 1998

KEUSCH GT: The rediscovery of Shiga toxin and its role in clinical disease. Jpn J Med Sci Biol 51(Suppl):S5, 1998

KHAN WA et al: Treatment of shigellosis: V. Comparison of azithromycin and ciprofloxacin. A double-blind, randomized, controlled trial. Ann Intern Med 126:697, 1997

―――― et al: Central nervous system manifestations of childhood shigellosis: Prevalence, risk factors, and outcome. Pediatrics 103:E18, 1999

KOTLOFF KL et al: Global burden of *Shigella* infection: Implications for vaccine development and implementation of control strategies. Bull World Health Organ 77:651, 1999

LINDBERG AA: Vaccination against enteric pathogens: From science to vaccine trials. Curr Opin Microbiol 1:116, 1998

Outbreaks of *Shigella sonnei* infection associated with eating fresh parsley—United States and Canada, July–August 1998. MMWR 48:285, 1999

SACK RB et al: Antimicrobial resistance in organisms causing diarrheal disease. Clin Infect Dis 24(Suppl 1):S102, 1997

SALAM MA et al: Randomised comparison of ciprofloxacin suspension and pivmecillinam for childhood shigellosis. Lancet 352:522, 1998

SANSONETTI PJ et al: Rupture of the intestinal epithelial barrier and mucosal invasion by *Shigella flexneri*. Clin Infect Dis 28:466, 1999

158   *Martin J. Blaser*

INFECTIONS DUE TO *CAMPYLOBACTER* AND RELATED SPECIES

DEFINITION   Bacteria of the genus *Campylobacter* and of the related genera *Arcobacter* and *Helicobacter* (Chap. 154) cause a variety of pyogenic infections. Although acute diarrheal illnesses are most common, these organisms may cause infections in virtually all parts of the body, especially in compromised hosts, and these infections may have late nonsuppurative sequelae. The designation *Campylobacter* comes from the Greek for "curved rod" and refers to the organism's vibrio-like morphology.

ETIOLOGY   Campylobacters are motile, non-spore-forming, curved gram-negative rods. Originally known as *Vibrio fetus*, these bacilli were reclassified as a new genus in 1973, after it was recognized that they were quite dissimilar to other vibrios. Since then, more than 15 species have been identified. These species are currently divided into three genera: *Campylobacter*, *Arcobacter*, and *Helicobacter*. Not all of the species are pathogens of humans. The human pathogens can be divided into two major groups: those that primarily cause diarrheal disease and those that cause extraintestinal infection. The principal diarrheal pathogen is *C. jejuni*, which accounts for 80 to 90% of all cases of recognized illness due to campylobacters. Other organisms that cause diarrheal disease include *C. coli*, *C. upsaliensis*, *C. lari*, and *C. fetus*. The major species causing extraintestinal illnesses is *C. fetus*; however, any of the diarrheal agents may cause systemic or localized infection as well. Neither aerobes nor strict anaerobes, these microaerophilic organisms are adapted for survival in the gastrointestinal mucous layer. This chapter will focus on *C. jejuni* and *C. fetus* as the major pathogens and prototypes for their groups; the key features of infection are listed by species (excluding *C. jejuni*, described in detail in the text below) in Table 158-1.

EPIDEMIOLOGY   Campylobacters are found in the gastrointestinal tract of many animals used for food (including poultry, cattle, sheep, and swine) and of many household pets (including birds, dogs, and cats). These microorganisms usually do not cause illness in their animal hosts. In most cases, campylobacters are transmitted to humans in raw or undercooked food products or through direct contact with infected animals. In the United States and other developed countries, ingestion of contaminated poultry that has not been sufficiently cooked is the most common means of acquiring infection (50 to 70% of cases). Other modes of transmission include ingestion of raw (unpasteurized) milk or untreated water, contact with infected household pets, travel to developing countries (campylobacters being among the causes of traveler's diarrhea; Chap. 131), and (occasionally) contact with an index case who is incontinent of stool.

Campylobacter infections are not rare. Several studies indicate that, in the United States, diarrheal disease due to campylobacters is more common than that due to *Salmonella* and *Shigella* combined. Infections occur throughout the year, but their incidence peaks during summer and early autumn. Persons of all ages are affected; however, attack rates for *C. jejuni* are highest among young children and young adults, while those for *C. fetus* are highest at the extremes of age. Systemic infections due to *C. fetus* (and to other *Campylobacter* and related species) are most common in compromised hosts. Persons at increased risk include those with AIDS, hypogammaglobulinemia, neoplasia, liver disease, diabetes mellitus, and generalized atherosclerosis as well as pregnant women. However, apparently healthy nonpregnant persons occasionally develop transient *Campylobacter* bacteremia as part of a gastrointestinal illness.

In developing countries, *C. jejuni* infections are hyperendemic, with the highest rates among children <2 years old. Infection rates fall with age, as does the illness-to-infection ratio; these observations suggest that frequent exposure to *C. jejuni* leads to the acquisition of immunity.

Table 158-1 Clinical Features Associated with Infection due to "Atypical" *Campylobacter* and Related Species Implicated as Causes of Human Illness

Species	Common Clinical Features	Less Common Clinical Features	Additional Information
Campylobacter coli	Fever, diarrhea, abdominal pain	Bacteremia[a]	Clinically indistinguishable from *C. jejuni*
Campylobacter fetus	Bacteremia,[a] sepsis, meningitis, vascular infections	Diarrhea, relapsing fevers	Not usually isolated from media containing cephalothin or incubated at 42°C
Campylobacter upsaliensis	Watery diarrhea, low-grade fever, abdominal pain	Bacteremia, abscesses	Difficult to isolate because of cephalothin susceptibility
Campylobacter lari	Abdominal pain, diarrhea	Colitis, appendicitis	Seagulls frequently colonized; organism often transmitted to humans via contaminated water
Campylobacter hyointestinalis	Watery or bloody diarrhea, vomiting, abdominal pain	Bacteremia	Causes proliferative enteritis in swine
Helicobacter fennelliae	Chronic mild diarrhea, abdominal cramps, proctitis	Bacteremia[a]	Best treated with fluoroquinolones
Helicobacter cinaedi	Chronic mild diarrhea, abdominal cramps, proctitis	Bacteremia[a]	Best treated with fluoroquinolones; identified in healthy hamsters
Campylobacter jejuni subspecies *doylei*	Diarrhea	Chronic gastritis, bacteremia[b]	Uncertain role as human pathogen
Arcobacter cryaerophila	Diarrhea	Bacteremia	Cultured under aerobic conditions
Arcobacter butzleri	Fever, diarrhea, abdominal pain, nausea	Bacteremia, appendicitis	Cultured under aerobic conditions; enzootic in nonhuman primates
Campylobacter sputorum	Pulmonary, perianal, groin, and axillary abscesses	Bacteremia	Three clinically relevant biovars: *C. sputorum* subspecies *sputorum*, *C. sputorum* subspecies *bubulus*, and *Campylobacter mucosalis*

[a] In immunocompromised hosts, especially HIV-infected persons.
[b] In children.

SOURCE: Adapted from Allos and Blaser.

PATHOLOGY AND PATHOGENESIS Many *C. jejuni* infections are subclinical, especially in partially immune hosts. Most illnesses occur within 2 to 4 days (range, 1 to 7 days) of exposure to the organism in food or water. The sites of tissue injury include the jejunum, ileum, and colon. Biopsies show an acute nonspecific inflammatory reaction, with neutrophils, monocytes, and eosinophils in the lamina propria, as well as damage to the epithelium, including loss of mucus, glandular degeneration, and crypt abscesses. Biopsy findings may be consistent with Crohn's disease or ulcerative colitis, but these "idiopathic" chronic inflammatory diseases should not be diagnosed unless infectious colitis, *specifically including* that due to infection with *Campylobacter*, has been ruled out.

The high frequency of *C. jejuni* infections and their severity and recurrence among hypogammaglobulinemic patients suggest that antibodies are important in protective immunity. The pathogenesis of infection is uncertain. Both the motility of the strain and its capacity to adhere to host tissues appear to favor disease, but classic enterotoxins and cytotoxins (although described) appear not to play any substantial role in tissue injury or disease production. The organisms have been visualized in the epithelium, albeit in low numbers. The documentation of a significant tissue response and occasionally of *C. jejuni* bacteremia further suggests that tissue invasion is clinically significant.

The pathogenesis of *C. fetus* infections is better defined. Virtually all clinical isolates of *C. fetus* possess a proteinaceous capsule-like structure (an S-layer) that renders the organism resistant to complement-mediated killing and opsonization. As a result, *C. fetus* can cause bacteremia and can seed sites beyond the intestinal tract. The ability of the organism to switch the S-layer proteins expressed, a phenomenon that results in antigenic variability, may contribute to the chronicity and high rate of recurrence of these infections in compromised hosts.

CLINICAL MANIFESTATIONS OF *C. JEJUNI* AND *C. FETUS* INFECTIONS The clinical features of infections due to all of the *Campylobacter* and related species causing enteric disease appear to be highly similar. There is often a prodrome, with fever, headache, myalgia, and/or malaise, 12 to 48 h before the onset of diarrheal symptoms. The most common symptoms of the intestinal phase are diarrhea, abdominal pain, and fever. The degree of diarrhea varies from several loose stools to grossly bloody stools; most patients presenting for medical attention have 10 or more bowel movements on the worst day of illness. Abdominal pain usually consists of cramp-

ing and may be the most prominent symptom. Pain usually is generalized but may become localized; *C. jejuni* infection may cause pseudoappendicitis. Fever may be the only initial manifestation of *C. jejuni* infection, a situation mimicking the early stages of typhoid fever. Febrile young children may develop convulsions. *Campylobacter* enteritis generally is self-limited; however, symptoms persist for longer than 1 week in 10 to 20% of patients seeking medical attention, and relapses occur in 5 to 10% of untreated patients.

C. fetus may cause a diarrheal illness similar to that due to *C. jejuni*, especially in normal hosts, or may cause either intermittent diarrhea or nonspecific abdominal pain without localizing signs. Sequelae are uncommon, and outcome is benign. *C. fetus* also may cause a prolonged relapsing systemic illness (with fever, chills, and myalgias) that has no obvious primary source; this manifestation is especially common in compromised hosts. Secondary seeding of an organ (e.g., meninges, brain, bone, urinary tract, or soft tissue) complicates the course, which may be fulminant. *C. fetus* infections have a tropism for vascular sites: endocarditis, mycotic aneurysm, and septic thrombophlebitis all may occur. Infection during pregnancy often leads to fetal death. *H. cinaedi* causes recurrent cellulitis with fever and bacteremia in immunocompromised hosts.

COMPLICATIONS Except in the case of infection with *C. fetus*, bacteremia is uncommon, developing most often in immunocompromised hosts and at the extremes of age. Three patterns of extraintestinal infection have been noted: (1) transient bacteremia in a normal host with enteritis (benign course, no specific treatment needed); (2) sustained bacteremia or focal infection in a normal host (bacteremia originating from enteritis, with patients responding well to antimicrobial therapy); and (3) sustained bacteremia or focal infection in a compromised host. Enteritis may not be clinically apparent. Antimicrobial therapy, possibly prolonged, is necessary for suppression or cure of the infection.

Campylobacter infections in patients with AIDS or hypogammaglobulinemia may be severe, persistent, and extraintestinal; relapse after cessation of therapy is common. Hypogammaglobulinemic patients also may develop osteomyelitis and an erysipelas-like rash.

Local suppurative complications of infection include cholecystitis, pancreatitis, and cystitis; distant complications include meningitis, endocarditis, arthritis, peritonitis, cellulitis, and septic abortion. All are rare. Hepatitis, interstitial nephritis, and the hemolytic-uremic syndrome occasionally complicate acute infection. Reactive arthritis and other rheumatologic complaints may develop several weeks after infection, especially in persons with the HLA-B27 phenotype. Guillain-Barré syndrome follows *Campylobacter* infections uncommonly (i.e., in 1 of every 1000 to 2000 cases). For certain *C. jejuni* serotypes, such as O19, Guillain-Barré syndrome may follow 1 in every 100 to 200 cases. Because of their high incidence, it is now estimated that *Campylobacter* infections may trigger 20 to 40% of all cases of Guillain-Barré syndrome.

LABORATORY FINDINGS In patients with *Campylobacter* enteritis, peripheral leukocyte counts reflect the severity of the inflammatory process. However, stools from nearly all *Campylobacter*-infected patients presenting for medical attention in the United States contain leukocytes or erythrocytes. Fecal smears should be treated with Gram's or Wright's stain and examined in all suspected cases. When the diagnosis of *Campylobacter* enteritis is suspected on the basis of findings indicating inflammatory diarrhea (fever, fecal leukocytes), clinicians can ask the laboratory to attempt the visualization of organisms with characteristic vibrioid morphology by direct microscopic examination of stools with Gram's staining or to use phase-contrast or dark-field microscopy to identify the organisms' characteristic "darting" motility. Confirmation of the diagnosis of *Campylobacter* infection is based on identification of an isolate from cultures of stool, blood, or another site. *Campylobacter*-specific media should be used to culture stools from all patients with inflammatory or bloody diarrhea. Since all *Campylobacter* species are fastidious, they will not be isolated unless selective media or other selective techniques are used. Not all media are equally useful for isolation of the broad array of campylobacters; therefore, failure to isolate campylobacters from stool does not entirely rule out their presence. The detection of the organisms in stool almost always implies infection; there is a brief period of postconvalescent fecal carriage and no commensalism in humans. In contrast, *C. sputorum* and related organisms found in the oral cavity are commensals with rare pathogenic significance.

DIFFERENTIAL DIAGNOSIS The symptoms of *Campylobacter* enteritis are not sufficiently unusual to distinguish this illness from that due to *Salmonella*, *Shigella*, or *Yersinia*, among other pathogens. The combination of fever and fecal leukocytes or erythrocytes is indicative of inflammatory diarrhea, and definitive diagnosis is based on culture or demonstration of the characteristic organisms on stained fecal smears. Similarly, extraintestinal *Campylobacter* illness is diagnosed by culture. Infection due to *Campylobacter* should be suspected in the setting of septic abortion and that due to *C. fetus* specifically in the setting of septic thrombophlebitis. It is important to reiterate that the presentation of *Campylobacter* enteritis may mimic that of ulcerative colitis or Crohn's disease, that *Campylobacter* enteritis is much more common than either of the latter (especially among young adults), and that biopsy may not distinguish among these entities. Thus a diagnosis of inflammatory bowel disease should not be made until *Campylobacter* infection has been ruled out, especially in persons with a history of foreign travel, significant animal contact, immunodeficiency, or practices incurring a high risk of transmission.

R_X **TREATMENT** Fluid and electrolyte replacement is central to the treatment of diarrheal illnesses (Chap. 131). Even among patients presenting for medical attention with *Campylobacter* enteritis, fewer than half will clearly benefit from specific antimicrobial therapy. Indications for such therapy include high fever, bloody diarrhea, severe diarrhea, persistence for more than 1 week, and worsening of symptoms. A 5- to 7-day course of erythromycin (250 mg orally four times daily or—for children—30 to 50 mg/kg per day, in divided doses) is the regimen of choice. Although no relevant clinical trials have been conducted, the in vitro susceptibility of *Campylobacter* species to macrolides such as clarithromycin and azithromycin suggests that these antibiotics also would be useful therapeutic agents. An alternative regimen for adults is ciprofloxacin (500 mg orally twice daily) or another fluoroquinolone for 5 to 7 days, but resistance to this class of agents

is increasing. Other alternatives include tetracycline and furazolidone. Use of antimotility agents, which may prolong the duration of symptoms and has been associated with toxic megacolon and with death, is not recommended.

For systemic infections, treatment with gentamicin (1.7 mg/kg intravenously every 8 h after a loading dose of 2 mg/kg), imipenem (500 mg intravenously every 6 h), or chloramphenicol (50 mg/kg intravenously each day in three or four divided doses) should be started empirically, but susceptibility testing should then be performed. Ciprofloxacin and amoxicillin/clavulanate are alternative agents for susceptible strains. In the absence of immunocompromise or endovascular infections, therapy should be administered for 14 days. For immunocompromised patients with systemic infections due to *C. fetus* and for patients with endovascular infections, prolonged therapy (for up to 4 weeks) is usually necessary.

PROGNOSIS Nearly all patients recover fully from *Campylobacter* enteritis, either spontaneously or after antimicrobial therapy. Volume depletion likely contributes to the few deaths that are reported. As stated above, occasional patients develop reactive arthritis or Guillain-Barré syndrome. Systemic infection with *C. fetus* is much more often fatal than that due to related species; this higher mortality reflects in part the population affected. Prognosis is dependent on the rapidity with which appropriate therapy is begun. Otherwise healthy hosts usually survive *C. fetus* infections without sequelae. Compromised hosts often have recurrent infections.

BIBLIOGRAPHY

ALLOS BM, BLASER MJ: *Campylobacter jejuni* and the expanding spectrum of related infections. Clin Infect Dis 20:1092, 1995

BLASER MJ et al: *Campylobacter* enteritis in the United States: A multicenter study. Ann Intern Med 98:360, 1983

LANG DR et al (eds): Development of Guillain-Barré syndrome following *Campylobacter* infection. J Infect Dis 176 (Suppl 2):S91, 1997

NACHAMKIN I et al (eds): *Campylobacter jejuni: Current Strategy and Future Trends.* Washington, American Society for Microbiology, 1992, pp 1–300

---

159   *Gerald T. Keusch, Matthew K. Waldor*

CHOLERA AND OTHER VIBRIOSES

Members of the genus *Vibrio* cause a number of important infectious syndromes. Classic among them is cholera, a devastating diarrheal disease caused by *V. cholerae* that has been responsible for seven global pandemics and much suffering over the past two centuries. Epidemic cholera remains a major public health concern and is dealt with at length in this chapter. Other vibrioses have also been described, including syndromes of diarrhea, soft tissue infection, or primary sepsis caused by additional named species in the genus *Vibrio*. These, too, are considered below.

All members of the genus are highly motile, facultatively anaerobic, curved gram-negative rods with one or more polar flagella. Except for *V. cholerae* and *V. mimicus*, all require salt for growth ("halophilic vibrios"). In nature, vibrios most commonly reside in tidal rivers and bays under conditions of moderate salinity. They proliferate in the summer months when water temperatures exceed 20°C. As might be expected, the illnesses they cause also increase in frequency during the warm months.

CHOLERA

DEFINITION Cholera is an acute diarrheal disease that can, in a matter of hours, result in profound, rapidly progressive dehydration and death. Accordingly, cholera gravis (the severe form of cholera) is a much-feared disease, particularly in its epidemic presentation. Fortunately, prompt aggressive fluid repletion and supportive care can obviate the high mortality that it has historically wrought. While the term *cholera* has occasionally been applied to any severely dehydrating secretory diarrheal illness, whether infectious in etiology or not, it has generally referred to disease caused by *V. cholerae* serogroup O1. In 1992, however, a new epidemic serogroup (O139) that causes epidemic cholera emerged on the Indian subcontinent and has since killed many thousands of people.

ETIOLOGY AND EPIDEMIOLOGY The species *V. cholerae* comprises a host of organisms classified on the basis of the carbohydrate determinants of their lipopolysaccharide (LPS) O antigens. Some 155 serogroups have now been recognized. They are divided into those that agglutinate in antisera to the O1 group antigen (*V. cholerae* O1) and those that do not (non-O1 *V. cholerae*). Although some non-O1 *V. cholerae* serogroups have occasionally caused sporadic outbreaks of diarrhea, serogroup O1 was, until the emergence of serogroup O139, the exclusive cause of epidemic cholera. *V. cholerae* O139 (also called *V. cholerae* Bengal) is discussed in greater detail below.

V. cholerae O1 exists in two biotypes, *classical* and *El Tor*, that are distinguished on the basis of a number of characteristics, including phage susceptibility and hemolysin production. Each biotype is further subdivided into two serotypes, termed *Inaba* and *Ogawa*. Serotyping is a useful tool in field epidemiologic studies. Newer molecular epidemiologic techniques, such as ribotyping and other gene-based methods, now make it possible to trace the source and origin of cholera strains from around the world.

The natural habitat of *V. cholerae* is coastal salt water and brackish estuaries, where the organism lives in close relation to plankton and where it may survive in a viable but nonculturable form. Humans become infected incidentally but, once infected, can act as vehicles for spread. Ingestion of water contaminated by human feces is the most common means of acquisition of *V. cholerae*. Consumption of contaminated food in the home, in restaurants, or from street vendors can also contribute to spread. There is no known animal reservoir. While the infectious dose is relatively high, it is markedly reduced in hypochlorhydric persons, in those using antacids, and when gastric acidity is buffered by a meal. Cholera is predominantly a pediatric disease in endemic areas, but it affects adults and children equally when newly introduced into a population. In endemic areas, the disease is more common in the summer and fall months. While this seasonality has not been explained fully, it may be due to environmental conditions that affect the multiplication of vibrios or to seasonal alterations in human behavior that affect contact with water. Asymptomatic infections are frequent and more common with the El Tor than the classical biotype. In endemic areas, children <2 years of age are less likely to develop severe cholera than are older children, perhaps because of passive immunity acquired from breast milk. For unexplained reasons, susceptibility to cholera is significantly influenced by ABO blood group status; those with type O blood are at greatest risk, while those with type AB are at least risk.

Cholera is native to the Ganges delta in the Indian subcontinent. Since 1817, seven global pandemics have occurred. The current (seventh) pandemic—the first due to the El Tor biotype—began in Indonesia in 1961 and spread throughout Asia as *V. cholerae* El Tor displaced the endemic classical strain in many areas. It briefly invaded Europe, but effective public health measures and the high level of sanitation combined to limit its impact. In the early 1970s, El Tor cholera exploded in Africa, causing major epidemics before becoming a persistent endemic problem. Its recent history in Africa has been punctuated by severe outbreaks, often fed by the chaos of war and genocide. Such was the case in the camps for Rwandan refugees set up in 1994 around Goma, Zaire. Tens of thousands of cases occurred and mortality was high. In 1995, the occurrence of hundreds of cases in Romania and the Black Sea states of the former Soviet Union demonstrated the potential of this organism to cause epidemics whenever public health measures break down.

Since 1973, sporadic endemic infections due to vibrios related to the seventh-pandemic strain have been recognized along the U.S. Gulf Coast of Louisiana and Texas. These infections are typically associated with the consumption of contaminated, locally harvested shellfish. Occasionally, cases in U.S. locations remote from the Gulf Coast have been linked to shipped-in Gulf Coast seafood.

Although the event was long expected, it was not until 1991 that the current cholera pandemic reached Latin America. Beginning along the Peruvian coast in January 1991, the disease was carried by fishermen to Ecuador and Colombia. It then spread in an explosive epidemic to virtually all of South and Central America and to Mexico (Fig. 159-1). About 400,000 cases were reported in the first year of the outbreak, and >1 million had been reported by the end of 1994. While the cumulative mortality rate has been <1%, the mortality rate approached 30% in the communities first affected, where a lack of familiarity with the disease led initially to the deployment of wholly ineffective treatment. Intensive education of health care providers and of the community at large has enhanced awareness of the disease and its appropriate management and has greatly diminished mortality. As it did in Africa two decades earlier, the epidemic El Tor strain proved capable of establishing itself in inland waters rather than in its classic niche of coastal salt waters; the organism has already become endemic in many of the Latin American countries into which it was recently introduced.

Cases linked to the Latin American epidemic have occurred in the United States. For example, 11 people in New York and New Jersey were infected in two separate outbreaks in 1991 after eating boiled crabmeat illegally transported by travelers from Ecuador. Although secondary spread of this strain has not taken place in the United States, these events underscore the need for vigilance among health care professionals, even in locations remote from an epidemic.

In October 1992, a large-scale outbreak of clinical cholera occurred in the port city of Madras and surrounding towns in southern India.

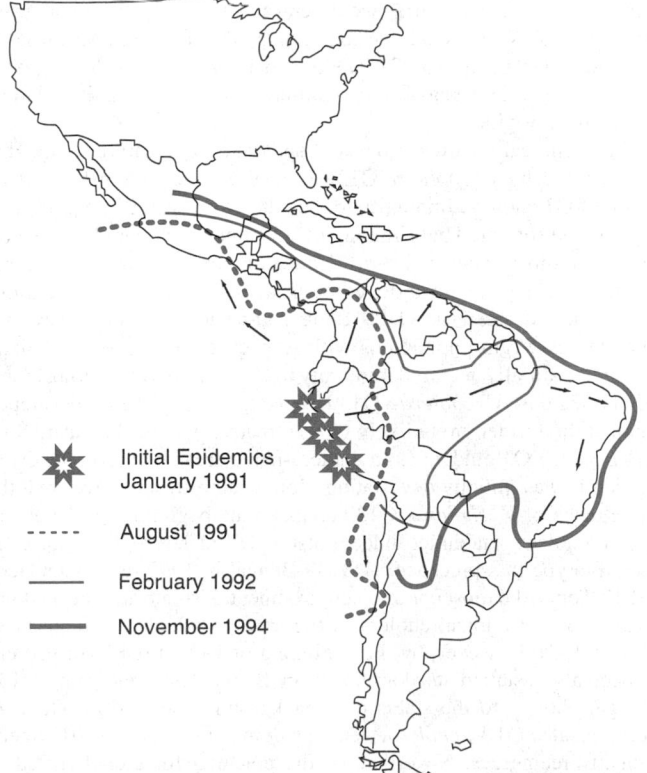

FIGURE 159-1 Spread of *Vibrio cholerae* O1 in the Americas, 1991–1994. *(Courtesy of Dr. Robert V. Tauxe, Centers for Disease Control and Prevention, Atlanta.)*

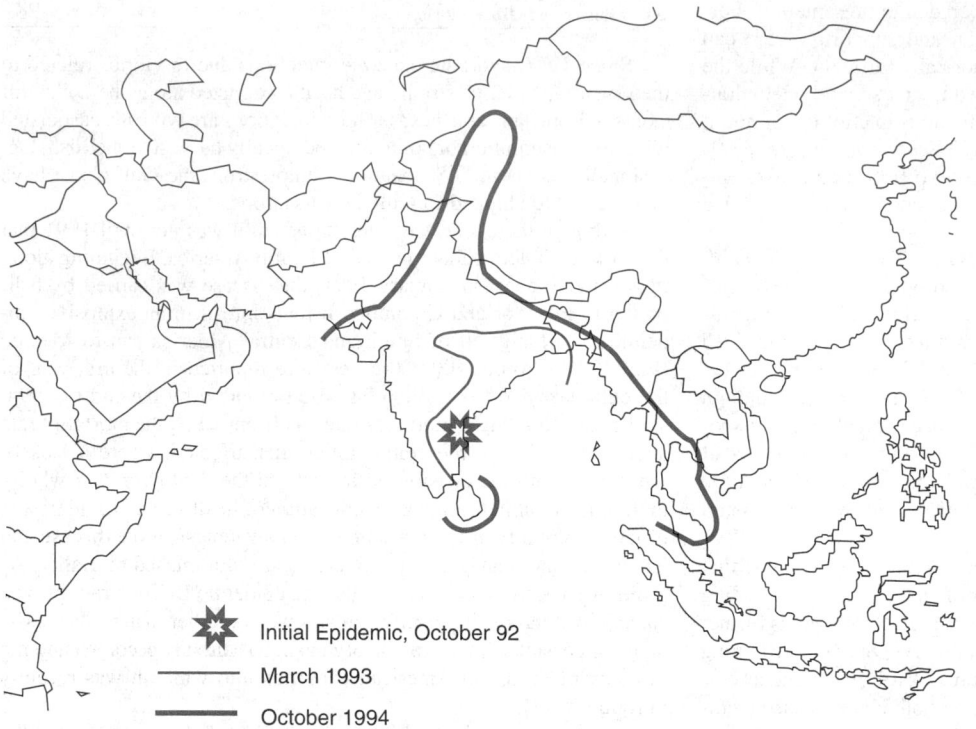

FIGURE 159-2 Spread of *Vibrio cholerae* O139 in the Indian subcontinent and elsewhere in Asia, 1992–1994. *(Courtesy of Dr. Robert V. Tauxe, Centers for Disease Control and Prevention, Atlanta.)*

Initial Epidemic, October 92

March 1993

October 1994

PATHOGENESIS In the final analysis, cholera is a toxin-mediated disease. Its characteristic watery diarrhea is due to the action of cholera toxin (CTX), a potent protein enterotoxin elaborated by the organism following its colonization of the small intestine. The bacterial properties that facilitate intestinal colonization are incompletely understood. For *V. cholerae* to colonize the small intestine and produce CTX, it must first recognize, contend with, and traverse several hostile environments. The first of these is the acidic milieu of the stomach. To elude the bactericidal effects of gastric acidity, *V. cholerae* relies, at least in part, on a relatively large inoculum size (compared to that needed for colonization by *Shigella*, for instance). The organism must next traverse the mucous layer lining the small bowel. *V. cholerae* chemotaxis and motility and a variety of proteases may allow the organism to traverse this gel covering the intestinal epithelium. Adherence to the intestinal epithelium is believed to be mediated by the toxin-coregulated pilus (TCP), so named because its synthesis is regulated in parallel with that of CTX. Studies of volunteers have established that TCP is essential for *V. cholerae* intestinal colonization. Other *V. cholerae* gene products known to be important in intestinal colonization of experimental animals include accessory colonization factors ABCD, a cell-associated hemagglutinin, iron and magnesium transport proteins, and purine and biotin biosynthesis enzymes.

CTX, TCP, and several other virulence factors, including accessory colonization factors and various outer-membrane proteins, are coordinately regulated by the *toxR* gene product. ToxR protein is a "master switch" that modulates the expression of virulence genes in response to signals that it senses within the environment of the host via a cascade of regulatory proteins. Coordinate regulation of virulence factor expression presumably enables the organism to tailor its repertoire of proteins to suit its needs as it passes from one microenvi-

The etiologic agent proved to be a novel strain of *V. cholerae* belonging neither to the O1 serogroup that typically causes epidemic cholera nor to any of the 137 other serogroups known at the time. This strain spread rapidly up and down the coast of the Bay of Bengal, reaching Bangladesh in December 1992. There alone, it caused more than 100,000 cases of cholera in the first 3 months of 1993. It subsequently spread across the Indian subcontinent and to neighboring countries, affecting Pakistan, Nepal, western China, Thailand, and Malaysia by the end of 1994 (Fig. 159-2). The organism has since been designated *V. cholerae* O139 Bengal in recognition of its novel O antigen and its geographic origin.

The clinical manifestations and epidemiologic features of the disease caused by *V. cholerae* O139 Bengal are indistinguishable from those of O1 cholera. Immunity to the latter, however, is not protective against the former. Thus, although O139 Bengal cholera has been restricted almost exclusively to O1-endemic areas, it has affected patients of all ages, with most cases in adults. Moreover, populations into which *V. cholerae* O139 Bengal has been introduced have responded as virgin populations with respect to severe, lethal cholera. Because naturally acquired immunity to *V. cholerae* O1 does not cross-protect against *V. cholerae* O139 Bengal, vaccines being developed against the former are unlikely to be effective against the latter.

Like the O1 epidemics in cholera-naive areas before it, the O139 epidemic was initially devastating. Some authorities believed that the emergence of *V. cholerae* O139 signaled the beginning of the eighth global cholera pandemic. Indeed, just as O1 El Tor replaced the classical biotype that preceded it, O139 Bengal in 1993 rapidly replaced O1 El Tor as the most common environmental isolate and the predominant cause of clinical cholera in the areas in which it had appeared (Fig. 159-3). However, by the beginning of 1994, O1 El Tor had unexpectedly resumed its dominance in Bangladesh, relegating O139 Bengal cholera to the status of a background endemic infection. In some locales O1 *V. cholerae* remains dominant; in others O139 periodically reemerges. Nevertheless, the potential for global spread of O139 Bengal was underscored by an intercontinental food-borne outbreak that occurred in early 1994 among American and British passengers on a cruise ship in Southeast Asia. Six of the 630 travelers became ill, their symptoms beginning only after they returned home.

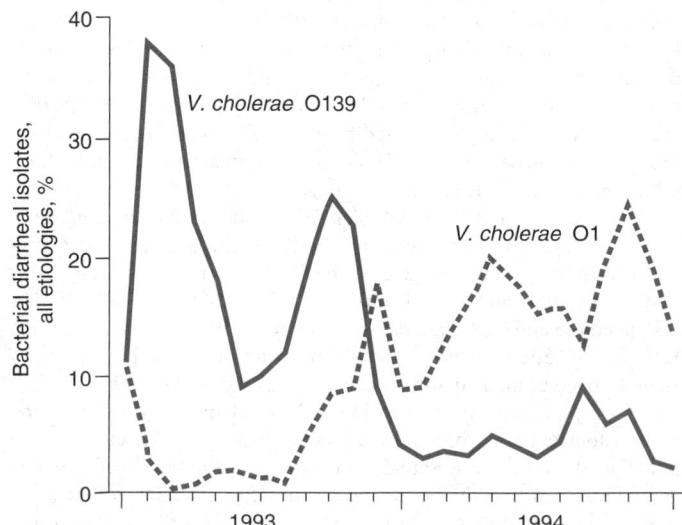

V. cholerae O139

V. cholerae O1

FIGURE 159-3 Isolations of *Vibrio cholerae* O1 and *V. cholerae* O139 in Bangladesh, 1993–1994, by month. *(Courtesy of Dr. John Albert and Dr. A.S.G. Faruque, International Centre for Diarrhoeal Disease Research, Bangladesh.)*

ronment to another. Coordinate regulation of virulence gene expression by a central sensor-effect protein like ToxR has become a paradigm for similar systems that have been discovered in a wide range of pathogenic bacteria.

Once established in the human small bowel, the organism produces CTX, which consists of a monomeric enzymatic moiety (the A subunit) and a pentameric binding moiety (the B subunit). The B pentamer binds to G_{M1} ganglioside, a glycolipid on the surface of jejunal epithelial cells that serves as the toxin receptor and makes possible the delivery of the A subunit to its cytosolic target. The activated A subunit (A_1) irreversibly transfers ADP-ribose from nicotinamide adenine dinucleotide to its specific target protein, the GTP-binding regulatory component of adenylate cyclase in intestinal epithelial cells. In this configuration, this G protein permanently upregulates the cyclase catalytic subunit; the result is the intracellular accumulation of high levels of cyclic AMP. In intestinal epithelial cells, cyclic AMP inhibits the absorptive sodium transport system in villus cells and activates the excretory chloride transport system in crypt cells, and these events lead to the accumulation of sodium chloride in the intestinal lumen. Since water moves passively to maintain osmolality, isotonic fluid accumulates in the lumen. When the volume of that fluid exceeds the capacity of the rest of the gut to resorb it, watery diarrhea results. Unless the wasted fluid and electrolytes are adequately replaced, shock (due to profound dehydration) and acidosis (due to loss of bicarbonate) follow.

Although perturbation of the adenylate cyclase pathway is the primary mechanism by which CTX causes excess fluid secretion, it is not the only one. Increasing evidence indicates that CTX also enhances intestinal secretion via prostaglandins and/or neural histamine receptors. It is possible that the redundancy of secretory mechanisms activated by CTX accounts for the profound diarrhea and dehydration characteristic of severe cholera.

The genes encoding CTX (*ctxAB*) are part of the genome of a bacteriophage designated CTXΦ. The receptor for this phage on the *V. cholerae* surface is the essential *V. cholerae* intestinal colonization factor TCP. Following infection of TCP+ *ctxAB*− *V. cholerae* cells, the CTXΦ genome stably integrates at a specific site on the *V. cholerae* chromosome. Since *ctxAB* is part of a mobile genetic element (CTXΦ), horizontal transfer of this bacteriophage may account for the emergence of new toxigenic *V. cholerae* serogroups. In addition, since the CTXΦ receptor TCP is a *V. cholerae* host colonization factor, it is possible that CTXΦ infection of TCP+ *ctxAB*− *V. cholerae* strains occurs primarily within the human intestine. Many of the other genes important for *V. cholerae* pathogenicity, including the genes encoding the biosynthesis of TCP, those encoding accessory colonization factors, and those regulating virulence gene expression, are clustered together on one of the two *V. cholerae* chromosomes. This cluster of virulence genes is referred to as the *V. cholerae pathogenicity island*. Similar clustering of virulence genes is found in other bacterial pathogens. It is believed that these pathogenicity islands have been acquired by horizontal gene transfer.

Molecular analysis of *V. cholerae* O139 Bengal has suggested the basis of its origin and the reasons it was able to cause an explosive epidemic of cholera. Both phenotypically and genotypically, O139 Bengal is closely related to the O1 El Tor strains of the seventh pandemic, and it seems to have arisen from them by horizontal gene transfer. It shares the virulence attributes and general pathogenic mechanisms of O1 vibrios, including possession of the same CTX prophage and the same TCP. *V. cholerae* O139 Bengal is in fact virtually identical to the seventh-pandemic strains of *V. cholerae* O1 El Tor except for two important differences: production of the novel O139 LPS and of an immunologically related O-antigen polysaccharide capsule. Both of these molecules are putative virulence factors, independently enhancing colonization in a murine infection model. The ability to produce the O139 LPS is due to a replacement of a 22-kb DNA segment encoding O1 antigen biosynthesis with a 35-kb segment containing the genes encoding O139 LPS and capsule biosynthesis. Encapsulation is not a feature of O1 strains and may explain the resistance of O139

strains to human serum in vitro as well as the occasional development of O139 bacteremia.

CLINICAL MANIFESTATIONS   After a 24- to 48-h incubation period, cholera begins with the sudden onset of painless watery diarrhea that may quickly become voluminous and is often followed shortly by vomiting. In severe cases, stool volume can exceed 250 mL/kg in the first 24 h. If fluids and electrolytes are not replaced, hypovolemic shock and death ensue. Fever is usually absent. Muscle cramps due to electrolyte disturbances are common. The stool has a characteristic appearance: a nonbilious, gray, slightly cloudy fluid with flecks of mucus, no blood, and a somewhat sweet, inoffensive odor. It has been called "rice-water" stool because of its resemblance to the water in which rice has been washed. Clinical symptoms parallel volume contraction: At losses of 3 to 5% of normal body weight, thirst develops; at 5 to 8%, postural hypotension, weakness, tachycardia, and decreased skin turgor are documented; and at >10%, oliguria, weak or absent pulses, sunken eyes (and, in infants, sunken fontanelles), wrinkled ("washerwoman") skin, somnolence, and coma are characteristic. Complications derive exclusively from the effects of volume and electrolyte depletion and include renal failure due to acute tubular necrosis. Thus, if the patient is adequately treated with fluid and salt, complications are averted and the process is self-limited, resolving in a few days.

Laboratory data usually reveal an elevated hematocrit (due to hemoconcentration) in nonanemic patients; mild neutrophilic leukocytosis; elevated levels of blood urea nitrogen and creatinine consistent with prerenal azotemia; normal sodium, potassium, and chloride levels; a markedly reduced bicarbonate level (<15 mmol/L); and an elevated anion gap (due to increases in serum lactate, protein, and phosphate). Arterial pH is usually low (about 7.2).

DIAGNOSIS   The clinical suspicion of cholera can be confirmed by the identification of *V. cholerae* in stool; however, the organism must be specifically sought. In experienced hands, it can be detected directly by dark-field microscopy on a wet mount of fresh stool, and its serotype can be discerned by immobilization with Inaba- or Ogawa-specific antiserum. Laboratory isolation of the organism requires the use of a selective medium. The best of these is thiosulfate–citrate–bile salts–sucrose (TCBS) agar, on which the organism grows as a flat yellow colony. If a delay in sample processing is expected, Carey-Blair transport medium and/or alkaline-peptone water-enrichment medium should be inoculated as well. In endemic areas there is little need for biochemical confirmation and characterization, although these tasks may be worthwhile in places where *V. cholerae* is an uncommon isolate. Standard microbiologic biochemical testing for Enterobacteriaceae will suffice for identification of *V. cholerae*. All vibrios are oxidase-positive. *V. cholerae* can be distinguished from the otherwise similar *V. mimicus* by its ability to ferment sucrose.

The yield of stool cultures for the diagnosis of *V. cholerae* infection declines late in the course of the illness or when effective antibacterial therapy is initiated. Although not generally evaluable in clinical laboratories, serum vibriocidal antibody titers can be used to confirm the diagnosis in non-cholera-endemic regions of the world. Monoclonal antibody–based diagnostic kits and methods based on the polymerase chain reaction and on DNA probes have been developed for *V. cholerae* O1 and O139 but are unlikely to become available in U.S. clinical laboratories.

℞ **TREATMENT**   Cholera is simple to treat; only the rapid and adequate replacement of fluids, electrolytes, and base is required. The mortality rate for appropriately treated disease is usually <1%. However, analysis of a large outbreak of cholera among airline travelers from an endemic country to the United States revealed frequent misdiagnoses by U.S. health professionals and poor appreciation on their part of the principles of management. Compounding these problems was the general unavailability of appropriate oral fluids. Even intravenous fluid therapy typically was not optimal.

It has been proved conclusively that fluid may be given orally. This approach takes advantage of the hexose-Na⁺ cotransport mechanism to move Na⁺ across the gut mucosa together with an actively transported molecule such as glucose. Since Na⁺ losses in the stool are high, a fluid containing Na⁺ at 90 mmol/L has been recommended by the World Health Organization (WHO) (Table 159-1). This amount of Na⁺ is higher than that needed to treat diarrhea due to most other causes. The solution is safe, even for infants, if its intake is alternated with the consumption of sodium-free fluids such as breast milk or water. For the sake of simplicity, WHO advises routine use of this single solution for diarrheal disease rather than attempts to choose among multiple formulations according to etiology.

Cereal-based formulations are receiving increased attention as alternative oral rehydration solutions. Because of their lower osmolarity, they may reduce stool output. A mixture with a lower sugar and salt content has also been evaluated in cholera patients, with favorable results. However, concerns have been raised over the safety of its use—in particular, whether it could cause significant hyponatremia in patients with moderate or severe diarrhea. Because commercial oral rehydration solutions also contain concentrations of glucose and sodium lower than those of the WHO formulation, they should not yet be used routinely to treat cholera.

For initial management of severely dehydrated patients, intravenous fluid replacement is preferable, if available. Because profound acidosis (pH < 7.2) is common in this group, Ringer's lactate is the best choice among commercial products (Table 159-2). It must be used with additional potassium supplements, preferably given by mouth. The total fluid deficit in severely dehydrated patients (≥10% of body weight) can be replaced safely within the first 4 h of therapy, half within the first hour. Thereafter, oral therapy can usually be initiated, with the goal of maintaining fluid intake equal to fluid output. However, patients with continued large-volume diarrhea may require prolonged intravenous treatment to keep up with gastrointestinal fluid losses. Severe hypokalemia can develop but will respond to potassium given either intravenously or orally. In the absence of adequate staff to monitor the patient's progress, the oral route of rehydration and potassium replacement is safer than the intravenous route and is physiologically regulated by thirst and urine output.

Although not necessary for cure, the use of an antibiotic to which the organism is susceptible will diminish the duration and volume of fluid loss and will hasten clearance of the organism from the stool. Single-dose tetracycline (2 g) or doxycycline (300 mg) is effective in adults but is not recommended for children under 8 years of age because of possible deposition in bone and developing teeth. Emerging drug resistance is an ever-present concern. For adults with cholera in areas where tetracycline resistance is prevalent, ciprofloxacin—either in a single dose (30 mg/kg, not to exceed a total dose of 1 g) or in a short course (15 mg/kg bid for 3 days, not to exceed a total daily dose of 1 g)—or erythromycin (a total of 40 mg/kg daily in three divided doses for 3 days) is a clinically effective substitute. Both drugs are

Table 159-1   Composition of World Health Organization Oral Rehydration Solution (ORS)[a,b]

Constituent	Concentration, mmol/L
Na⁺	90
K⁺	20
Cl⁻	80
Citrate[c]	10
Glucose	110

[a] Contains (per package, to be added to 1 L of drinking water): NaCl, 3.5 g; Na₃C₆H₅O₇·2H₂O, 2.9 g; KCl, 1.5 g; and glucose, 20 g.
[b] If prepackaged ORS is unavailable, a simple homemade alternative can be prepared by combining 5 g NaCl (about 1 level teaspoon) with either 50 g precooked rice cereal or 40 g sucrose in 1 L of drinking water. In that case, potassium must be supplied separately (e.g., in orange juice or coconut water).
[c] 10 mmol citrate per liter, which supplies 30 mmol HCO₃/L.

Table 159-2   Electrolyte Composition of Cholera Stool and of Intravenous Rehydration Solution

Substance	Concentration, mmol/L			
	Na⁺	K⁺	Cl⁻	Base
Stool				
Adult	135	15	90	30
Child	100	25	90	30
Ringer's lactate	130	4[a]	109	28

[a] Potassium supplements, preferably administered by mouth, are required to replace the usual potassium losses from stool.

highly effective in reducing total stool output, and each is significantly better than trimethoprim-sulfamethoxazole. Because of the high cost of quinolones, WHO recommends erythromycin as the first alternative to tetracycline. For children, furazolidone has been the recommended agent and trimethoprim-sulfamethoxazole the second choice. It is of note that *V. cholerae* O139 is often resistant to both of these drugs but is susceptible to quinolones, erythromycin, tetracycline, and ampicillin (among others). Because of cost and/or toxicity issues related to the other drugs, erythromycin is a good choice for pediatric cholera, especially where O139 Bengal is present. The efficacy of single-dose erythromycin therapy for cholera has not been demonstrated.

CONTROL   In outbreaks, efforts should first be made to identify case contacts and to treat incubating carriers. Next, epidemiologic studies should be undertaken to establish the modes of transmission to define the best strategy to interrupt them. Both the establishment of rehydration centers and instruction in rehydration techniques are essential to the reduction of mortality. Immunization in these circumstances is not an effective means of control.

PREVENTION   Provision of safe water and facilities for sanitary disposal of feces, improved nutrition, and attention to food preparation and storage in the household could significantly reduce the incidence of cholera. Much effort has been devoted to the development of an effective cholera vaccine over the past two decades, with a particular focus on oral vaccine strains. Traditional killed cholera vaccine given intramuscularly provides little protection to nonimmune subjects and predictably causes adverse effects, including pain at the injection site, malaise, and fever. The vaccine's limited efficacy is at least partially due to its failure to induce a local immune response at the intestinal mucosal surface.

Two types of oral cholera vaccines are under development. The first is a killed whole-cell (WC) vaccine. Two formulations of the killed WC vaccine have been prepared: one that also contains the nontoxic B subunit of CTX (WC/BS) and one composed solely of killed bacteria. In field trials in Bangladesh, both of the killed vaccines were compared with placebo and conferred ~50% protection over a 3-year evaluation period. The protective efficacy of WC/BS was superior to that of WC during the initial 8 months of follow-up (69 versus 41%) but equivalent or inferior thereafter. Immunity was relatively sustained in persons vaccinated at an age of >5 years but was not well sustained in younger vaccinees.

The second approach is that of a live attenuated vaccine strain developed, for example, by the isolation or creation of mutants lacking active CTX. Three criteria must be met in live vaccine design: The vaccine strain must induce protective immunity, it must be safe to administer, and it must be minimally reactogenic. *Safety criteria* include the vaccine strain's potential to regain virulence, either spontaneously or via horizontal gene transfer from environmental strains, as well as its potential to donate virulence genes to other strains. *Reactogenicity* refers to its potential to cause symptoms such as fever or diarrhea in vaccinees.

Strain CVD 103-HgR, an oral live cholera vaccine licensed for immunization of travelers in Europe, is derived from a classical biotype strain of *V. cholerae* by the deletion of the CTX A subunit gene and the insertion in the hemolysin gene of a mercury resistance marker.

This strain has been extensively tested in volunteers; although it is poorly excreted in the stool of human vaccinees, a single dose produces a significant increase in the titer of vibriocidal antibody in ~75% of recipients, including children between the ages of 2 and 4 years, with almost no reactogenicity. Studies in volunteers demonstrate that this vaccine is more effective against classical than against El Tor cholera. Unfortunately, in a large field trial in Indonesian children, this vaccine failed to induce protection against clinical cholera.

Other live attenuated vaccine candidate strains have been prepared from El Tor and O139 *V. cholerae*. In studies in volunteers, these vaccine strains have often exhibited significant reactogenicity whose cause (given the absence of active CTX) is unclear. Reactogenicity may result from the production of another toxic moiety (e.g., the hemagglutinin/protease or the RTX toxin) by the live attenuated strain. Alternatively, intestinal colonization itself may result in reactogenicity. These El Tor– and O139-derived live vaccine strains are therefore at least several years away from potential licensing. Because of the minimal efficacy of existing parenteral vaccines, cholera immunization is recommended for U.S. travelers only if it is mandated by the countries they plan to visit.

OTHER *VIBRIO* SPECIES

In recent years, the taxonomic, epidemiologic, pathophysiologic, and clinical features of vibrios that do not cause clinical cholera have become increasingly well understood. Ten human pathogens are currently recognized in the genus *Vibrio*. Included are species associated primarily with gastrointestinal illness (*V. parahaemolyticus*, non-O1 *V. cholerae*, *V. mimicus*, *V. fluvialis*, *V. hollisae*, and *V. furnissii*) and species associated primarily with soft tissue infections (*V. vulnificus*, *V. alginolyticus*, and *V. damsela*). In addition, *V. vulnificus* has emerged as a cause of primary sepsis in certain compromised hosts. Vibrios are abundant in coastal waters the world over and tend to concentrate in the tissues of filter-feeding mollusks. Under optimal conditions, some can double in number in as little as 9 min. Consequently, seawater and raw or undercooked shellfish are important sources of human infection (Table 159-3). Vibrios grow best at temperatures of 28°C to 44°C but not at all below 4°C or above 60°C. Most can be cultured on blood or MacConkey agar, each of which contains enough salt to support the growth of the halophilic organisms (≥0.5%). As with *V. cholerae*, TCBS is the best selective medium. The species can be differentiated in the laboratory by standard biochemical tests. The most important members of the group are *V. parahaemolyticus* and *V. vulnificus*. These and selected other species are considered below in greater detail.

SPECIES ASSOCIATED PRIMARILY WITH GASTROINTESTINAL ILLNESS *V. parahaemolyticus* First implicated as a cause of enteritis by Japanese workers in 1953, *V. parahaemolyticus* is now recognized as an important intestinal pathogen in many parts of the world. In one study from Japan, 24% of reported cases of food poisoning were attributed to this organism, presumably owing to the widespread consumption of raw seafood there. In the United States, *V. parahaemolyticus* has been responsible for several well-documented common-source outbreaks of diarrhea, typically linked to ingestion of undercooked or improperly handled seafood or of other foods that have been contaminated by seawater. Most reports have come from the Atlantic Coast, the Gulf of Mexico, and Hawaii. The organism is ubiquitous in marine environments and is able to grow in saline concentrations as high as 8 to 10%. The ability to cause hemolysis on Wagatsuma agar (known as the *Kanagawa phenomenon*) is closely linked to enteropathogenicity. In one study, 96.5% of isolates from patients with diarrhea were hemolytic versus only ~1% of iso-

Table 159-3 Features of Selected Noncholera Vibrioses

Organism	Vehicle or Activity	Host at Risk	Syndrome
V. parahaemolyticus	Shellfish, seawater	Normal	Gastroenteritis
	Seawater	Normal	Wound infection
Non-O1 *V. cholerae*	Shellfish, travel	Normal	Gastroenteritis
	Seawater	Normal	Wound infection, otitis media
V. vulnificus	Shellfish	Immunosuppressed[a]	Sepsis, secondary cellulitis
	Seawater	Normal	Wound infection, cellulitis
V. alginolyticus	Seawater	Normal	Wound infection, cellulitis, otitis
	Seawater	Burned, other immunosuppressed	Sepsis

[a] Especially with liver disease or hemochromatosis.

lates from seawater. Hemolysis is attributed to a 42-kDa heat-stable protein, the exact pathophysiologic role of which is uncertain. The mechanism by which *V. parahaemolyticus* causes diarrhea is not clear.

V. parahaemolyticus has been associated with two distinct gastrointestinal presentations. The more common is a syndrome of watery diarrhea, accompanied in most cases by abdominal cramps, nausea, and vomiting and in about one-quarter of cases by fever and chills. The incubation period ranges from 4 h to 4 days, and the symptomatic period lasts for a median of 3 days. The vast majority of North American cases have been of this type. The less common syndrome is one of dysentery, described in India and Bangladesh and characterized by severe abdominal cramps, nausea, vomiting, and bloody or mucoid stools. Most cases of either type are self-limited and require neither antimicrobial treatment nor hospitalization. Severe infections are associated with underlying diseases, including diabetes, preexisting liver disease, iron-overload states, or immunosuppression. The occasional severe case should be treated with fluid replacement and antibiotics, as described above for cholera. Death is very rare. There are no reliable differential diagnostic features. *V. parahaemolyticus* should be considered as a possible cause in all cases of diarrhea that can be epidemiologically linked to seafood consumption or to the sea itself.

In addition to gastrointestinal disease, *V. parahaemolyticus* is a rare cause of extraintestinal infections, including wound infections, otitis, and—very rarely—sepsis.

Non-O1 *V. cholerae* The heterogeneous non-O1 *V. cholerae* organisms are biochemically indistinguishable from *V. cholerae* O1 on routine testing but fail to agglutinate in O1 antiserum. While technically a non-O1 vibrio, *V. cholerae* O139 Bengal is not grouped with these pathogens because of its potential to cause epidemic cholera, as detailed above. Non-O1 *V. cholerae* strains have been responsible for several well-described food-borne outbreaks of gastroenteritis as well as for sporadic cases of otitis media, wound infection, and bacteremia. About half of all U.S. isolates are obtained from stool specimens. Like other vibrios, non-O1 *V. cholerae* organisms are widely distributed in marine environments; unlike most other vibrios, however, they require only trace amounts of NaCl to survive (i.e., they are nonhalophilic). Recognized U.S. cases invariably have been associated either with the consumption of raw oysters or with recent travel, typically to Mexico. The clinical spectrum of diarrheal disease caused by non-O1 *V. cholerae* is broad and likely reflects the heterogeneous virulence attributes of the group. Occasional isolates make a protein enterotoxin very similar to CTX. Others produce cytotoxins, hemolysins, or invasins.

Gastroenteritis due to non-O1 *V. cholerae* typically has an incubation period of <2 days. Stools may be copious and watery. On occasion, diarrhea may leave the patient severely dehydrated, as in cholera. Alternatively, the stools may be partly formed, less voluminous, and bloody or mucoid. Abdominal cramps, nausea, vomiting, and fever are often reported. In one series, 11% of patients were hospitalized; in another, the figure was 50%. The duration of illness ranges from about 2 to 7 days. As in cholera, patients with significant dehydration should be treated with oral or intravenous fluids. The role of antibiotics is uncertain.

Wound infection and otitis media each account for ~10% of non-O1 *V. cholerae* isolates. Bacteremia accounts for another 20%. Patients with extraintestinal infection often have a history of occupational or recreational exposure to seawater. Bacteremia is more likely to develop in the presence of liver disease. Extraintestinal infections should be treated with antibiotics. There is a paucity of information to guide the choice of a specific agent and schedule. Most strains are sensitive in vitro to tetracycline, chloramphenicol, and other agents.

SPECIES ASSOCIATED PRIMARILY WITH SOFT TISSUE INFECTION OR BACTEREMIA   *V. vulnificus*   Though it represents only a small minority of the *Vibrio* species found in nature (4% of Atlantic Coast isolates in one study), *V. vulnificus* is perhaps the most important cause of severe *Vibrio* infections in the United States (0.8 cases per 100,000 population in one study from Louisiana). Formerly included in the species *V. parahaemolyticus*, *V. vulnificus* was distinguished in the 1970s by its ability to ferment lactose and to cause distinct clinical syndromes. Like most vibrios, it proliferates in the warm summer months. It requires a saline environment for growth but prefers concentrations lower than those preferred by *V. parahaemolyticus* and *V. alginolyticus* (range, up to ~8%; optimal, ~1%). Infections in humans typically occur in coastal states between May and October and most often involve men over age 40. *V. vulnificus* has been linked unequivocally to two distinct syndromes: primary sepsis, typically in patients with antecedent liver disease, and primary wound infections, usually in people without underlying disease. Some authors have suggested that this organism causes gastroenteritis, but the evidence for this association is tenuous.

V. vulnificus is remarkably invasive in animal models. It is endowed with a number of virulence attributes, including an antiphagocytic capsule, serum resistance, a cytotoxin/hemolysin (the organism is Kanagawa-positive), collagenase, elastolytic protease, phospholipase, and siderophores. Its virulence, as measured by the 50% lethal dose in mice, is markedly enhanced under conditions of iron overload, a fact consonant with its propensity to infect patients with hemochromatosis.

Primary sepsis occurs most commonly in patients with cirrhosis or hemochromatosis but has also developed in patients with hematopoietic disorders or chronic renal insufficiency, in persons using immunosuppressive medications or alcohol, and (rarely) in individuals without apparent underlying disease. Most of those affected have ingested raw oysters within 2 days of onset (median incubation period, 16 h). The process begins precipitously with malaise, chills, fever (mean temperature, 39.8°C), and prostration. Hypotension develops in one-third of cases, often by the time of admission. Cutaneous manifestations, which develop in three-quarters of cases (usually by 36 h after onset), typically involve the extremities—lower more often than upper. A common sequence is the evolution of erythematous patches followed by ecchymoses, vesicles, and bullae. (Indeed, the presence of sepsis and bullous skin lesions suggests the diagnosis in an appropriate setting.) Necrosis and sloughing may occur. Laboratory study reveals leukopenia more often than leukocytosis, thrombocytopenia, and (occasionally) elevated levels of fibrin split products. *V. vulnificus* can be cultured from blood or cutaneous lesions.

Mortality approaches 50%, with most deaths due to uncontrolled sepsis. Accordingly, prompt treatment is critical and should include empirical antibiotic administration, aggressive debridement, and general supportive care. *V. vulnificus* is sensitive to a number of antimicrobials in vitro, including tetracycline, gentamicin, and third-generation cephalosporins. No compelling clinical data from studies of humans support the preferential use of any one of these agents. Tetracycline is demonstrably superior in a murine model and on that basis is considered the drug of choice (0.5 to 1 g intravenously every 12 h), either alone or in combination with gentamicin. The duration of therapy is guided by the clinical response.

Wound infections with *V. vulnificus* can develop in patients with or without underlying disease and invariably follow contact of seawater with either a prior or a fresh wound. The incubation period is brief (4 h to 4 days; mean, 12 h). The disease begins with swelling, erythema, and—in many cases—intense pain around the wound. Rapidly spreading cellulitis follows, with vesicular, bullous, or necrotic lesions developing in some instances. Metastatic events do not generally occur. Fever (median temperature, 38.9°C) and leukocytosis are demonstrable in most cases. The organism can be cultured from skin lesions and occasionally from blood. Prompt antibiotic therapy and debridement are usually curative.

V. alginolyticus   This species was first recognized as a human pathogen in 1973 and is now known to cause occasional wound, ear, and eye infections. It is the most salt-tolerant of the vibrios, able to grow in concentrations >10%. Most clinical isolates come from superinfected wounds, which presumably became contaminated at the beach. Infection varies in severity but is generally not serious and responds well to antibiotic therapy and drainage. A few reports have described otitis externa, otitis media, or conjunctivitis. Therapy with tetracycline is usually curative. *V. alginolyticus* is a rare cause of bacteremia in immunocompromised hosts.

BIBLIOGRAPHY

ALI A et al: *Vibrio vulnificus* sepsis in solid organ transplantation: A medical nemesis. J Heart Lung Transplant 14:598, 1995

BESSER RE et al: Diagnosis and treatment of cholera in the United States. Are we prepared? JAMA 272:1203, 1994

COLWELL RR: Global climate and infectious disease: The cholera paradigm. Science 274: 2025, 1996

FYFE M et al: Outbreak of *Vibrio parahaemolyticus* infections associated with eating raw oysters. MMWR 47:457, 1998

KARAOLIS DK et al: A *Vibrio cholerae* pathogenicity island associated with epidemic and pandemic strains. Proc Natl Acad Sci USA 95:3134, 1998

KHAN WA et al: Comparative trial of five antimicrobial compounds in the treatment of cholera in adults. Trans R Soc Trop Med Hyg 89:103, 1995

LACEY SW: Cholera: Calamitous past, ominous future. Clin Infect Dis 20:1409, 1995

LIN W et al: Identification of a *Vibrio cholerae* RTX toxin gene cluster that is tightly linked to the cholera toxin prophage. Proc Natl Acad Sci USA 96:1071, 1999

MEKALANOS JJ, SADOFF JC: Cholera vaccines: Fighting an ancient scourge. Science 265: 1387, 1994

MORRIS JG JR: Non-O1 *V. cholerae*: A look at the epidemiology of an occasional pathogen. Epidemiol Rev 12:179, 1990

NAFICY A et al: Treatment and vaccination strategies to control cholera in sub-Saharan refugee settings: A cost-effectiveness analysis. JAMA 279:521, 1998

RAUFMAN JP: Cholera. Am J Med 104:386, 1998

SHAPIRO R et al: The role of Gulf Coast oysters harvested in warmer months in *Vibrio vulnificus* infections in the United States, 1988–1996. J Infect Dis 178:752, 1998

TAYLOR DN et al: Cholera among Americans living in Peru. Clin Infect Dis 22:1108, 1996

WALDOR MK, MEKALANOS JJ: Lysogenic conversion by a filamentous phage encoding cholera toxin. Science 272:1910, 1996

——— et al: Emergence of a new cholera pandemic: Molecular analysis of virulence determinants in *Vibrio cholerae* O139 and development of a live vaccine prototype. J Infect Dis 170:278, 1994

——— et al: The *Vibrio cholerae* O139 serogroup antigen includes an O-antigen capsule and lipopolysaccharide virulence determinants. Proc Natl Acad Sci USA 91:11388, 1994

160   BRUCELLOSIS

M. Monir Madkour, Dennis L. Kasper

DEFINITION   Brucellosis is a zoonosis transmitted to humans from infected animals. Its clinical features are not disease specific. *Brucellosis* has many synonyms derived from the geographical regions in which the disease occurs (e.g., Mediterranean fever, Malta fever, Gibraltar fever, Cyprus fever); from the remittent character of its fever (e.g., undulant fever); or from its resemblance to malaria and typhoid (e.g., typhomalarial fever, intermittent typhoid).

ETIOLOGY Human brucellosis can be caused by any of four species: *Brucella melitensis* (the most common and most virulent cause of brucellosis worldwide) is acquired primarily from goats, sheep, and camels; *B. abortus* from cattle; *B. suis* from hogs; and *B. canis* from dogs. These small aerobic gram-negative bacilli are unencapsulated, nonmotile, non-spore-forming, facultative intracellular parasites that cause lifelong infection in animals. Brucellae are killed by boiling or pasteurization of milk and milk products. They survive for up to 8 weeks in unpasteurized, white, soft cheese made from goat's milk and are not killed by freezing. The organisms remain viable for up to 40 days in dried soil contaminated with infected-animal urine, stool, vaginal discharge, and products of conception and for longer periods in damp soil.

EPIDEMIOLOGY The global incidence of human brucellosis is not known because of the variable quality of disease reporting and notification systems in many countries. Worldwide, the only countries believed to be free of brucellosis are Norway, Sweden, Finland, Denmark, Iceland, Switzerland, the Czech and Slovak republics, Romania, the United Kingdom (including the Channel Islands), the Netherlands, Japan, Luxembourg, Cyprus, and Bulgaria; the U.S. Virgin Islands are also free of the disease. Reports indicate that, even in developed nations, the true incidence of brucellosis may be up to 26 times higher than official figures suggest. In the United States, about 200 new cases are reported every year; however, it is estimated that only 4 to 10% of cases are recognized and reported. Consumption of imported cheese, travel abroad, and occupation-related exposures are the most frequently identified sources of infection. In communities where brucellosis is endemic, the disease occurs in children and the family members of infected persons are at risk. Even in countries where animal brucellosis is controlled, the disease occasionally develops among farmers, meat-processing workers, veterinarians, and laboratory workers.

The *Brucella* organism is transmitted most commonly through the ingestion of untreated milk or milk products; raw meat (i.e., blood) and bone marrow have also been implicated. However, the organism can be contracted via inhalation during contact with animals, especially by children and by slaughterhouse, farm, and laboratory workers. Other routes of infection for at-risk workers include skin abrasion, autoinoculation, and conjunctival splashing. The organism has occasionally been transmitted from person to person through the placenta, during breast-feeding, and during sexual activity. Aerosolized *B. melitensis* is a classic agent of biological warfare.

PATHOGENESIS AND IMMUNITY Serum opsonizes *Brucella* organisms for ingestion by polymorphonuclear leukocytes and activated macrophages. Brucellae resist intracellular phagocytic killing by mechanisms such as the suppression of the myeloperoxide–hydrogen peroxide–halide system and the production of superoxide dismutase. The pathogen-phagocyte interaction plays a key role in determining the severity and outcome of brucellosis. The organisms surviving within and escaping from the phagocytes multiply and reach the bloodstream via the lymphatics, subsequently localizing in the liver, spleen, bones, kidneys, lymph nodes, heart valves, nervous system, and testes. In these organs, the bacteria are ingested by macrophages and survive by inhibition of phagosome-lysosome fusion. In infected tissues, inflammatory responses or noncaseating granulomas typically develop, and caseating granulomas and abscesses have been described.

Cytokines, including interleukin (IL) 1, IL-12, and tumor necrosis factor, appear to be important in host defense against *Brucella* infection. The smooth lipopolysaccharide (LPS) of *Brucella* is the major known virulence factor. Strains with rough LPS are more likely than those with smooth LPS to be lysed by nonimmune serum. In virulent strains, the foremost target for specific antibodies is the LPS. Serum IgM antibodies to LPS appear within 1 week after infection and are followed later by IgG and IgA. Titers of both IgM and IgG antibody fall after treatment, and failure of these titers to decline should prompt an evaluation for relapse or persistent infection.

CLASSIFICATION Brucellosis is classified according to whether or not the disease is active (i.e., symptoms or progressive tissue damage and significantly raised *Brucella* agglutinin levels with or without positive cultures) and whether or not there is localized infection. The state of activity and the site of localization have a significant impact on recommended treatment. Classification of brucellosis as acute, subacute, serologic, bacteremic, or of mixed types serves no purpose in diagnosis and management.

CLINICAL MANIFESTATIONS AND COMPLICATIONS Brucellosis is a systemic disease with protean manifestations. Its features may mimic those of other febrile illnesses. The incubation period lasts for about 1 to 3 weeks but may be as long as several months, depending on the virulence of the organisms, their route of entry, the infecting dose, and the host's preexisting health status. The onset of symptoms may be either abrupt (over 1 to 2 days) or gradual (≥ 1 week). The most common symptoms are fever, chills, diaphoresis, headaches, myalgia, fatigue, anorexia, joint and low-back pain, weight loss, constipation, sore throat, and dry cough. Physical examination often reveals no abnormalities, and patients can look deceptively well. Some patients, in contrast, are acutely ill, with pallor, lymphadenopathy, hepatosplenomegaly, arthritis, spinal tenderness, epididymoorchitis, rash, meningitis, cardiac murmurs, or pneumonia. The fever of brucellosis has no distinctive pattern but may exhibit diurnal variation, with normal temperatures in the morning and high temperatures in the afternoon and evening. Localization to an organ or a system may be evident at the onset of the disease. Table 160-1 lists the frequencies of key historic features, symptoms, and signs among 500 patients with brucellosis due to *B. melitensis*.

Bones and Joints Although monarticular septic arthritis occurs, 30 to 40% of patients have reactive asymmetric polyarthritis involving the knees, hips, shoulders, and sacroiliac and sternoclavicular joints.

Table 160-1 Relevant Historical Features, Symptoms, and Signs in 500 Patients with Brucellosis due to *Brucella melitensis*

Feature	No. of Patients (%)
History	
Animal contact	368 (74)
Raw milk/cheese ingestion	350 (70)
Raw liver ingestion	147 (29)
Family history of brucellosis	188 (38)
Symptom/Sign	
Fever	464 (93)
Chills	410 (82)
Sweats	437 (87)
Aches	457 (91)
Lack of energy	473 (95)
Joint and back pain	431 (86)
Arthritis	202 (40)
Spinal tenderness	241 (48)
Headache	403 (81)
Loss of appetite	388 (78)
Weight loss	326 (65)
Constipation	234 (47)
Abdominal pain	225 (45)
Diarrhea	34 (7)
Cough	122 (24)
Testicular pain/epididymoorchitis	62 (21[a])
Rash	72 (14)
Sleep disturbances	185 (37)
Ill appearance	127 (25)
Pallor	110 (22)
Lymphadenopathy	160 (32)
Splenomegaly	125 (25)
Hepatomegaly	97 (19)
Jaundice	6 (1)
Central nervous system abnormalities	20 (4)
Cardiac murmur	17 (3)
Pneumonia	7 (1)

[a] Among 290 males.

The total white cell count in synovial fluid ranges from 4000 to 40,000/mL, typically with about 60% polymorphonuclear leukocytes. The synovial fluid glucose concentration may be reduced and the protein concentration elevated; cultures of synovial fluid are positive in about 50% of cases.

Infection with *Brucella* organisms commonly causes osteomyelitis of the lumbar vertebrae, starting at the superior end plate (an area with a rich blood supply) and occasionally progressing to involve the entire vertebra, disk space, and adjacent vertebrae. Extraspinal *Brucella* osteomyelitis is rare. In *Brucella* septic arthritis and osteomyelitis, the peripheral white cell count is typically normal, while the erythrocyte sedimentation rate may be either normal or elevated.

Heart Cardiovascular complications of brucellosis include endocarditis, myocarditis, pericarditis, aortic root abscess, mycotic aneurysms, thrombophlebitis with pulmonary aneurysm, and pulmonary embolism. *Brucella* endocarditis may develop on valves previously damaged by rheumatic fever or congenital malformation but also occurs on previously normal valves. The clinical features are indistinguishable from those of endocarditis caused by other organisms (Chap. 126). Endocarditis is the leading cause of death in brucellosis, although the outcome of *Brucella* endocarditis has been more favorable in recent years because of advances in early diagnosis, antibiotic treatment, and cardiac surgery. Physicians who suspect brucellae as a cause of culture-negative endocarditis in patients with possible environmental exposure should notify the bacteriology laboratory performing the blood culture so that extended incubation, specific media, and biohazard precautions can be employed.

Respiratory Tract Brucellae can produce respiratory symptoms. A flulike illness with sore throat, tonsillitis, and dry cough is common and usually mild. Hilar and paratracheal lymphadenopathy, pneumonia, solitary or multiple pulmonary nodules, lung abscess, and empyema have been reported.

Gastrointestinal Tract and Hepatobiliary System Gastrointestinal manifestations of *Brucella* infection are generally mild and may include nausea, vomiting, constipation, acute abdominal pain, and/or diarrhea. Pathologic examination of the liver may reveal any of several changes, including noncaseating granulomas, suppurative abscesses, mononuclear cell infiltration, or hyperemia of the intestinal mucosa. Acute ileitis with inflammation of Peyer's patches and colitis have been reported. Hepatic and splenic enlargement may be documented in 15 to 20% of cases, and abscesses may develop in the liver and spleen. Infected ascites, pancreatitis, and cholecystitis have been reported. Mild jaundice may be evident, with elevated levels of bilirubin and hepatic enzymes.

Genitourinary Tract The various genitourinary infections attributed to brucellae include unilateral or bilateral epididymoorchitis, which is rarely associated with testicular abscess. Prostatitis, seminal vesiculitis, dysmenorrhea, amenorrhea, tuboovarian abscess, salpingitis, cervicitis, acute pyelonephritis, glomerulonephritis, and massive proteinuria have also been documented. *Brucella* organisms have been cultured from the urine in up to 50% of cases of genitourinary tract infection.

Central Nervous System Neurobrucellosis is uncommon but serious and includes meningitis, meningoencephalitis, multiple cerebral or cerebellar abscesses, ruptured mycotic aneurysms, myelitis, Guillain-Barré syndrome, cranial nerve lesions, hemiplegia, sciatica, myositis, and rhabdomyolysis. Papillitis, papilledema, retrobulbar neuritis, optic atrophy, and ophthalmoplegia due to lesions in cranial nerves III, IV, and VI may occur in *Brucella* meningoencephalitis. Cerebrospinal fluid (CSF) pressure is usually elevated; the fluid may appear clear, turbid, or hemorrhagic; the protein concentration and cell count (predominantly lymphocytes) are elevated; and the glucose concentration may be either reduced or normal. In *Brucella* meningitis, which can occur at any time during the course of the disease, the organism may be cultured from the CSF.

Other Manifestations Conjunctival splashing with live attenuated *B. abortus* vaccine (S19) during animal vaccination may cause conjunctivitis, keratitis, and corneal ulcers, with progression to systemic disease in some cases. Uveitis, optic neuritis, retinopathy, retinal detachment, and endophthalmitis may result from hematogenous spread.

Skin manifestations of brucellosis are uncommon. They include maculopapular eruptions, purpura and petechiae, chronic ulcerations, multiple cutaneous and subcutaneous abscesses, discharging sinuses, superficial thrombophlebitis, erythema nodosum, and pemphigus.

Brucellosis during human pregnancy can cause abortion or intrauterine fetal death. Brucellae have been isolated from the human placenta, fetus, and newborn.

The bone marrow of *Brucella*-infected patients frequently contains noncaseating granulomas. Among the hematologic complications of brucellosis are anemia, leukopenia, and thrombocytopenia.

Endocrinologic findings reported in brucellosis include thyroiditis with abscess formation, adrenal insufficiency, and the syndrome of inappropriate secretion of antidiuretic hormone.

DIAGNOSIS The combination of potential exposure, consistent clinical features, and significantly raised levels of *Brucella* agglutinin (with or without positive cultures of blood, body fluid, or tissues) confirms the diagnosis of active brucellosis. The organism's identity is confirmed by phage typing, DNA characterization, or metabolic profiling. Use of a CO_2 detection system (such as BACTEC; Becton Dickinson, Sparks, MD) for blood culture provides a more sensitive and rapid culture result than standard methods, with positivity usually apparent after only 2 to 5 days of incubation. Serum antibodies to *Brucella* can be detected by several methods, including standard tube agglutinins (STA), the 2-mercaptoethanol agglutination test, Coombs' test, enzyme-linked immunosorbent assay, and polymerase chain reaction (PCR). *B. abortus* antigens, which are commonly used for serologic tests, cross-react with *B. melitensis* and *B. suis* but not with *B. canis*. The specific antigen required for assay of antibodies to *B. canis* is not commercially available. *B. canis* antibody titers can be determined in the United States at the Centers for Disease Control and Prevention in Atlanta. A false-negative result in the STA may be obtained because of the prozone phenomenon, which can be avoided by testing of sera at both low and high dilutions.

In endemic areas a *Brucella* antibody titer of 1:320 or 1:640 is significant, while in nonendemic areas an antibody titer of 1:160 is considered significant. Detection of elevated levels of antibody to *Brucella* organisms in the absence of symptoms during the screening of potential blood donors is common in endemic areas. To establish a diagnosis in these regions, clinical and serologic evaluation should be repeated after 2 to 4 weeks and a further rise in titer sought. A high titer of specific IgM suggests recent exposure, while a high titer of specific IgG suggests active disease. Lower titers of IgG may indicate past exposure or treated infection.

Cooperation and consultation with a clinical microbiology laboratory are important when brucellosis is suspected. It may be necessary to observe culture bottles for up to 6 weeks before organisms become detectable. Subcultures should be prepared on duplicate blood agar plates (with and without an atmosphere of 10% CO_2) and special media (such as a blood- or serum-enriched peptone-based medium) or with a rapid CO_2 detection system. Patients whose blood or bone marrow is cultured are positive at one site or the other in 50 to 70% of cases. The peripheral white cell count is usually normal but may be low, with relative lymphocytosis. Thrombocytopenia and disseminated intravascular coagulation may be documented. Levels of hepatic enzymes and serum bilirubin may be raised.

Radiologic investigations aimed at detecting skeletal involvement include plain radiography, bone scintigraphy, computed tomography (CT), and magnetic resonance imaging (MRI). Bone scintigraphy is more sensitive than conventional radiography in detecting areas of spinal and extraspinal involvement, particularly in the early stage of infection. CT is useful for further evaluation of spinal lesions and of the extension of infection into the spinal canal. MRI is the modality of choice for the assessment of *Brucella* spondylitis and is more sensitive than scintigraphy or CT for demonstration of the extent of disease.

Plain lateral radiography of the spine may reveal bone sclerosis, with destruction and erosion of the superior end plate anteriorly. As the disease progresses, healing with osteophyte formation and reduction of disk space may take place. In *Brucella* septic monarthritis, plain radiography may show effusion and soft tissue swelling without bone or joint destruction. Scintigraphy may document increased uptake in sacroiliac joints or lumbar vertebrae, even when plain radiography gives normal results. MRI shows diffuse high-signal intensity of the affected vertebrae and may reveal narrowing of the spinal canal as well as loss of definition of the posterior aspect of the vertebrae.

℞ **TREATMENT**   Single-agent therapy for brucellosis has now been abandoned because of the high rates of failure and relapse and the potential development of antibiotic resistance. Relatively short courses (<8 weeks) of treatment with antibiotic combinations have similarly been associated with high rates of relapse. The combination of doxycycline and an aminoglycoside (gentamicin, streptomycin, or netilmicin) for 4 weeks followed by the combination of doxycycline and rifampin for 4 to 8 weeks is the most effective regimen. Doxycycline (which is preferred over tetracycline) is given orally in a dose of 100 mg twice daily. Gentamicin is given intramuscularly or as a slow intravenous infusion (3 to 5 mg/kg per day in divided doses every 8 h). Netilmicin (which is preferred to streptomycin) is given (intramuscularly to outpatients, intravenously to inpatients) in a dose of 2 mg/kg every 12 h; trough levels in plasma should be monitored regularly and maintained at ≤2 μg/mL. Streptomycin is given intramuscularly in a dose of 1 g once daily to patients under 45 years of age and in a dose of 0.5 to 0.75 g/d to older patients. Tetracycline is given orally in a dose of 250 mg every 6 h and rifampin as a single daily dose of 600 to 900 mg. An alternative regimen consists of the doxycycline/rifampin combination given for 8 to 12 weeks. The doxycycline/aminoglycoside combination is more effective than the doxycycline/rifampin combination in that rifampin reduces levels of doxycycline in plasma.

Patients with serious complications of brucellosis require urgent surgical and medical treatment. These complications include endocarditis, aortic root abscesses, mycotic aortic aneurysms, meningitis, cerebral or cerebellar abscesses, spinal or extraspinal osteomyelitis, and liver or splenic abscess. These patients should be hospitalized and given first a three-drug regimen—i.e., oral doxycycline with intravenous aminoglycoside and rifampin—for 4 weeks and then a two-drug regimen—i.e., doxycycline and rifampin—for 8 to 12 weeks. In instances of renal failure, doxycycline (at adjusted doses) can be used safely. In contrast, the use of aminoglycosides requires facilities for the monitoring of plasma levels; if such facilities are not available, then the doxycycline/rifampin combination should be administered for 8 to 12 weeks.

When used alone, fluoroquinolones (which exhibit good intracellular penetration and efficacy against *Brucella* organisms in vitro) have been associated with the development of quinolone resistance and with high rates of failure and relapse. At present, clinical data are inadequate for the formulation of recommendations regarding the combination of fluoroquinolones with doxycycline, rifampin, or streptomycin.

Third-generation cephalosporins (e.g., ceftriaxone), although active in vitro against brucellae when used alone, have also been associated with a high incidence of clinical failure and relapse. These agents may be useful in combination with other drugs for the treatment of *Brucella* meningitis.

In pregnancy, trimethoprim-sulfamethoxazole (TMP-SMZ) can be given in combination with rifampin for 8 to 12 weeks. The TMP-SMZ dosage appropriate for pregnant women is two or three tablets every 12 h (each tablet contains 80 mg of TMP and 400 mg of SMZ). Children below the age of 8 years can also be treated with rifampin and TMP-SMZ for 8 to 12 weeks, while older children should receive the same antibiotics as adults in the following doses: doxycycline, 100 mg/d orally; an aminoglycoside (gentamicin, 2 mg/kg per day in divided doses every 8 h); and rifampin, 15 mg/kg per day orally or by slow intravenous infusion. TMP-SMZ is given orally every 12 h in a dose that depends on the patient's age (birth to 6 months, 120 mg; 6 months to 6 years, 240 mg).

Within 4 to 14 days after the initiation of therapy, patients become afebrile and constitutional symptoms disappear. The enlarged liver and spleen return to their normal size within 2 to 4 weeks. An acute, intense flare-up of symptoms may follow the start of treatment, especially that with tetracyclines. This reaction is transient and does not necessitate the discontinuation of therapy. In endemic areas the coexistence of brucellosis and tuberculous spondylitis may result in a failure to respond to appropriate treatment. Treated patients whose infections are apparently cured should be followed clinically and serologically, with repeat blood cultures, every 3 to 6 months for 2 years.

PREVENTION   Efforts at prevention should be aimed at the source of infection. Immunization of animals and boiling or pasteurization of milk and milk products are important. Workers in the meat and dairy industries in the former Soviet Union, China, and France have been vaccinated; the vaccine (two injections given 2 weeks apart, each containing 1 mg of an insoluble fraction of phenol-extracted bacteria) markedly reduces the rate of infection. However, the vaccine induces fever in 6% of recipients and severe pain at the injection site in 16%. Moreover, immunity is short-lived, and vaccination should be repeated every 2 years. This vaccine is not used in the United States.

PROGNOSIS   Deaths attributable to brucellosis should be avoidable. Even before the discovery of antibiotics, the mortality rate was <2% and endocarditis was most frequently the cause of death. Morbidity due to brucellosis remains significant; its severity depends on the infecting *Brucella* species and is greatest with *B. melitensis*. Spinal damage, paraplegia, and other neurologic deficits may occur. Nerve deafness due to meningitis or secondary to treatment with streptomycin has been documented.

BIBLIOGRAPHY

BANNATYNE RM et al: Rapid diagnosis of *Brucella* bacteremia by using BACTEC 9240 system. J Clin Microbiol 35:673, 1997

CORBEL MJ: Recent advances in brucellosis. J Med Microbiol 46:101, 1997

FRANZ DR et al: Clinical recognition and management of patients exposed to biological warfare agents. JAMA 278:399, 1997

JIANG X, BALDWIN CL: Effect of cytokines on intracellular growth of *Brucella abortus*. Infect Immun 61:124, 1993

LIAUTARD JP et al: Interaction between professional phagocytes and *Brucella* spp. Microbiologia 12:197, 1996

MADKOUR MM: *Brucellosis*. London, Butterworths, 1989

——— et al: Osteoarticular brucellosis: Results of bone scintigraphy in 140 patients. Am J Roentgenol 150:1101, 1988

SIFUENTES RICON AM et al: Detection and differentiation of six *Brucella* species by PCR. Mol Med 3:734, 1997

SOLERA J et al: Doxycycline-rifampin versus doxycycline-streptomycin in treatment of human brucellosis due to *Brucella melitensis*. Antimicrob Agents Chemother 39: 2061, 1995

SOLERA L et al: Multivariate model for predicting relapse in human brucellosis. J Infect 36:85, 1998

161

Richard F. Jacobs

TULAREMIA

DEFINITION Tularemia is a zoonosis caused by *Francisella tularensis*, so named in 1974 in recognition of the contributions of Edward Francis. Humans of any age, sex, or race are universally susceptible to this systemic infection. Tularemia is primarily a disease of wild animals and persists in contaminated environments, ectoparasites, and animal carriers. Human infection is incidental and usually results from interaction with biting or blood-sucking insects, wild or domestic animals, or the environment. Tularemia is common in Arkansas, Oklahoma, and Missouri, where more than 50% of the cases in the United States occur. An increasing number of cases of tularemia have been reported from the Scandinavian countries, eastern Europe, and Siberia. The illness is characterized by various clinical syndromes, the most common of which consists of an ulcerative lesion at the site of inoculation, with regional lymphadenopathy and lymphadenitis. Systemic manifestations, including pneumonia, typhoidal tularemia, and fever without localizing findings, pose a greater diagnostic challenge.

ETIOLOGY AND EPIDEMIOLOGY *F. tularensis* is the etiologic agent of tularemia, which, with rare exceptions, is the only disease produced by this genus. The organism is a small, gram-negative, pleomorphic, nonmotile, non-spore-forming bacillus measuring 0.2 μm by 0.2 to 0.7 μm. Bipolar staining results in a coccoid appearance. The organism is a thinly encapsulated, nonpiliated strict aerobe that invades host cells.

In nature, *F. tularensis* is a hardy organism that persists for weeks or months in mud, water, and decaying animal carcasses. Dozens of biting and blood-sucking insects, especially ticks and tabanid flies, serve as vectors. Ticks and wild rabbits are the source for most of the human cases in the endemic areas of the southeastern United States and the Rocky Mountain states. In Utah, Nevada, and California, tabanid flies are the most common vectors. Animal reservoirs include wild rabbits, squirrels, birds, sheep, beavers, muskrats, and domestic dogs and cats.

The two main biovars of *F. tularensis*—*tularensis* (type A) and *palearctica* (type B)—are both found in the United States. Type A produces more serious disease in humans; without treatment, the associated fatality rate is approximately 5%. Type B produces a milder, often subclinical infection that is usually contracted from water or marine mammals. Although all strains appear serologically identical, individual strains may possess varying degrees of virulence. *F. tularensis* does not produce an exotoxin, but an endotoxin similar to that of other gram-negative bacilli has been identified. The progression of illness depends upon the organism's virulence, the inoculum size, the portal of entry, and the host's immune status.

Ticks pass the organism to their offspring via a transovarian route. The organism is found in tick feces but not in large quantities in tick salivary glands. In the United States, the disease can be carried by *Dermacentor andersoni* (Rocky Mountain wood tick), *D. variabilis* (American dog tick), *D. occidentalis* (Pacific coast dog tick), and *Amblyomma americanum* (Lone Star tick). *F. tularensis* is transmitted frequently during blood meals taken by embedded ticks following hours of attachment. It is the taking of a blood meal through a fecally contaminated field that transmits the organism. Tularemia is more common among men than among women. Person-to-person transmission is rare or nonexistent. Transmission of the organism by ticks and tabanid flies takes place mainly in the spring and summer. However, continued transmission in the winter months by trapped or hunted animals has been documented. The organism is extremely infectious. Biosafety level 2 is recommended for clinical laboratory work with material whose contamination is suspected, and biosafety level 3 is required for culture of the organism in large quantities.

PATHOGENESIS AND PATHOLOGY The most common portal of entry for human infection is through skin or mucous membranes, either directly—through the bite of ticks, other arthropods, or other animals—or via inapparent abrasions. Inhalation or ingestion of *F. tularensis* can also result in infection. Although more than 10^8 organisms are usually required to produce infection via the oral route (oropharyngeal or gastrointestinal tularemia), fewer than 50 organisms will result in infection when injected into the skin (ulceroglandular/glandular tularemia) or inhaled (pneumonia). After inoculation into the skin, the organism multiplies locally; within 2 to 5 days (range, 1 to 10 days), it produces an erythematous, tender, or pruritic papule. The papule rapidly enlarges and forms an ulcer with a black base (chancriform lesion). The bacteria spread to regional lymph nodes, producing lymphadenopathy (buboes), and, with bacteremia, may spread to distant organs.

Tularemia is characterized by mononuclear cell infiltration with pyogranulomatous pathology. The histopathologic findings can be quite similar to those in tuberculosis, although tularemia develops more rapidly. As a facultatively intracellular bacterium, *F. tularensis* can parasitize both phagocytic and nonphagocytic host cells and survive intracellularly for prolonged periods. In the acute phase of infection, the primary organs affected (skin, lymph nodes, liver, and spleen) include areas of focal necrosis, initially surrounded by polymorphonuclear leukocytes (PMNs). Subsequently, granulomas form, with epithelioid cells, lymphocytes, and multinucleated giant cells surrounded by areas of necrosis. These areas may resemble caseation necrosis but later coalesce to form abscesses.

Conjunctival inoculation can result in infection of the eye, with regional lymph node enlargement (preauricular lymphadenopathy, Parinaud's complex). Aerosolization and inhalation or hematogenous spread of organisms can result in pneumonia. In the lung, an inflammatory reaction—including foci of alveolar necrosis and cell infiltration (initially polymorphonuclear and later mononuclear) with granulomas—develops. Chest roentgenograms usually reveal bilateral patchy infiltrates rather than large areas of consolidation. Pleural effusions are common and may contain blood. Lymphadenopathy occurs in regions draining infected organs. Therefore, in pulmonary infection, mediastinal adenopathy may be evident, while patients with oropharyngeal tularemia develop cervical lymphadenopathy. In gastrointestinal or typhoidal tularemia, mesenteric lymphadenopathy may follow the ingestion of large numbers of organisms. The term *typhoidal tularemia* may be used to describe severe bacteremic disease, irrespective of the mode of transmission or portal of entry. Meningitis has been reported as a primary or secondary manifestation of bacteremia. Patients may also present with fever and no localizing signs.

IMMUNOLOGY Infection with *F. tularensis* stimulates the host to produce antibodies. However, this antibody response probably plays only a minor role in the containment of infection. In contrast, cell-mediated immunity, which develops over 2 to 4 weeks, plays a major role in containment and eradication of the infection. Macrophages, once activated, are capable of killing *F. tularensis*.

Immunospecific protection against tularemia can be afforded either by natural infection or by vaccination with live attenuated strains of *F. tularensis*. Killed vaccines, on the other hand, induce no protection against virulent *F. tularensis*. After natural infection or vaccination, serum antibodies to surface-exposed carbohydrate antigens predominate, whereas T cell determinants are located on membrane proteins beneath the bacterial capsule. T cell responses are thought to be due to priming by the organism. The anamnestic T cell response to *F. tularensis* seems to involve a multitude of microbial proteins, each with a distinct set of T cell determinants. A predominant role for CD4+ T cells is supported by the results of experiments in mice, which indicated that resistance to infection was restricted at the level of the MHC class II determinants. Humans primed to *F. tularensis* (like those primed to *Mycobacterium tuberculosis*) show a T_H1-like response. T cell proliferation is associated with the production of interleukin (IL) 2 and interferon γ but with little or no production of IL-4.

Investigations of neutrophils in cases of tularemia have suggested that PMNs are needed for defense against primary infection. PMNs may restrict the growth of *F. tularensis* before the organism becomes intracellular.

CLINICAL MANIFESTATIONS Tularemia often starts with a sudden onset of fever, chills, headache, and generalized myalgias and arthralgias (Table 161-1). This onset takes place when the organism penetrates the skin, is ingested, or is inhaled. An incubation period of 2 to 10 days is followed by the formation of an ulcer at the site of penetration, with local inflammation. The ulcer may persist for several months as organisms are transported via the lymphatics to the regional lymph nodes. These nodes enlarge and may become necrotic and suppurative. If the organism enters the bloodstream, widespread dissemination as well as signs and symptoms of endotoxemia may result.

In the United States, most patients with tularemia (75 to 85%) acquire the infection by inoculation of the skin. In adults, the most common localized form is inguinal/femoral lymphadenopathy; in children, it is cervical lymphadenopathy. About 20% of patients develop a generalized maculopapular rash, which occasionally becomes pustular. Erythema nodosum occurs infrequently. The clinical manifestations of tularemia have been divided into various syndromes, which are listed in Table 161-2.

Ulceroglandular/Glandular Tularemia These two forms of tularemia account for approximately 75 to 85% of cases. The predominant form in children involves cervical or posterior auricular lymphadenopathy and is usually related to tick bites on the head and neck. In adults, the most common form is inguinal/femoral lymphadenopathy resulting from insect and tick exposures on the lower limbs. In cases related to wild game, the usual portal of entry for *F. tularensis* is either an injury sustained while skinning or cleaning an animal carcass or a bite (usually on the hand). Epitrochlear lymphadenopathy/lymphadenitis is common in patients with bite-related injuries.

In ulceroglandular tularemia, the ulcer is erythematous, indurated, and nonhealing, with a punched-out appearance that lasts from 1 to 3 weeks. The papule may begin as an erythematous lesion that is tender or pruritic; it evolves over several days into an ulcer with sharply demarcated edges and a yellow exudate. The ulcer gradually develops a black base, and simultaneously the regional lymph nodes become tender and severely enlarged (Fig. 161-1). The affected lymph nodes may become fluctuant and drain spontaneously, but usually the con-

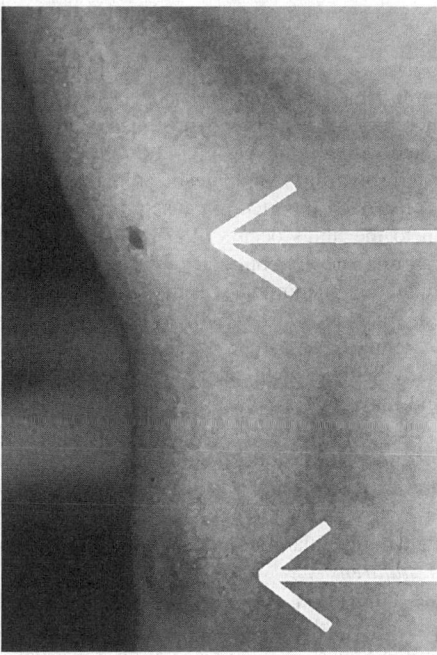

FIGURE 161-1 An ulcerative lesion *(lower arrow)* with adjacent lymphadenitis *(upper arrow)* on the lateral chest wall of a patient with ulceroglandular tularemia.

dition resolves with effective treatment. Late suppuration of lymph nodes has been described in up to 25% of patients with ulceroglandular/glandular tularemia. Examination of material taken from these late fluctuant nodes after successful antimicrobial treatment has revealed sterile necrotic tissue. In 5 to 10% of patients, the skin lesion may be inapparent, with lymphadenopathy plus systemic signs and symptoms the only physical findings. This clinical syndrome is designated *glandular tularemia*. Conversely, a tick or deerfly bite on the trunk may result in an ulcer without evident lymphadenopathy.

Oculoglandular Tularemia In about 1% of patients, the portal of entry for *F. tularensis* is the conjunctiva. Usually, the organism reaches the conjunctiva through contact with contaminated fingers. The inflamed conjunctiva is painful, with numerous yellowish nodules and pinpoint ulcers. Purulent conjunctivitis with regional lymphadenopathy (preauricular, submandibular, or cervical) is evident. Because of debilitating pain, the patient may seek medical attention before regional lymphadenopathy develops. Painful preauricular lymphadenopathy is unique to tularemia and distinguishes it from cat-scratch disease, tuberculosis, sporotrichosis, and syphilis. Corneal perforation may occur.

Oropharyngeal and Gastrointestinal Tularemia Rarely, tularemia follows the ingestion of contaminated undercooked meat, the oral inoculation of *F. tularensis* from the hands in association with the skinning and cleaning of animal carcasses, or the consumption of contaminated food or water. Oral inoculation may result in acute, exudative, or membranous pharyngitis associated with cervical lymphadenopathy or in ulcerative intestinal lesions associated with mesenteric lymphadenopathy, diarrhea, abdominal pain, nausea, vomiting, and gastrointestinal bleeding. Infected tonsils become enlarged and develop a yellowish-white pseudomembrane, which can be confused with that of diphtheria. The clinical severity of gastrointestinal tularemia varies from mild, unexplained, persistent diarrhea with no other symptoms to a rapidly fulminant, fatal disease. In fatal cases, the extensive intestinal ulceration found at autopsy suggests an enormous inoculum.

Pulmonary Tularemia Tularemia pneumonia presents as variable parenchymal infiltrates that are unresponsive to treatment with β-lactam antibiotics. Tularemia must be considered in the differential

Table 161-1 Clinical Presentation of Tularemia

| | Rate of Occurrence, % | |
Sign or Symptom	Children	Adults
Lymphadenopathy	96	65
Fever (≥38.3°C or ≥101°F)	87	21
Ulcer/eschar/papule	45	51
Myalgias/arthralgias	39	2
Headache	9	5
Cough	9	5
Pharyngitis	43	—
Diarrhea	43	—

SOURCE: Adapted from Jacobs and Narain (1985).

Table 161-2 Clinical Syndromes of Tularemia

| | Rate of Occurrence, % | |
Syndrome	Children	Adults
Ulceroglandular	45	51
Glandular	25	12
Pulmonary (pneumonia)	14	18
Oropharyngeal	4	—
Oculoglandular	2	—
Typhoidal	2	12
Unclassified	6	11

SOURCE: Adapted from Jacobs and Narain (1985).

diagnosis of atypical pneumonia in a patient with a history of travel to an endemic area. The disease can result from either inhalation of an infectious aerosol or spread to the lungs and pleura after bloodstream dissemination. Inhalation-related pneumonia has been described in laboratory workers after exposure to contaminated materials and is associated with a relatively high mortality rate. Exposure to *F. tularensis* in aerosols from live domestic animals or dead wildlife (including birds) has been reported to cause pneumonia. Hematogenous dissemination to the lungs occurs in 10 to 15% of cases of ulceroglandular tularemia and in about half of cases of typhoidal tularemia. Previously, tularemia pneumonia was thought to be a disease of older patients, but as many as 10 to 15% of children with clinical manifestations of tularemia have parenchymal infiltrates detected by chest roentgenography. Patients with pneumonia usually have a nonproductive cough and may have dyspnea or pleuritic chest pain. Roentgenograms of the chest usually reveal bilateral patchy infiltrates (described as ovoid or lobar densities), lobar parenchymal infiltrates, and cavitary lesions. Pleural effusions may have a predominance of mononuclear leukocytes or PMNs and sometimes red blood cells. Empyema may develop. Patients with tularemia pneumonia can have blood cultures positive for *F. tularensis*.

Typhoidal Tularemia   Once thought to represent up to 10% of all cases of tularemia, the typhoidal presentation is now considered rare in the United States. In this presentation, fever develops without apparent skin lesions or lymphadenopathy. In the absence of a history of possible contact with a vector, diagnosis can be extremely difficult. Blood cultures may be positive and patients may present with classic sepsis or septic shock in this acute systemic form of the infection. Typhoidal tularemia is usually associated with a huge inoculum or with a preexisting compromising condition. High continuous fevers, signs of endotoxemia, and severe headache are common findings. The patient may be delirious and may develop prostration and shock. If presumptive antibiotic therapy in culture-negative cases does not include an aminoglycoside, the mortality rate can approach 30%.

Other Manifestations   *F. tularensis* infection has been associated with meningitis, pericarditis, hepatitis, peritonitis, endocarditis, osteomyelitis, and sepsis and septic shock with rhabdomyolysis and acute renal failure. In the rare cases of tularemia meningitis, a predominantly lymphocytic response is demonstrated in cerebrospinal fluid.

DIFFERENTIAL DIAGNOSIS   When patients in endemic areas present with fever, chronic ulcerative skin lesions, and large tender lymph nodes, a diagnosis of tularemia should be made presumptively, and confirmatory diagnostic testing and appropriate therapy should be undertaken. When the possibility of tularemia is considered in a patient with this presentation in a nonendemic area, an attempt should be made to determine whether the individual has come into contact with a potential animal vector. The level of suspicion of tularemia should be especially high in hunters, trappers, game wardens, veterinarians, laboratory workers, and individuals with a history of exposure to an insect or another animal vector. However, up to 40% of patients with tularemia have no known history of epidemiologic contact with an animal vector.

The characteristic presentation of ulceroglandular tularemia does not pose a diagnostic problem, but a less classic progression of regional lymphadenopathy or glandular tularemia must be differentiated from other diseases. The skin lesion may resemble those seen in sporotrichosis; skin infection with *Staphylococcus aureus*, *Streptococcus pyogenes*, or *Mycobacterium marinum*; syphilis; anthrax; rat-bite fever (due to *Spirillum minus*); or rickettsiosis (scrub typhus). In the latter infections, regional lymphadenopathy is usually not as impressive as in tularemia. The lymphadenopathy of tularemia (especially glandular tularemia) must be differentiated from that of plague, lymphogranuloma venereum, and cat-scratch disease. In children, the differentiation from cat-scratch disease is made more difficult by the chronic papulovesicular lesion associated with *Bartonella henselae* infection (Chap. 163).

Oropharyngeal tularemia can resemble and must be differentiated from pharyngitis due to group A β-hemolytic streptococci, *Arcanobacterium haemolyticum*, or *Corynebacterium diphtheriae* as well as from infectious mononucleosis. Tularemia pneumonia may resemble any of the atypical pneumonias, including those due to various viruses, *Mycoplasma pneumoniae*, *Chlamydia pneumoniae*, *C. psittaci*, *Legionella pneumophila*, *Coxiella burnetii*, and (occasionally) *Histoplasma capsulatum*. Typhoidal tularemia may resemble typhoid fever, other *Salmonella* bacteremias, rickettsial infections (Rocky Mountain spotted fever, ehrlichiosis), brucellosis, infectious mononucleosis, acquired toxoplasmosis, miliary tuberculosis, sarcoidosis, and hematologic or reticuloendothelial malignancies.

LABORATORY DIAGNOSIS   Direct microscopic examination of polychromatically stained tissue smears or clinical specimens reveals *F. tularensis* organisms, singly and in groups, both intra- and extracellularly. Gram's staining of clinical or biopsy material is of little value, as the small, weakly staining organisms cannot be readily distinguished from the background. An indirect fluorescent antibody test with commercially available antisera can be useful, although false-positive results due to *Legionella* spp. have been reported.

The diagnosis of tularemia is most frequently confirmed by serologic testing. In the standard tube agglutination test, a single titer of $\geq$1:160 is interpreted as a presumptive positive result. A fourfold increase in titer between paired serum samples collected 2 to 3 weeks apart is considered diagnostic. False-negative serologic responses are obtained early in infection; up to 30% of patients infected for 3 weeks have sera that test negative. Late in infection, titers into the thousands are common, and titers of 1:20 to 1:80 may persist for years. A microagglutination test that may be as much as 100-fold more sensitive than the standard tube agglutination test has been described and is currently being used in many clinical microbiology laboratories. Enzyme-linked immunosorbent assays have proven useful for the detection of both antibodies and antigens. Analysis of urine for *F. tularensis* antigen has yielded promising results in clinical trials, but facilities for this type of analysis are not widely available. A skin test for delayed hypersensitivity to *F. tularensis* turns positive during the first week of illness and remains positive for years. The skin-test antigen, which is not commercially available, can boost titers of agglutinating antibody.

Culture and isolation of *F. tularensis* are difficult. In one study the organism was isolated in only 10% of more than 1000 human cases, 84% of which were confirmed by serology. The medium of choice is cysteine-glucose-blood agar. *F. tularensis* can be isolated directly from infected ulcer scrapings, lymph-node biopsy specimens, gastric washings, sputum, and blood cultures. Colonies are blue-gray, round, smooth, and slightly mucoid. On media containing blood, a small zone of α hemolysis usually surrounds the colony. Slide agglutination tests or direct fluorescent antibody tests with commercially available antisera can be applied directly to culture suspensions for identification.

The polymerase chain reaction (PCR) has been used to detect *F. tularensis* DNA. During a recent outbreak, a multiplex PCR was used to target 16S rRNA and to diagnose ulceroglandular tularemia with DNA extracted from wound swabs; the PCR result was positive in 29 (73%) of 40 serologically confirmed cases. However, this test has not been shown to be more sensitive than direct culture and at present remains a research tool.

TREATMENT   *F. tularensis* cannot be subjected to standardized antimicrobial susceptibility testing because the organism will not grow on the media used. A wide variety of antibiotics, including all β-lactam antibiotics and the newer cephalosporins, are ineffective for the treatment of this infection. Several studies indicated that third-generation cephalosporins were active against *F. tularensis* in vitro, but clinical case reports suggested a nearly universal failure rate of ceftriaxone in pediatric patients with tularemia. Although in vitro data indicate that imipenem may be active, therapy with imipenem, sulfanilamides, and macrolides is not presently recommended because of the lack of relevant clinical data. Fluoroquinolones have shown promise in terms of their relatively low toxicity and their potential for oral administration. Chloramphenicol and tetracycline have been successfully for treatment of the acute stages of tularemia but have been associated with higher relapse rates (up to 20%) than conventionally used agents.

Streptomycin, given intramuscularly at a dose of 7.5 to 10 mg/kg every 12 h, is considered the drug of choice for adults. In severe cases, 15 mg/kg every 12 h may be used for the first 48 to 72 h. Streptomycin is also considered the drug of choice for children; the appropriate dose is 30 to 40 mg/kg daily in two divided doses administered intramuscularly. In children, after a clinical response is demonstrated at 3 to 5 days, the dose can be reduced to 10 to 15 mg/kg daily in two divided doses. Therapy is typically continued for 7 to 10 days; however, in mild to moderate cases of tularemia in which the patient becomes afebrile within the first 48 to 72 h of streptomycin treatment, a 5- to 7-day course has been successful.

Gentamicin, at a dose of 1.7 mg/kg given intravenously or intramuscularly every 8 h, is also effective. The published experience in adults consists of two reports describing, respectively, nine and eight patients who were treated effectively with gentamicin. The eight patients in one of the reports all had fever before treatment, and all eight became afebrile within 24 to 72 h. In a recent pediatric study, other symptoms, such as tender lymphadenitis and pharyngitis, also responded within 24 to 72 h of the start of gentamicin therapy.

Virtually all strains of *F. tularensis* are susceptible to streptomycin and gentamicin. In successfully treated patients, defervescence usually occurs within 2 days, but skin lesions and lymph nodes may take 1 to 2 weeks to heal. When therapy is not initiated within the first several days of illness, defervescence may be delayed. Relapses are uncommon with streptomycin or gentamicin therapy. Late lymph-node suppuration, however, occurs in approximately 40% of children, regardless of the treatment received. These nodes have typically been found to contain sterile necrotic tissue without evidence of active infection. Patients with fluctuant nodes should receive several days of antibiotic therapy before drainage to minimize the risk to hospital personnel. Unlike streptomycin and gentamicin, tobramycin is ineffective in the treatment of tularemia and should not be used.

PROGNOSIS If tularemia goes untreated, symptoms usually last 1 to 4 weeks but may continue for months. The mortality rate from severe untreated infection (including all cases of untreated tularemia pneumonia and typhoidal tularemia) can be as high as 30%. However, the overall mortality rate for untreated tularemia is <8%. Mortality is <1% with appropriate treatment. Poor outcomes are often associated with long delays in diagnosis and treatment. Lifelong immunity usually follows tularemia.

PREVENTION The prevention of tularemia is based on avoidance of exposure to biting and blood-sucking insects, especially ticks and deerflies. An intradermal vaccine made from live attenuated *F. tularensis* is available from the Centers for Disease Control and Prevention. This vaccine is effective in reducing the frequency and severity of infection. Vaccination of high-risk individuals working with large quantities of cultured organisms is recommended. Others who come into contact with the organisms, such as veterinarians, hunters, or game wardens, should consider vaccination, particularly if they live in endemic areas. The avoidance of skinning wild animals, especially rabbits, and the wearing of gloves while handling animal carcasses decrease the risk of transmission. Use of insect repellents and preparations that prevent tick attachment as well as prompt removal of ticks can be helpful. Prophylaxis of tularemia has not proved effective in patients with embedded ticks or insect bites. However, in patients who are known to have been exposed to large quantities of organisms (e.g., in the laboratory) and who have incubating infection with *F. tularensis*, early treatment can prevent the development of significant clinical disease.

BIBLIOGRAPHY

CROSS JT, JACOBS RF: Tularemia: Treatment failures with outpatient use of ceftriaxone. Clin Infect Dis 17:976, 1993

ENDERLIN G et al: Streptomycin and alternative agents for the treatment of tularemia: Review of the literature. Clin Infect Dis 19:42, 1994

JACOBS RF, NARAIN JP: Tularemia in children. Pediatr Infect Dis J 2:487, 1983

——, ——: Tularemia in adults and children: A changing presentation. Pediatrics 76:818, 1985

LONG GW et al: Detection of *Francisella tularensis* in blood by polymerase chain reaction. J Clin Microbiol 31:152, 1993

SCHEEL O et al: Treatment of tularemia with ciprofloxacin. Eur J Microbiol Infect Dis 11: 447, 1992

SJOSTEDT A et al: Detection of *Francisella tularensis* in ulcers of patients with tularemia by PCR. J Clin Microbiol 35:1045, 1997

TAYLOR JP et al: Epidemiologic characteristics of human tularemia in the southwest-central states, 1981–1987. Am J Epidemiol 133:1032, 1991

162 *Grant L. Campbell, David T. Dennis*

PLAGUE AND OTHER *YERSINIA* INFECTIONS

PLAGUE

DEFINITION Plague is an acute, febrile, zoonotic disease caused by infection with *Yersinia pestis*. Although human cases are infrequent and are curable with antibiotics, plague is one of the most virulent and potentially lethal bacterial diseases known. The plague bacterium occurs in widely scattered foci in Asia, Africa, and the Americas, where its usual hosts are wild and peridomestic rodents. It is transmitted to humans typically by flea bite and less commonly by direct contact with infected animal tissues or by airborne droplet. The principal clinical forms of plague are bubonic, septicemic, and pneumonic. Although most cases are now sporadic, occurring singly or in small clusters, the potential for epidemic spread remains.

ETIOLOGIC AGENT *Y. pestis* is a gram-negative coccobacillus in the family Enterobacteriaceae. It is microaerophilic, nonmotile, nonsporulating, oxidase and urease negative, and biochemically unreactive. The organism is nonfastidious and infective for laboratory rodents. It grows well, if slowly, on routinely used microbiologic media (e.g., sheep blood agar, brain-heart infusion broth, and MacConkey agar). *Y. pestis* can multiply within a wide range of temperatures (−2°C to 45°C) and pH values (5.0 to 9.6), but optimal growth occurs at 28°C and at pH ~7.4. When incubated on agar plates at 37°C, colonies are pinpoint in size at 24 h and 1 to 2 mm in diameter at 48 h. The colonies are gray-white with irregular surfaces, described as having a "hammered-metal" appearance when viewed microscopically. In broth culture, *Y. pestis* grows without turbidity in clumps clinging to the sides of tubes. When stained with a polychromatic stain (e.g., Wayson or Giemsa), *Y. pestis* isolated from clinical specimens exhibits a characteristic bipolar appearance, often resembling closed safety pins. The bacterium is nonencapsulated but when grown at ≥30°C produces a plasmid-expressed immunogenic envelope glycoprotein, fraction 1 (F1).

HISTORIC BACKGROUND Plague's deadly epidemic potential is notorious and well documented. The Justinian pandemic (542 to 767 A.D.) spread from central Africa to the Mediterranean littoral and thence to Asia Minor, causing an estimated 40 million deaths. The second pandemic began in central Asia, was carried to Sicily by ship from Constantinople in 1347, and swept through Europe and the British Isles in successive waves over the next four centuries. At its height, it killed as many as a quarter of the affected population and became known as the Black Death. In the third (modern) pandemic, plague appeared in Yunnan, China, in the latter half of the nineteenth century; established itself in Hong Kong in 1894; and spread by ship to Bombay in 1896 and subsequently to major port cities throughout the world, including San Francisco and several other West Coast and Gulf Coast ports in the United States. The plague bacillus was first cultured by

Alexandre Yersin in Hong Kong in 1894. In 1898, Paul-Louis Simond, a French scientist sent to investigate epidemic bubonic plague in Bombay, identified the bacillus in the tissues of dead rats and proposed transmission by rat fleas. Waldemar Haffkine, also in Bombay at that time, developed a crude vaccine.

By 1910, plague had circled the globe and established itself in rodent populations on all inhabited continents other than Australia. After 1920, however, the spread of plague was largely halted by international regulations that mandated control of rats in harbors and inspection and rat-proofing of ships. Before the third pandemic subsided, it resulted in an estimated 26 million plague cases and more than 12 million deaths, the vast majority in India. By 1950, plague outbreaks around the world had become isolated, sporadic, and manageable with modern techniques of surveillance, flea and rat control, and antimicrobial treatment of patients. Plague has nearly disappeared from cities and now occurs mostly in rural and semirural areas, where it is maintained in various rodents and their fleas. In the United States, the last outbreak of urban plague occurred in Los Angeles in 1924 and 1925, and human cases since then have resulted from animal plague exposures in rural areas of western states.

Because of its pandemic history, plague remains one of three quarantinable diseases subject to international health regulations (the other two being cholera and yellow fever). The alarm that plague is still able to evoke was highlighted by the public panic over an exaggerated international response to purported outbreaks of bubonic and pneumonic plague in India in 1994. The plague bacillus is considered to have a high potential for use in biologic terrorism; the agent is available around the world, has been "weaponized" for airborne delivery, and would be expected to cause a high primary fatality rate as well as secondary spread among an affected population.

EPIDEMIOLOGY *Y. pestis* is maintained in enzootic cycles involving relatively resistant wild rodents and their fleas in mostly remote, lightly populated areas of Asia, Africa, and the Americas and in limited rural foci in extreme southeastern Europe near the Caspian Sea. Humans and other nonrodent mammals are incidental hosts. Enzootic transmission places humans at low risk, and cases are typically infrequent and sporadic. Epizootic transmission involving susceptible rodents and efficient flea vectors (both are amplifying hosts) results in local or even widespread depopulation of susceptible rodents and poses a more serious threat to humans than does enzootic transmission. In the United States, the principal epizootic hosts are various ground squirrels, prairie dogs, and chipmunks; a variety of burrowing rodents act as epizootic hosts in rural areas elsewhere in the world. *Y. pestis* occasionally spills over from wild rodents to rat species that inhabit cultivated fields and adjacent homes, villages, and towns. The organism can then be transported from towns to cities by these highly adaptable rats and their fleas. Urban plague is currently reported sporadically from a few countries such as Vietnam, Myanmar, and Madagascar.

Plague in populated areas is most likely to develop when sanitation is poor and rats are numerous—especially the common black or roof rat (*Rattus rattus*), its close relatives, and the larger brown sewer or Norway rat (*R. norvegicus*). A high mortality rate from plague in these susceptible rat populations forces their fleas to seek alternative hosts, including humans. The cosmopolitan oriental rat flea *Xenopsylla cheopis* and (in southern Africa and Brazil) the related species *X. brasiliensis* are efficient vectors of the plague bacillus among rats and are also efficient vectors to humans. *Y. pestis* can multiply to enormous numbers in the foregut (proventriculus) of these fleas, resulting in a bolus of organisms and clotted blood that blocks the passage of subsequent blood meals. This situation occurs only at temperatures of ≤28°C and depends on a single protease expressed by the plasminogen activator (*pla*) gene of a 9.5-kb plasmid of *Y. pestis*. Regurgitation by a "blocked" flea while it feeds facilitates transmission of the plague bacillus to the new host.

Except for large outbreaks of pneumonic plague in Manchuria in

the early part of the twentieth century, person-to-person respiratory transmission of plague during and since the third pandemic has occurred only sporadically and has been limited to clusters of close contacts of pneumonic plague patients, such as household members and caregivers. The 1994 outbreak of pneumonic plague in the city of Surat, India, although reported to be extensive, most likely involved fewer than 100 cases and 50 deaths; in 1998, a small outbreak of pneumonic plague occurred in the Ecuadoran Andes.

International health regulations require that national health authorities immediately report plague cases to the World Health Organization. From 1982 through 1996, 23,904 human plague cases and 2105 deaths (mortality, 9%) were reported by 24 countries. In the same 15-year period, the United States reported 212 plague cases (mean, 14 cases per year) and 27 deaths (mortality, 13%). Cases reported by the United States are confirmed by the plague laboratory of the Centers for Disease Control and Prevention (CDC). Animal plague occurs in 17 contiguous western states, extending from the Great Plains states and eastern Texas to the Pacific Coast; around 80% of human cases in this country now occur in New Mexico, Arizona, and Colorado and around 10% in California. Although plague in the United States is a rural disease, more than 50% of cases are thought to be caused by peridomestic exposures, especially in the southwestern states, where homes are often situated in natural surroundings that provide a favorable habitat for plague-susceptible animals (such as rock squirrels and wood rats) and their fleas. In the Sierra Nevadas of California and Nevada, epizootic plague in chipmunks and ground squirrels poses a risk to visitors in public parks. Hikers, campers, and hunters in natural areas throughout the western states are at a small but finite risk of exposure to plague, especially in the summer months.

Plague can be transmitted during the skinning and handling of carcasses of wild animals such as rabbits and hares, prairie dogs, wildcats, and coyotes. Such direct inoculation of mammal-adapted organisms is associated with primary septicemia and high mortality. Oropharyngeal plague can result from the ingestion of undercooked contaminated meat and perhaps from the manual transfer of infected fluids to the mouth during the handling of infected animal tissues.

Carnivores, including dogs and cats, can become infected with *Y. pestis* by eating infected rodents and perhaps by being bitten by fleas from infected rodents. Although clinical plague commonly develops in infected cats, it rarely does so in infected dogs, which thus do not directly expose humans to infection. However, both dogs and cats may transport infected fleas from rodent-infested areas to the home environment.

From 1950 through 1996, 387 plague cases were reported in the United States. Of the 376 evaluable cases, 322 cases (86%) presented as primary lymphadenitic (bubonic) plague, almost all of them thought to be associated with flea bites; 46 cases (12%) presented as primary septicemic plague, many of them following direct animal exposures; and 8 cases (2%) presented as primary pneumonic plague, 6 resulting from the inhalation of respiratory droplets released by infected cats and 2 from unknown sources. The last case of human-to-human plague transmission in the United States occurred in the Los Angeles outbreak of 1924/1925.

PATHOGENESIS AND PATHOLOGY *Y. pestis* is highly invasive and pathogenic. The mechanisms by which the organism causes disease are incompletely understood, but both chromosome- and plasmid-encoded gene products as well as altered cell-mediated immune responses are probably involved. Three plasmids encode for a variety of known or presumed virulence factors, including the F1 envelope antigen, which confers bacterial resistance to phagocytosis by polymorphonuclear leukocytes (PMNs) in vitro; a murine exotoxin; the V antigen, which is essential for virulence, may immunocompromise the host by suppressing the synthesis of interferon γ and tumor necrosis factor α, and stimulates protective immunity in laboratory animals; pesticin, a bactericidal protein of unknown function and importance; a protease that can activate plasminogen and degrade serum complement and that is thought to play a role in the dissemination of *Y. pestis* from peripheral sites of infection; a coagulase; and a fibri-

A lipopolysaccharide endotoxin, believed to be chromosomally encoded, is probably important in triggering the systemic inflammatory response syndrome and its complications.

Y. pestis organisms inoculated through the skin or mucous membranes usually invade superficial lymphatic vessels and are carried to regional lymph nodes, although direct bloodstream inoculation may take place. Mononuclear phagocytes, which can phagocytize *Y. pestis* organisms without destroying them, may play a role in dissemination of the infection to distant sites. Plague can involve almost any organ, and untreated plague generally results in widespread and massive tissue destruction. In the early stages, infected lymph nodes (buboes, Fig. 162-1) are characterized by edema and congestion without inflammatory infiltrates or apparent vascular injury. Fully developed buboes contain huge numbers of infectious plague organisms and show distorted or obliterated lymph node architecture with vascular destruction and hemorrhage, serosanguineous effusion, necrosis, and a mild neutrophilic infiltration. At this stage, the effusion often involves perinodal tissues. If several adjacent lymph nodes are involved, a boggy edematous mass can result.

Primary septicemic plague results from the direct inoculation of bacteria from infected fluids or tissues or from an infective flea bite in the apparent absence of a bubo; secondary septicemic plague occurs when lymphatic and other host defenses are breached and the plague bacillus multiplies within the bloodstream. In fatal septicemic plague, multifocal hepatic and splenic necrosis is common. Diffuse interstitial myocarditis with cardiac dilatation is sometimes found. If disseminated intravascular coagulation (DIC) ensues, vascular necrosis may lead to widespread cutaneous, mucosal, and serosal ecchymoses and petechiae. Acral gangrene sometimes develops.

Primary plague pneumonia generally begins as a lobular process and then extends by confluence, becoming lobar and then multilobar (Fig. 162-2). Plague organisms are typically most numerous in the alveoli. Secondary plague pneumonia begins more diffusely, with organisms usually most numerous in the interstitium. In untreated cases of both primary and secondary plague pneumonia, diffuse pulmonary hemorrhage, necrosis, and neutrophilic infiltration develop.

MANIFESTATIONS Plague is characterized by a rapid onset of fever and other systemic manifestations of gram-negative bacterial infection. If it is not quickly and correctly treated, plague can follow a toxic course, resulting in shock, multiple-organ failure, and death. In humans, the three principal forms of plague are bubonic, septicemic, and pneumonic. Bubonic plague, the most common form, is almost always caused by the bite of an infected flea but occasionally results

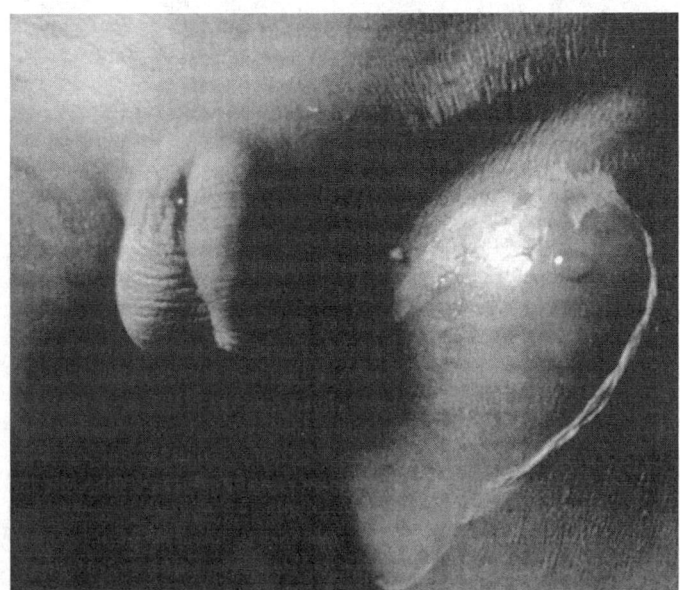

FIGURE 162-1 Left inguinal and femoral buboes, with surrounding edema and overlying desquamation.

from direct inoculation of infectious fluids. Septicemic and pneumonic plague can be either primary or secondary to metastatic spread. Unusual secondary forms include plague meningitis, endophthalmitis, and lymphadenitis at multiple sites. Primary plague pharyngitis has been documented by culture of organisms from throat swabs and can result from respiratory exposure or ingestion of contaminated meat.

Bubonic plague usually has an incubation period of 2 to 6 days, occasionally longer. Typically, the patient experiences chills; fever, with temperatures that rise within hours to $\geq 38°C$; myalgias; arthralgias; headache; and a feeling of weakness. Soon—usually within 24 h—the patient notices tenderness and pain in one or more regional lymph nodes proximal to the site of inoculation of the plague bacillus (Fig. 162-1). Because fleas often bite the legs, femoral and inguinal nodes are most commonly involved; axillary and cervical nodes are next most commonly affected. The enlarging bubo becomes progressively painful and tender, sometimes exquisitely so. The patient usually guards against palpation and limits movement, pressure, and stretch around the bubo. The surrounding tissue often becomes edematous, sometimes markedly so, and the overlying skin may be erythematous, warm, and tense. Inspection of the skin surrounding or distal to the bubo sometimes reveals the site of a flea bite marked by a small papule, pustule, eschar, or ulcer. A list of lymphadenitic conditions that could be confused with a plague bubo would include *Staphylococcus aureus* and group A β-hemolytic streptococcal infections, cat-scratch disease, and tularemia. The bubo of plague is distinguishable from lymphadenitis of most other causes, however, by its rapid onset, its extreme tenderness, the accompanying signs of toxemia, and the absence of cellulitis or obvious ascending lymphangitis.

Treated in the uncomplicated state with an appropriate antibiotic, bubonic plague usually responds quickly, with defervescence and alleviation of other systemic manifestations over 2 to 5 days. Buboes often remain enlarged and tender for a week or more after the initiation of treatment and can become fluctuant. Without effective antimicrobial treatment, patients with typical bubonic plague manifest an increasingly toxic state of fever, tachycardia, lethargy leading to prostration, agitation and confusion, and (occasionally) convulsions and delirium. Secondary plague sepsis may result in an alarmingly rapid and refractory cascade of DIC, bleeding, shock, and organ failure. Mild forms of bubonic plague, called *pestis minor*, have been described in South America and elsewhere; in these cases, the patients are ambulatory, are only mildly febrile, and have subacute buboes.

Septicemic plague is a progressive, overwhelming bacterial infection. Primary septicemia develops in the absence of apparent regional lymphadenitis, and the diagnosis of plague is often not suspected until preliminary blood culture results are reported to be positive by the laboratory. *Y. pestis*, however, can also be cultured from the blood of most bubonic plague patients, and bacteremia should be distinguished from septicemia, in which the patient is desperately ill and requires aggressive care. Patients with septicemic plague often present with gastrointestinal symptoms of nausea, vomiting, diarrhea, and abdominal pain, which may further confound the correct diagnosis. If not treated early with appropriate antibiotics, septicemic plague can be fulminant and fatal. In the United States in 1950 through 1996, 66 cases of septicemic plague and 18 deaths were reported, for a case-fatality rate of 27%. Petechiae, ecchymoses, bleeding from puncture wounds and orifices, and gangrene of acral parts are manifestations of DIC; refractory hypotension, renal shutdown, obtundation, and other signs of shock are preterminal events. Adult respiratory distress syndrome (ARDS), which can occur at any stage of septicemic plague, is sometimes confused with other conditions, such as hantavirus pulmonary syndrome.

Of all forms of the disease, pneumonic plague develops most rapidly and is most frequently fatal. The incubation period for primary pneumonic plague is rarely longer than 1 to 4 days. The onset is most often sudden, with chills, fever, headache, myalgias, weakness, and

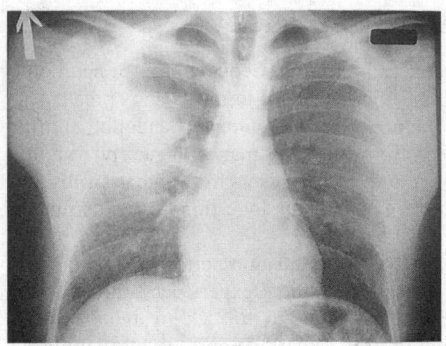
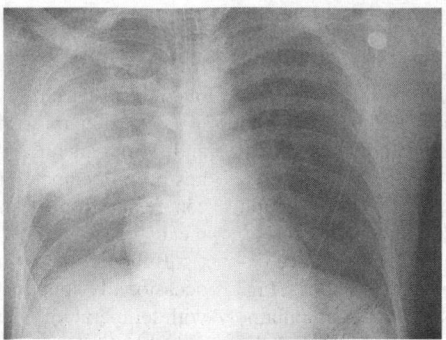
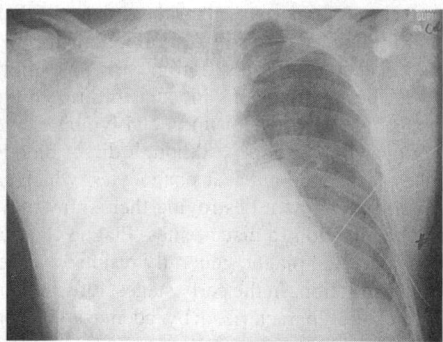

FIGURE 162-2 Sequential chest radiographs of a patient with fatal primary plague pneumonia. *Left:* Upright posteroanterior film taken at admission to hospital emergency department on third day of illness, showing segmental consolidation of right upper lobe. *Center:* Portable anteroposterior film taken 8 h after admission, showing extension of pneumonia to right middle and right lower lobes. *Right:* Portable anteroposterior film taken 13 h after admission (when patient had clinical adult respiratory distress syndrome), showing diffuse infiltration throughout right lung and patchy infiltration of left lower lung. A cavity later developed at the site of initial right upper lobe consolidation.

dizziness. Pulmonary signs, including cough, sputum production, chest pain, tachypnea, and dyspnea, typically arise on the second day of illness and may be accompanied by hemoptysis, increasing respiratory distress, cardiopulmonary insufficiency, and circulatory collapse. In primary plague pneumonia, the sputum is most often watery or mucoid, frothy, and blood-tinged, but it may become frankly bloody. Pulmonary signs in primary pneumonic plague may indicate involvement of a single lobe in the early stage, with rapidly developing segmental consolidation before bronchopneumonic spread to other lobes of the same and opposite lungs. Liquefaction necrosis and cavitation may occur early in areas of consolidation and may or may not leave significant residual scarring.

Secondary plague pneumonia manifests first as diffuse interstitial pneumonitis in which sputum production is scant; since the sputum is more likely to be inspissated and tenacious in character than the sputum found in primary pneumonia, it may be less infectious. In the United States in 1950 through 1996, 39 cases of secondary pneumonic plague and 8 cases of primary pneumonic plague were reported, with no known transmission to contacts and an overall case-fatality rate of 41%. Observers in the early twentieth century remarked on the relative lack of auscultatory findings, the usual presence of toxemia, and the frequency of sudden death in patients with pneumonic plague as compared to patients with other bacterial pneumonias.

Meningitis is an unusual manifestation of plague. In the United States, there were 12 meningitis cases among the 376 evaluable plague cases reported in 1950 through 1996. All cases of meningitis were complications of bubonic plague, and all patients survived. Although meningitis may be a part of the initial presentation of plague, its onset is often delayed and is a manifestation of insufficient treatment. Recent cases in the United States have occurred during the first and second weeks of antibiotic treatment for bubonic plague. Chronic relapsing meningeal plague over periods of weeks or even months was described in the preantibiotic era. The affected patients typically presented with fever, headache, meningismus, and pleocytosis.

Plague pharyngitis presents as fever, sore throat, cervical lymphadenitis, and headache and is often indistinguishable clinically from pharyngitis of other infectious etiologies. Caregivers working in plague-endemic areas must be alert to the possibility of plague to avoid misdiagnosis leading to delayed and/or inappropriate treatment.

LABORATORY FINDINGS AND DIAGNOSIS Since plague is a rare disease in the United States, a high index of clinical suspicion as well as the elicitation of a thorough clinical and epidemiologic history and a careful physical examination are required for timely diagnosis and prompt institution of specific therapy. When the diagnosis of plague is delayed or missed altogether, a high case-fatality rate results; infected travelers who seek medical care after they have left endemic areas (peripatetic plague cases) are at especially high risk. Plague must be considered in the differential diagnosis of sepsis in an otherwise-healthy person who has a history of recent travel to or res-

idence in the rural western United States. When the diagnosis of plague is being considered, close communication between clinicians and the diagnostic laboratory and between the diagnostic laboratory and a qualified reference laboratory is essential. Tests for plague are highly reliable when conducted by laboratory personnel experienced with *Y. pestis*, but such expertise is usually limited to selected reference laboratories, including state health department laboratories in some plague-endemic states and the CDC plague laboratory (Fort Collins, Colorado; tel. 970-221-6400).

When plague is suspected, specimens should be collected promptly for laboratory studies, chest roentgenograms should be obtained, and specific antimicrobial therapy should be initiated pending confirmation. Appropriate diagnostic specimens for smear and culture include citrated or heparinized whole blood from all patients with suspected plague, bubo aspirates from those with suspected buboes, sputum samples or tracheal aspirates from those with suspected pneumonic plague, and cerebrospinal fluid (CSF) from those with suspected plague meningitis. Since early buboes are often exquisitely tender and are seldom fluctuant or necrotic, these lesions usually require aspiration under local anesthesia following the injection of 1 to 2 mL of normal saline (sterile but nonbacteriostatic) into the bubo with a 20- to 22-gauge needle. A variety of appropriate culture media (including brain-heart infusion broth, sheep blood agar, and MacConkey agar) should be inoculated with a portion of each specimen. Moreover, for each specimen, at least one smear should be examined immediately with Wayson or Giemsa stain and at least one with Gram's stain; a smear should also be submitted for direct fluorescent antibody testing. An acute-phase serum specimen should be tested for antibody to *Y. pestis*; whenever possible, a convalescent-phase serum specimen collected 3 to 4 weeks later should also be tested. When a patient dies and plague is suspected, appropriate autopsy tissues for culture, direct fluorescent antibody testing, and immunohistochemical staining include buboes, all solid organs (especially liver, spleen, and lung), and bone marrow. If culture of such specimens is to be attempted, they should be sent to the laboratory either fresh or frozen on dry ice, not in preservatives or fixatives. If necessary, Cary-Blair or a similar medium can be used to transport *Y. pestis*—infected tissues.

Laboratory confirmation of plague depends on the isolation of *Y. pestis* from cultures of body fluids or tissues. Cultures of three blood samples taken over a 45-min period before treatment will usually result in isolation of the bacterium. *Y. pestis* strains are readily distinguished from those of the closely related species *Y. pseudotuberculosis* by differences in biochemical profile, temperature-dependent susceptibility to lysis by a *Y. pestis*—specific bacteriophage, and motility. Automated bacteriologic test systems can be used to assist in the identification of isolates as *Y. pestis*, but *Y. pestis* can be misidentified (e.g., as *Y. pseudotuberculosis*) or overlooked if these systems are improperly programmed.

In the absence of *Y. pestis* isolation, plague cases can be confirmed

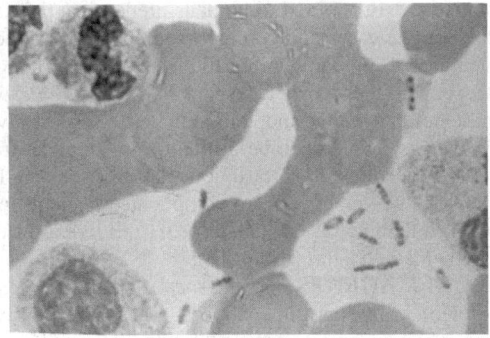

FIGURE 162-3 Peripheral blood smear from a patient with fatal plague septicemia and shock, showing characteristic bipolar-staining *Y. pestis* bacilli (Wright's stain, oil immersion).

either by the demonstration of seroconversion (a fourfold or greater titer rise) to *Y. pestis* F1 antigen in passive hemagglutination tests of acute- and convalescent-phase serum specimens or by detection of an antibody titer of >128 in a single serum sample from a patient with a plague-compatible illness who has not received plague vaccine. The specificity of a positive passive-hemagglutination test requires confirmation with the F1 antigen hemagglutination-inhibition test. A few plague patients seroconvert to F1 antigen as early as 5 days after the onset of illness. Most seroconvert between 1 and 2 weeks after onset; a few seroconvert 3 weeks or more after onset; and a few (<5%) fail to seroconvert at all. Early, specific antibiotic treatment may delay seroconversion by several weeks. After seroconversion, positive serologic titers diminish gradually over months to years. Enzyme-linked immunosorbent assays (ELISAs) for IgM and IgG antibodies to *Y. pestis* are replacing hemagglutination tests in some laboratories. Other new test methods include IgM antibody capture and competitive blocking for detection of antibody to F1.

Detection of F1 antigen in tissues or fluids by direct fluorescent antibody testing or by antigen capture is presumptive evidence of plague, as is an F1 antibody titer of >10 in a single serum sample from a patient with a plague-compatible illness who has not received plague vaccine. Visualization of characteristic bipolar bacilli in a Giemsa- or Wayson-stained smear constitutes supportive evidence of plague. Tularemia, especially the glandular, typhoidal, and pneumonic forms, can sometimes be confused clinically and epidemiologically with plague, but the results of microbiologic and serologic tests should readily distinguish these two diseases.

Patients with plague typically have white blood cell (WBC) counts of 15,000 to 25,000/μL, with a predominance of PMNs and a left shift. Leukemoid reactions with WBC counts as high as 100,000/μL can occur. Modest thrombocytopenia is usually documented, and fibrin-fibrinogen split products are often detected even in patients without frank DIC. Serum levels of aminotransferases and bilirubin may be elevated. Chest roentgenograms of patients with pneumonic plague usually show patchy bronchopneumonic infiltrates as well as lobar or segmental consolidation with or without confluence (Fig. 162-2); they occasionally show cavitation. Stained sputum samples usually contain PMNs and characteristic bipolar-staining bacilli. In *Y. pestis* septicemia, visualization of the characteristic bacilli in a routine blood smear or a buffy-coat smear is an uncommon but grave prognostic sign (Fig. 162-3). In patients with plague meningitis, pleocytosis with a predominance of PMNs is the rule, and the characteristic bacilli are usually visible in stained CSF smears.

℞ **TREATMENT** Left untreated, plague is fatal in more than 50% of cases of bubonic disease and in nearly all cases of septicemic and pneumonic disease. The overall mortality rate for plague cases in the United States since 1950 has been ~16%; deaths are almost always due to delays in seeking treatment, misdiagnosis, delays in the institution of treatment, or incorrect treatment. Rapid diagnosis and appropriate antimicrobial therapy are essential.

Guidelines for the treatment of plague are given in Table 162-1. Although streptomycin is the drug of choice, gentamicin is increasingly used for the treatment of plague in the United States because of its ready availability; it is probably as effective as streptomycin, although results of controlled studies in humans have not been published. Alternative antibiotics include the tetracyclines and chloramphenicol; these agents are usually given orally with initial loading doses but may be given intravenously to critically ill patients and to patients unable to tolerate oral medication. Penicillins, cephalosporins, and macrolides are suboptimal and should not be used. Doxycycline may be as effective as other tetracyclines or even more so, but comparative evaluations have not been made. Trimethoprim-sulfamethoxazole has been used successfully to treat bubonic plague but is not considered a first-line choice. Chloramphenicol is indicated for the treatment of plague meningitis, pleuritis, endophthalmitis, and myocarditis because of its superior tissue penetration; it is used alone or in combination with streptomycin. In general, antimicrobial treatment should be continued for 10 days or for at least 3 days after the patient has become afebrile and has made a clinical recovery. Patients initially given intravenous antibiotics may be switched to oral regimens upon clinical improvement. Such improvement is usually evident 2 or 3 days after the start of treatment, even though fever may continue for several days.

Consequences of delayed treatment of plague include DIC, ARDS, and other complications of gram-negative sepsis. Patients with these disorders require intensive monitoring and close physiologic support, as outlined elsewhere (Chaps. 117 and 265). Buboes may require surgical drainage. Abscessed nodes can cause recurrent fever in patients who have apparently recovered; this relation may be occult if intrathoracic or intraabdominal nodes are involved. Although *Y. pestis* is considered to be genetically stable, a multidrug-resistant strain was isolated from a plague patient in Madagascar. This strain exhibited resistance (mediated by a transferable plasmid) to all first-line antibiotics used for treatment of plague and to the principal alternatives used for treatment and prophylaxis.

PREVENTION AND CONTROL Persons at greatest risk for plague in the United States are those who live, work, and participate in outdoor recreational activities in areas of those western states in which plague is enzootic. Surveillance, education, and environmental management are the cornerstones of prevention and control. A network

Table 162-1 Guidelines for the Treatment of Plague

Drug	Daily Dosage	Interval, h	Route(s) of Administration
Streptomycin			
Adults	2 g	12	IM
Children	30 mg/kg	12	IM
Gentamicin			
Adults	3–5 mg/kg[a]	8	IM or IV
Children	6.0–7.5 mg/kg	8	IM or IV
Infants/neonates	7.5 mg/kg	8	IM or IV
Tetracycline			
Adults	2 g	6	PO or IV
Children ≥8 y	25–50 mg/kg	6	PO or IV
Doxycycline			
Adults	200 mg	12 or 24	PO or IV
Children ≥8 y	4 mg/kg	12 or 24	PO or IV
Oxytetracycline			
Adults	250–300 mg	8, 12, or 24	PO or IM
Children ≥8 y	15–25 mg/kg[b]	8, 12, or 24	PO or IM
Chloramphenicol			
Adults	50 mg/kg[c]	6	PO or IV
Children ≥1 y	50 mg/kg[c]	6	PO or IV

[a] Dosage should be reduced to 3 mg/kg daily as soon as clinically indicated.
[b] Maximum, 250 mg IM in a single daily dose.
[c] For meningitis, up to 100 (mg/kg)/d initially.

of biologists and public health specialists coordinates these activities through local and state health departments and the CDC. Personal protective measures include the avoidance of areas with known epizootic plague (which may be posted) and of sick or dead animals; the use of repellents, insecticides, and protective clothing when at risk of exposure to rodents' fleas; and the wearing of gloves when handling animal carcasses. Short-term antibiotic prophylaxis (Table 162-2) is recommended for persons known to have had direct contact with a patient with suspected or confirmed pneumonic plague and occasionally for persons who are unable to avoid an area where a plague outbreak is in progress or who may be caring for patients with plague. Patients in whom plague is suspected should be managed under isolation precautions for respiratory droplet transmission until pneumonia has been ruled out or until 48 h of specific antimicrobial therapy has been administered, after which universal precautions are adequate.

Rodent food (garbage, pet food) and habitats (brush piles, junk heaps, woodpiles) should be eliminated in domestic, peridomestic, and working environments; buildings and food stores should be rodent-proofed. The control of fleas with insecticides is a key public health measure in situations where epizootic plague activity places humans at high risk; this effort includes dusting and spraying of rodent burrows, rodent runs, and other sites where rodents and their fleas are found. In plague-endemic areas of the western United States, persons should keep their dogs and cats free of fleas and restrained. The decision to control plague by killing rodents should be left to public health authorities, and such a program should be carried out only in conjunction with effective flea control. Killing of rodents has no lasting benefit without environmental sanitation.

The previously used killed, whole-cell plague vaccine is no longer manufactured in the United States. Efforts are being made to develop improved vaccines in which the production of specific immunoprotective antibodies to *Y. pestis* is induced by recombinant antigens. In the United States, the indications for use of these newer vaccines would probably be similar to those for the previously available killed vaccine, which was mostly limited to protecting laboratory personnel who routinely worked with *Y. pestis* and some persons whose vocations brought them into regular contact with wild rodents and their fleas in areas with enzootic or epizootic plague. In addition, a vaccine might be useful in protecting selected military personnel and in responding to the possible use of *Y. pestis* as a weapon of bioterrorism.

OTHER *YERSINIA* INFECTIONS

DEFINITION   Yersiniosis is an uncommon bacterial zoonosis caused by infection with either of the two enteropathogenic *Yersinia* species: *Y. enterocolitica* or *Y. pseudotuberculosis*. Reservoir hosts of these bacteria include swine and other wild and domestic animals.

Table 162-2   Guidelines for Plague Prophylaxis

Drug	Daily Dosage	Interval, h	Route of Administration
Tetracycline			
Adults	1–2 g	6 or 12	PO
Children ≥8 y	25–50 mg/kg	6 or 12	PO
Doxycycline			
Adults	100–200 mg	12 or 24	PO
Children ≥8 y	2–4 mg/kg	12 or 24	PO
Trimethoprim-sulfamethoxazole			
Adults	320 mg[a]	12	PO
Children ≥2 mo	8 mg/kg[a]	12	PO

[a] Trimethoprim component.

These yersiniae are transmitted to humans predominantly via the oral route. Both sporadic cases and common-source outbreaks occur. The most frequent acute clinical manifestations are (1) enteritis or enterocolitis with self-limited diarrhea (especially with *Y. enterocolitica*), and (2) mesenteric adenitis and terminal ileitis (especially with *Y. pseudotuberculosis*), which can be difficult to distinguish from acute appendicitis. Septicemia and metastatic focal infections are less common. Some cases of yersiniosis are complicated by nonsuppurative, extraintestinal, inflammatory sequelae—e.g., reactive arthritis (Chap. 315) and erythema nodosum (Chap. 18).

ETIOLOGIC AGENTS   *Y. enterocolitica* and *Y. pseudotuberculosis* are pleomorphic gram-negative bacilli in the family Enterobacteriaceae. They are aerobic or facultatively anaerobic, motile at 25°C, nonmotile at 37°C, oxidase negative, urease positive, able to ferment glucose, unable to ferment lactose, and usually able to reduce nitrates. They grow well, if slowly, on nonselective media (e.g., blood agar) and on most of the routine media used to select for enteric bacteria (e.g., MacConkey agar). They can multiply within a wide temperature range (−1°C to 45°C). The most clinically and epidemiologically useful methods for identifying pathogenic *Y. enterocolitica* isolates are biotyping based on biochemical profiles and serotyping according to somatic O and H antigens. Six biotypes and more than 60 serotypes of *Y. enterocolitica* are recognized. A separate serotyping system for *Y. pseudotuberculosis* (also based on somatic antigens) has distinguished six major serotypes (I through VI) and their subtypes.

EPIDEMIOLOGY   *Y. enterocolitica* is distributed worldwide and has been isolated from soil, fresh water, contaminated foodstuffs (e.g., meat, milk, and vegetables), and a wide variety of wild and domestic animals, including mammals, birds, amphibians, fish, and shellfish. Many serotypes isolated from environmental sources, however, evidently are not human pathogens. Most human infections have been caused by *Y. enterocolitica* serotypes O:3, O:5, O:8, and O:9, which are primarily associated with wild and domestic mammals. The incidence of these infections and their sequelae is highest in Scandinavia and some other northern European countries, but this observation may be in part an artifact of underrecognition in other countries. Because many individuals with enteric *Y. enterocolitica* infection are asymptomatic or minimally symptomatic and do not seek medical attention, reliable population-based estimates of incidence are unavailable. However, in many clinical microbiology laboratories in recent decades, *Y. enterocolitica* has been the fourth most common bacterial pathogen isolated from patients' fecal specimens, trailing *Salmonella* (the most frequently isolated), *Campylobacter*, and *Shigella* species.

All age groups are susceptible to *Y. enterocolitica* infections, but the majority of cases of enterocolitis are in children aged 1 to 4. Moreover, these infections show a modest predilection for males. Mesenteric adenitis and terminal ileitis are most common among older children and young adults. Risk factors for *Y. enterocolitica* septicemia and metastatic focal infections include chronic liver disease, malignancy, diabetes mellitus, immunosuppressive therapy, alcoholism, malnutrition, advanced age, iron overload (see below), and hemolytic anemias (including the thalassemias). The nonsuppurative sequelae of yersiniosis are most common among adults. HLA-B27 is expressed in 70 to 80% of patients who develop reactive arthritis associated with yersiniosis. HLA-B27 is not a risk factor for *Yersinia*-induced erythema nodosum; females with this condition outnumber males by 2 to 1. In Europe, *Y. enterocolitica* infections are more common in the cooler months than in warmer weather. In North America, no consistent seasonal pattern has been documented.

For several decades, serotypes O:3 and O:9 have predominated among *Y. enterocolitica* isolates from patients in Europe. Serotype O:3 has also predominated in Canada and Japan. In the United States, serotype O:3 emerged in the 1980s to surpass serotype O:8 in frequency of isolation from patients. The incidence of *Yersinia*-induced nonsuppurative sequelae reportedly is 10 to 30% in Scandinavia and much lower in most other countries, including the United States. No

162   Plague, Other *Yersinia* Infections   **999**

convincing explanation for this observation has been confirmed, but reasonable possibilities include population genetic factors and geographic strain variation.

Common-source outbreaks of *Y. enterocolitica* enteritis have been traced to such vehicles as raw milk, contaminated pasteurized milk, and foods prepared with contaminated fresh water. In Belgium, the ingestion of ground raw pork (a regional custom) is a significant risk factor for sporadic infection with *Y. enterocolitica* serotypes O:3 and O:9. These serotypes commonly colonize the oral cavity and intestines of European swine, and *Y. enterocolitica* infection is an occupational risk of swine butchers in Europe. In the United States, sporadic cases and one outbreak of *Y. enterocolitica* O:3 infection have been associated with the preparation or ingestion of raw pork intestines (chitterlings). In some cases of yersiniosis, circumstantial evidence suggests transmission via contact with dogs and cats or their feces. Several nosocomial outbreaks of *Y. enterocolitica* infection have been described; fecal-oral transmission from person to person was suspected. Fecal-oral transmission among family members may also explain occasional secondary cases in households. In a prospective study of 50 children with *Y. enterocolitica* enteritis, fecal excretion of the organism persisted for an average of 27 days (range, 4 to 79 days) after the cessation of symptoms. A chronic carrier state, however, has not been demonstrated. *Y. enterocolitica* is a rare but often lethal cause of transfusion-associated septicemia. The explanation is that blood donors occasionally have transient, occult *Y. enterocolitica* bacteremia and that this organism can slowly multiply to high concentrations in blood refrigerated for at least 10 to 20 days.

The ecology of *Y. pseudotuberculosis* seems to parallel that of *Y. enterocolitica* closely. *Y. pseudotuberculosis* is also widespread in wild and domestic animals and is isolated from many environmental sources. Human infections with *Y. pseudotuberculosis*, however, appear to be rare. In North America and Europe, most such infections have been with serotype I, but outbreaks involving other serotypes have occurred in Japan and Scandinavia. Swine appear to be an important reservoir for pathogenic strains of *Y. pseudotuberculosis*.

PATHOGENESIS AND PATHOLOGY   Except in rare instances of transmission via contaminated blood products or direct cutaneous inoculation, the enteropathogenic yersiniae are thought to enter the host via the oral route. The 50% infectious dose in humans is uncertain but may be $\geq 10^9$. The incubation period averages 5 days (range, 1 to 11 days). Studies of animals have shown that the organisms initially invade the ileal epithelium, then are translocated via M cells into the lamina propria, and finally enter Peyer's patches, where they are able to replicate. They subsequently drain into the mesenteric lymph nodes, which undergo hyperplasia and from which the bacteria can be distributed systemically. The mesenteric lymph nodes can become intensely swollen and matted and are occasionally detected on physical examination as a tender right lower quadrant mass. Intestinal inflammation (most commonly of the distal ileum and less commonly of the ascending colon) develops and may be accompanied by mucosal ulcerations and by the shedding of PMNs and red blood cells into the intestinal lumen. In relatively severe cases, thrombosis of mesenteric blood vessels, intestinal hemorrhage, and necrosis can occur. In patients with enteropathogenic yersinial infections who undergo exploratory laparotomy, the appendix usually is histologically normal or shows only lymphoid hyperplasia, but frank suppuration is sometimes evident.

A plasmid of ~70 kb is essential for virulence of the enteropathogenic yersiniae because it encodes at least six *Yersinia* outer-membrane proteins, some of which confer to bacterial strains such properties as cytotoxicity; resistance to phagocytosis by PMNs; and the abilities to cause monocyte apoptosis (programmed cell death), to suppress the host's expression of tumor necrosis factor α, to interfere with platelet aggregation and host complement activation, and to dephosphorylate host proteins. A chromosomal gene (*inv*) encodes for the surface protein invasin, which is necessary for yersinial invasion of nonphagocytic host cells (e.g., epithelial cells) in vitro and which facilitates the translocation of bacteria across the intestinal epithelium. Both *Y. enterocolitica* and *Y. pseudotuberculosis* can express at least one protein superantigen that selectively stimulates the proliferation of T cells. Many strains of *Y. enterocolitica* produce a heat-stable enterotoxin that is similar to *Escherichia coli* enterotoxin. The cell walls of *Y. enterocolitica* and *Y. pseudotuberculosis* contain a lipopolysaccharide (endotoxin). The roles of superantigens, enterotoxin, and endotoxin in the pathogenesis of yersiniosis are unclear. Some *Yersinia* strains are unable to synthesize bacterial iron chelators called *siderophores*. However, they can exploit host-chelated iron stores and the drug deferoxamine (a siderophore produced by *Streptomyces pilosus*). Therefore, iron overload (e.g., caused by hemodialysis or multiple transfusions) and deferoxamine therapy appear to be independent risk factors for *Y. enterocolitica* bacteremia (especially that involving serotypes O:3 and O:9) and to a lesser degree for *Y. pseudotuberculosis* bacteremia.

Immunogenetic factors and cell-mediated immune responses are clearly involved in the pathogenesis of reactive arthritis following infection with the enteropathogenic yersiniae. As noted above, most patients with *Yersinia*-induced reactive arthritis express HLA-B27. In addition, *Y. pseudotuberculosis* shares at least one cross-reactive epitope with HLA-B27, and *Y. enterocolitica* infection alters the expression of serologic HLA-B27 epitopes on lymphocytes and monocytes. In patients with reactive arthritis following *Y. enterocolitica* infection, yersinial antigens are commonly detectable in synovial fluid cells in the apparent absence of whole organisms. Thus, it is unknown whether the arthritis results from occult bacterial persistence through self-tolerance of HLA-B27 with a failure of cross-reactive immune responses to yersiniae, from an immune response to common antigenic determinants shared by the bacteria and host HLA-B27 (i.e., molecular mimicry), or from other mechanisms. The pathogenesis of *Yersinia*-induced erythema nodosum is obscure.

In some assays, patients with Graves' disease have an increased prevalence of serum antibodies to *Y. enterocolitica*, and the immunoglobulins of patients recovering from *Y. enterocolitica* infections react with the human thyroid-stimulating hormone receptor. However, a link between *Y. enterocolitica* infection and the subsequent development of autoimmune thyroiditis has not been convincingly demonstrated.

MANIFESTATIONS   The principal clinical manifestations of *Y. enterocolitica* infection are enteritis, enterocolitis, mesenteric adenitis, and terminal ileitis. Less common manifestations include exudative pharyngitis, septicemia, metastatic focal infections, reactive polyarthritis, and erythema nodosum. When age groups are combined, the most common presentation of *Y. enterocolitica* infection is acute diarrhea from enteritis or enterocolitis. Low-grade fever and cramping abdominal pain occur in most cases, nausea and vomiting in 15 to 40%, hematochezia in up to 30%, and a generalized maculopapular skin rash in a few cases. Diarrhea persists for an average of 2 weeks (range, 1 day to many months), during which the frequency of bowel movements diminishes. Uncommonly, enteritis or enterocolitis can be complicated by severe abdominal pain and high fever. Rare (and sometimes fatal) complications include diffuse inflammation, ulceration, hemorrhage, and necrosis of the small bowel and colon; intestinal perforation; peritonitis; ascending cholangitis; mesenteric vein thrombosis; diverticulitis; toxic megacolon; and ileocecal intussusception.

The syndrome of mesenteric adenitis and terminal ileitis without diarrhea is easily confused with appendicitis. Low-grade fever and right lower quadrant pain, tenderness, guarding, and rebound tenderness are common. During six recognized common-source outbreaks in the United States, 10% of 444 patients with symptomatic undiagnosed *Y. enterocolitica* infections underwent laparotomy for suspected appendicitis; surgical incisions became infected with *Y. enterocolitica* in a few of these cases.

Acute pharyngitis and pharyngotonsillitis, with or without cervical adenitis or intestinal illness, are less common but potentially lethal manifestations of *Y. enterocolitica* infection, particularly in adults. *Y. enterocolitica* septicemia generally presents as a severe illness with fever and leukocytosis, often with abdominal pain and jaundice and without localized signs of infection. Metastatic focal *Y. enterocolitica* infections can occur with or without clinically apparent bacteremia and can affect almost any organ system. Examples include abscess formation (e.g., in liver, spleen, kidney, lung, skeletal muscle, lymph node, or cutaneous tissue), osteomyelitis, meningitis, peritonitis, urinary tract infection, pneumonia, empyema, endocarditis, pericarditis, mycotic aneurysm, septic arthritis, suppurative conjunctivitis, panophthalmitis, Parinaud's oculoglandular syndrome, and cutaneous pustules or bullae.

In Scandinavia, the incidence of reactive arthritis following *Y. enterocolitica* infection among adults is estimated to be at least 10%. About 80% of these patients have preceding symptoms such as fever, diarrhea, or abdominal pain. Typically, these symptoms precede the arthritis by 1 week and are of short duration. The most commonly affected joints are the knees and ankles, but other joints can be involved. Typically, multiple (two to eight) joints become involved sequentially and asymmetrically over a period of a few days to 2 weeks, after which no additional joints are affected. Monoarticular arthritis occurs less commonly. In two-thirds of cases, the acute arthritis remits spontaneously within 1 to 3 months. Chronic joint disease is documented in a minority of cases. A few HLA-B27-positive patients with *Y. enterocolitica*–induced arthritis have subsequent ankylosing spondylitis, but this development is best explained by the fact that HLA-B27 is a major risk factor for each of these diseases. Mild, self-limited myocarditis accompanies about 10% of cases of *Yersinia*-induced arthritis and can occur independently. Typical manifestations include cardiac murmurs and transient electrocardiographic abnormalities, such as prolongation of the PR interval and nonspecific ST-segment and T-wave changes. The syndrome of *Yersinia*-induced arthritis and carditis can be confused with acute rheumatic fever. In Scandinavia, erythema nodosum occurs in 15 to 20% of patients with yersiniosis, usually within a few days to 3 weeks after the onset of intestinal illness. Lesions typically are located on the lower extremities and resolve within 1 month. Less commonly reported nonsuppurative sequelae of *Y. enterocolitica* infections include reactive uveitis, iritis, conjunctivitis, urethritis, and glomerulonephritis. The complete triad of Reiter's syndrome (arthritis, conjunctivitis, and urethritis) is seen in 5 to 10% of patients with *Yersinia*-induced arthritis.

The most common clinical presentation of *Y. pseudotuberculosis* infection is fever and abdominal pain caused by mesenteric adenitis; diarrheal illness is less common than in *Y. enterocolitica* infection. Systemic manifestations, including septicemia, focal infections, reactive arthritis, and erythema nodosum, are generally similar to those associated with *Y. enterocolitica* infection. In addition, *Y. pseudotuberculosis* has been associated with a scarlet fever–like syndrome, acute interstitial nephritis, and hemolytic-uremic syndrome.

LABORATORY FINDINGS AND DIAGNOSIS Results of routine laboratory tests in most patients with yersiniosis are nonspecific. Leukocyte counts are usually normal or slightly elevated, often with a modest left shift. Standard microbiologic methods are sufficient to isolate *Y. enterocolitica* and *Y. pseudotuberculosis* from otherwise-sterile sites, such as blood, CSF, lymph node tissue, and peritoneal fluid, and from abscesses. Isolation of these organisms from feces is impeded by their slow growth and the overgrowth of normal fecal flora on culture media routinely used to select for enteric bacteria. When routine enteric media are used, the yield of yersinial isolates from feces is increased by incubation at 22 to 25°C for 48 h. The yield from feces and other grossly contaminated specimens can be further increased by the use of *Yersinia*-selective cefsulodin-Irgasan-novobiocin (CIN) agar

and by cold enrichment (i.e., inoculation of feces into buffered saline and incubation at 4°C for 2 to 4 weeks, with periodic plating onto enteric media). Because bacteriologic procedures designed to isolate yersiniae from feces are not considered cost-effective, many laboratories undertake them by special request only.

The results of serologic tests can be used to support a diagnosis of yersiniosis. Agglutination tests or ELISAs are used most commonly; immunoblotting has also been used. The existence of multiple serotypes makes routine serologic tests laborious; thus these tests are generally conducted only in research laboratories or large commercial laboratories. Since these tests are experimental and are neither standardized nor well validated, and since some strains of *Yersinia* cross-react with other bacteria (e.g., *Brucella*, *Salmonella*, and *Vibrio*) and with serum from some patients with thyroiditis, results should be interpreted with caution. In typical uncomplicated cases of yersiniosis, agglutinin titers begin to rise within the first week of illness, peak in the second week, and then gradually diminish and return to normal within 3 to 6 months, although agglutinating antibody may remain detectable for several years in some cases. Because an initial serum specimen is often collected a week or more after the onset of illness, when agglutinin titers are already high, it is usually impossible to document a fourfold or greater rise in titer between paired specimens (although a fourfold or greater fall in titer may be found). Immunohistologic techniques and polymerase chain reaction tests to detect yersinial antigens and DNA, respectively, in clinical specimens are experimental at this time.

In patients with *Yersinia*-induced reactive arthritis, synovial fluid is sterile and the leukocyte count ranges from a few hundred to 60,000/μL, with a majority of PMNs. The erythrocyte sedimentation rate is often >100 mm/h. Rheumatoid factor and antinuclear antibodies are usually absent. The diagnosis of *Yersinia*-induced reactive arthritis or other nonsuppurative inflammatory sequelae can be difficult, especially when triggering infections are asymptomatic or clinically mild or occur several weeks before the diagnosis is attempted. Because the isolation of a pathogenic *Yersinia* strain from feces is the most specific diagnostic test in such cases, it should be attempted. Since culture is of limited sensitivity in this clinical setting, a high index of suspicion and positive results of serologic tests for *Y. enterocolitica* or *Y. pseudotuberculosis* are usually required for diagnosis.

℞ TREATMENT The effectiveness of antimicrobial agents in the treatment of yersinial enteritis, enterocolitis, mesenteric adenitis, or terminal ileitis has not been established. These conditions are usually self-limited, and their treatment is symptom-based and supportive. In uncomplicated cases, diarrhea should be treated with fluid and electrolyte replacement, with the route of delivery dependent on clinical severity. Enteric precautions are advisable for patients hospitalized with yersinial diarrhea. In general, antimicrobial treatment should be reserved for patients with septicemia, metastatic focal infections, or immunosuppression and enterocolitis. Controlled clinical comparisons of antimicrobial agents in the treatment of severe cases of yersiniosis have not yet been conducted. In such cases, drug selection should ultimately be guided by clinical response and bacterial sensitivity patterns. Clinical isolates of *Y. enterocolitica* and *Y. pseudotuberculosis* are usually susceptible in vitro to aminoglycosides, third-generation cephalosporins, chloramphenicol, quinolones, tetracyclines, and trimethoprim-sulfamethoxazole. In laboratory animals infected with enteropathogenic yersiniae, the fluoroquinolones have exerted the strongest bactericidal effects in vivo; clinical experience with these drugs against these pathogens in humans is promising but limited. Because they produce β-lactamases, isolates typically are resistant to penicillin, ampicillin, carbenicillin, and first-generation and most second-generation cephalosporins. Optimal dosages and durations of therapy have not been established. Mortality from *Y. enterocolitica* septicemia currently is ~10% despite treatment. Focal extraintestinal infections may require at least 3 weeks of therapy. No role for antimicrobial agents in the management of the nonsuppurative inflammatory manifestations of yersiniosis has been established. Patients with reactive arthritis may benefit from treatment with nonsteroidal anti-inflammatory drugs, intraarticular steroid injections, and physical therapy.

PREVENTION AND CONTROL The importance of safe food-handling and food-preparation practices in the prevention of yersiniosis cannot be overemphasized. Caution is particularly warranted in the case of pork and other animal products. The consumption of raw or undercooked meats, especially pork, should be avoided. Increased efforts to prevent the spread of enteric pathogens in household, pet-care, day-care, and hospital settings and in the food industry would be likely to decrease the incidence of yersiniosis. Current regulations of the U.S. Food and Drug Administration require visual inspection of packed red cell units before transfusion, with the discarding of units in which bacterial contamination is suspected on the basis of darkening (reflecting decreased oxygen saturation and hemolysis). Since the risk is minimal, more specific measures to further decrease the likelihood of transfusion of *Y. enterocolitica*–contaminated blood products (e.g., limiting the period for which red cells can be stored before transfusion) are not considered cost-effective.

Yersiniosis is not routinely reportable to public health authorities in most jurisdictions. However, clinicians who suspect a common-source outbreak (e.g., because they have documented a familial case cluster or have diagnosed the disease in several apparently unrelated patients over a short period) or some other public health threat (e.g., because they have found occult *Y. enterocolitica* bacteremia in a recent blood donor) should consult promptly with local public health officials.

BIBLIOGRAPHY

PLAGUE

CENTERS FOR DISEASE CONTROL AND PREVENTION: Fatal human plague—Arizona and Colorado, 1996. MMWR 46:617, 1997

CORNELIS GR et al: The virulence plasmid of *Yersinia*, an antihost genome. Microbiol Mol Biol Rev 62:1315, 1998

DENNIS DT: Plague as an emerging disease, in *Emerging Infections 2*, WM Scheld et al (eds). Washington, DC, ASM Press, 1998, pp 169–183

GALIMAND M et al: Multidrug resistance in *Yersinia pestis* mediated by a transferable plasmid. N Engl J Med 337:677, 1997

INGLESBY TV et al: Plague as a biological weapon: Medical and public health management. Consensus statement of the Working Group on Civilian Biodefense. JAMA, 1999 (in press)

OTHER *YERSINIA* INFECTIONS

BOTTONE EJ: *Yersinia enterocolitica*: The charisma continues. Clin Microbiol Rev 10:257, 1997

RATSITORAHINA M et al: Epidemiological and diagnostic aspects of the outbreak of pneumonic plague in Madagascar. Lancet 355:111, 2000

STOLK-ENGELAAR VM, HOOGKAMP-KORSTANJE JA: Clinical presentation and diagnosis of gastrointestinal infections by *Yersinia enterocolitica* in 261 Dutch patients. Scand J Infect Dis 28:571, 1996

——— et al: In-vitro antimicrobial susceptibility of *Yersinia enterocolitica* isolates from stools of patients in the Netherlands from 1982–1991. J Antimicrob Chemother 36:839, 1995

WUORELA M et al: Monocytes that have ingested *Yersinia enterocolitica* serotype O:3 acquire enhanced capacity to bind to nonstimulated vascular endothelial cells via P-selectin. Infect Immun 67:726, 1999

YLI-KERTTULA T et al: Ten-year follow up study of patients from a *Yersinia pseudotuberculosis* III outbreak. Clin Exp Rheumatol 13:333, 1995

163 *Lucy Stuart Tompkins*

BARTONELLA INFECTIONS, INCLUDING CAT-SCRATCH DISEASE

Bartonella spp., including *B. bacilliformis*, *B. henselae*, *B. quintana*, and *B. clarridgeiae*, are tiny gram-negative bacilli that can adhere to and invade mammalian cells, including endothelial cells and erythrocytes. Previously classified as *Rochalimaea* spp. within the rickettsia group, *Bartonella* spp. have now been removed from the order Rickettsiales on the grounds that they are not obligate intracellular parasites. These agents cause a wide spectrum of clinical illnesses, including trench fever, cat-scratch disease (CSD), bacillary angiomatosis, endocarditis, Oroya fever, and verruga peruana. The pathologic manifestations of *Bartonella* disease vary with the immune status of the host.

OROYA FEVER AND VERRUGA PERUANA

DEFINITION AND ETIOLOGY Oroya fever and verruga peruana are caused by *B. bacilliformis*. Oroya fever is characterized by fever, profound anemia, and—unless antibiotic treatment is given—high mortality. The lesions referred to as verruga peruana may develop during the convalescent phase of Oroya fever or during chronic infection with *B. bacilliformis*. In 1885 Daniel Carrión, a Peruvian medical student, inoculated himself with blood from a patient with verruga peruana and subsequently died of Oroya fever, thus proving that both diseases are caused by a single agent.

EPIDEMIOLOGY Infection with *B. bacilliformis* follows the bite of the sandfly vector *Phlebotomus*, an insect found in the river valleys of the Andes Mountains at altitudes of 600 to 2500 m. Oroya fever develops in nonimmune individuals who are not residents of the endemic region, whereas verruga peruana occurs in persons who apparently have been exposed in the past, including those who have recently had Oroya fever. The infection has not been acquired in the United States.

PATHOLOGY During initial infection in the nonimmune host, *B. bacilliformis* cells adhere to erythrocytes and produce indentations in the cell membrane; the bacteria subsequently enter the erythrocytes and cause persistent deformation of the cytoskeleton. The parasitized erythrocytes are ultimately phagocytosed and destroyed. Although the life span of infected erythrocytes is markedly shortened, not all of this change can be attributed to the mechanical fragility induced by the internalization of bacteria. Decreased bone marrow erythropoiesis also contributes to anemia.

CLINICAL MANIFESTATIONS The onset of symptoms in Oroya fever may be either insidious or abrupt, after an incubation period of approximately 3 weeks. The subacute presentation may include low-grade fever, malaise, headache, and anorexia. Sudden-onset disease commences with high fever, chills, diaphoresis, headaches, and changes in mental status. These manifestations are followed by the sudden development of profound anemia, which is due to a marked decrease in erythrocyte numbers and is associated with macrocytic changes, poikilocytosis, Howell-Jolly bodies, nucleated erythrocytes, and immature myeloid cells. The leukocyte differential usually shifts to the left, although the total leukocyte count may be normal. The erythrocyte count may fall to extremely low levels. In eosin/thiazine-stained peripheral-blood smears, numerous microorganisms can be seen adhering to most erythrocytes.

During the acute phase, muscle and joint pain and headache may be severe; central nervous system changes include insomnia, delirium, and a decreased level of consciousness. Thrombocytopenic purpura may develop. If the patient survives, a convalescent phase ensues, characterized by the sudden disappearance of bacteria from blood smears, declining fever, and an increase in the erythrocyte count. Although much of the mortality associated with Oroya fever is due to profound anemia and toxicity, secondary bacterial infections (including salmonellosis and other enteric infections, malaria, and tuberculosis) are often an important contributing factor.

After convalescence from acute Oroya fever, verrugas may develop. These red or purple cutaneous lesions may be either tiny and sessile or large, pedunculated, and nodular. They bear a marked resemblance to the lesions of bacillary angiomatosis and to Kaposi's sarcoma.

DIAGNOSIS During acute infection, bacteria can be cultured from the blood on agar containing rabbit blood, with incubation at 28°C. The hallmark of verruga peruana is the formation of new blood vessels (angiogenesis) at the sites of bacterial replication.

℞ **TREATMENT** Oroya fever responds to a variety of antimicrobial agents, including chloramphenicol, tetracyclines, penicillin, and streptomycin. Chloramphenicol is used most often because of its efficacy against most *Salmonella* infections (as salmonellosis may develop intercurrently). Verruga peruana may respond similarly; however, failure to respond to therapy and relapse are common and require the reinstitution of prolonged therapy.

BACILLARY ANGIOMATOSIS

DEFINITION AND ETIOLOGY Bacillary angiomatosis was initially described as a condition occurring primarily in patients with AIDS and characterized by vascular cutaneous lesions resembling Kaposi's sarcoma. The disease can disseminate to involve virtually any organ system. Immunocompromised individuals, especially those infected with HIV, are at particularly high risk for bacillary angiomatosis, although in rare instances the patient is not obviously immunosuppressed. Both *B. henselae* and *B. quintana* (the infectious agent initially associated with trench fever) produce bacillary angiomatosis in persons with immunodeficiency.

EPIDEMIOLOGY Acquisition of *B. henselae* has been significantly associated with exposure to young cats infested with fleas (*Ctenocephalides felis*). Because a high percentage of cats are seropositive, it has been suggested that patients with HIV infection avoid exposure to these animals. The finding that a large proportion of cats with fleas have persistent asymptomatic *B. henselae* bacteremia suggests that the domestic cat is the animal reservoir of this microorganism. The flea may serve as a transmitting vector in the cross-infection of cats, but its role in human infection is not clear. Tick-associated cases of *B. henselae* bacteremia have been reported in healthy immunocompetent individuals.

Person-to-person transmission of *B. quintana* by the human body louse (*Pediculus humanis corporis*) was documented during World War I under conditions of poor personal hygiene and sanitation. Although lice are suspected of transmission, the reservoir of *B. quintana* has not been identified.

A case-control study revealed that *B. henselae* and *B. quintana* differ significantly in terms of epidemiologic risk factors. All cases of *B. henselae* infection were associated with exposure to cats and their fleas and occurred sporadically, whereas the cases of *B. quintana* infection occurred in clusters and were associated with low socioeconomic status, homelessness, and exposure to body lice. Direct transmission of *B. henselae* from cats to their owners, presumably through cutaneous trauma, was supported by the matching DNA fingerprint patterns of isolates from the two sources.

MICROBIOLOGY *B. henselae* can be demonstrated in tissue by Warthin-Starry staining. Clumps and clusters of pleomorphic bacilli appear as purple deposits in tissue stained with hematoxylin and eosin. Although the bacteria may be difficult to cultivate in the laboratory, they can eventually be isolated from cultures of blood and of material from other sites. Colonies develop after prolonged incubation (1 to 4 weeks) on blood-containing media and pit the agar; bacterial cells are gram-negative. *B. quintana* grows as a smooth, nonpitting colony on solid agar after prolonged incubation.

Classification of *B. henselae* was first accomplished when molecular techniques were used to analyze bacterial ribosomal genes extracted from tissue samples. Definitive identification of *Bartonella* spp. is based on sequence analysis of 16S ribosomal DNA.

PATHOGENESIS AND PATHOLOGY Bacillary angiomatosis is characterized by a lobular proliferation of new blood vessels (angiogenesis) and a neutrophilic inflammatory response to myriad bacilli located within collagen-rich microscopic and macroscopic nodules. The endothelial cells lining the vascular spaces have a typical epithelioid appearance, and the lesions may resemble Kaposi's sarcoma histopathologically, although the characteristic spindle cell of the latter disease is usually absent. The bacterial and eukaryotic host factors that elicit the pathologic response are unknown.

CLINICAL MANIFESTATIONS The skin lesions of bacillary angiomatosis (also called *epithelioid angiomatosis*) are vascular nodules, papules, or tumors that range from tiny lesions resembling cherry angiomas or pyogenic granulomas to large, pedunculated, exophytic masses (Fig. 163-1). Characteristically, the lesions are red or purple, resembling Kaposi's sarcoma; they may be surrounded by an epithelial collarette, may be located anywhere on the skin, and may involve mucous membranes. The overlying epidermis may be focally ulcerated, and the underlying bone may be invaded and destroyed.

Dissemination of *B. henselae* infection occurs primarily in patients with cellular immune defects. Clinical manifestations accompanying dissemination are often nonspecific and include persistent fever, abdominal pain, weight loss, and malaise. Although the liver, spleen, bone marrow, and lymph nodes are primarily affected, HIV-infected patients may also develop central nervous system abnormalities (including psychiatric disorders and brain lesions), which are responsive to antibiotic therapy. Skin lesions usually are not evident in disseminated infection. Involvement of the liver or spleen may produce bacillary peliosis hepatis. Patients with the latter condition may report localized pain on palpation of the abdomen. Nodular lesions of variable size can be demonstrated by computed tomography or magnetic resonance imaging, with or without contrast agents.

In a case-control study of bacillary angiomatosis (see "Epidemiology" above), only *B. henselae* was associated with hepatosplenic disease (peliosis hepatis) and displayed a predilection for the lymph nodes. *B. quintana*, in contrast, was associated with osseous and subcutaneous infection.

DIAGNOSIS The diagnosis of bacillary angiomatosis is based primarily on the typical histopathologic findings of angiomas in association with clumps of tiny bacilli revealed by Warthin-Starry silver stain. Infection due to *B. henselae* can also be established by culture or by identification of specific DNA sequences. *B. henselae* is most easily isolated from blood through a lysis-centrifugation system. Colonies may be detected on blood-containing agar (rabbit blood is preferred) incubated with 5 to 10% CO_2 at 37°C for 2 to 4 weeks. *B. quintana* may be isolated from BACTEC (Becton Dickinson, Sparks, MD) aerobic bottles containing resin. Isolation from skin lesions and other tissues is more difficult but should be attempted when feasible. Initial reports suggested that cocultivation with endothelial cell monolayers was necessary; however, isolation by direct plating onto freshly prepared agar media has also been successful. Bacilli picked from new colonies but not subcultured may not stain, even with acridine orange; they stain weakly with safranin. Identification of *B.*

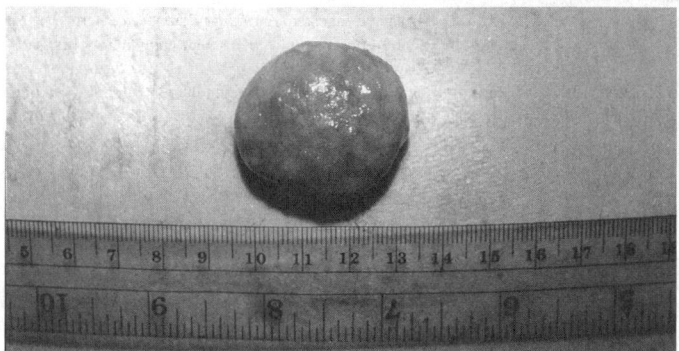

FIGURE 163-1 Characteristic skin lesion of bacillary angiomatosis in an HIV-positive young woman. This large, pedunculated tumor exhibits the typical angiomatous appearance. The patient was treated with oral erythromycin, with nearly complete resolution of the lesion; however, on discontinuation of antibiotic therapy after a 4-week course, the lesion recurred.

henselae and *B. quintana* is based primarily on cellular fatty-acid analysis and polymerase chain reaction (PCR)–based restriction fragment length polymorphism analysis. Definitive identification of *Bartonella* spp. depends on DNA sequence analysis of 16S ribosomal RNA genes. The diagnosis of CSD (see next section) can be made by specific serologic testing that detects *B. henselae*–specific antibodies, but the sensitivity and specificity of this method in patients with cutaneous and disseminated bacillary angiomatosis have not been determined.

DIFFERENTIAL DIAGNOSIS The differential diagnosis of cutaneous bacillary angiomatosis includes Kaposi's sarcoma, angiomas, and pyogenic granulomas. These conditions can be distinguished by histopathologic examination of biopsied material.

Cutaneous bacillary angiomatosis caused by *B. henselae* or *B. quintana* resembles verruga peruana, which is not seen outside of South America. In patients with AIDS, Kaposi's sarcoma lesions and bacillary angiomatosis may coexist.

℞ **TREATMENT** Cutaneous lesions have been treated with a wide variety of antimicrobial drugs, including macrolides, tetracyclines, and antituberculous agents; *B. henselae* is susceptible to most antibiotics in vitro. Erythromycin (2 g/d), given orally for 3 weeks, is usually effective, as are newer macrolides; however, relapse may require prolonged therapy (3 weeks to 2 months) with an antibiotic that reaches an intracellular compartment, such as a macrolide or doxycycline (200 mg/d). Patients with peliosis hepatis should be treated with intravenous antibiotics, and those with disseminated disease or bacteremia should be treated with a prolonged course (3 weeks to 2 months) of systemic antibiotic, such as a macrolide (e.g., erythromycin, 2 g/d). In a case-control study of bacillary angiomatosis, treatment with a macrolide was associated with a therapeutic response and sterile tissue samples and may have been protective, whereas treatment with trimethoprim-sulfamethoxazole, ciprofloxacin, penicillins, or cephalosporins had no protective effect. Cutaneous lesions may or may not regress spontaneously, perhaps depending on the status of the host's immunity. The safety of ciprofloxacin in pregnant or lactating women has not been established. No antimicrobial has been studied prospectively, and information on efficacy comes only from case reports.

CAT-SCRATCH DISEASE

DEFINITION AND ETIOLOGY Typical CSD is manifested by painful regional lymphadenopathy persisting for several weeks or months after a cat scratch. Occasionally, infection may disseminate and produce more generalized lymphadenopathy and systemic manifestations, which may be confused with the manifestations of lymphoma. *B. henselae* is the causative agent of CSD. There is no evidence that *B. quintana* causes CSD, and this microbe is not carried by cats. The role of *Afipia felis* (originally proposed as the agent of CSD) is unclear inasmuch as only a few cases are associated with its isolation. *B. henselae* remains the predominant species causing typical CSD. Several reports suggest that *B. clarridgeiae* may also cause feline lymphadenopathy.

EPIDEMIOLOGY Approximately 60% of cases of CSD in the United States occur in children. Exposure to bacteremic young cats that either are flea-infested or have been in contact with another cat carrying fleas poses a significant risk of infection. Most infections are caused by a scratch and only rare cases by a bite or by licking. Most cases occur in the warmer months, when fleas are active. Regions of the United States where fleas are endemic have higher rates of infection. The flea may serve to transmit infection between cats; it is not known whether humans can be infected through the bite of an infected flea.

CLINICAL MANIFESTATIONS A localized papule, progressing to a pustule that often crusts over, develops 3 to 5 days after a cat scratch. Tender regional lymphadenopathy develops within 1 to 2 weeks after inoculation; by this time, the papule may have healed spontaneously. Scratches are most often sustained on the hands or face, producing epitrochlear, axillary, pectoral, and cervical lymph node in-

volvement. The involved nodes occasionally become suppurative; bacterial superinfection with staphylococci or other cutaneous pathogens may develop. Although most patients do not have fever, systemic symptoms are frequent and include malaise, anorexia, and weight loss. Without treatment, lymphadenopathy persists for weeks or even months and may be confused with lymphatic malignancy. Other manifestations in apparently immunocompetent patients include encephalitis, seizures and coma (especially in children), meningitis, transverse myelitis, granulomatous hepatitis and splenitis, osteomyelitis, and disseminated infection. Conjunctival inoculation may cause Parinaud's oculoglandular syndrome, with conjunctivitis and preauricular lymphadenopathy.

PATHOLOGY The histopathologic hallmark of CSD is granulomatous inflammation with stellate necrosis but no evidence of angiogenesis. Thus, infection by *B. henselae* can produce two entirely different pathologic reactions, depending on the immune status of the host: CSD or bacillary angiomatosis.

DIAGNOSIS CSD should be suspected if the patient has a history of exposure to cats and develops lymphadenopathy and a skin lesion. The diagnosis can be confirmed by pathologic examination of the involved nodes. Tiny bacilli in clusters can sometimes be seen in biopsy samples stained with Warthin-Starry silver. The CSD skin test, in which lymph node material obtained from patients with CSD serves as an antigen, is no longer used for diagnosis because of concerns about the transmission of viral agents. A specific serologic test has been developed and may produce a positive result in 70 to 90% of patients with intact immunity. The identification of *B. henselae* 16S ribosomal RNA genes in biopsy material by PCR amplification with specific oligonucleotide primers can also be diagnostically useful; however, these methods are not yet commercially available. Cultures of lymph nodes, cerebrospinal fluid, or other tissues are rarely positive.

℞ **TREATMENT** Although CSD is generally self-limited, tender regional lymphadenopathy and systemic symptoms may be debilitating. Patients with encephalitis or other serious manifestations should be treated with antibiotics. A randomized, double-blind, placebo-controlled trial demonstrated significant clinical benefit of treatment with oral azithromycin for 5 days in cases of typical CSD (regimen for adults weighing >100 lb: one dose of 500 mg on day 1, 250 mg on days 2 through 5). Several reports suggest that aminoglycoside treatment (e.g., intravenous gentamicin at standard doses calculated to result in therapeutic levels) is effective in patients with encephalitis and other systemic infections. The oral agents that appear to be useful are those that also are most effective for the treatment of bacillary angiomatosis; they include ciprofloxacin, doxycycline, and azithromycin. Unlike bacillary angiomatosis, CSD responds to treatment with ciprofloxacin. The necessary duration of therapy is variable.

TRENCH FEVER

DEFINITION AND ETIOLOGY Trench fever was first described as a debilitating febrile illness associated with prolonged *B. quintana* bacteremia in soldiers fighting in Europe during World War I. Although not usually fatal, the illness accounted for substantial morbidity. In recent years, trench fever has reemerged in the United States and has been caused by either *B. henselae*—the agent of CSD and bacillary angiomatosis—or *B. quintana*.

EPIDEMIOLOGY Although trench fever was thought to have disappeared from the United States, recent cases have been diagnosed in homeless persons (*B. quintana*) and in persons bitten by ticks (*B. henselae*). During World War I, trench fever was transmitted from person to person by the human body louse. Transmission by ectoparasites is suspected in the recent cases of *B. quintana* infection but has not been firmly documented. Patients with trench fever have apparently normal immune defenses.

CLINICAL MANIFESTATIONS Trench fever is characterized by the sudden onset of headache, aseptic meningitis, persistent fever (which can be high-grade and is commonly paroxysmal), malaise, weight loss, and other nonspecific symptoms. Severe musculoskeletal pain is more common among immunocompetent than among immunocompromised patients. Bacteremia can persist for days or weeks, and relapses have followed short courses of antibiotic therapy. Localized findings are uncommon.

DIAGNOSIS Trench fever is diagnosed by the finding of sustained bacteremia. *B. henselae* and *B. quintana* grow slowly. Colonies develop on rabbit blood agar after 1 to 4 weeks of incubation under conditions of increased CO_2. Serologic tests for this disease have not yet been standardized.

℞ **TREATMENT** A prolonged course (4 weeks) of antimicrobial therapy may be required. Agents that can cross the mammalian cell membrane are most effective, including erythromycin (2 g/d) or azithromycin (500 mg/d). Data on the efficacy of these agents come from a limited number of case reports.

OTHER *BARTONELLA* INFECTIONS, INCLUDING CULTURE-NEGATIVE ENDOCARDITIS

The application of molecular methods to the detection of microorganisms that are difficult to cultivate in the laboratory has revealed new *Bartonella* spp. and has established *Bartonella* spp. as a cause of endocarditis cases previously classified as being of unknown etiology. *B. quintana* is the most frequently isolated *Bartonella* species in these cases. Two new species, *B. elizabethae* and *B. clarridgeiae*, as well as *B. henselae* have also been identified as agents of subacute and chronic endocarditis.

The diagnosis of *Bartonella* endocarditis is confirmed by blood cultures. Specific antibodies are produced; however, *B. quintana* infection may produce antibodies that cross-react with *Chlamydia pneumoniae*.

BIBLIOGRAPHY

ANDERSON BE, NEUMAN MA: *Bartonella* spp. as emerging human pathogens. Clin Microbiol Rev 10:203, 1997

BASS JW et al: Prospective randomized double blind placebo-controlled evaluation of azithromycin for treatment of cat-scratch disease. Pediatr Infect Dis J 17:447, 1998

BROUQUI P et al: Chronic *Bartonella quintana* bacteremia in homeless patients. N Engl J Med 340:184, 1999

CARITHERS HA: Cat scratch disease: An overview based on a study of 1,200 patients. Am J Dis Child 139:1124, 1985

COCKERELL DJ, LEBOIT PE: Bacillary angiomatosis: A newly characterized, pseudoneoplastic, infectious, cutaneous vascular disorder. J Am Acad Dermatol 22:501, 1990

KOEHLER JE, TAPPERO JW: *Rochalimaea henselae* infection: A new zoonosis with the domestic cat as reservoir. JAMA 271:531, 1994

——— et al: Molecular epidemiology of *Bartonella* infections in patients with bacillary angiomatosis. N Engl J Med 337:1876, 1997

PERKOCHA LA et al: Clinical and pathological features of bacillary peliosis hepatis in association with human immunodeficiency virus infection. N Engl J Med 323:148, 1990

REGNERY RL et al: Characterization of a novel *Rochalimaea* species, *R. henselae*, sp.nov., isolated from blood of a febrile, human immunodeficiency virus–positive patient. J Clin Microbiol 30:265, 1992

SPACH DH et al: *Bartonella (Rochalimaea) quintana* bacteremia in inner-city patients with chronic alcoholism. N Engl J Med 332:425, 1995

ZANGWILL KM et al: Cat scratch disease in Connecticut: Epidemiology, risk factors, and evaluation of a new diagnostic test. N Engl J Med 329:8, 1993

164   *Gavin Hart*

DONOVANOSIS

Donovanosis is a chronic, progressively destructive bacterial infection of the genital region that is generally regarded as sexually transmitted. The disease has been known by many other names, the most common of which are granuloma inguinale and granuloma venereum.

ETIOLOGY Donovanosis is caused by *Calymmatobacterium granulomatis*, an intracellular, gram-negative, pleomorphic, encapsulated (when mature) bacterium measuring 1.5 by 0.7 μm. *C. granulomatis* shares many morphologic and serologic characteristics and >99% homology at the nucleotide level with *Klebsiella* species that are pathogenic to humans. Polymerase chain reaction amplification of the *phoE* gene shows it to be closely related to that in *Klebsiella pneumoniae*, *K. rhinoscleromatis*, and *K. ozaenae*. Electron microscopy shows typical gram-negative morphology and a large capsule but no flagella. Filiform or vesicular protrusions occur on a corrugated cell wall.

EPIDEMIOLOGY Donovanosis is endemic among Aborigines in central Australia as well as in Papua New Guinea, southeastern India, southern Africa, and the Caribbean and adjacent areas of South America. In the first half of the twentieth century, the disease was endemic in parts of the United States (with an estimated 5000 to 10,000 cases in 1947); small epidemics still occur in this country and in other developed countries. Over 70% of cases involve persons 20 to 40 years of age. The infection is predominantly sexually transmitted, but extragenital skin lesions can follow transmission from concurrent genital lesions via the fingers or through other nonsexual contact, and autoinoculation may produce new lesions from contact with adjacent skin ("kissing" lesions). Infants born to infected mothers have acquired infection at birth.

The classification of donovanosis as a sexually transmitted disease (STD) has been disputed because of cases in young children and occasionally in sexually inactive individuals, transmission by direct body contact and via inanimate intermediaries, and the low and variable prevalence of donovanosis among sexual partners (0.4 to 52%). The dominance of sexual transmission is suggested by the combined factors of lesions predominantly affecting the genitalia, the highest prevalence among persons in age and socioeconomic groups that are most often affected by STDs, and the predictable occurrence of disease in visitors to areas of endemicity following sexual exposure.

CLINICAL MANIFESTATIONS The incubation period is usually 1 to 4 weeks but may extend to 1 year. Skin lesions have been detected in infants 6 weeks to 6 months after birth. The disease begins as one or more subcutaneous nodules that erode through the skin to produce clean, granulomatous, sharply defined, usually painless lesions (Fig. 164-1). These lesions, which bleed readily on contact, slowly enlarge. The genitalia are involved in 90% of cases, the inguinal region in 10%, and the anal region in 5 to 10%. Genital swelling, particularly of the labia, is a common feature and occasionally progresses to pseudoelephantiasis. Phimosis and paraphimosis are common local complications, and progressive erosion of affected tissues may completely destroy the penis or other organs. Less common clinical variants include a hypertrophic form (cauliflower- or wartlike lesions), a necrotic form (destructive lesions with foul-smelling exudate, often resembling amebiasis), and a sclerotic or cicatricial form, which has a dry base with extensive scar tissue.

Extragenital lesions occur in at least 6% of cases. Oral donovanosis, the most common extragenital manifestation, presents as pain or bleeding in the mouth, lesions on the lips, or extensive swelling of the gums and palate. Donovanosis may affect most bones, and sometimes many bones are affected at the same time; the tibia is involved in over 50% of such cases. Bony lesions are associated with constitutional symptoms (weight loss, fever, night sweats, and malaise) and

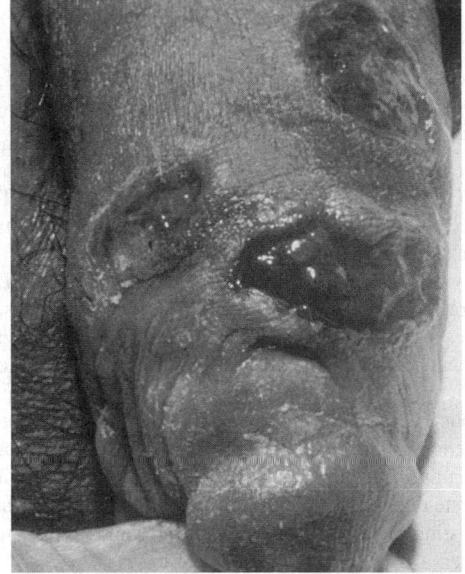

FIGURE 164-1 Multiple granulomatous lesions of the penis in a patient with donovanosis.

Table 164-1 The Most Effective Antibiotic Regimens for Treatment of Donovanosis[a]

Antibiotic	Oral Dosage
Tetracycline	500 mg qid
Doxycycline	100 mg bid
Trimethoprim-sulfamethoxazole	1 double-strength tablet (160 mg/800 mg) bid
Erythromycin	500 mg qid
Azithromycin	1 g weekly
Chloramphenicol	500 mg tid

[a] Patients should be examined weekly, and therapy should be continued until lesions have healed (3 to 5 weeks, except in severe cases).

are usually found in women. More than 50% of women have primary lesions on the cervix. Prompt pelvic examinations and early diagnosis are likely to substantially decrease the morbidity and mortality (a likely outcome in misdiagnosed spinal lesions) associated with extragenital donovanosis in women.

DIAGNOSIS **Laboratory Diagnosis** The preferred method involves demonstration of typical intracellular Donovan bodies within large mononuclear cells visualized in smears prepared from lesions or biopsy specimens. With typical beefy lesions, a small piece of tissue is removed with forceps and scalpel, and a crush impression of the deep surface is made on a glass slide. The smear is air-dried, heat-fixed, and stained with Giemsa, Leishman's, or Wright's stain. For dry, flat, or necrotic lesions, a punch-biopsy specimen should be obtained from the advancing edge. This specimen can be used to prepare a smear or embedded for histologic examination (with a silver stain). Histologic examination shows epithelial proliferation, often simulating neoplasia, with a heavy inflammatory infiltrate of plasma cells, some neutrophils, and few if any lymphocytes. The large mononuclear cells are 25 to 90 μm in diameter, with a vesicular or pyknotic nucleus. Up to 20 intracytoplasmic vacuoles contain pleomorphic Donovan bodies in either young uncapsulated forms (which often resemble closed safety pins) or mature capsulated forms. *C. granulomatis* has never been grown on artificial solid media but has been cultured in chicken embryonic yolk sacs, on human monocytes, and on human epithelial (HEp-2) cells. A sensitive and specific serologic test, based on indirect immunofluorescence, has been developed.

Differential Diagnosis Condylomata lata of secondary syphilis may be confused with donovanosis; however, these lesions usually appear as white or pale moist plaques in the anogenital area, whereas the lesions of donovanosis are usually bright red. Syphilis and donovanosis frequently coexist because syphilis is usually highly prevalent in areas where donovanosis is endemic; thus positive syphilis serology does not exclude a diagnosis of donovanosis. Condylomata lata subside within 1 week of treatment with benzathine penicillin (2.4 million units), whereas donovanosis lesions remain unchanged.

The necrotic form of donovanosis may resemble squamous cell carcinoma; likewise, cervical and vulvar lesions may closely resemble carcinoma. Penile amebiasis may resemble necrotic donovanosis but usually follows anal intercourse and is much less common than donovanosis in areas where the latter is endemic. Atypical clinical variants of chancroid, referred to as *pseudogranuloma inguinale*, have been described in patients seen at clinics in Atlanta. Disseminated donovanosis lesions of bones, particularly in the spine, can mimic tuberculosis. Lesions that produce draining sinuses near the jaw may simulate actinomycosis. The histologic findings of donovanosis must be distinguished from those of rhinoscleroma, leishmaniasis, and histoplasmosis. Genital ulcers are a risk factor for HIV acquisition in developing countries, and patients with donovanosis should be tested for HIV infection.

TREATMENT Table 164-1 shows the most effective regimens for treating donovanosis. Doxycycline is the first choice for therapy in developed countries. Erythromycin provides an effective option for pregnant patients, and azithromycin is an effective alternative that is more convenient to administer. Extensive lesions have been cured with oral azithromycin at a dosage of 500 mg/d, but the more convenient dose of 1 g weekly is also effective. Although chloramphenicol is the drug of choice in some developing countries, it is unlikely to be acceptable in developed countries because of bone marrow toxicity. Penicillin is not effective for treating donovanosis. Patients should be examined weekly, and therapy should be continued until lesions have healed (3 to 5 weeks, except in severe cases). If antibiotic therapy is stopped earlier, lesions often continue to heal, but the relapse rate is higher. If the lesions are unchanged after 2 weeks of treatment, an alternative antibiotic regimen should be used.

The treatment regimens just described are usually adequate in HIV-infected patients without immunosuppression, but an increasing failure rate has been reported in immunosuppressed patients, for whom daily administration of azithromycin is recommended if other regimens fail to elicit a response.

BIBLIOGRAPHY

CARTER J et al: Culture of the causative organism of donovanosis (*Calymmatobacterium granulomatis*) in HEp-2 cells. J Clin Microbiol 35:2915, 1997

HART G: Donovanosis (granuloma inguinale), in *Atlas of Infectious Diseases*, vol V: *Sexually Transmitted Diseases*, MF Rein (ed). Philadelphia, Churchill Livingstone, 1996, pp 17.1–17.10

————: Donovanosis. Clin Infect Dis 25:24, 1997

PATERSON DL: Disseminated donovanosis (granuloma inguinale) causing spinal cord compression: Case report and review of donovanosis involving bone. Clin Infect Dis 26:379, 1998

165 *Gregory A. Filice*

NOCARDIOSIS

The term *nocardiosis* refers to invasive disease associated with members of the genus *Nocardia*. Of the several distinctive syndromes, pneumonia and disseminated disease are most common. Others include cellulitis, lymphocutaneous syndrome, actinomycetoma, and keratitis.

MICROBIOLOGY Nocardiae are saprophytic aerobic actinomycetes that are common worldwide in soil, where they contribute to decay of organic matter. Nocardial taxonomy is complex and incompletely understood. Seven species have been associated with human disease: *N. asteroides*, *N. brasiliensis*, *N. otitidis-caviarum* (formerly *N. caviae*), *N. farcinica*, *N. nova*, *N. transvalensis*, and *N. pseudobrasiliensis*. *N. asteroides* is the species most commonly associated with invasive disease. *N. farcinica* is less common but tends to be virulent and prone to dissemination. The new species *N. pseudobrasiliensis* accounts for most cases of invasive disease previously attributed to *N. brasiliensis*. True *N. brasiliensis* isolates are usually associated with disease limited to the skin. *N. transvalensis* is generally associated with mycetoma or, in immunosuppressed persons, with pulmonary or systemic disease.

EPIDEMIOLOGY Approximately 1000 cases of nocardial infection are diagnosed annually in the United States, 85% of them pulmonary and/or systemic. The disease is more common among adults and males. Outbreaks, which are rare, have been associated with contamination of the hospital environment, solutions, or drug injection equipment. Person-to-person spread is not well documented. There is no known seasonality.

The risk of pulmonary or disseminated disease is greater than usual among people with deficient cell-mediated immunity, especially that associated with lymphoma, transplantation, or AIDS. In persons with AIDS, nocardiosis usually presents at a CD4+ lymphocyte concentration of $<250/\mu L$. Prophylaxis with sulfamethoxazole and trimethoprim appears to reduce the risk of nocardiosis in persons with AIDS or transplanted organs. Nocardiosis has also been associated with pulmonary alveolar proteinosis, tuberculosis and other mycobacterial diseases, and chronic granulomatous disease.

N. brasiliensis, *N. asteroides*, *N. otitidis-caviarum*, and *N. transvalensis* are associated with actinomycetoma. Cases occur mainly in tropical and subtropical regions, especially those of Mexico, Central and South America, Africa, and India. The most important risk factor is frequent contact with soil or vegetable matter.

PATHOLOGY AND PATHOGENESIS Pneumonia and disseminated disease are both thought to follow inhalation of fragmented bacterial mycelia. The characteristic histologic feature of nocardiosis is an abscess with extensive infiltration by neutrophils and prominent necrosis. Granulation tissue usually surrounds the lesions, but extensive fibrosis or encapsulation is uncommon. Actinomycetoma is characterized by suppurative inflammation with sinus tract formation. Granules—microcolonies composed of dense masses of bacterial filaments extending radially from a central core—are occasionally observed in histologic preparations. They are frequently found in discharges from lesions of actinomycetoma but almost never from lesions in other forms of nocardiosis.

Nocardiae have evolved a number of properties that enable them to survive within phagocytes, including neutralization of oxidants, prevention of phagosome-lysosome fusion, and prevention of phagosome acidification. Neutrophils phagocytose the organisms and limit their growth but do not kill them efficiently. Cell-mediated immunity is important for definitive control and elimination of nocardiae.

CLINICAL MANIFESTATIONS Respiratory Tract Disease Pneumonia is by far the most common respiratory tract nocardial disease. Nocardial pneumonia is typically subacute; symptoms have usually been present for days or weeks at presentation. The onset may be more acute in immunosuppressed patients. Cough is prominent and produces small amounts of thick, purulent sputum that is not malodorous. Fever, anorexia, weight loss, and malaise are common; dyspnea, pleuritic pain, and hemoptysis are less common. Remissions and exacerbations over several weeks are frequent.

Roentgenographic patterns are variable, but some characteristics are highly suggestive. Infiltrates vary in size and are typically of at least moderate density. Single or multiple nodules are common, sometimes suggesting metastatic tumors. Infiltrates and nodules tend to cavitate. Empyema is present in one-third of cases.

Nocardiosis may spread directly from the lungs to adjacent tissues. Pericarditis, mediastinitis, and the superior vena cava syndrome have all been reported. Spread through the chest wall is rare.

Nocardial laryngitis, tracheitis, and bronchitis are much less common than pneumonia. In the major airways, disease often presents as a nodular or granulomatous mass. A few cases of sinusitis have been reported.

Nocardiae are sometimes isolated from respiratory secretions of patients without apparent nocardial disease. Most of these patients have chronic pulmonary disease with abnormal airways or parenchyma.

Extrapulmonary Dissemination In half of all cases of pulmonary nocardiosis, disease appears outside the lungs. In one-fifth of cases of disseminated disease, lung disease is not apparent. The most common site of dissemination is the brain. Other common sites include the skin and supporting structures, kidneys, bone, and muscle, but almost any organ can be involved. Peritonitis and endocarditis have been reported. The typical manifestation of extrapulmonary dissemination is a subacute abscess. A minority of abscesses outside the lungs or central nervous system (CNS) form fistulae and discharge small amounts of pus. Nocardiae have been recovered from blood in a few cases of pneumonia or disseminated disease.

In CNS infections, brain abscesses are usually supratentorial, are often multiloculated, and may be single or multiple (Fig. 165-1). Brain abscesses tend to burrow into the ventricles or extend out into the subarachnoid space. The symptoms and signs are somewhat more indolent than those of other types of bacterial brain abscess. Meningitis is uncommon and is usually due to spread from a nearby brain abscess. Nocardiae are not easily recovered from cerebrospinal fluid (CSF).

Disease Following Transcutaneous Inoculation Disease following transcutaneous nocardial inoculation usually takes one of three forms: cellulitis, lymphocutaneous syndrome, or actinomycetoma. Cellulitis generally begins 1 to 3 weeks after a recognized breach of the skin, often with soil contamination. Subacute cellulitis with pain, swelling, erythema, and warmth develops over days to weeks. The lesions are usually firm and nonfluctuant. Disease may progress to involve underlying muscle, tendon, bones, or joints. Dissemination is rare. *N. asteroides* is common in colder climates, while *N. brasiliensis* predominates in warmer climates.

In the lymphocutaneous syndrome, there is typically a pyodermatous lesion at the site of inoculation, with central ulceration and purulent or honey-colored drainage. Subcutaneous nodules often appear along lymphatics that drain the primary lesion. The lymphangitic form closely resembles lymphocutaneous sporotrichosis (Chap. 208). Most cases of the lymphocutaneous syndrome are associated with *N. brasiliensis*.

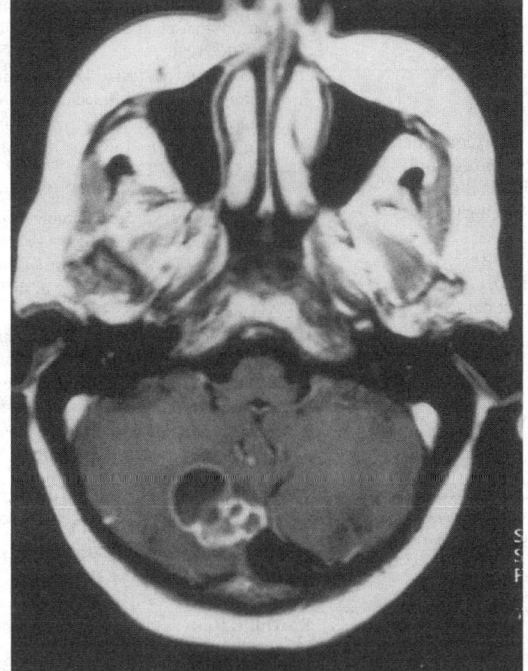

FIGURE 165-1 Nocardial abscesses in the right cerebellum. The appearance suggests one large abscess and multiple daughter abscesses.

Actinomycetoma usually begins with a nodular swelling, sometimes at a site of local trauma. Lesions typically develop on the feet or hands but may involve the posterior part of the neck, the upper back, the head, and other sites. The nodule eventually breaks down and a fistula appears. This fistula is soon accompanied by others. The fistulas tend to come and go, with new ones forming as old ones disappear. The discharge is serous or purulent, may be bloody, and often contains 0.1- to 2-mm white granules consisting of masses of mycelia. The lesions spread slowly along fascial planes to involve adjacent areas of skin, subcutaneous tissue, and bone. Over months or years, there may be extensive deformation of the affected part. Lesions involving soft tissues are only mildly painful; those affecting bones or joints are more so. Systemic symptoms are absent or minimal. Infection rarely disseminates from actinomycetoma, and lesions on the hands and feet usually cause only local disability. Lesions on the head, neck, and trunk can invade locally to involve deep organs and result in severe disability or death.

Keratitis *Nocardia* spp., usually *N. asteroides*, are uncommon causes of subacute keratitis. The infection usually follows eye trauma. Nocardial infection of lacrimal glands has been reported. Disease involving deeper eye structures is usually a manifestation of dissemination.

DIAGNOSIS The first step in diagnosis is examination of sputum or pus for crooked, branching, beaded, gram-positive filaments 1 μm wide and up to 50 μm long. Most nocardiae are acid-fast in direct smears if a weak acid is used for decolorization (e.g., in the modified Kinyoun, Ziehl-Neelsen, and Fite-Faraco methods). The organisms often take up silver stains. Nocardiae grow relatively slowly; colonies may take up to 2 weeks to appear and may not develop their characteristic appearance for up to 4 weeks. Several blood culture systems support nocardial growth. Yield is enhanced when blood cultures are incubated aerobically for up to 4 weeks and when blind subcultures are performed. Nocardial growth is so different from that of more common pathogens that the laboratory should be alerted when nocardiosis is suspected to maximize the likelihood of isolation. Since nocardiae are among the few aerobic microorganisms that use paraffin as a carbon source, paraffin baiting can be useful in isolating the organisms from mixed cultures.

In cases of pneumonia, sputum smears are often negative. Unless the diagnosis can be made in these cases by sampling lesions in other,

more accessible sites, bronchoscopy or lung aspiration is usually necessary. Transtracheal aspiration should be avoided, as it frequently leads to nocardial cellulitis in tissues around the puncture wound.

In patients with nocardial pneumonia, a careful history should be obtained and a thorough physical examination performed to evaluate the possibility of dissemination. Suggestive symptoms or signs should be pursued with further diagnostic tests. Computed tomography or magnetic resonance imaging of the head, with and without contrast material, should be undertaken if signs or symptoms suggest brain involvement. Many authorities recommend brain imaging in all cases of pulmonary or disseminated disease.

When clinically indicated, CSF or urine should be concentrated and then cultured. In actinomycetoma cases, granules should be sought in the discharge. Suspect particles should be washed in saline, examined microscopically, and cultured.

Isolation of nocardiae from sputum or blood occasionally represents colonization, transient infection, or contamination. In typical cases of respiratory tract colonization, Gram-stained specimens are negative and cultures are only intermittently positive. A positive sputum culture in an immunosuppressed patient usually reflects disease. When nocardiae are isolated from an immunocompetent patient without apparent nocardial disease, the patient should be observed carefully without treatment. A patient with a host-defense defect that increases the risk of nocardiosis should usually receive antimicrobial treatment.

Nocardia spp. are difficult to differentiate from one another with standard biochemical tests, and isolates from patients with systemic or severe disease should be sent to a reference laboratory for definitive identification and antimicrobial susceptibility testing. Susceptibility results, which help differentiate species, are of less certain clinical value but sometimes guide therapy in difficult cases.

In vitro, strains of *N. farcinica* differ from most in that they are usually resistant to cephalosporins and in one-fifth of cases are resistant to imipenem. *N. pseudobrasiliensis* strains often exhibit resistance to minocycline or amoxicillin/clavulanic acid and susceptibility to ciprofloxacin or clarithromycin. *N. transvalensis* displays increased resistance to many antimicrobial agents, including amikacin, tobramycin, cefotaxime, ceftriaxone, and amoxicillin/clavulanic acid. *N. nova* isolates appear to be susceptible to ampicillin and erythromycin in vitro but also produce β-lactamase constitutively or in the presence of a β-lactam.

Several presumptive diagnostic tests for nocardial infection have been studied, including tests for antibodies, nocardial metabolites, and nocardial DNA. None is ready for clinical use at this time.

TREATMENT Sulfonamides are the drugs of choice for nocardiosis (Table 165-1). Initially, 6 to 8 g of sulfadiazine or sulfisoxazole per day in four divided doses should be used. After disease is controlled, 4 g/d can be used to complete therapy. In difficult cases, sulfonamide levels should be measured and dosages adjusted to keep serum levels between 100 and 150 μg/mL. The combination of sulfamethoxazole (SMZ) and trimethoprim (TMP) is probably equivalent to sulfonamides; some authorities believe that the combination may in fact be more effective, but it also poses a modestly greater risk of hematologic toxicity. At the outset, 10 to 20 mg of TMP per kg and 50 to 100 mg of SMZ per kg should be given each day in two divided doses. Later, the daily doses can be decreased to as little as 5 mg/kg and 25 mg/kg, respectively. In persons with sulfonamide allergies, desensitization usually allows continuation of therapy with these effective and inexpensive drugs.

Minocycline is the best-established alternative oral drug and should be given in doses of 100 to 200 mg twice a day. Other tetracyclines are usually ineffective. *N. nova* infections can be treated with erythromycin (500 to 750 mg four times a day) and/or ampicillin (1 g four times a day), but other *Nocardia* spp. are often resistant to both drugs. Amoxicillin (500 mg) combined with clavulanic acid (125 mg), given three times a day, has been effective in a few cases but should

Table 165-1 Treatment for Nocardiosis

Disease	Duration	Drugs (Daily Dose)[a]
Pulmonary or systemic		**Systemic therapy**
Intact host defenses	6–12 mo	**Oral**
Deficient host defenses	12 mo[b]	1. Sulfonamides (6–8 g) or combination of
CNS disease	12 mo[c]	trimethoprim (10–20 mg/kg) and
Cellulitis, lympho-		sulfamethoxazole (50–100 mg/kg)
cutaneous syndrome	2 mo	2. Minocycline (200–400 mg)
Osteomyelitis, arthritis,		**Parenteral**
laryngitis, sinusitis	4 mo	1. Amikacin (10–15 mg/kg)
Actinomycetoma	6–12 mo after	2. Cefotaxime (6 g), ceftizoxime (6 g),
	clinical cure	ceftriaxone (2 g), imipenem (2 g)
Keratitis	**Topical:** Until apparent cure	1. Sulfonamide drops
		2. Amikacin drops
	Systemic: Until 2–4 mo after apparent cure	Drugs for systemic therapy as listed above

[a] For each category, choices are numbered in order of preference.

[b] In some patients with AIDS or chronic granulomatous disease, therapy for pulmonary or systemic disease must be continued indefinitely.

[c] If all apparent CNS disease has been excised, the duration of therapy may be reduced to 6 months.

be avoided in cases due to *N. nova*, in which clavulanate induces β-lactamase production. Ofloxacin (400 mg twice a day) and clarithromycin (500 mg twice a day) have each been successful in a few cases.

Amikacin, the best-established parenteral drug, is given in doses of 5 to 7.5 mg/kg every 12 h. Serum levels should be monitored with prolonged therapy in patients with diminished renal function and in the elderly. Newer β-lactam antibiotics, including cefotaxime, ceftizoxime, ceftriaxone, and imipenem, are usually effective. They may be less effective in some cases caused by *N. farcinica*.

In patients receiving immunosuppressive therapy, the regimen should be continued if necessary for treatment of an underlying disease or prevention of transplant rejection. In many cases, two or more antimicrobial agents have been used to treat nocardiosis, often in combinations including a sulfonamide or minocycline. Whether such therapy is better than monotherapy is not known, and combination therapy increases the risk of toxicity.

Surgical management of nocardial disease is similar to that of other bacterial diseases. Brain abscesses should be aspirated, drained, or excised if the diagnosis is unclear, if an abscess is large and accessible, or if an abscess fails to respond to chemotherapy. Abscesses that are small or inaccessible should be treated medically; in these cases, clinical improvement should be noticeable within 1 to 2 weeks. Brain imaging should be repeated to document the resolution of lesions, although abatement on images often lags behind clinical improvement.

Antimicrobial therapy usually suffices for nocardial actinomycetoma. In deep or extensive cases, drainage or excision of heavily involved tissue may facilitate healing, but structure and function should be preserved whenever possible.

Nocardial infections tend to relapse (particularly in patients with chronic granulomatous disease), and long courses of antimicrobial therapy are necessary. If disease is unusually extensive, if the patient is immunosuppressed, or if the response to therapy is slow, the recommendations in Table 165-1 should be exceeded.

The mortality rate for pulmonary or disseminated nocardiosis outside the CNS should be <5%. CNS disease carries a higher mortality rate. Patients should be followed carefully for at least 6 months after therapy has ended. Any child with nocardiosis and no known cause of immunosuppression should undergo tests to determine the adequacy of the phagocytic respiratory burst.

BIBLIOGRAPHY

BERKEY P, BODEY GP: Nocardial infection in patients with neoplastic disease. Rev Infect Dis 11:407, 1989

BROWN BA et al: Disseminated *Nocardia pesudobrasiliensis* infection in a patient with AIDS in Brazil. Clin Infect Dis 28:144, 1999

CHOUCIÑO C et al: Nocardial infections in bone marrow transplant recipients. Clin Infect Dis 23:1012, 1996

FILICE GA, NIEWOEHNER DE: Contribution of neutrophils and cell-mediated immunity to control of *Nocardia asteroides* in murine lungs. J Infect Dis 156:113, 1987

———, SIMPSON GL: Management of *Nocardia* infections, in *Current Clinical Topics in Infectious Diseases*, vol 5, JS Remington et al (eds). New York, McGraw-Hill, 1984

KONTOYIANNIS DP et al: *Nocardia* bacteremia. Report of 4 cases and review of the literature. Medicine 77:255, 1998

MINAMOTO GY, SORDILLO EM: Disseminated nocardiosis in a patient with AIDS: Diagnosis by blood and cerebrospinal fluid cultures. Clin Infect Dis 26:242, 1998

PALMER DL et al: Diagnostic and therapeutic considerations in *Nocardia asteroides* infection. Medicine 53:391, 1974

SATTERWHITE TK, WALLACE RJ JR: Primary cutaneous nocardiosis. JAMA 242:333, 1979

SMEGO RA Jr et al: Lymphocutaneous syndrome. A review of non-sporothrix causes. Medicine 78:38, 1999

TIGHT RR, BARTLETT MS: Actinomycetoma in the United States. Rev Infect Dis 3:1139, 1981

UTTAMCHANDANI RB et al: Nocardiosis in 30 patients with advanced human immunodeficiency virus infection: Clinical features and outcome. Clin Infect Dis 18:348, 1994

---

166 ACTINOMYCOSIS

Thomas A. Russo

Actinomycosis is an indolent, slowly progressive infection caused by anaerobic or microaerophilic bacteria, primarily of the genus *Actinomyces*, that colonize the mouth, colon, and vagina. Mucosal disruption may lead to infection at virtually any site in the body. The clinical presentations of actinomycosis are myriad; however, classic features include purulent foci surrounded by dense fibrosis that, over time, cross natural anatomic boundaries into contiguous structures, with the formation of fistulae and sinus tracts in some cases. In vivo growth of actinomycetes usually results in the formation of clumps called *grains* or *sulfur granules*. This infection is commonly confused with a neoplasm. Common in the preantibiotic era, actinomycosis has diminished in incidence, as has its timely recognition. Actinomycosis has been called "the most misdiagnosed disease," and it has been said that "no disease is so often missed by experienced clinicians." Thus this entity remains a diagnostic challenge. An awareness of the full spectrum of the disease will expedite its diagnosis and treatment and will minimize the unnecessary surgical interventions, morbidity, and mortality that are reported all too often.

ETIOLOGIC AGENTS Actinomycosis is most commonly caused by *A. israelii. A. naeslundii, A. odontolyticus, A. viscosus, A. meyeri, A. gerencseriae*, and *Propionibacterium propionicum* are established but less common causes of the disease. Most if not all actinomycotic infections are polymicrobial. *Actinobacillus actinomycetemcomitans, Eikenella corrodens*, Enterobacteriaceae, and species of *Fusobacterium, Bacteroides, Capnocytophaga, Staphylococcus*, and *Streptococcus* are commonly isolated with actinomycetes in various combinations, depending on the site of infection. The contribution of these other species to the pathogenesis of actinomycosis is uncertain.

An increasing number of bacterial species isolated from human clinical specimens have recently been classified as *Actinomyces*. Although their role in disease has not always been defined, *A. europaeus, A. neuii* subspecies *neuii, A. neuii* subspecies *anitratus, A. radingae*,

A. graevenitzii, and *A. turicensis* appear to be infrequent and often opportunistic human pathogens. The nature of the infections described to date does not clearly establish these agents as causes of the typical syndrome of actinomycosis.

EPIDEMIOLOGY The agents of actinomycosis are members of the normal oral flora and are often cultured from the bronchi, the gastrointestinal tract, and the female genital tract. Infection occurs throughout life, with a peak incidence in the middle decades. Males have a threefold higher incidence of infection, possibly because of poorer dental hygiene and/or more frequent trauma. Likely contributing factors to the decrease in the incidence of actinomycosis since the preantibiotic era include improved dental hygiene and the initiation of antimicrobial treatment early on—before the full development of the disease. Individuals who do not seek or have access to health care are undoubtedly at higher risk.

PATHOGENESIS AND PATHOLOGY A vital step in the development of actinomycosis is disruption of the mucosal barrier, which allows the actinomycetes to invade beyond their endogenous habitat in the mouth, lower gastrointestinal tract, and female genitourinary tract. Local infection, subsequent extension, and (in rare instances) distant hematogenous seeding may ensue. Initial acute inflammation is followed by the characteristic chronic, indolent phase. Lesions usually appear as single or multiple indurations. Central fluctuance, with pus containing neutrophils and sulfur granules, is virtually diagnostic of this disease (Fig. 166-1). The fibrous walls of the mass are typically described as "woody." The responsible bacterial and/or host factors have not yet been identified. Once established, actinomycosis spreads contiguously in a slow progressive manner, ignoring tissue planes. Given time, sinus tracts, which can spontaneously close and reopen, will form and extend to skin, adjacent organs, or bone. These unique features of actinomycosis mimic malignancy, with which it is often confused.

Foreign bodies appear to facilitate infection. This association most frequently involves intrauterine contraceptive devices (IUCDs). In addition, an increasing number of reports have described an association of actinomycosis with HIV infection, transplantation, and chemotherapy. Ulcerative mucosal infections (e.g., by herpes simplex virus or cytomegalovirus) and abnormalities in host defenses may facilitate the development of actinomycosis in the latter settings.

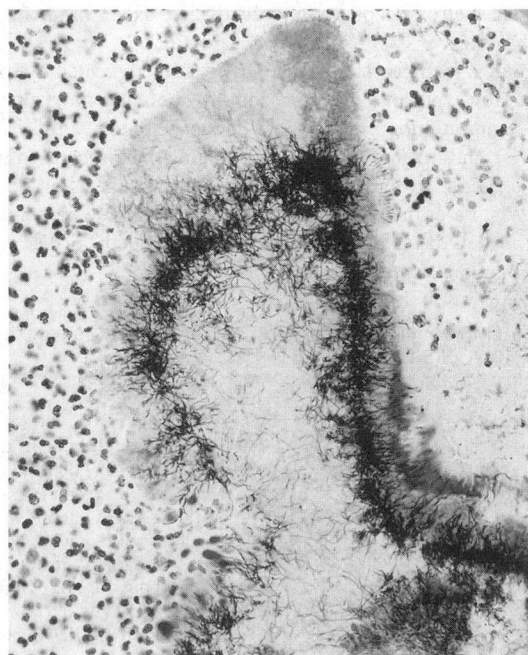

FIGURE 166-1 Actinomycotic sulfur granule surrounded by inflammatory cells. The delicate branched filaments of *Actinomyces* are surrounded by the proteinaceous eosinophilic coating of the granule (Slendore-Hoeppli phenomenon).

CLINICAL MANIFESTATIONS **Oral-Cervicofacial Disease** Actinomycosis occurs most frequently at an oral, cervical, or facial site, usually as a soft tissue swelling, abscess, or mass lesion that is often mistaken for a neoplasm. The angle of the jaw is generally involved, but a diagnosis of actinomycosis should be considered with any mass lesion or relapsing infection in the head and neck. Otitis, sinusitis, and canaliculitis can also develop. Pain, fever, and leukocytosis are variably reported. Contiguous extension to the cranium, cervical spine, or thorax is a potential sequela.

Thoracic Disease Thoracic actinomycosis usually follows an indolent progressive course, with involvement of the pulmonary parenchyma and/or the pleural space. Chest pain, fever, and weight loss are common. A cough, when present, is variably productive. The usual radiographic appearance is either a mass lesion or pneumonitis. Cavitary disease or hilar adenopathy may develop. More than 50% of cases include pleural thickening, effusion, or empyema. Rarely, pulmonary nodules or endobronchial lesions occur. Pulmonary lesions suggestive of actinomycosis may cross fissures or pleura; may involve the mediastinum, contiguous bone, or chest wall; or may be associated with a sinus tract. In the absence of these findings, thoracic actinomycosis is usually mistaken for a neoplasm or for pneumonitis due to more usual causes.

Mediastinal infection is uncommon, usually arising from thoracic extension but rarely resulting from perforation of the esophagus, from trauma, or from head and neck or abdominal disease. The structures within the mediastinum and the heart can be involved in various combinations; consequently, the possible presentations are diverse. Isolated disease of the breast has been described.

Abdominal Disease Abdominal actinomycosis poses a great diagnostic challenge. Months or years usually pass from the inciting event (e.g., appendicitis, diverticulitis, peptic ulcer disease, foreign-body perforation, bowel surgery, or ascension from IUCD-associated pelvic disease) to clinical recognition. Because of the flow of peritoneal fluid and/or the direct extension of primary disease, virtually any abdominal organ, region, or space can be involved. The disease usually presents as an abscess or a mass lesion that is often fixed to underlying tissue and mistaken for a tumor. Infiltrative disease with irregular contrast enhancement may be seen on computed tomography (CT). Sinus tracts to the abdominal wall or perianal region may develop. Recurrent disease or a wound or fistula that fails to heal (in the absence of inflammatory bowel disease) suggests actinomycosis.

Hepatic infection usually presents as single or multiple abscesses or masses. Isolated disease presumably develops via hematogenous seeding from cryptic foci. Presently available imaging and percutaneous techniques have resulted in improved diagnosis and treatment.

All levels of the urogenital tract can be infected. Renal disease usually presents as pyelonephritis and/or renal and perinephric abscess. Bladder involvement, usually due to extension of pelvic disease, may result in ureteral obstruction or fistulas to bowel, skin, or uterus.

Pelvic Disease Actinomycotic involvement of the pelvis occurs most commonly in association with an IUCD. Pelvic symptoms when an IUCD is in place or has recently been removed should prompt consideration of actinomycosis. Although the risk has not yet been quantified, it appears to be small. The disease rarely develops when the IUCD has been in place for <1 year, but the risk increases with time. Actinomycosis can also present months after the removal of the device. Symptoms are typically indolent; fever, weight loss, abdominal pain, and abnormal vaginal bleeding or discharge are the most common. The earliest stage of disease—often endometritis—commonly progresses to pelvic masses or a tuboovarian abscess (Fig. 166-2). Unfortunately, because the diagnosis is often delayed, a "frozen pelvis" mimicking malignancy or endometriosis can develop by the time of recognition.

An unresolved issue is whether the isolation of *Actinomyces*-like organisms (ALOs) from cultures of cervical or endometrial specimens

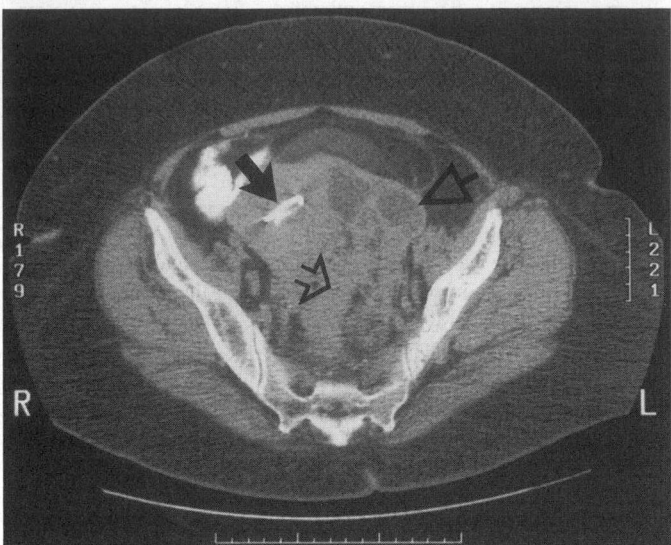

FIGURE 166-2 Computed tomogram showing pelvic actinomycosis associated with an intrauterine contraceptive device. The device is encased by endometrial fibrosis (*solid arrowhead*); also visible are paraendometrial fibrosis (*open arrow*) and an area of suppuration (*open arrowhead*).

or the detection of ALOs by immunofluorescence is correlated with IUCD-associated disease. A Papanicolaou smear may fail to detect ALOs even in the presence of active actinomycosis. Although the risk appears to be small, the consequences of infection are significant. Therefore, until more quantitative data become available, detection of ALOs or immunofluorescence-positive organisms in conjunction with symptoms that cannot be accounted for appears to warrant removal of the IUCD and—if advanced disease is excluded—initiation of a 14-day course of empirical treatment for possible early pelvic actinomycosis. The detection of ALOs or immunofluorescence-positive organisms in the absence of symptoms warrants education of the patient and close follow-up but not removal of the IUCD.

Central Nervous System Disease Actinomycosis of the central nervous system is rare. Single or multiple brain abscesses are most common. An abscess usually appears on CT as a ring-enhancing lesion with a thick wall that may be irregular or nodular. Meningitis, epidural or subdural space infection, and cavernous sinus syndrome have also been described.

Musculoskeletal Infection Actinomycotic infection of the bone is usually due to adjacent soft tissue infection but may be associated with trauma (e.g., fracture of the mandible) or hematogenous spread. Because of slow disease progression, new bone formation and bone destruction are seen concomitantly. Infection of an extremity is uncommon and is usually a result of trauma. Skin, subcutaneous tissue, muscle, and bone (with periostitis or acute or chronic osteomyelitis) are involved alone or in various combinations. Cutaneous sinus tracts frequently develop.

Disseminated Disease Hematogenous dissemination of disease from any location rarely results in multiple organ involvement. The lungs and liver are most commonly affected, with the presentation of multiple nodules mimicking disseminated malignancy. The clinical presentation may be surprisingly indolent given the extent of disease.

DIAGNOSIS The diagnosis of actinomycosis, particularly when it mimics malignancy, is rarely considered. All too often, the first mention of actinomycosis is by the pathologist after extensive surgery has been performed. Since medical therapy alone is often sufficient for cure, the challenge for the clinician is to consider the possibility of actinomycosis in time to diagnose it in the least invasive fashion and to avoid unnecessary surgery. Both fine-needle aspiration and biopsy are being used successfully to obtain clinical material for diagnosis,

as are CT- and ultrasound-guided aspirations or biopsies. The diagnosis is most commonly made by microscopic identification of sulfur granules; occasionally these granules, if sought, can be grossly identified from draining sinus tracts or other purulent material. Although sulfur granules are a defining characteristic of actinomycosis, granules are also found in mycetoma and botryomycosis; however, these entities can easily be differentiated from actinomycosis with appropriate histopathologic and microbiologic studies. Microbiologic identification of actinomycetes is possible in only a minority of cases and is often precluded by prior antimicrobial therapy. Therefore, for optimal yield, the avoidance of even a single dose of antibiotics is mandatory. Primary isolation usually requires 5 to 7 days but may take as long as 2 to 4 weeks. Immunofluorescence testing for *A. israelii*, *A. naeslundii*, and *P. propionicum* (available through the Centers for Disease Control and Prevention in Atlanta) has become a useful diagnostic alternative. Because these organisms are components of the normal oral and genital-tract flora, their identification in sputum, bronchial washings, and cervicovaginal secretions is of little significance in the absence of sulfur granules. *Actinomyces* can be detected in urine by means of appropriate staining and culture.

TREATMENT Actinomycosis must be treated with high doses of antimicrobials for a prolonged period. Although therapy needs to be individualized, the intravenous administration of 18 to 24 million units of penicillin for 2 to 6 weeks, followed by oral therapy with penicillin or amoxicillin for 6 to 12 months, is a reasonable guideline for serious infections. Less extensive disease, particularly that involving the oral-cervicofacial region, may require less intensive therapy. If therapy is extended beyond the point of resolution of measurable disease, the risk of relapse—a clinical hallmark of this infection—will be minimized. A similar approach is reasonable for immunocompromised patients, although refractory disease has been described in HIV-infected individuals. Antimicrobial agents whose use is supported by extensive clinical experience are listed in Table 166-1. Although the role played by "companion" microbes in actinomycosis is unclear, many isolates are pathogens in their own right, and a regimen covering these organisms during the initial treatment course is reasonable. Agents whose success has been reported anecdotally are ceftriaxone, ceftizoxime, imipenem, and ciprofloxacin. Drugs that should be avoided are metronidazole, aminoglycosides, oxacillin, dicloxacillin, and cephalexin.

Combined medical-surgical therapy is still advocated by some authorities. However, an increasing body of literature now supports an initial attempt at cure with medical therapy alone, even in extensive disease. CT and magnetic resonance imaging should be used to monitor the response to therapy. Percutaneous drainage is an additional option. When a critical location is involved (e.g., the epidural space, the central nervous system) or when suitable medical therapy fails, surgical intervention may be appropriate.

Table 166-1 Antibiotic Therapy for Actinomycosis: Regimens Supported by Extensive Clinical Experience

Agent	Dosage
Penicillin	18–24 million units/d IV q4h
	1–2 g/d PO q6h
Erythromycin	2–4 g/d IV q6h
	1–2 g/d PO q6h
Tetracycline	1–2 g/d PO q6h
Doxycycline	200 mg/d IV or PO q12–24h
Minocycline	200 mg/d IV or PO q12h
Clindamycin	2.7 g/d IV q8h
	1.2–1.8 g/d PO q6–8h

NOTE: Additional coverage for concomitant "companion" bacteria may be required. Controlled evaluations have not been performed. Regimens must be individualized according to the site and extent of infection. As a general rule, a maximal antimicrobial dose given parenterally for 2 to 6 weeks, followed by oral therapy, with a total duration of 6 to 12 months, optimizes the likelihood of cure.

BIBLIOGRAPHY

FIORINO AS: Intrauterine contraceptive device–associated actinomycotic abscess and *Actinomyces* detection on cervical smear. Obstet Gynecol 87:142, 1996

GOODMAN HM, CENTENO BA: Case records of the Massachusetts General Hospital, case 10-1992. N Engl J Med 326:692, 1992

RUSSO TA: Actinomycosis, in *Principles and Practice of Infectious Diseases*, 5th ed, GL Mandell et al (eds). New York, Churchill Livingstone, 1999

SMEGO RA, FOGLIA G: Actinomycosis. Clin Infect Dis 26:1255, 1998

| 167 | *Dennis L. Kasper* |

INFECTIONS DUE TO MIXED ANAEROBIC ORGANISMS

DEFINITIONS *Anaerobic* bacteria are organisms that require reduced oxygen tension for growth, failing to grow on the surface of solid media in 10% CO_2 in air. (In contrast, *microaerophilic* bacteria can grow in 10% CO_2 in air or under anaerobic or aerobic conditions, although they grow best in the presence of only a small amount of atmospheric oxygen, and *facultative* bacteria can grow in the presence or absence of air.) This chapter describes infections caused by non-sporulating anaerobic bacteria. In general, anaerobes associated with human infections are relatively aerotolerant. They can survive for as long as 72 h in the presence of oxygen, although generally they will not multiply in this environment. A far smaller number of pathogenic anaerobic bacteria (which are also part of the normal flora) die after brief contact with oxygen, even in low concentrations.

The nonsporulating anaerobic bacteria exist as components of the normal flora on the mucosal surfaces of humans and animals. The major reservoirs of these bacteria are the mouth, lower gastrointestinal tract, skin, and female genital tract. Among the constituents of the oral flora, anaerobes are the predominant commensal organisms, ranging in concentration from 10^9/mL in saliva to 10^{12}/mL in gingival scrapings. In the oral cavity, the ratio of anaerobic to aerobic bacteria ranges from 1:1 on the surface of a tooth to 1000:1 in the gingival crevice. Anaerobic bacteria are not found in appreciable numbers in the normal upper intestine until the distal ileum. In the colon, the proportion of anaerobes increases significantly, as does the overall bacterial count. For example, in the colon there are 10^{11} to 10^{12} organisms per gram of stool, with a ratio of anaerobes to aerobes of approximately 1000:1. In the female genital tract, there are approximately 10^9 organisms per milliliter of secretions, with a ratio of anaerobes to aerobes of approximately 10:1.

Hundreds of species of anaerobic bacteria have been identified as part of the normal flora of humans. Identification of as many as 500 different anaerobic species in fecal specimens reflects the diversity of the anaerobic flora. Despite the complex array of bacteria in the normal flora, relatively few species are isolated commonly from human infection.

Anaerobic infections occur when the harmonious relationship between the host and the bacteria is disrupted. Any site in the body is susceptible to infection with these indigenous organisms when a mucosal barrier or the skin is compromised by surgery, trauma, tumor, or ischemia or necrosis, which reduce local tissue redox potentials. Because the sites that are colonized by anaerobes contain many species of bacteria, disruption of anatomic barriers allows penetration of many organisms, resulting in mixed infections involving multiple species of anaerobes combined with facultative or microaerophilic organisms. Such mixed infections are seen in the head and neck (chronic sinusitis, chronic otitis media, Ludwig's angina, and periodontal abscesses). Brain abscesses and subdural empyema are the most frequent anaerobic infections of the central nervous system. Anaerobes are responsible for pleuropulmonary diseases such as aspiration pneumonia, necrotizing pneumonia, lung abscess, and empyema. These organisms also play an important role in various intraabdominal infections, such as peritonitis and intraabdominal and liver abscesses (Chap. 130). They are isolated frequently in female genital tract infections, such as salpingitis, pelvic peritonitis, tuboovarian abscess, vulvovaginal abscess, septic abortion, and endometritis (Chaps. 132 and 133). Anaerobic bacteria also are frequently found in infections of the skin, soft tissues, and bones and in bacteremia.

ETIOLOGY The major anaerobic gram-positive cocci that produce disease are *Peptostreptococcus* spp. The major species involved in infections are *Peptostreptococcus intermedius*, *P. micros*, *P. magnus*, *P. asaccharolyticus*, *P. anaerobius*, and *P. prevotii*. Clostridia are gram-positive rods that are isolated from wounds, abscesses, sites of abdominal infection, and blood; they are discussed in Chap. 145. The principal anaerobic gram-negative bacilli found in human infections are the members of the *Bacteroides* "family," which includes the *Bacteroides fragilis* group as well as *Fusobacterium*, *Prevotella*, and *Porphyromonas* spp. Another gram-negative rod, *Bilophila wadsworthia*, has been isolated from infected sites. Gram-positive anaerobic non-spore-forming bacilli are uncommon as etiologic agents of human infections. *Propionibacterium acnes*, a rare cause of foreign body infections, is one of the few non-clostridial gram-positive rods associated with infections.

The *B. fragilis* group contains the anaerobic pathogens most frequently isolated from clinical infections. Members of this group are part of the normal bowel flora; they include several distinct species, such as *B. fragilis*, *B. thetaiotaomicron*, *B. distasonis*, *B. vulgatus*, *B. uniformis*, and *B. ovatus*. (Ribosomal RNA analysis has shown that *B. distasonis* is more closely related to the genus *Porphyromonas* than it is to other *Bacteroides*.) Of this group, *B. fragilis* is the most important clinical isolate. However, *B. fragilis* is isolated from the normal fecal flora in lower numbers than other *Bacteroides* spp.

A second major group of phenotypically similar organisms is part of the indigenous oral flora. Thus these organisms are found at infected sites that can be seeded with oral microflora. Many of these species are pigment-producing bacteria previously classified as *Bacteroides melaninogenicus*. The nomenclature of this group has changed so that two distinct genera, *Prevotella* and *Porphyromonas*, are now recognized; these genera comprise several pathogenic species, including *Porphyromonas gingivalis*, *Porphyromonas asaccharolytica*, and *Prevotella oralis*. *Porphyromonas* and *Prevotella* spp. cause localized infections that can spread contiguously.

In female genital tract infections, organisms normally colonizing the vagina, such as *Prevotella bivia* and *Prevotella disiens*, are the most frequent isolates, although *B. fragilis* is not uncommon. The *Fusobacterium* species *Fusobacterium necrophorum*, *F. nucleatum*, and *F. varium*, which reside primarily in the oral cavity and the gastrointestinal tract, are also isolated from clinical infections, including necrotizing pneumonia and abscesses. *Bilophila wadsworthia* has been reported to cause serious infections, including bacteremia, necrotizing fasciitis, and abscesses; this organism is frequently resistant to several antimicrobials, including imipenem, cefoxitin, and other β-lactam agents.

Infections caused by anaerobic bacteria most frequently are due to more than one organism. These polymicrobial infections may be caused by one or several anaerobic species or by a combination of anaerobic organisms and microaerophilic or facultative bacteria acting synergistically.

Approach to the Patient

The physician must consider several points when approaching the patient with presumptive infection due to anaerobic bacteria.

1. Most of the organisms colonizing mucosal sites are harmless commensals; very few cause disease.
2. For anaerobes to cause tissue infection, they must spread beyond the normal mucosal barriers.

3. Conditions favoring the propagation of these bacteria, particularly a lowered oxidation-reduction potential, are necessary. These conditions exist at sites of trauma, tissue destruction, compromised vascular supply, and complications of preexisting infection, which produce necrosis.

4. There is a complex array of infecting flora. For example, as many as 12 different types of organisms can be isolated from a suppurative site.

5. Anaerobic organisms tend to be found in abscess cavities or in necrotic tissue. The failure of an abscess to yield organisms on routine culture is a clue that the abscess is likely to contain anaerobic bacteria. Often smears of this "sterile pus" are found to be teeming with bacteria when Gram's stain is applied. Malodorous pus suggests anaerobic infection. Although some facultative organisms, such as *Staphylococcus aureus*, are also capable of causing abscesses, abscesses in organs or deeper body tissues should call to mind anaerobic infection.

6. Gas is found in many anaerobic infections of deep tissues.

7. Some species (the best example being the *B. fragilis* group) require specific therapy. However, many synergistic infections can be cured with antibiotics directed at some but not all of the organisms involved. Antibiotic therapy, combined with debridement and drainage, disrupts the interdependent relationship among the bacteria, and some species that are resistant to the antibiotic do not survive without the coinfecting organisms.

8. Manifestations of disseminated intravascular coagulation are unusual in patients with purely anaerobic infection.

EPIDEMIOLOGY   Difficulties in the performance of appropriate cultures, contamination of cultures by aerobic bacteria or components of the normal flora, and the lack of readily available, reliable culture techniques have made it impossible to obtain accurate incidence or prevalence data. However, anaerobic infections are encountered frequently in hospitals with active surgical, trauma, and obstetric and gynecologic services. In some centers, anaerobic bacteria, particularly *B. fragilis*, account for approximately 4% of positive blood cultures.

PATHOGENESIS   Anaerobic bacterial infections usually occur when an anatomic barrier becomes disrupted and constituents of the local flora enter a site that was previously sterile. Because of the specific growth requirements of anaerobic organisms and their presence as commensals on mucosal surfaces, conditions must arise that allow these organisms to penetrate mucosal barriers and enter tissue with a lowered oxidation-reduction potential. Therefore, tissue ischemia, trauma, surgery, perforated viscus, shock, and aspiration provide environments conducive to the proliferation of anaerobes. In the case of a perforated viscus, hundreds of species of anaerobic bacteria are spilled into the peritoneal cavity, but many of these organisms are unable to survive because the highly vascularized tissue provides a sufficiently high redox potential. The entry of oxygen into the environment results in the selection of the more aerotolerant anaerobic organisms.

The ability of an organism to adhere to host tissues is important to the establishment of infection. Some oral species adhere to crevicular epithelium in the oral cavity. *Prevotella melaninogenica* actually attaches to other microorganisms; *P. gingivalis* is a common isolate in periodontal disease. These organisms have fimbriae that facilitate attachment. Some unencapsulated *Bacteroides* strains appear to be piliated, a characteristic that may account for their ability to adhere.

The most extensively studied virulence factor of the nonsporulating anaerobes is the polysaccharide capsule of *B. fragilis*. This polysaccharide possesses distinct biologic properties, such as the ability (owing to a unique zwitterionic motif of charged sugars) to promote abscess formation. Intraabdominal abscess induction is related to the capacity of the polysaccharide to stimulate the release of cytokines, in particular interleukin 8 (IL-8) and tumor necrosis factor α (TNF-α), from resident peritoneal cells. IL-8 results in the chemotaxis of polymorphonuclear neutrophils (PMNs) into the peritoneum, where they adhere to mesothelial cells induced by TNF-α to upregulate their expression of intercellular adhesion molecule 1 (ICAM-1). PMNs adherent to ICAM-1-expressing cells probably represent the nidus for an abscess. Prophylactic or therapeutic administration of the polysaccharide or a zwitterionic mimetic to experimental animals confers protection against abscess induction following challenge with intestinal microorganisms capable of inducing abscesses. This protection is mediated by T cells controlling cytokine release, which blocks the tissue response of abscess formation. Although abscesses constitute a host response that localizes and contains infecting bacteria, abscess formation in patients with sepsis often results in severe and chronic illness that requires surgical drainage in combination with antimicrobial therapy.

Anaerobic bacteria produce a number of exoproteins that are capable of enhancing the organisms' virulence. The collagenase produced by *P. gingivalis* may enhance tissue destruction. An enterotoxin has been identified in *B. fragilis* strains associated with diarrheal disease in animals and young children. This 20-kDa zinc-dependent metalloprotease reversibly alters the morphology of the tight junctional complexes of intestinal epithelial cells. Both *B. fragilis* and *P. melaninogenica* possess lipopolysaccharides (endotoxins) that are less biologically potent than endotoxins associated with aerobic gram-negative bacteria. This relative biologic inactivity may account for the lower frequency of disseminated intravascular coagulation and purpura in *Bacteroides* bacteremia than in facultative and aerobic gram-negative bacillary bacteremia.

CLINICAL MANIFESTATIONS   **Anaerobic Infections of the Mouth, Head, and Neck** (See also Chap. 30)   Infections of the mouth can arise from either the supragingival or the subgingival dental plaque. Supragingival plaque formation begins with the adherence of gram-positive bacteria to the tooth surface. This form of plaque is influenced by salivary and dietary components, oral hygiene, and local host factors. Once the supragingival plaque is established, the acquisition of pathogenic bacteria and an increase in the amount of plaque are responsible for the ultimate development of gingivitis. Early bacteriologic changes in the supragingival plaque initiate an inflammatory response in the gingiva, including edema, swelling, and increased gingival fluid, and cause the development of caries and endodontic (pulp) infections. In addition, these changes contribute to the subsequent pathogenic alteration in the subgingival plaque that arises from poor or inadequate oral hygiene.

Subgingival plaque is associated with periodontal disease and disseminated infection arising from the oral cavity. Bacteria that colonize the subgingival area are primarily anaerobic. The black-pigmented gram-negative anaerobic bacilli, principally *P. gingivalis* and *P. melaninogenica*, are the most important. Infections in this area are frequently mixed and involve both anaerobic and aerobic bacteria. After establishment of local infection either in root canals or in the periodontal area, infection may extend into the mandible, causing osteomyelitis to the maxillary sinuses; or to local tissues in the submandibular or submental spaces, depending on which teeth are involved. Periodontitis also may result in spreading infection that can involve adjacent bone or soft tissues.

Gingivitis   Gingivitis may become a necrotizing infection (trench mouth, Vincent's stomatitis). The onset of disease is usually sudden and is associated with tender bleeding gums, foul breath, and a bad taste. The gingival mucosa, especially the papillae between the teeth, becomes ulcerated and may be covered by a gray exudate, which is removable with gentle pressure. Patients may become systemically ill, developing fever, cervical lymphadenopathy, and leukocytosis. Occasionally, ulcerative gingivitis can spread to the buccal mucosa, the teeth, and the mandible or maxilla, resulting in widespread destruction of bone and soft tissue. This infection is termed *acute necrotizing ulcerative mucositis* (cancrum oris, noma). It destroys tissue rapidly, causing the teeth to fall out and large areas of bone—or even the whole mandible—to be sloughed. A strong putrid odor is frequently detected, although the lesions are not painful. The gangrenous lesions eventually heal, leaving large disfiguring defects. This infection is seen most commonly following a debilitating illness or in severely malnourished children. It has been known to complicate leukemia or to develop in individuals with a genetic deficiency of catalase.

Acute necrotizing infections of the pharynx These infections usually occur in association with ulcerative gingivitis. Symptoms include an extremely sore throat, foul breath, and a bad taste accompanied by fever and a sensation of choking. Examination of the pharynx demonstrates that the tonsillar pillars are swollen, red, ulcerated, and covered with a grayish membrane that peels easily. Lymphadenopathy and leukocytosis are common. The disease may last for only a few days or, if not treated, may persist for weeks. Lesions begin unilaterally but may spread to the other side of the pharynx or the larynx. Aspiration of the infected material by the patient can result in lung abscesses. Soft tissue infection of the oral-facial area may or may not be odontogenic. *Ludwig's angina*, a periodontal infection usually arising from the tissues surrounding the third molar, may produce submandibular cellulitis that results in marked local swelling of tissues, with pain, trismus, and superior and posterior displacement of the tongue. Submandibular swelling of the neck can impair swallowing and cause respiratory obstruction. In some cases, tracheotomy may be life-saving.

Fascial infections These infections arise from the spread of organisms originating in the upper airways to potential spaces formed by the fascial planes of the head and neck. Perimandibular space infection most commonly involves the submandibular, peritonsillar, and parapharyngeal spaces. Peritonsillar abscesses occur in association with pharyngitis. Complicated dental infections spread to the submandibular and buccal spaces. Entry of organisms by either portal can result in parapharyngeal space infections. Although there are few well-documented reports on the microbiology of these syndromes, anaerobes from the oral flora have been implicated in many cases. Fascial infections associated with *S. aureus* or *Streptococcus pyogenes* may arise from boils or impetigo, whereas anaerobes are associated with space infections either occurring spontaneously or arising from diseases of the mucous membranes or from dental manipulations.

Sinusitis and otitis The role of anaerobic bacteria in acute sinusitis may be underestimated because of improper collection of specimens. In a study of chronic sinusitis, anaerobic bacteria were found in 52% of specimens collected during external frontoethmoidotomy or radical antrotomy. Anaerobic bacteria are much more easily implicated in chronic suppurative otitis media than in acute otitis media. Purulent exudate from chronically draining ears has been found to contain anaerobes, particularly *Bacteroides* spp., in up to 50% of cases. *B. fragilis* has been isolated from up to 28% of patients with chronic otitis media.

Complications of anaerobic head and neck infections Contiguous craniad spread of these infections may result in osteomyelitis of the skull or mandible or in intracranial infections such as brain abscess and subdural empyema. Caudad spread can produce mediastinitis or pleuropulmonary infection. Hematogenous complications may also result from anaerobic infections of the head and neck. Bacteremia, which occasionally is polymicrobial, can lead to endocarditis or other distant infections. When infections spread to produce suppurative thrombophlebitis of the internal jugular vein, a destructive syndrome (*Lemierre's*)—with prolonged fever, bacteremia, septic emboli to both the lung and the brain, and multiple metastatic foci of suppurative infection—may develop. This syndrome has been reported with fusobacterial septicemia following exudative pharyngitis but has been uncommon in the antimicrobial era.

Central Nervous System Infections Brain abscesses are frequently associated with anaerobic bacteria (Chap. 372). If optimal bacteriologic techniques are employed, as many as 85% of brain abscesses yield anaerobic bacteria—most often anaerobic gram-positive cocci (especially peptostreptococci), which are followed in frequency by *Fusobacterium* and *Bacteroides* spp. Facultative or microaerophilic strep-

tococci and coliforms often are part of a mixed infecting flora in brain abscesses.

Pleuropulmonary Infections Anaerobic pleuropulmonary infections result from the aspiration of oropharyngeal contents, often in the context of an altered state of consciousness or an absent gag reflex. Four clinical syndromes are associated with anaerobic pleuropulmonary infection produced by aspiration: simple aspiration pneumonia, necrotizing pneumonia, lung abscess, and empyema.

Aspiration pneumonitis Aspiration pneumonitis must be distinguished from two other clinical syndromes associated with aspiration that are not of bacterial etiology. One syndrome results from aspiration of solids, usually food. Obstruction of major airways typically results in atelectasis and moderate nonspecific inflammation. Therapy consists of removal of the foreign body.

The second aspiration syndrome is more easily confused with bacterial aspiration. *Mendelson's* syndrome results from regurgitation of stomach contents and aspiration of chemical material, usually gastric juices. Pulmonary inflammation—including the destruction of the alveolar lining, with transudation of fluid into the alveolar space—occurs with remarkable rapidity. Typically this syndrome develops within hours, often following anesthesia when the gag reflex is depressed. The patient becomes tachypneic, hypoxic, and febrile. The leukocyte count may rise, and the chest x-ray may evolve suddenly from normal to a complete bilateral "whiteout" within 8 to 24 h. Sputum production is minimal. The pulmonary signs and symptoms can resolve quickly with symptom-based therapy or can culminate in respiratory failure, with the subsequent development of bacterial superinfection over a period of days. Antibiotic therapy is not indicated unless bacterial infection supervenes. The signs of bacterial infection include sputum production, persistent fever, leukocytosis, and clinical evidence of sepsis.

In contrast to these syndromes, bacterial aspiration pneumonia develops more slowly. It is seen in patients who are hospitalized and have a depressed gag reflex, impaired swallowing, or a tracheal or nasogastric tube; elderly patients; or those with transiently impaired consciousness in the wake of seizures, cerebrovascular accidents, or alcoholic blackouts. Patients who enter the hospital with this syndrome typically have been ill for several days and generally report low-grade fever, malaise, and sputum production. Usually the history reveals factors predisposing to aspiration, such as alcohol overdose or residence in a nursing home. Sputum characteristically is not malodorous unless the process has been under way for at least a week. A mixed bacterial flora with many PMNs is evident on Gram's staining; cultures are reliable only if contamination with the normal oral flora is avoided—that is, if specimens are obtained by transtracheal aspiration. In general, this procedure is not indicated in the evaluation of these patients. The most commonly encountered anaerobes in these infections are pigmented and nonpigmented *Prevotella* spp., *F. nucleatum*, *Peptostreptococcus* spp., and *Bacteroides* spp. Chest x-rays show consolidation in dependent pulmonary segments: in the basilar segments of the lower lobes if the patient has aspirated while upright and in either the posterior segment of the upper lobe (usually on the right side) or the superior segment of the lower lobe if the patient has aspirated while supine. The organisms isolated reflect the pharyngeal flora; *P. melaninogenica, Fusobacterium* spp., and anaerobic cocci are the most frequent isolates. The patient who aspirates in the hospital also may have a mixed infection involving enteric gram-negative rods.

Necrotizing pneumonitis This form of anaerobic pneumonitis is characterized by numerous small abscesses that spread to involve several pulmonary segments. The process can be indolent or fulminating. This syndrome is less common than either aspiration pneumonia or lung abscess and includes features of both types of infection.

Anaerobic lung abscesses These abscesses result from subacute anaerobic pulmonary infection. The clinical syndrome typically involves a history of constitutional symptoms, including malaise, weight loss, fever, chills, and foul-smelling sputum, perhaps over a period of weeks (Chap. 255). Patients who develop lung abscesses characteristically have dental infection and periodontitis, but lung abscesses in edentulous patients have been reported. Abscess cavities may be single or multiple and generally occur in dependent pulmonary segments. Anaerobic abscesses must be distinguished from those associated with tuberculosis, neoplasia, and other conditions. Oral anaerobes predominate, although *B. fragilis* is isolated in up to 10% of cases. *S. aureus* may be found as well.

Empyema　Empyema is a manifestation of long-standing anaerobic pulmonary infection. The clinical presentation, which includes the presence of foul-smelling sputum, resembles that of other anaerobic pulmonary infections. Patients may report pleuritic chest pain and marked chest-wall tenderness.

Empyema may be masked by overlying pneumonitis and should be considered especially in cases of persistent fever despite antibiotic therapy. Diligent physical examination and the use of ultrasound to localize a loculated empyema are important diagnostic tools. The collection of a foul-smelling exudate by thoracentesis is typical. Cultures of infected pleural fluid yield an average of 3.5 anaerobes and 0.6 facultative or aerobic bacterial species. Drainage is required. Defervescence, a return to a feeling of well-being, and resolution of the process may require several months.

Extension from a subdiaphragmatic infection also may result in anaerobic empyema. Septic pulmonary emboli may originate from intraabdominal or female genital tract infections and can produce anaerobic pneumonia.

Intraabdominal Infections　Enterotoxigenic *B. fragilis* has been associated with watery diarrhea in a small number of young children and adults. In case-control studies of children with undiagnosed diarrheal disease, enterotoxigenic *B. fragilis* was isolated from significantly more children with diarrhea than children in the control group. This organism may play a role in a small proportion of childhood diarrhea cases. Neutropenic enterocolitis (typhlitis) has been associated with anaerobic infection of the cecum but—in the setting of neutropenia (Chap. 85)—may involve the entire bowel. Patients usually present with fever; abdominal pain, tenderness, and distension; and watery diarrhea. The bowel wall is edematous with hemorrhage and necrosis. The primary pathogen is thought by some authorities to be *C. septicum*, but other clostridia and mixed anaerobic infections have also been implicated. More than 50% of patients developing early clinical signs can benefit from antibiotic therapy and bowel rest. Surgery is sometimes required to remove gangrenous bowel. →*See Chap. 130 for a complete discussion of intraabdominal infections.*

Pelvic Infections　The vagina of a healthy woman is one of the major reservoirs of anaerobic and aerobic bacteria. In the normal flora of the female genital tract, anaerobes outnumber aerobes by a ratio of approximately 10:1 and include anaerobic gram-positive cocci and *Bacteroides* spp. Anaerobes are isolated from most patients with genital tract infections not caused by a sexually transmitted pathogen. The major anaerobic pathogens are *B. fragilis, P. bivia, P. disiens, P. melaninogenica*, anaerobic cocci, and *Clostridium* spp. Anaerobes frequently are encountered in tuboovarian abscess, septic abortion, pelvic abscess, endometritis, and postoperative wound infection, particularly following hysterectomy. Although these infections are frequently mixed, involving both anaerobes and coliforms, pure anaerobic infections without coliform or other facultative bacterial species occur more often in pelvic than in intraabdominal sites and are characterized by drainage of foul-smelling pus or blood from the uterus, generalized uterine or local pelvic tenderness, and continued fever and chills. Suppurative thrombophlebitis of the pelvic veins may complicate the infections and lead to repeated episodes of septic pulmonary emboli.

Anaerobic bacteria have been thought to be contributing factors in the etiology of *bacterial vaginosis*. This syndrome of unknown etiology is characterized by a profuse malodorous discharge and an increase in the number of bacteria in the vagina, including *Gardnerella vaginalis, Prevotella* spp., *Mobiluncus* spp., peptostreptococci, and genital mycoplasmas. Anaerobic bacteria are thought to play a role in the etiology of pelvic inflammatory disease (Chap. 133), and several investigations have shown an association between bacterial vaginosis and the development of pelvic inflammatory disease.

Pelvic infections due to *Actinomyces* spp. have been associated with use of intrauterine devices (Chap. 166).

Skin and Soft Tissue Infections　Injury to skin, bone, or soft tissue by trauma, ischemia, or surgery creates a suitable environment for anaerobic infections. These infections are most frequently found in sites prone to contamination with feces or with upper airway secretions—for example, wounds associated with intestinal surgery, decubitus ulcers, or human bites. Anaerobic bacteria can be isolated in cases of crepitant cellulitis, synergistic cellulitis, or gangrene and necrotizing fasciitis (Chaps. 128 and 145). Moreover, these organisms have been isolated from cutaneous abscesses, rectal abscesses, and axillary sweat gland infections (hydradenitis suppurativa). Anaerobes are frequently cultured from foot ulcers in diabetic patients.

These soft tissue or skin infections are usually polymicrobial. A mean of 4.8 bacterial species are isolated, with a roughly 3:2 ratio of anaerobes to aerobes. The most frequently isolated organisms include *Bacteroides* spp., *Peptostreptococcus* spp., enterococci, *Clostridium* spp., and *Proteus* spp. The involvement of anaerobes in these types of infections is associated with a higher frequency of fever, foul-smelling lesions, gas in the tissues, or visible foot ulcer.

Anaerobic bacterial *synergistic gangrene (Meleney's gangrene)* is characterized by exquisite pain, redness, and swelling followed by induration. Erythema surrounds a central zone of necrosis. A granulating ulcer forms at the original center as necrosis and erythema extend outward. Symptoms are limited to pain; fever is not typical. These infections usually involve a combination of *Peptostreptococcus* spp. and *S. aureus*; the usual site of infection is an abdominal surgical wound or the area surrounding an ulcer on an extremity. Treatment includes surgical removal of necrotic tissue and antimicrobial administration.

Necrotizing fasciitis, a rapidly spreading destructive disease of the fascia, is usually attributed to group A streptococci but can also be caused by anaerobic bacteria, including *Peptostreptococcus* and *Bacteroides* spp. Gas may be found in the tissues. Similarly, myonecrosis can be associated with mixed anaerobic infection. *Fournier's gangrene* consists of cellulitis involving the scrotum, perineum, and anterior abdominal wall, with mixed anaerobic organisms spreading along deep external fascial planes and causing extensive loss of skin.

Bone and Joint Infections　Although *actinomycosis* (Chap. 166) accounts on a worldwide basis for most anaerobic infections in bone, organisms including *Peptostreptococcus* spp. or microaerophilic cocci, *Bacteroides* spp., *Fusobacterium* spp., and *Clostridium* spp. can also be found. These infections frequently arise adjacent to soft tissue infections. Hematogenous seeding of bone is uncommon. *Prevotella* and *Porphyromonas* spp. are detected in infections involving the maxilla and mandible, whereas *Clostridium* spp. have been reported as anaerobic pathogens in cases of osteomyelitis of the long bones following fracture or trauma. Fusobacteria have been isolated in pure culture from sites of osteomyelitis adjacent to the perinasal sinuses. *Peptostreptococcus* spp. and microaerophilic cocci have been reported as significant pathogens in infections involving the skull, mastoid, and prosthetic implants placed in bone. In patients with osteomyelitis (Chap. 129), the most reliable culture specimen is a bone biopsy sample free of normal uninfected skin and subcutaneous tissue. In patients with anaerobic osteomyelitis, a mixed flora is frequently isolated from a bone biopsy specimen.

In cases of anaerobic septic arthritis, the most common isolates are *Fusobacterium* spp. Most of the patients involved have uncontrolled peritonsillar infections progressing to septic cervical venous thrombophlebitis and resulting in hematogenous dissemination with a predilection for the joints. Unlike anaerobic osteomyelitis, anaerobic pyoarthritis in most cases is not polymicrobial and may be acquired hematogenously. Anaerobes are important pathogens in infections involving prosthetic joints; in these infections, the causative organisms

Bacteremia Transient bacteremia is a well-known event in healthy people whose anatomic mucosal barriers have been injured (e.g., during dental extractions or dental scaling). These bacteremic episodes, which are often due to anaerobes, have no pathologic consequences. However, anaerobic bacteria are found in cultures of blood from clinically ill patients when proper culture techniques are used. *B. fragilis* is the single most common anaerobic isolate from the bloodstream.

In recent years, the rate of isolation of anaerobic bacteria from blood cultures has been decreasing. Studies from the 1970s and early 1980s found that 10 to 15% of positive blood cultures yielded anaerobes, while more recent surveys have found rates as low as 4%. The cause of this change is unknown but may be related to the administration of antibiotic prophylaxis before intestinal surgery, the earlier recognition of localized infections, and the empirical use of broad-spectrum antibiotics for presumed infection.

Once the organism has been identified, both the portal of bloodstream entry and the underlying problem that probably led to seeding of the bloodstream can often be deduced from an understanding of the organism's normal site of residence. For example, mixed anaerobic bacteremia including *B. fragilis* usually implies colonic pathology with mucosal disruption from neoplasia, diverticulitis, or some other inflammatory lesion. The initial manifestations are determined by the portal of entry and reflect the localized condition. When bloodstream invasion occurs, patients can become extremely ill, with rigors and hectic fevers ranging up to 40.6°C (105°F). The clinical picture may be quite similar to that seen in sepsis involving aerobic gram-negative bacilli. Although other complications of anaerobic bacteremia, such as septic thrombophlebitis and septic shock, have been reported, the incidence of these complications in association with anaerobic bacteremia is low. Anaerobic bacteremia is potentially fatal and requires rapid diagnosis and appropriate therapy. Mortality appears to increase with the age of the patient (with reported rates of more than 66% among patients over 60 years old), with the isolation of multiple species from the bloodstream, and with the failure to surgically remove a focus of infection.

Endocarditis and Pericarditis (See also Chap. 126) Endocarditis due to anaerobes is uncommon. However, anaerobic streptococci, which are often classified incorrectly, are responsible for this disease more frequently than is generally appreciated. Gram-negative anaerobes are unusual causes of endocarditis. Anaerobes, particularly *B. fragilis* and *Peptostreptococcus* spp., are uncommonly found in infected pericardial fluids. Anaerobic pericarditis is associated with a mortality rate of >50%.

DIAGNOSIS Because of the time and difficulty involved in the isolation of anaerobic bacteria, diagnosis of anaerobic infections must frequently be based on presumptive evidence. Certain sites (such as avascular necrotic tissues) with lowered oxidation-reduction potential favor the diagnosis of an anaerobic infection. When infections occur in proximity to mucosal surfaces normally harboring an anaerobic flora, such as the gastrointestinal tract, female genital tract, or oropharynx, anaerobes should be considered as potential etiologic agents. A foul odor is often indicative of anaerobes, which produce certain organic acids as they proliferate in necrotic tissue. Although these odors are nearly pathognomonic for anaerobic infection, the absence of odor does not exclude an anaerobic etiology. Because anaerobes often coexist with other bacteria to cause mixed or synergistic infection, Gram's staining of exudate frequently reveals numerous pleomorphic cocci and bacilli suggestive of anaerobes. Sometimes these organisms have morphologic characteristics associated with specific species.

The presence of gas in tissues is highly suggestive, but not diagnostic, of anaerobic infection. When cultures of obviously infected sites yield no growth, streptococci only, or a single aerobic species (such as *Escherichia coli*) and Gram's staining reveals a mixed flora, the implication is that the anaerobic microorganisms failed to grow

because of inadequate transport and/or culture techniques. Failure of a patient to respond to antibiotics that are not active against anaerobes—for example, aminoglycosides and in some circumstances penicillin, cephalosporins, or tetracyclines—suggests anaerobic infection.

There are three critical steps in the diagnosis of anaerobic infection: (1) proper specimen collection; (2) rapid transport of the specimens to the microbiology laboratory, preferably in anaerobic transport media; and (3) proper handling of the specimens by the laboratory. Specimens must be collected by meticulous sampling of infected sites, with avoidance of contamination by the normal flora. When such contamination is likely, the specimen is unacceptable. Examples of specimens unacceptable for anaerobic culture include sputum collected by expectoration or nasal tracheal suction, bronchoscopy specimens, samples collected directly through the vaginal vault, urine collected by voiding, and feces. Specimens that can be cultured for anaerobes include blood, pleural fluid, transtracheal aspirates, pus obtained by direct aspiration from an abscess cavity, fluid obtained by culdocentesis, suprapubic bladder aspirates, cerebrospinal fluid, and lung puncture specimens.

Because even brief exposure to oxygen may kill some anaerobic organisms and result in failure to isolate them in the laboratory, air must be expelled from the syringe used to aspirate the abscess cavity, and the needle must be capped with a sterile rubber stopper. Proper precautions should be used in the handling of contaminated needles. Specimens can be injected into transport bottles containing a reduced medium or taken immediately in syringes to the laboratory for direct culture on anaerobic media. In general, swabs should not be used. If a swab must be used, it should be placed in a reduced semisolid carrying medium before transport to the laboratory. Delays in transport may lead to a failure to isolate anaerobes due to exposure to oxygen or overgrowth of facultative organisms, which may eliminate or obscure any anaerobes that are present. All clinical specimens from suspected anaerobic infections should be Gram-stained and examined for organisms with characteristic morphology. It is not unusual for organisms to be observed on Gram's staining but not isolated in culture. If purulent materials are found to be sterile or organisms are seen on Gram's staining but do not grow in the culture, the involvement of anaerobes should be suspected.

℞ **TREATMENT** Successful therapy for anaerobic infections requires the administration of a combination of appropriate antibiotics, surgical resection, debridement of devitalized tissues, and drainage. Perforations must be closed promptly, closed spaces drained, tissue compartments decompressed, and an adequate blood supply established. Abscess cavities should be drained as soon as fluctuation or localization occurs. Surgery was formerly required to establish drainage; however, computed tomography (CT), magnetic resonance imaging (MRI), and ultrasound now allow diagnostic radiologists to drain many abscess sites percutaneously.

Antibiotic Therapy and Resistance Decisions about the treatment of anaerobic infections with antibiotics are usually based on known resistance patterns in certain species, on the likelihood of encountering a given species in the case at hand, and on Gram's stain findings. Antibiotics active against *Bacteroides* spp., penicillin-resistant *Prevotella* and *Porphyromonas* spp., and *Fusobacterium* spp. can be grouped into four categories on the basis of their predicted activity against anaerobes (Table 167-1). (Nearly all the drugs listed have toxic side effects, which are described in detail in Chap. 137.) In many infections, anaerobes are mixed with coliforms and other facultative organisms. The best therapeutic regimens, therefore, are usually those active against both aerobic and anaerobic bacteria. The choice of empirical antibiotics for the anaerobes in mixed infections can nearly always be made reliably, since patterns of antimicrobial susceptibility are usually predictable (Chap. 137 and Table 167-1).

Antibiotic susceptibility testing of anaerobic bacteria has been difficult and controversial. Owing to the slow growth rate of many an-

Table 167-1   Antimicrobial Therapy for Infections Involving Commonly Encountered Anaerobic Gram-Negative Rods

Group 1 (<1% Resistance)	Group 2 (<15% Resistance)	Group 3 (Variable Resistance)	Group 4 (Resistance)
Metronidazole[a]	Clindamycin	Penicillin	Aminoglycosides
Ampicillin/ sulbactam	Cefoxitin	Cephalosporins	Quinolones
Ticarcillin/ clavulanic acid	High-dose antipseudomonal penicillins	Tetracycline	Monobactams
Piperacillin/ tazobactam		Vancomycin	
Imipenem		Erythromycin	
Meropenem			
Chloramphenicol[b]			
Clinafloxacin			

[a] Usually needs to be given in combination with aerobic bacterial coverage. For infections originating below the diaphragm, aerobic gram-negative coverage is essential. For infections from an oral source, aerobic gram-positive coverage is added. Metronidazole also is not active against *Actinomyces*, *Propionibacterium*, or other gram-positive non-spore-forming bacilli (e.g., *Eubacterium*, *Bifidobacterium*) and is unreliable against peptostreptococci.

[b] Chloramphenicol is probably not as effective as other group 1 antimicrobials in treating anaerobic infections.

aerobes, the lack of standardized testing methods and of clinically relevant standards for resistance, and the generally good results obtained with empirical therapy, susceptibility testing has been recommended only for the study of local or regional resistance patterns, for the prediction of the efficacy of new antibiotics, and for the management of selected patients.

Anaerobic gram-negative rods that are frequently resistant to penicillin are listed in Table 167-2. Clinically important *Bacteroides* spp. are essentially all resistant to penicillin. Failures of therapy are common when documented *Bacteroides* (especially *B. fragilis*) infection is treated with penicillin or first-generation cephalosporins. The number of antimicrobial agents effective against *Bacteroides* spp. has expanded, and there are currently several useful choices (Table 167-1). In general, cure rates of >80% can be attained in patients with *Bacteroides* infection by means of appropriate antimicrobial therapy and drainage.

Resistance to metronidazole has been reported only rarely in *Bacteroides* spp. This well-tolerated drug, which reaches significant levels in serum and also can be found at high concentrations in abscess cavities, should be considered first-line therapy against *Bacteroides* infection. However, if metronidazole is used to treat mixed anaerobic and aerobic infections, it is imperative that other appropriate antibiotics be used in conjunction. Metronidazole is inactive against aerobic and facultative bacteria, *Actinomyces* spp., and *Propionibacterium* spp.

Table 167-2   Frequency of Penicillin Resistance among Commonly Encountered Anaerobic Gram-Negative Rods

Organism	Frequency of Penicillin Resistance[a]
Bacteroides fragilis	High
Bacteroides thetaiotaomicron	High
Bacteroides ovatus	High
Bacteroides distasonis	High
Bacteroides vulgatus	High
Bilophila wadsworthia	High
Fusobacterium nucleatum	Low
Fusobacterium necrophorum	Low
Fusobacterium mortiferum	Low
Fusobacterium varium	Low
Prevotella spp.	Moderate
Porphyromonas spp.	Low

[a] High, >90% of strains; moderate, 5 to 90% of strains; low, <5% of strains.

The sensitivity of peptostreptococci to metronidazole is unpredictable, and penicillin remains the drug of choice.

If a patient fails to respond to one of the group 1 or group 2 drugs (Table 167-1), consideration should be given to alternative therapy and to determination of the resistance patterns among *Bacteroides* isolates. Although in vitro resistance of *Bacteroides* spp. to chloramphenicol has not been reported, this drug may not be as effective as other group 1 drugs. Ampicillin/sulbactam, ticarcillin/clavulanic acid, piperacillin/tazobactam, imipenem, and meropenem have been effective in the treatment of *B. fragilis* infection. Some newer fluoroquinolones, such as clinafloxacin, appear to be highly active against most anaerobes, including *B. fragilis*; however, ciprofloxacin and other earlier-generation quinolones should not be used as primary agents.

Treatment of Infections at Specific Sites   In clinical situations, specific regimens must be tailored to the initial site of infection. The duration of therapy also depends on the infection site; the reader is referred to specific chapters on sites of infection for recommendations.

β-Lactamase production has been reported in anaerobic strains that are usually isolated from infections originating above the diaphragm. Up to 60% of clinical isolates classified as *Prevotella* or *Porphyromonas* spp., non-*B. fragilis* species of *Bacteroides*, or *Fusobacterium* spp. reportedly produce β-lactamase (Table 167-2). The clinical significance of resistance in these organisms has been suggested by studies showing clindamycin to be superior to penicillin (which for many years was considered the therapeutic gold standard) for the treatment of lung abscesses. Presumably, the success of clindamycin is attributable to a broader spectrum of activity against oral anaerobes; thus, a combination of penicillin and metronidazole or another antibiotic combination that is active against both oral anaerobes and aerobes is likely to be as effective as clindamycin. Bronchoscopy in lung abscess is indicated only to rule out airway obstruction and does not enhance drainage; in any event, it should be delayed until the antimicrobial regimen has begun to affect the disease process so that the procedure does not spread the infection. Surgery is almost never indicated because of the danger of spilling the abscess contents into the lungs.

Although most oral anaerobic infections and most cases of anaerobic pneumonia still respond to penicillin therapy, some infections due to oral organisms fail to respond to this drug, and in these cases the use of a drug that is effective against penicillin-resistant anaerobes is recommended (Table 167-1). Life-threatening infections involving the anaerobic flora of the mouth, such as space infections of the head and neck, should be treated empirically as if penicillin-resistant anaerobes are involved. Less serious infections involving the oral microflora can be treated with penicillin alone; metronidazole can be added (or clindamycin can be substituted) if the patient responds poorly to penicillin therapy. Combinations of antibiotics used to treat mixed infections of oral origin must include drugs active against the gram-positive aerobic flora of the mouth.

Chloramphenicol has been used successfully against anaerobic central nervous system infections at doses of 30 to 60 mg/kg per day, with the exact dose depending on the severity of illness. However, penicillin G and metronidazole also cross the blood-brain barrier and are bactericidal for many anaerobic organisms (Chap. 372).

Anaerobic infections arising below the diaphragm (e.g., colonic and intraabdominal infections) must be treated specifically with agents active against *Bacteroides* spp. (see Table 167-1). In intraabdominal sepsis (Chap. 130), the use of antibiotics effective against penicillin-resistant anaerobes has clearly reduced the incidence of postoperative infections and serious infectious complications. Specifically, a drug from group 1 (Table 167-1) must be included for broad-spectrum coverage. Recommended doses for commonly used group 1 drugs are given in Table 167-3. Therapy for intraabdominal sepsis also must include drugs active against the gram-negative aerobic flora of the bowel. If the involvement of gram-positive bacteria such as enterococci is suspected, either ampicillin or vancomycin should be added.

Cases of anaerobic osteomyelitis in which a mixed flora is isolated from a bone biopsy specimen should be treated with a regimen that covers all the isolates. When an anaerobic organism is recognized as

Table 167-3 Doses and Schedules for Treatment of Serious Infections due to Commonly Encountered Anaerobic Gram-Negative Rods

First-Line Therapy	Dose	Schedule[a]
Metronidazole[b]	7.5 mg/kg	q6h
Ticarcillin/clavulanic acid	3.1 g	q4h
Piperacillin/tazobactam	3.375 g	q6h
Imipenem	0.5 g	q6h
Meropenem	1.0 g	q8h

[a] See disease-specific chapters for recommendations on duration of therapy.
[b] Should generally be used in conjunction with drugs active against aerobic or facultative organisms.
NOTE: All drugs are given by the intravenous route.

a major or sole pathogen infecting a joint, the duration of treatment should be similar to that used for arthritis caused by aerobic bacteria (Chap. 323). Therapy includes the management of underlying disease states, the administration of appropriate antimicrobial agents, temporary joint immobilization, percutaneous drainage of effusions, and usually the removal of infected prostheses or internal fixation devices. Surgical drainage and debridement procedures such as sequestrectomy are essential for the removal of necrotic tissue that can sustain anaerobic infections.

The outcome of anaerobic bacteremia has been shown to be significantly better in patients either initially given or switched to appropriate therapy based on known antibiotic susceptibilities.

Failure of Therapy Anaerobic infections that fail to respond to treatment or that relapse should be reassessed. Consideration should be given to additional surgical drainage or debridement. Superinfections with resistant gram-negative facultative or aerobic bacteria should be ruled out. The possibility of drug resistance must be entertained; if resistance is involved, repeated cultures may yield the pathogenic organism.

Supportive Measures Other supportive measures in the management of anaerobic infections include careful attention to fluid and electrolyte balance (since extensive local edema may lead to hypoalbuminemia); hemodynamic support for septic shock; immobilization of infected extremities; maintenance of adequate nutrition during chronic infections by parenteral hyperalimentation; relief of pain; and anticoagulation with heparin for thrombophlebitis. For patients with severe anaerobic infections of soft tissues, hyperbaric oxygen therapy is advocated by some experts, but its value has not been proven in controlled trials.

BIBLIOGRAPHY

APPELBAUM PC et al: β-Lactamase production and susceptibilities to amoxicillin, amoxicillin-clavulanate, ticarcillin, ticarcillin-clavulanate, cefoxitin, imipenem, and metronidazole of 320 non–*Bacteroides fragilis Bacteroides* isolates and 129 fusobacteria from 28 US centers. Antimicrob Agents Chemother 34:1546, 1990

FINEGOLD SM: Anaerobic bacteria: General concepts, in *Principles and Practice of Infectious Diseases*, 4th ed, GL Mandell et al (eds). New York, Churchill Livingstone, 1995

———: Overview of clinically important anaerobes. Clin Infect Dis 20:S205, 1995

FUCHS PC et al: In vitro activities of clinafloxacin against contemporary clinical bacterial isolates from 10 North American centers. Antimicrob Agents Chemother 42:1274, 1998

NICHOLS RL: Surgical infections: Prevention and treatment—1965 to 1995. Am J Surg 172:68, 1996

SALONEN JH et al: Clinical significance and outcome of anaerobic bacteremia. Clin Infect Dis 26:1413, 1998

SEARS CL et al: Enterotoxigenic *Bacteroides fragilis*. Clin Infect Dis 20:S142, 1995

SUMMANEN PH et al: *Bilophila wadsworthia* isolates from clinical specimens. Clin Infect Dis 20:S210, 1995

TZIANABOS AO et al: Structural features of polysaccharides that induce intra-abdominal abscesses. Science 262:416, 1993

Section 8
MYCOBACTERIAL DISEASES

168

Paul W. Wright, Richard J. Wallace, Jr.

ANTIMYCOBACTERIAL AGENTS

The physician is greatly challenged to provide optimal therapy for mycobacterial illnesses because of the advent of AIDS, the increase in both drug-susceptible and multidrug-resistant tuberculosis, and the plethora of new antibiotics with antimycobacterial potential. This chapter reviews the agents used for the treatment of tuberculosis, leprosy (Hansen's disease), and diseases caused by pathogenic nontuberculous mycobacteria, including *Mycobacterium avium-intracellulare*, *M. kansasii*, the rapidly growing mycobacteria, and *M. marinum*. The use of antimycobacterial agents in patients with renal or hepatic disease and in pregnant women is summarized in Table 168-1. The effects of major antimycobacterial agents on the levels, activity, and toxicity of other commonly used drugs are summarized in Table 168-2.

TUBERCULOSIS

Drugs used to treat tuberculosis are classified as first-line and second-line agents. *First-line essential* antituberculous agents are the most effective and are a necessary component of any short-course therapeutic regimen. The three drugs in this category are rifampin, isoniazid,

and pyrazinamide. The *first-line supplemental* agents, which are highly effective and infrequently toxic, include ethambutol and streptomycin. *Second-line* antituberculous drugs are clinically much less effective than first-line agents and much more frequently elicit severe reactions. These drugs are rarely used in therapy and then only by caregivers experienced with their use. They include para-aminosalicylic acid (PAS), ethionamide, cycloserine, kanamycin, amikacin, capreomycin, viomycin, and thiacetazone. *Newer* antituberculous drugs, which have not yet been placed in the above categories, include rifapentine, rifabutin, and the quinolones, especially ciprofloxacin, ofloxacin, and sparfloxacin.

FIRST-LINE ESSENTIAL DRUGS Rifampin Rifampin, a semisynthetic derivative of *Streptomyces mediterranei*, is considered the most important and potent antituberculous agent. It is also active against a wide spectrum of other organisms, including some gram-positive and gram-negative bacteria, *Legionella* spp., *M. kansasii*, and *M. marinum*.

Pharmacology Rifampin is a fat-soluble complex macrocyclic antibiotic that is absorbed readily after either oral or intravenous administration. Serum levels of 10 to 20 µg/mL follow a standard oral dose of 600 mg. Rifampin distributes well throughout most body tissues, including inflamed meninges. The fact that rifampin turns body fluids (urine, saliva, sputum, tears) to a red-orange color makes it simple and inexpensive to check on a patient's compliance with therapy. Rifampin is excreted primarily through the bile and the enterohepatic circulation, while 30 to 40% of a dose is excreted via the kidneys. The

Agent	Severe Hepatic Disease	Renal Disease: Creatinine Clearance Rate		Pregnancy[a]
		>30 mL/min	≤30 mL/min	
Azithromycin	No change	No change	?Decrease dose	No evidence of risk (B)
Clarithromycin	No change	No change	Decrease dose	Risk cannot be ruled out (C)
Ethambutol	No change	No change	Decrease dose	Risk cannot be ruled out (C)
Isoniazid	Avoid use or decrease dose	No change	Decrease dose	Risk cannot be ruled out (C)
Pyrazinamide	Avoid use or decrease dose	No change	Decrease dose[b]	Risk cannot be ruled out (C)[c]
Rifabutin	No change	No change	No change	No evidence of risk (B)
Rifampin	Avoid use or decrease dose	No change	No change	Risk cannot be ruled out (C)
Rifapentine	Avoid use or decrease dose	No change	No change	Risk cannot be ruled out (C)
Streptomycin	No change	Decrease dose	Decrease dose and frequency	Definite evidence of risk (D)

[a] Based on Food and Drug Administration pregnancy categories of A–D, X.
[b] Prudent but not absolutely necessary.
[c] Use in pregnancy is recommended by international organizations outside the United States.

drug is administered either twice weekly or daily at a dose of 600 mg for adults (10 mg/kg) and 10 to 20 mg/kg for children.

Mechanism of action   Rifampin has both intracellular and extracellular bactericidal activity. It blocks RNA synthesis by specifically binding and inhibiting DNA-dependent RNA polymerase. Susceptible strains of *M. tuberculosis* as well as *M. kansasii* and *M. marinum* are inhibited by ≤1 μg/mL.

Adverse effects (Table 168-3)   Rifampin is generally well tolerated; the most common adverse event is gastrointestinal upset. Patients with chronic liver disease, especially those with alcoholism and the elderly, appear to be at unusually high risk for the most serious adverse reaction: hepatitis. Other adverse effects of rifampin include rash (0.8%), hemolytic anemia (<1%), thrombocytopenia, and immunosuppression of unknown clinical importance. Rifampin is a potent inducer of the hepatic microsomal enzymes and thereby decreases the half-life of a number of drugs, including digoxin, warfarin, prednisone,

Table 168-2   Effects of Major Antimycobacterial Agents on Levels/Activity/Toxicity of Other Commonly Used Drugs[a]

Rifampin/rifapentine[b]
Acetaminophen (↓)
Antiarrhythmics (↓)
Anticonvulsants (↓)
Azole antifungals (↓)
Barbiturates (↓)
β Blockers (↓)
Calcium channel blockers (↓)
Chloramphenicol (↓)
Clarithromycin (↓)
Cyclosporine (↓)
Dapsone (↓)
Delavirdine (↓)
Diazepam (↓)
Digoxin (↓)
Doxycycline (↓)
Fluoroquinolones (↓)
Glucocorticoids (↓)
Halothane (↓)
Hormonal contraceptives (↓)
Narcotics (↓)
Oral hypoglycemics (↓)
Probenecid (↓)
Protease inhibitors (↓)
Quinidine (↓)
Theophylline (↓)
Tricyclic antidepressants (↓)
Warfarin (↓)
Zidovudine (↓)

Isoniazid
Alcohol (↑ in risk of hepatitis)
Carbamazepine (↑)
Diphenylhydantoin (↑)
Enflurane (↑ in risk of renal failure)
Warfarin (↑)
Clarithromycin
Astemizole (↑)
Carbamazepine (↑)
Digoxin (↑)
Rifabutin (↑)
Ritonavir (↓)
Terfenadine (↑)
Zidovudine (↓)

[a] The following antimycobacterial agents have no or minimal effects on other drugs: amikacin, azithromycin, capreomycin, ethambutol, streptomycin, pyrazinamide.
[b] Rifabutin, which induces the cytochrome P450 system, has the same effects (↓) as rifampin but to a lesser degree. All drugs whose half-life is decreased by rifampin induction of hepatic microsomal enzymes may be subject to the same effect when coadministered with rifabutin; however, this point has not yet been studied.

cyclosporine, methadone, oral contraceptives, clarithromycin, the HIV protease inhibitors, and quinidine (Table 168-2).

Resistance   Resistance to rifampin results from spontaneous point mutations that alter the β subunit of the RNA polymerase (*rpoB*) gene. Studies have shown that 96% of rifampin-resistant strains have a missense mutation within a 91-bp central core region of the gene. Rifampin-resistant strains of *M. leprae* have similar mutations that alter a single serine residue (Ser-425) in the same core region of the *rpoB* gene.

Isoniazid   Now considered the best antituberculous drug available after rifampin, isoniazid should be included in all tuberculosis treatment regimens unless the organism is resistant. Isoniazid is inexpensive, readily synthesized, available worldwide, highly selective for mycobacteria, and well tolerated, with only 5% of patients exhibiting adverse effects.

Mechanism of action   Isoniazid is the hydrazide of isonicotinic acid, a small water-soluble molecule that easily penetrates the cell. Its mechanism of action involves inhibition of mycolic acid cell-wall synthesis via oxygen-dependent pathways such as the catalase-peroxidase reaction. Isoniazid is bacteriostatic against resting bacilli and bactericidal against rapidly multiplying organisms, both extracellularly and intracellularly. The minimal inhibitory concentrations (MICs) of isoniazid for wild-type (untreated) strains of *M. tuberculosis* are <0.1 μg/mL, while those for *M. kansasii* are usually 0.5 to 2.0 μg/mL. The MICs of this drug for other mycobacteria are much higher.

Pharmacology   Both oral and intramuscular preparations of isoniazid are readily absorbed. A 300-mg oral dose generally produces peak serum levels of 3 to 5 μg/mL. Isoniazid diffuses well throughout the body and reaches therapeutic concentrations in serum, cerebrospinal fluid (CSF), and infected tissue, including caseous granulomas. Isoniazid is metabolized in the liver via acetylation and hydrolysis; its metabolites are excreted into the urine. The rate of acetylation is genetically controlled. The recommended daily dose for the treatment of tuberculosis in the United States is 5 mg/kg for adults and 10 to 20 mg/kg for children, with a maximal daily dose of 300 mg for both groups. (Tuberculosis organizations outside the United States have recommended 5 mg/kg daily for both groups.) For intermittent therapy (usually directly observed), a maximal dose of 900 mg twice or thrice weekly is used. Even in moderate or severe renal failure, the adult dose rarely needs to be reduced below 200 mg/d.

Adverse effects (Table 168-3)   The two most important adverse effects of isoniazid therapy are hepatotoxicity and peripheral neuropathy. Other adverse reactions are either rare or less significant and include rash (2%), fever (1.2%), anemia, acne, arthritic symptoms, a systemic lupus erythematosus–like syndrome, optic atrophy, seizures, and psychiatric symptoms. Isoniazid-associated hepatitis is idiosyncratic and increases in incidence with age. It occurs in 0.3% of treated persons under 35 years of age, 1.2% of those under 49 years of age, and 2.3% of those over 50 years of age. The risk of isoniazid-associated hepatitis is increased by daily alcohol consumption, concomitant

Table 168-3 Monitoring Side Effects of Common Antituberculous Drugs

Drug	Side Effect	Management
Rifampin	Rash	Observe patient
	Liver dysfunction	Monitor AST/limit alcohol consumption/monitor for hepatitis symptoms
	Flulike syndrome	Administer at least twice weekly/limit dose to 10 mg/kg (adults)
	Red-orange urine	Reassure patient
	Drug interactions	Consider monitoring drug levels when possible, especially with contraceptives, anticoagulants, and digoxin/avoid use with protease inhibitors
Isoniazid	Hepatitis	Monitor AST/limit alcohol consumption/monitor for hepatitis symptoms/educate patient/stop drug at first symptoms of hepatitis (nausea, vomiting, anorexia, flulike syndrome)
	Peripheral neuritis	Administer vitamin B$_6$
	Optic neuritis	Administer vitamin B$_6$
	Seizures	Administer vitamin B$_6$
Pyrazinamide	Hepatitis	Monitor AST/limit daily dosage to 15–30 mg/kg
	Hyperuricemia	Monitor uric acid level only in cases of gout or renal failure
Ethambutol	Optic neuritis	Use lower daily dose (15 mg/kg) when possible/monitor visual acuity (eye chart) and red-green color vision (Ishihara Color Book) monthly and with any visual complaint/educate patient/stop drug at first change in vision
Streptomycin, amikacin, capreomycin	Ototoxicity, renal toxicity	Limit dose and duration of therapy as much as possible/avoid daily therapy in patients >50 years old/monitor BUN and serum creatinine levels and possibly conduct audiometry before and as needed during therapy/question patient regularly about tinnitus, dizziness, vertigo, and decreased hearing/measure serum drug levels if possible/educate patient/stop drug at first development of adverse effect

NOTE: AST, aspartate aminotransferase; BUN, blood urea nitrogen.

rifampin administration, and slow isoniazid acetylation. Mortality rates from isoniazid-induced hepatitis have been reported to be 6 to 12%, but the real risk is certainly much lower: the reported rates were documented in high-risk patients who continued to take the drug despite progressive symptoms of hepatitis and without monitoring of liver enzyme levels. Liver enzymes are monitored in most settings among high-risk patients, and administration of the drug is discontinued at the onset of hepatitis. The American Thoracic Society (ATS) recommends that serum concentrations of aspartate aminotransferase (AST) or alanine aminotransferase (ALT) be determined at baseline in patients over 35 years of age who are receiving isoniazid for chemoprophylaxis, with monthly determinations thereafter. The benefit of such routine monitoring remains controversial, however. Measurement of the ALT or AST level is certainly mandatory whenever a patient notices the onset of symptoms suggestive of isoniazid-associated hepatitis (e.g., fever, anorexia, nausea, vomiting, and/or a flulike syndrome including fever and myalgias), and treatment should be discontinued until the relationship between therapy and symptoms is ascertained. Several studies have demonstrated that many patients with isoniazid intolerance can be desensitized. The ATS also recommends that discontinuation of isoniazid be strongly considered whenever an asymptomatic AST or ALT level exceeds 150 to 200 IU (three to five times the upper limit of normal) in high-risk patients whose baseline values were normal. In one study, only 11 (0.1%) of 11,141 patients had hepatotoxic reactions to isoniazid during preventive treatment.

Peripheral neuritis associated with isoniazid develops at a dose-dependent rate of 2 to 20% and probably relates to interference with pyridoxine (vitamin B$_6$) metabolism. This rate can be reduced to 0.2% with the prophylactic administration of 10 to 50 mg of pyridoxine daily.

Resistance   Isoniazid-resistant mutants of *M. tuberculosis* occur spontaneously at a rate of 1 in 10^5 to 10^6 organisms. The molecular sites of isoniazid resistance have been detailed. Almost all isoniazid-resistant strains have amino acid changes in the catalase-peroxidase gene (*katG*) or a two-gene locus known as *inhA*. Missense mutations or deletion of *katG* is also associated with reduced catalase and peroxidase activity. Primary isoniazid resistance is detected in 7% of untreated patients in native U.S. populations, but the percentage is much higher in many immigrant populations.

Pyrazinamide   A derivative of nicotinic acid, pyrazinamide is an important bactericidal drug used in short-course therapy for tuberculosis.

Pharmacology   Pyrazinamide is well absorbed after oral administration, with a plasma concentration range of 20 to 60 μg/mL 1 to 2 h after oral ingestion of 15 to 30 mg/kg, and is well distributed throughout the body. Levels in CSF are excellent, reaching 50 to 100% of levels in serum. The serum half-life of the drug is 9 to 11 h. Pyrazinamide is metabolized by at least two major pathways and one minor pathway in the liver; its several metabolites include pyrazinoic acid, 5-hydroxypyrazinamide, and 5-hydroxypyrazinoic acid.

Mechanism of action   Pyrazinamide is similar to isoniazid in its narrow spectrum of antibacterial activity, which essentially includes only *M. tuberculosis*. The drug is bactericidal to slowly metabolizing organisms located within the acidic environment of the phagocyte or caseous granuloma; it is active only at a pH of <6.0. Pyrazinamide is considered a prodrug and is converted by the tubercle bacillus to the active form pyrazinoic acid. The target for this compound, however, remains unknown. Susceptible strains of *M. tuberculosis* are inhibited by 20 μg/mL.

Adverse effects (Table 168-3)   At the high dosages used in the past, hepatotoxicity was a prominent complication of pyrazinamide therapy. However, at the currently recommended daily dosage of 15 to 30 mg/kg, with a maximum of 2 g (which can be given in one dose), the frequency of hepatotoxicity is no higher than that for concomitant isoniazid and rifampin therapy. Although pyrazinamide is recommended by international tuberculosis organizations for routine use in pregnancy, it is not recommended in the United States because of inadequate teratogenicity data. Hyperuricemia is a common adverse effect of pyrazinamide therapy whose incidence is probably reduced by concurrent rifampin therapy. Clinical gout is seen only rarely. Polyarthralgias are encountered fairly commonly but are not related to hyperuricemia.

Resistance   Resistance to pyrazinamide is associated with loss of pyrazinamidase activity such that pyrazinamide is no longer converted to pyrazinoic acid. More than 90% of isolates with MICs of >100 μg/mL have mutations in the *pncA* gene, which encodes for pyrazinamidase. All strains of *M. bovis* are naturally resistant to pyrazinamide and have a point mutation within the *pncA* gene.

FIRST-LINE SUPPLEMENTAL DRUGS Ethambutol   A derivative of ethylenediamine, ethambutol is a water-soluble compound that is active only against mycobacteria. Susceptible species include *M. tuberculosis*, *M. marinum*, *M. kansasii*, and *M. avium-intracellulare* (MAI). Among first-line drugs, ethambutol is the least potent against *M. tuberculosis*. It is used most often with rifampin for the treatment of tuberculosis in patients who cannot tolerate isoniazid or who are thought or known to be infected with isoniazid-resistant organisms.

Mechanism of action   Ethambutol is bacteriostatic against rapidly growing mycobacteria. Its primary mechanism of action appears to be inhibition of arabinosyltransferases that mediate the polymerization of arabinose into arabinogalactan within the cell wall.

Pharmacology   After oral administration, 75 to 80% of a dose of ethambutol is absorbed from the gastrointestinal tract. Serum levels peak at 2 to 4 μg/mL 2 to 4 h after a dose of 15 mg/kg. The drug's distribution throughout the body is adequate except in the CSF, where it reaches only low levels. However, ethambutol can reach CSF levels up to 50% as high as peak plasma levels when administered at a daily dose of 25 mg/kg to a patient with inflamed meninges. Almost all of the dose is excreted by the kidneys within 24 h of ingestion, either unchanged or as metabolites. The usual daily adult dosage of ethambutol is 25 mg/kg (which may be given in one dose) for the first 2 months, with a subsequent reduction to 15 mg/kg. In cases where pretreatment is necessary, the higher dose may be given for the duration. For intermittent therapy, the dosage is 50 mg/kg twice weekly or 30 mg/kg three times weekly. The dosage must be lowered for patients with renal insufficiency (a creatinine clearance rate of <25 mL/min) to prevent drug accumulation and toxicity.

Adverse effects (Table 168-3)   Ethambutol is usually well tolerated. Retrobulbar optic neuritis is the most serious adverse effect; axial or central neuritis—the only form reported in patients taking daily doses of <30 mg/kg—involves the papillomacular bundle of fibers and results in reduced visual acuity, central scotoma, and loss of the ability to see green. Symptoms of ocular toxicity typically develop several months after the initiation of therapy, but rapid-onset optic neuritis has been reported. The risk of optic neuritis depends on the dose and duration of therapy: this reaction develops in 5% of patients receiving a daily dose of 25 mg/kg but in fewer than 1% of patients given a daily dose of 15 mg/kg. Patients taking the lower dose should be tested at baseline and whenever there is a subjective visual change for visual acuity and red-green color discrimination. Patients taking the higher dose should be tested at baseline, monthly thereafter, and whenever there is a subjective visual change. Optic neuritis with associated visual loss is usually reversible, but recovery may take 6 months or longer.

Other adverse effects of ethambutol are infrequent. Hyperuricemia occurs but is usually asymptomatic. Optic neuritis is rare at the low dose in children; however, the use of ethambutol in very young children is problematic because visual complications are difficult to monitor.

Resistance   Resistance in *M. tuberculosis* relates to missense mutations in the *embB* gene that encodes for arabinosyltransferase. Such mutations have been found in 70% of resistant strains and involve amino acid residue 306 in approximately 90% of cases. Species of nontuberculous mycobacteria that are intrinsically resistant to ethambutol have variant amino acids in this region of the gene, while susceptible species have the same amino acid sequences as *M. tuberculosis*.

Streptomycin   An aminoglycoside isolated from *Streptomyces griseus*, streptomycin is available for intramuscular and intravenous administration only. In the United States, it is the least-used first-line supplemental drug for tuberculosis because of its toxicity, the difficulty in obtaining adequate CSF levels, and the inconvenience of its parenteral administration. In developing countries, however, streptomycin is frequently used because of its low cost. The drug is active against untreated strains of *M. tuberculosis*, *M. kansasii*, and *M. marinum* and against some strains of MAI at readily achievable serum levels.

Pharmacology   Serum levels of streptomycin peak at 25 to 40 μg/mL after a 1.0-g dose. Streptomycin is bactericidal for rapidly dividing extracellular mycobacteria but is ineffective in the acidic environment within the macrophage. It diffuses poorly into the meninges

and, in patients with meningitis, reaches CSF levels that are only 20% of serum levels.

The usual adult dose of streptomycin is 0.5 to 1.0 g (10 to 15 mg/kg) daily or five times per week; the pediatric dose is 20 to 40 mg/kg daily, with a maximum of 1 g/d. Because streptomycin is eliminated almost exclusively by the kidneys, the dosage must be lowered and the frequency of administration reduced (to only two or three times per week) in most patients over 50 years of age and in any patient with renal impairment.

Mechanism of action   Streptomycin inhibits protein synthesis by disruption of ribosomal function.

Adverse effects (Table 168-3)   Adverse reactions to streptomycin therapy occur in 10 to 20% of patients. Ototoxicity and renal toxicity are the most common and the most serious. Renal toxicity, usually manifested as nonoliguric renal failure, is less common with streptomycin than with other frequently used aminoglycosides, such as gentamicin. Ototoxicity involves both hearing loss and vestibular dysfunction. The latter is more common and includes loss of balance, vertigo, and tinnitus. Patients receiving streptomycin must be monitored carefully for these adverse effects. Less serious reactions include perioral paresthesia, eosinophilia, rash, and drug fever.

Resistance   Spontaneous resistance to streptomycin occurs in 1 in 10^5 to 10^7 organisms. In two-thirds of streptomycin-resistant strains of *M. tuberculosis*, mutations have been identified in one of two targets: a 16S rRNA gene (*rrs*) and the gene encoding ribosomal protein S12 (*rpsL*). Both targets are believed to be involved in streptomycin ribosomal binding. No mutational change has been identified in the other one-third of resistant isolates. Strains of *M. tuberculosis* that are resistant to streptomycin are not cross-resistant to capreomycin or amikacin.

SECOND-LINE DRUGS   Second-line and/or newer antituberculous agents are used either when tuberculosis is drug resistant or when first-line supplemental drugs are not available. The most important second-line drugs are discussed below in the general (descending) order of usefulness.

Capreomycin   Capreomycin, a complex cyclic polypeptide antibiotic derived from *Streptomyces capreolus*, is similar to streptomycin in terms of dosing, mechanism of action, pharmacology, and toxicity. It is administered only by the intramuscular route in doses of 10 to 15 mg/kg daily or five times per week (maximal daily dose, 1 g), with peak blood levels of 20 to 40 μg/mL. After 2 to 4 months, the dosage should be reduced to 1 g two or three times a week. Cross-resistance to kanamycin and amikacin—but not to streptomycin—is common. After streptomycin, capreomycin is the injectable drug of choice for tuberculosis.

Amikacin and Kanamycin   These well-known aminoglycosides are bactericidal to extracellular organisms. Kanamycin is rarely used because of its toxicity. Amikacin is active against *M. tuberculosis* and several of the nontuberculous species, including the rapidly growing mycobacteria, *M. scrofulaceum*, *M. leprae*, and *MAI*. The usual adult dosage is 10 to 15 mg/kg intramuscularly or intravenously three to five times per week. Resistance to both drugs relates to a single-base-pair change at position 1408 in the 16S ribosomal RNA gene.

Para-Aminosalicylic Acid   PAS, a calcium or sodium salt that inhibits the growth of *M. tuberculosis* by impairing folate synthesis, is rarely indicated for the treatment of tuberculosis because of its low level of antituberculous activity and its high level of gastrointestinal toxicity (manifesting as nausea, vomiting, and diarrhea). Enteric-coated PAS granules (4 g every 8 h) may be better tolerated than other formulations and produce higher therapeutic blood levels. PAS is well absorbed after oral administration but reaches only low concentrations in the CSF. The drug has a short half-life (1 h), and 80% of the dose is excreted in the urine.

Thiacetazone   Also called amithiozone, thiacetazone is not available in the United States but—because it is inexpensive and readily available—is widely used in the developing world as a single-tablet combination with isoniazid to treat tuberculosis. The usual daily dosage is 150 mg. Thiacetazone is structurally related to isoniazid but is bacteriostatic and more toxic. The World Health Organization advises against the use of thiacetazone by HIV-infected patients because of an unacceptably high rate of severe adverse (gastrointestinal) and fatal (skin) reactions.

Viomycin A complex basic polypeptide antibiotic, viomycin has properties similar to those of capreomycin, amikacin, and kanamycin and must be administered by intramuscular injection. Ninety percent of strains of multidrug-resistant *M. tuberculosis* are inhibited by viomycin levels of 1 to 10 μg/mL. Toxic effects are more common and severe than with other polypeptide antibiotics. This drug is not available in the United States.

Ethionamide Like isoniazid and pyrazinamide, ethionamide is a derivative of isonicotinic acid. This agent is bacteriostatic against metabolizing *M. tuberculosis* and some nontuberculous mycobacteria. It is most useful in therapy for multidrug-resistant tuberculosis. However, its use is severely limited by its toxicity and frequent side effects, which include intense gastrointestinal intolerance (anorexia, vomiting, and dysgeusia), serious neurologic reactions, reversible hepatitis (3% of cases), hypersensitivity reactions, and hypothyroidism. Ethionamide is well absorbed orally and is widely distributed throughout the body at sites including the CSF.

Cycloserine Cycloserine (D-4-amino-3-isoxazolidinone) is produced by *Streptomyces orchidaceus* and is active against a broad spectrum of bacteria, including *M. tuberculosis*. Cycloserine is well absorbed after oral administration and is widely distributed throughout the body fluids, including the CSF. Serious side effects limit the use of this drug and include psychosis (with suicide in some cases), seizures, peripheral neuropathy, headaches, somnolence, and allergic reactions. Cycloserine should not be given to patients with epilepsy, active alcohol abuse, severe renal insufficiency, or a history of depression or psychosis.

Newer Antituberculous Drugs A number of other drugs are being evaluated for their antituberculous activity. This group includes rifabutin, rifapentine, the newer fluorinated quinolones, amoxicillin/clavulanic acid, clofazimine, clarithromycin, and rifamycins not yet approved by the U.S. Food and Drug Administration (FDA), such as KRM-1648 (benzoxazinorifamycin).

Rifabutin Rifabutin, a semisynthetic rifamycin spiropiperidyl derivative, shares many characteristics with rifampin, including activity against *M. tuberculosis*. Rifabutin is also active against some strains of rifampin-resistant *M. tuberculosis* and is more active than rifampin against MAI and other nontuberculous mycobacteria. To date, rifabutin has been most useful in the prophylaxis of disseminated MAI infection and in the treatment of drug-resistant tuberculosis. Because it seems to exhibit more antituberculous activity than rifampin in vitro and in animals, its possible clinical advantages over rifampin are being evaluated. In a multinational trial in which either rifampin (600 mg/d) or rifabutin (150 mg/d) was administered in combination with isoniazid plus a 2-month regimen of pyrazinamide and ethambutol, the two rifamycins were equally effective and well tolerated in the treatment of newly diagnosed pulmonary tuberculosis. Rifabutin is recommended in place of rifampin for the treatment of HIV-positive individuals who are also taking a protease inhibitor.

PHARMACOLOGY The pharmacology of rifabutin is dramatically different from that of rifampin. Rifabutin is readily absorbed after a single oral dose of 300 mg and reaches peak serum levels (0.35 μg/mL) in 2 to 4 h. This lipophilic drug distributes best to tissues: tissue levels are 5 to 10 times higher than plasma levels. CSF concentrations are 30 to 70% of plasma levels in HIV-infected patients who have meningitis. The drug's slow clearance via hepatic metabolism and renal excretion results in a mean serum half-life of 45 h, which is much longer than the 3- to 5-h half-life of rifampin. Clarithromycin (but not azithromycin) and fluconazole appear to block the hepatic metabolism of rifabutin, with consequent increases in serum levels. When rifabutin is administered orally with food, its rate of absorption is slowed, but the extent of its absorption is unchanged. Adjustment of dosage is usually unnecessary in elderly patients and in patients with reduced hepatic or renal function.

MECHANISM OF ACTION In *Escherichia coli* and *Bacillus subtilis*, rifabutin inhibits DNA-dependent RNA polymerase in the same manner as rifampin. Its mode of action against mycobacteria is believed to be the same.

ADVERSE EFFECTS Most adverse effects of rifabutin are dose related and occur most frequently in patients receiving >300 mg/d. Discontinuation of therapy because of adverse drug reactions is reported in 16% of patients receiving rifabutin as opposed to 8% of those receiving a placebo. The most common symptoms are gastrointestinal; other reactions include rash, headache, asthenia, chest pain, myalgia, and insomnia. Like those taking rifampin, most patients taking rifabutin have discolored (orange to tan) urine and other body fluids. Less common adverse reactions include fever, chills, a flulike syndrome, hepatitis, *Clostridium difficile*–associated diarrhea, and a yellow skin discoloration ("pseudojaundice"). After a rifabutin dose of 450 to 600 mg in combination with clarithromycin, anterior uveitis is reported in up to 40% of patients; also common at these high doses are hyperpigmentation and the polymyalgia/arthralgia syndrome. All of these conditions are reversible when treatment is discontinued. Laboratory abnormalities include neutropenia, leukopenia, thrombocytopenia, and increased levels of liver enzymes.

Rifabutin induces the hepatic cytochrome P450 enzymes but does so much less strongly than rifampin. Drugs whose metabolism is enhanced by rifabutin include anticoagulants, quinidine, oral contraceptives, sulfonylureas, analgesics, dapsone, narcotics, glucocorticoids, clarithromycin, zidovudine, and cardiac glycosides.

RESISTANCE Resistance to rifabutin is attributable to the same mechanism as that to rifampin—i.e., mutations involving the *rpoB* gene. However, of the 14 mutant *rpoB* alleles that confer resistance to rifampin, only nine confer high-level resistance to rifabutin, while the remaining five result in only small changes in rifabutin MICs, which remain ≤0.5 μg/mL. The MIC of rifabutin for susceptible strains of *M. tuberculosis* is low (<0.06 μg/mL), and the drug is considered clinically active against partially resistant strains that are inhibited by plasma levels of ≤0.5 μg/mL. Thus rifabutin inhibits about one-quarter of rifampin-resistant strains of *M. tuberculosis*.

Rifapentine A semisynthetic cyclopentyl rifamycin antibiotic, rifapentine has received accelerated approval from the FDA for the treatment of tuberculosis. It is the first new drug approved for tuberculosis in 25 years in the United States. While similar to rifampin, rifapentine is lipophilic and longer acting—characteristics that enhance patient compliance; the drug can be administered at a dose of 600 mg once or twice weekly. It has antibacterial activity against *M. tuberculosis* but has undergone only minimal testing against nontuberculous mycobacteria. Rifapentine has not yet been approved for the treatment of patients with HIV disease because rifapentine/rifampin monoresistance frequently develops in HIV-positive patients receiving isoniazid plus rifapentine. Like rifampin, rifapentine is active against many nonmycobacterial organisms, including *Haemophilus influenzae*, *Bordetella pertussis*, *B. parapertussis*, *Brucella* spp., *Legionella* spp., *Neisseria* spp., streptococci, and staphylococci.

In a randomized comparative study, 672 Chinese patients received isoniazid plus either rifapentine or rifampin. The isoniazid/rifapentine group had a higher relapse rate (10% versus 5%) than the isoniazid/rifampin group. Nevertheless, this disadvantage was considered acceptable in light of the lower rate of adverse effects and less frequent administration in the isoniazid/rifapentine group.

PHARMACOLOGY Food enhances the oral absorption of rifapentine, while antacids impair its absorption. After oral administration with food, this drug reaches peak serum concentrations in 5 to 6 h and achieves a steady state in 10 days. The half-life of rifapentine and its active metabolite 25-desacetyl rifapentine is approximately 13 h. The drug is highly bound to serum protein (93 to 97%), and most of the administered dose is excreted via the liver (70%). Oral clearance is more rapid in males than in females (2.51 vs 1.69 L/h), but the clinical significance of this difference is unknown.

MECHANISM OF ACTION Rifapentine exerts its bactericidal effect by inhibiting DNA-dependent RNA polymerase in susceptible bacteria. The MICs of rifapentine for rifampin-susceptible strains of *M. tuberculosis* range from 0.03 to 0.12 μg/mL.

ADVERSE EFFECTS Rifapentine demonstrates an adverse-event pattern similar to that of rifampin. Both drugs are frequently associated with hyperuricemia when administered with pyrazinamide and with elevated hepatocellular enzyme levels in 3 to 4% of patients when administered with other antituberculous agents. Liver enzyme levels should be monitored in patients receiving rifapentine who already have elevated liver enzyme concentrations or known liver disease. Like rifampin, rifapentine causes an orange-red discoloration of body fluids, including urine, saliva, and tears, and stains contact lenses.

Rifapentine induces the hepatic cytochrome P450 enzymes CYP3A4 and 2C8/9. Current induction studies suggest that its potential for drug-drug interaction may be less than that of rifampin but greater than that of rifabutin. Other drugs potentially affected by concomitant administration of rifapentine are listed in Table 168-2.

Rifapentine is in category C for use in pregnancy (Table 168-1) because of its teratogenesis in rats and rabbits. There are insufficient data concerning use of this drug in pregnant and breast-feeding patients.

RESISTANCE Strains of *M. tuberculosis* resistant to rifapentine, rifampin, and rifabutin all involve spontaneous point mutations in the *rpoB* gene. All strains resistant to rifampin are also resistant to rifapentine.

Quinolones A surprisingly large number of fluorinated quinolones are being developed and studied as inhibitors of mycobacteria. Their mode of action presumably is the prevention of DNA synthesis through the inhibition of DNA gyrase. Ofloxacin, ciprofloxacin, sparfloxacin, and pefloxacin are active against many mycobacteria, including *M. tuberculosis*, *M. leprae*, *M. marinum*, *M. kansasii*, and *M. fortuitum*. These drugs are well absorbed orally, reach high serum levels, and distribute well to body tissues and fluids. While not approved for antituberculous therapy in the United States, ofloxacin—used in combination with isoniazid and rifampin for the treatment of pulmonary tuberculosis—has been as active and safe as ethambutol in initial trials. Adverse effects are relatively uncommon, occurring in 0.5 to 10% of cases and consisting mostly of benign reactions such as gastrointestinal intolerance, rashes, dizziness, and headache. However, more serious adverse effects are being reported and include confusion, seizures, interstitial nephritis, skin vasculitis, and acute renal failure.

Mycobacterial resistance to the fluoroquinolones develops rapidly. Its molecular basis is complex; only some strains exhibit missense mutations in the A subunit (*gyrA* gene) of DNA gyrase. Fluoroquinolone-resistant tuberculosis is a source of growing concern: 22 such cases were reported recently from New York City. Antituberculous therapy with quinolones should be reserved for patients with multidrug resistance or those who cannot tolerate first-line drugs.

LEPROSY (HANSEN'S DISEASE)

Therapy for leprosy remains difficult, especially in developing countries, because of the long course required, the high cost and low availability of most drugs, the frequency of adverse reactions to drugs, the acquisition of drug resistance, the difficulty of determining a disease end point or cure, and (given that *M. leprae* still cannot be grown in vitro) the difficulty of conducting susceptibility testing. While many drugs are active against *M. leprae*, efficacy in the treatment of leprosy has been established only for dapsone, rifampin, clofazimine, and ethionamide.

Rifampin Rifampin is considered the most active agent for the treatment of leprosy. Its worldwide use is limited only by its cost. This drug is markedly bactericidal against *M. leprae* and reduces the number of viable bacilli in the patient's tissues faster than any other available agent. Rifampin must be combined with other antileprosy drugs to forestall resistance. For cost reasons, the drug is given at a dose of 600 mg once a month (supervised) outside the United States, but it is given daily in the United States. For details on pharmacology, adverse events, and resistance, see relevant sections under "Tuberculosis."

Dapsone Dapsone (4,4'-diaminodiphenylsulfone) inhibits bacterial folic acid synthesis. It is now considered the second drug of choice (after rifampin) in most cases of Hansen's disease because of its ready availability, low cost, and low toxicity and the susceptibility of untreated strains of *M. leprae* to very low concentrations.

Pharmacology Dapsone is well absorbed orally and distributes well throughout the body. The usual daily dosage is 100 mg for adults and 0.9 to 1.4 mg/kg for children. Plasma concentrations peak within 1 to 3 h. The median elimination half-life is 22 h. Dapsone is cleared by acetylation in the liver, with genetic variation similar to that documented for the acetylation of isoniazid. The drug is 70% bound to plasma protein. Usual daily doses produce serum concentrations of 10 to 15 μg/mL, which far exceed the MIC for *M. leprae* (0.01 to 0.001 μg/mL).

Adverse effects Hemolysis and methemoglobinemia are common untoward reactions to dapsone. Patients should be screened for glucose-6-phosphate dehydrogenase deficiency to prevent drug-induced hemolysis. However, most patients tolerate dapsone therapy well with adequate clinical and laboratory supervision. Other side effects include gastrointestinal intolerance, headache, pruritus, peripheral neuropathies, nephritic syndrome, fever, and rash. In lepromatous and borderline lepromatous leprosy, erythema nodosum leprosum (ENL) may occur. This reaction may be difficult to distinguish from reactions of leprosy, including drug reactions and the infectious mononucleosis–like dapsone syndrome.

Clofazimine A phenazine iminoquinone dye, clofazimine is weakly bactericidal against *M. leprae*. It is useful in treating dapsone-resistant leprosy and may lessen the severity of ENL. Clofazimine's mode of action is not well understood, but the drug may inhibit DNA binding. It is absorbed orally and distributed to the fatty tissues and the reticuloendothelial system. Its serum half-life is about 60 to 70 days; only a small proportion of the dose is excreted daily into the urine or bile. Bactericidal activity is very slow and is evident for about 50 days after administration. The usual adult dosage is 50 to 100 mg/d, 100 mg three times a week, or (for treatment of ENL) 300 mg/d. Untoward effects include skin discoloration and, less commonly, gastrointestinal intolerance. Clofazimine was reported to be responsible for a case of cardiotoxicity induced via ventricular arrhythmia. Even though clofazimine-resistant disease has been reported only rarely when this agent is used alone, it should be used with other effective antibiotics. Clofazimine is active in vitro against some nontuberculous mycobacterial species, including MAI, *M. kansasii*, *M. simiae*, and *M. abscessus*.

Ethionamide While ethionamide (250 mg/d) has not been approved by the FDA for the treatment of leprosy, it is sometimes used in the United States in combination with rifampin (600 mg/d) to treat dapsone-resistant leprosy in patients who cannot accept the skin-depigmentation effect of clofazimine. Because resistance to ethionamide develops quickly when the drug is used alone, it must be used with other effective agents. Patients should be monitored closely for hepatotoxicity when taking ethionamide (especially in combination with rifampin), and treatment should be discontinued if the patient's ALT levels exceed 2.5 times the normal value. Prothionamide, a congener of ethionamide that is not available in the United States, has pharmacologic properties similar to those of ethionamide and is widely used throughout the world.

Other Agents A number of other drugs exhibit significant activity against *M. leprae*, but clinical experience with these agents is lacking. Thalidomide is now approved by the FDA for treatment of ENL. Although this drug may be useful in suppressing ENL, it acts as a tranquilizer, is extremely teratogenic, and should *never* be taken by anyone who is or may become pregnant. Physicians wishing to prescribe thalidomide must register with the System for Thalidomide Education and Prescription Safety (S.T.E.P.S.) at 1-888-423-5436 (Celgese Corporation).

The newer macrolide antibiotics (particularly clarithromycin), minocycline (a long-acting tetracycline), and a number of fluoroquinolones (including ofloxacin, sparfloxacin, and pefloxacin) have shown promising bactericidal activity against *M. leprae*. Ofloxacin and minocycline are being investigated with rifampin in short-course regimens for lepromatous disease. All of these newer leprosy drugs have low toxicity profiles, modes of action different from those of the established agents, and powerful bactericidal activity against *M. leprae*. However, their levels of bactericidal activity are lower than that of rifampin.

NONTUBERCULOUS MYCOBACTERIA

Although less pathogenic than *M. tuberculosis*, the nontuberculous mycobacteria can cause pulmonary, skin, bone and joint, lymph node, and soft tissue infection as well as disseminated disease in immunocompromised hosts, including patients with AIDS. MAI and *M. kansasii* are the two most common causes of nontuberculous mycobacterial pulmonary infection. Up to 40% of AIDS patients develop disseminated disease due to MAI.

Clarithromycin Clarithromycin (6-*O*-methylerythromycin) is a new macrolide that is similar to erythromycin in its mechanism of action. However, unlike erythromycin, it is well absorbed with or without meals and elicits little gastrointestinal intolerance at low doses. Clarithromycin distributes well into body tissues and fluids and is highly concentrated in macrophages. The drug is metabolized in the liver, and approximately 30% of a given dose is excreted in the urine. The dosage should be reduced if the creatinine clearance rate is ≤30 mL/min. Like erythromycin, clarithromycin binds with plasma proteins (65 to 70%) and can raise the levels of drugs such as theophylline and carbamazepine. As noted earlier, serum levels of clarithromycin are reduced by the concomitant administration of rifampin and to a lesser degree by that of rifabutin; clarithromycin treatment increases serum levels of rifabutin and some antihistamines (e.g., terfenadine), thus increasing their toxicity. Clarithromycin and (probably) azithromycin are the most active agents for the treatment of MAI infections; one of these drugs is considered an essential component of any regimens for this purpose. However, because of mutational drug resistance, clarithromycin should be given in combination with other agents, such as ethambutol and rifampin or rifabutin. The drug is also highly active against almost all other nontuberculous mycobacteria, including *M. marinum*, *M. kansasii*, *M. haemophilum*, *M. genavense*, *M. xenopi*, *M. abscessus*, *M. chelonae*, and most isolates of *M. fortuitum*. Standard antimycobacterial doses have been 500 mg twice daily; doses of 1000 mg twice daily have been associated with increased mortality among patients with AIDS and disseminated MAI disease. The more common side effects of high doses include nausea, vomiting, a bitter taste, and (occasionally) abnormal liver-function tests. Most side effects can be minimized by reducing the dose, usually by 50%. Clarithromycin is teratogenic in laboratory animals and is in category C for use in pregnancy (Table 168-1). Mutational resistance occurs in one in 10^8 to 10^9 organisms and develops rapidly with monotherapy, especially that for disseminated MAI disease. Resistance results from point mutations involving adenine at positions 2058 or 2059 in the 23S ribosomal binding site.

Azithromycin Azithromycin is a macrolide that belongs to the family of azalides. It reaches much lower serum levels than clarithromycin (usually ≤0.5 μg/mL) but attains high tissue and macrophage concentrations and has a longer half-life, which suggests the feasibility of intermittent therapy. It is involved in few drug interactions since it does not affect the cytochrome P450 system. The usual dose is 250 to 500 mg/d. No alteration in dose is required in renal failure. The most common side effects are gastrointestinal symptoms and reversible hearing loss. Azithromycin appears to be less active than clarithromycin for both pulmonary and disseminated MAI disease. Resistance

to azithromycin develops by the same mechanism as that to clarithromycin, with cross-resistance between the two macrolides.

THERAPY FOR SPECIFIC NONTUBERCULOUS MYCOBACTERIA MAI First-line antituberculous drugs are much less active against MAI than against *M. tuberculosis*. Therapy for MAI is controversial because of the lack of controlled clinical trials. In 1990 the ATS recommended the following four-drug regimen for MAI lung disease in HIV-negative patients: 18 to 24 months of isoniazid (300 mg), rifampin (600 mg), and ethambutol (25 mg/kg, then 15 mg/kg beginning in the third month), with intermittent streptomycin. However, two subsequent events—the demonstration of the dramatic activity of clarithromycin against both pulmonary and disseminated MAI infection and the introduction of rifabutin—have altered the therapeutic approach to MAI infection. In the 1997 ATS recommendations for MAI lung disease, clarithromycin (500 mg twice daily) now replaces isoniazid, and rifabutin (300 mg/d) is often used in place of rifampin. Therapy for pulmonary disease is generally given until cultures have been negative for 12 months.

For disseminated disease in AIDS, one of the newer macrolides (clarithromycin or azithromycin) and ethambutol (15 mg/kg) are considered essential components of any treatment regimen, with rifabutin (300 mg) a commonly used third drug in patients not taking a protease inhibitor for their HIV infection. Other alternative drugs include ciprofloxacin, streptomycin, and amikacin. Clofazimine appears to increase mortality and should be avoided. For the prophylaxis of disseminated MAI disease, rifabutin (300 mg/d), clarithromycin (500 mg twice daily), and azithromycin (1200 mg once weekly) have all been demonstrated to be effective in controlled or comparative clinical trials.

Mycobacterium kansasii *M. kansasii* is usually susceptible to most antituberculous drugs except for pyrazinamide. Current ATS recommendations for the treatment of *M. kansasii* pulmonary disease are 18 to 24 months of daily isoniazid (300 mg), rifampin (600 mg), and ethambutol (15 mg/kg). In patients taking protease inhibitors, rifabutin (150 mg) or clarithromycin (500 mg) twice daily should be substituted for rifampin. The potential advantages of the highly active rifabutin and the newer macrolides in immunocompetent patients have not been studied.

Rapidly Growing Mycobacteria *M. fortuitum*, *M. abscessus*, and *M. chelonae* account for more than 80% of cases of clinical disease due to rapidly growing mycobacteria. These organisms are resistant to antituberculous agents other than amikacin but are variably susceptible to several other antibiotics. Clarithromycin has dramatically changed the approach to therapy for infection with these organisms, as it inhibits all rapidly growing mycobacteria—except for 20% of *M. fortuitum* strains and most *M. smegmatis* strains—at concentrations of ≤4 μg/mL. Other drugs with good activity include amikacin (which inhibits 80 to 100% of strains), cefoxitin (80% of *M. abscessus* and *M. fortuitum* strains), doxycycline (50% of *M. fortuitum* strains), imipenem (100% of *M. fortuitum* strains, 70% of *M. chelonae* strains, and 70% of *M. abscessus* strains), the fluorinated quinolones ciprofloxacin and ofloxacin (100% of *M. fortuitum* strains), and sulfonamides (90% of *M. fortuitum* strains).

Mycobacterium marinum *M. marinum*, a photochromogen, is typically susceptible to minocycline, rifampin, ethambutol, clarithromycin, and trimethoprim-sulfamethoxazole and is resistant to isoniazid.

Mycobacterium haemophilum Infection due to *M. haemophilum* occurs most commonly as disseminated disease in immunocompromised patients with or without AIDS. This organism can cause bone and joint infection and skin infection. Isolates typically show in vitro resistance to most drugs but may be susceptible to rifampin, rifabutin, quinolones, and clarithromycin.

Mycobacterium xenopi In the United States, *M. xenopi* most often causes nosocomial infections; these infections most commonly occur in the environment of the hospital's hot-water system. In one study from Brooklyn, NY, *M. xenopi* was the second most common pathogenic nontuberculous mycobacterial species; of the 86 hospitalized patients from whom it was isolated, 41% were HIV-positive. Drug therapy for *M. xenopi* infection is difficult because in vitro drug sensitivity tests do not reliably predict clinical results. *M. xenopi* is often resistant to first-line antituberculous agents but susceptible to the newer macrolides, quinolones, streptomycin, and ethionamide.

Mycobacterium genavense *M. genavense* is a newly recognized organism that grows only in liquid media, such as Bactec 12B or 13A. This organism almost exclusively infects AIDS patients, causing disseminated disease and being isolated from blood, bone marrow, liver, lymph node, spleen, and intestinal cultures. The in vitro susceptibility profile of *M. genavense* has not been well established. Some isolates are susceptible to amikacin, clarithromycin, ofloxacin, rifampin, and rifabutin.

BIBLIOGRAPHY

ALANGADEN GJ, LERNER SA: The clinical use of fluoroquinolones for the treatment of mycobacterial disease. Clin Infect Dis 25:1213, 1997

ALCAIDE F et al: Role of *embB* in natural and acquired resistance to ethambutol in mycobacteria. Antimicrob Agents Chemother 41:2270, 1997

BROGDEN RN, FITTON A: Rifabutin: A review of its antimicrobial activity, pharmacokinetic properties and therapeutic efficacy. Drugs 47:983, 1994

KEUNG A et al: Single and multiple dose pharmacokinetics of rifapentine in man: Part II. Int J Tuberc Lung Dis 3:437, 1999

MCEVOY GK (ed): *AHFS Drug Information 1999*. Bethesda, MD, American Society of Health-System Pharmacists, 1999, pp 464–502

MUSSER JM: Antimicrobial agent resistance in mycobacteria: Molecular genetic insights. Clin Microbiol Rev 8:496, 1995

NOLAN CM et al: Hepatotoxicity associated with isoniazid preventive therapy: A 7-year survey from a public health tuberculosis clinic. JAMA 281:1014, 1999

SREEVATSAN S et al: Mutations associated with pyrazinamide resistance in *pncA* of *Mycobacterium tuberculosis* complex organisms. Antimicrob Agents Chemother 41:636, 1997

WALLACE RJ JR et al: American Thoracic Society statement: Diagnosis and treatment of disease caused by nontuberculous mycobacteria. Am J. Respir Crit Care Med 156: S1, 1997

WHO EXPERT COMMITTEE ON LEPROSY: Seventh report. Geneva, World Health Organization, 1998, Technical Report Series, No. 874

169 *Mario C. Raviglione, Richard J. O'Brien*

TUBERCULOSIS

AFB acid-fast bacilli	MDR multidrug-resistant
ARDS adult respiratory distress syndrome	MRI magnetic resonance imaging
BCG bacille Calmette-Guérin	NK natural killer
CDC Centers for Disease Control and Prevention	OT "old tuberculin"
	PAS para-aminosalicylic acid
CSF cerebrospinal fluid	PCR polymerase chain reaction
CT Computed tomography	PPD purified protein derivative
DTH delayed-type hypersensitivity	SIADH syndrome of inappropriate secretion of antidiuretic hormone
IFN-γ interferon γ	TNF-α tumor necrosis factor α
IL interleukin	WHO World Health Organization

DEFINITION Tuberculosis, one of the oldest diseases known to affect humans, is caused by bacteria belonging to the *Mycobacterium tuberculosis* complex. The disease usually affects the lungs, although in up to one-third of cases other organs are involved. If properly treated, tuberculosis caused by drug-susceptible strains is curable in virtually all cases. If untreated, the disease may be fatal within 5 years in more than half of cases. Transmission usually takes place through the airborne spread of droplet nuclei produced by patients with infectious pulmonary tuberculosis.

ETIOLOGIC AGENT Mycobacteria belong to the family Mycobacteriaceae and the order Actinomycetales. Of the pathogenic species belonging to the *M. tuberculosis* complex, the most frequent and important agent of human disease is *M. tuberculosis* itself. The complex includes *M. bovis* (the bovine tubercle bacillus, once an important cause of tuberculosis transmitted by unpasteurized milk and currently the cause of a small percentage of cases in developing countries), *M. africanum* (isolated in a small proportion of cases in West and Central Africa), and *M. microti* (the "vole" bacillus, a closely related but rarely encountered organism).

M. tuberculosis is a rod-shaped, non-spore-forming, thin aerobic bacterium measuring about 0.5 μm by 3 μm. Mycobacteria, including *M. tuberculosis*, do not stain readily and are often neutral on Gram's staining. However, once stained, the bacilli cannot be decolorized by acid alcohol, a characteristic justifying their classification as acid-fast bacilli (AFB). Acid fastness is due mainly to the organisms' high content of mycolic acids, long-chain cross-linked fatty acids, and other cell-wall lipids. Microorganisms other than mycobacteria that display some acid fastness include species of *Nocardia* and *Rhodococcus*, *Legionella micdadei*, and the protozoa *Isospora* and *Cryptosporidium*. In the mycobacterial cell wall, lipids (e.g., mycolic acids) are linked to underlying arabinogalactan and peptidoglycan. This structure is responsible for the very low permeability of the cell wall and thus for the ineffectiveness of most antibiotics against the organism. Another molecule in the mycobacterial cell wall, lipoarabinomannan, is involved in the pathogen-host interaction and facilitates the survival of *M. tuberculosis* within macrophages. The several proteins characteristic of *M. tuberculosis* include those in purified protein derivative (PPD) tuberculin, a precipitate of non-species-specific molecules obtained from filtrates of heat-sterilized, concentrated broth cultures. The complete genome sequence of *M. tuberculosis* comprises about 4000 genes and has a high guanine-plus-cytosine content. A large proportion of the genes are devoted to the production of enzymes involved in lipogenesis and lipolysis and of glycine-rich proteins that are probably responsible for antigenic variations.

EPIDEMIOLOGY Between 3.5 and 4 million new cases of tuberculosis—all forms (pulmonary and extrapulmonary), 90% of them from developing countries—were reported annually to the World Health Organization (WHO) in the late 1990s. However, because of a low level of case detection and incomplete notifications in many national programs, reported cases represent only a fraction of the total. It is estimated that 8 million new cases of tuberculosis occurred worldwide in 1997, 95% of them in developing countries of Asia (5 million), Africa (1.6 million), the Middle East (0.6 million), and Latin America (0.4 million). It is also estimated that nearly 2 million deaths from tuberculosis occurred in 1997, 98% of them in developing countries.

Beginning in the mid-1980s in many industrialized countries, the number of tuberculosis case notifications, which had been falling steadily, stabilized or even began to increase. This phenomenon was first noted in the United States but was soon observed in many European countries as well. A number of factors were implicated in the resurgence of tuberculosis in the United States in 1986 through 1992—most notably, immigration from countries with a high prevalence of tuberculosis; infection with HIV; emergence of multidrug-resistant (MDR) tuberculosis due to strains resistant at least to isoniazid and rifampin; and social problems such as poverty, homelessness, and drug abuse. In some areas (e.g., New York City), deterioration in the public health system and dismantling of tuberculosis management services also contributed to the worsening situation. With the implementation of stronger control programs, cases began to decrease in 1993. In 1998, 18,361 cases of tuberculosis (6.8 per 100,000 population) were reported to the U.S. Centers for Disease Control and Prevention (CDC)—a 31% decrease from the 1992 peak.

In the United States, tuberculosis is uncommon among young adults of European descent, who have only rarely been exposed to *M. tuberculosis* infection during recent decades. In contrast, because of a high risk in the past, the prevalence of *M. tuberculosis* infection is relatively high among elderly Caucasians, who remain at increased

COLOR ATLASES

I. Atlas of Cardiology

II. Atlas of Dermatology

   A. Common Skin Diseases and Lesions
   B. Cutaneous Neoplasms
   C. Pigmented Lesions—Benign and Malignant
   D. Infectious Disease and the Skin
   E. Immunologically Mediated Skin Disease
   F. Skin Manifestations of Internal Disease

III. Atlas of Endoscopic Findings

IV. Atlas of Funduscopic Findings

V. Atlas of Hematology

VI. Atlas of Diagnostic Microbiology

I. Atlas of Cardiology

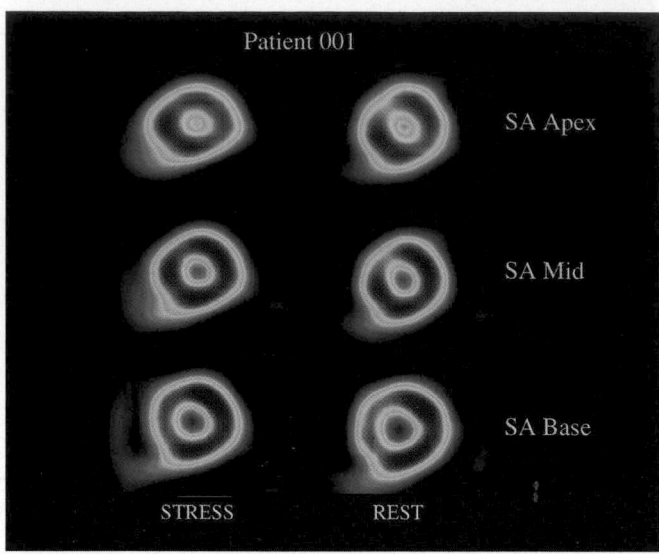

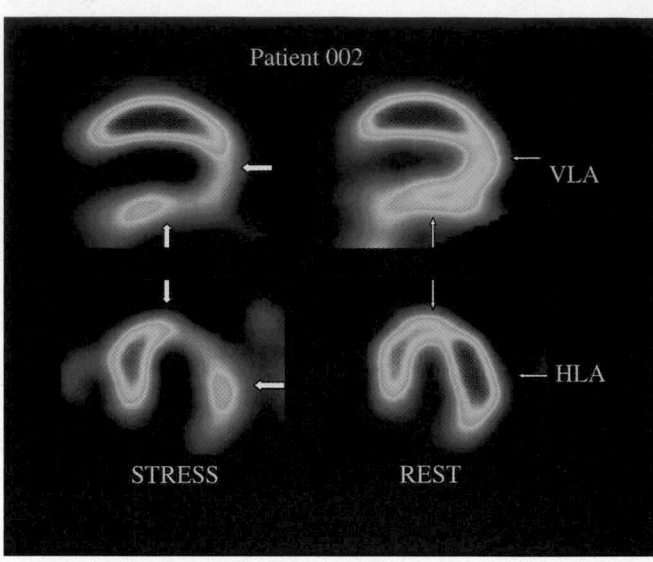

I-1A **Exercise sestamibi study** on a 71-year-old, white female with atypical angina. *Left:* stress images; *right:* rest images. The images are normal. There is even sestamibi update throughout the myocardium at rest and during stress. SA, short axis. Mid, middle of the left ventricle. VLA, vertical long axis. HLA, horizontal long axis.

I-1B **Exercise sestamibi study** on a 75-year-old male with a history of typical angina. *Left:* stress images; *right:* rest images. The stress images show a large defect involving the apex, lateral, and inferior walls (*thick arrows*), which improves at rest (*thin arrows*). Subsequent coronary angiography demonstrates severe three-vessel coronary artery disease.

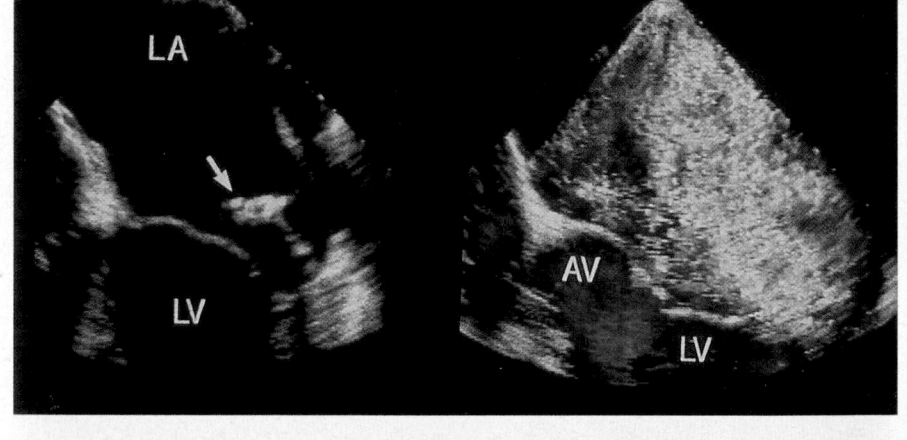

I-2 **Transesophageal echocardiographic view** of a patient with severe mitral regurgitation due to a flail posterior leaflet. The *arrow* points to the portion of the posterior leaflet that is unsupported and moves into the left atrium during systole. *Right:* color flow imaging demonstrating a large mosaic jet of mitral regurgitation during systole. LA, left atrium; LV, left ventricle; AV, aortic valve.

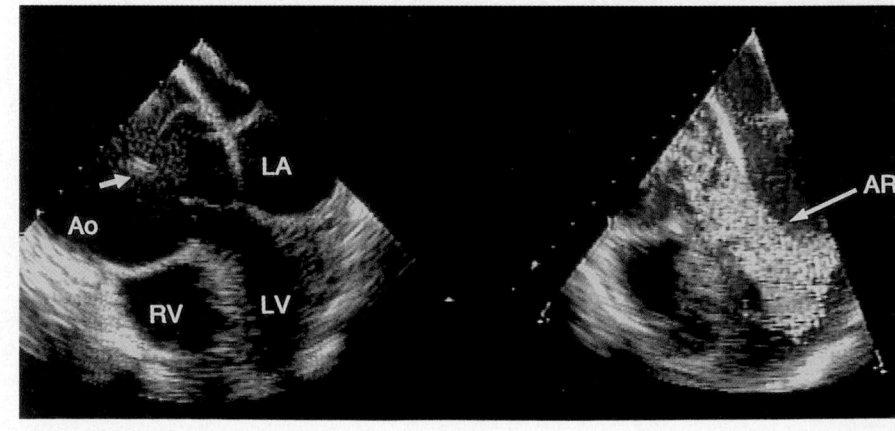

I-3 **Transesophageal echocardiographic view** of a patient with a dilated aorta, aortic dissection, and severe aortic regurgitation. The *arrow* points to the intimal flap that is seen in the dilated ascending aorta. *Left:* the long axis apex down view of the black and white two-dimensional image in diastole. *Right:* color flow imaging that demonstrates a large mosaic jet of aortic regurgitation. AO, aorta; RV, right ventricle; AR, aortic regurgitation.

II. Atlas of Dermatology

Stephen F. Templeton / Thomas J. Lawley

A. Common Skin Diseases and Lesions

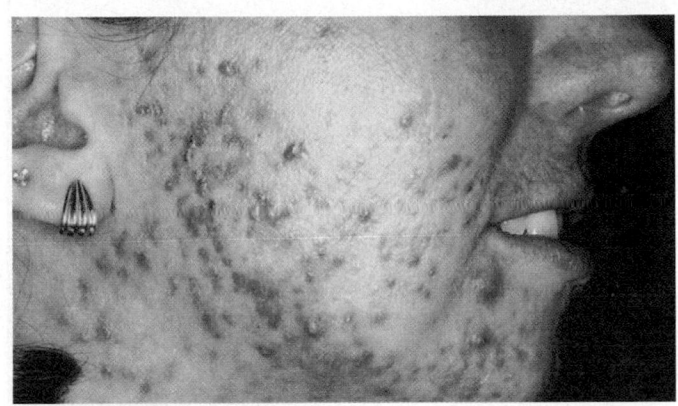

IIA-1 **Acne vulgaris** with inflammatory papules, pustules, and comedones

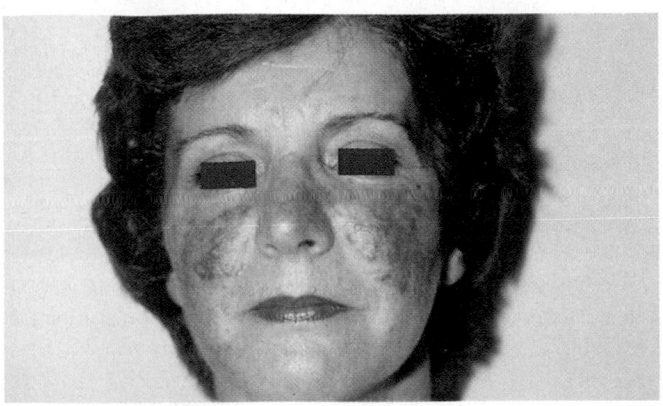

IIA-2 **Acne rosacea** with prominent facial erythema, telangiectasias, scattered papules, and small pustules.

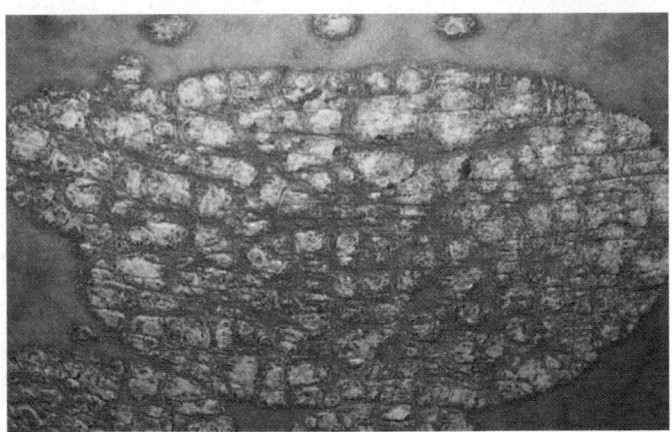

IIA-3 **Psoriasis** is characterized by small and large erythematous plaques with adherent silvery scale.

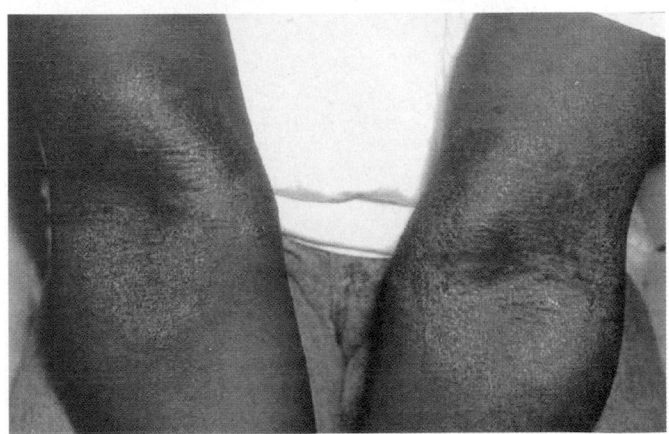

IIA-4 **Atopic dermatitis** with hyperpigmentation, lichenification, and scaling in the antecubital fossae.

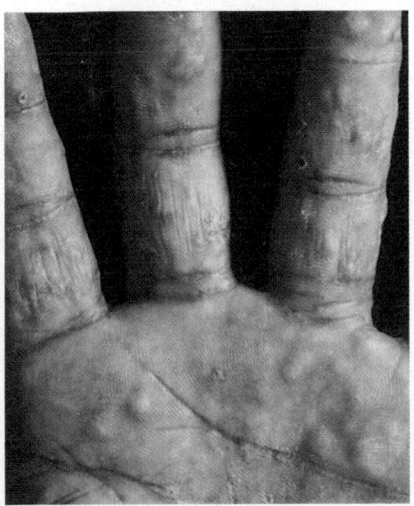

IIA-5 **Dyshidrotic eczema,** characterized by deep-seated vesicles and scaling on palms and lateral fingers, is often associated with an atopic diathesis.

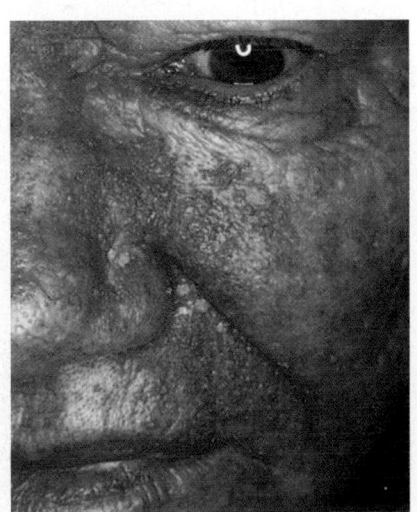

IIA-6 **Seborrheic dermatitis** showing central facial erythema with overlying greasy, yellowish scale.

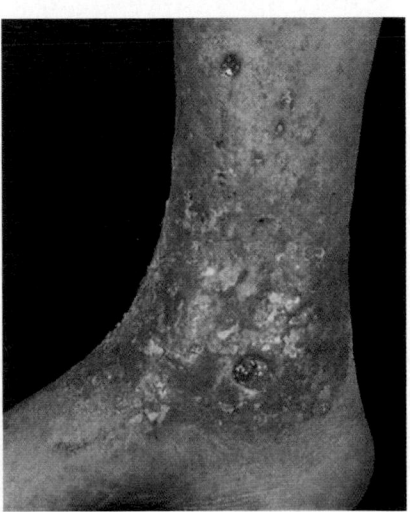

IIA-7 **Stasis dermatitis** showing erythematous, scaly, and oozing patches over the lower leg. Several stasis ulcers are also seen in this patient.

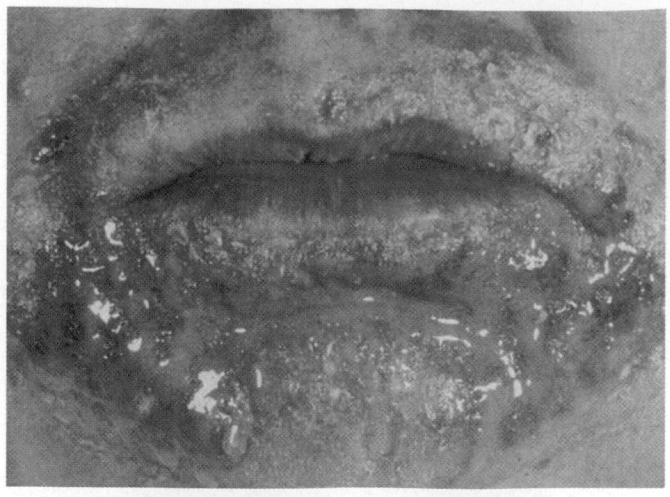

IIA-8A **Allergic contact dermatitis,** acute phase, with sharply demarcated, weeping, eczematous plaques in a perioral distribution.

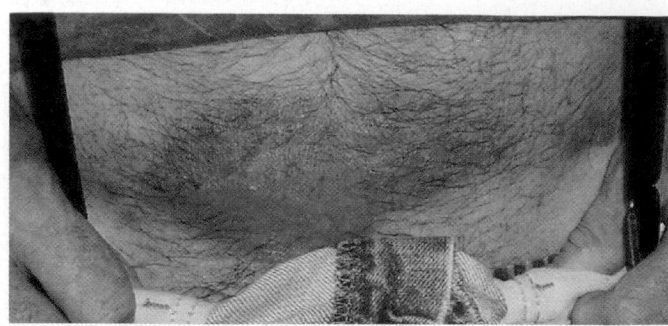

IIA-8B **Allergic contact dermatitis** to nickel, chronic phase demonstrating an erythematous, lichenified, weeping plaque on skin chronically exposed to a metal snap.

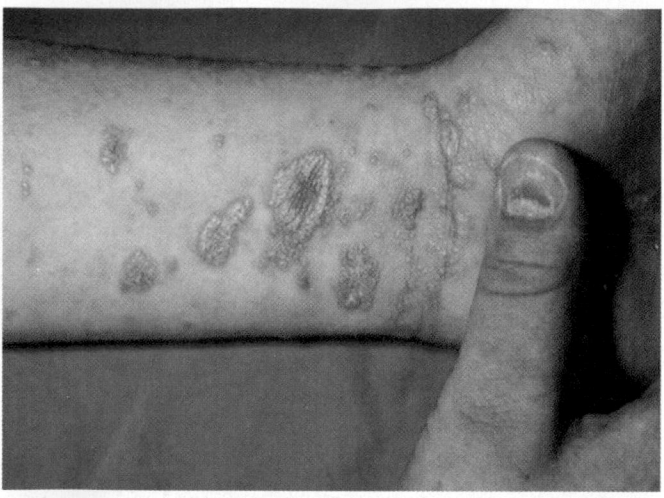

IIA-9 **Lichen planus** showing multiple flat-topped, violaceous papules and plaques. Nail dystrophy as seen in this patient's thumbnail may also be a feature.

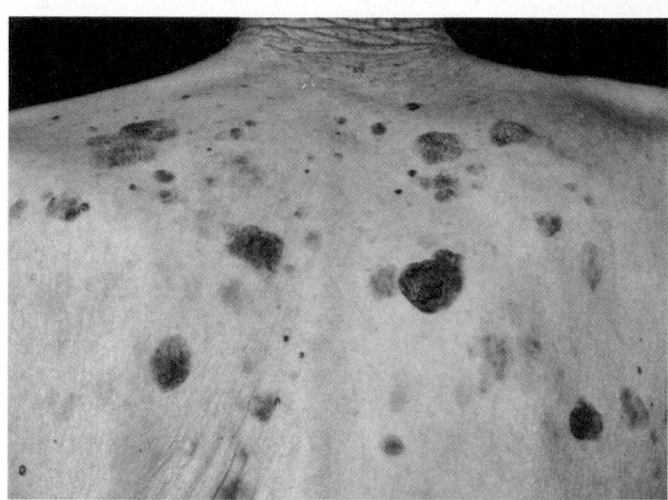

IIA-10 **Seborrheic keratoses** are seen as "stuck on," waxy, verrucous papules and plaques with a variety of colors ranging from light tan to black.

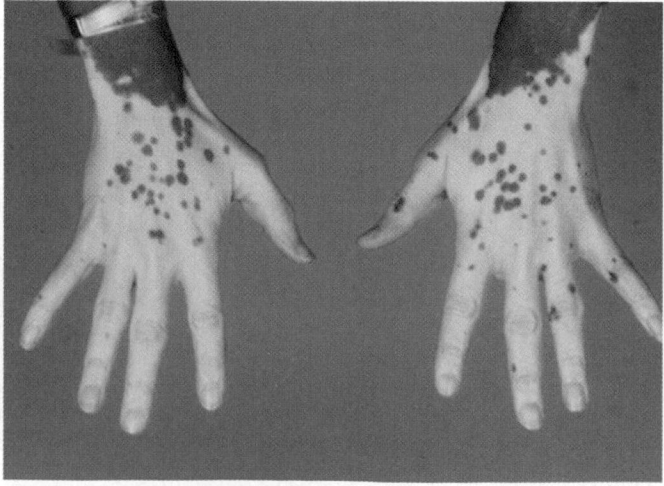

IIA-11 **Vitiligo** in a typical acral distribution demonstrating striking cutaneous depigmentation, as a result of loss of melanocytes.

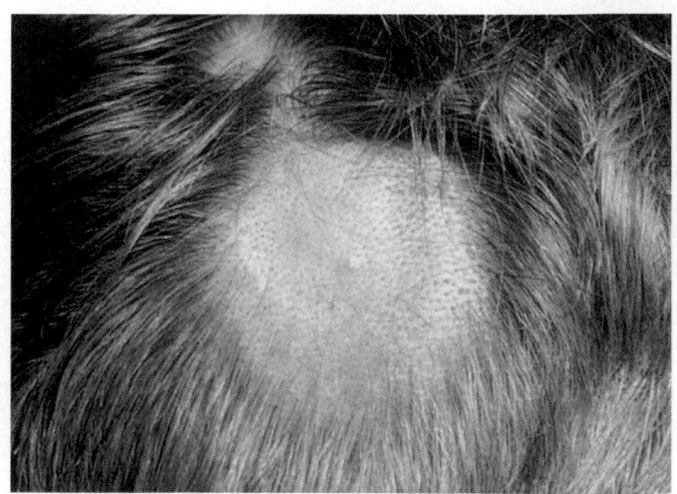

IIA-12 **Alopecia areata** characterized by a sharply demarcated circular patch of scalp completely devoid of hairs. Follicular orifices are preserved, indicating a nonscarring alopecia.

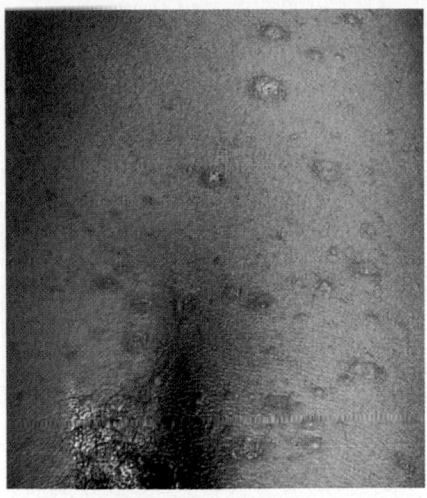

IIA-13 **Pityriasis rosea** Multiple round to oval erythematous patches with fine central scale are distributed along the skin tension lines on the trunk.

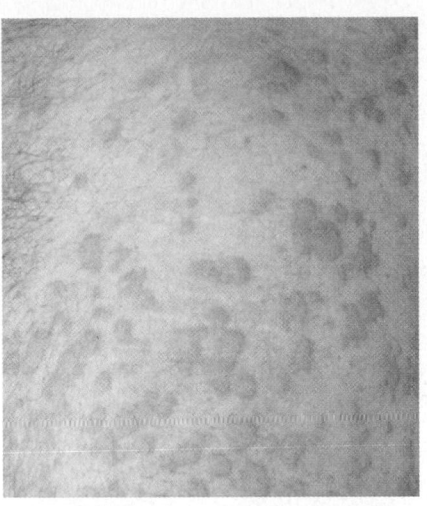

IIA-14A **Urticaria** showing characteristic discrete and confluent, edematous, erythematous papules and plaques.

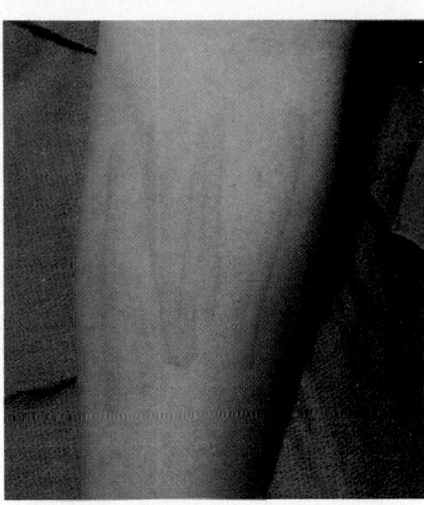

IIA-14B **Dermatographism** Erythema and whealing that developed after firm stroking of the skin.

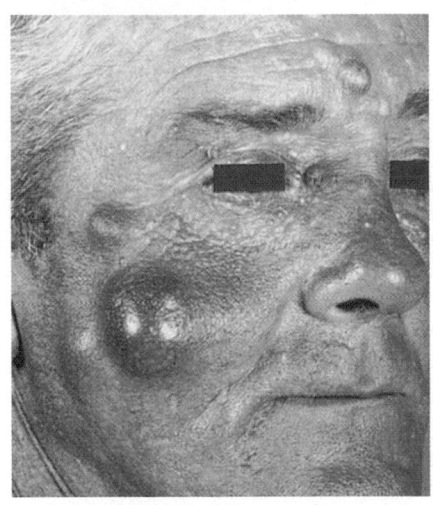

IIA-15 **Epidermoid cysts** Several inflamed and noninflamed firm, cystic nodules are seen in this patient. Often a patulous follicular punctum is observed on the overlying epidermal surface.

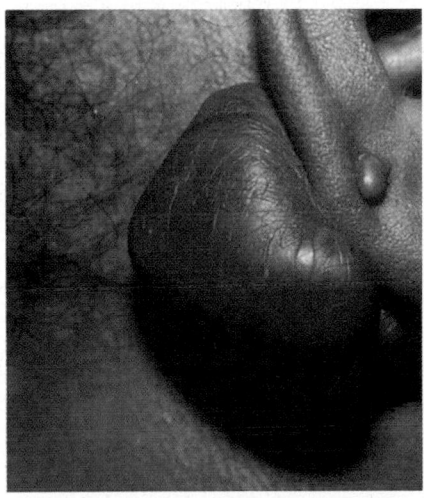

IIA-16 **Keloids** resulting from ear piercing, with firm exophytic flesh-colored to erythematous nodules of scar tissue.

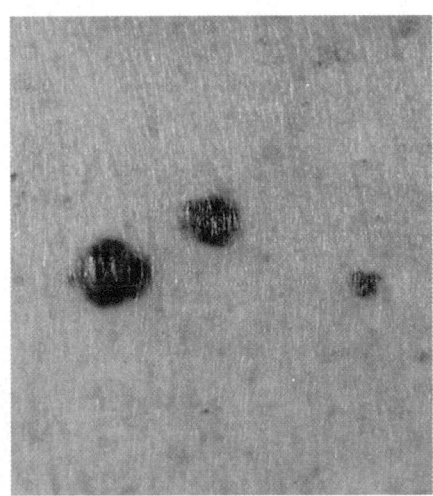

IIA-17 **Cherry hemangiomas** are very common and arise in middle-aged to older adults. They are characterized by multiple erythematous to dark purple papules usually located on the trunk.

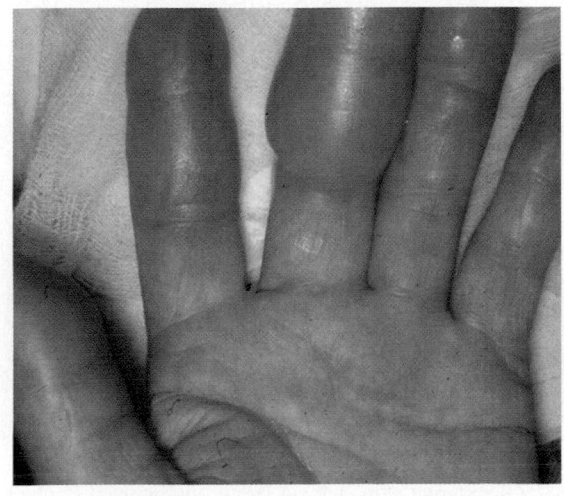

IIA-18 **Frostbite** with vesiculation, surrounded by edema and erythema.

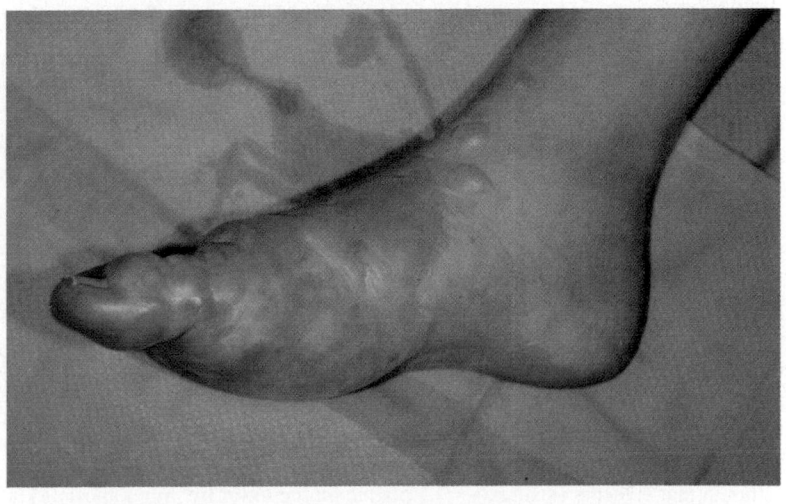

IIA-19 **Frostbite** with vesiculation, surrounded by edema and erythema.

B. Cutaneous Neoplasms

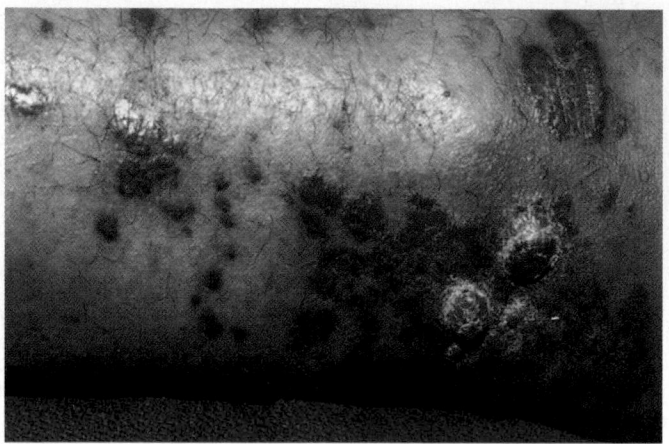

IIB-20 **Kaposi's sarcoma** in a patient with AIDS demonstrating patch, plaque, and tumor stages.

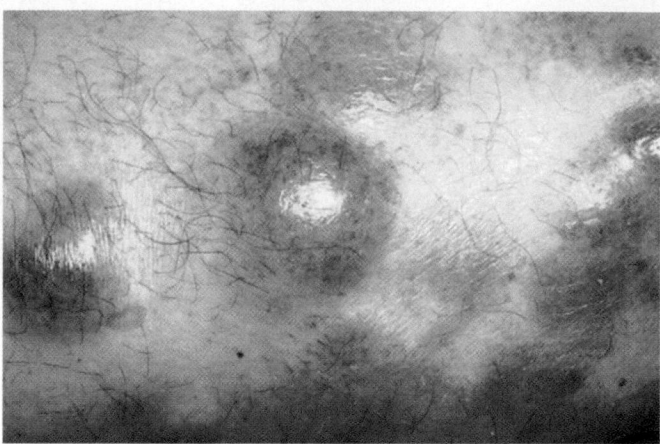

IIB-21 **Non-Hodgkin's lymphoma** involving the skin with typical violaceous, "plum-colored" nodules.

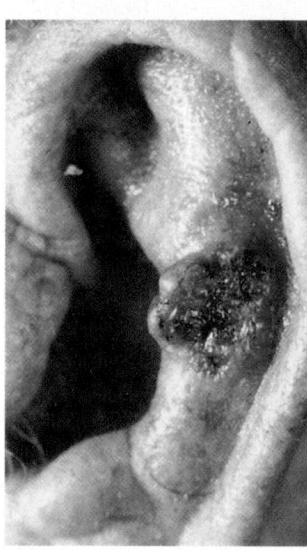

IIB-22 **Basal cell carcinoma** showing central ulceration and a pearly, rolled, telangiectatic tumor border.

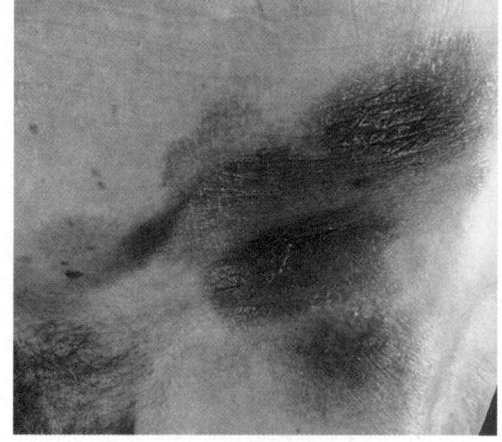

IIB-23 **Mycosis fungoides** is a cutaneous T cell lymphoma, and plaque stage lesions are seen in this patient.

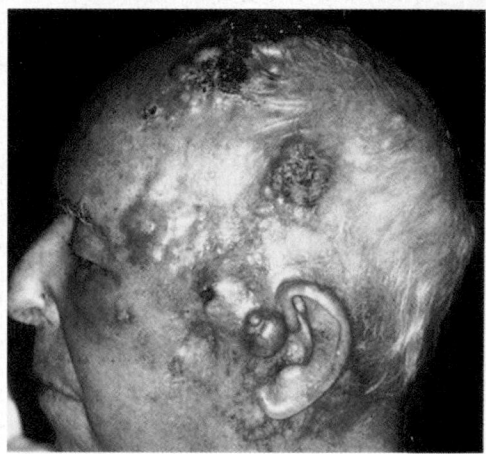

IIB-24 **Metastatic carcinoma** to the skin is characterized by inflammatory, often ulcerated dermal nodules.

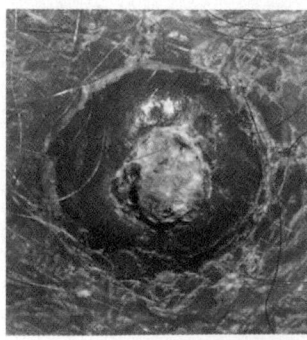

IIB-25 **Keratoacanthoma** is a low-grade squamous cell carcinoma that presents as an exophytic nodule with central keratinous debris.

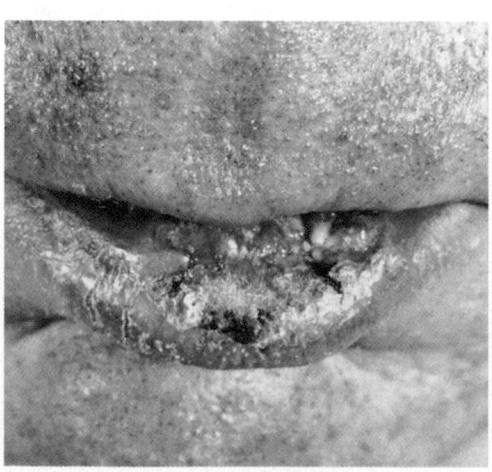

IIB-26 **Squamous cell carcinoma** seen here as a hyperkeratotic crusted and somewhat eroded plaque on the lower lip. Sun-exposed skin such as the head, neck, hands, and arms are other typical sites of involvement.

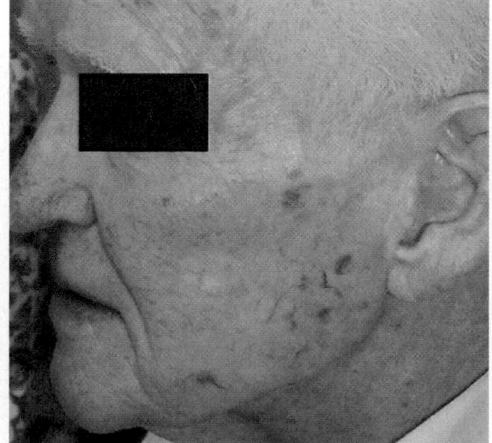

IIB-27 **Actinic keratoses** consists of hyperkeratotic erythematous papules and patches on sun-exposed skin. They arise in middle-aged to older adults and have some potential for malignant transformation.

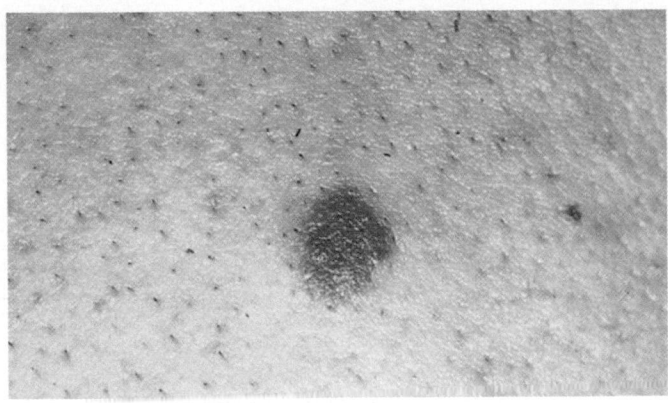

IIC-28 **Nevus** Nevi are benign proliferations of nevomelanocytes characterized by regularly shaped hyperpigmented macules or papules of a uniform color.

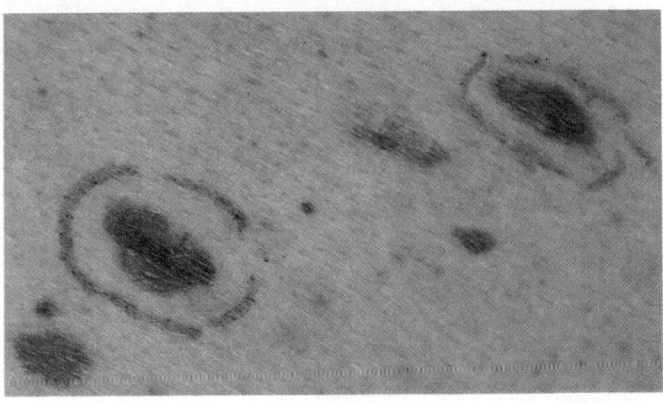

IIC-29 **Dysplastic nevi** are irregularly pigmented and shaped nevomelanocytic lesions which may be associated with familial melanoma.

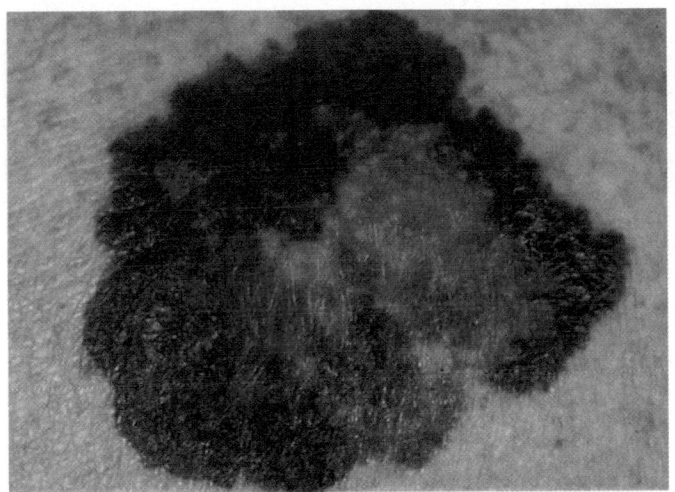

IIC-30 **Superficial spreading melanoma** is the most common type of malignant melanoma and demonstrates color variegation (black, blue, brown, pink, and white) and irregular borders.

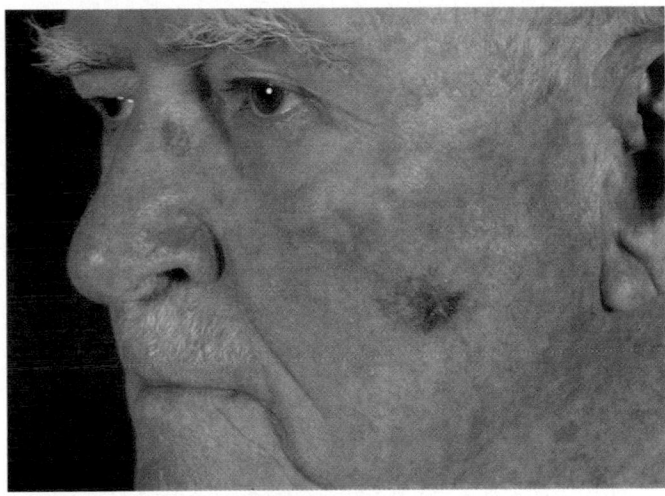

IIC-31 **Lentigo maligna melanoma** occurs on sun-exposed skin as a large, hyperpigmented macule or plaque with irregular borders and variable pigmentation.

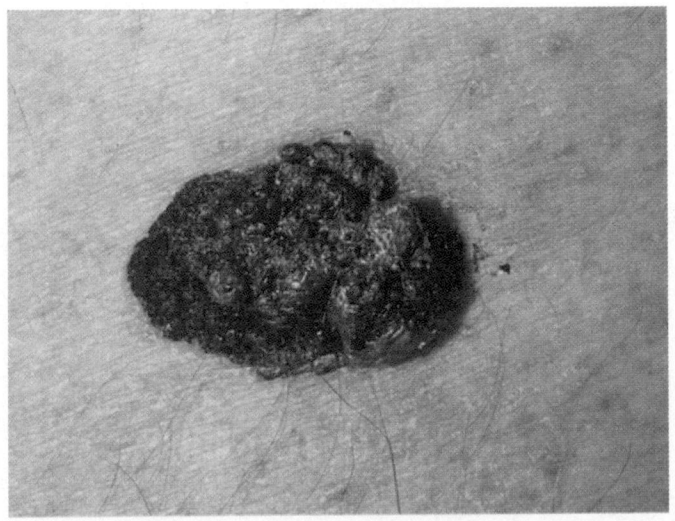

IIC-32 **Nodular melanoma** most commonly manifests itself as a rapidly growing, often ulcerated or crusted black nodule.

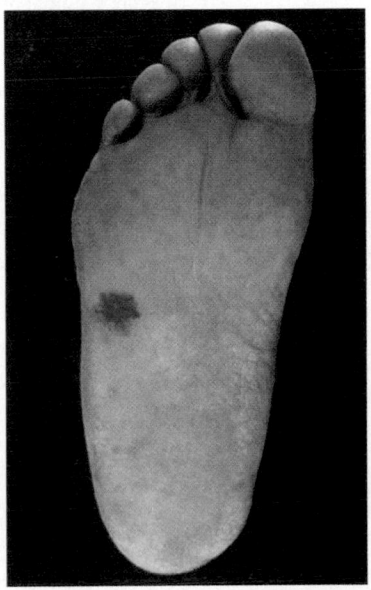

IIC-33 **Acral lentiginous melanoma** is more common in blacks, Asians, and Hispanics and occurs as an enlarging hyperpigmented macule or plaque on the palms and soles. Lateral pigment diffusion is present.

D. Infectious Disease and the Skin

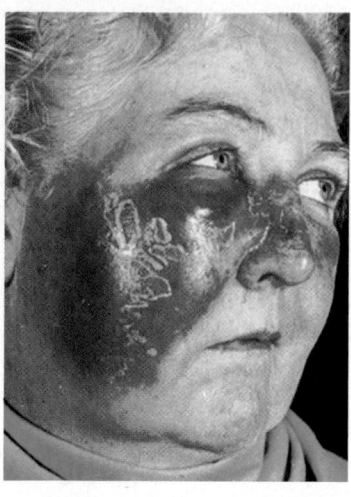

IID-34 **Erysipelas** is a streptococcal infection of the superficial dermis and consists of well-demarcated, erythematous, edematous, warm plaques.

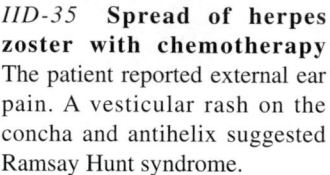

IID-35 **Spread of herpes zoster with chemotherapy** The patient reported external ear pain. A vesticular rash on the concha and antihelix suggested Ramsay Hunt syndrome.

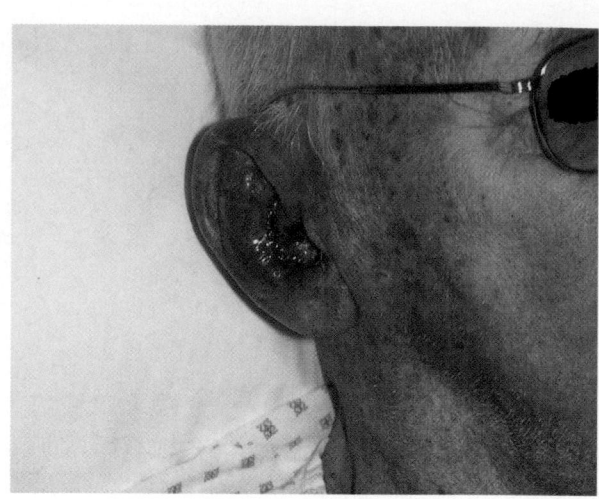

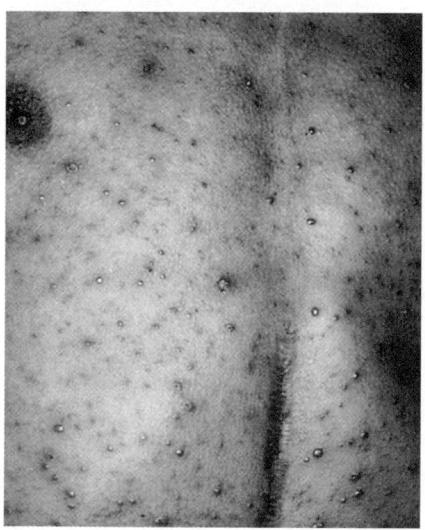

IID-36 **Varicella** showing numerous lesions in various stages of evolution: vesicles on an erythematous base, umbilicated vesicles, and crusts.

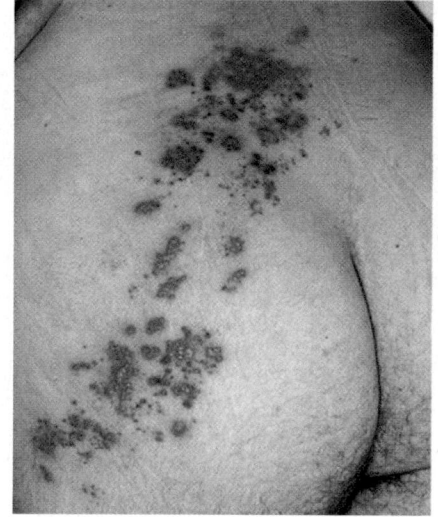

IID-37 **Herpes zoster** is seen in this HIV-infected patient as hemorrhagic vesicles and pustules on an erythematous base grouped in a dermatomal distribution.

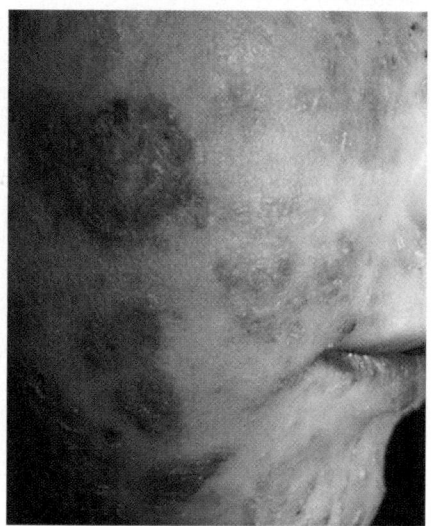

IID-38 **Impetigo contagiosa** is a superficial streptococcal or *Staphylococcus aureus* infection consisting of honey-colored crusts and erythematous weeping erosions. Occasionally, bullous lesions may be seen.

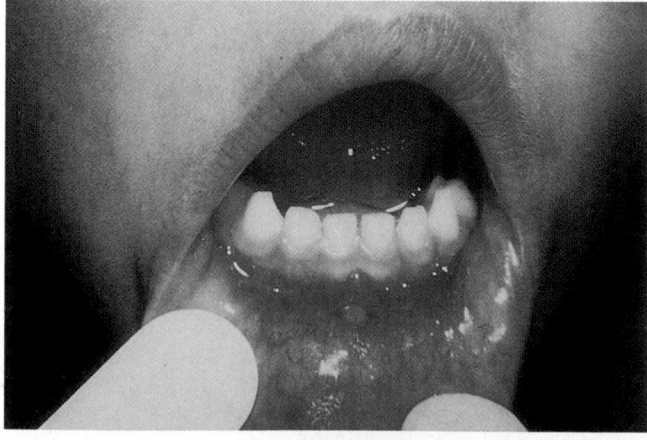

IID-39 **Tender vesicles and erosions** in the mouth of a patient with hand-foot-and-mouth disease.

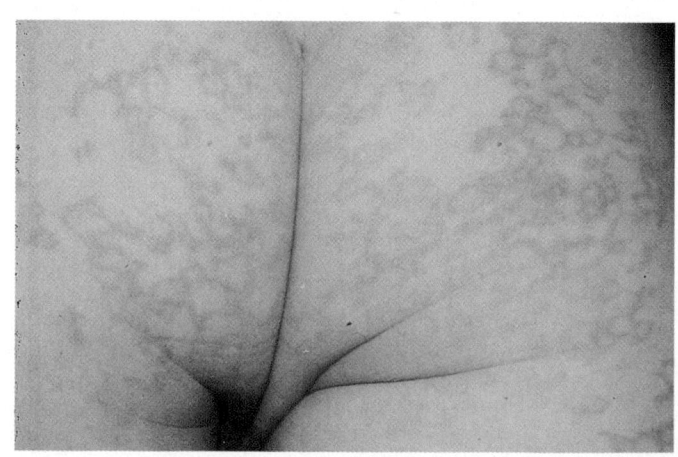

IID-40 **Lacy reticular rash of erythema infectiosum** (fifth disease).

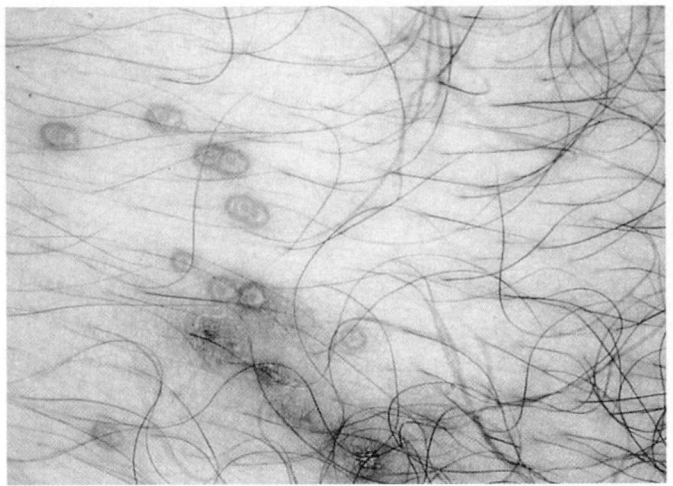

IID-41 **Molluscum contagiosum** is a cutaneous poxvirus infection characterized by multiple umbilicated flesh-colored or hypopigmented papules.

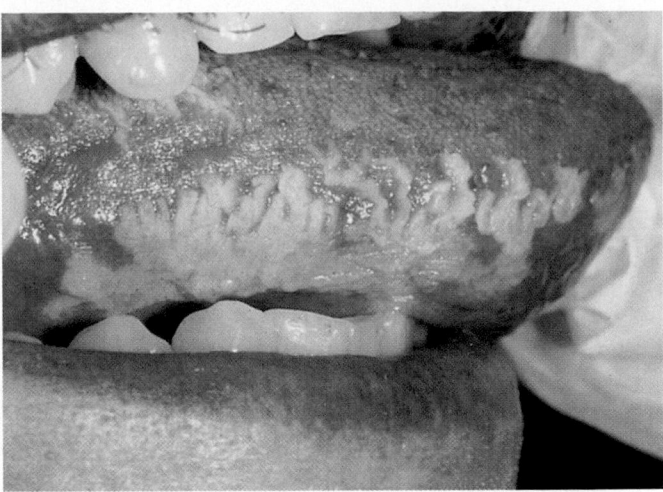

IID-42 **Oral hairy leukoplakia** often presents as white plaques on the lateral tongue and is associated with Epstein-Barr virus infection.

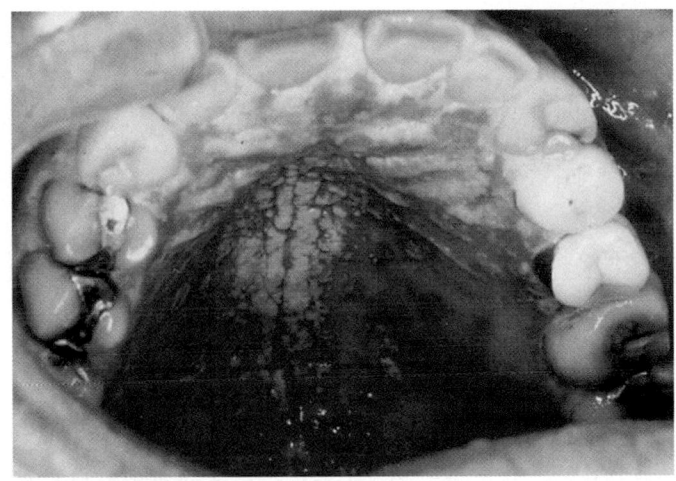

IID-43 **Pseudomembranous oral candidiasis** Adherent white, mucoid plaques with an erythematous halo seen here on the palate often indicate an immunocompromised state.

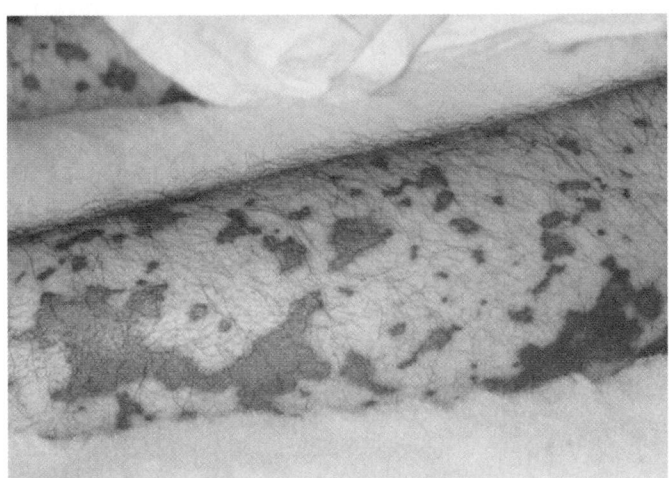

IID-44 **Fulminant meningococcemia** with extensive angular purpuric patches.

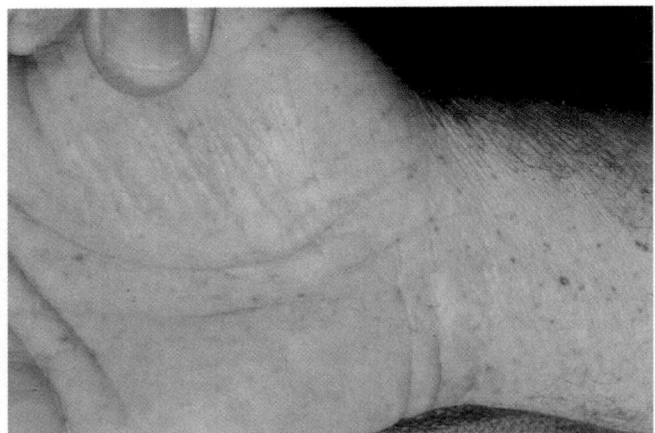

IID-45 **Rocky Mountain spotted fever** demonstrating pinpoint petechial lesions on the palm and volar aspect of the wrist.

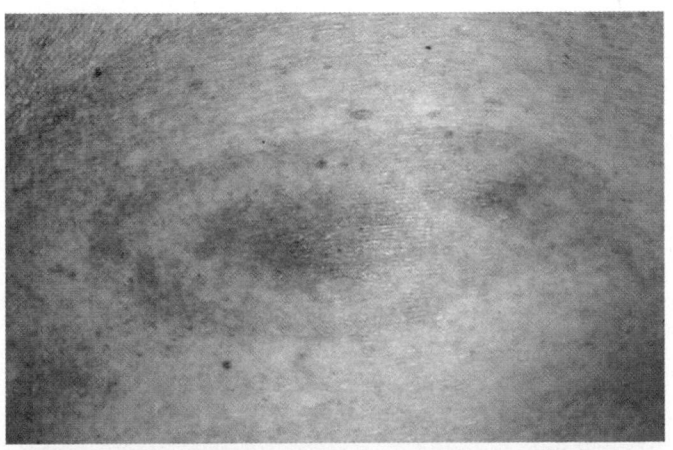

IID-46 **Erythema chronicum migrans** is the early cutaneous manifestation of Lyme disease and is characterized by erythematous annular patches, often with a central erythematous papule at the tick bite site.

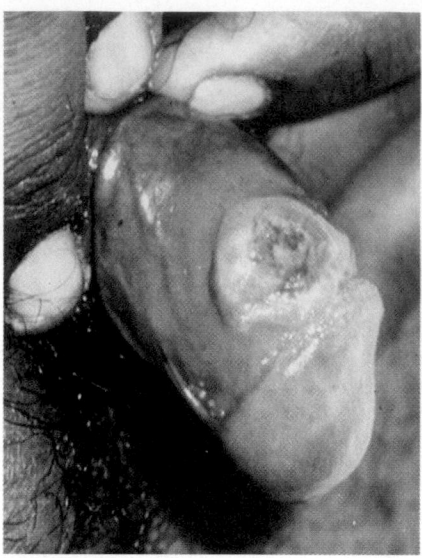

IID-47 **Primary syphilis** with a firm, nontender chancre.

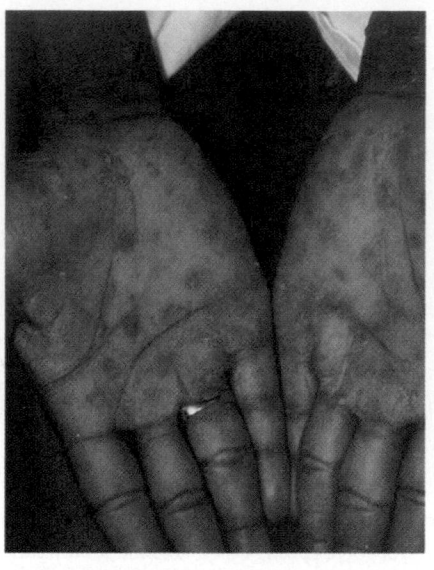

IID-48 **Secondary syphilis** commonly affects the palms and soles with scaling, firm, red-brown papules.

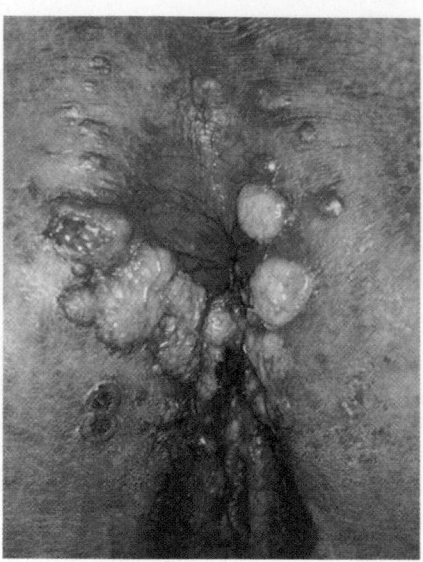

IID-49 **Condylomata lata** are moist, somewhat verrucous intertriginous plaques seen in secondary syphilis.

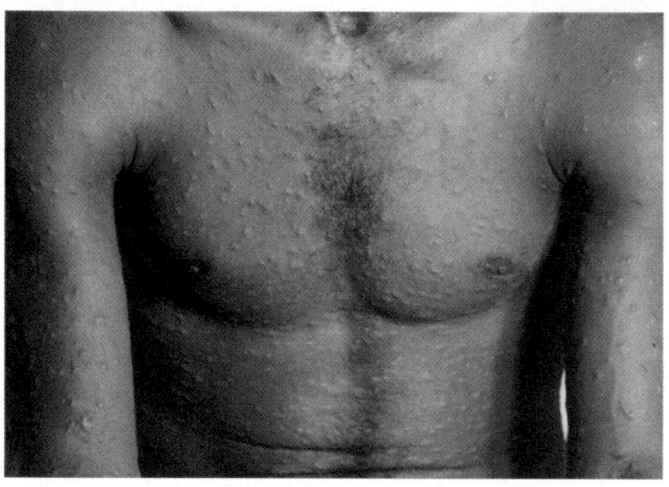

IID-50 **Secondary syphilis** demonstrating the papulosquamous truncal eruption.

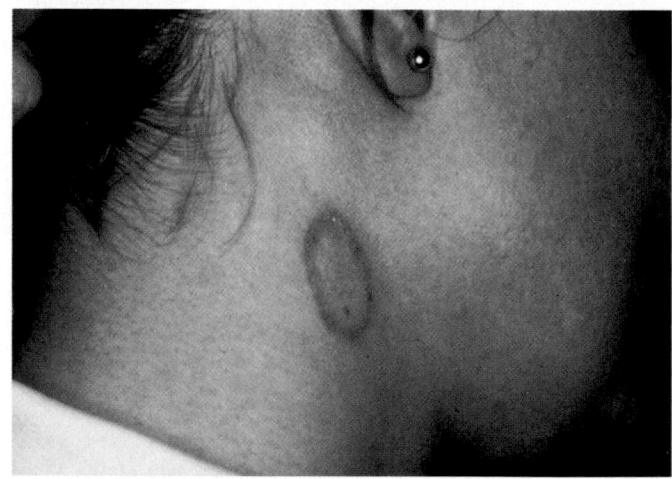

IID-51 **Tinea corporis** is a superficial fungal infection, seen here as an erythematous annular scaly plaque with central clearing.

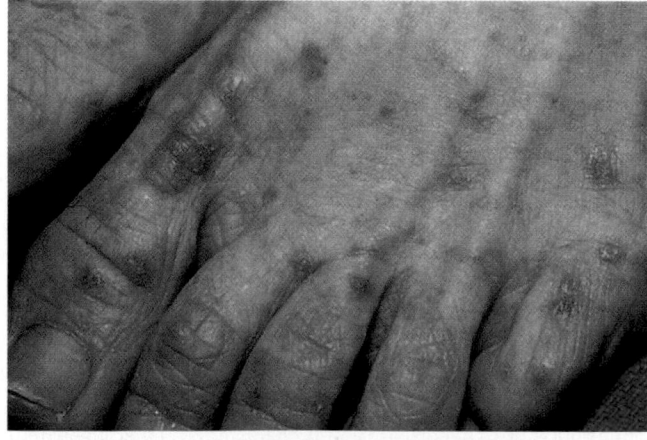

IID-52 **Scabies** showing typical scaling erythematous papules and few linear burrows.

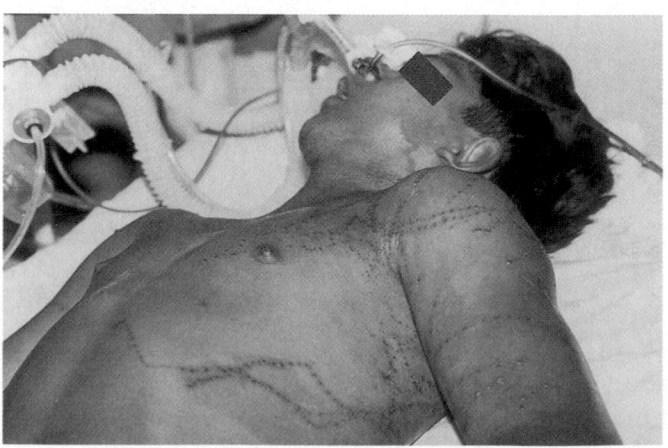

IID-53 **Skin lesions** caused by *Chironex fleckeri* sting.

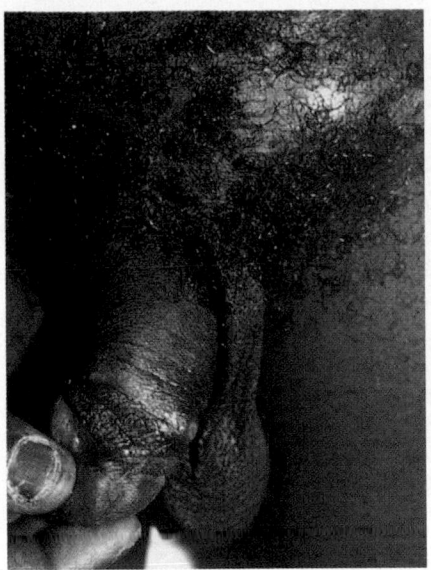

IID-54 **Chancroid** with characteristic penile ulcers and associated left inguinal adenitis (bubo).

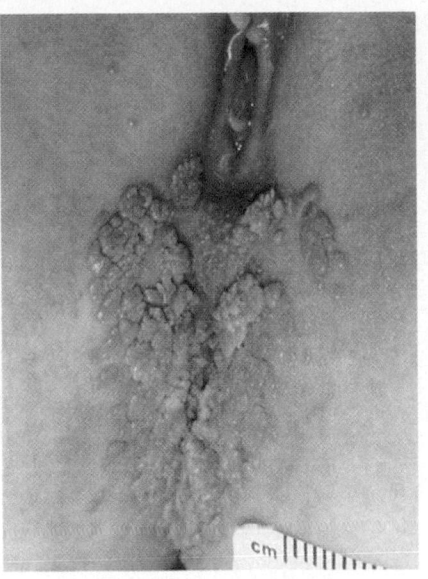

IID-55 **Condylomata acuminata** are lesions induced by human papillomavirus and in this patient are seen as multiple verrucous papules coalescing into plaques.

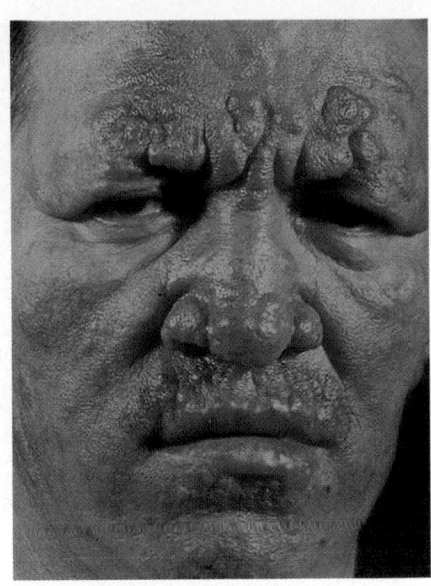

IID-56 **A patient with features of polar lepromatous leprosy;** multiple nodular skin lesions, particularly of the forehead, and loss of eyebrows.

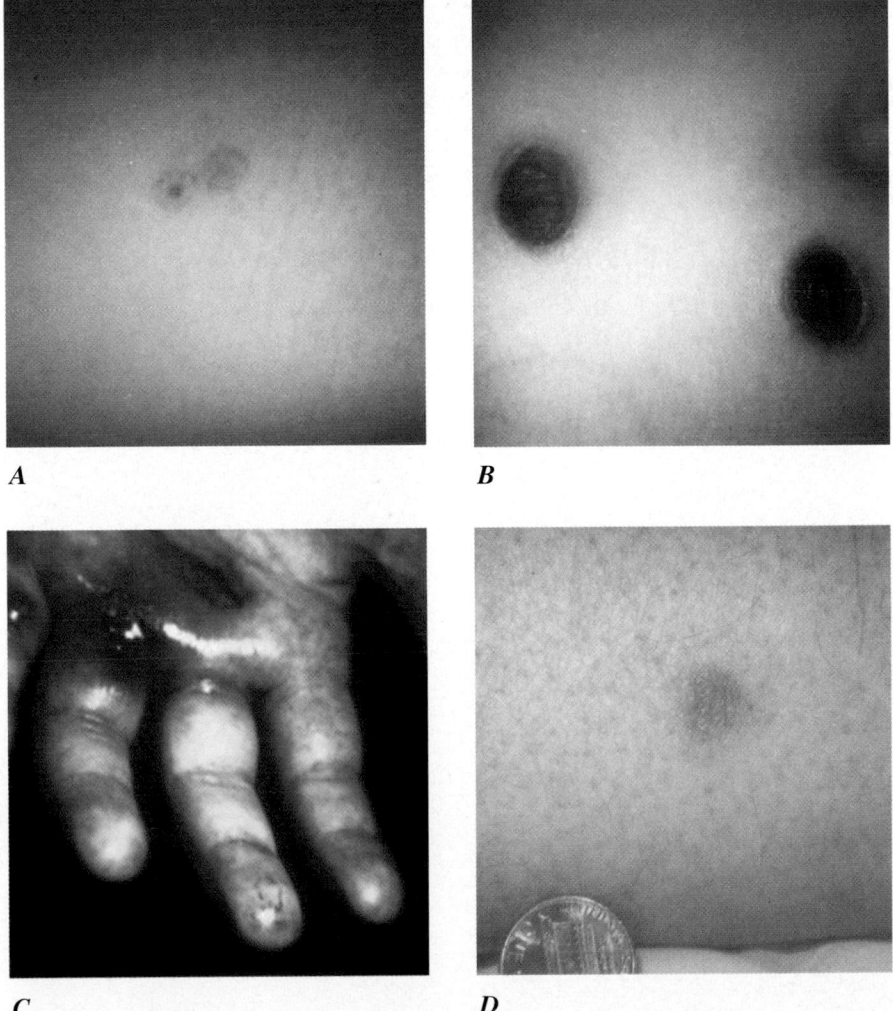

A

B

C

D

IID-57 **Skin lesions of neutropenic patients** *A.* Papules related to *Escherichia coli* bacteremia in a neutropenic patient with acute lymphocytic leukemia. *B.* The same lesion the following day. *C.* Ecthyma gangrenosum in a neutropenic patient with *Pseudomonas aeruginosa* bacteremia. *D.* Papule in a neutropenic patient with *Candida tropicalis* fungemia.

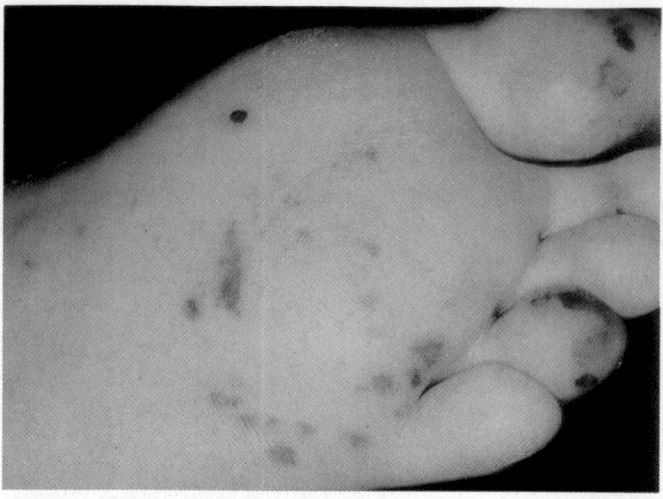

IID-58 **Septic emboli** with hemorrhage and infarction due to acute *Staphylococcus aureus* endocarditis.

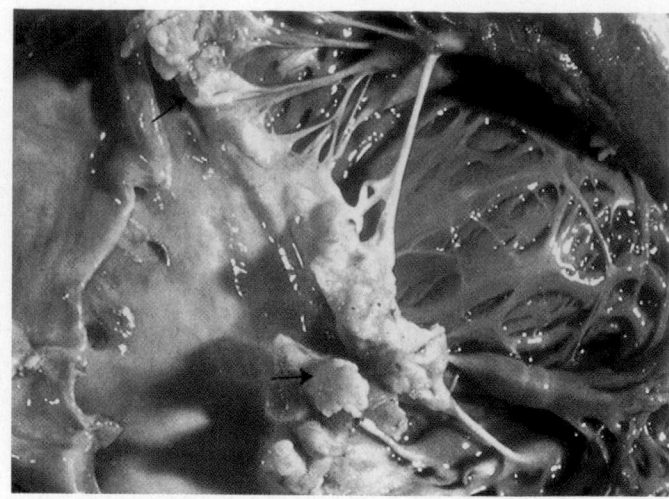

IID-59 Vegetations (*arrows*) due to viridans streptococcal endocarditis involving the mitral valve.

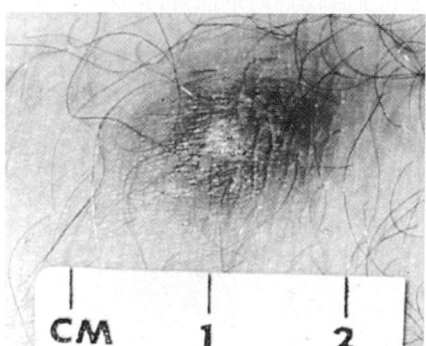

IID-60 **Disseminated gonococcemia** in the skin is seen as hemorrhagic papules and pustules with purpuric centers in an acral distribution.

E. Immunologically Mediated Skin Disease

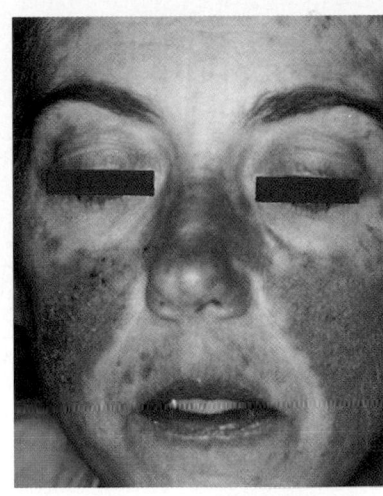

IIE-61A **Systemic lupus erythematosus** showing prominent, scaly, malar erythema. Involvement of other sun-exposed sites is also common.

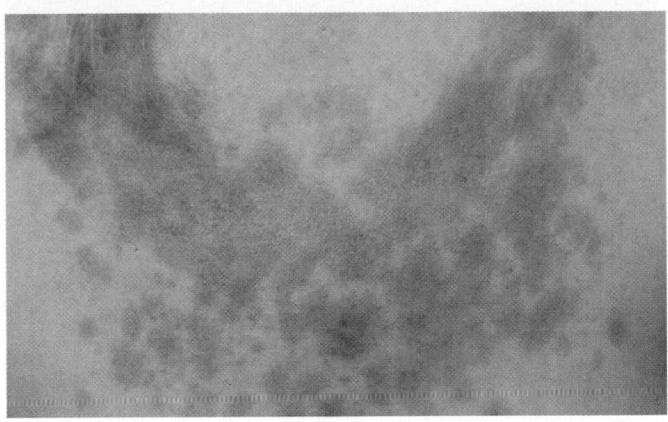

IIE-61B **Acute LE** on the upper chest demonstrating brightly erythematous and slightly edematous coalescence papules and plaques.

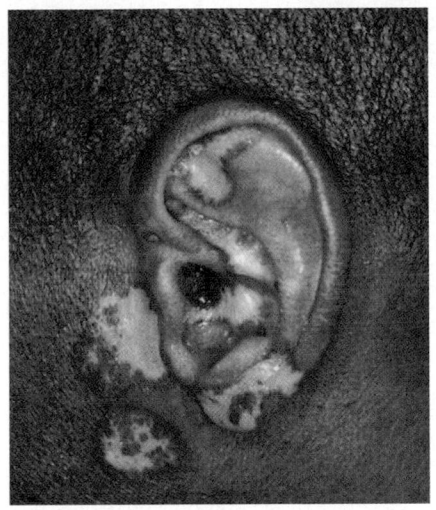

IIE-62 **Discoid lupus erythematosus** Violaceous, hyperpigmented, atrophic plaques, often with evidence of follicular plugging, which may result in scarring, are characteristic of this cutaneous form of lupus.

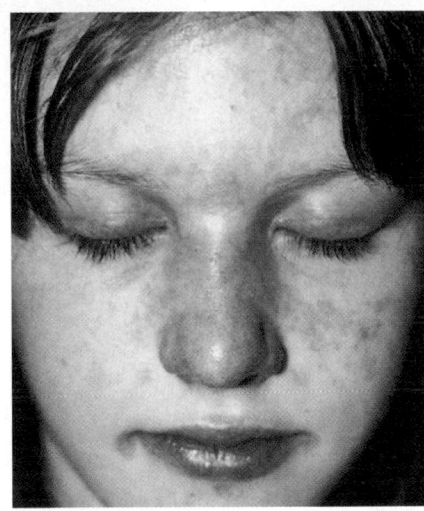

IIE-63 **Dermatomyositis** Periorbital violaceous erythema characterizes the classic heliotrope rash.

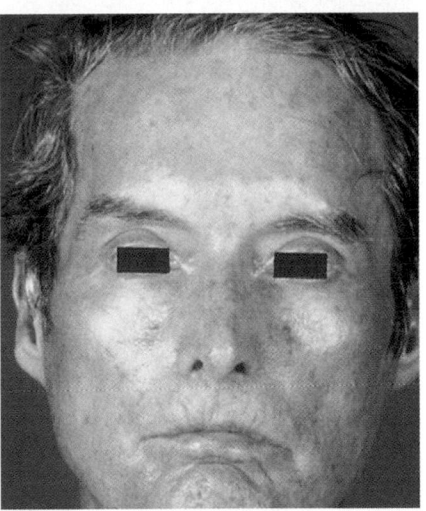

IIE-64 **Scleroderma** characterized by typical expressionless, mask-like facies.

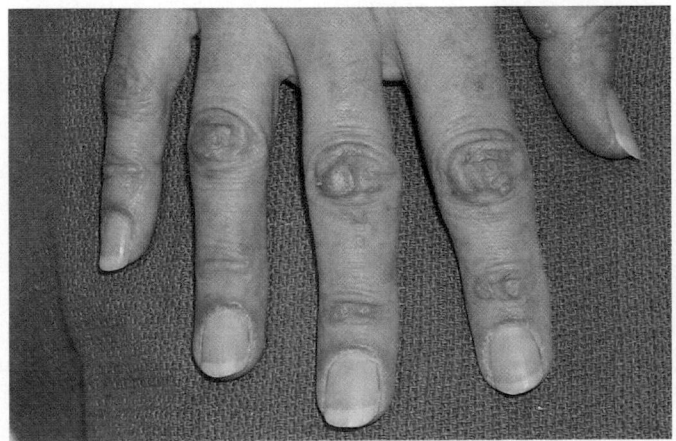

IIE-65 **Dermatomyositis** often involves the hands as erythematous flat-topped papules over the knuckles (Gottron's sign) and periungal telangiectasias.

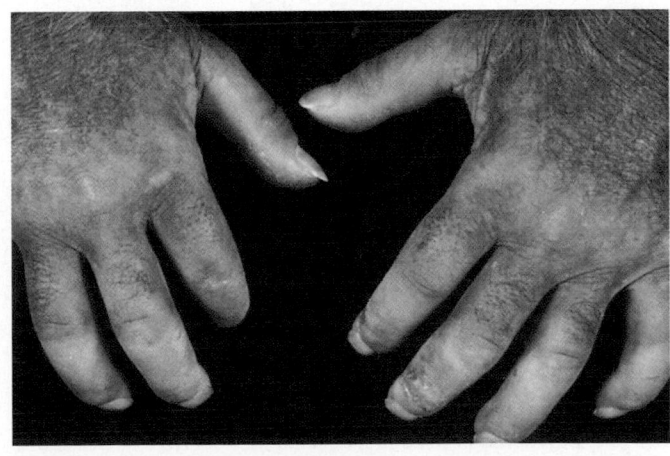

IIE-66 **Scleroderma** showing acral sclerosis and focal digital ulcers.

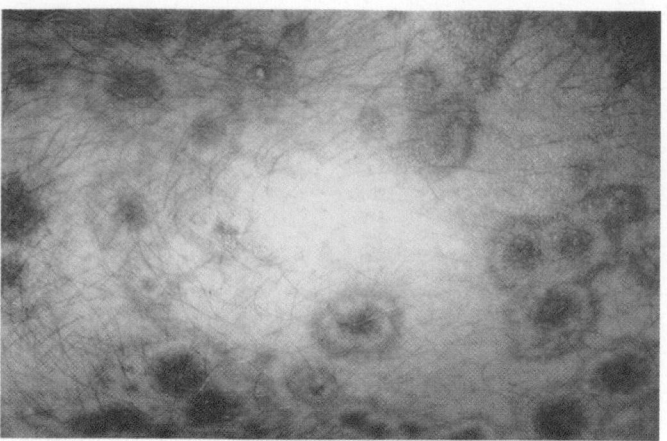

IIE-67 **Erythema multiforme** is characterized by multiple erythematous plaques with a target or iris morphology and usually represents a hypersensitivity reaction to drugs or infections (especially herpes simplex virus).

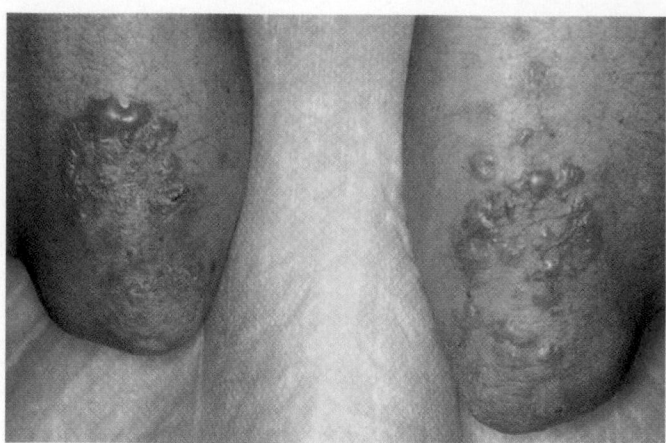

IIE-68 **Dermatitis herpetiformis** manifested by pruritic, grouped vesicles in a typical location. The vesicles are often excoriated and may occur on knees, buttocks, and posterior scalp.

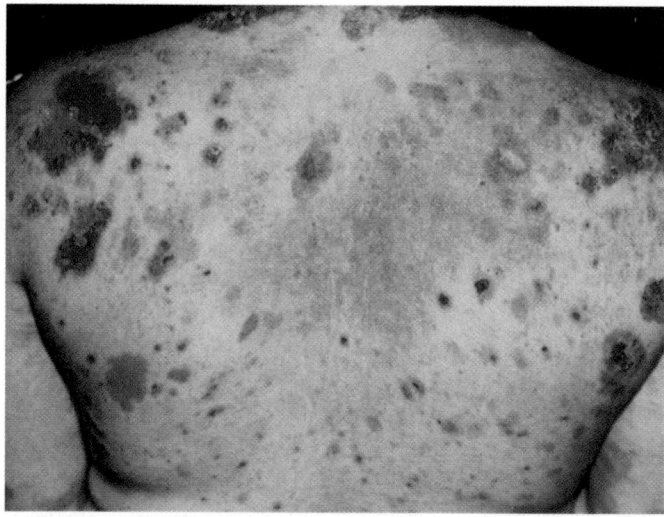

IIE-69A **Pemphigus vulgaris** demonstrating flaccid bullae that are easily ruptured, resulting in multiple erosions and crusted plaques.

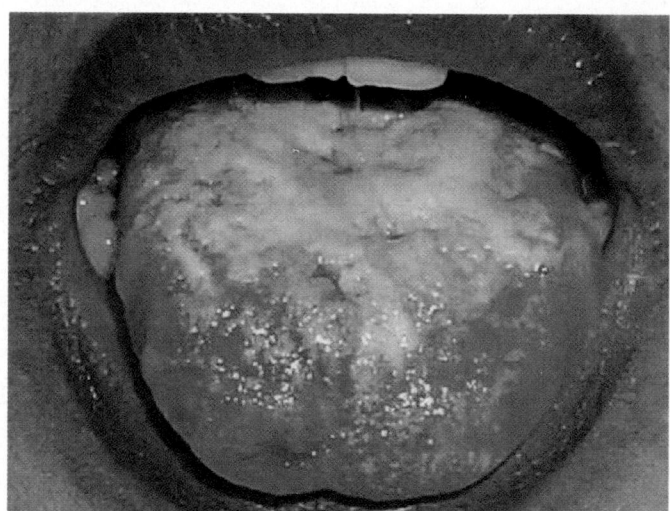

IIE-69B **Pemphigus vulgaris** almost invariably involves the oral mucosa and may present with erosions involving the gingiva, buccal mucosa, palate, posterior pharynx, or the tongue.

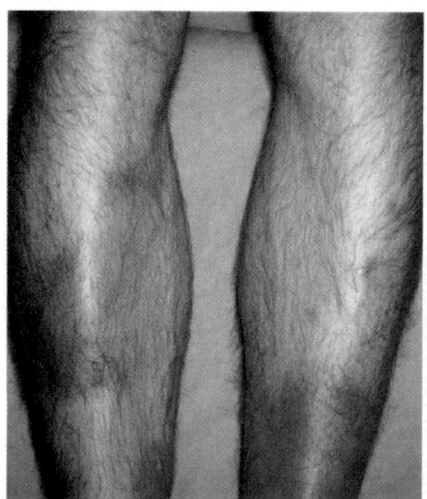

IIE-70 **Erythema nodosum** is a panniculitis characterized by tender deep-seated nodules and plaques usually located on the lower extremities.

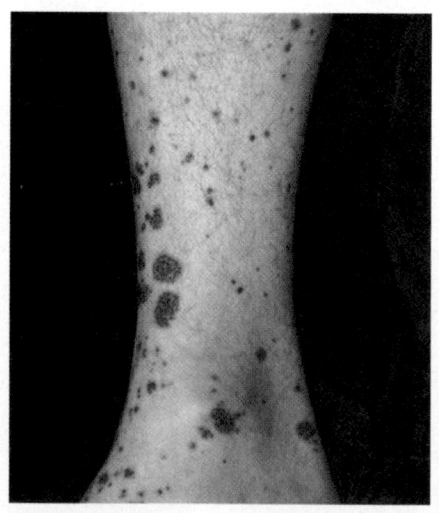

IIE-71 **Vasculitis** Palpable purpuric papules on the lower legs are seen in this patient with cutaneous small vessel vasculitis.

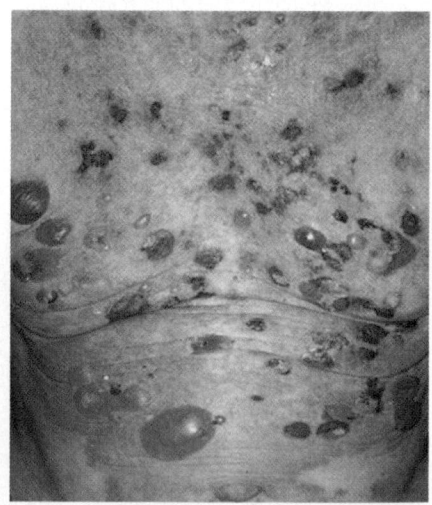

IIE-72 **Bullous pemphigoid** with tense vesicles and bullae on an erythematous, urticarial base.

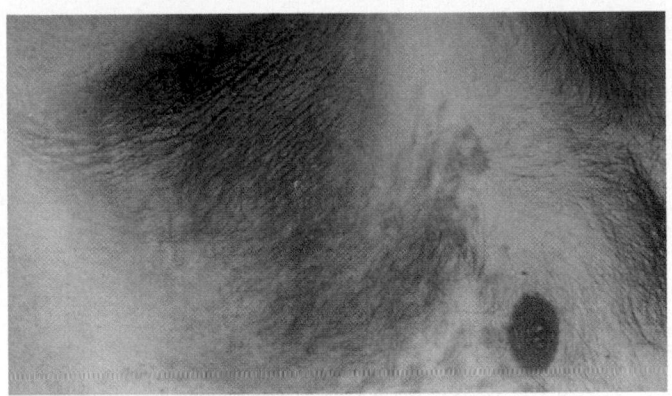

IIF-73 **Acanthosis nigricans** demonstrating typical hyperpigmented axillary plaques with a velvet-like, verrucous surface.

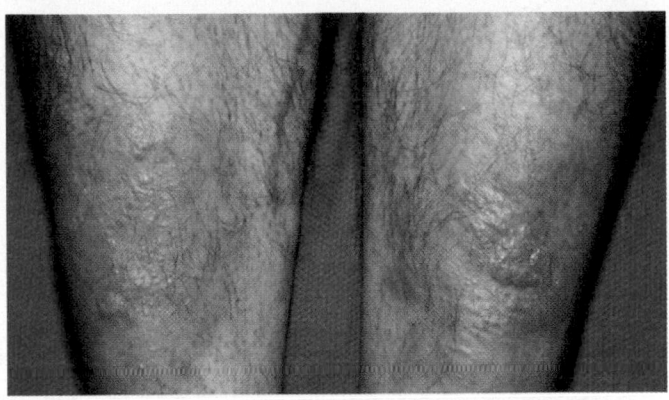

IIF-74 **Pretibial myxedema** manifesting as waxy, infiltrated plaques in a patient with Graves' disease.

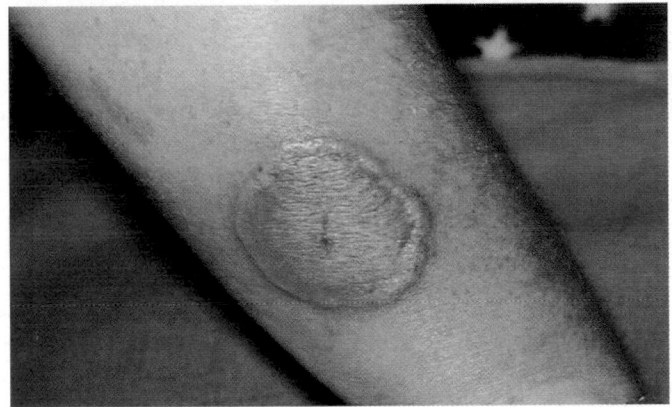

IIF-75 **Plaque of Sweet's syndrome** demonstrating an erythematous indurated plaque with a pseudo-vesicular border.

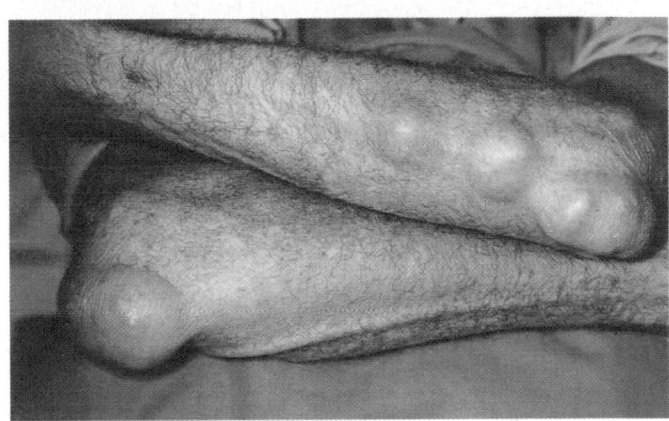

IIF-76 **Bilateral rheumatoid nodules** of the upper extremities.

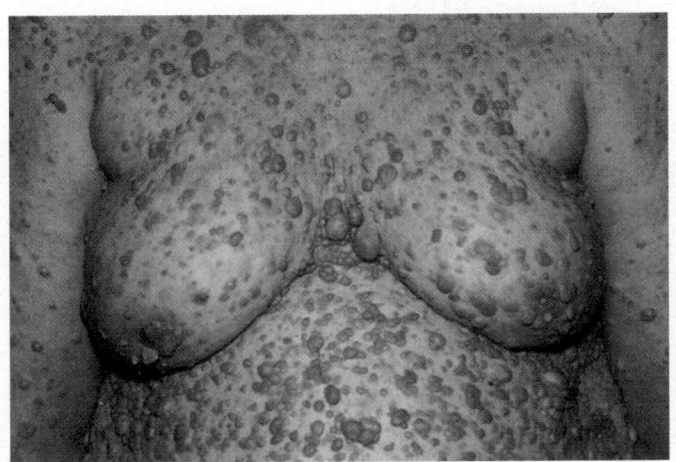

IIF-77 **Neurofibromatosis** demonstrating numerous flesh-colored cutaneous neurofibromas.

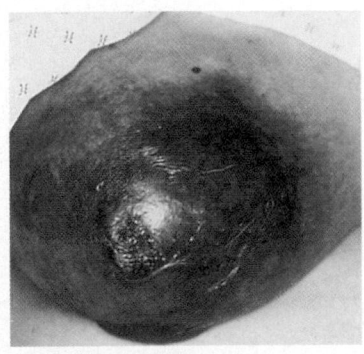

IIF-78 **Coumarin** necrosis showing cutaneous and subcutaneous necrosis of a breast. Other fatty areas such as buttocks and thighs are also common sites of involvement.

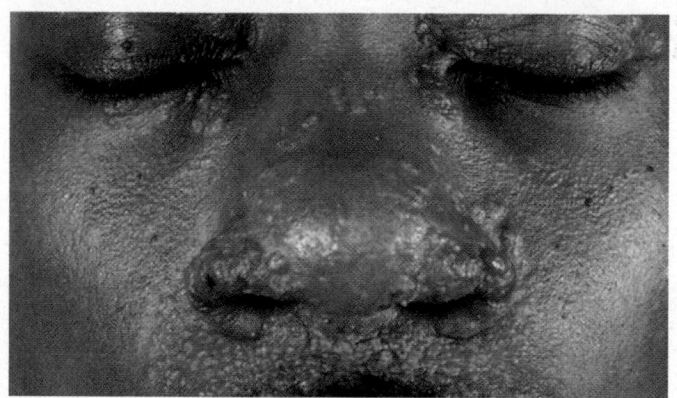

IIF-79A **Sarcoid** Infiltrated papules and plaques of variable color are seen in a typical paranasal and periorbital location.

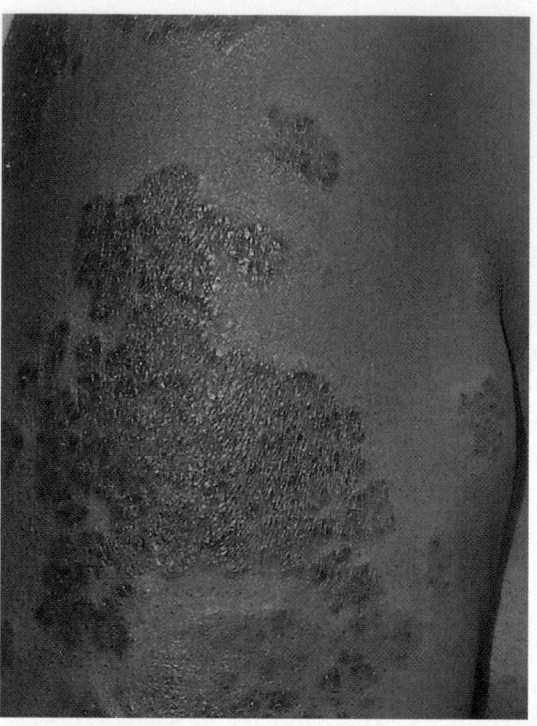

IIF-79B **Sarcoid** Infiltrated, hyperpigmented, and slightly erythematous coalescent papules and plaques on the upper arm.

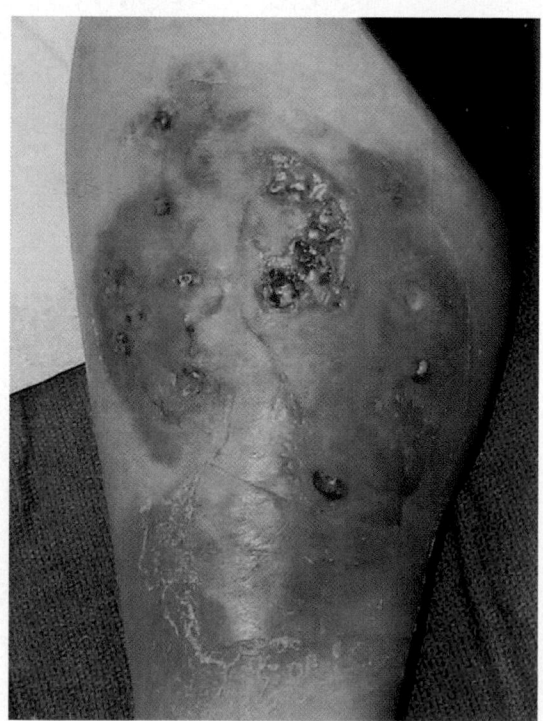

IIF-80 **Pyoderma gangrenosum** on the posterior-lateral aspect of the lower leg demonstrating multiple purulent draining ulcers on an infiltrated erythematous plaque.

III.   Atlas of Endoscopic Findings

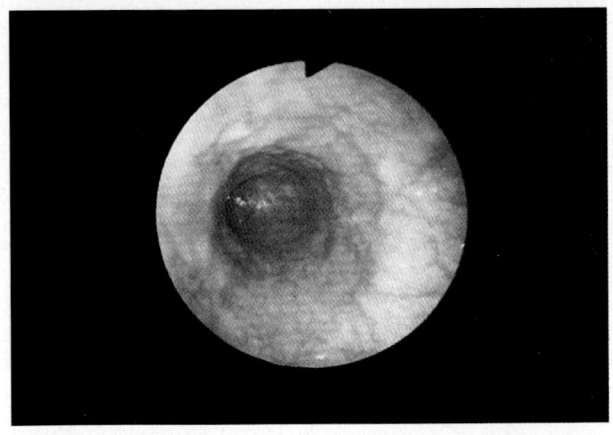

III-1   **Normal esophagus**   Fine vasculature can be seen.

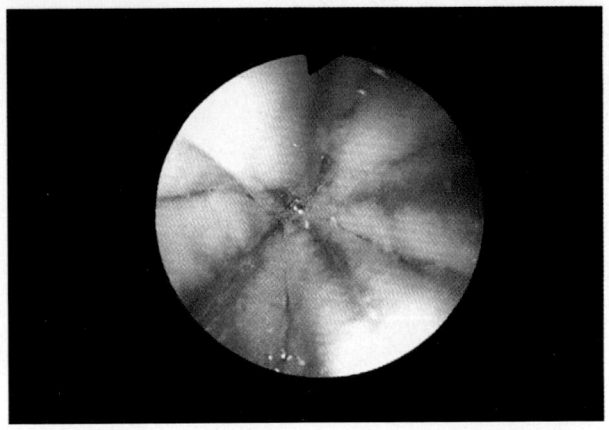

III-2   **Peptic regurgitant esophagitis**   Linear red streaks with a central white streak extend up the esophagus.

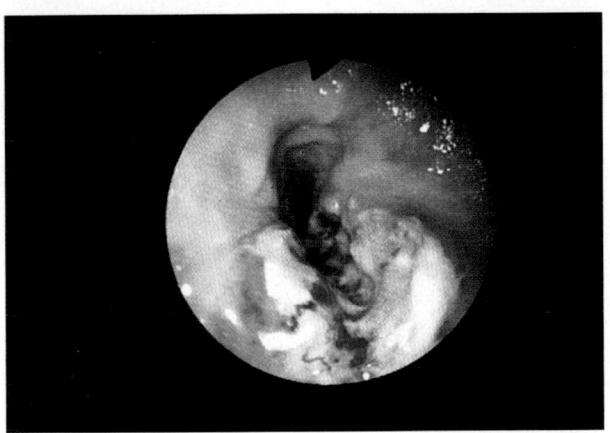

III-3   **Ulcerated squamous cell carcinoma,** with a depressed center, involving one wall of the esophagus.

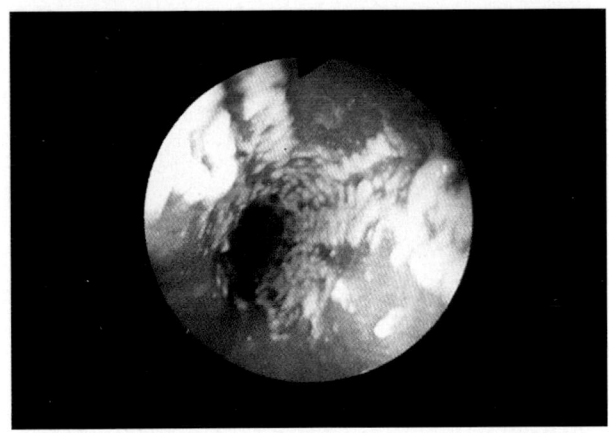

III-4   **Moniliasis of the esophagus**   A white exudate is seen with underlying erythematous mucosa.

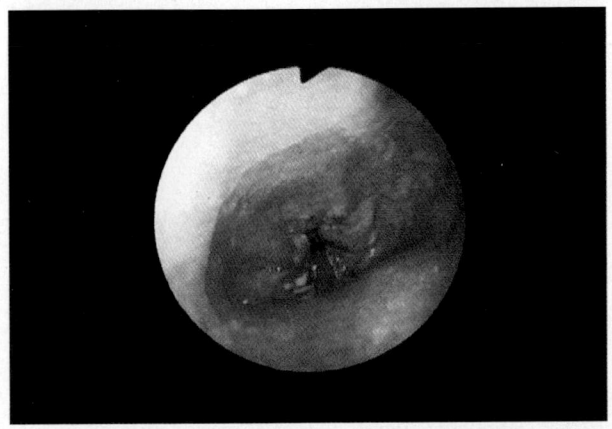

III-5   **Barrett's metaplasia of the esophagus with an adenocarcinoma**   The squamocolumnar junction is noted in the proximal esophagus. A mucosal irregularity in the center of the photograph was an adenocarcinoma.

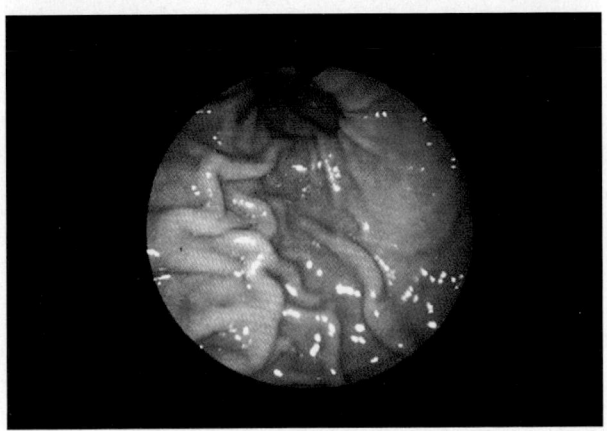

III-6   **Normal body of the stomach with rugal folds**

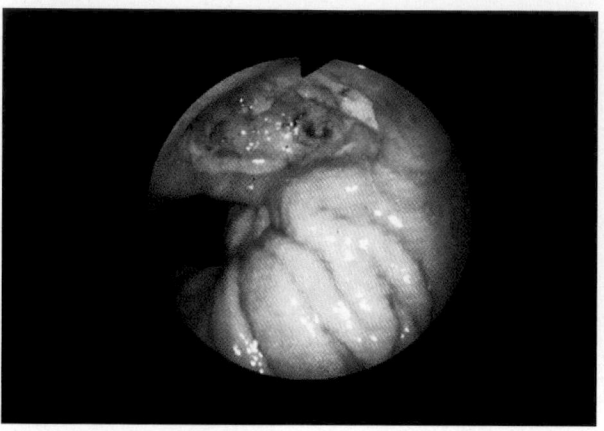

III-7 **Large, benign, lesser curve gastric ulcer** The folds end at the ulcer margin.

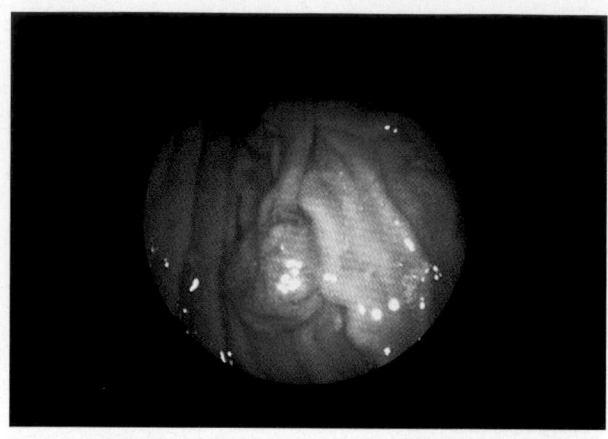

III-8 **Gastric polyp** The histologic type must be determined by excision and pathologic examination.

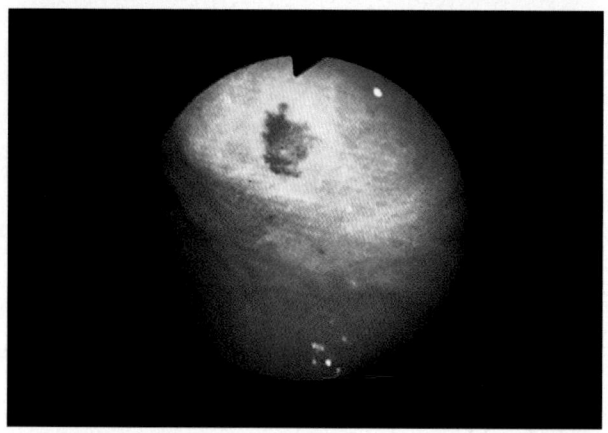

III-9 **Arteriovenus malformation of the gastric mucosa**

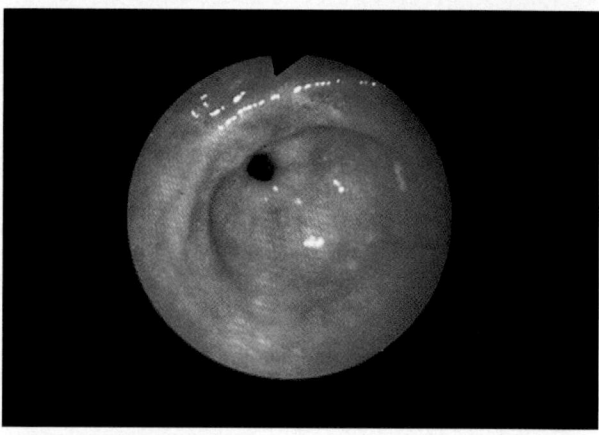

III-10 **Normal pylorus** Note the absence of gastric rugal folds in the antrum proximal to the pylorus.

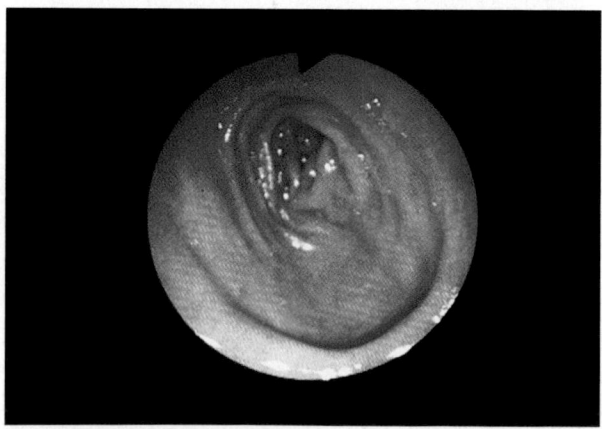

III-11 **Normal duodenal bulb**

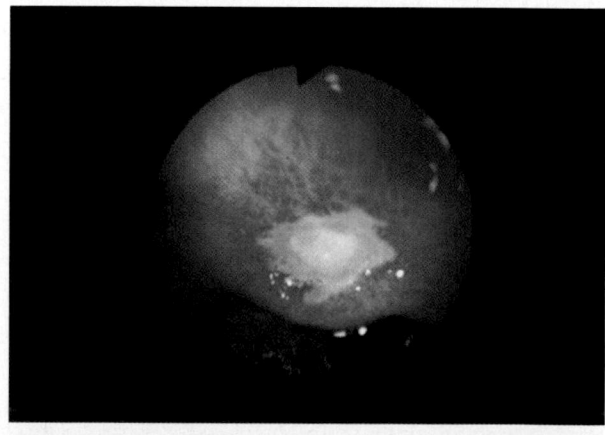

III-12 **Duodenal ulcer** A typical ulcer with a clean base is seen on the anterior surface of the duodenal bulb.

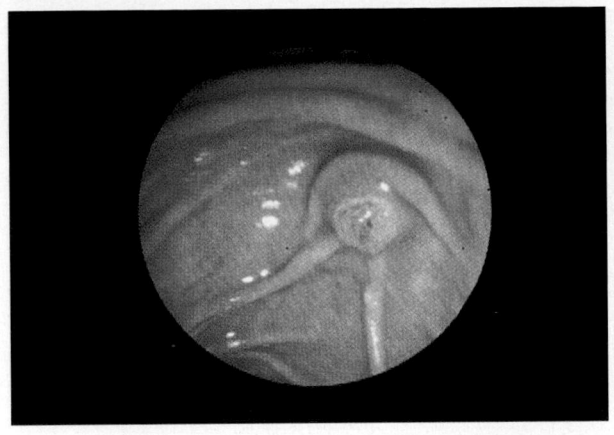

III-13 **Normal papilla of Vater** The fold pattern surrounding the papilla is normal; bile is seen adjacent to the papilla.

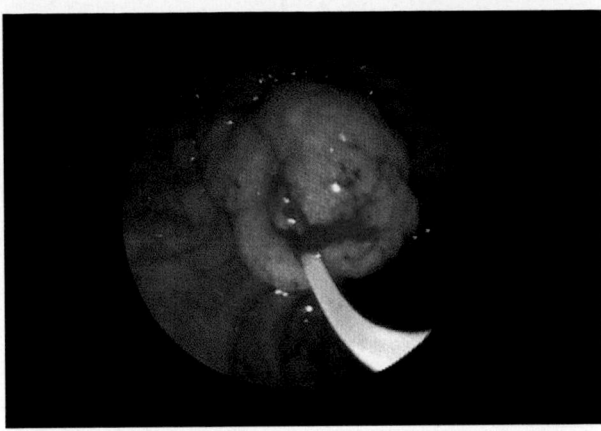

III-14 **Periampullary carcinoma** The mass at the papilla of Vater has been catheterized during ERCP.

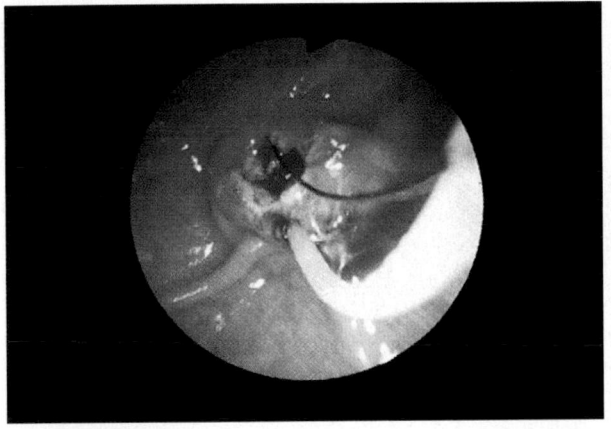

III-15 **Endoscopic papillotomy** A papillotome has been passed into the papilla, the wire bowed, and an incision made, with electrosurgical current, in the superior aspect of the papilla.

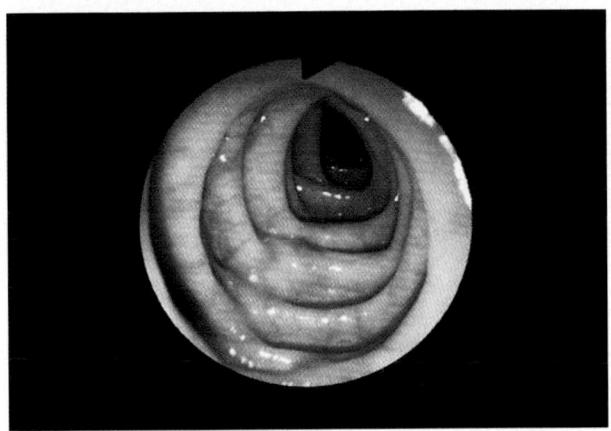

III-16 **Normal colon** Typical folds and vascular pattern can be seen.

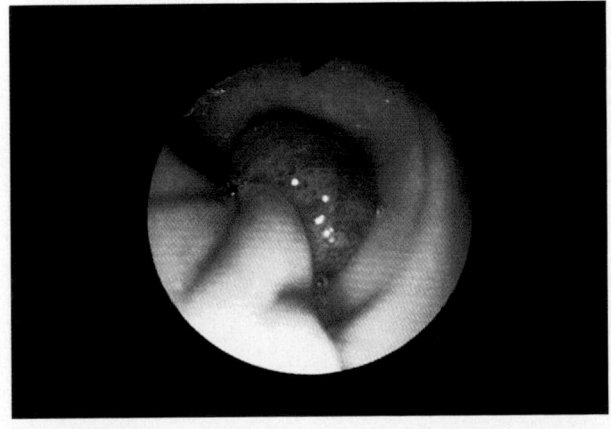

III-17 **Colonic adenomatous polyp** The polyp is erythematous; a stalk is seen covered with normal mucosa.

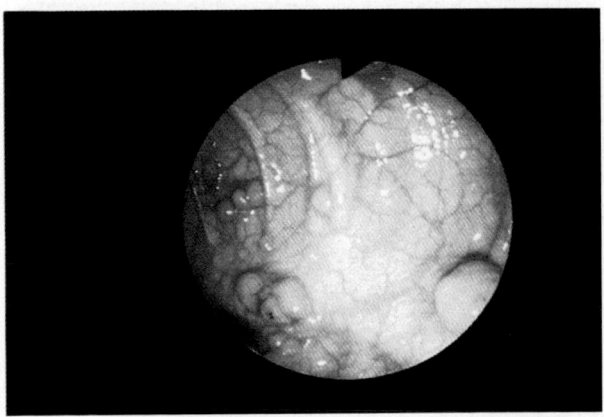

III-18 **Multiple, small, colonic adenomatous polyps in a case of familial polyposis coli** This colon must be removed to prevent the development of cancer.

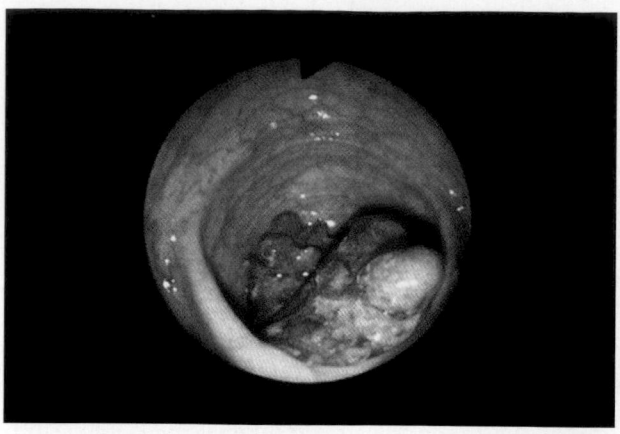

III-19 **Colon adenocarcinoma** The cancer is multilobed and growing into the lumen.

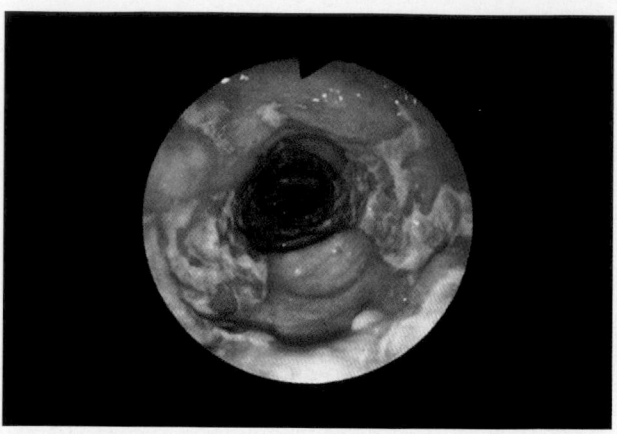

III-20 **Crohn's colitis** with linear, serpiginous, white-based ulcers surrounded by colonic mucosa which is relatively normal.

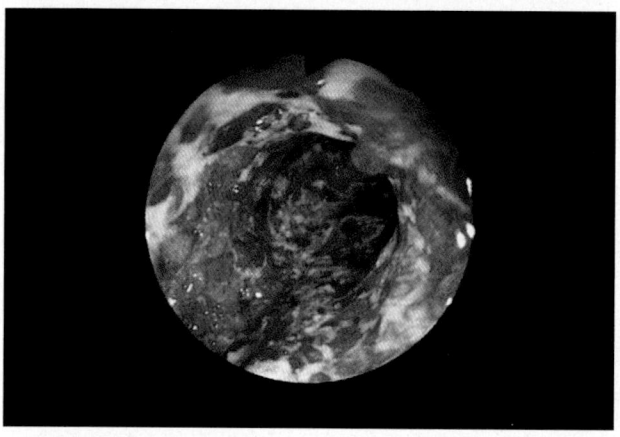

III-21 **Severe ulcerative colitis** with diffuse ulceration, bleeding, and exudation.

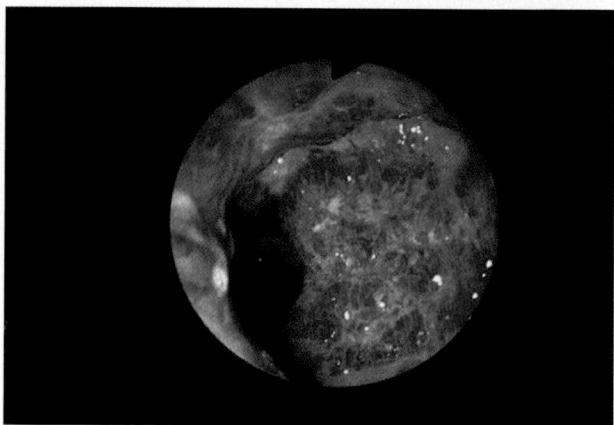

III-22 **Kaposi's sarcoma involving the colon in a patient with AIDS** The erythematous lesions involve most of the colonic mucosa in the photograph.

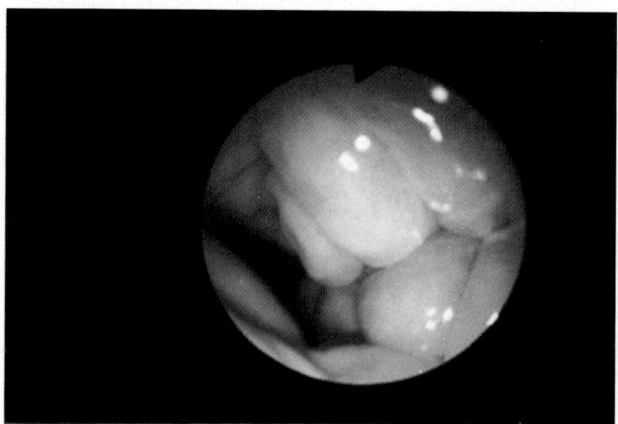

III-23 **Colonic varices** Multiple, serpiginous, subepithelial structures impinge on the colonic lumen.

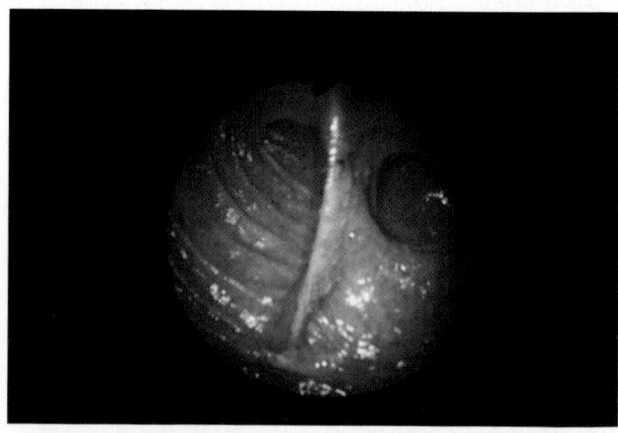

III-24 **Ileal pouch** The mucosa appears normal in this pouch reconstructed from ileum to provide a reservoir after total proctocolectomy and ileoanal anastomosis.

IV. Atlas of Funduscopic Findings

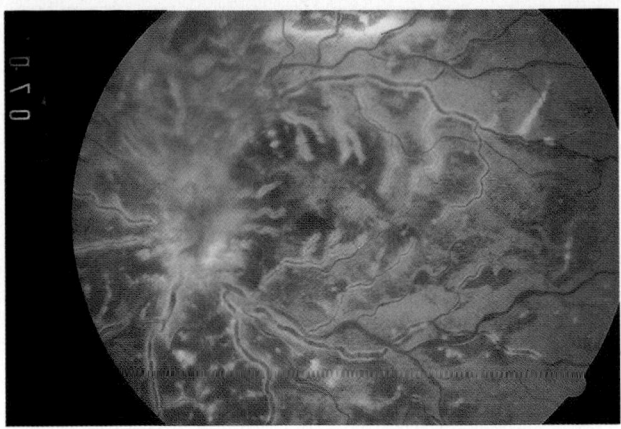

IV-1 **Retinal vasculitis, uveitis, and hemorrhage** in a 32-year-old woman with Crohn's disease. Note that the veins are frosted with a white exudate. Visual acuity improved from 20/400 to 20/20 following treatment with intravenous methylprednisolone.

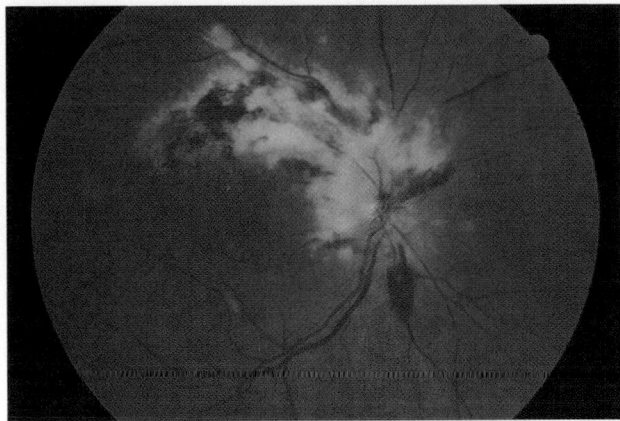

IV-2 **Cytomegalovirus** in a patient with AIDS appears as an arcuate zone of retinitis with hemorrhages and optic disc swelling. Often CMV is confined to the retinal periphery, beyond view of the direct ophthalmoscope.

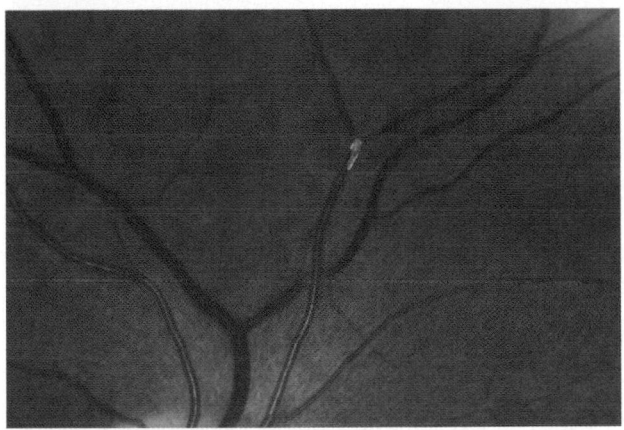

IV-3 **Hollenhorst plaque** lodged at the bifurcation of a retinal arteriole proves that a patient is shedding emboli from either the carotid artery, great vessels, or heart.

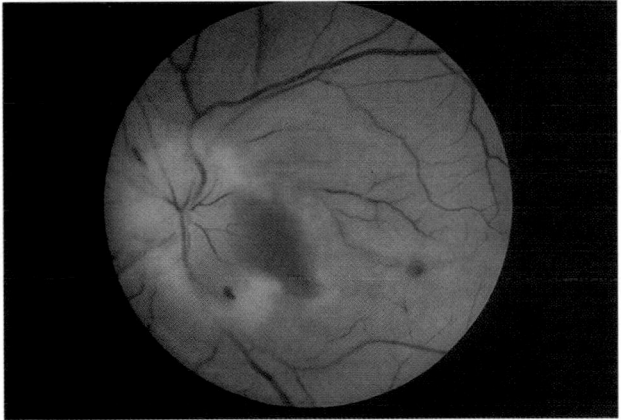

IV-4 **Central retinal artery occlusion** combined with ischemic optic neuropathy in a 19-year-old woman with an elevated titer of anticardiolipin antibodies. Note the orange dot (rather than cherry red) corresponding to the fovea and the spared patch of retina just temporal to the optic disc.

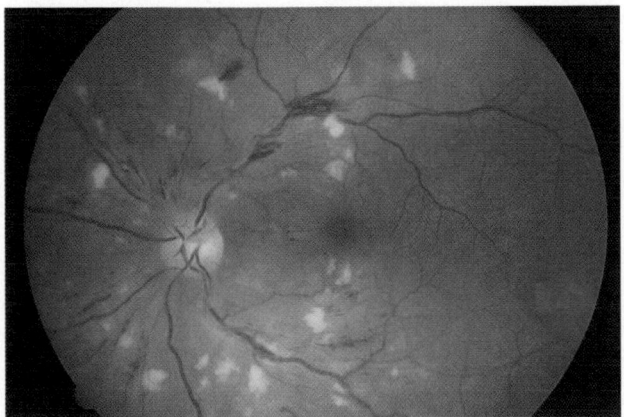

IV-5 **Hypertensive retinopathy** with scattered flame (splinter) hemorrhages and cotton wool spots (nerve fiber layer infarcts) in a patient with headache and a blood pressure of 234/120.

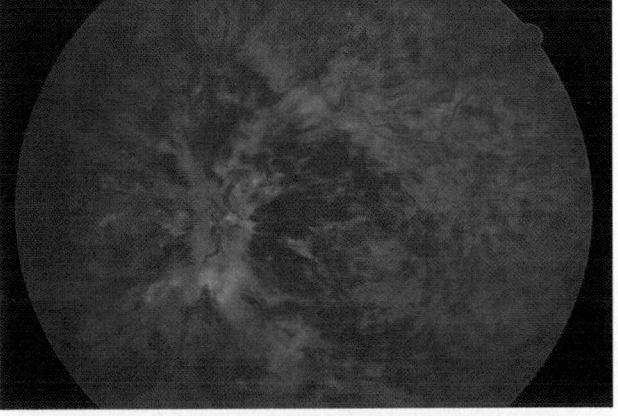

IV-6 **Central retinal vein occlusion** can produce massive retinal hemorrhage ("blood and thunder"), ischemia, and vision loss.

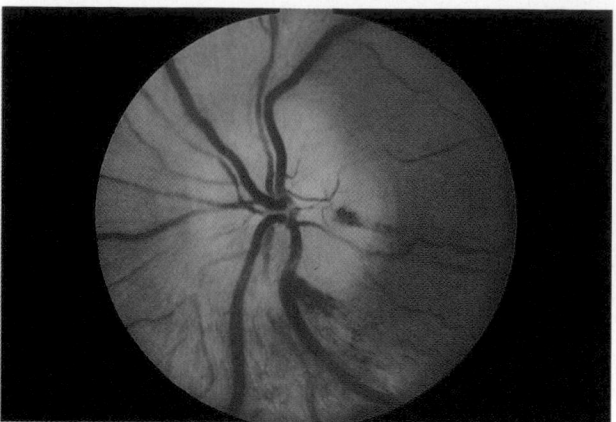

IV-7 **Anterior ischemic optic neuropathy** from temporal arteritis in a 78-year old woman with pallid disc swelling, hemorrhage, visual loss, myalgia, and an erythrocyte sedimentation rate of 86 mm/h..

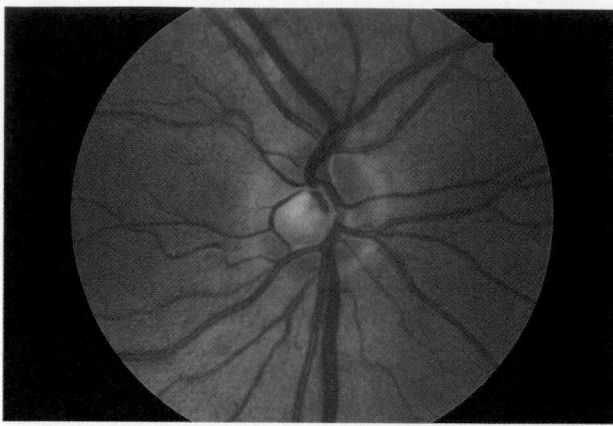

IV-8 **Retrobulbar optic neuritis** is characterized by a normal fundus examination initially, hence the rubric, "the doctor sees nothing, and the patient sees nothing." Optic atrophy develops after severe or repeated attacks.

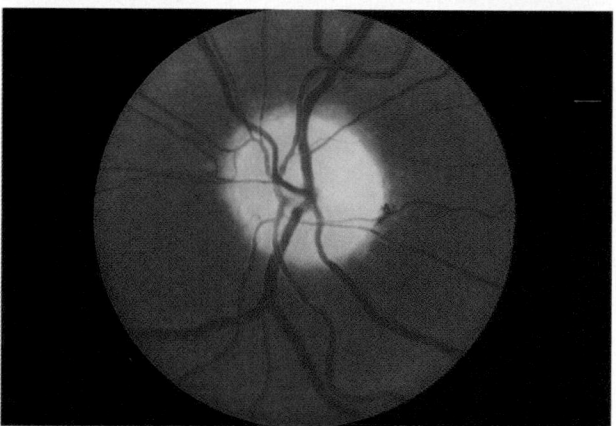

IV-9 **Optic atrophy** is not a specific diagnosis, but refers to the combination of optic disc pallor, arteriolar narrowing, and nerve fiber layer destruction produced by a host of eye diseases, especially optic neuropathies.

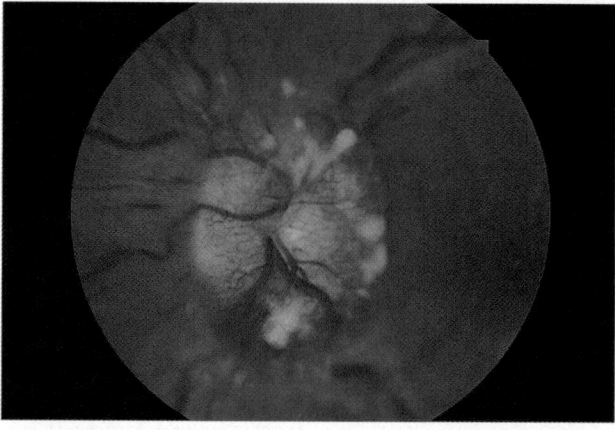

IV-10 **Papilledema** means optic disc edema from raised intracranial pressure. This obese young woman with pseudotumor cerebri was misdiagnosed as a migraineur until fundus examination was performed, showing optic disc elevation, hemorrhages, and cotton wool spots.

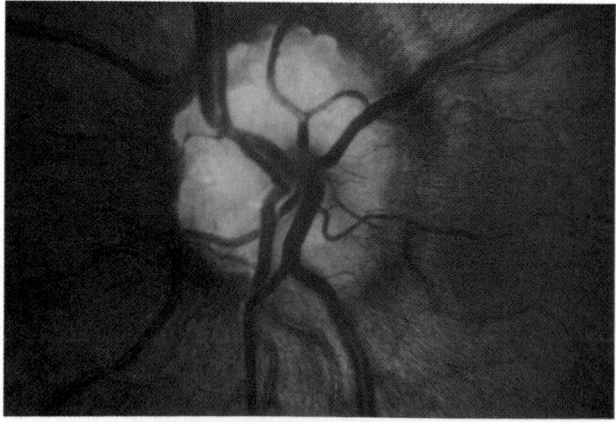

IV-11 **Optic disc drusen** are calcified deposits of unknown etiology within the optic disc. They are sometimes confused with papilledema.

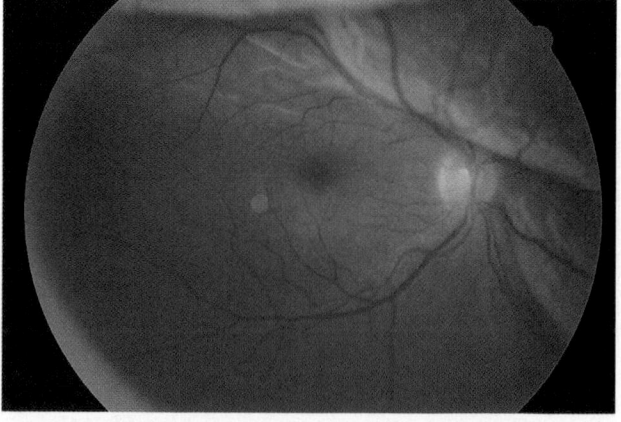

IV-12 **Retinal detachment** appears as an elevated sheet of retinal tissue with folds. In this patient the fovea was spared, so acuity was normal, but a superior detachment produced an inferior scotoma.

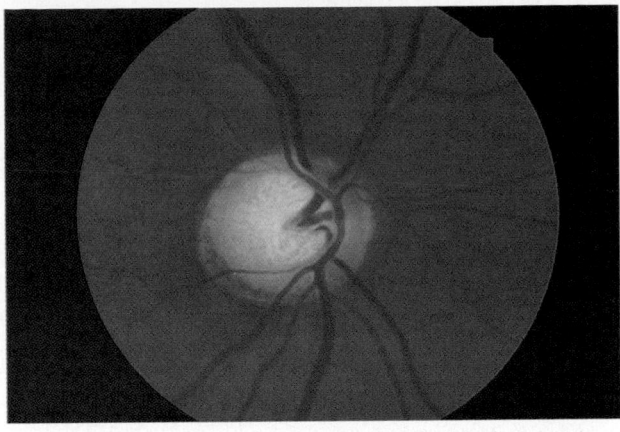

IV-13 **Glaucoma** results in "cupping" as the neural rim is destroyed and the central cup becomes enlarged and excavated. The cup-to-disc ratio is about 0.7/1.0 in this patient.

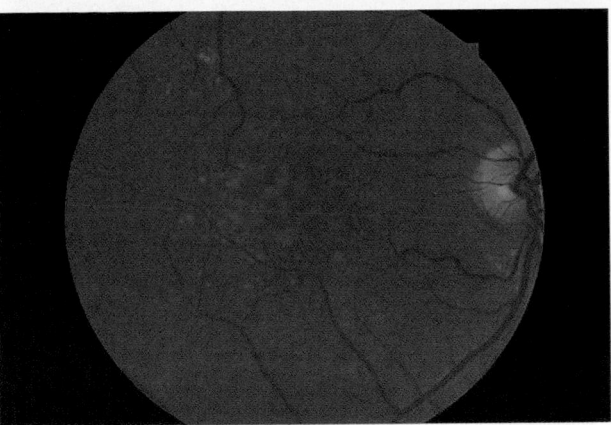

IV-14 **Age-related macular degeneration** begins with the accumulation of drusen within the macula. They appear as scattered yellow subretinal deposits.

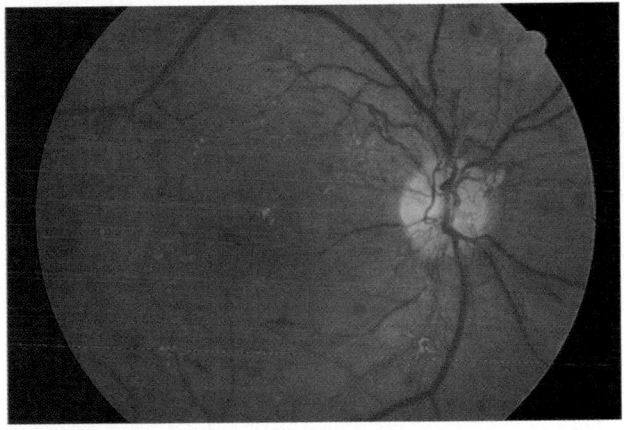

IV-15 **Diabetic retinopathy** results in scattered hemorrhages and yellow exudates. This patient has neovascular vessels proliferating from the optic disc, requiring urgent pan retinal laser photocoagulation.

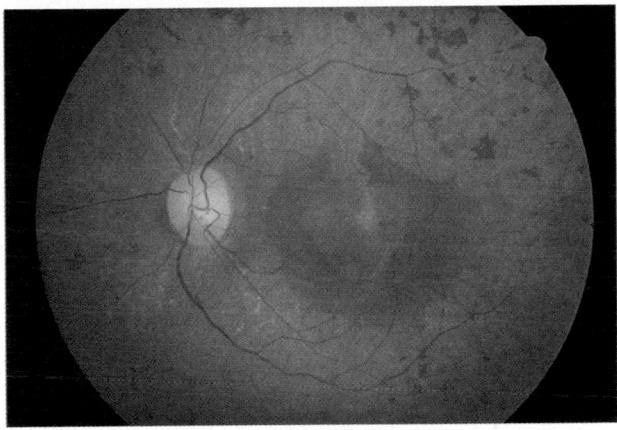

IV-16 **Retinitis pigmentosa** with black clumps of pigment in the retinal periphery known as "bone spicules." There is also atrophy of the retinal pigment epithelium, making the vasculature of the choroid easily visible.

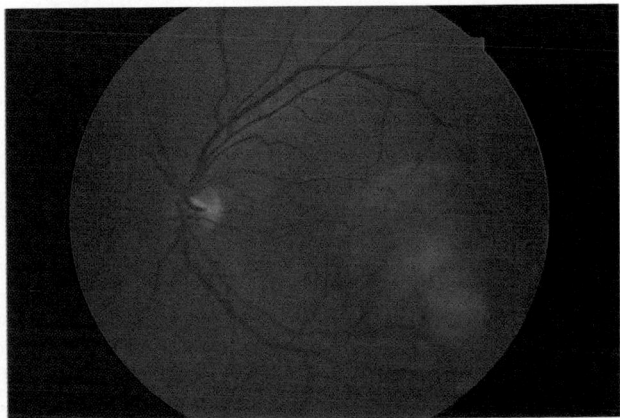

IV-17 **Melanoma of the choroid,** appearing as an elevated dark mass in the inferior temporal fundus, just encroaching upon the fovea.

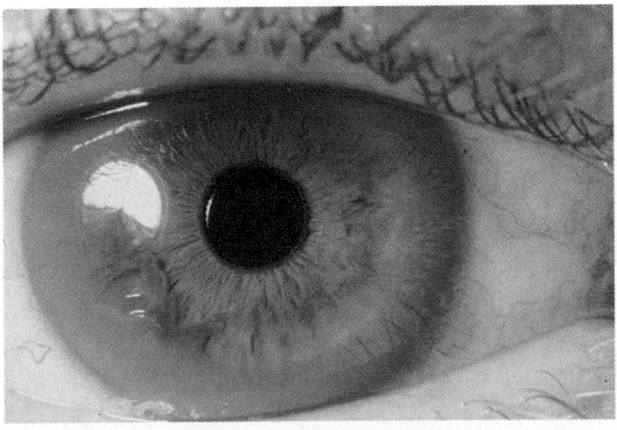

IV-18 **Kayser-Fleischer ring** develops in Wilson's disease from copper deposition in Descemet's membrane, producing brownish discoloration of the peripheral cornea. It should not be confused with the yellow-white lipid ring of arcus senilis, which is common in the elderly and occasionally signifies hyperlipidemia, especially when it appears at a young age.

V. Atlas of Hematology

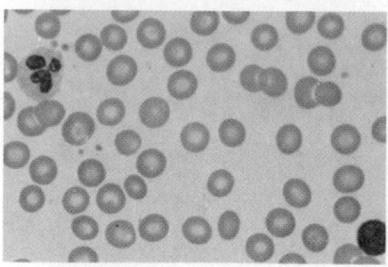

V-1 **Normal blood smear** Normal red blood cells are round, possess an area of central pallor, appear slightly smaller than the nucleus of a mature lymphocyte, and vary little in size (anisocytosis) or in shape (poikilocytosis).

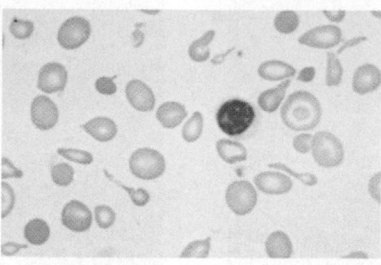

V-2 **β-Thalassemia intermedia** Microcytic and hypochromic red blood cells are seen that resemble the red blood cells of severe iron deficiency anemia shown in Fig. IV-4. Many elliptical and teardrop-shaped red blood cells are noted.

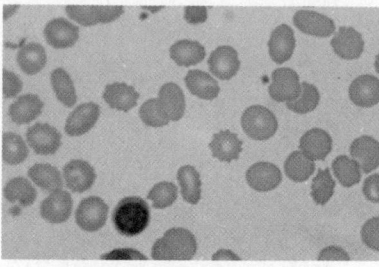

V-3 **Uremia** The red blood cells in uremia may acquire numerous, regularly spaced, small spiny projections. Such cells, called burr cells or echinocytes, are readily distinguishable from irregularly spiculated acanthocytes shown in Fig. V-27.

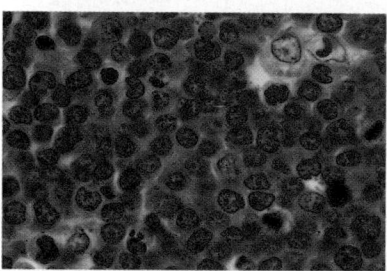

V-4 **Burkitt's lymphoma** The neoplastic cells are homogenous, medium-sized B cells with frequent mitotic figures, a morphologic correlate of high growth fraction. Reactive macrophages are scattered through the tumor and their pale cytoplasm in a background of blue-staining tumor cells gives the tumor a so-called "starry sky" appearance.

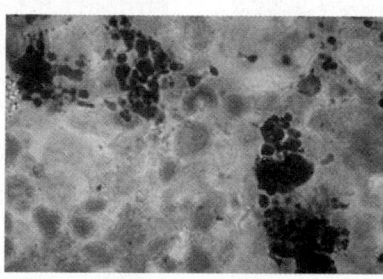

V-5 **Marrow iron stores** This marrow section is stained with Prussian blue. Iron takes up the stain and is concentrated in reticuloendothelial cells. This picture shows normal iron stores. In iron deficiency states, no stainable iron is detectable. In the anemia of chronic disease, iron is present but cytokines prevent its mobilization and utilization in heme synthesis.

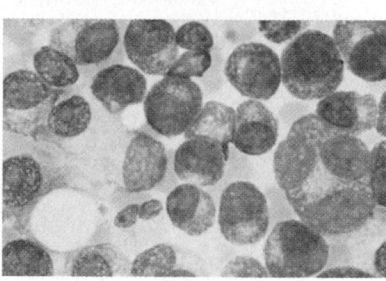

V-6 **Multiple myeloma (marrow)** The cells bear characteristic morphologic features of plasma cells, round or oval cells with an eccentric nucleus composed of coarsely clumped chromatin, a densely basophilic cytoplasm, and a perinuclear clear zone (hof) containing the Golgi apparatus. Binucleate and multinucleate malignant plasma cells also can be seen.

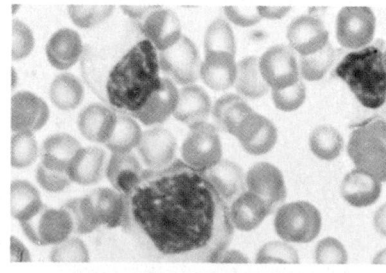

V-7 **Reactive lymphocytes (infectious mononucleosis)** Reactive lymphocytes are usually large and contain abundant cytoplasm. The nucleus may be eccentrically placed and may have irregular borders and indentations (not seen on this plate). The cytoplasm contains areas that stain a darker blue due to their increased content of RNA. The cytoplasm may be indented where it abuts against a red blood cell.

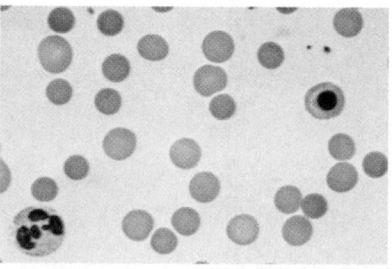

V-8 **Immunohemolytic anemia** Microspherocytes are seen on this blood smear along with several macrocytes with a slight purple tinge (polychromasia). The latter represent new red blood cells released early from the bone marrow. The microspherocytes seen in immunohemolytic anemia may be indistinguishable from the microspherocytes seen in hereditary spherocytosis (Fig. V-26).

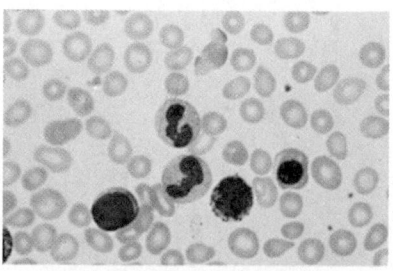

V-9 **Leukoerythroblastic smear** Teardrop-shaped red blood cells indicative of membrane damage from collagen fibers, a nucleated red blood cell indicative of premature release of erythroid precursors, and immature myeloid cells indicative of extramedullary hematopoiesis are noted. This peripheral blood smear is related to marrow fibrosis, either primary myelofibrosis or secondary myelophthisis.

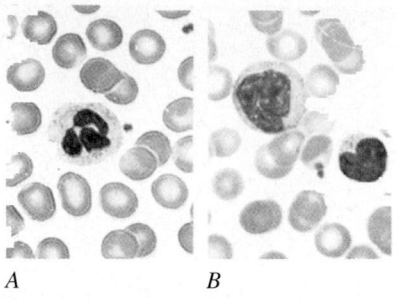

A   *B*

V-10 A. **Normal granulocyte** The normal granulocyte has a segmented nucleus with heavy, clumped chromatin; fine neutrophilic granules are dispersed throughout its cytoplasm. *B.* **Normal monocyte and lymphocyte** The normal monocyte is a large cell with an indented or folded nucleus containing loose, strand-like chromatin; the cytoplasm is a blue-gray color and usually contains fine azurophilic granules. The normal lymphocyte is a smaller cell. Its nucleus is usually round but may be indented, as in the cell shown in this plate. The nuclear chromatin has a smudgy appearance; the cytoplasm is blue.

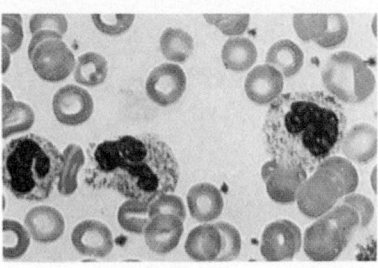

V-11 **Normal granulocyte precursors in marrow** The earliest granulocytic precursor (myeloblast) possesses a round nucleus with fine, punctate chromatin and one or more nucleoli; the cytoplasm is blue. As nuclear differentiation proceeds, the nucleoli disappear, the chromatin coarsens, and the nucleus becomes increasingly indented and finally segmented. As cytoplasmic differentiation proceeds, azurophilic granules appear and cytoplasm changes color from blue to the yellow-pink-gray hue of the mature granulocyte, and as this occurs the azurophilic granules become obscured by fine neutrophilic granules.

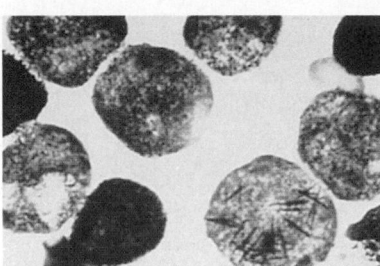

V-12 **Leukemic cell in acute promyelocytic leukemia** Note multiple Auer rods.

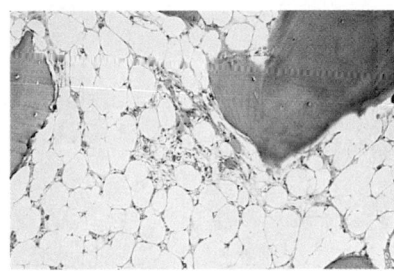

V-13 **Aplastic anemia** This marrow section shows only fat with nearly complete absence of hematopoietic tissue.

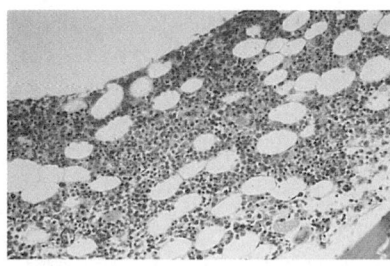

V-14 **Normal bone marrow biopsy** This a low power view of an H&E-stained section of normal marrow. Note that the nucleated cellular elements account for about 40 to 50 percent and the fat *(clear areas)* accounts for about 50 to 60 percent of the area.

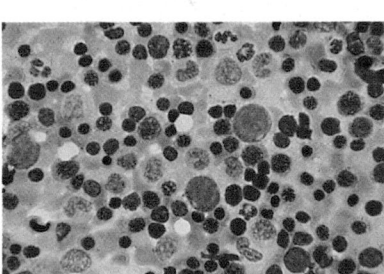

V-15 **Erythroid hyperplasia** This marrow section shows an increase in the fraction of cells in the erythroid lineage as might be seen in a healthy marrow compensating for acute blood loss or hemolysis. The E/G ratio is greater than 1/1.

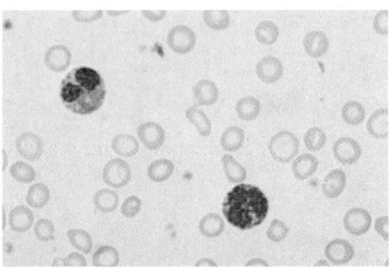

V-16 **Iron-deficiency anemia** In severe iron deficiency, the red blood cells are smaller than normal (microcytosis), and their central area of pallor is expanded (hypochromia) so that the cells appear to have only a thin rim of hemoglobin.

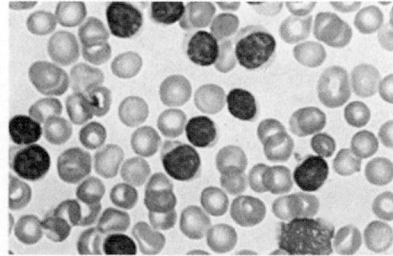

V-17 **Chronic lymphocytic leukemia** The peripheral WBC count is high due to increased numbers of small, well-differentiated lymphocytes. However, the leukemic lymphocytes are fragile, and substantial numbers of broken, smudged cells are usually also present on the blood smear.

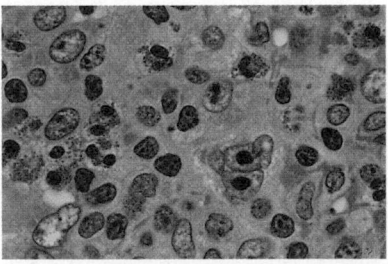

V-18 **Hodgkin's disease, mixed cellularity** A Reed-Sternberg cell is present near the center of the field; a large cell with a bilobed nucleus and prominent nucleoli. The majority of the cells are normal lymphocytes, neutrophils, and eosinophils that form a pleiomorphic cellular infiltrate.

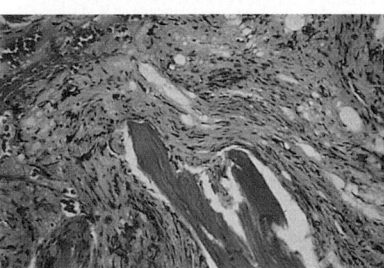

V-19 **Marrow fibrosis** This marrow section shows the marrow cavity replaced by fibrous tissue composed of reticulin fibers and collagen. When this fibrosis is due to a primary hematologic process, it is called *myelofibrosis*. When the fibrosis is secondary to a tumor or a granulomatous process, it is called *myelophthisis*.

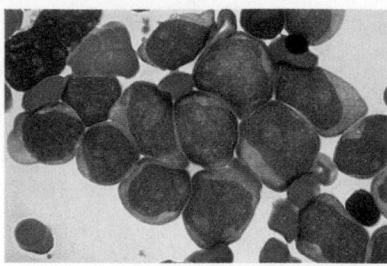

V-20 **Acute myelocytic leukemia** This marrow section shows sheets of primitive myeloblasts with numerous large nucleoli.

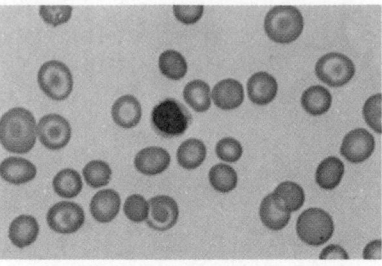

V-21 **Liver disease** Round macrocytes of rather uniform size are seen. Many of the macrocytes are also target cells.

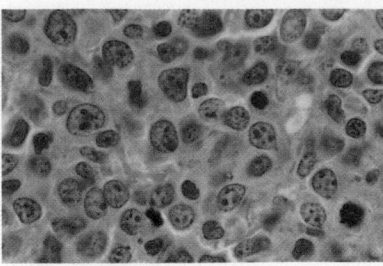

V-22 **Diffuse large B cell lymphoma** The neoplastic cells are large with vesicular nuclear chromatin and prominent nucleoli.

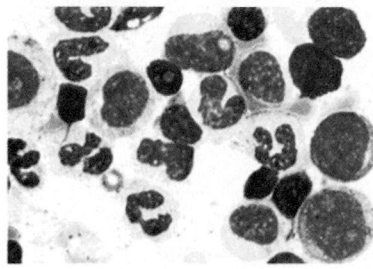

V-23 **Neutrophils with toxic granulation** In infection and other toxic states, azurophilic granules may become visible in mature granulocytes as coarse, dark-staining cytoplasmic granules.

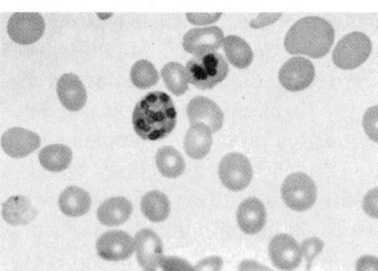

V-24 **Megaloblastic anemia** Oval macrocytes, well filled with hemoglobin, are admixed with lesser numbers of small teardrop-shaped red blood cells. Note also hypersegmented granulocyte.

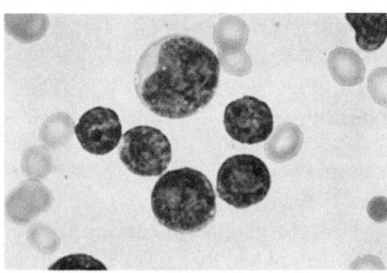

V-25 **Leukemic cells in acute lymphoblastic leukemia** characterized by round or convoluted nuclei, high nuclear/cytoplasmic ratio and absence of cytoplasmic granules.

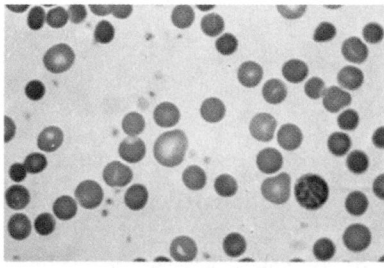

V-26 **Hereditary spherocytosis** Small, densely staining red blood cells are seen that have lost their central area of pallor (microsherocytes). Microspherocytes may also be found in other hemolytic disorders (Fig. V-8).

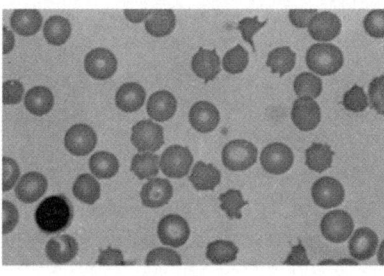

V-27 **Spur cell anemia** Spur cells are recognized as distorted red blood cells containing several irregularly distributed thornlike projections. Cells with this morphologic abnormality are also called acanthocytes.

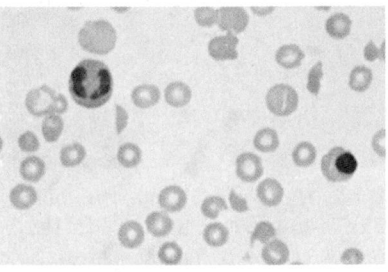

V-28 **Traumatic hemolysis** The helmet-shaped red blood cell and the small triangular-shaped red blood cells seen on this smear represent morphologic evidence of mechanical damage to red blood cells within the blood vessels.

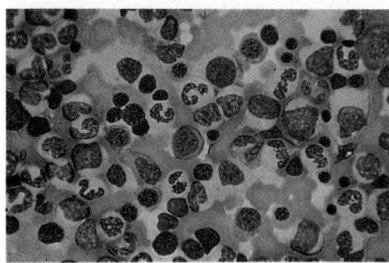

V-29 **Granulocytic hyperplasia** This marrow section shows an increase in the fraction of cells in the myeloid or granulocytic lineage as might be seen in a healthy marrow responding to infection. The E/G ratio is less than 1/3.

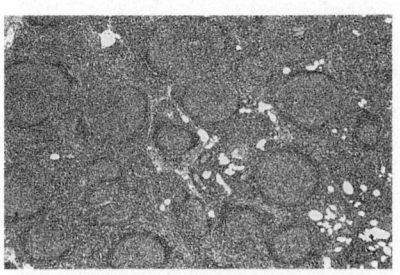

V-30 **Follicular lymphoma** The normal nodal architecture is effaced by nodular expansions of tumor cells. Nodules vary in size and mimic normal lymphoid follicles.

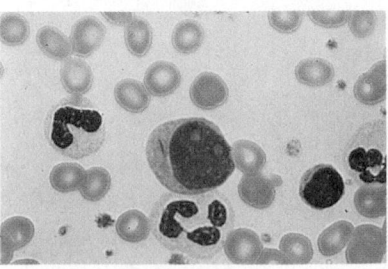

V-31 **Auer rod** This peripheral blood smear shows a myeloblast with a single Auer rod in the cytoplasm. Auer rods, when present, are usually seen in acute myelocytic leukemia.

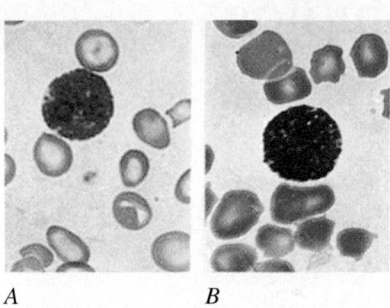

A   *B*

V-32 A. **Normal eosinophil** The eosinophil contains large, bright-orange granules; the nucleus is bilobed. *B.* **Basophil** The basophil contains large, purple-black granules that fill the cell and obscure the nucleus.

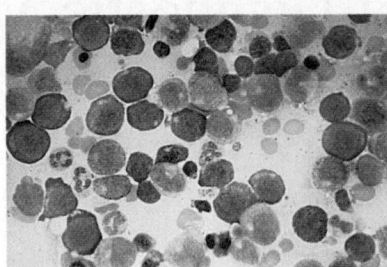

V-33 **Megaloblastic erythropoiesis** This marrow section demonstrates so-called nuclear-cytoplasmic dissociation; the cytoplasm of erythroblasts is filled with hemoglobin demonstrating nearly complete maturation while the nuclei have loose chromatin characteristic of more immature erythroid cells. The slow nuclear maturation is related to a decrease in DNA synthesis related to an insufficient supply of reduced folate to synthesize thymidylate. DNA synthesis inhibitors can produce this picture, as can folate and B$_{12}$ deficiency.

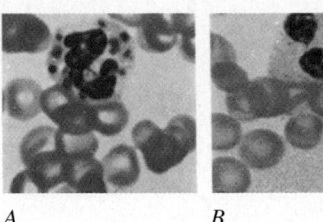

A   *B*

V-34 A. **Chédiak-Higashi anomaly** In this ultimately fatal disorder, the granulocytes contain huge cytoplasmic granules, formed from aggregation and fusion of azurophilic and specific granules. Large abnormal granules are found in other granule-containing cells throughout the body. *B.* **Pelger-Hüet anomaly** In this benign disorder, the majority of granulocytes are bilobed. The nucleus frequently has a spectacle-like or "pince-nez" configuration.

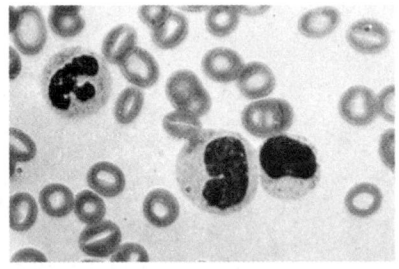

V-35 **Band with Döhle body** (center) Döhle bodies are discrete, blue-staining non-granular areas found in the periphery of the cytoplasm of the neutrophil in infections and other toxic states. They represent aggregates of rough endoplasmic reticulum.

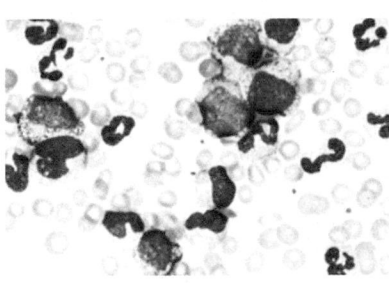

V-36 **Chronic granulocytic leukemia** The peripheral WBC count is high due to increased numbers of granulocytes and their precursors. The majority of the WBCs are segmented granulocytes or band forms, but myelocytes (as seen on this plate) and promyeloblasts (not seen on this plate) may also be found on review of the blood smear.

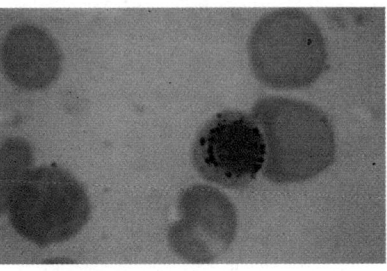

V-37 **Ringed sideroblast** Refractory anemia with ringed sideroblasts (RARS) is in the spectrum of myelodysplastic syndromes. This marrow Prussian blue stain shows an orthochromatic normoblast with a collar of blue granules surrounding the nucleus. The blue granules represent iron-laden mitochondria.

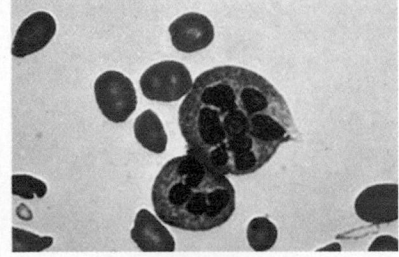

V-38 **Hypersegmentation** Frequent five-lobed granulocytes on a blood smear or granulocytes with more than five lobes are evidence of hypersegmentation, an important clue to the diagnosis of megaloblastic anemia.

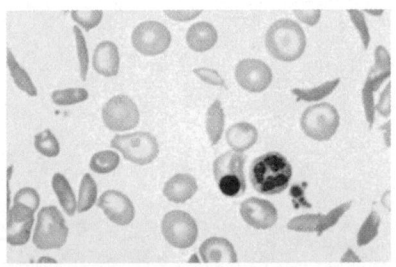

V-39 **Sickle cell anemia** The elongated and crescent-shaped red blood cells seen on this smear represent circulating irreversibly sickled cells. Target cells and a nucleated red blood cell are also seen.

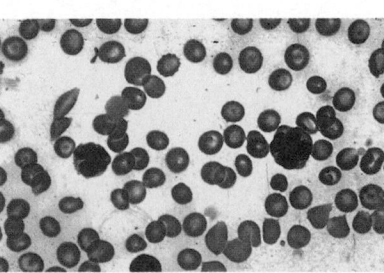

V-40 **Adult T cell leukemia/lymphoma** This peripheral blood smear reveals leukemia cells with the typical "flower-shaped" nucleus.

VI.   Atlas of Diagnostic Microbiology

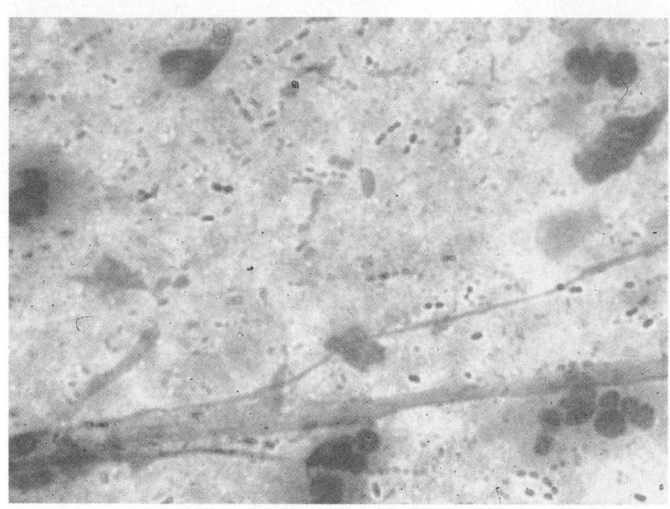

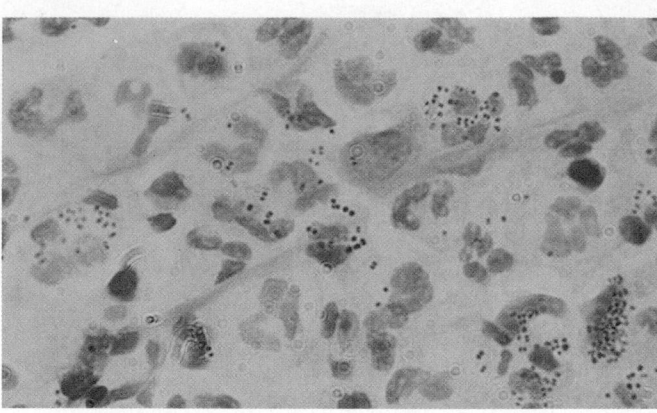

VI-1 **Gram-stained sputum** from a patient with acute purulent tracheobronchitis. Many polymorphonuclear neutrophils and a few macrophages are seen along with many gram-negative cocci, (*Moraxella catarrhalis*), a few of which appear as pairs. Nearly all organisms are cell associated and probably have been taken up by phagocytes, consistent with the notion that *Moraxella* is a lower-grade pathogen than organisms such as *Streptococcus pneumoniae*.

VI-2 The microbiologist can easily identify *Streptococcus pneumoniae* as the etiologic agent of pneumonia when microscopic examination of Gram-stained sputum specimen reveals this kind of picture.

Plates VI-3 through VI-33 are photomicrographs reproduced from "Benchaids for the Diagnosis of Malaria Infections," 2d ed, with the permission of the World Health Organization.

P. falciparum—thin film

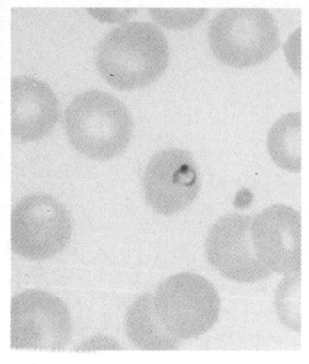

VI-3   Trophozoites–young

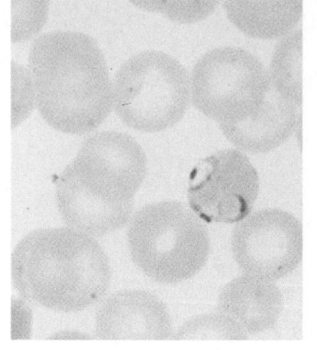

VI-4   Trophozoites–old

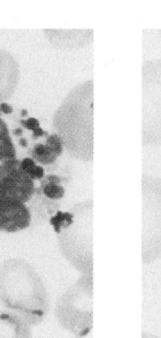

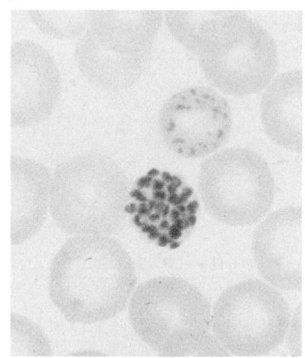

VI-5   Pigment in polymorphonuclear cell and trophozoites

VI-6   Schizonts–mature

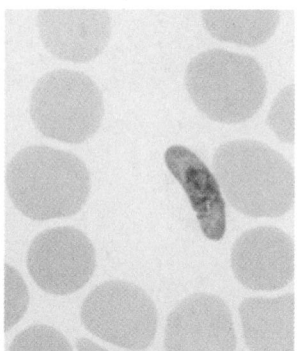

VI-7   Gametocytes–female

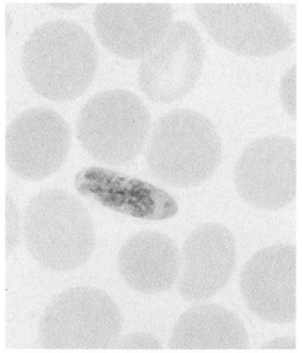

VI-8   Gametocytes–male

P. vivax—thin film

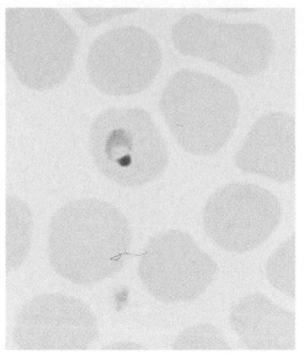

VI-9   Trophozoites–young

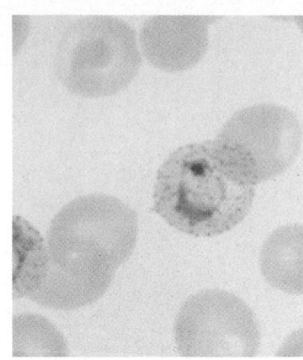

VI-10   Trophozoites–old

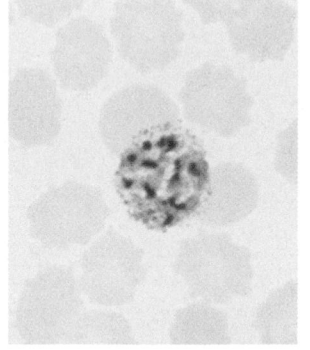

VI-11   Schizonts–mature

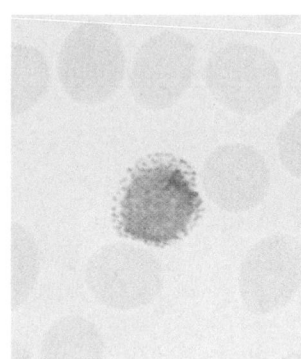

VI-12   Gametocytes–female

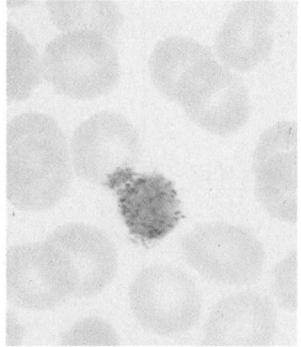

VI-13   Gametocytes–male

P. ovale—thin film

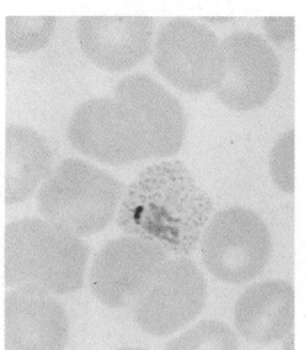

VI-14   Trophozoites–old

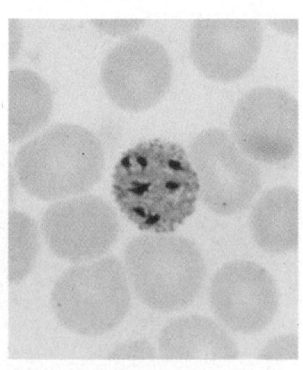

VI-15   Schizonts–mature

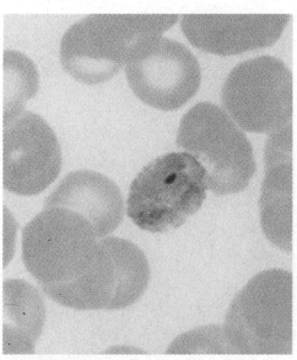

VI-16   Gametocytes–male

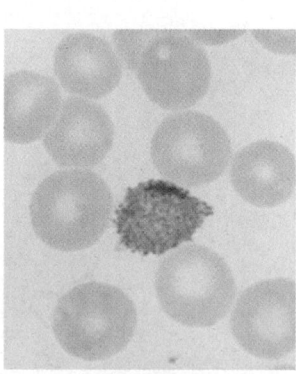

VI-17   Gametocytes–female

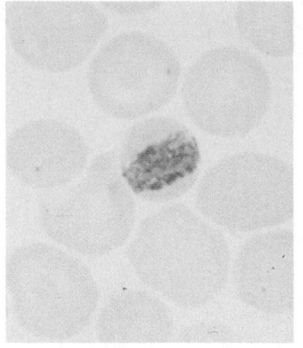

VI-18 Trophozoites–old

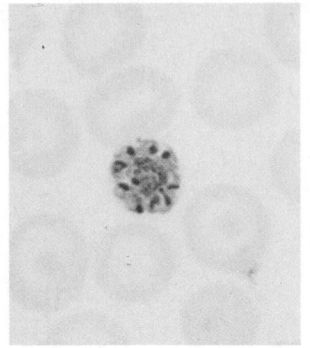

VI-19 Schizonts–mature

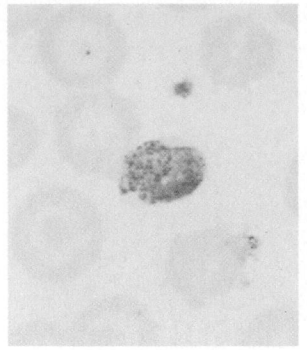

VI-20 Gametocytes–male

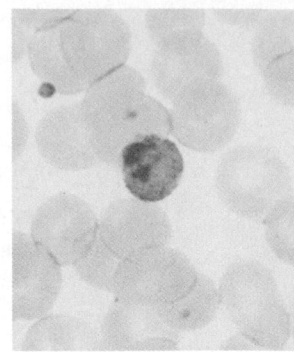

VI-21 Gametocytes–female

Babesia—thin film

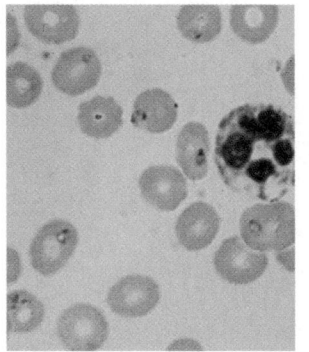

VI-22 Trophozoites

P. vivax—thick film

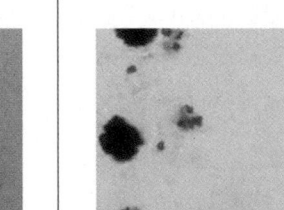

VI-25 Trophozoites

P. ovale—thick film

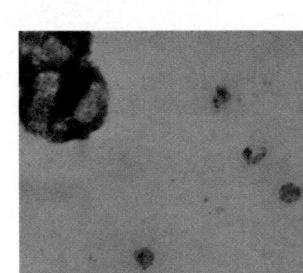

VI-28 Trophozoites

P. malariae—thick film

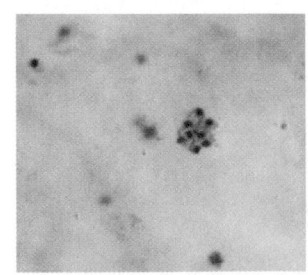

VI-31 Trophozoites

P. falciparum—thick film

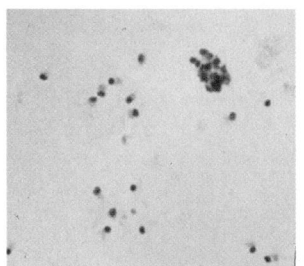

VI-23 Trophozoites

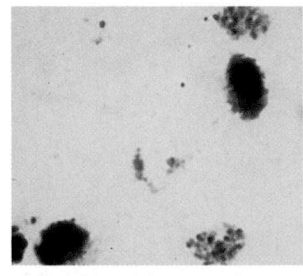

VI-26 Schizonts

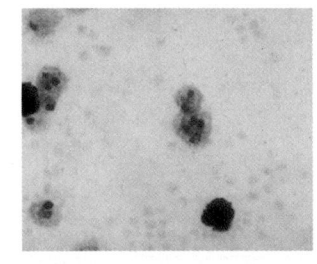

VI-29 Schizonts

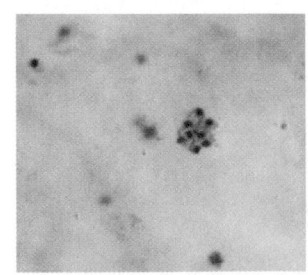

VI-32 Schizonts

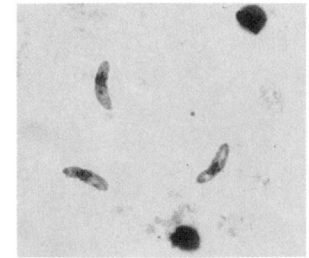

VI-24 Gametocytes

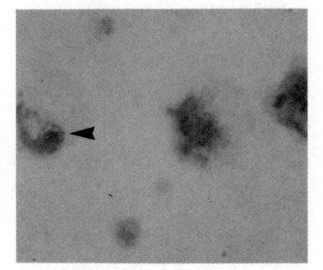

VI-27 Gametocytes

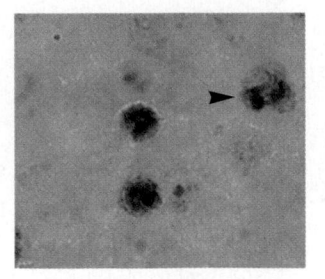

VI-30 Gametocytes

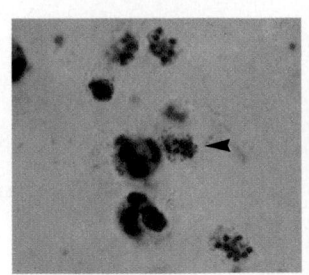

VI-33 Gametocytes

SOURCES OF PHOTOGRAPHS

I. CARDIOLOGY

R. Gibbons, MD I-1A, I-1B Exercise sestamibi study

II. DERMATOLOGY

L. Baden, MD IID-58 Septic emboli
Jean Bolognia, MD IIA-6 Seborrheic dermatitis; IIB-21 Non-Hodgkin's lymphoma
S. Wright Caughman, MD IIC-32 Nodular melanoma; IID-55 Condylomata acuminatum
Gregory Cox, MD IID-47 Primary syphilis
Daniel F. Danzl, MD IIA-18, IIA-19 Frostbite
Robert Gelber, MD IID-56 Polar lepromatous leprosy
Stephen E. Gellis, MD IID-39 Hand foot-and-mouth disease; IID 44 Fulminant meningococcemia
John Greenspan, PhD IID-42 Oral hairy leukoplakia; IID-43 Pseudomembranous oral candidiasis
Robert Hartman, MD IID-36 Varicella
A.W. Kerchner, MD IID-59 Veridans streptococcal endocarditis
James Krell, MD IIE-63 Dermatomyositis
Marilynne McKay, MD IIE-62 Discoid lupus erythematosus
V. Pranava Murthy, MD IID-53 Skin lesions
Daniel M. Musher, MD IID-60 Disseminated gonococcemia
Alvin Solomon, MD IIC-31 Lentigo maligna melanoma; IID-48 Secondary syphilis of the palms
Mary Spraker, MD IID-38 Impetigo contagiosa
Robert Swerlick, MD IIA-2 Acne rosacea; IIA-4 Atopic dermatitis; IIA-8B Allergic contact dermatitis; IIA-9 Lichen planus; IIA-12 Alopecia areata; IIA-14B Dermatographism; IIB-27 Actinic keratoses; IID-37 Disseminated herpes zoster; IID-45 Rocky Mountain spotted fever; IIE-61B Acute lupus erythematosus; IIE-63 Dermatomyositis; IIE-69B Pemphigus vulgaris; IIE-70 Erythema nodosum; IIE-71 Vasculitis; IIF-75 Sweet's syndrome; IIF-76 Rheumatoid nodules; IIF-79B Sarcoid; IIF-80 Pyoderma gangrenosum
Kalman Watsky, MD IIA-1 Acne vulgaris
Yale Resident's Slide Collection IID-41 Molluscum contagiosum; IID-46 Erythema chronicum migrans; IID-49 Condylomata lata; IIE-67 Erythema multiforme; IIE-72 Bullous pemphigoid
Kim Yancey, MD IIF-78 Coumarin necrosis

III. ENDOSCOPIC FINDINGS

FE Silverstein and **GN Tytgat** *Atlas of Gastrointestinal Endoscopy,* New York, Gower Medical Publishing, 1987. All photographs except III-12, III-23, III-24
GN Tytgat III-12; III-23; III-24

IV FUNDUSCOPIC FINDINGS

Jonathan C. Horton, MD, PhD IV-1 to IV-18

V. HEMATOLOGY

Robert S. Hillman, MD, and **Kenneth A. Ault, MD** *Hematology in General Practice,* New York, McGraw-Hill, 1995. Courtesy of the American Society of Hematology Slide Bank. V-30 to V-39
Elaine Jaffe, MD V-25 to V-29

VI. DIAGNOSTIC MICROBIOLOGY

Elil Renganathan, MD, WHO, Geneva VI-3 to VI-33

risk of developing active tuberculosis. Tuberculosis in the United States is also a disease of young adult members of the HIV-infected, immigrant, and disadvantaged/marginalized populations. Similarly, in Europe, tuberculosis has reemerged as an important public health problem, mainly as a result of cases among immigrants from high-prevalence countries.

In developing countries of Africa and Asia, tuberculosis trends over the past several decades are not entirely clear. However, in sub-Saharan African countries with reliable reporting systems, the recent spread of the HIV epidemic has been accompanied by doubling or tripling of the number of reported cases of tuberculosis during a period as short as 10 years. The growing number of young adults with *M. tuberculosis* infection has fueled the rates of active tuberculosis in many developing countries. Without greater control efforts, the annual incident cases of tuberculosis globally may increase by 40% between now and 2020.

From Exposure to Infection *M. tuberculosis* is most commonly transmitted from a patient with infectious pulmonary tuberculosis to other persons by droplet nuclei, which are aerosolized by coughing, sneezing, or speaking. The tiny droplets dry rapidly; the smallest (<5 to 10 μm in diameter) may remain suspended in the air for several hours and may gain direct access to the terminal air passages when inhaled. There may be as many as 3000 infectious nuclei per cough. In the past, a frequent source of infection was raw milk containing *M. bovis* from tuberculous cows. Other routes of transmission of tubercle bacilli, such as through the skin or the placenta, are uncommon and of no epidemiologic significance.

The probability of contact with a case of tuberculosis, the intimacy and duration of that contact, the degree of infectiousness of the case, and the shared environment of the contact are all important determinants of transmission. Several studies of close contacts have clearly demonstrated that tuberculosis patients whose sputum contains AFB visible by microscopy play the greatest role in the spread of infection. These patients often have cavitary pulmonary disease or tuberculosis of the respiratory tract (endobronchial or laryngeal tuberculosis) and produce sputa containing as many as 10^5 AFB/mL. Patients with sputum smear–negative/culture-positive tuberculosis are less infectious, and those with culture-negative pulmonary disease and extrapulmonary tuberculosis are essentially noninfectious. Crowding in poorly ventilated rooms is one of the most important factors in the transmission of tubercle bacilli, since it increases the intensity of contact with a case.

In short, the risk of acquiring *M. tuberculosis* infection is determined mainly by exogenous factors. Because of delays in seeking care and in diagnosis, it is estimated that up to 20 contacts will usually be infected by each AFB-positive case before detection in high-prevalence countries.

From Infection to Disease Unlike the risk of acquiring infection with *M. tuberculosis*, the risk of developing disease after being infected depends largely on endogenous factors, such as the individual's innate susceptibility to disease and level of function of cell-mediated immunity. Clinical illness directly following infection is classified as *primary tuberculosis* and is common among children up to 4 years of age. Although this form may be severe and disseminated, it is usually not transmissible. When infection is acquired later in life, the chance is greater that the immune system will contain it, at least temporarily. The majority of infected individuals who ultimately develop tuberculosis do so within the first year or two after infection. Dormant bacilli, however, may persist for years before being reactivated to produce *secondary* (or *postprimary*) *tuberculosis*, which is often infectious. Overall, it is estimated that about 10% of infected persons will eventually develop active tuberculosis. *Reinfection* of a previously infected individual, which is probably common in areas with high rates of tuberculosis transmission, may also favor the development of disease. Molecular typing and comparison of strains of *M. tuberculosis* have suggested that up to one-third of cases of active tuberculosis in U.S. inner-city communities are due to recent transmission rather than to reactivation of latent infection.

Age is an important determinant of the risk of disease after infection. Among infected persons, the incidence of tuberculosis is highest during late adolescence and early adulthood; the reasons are unclear. The incidence among women peaks at 25 to 34 years of age. In this age group rates among women are usually higher than those among men, while at older ages the opposite is true. The risk may increase in the elderly, possibly because of waning immunity and comorbidity.

A variety of diseases favor the development of active tuberculosis. The most potent risk factor for tuberculosis among infected individuals is clearly HIV co-infection, which suppresses cellular immunity. The risk that latent *M. tuberculosis* infection will proceed to active disease is directly related to the patient's degree of immunosuppression. In a study of HIV-infected, PPD-positive persons, this risk varied from 2.6 to 13.3 cases per 100 person-years and depended upon the CD4+ cell count. The risk of developing tuberculosis is significantly greater among HIV-infected than among HIV-uninfected hosts. Other conditions known to increase the risk of active tuberculosis among persons infected with tubercle bacilli include silicosis; lymphoma, leukemia, and other malignant neoplasms; hemophilia; chronic renal failure and hemodialysis; insulin-dependent diabetes mellitus; immunosuppressive treatment, including that administered for solid-organ transplantation; and conditions associated with malnutrition, such as gastrectomy and jejunoileal bypass surgery. Finally, the presence of old, self-healed, fibrotic tuberculous lesions constitutes a serious risk of active disease.

NATURAL HISTORY OF DISEASE Studies conducted in various countries before the advent of chemotherapy clearly showed that untreated tuberculosis is often fatal. About one-third of patients died within 1 year after diagnosis, and one-half within 5 years. Five-year mortality among sputum smear–positive cases was 65%. Of the survivors at 5 years, about 60% had undergone spontaneous remission, while the remainder were still excreting tubercle bacilli.

The introduction of effective chemotherapy has markedly affected the natural history of tuberculosis. With proper treatment, patients have a high chance of being cured. However, improper use of antituberculosis drugs, while reducing mortality, may also result in large numbers of chronic infectious cases, often with drug-resistant bacilli.

PATHOGENESIS AND IMMUNITY The interaction of *M. tuberculosis* with the human host begins when droplet nuclei containing microorganisms from infectious patients are inhaled. While the majority of inhaled bacilli are trapped in the upper airways and expelled by ciliated mucosal cells, a fraction (usually fewer than 10%) reach the alveoli. There, nonspecifically activated alveolar macrophages ingest the bacilli. Invasion of macrophages by mycobacteria may result in part from association of C2a with the bacterial cell wall followed by C3b opsonization of the bacteria and recognition by the macrophages. The balance between the bactericidal activity of the macrophage and the virulence of the bacillus (the latter being partially linked to the bacterium's lipid-rich cell wall and to its glycolipid capsule, both of which confer resistance to complement and free radicals of the phagocyte) determines the events following phagocytosis. The number of invading bacilli is also important.

Several genes thought to confer virulence to *M. tuberculosis* have been identified. *katG* encodes for catalase, an enzyme protective against oxidative stress; *rpoV* is the main sigma factor initiating transcription of several genes. Defects in these two genes result in loss of virulence. The *erp* gene, encoding a protein required for multiplication, also contributes to virulence. The effects of a highly virulent strain are exemplified by an outbreak of tuberculosis in two rural counties in Tennessee and Kentucky in 1994 through 1996. In this outbreak, both epidemiologic evidence of enhanced transmission with high rates of disease and accelerated growth of the strain in mice were documented.

Several observations suggest that genetic factors play a key role in innate nonimmune resistance to infection with *M. tuberculosis*. The existence of this resistance is suggested by the differing degrees of susceptibility to tuberculosis in different populations. In mice, a gene called *Nramp1* (natural resistance–associated macrophage protein 1) has a regulatory role in resistance/susceptibility to mycobacteria. The human homologue NRAMP1, cloned to chromosome 2q, may have a role in determining susceptibility to tuberculosis. In a study among West Africans, subjects heterozygous for two polymorphisms of NRAMP1 (INT4 and 3'UTR) had an apparently increased risk of tuberculosis, a finding suggesting that the susceptibility allele behaves as dominant.

In the initial stage of host-bacterium interaction, either the host's macrophages contain bacillary multiplication by producing proteolytic enzymes and cytokines or the bacilli begin to multiply. If the bacilli multiply, their growth quickly kills the macrophages, which lyse. Nonactivated monocytes attracted from the bloodstream to the site by various chemotactic factors ingest the bacilli released from the lysed macrophages. These initial stages of infection are usually asymptomatic.

About 2 to 4 weeks after infection, two additional host responses to *M. tuberculosis* develop: a tissue-damaging response and a macrophage-activating response. The *tissue-damaging response* is the result of a delayed-type hypersensitivity (DTH) reaction to various bacillary antigens; it destroys nonactivated macrophages that contain multiplying bacilli. The *macrophage-activating response* is a cell-mediated phenomenon resulting in the activation of macrophages that are capable of killing and digesting tubercle bacilli. Although both of these responses can inhibit mycobacterial growth, it is the balance between the two that determines the form of tuberculosis that will develop subsequently.

With the development of specific immunity and the accumulation of large numbers of activated macrophages at the site of the primary lesion, granulomatous lesions (tubercles) are formed. These lesions consist of lymphocytes and activated macrophages, such as epithelioid cells and giant cells. Initially, the newly developed tissue-damaging response is the only event capable of limiting mycobacterial growth within macrophages. This response, mediated by various bacterial products, not only destroys macrophages but also produces early solid necrosis in the center of the tubercle. Although *M. tuberculosis* can survive, its growth is inhibited within this necrotic environment by low oxygen tension and low pH. At this point, some lesions may heal by fibrosis and calcification, while others undergo further evolution.

Cell-mediated immunity is critical at this early stage. In the majority of infected individuals, local macrophages are activated when bacillary antigens processed by macrophages stimulate T lymphocytes to release a variety of lymphokines. These activated cells aggregate around the lesion's center and effectively neutralize tubercle bacilli without causing further tissue destruction. In the central part of the lesion, the necrotic material resembles soft cheese (*caseous necrosis*). Even when healing takes place, viable bacilli may remain dormant within macrophages or in the necrotic material for years or even throughout the patient's lifetime. These "healed" lesions in the lung parenchyma and hilar lymph nodes may later undergo calcification (*Ranke complex*).

In a minority of cases, the macrophage-activating response is weak, and mycobacterial growth can be inhibited only by intensified DTH reactions, which lead to tissue destruction. The lesion tends to enlarge further, and the surrounding tissue is progressively damaged. At the center of the lesion, the caseous material liquefies. Bronchial walls as well as blood vessels are invaded and destroyed, and cavities are formed. The liquefied caseous material, containing large numbers of bacilli, is drained through bronchi. Within the cavity, tubercle bacilli multiply well and spread into the airways and the environment through expectorated sputum.

In the early stages of infection, bacilli are usually transported by macrophages to regional lymph nodes, from which they disseminate widely to many organs and tissues. The resulting lesions may undergo the same evolution as those in the lungs, although most tend to heal. In young children with poor natural immunity, hematogenous dissemination may result in fatal miliary tuberculosis or tuberculous meningitis.

Cell-mediated immunity confers partial protection against *M. tuberculosis*, while humoral immunity has no defined role in protection. Two types of cells are essential: macrophages, which directly phagocytize tubercle bacilli, and T cells (mainly CD4+ lymphocytes), which induce protection through the production of lymphokines.

After infection with *M. tuberculosis*, alveolar macrophages secrete a number of cytokines: interleukin (IL) 1 contributes to fever; IL-6 contributes to hyperglobulinemia; and tumor necrosis factor α (TNF-α) contributes to the killing of mycobacteria, the formation of granulomas, and a number of systemic effects, such as fever and weight loss. Macrophages are also critical in processing and presenting antigens to T lymphocytes; the result is a proliferation of CD4+ lymphocytes, which are crucial to the host's defense against *M. tuberculosis*. Qualitative and quantitative defects of CD4+ T cells explain the inability of HIV-infected individuals to contain mycobacterial proliferation. Reactive CD4+ lymphocytes produce cytokines of the T_H1 pattern and participate in MHC class II–restricted killing of cells infected with *M. tuberculosis*. T_H1 CD4+ cells produce interferon γ (IFN-γ) and IL-2 and promote cell-mediated immunity. T_H2 cells produce IL-4, IL-5, and IL-10 and promote humoral immunity. The interplay of these various cytokines and their cross-regulation determine the host's response. The role of cytokines in promoting intracellular killing of mycobacteria has not been entirely elucidated. IFN-γ may induce release of nitric oxide, and TNF-α seems also to be important. Finally, the role of other cells, such as natural killer (NK) cells, "double-negative" CD4–CD8– cells, and γ/δ T cells, in protective immunity remains unclear.

M. tuberculosis possesses various protein antigens. Some are present in the cytoplasm and cell wall; others are secreted. That the latter are more important in eliciting a T lymphocyte response is suggested by experiments documenting the appearance of protective immunity in animals after immunization with live, protein-secreting mycobacteria. Among the antigens with a potential protective role are the 30-kDa (or 85B) and the ESAT-6 antigens. Protective immunity is probably the result of reactivity to a large number of different mycobacterial antigens.

Coincident with the appearance of immunity, DTH to *M. tuberculosis* develops. This reactivity is the basis of the PPD skin test, currently the only test that reliably detects *M. tuberculosis* infection in persons without symptoms. The cellular mechanisms responsible for PPD reactivity are related mainly to previously sensitized CD4+ lymphocytes, which are attracted to the skin-test site. There, they proliferate and produce cytokines.

In 1891, Robert Koch discovered components of *M. tuberculosis* in a concentrated liquid culture medium. Subsequently named "old tuberculin" (OT), this material was initially believed to be useful in the treatment of tuberculosis (although this idea was later disproved). It soon became clear that OT was capable of eliciting a skin reaction when injected subcutaneously into patients with tuberculosis. In 1932, Seibert and Munday purified this product by ammonium sulfate precipitation. The result was an active protein fraction known as tuberculin PPD. However, the complexity and diversity of the constituents of PPD rendered its standardization difficult. PPD-S, developed by Seibert and Glenn in 1941, was chosen as the international standard. Later, the WHO and UNICEF sponsored large-scale production of a master batch of PPD, termed RT23, and made it available for general use. The greatest limitation of PPD is its lack of mycobacterial species specificity, a property that is due to the large number of proteins in this product that are highly conserved in the various species of mycobacteria.

While DTH is associated with protective immunity (PPD-positive persons being less susceptible to a new *M. tuberculosis* infection than PPD-negative persons), it by no means guarantees protection against reactivation. In fact, severe cases of active tuberculosis are often accompanied by strongly positive skin-test reactions.

CLINICAL MANIFESTATIONS   Tuberculosis is usually classified as pulmonary or extrapulmonary. Before the recognition of HIV infection, more than 80% of all cases of tuberculosis were limited to the lungs. However, up to two-thirds of HIV-infected patients with tuberculosis may have both pulmonary and extrapulmonary disease or extrapulmonary disease alone.

Pulmonary Tuberculosis Pulmonary tuberculosis can be categorized as primary or postprimary (secondary).

Primary disease Primary pulmonary tuberculosis results from an initial infection with tubercle bacilli. In areas of high tuberculosis prevalence, this form of disease is often seen in children and is frequently localized to the middle and lower lung zones. The lesion forming after infection is usually peripheral and accompanied by hilar or paratracheal lymphadenopathy, which may not be detectable on chest radiography. In the majority of cases, the lesion heals spontaneously and may later be evident as a small calcified nodule (*Ghon lesion*).

In children and in persons with impaired immunity, such as those with malnutrition or HIV infection, primary pulmonary tuberculosis may progress rapidly to clinical illness. The initial lesion increases in size and can evolve in different ways. Pleural effusion, a frequent finding, results from the penetration of bacilli into the pleural space from an adjacent subpleural focus. In severe cases, the primary site rapidly enlarges, its central portion undergoes necrosis, and acute cavitation develops (progressive primary tuberculosis). Tuberculosis in young children is almost invariably accompanied by hilar or mediastinal lymphadenopathy due to the spread of bacilli from the lung parenchyma through lymphatic vessels. Enlarged lymph nodes may compress bronchi, causing obstruction and subsequent segmental or lobar collapse. Partial obstruction may cause obstructive emphysema, and bronchiectasis may also develop. Hematogenous dissemination, which is common and is often asymptomatic, may result in the most severe manifestations of primary *M. tuberculosis* infection. Bacilli reach the bloodstream from the pulmonary lesion or the lymph nodes and disseminate into various organs, where they may produce granulomatous lesions. Although healing frequently takes place, immunocompromised persons (e.g., patients with HIV infection and those recovering from measles) may develop miliary tuberculosis and/or tuberculous meningitis.

Postprimary disease Also called adult-type, reactivation, or secondary tuberculosis, postprimary disease results from endogenous reactivation of latent infection and is usually localized to the apical and posterior segments of the upper lobes, where the high oxygen concentration favors mycobacterial growth. In addition, the superior segments of the lower lobes are frequently involved. The extent of lung parenchymal involvement varies greatly, from small infiltrates to extensive cavitary disease. With cavity formation, liquefied necrotic contents are ultimately discharged into the airways, resulting in satellite lesions within the lungs that may in turn undergo cavitation. Massive involvement of pulmonary segments or lobes, with coalescence of lesions, produces tuberculous pneumonia. While up to one-third of untreated patients reportedly succumb to severe pulmonary tuberculosis within a few weeks or months after onset, others undergo a process of spontaneous remission or proceed along a chronic, progressively debilitating course ("consumption"). Under these circumstances, some pulmonary lesions become fibrotic and may later calcify, but cavities persist in other parts of the lungs. Individuals with such chronic disease continue to discharge tubercle bacilli into the environment. Most patients respond to treatment, with defervescence, decreasing cough, weight gain, and a general improvement in well-being within several weeks.

Early in the course of disease, symptoms and signs are often nonspecific and insidious, consisting mainly of fever and night sweats, weight loss, anorexia, general malaise, and weakness. However, in the majority of cases, cough eventually develops—perhaps initially nonproductive and subsequently accompanied by the production of purulent sputum. Blood streaking of the sputum is frequently documented. Massive hemoptysis may ensue as a consequence of the erosion of a fully patent vessel located in the wall of a cavity. Hemoptysis, however, may also result from rupture of a dilated vessel in a cavity (*Rasmussen's aneurysm*) or from aspergilloma formation in an old cavity. Pleuritic chest pain sometimes develops in patients with

subpleural parenchymal lesions but can also result from muscle strain due to persistent coughing. Extensive disease may produce dyspnea and (occasionally) adult respiratory distress syndrome (ARDS).

Physical findings are of limited use in pulmonary tuberculosis. Many patients have no abnormalities detectable by chest examination, while others have detectable rales in the involved areas during inspiration, especially after coughing. Occasionally, rhonchi due to partial bronchial obstruction and classic amphoric breath sounds in areas with large cavities may be heard. Systemic features include fever (often low-grade and intermittent) and wasting. In some cases, pallor and finger clubbing develop. The most common hematologic findings are mild anemia and leukocytosis. Hyponatremia due to the syndrome of inappropriate secretion of antidiuretic hormone (SIADH) has also been reported.

Extrapulmonary Tuberculosis In order of frequency, the extrapulmonary sites most commonly involved in tuberculosis are the lymph nodes, pleura, genitourinary tract, bones and joints, meninges, and peritoneum. However, virtually all organ systems may be affected. As a result of hematogenous dissemination in HIV-infected individuals, extrapulmonary tuberculosis is seen more commonly today than in the past.

Lymph-node tuberculosis (tuberculous lymphadenitis) The commonest presentation of extrapulmonary tuberculosis (being documented in more than 25% of cases), lymph-node disease is particularly frequent among HIV-infected patients. In the United States, children and women (particularly non-Caucasians) also seem to be especially susceptible. Lymph-node tuberculosis presents as painless swelling of the lymph nodes, most commonly at cervical and supraclavicular sites. Lymph nodes are usually discrete in early disease but may be inflamed and have a fistulous tract draining caseous material. Systemic symptoms are usually limited to HIV-infected patients, and concomitant lung disease may or may not be present. The diagnosis is established by fine-needle aspiration or surgical biopsy. AFB are seen in up to 50% of cases, cultures are positive in 70 to 80%, and histologic examination shows granulomatous lesions. Among HIV-infected patients, granulomas are usually not seen. Differential diagnosis includes a variety of infectious conditions as well as neoplastic diseases such as lymphomas or metastatic carcinomas (Chap. 63).

Pleural tuberculosis Involvement of the pleura is common in primary tuberculosis and results from penetration by a few tubercle bacilli into the pleural space. Depending on the extent of reactivity, the effusion may be small, remain unnoticed, and resolve spontaneously or may be sufficiently large to cause symptoms such as fever, pleuritic chest pain, and dyspnea. Physical findings are those of pleural effusion: dullness to percussion and absence of breath sounds. A chest radiograph reveals the effusion and, in no more than one-third of cases, also shows a parenchymal lesion. Thoracentesis is required to ascertain the nature of the effusion. The fluid is straw colored and at times hemorrhagic; it is an exudate with a protein concentration >50% of that in serum, a normal to low glucose concentration, a pH that is generally <7.2, and detectable white blood cells (usually 500 to 2500/mL). Neutrophils may predominate in the early stage, while mononuclear cells are the typical finding later. Mesothelial cells are generally rare or absent. AFB are very rarely seen on direct smear, but cultures may be positive for *M. tuberculosis* in up to one-third of cases. Needle biopsy of the pleura is often required for diagnosis and reveals granulomas and/or yields a positive culture in up to 70% of cases. This form of pleural tuberculosis responds well to chemotherapy and may resolve spontaneously.

Tuberculous empyema is a less common complication of pulmonary tuberculosis. It is usually the result of the rupture of a cavity, with delivery of a large number of organisms into the pleural space, or of a bronchopleural fistula from a pulmonary lesion. A chest radiograph may show pyopneumothorax with an air-fluid level. The effusion is purulent and thick and contains large numbers of lymphocytes. An acid-fast smear of pleural fluid is often found to be positive when examined by microscopy, as is culture of the pleural fluid. Surgical drainage is usually required as an adjunct to chemotherapy. Tuberculous empyema may result in severe pleural fibrosis and restrictive lung disease.

Tuberculosis of the upper airways Nearly always a complication of advanced cavitary pulmonary tuberculosis, tuberculosis of the upper airways may involve the larynx, pharynx, and epiglottis. Symptoms include hoarseness and dysphagia in addition to chronic productive cough. Findings depend on the site of involvement, and ulcerations may be seen on laryngoscopy. Acid-fast smear of the sputum is often positive, but biopsy may be necessary in some cases to establish the diagnosis. Cancer may have similar features but is usually painless.

Genitourinary tuberculosis Genitourinary tuberculosis accounts for about 15% of all extrapulmonary cases, may involve any portion of the genitourinary tract, and is usually due to hematogenous seeding following primary infection. Local symptoms predominate. Urinary frequency, dysuria, hematuria, and flank pain are common presentations. However, patients may be asymptomatic and the disease discovered only after severe destructive lesions of the kidneys have developed. Urinalysis gives abnormal results in 90% of cases, revealing pyuria and hematuria. The documentation of culture-negative pyuria in acidic urine raises the suspicion of tuberculosis. An intravenous pyelogram helps in diagnosis. Calcifications and ureteral strictures are suggestive findings. Culture of three morning urine specimens yields a definitive diagnosis in nearly 90% of cases. Severe ureteral strictures may lead to hydronephrosis and renal damage.

Genital tuberculosis is diagnosed more commonly in females than in males. In females, it affects the fallopian tubes and the endometrium and may cause infertility, pelvic pain, and menstrual abnormalities. Diagnosis requires biopsy or culture of specimens obtained by dilatation and curettage. In males, tuberculosis preferentially affects the epididymis, producing a slightly tender mass that may drain externally through a fistulous tract; orchitis and prostatitis may also develop. In almost half of cases of genitourinary tuberculosis, urinary tract disease is also present. Genitourinary tuberculosis responds well to chemotherapy.

Skeletal tuberculosis In the United States, tuberculosis of the bones and joints is responsible for about 10% of extrapulmonary cases. In bone and joint disease, pathogenesis is related to reactivation of hematogenous foci or to spread from adjacent paravertebral lymph nodes. Weight-bearing joints (spine, hips, and knees—in that order) are affected most commonly. Spinal tuberculosis (Pott's disease or tuberculous spondylitis) often involves two or more adjacent vertebral bodies. While the upper thoracic spine is the most common site of spinal tuberculosis in children, the lower thoracic and upper lumbar vertebrae are usually affected in adults. From the anterior superior or inferior angle of the vertebral body, the lesion reaches the adjacent body, also destroying the intervertebral disk. With advanced disease, collapse of vertebral bodies results in kyphosis (*gibbus*). A paravertebral "cold" abscess may also form. In the upper spine, this abscess may track to the chest wall as a mass; in the lower spine, it may reach the inguinal ligaments or present as a psoas abscess. Computed tomography (CT) or magnetic resonance imaging (MRI) reveals the characteristic lesion and suggests its etiology, although the differential diagnosis includes other infections and tumors. Aspiration of the abscess or bone biopsy confirms the tuberculous etiology, as cultures are usually positive and histologic findings highly typical. A catastrophic complication of Pott's disease is paraplegia, which is usually due to an abscess or a lesion compressing the spinal cord. Paraparesis due to a large abscess is a medical emergency and requires abscess drainage. Tuberculosis of the hip joints causes pain and limping; tuberculosis of the knee produces pain and swelling and sometimes follows trauma. If the disease goes unrecognized, the joints may be destroyed. Skeletal tuberculosis responds to chemotherapy, but severe cases may require surgery.

Tuberculous meningitis and tuberculoma Tuberculosis of the central nervous system accounts for about 5% of extrapulmonary cases. It is seen most often in young children but also develops in adults, especially those who are infected with HIV. Tuberculous meningitis results from the hematogenous spread of primary or postprimary pulmonary disease or from the rupture of a subependymal tubercle into the subarachnoid space. In more than half of cases, evidence of old pulmonary lesions or a miliary pattern is found on chest radiography. The disease may present subtly as headache and mental changes or acutely as confusion, lethargy, altered sensorium, and neck rigidity. Typically, the disease evolves over 1 or 2 weeks, a course longer than that of bacterial meningitis. Paresis of cranial nerves (ocular nerves in particular) is a frequent finding, and the involvement of cerebral arteries may produce focal ischemia. Hydrocephalus is common. Lumbar puncture is the cornerstone of diagnosis. In general, examination of the cerebrospinal fluid (CSF) reveals a high leukocyte count (usually with a predominance of lymphocytes but often with a predominance of neutrophils in the early stage), a protein content of 1 to 8 g/L (100 to 800 mg/dL), and a low glucose concentration; however, any of these three parameters can be within the normal range. AFB are seen on direct smear of CSF sediment in only 20% of cases, but repeated lumbar punctures increase the yield. Culture of CSF is diagnostic in up to 80% of cases. Imaging studies (CT and MRI) may show hydrocephalus and abnormal enhancement of basal cisterns or ependyma. If unrecognized, tuberculous meningitis is uniformly fatal. This disease responds to chemotherapy; however, neurologic sequelae are documented in 25% of treated cases, in most of which the diagnosis has been delayed. Clinical trials have demonstrated that patients treated with adjunctive glucocorticoids experience a significantly faster resolution of CSF abnormalities and elevated CSF pressure. Adjunctive glucocorticoids enhance survival and reduce the frequency of neurologic sequelae.

Tuberculoma, an uncommon manifestation of tuberculosis, presents as one or more space-occupying lesions and usually causes seizures and focal signs. CT or MRI reveals contrast-enhanced ring lesions, but biopsy is necessary to establish the diagnosis.

Gastrointestinal tuberculosis Any portion of the gastrointestinal tract may be affected by tuberculosis. Various pathogenetic mechanisms are involved: swallowing of sputum with direct seeding, hematogenous spread, or (although rarely today) ingestion of milk from cows affected by bovine tuberculosis. The terminal ileum and the cecum are the sites most commonly involved. Abdominal pain (at times similar to that associated with appendicitis), diarrhea, obstruction, hematochezia, and a palpable mass in the abdomen are common findings at presentation. Fever, weight loss, and night sweats are also frequent. With intestinal-wall involvement, ulcerations and fistulae may simulate Crohn's disease. Anal fistulae should prompt an evaluation for rectal tuberculosis. As surgery is required in most cases, the diagnosis can be established by histologic examination and culture of specimens obtained intraoperatively.

Tuberculous peritonitis follows either the direct spread of tubercle bacilli from ruptured lymph nodes and intraabdominal organs or hematogenous seeding. Nonspecific abdominal pain, fever, and ascites should raise the suspicion of tuberculous peritonitis. The coexistence of cirrhosis (Chap. 298) in patients with tuberculous peritonitis complicates the diagnosis. In tuberculous peritonitis, paracentesis reveals an exudative fluid with a high protein content and leukocytosis that is usually lymphocytic (although neutrophils occasionally predominate). The yield of direct smear and culture is relatively low; culture of a large volume of ascitic fluid can increase the yield, but peritoneal biopsy is often needed to establish the diagnosis.

Pericardial tuberculosis (tuberculous pericarditis) Due to direct progression of a primary focus within the pericardium, to reactivation of a latent focus, or to rupture of an adjacent lymph node, pericardial tuberculosis has often been a disease of the elderly in countries with low tuberculosis prevalence but develops frequently in HIV-infected patients. Case-fatality rates are as high as 40% in some series. The onset may be subacute, although an acute presentation, with fever, dull retrosternal pain, and a friction rub, is possible. An effusion eventually develops in many cases; cardiovascular symptoms and signs of cardiac tamponade may ultimately appear (Chap. 239). In the presence of effusion detected on chest radiography, tuberculosis must be suspected if the patient belongs to a high-risk population (HIV-infected, originating in a high-prevalence country), if there is evidence of previous tuberculosis or disease in other organs, or if echocardiography shows thick strands crossing the pericardial space. Diagnosis can be facilitated by pericardiocentesis under echocardiographic guidance. The pericardial fluid must be submitted for biochemical, cytologic, and microbiologic study. The effusion is exudative in nature, with a high count of leukocytes (predominantly mononuclear cells). Hemorrhagic effusion is frequent. Culture of the fluid reveals *M. tuberculosis* in about 30% of cases, while biopsy has a higher yield. Without treatment, pericardial tuberculosis is usually fatal. Even with treatment, complications may develop, including chronic constrictive pericarditis with thickening of the pericardium, fibrosis, and sometimes calcification, which may be visible on a chest radiograph. A course of glucocorticoid treatment is useful in the management of acute disease, reducing effusion, facilitating hemodynamic recovery, and thus decreasing mortality. Progression to chronic constrictive pericarditis, however, seems unaffected by such therapy.

Miliary or disseminated tuberculosis Miliary tuberculosis is due to hematogenous spread of tubercle bacilli. Although in children it is often the consequence of a recent primary infection, in adults it may be due to either recent infection or reactivation of old disseminated foci. Lesions are usually yellowish granulomas 1 to 2 mm in diameter that resemble millet seeds (thus the term *miliary*, coined by nineteenth-century pathologists).

Clinical manifestations are nonspecific and protean, depending on the predominant site of involvement. Fever, night sweats, anorexia, weakness, and weight loss are presenting symptoms in the majority of cases. At times, patients have a cough and other respiratory symptoms due to pulmonary involvement as well as abdominal symptoms. Physical findings include hepatomegaly, splenomegaly, and lymphadenopathy. Eye examination may reveal choroidal tubercles, which are pathognomonic of miliary tuberculosis, in up to 30% of cases. Meningismus occurs in fewer than 10% of cases.

A high index of suspicion is required for the diagnosis of miliary tuberculosis. Frequently, chest radiography reveals a miliary reticulonodular pattern (more easily seen on underpenetrated film), although no radiographic abnormality may be evident early in the course and among HIV-infected patients. Other radiologic findings include large infiltrates, interstitial infiltrates (especially in HIV-infected patients), and pleural effusion. A sputum smear is negative in 80% of cases. Various hematologic abnormalities may be seen, including anemia with leukopenia, neutrophilic leukocytosis and leukemoid reactions, and polycythemia. Disseminated intravascular coagulation has been reported. Elevation of alkaline phosphatase levels and other abnormal values in liver function tests are detected in patients with severe hepatic involvement. The PPD test may be negative in up to half of cases, but reactivity may be restored during chemotherapy. Bronchoalveolar lavage and transbronchial biopsy are more likely to permit bacteriologic confirmation, and granulomas are evident in liver or bone-marrow biopsy specimens from many patients. If it goes unrecognized, miliary tuberculosis is lethal; with proper treatment, however, it is amenable to cure.

A rare presentation seen in the elderly is *cryptic miliary tuberculosis*, which has a chronic course characterized by mild intermittent fever, anemia, and—ultimately—meningeal involvement preceding death. An acute septicemic form, *nonreactive miliary tuberculosis*, occurs very rarely and is due to massive hematogenous dissemination of tubercle bacilli. Pancytopenia is common in this form of disease, which is rapidly fatal. At postmortem examination, multiple necrotic but nongranulomatous ("nonreactive") lesions are detected.

Less common extrapulmonary forms Tuberculosis may cause chorioretinitis, uveitis, panophthalmitis, and painful hypersensitivity-related phlyctenular conjunctivitis. Tuberculous otitis is rare and presents as hearing loss, otorrhea, and tympanic membrane perforation. In the nasopharynx, tuberculosis may simulate Wegener's granulomatosis. Cutaneous manifestations of tuberculosis include primary infection due to direct inoculation, abscesses and chronic ulcers, scrofuloderma, lupus vulgaris, miliary lesions, and erythema nodosum. Adrenal tuberculosis is a manifestation of advanced disease presenting as signs of adrenal insufficiency. Finally, congenital tuberculosis results from transplacental spread of tubercle bacilli to the fetus or from ingestion of contaminated amniotic fluid. This rare disease affects the liver, spleen, lymph nodes, and various other organs.

HIV-Associated Tuberculosis Tuberculosis is an important opportunistic disease among HIV-infected persons worldwide. In developing countries of Africa, Southeast Asia, and Latin America, an estimated 10 million persons were coinfected as of 1997. In the United States, coinfection with HIV and *M. tuberculosis* is common in certain segments of the population, including drug users and some minorities. A person with skin test–documented *M. tuberculosis* infection who acquires HIV infection has a 3 to 15% annual risk of developing active tuberculosis.

The association between tuberculosis and HIV infection is supported by other epidemiologic observations. First, the rate of HIV seropositivity among patients with tuberculosis is several times higher than that among the general population: in African countries it reaches 60 to 70%. Second, marked increases in numbers of tuberculosis cases have been reported at locations hard hit by the HIV epidemic, such as large parts of Africa (including Kenya, Tanzania, and Malawi), northern Thailand, and New York City. Globally, the proportion of tuberculosis cases associated with HIV infection reached 8% in 1997.

HIV directly attacks the critical immune mechanisms involved in protection against tuberculosis. Tuberculosis can appear at any stage of HIV infection, but its presentation varies with the stage. When cell-mediated immunity is only partially compromised, pulmonary tuberculosis presents as a typical pattern of upper lobe infiltrates and cavitation, without significant lymphadenopathy or pleural effusion. In late stages of HIV infection, a primary tuberculosis–like pattern, with diffuse interstitial or miliary infiltrates, little or no cavitation, and intrathoracic lymphadenopathy, is more common. Overall, sputum smears may be positive less frequently among tuberculosis patients with HIV infection than among those without; thus the diagnosis of tuberculosis may be unusually difficult, especially in view of the variety of HIV-related pulmonary conditions mimicking tuberculosis.

As has been mentioned, extrapulmonary tuberculosis is common among HIV-infected patients. In various series studied in the United States and many developing countries, extrapulmonary tuberculosis—alone or in association with pulmonary disease—has been documented in 40 to 60% of all cases in HIV co-infected individuals. The most common forms are lymphatic, disseminated, pleural, and pericardial. Mycobacteremia and meningitis are also frequent, particularly in advanced HIV disease.

The diagnosis of tuberculosis in HIV-infected patients may be difficult not only because of the increased frequency of sputum-smear negativity (up to 40% in culture-proven pulmonary cases) but also because of atypical radiographic findings, a lack of classic granuloma formation in the late stages, and negative results in PPD skin tests. Delays in treatment may prove fatal. The response to short-course chemotherapy is similar to that in HIV-seronegative patients. However, adverse effects may be more pronounced, including severe or even fatal skin reactions to amithiozone (thiacetazone).

Exacerbations in symptoms, signs, and laboratory or radiographic manifestations of tuberculosis—termed *paradoxical reactions*—have been associated with the administration of highly active antiretroviral treatment (HAART) regimens. The presumed pathogenesis of paradoxical reactions is an immune response to antigens released as bacilli are killed by effective chemotherapy. In patients in whom antiretroviral therapy has recently been started, paradoxical reactions may be due to improving immune function. The first priority in the management of a possible paradoxical reaction is to ensure that the clinical syndrome does not represent a failure of tuberculosis treatment or the development of another infection. Mild paradoxical reactions can be managed with symptom-based treatment. More severe manifestations may necessitate discontinuation of antiretroviral therapy. Immuno-modulators, such as glucocorticoids, have been used to treat severe paradoxical reactions, although this practice has not been formally evaluated in clinical trials.

Recommendations for the prevention and treatment of tuberculosis in HIV-infected individuals have been published by the CDC.

DIAGNOSIS The key to the diagnosis of tuberculosis is a high index of suspicion. Diagnosis is not difficult with a high-risk patient—e.g., a homeless alcoholic who presents with typical symptoms and a classic chest radiograph showing upper lobe infiltrates with cavities. On the other hand, the diagnosis can easily be missed in an elderly nursing-home resident or a teenager with a focal infiltrate.

Often, the diagnosis is first entertained when the chest radiograph of a patient being evaluated for respiratory symptoms is abnormal. If the patient has no complicating medical conditions that favor immu-nosuppression, the chest radiograph may show the typical picture of upper lobe infiltrates with cavitation. The longer the delay between the onset of symptoms and the diagnosis, the more likely is the finding of cavitary disease. In contrast, immunosuppressed patients, including those with HIV infection, may have "atypical" findings on chest ra-diography—e.g., lower zone infiltrates without cavity formation.

AFB Microscopy A presumptive diagnosis is commonly based on the finding of AFB on microscopic examination of a diagnostic specimen such as a smear of expectorated sputum or of tissue (for example, a lymph node biopsy). Most modern laboratories processing large numbers of diagnostic specimens use auramine-rhodamine stain-ing and fluorescence microscopy. The more traditional method—light microscopy of specimens stained with Kinyoun or Ziehl-Neelsen basic fuchsin dyes—is satisfactory, although more time-consuming. For pa-tients with suspected pulmonary tuberculosis, three sputum specimens, preferably collected early in the morning, should be submitted to the laboratory for AFB smear and mycobacteriology culture. If tissue is obtained, it is critical that the portion of the specimen intended for culture not be put in formaldehyde. The use of AFB microscopy on urine or gastric lavage fluid is limited by the presence of mycobacterial commensals, which can cause false-positive results.

Mycobacterial Culture Definitive diagnosis depends on the iso-lation and identification of *M. tuberculosis* from a diagnostic speci-men—in most cases, a sputum specimen obtained from a patient with a productive cough. Specimens may be inoculated onto egg- or agar-based medium (e.g., Löwenstein-Jensen or Middlebrook 7H10) and incubated at 37°C under 5% CO_2. Because most species of mycobac-teria, including *M. tuberculosis*, grow slowly, 4 to 8 weeks may be required before growth is detected. Although *M. tuberculosis* may be presumptively identified on the basis of growth time and colony pig-mentation and morphology, a variety of biochemical tests have tradi-tionally been used to speciate mycobacterial isolates. In today's lab-oratories, the use of liquid media with radiometric growth detection (e.g., BACTEC-460) and the identification of isolates by nucleic acid probes or high-pressure liquid chromatography of mycolic acids have replaced the traditional methods of isolation on solid media and iden-tification by biochemical tests. These new methods have decreased the time required for isolation and speciation to 2 to 3 weeks. Other sys-tems for culture on liquid media with nonradiometric detection have become available.

Nucleic Acid Amplification Several test systems based on am-plification of mycobacterial nucleic acid are available. These systems permit the diagnosis of tuberculosis in as short a period as several hours. However, their applicability is limited by low sensitivity (lower than culture) and high cost. At present, these tests are approved by the U.S. Food and Drug Administration only for species identification on AFB-positive sputa. With further improvements in performance, these tests may also be useful for the diagnosis of patients with AFB-neg-ative pulmonary and extrapulmonary tuberculosis.

Radiographic Procedures As noted above, the initial suspicion of pulmonary tuberculosis is often based on abnormal chest radio-graphic findings in a patient with respiratory symptoms. Although the "classic" picture is that of upper lobe disease with infiltrates and cav-ities, virtually any radiographic pattern—from a normal film or a sol-itary pulmonary nodule to diffuse alveolar infiltrates in a patient with ARDS—may be seen. In the era of AIDS, no radiographic pattern can be considered pathognomonic.

PPD Skin Testing Skin testing with PPD is most widely used in screening for *M. tuberculosis* infection (see below). The test is of limited value in the diagnosis of active tuberculosis because of its low sensitivity and specificity. False-negative reactions are common in im-munosuppressed patients and in those with overwhelming tuberculo-sis. Positive reactions are obtained when patients have been infected with *M. tuberculosis* but do not have active disease and when persons have been sensitized by nontuberculous mycobacteria (Chap. 171) or bacille Calmette-Guérin (BCG) vaccination. Although BCG vaccine is not commonly used in the United States, many immigrants will have received it. In the absence of a history of BCG vaccination, a positive skin test may provide additional support for the diagnosis of tuber-culosis in culture-negative cases.

Drug Susceptibility Testing In general, the initial isolate of *M. tuberculosis* should be tested for susceptibility to the primary drugs used for treatment: isoniazid, rifampin, ethambutol, pyrazinamide, and streptomycin. In addition, drug susceptibility tests are mandatory when patients fail to respond to initial therapy or experience a relapse after the completion of treatment (see below). Susceptibility testing may be conducted directly (with the clinical specimen) or indirectly (with my-cobacterial cultures) on solid or liquid medium. Results are obtained most rapidly by direct susceptibility testing on liquid medium, with an average reporting time of 3 weeks. With indirect testing on solid media, results may not be available for 8 weeks or longer. Molecular methods for the rapid identification of drug resistance are becoming available. One of the most promising uses polymerase chain reaction (PCR) for the *rpoB* gene to detect resistance to rifampin.

Additional Diagnostic Procedures Other diagnostic tests may be used when pulmonary tuberculosis is suspected. Sputum induction by ultrasonic nebulization of hypertonic saline may be useful for pa-tients unable to produce a sputum specimen spontaneously. Fre-quently, patients with radiographic abnormalities that are consistent with other diagnoses (e.g., bronchogenic carcinoma) undergo fiber-optic bronchoscopy with bronchial brushings or transbronchial biopsy of the lesion. Bronchoalveolar lavage of a lung segment containing an abnormality may also be performed. In all cases, it is essential that specimens be submitted for AFB smear and mycobacterial culture. For the diagnosis of primary pulmonary tuberculosis in children, who often do not expectorate sputum, specimens from early-morning gastric lav-age may yield positive cultures.

Invasive diagnostic procedures are indicated for patients with sus-pected extrapulmonary tuberculosis. In addition to specimens of in-volved sites (e.g., CSF for tuberculous meningitis, pleural fluid and biopsy samples for pleural disease), bone marrow and liver biopsy and culture have a good diagnostic yield in disseminated (miliary) tuber-culosis, particularly in HIV-infected patients, who also have a high frequency of positive blood cultures.

In some cases, cultures will be negative, but a clinical diagnosis of tuberculosis will be supported by consistent epidemiologic evidence (e.g., a history of close contact with an infectious patient), a positive PPD skin test, and a compatible clinical and radiographic response to treatment. In the United States and other industrialized countries with low rates of tuberculosis, some patients with limited abnormalities on chest radiographs and sputum positive for AFB are infected with or-ganisms of the *M. avium* complex or *M. kansasii* (Chap. 171). Factors favoring the diagnosis of nontuberculous mycobacterial disease over tuberculosis include an absence of risk factors for tuberculosis, a neg-ative PPD skin test, and underlying chronic obstructive pulmonary disease.

Patients with HIV-associated tuberculosis pose several diagnostic problems, as noted above in the description of clinical manifestations. Moreover, HIV-infected patients with sputum culture–positive and AFB-positive tuberculosis may present with a normal chest radiograph. Thus, in a patient with HIV infection, the finding of a normal chest radiograph does not rule out the diagnosis of pulmonary tuberculosis. An additional consideration is that, among relatively severely immunosuppressed AIDS patients in Europe and North America, *M. avium* complex disease is more common than tuberculosis, usually presenting as a disseminated disease without pulmonary parenchymal involvement.

Adjunctive Diagnostic Tests A number of methods have been evaluated as adjuncts to standard laboratory diagnosis. The most thoroughly investigated is serologic diagnosis based on detection of antibody to a variety of mycobacterial antigens. However, tests with most of the target antigens have a low predictive value when used in a population with a presumably low probability of disease. Tests aimed at detection of mycobacterial antigen by serologic methods have generally not been sufficiently sensitive to be useful. Nonspecific tests, such as the measurement of adenine deaminase in pleural fluid, have been evaluated but have not gained acceptance.

℞ **TREATMENT** Chemotherapy for tuberculosis became possible with the discovery of streptomycin in the mid-1940s. Randomized clinical trials clearly indicated that the administration of streptomycin to patients with chronic tuberculosis reduced mortality and led to cure in the majority of cases. However, monotherapy with streptomycin was frequently associated with the development of resistance to streptomycin and the attendant failure of treatment. With the discovery of para-aminosalicylic acid (PAS) and isoniazid, it became axiomatic that cure of tuberculosis required the concomitant administration of at least two agents to which the organism was susceptible. Furthermore, early clinical trials demonstrated that a long period of treatment—i.e., 12 to 24 months—was required to prevent the recurrence of tuberculosis.

The introduction of rifampin in the early 1970s heralded the era of effective short-course chemotherapy, with a treatment duration of <12 months. The discovery that pyrazinamide, which was first used in the 1950s, augmented the potency of isoniazid/rifampin regimens led to the use of a 6-month course of this triple-drug regimen as standard therapy.

Drugs Five major drugs are considered the first-line agents for the treatment of tuberculosis: isoniazid, rifampin, pyrazinamide, ethambutol, and streptomycin (Table 169-1). The first four, which are usually given orally, are well absorbed, with peak serum levels at 2 to 4 h and nearly complete elimination within 24 h. These agents are recommended on the basis of their bactericidal activity (ability to rapidly reduce the number of viable organisms), their sterilizing activity (ability to kill all bacilli and thus sterilize the affected organ, measured in terms of the ability to prevent relapses), and their low rate of induction of drug resistance. Rifapentine and rifabutin, two drugs related to rifampin, are also available in the United States. →*For a detailed discussion of the drugs used for the treatment of tuberculosis, see Chap. 168.*

Because of a lower degree of efficacy and a higher degree of intolerability and toxicity, a num-

Table 169-1 Dosage Recommendations for Initial Treatment of Tuberculosis in Adults[a]

Drug	Dosage	
	Daily	Thrice Weekly[b]
Isoniazid	5 mg/kg, max. 300 mg	15 mg/kg, max. 900 mg
Rifampin	10 mg/kg, max. 600 mg	10 mg/kg, max. 600 mg
Pyrazinamide	15–30 mg/kg, max. 2 g	50–70 mg/kg, max. 3 g
Ethambutol	15–25 mg/kg	25–30 mg/kg
Streptomycin	15 mg/kg, max. 1 g	25–30 mg/kg, max. 1.5 g

[a] Dosages for children are similar, except that some authorities recommend higher doses of isoniazid (10–20 mg/kg daily; 20–40 mg/kg intermittent) and rifampin (10–20 mg/kg).
[b] Dosages for twice-weekly administration are the same, except for pyrazinamide (maximum, 4 g/d) and ethambutol (50 mg/kg).
SOURCE: Based on recommendations of the American Thoracic Society, Am J Respir Crit Care Med 149:1359, 1994, and the Centers for Disease Control, 1994.

ber of second-line drugs are used only for the treatment of patients with tuberculosis resistant to first-line drugs. Included in this group are the injectable drugs kanamycin, amikacin, and capreomycin and the oral agents ethionamide, cycloserine, and PAS. Recently, quinolone antibiotics have become the most commonly used second-line drugs. Of available agents, ofloxacin is the most widely used, but levofloxacin and sparfloxacin are the most active, although the latter drug is associated with high rates of photosensitization. Other second-line drugs include clofazimine, amithiozone (thiacetazone, widely used with isoniazid in less wealthy countries but not marketed in North America or Europe), and amoxicillin/clavulanic acid.

Regimens Short-course regimens are divided into an initial or bactericidal phase and a continuation or sterilizing phase. During the initial phase, the majority of the tubercle bacilli are killed, symptoms resolve, and the patient becomes noninfectious. The continuation phase is required to eliminate semidormant "persisters."

The treatment regimen of choice for virtually all forms of tuberculosis in both adults and children consists of a 2-month initial phase of isoniazid, rifampin, and pyrazinamide followed by a 4-month continuation phase of isoniazid and rifampin (Table 169-2). Except for patients who seem unlikely on epidemiologic grounds to be initially infected with a drug-resistant strain, ethambutol (or streptomycin)

Table 169-2 Recommended Regimens for the Treatment of Tuberculosis

Indication	Initial Phase		Continuation Phase	
	Duration, Months	Drugs	Duration, Months	Drugs
New smear- or culture-positive case	2	HRZE[a]	4	HR[a]
New culture-negative case	2	HRZE[a]	2 (or 4)	HR[a]
Pregnancy[b]	2	HRE	7	HR
Failure and relapse[c]	—		—	
Standardized re-treatment (susceptibility testing unavailable)	3	HRZES[d]	5	HRE
Resistance to H + R	Throughout (12–18)	ZE + Q + S (or another injectable agent[e])	—	—
Resistance to all first-line drugs	Throughout (24)	1 injectable agent[e] + 3 of these 4: ethionamide, cycloserine, Q, PAS	—	—
Intolerance or resistance to H	2[f]	RZE[f]	7	RE
Intolerance to R	2	HES(Z)	16	HE
Intolerance to Z	2	HRE	7	HR

[a] All drugs can be given daily or intermittently (three times weekly throughout or twice weekly after an initial phase of daily therapy).
[b] See also Table 168-1.
[c] Regimen is tailored according to the results of drug susceptibility tests.
[d] Streptomycin treatment should be discontinued after 2 months.
[e] Amikacin, kanamycin, or capreomycin. Treatment with all of these agents should be discontinued after 2 to 6 months, depending upon the patient's tolerance and response.
[f] RZE can be used throughout (for 6 months).
NOTE: H, isoniazid; R, rifampin; Z, pyrazinamide; E, ethambutol; S, streptomycin; Q, quinolone; PAS, para-aminosalicylic acid.

should be included in the regimen for the first 2 months or until the results of drug susceptibility testing become available. Treatment may be given daily throughout the course or intermittently (either three times weekly throughout the course or twice weekly following an initial phase of daily therapy). A continuation phase of once-weekly rifapentine and isoniazid appears to be effective for patients who have adhered to the initial-phase treatment and have negative sputum cultures at 2 months. Intermittent treatment is especially useful for patients whose therapy is being directly observed (see below). For patients with sputum culture–negative pulmonary tuberculosis, the duration of treatment may be reduced to a total of 4 months. Pyridoxine (10 to 25 mg/d) should be added to the regimen given to persons at high risk of vitamin deficiency (e.g., alcoholics; malnourished persons; pregnant and lactating women; and patients with conditions such as chronic renal failure, diabetes, and HIV infection or AIDS, which are also associated with neuropathy).

Lack of adherence to treatment regimens is recognized worldwide as the most important impediment to cure. Moreover, the mycobacterial strains infecting patients who do not adhere to the prescribed regimen are especially likely to develop acquired drug resistance. Both patient- and provider-related factors may affect compliance. Patient-related factors include a lack of belief that the illness is significant and/or that treatment will have a beneficial effect; the existence of concomitant medical conditions (notably substance abuse); lack of social support; and poverty, with attendant joblessness and homelessness. Provider-related factors that may promote compliance include the education and encouragement of patients, the offering of convenient clinic hours, and the provision of incentives such as bus tokens.

In addition to specific measures addressing noncompliance, two other strategic approaches are used: direct observation of treatment and provision of drugs in combined formulations. Because it is difficult to predict which patients will adhere to the recommended treatment, all patients should have their therapy directly supervised, especially during the initial phase. In the United States, personnel to supervise therapy are usually available through tuberculosis control programs of local public health departments. Supervision increases the proportion of patients completing treatment and greatly lessens the chances of relapse and acquired drug resistance. Combination products (e.g., isoniazid/rifampin and isoniazid/rifampin/pyrazinamide) are available and are strongly recommended as a means of minimizing the likelihood of prescription error and of the development of drug resistance (as the result of treatment with only one agent). In some formulations of these combination products, the bioavailability of rifampin has been found to be substandard. In North America and Europe, regulatory authorities ensure that combination products are of good quality; however, this type of monitoring cannot be assumed to take place in less affluent countries. Alternative regimens for patients who exhibit drug intolerance or adverse reactions are listed in Table 169-2. However, severe side effects prompting discontinuation of any of the first-line drugs and use of these alternative regimens are uncommon.

Monitoring the Response to Treatment   Bacteriologic evaluation is the preferred method of monitoring the response to treatment for tuberculosis. Patients with pulmonary disease should have their sputum examined monthly until cultures become negative. With the recommended 6-month regimen, more than 80% of patients will have negative sputum cultures at the end of the second month of treatment. By the end of the third month, virtually all patients should be culture-negative. In some patients, especially those with extensive cavitary disease and large numbers of organisms, AFB smear conversion may follow culture conversion. This phenomenon is presumably due to the expectoration and microscopic visualization of dead bacilli. When a patient's sputum cultures remain positive at or beyond 3 months, treatment failure and drug resistance should be suspected (see below). A sputum specimen should be collected at the end of treatment to document cure. If mycobacterial cultures are not practical, then monitoring by AFB smear examination should be undertaken at 2, 5, and 6 months. Smears positive after 5 months are indicative of treatment failure.

Bacteriologic monitoring of patients with extrapulmonary tuberculosis is more difficult and often is not feasible. In these cases, the response to treatment must be assessed clinically.

Monitoring of the response to treatment during chemotherapy by serial chest radiographs is not recommended, as radiographic changes may lag behind bacteriologic response and are not highly sensitive. After the completion of treatment, neither sputum examination nor chest radiography is recommended for follow-up purposes. However, a chest radiograph may be obtained at the end of treatment and used for comparative purposes should the patient develop symptoms of recurrent tuberculosis months or years later. Patients should be instructed to report promptly for medical assessment should they develop any such symptoms.

During treatment, patients should be monitored for drug toxicity (see also Table 168-3). The most common adverse reaction of significance is hepatitis. Patients should be carefully educated about the signs and symptoms of drug-induced hepatitis (e.g., dark urine, loss of appetite) and should be instructed to discontinue treatment promptly and see their health care provider should these symptoms occur. Although biochemical monitoring is not routinely recommended, all adult patients should undergo baseline assessment of liver function (e.g., measurement of levels of hepatic aminotransferases and serum bilirubin). Older patients, those with histories of hepatic disease, and those using alcohol daily should be monitored especially closely (i.e., monthly), with repeated measurements of aminotransferases, during the initial phase of treatment. Up to 20% of patients have small increases in aspartate aminotransferase (up to three times the upper limit of normal) that are accompanied by no symptoms and are of no consequence. For patients with symptomatic hepatitis and those with marked (five- to sixfold) elevations in aspartate aminotransferase, treatment should be stopped and drugs reintroduced one at a time after liver function has returned to normal.

Hypersensitivity reactions usually require the discontinuation of all drugs and rechallenge to determine which agent is the culprit. Because of the variety of regimens available, it is usually not necessary—although it is possible—to desensitize patients. Hyperuricemia and arthralgia caused by pyrazinamide can usually be managed by the administration of acetylsalicylic acid; however, pyrazinamide treatment should be stopped if the patient develops gouty arthritis. Individuals who develop autoimmune thrombocytopenia secondary to rifampin therapy should not receive the drug thereafter. Similarly, the occurrence of optic neuritis with ethambutol and the development of eighth-nerve damage with streptomycin are indications for permanent discontinuation of these respective drugs. Other common manifestations of drug intolerance, such as pruritus and gastrointestinal upset, can generally be managed without the interruption of therapy.

Treatment Failure and Relapse   As stated above, treatment failure should be suspected when a patient's sputum cultures remain positive after 3 months or when AFB smears remain positive after 5 months. In the management of such patients, it is imperative that the current isolate be tested for susceptibility to first- and second-line agents. When the results of susceptibility testing are expected to become available within a few weeks, changes in the regimen can be postponed until that time. However, if the patient's clinical condition is deteriorating, an earlier change in regimen may be indicated. A cardinal rule in the latter situation is always to add more than one drug at a time to a failing regimen: at least two and preferably three drugs that have never been used should be added. The patient may continue to take isoniazid and rifampin along with these new agents pending the results of susceptibility tests.

The mycobacterial strains infecting patients who experience a relapse after apparently successful treatment are less likely to have acquired drug resistance (see below) than are strains from patients in whom treatment has failed. However, if the regimen administered initially does not contain rifampin (and thus is not a short-course regimen), the probability of isoniazid resistance is high. Acquired resistance is uncommon among strains from patients who relapse after completing a short course of therapy. However, it is prudent to begin the treatment of all relapses with all five first-line drugs pending the results of susceptibility testing. In less affluent countries and other settings where facilities for culture and drug susceptibility testing are not available, a standard regimen should be used in all instances of relapse and treatment failure (Table 169-2).

Adjunctive Glucocorticoid Therapy The use of glucocorticoids for adjunctive treatment of tuberculosis is justified by their potent anti-inflammatory activity in a disease where host response plays a major role. There is a sound basis for using glucocorticoids in tuberculous meningitis and pericarditis to hasten clinical improvement (see above). Long-term benefits are limited to reduced mortality in effusive-constrictive pericarditis and decreased neurologic sequelae in meningitis. Studies have indicated that the usefulness of these agents in pleuritis may be less important than previously thought. There is not yet conclusive evidence that glucocorticoids produce benefits in patients with acute life-threatening pulmonary tuberculosis, including ARDS. In general, depending upon the urgency and severity of clinical conditions, prednisone may be administered at a daily dose of 20 to 60 mg for up to 6 weeks. In meningitis, dexamethasone (up to 12 mg/d) is the preferred drug; therapy continues for 4 to 6 weeks, with gradual tapering of the dose after the first 2 weeks. Rifampin interaction with glucocorticoids, resulting in accelerated metabolism and potential adrenal crisis, must be taken into account. Caution should be exercised in the use of glucocorticoids in HIV-infected patients.

Drug-Resistant Tuberculosis Strains of *M. tuberculosis* resistant to individual drugs arise by spontaneous point mutations in the mycobacterial genome, which occur at low but predictable rates. Because there is no cross-resistance among the commonly used drugs, the probability that a strain will be resistant to two drugs is the product of the probabilities of resistance to each drug and thus is low. The development of drug-resistant tuberculosis is invariably the result of monotherapy—i.e., the failure of the health care provider to prescribe at least two drugs to which tubercle bacilli are susceptible or of the patient to take properly prescribed therapy.

Drug-resistant tuberculosis may be either primary or acquired. *Primary* drug resistance is that in a strain infecting a patient who has not previously been treated. *Acquired* resistance develops during treatment with an inappropriate regimen. In North America and Europe, rates of primary resistance are generally low, and isoniazid resistance is most common. In the United States, while isoniazid resistance was stable at about 8% in 1993 through 1996, rates of MDR tuberculosis were declining. Resistance rates are higher among foreign-born and HIV-infected patients. Worldwide, MDR tuberculosis is a serious problem in some regions, especially in the former USSR and parts of Asia. As noted above, drug-resistant tuberculosis can be prevented by adherence to the principles of sound therapy: the inclusion of at least two bactericidal drugs to which the organism is susceptible (in practice, four drugs are commonly given in the initial phase) and the verification that patients complete the prescribed course.

Although the 6-month regimen described in Table 169-2 is highly effective for patients with initial isoniazid-resistant disease, it is prudent to extend treatment to 9 months and to include ethambutol throughout. Alternatively, rifampin, pyrazinamide, and ethambutol may be given for 6 months. For disease with high-level isoniazid resistance, isoniazid probably does not contribute to a successful outcome and can be omitted. MDR tuberculosis is more difficult to manage than is disease caused by a drug-susceptible organism, especially because resistance to other first-line drugs as well as to isoniazid and rifampin is common. For strains resistant to isoniazid and rifampin, combinations of ethambutol, pyrazinamide, and streptomycin (or, for those resistant to streptomycin as well, another injectable agent such as amikacin), given for 12 to 18 months in all and for at least 9 months after sputum culture conversion, may be effective. Many authorities would add a quinolone antibiotic to this regimen. For patients with bacilli resistant to all of the first-line agents, cure may be attained with a combination of four second-line drugs, including one injectable agent

(Table 169-2). The optimal duration of treatment in this situation is not known; however, a duration of up to 24 months is recommended. For patients with localized disease and sufficient pulmonary reserve, lobectomy or pneumonectomy may be helpful. Because the management of patients with MDR tuberculosis is complicated by both social and medical factors, care of these patients should be restricted to specialists and tuberculosis control programs.

Special Clinical Situations Although comparative clinical trials of treatment for extrapulmonary tuberculosis are limited, the available evidence indicates that most forms of disease can be treated with the 6-month regimen recommended for patients with pulmonary disease. The American Academy of Pediatrics recommends that children with bone and joint tuberculosis, tuberculous meningitis, or miliary tuberculosis receive a minimum of 12 months of treatment.

Treatment for tuberculosis may be complicated by underlying medical problems that require special consideration (see also Table 168-1). As a rule, patients with chronic renal failure should not receive aminoglycosides and should receive ethambutol only if serum levels can be monitored. Isoniazid, rifampin, and pyrazinamide may be given in the usual doses in cases of mild to moderate renal failure, but the dosages of isoniazid and pyrazinamide should be reduced for all patients with severe renal failure except those undergoing hemodialysis. Patients with hepatic disease pose a special problem because of the hepatotoxicity of isoniazid, rifampin, and pyrazinamide. Patients with severe hepatic disease may be treated with ethambutol and streptomycin and, if required, with isoniazid and rifampin under close supervision. The use of pyrazinamide by patients with liver failure should be avoided. Silicotuberculosis necessitates the extension of therapy by at least 2 months. Patients with HIV infection or AIDS appear to respond well to standard 6-month therapy, although treatment may need to be prolonged if the response is suboptimal. Rifampin, a powerful inducer of hepatic microsomal enzymes, shortens the half-life of HIV protease inhibitors and therefore is contraindicated for patients receiving these drugs; instead, these individuals should be given rifabutin (150 mg/d or 300 mg twice weekly) with either indinavir or nelfinavir. Studies have shown that total systemic drug exposure, especially for rifampin, is reduced in HIV-infected patients because of decreased bioavailability secondary to malabsorption. The clinical importance of this phenomenon remains unclear.

The regimen of choice for pregnant women (see also Table 168-1) is 9 months of treatment with isoniazid and rifampin supplemented by ethambutol for the first 2 months. When required, pyrazinamide may be given, although there are no data concerning its safety in pregnancy. Streptomycin is contraindicated because it is known to cause eighth-cranial-nerve damage in the fetus. Treatment for tuberculosis is not a contraindication to breast feeding; most of the drugs administered will be present in small quantities in breast milk, albeit at concentrations far too low to provide any therapeutic or prophylactic benefit to the child.

PREVENTION By far the best way to prevent tuberculosis is to diagnose infectious cases rapidly and administer appropriate treatment until cure. Additional strategies include BCG vaccination and preventive chemotherapy.

BCG Vaccination BCG was derived from an attenuated strain of *M. bovis* and was first administered to humans in 1921. Many BCG vaccines are available worldwide; all are derived from the original strain, but the vaccines vary in efficacy. In fact, estimates of efficacy from randomized, placebo-controlled trials have ranged from 80% to nil. A similar range of efficacy was found in recent observational studies (case-control, historic cohort, and cross-sectional) in areas where infants are vaccinated at birth. These studies also found higher rates of efficacy in the protection of infants and young children from relatively serious forms of tuberculosis, such as tuberculous meningitis and miliary tuberculosis.

BCG vaccine is safe and rarely causes serious complications. The local tissue response begins 2 to 3 weeks after vaccination, with scar formation and healing within 3 months. Side effects—most commonly, ulceration at the vaccination site and regional lymphadenitis—occur in 1 to 10% of vaccinated persons. Some vaccine strains have caused osteomyelitis in approximately one case per million doses administered. Disseminated BCG infection and death have occurred in 1 to 10 cases per 10 million doses administered, although this problem is restricted almost exclusively to persons with impaired immunity, such as children with severe combined immunodeficiency syndrome (SCIDS) or adults with HIV infection. BCG vaccination induces PPD reactivity, which tends to wane with time. The presence or size of PPD skin-test reactions after vaccination does not predict the degree of protection afforded.

BCG vaccine is recommended for routine use at birth in countries with high tuberculosis prevalence. However, because of the low risk of transmission of tuberculosis in the United States and the unreliable protection afforded by BCG, the vaccine has never been recommended for general use in the United States. Currently, vaccination should be considered for PPD-negative infants and children who reside in settings where the likelihood of *M. tuberculosis* transmission and subsequent infection is high, provided no other measures can be implemented (e.g., removing the child from the source of infection). BCG vaccination may also be considered for health care workers who are employed in settings where the risk of infection by MDR strains is high despite implementation of comprehensive tuberculosis control measures. The CDC has recommended that HIV-infected adults and children not receive BCG vaccine, although the WHO has recommended that asymptomatic HIV-infected children residing in tuberculosis-endemic areas receive BCG.

Treatment of Latent Tuberculosis Infection   A major component of tuberculosis control in the United States is the treatment of selected persons with latent tuberculosis infection to prevent active disease. This intervention (formerly called preventive chemotherapy or chemoprophylaxis) is based on the results of a large number of randomized, placebo-controlled clinical trials demonstrating that a 6- to 12-month course of isoniazid reduces the risk of active tuberculosis in infected people by ≥90%. Analysis of available data indicates that the optimal duration of treatment is 9 to 10 months. In the absence of reinfection, the protective effect is believed to be lifelong. Clinical trials have also shown that isoniazid reduces rates of tuberculosis among PPD-positive persons with HIV infection. Studies in HIV-infected patients have demonstrated the effectiveness of a shorter course of rifampin-based treatment.

In most cases, candidates for treatment of latent tuberculosis (Table 169-3) are identified by PPD skin testing of persons in defined high-risk groups. For skin testing, 5 tuberculin units of polysorbate-stabilized PPD should be injected intradermally into the volar surface of the forearm (Mantoux method). Multipuncture tests, which may be useful for screening large populations, are not recommended for this purpose; any positive reaction to a multipuncture test must be confirmed by Mantoux testing. Reactions are read at 48 to 72 h as the transverse diameter in millimeters of induration; the diameter of erythema is not considered. In some persons, PPD reactivity wanes with time but can be recalled by a second skin test administered 1 week or more after the first (i.e., two-step testing). For persons undergoing periodic PPD skin testing, such as health care workers and individuals admitted to long-term-care institutions, initial two-step testing may preclude subsequent misclassification of persons with boosted reactions as PPD converters.

The cutoff for a positive skin test (and thus for treatment) is related both to the probability that the reaction represents true infection and to the likelihood that the individual, if truly infected, will develop tuberculosis (Table 169-3). Thus positive reactions for close contacts of infectious cases, persons with HIV infection, and previously untreated persons whose chest radiograph is consistent with healed tuberculosis are defined as an area of induration 5 mm in diameter. A

Table 169-3   Tuberculin Reaction Size and Treatment of Latent Tuberculosis Infection

Risk Group	Tuberculin Reaction, mm
HIV-infected persons	≥5
Close contacts of tuberculosis patients	≥5[a]
Persons with fibrotic lesions on chest radiography	≥5
Recently infected persons (≤2 years)	≥10
Persons with high-risk medical conditions[b]	≥10
High-risk group, <35 years of age[c]	≥10
Low-risk group, <35 years of age[d]	≥15

[a] Tuberculin-negative contacts, especially children, should receive prophylaxis for 2 to 3 months after contact ends and should then be retested with PPD. Those whose results remain negative should discontinue prophylaxis. HIV-infected contacts should receive a full course of treatment regardless of PPD results.

[b] Includes diabetes mellitus, prolonged therapy with systemic glucocorticoids, other immunosuppressive therapy, some hematologic and reticuloendothelial diseases, injection drug use (with HIV seronegativity), end-stage renal disease, and clinical situations associated with rapid weight loss.

[c] Includes persons born in high-prevalence countries, members of medically underserved low-income populations, and residents of long-term-care facilities.

[d] Decision to treat should be based on individual considerations of risk/benefit.

10-mm cutoff is used to define positive reactions in most other at-risk persons. For persons with a very low risk of developing tuberculosis if infected, a cutoff of 15 mm is used. Persons with a history of BCG vaccination may receive treatment, especially if BCG was given many years before.

Some PPD-negative individuals are also candidates for treatment. Infants and children who have come into contact with infectious cases should be treated and should have a repeat skin test 2 or 3 months after contact ends. Those whose test results remain negative should discontinue treatment. HIV-infected persons who have been exposed to an infectious tuberculosis patient should receive treatment regardless of the PPD test result.

Isoniazid is administered at a daily dose of 5 mg/kg (up to 300 mg/d) for 9 months. On the basis of cost-benefit analyses, a 6-month period of treatment has been recommended in the past and may be considered for HIV-negative adults with normal chest radiographs when financial considerations are important. When supervised treatment is desirable and feasible, isoniazid may be given at a dose of 15 mg/kg (up to 900 mg) twice weekly. There are two recommended alternative regimens for adults: 2 months of daily rifampin plus pyrazinamide and 4 months of daily rifampin. Although the 2-month regimen may be associated with increased drug intolerance, it may be useful in situations where long courses of isoniazid have not been feasible (e.g., jails). Either regimen should be considered for persons who are likely to have been infected with an isoniazid-resistant strain.

Contraindications to treatment with isoniazid and pyrazinamide include active liver disease. Since the major adverse reaction to these drugs is hepatitis, persons at increased risk of toxicity (e.g., those abusing alcohol daily and those with a history of liver disease) should undergo baseline and then monthly assessment of liver function during treatment. All patients should be carefully educated about hepatitis and instructed to discontinue use of the drug immediately should any symptoms develop. Moreover, patients should be seen and questioned monthly during therapy about adverse reactions and should be given no more than 1 month's supply of drug at each visit.

It may be more difficult to ensure compliance when treating persons with latent infection than when treating those with active tuberculosis. If family members of active cases are being treated, compliance and monitoring may be easier. When feasible, twice-weekly supervised therapy may increase the likelihood of completion. As in active cases, the provision of incentives may also be helpful.

BASICS OF CONTROL   The highest priority in any tuberculosis control program is the prompt detection of cases and the provision of directly observed short-course chemotherapy to all tuberculosis patients, with emphasis on the cure of sputum smear–positive cases. In addition, in low-prevalence countries with adequate resources, screening of high-risk groups (such as immigrants from high-prevalence countries and HIV-seropositive persons) is recommended. Identification of active cases of tuberculosis should be followed by treatment. PPD-positive high-risk persons should be treated for latent infection. Contact investigation is an important component of efficient tuberculosis control. In the United States, a great deal of attention has been given to the transmission of tuberculosis (particularly in association with HIV infection) in institutional settings such as hospitals, homeless shelters, and prisons. Measures to limit such transmission include respiratory isolation of persons with suspected tuberculosis until they are proven to be noninfectious (i.e., by sputum AFB smear negativity), proper ventilation in rooms of patients with infectious tuberculosis, use of ultraviolet lights in areas of increased risk of tuberculosis transmission, and periodic screening of personnel who may come into contact with known or unsuspected cases of tuberculosis. In the past, radiographic surveys, especially those conducted with portable equipment and miniature films, were advocated for case finding. Today, however, the prevalence of tuberculosis in industrialized countries is sufficiently low that "mass miniature radiography" is not cost-effective. As mentioned above, current recommendations for the prevention and treatment of tuberculosis in HIV-infected individuals have been published by the CDC.

In high-prevalence countries, tuberculosis control programs should be based on the following key elements: (1) case detection through microscopic examination of sputum from patients who present to health care facilities with cough of >3 weeks' duration; (2) administration of standard short-course chemotherapy to all sputum smear-positive patients, with direct observation of drug ingestion; (3) establishment and maintenance of a system of regular drug supply; and (4) establishment and maintenance of an effective surveillance and treatment-monitoring system allowing an analysis of treatment outcomes (e.g., cure, completion of treatment without bacteriologic proof of cure, death, treatment failure, and default) in all cases registered.

BIBLIOGRAPHY

BERTHET FX et al: Attenuation of virulence by disruption of the *Mycobacterium tuberculosis erp* gene. Science 282:759, 1998

BREIMAN RF et al: Proceedings of the International Symposium on Tuberculosis Vaccine Development and Evaluation. Clin Infect Dis 30(Suppl 3):S199-322, 2000

CENTERS FOR DISEASE CONTROL AND PREVENTION: Guidelines for preventing the transmission of *Mycobacterium tuberculosis* in health-care facilities. MMWR 43(RR-13):1, 1994

————: Prevention and treatment of tuberculosis among patients infected with human immunodeficiency virus: Principles of therapy and revised recommendations. MMWR 47(RR-20):1, 1998

COLE ST et al: Deciphering the biology of *Mycobacterium tuberculosis* from the complete genome sequence. Nature 392:537, 1998

COLLINS DM: In search of tuberculosis virulence genes. Trends Microbiol 4:426, 1996

CROFTON J et al: *Guidelines for the Management of Drug-Resistant Tuberculosis*. Geneva, World Health Organization, 1997

DOOLEY DP et al: Adjunctive corticosteroid therapy for tuberculosis: A critical reappraisal of the literature. Clin Infect Dis 25:872, 1997

DYE C et al: Global burden of tuberculosis: Estimated incidence, prevalence, and mortality by country. JAMA 282:677, 1999

ELLNER JJ: The immune response in human tuberculosis—implications for tuberculosis control. J Infect Dis 176:1351, 1997

MOORE MM et al: Trends in drug-resistant tuberculosis in the United States, 1993–1996. JAMA 278:833, 1997

O'BRIEN RJ: Preventive therapy, in *Clinical Tuberculosis*, 2d ed, PDO Davies (ed). London, Chapman & Hall, 1998, pp 397–416

PABLOS-MÉNDEZ A et al: Global surveillance for antituberculosis-drug resistance, 1994–1997. N Engl J Med 338:1641, 1998

RAVIGLIONE MC et al: Assessment of worldwide tuberculosis control. Lancet 350:624, 1997

SCHLOSSBERG D: *Tuberculosis and Nontuberculous Mycobacterial Infections*, 4th ed. Philadelphia, Saunders, 1999

SCHOREY JS et al: A macrophage invasion mechanism of pathogenic mycobacteria. Science 277:1091, 1997

VALWAY SE et al: An outbreak involving extensive transmission of a virulent strain of *Mycobacterium tuberculosis*. N Engl J Med 338:633, 1998

WORLD HEALTH ORGANIZATION: *Treatment of Tuberculosis. Guidelines for National Programmes*. Geneva, World Health Organization, 1997

170 *Robert H. Gelber*

LEPROSY (HANSEN'S DISEASE)

Leprosy, first described in ancient Indian texts from the sixth century B.C., is a nonfatal, chronic infectious disease caused by *Mycobacterium leprae*, whose clinical manifestations are largely confined to the skin, peripheral nervous system, upper respiratory tract, eyes, and testes. The unique tropism of *M. leprae* for peripheral nerves (from large nerve trunks to microscopic dermal nerves) and certain immunologically mediated reactional states are the major causes of morbidity in leprosy. The propensity of the disease, when untreated, to result in certain characteristic deformities and the recognition in most cultures that the disease is communicable from person to person have resulted historically in a profound social stigma. Today, with early diagnosis and the institution of appropriate and effective antimicrobial therapy, patients can lead productive lives in the community, and deformities and other visible manifestations can largely be prevented.

ETIOLOGY *M. leprae* is an obligate intracellular bacillus (0.3 to 1 μm wide and 1 to 8 μm long) that is acid-fast, indistinguishable microscopically from other mycobacteria, ideally detected in tissue sections by a modified Fite stain, and without demonstrable strain variability. *M. leprae* produces no known toxins and is well adapted to penetrate and reside within macrophages, yet it may survive outside the body for 7 to 10 days. In untreated patients, only ~1% of *M. leprae* organisms are viable. The morphologic index, a measure of the number of acid-fast bacilli (AFB) in skin scrapings that stain uniformly bright, correlates with viability. The bacteriologic index, a logarithmic-scaled measure of the density of *M. leprae* in the dermis, may be as high as 4+ to 6+ in untreated patients, falling by one unit per year during effective therapy; the rate of fall is independent of the relative potency of effective antimicrobial therapy. A rising bacteriologic or morphologic index suggests relapse and perhaps—if the patient is being treated—drug resistance; the latter possibility can be confirmed or excluded in the mouse model.

The genome of *M. leprae* is only 3 million base pairs, two-thirds as large as that of *M. tuberculosis*. The bacterium's complex cell wall has a peptidoglycan backbone, which is linked to arabinogalactan and mycolic acids. Lipoarabinomannan is a key component of the cell membrane, and the outer capsule contains large amounts of an *M. leprae*–specific phenolic glycolipid (PGL-1), which is detected in serologic tests. In addition, highly conserved, usually immunogenic heat-shock proteins containing *M. leprae*–specific and mycobacterial cross-reactive epitopes are found in the cytoplasm and cell wall.

Among the mycobacteria, *M. leprae* is unique in exhibiting dopa oxidase activity and an acid-fastness that is pyridine-extractable. Although it was the first bacterium to be etiologically associated with human disease, *M. leprae* remains one of the few bacterial species that still has not been cultivated on artificial medium or tissue culture. The multiplication of *M. leprae* in mouse footpads (albeit limited, with a doubling time of ~2 weeks) has provided a means to evaluate antimicrobial agents, monitor clinical trials, and screen vaccines. *M. leprae* grows best in cooler tissues (the skin, peripheral nerves, anterior chamber of the eye, upper respiratory tract, and testes), sparing warmer areas of the skin (the axilla, groin, scalp, and midline of the back).

EPIDEMIOLOGY   Demographics Leprosy is almost exclusively a disease of the developing world, affecting areas of Asia, Africa, Latin America, and the Pacific. While Africa has the highest disease prevalence, Asia has the most cases. More than 80% of the world's cases occur in a few countries: India, China, Myanmar, Indonesia, Brazil, and Nigeria. Within endemic locales, the distribution of leprosy is quite uneven, with areas of high prevalence bordering on areas with little or no disease. In Brazil the majority of cases occur in the Amazon basin, while in Mexico leprosy is mostly confined to western states. Except as imported cases, leprosy is largely absent from the United States, Canada, and northwestern Europe. In the United States, ~4000 persons have leprosy and 100 to 200 new cases are reported annually, most of them in California, Texas, New York, and Hawaii among immigrants from Mexico, Southeast Asia, the Philippines, and the Caribbean.

The global prevalence of leprosy is difficult to assess, given that many of the locales with high prevalence lack a significant medical or public health infrastructure. Estimates range from 1.5 to 8 million affected individuals. The lower estimate includes only persons who have not completed chemotherapy, excluding those who may be physically or psychologically damaged from leprosy and who may yet relapse or develop certain immune-mediated reactions; the higher figure includes patients whose infections probably are already cured and many who have no leprosy-related deformity or disability. Although the figures on the worldwide prevalence of leprosy are debatable, it is generally agreed that the annual incidence of new cases is stable and approximates 600,000.

Leprosy is associated with poverty and rural residence. It appears not to be associated with AIDS, perhaps because of leprosy's long incubation period. Most people appear to be naturally immune to leprosy and do not develop disease manifestations following exposure. The time of peak onset is in the second and third decades of life. The most severe form, lepromatous leprosy, is twice as common among men as among women and is rarely encountered in children. The frequency of the polar forms of leprosy (see "Clinical, Histologic, and Immunologic Spectrum," below) in different countries varies widely and may in part be genetically determined; certain HLA associations are known for both lepromatous and tuberculoid leprosy (see below). In India and Africa, 90% of cases are tuberculoid; in Southeast Asia, 50% are lepromatous and 50% tuberculoid; and in Mexico, 90% are lepromatous.

Transmission *M. leprae* causes disease primarily in humans. However, in Texas and Louisiana, 15% of nine-banded armadillos are infected, and armadillo contact occasionally results in human disease. Following intravenous experimental inoculation of *M. leprae*, 60% of armadillos develop a heavy disseminated infection of the liver, spleen, lymph nodes, and skin; these experimental animals have been the source of vast quantities of *M. leprae* organisms for laboratory and clinical research.

The route of transmission of leprosy remains uncertain and may be multiple; nasal droplet infection, contact with infected soil, and even insect vectors have been considered the prime candidates. Aerosolized *M. leprae* can cause infection in immunosuppressed mice, and a sneeze from an untreated lepromatous patient may contain >10^{10} AFB. Furthermore, both IgA antibody to *M. leprae* and genes of *M. leprae*—demonstrable by polymerase chain reaction (PCR)—have been found in the nose of individuals without signs of leprosy from endemic areas and in 19% of occupational contacts of lepromatous patients.

Several lines of evidence implicate soil transmission of leprosy. (1) In endemic countries such as India, leprosy is primarily a rural and not an urban disease. (2) *M. leprae* products have been demonstrated to be resident in soil in endemic locales. (3) Direct dermal inoculation (e.g., during tattooing) may transmit *M. leprae*, and common sites of leprosy in children are the buttocks and thighs, suggesting that microinoculation of infected soil may transmit the disease.

Evidence for insect vectors of leprosy includes the demonstration that bedbugs and mosquitoes in the vicinity of leprosaria regularly harbor *M. leprae* and that experimentally infected mosquitoes can transmit infection to mice. Skin-to-skin contact is generally not considered an important route of transmission.

In endemic countries, ~50% of leprosy patients have a history of intimate contact with an infected person (often a household member),

while, for unknown reasons, leprosy patients in nonendemic locales can identify such contact only 10% of the time. Moreover, household contact with an infected lepromatous case carries an eventual risk of disease acquisition of ~10% in endemic areas as opposed to only 1% in nonendemic locales. Contact with a tuberculoid case carries a very low risk. Physicians and nurses caring for leprosy patients and the coworkers of these patients are not at risk for leprosy.

CLINICAL, HISTOLOGIC, AND IMMUNOLOGIC SPECTRUM The incubation period prior to manifestation of clinical disease can vary between 2 and 40 years, although it is generally 5 to 7 years in duration. Leprosy presents as a spectrum of clinical manifestations that have pathologic and immunologic counterparts. The spectrum from polar tuberculoid (TT) to borderline tuberculoid (BT) to borderline lepromatous (BL) to polar lepromatous (LL) disease is associated with an evolution from localized to more generalized disease manifestations, an increasing bacterial load, and loss of *M. leprae*–specific cellular immunity. Where a patient presents on the clinical spectrum largely determines prognosis, complications, reactional states, and the intensity of antimicrobial therapy required.

Tuberculoid Leprosy At the less severe end of the spectrum is tuberculoid leprosy, which encompasses TT and BT disease. In general, these forms of leprosy result in symptoms confined to the skin and peripheral nerves. The initial lesion of tuberculoid leprosy is often a hypopigmented macule that is sharply demarcated and hypesthetic. Later, the lesions enlarge by peripheral spread, and the margins become elevated and circinate or gyrate. The central area in turn becomes atrophic and depressed. Fully developed lesions are densely anesthetic and devoid of the normal skin organs (sweat glands and hair follicles). Patients eventually have one or more asymmetrically distributed, hypopigmented, anesthetic, nonpruritic, well-defined macules, often with an erythematous or raised border (Fig. 170-1). Skin lesions of tuberculoid leprosy vary in diameter from one to several centimeters and are often dry, scaly, and anhidrotic. Tuberculoid leprosy patients may also have asymmetric enlargement of one or a few peripheral nerves. Indeed, leprosy and certain rare hereditary neuropathies are the only human diseases associated with peripheral-nerve enlargement. Although any peripheral nerve may be enlarged (including small digital and supraclavicular nerves), those most commonly affected are the ulnar, posterior auricular, peroneal, and posttibial nerves, with associated hypesthesia and myopathy. At times, tuberculoid leprosy may present with only nerve-trunk involvement with no skin lesions; in such cases it is termed *neural leprosy*. TT leprosy may resolve spontaneously and is not associated with lepra reactions (see "Reactional States," below). BT leprosy does not heal spontaneously and may be associated with type 1 lepra reactions but not with erythema nodosum leprosum (ENL). TT leprosy is the most common form of the disease encountered in India and Africa but is virtually absent in Southeast Asia, where BT leprosy is frequent.

In TT leprosy the epidermis may be involved histologically, while

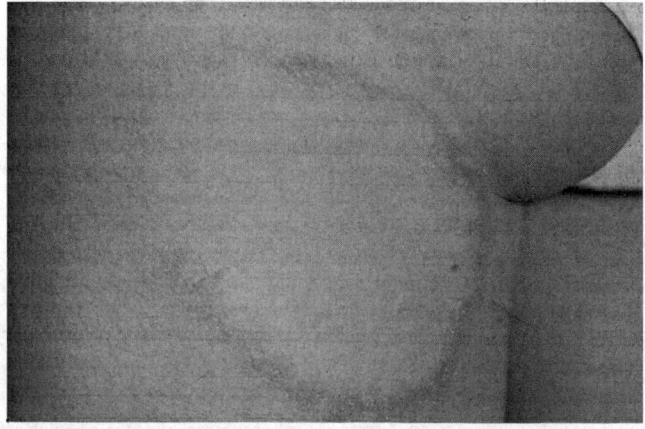

FIGURE 170-1 A skin lesion of tuberculoid leprosy: a well-demarcated, hypopigmented macule with an erythematous, slightly elevated border.

in all other forms of leprosy the epidermis and the superficial dermis are spared, with pathology confined to the deeper dermis. On hematoxylin and eosin staining, TT and BT lesions appear as well-defined noncaseating granulomas with many lymphocytes and Langhans' giant cells. In tuberculoid leprosy, T cells breach the perineurium, and destruction of Schwann cells and axons may be evident, resulting in fibrosis of the epineurium, replacement of the endoneurium with epithelial granulomas, and occasionally caseous necrosis. AFB are generally absent or few in number. Such invasion and destruction of nerves in the dermis by T cells are pathognomonic for leprosy.

Circulating lymphocytes from patients with tuberculoid leprosy readily recognize *M. leprae* and its constituent proteins, and patients have positive lepromin skin tests (see "Diagnosis" below). In tuberculoid leprosy tissue, there is a 2:1 predominance of helper CD4+ over CD8+ T lymphocytes. Tuberculoid tissues are rich in the mRNAs of the proinflammatory T_H1 family of cytokines: interleukin (IL) 2, interferon γ (IFN-γ), and IL-12; in contrast, IL 4, IL 5, and IL 10 mRNAs are scarce.

Lepromatous Leprosy At the more severe end of the leprosy spectrum is lepromatous disease, which encompasses the LL and BL forms. The initial skin lesions of lepromatous leprosy are skin-colored or slightly erythematous papules or nodules. In time, individual lesions grow in diameter up to 2 cm; new papules and nodules then appear and may coalesce. Patients later present with symmetrically distributed skin nodules, raised plaques, or diffuse dermal infiltration, which, when on the face, results in leonine facies. Late manifestations include loss of eyebrows (initially the lateral margins only; **see Plate IID-56**) and eyelashes, pendulous earlobes, and dry scaling skin, particularly on the feet. Almost exclusively found in western Mexico and the Caribbean is a form of lepromatous leprosy without visible skin lesions but with diffuse dermal infiltration and a demonstrably thickened dermis, termed *diffuse lepromatosis*. In lepromatous leprosy, nerve enlargement and damage tend to be symmetric, result from actual bacillary invasion, and are more insidious but ultimately more extensive than in tuberculoid leprosy. Patients with LL leprosy have symmetric acral distal peripheral neuropathy and a tendency toward symmetric nerve-trunk enlargement. They may also have signs and symptoms related to involvement of the upper respiratory tract, the anterior chamber of the eye, and the testes.

Dermatopathology in lepromatous leprosy is confined to the dermis and particularly affects the dermal appendages. Histologically, the dermis characteristically contains highly vacuolated cells (*foam cells*) otherwise found only in certain lipid-storage disorders. Indeed, on fat staining, these vacuoles are highly positive and are seen to include large amounts of *M. leprae*–associated cell wall lipids and the *M. leprae*–specific PGL-1. The dermis in lepromatous leprosy contains few lymphocytes and giant cells, and granulomas are absent. In LL leprosy, bacilli are numerous in the skin (as many as 10^9/g), where they are often found in large clumps (*globi*), and in peripheral nerves, where they initially invade Schwann cells, resulting in foamy degenerative myelination and axonal degeneration and later in Wallerian degeneration. In addition, bacilli are plentiful in circulating blood and in all organ systems except the lungs and the central nervous system. Nevertheless, patients are afebrile, and there is no evidence of major organ system dysfunction. The dermis contains more lymphocytes and fewer AFB and exhibits less vacuolization in BL than in LL leprosy.

In untreated LL patients, lymphocytes regularly fail to recognize either *M. leprae* or its protein constituents, and lepromin skin tests are negative (see "Diagnosis," below). This loss of protective cellular immunity appears to be antigen-specific, as patients are not unusually susceptible to opportunistic infections, cancer, or AIDS and maintain delayed-type hypersensitivity to *Candida*, *Trichophyton*, mumps, tetanus toxoid, and even purified protein derivative of tuberculin. At times, *M. leprae*–specific anergy is reversible with effective chemotherapy. In LL tissues, there is a 2:1 ratio of CD8+ to CD4+ T lymphocytes. LL tissues demonstrate a T_H2 cytokine profile, being rich in mRNAs for IL-4, IL-5, and IL-10 and poor in those for IL-2, IFN-γ, and IL-12. It appears that cytokines mediate a protective tissue response in leprosy, as injection of IFN-γ or IL-2 into lepromatous lesions causes a loss of AFB and histopathologic conversion toward a tuberculoid pattern. Macrophages of lepromatous leprosy patients appear to be functionally intact; circulating monocytes exhibit normal microbicidal function and responsiveness to IFN-γ.

LL and BL patients may develop type 2 lepra reactions (ENL; see "Reactional States," below), while BL patients (but not LL patients) can have type 1 lepra reactions.

Reactional States Lepra reactions comprise several common immunologically mediated inflammatory states that cause considerable morbidity. Some of these reactions precede diagnosis and the institution of effective antimicrobial therapy. Indeed, these reactions may precipitate presentation for medical attention and diagnosis; others occur after the initiation of appropriate chemotherapy. In the latter circumstances, patients often lose confidence in conventional therapy, perceiving that their leprosy is worsening. Only by warning patients of the potential for these reactions and describing their manifestations can physicians treating leprosy patients ensure continued credibility.

Type 1 lepra reactions (downgrading and reversal reactions) These reactions occur in almost half of patients with borderline forms of leprosy but not in patients with polar disease. Manifestations include classic signs of inflammation within previously involved macules, papules, and plaques and, on occasion, the appearance of new skin lesions, neuritis, and (less commonly) fever—generally low-grade. The nerve trunk most commonly involved in this process is the ulnar nerve at the elbow, which may be painful and exquisitely tender. If patients with affected nerves are not treated promptly with glucocorticoids (see below), irreversible nerve damage may result in as little as 24 h. The most dramatic manifestation is footdrop, which occurs when the peroneal nerve is involved.

When type 1 lepra reactions precede the initiation of appropriate antimicrobial therapy, they are termed *downgrading reactions*, and the case becomes histologically more lepromatous; when they occur after the initiation of therapy, they are termed *reversal reactions*, and the case becomes more tuberculoid. Reversal reactions often occur in the first months or years after the initiation of therapy but may also develop several years thereafter.

Edema is the most characteristic microscopic feature of type 1 lepra lesions, whose diagnosis is primarily clinical. Reversal reactions are typified by a T_H1 cytokine profile, with an influx of CD4+ helper cells and increased levels of IFN-γ and IL-2. In addition, type 1 reactions are associated with large numbers of T cells bearing γ/∂ receptors—a unique feature of leprosy.

Type 1 lepra reactions are best treated with glucocorticoids (e.g., prednisone, initially at doses of 40 to 60 mg/d). As the inflammation subsides, the glucocorticoid dose can be tapered, but steroid therapy must be continued for at least 3 months lest recurrence supervene. Because of the myriad toxicities of prolonged glucocorticoid therapy, the indications for its initiation are strictly limited to lesions whose intense inflammation poses a threat of ulceration; lesions at cosmetically important sites, such as the face; and the presence of neuritis. Mild to moderate lepra reactions that do not meet these criteria should be tolerated and glucocorticoid treatment withheld. Thalidomide is ineffective against type 1 lepra reactions; clofazimine (200 to 300 mg/d) is of questionable benefit but in any event is far less efficacious than glucocorticoids.

Type 2 lepra reactions (ENL) ENL occurs exclusively in patients near the lepromatous end of the leprosy spectrum, affecting nearly 50% of this group. Although ENL may precede leprosy diagnosis and initiation of therapy—sometimes, in fact, prompting the diagnosis—in 90% of cases it follows the institution of chemotherapy, generally within 2 years. The most common features of ENL are crops of painful erythematous papules that resolve spontaneously in a few days to a week but may recur; malaise; and fever that can be profound. However, patients may also experience symptoms of neuritis, lymphadenitis, uveitis, orchitis, and glomerulonephritis and may develop anemia, leukocytosis, and abnormal liver function tests, particularly increased aminotransferase levels. Individual patients may have either a single bout of ENL or chronic recurrent manifestations. Bouts may be either mild or severe and generalized; in rare instances, ENL results in death.

Skin biopsy of ENL papules reveals vasculitis or panniculitis, sometimes with many lymphocytes but characteristically with polymorphonuclear leukocytes as well.

Elevated levels of circulating tumor necrosis factor (TNF) have been demonstrated in ENL; thus TNF may play a central role in the pathobiology of this syndrome. ENL is thought to be a consequence of immune complex deposition, given its T_H2 cytokine profile and its high levels of IL-6 and IL-8. However, in ENL tissue, the presence of HLA Dr framework antigen of epidermal cells—considered a marker for a delayed-type hypersensitivity response—and evidence for higher levels of IL-2 and IFN-γ than are usually seen in polar lepromatous disease suggest an alternative mechanism.

Treatment must be individualized. If ENL is mild (i.e., without fever or other organ involvement, with occasional crops of only a few skin papules), it may be treated with antipyretics alone. However, in cases with many skin lesions, fever, malaise, and other tissue involvement, brief courses (1 to 2 weeks) of glucocorticoids (initially 40 to 60 mg/d) are often effective. With or without therapy, individual inflamed papules last for ≤1 week. Successful therapy is defined by the cessation of skin lesion development and the disappearance of other systemic signs and symptoms. If, despite two courses of glucocorticoid therapy, ENL appears to be recurring and persisting, treatment with thalidomide (100 to 300 mg nightly) should be initiated, with the dose depending on the initial severity of the reaction. Because even a single dose of thalidomide administered early in pregnancy may result in severe birth defects, including phocomelia, the use of this drug in the United States for the treatment of fertile females is tightly regulated and requires informed consent, prior pregnancy testing, and maintenance of birth control measures. Although the mechanism of thalidomide's dramatic action against ENL is not entirely clear, the drug's efficacy is probably attributable to its reduction of TNF levels and IgM synthesis and its slowing of polymorphonuclear leukocyte migration. After the reaction is controlled, lower doses of thalidomide (50 to 200 mg nightly) are effective in preventing relapses of ENL. Clofazimine in high doses (300 mg nightly) has some efficacy against ENL, but its use permits only a modest reduction of the glucocorticoid dose necessary for ENL control.

Lucio's phenomenon This unusual reaction is seen exclusively in patients from the Caribbean and Mexico who have the diffuse lepromatosis form of lepromatous leprosy, most often those who are untreated. Patients with this reaction develop recurrent crops of large, sharply marginated, ulcerative lesions—particularly on the lower extremities—that may be generalized and, when so, are frequently fatal as a result of secondary infection and consequent septic bacteremia. Histologically, the lesions are characterized by ischemic necrosis of the epidermis and superficial dermis, heavy parasitism of endothelial cells with AFB, and endothelial proliferation and thrombus formation in the larger vessels of the deeper dermis. Like ENL, the Lucio reaction is probably mediated by the immune complex. Neither glucocorticoids nor thalidomide is effective against this syndrome. Optimal wound care and therapy for bacteremia are indicated. Ulcers tend to be chronic and heal poorly. In severe cases, exchange transfusion may prove useful.

Nerve abscesses Patients with various forms of leprosy, but particularly those with the BT form, may develop abscesses of nerves (most commonly the ulnar) with an adjacent cellulitic appearance of the skin. In such conditions, the affected nerve is swollen and exquisitely tender. Although glucocorticoids may reduce signs of inflammation, rapid surgical decompression is necessary to prevent irreversible sequelae.

Complications • *The extremities* Complications of the extremities in leprosy patients are primarily a consequence of neuropathy leading to insensitivity and myopathy. Insensitivity affects fine touch, pain, and heat receptors but generally spares position and vibration appreciation. The most commonly affected nerve trunk is the ulnar nerve at the elbow, whose involvement results in clawing of the fourth and fifth fingers, loss of dorsal interosseous musculature in the affected hand, and loss of sensation in these distributions. Median nerve involvement in leprosy impairs thumb opposition and grasp, while radial nerve dysfunction, though rare in leprosy, leads to wristdrop. Tendon transfers can restore hand function but should not be performed until 6 months after the initiation of antimicrobial therapy and the conclusion of episodes of acute neuritis.

Plantar ulceration, particularly at the metatarsal heads, is probably the most frequent complication of leprous neuropathy. Plantar ulcers may become secondarily infected and lead to adjacent cellulitis and osteomyelitis. Because of the importance and critical integrity of the normal plantar fat pad, recurrent ulceration is unfortunately common once initial ulceration has occurred and the pad has been replaced by thin and less resilient fibrous scar tissue. The treatment of plantar ulceration includes debridement of devitalized and undermined tissue; discontinuation of weight-bearing, which may be accomplished by means of a total-contact cast or bed rest; and vigorous treatment of secondary infection, which most commonly is due to *Staphylococcus aureus*. Once healing takes place, walking must be limited, especially during the first week, with slow and progressive increases thereafter. Extra-depth shoes or individually fitted shoes with specially molded inserts are required to prevent recurrence.

Peroneal nerve palsies may result from leprosy itself or from one of its reactional states; the consequence is partial or complete footdrop, which causes an uneven distribution of weight on the plantar surface and hence a predilection to ulceration. Simple nonmetallic braces within the shoe may be useful, while tendon transfers can actually correct footdrop. Although uncommon, Charcot's joints, particularly of the foot and ankle, may result from leprosy.

The loss of distal digits in leprosy is a consequence of insensitivity, trauma, secondary infection, and—in lepromatous patients—a poorly understood and sometimes profound osteolytic process. Conscientious protection of the extremities during cooking and work and the early institution of therapy have substantially reduced the frequency and severity of distal digit loss in recent times.

The nose In lepromatous leprosy, bacillary invasion of the nasal mucosa can result in chronic nasal congestion and epistaxis. Saline nosedrops may relieve these symptoms. Long-untreated LL leprosy may further result in destruction of the nasal cartilage, with consequent saddle-nose deformity or anosmia (more common in the preantibiotic era than at present). Nasal reconstructive procedures can ameliorate significant cosmetic defects.

The eye Owing to cranial nerve palsies, lagophthalmus and corneal insensitivity may complicate leprosy, resulting in trauma, secondary infection, and (without treatment) corneal ulcerations and opacities. For patients with these conditions, eyedrops during the day and ointments at night provide some protection from such consequences. Furthermore, in LL leprosy, the anterior chamber of the eye is invaded by bacilli, and ENL may result in uveitis, with consequent cataracts and glaucoma. Thus leprosy is a major cause of blindness in the developing world. Slit-lamp evaluation of LL patients often reveals "corneal beading," representing globi of *M. leprae*.

The testes *M. leprae* invades the testes, while ENL may cause orchitis. Thus males with lepromatous leprosy often manifest mild to severe testicular dysfunction, with an elevation of luteinizing and follicle-stimulating hormones, decreased testosterone, and aspermia or hypospermia in 85% of LL patients but in only 25% of BL patients. LL patients may become impotent and infertile. Impotence is sometimes responsive to testosterone replacement.

Amyloidosis Secondary amyloidosis is a complication of LL leprosy and ENL that is encountered infrequently in the antibiotic era.

This complication may result in abnormalities of hepatic and particularly renal function.

DIAGNOSIS Leprosy most commonly presents with both characteristic skin lesions and skin histopathology. Thus the disease should be suspected when a patient from an endemic area has suggestive skin lesions or peripheral neuropathy; the diagnosis should be confirmed by histopathology. In tuberculoid leprosy, lesional areas—preferably the advancing edge—must be biopsied because normal-appearing skin does not have pathologic features. In lepromatous leprosy, nodules, plaques, and indurated areas are optimal biopsy sites, but biopsies of normal-appearing skin are also generally diagnostic. Lepromatous leprosy is associated with diffuse hyperglobulinemia, which may result in false-positive serologic tests (e.g., VDRL, RA, ANA) and therefore can cause diagnostic confusion. On occasion, tuberculoid lesions may not (1) appear typical, (2) be hypesthetic, and (3) contain granulomas but only nonspecific lymphocytic infiltrates. In such instances, two of these three characteristics are considered sufficient for a diagnosis. It is preferable to overdiagnose leprosy rather than to allow a patient to remain untreated.

IgM antibodies to PGL-1 are found in 95% of untreated lepromatous leprosy patients; the titer decreases with effective therapy. However, in tuberculoid leprosy—the form of disease most often associated with diagnostic uncertainty owing to the absence of AFB—patients have significant antibodies to PGL-1 only 60% of the time; moreover, in endemic locales, exposed individuals without clinical leprosy may harbor antibodies to PGL-1. Thus PGL-1 serology is of little diagnostic utility in tuberculoid leprosy. Heat-killed *M. leprae* (lepromin) has been used as a skin test reagent. It generally elicits a reaction in tuberculoid leprosy patients, may do so in individuals without leprosy, and gives negative results in lepromatous leprosy patients; consequently, it is likewise of little diagnostic value. Unfortunately, PCR of skin for *M. leprae*, although positive in LL and BL leprosy, yields negative results in 50% of tuberculoid leprosy cases, again offering little diagnostic assistance.

Included in the differential diagnosis of lesions that resemble leprosy are sarcoidosis, leishmaniasis, lupus vulgaris, lymphoma, syphilis, yaws, granuloma annulare, and various other disorders causing hypopigmentation. Sarcoidosis may result in perineural inflammation, but actual granuloma formation within dermal nerves is pathognomonic for leprosy. In lepromatous leprosy, sputum specimens may be loaded with AFB—a finding that can be inappropriately interpreted as representing pulmonary tuberculosis.

℞ **TREATMENT** **Active Agents** Established agents used to treat leprosy include dapsone (50 to 100 mg/d), clofazimine (50 to 100 mg/d, 100 mg three times weekly, or 300 mg monthly), and rifampin (600 mg daily or monthly). Of these drugs, only rifampin is bactericidal. The sulfones (folate antagonists), the foremost of which is dapsone, were the first antimicrobials found to be effective for the treatment of leprosy and are still the mainstay of therapy. With sulfone treatment, skin lesions resolve and numbers of viable bacilli in the skin are reduced. Although primarily bacteriostatic, dapsone monotherapy results in only a 10% resistance-related relapse rate; after ≥18 years of therapy and subsequent discontinuation, only another 10% of patients relapse, developing new, usually asymptomatic, shiny, "histoid" nodules. Dapsone is generally safe and inexpensive. Individuals with glucose-6-phosphate dehydrogenase deficiency who are treated with dapsone may develop severe hemolysis; those without this deficiency also have reduced red cell survival and a hemoglobin decrease averaging 1 g/dL. Dapsone's usefulness is limited occasionally by allergic dermatitis and rarely by the sulfone syndrome (including high fever, anemia, exfoliative dermatitis, and a mononucleosis-type blood picture). It must be remembered that rifampin induces microsomal enzymes, necessitating increased doses of medications such as glucocorticoids and oral birth control regimens. Clofazimine is often cosmetically unacceptable to light-skinned leprosy patients because it causes a red-black skin discoloration that accumulates, particularly in

lesional areas, and makes the patient's diagnosis obvious to members of the community.

Other antimicrobial agents active against *M. leprae* in animal models and at the usual daily doses used in clinical trials include ethionamide/prothionamide; the aminoglycosides streptomycin, kanamycin, and amikacin (but not gentamicin or tobramycin); minocycline; clarithromycin; and several fluoroquinolones, particularly ofloxacin. Next to rifampin, minocycline, clarithromycin, and ofloxacin appear to be most bactericidal for *M. leprae*, but these drugs have not been used extensively in leprosy control programs.

Choice of Regimens Antimicrobial therapy for leprosy must be individualized, depending on the clinical/pathologic form of the disease encountered. Tuberculoid leprosy, which is associated with a low bacterial burden and a protective cellular immune response, is the easier form to treat and can be reliably cured with a finite course of chemotherapy. In contrast, lepromatous leprosy may have a higher bacillary load than any other human bacterial disease, and the absence of a salutary T cell repertoire requires prolonged or even lifelong chemotherapy. Hence, careful classification of disease prior to therapy is important. In developed countries, clinical experience with leprosy classification is limited; fortunately, however, the resources needed for skin biopsy are highly accessible and pathologic interpretation is readily available. In developing countries, clinical expertise is greater, but it may now be waning as the care of leprosy patients is integrated into general health services. In addition, access to dermatopathology services is often limited. In such instances, skin smears may prove useful, but in many locales access to the resources needed for their preparation and interpretation may also be unavailable.

A reasoned approach to the treatment of leprosy is confounded by these and several other issues:

1. Even without therapy, TT leprosy may heal spontaneously, and prolonged dapsone monotherapy (even for LL leprosy) is generally curative in 80% of cases.
2. In tuberculoid disease, there are often no bacilli found in the skin prior to therapy, and thus there is no objective measure of therapeutic success. Furthermore, despite adequate treatment, TT and particularly BT lesions often resolve little or incompletely, while relapse and late type 1 lepra reactions can be difficult to distinguish.
3. LL leprosy patients commonly harbor viable persistent *M. leprae* organisms after prolonged intensive therapy; the propensity of these organisms to initiate clinical relapse is unclear. Because relapse in LL patients after discontinuation of rifampin-containing regimens usually begins only after 7 to 10 years, follow-up over the very long term is necessary to assess ultimate clinical outcomes.
4. Even though primary dapsone resistance is exceedingly rare and multidrug therapy is generally recommended (at least for lepromatous leprosy), there is a paucity of information from experimental animals and clinical trials on the optimal combination of antimicrobials, dosing schedule, or duration of therapy.

In 1982, the World Health Organization (WHO) made recommendations for "the chemotherapy of leprosy for control programs." These recommendations came on the heels of the demonstration of the relative success of long-term dapsone monotherapy and in the context of concerns about dapsone resistance. Other complicating considerations included the limited resources available for leprosy care in the very areas where it is most prevalent and the frustration and discouragement of patients and program managers with the previous requirement for lifelong therapy for many leprosy patients. The WHO delineated for the first time a finite duration of therapy for all forms of leprosy, and—given the prohibitive cost of daily rifampin treatment in developing countries—encouraged the monthly administration of this agent as part of a multidrug regimen.

Over the ensuing years, these WHO recommendations have been broadly implemented, and the duration of therapy required, particularly for lepromatous leprosy, has been progressively shortened. For treatment purposes, the WHO classifies patients as paucibacillary and multibacillary. Previously, patients without demonstrable AFB in the dermis were classified as paucibacillary and those with AFB as multibacillary. Currently, owing to the perceived unreliability of skin smears in the field, patients are classified as multibacillary if they have five or more skin lesions and as paucibacillary if they have fewer than five skin lesions. The WHO recommends that paucibacillary adults be treated with 100 mg of dapsone daily and 600 mg of rifampin monthly (supervised) for 6 months (Table 170-1). Multibacillary adults should be treated with 100 mg of dapsone plus 50 mg of clofazimine daily (unsupervised) and with 600 mg of rifampin plus 300 mg of clofazimine monthly (supervised). Originally, the WHO recommended that lepromatous patients be treated for 2 years or until smears became negative (generally in ~5 years); subsequently, the acceptable course was reduced to 1 year—a change that remains controversial in the absence of clinical trials.

Several factors, including an improved economic climate, the high relapse rates (20 to 40%, depending on the initial bacterial burden) among patients with lepromatous leprosy after WHO-recommended treatment, and the demonstrable lesional activity in fully half of tuberculoid leprosy patients after the completion of therapy, have caused many authorities to question the WHO recommendations and to favor a more intensive approach. This approach (Table 170-1) calls for tuberculoid leprosy to be treated with dapsone (100 mg/d) for 5 years and for lepromatous leprosy to be treated with rifampin (600 mg/d) for 3 years and with dapsone (100 mg/d) throughout life.

On effective antimicrobial therapy, new skin lesions and signs and symptoms of peripheral neuropathy cease appearing. Nodules and plaques of lepromatous leprosy noticeably flatten in 1 to 2 months and resolve in 1 or a few years, while tuberculoid skin lesions may disappear, improve, or remain relatively unchanged. Though the peripheral neuropathy of leprosy may improve somewhat in the first few months of therapy, rarely is it significantly ameliorated by treatment.

PREVENTION AND CONTROL   Vaccination at birth with bacille Calmette-Guérin (BCG) has proved variably effective in preventing leprosy, ranging from totally ineffective to 80% efficacious. The addition of heat-killed *M. leprae* to BCG does not increase vaccine efficacy. Because whole mycobacteria contain large amounts of lipids and carbohydrates that have proven in vitro to be immunosuppressive for lymphocytes and macrophages, *M. leprae* proteins may prove to be superior vaccines. Data from a mouse model support this possibility. Chemoprophylaxis with dapsone may reduce the number of cases of tuberculoid leprosy but not of lepromatous leprosy and hence is not recommended, even for household contacts. Because leprosy transmission appears to require close prolonged household contact, hospitalized patients need not be isolated.

BIBLIOGRAPHY

GELBER RH : Chemotherapy of lepromatous leprosy: Recent developments and prospects for the future. Eur J Clin Microbiol Infect Dis 13:942, 1994
———— et al: Vaccination of mice with a soluble protein fraction of *Mycobacterium leprae* provides consistent and long-term protection against *M. leprae* infection. Infect Immun 60:1840, 1992
JAMET P et al: Marchoux Chemotherapy Study Group. Relapse after long-term follow up of multibacillary patients treated by WHO multidrug regimen. Int J Lepr 63:195, 1995
MARCHOUX CHEMOTHERAPY STUDY GROUP: Relapses in multibacillary leprosy patients after stopping treatment with rifampicin-containing combined regimens. Int J Lepr 60:525, 1992
MODLIN RL, REA TH: Immunology of leprosy granulomas. Springer Semin Immunopathol 10:359, 1998
RIDLEY DS: Histological classification and the immunological spectrum of leprosy. Bull World Health Organ 51:451, 1974
SAMPAIO EP et al: Influence of thalidomide on the clinical and immunologic manifestations of erythema nodosum leprosum. J Infect Dis 168:408, 1993
SHEPARD CC: The experimental disease that follows injection of human leprosy bacilli into foot pads of mice. J Exp Med 112:445, 1960
WHO EXPERT COMMITTEE ON LEPROSY: Seventh Report. WHO Technical Report Series No. 874. Geneva, World Health Organization, 1998

171   *Bernard Hirschel*

INFECTIONS DUE TO NONTUBERCULOUS MYCOBACTERIA

Mycobacteria are slightly curved or straight, rod-shaped or coccoid bacilli traditionally identified by the property of acid-fastness: once stained, the organisms are not easily decolorized, even with acid-alcohol, because of the composition of their cell walls. The genetic relation of mycobacteria with one another is evidenced by their ribosomal RNA sequence homology, which can be used for diagnostic purposes.

Because of the overwhelming clinical importance of tuberculosis, mycobacteriologists have distinguished the *Mycobacterium tuberculosis* complex (consisting of *M. tuberculosis*, *M. bovis*, and *M. africanum*) from all other mycobacteria. Except for *M. leprae* (Chap. 170), the other mycobacteria are referred to as atypical mycobacteria, mycobacteria other than tuberculosis (MOTT), or nontuberculous mycobacteria (NTM). The most clinically important NTM are listed and described in Table 171-1. The isolation of NTM—or the lack thereof—from an individual patient or laboratory specimen must be interpreted with the following facts in mind:

1.   Some NTM require special media and/or growth conditions. The laboratory must be alerted and cultures for acid-fast bacilli requested if the diagnosis of these infections is not to be missed.

2.   NTM grow slowly. Even the so-called rapid growers take 3 to 7 days to form visible colonies on solid media, whereas slow-growing mycobacteria take weeks or do not grow at all on artificial media.

3.   The slow growth of mycobacteria complicates antibiotic susceptibility testing. During prolonged incubation, antibiotics may be degraded and disappear from the culture medium. Long delays reduce the clinical usefulness of whatever results are eventually obtained.

4.   Data on in vitro susceptibility correlate poorly with clinical results. For example, clarithromycin and azithromycin are highly and variably concentrated in tissues; consequently, the concentrations necessary for determining resistance are difficult to establish in vitro. Sensitivity testing, based on achievable serum levels, would have predicted that these drugs would have little efficacy in vivo; in fact, the opposite is true, both in animal models and in humans.

5.   In contrast to *M. tuberculosis*, NTM are ubiquitous in the en-

Table 170-1   Antimicrobial Regimens Recommended for the Treatment of Leprosy in Adults

Form of Leprosy	More Intensive Regimen	WHO Recommended Regimen (1982)
Tuberculoid (paucibacillary)	Dapsone (100 mg/d) for 5 years	Dapsone (100 mg/d, unsupervised) *plus* rifampin (600 mg/month, supervised) for 6 months
Lepromatous (multibacillary)	Rifampin (600 mg/d) for 3 years *plus* dapsone (100 mg/d) indefinitely	Dapsone (100 mg/d) *plus* clofazimine (50 mg/d), unsupervised; *and* rifampin (600 mg) *plus* clofazimine (300 mg) monthly (supervised) for 1 year

NOTE: See text for discussion and comparison of WHO recommendations and more intensive approach.

Table 171-1 The Most Important Nontuberculous Mycobacteria

| Mycobacterial Species | Disseminated Infections | Localized Infections | | Skin and Soft Tissue | Contaminant/ Commensal | Recommended Therapy | Percentage of Strains |
		Lung	Lymphadenitis				
M. abscessus	—	—	—	Typical, linked to surgery	Typical	Debridement; clarithromycin, clofazimine, amikacin	<1
M. avium	Typical in AIDS with CD4+ count of <50/μL; rare in other immunodeficiencies	See M. intracellulare	In children (rare)	In disseminated infection (rare)	Typical in sputum and feces	Clarithromycin,[a] ethambutol, rifabutin	30–50
M. celatum	AIDS (rare)	Rare	—	—	—	See M. avium	<1
M. chelonae	Rare	—	—	Typical, linked to surgery	Typical	See M. abscessus	<1
M. fortuitum	Rare	Rare	—	Typical	Typical	Amikacin, ciprofloxacin, sulfonamides, clofazimine, clarithromycin	1
M. genavense	Typical in AIDS	—	Rare	—	—	See M. avium	5
M. gordonae	Rare	—	—	Rare	Typical	—	10–30
M. haemophilum	Typical in AIDS and other immunodeficiencies	—	—	Typical in AIDS	—	See M. avium	<1
M. intracellulare	See M. avium	Cavities in CF or COPD[b]; lingular infection in normal hosts	In children (rare)	See M. avium	Possible in sputum	See M. avium	4–8
M. kansasii	In AIDS (rare)	Typical, resembling tuberculosis	Rare	Rare	Possible in sputum	Rifampin, isoniazid, ethambutol, clarithromycin, sulfonamides	2–4
M. malmoense	Rare	Rare	—	—	—	See M. avium	1–4
M. marinum	Rare	—	—	Typical	—	Trimethoprim-sulfamethoxazole[c]	1
M. scrofulaceum	Rare	Rare	Typical	—	—	See M. avium	1
M. simiae	In AIDS (rare)	Rare	—	—	Possible	See M. avium	1
M. szulgai	—	Rare	—	Typical	—	Rifampin, isoniazid, ethambutol	<1
M. xenopi	Rare	Rare	—	—	Typical	See M. avium	10–20

[a] Or azithromycin.
[b] CF, cystic fibrosis; COPD, chronic obstructive pulmonary disease.
[c] Or minocycline.

SOURCE: Data are from J Clin Microbiol 31:1882, 1993 (335 strains) and the Mycobacteriology Laboratory of the University Hospital in Geneva (1993–1994, 313 strains, Dr. P. Rohner).

vironment. Therefore, isolation of NTM from a site that is not normally sterile (such as sputum, urine, skin, or feces) does not constitute proof of disease. In Switzerland between 1983 and 1988, for example, only 23 of 513 HIV-negative patients with NTM isolates had clinically significant disease. Clusters of unusual isolates are more likely to suggest contamination—e.g., from tap water or bronchoscopy equipment—than to represent an epidemic of disease.

The original method for the classification of NTM, developed between 1950 and 1980, depends on speed of growth, morphology, and pigmentation of colonies on solid media as well as biochemical reactions. Although reliable and inexpensive, these procedures take a long time; a period of 12 weeks is often required for definitive identification. Of course, such delayed results are of little use in the care of patients.

The isolation of NTM from blood cultures requires the use of a special medium for lysis-centrifugation or broth culture. The lysis-centrifugation method (lysis of blood cells followed by centrifugation and plating of the pellet with the bacteria on solid medium) permits quantification of bacteremia; however, some mycobacteria (e.g., M. genavense) do not grow well on solid medium and will not be detected by this method. Culture in liquid broth, such as that used in the radiometric Bactec system, shortens the time needed to identify a positive culture but also precludes the study of colonial morphology and pigmentation. Molecular probes are now used for rapid identification of the most important species (M. avium, M. intracellulare, M. gordonae, M. kansasii, and the M. tuberculosis complex) in a positive culture; a color is produced upon hybridization of the probe to specific sequences of the mycobacterial ribosome.

Twenty years ago, the field of mycobacteriology was something of a backwater. Tuberculosis was incorrectly perceived as a disappearing problem, and NTM were causing only rare and chronic diseases. AIDS, however, has brought mycobacterial infections to the forefront of clinical medicine once more. HIV and M. tuberculosis make a volatile mixture, and disseminated infections with NTM are extremely frequent in the advanced stages of AIDS (Chap. 309). In this setting, it is fortunate that new molecular techniques based on DNA amplification accelerate diagnosis, identify common sources of infection, and reveal new types of NTM, while new antibiotics, such as the macrolides, the rifamycins, and the fluoroquinolones, offer improved options for treatment and prevention. In addition, highly active antiretroviral therapy (HAART) has had a dramatic impact. By preventing and reversing immunodeficiency, HAART (Chap. 309) also prevents and reverses NTM infections.

NTM INFECTIONS IN AIDS AND OTHER IMMUNODEFICIENCIES

DISSEMINATED INFECTIONS Etiology The majority of mycobacterial infections in immunocompromised hosts are caused by organisms belonging to the group referred to as the M. avium complex (MAC). This group has always been considered to include M. avium and M. intracellulare (designated by the abbreviation MAI) and in the past encompassed M. scrofulaceum as well (hence the abbreviation MAIS). With the development and marketing of diagnostic probes that distinguish M. avium from M. intracellulare, it has become clear that the vast majority of disseminated "MAC" infections in AIDS are actually caused by M. avium. Thus, from a microbiologic standpoint, this designation is now obsolete. However, it is still used in clinical practice and will be employed in that context herein.

M. genavense causes systemic infections similar to those caused by MAC organisms. *M. genavense* does not grow well in culture and may therefore be missed in some instances. However, in a series of nearly 200 disseminated NTM infections from Switzerland, 13% of cases were due to *M. genavense*. Other NTM, including *M. xenopi, M. simiae, M. scrofulaceum, M. malmoense,* and *M. celatum,* may also be involved in such cases. In addition, AIDS patients with localized NTM diseases (see "Localized Infections," below) often have positive blood cultures (e.g., patients with skin disease due to *M. haemophilum* or with lung disease due to *M. kansasii*).

Epidemiology and Host Factors Because gastrointestinal symptoms often predominate in NTM infection and because the intestinal submucosa is intensely involved, ingestion seems logical as a primary route of infection. Many environments and animals teem with NTM (especially MAC organisms), including swamps in the southeastern United States, swine almost everywhere, piped water in New England and in Finland, and soil from potted plants in San Francisco. Birds are frequently infected with *M. genavense*. Skin-test data and humoral antibody patterns point to widespread exposure. However, a direct connection of the environment to the patient is often lacking, and it is not always clear whether strains found in the environment are pathogenic in humans. In an exhaustive study of dietary factors, patients with NTM were found to have consumed more hard cheese than controls without NTM, but no NTM could be found in samples of cheese. At present, the epidemiologic evidence is not strong enough to serve as a basis for dietary recommendations in persons at high risk of NTM infection. There is no evidence for nosocomial spread of NTM from patient to patient; however, hospital hot-water systems have been suspected as the source of isolated clusters of cases. Whereas regional variations in the environmental frequency of NTM are striking, it is difficult to correlate these variations with the frequency of NTM infection among HIV-infected patients.

Disseminated infections with NTM occur almost exclusively in severely immunosuppressed patients, usually those with AIDS. Rarely, such infections are found in patients immunosuppressed for other reasons, including transplant recipients, and patients with leukemia (in particular, hairy cell leukemia) or lymphoma. Cases in children may suggest the presence of a congenital immunodeficiency disease, such as a deficiency in the receptors for interferon γ (IFN-γ) or interleukin (IL) 12. Finally, rare cases of dissemination occur in immunocompetent patients who have extensive pulmonary disease (see "NTM Infections in Immunocompetent Patients," below).

In patients with AIDS, the risk of NTM infection correlates well with the degree of depletion of CD4+ lymphocytes. Disseminated NTM disease is rare among patients with >100 CD4+ cells per microliter; however, among patients with <10 CD4+ lymphocytes per microliter, the actuarial probability of having a blood culture positive for NTM reaches 40% after 1 year. HAART has greatly diminished the overall incidence of NTM disease in AIDS. Current treatment recommendations suggest starting HAART when the CD4+ count falls below 500/μL. At these levels, NTM disease does not occur. In extremely immunosuppressed patients who start HAART, the CD4+ count typically rises above 100/μL within a few months; such patients are again unlikely to develop NTM disease.

Clinical Manifestations As has already been mentioned, disseminated infection with NTM is essentially a disease of advanced immunodeficiency. In HIV-infected patients, the median CD4+ lymphocyte count at the time of diagnosis is ~10/μL. Certainly, other diagnoses should be considered first when a patient with symptoms suggestive of NTM infection has >100 CD4+ cells per microliter. Prospective monthly blood cultures have shown that NTM bacteremia often causes few or no symptoms. In clinical practice, however, cultures are not performed if the patient is asymptomatic.

Disseminated NTM infection should be suspected on the basis of prolonged fever (sometimes of varying intensity—particularly at first—and accompanied by night sweats) and weight loss. Signs of abdominal involvement that may be evident on computed tomography or ultrasonography include enlargement of the liver and spleen and swelling of abdominal lymph nodes, which may result in diarrhea and/or abdominal pain. Anemia and leukopenia are frequently documented; although it is tempting to relate these abnormalities to infection of bone marrow by NTM, multiple factors are usually involved.

In short, the clinical picture of infection with NTM is not distinctive. Many other conditions, including abdominal lymphoma, the HIV wasting syndrome, *Salmonella* or *Campylobacter* infection, cryptosporidiosis, or microsporidiosis, may mimic (and coexist with) disseminated NTM infection. As stated earlier, suspicion of such infection should prompt a request for blood cultures.

Diagnosis Blood cultures on special media are the cornerstone of the diagnosis of NTM infection, both in patients with organ involvement and in those without. In most symptomatic patients, the intensity of mycobacteremia is such that most or all blood cultures are positive. Therefore, the performance of multiple, repetitive cultures at short intervals is not worthwhile. Rather, in clinical practice, two or three blood cultures are sufficient. In one study, the results of prospective cultures varied, and these variations (positive followed by negative or vice versa) were unrelated to symptom status. As mentioned above, liquid cultures (e.g., the Bactec system) are likely to become positive earlier (within 7 to 14 days) and are therefore preferred to cultures on solid medium. In patients infected with *M. genavense* or *M. xenopi* and in patients being treated for MAC infection, the interval to culture positivity may be much longer. In rare cases, organ involvement in NTM infection may be found to be widespread at autopsy despite multiple negative blood cultures during life.

Because the liver and bone marrow are often involved in disseminated NTM infection, the bacteria may be visible in acid-fast–stained biopsy samples from these sites. Presumptive diagnosis by examination of a biopsied liver specimen saves time. The yield has been as high as 50% in patients with clearly abnormal values in liver function tests. However, the yield of this method has been disappointing in patients with suspected NTM infection, negative blood cultures, and normal or nearly normal results in liver function tests.

℞ TREATMENT Compared with *M. tuberculosis*, NTM are of low virulence. NTM tend to affect severely immunosuppressed patients, who usually have many other medical problems. Treatment is complex, relies on the use of multiple drugs with numerous adverse effects, and may interfere with antiretroviral therapy.

The drugs used for the treatment of disseminated NTM infection are different from those used against tuberculosis (Table 171-1; Chaps. 168 and 169). In particular, isoniazid has little effect on MAC organisms. The best method for antibiotic sensitivity testing of NTM is controversial, and the question of what relation—if any—exists between in vitro resistance and treatment failure remains unanswered. From the clinician's viewpoint, growth inhibition in liquid cultures is preferred to other methods of sensitivity testing because the results become available within 7 days.

The agents most active against MAC organisms are the macrolides clarithromycin and azithromycin. Both of these drugs are well absorbed from the gastrointestinal tract and well concentrated in macrophages and tissues, where their levels exceed those in plasma by more than 10-fold. Given alone, either drug can render blood cultures negative in a substantial proportion of cases. However, resistance (due to a single point mutation in the gene coding for the large ribosomal subunit) invariably develops, and NTM reappear in the bloodstream.

A majority of MAC strains are sensitive to ethambutol, ciprofloxacin, clofazimine, amikacin, rifampin, and rifabutin; that is, the concentrations of these drugs attainable in serum are inhibitory in vitro. However, none of these drugs consistently reduces the intensity of mycobacteremia when used alone. The preferred regimen for treatment of disseminated NTM infections is the combination of rifabutin (300 to 600 mg/d), clarithromycin (1 g twice daily), and ethambutol (900 mg/d). In a randomized trial, this regimen was superior to the combination of rifampin, clofazimine, ciprofloxacin, and ethambutol, with more rapid resolution of bacteremia and increased survival. The higher dose of rifabutin was more effective but frequently caused uveitis. This side effect is of special concern when rifabutin is used in combination with ritonavir, which increases the concentration of a toxic metabolite. Among the HIV protease inhibitors, indinavir and nelfinavir may be used in combination with rifabutin.

The inclusion of intravenous amikacin in multidrug regimens has not conferred additional benefit. Nonetheless, this drug may be useful in certain cases—e.g., when resistance to clarithromycin develops or when severe gastrointestinal symptoms interfere with oral therapy. In addition, amikacin may prevent the emergence of resistance to clarithromycin when the two drugs are used concurrently.

It is not clear how long therapy needs to be administered. Older regimens did not eradicate MAC, and many experts recommended lifelong treatment. Unfortunately, multidrug regimens are often poorly tolerated. In patients whose symptoms have lessened, whose blood cultures have become negative, and whose CD4+ counts have recovered to >100/μL with HAART, it is reasonable to discontinue antimycobacterial treatment.

In vitro and in experimental animals, cytokines such as IL-12, granulocyte-macrophage colony-stimulating factor, and IFN-γ act synergistically with antibiotics against MAC. In a small-scale pilot trial including seven HIV-negative patients, IFN-γ was beneficial.

Encapsulation of many drugs into liposomes enhances their effect in animal models because both liposomes and MAC are ingested by macrophages. Relevant data from studies of humans are still scarce, however.

Disseminated infections caused by NTM other than MAC have been too rare for therapy to be evaluated in controlled trials. The presently recommended treatment for these infections is the same as that for disseminated MAC infections. In particular, *M. genavense* seems to be sensitive to clarithromycin and rifabutin.

Prevention As has been discussed, disseminated infection with MAC occurs almost exclusively in persons severely immunocompromised by HIV infection. Therefore, the best approach to the prevention of MAC infections is the prevention and reversal of immunodeficiency by HAART. In patients whose HIV is resistant to HAART and who are severely immunosuppressed, with CD4+ counts <100/μL, prophylaxis with rifabutin (300 mg/d), clarithromycin (500 mg once or twice daily), or azithromycin (1200 mg weekly) is likely to decrease the incidence of positive blood cultures by ~60%. Patients receiving prophylaxis have also had less fever, experienced less fatigue, and survived longer than patients not receiving prophylaxis. Although breakthrough bacteremia involving resistant organisms is a concern, this condition has not developed with rifabutin prophylaxis and is rare with clarithromycin. However, it is standard practice to rule out preexisting disseminated NTM infection (by blood culture) before starting prophylaxis.

LOCALIZED INFECTIONS Pulmonary Disease The significance of isolation of NTM from the airways of AIDS patients merits special discussion. In general, HIV-infected patients who have NTM in sputum or bronchoalveolar lavage fluid but have little evidence of lung damage require no treatment. *M. avium* only rarely causes significant pulmonary disease in AIDS; its isolation from sputum in the absence of radiographic changes is usually without clinical significance. In contrast, the isolation of *M. kansasii* from the lung is clinically significant: this organism causes a disease—often predominant in the upper lobes—that resembles pulmonary tuberculosis, with fever, cough, infiltrates, and cavities. Blood cultures are often positive. Drugs active against *M. tuberculosis*, such as rifampin (600 mg/d) and isoniazid (300 mg/d), are also effective against *M. kansasii*; treatment is generally continued for 18 to 24 months, although some data suggest that 12 months may be adequate.

Skin Disease MAC organisms, which frequently cause disseminated disease with positive blood cultures in AIDS, are also rarely associated with heterogeneous skin manifestations, such as nodules, ulcers, areas of erythema, pustules, abscesses, or panniculitis. Skin biopsies and blood cultures establish the diagnosis.

M. haemophilum In contrast to MAC organisms, *M. haemophilum* has a tendency to involve the skin, bones, joints, and lungs, although most patients also have positive blood cultures. Skin lesions are nodular, may ulcerate, and are disseminated. In the absence of specific data, treatment should follow the guidelines for MAC infection.

NTM INFECTIONS IN IMMUNOCOMPETENT PATIENTS

PULMONARY DISEASE Etiology The NTM most frequently causing pulmonary infections are *M. intracellulare*, *M. avium*, and *M. kansasii*. Many other species, such as *M. xenopi*, *M. malmoense*, and *M. interjectum*, can also be involved in these infections. Identification of the specific pathogen is important in the choice among the various therapeutic strategies. For example, *M. kansasii* responds to antituberculosis drugs, including isoniazid.

Epidemiology and Host Factors As has already been noted, NTM are ubiquitous in the environment, but their pathogenicity is low. Preexisting lung disease (e.g., chronic obstructive airway disease, cancer, previous tuberculosis, bronchiectasis, cystic fibrosis, and silicosis, with cavities and bronchiectases) is the main predisposing factor for pulmonary disease due to NTM.

Anecdotal evidence suggests that the proportion of patients without underlying lung pathology who are developing pulmonary disease due to NTM is increasing. These patients are usually elderly; many are women with pectus excavatum or scoliosis. In the latter elderly women, the lingula and the right middle lobes are particularly involved. Somewhat whimsically, the disease in these patients has been called "Lady Windermere syndrome" after the main character in Oscar Wilde's play *Lady Windermere's Fan*, who went to extremes to refrain from coughing.

Clinical Manifestations Most immunocompetent patients with pulmonary NTM infection present with chronic cough, low-grade fever, and malaise; some present with hemoptysis. These symptoms may be masked by those of the underlying disease process.

Diagnosis In contrast to the isolation of *M. tuberculosis*, of which even a single colony—whatever its origin—is clinically significant, the isolation of NTM from the sputum never in itself proves the existence of disease. NTM are frequently commensals and colonize both diseased and normal airways. Because treatment of NTM infection is complicated, it is important that the diagnosis be certain. The American Thoracic Society has formulated the following minimal guidelines for the diagnosis of pulmonary NTM disease: "evidence, such as an infiltrate visible on a chest roentgenogram, of disease, the cause of which has not been determined by careful clinical and laboratory studies, and . . . isolation of multiple colonies of the same strain of mycobacteria repeatedly, usually in the absence of other pathogens." For patients who have pulmonary infiltrates but not cavities, these criteria may not be specific enough; some patients are found to have cleared NTM after a 1-month trial of bronchial hygiene alone (inhalation of saline and bronchodilators to induce cough and sputum production). The detection by computed tomography of bronchiectases and nodular infiltrates in the same lobe may be particularly suggestive of NTM infection.

℞ **TREATMENT** Lung disease due to NTM may be managed by follow-up without treatment, by resection, or by drug therapy. No randomized trial has determined which is the best option. In retrospectively analyzed case series, patients undergoing surgery have had a better outcome than those treated only with drugs. However, selection bias has probably influenced these results since patients with extensive lung disease are poor candidates for surgery.

As in HIV-infected patients, immunocompetent patients with minimal disease do not need treatment at all. Likewise, NTM disease may present as a solitary pulmonary nodule that, once resected (to confirm or exclude a diagnosis of cancer), requires no further drug treatment.

Most other patients with pulmonary NTM disease are treated with antimicrobials; in addition, they may or may not undergo surgery. The drugs available for the treatment of infection with *M. avium* or *M. intracellulare* have already been discussed. The regimens recommended for disseminated MAC infection are preferred, although large doses of clarithromycin are often poorly tolerated by elderly patients. *M. intracellulare* may be easier to treat and eradicate than *M. avium*. In two small open studies, single-agent treatment with clarithromycin (500 mg twice daily) led to improvements detected by chest radiography and sputum culture.

Indications for surgery are difficult to establish but include a disappointing response to antibiotics, the presence of localized disease, and the absence of contraindications (especially impaired respiratory functions). Ideally, drug treatment should begin before surgery and should render the sputum negative by the time of the operation.

In contrast to MAC organisms, *M. kansasii* is predictably sensitive to antituberculosis agents. Treatment should consist of isoniazid (300 mg/d), rifampin (600 mg/d), and ethambutol (15 to 25 mg/kg per day). The optimal duration of therapy is unknown, but most patients have been treated for 18 to 24 months; 12 months may suffice. Sulfamethoxazole is recommended for the occasional patient whose infection relapses after *M. kansasii* becomes resistant to rifampin.

LYMPHADENITIS　NTM are among the causes of localized lymphadenitis. This disease occurs mostly in children between the ages of 1 and 5 years. Painless swelling of one node or a group of nodes usually affects the anterior cervical chain. Nodes may rapidly increase in size, with the formation of fistulas to the skin. *M. scrofulaceum* or MAC organisms most commonly cause NTM lymphadenitis, although many other species may be involved. Once tuberculosis has been excluded, the treatment of choice is excision without chemotherapy. When excision is dangerous because of proximity to the facial nerve, aspiration combined with chemotherapy may be effective.

SKIN DISEASE DUE TO NTM　**Swimming-Pool and Fish-Tank Granuloma**　Between 1 week and 2 months (usually 2 to 3 weeks) after contact with contaminated tropical fish tanks, swimming pools, or saltwater fish, a small violet nodule or pustule may appear at a site of minor trauma. This lesion may evolve to form a crusted ulcer or small abscess or may remain warty. Lesions are multiple and disseminated on occasion—particularly, but not exclusively, in immunosuppressed patients. The causative organism is *M. marinum*. The patient's clinical history, combined with the isolation of *M. marinum* after biopsy and culture, establishes the diagnosis. Lesions often heal spontaneously. In cases of persistence or dissemination, rifampin (300 to 600 mg/d) in combination with ethambutol (15 to 25 mg/kg per day), trimethoprim-sulfamethoxazole (160/800 mg twice daily), or minocycline (100 mg/d) may be tried for a period of at least 3 months.

Very rarely, a similar clinical picture is produced by *M. gordonae*, a frequently isolated but usually nonpathogenic species.

Buruli Ulcer　In many tropical areas throughout the world, *M. ulcerans* may cause an itching nodule on the arms or legs, which then breaks down to form a shallow ulcer of variable size. The course of this condition is usually prolonged. *M. ulcerans* is difficult to culture; plates need to be incubated at low temperature. Excision constitutes the usual therapy. Treatment with rifampin, clofazimine, or trimethoprim-sulfamethoxazole has met with variable success.

NTM INFECTIONS OF SOFT TISSUE, TENDONS, BONES, AND JOINTS　**Infections Linked to Injections and Surgery**　Occasionally, mycobacteria are isolated from nodular skin lesions of hospitalized patients, particularly those who are immunosuppressed; in some instances there is associated lymphatic spread. Many cases are linked to injection; diabetic patients are at especially high risk. In ophthalmology, mycobacteria may cause keratitis and corneal ulceration after surgery or injury. Epidemics of mycobacterial infection following cardiac surgery have been linked to contaminated ice packs and contaminated porcine heart valves. These infections are usually due to *M. fortuitum*, *M. chelonae*, or *M. abscessus*, which are referred to collectively as the *M. fortuitum* complex. These are the so-called rapidly growing mycobacteria: colonies on solid medium appear 3 to 7 days after inoculation. As organisms may fail to grow at 37°C, incubation at 30 to 33°C is recommended. These mycobacteria are notoriously resistant to most antituberculosis drugs. Debridement is best combined with administration of two or three of the antibiotics mentioned in Table 171-1.

Infections of Tendons, Joints, and Bones　In rare cases, mycobacteria invade deep tissues after direct inoculation, via contiguous spread from superficial sites of infection, or through the bloodstream. MAC organisms and *M. ulcerans* are most often cited in these instances. *M. szulgai* seems to be involved particularly frequently in olecranon bursitis.

BIBLIOGRAPHY

ABERG JA et al: Eradication of AIDS-related disseminated *Mycobacterium avium* complex infection after 12 months of antimycobacterial therapy combined with highly active antiretroviral therapy. J Infect Dis 178:1446, 1998

Diagnosis and treatment of disease caused by nontuberculous mycobacteria. Am Rev Respir Dis 142:940, 1990

NEWPORT MJ et al: A mutation in the interferon-gamma-receptor gene and susceptibility to mycobacterial infection. N Engl J Med 335:1941, 1996

SHAFRAN SD et al: A comparison of two regimens for the treatment of *Mycobacterium avium* complex bacteremia in AIDS: Rifabutin, ethambutol, and clarithromycin versus rifampin, ethambutol, clofazimine, and ciprofloxacin. Canadian HIV Trials Network Protocol 010 Study Group. N Engl J Med 335:377, 1996

TANAKA E et al: Effect of clarithromycin regimen for *Mycobacterium avium* complex pulmonary disease. Am J Respir Crit Care Med 160:866, 1999

VAN DER WERF TS et al: *Mycobacterium ulcerans* infection. Lancet 354:1013, 1999

WOLINSKY E: Mycobacterial lymphadenitis in children: A prospective study of 105 nontuberculous cases with long-term follow-up. Clin Infect Dis 20:954, 1995

YAMAZAKI Y et al: Markers indicating deterioration of pulmonary *Mycobacterium avium-intracellulare* infection. Am J Respir Crit Care Med 160:1851, 1999

Section 9
SPIROCHETAL DISEASES

172　*Sheila A. Lukehart*

SYPHILIS

DEFINITION　Syphilis, a chronic systemic infection caused by *Treponema pallidum* subspecies *pallidum*, is usually sexually trans-

mitted and is characterized by episodes of active disease interrupted by periods of latency. After an incubation period averaging 2 to 6 weeks, a primary lesion appears, often associated with regional lymphadenopathy. A secondary bacteremic stage, associated with generalized mucocutaneous lesions and generalized lymphadenopathy, is followed by a latent period of subclinical infection lasting many years. In about one-third of untreated cases, the tertiary stage is characterized by progressive destructive mucocutaneous, musculoskeletal, or parenchymal lesions; aortitis; or symptomatic central nervous system (CNS) disease.

172 Syphilis **1045**

ETIOLOGY The Spirochaetales include three genera that are pathogenic for humans and for a variety of other animals: *Leptospira*, which causes human leptospirosis; *Borrelia*, which causes relapsing fever and Lyme disease; and *Treponema*, which causes the diseases known as treponematoses. The genus *Treponema* includes *T. pallidum* subspecies *pallidum*, which causes venereal syphilis; *T. pallidum* subspecies *pertenue*, which causes yaws; *T. pallidum* subspecies *endemicum*, which causes endemic syphilis or bejel; and *T. carateum*, which causes pinta (Chap. 173). Other *Treponema* species found in the human mouth, genital mucosa, and gastrointestinal tract have no proven pathogenic role in human disease. These spirochetes can be confused with *T. pallidum* on dark-field examination. An oral treponeme that is very closely related to *T. pallidum* antigenically has been found to be significantly associated with periodontitis and acute necrotizing ulcerative gingivitis; its etiologic role in these gum diseases is unknown. None of the four pathogenic treponemes has yet been cultured in quantity. Until recently, the subspecies were distinguished primarily by the clinical syndromes they produce. Recent studies have identified molecular signatures that can differentiate *T. pallidum* subspecies *pallidum* from the other pathogenic *T. pallidum* subspecies by culture-independent, polymerase chain reaction (PCR)–based methods.

T. pallidum subspecies *pallidum* (hereafter referred to simply as *T. pallidum*), a thin delicate organism with 6 to 14 spirals and tapered ends, measures 6 to 15 μm in total length and 0.2 μm in width. The cytoplasm is surrounded by a trilaminar cytoplasmic membrane, which in turn is surrounded by a delicate peptidoglycan layer providing some structural rigidity. This layer is surrounded by a lipid-rich outer membrane that contains relatively few integral membrane proteins. Six endoflagella wind around the cell body in a space between the inner cell wall and the outer membrane and may be the elements responsible for motility.

The sequencing of the genome of *T. pallidum* has yielded information about the organism's metabolic capabilities. *T. pallidum* lacks the genes required to synthesize enzyme cofactors, fatty acids, and nucleotides de novo. In addition, it lacks genes encoding the enzymes of the Krebs cycle and oxidative phosphorylation. To compensate, the organism contains numerous genes predicted to code for transporters of amino acids, carbohydrates, and cations. In addition, the genome analyses and other studies have revealed the existence of a 12-member gene family (called *tpr*) that bears similarities to variable outer-membrane antigens of other spirochetes. Although the role of these encoded molecules has not yet been defined, the TprK antigen appears to be preferentially expressed and serves as a target of opsonic antibody.

The only known natural host for *T. pallidum* is the human. *T. pallidum* can infect many mammals, but only humans, higher apes, and a few laboratory animals regularly develop syphilitic lesions. Virulent strains of *T. pallidum* are grown and maintained in rabbits.

EPIDEMIOLOGY Nearly all cases of syphilis are acquired by sexual contact with infectious lesions (i.e., the chancre, mucous patch, skin rash, or condyloma latum). Less common modes of transmission include nonsexual personal contact and infection in utero or following blood transfusions.

The total number of cases of syphilis reported annually in the United States fell steadily from 575,593 in 1943 to a low of 64,621 in 1987—an 88% decrease—but then increased to 134,255 in 1990. The number of new cases of infectious syphilis reached a peak in 1947 and then fell to approximately 6000 in 1956; since then, a rather steady increase in infectious syphilis has been punctuated by four cycles of 7 to 10 years, each with a rapid rise and fall in incidence (with peaks in 1965, 1975, 1982, and 1990). Since 1990, the number of reported cases of infectious syphilis has again declined by >80%. In 1997, there were 8550 reported cases of primary and secondary syphilis and 46,540 cases of all stages.

The populations at highest risk for acquiring syphilis have changed. Between 1977 and 1982, approximately half of all patients with early syphilis in the United States were homosexual or bisexual

men. Largely because of changing sexual practices in this population due to the AIDS epidemic, this proportion has decreased. The most recent epidemic of syphilis predominantly involved African-American heterosexual men and women and occurred largely in urban areas, where infectious syphilis has been correlated significantly with the exchange of sex for "crack" cocaine. The incidence of syphilis peaks at 15 to 34 years of age. The reported incidence is much higher among African Americans than in other ethnic groups and is higher in urban than in rural areas; 80% of infectious syphilis cases are reported from 15% of the counties in the United States.

The incidence of congenital syphilis roughly parallels that of infectious syphilis in females. The number of reported cases of congenital syphilis in infants ≤1 year of age was lowest (107 cases) in 1978, when infectious syphilis was most prevalent among homosexual and bisexual men. The dramatic increase in the incidence of primary and secondary syphilis among women from 1986 to 1990 resulted in a proportionate increase in the number of infants born with congenital syphilis—to 3275 infants in 1991. The incidence of early syphilis among men and women has declined since 1991, as has the number of reported cases of congenital syphilis in infants (with 1049 cases in 1997). It is important to note, however, that the case definition for congenital syphilis was broadened in 1989 and now includes all live or stillborn infants delivered to women with untreated or inadequately treated syphilis at delivery.

Approximately one of every two individuals named as sexual contacts of persons with infectious syphilis becomes infected. Many sexual contacts will already have developed manifestations of syphilis when they are first seen, and about 30% of apparently uninfected contacts who are examined within 30 days of exposure actually have incubating infection and will later develop infectious syphilis if not treated. Thus, the identification and "epidemiologic" treatment of all recently exposed sexual contacts constitute an important aspect of syphilis control. Also important is the identification of infected persons by serologic testing of pregnant women, persons admitted to hospitals, military inductees, and persons undergoing examination in physicians' offices. Still controversial are laws and regulations requiring routine premarital serologic testing for syphilis, where—though national data are not available—the yield is undoubtedly lower.

NATURAL COURSE AND PATHOGENESIS OF UNTREATED SYPHILIS *T. pallidum* rapidly penetrates intact mucous membranes or microscopic abrasions in skin and within a few hours enters the lymphatics and blood to produce systemic infection and metastatic foci long before the appearance of a primary lesion. Blood from a patient with incubating or early syphilis is infectious. The generation time of *T. pallidum* during early active disease in vivo is estimated to be 30 to 33 h, and the incubation period of syphilis is inversely proportional to the number of organisms inoculated. The concentration of treponemes generally reaches at least 10^7 per gram of tissue before the appearance of a clinical lesion. On the basis of intradermal injection of graded doses of *T. pallidum* into eight volunteers, the 50% infectious dose was calculated to be 57 organisms. The median incubation period in humans (about 21 days) suggests an average inoculum of 500 to 1000 infectious organisms for naturally acquired disease. The incubation period (from inoculation until the primary lesion becomes discernible) rarely exceeds 6 weeks. Subcurative therapy during the incubation period may delay the onset of the primary lesion, but it is not certain that such treatment reduces the probability that symptomatic disease will ultimately develop.

The primary lesion appears at the site of inoculation, usually persists for 4 to 6 weeks, and then heals spontaneously. Histopathologic examination of primary lesions shows perivascular infiltration, chiefly by lymphocytes (including CD8+ and CD4+ cells), plasma cells, and macrophages, with capillary endothelial proliferation and subsequent obliteration of small blood vessels. The CD4+ infiltration displays a T_H1-type cytokine profile consistent with the activation of macrophages. At this time *T. pallidum* is demonstrable in the chancre in spaces between epithelial cells; within invaginations or phagosomes of epithelial cells, fibroblasts, plasma cells, and the endothelial cells of small capillaries; within lymphatic channels; and in the regional lymph nodes. Phagocytosis of organisms by activated macrophages ultimately causes their destruction, which results in spontaneous resolution of the chancre.

The generalized parenchymal, constitutional, and mucocutaneous manifestations of secondary syphilis usually appear about 6 to 8 weeks after healing of the chancre, although 15% of patients with secondary syphilis still have persisting or healing chancres. In other patients, secondary lesions may appear several months after the chancre has healed, and some patients may enter the latent stage without ever recognizing secondary lesions. The histopathologic features of secondary maculopapular skin lesions are hyperkeratosis of the epidermis; capillary proliferation with endothelial swelling in the superficial corium; and dermal papillae with transmigration of polymorphonuclear leukocytes and, in the deeper corium, perivascular infiltration by monocytes, plasma cells, and lymphocytes. Treponemes are found in many tissues, including the aqueous humor of the eye and the cerebrospinal fluid (CSF). Invasion of the CNS by *T. pallidum* occurs during the first weeks or months of infection, and CSF abnormalities are detected in as many as 40% of patients during the secondary stage. Clinical hepatitis and immune complex–induced membranous glomerulonephritis are relatively rare but recognized manifestations of secondary syphilis; liver function tests may yield abnormal results in up to a quarter of patients with early syphilis. Generalized nontender lymphadenopathy is noted in 85% of patients with secondary syphilis. The paradoxical appearance of secondary manifestations despite high titers of antibody (including immobilizing antibody) to *T. pallidum* is unexplained but may result from changes in expression of surface antigens. Secondary lesions subside within 2 to 6 weeks, and the infection enters the latent stage, which is detectable only by serologic testing. In the preantibiotic era, up to 25% of untreated patients experienced at least one generalized or localized mucocutaneous relapse, usually during the first year; therefore, identification and examination of sexual contacts are most important for patients with syphilis of <1 year's duration. Recurrent generalized rash is now rare.

In the preantibiotic era, about one-third of patients with untreated latent syphilis developed clinically apparent tertiary disease; today, in industrialized countries, specific treatment and coincidental therapy for early and latent syphilis have all but eliminated tertiary disease except for sporadic cases of neurosyphilis in persons infected with HIV. In the past, the most common type of tertiary disease was the gumma, a usually benign granulomatous lesion. Today, gummas are very uncommon. Cardiovascular syphilis, now also rare, is caused by obliterative small-vessel endarteritis, usually involving the vasa vasorum of the ascending aorta and resulting in aneurysm. Asymptomatic CNS involvement is demonstrable in up to 25% of patients with late latent syphilis. The factors that contribute to the development and progression of tertiary disease are unknown.

The course of untreated syphilis was studied retrospectively in a group of nearly 2000 patients with primary or secondary disease diagnosed clinically (the Oslo Study, 1891–1951) and prospectively in 431 African-American men with seropositive latent syphilis of 3 or more years' duration (the notorious Tuskegee Study, 1932–1972). In the Oslo Study, 24% of patients developed relapsing secondary lesions within 4 years, and 28% eventually developed one or more manifestations of tertiary syphilis. Cardiovascular syphilis, including aortitis, was detected in 10% of patients, none of whom had been infected before age 15; 7% of patients developed symptomatic neurosyphilis, and 16% developed benign tertiary syphilis (gummas of the skin, mucous membranes, and skeleton). Syphilis was the primary cause of death in 15% of men and 8% of women. Cardiovascular syphilis was documented in 35% of men and 22% of women who eventually came to autopsy. In general, serious late complications were nearly twice as common among men as among women.

The Tuskegee Study showed that the death rate among untreated African-American men with syphilis (25 to 50 years old) was 17% higher than that among uninfected subjects and that 30% of all deaths were attributable to cardiovascular or CNS syphilis. By far the most important factor in increased mortality was cardiovascular syphilis. Anatomic evidence of aortitis was found in 40 to 60% of autopsied subjects with syphilis (versus 15% of control subjects), while CNS syphilis was found in only 4%. Rates of hypertension were also higher among the infected subjects. The ethical issues eventually raised by this study, begun in the preantibiotic era but continuing into the early 1970s, had a major influence on the development of current guidelines for human medical experimentation, and the history of the study may still contribute to a reluctance of some African Americans to participate as subjects in clinical research.

These two studies both showed that about one-third of patients with untreated syphilis develop clinical or pathologic evidence of tertiary syphilis, that about one-fourth die as a direct result of tertiary syphilis, and that there is additional excess mortality not directly attributable to tertiary syphilis.

MANIFESTATIONS   Primary Syphilis   The typical primary chancre usually begins as a single painless papule that rapidly becomes eroded and usually becomes indurated, with a characteristic cartilaginous consistency on palpation of the edge and base of the ulcer (**see Plate IID-47**). In heterosexual men the chancre is usually located on the penis, whereas in homosexual men it is often found in the anal canal or rectum, in the mouth, or on the external genitalia. In women, common primary sites are the cervix and labia. Consequently, primary syphilis goes unrecognized in women and homosexual men more often than in heterosexual men.

Atypical primary lesions are common. The clinical appearance depends on the number of treponemes inoculated and on the immunologic status of the patient. A large inoculum produces a dark-field-positive ulcerative lesion in nonimmune volunteers but may produce a small dark-field-negative papule, an asymptomatic but seropositive latent infection, or no response at all in individuals with a history of syphilis. A small inoculum may produce only a papular lesion, even in nonimmune individuals. Therefore, syphilis should be considered even in the evaluation of trivial or atypical dark-field-negative genital lesions. The genital lesions that most commonly must be differentiated from those of primary syphilis include traumatic superinfected lesions, lesions of herpes simplex virus infection (Chap. 182), and lesions of chancroid (Chap. 149). *Primary genital herpes* may produce inguinal adenopathy, but the nodes are tender and the lesions consist of multiple painful vesicles, which later ulcerate and are often accompanied by systemic symptoms, including fever. *Recurrent genital herpes* typically begins with a unilateral cluster of painful vesicles, usually without associated adenopathy. *Chancroid* produces painful, superficial, exudative, nonindurated ulcers, more often multiple than in syphilis (**see Plate IID-54**); adenopathy is common, can be either unilateral or bilateral, is tender, and may be suppurative.

Regional lymphadenopathy usually accompanies the primary syphilitic lesion, appearing within 1 week of the onset of the lesion. The nodes are firm, nonsuppurative, and painless. Inguinal lymphadenopathy is bilateral and may occur with anal as well as with external genital chancres. Rectal chancres result in perirectal lymphadenopathy, while chancres of the cervix and vagina result in iliac or perirectal adenopathy. The chancre generally heals within 4 to 6 weeks (range, 2 to 12 weeks), but lymphadenopathy may persist for months.

Secondary Syphilis   The protean manifestations of the secondary stage usually include localized or diffuse symmetric mucocutaneous lesions and generalized nontender lymphadenopathy. The healing primary chancre is still present in 15% of cases. The skin rash consists of macular, papular, papulosquamous, and occasionally pustular syphilides; often more than one form is present simultaneously. The eruption may be very subtle. Approximately 25% of patients with a discernible rash of secondary syphilis may be unaware that they have dermatologic manifestations. Initial lesions are bilaterally symmetric, pale red or pink, nonpruritic, discrete, round macules that measure 5 to 10 mm in diameter and are distributed on the trunk and proximal extremities (**see Plate IID-50**). After several days or weeks, red papular lesions 3 to 10 mm in diameter also appear. These lesions, which may progress to necrotic lesions (resembling pustules) in association with increasing endarteritis and perivascular mononuclear infiltration, are distributed widely, frequently involve the palms and soles (**see Plate IID-48**), and may occur on the face and scalp. Tiny papular *follicular syphilides* involving hair follicles may result in patchy alopecia (alopecia areata), with loss of scalp hair, eyebrows, or beard in up to 5% of cases. Progressive endarteritis obliterans and ischemia result in superficial scaling of papules (*papulosquamous syphilides*) and eventually may lead to central necrosis (*pustular syphilides*).

In warm, moist, intertriginous body areas, including the perianal area, vulva, scrotum, inner thighs, axillae, and skin under pendulous breasts, papules can enlarge and become eroded to produce broad, moist, pink or gray-white, highly infectious lesions called *condylomata lata* (**see Plate IID-49**); these lesions develop in 10% of patients with secondary syphilis. Superficial mucosal erosions, called *mucous patches*, occur in 10 to 15% of patients and may involve the lips, oral mucosa, tongue (Fig. 172-1), palate, pharynx, vulva and vagina, glans penis, or inner prepuce. The typical mucous patch is a painless silver-gray erosion surrounded by a red periphery. During relapses of secondary syphilis, condylomata lata are particularly common, and skin lesions tend to be asymmetrically distributed and more infiltrated, resembling skin lesions of late syphilis. These characteristics may reflect increasing cellular immunity.

Constitutional symptoms that may accompany or precede secondary syphilis include sore throat (15 to 30%), fever (5 to 8%), weight loss (2 to 20%), malaise (25%), anorexia (2 to 10%), headache (10%), and meningismus (5%). *Acute meningitis* occurs in only 1 to 2% of cases, but numbers of cells and levels of protein in CSF are increased in ≥30% of cases. *T. pallidum* has been recovered from CSF during primary and secondary syphilis in 30% of cases; this finding is often but not always associated with other CSF abnormalities.

Less common complications of secondary syphilis include hepatitis, nephropathy, gastrointestinal involvement (hypertrophic gastritis, patchy proctitis, ulcerative colitis, or a rectosigmoid mass), arthritis, and periostitis. Ocular findings that suggest secondary syphilis include otherwise-unexplained pupillary abnormalities, optic neuritis, and a retinitis pigmentosa syndrome as well as the classic iritis (especially granulomatous iritis) or uveitis. The diagnosis of secondary syphilis is often considered only after the patient fails to respond to steroid therapy. Anterior uveitis has been reported in 5 to 10% of patients with secondary syphilis, and *T. pallidum* has been demonstrated in the aqueous humor from these patients. *Syphilitic hepatitis* is distinguished by an unusually high serum level of alkaline phosphatase and by a nonspecific histologic appearance that is unlike that of viral hepatitis

and includes moderate inflammation with polymorphonuclear leukocytes and lymphocytes, some hepatocellular damage, and no cholestasis. *Renal involvement* produces proteinuria associated with an acute nephrotic syndrome (or rarely with hemorrhagic glomerulonephritis) and is characterized by subepithelial electron-dense deposits and glomerular immune complexes—findings suggesting immune-complex glomerulonephritis.

Latent Syphilis Positive serologic tests for syphilis, together with a normal CSF examination and the absence of clinical manifestations of syphilis, indicate a diagnosis of latent syphilis. The diagnosis is often suspected on the basis of a history of primary or secondary lesions, a history of exposure to syphilis, or the delivery of an infant with congenital syphilis. A previous negative serologic test or a history of lesions or exposure may help establish the duration of latent infection. *Early latent* syphilis encompasses the first year after infection, while *late latent* syphilis (beginning ≥1 year after infection in the untreated patient) is associated with relative immunity to infectious relapse and with increasing resistance to reinfection. *T. pallidum* may still seed the bloodstream intermittently during this stage. Pregnant women with latent syphilis may infect the fetus in utero. Moreover, syphilis has been transmitted through the transfusion of blood from patients with latent syphilis of many years' duration. It was previously thought that untreated late latent syphilis had three possible outcomes: (1) it could persist throughout the lifetime of the infected individual, (2) it could end in the development of late syphilis, or (3) it could end with the spontaneous cure of infection, with reversion of serologic tests to negative. It is now apparent, however, that the more sensitive treponemal antibody tests rarely, if ever, become negative without treatment. About 70% of untreated patients with latent syphilis never develop clinically evident late syphilis, but the occurrence of spontaneous cure is in doubt.

Late Syphilis The slowly progressive inflammatory disease leading to tertiary manifestations begins early during the pathogenesis of syphilis, although these manifestations may not become clinically apparent for years. Early syphilitic aortitis becomes evident soon after secondary lesions subside, and patients who develop CSF abnormalities during the early stages of syphilis appear to be at highest risk of late neurologic complications.

Asymptomatic neurosyphilis CNS syphilis represents a continuum comprising early invasion, usually within the first weeks or months of infection, and asymptomatic involvement, which may or may not lead to neurologic manifestations. Traditionally, the diagnosis of asymptomatic neurosyphilis has been made in patients who lack neurologic symptoms and signs and who have CSF abnormalities including mononuclear pleocytosis, increased protein concentrations, or a reactive Venereal Disease Research Laboratory (VDRL) slide test. Such abnormalities are found in up to one-quarter of patients with untreated late latent syphilis, and it is these patients who are known to be at risk for neurologic complications. However, in primary and secondary syphilis, *T. pallidum* can be isolated from CSF of 40% of patients even in the absence of other CSF abnormalities. Although the therapeutic implications of these findings in early syphilis are uncertain, it seems appropriate to conclude that even patients with early syphilis who have such findings do indeed have asymptomatic neurosyphilis and should be treated for neurosyphilis. In patients with untreated asymptomatic neurosyphilis, the overall cumulative probability of progression to clinical neurosyphilis is about 20% in the first 10 years but increases with time; the likelihood is highest among patients with the greatest degree of pleocytosis or protein elevation. Patients with untreated latent syphilis and normal CSF probably run no risk of subsequent neurosyphilis.

Symptomatic neurosyphilis Although mixed features are common, the major clinical categories of symptomatic neurosyphilis include meningeal, meningovascular, and parenchymatous syphilis. The last category includes general paresis and tabes dorsalis. The onset of symptoms usually comes <1 year after infection for meningeal syph-

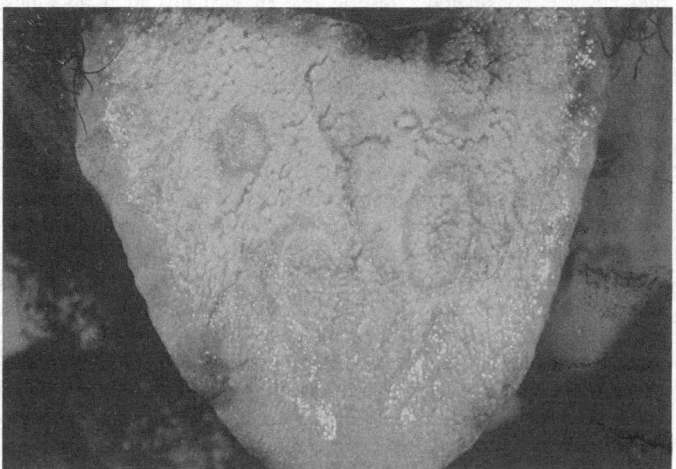

FIGURE 172-1 Mucous patches on the tongue of a patient with secondary syphilis. (*Courtesy of Ron Roddy.*)

ilis, at 5 to 10 years for meningovascular syphilis, at 20 years for general paresis, and at 25 to 30 years for tabes dorsalis. However, symptomatic neurosyphilis, particularly in the antibiotic era, often presents not as a classic picture but rather as mixed and subtle or incomplete syndromes.

Meningeal syphilis may involve either the brain or the spinal cord, and patients may present with headache, nausea, vomiting, neck stiffness, cranial nerve palsies, seizures, and changes in mental status. *Meningovascular syphilis* reflects diffuse inflammation of the pia and arachnoid together with evidence of focal or widespread arterial involvement of small, medium, or large vessels. The most common presentation is a stroke syndrome involving the middle cerebral artery of a relatively young adult; however, unlike the usual thrombotic or embolic stroke syndrome of sudden onset, meningovascular syphilis often becomes manifest after a subacute encephalitic prodrome (with headaches, vertigo, insomnia, and psychological abnormalities), which is followed by a gradually progressive vascular syndrome.

The manifestations of *general paresis* reflect widespread parenchymal damage and include abnormalities corresponding to the mnemonic *paresis*: *p*ersonality, *a*ffect, *r*eflexes (hyperactive), *e*ye (e.g., Argyll Robertson pupils), *s*ensorium (illusions, delusions, hallucinations), *i*ntellect (a decrease in recent memory and in the capacity for orientation, calculations, judgment, and insight), and *s*peech. *Tabes dorsalis* presents as symptoms and signs of demyelination of the posterior columns, dorsal roots, and dorsal root ganglia. Symptoms include ataxic wide-based gait and footslap; paresthesia; bladder disturbances; impotence; areflexia; and loss of position, deep pain, and temperature sensations. Trophic joint degeneration (Charcot's joints) and perforating ulceration of the feet can result from loss of pain sensation. The small, irregular Argyll Robertson pupil, a feature of both tabes dorsalis and paresis, reacts to accommodation but not to light. *Optic atrophy* also occurs frequently in association with tabes.

Cardiovascular syphilis Cardiovascular manifestations are attributable to endarteritis obliterans of the vasa vasorum, which provide the blood supply to large vessels. This condition produces medial necrosis with destruction of elastic tissue, particularly in the ascending and transverse segments of the aortic arch, resulting in uncomplicated aortitis, aortic regurgitation, saccular aneurysm, or coronary ostial stenosis. Symptoms appear from 10 to 40 years after infection. Cardiovascular complications occur more often and at an earlier age among men than among women and may be more common among African Americans than among whites. In the preantibiotic era, symptomatic cardiovascular complications developed in about 10% of persons with late untreated syphilis, and aortic regurgitation was two to four times as common as aneurysm. However, syphilitic aortitis was demonstrated at autopsy in about one-half of African-American men with untreated syphilis.

Linear calcification of the ascending aorta on chest x-ray films suggests asymptomatic syphilitic aortitis, as arteriosclerosis seldom produces this sign. Aortic dilation and a tambour quality to the sound of aortic closure are unreliable signs of aortitis. Syphilitic aneurysms—usually saccular, occasionally fusiform—do not lead to dissection. Approximately 1 in 10 aortic aneurysms of syphilitic origin involves the abdominal aorta, but these aneurysms tend to occur above the renal arteries, whereas arteriosclerotic abdominal aneurysms are usually found below the renal arteries. With increasing age, the nervous system is also affected in up to 40% of patients with cardiovascular syphilis.

Late lesions of the eyes Iritis associated with pain, photophobia, and dimness of vision or chorioretinitis occurs not only during secondary syphilis but also as a relatively common manifestation of late syphilis. Adhesions of the iris to the anterior lens may produce a fixed pupil, not to be confused with Argyll Robertson pupil.

Late benign syphilis (gumma) Gummas may be multiple or diffuse but are usually solitary lesions that range from microscopic size to several centimeters in diameter. From a histologic perspective, gum-

mas consist of a granulomatous inflammation with a central area of necrosis surrounded by mononuclear, epithelioid, and fibroblastic cells; occasional giant cells; and perivasculitis. Although rarely demonstrated microscopically, *T. pallidum* has reportedly been recovered from these lesions. The most commonly involved sites include the skin and skeletal system, the mouth and upper respiratory tract, the larynx, the liver, and the stomach; however, any organ may be involved. Gummas of the skin produce painless and indurated nodular, papulosquamous, or ulcerative lesions that form characteristic circles or arcs, with peripheral hyperpigmentation. Gummas are usually indolent and may heal spontaneously with scarring, but they may also be explosive in onset and are often destructive. These lesions may resemble those of many other chronic granulomatous conditions, including tuberculosis and sarcoidosis, leprosy, and deep fungal infections. Skeletal gummas most frequently involve the long bones of the legs, although any bone may be affected. Trauma may predispose a specific site to involvement. Presenting symptoms usually include focal pain and tenderness. Radiographic abnormalities with advanced gummas of bone include periostitis or destructive or sclerosing osteitis. Upper respiratory gummas can lead to perforation of the nasal septum or palate. Gummatous hepatitis may produce epigastric pain and tenderness as well as low-grade fever and may be associated with splenomegaly and anemia.

The histopathology and extensive tissue necrosis associated with gummas suggest delayed hypersensitivity to *T. pallidum*. Certain individuals appear to develop an exaggerated delayed-hypersensitivity response to *T. pallidum*, which presumably is mediated by sensitized T lymphocytes and macrophages. Because the histologic changes may be suggestive but are nonspecific, the diagnosis of late benign syphilis is confirmed by serologic testing and by therapeutic trial. Treatment with penicillin results in rapid healing of active gummatous lesions.

Congenital Syphilis Transmission of *T. pallidum* from a syphilitic woman to her fetus across the placenta may occur at any stage of pregnancy, but the lesions of congenital syphilis generally develop after the fourth month of gestation, when fetal immunologic competence begins to develop. This timing suggests that the pathogenesis of congenital syphilis depends on the immune response of the host rather than on a direct toxic effect of *T. pallidum*. The risk of infection of the fetus during untreated early maternal syphilis is estimated to be 75 to 95%, decreasing to about 35% for maternal syphilis of >2 years' duration. Adequate treatment of the mother before the 16th week of pregnancy should prevent fetal damage. Untreated maternal infection may result in a rate of fetal loss of up to 40% (with stillbirth more common than abortion because of the late onset of fetal pathology), prematurity, neonatal death, or nonfatal congenital syphilis. Among infants born alive, only fulminant congenital syphilis is clinically apparent at birth, and these babies have a very poor prognosis. The most common clinical problem is the healthy-appearing baby born to a mother with a positive serologic test. Routine serologic testing in early pregnancy is considered cost-effective in virtually all populations, even in areas with a low prenatal prevalence of syphilis. Where the prevalence of syphilis is high and when the patient is at high risk, syphilis serology should be repeated in the third trimester and at delivery.

The manifestations of congenital syphilis can be divided into three types according to their timing: (1) early manifestations, which appear within the first 2 years of life (often between 2 and 10 weeks of age), are infectious and resemble the manifestations of severe secondary syphilis in the adult; (2) late manifestations, which appear after 2 years and are noninfectious; and (3) residual stigmata. The earliest sign of congenital syphilis is usually rhinitis, or "snuffles" (23%), which is soon followed by other mucocutaneous lesions (35 to 41%). These may include bullae (syphilitic pemphigus), vesicles, superficial desquamation, petechiae, and (later) papulosquamous lesions, mucous patches, and condylomata lata. The most common early manifestations are bone changes (61%), including osteochondritis, osteitis, and periostitis. Hepatosplenomegaly (50%), lymphadenopathy (32%), anemia (34%), jaundice (30%), thrombocytopenia, and leukocytosis are common.

Neonatal congenital syphilis must be differentiated from other generalized congenital infections, including rubella, cytomegalovirus or herpes simplex virus infection, and toxoplasmosis, as well as from erythroblastosis fetalis. Neonatal death is usually due to pulmonary hemorrhage, secondary bacterial infection, or severe hepatitis.

Late congenital syphilis is that which remains untreated after 2 years of age. In perhaps 60% of cases, the infection remains subclinical; the clinical spectrum in the remainder of cases differs in certain respects from that of acquired late syphilis in the adult. For example, cardiovascular syphilis rarely develops in late congenital syphilis, whereas interstitial keratitis is much more common and occurs between the ages of 5 and 25. Other manifestations associated with interstitial keratitis are eighth-nerve deafness and recurrent arthropathy. Bilateral knee effusions are known as *Clutton's joints.* Asymptomatic neurosyphilis is present in about one-third of untreated patients, and clinical neurosyphilis occurs in one-quarter of untreated individuals over 6 years of age. Gummatous periostitis occurs between the ages of 5 and 20 and, as in nonvenereal endemic syphilis, tends to cause destructive lesions of the palate and nasal septum.

Characteristic stigmata include *Hutchinson's teeth*—centrally notched, widely spaced, peg-shaped upper central incisors—and "mulberry" molars—sixth-year molars with multiple, poorly developed cusps. The abnormal facies of patients with congenital syphilis include frontal bossing, saddle nose, and poorly developed maxillae. Saber shins, characterized by anterior tibial bowing, are rare. *Rhagades* are linear scars at the angles of the mouth and nose that are caused by secondary bacterial infection of the early facial eruption. Other stigmata include unexplained nerve deafness, old chorioretinitis, optic atrophy, and corneal opacities due to past interstitial keratitis.

LABORATORY EXAMINATIONS **Demonstration of the Organism** Dark-field microscopic examination of lesion exudate is useful in evaluating moist cutaneous lesions, such as the chancre of primary syphilis or the condylomata lata of secondary syphilis. The identification of a single characteristic motile organism by a trained observer is sufficient for diagnosis. Examination of oral lesions and anal ulcers by this method is not recommended, as it is difficult to differentiate *T. pallidum* from other spirochetes that may be present.

Most syphilis is diagnosed in settings where dark-field microscopy is not available. The direct fluorescent antibody *T. pallidum* (DFA-TP) test, an alternative available at central laboratories, uses fluorescein-conjugated polyclonal antitreponemal antibody for the detection of *T. pallidum* in fixed smears prepared from suspect lesions. More sensitive PCR tests have been developed but are available only in research laboratories.

T. pallidum can be found in tissue with appropriate silver stains, although these results should be interpreted with caution because artifacts resembling *T. pallidum* are often seen. Treponemes can be demonstrated more reliably in tissue by immunofluorescent or immunohistochemical methods using specific monoclonal or polyclonal antibodies to *T. pallidum.*

Serologic Tests for Syphilis There are two types of serologic tests for syphilis: nontreponemal and treponemal. Both types of tests are reactive in persons with any treponemal infection, including yaws, pinta, and endemic syphilis.

The nontreponemal tests measure IgG and IgM directed against a cardiolipin-lecithin-cholesterol antigen complex. The most widely used nontreponemal antibody tests for syphilis are the rapid plasma reagin (RPR) test, which can be automated (ART), and the VDRL slide test. In these tests, antibody is detected by the microscopic or macroscopic flocculation of the antigen suspension. The RPR test may be more expensive than the VDRL test, but it is easier to perform and uses unheated serum; it is the test of choice for rapid serologic diagnosis in a clinic or office setting. The VDRL test, however, remains the standard for use with CSF.

The RPR and VDRL tests are equally sensitive and may be used for initial screening or for quantitation of serum antibody. The titer reflects the activity of the disease. A fourfold or greater rise in titer may be seen during the evolution of early syphilis. VDRL titers usually

reach 1:32 or higher in secondary syphilis. A persistent fall of two dilutions (fourfold) or greater following treatment of early syphilis provides essential evidence of an adequate response to therapy. VDRL titers do not correspond directly to RPR titers, and sequential quantitative testing (as for response to therapy) must employ a single test.

Two standard treponemal tests are used for confirmation of reactive nontreponemal results: the fluorescent treponemal antibody–absorbed (FTA-ABS) test and the agglutination assays for antibodies to *T. pallidum.* The microhemagglutination assay for *T. pallidum* (MHA-TP) has been replaced by the Serodia TP-PA test (Fujirebio, Tokyo), which is more sensitive for primary syphilis. The *T. pallidum* hemagglutination test (TPHA) is widely used in Europe but is not available in the United States. Both the agglutination assays and the FTA-ABS tests are very specific and, when used for confirmation of positive nontreponemal tests, have a very high positive predictive value for the diagnosis of syphilis. However, even these tests give false-positive results at rates as high as 1 to 2% when used for the screening of normal populations. New enzyme-linked immunosorbent assays have also been approved as confirmatory tests.

The relative sensitivities of the VDRL test, the FTA-ABS test, and the MHA-TP in the various stages of untreated syphilis are shown in Table 172-1. The nontreponemal tests are nonreactive in about one-quarter of patients presenting with primary syphilis. In early primary syphilis, the detection of antibody can be maximized either by the performance of an FTA-ABS test or simply by repetition of a VDRL test after 1 to 2 weeks if the initial VDRL result is negative. All treponemal and nontreponemal tests are reactive during secondary syphilis, and a nonreactive result virtually excludes syphilis in a patient with otherwise-compatible mucocutaneous lesions. (Fewer than 1% of patients with secondary syphilis have a VDRL test that is nonreactive or weakly reactive with undiluted serum but is positive at higher serum dilutions—the *prozone phenomenon.*) While the nontreponemal tests will become nonreactive or will be reactive in lower titers following therapy for early syphilis, the treponemal tests often remain reactive after therapy and therefore are not helpful in determining the infection status of persons with past syphilis.

For practical purposes, most clinicians need to be familiar with the three uses of serologic tests for syphilis: (1) testing of large numbers of sera for screening or diagnostic purposes (e.g., the RPR or VDRL test), (2) quantitative measurement of the antibody titer to assess the clinical activity of syphilis or to monitor the response to therapy (e.g., the VDRL or RPR test), and (3) confirmation of the diagnosis of syphilis in a patient with a positive nontreponemal antibody test or with a suspected clinical diagnosis of syphilis (e.g., the FTA-ABS test or Serodia TP-PA).

For measurement of IgM in neonates in whom congenital syphilis is suspected, the syphilis Captia-M test (Trinity Biotech, Jamestown, NY) and the 19S IgM FTA-ABS test are available.

False-Positive Serologic Tests for Syphilis Because the antigen used in nontreponemal tests is found in other tissues, the tests may be reactive in persons without treponemal infection, although rarely do titers exceed 1:8 in such patients. In a population selected for screening because of clinical suspicion, history of exposure, or increased risk for

Table 172-1 Sensitivity of Serodiagnostic Tests in Untreated Syphilis

Test[a]	Mean Percentage Positive (Range) at Indicated Stage of Disease[b]			
	Primary	Secondary	Latent	Tertiary
VDRL	78 (74–87)	100	95 (88–100)	71 (37–94)
FTA-ABS	84 (70–100)	100	100	96
MHA-TP[c]	76 (69–90)	100	100	94

[a] The specificity for each of these tests is 97 to 99%.
[b] In CDC studies.
[c] The MHA-TP has recently been replaced by the Serodia TP-PA test. Early evaluations suggest that the TP-PA test is more sensitive than the MHA-TP in primary syphilis.
SOURCE: Modified from SA Larsen et al: Clin Microbiol Rev 8:1, 1995.

sexually transmitted infections, fewer than 1% of reactive tests are falsely positive. The modern VDRL and RPR tests are 97 to 99% specific, and false-positive reactions are now limited largely to those conditions listed in Table 172-2. False positivity is common among persons with autoimmune disorders. The prevalence of false-positive nontreponemal tests increases with advancing age; 10% of people over 70 years of age have false-positive reactions. In the patient with a false-positive nontreponemal test, syphilis is excluded by a nonreactive treponemal test.

Evaluation for Neurosyphilis Asymptomatic involvement of the CNS is detected by examination of CSF for pleocytosis, increased protein concentration, and VDRL activity. CSF abnormalities can be demonstrated in up to 40% of cases of primary or secondary syphilis and in 25% of cases of latent syphilis. In older asymptomatic seropositive individuals, the yield of lumbar puncture is relatively low. *T. pallidum* has been recovered by CSF inoculation into rabbits from up to 30% of patients with primary or secondary syphilis but rarely from those with latent syphilis. The demonstration of *T. pallidum* in CSF is often associated with other CSF abnormalities; however, organisms can be recovered from patients with otherwise-normal CSF. Before the advent of penicillin, the risk of developing clinical neurosyphilis was roughly proportional to the intensity of CSF changes in early syphilis. CSF examination is essential in the evaluation of any seropositive patient with neurologic signs and symptoms and is recommended for all patients with untreated syphilis of unknown duration or of >1 year's duration. The possibility of asymptomatic neurosyphilis in some patients with early disease is not addressed by these recommendations. Because standard therapy with penicillin G benzathine (benzathine benzylpenicillin) for early syphilis fails to result in treponemicidal levels in the CSF, some experts advise lumbar puncture in secondary and early latent syphilis, particularly in patients with HIV infection.

In short, lumbar puncture should be performed in the evaluation of latent syphilis of >1 year's duration, in suspected neurosyphilis, and in late complications other than symptomatic neurosyphilis (since asymptomatic neurosyphilis may coexist with other late complications). CSF examination is most clearly indicated in the following situations: neurologic signs or symptoms, treatment failure, a serum reagin titer ≥ 1:32, HIV antibody positivity, other evidence of active syphilis (e.g., aortitis, gumma, visual or hearing changes), or plans to administer nonpenicillin therapy.

The CSF VDRL test is highly specific but relatively insensitive and may be nonreactive even in cases of progressive symptomatic neurosyphilis. The degree of sensitivity is highest in meningovascular syphilis and paresis and is lower in asymptomatic neurosyphilis and tabes dorsalis. The unabsorbed FTA test on CSF is reactive far more often than the CSF VDRL test in all stages of syphilis, but FTA reactivity may reflect passive transfer of serum antibody into the CSF.

Table 172-2   Causes of False-Positive Reactions in Nontreponemal Serologic Tests for Syphilis

Cause	Rate of False-Positive Reactions, %[a]
ACUTE FALSE-POSITIVE REACTION (<6 MONTHS)	
Recent viral illness or immunization	1–2
Genital herpes	4.4
Human immunodeficiency virus infection	1–4
Malaria	11
Parenteral drug use	20–25
CHRONIC FALSE-POSITIVE REACTION (≥6 MONTHS)	
Aging	9–11
Autoimmune disorders	1–20
Systemic lupus erythematosus	11–20
Rheumatoid arthritis	5
Parenteral drug use	20–25

[a] Data were collected from a variety of published reports.

A nonreactive CSF FTA test, however, may be used to rule out neurosyphilis.

Evaluation for Syphilis in Patients Infected with HIV Because persons at highest risk for syphilis (inner-city populations, homosexually active men, and people in many developing countries) are also at increased risk for HIV infection, these two infections frequently coexist in the same patient. There is evidence that syphilis and other genital-ulcer diseases may be important risk factors for the acquisition and transmission of HIV infection.

The manifestations of syphilis may be altered in patients with concurrent HIV infection, and multiple cases of neurologic relapse following standard therapy have been reported in HIV-infected patients. *T. pallidum* has been isolated from the CSF of several patients after therapy for early syphilis with penicillin G benzathine. A recent multicenter U.S. study of early syphilis found similar therapeutic responses in persons with and without concurrent HIV infection, although the study lacked sufficient statistical power to exclude an effect of HIV and 41% of subjects were lost to follow-up. This investigation confirmed the high rate of CNS invasion in early syphilis and the persistence of *T. pallidum* after standard therapy: 11 of 43 HIV-infected patients and 21 of 88 HIV-uninfected patients had *T. pallidum* detectable in CSF before therapy; 7 of the 35 patients who underwent lumbar puncture after therapy (some HIV-infected and others uninfected) still had *T. pallidum* detectable in CSF.

The frequency of unusual clinical and laboratory manifestations of syphilis among patients co-infected with HIV is unknown. Such changes may be dependent on the stage of HIV infection and the degree of immunosuppression. There is no clear evidence that the sensitivity of serologic tests for syphilis or the serologic response to therapy in the vast majority of HIV-infected patients with early syphilis differs from the corresponding findings in patients not infected with HIV. Interpretation of serologic results should be the same for the two groups.

Persons with newly diagnosed HIV infection should be tested for syphilis. Some authorities, persuaded by reports of the persistence of *T. pallidum* in the CSF of HIV-infected persons after standard penicillin benzathine therapy for early syphilis, recommend examination of CSF for evidence of neurosyphilis for all co-infected patients, regardless of the clinical stage of syphilis, with treatment for neurosyphilis if CSF abnormalities are found or if CSF examination is not performed. Others do not recommend routine CSF examination for HIV-co-infected patients with early syphilis and believe that standard therapy is sufficient. Serologic testing after treatment is important for all patients with syphilis, particularly those also infected with HIV.

℞ **TREATMENT   Treatment of Acquired Syphilis** Penicillin G is the drug of choice for all stages of syphilis. *T. pallidum* is killed by very low concentrations of penicillin G, although a long period of exposure to penicillin is required because of the unusually slow rate of multiplication of the organism. The efficacy of penicillin for syphilis remains undiminished after 50 years of use. Other antibiotics effective in syphilis include the tetracyclines, erythromycin, and the cephalosporins. Aminoglycosides and spectinomycin inhibit *T. pallidum* only in very large doses, and the sulfonamides and the quinolones are inactive.

Serum levels of penicillin G of ≥0.03 μg/mL for at least 7 days are considered necessary for the cure of early syphilis. Recurrence rates for a given regimen increase as infection progresses from incubating to seronegative primary to seropositive primary to secondary to late syphilis. Therefore, it is probable, but unproven, that a longer duration of therapy is required to effect cure as the infection progresses. For these reasons, some authorities use more prolonged penicillin therapy than that recommended by the U.S. Public Health Service when treating secondary, latent, or late syphilis.

The treatment regimens recommended for syphilis are summarized in Table 172-3 and are discussed below.

Early syphilis Preventive (abortive, "epidemiologic") treatment is recommended for seronegative individuals without signs of syphilis who have been exposed to infectious syphilis within the previous 3 months. Before treatment is given, every effort should be made to establish a diagnosis by examination and serologic testing. *The regimens recommended for prevention are the same as those recommended for early syphilis.*

Penicillin G benzathine is the most widely used agent for the treatment of early syphilis (including primary, secondary, and early latent syphilis), although it is more painful on injection than penicillin G procaine. A single dose of 2.4 million units cures more than 95% of cases of primary syphilis. Because the drug's efficacy in secondary syphilis may be slightly lower, some physicians administer a second dose of 2.4 million units 1 week after the initial dose at this stage of disease. Clinical relapse can follow treatment with penicillin G benzathine in patients with both HIV infection and early syphilis. Because the risk of neurorelapse may be higher in HIV-infected patients, examination of CSF from HIV-seropositive individuals with syphilis of any stage is recommended by some experts; therapy appropriate for neurosyphilis should be given if there is any evidence of CNS syphilis.

For penicillin-allergic patients with early syphilis, a 2-week course of therapy with doxycycline or tetracycline is recommended. These regimens appear to be effective, although no well-controlled studies have been performed and poor compliance may be problematic. Although ceftriaxone and azithromycin have shown activity against *T. pallidum* in animals, human trials have not been of sufficient scope to permit the recommendation of either drug for any stage of syphilis.

Late latent and late syphilis (normal CSF) If CSF abnormalities are found, the patient should be treated for neurosyphilis. The recommended treatment for late latent syphilis with normal CSF, for cardiovascular syphilis, and for late benign syphilis (gumma) is penicillin G benzathine, 2.4 million units intramuscularly once a week for 3 successive weeks (7.2 million units total). Doxycycline or tetracycline (given for 1 month) offers an untested alternative for penicillin-allergic patients with latent or late syphilis and normal CSF. The clinical response to treatment for benign tertiary syphilis is usually impressive; however, responses to therapy for cardiovascular syphilis are not dramatic because aortic aneurysm and aortic regurgitation cannot be reversed by antibiotic treatment.

Neurosyphilis The 1998 neurosyphilis treatment guidelines of the Centers for Disease Control and Prevention (CDC) are presented in Table 172-3. Penicillin G benzathine, given in total doses of up to 7.2 million units to adults or 50,000 units per kilogram to infants, does not produce detectable concentrations of penicillin G in CSF, and asymptomatic neurosyphilis may relapse in patients treated with 2.4 million units; the risk may be higher in HIV-infected patients. Therefore, the use of penicillin G benzathine alone for the treatment of neurosyphilis is not recommended. On the other hand, administration of intravenous penicillin G in doses of ≥12 million units per day for 10 days or longer is thought to ensure treponemicidal concentrations of penicillin G in CSF and occasionally cures infection in patients who fail to respond to other therapy. The clinical response to penicillin therapy for meningeal syphilis is dramatic, but the response to treatment for parenchymal neurosyphilis is variable. In general, treatment of neurosyphilis in which damage has already been done may produce no clinical change but may arrest disease progression.

Several recent publications have reported neurologic relapse after high-dose intravenous penicillin therapy for neurosyphilis in HIV-infected patients. No alternative therapies have been explored, but careful follow-up is essential, and re-treatment is warranted in such patients.

No data support the use of antibiotics other than penicillin G for the treatment of neurosyphilis; however, some of the third-generation cephalosporins may deserve further evaluation. In patients with penicillin allergy demonstrated by skin testing, desensitization may be the best course (Chap. 126).

Management of syphilis in pregnancy Every pregnant woman should undergo a nontreponemal test at her first prenatal visit, and women at high risk of exposure should have a repeat test in the third trimester and at delivery. In the pregnant patient with presumed syphilis (evidenced by a reactive serology, with or without clinical manifestations) and with no history of treatment for syphilis, expeditious evaluation and initiation of treatment are essential. Therapy should be administered according to the stage of the disease, as for nonpregnant patients. Patients should be warned of the risk of a Jarisch-Herxheimer reaction, which may be associated with mild premature contractions but rarely results in premature delivery.

Penicillin is the only recommended therapy for syphilis in pregnancy. If the patient has a well-documented penicillin allergy, desensitization and penicillin treatment should be undertaken in a hospital according to the 1998 sexually transmitted diseases treatment guidelines issued by the CDC. After treatment, a quantitative nontreponemal test should be repeated monthly throughout pregnancy. Treated women whose titers rise fourfold or who do not show a fourfold decrease in titer in a 3-month period should be re-treated.

Evaluation and Management of Congenital Syphilis Newborn infants of mothers with reactive VDRL or FTA-ABS tests may themselves have reactive tests, whether or not they have become infected, because of transplacental transfer of maternal IgG antibody. Rising or persistent titers indicate infection, and the infant should be treated. Neonatal IgM antibody can be detected in cord or neonatal serum with the syphilis Captia-M or 19S IgM FTA-ABS test. Alternatively, monthly quantitative nontreponemal tests may be performed on asymptomatic infants born to women treated adequately with penicillin during pregnancy.

An infant should be treated at birth if the seropositive mother has received penicillin therapy in the third trimester, inadequate penicillin treatment, or therapy with a drug other than penicillin; if her treatment

Table 172-3   Recommendations for the Treatment of Syphilis[a]

Stage of Syphilis	Patients without Penicillin Allergy	Patients with Confirmed Penicillin Allergy
Primary, secondary, or early latent	Penicillin G benzathine (single dose of 2.4 million units IM, 1.2 million units in each buttock)	Tetracycline hydrochloride (500 mg PO qid) or doxycycline (100 mg PO bid) for 2 weeks

Late latent (or latent of uncertain duration), cardiovascular, or benign tertiary	Lumbar puncture
	  CSF normal: Penicillin G benzathine (2.4 million units IM weekly for 3 weeks)
	  CSF abnormal: Treat as neurosyphilis
		Lumbar puncture
		  CSF normal: Tetracycline hydrochloride (500 mg PO qid) or doxycycline (100 mg PO bid) for 4 weeks
		  CSF abnormal: Treat as neurosyphilis

Neurosyphilis (asymptomatic or symptomatic)	Aqueous penicillin G (18–24 million units/d IV, given in divided doses every 4 h) for 10–14 days *or* Aqueous penicillin G procaine (2.4 million units/d IM) plus oral probenecid (500 mg qid), both for 10–14 days	Desensitization and treatment with penicillin if allergy is confirmed by skin testing
Syphilis in pregnancy	According to stage	Desensitization and treatment with penicillin if allergy is confirmed by skin testing

[a] See text for discussion of syphilis therapy in HIV-infected individuals.
SOURCE: These recommendations are modified from those issued by the Centers for Disease Control and Prevention in 1998.

status is unknown; or if the infant may be difficult to follow. It is unwise to require proof of diagnosis before treatment in such cases. The CSF should be examined to obtain baseline values before treatment. Penicillin is the only recommended drug for syphilis in infants. The penicillin dosage used for the treatment of the patient with late congenital syphilis is calculated in the same way as for the infant, until dosage based on weight reaches that used for adult neurosyphilis. Specific recommendations for the treatment of infants are included in the CDC's 1998 guidelines.

Jarisch-Herxheimer Reaction   A dramatic though usually mild reaction consisting of fever (average temperature elevation, 1.5°C), chills, myalgias, headache, tachycardia, increased respiratory rate, increased circulating neutrophil count, and vasodilation with mild hypotension may follow the initiation of treatment for syphilis. This reaction occurs in approximately 50% of patients with primary syphilis, 90% of those with secondary syphilis, and 25% of those with early latent syphilis. The onset comes within 2 h of treatment, the temperature peaks at about 7 h, and defervescence takes place within 12 to 24 h. The reaction is more delayed in neurosyphilis, with fever peaking after 12 to 14 h. In patients with secondary syphilis, erythema and edema of the mucocutaneous lesions increase; occasionally, subclinical or early mucocutaneous lesions may first become apparent during the reaction. The pathogenesis of this reaction is undefined, although recent studies have demonstrated the induction of inflammatory mediators such as tumor necrosis factor by treponemal lipoproteins. Patients should be warned to expect such symptoms, which can be managed by bed rest and aspirin. Steroid and other anti-inflammatory therapy is not required for this mild transient reaction.

Follow-Up Evaluation of Responses to Therapy   The response of early syphilis to treatment should be determined by monitoring of the quantitative VDRL or RPR titer 1, 3, 6, and 12 months after treatment. More frequent serologic examination (1, 2, 3, 6, 9, and 12 months) is recommended for patients concurrently infected with HIV. Because the FTA-ABS and agglutination tests remain positive in most patients treated for seropositive syphilis, these tests are not useful in following the response to therapy. After successful treatment of seropositive first-episode primary or secondary syphilis, the VDRL titer progressively declines, becoming negative by 12 months in 40 to 75% of seropositive primary cases and in 20 to 40% of secondary cases. Patients with a history of syphilis have less rapid declines in titer and are less likely to become VDRL- or RPR-negative. If the VDRL test becomes negative or if VDRL titers drop to a fixed low value within 1 or 2 years, lumbar puncture is unnecessary since the CSF examination is almost invariably normal and there is little risk of subsequent neurosyphilis. However, if a VDRL titer ≥1:8 fails to fall by at least fourfold within 12 months, if the VDRL titer rises by fourfold, or if clinical symptoms persist or recur, re-treatment is indicated. Every effort should be made to differentiate treatment failure from reinfection, and the CSF should be examined. Patients in whom treatment failure is suspected, especially those with abnormal CSF, should be treated for neurosyphilis. If the patient remains seropositive but asymptomatic after such re-treatment, no further therapy is necessary. Patients treated for late latent syphilis frequently have low initial VDRL titers and may not have a fourfold drop after therapy with penicillin; about half of these patients remain seropositive (with low titers) for years after therapy. Re-treatment is not warranted unless the titer rises or signs and symptoms of syphilis appear.

The activity of neurosyphilis correlates best with the degree of CSF pleocytosis, and this measure provides the most sensitive index of response to treatment. CSF should be examined every 6 months for 3 years after the treatment of asymptomatic or symptomatic neurosyphilis or until CSF findings return to normal. An elevated CSF cell count falls to ≤10/μL in 3 to 12 months in 95% of adequately treated cases and becomes normal in all cases within 2 to 4 years. Elevated levels of CSF protein fall more slowly, and the CSF VDRL titer declines gradually over a period of several years.

Persistence of *T. pallidum*   The persistence of *T. pallidum* in the aqueous humor, CSF, lymph nodes, brain, inflamed temporal arteries, and other tissues after "adequate" penicillin treatment has been suggested by dark-field microscopy, immunofluorescent antibody and silver staining techniques, rabbit inoculation, and PCR. Because the data on persisting treponemes are scanty, no modification of the treatment recommendations seems warranted for HIV-uninfected persons. Adherence to recommendations regarding CSF examination before the selection of therapy should minimize the possibility that *T. pallidum* will persist in the CSF.

IMMUNITY TO AND PREVENTION OF SYPHILIS   About 60% of contacts of patients with primary and secondary syphilis become infected, with lower risk in contacts exposed to early latent syphilis. The rate of development of acquired resistance to *T. pallidum* after natural or experimental infection is related to the size of the antigenic stimulus, which depends on both the size of the infecting inoculum and the duration of infection before treatment. The role of serum antibody in conferring immunity to syphilis remains controversial. Passively administered antibody prevents or delays the appearance of clinical manifestations of syphilis in the rabbit model; it does not prevent infection. Cellular immunity is considered to be of major importance in the healing of early lesions and the control of syphilitic infection. The cellular infiltration of early lesions predominantly involves T lymphocytes and macrophages. The cytokine milieu of primary and secondary lesions is of the T_H1 type, consistent with the clearance of organisms by activated macrophages. Specific antibody enhances phagocytosis and is required for macrophage-mediated killing of *T. pallidum*.

Inability to cultivate pathogenic treponemes in vitro has hindered the analysis of treponemal antigens. Attempts to induce immunity to syphilis by vaccination have shown limited promise, although repeated injection of rabbits with γ-irradiated motile treponemes has conferred immunity to rechallenge. The outer membrane of *T. pallidum* contains few integral membrane proteins, and none has been definitively identified. Several newly described antigens of *T. pallidum*, including TprK, have induced partial immunity to challenge in the rabbit model, and syphilis vaccine development is being actively pursued.

ACKNOWLEDGMENT

The author wishes to acknowledge the substantive contributions of the former coauthor, Dr. King K. Holmes, to the content and organization of this chapter. His original framework continues to serve as the structure for this revision.

BIBLIOGRAPHY

CENTERS FOR DISEASE CONTROL AND PREVENTION : 1998 sexually transmitted diseases treatment guidelines. MMWR 47(RR-11):1, 1998

CENTURION-LARA A et al: The flanking region sequences of the 15-kDa lipoprotein gene differentiate pathogenic treponemes. J Infect Dis 177:1036, 1998

FLOOD JM et al: Neurosyphilis during the AIDS epidemic, San Francisco, 1985–1992. J Infect Dis 177:931, 1998

FRASER CM et al: Complete genome sequence of *Treponema pallidum*, the syphilis pirochete. Science 281:375, 1998

GORDON SM et al: The response of symptomatic neurosyphilis to high-dose intravenous penicillin G in patients with human immunodeficiency virus infection. N Engl J Med 331:1469, 1994

LUKEHART SA et al: Invasion of the central nervous system by *Treponema pallidum*: Implications for diagnosis and treatment. Ann Intern Med 109:855, 1988

MARRA CM et al: Resolution of serum and cerebrospinal fluid abnormalities after treatment of neurosyphilis: Influence of concomitant human immunodeficiency virus infection. Sex Transm Dis 23:184, 1996

MUSHER DM et al: Effect of human immunodeficiency virus infection on the course of syphilis and on the response to treatment. Ann Intern Med 113:872, 1990

RADOLF JD et al: Outer membrane ultrastructure explains the limited antigenicity of virulent *Treponema pallidum*. Proc Natl Acad Sci USA 86:2051, 1989

ROLFS RT et al: A randomized trial of enhanced therapy for early syphilis in patients with and without human immunodeficiency virus infection. N Engl J Med 337:307, 1997

ROMANOWSKI B et al: Serologic response to treatment of infectious syphilis. Ann Intern Med 114:1005, 1991

THOMAS JC et al: Syphilis in the South: Rural rates surpass urban rates in North Carolina. Am J Public Health 85:1119, 1995

WENDEL GD et al: Penicillin allergy and desensitization in serious infections during pregnancy. N Engl J Med 312:1229, 1985

ENDEMIC TREPONEMATOSES

The endemic, or nonvenereal, treponematoses are bacterial infections that are caused by close relatives of *Treponema pallidum* subspecies *pallidum*, the etiologic agent of venereal syphilis (Chap. 172). Yaws, pinta, and endemic syphilis are distinguished from venereal syphilis by mode of transmission, age of acquisition, geographic distribution, and clinical features. These infections are limited primarily to rural areas of developing nations and are seen in the United States and Europe only in recent immigrants from endemic regions. Much of our "knowledge" about the endemic treponematoses is based upon impressions and observations of health care workers who have visited endemic areas; virtually no well-designed studies of the natural history, diagnosis, or treatment of these infections have been conducted. A comparison of the treponemal infections is shown in Table 173-1.

EPIDEMIOLOGY The endemic treponematoses are chronic diseases acquired during childhood and, like syphilis, can cause severe late manifestations years after initial infection. These infections were very common in Africa, Asia, and South America when the World Health Organization (WHO) and UNICEF embarked on a highly successful mass eradication campaign. From 1952 to 1969, it is estimated that over 160 million people were examined for treponemal infections and over 50 million cases, contacts, and latent infections were treated. This categorical program is one of WHO's outstanding successes in that the prevalence of active yaws was reduced from >20% to <1% in many rural areas and endemic syphilis was eradicated in Bosnia. In the decades since the eradication programs, lack of focused surveillance and diversion of resources to other pressing needs have resulted in a resurgence of these infections in some regions, particularly in Africa. The estimated geographic distribution of the endemic treponematoses in the 1990s is shown in Fig. 173-1. In the early 1980s, WHO sponsored a series of regional meetings on the endemic treponematoses, and areas of resurgent yaws morbidity were identified in West Africa (Ivory Coast, Ghana, Togo, Benin) and extending into the Central African Republic and rural Democratic Republic of Congo (formerly Zaire). The prevalence of endemic syphilis is estimated to be >10% in some regions of Mali, Niger, Burkina Faso, and Senegal. In Asia and the western Pacific, yaws is still prevalent in Indonesia, Papua New Guinea, and the Solomon Islands; cases have also been identified in Laos and Kampuchea. In the Americas, foci of yaws persist in Haiti and other Caribbean islands, Peru, Colombia, Ecuador, Brazil, Guyana, and Surinam. Pinta is limited to Central America and northern South America, where it is found rarely and only in remote villages.

MICROBIOLOGY The etiologic agents of the endemic treponematoses are *T. pallidum* subspecies *pertenue* (yaws), *T. pallidum* subspecies *endemicum* (endemic syphilis), and *T. carateum* (pinta). These little-studied organisms are morphologically identical to *T. pallidum* subspecies *pallidum*, and no antigenic differences among the pathogenic treponemes have been identified to date. A controversy has existed about whether the treponematoses are caused by different organisms or by the same organism, with clinical manifestations and routes of transmission being defined by the climate of the region and the culture of the population. Three of the four organisms have been placed in the same species because of their genetic similarity; the fourth (*T. carateum*) remains a separate species simply because no organisms have been available for genetic studies. However, a molecular signature has been defined that can be used to differentiate *T. pallidum* subspecies *pallidum* from *T. pallidum* subspecies *pertenue* and *T. pallidum* subspecies *endemicum*, and unpublished studies have identified a number of distinct differences in the *tpr* gene family between venereal and nonvenereal treponemes. Whether these differ-

ences are related to the different clinical courses has not yet been determined.

CLINICAL FEATURES All of the treponemal infections are characterized by defined disease stages, with a localized primary lesion, disseminated secondary lesions, periods of latency, and possible late lesions. The stages are most clearly defined in venereal syphilis, while the primary and secondary manifestations are more frequently overlapping in yaws and endemic syphilis; the late manifestations of pinta are very mild relative to the destructive lesions of the other treponematoses. The current preference is to divide the clinical course of the endemic treponematoses into "early" and "late" stages.

The major clinical features that are thought to differ between venereal syphilis and the nonvenereal infections are the lack of congenital transmission and lack of central nervous system (CNS) involvement in the nonvenereal infections. It is not known whether these distinctions are accurate. Because of the high degree of genetic relatedness among the organisms, there is little biologic reason to think that *T. pallidum* subspecies *endemicum* and *T. pallidum* subspecies *pertenue* would be unable to cross the blood-brain barrier or to invade the placenta. These organisms obviously can disseminate from the site of primary infection to other tissues, and they can persist for decades. In this respect, they are like *T. pallidum* subspecies *pallidum*. Even if invasion of the placenta or the CNS occurs in endemic treponemal infection, there are a number of reasons that these manifestations might not have been recognized. The lack of recognized congenital infection may be due to the fact that the nonvenereal treponematoses are usually acquired during childhood. The degree of spirochetemia (the presumed source of placental and fetal infection) is greatly diminished during the latent stage, and by the time an infected girl becomes sexually mature, she would be at low risk for transplacental transmission. Neurologic involvement may not have been recognized in nonvenereal treponemal infection because of the lack of trained medical personnel in endemic regions, the lag of years to decades between acquisition of infection and possible CNS manifestations, or a low rate of symptomatic CNS disease. The lack of longitudinal studies in endemic areas makes conclusions about the natural history of these infections tenuous.

Some published evidence supports congenital transmission as well as cardiovascular, ophthalmologic, and CNS involvement in yaws. Although the case is strong, particularly for CNS involvement, most studies that have shown a relatively high incidence (average, 24.9%) of cerebrospinal fluid (CSF) abnormalities in patients with yaws were not controlled for other possible causes of CSF abnormalities, did not include treponeme-specific tests, or did not follow patients for resolution of abnormalities after antitreponemal therapy. Thus, while no firm conclusions can be drawn about the invasion of the CNS and placenta by the non-*pallidum* treponemes, it may be erroneous to accept unquestioningly the frequently repeated belief that these organisms fail to cause such manifestations.

Yaws Also known as *pian*, *framboesia*, or *bouba*, yaws is a chronic infection that is usually acquired in childhood and is caused by *T. pallidum* subspecies *pertenue*. The disease is characterized by the development of one or several primary lesions (called the "mother yaw"), followed by the appearance of multiple disseminated skin lesions. The early lesions may persist for many months, are infectious, and usually recur several times within the early years of infection. Late manifestations are destructive and can involve skin, bone, and joints.

The infection is transmitted by direct contact with infectious lesions, and transmission may be enhanced by disruption of the skin by insect bites or abrasions. Children with open lesions and without covering clothing are most likely to transmit infection during play or group sleeping. After an average incubation period estimated at 3 to 4 weeks, the first lesion begins as a papule, usually on an extremity, and then enlarges (particularly during moist warm weather) to become papillomatous or "raspberry-like" (thus the name "framboesia") (Fig. 173-2). Regional lymphadenopathy develops, and the lesion usually

Table 173-1 Comparison of the Treponemes and the Diseases They Cause

Feature	Venereal Syphilis	Yaws	Endemic Syphilis	Pinta
Organism	T. pallidum subspecies pallidum	T. pallidum subspecies pertenue	T. pallidum subspecies endemicum	T. carateum
Mode of transmission	Sexual, transplacental[a]	Skin-to-skin	Household contacts: mouth-to-mouth or via shared drinking/eating utensils; insect vector?	Skin-to-skin
Usual age of acquisition	Adulthood	Early childhood	Early childhood	Late childhood
Primary lesion	Cutaneous ulcer (chancre)	Papilloma, often ulcerative	Rarely seen	Nonulcerating papule with satellites, pruritic
Location	Genital, oral, anal	Extremities	Oral	Extremities, face
Secondary lesions	Mucocutaneous lesions; condylomata lata	Cutaneous papulosquamous lesions; osteoperiostitis	Florid mucocutaneous lesions (mucous patch, split papule, condyloma latum); osteoperiostitis	Pintides, pigmented, pruritic
Infectious relapses	~25%	Common	Unknown	None
Late complications	Gummas, cardiovascular and CNS involvement[b]	Destructive gummas of skin, bone, cartilage	Destructive gummas of skin, bone, cartilage	Nondestructive, dyschromic, achromic macules

[a] Because the nonvenereal treponematoses are usually acquired in childhood and treponemal bacteremia ceases with time, only in adult-onset venereal syphilis is there a reasonable likelihood that a woman will give birth to an infected child (see text).
[b] CNS involvement in the endemic treponematoses has been postulated by some investigators (see text).

patients and is manifested by gummas of the skin and long bone, hyperkeratoses of the palms and soles, osteitis and periostitis, and hydrarthrosis. The late gummatous lesions are characteristically very destructive and extensive. Destruction of the nose, maxilla, palate, and pharynx is termed *gangosa* and is similar to the destructive lesions seen in leprosy and leishmaniasis.

Endemic Syphilis Endemic syphilis, also called *bejel, siti, dichuchwa, njovera,* or *skerljevo,* is a chronic infection caused by *T. pallidum* subspecies *endemicum.* Like other endemic treponematoses, endemic syphilis is chronic and is acquired in childhood. The early lesions are primarily localized to the mucocutaneous and mucosal surfaces, and the infection may be transmitted by direct contact or by shared drinking and eating utensils. A role for insects in transmission has been suggested but is unproved. The initial lesion often goes unrecognized, and the first noticeable lesion is usually an intraoral mucous patch or a mucocutaneous lesion resembling the condylomata lata of secondary syphilis (Fig. 173-2). This eruption may last for months or even years, and treponemes can readily be demonstrated in early lesions. Periostitis and regional lymphadenopathy are common. After a variable period of latency, late manifestations may appear, including osseous and cutaneous gummas. Destructive gummas, osteitis, and gangosa are more common in endemic syphilis than in late yaws. Gummas of the

heals within 6 months; dissemination is thought to occur during the early weeks and months of infection. A generalized secondary eruption, accompanied by generalized lymphadenopathy, appears either concurrent with or following the primary lesion, may take several forms (macular, papular, or papillomatous), and may become secondarily infected with other bacteria. Painful papillomatous lesions on the soles of the feet result in a painful crablike gait ("crab yaws"), and periostitis may result in nocturnal bone pain and polydactylitis. All early skin lesions are infectious, and cutaneous relapses are common during the first 5 years. Late yaws is recognized in ~10% of untreated

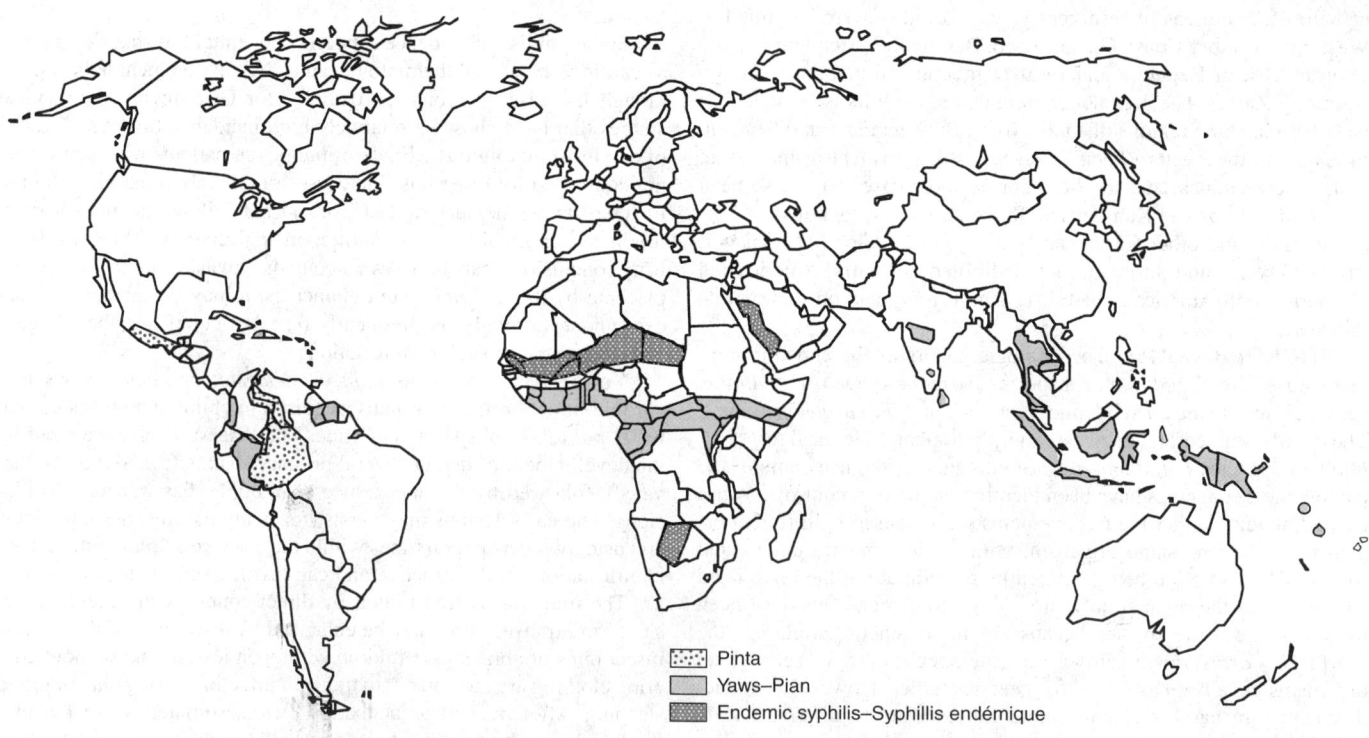

Pinta
Yaws–Pian
Endemic syphilis–Syphillis endémique

WHO 92522

FIGURE 173-1 Geographic distribution of endemic treponematoses in the 1990s. *(Courtesy of World Health Organization.)*

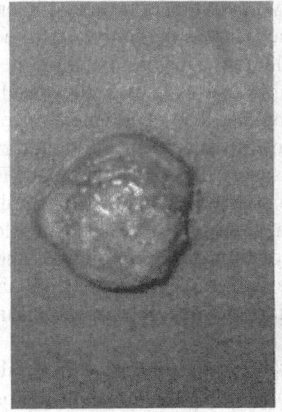
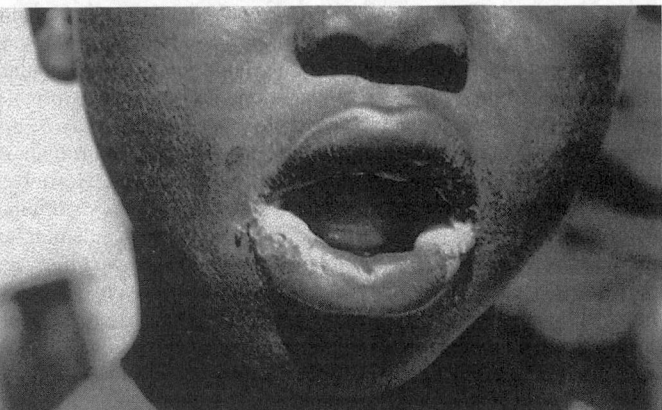
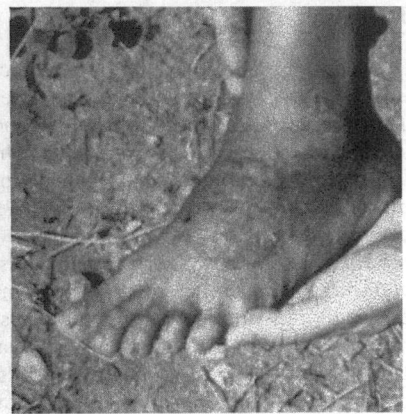

FIGURE 173-2 Clinical manifestations of endemic treponematoses. *Left*: Papillomatous primary lesions of yaws. *Center*: Split papules of early endemic syphilis. *Right*: Pigmented macules of pinta. *(From PL Perine et al.)*

nipples develop in women who have previously had endemic syphilis and who breast-feed infants with oral lesions. Thus, it appears that the late lesion may result from repeated exposure of a sensitized host.

Pinta Pinta (also called *mal del pinto, carate, azul*, or *purupuru*) is the most benign of the treponemal infections and is caused by *T. carateum*. This disease has three stages that are characterized by marked changes in skin color, but it does not appear to cause destructive lesions or to involve other tissues. Transmission occurs by direct contact, usually during late childhood. The initial papule is most often located on the extremities or face and is pruritic. After one to many months of infection, numerous disseminated secondary lesions (*pintides*) appear. These lesions are initially red but become deeply pigmented, ultimately turning a dark slate blue. The secondary lesions are infectious and highly pruritic and may persist for years. Late pigmented lesions are called *dyschromic macules* and contain treponemes. Over time, most pigmented lesions show varying degrees of depigmentation, becoming brown and eventually white and giving the skin a mottled appearance. The white achromic lesions are characteristic of the late stage.

DIAGNOSIS Diagnosis of the endemic treponematoses is based upon clinical manifestations and, when available, serologic testing. The same tests that are used for venereal syphilis (Chap. 172) become reactive during all treponemal infections, and there is no serologic test than can discriminate among the different infections. The nonvenereal treponemal infections should be considered in the evaluation of a reactive syphilis serology in any person who has immigrated from an endemic area.

℞ **TREATMENT** The recommended therapy for patients and their contacts is benzathine penicillin at a dose of 1.2 million units intramuscularly; that for children under 10 years of age is 600,000 units. This is half the dose recommended for patients and contacts with early venereal syphilis. There have been no controlled studies to show that the lower dose is effective in stopping relapse or progression to late disease. Definitive evidence of resistance to penicillin is lacking. However, because failure to heal existing lesions and frequent relapse following treatment for yaws have been described in Papua New Guinea, some health workers have suggested doubling the recommended dose of benzathine penicillin. Solely on the basis of experience with venereal syphilis, it is thought that doxycycline, tetracycline, and erythromycin (at doses appropriate for syphilis; Chap. 172) are therapeutic alternatives for patients allergic to penicillin. A Jarisch-Herxheimer reaction (Chap. 172) may follow treatment of endemic treponematoses.

CONTROL The endemic treponematoses can be controlled with inexpensive therapy. However, the often-remote locations of the affected populations limit availability of medical care. Although the mass treatment programs of three decades ago were widely successful,

time has shown that sustained control requires vigilance in regular screening and in the investigation of outbreaks—luxuries that are often impossible in countries with more pressing medical needs. There is concern that, as HIV spreads throughout developing countries, it may markedly affect the manifestations and transmission of the endemic treponematoses.

ACKNOWLEDGMENT
The author gratefully acknowledges the substantial contributions of Dr. Peter Perine, the author of previous editions of this chapter, to the framework of the current chapter and to our insight into these little-studied infections.

BIBLIOGRAPHY

BACKHOUSE JL et al: Failure of penicillin treatment of yaws on Karkar Island, Papua New Guinea. Am J Trop Med 59:388, 1998

CENTURION-LARA A et al: The flanking region sequences of the 15 kD lipoprotein gene differentiate pathogenic treponemes. J Infect Dis 177:1036, 1998

ENGELKENS HJH et al: Early yaws: A light microscopic study. Genitourin Med 66:264, 1990

——— et al: Endemic treponematosis. Part 1. Yaws. Int J Dermatol 30:77, 1991

PERINE PL et al: *Handbook of Endemic Treponematoses.* Geneva, World Health Organization, 1984

ROMÁN GC, ROMÁN LN: Occurrence of congenital, cardiovascular, visceral, neurologic, and neuro-ophthalmologic complications in late yaws: A theme for future research. Rev Infect Dis 8:760, 1986

---

174 *Peter Speelman*

LEPTOSPIROSIS

Leptospirosis is an infectious disease caused by pathogenic leptospires and characterized by a broad spectrum of clinical manifestations, varying from inapparent infection to fulminant, fatal disease. In its mild form, leptospirosis may present as an influenza-like illness with headache and myalgias. Severe leptospirosis, characterized by jaundice, renal dysfunction, and hemorrhagic diathesis, is referred to as *Weil's syndrome*.

ETIOLOGIC AGENTS Leptospires are spirochetes belonging to the order Spirochaetales and the family Leptospiraceae. Traditionally, the genus *Leptospira* comprised two species: the pathogenic *L. interrogans* and the free-living *L. biflexa*. Although seven species of pathogenic leptospires are now recognized on the basis of their DNA relatedness, it is more practical clinically and epidemiologically to use a classification based on serologic differences. The pathogenic leptospires are divided into serovars according to their antigenic composition. More than 200 serovars make up the 23 serogroups.

Leptospires are coiled, thin, highly motile organisms with hooked ends and two periplasmic flagella that permit burrowing into tissue. These organisms are 6 to 20 μm long and about 0.1 μm wide; they stain poorly but can be seen microscopically by dark-field examination and after silver impregnation staining. Leptospires require special media and conditions for growth; it may take weeks for cultures to become positive.

EPIDEMIOLOGY Leptospirosis is a zoonosis with a worldwide distribution that affects at least 160 mammalian species. Rodents, especially rats, are the most important reservoir, although other wild mammals, dogs, fish, and birds may also harbor these microorganisms. Leptospires establish a symbiotic relationship with their host and can persist in the renal tubules for years. Some serovars are associated with particular animals—e.g., icterohaemorrhagiae/copenhageni with rats, grippotyphosa with voles, hardjo with cattle, canicola with dogs, and pomona with pigs.

Transmission of leptospires may follow direct contact with urine, blood, or tissue from an infected animal or exposure to a contaminated environment; human-to-human transmission is rare. Since leptospires are excreted in the urine and can survive in water for many months, water is an important vehicle in their transmission. Epidemics of leptospirosis may result from exposure to flood waters contaminated by urine from infected animals, as has been reported from Nicaragua. Leptospirosis occurs most commonly in the tropics because the climate as well as the sometimes poor working and hygienic conditions favor the pathogen's survival.

Humans are not commonly infected with leptospires. However, in the United States, the 40 to 120 cases reported annually to the Centers for Disease Control and Prevention certainly represent a significant underestimation of the total number. Certain occupational groups are at especially high risk; included are veterinarians, agricultural workers, sewage workers, slaughterhouse employees, and workers in the fishing industry. Such individuals may acquire leptospirosis through direct exposure to or contact with contaminated water and soil. Leptospirosis has also been recognized in deteriorating inner cities where rat populations are expanding. One report described leptospirosis in urban residents of Baltimore who were sporadically exposed to rat urine.

In western countries, recreational exposure and domestic animal contact are also prominent sources of leptospirosis. Recreational water activities, such as canoeing, windsurfing, swimming, and waterskiing, place persons at risk for leptospirosis. Sometimes the infection is acquired during travel abroad. In a recent study in the Netherlands, 14% of patients with confirmed leptospirosis had acquired the infection while traveling in tropical countries, mostly in Southeast Asia. Transmission via laboratory accidents has been reported but is rare. Occasionally, leptospirosis develops after unanticipated immersion in contaminated water (e.g., in an automobile accident). Most cases occur in men, with a peak incidence during the summer and fall in western countries and during the rainy season in the tropics.

PATHOGENESIS The pathogenesis of leptospirosis is incompletely understood. Leptospires may enter the host through abrasions in the skin or through intact mucous membranes, especially the conjunctiva and the lining of the oro- and nasopharynx. Drinking of contaminated water may introduce leptospires through the mouth, throat, or esophagus. After entry of the organisms, leptospiremia develops, with subsequent spread to all organs. Multiplication takes place in blood and in tissues, and leptospires can be isolated from blood and cerebrospinal fluid (CSF) during the first 4 to 10 days of illness. It is not clear why the presence of leptospires in the CSF does not cause damage. All forms of leptospires can damage the wall of small blood vessels; this damage leads to vasculitis with leakage and extravasation of cells, including hemorrhages. The most important known pathogenic properties of leptospires are adhesion to cell surfaces and cellular toxicity.

Vasculitis is responsible for the most important manifestations of the disease. Although leptospires mainly infect the kidneys and liver, any organ may be affected. In the kidney, leptospires migrate to the interstitium, renal tubules, and tubular lumen, causing interstitial nephritis and tubular necrosis. Hypovolemia due to dehydration or altered capillary permeability may contribute to the development of renal failure. In the liver, centrilobular necrosis with proliferation of Kupffer cells may be found. However, severe hepatocellular necrosis is not a feature of leptospirosis. Pulmonary involvement is the result of hemorrhage and not of inflammation. Invasion of skeletal muscle by leptospires results in swelling, vacuolation of the myofibrils, and focal necrosis. In severe leptospirosis, vasculitis may ultimately impair the microcirculation and increase capillary permeability, resulting in fluid leakage and hypovolemia.

When antibodies are formed, leptospires are eliminated from all sites in the host except the eye, the proximal renal tubules, and perhaps the brain, where they may persist for weeks or months. The persistence of leptospires in the aqueous humor occasionally causes chronic or recurrent uveitis. The systemic immune response is effective in eliminating the organism but may also produce symptomatic inflammatory reactions. A rise in antibody titer coincides with the development of meningitis; this association suggests that an immunologic mechanism is responsible.

After the start of antimicrobial treatment for leptospirosis, a Jarisch-Herxheimer reaction similar to that seen in other spirochetal diseases may develop. Although frequently described in older publications, this reaction seems to be a rare event in leptospirosis and is certainly less frequent in this infection than in other spirochetal diseases.

CLINICAL MANIFESTATIONS It is important to try to obtain a history of exposure to contaminated materials. Serologic evidence of past inapparent infection is found in 15 to 40% of persons who have been exposed but have not become ill. In symptomatic cases of leptospirosis, clinical manifestations vary from mild to serious or even fatal. More than 90% of symptomatic persons have the relatively mild and usually anicteric form of leptospirosis, with or without meningitis. Severe leptospirosis with profound jaundice (Weil's syndrome) develops in 5 to 10% of infected individuals.

The incubation period is usually 1 to 2 weeks but ranges from 2 to 26 days. Typically, an acute leptospiremic phase is followed by an immune leptospiruric phase. The distinction between the first and second phases is not always clear, and milder cases do not always include the second phase.

Anicteric Leptospirosis Leptospirosis may present as an acute influenza-like illness, with fever, chills, severe headache, nausea, vomiting, and myalgias. Muscle pain, which especially affects the calves, back, and abdomen, is an important feature of leptospiral infection. Less common features include sore throat and rash. The patient usually has an intense headache (frontal or retroorbital) and sometimes develops photophobia. Mental confusion may be evident. Pulmonary involvement, manifested in most cases by cough and chest pain and in a few cases by hemoptysis, is not uncommon.

The most common finding on physical examination is fever with conjunctival suffusion. Less common findings include muscle tenderness, lymphadenopathy, pharyngeal injection, rash, hepatomegaly, and splenomegaly. The rash may be macular, maculopapular, erythematous, urticarial, or hemorrhagic. Mild jaundice may be present.

Most patients become asymptomatic within 1 week. After an interval of 1 to 3 days, the illness recurs in a number of cases. The start of this second (immune) phase coincides with the development of antibodies. Symptoms are more variable than during the first (leptospiremic) phase. Usually the symptoms last for only a few days, but occasionally they persist for weeks. Often the fever is less pronounced and the myalgias are less severe than in the leptospiremic phase. An important event during the immune phase is the development of aseptic meningitis. Although no more than 15% of all patients have symptoms and signs of meningitis, many patients may have CSF pleocytosis. Meningeal symptoms usually disappear within a few days but may persist for weeks. Similarly, pleocytosis generally disappears within 2 weeks but occasionally persists for months. Iritis, iridocyclitis, and chorioretinitis—late complications that may persist for years—can become apparent as early as the third week but often present several months after the initial illness. One epidemic of uveitis among patients with leptospirosis has been reported.

Severe Leptospirosis (Weil's Syndrome) Weil's syndrome, the most severe form of leptospirosis, is characterized by jaundice, renal dysfunction, hemorrhagic diathesis, and high mortality. This syndrome is frequently but not exclusively associated with infection due to serovar icterohaemorrhagiae/copenhageni. The onset of illness is no different from that of less severe leptospirosis; however, after 4 to 9 days, jaundice as well as renal and vascular dysfunction generally develop. Although some degree of defervescence may be noted after the first week of illness, a biphasic disease pattern like that seen in anicteric leptospirosis is lacking. The jaundice of Weil's syndrome, which can be profound and give an orange cast to the skin, is usually not associated with severe hepatic necrosis. Death is rarely due to liver failure. Hepatomegaly and tenderness in the right upper quadrant are usually detected. Splenomegaly is found in 20% of cases.

Renal failure may develop, often during the second week of illness. Hypovolemia and decreased renal perfusion contribute to the development of acute tubular necrosis with oliguria or anuria. Dialysis is sometimes required, although a fair number of cases can be managed without dialysis. Renal function may be completely regained.

Pulmonary involvement occurs frequently, resulting in cough, dyspnea, chest pain, and blood-stained sputum, and sometimes in hemoptysis or even respiratory failure. Hemorrhagic manifestations are seen in Weil's syndrome: epistaxis, petechiae, purpura, and ecchymoses are found commonly, while severe gastrointestinal bleeding and adrenal or subarachnoid hemorrhage are detected rarely.

Rhabdomyolysis, hemolysis, myocarditis, pericarditis, congestive heart failure, cardiogenic shock, adult respiratory distress syndrome, and multiorgan failure have all been described during severe leptospirosis.

LABORATORY AND RADIOLOGIC FINDINGS The kidneys are invariably involved in leptospirosis. Related findings range from urinary sediment changes (leukocytes, erythrocytes, and hyaline or granular casts) and mild proteinuria in anicteric leptospirosis to renal failure and azotemia in severe disease.

The erythrocyte sedimentation rate is usually elevated. In anicteric leptospirosis, peripheral leukocyte counts range from 3000 to 26,000/μL, with a left shift; in Weil's syndrome, leukocytosis is often marked. Mild thrombocytopenia occurs in up to 50% of patients and is associated with renal failure.

In contrast to patients with acute viral hepatitis, those with leptospirosis typically have elevated serum levels of bilirubin and alkaline phosphatase as well as mild increases (up to 200 U/L) in serum levels of aminotransferases. In Weil's syndrome, the prothrombin time may be prolonged but can be corrected with vitamin K. Levels of creatine phosphokinase, which are elevated in up to 50% of patients with leptospirosis during the first week of illness, may help to differentiate this infection from viral hepatitis.

When a meningeal reaction develops, polymorphonuclear leukocytes predominate initially and the number of mononuclear cells increases later. The protein concentration in the CSF may be elevated; CSF glucose levels are normal.

In severe leptospirosis, pulmonary radiographic abnormalities are more common than would be expected on the basis of physical examination. These abnormalities most frequently develop 3 to 9 days after the onset of illness. The most common radiographic finding is a patchy alveolar pattern that corresponds to scattered alveolar hemorrhage. Radiographic abnormalities most often affect the lower lobes in the periphery of the lung fields.

DIAGNOSIS A definite diagnosis of leptospirosis is based either on isolation of the organism from the patient or on seroconversion or a rise in antibody titer in the microscopic agglutination test (MAT).

For a presumptive diagnosis of leptospirosis, an antibody titer of ≥1: 100 in the MAT or a positive macroscopic slide agglutination test in the presence of a compatible clinical illness is required. Antibodies generally do not reach detectable levels until the second week of illness. The antibody response can be affected by early treatment.

The macroscopic slide agglutination test with killed antigen is useful for screening but is not specific. The MAT, which uses a battery of live leptospiral strains, and the enzyme-linked immunosorbent assay (ELISA), which uses a broadly reacting antigen, are the standard serologic procedures. These tests usually are available only in specialized laboratories and are used for the determination of the antibody titer and for the tentative identification of the serovar involved (thus the importance of using antigens representative of the serovars prevalent in the particular geographic area). Since cross-reactions occur frequently, however, it is often impossible to identify the infecting serovar. Serologic testing cannot be used as the basis for a decision about whether to start treatment.

In addition to the MAT and the ELISA, various other tests with diagnostic value have been developed. Some tests, such as an indirect hemagglutination test, a microcapsule agglutination test, and an IgM ELISA, are commercially available. Dot-ELISA, gold immunoblot, and polymerase chain reaction techniques have been developed but are not yet used for routine diagnosis.

Leptospires can be isolated from blood and/or CSF during the first 10 days of illness and from urine for several weeks beginning at around 1 week. Cultures may become positive after 2 to 4 weeks, with a range of 1 week to 4 months. Sometimes urine cultures remain positive for months or years after the start of illness. For isolation of leptospires from body fluids or tissues, Ellinghausen-McCullough-Johnson-Harris (EMJH) medium is useful; other possibilities are Fletcher medium and Korthoff medium. Specimens can be mailed to a reference laboratory for culture, since leptospires remain viable in anticoagulated blood (heparin, EDTA, or citrate) for up to 11 days. Isolation of leptospires is important since it is the only way the infecting serovar can be correctly identified. Dark-field examination of blood or urine frequently results in misdiagnosis and should not be used.

DIFFERENTIAL DIAGNOSIS Leptospirosis should be differentiated from other febrile illnesses associated with headache and muscle pain, such as malaria, enteric fever, viral hepatitis, dengue, *Hantavirus* infections, and rickettsial diseases. In light of the strong similarity in epidemiology and clinical presentation between leptospirosis and *Hantavirus* infections and given the reported occurrence of dual infections, it is advisable to conduct serologic testing for *Hantavirus* in cases of suspected leptospirosis. When patients have a flulike disease with disproportionately severe myalgia or aseptic meningitis, a diagnosis of leptospirosis should be considered.

TREATMENT The effectiveness of antimicrobial therapy for the mild febrile form of leptospirosis is controversial, but such treatment is indicated for more severe forms. Treatment should be initiated as early as possible; nevertheless, contrary to previous reports, treatment started after the first 4 days of illness is effective.

For severe cases of leptospirosis, intravenous administration of penicillin G, amoxicillin, ampicillin, or erythromycin is recommended (Table 174-1). In milder cases, oral treatment with tetracycline, doxycycline, ampicillin, or amoxicillin should be considered. Although several other antibiotics, including newer cephalosporins, are highly active against leptospires in vitro, no clinical experience has yet been gained with these drugs.

In rare cases, a Jarisch-Herxheimer reaction develops within hours after the start of antimicrobial therapy (see "Pathogenesis" above). Although so far the only effective mode of management is supportive, the role of antibodies to tumor necrosis factor in the treatment of this reaction deserves further study. A beneficial effect of the use of such antibodies for the modulation of the reaction has been demonstrated

Table 174-1   Treatment and Chemoprophylaxis of Leptospirosis

Purpose of Drug Administration	Regimen
Treatment	
Mild leptospirosis	Doxycycline, 100 mg orally bid
	or
	Ampicillin, 500–750 mg orally qid
	or
	Amoxicillin, 500 mg orally qid
Moderate/severe leptospirosis	Penicillin G, 1.5 million units IV qid
	or
	Ampicillin, 1 g IV qid
	or
	Amoxicillin, 1 g IV qid
	or
	Erythromycin, 500 mg IV qid
Chemoprophylaxis	Doxycycline, 200 mg orally once a week

NOTE: All regimens used for treatment are administered for 7 days.

in patients with louse-borne relapsing fever. Patients with severe leptospirosis and renal failure may require dialysis. Those with Weil's syndrome may need transfusions of whole blood and/or platelets. Intensive care may be necessary.

PROGNOSIS   Most patients with leptospirosis recover. Mortality is highest among patients who are elderly and those who have Weil's syndrome. Leptospirosis during pregnancy is associated with high fetal mortality. Long-term follow-up of patients with renal failure and hepatic dysfunction has documented good recovery of renal and hepatic function.

PREVENTION   Individuals who may be exposed to leptospires through their occupations or their involvement in recreational water activities should be informed about the risks. Measures for controlling leptospirosis include avoidance of exposure to urine and tissues from infected animals, vaccination of animals, and rodent control. The animal vaccine used in a given area should contain the serovars known to be present in that area. Unfortunately, some vaccinated animals still excrete leptospires in their urine. Vaccination of humans against a specific serovar prevalent in an area has been undertaken in some European and Asian countries and has proved effective. Chemoprophylaxis with doxycycline (200 mg once a week) has appeared to be efficacious in military personnel but is indicated only in rare instances of sustained short-term exposure.

BIBLIOGRAPHY

CHU KM et al: Identification of *Leptospira* species in the pathogenesis of uveitis and determination of clinical ocular characteristics in south India. J Infect Dis 177:1314, 1998

DUPONT H et al: Leptospirosis: Prognostic factors associated with mortality. Clin Infect Dis 25:720, 1997

FARR RW: Leptospirosis. Clin Infect Dis 21:1, 1995

O'NEILL KM et al: Pulmonary manifestations of leptospirosis. Rev Infect Dis 13:705, 1991

TREVEJO RT et al: Epidemic leptospirosis associated with pulmonary hemorrhage—Nicaragua. J Infect Dis 178:1457, 1998

VAN CREVEL R et al: Leptospirosis in travelers. Clin Infect Dis 19:132, 1994

VINETZ JM et al: Sporadic urban leptospirosis. Ann Intern Med 125:794, 1996

WATT G et al: Placebo-controlled trial of intravenous penicillin for severe and late leptospirosis. Lancet 1:433, 1988

——— et al: Skeletal and cardiac muscle involvement in severe, late leptospirosis. J Infect Dis 162:266, 1990

175   *David T. Dennis, Grant L. Campbell*

RELAPSING FEVER

DEFINITION   The term *relapsing fever* describes two distinct borrelial disease entities: louse-borne relapsing fever (LBRF) and tick-borne relapsing fever (TBRF). Both are characterized by recurrent acute episodes of spirochetemia and fever alternating with spirochetal clearance and apyrexia.

ETIOLOGY   The worldwide distribution of relapsing spirochetal fevers was recognized in the early part of the twentieth century, and the causative agents were shown to be transmitted by lice and ticks. *Borrelia recurrentis* was identified as the cause of LBRF; differing strains of borreliae causing TBRF were usually named according to the species of *Ornithodoros* tick responsible for their transmission (Table 175-1). Sequencing of both flagellin and 16S ribosomal RNA genes reveals homogeneity among LBRF strains and considerable heterogeneity between Old World and New World TBRF strains.

Relapsing-fever borreliae are gram-negative bacteria that belong to the family Spirochaetaceae. They are helical in shape and average 0.2 to 0.5 μm in width and 5 to 20 μm in length. They comprise an outer membrane, an intermediate peptidoglycan layer, and an inner cytoplasmic membrane, which encloses the protoplasmic cylinder. Periplasmic flagella (variable numbers have been described) are situated beneath the outer membrane. Relapsing-fever borreliae are slow-growing and microaerophilic; they grow best at 30 to 35°C. Both TBRF and LBRF spirochetes grow well in Barbour-Stoenner-Kelly (BSK II) medium.

Relapsing-fever borreliae are distinguished by remarkable antigenic variability and strain heterogeneity. New *Borrelia* serotypes spontaneously emerge at a high rate, resulting from a unique process of DNA rearrangement within genes located on linear plasmids. These genes code for variable major proteins (VMPs) found on the spirochete's outer-membrane surface. This antigenic variation, generated by sequential expression of previously silent *vmp* genes for serotype-specific VMPs, allows the borreliae to escape the immune response of the host and results in the relapse phenomenon characteristic of infection with these organisms. Borrelial *vmp* gene expression also varies between mammalian and arthropod hosts.

EPIDEMIOLOGY   **Louse-Borne Relapsing Fever**   Body lice (*Pediculus humanus* var. *corporis*) become infected with *B. recurrentis* by feeding on spirochetemic humans, the only reservoirs of infection. In lice, *B. recurrentis* spirochetes are found almost exclusively in the hemolymph; humans acquire infection when infected body lice are crushed and their fluids contaminate mucous membranes or breaks in the skin (such as abrasions caused by scratching of pruritic louse bites). Spirochetes are not transmitted directly by the bite of a louse (anterior station transmission) or by inoculation of louse feces (posterior station transmission). Lice have a life span of only a few weeks, feed at frequent intervals, and survive only a few days off the human host.

LBRF has severely affected military and civilian populations disrupted by war and other disasters. During the Industrial Revolution, the disease was common among slum dwellers, prisoners, and others living in impoverished, overcrowded, and unhygienic conditions. In the first half of the twentieth century, during periods of war and famine, both LBRF and louse-borne typhus were epidemic in eastern Europe, the Balkans, and the former Soviet Union. LBRF has disappeared from its former global range as improvements have been made in standards of living, sanitation, and hygiene; it is now an important disease only in northeastern Africa, especially the highlands of Ethiopia, where an estimated 10,000 cases occur annually. In Ethiopia, the disease affects mostly homeless men crowded together in unhygienic circumstances, especially during the cool rainy season, when it is more difficult for them to change and wash their clothing. LBRF has repeatedly spilled out of Ethiopia into neighboring Somalia and Sudan, especially affecting displaced persons. LBRF does not pose a significant risk to tourists or other casual visitors but can be acquired from lice by persons (such as relief workers) in intimate contact with those affected as well as through accidental needle stick or mucocutaneous contact with infected blood.

Tick-Borne Relapsing Fever Soft ticks (Argasidae, *Ornithodoros* spp.) transmit TBRF. The ticks become infected by feeding on spirochetemic hosts. Except for *B. duttoni* (a prominent cause of TBRF in sub-Saharan Africa), TBRF borreliae are zoonotic disease agents found naturally in rodents (rats, mice, chipmunks, and squirrels) and in lagomorphs (rabbits and hares). The spirochetes are transmitted by ticks to humans and animals via saliva and excretory fluids when the tick feeds. Infection in ticks is transmitted vertically from one stage to the next; in some species, infection is transmitted transovarially over several generations. Soft ticks are hardy and can survive for 10 years or more with only an occasional blood meal. These ticks feed painlessly, relatively quickly (for 20 to 45 min), and usually at night while hosts are sleeping. Thus patients with TBRF are often unaware of tick exposures.

TBRF borreliae are widely distributed throughout the world. Human infection with these organisms is generally underrecognized and underreported. TBRF is most highly endemic in sub-Saharan Africa but is also found in countries of the Mediterranean littoral, Middle Eastern states, southern Russia, the Indian subcontinent, and China. In the United States, this disease occurs west of the Mississippi River, especially in mountainous areas, where *B. hermsii* is the causative agent. TBRF is reported at low frequency throughout Latin America. The disease typically occurs sporadically or in small—often familial—clusters. Infected soft ticks may cause repeated infections among persons living or sleeping in the same dwelling. In sub-Saharan Africa, *O. moubata*, the vector of *B. duttoni*, infests native huts and rest houses, hiding in crevices of floors and walls during the day and emerging at night to feed on sleeping inhabitants. In the United States, *B. hermsii* infections most often occur during spring and summer months among persons sleeping in rustic mountain cabins. Infections of humans are sometimes precipitated by the disappearance of rodents (e.g., as a result of epizootic plague) that nest in foundations, wall spaces, and attics and that serve as the usual maintenance hosts for *O. hermsi* ticks. Outbreaks caused by *B. hermsii* have taken place among persons staying in cabins along the north rim of the Grand Canyon and in the mountains of California, Idaho, and Colorado. Rodent-infested caves in southwestern states are associated with occasional cases of relapsing fever caused by *B. turicatae*.

PATHOGENESIS AND PATHOLOGY In humans, relapsing-fever borreliae penetrate the skin or mucous membranes, multiply in the blood, and circulate in great numbers during febrile periods. The organisms also may be found in the liver, spleen, central nervous sys-

Table 175-1 Characteristics and Distribution of Louse-Borne and Tick-Borne Borreliae

Borrelia Species	Arthropod Vector	Animal Reservoir	Disease Distribution	Type(s) of Relapsing Fever
B. recurrentis[a]	*Pediculus humanus* var. *corporis*	Humans	Northeastern Africa	Louse-borne, epidemic
B. duttoni	*Ornithodoros moubata*	Humans	Central, eastern, southern Africa	East African tick-borne, endemic
B. hispanica	*O. erraticus* (large variety)	Rodents	Spain, Portugal, Morocco, Algeria, Tunisia	Hispano-African tick-borne
B. crocidurae, *B. merionesi,* *B. microti,* *B. dipodilli*	*O. erraticus* (small variety)	Rodents	Morocco, Libya, Egypt, Iran, Turkey, Senegal, Kenya	North African tick-borne
B. persica	*O. tholozani[b]*	Rodents	From western China and Kashmir to Iraq and Egypt, former USSR, India	Asiatic-African tick-borne
B. caucasica	*O. verrucosus*	Rodents	Caucasus to Iraq	Caucasian tick-borne
B. latyschewii	*O. tartakovskyi*	Rodents	Iran, Central Asia	Caucasian tick-borne
B. hermsii	*O. hermsi*	Rodents	Western United States	American tick-borne
B. turicatae	*O. turicata*	Rodents	Southwestern United States	American tick-borne
B. parkeri	*O. parkeri*	Rodents	Western United States	American tick-borne
B. mazzotti	*O. talaje[c]*	Rodents	Southern United States, Mexico, Central and South America	American tick-borne
B. venezuelensis	*O. rudis[d]*	Rodents	Central and South America	American tick-borne

[a] Synonyms: *B. obermeyeri, B. novyi.*
[b] Synonyms: *O. papillipes, O. crossi?*
[c] Synonym: *O. dugesi?*
[d] Synonym: *O. venezuelensis.*
SOURCE: From Burgdorfer and Schwan.

tem, bone marrow, and other tissues and may be sequestered at these sites during periods of remission. The severity of disease is positively related to spirochete density in the blood. Even though the pathophysiologic manifestations of the disease resemble responses to endotoxin, and although plasma from some patients with relapsing fever coagulates *Limulus* amebocyte lysates, borreliae and other spirochetes have not been shown to express a true lipopolysaccharide (endotoxin) molecule. Infection with *B. recurrentis* does, however, activate protein mediators of inflammation, such as Hageman factor, prekallikrein, and proteins of the complement system; furthermore, a spirochetal heat-stable pyrogenic factor stimulates mononuclear phagocytes to express increased amounts of leukocyte pyrogen and thromboplastin.

The Jarisch-Herxheimer reaction in patients with LBRF is associated with a release of various cytokines into the plasma, including interleukin 6, interleukin 8, C-reactive protein, and enormous amounts of tumor necrosis factor α (TNF-α). Pretreatment of LBRF patients with antibody to TNF-α suppresses the Jarisch-Herxheimer reactions that follow penicillin treatment and reduces the plasma concentrations of certain other cytokines.

Findings at autopsy of patients with relapsing fever most often include hepatosplenomegaly and variable edema and swelling of other organs, such as the brain, lungs, and kidneys. On microscopic examination, the spleen is congested and contains multiple microabscesses composed of mononuclear cells that replace the white pulp, the myocardium displays diffuse histiocytic inflammation and interstitial edema, and the liver has areas of midzonal necrosis. Petechial hemorrhages are commonly evident over the surfaces of the meninges, pleura, heart, spleen, liver, kidneys, and mesentery. Subcapsular and parenchymal hemorrhagic infarcts of the spleen, heart, liver, and brain are sometimes grossly visible. Icterus is a common finding in severe and fatal cases of relapsing fever.

CLINICAL MANIFESTATIONS The clinical manifestations of LBRF and TBRF are similar. The mean incubation period is 7 days (range, 2 to 18 days), and the onset of illness is sudden, with fever, headache, shaking chills, sweats, myalgias, and arthralgias. The arthralgia of relapsing fever can be severe, involving small and large joints, but there is no evidence of arthritis. Dizziness, nausea, and vomiting are common. Sleep may be difficult and is sometimes accompanied by disturbing dreams. The patient is coherent but withdrawn, thirsty, and disinterested in food and other outside stimuli. The fever is high from the first, with a usual temperature of ≥40°C (≥104°F); fever is most often irregular in pattern and is sometimes accompanied by delirium. Patients become progressively prostrate as the disease advances. The pulse is rapid and the patient is mildly tachypneic. Meningism may be found. The conjunctivae are often injected, and the patient usually exhibits photophobia. The sclerae are sometimes icteric, most commonly in the later stages of illness. The mucous membranes are often dry, and the patient is usually dehydrated. Scattered petechiae develop on the trunk, extremities, and mucous membranes in one-third or more of patients with LBRF and in fewer patients with TBRF. A nonproductive cough is common, but chest sounds are usually normal; pleuritic pain and an accompanying pleuritic rub are sometimes noted. Cardiac findings are compatible with a high-output state; tachycardia and summation gallop are common. Tender enlargement of the spleen and liver frequently characterizes the acute phase of illness.

Epistaxis and blood-tinged sputum are common complications, and gastrointestinal and central nervous system hemorrhage can occur. Because of this coagulopathy, one LBRF outbreak in southern Sudan was thought to be viral hemorrhagic fever. Other complications of variable incidence include iridocyclitis, optic neuritis, meningitis, coma, isolated cranial-nerve palsy, pneumonitis, myocarditis, and rupture of the spleen. Infection during pregnancy can result in spontaneous abortion, stillbirth, or neonatal infection. Life-threatening complications are unusual in otherwise healthy persons given supportive care, especially if the illness is diagnosed and treated early.

Without treatment, symptoms intensify over a 2- to 7-day period (average, 5 days in LBRF and 3 days in TBRF), ending in a spontaneous crisis during which spirochetes disappear from the circulation. Treatment with one of the rapidly acting antibiotics, such as erythromycin, a tetracycline, or chloramphenicol, regularly precipitates a Jarisch-Herxheimer reaction within 1 to 4 h. The severity of this reaction is positively correlated with the density of spirochetes in the blood at the time of treatment. In the first phase of the crisis or reaction (the *chill phase*), rigors and rising fever are accompanied by an increasing metabolic rate, alveolar hyperventilation, high cardiac output, increasing peripheral vascular resistance, and decreased pulmonary arterial pressure. The body temperature commonly rises to ≥41°C (≥105.8°F). This high fever is accompanied often by agitation and confusion and sometimes by delirium. Fever can be partially controlled by the use of a cooling blanket and ice packs and by sponging of the patient with tepid water and alcohol. The chill phase terminates after 10 to 30 min, giving way to a *flush phase* characterized by a fall in body temperature, drenching sweats, and sometimes (more commonly in LBRF) a potentially dangerous fall in systemic arterial pressure and rise in pulmonary arterial pressure. Although cardiac output is maintained at high levels, the effective circulating blood volume decreases as peripheral vascular resistance falls. Vital signs must be monitored carefully during this period of the reaction, which usually lasts ≤8 h. Clinical and electrocardiographic evidence of myocarditis and myocardial dysfunction includes a prolonged QT$_c$ interval, a third heart sound (S$_3$), elevated central venous pressure, arterial hypotension, and pulmonary edema.

The crisis is followed by a period of exhaustion, sleep, and an uneventful recovery. Not uncommonly, in the first week of convalescence, patients experience 1 or 2 days of mild fever unassociated with detectable spirochetemia. In untreated patients, spirochetemia and symptoms may recur after a period of several days or weeks (average

interval to first relapse, 9 days in LBRF and 7 days in TBRF). Only one or two relapses characteristically occur in untreated patients with LBRF, whereas as many as 10 (average, three) can occur in untreated patients with TBRF. In most cases, the illness becomes shorter and milder and the afebrile intervals longer with each relapse. Because of the great antigenic variation among *Borrelia* strains, infection confers only partial immunity, and repeated infections of the same individual have been recorded.

Diseases that should be considered in the differential diagnosis of relapsing fever or that may complicate relapsing fever include typhus fever, typhoid, nontyphoid salmonellosis, malaria, dengue and other arboviral illnesses, tuberculosis, leptospirosis, and viral hemorrhagic fevers. In the United States, the geographic distribution of Colorado tick fever overlaps that of TBRF, and the two diseases have similar manifestations early in their courses.

LABORATORY FINDINGS AND DIAGNOSIS　The diagnosis of relapsing fever is confirmed most easily by the detection of spirochetes in blood, bone marrow aspirates, or cerebrospinal fluid. Motile spirochetes can be seen when fresh blood is examined by darkfield microscopy; and fixed organisms are clearly visible in Wright-, Giemsa-, or acridine orange-stained preparations of thin or dehemoglobinized thick smears of peripheral blood or buffy-coat preparations (Fig. 175-1). Organisms are found in blood taken during periods of fever preceding the crisis; smears from ≥70% of patients with LBRF and from fewer patients with TBRF are positive. In reference laboratories, relapsing-fever spirochetes are cultured from blood by the inoculation of BSK II medium or by the intraperitoneal inoculation of immature laboratory mice. The detection of agglutinins against *Proteus* OX-K (Weil-Felix reaction) in convalescent-phase serum supports the diagnosis. Serum antibodies to *Borrelia* can be detected by enzyme immunoassays, but these tests are unstandardized and subject to insensitivity due to antigenic variations among strains. Serologic cross-reactions occur with other spirochetes, including *B. burgdorferi* (the agent of Lyme disease) and *Treponema pallidum*.

Other laboratory findings in relapsing fever are generally nonspecific. The leukocyte count is normal or moderately elevated, with an unremarkable cell differential. Serum bilirubin levels are generally only slightly elevated. Thrombocytopenia (mean platelet count, about 50,000/μL) is evident in patients with LBRF during the acute phase of the illness; platelet counts rebound during early convalescence. Prothrombin and partial thromboplastin times are moderately prolonged during acute illness, as are standardized bleeding times. Fibrinogen concentrations in the blood are normal, and fibrinolysis is mild or absent. Results of the Rumpel-Leede tourniquet test are negative, despite the presence of petechiae.

℞ TREATMENT　Relapsing-fever borreliae are exquisitely sensitive to antibiotics. Treatment with erythromycin, a tetracycline, chloramphenicol, or penicillin produces rapid clearance of spirochetes and a remission of symptoms (Table 175-2). Although a single dose of erythromycin, a tetracycline, or chloramphenicol is highly effective in the treatment of LBRF, less is known about the efficacy of single-dose treatment of TBRF. Empirical treatment of TBRF for 7 days is therefore recommended to reduce the risk of persisting or relapsing borreliosis. For children <8 years of age and for pregnant women, erythromycin and penicillin are the preferred drugs.

The use of delayed-release intramuscular penicillin may prolong or delay the clearance of spirochetes and thereby attenuate the accompanying Jarisch-Herxheimer reaction, but this response is not predictable; furthermore, single-dose penicillin treatment sometimes results in relapse of spirochetemia and symptoms. Glucocorticoids and nonsteroidal anti-inflammatory agents do not prevent or significantly modify the cardiopulmonary disturbances of the Jarisch-Herxheimer reaction, although hydrocortisone and acetaminophen given at the same time as antibiotics reduce peak body temperature. Although pretreatment with antibody to TNF-α may moderate the Jarisch-Herxheimer reaction in treated patients with LBRF, its widespread use in LBRF is

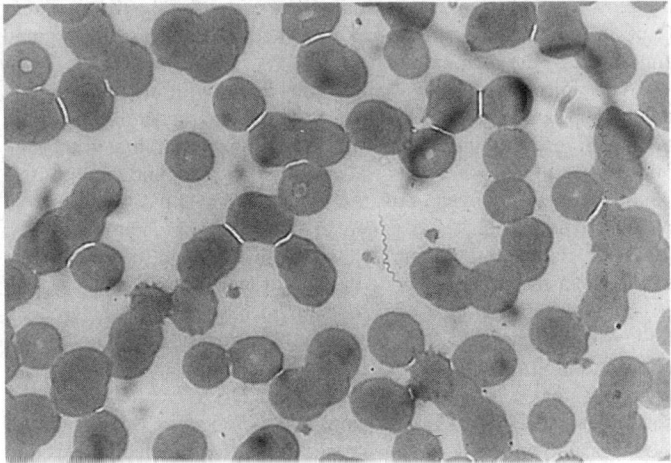

FIGURE 175-1 Photomicrograph of tick-borne relapsing fever spirochete (*B. hermsii*) in Wright's-Giemsa-stained peripheral blood film.

impractical and its use in TBRF (whose treatment is associated with a relatively mild Jarisch-Herxheimer reaction) is not warranted. Close monitoring of fluid balance, arterial and venous pressures, and myocardial function is advised in supportive management of the Jarisch-Herxheimer reaction in patients with LBRF.

The management of patients with myocardial dysfunction requires caution in the administration of intravenous fluids and, in some cases, rapid digitalization. Bleeding is not controlled by heparin, and clinical studies do not suggest that disseminated intravascular coagulopathy is important. Vitamin K and other soluble vitamins are sometimes given to counter dietary deficiencies in patients with LBRF. Because postural hypotension is often pronounced during the acute phase of relapsing fever and in the early stage of recovery, patients should be assisted when arising from bed.

Untreated LBRF has a high case-fatality rate, especially among persons in otherwise poor health, such as those in famine-affected populations. The fatality rate among treated persons is usually <5%. In general, TBRF is a milder disease than LBRF: the spontaneous crisis and the Jarisch-Herxheimer reactions are less pronounced and the case-fatality rates are lower for TBRF than for LBRF.

PREVENTION AND CONTROL LBRF can be prevented by elimination of circumstances that promote louse infestation (crowding, poverty, homelessness, poor personal hygiene), by use of practices that eliminate or reduce numbers of body lice (washing clothes, drying clothes in direct sunlight, changing clothes at frequent intervals), and by application of acaricides. Secondary complications and the spread of infection can be prevented by early case detection and treatment of

Table 175-2 Antibiotic Treatment of Louse-Borne and Tick-Borne Relapsing Fever in Adults

Medication	Louse-Borne Relapsing Fever (Single Dose)	Tick-Borne Relapsing Fever (7-Day Schedule)
Oral		
Erythromycin	500 mg	500 mg q6h
Tetracycline	500 mg	500 mg q6h
Doxycycline	100 mg	100 mg q12h
Chloramphenicol	500 mg	500 mg q6h
Parenteral[a]		
Erythromycin	500 mg	500 mg q6h
Tetracycline	250 mg	250 mg q6h
Doxycycline	100 mg	100 mg q12h
Chloramphenicol	500 mg	500 mg q6h
Penicillin G (procaine)	600,000 IU	600,000 IU daily

[a] For tick-borne relapsing fever, parenteral therapy is used only until oral treatment is tolerated.

infected persons and close contacts. Historically, outbreaks of LBRF have been controlled by mass delousing. In situations like those in refugee camps, individuals, their clothes, and their bedding should be deloused with appropriate acaricides, such as 0.5% permethrin dust. Impregnation of clothing with liquid permethrin, a residual acaricide, can provide long-term protection against infestation. In outbreaks of fever that involve louse-infested populations, empirical single-dose treatment with doxycycline will be effective against typhus as well as LBRF. *B. recurrentis* has a fragile life cycle and is eradicable.

TBRF can be prevented by the avoidance of rodent- and tick-infested dwellings and infested natural sites. Limiting rodent access to the foundations and attics of homes and vacation cabins and eliminating harborage for rodents in and around these dwellings reduce the potential for tick exposure. Rodents and rodent nests should be removed from infested buildings and their surroundings. Tick harborages of infested buildings or other circumscribed sites, such as rodent burrows and nests in hollow logs surrounding dwellings and in rodent-infested caves, can be chemically treated by pest-control specialists using various acaricides, such as carbaryl, diazinon, chlorpyrifos, pyrethrins, and malathion. Persons who enter tick-infested sites can protect themselves by wearing clothing that denies ticks access to the skin, by applying repellents to exposed skin and to clothing, and by applying an acaricide containing permethrin to clothing. Reporting of suspected cases of relapsing fever to public health authorities is important so that an epidemiologic investigation and control measures can be initiated promptly.

BIBLIOGRAPHY

BARBOUR AG: Antigenic variation of relapsing fever *Borrelia* species. Annu Rev Microbiol 44:155, 1990

BURGDORFER W, SCHWAN TG: *Borrelia*, in *Manual of Clinical Microbiology 6*, PR Murray et al (eds). Washington, DC, American Society for Microbiology, 1995, pp 626–635

CADAVID D, BARBOUR AG: Neuroborreliosis during relapsing fever: Review of clinical manifestations, pathology, and treatment of infections in humans and experimental animals. Clin Infect Dis 26:151, 1998

CUTLER SJ et al: *Borrelia recurrentis* characterization and comparison with relapsing fever, Lyme-associated, and other *Borrelia* spp. Int J Syst Bacteriol 47:958, 1997

DWORKIN MS et al: Tick-borne relapsing fever in the northwestern United States and southwestern Canada. Clin Infect Dis 26:122, 1998

FEKADE D et al: Prevention of Jarisch-Herxheimer reactions by treatment with antibodies against tumor necrosis factor α. N Engl J Med 335:311, 1996

HORTON JM, BLASER MJ: The spectrum of relapsing fever in the Rocky Mountains. Arch Intern Med 145:871, 1985

PERINE PL, TEKLU B: Antibiotic treatment of louse-borne relapsing fever in Ethiopia: A report of 377 cases. Am J Trop Med Hyg 32:1096, 1983

SPACH DH et al: Tick-borne diseases in the United States. N Engl J Med 329:936, 1993

176 LYME BORRELIOSIS

Allen C. Steere

DEFINITION Lyme borreliosis, a tick-transmitted spirochetal illness, usually begins with a characteristic expanding skin lesion, erythema migrans (EM; stage 1, localized infection). After several days or weeks, the spirochete may spread hematogenously to many different sites (stage 2, disseminated infection). Possible manifestations of disseminated infection include secondary annular skin lesions, meningitis, cranial or peripheral neuritis, carditis, atrioventricular nodal block, or migratory musculoskeletal pain. Months to years later (usually after periods of latent infection), intermittent or chronic arthritis, chronic encephalopathy or polyneuropathy, or acrodermatitis may develop (stage 3, persistent infection). Most patients experience early symptoms of the illness during the summer, but the infection may not become symptomatic until it progresses to stage 2 or 3. Despite regional variations, the basic stages of the illness are similar worldwide.

ETIOLOGIC AGENT   *Borrelia burgdorferi*, the causative agent of the disease, is a fastidious, microaerophilic bacterium. The organism contains many immunogenic proteins, including a number of differentially expressed lipoproteins, most of which are encoded by plasmid DNA. The spirochete grows best at 33°C in a complex liquid medium called Barbour, Stoenner, Kelly (BSK) medium. Culture of the organism from clinical specimens (except for biopsy samples of skin at sites of EM or acrodermatitis) has been difficult. Three groups of pathogenic *B. burgdorferi* organisms, together referred to as *B. burgdorferi sensu lato*, have been identified, and more groups surely exist. To date, North American strains have belonged to the first group, *B. burgdorferi sensu stricto*. Although all three of the identified groups have been found in Europe and Asia, most isolates there have been strains of group 2 (*B. garinii*) or group 3 (*B. afzelii*). These differences may well account for the clinical variations in the disease in different geographic regions.

EPIDEMIOLOGY   The distribution of Lyme borreliosis correlates closely with the geographic ranges of ticks of the *Ixodes ricinus* complex: *I. scapularis* (also called *I. dammini*), *I. pacificus*, *I. ricinus*, and *I. persulcatus*. *I. scapularis* is the principal vector in the northeastern United States from Massachusetts to Maryland and in the midwestern states of Wisconsin and Minnesota. Surveys in these regions have documented infection in at least 20% of *I. scapularis* ticks; most cases of Lyme disease in the United States have occurred in these areas. *I. pacificus* is the vector in the western states of California and Oregon. The disease is acquired throughout Europe (from Great Britain to Scandinavia to European Russia), where *I. ricinus* is the vector, and in Asian Russia, China, and Japan, where *I. persulcatus* is the vector. These ticks transmit other diseases that may have similar symptoms. In the United States, *I. scapularis* also transmits babesiosis and ehrlichiosis; in Europe and Asia, *I. ricinus* and *I. persulcatus* also transmit tick-borne encephalitis.

Ticks of the *I. ricinus* complex feed once during each of the three stages of their usual 2-year life cycle. Typically, larval ticks take one blood meal in the late summer, nymphs feed during the following spring and early summer, and adults feed during autumn. For *I. scapularis* in the northeast, the white-footed mouse is the preferred host of the immature larval and nymphal ticks. It is critical that both of the tick's immature stages feed on the same host, because the life cycle of the spirochete depends on horizontal transmission: in early summer from infected nymphs to mice and in late summer from infected mice to larvae, which then molt to become the infected nymphs that will begin the cycle again the following year. It is the tiny nymphal tick that is primarily responsible for transmission of the disease to humans during the early summer months. White-tailed deer, which are not involved in the life cycle of the spirochete, are the preferred host for the adult stage of *I. scapularis* and seem to be critical to the tick's survival. The adult tick occasionally transmits the spirochete to humans during the fall, but at this stage the tick is considerably larger and easier to recognize.

Lyme disease is now the most common vector-borne infection in the United States. Since surveillance was begun in 1982, more than 100,000 cases have been reported to the Centers for Disease Control and Prevention (CDC); during the 1990s, more than 10,000 new cases have been reported each summer. Cases have been noted in 48 states, but the life cycle of *B. burgdorferi* has been identified in only 19 states. Cases have occurred in association with hiking, camping, or hunting trips and with residence in wooded or rural areas. Persons of all ages and both sexes are affected.

PATHOGENESIS   To maintain its complex enzootic cycle, *B. burgdorferi* must adapt to two markedly different environments: the tick and the mammalian host. The spirochete expresses outer-surface proteins A and B (OspA and OspB) in the midgut of the tick, whereas OspC is upregulated as the organism travels to the tick's salivary gland and thence to the mammalian host.

After injection into the human skin, *B. burgdorferi* may migrate outward, producing EM, and may spread hematogenously to other organs. Spread within the human host is probably facilitated through binding to the spirochete's surface by human plasminogen and urokinase-type plasminogen activator, which activates plasmin, a potent protease. The spirochete can adhere to many types of mammalian cells; it binds specifically to certain ubiquitous host integrin receptors in the extracellular matrix, to vitronectin and fibronectin, and to matrix glycosaminoglycans. *B. burgdorferi* seems to have a particular tropism for tissues of the skin, nervous system, atrioventricular node, and joints, from all of which it has been cultured, seen in histologic sections, or (more commonly) detected (via its DNA) by the polymerase chain reaction (PCR). These findings and the response of all stages of the disease to antibiotic therapy suggest that the organism persists in affected tissues throughout the illness, but the mechanisms of persistent infection are not yet clear.

The immune response in Lyme disease develops gradually. After the first several weeks of infection, mononuclear cells generally exhibit heightened responsiveness to *B. burgdorferi* antigens, and evidence of B cell hyperactivity is found, including elevated total serum IgM levels, cryoprecipitates, and circulating immune complexes. Titers of specific IgM antibody to *B. burgdorferi* peak between the third and sixth week after disease onset. The specific IgG response develops gradually over months, with response to an increasing array of 12 or more spirochetal polypeptides and maximal expansion during the period of arthritis. The spirochete is a potent inducer of proinflammatory cytokines, including tumor necrosis factor α and interleukin 1β. Histologic examination of all affected tissues reveals an infiltration of lymphocytes and plasma cells with some degree of vascular damage (including mild vasculitis or hypervascular occlusion), suggesting that the spirochete may have been present in or around blood vessels.

CLINICAL MANIFESTATIONS   Early Infection: Stage 1 (Localized Infection)   After an incubation period of 3 to 32 days, EM, which occurs at the site of the tick bite, usually begins as a red macule or papule that expands slowly to form a large annular lesion, most often with a bright red outer border and partial central clearing (**Plate IID-46**). Because of the small size of ixodid ticks, most patients do not remember the preceding tick bite. The center of the lesion sometimes becomes intensely erythematous and indurated, vesicular, or necrotic. In other instances, the expanding lesion remains an even, intense red; several red rings are found within an outside ring; or the central area turns blue before the lesion clears. Although EM can be located anywhere, the thigh, groin, and axilla are particularly common sites. The lesion is warm but not often painful. Perhaps as many as 25% of patients do not exhibit this characteristic skin manifestation.

Early Infection: Stage 2 (Disseminated Infection)   Within days or weeks after the onset of EM, the organism often spreads hematogenously to many sites. In these cases patients frequently develop secondary annular skin lesions similar in appearance to the initial lesion. Skin involvement is commonly accompanied by severe headache, mild stiffness of the neck, fever, chills, migratory musculoskeletal pain, arthralgias, and profound malaise and fatigue. Less common manifestations include generalized lymphadenopathy or splenomegaly, hepatitis, sore throat, nonproductive cough, conjunctivitis, iritis, or testicular swelling. Except for fatigue and lethargy, which are often constant, the early signs and symptoms of Lyme disease are typically intermittent and changing. Even in untreated patients, the early symptoms usually become less severe or disappear within several weeks.

Symptoms suggestive of meningeal irritation may develop early in Lyme disease when EM is present but usually are not associated with cerebrospinal fluid (CSF) pleocytosis or an objective neurologic deficit. After several weeks or months, about 15% of untreated patients develop frank neurologic abnormalities, including meningitis, subtle encephalitic signs, cranial neuritis (including bilateral facial palsy), motor or sensory radiculoneuropathy, mononeuritis multiplex, or myelitis—alone or in various combinations. In the United States, the usual pattern consists of fluctuating symptoms of meningitis accompanied by facial palsy and peripheral radiculoneuropathy. Lymphocytic pleocytosis (about 100 cells per microliter) is found in CSF, often along with elevated protein levels and normal or slightly low glucose concentrations. In Europe and Asia, the first neurologic sign is characteristically radicular pain, which is followed by the development of CSF pleocytosis (called *Bannwarth's syndrome*), but meningeal or encephalitic signs are frequently absent. These early neurologic abnormalities usually resolve completely within months, but chronic neurologic disease may occur later.

Within several weeks after the onset of illness, about 8% of patients develop cardiac involvement. The most common abnormality is a fluctuating degree of atrioventricular block (first-degree, Wenckebach, or complete heart block). Some patients have more diffuse cardiac involvement, including electrocardiographic changes indicative of acute myopericarditis, left ventricular dysfunction evident on radionuclide scans, or (in rare cases) cardiomegaly or pancarditis. Cardiac involvement usually lasts for only a few weeks but may recur. Chronic cardiomyopathy caused by *B. burgdorferi* has been reported in Europe.

During this stage, musculoskeletal pain is common. The typical pattern consists of migratory pain in joints, tendons, bursae, muscles, or bones (usually without joint swelling) lasting for hours or days and affecting one or two locations at a time.

Late Infection: Stage 3 (Persistent Infection) Months after the onset of infection, about 60% of patients in the United States who have received no antibiotic treatment develop frank arthritis. The typical pattern comprises intermittent attacks of oligoarticular arthritis in large joints (especially the knees), lasting for weeks to months in a given joint. Small joints and periarticular sites also may be affected, primarily during early attacks. The number of patients who continue to have recurrent attacks decreases each year. However, in a small percentage of cases, involvement of large joints—usually one or both knees—becomes chronic and may lead to erosion of cartilage and bone. These patients have a higher frequency of the class II major histocompatibility complex alleles associated with rheumatoid arthritis, particularly HLA-DRBI*0401 or *0101 alleles, than patients with brief Lyme arthritis or normal control subjects. Moreover, they may have persistent arthritis for months or even several years after the apparent eradication of spirochetes from the joints with antibiotic therapy. In these genetically susceptible individuals, autoimmunity may develop within the proinflammatory milieu of the joints because of molecular mimicry between the dominant T cell epitope of OspA and human lymphocyte function–associated antigen 1 (hLFA-1).

White cell counts in joint fluid range from 500 to 110,000/μL (average, 25,000/μL); most of these cells are polymorphonuclear leukocytes. Tests for rheumatoid factor or antinuclear antibodies usually give negative results. Examination of synovial biopsy samples reveals fibrin deposits, villous hypertrophy, vascular proliferation, microangiopathic lesions, and a heavy infiltration of lymphocytes and plasma cells.

Although less common, chronic neurologic involvement may also become apparent months or years after the onset of infection, sometimes following long periods of latent infection. The most common form of chronic central nervous system involvement is subtle encephalopathy affecting memory, mood, or sleep and often accompanied by axonal polyneuropathy manifested as either distal paresthesia or spinal radicular pain. Patients with encephalopathy frequently have evidence of memory impairment in neuropsychological tests and abnormal results in CSF analyses. In cases with polyneuropathy, electromyography generally shows extensive abnormalities of proximal and distal nerve segments. Encephalomyelitis or leukoencephalitis, a rare manifestation of Lyme borreliosis reported primarily in Europe, is a severe neurologic disorder that may include spastic paraparesis, upper motor-neuron bladder dysfunction, and lesions in the periventricular white matter. The prolonged course of chronic neuroborreliosis following periods of latent infection is reminiscent of tertiary neurosyphilis.

Acrodermatitis chronica atrophicans, the late skin manifestation of the disorder, has been associated primarily with *B. afzelii* infection in Europe and Asia. It has been observed primarily in elderly women. The skin lesions, which are usually found on the acral surface of an arm or leg, begin insidiously with reddish-violaceous discoloration; they become sclerotic or atrophic over a period of years.

DIAGNOSIS Lyme disease is usually diagnosed by the recognition of a characteristic clinical picture with serologic confirmation. Although serologic testing may yield negative results during the first several weeks of infection, most patients have a positive antibody response to *B. burgdorferi* after that time. The limitation of serologic tests is that they do not clearly distinguish between active and inactive infection. Patients with previous Lyme disease—particularly in cases progressing to late stages—often remain seropositive for years, even after adequate antibiotic treatment. In addition, some patients are seropositive because of asymptomatic infection. If these individuals subsequently develop another illness, the positive serologic test for Lyme disease may cause diagnostic confusion. On the other hand, a few patients who receive inadequate antibiotic therapy during the first several weeks of infection develop subtle joint or neurologic symptoms but are seronegative. The important point is that seronegative Lyme disease is usually a mild, attenuated illness.

For serologic analysis in Lyme disease, the CDC recommends a two-step approach in which samples are first tested by enzyme-linked immunosorbent assay (ELISA) and equivocal or positive results are then tested by western blotting. During the first month of infection, both IgM and IgG responses to the spirochete should be determined, preferably in both acute- and convalescent-phase serum samples. Approximately 20 to 30% of patients have a positive response detectable in acute-phase samples, whereas about 70 to 80% have a positive response during convalescence (2 to 4 weeks later). After that time, the great majority of patients continue to have a positive IgG antibody response, and a single test (that for IgG) is usually sufficient. In persons with illness of longer than 1 month's duration, a positive IgM test result alone is likely to be false-positive; therefore, a positive IgM test should not be used to support the diagnosis in such patients. According to current criteria adopted by the CDC, an IgM western blot is considered positive if two of the following three bands are present: 23, 39, and 41 kDa. However, the combination of the 23- and 41-kDa bands may still represent a false-positive result. An IgG blot is considered positive if 5 of the following 10 bands are present: 18, 23, 28, 30, 39, 41, 45, 58, 66, and 93 kDa.

Because serologic tests do not distinguish between active and inactive infection, tests that detect the spirochete directly are being researched. *B. burgdorferi* may be cultured from skin lesions of patients with the disorder, but its culture from other sites has been a low-yield proposition. Detection of spirochetal DNA by PCR may serve as a substitute for culture in cases of Lyme arthritis. In one study, *B. burgdorferi* DNA was detected in synovial fluid samples from 75 (85%) of 88 patients and in none of 64 control samples. However, the sensitivity of PCR determinations in CSF from patients with neuroborreliosis has been much lower. There seems to be little if any role for PCR in the detection of *B. burgdorferi* DNA in blood or urine samples.

DIFFERENTIAL DIAGNOSIS Classic EM is a slowly expanding erythema with partial central clearing. If the lesion expands little, it may represent the red papule of an uninfected tick bite. If the lesion expands rapidly, it may represent cellulitis (e.g., streptococcal cellulitis) or an allergic reaction, perhaps to tick saliva. Patients with secondary annular lesions may be thought to have erythema multiforme, but neither the development of blistering mucosal lesions nor the involvement of the palms or soles is a feature of *B. burgdorferi* infection. In the southeastern United States, an EM-like skin lesion, sometimes with mild systemic symptoms, may be associated with *Am-*

blyomma americanum tick bites, but the cause of this illness has not yet been identified.

Later in the infection, the most common problem in diagnosis is to mistake Lyme disease for chronic fatigue syndrome or fibromyalgia. This difficulty is compounded by the fact that a small percentage of patients do in fact develop these chronic pain or fatigue syndromes in association with or soon after Lyme disease. Compared with Lyme disease, chronic fatigue syndrome (Chap. 384) or fibromyalgia tends to produce more generalized and disabling symptoms, including marked fatigue, severe headache, diffuse musculoskeletal pain, multiple symmetric tender points in characteristic locations, pain and stiffness in many joints, diffuse dysesthesia, difficulty with concentration, and sleep disturbances. Patients with chronic fatigue syndrome or fibromyalgia lack evidence of joint inflammation; they have normal results in neurologic tests; and they usually have a greater degree of anxiety and depression than patients with chronic neuroborreliosis.

℞ **TREATMENT** As outlined in the algorithm in Fig. 176-1, the various manifestations of Lyme disease can usually be treated successfully with orally administered antibiotics; the exceptions are objective neurologic abnormalities and third-degree atrioventricular heart block, which seem to require intravenous therapy. For early Lyme disease, doxycycline is effective in men and in nonpregnant women. An advantage of this regimen is that it is also effective against the agent of human granulocytic ehrlichiosis, which is transmitted by the same tick that transmits the Lyme disease agent. Amoxicillin, cefuroxime axetil, and erythromycin or its congeners are second-, third-, and fourth-choice alternatives, respectively. In children, amoxicillin is effective (not more than 2 g/d); in cases of penicillin allergy, cefuroxime axetil or erythromycin may be used. For patients with infection localized to the skin, a 20-day course of therapy is generally sufficient;

in contrast, for patients with disseminated infection, a 30-day course is recommended. Approximately 15% of patients experience a Jarisch-Herxheimer-like reaction during the first 24 h of therapy.

These oral antibiotic regimens, when given for 30 to 60 days, are effective for the treatment of Lyme arthritis. However, the response to oral therapy may be slower than that to intravenous therapy. In the small percentage of patients with arthritis in whom arthritic symptoms persist for months or even years after the apparent eradication of spirochetes from the joints with antimicrobial therapy, treatment with anti-inflammatory agents or synovectomy may be successful.

For objective neurologic abnormalities (with the possible exception of facial palsy alone), parenteral antibiotic therapy seems to be necessary. Intravenous ceftriaxone, given for 4 weeks, is most commonly used for this purpose, but intravenous cefotaxime or intravenous penicillin G for the same duration may also be effective. In patients with high-degree atrioventricular block or a PR interval of greater than 0.3 s, intravenous therapy for at least part of the course and cardiac monitoring are recommended. Prior to the use of antibiotics for the treatment of Lyme disease, the degree of heart block was found to decrease rapidly with prednisone (40 to 60 mg/d). Although rarely used today, glucocorticoids may be of benefit in patients with complete heart block or congestive heart failure if antimicrobial therapy alone does not result in improvement within 24 h.

It is unclear how and whether asymptomatic infection should be treated, but patients with such infection are often given a course of oral antibiotics. The appropriate treatment for Lyme disease during pregnancy is also unclear. Because the risk of maternal-fetal transmission seems to be very low, standard therapy for the documented stage and manifestation of the illness may be sufficient. Relapse may follow the use of any of the antibiotic regimens for Lyme disease, and a second course of therapy may be necessary. On the other hand, in patients who develop chronic fatigue syndrome or fibromyalgia after Lyme disease, further antibiotic therapy does not seem to be of benefit.

The risk of infection with *B. burgdorferi* after a recognized tick bite is so low that antibiotic prophylaxis is not routinely indicated. However, if the tick is engorged, if follow-up is difficult, or if the patient is quite anxious, therapy with amoxicillin or doxycycline for 10 days is likely to prevent Lyme disease.

PROGNOSIS The response to treatment is best early in the disease. Later treatment of Lyme borreliosis is still effective, but convalescence may be longer. Eventually, most patients recover with minimal or no residual deficits.

ALGORITHM FOR TESTING AND THERAPY According to guidelines recently published by the American College of Physicians, empirical antibiotic therapy without serologic testing is recommended for patients with a high pretest probability of Lyme disease (such as those with EM); two-step testing (by ELISA and, if positive, by western blot) is recommended for patients with an intermediate pretest probability (such as those with recurrent oligoarticular arthritis); and neither testing nor treatment is recommended for patients with a low pretest probability (such as those with nonspecific symptoms of myalgias, arthralgias, or fatigue).

REINFECTION Reinfection may occur after EM when patients are treated with antimicrobial agents. In such cases, the immune response is not adequate to provide protection from subsequent infection. However, patients who develop an expanded immune response to the spirochete over a period of months (such as those with Lyme arthritis) have protective immunity for a period of years and do not acquire the infection again.

VACCINATION A vaccine is now available for the prevention of Lyme disease in the United States. It consists of a recombinant outer-surface lipoprotein A (L-OspA) with adjuvant. High-titered antibody to OspA is necessary for protection. In a phase 3 efficacy trial in which subjects were given three doses of vaccine or placebo on a 0-, 1-, and 12-month schedule, vaccine efficacy in preventing definite cases of Lyme disease was 49% during the first year (after two doses)

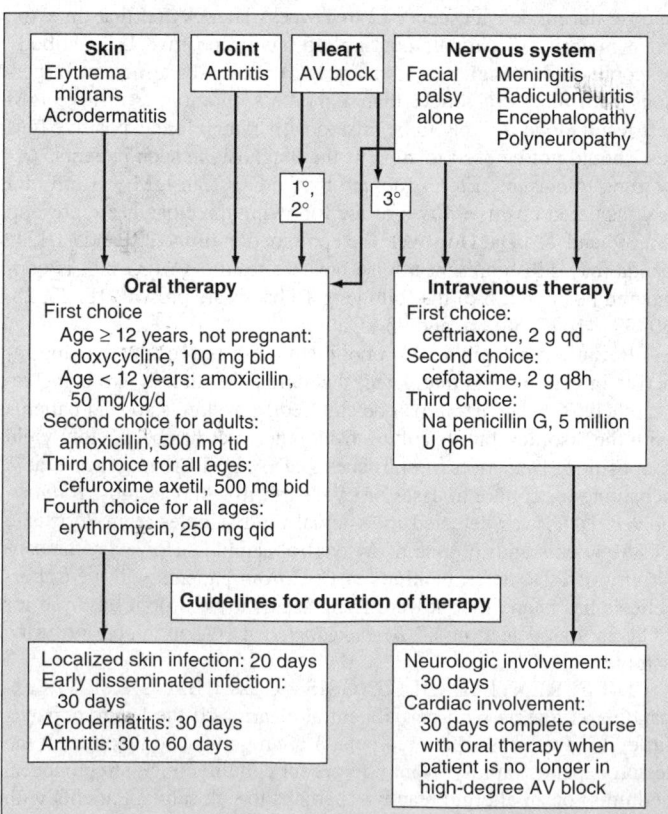

FIGURE 176-1 Algorithm for the treatment of the various acute or chronic manifestations of Lyme borreliosis. Relapse may occur with any of these regimens, and a second course of treatment may be necessary. AV, atrioventricular.

and 76% in year 2 (after three doses). Equivalent antibody titers may be obtained if the three doses are given on a 0-, 1-, and 2-month schedule. The third dose should be given in April so that the vaccine recipient will have peak antibody titers during the summer tick-transmission season. Although long-term data are not yet available, yearly booster injections may be necessary. Vaccine injection may cause a mild to moderate local or systemic reaction usually lasting for only a few days. Vaccination should be considered for individuals who live in areas that are highly endemic for the infection and who have frequent exposure to tick habitats.

BIBLIOGRAPHY

BARBOUR AG, HAYES SF: Biology of *Borrelia* species. Microbiol Rev 50:381, 1986

DATTWYLER RJ et al: Ceftriaxone compared with doxycycline for the treatment of acute disseminated Lyme disease. N Engl J Med 337:289, 1997

DRESSLER F et al: Western blotting in the serodiagnosis of Lyme disease. J Infect Dis 167:392, 1993

LOGIGIAN EL et al: Chronic neurologic manifestations of Lyme disease. N Engl J Med 323:1438, 1990

NOCTON JJ et al: Detection of *Borrelia burgdorferi* DNA by polymerase chain reaction in synovial fluid in Lyme arthritis. N Engl J Med 330:229, 1994

RAHN DW, MALAWISTA SE: Lyme disease: Recommendations for diagnosis and treatment. Ann Intern Med 114:472, 1991

STEERE AC: Lyme disease. N Engl J Med 321:586, 1989

―――― et al: Vaccination against Lyme disease with recombinant *Borrelia burgdorferi* outer-surface lipoprotein A with adjuvant. N Engl J Med 339:209, 1998

Section 10
RICKETTSIA, MYCOPLASMA, AND *CHLAMYDIA*

David Walker, Didier Raoult, J. Stephen Dumler, Thomas Marrie

RICKETTSIAL DISEASES

The rickettsiae make up a family of gram-negative coccobacilli and short bacilli that grow strictly in eukaryotic cells. Characteristics of these organisms include their obligately intracellular location and persistence. The pathogenic rickettsiae move through mammalian reservoirs; they are transmitted by insect or tick vectors. Except for louse-borne typhus, humans are incidental hosts. Among rickettsiae, *Coxiella burnetii* (the agent of Q fever) is notorious for its ability to survive for an extended period outside of the reservoir or vector and for its extreme infectiousness: inhalation of a single microorganism can cause pneumonia. Clinical infections with rickettsiae can be classified into five general groups: (1) tick- and gamasid mite–borne, spotted fever group (SFG) rickettsial diseases; (2) flea- and louse-borne typhus group rickettsial diseases; (3) chigger-borne scrub typhus; (4) ehrlichioses; and (5) Q fever. The rickettsiae that cause spotted fevers, typhus, and scrub typhus are listed along with their vectors, geographic ranges, and associated diseases in Table 177-1.

TICK- AND MITE-BORNE SPOTTED FEVERS

ROCKY MOUNTAIN SPOTTED FEVER Rocky Mountain spotted fever (RMSF), the most severe of the rickettsial diseases, is caused by *Rickettsia rickettsii*. This organism possesses two major immunodominant surface-exposed proteins, rOmpA and rOmpB, which have species-specific conformational epitopes. rOmpA functions as an adhesin for the host cell; rOmpB, the most abundant outer-membrane protein, shares genetic sequences and limited antigens with typhus group rickettsiae. This small (0.3 μm by 1.0 μm) bacillus has a gram-negative cell wall structure; its lipopolysaccharide shares antigens mainly within the SFG and is not endotoxic in the quantities found in human infections.

Discovered in the American West in the late nineteenth century, RMSF is at present documented in 48 states, Canada, Mexico, Costa Rica, Panama, Colombia, and Brazil. It is transmitted by *Dermacentor variabilis*, the American dog tick, in the eastern two-thirds of the United States and California; by *D. andersoni*, the Rocky Mountain wood tick, in the western United States; by *Rhipicephalus sanguineus*

in Mexico; and by *Amblyomma cajennense* in Central and South America. Maintained principally by transovarian transmission from one generation of ticks to the next, *R. rickettsii* can be acquired by uninfected ticks through the ingestion of a blood meal from rickettsemic small mammals.

Humans become infected during the active season of the vector tick species. In northern areas, cases occur mainly in the spring; in warmer southern states, most cases occur from May to September, although some cases are reported in the winter. Although 4% of *D. variabilis* ticks contain rickettsiae, the vast majority of these are non-pathogenic species such as *R. montana* and *R. bellii*. The likelihood of an individual tick's containing *R. rickettsii* is remote. From 1988 to 1997, the reported incidence of RMSF has been in the range of 0.16 to 0.26 cases per 100,000 population in the United States. This rate is probably an underestimate, since the diagnosis is difficult and reporting incomplete. The 5- to 9-year-old age group has the highest incidence. The mortality rate was 20 to 25% in the preantibiotic era and now remains at about 5% because of delayed diagnosis and treatment. The case-fatality ratio is higher for males than females and increases with each decade of life above age 20.

Pathogenesis *R. rickettsii* organisms are inoculated into the dermis along with secretions of the tick's salivary glands after ≥6 h of feeding. Rickettsiae spread lymphohematogenously throughout the body, attach via rOmpA to the endothelial cell membrane, and induce their own engulfment. Once intracellularly located, they escape rapidly from the phagosome, replicate in the cytosol by binary fission, and spread from cell to cell, propelled by polar polymerization of the host cell's actin. The result is numerous foci of contiguous infected endothelial cells that are extensive enough to manifest clinically after a dose-dependent incubation period of approximately 1 week (range, 2 to 14 days). *R. rickettsii* is more invasive than other rickettsiae, routinely spreading to infect vascular smooth-muscle cells. Despite frequent statements to the contrary, occlusive thrombosis and ischemic necrosis are not the fundamental pathologic basis for tissue and organ injury in RMSF. Instead, increased vascular permeability, with resulting edema, hypovolemia, and ischemia, is responsible. Indeed, immunohistologic studies of severely infected humans and animals have demonstrated numerous zones of infected endothelium, only a small proportion of which contain thrombi. The thrombi are usually located to one side of the lumen, which is not occluded. These hemostatic plugs appear to be an appropriate host response rather than a pathogenic process. Consumption of platelets results in thrombocytopenia

Table 177-1   Features of Selected Rickettsial Infections

Disease	Organism	Vector(s)	Geographic Range	Incubation Period	Duration
Rocky Mountain spotted fever	*Rickettsia rickettsii*	*Dermacentor andersoni* *D. variabilis* *Amblyomma cajennense* *Rhipicephalus sanguineus*	United States United States Central/South America Mexico	2–14 days	10–20 days
Mediterranean spotted fever[a]	*R. conorii*	*R. sanguineus*	Southern Europe, Africa, Middle East, Central Asia	5–7 days	7–14 days
Rickettsialpox[a]	*R. akari*	*Liponyssoides sanguineus*	United States, Ukraine, Slovenia	10–17 days	3–11 days
Epidemic typhus	*R. prowazekii*	*Pediculus humanus corporis*	Worldwide	7–14 days	10–18 days
Brill-Zinsser disease	*R. prowazekii*	—[b]	Worldwide	Years	7–11 days
Murine typhus	*R. typhi*	*Xenopsylla cheopis*	Worldwide	8–16 days	8–16 days
Murine typhus	*R. felis*	*Ctenocephalides felis*	Southern Texas, California, Mexico	8–16 days	8–16 days
Scrub typhus[a]	*Orientia tsutsugamushi*	*Leptotrombidium deliense*	Asia, Australia, New Guinea, Pacific Islands	9–18 days	6–21 days

[a] Eschar is usually present at the bite site.
[b] Brill-Zinsser disease represents a recrudescence of latent epidemic typhus.
NOTE: Rocky mountain spotted fever and epidemic typhus often manifest as severe illness, while scrub typhus sometimes does so; murine typhus and Mediterranean spotted fever cause moderately severe illness; and Brill-Zinsser disease and rickettsialpox usually cause mild illness. The rash in Rocky Mountain spotted fever spreads from the extremities to the trunk and face; palms and soles may also be involved. All other rickettsial diseases listed above have a rash that starts on the trunk and spreads to the extremities. The palms and soles are also involved in Mediterranean spotted fever.

in 32 to 52% of patients, but disseminated intravascular coagulation with hypofibrinogenemia is rare. Activation of platelets, generation of thrombin, and activation of the fibrinolytic system all appear to be homeostatic physiologic responses to endothelial injury.

Clinical Manifestations   Early in the illness, when medical attention usually is first sought, RMSF is difficult to distinguish from many self-limiting viral illnesses. Fever, headache, malaise, myalgia, nausea, vomiting, and anorexia are the most frequent symptoms during the first 3 days. The patient becomes progressively more ill as vascular infection and injury advance. In one large series, only one-third of patients were diagnosed with presumptive RMSF early in the clinical course and treated appropriately as outpatients. In the tertiary care setting, RMSF is all too often recognized only when its late severe manifestations, developing at the end of the first week or in the second week of illness in patients without appropriate treatment, prompt admission to the intensive care unit.

The progressive nature of the infection is clearly manifested in the skin. Rash is evident in only 14% of patients on the first day of illness and in only 49% during the first 3 days. Macules (1 to 5 mm) appear first on the wrists and ankles and then on the remainder of the extremities and the trunk. Later, more severe vascular damage results in frank hemorrhage at the center of the maculopapule, a petechia that does not disappear upon compression (**Plate IID-45**). This sequence of events is sometimes delayed or aborted by effective treatment. In fact, rash appears on day 6 or later in 20% of cases and does not appear at all in 9 to 16% of cases, including some with severe visceral lesions that result in death. Petechiae occur in 41 to 59% of cases, appearing on or after day 6 in 74% of cases that include a rash. Involvement of the palms and soles, often considered diagnostically important, usually occurs relatively late in the course (after day 5 in 43% of cases) and does not occur at all in 18 to 64% of cases.

The microcirculation, both systemic and pulmonary, is the target of intracellular rickettsial infection, and the clinical manifestations reflect the ensuing vascular changes. Widespread increased vascular permeability results in edema, decreased plasma volume, hypoalbuminemia, reduced serum oncotic pressure, and prerenal azotemia. Hypotension occurs in 17% of cases. Extensive infection of the pulmonary microcirculation is associated with noncardiogenic pulmonary edema. Cardiac involvement is most frequently manifested as dysrhythmia, which is detected in 7 to 16% of cases. Pulmonary involvement, often a major factor in fatal cases, is observed in 17% of cases, of which 12% are considered to represent severe respiratory disease and 8% require mechanical ventilation.

Central nervous system (CNS) involvement is the other important determinant of the outcome of RMSF. Encephalitis, presenting as confusion or lethargy, is apparent in 26 to 28% of cases. Progressively severe encephalitis manifests as stupor or delirium in 21 to 26% of cases, as ataxia in 18%, as coma in 9 to 10%, and as seizures in 8%. Cranial nerve palsy, hearing loss, severe vertigo, nystagmus, dysarthria, aphasia, unilateral corticospinal signs, ankle clonus, extensor toe signs, hyperreflexia, spasticity, fasciculations, athetosis, neurogenic bladder, hemiplegia, paraplegia, and complete paralysis have been reported. Meningoencephalitis results in cerebrospinal fluid (CSF) pleocytosis in 34 to 38% of cases; usually there are 10 to 100 cells per microliter with a mononuclear predominance, but occasionally there are more than 100 cells per microliter and a polymorphonuclear predominance. The CSF protein concentration is increased in 30 to 35% of cases, but the CSF glucose concentration is usually normal.

Renal failure, which occurs in more severely ill patients, is often reversible with rehydration. However, in the most severe cases, shock results in acute tubular necrosis–induced renal failure, which often requires hemodialysis.

Hepatic injury is manifested in 38% of cases as mildly or moderately increased serum aminotransferase concentrations and is due to focal death of individual hepatocytes, but hepatic failure does not occur. Jaundice is recognized in 8 to 9% of cases and an elevated serum bilirubin concentration in 18 to 30%. Marked hyperbilirubinemia occasionally occurs, probably as a consequence of both hemolysis and hepatocytic injury.

Bleeding is a potentially life-threatening effect of severe vascular damage. Anemia develops in 30% of cases and is severe enough to require red blood cell transfusions in 11%. Blood is detected in the stools or vomitus of 10% of patients, and death has followed massive upper gastrointestinal hemorrhage.

Other characteristic clinical laboratory findings include a normal white blood cell count with increased numbers of immature myeloid cells, increased plasma levels of proteins of the acute-phase response (C-reactive protein, fibrinogen, ferritin, and others), and hyponatremia (in 56% of cases) due to the appropriate secretion of antidiuretic hormone in response to the hypovolemic state. Skeletal muscle injury, clinically manifested as myositis, has been documented in several individual cases by the detection of marked elevations in serum creatine kinase or of histopathologic evidence of vascular injury in skeletal muscle and multifocal rhabdomyonecrosis. Ocular involvement includes conjunctivitis in 30% of cases and retinal vein engorgement, flame hemorrhages, arterial occlusion, and papilledema with normal CSF pressure in some instances.

In untreated cases, death usually occurs 8 to 15 days after the onset of illness. A rare presentation, fulminant RMSF, is fatal within 5 days after onset. This fulminant presentation has been associated with RMSF in black males who have glucose-6-phosphate dehydrogenase (G6PD) deficiency and is thought to be related to an undefined effect of hemolysis on the rickettsial infection. Although survivors of RMSF usually appear to return to their previous state of health, permanent sequelae, including neurologic deficits and amputation of gangrenous extremities, may follow severe illness.

Diagnosis The diagnosis of RMSF during the acute stage is more difficult than is generally appreciated. Clinical and epidemiologic considerations are more important than laboratory features early in the illness. The most important epidemiologic factor is a history of exposure within the 12 days preceding disease onset to a potentially tick-infested environment during a season of possible tick activity. However, only 60% of patients actually recall being bitten by a tick during the incubation period.

The differential diagnosis for early clinical manifestations of RMSF (fever, headache, and myalgia without a rash) includes influenza, enteroviral infection, infectious mononucleosis, viral hepatitis, leptospirosis, typhoid fever, gram-negative or -positive bacterial sepsis, human monocytic or granulocytic ehrlichiosis, murine typhus, sylvatic flying-squirrel typhus, and rickettsialpox. Enterocolitis may be suggested by nausea, vomiting, and abdominal pain; prominence of abdominal tenderness has resulted in exploratory laparotomy. CNS involvement may masquerade as bacterial and viral meningoencephalitis, with seizures, coma, neurologic signs, and CSF abnormalities. Cough, pulmonary signs, and chest roentgenographic opacities may lead to a diagnostic consideration of bronchitis or pneumonia.

During the first 3 days of illness, only 3% of patients exhibit the classic triad of fever, rash, and history of tick exposure. When a rash appears, a diagnosis of RMSF should certainly be considered. However, many illnesses considered in the differential diagnosis may also be associated with a rash, including rubeola, rubella, meningococcemia, disseminated gonococcal infection, secondary syphilis, toxic shock syndrome, drug hypersensitivity, idiopathic thrombocytopenic purpura, thrombotic thrombocytopenic purpura, Kawasaki syndrome, and immune complex vasculitis. The converse is also true: any person in an endemic area with a provisional diagnosis of one of the above illnesses may have RMSF.

The most common serologic test for confirmation of the diagnosis is the indirect immunofluorescence assay. Between 7 and 10 days after onset, a diagnostic titer of ≥1:64 is usually detectable. Latex agglutination and a solid-state enzyme immunoassay are also available commercially. Latex agglutination usually yields a diagnostic titer of ≥1: 128 at 7 to 9 days after onset. The sensitivity and specificity of the indirect immunofluorescence assay are 94 to 100% and 100%, respectively, and the latex agglutination test has a sensitivity of 71 to 94% and a specificity of 96 to 99%. The performance of the solid-state immunoassay has not been reported. It is important to understand that serologic tests for RMSF are usually negative at the time of presentation for medical care and that treatment should not be delayed while a positive serologic result is awaited.

The only diagnostic test that is useful during the acute illness is immunohistologic examination (immunofluorescence or immunoenzyme staining) of a cutaneous biopsy of a rash lesion for *R. rickettsii*. Examination of a 3-mm punch biopsy of such a lesion is 70% sensitive

and 100% specific. Polymerase chain reaction (PCR) amplification and detection of *R. rickettsii* DNA in peripheral blood is an insensitive approach except in the preterminal state; rickettsiae are present in large quantities in heavily infected foci of endothelial cells but in relatively low quantities in the circulation. Cultivation of rickettsiae in cell culture is technically feasible but is seldom undertaken because of biohazard and technologic concerns.

℞ **TREATMENT** The drug of choice for the treatment of both children and adults with RMSF is doxycycline, except when the patient is pregnant or allergic to the drug. Doxycycline is administered orally (or, in the presence of coma or vomiting, intravenously) at 200 mg/d in two divided doses. For children with RMSF reinfection, up to five courses of doxycycline may be administered with minimal risk of dental staining. Other regimens include oral tetracycline (25 to 50 mg/kg per day) in four divided doses. β-Lactam antibiotics, erythromycin, and aminoglycosides have no role in the treatment of RMSF, and sulfa-containing drugs are likely to exacerbate this infection. There is not enough clinical experience to comment on the use of fluoroquinolones in this setting. The most seriously ill patients are managed in intensive care units, with careful administration of fluids to achieve optimal tissue perfusion without precipitating noncardiogenic pulmonary edema. In some severely ill patients, hypoxemia requires intubation and mechanical ventilation; oliguric or anuric acute renal failure requires hemodialysis; seizures necessitate the use of antiseizure medication; anemia or severe hemorrhage necessitates transfusions of packed red blood cells; and bleeding with severe thrombocytopenia requires platelet transfusions. Heparin is not a useful component of treatment, and there is no evidence that glucocorticoids, although frequently administered, affect outcome.

Prevention Avoidance of tick bites is the only available preventive approach. Protective clothing and tick repellents, which could reduce the risk, are seldom actually used. After possible tick exposure, it is wise to inspect the body once or twice a day and remove ticks before they can inoculate rickettsiae.

MEDITERRANEAN SPOTTED FEVER (BOUTONNEUSE FEVER) AND OTHER SPOTTED FEVERS The etiologic agent of Mediterranean spotted fever, *R. conorii*, is prevalent in southern Europe (below the 45th parallel), all of Africa, and southwestern and south-central Asia. The tick vector and reservoir is *R. sanguineus*, the dog brown tick. The name of this disease varies with the region in which it occurs; examples include Kenya tick typhus, Indian tick typhus, Israeli spotted fever, and Astrakhan spotted fever. Whatever the designation, the disease is characterized by a high fever, rash, and—in most geographic locales—an inoculation eschar (*tâche noire*) at the site of the tick bite. A severe form of the disease, associated with a 50% mortality rate, has been observed in patients with diabetes, alcoholism, or heart failure.

African tick-bite fever, which is caused by *R. africae* and has been recognized since the beginning of the twentieth century, was first documented in the modern era in Zimbabwe in 1992. The disease occurs in rural areas and follows bites by ticks of cattle and wild animals. *R. africae* is prevalent in *Amblyomma hebraeum* and *A. variegatum* ticks, which readily feed on humans. Cases have been confirmed not only in Zimbabwe but also in Tanzania and South Africa, and the disease is prevalent in the Caribbean islands of Guadeloupe. The incubation period is 7 days. The illness is mild and consists of headache, fever, eschar at the tick bite site, and regional lymphadenopathy. *Amblyomma* ticks often feed in groups, and several ticks may be found on one patient, with the subsequent development of multiple eschars. Rash is frequently lacking or transient and may be vesicular. African tick-bite fever is the most prevalent rickettsiosis worldwide, and, as tourism to sub-Saharan Africa increases, it is expected that more cases will be seen in non-African countries.

Rickettsia japonica causes *Japanese spotted fever* or *Oriental spot-*

Disease	Laboratory Diagnosis	Treatment
Mediterranean spotted fever Japanese or Oriental spotted fever Queensland tick typhus Flinders Island spotted fever African tick-bite fever	Isolation of rickettsiae by shell-vial culture; serology, IFA[a] (IgM, ≥1:64; or IgG, ≥1:128); PCR[a] amplification of DNA from tissue specimens (especially for *R. japonica*)	Doxycycline (100 mg bid PO for 1–5 days) *or* Ciprofloxacin (750 mg bid PO for 5 days) *or* Chloramphenicol (500 mg qid PO for 7–10 days) *or* (in pregnancy) Josamycin[b] (3 g/d PO for 5 days)
Rickettsialpox	IFA: seroconversion to a titer of ≥1:64 or a single titer of ≥1:128; cross-adsorption to eliminate antibodies to shared antigens necessary for a specific diagnosis of the spotted fever rickettsial species	Doxycycline (100 mg bid PO for 1–5 days) *or* Ciprofloxacin (750 mg bid PO for 5 days) *or* Chloramphenicol (500 mg qid PO for 7–10 days) *or* (in pregnancy) Josamycin[b] (3 g/d PO for 5 days)
Endemic (murine) typhus	IFA: fourfold rise to a titer of ≥1:64 or a single titer of ≥1:128; immunohistology: skin biopsy; PCR amplification of *R. typhi* or *R. felis* DNA from blood; dot ELISA[a] and immunoperoxidase methods also available	Doxycycline (100 mg bid PO for 7–15 days) *or* Chloramphenicol (500 mg qid PO for 7–15 days)
Epidemic typhus	IFA: titer of ≥1:128; necessary to use clinical and epidemiologic data to distinguish among louse-borne epidemic typhus, flying-squirrel typhus, and Brill-Zinsser disease	Doxycycline (200 mg PO as a single dose or until patient is afebrile for 24 h)
Scrub typhus	IFA: titer of ≥1:200; PCR amplification of *O. tsutsugamushi* DNA from blood of febrile patients	Doxycycline (100 mg bid PO for 7–15 days)[c] *or* Chloramphenicol (500 mg qid PO for 7–15 days *or* (for children) Chloramphenicol (150 mg/kg per day for 5 days)

[a] IFA, indirect immunofluorescence assay; PCR, polymerase chain reaction; ELISA, enzyme-linked immunosorbent assay.
[b] Not approved by the U.S. Food and Drug Administration.
[c] Azithromycin is more effective than doxycycline in vitro against both doxycycline-susceptible and doxycycline-resistant strains of *O. tsutsugamushi*.

ted fever. Patients present with fever, cutaneous eruption, and an inoculation eschar. In Australia, two spotted fevers have been described. *Queensland tick typhus* is due to *R. australis* and is transmitted by *Ixodes holocyclus*. The skin rash in this disease is usually maculopapular but is sometimes vesicular, and there is an inoculation eschar. *Flinders Island spotted fever*, observed on an island close to Tasmania, is due to *R. honei*. In France, a case of *atypical Lyme disease* caused by *R. slovaca* and two cases of infection with *R. mongolotimonae* have been reported.

Diagnosis The diagnosis of these tick-borne spotted fevers is based on clinical and epidemiologic findings and is confirmed by cell-culture isolation of rickettsiae, by PCR of skin biopsies (a method not available in most laboratories), or by serology. The identification of specific species requires cross-adsorption (Table 177-2). In an endemic area, patients presenting with fever, rash, and/or a skin lesion consisting of a black necrotic area or a crust surrounded by erythema should be considered to have one of these rickettsial spotted fevers.

TREATMENT See Table 177-2.

RICKETTSIALPOX Rickettsialpox was first described in 1946 by a general practitioner in New York City and soon afterwards was shown to be caused by a distinct species, *R. akari*. This organism was isolated from mice and their mites (*Liponyssoides sanguineus*), which maintain the organisms by transovarian transmission. *R. akari* shares lipopolysaccharide antigens with other members of the SFG.

Epidemiology More than 100 cases of rickettsialpox were diagnosed annually in the northeastern United States in the late 1940s and the 1950s, and outbreaks occurred in the Ukraine in the 1950s. However, few cases are diagnosed currently. Recently, a culture-confirmed case of rickettsialpox was documented in southern Europe. This case was initially misdiagnosed as Mediterranean spotted fever on the basis of the development of serum antibodies cross-reactive with *R. conorii*. Cases have also been reported in Arizona, Utah, and Ohio.

Clinical Manifestations A papule forms at the site of the mite bite. This lesion develops a central vesicle that becomes a 1- to 2.5-cm painless black crusted eschar surrounded by an erythematous halo. Enlargement of the lymph nodes draining the region of the eschar suggests initial lymphogenous spread. After a 10-day incubation period, during which the eschar and regional lymphadenopathy frequently go unnoticed, the onset of illness is marked by malaise, chills, fever, headache, and myalgia. A macular rash appears 2 to 6 days after onset and evolves sequentially into papules, vesicles, and crusts that heal without scarring. In some cases the rash remains macular or maculopapular. Some patients suffer nausea, vomiting, abdominal pain, cough, conjunctivitis, or photophobia. Untreated rickettsialpox is not fatal, with fever lasting 6 to 10 days.

Diagnosis and Treatment See Table 177-2.

FLEA- AND LOUSE-BORNE RICKETTSIAL DISEASES

ENDEMIC MURINE TYPHUS (FLEA-BORNE) Murine typhus was postulated to be a distinct disease, with rats as the reservoir and fleas as the vector, by Maxcy in 1926. Dyer isolated the etiologic agent, *R. typhi*, from rats and fleas in 1931. By the end of World War II, murine typhus was known to be a global disease. A novel typhus group *Rickettsia* has now been shown to be maintained vertically in cat fleas and to cause human infection. This flea-transmitted species, *R. felis*, reportedly contains antigens most closely resembling typhus group rickettsiae but genetically is an SFG organism. *R. felis* has been found in 4% of cat fleas and in 33% of opossums collected in the vicinity of human murine typhus–like cases in southern Texas.

Epidemiology *R. typhi* is maintained in mammalian host/flea cycles, with rats (*Rattus rattus* and *R. norvegicus*) and the Oriental rat flea (*Xenopsylla cheopis*) as the classic zoonotic niche. Fleas acquire *R. typhi* from rickettsemic rats and carry the organism throughout the rest of their lifespan. Nonimmune rats and humans are infected when rickettsia-laden flea feces are "scratched" into pruritic bite lesions; less frequently, the flea bite itself transmits the organisms. Yet another possible route of transmission is the inhalation of aerosolized flea feces. Infected rats appear healthy, although they are rickettsemic for approximately 2 weeks.

Currently, fewer than 100 cases of endemic typhus are reported annually in the United States. These cases occur mainly in southern Texas and southern California, where the classic rat-flea cycle is absent and an opossum–cat flea (*Ctenocephalides felis*) cycle is prominent. Although *X. cheopis* fleas are inefficient at the transovarian maintenance of *R. felis*, cat fleas are highly effective at vertical transmission of this organism, whose natural occurrence has been detected in fleas in California, Texas, and Oklahoma. Infected opossums and cat fleas as well as a case of human infection were reported from Corpus Christi, Texas, in the same environment where humans, opossums, and cat fleas are infected with *R. typhi*. Cases of endemic typhus occur year-round, mainly in warm (often coastal) areas. This infection has also been reported from Greece, Spain, and Indonesia. The peak prevalence in southern Texas is from April through June and elsewhere is during the warm months of summer and early fall. Patients seldom recall a flea bite or exposure to fleas, although exposure to animals such as cats, opossums, raccoons, skunks, and rats is reported by nearly 40% of those who are questioned.

Clinical Manifestations The incubation period of experimental murine typhus in volunteers averages 11 days, with a range of 8 to 16 days. Close observation during this period reveals prodromal symptoms of headache, myalgia, arthralgia, nausea, and malaise developing 1 to 3 days before the abrupt onset of chills and fever. Nearly all patients experience nausea and vomiting early in the illness.

The duration of untreated illness averages 12 days, with a range of 9 to 18 days. Rash is present in only 13% of patients at the time of presentation for medical care (usually about 4 days after onset of symptoms), appearing an average of 2 days later in half of the remaining patients and never appearing in the other half. The initial macular rash is often detected by careful inspection of the axilla or the inner surface of the arm. Subsequently, the rash becomes maculopapular, involving the trunk more often than the extremities; it is seldom petechial and rarely involves the face, palms, or soles. A rash is detected in only 20% of patients with dark brown or black skin.

Pulmonary involvement is frequently prominent in murine typhus; 35% of patients have a hacking, nonproductive cough, and 23% of patients who undergo chest radiography have pulmonary densities due to interstitial pneumonia, pulmonary edema, and pleural effusions. Bibasilar rales are the most common pulmonary sign. Less common clinical symptoms and signs include abdominal pain, confusion, stupor, seizures, ataxia, coma, and jaundice. Clinical laboratory studies frequently reveal anemia and leukopenia early in the course, leukocytosis late in the course, thrombocytopenia, hyponatremia, hypoalbuminemia, mildly increased serum levels of hepatic aminotransferases, and prerenal azotemia. Complications may include respiratory failure requiring intubation and mechanical ventilation, hematemesis, cerebral hemorrhage, and hemolysis (in patients with G6PD deficiency and some hemoglobinopathies). The illness is severe enough to necessitate the admission of 10% of hospitalized patients to an intensive care unit. Greater severity is generally associated with old age, underlying disease, and treatment with a sulfa drug; the case-fatality rate is 1%. In a study of children with murine typhus, 50% suffered only nocturnal fevers, feeling well enough for active daytime play.

Diagnosis and Treatment See Table 177-2.

EPIDEMIC TYPHUS (LOUSE-BORNE) Epidemic typhus due to infection with *R. prowazekii* is transmitted by the human body louse (*Pediculus humanus corporis*), which lives on clothes and is found in poor hygienic conditions (especially in jails, where the disease it causes is called *jail fever*) and usually in cold areas. Lice acquire *R. prowazekii* when they ingest a blood meal from a rickettsemic patient. The rickettsiae multiply in the midgut epithelial cells of the louse and spill over into the louse feces. The infected louse defecates during its blood meal, and the patient autoinoculates the organisms by scratching. The fact that the louse abandons dead hosts and patients with high fever (>40°C) improves its efficiency as a vector. Since the louse does not pass *R. prowazekii* to its offspring, the disease is usually spread from person to person by the louse-borne route. Lice die within 1 to 2 weeks after infection, turning red just prior to death—hence the name *red louse disease*. This epidemic form of typhus is related to poverty, cold weather, war, and disasters and is currently prevalent in mountainous areas of Africa, South America, and Asia. A large outbreak involving 100,000 people in refugee camps in Burundi occurred in 1997, a small focus was reported in Russia for the first time in 1998, and sporadic cases have been reported from Algeria and from Peru. The global reemergence of the disease is due to proliferation of body lice. In the United States, sporadic cases of epidemic typhus are transmitted by flying-squirrel fleas. Eastern flying-squirrel (*Glaucomys volans*) lice and fleas have been found to be infected with *R. prowazekii*. The flying-squirrel fleas occasionally bite humans.

Brill-Zinsser disease is a recrudescent, mild form of epidemic typhus occurring years after the acute disease, probably as a result of immunosuppression or old age. Nathan Brill first identified recrudescent typhus in New York in 1898. In 1933 Hans Zinsser noted that more than 90% of patients with recrudescent typhus had emigrated from typhus-endemic areas of Europe. Strains of *R. prowazekii* indistinguishable from classic strains were isolated from patients with recrudescent typhus. Furthermore, *R. prowazekii* was isolated from the lymph nodes of patients undergoing elective surgery who had had typhus years earlier. Thus the typhus rickettsiae can remain dormant for years and can reactivate with waning immunity.

Clinical Manifestations After an incubation period of 1 week, the onset of illness is abrupt, with prostration, severe headache, and rapidly rising fever of 38.8 to 40.0°C (102 to 104°F). Cough is frequently prominent, occurring in 70% of patients. Myalgias are usually severe. In the outbreak in Burundi, the disease was referred to as *sutama* ("crouching"), the myalgias being so severe that patients crouched in an attempt to alleviate the pain. A rash begins on the upper trunk, usually on the fifth day, and then becomes generalized, involving all of the body except the face, palms, and soles. Initially, this rash is macular; without treatment, it becomes maculopapular, petechial, and confluent. The rash is frequently absent or not detected on black skin in Africa, where 60% of patients have *spotless epidemic typhus*. Photophobia, with considerable conjunctival injection and eye pain, is frequent. The tongue may be dry, brown, and furred. Confusion and coma are common. Skin necrosis and gangrene of the digits as well as interstitial pneumonia have been noted in severe cases. Untreated disease is fatal in 7 to 40% of cases, with outcome depending primarily on the condition of the host. Patients with untreated infections develop renal insufficiency and multiorgan involvement in which neurologic manifestations are frequently prominent. Overall, 12% of patients with epidemic typhus have neurologic involvement. North American *R. prowazekii* infection transmitted by flying-squirrel ectoparasites is a milder illness; whether this milder disease is due to host factors (e.g., better health status) or organism factors (e.g., attenuated virulence) is unknown.

Prevention Prevention of epidemic typhus involves control of body lice. Clothes should be changed regularly, and insecticides should be used every 6 weeks to control the louse population.

Diagnosis and Treatment See Table 177-2. Epidemic typhus is sometimes misdiagnosed as typhoid fever in tropical countries.

SCRUB TYPHUS

The etiologic agent of scrub typhus is a small, obligately intracellular bacterium of the family Rickettsiaceae that differs substantially from other family members in its genetic makeup and in the composition of its cell wall (which, for example, lacks lipopolysaccharide and peptidoglycan). Consequently, this organism has been classified as a species in a separate genus, *Orientia tsutsugamushi*.

O. tsutsugamushi is maintained in nature by transovarian transmission in trombiculid mites, mainly of the genus *Leptotrombidium*. After hatching, infected larval mites (chiggers, the only stage that feeds on an animal host) inoculate organisms into the skin while feeding. Scrub typhus is found in environments that harbor the infected chiggers, particularly areas of heavy scrub vegetation—e.g., where the forest is regrowing after being cleared and along riverbanks. Infections occur during the wet season, when the mites lay their eggs. The disease is endemic in eastern and southern Asia, northern Australia, and islands of the western Pacific Ocean. Scrub typhus is also found in tropical areas of India, Sri Lanka, Bangladesh, Myanmar, Thailand, Malaysia, Laos, Vietnam, Kampuchea, China, Taiwan, the Philippines, Indonesia, Papua New Guinea, northern Australia, and islands of the South Pacific Ocean; in temperate areas of Japan, Korea, far-eastern Russia, Tadzhikistan, the mountains of northern India, Pakistan, and Nepal; and in nontropical areas of China, such as Tibet and Shangdong Province. Those infected include indigenous rural workers, residents of suburban areas, and westerners visiting endemic areas for professional or recreational purposes. Infections are more prevalent than the number of clinical diagnoses would suggest; in some areas more than 3% of the population is infected or reinfected each month. Immunity wanes over 1 to 3 years, and there is remarkable antigenic diversity.

Clinical Manifestations   The illness varies in severity from mild and self-limiting to fatal. After an incubation period of 6 to 21 days (usually 8 to 10 days), the onset of disease is characterized by fever, headache, myalgia, cough, and gastrointestinal symptoms. Some patients develop no further signs or symptoms and recover spontaneously after a few days. The classic case description includes an eschar at the site of chigger feeding, regional lymphadenopathy, and a maculopapular rash—signs that are seldom observed in indigenous patients. Fewer than 50% of westerners develop an eschar, and fewer than 40% develop a rash (on day 4 to 6 of illness). Severe cases typically include prominent encephalitis and interstitial pneumonia as key features of vascular injury. Severe illness in persons with G6PD deficiency has been accompanied by hemolysis. The case-fatality rate for untreated classic cases is 7% but would probably be lower if all relatively mild cases (which are underdiagnosed) were included.

Diagnosis and Treatment   See Table 177-2. One report has described cases of scrub typhus in Thailand that do not respond to treatment with doxycycline or chloramphenicol.

EHRLICHIOSES

Ehrlichiae are small, obligately intracellular bacteria with a gram-negative-type cell wall that grow in cytoplasmic vacuoles to form clusters called *morulae* (Fig. 177-1). Two distinct *Ehrlichia* species cause human infections that can be severe and frequent (Table 177-3). *E. chaffeensis*, the agent of human monocytotropic ehrlichiosis (HME), infects predominantly mononuclear phagocytic cells in tissues and blood monocytes. A member of the *E. phagocytophila* group that infects cells of myeloid lineage is the agent of human granulocytotropic ehrlichiosis (HGE). Both *E. chaffeensis* and *E. phagocytophila* are tick-borne but are transmitted by distinct vectors with little geographic overlap. *E. ewingii* is a newly recognized agent of human ehrlichiosis. Identified in four patients to date by means of a broad-range PCR assay, *E. ewingii* has previously been reported as a cause of granulocytotropic ehrlichiosis in dogs.

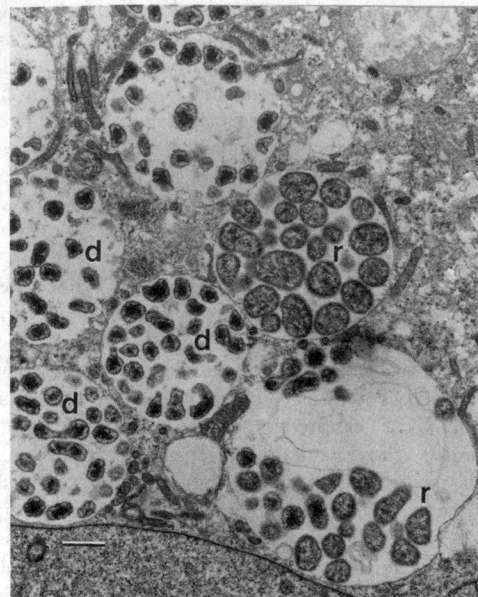

FIGURE 177-1   *Ehrlichia chaffeensis* microcolonies (morulae) within cytoplasmic vacuoles manifest as two morphologic forms: reticulate cells (r) and dense-core cells (d). Bar = 1 μm. *(Courtesy of Dr. Vsevolod L. Popov.)*

Ehrlichiae were discovered by veterinarians during the investigation of hemolytic anemia of cattle before 1910. Researchers thereafter discerned that "marginal points" within erythrocytes were infectious and named the agent *Anaplasma marginale*. Subsequently, several other species now known as ehrlichiae were detected as veterinary infectious agents, including *Cowdria ruminantium*, *E. canis*, *E. phagocytophila*, and *E. risticii*. In 1953, *E. sennetsu* was identified in humans with mononucleosis-like syndromes in Japan.

The current taxonomic positions are determined by nucleic acid sequences of conserved and unique genes among these species. By analysis of 16S ribosomal RNA sequences, the genus and related organisms can be divided into two major clades: the *E. canis* group (including *E. chaffeensis*) and the *E. phagocytophila* group (including *E. equi* and the agent of HGE). The *E. sennetsu* group is as distantly related to both of these clades as it is to the genus *Rickettsia* and is not tick-borne. Given the lack of transovarian transmission in ticks, the natural maintenance of the tick-borne ehrlichiae clearly depends in part upon transient or persistent infections in wild and feral mam-

Table 177-3   Comparison of Two Human Ehrlichioses: Human Monocytotropic Ehrlichiosis (HME) and Human Granulocytotropic Ehrlichiosis (HGE)

Variable	HME	HGE
Etiologic agent	*E. chaffeensis*	*E. phagocytophila* group
Tick vector(s)	*Amblyomma americanum*, *Dermacentor variabilis* (dog tick)	*Ixodes scapularis* (deer tick), *I. ricinus*, *I. pacificus*
Seasonality	April through September	Year-round (peak: May, June, and July
Major target cell	Monocyte	Granulocyte
Morulae seen	Rarely	Frequently
Antigen used in IFA test	*E. chaffeensis*	HGE strains
Diagnostic titer	Fourfold rise or a single titer of ≥1:128; cutoff for negative titer, 1:64	Fourfold rise; cutoff for negative titer, 1:80
Treatment of choice	Doxycycline	Doxycycline
Mortality	2–3%	<1%

NOTE: IFA, indirect immunofluorescence assay.

malian reservoirs. Thus, these bacteria are propagated by horizontal transmission that relies upon a tick-mammal-tick cycle; humans are inadvertently infected when they impinge upon the natural habitats occupied by the ticks and the reservoir hosts.

HUMAN MONOCYTOTROPIC EHRLICHIOSIS **Epidemiology** Infections caused by *E. chaffeensis* have been documented in more than 500 cases reported to the Centers for Disease Control and Prevention (CDC). However, since HME is not a reportable disease in most states, this figure is a gross underestimate. Most infections have been identified in the south-central, southeastern, and mid-Atlantic states, but cases have also been recognized in California, the Pacific northwest, New England, Europe, and Africa. The vector is the Lone Star tick (*Amblyomma americanum*), which in all its life stages feeds upon white-tailed deer, a major reservoir host. Dogs have been discovered to be subclinically infected and may also be an important reservoir. Tick bites and exposures are reported by patients, frequently in rural areas and especially in the months May through July. The median age of HME patients is 44 years, and 75% of the affected individuals are male; however, severe and fatal infections in children are also well recognized.

Clinical Manifestations *E. chaffeensis* is inoculated into the dermal blood pool created by the feeding tick and subsequently disseminates via the blood to tissues. After a median incubation period of 8 days, illness develops; only about one-third of individuals who seroconvert develop a consistent clinical illness. The classic clinical manifestations are not specific and include fever (97% of cases), headache (81%), myalgia (68%), and malaise (84%); less frequently observed are gastrointestinal involvement (nausea, vomiting, diarrhea; 25 to 68%), cough (25%), rash (36% overall, 6% at presentation), and confusion (20%). HME may be severe: 62% of patients with documented cases are hospitalized, and about 2% die. Severe complications include a toxic shock–like or septic shock–like syndrome, respiratory insufficiency and adult respiratory distress, meningoencephalitis, fulminant infection (in immunocompromised patients), severe opportunistic and nosocomial infections, and hemorrhage. Laboratory findings may be of value in the differential diagnosis; 60 to 74% of patients with HME have leukopenia (initially lymphopenia, later neutropenia), 72% have thrombocytopenia, and nearly 90% have elevations in serum levels of hepatic aminotransferases. With effective therapy, rebound lymphocytosis is common. In spite of abnormal blood counts, examinations reveal hypercellular bone marrow, and noncaseating granulomas may be present. Vasculitis is not a component of HME.

Diagnosis Because HME can be rapidly fatal, empirical antibiotic therapy should be instituted on the basis of a clinical diagnosis. This diagnosis may be suggested by fever in the setting of known tick exposure during the preceding 3 weeks, leukopenia and/or thrombocytopenia, and increased aminotransferase concentrations in serum. Morulae are rarely demonstrated in peripheral blood smears unless an intensive examination is performed; even then, an experienced microscopist is required. The active phase of HME may be diagnosed by PCR amplification of *E. chaffeensis* nucleic acids from EDTA-anticoagulated blood obtained before the start of doxycycline therapy. Retrospective serologic diagnosis requires a consistent clinical picture and detection of a fourfold increase in *E. chaffeensis* antibody titer (to ≥1:64) by indirect immunofluorescence in paired serum samples obtained approximately 30 days apart. It must be underscored that separate specific diagnostic tests for HME and HGE are necessary.

℞ **TREATMENT** Tetracycline is effective therapy for HME. Either tetracycline (250 to 500 mg given orally every 6 h) or doxycycline (100 mg given orally or intravenously twice daily) is associated with a lowered rate of hospitalization and a shortened duration of fever. The use of chloramphenicol is controversial, and *E. chaffeensis* is not susceptible to this drug in vitro. While a few reports document the persistence of *E. chaffeensis* in humans after the acute phase of illness, such persistence is very infrequent; most patients are cured after relatively short courses of tetracycline therapy (continuing for 3 to 5 days after defervescence).

Prevention HME is prevented by the avoidance of ticks in endemic areas. The use of protective clothing and tick repellents, careful tick searches after exposures, and prompt removal of attached ticks markedly diminish risk.

HUMAN GRANULOCYTOTROPIC EHRLICHIOSIS **Epidemiology** As of 1995, approximately 150 cases of HGE had been documented in 11 states (mostly in the upper midwest and the northeast), with a distribution similar to that of Lyme disease. Most cases have been identified within the range of various *I. ricinus*–complex ticks, particularly *I. scapularis*. White-footed deer mice in the United States and red deer in Europe appear to play a role in maintaining HGE in nature. The incidence of HGE peaks in May, June, and July, but the disease may occur throughout the year in conjunction with human exposure to *Ixodes* ticks. HGE affects predominantly males (79%) and older persons (median age, 58 years).

Clinical Manifestations Because of high seroprevalence rates in endemic regions, it seems likely that only a minority of infected individuals develop clinical manifestations. The incubation period for HGE varies between 4 and 8 days, and the disease manifests as fever (94 to 100% of cases), myalgia (78 to 98%), headache (61 to 85%), and malaise (98%)—findings suggestive of an influenza-like illness. A minority of patients develop gastrointestinal involvement, including nausea, vomiting, or diarrhea (22 to 39%); rash (2 to 11%); cough (27%); and confusion (17%). Severe complications occur most often in the elderly, but even children may be severely affected. Respiratory insufficiency, with adult respiratory distress syndrome, a toxic shock–like syndrome, and life-threatening opportunistic infections, are the most worrisome complications. Meningoencephalitis has not yet been conclusively recognized with HGE. The case-fatality rate is probably <1%, but nearly 7% of ill patients may require intensive care. As in HME, laboratory findings are of great assistance; most patients develop leukopenia and/or thrombocytopenia with increased serum levels of hepatic aminotransferases. The pancytopenia observed in HGE presumably relates to sequestration or destruction of platelets and leukocytes, since the bone marrow is ordinarily normo- or hypercellular. Vasculitis is not a component of HGE. Unlike HME, HGE is not associated with granulomas. While clear evidence exists for co-infections with *Borrelia burgdorferi* and *Babesia microti*, which are transmitted by the same tick vector(s), there is little evidence of comorbidity or of a persistent or chronic phase for HGE.

Diagnosis HGE should be included in the differential diagnosis for patients who have been exposed to ticks and who develop an influenza-like illness during the season of *Ixodes* tick activity (May through December). The concurrent detection of thrombocytopenia, leukopenia, and/or elevations in serum aminotransferase activities further increases the likelihood of HGE. A substantial proportion of patients with HGE develop serologic reactions considered diagnostic of Lyme disease in the absence of clear clinical findings consistent with that diagnosis. Thus, HGE should be considered in the differential diagnosis of atypical severe presentations of Lyme disease. Although not highly sensitive, a thorough peripheral blood film examination for morulae in neutrophils may identify 20 to 75% of infections. PCR on EDTA-anticoagulated blood collected before initiation of tetracycline therapy from patients with active disease is a sensitive and specific method for early confirmation. Serodiagnosis is based mostly upon the retrospective demonstration of a fourfold increase in *E. phagocytophila* group antibody titer to a minimum of 1:80 in paired sera obtained approximately 1 month apart. IgM antibodies may be detected in many patients within the first 1.5 months after illness. Approximately 15 to 40% of infected persons have a detectable antibody titer at presentation, but, in regions where seroprevalence is high, a single acute-phase polyvalent titer may be misleading.

TREATMENT   Doxycycline (100 mg given orally twice daily) is an effective therapeutic agent, while rifampin has been associated with clinical improvement in pregnant patients with HGE. In vitro studies suggest a role for trovafloxacin, but no prospective studies of any therapy for HGE have been conducted. Most treated patients defervesce within 24 to 48 h.

Prevention   Prevention of HGE requires tick avoidance. The Lyme disease vaccine offers no protection against HGE, and no other vaccine is available.

Q FEVER

Q fever results from infection with *C. burnetii*. This small gram-negative microorganism (0.2 μm by 0.7 μm) exists in two antigenic forms: phase I and phase II. When *C. burnetii* is passaged in cell cultures or embryonated eggs, its lipopolysaccharide undergoes truncation that results in an antigenic change called *phase variation*. The phase I form is extremely infectious and exists in humans and other animals. Passage in cell culture or embryonated eggs results in a shift to the phase II form, which is avirulent. The ability of *C. burnetii* to form spores allows the organism to survive in harsh environments. Indeed, it can survive for more than 40 months in skim milk at room temperature and is readily recovered from soil up to 1 month after contamination. Three different plasmids have been described in various isolates of *C. burnetii*. Q fever encompasses two broad clinical syndromes: acute and chronic infection. It is likely that the host's immune response (rather than characteristics of the infecting strain) determines whether or not chronic Q fever develops.

Epidemiology   Q fever is a zoonosis. The primary sources of human infection are infected cattle, sheep, and goats. However, infected cats, rabbits, and dogs have also been shown to transmit *C. burnetii* to humans. The extensive wildlife reservoir for *C. burnetii* includes mammals, birds, and ticks. In the infected female mammal, *C. burnetii* localizes to the uterus and the mammary glands. Infection is reactivated during pregnancy, and high concentrations of *C. burnetii* are found in the placenta. At parturition, *C. burnetii* is dispersed as an aerosol, and infection follows inhalation of aerosolized organisms by a susceptible host. Infected female animals shed the organism in milk for weeks to months after parturition. In rare instances, human-to-human transmission has followed delivery of an infant to an infected woman or autopsy on an infected individual. *C. burnetii* has been transmitted via blood transfusion. Those at risk for Q fever are abattoir workers, veterinarians, and other individuals who vocationally or avocationally come into contact with infected animals. Exposure to infected newborn animals or to infected products of conception poses the highest risk. Sexual transmission has been demonstrated experimentally in mice, as has transmission during artificial insemination in cattle. Whether *C. burnetii* is sexually transmitted among humans is not yet known. While the experimental evidence on this point is contradictory, the ingestion of contaminated milk in some areas is probably a major route of transmission to humans.

Infections due to *C. burnetii* occur in most countries. Indeed, the only areas known to be free of *C. burnetii* are New Zealand and Antarctica. The primary manifestation of acute Q fever differs from place to place: It is pneumonia in Nova Scotia (Canada) and granulomatous hepatitis in Marseille (France), while both of these manifestations are seen in the Basque country of Spain. These differences may reflect the route of infection; i.e., the ingestion of contaminated milk may result in hepatitis and the inhalation of contaminated aerosols in pneumonia.

Clinical Manifestations • *Acute Q fever*   The incubation period for acute Q fever ranges from 3 to 30 days. The clinical presentations include flulike syndromes, prolonged fever, pneumonia, hepatitis, pericarditis, myocarditis, meningoencephalitis, and infection during pregnancy. The symptoms of acute Q fever are nonspecific; common among them are fever, extreme fatigue, and severe headache. Other symptoms include chills, sweats, nausea, vomiting, and diarrhea, which occur in 5 to 20% of patients. Cough develops in about half of patients with Q fever pneumonia. Neurologic manifestations of acute Q fever are uncommon; however, in one outbreak in the West Midlands, United Kingdom, 23% of 102 patients had neurologic signs and symptoms as the major manifestation. A nonspecific rash may be evident in 4 to 18% of patients. The white blood cell count is usually normal. Thrombocytopenia is detected in about 25% of patients, and reactive thrombocytosis [with platelet counts of up to 1 million/μL (1×10^{12}/L)] frequently develops during recovery. This thrombocytosis may account for cases of deep vein thrombophlebitis complicating acute Q fever in some series. Uncommon manifestations of acute Q fever include optic neuritis, extrapyramidal neurologic disease, Guillain-Barré syndrome, inappropriate secretion of antidiuretic hormone, epididymitis, orchitis, priapism, hemolytic anemia, mediastinal lymphadenopathy mimicking lymphoma, pancreatitis, erythema nodosum, and mesenteric panniculitis. Chest radiography may show an opacity that is indistinguishable from those seen in pneumonia of other etiologies. Multiple rounded opacities are common; in the appropriate epidemiologic setting, they are highly suggestive of Q fever pneumonia. However, right-sided endocarditis resulting in septic pulmonary emboli can produce the same radiographic appearance.

Chronic Q fever   Chronic Q fever, which is uncommon, almost always implies endocarditis. This infection usually occurs in patients with previous valvular heart disease, immunosuppression, or chronic renal insufficiency. Fever is usually absent or low grade. Patients may have nonspecific symptoms for up to 1 year before diagnosis. Valvular vegetations have been seen in only 12% of patients with transthoracic echocardiograms, but the rate of detection may be higher with the use of transesophageal echocardiography. A high index of suspicion is necessary for a correct diagnosis. The disease should be suspected in all patients with culture-negative endocarditis. In addition, all patients with valvular heart disease and an unexplained purpuric eruption, renal insufficiency, stroke, and/or progressive heart failure should be tested for *C. burnetii* infection. Patients with chronic Q fever have hepatomegaly and/or splenomegaly. These two findings, especially in combination with positive rheumatoid factor, high erythrocyte sedimentation rate, high C-reactive protein level, and/or increased γ-globulin concentrations (up to 60 to 70 g/L), suggest this diagnosis. Other manifestations of chronic Q fever include infection of vascular prostheses, aneurysms, and bone.

Diagnosis   *C. burnetii* can be isolated from buffy-coat blood samples or tissue specimens by a shell-vial technique; however, most laboratories are not permitted to attempt the isolation of *C. burnetii* since it is considered highly infectious. PCR can be used to amplify *C. burnetii* DNA from tissue or biopsy specimens. This technique can also be used on paraffin-embedded tissues. Serology, however, is the most commonly used diagnostic tool. Three techniques are available: complement fixation, indirect immunofluorescence, and enzyme-linked immunosorbent assay. Indirect immunofluorescence is sensitive and specific and is the method of choice. Rheumatoid factor should be adsorbed from the specimen before testing. An IgG titer of ≥1:800 to phase I antigen is suggestive of chronic Q fever. In almost all instances of chronic Q fever, the antibody titer to phase I antigen is much higher than that to phase II antigen. The reverse is true in acute Q fever. In addition, in acute Q fever, it is usually possible to demonstrate a fourfold rise in titer between acute- and convalescent-phase serum samples.

TREATMENT   Treatment of acute Q fever with doxycycline (100 mg twice daily for 14 days) is usually successful. Quinolones are also effective. Treatment of chronic Q fever should include at least two antibiotics active against *C. burnetii*. The combination of rifampin and doxycycline has been used with success. For chronic infection, doxycycline should be given as 100 mg twice daily and rifampin as 300 mg once daily. The optimal duration of antibiotic therapy for chronic Q fever remains undetermined. We recommend a minimum of 3 years of treatment, with discontinuation only if the phase I IgA antibody titer is ≤1:50 and the IgG phase I titer is ≤1:200. Another therapeutic option under investigation is the combination of doxycycline (100 mg twice daily) with hydroxychloroquine (600 mg once daily). With this combination, therapy can be completed in 18 months. It is necessary to monitor hydroxychloroquine levels and to adjust the dosage to maintain a plasma concentration of 0.8 to 1.2 μg/mL. In vitro, the addition of 1 mg of hydroxychloroquine/mL renders doxycycline bactericidal for *C. burnetii*.

Prevention A vaccine has been shown to be effective in preventing Q fever in abattoir workers in Australia.

BIBLIOGRAPHY

ARCHIBALD LK, SEXTON DJ: Long-term sequelae of Rocky Mountain spotted fever. Clin Infect Dis 20:1122, 1995

BAKKEN JS et al: Human granulocytic ehrlichiosis in the upper midwest United States. A new species emerging? JAMA 272:212, 1994

BULLER RS et al: *Ehrlichia ewingii*, a newly recognized agent of human ehrlichiosis. N Engl J Med 341:148, 1999

DALTON MJ et al: National surveillance for Rocky Mountain spotted fever, 1981–1982: Epidemiologic summary and evaluation of risk factors for fatal outcome. Am J Trop Med Hyg 52:405, 1995

DUMLER JS, BAKKEN JS: Human ehrlichioses. Newly recognized infections transmitted by ticks. Annu Rev Med 49:201, 1998

—— et al: Clinical and laboratory features of murine typhus in south Texas, 1980 through 1987. JAMA 266:1365, 1991

FOURNIER PE et al: Outbreak of *Rickettsia africae* infections in participants of an adventure race from South Africa. Clin Infect Dis 27:316, 1998

HELMICK CG et al: Rocky Mountain spotted fever: Clinical, laboratory, and epidemiological features of 262 cases. J Infect Dis 150:480, 1984

KASS EM et al: Rickettsial pox in a New York City hospital, 1980–1989. N Engl J Med 331:1612, 1994

RAOULT D et al: Outbreak of epidemic typhus associated with trench fever in Burundi. Lancet 352:353, 1998

—— et al: Treatment of Q fever endocarditis. Comparisons of 2 regimens containing doxycycline and ofloxacin or hydroxychloroquine. Arch Intern Med 159:167, 1999

RIKIHISA Y: The tribe *Ehrlichieae* and ehrlichial diseases. Clin Microbiol Rev 4:286, 1991

STRICKMAN D et al: In vitro effectiveness of azithromycin against doxycycline-resistant and -susceptible strains of *Rickettsia tsutsugamushi*, etiologic agent of scrub typhus. Antimicrob Agents Chemother 39:2406, 1995

178 *William M. McCormack*

MYCOPLASMA INFECTIONS

Mycoplasmas, the smallest free-living organisms known, are prokaryotes that are bounded only by a plasma membrane. Their lack of a cell wall is associated with cellular pleomorphism and resistance to cell wall–active antimicrobial agents, such as penicillins and cephalosporins. The organisms' small genome limits biosynthesis and explains the difficulties encountered with in vitro cultivation. Mycoplasmas typically colonize mucosal surfaces of the respiratory and urogenital tracts of many animal species. Sixteen species of mycoplasmas have been recovered from humans. Most are commensals. *Mycoplasma pneumoniae* causes upper and lower respiratory tract infections. *M. genitalium* and *Ureaplasma urealyticum* are established causes of urethritis and have been implicated in other genital conditions. *M. hominis* and *U. urealyticum* are part of the complex microbial flora of bacterial vaginosis.

MECHANISMS OF PATHOGENICITY

Adherence of mycoplasmas to the surface of the host cell is necessary for colonization and infection. Some pathogenic mycoplasmas are

flask-shaped, with specialized tips that enhance adherence. *M. pneumoniae* adheres via a network of interactive adhesins and accessory proteins and produces hydrogen peroxide, which may cause injury to host cells. *M. hominis* metabolizes arginine, with the production of potentially cytotoxic amounts of ammonia. Ureaplasmas have been placed in a separate genus because of their unique urease activity; the metabolism of urea also produces ammonia. *M. pneumoniae* may evoke IgM autoantibodies that agglutinate human erythrocytes at 4°C. These cold agglutinins can cause anemia and other complications.

MYCOPLASMA PNEUMONIAE

EPIDEMIOLOGY *M. pneumoniae* causes upper and lower respiratory tract symptoms in all age groups, with the highest attack rates in 5- to 20-year-olds. The infection is acquired by inhalation of aerosols. The incubation period is 2 to 3 weeks, considerably longer than that of most other respiratory infections. Although epidemics have taken place in closed populations, such as schools and military installations, most cases occur sporadically or in families. In families, cases typically occur serially, with 2- to 3-week intervals between cases. Infections in adults are often the result of contact with children.

Infection with *M. pneumoniae* is worldwide. Cases occur throughout the year, with epidemics every few years. Some studies have noted an increase in the number of cases during the autumn months in temperate climates. Although pneumonia is the classic presentation, nonpneumonic infection is considerably more common. In very young children, most infections result only in upper respiratory symptoms, whereas children >5 and adults may have bronchitis and pneumonia.

CLINICAL PRESENTATION After a prolonged incubation period, fever and constitutional symptoms develop along with headache and cough, both of which can be prominent and distressing. Symptoms typically progress less rapidly than those of viral respiratory tract infections. In the minority (perhaps 5 to 10%) of infected individuals who develop tracheobronchitis or pneumonia, cough becomes more prominent. Sputum, if produced at all, is usually white and may be tinged with blood. The temperature seldom rises above 38.9 to 39.4°C (102 to 103°F). Shaking chills, myalgias, and gastrointestinal symptoms (e.g., nausea, vomiting, and diarrhea) are unusual. Chest muscle soreness may result from frequent and prolonged coughing, but true pleuritic pain is uncommon.

Pharyngeal injection is often noted. Cervical lymph node enlargement is unusual. Bullous myringitis is a unique but uncommon manifestation. As in other "atypical" pneumonias, findings on auscultation of the lung may be normal or nearly normal despite striking radiographic abnormalities. Pleural effusions develop in <20% of patients.

M. pneumoniae infection may be particularly severe in patients who have sickle cell disease and other hemoglobin S–related hemoglobinopathies. The functional asplenia seen in sickle cell disease may contribute to severe mycoplasmal disease as it does in pneumococcal infection. Severe respiratory distress and large pleural effusions may occur. Digital necrosis has been seen in patients with sickle cell disease who develop very high titers of cold agglutinins.

EXTRAPULMONARY MANIFESTATIONS A broad array of extrapulmonary abnormalities have been associated with *M. pneumoniae* infection. Although these events are unusual, they complicate other respiratory diseases even more rarely and often provide the only clue that an otherwise unremarkable respiratory infection may be mycoplasmal.

Erythema multiforme (Stevens-Johnson syndrome; **see Plate IIE-67**) typically occurs in young male patients with *M. pneumoniae* infection. Other dermatologic manifestations, such as maculopapular and vesicular exanthems, erythema nodosum, and urticaria, have been reported, but none is as clearly linked to *M. pneumoniae* as is erythema multiforme.

Cardiac abnormalities reported in conjunction with *M. pneumoniae* infection include myocarditis and pericarditis, which may result in abnormalities of conduction. Of the wide variety of neurologic conditions associated with *M. pneumoniae*, most have been documented in case reports, where establishment of a cause-and-effect relationship is problematic. Central nervous system abnormalities that have been associated with *M. pneumoniae* include encephalitis, cerebellar ataxia, Guillain-Barré syndrome, transverse myelitis, and peripheral neuropathies. Arthralgias are not unusual in patients who have mycoplasmal pneumonia; mycoplasmal arthritis is rare except in patients who have hypogammaglobulinemia. Hematologic abnormalities associated with *M. pneumoniae* include hemolytic anemia and coagulopathies.

The pathogenesis of the extrapulmonary manifestations of *M. pneumoniae* infection is controversial. Occasional reports have described the identification of *M. pneumoniae* or its nucleic acids in involved tissues. The fact that most attempts at detection have been negative, however, suggests that these extrapulmonary complications have an immunologic basis. Mycoplasmas, including *M. pneumoniae*, can nonspecifically stimulate B lymphocytes. *M. pneumoniae*–infected individuals can develop autoantibodies, including those reactive with brain, heart, and muscle.

DIAGNOSIS Most infections with *M. pneumoniae* are not diagnosed, as they are indistinguishable from upper and lower respiratory tract infections caused by myriad other viral and bacterial pathogens. When the diagnosis is suspected, it is usually because illness is prolonged or extrapulmonary manifestations develop. The white blood cell count is generally somewhat elevated, with few immature cells. Gram's stain of sputum shows leukocytes without a predominance of any bacterial morphologic type. Since *M. pneumoniae* lacks a cell wall, it cannot be detected on Gram's stain. In patients who have pneumonia, the chest radiograph may show reticulonodular or interstitial infiltration, primarily in the lower lobes. As in other "atypical" pneumonias, radiographic abnormalities may be more prominent than would be predicted by auscultation of the chest.

M. pneumoniae can be grown on artificial media, but the process is exacting, requires special media, and takes upwards of 2 weeks. Thus, mycoplasmal cultures do not provide timely information to aid in patient management. The same, unfortunately, is true of serologic diagnosis. Specific antibodies can be detected by enzyme-linked immunoassays, indirect immunofluorescence, or complement fixation but do not develop early enough to guide decisions regarding treatment. As with most serologic tests, examination of paired acute- and convalescent-phase serum specimens is required for good sensitivity and specificity.

Cold agglutinins are nonspecific but develop within the first 7 to 10 days in more than half of patients with *M. pneumoniae* pneumonia and may be detectable when the patient presents to a health care provider. In a patient with a compatible clinical picture, a cold agglutinin titer of ≥1:32 supports the diagnosis of mycoplasmal pneumonia. Cold agglutinin determinations are readily available from diagnostic laboratories. The test can also be performed at the bedside by the addition of 1 mL of the patient's blood to a tube containing anticoagulant (e.g., a tube used to collect blood for determination of prothrombin activity). Before cooling, the nonaggregated red blood cells coat the sides of the inverted tube. The blood is cooled to 4°C when the tube is placed in an ice bath for 3 to 5 min or in a standard refrigerator. In a positive test, clumps of red blood cells can be observed when the tube is inverted. Rewarming of the sample to 37°C in an incubator or by exposure to body heat should reverse the agglutination. A positive "bedside" cold agglutinin test is equivalent to a laboratory titer of ≥1:64.

The lack of sensitive, specific, and timely diagnostic tests has prompted the development of a variety of antigen detection tests that do not involve serology or the cultivation of live organisms. Such tests include antigen capture, indirect enzyme immunoassays, DNA probing, and nucleic acid amplification. Since many viral and bacterial infections result in clinical presentations similar to that caused by *M. pneumoniae*, examination of specimens for single antigens is unlikely to be useful. Rather, tests that examine an individual specimen for multiple antigens are needed. Multiplex nucleic acid amplification tests that examine a single throat swab or sputum sample for all of the most likely causative microorganisms are feasible with current technology. Prototype multiplex polymerase chain reaction (PCR) assays have already been developed. If such tests become available clinically, more precise etiologic diagnosis of upper and lower respiratory tract infections will be possible.

℞ **TREATMENT** Because most mycoplasmal infections are not specifically diagnosed, management is directed at one of two syndromes: upper respiratory tract infection or community-acquired pneumonia. Upper respiratory infections, whether caused by viruses or by *M. pneumoniae*, do not require antimicrobial treatment. Community-acquired pneumonia (Chap. 255) may be caused by bacteria such as *Streptococcus pneumoniae* and *Haemophilus influenzae* or by "atypical" agents such as *Chlamydia pneumoniae*, *Legionella pneumophila*, and *M. pneumoniae*. Recommended treatment regimens include a third-generation cephalosporin, such as intravenous ceftriaxone (1.0 g/d) or cefotaxime (1.0 g every 8 h), that is active against the conventional bacterial pathogens plus intravenous or oral erythromycin (500 mg four times a day) to cover atypical microorganisms. Newer agents that have antimicrobial activity against both conventional and atypical causes of community-acquired pneumonia may be prescribed as monotherapy. These drugs include oral clarithromycin (500 mg twice a day), intravenous or oral azithromycin (500 mg once daily), and intravenous or oral levofloxacin (500 mg once daily). Treatment of documented *M. pneumoniae* pneumonia is usually continued for 14 to 21 days.

Pneumonia due to *M. pneumoniae* is usually self-limited and is seldom life-threatening. Effective antimicrobial agents do shorten the duration of illness and, by reducing coughing, may conceivably render the patient less infectious. Although symptoms are alleviated by antimicrobial treatment, the organism usually is not eradicated. Cultures positive for *M. pneumoniae* may persist for months despite effective antimicrobial treatment. The beneficial effects, if any, of such treatment on extrapulmonary manifestations of *M. pneumoniae* infection are unknown.

GENITAL MYCOPLASMAS (See also Chap. 132)

EPIDEMIOLOGY *M. hominis* and *U. urealyticum* are the most prevalent genital mycoplasmas. Infants may become colonized with one or both of these organisms during passage through a colonized birth canal. Neonatal colonization tends not to persist. Only about 10% of prepubertal girls and even fewer prepubertal boys are colonized with ureaplasmas. After puberty, colonization occurs mainly as a result of sexual activity. Among adults, disadvantaged populations have higher colonization rates. Ureaplasmas can be cultured from the vaginas of ~80% of women cared for in public clinics and about half of women cared for by private obstetricians and gynecologists. Similarly, vaginal *M. hominis* is found in 50% of women attending public clinics and in ~20% of private patients. Men have somewhat lower rates of genital colonization than women. Nonetheless, both *U. urealyticum* and *M. hominis* are frequently detected in genital specimens from healthy, sexually experienced adults. Evaluation of the role of these organisms in human disease must take into account their high prevalence among healthy people.

M. fermentans colonizes both the respiratory and genital tracts in >20% of adults. There is no convincing evidence that *M. fermentans* causes human disease; although it had been implicated as a possible determinant of HIV-1 disease progression, more recent data do not support such a role. *M. genitalium* is a fastidious organism that is difficult to cultivate. PCR studies have identified the organism more successfully. Little is known about the epidemiology of *M. genitalium*.

ASSOCIATION WITH HUMAN DISEASE **Nongonococcal Urethritis** *Chlamydia trachomatis* is the organism most firmly implicated in the etiology of nongonococcal urethritis (NGU). There is no doubt that both *U. urealyticum* and *M. genitalium* also cause some cases of NGU. The ubiquity of ureaplasmas among men who do not have urethritis and the difficulty of identifying *M. genitalium* do not allow precise estimation of the proportion of cases of NGU caused by each of these mycoplasmas. *U. urealyticum* and *M. genitalium* do, however, appear to cause most of the nonchlamydial cases.

Epididymitis and Prostatitis Ureaplasmas may be an occasional cause of epididymitis. *M. hominis* has not been implicated in this disease. Neither organism has been convincingly associated with prostatitis.

Pelvic Inflammatory Disease (PID) (See also Chap. 133) *M. hominis* and *U. urealyticum* are both prominent components of the complex microbial flora of bacterial vaginosis. Since bacterial vaginosis is associated with PID, it is difficult to determine whether either organism plays an independent role in this condition. Although *M. genitalium* is not associated with bacterial vaginosis, preliminary studies have linked it to PID in women who are not infected with either *Neisseria gonorrhoeae* or *C. trachomatis*.

Disorders of Reproduction Ureaplasmas have been considered as causes of involuntary infertility in both men and women, but there is no convincing evidence for such an association. These organisms have been associated with chorioamnionitis and late abortion. Given the close association of ureaplasmas with bacterial vaginosis, a condition that is strongly associated with chorioamnionitis and late abortion, it is difficult to define an independent role for ureaplasmas in this condition. In infants of very low birthweight, ureaplasmas have been shown to cause pneumonia and chronic lung disease.

Extragenital Infections Sexually acquired reactive arthritis and Reiter's disease may be triggered by ureaplasmas, although *C. trachomatis* is the usual triggering agent. Patients who have hypogammaglobulinemia may develop chronic arthritis due to ureaplasmas and some other mycoplasmal species. *M. hominis* has been identified in patients with postthoracotomy sternal wound infection and in rare instances of prosthetic heart valve and prosthetic joint infection.

DIAGNOSIS There is seldom any reason to examine specimens from the lower genital tract (vagina, male urethra) for mycoplasmas. The ubiquity of the organisms among healthy individuals makes a positive result uninterpretable. The organisms should be sought only in specimens from normally sterile areas, such as joint fluid with evidence of inflammation and cultures negative for conventional microorganisms.

M. hominis can replicate in many routine blood culture media without changing the appearance of the media. *M. hominis* forms nonhemolytic pinpoint colonies on blood agar; organisms cannot be visualized in gram-stained smears of these colonies. Neither *U. urealyticum* nor *M. genitalium* will grow in ordinary microbiologic media.

Microbiologic diagnosis of genital mycoplasmal infection requires specially prepared media and is beyond the capability of all but reference and research laboratories. Nucleic acid amplification tests such as PCR have been developed and may become commercially available.

℞ **TREATMENT** Ureaplasmas, *M. genitalium*, and *M. hominis* are usually susceptible to tetracyclines (e.g., doxycycline). Tetracycline-resistant ureaplasmas can be treated with erythromycin, while tetracycline-resistant strains of *M. hominis* respond to treatment with clindamycin. As noted above, a specific microbiologic diagnosis of mycoplasmal infection is seldom made. Appropriate treatment provides antimicrobial coverage for the organisms that cause the particular syndrome. Accordingly, NGU is treated with doxycycline (100 mg orally twice a day for 7 days) or azithromycin (1.0 g as a single oral dose) to provide activity against *C. trachomatis*, *U. urealyticum*, and *M. genitalium*. Recommended regimens for the treatment of PID provide antimicrobial activity against gonococci, chlamydiae, and anaerobes as well as genital mycoplasmas.

BIBLIOGRAPHY

ALEXANDER ER et al: Pneumonia due to *Mycoplasma pneumoniae*. N Engl J Med 275:131, 1966

BASEMAN JB, TULLY JG: Mycoplasmas: Sophisticated, reemerging, and burdened by their notoriety. Emerg Infect Dis 3:21, 1997

GRONDAHL B et al: Rapid identification of nine microorganisms causing acute respiratory tract infections by single-tube multiplex reverse transcription-PCR: Feasibility study. J Clin Microbiol 37:1, 1999

MURRAY HW et al: The protean manifestations of *Mycoplasma pneumoniae* in adults. Am J Med 58:229, 1975

TAYLOR-ROBINSON D, FURR PM: Update on sexually transmitted mycoplasmas. Lancet 351(Suppl 3):12, 1998

179 *Walter E. Stamm*

CHLAMYDIAL INFECTIONS

DFA	direct immunofluorescent antibody	MPC	mucopurulent cervicitis
ELISA	enzyme-linked immunosorbent assay	NGU	nongonococcal urethritis
		PCR	polymerase chain reaction
HSV	herpes simplex virus	PGU	postgonococcal urethritis
LGV	lymphogranuloma venereum	PID	pelvic inflammatory disease
micro-IF	microimmunofluorescence	STDs	sexually transmitted diseases

The genus *Chlamydia* contains three species that infect humans: *Chlamydia psittaci*, *C. trachomatis*, and *C. pneumoniae* (formerly the TWAR agent). *C. psittaci* is widely distributed in nature, producing genital, conjunctival, intestinal, or respiratory infections in many mammalian and avian species. Genital infections with *C. psittaci* have been well characterized in several species and cause abortion and infertility. Although mammalian strains of *C. psittaci* are not known to infect humans, avian strains occasionally do so, causing pneumonia and the systemic illness known as *psittacosis*.

C. pneumoniae is a fastidious chlamydial species that appears to be a common cause of upper respiratory tract infection and pneumonia, primarily in children and young adults, and is a cause of recurrent respiratory infections in older adults. Studies have also linked *C. pneumoniae* infection to atherosclerotic cardiovascular disease and perhaps to asthma and sarcoidosis. No animal reservoir has been identified for *C. pneumoniae*; it appears to be an exclusively human pathogen spread via the respiratory route through close personal contact. To date, all strains of *C. pneumoniae* studied have been serologically homologous.

C. trachomatis is also an exclusively human pathogen and was identified as the cause of trachoma in the 1940s. Since then, *C. trachomatis* has been recognized as a major cause of sexually transmitted and perinatal infection.

Chlamydiae are obligate intracellular bacteria that are classified in their own order (Chlamydiales). They possess both DNA and RNA, have a cell wall and ribosomes similar to those of gram-negative bacteria, and are inhibited by antibiotics such as tetracycline.

A unique feature of all chlamydiae is their complex reproductive cycle. Two forms of the microorganism—the extracellular elementary body and the intracellular reticulate body—participate in this cycle. The elementary body is adapted for extracellular survival and is the infective form transmitted from one person to another. Elementary bodies attach to susceptible target cells (usually columnar or transitional epithelial cells) and enter the cells inside a phagosome. Within 8 h of cell entry, the elementary bodies reorganize into reticulate bodies, which are adapted to intracellular survival and multiplication. They undergo binary fission, eventually producing numerous replicates contained within the intracellular membrane-bound "inclusion body," which occupies much of the infected host cell. Chlamydial inclusions resist lysosomal fusion until late in the developmental cycle. After 24 h, the reticulate bodies condense and form elementary bodies still contained within the inclusion. The inclusion then ruptures, releasing elementary bodies from the cell to initiate infection of adjacent cells or transmission to another person.

Studies with monoclonal antibodies to and nucleotide sequencing of the major outer-membrane protein have delineated at least 20 serotypes of *C. trachomatis*. According to the classification of Wang and Grayston, strains associated with trachoma have generally been those of the A, B, Ba, and C serovars, while serovars D through K have largely been associated with sexually transmitted and perinatally acquired infections. Serovars L$_1$, L$_2$, and L$_3$ produce lymphogranuloma venereum (LGV) and hemorrhagic proctocolitis. The LGV strains demonstrate unique biologic behavior in that they are more invasive than the other serovars, produce disease in lymphatic tissue, grow readily in cell culture systems and macrophages, and are fatal when inoculated intracerebrally into mice and monkeys. Non-LGV strains of *C. trachomatis* characteristically produce infections involving the superficial columnar epithelium of the eye, genitalia, and respiratory tract.

C. trachomatis has been reported as an infrequent cause of endocarditis, peritonitis, pleuritis, and possibly periappendicitis and may occasionally cause respiratory infections in older children and adults. Some immunosuppressed patients with pneumonia have had either serologic or cultural evidence of *C. trachomatis* infection, but more data are necessary to define a pathogenic role for *Chlamydia* in these patients.

SEXUALLY TRANSMITTED AND PERINATAL INFECTIONS DUE TO *C. TRACHOMATIS*

SPECTRUM OF *C. TRACHOMATIS* GENITAL INFECTIONS Genital infections caused by *C. trachomatis* represent the most common bacterial sexually transmitted diseases (STDs) in the United States. An estimated 4 million cases occur each year. In adults, the clinical spectrum of sexually transmitted *C. trachomatis* infections parallels that of gonococcal infection. Both infections have been associated with urethritis, proctitis, and conjunctivitis in both sexes; with epididymitis in men; and with mucopurulent cervicitis (MPC), acute salpingitis, bartholinitis, and the Fitz-Hugh–Curtis syndrome (perihepatitis) in women. Moreover, both types of infection can be associated with septic arthritis. In general, however, chlamydial infections produce fewer symptoms and signs than corresponding gonococcal infections at the same anatomic site; in fact, chlamydial infections are often totally asymptomatic. Increasing evidence suggests that many chlamydial infections of the genital tract, especially in women, persist for months without producing symptoms. Simultaneous infection with *C. trachomatis* often occurs in women with cervical gonococcal infection and in heterosexual men with gonococcal urethritis.

EPIDEMIOLOGY Infections due to *C. trachomatis* are now reportable in the United States, and national incidence data show steadily rising numbers of reported infections, undoubtedly reflecting both increased testing and increased reporting. Most testing has focused upon women to date, and thus the reported incidence is severalfold greater in women than in men; this difference likely represents a surveillance artifact.

The age of peak incidence of genital *C. trachomatis* infections, as of other sexually transmitted infections, is the late teens and early twenties. The prevalence of chlamydial urethral infection among young men is at least 3 to 5% for those seen in general medical settings or in urban high schools, >10% for asymptomatic soldiers undergoing routine physical examination, and 15 to 20% for heterosexual men seen in STD clinics. In areas where chlamydial control programs have been implemented, prevalence may be markedly reduced. In short, prevalence varies widely with the population group studied and with the geographic locale. The ratio of chlamydial to gonococcal urethritis is highest for heterosexual men and for those of high socioeconomic status and is lowest for homosexual men and indigent populations.

The prevalence of cervical infection among women is approxi-

mately 5% for asymptomatic college students and prenatal patients in the United States, >10% for women seen in family planning clinics, and >20% for women seen in STD clinics. As in men, prevalence varies substantially by geographic locale. However, substantial prevalences (~8%) of asymptomatic chlamydial infection were recently demonstrated in young female military recruits from all parts of the United States. In this country, the prevalence of *C. trachomatis* in the cervix of pregnant women is 5 to 10 times higher than that of *Neisseria gonorrhoeae*. The prevalence of genital infection with either agent is highest among individuals who are between the ages of 18 and 24, single, and non-Caucasian (e.g., black or hispanic). Recurrent chlamydial infections occur frequently in these same risk groups, often acquired from untreated sexual partners. Oral contraceptive pill use and the presence of cervical ectopy also confer an increased risk of chlamydial infection. The proportion of infections that are asymptomatic appears to be higher for *C. trachomatis* than for *N. gonorrhoeae*, and symptomatic *C. trachomatis* infections are clinically less severe. Mild or asymptomatic chlamydial infections of the fallopian tubes nonetheless cause ongoing tubal damage and infertility. Furthermore, because the total number of *C. trachomatis* infections exceeds the total number of *N. gonorrhoeae* infections in industrialized countries, the total morbidity caused by *C. trachomatis* genital infections in these countries equals or exceeds that caused by *N. gonorrhoeae*. The prevalence of *C. trachomatis* is higher than that of *N. gonorrhoeae* in industrialized countries, in part because measures such as treatment of sex partners and routine cultures for case detection in asymptomatic individuals have been applied much more effectively to the control of gonorrhea than to the control of *C. trachomatis* infection.

PATHOGENESIS *C. trachomatis* preferentially infects the columnar epithelium of the eye and the respiratory and genital tracts. The infection induces an immune response but often persists for months or years in the absence of antimicrobial therapy. Serious sequelae often occur in association with repeated or persistent infections. The precise mechanism through which repeated infection elicits an inflammatory response that leads to tubal scarring and damage in the female upper genital tract is not yet clear. One antigen, the chlamydial 60-kDa heat-shock protein, may be involved in inducing the pathologic immune response or may elicit antibodies that cross-react with human heat-shock proteins. The recent sequencing of the chlamydial genome may soon offer further insights into the pathogenic mechanisms of *C. trachomatis*.

CLINICAL MANIFESTATIONS Nongonococcal and Postgonococcal Urethritis Nongonococcal urethritis (NGU) is a diagnosis of exclusion that is applied to men with symptoms and/or signs of urethritis who do not have gonorrhea. Postgonococcal urethritis (PGU) refers to nongonococcal urethritis developing in men 2 to 3 weeks after treatment of gonococcal urethritis with single doses of agents such as amoxicillin or cephalosporins that lack sufficient activity against chlamydiae. Since current treatment regimens for gonorrhea also include tetracycline, doxycycline, or azithromycin for possible concomitant chlamydial infection, both the incidence of PGU and the causative role of chlamydiae in this syndrome have declined. *C. trachomatis* causes 20 to 40% of cases of NGU in heterosexual men but is less commonly isolated from homosexual men with this syndrome. The cause of most of the remaining cases is uncertain; considerable evidence suggests that *Ureaplasma urealyticum* causes many cases of NGU, while *Trichomonas vaginalis* and herpes simplex virus (HSV) cause some cases.

NGU is diagnosed by documentation of a leukocytic urethral exudate and by exclusion of gonorrhea by Gram's staining or culture. *C. trachomatis* urethritis is generally less severe than gonococcal urethritis, although in an individual patient these two forms of urethritis cannot be reliably differentiated solely on clinical grounds. Symptoms include urethral discharge (often whitish and mucoid rather than frankly purulent), dysuria, and urethral itching. Physical examination may reveal meatal erythema and tenderness and a urethral exudate that is often demonstrable only by stripping of the urethra.

At least one-third of males with *C. trachomatis* urethral infection have no demonstrable signs or symptoms of urethritis. Use of nucleic acid amplification assays on first-void urine specimens to diagnose chlamydial infections in men has facilitated more broadly based testing for asymptomatic infection in males. As a result, asymptomatic chlamydial urethritis has been demonstrated in 5 to 10% of sexually active adolescent males screened in school-based clinics or community centers. Such patients generally have first-glass pyuria (≥ 15 leukocytes per $400\times$ microscopic field in the sediment of first-void urine), a positive leukocyte esterase test, or an increased number of leukocytes on Gram-stained smear prepared from a urogenital swab inserted 1 to 2 cm into the anterior urethra. For the enumeration of leukocytes, the smear is first scanned at low power to identify areas of the slide containing the highest concentration of leukocytes. These areas are then examined under oil immersion ($1000\times$). An average of four or more leukocytes in at least three of five $1000\times$ (oil-immersion) fields is indicative of urethritis and correlates with the recovery of *C. trachomatis*. To differentiate between true urethritis and functional symptoms among symptomatic patients or to make a presumptive diagnosis of *C. trachomatis* infection in a "high-risk" but asymptomatic man (e.g., male patients in STD clinics, sex partners of women with nongonococcal salpingitis or MPC, fathers of children with inclusion conjunctivitis), the examination of an endourethral specimen for increased leukocytes is useful if specific diagnostic tests for chlamydiae are not available. Alternatively, noninvasive screening for urethritis can be accomplished by testing of a first-void urine sample for pyuria, either by microscopy or by the leukocyte esterase test. Urine can also be directly tested for chlamydiae or gonococci by DNA amplification methods, as described below.

Epididymitis *C. trachomatis* is the foremost cause of epididymitis in sexually active heterosexual men under 35 years of age, accounting for about 70% of cases. *N. gonorrhoeae* causes most of the remaining cases, and some men have simultaneous infections with both pathogens, usually accompanied by asymptomatic urethritis as defined above. In homosexual men, sexually transmitted coliform infection acquired via rectal intercourse may cause epididymitis. Coliform bacteria and *Pseudomonas aeruginosa*, usually in association with preceding urologic instrumentation or surgery, are the most common causes of epididymitis in men over 35. Men with epididymitis typically present with unilateral scrotal pain, fever, and epididymal tenderness or swelling on examination. The illness may be mild enough to treat on an outpatient basis with oral antibiotics or severe enough to require hospitalization and parenteral therapy. Testicular torsion should be excluded promptly by radionuclide scan, Doppler flow study, or surgical exploration in a teenager or young adult who presents with acute unilateral testicular pain without urethritis. The possibility of testicular tumor or chronic infection (e.g., tuberculosis) should be excluded when a patient with unilateral intrascrotal pain and swelling does not respond to appropriate antimicrobial therapy.

Reiter's Syndrome Reiter's syndrome consists of conjunctivitis, urethritis (or cervicitis in females), arthritis, and characteristic mucocutaneous lesions (Chap. 315). *C. trachomatis* has been recovered from the urethra of up to 70% of men with untreated nondiarrheal Reiter's syndrome and associated urethritis. In the absence of overt urethritis, it is important to exclude subclinical urethritis in the men in whom this diagnosis is suspected.

The pathogenesis of Reiter's syndrome remains obscure. However, since more than 80% of affected patients have the HLA-B27 phenotype and since other mucosal infections (with *Salmonella*, *Shigella*, or *Campylobacter*, for example) produce an identical syndrome, chlamydial infection is thought to initiate an aberrant and hyperactive immune response that produces inflammation at the involved target organs in these genetically predisposed individuals. Evidence of exaggerated cell-mediated and humoral immune responses to chlamydial antigens in Reiter's syndrome supports this hypothesis. The presumptive demonstration of chlamydial elementary bodies and chlamydial DNA in the joint fluid and synovial tissue of patients with Reiter's syndrome suggests that chlamydiae may actually spread from genital to joint tissues in these patients, perhaps in macrophages.

Proctitis *C. trachomatis* strains of either the genital immunotypes D through K or the LGV immunotypes cause proctitis in homosexual men who practice receptive anorectal intercourse. In the United States, the vast majority of cases are due to immunotypes D through K and present either as asymptomatic infection or as mild proctitis not unlike gonococcal proctitis. These infections may develop in heterosexual women as well. Patients present with mild rectal pain, mucous discharge, tenesmus, and (occasionally) bleeding. Nearly all have neutrophils in their rectal Gram's stain. Anoscopy in these non-LGV cases of chlamydial proctitis reveals mild, patchy mucosal friability and mucopurulent discharge, and the disease process is limited to the distal rectum. LGV strains produce more severe ulcerative proctitis or proctocolitis that can be confused clinically with HSV proctitis (severe rectal pain, bleeding, discharge, and tenesmus) and that histologically resembles Crohn's disease in that giant cell formation and granulomas can be seen (Chap. 287). In the United States, these cases occur almost exclusively in homosexual men.

Mucopurulent Cervicitis Although many women with *C. trachomatis* infection of the cervix have no symptoms or signs, a careful speculum examination reveals evidence of MPC in 30 to 50% of cases. As is discussed more fully in Chap. 133, MPC is associated with yellow mucopurulent discharge from the endocervical columnar epithelium and with ≥ 20 neutrophils per $1000\times$ microscopic field within strands of cervical mucus on a thinly smeared, Gram-stained preparation of endocervical exudate. Other characteristic findings include edema of the zone of cervical ectopy and a propensity of the mucosa to bleed on minor trauma—e.g., when specimens are collected with a swab. A Pap smear shows increased numbers of neutrophils as well as a characteristic pattern of mononuclear inflammatory cells, including plasma cells, transformed lymphocytes, and histiocytes. Cervical biopsy shows a predominantly mononuclear cell infiltrate of the subepithelial stroma, often with follicular cervicitis.

Pelvic Inflammatory Disease (PID) (See also Chap. 133) *C. trachomatis* plays an important causative role in salpingitis. Infection with *C. trachomatis* has been demonstrated in laparoscopically verified salpingitis, the organism has been recovered from the fallopian tubes in the absence of other pathogens, and serologic evidence of recent *C. trachomatis* infection has been found in women with PID. In the United States, *C. trachomatis* has been identified in the fallopian tubes or endometrium of up to 50% of women with PID, and its role as an important etiologic agent in this syndrome is well accepted.

PID occurs via ascending intraluminal spread of *C. trachomatis* from the lower genital tract. MPC is thus followed by endometritis, endosalpingitis, and finally pelvic peritonitis. Evidence of MPC is usually found in women with laparoscopically verified salpingitis. Similarly, endometritis, demonstrated by endometrial biopsy showing plasma cell infiltration of the endometrial epithelium, is documented in most women with laparoscopically verified chlamydial (or gonococcal) salpingitis. Chlamydial endometritis can also occur in the absence of clinical evidence of salpingitis: approximately 40 to 50% of women with MPC have plasma cell endometritis. Histologic evidence of endometritis has been correlated with an "endometritis syndrome" consisting of vaginal bleeding, lower abdominal pain, and uterine tenderness in the absence of adnexal tenderness. It is not known what proportion of women who have chlamydial endometritis without adnexal tenderness also have salpingitis. However, chlamydial salpingitis produces milder symptoms than does gonococcal salpingitis and may be associated with less marked adnexal tenderness. Mild adnexal or uterine tenderness in sexually active women with cervicitis suggests PID.

Infertility associated with fallopian-tube scarring has been strongly linked to antecedent *C. trachomatis* infection in serologic studies. Since many infertile women with tubal scarring and antichlamydial antibody have no history of PID, it appears that subclinical tubal infection ("silent salpingitis") may produce scarring. Studies in animals and humans with salpingitis and tubal scarring suggest the continuing presence of persistent, slowly replicating chlamydial infection in tubal tissue. Ectopic pregnancy, which occurs in more than 70,000 women in the United States annually, is also thought to be related to *Chlamydia*-induced tubal scarring in many cases. While the pathogenesis of *Chlamydia*-induced tubal scarring remains poorly understood, antibodies to the chlamydial 60-kDa heat-shock protein have been correlated with tubal infertility, ectopic pregnancy, and Fitz-Hugh–Curtis syndrome (see below). Thus this antigen may initiate an immune-mediated process that ultimately damages the fallopian tube. Host genetic susceptibility, as defined by HLA type, may also play an important role.

Perihepatitis, or the Fitz-Hugh–Curtis syndrome, was originally described as a complication of gonococcal PID. However, cultural and/or serologic evidence of *C. trachomatis* infection is found in three-quarters of women with this syndrome. *C. trachomatis* has also been cultured from exudate on the hepatic capsule in laparoscopically verified cases. This syndrome should be suspected whenever a young, sexually active woman presents with an illness resembling cholecystitis (fever and right-upper-quadrant pain of subacute or acute onset). Symptoms and signs of salpingitis may be minimal. High titers of antibodies to *C. trachomatis* are generally present.

Urethral Syndrome in Women   In the absence of infection with uropathogens such as coliforms or *Staphylococcus saprophyticus*, *C. trachomatis* is the pathogen most commonly isolated from college women with dysuria, frequency, and pyuria (Chap. 280). *Chlamydia* can also be isolated from the urethra of women without symptoms of urethritis, and up to 25% of female STD clinic patients with chlamydial urogenital infection have cultures positive for *C. trachomatis* from the urethra only.

C. trachomatis Infection in Pregnancy   *C. trachomatis* in pregnancy has been associated in some studies (but not in others) with premature delivery and with postpartum endometritis. Whether these complications are in part attributable to *C. trachomatis* is not clear.

PERINATAL INFECTIONS: INCLUSION CONJUNCTI-VITIS AND PNEUMONIA   **Epidemiology**   Studies in the United States have demonstrated that 5 to 25% of pregnant women have *C. trachomatis* infections of the cervix. In these studies, approximately one-half to two-thirds of children exposed during birth have acquired *C. trachomatis* infection. Roughly half of the infected infants (or 25% of the group exposed) have developed clinical evidence of inclusion conjunctivitis. In addition to infecting the eye, *C. trachomatis* has been isolated frequently and persistently from the nasopharynx, rectum, and vagina of such infants, occasionally for periods exceeding 1 year in the absence of treatment. Pneumonia develops in about 10% of children infected perinatally, and otitis media may in some cases result from perinatally acquired chlamydial infection.

Inclusion Conjunctivitis of the Newborn (Neonatal Chlamydial Conjunctivitis)   Neonatal chlamydial conjunctivitis has an acute onset 5 to 14 days after birth and often produces a profuse mucopurulent discharge. However, it is impossible to differentiate chlamydial conjunctivitis from other forms of neonatal conjunctivitis (such as that due to *N. gonorrhoeae*, *Haemophilus influenzae*, *Streptococcus pneumoniae*, or HSV) on clinical grounds; instead, laboratory diagnosis is required. Inclusions within epithelial cells are often detected in Giemsa-stained conjunctival smears, but these smears are considerably less sensitive than cultures, antigen detection tests, or nucleic acid hybridization tests for chlamydiae. Gram-stained smears may show gonococci or occasional small gram-negative coccobacilli in *Haemophilus* conjunctivitis, but smears should be accompanied by cultures for these agents.

Infant Pneumonia   *C. trachomatis* causes a distinctive pneumonia syndrome in infants. Recent epidemiologic studies have linked chlamydial pulmonary infection in infants with increased occurrence of subacute lung disease (bronchitis, asthma, wheezing) in later childhood.

LYMPHOGRANULOMA VENEREUM   **Definition**   LGV is a sexually transmitted infection caused by *C. trachomatis* strains of the L$_1$, L$_2$, and L$_3$ serovars. In the United States, most cases are caused by L$_2$ organisms. Acute LGV in heterosexual men is characterized by a transient primary genital lesion followed by multilocular suppurative regional lymphadenopathy. Women, homosexual men, and—in occasional instances—heterosexual men may develop hemorrhagic proctitis with regional lymphadenitis. Acute LGV is almost always associated with systemic symptoms such as fever and leukocytosis but is rarely associated with systemic complications such as meningoencephalitis. After a latent period of years, late complications include genital elephantiasis due to lymphatic involvement; strictures; and fistulas of the penis, urethra, and rectum.

Epidemiology   LGV is usually sexually transmitted, but occasional transmission by nonsexual personal contact, fomites, or laboratory accidents has been documented. Laboratory work involving the creation of aerosols of LGV organisms (e.g., sonication, homogenization) must be conducted only with appropriate measures for biologic containment.

The peak incidence of LGV corresponds to the age of greatest sexual activity: the second and third decades of life. The worldwide incidence of LGV is falling, but the disease is still endemic and a major cause of morbidity in Asia, Africa, South America, and parts of the Caribbean. In the Bahamas, an apparent outbreak of LGV has been described in association with a concurrent increase in heterosexual infection with HIV. However, only 186 cases were reported in the United States in 1995, for a rate of 0.1 case per 100,000 population.

The frequency of infection following exposure is believed to be much lower than that for gonorrhea and syphilis. Early manifestations are recognized far more often in men than in women, who usually present with late complications. In the United States, where the reported male-to-female ratio of cases is 3.4:1, most cases have involved homosexually active men and persons returning from abroad (travelers, sailors, and military personnel). The main reservoir of infection, although it has not been directly demonstrated, is presumed to be asymptomatically infected individuals.

Clinical Manifestations   In heterosexuals, a *primary genital lesion* develops from 3 days to 3 weeks after exposure. It is a small, painless vesicle or nonindurated ulcer or papule located on the penis in men and on the labia, posterior vagina, or fourchette in women. The primary lesion is noticed by fewer than one-third of men with LGV and only rarely by women. It heals in a few days without scarring and, even when noticed, is usually recognized as LGV only in retrospect. LGV strains of *C. trachomatis* have occasionally been recovered from genital ulcers and from the urethra of men and the endocervix of women who present with inguinal adenopathy; these areas may be the primary site of infection in some cases.

In women and homosexual men, *primary anal* or *rectal infection* develops after receptive anorectal intercourse. In women, rectal infection with LGV (or non-LGV) strains of *C. trachomatis* presumably can also arise by the contiguous spread of infected secretions along the perineum (as in rectal gonococcal infections in women) or perhaps by spread to the rectum via the pelvic lymphatics.

From the site of the primary urethral, genital, anal, or rectal infection, the organism spreads via the regional lymphatics. Penile, vulvar, or anal infection can lead to inguinal and femoral lymphadenitis. Rectal infection produces hypogastric and deep iliac lymphadenitis. Upper vaginal or cervical infection results in enlargement of the obturator and iliac nodes.

The most common presenting picture in heterosexual men is the *inguinal syndrome*, which is characterized by painful inguinal lymphadenopathy beginning 2 to 6 weeks after presumed exposure; in rare instances, the onset comes after a few months. The inguinal adenopathy is unilateral in two-thirds of cases, and palpable enlargement of the iliac and femoral nodes is often evident on the same side as the enlarged inguinal nodes. The nodes are initially discrete, but progressive periadenitis results in a matted mass of nodes that becomes fluctuant and suppurative. The overlying skin becomes fixed, inflamed, and thin and finally develops multiple draining fistulas. Extensive enlargement of chains of inguinal nodes above and below the inguinal ligament ("the sign of the groove") is not specific and, although not uncommon, is documented in only a minority of cases. On histologic examination, infected nodes are initially found to have characteristic small stellate abscesses surrounded by histiocytes. These abscesses coalesce to form large, necrotic, suppurative foci. Spontaneous healing usually takes place after several months; inguinal scars or granulomatous masses of various sizes persist for life. Massive pelvic lymphadenopathy in women or homosexual men may lead to exploratory laparotomy.

As cultures and serologic tests for *C. trachomatis* are being used more often, increasing numbers of cases of LGV proctitis are being recognized in homosexual men. Such patients present with anorectal pain and mucopurulent, bloody rectal discharge. Although these patients may complain of diarrhea, they are often referring not to diarrhea but rather to frequent, painful, unsuccessful attempts at defecation (tenesmus). Sigmoidoscopy reveals ulcerative proctitis or proctocolitis, with purulent exudate and mucosal bleeding. The histopathologic findings in the rectal mucosa include granulomas with giant cells, crypt abscesses, and extensive inflammation. These clinical, sigmoidoscopic, and histopathologic findings may closely resemble those of Crohn's disease of the rectum.

Constitutional symptoms are common during the stage of regional lymphadenopathy and, in cases of proctitis, may include fever, chills, headache, meningismus, anorexia, myalgias, and arthralgias. These findings in the presence of lymphadenopathy are sometimes mistakenly interpreted as representing malignant lymphoma. Other systemic complications are infrequent but include arthritis with sterile effusion, aseptic meningitis, meningoencephalitis, conjunctivitis, hepatitis, and erythema nodosum. Chlamydiae have been recovered from the cerebrospinal fluid and in one case were isolated from the blood of a patient with severe constitutional symptoms—a result indicating the dissemination of infection. Laboratory-acquired infections suspected of being due to the inhalation of aerosols have been associated with mediastinal lymphadenitis, pneumonitis, and pleural effusion.

Complications of untreated anorectal infection include perirectal abscess; fistula in ano; and rectovaginal, rectovesical, and ischiorectal fistulas. Secondary bacterial infection probably contributes to these complications. Rectal stricture is a late complication of anorectal infection and usually develops 2 to 6 cm from the anal orifice—i.e., at a site within reach on digital rectal examination. Proximal extension of the stricture for several centimeters may lead to a mistaken clinical and radiographic diagnosis of carcinoma.

A small percentage of cases of LGV in men present as chronic progressive infiltrative, ulcerative, or fistular lesions of the penis, urethra, or scrotum. Associated lymphatic obstruction may produce elephantiasis. When urethral stricture occurs, it usually involves the posterior urethra and causes incontinence or difficulty with urination.

APPROACH TO THE DIAGNOSIS AND TREATMENT OF *C. TRACHOMATIS* GENITAL INFECTIONS

Four types of laboratory procedure are available to confirm *C. trachomatis* infection: direct microscopic examination of tissue scrapings for typical intracytoplasmic inclusions or elementary bodies; isolation of the organism in cell culture; detection of chlamydial antigens or nucleic acid by immunologic or hybridization methods; and detection of antibody in serum or in local secretions.

Except in conjunctivitis, direct microscopic examination of Giemsa-stained cell scrapings for typical inclusions has an unacceptably low degree of sensitivity, and false-positive interpretations by inexperienced observers are common. Even for conjunctivitis, this approach has been replaced by direct fluorescent antibody staining of conjunctival smears to identify chlamydial elementary bodies with specific monoclonal antibodies (see below).

Cell culture techniques for isolation of *C. trachomatis* are available in most large medical centers but not in other clinical settings. In addition to limited availability, other disadvantages of cell culture include its low and variable level of sensitivity (60 to 80%), its requirement for rigorous transport conditions, and its high cost and technically demanding nature. Therefore, nonculture alternatives involving antigen detection or nucleic acid hybridization have been developed. In the direct immunofluorescent antibody (DFA) slide test, potentially infected genital or ocular secretions are smeared onto a slide, fixed, and stained with fluorescein-conjugated monoclonal antibody specific for chlamydial antigens. The observation of fluorescing elementary bodies confirms the diagnosis. Compared with culture, this test is 70 to 85% sensitive, and it is quite specific when used for confirmation of urethral, cervical, or ocular infection in high-risk patients with suspected *C. trachomatis* infection. The sensitivity and specificity of the test depend directly upon the skill of the microscopist. The apparently lower sensitivity of the test in low-risk populations, along with its relatively labor-intensive nature, limits its value as a screening tool.

Enzyme-linked immunosorbent assay (ELISA) techniques for the detection of chlamydial antigens provide another alternative to culture. The reported sensitivity and specificity of these tests for genital infections (as compared with culture) have been 60 to 80% and 97 to 99%, respectively, in high-risk populations. Sensitivities have generally been higher in cervical infection and lower in urethritis among males. Like the DFA slide test, the ELISA is less sensitive and less specific in low-prevalence populations and largely asymptomatic patients. ELISAs are better suited to screening than is DFA because large numbers of specimens can easily be processed.

Assays with nucleic acid probes have also been developed for chlamydial diagnosis. One such test uses DNA-RNA hybridization and appears to be approximately equal to the best ELISAs in terms of sensitivity and specificity. Nucleic acid probes have also been developed for use in amplification assays such as ligase chain reaction and polymerase chain reaction (PCR). These tests are now the most sensitive chlamydial diagnostic methods available, being the first nonculture assays actually to surpass culture itself in sensitivity. In addition, the ability of these tests to detect chlamydial genes in urine with a high degree of sensitivity and specificity allows their use with urine specimens rather than with conventional urethral and cervical swabs for the first time. The use of urine specimens is particularly appealing for public-health chlamydial screening programs because of the ease of sample collection, even in community-based settings.

Serologic tests are of limited usefulness in the diagnosis of chlamydial oculogenital infections. The complement fixation test with heat-stable, genus-specific antigen has been used with some success to diagnose LGV but is insensitive in infections due to non-LGV strains of *C. trachomatis*. The microimmunofluorescence (micro-IF) test with *C. trachomatis* antigens is more sensitive but is generally available only in research laboratories. The test measures antibodies by serovar specificity and by immunoglobulin class (IgM, IgG, IgA, secretory IgA) in both serum and local secretions. Serologic diagnosis by the micro-IF test may be useful in infant pneumonia (in which high-titer IgM antibody and/or fourfold rises in titer are often demonstrated), in chlamydial salpingitis (especially Fitz-Hugh–Curtis syndrome), and in LGV. In all of these more invasive syndromes, high antibody levels are present.

Table 179-1 summarizes the diagnostic tests of choice for patients with suspected *C. trachomatis* infection. With few exceptions, the most suitable method for diagnosis is demonstration of the agent by either cell culture or one of the newer nonculture techniques. Selection of the most appropriate of these tests often depends upon local availability and expertise. However, it is clear that, in most settings and for most purposes, sensitivity and specificity will be greatest with nucleic acid amplification techniques. For patients to whom medicolegal considerations may apply (victims of sexual or child abuse), cultures or nucleic acid amplification methods should always be used. Since *C. trachomatis* is an intracellular pathogen, adequate specimens for chlamydial diagnostic testing must include epithelial cells. Cultures or

Table 179-1 Diagnostic Tests for Sexually Transmitted and Perinatal *Chlamydia trachomatis* Infection

Infection	Suggestive Signs/Symptoms	Presumptive Diagnosis[a]	Confirmatory Test of Choice
MEN			
NGU, PGU	Discharge, dysuria	Gram's stain with >4 neutrophils per oil-immersion field; no gonococci	Urethral culture or nonculture test for *C. trachomatis*; urine PCR or LCR for *C. trachomatis*
Epididymitis	Unilateral intrascrotal swelling, pain, tenderness; fever; NGU	Gram's stain with >4 neutrophils per oil-immersion field; no gonococci; urinalysis with pyuria	Urethral culture or nonculture test for *C. trachomatis*; urine PCR or LCR for *C. trachomatis*
WOMEN			
Cervicitis	Mucopurulent cervical discharge, bleeding and edema of the zone of cervical ectopy	Cervical Gram's stain with ≥20 neutrophils per oil-immersion field in cervical mucus	Cervical culture or nonculture test for *C. trachomatis*; urine PCR or LCR for *C. trachomatis*
Salpingitis	Lower abdominal pain, cervical motion tenderness, adnexal tenderness or masses	*C. trachomatis* always potentially present in salpingitis	Cervical culture or nonculture test for *C. trachomatis*; urine PCR or LCR for *C. trachomatis*
Urethritis	Dysuria and frequency without urgency or hematuria	MPC; sterile pyuria; negative routine urine culture	Urethral and cervical cultures or nonculture test for *C. trachomatis*; urine PCR or LCR for *C. trachomatis*
ADULTS OF EITHER SEX			
Proctitis	Rectal pain, discharge, tenesmus, bleeding; history of receptive anorectal intercourse	Negative gonococcal culture and Gram's stain; at least 1 neutrophil per oil-immersion field in rectal Gram's stain	Rectal culture or direct immunofluorescence test for *C. trachomatis*
Reiter's syndrome	NGU, arthritis, conjunctivitis, typical skin lesions	Gram's stain with >4 neutrophils per oil-immersion field; lack of gonococci indicative of NGU	Urethral culture or nonculture test for *C. trachomatis*
LGV	Regional adenopathy, primary lesion, proctitis, systemic symptoms	None	Isolation of LGV strain from node or rectum, occasionally from urethra or cervix; LGV CF titer, ≥1:64; micro-IF titer, ≥1:512
NEONATES			
Conjunctivitis	Purulent conjunctival discharge 6 to 18 days postdelivery	Negative culture and Gram's stain for gonococci, *Haemophilus* spp., pneumococci, staphylococci	Conjunctival culture or nonculture test for *C. trachomatis*; Giemsa-stained scraping of conjunctival material capable of providing more rapid diagnosis but less sensitive
Infant pneumonia	Afebrile, staccato cough, diffuse rales, bilateral hyperinflation, interstitial infiltrates	None	Chlamydial culture of sputum, pharynx, eye, rectum; micro-IF antibody to *C. trachomatis*—fourfold change in IgG or IgM antibody titer

[a] A presumptive diagnosis of chlamydial infection is often made in the syndromes listed when gonococci are not found. A positive test for *Neisseria gonorrhoeae* does not exclude the involvement of *C. trachomatis*, which often is present in patients with gonorrhea.

NOTE: CF, complement-fixing; LCR, ligase chain reaction; LGV, lymphogranuloma venereum; micro-IF, microimmunofluorescence; MPC, mucopurulent cervicitis; NGU, nongonococcal urethritis; PCR, polymerase chain reaction; PGU, postgonococcal urethritis.

nonculture tests of pus are less often positive. In urethritis, a thin-shafted urogenital swab should be inserted at least 2 cm into the urethra to obtain an appropriate specimen. Although cultures of urine for chlamydiae are less sensitive than urethral cultures, studies suggest that nucleic acid amplification testing of a first-void urine specimen from men is a more sensitive and less painful diagnostic alternative to the more invasive urethral swab–based tests, culture, or antigen detection tests. The first 30 mL of voided urine should be collected for testing. When a cervical sample is collected, the external os should first be cleaned of debris and purulent material; a plastic-shafted swab should then be inserted into the cervix, rotated slowly several times, and withdrawn. For the diagnosis of urogenital (cervical or urethral) infections in women, testing of a first-void urine specimen by nucleic acid amplification methods is at least as sensitive as testing of a cervical swab. When conjunctival specimens are sought, the epithelium should be swabbed to remove cells rather than just purulent material. All specimens for chlamydial culture should be placed immediately into transport medium and then either refrigerated (if they will reach the laboratory within 12 to 18 h) or frozen at −70°C (if longer storage is anticipated). A major advantage of the nonculture diagnostic techniques is their less rigid transport requirements; neither refrigeration nor rapid transport is needed.

From a public health viewpoint, the most effective use of chlamydial diagnostic testing has not been unequivocally established and varies with the clinical population, local resources, and laboratory expertise. Since chlamydial diagnostic testing has become more widely available and is now more sensitive and specific than in the past, its

use for specific diagnosis in patients with suspected chlamydial syndromes (such as MPC, NGU, and PID) and their partners should be promoted. High priority should be given to the screening of asymptomatic high-risk women who would not otherwise receive treatment for presumptive chlamydial infection, especially those seen in high-risk settings (e.g., STD clinics or abortion clinics) and those with a high-risk profile (e.g., sexually active and ≤21 years of age, new sex partner within the preceding 2 months, or more than one current sex partner). Similar screening programs should be used to detect and treat asymptomatic urethritis in high-risk adolescent males. Where implemented, screening programs of this type have been associated with reductions in the prevalence of chlamydial infection and of its complications, such as PID.

ANTIMICROBIAL SUSCEPTIBILITY In laboratory tests that evaluate the growth of chlamydiae in cell cultures, the tetracyclines, erythromycin, rifampin, certain fluoroquinolones (especially ofloxacin), and the macrolide azithromycin are all highly active against these organisms. Sulfonamides and clindamycin are also active against *C. trachomatis*, but to a lesser degree. Penicillin and ampicillin suppress chlamydial multiplication but do not eradicate the organism in vitro. The cephalosporins appear to be relatively ineffective against *C. trachomatis*. Streptomycin, gentamicin, neomycin, kanamycin, vancomycin, ristocetin, spectinomycin, and nystatin are not effective at concentrations inhibitory for most bacteria and fungi. There does not appear to be much strain-to-strain variation in susceptibility to antibiotics, and no clinically significant antimicrobial resistance in chlamydiae has been described. Thus antimicrobial susceptibility testing is not needed in the routine management of patients with chlamydial infection, even recurrent infection.

TREATMENT Until the introduction of azithromycin, chlamydial infections could not be eradicated by single-dose or short-term antimicrobial regimens. In most uncomplicated infections in adults, 7 days of treatment with doxycycline or tetracycline have to be given for genital infections, but a 2-week course of therapy is recommended for complicated chlamydial infections (e.g., PID, epididymitis) and at least a 3-week course for LGV. Failure of treatment of genital infections with a tetracycline usually indicates poor compliance or reinfection rather than the involvement of a drug-resistant strain.

Therapy for *C. trachomatis* urethritis is more efficacious than therapy for nonchlamydial NGU. *C. trachomatis* is eradicated from the urethra in nearly all cases by treatment with tetracycline hydrochloride (500 mg qid for 7 days) or doxycycline (100 mg by mouth bid for 7 days).

Eradication of *C. trachomatis* from the cervix by tetracycline, doxycycline, and erythromycin, with doses and durations similar to those specified above for urethritis, has been demonstrated. Erythromycin base (500 mg qid for 10 to 14 days) is the regimen of choice for pregnant women with *C. trachomatis* infection. Amoxicillin (500 mg tid for 10 days) has also been used successfully in pregnant women. Tetracycline hydrochloride (500 mg qid) or doxycycline (100 mg bid) for 14 days produces clinical and microbiologic cure of epididymitis and PID associated with *C. trachomatis* infection, but in this situation a tetracycline should always be used together with a drug that is highly effective against gonorrhea.

Azithromycin is highly active against *C. trachomatis*, exhibits prolonged bioavailability, is concentrated intracellularly, and has offered the prospect of single-dose therapy for chlamydial infection for the first time. In comparative trials, a 1-g single dose of azithromycin has been as effective as 7 days of doxycycline for uncomplicated chlamydial infection. Azithromycin causes fewer adverse gastrointestinal reactions than do older macrolides such as erythromycin. The single-dose regimen of azithromycin has great appeal for the treatment of patients with uncomplicated chlamydial infection (especially those without symptoms and those with a likelihood of poor compliance) and of sexual partners of infected patients. These advantages must be weighed against the considerably greater cost of azithromycin than of doxycycline. Whenever possible, the single 1-g dose should be given as directly observed therapy. Although not approved by the U.S. Food and Drug Administration, the 1-g single-dose regimen of azithromycin appears to be safe and effective in the treatment of pregnant women.

Of the newer fluoroquinolones, ofloxacin (300 mg by mouth bid for 7 days) has been shown to be as effective as doxycycline for the treatment of chlamydial infection and appears to be safe and well tolerated. It cannot be used in pregnancy.

Treatment of Sex Partners The continued high prevalence of chlamydial infections in most parts of the United States is due primarily to the failure to diagnose—and therefore treat—patients with symptomatic or asymptomatic infection and their sex partners. *C. trachomatis* urethral or cervical infection has been well documented in a high proportion of the sex partners of patients with NGU, epididymitis, Reiter's syndrome, salpingitis, or endocervicitis. If possible, confirmatory laboratory tests for *Chlamydia* should be undertaken in these individuals, but even those without evidence of clinical disease who have recently been exposed to proven or possible chlamydial infection (e.g., NGU) should be offered therapy.

Treatment of Neonates and Infants In neonates with conjunctivitis or infants with pneumonia, erythromycin ethylsuccinate or estolate can be given orally in a dose of 50 mg/kg per day, preferably in four divided doses, for 2 weeks. Careful attention must be given to compliance with therapy—a frequent problem. Relapses of eye infection are common following treatment with topical erythromycin or tetracycline ophthalmic ointment and may also occur after oral erythromycin therapy. Thus follow-up cultures should be performed after

treatment. Both parents should be examined for *C. trachomatis* infection and, if diagnostic testing is not readily available, should be treated with doxycycline or azithromycin.

PREVENTION Efforts to develop a vaccine for chlamydial infection have not yet been successful. Early diagnosis and treatment shorten the duration of infectiousness of the carrier and therefore constitute primary prevention of chlamydial infection. By the early 1990s, one of the 10 regions of the United States (Region X, the Pacific Northwest) had formally undertaken a chlamydial control program involving widespread screening of women attending family planning clinics. Approximately 500,000 tests per year were conducted at 150 such clinics throughout the region in women meeting the criteria for high risk. Within 5 years, the prevalence of chlamydial infection had been reduced by >30% in this population. While other regions of the United States have now initiated similar programs, many family planning and STD clinics still do not offer chlamydial testing. The availability of highly sensitive and specific diagnostic tests that can be done with urine specimens and of single-dose therapy makes it feasible to mount an effective chlamydial control program nationwide, with screening of high-risk persons both in traditional health care settings and in novel community- and school-based settings.

TRACHOMA AND ADULT INCLUSION CONJUNCTIVITIS

DEFINITION Trachoma is a chronic conjunctivitis associated with infection by *C. trachomatis* serovar A, B, Ba, or C. It has been responsible for an estimated 20 million cases of blindness throughout the world and remains an important cause of preventable blindness. Inclusion conjunctivitis is an acute ocular infection caused by sexually transmitted *C. trachomatis* strains (usually serovars D through K) in adults exposed to infected genital secretions and in their newborn offspring.

EPIDEMIOLOGY Epidemiologically, two types of eye disease are caused by *C. trachomatis*. In trachoma-endemic areas where the classic eye disease is seen, transmission is from eye to eye via hands, flies, towels, and other fomites and usually involves serovar A, B, Ba, or C. In nonendemic areas, organisms of serovars D through K can be transmitted from the genital tract to the eye, usually causing only the inclusion conjunctivitis syndrome, occasionally with keratitis. Rarely, the eye disease acquired in this way progresses, with the development of pannus and scars similar to those seen in endemic trachoma. These cases may be referred to as paratrachoma to differentiate them epidemiologically from eye-to-eye-transmitted endemic trachoma.

The worldwide incidence and severity of trachoma have decreased dramatically during the past 35 years, mainly as a result of improving hygienic and economic conditions. Endemic trachoma is still the major cause of preventable blindness in northern Africa, sub-Saharan Africa, the Middle East, and parts of Asia. The endemic disease is transmitted primarily through close personal contact, particularly among young children in rural communities with limited water supplies. In endemic areas, trachoma is associated with repeated exposure and reinfection, but the infection can also become chronic and persistent. In the United States a mild form of endemic trachoma still occurs in Mexican Americans as well as in immigrants from areas where trachoma is endemic. Acute relapse of old trachoma occasionally follows treatment with cortisone eye ointment or develops in very old persons who were exposed in their youth.

CLINICAL MANIFESTATIONS Both endemic trachoma and adult inclusion conjunctivitis present initially as a conjunctivitis characterized by small lymphoid follicles in the conjunctiva. In regions with hyperendemic classic blinding trachoma, the disease usually starts insidiously before the age of 2 years. Reinfection is common and probably contributes to the pathogenesis of trachoma. Studies using PCR techniques indicate that chlamydial DNA is often present in the ocular secretions of patients with trachoma, even in the absence of positive cultures. Thus persistent infection may be more common than was previously thought.

The cornea becomes involved, with inflammatory leukocytic infiltrations and superficial vascularization (pannus formation). As the inflammation continues, conjunctival scarring eventually distorts the eyelids, causing them to turn inward so that the inturned lashes constantly abrade the eyeball (trichiasis and entropion); eventually the corneal epithelium is abraded and may ulcerate, with subsequent corneal scarring and blindness. Destruction of the conjunctival goblet cells, lacrimal ducts, and lacrimal gland may produce a "dry-eye" syndrome, with resultant corneal opacity due to drying (xerosis) or secondary bacterial corneal ulcers.

Communities with blinding trachoma often experience seasonal epidemics of conjunctivitis due to *H. influenzae* that contribute to the intensity of the inflammatory process. In such areas the active infectious process usually resolves spontaneously in affected persons between 10 and 15 years of age, but the conjunctival scars continue to shrink, producing trichiasis and entropion and subsequent corneal scarring in adults. In areas with milder and less prevalent disease, the process may be much slower, with active disease continuing into adulthood; blindness is rare in these cases.

Eye infection with genital *C. trachomatis* strains in sexually active young adults presents as the acute onset of unilateral follicular conjunctivitis and preauricular lymphadenopathy similar to that seen in acute adenovirus or herpesvirus conjunctivitis. If untreated, the disease may persist for 6 weeks to 2 years. It is frequently associated with corneal inflammation in the form of discrete opacities ("infiltrates"), punctate epithelial erosions, and minor degrees of superficial corneal vascularization. Very rarely, conjunctival scarring and eyelid distortion occur, particularly in patients treated for many months with topical glucocorticoids. Recurrent eye infections develop most often in patients whose sexual consorts are not treated with antimicrobials.

DIAGNOSIS   The clinical diagnosis of classic trachoma can be made if two of the following signs are present:

1. Lymphoid follicles on the upper tarsal conjunctiva
2. Typical conjunctival scarring
3. Vascular pannus
4. Limbal follicles or their sequelae, Herbert's pits

The clinical diagnosis of endemic trachoma should be confirmed by laboratory tests in children with more marked degrees of inflammation. Intracytoplasmic chlamydial inclusions are found in 10 to 60% of Giemsa-stained conjunctival smears in such populations, but isolation in cell cultures, newer antigen detection testing, or chlamydial PCR is more sensitive. Follicular conjunctivitis in adult Europeans or Americans living in trachomatous regions is rarely due to trachoma.

Sporadic cases of adult inclusion conjunctivitis must be differentiated from keratoconjunctivitis due to adenovirus or HSV and from bacterial conjunctivitis during the first 15 days after onset; later, they must be distinguished from other forms of chronic follicular conjunctivitis. Demonstration of chlamydiae by Giemsa- or immunofluorescent-stained smears, by isolation in cell cultures, or by newer nonculture tests constitutes definitive evidence of infection. Genital examination and tests for genital chlamydial infection are indicated. Serum antibody does not constitute evidence of chlamydial eye infection since many sexually active adults have acquired serum antibody from genital infection.

TREATMENT   Public health control programs for endemic trachoma have consisted of the mass application of tetracycline or erythromycin ointment to the eyes of all children in affected communities for 21 to 60 days or on an intermittent schedule. These programs also include surgical correction of inturned eyelids by a mobile surgical team that visits each locale. Single-dose azithromycin therapy is now being evaluated as an alternative method of mass antibiotic treatment for trachoma in young children and pregnant women.

Adult inclusion conjunctivitis responds well to treatment with full doses of systemic tetracycline or erythromycin for 3 weeks. Treatment of all sexual consorts of the patient simultaneously is also necessary to prevent ocular reinfection and to avoid genital disease due to chlamydial infection. Topical antibiotic treatment is not required for patients who receive systemic antibiotics.

PREVENTION   Efforts to develop a trachoma vaccine have not yet been successful. General hygienic measures associated with improved living standards are effective in the elimination of endemic trachoma. An adequate water supply for personal cleanliness may be a key factor. In some areas the reduction of numbers of flies in the household is important.

PSITTACOSIS

DEFINITION   Psittacosis is primarily an infectious disease of birds and mammals that is caused by *C. psittaci*. Transmission of infection from birds to humans results in a febrile illness characterized by pneumonitis and systemic manifestations. Inapparent infections or mild influenza-like illnesses may also occur. The term *ornithosis* is sometimes applied to infections contracted from birds other than parrots or parakeets, but *psittacosis* is the preferred generic term for all forms of the disease.

EPIDEMIOLOGY   Almost any avian species can harbor *C. psittaci*. Psittacine birds (parrots, parakeets, budgerigars) are most commonly infected, but human cases have been traced to contact with pigeons, ducks, turkeys, chickens, and many other birds. Psittacosis may be considered an occupational disease of pet-shop owners, poultry workers, pigeon fanciers, taxidermists, veterinarians, and zoo attendants. During the past 20 years, there has been an increase in incidence, with cases and outbreaks occurring primarily among employees of poultry-processing plants. It is suspected that many cases go undiagnosed and unreported. The disease appears to be especially common in England, where budgerigars are popular household pets and where restrictions on the importation of these birds have been eased.

The agent is present in nasal secretions, excreta, tissues, and feathers of infected birds. Although the disease can be fatal, infected birds frequently show only minor evidence of illness, such as ruffled feathers, lethargy, and anorexia. Asymptomatic avian carriers are common, and complete recovery may be followed by continued shedding of the organism for many months.

Psittacosis is almost always transmitted to humans by the respiratory route. On rare occasions the disease may be acquired from the bite of a pet bird. Prolonged contact is not essential for transmission of the disease; a few minutes spent in an environment previously occupied by an infected bird has resulted in human infection. In one outbreak, gardening rather than direct exposure to birds was associated with infection. A psittacosis-like agent has been transmitted among hospital personnel, with severe and sometimes fatal infections. There is evidence that these "human" strains are more virulent than avian organisms. There is no record of infection acquired by the ingestion of poultry products.

PATHOGENESIS   The psittacosis agent gains entrance to the body through the upper part of the respiratory tract, spreads via the bloodstream, and eventually localizes in the pulmonary alveoli and in the reticuloendothelial cells of the spleen and liver. Invasion of the lung probably takes place by way of the bloodstream rather than by direct extension from the upper air passages. A lymphocytic inflammatory response occurs on both the interstitial and the respiratory surfaces of the alveoli as well as in the perivascular spaces. The alveolar walls and interstitial tissues of the lung are thickened, edematous, necrotic, and occasionally hemorrhagic. Histologic examination of the affected areas reveals alveolar spaces filled with fluid, erythrocytes, and lymphocytes. The picture is not pathognomonic of psittacosis unless macrophages containing characteristic cytoplasmic inclusion bod-

epithelium of the bronchi and bronchioles usually remains intact.

CLINICAL MANIFESTATIONS The clinical manifestations and course of psittacosis are extremely variable. After an incubation period of 7 to 14 days or longer, the disease may start abruptly with shaking chills and fever, with temperatures ranging as high as 40.5°C (105°F); however, the onset is often gradual, with fever increasing over a 3- to 4-day period. Headache is almost always a prominent symptom; it is usually diffuse and excruciating and is often the patient's chief complaint.

Many patients present with a dry hacking cough that is usually nonproductive, but small amounts of mucoid or bloody sputum may be raised as the disease progresses. Cough may begin early in the course of the disease or as late as 5 days after the onset of fever. Chest pain, pleurisy with effusion, or a friction rub may all occur but are rare. Pericarditis and myocarditis have been reported. Most patients have a normal or slightly increased respiratory rate; marked dyspnea with cyanosis occurs only in severe psittacosis with extensive pulmonary involvement. In psittacosis, as in mycoplasmal pneumonias, the physical signs of pneumonitis tend to be less prominent than symptoms and x-ray findings would suggest. The initial examination may reveal fine sibilant rales, or clinical evidence of pneumonia may be completely lacking. Rales usually become audible and more numerous as the illness progresses. Signs of frank pulmonary consolidation are usually absent. Symptoms of upper respiratory tract infection are not prominent, although mild sore throat, pharyngitis, and cervical adenopathy are often documented; on occasion, the last may be the only manifestation of illness. Epistaxis is encountered early in the course of nearly one-fourth of cases. Photophobia is also a common complaint.

Patients often report generalized myalgia, and spasm and stiffness of the muscles of the back and neck may lead to an erroneous diagnosis of meningitis. Lethargy, mental depression, agitation, insomnia, and disorientation have been prominent features of the illness in some epidemics but not in others; delirium and stupor develop near the end of the first week in severe cases. Occasional patients are comatose when first seen, and the diagnosis of psittacosis may be elusive in these cases. Gastrointestinal manifestations such as abdominal pain, nausea, vomiting, or diarrhea are noted in some cases; constipation and abdominal distention sometimes occur as late complications. Icterus, the result of severe hepatic involvement, is a rare and ominous finding. A faint macular rash (Horder's spots) resembling the rose spots of typhoid fever has been described.

Patients without cough or other clinical evidence of respiratory involvement present with fever of unknown origin (Chap. 125). The pulse rate is slow in relation to the fever. When splenomegaly is noted in a patient with acute pneumonitis, psittacosis should be considered; the reported incidence of splenomegaly in this disease ranges from 10 to 70%. Nontender hepatic enlargement also occurs, but jaundice is rare. Thrombophlebitis is not unusual during convalescence; indeed, pulmonary infarction is sometimes a late complication and may be fatal.

In untreated cases of psittacosis, sustained or mildly remittent fever persists for 10 days to 3 weeks or occasionally for as long as 3 months. Over this period, the respiratory manifestations gradually abate. Psittacosis contracted from parrots or parakeets is more likely to be a severe, prolonged illness than infection acquired from pigeons or barnyard fowl. Relapses occur but are rare. Occasional patients develop endocarditis, and *C. psittaci* infection should be considered in cases of culture-negative endocarditis. Secondary bacterial infections are uncommon. Immunity to reinfection is probably permanent.

LABORATORY FINDINGS The chest x-ray in psittacosis is nonspecific and may show pneumonic lesions that are usually patchy in appearance but can be hazy, diffuse, homogeneous, lobar, atelectatic, wedge-shaped, nodular, or miliary. The white blood cell count is normal or moderately decreased in the acute phase of the disease but may rise in convalescence. The erythrocyte sedimentation rate frequently is not elevated. Transient proteinuria is common. The cerebrospinal fluid sometimes contains a few mononuclear cells but is otherwise normal. Despite hepatomegaly, the results of liver function tests are generally normal or mildly elevated.

The diagnosis can be confirmed only by isolation of the causative microorganism or by serologic studies. The agent is present in the blood during the acute phase of the disease and in the bronchial secretions for weeks or sometimes years after infection, but it is difficult to isolate. Further, the organism is hazardous to work with in the laboratory, and most clinical laboratories do not offer culture for *C. psittaci*. Thus psittacosis is most readily diagnosed by the demonstration of a rising titer of complement fixation antibody in the serum of a patient with a compatible clinical syndrome. Both an acute-phase and a convalescent-phase specimen should always be tested. *C. trachomatis*, *C. psittaci*, and *C. pneumoniae* all share a genus-specific "group" antigen, which is the basis of the complement fixation test. Thus acute infections with *C. trachomatis* or *C. pneumoniae* can also produce titer rises in this test. However, these three species have different major outer-membrane proteins that are the principal antigens in the micro-IF test. If there is doubt as to the interpretation of the complement fixation test, the micro-IF test can be used to differentiate among these antigens. The prompt initiation of treatment with tetracycline has been shown to delay an antibody rise in convalescence for several weeks or months.

DIFFERENTIAL DIAGNOSIS A history of exposure to birds may be the only clinical basis for differentiating psittacosis from a variety of infectious and noninfectious febrile disorders. The list of pulmonary diseases that may be confused with psittacosis includes *Mycoplasma* pneumonia, *C. pneumoniae* pneumonia, legionellosis, viral pneumonia, Q fever, coccidioidomycosis, tuberculosis, enterovirus infection, carcinoma of the lung with bronchial obstruction, and common bacterial pneumonias. In the early stages, before pneumonitis appears, psittacosis may be mistaken for influenza, typhoid fever, miliary tuberculosis, or infectious mononucleosis.

TREATMENT The tetracyclines are consistently effective in the treatment of psittacosis. Defervescence and alleviation of symptoms usually take place within 24 to 48 h after the institution of therapy with 2 g daily in four divided doses. To avoid relapse, treatment should probably be continued for at least 7 to 14 days after defervescence. In severe cases, hospitalization and pulmonary intensive care may be indicated. Sulfonamides are not active against *C. psittaci*. Erythromycin can be used in patients allergic to or intolerant of tetracyclines.

C. PNEUMONIAE INFECTIONS

A third chlamydial species that causes disease in humans, *C. pneumoniae*, has been described in the past two decades. *C. pneumoniae* can be distinguished from the other two species on the basis of DNA hybridization and elementary body morphology. Although *C. pneumoniae* can be grown in a variety of cell cultures, it is considerably more difficult to culture than other chlamydiae, especially from clinical specimens. HL cells appear to be the most effective cell line for isolation of *C. pneumoniae*.

Knowledge of the epidemiology of *C. pneumoniae* infections has been derived primarily from serologic studies. Infections begin to occur in late childhood, achieve peak incidence in young adults, but continue throughout adult life. Seroprevalence in the many adult populations that have been tested throughout the world exceeds 40%—a figure suggesting that *C. pneumoniae* infections are ubiquitous. Secondary episodes (reinfections) appear to occur commonly in older adults throughout life. *C. pneumoniae* also produces epidemics of pneumonia and respiratory illness, especially in close residential quarters such as military barracks. The incidence of infections outside of epidemics remains poorly defined. Transmission appears to be from person to person, probably primarily in schools and family units.

Little is known about the pathogenesis of *C. pneumoniae* infection. The infection begins in the upper respiratory tract and in many persons is a long-lived asymptomatic condition of the upper respiratory mucosal surfaces. However, in at least some individuals, the organism is transported to distant sites—perhaps within macrophages—since evidence exists for replication within arteries and synovial membranes of joints. A *C. pneumoniae* outer-membrane protein may induce host immune responses whose cross-reaction with human proteins results in an autoimmune reaction.

The clinical spectrum of *C. pneumoniae* infection includes acute pharyngitis, sinusitis, bronchitis, and pneumonitis, primarily in young adults. The clinical manifestations of primary infection appear to be more severe and prolonged than those of reinfection. The pneumonitis resembles that of *M. pneumoniae* pneumonia in that leukocytosis is frequently lacking and patients often have prominent antecedent upper respiratory tract symptoms, fever, nonproductive cough, a mild to moderate degree of illness, minimal findings on chest auscultation, and small segmental infiltrates on chest x-ray. In elderly patients, pneumonia due to *C. pneumoniae* can be especially severe and may necessitate hospitalization and respiratory support.

Epidemiologic studies have demonstrated an association between serologic evidence of *C. pneumoniae* infection and atherosclerotic disease of the coronary and other arteries. In addition, *C. pneumoniae* has been identified in atherosclerotic plaques by electron microscopy, DNA hybridization, and immunocytochemistry. Recently, the organism has been recovered in culture from atheromatous plaque—a result indicating the presence of viable replicating bacteria in vessels. Evidence from animal models supports the hypothesis that *C. pneumoniae* infection of the upper respiratory tract is followed by recovery of the organism from atheromatous lesions in the aorta and that the infection accelerates the process of atherosclerosis, especially in hypercholesterolemic animals. Antimicrobial treatment of the infected animals reverses the increased risk of atherosclerosis. In humans, two small trials in patients with unstable angina or recent myocardial infarction also suggested that antibiotics reduce subsequent untoward cardiac events. Larger trials have been initiated to determine more definitively whether antibiotics affect the risk of atherosclerosis.

Diagnosis of *C. pneumoniae* infection is currently difficult because cell culture techniques are not available for routine clinical use and nonculture tests using antigen detection methods or DNA probes have not been developed for commercial use. Acute- and convalescent-phase sera can be tested for chlamydial complement fixation antibody to make a retrospective diagnosis. However, this test does not distinguish *C. pneumoniae* infection from infection due to *C. trachomatis* or *C. psittaci*. Although controlled treatment trials have not been conducted, *C. pneumoniae* is inhibited in vitro by erythromycin and tetracycline. Recommended therapy consists of 2 g per day of either agent for 10 to 14 days. Other macrolides, such as azithromycin, and some fluoroquinolones, such as levofloxacin, also appear to be effective.

BIBLIOGRAPHY

BACHMAIER K et al: *Chlamydia* infections and heart disease linked through antigenic mimicry. Science 283:1335, 1999

CENTERS FOR DISEASE CONTROL AND PREVENTION: Recommendations for the prevention and management of *Chlamydia trachomatis* infections, 1993. MMWR 42(RR-12):1, 1993

COULTS II et al: Clinical and radiographic features of psittacosis infection. Thorax 40:530, 1985

GILBERT DN, GRAYSTON JT (eds): The potential etiologic role of *Chlamydia pneumoniae* in atherosclerosis: A multidisciplinary meeting to promote collaborative research. J Infect Dis 181(Suppl 3):S383, 2000

GRAYSTON JT: Infections caused by *Chlamydia pneumoniae*, strain TWAR. Clin Infect Dis 15:757, 1992

HOLMES KK, STAMM WE: Lower genital tract infections in women: Cystitis, urethritis, vulvovaginitis, and cervicitis, in *Sexually Transmitted Diseases*, 3d ed, KK Holmes et al (eds). New York, McGraw-Hill, 1999

MARRAZZO JM, STAMM WE: New approaches to the diagnosis, treatment, and prevention of chlamydial infection. Curr Clin Top Infect Dis 18:37, 1998

—— et al: Community-based urine screening for *Chlamydia trachomatis* with a ligase chain reaction assay. Ann Intern Med 127:796, 1997

MUHLESTEIN JB: Bacterial infections and atherosclerosis. J Investig Med 46:396, 1998

SCHOLES D et al: Prevention of pelvic inflammatory disease by screening for cervical chlamydial infection. N Engl J Med 334:1362, 1996

STAMM WE: Expanding efforts to prevent chlamydial infection. N Engl J Med 339:768, 1998

——: *Chlamydia trachomatis* infections in adults, in *Sexually Transmitted Diseases*, 3d ed, KK Holmes et al (eds). New York, McGraw-Hill, 1999

—— et al: Azithromycin for empirical treatment of the nongonococcal urethritis syndrome in men. A randomized double-blind study. JAMA 274:545, 1995

Section 11
VIRAL DISEASES

180   *Fred Wang, Elliott Kieff*

MEDICAL VIROLOGY

AAV	adeno-associated virus	HSV	herpes simplex virus
CMV	cytomegalovirus	HTLV	human T-lymphotropic virus
CSF	cerebrospinal fluid	IFN	interferon
EBV	Epstein-Barr virus	IL	interleukin
ELISAs	enzyme-linked immunosorbent assays	KSHV	Kaposi's sarcoma–associated herpesvirus
HBV	hepatitis B virus	MHC	major histocompatibility complex
HCV	hepatitis C virus		
HDV	hepatitis D virus	NK	natural killer
HHV	human herpesvirus	TNF	tumor necrosis factor
HPVs	human papillomaviruses	VZV	varicella-zoster virus

DEFINING A VIRUS

Viruses consist of a nucleic acid surrounded by one or more proteins. Some viruses also have an outer-membrane envelope. Viruses differ from other replicating organisms in that they do not have ribosomes or enzymes for high-energy phosphate generation or for protein, carbohydrate, or lipid metabolism. Viruses are obligate intracellular parasites—that is, they require cells in order to replicate. Typically, viral nucleic acids encode proteins necessary for replicating and packaging the nucleic acids into new viral particles.

Viruses differ from viroids, prions, and virusoids. *Virusoids* are nucleic acids that depend on helper viruses to package the nucleic acids into virus-like particles. *Viroids* are simply molecules of naked, cyclical, mostly double-stranded, small RNAs and appear to be restricted to plants, in which they spread from cell to cell and are replicated by cellular RNA polymerase II. *Prions* (Chap. 375) are protein molecules that can spread from cell to cell and effect changes in the structure of their normal counterparts (cellular proteins). Prions have been implicated in neurodegenerative conditions such as Creutzfeldt-Jakob disease, kuru, and Gerstmann-Sträussler disease. Prions have also been implicated in neurodegeneration associated with human infection with bovine spongiform encephalopathy ("mad cow disease").

VIRAL STRUCTURE

Viruses have from a few to 200 genes. These genes may be embodied in a single-strand or double-strand DNA genome or in a single-strand sense, a single-strand or segmented antisense, or a double-strand segmented RNA genome. Sense-strand RNA genomes can be translated directly into protein. Sense and antisense genomes are also referred to as positive-strand and negative-strand genomes, respectively. The viral nucleic acid is usually associated with one or more virus-encoded nucleoproteins in the core of the viral particle. The viral nucleic acid is almost always enclosed in a protein shell called a *capsid*. Because of the limited genetic complexity of viruses, their capsids are usually composed of multimers of identical capsomers. Capsomers are in turn composed of one or a few proteins. Capsids have icosahedral or helical symmetry. Icosahedral structures approximate spheres but have two-, three-, and fivefold axes of symmetry, while helical structures have only a twofold axis of symmetry. The entire structural unit of nucleic acid, nucleoprotein(s), and capsid is called a *nucleocapsid*. Many human viruses have a simple nucleocapsid structure. For these viruses, the outer surface of the capsid mediates contact with uninfected cells. Other viruses are more complex and have an outer envelope that is derived from membranes of the infected cell. The piece of infected cell membrane that becomes the viral envelope has usually been modified during infection by the insertion of virus-encoded glycoproteins. These glycoproteins usually mediate contact of enveloped viruses with uninfected cells. Enveloped viruses frequently have matrix or tegument proteins that fill the space between the nucleocapsid and the envelope. In general, enveloped viruses are sensitive to solvents and nonionic detergents that can disrupt the envelope, while viruses that consist only of nucleocapsids are usually more resistant. The schematic diagram of a large and complex herpesvirus shown in Fig. 180-1 illustrates the components of a complicated DNA virus. Prototypical pathogenic human viruses are listed in Table 180-1. The relative sizes and structures of typical pathogenic human viruses are shown in Fig. 180-2.

TAXONOMY OF PATHOGENIC HUMAN VIRUSES

As is apparent from Table 180-1 and Fig. 180-2, the classification of viruses into orders and families is based on nucleic acid composition, nucleocapsid size and symmetry, and envelopment status. Viruses of a single family have similar types of genomes and are morphologically similar in electron micrographs. Further subclassification into genus is dependent on similarities in epidemiology and biologic effects and on the degree of colinear nucleic acid sequence homology. In general, each human virus has a common name related to its pathologic effects or the circumstances of its discovery and a formal species name assigned by the International Committee on Taxonomy of Viruses. The latter designation consists of the name of the host followed by the family or genus of the virus and a number. This dual terminology has created a confusing situation in which viruses are referred to and referenced by either name—e.g., varicella-zoster virus (VZV) or human herpesvirus (HHV) 3.

VIRAL INFECTION IN VITRO

STAGES OF INFECTION At the cellular level, viral infection proceeds in stages.

Viral Interactions at the Cell Surface First, virus adsorbs to a receptor on the cell surface. Adsorption is the consequence of a molecular interaction of a viral surface protein with a molecule on the

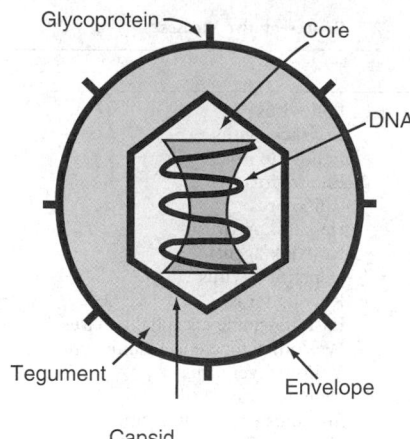

FIGURE 180-1 Schematic diagram of an enveloped herpesvirus with an icosahedral nucleocapsid. The approximate respective dimensions of the nucleocapsid and the enveloped particles are 110 nm and 180 nm. The capsid is composed of 162 capsomeres: 150 with sixfold and 12 with fivefold axes of symmetry.

cell's plasma membrane. For example, a poliovirus capsid protein binds to a cell plasma-membrane protein of the immunoglobulin superfamily type; a rhinovirus capsid protein binds to intracellular adhesion molecule 1; an echovirus capsid protein binds to an integrin; the influenza A virus envelope hemagglutinin protein binds to sialic acid; the HIV envelope glycoprotein binds to CD4 and then engages one of several chemokine receptors that function as coreceptors for the virus; the herpes simplex virus (HSV) envelope glycoproteins bind to heparan sulfate on cell surfaces and then engage one of several immunoglobulin superfamily or tumor necrosis factor (TNF) receptors; and an Epstein-Barr virus (EBV) glycoprotein binds to the B lymphocyte complement receptor CD21. Adsorption characteristically proceeds almost as well at 4°C as at 37°C, and adsorbed virus can still be neutralized by antibody. Adsorption frequently initiates changes in virion surface proteins that result in destabilization and preparation for the next stage of entry into the cell.

After adsorption, viruses penetrate through or fuse with the cell membrane, lose their sensitivity to neutralizing antibody, and become uncoated as they enter the cytoplasm. For all viruses, penetration and uncoating result in viral nucleocapsid or nucleoprotein entry into the cytoplasm. Penetration and uncoating as well as subsequent steps in viral replication depend on the cell's energy metabolism and on biochemical changes in the cell's plasma membrane and cytoskeleton. Therefore, penetration proceeds slowly at temperatures <37°C. Viruses use various strategies to penetrate and enter cells. Interaction of the viral surface protein with a cellular receptor can induce changes in viral glycoproteins or capsid proteins and in cell-surface proteins, with consequent penetration. The interaction of multiple protein molecules on the viral surface with multiple molecules on the cell-surface receptor may induce receptor aggregation at the site of viral adsorption. Receptor aggregation can trigger signaling events within the cytoplasm and changes in the plasma membrane. The cell frequently misperceives that the receptor has encountered its "normal ligand," and the aggregated receptor is internalized with the attached virus through an endocytic process that involves clathrin-coated pits. Endocytosis is important in the entry of viruses as diverse as picornaviruses, influenza viruses, HIV, adenoviruses, and herpesviruses. In many cases, entry of the virus into the cytoplasm depends on acidification of the viral endosome.

One of the best-studied examples of the effect of low pH on viral penetration is influenza virus. Influenza hemagglutinin mediates adsorption, receptor aggregation, and endocytosis. In low-pH endosomes, changes in the conformation of the hemagglutinin expose am-

Table 180-1 Virus Families Pathogenic for Humans

Family	Representative Viruses	Type of RNA/DNA	Lipid Envelope
RNA VIRUSES			
Picornaviridae	Poliovirus Coxsackievirus Echovirus Enterovirus Rhinovirus Hepatitis A virus	(+) RNA	No
Caliciviridae	Norwalk agent Hepatitis E virus	(+) RNA	No
Togaviridae	Rubella virus Eastern equine encephalitis virus Western equine encephalitis virus	(+) RNA	Yes
Flaviviridae	Yellow fever virus Dengue virus St. Louis encephalitis virus Hepatitis C virus Hepatitis G virus	(+) RNA	Yes
Coronaviridae	Coronavirus	(+) RNA	Yes
Rhabdoviridae	Rabies virus Vesicular stomatitis virus	(−) RNA	Yes
Filoviridae	Marburg virus Ebola virus	(−) RNA	Yes
Paramyxoviridae	Parainfluenza virus Respiratory syncytial virus Newcastle disease virus Mumps virus Rubeola (measles) virus	(−) RNA	Yes
Orthomyxoviridae	Influenza A, B, and C viruses	(−) RNA, 8 segments	Yes
Bunyaviridae	Hantavirus California encephalitis virus Sandfly fever virus	(−) RNA, 3 circular segments	Yes
Arenaviridae	Lymphocytic choriomeningitis virus Lassa fever virus South American hemorrhagic fever virus	(−) RNA, 2 circular segments	Yes
Reoviridae	Rotavirus Reovirus Colorado tick fever virus	ds RNA, 10–12 segments	No
Retroviridae	Human T-lymphotropic virus types I and II Human immunodeficiency virus types 1 and 2	(+) RNA, 2 identical segments	Yes
DNA VIRUSES			
Hepadnaviridae	Hepatitis B virus	ds DNA with ss portions	Yes
Parvoviridae	Parvovirus B19	ss DNA	No
Papovaviridae	Human papillomavirus JC virus BK virus	ds DNA	No
Adenoviridae	Human adenovirus	ds DNA	No
Herpesviridae	Herpes simplex virus types 1 and 2[a] Varicella-zoster virus[b] Epstein-Barr virus[c] Cytomegalovirus[d] Human herpesvirus 6 Human herpesvirus 7 Kaposi's sarcoma–associated herpesvirus[e]	ds DNA	Yes
Poxviridae	Variola (smallpox) virus Orf virus Molluscum contagiosum virus	ds DNA	Yes

[a] Also called human herpesvirus (HHV) 1 and 2, respectively.
[b] Also called HHV-3.
[c] Also called HHV-4.
[d] Also called HHV-5.
[e] Also called HHV-8.
ABBREVIATIONS: ds, double-strand; ss, single-strand.

fluenza virus, the M2 membrane protein also plays a key role in the uncoating of the viral envelope by providing an ion channel in the envelope. Fusion of viral and cell membranes results in the mixture of viral envelope lipids and proteins with cell membrane lipids and proteins and the penetration of the influenza nucleocapsid into the cytoplasm. Little is known about the details of the fusion processes or the subsequent biochemical interactions. With more complex viruses, such as herpesviruses, different glycoproteins interact with different receptors on different cell types or on different surfaces of polarized epithelial cells. Viral glycoproteins other than the protein that mediates initial adsorption may be critical in mediating envelope fusion with cell membranes.

Viral Gene Expression and Replication
After uncoating and release of viral nucleoprotein into the cytoplasm, the viral genome is transported to a site for expression and replication. In order to produce infectious progeny, viruses must (1) replicate their nucleic acid, (2) produce structural proteins, and (3) assemble the nucleic acid and proteins into progeny virions. Different viruses use different strategies and gene repertoires to accomplish these goals. DNA viruses (except for poxviruses) replicate their nucleic acid and assemble into nucleocapsid complexes in the cell nucleus. RNA viruses (except for influenza viruses) transcribe and replicate their nucleic acid and assemble entirely in the cytoplasm. Thus, the replication strategies of DNA and RNA viruses are presented separately below. Positive-strand and negative-strand RNA viruses are discussed separately. Medically important viruses of each group are used for illustrative purposes.

Positive-strand RNA viruses Medically important positive-strand RNA viruses include picornaviruses, flaviviruses, togaviruses, and caliciviruses. Genomic RNA from positive-strand RNA viruses is released into the cytoplasm without associated enzymes. Cell ribosomes recognize and associate with an internal ribosome entry sequence in the viral genomic RNA and translate a polyprotein that is a fusion of many or all of the viral proteins. The viral RNA polymerase and other viral proteins are cleaved from the polyprotein by protease components of the polyprotein. Antigenomic RNA is then transcribed from the genomic RNA template. Positive-strand genomes and mRNAs are next transcribed from the antigenomic RNA by the viral RNA polymerase. Positive-strand genomic RNA is encapsidated in the cytoplasm.

Negative-strand RNA viruses Medically important negative-strand RNA viruses include rhabdoviruses, filoviruses, paramyxoviruses, and bunyaviruses. Negative-strand RNA virus genomes are released into the cytoplasm with an associated RNA polymerase and one or more accessory proteins. Except for influenza viruses, negative-strand RNA viruses replicate entirely in the cytoplasm. The viral RNA polymerase transcribes messenger RNAs (mRNAs) as well as full-length antigenomic RNA, which is the template for replication of ge-

phipathic domains that interact chemically with the cell membrane and initiate fusion of the viral and cellular membranes. Data indicate that the HIV envelope glycoprotein undergoes similar conformational changes after interaction with CD4 and chemokine receptors. For in-

nomic RNA. The mRNAs encode for RNA polymerase and accessory factors as well as for viral structural proteins. Influenza virus is an unusual negative-strand RNA virus that transcribes its mRNAs and antigenic RNAs in the cell's nucleus. The influenza genome RNA snatches cellular mRNA cap sequences to enhance translation of viral mRNAs and uses cell splicing machinery to encode additional viral mRNAs. All negative-strand RNA viruses, including influenza viruses, assemble in the cytoplasm.

Double-strand segmented RNA viruses These viruses, which are taxonomically grouped in the reovirus family, have 10 to 12 RNA segments that make up their genome. The medically important viruses in this group are rotaviruses and Colorado tick fever virus. Reovirus virions include an RNA polymerase complex. Reoviruses replicate and assemble in the cytoplasm.

DNA viruses Medically important DNA viruses include parvoviruses, papovaviruses, human papillomaviruses (HPVs), adenoviruses, herpesviruses, and poxviruses. Other than poxviruses, most DNA viruses must get to the cell's nucleus for DNA transcription by cellular RNA polymerase II. For example, after receptor binding and fusion, herpesvirus nucleocapsids are released into the cytoplasm along with tegument proteins. The complex is then transported along microtubules to nuclear pores, and the DNA is released into the nucleus.

Transcriptional regulation and mRNA processing for nuclear DNA viruses depend on both viral and cellular proteins. For herpesviruses, the viral tegument protein can activate transcription of viral immediate-early genes, a class of genes expressed immediately after infection. Transcription of immediate-early genes requires the virus tegument protein and preexisting cellular transcription factors. One of the key preexisting cellular factors for HSV-1 immediate-early gene transcription is docked in the cytoplasm in neurons; this fact may explain why HSV-1 goes into a latent state in neurons.

Transcription is often regulated into an organized cascade of viral gene expression. Herpesvirus immediate-early genes turn on the promoters for early genes. Other DNA viruses are not as dependent on transactivators encoded from the viral genome for early-gene transcription. Most early genes encode proteins that are necessary for viral DNA synthesis and for the turn-on of late-gene transcription. Late genes encode mostly viral structural proteins or viral proteins necessary for the assembly and egress of the virus from the infected cell. Late-gene transcription is continuously dependent on DNA replication. Therefore, inhibitors of DNA replication also stop late-gene transcription.

Each DNA virus family uses unique mechanisms for replicating its DNA. Herpesvirus DNAs are linear in the virion but circularize in the infected cell. In lytic virus infection, circular herpesvirus genomes are replicated into linear concatemers through a "rolling-circle" mechanism. Herpesviruses encode a DNA polymerase and at least six other viral proteins necessary for viral DNA replication; these viruses also encode several enzymes that increase the pool of precursor deoxynucleotide triphosphates. Adenovirus genomes are linear in the virion and are replicated into complementary linear copies by a virus-encoded DNA polymerase and an initiator protein complex. The double-strand circular papovavirus genomes are replicated into progeny circular DNA molecules by cellular DNA replication enzymes. Two viral early proteins contribute to viral DNA replication and to the persistence of papovavirus DNA in latently infected cells. Other early papovavirus proteins stimulate cells to remain in cycle, thus facilitating viral DNA replication. Occasionally, HPVs integrate into the host chromosome; overexpression of viral early proteins and excessive stimulation of cellular growth result. Sometimes the consequence is the development of malignancies such as cervical cancer (see "Persistent Viral Infections and Cancer," below). Parvoviruses are the smallest DNA viruses:

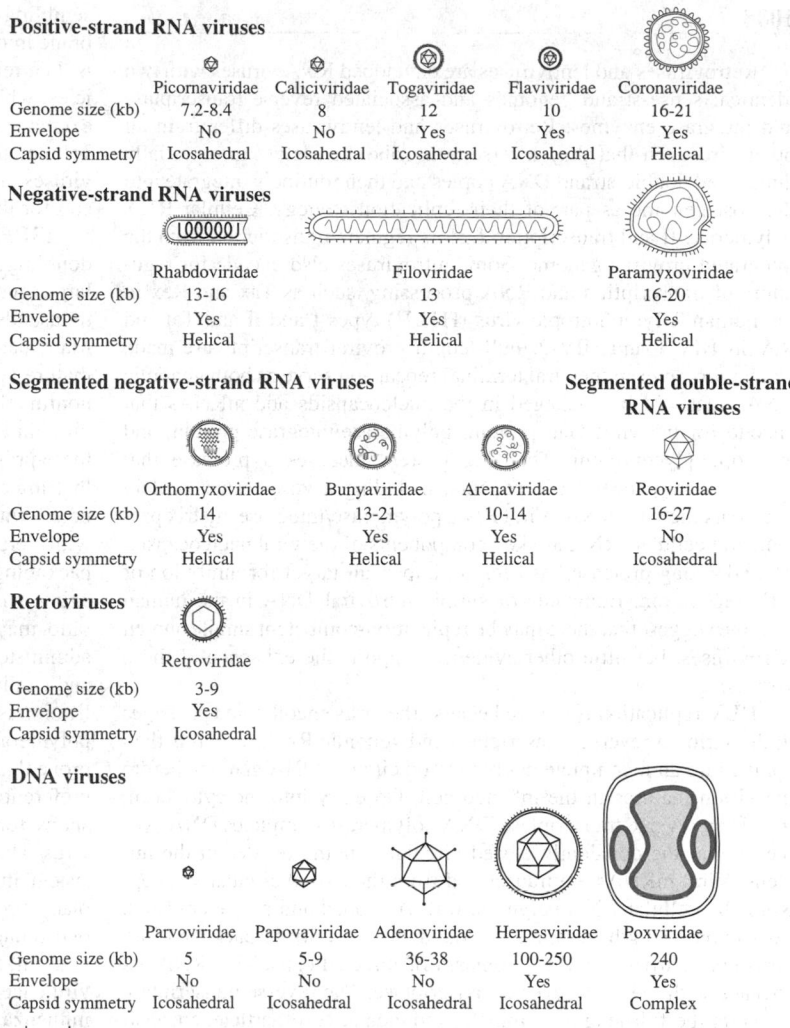

Positive-strand RNA viruses

	Picornaviridae	Caliciviridae	Togaviridae	Flaviviridae	Coronaviridae
Genome size (kb)	7.2–8.4	8	12	10	16–21
Envelope	No	No	Yes	Yes	Yes
Capsid symmetry	Icosahedral	Icosahedral	Icosahedral	Icosahedral	Helical

Negative-strand RNA viruses

	Rhabdoviridae	Filoviridae	Paramyxoviridae
Genome size (kb)	13–16	13	16–20
Envelope	Yes	Yes	Yes
Capsid symmetry	Helical	Helical	Helical

Segmented negative-strand RNA viruses | **Segmented double-strand RNA viruses**

	Orthomyxoviridae	Bunyaviridae	Arenaviridae	Reoviridae
Genome size (kb)	14	13–21	10–14	16–27
Envelope	Yes	Yes	Yes	No
Capsid symmetry	Helical	Helical	Helical	Icosahedral

Retroviruses

	Retroviridae
Genome size (kb)	3–9
Envelope	Yes
Capsid symmetry	Icosahedral

DNA viruses

	Parvoviridae	Papovaviridae	Adenoviridae	Herpesviridae	Poxviridae
Genome size (kb)	5	5–9	36–38	100–250	240
Envelope	No	No	No	Yes	Yes
Capsid symmetry	Icosahedral	Icosahedral	Icosahedral	Icosahedral	Complex

⊢——⊣
100 nm

FIGURE 180-2 Schematic diagrams of the major virus families including species that infect humans. The viruses are grouped by genome type and are drawn approximately to scale. Prototype viruses of each family that cause human disease are listed in Table 180-1.

their genomes are half the size of the papovavirus genomes and include only two genes. Parvoviruses have negative single-strand DNA genomes. The replication of autonomous parvoviruses, such as B19, depends on cellular DNA replication and requires the virus-encoded Rep protein. Other parvoviruses, such as adeno-associated virus (AAV), are not autonomous and require helper viruses of the adenovirus or herpesvirus family for their replication. AAV has been touted as a potentially safe human gene vector because its Rep protein causes its integration at a single chromosomal site.

Poxviruses are the largest DNA viruses and are unique among these viruses in replicating and assembling in the cytoplasm. Poxviruses encode transcription factors and an RNA polymerase as well as enzymes for RNA capping and polyadenylation and for DNA synthesis. Poxvirus DNA also has a unique structure. The two strands of the double-strand linear DNA are covalently linked at the ends so that the genome is also a covalently closed single-strand circle. In addition, there are inverted repeats at the ends of the DNA. During DNA replication, the genome is cleaved within the terminal inverted repeat, and the inverted repeats self-prime complementary-strand synthesis by the virus-encoded DNA polymerase. Like herpesviruses, poxviruses encode several enzymes that increase deoxynucleotide triphosphate precursor levels and thus facilitate viral DNA synthesis.

Viruses with both RNA and DNA genomes Retroviruses, lentiviruses, and hepatitis B virus (HBV) are not purely RNA or DNA viruses.

Retroviruses and lentiviruses are enveloped RNA viruses with two identical sense-strand genomes and associated reverse transcriptase and integrase enzymes. Retroviruses and lentiviruses differ from all other viruses in that they reverse-transcribe themselves into partially duplicated double-strand DNA copies and then routinely integrate into the host genome as part of their replication strategy. Cellular RNA polymerase II and transcription factors regulate transcription from the integrated provirus genome. Some retroviruses also encode for regulators of transcription and RNA processing, such as Tax and Rex in the human T-lymphotropic virus (HTLV) types I and II and Tat and Rev in HIV-1 and HIV-2. Full-length proviral transcripts are made from a promoter in the viral terminal repeat and serve as both genomic RNAs that will be packaged in the nucleocapsids and mRNAs that encode for the viral Gag protein, polymerase/integrase protein, and envelope glycoprotein. The Gag protein includes a protease that cleaves it into several components, including a viral matrix protein that coats the viral RNA. Viral RNA polymerase/integrase, matrix protein, and cellular tRNA are key components of the viral nucleocapsid. The HIV Gag protease has been an important target for inhibition of HIV replication. Remnants of simple retroviral DNA in the human genome suggest that there may be replication-competent simple human retroviruses, but little other evidence supports the existence of these viruses.

HBV replication is unique because the virus encodes and packages in the virion a reverse transcriptase and genomic RNA, which is then copied into an incomplete double-strand circular DNA genome before the virion matures in the infected cell. On entry into the cytoplasm, the virion reverse transcriptase/DNA polymerase completes DNA synthesis, and the covalently closed circular genome resides in the nucleus. Viral mRNAs are transcribed from the closed circular viral episome by cellular RNA polymerase II. A capped and polyadenylated, full-genome-length, terminally redundant transcript is packaged into virus core particles in the cytoplasm of infected cells. This RNA associates with the viral reverse transcriptase. The reverse transcriptase converts the full-length, terminally redundant, core-particle, encapsidated RNA genome into partially double-strand DNA. HBV is believed to mature by budding through the cell's plasma membrane, which has been modified by the insertion of viral surface antigen protein.

Viral Assembly and Egress For most viruses, nucleic acid and structural protein synthesis are accompanied by the assembly of protein and nucleic acid complexes. The assembly and egress of mature infectious virus mark the end of the eclipse phase of infection, during which infectious virus cannot be recovered from the infected cell. Nucleic acids from RNA viruses and poxviruses assemble into nucleocapsids in the cytoplasm. For all DNA viruses except poxviruses, viral DNA assembles into nucleocapsids in the nucleus. In general, the capsid proteins of viruses with icosahedral nucleocapsids can self-assemble into densely packed and highly ordered capsid structures. Herpesviruses require an assemblin protein as a scaffold for capsid assembly. Viral nucleic acid then spools into the assembled capsid. For herpesviruses, a full unit of the viral DNA genome is packaged into the capsid, and a capsid-associated nuclease cleaves the viral DNA at both ends. In the case of viruses with helical nucleocapsids, the protein component appears to assemble around the nucleic acid, which contributes to capsid organization.

Viruses must egress from the infected cell and not bind back to its plasma membrane. In many cases, enveloped viruses simply egress and acquire their envelope by budding through the cell's plasma membrane. Excess viral membrane glycoproteins are synthesized to saturate cell receptors and facilitate viral egress. Some viruses encode membrane proteins with enzymatic activity for receptor destruction. Influenza virus, for example, encodes a glycoprotein with neuraminidase activity, which destroys sialic acid on the infected cell's plasma membrane. Herpesvirus nucleocapsids acquire their initial envelope by assembling in the nucleus and then budding through the nuclear membrane into the endoplasmic reticular space. The enveloped herpesvirus is then released from the cell either by maturation in cytoplasmic vesicles, which fuse with the plasma membrane and release the virus by exocytosis, or by "de-envelopment" into the cytoplasm and "re-envelopment" at the plasma membrane. In most instances, nonenveloped viruses appear to depend on the death and dissolution of the infected cell for their release.

FIDELITY OF VIRAL REPLICATION Cells grow by doubling their genome and dividing, whereas viruses typically make large quantities of viral nucleic acid and structural proteins, and thousands of progeny may be produced from a single infected cell. Many particles partially assemble and never mature into virions. Many mature-appearing virions are imperfect and have only incomplete or nonfunctional genomes. Despite the inefficiency of assembly, a typical virus-infected cell releases 10 to 1000 infectious progeny. Some of these progeny may contain genomes that differ from those of the virus that infected the cell. Smaller, "defective" virus genomes have been noted with the replication of many RNA and DNA viruses. Virions with defective genomes can be produced in large numbers through packaging of incompletely synthesized nucleic acid. Adenovirus packaging is notoriously inefficient, and a high particle-to-infectious virus ratio may limit the amount of recombinant adenovirus that can be administered for gene therapy. Mutant viral genomes are also produced and can be of medical significance. In general, viral nucleic acid replication is more error-prone than cellular nucleic acid replication. RNA polymerases and reverse transcriptases are intrinsically more error-prone than DNA polymerases. Mutant viruses can be virulent and may preferentially cause disease through evasion of the host immune response or through resistance to antiviral drugs. Persistent hepatitis C virus (HCV) infection appears to be due to genome mutation and persistent immune escape. Changes in viral nucleic acid can also take place through infection by and recombination or reassortment between two related viruses in a single cell. While this occurrence is highly unusual, the changes could be substantial and could significantly alter virulence or epidemiology. Reassortment of an avian or mammalian influenza A hemagglutinin gene into a human influenza background is believed to play a role in the emergence of new epidemic influenza A strains.

VIRAL GENES NOT REQUIRED FOR VIRAL REPLICATION Viruses frequently have genes encoding proteins that are not directly involved in replication or packaging of the viral nucleic acid, in virion assembly, or in regulation of the transcription of viral genes involved in those processes. Most of these proteins fall into four classes: (1) proteins that directly or indirectly alter cell growth; (2) proteins that inhibit cellular DNA, RNA, or protein synthesis so that viral mRNA can be efficiently transcribed or translated; (3) proteins that promote the cell's survival or inhibit apoptosis so that progeny virus can mature and escape from the infected cell; and (4) proteins that downregulate host inflammatory or immune responses so that virus infection can proceed in an infected person to the maximum extent consistent with virus survival and efficient transmission to a new host. More complex viruses of the poxvirus or herpesvirus family encode many proteins that serve these functions. Some of these viral proteins have motifs similar to those of cell proteins, while others are quite novel. Virology has increasingly focused on these more sophisticated strategies evolved by viruses to permit the establishment of long-term infection in humans and other animals. These strategies often provide unique insights into the control of cell growth, cell survival, macromolecular synthesis, proteolytic processing, immune or inflammatory suppression, immune resistance, cytokine mimicry, or cytokine blockade.

HOST RANGE The concept of host range was originally based on the cell types in which a virus replicated in tissue culture. For the most part, the host range is limited by specific cell-surface proteins required for viral adsorption or penetration. Another common basis for host-range limitation is transcription from viral promoters. Most

DNA viruses depend not only on cellular RNA polymerase II and the basal components of the cellular transcription complex but also on activated components and transcriptional accessory factors, both of which differ among differentiated tissues, among cells at various phases of the cell cycle, and between resting and cycling cells.

The concept of host range for virus infection in humans includes these factors and others since (1) most viruses infect more than one cell type in vivo and (2) the virus life cycle and extent of viral replication can be affected by the differentiation and activated state of a given cell type. This point is particularly relevant for human papovavirus, herpesvirus, and lentivirus infections, in which vigorous replication during initial infection may be followed by quiescent or latent infection—a situation that allows the virus to persist.

VIRAL CYTOPATHIC EFFECTS AND INHIBITORS OF APOPTOSIS The replication of almost all viruses has adverse effects on the infected cell, inhibiting cellular synthesis of DNA, RNA, or proteins. This inhibitory effect probably stems from the viruses' need to prevent or limit nonspecific, innate host resistance factors, including interferon (IFN). Most commonly, viruses specifically inhibit host protein synthesis by attacking a component of the translational initiation complex—frequently, a component that is not required for efficient translation of viral RNAs. Poliovirus protease 2A, for example, cleaves a cellular component of the complex that ordinarily facilitates translation of cell mRNAs by interacting with their 5′ cap structure. Poliovirus RNA is efficiently translated without a 5′ cap since it has an internal ribosome entry sequence. Influenza virus inhibits the processing of mRNA by snatching 5′ cap structures from nascent cellular RNAs and using them as primers in the synthesis of viral mRNA. HSV has a virion tegument protein that inhibits cellular mRNA translation.

Apoptosis is the expected consequence of virus-induced inhibition of cellular macromolecular synthesis and viral nucleic acid replication. While the induction of apoptosis may be important for the release of some viruses (particularly nonenveloped viruses), many viruses have acquired genes or parts of genes that enable them to forestall infected-cell apoptosis. This delay may be advantageous in allowing the completion of viral replication. Adenoviruses and herpesviruses encode analogues of the cellular Bc12 protein, which blocks mitochondrial enhancement of proapoptotic stimuli. Poxviruses and some herpesviruses encode caspase inhibitors. Many viruses, including HPVs and adenoviruses, encode proteins that inhibit p53 or its downstream proapoptotic effects.

VIRAL INFECTION IN VIVO

The capsid and envelope of a virus protect its genome and permit its transmission from cell to cell and to prospective hosts. Most common viral infections are spread by aerosolized particles, by ingestion of contaminated water or food, or by direct contact. In all these situations, infection begins on an epithelial or mucosal surface and spreads along it or from it to deeper tissues. Infection may then spread through the body via the bloodstream, lymphatics, or neural circuits. Parenteral inoculation also serves to transmit some viral infections among humans or from animals (including insects) to humans.

PRIMARY INFECTION The first (primary) episode of viral infection usually lasts from several days to several weeks. During this period, the concentration of virus at sites of infection rises and then falls, usually to unmeasurable levels. The rate at which the intensity of viral infection rises and falls at a given site depends on the accessibility of that organ or tissue to both the virus and systemic immune effectors, the intrinsic ability of the virus to replicate at that site, and endogenous nonspecific and specific resistance. Typically, infections with enterovirus, mumps virus, measles virus, rubella virus, rotavirus, influenza virus, adenovirus, HSV, and VZV are cleared from almost all sites within 3 to 4 weeks. Some of these viruses are especially proficient in altering or evading the innate and acquired immune responses; thus primary infection with these viruses can last for several

months. Characteristically extending beyond several weeks are primary infections due to HBV, HCV, hepatitis D virus (HDV), EBV, cytomegalovirus (CMV), HIV, HPV, and molluscum contagiosum virus. For some of these viruses (e.g., HPV, HBV, HCV, HDV, and molluscum contagiosum virus), the primary phase of infection is almost indistinguishable from the persistent phase.

Disease manifestations usually arise as a consequence of viral replication at a specific site but do not necessarily correlate with levels of replication at that site. For example, the clinical manifestations of limited infection with poliovirus, enterovirus, rabies virus, measles virus, mumps virus, or HSV in neural cells are severe relative to the level of viral replication at mucosal surfaces. Similarly, significant morbidity may accompany in utero fetal infection with rubella virus or CMV.

Primary infections are cleared by specific and nonspecific immune responses. Thereafter, an immunocompetent host is usually immune to the disease manifestations of reinfection by the same virus. Immunity may not prevent transient surface colonization on reexposure, or even persistent colonization.

PERSISTENT AND LATENT INFECTIONS Relatively few viruses cause persistent or latent infections. HBV, HCV, rabies virus, measles virus, HIV, HTLV, HPV, herpesviruses, and some poxviruses are notable exceptions. The mechanisms for persistent infection vary widely. In persistent HCV infection and to a lesser extent in HIV infection, the high mutation rates in viral genome replication significantly facilitate persistent infection, continuously yielding mutant viruses that have lost antigenic determinants to which the host has developed effective immune responses. HIV is directly immunosuppressive, depleting CD4+ T lymphocytes and compromising CD8+ cytotoxic T cell immune responsiveness. Moreover, HIV encodes a Nef protein that downmodulates major histocompatibility complex (MHC) class I expression, rendering HIV-infected cells partially resistant to immune CD8+ cytolysis. The high mutation rate and the magnitude of virus load conspire to promote persistent infection with drug-resistant HIV mutants.

In contrast, herpesviruses and papovaviruses have much lower mutation rates. Their persistence is due to their ability to establish latent infection and to reactivate from latency. In this instance, *latency* is defined as a state of infection with a full viral genome replicated by cellular DNA polymerase in conjunction with the cell genome; there is no expression of viral genes associated with lytic infection and therefore no production of infectious virus. For HPVs, latently infected basal epithelial cells replicate. Some of the progeny cells provide a stable supply of latently infected basal cells, while others go on to squamous differentiation and in the process become permissive for lytic virus infection. For herpesviruses, latent infection is established in nonreplicating neural cells (HSV and VZV) and in replicating cells of early hematopoietic lineages [EBV and probably CMV, HHV-6, HHV-7, and Kaposi's sarcoma–associated herpesvirus (KSHV, also known as HHV-8)]. Reactivation from neural latency appears to be an intermittent process provoked by external stimuli, whereas reactivation from hematopoietic precursors appears to be a more continuous process. In their latent stage, HPV and herpesvirus genomes are hidden from the normal immune response. It is still not fully understood how latent and reactivated HPV and herpesvirus infections escape immediate and effective immune responses in highly immune hosts. HPV, HSV, and VZV may be somewhat protected because of their replication in middle and upper layers of the squamous epithelium. HSV and CMV are also known to encode proteins that downregulate MHC class I expression and antigenic peptide presentation on infected cells, thereby enabling these cells to escape CD8+ T lymphocyte cytotoxicity. Latent infection and intermittent reactivation perpetuate HPV and herpesvirus infections in human populations by allowing the viruses to persist in immune hosts and to be transmitted to the next generation of naive hosts.

Like other poxviruses, molluscum contagiosum virus cannot establish latent infection but rather causes persistent infection in hypertrophic lesions that last for months or years. This virus encodes a chemokine homologue that probably blocks inflammatory responses and an MHC class I analogue that may block cytotoxic T lymphocyte attack.

PERSISTENT VIRAL INFECTIONS AND CANCER

Persistent viral infection is estimated to be the root cause of as many as 20% of human malignancies. For the most part, cancer is an accidental and highly unusual or long-term effect of infection with oncogenic human viruses. In these malignancies, viral infection is a critical and ultimately determinative early step, and an unusual virus-infected cell undergoes the subsequent genetic changes that permit the enhanced autonomous growth and survival characteristic of a malignant cell. Most hepatocellular carcinoma is now believed to be caused by chronic inflammatory, immune, and regenerative responses to HBV or HCV infection. Epidemiologic data firmly link HBV and HCV infection to hepatocellular carcinoma, and studies in murine experimental models indicate that chronic liver injury and repair induced by virus-encoded proteins can result in hepatocellular cancer. In rare instances, HBV DNA integrates into cellular DNA—an event that probably contributes to the development of some tumors.

Almost all cervical carcinoma is caused by long-term persistent replication of "high-risk" genital HPV strains. An infrequent consequence of persistent HPV replication is the integration of a small fragment of the HPV genome encoding the HPV E6 and E7 proteins into chromosomal DNA. Overexpression of these proteins of HPV type 16 or 18 eliminates at least two major tumor-suppressive mechanisms in the infected cell and causes profound changes in cellular growth and survival. Nevertheless, subsequent chromosomal changes must occur over ensuing cycles of cell growth if a sufficiently malignant cell is to invade the surrounding tissues.

Similarly, long-term EBV infection and expression of the EBV oncogene LMP1 in a clone of latently infected epithelial cells appears to be a critical early step in the evolution of anaplastic nasopharyngeal carcinoma, a common malignancy in Chinese and North African populations. High-level LMP1 expression is a hallmark of many cases of Hodgkin's disease. Among younger age groups, >50% of Hodgkin's disease tumors are clonally derived from an EBV-infected cell. The HTLV-I Tax and Rex proteins appear to be critical to the initiation of cutaneous adult T cell lymphoma/leukemias that may occur long after primary HTLV-I infection.

A new EBV-related herpesvirus, KSHV, was identified in a search for the postulated sexually transmitted etiologic agent of Kaposi's sarcoma in HIV-infected individuals. Molecular data confirm the presence of KSHV DNA in all Kaposi's tumors, including those associated with HIV infection, transplantation, and familial transmission.

Evidence supporting a causal role of viral infection in these malignancies includes epidemiologic data, the presence of viral DNA in all tumor cells, the ability of the viruses to transform human cells in culture, the results of in vitro assays for transforming effects of specific viral genes on cell growth, and pathologic data indicating the expression of transforming viral genes in premalignant or malignant cells in vivo.

EBV is a unique example of a human virus that relies on the normal immune response to contain the potentially unrestrained growth of infected B lymphocytes. In the initial stages of normal primary EBV infection, EBV "latently" infects B lymphocytes and expresses at least eight viral proteins that cause continuous cell proliferation. The infected cells grow indefinitely in vitro or in T cell–deficient mice. Most of the viral proteins are highly antigenic, and these virus-infected cells, which can transiently constitute 10% of the circulating B lymphocyte population, are met with an overwhelming helper and cytotoxic T cell response during primary infection. The number of virus-infected cells then falls rapidly, and the one EBV-infected cell in a million that persists does not express most of the viral proteins that cause B cell proliferation. These persisting cells are the site of normal latent infection. Breakthrough growth of the EBV-infected B lymphocytes almost never occurs in immunocompetent hosts. However, in immunosuppressed AIDS patients or organ transplant recipients, EBV-infected B lymphocytes expressing the full set of growth-transforming genes may grow, uncontrolled by the immune system, and cause self-sustained and potentially fatal lymphoproliferative disease. Clinical investigation has resulted in novel strategies for treating these virus-induced malignancies by increasing T cell responsiveness through ex vivo expansion and readministration of EBV-specific T cells and by attacking the proliferating B cells with antibody coupled to toxins.

RESISTANCE TO VIRAL INFECTIONS

Resistance to viral infection is initially provided by factors that are not virus-specific. Physical protection is afforded by the cornified layers of the skin and by mucous secretions that continuously sweep over mucosal surfaces. Once the first cell is infected, viral infection induces IFNs, which are important local resistance factors. Viral infection may also cause the release of other cytokines from infected cells. Viral protein epitopes expressed on the cell surface in the context of MHC class I and II HLA proteins attract T cells with appropriate receptors. Cytokines, inflammatory agents, and antigens released by virus-induced cell death attract inflammatory cells, dendritic cells, granulocytes, natural killer (NK) cells, and B lymphocytes to the sites of initial infection. IFNs and NK cells are particularly important in containing viral infection for the first several days. Granulocytes and macrophages are also important in the phagocytosis and degradation of viruses, especially after an initial antibody response.

Some 7 to 10 days after infection, virus-specific antibody responses, virus-specific HLA class II–restricted CD4+ helper T lymphocyte responses, and virus-specific HLA class I–restricted CD8+ cytotoxic T lymphocyte responses are detected. These responses, whose magnitude typically increases over the second and third weeks of infection, are important in rapid recovery. Between the second and third weeks of infection, the antibody type usually changes from IgM to IgG, and IgA antibody is detected at initially infected mucosal surfaces. Antibody may directly neutralize virus by binding to its surface and preventing its adsorption or penetration. Complement usually enhances virus neutralization. Antibody and complement can also lyse virus-infected cells that express viral proteins on their surface. A cell infected with an enveloped virus usually expresses viral envelope glycoprotein components on its surface and is thus rendered subject to destruction by antibodies and complement.

The antibody and CD4+/CD8+ T lymphocyte responses tend to persist for several months after primary infection. Antibody-producing lymphocytes persist in small numbers as memory cells and begin to proliferate rapidly in response to a second infection, providing an early barrier to reinfection with the same virus. Immunologic memory for T cell responses appears to be less long-lived, and redevelopment of T cell immunity may take longer than secondary antibody responses, particularly when many years have elapsed between primary infection and reexposure.

Some viruses have genes that alter innate and acquired host defenses. Adenoviruses encode small RNAs that inhibit IFN shutoff of infected-cell protein synthesis. Adenovirus E1A inhibits IFN-mediated changes in cell gene transcription. Adenovirus E3 proteins prevent TNF-induced cytolysis and block HLA class I antigen synthesis by the infected cell. HSV ICP47 and CMV US11 block class I antigen presentation. EBV encodes an interleukin (IL) 10 homologue that inhibits NK and T cell responses. Vaccinia virus B15R is an IL-1 receptor decoy. Vaccinia virus B8R is a soluble TNF receptor that blocks the effects of TNF. Vaccinia virus CrmA inhibits the ability of CD8+ cytotoxic cells to kill virus-infected cells. Some poxviruses and herpesviruses encode blockers of chemokines and thereby inhibit cellular inflammatory responses. The adoption of these strategies by viruses highlights the importance of these host resistance factors in containing viral infection as well as that of redundancy in host resistance. The ultimate success of a virus requires a live host to help it disseminate.

Much has been written about the role of specific aspects of the host immune response in containment of specific virus infections. Certainly, T lymphocyte disorders are associated with severe primary and reactivated herpesvirus infections, and antibody responses are important in resistance to many RNA virus infections. However, antibody responses are also important in resistance to herpesvirus infections, as is exemplified by the utility of immunoglobulin therapy in early amelioration of these infections. T lymphocyte responses play a significant role in resistance to RNA virus infections, as is illustrated by the presence of cytotoxic T cells specific for influenza virus nucleoprotein.

Host resistance does not come without a price. Clearly, aspects of the host response contribute to the pathophysiologic manifestations and symptoms of viral infection. Inflammation at sites of viral infection can increase rates of local cell death. Immune responses to viral infection can target related epitopes on normal cells. While such effects have been demonstrated in experimental models, their role in the autoimmune manifestations of primary or recurrent human viral infections is uncertain.

INTERFERONS All human cells can synthesize IFN-α or -β in response to viral infection. The IFN response is usually induced by the presence of double-strand viral RNA, which can be made by both RNA and DNA viruses. IFN-γ is not directly related to IFN-α or -β and is produced mainly by NK cells and by immune T lymphocytes responding to IL-12. IFN-α and -β bind to the IFN-α receptor, while IFN-γ binds to a different but related receptor. Both receptors signal through receptor-associated JAK kinases and other cytoplasmic proteins, including "STAT" proteins. These proteins are tyrosine phosphorylated by JAK kinases, translocate to the nucleus, and transactivate promoters for specific cell genes. Three types of antiviral effects are induced by IFN at the transcriptional level. The first effect is attributable to the induction of 2'-5' oligo(A) synthetases, which require double-strand RNA for their activation. Activated synthetase polymerizes oligo(A) and thereby activates RNAse L, which in turn degrades single-strand RNA. The second effect takes place through the induction of PKR, a serine and threonine kinase that is also activated by double-strand RNA. PKR phosphorylates and negatively regulates the translational initiation factor eIF2-α, shutting down protein synthesis in the infected cell. A third effect is initiated through the induction of Mx proteins, a family of GTPases that is particularly important in inhibiting influenza virus and vesicular stomatitis virus replication. None of these IFN effects is directed specifically against the virus; infected-cell RNA and protein synthesis are globally inhibited. IFN probably contributes to the death of the infected cell.

DIAGNOSTIC VIROLOGY A wide variety of methods are now used to diagnose viral infection, but serology and viral isolation in tissue culture remain the backbone of diagnostic virology. Acute- and convalescent-phase sera with rising antibody titers to virus-specific antigens and a shift from IgM to IgG antibodies are generally accepted as diagnostic of acute viral infection. Traditionally, virus-specific antibodies have been detected by hemadsorption, hemagglutination, or indirect immunofluorescence. Immunofluorescence assays use fixed virus-infected cells as a target for serum antibodies. Hemadsorption and hemagglutination assays measure the ability of serum antibodies to the hemagglutinin proteins of RNA viruses to inhibit virus-induced adsorption or agglutination. Serologic diagnosis is based on a greater-than-fourfold rise in IgG antibody concentration when acute- and convalescent-phase serum samples are analyzed at the same time. A simultaneous fall in IgM antibody confirms recent primary viral infection. Immunofluorescence, hemadsorption, and hemagglutination assays are labor-intensive and are being replaced by enzyme-linked immunosorbent assays (ELISAs). ELISAs generally use specific viral proteins purified from virus-infected cells or produced by recombinant DNA technology. These viral antigens are attached to a solid phase, where they can be incubated with serum, washed to eliminate nonspecific antibodies, and reacted with an enzyme-linked reagent to detect human IgG or IgM antibody specifically adhering to the viral antigen on the solid phase. The amount of antibody can then be quantitated by the intensity of a color reaction mediated by the linked enzyme. ELISAs can be automated and can have enhanced sensitivity. Western blots measure antibody to multiple viral proteins

simultaneously. The proteins are separated by size and transferred to an inert membrane, where they are incubated with serum antibodies. Western blots have an internal specificity control, since the level of reactivity for viral proteins can be compared with that for cellular proteins in the same sample. Western blots are a useful confirmatory test but require individual evaluation and are inherently difficult to quantitate.

Viral isolation in tissue culture is dependent on the infection of susceptible cells and amplification through viral replication in infected cells. Virus growing in tissue culture cells can frequently be identified by its effect under light microscopy. For example, HSV produces a typical cytopathic effect in rabbit kidney cells within 3 days. Other viral cytopathic effects may not be as diagnostically useful. Identification may require confirmation by staining with virus-specific monoclonal antibodies. Viruses growing in tissue culture can also be identified by hemadsorption, by interference (e.g., rubella virus–infected cells resist lysis by echovirus), or by electron microscopy (assuming that the specimen has altered cell morphology, as observed by ordinary light microscopy).

The efficiency and speed of virus identification can be enhanced by combining short-term culture with immune detection. In assays with "shell vials" of tissue culture cells growing on a coverslip, viral infection can be detected by staining of the culture with a monoclonal antibody to a specific viral protein expressed early in viral replication. Thus, virus-infected cells can be detected within hours or days of inoculation—before the several rounds of infection that would be required to produce a visible cytopathic effect.

The sensitivity of virus isolation depends on the collection of specimens from the appropriate site and the rapid transport of these specimens in the appropriate medium to the virology laboratory. Rapid transport maintains viral viability and limits bacterial and fungal overgrowth. Lipid-enveloped viruses are generally much more sensitive to freezing and thawing than nonenveloped viruses. The most appropriate site for culture depends on the pathogenesis of the virus in question. Nasopharyngeal, tracheal, or endobronchial aspirates are most appropriate for the identification of respiratory viruses. Sputum cultures generally are not appropriate because bacterial contamination and viscosity threaten tissue-culture cell viability. Aspirates of vesicular fluid are useful for isolation of HSV and VZV. Nasopharyngeal aspirates and stool specimens may be useful when the patient has fever and a rash and an enteroviral infection is suspected. Adenoviruses can be cultured from the urine of patients with hemorrhagic cystitis. CMV can frequently be isolated from cultures of urine or buffy coat. Biopsy material can be effectively cultured when viruses infect major organs, as in HSV encephalitis or adenovirus pneumonia. Unlike serology, the isolation of a virus does not establish the time of primary infection. Many viruses persistently or intermittently colonize normal human mucosal surfaces. Saliva is not infrequently positive for herpesviruses, and 1% of normal urine samples are positive for CMV. Isolations from blood, cerebrospinal fluid (CSF), or biopsy specimens are more often diagnostic of significant virus infection.

Another method aimed at increasing the speed of viral diagnosis is direct antigen testing. Virus-infected cells obtained directly from the patient are detected by staining with virus-specific monoclonal antibodies; for example, epithelial cells obtained by nasopharyngeal aspiration can be stained with a variety of monoclonal antibodies to respiratory viruses. The Tzanck preparation used to detect multinucleated giant cells in HSV- or VSV-induced lesions was the predecessor of these direct antigen tests and can be enhanced by the use of HSV- or VZV-specific monoclonal antibodies. Similarly, monoclonal antibodies can be applied to histopathology specimens to identify virus-infected cells.

Advances in nucleic acid technology are revolutionizing diagnostic virology. The speed and sensitivity of tests that directly amplify minute amounts of viral nucleic acids present in specimens mean that detection no longer depends on viable virus and its replication. For

FIELDS BN et al (eds): *Virology*, 3d ed. New York, Raven, 1996
LENNETTE EH, SMITH TF (eds): *Laboratory Diagnosis of Viral Infections.* New York, Marcel Dekker, 1999
PLOEGH HL: Viral strategies of immune evasion. Science 280:248, 1998
ROULSTON A et al: Viruses and apoptosis. Annu Rev Microbiol 53:577, 1999
SENKEVICH T et al: Genome sequence of a human tumorigenic poxvirus: Prediction of specific host response-evasion genes. Science 273:813, 1996

example, amplification and detection of HSV nucleic acids leaking into the CSF of patients with HSV encephalitis can be more sensitive than culture of virus from CSF. The extreme sensitivity of these tests can be a problem, since trivial amounts of contamination can lead to false-positive results. In addition, detection of viral nucleic acids does not necessarily indicate virus-induced disease, especially in cases where viruses (e.g., herpesviruses) can cause persistent asymptomatic infection.

Measurement of the amount of viral RNA or DNA in peripheral blood is becoming an important means for determining which patients are at increased risk for virus-induced disease and for evaluating clinical responses to antiviral chemotherapy. Direct staining with CMV-specific monoclonal antibodies to quantitate virus-infected cells in the peripheral blood or CMV antigenemia can be useful in identifying which immunosuppressed patients may be at risk for CMV-induced disease. New CMV assays using nucleic acid technologies for the same purpose have been approved for clinical use. RNA viral-load measurements by nucleic acid technologies are now routinely used in AIDS patients to evaluate responses to an increasing number of antiviral agents. Viral-load measurements may also be useful for evaluating the treatment of patients with HBV and HCV infections.

The use of antiviral agents for the treatment of herpesvirus and HIV infections has been highly effective. However, the emergence of drug-resistant HIV strains in treated patients can limit efficacy in some cases. The increased number of antiviral agents and drug classes with different viral targets has made the identification of drug-resistant viruses clinically relevant, especially for HIV infection. Drug resistance in herpesviruses is a more unusual problem.

Viral genotyping is a new and faster method for the identification of drug-resistant viruses. Rising viral loads despite antiviral chemotherapy may indicate emergence of resistant HIV strains. Resistance to reverse transcriptase or protease inhibitors has been associated with specific mutations in the reverse transcriptase or protease genes. Identification of these mutations by polymerase chain reaction amplification and nucleic acid sequencing can be clinically useful for determining which antiviral agents may still be effective. Genotyping of HCV may also help identify patients who can benefit from combination chemotherapy.

Viral phenotyping may also be useful for identifying resistant viruses associated with new or unrecognized genetic mutations. These labor-intensive assays are not routinely available, but technical advances and continued evolution of drug-resistant viruses may make these tests more clinically relevant in the near future.

IMMUNIZATION FOR THE PREVENTION OF VIRAL INFECTIONS   Viral vaccines were among the outstanding accomplishments of twentieth-century science. The scourge of smallpox has been eradicated. Poliovirus eradication may soon follow. Rabies and measles can be contained or eliminated. Excess mortality due to influenza virus epidemics can be contained, and the threat of influenza pandemics has decreased. Widespread HBV vaccination has dramatically lessened the frequency of acute and chronic hepatitis and is expected to lead to a dramatic decrease in the incidence of hepatocellular carcinoma. The ease with which some viruses are attenuated in tissue culture has led to widespread immunization against rubella, measles, mumps, and chickenpox. Recombinant DNA-based strategies will make it possible to prevent severe infections with many other viruses by using purified proteins or genetically engineered live virus vaccines. Unfortunately, there are limits to these prospects. The evolutionary divergence of HIV and HCV, for example, complicates the development of highly effective immunogens for the prevention of infection with these agents. Modestly effective immunogens that incorporate multiple B and T cell epitopes may prove useful for low-level exposures.

BIBLIOGRAPHY

DURANT J et al: Drug resistance genotyping in HIV-1 therapy: The VIRADAPT randomised controlled trial. Lancet 353:2195, 1999

| **181** | *Raphael Dolin* |

ANTIVIRAL CHEMOTHERAPY, EXCLUDING ANTIRETROVIRAL DRUGS

ALT	alanine aminotransferase	HCV	hepatitis C virus
CMV	cytomegalovirus	HHV	human herpesvirus
CSF	cerebrospinal fluid	HSV	herpes simplex virus
EBV	Epstein-Barr virus	IFN	interferon
FDA	Food and Drug Administration	RSV	respiratory syncytial virus
HBeAg	hepatitis B e antigen	VZV	varicella-zoster virus
HBV	hepatitis B virus		

The development of drugs for antiviral chemotherapy and chemoprophylaxis is a relatively recent but now very active area of biomedical research. Significant progress has been made in recent years on new drugs for several viral infections. Despite these advances, the field of antiviral therapy—both the number of antiviral drugs and our understanding of their optimal use—continues to lag behind the field of antibacterial drug treatment, in which more than 60 years of experience have now been accumulated.

The development of antiviral drugs poses several challenges. Viruses replicate intracellularly and often employ host cell enzymes, macromolecules, and organelles for synthesis of viral particles. Therefore, useful antiviral compounds must discriminate between host and viral functions with a high degree of specificity; agents without such selectivity are likely to be too toxic for clinical use.

The development of laboratory assays to assist clinicians in the appropriate use of antiviral drugs is also in its infancy. Phenotypic and genotypic assays for resistance to antiviral drugs are becoming more widely available, and correlations of laboratory results with clinical outcomes in various settings are beginning to be defined. Of particular note has been the development of highly sensitive and specific methods to measure the concentration of virus in blood (*virus load*), which permit direct assessment of the antiviral effect of a given drug regimen in the host. Virus load measurements have been useful in recognizing the risk of disease progression in patients with certain viral infections and in identifying patients in whom antiviral chemotherapy might be of greatest benefit. Like any in vitro laboratory test, these tests yield results that are highly dependent on (and likely to vary with) the laboratory techniques employed.

Information regarding the pharmacokinetics of some antiviral drugs, particularly in diverse clinical settings, is limited. Assays to measure the concentrations of these drugs, especially of their active moieties within cells, are not widely available. Thus, there are relatively few guidelines for adjusting dosages of antiviral agents to maximize antiviral activity and minimize toxicity. Clinical use of antiviral drugs must therefore be accompanied by particular vigilance with regard to unanticipated adverse effects.

Like that of other infections, the course of viral infections is profoundly affected by an interplay of the pathogen with a complex set of host defenses. The presence or absence of preexisting immunity and the ability to mount humoral and/or cell-mediated immune responses are important determinants of the outcome of viral infections. The state of the host's defenses needs to be considered when antiviral agents are utilized or evaluated.

As with any therapy, the optimal use of antiviral compounds requires a specific and timely diagnosis. For some viral infections, such as herpes zoster, the clinical manifestations are so characteristic that a diagnosis can be made on clinical grounds alone. For other viral infections, such as influenza A, epidemiologic information (e.g., the documentation of a community-wide outbreak) can be used to make a presumptive diagnosis with a high degree of accuracy. However, for most other viral infections, including herpes simplex encephalitis, cytomegaloviral infections other than retinitis, and enteroviral infections, diagnosis on clinical grounds alone cannot be accomplished with certainty. For such infections, rapid viral diagnostic techniques are of great importance. Considerable progress has been made in recent years in the development of such tests, which are now widely available for a number of viral infections.

Despite these complexities, the efficacy of a number of antiviral compounds has been clearly established in rigorously conducted and controlled studies. As summarized in Table 181-1, this chapter reviews the antiviral drugs that are currently approved or are likely to be considered for approval in the near future for use against viral infections other than those caused by HIV. Antiretroviral drugs are reviewed in Chap. 309.

ANTIVIRAL DRUGS ACTIVE AGAINST RESPIRATORY INFECTIONS

AMANTADINE AND RIMANTADINE Amantadine and the closely related compound rimantadine are primary symmetric amines. Their antiviral activity is limited to influenza A viruses, whose replication they inhibit by interfering with the uncoating of virus after infection of the cell. This interference is attributable to the agents' interaction with the influenza A M2 matrix protein, during which the ion channel function of M2 is inhibited. A substitution of a single amino acid in the M2 protein can result in a virus that is resistant to amantadine and rimantadine.

Amantadine and rimantadine have been demonstrated to be effective in the prophylaxis of influenza A in large-scale studies of young adults and in less extensive studies of children and elderly subjects. In such studies, efficacy rates of 55 to 80% in the prevention of influenza-like illness were noted, and even higher rates were reported when virus-specific attack rates were calculated. Amantadine and rimantadine have also been demonstrated to be effective in the treatment of influenza A infection in studies involving predominantly young adults and, to a lesser extent, children. Administration of these compounds within 24 to 72 h after the onset of illness has resulted in a reduction of the duration of signs and symptoms by ~50% from that in a placebo-treated group. The effect on signs and symptoms of illness is superior to that of commonly used antipyretic-analgesics. Only anecdotal reports are available concerning the efficacy of amantadine or rimantadine in the prevention or treatment of complications of influenza (e.g., pneumonia).

Amantadine and rimantadine are available only in oral formulations and are ordinarily administered to adults once or twice daily in a dose of 100 to 200 mg/d. Despite their structural similarities, the pharmacokinetics of the two compounds are different. Amantadine is not metabolized and is excreted almost entirely by the kidney, with a half-life of 12 to 17 h and peak plasma concentrations of 0.4 μg/mL. Rimantadine is extensively metabolized to hydroxylated derivatives and has a half-life of 30 h. Only 30 to 40% of an orally administered dose is recovered in the urine. The peak plasma levels of rimantadine are approximately half those of amantadine, but rimantadine is concentrated in respiratory secretions to a greater extent than amantadine. For prophylaxis, the compounds must be administered daily for the period at risk (i.e., the peak duration of the outbreak). For therapy, amantadine or rimantadine is generally administered for 5 to 7 days.

Although these compounds are generally well tolerated, 5 to 10% of amantadine recipients experience mild central nervous system side effects consisting primarily of dizziness, anxiety, insomnia, and dif-

ficulty in concentrating. These effects are rapidly reversible upon cessation of the drug's administration. At a dose of 200 mg/d, rimantadine is better tolerated than amantadine; in a large-scale study of young adults, adverse effects were no more frequent among rimantadine recipients than among placebo recipients. Seizures and worsening of congestive heart failure have also been reported in patients treated with amantadine, although a causal relationship has not been established. The dosage of amantadine should be reduced to ≤100 mg/d in patients with renal insufficiency [i.e., a creatinine clearance (Cr_{Cl}) rate of <50 mL/min] and in the elderly. A rimantadine dose of 100 mg/d should be used for patients with a Cr_{Cl} of <10 mL/min and in the elderly. Resistance to amantadine and rimantadine can be induced readily in vitro. The emergence and probable transmission of virus resistant to these drugs have also been noted in vivo after their use for the treatment of children or adults. In the United States, both amantadine and rimantadine are approved for the prophylaxis and treatment of influenza A in adults and for prophylaxis in children. Amantadine is also approved for the treatment of influenza A in children.

RIBAVIRIN Ribavirin is a synthetic nucleoside analogue that inhibits a wide range of RNA and DNA viruses. The mechanism of action of ribavirin is not completely defined and may be different for different groups of viruses. Ribavirin-5'-monophosphate blocks the conversion of inosine-5'-monophosphate to xanthosine-5'-monophosphate and interferes with the synthesis of guanine nucleotides as well as that of both RNA and DNA. Ribavirin-5'-monophosphate also inhibits capping of virus-specific messenger RNA in certain viral systems. In studies demonstrating the effectiveness of ribavirin, the compound has been administered as a small-particle aerosol. It has been used to treat respiratory syncytial virus (RSV) infections in infants and—less extensively—to treat parainfluenza virus infections in children and influenza A and B virus infections in young adults. In infants with RSV infection who were given ribavirin by continuous aerosol for 3 to 6 days, illness and lower respiratory tract signs resolved more rapidly and arterial oxygen desaturation was less pronounced than in placebo-treated groups. Ribavirin has also had a beneficial clinical effect in infants with RSV infection who require mechanical ventilation. Aerosolized ribavirin has been administered to older children and adults with severe RSV and parainfluenza virus infections (including immunosuppressed patients), but the benefit of this treatment, if any, is unclear. In RSV infections, ribavirin is often given in combination with immunoglobulins.

Orally administered ribavirin has not been effective in the treatment of influenza A virus infections. Intravenous or oral ribavirin has reduced mortality among patients with Lassa fever; it has been particularly effective in this regard when given within the first 6 days of illness. Intravenous ribavirin has been reported to be of clinical benefit in the treatment of hemorrhagic fever with renal syndrome caused by Hantaan virus and as therapy for Argentinian hemorrhagic fever. Moreover, oral ribavirin has been recommended for the treatment and prophylaxis of Congo-Crimean hemorrhagic fever. Intravenous ribavirin is being evaluated as therapy for the hemorrhagic fever with pulmonary syndrome caused by newly described hantaviruses in the United States. Oral administration of ribavirin reduces serum aminotransferase levels in patients with chronic hepatitis C virus (HCV) infection; since it appears not to reduce serum HCV RNA levels, the mechanism of this effect is unclear. Given in doses of 1000 to 1200 mg/d in combination with interferon (IFN) α (see below), ribavirin has been approved for the treatment of patients with chronic HCV infection.

Large doses of ribavirin administered orally (800 to 1000 mg/d) have been associated with reversible hematopoietic toxicity. This effect has not been observed with aerosolized ribavirin, apparently because little drug is absorbed systemically. Aerosolized administration of ribavirin is generally well tolerated but occasionally is associated with bronchospasm, rash, or conjunctival irritation. Aerosolized ribavirin has been licensed for treatment of RSV infection in infants and

Table 181-1 Antiviral Chemotherapy and Chemoprophylaxis

Infection	Drug	Route	Dosage	Comment
Influenza A and B Prophylaxis	Amantadine or rimantadine (influenza A only)	Oral	Adults: 200 mg/d for period at risk Children ≤9 yrs: 5 mg/kg per day (maximum, 150 mg/d)	Therapy must continue for duration of outbreak. Dosage should be reduced (more for amantadine) in patients with renal failure and the elderly. Drugs can be administered along with vaccine.
Treatment	Zanamivir	Inhaled orally	10 mg q12h for 5 days in adults and children ≥7 years old	Zanamivir and oseltamivir reduce symptoms by 1.0–1.5 and 1.3 days, respectively, in uncomplicated disease when started within 2 days of onset and are under study in complicated disease. Zanamivir may exacerbate bronchospasm in patients with asthma. Oseltamivir's side effects of nausea and vomiting can be reduced in frequency by administration with food. Both amantadine and rimantadine are effective in uncomplicated influenza. Neither has been thoroughly studied in complicated cases (e.g., pneumonia).
	Oseltamivir	Oral	75 mg bid for 5 days in adults	
	Amantadine (influenza A only)	Oral	100–200 mg/d in adults and dosage for children as above for 5–7 days	
	Rimantadine (influenza A only)	Oral	100–200 mg/d for 5–7 days in adults	
RSV infection	Ribavirin	Small-particle aerosol	Administered continuously from reservoir containing 20 mg/mL for 3–6 days	Ribavirin is used for treatment of infants and young children hospitalized with RSV pneumonia and bronchiolitis.
CMV retinitis in immunocompromised host	Ganciclovir	IV	5 mg/kg bid for 14–21 days; then 5 mg/kg per day as maintenance dose	Both ganciclovir and foscarnet are licensed for treatment of CMV retinitis in immunosuppressed patients, including those with AIDS. They are also used for colitis, pneumonia, or ''wasting'' syndromes associated with CMV and for prevention of CMV disease in transplant recipients. Foscarnet is not myelosuppressive and is active against acyclovir- and ganciclovir-resistant herpesviruses.
		Oral	1 g tid as maintenance dose	
	Foscarnet	IV	60 mg/kg q8h for 14–21 days; then 90–120 mg/kg per day as maintenance dose	
	Cidofovir	IV	5 mg/kg twice weekly for 2 weeks, then once weekly; given with probenecid	
Varicella Immunocompetent host	Acyclovir	Oral	20 mg/kg (maximum, 800 mg) 4 or 5 times daily for 5 days	Treatment confers modest clinical benefit when administered within 24 h of rash onset.
Immunocompromised host	Acyclovir	IV	500 mg/m² q8h for 7 days	A change to oral valacyclovir can be considered once fever has subsided and there is no evidence of visceral involvement.
Herpes simplex encephalitis	Acyclovir	IV	10 mg/kg q8h for 10–14 days	Results are optimal when therapy is initiated early. Some authorities treat for 21 days to prevent relapses.
Neonatal herpes simplex	Acyclovir	IV	10 mg/kg q8h for 14–21 days	Serious morbidity is frequent despite therapy. Prolonged oral administration of acyclovir after initial IV therapy has been suggested because of long-term sequelae associated with cutaneous recurrences of HSV infection.
Genital herpes simplex Primary (treatment)	Acyclovir	IV	5 mg/kg q8h for 5–10 days	The IV route is preferred for infections severe enough to warrant hospitalization or with neurologic complications.
		Oral	200 mg 5 times daily for 10 days	The oral route is preferred for patients whose condition does not warrant hospitalization. Adequate hydration must be maintained.
		Topical	5% ointment; 4–6 applications daily for 7–10 days	Topical use—largely supplemented by oral therapy—may obviate systemic administration to pregnant women. Systemic symptoms and untreated areas are not affected.
	Valacyclovir	Oral	1 g bid for 10 days	Valacyclovir appears to be as effective as acyclovir but can be administered less frequently.
	Famciclovir	Oral	250 mg bid for 5–10 days[a]	Famciclovir appears to be similar in effectiveness to acyclovir.
Recurrent (treatment)	Acyclovir	Oral	200 mg 5 times daily for 5 days	Clinical effect is modest and is enhanced if therapy is initiated early. Treatment does not affect recurrence rates.
	Famciclovir	Oral	125 mg bid for 5 days	
	Valacyclovir	Oral	500 mg bid for 5 days	

(continued)

Table 181-1—(continued)

Infection	Drug	Route	Dosage	Comment
Recurrent (suppression)	Acyclovir Valacyclovir Famciclovir	Oral Oral Oral	400 mg bid for ≥12 months 500–1000 mg daily 125–250 mg bid	Suppressive therapy is recommended only for patients with at least 6–10 recurrences per year. "Breakthrough" occasionally takes place, and asymptomatic shedding of virus occurs. The need for suppressive therapy should be reevaluated after 1 year. Experience with >1 year of valacyclovir or famciclovir therapy is limited.
Mucocutaneous herpes simplex in immunocompromised host Treatment	Acyclovir	IV Oral Topical	250 mg/m² q8h for 7 days 400 mg 5 times daily for 10 days 5% ointment; 4–6 applications daily for 7 days or until healed	Choice of IV or oral route depends on severity of infection and patient's ability to take oral medication. Oral or IV treatment has supplanted topical therapy except for small, easily accessible lesions. Foscarnet is used for acyclovir-resistant viruses.
	Valacyclovir Famciclovir	Oral Oral	1 g tid for 7 days[a] 500 mg bid for 4 days[a]	
Prevention of recurrences during intense immunosuppression	Acyclovir Valacyclovir Famciclovir	Oral IV Oral Oral	200 mg qid 5 mg/kg q12h 1 g tid[a] 500 mg bid[a]	Treatment is administered during periods when intense immunosuppression is expected—e.g., during antitumor chemotherapy or after transplantation—and is usually continued for 2–3 months.
Herpes simplex orolabialis (recurrent)	Penciclovir	Topical	1.0% cream applied q2h during waking hours for 4 days	Treatment shortens healing time and symptoms by 0.5–1.0 day (compared with placebo).
Herpes simplex keratitis	Trifluridine	Topical	1 drop of 1% ophthalmic solution q2h while awake (maximum, 9 drops daily)	Therapy should be undertaken in consultation with an ophthalmologist.
	Vidarabine	Topical	0.5-in. ribbon of 3% ophthalmic ointment 5 times daily	
Herpes zoster Immunocompromised host	Acyclovir Famciclovir	IV Oral Oral	500 mg/m² q8h for 7 days 800 mg 5 times daily for 7 days 500 mg tid for 10 days[a]	Effectiveness in localized zoster is most marked when treatment is given early. Foscarnet may be used for VZV infections that are resistant to acyclovir.
Immunocompetent host	Valacyclovir	Oral	1 g tid for 7 days	Valacyclovir may be more effective than acyclovir for pain relief; otherwise, it has a similar effect on cutaneous lesions and should be given within 72 h of rash onset.
	Famciclovir	Oral	500 mg q8h for 7 days	The duration of postherpetic neuralgia is shorter than with placebo. Famciclovir showed overall efficacy similar to that of acyclovir in a comparative trial. It should be given ≤72 h of rash onset.
	Acyclovir	Oral	800 mg 5 times daily for 7–10 days	Acyclovir causes faster resolution of skin lesions than placebo and provides some relief of acute symptoms if given within 72 h of rash onset. Combined with tapering doses of prednisone, acyclovir improves quality-of-life outcomes.
Herpes zoster ophthalmicus	Acyclovir	Oral	600 mg 5 times daily for 10 days	Treatment reduces ocular complications, including ocular keratitis and uveitis.
Condyloma acuminatum	IFN-α2b	Intralesional	1 million units per wart (maximum of 5) thrice weekly for 3 weeks)	Intralesional treatment frequently results in regression of warts, but lesions often recur. Parenteral administration may be useful if lesions are numerous.
	IFN-αn3	Intralesional	250,000 units per wart (maximum of 10) twice weekly for up to 8 weeks	
Chronic hepatitis B	IFN-α2b	SC or IM	5 million units daily or 10 million units thrice weekly for 24 weeks	Hepatitis B e antigen and DNA are eliminated in 33–37% of cases. Histopathologic improvement is also seen.
	Lamivudine	Oral	100 mg/d for 1 year	Resistance develops in 15–36% of recipients.
Chronic hepatitis C	IFN-α2a or -α2b	SC or IM	3 million units thrice weekly for 12–18 months	A return of alanine aminotransferase levels to normal is documented in 54% of recipients but is sustained in only 28%. Improvement in liver histopathology is seen.

(continued)

Table 181-1   Antiviral Chemotherapy and Chemoprophylaxis—(continued)

Infection	Drug	Route	Dosage	Comment
	IFN-α2b/ribavirin	SC or IM/oral	3 million units thrice weekly/ 1000–1200 mg daily for 6–12 months	Combination therapy results in an increase in sustained responses (to 40–50% of recipients).
	IFN alfacon	SC	9–15 μg thrice weekly for 6–12 months	Doses of 9 and 15 μg are equivalent to IFN-α2a or -α2b doses of 3 million units and 5 million units, respectively.
Chronic hepatitis D	IFN-α2a or -α2b	SC or IM	5 million units daily or 10 million units thrice weekly for 6–12 months	The optimal regimen and duration of therapy have not been established. Responses are usually not sustained when therapy is stopped.

a Not approved for this indication by the U.S. Food and Drug Administration.
NOTE: CMV, cytomegalovirus; HSV, herpes simplex virus; IFN, interferon; RSV, respiratory syncytial virus; VZV, varicella-zoster virus.

should be administered under close supervision—particularly in the setting of mechanical ventilation, where precipitation of the drug is possible. Health care workers exposed to the drug have experienced minor toxicity, including eye and respiratory tract irritation. Because ribavirin is mutagenic, teratogenic, and embryotoxic, its use is generally contraindicated in pregnancy. Its administration as an aerosol poses a risk to pregnant health care workers.

ZANAMIVIR AND OSELTAMIVIR   Influenza viral neuraminidase is essential for release of the virus from infected cells and for its subsequent spread throughout the respiratory tract of the infected host. The enzyme cleaves terminal sialic acid residues, thus destroying the cellular receptors recognized by the viral hemagglutinin. Zanamivir, a sialic acid analogue, is a highly active and specific inhibitor of the neuraminidases of influenza A and B viruses. Oseltamivir is another neuraminidase inhibitor that is a transition-state analogue of sialic acid cleavage. Its antineuraminidase activity is similar to that of zanamivir. Oseltamivir phosphate is an ethyl ester prodrug that is converted to oseltamivir carboxylate by esterases in the liver. Both zanamivir and oseltamivir act through competitive and reversible inhibition of the active site of influenza A and B viral neuraminidases and have relatively little effect on mammalian cell enzymes. As would be expected from their different mechanisms of action, zanamivir and oseltamivir are active against strains of influenza A virus that are resistant to amantadine and rimantadine.

Zanamivir has low oral bioavailability. It is inhaled orally via a hand-held inhaler. By this route, ~15% of the dose is deposited in the lower respiratory tract, and low plasma levels of the drug are detected. Orally administered oseltamivir has an oral bioavailability of >60% and a plasma half-life of 7 to 9 h. The drug is excreted unmetabolized, primarily by the kidney.

Intranasal inhaled zanamivir is generally well tolerated. The most frequent toxicities encountered with orally administered oseltamivir are nausea, gastrointestinal discomfort, and (less commonly) vomiting. Gastrointestinal discomfort is usually transient and is less likely if the drug is administered with food. No serious clinical or laboratory toxicities have yet been reported with zanamivir or oseltamivir in clinical trials.

Inhaled zanamivir and orally administered oseltamivir have been effective in the treatment of naturally occurring influenza A or B in otherwise healthy adults. In placebo-controlled studies, illness has been shortened by 1 to 1.5 days of therapy with either of these drugs. Once-daily inhaled zanamivir or orally administered oseltamivir provides effective prophylaxis against laboratory-documented influenza A–associated illness. The emergence of viruses resistant to zanamivir or oseltamivir appears to be infrequent in clinical studies carried out thus far.

As of this writing, zanamivir and oseltamivir have been approved by the U.S. Food and Drug Administration (FDA) for treatment of influenza in adults (and—in the case of zanamivir—in children ≥7 years of age) who have been symptomatic for ≤2 days. Indications for prophylactic use are under review.

ANTIVIRAL DRUGS ACTIVE AGAINST HERPESVIRUS INFECTIONS

ACYCLOVIR AND VALACYCLOVIR   Acyclovir is a highly potent and selective inhibitor of the replication of certain herpesviruses, including herpes simplex virus (HSV) types 1 and 2, varicella-zoster virus (VZV), and Epstein-Barr virus (EBV). It is relatively ineffective in the treatment of human cytomegalovirus (CMV) infections; however, some studies have indicated its effectiveness in the prevention of CMV-associated disease in immunosuppressed patients. Valacyclovir, the L-valyl ester of acyclovir, is converted almost entirely to acyclovir after oral administration. Valacyclovir has pharmacokinetic advantages over orally administered acyclovir: it exhibits significantly greater oral bioavailability, results in higher blood levels, and can be given less frequently than acyclovir.

The high degree of selectivity of acyclovir is related to its mechanism of action, which requires that the compound first be phosphorylated to acyclovir monophosphate. This phosphorylation occurs efficiently in herpesvirus-infected cells by means of a virus-coded thymidine kinase. In uninfected mammalian cells, little phosphorylation of acyclovir occurs, and the drug is therefore concentrated in herpesvirus-infected cells. Acyclovir monophosphate is subsequently converted by host cell kinases to a triphosphate that is a potent inhibitor of virus-induced DNA polymerase but has relatively little effect on host cell DNA polymerase. Acyclovir triphosphate can also be incorporated into viral DNA, with early chain termination.

Acyclovir is available in intravenous, oral, and topical forms, while valacyclovir is available in an oral formulation. Intravenous acyclovir is markedly effective in the treatment of mucocutaneous HSV infections in immunocompromised hosts, reducing time to healing, duration of pain, and virus shedding. When administered prophylactically during periods of intense immunosuppression (e.g., related to chemotherapy for leukemia or transplantation) and before the development of lesions, intravenous acyclovir reduces the frequency of HSV-associated disease. After prophylaxis is discontinued, HSV lesions recur. Intravenous acyclovir is also effective in the treatment of HSV encephalitis; two comparative trials have indicated that acyclovir is more effective than vidarabine for this indication (see below). Because VZV is generally less sensitive to acyclovir than is HSV, higher doses of acyclovir must be used to treat VZV infections. In immunocompromised patients with herpes zoster, intravenous acyclovir reduces the frequency of cutaneous dissemination and visceral complications and—in one comparative trial—was more effective than vidarabine. Acyclovir, administered orally at doses of 800 mg five times a day, had a modest beneficial effect on localized herpes zoster lesions in both immunocompromised and immunocompetent patients. Combination of acyclovir with a tapering regimen of prednisone appeared to be more effective than acyclovir alone in terms of quality-of-life outcomes in immunocompetent herpes zoster patients over age 50. A comparative study of acyclovir (800 mg orally five times daily) and valacyclovir (1 g orally tid) in immunocompetent patients with herpes zoster indicated that the latter drug may be more effective in eliciting the resolution of zoster-associated pain. Orally administered acyclovir (600 mg five times a day) reduced complications of herpes zoster ophthalmicus in a placebo-controlled trial.

In normal children with chickenpox, acyclovir—administered at 20 mg/kg qid, up to a maximum of 800 mg qid, within 24 h of the onset of rash—resulted in a modest overall clinical benefit. Intravenous acyclovir has also been reported to be effective in the treatment of immunocompromised children with chickenpox.

The most widespread use of acyclovir is in the treatment of genital HSV infections. Intravenous or oral acyclovir or oral valacyclovir has shortened the duration of symptoms, reduced virus shedding, and accelerated healing when employed for the treatment of primary genital HSV infections. Oral acyclovir and valacyclovir have also had a modest effect in treatment of recurrent genital HSV infections. However, the failure of treatment of either primary or recurrent disease to reduce the frequency of subsequent recurrences has indicated that acyclovir is ineffective in eliminating latent infection. Chronic oral administration of acyclovir for periods of 1 to 6 years or longer or of valacyclovir for up to 1 year has reduced the frequency of recurrences markedly during therapy; once the drug is discontinued, lesions recur. In AIDS patients, chronic or intermittent administration of acyclovir has been associated with the development of HSV and VZV strains resistant to the action of the drug and with clinical failures. The most common mechanism of resistance is a deficiency of the virus-induced thymidine kinase. Patients with HSV or VZV infections resistant to acyclovir have frequently responded to foscarnet.

With the availability of the oral and intravenous forms, there are few indications for topical acyclovir, although treatment with this formulation has been modestly beneficial in primary genital HSV infections and in mucocutaneous HSV infections in immunocompromised hosts.

Overall, acyclovir is remarkably well tolerated and is generally free of toxicity. The most frequently encountered form of toxicity is renal dysfunction, particularly after rapid intravenous administration or with inadequate hydration. Central nervous system changes, including lethargy and tremors, are occasionally reported, primarily in immunosuppressed patients. However, whether these changes are related to acyclovir, to concurrent administration of other therapy, or to underlying infection remains unclear. Acyclovir is excreted primarily unmetabolized by the kidney, via both glomerular filtration and tubular secretion. Approximately 15% of a dose of acyclovir is metabolized to 9-[(carboxymethoxy)methyl]guanine or other minor metabolites. Reduction in dosage is indicated in patients with a Cr_{Cl} of <50 mL/ min per 1.73 m². The half-life of acyclovir is ~3 h in normal adults, and the peak plasma concentration after a 1-h infusion of a dose of 5 mg/kg is 9.8 μg/mL. Approximately 22% of an orally administered acyclovir dose is absorbed, and peak plasma concentrations of 0.3 to 0.9 μg/mL are attained after administration of a 200-mg dose. Acyclovir penetrates relatively well into the cerebrospinal fluid (CSF), with concentrations approaching half of those found in plasma.

Acyclovir causes chromosomal breakage at high doses, but its administration to pregnant women has not been associated with fetal abnormalities. Nonetheless, the potential risks and benefits of acyclovir should be carefully assessed before the drug is used in pregnancy.

Valacyclovir exhibits three to five times greater bioavailability than acyclovir. The concentration-time curve for valacyclovir, given as 1 g orally tid, is similar to that for acyclovir, given as 5 mg/kg intravenously every 8 h. The safety profiles of valacyclovir and acyclovir are similar, although thrombotic thrombocytopenic purpura/hemolytic-uremic syndrome has been reported in immunocompromised patients who have received high doses of valacyclovir. Valacyclovir is approved for the treatment of herpes zoster and for initial and recurrent episodes of genital HSV infections in immunocompetent adults as well as for suppressive treatment of genital herpes. It is being studied for use against other herpesvirus infections in various clinical settings.

CIDOFOVIR Cidofovir is a phosphonate nucleotide analogue of cytosine. Its major use is in CMV infections, particularly retinitis, but it is active against a broad range of herpesviruses, including HSV, human herpesvirus (HHV) type 6, HHV-8, and certain other DNA viruses such as polyomaviruses, papillomaviruses, and adenoviruses. Cidofovir does not require initial phosphorylation by virus-induced kinases; the drug is phosphorylated by host cell enzymes to cidofovir diphosphate, which is a competitive inhibitor of viral DNA polymerases and, to a lesser extent, of host cell DNA polymerases. Incorporation of cidofovir diphosphate slows or terminates nascent DNA chain elongation. Cidofovir is active against HSV isolates that are resistant to acyclovir because of absent or altered thymidine kinase and against CMV isolates that are resistant to ganciclovir because of UL97 mutations. Cidofovir is usually active against foscarnet-resistant CMV, although cross-resistance to foscarnet as well as to ganciclovir has been described.

Cidofovir has poor oral availability and is administered intravenously. It is excreted primarily by the kidney and has a plasma half-life of 2.6 h. Cidofovir diphosphate's intracellular half-life of >48 h is the basis for the recommended dosing regimen of 5 mg/kg twice a week for the initial 2 weeks and then 5 mg/kg once a week. The major toxic effect of cidofovir is proximal renal tubular injury, as manifested by elevated serum creatinine levels and proteinuria. The risk of nephrotoxicity can be reduced by vigorous saline hydration and by concomitant oral administration of probenecid. Neutropenia, rashes, and gastrointestinal tolerance may also occur.

Intravenous cidofovir has been approved for the treatment of CMV retinitis in AIDS patients who are intolerant of ganciclovir or foscarnet or in whom those drugs have failed. In a controlled study, a maintenance dosage of 5 mg/kg a week administered to AIDS patients reduced the progression of CMV retinitis from that seen at 3 mg/kg. Intravenous cidofovir has been reported anecdotally to be effective therapy for acyclovir-resistant mucocutaneous HSV infections. Likewise, topically administered cidofovir is reportedly beneficial against these infections in HIV patients; it is also being studied for the treatment of anogenital warts. Intravenous cidofovir is being evaluated as therapy for progressive multifocal leukoencephalopathy and for Kaposi's sarcoma. An ophthalmic formulation is being studied as treatment for adenoviral keratoconjunctivitis. Intravitreal cidofovir has been used to treat CMV retinitis but has been associated with significant toxicity.

FOMIVIRSEN Fomivirsen is the first antisense oligonucleotide approved by the U.S. Food and Drug Administration (FDA) for therapy in humans. This phosphorothioate oligonucleotide, 21 nucleotides in length, inhibits CMV replication through interaction with CMV messenger RNA. Fomivirsen is complementary to messenger transcripts of the major immediate early region 2 (IE2) of CMV, which codes for proteins regulating viral gene expression. In addition to its antisense mechanism of action, fomivirsen may exert activity against CMV through inhibition of viral adsorption to cells as well as direct inhibition of viral replication. Because of its different mechanism of action, fomivirsen is active against CMV isolates that are resistant to nucleoside or nucleotide analogues, such as ganciclovir, foscarnet, or cidofovir.

Fomivirsen has been approved for intravitreal administration in the treatment of CMV retinitis in AIDS patients who have failed to respond to other treatments or cannot tolerate them. Injections of 330 mg every 2 weeks have resulted in significant reductions in the rate of progression of CMV retinitis. The major toxicity is ocular inflammation, including vitritis and iritis, which usually responds to topically administered glucocorticoids.

GANCICLOVIR An analogue of acyclovir, ganciclovir is active against HSV and VZV and is markedly more active than acyclovir against CMV. Ganciclovir triphosphate inhibits CMV DNA polymerase and can be incorporated into CMV DNA, whose elongation it eventually terminates. In HSV- and VZV-infected cells, ganciclovir is phosphorylated by virus-encoded thymidine kinases; in CMV-infected cells, it is phosphorylated by a viral kinase encoded by the UL97 gene. Ganciclovir triphosphate is present in tenfold higher concentrations in CMV-infected cells than in uninfected cells. Ganciclovir is approved for the treatment of CMV retinitis in immunosuppressed patients and for the prevention of CMV disease in transplant recipients. It is widely used for the treatment of other CMV-associated syndromes, including pneumonia, esophagogastrointestinal infections, hepatitis, and "wasting" illness.

Ganciclovir is available for intravenous or oral administration. Because its oral bioavailability is low (5 to 9%), relatively large doses (1 g tid) must be administered by this route. Oral bioavailability is enhanced if the drug is administered with food, as recommended. The serum half-life of ganciclovir is 3.5 h after intravenous administration and 4.5 h after oral administration. The drug is excreted primarily by the kidney in unmetabolized form, and its dosage should be reduced in cases of renal failure. The most commonly employed dosage for initial therapy—5 mg/kg intravenously every 12 h for 14 to 21 days— is followed by a maintenance dose of 5 mg/kg intravenously per day or 5 times per week, possibly for as long as immunosuppression persists. Oral ganciclovir is approved as an alternative to the intravenous preparation in maintenance therapy for CMV retinitis, where it appears to be somewhat less effective although more convenient than intravenous therapy. Intraocular ganciclovir, given by either intravitreal injection or intraocular implantation, has also been used to treat CMV retinitis.

Ganciclovir is effective as prophylaxis against CMV-associated disease in organ and bone marrow transplant recipients. Oral ganciclovir administered prophylactically to AIDS patients with CD4+ counts of <100/μL provided protection against the development of CMV retinitis in one large-scale study and was subsequently approved for that indication. However, the long-term benefits of this approach to prophylaxis are unestablished, and most experts do not recommend the use of oral ganciclovir for that purpose.

The administration of ganciclovir has been associated with profound bone marrow suppression, particularly neutropenia, which significantly limits the drug's use in many patients. Bone marrow toxicity is potentiated when other bone marrow suppressants, such as zidovudine, are used concomitantly.

Resistance has been noted in CMV isolates obtained after therapy with ganciclovir, especially in patients with AIDS. Such resistance may develop through a mutation in either the viral UL97 gene or the viral DNA polymerase. Ganciclovir-resistant isolates are usually sensitive to foscarnet (see below).

FAMCICLOVIR AND PENCICLOVIR Famciclovir is the diacetyl 6-deoxyester of the guanosine analogue penciclovir. Famciclovir is well absorbed orally, with a bioavailability of 77%, and is rapidly converted by deacetylation and oxidation to penciclovir. Penciclovir's spectrum of activity and mechanism of action are similar to those of acyclovir; thus penciclovir is not active against acyclovir-resistant viruses. Penciclovir is phosphorylated initially by a virus-encoded thymidine kinase and subsequently by cellular kinases to penciclovir triphosphate, which inhibits HSV-1, HSV-2, and VZV DNA polymerases as well as hepatitis B virus (HBV). The serum half-life of penciclovir is 2 h, but the intracellular half-life of penciclovir triphosphate is 7 to 20 h—markedly longer than that of acyclovir triphosphate. Penciclovir is eliminated primarily in the urine by both glomerular filtration and tubular secretion. The usually recommended dosage interval should be adjusted for renal insufficiency.

Clinical trials involving immunocompetent adults with herpes zoster showed that famciclovir was superior to placebo in eliciting the resolution of skin lesions and virus shedding and in shortening the duration of postherpetic neuralgia; moreover, it was at least as effective as acyclovir administered orally at a dose of 800 mg five times daily. Famciclovir was also effective in the treatment of herpes zoster in immunosuppressed patients. Clinical trials have demonstrated its effectiveness in suppression of genital HSV infections for up to 1 year and in the treatment of initial and recurrent episodes of genital herpes. Famciclovir is effective as therapy for mucocutaneous HSV infections in HIV-infected patients. Application of a 1% penciclovir cream reduces the duration of signs and symptoms of herpes labialis in immunocompetent patients (by 0.5 to 1.0 day) and has been approved for that purpose by the FDA. Famciclovir is generally well tolerated, with occasional headache, nausea, and diarrhea reported in frequencies similar to those among placebo recipients. The administration of high doses of famciclovir for 2 years was associated with an increased incidence of mammary adenocarcinomas in female rats, but the clinical significance of this effect is unknown. Intravenous penciclovir is being investigated for the treatment of mucocutaneous HSV infections in immunosuppressed patients.

FOSCARNET Foscarnet (phosphonoformic acid) is a pyrophosphate-containing compound that potently inhibits herpesviruses, including CMV. This drug inhibits DNA polymerases at the pyrophosphate binding site at concentrations that have relatively little effect on cellular polymerases. Foscarnet does not require phosphorylation to exert its antiviral activity and is therefore active against HSV and VZV isolates that are resistant to acyclovir because of deficiencies in thymidine kinase as well as against most ganciclovir-resistant strains of CMV. Foscarnet also inhibits the reverse transcriptase of HIV and is active against HIV in vivo.

Foscarnet is poorly soluble and must be administered intravenously via an infusion pump in a dilute solution over 1 to 2 h. The plasma half-life of foscarnet is 3 to 5 h and increases with decreasing renal function, since the drug is eliminated primarily by the kidneys. It has been estimated that 10 to 28% of a dose may be deposited in bone, where it can persist for months. The most common initial dosage of foscarnet—60 mg/kg every 8 h for 14 to 21 days—is followed by a maintenance dose of 90 to 120 mg/kg once a day.

Foscarnet is approved for the treatment of CMV retinitis in patients with AIDS and of acyclovir-resistant mucocutaneous HSV infections. In a comparative clinical trial, the drug appeared to be about as efficacious as ganciclovir against CMV retinitis but was associated with a longer survival period, possibly because of its anti-HIV activity. Intraocular foscarnet has been used to treat CMV retinitis. Foscarnet has also been employed to treat acyclovir-resistant HSV and VZV infections as well as ganciclovir-resistant CMV infections, although resistance to foscarnet has been reported in CMV isolates obtained during therapy.

The major form of toxicity associated with foscarnet is renal impairment. Thus renal function should be monitored closely, particularly during the initial phase of therapy. Since foscarnet binds divalent metal ions, hypocalcemia, hypomagnesemia, hypokalemia, and hypo- or hyperphosphatemia can develop. Saline hydration and slow infusion appear to protect the patient against nephrotoxicity and electrolyte disturbances. Although hematologic abnormalities have been documented (most commonly anemia), foscarnet is not generally myelosuppressive and may be administered concomitantly with myelosuppressive medications such as zidovudine.

IDOXURIDINE Idoxuridine inhibits the replication of herpesviruses and poxviruses. It was formerly used systemically to treat herpesvirus infections, but, because of associated toxicity and lack of proven efficacy, its systemic use has largely been abandoned. Topical idoxuridine is effective in the treatment of HSV keratitis, particularly in superficial infections, but has been supplanted by topically applied trifluridine and vidarabine (see below).

TRIFLURIDINE Trifluridine is a pyrimidine nucleoside active against HSV-1, HSV-2, and CMV. Trifluridine monophosphate irreversibly inhibits thymidylate synthetase, and trifluridine triphosphate inhibits viral and, to a lesser extent, cellular DNA polymerases. Because of systemic toxicity, its use is limited to topical therapy. Trifluridine is approved for treatment of HSV keratitis, for which trials have shown that it is more effective than topical idoxuridine but similarly effective to topical vidarabine. The drug has benefited some patients with HSV keratitis who have failed to respond to idoxuridine or vidarabine. Topical application of trifluridine to sites of acyclovir-resistant HSV mucocutaneous infections has also been beneficial in some cases.

VIDARABINE Vidarabine is a purine nucleoside analogue with activity against HSV-1, HSV-2, VZV, and EBV. Vidarabine inhibits viral DNA synthesis through its $5'$-triphosphorylated metabolite, although its precise molecular mechanisms of action are not completely understood. Intravenously administered vidarabine has been shown to be effective in the treatment of herpes simplex encephalitis, mucocutaneous HSV infections and herpes zoster in immunocompromised patients and of neonatal HSV infections. Its use has been supplanted by intravenous acyclovir, which is more effective and easier to administer. Production of the intravenous preparation has been discontinued by the manufacturer, but vidarabine is available as an ophthalmic ointment, which is effective in the treatment of HSV keratitis.

OTHER ANTIVIRAL DRUGS *Lamivudine* is a pyrimidine nucleoside analogue that is used primarily in combination therapy against HIV infection (Chap. 309). It is also active against HBV through inhibition of the viral DNA polymerase and has been approved for the treatment of chronic HBV infection. In one study, at doses of 100 mg/d for ≥ 1 year, lamivudine was well tolerated and resulted in suppression of HBV DNA levels, normalization of serum aminotransferase levels in most patients, and reduction of hepatic inflammation and fibrosis. Loss of hepatitis B e antigen (HBeAg) occurred in a minority of patients. Resistance to lamivudine developed in 15 to 36% of patients treated for 1 year and was associated with changes in the YMDD motif of HBV DNA polymerase. This is an important limitation of monotherapy with the drug. Studies of lamivudine as a component of combination therapy for hepatitis B are under way. Lamivudine also appears to be useful in the prevention or suppression of HBV infection associated with liver transplantation.

Lobucavir is a synthetic cyclobutane nucleoside analogue with activity against a broad range of herpesviruses, HIV, and HBV. It is currently under investigation in clinical trials. Its mechanism of action is through inhibition of viral DNA synthesis. Lobucavir is initially phosphorylated by virus-induced kinases, and lobucavir triphosphate is a potent inhibitor of HSV, CMV, and HBV DNA polymerases. Lobucavir can be administered orally or intravenously. It is excreted largely unmetabolized via the kidney and has a plasma half-life of 2 h after intravenous administration. Its oral availability is dose-dependent, ranging from 25 to 40% at doses of ≤ 200 mg and decreasing at higher doses. The preclinical toxicity profile of lobucavir appears to be similar to that of ganciclovir. However, neutropenia has been uncommonly encountered in studies in humans. Aminotransferase elevations have been documented after intravenous and (less commonly) oral administration. The most frequent adverse effects after oral administration are headache, insomnia, and gastrointestinal discomfort. In clinical trials to date, oral lobucavir has demonstrated antiviral effects in CMV- and HBV-infected patients as well as clinical benefits against HSV infections in immunocompetent patients. Short-term (1-month) oral administration of 200 mg of lobucavir bid or qid reduced serum HBV DNA levels in chronically infected patients. HBV DNA levels returned to pretreatment values when the drug was stopped, and studies of longer-term administration are under way. Lobucavir is under clinical investigation for use in HIV infection and in several herpesvirus infections.

Pleconaril is an investigational drug in vitro against picornavirus replication, including over 90% of the most commonly isolated enterovirus types and 80% of rhinovirus serotypes. Its mechanism of action is through binding to a specific hydrophobic pocket in the viral capsid, which prevents attachment and/or uncoating of the virus. Pleconaril is poorly water soluble and is formulated as an oral suspension. After oral administration of 200- and 400-mg doses to adults, peak plasma concentrations are 1.1 and 2.4 $\mu g/mL$, respectively, and the terminal plasma half-life is 25 h. Pleconaril is generally well tolerated; the most frequently reported adverse effects are headache, nausea, diarrhea, and gastrointestinal discomfort, which have occurred at rates

similar to those among placebo recipients. Orally administered pleconaril, given before and after experimental infection of healthy volunteers with coxsackievirus A21, reduced peak viral titers by >100-fold and decreased the subsequent rate of development of illness. Pleconaril treatment of adults with enteroviral meningitis decreased the overall duration of illness and headache and reduced the use of analgesics from that by placebo recipients. Clinical studies of pleconaril in other enterovirus-induced diseases are in progress.

INTERFERONS

Interferons are cytokines that exhibit a broad spectrum of antiviral activities as well as immunomodulating and antiproliferative properties. The IFNs are not available for oral administration but must be given intramuscularly, subcutaneously, or intravenously. Early studies with human leukocyte IFN demonstrated an effect in the prophylaxis of experimentally induced rhinovirus infections in humans and in the treatment of VZV infections in immunosuppressed patients. DNA recombinant technology has made available highly purified α, β, and γ IFNs that have been evaluated in a variety of viral infections. Results of such trials have confirmed the effectiveness of intranasally administered IFN in the prophylaxis of rhinovirus infections, although its use has been associated with nasal mucosal irritation. Studies have also demonstrated a beneficial effect of intralesionally or systemically administered IFNs on genital warts. The effect of systemic administration consists primarily of a reduction in the size of lesions, and this mode of therapy may be useful in individuals who have numerous warts that cannot easily be treated by individual intralesional injection. However, lesions frequently recur after intralesional or systemic IFN therapy is discontinued.

Interferons have undergone extensive study in the treatment of chronic HBV infection. The administration of IFN-α2b (5 million units daily for 16 weeks) to patients with stable chronic HBV infection resulted in loss of markers of HBV replication, such as HBeAg and HBV DNA, in 33 to 37% of cases; 10 to 20% of patients also became negative for hepatitis B surface antigen. In >80% of patients who lose HBeAg and HBV DNA markers, serum aminotransferases return to normal levels, and both short- and long-term improvements in liver histopathology have been described. Predictors of a favorable response to therapy include low pretherapy levels of HBV DNA, high pretherapy serum levels of alanine aminotransferase (ALT), a short duration of chronic HBV infection, and active liver histopathology. Poor responses are seen in immunosuppressed patients, including those with HIV infection. Adverse effects of the above dose of IFN are common and include fever, chills, myalgia, fatigue, neurotoxicity (primarily manifested as somnolence and confusion), and leukopenia. Approximately 25% of patients receiving a daily dose of 5 million units require dose reduction, but fewer than 5% require discontinuation of therapy.

Several IFN preparations, including α2a, α2b, alfacon-1, and αm1 (lymphoblastoid), have been studied as therapy for chronic HCV infections. A variety of regimens have been employed, of which the most common is IFN-α2b or -α2a at 3 million units three times per week for 12 months. A complete biochemical response, defined as a return to normal serum ALT values at the end of treatment, has been documented in ~54% of patients. In addition, liver biopsies have shown decreases in lobular and periportal inflammation. However, relapse has occurred in approximately half of all cases upon discontinuation of therapy, so that sustained responses were documented in 28% of cases. The addition of oral ribavirin to IFN-α2b—either as initial therapy or after failure of interferon therapy alone—resulted in significantly higher rates of sustained response (40 to 50%) than were obtained with monotherapy. Prognostic factors for a favorable response include an age of <45 years, a short duration of disease, low levels of HCV RNA, and infection with HCV genotypes other than 1. IFN alfacon, a synthetic "consensus" α interferon, appears to produce response rates similar to those elicited by IFN-α2a or -α2b and has recently been approved in the United States for the treatment of chronic hepatitis C.

Treatment of chronic hepatitis D with IFN-α apparently requires higher doses (5 million units daily or 10 million units three times per week) and is less effective than treatment of chronic hepatitis B or C. After 12 months of therapy, biochemical and virologic responses were detected in $\geq$50% of patients, but few responses were sustained once therapy was stopped.

BIBLIOGRAPHY

BALFOUR HH: Antiviral drugs. N Engl J Med 340:1255, 1999

CRUMPACKER CS: Ganciclovir. N Engl J Med 335:721, 1996

DOLIN R et al: A controlled trial of amantadine and rimantadine in the prophylaxis of influenza A infection. N Engl J Med 307:580, 1982

HALL CB et al: Aerosolized ribavirin treatment of infants with respiratory syncytial viral infection: A randomized double-blind study. N Engl J Med 308:1443, 1983

LALEZARI JP et al: Randomized controlled study of the safety and efficacy of intravenous cidofovir for the treatment of relapsing cytomegalovirus retinitis in patients with AIDS. J AIDS 17:339, 1998

POYNARD T et al: Meta-analysis of interferon randomized trials in the treatment of viral hepatitis C: Effect of dose and duration. Hepatology 24:778, 1996

REICHMAN RC et al: Treatment of condyloma acuminatum with three different interferons administered intralesionally: A double-blind, placebo-controlled trial. Ann Intern Med 108:675, 1988

WHITLEY RJ et al: Herpes simplex encephalitis: Adenine arabinoside versus acyclovir therapies. N Engl J Med 314:144, 1986

WONG DKH et al: Effect of alpha-interferon treatment in patients with hepatitis B e antigen–positive chronic hepatitis B. Ann Intern Med 119:312, 1993

Section 12
DNA VIRUSES

182 *Lawrence Corey*

HERPES SIMPLEX VIRUSES

DEFINITION Herpes simplex viruses (HSV-1, HSV-2; *Herpesvirus hominis*) produce a variety of infections involving mucocutaneous surfaces, the central nervous system (CNS), and—on occasion—visceral organs. The advent of effective chemotherapy for HSV infections has made prompt recognition of these syndromes even more clinically important than in the past.

ETIOLOGIC AGENT The genome of HSV is a linear, double-stranded DNA molecule (molecular weight, $\sim$100 $\times$ 10^6) that encodes more than 75 gene products. The genomic structures of the two HSV subtypes are similar, and the overall sequence homology between HSV-1 and HSV-2 is $\sim$50%. The homologous sequences are distributed over the entire genome map, and most of the polypeptides specified by one viral type are antigenically related to polypeptides of the other viral type. Many type-specific regions unique to HSV-1 and HSV-2 proteins do exist, however, and a number of them appear to be important in host immunity. These type-specific regions have been used to develop serologic assays that distinguish between the two viral subtypes. Restriction endonuclease analysis of viral DNA can be used to distinguish between the two subtypes and among strains of each subtype. The variability of nucleotide sequences from clinical strains of HSV-1 and HSV-2 is such that HSV isolates obtained from two individuals can be differentiated by restriction enzyme patterns unless the isolates are from epidemiologically related sources, such as sexual partners, mother-infant pairs, or persons involved in a common-source outbreak.

The viral genome is packaged in a regular icosahedral protein shell (capsid) composed of 162 capsomers. The outer covering of the virus is a lipid-containing membrane (envelope) derived from modified cell membrane and acquired as the DNA-containing capsid buds through the inner nuclear membrane of the host cell. Between the capsid and lipid bilayer of the envelope is the tegument. Viral replication has both nuclear and cytoplasmic phases. The initial steps of replication include attachment, fusion between the viral envelope and the cell membrane to liberate the nucleocapsid into the cytoplasm of the cell, and disassembly of the nucleocapsid to release the viral DNA. Replication of HSV is highly regulated. After fusion of the virion envelope with the host cell membrane, several viral proteins are released from the HSV virion. Some shut off host protein synthesis (by increasing cellular RNA degradation), while others "turn on" transcription of early genes of HSV replication. These early gene products, designated α *genes*, are required for synthesis of the subsequent polypeptide group, the β polypeptides, many of which are regulatory proteins and enzymes required for DNA replication. Most current antiviral drugs interfere with β proteins, such as the viral DNA polymerase enzyme. The third (γ) class of HSV genes requires viral DNA replication for expression and constitutes most of the structural proteins specified by the virus.

After replication of the viral genome and synthesis of structural proteins, nucleocapsids are assembled in the nucleus of the cell. Envelopment occurs as the nucleocapsids bud through the inner nuclear membrane into the perinuclear space. In some cells, viral replication in the nucleus forms two types of inclusion bodies: type A basophilic Feulgen-positive bodies that contain viral DNA and an eosinophilic inclusion body that is devoid of viral nucleic acid or protein and represents a "scar" of viral infection. Virions are then transported via the endoplasmic reticulum and the Golgi apparatus to the cell surface.

HSV infection of some neuronal cells does not result in cell death. Instead, viral genomes are maintained by the cell in a repressed state compatible with survival and normal activities of the cell, a condition called *latency*. Latency is associated with transcription of only a limited number of virus-encoded proteins. Subsequently, the viral genome may become activated, resulting in the normal pattern of regulated viral gene expression, replication, and release of HSV. The release of virus from the neuron and its subsequent entry into epithelial cells result in viral replication. This process is termed *reactivation*. Whereas infectious virus rarely can be recovered from sensory or autonomic nervous system ganglia dissected from cadavers, maintenance and growth of the neural cells in tissue culture result in production of infectious virions (*explantation*) and in subsequent permissive infection of susceptible cells (*cocultivation*). The fact that HSV replication was first detected in neurons during reactivation in vitro suggested that the neuron harbors the latent virus in vivo. Viral DNA and RNA have since been found in neural tissue at times when infectious virus cannot be isolated. Two RNA "latency-associated" transcripts that overlap the immediate early (α) gene products, called ICP-O, are found in abundance in the nuclei of latently infected neurons. These latency-associated transcripts code proteins in an antisense direction. Deletion mutants of this region that can become latent have been made. However, the efficiency of their later reactivation is reduced; thus, the antisense transcripts may play a role in maintaining rather than in establishing latency. At present, the molecular mechanisms of the latency of HSV-1 and HSV-2 are not well understood, and strategies to interrupt latency or to maintain molecular latency in neurons are not available.

Exposure to HSV at mucosal surfaces or abraded skin sites permits entry of the virus and initiation of its replication in cells of the epidermis and dermis. Investigators have identified several cell receptors that are ligands for HSV attachment proteins. Studies to define how these receptors influence viral replication and pathogenesis are under way. Initial HSV infection is often subclinical—i.e., without clinically apparent lesions. Both clinical acquisition and subclinical acquisition are associated with sufficient viral replication to permit infection of either sensory or autonomic nerve endings. On entry into the neuronal cell, the virus—or, more likely, the nucleocapsid—is transported intraaxonally to the nerve cell bodies in ganglia. In humans, the interval from inoculation of virus in peripheral tissue to spread to the ganglia is unknown. During the initial phase of infection, viral replication occurs in ganglia and contiguous neural tissue. Virus then spreads to other mucosal skin surfaces through centrifugal migration of infectious virions via peripheral sensory nerves. This mode of spread helps explain the large surface area involved, the high frequency of new lesions distant from the initial crop of vesicles that is characteristic in patients with primary genital or oral-labial HSV infection, and the recovery of virus from neural tissue distant from neurons innervating the inoculation site. Contiguous spread of locally inoculated virus also may take place and allow further mucosal extension of disease.

After the resolution of primary disease, infectious HSV can no longer be recovered in the ganglia. However, viral DNA can be found in 10 to 50% of ganglion cells in the anatomic region of the initial infection. Only ~1% of such cells express latency-associated transcripts of RNA detectable by current techniques. The mechanisms controlling the reactivation of HSV infection are unknown. Alterations in cellular transcripts that "maintain" latency are suspected, and several cellular protein kinases are under investigation. Experimentally, ultraviolet light, systemic and local immunosuppression, and trauma to the skin or ganglia are associated with reactivation.

Analysis of the DNA from sequentially isolated strains of HSV or from isolates from multiple infected ganglia in any one individual has revealed identical restriction endonuclease patterns in most persons. Occasionally (most frequently in immunocompromised persons), multiple strains of the same viral subtype are detected in one individual. This finding suggests that exogenous infection with different strains of the same subtype is possible although very uncommon.

IMMUNITY Host responses to infection with HSV influence the acquisition of disease, the severity of infection, resistance to the development of latency, the maintenance of latency, and the frequency of recurrences. Both antibody-mediated and cell-mediated reactions are clinically important. Immunocompromised patients with defects in cell-mediated immunity experience more severe and more extensive HSV infections than those with deficits in humoral immunity, such as agammaglobulinemia. Experimental ablation of lymphocytes indicates that T cells play a major role in preventing lethal disseminated disease, although antibodies help reduce virus titers in neural tissue. Some of the clinical manifestations of HSV disease appear to be related to the host immune response (e.g., stromal opacities associated with recurrent herpetic keratitis). The surface viral glycoproteins have been shown to be antigens recognized by antibodies mediating neutralization and immune-mediated cytolysis (antibody-dependent cell-mediated cytotoxicity). Monoclonal antibodies specific for each of the known viral glycoproteins have, in experimental infections, conferred protection against subsequent neurologic disease or ganglionic latency. However, the use of subunit glycoprotein vaccines in humans has not been successful in reducing acquisition of infection, despite high titers of type-specific antibodies. Multiple cell populations, including natural killer cells, macrophages, a variety of T lymphocytes, and lymphokines generated by these cells, play a role in host defenses against HSV infections. In animals, passive transfer of primed lymphocytes confers protection from subsequent challenge. Maximum protection usually requires the activation of multiple T cell subpopulations, including cytotoxic T cells and T cells responsible for delayed hypersensitivity. The latter cells may confer protection by the antigen-stim-

ulated release of lymphokines (e.g., interferons), which may have a direct antiviral effect and may activate and enhance a variety of specific and nonspecific effector cells. Increasing evidence suggests that HSV-specific CD8+ T cell responses are critical for clearance of virus from lesions. In addition, immunosuppressed patients with frequent and prolonged HSV lesions have fewer functional CD8+ T cells directed at HSV. The HSV virion contains a gene called unique long gene no. 12 (UL-12) that can bind to the cellular transporter-activating protein TAP-1 and reduce the ability of this protein to bind HSV peptides to HLA class I, thereby reducing recognition of viral proteins by cytotoxic T cells of the host. This effect can be overcome by the addition of interferon γ, but this requires 24 to 48 h; thus, the virus has time to replicate and invade other host cells. Prior HSV-1 infection does not appear to reduce the frequency of acquisition of HSV-2 as measured by seroconversion. However, persons with prior HSV-1 infection who acquire HSV-2 appear to have a greater frequency of subclinical acquisition. These data suggest that type-specific immune responses are central to the control of HSV infection.

EPIDEMIOLOGY Seroepidemiologic studies have documented HSV infections worldwide. Much of the humoral immune response to HSV is to type-common antigenic determinants. Serologic assays with whole-virus antigen preparations, such as complement fixation, neutralization, indirect immunofluorescence, passive hemagglutination, radioimmunoassay, and enzyme-linked immunosorbent assay, do not reliably distinguish between the two viral subtypes. Such assays are useful for differentiating uninfected (seronegative) persons from those with past HSV-1 or HSV-2 infection, but they do not reliably distinguish between the two subtypes. Serologic assays that identify antibodies to type-specific surface proteins of the two subtypes have been developed. These assays, which are based on the demonstration of antibodies to type-specific epitopes of the virus, can reliably distinguish between the human antibody responses to HSV-1 and HSV-2. The most commonly used assays are those that measure antibodies to glycoprotein G of HSV-1 (gG1) and HSV-2 (gG2). A western blot assay that can detect several HSV type-specific proteins can also be used.

Infection with HSV-1 is acquired more frequently and earlier than infection with HSV-2. More than 90% of adults have antibodies to HSV-1 by the fifth decade of life. In populations of low socioeconomic status, most persons acquire HSV-1 infection before the third decade of life.

Antibodies to HSV-2 are not detected routinely until puberty. Antibody prevalence rates correlate with past sexual activity and vary greatly among different population groups. Serosurveys indicate that nearly 22% of the United States population has antibodies to HSV-2—a 30% increase in the past 12 years. In most routine obstetric and family planning clinics, 25% of women have HSV-2 antibodies, although only 10% report a history of genital lesions. As many as 50% of heterosexual adults attending sexually transmitted disease clinics have antibodies to HSV-2. Antibody prevalence rates average about 5% higher among women than among men. Several studies suggest that much of this "asymptomatic" infection is largely unrecognized in that when "asymptomatic" seropositive persons are shown pictures of genital lesions, >60% subsequently identify episodes of symptomatic reactivation. Most important, these asymptomatic seropositive persons with reactivation shed virus on mucosal surfaces as frequently as those with symptomatic disease. The large reservoir of unidentified carriers of HSV-2 and the frequent asymptomatic reactivation of virus from the genital tract have fostered the continued spread of genital herpes throughout the world. HSV-2 infection is an independent risk factor for the acquisition and transmission of infection with HIV type 1. Among coinfected persons, HIV-1 virions can be shed from herpetic lesions of the genital region. This shedding may facilitate the spread of HIV through sexual contact.

HSV infections occur throughout the year. The incubation period ranges from 1 to 26 days (median, 6 to 8 days). Transmission can result from contact with persons with active ulcerative lesions or with persons without clinical manifestations of infection who are shedding HSV or on whose mucosal surfaces the virus is replicating. Studies using the polymerase chain reaction (PCR) have shown that HSV reactivation on mucosal surfaces is much more frequent than previously recognized. Among immunocompetent adults, HSV-2 can be isolated from the genital tract on 2 to 3% of days, and HSV DNA can be detected on 20 to 30% of days. Corresponding figures for HSV-1 in oral secretions are similar. Shedding rates are highest during the initial years of acquisition and may be as high as 30 to 50% of days during this period. Immunosuppressed patients shed HSV on mucosal sites at even higher frequency (20 to 50% of days). Daily antiviral chemotherapy can markedly reduce shedding rates. These data indicate that potential exposure to HSV from sexual or other close contact (kissing, sharing of glasses or silverware) is more common than has been thought. These shedding-rate data are consistent with the high seroprevalence of HSV infections worldwide.

CLINICAL SPECTRUM HSV has been isolated from nearly all visceral or mucocutaneous sites. The clinical manifestations and course of HSV infection depend on the anatomic site involved, the age and immune status of the host, and the antigenic type of the virus. Primary HSV infections (i.e., first infections with either HSV-1 or HSV-2 in which the host lacks HSV antibodies in acute-phase serum) are frequently accompanied by systemic signs and symptoms, involve both mucosal and extramucosal sites, and have a longer duration of symptoms, a longer duration of virus isolation from lesions, and a higher rate of complications than recurrent episodes of disease. Both viral subtypes can cause genital and oral-facial infections, and the infections caused by the two subtypes are clinically indistinguishable. However, the frequency of reactivation of infection is influenced by anatomic site and virus type. Genital HSV-2 infection is twice as likely to reactivate and recurs 8 to 10 times more frequently than genital HSV-1 infection. Conversely, oral-labial HSV-1 infection recurs more frequently than oral-labial HSV-2 infection. Asymptomatic shedding rates follow the same pattern.

Oral-Facial Infections Gingivostomatitis and pharyngitis are the most frequent clinical manifestations of first-episode HSV-1 infection, while recurrent herpes labialis is the most frequent clinical manifestation of reactivation HSV infection. HSV pharyngitis and gingivostomatitis usually result from primary infection and are most commonly seen in children and young adults. Clinical symptoms and signs, which include fever, malaise, myalgias, inability to eat, irritability, and cervical adenopathy, may last from 3 to 14 days. Lesions may involve the hard and soft palate, gingiva, tongue, lip, and facial area. HSV-1 or HSV-2 infection of the pharynx usually results in exudative or ulcerative lesions of the posterior pharynx and/or tonsillar pillars. Lesions of the tongue, buccal mucosa, or gingiva may occur later in the course in one-third of cases. Fever lasting from 2 to 7 days and cervical adenopathy are common. It can be difficult to differentiate HSV pharyngitis clinically from bacterial pharyngitis, *Mycoplasma pneumoniae* infections, and pharyngeal ulcerations of noninfectious etiologies (e.g., Stevens-Johnson syndrome). No substantial evidence suggests that reactivation oral-labial HSV infection is associated with symptomatic recurrent pharyngitis.

Reactivation of HSV from the trigeminal ganglia may be associated with asymptomatic virus excretion in the saliva, development of intraoral mucosal ulcerations, or herpetic ulcerations on the vermilion border of the lip or external facial skin. About 50 to 70% of seropositive patients undergoing trigeminal nerve root decompression and 10 to 15% of those undergoing dental extraction develop oral-labial HSV infection a median of 3 days after these procedures.

In immunosuppressed patients, infection may extend into mucosal and deep cutaneous layers. Friability, necrosis, bleeding, severe pain, and inability to eat or drink may result. The lesions of HSV mucositis are clinically similar to mucosal lesions caused by cytotoxic drug therapy, trauma, or fungal or bacterial infections. Persistent ulcerative

HSV infections are among the most common infections in patients with AIDS. HSV and *Candida* infections often occur concurrently. Systemic antiviral therapy speeds the rate of healing and relieves the pain of mucosal HSV infections in immunosuppressed patients. The frequency of HSV reactivation during the early phases of transplantation or induction chemotherapy is high (50 to 90%), and prophylactic systemic antivirals such as intravenous acyclovir or penciclovir are used to reduce reactivation rates. Patients with atopic eczema also may develop severe oral-facial HSV infections (eczema herpeticum), which may rapidly come to involve extensive areas of skin and occasionally disseminate to visceral organs. Extensive eczema herpeticum has resolved promptly with the administration of intravenous acyclovir. Erythema multiforme (EM) also may be associated with HSV infections (**Plate IIE-67**); some evidence suggests that HSV infection is the precipitating event in ~75% of cases of cutaneous EM. HSV antigen has been demonstrated both in circulatory immune complexes and in skin lesion biopsy samples from these patients. Patients with severe HSV-associated EM are candidates for chronic suppressive oral antiviral therapy.

HSV-1 has been implicated in the etiology of Bell's palsy (flaccid paralysis of the mandibular portion of the facial nerve). Whether antiviral chemotherapy can alter the clinical course and complications of this infection is unclear.

Genital Infections First-episode primary genital herpes is characterized by fever, headache, malaise, and myalgias. Pain, itching, dysuria, vaginal and urethral discharge, and tender inguinal lymphadenopathy are the predominant local symptoms. Widely spaced bilateral lesions of the external genitalia are characteristic. Lesions may be present in varying stages, including vesicles, pustules, or painful erythematous ulcers. The cervix and urethra are involved in >80% of women with first-episode infections. First episodes of genital herpes in patients who have had prior HSV-1 infection are associated with less frequent systemic symptoms and faster healing than primary genital herpes. The clinical courses of acute first-episode genital herpes among patients with HSV-1 and HSV-2 infections are similar. However, the recurrence rates of genital disease differ with the viral subtype: the 12-month recurrence rates among patients with first-episode HSV-2 and HSV-1 infections are ~90% and ~55%, respectively (median number of recurrences, 4 and <1, respectively). Recurrence rates for genital HSV-2 infections vary greatly among individuals and over time within the same individual. HSV has been isolated from the urethra and urine of men and women without external genital lesions. A clear mucoid discharge and dysuria are characteristics of symptomatic HSV urethritis. HSV has been isolated from the urethra of 5% of women with the dysuria-frequency syndrome. Occasionally, HSV genital tract disease is manifested by endometritis and salpingitis in women and by prostatitis in men. About 15% of cases of HSV-2 acquisition are associated with these nonlesional clinical syndromes, such as aseptic meningitis, cervicitis, or urethritis.

Both HSV-1 and HSV-2 can cause symptomatic or asymptomatic rectal and perianal infections. HSV proctitis is usually associated with rectal intercourse. However, subclinical perianal shedding of HSV is detected both in heterosexual men and in women who report no rectal intercourse. This phenomenon is due to the establishment of latency in the sacral dermatome from prior genital tract infection, with subsequent reactivation in epithelial cells in the perianal region. Such reactivations are often subclinical. Symptoms of HSV proctitis include anorectal pain, anorectal discharge, tenesmus, and constipation. Sigmoidoscopy reveals ulcerative lesions of the distal 10 cm of the rectal mucosa. Rectal biopsies show mucosal ulceration, necrosis, polymorphonuclear and lymphocytic infiltration of the lamina propria, and (in occasional cases) multinucleated intranuclear inclusion–bearing cells. Perianal herpetic lesions are also found in immunosuppressed patients receiving cytotoxic therapy. Extensive perianal herpetic lesions and/or HSV proctitis is common among patients with HIV infection.

Herpetic Whitlow Herpetic whitlow—HSV infection of the finger—may occur as a complication of primary oral or genital herpes by inoculation of virus through a break in the epidermal surface or by direct introduction of virus into the hand through occupational or some other type of exposure. Clinical signs and symptoms include the abrupt onset of edema, erythema, and localized tenderness of the infected finger. Vesicular or pustular lesions of the fingertip that are indistinguishable from lesions of pyogenic bacterial infection are seen. Fever, lymphadenitis, and epitrochlear and axillary lymphadenopathy are common. The infection may recur. Prompt diagnosis (to avoid unnecessary and potentially exacerbating surgical therapy and/or transmission) is essential. Antiviral chemotherapy (to speed the healing of the process) is usually recommended (see below).

Herpes Gladiatorum   HSV may infect almost any area of skin. Mucocutaneous HSV infections of the thorax, ears, face, and hands have been described among wrestlers. Transmission of these infections is facilitated by trauma to the skin sustained during wrestling. Prompt diagnosis and therapy are required to contain the spread of this infection.

Eye Infections   HSV infection of the eye is the most frequent cause of corneal blindness in the United States. HSV keratitis presents with an acute onset of pain, blurring of vision, chemosis, conjunctivitis, and characteristic dendritic lesions of the cornea. Use of topical glucocorticoids may exacerbate symptoms and lead to involvement of deep structures of the eye. Debridement, topical antiviral treatment, and/or interferon therapy hastens healing. However, recurrences are common, and the deeper structures of the eye may sustain immunopathologic injury. Stromal keratitis due to HSV appears to be related to T cell–dependent destruction of deep corneal tissue. An HSV-1 epitope that is autoreactive with T cell–targeting corneal antigens has been postulated to be a factor in this infection. Chorioretinitis, usually a manifestation of disseminated HSV infection, may occur in neonates or in patients with HIV infection. HSV and varicella-zoster virus can cause acute necrotizing retinitis as an uncommon but severe manifestation.

Central and Peripheral Nervous System Infections   HSV accounts for 10 to 20% of all cases of sporadic viral encephalitis in the United States. The estimated incidence is about 2.3 cases per million persons per year. Cases are distributed throughout the year, and the age distribution appears to be biphasic, with peaks at 5 to 30 and >50 years of age. Subtype 1 virus causes >95% of cases of HSV encephalitis.

The pathogenesis of HSV encephalitis varies. In children and young adults, primary HSV infection may result in encephalitis; presumably, exogenously acquired virus enters the CNS by neurotropic spread from the periphery via the olfactory bulb. However, most adults with HSV encephalitis have clinical or serologic evidence of mucocutaneous HSV-1 infection before the onset of the CNS symptoms. In ~25% of the cases examined, the HSV-1 strains from the oropharynx and brain tissue of the same patient differ; thus some cases may result from reinfection with another strain of HSV-1 that reaches the CNS. Two theories have been proposed to explain the development of actively replicating HSV in localized areas of the CNS in persons whose ganglionic and CNS isolates are similar. Reactivation of latent HSV-1 infection in trigeminal or autonomic nerve roots may be associated with extension of virus into the CNS via nerves innervating the middle cranial fossa. HSV DNA has been demonstrated by DNA hybridization in brain tissue obtained at autopsy—even from healthy adults. Thus, reactivation of long-standing latent CNS infection may be another mechanism for the development of HSV encephalitis.

The clinical hallmark of HSV encephalitis has been the acute onset of fever and focal neurologic (especially temporal-lobe) symptoms. Clinical differentiation of HSV encephalitis from other viral encephalitides, focal infections, or noninfectious processes is difficult. The most sensitive noninvasive method for early diagnosis of HSV encephalitis is the demonstration of HSV DNA in cerebrospinal fluid (CSF) by PCR. Although titers of CSF and serum antibodies to HSV increase in most cases of HSV encephalitis, they rarely do so earlier than 10 days into the illness and therefore, while useful retrospectively, are generally not helpful in establishing an early clinical diagnosis. Demonstration of HSV antigen, HSV DNA, or HSV replication in

brain tissue obtained by biopsy is highly sensitive and has a low complication rate; examination of such tissue also provides the best opportunity to identify alternative, potentially treatable causes of encephalitis. Antiviral chemotherapy reduces the rate of death from HSV encephalitis. Intravenous acyclovir is more effective than vidarabine. Even with therapy, however, neurologic sequelae are frequent, especially in persons over 35 years of age. Most authorities recommend the administration of intravenous acyclovir to patients with presumed HSV encephalitis until the diagnosis is confirmed or an alternative diagnosis is made.

HSV has been isolated from the CSF of 0.5 to 3% of patients presenting to the hospital with aseptic meningitis. HSV meningitis, which is usually seen in association with primary genital HSV infection, is an acute, self-limited disease manifested by headache, fever, and mild photophobia and lasting from 2 to 7 days. Lymphocytic pleocytosis in the CSF is characteristic. Neurologic sequelae of HSV meningitis are rare. HSV is the most commonly identified cause of recurrent lymphocytic meningitis (Mollaret's meningitis). Demonstration of HSV antibodies in CSF or persistence of HSV DNA in CSF can establish the diagnosis. Daily administration of antiviral therapy aimed at reducing the likelihood of clinical HSV reactivation has been successful in such cases.

Autonomic nervous system dysfunction, especially of the sacral region, has been reported in association with both HSV and varicella-zoster virus infections. Numbness, tingling of the buttocks or perineal areas, urinary retention, constipation, CSF pleocytosis, and (in males) impotence may occur. Symptoms appear to resolve slowly over days to weeks. Occasionally, hypesthesia and/or weakness of the lower extremities may persist for many months. Rarely, transverse myelitis manifested by a rapidly progressive symmetric paralysis of the lower extremities or a Guillain-Barré syndrome may follow HSV infection. Similarly, peripheral nervous system involvement (Bell's palsy) or cranial polyneuritis also may be related to reactivation of HSV-1 infection. Transitory hypesthesia of the area of skin innervated by the trigeminal nerve and vestibular system dysfunction as measured by electronystagmography are the predominant signs of disease. Studies to determine whether antiviral chemotherapy may abort these signs or reduce their frequency and severity are unavailable.

Visceral Infections   HSV infection of visceral organs usually results from viremia, and multiple-organ involvement is common. Occasionally, however, the clinical manifestations of HSV infection involve only the esophagus, lung, or liver. HSV esophagitis may result from direct extension of oral-pharyngeal HSV infection into the esophagus or may occur de novo by reactivation and spread of HSV to the esophageal mucosa via the vagus nerve. The predominant symptoms of HSV esophagitis are odynophagia, dysphagia, substernal pain, and weight loss. There are multiple oval ulcerations on an erythematous base with or without a patchy white pseudomembrane. The distal esophagus is most commonly involved. With extensive disease, diffuse friability may spread to the entire esophagus. Neither endoscopic nor barium examination can differentiate HSV esophagitis from *Candida* esophagitis or from esophageal ulcerations due to thermal injury, radiation, or corrosives. Endoscopically obtained secretions for cytologic examination and culture provide the most useful material for diagnosis. Systemic antiviral chemotherapy usually reduces symptoms and heals esophageal ulcerations.

HSV pneumonitis is uncommon except in severely immunosuppressed patients and may result from extension of herpetic tracheobronchitis into lung parenchyma. Focal necrotizing pneumonitis usually ensues. Hematogenous dissemination of virus from sites of oral or genital mucocutaneous disease also may occur and produce bilateral interstitial pneumonitis. Bacterial, fungal, and parasitic pathogens are commonly present in HSV pneumonitis. The mortality rate from untreated HSV pneumonia in immunosuppressed patients is high (>80%). HSV has also been isolated from the lower respiratory tract of persons with adult respiratory distress syndrome (ARDS). However, the relationship between the isolation of HSV and the pathogenesis of ARDS is unclear.

HSV is an uncommon cause of hepatitis in immunocompetent patients. HSV infection of the liver is associated with fever, abrupt elevations of bilirubin and serum aminotransferase levels, and leukopenia (<4000 white blood cells per microliter). Disseminated intravascular coagulation also may develop.

Other reported complications of HSV infection include monarticular arthritis, adrenal necrosis, idiopathic thrombocytopenia, and glomerulonephritis. Disseminated HSV infection in immunocompetent patients is rare. In immunocompromised, burned, or malnourished patients, HSV occasionally disseminates to other visceral organs, such as the adrenal glands, pancreas, small and large intestines, and bone marrow. Rarely, primary HSV infection in pregnancy disseminates and may be associated with the death of both mother and fetus. This uncommon event is usually related to the acquisition of primary infection in the third trimester.

Neonatal HSV Infection Neonates (infants younger than 6 weeks) have the highest frequency of visceral and/or CNS infection of any HSV-infected patient population. Without therapy, the overall rate of death from neonatal herpes is 65%; fewer than 10% of neonates with CNS infection develop normally. Although skin lesions are the most commonly recognized features of disease, many infants do not develop lesions until well into the course of disease. Neonatal infection is usually acquired perinatally from contact with infected genital secretions at the time of delivery. Congenitally infected infants have been reported. In most series, 30% of neonatal HSV infections are due to HSV-1 and 70% to HSV-2. The risk of developing neonatal HSV infection is 10 times higher for an infant born to a mother who has recently acquired HSV than for other infants. Guidelines to evaluate routine serologic testing for HSV in pregnancy are being drafted and will serve as a basis on which to counsel "susceptible" (HSV-2-uninfected) women regarding the dangers of unprotected coitus and HSV-2 infection near term. Neonatal HSV-1 infections may also be acquired through postnatal contact with immediate family members who have symptomatic or asymptomatic oral-labial HSV-1 infection or through nosocomial transmission within the hospital. Antiviral chemotherapy has reduced the rate of death from neonatal herpes to 25%. However, the rate of morbidity, especially in infants with HSV-2 infection involving the CNS, is still very high.

DIAGNOSIS Both clinical and laboratory criteria are useful for establishing the diagnosis of HSV infections. A clinical diagnosis can be made accurately when characteristic multiple vesicular lesions on an erythematous base are present. However, it is increasingly being recognized that herpetic ulcerations may clinically resemble skin ulcerations of other etiologies. Mucosal HSV infections may also present as urethritis or pharyngitis without cutaneous lesions. Thus, laboratory studies to confirm the diagnosis and to guide therapy are recommended. Staining of scrapings from the base of the lesions with Wright's, Giemsa's (Tzanck preparation), or Papanicolaou's stain demonstrates characteristic giant cells or intranuclear inclusions of herpesvirus infection. These cytologic techniques are often useful as quick office procedures to confirm the diagnosis. Limitations of the cytologic method are that it does not differentiate between HSV and varicella-zoster virus infections, that it is relatively insensitive, and that the correct identification of giant cells requires experience.

HSV infection is best confirmed in the laboratory by isolation of virus in tissue culture or by demonstration of HSV antigens or DNA in scrapings from lesions. HSV causes a discernible cytopathic effect in a variety of cell culture systems, and most specimens can be identified within 48 to 96 h after inoculation. Spin-amplified culture with subsequent staining for HSV antigen has shortened the time needed to identify HSV to <24 h. The sensitivity of viral isolation depends on the stage of lesions (with higher sensitivity in vesicular than in ulcerative lesions), on whether the patient has a first or a recurrent episode of the disease (with higher sensitivity in first than in recurrent episodes), and on whether the sample is from an immunosuppressed or an immunocompetent patient (with more antigen in immunosuppressed patients). Antigen detection procedures have approached viral isolation in terms of sensitivity in detecting HSV in genital or oral-labial lesions; however, antigen detection appears to be only ~50% as sensitive as viral isolation for the identification of HSV in cervical or salivary secretions of asymptomatic patients. PCR techniques appear to be more sensitive for HSV than viral isolation, especially for the diagnosis of CNS infections and for the detection of HSV as a cause of late-stage ulcerative lesions. Laboratory confirmation permits subtyping of the virus; information on subtype may be useful epidemiologically and may help to predict the frequency of reactivation after first-episode oral-labial or genital HSV infection.

Acute- and convalescent-phase serum can be useful in demonstrating seroconversion during primary HSV-1 or HSV-2 infection. However, only 5% of patients with recurrent mucocutaneous HSV infections have a fourfold or greater rise in titer of antibody to HSV in the interval between the collection of the first and second samples. Serologic assays, especially type-specific assays, should be used to identify asymptomatic carriers of HSV-1 or HSV-2 infection.

Several studies have shown that persons seropositive for HSV-2 to whom the clinical manifestations of HSV have been explained are able to identify symptomatic reactivations. Individuals seropositive for HSV-2 should be told about the high frequency of subclinical reactivation in mucosal surfaces not visible to the eye (e.g., cervix, urethra, perianal skin) or in microscopic ulcerations that may not be clinically symptomatic. Transmission of infection during such episodes is well established. HSV-2-seropositive persons should be educated about the high likelihood of subclinical shedding and the role condoms (male or female) may play in reducing transmission. Chronic antiviral therapy is being studied as a means of reducing the transmission of infection.

TREATMENT Many aspects of mucocutaneous and visceral HSV infections are amenable to antiviral chemotherapy. For mucocutaneous infections, acyclovir and its congeners famciclovir and valacyclovir have been the mainstay of therapy. Several antiviral agents are available for topical use in HSV eye infections: idoxuridine, trifluorothymidine, topical vidarabine, and cidofovir. For HSV encephalitis and neonatal herpes, intravenous acyclovir is the treatment of choice.

All licensed antivirals for HSV inhibit the viral DNA polymerase. One class of drugs, typified by the drug acyclovir, is made up of substrates for the HSV enzyme thymidine kinase. Acyclovir, ganciclovir, famciclovir, and valacyclovir are all selectively phosphorylated to the monophosphate form in virus-infected cells. Cellular enzymes convert the monophosphate form of the drug to the triphosphate, which is then incorporated into the viral DNA chain.

Acyclovir is the most frequently used agent for the treatment of HSV infections and is available in intravenous, oral, and topical formulations. Famciclovir, the oral formulation of penciclovir, is clinically effective in the treatment of a variety of HSV-1 and HSV-2 infections. Intravenous penciclovir is also available. Valacyclovir is the valyl ester of acyclovir and has greater bioavailability than acyclovir. Ganciclovir has activity against both HSV-1 and HSV-2; however, it is more toxic than acyclovir, valacyclovir, and famciclovir and is generally not recommended for the treatment of HSV infections.

All three compounds—acyclovir, valacyclovir, and famciclovir—have proven effective in shortening the duration of symptoms and lesions of mucocutaneous HSV infections in both immunocompromised and immunocompetent patients (Table 182-1). Intravenous and oral formulations prevent reactivation of HSV in seropositive immunocompromised patients during induction chemotherapy or in the period immediately after bone marrow or solid organ transplantation. Chronic daily suppressive therapy reduces the frequency of reactivation disease among patients with frequent genital or oral-labial herpes.

Intravenous acyclovir (30 mg/kg per day, given as a 10-mg/kg infusion over 1 h at 8-h intervals) is effective in reducing rates of death and morbidity from HSV encephalitis. Early initiation of therapy is a

Table 182-1   Antiviral Chemotherapy for HSV Infection

Mucocutaneous HSV infections

Infections in immunosuppressed patients

Acute symptomatic first or recurrent episodes: IV acyclovir (5 mg/kg q8h) or oral acyclovir (400 mg qid for 7–10 days) relieves pain and speeds healing.

Suppression of reactivation disease: IV acyclovir (5 mg/kg q12h) or oral acyclovir (400–800 mg 3–5 times per day) prevents recurrences during high-risk periods, e.g., the immediate posttransplantation period. In HIV-infected persons, oral famciclovir (500 mg bid) or valacyclovir (500 mg bid) is also effective.

Genital herpes

First episodes: Oral acyclovir (200 mg 5 times per day or 400 mg tid) is given. Oral valacyclovir (1000 mg bid) or famciclovir (250 mg tid) for 10–14 days is effective. IV acyclovir (5 mg/kg q8h for 5 days) is given for severe disease or neurologic complications such as aseptic meningitis.

Symptomatic recurrent genital herpes: Oral acyclovir (200 mg 5 times per day or 400 mg tid for 5 days), valacyclovir (500 mg bid), or famciclovir (125 mg bid) is effective in shortening lesion duration and viral excretion time.

Suppression of recurrent genital herpes: Oral acyclovir (200-mg capsules; 400 mg bid or 800 mg qd), famciclovir (250 mg bid), or valacyclovir (250 or 500 mg bid or 1000 mg qd) prevents symptomatic reactivation.

Oral-labial HSV infections

First episode: Oral acyclovir (200 mg) is given 4 or 5 times per day. Famciclovir (250 mg bid) or valacyclovir (1000 mg bid) has been used clinically.

Recurrent episodes: Topical penciclovir cream is effective in speeding the healing of oral-labial HSV. Topical acyclovir cream is licensed in Europe. The ointment formulation of acyclovir available in the U.S. has no clinical benefit. Oral valacyclovir has some benefit. Oral acyclovir has minimal benefit.

Suppression of reactivation of oral-labial HSV: Oral acyclovir (400 mg bid), if started before exposure and continued for the duration of exposure (usually 5–10 days), prevents reactivation of recurrent oral-labial HSV infection associated with severe sun exposure.

Herpetic whitlow: Oral acyclovir (200 mg) is given 5 times daily for 7–10 days.

HSV proctitis: Oral acyclovir (400 mg 5 times per day) is useful in shortening the course of infection. In immunosuppressed patients or in patients with severe infection, IV acyclovir (5 mg/kg q8h) may be useful.

Herpetic eye infections: In acute keratitis, topical trifluorothymidine, vidarabine, idoxuridine, acyclovir, penciclovir, and interferon are all beneficial. Debridement may be required; topical steroids may worsen disease.

CNS HSV infections

HSV encephalitis: Intravenous acyclovir (10 mg/kg q8h; 30 mg/kg per day) for 10 days is preferred.

HSV aseptic meningitis: No studies of systemic antiviral chemotherapy exist. If therapy is to be given, IV acyclovir (15–30 mg/kg per day) should be used.

Autonomic radiculopathy: No studies are available.

Neonatal HSV infections: Acyclovir (60 mg/kg per day, divided into 3 doses) is given. The recommended duration of treatment is 21 days.

Visceral HSV infections

HSV esophagitis: IV acyclovir (5 mg/kg q8h) is given. In some patients with milder forms of immunosuppression, oral therapy with valacyclovir or famciclovir is effective.

HSV pneumonitis: No controlled studies exist. IV acyclovir (15 mg/kg per day) should be considered.

Surgical prophylaxis: IV acyclovir (5 mg/kg q12h) or oral acyclovir (800 mg bid), famciclovir (250 mg bid), or valacyclovir (500 mg bid) is given 2–3 days before laser resurfacing or other neurologic procedures.

Disseminated HSV infections: No controlled studies exist. Intravenous acyclovir nevertheless should be tried. No definite evidence indicates that therapy decreases the risk of death.

Erythema multiforme associated with HSV: Anecdotal observations suggest that oral acyclovir (400 mg bid or tid) suppresses erythema multiforme.

Infections due to acyclovir-resistant HSV: Foscarnet (40 mg/kg IV q8h) should be given until lesions heal. The optimal duration of therapy and the usefulness of its continuation to suppress lesions are unclear. Some patients may benefit from cutaneous application of trifluorothymidine or 5% cidofovir gel.

critical factor in outcome. The major side effect associated with intravenous acyclovir is transient renal insufficiency, usually due to crystallization of the compound in the renal parenchyma. This adverse reaction can be avoided if the medication is given slowly over 1 h and the patient is well hydrated. Because CSF levels of acyclovir average only 30 to 50% of plasma levels, the dosage of acyclovir used for treatment of CNS infection (30 mg/kg per day) is double that used for treatment of mucocutaneous or visceral disease (15 mg/kg per day).

Acyclovir-resistant strains of HSV have been identified. Most of these strains have an altered substrate specificity for phosphorylating acyclovir. Thus, cross-resistance to famciclovir and valacyclovir is usually found. Occasionally, an isolate with altered thymidine kinase (TK) specificity arises and is sensitive to famciclovir but not to acyclovir. In some patients infected with TK-deficient virus, higher doses of acyclovir are associated with clearing of lesions. In others, clinical disease progresses despite high-dose therapy. Almost all clinically significant acyclovir resistance has been seen in immunocompromised patients, and HSV-2 isolates are more often resistant than HSV-1 strains. A study by the Centers for Disease Control and Prevention indicated that ~5% of isolates from HIV-positive persons exhibit some degree of in vitro resistance to acyclovir. Isolation of HSV from persisting lesions despite adequate dosages and blood levels of acyclovir should raise the suspicion of acyclovir resistance. Therapy with the antiviral drug foscarnet is useful (Chap. 181). Because of its toxicity and cost, this drug is usually reserved for patients with extensive mucocutaneous infections. Cidofovir is a nucleotide analogue and exists as a phosphonate or monophosphate form. Most TK-deficient strains of HSV are sensitive to cidofovir. Cidofovir ointment speeds healing of acyclovir-resistant lesions. No well-controlled trials of systemic cidofovir have been reported. True TK-negative variants of HSV appear to have a reduced capacity to spread because of altered neurovirulence—a feature important in the relatively infrequent presence of such strains in immunocompetent populations, even with increasing use of antivirals.

PREVENTION   The large reservoir of persons with asymptomatic HSV-1 and HSV-2 infections indicates that the success of efforts to control HSV disease through suppressive antiviral chemotherapy and/or educational programs will be limited. Rather, control of HSV infection will require the prevention of infection—a goal most likely to be attained by vaccination. Several candidate vaccines are under investigation, and the prevention of HSV infection has been assigned a high public health priority.

Barrier forms of contraception, especially condoms, decrease the likelihood of transmission of HSV infection, especially during periods of asymptomatic viral excretion. When lesions are present, HSV infection may be transmitted by skin-to-skin contact despite the use of a condom. Nevertheless, the available data suggest that consistent condom use is an effective means of reducing the risk of genital HSV-2 transmission. Prevention of neonatal HSV requires the prevention of acquisition of HSV in the third trimester of pregnancy. Identification of women or couples susceptible to acquisition of HSV in pregnancy through serologic screening is receiving increasing attention, and such screening is being used with increasing frequency.

BIBLIOGRAPHY

BENEDETTI J et al: Clinical reactivation of genital herpes simplex virus infection decreases in frequency over time. Ann Intern Med 131:14, 1999

BLOWER SM et al: Predicting and preventing the emergence of antiviral drug resistance in HSV-2. Nat Med 4:673, 1998

BROWN ZA et al: The acquisition of herpes simplex virus during pregnancy. N Engl J Med 337:509, 1997

COREY L, SPEAR P: Infections with herpes simplex viruses. N Engl J Med 314:686, 1986

FLEMING DT et al: Herpes simplex virus type 2 in the United States, 1976 to 1994. N Engl J Med 337:1105, 1997

LANGENBERG AGM et al: A prospective study of new infections with herpes simplex virus type 1 and herpes simplex virus type 2. N Engl J Med 341:1532, 1999

Mertz GJ et al: Oral famciclovir for the suppression of recurrent genital herpes simplex virus infection in women. Arch Intern Med 157:334, 1997

Reitano M et al: Valaciclovir for the suppression of recurrent genital herpes simplex virus infection: A large-scale dose range–finding study. J Infect Dis 178:602, 1998

Schacker T et al: Frequent recovery of HIV-1 from genital herpes simplex virus lesions in HIV-1-infected men. JAMA 280:61, 1998

Wald A et al: Suppression of subclinical shedding of herpes simplex virus type 2 with acyclovir. Ann Intern Med 124:8, 1996

——— et al: Frequent genital herpes simplex virus 2 shedding in immunocompetent women: Effect of acyclovir treatment. J Clin Invest 99:1092, 1997

Whitley RJ et al: Herpes simplex virus infections of the central nervous system: Therapeutic and diagnostic considerations. Clin Infect Dis 20:414, 1995

——— et al: Herpes simplex viruses. Clin Infect Dis 26:541, 1998

Zhao ZS et al: Molecular mimicry by herpes simplex virus-type 1: Autoimmune disease after viral infection. Science 279:1344, 1998

183   Richard J. Whitley

VARICELLA-ZOSTER VIRUS INFECTIONS

DEFINITION   Varicella-zoster virus (VZV) causes two distinct clinical entities: varicella (chickenpox) and herpes zoster (shingles). Chickenpox, a ubiquitous and extremely contagious infection, is usually a benign illness of childhood characterized by an exanthematous vesicular rash. With reactivation of latent VZV (which is most common after the sixth decade of life), herpes zoster presents as a dermatomal vesicular rash, usually associated with severe pain.

ETIOLOGY   A clinical association between varicella and herpes zoster has been recognized for nearly 100 years. Early in the twentieth century, similarities in the histopathologic features of skin lesions resulting from varicella and herpes zoster were demonstrated. Viral isolates from patients with chickenpox and herpes zoster produced similar alterations in tissue culture—specifically, the appearance of eosinophilic intranuclear inclusions and multinucleated giant cells. These results suggested that the viruses were biologically similar. Restriction endonuclease analyses of viral DNA from a patient with chickenpox who subsequently developed herpes zoster verified the molecular identity of the two viruses responsible for these different clinical presentations.

VZV is a member of the family Herpesviridae, sharing with other members such structural characteristics as a lipid envelope surrounding a nucleocapsid with icosahedral symmetry, a total diameter of approximately 180 to 200 nm, and centrally located double-stranded DNA that is about 125,000 bp in length.

PATHOGENESIS AND PATHOLOGY   Primary Infection Transmission is most likely to take place by the respiratory route; the subsequent localized replication of the virus at an undefined site (presumably the nasopharynx) leads to seeding of the reticuloendothelial system and ultimately to the development of viremia. Viremia in patients with chickenpox is reflected in the diffuse and scattered nature of the skin lesions and can be verified in selected cases by the recovery of VZV from the blood. Vesicles involve the corium and dermis, with degenerative changes characterized by ballooning, the presence of multinucleated giant cells, and eosinophilic intranuclear inclusions. Infection may involve localized blood vessels of the skin, resulting in necrosis and epidermal hemorrhage. With the evolution of disease, the vesicular fluid becomes cloudy because of the recruitment of polymorphonuclear leukocytes and the presence of degenerated cells and fibrin. Ultimately, the vesicles either rupture and release their fluid (which includes infectious virus) or are gradually reabsorbed.

Recurrent Infection   The mechanism of reactivation of VZV that results in herpes zoster is unknown. Presumably, the virus infects the dorsal root ganglia during chickenpox, where it remains latent until reactivated. Histopathologic examination of representative dorsal root ganglia during active herpes zoster demonstrates hemorrhage, edema, and lymphocytic infiltration.

Active replication of VZV in other organs, such as the lung or the brain, can occur during either chickenpox or herpes zoster but is uncommon in the immunocompetent host. Pulmonary involvement is characterized by interstitial pneumonitis, multinucleated giant cell formation, intranuclear inclusions, and pulmonary hemorrhage. Central nervous system (CNS) infection leads to histopathologic evidence of perivascular cuffing similar to that encountered in measles and other viral encephalitides. Focal hemorrhagic necrosis of the brain, characteristic of herpes simplex virus encephalitis, is uncommon in VZV infection.

EPIDEMIOLOGY AND CLINICAL MANIFESTATIONS Chickenpox   Humans are the only known reservoir for VZV. Chickenpox is highly contagious, with an attack rate of at least 90% among susceptible (seronegative) individuals. Persons of both sexes and all races are infected equally often. The virus is endemic in the population at large; however, it becomes epidemic among susceptible individuals during seasonal peaks—namely, late winter and early spring in the temperate zone. Children between the ages of 5 and 9 are most commonly affected and account for 50% of all cases. Most other cases involve children aged 1 to 4 and those aged 10 to 14. Approximately 10% of the population of the United States over the age of 15 is susceptible to infection.

The incubation period of chickenpox ranges between 10 and 21 days but is usually between 14 and 17 days. Secondary attack rates in susceptible siblings within a household are between 70 and 90%. Patients are infectious approximately 48 h prior to the onset of the vesicular rash, during the period of vesicle formation (which generally lasts 4 to 5 days), and until all vesicles are crusted.

Clinically, chickenpox presents as a rash, low-grade fever, and malaise, although a few patients develop a prodrome 1 to 2 days before onset of the exanthem. In the immunocompetent patient, this is usually a benign illness that is associated with lassitude and with body temperatures of 37.8 to 39.4°C (100 to 103°F) of 3 to 5 days' duration. The skin lesions—the hallmark of the infection—include maculopapules, vesicles, and scabs in various stages of evolution (**Plate IID-36**). These lesions, which evolve from maculopapules to vesicles over hours to days, appear on the trunk and face and rapidly spread to involve other areas of the body. Most are small and have an erythematous base with a diameter of 5 to 10 mm. Successive crops appear over a 2- to 4-day period. Lesions also can be found on the mucosa of the pharynx and/or the vagina. Their severity varies from one person to another. Some individuals have very few lesions, while others have as many as 2000. Younger children tend to have fewer vesicles than older individuals. Secondary and tertiary cases within families are associated with a relatively large number of vesicles. Immunocompromised patients—both children and adults, particularly those with leukemia—have lesions (often with a hemorrhagic base) that are more numerous and take longer to heal than those of immunocompetent patients. Immunocompromised individuals are also at greater risk for visceral complications, which occur in 30 to 50% of cases and are fatal 15% of the time.

The most common infectious complication of varicella is secondary bacterial superinfection of the skin, which is usually caused by *Streptococcus pyogenes* or *Staphylococcus aureus*. This complication may result from excoriation of skin lesions after scratching. Gram's staining of skin lesions should help clarify the etiology of unusually erythematous and pustulated lesions.

The most common extracutaneous site of involvement in children is the CNS. The syndrome of acute cerebellar ataxia and meningeal irritation generally appears around 21 days after the onset of the rash and rarely develops in the preeruptive phase. The cerebrospinal fluid (CSF) contains lymphocytes and elevated levels of protein. CNS involvement is a benign complication of VZV infection in children and generally does not require hospitalization. Aseptic meningitis, encephalitis, transverse myelitis, Guillain-Barré syndrome, and Reye's syndrome also can occur. Encephalitis is reported in 0.1 to 0.2% of children with chickenpox. Other than supportive care, no specific therapy is available for patients with CNS involvement.

Varicella pneumonia is the most serious complication following chickenpox, developing more commonly in adults (up to 20% of cases) than in children. It usually has its onset 3 to 5 days into the illness and is associated with tachypnea, cough, dyspnea, and fever. Cyanosis, pleuritic chest pain, and hemoptysis are frequent. Roentgenographic evidence of disease consists of nodular infiltrates and interstitial pneumonitis. Resolution of pneumonitis parallels improvement of the skin rash; however, patients may have persistent fever and compromised pulmonary function for weeks.

Other complications of chickenpox include myocarditis, corneal lesions, nephritis, arthritis, bleeding diatheses, acute glomerulonephritis, and hepatitis. Hepatic involvement, distinct from Reye's syndrome and usually asymptomatic, is common in chickenpox and is usually characterized by elevated levels of liver enzymes, particularly aspartate and alanine aminotransferases.

Perinatal varicella is associated with a high mortality rate when maternal disease develops within 5 days before delivery or within 48 h thereafter. Because the newborn does not receive protective transplacental antibodies and has an immature immune system, the illness may be unusually severe. The reported mortality rate has been as high as 30% in this group. Congenital varicella, with clinical manifestations of limb hypoplasia, cicatricial skin lesions, and microcephaly at birth, is extremely uncommon.

Herpes Zoster Herpes zoster, a sporadic disease, is the consequence of reactivation of latent VZV from the dorsal root ganglia. Most patients have no history of recent exposure to other individuals with VZV infection. Herpes zoster occurs at all ages, but its incidence is highest (5 to 10 cases per 1000 persons) among individuals in the sixth through the eighth decades of life. Recurrent herpes zoster is exceedingly rare except in immunocompromised hosts, especially those with AIDS.

Herpes zoster, also called shingles, is characterized by a unilateral vesicular eruption within a dermatome, often associated with severe pain. The dermatomes from T3 to L3 are most frequently involved. If the ophthalmic branch of the trigeminal nerve is involved, zoster ophthalmicus results. The factors responsible for the reactivation of VZV are not known. In children reactivation is usually benign, whereas in adults it can be debilitating. The continuum of pain from onset to resolution is known as *zoster-associated pain*. The onset of disease is heralded by pain within the dermatome that may precede lesions by 48 to 72 h; an erythematous maculopapular rash evolves rapidly into vesicular lesions. In the normal host, these lesions may remain few in number and continue to form only for a period of 3 to 5 days. The total duration of disease is generally between 7 and 10 days; however, it may take as long as 2 to 4 weeks for the skin to return to normal. In a few patients, characteristic localization of pain to a dermatome with serologic evidence of herpes zoster has been reported in the absence of skin lesions. When branches of the trigeminal nerve are involved, lesions may appear on the face, in the mouth, in the eye, or on the tongue. In the Ramsay Hunt syndrome (**Plate IID-35**), pain and vesicles appear in the external auditory canal, and patients lose their sense of taste in the anterior two-thirds of the tongue while developing ipsilateral facial palsy. The geniculate ganglion of the sensory branch of the facial nerve is involved.

The most debilitating complication of herpes zoster, in both the normal and the immunocompromised host, is pain associated with acute neuritis and postherpetic neuralgia. Postherpetic neuralgia is uncommon in young individuals; however, at least 50% of patients over age 50 with zoster report some degree of pain in the involved dermatome months after the resolution of cutaneous disease. Changes in sensation in the dermatome, resulting in either hypo- or hyperesthesia, are common.

CNS involvement may follow localized herpes zoster. Many pa-

tients without signs of meningeal irritation have CSF pleocytosis and moderately elevated levels of CSF protein. Symptomatic meningoencephalitis is characterized by headache, fever, photophobia, meningitis, and vomiting. A rare manifestation of CNS involvement is granulomatous angiitis with contralateral hemiplegia, which can be diagnosed by cerebral arteriography. Other neurologic manifestations include transverse myelitis with or without motor paralysis.

Like chickenpox, herpes zoster is more severe in the immunocompromised host than in the normal individual. Lesions continue to form for over a week, and scabbing is not complete in most cases until 3 weeks into the illness. Patients with Hodgkin's disease and non-Hodgkin's lymphoma are at greatest risk for progressive herpes zoster. Cutaneous dissemination (**Plate IID-37**) develops in about 40% of these patients. Among patients with cutaneous dissemination, the risk of pneumonitis, meningoencephalitis, hepatitis, and other serious complications is increased by 5 to 10%. However, even in immunocompromised patients, disseminated zoster is rarely fatal.

Patients who have received a bone marrow transplant are at particularly high risk of VZV infection. Thirty percent of cases of posttransplantation VZV infection occur within 1 year (50% of these within 9 months); 45% of the patients involved have cutaneous or visceral dissemination. The mortality rate in this situation is 10%. Postherpetic neuralgia, scarring, and bacterial superinfection are especially frequent in VZV infections occurring within 9 months of transplantation. Among infected patients, concomitant graft-versus-host disease increases the chance of dissemination and/or death.

DIFFERENTIAL DIAGNOSIS The diagnosis of chickenpox is not difficult. The characteristic rash and a history of recent exposure should lead to a prompt diagnosis. Other viral infections that can mimic chickenpox include disseminated herpes simplex virus infection in patients with atopic dermatitis and the disseminated vesiculopapular lesions sometimes associated with coxsackievirus infection, echovirus infection, or atypical measles. However, these rashes are more commonly morbilliform with a hemorrhagic component rather than vesicular or vesiculopustular. Rickettsialpox can be confused with chickenpox; however, it can be distinguished easily by detection of the "herald spot" at the site of the mite bite and the development of a more pronounced headache. Serologic testing is also useful in differentiating rickettsialpox from varicella.

Unilateral vesicular lesions in a dermatomal pattern should lead rapidly to the diagnosis of herpes zoster, although the occurrence of shingles without a rash has been reported. Both herpes simplex virus infections and coxsackievirus infections can cause dermatomal vesicular lesions. Supportive diagnostic virology and fluorescent staining of skin scrapings with monoclonal antibodies are helpful in ensuring the proper diagnosis. In the prodromal stage of herpes zoster, the diagnosis can be exceedingly difficult and may be made only after lesions have appeared or by retrospective serologic assessment.

LABORATORY FINDINGS Unequivocal confirmation of the diagnosis is possible only through the isolation of VZV in susceptible tissue-culture cell lines, the demonstration of either seroconversion or a fourfold or greater rise in antibody titer between convalescent- and acute-phase serum specimens, or the detection of VZV DNA by polymerase chain reaction (PCR). A rapid impression can be obtained by a Tzanck smear, with scraping of the base of the lesions in an attempt to demonstrate multinucleated giant cells, although the sensitivity of this method is low (about 60%). PCR technology for the detection of viral DNA in vesicular fluid is available in a limited number of diagnostic laboratories. Direct immunofluorescent staining of cells from the lesion base or detection of viral antigens by other assays (such as the immunoperoxidase assay) is also useful, although these tests are not commercially available. The most frequently employed serologic tools for assessing host response are the immunofluorescent detection of antibodies to VZV membrane antigens, the fluorescent antibody to membrane antigen (FAMA) test, immune adherence hemagglutination, and enzyme-linked immunosorbent assay (ELISA). The FAMA test and the ELISA appear to be the most sensitive.

PROPHYLAXIS While chickenpox in the otherwise healthy host is relatively benign, it can cause morbidity and death. Furthermore, the parents of a child with chickenpox often lose a significant amount of time from work. A live attenuated varicella vaccine has been licensed and is recommended for administration to all immunocompetent children and adults at risk of infection.

The immunocompromised individual is at significant risk for developing progressive varicella; modalities of prevention include passive immunization or experimental administration of the same live attenuated vaccine used in the immunocompetent child. Immune prophylaxis can consist of the administration of specific zoster immune globulin (ZIG) derived from patients with herpes zoster, varicella-zoster immune globulin (VZIG), or the intravenous formulation of zoster immune plasma (ZIP). Both ZIG and VZIG should be given within 96 h (preferably within 72 h) of exposure to ensure efficacy. It is likely that ZIP can be given somewhat later. Indications for the administration of VZIG are summarized in Table 183-1.

℞ **TREATMENT** Medical management of chickenpox in the immunologically normal host is directed toward the prevention of avoidable complications. Obviously, good hygiene includes daily bathing and soaks. Secondary bacterial infection of the skin can be avoided by meticulous skin care, particularly with close cropping of fingernails. Pruritus can be decreased with topical dressings or the administration of antipruritic drugs. Tepid water baths and wet compresses are better than drying lotions for the relief of itching. Aluminum acetate soaks for the management of herpes zoster can be both soothing and cleansing. Administration of aspirin to children with chickenpox should be avoided because of the association of aspirin derivatives with the development of Reye's syndrome. Acyclovir therapy (800 mg by mouth five times daily for 5 to 7 days) is recommended for adolescents and adults with chickenpox of ≤24 h duration. Likewise, acyclovir therapy may be of benefit to children <12 years of age if initiated early in the disease (<24 h) at a dose of 20 mg/kg every 6 h.

Patients with herpes zoster benefit from oral antiviral therapy, as evidenced by accelerated healing of lesions and resolution of zoster-associated pain with acyclovir, valacyclovir, or famciclovir. Acyclovir,

now off patent, is administered at a dosage of 800 mg five times daily for 7 to 10 days. Famciclovir, the prodrug of penciclovir, is at least as effective as acyclovir and perhaps more so. One study showed twofold faster resolution of postherpetic neuralgia in famciclovir-treated patients with zoster than in recipients of placebo. The dose is 500 mg by mouth three times daily for 7 days. Valacyclovir, the prodrug of acyclovir, accelerates healing and resolution of zoster-associated pain more promptly than acyclovir. The dose is 1 g by mouth three times daily for 5 to 7 days. Both famciclovir and valacyclovir offer the advantage of a lower dosing frequency than acyclovir.

In the immunocompromised host, both chickenpox and herpes zoster (including disseminated disease) should be treated with intravenous acyclovir, which reduces the occurrence of visceral complications but has no effect on healing of skin lesions or pain. The dose is 10 to 12.5 mg/kg every 8 h for 7 days. Oral acyclovir therapy is not recommended for the treatment of VZV infections in immunocompromised patients. Concomitant with the administration of intravenous acyclovir, it is desirable to attempt to wean these patients from immunosuppressive treatment.

Patients with varicella pneumonia may require removal of bronchial secretions and ventilatory support. Persons with zoster ophthalmicus should be referred immediately to an ophthalmologist. Therapy for this condition consists of the administration of analgesics for severe pain and the use of atropine. Acyclovir accelerates healing.

The management of acute neuritis and/or postherpetic neuralgia can be particularly difficult. In addition to the judicious use of analgesics, ranging from nonnarcotics to narcotic derivatives, drugs such as gabapentin, amitriptyline hydrochloride, and fluphenazine hydrochloride have been reported to be beneficial for pain relief. In one study, glucocorticoid therapy administered early in the course of localized herpes zoster significantly accelerated such quality-of-life improvements as a return to usual activity and termination of analgesia. The dose of prednisone administered orally was 60 mg/d on days 1 through 7, 30 mg/d on days 8 through 14, and 15 mg/d on days 15 through 21. This regimen is appropriate only for relatively healthy elderly persons who have moderate or severe pain at presentation. Patients with osteoporosis, diabetes mellitus, glycosuria, or hypertension may not be appropriate candidates. Glucocorticoids should not be used without concomitant antiviral therapy.

BIBLIOGRAPHY

BEUTNER KR et al: Valacyclovir compared with acyclovir for improved therapy for herpes zoster in immunocompetent adults. Antimicrob Agents Chemother 39:1547, 1995

DUNKLE LM et al: A controlled trial of acyclovir for chickenpox in normal children. N Engl J Med 325:1539, 1991

IZURIETA HS et al: Postlicensure effectiveness of varicella vaccine during an outbreak in a child care center. JAMA 278:1495, 1997

LOCKSLEY RM et al: Infection with varicella-zoster virus after marrow transplantation. J Infect Dis 152:1172, 1985

ROWBOTHAM M et al: Gabapentin for the treatment of postherpetic neuralgia. A randomized controlled trial. JAMA 280:1837, 1998

SHEPP D et al: Treatment of varicella-zoster virus in severely immunocompromised patients: A randomized comparison of acyclovir and vidarabine. N Engl J Med 314:208, 1987

TYRING S et al: Famciclovir for the treatment of acute herpes zoster. Effects on acute disease and postherpetic neuralgia: A randomized, double-blind, placebo-controlled trial. Ann Intern Med 123:89, 1995

WEIBEL RE et al: Live attenuated varicella virus vaccine: Efficacy trial in healthy children. N Engl J Med 310:1409, 1984

WHITLEY RJ et al: Early vidarabine therapy to control the complications of herpes zoster in immunosuppressed patients. N Engl J Med 307:971, 1982

—— et al: Disseminated herpes zoster in the immunocompromised host: A comparative trial of acyclovir and vidarabine. J Infect Dis 165:450, 1992

—— et al: Acyclovir with and without prednisone for the treatment of herpes zoster: A randomized, placebo-controlled trial. Ann Intern Med 125:376, 1996

WOOD MJ et al: A randomized trial of acyclovir for 7 days or 21 days with and without prednisolone for treatment of acute herpes zoster. N Engl J Med 330:896, 1994

Table 183-1   Recommendations for VZIG Administration

Exposure criteria
1. Both exposure to person with chickenpox or zoster as
   a. Continuous household contact
   b. Playmate for >1 h indoors
   c. Hospital contact (same room or prolonged face-to-face)
   d. Mother (see 3 below)
2. And time elapsed ≤96 h (preferably ≤72 h)

Candidates (provided they have significant exposure) include
1. Immunocompromised susceptible children
2. Immunocompetent susceptible adolescents (≥15 years old) and adults, especially pregnant women
3. Newborn infants of mothers with onset of chickenpox <5 days before or <2 days after delivery
4. Hospitalized premature infants
   a. ≥28 weeks of gestation when mother has no history of chickenpox
   b. <28 weeks of gestation and/or birth weight of ≤1000 g, regardless of maternal history

SOURCE: Adapted from American Academy of Pediatrics, in Red Book, Report of the Committee on Infectious Diseases, G Peter (ed), Elk Grove Village, IL, American Academy of Pediatrics, 1997.

184

Jeffrey I. Cohen

EPSTEIN-BARR VIRUS INFECTIONS, INCLUDING INFECTIOUS MONONUCLEOSIS

DEFINITION   Epstein-Barr virus (EBV) is the cause of heterophile-positive infectious mononucleosis (IM), which is characterized by fever, sore throat, lymphadenopathy, and atypical lymphocytosis. EBV is also associated with several human tumors, including nasopharyngeal carcinoma, Burkitt's lymphoma, Hodgkin's disease, and—in patients with immunodeficiencies (including AIDS)—B cell lymphoma. The virus, a member of the family Herpesviridae, consists of a linear, double-stranded DNA core surrounded by an icosahedral nucleocapsid and by the viral envelope, which contains glycoproteins. The two types of EBV that are widely prevalent in nature are not distinguishable by conventional serologic tests.

EPIDEMIOLOGY   EBV infections occur worldwide. These infections are most common in early childhood, with a second peak during late adolescence. By adulthood, more than 90% of individuals have been infected and have antibodies to the virus. IM is usually a disease of young adults. In lower socioeconomic groups and in areas of the world with lower standards of hygiene (e.g., developing countries), EBV tends to infect children at an early age, and symptomatic IM is uncommon. In areas with higher standards of hygiene (e.g., the United States), infection with EBV is often delayed until adulthood, and IM is more prevalent.

EBV is spread by contact with oral secretions. The virus is frequently transmitted from asymptomatic adults to infants and among young adults by transfer of saliva during kissing. Transmission by less intimate contact is rare. EBV has been transmitted by blood transfusion and by bone marrow transplantation. Studies indicate that more than 90% of asymptomatic seropositive individuals shed the virus in oropharyngeal secretions.

PATHOGENESIS   EBV is transmitted by salivary secretions. The virus infects the epithelium of the oropharynx and the salivary glands and is shed from these cells. While B cells may become infected after contact with epithelial cells, studies suggest that lymphocytes in the tonsillar crypts can be infected directly. The virus then spreads through the bloodstream. The proliferation and expansion of EBV-infected B cells along with reactive T cells during IM result in enlargement of lymphoid tissue. Polyclonal activation of B cells leads to the production of antibodies to host-cell and viral proteins. During the acute phase of IM, up to 1 in every 100 B cells in the peripheral blood is infected by EBV, while after recovery, about 1 in every million B cells is infected. During IM there is an inverted CD4+/CD8+ T cell ratio. The percentage of CD4+ T cells decreases, while there are large clonal expansions of CD8+ T cells; up to 40% of CD8+ T cells are directed against EBV antigens during acute infection. Data suggest that memory B cells, not epithelial cells, are the reservoir for EBV in the body. Shedding of EBV from the oropharynx stops but the virus persists in B cells when patients are treated with acyclovir.

The EBV receptor (CD21), present on the surface of B cells and epithelial cells, is also the receptor for the C3d component of complement. EBV infection of epithelial cells results in viral replication and production of virions. When B cells are infected by EBV in vitro, they become transformed and can proliferate indefinitely. During latent infection of B cells, only the EBV nuclear antigens (EBNAs), latent membrane proteins (LMPs), and small EBV RNAs are expressed in vitro. EBV-transformed B cells secrete immunoglobulin; only a small fraction of cells produce virus.

Cellular immunity is more important than humoral immunity in controlling EBV infection. In the initial phase of infection, suppressor T cells, natural killer cells, and nonspecific cytotoxic T cells are important in controlling the proliferation of EBV-infected B cells. Levels of markers of T cell activation and serum interferon γ are elevated.

Later in infection, HLA-restricted cytotoxic T cells that recognize EBNAs and LMPs and destroy EBV-infected cells are generated. Studies have shown that one of the late genes expressed during EBV replication, *BCRF1*, is a homologue of interleukin 10 and can inhibit the production of interferon γ by mononuclear cells in vitro. In addition, EBNA-1 inhibits antigen processing.

If T cell immunity is compromised, EBV-infected B cells may begin to proliferate. When EBV is associated with lymphoma, virus-induced proliferation is but one step in a multistep process of neoplastic transformation. In many EBV-containing tumors, LMP-1 mimics members of the tumor necrosis factor receptor family (e.g., CD40), transmitting growth-proliferating signals.

CLINICAL MANIFESTATIONS   Most EBV infections in infants and young children either are asymptomatic or present as mild pharyngitis with or without tonsillitis. In contrast, up to 75% of infections in adolescents present as IM.

Signs and Symptoms   The incubation period for IM in young adults is about 4 to 6 weeks. A prodrome of fatigue, malaise, and myalgia may last for 1 to 2 weeks before the onset of fever, sore throat, and lymphadenopathy. Fever is usually low-grade and is most common in the first 2 weeks of the illness; however, it may persist for over a month. Common signs and symptoms are listed along with their frequencies in Table 184-1. Lymphadenopathy and pharyngitis are most prominent during the first 2 weeks of the illness, while splenomegaly is more prominent during the second and third weeks. Lymphadenopathy most often affects the posterior cervical nodes but may be generalized. Enlarged lymph nodes are frequently tender and symmetric but are not fixed in place. Pharyngitis, often the most prominent sign, can be accompanied by enlargement of the tonsils with an exudate resembling that of streptococcal pharyngitis. A morbilliform or papular rash, usually on the arms or trunk, develops in about 5% of cases. Most patients treated with ampicillin develop a macular rash; this rash is not predictive of future adverse reactions to penicillins. Erythema nodosum and erythema multiforme have also been described (Chap. 57). Most patients have symptoms for 2 to 4 weeks, but malaise and difficulty concentrating can persist for months.

Symptomatic IM is uncommon in infants and young children. IM in the elderly presents relatively often as nonspecific symptoms, including prolonged fever, fatigue, myalgia, and malaise; in contrast, pharyngitis, lymphadenopathy, splenomegaly, and atypical lymphocytes are relatively rare in elderly patients.

Laboratory Findings   The white blood cell count is usually elevated and peaks at 10,000 to 20,000/μL during the second or third week of illness. Lymphocytosis is usually demonstrable, with more than 10% atypical lymphocytes. The latter cells are enlarged lympho-

Table 184-1   Signs and Symptoms of Infectious Mononucleosis

Manifestation	Median Percentage of Patients (Range)
Symptoms	
Sore throat	75 (50–87)
Malaise	47 (42–76)
Headache	38 (22–67)
Abdominal pain, nausea, or vomiting	17 (5–25)
Chills	10 (9–11)
Signs	
Lymphadenopathy	95 (83–100)
Fever	93 (60–100)
Pharyngitis or tonsillitis	82 (68–90)
Splenomegaly	51 (43–64)
Hepatomegaly	11 (6–15)
Rash	10 (0–25)
Periorbital edema	13 (2–34)
Palatal enanthem	7 (3–13)
Jaundice	5 (2–10)

Table 184-2 Serologic Features of EBV-Associated Diseases

Condition	Heterophile	Anti-VCA		Anti-EA		Anti-EBNA
		IgM	IgG	EA-D	EA-R	
Acute infectious mononucleosis	+	+	++	+	−	−
Convalescence	±	−	+	−	±	+
Past infection	−	−	+	−	−	+
Reactivation with immunodeficiency	−	−	++	+	+	±
Burkitt's lymphoma	−	−	+++	±	++	+
Nasopharyngeal carcinoma	−	−	+++	++	±	+

Result in Indicated Test[a]

[a] VCA, viral capsid antigen; EA, early antigen; EA-D antibody, antibody to early antigen, diffuse pattern in nucleus and cytoplasm of infected cells; EA-R antibody, antibody to early antigen, restricted to the cytoplasm; and EBNA, Epstein-Barr nuclear antigen.

SOURCE: Adapted from Okano, 1988.

cytes that have abundant cytoplasm, vacuoles, and indentations of the cell membrane. CD8+ cells predominate among the atypical lymphocytes. Low-grade neutropenia and thrombocytopenia are common during the first month of illness. Liver function is abnormal in more than 90% of cases. Serum levels of aminotransferases and alkaline phosphatase are usually mildly elevated; the serum concentration of bilirubin is elevated in about 40% of cases.

Complications Most cases of IM are self-limited. Deaths are very rare and most often are due to central nervous system (CNS) complications, splenic rupture, upper airway obstruction, or bacterial superinfection.

When CNS complications develop, they usually do so during the first 2 weeks of EBV infection; in some patients, especially children, they are the only clinical manifestations of IM. Heterophile antibodies and atypical lymphocytes may be absent. Meningitis and encephalitis are the most common neurologic abnormalities, and patients may present with headache, meningismus, or cerebellar ataxia; acute hemiplegia and psychosis have also been described. The cerebrospinal fluid (CSF) contains mainly lymphocytes, with occasional atypical lymphocytes. Most cases resolve without neurologic sequelae. Acute EBV infection has also been associated with cranial nerve palsies (especially ones involving cranial nerve VII), Guillain-Barré syndrome, acute transverse myelitis, and peripheral neuritis.

Autoimmune hemolytic anemia occurs in about 2% of cases during the first 2 weeks. In most cases the anemia is Coombs'-test positive, with cold agglutinins directed against the i red blood cell antigen. Most patients with hemolysis have mild anemia that lasts for 1 or 2 months, but some patients have severe disease with hemoglobinuria and jaundice. Nonspecific antibody responses may also include rheumatoid factor, antinuclear antibodies, anti–smooth muscle antibodies, antiplatelet antibodies, and cryoglobulins. IM has been associated with red-cell aplasia, severe granulocytopenia, thrombocytopenia, pancytopenia, and hemophagocytic syndrome. The spleen ruptures in fewer than 0.5% of cases. Splenic rupture is more common among males than among females and may be manifest as abdominal pain, referred shoulder pain, or hemodynamic compromise.

Hypertrophy of lymphoid tissue in the tonsils or adenoids can result in upper airway obstruction, as can inflammation and edema of the epiglottis, pharynx, or uvula. About 10% of patients with IM develop streptococcal pharyngitis after their initial sore throat resolves.

Other rare complications associated with acute EBV infection include hepatitis (which can be fulminant), myocarditis or pericarditis with electrocardiographic changes, pneumonia with pleural effusion, interstitial nephritis, genital ulcerations, and vasculitis.

OTHER DISEASES ASSOCIATED WITH EBV INFECTION EBV-associated lymphoproliferative disease has been described in patients with congenital or acquired immunodeficiency, including those with severe combined immunodeficiency or AIDS, recipients of bone marrow transplants, and recipients of organ transplants who are receiving immunosuppressive drugs (especially cyclosporine). Proliferating EBV-infected B cells infiltrate lymph nodes and

multiple organs, and patients present with fever and lymphadenopathy or gastrointestinal symptoms. Pathologic studies show B cell hyperplasia or poly- or monoclonal lymphoma. The X-linked lymphoproliferative syndrome (Duncan's disease) is a recessive disorder of young boys who have a normal response to childhood infections but develop fatal lymphoproliferative disorders after infection with EBV. The gene mutated in this syndrome, SAP or SH2D1A, has been identified; its product binds to a protein that mediates interactions of B and T cells. Most patients with this syndrome die of acute IM; others develop hypogammaglobulinemia, malignant B cell lymphomas, aplastic anemia, or agranulocytosis. IM has also proved fatal to some patients with no obvious preexisting immune abnormality.

Oral hairy leukoplakia (**Plate IID-42**) is an early manifestation of infection with HIV in adults (Chap. 309). Most patients present with raised, white corrugated lesions on the tongue (and occasionally on the buccal mucosa) that contain EBV DNA. Children infected with HIV can develop lymphoid interstitial pneumonitis; EBV DNA is often found in lung tissue from these patients.

Patients with the chronic fatigue syndrome may have titers of antibody to EBV that are elevated but are not significantly different from those in healthy EBV-seropositive adults. While some patients have malaise and fatigue that persist for weeks or months after IM, persistent EBV infection is not a cause of the chronic fatigue syndrome. Chronic active EBV infection is very rare and is distinct from the chronic fatigue syndrome. The affected patients have an illness lasting more than 6 months with markedly elevated titers of antibody to EBV and evidence of organ involvement, including hepatosplenomegaly, lymphadenopathy, and pneumonitis, uveitis, or neurologic disease.

EBV is associated with several malignancies. About 15% of cases of Burkitt's lymphoma in the United States and about 90% of those in Africa are associated with EBV (Chap. 112). African patients with Burkitt's lymphoma have high levels of antibody to EBV, and their tumor tissue usually contains viral DNA. EBV-containing Burkitt's lymphoma also occurs in patients with AIDS. Anaplastic nasopharyngeal carcinoma is uniformly associated with EBV; the affected tissues contain viral DNA and antigens. Patients with nasopharyngeal carcinoma often have elevated titers of antibody to EBV (Chap. 87).

EBV has been associated with Hodgkin's disease, especially the mixed-cellularity type (Chap. 112). Patients with Hodgkin's disease often have elevated titers of antibody to EBV, and in about half of cases viral DNA and antigens are found in Reed-Sternberg cells. In some cases, EBV DNA has been detected in tonsillar carcinoma, angioimmunoblastic lymphadenopathy, angiocentric nasal NK/T cell immunoproliferative lesions, T cell lymphoma, thymoma, gastric carcinoma, and CNS lymphoma from patients with no underlying immunodeficiency. Studies have demonstrated viral DNA in leiomyosarcomas from AIDS patients and in smooth-muscle tumors from organ transplant recipients. Virtually all CNS lymphomas in AIDS patients are associated with EBV.

DIAGNOSIS Serologic Testing The heterophile test is used for the diagnosis of IM in children and adults (Table 184-2). Heterophile antibody is an IgM antibody that does not bind EBV proteins. In the test for this antibody, human serum is absorbed with guinea pig kidney, and the heterophile titer is defined as the greatest serum dilution that agglutinates sheep, horse, or cow erythrocytes. A titer of 40-fold or greater is diagnostic of acute EBV infection in a patient who has symptoms compatible with IM and atypical lymphocytes. Tests for heterophile antibodies are positive in 40% of patients with IM during the first week of illness and in 80 to 90% during the third week. Therefore, repeated testing may be necessary, especially if the initial test is performed early. Tests usually remain positive for 3 months after the onset of illness, but heterophile antibodies can persist for up to 1 year. These antibodies usually are not detectable in children <5 years of age, in the elderly, or in patients presenting with symptoms not typical of IM. The commercially available monospot test for heterophile antibodies is somewhat more sensitive than the classic heterophile test. False-positive results in the monospot test are more common in children and in patients with other viral infections.

EBV-specific antibody testing is used for patients with suspected acute EBV infection who lack heterophile antibodies and for patients with atypical infections. Serologic tests are particularly useful in young children, who often do not develop heterophile antibodies. Titers of IgM and IgG antibodies to viral capsid antigen (VCA) are elevated in the serum of more than 90% of patients at the onset of disease. IgM antibody to VCA is useful for the diagnosis of acute IM because it is present at elevated titers only during the first 2 months of the disease; in contrast, IgG antibody to VCA is often used to assess exposure to EBV in the past because it persists for life.

Antibodies to early antigens (EAs) are found either in a diffuse pattern in the nucleus and cytoplasm of infected cells (EA-D antibody) or restricted to the cytoplasm (EA-R antibody). These antibodies are detectable 3 to 4 weeks after the onset of symptoms in patients with IM. About 70% of individuals with IM, especially those with relatively severe disease, have EA-D antibodies during the course of their illness. These antibodies usually persist for only 3 to 6 months. Levels of EA-D antibodies are also elevated in patients with nasopharyngeal carcinoma or chronic active EBV infection. EA-R antibodies are only occasionally detected in patients with IM but are often found at elevated titers in patients with African Burkitt's lymphoma or chronic active EBV infection.

IgA antibodies to EBV antigens have proved useful for the identification of patients with nasopharyngeal carcinoma and of persons at high risk for the disease. Seroconversion to EBNA positivity is also useful for the diagnosis of acute infection with EBV. Antibodies to EBNA are detectable relatively late (3 to 6 weeks after the onset of symptoms) in nearly all cases of acute EBV infection and persist for the lifetime of the patient. These antibodies may be lacking in immunodeficient patients and in those with chronic active EBV infection.

Other Studies Detection of EBV DNA, RNA, or proteins has been valuable in demonstrating the association of the virus with various malignancies. The polymerase chain reaction has been used to detect EBV DNA in the CSF of some AIDS patients with lymphomas and to monitor the amount of EBV DNA in the blood of patients with lymphoproliferative disease. Culture of EBV from throat washings or blood is not helpful in the diagnosis of acute infection, since EBV commonly persists in the oropharynx and in B cells for the lifetime of the infected individual.

Differential Diagnosis The differential diagnosis of IM and atypical lymphocytosis includes acute infection with cytomegalovirus, *Toxoplasma*, HIV, human herpesvirus 6, and hepatitis viruses as well as drug hypersensitivity reactions. Cytomegalovirus is the most common cause of heterophile-negative mononucleosis, usually involves older patients, and is associated with a lower frequency of sore throat, splenomegaly, and lymphadenopathy than IM due to EBV. Other diseases that share some of the features of IM include rubella, acute infectious lymphocytosis in children, and lymphoma or leukemia.

℞ **TREATMENT** Therapy for IM consists of supportive measures, with rest and analgesia. Excessive physical activity during the first month should be avoided to reduce the possibility of splenic rupture. If splenic rupture occurs, splenectomy is required. Glucocorticoid therapy is not indicated for uncomplicated IM and in fact may predispose to bacterial superinfection. Prednisone (40 to 60 mg/d for 2 to 3 days, with subsequent tapering of the dose over 1 to 2 weeks) has been used for the prevention of airway obstruction in patients with severe tonsillar hypertrophy, for autoimmune hemolytic anemia, and for severe thrombocytopenia. Glucocorticoids have also been used in

a few selected patients with severe malaise and fever and in patients with severe CNS or cardiac disease.

Acyclovir has had no significant clinical impact on IM in controlled trials. In one study, the combination of acyclovir and prednisolone had no significant effect on the duration of symptoms of IM. Acyclovir, at a dosage of 400 to 800 mg five times daily, has been effective for the treatment of oral hairy leukoplakia (despite common relapses) and some cases of chronic active EBV disease. This agent generally has not been beneficial for patients with lymphoproliferative syndromes. When possible, therapy for EBV lymphoproliferative disease should be directed toward the reduction of immunosuppressive medication. New therapies, including the use of interferon α and the infusion of donor T cells or EBV-specific cytotoxic T cells, are being studied.

The isolation of patients with IM is unnecessary. Vaccines directed against the major EBV glycoprotein have been effective in animal studies and are currently undergoing small-scale clinical trials.

BIBLIOGRAPHY

AUWAERTER PG: Infectious mononucleosis in middle age. JAMA 281:454, 1999

COHEN JI: Epstein-Barr virus and the immune system—hide and seek. JAMA 278:510, 1997

———: Epstein-Barr virus lymphoproliferative disease associated with acquired immunodeficiency. Medicine 70:137, 1991

HESLOP HE et al: Long-term restoration of immunity against Epstein-Barr virus infection by adoptive transfer of gene-modified virus-specific T lymphocytes. Nat Med 2:551, 1996

LIEBOWITZ D: Epstein-Barr virus and a cellular signaling pathway in lymphomas from immunosuppressed patients. N Engl J Med 338:1413, 1998

OKANO M et al: Epstein-Barr virus and human diseases: Recent advances in diagnosis. Clin Microbiol Rev 1:300, 1988

PAPADOPOULOS EB et al: Infusions of donor leukocytes to treat Epstein-Barr virus-associated lymphoproliferative disorders after allogeneic bone marrow transplantation. N Engl J Med 330:1185, 1994

PATHMANATHAN R et al: Clonal proliferations of cells infected with Epstein-Barr virus in proliferative lesions related to nasopharyngeal carcinoma. N Engl J Med 333:693, 1995

RICKINSON AB, KIEFF E: Epstein-Barr virus, in *Fields Virology,* 3d ed, BN Fields et al (eds). Philadelphia, Lippincott-Raven, 1996

SAYOS J et al: The X-linked lymphoproliferative-disease gene product SAP regulates signals induced through the co-receptor SLAM. Nature 395:462, 1998

STRAUS SE: Epstein-Barr virus infections: Biology, pathogenesis, and management. Ann Intern Med 118:45, 1993

TYNELL E et al: Acyclovir and prednisolone treatment of acute infectious mononucleosis: A multicenter, double blind, placebo-controlled study. J Infect Dis 174:324, 1996

---

185   *Martin S. Hirsch*

CYTOMEGALOVIRUS AND HUMAN HERPESVIRUS TYPES 6, 7, AND 8

CYTOMEGALOVIRUS

DEFINITION Cytomegalovirus (CMV), which was initially isolated from patients with congenital cytomegalic inclusion disease, is now recognized as an important pathogen in all age groups. In addition to inducing severe birth defects, CMV causes a wide spectrum of disorders in older children and adults, ranging from an asymptomatic, subclinical infection to a mononucleosis syndrome in healthy individuals to disseminated disease in immunocompromised patients. Human CMV is one of several related species-specific viruses that cause similar diseases in various animals. All are associated with the production of characteristic enlarged cells—hence the name *cytomegalovirus*.

CMV is a member of the β-herpesvirus group and has double-

Table 185-1 CMV in the Immunocompromised Host

Population	Risk Factors	Principal Syndromes	Treatment	Prevention
Fetus	Primary maternal infection/early pregnancy	Cytomegalic inclusion disease	None	Avoidance of exposure
Organ transplant recipient	Seropositive donor, seronegative recipient; intensive immunosuppression, particularly with antilymphocyte globulins, cyclosporine	Febrile leukopenia; pneumonia; gastrointestinal disease	Ganciclovir	Donor matching; CMV immunoglobulin; ganciclovir or high-dose acyclovir
Bone marrow transplant recipient	Graft-vs.-host disease; older age; seropositive recipient; viremia	Pneumonia; gastrointestinal disease	Ganciclovir plus CMV immunoglobulin	Ganciclovir or high-dose acyclovir
Person with AIDS	<100 CD4+ cells per microliter; CMV seropositivity	Retinitis; gastrointestinal disease; neurologic disease	Foscarnet, ganciclovir, or cidofovir	Oral ganciclovir

stranded DNA, a protein capsid, and a lipoprotein envelope. Like other herpesviruses, CMV demonstrates icosahedral symmetry, replicates in the cell nucleus, and can cause either a lytic and productive or a latent infection. CMV can be distinguished from other herpesviruses by certain biologic properties, such as host range and type of cytopathology induced. Viral replication is associated with the production of large intranuclear inclusions and smaller cytoplasmic inclusions. The virus appears to replicate in a variety of cell types in vivo; in tissue culture it grows preferentially in fibroblasts. Although there is little evidence that CMV is oncogenic in vivo, the virus does transform fibroblasts in rare instances, and genomic transforming fragments have been identified.

EPIDEMIOLOGY CMV has a worldwide distribution. Approximately 1% of newborns in the United States are infected with CMV, and the percentage is higher in many less developed countries. Communal living and poor personal hygiene facilitate early spread. Perinatal and early childhood infections are common. Virus may be present in milk, saliva, feces, and urine. Transmission of CMV has been identified among young children in day-care centers and has been traced from infected toddler to pregnant mother to developing fetus. When an infected child introduces CMV into a household, 50% of susceptible family members seroconvert within 6 months.

The virus is not readily spread by casual contact but requires repeated or prolonged intimate exposure for transmission. In late adolescence and young adulthood, CMV is often transmitted sexually, and asymptomatic viral carriage in semen or cervical secretions is common. CMV antibody is present at detectable levels in nearly 100% of female prostitutes and sexually active homosexual men. Sexually active adults may harbor several strains of CMV simultaneously. Transfusion of whole blood or certain blood products containing viable leukocytes may also transmit CMV, with a frequency of 0.14 to 10% per unit transfused.

Once infected, an individual probably carries CMV for life. The infection usually remains latent. However, CMV reactivation syndromes develop frequently when T lymphocyte–mediated immunity is compromised—for example, after organ transplantation or in association with lymphoid neoplasms and certain acquired immunodeficiencies (in particular, infection with HIV; Chap. 309). Most primary CMV infections in organ transplant recipients (Chap. 136) result from transmission of the virus in the graft itself. In CMV-seropositive transplant recipients, infection results from reactivation of latent virus or, less commonly, from reinfection by a new strain of CMV. CMV infection may be associated with coronary artery stenosis following heart transplantation or coronary angioplasty, but this association requires further validation.

PATHOGENESIS Congenital CMV infection can result from either primary or reactivation infection of the mother. However, clinical disease in the fetus or newborn is almost exclusively related to primary maternal infection (Table 185-1). The factors determining the severity of congenital infection are unknown; a deficient capacity to produce precipitating antibodies and to mount T cell responses to CMV is associated with relatively severe disease.

Primary infection in late childhood or adulthood is often associated with a vigorous T lymphocyte response that may contribute to the development of a mononucleosis syndrome similar to that observed following Epstein-Barr virus (EBV) infection (Chap. 184). The hallmark of such infection is the appearance of atypical lymphocytes in the peripheral blood; these cells are predominantly activated CD8+ T lymphocytes. Polyclonal activation of B cells by the virus contributes to the development of rheumatoid factors and other autoantibodies during CMV mononucleosis.

Once acquired by symptomatic or asymptomatic primary infection, CMV persists indefinitely in tissues of the host. The sites of persistent or latent infection are unclear but probably include multiple cell types and various organs. Transmission following blood transfusion or organ transplantation is due to silent infections in these tissues. Autopsy studies suggest that salivary glands and bowel may be areas of latent infection.

If the host's T cell responses become compromised by disease or by iatrogenic immunosuppression, latent virus can be reactivated to cause a variety of syndromes. Chronic antigenic stimulation in the presence of immunosuppression (for example, following tissue transplantation) appears to be an ideal setting for CMV activation and CMV-induced disease. Certain particularly potent suppressants of T cell immunity, such as antithymocyte globulin, are associated with a high rate of clinical CMV syndromes, which may follow either primary or reactivation infection. CMV may itself contribute to further T lymphocyte hyporesponsiveness, which often precedes superinfection with other opportunistic pathogens, such as *Pneumocystis carinii*. CMV and *P. carinii* are frequently found together in immunosuppressed patients with severe interstitial pneumonia. CMV may function as a cofactor to activate latent HIV infection.

PATHOLOGY Cytomegalic cells in vivo (presumed to be infected epithelial cells) are two to four times larger than surrounding cells and often contain an 8- to 10-μm intranuclear inclusion that is eccentrically placed and is surrounded by a clear halo, producing an "owl's eye" appearance. Smaller granular cytoplasmic inclusions are demonstrated occasionally. Cytomegalic cells are found in a wide variety of organs, including salivary gland, lung, liver, kidney, intestine, pancreas, adrenal gland, and the central nervous system.

The cellular inflammatory response to infection consists of plasma cells, lymphocytes, and monocyte-macrophages. Granulomatous reactions occasionally develop, particularly in the liver. Immunopathologic reactions may contribute to CMV disease. Immune complexes have been detected in infected infants, sometimes in association with CMV-related glomerulopathies. Immune-complex glomerulopathy has been observed in some CMV-infected patients after renal transplantation.

CLINICAL MANIFESTATIONS Congenital CMV Infection Fetal infections range from inapparent to severe and disseminated. Cytomegalic inclusion disease develops in approximately 5% of infected fetuses and is seen almost exclusively in infants born to mothers who develop primary infections during pregnancy. Petechiae, hepatosplenomegaly, and jaundice are the most common presenting features (60 to 80% of cases). Microcephaly with or without cerebral calcifications, intrauterine growth retardation, and prematurity are reported in 30 to 50% of cases. Inguinal hernias and chorioretinitis are less common. Laboratory abnormalities include elevated alanine aminotransferase levels, thrombocytopenia, conjugated hyperbilirubinemia, hemolysis, and elevated cerebrospinal fluid protein levels. The prognosis for severely infected infants is poor; the mortality rate is 20 to 30%, and few of the patients who survive escape intellectual or hearing difficulties in later years. The differential diagnosis of cytomegalic inclusion disease in infants includes syphilis, rubella, toxoplasmosis, infection with herpes simplex virus or enterovirus, and bacterial sepsis.

Most congenital CMV infections are clinically inapparent at birth. Between 5 and 25% of asymptomatically infected infants develop significant psychomotor, hearing, ocular, or dental abnormalities over the next several years.

Perinatal CMV Infection The newborn may acquire CMV at the time of delivery by passage through an infected birth canal or by postnatal contact with maternal milk or other secretions. Approximately 40 to 60% of infants who are breast-fed for longer than 1 month by seropositive mothers become infected. Iatrogenic transmission also can result from neonatal blood transfusion. Screening of blood products before they are transfused into low-birth-weight seronegative infants or into seronegative pregnant women decreases the risk of infection.

The great majority of infants infected at or after delivery remain asymptomatic. However, protracted interstitial pneumonitis has been associated with perinatally acquired CMV infection, particularly in premature infants, and occasionally has been accompanied by infection with *Chlamydia trachomatis*, *P. carinii*, or *Ureaplasma urealyticum*. Poor weight gain, adenopathy, rash, hepatitis, anemia, and atypical lymphocytosis may also be found, and CMV excretion often persists for months or years.

CMV Mononucleosis The most common clinical manifestation of CMV infection in normal hosts beyond the neonatal period is a heterophil antibody–negative mononucleosis syndrome. This manifestation may develop spontaneously or may follow the transfusion of leukocyte-containing blood products. Although the syndrome occurs at all ages, it most often involves sexually active young adults. Incubation periods range from 20 to 60 days, and the illness generally lasts for 2 to 6 weeks. Prolonged high fevers, sometimes accompanied by chills, profound fatigue, and malaise, characterize this disorder. Myalgias, headache, and splenomegaly are frequent, but in CMV mononucleosis (as opposed to infectious mononucleosis caused by EBV), exudative pharyngitis and cervical lymphadenopathy are rare. Occasional patients develop rubelliform rashes, often after exposure to ampicillin. Less commonly observed are interstitial or segmental pneumonia, myocarditis, pleuritis, arthritis, and encephalitis. In rare cases, Guillain-Barré syndrome complicates CMV mononucleosis. The characteristic laboratory abnormality is relative lymphocytosis in peripheral blood, with more than 10% atypical lymphocytes. Total leukocyte counts may be low, normal, or markedly elevated. Although significant jaundice is uncommon, serum aminotransferase and alkaline phosphatase levels are often moderately elevated. Heterophil antibodies are absent; however, transient immunologic abnormalities are common and may include the presence of cryoglobulins, rheumatoid factors, cold agglutinins, and antinuclear antibodies. Hemolytic anemia, thrombocytopenia, and granulocytopenia complicate recovery in rare instances.

Most patients recover without sequelae, although postviral asthenia may persist for months. The excretion of CMV in urine, genital secretions, and/or saliva often continues for months or years. Rarely, CMV infection is fatal in immunocompetent hosts; even when such patients survive, they can have recurrent episodes of fever and malaise that are sometimes associated with autonomic nervous system dysfunction (e.g., attacks of sweating or flushing).

CMV Infection in the Immunocompromised Host (See also Table 185-1) CMV appears to be the most common and important viral pathogen complicating organ transplantation (Chap. 136). In recipients of kidney, heart, lung, and liver transplants, CMV induces a variety of syndromes, including fever and leukopenia, hepatitis, pneumonitis, esophagitis, gastritis, colitis, and retinitis. CMV disease may be an independent risk factor for both graft loss and death. The period of maximal risk is between 1 and 4 months after transplantation, although retinitis may be a later complication. The risk of disease appears to be greater after primary infection than after reactivation. In addition, molecular studies indicate that seropositive transplant recipients are susceptible to reinfection with donor-derived, genotypically variant CMV, and such infection often results in disease. Reactivation infection, although frequent, is less likely than primary infection to be important clinically. Clinical disease is related to various factors, such as the degree of immunosuppression; patients receiving certain immunosuppressive agents, such as antithymocyte globulin, appear to be more likely to have severe infections than those receiving other agents, such as cyclosporine. The transplanted organ is particularly vulnerable as a target for CMV infection; thus, there is a tendency for CMV hepatitis to follow liver transplantation and for CMV pneumonitis to follow lung transplantation.

CMV pneumonia occurs in 15 to 20% of bone marrow transplant recipients, with a case-fatality rate of 84 to 88%. The risk is greatest between 5 and 13 weeks after transplantation, and the several risk factors identified include certain types of immunosuppressive therapy, acute graft-versus-host disease, older age, viremia, and seropositivity before transplantation.

CMV is recognized as an important pathogen in patients with advanced HIV infection (Chap. 309), in whom it often causes retinitis or disseminated disease, particularly when peripheral-blood CD4+ cell counts fall below 50 to $100/\mu L$. As treatment for underlying HIV infection has improved, the incidence of serious CMV infections (e.g., retinitis) has decreased. However, institution of highly active antiretroviral regimens sometimes leads to acute flare-ups of CMV retinitis during the first few weeks of therapy.

Syndromes produced by CMV in the immunocompromised host often begin with prolonged fever, malaise, anorexia, fatigue, night sweats, and arthralgias or myalgias. Liver function abnormalities, leukopenia, thrombocytopenia, and atypical lymphocytosis may be observed during these episodes. The development of tachypnea, hypoxia, and unproductive cough signals respiratory involvement. Radiologic examination of the lung often demonstrates bilateral interstitial or reticulonodular infiltrates, which begin in the periphery of the lower lobes and spread centrally and superiorly; localized segmental, nodular, or alveolar patterns are less common. The differential diagnosis includes infection with *P. carinii*; infections due to other viral, bacterial, or fungal pathogens; pulmonary hemorrhage; and injury secondary to irradiation or to treatment with cytotoxic drugs.

Gastrointestinal CMV involvement may be localized or extensive and almost exclusively affects compromised hosts. Ulcers of the esophagus, stomach, small intestine, or colon may result in bleeding or perforation. CMV infection may lead to exacerbations of underlying ulcerative colitis. Hepatitis occurs frequently, particularly following liver transplantation, and CMV-associated acalculous cholecystitis and adrenalitis have been described.

CMV rarely causes meningoencephalitis in otherwise healthy individuals. Two forms of CMV encephalitis are seen in patients with AIDS. One resembles HIV encephalitis and presents as progressive dementia; the other is a ventriculoencephalitis characterized by cranial-nerve deficits, nystagmus, disorientation, lethargy, and ventriculomegaly. In immunocompromised patients, CMV can also cause subacute progressive polyradiculopathy, which is often reversible if recognized and treated promptly.

CMV retinitis is an important cause of blindness in immunocompromised patients, particularly patients with advanced AIDS (Chap. 309). Early lesions consist of small, opaque, white areas of granular retinal necrosis that spread in a centrifugal manner and are later accompanied by hemorrhages, vessel sheathing, and retinal edema (see **Plate IV-2**). CMV retinopathy must be distinguished from that due to other conditions, including toxoplasmosis, candidiasis, and herpes simplex virus infection.

Fatal CMV infections are often associated with persistent viremia and the involvement of multiple organ systems. Progressive pulmonary infiltrates, pancytopenia, hyperamylasemia, and hypotension are characteristic features that are frequently found in conjunction with a terminal bacterial, fungal, or protozoan superinfection. Extensive adrenal necrosis with CMV inclusions is often documented at autopsy, as is CMV involvement of many other organs.

DIAGNOSIS   The diagnosis of CMV infection usually cannot be made reliably on clinical grounds alone. Isolation of the virus or detection of CMV antigens or DNA from appropriate clinical specimens, together with demonstration of a fourfold or greater rise in antibody titers or persistently elevated antibody titers, is the preferred diagnostic approach. Virus excretion or viremia is readily detected by culture of appropriate specimens on human fibroblast monolayers. If viral titers are high, as is frequently the case in congenital disseminated infection or in patients with AIDS, characteristic cytopathic effects may be detected within a few days. However, in some situations—such as CMV mononucleosis—viral titers are low, and cytopathic effects may take several weeks to appear. Many laboratories expedite diagnosis with an overnight tissue-culture method (shell vial assay) involving centrifugation and an immunocytochemical detection technique employing monoclonal antibodies to an immediate-early CMV antigen. Isolation of virus from urine or saliva does not, by itself, constitute proof of acute infection, since excretion from these sites may continue for months or years after illness. Detection of CMV viremia is a better predictor of acute infection.

Detection of CMV antigens (pp65) in peripheral-blood leukocytes or of CMV DNA in blood or tissues may hasten the diagnosis of CMV disease in certain populations, including organ transplant recipients and persons with AIDS. Such assays may yield a positive result several days earlier than culture methods. The detection of CMV DNA in cerebrospinal fluid by the polymerase chain reaction is useful in the diagnosis of CMV encephalitis or polyradiculopathy.

A variety of serologic assays are available to detect increases in titers of antibody to CMV antigens. An increased antibody level may not be detectable for up to 4 weeks after primary infection, and titers often remain high for years after infection. For this reason, single-sample antibody determinations are of no value in assessing the acuteness of infection. Detection of CMV-specific IgM is sometimes useful in the diagnosis of recent or active infection; circulating rheumatoid factors may result in occasional false-positive IgM tests.

℞ **TREATMENT**   Several prophylactic measures are useful for the prevention of CMV infection in patients at high risk. The use of blood from seronegative donors or of blood that has been frozen, thawed, and deglycerolized greatly decreases the rate of transfusion-associated transmission of CMV. Similarly, matching of organ or bone marrow transplants by CMV serology, using organs only from seronegative donors for seronegative recipients, reduces rates of primary infection following transplantation. Both live attenuated and CMV subunit vaccines have been evaluated, but neither is close to approval for general use.

CMV immune globulin has been reported to reduce rates of occurrence of CMV-associated syndromes and of fungal or parasitic superinfections among seronegative renal transplant recipients. Studies in bone marrow transplant recipients have produced conflicting results. Prophylactic acyclovir has been demonstrated to reduce rates of CMV infection and disease in certain seronegative renal transplant recipients; acyclovir is not effective in the treatment of active CMV disease, however.

Ganciclovir is a guanosine derivative that has considerably more activity against CMV than its congener acyclovir. After intracellular conversion by a viral phosphotransferase encoded by CMV gene re-

gion UL97, ganciclovir triphosphate is a selective inhibitor of CMV DNA polymerase. Several clinical studies have indicated response rates of 70 to 90% among patients with AIDS given ganciclovir for the treatment of CMV retinitis or colitis. In bone marrow transplant recipients with CMV pneumonia, ganciclovir is less effective when given alone, but it elicits a favorable clinical response 50 to 70% of the time when it is combined with CMV immune globulin. Prophylactic or suppressive ganciclovir may be useful in high-risk bone marrow or organ transplant recipients (e.g., those who are CMV-seropositive before transplantation or who are CMV culture–positive afterward). In many patients with AIDS, persistently low CD4+ cell counts, and CMV disease, clinical and virologic relapses occur promptly if treatment with ganciclovir is discontinued. Therefore, prolonged maintenance regimens are recommended for such patients. Resistance to ganciclovir is common among patients treated for more than 3 months and is usually related to mutations in the CMV UL97 gene.

Ganciclovir therapy for CMV retinitis consists of a 14- to 21-day induction course (5 mg/kg intravenously twice a day) followed by a prolonged intravenous or oral maintenance regimen. For parenteral maintenance, the dose is 5 mg/kg daily or 6 mg/kg 5 days per week. Peripheral-blood neutropenia develops in 16 to 29% of treated patients but is often ameliorated by granulocyte or granulocyte-macrophage colony-stimulating factor. Oral ganciclovir at a high dose (3 g/d) can also be used for maintenance, although the blood levels achieved are insufficient for acute induction regimens. Although progression (as assessed by funduscopy) is more rapid with oral than with intravenous ganciclovir maintenance (mean time to progression, 68 vs. 96 days; $p = .03$), the ease of administration and reduced toxicity of the oral preparation may make it an acceptable alternative for some patients who do not have sight-threatening central retinitis. The use of oral ganciclovir as prophylaxis in high-risk AIDS patients (i.e., those with CD4+ cell counts of $<100/\mu L$) has been studied in two placebo-controlled trials, with somewhat contradictory results.

Foscarnet (sodium phosphonoformate) also acts against CMV infection by inhibiting viral DNA polymerase. Because this agent does not require phosphorylation to be active, it is also effective against most ganciclovir-resistant CMV isolates. A comparative trial of foscarnet and ganciclovir in 234 patients with AIDS and CMV retinitis demonstrated equivalent activity against retinitis but longer survival (12.6 vs. 8.5 months) in the foscarnet group. Although the reasons for the latter difference are unclear, the antiretroviral activity of foscarnet and the greater use of zidovudine by foscarnet recipients are strong possibilities. Foscarnet is less well tolerated than ganciclovir and causes considerable toxicity, including renal dysfunction, hypomagnesemia, hypokalemia, hypocalcemia, genital ulcers, dysuria, nausea, and paresthesia. Moreover, foscarnet administration requires the use of an infusion pump and close clinical monitoring. With aggressive hydration and dose adjustments for renal dysfunction, the toxicity of foscarnet can be reduced. The use of foscarnet should be avoided when a saline load cannot be tolerated (e.g., in cardiomyopathy). The approved induction regimen is 60 mg/kg every 8 h for 2 weeks, although 90 mg/kg every 12 h is equally effective and no more toxic. Maintenance infusions should deliver 90 to 120 mg/kg once daily; no oral preparation is available. Foscarnet-resistant viruses may emerge during extended therapy.

Ganciclovir may also be administered via a slow-release pellet sutured into the eye. Although this intraocular device provides good local protection, contralateral eye disease and disseminated disease are not affected, and early retinal detachment is possible. A combination of intraocular and systemic therapy may be better than the intraocular implant alone.

Cidofovir is a nucleotide analogue with a long intracellular half-life that allows intermittent intravenous administration. Induction regimens of 5 mg/kg weekly for 2 weeks are followed by maintenance regimens of 3 to 5 mg/kg every 2 weeks. Cidofovir can cause severe nephrotoxicity through dose-dependent proximal tubular cell injury;

however, this adverse effect can be ameliorated somewhat by saline hydration and probenecid.

HUMAN HERPESVIRUS TYPES 6, 7, AND 8

Human herpesvirus (HHV) type 6 was first isolated in 1986 from peripheral-blood leukocytes of six persons with various lymphoproliferative disorders. The virus has a worldwide distribution, and two genetically distinct variants (HHV-6A and HHV-6B) are now recognized.

Infection with HHV-6 frequently develops during infancy as maternal antibody wanes. Congenital infections have also been described. HHV-6 (mostly variant B) can cause exanthem subitum (roseola infantum), a common illness characterized by fever with subsequent rash. HHV-6 is also a major cause of febrile seizures without rash during infancy. In older age groups, HHV-6 has been associated with mononucleosis syndromes, focal encephalitis, and (in immunocompromised hosts) pneumonitis and disseminated disease. In transplant recipients, HHV-6 infection may be associated with graft dysfunction. As many as 80% of adults are seropositive for HHV-6. The virus may be transmitted by saliva and possibly by genital secretions. There is no established treatment or vaccine.

HHV-7 was isolated in 1990 from T lymphocytes from the peripheral blood of a healthy 26-year-old man. Other isolates have since been obtained. It appears that the virus is frequently acquired during childhood and is frequently present in the saliva of healthy adults. No human disease has yet been definitively linked to HHV-7, although some cases of exanthem subitum and other childhood febrile illnesses have been associated with HHV-7 infection. An association has been made between HHV-7 and pityriasis rosea, but further studies must confirm this relationship.

Unique herpesvirus-like DNA sequences were reported during 1994 and 1995 in tissues derived from Kaposi's sarcoma and body cavity–based lymphoma occurring in patients with AIDS. When subjected to representational-difference analyses, more than 90% of Kaposi's sarcoma tissue samples were found to contain these sequences, whereas appropriate control tissues did not. The same herpesvirus-like DNA sequences have been reported in Kaposi's sarcoma tissue from non-AIDS patients, in a subgroup of AIDS-related B-cell body cavity–based lymphomas, and in lymph nodes from patients with multicentric Castleman's disease (a condition also known as angiofollicular lymph node hyperplasia, giant lymph node hyperplasia, lymphoid hamartoma, and follicular lymphoreticuloma, which is especially aggressive and frequently fatal). Approximately 15% of non–Kaposi's sarcoma tissue specimens from patients with AIDS contain these herpesvirus-like sequences, which have also been found in semen from both AIDS and non-AIDS patients. The virus has been propagated in cell culture and named HHV-8; it is also referred to as Kaposi's sarcoma–associated herpesvirus. Several serologic assays suggest a low rate of background positivity (0 to 29%) among HIV-negative blood donors but a high rate of positivity (>80%) among patients with Kaposi's sarcoma. The etiologic role of HHV-8 in Kaposi's sarcoma and other diseases remains to be established, although HHV-8 seroconversion during HIV infection appears to be highly predictive of the development of Kaposi's sarcoma.

BIBLIOGRAPHY

ADAMS O et al: Congenital infection with human herpesvirus 6. J Infect Dis 178:544, 1998

ADLER SP et al: Prior infection with cytomegalovirus is not a major risk factor for angiographically demonstrated coronary artery atherosclerosis. J Infect Dis 177:209, 1998

ANDERS HJ, GOEBEL F: Cytomegalovirus polyradiculopathy in patients with AIDS. Clin Infect Dis 27:345, 1998

CESARMAN E et al: Kaposi's sarcoma–associated herpesvirus-like DNA sequences in AIDS-related body-cavity-based lymphomas. N Engl J Med 332:1186, 1995

CONE RU et al: Human herpesvirus 6 infections after bone marrow transplantation: Clinical and virologic manifestations. J Infect Dis 179:311, 1999

DE OTERO J et al: Cytomegalovirus disease as a risk factor for graft loss and death after orthotopic liver transplantation. Clin Infect Dis 26:865, 1998

DRAGO F et al: Human herpesvirus 7 in patients with pityriasis rosea. Electron microscopy investigations and polymerase chain reaction in mononuclear cells, plasma and skin. Dermatology 196:275, 1997

EDDLESTON M et al: Severe cytomegalovirus infection in immunocompetent patients. Clin Infect Dis 24:52, 1997

JABS DA et al: Cytomegalovirus retinitis and viral resistance: Ganciclovir resistance. J Infect Dis 177:770, 1998

JACOBSON MA: Treatment of cytomegalovirus retinitis in patients with the acquired immunodeficiency syndrome. N Engl J Med 337:105, 1997

LAUTENSCHLAGER I et al: Human herpesvirus-6 infection after liver transplantation. Clin Infect Dis 26:702, 1998

McCUTCHAN JA: Cytomegalovirus infections of the nervous system in patients with AIDS. Clin Infect Dis 20:747, 1995

RENWICK N et al: Seroconversion for human herpesvirus 8 during HIV infection is highly predictive of Kaposi's sarcoma. AIDS 12:2481, 1998

SPECTOR SA et al: Plasma cytomegalovirus (CMV) DNA load predicts CMV disease and survival in AIDS patients. J Clin Invest 101:497, 1998

WALMSLEY S et al: Predictive value of cytomegalovirus (CMV) antigenemia and digene hybrid capture DNA assays for CMV disease in human immunodeficiency virus–infected patients. Clin Infect Dis 27:573, 1998

WALSH JC et al: Increasing survival in AIDS patients with cytomegalovirus retinitis treated with combination antiretroviral therapy including protease inhibitors. AIDS 12:613, 1998

WHITLEY RJ et al: Guidelines for the treatment of cytomegalovirus diseases in patients with AIDS in the era of potent antiretroviral therapy. Recommendations of an international panel. Arch Intern Med 158:957, 1998

186 *Fred Wang*

SMALLPOX, VACCINIA, AND OTHER POXVIRUSES

Two poxviruses, smallpox virus and molluscum contagiosum virus, cause natural disease in humans, and other poxviruses are associated with zoonotic infections. Monkeypox virus and smallpox virus typically cause systemic disease with rash, whereas the other poxviruses cause localized skin lesions. Poxviruses are the only DNA viruses that replicate in the cytoplasm, where accumulated viral particles form eosinophilic inclusions, or Guarnieri bodies, visible by light microscopy. Many poxvirus genes interfere with different aspects of the host immune response and provide important insights into the pathogenesis and virulence of viral infection. Genetically engineered vaccinia and avipoxviruses offer great promise as potential vectors for vaccination against other diseases.

SMALLPOX

The last case of endemic smallpox was reported in 1977 from Somalia. In 1980 the World Health Organization officially declared that smallpox had been eliminated worldwide as a result of a global vaccination and eradication program. Important features that contributed to the unique success of this vaccine program included (1) universal interest in eliminating this costly disease with high morbidity and mortality, (2) the infection's long incubation period and low level of communicability, (3) the ease of diagnosis of skin lesions by characteristic histology or antigen detection, (4) the fact that humans were the sole reservoir of the infection, (5) the absence of a carrier state, and (6) the availability of an effective live-virus vaccine that could readily be delivered to less developed countries because of its resistance to chemicals, temperature changes, and drying. The only known remaining repositories of smallpox virus reside in two research laboratories (located in the United States and Russia), and the issue of whether these last samples should be maintained or destroyed remains controversial.

Before the eradication of smallpox, variola virus existed as two related strains: *variola major* (smallpox), with a case-mortality rate of 20 to 50%, and *variola minor* (alastrim), which caused a clinically milder form of smallpox with a mortality of <1%. The clinical presentation of smallpox is now primarily of historic note. However, the threat of biologic terrorism means that smallpox remains a remote possibility in the differential diagnosis of a vesicular exanthem. Fever and macular rash appear after an average incubation period of 12 days, with a progression to typical vesicular and pustular lesions over 1 to 2 weeks. Rash generally appears first on the face, oral mucosa, and arms, with relative sparing of the trunk. Smallpox lesions may be confused with common chickenpox (varicella-zoster) infection but tend to be more diffuse, peripheral, and uniform in their stage of development. Polymerase chain reaction promises to be more useful than traditional electron microscopy or virus isolation for confirming variola or other poxvirus infections.

VACCINIA

The origin of vaccinia virus—the virus used for vaccination against smallpox—is uncertain, but it was probably derived from cowpox virus, variola virus, or a hybrid of the two. It is now a laboratory virus with no natural host. Experience has proven the effectiveness of live vaccinia virus vaccine, although its efficacy and safety were not established in controlled studies. Percutaneous administration of vaccinia virus vaccine results in protective cellular and humoral immune responses in >95% of primary vaccinees. Formation of a pustule and scab at the site of inoculation is indicative of immunity; because immunity wanes after 10 to 20 years, revaccination every 10 years is recommended for continued protection. Routine smallpox vaccination was discontinued in 1971 and has not been required for international travel since 1982. However, the development of recombinant vaccinia viruses for potential use in vaccines against other infectious agents or as immunotherapy against malignant diseases has led to the recommendation that laboratory and health care employees working directly with vaccinia virus vectors be considered for vaccination. Selected groups that may be exposed to poxviruses (e.g., some military personnel and individuals who work with animals) are also vaccinated.

The most frequent adverse complication of vaccination is inadvertent inoculation (usually autoinoculation) at other sites. More serious complications, which are more common among primary vaccinees and infants than among revaccinees and adults, include (1) generalized vaccinia in otherwise healthy individuals, which is generally self-limited; (2) eczema vaccinatum, which consists of disseminated cutaneous lesions in highly susceptible patients with eczema or other chronic skin diseases and is occasionally severe or even fatal; (3) progressive vaccinia (vaccinia necrosum), which is a severe, potentially fatal illness occurring in patients with immunodeficiency, whether congenital, acquired (e.g., via leukemia or lymphoma), iatrogenic (e.g., via chemotherapy or glucocorticoid treatment), or HIV induced; and (4) postinfectious encephalitis, which is rare (3 cases per million primary vaccinees) but can be fatal in 15 to 25% of cases and can leave 25% of patients with permanent neurologic sequelae. Since vaccinees can transmit vaccinia virus to susceptible individuals, vaccination is contraindicated if the proposed recipient or his or her household contacts have eczema, are immunocompromised, or are pregnant. Vaccinia immune globulin (0.6 mL/kg) derived from the plasma of vaccinated persons may be useful for the treatment of severe generalized vaccinia, eczema vaccinatum, progressive vaccinia, and ocular vaccinia resulting from inadvertent inoculation but is of no value for the treatment of postinfectious encephalitis.

MOLLUSCUM CONTAGIOSUM

Molluscum contagiosum is generally a benign disease characterized by pearly, flesh-colored, umbilicated skin lesions 2 to 5 mm in di-

ameter (**Plate IID-41**). A relative lack of inflammation and necrosis distinguishes these proliferative lesions from other poxvirus lesions. The infection can be transmitted by close contact, including sexual intercourse. Swimming pools are a common vector for transmission. Atopy and compromise of skin integrity can increase the risk of infection. Lesions can be found anywhere on the body except the palms and soles and may be associated with an eczematous rash. In most cases the disease is self-limited and has no systemic complications. Molluscum contagiosum develops especially often in association with the advanced stages of HIV infection, with a prevalence of 5 to 18% among HIV-infected patients (Chap. 309). The disease is often more generalized, severe, and persistent in AIDS patients than in other groups, frequently involving the face and upper body. Extensive molluscum contagiosum has also been reported in conjunction with other types of immunodeficiency.

The diagnosis of molluscum contagiosum can be made by histologic demonstration of cytoplasmic eosinophilic inclusions characteristic of poxvirus replication. This virus cannot be propagated in vitro, but electron microscopy and molecular studies can be used for its identification.

There is no specific systemic treatment for molluscum contagiosum, but a variety of techniques for physical ablation have been used. Molluscum contagiosum may respond to effective control of HIV infection with highly active antiretroviral therapy. Cidofovir is also being investigated for potential clinical use against molluscum contagiosum.

MONKEYPOX VIRUS AND OTHER POXVIRUSES

Monkeypox virus naturally infects nonhuman primates in the tropical rain forests of western and central Africa and can infect humans who come into direct contact with infected animals. Human disease is rare and is characterized by a systemic illness and vesicular rash similar to those of variola. A large outbreak of monkeypox occurred between February 1996 and October 1997 in central Africa, with a case-fatality ratio of 3%; a prolonged period of active cases, suggesting a potential for sustained person-to-person transmission; and a high proportion of younger patients, suggesting the possible consequences of discontinued smallpox vaccination. Clinical presentations were occasionally confused with the more common varicella-zoster virus infection.

Other poxviruses can cause localized vesicular lesions when humans come into direct contact with infected animals. These viruses include cowpox virus (rodents, cats); milkers' node virus (cows); buffalopox virus (buffaloes); bovine papular stomatitis virus (cows); and orf virus, which is also known as contagious pustular dermatitis virus (sheep, goats).

BIBLIOGRAPHY

BERTHISTLE K, CARRINGTON D: Molluscum contagiosum virus. J Infect 34:21, 1997

BREMAN JG, HENDERSON D: Poxvirus dilemmas—monkeypox, smallpox, and biologic terrorism. N Engl J Med 339:556, 1998

CATTELAN AM et al: A complete remission of recalcitrant molluscum contagiosum in an AIDS patient following highly active antiretroviral therapy. J Infect 38:58, 1999

FRANZ DR et al: Clinical recognition and management of patients exposed to biological warfare agents. JAMA 278:399, 1997

Human monkeypox—Kasai Oriental, Zaire, 1996–1997. MMWR 46:304, 1997

PAOLETTI E: Applications of pox virus vectors to vaccination: An update. Proc Natl Acad Sci USA 93:11349, 1996

SENKEVICH TG et al: Genome sequence of a human tumorigenic poxvirus: Prediction of specific host response-evasion genes. Science 273:813, 1996

SMITH GL et al: Vaccinia virus immune evasion. Immunol Rev 159:137, 1997

TARTAGLIA J et al: Canarypox virus–based vaccines: Prime-boost strategies to induce cell-mediated and humoral immunity against HIV. AIDS Res Hum Retroviruses 3: S291, 1998

Vaccinia (smallpox) vaccine. Recommendations of the Immunization Practices Advisory Committee (ACIP). MMWR 40:1, 1991

ZABAWSKI EJ, COCKERELL CJ: Topical and intralesional cidofovir: A review of pharmacology and therapeutic effects. J Am Acad Dermatol 39:741, 1998

187

PARVOVIRUS

DEFINITION The parvovirus group includes several species-specific viruses of animals. One parvovirus, designated B19, is known to be a human pathogen. B19 is a small (diameter, 20 to 25 nm), icosahedral, nonenveloped, single-stranded DNA virus with an outer capsid formed by two structural proteins. Individual virus particles contain DNA strands of positive or negative polarity. The virus is stable and retains infectivity after incubation at 60°C for 16 h. It has failed to grow in conventional cell culture lines and animal model systems but does replicate in vitro in erythroid progenitor cells derived from human bone marrow, umbilical cord, peripheral blood, or fetal liver sources.

During the 1980s, it was discovered that B19 causes a variety of disorders ranging from erythema infectiosum and acute arthropathy in otherwise healthy hosts to transient aplastic crisis and chronic anemia in compromised patients to fetal infection manifested by death or hydrops fetalis. Many of the severe manifestations of B19 viremia relate to the propensity of the virus to infect and lyse erythroid precursor cells in the bone marrow. The name B19 is derived from the code number of the human serum in which the virus was discovered.

PATHOGENESIS Two studies of adult volunteers have provided a basis for understanding the pathogenesis of B19 infection, which has two phases. The first phase is characterized by viremia that develops approximately 6 days after intranasal inoculation of B19 into susceptible individuals who lack serum antibodies to the virus. The viremia lasts about 1 week; its clearance is correlated with the development of IgM antibodies to B19, which remain detectable for up to a few months. IgG antibodies develop several days later and persist indefinitely. Nonspecific systemic symptoms lasting 2 or 3 days occur early during the viremic phase; these symptoms include headache, malaise, myalgia, fever, chills, and pruritus and are accompanied by reticulocytopenia and excretion of the virus from the respiratory tract. Several days after the onset of symptoms, a clinically insignificant decline in hemoglobin concentration is noted; the decreased level is maintained for 7 to 10 days, during which time examination of bone marrow samples reveals a marked depletion of erythroid precursor cells. Transient mild lymphopenia, neutropenia, and a drop in platelet count also may be found. A second phase of illness begins around 17 or 18 days after virus inoculation (after the clearance of viremia, the cessation of viral shedding in throat secretions, and the resolution of reticulocytopenia). This illness mimics erythema infectiosum in adults, with 2 or 3 days of fine maculopapular rash accompanied by arthralgias and arthritis that last another 1 or 2 days. This phase occurs in the presence of rising serum titers of antibody to B19.

The studies just described indicate that B19 disease in the otherwise *healthy host*, manifested by self-limited erythema infectiosum and/or arthropathy, is almost certainly an immune-complex disorder. This concept is supported by the induction of erythema infectiosum through the infusion of immunoglobulins into chronically viremic patients. In contrast, B19 disease in the *compromised host* (chronic hemolytic disease or immunodeficiency syndromes) is often serious, resulting from the destruction by B19 of erythroid precursor cells. Normal hosts can tolerate 7 to 10 days of shutoff of erythropoiesis; however, patients with hemolytic disease who require increased production of erythrocytes do not tolerate erythroid cell destruction and thus usually develop severe transient aplastic crisis. Patients who are immunodeficient may fail to clear B19 viremia, the results being persistent infection of red blood cells and chronic severe anemia. The fetus requires a higher level of red cell production than do adults and has an immature immune system; both these factors could explain B19-induced hydrops fetalis.

B19 binds specifically to a cellular receptor, erythrocyte P antigen; this specific binding explains the tropism of B19 for erythroid progenitor cells, particularly pronormoblasts and normoblasts. The few persons who lack P antigen cannot be infected with B19.

EPIDEMIOLOGY Although B19 infections occur year-round, they appear most commonly as outbreaks of erythema infectiosum in schools during winter and spring months. Between 20 and 60% of children in outbreaks are symptomatic, and many are asymptomatically infected. Seroepidemiologic studies indicate that approximately half of adults possess serum antibodies to B19. Antibody prevalence (reflecting prior exposure and probable immunity to the virus) rises rapidly between the ages of 5 and 18 years and continues to increase with age—a pattern probably indicating ongoing exposure during adulthood. B19 can be detected in throat swabbings, respiratory tract secretions, and serum, and its detection at these sites probably correlates with infectiousness. Thus, patients with transient aplastic crisis are highly infectious. Their infectivity has been firmly documented as the source of one well-defined nosocomial outbreak of erythema infectiosum among nurses. In contrast, individuals with erythema infectiosum are much less infectious. The usual route of viral transmission under natural conditions is unknown but may be respiratory or through direct contact. B19 can be transmitted during therapy with clotting factor concentrate, even after exposure to detergent, steam, or dry heat.

CLINICAL MANIFESTATIONS   **Erythema Infectiosum** Erythema infectiosum is the most common manifestation of B19 infection and occurs predominantly in children. This entity is also called *fifth disease* because it was classified in the late nineteenth century as the fifth in a series of six exanthems of childhood. Normally a mild illness, erythema infectiosum typically presents as a facial rash with a "slapped-cheek" appearance that is sometimes preceded by low-grade fever. The rash may develop quickly on the arms and legs and usually has a lacy, reticular, erythematous appearance **(Plate IID-40)**. The trunk, palms, and soles are less commonly involved. Occasionally, the rash appears with maculopapular, morbilliform, vesicular, purpuric, or pruritic characteristics. The typical rash resolves in about a week but can recur intermittently for several weeks, particularly after stress, exercise, exposure to sunlight, bathing, or change in environmental temperature. Arthralgia and arthritis are uncommon among children but are frequent among adults, in whom the rash is often absent or nonspecific, with a lack of the characteristic facial erythema.

Arthropathy B19 infection in adults most commonly presents as acute arthralgias and arthritis, sometimes accompanied by rash. The arthritis is characteristically symmetric and peripheral, involving the wrists, hands, and knees most frequently. It normally resolves in about 3 weeks and is nondestructive. However, a small percentage of patients have arthritis persisting for months or even (in rare cases) for years. It is not known whether these individuals have persistent infection or an abnormal immune response to the virus.

Transient Aplastic Crisis B19 infection is the cause in most instances of transient aplastic crisis developing suddenly in patients with chronic hemolytic disease. Nearly all hemolytic conditions can be affected by B19 infection, including sickle cell disease, erythrocyte enzyme deficiencies, hereditary spherocytosis, thalassemias, paroxysmal nocturnal hemoglobinuria, and autoimmune hemolysis. B19-induced aplastic crisis also can occur in the setting of acute blood loss. Patients present with weakness, lethargy, pallor, and severe anemia, a syndrome often preceded by a few days of nonspecific symptoms. These patients have intense reticulocytopenia lasting 7 to 10 days, and their bone marrow contains no erythroid precursor cells despite a normal myeloid series. Transient aplastic crisis can produce life-threatening anemia and may require urgent transfusion therapy. Unlike patients with erythema infectiosum or arthropathy, those with transient aplastic crisis are viremic and can readily transmit B19 infection to other people.

Chronic Anemia in Immunodeficient Patients Immunodeficient patients may be unable to eliminate B19 infection, probably because they cannot produce adequate levels of virus-specific IgG antibodies. The result is persistent infection with destruction of erythroid precursor cells in the bone marrow and chronic transfusion-dependent anemia. This condition has been described occasionally in patients with immunodeficiency related to infection with HIV, congenital immunodeficiencies, and acute lymphoblastic leukemia during maintenance chemotherapy as well as in recipients of bone marrow, heart, liver, and renal transplants. In addition, some cases of idiopathic pure red-cell aplasia probably are caused by persistent B19 infection. B19-induced chronic anemia may be the presenting finding of an otherwise unrecognized immunodeficiency. Chronic anemia may fluctuate in intensity over time and may be cured or controlled by immunoglobulin therapy. Both the spectrum of immunodeficiencies associated with B19-induced chronic anemia and the frequency of the association remain to be determined.

Fetal and Congenital Infection Maternal B19 infections usually do not adversely affect the fetus. More often than not, in fact, the fetus remains uninfected. Therefore, couples in which the pregnant woman is infected should be counseled as to the relatively low risk of fetal infection. It is estimated that fewer than 10% of maternal B19 infections in the first 20 weeks of pregnancy lead to fetal death; when fetal death does occur, it is usually attributable to the development of nonimmune hydrops fetalis, wherein the fetus succumbs to severe anemia and congestive heart failure. In these instances, B19 can be detected in fetal tissues, with predominant infection of erythroblasts. Pregnant women with known exposure to B19 should have their serum monitored for IgM antibodies to the virus and for elevated levels of α-fetoprotein and human chorionic gonadotropin; ultrasonic examinations of the fetus for hydrops should also be conducted. Some hydropic fetuses survive B19 infection and appear normal at delivery. Rarely, fetal infection with hydrops results in congenital anemia and hypogammaglobulinemia that is unresponsive to immunoglobulin therapy.

Possible Clinical Associations Case studies suggest a link—as yet inconclusive—between B19 and several rheumatic diseases, most notably rheumatoid arthritis but also vasculitis (including polyarteritis, Wegener's granulomatosis, and giant cell arteritis), lupus erythematosus, dermatomyositis, and juvenile rheumatoid arthritis. Other unproven associations include those involving multiple systems: cardiac (myocarditis), hematologic (hemophagocytic syndrome, idiopathic thrombocytopenic purpura), hepatic (fulminant hepatitis), neurologic (meningoencephalitis), and respiratory (pneumonia).

DIAGNOSIS Diagnosis most commonly relies on measurements of B19-specific IgM and IgG antibodies, which can be detected with commercially available immunoassay kits. The virus, its DNA, or its antigens are also detected in the serum or infected tissues of some patients. Acute infection can be proven by B19-compatible symptoms and the presence of IgM antibodies or virus itself, whereas past infection is documented by IgG antibodies. Individuals with erythema infectiosum and acute arthropathy usually have IgM antibodies without detectable virus in serum. Those with transient aplastic crisis may have IgM antibodies but typically possess high titers of virus and its DNA in serum; the bone marrow of these patients shows characteristic giant pronormoblasts and hypoplasia. Immunodeficient patients with anemia often lack readily detectable antibodies but have viral particles and DNA in serum. Fetal infection may be recognized by hydrops fetalis and the presence of B19 DNA in amniotic fluid or fetal blood in association with maternal IgM antibodies to B19.

℞ **TREATMENT** Erythema infectiosum usually requires no treatment; the same is true for many cases of arthropathy. More severe cases of arthritis, particularly those involving chronic symptoms, can be treated with nonsteroidal anti-inflammatory agents. Transient aplastic crisis is usually treated with erythrocyte transfusions. In immunodeficient anemic patients, B19 infection should be treated with commercial intravenous immunoglobulin, which is known to contain IgG antibodies to B19. This therapy controls and may cure B19 infection.

PROPHYLAXIS Prophylaxis of B19 infection with immunoglobulin should be considered for patients with chronic hemolysis or immunodeficiency and for pregnant women. The risk of infection for these persons may be reduced by hand washing before eating or after contact with respiratory or other secretions when B19 is known to be present in a community. Patients with transient aplastic crisis or chronic B19 infection (but not those with erythema infectiosum or arthropathy) pose a serious risk for nosocomial transmission of infection. They should be hospitalized in a private room with contact and respiratory isolation precautions. It is not known whether pre- or postexposure administration of immunoglobulin prevents infection. No vaccine for B19 is currently available; however, a baculovirus-infected insect cell line that expresses noninfectious immunogenic B19 capsid proteins is being evaluated to determine an optimal regimen for use as a vaccine.

BIBLIOGRAPHY

ABKOWITZ JL et al: Clinical relevance of parvovirus B19 as a cause of anemia in patients with human immunodeficiency virus infection. J Infect Dis 176:269, 1997

ANDERSON LJ, YOUNG NS (eds): *Monographs in Virology,* vol 20: *Human Parvovirus B19.* Basel, Karger, 1997

ANDERSON MJ et al: Experimental parvoviral infection in humans. J Infect Dis 152:257, 1985

BROWN KE et al: Resistance to parvovirus B19 infection due to lack of virus receptor (erythrocyte P antigen). N Engl J Med 330:1192, 1994

CENTERS FOR DISEASE CONTROL AND PREVENTION: Risks associated with human parvovirus B19 infection. MMWR 38:81, 1989

KURTZMAN G et al: Pure red-cell aplasia of 10 years' duration due to persistent parvovirus B19 infection and its cure with immunoglobulin therapy. N Engl J Med 321:519, 1989

MILLER E et al: Immediate and long term outcome of human parvovirus B19 infection in pregnancy. Br J Obstet Gynaecol 105:174, 1998

NAIDES SJ et al: Rheumatologic manifestations of human parvovirus B19 infection in adults: Initial two-year clinical experience. Arthritis Rheum 33:1297, 1990

PLUMMER FA et al: An erythema infectiosum–like illness caused by human parvovirus infection. N Engl J Med 313:74, 1985

SOKAL EM et al: Acute parvovirus B19 infection associated with fulminant hepatitis of favourable prognosis in young children. Lancet 352:1739, 1998

TAKAHASHI Y et al: Human parvovirus B19 as a causative agent for rheumatoid arthritis. Proc Natl Acad Sci USA 95:8227, 1998

188 *Richard C. Reichman*

HUMAN PAPILLOMAVIRUSES

DEFINITION Human papillomaviruses (HPVs) selectively infect the epithelium of the skin and mucous membranes. These infections may be asymptomatic, produce warts, or be associated with a variety of benign and malignant neoplasias.

ETIOLOGIC AGENT Papillomaviruses are members of the *Papillomavirus* genus of the family Papovaviridae. They are nonenveloped, measure 50 to 55 nm in diameter, have icosahedral capsids composed of 72 capsomeres, and contain a double-stranded circular DNA genome of about 7900 base pairs. The genomic organization of all papillomaviruses is similar and consists of an early (E) region, a late (L) region, and a noncoding upstream regulatory region. Oncogenic HPV types can immortalize human keratinocytes, and this activity has been mapped to products of early genes E6 and E7. E6 protein facilitates the degradation of the p53 tumor suppressor protein, and E7 protein binds the retinoblastoma gene product and related proteins. The E1 and E2 proteins modulate viral DNA replication and regulate gene expression. The L1 gene codes for the major capsid protein, which makes up 80% of the virion mass. L2 codes for a minor capsid protein. Type-specific conformational antigenic determinants are located on the virion surface. Papillomavirus types are distinguished from one another by the degree of nucleic acid sequence homology. Distinct types share fewer than 90% of their DNA sequences in L1. More than 80 types of HPV are recognized, and individual types are associated with specific clinical manifestations (Table 188-1). HPVs are species-specific and have not been propagated in tissue culture or in common experimental animals. However, HPV types 1, 6, 11, 16, 40, and 83 have been produced in human tissues implanted in immunodeficient mice.

EPIDEMIOLOGY There are few good studies of the incidence or prevalence of warts in well-defined human populations. Common warts (verruca vulgaris) are found in as many as 25% of some groups and are most prevalent among young children. Plantar warts (verruca plantaris) are also widely prevalent; they occur most often among adolescents and young adults. Condyloma acuminatum (anogenital warts) is one of the most common sexually transmitted diseases in the United States. HPV infection of the uterine cervix produces the squamous cell abnormalities most frequently detected on Papanicolaou smears.

Most genital HPV infections are transmitted through direct contact with infectious lesions. Close personal contact is also assumed to play a role in the transmission of most cutaneous warts; the importance of fomites in this setting is not clear. Minor trauma at the site of inoculation may facilitate transmission. Recurrent respiratory papillomatosis in young children is an uncommon disease that is acquired from maternal genital tract infection; in adults, the disease may be transmitted through orogenital sexual contact.

HPV infection has been strongly associated with the development of dysplasia and cancer of the uterine cervix. More than 95% of cervical cancers contain DNA of oncogenic (high-risk) HPV types, such as 16, 18, and 31. HPV DNA is also present in the precursor lesions of cervical cancer, known as cervical intraepithelial neoplasias. Such lesions containing DNA of oncogenic HPV types are more likely to progress than those associated with low-risk types, such as 6 and 11. HPV DNA is transcribed in tumor tissues; many epidemiologic studies

have confirmed a relation between HPV infection (with or without cofactors) and the development of cervical cancer, although most cervical HPV infections are self-limited. Infection with specific HPV types has also been associated with squamous cell carcinomas and dysplasias of the penis, anus, vagina, and vulva. In patients with epidermodysplasia verruciformis, squamous cell cancers develop frequently at sites infected with specific HPV types, including 5 and 8.

Serologic studies with virus-like particles as antigens have demonstrated type-specific antibodies in most patients with HPV genital tract infections.

CLINICAL MANIFESTATIONS The clinical manifestations of HPV infection depend on the location of the lesions and the type of virus. Common warts usually occur on the hands as flesh-colored to brown, exophytic, hyperkeratotic papules. Plantar warts may be quite painful; they can be differentiated from calluses by paring of the surface to reveal thrombosed capillaries. Flat warts (verruca plana) are most common among children and occur on the face, neck, chest, and flexor surfaces of the forearms and legs.

Anogenital warts develop on the skin and mucosal surfaces of the external genitalia and perianal areas (**Plate IID-55**). Among circumcised men, warts are most commonly found on the penile shaft. Lesions commonly occur at the urethral meatus and may extend proximally. Perianal warts are common among homosexual men but develop in heterosexual men as well. In women, warts appear first at the posterior introitus and adjacent labia. They then spread to other parts of the vulva and commonly involve the vagina and cervix. These lesions may be present without external warts. The differential diagnosis of anogenital warts includes condylomata lata of secondary syphilis, molluscum contagiosum, hirsutoid papillomatosis (pearly penile papules), fibroepitheliomas, and a variety of benign and malignant mucocutaneous neoplasms. Respiratory papillomatosis in young children may be life-threatening and presents as hoarseness, stridor, or respiratory distress. The disease in adults is usually milder.

Immunosuppressed patients, particularly those undergoing organ transplantation, often develop pityriasis versicolor–like lesions, from which DNA of several HPV types has been extracted. Occasionally, such lesions appear to undergo malignant transformation. Patients infected with HIV frequently have severe clinical manifestations of HPV infection and appear to be at unusually high risk for cervical and anal malignancies. HPV disease in patients with HIV infection is difficult to treat and often recurs.

Epidermodysplasia verruciformis is a rare autosomal recessive disease characterized by the inability to control HPV infection. Patients are often infected with unusual HPV types and frequently develop cutaneous squamous cell malignancies, particularly in sun-exposed areas. The lesions resemble flat warts or macules similar to those of pityriasis versicolor.

The complications of warts include itching and occasionally bleeding. In rare cases warts become secondarily infected with bacteria or fungi. Large masses of warts may cause mechanical problems, such as obstruction of the birth canal. Dysplasias of the uterine cervix are generally asymptomatic until frank carcinoma develops. Patients with anogenital HPV disease may develop serious psychological symptoms due to anxiety or depression over this condition.

PATHOGENESIS The incubation period of HPV disease is usually 3 to 4 months, with a range of 1 month to 2 years. All types of squamous epithelium can be infected by HPV, and the gross and histologic appearances of individual lesions vary with the site of infection and the type of virus. The replication of HPV begins with the infection of basal cells. As cellular differentiation proceeds, HPV DNA replicates and is transcribed. Ultimately, virions are assembled in the nucleus and released when keratinocytes are shed. This process is associated with proliferation of all epidermal layers except the basal layer and produces acanthosis, parakeratosis, and hyperkeratosis. Koilocytes, large round cells with pyknotic nuclei, appear in the granular layer. Histologically normal epithelium may contain HPV DNA,

Table 188-1 Correlation of Human Papillomavirus Type with Disease

Disease	Associated HPV Types
Plantar warts	1,[a] 2,[a] 4, 63
Common warts	1,[a] 2,[a] 4, 26, 27, 29, 41,[b] 57, 65, 77
Common warts of meat handlers	1, 2,[a] 3, 4, 7,[a] 10, 28
Flat warts	3,[a] 10,[a] 27, 38, 41,[b] 49, 75, 76
Intermediate warts	10,[a] 26, 28
Epidermodysplasia verruciformis	2,[a] 3,[a] 5,[ab] 8,[ab] 9,[a] 10,[a] 12,[a] 14,[ab] 15,[a] 17,[ab] 19, 20,[b] 21, 22, 23, 24, 25, 36, 37, 38,[b] 47, 50
Condyloma acuminatum	6,[a] 11,[a] 30,[b] 42, 43, 44, 45,[b] 51,[b] 54, 55, 70
Intraepithelial neoplasias	
Unspecified	30,[b] 34, 39,[b] 40, 53, 57, 59, 61, 62, 64, 66,[b] 67, 69, 71
Low-grade	6,[a] 11,[a] 16,[b] 18,[b] 31,[b] 33,[b] 35,[b] 42, 43, 44, 45,[b] 51,[b] 52,[b] 74
High-grade	6, 11, 16,[ab] 18,[ab] 31,[b] 33,[b] 34, 35,[b] 39,[b] 42, 44, 45,[b] 51,[b] 52,[b] 56,[b] 58,[b] 66[b]
Bowen's disease	16,[ab] 31,[b] 34
Bowenoid papulosis	16,[ab] 34, 39,[b] 42, 45,[b] 55
Cervical carcinoma	16,[ab] 18,[ab] 31,[b] 33,[b] 35,[b] 39,[b] 45,[b] 51,[b] 52,[b] 56,[b] 58,[b] 66,[b] 68, 70
Laryngeal papillomas	6,[a] 11[a]
Focal epithelial hyperplasia of Heck	13,[a] 32[a]
Conjunctival papillomas	6,[a] 11,[a] 16[ab]
Others	6, 11, 16,[b] 30,[b] 33,[b] 36, 37 38,[b] 41,[b] 48,[b] 60, 72, 73

[a] Most common associations.
[b] High malignant potential.
NOTE: Additional information on new HPV types can be found on the HPV Sequence Data Base through the Internet (hpv-web.lanl.gov).

and residual DNA after treatment can be associated with recurrent disease.

Episomal HPV DNA is present in the nuclei of infected cells in benign lesions caused by the virus. However, in severe dysplasias and cancers, HPV DNA is generally integrated, with disruption of the E1/E2 open reading frames. This disruption leads to upregulation of E6 and E7 and subsequent interference with cellular tumor suppressor proteins.

Host defense responses to HPV infection are incompletely understood, and immune correlates of protection from infection and resolution of disease have not been established. Because patients with defects in cell-mediated immune responses, including transplant recipients and patients with HIV infection, frequently develop severe HPV disease, such responses are probably important for the control of virus replication. Histologic studies demonstrating an epidermal lymphomonocytic infiltrate in resolving warts suggest that local immunity may be of particular importance in the resolution of disease. HPV infection can also elicit a serologic response, and antibodies to the viral capsid have been found in sera from patients with anogenital warts, cutaneous warts, and respiratory papillomatosis. Antibodies to E-region proteins, most notably E7, have been detected among patients with cervical carcinoma. Vaccine studies in animals have shown that production of neutralizing antibodies can be associated with protection from papillomavirus infection.

DIAGNOSIS   Most warts that are visible to the naked eye can be diagnosed correctly by history and physical examination alone. The use of a colposcope is invaluable in assessing vaginal and cervical lesions and is helpful in the diagnosis of oral and cutaneous HPV disease as well. Papanicolaou smears prepared from cervical scrapings often show cytologic evidence of HPV infection. Persistent or atypical lesions should be biopsied and examined by routine histologic methods. The most sensitive and specific methods of virologic diagnosis entail the use of techniques such as the polymerase chain reaction or the hybrid capture assay to detect HPV nucleic acids and to identify specific virus types. Serologic techniques to diagnose HPV infection are not helpful in individual cases and are not widely available.

℞ **TREATMENT**   Decisions regarding the initiation of therapy should be made with the knowledge that currently available modes of treatment are not completely effective and some have significant side effects. In addition, treatment may be expensive, and many HPV lesions resolve spontaneously. Frequently used therapies include cryosurgery, application of caustic agents, electrodesiccation, surgical excision, and ablation with a laser. Topical antimetabolites such as 5-fluorouracil also have been used. Both failure and recurrence

have been well documented with all of these methods of treatment. Cryosurgery is the initial treatment of choice for condyloma acuminatum. Topically applied podophyllum preparations as well as podofilox may also be used. Various interferon preparations have been used with modest success in the treatment of respiratory papillomatosis and condyloma acuminatum. A topically applied interferon inducer, imiquimod, is also of benefit in the treatment of condyloma acuminatum. The diagnosis and management of anogenital dysplasias and of internal anogenital warts require special skills and resources, and patients with such lesions should be referred to a qualified specialist.

No effective methods for the prevention of HPV infections are available at present other than the avoidance of contact with infectious lesions. Barrier methods of contraception may be helpful in preventing the transmission of condyloma acuminatum and other HPV-associated diseases of the genital tract. Vaccines consisting of virus-like particles can prevent papillomavirus disease in some animal models and have been shown to induce neutralizing antibodies in phase 1 studies in humans. More extensive clinical trials of these preparations are under way.

BIBLIOGRAPHY

BONNEZ W, REICHMAN RC: Papillomaviruses, in *Principles and Practice of Infectious Diseases*, 5th ed, GL Mandell et al (eds). Churchill Livingstone, New York, 2000

—— et al: Isolation and propagation of human papillomavirus type 16 in human xenografts implanted in the severe combined immunodeficiency mouse. J Virol 72: 5256, 1998

BROWN DR et al: Nucleotide sequence and characterization of human papillomavirus type 83, a novel genital papillomavirus. Virology 260:165, 1999

FRISCH M et al: Sexually transmitted infection as a cause of anal cancer. N Engl J Med 337:1350, 1997

GALLOWAY DA: Is vaccination against human papillomavirus a possibility? Lancet 351(Suppl 3):22, 1998

HAGENSEE ME et al: Seroprevalence of human papillomavirus types 6 and 16 capsid antibodies in homosexual men. J Infect Dis 176:625, 1997

HO GY et al: Natural history of cervicovaginal papillomavirus infection in young women. N Engl J Med 338:423, 1998

LUQUE AE et al: Association of human papillomavirus infection and disease with magnitude of human immunodeficiency virus type 1 (HIV-1) RNA plasma level among women with HIV-1 infection. J Infect Dis 179:1405, 1999

NOBBENHUIS MAE et al: Relation of human papillomavirus status to cervical lesions and consequences for cervical-cancer screening: A prospective study. Lancet 354:20, 1999

NORTHFELT DW et al: Anal neoplasia. Pathogenesis, diagnosis, and management. Hematol Oncol Clin North Am 10:1177, 1996

REICHMAN RC et al: A phase I study of a recombinant virus-like particle vaccine against human papillomavirus type 11 in healthy adult volunteers, in *Proceedings of the 38th Interscience Conference on Antimicrobial Agents and Chemotherapy*. Washington, DC, American Society of Microbiology, 1998, abstract 330

WIDEROFF L et al: Epidemiologic determinants of seroreactivity to human papillomavirus (HPV) type 16 virus-like particles in cervical HPV-16 DNA-positive and -negative women. J Infect Dis 174:937, 1996

Section 13
DNA AND RNA RESPIRATORY VIRUSES

| 189 | *Raphael Dolin* |

COMMON VIRAL RESPIRATORY INFECTIONS

GENERAL CONSIDERATIONS   Acute viral respiratory illnesses are among the most common of human diseases, accounting for one-half or more of all acute illnesses. The incidence of acute respiratory disease in the United States is from 3 to 5.6 cases per

person per year. The rates are highest among children under 1 year old (6.1 to 8.3 cases per year) and remain high until age 6, when a progressive decrease begins. Adults have 3 to 4 cases per person per year. Morbidity from acute respiratory illnesses accounts for 30 to 50% of time lost from work by adults and for 60 to 80% of time lost from school by children. The use of antibacterial agents to treat viral respiratory infections represents a major source of abuse of that category of drugs.

It has been estimated that two-thirds to three-fourths of cases of acute respiratory illnesses are caused by viruses. More than 200 antigenically distinct viruses from 8 different genera have been reported to cause acute respiratory illness, and it is likely that additional agents will be described in the future. The vast majority of these viral infections involve the upper respiratory tract, but lower respiratory tract disease can also develop, particularly in younger age groups and in certain epidemiologic settings.

The illnesses caused by respiratory viruses traditionally have been divided into multiple distinct syndromes, such as the "common cold," pharyngitis, croup (laryngotracheobronchitis), tracheitis, bronchiolitis, bronchitis, and pneumonia. Each of these general categories of illnesses has a certain epidemiologic and clinical profile; for example, croup occurs exclusively in very young children and has a characteristic clinical course. Some types of respiratory illnesses are more likely to be associated with certain viruses (e.g., the common cold with rhinoviruses), while others occupy characteristic epidemiologic niches (e.g., adenovirus infections in military re-

Table 189-1 Illnesses Associated with Respiratory Viruses

Virus	Frequency of Respiratory Syndromes		
	Most Frequent	Occasional	Infrequent
Rhinoviruses	Common cold	Exacerbation of chronic bronchitis and asthma	Pneumonia in children
Coronaviruses	Common cold	Exacerbation of chronic bronchitis and asthma	Pneumonia and bronchiolitis
Respiratory syncytial virus	Pneumonia and bronchiolitis in young children	Common cold in adults	Pneumonia in elderly and immunosuppressed patients
Parainfluenza viruses	Croup and lower respiratory tract disease in young children	Pharyngitis and common cold	Tracheobronchitis in adults; lower respiratory tract disease in immunosuppressed patients
Adenoviruses	Common cold and pharyngitis in children	Outbreaks of acute respiratory disease in military recruits[a]	Pneumonia in children; lower respiratory tract and disseminated disease in immunosuppressed patients
Influenza A viruses	Influenza[b]	Pneumonia and excess mortality in high-risk patients	Pneumonia in healthy individuals
Influenza B viruses	Influenza[b]	Rhinitis and pharyngitis alone	Pneumonia
Enteroviruses	Acute undifferentiated febrile illnesses[c]	Rhinitis and pharyngitis	Pneumonia
Herpes simplex viruses	Gingivostomatitis in children; pharyngotonsillitis in adults	Tracheitis and pneumonia in immunocompromised patients	Disseminated infection in immunocompromised patients

[a] Serotypes 4 and 7.
[b] Fever, cough, myalgia, malaise.
[c] May or may not have a respiratory component.

cruits). The syndromes most commonly associated with infections with the major respiratory virus groups are summarized in Table 189-1. Most respiratory viruses clearly have the potential to cause more than one type of respiratory illness, and frequently features of several types of illness are found in the same patient. Moreover, the clinical illnesses induced by these viruses are rarely sufficiently distinctive to permit an etiologic diagnosis on clinical grounds alone, although the epidemiologic setting increases the likelihood that one group of viruses rather than another is involved. In general, laboratory methods must be relied on to establish a specific viral diagnosis.

This chapter reviews viral infections caused by five of the major groups of respiratory viruses: rhinoviruses, coronaviruses, respiratory syncytial viruses, parainfluenza viruses, and adenoviruses. Influenza viruses, which are a major cause of mortality as well as morbidity, are reviewed in Chap. 190. Herpesviruses, which occasionally cause pharyngitis and which also cause lower respiratory tract disease in immunosuppressed patients, are reviewed in Chap. 182. Enteroviruses, which account for occasional respiratory illnesses during the summer months, are reviewed in Chap. 193.

RHINOVIRUS INFECTIONS

ETIOLOGIC AGENT Rhinoviruses are members of the Picornaviridae family, small (15 to 30 nm) nonenveloped viruses that contain a single-stranded RNA genome. In contrast to other members of the picornavirus family, such as enteroviruses, rhinoviruses are acid-labile and are almost completely inactivated at pH ≤ 3. Rhinoviruses grow preferentially at 33° to 34°C—the temperature of the human nasal passages—rather than at the higher temperature (37°C) of the lower respiratory tract. One hundred distinct serotypes and one subtype of rhinovirus are recognized.

EPIDEMIOLOGY Rhinoviruses are a major cause of the common cold and have been isolated from 15 to 40% of adults with common cold–like illnesses. Overall rates of infection with rhinoviruses are higher among infants and young children and decrease with increasing age. Rhinovirus infections occur throughout the year, with seasonal peaks in early fall and spring in temperate climates. Rhino-

virus infections are most often introduced into families by preschool or grade-school children younger than 6 years old. Between 25 and 70% of initial illnesses in family settings are followed by secondary cases, with the highest attack rates among the youngest siblings at home. Attack rates also increase with family size.

Rhinoviruses appear to spread through direct contact with infected secretions, usually respiratory droplets. In some studies of volunteers, transmission was most efficient by hand-to-hand contact, with subsequent self-inoculation of the conjunctival or nasal mucosa. In other studies, transmission by large- or small-particle aerosol was demonstrated. Virus also can be recovered from plastic surfaces inoculated 1 to 3 h previously; this observation suggests that environmental surfaces contribute to transmission. In studies of married couples in which neither partner had detectable serum antibody, transmission was associated with prolonged contact (122 h or more) during a 7-day period. Transmission was infrequent unless virus was recoverable from the donor's hands and nasal mucosa, at least 1000 $TCID_{50}$ of virus was present in nasal washes from the donor, and the donor was at least moderately symptomatic with the "cold." Despite anecdotal observations, exposure to cold temperatures, fatigue, or sleep deprivation has not been associated with increased rates of rhinovirus-induced illness in volunteers.

Infection with rhinoviruses is worldwide in distribution. By the time they reach adulthood, nearly all individuals have neutralizing antibodies to multiple serotypes, although the prevalence of antibody to any one serotype varies widely. Multiple serotypes circulate simultaneously, and generally no single serotype or group of serotypes has been more prevalent than the others.

PATHOGENESIS Rhinoviruses infect cells through attachment to specific cellular receptors; most serotypes attach to intercellular adhesion molecule 1, while a few use low-density lipoprotein as the cellular receptor. Relatively limited information is available on the histopathology and pathogenesis of acute rhinovirus infections in humans. Examination of biopsy specimens obtained during experimentally induced and naturally occurring illness indicates that the nasal mucosa is edematous, is often hyperemic, and—during acute illness—is covered by a mucoid discharge. There is a mild infiltrate with inflammatory cells, including neutrophils, lymphocytes, plasma cells, and eosinophils. Mucus-secreting glands in the submucosa appear hyperactive; the nasal turbinates are engorged, a condition that may lead to obstruction of nearby openings of sinus cavities. Several mediators, such as bradykinin, lysylbradykinin, prostaglandins, histamine, and interleukins 1, 6, and 8, have been linked to the development of signs and symptoms in rhinovirus-induced colds.

The incubation period for rhinovirus illness is short, generally 1 or 2 days. Virus shedding coincides with the onset of illness or may begin shortly before symptoms develop. The mechanisms of immunity to rhinovirus are not well worked out. In some studies, the presence of homotypic antibody has been associated with significantly reduced rates of subsequent infection and illness, but data conflict regarding the relative importance of serum and local antibody in protection from rhinovirus infection.

CLINICAL MANIFESTATIONS   The most common clinical manifestations of rhinovirus infections are those of the common cold. Illness usually begins with rhinorrhea and sneezing accompanied by nasal congestion. The throat is frequently sore, and in some cases sore throat is the initial complaint. Systemic signs and symptoms, such as malaise and headache, are mild or absent, and fever is unusual. Illness generally lasts for 4 to 9 days and resolves spontaneously without sequelae. In children, bronchitis, bronchiolitis, and bronchopneumonia have been reported; nevertheless, it appears that rhinoviruses are not major causes of lower respiratory tract disease in children. Rhinoviruses may cause exacerbations of asthma and chronic pulmonary disease in adults. The vast majority of rhinovirus infections resolve without sequelae, but complications related to obstruction of the eustachian tubes or sinus ostia, including otitis media or acute sinusitis, can develop.

DIAGNOSIS   Although rhinoviruses are the most frequently recognized cause of the common cold, similar illnesses are caused by a variety of other viruses, and the etiologic diagnosis cannot be made on clinical grounds alone. Rather, rhinovirus infection is diagnosed by isolation of the virus from nasal washes or nasal secretions in tissue culture. In practice, this procedure is rarely undertaken because of the benign, self-limited nature of the illness. Given the many serotypes of rhinovirus, diagnosis by serum antibody tests is currently impractical. Likewise, common laboratory tests, such as white cell count and sedimentation rate, are not helpful.

℞ **TREATMENT**   Rhinovirus infections are generally mild and self-limited, so treatment is not usually necessary. Therapy in the form of antihistamines and nonsteroidal anti-inflammatory drugs may be beneficial in patients with particularly pronounced symptoms, and reduction of activity is prudent in instances of significant discomfort or fatigability. Antibacterial agents should be used only if bacterial complications such as otitis media or sinusitis develop. Specific antiviral therapy is not available. Application of interferon sprays intranasally has been effective in the prophylaxis of rhinovirus infections but is also associated with local irritation of the nasal mucosa. Prevention of rhinovirus infection by antibodies directed against rhinovirus receptors or by the soluble purified receptors themselves is under study. Experimental vaccines to certain rhinovirus serotypes have been prepared, but their usefulness is questionable because of the myriad serotypes and the uncertainty about mechanisms of immunity. Thorough hand washing, environmental decontamination, and protection against autoinoculation may help to reduce rates of transmission of infection.

CORONAVIRUS INFECTIONS

ETIOLOGIC AGENT   Coronaviruses are pleomorphic, single-stranded RNA viruses that measure 80 to 160 nm in diameter. The name derives from the crownlike appearance produced by the club-shaped projections that stud the viral envelope. Coronaviruses that infect humans fall into two distinct antigenic groups (I and II), which are represented by prototype isolates 229E and OC43. Coronaviruses are fastidious and are difficult to culture in vitro. Some strains will grow only in human tracheal organ cultures rather than in tissue culture.

EPIDEMIOLOGY   Only limited seroepidemiologic studies of coronavirus infections have been conducted. Seroprevalence studies of strains 229E and OC43 have demonstrated the presence of serum antibodies at rates ranging from 12% to >80% in various populations. Overall, coronaviruses account for 10 to 20% of common colds. Coronavirus infections appear to be particularly prevalent in late fall, winter, and early spring—times when rhinovirus infections are less common. A cyclical pattern has been suggested for outbreaks of infection with strains OC43 and 229E, with outbreaks occurring every 2 to 4 years.

CLINICAL MANIFESTATIONS   The clinical features of illness caused by coronaviruses are similar to those of illness caused by rhinoviruses. In studies of volunteers, the mean incubation period of illness induced by coronaviruses (3 days) is somewhat longer than that of illness caused by rhinoviruses, and the duration of illness is somewhat shorter (mean, 6 to 7 days). In some studies, the amount of nasal discharge was somewhat greater in colds induced by coronaviruses than in those induced by rhinoviruses. Coronaviruses have been recovered from infants with pneumonia and from military recruits with lower respiratory tract disease and have been associated with worsening of chronic bronchitis. However, the overall significance of coronaviruses in lower respiratory tract disease in humans remains unclear.

℞ **TREATMENT**   The approach to the treatment of common colds caused by coronaviruses is similar to that discussed above for rhinovirus-induced illnesses. Because of uncertainty regarding the number and relative importance of coronavirus subgroups and the mechanisms of immunity, vaccines against coronaviruses have not been developed.

RESPIRATORY SYNCYTIAL VIRUS INFECTIONS

ETIOLOGIC AGENT   Respiratory syncytial virus (RSV) is a member of the Paramyxoviridae family and comprises the genus *Pneumovirus*. RSV, an enveloped virus approximately 150 to 300 nm in diameter, is so named because its replication in vitro leads to the fusion of neighboring cells into large multinucleated syncytia. The single-stranded RNA genome codes for 10 virus-specific proteins. Viral RNA is contained in a helical nucleocapsid surrounded by a lipid envelope bearing two glycoproteins: the G protein, by which the virus attaches to cells, and the F (fusion) protein, which facilitates entry of the virus into the cell by fusing host and viral membranes. RSV was once considered to be of a single antigenic type, but two distinct groups (A and B) and multiple subtypes within each group have now been described. Antigenic diversity is reflected by differences in the G protein, while the F protein is highly conserved. The epidemiologic significance of the antigenic diversity is under investigation. Both antigenic groups can circulate simultaneously in outbreaks, although the relative proportions of each vary.

EPIDEMIOLOGY   RSV is the major respiratory pathogen of young children and the foremost cause of lower respiratory disease in infants. Infection with RSV is seen throughout the world in annual epidemics that occur in late fall, winter, or spring and last up to 5 months. The virus is rarely encountered during the summer. Rates of illness are highest among infants between 1 and 6 months of age, peaking between 2 and 3 months of age. The attack rates among susceptible infants and children are extraordinarily high, approaching 100% in settings such as day-care centers where large numbers of susceptible infants are present. RSV accounts for 20 to 25% of hospital admissions of young infants and children for pneumonia and for up to 75% of cases of bronchiolitis in this age group. It has been estimated that more than half of infants who are at risk will become infected during an RSV epidemic.

189   Common Viral Respiratory Infections   **1123**

In older children and adults, reinfection with RSV is frequent but disease is milder than in infancy. A common cold–like syndrome is the illness most commonly associated with RSV infection in adults. Severe lower respiratory tract disease with pneumonitis can occur in elderly (often institutionalized) adults and in patients with immuno-compromising disorders or treatment, including recipients of bone-marrow and solid-organ transplants. RSV is also an important noso-comial pathogen; during an outbreak, it can infect pediatric patients and up to 25 to 50% of the staff on pediatric wards. The spread of virus among families is efficient: up to 40% of siblings may become infected when RSV is introduced into the family setting.

RSV is transmitted primarily by close contact with contaminated fingers or fomites and by self-inoculation of the conjunctiva or anterior nares. Virus also may be spread by coarse aerosols produced by cough-ing or sneezing, but it is inefficiently spread by fine-particle aerosols. The incubation period is ~4 to 6 days, and virus shedding may last for ≥2 weeks in children and for shorter periods in adults.

PATHOGENESIS   Little is known about the histopathology of minor RSV infection. Severe bronchiolitis or pneumonia is character-ized by necrosis of the bronchiolar epithelium and a peribronchiolar infiltrate of lymphocytes and mononuclear cells. Interalveolar thick-ening and filling of alveolar spaces with fluid can also be found. The characteristics of the immune response to RSV are not well elucidated. Because reinfection occurs frequently and is often associated with ill-ness, the immunity that develops after single episodes of infection clearly is not complete or long-lasting. However, the cumulative effect of multiple reinfections is to temper subsequent disease and to provide some temporary measure of protection against infection. Studies of experimentally induced disease in healthy volunteers indicate that the presence of nasal IgA neutralizing antibody correlates more closely with protection than does the presence of serum antibody. Studies in infants, however, suggest that maternally acquired antibody provides some protection from lower respiratory tract disease, although illness can be severe even in infants who have moderate levels of maternally derived serum antibody. The relatively severe disease observed in im-munosuppressed patients and experimental animal models indicates that cell-mediated immunity is an important mechanism of host de-fense against RSV. Evidence suggests that class I MHC-restricted cy-totoxic T cells may be particularly important in this regard.

CLINICAL MANIFESTATIONS   RSV infection leads to a wide spectrum of respiratory illnesses. In infants, 25 to 40% of infec-tions result in lower respiratory tract involvement, including pneu-monia, bronchiolitis, and tracheobronchitis. In this age group, illness begins most frequently with rhinorrhea, low-grade fever, and mild sys-temic symptoms, often accompanied by cough and wheezing. Most patients recover gradually over 1 to 2 weeks. In more severe illness, tachypnea and dyspnea develop, and eventually frank hypoxia, cya-nosis, and apnea can ensue. Physical examination may reveal diffuse wheezing, rhonchi, and rales. Chest radiography shows hyperexpan-sion, peribronchial thickening, and variable infiltrates ranging from diffuse interstitial infiltrates to segmental or lobar consolidation. Ill-ness may be particularly severe in children born prematurely and in those with congenital cardiac disease, bronchopulmonary dysplasia, nephrotic syndrome, or immunosuppression. One study documented a 37% mortality rate for infants with RSV pneumonia and congenital cardiac disease.

In adults, the most common symptoms of RSV infection are those of the common cold, with rhinorrhea, sore throat, and cough. Illness is occasionally associated with moderate systemic symptoms such as malaise, headache, and fever. RSV also has been reported to cause lower respiratory tract disease with fever in adults, including severe pneumonia in the elderly. RSV pneumonia can be a significant cause of morbidity and mortality in patients (particularly children) under-going bone-marrow and solid-organ transplantation.

LABORATORY FINDINGS AND DIAGNOSIS   The diag-nosis of RSV infection can be suspected on the basis of a suggestive epidemiologic setting—that is, severe illness among infants during an outbreak of RSV in the community. Infections in older children and adults cannot be differentiated with certainty from those caused by other respiratory viruses. The specific diagnosis is established by iso-lation of RSV from respiratory secretions, including sputum, throat swabs, or nasopharyngeal washes. Virus is detected in tissue culture and is identified specifically through immunologic reactions detected by immunofluorescence, enzyme-linked immunosorbent assay (ELISA), or other techniques. Immunofluorescence microscopy of na-sal scrapings or washings provides a rapid diagnosis. Serologic tests that depend on fourfold or greater rises in complement-fixing or neu-tralizing antibody titers are useful for diagnosis in older children and adults but are less sensitive in children under 4 months of age. ELISA is more sensitive than complement-fixation or neutralization tests in the detection of serum antibody. Serologic diagnosis requires com-parison of acute- and convalescent-phase serum specimens and is therefore not useful during acute illness.

TREATMENT   Treatment of upper respiratory tract RSV in-fection is aimed primarily at the alleviation of symptoms and is similar to that for other viral infections of the upper respiratory tract. For lower respiratory tract infections, respiratory therapy, including hydration, suctioning of secretions, and administration of humidified oxygen and antibronchospastic agents, is given as needed. In severe hypoxia, intubation and ventilatory assistance may be required. Stud-ies of infants with RSV infection who were given aerosolized ribavirin, a nucleoside analogue active in vitro against RSV, have demonstrated a beneficial effect on the resolution of lower respiratory tract illness, including alleviation of blood-gas abnormalities. Treatment with ri-bavirin is recommended for infants who are severely ill or who are at high risk for complications of RSV infection; included are premature infants and those with bronchopulmonary dysplasia, congenital heart disease, or immunosuppression. The effects of ribavirin in adults with RSV pneumonia have not been established. The monthly administra-tion of human immunoglobulin with high titers of antibody to RSV (RSVIG) or of a chimeric mouse-human IgG antibody to RSV (palivizumab) has been approved as prophylaxis against RSV for chil-dren younger than 2 years of age who have bronchopulmonary dys-plasia or were born prematurely.

Considerable interest exists in the development of vaccines against RSV. Inactivated whole-virus vaccines have been ineffective; in one study, they actually potentiated the disease in infants. Other ap-proaches include immunization with purified F and G surface glyco-proteins of RSV or generation of stable, live attenuated virus vaccines. In settings such as pediatric wards where rates of transmission are high, barrier methods for the protection of hands and conjunctivae may be useful in reducing the spread of virus.

PARAINFLUENZA VIRUS INFECTIONS

ETIOLOGIC AGENT   Parainfluenza viruses belong to the Paramyxoviridae family, are 150 to 250 nm in diameter, are enveloped, and contain a single-stranded RNA genome. The envelope is studded with two glycoproteins: one possesses both hemagglutinin and neu-raminidase activity and the other contains fusion activity. The viral RNA genome is enclosed in a helical nucleocapsid and codes for seven or eight virus-specific proteins. All four distinct serotypes of parain-fluenza viruses share certain antigens with other members of the Paramyxoviridae family, including mumps and Newcastle disease viruses.

EPIDEMIOLOGY   Parainfluenza viruses are distributed throughout the world; infection with type 4 (subtypes 4A and 4B) has been reported less widely, probably because type 4 is more difficult to grow in tissue culture. Infection is acquired in early childhood, so that by 8 years of age most children have antibodies to serotypes 1, 2, and 3. Types 1 and 2 cause epidemics during the fall, primarily in odd-numbered years. Type 3 infection has been detected during all seasons of the year, but epidemics have occurred annually in the spring.

The contribution of parainfluenza infections to respiratory disease varies with both the location and the year. In studies conducted in the United States, parainfluenza virus infections have accounted for 4.3 to 22% of respiratory illnesses in children. In adults, parainfluenza infections are generally mild and account for fewer than 5% of respiratory illnesses. The major importance of parainfluenza viruses is as a cause of respiratory illness in young children, in whom they rank second only to RSV as causes of lower respiratory tract illness. Parainfluenza virus type 1 is the most frequent cause of croup (laryngotracheobronchitis) in children, while serotype 2 causes similar, although generally less severe, disease. Type 3 is an important cause of bronchiolitis and pneumonia in infants, while illnesses associated with type 4 have generally been mild. Unlike types 1 and 2, type 3 frequently causes illness during the first month of life, when passively acquired maternal antibody is still present. Parainfluenza viruses are spread through infected respiratory secretions, primarily by person-to-person contact and/or by large droplets. The incubation period has varied from 3 to 6 days in experimental infections but may be somewhat shorter for naturally occurring disease in children.

PATHOGENESIS Immunity to parainfluenza viruses is incompletely understood, but evidence suggests that immunity to infections with serotypes 1 and 2 is mediated by local IgA antibodies in the respiratory tract. Passively acquired serum neutralizing antibodies also confer some protection against infection with types 1, 2, and—to a lesser degree—3. Studies in experimental animal models and in immunosuppressed patients suggest that cell-mediated immunity may also be important in parainfluenza virus infections.

CLINICAL MANIFESTATIONS Parainfluenza virus infections occur most frequently among children, in whom initial infection with serotype 1, 2, or 3 is associated with an acute febrile illness 50 to 80% of the time. Children may present with coryza, sore throat, hoarseness, and cough that may or may not be croupy. In severe croup, fever persists, with worsening coryza and sore throat. A brassy or barking cough may progress to frank stridor. Most children recover over the next 1 or 2 days, although progressive airway obstruction and hypoxia ensue occasionally. If bronchiolitis or pneumonia develops, progressive cough accompanied by wheezing, tachypnea, and intercostal retractions may occur. In this setting, sputum production increases modestly. Physical examination shows nasopharyngeal discharge and oropharyngeal injection, along with rhonchi, wheezes, or coarse breath sounds. Chest x-rays can show air trapping and occasionally interstitial infiltrates.

In older children and adults, parainfluenza infections tend to be milder, presenting most frequently as a common cold or as hoarseness, with or without cough. Lower respiratory tract involvement in older children and adults is uncommon, but tracheobronchitis in adults has been reported. Severe, prolonged, and even fatal parainfluenza infection has been reported in children and adults with severe immunosuppression, including bone-marrow and solid-organ transplant recipients.

LABORATORY FINDINGS AND DIAGNOSIS The clinical syndromes caused by parainfluenza viruses (with the possible exception of croup in young children) are not sufficiently distinctive to be diagnosed on clinical grounds alone. A specific diagnosis is established by detection of virus in respiratory tract secretions, throat swabs, or nasopharyngeal washings. Virus is detected by growth in tissue culture (either by hemagglutination or by a cytopathic effect), by immunofluorescence of viral antigens in exfoliated cells from the respiratory tract, or by ELISA. Polymerase chain reaction assays have also been developed. Serologic diagnosis is based on a fourfold or greater rise in antibody titer, as detected by hemagglutination inhibition or by complement-fixation or neutralization tests in acute- and convalescent-phase specimens. However, as frequent heterotypic responses occur among the parainfluenza serotypes, the serotype causing illness often cannot be identified by serologic techniques alone.

Acute epiglottitis caused by *Haemophilus influenzae* type b must be differentiated from viral croup. Influenza A virus also is a common cause of croup during epidemic periods.

℞ TREATMENT For upper respiratory tract illness, symptoms can be treated as discussed for other viral respiratory tract illnesses. If complications such as sinusitis, otitis, or superimposed bacterial bronchitis develop, appropriate antibiotics should be administered. Mild cases of croup should be treated with bed rest and moist air generated by vaporizers. More severe cases require hospitalization and close observation for the development of respiratory distress. If acute respiratory distress develops, humidified oxygen and intermittent racemic epinephrine are usually administered. Aerosolized or systemically administered glucocorticoids are beneficial; the latter have a more profound effect. No specific antiviral therapy is available, although ribavirin is active against parainfluenza viruses in vitro and anecdotal reports describe its use clinically. Effective vaccines against parainfluenza viruses have not been developed.

ADENOVIRUS INFECTIONS

ETIOLOGIC AGENT Adenoviruses are complex DNA viruses that measure 70 to 80 nm in diameter. Human adenoviruses belong to the genus *Mastadenovirus*, which includes at least 47 serotypes. Adenoviruses have a characteristic morphology consisting of an icosahedral shell composed of 20 equilateral triangular faces and 12 vertices. The protein coat (capsid) consists of hexon subunits with group-specific and type-specific antigenic determinants and penton subunits at each vertex primarily containing group-specific antigens. A fiber with a knob at the end projects from each penton; this fiber contains type-specific and some group-specific antigens. Human adenoviruses have been divided into six subgenera (A through F) on the basis of the homology of DNA genomes and other properties. The adenovirus genome is a linear double-stranded DNA that codes for structural and nonstructural polypeptides. The replicative cycle of adenovirus may result either in lytic infection of cells or in the establishment of a latent infection (primarily involving lymphoid cells). Some adenovirus types can induce oncogenic transformation, and tumor formation has been observed in rodents; however, despite intensive investigation, adenoviruses have not been associated with tumors in humans.

EPIDEMIOLOGY Adenovirus infections most frequently affect infants and children. Infections occur throughout the year but are most common from fall to spring. Adenoviruses account for 3 to 5% of acute respiratory infections in children but for fewer than 2% of respiratory illnesses in civilian adults. Nearly 100% of adults have serum antibody to multiple serotypes—a finding indicating that infection is common in childhood. Types 1, 2, 3, and 5 are the most frequent isolates from children. Certain adenovirus serotypes—particularly 4 and 7 but also 3, 14, and 21—are associated with outbreaks of acute respiratory disease in military recruits in winter and spring. Adenovirus infection can be transmitted by inhalation of aerosolized virus, by inoculation of virus into conjunctival sacs, and probably by the fecal-oral route as well. Type-specific antibody generally develops after infection and is associated with protection against infection with the same serotype.

CLINICAL MANIFESTATIONS In children, adenoviruses cause a variety of clinical syndromes. The most common is an acute upper respiratory tract infection, with prominent rhinitis. On occasion, lower respiratory tract disease, including bronchiolitis and pneumonia, also develops. Adenoviruses, particularly types 3 and 7, cause pharyngoconjunctival fever, a characteristic acute febrile illness of children that occurs in outbreaks, most often in summer camps. The syndrome is marked by bilateral conjunctivitis in which the bulbar and palpebral conjunctivae have a granular appearance. Low-grade fever is frequently present for the first 3 to 5 days, and rhinitis, sore throat, and cervical adenopathy develop. The illness generally lasts for 1 to 2 weeks and resolves spontaneously. Febrile pharyngitis without conjunctivitis also has been associated with adenovirus infection. Adenoviruses have been isolated from cases of whooping cough with or without *Bordetella pertussis;* the significance of adenovirus in that disease is unknown.

In adults, the most frequently reported illness has been acute respiratory disease caused by adenovirus types 4 and 7 in military recruits. This illness is marked by a prominent sore throat and the gradual onset of fever, which often reaches 39°C (102.2°F) on the second or third day of illness. Cough is almost always present, and coryza and regional lymphadenopathy are frequently seen. Physical examination may show pharyngeal edema, injection, and tonsillar enlargement with little or no exudate. If pneumonia has developed, auscultation and x-ray of the chest may indicate areas of patchy infiltration.

Adenoviruses have been associated with a number of non–respiratory tract diseases, including acute diarrheal illness caused by types 40 and 41 in young children and hemorrhagic cystitis caused by types 11 and 21. Epidemic keratoconjunctivitis, caused most frequently by types 8, 19, and 37, has been associated with contaminated common sources such as ophthalmic solutions and roller towels. Adenoviruses also have been implicated in disseminated disease and pneumonia in immunosuppressed patients, including recipients of solid-organ or bone-marrow transplants and patients with AIDS. In the latter group, high-numbered and intermediate serotypes have been isolated, usually in the setting of low CD4+ counts, but their isolation frequently has not been clearly linked to disease manifestations. Adenovirus nucleic acids have been detected in myocardial cells from patients with "idiopathic" myocardiopathies, and adenoviruses have been suggested as causative agents in some cases.

LABORATORY FINDINGS AND DIAGNOSIS Adenovirus infection should be suspected in the epidemiologic setting of acute respiratory disease in military recruits and in certain of the clinical syndromes (such as pharyngoconjunctival fever or epidemic keratoconjunctivitis) in which outbreaks of characteristic illnesses occur. In most cases, however, illnesses caused by adenovirus infection cannot be differentiated from those caused by a number of other viral respiratory agents and *Mycoplasma pneumoniae*. A definitive diagnosis of adenovirus infection is established by culture or detection of the virus by means of ELISA or nucleic acid hybridization from sites such as the conjunctiva and oropharynx or from sputum, urine, or stool. Virus may be detected in tissue culture by cytopathic changes and specifically identified by immunofluorescence or other immunologic techniques. Adenovirus types 40 and 41, which have been associated with diarrheal disease in children, require special tissue-culture cells for isolation, and these serotypes are most commonly detected by direct ELISA of stool. Serum antibody rises can be demonstrated by complement-fixation or neutralization tests, ELISA, radioimmunoassay, or (for those adenoviruses that hemagglutinate red cells) hemagglutination inhibition tests.

℞ **TREATMENT** Only symptom-based treatment and supportive therapy are available for adenovirus infections, and no clinically useful antiviral compounds have been identified. Live vaccines have been developed against adenovirus types 4 and 7 and have been used to control illness in military recruits. These vaccines consist of live, unattenuated virus administered in enteric-coated capsules. Infection of the gastrointestinal tract with types 4 and 7 does not cause disease but stimulates local and systemic antibodies that are protective against subsequent acute respiratory disease due to those serotypes. Vaccines prepared from purified subunits of adenovirus are being investigated. Adenoviruses are also being studied as live-virus vectors for the delivery of vaccine antigens and for gene therapy.

BIBLIOGRAPHY

RHINOVIRUSES

GWALTNEY JM: Rhinoviruses, in *Principles and Practice of Infectious Diseases*, 5th ed, GF Mandell et al (eds). New York, Saunders, 2000, pp 1940–1948

MAKELA MJ et al: Viruses and bacteria in the etiology of the common cold. J Clin Microbiol 36:539, 1998

ROSSMAN MG et al: Structure of a human common cold virus and functional relationships to other picornaviruses. Nature 317:145, 1985

TYRRELL DAJ: A view from the Common Cold Unit. Antiviral Res 18:105, 1992

CORONAVIRUSES

LAI MMC: Coronavirus: Organization, replication, and expression of genome. Annu Rev Microbiol 44:303, 1990

LARSON HE et al: Isolation of rhinoviruses and coronaviruses from 38 colds in adults. J Med Virol 5:221, 1980

MCINTOSH K: Coronaviruses, in *Virology*, 3d ed, BN Fields (ed). New York, Raven, 1995, pp 1095–1103

RESPIRATORY SYNCYTIAL VIRUS

ANDERSON LJ et al: Multicenter study of strains of respiratory syncytial virus. J Infect Dis 163:687, 1991

CANE PA et al: Molecular epidemiology of human respiratory syncytial virus. Semin Virol 6:371, 1995

CHANOCK RM et al: Serious respiratory tract disease caused by respiratory syncytial virus: Prospects for improved therapy and effective immunization. Pediatrics 90:137, 1992

COMMITTEE ON INFECTIOUS DISEASES: Use of ribavirin in the treatment of respiratory syncytial virus infection. Pediatrics 92:501, 1993

ENGLUND JA et al: Respiratory syncytial virus infection in immunocompromised adults. Ann Intern Med 109:203, 1988

GLEZEN WP et al: Risk of primary infection and reinfection with respiratory syncytial virus. Am J Dis Child 140:543, 1986

PARAINFLUENZA VIRUSES

DENNY FW et al: Croup: An 11 year study in a pediatric practice. Pediatrics 71:871, 1983

REED G et al: Epidemiology and clinical impact of parainfluenza virus infections in otherwise healthy infants and young children <5 years old. J Infect Dis 175:807, 1997

WRIGHT PF: Parainfluenza viruses, in *Viral Infections of the Respiratory Tract*, R Dolin, PF Wright (eds). New York, Marcel Dekker, 1999

ADENOVIRUSES

BAUM SG: Adenoviruses, in *Principles and Practice of Infectious Diseases*, 5th ed, GF Mandell et al (eds). New York, Saunders, 2000, pp 1624–1629

CRAWFORD-MIKSZU XX et al: Seroepidemiology of new AIDS-associated adenoviruses among the San Francisco Men's Health Study. J Med Virol 50:230, 1996

HIERHOLZER JC: Adenoviruses in the immunocompromised host. Clin Microbiol Rev 5:262, 1992

ROSE HM et al: Adenoviral infection in military recruits. Arch Environ Health 21:356, 1970

190 *Raphael Dolin*

INFLUENZA

DEFINITION Influenza is an acute respiratory illness caused by infection with influenza viruses. The illness affects the upper and/or lower respiratory tract and is often accompanied by systemic signs and symptoms such as fever, headache, myalgia, and weakness. Outbreaks of illness of variable extent and severity occur nearly every winter. Such outbreaks result in significant morbidity in the general population and in increased mortality rates among certain high-risk patients, mainly as a result of pulmonary complications.

ETIOLOGIC AGENT Influenza viruses are members of the Orthomyxoviridae family. Influenza A and B viruses constitute one genus, and influenza C viruses make up the other. The designation of influenza viruses as type A, B, or C is based on antigenic characteristics of the nucleoprotein (NP) and matrix (M) protein antigens. Influenza A viruses are further subdivided (subtyped) on the basis of the surface hemagglutinin (H) and neuraminidase (N) antigens (see below); individual strains are designated according to the site of origin, isolate number, year of isolation, and subtype—for example, influenza A/Sydney/5/97 (H3N2). Influenza B and C viruses are similarly designated, but H and N antigens from these viruses do not receive subtype designations, since intratypic variations in influenza B antigens are less extensive than those in influenza A viruses and may not occur with influenza C virus.

Most of the information on the molecular biology of influenza viruses has come from studies of influenza A viruses; less is known about the replicative cycle of influenza B and C viruses. Morphologically, influenza viruses A, B, and C are similar. The virions are irregularly shaped spherical particles, 80 to 120 nm in diameter, and have a lipid envelope from the surface of which the H and N glycoproteins project (Fig. 190-1). The hemagglutinin is the site by which virus binds to cell receptors, whereas the neuraminidase degrades the receptor and probably plays a role in the release of virus from infected cells after replication has taken place. Influenza viruses enter cells by receptor-mediated endocytosis, forming a virus-containing endosome. The viral hemagglutinin mediates fusion of the endosomal membrane with the virus envelope, and viral nucleocapsids are subsequently released into the cytoplasm. Antibodies to the H antigen are the major determinants of immunity to influenza virus, while those to the N antigen limit viral spread and contribute to reduction of the infection. The inner surface of the lipid envelope contains the M proteins M1 and M2, the functions of which are incompletely understood but which may be involved in virus assembly and in stabilization of the lipid envelope. The virion also contains the NP antigen, which is associated with the viral genome, as well as three polymerase (P) proteins that are essential for transcription and synthesis of viral RNA. Two nonstructural (NS) proteins of unknown function are also present in infected cells.

The genomes of influenza A and B viruses consist of eight single-stranded RNA segments, which code for the structural and nonstructural proteins. Because the genome is segmented, the opportunity for reassortment of genes during infection is high, and reassortment occurs frequently during infection of cells with more than one influenza A virus.

EPIDEMIOLOGY Influenza outbreaks are recorded virtually every year, although their extent and severity vary widely. Localized outbreaks take place at variable intervals, usually every 1 to 3 years. Except for the past two decades, global epidemics or pandemics have occurred approximately every 10 to 15 years since the 1918–1919 pandemic (Table 190-1).

The most extensive and severe outbreaks are caused by influenza A viruses. In part, this predominance is a result of the remarkable propensity of the H and N antigens of influenza A virus to undergo periodic antigenic variation. Major antigenic variations are referred to as *antigenic shifts*, which may be associated with pandemics and are restricted to influenza A viruses. Minor variations are called *antigenic drifts*. These antigenic changes may involve the hemagglutinin alone or both the hemagglutinin and the neuraminidase. In human infections,

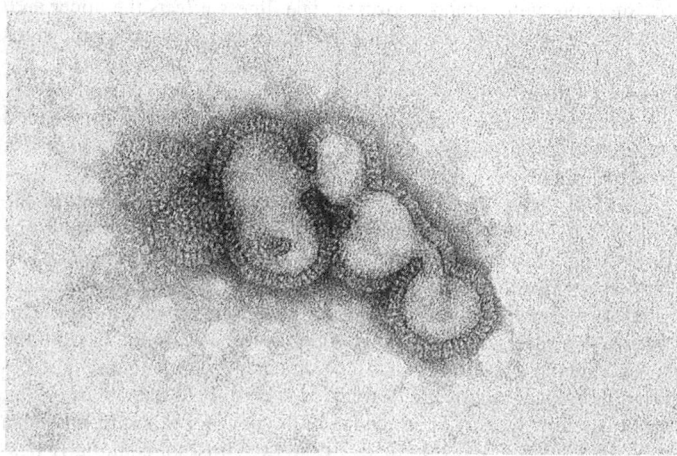

FIGURE 190-1 An electron micrograph of influenza virus (×143,000). *(From R Dolin, Am Fam Phys 14:74, 1976.)*

Table 190-1 Emergence of Antigenic Subtypes of Influenza A Virus Associated with Pandemic or Epidemic Disease

Years	Subtype	Extent of Outbreak
1889–90	H2N8[a]	Severe pandemic
1900–03	H3N8[a]	?Moderate epidemic
1918–19	H1N1[b] (formerly HswN1)	Severe pandemic
1933–35	H1N1[b] (formerly H0N1)	Mild epidemic
1946–47	H1N1	Mild epidemic
1957–58	H2N2	Severe pandemic
1968–69	H3N2	Moderate pandemic
1977–78[c]	H1N1	Mild pandemic

[a] As determined by retrospective serologic survey of individuals alive during those years (''seroarcheology'').
[b] Hemagglutinins formerly designated as Hsw and H0 are now classified as variants of H1.
[c] From this time until the present (1999–2000), viruses of the H1N1 and H3N2 subtypes have circulated either in alternating years or concurrently.

three major antigenic subtypes of hemagglutinins (H1, H2, and H3) and two of neuraminidases (N1 and N2) have been recognized. The hemagglutinins formerly designated as H0 and Hsw are now classified as variants of H1. An example of an antigenic shift involving both the hemagglutinin and the neuraminidase is that of 1957, when the predominant influenza A virus subtype shifted from H1N1 to H2N2; this shift resulted in a severe pandemic, with an estimated 70,000 excess deaths (i.e., deaths in excess of the number expected without an influenza epidemic) in the United States alone. In 1968, an antigenic shift involving only the hemagglutinin occurred (H2N2 to H3N2); the subsequent pandemic was less severe than that of 1957. In 1977, an H1N1 virus emerged and caused a pandemic that primarily affected younger individuals (i.e., those born after 1957). As can be seen in Table 190-1, H1N1 viruses circulated from 1918 to 1956; thus, individuals born prior to 1957 would be expected to have some degree of immunity to H1N1 viruses. During most outbreaks of influenza A, a single subtype has circulated at a time. However, since 1977, H1N1 and H3N2 viruses have circulated simultaneously, resulting in outbreaks of varying severity. In some outbreaks, influenza B viruses have also circulated simultaneously with influenza A viruses.

The origin of pandemic strains is unknown. Given the marked differences between the primary structures of the hemagglutinins of different subtypes of influenza A viruses (H1, H2, and H3), it seems unlikely that antigenic shifts result from spontaneous mutations in the hemagglutinin gene. Because the segmented genome of influenza viruses may result in high rates of reassortment, it has been suggested that pandemic strains may emerge by reassortment of genes between human and animal viruses. There was concern that such reassortment might have occurred in 1997 in Hong Kong, where cases of infection caused by influenza virus A/H5N1 were detected in humans during an extensive outbreak of avian influenza A/H5N1 in poultry. However, only a few cases of A/H5N1 influenza in humans were documented, and the infection did not spread into the community. Influenza B viruses do not have an animal reservoir and do not undergo antigenic shifts, although they do undergo antigenic drift.

Pandemics provide the most dramatic evidence of the impact of influenza. However, illnesses that occur between pandemics account for greater total mortality and morbidity, albeit over a longer period. From 1972 through the present, influenza has been associated with at least 20,000 excess deaths during more than half of the interpandemic epidemics in the United States; more than 40,000 influenza-associated deaths occurred in each of three of these epidemics. Influenza A viruses that circulate between pandemics demonstrate antigenic drifts in the H antigen. These antigenic drifts apparently result from point mutations involving the RNA segment that codes for the hemagglutinin. Epidemiologically significant strains—that is, those with the potential to cause widespread outbreaks—exhibit changes in amino acids in at least two of the major antigenic sites in the hemagglutinin molecule. Since two point mutations are unlikely to occur simultaneously, it is believed that antigenic drifts result from point mutations occurring sequentially during the spread of virus from person to person. Antigenic drifts have been reported nearly annually since 1977 for H1N1 viruses and since 1968 for H3N2 viruses.

Influenza A epidemics begin abruptly, peak over a 2- to 3-week period, generally last for 2 to 3 months, and often subside almost as rapidly as they began. The first indication of influenza activity in a community is an increase in the number of children with febrile respiratory illnesses who present for medical attention. This increase is followed by increases in rates of influenza-like illnesses among adults and eventually by an increase in hospital admissions for patients with pneumonia, worsening of congestive heart failure, and exacerbations of chronic pulmonary disease. Rates of absence from work and school also rise at this time. An increase in the number of deaths caused by pneumonia and influenza is generally a late observation in an outbreak. Attack rates have been highly variable from outbreak to outbreak but most commonly are in the range of 10 to 20% of the general population. During the pandemic of 1957, it was estimated that the attack rate of clinical influenza exceeded 50% in urban populations and that an additional 25% or more of individuals in these populations may have been subclinically infected with influenza A virus. Among institutionalized populations and in semiclosed settings with a large number of susceptible individuals, even higher attack rates have been reported.

Epidemics of influenza occur almost exclusively during the winter months in the temperate zones of the northern and southern hemispheres. In those locations, it is highly unusual to detect influenza A virus at other times, although serologic rises or even outbreaks have been noted rarely during warm-weather months. In contrast, influenza virus infections occur throughout the year in the tropics. Where or how influenza A virus persists between outbreaks in temperate zones is unknown. It is possible that influenza A viruses are maintained in the human population on a worldwide basis by person-to-person transmission and that large population clusters support a low level of interepidemic transmission. Alternatively, human strains may persist in animal reservoirs. Convincing evidence to support either explanation is not available. In the modern era, rapid transportation may contribute to the transmission of viruses among widespread geographic locales.

The factors that result in the inception and termination of outbreaks of influenza are incompletely understood. A major determinant of the extent and severity of an outbreak is the level of immunity in the population at risk. With the emergence of an antigenically novel influenza virus to which little or no antibody is present in a community, extensive outbreaks may occur. When the absence of antibody is worldwide, epidemic disease may spread around the globe, resulting in a pandemic. Such pandemic waves can continue for several years, until immunity in the population reaches a high level. In the years following pandemic influenza, antigenic drifts among influenza viruses result in outbreaks of variable severity in populations with high levels of immunity to the pandemic strain that circulated earlier. This situation persists until another antigenically novel pandemic strain emerges. On the other hand, outbreaks sometimes end despite the persistence of a large pool of susceptible individuals in the population.

Occasionally, the emergence of a significantly different antigenic variant will result only in a localized outbreak. The swine influenza outbreak of 1976 in the United States, caused by an A/H1N1 virus antigenically similar to the virus that circulated in 1918–1919, may be an example, although this outbreak may have represented simply the introduction of a swine influenza virus into a crowded human population without spread beyond that setting. The cluster of human infections with influenza A/H5N1 in Hong Kong in 1997 may also be an example of this phenomenon. It has been suggested that certain viruses, such as recently circulating A/H1N1 strains, may be intrinsically less virulent and cause less severe disease than other variants, even in immunologically virgin subjects. If so, then other (undefined) factors besides the level of preexisting immunity must play a role in the epidemiology of influenza.

Influenza B virus causes outbreaks that are generally less extensive and are associated with less severe disease than those caused by influenza A virus. The hemagglutinin and neuraminidase of influenza B virus undergo less frequent and less extensive variation than those of influenza A viruses; this characteristic may account, in part, for the lesser extent of disease. Influenza B outbreaks are seen most frequently in schools and military camps, although outbreaks in institutions in which elderly individuals reside have also been noted on occasion. The most serious complication of influenza B virus infection is Reye's syndrome (Chap. 300). Influenza C virus has only infrequently been associated with human disease, although the wide prevalence of serum antibody to this virus indicates that asymptomatic infection may be common.

The morbidity and mortality caused by influenza outbreaks continue to be substantial. Most individuals who die in this setting have underlying diseases that place them at high risk for complications of influenza. Excess hospitalizations for adults with high-risk medical conditions have ranged from 20 to 1000 per 100,000 during recent outbreaks of influenza. The most prominent high-risk conditions are chronic cardiac and pulmonary diseases as well as old age. Mortality among individuals with chronic metabolic, renal, and certain immunosuppressive diseases has also been elevated, although lower than that among patients with chronic cardiopulmonary diseases. The morbidity attributable to influenza in the general population is considerable. For each of three outbreaks in the United States that were studied during the 1960s, estimated direct and indirect economic costs ranged from $1.5 to $3.5 billion; today such costs would obviously be much greater.

PATHOGENESIS The initial event in influenza is infection of the respiratory epithelium with influenza virus acquired from respiratory secretions of acutely infected individuals. In all likelihood, transmission occurs via aerosols generated by coughs and sneezes, although hand-to-hand contact, other personal contact, and even fomite transmission may take place. Experimental evidence suggests that infection by a small-particle aerosol (particle diameter, $<10\ \mu m$) is more efficient than that by larger droplets. Initially, viral infection involves the ciliated columnar epithelial cells, but it also may involve other respiratory tract cells, including alveolar cells, mucous gland cells, and macrophages. In infected cells, virus replicates within 4 to 6 h, after which infectious virus is released to infect adjacent or nearby cells. In this way, infection spreads from a few foci to a large number of respiratory cells over several hours. In experimentally induced infection, the incubation period of illness has ranged from 18 to 72 h, depending on the size of the virus inoculum. Histopathologic study reveals degenerative changes, including granulation, vacuolization, swelling, and pyknotic nuclei, in infected ciliated cells. The cells eventually become necrotic and desquamate; in some areas, previously columnar epithelium is replaced by flattened and metaplastic epithelial cells. The severity of illness is correlated with the quantity of virus shed in secretions; thus, the degree of viral replication itself may be an important factor in pathogenesis. Despite the frequent development of systemic signs and symptoms such as fever, headache, and myalgias, influenza virus has only rarely been detected in extrapulmonary sites (including the bloodstream). Evidence suggests that the pathogenesis of systemic symptoms in influenza may be related to the induction of certain cytokines, particularly tumor necrosis factor α and interleukin 6.

The host response to influenza infections involves a complex interplay of humoral antibody, local antibody, cell-mediated immunity, interferon, and other host defenses. Serum antibody responses, which can be detected by the second week after primary infection, are measured by a variety of techniques: hemagglutination inhibition (HI), complement fixation (CF), neutralization, enzyme-linked immunosorbent assay (ELISA), and antineuraminidase antibody assay. Antibodies directed against the hemagglutinin appear to be the most important mediators of immunity; in several studies, HI titers of ≥ 40 have been associated with protection from infection. Secretory antibodies produced in the respiratory tract are predominantly of the IgA class and also play a major role in protection against infection. Secretory antibody neutralization titers of ≥ 4 have also been associated with protection. A variety of cell-mediated immune responses, both antigen-specific and antigen-nonspecific, can be detected early after infection and depend on the prior immune status of the host. These responses include T-cell proliferative, T-cell cytotoxic, and natural killer cell activity. Interferons have been detected in respiratory secretions shortly after the shedding of virus has begun, and rises in interferon titers coincide with decreases in virus shedding.

The host defense factors responsible for cessation of virus shedding and resolution of illness have not been defined specifically. Virus shedding generally stops within 2 to 5 days after symptoms first appear, at a time when serum and local antibody responses often are not detectable by conventional techniques (although antibody rises may be detected earlier by use of highly sensitive techniques, particularly in individuals with previous immunity to the virus). It has been suggested that interferon, cell-mediated immune responses, and/or nonspecific inflammatory responses are important in the resolution of illness.

MANIFESTATIONS　Influenza has most frequently been described as an illness characterized by the abrupt onset of systemic symptoms, such as headache, feverishness, chills, myalgia, or malaise, and accompanying respiratory tract signs, particularly cough and sore throat. In many cases, the onset is so abrupt that patients can recall the precise time they became ill. A typical case of naturally occurring influenza is depicted in Fig. 190-2. However, the spectrum of clinical presentations is wide, ranging from a mild, afebrile respiratory illness similar to the common cold (with either a gradual or an abrupt onset) to severe prostration with relatively few respiratory signs and symptoms. In most of the cases that come to a physician's attention, the patient has a fever, with temperatures of 38° to 41°C (100.4° to 105.8°F). A rapid temperature rise within the first 24 h of illness is generally followed by a gradual defervescence over a 2- to 3-day period, although, on occasion, fever may last for as long as a week. Patients report a feverish feeling and chilliness, but true rigors are rare. Headache, either generalized or frontal, is often particularly troublesome. Myalgias may involve any part of the body but are most common in the legs and lumbosacral area. Arthralgias may also develop.

Respiratory complaints often become more prominent as systemic

symptoms subside. Many patients have a sore throat or persistent cough, which may last for a week or more and which is often accompanied by substernal discomfort. Ocular signs and symptoms include pain on motion of the eyes, photophobia, and burning of the eyes.

Physical findings are usually minimal in cases of uncomplicated influenza. Early in the illness, the patient appears flushed and the skin is hot and dry, although diaphoresis and mottled extremities are sometimes evident, particularly in older patients. Examination of the pharynx may yield surprisingly unremarkable results despite a severe sore throat, but injection of the mucous membranes and postnasal discharge are apparent in some cases. Mild cervical lymphadenopathy may be noted, especially in younger individuals. The results of chest examination are largely negative in uncomplicated influenza, although rhonchi, wheezes, and scattered rales have been reported with variable frequency in different outbreaks. Frank dyspnea, hyperpnea, cyanosis, diffuse rales, and signs of consolidation are indicative of pulmonary complications. Patients with apparently uncomplicated influenza have been reported to have a variety of mild ventilatory defects and increased alveolar-capillary diffusion gradients; thus, subclinical pulmonary involvement may be more frequent than is appreciated.

In uncomplicated influenza, the acute illness generally resolves over a 2- to 5-day period, and most patients have largely recovered in 1 week. In a significant minority (particularly the elderly), however, symptoms of weakness or lassitude (postinfluenzal asthenia) may persist for several weeks and may prove troublesome for persons who wish to resume their full level of activity promptly. The pathogenetic basis for this asthenia is unknown, although pulmonary function abnormalities may persist for several weeks after uncomplicated influenza.

COMPLICATIONS　The most common complication of influenza is pneumonia: "primary" influenza viral pneumonia, secondary bacterial pneumonia, or mixed viral and bacterial pneumonia. Primary influenza viral pneumonia is the least common but most severe of the pneumonic complications. It presents as acute influenza that does not resolve but instead progresses relentlessly, with persistent fever, dyspnea, and eventual cyanosis. Sputum production is generally scanty, but the sputum can contain blood. Few physical signs may be evident early in the illness. In more advanced cases, diffuse rales may be noted, and chest x-ray findings consistent with diffuse interstitial infiltrates and/or acute respiratory distress syndrome may be present. In such cases, arterial blood-gas determinations show marked hypoxia. Viral cultures of respiratory secretions and lung parenchyma, especially if samples are taken early in illness, yield high titers of virus. In fatal cases of primary viral pneumonia, histopathologic examination reveals a marked inflammatory reaction in the alveolar septa, with edema and infiltration by lymphocytes, macrophages, occasional plasma cells, and variable numbers of neutrophils. Fibrin thrombi in alveolar capillaries, along with necrosis and hemorrhage, have also been noted. Eosinophilic hyaline membranes can be found lining alveoli and alveolar ducts.

Primary influenza viral pneumonia has a predilection for individuals with cardiac disease, particularly those with mitral stenosis, but has also been reported in otherwise healthy young adults as well as in older individuals with chronic pulmonary disorders. In some epidemics of influenza (notably those of 1918 and 1957), pregnancy increased the risk of primary influenza pneumonia.

Secondary bacterial pneumonia follows acute influenza. Improvement of the patient's condition over 2 to 3 days is followed by a reappearance of fever along with clinical signs and symptoms of bacterial pneumonia, including cough, production of purulent sputum, and physical and x-ray signs of consolidation. The most common bacterial pathogens in this setting are *Streptococcus pneumoniae*, *Staphylococcus aureus*, and *Haemophilus influenzae*—organisms that can colonize the nasopharynx and that cause infection in the wake of changes in bronchopulmonary defenses. The etiology can often be determined by Gram's staining and culture of an appropriately obtained sputum specimen. Secondary bacterial pneumonia occurs most frequently in high-risk individuals with chronic pulmonary and cardiac disease and

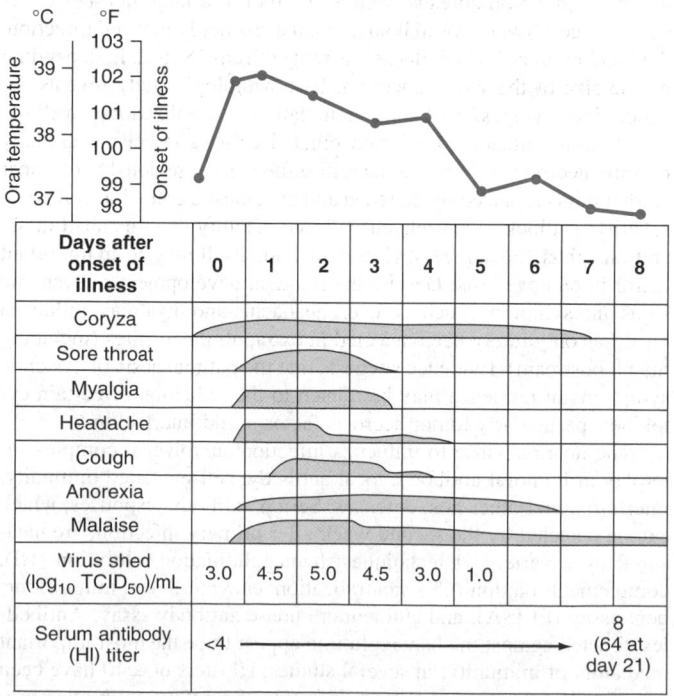

FIGURE 190-2　Clinical characteristics of a naturally occurring case of influenza A in an otherwise healthy 28-year-old man. *(From R Dolin, Am Fam Phys 14:74, 1976.)*

in elderly individuals. Patients with secondary bacterial pneumonia often respond to antibiotic therapy when it is instituted promptly.

Perhaps the most common pneumonic complications during outbreaks of influenza have mixed features of viral and bacterial pneumonia. Patients may experience a gradual progression of their acute illness or may show transient improvement followed by clinical exacerbation, with eventual manifestation of the clinical features of bacterial pneumonia. Sputum cultures may contain both influenza A virus and one of the bacterial pathogens described above. Patchy infiltrates or areas of consolidation may be detected by physical examination and chest x-ray. Patients with mixed viral and bacterial pneumonia generally have less widespread involvement of the lung than those with primary viral pneumonia, and their bacterial infections may respond to appropriate antibiotics. Mixed viral and bacterial pneumonia occurs primarily in patients with chronic cardiovascular and pulmonary diseases.

Other pulmonary complications associated with influenza include worsening of chronic obstructive pulmonary disease and exacerbation of chronic bronchitis and asthma. In children, influenza infection may present as croup.

In addition to the pulmonary complications of influenza, a number of extrapulmonary complications may occur. These include *Reye's syndrome*, a serious complication in children that is associated with influenza B and to a lesser extent with influenza A virus infection as well as with varicella-zoster virus infection. An epidemiologic association between Reye's syndrome and aspirin therapy for the antecedent viral infection has been noted, and the incidence of Reye's syndrome has decreased markedly with widespread warnings regarding the use of aspirin by children with acute viral respiratory infections. A detailed description of Reye's syndrome is found in Chap. 300.

Myositis, rhabdomyolysis, and myoglobinuria are occasional complications of influenza infection. Although myalgias are exceedingly common in influenza, true myositis is rare. Patients with acute myositis have exquisite tenderness of the affected muscles, most commonly in the legs, and may not be able to tolerate even the slightest pressure, such as the touch of bedsheets. In the most severe cases, there is frank swelling and bogginess of muscles. Serum levels of creatine phosphokinase and aldolase are markedly elevated, and an occasional patient has developed renal failure from myoglobinuria. The pathogenesis of influenza-associated myositis is also unclear, although the presence of influenza virus in affected muscles has been reported.

Myocarditis and pericarditis were reported in association with influenza virus infection during the 1918–1919 pandemic; these reports were based largely on histopathologic findings, and these complications have been reported only infrequently since that time. Electrocardiographic changes during acute influenza are common among patients who have cardiac disease but have been ascribed most often to exacerbations of the underlying cardiac disease rather than to direct involvement of the myocardium with influenza virus.

Central nervous system (CNS) diseases, including encephalitis, transverse myelitis, and Guillain-Barré syndrome, have been reported during influenza. The etiologic relationship of influenza virus to such CNS illnesses remains unestablished. Toxic shock syndrome caused by *S. aureus* infection following acute influenza infection has also been reported (Chap. 139).

In addition to complications involving the specific organ systems described above, influenza outbreaks include a number of cases in which elderly and other high-risk individuals develop influenza and subsequently experience a gradual deterioration of underlying cardiovascular, pulmonary, or renal function—changes that occasionally are irreversible and lead to death. These fatalities contribute to the overall excess mortality associated with influenza A outbreaks.

LABORATORY FINDINGS AND DIAGNOSIS Laboratory diagnosis is accomplished during acute influenza by isolation of the virus from throat swabs, nasopharyngeal washes, or sputum. Virus is usually detected in tissue culture or less commonly is found in the amniotic cavity of chick embryos within 48 to 72 h after inoculation. The rapid viral diagnostic tests now available detect viral nucleoprotein or neuraminidase with high specificity and sensitivities of 57 to 81% compared with tissue culture. Viral nucleic acids have been detected in clinical samples by reverse transcriptase polymerase chain reaction. The type of influenza virus (A or B) may be determined by either immunofluorescence or HI techniques, and the hemagglutinin subtype of influenza A virus (H1, H2, or H3) may be identified by HI with use of subtype-specific antisera. Serologic methods for diagnosis require comparison of antibody titers in sera obtained during the acute illness with those in sera obtained 10 to 14 days after the onset of illness and are useful primarily in retrospect. Fourfold or greater titer rises as detected by HI or CF or significant rises as measured by ELISA are diagnostic of acute infection. CF tests are generally less sensitive than other serologic techniques, but, as they detect type-specific antigens, they may be particularly useful when subtype-specific reagents are not available.

Other laboratory tests are generally not helpful in making a specific diagnosis of influenza virus infection. Leukocyte counts are variable, frequently being low early in illness and normal or slightly elevated later. Severe leukopenia has been described in overwhelming viral or bacterial infection, while leukocytosis with more than 15,000 cells/μL raises the suspicion of secondary bacterial infection.

DIFFERENTIAL DIAGNOSIS On clinical grounds alone, an individual case of influenza may be difficult to differentiate from an acute respiratory illness caused by any of a variety of respiratory viruses or by *Mycoplasma pneumoniae*. Severe streptococcal pharyngitis or early bacterial pneumonia may mimic acute influenza, although bacterial pneumonias generally do not run a self-limited course. Purulent sputum in which a bacterial pathogen can be detected by Gram's staining is an important diagnostic feature in bacterial pneumonia. The fact that influenza occurs in characteristic outbreaks during the winter months may facilitate a clinical diagnosis. When local health authorities indicate that influenza is present in the community, an acute febrile respiratory illness can be attributed to influenza with a high degree of certainty, particularly if the typical features of abrupt onset and systemic symptoms are present.

TREATMENT In uncomplicated cases of influenza, symptom-based therapy with acetaminophen for the relief of headache, myalgia, and fever may be considered, but the use of salicylates should be avoided in children below 18 years of age because of the possible association of salicylates with Reye's syndrome. Since cough is ordinarily self-limited, treatment with cough suppressants generally is not indicated, although codeine-containing compounds may be employed if the cough is particularly troublesome. Patients should be advised to rest and maintain hydration during acute illness and should return to full activity only gradually after the illness has resolved, especially if the illness has been severe.

Specific antiviral therapy is available for influenza: amantadine and rimantadine for influenza A and the neuraminidase inhibitors zanamivir and oseltamivir for both influenza A and influenza B. If begun within 48 h of the onset of illness, treatment with amantadine or rimantadine has reduced the duration of systemic and respiratory symptoms of influenza by ~50%. From 5 to 10% of individuals who receive amantadine experience mild CNS side effects, primarily jitteriness, anxiety, insomnia, or difficulty in concentrating. These side effects disappear promptly upon cessation of the drug. Rimantadine appears to be equally efficacious and is associated with less frequent CNS side effects than is amantadine. In adults, the usual dose of amantadine or rimantadine is 200 mg/d for 3 to 7 days. Since both drugs are excreted via the kidney, the dose should be reduced to ≤100 mg/d in elderly patients and patients with renal insufficiency. Zanamivir, inhaled orally at a dose of 10 mg twice a day for 5 days, or oseltamivir, ingested orally at a dose of 75 mg twice a day for 5 days, has reduced the duration of signs and symptoms of influenza by 1 to 1.5 days if treatment is started within 2 days of the onset of illness. Zanamivir may exacerbate bronchospasm in asthmatic patients, and oseltamivir has been associated with nausea and vomiting, whose frequency can be reduced by drug administration with food. Currently, only amantadine and zanamivir are approved in the United States for treatment of children (the latter for use in children ≥7 years old). Ribavirin, a nucleoside analogue with activity against a variety of viral agents, has been reported to be effective against both influenza A and influenza B virus infections when administered as an aerosol, although it is relatively ineffective when administered orally.

Studies demonstrating the therapeutic efficacy of antiviral compounds in influenza have primarily involved young adults with uncomplicated disease; it is not known whether such compounds are effective in the treatment of complications such as influenza pneumonia. Therapy for primary influenza pneumonia is directed at maintaining oxygenation and is most appropriately undertaken in an intensive care unit, with aggressive respiratory and hemodynamic support as needed. Bypass membrane oxygenators have been employed in this setting with variable results. When an acute respiratory distress syndrome develops, fluids must be administered cautiously, with close monitoring of blood gases and hemodynamic function.

Antibacterial drugs should be reserved for the therapy of bacterial complications of acute influenza, such as secondary bacterial pneumonia. The choice of antibiotics should be guided by Gram's staining and culture of appropriate specimens of respiratory secretions, such as sputum or transtracheal aspirates. If the etiology of a case of bacterial pneumonia is unclear from an examination of respiratory secretions, empirical antibiotics effective against the most common bacterial pathogens in this setting (*S. pneumoniae*, *S. aureus*, and *H. influenzae*) should be selected (Chaps. 138, 139, and 149).

PROPHYLAXIS   The major public health measure for prevention of influenza has been the use of inactivated influenza vaccines derived from influenza A and B viruses that circulated during the previous influenza season. If the vaccine virus and the currently circulating viruses are closely related, 50 to 80% protection against influenza would be expected. Presently available vaccines have been highly purified and are associated with few reactions. Up to 5% of individuals experience low-grade fever and mild systemic symptoms 8 to 24 h after vaccination, and up to one-third develop mild redness or tenderness at the vaccination site. Since the vaccine is produced in eggs, individuals with true hypersensitivity to egg products either should be desensitized or should not be vaccinated. Although the 1976 swine influenza vaccine appears to have been associated with an increased frequency of Guillain-Barré syndrome, influenza vaccines administered since 1976 generally have not been. Possible exceptions were noted during the 1992–1993 and 1993–1994 influenza seasons, when there may have been an excess risk of Guillain-Barré syndrome of slightly more than one case per million among vaccine recipients. However, the overall health risk following influenza outweighs the potential risk associated with vaccination. Investigational live attenuated ("cold-adapted") influenza A and B vaccines also have been developed and have been highly effective in preventing influenza in studies in adults and children. Such vaccines are administered intranasally and stimulate local antibody production more efficiently than conventional inactivated vaccines.

The U.S. Public Health Service recommends influenza vaccination for any individual >6 months of age who is at an increased risk for complications of influenza. Included are individuals with chronic cardiovascular or pulmonary disorders (including asthma) and residents of nursing homes and other chronic-care facilities. Other populations for whom the vaccine is recommended include healthy individuals >65 years of age and individuals who have required regular medical attention for diabetes mellitus, renal disease, hemoglobinopathies, or immunosuppression. Individuals who provide care for high-risk pa-

tients or who come into frequent contact with such patients, including household members, should also receive vaccine to reduce the likelihood of transmission of infection. Vaccination is recommended for women who will be in the second or third trimester of pregnancy during the influenza season and for individuals 6 months to 18 years of age who are receiving long-term aspirin therapy and may be at risk for Reye's syndrome. Since commercially available vaccines are inactivated ("killed"), they may be administered safely to immunocompromised patients. Influenza vaccination is not associated with exacerbations of chronic nervous-system diseases such as multiple sclerosis. Vaccine should be administered early in the autumn before influenza outbreaks occur and should be repeated annually to maintain immunity against the most current influenza virus strains.

Of the vaccines currently available (inactivated whole-virus vaccine, subvirion vaccine, and purified surface-antigen vaccine), only the "split-virus" preparations (i.e., the subvirion and purified surface-antigen vaccines) should be given to children <13 years old, since the whole-virus preparations have been associated with higher rates of adverse reactions in this age group.

Studies have shown amantadine and rimantadine to be 70 to 100% effective in the prophylaxis of illness associated with influenza A virus infection. Such prophylaxis is most likely to be used for high-risk individuals who have not received influenza vaccine or in a situation where the vaccines previously administered are relatively ineffective because of antigenic changes in the circulating virus. During an outbreak, amantadine or rimantadine can be administered simultaneously with inactivated vaccine, since neither drug interferes with an immune response to the vaccine. In fact, there is evidence that the protective effects of amantadine and vaccine may be additive. Amantadine has also been employed to control nosocomial outbreaks of influenza A. For prophylaxis, administration of amantadine or rimantadine should be instituted promptly when influenza A activity is detected and must be continued daily for the duration of the outbreak. The dosage most frequently employed has been 200 mg/d for adults, but the dose should be reduced for patients with renal insufficiency and for the elderly. Viruses resistant to both amantadine and rimantadine can emerge quickly after therapy with these drugs, and the possible transmission of these resistant viruses has been reported. The neuraminidase inhibitors zanamivir and oseltamivir have also been reported to be highly effective in the prophylaxis of influenza A and offer the advantage of efficacy against influenza B as well. They are currently under review for use as prophylaxis. As with amantadine and rimantadine, the neuraminidase inhibitors must be administered daily to maintain prophylaxis.

BIBLIOGRAPHY

BELSHE RB et al: The efficacy of live attenuated, cold adapted trivalent, intranasal influenza vaccine in children. N Engl J Med 38:1405, 1998

CENTERS FOR DISEASE CONTROL AND PREVENTION: Prevention and control of influenza. MMWR 47(RR–6):1, 1998

DOLIN R et al: A controlled trial of amantadine and rimantadine in the prophylaxis of influenza A infection. N Engl J Med 307:580, 1982

GLEZEN WP: Serious morbidity and mortality associated with influenza epidemics. Epidemiol Rev 4:25, 1982

GROSS PA et al: Association of influenza immunization with reduction in mortality in an elderly population: A prospective study. Arch Intern Med 148:562, 1988

HAYDEN FG et al: Use of the selective oral neuraminidase inhibitor oseltamivir to prevent influenza. N Engl J Med 341:1336, 1999

—— et al: Use of the oral neuraminidase inhibitor oseltamivir in experimental human influenza: Randomized controlled trials for prevention and treatment. JAMA 282:1240, 1999

MIST (MANAGEMENT OF INFLUENZA IN THE SOUTHERN HEMISPHERE TRIALISTS) STUDY GROUP: Randomized trial of efficacy and safety of inhaled zanamivir in treatment of influenza A and B infections. Lancet 352:1871, 1998

MURPHY BR, WEBSTER RG: Orthomyxoviruses, in *Virology*, 3d ed, BN Fields (ed). New York, Raven Press, 1995, pp 1091–1152

SIMONSEN L et al: Pandemic vs epidemic mortality: A pattern of changing age distribution. J Infect Dis 178:53, 1998

191 *Anthony S. Fauci, Dan L. Longo*

THE HUMAN RETROVIRUSES

The retroviruses, which make up a large family (Retroviridae), infect mainly vertebrates. They have a unique replication cycle whereby their genetic information is encoded by RNA rather than DNA. Retroviruses contain an RNA-dependent DNA polymerase (a reverse transcriptase) that directs the synthesis of a DNA form of the viral genome after infection of a host cell. The designation *retrovirus* denotes that information in the form of RNA is transcribed into DNA in the host cell—a sequence that overturned a central dogma of molecular biology: that information passes unidirectionally from DNA to RNA to protein. The observation that RNA was the source of genetic information in the causative agents of certain animal tumors led to a number of paradigm-shifting biologic insights regarding not only the direction of genetic-information passage but also the viral etiology of certain cancers and the concept of oncogenes as normal host genes scavenged and altered by a viral vector.

The family Retroviridae includes three subfamilies (Table 191-1): Oncovirinae, of which human T-cell lymphotropic virus (HTLV) type I is the most important in humans; Lentivirinae, of which HIV is the most important in humans; and Spumavirinae, the "foamy" viruses, named for the pathologic appearance of infected cells. A number of spumaviruses have been isolated from humans; however, they are not associated with any known disease and therefore are not discussed further in this chapter.

The wide variety of interactions of a retrovirus with its host range from completely benign events (e.g., silent carriage of endogenous retroviral sequences in the germ-line genome of many animal species) to rapidly fatal infections (e.g., exogenous infection with an oncogenic virus such as Rous sarcoma virus in chickens). The ability of retroviruses to acquire and alter the structure and function of host cell sequences has revolutionized our understanding of molecular carcinogenesis. The viruses can insert into the germ-line genome of the host cell and behave as a transposable or movable genetic element. They can activate or inactivate genes near the site of integration into the genome. They can rapidly alter their own genome by recombination and mutation under selective environmental stimuli.

Most human viral diseases occur as a consequence of either tissue destruction by the virus itself or the host's response to the virus. Although these mechanisms are operative in retroviral infections, retroviruses have additional mechanisms of inducing disease, including the malignant transformation of an infected cell and the induction of an immunodeficiency state that leads to opportunistic diseases (infections and neoplasms; Chap. 309).

STRUCTURE AND LIFE CYCLE
Despite the wide range of biologic consequences of retroviral infection, all retroviruses are similar in structure, genome organization, and mode of replication. Retroviruses are 70 to 130 nm in diameter and have a lipid-containing envelope surrounding an icosahedral capsid with a dense inner core. The core contains two identical copies of the single-stranded RNA genome. The RNA molecules are 8 to 10 kb long and are complexed with reverse transcriptase and tRNA. Other viral proteins, such as integrase, are also components of the virion particle. The RNA has features usually found in mRNA: a cap site at the 5′ end of the molecule, which is important in the initiation of mRNA translation, and a polyadenylation site at the 3′ end, which influences mRNA turnover (i.e., messages with shorter polyA tails turn over faster than messages with longer polyA tails). However, the retroviral RNA is not translated; instead it is transcribed into DNA. The DNA form of the retroviral genome is called a *provirus*.

The replication cycle of retroviruses proceeds in two phases (Fig. 191-1). In the first phase, the virus enters the cytoplasm after binding to a specific cell surface receptor (with HIV, a cell-surface coreceptor is also utilized for binding and entry); the viral RNA and reverse transcriptase synthesize a double-stranded DNA version of the RNA template; and the provirus moves into the nucleus and integrates into the host cell genome. This proviral integration is permanent. Although some animal retroviruses integrate into a single specific site of the host genome in every infected cell, the four known pathogenic human retroviruses (HTLV-I, HTLV-II, HIV-1, and HIV-2) integrate randomly. This first phase of replication depends entirely on gene products in the virus. The second phase includes the synthesis and processing of viral genomes, mRNAs, and proteins using host cell machinery, often under the influence of viral gene products. Virions are assembled and released from the cell by budding from the membrane; host cell membrane proteins are frequently incorporated into the envelope of the virus. Proviral integration occurs during the S phase of the cell cycle; thus, in general, nondividing cells are resistant to retroviral infection. Only the lentiviruses are able to infect nondividing cells. Once a host is infected, it is infected for life.

Retroviral genomes include both coding and noncoding sequences (Fig. 191-2). In general, noncoding sequences are important recognition signals for DNA or RNA synthesis or processing events and are located in the 5′ and 3′ terminal regions of the genome. All retroviral genomes are terminally redundant, containing identical sequences called *long terminal repeats* (LTRs). The ends of the retroviral RNA genome differ slightly in sequence from the integrated retroviral DNA. In the latter, the LTR sequences are repeated in both the 5′ and the 3′ terminus of the virus. The LTRs contain sequences involved in initiating the expression of the viral proteins, the integration of the provirus, and the polyadenylation of viral RNAs. The primer binding site, which is critical for the initiation of reverse transcription, and the viral

Table 191-1 Classification of Retroviruses: The Family Retroviridae

Subfamily, Group[a]	Example	Feature
Oncovirinae (oncogenic viruses)		
Avian leukosis	Rous sarcoma virus	Contains *src* oncogene
Mammalian C-type	Abelson leukemia virus	Contains *abl* oncogene
B-type	Murine mammary tumor virus	Can be endogenous or exogenous
D-type	Mason-Pfizer monkey virus	—
HTLV-BLV	HTLV-I	Causes T-cell lymphoma and neurologic disease
Lentivirinae (slow viruses)	HIV-1, HIV-2	Causes AIDS
	Visna virus	Causes lung and brain diseases in sheep
	Feline immunodeficiency virus	Causes immunodeficiency in cats
Spumavirinae (foamy viruses)	Simian foamy virus, human foamy virus	Causes no known disease

[a] The Oncovirinae were originally grouped into types A–D on the basis of morphologic features (size, core location, budding) under electron microscopy; however, this system has been replaced by groupings based on relationships of genome structure and sequence.

NOTE: HTLV, human T-lymphotropic virus; BLV, bovine leukemia virus.

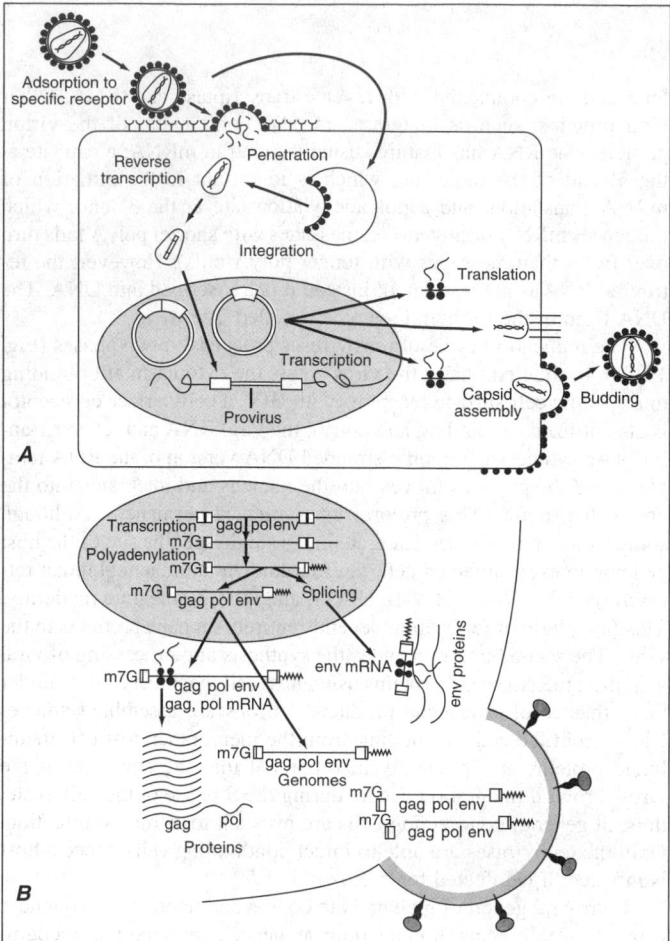

FIGURE 191-1 The life cycle of retroviruses. *A.* Overview of virus replication. The retrovirus enters a target cell by binding to a specific cell-surface receptor; once the virus is internalized, its RNA is released from the nucleocapsid and is reverse-transcribed into proviral DNA. The provirus is inserted into the genome and then transcribed into RNA; the RNA is translated; and virions assemble and are extruded from the cell membrane by budding. *B.* Overview of retroviral gene expression. The provirus is transcribed, capped, and polyadenylated. Viral RNA molecules then have one of three fates: They are exported to the cytoplasm, where they are packaged as the viral RNA in infectious viral particles; they are spliced to form the message for the envelope polyprotein; or they are translated into Gag and Pol proteins. Most of the messages for the Pol protein fail to initiate Pol translation because of a stop codon before its initiation; however, in a fraction of the messages, the stop codon is missed and the Pol proteins are translated. *(Modified from JM Coffin, in BN Fields, DM Knipe (eds): Fields Virology. New York, Raven, 1990.)*

packaging sequences are located outside the LTR sequences. The coding regions include the *gag* (group-specific antigen, core protein), *pol* (RNA-dependent DNA polymerase), and *env* (envelope) genes. The *gag* gene encodes a precursor polyprotein that is cleaved to form three to five capsid proteins; a fraction of the Gag precursor proteins also contain a protease responsible for cleaving the Gag and Pol polyproteins. A Gag-Pol polyprotein gives rise to the protease that is responsible for cleaving the Gag-Pol polyprotein. The *pol* gene encodes three proteins: the reverse transcriptase, the integrase, and the protease. The reverse transcriptase functions to copy the viral RNA into the double-stranded DNA provirus, which can attach to the host cell DNA via the action of integrase. The protease functions to cleave the Gag-Pol polyprotein into smaller protein products. The *env* gene encodes the envelope glycoproteins: one protein that binds to specific surface receptors and determines what cell types can be infected and a smaller

transmembrane protein that anchors the complex to the envelope. The cartoon in Fig. 191-3 shows how the retroviral gene products make up the virus structure.

HTLVs have a region between *env* and the 3' LTR that encodes at least two proteins in overlapping reading frames; Tax, a 40-kD protein that does not bind to DNA but induces the expression of host cell transcription factors that alter host cell gene expression; and Rex, a 27-kD protein that regulates the expression of viral mRNAs. These two proteins are produced from messages that are similar but that are spliced differently from overlapping but distinct exons.

The lentiviruses in general, and HIV-1 and -2 in particular, contain a larger genome than other pathogenic retroviruses. They contain an untranslated region between *pol* and *env* that encodes portions of several proteins, varying with the reading frame into which the mRNA is spliced. Tat is a 14-kD protein that augments the expression of virus from the LTR. The Rev protein of HIV-1, similar to the Rex protein of HTLV, regulates RNA splicing and/or RNA transport. The Nef protein downregulates CD4, the cellular receptor for HIV; alters host T cell activation pathways; and enhances viral infectivity. The Vif protein is necessary for the proper assembly of the HIV nucleoprotein core in many types of cells; without Vif, proviral DNA is not efficiently produced in these infected cells. Vpr, Vpu (HIV-1 only), and Vpx (HIV-2 only) are viral proteins encoded by translation of the same message in different reading frames. As noted above, oncogenic retroviruses depend on cell proliferation for their replication; lentiviruses can infect nondividing cells, largely owing to effects mediated by Vpr. Vpr facilitates transport of the provirus into the nucleus and can induce other cellular changes, such as G2 growth arrest and differentiation of some target cells. Vpx is structurally related to Vpr, but its functions are not fully defined. Vpu promotes the degradation of CD4 in the endoplasmic reticulum and stimulates the release of virions from infected cells.

Retroviruses can be either exogenously acquired by infection with a virion capable of replication or transmitted in the germ line as endogenous virus. Endogenous retroviruses are often replication-defective. The human genome contains endogenous retroviral sequences, but there are no known replication-competent endogenous retroviruses in humans.

In general, viruses that contain only the *gag*, *pol*, and *env* genes either are not pathogenic or take a long time to induce disease because the pathogenesis of neoplastic transformation relies on the chance integration of the provirus at a spot in the genome that will result in the expression of a cellular gene (proto-oncogene) that becomes transforming by virtue of its unregulated expression. For example, avian leukosis virus causes B cell leukemia by inducing the expression of *myc*. Some retroviruses possess captured and altered cellular genes near their integration site, and these viral oncogenes are capable of transforming the infected host cell. Viruses that have oncogenes often have lost a portion of their genome that is required for replication. Such viruses need helper viruses to reproduce, a feature that may explain why these acute transforming retroviruses are rare in nature. All human retroviruses identified to date are exogenous and are not acutely transforming (that is, they lack a transforming oncogene).

These remarkable properties of retroviruses have led to experimental efforts to use them as vectors to insert specific genes into particular cell types, a process known as *gene therapy* or *gene transfer*. The process could be used to repair a genetic defect or to introduce a new property that could be used therapeutically; for example, a gene (e.g., thymidine kinase) that would make a tumor cell susceptible to killing by a drug (e.g., ganciclovir) could be inserted. One source of concern about the use of retroviral vectors in humans is that replication-competent viruses might rescue endogenous retroviral replication, with unpredictable results. This concern is not merely hypothetical: The detection of proteins encoded by endogenous retroviral sequences on the surface of cancer cells implies that the genetic events leading to the cancer were able to activate the synthesis of these usually silent genes.

HUMAN T-CELL LYMPHOTROPIC VIRUS

HTLV-I was isolated in 1980 from a T-cell lymphoma cell line from a patient originally thought to have cutaneous T cell lymphoma. Later it became clear that the patient had a distinct form of lymphoma (originally reported in Japan) called *adult T cell leukemia/lymphoma* (ATL). Serologic data have determined that HTLV-I is the cause of at least two important diseases: ATL and tropical spastic paraparesis, also called *HTLV-I–associated myelopathy* (HAM). HTLV-I may also play a role in infective dermatitis and uveitis syndromes.

Two years after the isolation of HTLV-I, HTLV-II was isolated from a patient with an unusual form of hairy cell leukemia that affected T cells. Although early epidemiologic studies of HTLV-II failed to reveal a consistent disease association, more recent studies suggest an association of HTLV-II with human disease (see "Associated Diseases" under "Features of HTLV-II Infection," below), particularly among injection drug users.

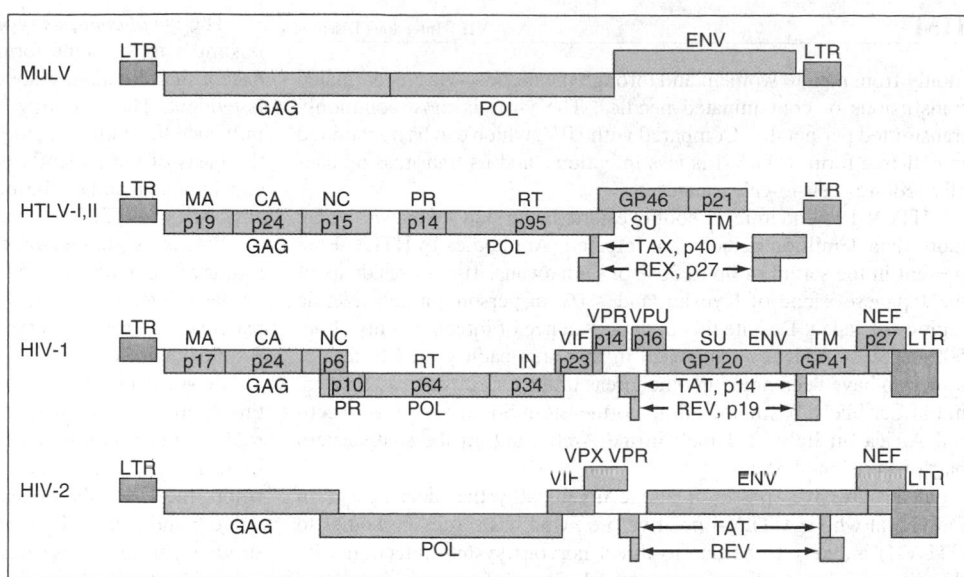

FIGURE 191-2 Genomic structure of retroviruses. The murine leukemia virus MuLV has the typical three structural genes: *gag*, *pol*, and *env*. The *gag* region gives rise to three proteins: matrix (MA), capsid (CA), and nucleic acid–binding (NC) proteins. The *pol* region encodes both a protease (PR) responsible for cleaving the viral polyproteins and a reverse transcriptase (RT). In addition, HIV *pol* encodes an integrase (IN). The *env* region encodes a surface protein (SU) and a small transmembrane protein (TM). The human retroviruses have additional gene products translated in each of the three possible reading frames. HTLV-I and HTLV-II have *tax* and *rex* genes with exons on either side of the *env* gene. HIV-1 and HIV-2 have six accessory gene products: *tat*, *rev*, *vif*, *nef*, *vpr*, and either *vpu* (in HIV-1) or *vpx* (in HIV-2). The genes for these proteins are located mainly between the *pol* and *env* genes.

BIOLOGY AND MOLECULAR BIOLOGY

Because the biology of HTLV-I and that of HTLV-II are similar, the following discussion will focus on HTLV-I.

The cellular receptor for HTLV-I has not yet been identified, but it maps to chromosome 17. Generally, only T cells are productively infected, but infection of B cells and other cell types is occasionally detected. The most common outcome of HTLV-I infection is latent carriage of randomly integrated provirus in CD4+ T cells. HTLV-I does not contain an oncogene and does not insert into a unique site in the genome. Indeed, most infected cells express no viral gene products. The only viral gene product that is routinely expressed in tumor cells transformed by HTLV-I in vivo is *tax*, and even *tax* is not expressed in the tumor cells of many ATL patients. Cells transformed in vitro, by contrast, actively transcribe HTLV-I RNA and produce infectious virions. Most HTLV-I–transformed cell lines are the result of the infection of a normal host T cell in vitro. It is difficult to establish cell lines derived from authentic ATL cells.

Although *tax* does not itself bind to DNA, it does induce the expression of a wide range of host-cell gene products, including transcription factors (especially *c-rel*, *ets*-1 and -2, and members of the *fos/jun* family), cytokines [e.g., interleukin (IL) 2, granulocyte-macrophage colony-stimulating factor, and tumor necrosis factor (TNF)], and membrane proteins and receptors [major histocompatibility (MHC) molecules and IL-2 receptor α]. The genes activated by *tax* are generally controlled by transcription factors of the *c-rel* and cyclic AMP response element binding (CREB) protein families. It is unclear how this induction of host gene expression leads to neoplastic transformation. Induction of a cytokine-autocrine loop has been proposed; however, IL-2 is not the crucial cytokine. The involvement of IL-4, IL-7, and IL-15 has been proposed.

In light of the irregular expression of *tax* in ATL cells, it has been suggested that *tax* is important in the early phases of transformation but is not essential for the maintenance of the transformed state. As is clear from the epidemiology of HTLV-I infection, transformation of an infected cell is a rare event and may depend on heterogeneous second, third, or fourth genetic hits. No consistent chromosomal abnormalities have been described in ATL; however, individual cases

with *p53* mutations and translocations involving the T cell receptor genes on chromosome 14 have been reported. *Tax* may repress certain DNA repair enzymes, permitting the accumulation of genetic damage that would normally be repaired. However, the molecular pathogenesis of HTLV-I–induced neoplasia is not fully understood.

FEATURES OF HTLV-I INFECTION   Epidemiology

HTLV-I infection is transmitted in at least three ways: from mother to child, especially in breast milk; through sexual activity, more com-

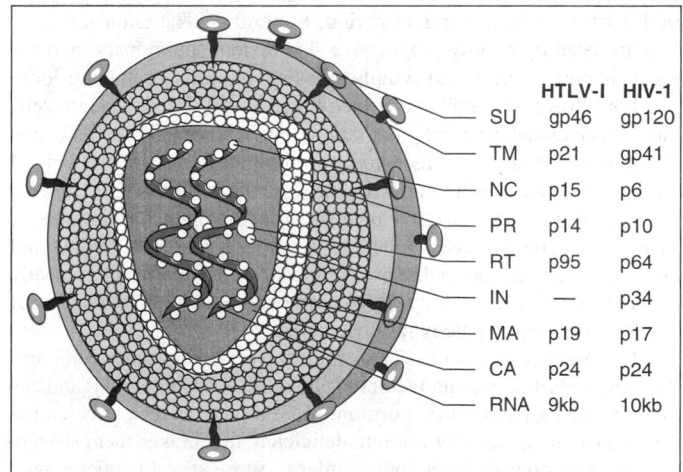

	HTLV-I	HIV-1
SU	gp46	gp120
TM	p21	gp41
NC	p15	p6
PR	p14	p10
RT	p95	p64
IN	—	p34
MA	p19	p17
CA	p24	p24
RNA	9kb	10kb

FIGURE 191-3 Schematic structure of human retroviruses. The surface glycoprotein (SU) is responsible for binding to receptors of host cells. The transmembrane protein (TM) anchors SU to the virus. NC is a nucleic acid–binding protein found in association with the viral RNA. A protease (PR) cleaves the polyproteins encoded by the *gag*, *pol*, and *env* genes into their functional components. RT is reverse transcriptase, and IN is an integrase present in some retroviruses (e.g., HIV-1) that facilitates insertion of the provirus into the host genome. MA is a Gag protein closely associated with the lipid of the envelope. The capsid protein (CA) forms the major internal structure of the virus, the core shell.

monly from men to women; and through the blood—via contaminated transfusions or contaminated needles. The virus is most commonly transmitted perinatally. Compared with HIV, which can be transmitted in cell-free form, HTLV-I is less infectious, and its transmission usually requires cell-to-cell contact.

HTLV-I is endemic in southwestern Japan and Okinawa, where more than 1 million persons are infected. Antibodies to HTLV-I are present in the serum of up to 35% of Okinawans, 10% of residents of the Japanese island of Kyushu, and <1% of persons in nonendemic regions of Japan. Despite this high prevalence of infection, only about 500 cases of ATL are diagnosed in this area each year. Clusters of infection have been noted in other areas of the Orient, such as Taiwan; in the Caribbean basin, including northeastern South America; in central Africa; in Italy; in Israel; in the Arctic; and in the southeastern part of the United States.

A progressive spastic or ataxic myelopathy that develops in an individual who is HTLV-I positive (i.e., who has serum antibodies to HTLV-I) is likely to be due to direct nervous system infection with the virus; a similar disorder may result from infection with HIV or HTLV-II. In rare instances, patients with HAM are seronegative but have detectable antibody to HTLV-I in the cerebrospinal fluid (CSF).

The cumulative lifetime risk of developing ATL is 2% among HTLV-I–infected patients; a similar risk is projected for HAM. The distribution of the two diseases overlaps the distribution of HTLV-I, with >95% of affected patients showing serologic evidence of HTLV-I infection. The latent period between infection and the emergence of disease is 20 to 30 years for ATL. For HAM, the median latency period is about 3.3 years (range, 4 months to 30 years). The development of ATL is rare among persons infected by blood products; however, ~20% of patients with HAM acquire HTLV-I from contaminated blood.

Associated Diseases • *ATL* Four clinical types of HTLV-I–induced neoplasia have been described: acute, lymphomatous, chronic, and smoldering. All of these tumors are monoclonal proliferations of CD4+ post-thymic T cells with clonal proviral integrations and clonal T-cell receptor gene rearrangements.

About 60% of patients who develop malignancy have classic *acute* ATL, which is characterized by a short clinical prodrome (~2 weeks between the first symptoms and the diagnosis) and an aggressive natural history (median survival period, 6 months). The clinical picture is dominated by rapidly progressive skin lesions, pulmonary involvement, hypercalcemia, and lymphocytosis with cells containing lobulated or "flower-shaped" nuclei (**see Plate V-40**). The malignant cells have monoclonal proviral integrations and express CD4, CD3, and CD25 (low-affinity IL-2 receptors) on their surface. Serum levels of CD25 can be used as a tumor marker. Anemia and thrombocytopenia are rare. The skin lesions may be difficult to distinguish from those in mycosis fungoides. Lytic bone lesions, which are common, do not contain tumor cells but rather are composed of osteolytic cells, usually without osteoblastic activity. Despite the leukemic picture, bone marrow involvement is patchy in most cases.

The hypercalcemia of ATL is multifactorial; the tumor cells produce osteoclast-activating factors (TNF-α, IL-1, lymphotoxin) and can also produce a parathyroid hormone–like molecule. The affected patients have an underlying immunodeficiency that makes them susceptible to opportunistic infections similar to those seen in patients with AIDS (Chap. 309). The pathogenesis of the immunodeficiency is unclear. Pulmonary infiltrates in ATL patients reflect leukemic infiltration half the time and opportunistic infections with organisms such as *Pneumocystis carinii* and other fungi the other half. Gastrointestinal symptoms are nearly always related to opportunistic infection. Serum concentrations of lactate dehydrogenase (LDH) and alkaline phosphatase are often elevated. About 10% of patients have leptomeningeal involvement leading to weakness, altered mental status, paresthesia, and/or headache. Unlike other forms of central nervous system (CNS) lymphoma, ATL may be accompanied by normal CSF protein levels. The diagnosis depends on finding ATL cells in the CSF (Chap. 112).

The *lymphomatous* type of ATL occurs in ~20% of patients and is similar to the acute form in its natural history and clinical course, except that circulating abnormal cells are rare and lymphadenopathy is evident. The histology of the lymphoma is variable but does not influence the natural history. In general, the diagnosis is suspected on the basis of the patient's birthplace and the presence of skin lesions and hypercalcemia. The diagnosis is confirmed by the detection of antibodies to HTLV-I in serum.

Patients with the *chronic* form of ATL generally have normal serum levels of calcium and LDH and no involvement of the CNS, bone, or gastrointestinal tract. The median duration of survival for these patients is 2 years. In some cases, chronic ATL progresses to the acute form of the disease.

Fewer than 5% of patients have the *smoldering* form of ATL. In this form, the malignant cells have monoclonal proviral integration; <5% of peripheral-blood cells exhibit typical morphologic abnormalities; hypercalcemia, adenopathy, and hepatosplenomegaly do not develop; the CNS, the bones, and the gastrointestinal tract are not involved; and skin and pulmonary lesions may be present. The median survival period of this small subset of patients appears to be ≥5 years.

HAM (tropical spastic paraparesis) In contrast to ATL, in which there is a slight predominance of male patients, HAM affects females disproportionately. HAM resembles multiple sclerosis in certain ways (Chap. 371). The onset is insidious. Symptoms include weakness or stiffness in one or both legs, back pain, and urinary incontinence. Sensory changes are usually mild, but peripheral neuropathy may develop. The disease generally takes the form of slowly progressive and unremitting thoracic myelopathy; one-third of patients are bedridden within 10 years of diagnosis, and one-half are unable to walk unassisted by this point. Patients display spastic paraparesis or paraplegia with hyperreflexia, ankle clonus, and extensor plantar responses. Cognitive function is usually spared; cranial nerve abnormalities are unusual.

Magnetic resonance imaging (MRI) reveals lesions in both the white matter and the paraventricular regions of the brain as well as in the spinal cord. Pathologic examination of the spinal cord shows symmetric degeneration of the lateral columns, including the corticospinal tracts; some cases involve the posterior columns as well. The spinal meninges and cord parenchyma contain an inflammatory infiltrate with myelin destruction.

HTLV-I is not usually found in cells of the CNS but may be detected in a small population of lymphocytes present in the CSF. In general, HTLV-I replication is greater in HAM than in ATL, and patients with HAM have a stronger immune response to the virus. Antibodies to HTLV-I are present in the serum and appear to be produced in the CSF of HAM patients, where titers are often higher than in the serum. The pathophysiology of HAM may involve the induction of autoimmune destruction of neural cells by T cells with specificity for viral components such as Tax or Env proteins. One theory is that susceptibility to HAM may be related to the presence of human leukocyte antigen (HLA) alleles capable of presenting viral antigens in a fashion that leads to autoimmunity. Insufficient data are available to confirm an HLA association.

Other putative HTLV-I–related diseases In areas where HTLV-I is endemic, diverse inflammatory and autoimmune diseases have been attributed to the virus, including uveitis, dermatitis, pneumonitis, rheumatoid arthritis, and polymyositis. However, a causal relationship between HTLV-I and these illnesses has not been rigorously established.

Prevention Women in endemic areas should not breast-feed their children, and blood donors should be screened for serum antibodies to HTLV-I. As in the prevention of HIV infection, the practice of safe sex and the avoidance of needle sharing are important.

℞ **TREATMENT** For the small number of patients who develop HTLV-I–related disease, therapies are not curative. In patients with the acute and lymphomatous types of ATL, the disease progresses rapidly. Hypercalcemia is generally controlled by glucocorticoid administration and cytotoxic therapy directed against the neoplasm. The tumor is highly responsive to combination chemotherapy that is employed against other forms of lymphoma; however, patients are susceptible to overwhelming bacterial and opportunistic infections, and ATL relapses within 4 to 10 months after remission in most patients. The combination of interferon α and zidovudine may extend survival. Because viral replication is not clearly associated with ATL progression, zidovudine is probably effective through its cytotoxic effects (as a chain-terminating thymidine analogue) rather than its antiviral effects. An experimental approach using an yttrium 90–labeled antibody to the IL-2 receptor appears promising but is not widely available. Patients with the chronic or smoldering form of ATL may be managed with an expectant approach: Treat any infections, and watch and wait for signs of progression to acute disease.

Patients with HAM may obtain some benefit from the use of glucocorticoids to reduce inflammation. Antiretroviral regimens have not been effective. In one study, danazol (200 mg tid) produced significant neurologic improvement in five of six treated patients, with resolution of urinary incontinence in two cases, decreased spasticity in three, and the restoration of the ability to walk after confinement to a wheelchair in two. Physical therapy and rehabilitation are important components of management.

FEATURES OF HTLV-II INFECTION **Epidemiology** HTLV-II is endemic in certain Native American tribes. It is generally considered to be a New World virus that was brought from Asia to the Americas 10,000 to 40,000 years ago during the migration of infected populations across the Bering land bridge.

The mode of transmission of HTLV-II is probably the same as that of HTLV-I (see above). HTLV-II may be less readily transmitted sexually than HTLV-I.

Studies of large cohorts of injection drug users with serologic assays that reliably distinguish HTLV-I from HTLV-II indicate that the vast majority of HTLV-positive subjects are infected with HTLV-II. The seroprevalence of HTLV in a cohort of 7841 injection drug users from drug treatment centers in Baltimore, Chicago, Los Angeles, New Jersey (Asbury Park and Trenton), New York City (Brooklyn and Harlem), Philadelphia, and San Antonio was 20.9%, with >97% of cases due to HTLV-II. The seroprevalence of HTLV-II was higher in the Southwest and the Midwest than in the Northeast. In contrast, the seroprevalence of HIV-1 was higher in the Northeast than in the Southwest or the Midwest. Approximately 3% of the cohort members were infected with both HTLV-II and HIV-1. The seroprevalence of HTLV-II increased linearly with age. Women were significantly more likely to be infected with HTLV-II than were men; the virus is thought to be more efficiently transmitted from male to female than from female to male.

Associated Diseases Although HTLV-II was isolated from a patient with a T cell variant of hairy cell leukemia, this virus has not been consistently associated with a particular disease and in fact has been thought of as "a virus searching for a disease." However, evidence is accumulating that HTLV-II may play a role in certain neurologic, hematologic, and dermatologic diseases. These data require confirmation, particularly in light of the previous confusion regarding the relative prevalences of HTLV-I and HTLV-II among injection drug users.

Prevention Avoidance of needle sharing, safe-sex practices, screening of blood (by assays for HTLV-I, which also detect HTLV-II), and avoidance of breast-feeding by infected women are important principles in the prevention of spread of HTLV-II.

HUMAN IMMUNODEFICIENCY VIRUS

HIV-1 and HIV-2 are members of the lentivirus subfamily of Retroviridae and are the only lentiviruses known to infect humans. The lentiviruses are slow-acting by comparison with viruses that cause acute infection (e.g., influenza virus) but not by comparison with other retroviruses. The features of acute primary infection with HIV resemble those of more classic acute infections. The characteristic chronicity

of HIV disease is consistent with the designation *lentivirus*. →*For a detailed discussion of HIV, see Chap. 309.*

BIBLIOGRAPHY

BLATTNER WA: Human retroviruses: Their role in cancer. Proc Assoc Am Physicians 111:563, 1999
DECOCK KM et al: Prevention of mother-to-child HIV transmission in resource-poor countries: Translating research into policy and practice. JAMA 283:1175, 2000
FAUCI AS: The AIDS epidemic—considerations for the 21st century. N Engl J Med 341:1046, 1999
HARRINGTON WJ JR et al: Tropical spastic paraparesis/HTLV-I-associated myelopathy (TSP/HAM): Treatment with an anabolic steroid danazol. AIDS Res Hum Retroviruses 7:1031, 1991
HOLLSBERG P, HAFLER DA: Pathogenesis of diseases induced by human lymphotropic virus type I infection. N Engl J Med 328:1173, 1993
MURPHY RL (Chairman): Critical issues surrounding treatment in the era of active antiretroviral therapeutics: Proceedings of a Northwestern University Medical School Conference. Clin Infect Dis 30(Suppl 2):S95–197, 2000
NEUVEUT C, JEANG KT: HTLV-I Tax and cell cycle progression. Prog Cell Cycle Res 4:157, 2000
POIESZ BJ et al: Detection and isolation of type C retrovirus particles from fresh and cultured lymphocytes of a patient with cutaneous T-cell lymphoma. Proc Natl Acad Sci USA 77:7415, 1980
TOBINAI K: Adult T-cell leukemia, in *Clinical Oncology*, 2d ed, MD Abeloff et al (eds). New York, Churchill-Livingstone, 2000, p 2748
TRONO D: HIV accessory proteins: Leading roles for the supporting cast. Cell 82:189, 1995
YAO J, WIGDAHL B: Human T-cell lymphotropic virus type I genomic expression and impact on intracellular signaling pathways during neurodegenerative disease and leukemia. Front Biosci 5:D138, 2000

192 *Harry B. Greenberg*

VIRAL GASTROENTERITIS

In less developed countries, acute infectious diarrheal disease is a leading cause of morbidity in all age groups and of mortality in infants and young children. In developed countries, acute diarrheal illness remains an important cause of morbidity among both children and adults. Two distinct groups of viruses—the rotaviruses and the enteric caliciviruses, such as Norwalk virus—as well as a variety of bacterial pathogens (Chap. 131) have emerged as important etiologic agents of gastroenteritis. The rotaviruses are primarily pathogens of young children. The Norwalk and related enteric caliciviruses affect adults as well as children. Several important gastrointestinal viruses are characterized in Table 192-1 and depicted in Fig. 192-1.

ROTAVIRUS **Classification and Characterization** Rotaviruses are members of the Reoviridae family. The rotavirus virion consists of a 100-nm triple-shelled icosahedral capsid surrounding a genome composed of 11 segments of double-stranded RNA. Several genetically distinct groups of rotaviruses (groups A, B, C, etc.) have been identified, but group A strains account for the great majority of illnesses in humans. With only one exception, the rotavirus gene segments are monocistronic. The virus has two surface proteins (VP4 and VP7), both of which are involved in viral neutralization. The major internal capsid protein (VP6) is the target of cross-reactive antibody to different virus strains. This protein also appears to induce protective immunity, although the mechanism is not clear. Because rotaviruses have a segmented genome, they are capable of undergoing gene reassortment at high frequency. The role of gene reassortment in generating rotavirus antigenic diversity is not known. In immunocompetent humans and animals, rotavirus infection is characterized by replication that is localized almost exclusively in the epithelial cells of the small intestine.

Epidemiology Rotavirus infection occurs worldwide. By the age of 3 years, virtually every individual has been infected by rotaviruses

Table 192-1 Characteristics of Several Gastrointestinal Viruses

Virus Type	Genome Structure	Major Risk Groups	Seasonality	Diagnostic Tests[a]	Treatment
Rotavirus (group A)	Double-stranded segmented RNA	Children <3 years	Winter	ELISA	1. Oral rehydration 2. Vaccination
Adenovirus (types 40, 41)	Double-stranded DNA	Children <3 years	Year-round	ELISA	Oral rehydration
Caliciviruses (genogroup III, SLVs)	Plus-sense single-stranded RNA	Young children	Unknown	Experimental and EM	Oral rehydration
Astrovirus	Plus-sense single-stranded RNA	Young children ?Immunocompromised individuals	Winter	Experimental and EM	Oral rehydration
Norwalk-like viruses (genogroups I, II)	Plus-sense single-stranded RNA	Children and adults, epidemics	Winter	Experimental and EM	Oral rehydration
Parvovirus[b]	Single-stranded DNA	No enteric disease	Year-round	EM	None needed
Picornavirus[c] (enterovirus)	Plus-sense single-stranded RNA	Usually no enteric disease	Depends on strain	Culture and EM	None needed
Coronavirus	Plus-sense single-stranded RNA, enveloped	Unknown, no well-characterized enteric disease	Unknown	EM	None

[a] ELISA, enzyme-linked immunosorbent assay; EM, electron microscopy.
[b] See also Chap. 187.
[c] See also Chap. 193.

at least once. Most rotavirus infections are subclinical or cause mild gastrointestinal illnesses that do not require hospitalization. The first infection is the most likely to be symptomatic; subsequent infections are often mild or asymptomatic. In areas with a temperate climate, rotavirus infection is seasonal, occurring in the colder winter months. In the United States, the annual seasonal rotavirus epidemic tends to spread from west to east, starting in California and ending in New England. In tropical areas, rotavirus infection tends to occur throughout the year, with some increase in incidence during the cooler rainy season.

Rotaviruses are the single most important cause of severe dehydrating diarrhea in infants and children <3 years old in both developed and less developed countries; they account for 25 to 50% of all cases of diarrhea requiring hospitalization or intensive rehydration therapy. During a rotavirus outbreak in a temperate climate, this percentage can be as high as 80%. In the United States, between 5 and 10% of all diarrheal episodes among children under the age of 5 years are caused by rotavirus. Infection due to rotavirus accounts for ~500,000 physician visits per year in the United States. Although severe rotavirus infections are confined primarily to infants and young children, these agents are frequently associated with mild diarrhea in adults, particularly family members of affected infants, geriatric patients, and immunocompromised hosts. They are responsible for up to 10% of cases of traveler's diarrhea (Chap. 131). Rotaviruses also may cause occasional cases of acute and chronic diarrhea in patients with AIDS.

Rotavirus serotypes have been defined by the antigenicity of both VP4 (P serotype) and VP7 (G serotype). At least 14 distinct G serotypes of rotavirus have been described, but only four types are commonly encountered in the United States. At least 20 P serotypes have been identified to date, of which only two are common among children in this country. The relationship of the frequency of infection with these multiple serotypes to host immune status is unclear. It does appear, however, that infection with one or two serotypes induces some degree of heterotypic immunity to severe disease.

A large variety of mammalian and avian species can be infected by rotavirus, but these animal rotavirus strains do not frequently cause disease in humans. Rotaviruses are shed in very large numbers in the stool (up to 10^{10} particles per gram of feces). Although transmission presumably takes place via the fecal-oral route, rotavirus infection spreads with great efficacy in developed as well as less developed countries.

Pathophysiology Rotavirus infects and kills the mature villus tip cells of the small intestine. The mature epithelial cells are replaced by immature absorptive cells that cannot absorb carbohydrates or other nutrients efficiently. Rotavirus infection thus leads to osmotic diarrhea due to nutrient malabsorption. Changes in intracellular cyclic adenosine monophosphate or guanosine monophosphate are not involved in the etiology of rotavirus diarrhea. Rotavirus also encodes a nonstructural protein (NSP4) that appears to function as an enterotoxin during infection. It is not known whether immunity to NSP4 plays a role in protection or disease resolution.

Manifestations The manifestations of rotavirus infection range from subclinical infection through mild diarrhea to severe, occasionally fatal dehydrating illness. Most information concerning the signs and symptoms of rotavirus infection has been derived from studies of hospitalized young children. The onset of illness is usually abrupt. More than 80% of affected children develop vomiting followed by diarrhea. About one-third of hospitalized children have a temperature of >39°C (>102.2°F). Mucus is commonly found in the stool, but white and red blood cells are present in the stool in fewer than 15% of cases.

Rotavirus infection frequently occurs in conjunction with respiratory tract symptoms, but there is little evidence to indicate that rotavirus replicates in the respiratory tract. Rotavirus infection has been observed in association with a wide variety of other clinical syndromes, including sudden infant death syndrome, Reye's syndrome, encephalitis, aseptic meningitis, pneumonia, exanthema subitum, Kawasaki's syndrome, necrotizing enterocolitis, intussusception, Schönlein-Henoch purpura, hemolytic-uremic syndrome, disseminated intravascular coagulation, and Crohn's disease. The etiologic relationship between these clinical syndromes and rotavirus infection is probably coincidental rather than causal. Rotavirus infection may be especially severe or even fatal in immunocompromised children.

Clinical Immunity Relative immunity to rotavirus illness is acquired early in childhood, after one or two natural infections. Subclinical infections in neonates have been shown to protect these children against severe rotavirus gastroenteritis for up to 3 years. Immunity is not complete, and adults with low levels of antibody can be symptomatically infected. Local humoral immunity appears to be the critical determinant in protection, and cellular immune mechanisms seem to be involved as well.

Diagnosis Because rotavirus is shed in large amounts in the stool, detection is relatively easy. Various specific and highly sensitive commercial immunoassays are available to detect rotavirus antigen in fecal specimens. DNA probe diagnosis appears to be sensitive and specific, as do polymerase chain reaction (PCR)–based assays, but these detection methods have been used primarily for research purposes. No particular signs or symptoms are pathognomonic for rotavirus infection, but this infection is more frequently associated with severe dehydration than are infections caused by other enteric bacterial or viral pathogens.

℞ **TREATMENT** Although rotavirus diarrhea appears to be caused primarily by intestinal epithelial-cell lysis and death, it can be adequately managed with standard oral rehydration therapy. Only rarely is intravenous rehydration required. Since rotavirus infections have persisted in developed countries with advanced sanitation facilities and widely available clean water, it is unlikely that these infections will prove to be preventable by hygienic measures alone. Progress with a number of candidate live attenuated vaccines suggests that prevention through vaccination may be feasible. In 1998, a multivalent rotavirus vaccine was licensed for use in children under the age of 6 months in the United States. The vaccine virus was a live attenuated animal rotavirus containing genes encoding the four human G serotypes most common in the United States. The licensed vaccine was administered orally as three doses and was highly effective in preventing severe rotavirus illness. Reports of intussusception associated with the administration of rotavirus vaccine have been published; further studies are required to define the relative risk. However, because of the apparent association with intussusception, this first rotavirus vaccine has been withdrawn from use.

NORWALK AND RELATED ENTERIC CALICIVIRUSES Classification and Characterization Various round 27- to 32-nm particles, some with clearly defined ultrastructure, have been identified in the stools of individuals with acute nonbacterial gastroenteritis. In the past, these agents have been difficult to classify because they are shed in the stool in small amounts for only a few days and have not been adapted to cell culture or to animal models. The Norwalk virus is the most extensively studied and best-characterized member of this group of enteric caliciviruses, which also in-

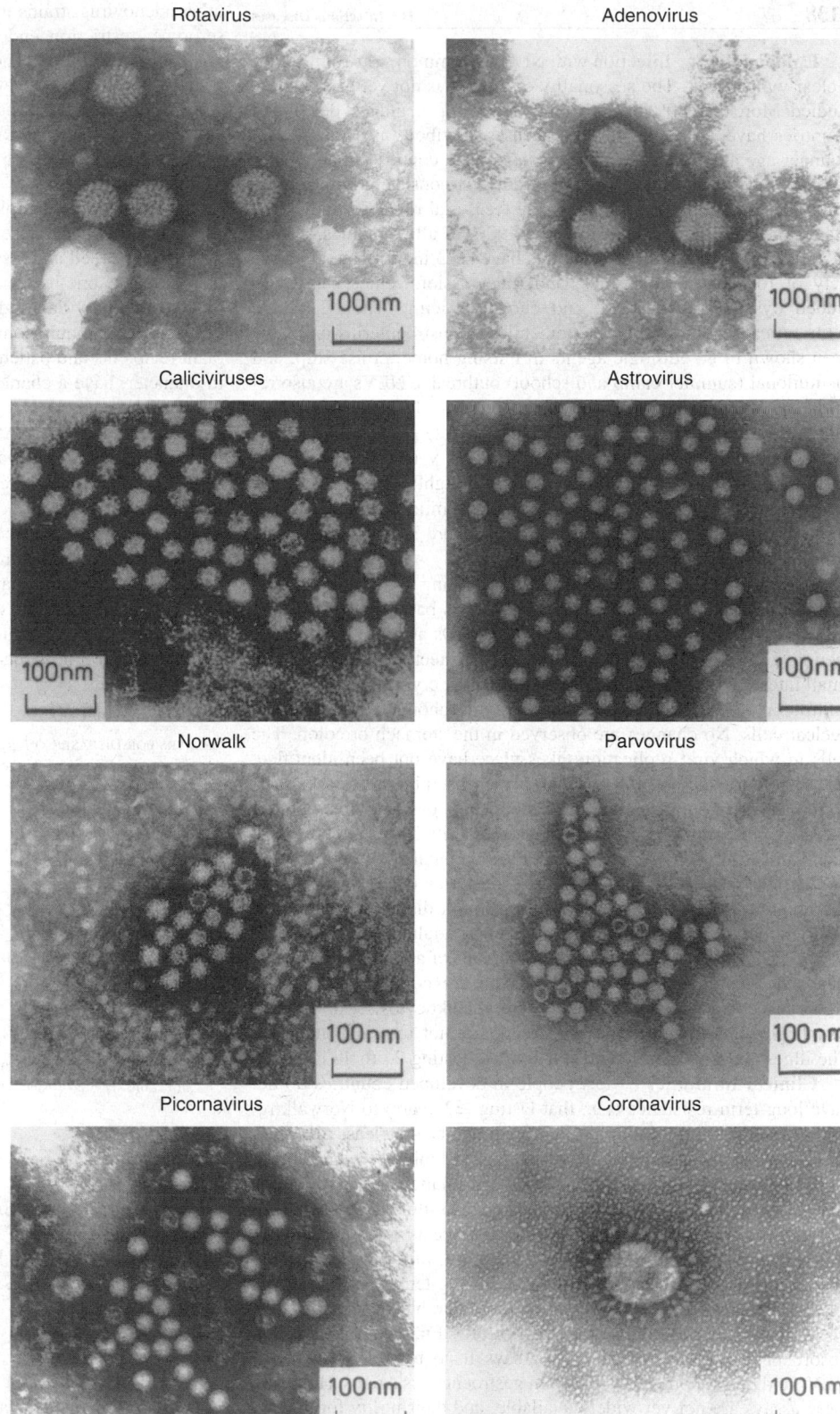

FIGURE 192-1 Electron micrographs of selected viruses found in the intestine. *(From S Monroe et al: J Med Virol 33:193, 1991, with permission.)*

cludes such serologically or genetically distinct viruses as Hawaii virus, Snow Mountain virus, Southampton virus, Lordsdale virus, Mexico virus, Sapporo virus, and a number of agents described as calicivirus-like. Molecular biologic studies have shown that all these viruses have a protein structure similar to that of typical caliciviruses, with a single structural protein of ~60 kDa. The genomes of Norwalk virus and numerous related viruses have been cloned and sequenced.

The genomes are plus-stranded RNA molecules of ~7.5 kb. On the basis of these molecular biologic studies, the human enteric caliciviruses can be divided into two groups: the Norwalk-like viruses (NLVs) and the Sapporo-like viruses (SLVs). The SLVs have a more typical calicivirus-like ultrastructure and cause diarrhea in young children. Unlike the NLVs, the SLVs may not cause frequent epidemics in adults.

Epidemiology Infection with NLVs is common year-round, with a clear winter peak. The seasonality of SLVs has not yet been widely studied. More than 80% of adults in both developed and less developed countries have antibodies to these viruses. Antibody is acquired at a younger age among children in less developed countries than among those in developed areas; this observation is consistent with the assumption that NLVs are spread by the fecal-oral route. In the United States, the NLVs are responsible for ~90% of all epidemics of non-bacterial gastroenteritis. These agents have been incriminated in a variety of food-borne epidemics, and transmission vehicles have included oysters, green salad, and chocolate icing. The NLVs are common causes of waterborne epidemics of gastroenteritis and have been shown to be etiologic agents in nursing home, cruise ship, and institutional (summer camp and school) outbreaks. NLVs are also responsible for a small proportion of cases of traveler's diarrhea. NLV infection is a common cause of mild to moderate childhood diarrhea.

In less developed countries, the role of NLV infection in the etiology of diarrhea in adults has not been thoroughly investigated. Preliminary studies indicate that NLVs can cause mild diarrhea in young children, but they do not appear to cause severe illness in infants in either developed or less developed countries.

Pathophysiology Information concerning the pathologic changes induced by the enteric caliciviruses is based almost entirely on a few studies of volunteers during the 1970s and 1980s. After infection with Norwalk or Hawaii virus, the architecture of the proximal small intestine is altered, with villus shortening, crypt hyperplasia, and infiltration of the lamina propria by polymorphonuclear and mononuclear cells. No changes are observed in the stomach or colon. The cells in which viral replication takes place have not been identified. The histologic alterations are accompanied by mild steatorrhea, carbohydrate malabsorption, and decreased levels of some brush border enzymes. No changes in adenylate cyclase activity have been observed.

Manifestations Norwalk illness has an incubation period of 18 to 72 h. The disease is characterized by the abrupt onset of nausea and abdominal cramps followed by vomiting and/or diarrhea. Vomiting is reported more frequently for children than for adults. Low-grade fever [>37.5° C (>99.5° F)] develops in about half of affected individuals. Headache, myalgias, and abdominal pain are common. The white blood cell count is normal; rarely, there is leukocytosis with relative lymphopenia. Red and white blood cells are not found in the stool. The illness is usually mild and self-limited, lasting 24 to 48 h.

Clinical Immunity Most people in developed countries do not have long-term resistance (i.e., that lasting ≥2 years) to Norwalk reinfection. Short-term (several-month) immunity—at least to homotypic challenge—does appear to develop. In volunteers challenged with Norwalk agent, there is a paradoxical relationship between the level of antibody to NLVs and susceptibility to illness: Low levels of Norwalk antibody in the serum and intestine are associated with clinical resistance to illness. It appears, therefore, that immune mechanisms are not the primary determinants of long-term protection from NLVs. Immunity to the SLVs may be more durable.

Diagnosis, Treatment, and Prevention Enzyme-linked immunosorbent assays and PCR-based assays have been developed for NLVs and several other 27- to 32-nm gastroenteritis agents. However, these assays are not yet widely available, and their utility for general diagnosis has not been tested. Because Norwalk illness is acute and self-limited, treatment is not usually required. In the rare case of severe vomiting or diarrhea, oral or intravenous rehydration is indicated. Because long-term immunity to the NLVs does not usually follow natural infection, the role of vaccination may be limited to specific settings (e.g., the military). Recombinant NLV particles have been produced and are capable of inducing an immune response when administered orally to volunteers.

MISCELLANEOUS ENTERIC VIRAL PATHOGENS *Enteric adenoviruses* are a minor cause of diarrheal illness in infants and children, accounting for 10% of cases. These viruses differ from other adenovirus strains in a variety of ways, including neutralization serotype, restriction endonuclease digestion pattern, and ability to grow in tissue culture. The role of enteric adenovirus illness in adults or in persons in less developed countries is not known.

Several strains of antigenically distinct rotaviruses, presently called *atypical rotaviruses* or *groups B and C rotaviruses*, have been identified as the cause of occasional episodes of diarrhea in humans and animals.

Preliminary epidemiologic studies have indicated that *astroviruses* are a fairly frequent cause of mild to moderate diarrhea in young children in developed and less developed countries, accounting for about one-quarter to one-half as much illness as group A rotaviruses. Moreover, preliminary data indicate that astroviruses are a common cause of diarrhea in immunocompromised hosts, such as bone marrow transplant recipients and patients with AIDS. Astroviruses are 27 to 32 nm in diameter, have a characteristic icosahedral ultrastructure, and contain a plus-stranded RNA genome with a size of ~7.0 kb and a unique genomic organization. At least seven distinct serotypes have been identified. The current availability of sensitive and specific diagnostic assays should allow more complete assessment of the importance of these agents.

Coronaviruses are frequent causes of diarrheal disease in a variety of animals. Using electron microscopy, several investigators have identified putative coronavirus-like particles in the stools of patients with diarrhea. In most cases, however, these particles do not have the typical morphologic features of coronaviruses and may represent bacterial breakdown products or cellular fragments.

BIBLIOGRAPHY

CENTERS FOR DISEASE CONTROL AND PREVENTION: Intussusception among recipients of rotavirus vaccine—United States, 1998–1999. MMWR 48:577, 1999

JIANG X et al: Sequence and genomic organization of Norwalk virus. Virology 195:51, 1993

JOENSUU J et al: Prolonged efficacy of rhesus-human reassortant rotavirus vaccine. Pediatr Infect Dis J 17:427, 1998

NOEL JS et al: Identification of a distinct common strain of "Norwalk-like viruses" having a global distribution. J Infect Dis 179:1334, 1999

PANG XL et al: Human calicivirus-associated sporadic gastroenteritis in Finnish children less than two years of age followed prospectively during a rotavirus vaccine trial. Pediatr Infect Dis J 18:420, 1999

PARASHAR UD et al: Hospitalizations associated with rotavirus diarrhea in the United States, 1993 through 1995: Surveillance based on the new ICD-9-CM rotavirus specific diagnostic code. J Infect Dis 177:13, 1998

PÉREZ-SCHAEL I et al: Efficacy of the rhesus rotavirus-based quadrivalent vaccine in infants and young children in Venezuela. N Engl J Med 337:1181, 1997

VELAZQUEZ FR et al: Rotavirus infection in infants as protection against subsequent infections. N Engl J Med 335:1022, 1996

193 *Jeffrey I. Cohen*

ENTEROVIRUSES AND REOVIRUSES

ENTEROVIRUSES

CLASSIFICATION AND CHARACTERIZATION Enteroviruses are so named because of their ability to multiply in the gastrointestinal tract. Despite their name, these viruses are not a prominent cause of gastroenteritis. Enteroviruses encompass 64 human serotypes: 3 serotypes of poliovirus, 23 serotypes of coxsackievirus A, 6 serotypes of coxsackievirus B, 28 serotypes of echovirus, and enteroviruses 68 through 71.

Human enteroviruses contain a single-stranded RNA genome surrounded by an icosahedral capsid comprising four viral proteins. These viruses have no lipid envelope and are stable in acidic environments, including the stomach. They are resistant to inactivation by standard disinfectants (e.g., alcohol, detergents) and can persist for days at room temperature.

PATHOGENESIS AND IMMUNITY Much of what is known about the pathogenesis of enteroviruses has been derived from studies of poliovirus infection. After ingestion, poliovirus is thought to infect epithelial cells in the mucosa of the gastrointestinal tract and then to spread to and replicate in the submucosal lymphoid tissue of the tonsils and Peyer's patches. The virus next spreads to the regional lymph nodes, a viremic phase ensues, and the virus replicates in organs of the reticuloendothelial system. In some cases, a second viremia occurs and the virus replicates further in various tissues, sometimes causing symptomatic disease.

It is uncertain whether poliovirus reaches the central nervous system (CNS) during viremia or whether it also spreads via peripheral nerves. Since viremia precedes the onset of neurologic disease in humans and in experimentally infected chimpanzees, it has been assumed that the virus enters the CNS via the bloodstream. The poliovirus receptor is a member of the immunoglobulin superfamily. Poliovirus infection is limited to primates, largely because of the ability of their cells to express the viral receptor. Studies demonstrating the poliovirus receptor in the end-plate region of muscle at the neuromuscular junction suggest that if the virus enters the muscle during viremia, it could travel across the neuromuscular junction up the axon to the anterior horn cells. Studies of monkeys or transgenic mice expressing the poliovirus receptor show that, after intramuscular injection, poliovirus does not reach the spinal cord if the sciatic nerve is cut. Taken together, these findings suggest that poliovirus can spread directly from muscle to the CNS by neural pathways. The receptor for echovirus types 1 and 8 is VLA-2 integrin, that for echovirus 7 is CD55, and that for coxsackievirus B is CAR (also used by adenovirus).

Poliovirus can usually be cultured from the blood 3 to 5 days after infection, before the development of neutralizing antibodies. While viral replication at secondary sites begins to slow 1 week after infection, it continues in the gastrointestinal tract. Poliovirus is shed from the oropharynx for up to 3 weeks after infection and from the gastrointestinal tract for as long as 12 weeks; immunodeficient patients can shed poliovirus for more than 1 year. During replication in the gastrointestinal tract, attenuated oral poliovirus can mutate, reverting to a more neurovirulent phenotype within a few days. The clinical significance of this increased neurovirulence is unknown.

Humoral and secretory immunity in the gastrointestinal tract is important for the control of enterovirus infections. Enteroviruses induce specific IgM, which usually persists for < 6 months, and specific IgG, which persists for life. Capsid protein VP1 is the predominant target of neutralizing antibody, which generally confers lifelong protection against subsequent disease caused by the same serotype but does not prevent infection or virus shedding. Enteroviruses also induce cellular immunity, but the importance of this mechanism in limiting infection is uncertain. Patients with impaired cellular immunity are not known to develop unusually severe disease when infected with enteroviruses. In contrast, the severe infections in patients with agammaglobulinemia emphasize the importance of humoral immunity in controlling enterovirus infections. IgA antibodies are important in reducing poliovirus replication in and shedding from the gastrointestinal tract. Breast milk contains IgA specific for enteroviruses and can protect humans from infection.

EPIDEMIOLOGY Enteroviruses have a worldwide distribution. More than 50% of nonpoliovirus enterovirus infections and more than 90% of poliovirus infections are subclinical. When symptoms do develop, they are usually nonspecific and occur in conjunction with fever; only a minority of infections are associated with specific clinical syndromes. The incubation period for most enterovirus infections ranges from 2 to 14 days but usually is less than a week.

Enterovirus infection is more common in socioeconomically disadvantaged areas, especially in those where conditions are crowded and in tropical areas where hygiene is poor. Infection is most common among infants and young children; serious illness develops most often during the first few days of life and in older children and adults. In developing countries, where children are infected at an early age, poliovirus infection has less often been associated with paralysis; in countries with better hygiene, older children and adults are more likely to be seronegative, become infected, and develop paralysis. Passively acquired maternal antibody reduces the risk of symptomatic infection in neonates. Young children are the most frequent shedders of enteroviruses and are usually the index cases in family outbreaks. In temperate climates, enterovirus infections occur most often in the summer and fall; no seasonal pattern is apparent in the tropics.

Most enteroviruses are transmitted primarily by the fecal-oral route from fecally contaminated fingers or inanimate objects. Patients are most infectious shortly before and after the onset of symptomatic disease, when virus is present in the stool and throat. The ingestion of virus-contaminated food or water can also cause disease. Certain enteroviruses (such as enterovirus 70, which causes acute hemorrhagic conjunctivitis) can be transmitted by direct inoculation from the fingers to the eye. Airborne transmission is important for some viruses that cause respiratory tract disease, such as coxsackievirus A21. Enteroviruses can be transmitted across the placenta from mother to fetus, causing severe disease in the newborn. The transmission of enteroviruses through blood transfusions or insect bites has not been documented. Nosocomial spread of coxsackievirus and echovirus has taken place in hospital nurseries.

DIAGNOSIS Isolation of enterovirus in cell culture is the most common procedure for the diagnosis of infection. While cultures of stool, nasopharyngeal, or throat samples from patients with enterovirus diseases are often positive, isolation of the virus from these sites does not prove that it is directly associated with disease because these sites are frequently colonized for weeks in patients with subclinical infections. Isolation of virus from the throat is more likely to be associated with disease than isolation from the stool since virus is shed for shorter periods from the throat. Cultures of cerebrospinal fluid (CSF), serum, fluid from body cavities, or tissues are positive less frequently, but a positive result is indicative of disease caused by enterovirus. In some cases the virus can be isolated only from the blood or only from the CSF; therefore, it is important to culture multiple sites. Cultures are more likely to be positive earlier than later in the course of infection. Most human enteroviruses can be detected within a week after inoculation of cell cultures. Cultures may be negative because of the presence of neutralizing antibody, lack of susceptibility of the cells used, or inappropriate handling of the specimen. Coxsackievirus A may require inoculation into special cell-culture lines or into suckling mice.

Identification of the serotype of an enterovirus is useful primarily for epidemiologic studies and, with a few exceptions, has little clinical utility. It is important to identify serious infections with enterovirus during epidemics and to distinguish the vaccine strain of poliovirus from the other enteroviruses in the throat or in the feces. Stool and throat samples for culture as well as acute- and convalescent-phase serum specimens should be obtained from all patients with suspected poliomyelitis. In the absence of a positive CSF culture, a positive culture of stool obtained within the first 2 weeks after the onset of symptoms is most often used to confirm the diagnosis of poliomyelitis. If poliovirus is isolated, it should be sent to the Centers for Disease Control and Prevention (CDC) in Atlanta for identification as either a wild-type or a vaccine virus.

The polymerase chain reaction (PCR) has been used to amplify viral nucleic acid from CSF, serum, urine, throat swabs, and tissues. A single pair of PCR primers can detect more than 92% of the serotypes that infect humans. With the proper controls, PCR of the CSF is highly sensitive ($\geq$95%) and specific (>80%) and is more rapid than culture. PCR of serum is also highly sensitive and specific in the diagnosis of disseminated disease. PCR may be particularly helpful for the diagnosis and follow-up of enterovirus disease in immunodeficient patients receiving immunoglobulin therapy, whose viral cultures may be negative. Antigen detection and hybridization of enterovirus sequences in human tissues with a specific probe are additional options, but these techniques are generally less sensitive than PCR.

Serologic diagnosis of enterovirus infection is limited by the large number of serotypes and the lack of a common antigen. Demonstration of seroconversion may be useful in rare cases for confirmation of culture results, but serologic testing is usually limited to epidemiologic studies. Serum should be collected and frozen soon after the onset of disease and again about 4 weeks later. Measurement of neutralizing titers is the most accurate method for antibody determination; measurement of complement-fixation titers is usually less sensitive. Titers of virus-specific IgM are elevated in both acute and chronic infection.

℞ **TREATMENT** Most enterovirus infections are mild and resolve spontaneously; however, intensive supportive care may be needed for cardiac, hepatic, or CNS disease. Intravenous, intrathecal, or intraventricular immunoglobulin has been used with apparent success for the treatment of chronic enterovirus meningoencephalitis and dermatomyositis in patients with hypo- or agammaglobulinemia. The disease may stabilize or resolve during therapy; however, some patients decline inexorably despite therapy. Intravenous administration of immunoglobulin with high titers of antibody to the infecting virus has been successful in the treatment of some cases of life-threatening infection in neonates, who may not have maternally acquired antibody. In one trial involving neonates with enterovirus infections, immunoglobulin containing very high titers of antibody to the infecting virus reduced rates of viremia; however, the study was too small to show a substantial clinical benefit. Oral pleconaril, a capsid-binding antiviral agent, reduced symptoms in a placebo-controlled trial of enteroviral aseptic meningitis and in a challenge study with coxsackievirus. This drug is available for compassionate use in patients with certain severe enterovirus infections. Glucocorticoids are contraindicated.

Good hand-washing practices and the use of gowns and gloves are important in limiting nosocomial transmission of enteroviruses during epidemics. Enteric precautions are indicated for 7 days after the onset of enterovirus infections.

POLIOVIRUS **Manifestations** Most infections with poliovirus are asymptomatic. After an incubation period of 3 to 6 days, about 5% of patients present with a minor illness (abortive poliomyelitis) manifested by fever, malaise, sore throat, anorexia, myalgias, and headache. This condition usually resolves in 3 days. About 1% of patients present with aseptic meningitis (nonparalytic poliomyelitis). Examination of CSF reveals lymphocytic pleocytosis, a normal glucose level, and a normal or slightly elevated protein level; CSF polymorphonuclear leukocytes may be present early. In some patients, especially children, malaise and fever precede the onset of aseptic meningitis.

The least common presentation is that of paralytic disease. After one or several days, signs of aseptic meningitis are followed by severe back, neck, and muscle pain and by the rapid or gradual development of motor weakness. In some cases the disease appears to be biphasic, with aseptic meningitis followed first by apparent recovery but then (1 or 2 days later) by the return of fever and the development of paralysis; this form is more common among children than among adults. Weakness is generally asymmetric, is proximal more than distal, and may involve the legs (most commonly); the arms; or the abdominal, thoracic, or bulbar muscles. Paralysis develops during the febrile phase of the illness and usually does not progress after defervescence. Urinary retention may also occur. Examination reveals weakness, fasciculations, decreased muscle tone, and reduced or absent reflexes in affected areas. Transient hyperreflexia sometimes precedes the loss of reflexes. Patients frequently report sensory symptoms, but objective sensory testing usually yields normal results. Bulbar paralysis may lead to dysphagia, difficulty in handling secretions, or dysphonia. Respiratory insufficiency due to aspiration, involvement of the respiratory center in the medulla, or paralysis of the phrenic or intercostal nerves may develop, and severe medullary involvement may lead to circulatory collapse. Most patients with paralysis recover some function weeks to months after infection. About two-thirds of patients have residual neurologic sequelae.

Paralytic disease is more common among older individuals, pregnant women, and persons exercising strenuously or undergoing trauma at the time of CNS symptoms. Tonsillectomy predisposes to bulbar poliomyelitis, and intramuscular injections increase the risk of paralysis in the involved limb(s).

At present, the only cases of poliomyelitis in the United States are due to live poliovirus vaccine; of the four cases reported in the United States in 1997 and 1998, three occurred in recipients of the first or second dose of oral poliovirus vaccine (OPV), and one occurred in an adult contact of a recipient of OPV. The median interval from vaccination to the onset of symptoms is usually 3 weeks. About 5% of the cases of poliomyelitis associated with vaccine occur in members of the community who have had no known direct contact with vaccinees. About 15% of all cases of vaccine-associated poliomyelitis involve immunodeficient children or adults, most of whom have hypo- or agammaglobulinemia. In these patients the median interval between vaccination and the onset of symptoms is 6 weeks, but disease can develop up to 6 months after vaccination. The risk of developing poliomyelitis after oral vaccination is estimated at 1 case per 2.5 million doses administered. The risk of developing paralytic disease after oral vaccination is about 2000 times higher among immunodeficient patients than among immunocompetent children.

The *postpolio syndrome* presents as a new onset of weakness, fatigue, fasciculations, and pain with additional atrophy of the muscle group involved during the initial paralytic disease 20 to 40 years earlier. The syndrome is more common among women and with increasing time after acute disease. The onset is insidious, and weakness occasionally extends to muscles that were not involved during the initial illness. The prognosis is generally good; progression to further weakness is usually slow, with plateau periods that range from 1 to 10 years. The postpolio syndrome is thought to be due to progressive dysfunction and loss of motor neurons that compensated for the neurons lost during the original infection and not to persistent or reactivated poliovirus infection.

Prevention and Eradication (See also Chap. 122) After a peak of 57,879 cases of poliomyelitis in the United States in 1952, the introduction of inactivated vaccine in 1955 and of oral vaccine in 1961 ultimately eradicated disease due to wild-type poliovirus in the western hemisphere. Such disease has not been documented in the United States since 1979, when cases occurred among religious groups who had declined immunization. In the western hemisphere, paralysis due to wild-type poliovirus was last documented in 1991.

In 1988, the World Health Organization adopted a resolution to eradicate poliomyelitis by the year 2000. From 1988 to 1997, the number of cases worldwide decreased by 89%, with about 6227 cases reported from 46 countries in 1998. More than 80% of the world's cases of confirmed polio in 1998 occurred in India, Pakistan, Bangladesh, and Nigeria. Polio is a source of concern for unimmunized or partially immunized travelers to these regions. Outbreaks of polio in Europe and North America have been traced to cases imported from the Indian subcontinent. Clearly, global eradication of polio is necessary to eliminate the risk of importation of wild-type virus. Outbreaks are thought to have been facilitated by suboptimal rates of vaccination, isolated pockets of unvaccinated children, poor sanitation and crowding, improper vaccine-storage conditions, and a reduced level of response to one of the serotypes in the vaccine.

For the development of live OPV containing all three poliovirus serotypes, wild-type virus was attenuated by passage in monkey kidney cell cultures. OPV strains differ from the wild-type strains in a limited number of nucleotide changes (i.e., fewer than 60). Multiple doses are required to ensure infection and development of immunity to all three serotypes. While intramuscular injections of other vaccines (live or attenuated) can be given concurrently with OPV, unnecessary intramuscular injections should be avoided during the first month after vaccination because they increase the risk of vaccine-associated paralysis. Inactivated poliovirus vaccine is generated by formalin inac-

1. Routine primary poliovirus vaccination is not indicated for unvaccinated adults residing in the United States, except for:
    a. travelers to areas where poliovirus is or may be epidemic or endemic;
    b. members of communities or population groups with disease caused by wild-type polioviruses;
    c. laboratory workers handling specimens that may contain wild-type polioviruses;
    d. health care workers in close contact with patients who may be excreting wild-type polioviruses;
    e. persons whose children will be receiving OPV.
2. Three doses of IPV are recommended for adults who need to be immunized.

ABBREVIATIONS: IPV, inactivated poliovirus vaccine; OPV, oral poliovirus vaccine.
SOURCE: Modified from 1997 Redbook, Report of the Committee on Infectious Diseases.

tivation of the three serotypes of live poliovirus. Since 1988 an enhanced-potency inactivated poliovirus vaccine (IPV) has been available in the United States.

OPV and IPV induce antibodies that persist for at least 5 years. Both vaccines induce IgG and IgA antibodies. Compared with recipients of IPV, recipients of OPV shed less virus and less frequently develop reinfection with wild-type virus after exposure to poliovirus. Although IPV is safe and efficacious, OPV offers the advantages of ease of administration, lower cost, and induction of intestinal immunity resulting in a reduction in the risk of community transmission of wild-type virus. Because of progress toward global eradication of polio (with a reduced risk of imported cases) and the continued occurrence of cases of vaccine-associated polio, the CDC recommended in 1997 that children receive a sequential schedule of two doses of IPV followed by two doses of OPV or a four-dose schedule of IPV alone. To further reduce the risk of vaccine-associated polio, the Advisory Committee for Immunization Practices recommended (in June 1999) an all-IPV regimen for childhood poliovirus vaccination. Beginning in January 2000, children should receive IPV at 2, 4, and 6 to 18 months and 4 to 6 years of age. OPV will be used only in special circumstances: (1) for mass immunization campaigns to control outbreaks of polio; (2) for vaccination of unimmunized children who will be traveling to a polio-endemic area within 4 weeks; and (3) for children whose parents do not accept an all-IPV regimen. The latter children should receive at least two doses of IPV before receiving OPV. The risk of vaccine-associated polio should be discussed before administering OPV. Recommendations for vaccination of adults are listed in Table 193-1.

COXSACKIEVIRUS, ECHOVIRUS, AND OTHER ENTEROVIRUSES   An estimated 5 to 10 million cases of symptomatic enterovirus disease occur in the United States each year. Enteroviruses are the most common cause of aseptic meningitis and nonspecific febrile illnesses of neonates. Certain clinical syndromes are more likely to be caused by certain serotypes (Table 193-2), but there is much overlap. From 1970 to 1983, 70% of enterovirus infections were caused by only 10 of the 64 human serotypes. Echoviruses 9 and 11 alone accounted for 24% of recognized enterovirus infections; echoviruses 4, 6, and 30 and coxsackieviruses A9 and B2 through B5 accounted for 46%.

Nonspecific Febrile Illness (Summer Grippe)   The most common clinical manifestation of enterovirus infection is a nonspecific febrile illness. After an incubation period of 3 to 6 days, patients present with an acute onset of fever, malaise, and headache. Occasional cases are associated with upper respiratory symptoms, and some cases include nausea and vomiting. Symptoms often last for 3 to 4 days, and most cases resolve in a week. While infections with other respiratory viruses occur more of-

ten from late fall to early spring, enterovirus febrile illness frequently occurs in the summer and early fall.

Generalized Disease of the Newborn   Most serious enterovirus infections in infants develop during the first week of life, although severe disease can occur up to 3 months of age. Neonates often present with an illness resembling bacterial sepsis, with fever, irritability, and lethargy. Laboratory abnormalities include leukocytosis with a left shift, thrombocytopenia, elevated values in liver function tests, and CSF pleocytosis. The illness can be complicated by myocarditis and hypotension, fulminant hepatitis and disseminated intravascular coagulation, meningitis or meningoencephalitis, or pneumonia. It may be difficult to distinguish enterovirus infection from bacterial sepsis, although a history of a recent virus-like illness in the mother provides a clue.

Aseptic Meningitis and Encephalitis   Enteroviruses are the cause of up to 90% of cases of aseptic meningitis in children and young adults in which an etiologic agent can be identified. Patients with aseptic meningitis typically present with an acute onset of fever, chills, headache, photophobia, and pain on eye movement. Nausea and vomiting are also common. Examination reveals meningismus without localizing neurologic signs; drowsiness or irritability may also be apparent. In some cases, a febrile illness may be reported that remits but returns several days later in conjunction with signs of meningitis. Other systemic manifestations may provide clues to an enteroviral cause, including diarrhea, myalgias, rash, pleurodynia, myocarditis, and herpangina. Examination of the CSF invariably reveals pleocytosis; early in the course, polymorphonuclear leukocytes may be present or even predominant, raising the possibility of bacterial or other nonviral causes of meningitis. Partially treated bacterial meningitis may be particularly difficult to exclude in some instances. A useful rule is that the CSF cell count in enteroviral meningitis shows a shift to lymphocytic predominance within 24 h of presentation, and the total count generally does not exceed 1000 cells/μL. Additional CSF findings consist of a normal glucose content and a normal or only slightly elevated (by $\leq$100 mg/mL) level of protein. Enteroviruses and mumps virus may produce a similar picture of meningitis; a low CSF glucose level suggests mumps, whereas a normal CSF glucose level and transient CSF polymorphonuclear pleocytosis suggest enterovirus infection. Symptoms ordinarily resolve within a week, although CSF abnormalities can persist for several weeks. Enteroviral meningitis is often more severe in adults than in children. Neurologic sequelae are rare, and most patients have an excellent prognosis.

Enteroviral encephalitis is much less common than enteroviral aseptic meningitis. Occasional highly inflammatory cases of enteroviral meningitis may be complicated by a mild form of encephalitis that is recognized on the basis of progressive lethargy, disorientation, and sometimes seizures. Less commonly, severe primary encephalitis may develop. It is estimated that 10 to 20% of cases of viral encephalitis are due to enteroviruses. Immunocompetent patients generally have a good prognosis.

Table 193-2   Manifestations Commonly Associated with Enterovirus Serotypes

Manifestation	Serotype(s) of Indicated Virus	
	Coxsackievirus	Echovirus (E) and Enterovirus (Ent)
Aseptic meningitis	A2, 4, 7, 9, 10; B1-5	E4, 6, 7, 9, 11, 16, 18, 19, 30, 33; Ent70, 71
Exanthem	A4, 5, 9, 10, 16; B1, 3-5	E4-7, 9, 11, 16-19, 25, 30; Ent71
Generalized disease of the newborn	B2-5	E4-6, 9, 11, 14, 16, 19
Hand-foot-and-mouth disease	A5, 7, 9, 10, 16; B2, 5	Ent71
Herpangina	A1-10, 16, 22; B1-5	E6, 9, 11, 16, 17, 25; Ent71
Myocarditis, pericarditis	A4, 9, 16; B1-5	E6, 9, 11
Paralysis	A4, 7, 9; B1-5	E2, 4, 6, 9, 11, 30; Ent70, 71
Pleurodynia	A1, 2, 4, 6, 9, 10, 16; B1-6	E1-3, 6, 7, 9, 11, 12, 14, 16, 19, 24, 25, 30
Pneumonia	A9, 16; B1-5	E6, 7, 9, 11, 12, 19, 20, 30; Ent68, 71

Patients with hypo- or agammaglobulinemia or severe combined immunodeficiency may develop chronic meningitis or encephalitis; about half of these patients have a dermatomyositis-like syndrome, with peripheral edema, rash, and myositis. They may also have chronic hepatitis. Patients may develop neurologic disease while receiving gamma globulin replacement therapy. Echoviruses (especially echovirus 11) are the most common pathogens in this situation.

Paralytic disease due to enteroviruses other than poliovirus occurs sporadically and is usually less severe than poliomyelitis. Most cases are due to enterovirus 70 or 71 or to coxsackievirus A7 or A9. Guillain-Barré syndrome is also associated with enterovirus infection. While some studies have suggested a link between enteroviruses and the chronic fatigue syndrome, most recent studies have not demonstrated such an association.

Pleurodynia (Bornholm Disease) Patients with pleurodynia present with an acute onset of fever and spasms of pleuritic chest or upper abdominal pain. Chest pain is more frequent in adults, and abdominal pain is more common in children. Paroxysms of severe, knifelike pain usually last 15 to 30 min and are associated with diaphoresis and tachypnea. Fever peaks within an hour after the onset of paroxysms and subsides when pain resolves. The involved muscles are tender to palpation, and a pleural rub may be detected. The white blood cell count and chest x-ray are usually normal. Most cases are due to coxsackievirus B and occur during epidemics. Symptoms resolve in a few days, and recurrences are rare. Treatment includes the administration of nonsteroidal anti-inflammatory agents or the application of heat to the affected muscles.

Myocarditis and Pericarditis Enteroviruses are estimated to cause up to one-third of cases of acute myocarditis. Coxsackievirus B and its RNA have been detected in pericardial fluid and myocardial tissue in some cases of acute myocarditis and pericarditis. Most cases of enteroviral myocarditis or pericarditis occur in newborns, adolescents, or young adults. More than two-thirds of patients are male. Patients often present with an upper respiratory tract infection that is followed by fever, chest pain, dyspnea, arrhythmias, and occasionally heart failure. A pericardial friction rub is documented in half of cases, and the electrocardiogram shows ST segment elevations or ST- and T-wave abnormalities. Serum levels of myocardial enzymes are often elevated. Neonates commonly have severe disease, while most older children and adults recover completely. Up to 10% of cases progress to chronic dilated cardiomyopathy. Chronic constrictive pericarditis may also be a sequela.

Exanthems Enterovirus infection is the leading cause of exanthems in children in the summer and fall. While exanthems are associated with many enteroviruses, certain types have been linked to specific syndromes. Echoviruses 9 and 16 have frequently been associated with exanthem and fever. Rashes may be discrete (rubelliform) or confluent (morbilliform), beginning on the face and spreading to the trunk and extremities. Echovirus 9 is the most common cause of rubelliform rash. Unlike the rash of rubella, the enteroviral rash occurs in the summer and is not associated with lymphadenopathy. Roseola-like rashes develop after defervescence, with macules and papules on the face and trunk. The Boston exanthem, caused by echovirus 16, is a roseola-like rash that often affects multiple members of a family. A variety of other rashes have been associated with enteroviruses, including erythema multiforme and vesicular, urticarial, petechial, or purpuric lesions. Enanthems also occur, including lesions that resemble the Koplik's spots seen with measles.

Hand-Foot-and-Mouth Disease After an incubation period of 4 to 6 days, patients with hand-foot-and-mouth disease present with fever, anorexia, and malaise; these manifestations are followed by the development of sore throat and vesicles (**Plate IID-39**) on the buccal mucosa and often on the tongue and then by the appearance of tender vesicular lesions on the dorsum of the hands, sometimes with involvement of the palms. The vesicles may form bullae and quickly ulcerate. About one-third of patients also have lesions on the palate,

uvula, or tonsillar pillars, and one-third have a rash on the feet (including the soles) or on the buttocks. The disease is highly infectious, with attack rates of close to 100% among young children. The lesions usually resolve in 1 week. Most cases are due to coxsackievirus A16 or enterovirus 71.

An epidemic of enterovirus 71 infection in Taiwan in 1998 resulted in thousands of cases of hand-foot-and-mouth disease or herpangina. Severe complications included CNS disease, myocarditis, and pulmonary hemorrhage. About 90% of those who died were children ≤5 years old, and these deaths were associated with pulmonary edema or pulmonary hemorrhage. CNS disease included aseptic meningitis, flaccid paralysis (similar to poliomyelitis), or rhombencephalitis with myoclonus and tremor or ataxia. The mean age of patients with CNS complications was 2.5 years, and magnetic resonance imaging in cases with encephalitis usually showed brain-stem lesions.

Herpangina Herpangina is usually caused by coxsackievirus A and presents as acute-onset fever, sore throat, dysphagia, and grayish-white papulovesicular lesions on an erythematous base that ulcerate. The lesions can persist for weeks; are present on the soft palate, anterior pillars of the tonsils, and uvula; and are concentrated in the posterior portion of the mouth. In contrast to herpes stomatitis, enteroviral herpangina is not associated with gingivitis. Acute lymphonodular pharyngitis associated with coxsackievirus A10 presents as white or yellow nodules surrounded by erythema in the posterior oropharynx. The lesions do not ulcerate.

Acute Hemorrhagic Conjunctivitis Patients with acute hemorrhagic conjunctivitis present with an acute onset of severe eye pain, blurred vision, photophobia, and watery discharge from the eye. Examination reveals edema, chemosis, and subconjunctival hemorrhage and often shows punctate keratitis and conjunctival follicles as well. Preauricular adenopathy is often found. Epidemics and nosocomial spread have been associated with enterovirus 70 and coxsackievirus A24. Systemic symptoms, including headache and fever, develop in 20% of cases, and recovery is usually complete in 10 days. The sudden onset and short duration of the illness help to distinguish acute hemorrhagic conjunctivitis from other ocular infections such as those due to adenovirus and *Chlamydia*. Paralysis has been associated with some cases of acute hemorrhagic conjunctivitis due to enterovirus 70 during epidemics.

Other Manifestations Enteroviruses are an infrequent cause of childhood pneumonia and the common cold. Coxsackievirus B has been isolated at autopsy from the pancreas of a few children presenting with insulin-dependent diabetes mellitus; however, most attempts to isolate the virus have been unsuccessful. Other diseases that have been associated with enterovirus infection include bronchitis, bronchiolitis, croup, infectious lymphocytosis, polymyositis, acute arthritis, and acute nephritis.

REOVIRUSES

Reoviruses are double-stranded RNA viruses encompassing three serotypes. Serologic studies indicate that most humans are infected with reoviruses during childhood; however, it has been difficult to establish a definite link of reovirus infection with a particular disease. It is likely that most infections either are asymptomatic or cause very mild disease. One outbreak of reovirus infection in children resulted in minor upper respiratory tract symptoms. Reovirus is considered a rare cause of mild gastroenteritis in infants and children. Speculation regarding an association of reovirus type 3 with idiopathic neonatal hepatitis and extrahepatic biliary atresia is based on an elevated prevalence of antibody to reovirus among some of these patients, detection of viral RNA by PCR in hepatobiliary tissues in some studies, and detection of virus in the porta hepatis in one case.

BIBLIOGRAPHY

ABZUG MJ et al: Neonatal enterovirus infection: Virology, serology, and effects of intravenous immune globulin. Clin Infect Dis 20:1201, 1995

AHMED A et al: Clinical utility of the polymerase chain reaction for diagnosis of enteroviral meningitis in infancy. J Pediatr 131:393, 1997

CHEN RT et al: Seroprevalence of antibody against poliovirus in inner-city preschool children: Implications for vaccination policy in the United States. JAMA 275:1639, 1996

COCHI SL et al (eds): *Global Poliomyelitis Eradication Initiative: Status Report.* J Infect Dis 175(Suppl 1):S1–S292, 1997

DALAKAS MC et al: The postpolio syndrome: Advances in the pathogenesis and treatment. Ann NY Acad Sci 753:1, 1995

HO M et al: An epidemic of enterovirus 71 infection in Taiwan. N Engl J Med 341:929, 1999

HUANG C-C et al: Neurologic complications in children with enterovirus 71 infection. N Engl J Med 341:936, 1999

MCKINNEY R et al: Chronic enteroviral meningoencephalitis in agammaglobulinemic patients. Rev Infect Dis 9:334, 1987

PREVOTS DR et al: Poliomyelitis prevention in the United States: New recommendations for routine childhood vaccination place greater reliance on inactivated poliovirus vaccine. Pediatr Ann 26:378, 1997

ROTBART HA (ed): *Human Enterovirus Infections.* Washington, DC, ASM Press, 1995

ROTBART HA et al: Treatment of human enterovirus infections. Antiviral Res 38:1, 1998

STREBEL PM et al: Intramuscular injections within 30 days of immunization with oral poliovirus vaccine—a risk factor for vaccine-associated paralytic poliomyelitis. N Engl J Med 332:500, 1995

194   *Anne Gershon*

MEASLES (RUBEOLA)

DEFINITION   Measles (rubeola) is a highly contagious, acute, exanthematous respiratory disease with a characteristic clinical picture and pathognomonic enanthem. A successful live attenuated measles vaccine became available in 1963 in the United States and elsewhere, and measles is now an unusual disease in most developed countries where this vaccine is widely used. However, measles continues to occur sporadically in mini-epidemics in the United States, and major epidemics in developing nations make this disease a persistent cause of childhood morbidity and mortality.

ETIOLOGIC AGENT   Measles virus is a member of the genus *Morbillivirus* and the family Paramyxoviridae. It is closely related to the viruses causing canine and porcine distemper, rinderpest of cattle, and *peste des petits ruminants* of goats and sheep. There is only one antigenic type. Measles virions are pleomorphic spherical structures having a diameter of 100 to 250 nm and consisting of six proteins. The inner capsid is composed of a coiled helix of RNA and three proteins, and the outer envelope consists of a matrix protein bearing two types of short surface-glycoprotein projections or peplomers. One peplomer is a conical hemagglutinin (H) and the other a dumbbell-shaped fusion (F) protein. The genome has been sequenced, and it is thereby possible to distinguish vaccine-type measles virus from the wild type. In addition, genetic variability of wild-type measles virus occurs; eight genotypes have been identified.

EPIDEMIOLOGY   Measles has a worldwide distribution; humans are the only natural hosts, although other primates can be experimentally infected. During the prevaccination era in the United States, measles epidemics occurred every 2 to 5 years in the winter and spring. In an epidemic year, roughly half a million measles cases were reported; 99% of adults had serologic evidence of previous measles infection. After the live attenuated vaccine became available, the number of cases reported to the Centers for Disease Control and Prevention (CDC) fell, with a nadir of 1497 cases in 1983. After an upsurge to more than 27,000 cases (with 89 deaths) in 1990, the disease was once more brought under control (with only 312 cases reported to the CDC in 1993), in part through the routine administration of two doses of vaccine. The foremost reason for the resurgence of measles was failure to immunize infants and young children, especially in inner-city areas. Primary vaccine failure (documented in about 5% of individuals) and secondary vaccine failure or waning immunity accounted for some cases.

In recent years the majority of cases of measles have involved preschool children. Between 1993 and 1996, fewer than 1000 cases were reported annually in the United States; in 1995 there were 309 reported cases, and in 1996 there were 508. Molecular studies indicated interruption of transmission of indigenous measles in 1993. Most cases have since resulted from international importations of the virus. Mortality is highest among children under 2 years of age and among adults. Patients with impaired cell-mediated immunity are at especially high risk for severe or even fatal measles. The measles-associated mortality rate in the United States is about 0.3%; in developing countries, mortality frequently exceeds 1% and sometimes approaches 10%.

Measles virus is transmitted by respiratory secretions, predominantly through exposure to aerosols but also through direct contact with larger droplets. Patients are contagious from 1 or 2 days before the onset of symptoms until 4 days after the appearance of the rash. Infectivity peaks during the prodromal phase. The mean intervals from infection to onset of symptoms and to appearance of rash are 10 and 14 days, respectively.

PATHOGENESIS AND PATHOLOGY   Measles virus invades the respiratory epithelium and spreads via the bloodstream to the reticuloendothelial system, from which it infects all types of white blood cells, thereby establishing infection of the skin, respiratory tract, and other organs. Both viremia and viruria develop. Multinucleated giant cells with inclusion bodies in the nucleus and cytoplasm (Warthin-Finkeldey cells) are found in respiratory and lymphoid tissues and are pathognomonic for measles. Direct invasion of T lymphocytes and increased levels of suppressive cytokines, such as interleukin 4, may play a role in the temporary depression of cellular immunity that accompanies and transiently follows measles. The major infected cell in the blood is the monocyte. Infection of the entire respiratory tract accounts for the characteristic cough and coryza of measles and for the less frequent manifestations of croup, bronchiolitis, and pneumonia. Generalized damage to the respiratory tract, with resultant loss of cilia, predisposes to secondary bacterial infections such as pneumonia and otitis media.

Specific antibodies are not detectable before the onset of rash. Cellular immunity (consisting of cytotoxic T cells and possibly natural killer cells) plays a prominent role in host defense, and patients who are deficient in cellular immunity are at high risk for severe measles. Children with isolated agammaglobulinemia are not at increased risk. Immune reactions to the virus in the endothelial cells of dermal capillaries play a substantial role in the development of Koplik's spots (the pathognomonic enanthem) as well as in that of rash; in immunodeficient hosts, measles may be severe despite the absence of these manifestations. Measles antigens have been demonstrated in involved skin during early stages of the illness.

Pathologic changes in measles encephalitis include focal hemorrhage, congestion, and perivascular demyelination. Measles virus is rarely isolated from cerebrospinal fluid (CSF) in cases of encephalitis, which are thought to be due to the interaction of virus-infected cells with local cellular immune factors.

CLINICAL MANIFESTATIONS   Measles begins with a 2- to 4-day respiratory prodrome of malaise, cough, coryza, conjunctivitis with lacrimation, nasal discharge, and increasing fever [with temperatures as high as 40.6°C (105°F), probably reflecting secondary viremia]. At this stage of the illness, in which the rash has not yet developed, influenza may be suspected. Just before the onset of the rash, Koplik's spots appear as 1- to 2-mm blue-white spots on a bright red background. Without adequate illumination for examination, they may be overlooked. Koplik's spots are typically located on the buccal mucosa alongside the second molars and may be extensive; they are not associated with any other infectious disease. The spots wane after the onset of rash and soon disappear. The entire buccal and inner labial mucosa may be inflamed, and the lips may be reddened.

The characteristic erythematous, nonpruritic, maculopapular rash of measles begins at the hairline and behind the ears, spreads down the trunk and limbs to include the palms and soles, and often becomes confluent. At this time, the patient is at the most severe point of the illness. By the fourth day, the rash begins to fade in the order in which it appeared. Brownish discoloration of the skin and desquamation may occur later. Fever usually resolves by the fourth or fifth day after the onset of rash; prolonged fever suggests a complication of measles. Lymphadenopathy, diarrhea, vomiting, and splenomegaly are common features. The chest x-ray may be abnormal, even in uncomplicated measles, because of the propensity of this virus to invade the respiratory tract. The entire illness usually lasts about 10 days. The disease tends to be more severe in adults than in children, with higher fever, more prominent rash, and a higher incidence of complications.

Milder forms of the illness with less intense symptoms and a milder rash, termed *modified measles*, may occur in individuals with preexisting partial immunity induced by active or passive vaccination. These patients include infants under 1 year of age who retain some proportion of passively acquired maternal antibodies. On occasion, individuals with a history of immunization may develop modified measles.

COMPLICATIONS   The complications of measles can conveniently be divided into three groups, according to the site involved: the respiratory tract, the central nervous system (CNS), and the gastrointestinal tract. Respiratory tract involvement, manifested as laryngitis, croup, or bronchitis, occurs in the majority of cases of uncomplicated measles. In young children, otitis media is the most common complication. Pneumonia is a frequent reason for hospitalization, especially of adults. The pneumonia is of viral origin in the majority of cases, but secondary bacterial infection (most commonly caused by streptococci, pneumococci, or staphylococci) also takes place with some frequency. Primary giant cell (Hecht's) pneumonia is most often documented in immunocompromised and/or malnourished patients.

Encephalographic abnormalities in the absence of symptoms of CNS disease are extremely frequent in measles. Symptomatic CNS disease, with fever, headache, drowsiness, coma, and/or seizures, occurs in about 1 case in 1000. Symptoms usually begin within days after the onset of rash but occasionally appear for the first time several weeks later. About 10% of patients do not survive acute measles encephalitis; a significant percentage of surviving patients develop permanent sequelae, such as mental retardation or epilepsy. Most cases appear to result from an immune-mediated response to myelin proteins (postinfectious encephalomyelitis) and not directly from viral infection of the CNS (Chap. 371). Rarely, transverse myelitis follows measles. Immunocompromised patients are at risk for progressive fatal encephalitis 1 to 6 months after measles; in some cases, even though prior measles has not been recognized, the virus is identified at autopsy. Subacute sclerosing panencephalitis (SSPE)—a protracted, chronic, extremely rare form of measles encephalitis—sometimes follows measles and is particularly common among children who have measles before the age of 2 years (Chap. 373). SSPE has virtually disappeared in the United States as a result of widespread vaccination. Typically, progressive dementia evolves over several months. SSPE is thought to be due to a complex interaction of the host with defective measles virus. It is associated with extremely high levels of antibodies to measles virus in the blood and CSF.

Gastrointestinal complications of measles include gastroenteritis, hepatitis, appendicitis, ileocolitis, and mesenteric adenitis. It is not uncommon to detect high levels of alanine and aspartate aminotransferases in the absence of gastrointestinal signs such as jaundice.

Other, rare complications include myocarditis, glomerulonephritis, and postinfectious thrombocytopenic purpura. Measles can exacerbate preexisting tuberculosis, presumably through depression of cellular immunity induced by the virus. Natural measles and immunization against measles can result in tuberculin skin-test anergy lasting for about 1 month.

ATYPICAL MEASLES   An atypical form of measles has been reported in individuals who received formalin-inactivated measles vaccine (used in the United States from 1963 through 1967 and in Canada until 1970) and subsequently were exposed to measles virus. After a several-day prodrome of fever, myalgia, and headache, the rash appears. Unlike the rash of typical measles, that of atypical measles begins peripherally and moves centrally; it can be urticarial, maculopapular, hemorrhagic, and/or vesicular. Fever is usually high and is accompanied by edema of the extremities, interstitial pulmonary infiltrates, hepatitis, and (on occasion) pleural effusion. The differential diagnosis often includes Rocky Mountain spotted fever, Henoch-Schönlein purpura, meningococcemia, drug allergy, toxic shock syndrome, and varicella. Despite the severity of atypical measles, patients invariably recover after a convalescence that may be prolonged. Measles virus is not isolated from these patients, and they do not spread the virus to others. This disease is believed to be due to hypersensitivity to measles virus induced by the inactivated vaccine. Formalin inactivation destroys the antigenicity of the F protein, antibodies to which are important in preventing spread of the virus from one cell to another. The role of cellular immunity in this process is unknown. Extremely high convalescent titers of antibody to measles virus (e.g., 1:1,000,000) are diagnostic of atypical measles. To prevent this syndrome, adults who received formalin-inactivated measles vaccine should be reimmunized with at least one dose of live attenuated measles vaccine. Since inactivated measles vaccine has not been available for more than 25 years, atypical measles has now virtually disappeared.

MEASLES IN THE IMMUNOCOMPROMISED HOST   Patients with defects in cell-mediated immunity are at risk for severe protracted and fatal measles. Included in this category are patients with congenital cellular immune defects or malignancy, recipients of immunosuppressive therapy, or persons infected with HIV. In these patients, measles may not be accompanied by a rash. Complications are primary measles (giant cell) pneumonia, progressive encephalitis beginning weeks to months after initial infection, and (in HIV-infected patients) progression to AIDS.

MEASLES IN ADULTS   Measles is naturally a disease of childhood and, like many other viral infections, is more severe in adults than in children. About 3% of young adults with measles develop primary viral pneumonia and require hospitalization. Hepatitis and bronchospasm are more common among adults with measles than among children, and the rash is more severe and more confluent in adults. Bacterial superinfection is more common among adults, more than one-third of whom develop respiratory complications such as otitis media, sinusitis, and pneumonia. Adults may develop measles because they were never immunized or (more rarely) because their vaccine-induced immunity has waned. Very low titers of antibody to measles virus have been associated with lack of protection.

LABORATORY FINDINGS   Lymphopenia and neutropenia are common in measles and may be due to invasion of leukocytes by the virus, with subsequent cell death. Leukocytosis may herald a bacterial superinfection. Patients with measles encephalitis usually have an elevated protein concentration in CSF as well as lymphocytosis. A specific diagnosis of measles can be made quickly by immunofluorescent staining of a smear of respiratory secretions for measles antigen; monoclonal antibodies conjugated to fluorescein are commercially available for this purpose. Secretions can also be examined microscopically for multinucleated giant cells. Measles virus can be isolated from respiratory secretions or urine and rapidly identified in tissue culture with fluorescein-labeled monoclonal antibodies. Measles virus RNA has been demonstrated by diagnostic reverse-transcription polymerase chain reaction. A number of serologic tests are available for the diagnosis of measles; however, a serologic diagnosis cannot necessarily be made quickly since both acute- and convalescent-phase sera are usually tested, ideally at the same time. The older hemagglutination inhibition test has been replaced by enzyme immunoassay (EIA), which is more sensitive and simpler to perform. EIA can be used to measure specific IgM and thus to diagnose measles on the basis of an acute-phase serum sample alone. Specific IgM antibodies are detectable within 1 to 2 days after the appearance of rash, and the IgG titer rises significantly after 10 days. As already mentioned, atypical measles and SSPE are associated with extremely high titers of antibody.

DIFFERENTIAL DIAGNOSIS Classic measles—with Koplik's spots, cough, coryza, conjunctivitis, and a rash beginning on the head—is easily diagnosed on clinical grounds. Modified measles is more difficult to diagnose clinically since one or more characteristic signs may be lacking. The differential diagnosis of measles includes Kawasaki's syndrome, scarlet fever, infectious mononucleosis, toxoplasmosis, drug eruption, and *Mycoplasma pneumoniae* infection. Most of these conditions can be identified by either culture or serologic assay. In the differential diagnosis of measles, attention should be paid to the current epidemiology of the disease in the community and to the patient's history of measles vaccination and foreign travel.

PREVENTION The development of live attenuated measles vaccine by Enders and his colleagues was a milestone in American medicine. This vaccine, used in the United States for the routine immunization of children since 1963, induces seroconversion in about 95% of recipients and probably confers lifelong protection. Waning immunity to measles after immunization has been documented only on rare occasions. For the past 25 years, measles vaccine has been available as the combination vaccine measles-mumps-rubella (MMR); MMR vaccine should be administered to children between the ages of 12 and 15 months. (Vaccination at 12 months is preferred for infants whose mothers were immunized against measles in childhood. These mothers have lower antibody titers than women who have had natural measles, and their infants correspondingly have transplacental antibodies of lower titer and shorter duration.) A second dose of MMR vaccine is recommended for school-aged children at 4 to 12 years of age. This two-dose policy was developed in the late 1980s in response to measles outbreaks in the United States. Since the institution of the two-dose regimen and the increased effort to immunize all children, measles has again become an unusual disease in the United States. Regional guidelines that reflect the current local epidemiology of measles should be followed.

Older susceptible persons should also be immunized. Individuals should be considered susceptible to measles unless they have documentation of physician-diagnosed measles or of the receipt of two doses of vaccine, have laboratory evidence of measles immunity, or were born before 1957. Rarely, individuals born before 1957 develop measles, and those who are at risk of exposure to measles (e.g., health workers, teachers, and international travelers) should be tested for measles antibody and immunized if necessary. Approximately 10% of healthy vaccinees develop a fever, with temperatures up to 39.4°C (103°F), 5 to 7 days after vaccination; this fever lasts 1 to 5 days and is accompanied by a transient rash. Individuals previously immunized only with killed vaccine are considered susceptible and should receive at least one dose—and preferably two doses—of MMR vaccine. Transient adverse reactions in these individuals include fever, malaise, and redness and swelling at the injection site.

Because of the severity of measles in this group and the lack of reported problems following vaccination, children with asymptomatic HIV infection should receive MMR vaccine; those with severe immunosuppression (<15% CD4 lymphocytes) should not. A case of fatal measles due to vaccine-type virus was reported in a college student with AIDS. Measles vaccine is contraindicated for persons with impaired cell-mediated immunity, for pregnant women, and for persons with a history of anaphylaxis due to egg protein or neomycin. Minor illnesses, with or without fever and a history of convulsions, are not contraindications to vaccination. Vaccination should be deferred for 6 to 11 months after the receipt of immune globulin or of blood products containing antibodies and for at least 3 months after the discontinuation of immunosuppressive treatment. Vaccine failures have been ascribed to faulty storage of the preparation used, immunization of infants with preexisting (maternally derived) antibodies, and simultaneous administration of measles vaccine and immune globulin.

Children and adults who are susceptible to measles and are exposed to the disease should receive postexposure prophylaxis. Standard immune globulin, given intramuscularly within 6 days of exposure, can exert a protective or modifying effect; the earlier it is given, the better the outcome. The dose is 0.25 mL/kg for healthy persons and 0.5 mL/kg for immunocompromised persons, with a maximum dose of 15 mL. Immune globulin is particularly strongly indicated for susceptible household contacts, especially those less than 1 year of age, and for immunocompromised persons. HIV-infected persons, particularly those with severe immunosuppression, should be given immune globulin after exposure, regardless of their measles immune status and whether or not they are receiving intravenous immunoglobulin. Vaccination within 72 h of exposure may also provide protection against clinical measles, but this strategy is contraindicated as postexposure prophylaxis for immunocompromised individuals. Vaccine and immune globulin should not be given concurrently.

℞ **TREATMENT** Therapy for measles is largely supportive and symptom-based. Patients with otitis media and pneumonia should be given standard antibiotics. Patients with encephalitis need supportive care, including observation for increased intracranial pressure. Controlled trials suggest clinical benefit from high doses of vitamin A in severe or potentially severe measles, especially in children under the age of 2 years. A dose of 50,000 IU is used for infants age 1 to 6 months, 100,000 IU for infants age 7 to 12 months, and 200,000 IU for children over 1 year. A single dose is administered on two consecutive days. Transient vomiting and headache may be associated with the administration of vitamin A. Ribavirin is effective against measles virus in vitro and may be considered for use in immunocompromised individuals.

BIBLIOGRAPHY

CENTERS FOR DISEASE CONTROL AND PREVENTION: Measles, mumps, and rubella—vaccine use and strategies for elimination of measles, rubella, and congenital rubella syndrome and control of mumps. MMWR 47:1, 1998

EBERHART-PHILLIPS JE et al: Measles in pregnancy: A descriptive study of 58 cases. Obstet Gynecol 82:797, 1993

FORNI AL et al: Severe measles pneumonitis in adults: Evaluation of clinical characteristics and therapy with intravenous ribavirin. Clin Infect Dis 19:454, 1994

GREMILLION DH et al: Measles pneumonia in young adults. An analysis of 106 cases. Am J Med 71:539, 1981

HUSSEY GD et al: A randomized, controlled trial of vitamin A in children with severe measles. N Engl J Med 323:160, 1990

KAPLAN LJ et al: Severe measles in immunocompromised patients. JAMA 267:1237, 1992

LA BOCCETTA AC et al: Measles encephalitis. Report of 61 cases. Am J Dis Child 107:247, 1964

MARKOWITZ LE et al: Duration of live measles vaccine–induced immunity. Pediatr Infect Dis J 9:101, 1990

PELTOLA H et al: The elimination of indigenous measles, mumps, and rubella from Finland by a 12-year, two-dose vaccination program. N Engl J Med 331:1397, 1994

SMARON MF et al: Diagnosis of measles by fluorescent antibody and culture of nasopharyngeal secretions. J Virol Methods 33:223, 1991

TAKAHASHI H et al: Detection and comparison of viral antigens in measles and rubella rashes. Clin Infect Dis 22:36, 1996

195   *Anne Gershon*

RUBELLA (GERMAN MEASLES)

DEFINITION Rubella is an acute viral infection of children and adults that characteristically includes rash, fever, and lymphadenopathy and has a broad spectrum of other possible manifestations. However, a high percentage of rubella infections in both children and adults are subclinical. In addition, the illness can resemble a mild attack of measles (rubeola) and can cause arthritis, especially in adults. Rubella during pregnancy can lead to fetal infection, with the production of a significant constellation of malformations (*congenital rubella syndrome*) in a high proportion of infected fetuses.

ETIOLOGIC AGENT Rubella virus, a togavirus, is the only member of the *Rubivirus* genus and is closely related to the alphaviruses. Unlike these agents, however, it does not require a vector for transmission. Moreover, there is no RNA sequence homology between rubella virus and the alphaviruses.

The rubella virion is composed of an inner icosahedral capsid of RNA and protein that is surrounded by a lipid-containing envelope with a diameter of about 60 nm. The structural proteins associated with rubella virus are E1 and E2 (transmembrane envelope glycoproteins) and C (the capsid protein that surrounds the viral RNA). Only one serotype has been identified.

EPIDEMIOLOGY In the United States during the prevaccine era, rubella was most common in the spring and most often affected school-age children; only 80 to 90% of adults were immune; and major epidemics occurred every 6 to 9 years. The most recent epidemic in the United States occurred in 1964 to 1965, when there were more than 12 million reported cases of postnatal rubella and more than 20,000 cases of the congenital rubella syndrome. Since the introduction of live attenuated rubella vaccine in 1969, there have been no epidemics; limited outbreaks have been reported in settings where susceptible individuals come into close contact with one another (e.g., schools and workplaces). In 1996, only 213 cases of postnatally acquired rubella—most of them in young adults—and 2 confirmed cases of congenital rubella syndrome were reported to the Centers for Disease Control and Prevention (CDC).

Whether symptomatic or subclinical, rubella is contagious, albeit less so than measles. Its incubation period is 18 days on average, with a range of 12 to 23 days. The virus, which is spread in droplets shed in respiratory secretions, infects the respiratory tract and then the bloodstream. In postnatally acquired infections, rubella virus is shed during the prodromal phase of the illness, and shedding from the pharynx can continue for about a week after onset. Despite high titers of specific neutralizing antibodies, infants with congenital rubella may excrete rubella virus from the respiratory tract and in the urine until the age of 2 years. This excretion raises important issues related to infection control in hospital and day-care settings. Persons recently immunized with live attenuated rubella vaccine do not transmit the vaccine virus to others, although low titers of rubella virus may be detected transiently in the pharynx.

After an attack of rubella, specific antibodies and cell-mediated immunity develop and probably play a significant role in protection against future disease. Asymptomatic reinfection at the level of the respiratory tract is common upon reexposure to the virus but is rarely if ever associated with viremia.

Rubella virus has been cultured from respiratory secretions during reinfection. Fetal infection may occur during maternal reinfection but is acknowledged to be extremely rare because of the absence of maternal viremia under these circumstances. Viremia following reinfection of individuals immunized against rubella is also rare. Thus the current level of congenital rubella in the United States is exceedingly low.

PATHOGENESIS AND PATHOLOGY Little is known about the microscopic pathology of postnatally acquired rubella since the disease is invariably self-limited. Like that of measles, the rash of rubella is immunologically mediated; its onset coincides with the development of specific antibodies. Viremia can be demonstrated for about a week before and ends within a few days after the onset of rash.

The cause of the damage to cells and organs in congenital rubella is not well understood. Proposed mechanisms of fetal damage include mitotic arrest of cells, tissue necrosis without inflammation, and chromosomal damage. The growth of the fetus may be retarded. Other findings may include decreased numbers of megakaryocytes in the bone marrow, extramedullary hematopoiesis, and interstitial pneumonia.

CLINICAL MANIFESTATIONS Postnatally Acquired Rubella Infection acquired after birth usually results in an extremely mild or subclinical illness. A prodromal phase is uncommon in children; adults may have more severe disease, with a brief prodrome of malaise, fever, and anorexia. The foremost symptoms of postnatally acquired rubella include posterior auricular, cervical, and suboccipital lymphadenopathy; fever; and rash. The rash often begins on the face and spreads down the body. It is maculopapular but not confluent, is sometimes accompanied by mild coryza and conjunctivitis, and generally lasts for 3 to 5 days. A petechial enanthem on the soft palate, designated *Forschheimer spots*, may occur but is not specific for rubella. Fever may be absent entirely or may be present for only several days in the early phase of the illness.

Complications of postnatally acquired rubella are uncommon; bacterial superinfection is rare. One particularly troublesome complication is seen almost exclusively in women: arthritis, most frequently involving the fingers, wrists, and/or knees, develops as the rash is appearing and may take several weeks to resolve. Chronic arthritis resulting from rubella is extremely rare. Rubella virus has been isolated from joint fluid during acute rubella arthritis and from peripheral blood in chronic rubella arthritis.

Another complication of postnatally acquired rubella is hemorrhage due to both thrombocytopenia and vascular damage, which occurs in 1 of every 3000 patients. Thrombocytopenia may last for weeks or months; it can have long-term consequences if there is bleeding into organs such as the eye or the brain.

Both children and adults may develop encephalitis after rubella; the incidence is about five times lower than that of encephalitis following measles. Adults are more likely than children to develop encephalitis; the mortality rate from this complication is 20 to 50%. Mild hepatitis is an unusual complication. Immunosuppressed patients are not at increased risk for rubella as they are for measles.

Congenital Rubella Maternal infection in early pregnancy can lead to fetal infection, with resultant congenital rubella. The classic signs of congenital rubella are cataract, heart disease, and deafness, but a myriad of other defects have been reported. These abnormalities include signs and symptoms that are transient, such as low birth weight, thrombocytopenia, hepatosplenomegaly, jaundice, and pneumonia; those that are permanent, such as deafness, pulmonic stenosis, patent ductus arteriosus, glaucoma, and cataract; and those that are developmental, such as mental retardation, diabetes mellitus, and behavioral disorders.

The most important factor in the pathogenicity of rubella virus for the fetus is gestational age at the time of infection. Maternal infection during the first trimester leads to fetal infection in about 50% of cases; maternal infection early in the second trimester leads to fetal infection in about one-third of cases. Fetal malformations not only are more common after maternal infection in the first trimester but also tend to be more severe and to involve more organ systems. While a fetus infected in the fourth week of gestation may develop many problems, one infected later (e.g., in the 20th week) may have isolated deafness as the only symptom.

DIAGNOSIS Since postnatally acquired rubella is such a mild disease and since many cases are subclinical, diagnosis on clinical grounds can be difficult. Other diseases that may mimic rubella include toxoplasmosis, scarlet fever, modified measles, roseola, fifth disease (erythema infectiosum due to parvovirus B19), and enteroviral infection. Routine laboratory tests usually reveal leukopenia and atypical lymphocytes.

The isolation of rubella virus in cell cultures of throat samples, urine, or other secretions is difficult and expensive but is sometimes undertaken. This technique is most useful when congenital rubella is suspected. A laboratory diagnosis is more often made serologically. The most commonly used test is an enzyme-linked immunosorbent assay (ELISA) for IgG and IgM antibodies. Acute rubella is diagnosed by the documentation of a fourfold or greater rise in the titer of IgG antibodies in paired acute- and convalescent-phase serum specimens or by the detection of rubella-specific IgM antibodies in one serum specimen. However, false-negative and -positive IgM reactions are sometimes obtained. Moreover, true-positive IgM reactions can be obtained in both primary infection and reinfection. Congenital rubella is diagnosed by the isolation of rubella virus, the detection of IgM antibodies in a single serum sample, and/or the documentation of either the persistence of rubella antibodies in serum beyond 1 year of age or a rising antibody titer anytime during infancy in an unvaccinated child. Biopsied tissues and/or blood and cerebrospinal fluid have also been used for the demonstration of rubella antigens with monoclonal antibodies and for the detection of rubella RNA by in situ hybridization and polymerase chain reaction.

PREVENTION Live attenuated rubella vaccine was licensed in 1969, 7 years after the virus was first isolated in culture. This vaccine was developed as a strategy to prevent congenital rubella by ensuring that very few pregnant women would be susceptible and that there would be little circulating wild-type virus. Rubella vaccine induces seroconversion in more than 95% of recipients. Since its licensure, there have been no major epidemics in the United States, and the number of cases has declined by 98%. The vaccine currently licensed in the United States, RA 27/3, is propagated in human diploid cells and is more immunogenic (particularly with regard to the stimulation of secretory immunity) than previously licensed vaccines. The present vaccination strategy, developed in part when measles was not being adequately controlled, is to immunize all infants at 12 to 15 months of age with measles-mumps-rubella (MMR) vaccine and to administer a second dose at 4 to 12 years of age. Rubella vaccine may also be administered to anyone who is thought to be susceptible to the infection and is not pregnant; it is particularly important that hospital workers of either sex be immune to rubella so that nosocomial transmission is avoided. While there has been little change in the prevalence of immunity to rubella among women of childbearing age (about 80%), the incidence of congenital rubella is extremely low—about 10 cases annually. It is likely that, although antibody may be undetectable years after immunization, protection against infection—possibly due to cell-mediated immunity—is the rule. At present, there is little if any evidence of significant waning of clinically important immunity to rubella with time.

On occasion, rubella vaccine may cause arthralgia or arthritis, especially in young women. Very rarely, rubella vaccination results in chronic arthritis; however, even cases of frank arthritis in vaccinees are self-limited, lasting only about 1 week.

After investigation of a series of more than 400 women who were inadvertently immunized during pregnancy and who carried their infants to term, the CDC has concluded that vaccine-type rubella virus either does not cause the congenital rubella syndrome at all or does so at an incidence too low to be detected. Nonetheless, rubella vaccine is contraindicated for use in pregnant women, and it is recommended that pregnancy be avoided for at least 3 months after rubella vaccination. It is acceptable for rubella-susceptible children whose mothers are also susceptible to be immunized, since vaccinated individuals do not shed rubella virus or transmit it to susceptible individuals. Although it is recommended that rubella vaccine not be given to immunosuppressed persons, the vaccine is given to children infected with HIV. No adverse effects of rubella vaccine have been reported in immunocompromised patients.

℞ **TREATMENT** There is no specific therapy for rubella. At one time, immune globulin was used in an effort to prevent congenital rubella when pregnant women became infected. However, since administration of immune globulin did not prevent maternal viremia, this approach was discarded. Treatment is given for symptoms such as fever, arthralgia, and arthritis.

BIBLIOGRAPHY

BOSMA TJ et al: Use of PCR for prenatal and postnatal diagnosis of congenital rubella. J Clin Microbiol 33:2881, 1995

CENTERS FOR DISEASE CONTROL AND PREVENTION: Measles, mumps, and rubella—vaccine use and strategies for elimination of measles, rubella, and congenital rubella syndrome and control of mumps. MMWR 47:1, 1998

CHANTLER JK et al: Persistent rubella virus infection associated with chronic arthritis in children. N Engl J Med 313:1117, 1985

CUSI MG et al: Serological evidence of reinfection among vaccinees during rubella outbreak. Lancet 336:1071, 1991

FREY TK et al: Molecular analysis of rubella virus epidemiology across three continents, North America, Europe, and Asia. J Infect Dis 178:642, 1998

GREGG NM: Congenital cataract following German measles in the mother. Trans Ophthalmol Soc Aust 3:35, 1941

HERRMANN KL: Available rubella serologic tests. Rev Infect Dis 7:S108, 1985

HORSTMANN D et al: Persistence of vaccine-induced immune responses to rubella. Rev Infect Dis 7:S80, 1985

MELLINGER AK et al: High incidence of congenital rubella syndrome after a rubella outbreak. Pediatr Infect Dis J 14:573, 1995

TOWNSEND JJ et al: Progressive rubella panencephalitis: Late onset after congenital rubella. N Engl J Med 292:990, 1975

WEIBEL RE, BENOR DE: Chronic arthropathy and musculoskeletal symptoms associated with rubella vaccines: A review of 124 claims submitted to the National Vaccine Injury Compensation Program. Arthritis Rheum 39:1529, 1996

196 Anne Gershon

MUMPS

DEFINITION Mumps is an acute, systemic, communicable viral infection whose most distinctive feature is swelling of one or both parotid glands. Involvement of other salivary glands, the meninges, the pancreas, and the gonads is also common.

ETIOLOGIC AGENT Mumps virus, a paramyxovirus, is pleomorphic and has a diameter ranging from 100 to 600 nm. The virion is composed of RNA and five proteins. The RNA is surrounded by an envelope with glycoprotein projections. There are two envelope glycoproteins—a hemagglutinin-neuraminidase (HN) and a hemolysis cell fusion antigen (F)—as well as a matrix envelope protein (M). There are two internal components: a nucleocapsid protein (NP) and an RNA polymerase protein. There is only one antigenic type of mumps virus.

EPIDEMIOLOGY After the introduction of mumps vaccine in 1967, the incidence of clinical mumps declined significantly in the United States. In 1968 (before widespread immunization), 185,691 cases of mumps were reported in this country. The 906 cases reported in 1995 represent a reduction in the number of cases by >99% from prevaccine levels; this is the lowest number of cases ever reported in a year. Before widespread vaccination, the incidence of mumps was highest in the winter and spring, with epidemics every 2 to 5 years. At that time, mumps was principally a disease of childhood, although today more than 50% of cases occur in young adults. Epidemics tended to occur in confined populations, such as those in schools and the military services.

The incubation period of mumps generally ranges from 14 to 18 days, with extremes of 7 and 23 days. However, because a contact may be shedding virus before the onset of clinical disease or (like one-third of patients) may have subclinical infection, the incubation period in individual cases is often uncertain. One attack of mumps usually confers lifelong immunity. Long-term immunity is also associated with immunization.

PATHOGENESIS Mumps virus is transmitted by droplet nuclei, saliva, and fomites. Replication of the virus in the epithelium of the upper respiratory tract leads to viremia, which is followed by infection of glandular tissues and/or the central nervous system (CNS).

Little is known of the pathology of mumps since the disease is rarely fatal. The affected glands contain perivascular and interstitial mononuclear cell infiltrates with prominent edema. Necrosis of acinar and epithelial duct cells is evident in the salivary glands and in the germinal epithelium of the seminiferous tubules.

CLINICAL MANIFESTATIONS The prodrome of mumps consists of fever, malaise, myalgia, and anorexia. Parotitis, if it develops, usually does so within the next 24 h but may be delayed for as long as a week; it is generally bilateral, although the onset on the two sides may not be synchronous and at times only one side is affected. The submaxillary and sublingual glands are involved less often than the parotid and are almost never involved alone. Swelling of the parotid is accompanied by tenderness and obliteration of the space between the ear lobe and the angle of the mandible. The patient frequently reports an earache and finds it difficult to eat, swallow, or talk. Glandular swelling increases for a few days and then gradually subsides, disappearing within a week. The orifice of Stensen's duct is commonly red and swollen. Presternal pitting edema has been described in about 5% of mumps cases, often in association with submandibular adenitis.

Other than parotitis, orchitis is the most common manifestation of mumps among postpubertal males, developing in about 20% of cases. The testis is painful and tender and is enlarged to several times its normal size; accompanying fever is common. Later, testicular atrophy develops in half of the affected men. Since orchitis is bilateral in fewer than 15% of cases, sterility after mumps is rare. Oophoritis in women—far less common than orchitis in men—may cause lower abdominal pain but does not lead to sterility.

Aseptic meningitis, which may develop before, during, after, or in the absence of parotitis, is a common manifestation of mumps in both children and adults. Symptoms include stiff neck, headache, and drowsiness. Pleocytosis of the cerebrospinal fluid (CSF), with up to 1000 cells/μL, may develop in up to 50% of cases of clinical mumps, but clinical signs of meningeal irritation are documented in only 5 to 25% of cases. Within the first 24 h, polymorphonuclear leukocytes may predominate in CSF, but by the second day nearly all the cells are lymphocytes. The glucose level in CSF may be abnormally low, and this finding may arouse suspicion of bacterial meningitis. Aseptic meningitis due to mumps without parotitis is indistinguishable clinically from that caused by other viruses. Mumps meningitis is almost invariably self-limited, although cranial nerve palsies have occasionally led to permanent sequelae, particularly deafness. More rarely, mumps virus may cause encephalitis, which presents as high fever with marked changes in the level of consciousness and frequently results in permanent sequelae in survivors. Other CNS problems occasionally associated with mumps include cerebellar ataxia, facial palsy, transverse myelitis, Guillain-Barré syndrome, and aqueductal stenosis leading to hydrocephalus.

Mumps pancreatitis, which may present as abdominal pain, is difficult to diagnose because an elevated serum amylase level can be associated with either parotitis or pancreatitis. Other unusual complications of mumps include myocarditis, mastitis, thyroiditis, nephritis, arthritis, and thrombocytopenic purpura. An excessive number of spontaneous abortions are associated with gestational mumps when the disease occurs during the first trimester. Mumps in pregnancy does not lead to premature birth or fetal malformations.

DIFFERENTIAL DIAGNOSIS The diagnosis of mumps is made easily in patients with acute bilateral parotitis and a history of recent exposure. When parotitis is unilateral or absent or when sites other than the parotid gland are involved, laboratory diagnosis is required (see below).

The myriad causes of bilateral parotid swelling other than mumps virus include infection with other viruses, such as parainfluenza virus type 3, coxsackieviruses, and influenza A virus; metabolic diseases, such as diabetes mellitus and uremia; and drugs, such as phenylbutazone and thiouracil. Unilateral parotid swelling can result from a tumor, a cyst, or a ductal obstruction due to stones or strictures. Other conditions associated with chronic parotid swelling include sarcoidosis, Sjögren's syndrome, and infection with HIV. Suppurative parotitis, usually caused by *Staphylococcus aureus*, is most often unilateral.

Other entities should be considered when manifestations consistent with mumps appear in organs other than the parotid. Testicular torsion may produce a painful scrotal mass resembling that seen in mumps orchitis. Other viruses (e.g., enteroviruses) may cause aseptic meningitis that is clinically indistinguishable from that due to mumps virus.

LABORATORY DIAGNOSIS Mumps virus is readily isolated after inoculation of appropriate clinical specimens into a variety of host systems, such as rhesus monkey kidney cells and human embryonic lung fibroblasts. The virus can be rapidly identified by the use of cells grown in shell vials and of fluorescein-labeled monoclonal antibodies. Mumps virus may be recovered from saliva, throat, and urine during the first few days of illness and from the CSF of patients with mumps meningitis. Shedding of virus in the urine may persist for as long as 2 weeks. No particular peripheral blood cell count is characteristic of mumps.

Highly sensitive enzyme-linked immunosorbent assays are useful for diagnosis of mumps and for determination of susceptibility to the disease. Acute mumps can be diagnosed either by the examination of acute- and convalescent-phase sera for a significant increase in IgG antibody titer or by the demonstration of specific IgM in one serum specimen. Use of a skin-test antigen to assess immunity to mumps has been replaced by serologic testing.

PREVENTION Live attenuated mumps vaccine (Jeryl Lynn strain) induces antibodies that protect against infection in more than 95% of cases. The subcutaneously administered vaccine may be given to children older than 1 year but is not recommended for younger infants because of the potential for interference by passive maternal antibodies. Mumps vaccine is usually administered as part of the measles-mumps-rubella (MMR) vaccine at the age of 12 to 15 months and again at 4 to 12 years of age. This MMR vaccine is also recommended for susceptible older children, adolescents, and adults, particularly adolescent males who have not had mumps. For these patients, either MMR or monovalent mumps vaccine may be given; two doses are preferred. Inadvertent immunization of individuals who are already immune is not associated with significant adverse reactions. Mumps vaccine is not recommended for pregnant women, for patients receiving glucocorticoids, or for other immunocompromised hosts. However, children with HIV infection who are not severely immunocompromised can safely be immunized against mumps; MMR vaccine is usually used for this purpose (Chap. 194).

℞ **TREATMENT** Therapy for parotitis and other manifestations of mumps is symptom-based. The administration of analgesics and the application of warm or cold compresses to the parotid area may be helpful. Mumps immune globulin is of no value in the prophylaxis or treatment of established disease. Testicular pain may be minimized by the local application of cold compresses and gentle support for the scrotum. Anesthetic blocks may also be used. Neither the administration of glucocorticoids nor incision of the tunica albuginea is of proven value for the treatment of severe orchitis. Anecdotal information on a small number of patients with orchitis suggests that administration of interferon α may be helpful.

BIBLIOGRAPHY

BROWN E et al: The Urabe AM9 mumps vaccine is a mixture of viruses differing at amino acid 335 of the hemagglutinin-neuraminidase gene with one form associated with disease. J Infect Dis 174:619, 1996

CENTERS FOR DISEASE CONTROL AND PREVENTION: Update on adult immunization: Recommendations of the Immunization Practices Advisory Committee (ACIP). MMWR 40:22, 1991

———: Measles, mumps, and rubella—vaccine use and strategies for elimination of measles, rubella, and congenital rubella syndrome and control of mumps. MMWR 47:1, 1998

CHAUDARY S et al: Fulminant mumps myocarditis. Ann Intern Med 110:569, 1989

GUT JP et al: Symptomatic mumps reinfections. J Med Virol 45:17, 1995

HAREL L et al: Mumps arthritis in children. Pediatr Infect Dis J 9:928, 1990

HERSH BS et al: Mumps outbreak in a highly vaccinated population. J Pediatr 119:187, 1991

LYON RP et al: Mumps epididymo-orchitis: Treatment by anesthetic block of the spermatic cord. JAMA 196:736, 1966

MCDONALD JC et al: Clinical and epidemiologic features of mumps encephalitis and possible causes of vaccine-related disease. Pediatr Infect Dis J 8:751, 1989

RUTHER U et al: Successful interferon-alpha 2 therapy for a patient with acute mumps orchitis. Eur Urol 27:174, 1995

197

RABIES VIRUS AND OTHER RHABDOVIRUSES

RABIES VIRUS

DEFINITION Rabies is an acute viral disease of the central nervous system (CNS) that affects all mammals and that is transmitted by infected secretions, usually saliva. Most exposures to rabies are through the bite of an infected animal, but on occasion contact with a virus-containing aerosol or the ingestion or transplantation of infected tissues may initiate the disease process.

ETIOLOGY The rabies virus is a bullet-shaped, enveloped, single-stranded RNA virus that is 75 to 80 nm in diameter and belongs to the genus *Lyssavirus* within the rhabdovirus family. The envelope glycoproteins of rabies viruses are arranged in knoblike structures that cover the surface of the virion. Genetic and phenotypic analyses of the envelope have been used to detail the molecular epidemiology and spread of unique variants within animal species. The viral glycoproteins bind to acetylcholine receptors, contribute to the neurovirulence of rabies virus, elicit neutralizing and hemagglutination-inhibiting antibodies, and stimulate cytotoxic T cell immunity. The nucleocapsid antigen induces a complement-fixing antibody as well as T helper cell reactivity. Neutralizing antibodies to the surface glycoproteins appear to be protective and are directed at conformational epitopes of the viral envelope glycoprotein. The antibodies to rabies virus used in diagnostic immunofluorescence assays are generally directed against the nucleocapsid antigens. Isolates of rabies virus from different animal species and locales differ in their antigenic and biologic properties. These variations may account for differences in virulence between isolates. Interferon is induced by rabies virus, particularly in those tissues with high virus concentrations, and may play some role in retarding progressive infection.

EPIDEMIOLOGY Rabies is found in animals in all regions of the world except Australasia and Antarctica. Rabies exists in two epidemiologic forms: *urban rabies*, propagated chiefly by unimmunized domestic dogs and cats, and *sylvatic rabies*, propagated by skunks, foxes, raccoons, mongooses, wolves, and bats. Infection in domestic animals usually represents a "spillover" from sylvatic reservoirs of infection. Human infection occurs through contact with unimmunized domestic animals or from exposure to wild animals in locales where rabies is enzootic or epizootic. The worldwide incidence of rabies is estimated at more than 30,000 cases per year. Southeast Asia, the Philippines, Africa, the Indian subcontinent, and tropical South America are areas where the disease is especially common. In some endemic areas, 1 to 2% of autopsies yield evidence of rabies. Increased spread of terrestrial rabies (i.e., rabies in animals that walk on the ground rather than rabies in animals that fly) and increased travel to countries where urban rabies exists have made the recognition of clinical rabies and its prevention of increasing importance. While focal epidemics of terrestrial rabies have occurred in the United States and Europe, human rabies is uncommon, largely because of successful domestic-animal vaccination programs. Since 1980, 36 human cases of rabies have been diagnosed in the United States; 58% of these cases were associated with exposure to bats, while one-third were acquired through dog bites sustained outside the United States. Most persons with proven clinical rabies in this country report no history of an animal bite. More than one-third of recent cases have been diagnosed post-mortem.

In most areas of the world, the dog is the most important vector of rabies virus for humans. However, the wolf (in eastern Europe and Arctic regions), the mongoose (in South Africa and the Caribbean), the fox (in western Europe), and the vampire bat (in Latin America) may also be prominent vectors. Although rabies in wildlife is common throughout both the developed and the undeveloped world, most cases of postexposure prophylaxis are associated with domesticated animals such as dogs and cats. In the United States, local governments are charged with initiating and maintaining programs for rabies vaccination of all dogs, cats, and ferrets. Rodents and lagomorphs are rarely infected with rabies virus. Several cases of human-to-human transmission of rabies through corneal transplantation have also been documented. Bite and nonbite exposures to infected humans could theoretically transmit rabies. Because of delayed diagnosis, postexposure prophylaxis of health care workers and close contacts of cases is common.

PATHOGENESIS The first event in rabies is the introduction of live virus through the epidermis or onto a mucous membrane. Initial viral replication appears to occur within striated muscle cells at the site of inoculation. The peripheral nervous system is exposed at the neuromuscular and/or neurotendinous spindles of unmyelinated sensory nerve cell endings. The virus then spreads centripetally up the nerve to the CNS, probably via peripheral nerve axoplasm, at a rate of ~3 mm/h. Viremia has been documented in experimental conditions but is thought not to play a role in naturally acquired disease. Once the virus reaches the CNS, it replicates almost exclusively within the gray matter and then passes centrifugally along autonomic nerves to other tissues—the salivary glands, adrenal medulla, kidneys, lungs, liver, skeletal muscles, skin, and heart. Passage of the virus into the salivary glands and viral replication in mucinogenic acinar cells facilitate further transmission via infected saliva. The incubation period of rabies is exceedingly variable, ranging from 7 days to >1 year (mean, 1 to 2 months) and apparently depending on the amount of virus introduced, the amount of tissue involved, host defense mechanisms, and the actual distance that the virus has to travel from the site of inoculation to the CNS. Rates of infection and mortality are highest from bites on the face, intermediate from bites on the hands and arms, and lowest from bites on the legs. Cases of human rabies with an extended incubation period (2 to 7 years) have been reported, but they are rare. Host immune responses and viral strains also influence disease expression.

The neuropathology of rabies resembles that of other viral diseases of the CNS: hyperemia, varying degrees of chromatolysis, nuclear pyknosis, and neuronophagia of the nerve cells; infiltration by lymphocytes and plasma cells of the Virchow-Robin space; microglial infiltration; and parenchymal areas of nerve cell destruction. In experimental animal models, adenohypophyseal infection with rabies virus, with reduction in growth hormone and vasopressin release, is common. The most characteristic pathologic finding of rabies in the CNS is the formation of cytoplasmic inclusions called *Negri bodies* within neurons. Each eosinophilic mass measures ~10 nm and is made up of a finely fibrillar matrix and rabies virus particles. Negri bodies are distributed throughout the brain, particularly in Ammon's horn, the cerebral cortex, the brainstem, the hypothalamus, the Purkinje cells of the cerebellum, and the dorsal spinal ganglia. Negri bodies are not demonstrated in at least 20% of cases of rabies, and their absence from brain material does not rule out the diagnosis.

CLINICAL MANIFESTATIONS The clinical manifestations of rabies can be divided into four stages: (1) a nonspecific prodrome, (2) an acute encephalitis similar to other viral encephalitides, (3) a profound dysfunction of brainstem centers that produces the classic features of rabies encephalitis, and (4) death or, in rare cases, recovery.

The prodromal period usually lasts 1 to 4 days and is marked by fever, headache, malaise, myalgias, increased fatigability, anorexia, nausea and vomiting, sore throat, and a nonproductive cough. The prodromal symptom suggestive of rabies is the complaint of paresthesia and/or fasciculations at or around the site of inoculation of virus. These sensations, which may be related to the multiplication of virus in the dorsal root ganglion of the sensory nerve supplying the area of the bite, are reported by 50 to 80% of patients.

The encephalitic phase is usually ushered in by periods of excessive motor activity, excitation, and agitation. Confusion, hallucinations, combativeness, bizarre aberrations of thought, muscle spasms, meningismus, opisthotonic posturing, seizures, and focal paralysis soon appear. Characteristically, the periods of mental aberration are interspersed with completely lucid periods, but as the disease progresses the lucid periods get shorter until the patient lapses into coma. Hyperesthesia, with excessive sensitivity to bright light, loud noise, touch, and even gentle breezes, is very common. On physical examination, the temperature may be found to be as high as 40.6°C (105°F). Abnormalities of the autonomic nervous system include dilated irregular pupils; increased lacrimation, salivation, and perspiration; and postural hypotension. Evidence of upper motor neuron paralysis, with weakness, increased deep tendon reflexes, and extensor plantar responses, is the rule. Paralysis of the vocal cords is common. Unfortunately, the presenting signs and symptoms of rabies are indistinguishable from those of other viral and neurologic diseases. Thus delays in diagnosis are frequent. The presence of hydrophobia or aerophobia (seen in about two-thirds of recent cases) increases the likelihood of antemortem diagnosis.

The manifestations of brainstem dysfunction begin shortly after the onset of the encephalitic phase. Cranial nerve involvement causes diplopia, facial palsies, optic neuritis, and the characteristic difficulty with deglutition. The combination of excessive salivation and difficulty in swallowing produces the traditional picture of "foaming at the mouth." Hydrophobia, the painful, violent, involuntary contraction of the diaphragmatic, accessory respiratory, pharyngeal, and laryngeal muscles initiated by swallowing liquids, is seen in ~50% of cases. Involvement of the amygdaloid nucleus may result in priapism and spontaneous ejaculation. The patient lapses into coma, and involvement of the respiratory center produces an apneic death. The prominence of early brainstem dysfunction distinguishes rabies from other viral encephalitides and accounts for the rapid downhill course. The median period of survival after the onset of symptoms is 4 days, with a maximum of 20 days, unless artificial supportive measures are instituted.

If intensive respiratory support is used, a number of late complications may appear. These include inappropriate secretion of antidiuretic hormone, diabetes insipidus, cardiac arrhythmias, vascular instability, adult respiratory distress syndrome, gastrointestinal bleeding, thrombocytopenia, and paralytic ileus. Recovery is very rare and, when it occurs, gradual.

Rabies may also present as an ascending paralysis resembling the Landry/Guillain-Barré syndrome (dumb rabies, *rage tranquille*). Initially, this clinical pattern was reported most frequently among persons given postexposure rabies prophylaxis after being bitten by vampire bats. Paralytic rabies also occurs in Southeast Asia among persons with canine exposures.

The difficulty of diagnosing rabies associated with ascending paralysis is illustrated by cases of person-to-person transmission of the virus by tissue transplantation. Corneal transplants from donors who died of presumed Landry/Guillain-Barré syndrome produced clinical rabies in and caused the deaths of the recipients. Retrospective pathologic examinations of the brains of recipients demonstrated Negri bodies, and rabies virus was subsequently isolated from each donor's frozen eye.

LABORATORY FINDINGS   Early in the disease, hemoglobin values and routine blood chemistry results are normal; abnormalities develop as hypothalamic dysfunction, gastrointestinal bleeding, and other complications ensue. The peripheral white blood cell count is usually slightly elevated (12,000 to 17,000/μL) but may be normal or as high as 30,000/μL.

The specific diagnosis of rabies depends on (1) the isolation of virus from infected secretions [saliva or, rarely, cerebrospinal fluid (CSF)] or tissue (brain), (2) the serologic demonstration of acute infection, (3) the detection of viral antigen in infected tissue (e.g., corneal impression smears, skin biopsies, or brain), or (4) the detection of viral nucleic acid (RNA) by polymerase chain reaction (PCR). A reference laboratory evaluating antemortem samples can confirm rabies with high sensitivity and specificity. Isolation of virus from saliva,

demonstration of viral nucleic acid in saliva, or detection of viral antigen in a nuchal skin biopsy specimen is most sensitive. Examination of corneal epithelium specimens appears less sensitive. In the unvaccinated person, demonstration of rabies antibodies in serum or CSF may be useful, although such antibodies may not appear until late in the course of disease. Samples of brain obtained at postmortem examination or brain biopsy should be subjected to (1) mouse inoculation studies for virus isolation, (2) fluorescent antibody (FA) staining for viral antigen, and (3) histologic and/or electron microscopic examination for Negri bodies or reverse transcription PCR for rabies virus RNA.

Postexposure rabies prophylaxis rarely elicits CSF neutralizing antibody to rabies virus. If present after prophylaxis, such antibody is usually found at a low titer (<1:64), whereas CSF titers in human rabies may vary from 1:200 to 1:160,000.

DIFFERENTIAL DIAGNOSIS   There is little to distinguish rabies from other viral encephalitides. The most helpful clue to the diagnosis is a history of a bite or other salivary exposure to a potentially infected animal. As bite exposures are infrequent among U.S. cases, a history of relatively recent travel to a rabies-endemic area should be sought. Other problems to be considered in the differential diagnosis include hysterical reactions to animal bites (pseudohydrophobia), Landry/Guillain-Barré syndrome, poliomyelitis, and allergic encephalomyelitis developing in response to rabies vaccine; this last problem is usually associated with receipt of nerve tissue–derived vaccine and usually begins 1 to 4 weeks after vaccination.

℞ **TREATMENT   Postexposure Prophylaxis**   (See Fig. 197-1) Although rabies among humans is rare in the United States, each year ~35,000 persons receive postexposure prophylaxis. The decision to initiate postexposure prophylaxis should include the following considerations: (1) whether the individual came into physical contact with saliva or another substance likely to contain rabies virus, (2) whether rabies is known or suspected in the species and area associated with

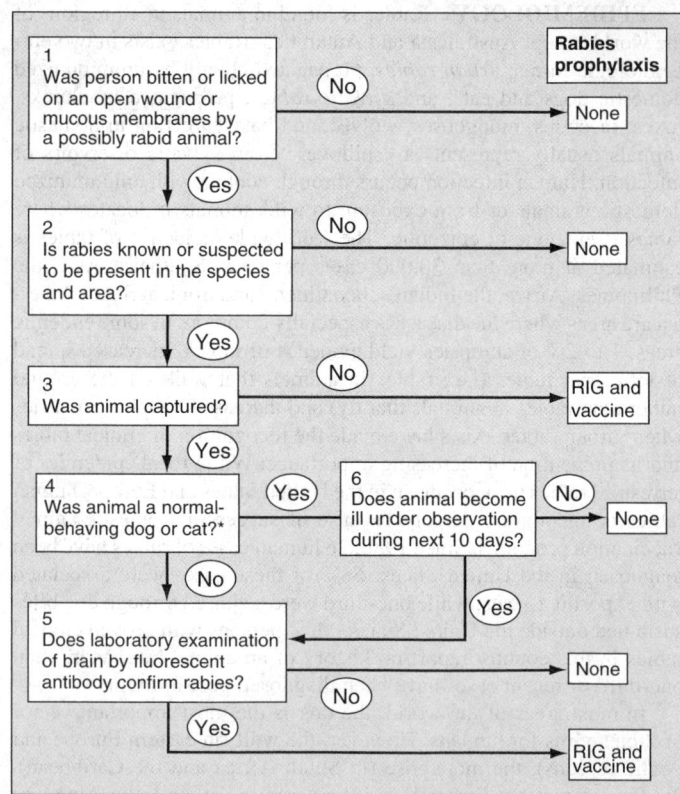

FIGURE 197-1 Postexposure rabies prophylaxis algorithm. *Instances of exposure to livestock or to normal-behaving, unvaccinated dogs or cats should be considered individually, and local and state public health officials should be consulted.

the exposure (e.g., all persons within the continental United States bitten by a bat that escapes should receive postexposure prophylaxis), and (3) the circumstances surrounding the exposure (e.g., whether the bite was provoked or unprovoked). Bites associated with the feeding of an animal are considered to have been provoked.

If rabies is known or suspected to be present in the animal species involved in a human exposure, the implicated animal should be captured if possible. Any wild animal involved in a rabies exposure; any ill, unvaccinated, or stray domestic animal involved in a rabies exposure; and any animal inflicting an unprovoked bite, exhibiting abnormal behavior, or suspected of being rabid should be humanely killed. The animal's head should be sent immediately to an appropriate laboratory for rabies FA examination. If examination of the brain by the FA technique gives negative results, it can be assumed that the saliva contains no virus, and the exposed person need not be treated. Persons exposed to wild animals that subsequently escape, that are capable of carrying rabies (bats, skunks, coyotes, foxes, raccoons, etc.), and that inhabit an area where rabies is known or suspected to be present should undergo both passive and active immunization against rabies (see below) as soon as possible after exposure.

In an area in which feline or canine rabies is not prevalent, a healthy biting dog, cat, or ferret can be confined and observed for 10 days. Persons in such an area should not begin a course of prophylaxis unless the animal develops clinical signs of rabies. If the animal becomes ill or behaves abnormally during the observation period, it should be killed for FA examination. Experimental and epidemiologic evidence suggests that animals that remain healthy for 10 days after a bite will not have transmitted rabies virus at the time of the bite. In areas of high endemicity for canine rabies, immediate examination of the animal's brain, especially in the case of a severe bite, may be warranted. Bites of rodents, rabbits, and hares almost never require antirabies postexposure prophylaxis. Unless the exposed person can rule out a bite, scratch, or mucous membrane exposure, postexposure prophylaxis should be considered after direct contact between a human and a bat.

Postexposure prophylaxis of rabies includes rigorous cleansing and treatment of the wound and the administration of rabies vaccine together with antirabies immunoglobulin. Postexposure prophylaxis should be initiated as soon as possible after exposure. As the incubation period of rabies is quite variable, postexposure prophylaxis should be begun as long as clinical signs of rabies are not present.

1. *Wound cleansing and treatment.* Thorough cleansing and treatment of the bite wound constitute an important component of rabies prevention. The wound should be scrubbed with soap and then flushed with water. Both mechanical cleansing and chemical cleansing are important. Quaternary ammonium compounds such as 1 to 4% benzalkonium chloride, 1% cetrimonium bromide, or povidone-iodine solutions should be utilized. Tetanus toxoid and antibiotic prophylaxis should be administered as needed.

2. *Passive immunization with antirabies antiserum of either equine or human origin.* Postexposure antirabies vaccination should include the administration of both passive antibody and vaccine, except when the individual has previously received preexposure prophylaxis. Human rabies immune globulin (RIG) is preferred because equine antiserum may cause serum sickness. RIG is administered only once, at the beginning of the postexposure prophylaxis regimen. The recommended dose of RIG is 20 IU/kg. The dose of equine antiserum is 40 units/kg. The full dose should be thoroughly infiltrated into the area around the wound and into the wound itself. Any remaining portion of the dose is injected intramuscularly at a site distant from the vaccine.

3. *Active immunization with antirabies vaccine.* Three rabies vaccines are available in the United States: (1) human diploid cell vaccine (HDCV), which can be given either intramuscularly or intradermally; (2) rabies vaccine absorbed (RVA); and (3) purified chick embryo cell vaccine. The latter two vaccines are administered intramuscularly. Each vaccine is derived from a different strain of rabies virus and prepared in a slightly different formulation. The three vac-

cines are considered equally efficacious and safe, and any of the three can be administered in conjunction with RIG. Five 1-mL doses of HDCV are given intramuscularly, preferably in the deltoid or anterolateral thigh area: the gluteal area should not be utilized. The five doses of HDCV should be administered within 28 days on the following schedule: days 0, 3, 7, 14, and 28. The World Health Organization also recommends 21- and 90-day injections. Severe reactions to these vaccines are uncommon. Immediate hypersensitivity responses, such as urticaria, have been reported in ~1 of every 650 recipients. Systemic reactions, such as fever, headache, and nausea, are generally mild and are reported in 1 to 4% of recipients. Local reactions, such as swelling, erythema, and induration at the injection site, occur in 15 to 20% of vaccinees. Guillain-Barré syndrome has been reported but appears to be quite rare.

In the developing world, several other effective rabies vaccines have been licensed and used extensively. They include vaccines made in chick embryonic cells, primary hamster cells, Vero cells, and duck embryonic cells. As some of these preparations are somewhat less immunogenic than the vaccines approved by the U.S. Food and Drug Administration (FDA), evaluation of serum antibodies after immunization is suggested by some authorities.

The combination of RIG and HDCV elicits high titers of neutralizing antibodies in almost all recipients. Only rarely has this regimen proved unsuccessful in preventing the development of rabies. None of the patients in whom rabies was diagnosed in the United States between 1980 and 1996 had received postexposure prophylaxis. Administration of vaccine alone appears to be associated with a higher failure rate than use of the combination, especially in severe bite exposures. Because of cost, postexposure prophylaxis consisting of intradermal injections of rabies vaccine is being used increasingly in the developing world. The combination of RIG plus 0.1-mL intradermal doses of HDCV at eight sites on day 0, four sites on day 7, and one site on days 28 and 91 produces good antibody responses and has had excellent clinical results. Alternatively, the World Health Organization has approved a regimen of two 0.1-mL doses at two intradermal sites on days 0, 3, and 7 and a 0.1-mL intradermal injection at a single site on days 21 and 90. The FDA has not approved the intradermal route for postexposure prophylaxis.

Preexposure Prophylaxis Individuals at high risk of contact with rabies virus, including veterinarians, cave explorers, laboratory workers, and animal handlers, should receive preexposure prophylaxis with rabies vaccine. Three 1-mL intramuscular or three 0.1-mL intradermal injections of HDCV on days 0, 7, and 21 or 28 should be administered. Concomitant chloroquine administration interferes with the antibody response to rabies vaccine. Depending on the level of risk, serologic testing should be done at 6-month to 2-year intervals.

An immune complex reaction consisting of urticaria, arthralgia, arthritis, angioedema, and systemic symptoms has been reported in up to 6% of persons receiving intramuscular booster doses of HDCV. This reaction is self-limited and appears to be associated with the presence of β-propiolactone-altered human serum albumin in the vaccine and the development of IgE antibodies to this antigen.

Persons who work in high-risk areas should undergo periodic measurement of antibodies. When neutralizing titers fall below 1:5, booster doses should be given. Booster doses may be administered as a single 1-mL intramuscular or 0.1-mL intradermal injection. Postexposure prophylaxis in individuals previously given preexposure prophylaxis consists of two intramuscular doses of HDCV on days 0 and 3. RIG is not given in these situations.

MOKOLA VIRUS

Mokola virus was first isolated from wild shrews captured in Nigeria and was shown to be related morphologically and serologically to rabies virus. The subsequent isolation of the virus from cats in South Africa suggested a wider prevalence of the agent than had previously been expected. Only two cases of clinical infection have been reported; both were in children. One patient had a nonfatal illness characterized by fever, pharyngitis, and convulsions; Mokola virus was recovered from CSF. In the second patient, fever with cough and vomiting was followed within several days by drowsiness, confusion, and generalized flaccid weakness. The CSF was normal. The patient progressed to deep coma and died within 10 days of onset. Mokola virus was isolated from the brain, and examination of histopathologic sections revealed finely granular cytoplasmic inclusions that were distinguishable from Negri bodies in many neurons.

VESICULAR STOMATITIS VIRUS

Vesicular stomatitis is a viral illness of animals that occasionally affects humans. It presents as an acute, self-limited, influenza-like disease. The disease in animals is found in the United States and South America and affects chiefly domestic cattle, horses, swine, wild deer, raccoons, skunks, and bobcats.

In animals, vesicular stomatitis is characterized by the development of vesicles on the oral mucosa, particularly the tongue; the udders; and the heels. The mode of spread is probably by direct contact; however, epidemics tend to occur in warm weather, and isolation of the virus from *Phlebotomus* sandflies in Panama and *Aedes* species in New Mexico suggests that these insects may be vectors. Two distinct serotypes, New Jersey and Indiana, have been recognized, and most outbreaks in North America have been attributed to the New Jersey strain.

In humans, vesicular stomatitis is most common among laboratory workers. In one report, three-fourths of laboratory personnel handling experimentally infected animals or manipulating the virus developed neutralizing antibodies. The disease is also transmissible, however, under natural conditions among workers having direct contact with infected animals, especially cattle. An incubation period ranging from 1 to 6 days is followed by the sudden onset of fever [with temperatures of up to 40°C (104°F)], chills, profuse sweating, myalgias, malaise, headache, and pain on ocular movement. One-third to one-half of patients have a sore throat and cervical and/or submandibular adenopathy. Small raised vesicular lesions may appear on the buccal mucosa. Conjunctivitis and coryza are evident in ~20% of cases. Occasionally, small subcorneal, intraepithelial vesicles appear on the fingers, usually in association with direct inoculation of the virus. Symptoms generally last 3 to 4 days, but occasionally the course is diphasic. Inapparent infection is common: among laboratory workers with serologic evidence of infection, only about one-half report symptoms. In some areas of Panama, 17 to 35% of the population have neutralizing antibodies to vesicular stomatitis virus.

The differential diagnosis includes hand-foot-and-mouth disease, herpangina, primary herpetic pharyngitis and other mucocutaneous syndromes, and influenza. The virus is not commonly isolated from patients. However, a rise in titer of complement-fixation and/or neutralizing antibody to vesicular stomatitis virus between acute- and convalescent-phase sera helps to confirm the diagnosis. Treatment is nonspecific.

BIBLIOGRAPHY

ADVISORY COMMITTEE ON IMMUNIZATION PRACTICES (ACIP): Human rabies prevention—United States, 1999. MMWR 48:RR-1,1999

Case records of the MGH 21-1998: A 32-year-old woman with pharyngeal spasms and paresthesia after a dog bite. N Engl J Med 339:105, 1998

Compendium of animal rabies control 1999. MMWR 48:RR-31-9, 1999

DIETZSCHOLD B et al: Human diploid cell culture rabies vaccine (HDCV) and purified chick embryo cell culture (PCEC) both confer protective immunity against infection with the silver fixed rabies virus strain (SH BRV). Vaccine 16:1656, 1998

FISHBEIN DB, ROBINSON LE: Current concepts. Rabies. N Engl J Med 329:1632, 1993

JAVADI MA et al: Transmission of rabies by corneal graft. Cornea 15:431, 1996

NOAH DL et al: Epidemiology of human rabies in the United States, 1980 to 1996. Ann Intern Med 128:922, 1998

PAPE WS et al: Risk for rabies transmission from encounters with bats, Colorado 1977–1996. Emerg Infect Dis 5:433, 1999

SMITH JS: New aspects of rabies with emphasis on epidemiology, diagnosis, and prevention of the disease in the United States. Clin Microbiol Rev 9:166, 1996

STRADY A et al: Antibody persistence following preexposure regimens of cell-culture rabies vaccines: 10-year follow-up and proposal for a new booster policy. J Infect Dis 177:1290, 1998

TANTAWICHIEN T et al: Antibody response after a far site intradermal booster vaccination with cell culture rabies vaccine. Clin Infect Dis 28:1100, 1999

198 C. J. Peters

INFECTIONS CAUSED BY ARTHROPOD- AND RODENT-BORNE VIRUSES

Most viral infections that come to medical attention in office or hospital practice in the developed countries are caused by viruses that can be latent in the human host, such as the herpesviruses, or by viruses that are continuously transmitted among humans, such as measles virus, influenza virus, and HIV. However, some other viruses are transmitted in nature without regard to humans and only incidentally infect and produce disease in humans; in addition, a few agents are regularly spread among humans by arthropods. Most of these viruses either are maintained by arthropods or chronically infect rodents. Obviously, the mode of transmission is not a rational basis for taxonomic classification. Indeed, zoonotic viruses from at least seven virus families act as significant human pathogens (Table 198-1). The virus families differ fundamentally from one another in terms of morphology, replication mechanisms, and genetics. Information on a virus's membership in a family or genus is enlightening with regard to maintenance strategies, sensitivity to antivirals, and some aspects of pathogenesis but does not necessarily predict which clinical syndromes—if any—the virus will cause in humans.

FAMILIES OF ARTHROPOD- AND RODENT-BORNE VIRUSES The Arenaviridae The Arenaviridae are spherical, 110- to 130-nm particles that bud from the cell's plasma membrane and utilize ambisense RNA genomes with two segments for replication. There are two main phylogenetic branches of Arenaviridae: the Old World viruses, such as Lassa fever and lymphocytic choriomeningitis (LCM) viruses, and the New World viruses, including those causing the South American hemorrhagic fevers (HFs). Arenaviruses persist in nature by chronically infecting rodents with a striking one-virus–one-rodent species relationship. These rodent infections result in long-term virus excretion and perhaps in lifelong viremia; vertical infection is common with some arenaviruses. Humans become infected through the inhalation of aerosols containing arenaviruses, which are then deposited in the terminal air passages, and probably also through close contact with rodents and their excreta, which results in the contamination of mucous membranes or breaks in the skin.

The Bunyaviridae The family Bunyaviridae includes four medically significant genera. All of these spherical viruses have three negative-sense RNA segments maturing into 90- to 120-nm particles in the Golgi complex and exiting the cell by exocytosis. Viruses of the genus *Bunyavirus* are largely mosquito-borne and have a viremic vertebrate intermediate host; many are also transovarially transmitted in their specific mosquito host. One serologic group also uses biting midges as vectors. Sandflies or mosquitoes are the vectors for the genus *Phlebovirus* (named after phlebotomus fever or sandfly fever, the best-known disease associated with the genus), while ticks serve as vectors for the genus *Nairovirus*. Viruses of both of these genera are also associated with vertical transmission in the arthropod host and with horizontal spread through viremic vertebrate hosts. The genus

Table 198-1 Major Zoonotic Virus Families and Some Characteristics of Typical Members

Family	Genus or Group	Syndrome(s): Typical Viruses	Maintenance Strategy
Arenaviridae	Old World complex	FM, E: Lymphocytic choriomeningitis virus HF: Lassa fever virus	Chronic infection of rodents, often with persistent viremia; vertical transmission common
	New World or Tacaribe complex	HF: South American HF viruses (Machupo, Junin, Guanarito, Sabia)	Chronic infection of rodents, sometimes with persistent viremia; vertical infection may occur
Bunyaviridae	*Bunyavirus*	E: California serogroup viruses (La Crosse, Jamestown Canyon, California encephalitis)	Mosquito-vertebrate cycle; transovarial transmission in mosquito common
		FM: Bunyamwera, group C, Tahyna viruses	
		FM: Oropouche virus	Transmitted by *Culicoides*
	Phlebovirus	FM: Sandfly fever, Toscana viruses	Sandfly transmission between vertebrates, with prominent transovarial component in sandfly
		FM: Punta Toro virus	
		HF, FM, E: Rift Valley fever virus	Mosquito-vertebrate transmission, with transovarial component in mosquito
	Nairovirus	HF: Crimean Congo HF virus	Tick-vertebrate, with transovarial transmission in tick
	Hantavirus	HF: Hantaan, Dobrava, Puumala viruses	Rodent reservoir; chronic virus shedding, but chronic viremia unknown
		HF: Sin Nombre and related hantaviruses	Sigmodontine rodent reservoir
Filoviridae[a]		HF: Marburg viruses, Ebola viruses (4 subtypes)	Unknown
Flaviviridae	*Flavivirus* (mosquito-borne)	HF: Yellow fever virus	Mosquito-vertebrate; transovarial rare
		FM, HF: Dengue viruses (4 subtypes)	
		E: St. Louis, Japanese, West Nile, and Murray Valley encephalitis viruses; Rocio viruses	
	Flavivirus (tick-borne)	E: Central European tick-borne encephalitis, Russian spring-summer encephalitis, Powassan viruses	Tick-vertebrate
		HF: Omsk HF, Kyasanur Forest disease viruses	
Reoviridae	*Coltivirus*	FM, E: Colorado tick fever virus	Tick-vertebrate
	Orbivirus	FM, E: Orungo, Kemerova viruses	Arthropod-vertebrate
Rhabdoviridae[b]	*Vesiculovirus*	FM: Vesicular stomatitis virus (Indiana, New Jersey); Chandipura, Piry viruses	Sandfly-vertebrate, with prominent transovarial component in sandfly
Togaviridae	*Alphavirus*	AR: Sindbis, chikungunya, Mayaro, Ross River, Barmah Forest viruses	Mosquito-vertebrate
		E: Eastern, western, and Venezuelan equine encephalitis viruses	

[a] The Filoviridae are discussed in Chap. 199.
[b] The Rhabdoviridae are discussed in Chap. 197.

NOTE: Abbreviations refer to the disease syndrome most commonly associated with the virus: FM, fever, myalgia; AR, arthritis, rash; E, encephalitis; HF, hemorrhagic fever.

Hantavirus is unique among the Bunyaviridae in that it is not transmitted by arthropods but is maintained in nature by rodent hosts that chronically shed virus. Like the arenaviruses, the hantaviruses usually display striking virus-rodent species specificity. Hantaviruses do not cause chronic viremia in their rodent host and are transmitted only horizontally from rodent to rodent.

Other Families The Flaviviridae are positive-sense, single-stranded RNA viruses that form particles of 40 to 50 nm in the endoplasmic reticulum. The flaviviruses discussed here are from the genus *Flavivirus* and make up two phylogenetically and antigenically distinct divisions transmitted among vertebrates by mosquitoes and ticks, respectively. The mosquito-borne viruses fall into phylogenetic groups that include yellow fever virus, the four dengue viruses, and encephalitis viruses, while the tick-borne group encompasses a geographically varied spectrum of species, some of which are responsible for encephalitis or for hemorrhagic disease with encephalitis. The Reoviridae are double-stranded RNA viruses with multisegmented genomes. These 80-nm particles are the only viruses discussed in this chapter that do not have a lipid envelope and thus are insensitive to detergents. The Togaviridae have a single positive strand RNA genome and bud particles of ~60 to 70 nm from the plasma membrane. The togaviruses discussed here are all members of the genus *Alphavirus* and are transmitted among vertebrates by mosquitoes in their natural cycle.→*The Filoviridae and the Rhabdoviridae are discussed in Chaps. 199 and 197, respectively.*

PROMINENT FEATURES OF ARTHROPOD- AND RODENT-BORNE VIRUSES Although this chapter discusses the major features of selected arthropod- and rodent-borne viruses, it does not deal with more than 500 other distinct recognized zoonotic viruses, about one-fourth of which infect humans. Zoonotic viruses are undergoing genetic evolution, "new" zoonotic viruses are being discovered, and the epidemiology of zoonotic viruses is continuing to evolve

through environmental changes affecting vectors, reservoirs, and humans. These zoonotic viruses are most numerous in the tropics but are also found in temperate and frigid climates. Their distribution and seasonal activity may be variable and often depend largely on ecologic conditions such as rainfall and temperature, which in turn affect the density of vectors and reservoirs and the development of infection therein.

Maintenance and Transmission Arthropod-borne viruses infect their vectors after the ingestion of a blood meal from a viremic vertebrate. The vectors then develop chronic, systemic infection as the viruses penetrate the gut and spread throughout the body. The viruses eventually reach the salivary glands during a period that is referred to as *extrinsic incubation* and that typically lasts 1 to 3 weeks in mosquitoes. At this point an arthropod is competent to continue the chain of transmission by infecting another vertebrate when a subsequent blood meal is taken. The arthropod generally is unharmed by the infection, and the natural vertebrate partner usually has only transient viremia with no overt disease. An alternative mechanism for virus maintenance in its arthropod host is transovarial transmission, which is common among members of the family Bunyaviridae.

Rodent-borne viruses such as the hantaviruses and arenaviruses are maintained in nature by chronic infection transmitted between rodents. As in arthropod-borne virus cycles, there is usually a high degree of rodent-virus specificity, and there is no overt disease in the reservoir/vector.

Epidemiology The distribution of arthropod- and rodent-borne viruses is restricted by the areas inhabited by their reservoir/vectors and provides an important clue in the differential diagnosis. Table 198-2 shows the approximate geographic distribution of the most important of these viruses. Members of each family, each genus, and even each serologically related group usually occur in each area but may not be pathogenic in all areas or may not be a commonly rec-

Table 198-2   Geographic Distribution of Some Important and Commonly Encountered Human Zoonotic Viral Diseases

Area	Arenaviridae	Bunyaviridae	Flaviviridae	Rhabdoviridae	Togaviridae
North America	Lymphocytic chorio-meningitis	La Crosse, Jamestown Canyon, California encephalitis; hantavirus pulmonary syndrome	St. Louis, Powassan encephalitis; dengue	Vesicular stomatitis	Eastern, western equine encephalitis
South America	Bolivian, Argentine, Venezuelan, and Brazilian HF ; lymphocytic choriomeningitis	Oropouche, group C, Punta Toro infection; hantavirus pulmonary syndrome	Yellow fever, dengue, Rocio virus infection	Vesicular stomatitis, Piry virus infection	Mayaro virus infection, Venezuelan equine encephalitis
Europe	Lymphocytic chorio-meningitis	Tahyna, Toscana, sandfly fever, HF with renal syndrome	West Nile, Central European tick-borne, Russian spring-summer encephalitis	—	Sindbis virus infection
Middle East	—	Sandfly fever, Crimean Congo HF	West Nile encephalitis, dengue	—	—
Eastern Asia	—	Sandfly fever; Hantaan, Seoul virus infection	Dengue; Japanese, Russian spring-summer encephalitis; Omsk HF	Chandipura virus infection	—
Southwestern Asia	—	Sandfly fever, Crimean Congo HF	West Nile, Japanese encephalitis; dengue; Kyasanur Forest disease	—	Chikungunya
Southeast Asia	—	Seoul virus infection	Japanese encephalitis, dengue	—	Chikungunya
Africa	Lassa fever	Bunyamwera virus infection, Rift Valley fever	Yellow fever, dengue	—	Sindbis virus infection, chikungunya
Australia	—	—	Murray Valley encephalitis, dengue		Ross River, Barmah Forest virus infection

NOTE: HF, hemorrhagic fever.

ognized cause of disease in all areas and so may not be included in the table. Although there is generally no overt disease in the vertebrate reservoirs, disease in nonhuman target species may be a useful diagnostic clue, and serologic testing of selected animals may be a useful way to monitor virus circulation.

Most of these diseases are acquired in a rural setting; a few have urban vectors. Seoul, sandfly fever, and Oropouche viruses are examples of urban viruses, but the most notable are yellow fever, dengue, and chikungunya viruses, which are transmitted between humans with the mosquito *Aedes aegypti* as a principal or alternate vector. A history of mosquito bite has little diagnostic significance in the individual; a history of tick bite is more diagnostically specific. Rodent exposure is often reported by persons infected with an arenavirus or a hantavirus but again has little specificity. Indeed, aerosols may infect persons who have no recollection of having even seen rodents.

Syndromes Human disease caused by arthropod- and rodent-borne viruses is often subclinical. The spectrum of possible responses to infection is wide, and our knowledge of the outcome of most of these infections is limited. The usual disease syndromes associated with these viruses have been grouped into four categories: fever and myalgia, arthritis and rash, encephalitis, and hemorrhagic fever. Although for the purposes of this discussion most viruses have been placed in a single group, the categories often overlap. For example, West Nile and Venezuelan equine encephalitis viruses are discussed as encephalitis viruses, but during epidemics they may cause many cases of milder febrile syndromes and relatively uncommon cases of encephalitis. Similarly, Rift Valley fever virus is best known as a cause of HF, but the attack rates for febrile disease are far higher, and encephalitis is occasionally seen as well. LCM virus is classified as a cause of fever and myalgia because this syndrome is its most common disease manifestation and, even when central nervous system (CNS) disease occurs, it is usually mild and is preceded by fever and myalgia. Dengue virus infection is considered as a cause of fever and myalgia (dengue fever) because this is by far the most common manifestation worldwide and is the syndrome most likely to be seen in the United

States; however, dengue HF is also discussed in the HF section because of its complicated pathogenesis and importance in pediatric practice in certain areas of the world.

Diagnosis Laboratory diagnosis is required in any given case, although epidemics occasionally provide clinical and epidemiologic clues on which an educated guess as to etiology can be based. For most arthropod- and rodent-borne viruses, acute-phase serum samples (collected within 3 or 4 days of onset) have yielded isolates, and paired sera have been used to demonstrate rising antibody titers by a variety of tests. Intensive efforts to develop rapid tests for HF have resulted in an antigen-detection enzyme-linked immunosorbent assay (ELISA) and an IgM-capture ELISA that can provide a diagnosis based on a single serum sample within a few hours and are particularly useful in severe cases. More sensitive reverse transcription polymerase chain reaction (RT-PCR) tests may yield diagnoses based on samples without detectable antigen and may also provide useful genetic information about the virus. Preliminary data suggest that similar tests applied to some fever-myalgia syndromes would give positive results if developed further. Hantavirus infections differ from others discussed here in that severe acute disease is immunopathologic; patients present with serum IgM that serves as the basis for a sensitive and specific test. Every ELISA must include a control incorporating a negative antigen with each serum sample tested; the frequent failure to include such a control has resulted in numerous false-positive results in diagnostic tests.

At the time of diagnosis, patients with encephalitis are generally no longer viremic or antigenemic and usually do not have virus in cerebrospinal fluid (CSF). In this situation, the value of serologic methods and RT-PCR is being validated. IgM capture is increasingly being used for the simultaneous testing of serum and CSF. IgG ELISA or classic serology is useful in the evaluation of past exposure to the viruses, many of which circulate in areas with a minimal medical infrastructure and sometimes cause mild or subclinical infection.

The remainder of this chapter offers general descriptions of the broad syndromes caused by arthropod- and rodent-borne viruses and then addresses specific differences between diseases. It is important to remember that most of the diseases under consideration have not been studied in detail with modern medical approaches and thus available data may be incomplete or biased.

FEVER AND MYALGIA

Fever and myalgia constitute the syndrome most commonly associated with zoonotic virus infection. Many of the numerous viruses belonging to the families listed in Table 198-1 probably cause this syndrome, but several viruses have been selected for inclusion in the table because of their prominent associations with the syndrome and their biomedical importance.

The syndrome typically begins with the abrupt onset of fever, chills, intense myalgia, and malaise. Patients may also report joint pains, but no true arthritis is detectable. Anorexia is characteristic and may be accompanied by nausea or even vomiting. Headache is common and may be severe, with photophobia and retroorbital pain. Physical findings are minimal and are usually confined to conjunctival injection with pain on palpation of muscles or the epigastrium. The duration of symptoms is quite variable but generally is 2 to 5 days, with a biphasic course in some instances. The spectrum of disease varies from subclinical to temporarily incapacitating.

Less constant findings include a maculopapular rash. Epistaxis may occur but does not necessarily indicate a bleeding diathesis. A minority of the cases caused by some viruses are known or suspected to include aseptic meningitis, but this diagnosis is difficult in remote areas, given the patients' photophobia and myalgia as well as the lack of opportunity to examine the CSF. Although pharyngitis may be noted or radiographic evidence of pulmonary infiltrates found in some cases, these viruses are not primary respiratory pathogens. The differential diagnosis includes anicteric leptospirosis, rickettsial diseases, and the early stages of other syndromes discussed in this chapter. These diseases are often described as "flulike," but the usual absence of cough and coryza makes influenza an unlikely confounder except at the earliest stages.

Complete recovery is generally the outcome in this syndrome, although prolonged asthenia and nonspecific symptoms have been described in some cases, particularly after infection with LCM or dengue virus. Treatment is supportive, with aspirin avoided because of the potential for exacerbated bleeding and Reye's syndrome. Efforts at prevention are best based on vector control, which, however, may be expensive or impossible. For mosquito control, destruction of breeding sites is generally the most economically and environmentally sound approach; spraying to kill adult mosquitoes and thus to reduce their numbers transiently may have a preventive role in selected settings but has not been notably effective in the past. Measures taken by the individual to avoid the vector can be valuable. Avoiding the vector's habitat and times of peak activity, preventing the vector from entering dwellings by using screens or other barriers, judiciously applying arthropod repellents such as diethyltoluamide (DEET) to the skin, and wearing permethrin-impregnated clothing are all possible approaches, depending on the vector and its habits.

LYMPHOCYTIC CHORIOMENINGITIS LCM is transmitted from the common house mouse (*Mus musculus*) to humans by aerosols of excreta and secreta. LCM virus, an arenavirus, is maintained in the mouse mainly by vertical transmission from infected dams. The vertically infected mouse remains viremic for life, with high concentrations of virus in all tissues. Infected colonies of pet hamsters have also served as a link to humans. LCM virus is widely used in immunology laboratories as a model of T cell function and can silently infect cell cultures and passaged tumor lines, resulting in infections among scientists and animal caretakers. Patients with LCM may have a history of residence in rodent-infested housing or other exposure to rodents. An antibody prevalence of ~5 to 10% has been reported in adults from the United States, Argentina, and endemic areas of Germany.

LCM differs from the general syndrome of fever and myalgia in that its onset is gradual. Among the conditions occasionally associated with LCM are orchitis, transient alopecia, arthritis, pharyngitis, cough, and maculopapular rash. An estimated one-fourth of patients or fewer suffer a febrile phase of 3 to 6 days and then, after a brief remission, develop renewed fever accompanied by severe headache, nausea and vomiting, and meningeal signs lasting for about a week. These patients virtually always recover fully, as do the uncommon patients with clear-cut signs of encephalitis. Recovery may be delayed by transient hydrocephalus.

During the initial febrile phase, leukopenia and thrombocytopenia are common and virus can usually be isolated from blood. During the CNS phase of the illness, virus may be found in the CSF, but antibodies are present in blood. The pathogenesis of LCM is thought to resemble that following direct intracranial inoculation of the virus into adult mice; the onset of the immune response leads to T cell–mediated immunopathologic meningitis. During the meningeal phase, CSF mononuclear-cell counts range from the hundreds to the low thousands per microliter, and hypoglycorrhachia is found in one-third of cases. The IgM-capture ELISA of serum and CSF is usually positive; RT-PCR assays have been developed for application to CSF.

Infection with LCM virus should be suspected in acutely ill febrile patients with marked leukopenia and thrombocytopenia. In cases of aseptic meningitis, any of the following should suggest LCM: well-marked febrile prodrome, adult age, autumn seasonality, low CSF glucose levels, or CSF mononuclear cell counts $>1000/\mu L$.

In pregnant women, LCM virus infection may lead to fetal invasion with consequent congenital hydrocephalus and chorioretinitis. Since the maternal infection may be mild, consisting of only a short febrile illness, antibodies to the virus should be sought in both the mother and the fetus in suspicious circumstances, particularly TORCH-negative neonatal hydrocephalus. [TORCH is a battery of tests encompassing *t*oxoplasmosis, *o*ther conditions (congenital syphilis and viruses), *r*ubella, *c*ytomegalovirus, and *h*erpes simplex virus.]

BUNYAMWERA VIRUS INFECTION The mosquito-transmitted Bunyamwera serogroup viruses are found on every continent except Australia and Antarctica. Bunyamwera virus and its close relative Ilesha virus commonly cause febrile disease in Africa. Other related viruses are implicated in such disease in Southeast Asia (Batai virus), Europe (Calovo virus), and South America (Wyeomyia virus). In North America, Cache Valley virus has been implicated in febrile human disease and in rare instances of more serious systemic illness; the presence of serum antibodies to this virus may be associated with congenital malformations. In Central America, the closely related Fort Sherman virus causes the fever-myalgia syndrome.

GROUP C VIRUS INFECTION The group C viruses include at least 11 agents transmitted by mosquitoes in neotropical forests. These agents are among the most common causes of arboviral infection in humans entering American jungles and cause acute febrile disease.

TAHYNA VIRUS INFECTION This California serogroup virus (see discussion of California encephalitis, below) occurs in central and western Europe, and related viruses are emerging in Russia. The significance of Tahyna virus in human health has been studied only in the Czech and Slovak Republics; there, the virus was found to be a prominent cause of febrile disease, in some cases causing pharyngitis, pulmonary syndromes, and aseptic meningitis. The potential for arboviruses to be unexpectedly involved in such cases in areas of high mosquito prevalence needs to be kept in mind.

OROPOUCHE FEVER Oropouche virus is transmitted in Central and South America by a biting midge, *Culicoides paraensis*, which often breeds to high density in cacao husks and other vegetable detritus found in towns and cities. Explosive epidemics involving thousands of cases have been reported from several towns in Brazil and Peru. Rash and aseptic meningitis have been detected in a number of cases.

SANDFLY FEVER   The sandfly *Phlebotomus papatasi* transmits sandfly fever. Female sandflies may be infected by the oral route as they take a blood meal and may transmit the virus to offspring when they lay their eggs after a second blood meal. This prominent transovarial pattern was the first to be recognized among dipterans and complicates virus control. A previous designation for sandfly fever, "3-day fever," instructively describes the brief, debilitating course associated with this essentially benign infection. There is neither a rash nor CNS involvement, and complete recovery is the rule.

Sandfly fever is found in the circum-Mediterranean area, extending to the east through the Balkans into China as well as into the Middle East and southwestern Asia. The vector is found in both rural and urban settings and is known for its small size, which enables it to penetrate standard mosquito screens and netting, and for its short flight range. Epidemics have been described in the wake of natural disasters and wars. In parts of Europe, sandfly populations and virus transmission were greatly reduced by the extensive residual spraying conducted after World War II to control malaria, and the incidence continues to be low. A common pattern of disease in endemic areas consists of high attack rates among travelers and military personnel with little or no disease in the local population, who are protected after childhood infection. In addition to the two well-characterized, non-cross-protective Sicilian and Naples virus species, more than 30 related phleboviruses are transmitted by sandflies and mosquitoes, but most are of unknown significance in terms of human health.

TOSCANA VIRUS DISEASE   Toscana virus is a *Phlebovirus* (family Bunyaviridae) transmitted primarily by the circum-Mediterranean sandfly *P. perniciosus*. The vertebrate amplifying host, if one exists, is unknown. Toscana virus infection is common during the summer among rural residents and vacationers; a number of cases have been identified in travelers returning to Germany and Scandinavia. The disease may manifest as an uncomplicated febrile illness but is often associated with aseptic meningitis, with virus isolated from the CSF.

PUNTA TORO VIRUS DISEASE   Of the several phleboviruses that are associated with New World sandflies and infect humans, Punta Toro virus is the best known. The disease caused by this virus is clinically similar to but epidemiologically different from that caused by the Naples or Sicilian sandfly fever viruses. Punta Toro virus infections are sporadic and are acquired in the tropical forest, where the vectors rest on tree buttresses. Epidemics have not been reported, but antibody prevalences among inhabitants of villages in the endemic areas indicate a cumulative lifetime exposure rate of >50%.

DENGUE FEVER   All four distinct dengue viruses (dengue 1–4) have *A. aegypti* as their principal vector, and all cause a similar clinical syndrome. In rare cases, second infection with a serotype of dengue virus different from that involved in the primary infection leads to dengue HF with severe shock (see below). Sporadic cases are seen in the settings of endemic transmission and epidemic disease. Year-round transmission between latitudes 25°N and 25°S has been established, and seasonal forays of the viruses to points as far north as Philadelphia are thought to have taken place in the United States. With increasing spread of the vector mosquito throughout the tropics and subtropics, large areas of the world have become vulnerable to the introduction of dengue viruses, particularly through air travel by infected humans, and both dengue fever and the related dengue HF are becoming increasingly common. Conditions favorable to dengue transmission exist in the southern United States, and bursts of dengue fever activity are to be expected in this region, particularly along the Mexican border, where water may be stored in containers and *A. aegypti* numbers may therefore be greatest: this mosquito, which is also an efficient vector of the yellow fever and chikungunya viruses, typically breeds near human habitation, using relatively fresh water from sources such as water jars, vases, discarded containers, coconut husks, and old tires. *A. aegypti* usually inhabits dwellings and bites during the day.

After an incubation period of 2 to 7 days, the typical patient experiences the sudden onset of fever, headache, retroorbital pain, and back pain along with the severe myalgia that gave rise to the colloquial designation "break-bone fever." There is often a macular rash on the first day as well as adenopathy, palatal vesicles, and scleral injection. The illness may last a week, with additional symptoms usually including anorexia, nausea or vomiting, marked cutaneous hypersensitivity, and—near the time of defervescence—a maculopapular rash beginning on the trunk and spreading to the extremities and the face. Epistaxis and scattered petechiae are often noted in uncomplicated dengue, and preexisting gastrointestinal lesions may bleed during the acute illness.

Laboratory findings include leukopenia, thrombocytopenia, and, in many cases, serum aminotransferase elevations. The diagnosis is made by IgM ELISA or paired serology during recovery or by antigen-detection ELISA or RT-PCR during the acute phase. Virus is readily isolated from blood in the acute phase if mosquito inoculation or mosquito cell culture is used.

COLORADO TICK FEVER   Several hundred cases of Colorado tick fever are reported annually in the United States. The infection is acquired between March and November through the bite of an infected *Dermacentor andersoni* tick in mountainous western regions at altitudes of 1200 to 3000 m (4000 to 10,000 ft). Small mammals serve as the amplifying host. The most common presentation consists of fever and myalgia; meningoencephalitis is not uncommon, and hemorrhagic disease, pericarditis, myocarditis, orchitis, and pulmonary presentations are also reported. Rash develops in a substantial minority of cases. The disease usually lasts 7 to 10 days and is often biphasic. The most important differential diagnostic considerations since the beginning of the twentieth century have been Rocky Mountain spotted fever and tularemia.

Infection of erythroblasts and other marrow cells by Colorado tick fever virus results in the appearance and persistence (for several weeks) of erythrocytes containing the virus. This feature, detected in smears stained by immunofluorescence, can be diagnostically helpful. The clinical laboratory detects leukopenia and thrombocytopenia.

ORBIVIRUS INFECTION   The orbiviruses encompass many human and veterinary pathogens. For example, Orungo virus is widely transmitted by mosquitoes in tropical Africa and causes febrile disease in humans. The Kemerova complex includes the Kemerova, Lipovnik, and Tribec viruses of Russia and central Europe; these viruses are transmitted by ticks and are associated with febrile and neurologic disease.

VESICULAR STOMATITIS   See Chap. 197.

ENCEPHALITIS

Arboviral encephalitis is a seasonal disease, commonly occurring in the warmer months. Its incidence varies markedly with time and place, depending on ecologic factors. The causative viruses differ substantially in terms of case-infection ratio (i.e., the ratio of clinical to subclinical infection), mortality, and residua (Table 198-3). Humans are not an important amplifier of these viruses.

All the viral encephalitides discussed in this section have a similar pathogenesis as far as is known. An infected arthropod ingests a blood meal from a human and infects the host. The initial period of viremia is thought to originate most commonly from the lymphoid system. Viremia leads to CNS invasion, presumably through infection of olfactory neuroepithelium with passage through the cribiform plate or through infection of brain capillaries and multifocal entry into the CNS. During the viremic phase, there may be little or no recognized disease except in the case of tick-borne flaviviral encephalitis, in which there may be a clearly delineated phase of fever and systemic illness. The disease process in the CNS arises partly from direct neuronal infection and subsequent damage and partly from edema, inflammation, and other indirect effects. The usual pathologic picture is one of focal necrosis of neurons, inflammatory glial nodules, and perivascular lymphoid cuffing; the severity and distribution of these abnormalities

Table 198-3 Prominent Features of Arboviral Encephalitis

Virus	Natural Cycle	Incubation Period, Days	Annual No. of Cases	Case-to-Infection Ratio	Age of Cases	Case-Fatality Rate, %	Residua
La Crosse	*Aedes triseriatus*–chipmunk (transovarial component in mosquito also important)	~3–7	70 (U.S.)	<1:1000	<15 years	<0.5	Recurrent seizures in ~10%; severe deficits in rare cases; decreased school performance and behavioral change suspected in small proportion
St. Louis	*Culex tarsalis, C. pipiens, C. quinquefasciatus*–birds	4–21	85, with hundreds to thousands in epidemic years (U.S.)	<1:200	Milder cases in the young; more severe cases in adults >40 years old, particularly the elderly	7	Common in the elderly
Japanese	*Culex tritaeniorhyncus*–birds	5–15	>25,000	1:200 300	All ages; children in highly endemic areas	20–50	Common (approximately half of cases); may be severe
West Nile	*Culex* mosquitoes–birds	3–6	?	Very low	Mainly the elderly and children	—	Uncommon
Central European	*Ixodes ricinus*–rodents, insectivores	7–14	Thousands	1:12	All ages; milder in children	1–5	20%
Russian spring-summer	*I. persulcatus*–rodents, insectivores	7–14	Hundreds	—	All ages; milder in children	20	Approximately half of cases; often severe; limb-girdle paralysis
Powassan	*I. cookei*–wild mammals	~10	~1 (U.S.)	—	All ages; some predilection for children	~10	Common (approximately half of cases)
Eastern equine	*Culiseta melanura*–birds	~5–10	5 (U.S.)	1:40 adult 1:17 child	All ages; predilection for children	50–75	Common
Western equine	*Culex tarsalis*–birds	~5–10	~20 (U.S.)	1:1000 adult 1:50 child 1:1 infant	All ages; predilection for children <2 years old (increased mortality in elderly)	3–7	Common only among infants < 1 year old
Venezuelan equine (epidemic)	Unknown (multiple mosquito species and horses in epidemics)	1–5	?	1:250 adult 1:25 child (approximate)	All ages; predilection for children	~10	—

vary with the infecting virus. Involved areas display the "luxury perfusion" phenomenon, with normal or increased total blood flow and low oxygen extraction.

The typical patient presents with a prodrome of nonspecific constitutional symptoms, including fever, abdominal pain, vertigo, sore throat, and respiratory symptoms. Headache, meningeal signs, photophobia, and vomiting follow quickly. Involvement of deeper structures may be signaled by lethargy, somnolence, and intellectual deficit (as disclosed by the mental status examination or failure at serial 7 subtraction); more severely affected patients will be obviously disoriented and may be comatose. Tremors, loss of abdominal reflexes, cranial nerve palsies, hemiparesis, monoparesis, difficulty in swallowing, and frontal lobe signs are all common. Convulsions and focal signs may be evident early or may appear during the course of the disease. Some patients present with an abrupt onset of fever, convulsions, and other signs of CNS involvement. The results of human infection range from no significant symptoms through febrile headache to aseptic meningitis and finally to full-blown encephalitis; the proportions and severity of these manifestations vary with the infecting virus.

The acute encephalitis usually lasts from a few days to as long as 2 to 3 weeks, but recovery may be slow, with weeks or months required for the return of maximal recoupable function. Common complaints during recovery include difficulty concentrating, fatigability, tremors, and personality changes. The acute illness requires management of a comatose patient who may have intracranial pressure elevations, inappropriate secretion of antidiuretic hormone, respiratory failure, and convulsions. There is no specific therapy for these viral encephalitides. The only practical preventive measures are vector management and personal protection against the arthropod transmitting the virus; for

Japanese encephalitis or tick-borne encephalitis, vaccination should be considered in certain circumstances (see relevant sections below).

The diagnosis of arboviral encephalitis depends on the careful evaluation of a febrile patient with CNS disease, with rapid identification of treatable herpes simplex encephalitis, ruling out of brain abscess, exclusion of bacterial meningitis by serial CSF examination, and performance of laboratory studies to define the viral etiology. Leptospirosis, neurosyphilis, Lyme disease, cat-scratch fever, and newer viral encephalitides such as Nipah virus infection from Malaysia should be considered. The CSF examination usually shows a modest cell count—in the tens or hundreds or perhaps a few thousand. Early in the process, a significant proportion of these cells may be polymorphonuclear leukocytes, but usually there is a mononuclear cell predominance. CSF glucose levels are usually normal. There are exceptions to this pattern of findings. In eastern equine encephalitis, for example, polymorphonuclear leukocytes may predominate during the first 72 h of disease and hypoglycorrhachia may be detected. In LCM, lymphocyte counts may be in the thousands, and the glucose concentration may be diminished. Experience with imaging studies is still evolving; clearly, however, both computed tomography (CT) and magnetic resonance imaging (MRI) may be normal except for evidence of preexisting conditions or sometimes may suggest diffuse edema. Several patients with eastern equine encephalitis have had focal abnormalities, and individuals with severe Japanese encephalitis have presented with bilateral thalamic lesions that have often been hemorrhagic. Electroencephalography usually shows diffuse abnormalities and is not directly helpful.

A humoral immune response is usually detectable at or near the onset of disease. Both serum and CSF should be examined for IgM antibodies. Virus generally cannot be isolated from blood or CSF, although Japanese encephalitis virus has been recovered from CSF in severe cases. Virus can be obtained from and viral antigen is present in brain tissue, although its distribution may be focal.

CALIFORNIA, LA CROSSE, AND JAMESTOWN CANYON VIRUS ENCEPHALITIS The isolation of California encephalitis virus established the California serogroup of viruses as a cause of encephalitis, and its use as a diagnostic antigen led to the description of many cases of "California encephalitis." In fact, however, this virus has been implicated in only a few cases of encephalitis, and the serologically related La Crosse virus is the major cause of encephalitis among viruses in the California serogroup. "California encephalitis" due to La Crosse virus infection is most commonly reported from the upper Midwest but is also found in other areas of the central and eastern United States, most often in West Virginia, Tennessee, North Carolina, and Georgia. The serogroup includes 13 other viruses, some of which may also be involved in human disease that is misattributed because of the complexity of the group's serology; these viruses include the Jamestown Canyon, snowshoe hare, Inkoo, and Trivittatus viruses, all of which have *Aedes* mosquitoes as their vector and all of which have a strong element of transovarial transmission in their natural cycles.

The mosquito vector of La Crosse virus is *A. triseriatus*. In addition to a prominent transovarial component of transmission, a mosquito can also become infected through feeding on viremic chipmunks and other mammals as well as through venereal transmission from another mosquito. The mosquito breeds in sites such as tree holes and abandoned tires and bites during daylight hours; these findings correlate with the risk factors for cases: recreation in forested areas, residence at the forest's edge, and the presence of abandoned tires around the home. Intensive environmental modification based on these findings has reduced the incidence of disease in a highly endemic area in the Midwest. Most cases occur from July through September. The Asian tiger mosquito, *A. albopictus*, efficiently transmits the virus to mice and also transmits the agent transovarially in the laboratory; this aggressive anthropophilic mosquito has the capacity to urbanize, and its possible impact on transmission to humans is of concern.

An antibody prevalence of ≥20% in endemic areas indicates that infection is common, but CNS disease has been recognized primarily in children <15 years of age. The illness varies from a picture of aseptic meningitis accompanied by confusion to severe and occasionally fatal encephalitis. Although there may be prodromal symptoms, the onset of CNS disease is sudden, with fever, headache, and lethargy often joined by nausea and vomiting, convulsions (in one-half of patients), and coma (in one-third of patients). Focal seizures, hemiparesis, tremor, aphasia, chorea, Babinski's sign, and other evidence of significant neurologic dysfunction are common, but residua are not. Perhaps 10% of patients have recurrent seizures in the succeeding months. Other serious sequelae are rare, although a decrease in scholastic standing has been reported and mild personality change has occasionally been suggested. Treatment is supportive over a 1- to 2-week acute phase during which status epilepticus, cerebral edema, and inappropriate secretion of antidiuretic hormone are important concerns. Ribavirin has been used in severe cases, and a clinical trial of this drug is under way.

The blood leukocyte count is commonly elevated, sometimes reaching levels of 20,000/μL, and there is usually a left shift. CSF cell counts are typically 30 to 500/μL with a mononuclear cell predominance (although 25 to 90% of cells are polymorphonuclear in some cases). The protein level is normal or slightly increased, and the glucose level is normal. Specific virologic diagnosis based on IgM-capture assays of serum and CSF is efficient. The only human anatomic site from which virus has been isolated is the brain.

Jamestown Canyon virus has been implicated in several cases of encephalitis in adults; in these cases the disease was usually associated with a significant respiratory illness at onset. Human infection with this virus has been documented in New York, Wisconsin, Ohio, Mich-

igan, Ontario, and other areas of North America where the vector mosquito, *A. stimulans*, feeds on its main host, the white-tailed deer.

ST. LOUIS ENCEPHALITIS St. Louis encephalitis virus is transmitted between *Culex* mosquitoes and birds. This virus causes low-level endemic infection among rural residents of the western and central United States, where *C. tarsalis* is the vector (see "Western Equine Encephalitis," below), but the more urbanized mosquito species *C. pipiens* and *C. quinquefasciatus* have been responsible for epidemics resulting in hundreds or even thousands of cases in cities of the central and eastern United States. Most cases occur in June through October. The urban mosquitoes breed in accumulations of stagnant water and sewage with high organic content and readily bite humans in and around houses at dusk. The elimination of open sewers and trash-filled drainage systems is expensive and may not be possible, but screening of houses and implementation of personal protective measures may be an effective approach for individuals. The rural vector is most active at dusk and outdoors; its bites can be avoided by modification of activities and use of repellents.

Disease severity increases with age: infections that result in aseptic meningitis or mild encephalitis are concentrated in children and young adults, while severe and fatal cases primarily affect the elderly. Infection rates are similar in all age groups; thus the greater susceptibility of older persons to disease is a biologic consequence of aging. The disease has an abrupt onset, sometimes following a prodrome, and begins with fever, lethargy, confusion, and headache. In addition, nuchal rigidity, hypotonia, hyperreflexia, myoclonus, and tremor are common. Severe cases can include cranial nerve palsies, hemiparesis, and convulsions. Patients often complain of dysuria and may have viral antigen in urine as well as pyuria. The overall mortality is generally ~7% but may reach 20% among patients over the age of 60. Recovery is slow. Emotional lability, difficulties in concentration and memory, asthenia, and tremor are commonly prolonged in older patients.

The CSF of patients with St. Louis encephalitis usually contains tens to hundreds of cells, with a lymphocytic predominance and a normal glucose level. Leukocytosis with a left shift is often documented.

JAPANESE ENCEPHALITIS Japanese encephalitis virus is found throughout Asia, including far eastern Russia, Japan, China, India, Pakistan, and Southeast Asia, and causes occasional epidemics on western Pacific islands. The virus has been detected in the Torres Strait islands, and a human encephalitis case has been identified on the nearby Australian mainland. This flavivirus is particularly common in areas where irrigated rice fields attract the natural avian vertebrate hosts and provide abundant breeding sites for mosquitoes such as *C. tritaeniorhyncus*, which transmit the virus to humans. Additional amplification by pigs, which suffer abortion, and horses, which develop encephalitis, may be significant as well. Vaccination of these additional amplifying hosts may reduce the transmission of the virus. An effective, formalin-inactivated vaccine purified from mouse brain is produced in Japan and licensed for human use in the United States. It is given on days 0, 7, and 30 or—with some sacrifice in serum neutralizing titer—on days 0, 7, and 14. Vaccination is indicated for summer travelers to rural Asia, where the risk of clinical disease may be 0.05 to 2.1/10,000 per week. The severe and often fatal disease reported in expatriates must be balanced against the 0.1 to 1% chance of a late systemic or cutaneous allergic reaction. These reactions are rarely fatal but may be severe and have been known to begin 1 to 9 days after vaccination, with associated pruritus, urticaria, and angioedema. Live attenuated vaccines are being used in China but are not recommended in the United States at this time.

WEST NILE VIRUS INFECTION West Nile virus is transmitted among wild birds by *Culex* mosquitoes in Africa, the Middle East, southern Europe, and Asia. It is a frequent cause of febrile disease without CNS involvement, but it occasionally causes aseptic meningitis and severe encephalitis; these serious infections are particularly common among children and the elderly. The febrile-myalgic syndrome caused by West Nile virus differs from many others by the frequent appearance of a maculopapular rash concentrated on the trunk and lymphadenopathy. Headache, ocular pain, sore throat, nausea and vomiting, and arthralgia (but not arthritis) are common accompaniments. In addition, the virus has been implicated in severe and fatal hepatic necrosis in Africa.

In 1996 West Nile virus caused more than 300 cases of CNS disease, with 10% mortality, in the Danube flood plain, including Bucharest. In 1999 the virus appeared in New York City and other areas of the northeastern United States, causing more than 60 cases of aseptic meningitis or encephalitis among humans as well as die-offs among crows, exotic zoo birds, and other avians. The encephalitis was most severe among the elderly and was often associated with notable muscle weakness and even with flaccid paralysis. The virus, thought to have been transmitted in New York City by the ubiquitous *C. pipiens* mosquito, returned to larger areas of the northeastern United States in the summer of 2000 and threatens to spread farther in the Americas via bird migration.

West Nile virus falls into the same phylogenetic group of flaviviruses as St. Louis and Japanese encephalitis viruses, as do Murray Valley and Rocio viruses. The latter two viruses are both maintained in mosquitoes and birds and produce a clinical picture resembling that of Japanese encephalitis. Murray Valley virus has caused occasional epidemics and sporadic cases in Australia. Rocio virus caused recurrent epidemics in a focal area of Brazil in 1975 to 1977 and then virtually disappeared.

CENTRAL EUROPEAN TICK-BORNE ENCEPHALITIS AND RUSSIAN SPRING-SUMMER ENCEPHALITIS

A spectrum of tick-borne flaviviruses has been identified across the Eurasian land mass. Many are known mainly as agricultural pathogens (e.g., louping ill virus in the United Kingdom). From Scandinavia to the Urals, central European tick-borne encephalitis is transmitted by *Ixodes ricinus*. Human cases occur between April and October, with a peak in June and July. A related and more virulent virus is that of Russian spring-summer encephalitis, which is associated with *I. persulcatus* and is distributed from Europe across the Urals to the Pacific Ocean. The ticks transmit the disease primarily in the spring and early summer, with a lower rate of transmission later in summer. Small mammals are the vertebrate amplifiers for both viruses. The risk varies by geographic area and can be highly localized within a given area; human cases usually follow outdoor activities or consumption of raw milk from infected goats or other infected animals.

After an incubation period of 7 to 14 days or perhaps longer, the central European viruses classically result in a febrile-myalgic phase that lasts for 2 to 4 days and is thought to correlate with viremia. A subsequent remission for several days is followed by the recurrence of fever and the onset of meningeal signs. The CNS phase varies from mild aseptic meningitis, which is more common among younger patients, to severe encephalitis with coma, convulsions, tremors, and motor signs lasting for 7 to 10 days before improvement begins. Spinal and medullary involvement can lead to typical limb-girdle paralysis and to respiratory paralysis. Most patients recover, only a minority with significant deficits. Infections with the far eastern viruses generally run a more abrupt course. The encephalitic syndrome caused by these viruses sometimes begins without a remission and has more severe manifestations than the European syndrome. Mortality is high, and major sequelae—most notably, lower motor neuron paralyses of the proximal muscles of the extremities, trunk, and neck—are common.

In the early stage of the illness, virus may be isolated from the blood. In the CNS phase, IgM antibodies are detectable in serum and/or CSF. Thrombocytopenia sometimes develops during the initial febrile illness, which resembles the early hemorrhagic phase of some other tick-borne flaviviral infections, such as Kyasanur Forest disease. Other tick-borne flaviviruses are less common causes of encephalitis, including louping ill virus in the United Kingdom and Powassan virus.

There is no specific therapy for infection with these viruses. However, effective alum-adjuvanted, formalin-inactivated vaccines are produced in Austria, Germany, and Russia. Two doses of the Austrian vaccine separated by an interval of 1 to 3 months appear to be effective in the field, and antibody responses are similar when vaccine is given

on days 0 and 14. Other vaccines have elicited similar neutralizing antibody titers. Since rare cases of postvaccination Guillain-Barré syndrome have been reported, vaccination should be reserved for persons likely to experience rural exposure in an endemic area during the season of transmission. Cross-neutralization for the central European and far eastern strains has been established, but there are no published field studies on cross-protection of formalin-inactivated vaccines. Because 0.2 to 4% of ticks in endemic areas may be infected, tick bites raise the issue of immunoglobulin prophylaxis. Prompt administration of high-titered specific preparations should probably be undertaken, although no controlled data are available to prove the efficacy of this measure. Immunoglobulin should not be administered late because of the risk of antibody-mediated enhancement.

POWASSAN ENCEPHALITIS

Powassan virus is a member of the tick-borne encephalitis virus complex and is transmitted by *I. cookei* among small mammals in eastern Canada and the United States, where it has been responsible for 20 recognized cases of human disease. Other ticks may transmit the virus in a wider geographic area, and there is some concern that *I. scapularis* (also called *I. dammini*), a competent vector in the laboratory, may become involved as it becomes more prominent in the United States. Patients with Powassan encephalitis—often children—present in May through December after outdoor exposure and an incubation period thought to be about 1 week. Powassan encephalitis is severe, and sequelae are common.

EASTERN EQUINE ENCEPHALITIS

Eastern equine encephalitis is found primarily within endemic swampy foci along the eastern coast of the United States, with a few inland foci as far removed as Michigan. Human cases present from June through October, when the bird–*Culiseta* mosquito cycle spills over into other mosquito species such as *A. sollicitans* or *A. vexans*, which are more likely to bite mammals. There is concern over the potential role of the introduced anthropophilic mosquito species *A. albopictus*, which has been found to be naturally infected and is an effective vector in the laboratory. Horses are a common target for the virus; if not vaccinated, they serve as a harbinger of human disease but probably do not play a significant role in amplification of the virus.

Eastern equine encephalitis is one of the most destructive of the arboviral conditions, with a brusque onset, rapid progression, high mortality, and frequent residua. This severity is reflected in the extensive necrotic lesions and polymorphonuclear infiltrates found at postmortem examination of the brain and the acute polymorphonuclear CSF pleocytosis often occurring during the first 1 to 3 days of disease. In addition, leukocytosis with a left shift is a common feature. A formalin-inactivated vaccine has been used to protect laboratory workers but is not generally available or applicable.

WESTERN EQUINE ENCEPHALITIS

The primary maintenance cycle for western equine encephalitis virus in the United States is between *C. tarsalis* and birds, principally sparrows and finches. Equines and humans become infected, and both species suffer encephalitis without amplifying the virus in nature. St. Louis encephalitis is transmitted in a similar cycle in the same region but causes human disease about a month earlier than the period (July through October) in which western equine encephalitis virus is active. Large epidemics of western equine encephalitis took place in the western and central United States and Canada during the 1930s to 1950s, but in recent years the disease has been uncommon. There were 41 reported cases in the United States in 1987 but only 4 reported cases from 1988 to 1995. This decline in incidence may reflect in part the integrated approach to mosquito management that has been employed in irrigation projects and the increasing use of agricultural pesticides; it almost certainly reflects the increased tendency for humans to be indoors behind closed windows at dusk, the peak period of biting by the major vector.

Western equine encephalitis virus causes a typical diffuse viral encephalitis with an increased attack rate and increased morbidity in the young, particularly children <2 years old. In addition, mortality is high among the young and the very elderly. One-third of individuals who have convulsions during the acute illness have subsequent seizure activity. Infants <1 year old—particularly those in the first months of life—are at serious risk of motor and intellectual damage. Twice as many males as females develop clinical encephalitis after 5 to 9 years of age; this difference may be related to greater outdoor exposure of boys to the vector but is also likely due in part to biologic differences. A formalin-inactivated vaccine has been used to protect laboratory workers but is not generally available or applicable.

VENEZUELAN EQUINE ENCEPHALITIS   There are six known types of virus in the Venezuelan equine encephalitis complex. An important distinction is between the "epizootic" viruses (subtypes IAB and IC) and the "enzootic" viruses (subtypes ID to IF and types II to VI). The epizootic viruses have an unknown natural cycle but periodically cause extensive epidemics in equines and humans in the Americas. These epidemics rely on the high-level viremia in horses and mules that results in the infection of several species of mosquitoes, which in turn infect humans and perpetuate virus transmission. Humans also have high-level viremia but probably are not important in virus transmission. Enzootic viruses are found primarily in humid tropical forest habitats and are maintained between *Culex* mosquitoes and rodents; these viruses cause human disease but are not pathogenic for horses and do not cause epizootics.

Epizootics of Venezuelan equine encephalitis occurred repeatedly in Venezuela, Colombia, Ecuador, Peru, and other South American countries at intervals of ≤10 years from the 1930s until 1969, when a massive epizootic spread throughout Central America and Mexico, reaching southern Texas in 1972. Genetic sequencing of the virus from the 1969 to 1972 outbreak suggested that it originated from residual "un-inactivated" virus in veterinary vaccines. The outbreak was terminated in Texas with the use of a live attenuated vaccine (TC-83) originally developed for human use by the U.S. Army; this virus was then used for further production of inactivated veterinary vaccines. No further epizootic disease was identified until 1995 and subsequently, when additional epizootics took place in Colombia, Venezuela, and Mexico. The viruses involved in these epizootics as well as previously epizootic subtype IC viruses have been shown to be close phylogenetic relatives of known enzootic subtype ID viruses. This finding suggests that active evolution and selection of epizootic viruses are under way in northern South America.

During epizootics, extensive human infection is the rule, with clinical disease in 10 to 60% of infected individuals. Most infections result in notable acute febrile disease, while relatively few result in encephalitis. A low rate of CNS invasion is supported by the absence of encephalitis among the many infections resulting from exposure to aerosols in the laboratory or from vaccine accidents. The most recent large epizootic of Venezuelan equine encephalitis occurred in Colombia and Venezuela in 1995; of the more than 85,000 clinical cases, 4% (with a higher proportion among children than adults) included neurologic symptoms and 300 ended in death.

Enzootic strains of Venezuelan equine encephalitis virus are common causes of acute febrile disease, particularly in areas such as the Florida Everglades and the humid Atlantic coast of Central America. Encephalitis has been documented only in the Florida infections; the three cases were caused by type II enzootic virus, also called *Everglades virus*. All three patients had preexisting cerebral disease. Extrapolation from the rate of genetic change suggests that Everglades virus may have been introduced into Florida <200 years ago and that it is most closely related to the ID subtypes that appear to have given evolutionary rise to the epizootic strains active in South America.

The prevention of epizootic Venezuelan equine encephalitis depends on vaccination of horses with the attenuated TC-83 vaccine or with an inactivated vaccine prepared from that strain. Humans can be protected with similar vaccines, but the use of such products is restricted to laboratory personnel because of reactogenicity and limited availability. In addition, wild-type virus and perhaps TC-83 vaccine may have some degree of fetal pathogenicity. Enzootic viruses are genetically and antigenically different from epizootic viruses, and protection against the former with vaccines prepared from the latter is relatively ineffective.

ARTHRITIS AND RASH

True arthritis is a common accompaniment of several viral diseases, such as rubella (caused by a non-alphavirus togavirus), parvovirus B19 infection, and hepatitis B; it is an occasional accompaniment of infection due to mumps virus, enteroviruses, herpesviruses, and adenoviruses. It is not generally appreciated that the alphaviruses are also common causes of arthritis. In fact, the alphaviruses discussed below all cause acute febrile diseases accompanied by the development of true arthritis and a maculopapular rash. Rheumatic involvement includes arthralgia alone, periarticular swelling, and (less commonly) joint effusions. Most of these diseases are less severe and have fewer articular manifestations in children than in adults. In temperate climates, these are summer diseases. No specific therapy or licensed vaccines exist.

SINDBIS VIRUS INFECTION   Sindbis virus is transmitted among birds by mosquitoes. Infections with the northern European strains of this virus (which cause, for example, Pogosta disease in Finland, Karelian fever in the independent states of the former Soviet Union, and Okelbo disease in Sweden) and with the genetically related southern African strains are particularly likely to result in the arthritis-rash syndrome. Exposure to a rural environment is commonly associated with this infection, which has an incubation period of <1 week.

The disease begins with rash and arthralgia. Constitutional symptoms are not marked, and fever is modest or lacking altogether. The rash, which lasts about a week, begins on the trunk, spreads to the extremities, and evolves from macules to papules that often vesiculate. The arthritis of this condition is multiarticular, migratory, and incapacitating, with resolution of the acute phase in a few days. Wrists, ankles, phalangeal joints, knees, elbows, and—to a much lesser extent—proximal and axial joints are involved. Persistence of joint pains and occasionally of arthritis is a major problem and may go on for months or even years despite a lack of deformity.

CHIKUNGUNYA VIRUS INFECTION   It is likely that chikungunya virus ("that which bends up") is of African origin and is maintained among nonhuman primates on that continent by *Aedes* mosquitoes of the subgenus *Stegomyia* in a fashion similar to yellow fever virus. Like yellow fever virus, chikungunya virus is readily transmitted among humans in urban areas by *A. aegypti*. The *A. aegypti*–chikungunya virus transmission cycle has also been introduced into Asia, where it poses a prominent health problem. The disease is endemic in rural areas of Africa, and intermittent epidemics take place in towns and cities of Africa and Asia. Chikungunya is one more reason (in addition to dengue and yellow fever) that *A. aegypti* must be controlled.

Full-blown disease is most common among adults, in whom the clinical picture may be dramatic. The brusque onset follows an incubation period of 2 to 3 days. Fever and severe arthralgia are accompanied by chills and constitutional symptoms such as headache, photophobia, conjunctival injection, anorexia, nausea, and abdominal pain. Migratory polyarthritis mainly affects the small joints of the hands, wrists, ankles, and feet, with lesser involvement of the larger joints. Rash may appear at the outset or several days into the illness; its development often coincides with defervescence, which takes place around day 2 or day 3 of disease. The rash is most intense on the trunk and limbs and may desquamate. Petechiae are occasionally seen, and epistaxis is not uncommon, but this virus is not a regular cause of the HF syndrome, even in children. A few patients develop leukopenia. Elevated levels of aspartate aminotransferase (AST) and C-reactive protein have been described, as have mildly decreased platelet counts. Recovery may require weeks. Some older patients continue to suffer from stiffness, joint pain, and recurrent effusions for several years; this persistence may be especially common in HLA-B27 patients. An investigational live attenuated vaccine has been developed but requires further testing.

A related virus, O'nyong-nyong, caused a major epidemic of arthritis and rash involving at least 2 million people as it moved across eastern and central Africa in the 1960s. After its mysterious emergence, the virus virtually disappeared, leaving only occasional evidence of its persistence in Kenya until a transient resurgence of epidemic activity in 1997.

MAYARO FEVER Mayaro virus is maintained in the forests of the Americas by *Haemagogus* mosquitoes and nonhuman primates. It causes a frequently endemic and sometimes epidemic infection of humans and appears to produce a syndrome resembling chikungunya.

EPIDEMIC POLYARTHRITIS (ROSS RIVER VIRUS INFECTION) Ross River virus has caused epidemics of distinctive clinical disease in Australia since the beginning of the twentieth century and continues to be responsible for thousands of cases in rural and suburban areas annually. The virus is transmitted by *A. vigilax* and other mosquitoes, and its persistence is thought to involve transovarial transmission. No definitive vertebrate host has been identified, but several mammalian species, including wallabies, have been suggested. Endemic transmission has also been documented in New Guinea, and in 1979 the virus swept through the eastern Pacific Islands, causing hundreds of thousands of illnesses. The virus was carried from island to island by infected humans and was believed to have been transmitted among humans by *A. polynesiensis* and *A. aegypti*.

The incubation period is 7 to 11 days long, and the onset of illness is sudden, with joint pain usually ushering in the disease. The rash generally develops coincidentally or follows shortly but in some cases precedes joint pains by several days. Constitutional symptoms such as low-grade fever, asthenia, myalgia, headache, and nausea are not prominent and indeed are absent in many cases. Most patients are incapacitated for considerable periods by joint involvement, which interferes with sleeping, walking, and grasping. Wrist, ankle, metacarpophalangeal, interphalangeal, and knee joints are the most commonly involved, although toes, shoulders, and elbows may be affected with some frequency. Periarticular swelling and tenosynovitis are common, and one-third of patients have true arthritis. Only half of all arthritis patients can resume normal activities within 4 weeks, and 10% still must limit their activity at 3 months. Occasional patients are symptomatic for 1 to 3 years but without progressive arthropathy. Aspirin and nonsteroidal anti-inflammatory drugs are effective for the treatment of symptoms.

Clinical laboratory values are normal or variable in Ross River virus infection. Tests for rheumatoid factor and antinuclear antibodies are negative, and the erythrocyte sedimentation rate is acutely elevated. Joint fluid contains 1000 to 60,000 mononuclear cells per microliter, and Ross River virus antigen is demonstrable in macrophages. IgM antibodies are valuable in the diagnosis of this infection, although they occasionally persist for years. The isolation of the virus from blood by mosquito inoculation or mosquito cell culture is possible early in the illness. Because of the great economic impact of annual epidemics in Australia, an inactivated vaccine is being developed and has been found to be protective in mice.

Perhaps because of the local interest in arboviruses in general and in Ross River virus in particular, other arthritogenic arboviruses have been identified in Australia, including Gan Gan virus, a member of the family Bunyaviridae; Kokobera virus, a flavivirus; and Barmah Forest virus, an alphavirus. The last virus is a common cause of infection and must be differentiated from Ross River virus by specific testing.

HEMORRHAGIC FEVERS

The viral HF syndrome is a constellation of findings based on vascular instability and decreased vascular integrity. An assault, direct or indirect, on the microvasculature leads to increased permeability and (particularly when platelet function is decreased) to actual disruption and local hemorrhage. Blood pressure is decreased, and in severe cases shock supervenes. Cutaneous flushing and conjunctival suffusion are examples of common, observable abnormalities in the control of local circulation. The hemorrhage is inconstant and is in most cases an indication of widespread vascular damage rather than a life-threatening loss of blood volume. Disseminated intravascular coagulation is occasionally found in any severely ill patient with HF but is thought to occur regularly only in the early phases of HF with renal syndrome, Crimean Congo HF, and perhaps some cases of filovirus HF. In some viral HF syndromes, specific organs may be particularly impaired, such as the kidney in HF with renal syndrome, the lung in hantavirus pulmonary syndrome, or the liver in yellow fever, but in all these diseases the generalized circulatory disturbance is critically important.

The pathogenesis of HF is poorly understood and varies among the viruses regularly implicated in the syndrome, which number more than a dozen. In some cases direct damage to the vascular system or even to parenchymal cells of target organs is important, whereas in others soluble mediators are thought to play the major role. The acute phase in most cases of HF is associated with ongoing virus replication and viremia. Exceptions are the hantavirus diseases and dengue HF/dengue shock syndrome (DHF/DSS), in which the immune response plays a major pathogenic role.

The HF syndromes all begin with fever and myalgia, usually of abrupt onset. Within a few days the patient presents for medical attention because of increasing prostration that is often accompanied by severe headache, dizziness, photophobia, hyperesthesia, abdominal or chest pain, anorexia, nausea or vomiting, and other gastrointestinal disturbances. Initial examination often reveals only an acutely ill patient with conjunctival suffusion, tenderness to palpation of muscles or abdomen, and borderline hypotension or postural hypotension, perhaps with tachycardia. Petechiae (often best visualized in the axillae), flushing of the head and thorax, periorbital edema, and proteinuria are common. Levels of AST are usually elevated at presentation or within a day or two thereafter. Hemoconcentration from vascular leakage, which is usually evident, is most marked in hantavirus diseases and in DHF/DSS. The seriously ill patient progresses to more severe symptoms and develops shock and other findings typical of the causative virus. Shock, multifocal bleeding, and CNS involvement (encephalopathy, coma, convulsions) are all poor prognostic signs.

One of the major diagnostic clues is travel to an endemic area within the incubation period for a given syndrome (Table 198-4). Except for Seoul, dengue, and yellow fever virus infections, which have urban vectors, travel to a rural setting is especially suggestive of a diagnosis of HF.

Early recognition is important because of the need for virus-specific therapy and supportive measures, including prompt, atraumatic hospitalization; judicious fluid therapy that takes into account the patient's increased capillary permeability; administration of cardiotonic drugs; use of pressors to maintain blood pressure at levels that will support renal perfusion; treatment of the relatively common secondary bacterial infections; replacement of clotting factors and platelets as indicated; and the usual precautionary measures used in the treatment of patients with hemorrhagic diatheses. Disseminated intravascular coagulation should be treated only if clear laboratory evidence of its existence is found and if laboratory monitoring of therapy is feasible; there is no proven benefit of such therapy. The available evidence suggests that HF patients have a decreased cardiac output and will respond poorly to fluid loading as it is often practiced in the treatment of shock associated with bacterial sepsis. Specific therapy is available for several of the HF syndromes. In addition, several diseases considered in the differential diagnosis—malaria, shigellosis, typhoid, leptospirosis, relapsing fever, and rickettsial disease—are treatable and potentially lethal. Strict barrier nursing and other precautions against infection of medical staff and visitors are indicated in HF except that due to hantaviruses, yellow fever, Rift Valley fever, and dengue.

LASSA FEVER Lassa virus is known to cause endemic and epidemic disease in Nigeria, Sierra Leone, Guinea, and Liberia, al-

Table 198-4 Viral Hemorrhagic Fever (HF) Syndromes and Their Distribution

Disease	Incubation Period, Days	Case-Infection Ratio	Case-Fatality Rate, %	Geographic Range	Target Population
Lassa fever	5–16	Mild infections probably common	15	West Africa	All ages, both sexes
South American HF	7–14	Most infections (more than half) result in disease	15–30	Selected rural areas of Bolivia, Argentina, Venezuela, and Brazil	Bolivia: Men in countryside; all ages, both sexes in villages. Argentina: All ages, both sexes; excess exposure and disease in men. Venezuela: All ages, both sexes
Rift Valley fever	2–5	~1:100 (most infections result in fever and myalgia)	~50	Sub-Saharan Africa, Madagascar, Egypt	All ages, both sexes; more often diagnosed in men; preexisting liver disease may predispose
Crimean Congo HF	3–12	≧1:5 or higher	15–30	Africa, Middle East, Balkans, southern region of former Soviet Union, western China	All ages, both sexes; men more exposed in some settings
HF with renal syndrome	9–35	Hantaan, >1:1.25; Puumala, 1:20	5–15, Hantaan; <1, Puumala	Worldwide, depending on rodent reservoir	Excess of male patients (partly due to greater exposure); mainly adults
Hantavirus pulmonary syndrome	~7–28	Very high	40–50	Americas	Excess of male patients due to some occupational exposure; mainly adults
Marburg or Ebola HF	3–16	High	25–90	Sub-Saharan Africa	All ages, both sexes; children less exposed
Yellow fever	3–6	1:2–1:20	20	Africa, South America	All ages, both sexes; adults more exposed in jungle setting; preexisting flavivirus immunity may cross-protect
Dengue HF/dengue shock syndrome	2–7	1:10,000, nonimmune; 1:100, heterologous immune	<1 with supportive treatment	Tropics and subtropics worldwide	Predominantly children; previous heterologous dengue infection predisposes to HF
Kyasanur Forest/ Omsk HF	3–8	Variable	0.5–10	Mysore State, India/ western Siberia	Variable

though it is probably more widely distributed in West Africa. This virus and its relatives exist elsewhere in Africa, but their health significance is unknown. Like other arenaviruses, Lassa virus is spread to humans by small-particle aerosols from chronically infected rodents and may also be acquired during the capture or eating of these animals. It can be transmitted by close person-to-person contact. The virus is often present in urine during convalescence and is suspected to be present in seminal fluid early in recovery. Nosocomial spread has occurred but is uncommon if proper sterile parenteral techniques are used. People of all ages and both sexes are affected; the incidence of disease is highest in the dry season, but transmission takes place year-round. In countries where Lassa virus is endemic, Lassa fever can be a prominent cause of febrile disease. For example, in one hospital in Sierra Leone, laboratory-confirmed Lassa fever is consistently responsible for one-fifth of admissions to the medical wards. There are probably tens of thousands of Lassa fever cases annually in West Africa alone.

The average case has a gradual onset (among the HF agents, only the arenaviruses are typically associated with a gradual onset) that gives way to more severe constitutional symptoms and prostration. Bleeding is seen in only ~15 to 30% of cases. A maculopapular rash is often noted in light-skinned Lassa patients. Effusions are common, and male-dominant pericarditis may develop late. The fetal death rate is 92% in the last trimester, when maternal mortality is also increased from the usual 15% to 30%; these figures suggest that interruption of the pregnancy of infected women should be considered. White blood cell counts are normal or slightly elevated, and platelet counts are normal or somewhat low. Deafness coincides with clinical improvement in ~20% of cases and is permanent and bilateral in some. Reinfection may occur but has not been associated with severe disease.

High-level viremia or a high serum concentration of AST statistically predicts a fatal outcome. Thus patients with an AST level of >150 IU/mL should be treated with intravenous ribavirin. This antiviral nucleoside analogue appears to be effective in reducing mortality from rates among retrospective controls, and its only major side effect is reversible anemia that usually does not require transfusion. The drug should be given by slow intravenous infusion in a dose of 32 mg/kg; this dose should be followed by 16 mg/kg q6h for 4 days and then by 8 mg/kg q8h for 6 days.

SOUTH AMERICAN HF SYNDROMES (ARGENTINE, BOLIVIAN, VENEZUELAN, AND BRAZILIAN) These diseases are similar to one another clinically, but their epidemiology differs with the habits of their rodent reservoirs and the interactions of these animals with humans (Table 198-4). Person-to-person or nosocomial transmission is rare but has occurred.

The basic disease resembles Lassa fever with two marked differences. First, thrombocytopenia—often marked—is the rule, and bleeding is quite common. Second, CNS dysfunction is much more common than in Lassa fever and is often manifest by marked confusion, tremors of the upper extremities and tongue, and cerebellar signs. Some cases follow a predominantly neurologic course, with a poor prognosis. The clinical laboratory is helpful in diagnosis since thrombocytopenia, leukopenia, and proteinuria are typical findings.

Argentine HF is readily treated with convalescent-phase plasma given within the first 8 days of illness. In the absence of passive antibody therapy, intravenous ribavirin in the dose recommended for Lassa fever is likely to be effective in all the South American HF syndromes. The transmission of the disease from men convalescing from Argentine HF to their wives suggests the need for counseling of arenavirus HF patients concerning the avoidance of intimate contacts for several weeks after recovery. A safe, effective, live attenuated vaccine exists for Argentine HF. In experimental animals, this vaccine is cross-protective against the Bolivian HF virus.

RIFT VALLEY FEVER   This mosquito-borne virus is also a pathogen of domestic animals such as sheep, cattle, and goats. It is maintained in nature by transovarial transmission in floodwater *Aedes* mosquitoes and presumably also has a vertebrate amplifier. Epizootics and epidemics occur when sheep or cattle become infected during particularly heavy rains; developing high-level viremia, these animals infect many different species of mosquitoes. Remote sensing via satellite can detect the ecologic changes associated with high rainfall that predict the likelihood of Rift Valley fever transmission; it can also detect the special depressions from which the floodwater *Aedes* mosquito vectors emerge. In addition, the virus is infectious when transmitted by contact with blood or aerosols from domestic animals or their abortuses. The slaughtered meat is not infectious; anaerobic glycolysis in postmortem tissues results in an acidic environment that rapidly inactivates Bunyaviridae such as Rift Valley fever virus and Crimean-Congo HF virus. The natural range of Rift Valley fever virus is confined to sub-Saharan Africa, where its circulation is markedly enhanced by substantial rainfall such as that which occurred during the El Niño phenomenon of 1997. The virus has also been found in Madagascar and has been introduced into Egypt, where it caused major epidemics in 1977 to 1979, 1993, and subsequently. Neither person-to-person nor nosocomial transmission has been documented.

Rift Valley fever virus is unusual in that it causes at least four different clinical syndromes. Most infections are manifested as the febrile-myalgic syndrome. A small proportion result in HF with especially prominent liver involvement. Perhaps 10% of otherwise mild infections lead to retinal vasculitis; funduscopic examination reveals edema, hemorrhages, and infarction, and some patients have permanently impaired vision. A small proportion of cases (<1 in 200) are followed by typical viral encephalitis. One of the complicated syndromes does not appear to predispose to another.

There is no proven therapy for any of the syndromes described above. The sensitivity of animal models of Rift Valley fever to antibody or ribavirin therapy suggests that either could be given intravenously to persons with HF. Both retinal disease and encephalitis occur after the acute febrile syndrome has ended and serum neutralizing antibody has developed—events suggesting that only supportive care need be given. Epidemic disease is best prevented by vaccination of livestock. The established ability of this virus to propagate after an introduction into Egypt suggests that other potentially receptive areas, including the United States, should have a response ready for such an eventuality. It seems likely that this disease, like Venezuelan equine encephalitis, can be controlled only with adequate stocks of an effective live attenuated vaccine, and there are no such global stocks. A formalin-inactivated vaccine confers immunity to humans, but quantities are limited and three injections are required; this vaccine is recommended for exposed laboratory workers and for veterinarians working in sub-Saharan Africa.

CRIMEAN CONGO HF   This severe HF syndrome has a wide geographic distribution, potentially being found wherever ticks of the genus *Hyalomma* occur (Table 198-4). The propensity of these ticks to feed on domestic livestock and certain wild mammals means that veterinary serosurveys are the most effective mechanism for the surveillance of virus circulation in a region. Human infection is acquired via a tick bite or during the crushing of infected ticks. Domestic animals do not become ill but do develop viremia; thus there is danger

of infection at the time of slaughter and for a brief interval thereafter (through contact with hides or carcasses). Cases have followed sheep shearing. An epidemic in South Africa was associated with slaughter of tick-infested ostriches. Nosocomial epidemics are common and are usually related to extensive blood exposure or needle sticks.

Although generally similar to other HF syndromes, Crimean Congo HF causes extensive liver damage, resulting in jaundice in some cases. Clinical laboratory values indicate disseminated intravascular coagulation and show elevations in AST, creatine phosphokinase, and bilirubin. Patients with fatal cases generally have more marked changes, even in the early days of illness, and also develop leukocytosis rather than leukopenia. Thrombocytopenia is also more marked and develops earlier in cases with a fatal outcome.

No controlled trials have been performed with intravenous ribavirin, but clinical experience and retrospective comparison of patients with ominous clinical laboratory values suggest that ribavirin is efficacious and should be given. No human or veterinary vaccines are recommended.

HF WITH RENAL SYNDROME   This disease, the first to be identified as an HF, is widely distributed over Europe and Asia; the major causative viruses and their rodent reservoirs on these two continents are Puumala virus (bank vole, *Clethrionomys glareolus*) and Hantaan virus (striped field mouse, *Apodemus agrarius*), respectively. Other potential causative viruses exist, including Dobrava virus (yellow-necked field mouse, *A. flavicollus*), which causes severe HF with renal syndrome in the Balkans. Seoul virus is associated with the Norway or sewer rat, *Rattus norvegicus*, and has a worldwide distribution through the migration of the rodent; it is associated with mild or moderate HF with renal syndrome in Asia, but in many areas of the world the human disease has been difficult to identify. Most cases occur in rural residents or vacationers; the exception is Seoul virus disease, which may be acquired in an urban or rural setting or from contaminated laboratory rat colonies. Classic Hantaan disease in Korea (Korean HF) and in rural China (epidemic HF) is most common in spring and fall and is related to rodent density and agricultural practices. Human infection is acquired primarily through aerosols of rodent urine, although virus is also present in saliva and feces. Patients with hantavirus diseases are not infectious. HF with renal syndrome is the most important form of HF today, with more than 100,000 cases of severe disease in Asia annually and milder Puumala infections numbering in the thousands as well.

Severe cases of HF with renal syndrome caused by Hantaan virus evolve in identifiable stages: the febrile stage with myalgia, lasting 3 to 4 days; the hypotensive stage, often associated with shock and lasting from a few hours to 48 h; the oliguric stage with renal failure, lasting 3 to 10 days; and the polyuric stage with diuresis and hyposthenuria.

The *febrile period* is initiated by the abrupt onset of fever, headache, severe myalgia, thirst, anorexia, and often nausea and vomiting. Photophobia, retroorbital pain, and pain on ocular movement are common, and the vision may become blurred with ciliary body inflammation. Flushing over the face, the V area of the neck, and the back are characteristic, as are pharyngeal injection, periorbital edema, and conjunctival suffusion. Petechiae often develop in areas of pressure, the conjunctivae, and the axillae. Back pain and tenderness to percussion at the costovertebral angle reflect massive retroperitoneal edema. Laboratory evidence of mild to moderate disseminated intravascular coagulation is present. Other laboratory findings include proteinuria and an active urinary sediment.

The *hypotensive phase* is ushered in by falling blood pressure and sometimes by shock. The relative bradycardia typical of the febrile phase is replaced by tachycardia. Kinin activation is marked. The rising hematocrit reflects increasing vascular leakage. Leukocytosis with a left shift develops, and thrombocytopenia continues. Atypical lymphocytes—which in fact are activated CD8+ and to a lesser extent CD4+ T cells—circulate. Proteinuria is marked, and the urine's specific gravity falls to 1.010. The renal circulation is congested and compromised from local and systemic circulatory changes resulting in necrosis of tubules, particularly at the corticomedullary junction, and oliguria.

During the *oliguric phase*, hemorrhagic tendencies continue, probably in large part because of uremic bleeding defects. The oliguria persists for 3 to 10 days before renal function returns and marks the onset of the *polyuric stage*, which carries the danger of dehydration and electrolyte abnormalities.

Mild cases of HF with renal syndrome may be much less stereotypical. The presentation may include only fever, gastrointestinal abnormalities, and transient oliguria followed by hyposthenuria.

HF with renal syndrome should be suspected in patients with rural exposure in an endemic area. Prompt recognition of the disease will permit rapid hospitalization and expectant management of shock and renal failure. Useful clinical laboratory parameters include leukocytosis, which may be leukemoid and is associated with a left shift; thrombocytopenia; and proteinuria. Mainstays of therapy are the management of shock, reliance on pressors, modest crystalloid infusion, intravenous use of human serum albumin, and treatment of renal failure with prompt dialysis for the usual indications. Hydration may result in pulmonary edema, and hypertension should be avoided because of the possibility of intracranial hemorrhage. Use of intravenous ribavirin has reduced mortality and morbidity in severe cases provided treatment is begun within the first 4 days of illness. The case-fatality ratio may be as high as 15% but with proper therapy should be <5%. Sequelae have not been definitely established, but there is a correlation in the United States between chronic hypertensive renal failure and the presence of antibodies to Seoul virus.

Infections with Puumala virus, the most common cause of HF with renal syndrome in Europe, result in a much attenuated picture but the same general presentation. The syndrome may be referred to by its former name, *nephropathia epidemica*. Bleeding manifestations are found in only 10% of cases, hypotension rather than shock is usually seen, and oliguria is present in only about half of patients. The dominant features may be fever, abdominal pain, proteinuria, mild oliguria, and sometimes blurred vision or glaucoma followed by polyuria and hyposthenuria in recovery. Mortality is <1%.

The diagnosis is readily made by IgM-capture ELISA, which should be positive at admission or within 24 to 48 h thereafter. The isolation of virus is difficult, but RT-PCR of a blood clot collected early in the clinical course or of tissues obtained postmortem will give positive results. Such testing is usually undertaken only if definitive identification of the infecting viral species is required or if molecular epidemiologic questions exist.

HANTAVIRUS PULMONARY SYNDROME   Hantavirus pulmonary syndrome was discovered in 1993, but retrospective identification of cases by immunohistochemistry (1978) and serology (1959) support the idea that it is a recently discovered rather than a truly new disease. The causative viruses are hantaviruses of a distinct phylogenetic lineage that is associated with the rodent subfamily Sigmodontinae. Sin Nombre virus chronically infects the deer mouse (*Peromyscus maniculatus*) and is the most important virus causing hantavirus pulmonary syndrome in the United States. The disease is also caused by a Sin Nombre virus variant from the white-footed mouse (*P. leucopus*), by Black Creek Canal virus (*Sigmodon hispidus*, the cotton rat), and by Bayou virus (*Oryzomys palustris*, the rice rat). Several other related viruses cause the disease in South America, but Andes virus is unusual in that it, alone among hantaviruses, has been implicated in human-to-human transmission. The disease is linked to rodent exposure and particularly affects rural residents living in dwellings permeable to rodent entry or working at occupations that pose a risk of rodent exposure. Each rodent species has its own particular habits; in the case of the deer mouse, these behaviors include living in and around human habitation.

The disease begins with a prodrome of about 3 to 4 days (range,

1 to 11 days) comprising fever, myalgia, malaise, and often gastrointestinal disturbances such as nausea, vomiting, and abdominal pain. Dizziness is common and vertigo occasional. Severe prodromal symptoms bring some individuals to medical attention, but patients are usually recognized as the cardiopulmonary phase begins. Typically, there is slightly lowered blood pressure, tachycardia, tachypnea, mild hypoxemia, and early radiographic signs of pulmonary edema. Physical findings in the chest are often surprisingly scant. The conjunctival and cutaneous signs of vascular involvement seen in other types of HF are absent. During the next few hours, decompensation may progress rapidly to severe hypoxemia and respiratory failure. Most patients surviving the first 48 h of hospitalization are extubated and discharged within a few days, with no apparent residua.

Management during the first few hours after presentation is critical. The goal is to prevent severe hypoxemia by oxygen therapy and, if needed, intubation and intensive respiratory management. During this period, hypotension and shock with increasing hematocrit invite aggressive fluid administration, but this intervention should be undertaken with great caution. Because of low cardiac output with myocardial depression and increased pulmonary vascular permeability, shock should be managed expectantly with pressors and modest infusion of fluid guided by the pulmonary capillary wedge pressure. Mild cases can be managed by frequent monitoring and oxygen administration without intubation. Many patients require intubation to manage hypoxemia and also develop shock. Mortality remains at ~30 to 40% with good management. The antiviral drug ribavirin inhibits the virus in vitro but did not have a marked effect on patients treated in an open-label study.

During the prodrome, the differential diagnosis of hantavirus pulmonary syndrome is difficult, but by the time of presentation or within 24 h thereafter, a number of diagnostically helpful clinical features become apparent. Cough is not usually present at the outset but may develop later. Interstitial edema is evident on the chest x-ray. Later, bilateral alveolar edema with a central distribution develops in the setting of a normal-sized heart; occasionally, the edema is initially unilateral. Pleural effusions are often visualized. Thrombocytopenia, circulating atypical lymphocytes, and a left shift (often with leukocytosis) are almost always evident; thrombocytopenia has been a particularly important early clue. Hemoconcentration, proteinuria, and hypoalbuminemia should also be sought. Although thrombocytopenia virtually always develops and prolongation of the partial thromboplastin time is the rule, clinical evidence for coagulopathy or laboratory indications of disseminated intravascular coagulation are found in only a minority of cases, usually in severely ill patients. Severely ill patients also have acidosis and elevated serum levels of lactate. Mildly increased values in renal function tests are common, but patients with severe cases often have markedly elevated concentrations of serum creatinine; some of the viruses other than Sin Nombre virus have been associated with more kidney involvement, but few such cases have been studied. The differential diagnosis includes abdominal surgical conditions and pyelonephritis as well as rickettsial disease, sepsis, meningococcemia, plague, tularemia, influenza, and relapsing fever.

A specific diagnosis is best made by IgM testing of acute-phase serum, which has yielded positive results even in the prodrome. Tests using a Sin Nombre virus antigen detect the related hantaviruses causing the pulmonary syndrome in the Americas. Occasionally, heterologous viruses will react only in the IgG ELISA, but this finding is highly suspicious given the very low seroprevalence of these viruses in normal populations. RT-PCR is usually positive when used to test blood clots obtained in the first 7 to 9 days of illness as well as tissues; this test is useful in identifying the infecting virus in areas outside the home range of the deer mouse and in atypical cases.

YELLOW FEVER   Yellow fever virus caused major epidemics in the Americas, Africa, and Europe before the discovery of mosquito transmission in 1900 led to its control through attacks on its urban vector, *A. aegypti*. Only then was it found that a jungle cycle also existed in Africa, involving other *Aedes* mosquitoes and monkeys, and that colonization of the New World with *A. aegypti*, originally an African species, had established urban yellow fever as well as an independent sylvatic yellow fever cycle in American jungles involving *Haemagogus* mosquitoes and New World monkeys. Today, urban yellow fever transmission occurs only in some African cities, but the threat exists in the great cities of South America, where reinfestation by *A. aegypti* has taken place and dengue transmission by the same mosquito is common. As late as 1905, New Orleans suffered more than 3000 cases with 452 deaths from "yellow jack." Despite the existence of a highly effective and safe vaccine, several hundred jungle yellow fever cases occur annually in South America, and thousands of jungle and urban cases occur each year in Africa.

Yellow fever is a typical HF accompanied by prominent hepatic necrosis. A period of viremia, typically lasting 3 or 4 days, is followed by a period of "intoxication." During the latter phase in severe cases, the characteristic jaundice, hemorrhages, black vomit, anuria, and terminal delirium occur, perhaps related in part to extensive hepatic involvement. Blood leukocyte counts may be normal or reduced and are often high in terminal stages. Albuminuria is usually noted and may be marked; as renal function fails in terminal or severe cases, the level of blood urea nitrogen rises proportionately. Abnormalities detected in liver function tests range from modest elevations of AST levels in mild cases to severe derangement.

Urban yellow fever can be prevented by the control of *A. aegypti*. The continuing sylvatic cycle requires vaccination of all visitors to areas of potential transmission. With few exceptions (in the very young and the elderly), reactions to vaccine are minimal; immunity is provided within 10 days and lasts for at least 10 years. An egg allergy dictates caution in vaccine administration. Although there are no documented harmful effects of the vaccine on the fetus, pregnant women should be immunized only if they are definitely at risk of yellow fever exposure. Since vaccination has been associated with several cases of encephalitis in children under 6 months of age, it should be delayed until after 12 months of age unless the risk of exposure is very high. Timely information on changes in yellow fever distribution and yellow fever vaccine requirements can be obtained from Health Information for Travelers, Centers for Disease Control and Prevention, Atlanta, GA 30333; by fax request (404-332-4565; document number 220022#); by phone (404-332-4559); or on the World-Wide Web at www.cdc.gov.

DENGUE HEMORRHAGIC FEVER/DENGUE SHOCK SYNDROME A syndrome of HF noted in the 1950s among children in the Philippines and Southeast Asia was soon associated with dengue virus infections, particularly those occurring against a background of previous exposure to another serotype. The transient heterotypic protection after dengue virus infection is replaced within several weeks by the potential for heterotypic infection resulting in typical dengue fever (see above) or—uncommonly—for enhanced disease (secondary DHF/DSS). In rare instances, primary dengue infections lead to an HF syndrome, but much less is known about pathogenesis in this situation. In the past 20 years, *A. aegypti* has progressively reinvaded Latin America and other areas, and frequent travel by infected individuals has introduced multiple strains of dengue virus from many geographic areas. Thus the pattern of hyperendemic transmission of multiple dengue serotypes has now been established in the Americas and the Caribbean and has led to the emergence of DHF/DSS as a major problem there as well. Millions of dengue infections, including many thousands of cases of DHF/DSS, occur annually. The severe syndrome is unlikely to be seen in U.S. citizens since few children have the dengue antibodies that can trigger the pathogenetic cascade when a second infection is acquired.

Macrophage/monocyte infection is central to the pathogenesis of dengue fever and to the origin of DHF/DSS. Previous infection with a heterologous dengue-virus serotype may result in the production of nonprotective antiviral antibodies that nevertheless bind to the virion's surface and through interaction with the Fc receptor focus secondary dengue viruses on the target cell, the result being enhanced infection. The host is also primed for a secondary antibody response when viral antigens are released and immune complexes lead to activation of the classic complement pathway, with consequent phlogistic effects. Cross-reactivity at the T cell level results in the release of physiologically active cytokines, including interferon γ and tumor necrosis factor α. The induction of vascular permeability and shock depends on multiple factors, including the following:

1. *Presence of enhancing and nonneutralizing antibodies*—Transplacental maternal antibody may be present in infants <9 months old, or antibody elicited by previous heterologous dengue infection may be present in older individuals. T cell reactivity is also intimately involved.
2. *Age*—Susceptibility to DHF/DSS drops considerably after 12 years of age.
3. *Sex*—Females are more often affected than males.
4. *Race*—Caucasians are more often affected than blacks.
5. *Nutritional status*—Malnutrition is protective.
6. *Sequence of infection*—For example, serotype 1 followed by serotype 2 seems to be more dangerous than serotype 4 followed by serotype 2.
7. *Infecting serotype*—Type 2 is apparently more dangerous than other serotypes.

In addition, there is considerable variation among strains of a given serotype, with Southeast Asian serotype 2 strains having more potential to cause DHF/DSS than others.

Dengue HF is identified by the detection of bleeding tendencies (tourniquet test, petechiae) or overt bleeding in the absence of underlying causes such as preexisting gastrointestinal lesions. Dengue shock syndrome, usually accompanied by hemorrhagic signs, is much more serious and results from increased vascular permeability leading to shock. In mild DHF/DSS, restlessness, lethargy, thrombocytopenia (<100,000/μL), and hemoconcentration are detected 2 to 5 days after the onset of typical dengue fever, usually at the time of defervescence. The maculopapular rash that often develops in dengue fever may also appear in DHF/DSS. In more severe cases, frank shock is apparent, with low pulse pressure, cyanosis, hepatomegaly, pleural effusions, ascites, and in some cases severe ecchymoses and gastrointestinal bleeding. The period of shock lasts only 1 or 2 days, and most patients respond promptly to close monitoring, oxygen administration, and infusion of crystalloid or—in severe cases—colloid. The case-fatality rates reported vary greatly with case ascertainment and the quality of treatment; however, most DHF/DSS patients respond well to supportive therapy, and overall mortality in an experienced center in the tropics is probably as low as 1%.

A virologic diagnosis can be made by the usual means, although multiple flavivirus infections lead to a broad immune response to several members of the group, and this situation may result in a lack of virus specificity of the IgM and IgG immune responses. A secondary antibody response can be sought with tests against several flavivirus antigens to demonstrate the characteristic wide spectrum of reactivity.

The key to control of both dengue fever and DHF/DSS is the control of *A. aegypti*, which also reduces the risk of urban yellow fever and chikungunya virus circulation. Control efforts have been handicapped by the presence of nondegradable tires and long-lived plastic containers in trash repositories, insecticide resistance, urban poverty, and an inability of the public health community to mobilize the populace to respond to the need to eliminate mosquito breeding sites. Live attenuated dengue vaccines are in the late stages of development and have produced promising results in early tests. Whether vaccines can provide safe, durable immunity to an immunopathologic disease such as DHF/DSS in endemic areas is an issue that will have to be tested, but it is hoped that vaccination will reduce transmission to negligible levels.

KYASANUR FOREST DISEASE AND OMSK HEMORRHAGIC FEVER Kyasanur Forest virus and Omsk HF virus are geographically restricted, tick-borne flaviviruses that cause a syndrome of viral HF during a wave of viremia and that may also enter the CNS to cause subsequent viral encephalitis (see discussion of tick-borne encephalitis above). There is no therapy for these infections, but an inactivated vaccine has been used in India against Kyasanur Forest disease. A new and related virus isolate has been obtained from butchers with HF in the Middle East; the implication is that there are more agents in this group.

FILOVIRUS HEMORRHAGIC FEVER　See Chap. 199.

BIBLIOGRAPHY

ZOONOTIC VIRUSES

CALISHER CH: Medically important arboviruses of the United States and Canada. Clin Microbiol Rev 7:89, 1994

TSAI TF: Arboviral infections in the US. Infect Dis Clin North Am 5:73, 1991

HEMORRHAGIC FEVERS

CENTERS FOR DISEASE CONTROL AND PREVENTION: Management of patients with suspected viral hemorrhagic fever. MMWR 37(S-3):1, 1988

———: Update: Management of patients with suspected viral hemorrhagic fever—United States. MMWR 44:475, 1995

PETERS CJ et al: Management of patients infected with high-hazard viruses. Arch Virol 11(Suppl):141, 1996

——— et al: Pathogenesis of viral hemorrhagic fevers, in *Viral Pathogenesis*, N Nathanson et al (eds). Philadelphia, Lippincott-Raven, 1996

ARENAVIRUSES

BARRY M et al: Treatment of a laboratory-acquired Sabiá virus infection. N Engl J Med 333:294, 1995

ENRIA D, MAIZTEGUI JI: Antiviral treatment of Argentine hemorrhagic fever. Antiviral Res 23:23, 1994

——— et al: Arenaviruses, in *Tropical Infectious Diseases: Principles, Pathogens, & Practice*, RL Guerrant et al (eds). New York, Saunders, 1999, pp 1189–1212

JOHNSON KM et al: Clinical virology of Lassa fever in hospitalized patients. J Infect Dis 155:456, 1987

MCCORMICK JB et al: A case-control study of the clinical diagnosis and course of Lassa fever. J Infect Dis 155:445, 1987

SALAS R et al: Venezuelan hemorrhagic fever. Lancet 338:1033, 1991

BUNYAVIRIDAE

ANTONIADIS A et al: Direct genetic detection of Dobrava virus in Greek and Albanian haemorrhagic fever with renal syndrome (HFRS) patients. J Infect Dis 174:407, 1996

BRUNO P et al: The protean manifestations of hemorrhagic fever with renal syndrome. A retrospective review of 26 cases from Korea. Ann Intern Med 113:385, 1990

DUCHIN JS et al: Hantavirus pulmonary syndrome: A clinical description of 17 patients with a newly recognized disease. N Engl J Med 330:949, 1994

HUGGINS JW et al: Prospective, double-blind, concurrent, placebo controlled clinical trial of intravenous ribavirin therapy of hemorrhagic fever with renal syndrome. J Infect Dis 164:1119, 1991

KETAI LH et al: Hantavirus pulmonary syndrome (HPS): Radiographic findings in 16 patients. Radiology 191:665, 1994

LAUGHLIN LW et al: Epidemic Rift Valley fever in Egypt: Observations of the spectrum of human illness. Trans R Soc Trop Med Hyg 73:630, 1979

PETERS CJ: Hantavirus pulmonary syndrome in the Americas, in *Emerging Infections II*, WM Scheld et al (eds). Washington, DC, ASM Press, 1998, pp 17–64

———, LEDUC JW: Bunyaviridae: Bunyaviruses, phleboviruses, and related viruses, in *Textbook of Human Virology*, 2d ed, R Belshe (ed). St Louis, Mosby Year Book, 1991, pp 571–614

SEXTON DJ et al: Life-threatening Cache Valley virus infection. N Engl J Med 336:547, 1997

SWANEPOEL R et al: Epidemiologic and clinical features of Crimean-Congo hemorrhagic fever in South Africa. Am J Trop Med Hyg 6:120, 1987

——— et al: The clinical pathology of Crimean-Congo hemorrhagic fever. Rev Infect Dis 11(Suppl 4):S794, 1989

ZAKI SR: Hantavirus-associated diseases, in *The Pathology of Infectious Diseases*, DH Connor et al (eds). Stamford, CT, Appleton & Lange, 1997

FLAVIVIRUSES

BARROS MLB, BOECKEN G: Jungle yellow fever in the central Amazon. Lancet 348:969, 1996

HALSTEAD SB: Antibody, macrophages, dengue virus infection, shock, and hemorrhage: A pathogenic cascade. Rev Infect Dis 11(Suppl 4):S830, 1989

KURANE I et al: Immunopathologic mechanisms of dengue hemorrhagic fever and dengue shock syndrome. Arch Virol 9:59, 1994

LUBY JP: St. Louis encephalitis, Rocio encephalitis, and West Nile fever, in *Kass Hand-*
book of Infectious Diseases. Exotic Viral Infections, JS Porterfield (ed). New York, Chapman and Hall, 1995, pp 183–202

MONATH TP, HEINZ FX: Flaviviruses, in *Fields Virology*, 3d ed, BN Fields et al (eds). Philadelphia, Lippincott-Raven, 1996, pp 961–1034

TSAI T, YU XX: Japanese encephalitis vaccines, in *Vaccines*, 2d ed, SW Plotkin and E Mortimer (eds). Philadelphia, WB Saunders, 1994, pp 671–713

——— et al: West Nile encephalitis epidemic in southeastern Romania. Lancet 352:767, 1998

WALDVOGEL K et al: Severe tick-borne encephalitis following passive immunization. Eur J Pediatr 155:775, 1996

REOVIRUSES

EMMONS RW: Colorado tick fever, in *Handbook Series of Zoonoses, Section B: Viral Zoonoses, vol 1*, GW Beran (ed). Boca Raton, FL, CRC Press, 1981, pp 113–124

MONATH TP, GUIRAKHOO F: Orbiviruses and coltiviruses, in *Fields Virology*, 3d ed, BN Fields et al (eds). Philadelphia, Lippincott-Raven, 1996, pp 1735–1766

TOGAVIRUSES

FRASER JRE: Epidemic polyarthritis and Ross River virus disease. Clin Rheum Dis 12:369, 1986

JOHNSTON RE, PETERS CJ: Alphaviruses, in *Fields Virology*, 3d ed, BN Fields et al (eds). Philadelphia, Lippincott-Raven, 1996, pp 843–898

MACKENZIE JS: Mosquito-borne viruses and epidemic polyarthritis. Med J Aust 164:90, 1996

PHILLIPS DA et al: Clinical and subclinical Barmah Forest virus infection in Queensland. Med J Aust 152:463, 1990

RIVAS F et al: Epidemic Venezuelan equine encephalitis in La Guajira, Colombia, 1995. J Infect Dis 175:828, 1997

199　*C. J. Peters*

FILOVIRIDAE (MARBURG AND EBOLA VIRUSES)

DEFINITION　Both Marburg virus and Ebola virus cause an acute febrile illness associated with high mortality. This illness is characterized by multisystem involvement that begins with the abrupt onset of headache, myalgias, and fever and proceeds to prostration, rash, shock, and often bleeding manifestations. Epidemics usually begin with a single case acquired from an unknown reservoir in nature and spread mainly through close contact with sick persons or their body fluids, either in the home or at the hospital.

ETIOLOGY　The family Filoviridae comprises two antigenically and genetically distinct viruses: Marburg virus and Ebola virus. Ebola virus has four readily distinguishable subtypes named for their original site of recognition (Zaire, Sudan, Cote d'Ivoire, and Reston). Except for Ebola virus subtype Reston, all the Filoviridae are African viruses that cause severe and often fatal disease in humans. The Reston virus, which has been exported from the Philippines on several occasions, has caused fatal infections in monkeys but only subclinical infections in humans. Different isolates of the four Ebola subtypes made over time and space exhibit remarkable sequence conservation, indicating marked genetic stability in their selective niche. Typical filovirus particles contain a single linear, negative-sense, single-stranded RNA arranged in a helical nucleocapsid. The virions are 790 to 970 nm in length; they may also appear in elongated, contorted forms. The lipid envelope confers sensitivity to lipid solvents and common detergents. The viruses are largely destroyed by heat (60°C, 30 min) and by acidity but may persist for weeks in blood at room temperature. The surface glycoprotein self-associates to form the virion surface spikes, which presumably mediate attachment to cells and fusion. The glycoprotein's high sugar content may contribute to its low capacity to elicit neutralizing antibodies. A smaller form of the glycoprotein, bearing many of its antigenic determinants, is produced by in vitro–infected cells and is found in the circulation in human disease; it has been speculated that this circulating soluble protein may suppress the immune response to the virion surface protein or block antiviral effector mechanisms. Both Marburg virus and Ebola virus are biosafety

EPIDEMIOLOGY Marburg virus was first identified in Germany in 1967, when infected African green monkeys (*Cercopithecus aethiops*) imported from Uganda transmitted the agent to vaccine-laboratory workers. Of the 25 human cases acquired from monkeys, 7 ended in death. The six secondary cases were associated with close contact or parenteral exposure. Secondary spread to the wife of one patient was documented, and virus was isolated from the husband's semen despite the presence of circulating antibodies. Subsequently, isolated cases of Marburg virus infection have been reported from eastern and southern Africa, with limited spread.

In 1999, repeated transmission of Marburg virus to workers in a gold mine in eastern Democratic Republic of Congo was documented. The secondary spread of the virus among patients' families was more extensive than previously noted, resembling that of Ebola virus and emphasizing the importance of hygiene and proper barrier nursing in the epidemiology of these viruses in Africa.

In 1976, epidemics of severe hemorrhagic fever (550 human cases) occurred simultaneously in Zaire and Sudan, and Ebola virus was found to be the etiologic agent. Later, it was shown that different subtypes of virus—associated with 90% and 50% mortality, respectively—caused the two epidemics. Both epidemics were associated with interhuman spread (particularly in the hospital setting) and the use of unsterilized needles and syringes, a common practice in developing-country hospitals. The epidemics dwindled as the clinics were closed and people in the endemic area increasingly shunned affected persons and avoided traditional burial practices.

The Zaire subtype of Ebola virus recurred in a major epidemic (317 cases, 88% mortality) in Democratic Republic of Congo in 1995 and in smaller epidemics in Gabon in 1994–1996. Mortality was high, transmission to caregivers and others who had direct contact with body fluids was common, and poor hygiene in hospitals exacerbated spread. In the Congo epidemic, an index case was infected in Kikwit in January 1995. The epidemic smoldered until April, when intense nosocomial transmission forced closure of the hospitals; samples were finally sent to the laboratory for Ebola testing, which yielded positive results within a few hours. International assistance, with barrier nursing instruction and materials, was provided; nosocomial transmission ceased, hospitals reopened, and patients were segregated to prevent intrafamilial spread. The last case was reported in June 1995.

Three separate emergences of Ebola virus (subtype Zaire) were detected in Gabon from 1994 through 1996, all associated with deep forest exposure and subsequent familial and nosocomial transmission. In the 1996 episode, a physician exposed to Ebola-infected patients traveled to South Africa with a fever; a nurse who assisted in a cutdown on the physician developed Ebola hemorrhagic fever and died in spite of intensive care. The index patient was identified retrospectively on the basis of serum antibodies and virus isolation from semen. Thus, distant transport of Ebola virus is an established risk, and limited nosocomial spread is possible even under hygienic conditions.

The Reston subtype of Ebola virus was first seen in the United States in 1989, when it caused a fatal, highly transmissible disease among cynomolgus macaques imported from the Philippines and quarantined in Reston, VA, pending distribution to biomedical researchers. This and other appearances of the Reston virus have been traced to a single export facility in the Philippines, but no source in nature has been established.

Epidemiologic studies (including a specific search in the Kikwit epidemic) have failed to yield evidence for an important role of airborne particles in human disease. This lack of epidemiologic evidence is surprising and seems to conflict with the viruses' classification as biosafety level 4 pathogens based in part on their aerosol infectivity and with formal laboratory assessments showing a high degree of aerosol infectivity for monkeys. Sick humans apparently do not usually generate sufficient amounts of infectious aerosols to pose a significant hazard to those around them.

Available evidence points to a nonprimate reservoir for these viruses, but an intensive search has failed to elucidate what this reservoir might be. Speculation has centered on a possible role for bats, but that hypothesis has arisen in part merely because of the ubiquity of bats when sought in affected areas and the frustration of researchers in identifying a source of virus.

PATHOLOGY AND PATHOGENESIS In humans and in animal models, Ebola and Marburg viruses replicate well in virtually all cell types, including endothelial cells, macrophages, and parenchymal cells of multiple organs. Viral replication is associated with cellular necrosis both in vivo and in vitro. Significant findings at the light-microscopic level include liver necrosis with Councilman bodies (intracellular inclusions that correlate with extensive collections of viral nucleocapsids), interstitial pneumonitis, cerebral glial nodules, and small infarcts. Antigen and virions are abundant in fibroblasts, interstitium, and (to a lesser extent) the appendages of the subcutaneous tissues in fatal cases; escape through small breaks in the skin or possibly through sweat glands may occur and, if so, may be correlated with the established epidemiologic risk of close contact with patients and the touching of the deceased. Inflammatory cells are not prominent, even in necrotic areas.

In addition to sustaining direct damage from viral infection, patients infected with Ebola virus (Zaire subtype) have high circulating levels of proinflammatory cytokines, which presumably contribute to the severity of the illness. In fact, the virus interacts intimately with the cellular cytokine system. It is resistant to the antiviral effects of interferon α, although this mediator is amply induced. Viral infection of endothelial cells selectively inhibits the expression of MHC class I molecules and blocks the induction of several genes by the interferons. In addition, glycoprotein expression inhibits αV integrin expression, an effect that has been shown in vitro to lead to detachment and subsequent death of endothelial cells.

Acute infection is associated with high levels of circulating virus and viral antigen. Clinical improvement takes place when viral titers decrease concomitantly with the onset of a virus-specific immune response, as detected by enzyme-linked immunosorbent assay (ELISA) or fluorescent antibody test. In fatal cases, there is usually little evidence of an antibody response and there is extensive depletion of spleen and lymph nodes. Recovery is apparently mediated by the cellular immune response: convalescent-phase plasma has little in vitro virus-neutralizing capacity and is not protective in passive transfer experiments in monkey and guinea pig models.

CLINICAL MANIFESTATIONS After an incubation period of ~7 to 10 days (range, 3 to 16 days), the patient abruptly develops fever, severe headache, malaise, myalgia, nausea, and vomiting. Continued fever is joined by diarrhea (often severe), chest pain (accompanied by cough), prostration, and depressed mentation. In light-skinned patients (and less often in blacks), a maculopapular rash appears around day 5 to 7 and is followed by desquamation. Bleeding may begin about this time and is apparent from any mucosal site and into the skin. In some epidemics, fewer than half of patients have had overt bleeding, and this manifestation has been absent even in some fatal cases. Additional findings include edema of the face, neck, and/or scrotum; hepatomegaly; flushing; conjunctival injection; and pharyngitis. Around 10 to 12 days after the onset of disease, the sustained fever may break, with improvement and eventual recovery of the patient. Recrudescence of fever may be associated with secondary bacterial infections or possibly with localized virus persistence. Late hepatitis, uveitis, and orchitis have been reported, with isolation of virus from semen or detection of polymerase chain reaction (PCR) products in vaginal secretions for several weeks.

LABORATORY FINDINGS Leukopenia is common early on; neutrophilia has its onset later. Platelet counts fall below (sometimes much below) 50,000/μL. Laboratory evidence of disseminated intravascular coagulation may be found, but its clinical significance and the need for therapy are controversial. Serum levels of alanine and aspartate aminotransferases (particularly the latter) rise progressively, and jaundice develops in some cases. The serum amylase level may be elevated, and this elevation may be associated with abdominal pain suggesting pancreatitis. Proteinuria is usual; decreased kidney function is proportional to shock.

DIAGNOSIS   Most patients acutely ill with Ebola or Marburg viruses have high concentrations of virus in blood. Antigen-detection ELISA is a sensitive, robust diagnostic modality. Virus isolation and reverse transcriptase PCR are also effective and provide additional sensitivity in some cases. Patients who are recovering develop IgM and IgG antibodies that are best detected by ELISA but are also reactive in the less specific fluorescent antibody test. Skin biopsies are an extremely useful adjunct in postmortem diagnosis of Ebola and, to a lesser extent, Marburg virus infections because of the presence of large amounts of viral antigen, the relative safety of obtaining the sample, and the freedom from cold-chain requirements for formalin-fixed tissues.

R_x **TREATMENT**   No virus-specific therapy is available, and, given the extensive viral involvement in fatal cases, supportive treatment may not be as useful as was once hoped. Vigorous treatment of shock should take into account the likelihood of vascular leak in the pulmonary and systemic circulation and of myocardial functional compromise. The membrane fusion mechanism of Ebola resembles that of retroviruses, and the identification of "fusogenic" sequences

suggests that inhibitors of cell entry may be developed. Despite the poor neutralizing capacity of polyclonal convalescent-phase sera, phage display of immunoglobulin mRNA from convalescent bone marrow has produced monoclonal antibodies that have in vitro neutralizing capacity and mediate protection in guinea pig models.

PREVENTION   No vaccine is available, but barrier nursing precautions in African hospitals can greatly decrease the spread of the virus beyond the index case and thus prevent epidemics of filoviruses and other agents as well.

BIBLIOGRAPHY

HARCOURT BH et al: Ebola virus selectively inhibits responses to interferons, but not to IL-1beta in endothelial cells. J Virol 73:3491, 1999

KLENK HD (ed): Marburg and Ebola viruses. Curr Top Microbiol Immunol 235:1, 1999

MALASHKEVICH VN et al: Core structure of the envelope glycoprotein GP2 from Ebola virus at 1.9-Å resolution. Proc Natl Acad Sci USA 96:2662, 1999

MARTINI GA, SIEGERT R (eds): *Marburg Virus Disease.* Berlin, Springer-Verlag, 1971, pp 1–230

PATTYN SR (ed): *Ebola Virus Haemorrhagic Fever.* Amsterdam, Elsevier/North-Holland, 1978, pp 1–436 (Also available at www.itg.be/ebola)

PETERS CJ, LEDUC JW: An introduction to Ebola: The virus and the disease. J Infect Dis 179(Suppl 1): Six, 1999 (Also available at www.journals.uchicago.edu/JID/)

WORLD HEALTH ORGANIZATION: Ebola haemorrhagic fever in Zaire, 1976. Report of an international commission. Bull World Health Organ 56:271, 1978

————: Ebola haemorrhagic fever in Sudan, 1976. Report of a World Health Organization International Study Team. Bull World Health Organ 56:247, 1978

Section 15
FUNGAL AND ALGAL INFECTIONS

200   *John E. Bennett*

DIAGNOSIS AND TREATMENT OF FUNGAL INFECTIONS

MYCOLOGY FUNDAMENTALS

Fungi can appear microscopically as either rounded, budding forms (yeastlike organisms) or hyphae (molds). Yeastlike colonies are smooth, while mold colonies are fuzzy; fungi that grow as yeasts include species of *Candida* and *Cryptococcus*, while fungi that grow as molds include species of *Aspergillus*, *Rhizopus*, and dermatophytes (ringworm fungi). The fungi that cause histoplasmosis, blastomycosis, sporotrichosis, coccidioidomycosis, and paracoccidioidomycosis are called *dimorphic* ("having two forms") because they are spherical in tissue but grow like molds when cultured at room temperature. *Candida* species other than *Candida glabrata* appear in tissue as both budding yeasts and tubular elements called *pseudohyphae*. *Pneumocystis carinii* is closer to fungi than to parasites by ribosomal sequences (Chap. 209). Because the drugs used to treat *Pneumocystis* pneumonia are also used to treat parasitic or bacterial infections, those drugs will not be discussed in this chapter.

Many fungi can form two different types of spores and are given different names, depending on the spore-bearing structures. When the spores are produced by mitosis, the fungus is said to be an *anamorph*, or to be in the imperfect state. Many fungi can have different sporulating structures in which genetic recombination occurs, often as a result of coculture with a strain of the opposite mating type. A fungus producing those distinctive spores is said to be a *teleomorph*, or to be in the perfect state. Diagnostic laboratories usually use the name of

the anamorph because they do not use culture conditions that would produce the teleomorph. One exception is *Scedosporium apiospermum*, which is often observed as a teleomorph in the diagnostic laboratory and identified as *Pseudallescheria boydii*.

Most fungi that are pathogenic for humans are saprophytes in nature; they cause infection when airborne spores reach the lung or paranasal sinus or when hyphae or spores are accidentally inoculated into the skin or cornea. Acquisition of infection from another person or an animal has been reported in the case of ringworm but is very rare in other mycoses. Thus, hospitalized patients with fungal infections do not require special isolation. Most fungi infect hosts preferentially by one route and only infrequently by other routes. For example, the agents of ringworm, pityriasis versicolor, and piedra infect the epidermis and its appendages. Sporotrichosis and mycetoma usually arise from subcutaneous inoculation. Inhalation is the route of inoculation for the agents of most deep mycoses. Ingestion of fungi rarely causes infection; *Candida albicans*, a normal commensal in the mouth and intestine, reaches deeper tissues only when mucosal or cutaneous barriers are breached by disease, surgery, trauma, or catheterization. Histoplasmosis, blastomycosis, coccidioidomycosis, and paracoccidioidomycosis have been called "endemic" mycoses to emphasize their restricted geographic distribution. Some fungi, such as *Aspergillus*, are said to be opportunists in that they usually infect hosts with compromised immunity. This distinction is relative, not absolute.

Immunity after exposure to fungi may confer partial protection against reinfection. Residents of areas in which mycoses are endemic are less subject to infection than are newcomers. Predisposing factors are helpful in defining host defense. Immunoglobulin deficiencies do not appear to predispose to any mycosis, whereas neutropenia is common among patients who develop invasive aspergillosis or deep candidiasis. Cell-mediated immunity appears to be of paramount importance in most other deep mycoses.

Many fungi can be identified to the genus or even the species level by microscopic examination of smears or biopsy specimens. Calcofluor white staining with fluorescence microscopy is a sensitive technique for smears of sputum, bronchoalveolar lavage fluid, or pus. India ink smear remains the method of choice for detecting cryptococci in cerebrospinal fluid (CSF). *Candida* yeast cells and pseudohyphae are the only fungi that are usually gram-positive on smears. For other fungi, Gram's staining is distinctly suboptimal. For histopathology slides, Gomori methenamine silver and a neutral counterstain are preferred.

The method used has a marked effect on the rapidity and sensitivity of blood cultures for fungi except in the case of *Candida* species, which are relatively easy to grow. For most other fungi, concentration of the blood by lysis centrifugation and culture on solid medium constitute the optimal technique. Commercially available nucleic acid hybridization techniques can speed the identification of slow-growing molds, such as *Histoplasma capsulatum* and *Coccidioides immitis*. Serology has limited value, but testing of serum or CSF for cryptococcal antigen or antibody to *C. immitis* can be diagnostic. Detection of *Histoplasma* antigen in urine or serum is helpful in diagnosis and in following the results of treatment for disseminated histoplasmosis. Skin testing with fungal antigens is not useful in detecting active infection.

ANTIFUNGAL THERAPY

TOPICAL AGENTS Imidazoles and Triazoles (See also "Systemic Antifungals," below) These synthetic compounds act by inhibiting ergosterol synthesis in the fungal cell wall and, when given topically, may cause direct damage to the fungal cytoplasmic membrane. The imidazoles available for cutaneous application include clotrimazole, econazole, ketoconazole, sulconazole, oxiconazole, and miconazole. Vaginal formulations include four imidazoles (miconazole, clotrimazole, tioconazole, and butoconazole) and one triazole (terconazole). As yet, no substantial differences in the efficacy of or local intolerance to the various topical azoles have become apparent. All are effective in the treatment of cutaneous candidiasis, tinea (pityriasis) versicolor, and mild to moderately severe ringworm of the glabrous skin. Vaginal formulations are effective for vulvovaginal candidiasis. Clotrimazole is poorly absorbed from the gastrointestinal tract, but the oral troche is useful as a topical treatment for oral and esophageal candidiasis.

Polyene Macrolide Antibiotics These broad-spectrum antifungal agents combine with sterol in the fungal cytoplasmic membrane, increasing membrane permeability. Topically, they are not active against ringworm but are effective against candidiasis of the skin and mucous membranes. Nystatin and amphotericin B suspensions are effective in oral thrush, and vaginal troches are effective in vulvovaginal candidiasis. Both nystatin and amphotericin B are available in topical preparations for cutaneous candidiasis.

Other Topical Antifungals Ciclopirox olamine, haloprogin, terbinafine, and naftifine have the same clinical spectrum among the cutaneous mycoses as the imidazoles. Tolnaftate and undecylenic acid are effective against ringworm but not candidiasis. Keratolytic agents, such as salicylic acid, are helpful as accessory drugs for some hyperkeratotic skin lesions.

SYSTEMIC ANTIFUNGALS Griseofulvin Griseofulvin is a useful drug in the treatment of certain kinds of ringworm; however, it is ineffective in the treatment of candidiasis. The microcrystalline and ultramicrocrystalline preparations differ in dose but not in efficacy. Absorption of both is enhanced when the drug is ingested with fat-containing foods. Griseofulvin interacts with phenobarbital and coumarin-type anticoagulants.

Terbinafine Oral terbinafine (250 mg once daily) is at least as effective as itraconazole and more effective than griseofulvin in onychomycosis and ringworm. Treatment duration ranges from 3 months for fingernails to 6 months for toenails. Gastrointestinal distress is the most common side effect. Rash, hepatitis, and pancytopenia have oc-

curred, but serious adverse effects have been uncommon. Terbinafine decreases cyclosporine levels. Cimetidine increases and rifampin decreases terbinafine levels in blood.

Imidazoles and Triazoles • *General features* The azole antifungals include imidazoles and triazoles. Fluconazole, itraconazole, and investigational azoles are all triazoles, so named because they have three nitrogens in the ring structure. This class has less impact on human hormonal synthesis and less hepatotoxicity than the only widely used systemic imidazole, ketoconazole. Itraconazole has many structural features in common with ketoconazole; however, it has a broader spectrum of activity and has largely replaced ketoconazole.

Reported interactions of itraconazole and fluconazole with other drugs are listed in Table 200-1. Ketoconazole interactions (not listed) appear to be the same as those listed for itraconazole. Azole interactions with any one class of drugs, such as benzodiazepines, HMG-CoA reductase inhibitors, or drugs that decrease gastric acidity, should be considered to apply to all drugs of that class until proven otherwise. Fluconazole differs substantially from itraconazole: unlike that of itraconazole, the absorption of fluconazole is independent of food or gastric acid, and fluconazole has much less effect on the hepatic metabolism of other drugs than does itraconazole. High fluconazole blood levels engendered by azotemia or by dosages above those used in pharmacologic studies may lead to new and profound drug interactions.

All azoles have the potential for embryotoxicity and teratogenicity. In fact, it seems likely that azoles should not be given during pregnancy without a discussion of the serious risks and possible benefits with the mother. Four infants born to mothers taking at least 400 mg of fluconazole daily for coccidioidal meningitis have had severe bone, craniofacial, or cardiac abnormalities. Similarity of these abnormalities to those in pregnant animals given fluconazole suggests that fluconazole caused the defects.

Table 200-1   Interactions of Itraconazole and Fluconazole with Other Drugs

Interaction, Drug(s)	Intraconazole	Fluconazole
Azole increases blood level of other drug		
Antihistamines (nonsedating astemizole, terfenadine)	+	0
Antimetabolites (busulfan, vincristine, vinblastine)	+	0
Benzodiazepines (midazolam, triazolam)	+	0
Calcium channel inhibitors (felodipine)	+	0
Cisapride	+	0
Cyclosporine	+	+
Digoxin	+	0
HMG-CoA reductase inhibitors (lovastatin, simvastatin)	+	?
Phenytoin	+	+
Prednisolone	±[a]	0
Protease inhibitors (indinavir, ritonavir)	+	0
Quinidine	+	?
Sulfonylureas (glipizide, glyburide, tolbutamide)	+	+
Tacrolimus	+	?
Warfarin	±	±
Other drug decreases azole blood level		
Antacids (simultaneous administration)	+	0
Carbamazepine	+	0
H₂ receptor antagonists (cimetidine, ranitidine, famotidine, nizatidine)	+	0
Isoniazid	+	0
Phenobarbital	+	0
Phenytoin	+	0
Proton pump inhibitors (omeprazole, lansoprazole)	+	0
Rifampin, rifabutin	+	±

[a] The symbol "±" indicates that interaction is variable but is more likely with a high azole blood concentration.

Itraconazole Itraconazole is useful in the treatment of blasto-mycosis, histoplasmosis, candidiasis, coccidioidomycosis, sporotri-chosis, pseudallescheriasis, onychomycosis, ringworm, tinea versi-color, and some cases of aspergillosis. Its efficacy in mycoses of the central nervous system has been modest at best. Almost no bioactive drug appears in urine. Itraconazole is metabolized in the liver, with the hydroxy metabolite accounting for at least half of the antifungal activity in serum. Food increases absorption of itraconazole capsules by about threefold but substantially reduces absorption of the cyclo-dextrin suspension. Ability of the suspension to exert a topical as well as a systemic effect probably accounts for its improved efficacy in oropharyngeal candidiasis. The usual dosage of either oral itraconazole formulation is 100 to 200 mg once daily for oropharyngeal and esoph-ageal candidiasis. For deep infections, itraconazole capsules are given at an initial dosage of 600 to 800 mg daily for 3 days and a subsequent dosage of 200 to 400 mg once daily continued for 6 to 12 months. Itraconazole blood levels are helpful in documenting absorption of oral itraconazole when the drug is used for the treatment of deep mycoses. An intravenous formulation is commercially available and should be considered for initial therapy in hospitalized patients in whom itra-conazole absorption may be suboptimal. Immunosuppressed patients with rapidly progressing pseudallescheriasis, an infection that does not respond to amphotericin B, are candidates for intravenous itraconazole treatment.

Fluconazole This triazole can be administered in tablet form, as a suspension, or as an intravenous infusion. With a half-life of about 31 h, fluconazole can be given once a day. Approximately 80% of the drug is excreted unchanged in the urine. Patients with creatinine clear-ance rates of 21 to 50 mL/min and 11 to 20 mL/min should have their fluconazole doses reduced by 50 and 75%, respectively. The drug pen-etrates the CSF and other body fluids very well.

Nausea and abdominal distress are the most common forms of dose-limiting fluconazole toxicity. An allergic rash may develop and is particularly common among patients infected with HIV. Fatal cases of Stevens-Johnson syndrome have been described in the HIV-infected population. Alopecia commonly follows prolonged administration of ≥400 mg daily but resolves when therapy is discontinued. Rare cases of anaphylaxis, hepatic necrosis, and neutropenia have been described.

Fluconazole is useful in the treatment of oropharyngeal and esoph-ageal candidiasis in adults. A single 150-mg tablet is effective in vul-vovaginal candidiasis. Catheter-acquired candidemia in the immuno-competent host responds to 400 mg of fluconazole daily in conjunction with the removal of the infected catheter. Treatment should be contin-ued for 10 to 14 days after the patient has become afebrile. Fluconazole is also effective in initial and maintenance therapy for cryptococcal meningitis in patients with AIDS, although most of these patients should initially receive a 2-week course of intravenous amphotericin B. Patients with coccidioidal meningitis can often be given fluconazole rather than intrathecal amphotericin B as maintenance therapy.

The incidence of deep candidiasis among recipients of allogeneic bone marrow transplants can be reduced by the administration of flu-conazole (400 mg daily) for 75 days after initiation of the transplan-tation-preparative regimen. Prophylaxis in other neutropenic patients has not appeared useful. Fluconazole (200 mg daily) reduced the in-cidence of cryptococcosis and mucosal candidiasis among AIDS pa-tients whose CD4+ cell counts were $<200/\mu L$ and was particularly effective among those with counts of $<50/\mu L$. However, this regimen is not recommended because it does not reduce mortality, is expensive, and can lead to drug resistance.

Fluconazole is less effective than itraconazole in blastomycosis, histoplasmosis, and sporotrichosis. The drug is not active in aspergil-losis or mucormycosis.

Amphotericin B A colloidal deoxycholate complex of the polyene drug amphotericin B is available for intravenous or intrathecal administration. In-line filters with a 0.22-μm pore diameter may trap some of the colloid. The catabolism of amphotericin B is extremely slow and is not influenced by renal failure, hepatic failure, or hemo-dialysis. The drug's penetration into CSF and vitreous humor is poor; however, the concentrations in pleural, peritoneal, and articular exu-dates are adequate for many mycoses. Histoplasmosis, blastomycosis, paracoccidioidomycosis, candidiasis, and cryptococcosis are the most responsive mycoses; coccidioidomycosis, extraarticular sporotri-chosis, aspergillosis, and mucormycosis are less responsive; and chro-moblastomycosis, mycetoma, and pseudallescheriasis respond little, if at all. The usual course is 0.5 to 0.7 mg/kg daily for 8 to 10 weeks. Infusions are generally given in 5% dextrose over 2 to 4 h.

Initial doses of amphotericin B occasionally cause marked febrile reactions that may be poorly tolerated by adult patients with limited cardiac or pulmonary function. It may be prudent to give such patients an initial 1-mg test dose followed by rapidly escalating doses, de-pending on tolerance. Premedication with aspirin or acetaminophen or the addition of hydrocortisone (25 mg) to the infusion decreases chills and fever. Azotemia during treatment is usual, the extent depending on the daily dose. Saline infusions have been advocated to reduce azotemia. Permanent loss of renal function is related to the total dose of amphotericin B; this condition is generally noted in adults who have received >3 g. Other side effects include anemia, hypoka-lemia, renal tubular acidosis, nausea, anorexia, weight loss, phlebitis, and occasionally hypomagnesemia. Intrathecal amphotericin B has been used in coccidioidal meningitis and refractory cryptococcal meningitis, although this therapy is associated with considerable toxicity.

Three lipid formulations of amphotericin B are commercially available in the United States: amphotericin B lipid complex (ABLC), amphotericin B colloidal dispersion (ABCD), and liposomal ampho-tericin B (L-AB). All cause less nephrotoxicity than the older ampho-tericin B deoxycholate complex (ABD). Acute, febrile infusion-related reactions occur with all three lipid formulations but are most severe with ABCD. The recommended duration for initial infusions of ABCD is 1 mg/kg per hour, somewhat slower than the 2-h duration of ABLC or L-AB infusions, with the intent of decreasing febrile reactions. Pre-medication with acetaminophen is also an option. Use of these re-markably expensive formulations should be confined to patients who cannot tolerate the nephrotoxicity of ABD. Although the lipid for-mulations are also approved for patients failing to respond to ABD, there is no indication that these formulations are more effective than ABD for any mycosis.

Flucytosine Flucytosine (5-fluorocytosine) is a synthetic oral drug useful in cryptococcosis, candidiasis, and chromoblastomycosis. Within the fungal cell, flucytosine is converted to the antimetabolite 5-fluorouracil. Drug resistance appears rather rapidly when flucytosine is used alone. For this reason, the drug is generally used in combination with amphotericin B. The usual dose of flucytosine is 25 to 37.5 mg/ kg every 6 h. Flucytosine is well absorbed from the gastrointestinal tract. The drug penetrates well into the CSF and is excreted unchanged in the urine. Even modest reductions in renal function may elevate flucytosine blood levels into the toxic range (≥100 to 125 μg/mL). Elevated levels are associated with a significant incidence of neutro-penia and thrombocytopenia and also seem to predispose to colitis, the other major toxic effect of this drug. Hepatotoxicity is idiosyncratic and uncommon. An allergic rash may develop.

BIBLIOGRAPHY

BOWDEN RA et al: Phase 1 study of amphotericin B colloidal dispersion for the treatment of invasive fungal infections after bone marrow transplant. J Infect Dis 173:1208, 1996

DISMUKES WE: Introduction to antifungal drugs. Clin Infect Dis 30:653, 2000

KWON-CHUNG KJ, BENNETT JE: *Medical Mycology*. Philadelphia, Lea & Febiger, 1992

MANGINO JE, PAPPAS PG: Itraconazole for the treatment of histoplasmosis and blasto-mycosis. Int J Antimicrob Agents 5:219, 1995

PAPPAS PG et al: Alopecia associated with fluconazole therapy. Ann Intern Med 123:354, 1995

POWDERLY WG et al: A randomized trial comparing fluconazole with clotrimazole troches for the prevention of fungal infections in patients with advanced human immunode-ficiency virus infection. N Engl J Med 332:700, 1995

REX J et al: A randomized trial comparing fluconazole with amphotericin B for the treatment of candidemia in patients with neutropenia. N Engl J Med 331:1325, 1994

SLAVIN MA et al: Efficacy and safety of fluconazole prophylaxis for fungal infections after marrow transplantation—a prospective, randomized, double-blind trial. J Infect Dis 171:1545, 1995

SOBEL JD: Practice guidelines for the treatment of fungal infections. Clin Infect Dis 30: 652, 2000

VAN DER HORST CM et al: Treatment of cryptococcal meningitis associated with the acquired immunodeficiency syndrome. N Engl J Med 337:15, 1997

WHITE MH et al: Randomized, double-blind clinical trial of amphotericin B colloidal dispersion vs amphotericin B in the empirical treatment of fever and neutropenia. Clin Infect Dis 27:296, 1998

WONG-BERINGER A et al: Lipid formulations of amphotericin B: Clinical efficacy and toxicities. Clin Infect Dis 27:603, 1998

201

John E. Bennett

HISTOPLASMOSIS

ETIOLOGIC AGENT *Histoplasma capsulatum* is a dimorphic fungus that grows as a mold in nature or on Sabouraud's agar at room temperature. Hyphae bear both large and small spores, which are used for identification. Nucleic acid hybridization can also be used to identify the organism in culture. *H. capsulatum* grows as a small budding yeast in host tissue and on enriched agar, such as blood cysteine glucose, at 37°C. Despite its name, the fungus is unencapsulated. Coculture of isolates with opposite mating types can produce different sporulating structures in which genetic recombination occurs. When these structures, referred to as a *teleomorph* or the *perfect state*, are seen in culture, the name *Ajellomyces capsulatus* is used.

EPIDEMIOLOGY Infection with *H. capsulatum* has been encountered in many areas of the world but is much more frequent in certain areas. Within the United States, infection is most common in the southeastern, mid-Atlantic, and central states. Endemicity is probably contingent on the availability of proper conditions in nature for growth of the fungus. *H. capsulatum* prefers moist surface soil, particularly soil enriched by droppings of certain birds and bats. The fungus has been isolated repeatedly from such sites, and many case clusters have occurred 5 to 18 days after the exposure of groups of people to dust while (for example) cleaning dirt-floored chicken coops; raking soil beneath bird-roosting sites; exploring caves; and cleaning, remodeling, or demolishing old buildings. Skin-test reactivity in many endemic areas indicates that ≥80% of residents over age 16 have been exposed.

PATHOGENESIS AND PATHOLOGY Microconidia, or small spores, of *H. capsulatum* are small enough to reach the alveoli on inhalation and are transformed there to budding forms. With time, an intense granulomatous reaction occurs. Caseation necrosis or calcification may mimic tuberculosis. In children, the primary infection usually heals completely but may leave spotty calcification in the hilar nodes or lung. Transient dissemination may leave calcified granulomas in the spleen. In adults, a rounded mass of scar tissue, with or without central calcification, may remain in the lung. This mass has been called a *histoplasmoma*. Previous exposure is thought to confer some protection against reinfection, but infection in persons with prior positive skin tests clearly has occurred.

In a small proportion of patients, histoplasmosis becomes a progressive, potentially fatal infection. The disease occurs either as chronic fibrocavitary pneumonia or, less commonly, as disseminated infection. Patients with either form lack a history of acute primary pulmonary histoplasmosis. Chronic pulmonary infection favors otherwise healthy males over the age of 40. A history of cigarette use or the presence of emphysema is elicited from nearly all patients with chronic progressive pulmonary histoplasmosis. An acute, rapidly fatal

disseminated infection is most likely to be encountered among young children and immunosuppressed patients, including those with AIDS. A more chronic but equally lethal disseminated infection is more common among previously healthy adults.

CLINICAL MANIFESTATIONS The vast majority of infections are either asymptomatic or mild, and the diagnosis is elusive. Cough, fever, malaise, and chest x-ray findings of hilar adenopathy with or without one or more areas of pneumonitis are typical features. Erythema nodosum and erythema multiforme have been reported in a few outbreaks. Hilar adenopathy may cause temporary compression of the right-middle-lobe bronchus in children and young adults. Subacute pericarditis may develop, probably by extension from contiguous lymph nodes. Rarely, hilar nodes undergo a caseous, granulomatous reaction with perinodal fibrosis. Mediastinal structures become encased by progressive fibrosis, and compression of the pulmonary veins, superior vena cava, pulmonary arteries, and esophagus may take place over many years. Late in mediastinal disease, only rare nonviable *Histoplasma* cells can be found in caseous residua of lymph nodes.

Chronic pulmonary histoplasmosis is characterized by a gradual onset (over weeks or months) of increasing productive cough, weight loss, and sometimes night sweats. Chest x-ray reveals uni- or bilateral fibronodular apical infiltrates. Approximately one-third of cases stabilize or improve spontaneously early in the course. The remainder progress insidiously. Retraction and cavitation of the upper lobes occur, with spread to the apex of the lower lobes and other areas of the lung. Emphysema and bulla formation further compromise pulmonary function. Death from cor pulmonale, bacterial pneumonia, or histoplasmosis occurs after months or years.

Acute disseminated histoplasmosis may be mistaken for miliary tuberculosis (Chap. 169). Common findings include fever, emaciation, hepatosplenomegaly, lymphadenopathy, jaundice, anemia, leukopenia, and thrombocytopenia. A high index of suspicion is necessary in patients with AIDS, in whose cases there may be other explanations for the abnormalities caused by disseminated histoplasmosis. All these features may be noted in chronic dissemination as well, but chronic disease tends to be more localized. Indurated ulcers of the mouth, tongue, nose, or larynx are reported in about one-fourth of cases. Other focal findings include granulomatous hepatitis, Addison's disease, gastrointestinal ulceration, endocarditis, and chronic meningitis. Chest x-ray abnormalities are evident in half of cases and characteristically consist of discrete nodules or a miliary pattern.

Infection with *H. capsulatum* var. *duboisii* is rare outside of Africa. The yeast form is larger in tissue than that of *H. capsulatum* var. *capsulatum*. Clinical manifestations resemble those of blastomycosis more than those of histoplasmosis in that skin and bone lesions are very common.

DIAGNOSIS Culture of the etiologic organism is the preferred method for diagnosis of histoplasmosis but is often difficult. Blood cultures are best done by the lysis-centrifugation technique, with plates held at 30°C for at least 2 weeks. Approximately 15 mL of blood should be cultured from adults. Routine blood cultures in broth are generally unsuitable. Cultures of bone marrow, mucosal lesions, liver, and bronchoalveolar lavage fluid are diagnostically useful in disseminated histoplasmosis. Sputum culture is the preferred method for the diagnosis of chronic pulmonary histoplasmosis. However, growth may require 2 to 4 weeks to become visible, and other organisms may overgrow the plate. Diagnosis based on Giemsa-stained smears of blood or bronchoalveolar lavage fluid or on methenamine silver staining of infected lung, bone marrow, lymph node, or mucosal lesions requires considerable expertise, although these techniques yield results rapidly and provide specimens that can easily be sent to a referral laboratory. Organisms may be very scanty in lesions with marked caseous necrosis. An assay for *Histoplasma* antigen in blood or urine is commercially available and is useful both for diagnosis and for monitoring of the response to therapy in patients with AIDS who have disseminated infection. Diagnosis by antigen detection requires confirmation by culture or histopathology because false-positive results have occasionally been obtained. Tests for antibody to *H. capsulatum* have been of limited value in diagnosis. Histoplasmin skin testing has proven useful in epidemiologic studies but not in clinical diagnosis. Neither skin testing nor serology has been predictive of histoplasmosis in patients infected with HIV.

℞ TREATMENT Acute pulmonary histoplasmosis requires no therapy. Oral itraconazole (200 mg/d) can be given to shorten the course of illness, although this effect has not been proven. Patients with mediastinal fibrosis may benefit from surgery, but their ultimate prognosis is poor. All patients with disseminated or chronic fibronodular pulmonary histoplasmosis should receive chemotherapy. Intravenous amphotericin B (0.6 mg/kg daily) is the drug of choice for the initial treatment of patients with disseminated histoplasmosis who are severely ill or immunosuppressed or whose infection involves the central nervous system; the regimen can be changed to itraconazole (200 mg twice daily) once clinical improvement is evident in these patients. Measuring itraconazole trough blood levels should be considered in those patients (e.g., patients with AIDS) who may not be absorbing the drug well (Chap. 200). Itraconazole suspension, taken fasting, is better absorbed than the capsule formulation. Fluconazole is reliably absorbed, even in patients taking drugs to block gastric acid secretion, but at doses up to 400 mg/d has been less effective in treatment of chronic pulmonary or disseminated histoplasmosis. Patients with AIDS whose disseminated histoplasmosis has responded to 10 weeks of therapy should receive itraconazole (200 mg/d) for life to prevent relapse. It remains unknown whether patients with a sustained response to highly active antiretroviral therapy can discontinue maintenance therapy with itraconazole.

Immunocompetent patients can initially be given itraconazole (200 mg twice daily) and are generally treated for 6 to 12 months. Ketoconazole (400 to 800 mg once daily) can be used instead of itraconazole for the treatment of immunocompetent patients without central nervous system disease when the lower cost is more important than the higher incidence of side effects. Alternatively, immunocompetent patients can be given a 10-week course of amphotericin B (0.5 mg/kg daily).

Long-term maintenance therapy with an azole is not recommended for patients other than those with AIDS. However, relapse of chronic pulmonary and disseminated histoplasmosis is not rare and warrants careful follow-up for 1 year after therapy.

BIBLIOGRAPHY

GOODWIN RA et al: Histoplasmosis in normal hosts. Medicine 60:231, 1981

HECHT FM et al: Itraconazole maintenance treatment for histoplasmosis in AIDS: A prospective, multicenter trial. J Acquir Immune Defic Syndr 16:100, 1997

PEDDI VR et al: Disseminated histoplasmosis in renal allograft recipients. Clin Transplant 10:160, 1996

RAYMOND LW et al: Scars without wounds: Spectrum of delayed manifestations of histoplasmosis outside of the endemic area. Crit Rev Diagn Imaging 14:37, 1980

WHEAT J: Histoplasmosis. Experience during outbreaks in Indianapolis and review of the literature. Medicine (Baltimore) 76:339, 1997

——— et al: Disseminated histoplasmosis in the acquired immune deficiency syndrome: Clinical findings, diagnosis and treatment, and review of the literature. Medicine 69: 361, 1990

——— et al: Prevention of relapse of histoplasmosis with itraconazole in patients with the acquired immunodeficiency syndrome. Ann Intern Med 118:610, 1993

——— et al: Endemic mycoses in AIDS: A clinical review. Clin Microbiol Rev 8:146, 1995

——— et al: Itraconazole treatment of disseminated histoplasmosis in patients with the acquired immunodeficiency syndrome. Am J Med 98:336, 1995

——— et al: Practice guidelines for the management of patients with histoplasmosis. Clin Infect Dis 30:688, 2000

202 *John E. Bennett*

COCCIDIOIDOMYCOSIS

ETIOLOGIC AGENT *Coccidioides immitis* has two forms, growing as a white fluffy mold on most culture media but as a nonbudding spherical form (a spherule) in host tissue or under special conditions. The organism reproduces in host tissue by forming small endospores within mature spherules. After rupture of the spherule, the released endospores enlarge, become spherules, and repeat the cycle. The fungus is identified by its appearance and by the formation of thick-walled, barrel-shaped spores, called *arthrospores*, in the hyphae of the mold form.

EPIDEMIOLOGY, PATHOGENESIS, AND PATHOLOGY *C. immitis* is a soil saprophyte found in certain arid regions of the United States, Mexico, Central America, and South America. Within the United States, most cases of infection with *C. immitis* are acquired in California, Arizona, and western Texas. A few cases are acquired by exposure to fomites from endemic areas (e.g., in cotton bales).

Infection in humans and animals results from inhalation of windborne arthrospores from soil sites. This primary pulmonary infection is symptomatic in only 40% of cases, with symptoms ranging from a mild influenza-like illness to severe pneumonia. Mild self-limited infections may come to medical attention because of case clusters or hypersensitivity reactions: erythema nodosum, erythema multiforme, toxic erythema, arthralgia, arthritis, conjunctivitis, or episcleritis. Case clusters occur 10 to 14 days after a group of susceptible individuals is exposed to dust in an endemic area through such activities as archaeologic excavation, rock hunting, military maneuvers, or construction work. Windstorms can carry spores to adjacent nonendemic areas and cause case clusters. The usual course of primary pneumonia is complete healing, although an area of pneumonitis (detected on radiographs) may heal by the formation of a coinlike lesion called a *coccidioidoma*. Less commonly, a single thin-walled cavity remains as a chronic sequela in the area of consolidation. Alternatively, an area of consolidation may persist as chronic pneumonia or progress to fibronodular cavitary disease.

Pleural effusion may be the only manifestation of primary infection. Spontaneous healing of this form is common.

An uncommon but dreaded complication of coccidioidomycosis is dissemination beyond the lung and hilar lymph nodes. Dissemination is especially frequent among blacks, Filipinos, Native Americans, Mexican-Americans, pregnant women, and immunosuppressed patients, including those with AIDS.

C. immitis incites a chronic granulomatous reaction in host tissue, often with caseation necrosis. Lung and hilar node lesions may show calcification. Both IgM and IgG antibodies to *C. immitis* are induced by infection, but neither type of antibody appears to be protective. The amount of specific IgG antibody is a rough measure of the antigenic mass (i.e., of the intensity of infection), and a high titer is a poor prognostic sign. Appearance of delayed hypersensitivity to antigens of *C. immitis* is most common in clinical forms of disease with a good prognosis, such as self-limited primary pulmonary disease. In skin tests for *Coccidioides* antigens, about half of patients with disseminated disease have negative results that portend a poor outcome.

CLINICAL MANIFESTATIONS Symptomatic primary pulmonary infection is manifested by fever, cough, chest pain, malaise, and sometimes the hypersensitivity reactions listed above. Chest radiographs may show an infiltrate, hilar adenopathy, or pleural effusion. Mild peripheral-blood eosinophilia may be found. Spontaneous improvement begins after several days to 2 weeks of illness and usually culminates in complete recovery.

The symptoms of a chronic thin-walled cavity include cough or hemoptysis in half of cases; the other half are asymptomatic. Chronic progressive pulmonary coccidioidomycosis causes cough, sputum production, variable degrees of fever, and weight loss. The first indications of dissemination usually appear during primary infection. Reactivation with dissemination in later years occurs occasionally, especially if Hodgkin's disease, non-Hodgkin's lymphoma, renal transplantation, AIDS, or immunosuppression of some other etiology has supervened. Dissemination should be suspected when fever, malaise, hilar or paratracheal lymphadenopathy, elevated sedimentation rate, and high complement fixation titers signal abnormal persistence in patients with primary pulmonary coccidioidomycosis. With time, lesions appear in the bone, skin, subcutaneous tissue, meninges, joints, and other sites. Chronic meningitis presents as headache of indolent onset, with or without other signs of disseminated coccidioidomycosis. Cultures and smears of cerebrospinal fluid (CSF) are most often negative, but antibody is usually detectable in CSF by complement fixation. Skin lesions are indolent and maculopapular; soft tissue and bony lesions contain pus and may present as a draining sinus. Without treatment, disseminated coccidioidomycosis progresses to death over weeks to years.

Disseminated coccidioidomycosis can progress rapidly in patients with advanced HIV infection. Fever with skin or bone lesions may be the first sign. Those who present with diffuse pulmonary infiltrates have a poor prognosis. Blood cultures are positive late in the disease, if at all.

DIAGNOSIS When coccidioidomycosis is suspected, sputum, urine, and pus should be examined for *C. immitis* by wet smear and culture. *The laboratory request should indicate clearly that coccidioidomycosis is suspected, because the mold form must be handled with extreme care to prevent infection of laboratory personnel.* On biopsy, smaller spherules must be distinguished from nonbudding forms of *Blastomyces* and *Cryptococcus*, but the appearance of the mature spherule is diagnostic.

Serologic tests are very helpful in the diagnosis of coccidioidomycosis. Latex agglutination and agar gel diffusion tests are useful in screening sera for antibody to *Coccidioides*. The complement fixation test is used for CSF determinations and for the confirmation and quantitation of serum antibody detected by screening tests. The number of cases with a positive complement fixation test depends on the severity of disease and on the laboratory performing the test. Positive tests are least common among patients with solitary pulmonary cavities or primary pulmonary infection, while sera from patients with disseminated disease in multiple organs are nearly all positive. Seroconversion is helpful in primary pulmonary coccidioidomycosis but may not occur for up to 8 weeks after onset. A positive complement fixation test of unconcentrated CSF is diagnostic of meningitis. Rarely, a parameningeal focus causes a positive complement fixation test of CSF.

Conversion of the skin test from negative to positive (≥ 5 mm of induration at 24 or 48 h) with spherulin may take place between days 3 and 21 of symptoms in primary pulmonary coccidioidomycosis. Skin testing can be helpful in epidemiologic studies, such as investigations of case clusters or the definition of endemic areas. The utility of skin testing as a diagnostic tool is limited by the persistence of positive tests resulting from remote exposures to *Coccidioides* and by the frequency of negative skin tests among patients with either thin-walled cavities or disseminated coccidioidomycosis. A positive skin test has not predicted dissemination in HIV-infected patients. The presence of complement-fixing antibody to *C. immitis* in AIDS patients should prompt a search for active infection.

TREATMENT Primary pulmonary coccidioidomycosis usually resolves spontaneously. Some physicians give a few weeks of treatment with intravenous amphotericin B or itraconazole to patients with unusually severe or protracted primary infection in the hope of aborting disseminated or chronic pulmonary disease.

Patients with severe or rapidly progressing disseminated coccidioidomycosis are first given intravenous amphotericin B at a dose of 0.5 to 0.7 mg/kg daily. Patients whose condition improves after 2 to 3 months of treatment with amphotericin B or who have more indolent disseminated infection are given itraconazole (200 mg twice daily) or fluconazole (400 to 600 mg/d). These oral agents are useful for long-term suppression of infection, and treatment should be continued for years. Patients with coccidioidal meningitis usually are initially given fluconazole (400 to 800 mg/d) but may require intrathecal amphotericin B. Hydrocephalus is a frequent complication of uncontrolled meningitis. Surgical debridement of bone lesions or drainage of abscesses can be helpful. The prognosis for ultimate cure of disseminated coccidioidomycosis is guarded.

Resection of chronic progressive pulmonary lesions is a helpful adjunct to chemotherapy when infection is confined to the lung and to one lobe. A single thin-walled cavity tends to close spontaneously and ordinarily is not resected. Such a cavity responds poorly to chemotherapy.

BIBLIOGRAPHY

CATANZARO A et al: Fluconazole in the treatment of chronic pulmonary and nonmeningeal disseminated coccidioidomycosis. Am J Med 98:249, 1995

FISH DG et al: Coccidioidomycosis during human immunodeficiency virus infection. A review of 77 patients. Medicine 69:384, 1990

GALGIANI JN: Coccidioidomycosis: A regional disease of national importance. Rethinking approaches for control. Ann Intern Med 130:293, 1999

——— et al: Practice guidelines for the treatment of coccidioidomycosis. Clin Infect Dis 30:658, 2000

KIM K et al: Chronic pulmonary coccidioidomycosis: Computed tomographic and pathologic findings in 18 patients. Can Assoc Rad J 49:401, 1998

KIRKLAND TN, FIERER J: Coccidioidomycosis: A reemerging infectious disease. Emerg Infect Dis 2:192, 1996

SCHNEIDER E et al: A coccidioidomycosis outbreak following the Northridge, California, earthquake. JAMA 277:904, 1997

203   *John E. Bennett*

BLASTOMYCOSIS

ETIOLOGIC AGENT *Blastomyces dermatitidis* is a dimorphic fungus that grows at room temperature as a white or tan mold but grows within the host or at 37°C as budding, round yeastlike cells. The fungus can be identified on the basis of its appearance, its dimorphism, the small spores borne on hyphae of the mold form, or the results of nucleic acid hybridization. When isolates of the two opposite mating types are grown close together on special culture medium, such as yeast extract or soil extract agar, sporulating structures that characterize the perfect state (teleomorph), called *Ajellomyces dermatitidis*, appear.

EPIDEMIOLOGY The infection is restricted by geography and age. Blastomycosis is uncommon in any locality, but most cases occur in the southeastern, central, and mid-Atlantic areas of the United States, with occasional cases in other localities in the United States and Canada. Cases have also been encountered in Africa, Mexico, Central America, and (rarely) South America. Most patients are between 20 and 69 years old. The male-to-female ratio is about 10:1. There is no occupational predisposition to the development of blastomycosis.

PATHOGENESIS AND PATHOLOGY Infection with *B. dermatitidis* appears to be acquired by inhalation of the fungus from soil, decomposed vegetation, or rotting wood. Several case clusters have resulted from participation in recreational activities in wooded areas along waterways. Infection is not transmissible from person to person. The initial pulmonary infection may either heal spontaneously or become chronic. Spread to other portions of the lung, cavitation, or endobronchial lesions may be found in patients with chronic disease.

Whether or not the lung lesion resolves spontaneously, infection commonly spreads hematogenously to the skin, subcutaneous tissue, bone, prostate, epididymis, or mucosa of the nose, mouth, or larynx. Less commonly, infection spreads to the brain, meninges, liver, lymph nodes, or spleen. Dissemination may not be evident for weeks or years after the appearance of the lung lesion. Progressive infection is only rarely attributable to an underlying disease, to HIV infection, or to immunosuppressive treatment. The inflammatory response includes lymphocytes, giant cells, and neutrophils. Pseudoepitheliomatous hyperplasia may be striking and may lead to a mistaken diagnosis of squamous cell carcinoma.

CLINICAL MANIFESTATIONS   A few patients have acute, self-limited pneumonia. Fever, productive cough, myalgia, and malaise usually resolve within a month. Pulmonary infiltrates clear slowly as *B. dermatitidis* disappears from the sputum.

In the vast majority of patients, blastomycosis has an indolent onset and a chronically progressive course. Fever, cough, weight loss, lassitude, skin lesions, and chest ache are common. Skin lesions favor exposed areas and enlarge over many weeks from pimples to well-circumscribed, verrucous, crusted, or ulcerated lesions. Pain and regional lymphadenopathy are minimal. Large chronic lesions may undergo central healing with scarring and contracture. Mucous membrane lesions resemble squamous cell carcinoma. Chest x-ray findings are abnormal in two-thirds of patients, with one or more pneumonic or nodular infiltrates. Calcification, hilar adenopathy, and large pleural effusions are rare. Osteolytic lesions may be found in nearly any bone and present as a cold abscess or a draining sinus. Extension to a contiguous joint may cause indolent swelling, pain, and restricted motion. Prostatic and epididymal lesions clinically resemble those of tuberculosis.

DIAGNOSIS   The diagnosis of blastomycosis is made by demonstration of the fungus in a culture of sputum, pus, or urine. An expert can diagnose blastomycosis on the basis of the appearance of the organism in wet smear or histopathologic section. The fungus may be visible in a sputum cytology smear but is easily overlooked.

℞ **TREATMENT**   A few patients have developed only transitory lung lesions, but no guidelines are known to distinguish these patients from those whose disease will progress locally or disseminate. Therefore, every patient should receive treatment. Intravenous amphotericin B is the drug of choice for patients with rapidly progressive infections, severe illness, or central nervous system lesions. Skin and noncavitary lung lesions should be treated for about 8 to 10 weeks. The recommended total dose for an adult is about 2 g. Cavitary lung disease or infection extending beyond the lung and skin should be treated for about 10 to 12 weeks with ≥2.5 g.

Oral itraconazole (200 mg twice daily with food) is the drug of choice for the treatment of patients who have indolent nonmeningeal blastomycosis of mild to moderate severity and who take the drug reliably. Therapy with itraconazole is continued for 6 to 12 months.

The mortality rate in appropriately treated cases is ≤15%.

BIBLIOGRAPHY

BAUMGARDNER DJ et al: Epidemiology of blastomycosis in a region of high endemicity in north-central Wisconsin. Clin Infect Dis 15:629, 1992

BRADSHER RW: Blastomycosis: Fungal infections of the lung. Update 1989. Semin Respir Infect 5:105, 1990

CHAPMAN SW et al: Endemic blastomycosis in Mississippi: Epidemiological and clinical studies. Semin Respir Infect 12:219, 1997

——— et al: Practice guidelines for the management of patients with blastomycosis. Clin Infect Dis 30:679, 2000

MANGINO JE, PAPPAS PG: Itraconazole for the treatment of histoplasmosis and blastomycosis. Int J Antimicrob Agents 5:219, 1995

PAPPAS PG et al: Blastomycosis in immunocompromised patients. Medicine 72:311, 1993

SACCENTE M et al: Vertebral blastomycosis with paravertebral abscess: Report of eight cases and review of the literature. Clin Infect Dis 26:413, 1998

204

John E. Bennett

CRYPTOCOCCOSIS

ETIOLOGIC AGENT   Cryptococcosis is an infection caused by the yeastlike fungus *Cryptococcus neoformans*. This fungus reproduces by budding and forms round, yeastlike cells. Within the host and on certain culture media, a large polysaccharide capsule surrounds each yeast cell. The fungus grows well in smooth, creamy-white colonies on Sabouraud's or other simple media at 20 to 37°C. Identification of the organism is based on gross and microscopic appearance, biochemical test results, and growth at 37°C. The results of nucleic acid hybridization or the formation of brown pigment on Niger seed agar can also be used for identification.

The fungus has four capsular serotypes, designated A, B, C, and D. There are also two mating types. Coculture of opposite mating types creates a transient diploid state called *Filobasidiella neoformans* var. *neoformans* for serotypes A and D and *F. neoformans* var. *bacillispora* for serotypes B and C. Organisms not cultured under mating conditions are designated *C. neoformans* var. *neoformans* for serotypes A and D and *C. neoformans* var. *gattii* for serotypes B and C; a simple color medium distinguishes the two varieties.

EPIDEMIOLOGY   Weathered pigeon droppings commonly contain serotype A or D (*C. neoformans* var. *neoformans*). *C. neoformans* var. *gattii* has been isolated from the litter around trees of the species *Eucalyptus camaldulensis* and *E. tereticornis*. Eucalyptus isolates have so far typed as serotype B. The distribution of these eucalyptus species in Australia corresponds to the distribution of infections due to *C. neoformans* var. *gattii* in that country. The high prevalence of these trees in other subtropical climates has been postulated to explain the relative restriction of such infections to warm climates.

Cryptococcosis due to *C. neoformans* var. *neoformans* is a common complication of late infection with HIV. The incidence appears to be declining in some areas of the United States, probably as a result of highly active antiretroviral therapy and use of fluconazole for oropharyngeal candidiasis. Patients who have undergone solid-organ transplantation or glucocorticoid therapy and those with sarcoidosis are also at increased risk for infections with *C. neoformans* var. *neoformans*. Almost all such infections are caused by serotype A, although serotype D occurs in up to 20% of cases in Western Europe. Infections with var. *gattii* have been rare among AIDS patients and other immunocompromised patients, even in subtropical climates, where var. *gattii* infection occurs in previously healthy individuals.

Animals, particularly cats, can acquire cryptococcosis but have not transmitted the infection to other animals or to humans. The source from which humans acquire the infection is unknown, with the rare exception of cases acquired through a transplanted cornea, kidney, or other solid organ. Cryptococcosis is rare before puberty.

PATHOGENESIS AND PATHOLOGY   Infection is thought to be acquired by inhalation of fungus into the lungs. Pulmonary infection has a tendency toward spontaneous resolution and is frequently asymptomatic. Silent hematogenous spread to the brain leads to clusters of cryptococci in the perivascular areas of cortical gray matter, in the basal ganglia, and, to a lesser extent, in other areas of the central nervous system. The inflammatory response around these foci is usually scant. In the more chronic cases, a dense basilar arachnoiditis is typical. Lung lesions are characterized by intense granulomatous inflammation. Cryptococci are best seen in tissue by staining with methenamine silver or periodic acid–Schiff. Although a strongly positive result on mucicarmine staining of tissue is diagnostic, staining varies from intense to absent.

CLINICAL MANIFESTATIONS   Most patients have *meningoencephalitis* at the time of diagnosis. This form of the infection is invariably fatal without appropriate therapy; death occurs any time from 2 weeks to several years after the onset of symptoms. Early manifestations include headache, nausea, staggering gait, dementia, irritability, confusion, and blurred vision. Both fever and nuchal rigidity are often mild or lacking. Papilledema is evident in one-third of cases at the time of diagnosis. Cranial nerve palsies, typically asymmetric, occur in about one-fourth of cases. Other lateralized signs are rare. With progression of the infection, deepening coma and signs of brainstem compression appear. Autopsy often reveals cerebral edema in more acute cases and hydrocephalus in more chronic cases.

Pulmonary cryptococcosis causes chest pain in about 40% of patients and cough in 20%. The chest x-ray shows one or more dense infiltrates, which are often well circumscribed. Cavitation, pleural effusions, and hilar adenopathy are infrequent. Calcification is not evident, and fibrotic stranding is rarely noticeable.

Ten percent of patients with cryptococcosis have skin lesions, and the vast majority of patients with skin lesions have disseminated infection. One or a few asymptomatic tiny papular lesions appear and slowly enlarge; they display a tendency toward central softening leading to ulceration. Osteolytic lesions occur in 4% of cases and usually present as a cold abscess. Rare manifestations of cryptococcosis include prostatitis, endophthalmitis, hepatitis, pericarditis, endocarditis, and renal abscess.

DIAGNOSIS Fever and headache in a patient with AIDS or with risk factors for HIV infection suggest the possibility of cryptococcosis, toxoplasmosis, or central nervous system lymphoma. Evidence of a focal lesion on magnetic resonance imaging is unusual in cryptococcosis. Most cryptococcal cerebral mass lesions occur in patients infected with *C. neoformans* var. *gattii* who also have meningitis. In patients without AIDS, meningitis due to *C. neoformans* resembles that due to *Mycobacterium tuberculosis*, *Histoplasma capsulatum*, *Coccidioides immitis*, or metastatic cancer. Lumbar puncture is the single most useful diagnostic test. An india ink smear of centrifuged cerebrospinal fluid (CSF) sediment reveals encapsulated yeast in more than half of cases, although artifacts can cause confusion. In patients without AIDS, levels of glucose in CSF are reduced in half of all cases; protein levels are usually increased; and lymphocytic pleocytosis is usually found. CSF abnormalities are less pronounced in patients with AIDS, although india ink smear is more often positive.

Approximately 90% of patients with cryptococcal meningoencephalitis, including all those with a positive CSF smear, have capsular antigen detectable in CSF or serum by latex agglutination. An enzyme immunoassay for cryptococcal antigen is also available. Occasional false-positive results in the above tests make culture the definitive diagnostic test and have prevented serum antigen from being a useful screening test in asymptomatic patients with AIDS. *C. neoformans* is often present in urine from patients with meningoencephalitis. Fungemia occurs in 10 to 30% of patients and is particularly common among patients with AIDS.

Pulmonary cryptococcosis mimics malignancy with regard to radiographic findings and symptoms. Sputum culture is positive in only 10% of cases, and serum antigen tests are positive in only one-third. Occasionally, *C. neoformans* appears in one or more sputum specimens as an endobronchial saprophyte. Biopsy is usually required for diagnosis.

Cutaneous cryptococcosis may be mistaken for a comedo, basal cell carcinoma, or sarcoidosis. In patients with AIDS, skin lesions may be numerous and are sometimes mistaken for molluscum contagiosum. Biopsy reveals myriad cryptococci. Osseous cryptococcosis resembles tuberculosis.

TREATMENT Patients with AIDS and cryptococcosis are treated initially with intravenous amphotericin B (0.7 mg/kg daily) for at least 2 weeks and until their clinical condition is stable; thereafter, they receive fluconazole. The addition of flucytosine (25 mg/kg every 6 h) to amphotericin B for 2 weeks has minimal impact on morbidity and mortality. After treatment with amphotericin B, fluconazole (400 mg) is given once daily. Daily doses of 800 mg have

been used with marginal changes in toxicity or efficacy. The addition of flucytosine to fluconazole increases gastrointestinal intolerance. After infection is controlled, treatment with a smaller dose of fluconazole (200 mg/d) is continued indefinitely. Itraconazole is less effective than fluconazole for maintenance therapy. It is not yet known whether patients whose CD4+ T lymphocyte counts have exhibited a sustained rise in response to antiretroviral therapy can safely discontinue fluconazole maintenance therapy.

In patients without AIDS, the therapeutic goal is to cure the infection, not merely to control its symptoms. A single intensive course is given until cultures from all previously positive sites (particularly CSF) become convincingly negative. Normalization of the glucose level in lumbar CSF is desirable, but complete clearing of CSF or serum antigen during therapy is not essential. Amphotericin B (0.6 to 0.7 mg/kg daily for ≥10 weeks) is the best-studied regimen. Flucytosine has been added to amphotericin B to accelerate the culture response, but grave toxicity can result unless flucytosine blood levels are kept below 100 μg/mL. Case reports have described patients without HIV infection who have responded to fluconazole or liposomal amphotericin B, but the dose and duration of treatment required to cure cryptococcal meningitis are undefined. Amphotericin B lipid complex and amphotericin B colloidal dispersion are not recommended pending further study.

Hydrocephalus may be the presenting manifestation or a later complication of cryptococcosis. Blindness, dementia, and personality change are among the other sequelae. Daily lumbar puncture or CSF shunting has been advocated—in the hope of averting permanent blindness—for patients with marked cerebral edema who have incipient blurred vision.

Patients with extraneural cryptococcosis most often require treatment with intravenous amphotericin B, with or without flucytosine. Observation or excision of lesions may suffice for some patients who have previously been healthy; who have a single focus in lung, skin, or bone; and who have no cryptococci in CSF, urine, or blood.

PREVENTION Fluconazole (200 mg/d) has been shown to decrease the incidence of cryptococcosis in HIV-infected patients with CD4+ cell counts of <200/μL and particularly in those with counts of <50/μL. Weekly fluconazole has not provided this protection. Daily fluconazole has not conferred a survival advantage; in light of its cost and the currently low incidence of cryptococcosis in patients with AIDS in the United States, prophylaxis is strongly discouraged.

BIBLIOGRAPHY

MEYOHAS M-C et al: Pulmonary cryptococcosis: Localized and disseminated infections in 27 patients with AIDS. Clin Infect Dis 21:628, 1995

MURAKAWA GJ et al: Cutaneous *Cryptococcus* infection and AIDS: Report of 12 cases and review of the literature. Arch Dermatol 132:545, 1996

POWDERLY WG et al: Measurement of cryptococcal antigen in serum and cerebrospinal fluid: Value in the management of AIDS-associated cryptococcal meningitis. Clin Infect Dis 18:789, 1994

——— et al: A randomized trial comparing fluconazole with clotrimazole troches for the prevention of fungal infections in patients with advanced human immunodeficiency virus infection. NIAID AIDS Clinical Trials Group. N Engl J Med 332:700, 1995

REX JR et al: Catastrophic visual loss due to *Cryptococcus neoformans* meningitis. Medicine 72:207, 1993

SAAG MS et al: A comparison of itraconazole versus fluconazole as maintenance therapy for AIDS-associated cryptococcal meningitis. Clin Infect Dis 28:291, 1999

——— et al: Practice guidelines for the management of cryptococcal disease. Clin Infect Dis 30:710, 2000

SPEED B, DUNT D: Clinical and host differences between infections with the two varieties of *Cryptococcus neoformans*. Clin Infect Dis 21:28, 1995

VAN DER HORST CM et al: Treatment of cryptococcal meningitis associated with the acquired immunodeficiency syndrome. NIAID Mycoses Study Group and AIDS Clinical Trials Group. N Engl J Med 337:15, 1997

205　*John E. Bennett*

CANDIDIASIS

ETIOLOGIC AGENTS　*Candida albicans* is the most common cause of mucosal candidiasis and is responsible for about half of all cases of candidemia in hospitalized patients. A small proportion of *C. albicans* isolates have been transferred to a new species, *C. dubliniensis*. *C. tropicalis*, *C. parapsilosis*, *C. guilliermondii*, *C. glabrata* (formerly *Torulopsis glabrata*), *C. krusei*, and a few other *Candida* species also cause potentially fatal bloodstream infection. Many of these non-*albicans* species can enter the bloodstream through an intravascular catheter. *Candida* species, taken together, are the fifth most common cause of nosocomial bloodstream infections in the United States.

All *Candida* species pathogenic for humans are also encountered as commensals of humans, particularly in the mouth, stool, and vagina. These species grow rapidly at 25° to 37°C on simple media as oval, budding cells. In special culture media and in tissue, hyphae or elongated branching structures called *pseudohyphae* are formed. *C. glabrata* differs from other members of the genus in that it forms no true hyphae or pseudohyphae in vitro or in infected tissue. *C. albicans* and *C. dubliniensis* can be identified presumptively by their ability to form germ tubes in serum or by the formation of thick-walled large spores called *chlamydospores*. Final identification of all *Candida* species requires biochemical tests.

PATHOGENESIS　Candidiasis is often preceded by increased colonization of the mouth, vagina, and stool with *Candida* due to broad-spectrum antibiotic therapy. Additional local and systemic factors favor infection. Oropharyngeal thrush is particularly likely to occur in neonates and in patients with diabetes mellitus, HIV infection, or dentures. Vulvovaginal candidiasis (Chap. 132) is especially common in the third trimester of pregnancy. *Candida* from the perineum can enter the urinary tract via an indwelling bladder catheter. Cutaneous candidiasis most often involves macerated skin, such as that in the diapered area of infants, under pendulous breasts, or on hands constantly in water or covered by occlusive gloves. *Candida* can pass from the colonized surface into deep tissue when the integrity of the mucosa or skin is violated, as, for example, by perforation of the gastrointestinal tract through trauma, surgery, or peptic ulceration or by mucosal damage due to cytotoxic agents used for cancer chemotherapy. Although *Candida* is not normally a resident of the skin, secretions from the mouth, rectum, or vagina as well as drainage from surgical wounds or tracheostomy sites can contaminate the hub or skin site of a catheter in an umbilical or central vein. Intravenous drug abuse or third-degree burns can also provide a skin portal for *Candida* that can lead to deep candidiasis. Once *Candida* has passed the integumentary barrier, very low birth weight (in neonates) and neutropenia or glucocorticoid therapy (in any patient) markedly compromise host defense. Hematogenous seeding is particularly evident in the retina, kidney, spleen, and liver.

CLINICAL MANIFESTATIONS　*Oral thrush* presents as discrete and confluent adherent white plaques on the oral and pharyngeal mucosa, particularly in the mouth and on the tongue. These lesions are usually painless, but fissuring at the corners of the mouth can be painful. Unexplained oropharyngeal thrush raises the possibility of HIV infection. Oral thrush is common in acute HIV infection and becomes increasingly common as the CD4+ cell count falls. At CD4+ counts <50/μL, esophageal thrush also becomes common. HIV infection appears not to be an independent risk factor for vulvovaginal thrush.

Cutaneous candidiasis presents as red macerated intertriginous areas, paronychia, balanitis, or pruritus ani. Candidiasis of the perineal

and scrotal skin may be accompanied by discrete pustular lesions on the inner aspects of the thighs. *Chronic mucocutaneous candidiasis* or *candidal granuloma* typically presents as circumscribed hyperkeratotic skin lesions, crumbling dystrophic nails, partial alopecia in areas of scalp lesions, and both oral and vaginal thrush. Systemic infection is very rare, but disfigurement of the face and hands can be severe. Other findings may include chronic epidermophytosis, dental dysplasia, and hypofunction of the parathyroid, adrenal, or thyroid gland. A variety of defects in T cell function have been described in these patients. Vulvovaginal thrush (Chap. 132) causes pruritus, discharge, and sometimes pain on intercourse or urination. Speculum examination reveals an inflamed mucosa and a thin exudate, often with white curds.

Esophageal candidiasis is often asymptomatic but can cause substernal pain or a sense of obstruction on swallowing. Most lesions are in the distal third of the esophagus and appear on endoscopy as areas of redness and edema, focal white patches, or ulcers. Biopsy or brushing is required for diagnosis and for detection of concomitant infections, particularly herpes simplex in patients with hematologic malignancies and cytomegalovirus infection in AIDS patients. Esophagography (barium swallow) is diagnostically insensitive but may reveal spasm or mucosal irregularities. *Candida* esophagitis can cause bleeding and impaired alimentation. Hematogenous dissemination from the esophagus probably occurs in some neutropenic patients but is rarely reported in HIV-infected patients.

Candida can cause cystitis, pyelitis, or renal papillary necrosis in an obstructed urinary tract. When a colonized urinary tract is operated on or instrumented, candidemia may result. However, most patients with *Candida* cultured from the urine simply have bladder colonization from a Foley catheter or a sizable volume of residual urine. Contamination of a voided midstream specimen by vaginal *Candida* is also common.

Candidemia originating from an intravascular catheter may clear in the immunocompetent patient when the catheter is removed. Focal seeding of the retina can take place even if candidemia clears and the patient becomes afebrile. Unilateral or bilateral small white retinal exudates appear within 2 weeks of the onset of candidemia. Lesions may regress spontaneously or enlarge slowly. The vitreous humor becomes cloudy, and the patient notices blurring, ocular pain, or a scotoma. Retinal detachment, vitreous abscess, and extension to the anterior chamber can occur over the ensuing weeks. These retinal lesions, present in ~10% of nonneutropenic patients with candidemia, are the principal reason that systemic antifungal therapy is recommended for all patients with candidemia. Funduscopy should be performed to be certain that retinal lesions, if present, resolve completely. Most cases with ocular involvement have occurred in nonneutropenic patients. In contrast, so-called hepatosplenic candidiasis is usually recognized in patients with acute leukemia who are recovering from profound neutropenia. This entity, better called *chronic disseminated candidiasis*, originates from intestinal seeding of the portal and venous circulation. Fever, modestly elevated serum concentrations of alkaline phosphatase, and multiple small abscesses evident on ultrasonography, magnetic resonance imaging, or computed tomography of the liver, spleen, or kidney suggest the diagnosis. During acute candidemia in neutropenic patients, small erythematous papules may appear anywhere on the skin **(Plate IID-57D)**. If the patient does not expire promptly from disseminated candidiasis, the lesions will develop a necrotic center. Painful muscle lesions may also be found. Punch biopsy of a skin lesion helps distinguish this extremely grave condition from *Malassezia* folliculitis, a similar-appearing but benign condition that can involve the cape area of the chest or the extremities of a sweaty febrile patient.

Hematogenous seeding in the neutropenic patient is occasionally visible radiologically as tiny pulmonary nodules. *Candida* pneumonia, apart from hematogenous candidiasis, is very rare. Organisms seeding a native or prosthetic cardiac valve originate principally from central venous catheters; occasionally, valvular seeding is encountered in intravenous drug abusers. Emboli to large arteries, such as the iliac or femoral artery, are characteristic. Intravenous injection of impure

endophthalmitis and purulent folliculitis, sometimes accompanied by vertebral osteomyelitis. This diffuse folliculitis favors hairy areas, including the scalp and bearded facial skin.

Candida can cause indolent arthritis, most commonly of the knee, in patients who have received glucocorticoid injections into the joint, in patients who are immunosuppressed, and in low-birth-weight neonates. Prosthetic joints may become infected during implantation. Scanty growth of *Candida* from joint fluid can cause the laboratory to incorrectly dismiss the organism as a contaminant.

Hematogenous dissemination can lead to brain abscess or chronic meningitis. Diagnosis of infections of ventriculoperitoneal shunts is difficult because symptoms are indolent and cultures of lumbar fluid are usually sterile.

DIAGNOSIS Demonstration of pseudohyphae on wet smear with confirmation by culture is the procedure of choice for diagnosing superficial candidiasis. Scrapings for the smear may be obtained from skin, nails, and oral and vaginal mucosa. Culture alone is not diagnostic; however, recovery of *Candida* species from multiple superficial sites in immunosuppressed patients may portend visceral invasion.

Deeper lesions due to *Candida* may be diagnosed by histologic section of biopsy specimens or by culture of cerebrospinal fluid, blood, joint fluid, or surgical specimens. Blood cultures are useful in the diagnosis of *Candida* endocarditis and intravenous catheter–induced sepsis but are positive less often in other forms of disseminated disease. Serologic tests for antibody or antigen are not useful.

℞ **TREATMENT** Cutaneous candidiasis of macerated areas responds to measures that reduce moisture and chafing plus topical application of an antifungal agent in a nonocclusive base. Nystatin powder or a cream containing ciclopirox or an azole is useful. Clotrimazole, miconazole, econazole, ketoconazole, sulconazole, and oxiconazole are available as creams or lotions. *Candida* vulvovaginitis responds better to an azole than to nystatin suppositories. There is little difference in efficacy among miconazole, clotrimazole, tioconazole, butoconazole, and terconazole vaginal formulations. Systemic treatment of *Candida* vulvovaginitis with a single 150-mg capsule of fluconazole is more convenient than topical treatment but also poses a higher risk of adverse effects. Clotrimazole troches, used five times a day, are more effective in oral and esophageal candidiasis than nystatin suspension. Oral fluconazole (100 to 200 mg once daily) is more convenient and more effective in esophagitis than clotrimazole troches. Esophagitis not responding to fluconazole may warrant repeat endoscopy to exclude other conditions. Itraconazole suspension (100 to 200 mg/d) alleviates *Candida* esophagitis in some patients in whom fluconazole treatment fails. Amphotericin B suspension has limited use but can be tried in patients whose oropharyngeal candidiasis does not respond to azoles.

Management of recurrent oropharyngeal candidiasis in the HIV-infected patient presents special problems. Patients with CD4+ cell counts <100/μL who have received prolonged fluconazole therapy are at risk of developing azole resistance, requiring an increased dose to mount a response, relapsing early, and eventually failing to respond well to any dose of fluconazole. The increasing azole resistance in this population suggests that HIV-infected patients with oropharyngeal candidiasis should be treated for each individual episode and that only when episodes become intolerably frequent should weekly or daily preventive therapy be given and even then at the lowest dose required to maintain remission. In contrast, AIDS patients with *Candida* esophagitis are so prone to relapse that preventive therapy with fluconazole is recommended for all proven cases. Most HIV-infected patients with azole-resistant oropharyngeal candidiasis also have esophagitis. Nearly all patients with azole-resistant oropharyngeal or esophageal candidiasis respond to intravenous amphotericin B (0.3 to 0.5 mg/kg daily) but relapse promptly after the completion of therapy.

Bladder thrush responds to bladder irrigations with amphotericin B (50 μg/mL for 5 days). If no bladder catheter is in place, oral fluconazole can be used to control candiduria. In all forms of superficial candidiasis, relapse after successful treatment is common unless the underlying factor can be eliminated.

Intravenous amphotericin B is the drug of choice in disseminated candidiasis. The deoxycholate formulation is usually given at a dosage of 0.5 to 0.7 mg/kg daily. Open, noncomparative studies of the lipid formulations of amphotericin B have suggested that they may be useful in disseminated candidiasis, but the optimal dose and formulation remain unknown. Fluconazole in an adult dose of 100 mg/d is probably the drug of choice for chronic mucocutaneous candidiasis.

In immunocompetent patients with intravenous catheter–acquired *C. albicans* fungemia, the catheter should be removed in conjunction with the administration of either fluconazole (400 mg/d) or amphotericin B (0.5 mg/kg daily). Patients with suppurative phlebitis of a peripheral vein should have the infected portion of the vein excised. Therapy for candidemia is continued for 2 weeks after the patient becomes afebrile. The *Candida* species involved should be considered in choosing between fluconazole and amphotericin B. *C. krusei* and *C. inconspicua* are rare causes of candidemia but are resistant to fluconazole in vitro. *C. glabrata* exhibits intermediate susceptibility to fluconazole, but too few cases have been studied to determine whether candidemia involving that species will respond as well to fluconazole as to amphotericin B. Strains of *C. lusitaniae* resistant to amphotericin B but susceptible to azoles have been encountered. Intravenous amphotericin B, with or without flucytosine, is the preferred treatment for *Candida* endophthalmitis, although cures have been reported with fluconazole. Pars plana vitrectomy may facilitate diagnosis and cure when a *Candida* vitreous abscess is present. Injection of amphotericin B into the vitreous humor can also be helpful.

Injection of amphotericin B into an infected joint, pleural cavity, or peritoneum is rarely indicated. Removal of prostheses, including prosthetic joints, cardiac valves, peritoneal dialysis catheters, and central venous catheters, is usually essential. Collections of pus, such as those in the postoperative abdomen, need to be drained surgically or by percutaneous, computed tomography–guided catheterization; an exception relates to the numerous small abscesses in liver, spleen, or kidney in chronic disseminated candidiasis, which cannot be drained effectively and require prolonged antifungal therapy. In general, treatment should continue until the patient with chronic disseminated candidiasis has been afebrile and nonneutropenic for at least 2 weeks. Defects may persist on imaging studies long after cure. Relapse during another episode of neutropenia is common unless the patient is receiving amphotericin B. Repeat cytotoxic therapy or even bone marrow transplantation can be undertaken in patients with prior chronic disseminated candidiasis, but amphotericin B should be given prophylactically during neutropenia.

Fluconazole can decrease the incidence of deep candidiasis in recipients of allogeneic bone marrow transplants when 400 mg is given daily until engraftment. Although the incidence of superficial candidiasis is also decreased by fluconazole prophylaxis, superficial infection can be readily detected and treated. Aspergillosis is not prevented by prophylactic fluconazole. Studies of leukemic and other neutropenic patients have found no beneficial effect of prophylactic fluconazole.

BIBLIOGRAPHY

BENOIT D et al: Management of candidal thrombophlebitis of the central veins: Case report and review. Clin Infect Dis 26:393, 1998

CASADO JL et al: Candidal meningitis in HIV-infected patients: Analysis of 14 cases. Clin Infect Dis 25:673, 1997

DONAHUE SP et al: Intraocular candidiasis in patients with candidemia. Clinical implications derived from a prospective multicenter study. Ophthalmology 101:1302, 1994

EDWARDS JE et al: International Conference for the Development of a Consensus on the Management and Prevention of Severe Candidal Infections. Clin Infect Dis 25:43, 1997

MELGAR GR et al: Fungal prosthetic valve endocarditis in 16 patients. An 11-year experience in a tertiary care hospital. Medicine 76:94, 1997

NGUYEN MH et al: *Candida* prosthetic valve endocarditis: Prospective study of six cases and review of the literature. Clin Infect Dis 22:262, 1996

ODDS FC: *Candida and Candidosis.* Philadelphia, Saunders, 1988

PFALLER MA et al: National surveillance of nosocomial bloodstream infection due to *Candida albicans*: Frequency of occurrence and antifungal susceptibility in the SCOPE Program. Diagn Microbiol Infect Dis 31:327, 1998

REX JH et al: A randomized trial comparing fluconazole with amphotericin B for the treatment of candidemia in patients without neutropenia. N Engl J Med 331:1325, 1994

——— et al: Practice guidelines for the treatment of candidiasis. Clin Infect Dis 30:662, 2000

SLAVIN MA et al: Efficacy and safety of fluconazole prophylaxis for fungal infections after marrow transplantation—a prospective, randomized, double-blind study. J Infect Dis 171:1545, 1995

SOBEL JD et al: Vulvovaginal candidiasis: Epidemiologic, diagnostic, and therapeutic considerations. Am J Obstet Gynecol 178:203, 1998

THALER M et al: Hepatic candidiasis in cancer patients: The evolving picture of the syndrome. Ann Intern Med 198:88, 1988

WILCOX CM et al: A randomized, double-blind comparison of itraconazole oral solution and fluconazole tablets in the treatment of esophageal candidiasis. J Infect Dis 176:227, 1997

206   *John E. Bennett*

ASPERGILLOSIS

ETIOLOGIC AGENTS   *Aspergillus fumigatus* is the most common cause of aspergillosis, but *A. flavus, A. niger,* and several other species can also cause disease. *Aspergillus* is a mold with septate hyphae about 2 to 4 μm in diameter. The fungus is identified by its gross and microscopic appearance in culture.

PATHOGENESIS AND PATHOLOGY   All the common species of *Aspergillus* that cause disease in humans are ubiquitous in the environment, growing on dead leaves, stored grain, compost piles, hay, and other decaying vegetation. Inhalation of *Aspergillus* spores must be extremely common, but disease is rare. Invasion of lung tissue is confined almost entirely to immunosuppressed patients, in roughly 90% of whom two of the following three conditions will be operative: a granulocyte count in peripheral blood of $<500/\mu$L, treatment with supraphysiologic doses of adrenal glucocorticoids, and a history of treatment with cytotoxic drugs such as cyclosporine. Invasive aspergillosis is an occasional complication of AIDS. *Aspergillus* infection is characterized by hyphal invasion of blood vessels, thrombosis, necrosis, and hemorrhagic infarction. Chronic granulomatous disease of childhood also predisposes to invasive pulmonary aspergillosis, but in that situation the inflammatory response is a pyogranuloma and blood vessel invasion is rare.

Massive inhalation of *Aspergillus* spores by healthy persons can lead to acute, diffuse, self-limited pneumonitis. Epithelioid granulomas with giant cells and central pyogenic areas containing hyphae are detected in these cases. Spontaneous recovery taking several weeks is the usual course.

Aspergillus can colonize the damaged bronchial tree, pulmonary cysts, or cavities of patients with underlying lung disease. Balls of hyphae within cysts or cavities (aspergillomas), usually in the upper lobe, may reach several centimeters in diameter and may be visible on chest x-ray. Tissue invasion does not occur. The term *allergic bronchopulmonary aspergillosis* denotes the condition of patients with preexisting asthma who have eosinophilia, IgE antibody to *Aspergillus*, and fleeting pulmonary infiltrates from bronchial plugging.

CLINICAL MANIFESTATIONS   *Endobronchial saprophytic pulmonary aspergillosis* presents as chronic productive cough, often with hemoptysis, in a patient with prior chronic lung disease, such as tuberculosis, sarcoidosis, bronchiectasis, or histoplasmosis. *Aspergillus* may be spread from its endocavitary or endobronchial site to the pleura during the course of bacterial lung abscess or surgery. Patients reported to have chronic necrotizing *Aspergillus* pneumonia appear in most instances to have had saprophytic endobronchial colonization and a pulmonary process attributable to another disease, with or without superimposed bacterial infections. Patients with chronic pneumonia and *Aspergillus* in the sputum should be assumed to have either pneumonia of a different etiology (e.g., histoplasmosis) or *Aspergillus* pneumonia with underlying immunosuppression (e.g., chronic granulomatous disease or infection with HIV).

Invasive aspergillosis in the immunocompromised host presents as an acute, rapidly progressive, densely consolidated pulmonary infiltrate and is most common among patients with acute leukemia and recipients of tissue transplants. Infection progresses by direct extension across tissue planes and by hematogenous dissemination to lung, brain, and other organs. Computed tomography (CT) has been particularly valuable in suggesting the diagnosis of invasive pulmonary aspergillosis in patients with neutropenia. The earliest CT finding is one or more small pulmonary nodules. As a nodule enlarges, the dense central core of infarcted tissue becomes surrounded by edema or hemorrhage, forming a hazy rim called the *halo sign*. This rim disappears in a few days as the dense core enlarges. When bone marrow function recovers, the infarcted central core cavitates, creating the *crescent sign*. *Aspergillus* may invade immunosuppressed patients through the skin at a site of minor trauma or through the upper airway mucosa. Early lesions in the nose should be sought in patients with neutropenia who have fever and minimal epistaxis. Scarlet-red patches of the mucosa rapidly become necrotic and white, then black. Rapid extension into the adjacent paranasal sinus, orbit, or face is usual, with or without the appearance of lung lesions.

Aspergillus sinusitis in immunocompetent patients may take three forms. A ball of hyphae may form in a chronically obstructed paranasal sinus, without tissue invasion. Much less commonly, a chronic, fibrosing granulomatous inflammation associated with *Aspergillus* hyphae within tissue may begin in the sinus and spread slowly to the orbit and the brain. *Aspergillus* is also a cause of allergic fungal sinusitis, but dark-walled fungi (e.g., *Cladosporium, Alternaria*) are more common in this setting. Patients usually have a history of chronic allergic rhinitis, sometimes with nasal polyps, but are otherwise healthy, presenting with painless proptosis, nasal obstruction, or dull aching pain. On CT or magnetic resonance imaging, a solid soft tissue mass pushing out the lateral wall of the ethmoid sinus or the medial wall of the maxillary sinus may be detected. On sinus exploration, the mucosa is found to be thickened and inflamed but intact. Within the sinus cavity, sticky mucopus with strands of neutrophils, eosinophils, Charcot-Leyden crystals, and occasional hyphae can be found.

Aspergillosis in HIV-infected patients most commonly involves the lung, presenting as fever, cough, and dyspnea. Typically, the CD4 cell count is below $50/\mu$L. Roughly half of these patients have neutropenia or have recently been treated with glucocorticoids. Bilateral diffuse or focal pulmonary infiltrates with a tendency to cavitate constitute the most common radiologic manifestation. Well-localized, white, necrotic pseudomembranes full of hyphae or ulcers may develop in the trachea or the major bronchi. Progression of bronchitis to pneumonia is usual, but hematogenous dissemination is uncommon. Either allergic or invasive *Aspergillus* sinusitis can occur in HIV-infected patients; the allergic form can develop even at CD4 cell counts above $50/\mu$L.

The growth of *Aspergillus* on cerumen and detritus within the external auditory canal is termed *otomycosis*. Trauma to the cornea may cause *Aspergillus* keratitis. Endophthalmitis follows the introduction of *Aspergillus* into the globe by trauma or surgery. *Aspergillus* may infect intracardiac or intravascular prostheses.

DIAGNOSIS   The repeated isolation of *Aspergillus* from sputum or the demonstration of hyphae in sputum or bronchoalveolar lavage fluid suggests endobronchial colonization or infection. Even a single isolation of *Aspergillus* from the sputum of a neutropenic patient with pneumonia, particularly a child or a nonsmoker, suggests the diagnosis of invasive aspergillosis. In patients with advanced AIDS, fever, and cough, the isolation of *Aspergillus* from respiratory secretions raises the possibility of aspergillosis and thus should prompt bronchoscopy. Fungus ball of the lung is usually detectable by chest x-ray. IgG antibody to *Aspergillus* antigens is demonstrable in the serum of many colonized patients and of virtually all patients with fungus ball.

Biopsy is usually required for the diagnosis of invasive aspergillosis of the lung, nose, paranasal sinus, bronchi, or sites of dissemination. Blood cultures are rarely positive, even in patients with infected cardiac valves (native or prosthetic). Detection of galactomannan antigen in serum suggests the diagnosis, but false-positives are frequent, particularly in children. *Aspergillus* hyphae can be identified presumptively by histology, but culture is required for confirmation and for determination of the species. Only culture can reliably distinguish aspergillosis from pseudallescheriasis; drug therapy for these two diseases differs.

R_X TREATMENT   Patients with severe hemoptysis due to fungus ball of the lung may benefit from lobectomy. Poor pulmonary function in residual lung and dense pleural adhesions around the lesion can complicate the resection. Systemic chemotherapy is of no value in endobronchial or endocavitary aspergillosis.

Treatment with intravenous amphotericin B (1.0 to 1.5 mg/kg daily) has resulted in the arrest or cure of invasive aspergillosis when immunosuppression is not severe. Liposomal amphotericin B at daily doses of 1 to 4 mg/kg has given results that seem roughly comparable to those obtained with amphotericin B deoxycholate. Itraconazole (200 mg twice daily) is useful in some less immunosuppressed patients with indolent or slowly progressive invasive aspergillosis. Surgery is the only treatment needed for fungus ball of the sinus and for allergic fungal sinusitis. Antifungal therapy has little effect on either entity if used alone, but chronic suppressive therapy has been begun postoperatively for relapse of allergic fungal sinusitis. The prognosis for cure of invasive aspergillosis in the paranasal sinus is very poor when the patient has profound and unremitting neutropenia. The prognosis is better in less immunosuppressed patients.

BIBLIOGRAPHY

DENNING DW: Invasive aspergillosis. Clin Infect Dis 26:781, 1998

LOGAN PM et al: Invasive aspergillosis of the airways: Radiographic, CT and pathologic findings. Radiology 193:383, 1994

LOTHLOLARY O et al: Invasive aspergillosis in patients with acquired immunodeficiency syndrome: Report of 33 cases. Am J Med 95:177, 1993

SHIRAKUSA T et al: Surgical treatment of pulmonary aspergilloma and *Aspergillus* empyema. Ann Thorac Surg 48:779, 1989

STEVENS DA et al: Practice guidelines for diseases caused by *Aspergillus*. Clin Infect Dis 30:696, 2000

TALBOT GH et al: Invasive *Aspergillus* rhinosinusitis in patients with acute leukemia. Rev Infect Dis 13:219, 1991

WALD A et al: Epidemiology of *Aspergillus* infections in a large cohort of patients undergoing bone marrow transplantation. J Infect Dis 175:1459, 1997

207 *John E. Bennett*

MUCORMYCOSIS

ETIOLOGIC AGENTS   Species of *Rhizopus, Rhizomucor,* and *Cunninghamella* are the most common causes of mucormycosis, but species of *Apophysomyces, Saksenaea, Mucor,* and *Absidia* also are occasionally responsible for this infection. The organism in tissue is composed of broad, rarely septate hyphae of uneven diameter (6 to 50 μm). The organisms are inexplicably difficult to grow from infected tissue. When growth does take place, it is rapid and profuse on most media at room temperature. Identification is based on the gross and microscopic appearance of the mold.

Zygomycosis is a term that includes mucormycosis and entomophthoramycosis. The latter is a tropical infection of the subcutaneous tissue or paranasal sinuses caused by species of *Basidiobolus* and *Conidiobolus,* respectively.

EPIDEMIOLOGY AND PATHOLOGY   *Rhizopus* and *Rhizomucor* species are ubiquitous, appearing on decaying vegetation, dung, and foods of high sugar content. Mucormycosis is uncommon and is largely confined to patients with serious preexisting diseases. Mucormycosis originating in the paranasal sinuses and nose predominantly affects patients with poorly controlled diabetes mellitus. Patients who have undergone organ transplantation, who have a hematologic malignancy, or who are receiving long-term deferoxamine therapy are predisposed to mucormycosis of either sinus or lung. Gastrointestinal mucormycosis occurs in a variety of conditions, including uremia, severe malnutrition, and diarrheal diseases. The infection is acquired from nature, with no person-to-person spread. In all forms of mucormycosis, vascular invasion by hyphae is a prominent feature. Ischemic or hemorrhagic necrosis is the foremost histologic finding.

CLINICAL MANIFESTATIONS   Mucormycosis originating in the nose and paranasal sinuses produces a characteristic clinical picture. Low-grade fever, dull sinus pain, and sometimes nasal congestion or a thin, bloody nasal discharge are followed in a few days by double vision, increasing fever, and obtundation. Examination reveals a unilateral generalized reduction of ocular motion, chemosis, and proptosis. The nasal turbinates on the involved side may be dusky red or necrotic. A sharply delineated area of necrosis, strictly respecting the midline, may appear in the hard palate. The skin of the cheek may become inflamed. Fungal invasion of the globe or ophthalmic artery leads to blindness. Opacification of one or more sinuses is detected by computed tomography (CT) or by magnetic resonance imaging (MRI). Carotid arteriography may show invasion or obstruction of the carotid siphon. Coma is due to direct invasion of the frontal lobe. Early symptoms mimic those of bacterial sinusitis. Clouding of the sensorium may be attributed to diabetic acidosis. Cavernous sinus thrombosis may be considered when orbital invasion occurs. Without treatment, the patient may die after an interval ranging from a few days to a few weeks.

Pulmonary mucormycosis manifests as progressive severe pneumonia accompanied by high fever and toxicity. The necrotic center of large infiltrates may cavitate. Hematogenous spread to other areas of the lung, as well as to the brain and other organs, is common. Survival beyond 2 weeks is unusual. Gastrointestinal invasion presents as one or more ulcers that tend to perforate. Hematogenous dissemination can originate from the gastrointestinal tract, lung, or paranasal sinuses. Sometimes no portal of entry can be found.

DIAGNOSIS   CT or MRI is very helpful in assessing the extent of sinusitis before surgery and in evaluating the patient afterward. CT is better for detecting bony erosion; MRI better visualizes extension into the frontal lobe or carotid artery in the siphon. Lesions of the lung and craniofacial structures are best diagnosed by biopsy and histologic section. Cultural confirmation should be attempted. Wet smear of crushed tissue can provide a rapid diagnosis. Cultures of blood and cerebrospinal fluid are negative. Smear and culture of sputum may be positive during cavitation of a lung lesion.

R_X TREATMENT   Regulation of diabetes mellitus and a decrease in the dose of immunosuppressive drugs facilitate the treatment of mucormycosis. Extensive debridement of craniofacial lesions appears to be very important. Orbital exenteration may be required. Intravenous amphotericin B is clearly of value in craniofacial mucormycosis and should be employed in the other forms of mucormycosis as well. The maximal tolerated doses are given until progression is halted. With the deoxycholate formulation, 1 to 1.5 mg/kg daily is indicated. Therapy is continued for a total of 10 to 12 weeks. Azoles are of no value. Appropriate management results in cure of about half of craniofacial infections. The survival of patients with pulmonary, gastrointestinal, or disseminated mucormycosis is rare.

BIBLIOGRAPHY

GALETTA SL et al: Rhinocerebral mucormycosis: Management and survival after carotid occlusion. Ann Neurol 28:103, 1990

HOLLAND J: Emerging zygomycoses of humans: *Saksenaea vasiformis* and *Apophysomyces elegans*. Curr Top Med Mycol 8:27, 1997

MCADAMS HP et al: Pulmonary mucormycosis: Radiologic findings in 32 cases. Am J Radiol 168:1541, 1997

PETERSON KL et al: Rhinocerebral mucormycosis: Evolution of the disease and treatment options. Laryngoscope 107:855, 1997

SINGH N et al: Invasive gastrointestinal zygomycosis in a liver transplant recipient: Case report and review of zygomycosis in solid-organ transplant recipients. Clin Infect Dis 20:617, 1995

TEDDER M et al: Pulmonary mucormycosis: Results of medical and surgical therapy. Ann Thorac Surg 57:1044, 1994

208   John E. Bennett

MISCELLANEOUS MYCOSES AND ALGAL INFECTIONS

CHROMOBLASTOMYCOSIS This chronic subcutaneous mycosis, rarely seen in the United States, presents as a verrucoid, ulcerated, or crusted skin lesion. The disease follows the introduction of any of several fungi into subcutaneous tissue by thorns or bits of vegetation. The infection spreads over ensuing months and years to contiguous tissue, causing few symptoms. The appearance of thick-walled, dark-colored, rounded forms ("copper pennies") in histopathologic section is diagnostic. Surgical excision is the treatment of choice. Itraconazole has ameliorated some relatively small and incompletely excised lesions.

DERMATOPHYTOSIS **Definition** Dermatophytosis, also known as ringworm or tinea, is a chronic fungal infection of the skin, hair, or nails.

Etiology Species of *Trichophyton*, *Microsporum*, and *Epidermophyton* are called *dermatophytes*. These organisms grow in and remain confined to the keratinous structures of the body. Other mycoses, such as candidiasis, pityriasis versicolor, and tinea nigra, sometimes include fungal invasion of keratinous structures but traditionally are not called dermatophytoses.

Pathology and Pathogenesis Dermatophyte species are referred to as *anthropophilic*, *zoophilic*, or *geophilic*, depending on whether their usual reservoir in nature appears to be humans, animals, or soil, respectively. The infectivity of organisms from all these sources is low, and outbreaks are largely confined to occasional clusters of cases of scalp infection in children. Acquisition of a dermatophytosis appears to be favored by minor trauma, maceration, and poor hygiene of the skin. Infection does not seem to confer solid immunity: Repeated infection with the same species is common, particularly with anthropophilic species. The infrequency of scalp infection among adults has been attributed to local factors rather than immunity.

Invasion of the stratum corneum by dermatophytes may cause inflammation that is either mild or (particularly with zoophilic fungi) intense. Shedding of the stratum corneum is increased by inflammation. To the extent that fungal growth cannot keep up with shedding, inflammation may help terminate infection. Conversely, infection is probably favored when shedding is reduced by treatment with glucocorticoids and cytotoxic drugs. Antifungal drugs interfere with the ability of fungal growth to keep up with shedding.

Clinical Manifestations The disease varies with the site of infection and the fungal species involved. Foot infection (athlete's foot, tinea pedis) may present as fissuring of the toe webs, scaling of the plantar surfaces, or vesicles around the toe webs and soles. Interdigital lesions may be pruritic or, when bacterial superinfection occurs, may be painful. Hand infection is less common but resembles foot infection.

Scalp dermatophytosis (tinea capitis) is characterized by areas of alopecia and scaling. In so-called endothrix infection, the hair shaft breaks off at the skin surface, leaving the hairs visible as black dots in the scalp. Some forms of scalp infection include an area of intense boggy suppuration called a *kerion*.

Dermatophytosis of the glabrous skin (tinea corporis, **Plate IID-51**) presents as circumscribed lesions with a wide variety of appearances, including scales, vesicles, and pustules. Inflammation may be minimal or intense. Central healing of less inflamed lesions may take place. The serpiginous border of inflammation is the source of the name *ringworm*.

Dermatophytosis of the bearded area (tinea barbae) appears as a pustular folliculitis. Onychomycosis (tinea unguium) presents as a white discoloration of the nails or as thickening, chalkiness, and crumbling of the nails. Peeling and fissuring of paronychial nail folds or keratotic debris under the nail edge also may be evident.

Diagnosis Discolored hairs, scales, and keratotic debris under infected nails should be collected for KOH smear and culture. In the scraping of skin lesions, a drop of water on the skin site may keep the removed scales from flying off and thus may aid in their collection. Culture is important in distinguishing dermatophytes from *Candida* and fungal saprophytes growing in keratinaceous debris.

TREATMENT Noninflammatory lesions of the trunk, groin, hands, and feet usually respond to twice-daily applications of clotrimazole, miconazole, ketoconazole, econazole, naftifine, terbinafine, or ciclopirox olamine cream. Hyperkeratotic lesions of the palms and soles respond slowly to these agents and may benefit from Whitfield's ointment initially to thin the keratin. Ointment should not be used between the toes, in the groin, or in the gluteal crease because maceration promotes bacterial infection.

Ringworm that is moderately severe, that is unresponsive to topical therapy, or that involves the scalp, nails, or bearded area should be treated systemically. Once-daily therapy with itraconazole (200 mg), terbinafine (250 mg), microcrystalline griseofulvin (500 mg), or ultramicrocrystalline griseofulvin (375 mg) is effective. Treatment must be continued until all infected keratin is gone. Cutting off infected hair and cleansing interdigital webs can expedite cure. Secondary bacterial infection of the foot may require soaks or antibacterial agents. The likelihood of relapse of dermatophyte foot infections may be decreased by keeping the feet clean and dry. For nail infections, itraconazole or terbinafine is preferred. In distal subungual onychomycosis, a single course of either drug results in initial improvement in half of patients, of whom half relapse. Results are better with fingernails than with toenails and for more distal rather than lateral nail involvement. To save money, itraconazole can be given as a double dose (400 mg) for 1 week each month with only marginal loss of efficacy. The duration of therapy is 2 to 3 months for fingernails and 4 to 6 months for toenails.

PROTOTHECOSIS *Prototheca* species are ubiquitous achlorophyllic algae that enter the skin through contaminated wounds and cause localized infections in the olecranon bursa, skin, subcutaneous tissue, tendon sheaths, or deeper tissue. Diagnosis is based on culture or histopathologic demonstration of sporangia with endospores in tissue. Surgical debridement and treatment with intravenous amphotericin B are useful.

FUSARIOSIS *Fusarium* species can cause localized or hematogenously disseminated infection. Localized infection results from contaminated wounds. Almost all patients with hematogenously disseminated infection are severely immunosuppressed and profoundly neutropenic. Skin lesions occur in two-thirds of patients. Several painful red indurated lesions appear on the extremities or sometimes the trunk. These lesions often develop an ecchymotic center that ulcerates. A portal of infection is not usually apparent. Blood cultures have been positive in 59% of cases. Amphotericin B is probably the drug of choice for the treatment of fusariosis, but recovery depends on the diminution of neutropenia.

MALASSEZIA INFECTION (PITYRIASIS) *Malassezia furfur* is part of the normal flora of the human skin but can cause tinea (pityriasis) versicolor or catheter-acquired sepsis. Tinea versicolor appears as asymptomatic, well-delineated, hyperpigmented or hypopigmented macules centered on the upper trunk and upper arms. Confluent lesions may cover large areas, making the border difficult to find. A fine "branny" scale or folliculitis is sometimes visible. When examined microscopically by KOH mount, skin sections are seen to contain characteristic round and elongated cells. On inspection with Wood's light, lesions either do not fluoresce or appear yellow-green. *Erythrasma* resembles tinea versicolor but is characterized by gram-positive bacilli on smear and coral-red fluorescence. Azole creams are effective for the treatment of small areas of tinea versicolor; however, the application of selenium sulfide shampoo (Selsun) for 10 min daily, followed by showering to remove the shampoo, is more practical for large areas. Itraconazole is also effective. Catheter-acquired sepsis due to *M. furfur* develops in patients (particularly neonates) receiving intravenous lipid. The organism requires special culture conditions for growth, and the infection is cured by catheter removal.

MYCETOMA Etiology *Actinomycetoma* refers to infection by actinomycetes of the genera *Nocardia, Nocardiopsis, Streptomyces,* and *Actinomadura. Eumycetoma* is caused by true fungi of many different genera. The predominant agent varies with the locality.

Pathogenesis and Pathology The pathogens live in the soil and enter the skin through minor trauma. The most common site of infection is the foot. The infection runs a relentless course over many years, with destruction of contiguous bone and fascia. Grains are found in purulent foci surrounded by fibrosis and a mononuclear cell inflammatory response.

Clinical Manifestations Mycetoma is a chronic suppurative infection originating in subcutaneous tissue and characterized by the presence of grains, which are tightly clumped colonies of the causative agent. The infected site is characterized by painless swelling, woody induration, and sinus tracts that discharge pus intermittently. Systemic symptoms do not develop, and spread to distant sites in the body does not take place.

Diagnosis Although the clinical picture is characteristic, mycetoma is sometimes confused with chronic osteomyelitis or botryomycosis. The diagnosis requires demonstration of grains in pus from the draining sinus or in biopsy sections. Many histologic sections may need to be examined to locate a grain.

> **℞ TREATMENT** Actinomycetoma may respond to prolonged combination chemotherapy—e.g., with streptomycin and either dapsone or trimethoprim-sulfamethoxazole. Eumycetoma rarely responds to chemotherapy; some cases caused by *Madurella mycetomatis* have appeared to respond to ketoconazole or itraconazole.

PARACOCCIDIOIDOMYCOSIS Etiology Formerly called *South American blastomycosis,* this mycosis is caused by *Paracoccidioides brasiliensis.* A dimorphic fungus, *P. brasiliensis* grows as a budding yeast in tissue but may be grown as either a yeast or a mold on culture medium. The organism is identified by its gross and microscopic appearance.

Pathogenesis and Pathology Infection is thought to be acquired by inhalation of spores from environmental sources, possibly soil. Pulmonary infection produces few symptoms initially. Hematogenous spread to the mucous membranes of the mouth and nose, the lymph nodes, and other sites causes patients to seek medical attention. In fatal cases, the infection spreads to the adrenals, the gastrointestinal tract, and many other viscera.

Clinical Manifestations Common signs include indurated ulcers of the mouth, oropharynx, larynx, and nose; enlarged and draining lymph nodes; lesions of the skin and genitalia; and productive cough, weight loss, dyspnea, and sometimes fever. Paracoccidioidomycosis is acquired only in South America, Central America, and Mexico, but its extreme indolence may delay its recognition until many years after

the patient has left the endemic area. Chest radiography most often shows bilateral patchy pneumonia.

Diagnosis Cultures of sputum, pus, and mucosal lesions are often diagnostic. The diagnosis can be made by smear or histologic section, although confirmation by culture is preferable. Serologic tests are useful in suggesting the diagnosis and monitoring the response to therapy.

> **℞ TREATMENT** Relatively mild cases of paracoccidioidomycosis may be cured by 1 year of treatment with oral ketoconazole or itraconazole (200 to 400 mg daily). More advanced cases are treated with intravenous amphotericin B followed by itraconazole.

PHAEOHYPHOMYCOSIS This is the name given to infections caused by fungi with dark-walled hyphae, excluding those given conventional names like chromoblastomycosis. Although an extraordinary variety of fungi and clinical syndromes are encompassed by this definition, most patients have brain abscess, subcutaneous abscess, or allergic fungal sinusitis. Most of the brain abscesses are due to *Cladophialophora bantiana, Ochroconis gallopavum, Exophiala dermatitidis, Bipolaris* species, and *Ramichloridium mackenziei.* Patients are previously healthy. Subcutaneous abscesses are usually single, arise at the site of minor trauma, and occur in both immunosuppressed and immunocompetent individuals. A large number of dematiaceous (dark-walled) mold species cause subcutaneous phaeohyphomycosis as well as allergic fungal sinusitis. The latter entity develops in patients with allergic rhinitis and presents as an expanding mucoid mass in one or more paranasal sinuses. The tenacious mucus contains eosinophils, Charcot-Leyden crystals, and occasional hyphae. Surgical excision of phaeohyphomycotic lesions is important. Antifungal therapy may retard recurrences but is of little value unless surgical excision has been performed.

PSEUDALLESCHERIASIS Etiology Also called *Petriellidium boydii, Pseudallescheria boydii* is a mold frequently found in soil. When the fungus is isolated in the imperfect state, it is called *Scedosporium apiospermum.*

Pathogenesis and Pathology Wind-borne spores of *P. boydii,* arising from the soil, are the presumed source of infection. The fungus grows as a mold within tissue, causing necrosis and abscess formation.

Clinical Manifestations *P. boydii* resembles *Aspergillus* in its ability to colonize the endobronchial tree, to form fungus balls in the lungs or paranasal sinuses, and to invade the cornea or globe of the eye, the soft tissues, the joints, or the bones after trauma or surgery and in its propensity to invade the lungs and paranasal sinuses of immunosuppressed hosts, including patients with AIDS. Hyphae of *P. boydii* in tissue may be difficult to distinguish from those of *Aspergillus.* Infection with *P. boydii* is much less common than that with *Aspergillus.* Intravascular hyphae, a hallmark of invasive aspergillosis, are also found in pseudallescheriasis. Near-drowning in polluted water has led to severe *P. boydii* pneumonia, often with dissemination and fatal brain abscesses.

Diagnosis Demonstration of hyphae in tissue and culture confirmation are required for diagnosis.

> **℞ TREATMENT** Itraconazole at the maximal tolerated doses is the regimen of choice. Surgical drainage or debridement can be helpful. The prognosis is poor.
> *Scedosporium prolificans,* a fungus closely related to *P. boydii,* has caused infections in bones, joints, or soft tissue, usually after trauma. These infections have responded to surgical debridement. Disseminated infection with *S. prolificans* in immunosuppressed patients has been fatal. The response to treatment with all antifungal agents has been poor.

SPOROTRICHOSIS Etiology *Sporothrix schenckii* lives as a saprophyte on plants in many areas of the world. In nature and on culture at room temperature, the fungus grows as a mold; within host tissue or at 37°C on enriched media, it grows as a budding yeast. It is identified by its appearance in mold and yeast forms.

Pathogenesis and Pathology　Infection results from the inoculation of *S. schenckii* into subcutaneous tissue through minor trauma. Nursery workers, florists, and gardeners acquire the illness from roses, sphagnum moss, and other plants. Infection may be limited to the site of inoculation (plaque sporotrichosis) or extend along proximal lymphatic channels (lymphangitic sporotrichosis). Spread beyond an extremity—the usual site of infection—is rare, and hematogenous dissemination from the skin remains unproven. The portal for osteoarticular, pulmonary, and other extracutaneous forms of sporotrichosis is unknown but is likely the lung.

Untreated sporotrichosis persists for months. The inflammatory response includes both the clustering of neutrophils and a marked granulomatous response with epithelioid cells and giant cells.

Clinical Manifestations　In lymphangitic sporotrichosis, which is by far the most common manifestation, a nearly painless red papule forms at the site of inoculation. Over the next several weeks, similar nodules form along proximal lymphatic channels. The nodules intermittently discharge small amounts of pus. Ulceration may occur. The proximal extension of these lesions, often with skip areas, is quite distinctive but may be mimicked by lesions of *Nocardia brasiliensis*, *Mycobacterium marinum*, or (in rare cases) *Leishmania brasiliensis* or *Mycobacterium kansasii*.

Plaque sporotrichosis manifests as a nontender red maculopapular granuloma confined to the site of inoculation. Osteoarticular sporotrichosis presents as mono- or polyarticular arthritis of indolent onset and progression over months or years, involving the elbows, knees, wrists, ankles, and (rarely) smaller joints of the extremities. Periarticular bone develops areas of demineralization detectable on x-ray, and draining sinuses may appear over joints and bursae. Hematogenous spread to the skin may take place during polyarticular disease, but none of the skin lesions shows lymphangitic spread. Immunosuppression, including that due to advanced infection with HIV, predisposes to hematogenous spread. Pulmonary sporotrichosis usually presents as a single chronic cavitary upper-lobe lung lesion. Chronic meningitis can develop in the absence of skin or lung lesions. *S. schenckii* is difficult to recover from cerebrospinal fluid.

Diagnosis　Culture of pus, joint fluid, sputum, or a skin biopsy specimen is the preferred method of diagnosis. The appearance of *S. schenckii* in tissue is quite variable. In skin lesions, the organisms are hard to find.

℞ TREATMENT　Cutaneous sporotrichosis can be cured with a saturated solution of potassium iodide given orally in increasing divided doses of up to 4.5 to 9 mL/d for adults, as tolerated. Gastrointestinal disturbance or acneiform rash over the cape area and face is common, but therapy should be continued for 1 month after the resolution of all lesions. Itraconazole (100 to 200 mg daily) is an effective and better-tolerated alternative. Extracutaneous sporotrichosis rarely responds to iodides, but more than half of cases have been cured by prolonged courses of intravenous amphotericin B. Itraconazole (200 mg once or twice daily) is effective in some cases of extracutaneous sporotrichosis.

TRICHOSPORONOSIS　A recent change in taxonomy of the genus *Trichosporon* has moved most of the agents causing deep infections from *T. beigelii* into the species *T. asahii*, with a few categorized as *T. mucoides*. White piedra of the scalp is caused by *T. ovoides* and that of the pubic hair by *T. inkin*. *T cutaneum* and *T. asteroides* cause superficial infections. Most of what is currently known about *Trichosporon* infections is not species specific, so the following description refers to *T. beigelii*. *T. capitatum*, which causes disseminated infection in patients with neutropenia, was previously reclassified as *Blastoschizomyces capitatus* and will not be covered here.

T. beigelii can colonize the human gastrointestinal tract and skin and can enter the bloodstream of patients with severe neutropenia through an inapparent source. Hematogenously disseminated infection is manifested by fever and often by the development of several erythematous or purpuric tender papules anywhere on the body. Lesions can form large, tense hemorrhagic bullae. In some patients, native or prosthetic cardiac valves become infected. In tissue, hyphae and yeast-like cells are seen. Amphotericin B is probably the drug of choice for treatment, but recovery is dependent on the return of bone marrow function.

BIBLIOGRAPHY

BARBER GR et al: Catheter-related *Malassezia furfur* fungemia in immunocompromised patients. Am J Med 95:365, 1993

BOUTATI EI, ANAISSIE EJ: *Fusarium*, a significant emerging pathogen in patients with hematologic malignancy: Ten years' experience at a cancer center and implications for management. Blood 90:999, 1997

CAREY WP et al: Cutaneous protothecosis in a patient with AIDS and severe functional defect: Successful therapy with amphotericin B. Clin Infect Dis 25:1265, 1997

DUONG TA: Infection due to *Penicillium marneffei*, an emerging pathogen: Review of 155 reported cases. Clin Infect Dis 23:125, 1996

ENGLAND DM, HOCHHOLZER L: Adiaspiromycosis: An unusual fungal infection of the lung. Am J Surg Pathol 17:876, 1993

HAY RJ et al: Mycetoma. J Med Vet Mycol 30(Suppl 1):41, 1992

KAUFFMAN CA et al: Practice guidelines for the management of patients with sporotrichosis. Clin Infect Dis 30:684, 2000

MARCON MJ, POWELL DA: Human infections due to *Malassezia* spp. Clin Microbiol Rev 5:101, 1992

MEYER RD et al: Fungal sinusitis in patients with AIDS: Report of 4 cases and review of the literature. Medicine 73:69, 1994

NARANJO MS et al: Treatment of paracoccidioidomycosis with itraconazole. J Med Vet Mycol 28:67, 1990

REIDY JJ et al: Infection of the conjunctiva by *Rhinosporidium seeberi*. Surv Ophthalmol 41:409, 1997

RESTREPO A: Treatment of tropical mycoses. J Am Acad Dermatol 31:S91, 1994

RINALDI MG: Phaeohyphomycosis. Dermatol Clin 14:147, 1996

RUXIN TA et al: *Pseudallescheria boydii* in an immunocompromised host: Successful treatment with debridement and itraconazole. Arch Dermatol 132:382, 1996

SUGITA T et al: Taxonomic position of deep-seated, mucosa associated, and superficial isolates of *Trichosporon cutaneum* from trichosporonosis patients. J Clin Microbiol 33:1368, 1995

SUPPARATPINYO K et al: A controlled trial of itraconazole to prevent relapse of *Penicillium marneffei* infection in patients infected with the human immunodeficiency virus. N Engl J Med 339:1739, 1998

SUTTON DA et al: U.S. case report of cerebral phaeohyphomycosis caused by *Ramichloridium obovoideum* (*R. mackenziei*): Criteria for identification, therapy, and review of other known dematiaceous neurotropic taxa. J Clin Microbiol 36:708, 1998

VARTIVARIAN SE et al: Emerging fungal pathogens in immunocompromised patients: Classification, diagnosis, and management. Clin Infect Dis 17(Suppl 2):487, 1993

WINN RE et al: Systemic sporotrichosis treated with itraconazole. Clin Infect Dis 17:210, 1993

209　*Peter D. Walzer*

PNEUMOCYSTIS CARINII INFECTION

DEFINITION AND DESCRIPTION　*Pneumocystis carinii* is an opportunistic pathogen whose natural habitat is the lung. The organism is an important cause of pneumonia in the compromised host.

Although the taxonomic status of *P. carinii* has long been controversial, molecular studies during the past decade have clearly placed the organism among the fungi. This classification is based on analysis of gene sequences for ribosomal RNA, mitochondrial proteins, and major enzymes. The cell wall of *P. carinii* contains β-1,3-glucan; drugs that inhibit β-glucan synthesis in fungi are highly active against *P. carinii* in animal models. However, in contrast to most fungi, *P. carinii* lacks ergosterol and is not susceptible to antifungal drugs that inhibit ergosterol synthesis.

Study of the basic biology of *P. carinii* has been severely hampered by the lack of a reliable in vitro cultivation system. Major developmental stages of the organism include the small (1- to 4-μm) pleomorphic trophozoite or trophic form; the 5- to 8-μm cyst, which has a thick cell wall and contains up to eight intracystic bodies; and the precyst, an intermediate stage. The life cycle of *P. carinii* probably involves asexual replication by the trophic form and sexual reproduction by the cyst, which ends in release of the intracystic bodies; an intracellular stage has not been identified. Ultrastructurally, *P. carinii* has a primitive organelle system, but little is known about its metabolism.

P. carinii contains two prominent antigen groups. The 95- to 140-kDa major surface glycoprotein (MSG) complex represents a family of proteins encoded by multiple genes. The MSG complex is highly immunogenic, contains shared and species-specific antigenic determinants, and exhibits protective B and T cell epitopes in animal models. The MSG complex plays a pivotal role in the host-parasite relationship in *P. carinii* infection. It facilitates adherence to host proteins via extracellular matrix proteins, surfactant proteins, and the mannose receptor; and its ability to undergo antigenic variation may represent a mechanism by which *P. carinii* evades the host immune response. The other antigen, which migrates as a band of 35 to 55 kDa, is the most common antigen recognized by the host and thus may serve as a marker of infection.

EPIDEMIOLOGY   *P. carinii* has a worldwide distribution among humans and has been detected in a variety of animals. The organisms found in these hosts are morphologically identical, but recent studies have revealed a high degree of genetic diversity and host specificity. Serologic surveys indicate that most healthy children have been exposed to the organism by 3 to 4 years of age. Animal model experiments have demonstrated that *P. carinii* is transmitted by the airborne route. Person-to-person transmission has been suggested by the occurrence of outbreaks of pneumocystosis among institutionalized debilitated infants and in hospitals caring for immunosuppressed patients. On the basis of animal studies, the incubation period is thought to be 4 to 8 weeks.

PATHOGENESIS AND PATHOLOGY   The host factors that predispose to the development of pneumocystosis involve defects in cellular and humoral immunity. People at risk for the disease include patients infected with HIV; persons receiving immunosuppressive therapy (particularly glucocorticoids) for cancer, organ transplantation, and other disorders; children with primary immunodeficiency diseases; and premature malnourished infants. The central role of CD4+ cells in host resistance to *P. carinii* has been shown by research in experimental animals and by studies that have correlated the risk of pneumocystosis in HIV-infected patients with CD4+ cell counts. Evidence supporting the importance of impaired humoral immunity consists of the occurrence of pneumocytosis in patients and animals with B cell defects and the beneficial effect of passively administered antibodies.

The principal host effector cells against *P. carinii* are alveolar macrophages, which ingest and kill the organism, releasing a variety of inflammatory mediators. Tumor necrosis factor α and interleukin (IL) 1 are important in the early host defenses against *P. carinii*, but the role of other cytokines is less clear. Recent evidence suggests that HIV alters the mannose receptor–mediated binding and phagocytosis of *P. carinii*.

After being inhaled, *P. carinii* takes up residence in the alveoli, where it attaches tightly to type I cells but maintains an extracellular existence. In some cases, the organism remains in the host for long periods, and pneumonia develops by reactivation of latent infection; in other cases, pneumonia arises from a new bout of infection. As the immune system of the host becomes compromised, *P. carinii* organisms propagate and gradually fill the alveoli. This scenario is accompanied by a complex series of events that result in increased alveolar-capillary permeability and damage to type I cells. Surfactant abnormalities include a fall in bronchoalveolar lavage (BAL) fluid phospholipids and an increase in surfactant proteins A and D. Contri-

butions of the host inflammatory response to lung injury are suggested by the correlation of increased IL-8 levels and neutrophil counts in BAL fluid from patients with relatively severe disease.

On lung sections stained with hematoxylin and eosin, the alveoli are filled with a typical foamy, vacuolated exudate. Severe disease may include interstitial edema, fibrosis, and hyaline membrane formation. The host inflammatory changes usually consist of hypertrophy of alveolar type II cells, a typical reparative response, and a mild mononuclear cell interstitial infiltrate. Malnourished infants display an intense plasma cell infiltrate that gave the disease its early name: interstitial plasma cell pneumonia.

CLINICAL FEATURES   Patients with *P. carinii* pneumonia develop dyspnea, fever, and nonproductive cough. Symptoms in non-HIV-infected patients often begin after the glucocorticoid dose has been tapered and typically last 1 to 2 weeks. HIV-infected patients are usually ill for several weeks or longer and have relatively subtle manifestations. However, the clinical picture in individual patients is quite variable, and a high index of suspicion and elicitation of a careful history are key factors in early detection.

Physical findings include tachypnea, tachycardia, and cyanosis, but lung auscultation reveals few abnormalities. The white blood cell count is variable and is usually governed by the patient's underlying disease. Assessment of arterial blood gases demonstrates hypoxia, an increased alveolar-arterial oxygen gradient ($PA_{O_2} - Pa_{O_2}$), and respiratory alkalosis. There also may be changes in pulmonary function test values (diffusing capacity) and increased uptake with nuclear imaging techniques (gallium scan). Elevated serum concentrations of lactate dehydrogenase (LDH) have been reported; they probably reflect lung parenchymal damage but are not specific to *P. carinii* infection. In general, laboratory abnormalities are less severe in HIV-infected patients than in non-HIV-infected patients.

The classic findings on chest radiography consist of bilateral diffuse infiltrates beginning in the perihilar regions (Fig. 209-1), but various atypical manifestations (nodular densities, cavitary lesions) have also been reported. Patients who receive aerosolized pentamidine have an increased frequency of upper-lobe infiltrates and pneumothorax. Early in the course of pneumocystosis, the chest radiograph may be normal.

Although *P. carinii* usually remains confined to the lungs, cases of disseminated infection have occurred in both HIV-infected and non-HIV-infected patients. One risk factor for extrapulmonary spread in patients with HIV is the administration of aerosolized pentamidine. The most common sites of extrapulmonary involvement are the lymph

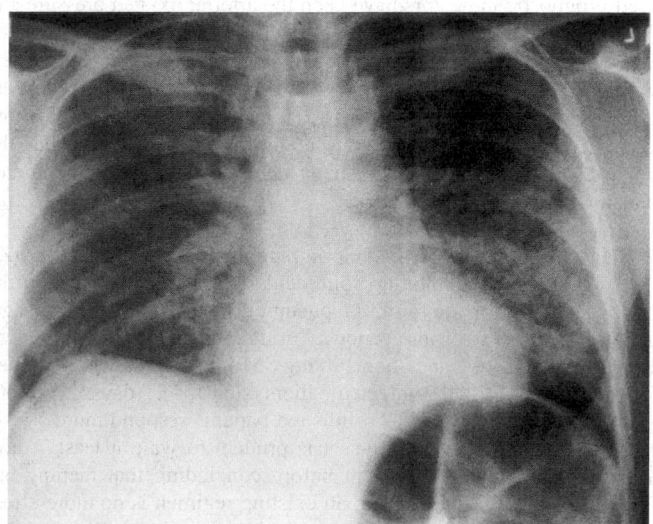

FIGURE 209-1 Chest radiograph depicting diffuse infiltrates in an HIV-infected patient with pneumocystosis.

nodes, spleen, liver, and bone marrow. Clinical manifestations range from incidental findings at autopsy to specific organ involvement. Histopathologic examination reveals the presence of *P. carinii* and the characteristic associated foamy material. Treatment for the extrapulmonary forms of pneumocystosis is the same as that for pneumonia.

DIAGNOSIS Because the clinical picture of *P. carinii* infection can be produced by many other infectious and noninfectious agents, the diagnosis must be based on specific identification of the organism. A definitive diagnosis is made by histopathologic staining. Traditional stains have included reagents such as methenamine silver, toluidine blue, and cresyl echt violet, which selectively stain the wall of *P. carinii* cysts, and reagents such as Wright-Giemsa, which stain the nuclei of all developmental stages. Other reagents include nonspecific fluorochrome stains (calcofluor white) and Papanicolaou's stain. Immunofluorescence with monoclonal antibodies is more sensitive than histologic staining but is also more expensive. DNA amplification by the polymerase chain reaction offers the greatest sensitivity and may find a place in the routine diagnosis of *P. carinii* when commercial kits become available.

The successful diagnosis of pneumocystosis depends upon the collection of proper specimens. In general, the yield from different diagnostic procedures is higher in HIV-infected patients than in non-HIV-infected patients because of the higher organism burden in the former group. Sputum induction has gained popularity as a simple, noninvasive technique; this procedure requires trained and dedicated personnel, and its success has varied at different institutions. Fiberoptic bronchoscopy with BAL, which is more sensitive than sputum induction, remains the mainstay of *P. carinii* diagnosis. This procedure also provides information about the organism burden, the host inflammatory response, and the presence of other opportunistic infections. Transbronchial biopsy and open lung biopsy, which are the most invasive procedures, are reserved for situations in which a diagnosis cannot be made by BAL.

COURSE AND PROGNOSIS In the typical case of untreated *P. carinii* pneumonia, progressive respiratory embarrassment leads to death. Therapy is most effective when instituted early in the course of the disease, before there is extensive alveolar damage. If induced sputum is nondiagnostic and BAL cannot be performed in a timely manner, it is reasonable to begin empiric therapy with drugs active against *P. carinii*. However, this practice does not obviate the need for a specific etiologic diagnosis. With improvements in management, the case-fatality rate has been lowered to about 15% in HIV-infected patients but remains high (40%) in non-HIV-infected patients. The most widely used prognostic indicators have been the arterial oxygen pressure and the alveolar-arterial oxygen gradient. Other factors that may influence survival include neutrophil counts and IL-8 levels in BAL fluid, chest radiographic abnormalities, serum LDH and albumin levels, and the expertise of the hospital in caring for patients with HIV infection. Concurrent pulmonary infections complicate management, but the presence of cytomegalovirus usually does not affect the outcome of pneumocystosis.

℞ TREATMENT Trimethoprim-sulfamethoxazole (TMP-SMZ), which acts by inhibiting folic acid synthesis, is considered the drug of choice for all forms of pneumocystosis. The daily dosage, administered orally or intravenously in three or four divided doses, is 15 to 20 mg TMP/kg and 75 to 100 mg SMZ/kg. Therapy is continued for 14 days in non-HIV-infected patients and for 21 days in persons infected with HIV. Since HIV-infected patients respond more slowly than non-HIV-infected patients, it is prudent to wait at least 7 days after the initiation of treatment before concluding that therapy has failed. The addition of drugs to an existing regimen is no more effective than switching regimens and may increase the risk of toxicity. TMP-SMZ is well tolerated by non-HIV-infected patients, but more than half of HIV-infected patients experience serious adverse reactions, including fever, rash, neutropenia, thrombocytopenia, hepatitis, and hyperkalemia.

Several alternative regimens are available for the treatment of mild to moderate cases of *P. carinii* pneumonia: TMP (15 mg/kg per day orally) plus dapsone (100 mg/d orally), clindamycin (600 mg every 6 h intravenously or 300 to 450 mg every 6 h orally) plus primaquine (15 to 30 mg of base per day orally), or atovaquone alone (750 mg twice daily orally). Dapsone and primaquine should be used with caution in patients with glucose-6-phosphate dehydrogenase deficiency.

Two alternative drugs are available for the treatment of moderate to severe forms of pneumocystosis. Pentamidine, which has been used against *P. carinii* for many years, is administered as a single daily dose of 4 mg/kg by slow intravenous infusion. Pentamidine is highly toxic; its major side effects are hypotension, cardiac arrhythmias, dysglycemias, azotemia, electrolyte changes, and neutropenia. Trimetrexate is administered intravenously as a single daily dose of 45 mg/m^2; in conjunction with trimetrexate therapy, folinic acid is given orally or intravenously at a dose of 20 mg/m^2 every 6 h to prevent bone marrow suppression.

Patients with HIV frequently experience deterioration in respiratory function shortly after receiving anti–*P. carinii* drugs. Several studies have shown that the administration of glucocorticoids to patients with HIV and moderate to severe pneumocystosis (a P_{O_2} of ≤70 mmHg or a $PA_{O_2} - Pa_{O_2}$ of ≥35 mmHg) can prevent this problem and improve the rate of survival. The administration of steroids should be started early in the course of the illness (usually when antimicrobial drugs are begun) for maximal benefit; the recommended regimen is 40 mg of prednisone orally twice daily on days 1 to 5, 40 mg/d on days 6 to 10, and 20 mg/d on days 11 to 20. This regimen has generally proven to be safe despite concern about its effects on other opportunistic infections. The use of steroids as adjunctive therapy in HIV-infected patients with mild pneumocystosis or in non-HIV-infected patients remains to be evaluated.

PREVENTION Primary prophylaxis is indicated for HIV-infected patients at high risk of developing pneumocystosis—that is, those who have CD4+ cell counts of <200/μL, unexplained fever [>37.8°C (100° F)] for ≥2 weeks, or a history of oropharyngeal candidiasis. Guidelines for the administration of primary prophylaxis to other immunocompromised hosts are less clear. Secondary prophylaxis is indicated for all patients who have recovered from *P. carinii* pneumonia. Among HIV-infected patients, the risk of recurrent episodes of pneumocystosis is high and lifelong; among non-HIV-infected patients, the risk is lower and exists for as long as the immunosuppressive condition persists.

Several antimicrobial drugs are effective in preventing pneumocystosis, although some concern has been raised about possible resistance. One double-strength tablet of TMP-SMZ (160 mg TMP, 800 mg SMZ) per day is the prophylactic regimen of choice. The major limitation of TMP-SMZ treatment is the high frequency of adverse reactions among HIV-infected patients. Recommended alternative regimens include TMP-SMZ at a reduced dose (80 mg TMP, 400 mg SMZ) or frequency (3 times per week), dapsone alone at a daily oral dose of 100 mg, dapsone at a dose of 50 mg/d combined with weekly oral doses of pyrimethamine (50 mg) and folinic acid (25 mg), pentamidine at a monthly dose of 300 mg administered by Respigard nebulizer, and atovaquone at an oral dose of 1500 mg/d.

Although there are no specific recommendations for preventing the spread of *P. carinii* in health care facilities, it seems prudent to prevent direct contact between patients with pneumocystosis and other susceptible hosts.

BIBLIOGRAPHY

BENEFIELD TL et al: Prognostic value of interleukin-8 in AIDS-associated *Pneumocystis carinii* pneumonia. Am J Respir Crit Care Med 151:1058, 1995

HORNER RD et al: Relationship between procedures and health insurance for critically ill patients with *Pneumocystis carinii* pneumonia. Am J Respir Crit Care Med 152:1435, 1995

KAZANJIAN P et al: *Pneumocystis carinii* mutations associated with sulfa and sulfone prophylaxis failures in AIDS patients. AIDS 12:873, 1998

KOZIEL H et al: Reduced binding and phagocytosis of *Pneumocystis carinii* by alveolar macrophages from persons infected with HIV-1 correlates with mannose receptor down regulation. J Clin Invest 102:1322, 1998

LIMPER AH et al: Interactions of parasite and host epithelial cell cycle regulation during *Pneumocystis carinii* pneumonia. J Lab Clin Med 130:132, 1997

SAFRIN S et al: Comparison of three regimens for treatment of mild to moderate *Pneumocystis carinii* pneumonia in patients with AIDS. Ann Intern Med 124:792, 1996

STRINGER JR, WALZER PD: Molecular biology and epidemiology of *Pneumocystis carinii* infection in AIDS. AIDS 10:561, 1996

THEUS SA et al: Adoptive transfer of lymphocytes sensitized to the major surface glycoprotein of *Pneumocystis carinii* confers protection in the rat. J Clin Invest 95:2587, 1995

US PUBLIC HEALTH SERVICE/INFECTIOUS DISEASES SOCIETY OF AMERICA: Guidelines for the prevention of opportunistic infections in persons infected with human immunodeficiency virus: A summary. MMWR 46(RR-12):1, 1997

WALZER PD: Immunological features of *Pneumocystis carinii* infection in humans. Clin Diagn Lab Immunol 6:149, 1999

Section 16
PROTOZOAL AND HELMINTHIC INFECTIONS: GENERAL CONSIDERATIONS

Peter F. Weller

APPROACH TO THE PATIENT WITH PARASITIC INFECTION

Because diverse parasitic organisms may infect humans, a range of factors are germane to an assessment of the possible parasitic etiology of a patient's disease. These factors include issues related to the patient's history, immune status, and presenting clinical and laboratory characteristics, especially eosinophilia. Complementing historical information, a full clinical evaluation and laboratory testing provide additional data to direct the assessment for parasitic infection. The specific tests required, ranging from standard blood biochemical assays to imaging of selected organs, are dictated by the nature of the patient's illness. Additional diagnostic testing for parasitic infections (Chap. 211) completes the evaluation.

HISTORY   Geographic History   The history can provide valuable information about potential exposures to parasitic infections. A history of travel to, residence or work in, or immigration from areas of the world in which various parasites not endemic in the United States are encountered offers a clue to possible parasitic or other infectious etiologies of a patient's disease (Chap. 123). Some parasitic infections may become manifest early after a traveler's return home; paramount among these in terms of preventable mortality is malaria. If a patient has been in a region of the world where malaria is endemic (even only briefly, as in an airport layover), fever mandates a consideration of malaria, whether or not malaria chemoprophylaxis has been used. Falciparum malaria, which in a nonimmune patient may progress rapidly to serious and even life-threatening consequences (Chap. 214), is a potential medical emergency and must be considered at the initial evaluation, even if symptoms and fever patterns are suggestive of less specific flulike or gastrointestinal illness. Rarely, malaria transmission has been reported within the United States.

For patients with a history of recent travel, the onset of gastrointestinal symptoms only after return suggests protozoal diseases characterized by a 1- to 2-week delay between acquisition and appearance of symptoms—notably, giardiasis, cyclosporiasis, and cryptosporidiosis (Chap. 218). Gastrointestinal symptoms lasting longer than a week also suggest protozoan etiologies, including giardiasis, amebiasis, and cyclosporiasis. For patients who have traveled less recently, information on the specific countries and the types of regions (urban or rural) visited and on the nature and duration of the visit, whether for general tourism or for activities related to specific occupations, is helpful in concert with presenting clinical features and hematologic and other laboratory findings. Diseases that may become manifest only some years after an individual leaves an endemic region include schistosomiasis, some forms of filariasis, strongyloidiasis, echinococcosis, and cysticercosis.

For the illnesses of patients who have never left the United States, various parasitic etiologies should be considered, depending on the presenting disease. Trichomoniasis, trichinellosis, strongyloidiasis, giardiasis, cryptosporidiosis, cyclosporiasis, echinococcosis, and pinworm are among the parasitic infections endemic in settings within the United States. Diseases that are more frequent where there is fecal contamination of soil or other environmental sites include hookworm, ascariasis, trichuriasis, amebiasis, and strongyloidiasis; dermal exposure, as by walking barefoot on soil contaminated with parasitic larvae, predisposes residents of such an area as well as travelers to the acquisition of cutaneous larva migrans, hookworm, and strongyloidiasis.

Dietary History   If more than one patient develops similar symptoms in a given situation, common-source water- or foodborne diseases (giardiasis, cryptosporidiosis, cyclosporiasis) should be considered. Waterborne infections are more likely to be acquired from surface water supplies, ranging from mountain streams to municipal reservoirs. Likewise, attention to dietary history may be helpful. Trichinellosis should be considered when the patient may have consumed contaminated pork, bear, walrus, or other meat from carnivores. Ingestion of undercooked fish predisposes to anisakiasis and to infection with other fish-dwelling nematodes, tapeworms (*Diphyllobothrium latum*), or flukes (*Nanophyetus salmincola*). Ingestion of snails or of produce contaminated with land snails can lead to infection with *Angiostrongylus cantonensis* (eosinophilic meningitis; Chap. 219). Ingestion of more exotic animal foodstuffs, including snakes, can result in the transmission of gnathostomiasis (Chap. 219). For children with a propensity for pica, ingestion of soil containing *Toxocara* eggs may lead to visceral larva migrans. Consumption of ground-grown vegetables, including those shipped in from distant fields contaminated with human feces, provides an opportunity for the ingestion of nematode eggs of *Ascaris lumbricoides* or *Trichuris trichiura*.

Other Exposure Histories   An antecedent blood transfusion raises the possibility of malaria (especially that due to *Plasmodium malariae* or *P. falciparum*), babesiosis, or Chagas' disease. A history of wading or swimming in fresh water is germane to the acquisition of schistosomiasis or avian schistosome dermatitis. Fresh water may be a source of infection with free-living amebae, and these protozoa may cause meningoencephalitis or ocular infections. Arthropod vector–borne parasitic infections include malaria and lymphatic filariasis (carried by mosquitoes) and babesiosis (carried by ticks); the latter is transmitted in some regions of the United States.

Residence in an institutional setting where fecal-oral hygiene may be imperfect raises the possibility of giardiasis, cryptosporidiosis, or strongyloidiasis. Child-care centers provide opportunities for young children and their family members to acquire giardiasis, cryptosporidiosis, and pinworm infections. Trichomoniasis is transmitted sexually;

giardiasis, cryptosporidiosis, amebiasis, and strongyloidiasis can be transmitted during anal intercourse or oral-anal contact.

IMMUNE STATUS The patient's immune status is relevant in determining which parasitic infections need to be considered. In patients infected with HIV-1, especially those with depressed CD4+ lymphocyte counts, specific protozoan diseases may develop opportunistically. These infections include toxoplasmosis, isosporiasis, cyclosporiasis, cryptosporidiosis, visceral leishmaniasis, American trypanosomiasis, microsporidiosis, and infections with free-living amebae (*Acanthamoeba* and related genera). In individuals infected with human T-lymphotropic virus type 1, strongyloidiasis is a prominent consideration. Patients who are asplenic are at risk not only for overwhelming infections due to encapsulated bacteria but also for fulminant infections caused by intraerythrocytic protozoa, including malaria and babesiosis. Patients with hypogammaglobulinemia or cystic fibrosis may develop refractory giardiasis. In patients developing symptoms of enterocolitis while receiving glucocorticoids, the possibility of an exacerbation of unsuspected strongyloidiasis or amebic colitis should be considered.

EOSINOPHILIA Eosinophilia may offer a hematologic clue to the presence of some parasites. Only two protozoan parasites have been associated with eosinophilia: *Isospora belli* and, on occasion, *Dientamoeba fragilis*. The detection of eosinophilia generally mandates a consideration of the multicellular helminthic parasites that characteristically elicit interleukin 5–mediated eosinophilia. (Helminth-elicited eosinophilia, however, may be suppressed by glucocorticoid therapy or by intercurrent bacterial or viral infections.) The magnitude of eosinophilia tends to correlate with the extent of tissue invasion by helminths. Marked blood eosinophilia (more than 3000 eosinophils per microliter) develops during the early transpulmonary migration of intestinal nematodes, including *Ascaris* and hookworms, at a time when eggs (whose presence confirms the diagnosis) have not yet been produced in the intestinal tract.

Eosinophilia is also marked in the early stages of fluke infections, including schistosomiasis (Katayama fever), paragonimiasis, clonorchiasis, and fascioliasis; during the stage of muscle invasion in trichinellosis; during tissue migration of adult worms in loiasis and gnathostomiasis; and with heavy infections in visceral larva migrans. Eosinophilia persisting for more than a year may be indicative of hookworm infection, strongyloidiasis, visceral larva migrans (especially in children), filarial infection (including onchocerciasis, loiasis, and tropical pulmonary eosinophilia), fluke infections (including schistosomiasis, fascioliasis, clonorchiasis, and paragonimiasis), and cysticercosis. Leakage of fluids from echinococcal cysts can cause intermittent increases in eosinophilia.

Eosinophilia sometimes provides the only clue to the presence of helminthic infection and should prompt an evaluation for such infection. Serologic testing for schistosomiasis, filariasis, visceral larva migrans, and strongyloidiasis will be helpful in an assessment for some of the diseases most likely to elicit eosinophilia. Serologic evaluation for strongyloidiasis is especially important since autoinfection may permit persistence of the organisms for decades and put the patient at risk for disseminated disease if immunosuppressive glucocorticoids are later administered for any reason.

BIBLIOGRAPHY

GYORKOS TW et al: Intestinal parasite infection in the Kampuchean refugee population 6 years after resettlement in Canada. J Infect Dis 166:413, 1992

JONES JL et al: Surveillance for AIDS-defining opportunistic illnesses, 1992–1997. MMWR Surveill Summ 48(SS-2):1, 1999

KAPPUS KD et al: Intestinal parasitism in the United States: Update on a continuing problem. Am J Trop Med Hyg 50:705, 1994

KARP CL, NEVA FA: The human immunodeficiency virus and tropical infectious disease coinfection, in *Tropical Infectious Diseases: Principles, Pathogens and Practice*, RL Guerrant et al (eds). Philadelphia, Churchill Livingstone, 1999, pp 1586–1630

LEVY DA et al: Surveillance for waterborne-disease outbreaks—United States, 1995–1996. MMWR Surveill Summ 47(SS-5):1, 1998

LIBMAN MD et al: Screening for schistosomiasis, filariasis, and strongyloidiasis among expatriates returning from the tropics. Clin Infect Dis 17:353, 1993

SVENSON JE et al: Imported malaria. Clinical presentation and examination of symptomatic travelers. Arch Intern Med 155:861, 1995

WILSON ME, WELLER PF: Eosinophilia, in *Tropical Infectious Diseases: Principles, Pathogens and Practice*, RL Guerrant et al (eds). Philadelphia, Churchill Livingstone, 1999, pp 1400–1419

211 | *Charles E. Davis*

LABORATORY DIAGNOSIS OF PARASITIC INFECTIONS

The cornerstone for the diagnosis of parasitic infections is a thorough history of the patient's illness. Epidemiologic aspects of the illness are especially important because the risks of acquiring many parasites are closely related to occupation, recreation, or travel to areas of high endemicity. Without a basic knowledge of the epidemiology and life cycles of the major parasites, it is difficult to approach the diagnosis of parasitic infections systematically. Accordingly, the medical classification of important human parasites in this chapter emphasizes their geographic distribution, their transmission, and the anatomic location and stages of their life cycle in humans. The text and tables are intended to serve as a guide to the correct diagnostic procedures for the major parasitic infections and to direct the reader to other chapters that contain more comprehensive information about each infection. Tables 211-1, 211-2, and 211-3 summarize the geographic distributions, the anatomic locations, and the laboratory methods employed for the diagnosis of flatworm, roundworm, and protozoal infections, respectively.

In addition to selecting the correct diagnostic procedures, physicians must counsel their patients to ensure that specimens are collected properly and arrive at the laboratory promptly. For example, the diagnosis of bancroftian filariasis is unlikely to be confirmed by the laboratory unless blood is drawn near midnight, when the nocturnal microfilariae are active. Laboratory personnel and surgical pathologists should be notified in advance when a parasitic infection is suspected. Continuing interaction with the laboratory staff and the surgical pathologists increases the likelihood that parasites in body fluids or biopsy specimens will be examined carefully by the most capable individuals.

INTESTINAL PARASITES Most helminths and protozoa exit the body in the fecal stream. The patient or the patient's attendant should be instructed to collect feces in a clean cardboard container and to record the time of collection on the container. Contamination with water, which could contain free-living protozoa, or with urine should be avoided. Fecal samples should be collected before ingestion of barium or other contrast agents for radiologic procedures and before treatment with antidiarrheal agents and antacids, because these substances change the consistency of the feces and interfere with microscopic detection of parasites. Because of the cyclic shedding of most parasites in the feces, a minimum of three samples collected on alternate days should be examined. When delays in transport to the laboratory are unavoidable or specimens must be shipped by mail, fecal samples should be kept in polyvinyl alcohol to preserve protozoal trophozoites. Refrigeration will also preserve trophozoites for a few hours and protozoal cysts and helminthic ova for several days.

Analysis of fecal samples consists of both a macroscopic and a microscopic examination. Watery or loose stools are more likely to contain protozoal trophozoites, but protozoal cysts and all stages of helminths may be found in formed feces. If adult worms or tapeworm segments are observed, they should be transported promptly to the laboratory or washed and preserved in fixative for later examination. The only tapeworm with motile segments is *Taenia saginata*, the beef tapeworm, which patients sometimes bring to the physician. Motility is an important distinguishing characteristic, because the ova of *T.*

Table 211-1 Flatworm Infections

Parasite	Geographic Distribution	Intermediate (Transmission)	Definitive	Parasite Stage	Body Fluid or Tissue	Serologic Tests	Other
TAPEWORMS (CESTODES)							
Intestinal tapeworms							
Taenia saginata (beef tapeworm)	Worldwide	Beef	Humans	Ova, segments	Feces	—	Motile segments
Hymenolepis nana (dwarf tapeworm)	Worldwide	Grain beetles	Humans, mice[a]	Ova	Feces	—	—
Diphyllobothrium latum (fish tapeworm)	Worldwide	Copepods–fish[c]	Humans, other mammals	Ova, segments	Feces	—	Megaloblastic anemia in 1%
T. solium[b] (pork tapeworm)	Worldwide	Swine	Humans	Ova, segments	Feces	WB	Especially Mexico, Central and South America, Africa
Somatic tapeworms							
Echinococcus granulosus (hydatid disease)	Sheep-raising and hunting areas	Sheep, camels, humans, others	Dogs	Hydatid	Lung, liver	WB, EIA	Chest radiography, CT, MRI
E. multilocularis (hydatid disease)	Subarctic areas	Rodents, humans	Foxes, dogs, cats	Hydatid	Liver	—	May resemble cholangiocellular carcinoma
T. solium[b] (pork tapeworm)	Worldwide	Swine, humans	Humans	Cysticercus	Muscles, CNS	WB	CT, MRI, radiography
FLUKES (TREMATODES)							
Intestinal flukes							
Fasciolopsis buski	China, India	Snails–water chestnuts	Humans	Ova	Feces	—	—
Heterophyes heterophyes	Far East, India	Snails–fish	Humans	Ova	Feces	—	—
Metagonimus yokogawai	Focal in Europe and North Africa	Snails–fish	Humans	Ova	Feces	—	—
Liver flukes							
Clonorchis sinensis	China, Southeast Asia	Snails–fish	Humans	Ova	Feces, bile	—	Recurrent bacterial cholangitis
Fasciola hepatica	Sheep-raising areas	Snails–watercress	Humans, sheep	Ova	Feces,[d] bile	—	Cirrhosis, portal hypertension
Lung flukes							
Paragonimus spp.	Orient, Africa, South America	Snails–crabs/crayfish	Humans, other mammals	Adults, ova	Lung, sputum, feces	WB	Chest radiography, CT, MRI
Blood flukes							
Schistosoma mansoni	Africa, Central and South America, West Indies	Snails	Humans	Ova, adults	Feces	EIA, WB	Rectal snips, liver biopsy
S. haematobium	Africa	Snails	Humans	Ova, adults	Urine	WB	Liver, urine, or bladder biopsy
S. japonicum	Far East	Snails	Humans	Ova, adults	Feces	WB	Liver biopsy

[a] Larvae also can mature in intestinal villi of humans and mice.

[b] *T. solium* can cause either intestinal infections or cysticercosis. Its ova are identical to those of *T. saginata*; scolices and segments of the two species differ.

[c] When there are two intermediate hosts, the first is separated from the second by a dash. Definitive hosts are infected by the second intermediate host.

[d] Ova seldom reach the fecal stream during acute disease.

NOTE: WB, western blot; CT, computed tomography; MRI, magnetic resonance imaging; CNS, central nervous system; EIA, enzyme immunoassay. Serologic tests listed in Tables 211-1, 211-2, and 211-3 are available from the Centers for Disease Control and Prevention, Atlanta, GA.

saginata and *T. solium*, the cause of cysticercosis, are morphologically indistinguishable.

Microscopic examination of feces (Table 211-4) is not complete until direct wet mounts have been evaluated and concentration techniques as well as permanent stains have been applied. Before accepting a report of negativity for ova and parasites as final, the physician should insist that the laboratory undertake each of these procedures. Some intestinal parasites are more readily detected in material other than feces. For example, use of the string test (or one of its commercial substitutes) to sample duodenal contents is sometimes necessary to detect *Giardia lamblia*, *Cryptosporidium*, and *Strongyloides* larvae. Use of the "Scotch tape" technique to detect pinworm ova on the perianal skin sometimes also reveals ova of *T. saginata*

deposited perianally when the motile segments disintegrate (Table 211-4).

Two routine solutions are used to make wet mounts for the identification of the various life stages of helminths and protozoa: physiologic saline for trophozoites, cysts, ova, and larvae and dilute iodine solution for protozoal cysts and ova. Iodine solution must never be used to examine specimens for trophozoites because it kills the parasites and thus eliminates their characteristic motility.

The two most common concentration procedures for detecting small numbers of cysts and ova are formalin-ether sedimentation and zinc sulfate flotation. The formalin-ether technique is preferable, because all parasites sediment but not all float. Slides permanently stained for trophozoites should be prepared before concentration. Ad-

Table 211-2 Roundworm Infections

Parasite	Geographic Distribution	Life-Cycle Hosts Intermediate (Transmission)	Definitive	Diagnosis Parasite Stage	Body Fluid or Tissue	Serologic Tests	Other
INTESTINAL ROUNDWORMS							
Enterobius vermicularis (pinworm)	Temperate and tropical zones	Fecal-oral	Humans	Ova	Perianal skin	—	"Scotch tape" test
Trichuris trichiura (whipworm)	Temperate and tropical zones	Soil, fecal-oral	Humans	Ova	Feces	—	Rectal prolapse
Ascaris lumbricoides (roundworm of humans)	Temperate and tropical zones	Soil, fecal-oral	Humans	Ova	Feces	—	Sx of pulmonary migration
Ancylostoma duodenale (Old World hookworm)	Eurasia, Africa, Pacific	Soil→skin	Humans	Ova/larvae	Feces	—	Sx of pulmonary migration, anemia
Necator americanus (New World hookworm)	U.S., Africa, worldwide	Soil→skin	Humans	Ova/larvae	Feces	—	Sx of pulmonary migration, anemia
Strongyloides stercoralis (strongyloidiasis)	Moist tropics and subtropics	Soil→skin	Humans	Larvae	Feces, sputum, duodenal fluid	EIA	Dissemination in immunodeficiency
TISSUE ROUNDWORMS							
Trichinella spiralis (trichinosis)	Worldwide	Swine/humans	Swine/humans	Larvae	Muscle	BF, EIA	Muscle biopsy
Wuchereria bancrofti (filariasis)	Coastal areas in tropics and subtropics	Mosquitoes	Humans	Microfilariae	Blood, lymph nodes	—	Nocturnal periodicity[a]
Brugia malayi (filariasis)	Asia, Indian subcontinent	Mosquitoes	Humans	Microfilariae	Blood	—	Nocturnal
Loa loa (African eye worm)	West and Central Africa	Mango flies (*Chrysops*)	Humans	Microfilariae	Blood	—	May be visible in eye, diurnal
Onchocerca volvulus (river blindness)	Africa, Mexico, Central and South America	Blackflies	Humans	Adults/larvae	Skin/eye	—	Examine nodules or skin snips
Dracunculus medinensis (guinea worm)	Africa	*Cyclops*	Humans	Adults/larvae	Skin		May be visible in lesion
LARVA MIGRANS SYNDROMES							
Ancylostoma braziliense (creeping eruption)	Tropical and temperate zones	Soil→skin	Dogs/cats, humans	Larvae	Skin	—	Dog and cat hookworm
Toxocara canis and *cati* (visceral larva migrans)	Tropical and temperate zones	Soil, fecal-oral	Dogs/cats, humans	Larvae	Viscera, CNS, eye	EIA[b]	Also caused by roundworms of other species

[a] Blood should be drawn at midnight, except for infection acquired in the South Pacific.
[b] The presence of hemagglutinins is a useful clue.

NOTE: BF, bentonite flocculation; Sx, signs/symptoms; EIA, enzyme immunoassay; CNS, central nervous system.

ditional slides stained for cysts and ova may be made from the concentrate.

In many instances, especially in the differentiation of *Entamoeba histolytica* from other amebas, identification of parasites from wet mounts or concentrates must be considered tentative. Permanently stained smears allow study of the cellular detail necessary for definitive identification. The iron-hematoxylin stain is excellent for critical work, but trichrome staining, which can be completed in 1 h, is a satisfactory alternative that also reveals parasites in specimens preserved in polyvinyl alcohol fixative.

BLOOD AND TISSUE PARASITES Invasion of tissue by protozoa and helminths renders the choice of diagnostic techniques more difficult. For example, physicians must understand that aspiration of an amebic liver abscess rarely reveals *E. histolytica* because the trophozoites are located primarily in the abscess wall. They must remember that the urine sediment offers the best opportunity to detect *Schistosoma haematobium* in the Ethiopian youngster or the American traveler who returns from Africa with hematuria (Table 211-5). Tables 211-1, 211-2, and 211-3, which offer a quick guide to the geographic distribution and anatomic locations of the major tissue parasites,

should help the physician to select the appropriate body fluid or biopsy site for microscopic examination. Tables 211-5, 211-6, and 211-7 provide additional information about the identification of parasites in samples from specific anatomic locations. The laboratory procedures for detection of parasites in other body fluids are similar to those used in the examination of feces. The physician should insist on wet mounts, concentration techniques, and permanent stains for all body fluids. The trichrome or iron-hematoxylin stain is satisfactory for all tissue helminths in body fluids other than blood, but microfilarial worms and blood protozoa are more easily visualized when stained with Giemsa or Wright's stain.

The most common parasites detected in Giemsa-stained blood smears are the plasmodia, microfilariae, and African trypanosomes (Table 211-5). Most patients with Chagas' disease present in the chronic phase, when *Trypanosoma cruzi* is no longer microscopically detectable in blood smears. Wet mounts are sometimes more sensitive than stained smears for the detection of microfilariae and African trypanosomes because these active parasites cause noticeable movement of the erythrocytes in the microscopic field. Nuclepore filtration of blood facilitates the detection of microfilariae. The intracellular amas-

Table 211-3 Protozoal Infections

Parasite	Geographic Distribution	Life-Cycle Hosts Intermediate (Transmission)	Life-Cycle Hosts Definitive	Parasite Stage	Diagnosis Body Fluid or Tissue	Diagnosis Serologic Tests	Diagnosis Other
INTESTINAL PROTOZOANS							
Entamoeba histolytica (amebiasis)	Worldwide, especially tropics	Fecal-oral	Humans	Troph, cyst	Feces, liver	EIA, ID, antigen detection	Ultrasound, liver CT, PCR
Giardia lamblia (giardiasis)	Worldwide	Fecal-oral	Humans	Troph, cyst	Feces	Antigen detection	String test
Isospora belli	Worldwide	Fecal-oral	Humans	Oocyst	Feces	—	Acid-fast
Cryptosporidium	Worldwide	Fecal-oral	Humans, other animals	Oocyst	Feces	Antigen detection	Acid-fast, biopsy, PCR
Cyclospora cayetanensis	Worldwide?	Fecal-oral	Humans, other animals?	Oocyst	Feces	—	Modified safranin, epifluorescence, PCR
Enterocytozoon bieneusi (microsporidiosis)	Worldwide?	?	Animals, humans	Spore	Feces	—	Modified trichrome, biopsy, PCR
FREE-LIVING AMEBAS							
Naegleria	Worldwide	Warm water	Humans	Troph, cyst	CNS, nares	—	Biopsy, nasal swab
Acanthamoeba	Worldwide	Soil, water	Humans	Troph, cyst	CNS, skin, cornea	—	Biopsy, scrapings
BLOOD AND TISSUE PROTOZOANS							
Plasmodium spp. (malaria)	Subtropics and tropics	Mosquitoes	Humans	Asexual	Blood	Limited use	PCR
Babesia microti (babesiosis)	U.S., especially New England	Ticks	Rodents, humans	Asexual	Blood	IIF	Animal spp. in asplenia, PCR
Trypanosoma rhodesiense (African sleeping sickness)	Sub-Saharan East Africa	Tsetse flies	Humans, herbivores	Tryp	Blood, CSF	Card agglutination, IIF[a]	Also chancre, lymph nodes
T. gambiense (African sleeping sickness)	Sub-Saharan West Africa	Tsetse flies	Humans, swine	Tryp	Blood, CSF	Card agglutination, IIF[a]	Also chancre, lymph nodes
T. cruzi (Chagas' disease)	Mexico→South America	Reduviid bugs (triatomes)	Humans, dogs, wild animals	Amastigote, tryp	Multiple organs/blood	IIF	Reactivation in immunosuppression
Leishmania tropica, etc.	Widespread in tropics and subtropics	Sandflies (*Phlebotomus*)	Humans, dogs, rodents	Amastigote	Skin	IFA[b]	Biopsy, scraping, culture
L. braziliensis (mucocutaneous)	Mexico→South America	Sandflies (*Lutzomyia*)	Humans, dogs, rodents	Amastigote	Skin, mucous membranes	IFA[b]	Biopsy, scraping, culture
L. donovani (kala-azar)	Widespread in tropics and subtropics	Sandflies (*Phlebotomus*)	Humans, dogs, wild animals	Amastigote	RE system	IFA[b]	Biopsy, culture
Toxoplasma gondii (toxoplasmosis)	Worldwide	Humans, other mammals	Cats	Cyst, troph	CNS, eye, muscles, other	EIA, IIF	Reactivation in immunosuppression

[a] Card agglutination provided to endemic countries by the World Health Organization; contact the CDC.

[b] Limited specificity. Most sensitive for *L. donovani* (kala-azar).

NOTE: ID, immunodiffusion by commercial kit (not available from the CDC); CT, computed tomography; troph, trophozoite; tryp, trypomastigote form; IIF, indirect immunofluorescence; RE, reticuloendothelial; PCR, polymerase chain reaction; EIA, enzyme immunoassay; CNS, central nervous system; IFA, indirect fluorescent antibody.

tigote forms of *Leishmania* spp. and *T. cruzi* can sometimes be visualized in stained smears of peripheral blood, but aspirates of the bone marrow, liver, and spleen are the best sources for microscopic detection and culture of *Leishmania* in kala-azar and of *T. cruzi* in chronic Chagas' disease.

The diagnosis of malaria and the critical distinction among the various *Plasmodium* spp. are made by microscopic examination of stained thick and thin blood films (Table 211-6; **Plates VI-3 through VI-33**). Most malariologists prefer Giemsa stain because of its overall high quality, suitability for staining of both thick and thin smears, and stability in tropical climates. Wright's stain can produce high-quality thin smears and is widely used in the Americas, but it deteriorates rapidly in the tropics because its methanol base is highly hygroscopic. Specimens of capillary or venous blood should be obtained every 4 to 12 h until a diagnosis is established. The thin smear is made on clean slides exactly like a blood film for a white blood cell differential. The thick film is made by placing one drop of blood on the slide and stirring it in a circular motion to a diameter of about 2 cm. The erythrocytes in the thick film are lysed with water, but the thin film is fixed in methanol to preserve erythrocyte morphology.

Although most tissue parasites stain with the traditional hematoxylin and eosin, surgical biopsy specimens should also be stained with appropriate special stains. The surgical pathologist who is accustomed to applying silver stains for *Pneumocystis carinii* to induced sputum and transbronchial biopsies may have to be reminded to examine wet mounts and iron-hematoxylin–stained preparations of pulmonary specimens for helminthic ova and *E. histolytica*. The clinician should also be able to advise the surgeon and pathologist about optimal techniques for the identification of parasites in specimens obtained by certain specialized minor procedures (Table 211-7). For example, the excision of skin snips for the diagnosis of onchocerciasis, the collection of rectal snips for the diagnosis of schistosomiasis, and punch biopsy of skin lesions for the identification and culture of cutaneous and mucocutaneous species of *Leishmania* are simple procedures, but the diagnosis can be missed if the specimens are improperly obtained or processed.

NONSPECIFIC TESTS Eosinophilia is a common accompaniment of infections with most of the tissue helminths; absolute numbers of eosinophils may be high in trichinosis and the migratory phases of filariasis (Table 211-8). Intestinal helminths provoke eosinophilia

1189

Table 211-4   Laboratory Diagnosis of Parasites Found in Feces[a]

Parasites and Fecal Stages	Alternative Diagnostic Procedures
TAPEWORMS (CESTODES)	
Taenia saginata ova and segments	Perianal "Scotch tape" test for ova
Hymenolepis nana ova	None
Diphyllobothrium ova and segments	None
T. solium ova and segments	Serology; brain biopsy for neurocysticercosis
FLUKES (TREMATODES)	
Fasciolopsis buski ova	None
Heterophyes heterophyes ova	None
Metagonimus yokogawai ova	None
Clonorchis (Opisthorchis) sinensis ova	Examination of bile for ova and adults in cholangitis
Fasciola hepatica ova	Examination of bile for ova and adults in cholangitis
Paragonimus spp. ova	Serology; sputum; biopsy of lung or brain for ova
Schistosoma ova	Serology for all; rectal snips (especially for *S. mansoni*), urine (*S. haematobium*), liver biopsy and liver ultrasound
ROUNDWORMS	
Enterobius vermicularis ova and adults	Perianal "Scotch tape" test for ova and adults
Trichuris trichiura ova	None
Ascaris lumbricoides ova and adults	Examination of sputum for larvae in lung disease
Hookworm ova and occasional larvae	Examination of sputum for larvae in lung disease
Strongyloides larvae	Duodenal aspirate or jejunal biopsy; serology; sputum or lung biopsy for filariform larvae in disseminated disease
Capillaria philippinensis ova[b]	None
PROTOZOANS	
Entamoeba histolytica trophozoites and cysts	Serology; liver biopsy for trophozoites
Giardia lamblia trophozoites and cysts	Duodenal aspirate or jejunal biopsy[c]
Isospora belli oocysts	Duodenal aspirate or jejunal biopsy[c]
Cryptosporidium oocysts	Duodenal aspirate or jejunal biopsy[c]
Enterocytozoon bieneusi spores	Duodenal aspirate or jejunal biopsy[c]

[a] Stains and concentration techniques are discussed in the text.
[b] Can be confused with *T. trichiura*.
[c] Commercial string test or Crosby capsule is satisfactory; *Isospora* and *Cryptosporidium* are acid-fast.

only during pulmonary migration of the larval stages. Eosinophilia is not a manifestation of protozoal infections, with the possible exceptions of those due to *Isospora* and *Dientamoeba fragilis*.

Like the hypochromic, microcytic anemia of heavy hookworm infections, other nonspecific laboratory abnormalities may suggest parasitic infection in patients with appropriate geographic and/or environmental exposures. Biochemical evidence of cirrhosis or an abnormal urine sediment in an African immigrant certainly raises the possibility of schistosomiasis, and anemia and thrombocytopenia in a febrile traveler or immigrant are among the hallmarks of malaria. Computed tomography and magnetic resonance imaging also contribute to the diagnosis of infections with many tissue parasites and have become invaluable adjuncts in the diagnosis of neurocysticercosis and cerebral toxoplasmosis.

ANTIBODY AND ANTIGEN DETECTION Useful antibody assays for many of the important tissue parasites are available; those listed in Table 211-9 can be obtained from the Centers for Disease Control and Prevention (CDC) in Atlanta. The results of most

serologic tests not listed in the tables and not offered by the CDC should be interpreted with caution.

The value of antibody assays is limited in the case of the filarial worms and plasmodia. The detection of antibody to plasmodia is of limited use for establishing the diagnosis of malaria in individual patients because diagnostic titers develop slowly and the tests must be sent to the CDC. Filarial antigens cross-react with those from other nematodes, and antibody assays do not distinguish between past and current infection. In contrast, a negative result in an American or European traveler virtually rules out the diagnosis of bancroftian or brugian filariasis. Promising new assays for filarial antigens and antibodies in lymphatic filariasis are not yet available in commercial kits or from the CDC.

Despite these specific limitations, the restricted geographic distribution of many tropical parasites increases the diagnostic usefulness of antibody detection in travelers from industrialized countries. On the other hand, a large proportion of the world has been exposed to *Toxoplasma gondii*, and the presence of IgG antibody does not constitute proof of active disease.

Fewer antibody assays are available for the diagnosis of infection with intestinal parasites. Cross-reactivity and lack of efficient cultivation techniques, along with the ability to establish diagnoses without invasive procedures, have discouraged intensive investigation of these methods. *E. histolytica* is the major exception. Sensitive, specific serologic tests are invaluable in the diagnosis of amebiasis. Commercial kits for the detection of antigen by enzyme-linked immunosorbent assay or of whole organisms by fluorescent antibody assay are now available for several protozoan parasites (Table 211-9).

Table 211-5   Identification of Parasites in Blood and Other Body Fluids

Body Fluid, Parasite	Enrichment/Stain	Culture Technique
BLOOD		
Plasmodium spp.	Thick and thin smears/Giemsa or Wright's	Not useful for diagnosis
Leishmania spp.	Buffy coat/Giemsa	Media available from CDC
African trypanosomes[a]	Buffy coat, anion column/wet mount and Giemsa	Mouse or rat inoculation[b]
Trypanosoma cruzi[c]	As for African species	As above and xenodiagnosis
Toxoplasma gondii Microfilariae[d]	Buffy coat/Giemsa Nuclepore filtration/wet mount and Giemsa	Fibroblast cell lines None
URINE[e]		
Schistosoma haematobium	Centrifugation/wet mount	None
Microfilariae (in chyluria)	As for blood	None
SPINAL FLUID		
African trypanosomes	Centrifugation, anion column/wet mount and Giemsa	As for blood
Naegleria fowleri	Centrifugation/wet mount and Giemsa or trichrome	Nonnutrient agar overlaid with *Escherichia coli*

[a] *Trypanosoma rhodesiense* and *T. gambiense*.
[b] Inject mice intraperitoneally with 0.2 mL of whole heparinized blood (0.5 mL for rats). After 5 days, tail blood should be checked daily for trypanosomes as described above.
[c] Detectable in blood by conventional techniques only during acute disease. Xenodiagnosis is successful in about 50% of patients with chronic Chagas' disease.
[d] Day (1000–1400 h) and night (2200–0200 h) blood should be drawn to maximize the chance of detecting *Wuchereria* (nocturnal except for Pacific strains), *Brugia* (nocturnal), and *Loa loa* (diurnal).
[e] *Trichomonas vaginalis* is often detectable in urine, but examination of vaginal secretions is probably the preferable technique.

Table 211-6 Differential Diagnosis of *Plasmodium* Spp. in Blood Smears[a]

Feature	*P. falciparum*	*P. vivax*	*P. malariae*	*P. ovale*
FEATURE OF RED CELLS				
Size	All sizes	Large (young)	Small (old)	Large (young)
Shape	Round; may be crenated	Round or oval	Round	Round or pear-shaped, fimbriated
Stippling	Maurer's clefts: large, red (up to 20)	Schüffner's dots: numerous, small, red	None	Schüffner's dots
FEATURE OF PARASITE				
Ring trophozoites	Threadlike, multiple infections, double chromatin dots, accolé forms[b]	Thicker	Compact	Compact
Mature trophozoites	Absent	Ameboid, may fill cell	More regular, smaller band forms[c]	Less ameboid and smaller than those of *P. vivax*
Schizonts	Absent	12 to 24 merozoites	8 to 12 merozoites, often rosetted around pigment	8 to 12 merozoites
Gametocytes	Banana-shaped, central chromatin (female) or diffuse (male)	Round, fills cell, pigment often central	Round, large, coarse pigment	Smaller and oval, but similar to those of *P. vivax*
DIAGNOSTIC KEYS				
	Gametocyte, multiple rings, double chromatin dots, accolé forms, heavy infections	Schizont, large RBCs, ameboid forms	Schizont, small RBCs, band forms	Schizont and large RBCs, pear-shaped, fimbriated RBCs

[a] See Plates VI-3 through VI-33.
[b] At periphery of RBCs; may be flattened into rod shape.
[c] Stretch across RBCs, but not banana-shaped.
NOTE: RBCs, red blood cells.

MOLECULAR TECHNIQUES DNA hybridization with probes that are repeated many times in the genome of a specific parasite and amplification of a specific DNA fragment by the polymerase chain reaction (PCR) are promising techniques for the diagnosis of parasitic infections. Although molecular techniques for the detection of many parasites are already being used in insect vectors, animal models, and human trials, few are available for routine use in patients at this time. The only available commercial kit is that for the identi-

Table 211-7 Minor Procedures for Diagnosis of Parasitic Infections

Procedure	Parasite(s) and Stage
Skin snips: Lift skin with a needle and excise about 1 mg to a depth of 0.5 mm from several sites. Weigh each sample, place it in 0.5 mL of saline for 4 h, and examine wet mounts and Giemsa stains of the saline either directly or after filtration. Count microfilariae.[a]	*Onchocerca volvulus* and *Mansonella streptocerca* microfilariae
Biopsies of subcutaneous nodules: Stain routine histopathologic sections and impression smears with Giemsa.	*Loa loa* adults and *O. volvulus* adults and microfilariae
Muscle biopsies: Excise about 1.0 g of deltoid or gastrocnemius muscle and squash between two glass slides for direct microscopic examination.	*Trichinella spiralis* larvae (and perhaps *Taenia solium* cysticerci)
Rectal snips: From four areas of mucosa take 2-mg snips, tease onto a glass slide, and flatten with a second slide before examining directly at 10×. Preparations may be fixed in alcohol or stained.	*Schistosoma* ova of all species, but especially *S. mansoni*
Aspirate of chancre or lymph node[b]: Aspirate center with 18-gauge needle, place a drop on a slide, and examine for motile forms. An otherwise insufficient volume of material may be stained with Giemsa.	*Trypanosoma gambiense* and *T. rhodesiense* trypomastigotes
Corneal scrapings: Obtain sample from ophthalmologist for immediate Giemsa staining and culture on nutrient agar overlaid with *Escherichia coli*.	*Acanthamoeba* spp. trophozoites or cysts
Swabs, aspirates, or punch biopsies of skin lesions: Obtain specimen from margin of lesion for Giemsa staining of impression smears, and section and culture on special media from CDC.	Cutaneous and mucocutaneous *Leishmania* spp.

[a] Counts of >100/mg are associated with significant risk of complications.
[b] Lymph node aspiration is contraindicated in some infections and should be used judiciously.

Table 211-8 Parasites Frequently Associated with Eosinophilia[a]

Parasite	Comment
TAPEWORMS (CESTODES)	
Echinococcus granulosus	When hydatid cyst leaks
Taenia solium	During muscle encystation and in CSF with neurocysticercosis
FLUKES (TREMATODES)	
Paragonimus spp.	Uniformly high in acute stage
Fasciola hepatica	May be high in acute stage
Clonorchis (Opisthorchis) sinensis	Variable
Schistosoma mansoni	50% of infected travelers
S. haematobium	25% of infected travelers
S. japonicum	Up to 6000/μL in acute infection
ROUNDWORMS	
Ascaris lumbricoides	During larval migration
Hookworm species	During larval migration
Strongyloides stercoralis	Profound during migration and early years of infection
Trichinella spiralis	Up to 7000/μL
Filarial species[b]	Varies but can reach 5000 to 8000/μL
Toxocara spp.	>3000/μL
Ancylostoma braziliense	With extensive cutaneous eruption
Gnathostoma spinigerum	In visceral larva migrans and eosinophilic meningitis
Angiostrongylus cantonensis	In eosinophilic meningitis
A. costaricensis	During larval migration in mesenteric vessels
POSSIBLE PROTOZOAL CAUSES	
Isospora belli	A few reports of profound eosinophilia
Dientamoeba fragilis	Possible pathogenicity and eosinophilia

[a] Virtually every helminth has been associated with eosinophilia. This table includes both common and uncommon parasites that frequently elicit eosinophilia during infection.
[b] *Wuchereria bancrofti*, *Brugia* spp., *Loa loa*, and *Onchocerca volvulus*.

Table 211-9 Serologic and Molecular Tests for Parasitic Infections

Parasite, Infection	Antibody	Antigen or DNA/RNA
TAPEWORMS		
Echinococcosis	WB, EIA	
Cysticercosis	WB	
FLUKES		
Paragonimiasis	WB	
Schistosomiasis	EIA, WB	
ROUNDWORMS		
Strongyloidiasis	EIA	
Trichinellosis	BF, EIA	
Toxocariasis	EIA	
PROTOZOANS		
Amebiasis	EIA	EIA, PCR
Giardiasis		EIA, IIF, DFA
Cryptosporidiosis		IIF, EIA, DFA, PCR
Malaria (all species)	IIF[a]	PCR
Babesiosis	IIF	PCR
Chagas' disease	IIF	
Leishmaniasis	IIF	
Toxoplasmosis	IIF, EIA (IgM)	
Microsporidiosis		PCR
Cyclosporiasis		PCR

[a] Of limited use for management of acute disease.
NOTE: BF, bentonite flocculation; EIA, enzyme immunoassay; WB, western blot; IIF, indirect immunofluorescence; DFA, direct fluorescent antibody; PCR, polymerase chain reaction. All antibody tests listed are available from the CDC. Antigen and parasite detection kits are available commercially. The PCRs listed are those currently available from the CDC.

fication of *Trichomonas vaginalis* by hybridization of secretions from vaginal swabs with synthetic oligonucleotide probes. The CDC will perform PCR for microsporidia, cryptosporidia, *Cyclospora*, and *E. histolytica* on stools (frozen or fixed in either potassium dichromate or ethanol) and on biopsy and bronchoalveolar lavage samples (fixed in methanol or ethanol). For *Plasmodium* and *Babesia*, PCR is performed on blood treated with EDTA or collected in IsoCode Stix (Schleicher and Schuell).

BIBLIOGRAPHY

EBERHARD M et al: Laboratory diagnosis of *Cyclospora* infections. Acta Pathol Lab Med 121:792, 1997

FLECK SL, MOODY AH: *Diagnostic Techniques in Medical Parasitology.* London, Wright, 1988

GARCIA LS et al: Diagnosis of parasitic infections: Collection, processing, and examination of specimens, in *Manual of Clinical Microbiology,* 6th ed, PR Murray et al (eds). Washington, DC, ASM Press, 1995, pp 1145–1158

HAQUE R et al: Comparison of PCR, isoenzyme analysis, and antigen detection for diagnosis of *Entamoeba histolytica* infection. J Clin Microbiol 36:449, 1998

MOLYNEUX DH: Vector-borne parasitic diseases—an overview of recent changes. Int J Parasitol 28:927, 1998

TOMECKI JK (ed): *Dermatologic Clinics, Systemic Mycoses and Parasitic Diseases.* Philadelphia, Saunders, 1989, vol 7

WEBER R et al: Improved light-microscopical detection of microsporidia spores in stool and duodenal aspirates. N Engl J Med 326:161, 1992

WELLER PF: Eosinophilia in travelers. Med Clin North Am 76:1413, 1992

WILSON M et al: Evaluation of six commercial kits for detection of human immunoglobulin M antibodies to *Toxoplasma gondii*. J Clin Microbiol 35:3112, 1997

——— et al: Clinical immunoparasitology, in *Manual of Clinical Laboratory Immunology,* 5th ed, NR Rose et al (eds). Washington, DC, ASM Press, 1997, pp 575–584

212 *Thomas A. Moore*

THERAPY FOR PARASITIC INFECTIONS

Over the last few decades, the reach of some parasitic diseases such as malaria has extended because of factors such as deforestation, population shifts, global warming, and other climatic events (e.g., "El Niño"). Efforts to combat this trend are complicated by the development and spread of drug resistance among parasites and the limited introduction of new antiparasitic agents. However, significant advances toward the reduction of the burden of parasitic disease have been made. The generous donation of ivermectin and albendazole for global eradication programs has improved the health of countless individuals and offers the promise of disease eradication. The expanded use of traditionally nonparasitic agents, such as amphotericin B for visceral leishmaniasis, has offered hope against the specter of drug resistance. The introduction of newer agents, such as triclabendazole, also appears promising.

Currently recommended treatment options for most parasitic diseases of humans are listed in Table 212-1. A brief summary of some of the agents can be found below; each agent is listed by its generic name. Many of the agents are approved by the Food and Drug Administration (FDA) but are considered investigational for the treatment of certain infections; these drugs are marked accordingly in Table 212-1. Drugs marked in the text with an asterisk (*) are available only through the Centers for Disease Control and Prevention (CDC) Drug Service (telephone: 404-639-3670). Other drugs, marked with a dagger (†), are available only through the manufacturer; contact information for these manufacturers may be available from the CDC. Information on dosing in children and pregnant women can be obtained in the references at the end of the chapter.

Albendazole This benzimidazole derivative has recently become generally available and is active against a broad range of helminths and protozoa. All benzimidazoles act by binding to free β-tubulin, inhibiting the polymerization of tubulin and the microtubule-dependent uptake of glucose. In helminths, the result is the depletion of glycogen stores, but this fundamental disruption of cellular metabolism also offers treatment for a wide range of parasitic diseases. Like all benzimidazoles, albendazole is poorly absorbed from the gastrointestinal tract. However, since the active metabolite attains higher serum and cyst concentrations than mebendazole, it is more effective against echinococcal disease. Significant adverse reactions are usually limited to prolonged use and include abdominal pain and reversible hepatic dysfunction. Rarely, leukopenia and reversible alopecia occur. Albendazole is contraindicated in early pregnancy.

Artesunate and Artemether Artesunate, artemether, and the parent compound artemisinin are sesquiterpene lactones derived from the wormwood plant *Artemisia annua*. These agents have become first-line treatments for severe falciparum malaria in some areas of the world where drug resistance is a major problem. They are rapidly effective against the asexual blood forms of *Plasmodium* spp., including multidrug-resistant *P. falciparum*, but they are not active against intrahepatic forms. Their mechanism of action is not completely understood, but they are believed to act by converting to free radicals and other intermediates in the presence of intraparasitic iron; the result is alkylation of parasite proteins or membrane damage. Artemisinin derivatives presently show no cross-resistance with known antimalarials and thus are important for treating severe malaria in areas of multidrug resistance. However, long treatment courses are required and, when these agents are used alone, recrudescence may occur. Artemisinin and its derivatives are cleared rapidly from the circulation, and their short half-lives limit their use for prophylaxis. Adverse events are usually infrequent and mild and include drug fever and contact dermatitis. Animal data suggest that neurotoxicity can develop if the compounds are administered chronically, and cerebellar dysfunction

Table 212-1   General Recommendations for the Treatment of Parasitic Infections

Infection: Organism (See Also Chapter[a])	Treatment of Choice	Alternative Treatment
Amebiasis: *Entamoeba histolytica* (213)		
Asymptomatic infection	Paromomycin 500 mg PO tid for 10 days	Iodoquinol 650 mg PO tid for 20 days
Intestinal disease	Metronidazole 750 mg PO or IV tid for 5–10 days *plus* luminal agent as for asymptomatic infection	Tinidazole 2 g PO once *plus* luminal agent as for asymptomatic infection
Hepatic abscess	Metronidazole 750 mg PO or IV tid for 5–10 days *plus* luminal agent as for asymptomatic infection	Tinidazole 2 g PO once (repeat as needed) *plus* luminal agent as for asymptomatic infection
Amebic Meningoencephalitis: *Naegleria fowleri* (213)	Amphotericin B[b] 1 mg/kg per day IV; duration of treatment uncertain; benefit of adding rifampin 600 mg PO bid uncertain	—
Angiostrongyliasis (219)		
Angiostrongylus cantonensis	Supportive therapy with serial lumbar punctures and glucocorticoids as needed; benefit of medical therapy unclear	—
A. costaricensis	Thiabendazole[b] 25 mg/kg PO tid for 3 days (max 3 g/d); repeat 3 times within 3 weeks	—
Anisakiasis: *Anisakis, Pseudoterranova* spp. (220)	Surgical or endoscopic removal, if possible	—
Ascariasis: *Ascaris lumbricoides* (220)	Albendazole[b] 400 mg PO once	Mebendazole 100 mg PO bid for 3 days or 500 mg once, *or* pyrantel pamoate 11 mg/kg PO once (max 1 g)
Babesiosis: *Babesia* spp. (214)	Clindamycin[b] 1.2 g IV bid or 600 mg PO tid for 7–10 days *plus* quinine 650 mg PO tid for 7–10 days; consider exchange transfusion for critically ill patients	Atovaquone[b] 750 mg PO bid for 7–10 days *plus* azithromycin[b] 0.5–1 g/d PO for 7–10 days, *or* quinine 650 mg PO tid for 7–10 days *plus* azithromycin[b] 0.5–1 g/d PO for 7–10 days
Balantidiasis: *Balantidium coli* (218)	Tetracycline[b] 500 mg PO qid for 10 days, *or* doxycycline[b] 100 mg PO bid for 10 days	Metronidazole[b] 750 mg PO tid for 5 days, *or* iodoquinol[b] 650 mg PO tid for 20 days
Capillariasis: *Capillaria philippinensis* (220)	Albendazole[b] 400 mg/d PO for 10 days	Mebendazole[b] 200 mg PO bid for 20 days
Cestode Infections (223)		
Intestinal stage (adults)		
Diphyllobothrium latum, Dipylidium caninum, Taenia saginata, T. solium	Praziquantel[b] 5–10 mg/kg PO once	—
Hymenolepis nana	Praziquantel 25 mg/kg PO once	—
Tissue stage (larvae)		
Cysticercosis: *T. solium*[c]	Praziquantel 50–60 mg/kg per day PO in 3 divided doses for 15 days, with glucocorticoids and cimetidine for CNS lesions; *or* praziquantel 25 mg/kg PO q2h for 3 doses followed by dexamethasone 10 mg IM 4 h later and 10 mg/d IM for the next 2 days	Albendazole 7.5 mg/kg PO q12h for 8 days, with dexamethasone 10 mg/d IM for the first 4 days for CNS lesions
Echinococcosis		
Echinococcus granulosus	PAIR[d] or surgical excision *plus* albendazole 15 mg/kg per day for at least 4 days before procedure and continued for at least 4 weeks afterward; for uncomplicated lesions, albendazole 400 mg PO bid for 12 weeks (repeat as needed)	Mebendazole 40–50 mg/d PO for 3–6 months, repeat as needed
E. multilocularis	Surgical resection *plus* albendazole 400 mg PO bid for up to 2 years	—
Cryptosporidiosis: *Cryptosporidium parvum* (218)	Supportive care in normal hosts; paromomycin[b] 500–750 mg PO qid may be effective in HIV-infected patients	Nitazoxanide[b] 500 mg PO bid for 7 days
Cutaneous Larva Migrans: *Ancylostoma* spp. (219)	Ivermectin[b] 150–200 µg/kg PO once, *or* thiabendazole 25 mg/kg PO bid or 10% suspension topically for 2–5 days	Albendazole[b] 200 mg PO bid for 2–7 days
Cyclosporiasis: *Cyclospora cayetanensis* (218)	Trimethoprim-sulfamethoxazole[b] 160/800 mg PO bid for 7 days	—
Dientamebiasis: *Dientamoeba fragilis* (218)	Paromomycin[b] 10 mg/kg PO tid for 7 days	Iodoquinol 650 mg PO tid for 20 days, *or* tetracycline[b] 500 mg PO qid for 10 days
Dracunculiasis: *Dracunculus medinensis* (221)	Worm removal *plus* metronidazole[b] 250 mg PO tid for 10 days	Worm removal *plus* thiabendazole 25 mg/kg PO bid/tid for 3 days
Enterobiasis: *Enterobius vermicularis* (220)	Mebendazole 100 mg PO once, repeat in 2 weeks	Albendazole[b] 400 mg PO once, repeat in 2 weeks; *or* pyrantel pamoate 11 mg/kg once (max 1 g), repeat in 2 weeks
Filariasis (221)		
Lymphatic filariasis: *Wuchereria bancrofti, Brugia* spp.[e]	DEC[f] 2 mg/kg PO tid for 12 days[g]	Albendazole[b] 400 mg PO bid for 21 days (macrofilaricidal only)
Tropical pulmonary eosinophilia: *W. bancrofti, Brugia* spp.	DEC 2 mg/kg PO tid for 14 days	—
Loiasis: *Loa loa*		
Microfilariae present in concentrated blood[e]	Prednisone 40–60 mg/d followed by DEC 0.5 mg/kg per day; if well tolerated, taper prednisone and gradually increase DEC dose to 8–10 mg/kg per day for 21 days	—

(continued)

Infection: Organism (See Also Chapter[a])	Treatment of Choice	Alternative Treatment
Microfilariae absent in concentrated blood[h]	DEC 8–10 mg/kg per day (divided into 3 doses) PO for 21 days	—
Mansonellosis		
Mansonella ozzardi	Ivermectin 6 mg PO once	
M. perstans	DEC as for loiasis; no treatment has been proven completely effective	Mebendazole 100 mg PO bid for 30 days, *or* albendazole 400 mg PO bid for 10 days
M. streptocerca	Ivermectin[b] 150 μg/kg PO once	DEC 2 mg/kg PO tid for 14–21 days
Onchocerciasis: *Onchocerca volvulus*	Ivermectin 150 μg/kg once, repeat every 6–12 months; onchocercal nodules on head should be surgically excised	—
Flukes (222)		
Biliary duct-dwelling flukes: *Clonorchis sinensis, Opisthorchis* spp.	Praziquantel 25 mg/kg PO tid for 1 day	Albendazole[b] 400 mg PO bid for 7 days
Liver-dwelling flukes		
Fasciola hepatica	Triclabendazole 10 mg/kg PO once	Bithionol 30–50 mg/kg PO qod for 10–15 doses
Metorchis conjunctus	Praziquantel[b] 25 mg/kg PO tid for 1 day	—
Intestine-dwelling flukes		
Fasciolopsis buski, Heterophyes heterophyes, Metagonimus yokogawai, Echinostoma spp.	Praziquantel[b] 25 mg/kg PO tid for 1 day	—
Nanophyetus salmincola	Praziquantel[b] 20 mg/kg PO tid for 1 day	—
Lung-dwelling flukes: *Paragonimus* spp.	Praziquantel[b] 25 mg/kg PO tid for 2 days	Triclabendazole 10 mg/kg PO bid for 1 day
Giardiasis: *Giardia lamblia* (218)	Metronidazole[b] 250 mg PO tid for 5 days	Tinidazole 2 g PO once, *or* furazolidone 100 mg PO qid for 7–10 days, *or* paromomycin[b] 10 mg/kg PO tid for 7 days, *or* albendazole 400 mg/d PO for 5 days, *or* quinacrine 100 mg PO tid for 5 days
Gnathostomiasis: *Gnathostoma spinigerum* (219)	Albendazole[b] 400–800 mg/d PO for 21 days	Surgical removal if possible
Hookworm: *Ancylostoma duodenale, Necator americanus* (220)	Mebendazole 100 mg PO bid for 3 days or 500 mg PO once	Albendazole[b] 400 mg PO once
Isosporiasis: *Isospora belli* (218)	Trimethoprim-sulfamethoxazole[b] 160/800 mg PO qid for 10 days, then bid for 3 weeks	Pyrimethamine 50–75 mg/d PO for 3 weeks
Leishmaniasis: *Leishmania donovani, L. major, L. infantum, L chagasi, L mexicana, L. tropica, Viannia* spp. (215)		
Cutaneous leishmaniasis	Sodium stibogluconate *or* meglumine antimonate 20 mg Sb/kg per day IV or IM for 20 days	Pentamidine 3 mg/kg IV or IM qod for 4 doses or 2 mg/kg qod for 7 doses, *or* amphotericin B[b] 0.5–1 mg/kg IV qod or qd to a total dose of 20 mg/kg
Mucosal leishmaniasis	Sodium stibogluconate *or* meglumine antimonate 20 mg Sb/kg per day IV or IM for 28 days	Amphotericin B[b] 1 mg/kg IV qod or qd to a total dose of 20–40 mg/kg, *or* pentamidine 2–4 mg/kg IV or IM qod or 3 times weekly for ≥15 doses
Visceral leishmaniasis	Sodium stibogluconate *or* meglumine antimonate 20 mg Sb/kg per day IV or IM for 28 days, *or* lipid-complexed amphotericin B 2–5 mg/kg per day (total dose 15–40 mg/kg)[i]	Amphotericin B[b] deoxycholate 0.5–1 mg/kg IV qod or qd to a total dose of 15–20 mg/kg, *or* pentamidine 4 mg/kg qod or 3 times weekly for 15–30 doses
Malaria: *Plasmodium vivax, P. falciparum, P. ovale, P. malariae* (214)		
Severe malaria (parenteral therapy)	Quinidine gluconate 10 mg base/kg (max 600 mg) by continuous infusion over 1–2 h followed by 0.02 mg/kg per min, until patient can take oral therapy; consider exchange transfusion in critically ill patients	Artesunate 2.4 mg/kg IV or IM followed by 1.2 mg/kg at 12 and 24 h, then daily; *or* artemether 3.2 mg/kg IM, then 1.6 mg/kg per day
Uncomplicated malaria (oral therapy)		
All *except* chloroquine-resistant *Plasmodium* spp.	Chloroquine phosphate 10 mg base/kg followed by 10 mg/kg at 24 h and 5 mg/kg at 48 h or by 5 mg/kg at 12, 24, and 36 h (total dose, 25 mg/kg); treatment of infections due to *P. vivax* or *P. ovale* should be followed by radical cure	—
Chloroquine-resistant *P. falciparum*	Quinine sulfate 10 mg salt/kg tid for 7 days *plus* tetracycline[b] 4 mg/kg qid or doxycycline[b] 3 mg/kg per day for 7 days	Mefloquine 15 mg base/kg PO once for semi-immunes or followed 8–12 h later by second dose of 10 mg/kg for nonimmunes or in areas with mefloquine resistance; *or* atovaquone 1 g/d for 3 days *plus* either proguanil 400 mg/d for 3 days or doxycycline[b] 100 mg bid for 3 days; *or* artesunate 4 mg/kg per day for 3 days *plus* mefloquine 1.25 g once; *or* halofantrine 500 mg qid for 3 doses, repeat in 1 week

(continued)

Table 212-1—*(continued)*

Infection: Organism (See Also Chapter[a])	Treatment of Choice	Alternative Treatment
Chloroquine-resistant *P. vivax*	Quinine sulfate 650 mg PO q8h for 3–7 days *plus* either doxycycline[b] 100 mg PO bid for 7 days or pyrimethamine/sulfadoxine 3 tablets once on last day of quinine; treatment should be followed by radical cure	Mefloquine 1.25 g PO once
Radical cure (*P. vivax* and *P. ovale* only)	Primaquine phosphate 26.3 mg (15 mg base)/d for 14 days, or 79 mg (45 mg base)/week for 8 weeks	—
Microsporidiosis (218)		
Ocular: *Encephalitozoon hellem, E. cuniculi, Vittaforma corneae*	Albendazole[b] 400 mg PO bid for 4 weeks, repeat as needed	—
Intestinal: *Enterocytozoon bieneusi, Encephalitozoon intestinalis*	Albendazole[b] 400 mg PO bid for 3 weeks, repeat as needed	—
Disseminated: *E. hellem, E. cuniculi, E. intestinalis, Pleistophora* spp.	Albendazole[b] 400 mg PO bid; duration of therapy uncertain	—
Schistosomiasis (222)		
Schistosoma haematobium	Praziquantel 20 mg/kg PO bid for 1 day	Metrifonate 7.5–10 mg/kg PO once every other week for 3 doses
S. japonicum, S. mekongi	Praziquantel 20 mg/kg PO tid for 1 day	—
S. mansoni	Praziquantel 20 mg/kg PO bid for 1 day	Oxamniquine 15 mg/kg PO once for disease acquired in the western hemisphere; 15 mg/kg PO bid for 2 days for disease acquired in Africa or the Middle East
Strongyloidiasis: *Strongyloides stercoralis* (220)	Ivermectin 200 μg/kg per day PO for 1–2 days; in hyperinfection syndrome, continue treatment until parasites are eradicated	Albendazole 400 mg/d PO for 3 days, *or* thiabendazole 25 mg/kg PO bid (max 3 g/d) for 2 days
Toxoplasmosis: *Toxoplasma gondii* (217)		
Acute infection or relapse	Pyrimethamine 200 mg PO once, then 50–75 mg/d PO *plus* sulfadiazine 4–6 g/d in 4 divided doses *plus* folinic acid 10 mg/d PO for 6 weeks; adjunctive therapy with prednisone 80–120 mg/d PO is indicated in ocular disease	Pyrimethamine 200 mg PO once, then 50–75 mg/d PO *plus* folinic acid 10 mg/d PO *plus* either clindamycin 1.2–4.8 g/d IV or atovaquone 750 mg PO qid for 6 weeks
Infection in pregnancy	Spiramycin 10–15 mg/kg IV tid until delivery; if fetal infection is suspected or confirmed, treat after first trimester for immunocompetent patients	—
Trichinellosis: *Trichinella* spp. (219)	Glucocorticoids (for severe symptoms) *plus* albendazole[b] 400 mg PO bid for 8 days	Mebendazole[b] 200–300 mg PO tid for 3 days, then 400–500 mg PO tid for 10 days; *or* thiabendazole[b] 25 mg/kg PO bid (max 3 g) for 7 days
Trichomoniasis: *Trichomonas vaginalis* (218)	Metronidazole 2 g PO once or 250 mg PO tid for 7 days	Tinidazole 2 g PO once
Trichostrongyliasis: *Trichostrongylus* spp. (220)	Albendazole[b] 400 mg PO once	Mebendazole[b] 100 mg PO bid for 3 days
Trichuriasis: *Trichuris trichiura* (220)	Albendazole[b] 400 mg PO once	Mebendazole 100 mg PO bid for 3 days or 500 mg PO once
Trypanosomiasis (216)		
Chagas' disease: *Trypanosoma cruzi*	Nifurtimox 2–2.5 mg/kg PO qid for 90–120 days	Benznidazole 5 mg/kg per day PO for 60–90 days
Sleeping sickness		
West African trypanosomiasis: *T. brucei gambiense*		
Stage 1	Suramin 1 g IV on days 1, 3, 7, 14, and 21	Eflornithine 100 mg IV qid for 2 weeks, then 300 mg/kg per day PO for 3–4 weeks; *or* pentamidine[b] 4 mg/kg per day IV or IM for 10 days
Stage 2	Eflornithine 100 mg IV qid for 2 weeks, then 300 mg/kg/d PO for 3–4 weeks	—
East African trypanosomiasis: *T. brucei rhodesiense*		
Stage 1	Suramin 1 g IV on days 1, 3, 7, 14, and 21	Pentamidine[b] 4 mg/kg per day IV or IM for 10 days, *or* melarsoprol 2–3.6 mg/kg per day IV in 3 divided doses for 3 days
Stage 2	Melarsoprol 2–3.6 mg/kg per day IV in 3 divided doses for 3 days	Tryparsamide 30 mg/kg (max 2 g) *plus* suramin 10 mg/kg IV every 5 days, to a total of 12 doses of each drug
Visceral Larva Migrans: *Toxocara* spp. (219)	Supportive therapy; glucocorticoids as needed	DEC 2 mg/kg PO tid for 7–10 days, *or* albendazole[b] 400 mg PO bid for 3–5 days, *or* mebendazole[b] 100–200 mg PO bid for 5 days

[a] See also the indicated chapters on specific parasitic diseases, which present more detailed information on topics such as alternative regimens, contraindications, and adverse reactions.

[b] Not specifically approved by the U.S. Food and Drug Administration (FDA) for use in this infection.

[c] Surgery indicated for ocular and spinal lesions.

[d] Percutaneous aspiration, infusion of scolicidal agents, and reaspiration.

[e] Apheresis before treatment may be beneficial to heavily infected individuals.

[f] Diethylcarbamazine.

[g] Coinfection with *Onchocerca volvulus* or *Loa loa* must be ruled out before initiation of therapy because of potentially fatal adverse effects.

[h] When microfilariae are absent from concentrated blood, coinfection with *O. volvulus* must be ruled out before initiation of therapy because of potentially adverse effects (Mazzotti reaction).

[i] See Table 215-2 for detailed information on regimens approved by the FDA.

has been reported in persons treated with artesunate. These drugs are not available in the United States.

Amphotericin B Amphotericin exerts its effect by inserting itself into the cytoplasmic membrane of the organism and binding sterols, causing membrane permeability. Amphotericin B deoxycholate, a lipophilic polyene drug, is an effective agent for the treatment of leishmaniasis and amebic meningoencephalitis due to *Naegleria* spp., but its use is associated with significant nephrotoxicity and occasional allergic reactions. Three lipid-complexed formulations of amphotericin B have been released: amphotericin B colloidal dispersion (ABCD), amphotericin B lipid complex (ABLC), and liposomal amphotericin B. These agents are effective against antimony-resistant visceral leishmaniasis and offer the benefits of shorter courses and less toxicity.

Atovaquone Atovaquone is a hydroxynaphthoquinone that exerts its broad-spectrum antiprotozoal activity via inhibition of parasite mitochondrial electron transport. Although it has relatively poor bioavailability, atovaquone exhibits potent activity against toxoplasmosis when used with pyrimethamine. When combined with proguanil or doxycycline, it is effective for both treatment and prophylaxis of malaria. Side effects are rare but can include nausea and a maculopapular rash.

Azithromycin An azalide antibiotic, azithromycin has been used to treat a number of protozoal infections such as babesiosis, malaria, toxoplasmosis, and cryptosporidiosis. Azithromycin acts by inhibiting protein synthesis; in apicomplexan parasites, this inhibition occurs in the plastid. Most adverse reactions are gastrointestinal (diarrhea, nausea, abdominal pain) and uncommon and rarely require discontinuation of the drug.

Benznidazole This oral nitroimidazole derivative is used to treat acute Chagas' disease, and cure rates of 80 to 90% have been recorded. Benznidazole acts by generating oxygen radicals to which the parasite is more sensitive than mammalian cells because of a relative deficiency in antioxidant enzymes. Adverse effects are frequent and include rashes, nausea, paresthesias, and leukopenia. The safety of benznidazole in early pregnancy has not been established, but the drug should be used immediately after the first trimester to prevent congenital transmission. Benznidazole is currently unavailable in the United States.

Bithionol* Bithionol is a phenolic substance structurally related to hexachlorophene. Its antihelminthic activity is poorly understood, but the agent is believed to inhibit oxidative phosphorylation. Bithionol is no longer manufactured. A dwindling supply is available from the CDC for treatment of fascioliasis and paragonimiasis. The drug's distribution is limited to physicians treating patients with one of these diseases who are unable to use praziquantel because of previous idiosyncratic or allergic reactions or in whom a course of praziquantel has failed to eradicate infection. Significant side effects are common and include abdominal pain, diarrhea, and urticaria.

Chloroquine The best-known of the 4-aminoquinolines, chloroquine has marked, rapid schizonticidal and gametocidal activity against blood forms of *P. ovale* and *P. malariae* and against susceptible strains of *P. vivax* and *P. falciparum*. It is not active against intrahepatic forms (*P. vivax* and *P. ovale*). Chloroquine is concentrated in the acidic food vacuoles of intraerythrocytic parasites, where it reaches levels 600-fold higher than plasma levels. The drug inhibits a parasite heme polymerase that protects the parasite from the membrane-damaging byproducts of hemoglobin degradation; as a result of this inhibition, the parasite is effectively killed with its own metabolic waste. Chloroquine resistance appears to arise as a result of a decreased level of chloroquine uptake. This drug is safe for use in pregnancy. Adverse reactions include pruritus, transient headaches, and nausea.

Clindamycin This macrolide is an effective adjunct for the treatment of several protozoal infections, including toxoplasmosis, malaria,

and babesiosis. The most significant potential adverse reaction is the development of *Clostridium difficile*–associated diarrhea. When administered with quinine, clindamycin is active against drug-resistant falciparum malaria; this combination is the therapy of choice for babesiosis.

Diethylcarbamazine* A piperazine derivative with a long history of successful use, this drug remains the treatment of choice for lymphatic filariasis and loiasis and has also been used for visceral larva migrans. Diethylcarbamazine exerts effects on helminths, including immobilization due to a decrease in muscle activity, disruption of microtubule formation, and alteration of helminthic surface membranes resulting in enhanced killing by the host's immune system. In addition, this agent enhances adherence properties of eosinophils. It is safe for use in pregnancy and well tolerated. Significant adverse events associated with the drug, including encephalopathy and death, are attributable to the parasite burden, which is best assessed by the degree of microfilaremia. Use in patients with onchocerciasis can precipitate a Mazzotti reaction with pruritus, fever, and arthralgias. Untoward effects produced directly by diethylcarbamazine usually involve the gastrointestinal tract and are dose-related.

Eflornithine (Difluoromethylornithine, DFMO)† This ornithine derivative has specific activity against all stages of infection with *Trypanosoma brucei gambiense* and acts by irreversibly inhibiting ornithine decarboxylase—an enzyme critical to the formation of polyamines, which are essential to trypanosomatids. Eflornithine readily crosses the blood-brain barrier and is excreted mainly by the kidneys. Its use is contraindicated in pregnancy. Adverse reactions, which are usually mild and reversible, include pancytopenia, diarrhea, and transient hearing loss.

Furazolidone This nitrofuran derivative, which is an effective alternative agent for the treatment of giardiasis, acts by damaging parasite DNA. Since it is the only agent active against *Giardia* that is available in liquid form, it is often used to treat young children. Side effects include allergic reactions, nausea, vomiting, and disulfiram-like reactions when ingested with alcohol. Because hemolytic anemia due to glutathione instability can occur, furazolidone treatment is contraindicated in mothers who are breast-feeding and in neonates.

Halofantrine An oral alternative drug for treatment of malaria due to chloroquine-resistant *P. falciparum*, this 9-phenanthrenemethanol is one of three classes of arylaminoalcohols first identified as potential antimalarial agents by the World War II Malaria Chemotherapy Program. Its activity is believed to be similar to that of chloroquine. Halofantrine is generally well tolerated; the most commonly reported adverse effects are abdominal pain and diarrhea. The incidence of pruritus is lower than that with chloroquine. Halofantrine causes dose-related prolongation of the PR and QT intervals, and its use is contraindicated in persons who have cardiac disease or who have taken mefloquine in the preceding 3 weeks. Halofantrine treatment is also contraindicated in pregnant and lactating women. The drug is currently unavailable in the United States.

Iodoquinol This hydroxyquinoline is an effective luminal agent for the treatment of amebiasis, balantidiasis, and infection with *Dientamoeba fragilis*. Its mechanism of action is unknown. Adverse effects include headache, diarrhea, nausea, vomiting, abdominal pain, pruritus, fever, seizures, and encephalopathy. Most serious are the reactions related to prolonged high-dose therapy, which should not occur if the dosage regimens recommended in Table 212-1 are followed. Because the drug contains iodine, it should be used with caution in patients with thyroid disease.

Ivermectin This derivative of avermectin is used to treat infections caused by a wide range of helminths. It is the drug of choice for the treatment of onchocerciasis, strongyloidiasis, and cutaneous larva migrans. While active against the intestinal helminths *Ascaris lumbricoides* and *Enterobius vermicularis*, it is variably effective in trichuriasis and ineffective against hookworms. Recent data suggest that ivermectin acts by opening neuromuscular membrane-associated glutamate-dependent chloride channels (unique to nematodes and arthropods)—an event resulting in an influx of chloride ions, worm paralysis, and subsequent death by immune or other mechanisms. Ivermectin is generally safe, easy to administer, and well tolerated, but encephalopathy and occasional deaths have been reported when the drug is given to persons with high burdens of *Loa loa* microfilaremia. Ivermectin is not approved for use during pregnancy.

Mebendazole   This benzimidazole derivative is widely used for treatment of intestinal helminths and exhibits activity against *Echinococcus granulosus*. Benzimidazoles block parasite microtubule assembly and glucose uptake. Because mebendazole is poorly absorbed, its incidence of side effects is low, but its usefulness in treating tissue helminths is limited. Transient abdominal pain and diarrhea sometimes occur, usually in persons with massive parasite burdens. The use of mebendazole is contraindicated in pregnancy.

Mefloquine   Like quinine and chloroquine, this quinoline is active only against the asexual erythrocytic stages of malarial parasites. The mode of action of mefloquine is similar to that of chloroquine, but mefloquine is not concentrated so extensively in the food vacuole and may act on alternative targets in the parasite. Taken as a single dose, it is the preferred drug for prophylaxis of chloroquine-resistant malaria; high doses can be used for treatment. The development of drug-resistant strains of *P. falciparum* in parts of Africa and Southeast Asia is ominous, but mefloquine is still an effective drug in most of the world. It is well tolerated by most persons, but its safety in pregnancy is unknown. Adverse effects are usually dose-related and include nausea and dizziness. Psychosis and seizures occur rarely, but treatment of patients with neuropsychiatric conditions warrants caution. Concomitant use of quinine, quinidine, or drugs causing β-adrenergic blockade may produce electrocardiographic disturbances or cardiac arrest.

Melarsoprol*   This trivalent arsenical is used for the treatment of late-stage East African trypanosomiasis and is not uniformly effective. The drug enters the parasite via an adenosine transporter; resistant strains lack this transport system. Arsenicals react avidly with sulfhydryl groups on proteins and inhibit their function. This is the likely mechanism of action and the cause of the severe adverse effects commonly seen. Encephalopathy is the most serious side effect, usually occurring within 4 days of the initiation of therapy and resulting in death in 6% of recipients.

Metrifonate   This organophosphorus compound has selective activity against *Schistosoma haematobium*. It is partially metabolized to 2,2-dimethyldichlorovinyl phosphate (DDVP), a highly active chemical that irreversibly inhibits the acetylcholinesterase enzyme. Schistosomal cholinesterase is more susceptible to this metabolite than is the corresponding human enzyme. Metrifonate's exact mechanism of action is uncertain, but it is believed to inhibit tegumental acetylcholine receptors that mediate glucose transport. Although the drug is well tolerated, recipients experience a transient decrease in plasma cholinesterase activity and should not be exposed to neuromuscular blocking agents or organophosphate insecticides for at least 48 h after treatment. Metrifonate's safety in pregnancy is not established. The drug is currently unavailable in the United States.

Metronidazole   Of the nitroimidazoles, only metronidazole has been licensed in the United States. This drug has FDA approval only for the treatment of amebiasis and trichomoniasis, although it is currently the drug of choice for giardiasis and trichomoniasis and is an alternative agent for balantidiasis. Metronidazole is reduced by anaerobic metabolism, and the metabolite acts as an electron sink, depriving anaerobes of reducing equivalents. Covalent binding or other interactions of intermediate metabolites of metronidazole with parasite macromolecules may partly explain the efficacy of this agent. Its benefit in dracunculiasis appears to be due to a reduction in inflammation rather than to any specific antihelminthic effect. Metronidazole is generally well tolerated despite common side effects such as nausea, headache, and a metabolic aftertaste. Alcohol should be avoided due to disulfiram-like effects. Although metronidazole has not been approved

or recommended for use during pregnancy, it has not been associated with birth defects.

Nifurtimox*   This nitrofuran compound is an effective oral agent for the treatment of acute Chagas' disease. Intracellular reduction followed by auto-oxidation yielding oxygen radicals has been suggested as the mode of action of nifurtimox on *Trypanosoma cruzi* and as the basis of its toxicity in humans. Prolonged use is required, but the course may have to be interrupted due to drug toxicity, which develops in 40 to 70% of recipients. Adverse reactions are common, dose-related, and reversible. They include nausea, vomiting, abdominal pain, insomnia, seizures, and polyneuritis. Nifurtimox should be avoided in early pregnancy.

Nitazoxanide†   This 5-nitrothiazole compound appears to be a safe and effective alternative agent for the treatment of cryptosporidiosis. Its mechanism of action is unknown. It is currently available only from Romark Laboratories in the United States.

Oxamniquine   This tetrahydroquinoline derivative is an effective alternative agent for the treatment of schistosomiasis, although susceptibility to this drug exhibits regional variation. In treated adult schistosomes, oxamniquine produces marked tegumental alterations similar to those seen with praziquantel but less rapid (evident 4 to 8 days after treatment). Patients should be warned that their urine may have an intense orange-red color. Side effects are uncommon and usually mild, although hallucinations and seizures have been reported. Oxamniquine has not been shown to be teratogenic or embryotoxic, but its use in pregnancy has not been approved.

Paromomycin   This aminoglycoside is an effective oral agent for the treatment of infections due to intestinal protozoa. Like other aminoglycosides, it is poorly absorbed after oral administration and binds to the 30S ribosomal RNA in the aminoacyl-tRNA site, resulting in inhibition of protein synthesis. Paromomycin is well tolerated and safe for use in pregnancy.

Pentamidine Isethionate   This diamine is an effective alternative agent for some forms of leishmaniasis and trypanosomiasis. While its mechanism of action remains undefined, it is known to exert a wide range of effects, including interaction with trypanosomal kinetoplast DNA, interference with polyamine synthesis through a decrease in the activity of ornithine decarboxylase, and inhibition of RNA polymerase, ribosomal function, and the synthesis of nucleic acids and proteins. Adverse reactions are common and include hypotension, pancreatitis, hypoglycemia, arrhythmias, and reversible renal failure.

Praziquantel   This heterocyclic prazino-isoquinoline derivative is highly active against a broad spectrum of trematodes and cestodes. It disrupts the parasite tegument, resulting in contracture with loss of adherence to host tissues and ultimately disintegration or expulsion. Drug levels are reduced by concomitantly administered glucocorticoids, but cimetidine can be used to offset this problem. Praziquantel is generally well tolerated, but seizures may result in persons with neurocysticercosis. Patients with schistosomiasis who have heavy parasite burdens may develop abdominal discomfort, nausea, headache, dizziness, and drowsiness. Although praziquantel has not been shown to be mutagenic, teratogenic, or embryotoxic, it is preferable to delay treatment until after delivery unless immediate intervention is essential. Because praziquantel is excreted in breast milk, it is recommended that women not nurse on the day(s) of drug administration or for 72 h thereafter.

Primaquine Phosphate   This drug is the only agent available for eradication of the hepatic stage of malarial parasites. In order to be effective, it must be metabolized by the host. Although their parasiticidal activity remains unclear, the metabolites are believed to affect both pyrimidine synthesis and the mitochondrial electron transport chain. The major adverse effect of this drug is acute hemolysis in patients with glucose-6-phosphate dehydrogenase (G6PD) deficiency. Primaquine phosphate is otherwise well tolerated. Its use in pregnancy is contraindicated.

Proguanil (Chloroguanide) This agent, which inhibits plasmodial dihydrofolate reductase, is used with atovaquone for oral treatment of uncomplicated malaria or with chloroquine for prophylaxis in parts of Africa without widespread chloroquine-resistant *P. falciparum*. Proguanil is quite well tolerated at the usually prescribed doses, but higher doses can produce nausea, vomiting, abdominal pain, and diarrhea. It is not available in the United States.

Pyrantel Pamoate This safe, well-tolerated, and inexpensive pyrimidine derivative depolarizes the neuromuscular junctions of most intestinal nematodes, resulting in irreversible paralysis and allowing natural expulsion of the worms with the host's feces. The drug is poorly absorbed from the gastrointestinal tract and is usually effective in a single dose. It has minimal toxicity at the oral doses used to treat intestinal helminthic infection.

Pyrimethamine When combined with short-acting sulfonamides, this diaminopyrimidine is effective in malaria, toxoplasmosis, and isosporiasis. Unlike mammalian cells, the parasites that cause these infections cannot utilize preformed pyrimidines obtained through salvage pathways but rather rely completely on de novo synthesis of pyrimidines, for which folate derivatives are essential cofactors.

Pyrimethamine-sulfadoxine is an effective adjunctive agent for the oral treatment of uncomplicated malaria due to chloroquine-resistant organisms. However, its usefulness as a first-line agent is limited by the development of resistant strains of *P. falciparum* and *P. vivax*.

When combined with sulfadiazine, pyrimethamine is the treatment of choice for toxoplasmosis, but the duration of the required course of therapy often results in the development of folate deficiency requiring folinic acid supplementation. Sulfadiazine crystals can cause hematuria, and allergic drug reactions due to sulfadiazine often require a switch to clindamycin.

Quinacrine* Quinacrine is the only drug approved by the FDA for the treatment of giardiasis. It is not commercially available but can be obtained from alternative sources through the CDC Drug Service. Quinacrine intercalates into parasite DNA and inhibits nucleic acid synthesis. Side effects are common and include nausea and vomiting, headache, and skin discoloration. Alcohol is best avoided due to a disulfiram-like effect.

Quinine and Quinidine When combined with another agent, the cinchona alkaloid quinine is effective for the oral treatment of both uncomplicated malaria due to chloroquine-resistant strains and babesiosis. Quinine acts rapidly against the asexual blood stages of all forms of human malaria. For severe malaria, only quinidine (the dextroisomer of quinine) is available in the United States. Its use requires cardiac monitoring, and dose reduction is necessary in persons with severe renal impairment. Both quinine and quinidine can produce hypoglycemia. Symptoms of cinchonism (tinnitus, headache, nausea, and visual disturbances) are dose-related and reversible.

Spiramycin† This macrolide antibiotic is used to treat acute toxoplasmosis in pregnancy and congenital toxoplasmosis. Although not yet licensed in the United States, it is available through the FDA. Complications of treatment are rare but can include life-threatening ventricular arrhythmias in neonates.

Sodium Stibogluconate* and Meglumine Antimonate These pentavalent antimony compounds are first-line agents for the treatment of all forms of leishmaniasis. Despite their use in leishmaniasis for almost 100 years, their mechanism of action against *Leishmania* spp. remains unknown. Presumably, the compounds interfere with parasite metabolism. The drugs are taken up by the reticuloendothelial system, and their activity against *Leishmania* spp. may be enhanced by this localization. Resistance is a major problem in some areas of the world. Side effects are common and generally reversible but require temporary interruption of therapy in many cases. Chemical pancreatitis is almost universal, although it is often asymptomatic. In rare instances, pentavalent antimony compounds produce prolongation of the QT interval, and sudden death due to arrhythmia or cardiac failure has been reported. Arthralgias, myalgias, and headaches occur frequently. Since the drugs' safety in pregnancy has not been established, their use should be avoided if possible in pregnant women. These agents may be used in children >18 months of age.

Suramin* This derivative of urea is the drug of choice for the early stage of African trypanosomiasis. The drug acts by forming stable complexes with proteins, inhibiting multiple enzymes. Suramin has a variety of potentially severe side effects, including anaphylaxis, exfoliative dermatitis, paresthesias, photophobia, and renal dysfunction.

Tetracycline and Doxycycline These antibiotics are useful in the treatment of balantidiasis and *D. fragilis* infection as well as in the oral treatment of uncomplicated malaria due to chloroquine-resistant strains. The tetracyclines inhibit protein synthesis in prokaryotic ribosomes, and they probably have the same activity in parasites. Potential side effects in adults include nausea, vomiting, and photosensitivity dermatitis. Because they can impair normal development of bones and teeth, tetracyclines are contraindicated in pregnant women and children <8 years of age.

Thiabendazole This benzimidazole derivative is a potent antihelminthic agent, but its use in strongyloidiasis and other infections is limited by frequent, severe side effects. Patients most often report dizziness, headache, nausea, and vomiting. Less commonly, hepatitis and severe hypersensitivity reactions develop. The drug's mechanism of action is similar to that of other benzimidazoles. Treatment with thiabendazole is contraindicated in pregnancy.

Tinidazole This nitroimidazole is effective for the treatment of amebiasis, giardiasis, and trichomoniasis. Its mechanism of action and side effects are similar to those seen with metronidazole, but adverse events appear to be less frequent and severe with tinidazole. In addition, tinidazole is potentially curative in a single dose. This agent is currently unavailable in the United States.

Triclabendazole This benzimidazole is effective against paragonimiasis and all stages of *Fasciola hepatica*, a trematode with inherent resistance to praziquantel. The sulfoxide metabolite, which is believed to be responsible for the drug's activity, binds to fluke tubulin and disrupts microtubule-based processes. Triclabendazole is safe and well tolerated and offers single-dose cure. It is currently unavailable in the United States.

Trimethoprim-Sulfamethoxazole This synergistic antifolate compound is active against cyclosporiasis, isosporiasis, and encephalitis due to *Toxoplasma gondii*. Trimethoprim is a dihydrofolate reductase inhibitor whose effect is enhanced by sulfamethoxazole. Adverse effects, which can be severe, are usually attributable to the sulfonamide component and involve allergic skin reactions, bone marrow suppression, and hemolysis.

BIBLIOGRAPHY

ABRAMOWICZ M (ed): Drugs for parasitic infections. Med Lett Drugs Ther 40:1, 2000

LIU LX, WELLER PF: Antiparasitic drugs. N Engl J Med 334:1178, 1996

MOORE TA, NASH TE: Tissue Nematodes, in *Current Therapy of Infectious Disease*, 2d ed, D Schlossberg (ed). St. Louis, Mosby, 2000, pp 660–665

ROSENBLATT JE: Antiparasitic agents. Mayo Clin Proc 74:1161, 1999

WORLD HEALTH ORGANIZATION: *Model Prescribing Information: Drugs Used in Parasitic Diseases*, 2d ed. Geneva, WHO, 1995

213 | *Sharon L. Reed*

AMEBIASIS AND INFECTION WITH FREE-LIVING AMEBAS

AMEBIASIS

DEFINITION Amebiasis is an infection with the intestinal protozoan *Entamoeba histolytica*. About 90% of infections are asymptomatic, and the remaining 10% produce a spectrum of clinical syndromes ranging from dysentery to abscesses of the liver or other organs.

LIFE CYCLE AND TRANSMISSION *E. histolytica* is acquired by ingestion of viable cysts from fecally contaminated water, food, or hands. Food-borne exposure is most prevalent and is particularly likely when food handlers are shedding cysts or food is being grown with feces-contaminated soil, fertilizer, or water. Less common means of transmission include contaminated water, oral and anal sexual practices, and—in rare instances—direct rectal inoculation through colonic irrigation devices. Motile trophozoites are released from cysts in the small intestine and, in most patients, remain as harmless commensals in the large bowel. After encystation, infectious cysts are shed in the stool and can survive for several weeks in a moist environment. In some patients, the trophozoites invade either the bowel mucosa, causing symptomatic colitis, or the bloodstream, causing distant abscesses of the liver, lungs, or brain. The trophozoites may not encyst in patients with active dysentery, and motile hematophagous trophozoites are frequently present in fresh stools. Trophozoites are rapidly killed by exposure to air or stomach acid, however, and therefore cannot cause infection.

EPIDEMIOLOGY About 10% of the world's population is infected with *Entamoeba*, the majority with noninvasive *Entamoeba dispar*. Amebiasis results from infection with *E. histolytica* and is the third most common cause of death from parasitic disease (after schistosomiasis and malaria). Areas of highest incidence (due to inadequate sanitation and crowding) include most developing countries in the tropics, particularly Mexico, India, and nations of Central and South America, tropical Asia, and Africa. The main groups at risk in developed countries are travelers, recent immigrants, homosexual men, and inmates of institutions.

The wide spectrum of clinical disease is caused in part by infection with the two different species of *Entamoeba*. Isolates of *E. histolytica* from patients with invasive amebiasis have unique isoenzymes, surface antigens, DNA markers, and virulence properties and now are recognized as a distinct species from the noninvasive *E. dispar*.

Most asymptomatic carriers, including homosexual men and AIDS patients, harbor *E. dispar* and have self-limited infections. These observations suggest that *E. dispar* is incapable of causing invasive disease, since *Cryptosporidium* and *Isospora belli*, which also cause only self-limited illnesses in immunocompetent people, cause devastating diarrhea in patients with AIDS. However, host factors play a role as well. In one study, 10% of asymptomatic patients who were colonized with *E. histolytica* went on to develop amebic colitis, while the rest remained asymptomatic and cleared the infection within 1 year.

PATHOGENESIS AND PATHOLOGY Both trophozoites (Fig. 213-1) and cysts (Fig. 213-2) are found in the intestinal lumen, but only trophozoites of *E. histolytica* invade tissue. The trophozoite is 20 to 60 μm in diameter and contains vacuoles and a nucleus with a characteristic central karyosome. In animals, depletion of intestinal mucus, diffuse inflammation, and disruption of the epithelial barrier occur before trophozoites actually come into contact with the colonic mucosa. Trophozoites attach to colonic mucus and epithelial cells by a galactose-inhibitable lectin. The earliest intestinal lesions are mi-

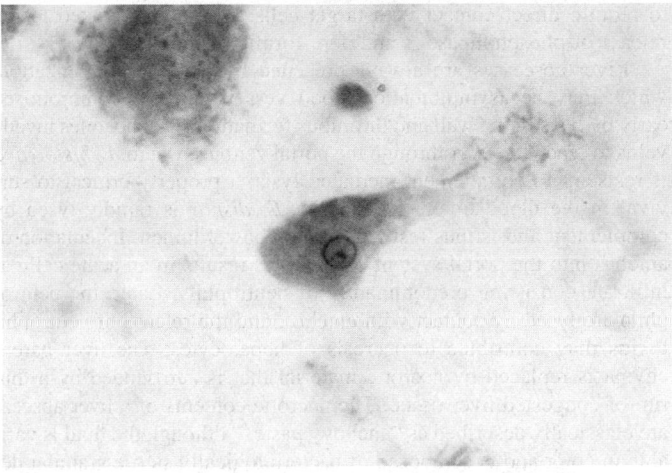

FIGURE 213-1 Trophozoite of *E. histolytica* demonstrating a single nucleus with a central, dotlike karyosome (trichrome stain).

croulcerations of the mucosa of the cecum, sigmoid colon, or rectum that release erythrocytes, inflammatory cells, and epithelial cells. Proctoscopy reveals small ulcers with heaped up margins and normal intervening mucosa. Submucosal extension of ulcerations under viable-appearing surface mucosa causes the classic "flask-shaped" ulcer containing trophozoites at the margins of dead and viable tissues. Although neutrophilic infiltrates may accompany the early lesions in animals, human intestinal infection is marked by a paucity of inflammatory cells, probably in part because of the killing of neutrophils by trophozoites. Treated ulcers characteristically heal with little or no scarring. Occasionally, however, full-thickness necrosis and perforation occur.

Rarely, intestinal infection results in the formation of a mass lesion, or *ameboma*, in the bowel lumen. The overlying mucosa is usually thin and ulcerated, while other layers of the wall are thickened, edematous, and hemorrhagic; this condition results in exuberant formation of granulation tissue with little fibrous-tissue response.

A number of virulence factors have been linked to the ability of *E. histolytica* to invade through the interglandular epithelium. One is an extracellular cysteine proteinase that degrades collagen, elastin, secretory IgA, and the anaphylatoxins C3a and C5a. Other enzymes may

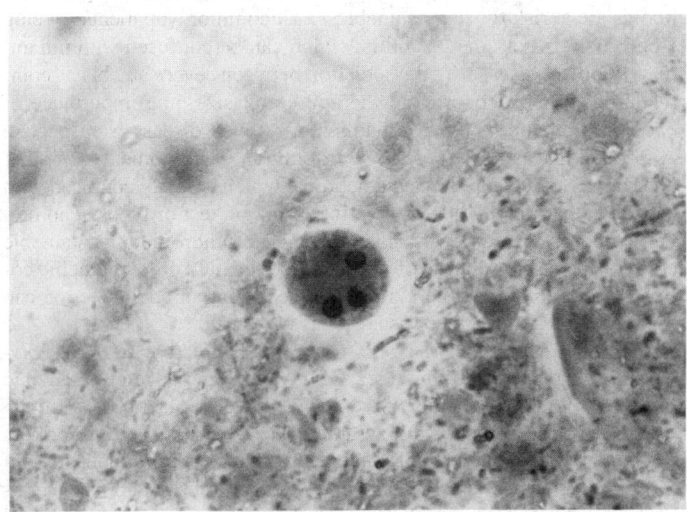

FIGURE 213-2 Cyst of *E. histolytica* showing three of the four nuclei (trichrome stain).

disrupt glycoprotein bonds between mucosal epithelial cells in the gut. Amebas can lyse neutrophils, monocytes, lymphocytes, and cells of colonic and hepatic cell lines. The cytolytic effect of amebas appears to require direct contact with target cells and may be linked to the release of phospholipase A and pore-forming peptides.

Liver abscesses are always preceded by intestinal colonization, which may be asymptomatic. Blood vessels may be compromised early by lysis of the wall and thrombus formation. Trophozoites invade veins to reach the liver through the portal venous system. *E. histolytica* is resistant to complement-mediated lysis, a property critical to survival in the bloodstream. In contrast, *E. dispar* is rapidly lysed by complement and is thus restricted to the bowel lumen. Inoculation of amebas into the portal system of hamsters results in an acute cellular infiltrate consisting predominantly of neutrophils. Later, the neutrophils are lysed by contact with amebas, and the release of neutrophil toxins may contribute to necrosis of hepatocytes. The liver parenchyma is replaced by necrotic material that is surrounded by a thin rim of congested liver tissue. The necrotic contents of a liver abscess are classically described as "anchovy paste," although the fluid is variable in color and is composed of bacteriologically sterile granular debris with few or no cells. Amebas, if seen, tend to be found near the capsule of the abscess.

Clinical infection does not induce immunity to recurrent colonization with *E. histolytica*, but repeated episodes of colitis or liver abscess are unusual. Antibody is not protective; titers correlate with the length of illness rather than with the severity of disease. Studies of animals suggest that cell-mediated immunity may be important for protection, although patients with AIDS appear not to be predisposed to more severe disease.

CLINICAL SYNDROMES   **Intestinal Amebiasis**   The most common type of amebic infection is asymptomatic cyst passage. Even in highly endemic areas, most patients harbor *E. dispar*.

Symptomatic amebic colitis develops 2 to 6 weeks after the ingestion of infectious cysts. Lower abdominal pain and mild diarrhea develop gradually and are followed by malaise, weight loss, and diffuse lower abdominal or back pain. Cecal involvement may mimic acute appendicitis. Patients with full-blown dysentery may pass 10 to 12 stools per day. The stools contain little fecal material and consist mainly of blood and mucus. In contrast to those with bacterial diarrhea, fewer than 40% of patients with amebic dysentery are febrile. Virtually all patients have heme-positive stools.

More fulminant intestinal infection, with severe abdominal pain, high fever, and profuse diarrhea, is rare and occurs predominantly in children. Patients may develop toxic megacolon, in which there is severe bowel dilation with intramural air. Patients receiving glucocorticoids are at risk for severe amebiasis. Uncommonly, patients develop a chronic form of amebic colitis, which can be confused with inflammatory bowel disease. The association between severe amebiasis complications and glucocorticoid therapy emphasizes the importance of excluding amebiasis when inflammatory bowel disease is suspected. An occasional patient presents with only an asymptomatic or tender abdominal mass caused by an ameboma, which is easily confused with cancer on barium studies. A positive serologic test or biopsy can prevent unnecessary surgery in this setting. The syndrome of postamebic colitis—persistent diarrhea following documented cure of amebic colitis—is controversial; no evidence of recurrent amebic infection can be found, and re-treatment usually has no effect.

Amebic Liver Abscess   Extraintestinal infection by *E. histolytica* most often involves the liver. Of travelers who develop an amebic liver abscess after leaving an endemic area, 95% do so within 5 months. Young patients with an amebic liver abscess are more likely than older patients to present in the acute phase with prominent symptoms of <10 days duration. Most patients are febrile and have right-upper-quadrant pain, which may be dull or pleuritic in nature and radiate to the shoulder. Point tenderness over the liver and right-sided pleural effusion are common. Jaundice is rare. Although the initial site

of infection is the colon, fewer than one-third of patients with an amebic abscess have active diarrhea. Older patients from endemic areas are more likely to have a subacute course lasting 6 months, with weight loss and hepatomegaly. About one-third of patients with chronic presentations are febrile. Thus, the clinical diagnosis of an amebic liver abscess may be difficult to establish because the symptoms and signs are often nonspecific. Since 10 to 15% of patients present only with fever, amebic liver abscess must be considered in the differential diagnosis of fever of unknown origin (Chap. 125).

Complications of Amebic Liver Abscess   Pleuropulmonary involvement, which is reported in 20 to 30% of patients, is the most frequent complication of amebic liver abscess. Manifestations include sterile effusions, contiguous spread from the liver, and rupture into the pleural space. Sterile effusions and contiguous spread usually resolve with medical therapy, but frank rupture into the pleural space requires drainage. A hepatobronchial fistula may cause cough productive of large amounts of necrotic material that may contain amebas. This dramatic complication carries a good prognosis. Abscesses that rupture into the peritoneum may present as an indolent leak or an acute abdomen and require both percutaneous catheter drainage and medical therapy. Rupture into the pericardium, usually from abscesses of the left lobe of the liver, carries the gravest prognosis; it can occur during medical therapy and requires surgical drainage.

Other Extraintestinal Sites   The genitourinary tract may become involved by direct extension of amebiasis from the colon or by hematogenous spread of the infection. Painful genital ulcers, characterized by a punched-out appearance and profuse discharge, may develop secondary to extension from either the intestine or the liver. Both these conditions respond well to medical therapy. Cerebral involvement has been reported in fewer than 0.1% of patients in large clinical series. Symptoms and prognosis depend on the size and location of the lesion.

DIAGNOSTIC TESTS   **Laboratory Diagnosis**   Stool examinations, serologic tests, and noninvasive imaging of the liver are the most important procedures in the diagnosis of amebiasis. Fecal findings suggestive of amebic colitis include a positive test for heme, a paucity of neutrophils, and the presence of Charcot-Leyden crystal protein (double pyramid-shaped crystals normally found in the cytoplasm of eosinophils). The definitive diagnosis of amebic colitis is made by the demonstration of hematophagous trophozoites of *E. histolytica* (Fig. 213-1). Because trophozoites are killed rapidly by water, drying, or barium, it is important to examine at least three fresh stool specimens. Examination of a combination of wet mounts, iodine-stained concentrates, and trichrome-stained preparations of fresh stool and concentrates for cysts (Fig. 213-2) or trophozoites (Fig. 213-1) confirms the diagnosis in 75 to 95% of cases. Cultures of amebas are more sensitive but are not routinely available. If stool examinations are negative, sigmoidoscopy with biopsy of the edge of ulcers may increase the yield, but this procedure is dangerous during fulminant colitis because of the risk of perforation. Trophozoites in a biopsy specimen from a colonic mass confirm the diagnosis of ameboma, but trophozoites are rare in liver aspirates. Accurate diagnosis requires experience, since the trophozoites may be confused with neutrophils and the cysts must be differentiated morphologically from *Entamoeba hartmanni*, *Entamoeba coli*, and *Endolimax nana*, which do not cause clinical disease and do not warrant therapy. Unfortunately, the cysts of *E. histolytica* cannot be distinguished microscopically from those of *E. dispar*. Therefore, the microscopic diagnosis of *E. histolytica* can be made only by the detection of *Entamoeba* trophozoites that have ingested erythrocytes (Fig. 213-1). Diagnostic tests based on the detection of the galactose-inhibitable lectin of *E. histolytica* are now available and compare favorably with the polymerase chain reaction and with isolation in culture followed by isoenzyme analysis in terms of sensitivity.

Serology is an important addition to the methods used for the parasitologic diagnosis of invasive amebiasis. Kits for the performance of agar gel diffusion assays and ELISAs are commercially available, and the results of these tests are positive in more than 90% of patients with colitis, amebomas, or liver abscess. Positive results in conjunction with the appropriate clinical syndrome suggest active disease because serologic findings usually revert to negative within 6 to 12 months. Even in highly endemic areas such as South Africa, fewer than 10% of asymptomatic individuals have a positive amebic serology. The interpretation of the indirect hemagglutination test is more difficult because titers may remain positive for as long as 10 years.

Up to 10% of patients with acute amebic liver abscess may have negative serologic findings; in suspected cases with an initially negative result, testing should be repeated in a week. In contrast to carriers of *E. dispar*, most asymptomatic carriers of *E. histolytica* develop antibodies. Thus, serologic tests are helpful in assessing the risk of invasive amebiasis in asymptomatic, cyst-passing individuals in non-endemic areas. Serologic tests also should be performed in patients with ulcerative colitis before the institution of glucocorticoid therapy to prevent the development of severe colitis or toxic megacolon owing to unsuspected amebiasis.

Routine hematology and chemistry tests are usually not very helpful in the diagnosis of invasive amebiasis. About three-fourths of patients with an amebic liver abscess have leukocytosis ($>$10,000 cells/μL); this condition is particularly likely if symptoms are acute or complications have developed. Invasive amebiasis does not elicit eosinophilia. Anemia, if present, is usually multifactorial. Even with large liver abscesses, liver enzyme levels are normal or minimally elevated. The alkaline phosphatase level is most often elevated and may remain so for months. Aminotransferase elevations suggest acute disease or a complication.

Radiographic Studies Radiographic barium studies are potentially dangerous in acute amebic colitis. Amebomas are usually identified first by a barium enema, but biopsy is necessary for differentiation from carcinoma.

Radiographic techniques such as ultrasonography, computed tomography (Fig. 213-3), and magnetic resonance imaging are all useful for detection of the round or oval hypoechoic cyst. More than 80% of patients who have had symptoms for $>$10 days have a single abscess of the right lobe of the liver. Approximately 50% of patients who have had symptoms for $<$10 days have multiple abscesses. Findings associated with complications include large abscesses ($>$10 cm) in the superior part of the right lobe, which may rupture into the pleural space; multiple lesions, which must be differentiated from pyogenic abscesses; and lesions of the left lobe, which may rupture into the pericardium. Because abscesses resolve slowly and may increase in size in patients who are responding clinically to therapy, frequent follow-up ultrasonography may prove confusing. Complete resolution of a liver abscess within 6 months can be anticipated in two-thirds of patients, but 10% may have persistent abnormalities for a year.

DIFFERENTIAL DIAGNOSIS The differential diagnosis of intestinal amebiasis includes bacterial diarrheas caused by *Campylobacter*; enteroinvasive *Escherichia coli*; and *Shigella*, *Salmonella*, and *Vibrio* species. Although the typical patient with amebic colitis has less prominent fever than in these other conditions as well as heme-positive stools with few neutrophils, correct diagnosis requires bacterial cultures, microscopic examination of stools, and amebic serologic testing. As has already been mentioned, amebiasis must be ruled out in any patient thought to have inflammatory bowel disease.

Because of the variety of presenting signs and symptoms, amebic liver abscess can easily be confused with pulmonary or gallbladder disease or with any febrile illness with few localizing signs, such as malaria or typhoid fever. The diagnosis should be considered in members of high-risk groups who have recently traveled outside the United States and in inmates of institutions. Once radiographic studies have identified an abscess in the liver, the most important differential diagnosis is between amebic and pyogenic abscess. Patients with pyogenic abscess typically are older and have a history of underlying bowel disease or recent surgery. Amebic serology is helpful, but aspiration of the abscess, with Gram's staining and culture of the material, may be required for differentiation of the two diseases.

℞ **TREATMENT Intestinal Disease** The drugs used to treat amebiasis can be classified according to their primary site of action. Luminal amebicides are poorly absorbed and reach high concentrations in the bowel, but their activity is limited to cysts and trophozoites close to the mucosa. Only two luminal drugs are available in the United States: iodoquinol and paromomycin (Table 213-1). Indications for the use of luminal agents include eradication of cysts in patients with colitis or a liver abscess and treatment of asymptomatic carriers. The majority of asymptomatic individuals who pass cysts are colonized with *E. dispar*, which does not warrant specific therapy. However, unless the presence of *E. dispar* can be proven by specific antigen detection tests and the lack of an antibody response, it may be prudent to treat asymptomatic individuals who pass cysts.

Tissue amebicides reach high concentrations in the blood and tissue after oral or parenteral administration. The development of nitro-imidazole compounds, especially metronidazole, was a major advance in the treatment of invasive amebiasis. Patients with amebic colitis should be treated with intravenous or oral metronidazole (750 mg three times daily for 5 to 10 days). Side effects include nausea, vomiting, abdominal discomfort, and a disulfiram-like reaction. Other imidazole compounds, such as tinidazole and ornidazole, are as effective but are

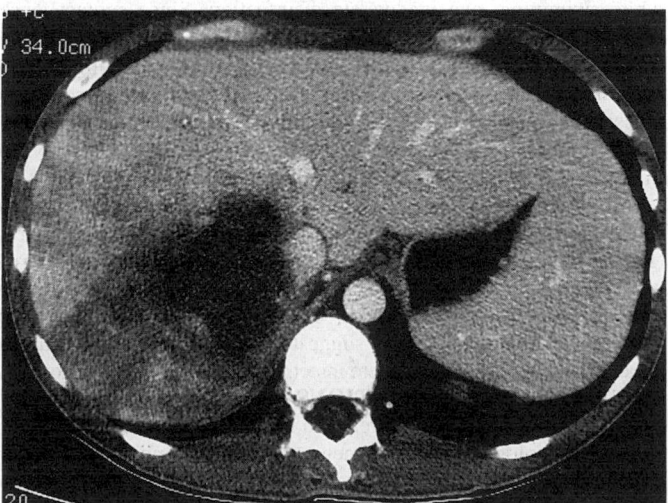

FIGURE 213-3 Abdominal computed tomography scan of a large amebic abscess of the right lobe of the liver. *(Courtesy of the Department of Radiology, UCSD Medical Center, San Diego.)*

Table 213-1 Drug Therapy for Amebiasis

Drug	Dosage
ASYMPTOMATIC CARRIER (LUMINAL AGENTS)	
Iodoquinol (650-mg tablets)	650 mg tid for 20 days
Paromomycin (250-mg tablets)	500 mg tid for 10 days
ACUTE COLITIS	
Metronidazole (250- or 500-mg tablets)	750 mg PO or IV tid for 5 to 10 days
plus	
Luminal agent as above	
AMEBIC LIVER ABSCESS	
Metronidazole	750 mg PO or IV tid for 5 to 10 days
Tinidazole[a]	2 g PO
Ornidazole[a]	2 g PO
plus	
Luminal agent as above	

[a] Not available in the United States.

not available in the United States. All patients should also receive a full course of therapy with a luminal agent, since metronidazole does not eradicate cysts. Resistance to metronidazole has not been identified. Relapses are not uncommon and probably represent reinfection or failure to eradicate amebas from the bowel because of an inadequate dosage or duration of therapy.

Amebic Liver Abscess　Metronidazole is the drug of choice for amebic liver abscess. The usefulness of nitroimidazoles in single-dose or abbreviated regimens is important in endemic areas where access to hospitalization is limited. With early diagnosis and therapy, mortality from uncomplicated amebic liver abscess is <1%. The second-line therapeutic agents emetine and chloroquine should be avoided if possible because of the potential cardiovascular and gastrointestinal side effects of the former and the higher relapse rates with the latter. There is no evidence that combined therapy with two drugs is more effective than the single-drug regimen. Studies of South Africans with liver abscesses demonstrated that 72% of patients without intestinal symptoms had bowel infection with *E. histolytica*; thus, all treatment regimens should include a luminal agent to eradicate cysts and prevent further transmission. Amebic liver abscess recurs rarely.

Aspiration of Liver Abscesses　More than 90% of patients respond dramatically to metronidazole therapy with decreases in both pain and fever within 72 h. Indications for aspiration of liver abscesses are (1) the need to rule out a pyogenic abscess, particularly in patients with multiple lesions; (2) the failure to respond clinically in 3 to 5 days; (3) the threat of imminent rupture; and (4) the prevention of rupture of left-lobe abscesses into the pericardium. There is no evidence that aspiration, even of large abscesses (up to 10 cm), accelerates healing. Percutaneous drainage may be successful even if the liver abscess has already ruptured. Surgery should be reserved for instances of bowel perforation and rupture into the pericardium.

PREVENTION　Amebic infection is spread by ingestion of food or water contaminated with cysts. Since an asymptomatic carrier may excrete up to 15 million cysts per day, prevention of infection requires adequate sanitation and eradication of cyst carriage. In high-risk areas, infection can be minimized by the avoidance of unpeeled fruits and vegetables and the use of bottled water. Because cysts are resistant to readily attainable levels of chlorine, disinfection by iodination (tetraglycine hydroperiodide) is recommended. There is no effective prophylaxis.

INFECTION WITH FREE-LIVING AMEBAS

EPIDEMIOLOGY　Free-living amebas of the genera *Acanthamoeba*, *Naegleria*, and *Balamuthia* are distributed throughout the world and have been isolated from a wide variety of fresh and brackish water, including that from lakes, taps, hot springs, swimming pools, and heating and air-conditioning units, and even from the nasal passages of healthy children. Encystation may protect the protozoa from desiccation and food deprivation. The persistence of *Legionella pneumophila* in water supplies may be attributable in part to chronic infection of free-living amebas, particularly *Naegleria*.

NAEGLERIA **INFECTIONS**　Primary amebic meningoencephalitis caused by *Naegleria fowleri* follows the aspiration of water contaminated with trophozoites or cysts or the inhalation of contaminated dust, leading to invasion of the olfactory neuroepithelium. After an incubation period of 2 to 15 days, severe headache, high fever, nausea, vomiting, and meningismus develop. Photophobia and palsies of the third, fourth, and sixth cranial nerves are common. Rapid progression to seizures and coma may follow, and most patients die within a week. Infection is most common in otherwise healthy children or young adults, who often report recent swimming in lakes or heated swimming pools.

Diagnosis depends on the detection of motile trophozoites in wet mounts of fresh spinal fluid. Other laboratory findings resemble those for fulminant bacterial meningitis, with elevated intracranial pressure, high white blood cell counts (up to 20,000 cells/μL), and elevated protein concentrations and low glucose levels in cerebrospinal fluid. The diagnosis should be considered in any patient who has purulent meningitis without evidence of bacteria on Gram's staining, antigen detection assay, and culture. The prognosis is uniformly poor. Only four survivors, treated with high-dose amphotericin B and rifampin, have been reported. Antibodies to *Naegleria* spp. have been detected in normal adults; serologic testing is not useful in the diagnosis of acute infection.

ACANTHAMOEBA **INFECTIONS**　**Granulomatous Amebic Encephalitis**　Infection with *Acanthamoeba* species follows a more indolent course and occurs typically in chronically ill or debilitated patients. Risk factors include lymphoproliferative disorders, chemotherapy, glucocorticoid therapy, lupus erythematosus, and AIDS. Infection usually reaches the central nervous system hematogenously from a primary focus in the sinuses, skin, or lungs. In the central nervous system, the onset is insidious, and the syndrome often mimics a space-occupying lesion. Altered mental status, headache, and stiff neck may be accompanied by focal findings such as cranial nerve palsies, ataxia, and hemiparesis. In the United States, cutaneous ulcers or hard nodules containing amebas were detected in 8 of 13 AIDS patients with disseminated *Acanthamoeba* infection.

Examination of the cerebrospinal fluid for trophozoites may be diagnostically helpful, but lumbar puncture may be contraindicated because of increased intracerebral pressure. Computed tomography frequently reveals cortical and subcortical lesions of decreased density consistent with embolic infarcts. In other patients, multiple enhancing lesions with edema may mimic the computed tomographic appearance of toxoplasmosis. Demonstration of the trophozoites and cysts of *Acanthamoeba* on wet mounts or in biopsy specimens establishes the diagnosis. Culture on nonnutrient agar plates seeded with *Escherichia coli* may also be helpful. Fluorescein-labeled antiserum is available from the Centers for Disease Control and Prevention (CDC) for the detection of protozoa in biopsy specimens. At least nine cases of granulomatous amebic encephalitis have been reported in patients with AIDS, in whom the disease may have an accelerated course (with survival for only 3 to 40 days) because of their difficulty in forming granulomas. Although studies in animals suggest that rifampin may be useful, the infection is almost uniformly fatal.

Keratitis　The incidence of keratitis caused by *Acanthamoeba* has increased in the past 20 years, in part as a result of improved diagnosis. The first of these infections to be recognized were associated with trauma to the eye and exposure to contaminated water. At present, most infections are linked to extended-wear contact lenses. Risk factors include the use of homemade saline, the wearing of lenses while swimming, and inadequate disinfection. Since contact lenses presumably cause microscopic trauma, the early corneal findings may be nonspecific. The first symptoms usually include tearing and the painful sensation of a foreign body. Once infection is established, progression is rapid; the characteristic clinical sign is an annular, paracentral corneal ring representing a corneal abscess. Deeper corneal invasion and loss of vision may follow.

The differential diagnosis includes bacterial, mycobacterial, and herpetic infection. The irregular polygonal cysts of *Acanthamoeba* (Fig. 213-4) may be identified in corneal scrapings or biopsy material, and trophozoites can be grown on special media. Cysts are resistant to available drugs, and the results of medical therapy have been disappointing. Some reports have suggested partial responses to propamidine isethionate eyedrops. Severe infections usually require keratoplasty.

BALAMUTHIA **INFECTIONS**　*Balamuthia mandrillaris*, a free-living ameba previously referred to as a leptomyxid ameba, is an important etiologic agent of amebic meningoencephalitis in immunocompetent hosts. The course is typically subacute, with focal neurologic signs, fever, seizures, and headaches leading to death within 1 week to several months after onset. Examination of cerebrospinal fluid reveals mononuclear pleocytosis, elevated protein levels, and normal to low glucose concentrations. Multiple hypodense lesions are usually

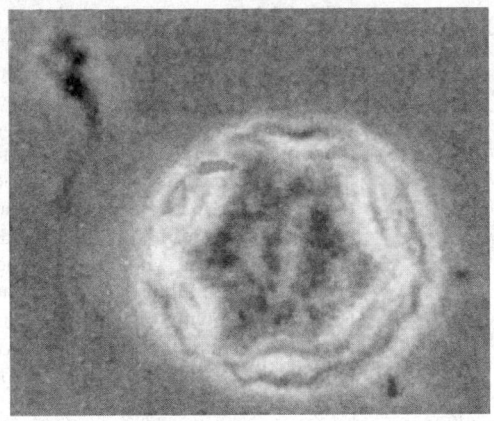

FIGURE 213-4 Double-walled cyst of *Acanthamoeba castellani*, as seen by phase-contrast microscopy. *[From DJ Krogstad et al, in A Balows et al (eds): Manual of Clinical Microbiology, 5th ed. Washington, DC, American Society for Microbiology, 1991.]*

detected with imaging studies. The diagnosis is almost always made post-mortem, and specific identification may require immunofluorescence with antibodies from the CDC to differentiate the trophozoites from *Acanthamoeba*.

BIBLIOGRAPHY

AMEBIASIS

HAQUE R et al: Comparison of PCR, isoenzyme analysis, and antigen detection for diagnosis of *Entamoeba histolytica* infection. J Clin Microbiol 36:449, 1998

IRUSEN EM et al: Asymptomatic intestinal colonization by pathogenic *Entamoeba histolytica* in amebic liver abscess: Prevalence, response to therapy, and pathogenic potential. Clin Infect Dis 14:889, 1992

PETRI WA: Amebiasis and the *Entamoeba histolytica* Gal/GalNAc lectin: From bench to bedside. J Invest Med 44:24, 1996

———, SINGH U: Diagnosis and management of amebiasis. Clin Infect Dis 29:1117, 1999

QUE X, REED SL: The role of extracellular cysteine proteinases in pathogenesis of *Entamoeba histolytica* invasion. Parasitol Today 13:190, 1997

REED SL et al: *Entamoeba histolytica* infection and AIDS. Am J Med 90:269, 1991

STANLEY SL: Progress toward development of a vaccine for amebiasis. Clin Microbiol Rev 10:637, 1997

THOMPSON JE et al: Amebic liver abscess: A therapeutic approach. Rev Infect Dis 7:171, 1985

ACANTHAMOEBA, *NAEGLERIA*, AND *BALAMUTHIA*

DENNEY CF et al: Amebic meningoencephalitis caused by *Balamuthia mandrillaris*: Case report and review. Clin Infect Dis 25:1354, 1997

LARKIN DFP : *Acanthamoeba* keratitis. Int Ophthalmol Clin 31:163, 1991

MARTINEZ AJ, VISVESVARA GS: Free-living, amphizoic and opportunistic amebas. Brain Pathol 7:583, 1997

SISON JP et al: Disseminated *Acanthamoeba* infection in patients with AIDS: Case reports and review. Clin Infect Dis 20:1207, 1995

214 Nicholas J. White, Joel G. Breman

MALARIA AND BABESIOSIS: DISEASES CAUSED BY RED BLOOD CELL PARASITES

"Humanity has but three great enemies: Fever, famine and war; of these by far the greatest, by far the most terrible, is fever."

William Osler

MALARIA

Malaria is a protozoan disease transmitted by the bite of infected *Anopheles* mosquitoes. It is the most important of the parasitic diseases of humans, with transmission in 103 countries affecting more than 1 billion people and causing between 1 and 3 million deaths each year. Malaria has now been eradicated from North America, Europe, and Russia but, despite enormous control efforts, has resurged in many parts of the tropics. Added to this resurgence are the increasing problems of drug resistance of the parasite and insecticide resistance of the vectors. Occasional local transmission following importation of malaria has occurred recently in several southern and eastern areas of the United States and in Europe, indicating the continual danger to nonmalarious countries. Malaria remains today, as it has been for centuries, a heavy burden on tropical communities, a threat to nonendemic countries, and a danger to travelers.

ETIOLOGY AND PATHOGENESIS Four species of the genus *Plasmodium* cause nearly all malarial infections in humans (although rare infections involve species normally affecting other primates). These are *P. falciparum*, *P. vivax*, *P. ovale*, and *P. malariae* (Table 214-1). Almost all deaths are caused by falciparum malaria. Human infection begins when a female anopheline mosquito inoculates plasmodial sporozoites from its salivary gland during a blood meal (Fig. 214-1). These microscopic motile forms of the malarial parasite are carried rapidly via the bloodstream to the liver, where they invade hepatic parenchymal cells and begin a period of asexual reproduction. By this amplification process (known as intrahepatic or pre-erythrocytic schizogony or merogony), a single sporozoite eventually may produce 10,000 to more than 30,000 daughter merozoites. The swollen liver cell eventually bursts, discharging motile merozoites into the bloodstream; at this point the symptomatic stage of the infection begins. In *P. vivax* and *P. ovale* infections, a proportion of the intrahepatic forms do not divide immediately but remain dormant for months to years before reproduction begins. These dormant forms, or hypnozoites, are the cause of the relapses that characterize infection with these two species.

After entry into the bloodstream, merozoites rapidly invade erythrocytes and become trophozoites. Attachment is mediated via a specific erythrocyte surface receptor. In the case of *P. vivax*, this receptor is related to the Duffy blood-group antigen Fy^a or Fy^b. Most West Africans and people with origins in that region carry the Duffy-negative FyFy phenotype and are therefore resistant to *P. vivax* malaria. During the early stage of intraerythrocytic development, the small "ring forms" of the four parasitic species appear similar under light microscopy. As the trophozoites enlarge, species-specific characteristics become evident, pigment becomes visible, and the parasite assumes an irregular or ameboid shape. By the end of the 48-h intraerythrocytic life cycle (72 h for *P. malariae*), the parasite has consumed nearly all the hemoglobin and grown to occupy most of the red cell. Multiple nuclear divisions take place (merogony), and the red cell ruptures to release 6 to 30 daughter merozoites, each capable of invading a new red cell and repeating the cycle. The disease in human beings is caused by the direct effects of red cell invasion and destruction by the asexual parasite and the host's reaction. After a series of asexual cycles (*P. falciparum*) or immediately (*P. vivax*, *P. ovale*, *P. malariae*), some of the parasites develop into morphologically distinct long-lived sexual forms (gametocytes) that can transmit malaria.

After being ingested in the blood meal of a biting female anopheline mosquito, the male and female gametocytes form a zygote in the insect's midgut. This zygote matures into an ookinete, which penetrates and encysts in the mosquito's gut wall. The resulting oocyst expands by asexual division until it bursts to liberate myriad motile sporozoites, which then migrate in the hemolymph to the salivary gland of the mosquito to await inoculation into another human at the next feeding.

EPIDEMIOLOGY Malaria occurs throughout most of the tropical regions of the world (Fig. 214-2). *P. falciparum* predominates in Africa, New Guinea, and Haiti; *P. vivax* is more common in Central America and the Indian subcontinent. The prevalence of these two

Table 214-1 Characteristics of *Plasmodium* Species Infecting Humans

Characteristic	Finding for Indicated Species			
	P. falciparum	*P. vivax*	*P. ovale*	*P. malariae*
Duration of intrahepatic phase (days)	5.5	8	9	15
Number of merozoites released per infected hepatocyte	30,000	10,000	15,000	15,000
Duration of erythrocytic cycle (hours)	48	48	50	72
Red cell preference	Younger cells (but can invade cells of all ages)	Reticulocytes	Reticulocytes	Older cells
Morphology	Usually only ring forms[a]; banana-shaped gametocytes	Irregularly shaped large rings and trophozoites; enlarged erythrocytes; Schüffner's dots	Infected erythrocytes, enlarged and oval; Schüffner's dots	Band or rectangular forms of trophozoites common
Pigment color	Black	Yellow-brown	Dark brown	Brown-black
Ability to cause relapses	No	Yes	Yes	No

[a] Parasitemia sometimes exceeds 2% with multiple infections of a single erythrocyte.

species is approximately equal in South America, eastern Asia, and Oceania. *P. malariae* is found in most endemic areas, especially throughout sub-Saharan Africa, but is much less common than the other species mentioned. *P. ovale* is relatively unusual outside of Africa and, where it is found, comprises <1% of isolates.

The epidemiology of malaria is complex and may vary considerably even within relatively small geographic areas. Endemicity traditionally has been defined in terms of parasitemia rates or palpable-spleen rates in children 2 to 9 years of age as hypoendemic (<10%), mesoendemic (11 to 50%), hyperendemic (51 to 75%), and holoendemic (>75%). In holo- and hyperendemic areas—e.g., certain regions of tropical Africa or coastal New Guinea, where there is intense *P. falciparum* transmission and there can be more than one human bite per infected mosquito per day—people are infected repeat-edly throughout their lives. Here, morbidity and mortality during childhood are considerable. Immunity against disease is hard won in these areas, and the young-childhood burden of disease is high; by adulthood, however, most malarial infections are asymptomatic. This situation, with frequent year-round infection, is termed *stable transmission* and generally occurs where there is holo- and hyperendemicity. In areas where transmission is low, erratic, or focal, full protective immunity is not acquired, and symptomatic disease may occur at all ages. This situation usually exists in hypoendemic areas and is termed *unstable transmission*. Even in areas with stable transmission, there is often an increased incidence coinciding with increased mosquito breeding during the rainy season. Malaria behaves like an epidemic disease in some areas, particularly those with unstable malaria, such as northern India, Sri Lanka, Southeast Asia, Ethiopia, southern Africa, and Madagascar. An epidemic can develop when there are changes in environmental, economic, or social conditions, such as heavy rains following drought or migrations (usually of refugees or workers) from a nonmalarious region to an area of high transmission; a breakdown in malaria control and prevention services can intensify epidemic conditions. This situation usually results in considerable mortality among all age groups.

The principal determinants of the epidemiology of malaria are the number (density), the human-biting habits, and the longevity of the anopheline mosquito vectors. Not all anophelines can transmit malaria, and those that do vary considerably in their efficiency as malaria vectors. More specifically, the transmission of malaria is directly proportional to the density of the vector, the square of the number of human bites per day per mosquito, and the tenth power of the probability of the mosquito's surviving for 1 day. Mosquito longevity is particularly important, because the portion of the parasite's life cycle that takes place within the mosquito—from gametocyte ingestion to subsequent inoculation (sporogony)—lasts for 8 to 30 days, depending on ambient temperature; thus, to transmit malaria, the mosquito must survive for longer than 7 days. In general, at temperatures below 16 to 18°C, sporogony is not completed and transmission does not occur. Therefore, the most effective mosquito vectors of malaria are those such as *A. gambiae*, which are long-lived, occur in high densities in tropical climates, breed readily, and bite humans in preference to other animals. The entomologic inoculation rate—the number of sporozoite-positive mosquito bites per year—is the most common measure of malarial transmission and varies from <1 in some parts of Latin America and Southeast Asia to >300 in parts of tropical Africa.

ERYTHROCYTE CHANGES IN MALARIA After invading an erythrocyte, the growing parasite progressively consumes and degrades intracellular proteins, principally hemoglobin. The potentially toxic heme is polymerized to biologically inert hemozoin, or malaria pigment. The parasite also alters the red cell membrane by changing its transport properties, exposing cryptic surface antigens, and inserting new parasite-derived proteins. The red cell becomes more irregular in shape, more antigenic, and less deformable.

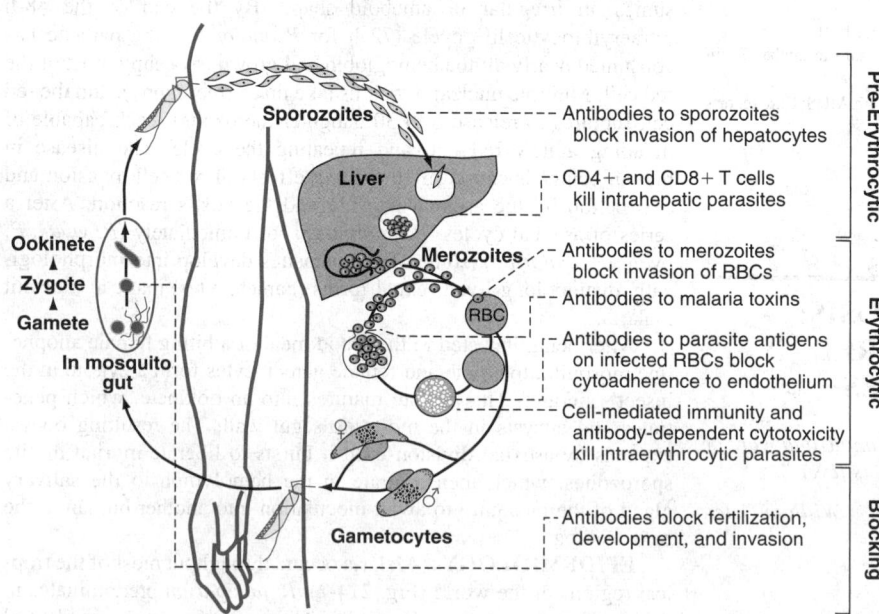

FIGURE 214-1 The malaria transmission cycle.

In *P. falciparum* infections, membrane protuberances appear on the erythrocyte's surface in the second 24 h of the asexual cycle. These "knobs" extrude a high-molecular-weight, antigenically variant, strain-specific, adhesive protein (PfEMP1) that mediates attachment to receptors on venular and capillary endothelium—an event termed *cytoadherence*. Several receptors have been identified, of which intercellular adhesion molecule 1 is probably the most important in the brain, chondroitin sulfate B in the placenta, and CD36 in most other organs. Thus the infected erythrocytes stick inside the small blood vessels. At the same stage, these *P. falciparum*–infected red cells may also adhere to uninfected red cells to form rosettes. The processes of cytoadherence and rosetting are central to

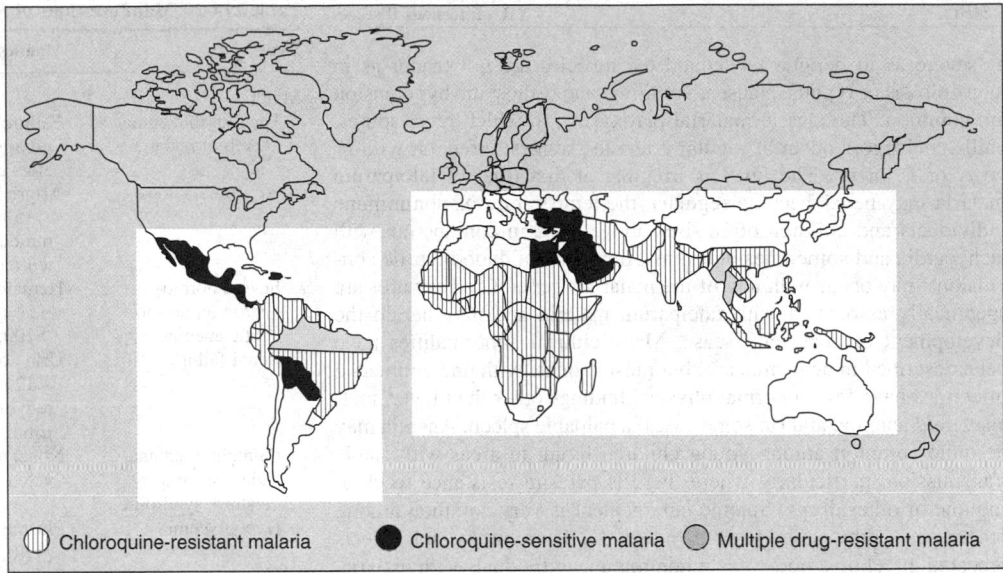

FIGURE 214-2 Worldwide distribution of malaria and drug-resistant *Plasmodium falciparum*, 1999.

Chloroquine-resistant malaria   Chloroquine-sensitive malaria   Multiple drug-resistant malaria

the pathogenesis of falciparum malaria. They result in the sequestration of red cells containing mature forms of the parasite in vital organs (particularly the brain), where they interfere with microcirculatory flow and metabolism. Sequestered parasites continue to develop out of reach of the principal host defense mechanism: splenic processing and filtration. As a consequence, only the younger ring forms of the asexual parasites are seen in the peripheral blood in falciparum malaria, and the level of peripheral parasitemia underestimates the true number of parasites within the body. Severe malaria is also associated with reduced deformability of the uninfected erythrocytes, which compromises their passage through the partially obstructed capillaries and venules and shortens red cell survival.

In the other three "benign" malarias, sequestration does not occur, and all stages of the parasite's development are evident on peripheral blood smears. Whereas *P. vivax*, *P. ovale*, and *P. malariae* show a marked predilection for either old red cells or reticulocytes and produce a level of parasitemia seldom exceeding 2%, *P. falciparum* can invade erythrocytes of all ages and may be associated with very high levels of parasitemia.

HOST RESPONSE Initially, the host responds to plasmodial infection by activating nonspecific defense mechanisms. Splenic immunologic and filtrative clearance functions are augmented in malaria, and the removal of both parasitized and uninfected erythrocytes is accelerated. The parasitized cells escaping splenic removal are destroyed when the schizont ruptures. The material released induces the activation of macrophages and the release of proinflammatory mononuclear cell–derived cytokines, which cause fever and exert other pathologic effects. Temperatures of ≥40°C damage mature parasites; in untreated infections, the effect of such temperatures is to synchronize further the parasitic cycle with eventual production of the regular fever spikes and rigors that originally served to characterize the different malarias. These regular fever patterns (tertian, every 2 days; quartan, every 3 days) are seldom seen in patients who receive prompt and effective antimalarial treatment.

The geographic distributions of sickle cell disease, thalassemia, and glucose-6-phosphate dehydrogenase (G6PD) deficiency closely resemble that of malaria before the introduction of control measures. This observation suggests that these genetic disorders confer protection against death from falciparum malaria. For example, HbA/S heterozygotes (sickle cell trait) have a sixfold reduction in the risk of dying from severe falciparum malaria. This decrease in risk appears to be related to impaired parasite growth at low oxygen tensions. In Melanesia, children with α-thalessemia appear to have more frequent malaria (both vivax and falciparum) in the early years of life, and this pattern of infection appears to protect against severe disease. In Melanesian ovalocytosis, rigid erythrocytes resist merozoite invasion and the intraerythrocytic milieu is hostile.

The specific immune response to malaria eventually controls the infection and, with exposure to sufficient strains, confers protection from high-level parasitemia and disease but not from infection. As a result of this state of infection without illness (premunition), asymptomatic parasitemia is common among adults and older children living in regions with stable and intense transmission (i.e., holo- or hyperendemic areas). Immunity is specific for both the species and the strain of infecting malarial parasite. Both humoral immunity and cellular immunity are necessary for protection, but the mechanisms of each are incompletely understood (Fig. 214-1). Immune individuals have a polyclonal increase in serum levels of IgM, IgG, and IgA, although much of this antibody is unrelated to protection. Antibodies to a variety of parasitic antigens presumably act in concert to limit in vivo replication of the parasite. In the case of falciparum malaria, the most important of these is the antigenically variant protein PfEMP1 mentioned above. Passively transferred IgG from immune adults has been shown to reduce levels of parasitemia in children, and passive transfer of maternal antibody contributes to the relative protection of infants from severe malaria in the first months of life. This complex immunity to disease is lost when a person lives outside an endemic area for several months or longer.

Several factors retard the development of cellular immunity to malaria. These factors include the absence of major histocompatibility antigens on the surface of infected red cells, which precludes direct T cell recognition; malaria antigen–specific immune unresponsiveness; and the enormous strain diversity of malarial parasites along with the ability of the parasites to express immunodominant variant antigens on the erythrocyte surface that change during the period of infection. Strain diversity also has an impact on the heterogeneity of the humoral antibody response. Immunity to all strains is never achieved. Parasites may persist in the blood for months (or, in the case of *P. malariae*, for many years) if treatment is not given. The complexity of the immune response in malaria, the sophistication of the parasites' evasion mechanisms, and the lack of a good in vitro correlate with clinical immunity have all slowed progress toward an effective vaccine.

CLINICAL FEATURES The first symptoms of malaria are nonspecific; the lack of a sense of well-being, headache, fatigue, abdominal discomfort, and muscle aches followed by fever are all similar to the symptoms of a minor viral illness. In some instances, a prominence of headache, chest pain, abdominal pain, arthralgia, myalgia, or diarrhea may suggest another diagnosis. Although headache may be severe in malaria, there is no neck stiffness or photophobia resembling that in meningitis. While myalgia may be prominent, it is not usually as severe as in dengue fever, and the muscles are not tender as in leptospirosis or typhus. Nausea, vomiting, and orthostatic hypotension are common. The classic malarial paroxysms, in which fever spikes, chills, and rigors occur at regular intervals, suggest infection with *P. vivax* or *P. ovale*. The fever is irregular at first (that of falciparum malaria may never become regular); the temperature of nonimmune individuals and children often rises above 40°C in conjunction with tachycardia and sometimes delirium. Although childhood febrile convulsions may occur with any of the malarias, generalized seizures are specifically associated with falciparum malaria and may herald the development of cerebral disease. Many clinical abnormalities have been described in acute malaria, but most patients with uncomplicated infections have few abnormal physical findings other than fever, malaise, mild anemia, and (in some cases) a palpable spleen. Anemia may be quite common among young children living in areas with stable transmission, particularly where there is parasite resistance to chloroquine or other drugs. Splenic enlargement is very common among otherwise-healthy individuals in malaria-endemic areas and reflects repeated infections; however, in nonimmune individuals with malaria, the spleen takes several days to become palpable. Slight enlargement of the liver is also common, particularly in young children. Mild jaundice is common in adults; it may develop in patients with otherwise uncomplicated falciparum malaria and usually resolves over 1 to 3 weeks. Malaria is not associated with a rash like those seen in meningococcal septicemia, typhus, enteric fever, viral exanthems, and drug reactions. Petechial hemorrhages in the skin or mucous membranes—features of viral hemorrhagic fevers and leptospirosis—develop only rarely in severe falciparum malaria.

Severe Falciparum Malaria Appropriately treated, uncomplicated falciparum malaria carries a mortality rate of ~0.1%. However, once vital organ dysfunction occurs or the proportion of erythrocytes infected increases to >3%, mortality rises steeply. The major manifestations of severe falciparum malaria are shown in Table 214-2.

Cerebral malaria Coma is a characteristic and ominous feature of falciparum malaria and, despite treatment, is associated with death rates of ~20% among adults and 15% among children. Lesser degrees of obtundation, delirium, and abnormal behavior should also be taken very seriously. The onset may be gradual or sudden following a convulsion.

Cerebral malaria manifests as diffuse symmetric encephalopathy; focal neurologic signs are unusual. Although some passive resistance to head flexion may be detected, signs of meningeal irritation are lacking. The eyes may be divergent and a pout reflex is common, but other primitive reflexes are usually absent. The corneal reflexes are preserved except in deep coma. Muscle tone may be either increased or decreased. The tendon reflexes are variable, and the plantar reflexes may be flexor or extensor; the abdominal and cremasteric reflexes are absent. Flexor or extensor posturing may be documented. Approximately 15% of patients have retinal hemorrhages; with pupillary dilatation and indirect ophthalmoscopy, this figure increases to 30 to 40%. Other abnormalities include discrete spots of retinal opacification (30 to 60%), papilledema (8% of children, rare in adults), cotton wool spots (<5%), and decolorization of a retinal vessel or segment of vessel (occasional cases). Convulsions, usually generalized and often repeated, occur in up to 50% of children with cerebral malaria. More covert seizure activity is common, particularly in children, and may manifest as repetitive tonic-clonic eye movements. Whereas adults rarely suffer neurologic sequelae, ~10% of children surviving cerebral malaria—especially those with hypoglycemia, severe anemia, repeated seizures, and deep coma—have some residual neurologic deficit when they regain consciousness; hemiplegia, cerebral palsy, cortical blindness, deafness, and impaired cognition and learning—all of varying duration—have been reported.

Hypoglycemia An important and common complication of severe malaria, hypoglycemia is associated with a poor prognosis and is particularly problematic in children and pregnant women. Hypogly-

Table 214-2 Manifestations of Severe Falciparum Malaria

Signs	Manifestations
Major	
Unarousable coma/ cerebral malaria	Failure to localize or respond appropriately to noxious stimuli; coma persisting for >30 min after generalized convulsion
Acidemia/acidosis	Arterial pH <7.25 or plasma bicarbonate level of <15 mmol/L; venous lactate level of >15 mmol/L manifests as labored deep breathing, often termed "respiratory distress"
Severe normochromic, normocytic anemia	Hematocrit of <15% or hemoglobin level of <50 g/L (<5 g/dL) with parasitemia level of >100,000/μL
Renal failure	Urine output (24 h) of <400 mL in adults or <12 mL/kg in children; no improvement with rehydration; serum creatinine level of >265 μmol/L (>3.0 mg/dL)
Pulmonary edema/ adult respiratory distress syndrome	Noncardiogenic pulmonary edema, often aggravated by overhydration
Hypoglycemia	Plasma glucose level of <2.2 mmol/L (<40 mg/dL)
Hypotension/shock	Systolic blood pressure of <50 mmHg in children 1–5 years or <80 mmHg in adults; core/ skin temperature difference of >10°C
Bleeding/disseminated intravascular coagulation	Significant bleeding and hemorrhage from the gums, nose, and gastrointestinal tract and/or evidence of disseminated intravascular coagulation
Convulsions	More than two generalized seizures in 24 h
Hemoglobinuria[a]	Macroscopic black, brown, or red urine; not associated with effects of oxidant drugs and red blood cell enzyme defects (such as G6PD deficiency)
Other	
Impaired consciousness	Obtunded but arousable
Extreme weakness	Prostration
Hyperparasitemia	Parasitemia level of >5% in nonimmune patients
Jaundice	Serum bilirubin level of >50 mmol/L (>3.0 mg/dL)

[a] Hemoglobinuria may occur in uncomplicated malaria.
NOTE: G6PD, glucose-6-phosphate dehydrogenase.

cemia in malaria results from a failure of hepatic gluconeogenesis and an increase in the consumption of glucose by both host and parasite. To compound the situation, quinine and quinidine—drugs used commonly for the treatment of severe chloroquine-resistant malaria—are powerful stimulants of pancreatic insulin secretion. Hyperinsulinemic hypoglycemia is especially troublesome in pregnant women receiving quinine treatment. In severe disease, the clinical diagnosis of hypoglycemia is difficult: the usual physical signs (sweating, gooseflesh, tachycardia) are absent, and the neurologic impairment caused by hypoglycemia cannot be distinguished from that caused by malaria.

Lactic acidosis Lactic acidosis commonly coexists with hypoglycemia in patients with malaria and is an important contributor to death from severe malaria. In adults, coexisting renal impairment often compounds the acidosis. Acidotic breathing, sometimes called respiratory distress, is a sign of poor prognosis. It is often followed by circulatory failure refractory to volume expansion or inotropic drugs or by respiratory arrest. The plasma concentrations of bicarbonate or lactate are the best biochemical prognosticators in severe malaria. Lactic acidosis is caused by the combination of anaerobic glycolysis in tissues where sequestered parasites interfere with microcirculatory flow, lactate production by the parasites, and a failure of hepatic and renal lactate clearance. The prognosis of lactic acidosis is poor.

Noncardiogenic pulmonary edema Adults with severe falciparum malaria may develop noncardiogenic pulmonary edema even after several days of antimalarial therapy. This manifestation may also develop in otherwise-uncomplicated vivax malaria, where recovery is usual. The pathogenesis of this variant of the adult respiratory distress syndrome is unclear. The mortality rate is >80%. This condition can be aggravated by overly vigorous administration of intravenous fluid.

Renal impairment Renal impairment is common among adults with severe falciparum malaria but rare among children. The pathogenesis of renal failure is unclear but may be related to erythrocyte sequestration interfering with renal microcirculatory flow and metabolism. Clinically and pathologically, this syndrome manifests as acute tubular necrosis; renal cortical necrosis never develops. Mortality in the initial phase of hypercatabolic acute renal failure is high; in survivors, urine flow resumes in a median of 4 days, and serum creatinine levels return to normal in a mean of 17 days (Chap. 269). Dialysis or hemofiltration considerably enhances the likelihood of a patient's survival.

Hematologic abnormalities Anemia results from accelerated red cell destruction and removal by the spleen in conjunction with ineffective erythropoiesis. In severe malaria, both infected and uninfected red cells show reduced deformability, which correlates with prognosis and development of anemia. Splenic clearance of cells is also increased. In nonimmune individuals and in areas with unstable transmission, anemia can develop rapidly and transfusion is often required. In many areas of Africa, children may develop severe anemia as a result of repeated malarial infections. Anemia is a common consequence of antimalarial drug resistance, which results in repeated or continued infection.

Slight coagulation abnormalities are common in falciparum malaria, and mild thrombocytopenia is usual. As mentioned above, fewer than 5% of patients with severe malaria have significant bleeding with evidence of disseminated intravascular coagulation. Hematemesis, presumably from stress ulceration or acute gastric erosions, may also occur.

Liver dysfunction Mild hemolytic jaundice is common in malaria. Severe jaundice is associated with *P. falciparum* infections, is more common among adults than among children, and results from hemolysis, hepatocyte injury, and cholestasis. When accompanied by other vital organ dysfunction (often renal impairment), liver dysfunction carries a poor prognosis. Hepatic dysfunction contributes to hypoglycemia, lactic acidosis, and impaired drug metabolism.

Other complications Aspiration pneumonia following convulsions is an important cause of death in cerebral malaria. Chest infections and catheter-induced urinary tract infections are common among patients who are unconscious for >3 days. Septicemia may complicate severe malaria; in endemic areas *Salmonella* bacteremia has been associated specifically with *P. falciparum* infections.

Malaria in Pregnancy In hyper- and holoendemic areas, falciparum malaria in primi- and secundigravid women is associated with low birth weight (average reduction, ~170 g) and consequently increased infant and childhood mortality. In general, infected mothers in areas of stable transmission remain asymptomatic despite intense parasitization of the placenta due to sequestration of parasitized erythrocytes in the placental microcirculation. Maternal HIV infection predisposes pregnant women to a higher prevalence of malaria and parasite density and predisposes their newborns to congenital malaria infection and low birth weight.

In areas with unstable transmission of malaria, pregnant women are prone to severe infections and are particularly vulnerable to high-level parasitemia with anemia, hypoglycemia, and acute pulmonary edema. Fetal distress, premature labor, and stillbirth or low birth weight are common results. Congenital malaria occurs in fewer than 5% of newborns whose mothers are infected and is related directly to the parasite density in maternal blood and in the placenta. *P. vivax* malaria in pregnancy is also associated with a reduction in birth weight (average, 100 g), but, in contrast with the situation in falciparum malaria, this effect is greater in multigravid than in primigravid women.

Malaria in Children Most of the estimated 1 to 3 million persons who die of falciparum malaria each year are young African children. Convulsions, coma, hypoglycemia, metabolic acidosis, and severe anemia are relatively common among children with severe malaria, whereas deep jaundice, acute renal failure, and acute pul-

monary edema are unusual. Severely anemic children may present with labored deep breathing, which in the past has been attributed incorrectly to "anemic congestive cardiac failure" but is in fact usually caused by metabolic acidosis, often compounded by hypovolemia. In general, children tolerate antimalarial drugs well and respond rapidly to treatment.

Transfusion Malaria Malaria can be transmitted by blood transfusion, needle-stick injury, sharing of needles by infected drug addicts, or organ transplantation. The incubation period in these settings is often short because there is no preerythrocytic stage of development. The clinical features and management of these cases are the same as for naturally acquired infections, although falciparum malaria tends to be especially severe in drug addicts. Radical chemotherapy with primaquine is unnecessary for *P. vivax* and *P. ovale* infections.

CHRONIC COMPLICATIONS OF MALARIA **Tropical Splenomegaly (Hyperreactive Malarial Splenomegaly)** Chronic or repeated malarial infections produce hypergammaglobulinemia; normochromic, normocytic anemia; and, in certain situations, splenomegaly. Some residents of malaria-endemic areas in tropical Africa and Asia exhibit an abnormal immunologic response to repeated infections that is characterized by massive splenomegaly, hepatomegaly, marked elevations in serum titers of IgM and malarial antibody, hepatic sinusoidal lymphocytosis, and (in Africa) peripheral B cell lymphocytosis. This syndrome has been associated with the production of cytotoxic IgM antibodies to suppressor (CD8+) lymphocytes, antibodies to CD5+ T cells, and an increase in the ratio of CD4+ T cells to CD8+ T cells. It is believed that these events lead to uninhibited B cell production of IgM and the formation of cryoglobulins (IgM aggregates and immune complexes). This immunologic process stimulates reticuloendothelial hyperplasia and clearance activity and eventually produces splenomegaly. Patients with hyperreactive malarial splenomegaly (HMS) present with an abdominal mass or a dragging sensation in the abdomen and occasional sharp abdominal pains suggesting perisplenitis. Anemia and some degree of pancytopenia are usually evident, but in many cases malarial parasites cannot be found in peripheral blood smears. Vulnerability to respiratory and skin infections is increased; many patients die of overwhelming sepsis. Persons with HMS who are living in endemic areas should receive antimalarial chemoprophylaxis: the results are usually good. In nonendemic areas, treatment is advised. In some cases refractory to therapy, clonal lymphoproliferation may develop and then evolve into a malignant lymphoproliferative disorder.

Quartan Malarial Nephropathy Chronic or repeated infections with *P. malariae*, and possibly other malarial species, may cause soluble immune-complex injury to the renal glomeruli, resulting in the nephrotic syndrome. Other, unidentified factors must contribute to this process since only a very small proportion of infected patients develop renal disease. The histologic appearance is that of focal or segmental glomerulonephritis with splitting of the capillary basement membrane. Subendothelial dense deposits are seen on electron microscopy, and immunofluorescence reveals deposits of complement and immunoglobulins; in samples of renal tissue from children, *P. malariae* antigens are often visible. A coarse-granular pattern of basement membrane immunofluorescent deposits (predominantly IgG3) with selective proteinuria carries a better prognosis than a fine-granular, predominantly IgG2 pattern with nonselective proteinuria. Quartan nephropathy usually responds poorly to treatment with either antimalarial agents or glucocorticoids and cytotoxic drugs.

Burkitt's Lymphoma and Epstein-Barr Virus Infection It is possible that malaria-related immunosuppression provokes infection with lymphoma viruses. Burkitt's lymphoma is strongly associated with Epstein-Barr virus. The prevalence of this childhood tumor is high in malarious areas of Africa.

DIAGNOSIS **Demonstration of the Parasite** The diagnosis of malaria rests on the demonstration of asexual forms of the parasite in peripheral blood smears subjected to Romanovsky staining. Following a negative blood smear, repeat smears should be made if there is a high degree of suspicion. Giemsa at pH 7.2 is preferred; Wright's, Field's, or Leishman's stain can also be used. Both thin and thick blood smears should be examined (**See Plates VI-3 through VI-21 and VI-23 through VI-33).**

The thin blood smear should be rapidly air-dried, fixed in anhydrous methanol, and stained, and the red cells in the tail of the film should then be examined under oil immersion. The level of parasitemia is expressed as the number of parasitized erythrocytes among 1000 cells, and this figure is converted to the number of parasitized erythrocytes per microliter. Simple, sensitive, and specific antibody–based diagnostic stick or card tests that detect *P. falciparum*–specific, histidine-rich protein (HRP) 2 or lactate dehydrogenase antigens in fingerprick blood samples have been introduced. Some of these tests carry a second antibody, which allows falciparum malaria to be distinguished from the less dangerous malarias. The relationship between parasitemia and prognosis is complex; in general, patients with $>10^5$ parasites per microliter are at increased risk of dying, but nonimmune patients may die with much lower counts and semi-immune persons may tolerate parasitemia levels many times higher with only minor symptoms. In severe malaria, a poor prognosis is indicated by a predominance of more mature *P. falciparum* parasites (i.e., $>20\%$ of parasites with visible pigment), by the presence of circulating schizonts in the peripheral blood film, or by the presence of phagocytosed malarial pigment in $>5\%$ of neutrophils. Gametocytes may remain evident for several days after treatment has begun; unless trophozoites are also visible on the blood film, their presence does not constitute evidence of drug resistance.

The thick blood film should be of uneven thickness. The smear should be dried thoroughly and stained without fixing. As many layers of erythrocytes overlie one another and are lysed during the staining procedure, the thick film has the advantage of concentrating the parasites (by 20- to 40-fold compared with a thin blood film) and thus increasing diagnostic sensitivity. Both parasites and white cells are counted, and the number of parasites per unit volume is calculated from the total leukocyte count. Alternatively, a white count of 8000/μL is assumed. A minimum of 200 white cells should be counted. Interpretation of thick films requires some experience because artifacts are common. Before a thick smear is judged to be negative, 100 to 200 fields should be examined under oil immersion. Phagocytosed malarial pigment is sometimes seen inside peripheral blood monocytes or polymorphonuclear leukocytes and may provide a clue to recent infection if malarial parasites are not detectable. After the clearance of the parasites, malarial pigment is often evident for several days in peripheral blood phagocytes, bone marrow aspirates, or smears of fluid expressed after intradermal puncture. Staining of parasites with the fluorescent dye acridine orange allows more rapid diagnosis of cases in which the level of parasitemia is low.

Laboratory Findings Normochromic, normocytic anemia is usually documented. The leukocyte count is generally low to normal, although it may be raised in very severe infections. The erythrocyte sedimentation rate, degree of plasma viscosity, and level of C-reactive protein are high. The platelet count is usually reduced to $\sim10^5/\mu$L. Severe infections may be accompanied by prolonged prothrombin and partial thromboplastin times and by severe thrombocytopenia. Levels of antithrombin III are reduced even in mild infection. In uncomplicated malaria, plasma concentrations of electrolytes, blood urea nitrogen, and creatinine are usually normal. Findings in severe malaria may include metabolic acidosis, with low plasma concentrations of glucose, sodium, bicarbonate, calcium, phosphate, and albumin together with elevations in lactate, blood urea nitrogen, creatinine, urate, muscle and liver enzymes, and conjugated and unconjugated bilirubin. Hypergammaglobulinemia is usual in immune and semi-immune subjects, and urinalysis generally gives normal results. In adults and children with cerebral malaria, the mean opening pressure at lumbar puncture is ~160 mm of cerebrospinal fluid (CSF); the CSF is usually normal or

has a slightly elevated total protein level [<1.0 g/L (100 mg/dL)] and cell count ($<20/\mu$L).

PREVENTION In most of the tropics, the eradication of malaria is not yet feasible because of the widespread distribution of *Anopheles* breeding sites; the great number of infected persons; and inadequacies in resources, infrastructure, and control programs. Where possible, the disease is contained by judicious use of insecticides to kill the mosquito vector, rapid diagnosis and appropriate patient management, and administration of chemoprophylaxis to high-risk groups. Malaria researchers are intensifying their efforts to better understand parasite-human-mosquito-environmental interactions and develop more effective control and prevention interventions. Despite the enormous investment in efforts to develop a malaria vaccine, no safe, effective, long-lasting vaccine is likely to be available for general use in the near future (Chap. 122). While there is promise for one or more malaria vaccines on the more distant horizon, prevention and control measures continue to rely on antivector and drug use strategies.

Personal Protection Against Malaria Simple measures to reduce the frequency of mosquito bites in malarious areas are very important. These measures include the avoidance of exposure to mosquitoes at their peak feeding times (usually dusk and dawn, but also throughout the night) and the use of insect repellents, suitable clothing, and insecticide-impregnated bed nets. Widespread use of bed nets, particularly those treated with residual pyrethroids, reduces the incidence of malaria and has been shown to reduce mortality in western and eastern Africa.

Chemoprophylaxis (Table 214-3) Few areas of therapeutics are as controversial as antimalarial drug prophylaxis. Recommendations for prophylaxis depend on knowledge of local patterns of plasmodial drug sensitivity and the likelihood of acquiring malarial infection. Chemoprophylaxis is never entirely reliable, and malaria should always be considered in the differential diagnosis of fever in patients who have traveled to endemic areas, even if they are taking prophylactic antimalarial drugs.

Pregnant women traveling to malarious areas should be warned about the potential risks. All pregnant women at risk in endemic areas should be encouraged to attend regular antenatal clinics and should receive either prophylaxis with chloroquine or proguanil (chloroguanide) or intermittent treatment with pyrimethamine-sulfadoxine, provided there is not high-level resistance to these drugs. In addition, antimalarial prophylaxis should be considered for children between the ages of 3 months and 4 years in areas where malaria causes high childhood mortality; such prophylaxis may not be logistically or economically feasible in many countries. Children born to nonimmune mothers in endemic areas (usually expatriates moving to these areas) should receive prophylaxis from birth.

Travelers should start taking antimalarial drugs at least 1 week before departure so that any untoward reactions can be detected and therapeutic antimalarial blood concentrations will be present when needed. Antimalarial prophylaxis should continue for 4 weeks after the traveler has left the endemic area.

Mefloquine has become the antimalarial prophylactic agent of choice for much of the tropics because it is usually effective against multidrug-resistant falciparum malaria and is reasonably well tolerated. Mild nausea, dizziness, fuzzy thinking, disturbed sleep patterns, and malaise are relatively common. Approximately 1 in every 10,000 recipients develops an acute reversible neuropsychiatric reaction manifested by confusion, psychosis, convulsions, or encephalopathy. The role of mefloquine prophylaxis in pregnancy remains uncertain; in studies in Africa, mefloquine prophylaxis was found to be effective and safe during pregnancy. However, in one study from Thailand, treatment of malaria with mefloquine was associated with an increased risk of stillbirth.

Daily administration of doxycycline is an effective alternative to mefloquine that also exhibits some causal (preerythrocytic) prophylactic activity. Doxycycline is generally well tolerated but may cause vulvovaginal thrush, diarrhea, and photosensitivity and cannot be used by children <8 years old or by pregnant women. The combination drug atovaquone-proguanil hydrochloride (3.75/1.5 mg/kg, or 250/100 mg daily, adult dose) has recently been shown to be a very effective alternate to mefloquine chemoprophylaxis in drug-resistant areas. This drug must be taken with food or a milky drink because it is highly lipophilic: it is well-tolerated by adults and children.

Chloroquine remains the drug of choice for the prevention of infection with drug-sensitive *P. falciparum* and with the other human malarial species (although chloroquine-resistant *P. vivax* has been reported from parts of eastern Asia, Oceania, and South America). Unfortunately, there are few areas of the world with chloroquine-sensitive *P. falciparum*. Chloroquine is generally well tolerated, although some patients are unable to take the drug because of malaise, headache, or (in dark-skinned patients) pruritus. A concomitant filarial infection may provoke or aggravate chloroquine-induced pruritus. Chloroquine is considered safe in pregnancy. With chronic administration for >5 years, a characteristic dose-related retinopathy may develop, but this condition is rare at the doses used for antimalarial prophylaxis. Idiosyncratic or allergic reactions are also rare. Skeletal and cardiac myopathy are potential problems with protracted prophylactic use; they occur most often at the high doses used in the treatment of rheumatoid arthritis. Neuropsychiatric reactions and skin rashes are unusual. Amodiaquine, a related aminoquinoline, is associated with a high risk of agranulocytosis (~1 person in 2000 with continuous use) and should not be used for prophylaxis.

Table 214-3 Prophylaxis and Self-Treatment for Malaria

Drug	Usage	Adult Dosage	Child Dosage
Prophylaxis			
Mefloquine	Used in areas where chloroquine-resistant malaria has been reported	228 mg of base (250 mg of salt) orally, once/week[a]	<15 kg: 4.6 mg of base/kg (5 mg of salt/kg) 15–19 kg: ¼ tablet/week 20–30 kg: ½ tablet/week 31–45 kg: ¾ tablet/week >45 kg: 1 tablet/week
Doxycycline[b]	Used as alternative to mefloquine	100 mg orally, once/day	>8 years of age: 2 mg/kg per day orally; maximum dose, 100 mg/d
Chloroquine	Used in areas where chloroquine-resistant malaria has *not* been reported	300 mg of base (500 mg of salt) orally, once/week	5 mg of base/kg (8.3 mg of salt/kg) orally, once/week; maximum dose, 300 mg of base
Proguanil (not available in U.S.)	Used simultaneously *with* chloroquine as alternative to mefloquine or doxycycline	200 mg orally, once/day, in combination with weekly chloroquine	<2 years: 50 mg/d 2–6 years: 100 mg/d 7–10 years: 150 mg/d >10 years: 200 mg/d
Primaquine[c]	Used for travelers only after testing for G6PD deficiency; postexposure prevention for relapsing malaria or prophylaxis	Postexposure: 15 mg of base (26.3 mg of salt) orally, once/day for 14 days Prophylaxis: 30 mg of base daily	0.3 mg of base/kg (0.5 mg of salt/kg) orally, once/day for 14 days
Atovaquone-proguanil[c]	Used as alternative to mefloquine	250/100 mg orally once/day	11–20 kg 62.5 mg/100 mg 21–30 kg 125 mg/50 mg 31–40 kg 187.5 mg/75 mg >40 kg 250 mg/100 mg
Self-treatment			
Pyrimethamine-sulfadoxine[d]	In areas with chloroquine-resistant malaria, should be carried during travel by persons taking mefloquine or doxycycline	3 tablets (75 mg of pyrimethamine and 1500 mg of sulfadoxine) orally, as a single dose	5–10 kg: ½ tablet 11–20 kg: 1 tablet 21–30 kg: 1½ tablets 31–45 kg: 2 tablets >45 kg: 3 tablets

[a] Tablets manufactured outside the United States contain 250 mg of base.
[b] Not in pregnant women or children <8 years old.
[c] Primaquine and atovaquone-proguanil have both proved safe and effective for antimalarial chemoprophylaxis in areas with chloroquine-resistant falciparum malaria, but more data are needed, particularly in children. These drugs should not be used in pregnancy.
[d] Regimen is used for treatment only, *not* prophylaxis.

In the past, the dihydrofolate reductase inhibitors pyrimethamine and proguanil (chloroguanide) have been administered widely, but resistant strains of both *P. falciparum* and *P. vivax* have limited their use. Whereas antimalarial quinolines such as chloroquine act on the erythrocyte stage of parasitic development, the dihydrofolate reductase inhibitors also inhibit preerythrocytic growth in the liver (causal prophylaxis) and development in the mosquito (sporonticidal activity). Proguanil is safe and well tolerated, although mouth ulceration occurs in ~8% of persons using this drug; it is considered safe for antimalarial prophylaxis in pregnancy. The prophylactic use of the combination of pyrimethamine and sulfadoxine is not recommended because of an unacceptable incidence of severe toxicity, principally exfoliative dermatitis and other skin rashes, agranulocytosis, hepatitis, and pulmonary eosinophilia. The combination of pyrimethamine with dapsone (0.2/1.5 mg/kg weekly; 25/200 mg maximum) is a second-line alternative available in some countries and can be used in areas with chloroquine-resistant *P. falciparum*. This combination is generally well tolerated; however, resistance is increasing, and dapsone may cause methemoglobinemia and allergic reactions and (at higher doses) may pose a significant risk of agranulocytosis. Primaquine (0.5 mg/kg, or 30 mg daily) has also proved safe and effective in clinical trials in drug-resistant areas and can be considered when all other options are containdicated. Proguanil and the pyrimethamine-dapsone combination are not available in the United States.

Because of the increasing spread and intensity of plasmodial resistance to chloroquine in Africa and other areas of the world (Fig. 214-2), the Centers for Disease Control and Prevention (CDC; www.cdc.gov/travel/index.htm), which recommends a weekly dose of mefloquine for all travelers, maintains an updated 24-h travel and malaria information audiotape that can be accessed by touch-tone telephone (888-232-3228). Regional and disease-specific documents may be requested from the CDC Fax Information Service (888-232-3299). Consultation for the evaluation of prophylaxis failures or treatment of malaria can be obtained from state and local health departments and the CDC (770-488-7788).

℞ **TREATMENT** When a patient in or from a malarious area presents with fever, thick and thin blood smears should be prepared and examined immediately to confirm the diagnosis and identify the species of infecting parasite. Repeat blood smears should be performed at least every 12 h for 2 days if the first smears are negative. Patients with severe malaria or those unable to take oral drugs should receive parenteral antimalarial therapy. If there is any doubt about the resistance status of the infecting organism, then quinine or quinidine should be given. Several drugs are available for oral treatment, and the choice of drug depends on the likely sensitivity of the infecting parasites. Despite recent evidence of chloroquine resistance in *P. vivax* (from parts of Indonesia, Oceania, and Brazil), chloroquine remains the treatment of choice for the "benign" human malarias (*P. vivax*, *P. ovale*, *P. malariae*). Characteristics of various antimalarial agents are shown in Table 214-4, and drug regimens approved by the U.S. Food and Drug Administration are detailed in Table 214-5. The avail-

Table 214-4 Properties of Antimalarial Drugs

Drug(s)	Pharmacokinetic Properties	Antimalarial Activity	Minor Toxicity	Major Toxicity
Quinine, quinidine	Good oral and IM absorption (quinine); Cl and V_d reduced, but plasma protein binding (principally to $\propto 1$ acid glycoprotein) increased (90%) in malaria; quinine $t_{1/2}$: 16 h in malaria, 11 h in healthy persons; quinidine $t_{1/2}$: 13 h in malaria, 8 h in healthy persons	Acts mainly on trophozoite blood stage; kills gametocytes of *P. vivax, P. ovale,* and *P. malariae*; no action on liver stages	*Common:* "Cinchonism": tinnitus, high-tone hearing loss, nausea, vomiting, dysphoria, postural hypotension; ECG QT_c interval prolongation (quinine usually by <10% but quinidine by up to 25%) *Rare:* Diarrhea, visual disturbance, rashes *Note:* Very bitter taste	*Common:* Hypoglycemia *Rare:* Hypotension, blindness, deafness, cardiac arrhythmias, thrombocytopenia, hemolysis, hemolytic-uremic syndrome, vasculitis, cholestatic hepatitis, neuromuscular paralysis *Note:* Quinidine more cardiotoxic
Chloroquine	Good oral absorption, very rapid IM and SC absorption; complex pharmacokinetics; enormous Cl and V_d (unaffected by malaria); blood concentration profile determined by distribution processes in malaria; $t_{1/2}$: 1–2 months	As for quinine but acts slightly earlier in asexual cycle	*Common:* Nausea, dysphoria, pruritus in dark-skinned patients, postural hypotension *Rare:* Accommodation difficulties, rash *Note:* Bitter taste, well tolerated	*Acute:* Hypotensive shock (parenteral), cardiac arrhythmias, neuropsychiatric reactions *Chronic:* Retinopathy (cumulative dose, >100 g), skeletal and cardiac myopathy
Mefloquine	Adequate oral absorption; no parenteral preparation; $t_{1/2}$: 14–20 days (shorter in malaria)	As for quinine	Nausea, giddiness, dysphoria, fuzzy thinking, sleeplessness, nightmares, sense of dissociation	Neuropsychiatric reactions, convulsions, encephalopathy
Tetracycline, doxycycline[a]	Excellent absorption; $t_{1/2}$: 8 h for tetracycline, 18 h for doxycycline	Weak antimalarial activity; should not be used alone for treatment	Gastrointestinal intolerance, deposition in growing bones and teeth, photosensitivity, moniliasis, benign intracranial hypertension	Renal failure in patients with impaired renal function (tetracycline)
Halofantrine[b]	Highly variable absorption related to fat intake; $t_{1/2}$: 1–3 days (active desbutyl metabolite $t_{1/2}$: 3–7 days)	As for quinine	Diarrhea	Cardiac conduction disturbances; atrioventricular block; ECG QT_c interval prolongation; potentially lethal ventricular tachyarrhythmias
Artemisinin and derivatives (artemether, artesunate)	Good oral absorption, variable absorption of IM artemether; artesunate and artemether biotransformed to active metabolite dihydroartemisinin; all drugs eliminated rapidly; $t_{1/2}$: <1 h	Broader stage specificity and more rapid than other drugs; no action on liver stages	Reduction in reticulocyte count; fever; allergy	Neurotoxicity of oil-based IM preparations reported in animals, but no evidence in humans
Pyrimethamine	Good oral absorption, variable IM absorption; $t_{1/2}$: 4 days	For blood stages, acts mainly on mature forms; causal prophylactic	Well tolerated	Megaloblastic anemia, pancytopenia, pulmonary infiltration
Proguanil (chloroguanide)	Good oral absorption; biotransformed to active metabolite cycloguanil; $t_{1/2}$: 16 h	Causal prophylactic; not used alone for treatment	Well tolerated; mouth ulcers and rare alopecia	Megaloblastic anemia in renal failure
Primaquine	Complete oral absorption; active compound not known; $t_{1/2}$: 7 h	Radical cure; eradicates hepatic forms of *P. vivax* and *P. ovale*; kills gametocytes of *P. falciparum*	Nausea, vomiting, diarrhea, abdominal pain, hemolysis, methemoglobinemia	Massive hemolysis in subjects with severe G6PD deficiency
Atovaquone	Highly variable absorption related to fat intake; $t_{1/2}$: 30–70 h	Acts mainly on trophozoite blood stage	None identified	—
Lumefantrine	Highly variable absorption related to fat intake; $t_{1/2}$: 3–4 days	As for quinine	None identified	—

[a] Tetracycline and doxycycline should not be given to pregnant women or to children <8 years of age.

[b] Halofantrine should not be used by patients with long ECG QT_c intervals or known conduction disturbances or by those taking drugs that may affect ventricular repolarization, e.g., quinidine, quinine, mefloquine, chloroquine, neuroleptics, antiarrhythmics, tricyclic antidepressants, terfenadine, or astemizole.

ABBREVIATIONS: Cl, systemic clearance; V_d, total apparent volume of distribution; IM, intramuscular; SC, subcutaneous; ECG, electrocardiogram; G6PD, glucose-6-phosphate dehydrogenase.

ability of antimalarial drugs varies considerably between countries. Many of the drugs used to treat malaria in endemic areas are not available in temperate countries such as the United States.

Severe Malaria Because of resistance, chloroquine can no longer be relied upon in most countries for the treatment of severe malaria. The antiarrhythmic quinidine gluconate is as effective as quinine and, as it is more readily available, has replaced quinine for the treatment of malaria in the United States. The administration of quinidine must be closely monitored if dysrrhythmias and hypotension are to be avoided. Total plasma levels in excess of 8 μg/mL, a QT_c interval of >0.6 s, or QRS widening beyond 25% of baseline are indications for slowing infusion rates. If arrhythmia or saline-unresponsive hypotension develops, treatment with this drug should be discontinued. Quinine is safer than quinidine; cardiovascular monitoring is not required except when the recipient has cardiac disease. In some areas of Asia, the Chinese drugs derived from artemisinin (artemether and artesunate) have become first-line treatments for severe malaria. These agents are rapidly effective against multidrug-resistant falciparum malaria and are at least as effective as and safer than quinine or quinidine. They are not available in the United States.

Severe falciparum malaria constitutes a medical emergency requiring intensive nursing care and careful management. The patient should be weighed and, if comatose, placed on his or her side. Frequent evaluation of the patient's condition is essential. Ancillary drugs such as high-dose glucocorticoids, urea, heparin, and dextran are of no value.

Parenteral antimalarial treatment should be started as soon as possible. An initial loading dose should be given so that therapeutic concentrations are reached as soon as possible. Both quinine and quinidine will cause dangerous hypotension if injected rapidly; when given intravenously, they must be administered carefully by rate-controlled infusion only. The optimal therapeutic range for quinine and quinidine in severe malaria is not known with certainty, but total plasma concentrations of 8 to 15 mg/mL for quinine and 3.5 to 8.0 mg/mL for quinidine are effective and do not cause serious toxicity. The systemic clearance and apparent volume of distribution of these alkaloids are markedly reduced and plasma protein binding is increased in severe malaria, so that the blood concentrations attained with a given dose are higher. If the patient remains seriously ill or in acute renal failure for >2 days, the maintenance doses of quinine or quinidine should be reduced by 30 to 50% to prevent toxic accumulation of the drugs. The initial doses should never be reduced. If one of the artemisinin derivatives or chloroquine is given, dose reductions are unnecessary, even in renal failure. Exchange transfusion should be considered for severely ill patients, although the precise indications for this procedure have not been agreed upon. It has been recommended that—if safe and feasible—exchange should be considered for parasitemia levels of 5 to 15% and is indicated for parasitemia levels of >15%. The role of prophylactic intramuscular phenobarbital in preventing convulsions in cerebral malaria also remains uncertain.

Table 214-5   Recommended Therapeutic Doses of Antimalarial Drugs

Drug	Uncomplicated Malaria (Oral)	Severe Malaria[a] (Parenteral)
Chloroquine	10 mg of base/kg followed by 10 mg/kg at 24 h and 5 mg/kg at 48 h *or* by 5 mg/kg at 12, 24, and 36 h (total dose, 25 mg/kg); for *P. vivax* or *P. ovale*, primaquine (0.25 mg of base/kg per day for 14 days[c]) added for radical cure	10 mg of base/kg by constant-rate infusion over 8 h followed by 15 mg/kg over 24 h *or* by 3.5 mg of base/kg by IM or SC injection every 6 h (total dose, 25 mg/kg)[b]
Sulfadoxine/pyrimethamine	25/1.25 mg/kg, single oral dose (3 tablets for adults)	—
Mefloquine	15 mg/kg followed 8–12 h later by second dose of 10 mg/kg	—
Quinine	10 mg of salt/kg q8h for 7 days combined with tetracycline[d] (4 mg/kg qid) or doxycycline (3 mg/kg once daily) or clindamycin (10 mg/kg bid) for 7 days	20 mg of salt/kg by IV infusion over 4 h[e] followed by 10 mg/kg infused over 2–8 h every 8 h
Quinidine gluconate	—	10 mg of base/kg by constant-rate infusion over 1–2 h followed by 0.02 mg/kg per min, with ECG monitoring[f]
Artesunate	In combination with 25 mg of mefloquine/kg, 12 mg/kg given in divided doses over 3–5 days (e.g., 4 mg/kg for 3 days or 4 mg/kg followed by 2 mg/kg per day for 4 days); if used alone, give for 7 days (usually 4 mg/kg initially followed by 2 mg/kg daily)	2.4 mg/kg IV or IM stat followed by 1.2 mg/kg at 12 and 24 h and then daily
Artemether	Same regimen as for artesunate	3.2 mg/kg IM stat followed by 1.6 mg/kg per day
Atovaquone-proguanil	For adults >40 kg, each dose comprises 4 tablets (each containing atovaquone 250 mg and proguanil 100 mg) taken once daily for 3 days with food	—
Artemether-lumefantrine	For adults ≥35 kg, each dose comprises 4 tablets (each containing artemether 20 mg and lumefantrine 120 mg) at 0, 8, 24, and 48 h (semi-immunes) or at 0, 8, 24, 36, 48, and 60 h (nonimmunes) taken after food	—

[a] Oral treatment should be substituted for parenteral therapy as soon as the patient can take tablets by mouth.
[b] Chloroquine-resistant *P. falciparum* is now very widespread.
[c] In Oceania and Southeast Asia, the dose should be 0.33 to 0.5 mg of base/kg. This regimen should not be used in patients with severe variants of G6PD deficiency.
[d] Neither tetracycline nor doxycycline should be given to pregnant women or to children <8 years old.
[e] Alternatively, infusion of 7 mg of salt/kg over 30 min can be followed by 10 mg of salt/kg over 4 h.
[f] Some authorities recommend a lower dose of intravenous quinidine: 6.2 mg of base/kg over 1–2 h followed by 0.0125 mg/kg per min.
NOTE: In severe malaria, quinine or quinidine should be used if there is any doubt about the infecting strain's sensitivity to chloroquine.
ABBREVIATIONS: IM, intramuscular; SC, subcutaneous; IV, intravenous; ECG, electrocardiogram; G6PD, glucose-6-phosphate dehydrogenase.

When the patient is unconscious, the blood glucose level should be measured every 4 to 6 h, and values below 2.2 mmol/L (40 mg/dL) should prompt treatment with intravenous dextrose. All patients treated with intravenous quinine or quinidine should receive a continuous infusion of 5 to 10% dextrose. The parasite count and hematocrit level should be measured every 6 to 12 h. Anemia develops rapidly; if the hematocrit falls below 20%, then whole blood (preferably fresh) or packed cells should be transfused slowly, with careful attention to circulatory status. Renal function should be checked daily. Judicious use of small doses of a diuretic to prevent fluid overload may be needed, particularly in the elderly. Children presenting with severe anemia and acidotic breathing are often hypovolemic; in this situation, resuscitation with crystalloids or blood is indicated. Accurate assessment is vital. Management of fluid balance is difficult in severe malaria, particularly in adults, because of the thin dividing line between overhydration (leading to pulmonary edema) and underhydration (contributing to renal impairment). If necessary, pulmonary artery occlusion pressures should be measured and maintained in the low-normal range. As soon as the patient can take fluids, oral therapy should be substituted for parenteral treatment.

Uncomplicated Malaria Infections due to *P. vivax*, *P. malariae*, *P. ovale*, and known sensitive strains of *P. falciparum* should be treated with oral chloroquine (total dose, 25 mg of base/kg). In Africa,

1211

chloroquine-resistant strains are usually sensitive to sulfadoxine/pyrimethamine. Where there is resistance to the latter combination, either (1) quinine plus tetracycline or doxycycline (or clindamycin) or (2) mefloquine should be used; tetracycline and doxycycline cannot be given to pregnant women or to children <8 years of age. Oral quinine is extremely bitter and regularly produces cinchonism comprising tinnitus, high-tone deafness, nausea, vomiting, and dysphoria. Compliance is poor with the required 5- to 7-day regimens of this drug. Mefloquine should be given at a total dosage of 25 mg/kg (15 mg/kg followed 8 to 12 h later by 10 mg/kg) and, where available and approved for use, combined with artesunate or artemether (4 mg/kg per day for 3 days). Although significant resistance to mefloquine has been documented in Thailand, Burma, Vietnam, and Cambodia, this agent is usually effective against multidrug-resistant strains of *P. falciparum* outside these areas. Artemether-lumefantrine and atovaquone-proguanil are recently introduced, well-tolerated antimalarial drugs used in 3-day regimens. They are both effective against multidrug-resistant falciparum malaria.

Patients should be monitored for vomiting for 1 h after the administration of any oral antimalarial drug. Symptom-based treatment, with tepid sponging and acetaminophen administration, lowers fever and thereby reduces the patient's propensity to vomit these drugs. Minor central nervous system reactions (nausea, dizziness, sleep disturbances) are common. The incidence of serious adverse neuropsychiatric reactions to mefloquine treatment is ~1 in 1000 in Asia but may be as high as 1 in 200 among Africans and Caucasians. All the antimalarial quinolines (chloroquine, mefloquine, and quinine) exacerbate the orthostatic hypotension associated with malaria, and all are tolerated better by children than by adults. Pregnant women, young children, patients unable to tolerate oral therapy, and nonimmune subjects (e.g., travelers) with suspected malaria should be evaluated carefully and hospitalization considered. If there is any doubt as to the identity of the infecting malarial species, treatment for falciparum malaria should be given. A negative blood smear does not rule out malaria; thick blood films should be checked 1 and 2 days later to exclude the diagnosis. Nonimmune subjects receiving treatment for malaria should have daily parasite counts performed until negative thick films indicate clearance of the parasite. If the level of parasitemia does not fall below 25% of the admission value in 48 h or if parasitemia has not cleared by 7 days (and compliance is assured), drug resistance is likely and the regimen should be changed. Quinine (or quinidine) and tetracycline should be reserved for multidrug-resistant infections, but if falciparum malaria has been contracted in an area of known drug sensitivity, then treatment with chloroquine, sulfadoxine/pyrimethamine, or mefloquine is preferable because these agents are better tolerated and simpler to administer.

Primaquine (0.3 mg of base/kg; 15 mg of base, adult dose) should be given daily for 14 days to patients with *P. vivax* or *P. ovale* infections after laboratory tests for G6PD deficiency have proved negative. A dose of 22.5 to 30 mg for an adult is recommended for infections acquired in Southeast Asia and Oceania. If the patient has a mild variant of G6PD deficiency, primaquine can be given in a dose of 0.6 mg of base/kg (45 mg maximum) once weekly for 8 weeks.

PREVENTING DRUG RESISTANCE   In much of the tropics, drug-resistant *P. falciparum* is increasing in distribution, frequency, and intensity. There is a growing belief among malariologists that, to prevent resistance, falciparum malaria should no longer be treated with single drugs in endemic areas; the same rationale has been applied in the treatment of tuberculosis and HIV/AIDS. This strategy is based upon simultaneous use of two or more drugs with different modes of action: one, an artemisinin derivative (artesunate, artemether, or dihydroartemisinin), given for 3 days; and the other, a slower-acting antimalarial. In areas where *P. falciparum* is still sensitive, chloroquine is used as the second drug; where there is low-grade chloroquine resistance (e.g., many areas of Africa), either amodiaquine or sulfadox-

ine/pyrimethamine can be used in combination with the artemisinin derivative. Where there is also resistance to sulfadoxine/pyrimethamine, the combinations artesunate plus mefloquine, artemether plus lumefantrine, or quinine plus tetracycline or clindamycin can be considered (although tetracycline cannot be given to pregnant women or to children <8 years of age). Atovaquone/proguanil, which is also effective against drug-resistant malaria, can also be combined with artesunate to prevent the emergence of resistance. While significant resistance to mefloquine occurs in Thailand, Burma, and Cambodia, the mefloquine/artesunate combinations are still reliably effective in these areas. The artemisinin derivatives and lumefantrine (all unlicensed in the United States) and atovaquone-proguanil are tolerated well with no significant adverse effects.

COMPLICATIONS   Acute Renal Failure   If the level of blood urea nitrogen or creatinine rises despite adequate rehydration, fluid administration should be restricted to prevent volume overload. The indications for dialysis are the same as those in other forms of hypercatabolic acute renal failure (Chap. 269). Even with adequate peritoneal dialysis, secondary bacterial infections are common in the tropics, and hemodialysis or hemofiltration is preferable. Some patients pass small volumes of urine sufficient to allow control of fluid balance; these cases can be managed conservatively if other indications for dialysis do not arise. Renal function usually improves within days, but full recovery may take weeks.

Acute Pulmonary Edema   Patients should be positioned at 45° and given oxygen and intravenous diuretics. Pulmonary artery occlusion pressures may be normal, indicating increased pulmonary capillary permeability. Positive pressure ventilation should be started early if the immediate measures fail (Chap. 233).

Hypoglycemia   An initial slow injection of 50% dextrose (0.5 g/kg) should be followed by an infusion of 10% dextrose (0.10 g/kg per hour). The blood glucose level should be checked regularly thereafter, as recurrent hypoglycemia is common, particularly in patients receiving quinine or quinidine. In severely ill patients, hypoglycemia commonly occurs together with metabolic (lactic) acidosis and carries a poor prognosis.

Other Complications   Patients who develop spontaneous bleeding should be given fresh blood and intravenous vitamin K. Convulsions should be treated with intravenous or rectal benzodiazepines and, if necessary, respiratory support. Aspiration pneumonia should be suspected in any unconscious patient with convulsions, particularly with persistent hyperventilation; intravenous antimicrobial agents and oxygen should be administered, and pulmonary toilet should be undertaken. Treatment for systemic *Salmonella* and other infections common in African children with falciparum malaria should be considered. Hypoglycemia or gram-negative septicemia should be suspected when the condition of any patient suddenly deteriorates for no obvious reason during antimalarial treatment.

BABESIOSIS

Babesiosis is a protozoan disease of animals that is transmitted by ticks; humans are infected incidentally and initially develop a nonspecific febrile illness. *Babesia* organisms enter red blood cells and resemble malarial parasites morphologically, thus posing a diagnostic problem.

ETIOLOGY AND NATURAL CYCLE   Of the more than 100 species of *Babesia*, *B. microti* and *B. divergens* are the two that cause most human infections. Ixodid (hard-bodied) ticks, in particular *Ixodes scapularis* (*I. dammini*) and *I. ricinus*, are the vectors of the parasite. Ticks ingest *Babesia* while feeding, and the parasite multiplies within the tick's gut wall. The organisms then spread to the salivary glands; their inoculation into a vertebrate host by a tick larva, nymph, or adult completes the cycle of transmission. Asexual reproduction of *Babesia* within red blood cells produces two or four parasites.

EPIDEMIOLOGY   While *Babesia* infections in wild and domestic animals are distributed globally, almost all *B. microti* infections in the United States occur along the northeastern coast, including Nantucket Island, Martha's Vineyard, and Cape Cod in Massachusetts; Block Island in Rhode Island; Long Island, Shelter Island, and Fire Island in New York; and the nearby mainland, including Connecticut. Cases also have been reported from Wisconsin, Minnesota, Virginia, Maryland, Georgia, and Mexico. *Babesia* isolates from patients in Washington and California have been characterized as WA-1-type parasites, a category that is genetically and antigenically distinct from *B. microti*. A strain isolated in Missouri differs from these isolates, suggesting that babesiosis may be an "emerging infection." The deer tick, *I. scapularis*, is the vector associated with *B. microti*. In Europe, *B. divergens* has been responsible for the majority of the 22 reported cases of babesiosis; Yugoslavia, Russia, France, the United Kingdom, and Ireland have accounted for most of these infections.

Transfusions are another source of babesiosis. In the more than 20 transfusion-associated cases reported, parasites were uncommonly detected in blood donors, but serologic testing of their blood for *Babesia* gave positive results.

Infections with *B. divergens* have occurred sporadically in previously splenectomized patients in several countries in Europe. *I. ricinus* is probably the vector in these cases, as it is for the transmission of this organism among cattle. The infected persons were predisposed to illness by their asplenic status.

I. scapularis feeds on rodents as a larva and a nymph and on deer as an adult; nymphs are abundant during the spring and summer and feed on humans readily. In some endemic areas, the seroprevalence in the human population may be >2%. This figure indicates that asymptomatic infection is more frequent than is generally thought.

CLINICAL PRESENTATION The incubation period for *B. microti* infection is about 1 to 4 weeks. Immunosuppressed patients, splenectomized individuals, and the elderly have the most severe illness. The clinical presentation varies widely; symptoms and signs include a gradual onset of irregular fever, chills, sweating, muscle pain, and fatigue. Mild hepatosplenomegaly and mild hemolytic anemia may develop. The level of parasitemia may exceed 10%. The illness may continue for weeks or months.

Patients infected with *B. divergens* have a more severe illness, with a rapid onset of chills, fever, nausea, vomiting, and hemolytic anemia progressing to jaundice, hemoglobinemia, and renal failure. *B. divergens* infections are often fatal.

DIAGNOSIS Whether or not they have a history of exposure to ticks or tick bites, febrile persons living in endemic areas should have Giemsa-stained thick and thin blood films (**see Plate VI-22**) examined for small intraerythrocytic parasites. *B. microti* appears as a small ring form resembling *P. falciparum*. Unlike infection with *Plasmodium*, however, that with *Babesia* does not cause the production of pigment in parasites, nor are schizonts or gametocytes formed. Dividing within red blood cells, *B. microti* can form four daughter parasites attached by strands of cytoplasm; these "tetrad" forms are seen infrequently in human blood films but are a distinguishing feature. An indirect immunofluorescence antibody test is useful for the diagnosis of infection with *B. microti* but does not replace the blood smear. The serum antibody titer rises 2 to 4 weeks after the onset of illness and then wanes over 6 to 12 months; cross-reactions can occur with other species of *Babesia* and *Plasmodium*.

About 50% of patients infected with *B. microti* have antibody to *Borrelia burgdorferi*, the agent of Lyme disease (Chap. 176); this figure varies with the geographic area. The occurrence of mixed infections is not surprising since both organisms are transmitted by *I. scapularis*. This tick species is also a potential vector of human granulocytic ehrlichiosis; the same tick may carry more than one tickborne disease. Intraperitoneal inoculation of blood from patients with babesiosis into hamsters or gerbils results in detectable parasitemia within 2 to 4 weeks.

℞ **TREATMENT** *B. microti* infections in patients with intact spleens are often self-limiting without treatment, although symptoms may persist for months with or without treatment. Because silent parasitemia may have prolonged symptoms and signs, treatment is advised for all patients infected with *Babesia*. Treatment with the combination of quinine sulfate (650 mg of salt orally tid) plus clindamycin (600 mg orally tid or 1.2 g parenterally bid) for 7 to 10 days is usually effective but may not always eliminate parasites. The pediatric dose is 20 to 40 mg/kg per day for quinine sulfate and 25 mg/kg per day for clindamycin, both given in three divided doses over 7 to 10 days. Atovaquone suspension (750 mg bid) plus azithromycin (500 to 1000 mg/d) may be effective when quinine and clindamycin fail. Especially severe infections with high-level *B. microti* parasitemia in asplenic patients have been successfully treated with exchange transfusions in addition to quinine and clindamycin.

BIBLIOGRAPHY

BAIRD JK et al: Primaquine for prophylaxis against malaria among nonimmune transmigrants in Irian Jaya, Indonesia. Am J Trop Med Hyg 52:479, 1995

CENTERS FOR DISEASE CONTROL AND PREVENTION: *Health Information for International Travel, 1999–2000.* Atlanta, Department of Health and Human Services, 1999

GARNHAM PCC: Malaria parasites of man: Life cycles and morphology (excluding ultrastructure) in malaria, in *Principles and Practice of Malariology*, WH Wernsdorfer, I McGregor (eds). Edinburgh, Churchill Livingstone, 1988, pp 61–96

GELFAND JA, CALLAHAN MV: Babesiosis. Curr Clin Top Infect Dis 18:201, 1998

HERWALDT BL et al: Babesiosis in Wisconsin: A potentially fatal disease. Am J Trop Med Hyg 53:146, 1995

HOFFMAN SL, MILLER LH: Perspectives on malaria vaccine development, in *Malaria Vaccine Development*, SL Hoffman (ed). Washington, DC, ASM Press, 1996, pp 1–13

KRAUSE PJ et al: Persistent parasitemia after acute babesiosis. N Engl J Med 339:160, 1998

NEWTON P, WHITE N: Malaria: New developments in treatment and prevention. Annu Rev Med 50:179, 1999

PASLOSKE BL, HOWARD RJ: Malaria, the red cell and the endothelium. Annu Rev Med 45:283, 1994

SHANKS GD: Malaria prevention and prophylaxis, in *Bailliere's Clinical Infectious Diseases*, vol 2-2, G Pasvol (ed). London, Bailliere Tindall, 1995, pp 331–349

SNOW RW: Estimating mortality, morbidity and disability due to malaria among Africa's non-pregnant population. Bull World Health Org 77:624, 1999

STEKETEE RW et al: Impairment of a pregnant woman's acquired ability to limit *Plasmodium falciparum* by infection with human immunodeficiency virus type-1. Am J Trop Med Hyg 55(Suppl):43, 1996

WHITE NJ: The treatment of malaria. N Engl J Med 335:800, 1996

———: Malaria pathophysiology, in *Malaria: Parasite Biology, Pathogenesis, Protection*, I. Sherman (ed). Washington, DC, ASM Press, 1998, pp 371–385

WORLD HEALTH ORGANIZATION: Control of tropical diseases. Severe and complicated malaria. Trans R Soc Trop Med Hyg 84(Suppl 2):1, 1990

215 *Barbara L. Herwaldt*

LEISHMANIASIS

OVERVIEW

DEFINITION The term *leishmaniases* refers collectively to various clinical syndromes caused by obligate intracellular protozoa of the genus *Leishmania* (order Kinetoplastida). Leishmaniasis is endemic in diverse ecologic settings in the tropics, the subtropics, and southern Europe that range from deserts to rain forests and from rural to periurban areas. It typically is a vector-borne zoonosis, with rodents and canids as common reservoir hosts and humans as incidental hosts. In humans, visceral, cutaneous, and mucosal leishmaniasis result from infection of macrophages throughout the mononuclear-phagocyte system, in the skin, and in the naso-oropharyngeal mucosa, respectively. Current challenges include the emergence of leishmaniasis in new geographic areas and host populations (e.g., visceral leishmaniasis in persons infected with HIV) as well as the need for field-applicable, rapid diagnostic tests and for effective, safe, and affordable oral therapies, control measures, and immunoprophylactic agents.

Table 215-1 Major *Leishmania* Species That Cause Disease in Humans

Species[a]	Clinical Syndrome[b]	Geographic Distribution
SUBGENUS *LEISHMANIA*		
L. donovani complex		
L. donovani	VL (PKDL, OWCL)	China, Indian subcontinent, southwestern Asia, Ethiopia, Kenya, Sudan; possibly sporadic in sub-Saharan Africa
L. infantum	VL (OWCL)	China, central and southwestern Asia, Middle East, southern Europe, North Africa, Ethiopia, Sudan; sporadic in sub-Saharan Africa
L. chagasi	VL (NWCL)	Central and South America
L. mexicana complex		
L. mexicana	NWCL (DCL)	Texas, Mexico, Central and South America
L. amazonensis	NWCL (ML, DCL, VL)	Panama and South America
L. tropica	OWCL (VL)[c]	Central Asia, India, southwestern Asia, Middle East, Turkey, Greece, North Africa, Ethiopia, Kenya, Namibia
L. major	OWCL[d]	Central Asia, India, southwestern Asia, Middle East, Turkey, North Africa, Sahel region of north-central Africa, Ethiopia, Sudan, Kenya
L. aethiopica	OWCL (DCL)	Ethiopia, Kenya
SUBGENUS *VIANNIA*		
L. (V.) braziliensis	NWCL (ML)	Central and South America
L. (V.) guyanensis	NWCL (ML)	South America
L. (V.) panamensis	NWCL (ML)	Central America, Venezuela, Colombia, Ecuador, Peru
L. (V.) peruviana	NWCL[e]	Peru (western slopes of Andes)

[a] Species other than those listed here have been reported to infect humans.

[b] Abbreviations: VL, visceral leishmaniasis; PKDL, post–kala-azar dermal leishmaniasis; OWCL, Old World cutaneous leishmaniasis; NWCL, New World (American) cutaneous leishmaniasis; DCL, diffuse cutaneous leishmaniasis; ML, mucosal leishmaniasis. Clinical syndromes less frequently associated with the various species are shown in parentheses.

[c] *L. tropica* also causes leishmaniasis recidivans and viscerotropic leishmaniasis.

[d] *L. major*–like organisms also cause New World cutaneous leishmaniasis.

[e] The cutaneous leishmaniasis syndrome caused by this species is called *uta*.

ETIOLOGY The organisms that cause the various forms of leishmaniasis in humans are listed in Table 215-1. Visceral leishmaniasis is typically but not exclusively caused by organisms of the *Leishmania donovani* complex; Old World cutaneous leishmaniasis by *L. tropica*, *L. major*, and *L. aethiopica*; New World (or American) cutaneous leishmaniasis by organisms of the *L. mexicana* complex and the *Viannia* subgenus; and mucosal leishmaniasis by some organisms in the *Viannia* subgenus.

LIFE CYCLE *Leishmania* parasites are transmitted by the bite of female phlebotomine sandflies [genus *Phlebotomus* (Old World) or *Lutzomyia* (New World)]. As the flies attempt to feed, they regurgitate the parasite's flagellated promastigote stage into the skin of mammalian hosts. Promastigotes attach to receptors on macrophages, are phagocytized, and transform within phagolysosomes into the nonflagellated amastigote stage, which multiplies by binary fission. After rupture of infected macrophages, amastigotes are phagocytized by other macrophages. If ingested by feeding sandflies, amastigotes transform back into promastigotes, which require at least 7 days to become infective.

IMMUNOLOGY Advances in the understanding of the immunology of leishmaniasis have made this parasitic disease the paradigm for studies of the T cell subsets and cytokines that govern resistance and susceptibility to intracellular pathogens. The paradigm is best demonstrated in murine *L. major* infection. In inbred mice, production of interferon γ (IFN-γ) by T_H1 and natural killer cells confers resistance. Interleukin (IL)12 induces naive T cells to differentiate into T_H1 cells and induces T cells and natural killer cells to produce IFN-γ. In contrast, expansion of IL-4-producing T_H2 cells mediates susceptibility.

Not all aspects of leishmaniasis in mice, whose susceptibility to leishmanial infection is genetically determined, apply to human infection, for which the genetic determinants are being investigated. However, a consistent principle is that healing and resistance to reinfection are associated with expanding numbers of *Leishmania*-specific T_H1 cells, production of IFN-γ, and activation of macrophages to kill intracellular amastigotes. In human visceral leishmaniasis, IL-10 appears to be associated with pathology; in addition, IL-4 may contribute to progression of disease.

GENERAL DIAGNOSTIC PRINCIPLES Definitive diagnosis of leishmaniasis requires demonstration of the parasite. To identify amastigotes by light-microscopic examination, the specimen obtained from an infected site (e.g., thin smear, histologic section) should be stained with Giemsa or another Romanovsky stain and presumptive amastigotes (2 to 4 μm in diameter) examined under oil immersion for the presence of a nucleus and a rod-shaped kinetoplast (Fig. 215-1); the latter is a specialized mitochondrial structure that contains extranuclear DNA. Other means of parasitologic confirmation include in vitro culture (e.g., on Novy-MacNeal-Nicolle medium), animal inoculation, and use of molecular techniques that are under investigation (e.g., polymerase chain reaction).

The *Leishmania* species that infect humans are morphologically similar. They can be distinguished by isoenzyme analysis of cultured promastigotes, determination of monoclonal antibody specificity, or various molecular methods.

Indirect immunologic methods for diagnosis include serologic assays and tests for *Leishmania*-specific cell-mediated immunity (e.g., skin testing for delayed-type hypersensitivity reactions). The usefulness of such methods depends in part on the clinical syndrome (see below). Traditional serologic assays (e.g., indirect immunofluorescent antibody testing) do not reliably distinguish past from current infec-

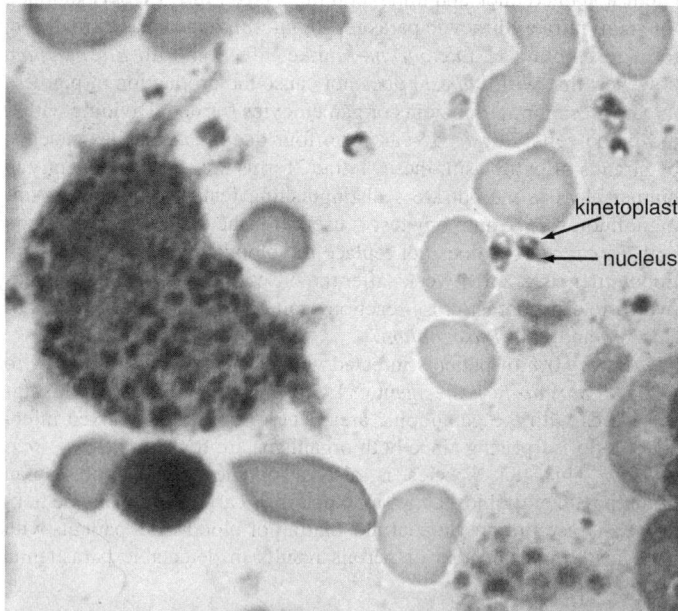

FIGURE 215-1 Amastigotes (the tissue form of the *Leishmania* parasite) in a bone marrow specimen from a patient with visceral leishmaniasis. Each amastigote has a nucleus and kinetoplast. The extracellular amastigotes probably were released from mononuclear phagocytes during specimen manipulation.

tion, and no leishmanin skin-test preparation has been approved for use in the United States. Advances in molecular methods (e.g., production of recombinant/synthetic antigens) may lead to the development of better diagnostic techniques.

GENERAL THERAPEUTIC PRINCIPLES For a given case of leishmaniasis, it is important to consider whether the patient's illness could result in substantial morbidity or in death and therefore requires expeditious treatment with a regimen that generally is highly effective. For decades, the pentavalent antimonial (Sb^V) compounds sodium stibogluconate and meglumine antimonate have been the mainstays of antileishmanial therapy (Table 215-2). Toxicity (with such manifestations as myalgia, arthralgia, fatigue, elevated amino-

transferase levels, chemical pancreatitis, and electrocardiographic abnormalities) becomes increasingly common as the course of treatment progresses but usually does not limit therapy and is reversible.

The traditional parenteral alternatives to Sb^V—amphotericin B and pentamidine isethionate—are generally considered more apt to induce serious or irreversible toxicity (e.g., nephrotoxicity). However, these agents are being advocated for use in some situations (see below; Table 215-2), in part because of the benefits of new formulations (e.g., lipid formulations of amphotericin B) or dosage regimens of these drugs and the decreasing effectiveness of Sb^V in some settings. Many other agents have been touted as alternatives or adjuncts to Sb^V, often on the basis of suboptimal data. Some of these agents may be useful in certain situations, with one caveat: even the results of well-conducted clinical trials are not always generalizable to the treatment of patients in other settings. Most of the nonparenteral agents evaluated to date have at best modest activity against some of the *Leishmania* species.

PREVENTION AND CONTROL The transmission of *Leishmania* species typically is focal, with local "hot spots," in part because of the limited flight range of sandflies; these insects have a short, hopping flight style and usually remain within a few hundred meters of their breeding site. They rest in dark, moist places in habitats ranging from deserts to rain forests; peridomestic sandflies rest in debris or rubble near buildings.

Personal protective measures include the avoidance of outdoor activities when sandflies are most active (dusk to dawn); the use of mechanical barriers such as screens and bed-nets that keep out sandflies, which are about one-third the size of mosquitoes; the wearing of protective clothing; and the application of insect repellent to exposed skin. Impregnation of clothing, bed-nets, and screens with permethrin may also be useful, as may spraying of dwellings with residual-action insecticide. Vaccine strategies are being investigated. Treatment of human cases is an effective control measure only where humans are the primary reservoirs of infection. Vector control and elimination of reservoir hosts may be useful in select settings—for example, where transmission is intra- or peridomiciliary.

VISCERAL LEISHMANIASIS

More than 90% of the world's cases of visceral leishmaniasis occur in Bangladesh, northeastern India (particularly Bihar State), Nepal, Sudan, and northeastern Brazil. The causative species typically are those of the *L. donovani* complex (Table 215-1). The organisms can be transmitted not only by sandflies but also congenitally and parenterally (e.g., through blood transfusions or sharing of needles). Infection begins in macrophages at the inoculation site (e.g., in dermal macrophages at the site of a sandfly bite) and disseminates throughout the mononuclear-phagocyte system in the context of both specific (i.e., to leishmanial antigens) and nonspecific (e.g., to tuberculin) anergy.

CLINICAL MANIFESTATIONS Visceral infection can remain subclinical or become symptomatic, with an acute, subacute, or chronic course. In some settings, inapparent infections far outnumber clinically apparent ones; malnutrition is among the risk factors for the development of disease. The incubation period usually ranges from weeks to months but can be as long as years. Whereas the general term *visceral leishmaniasis* covers a broad spectrum of severity and manifestations, the term *kala-azar* (Hindi for "black fever," indicating that the skin of some patients turns gray) generally conjures up the classic image of profoundly cachectic, febrile patients who are heavily infected with parasites and have life-threatening disease. Splenomegaly (with the spleen most often soft and nontender) typically is more impressive than hepatomegaly, and the spleen can in fact be massive; both splenomegaly and hepatomegaly result from reticuloendothelial cell hyperplasia. Peripheral lymphadenopathy is common in some settings, including Sudan.

The abnormal laboratory findings associated with advanced dis-

Table 215-2 Drug Regimens for Treatment of Leishmaniasis[a]

Clinical Syndrome, Drug	Route of Administration	Regimen
VISCERAL LEISHMANIASIS		
First-line		
Pentavalent antimony[b]	IV, IM	20 mg Sb^V/kg qd for 28 days
Amphotericin B, lipid formulation[c]	IV	2–5 mg/kg qd (total: usually ~15–21 mg/kg)
Alternatives		
Amphotericin B (deoxycholate)	IV	0.5–1 mg/kg qod or qd (total: usually ~15–20 mg/kg)
Paromomycin sulfate[d]	IV, IM	15–20 mg/kg qd for ~21 days
Pentamidine isethionate	IV, IM	4 mg/kg qod or thrice weekly for ~15–30 doses
CUTANEOUS LEISHMANIASIS		
First-line		
Pentavalent antimony[b]	IV, IM	20 mg Sb^V/kg qd for 20 days
Parenteral alternatives		
Pentamidine isethionate	IV, IM	3 mg/kg qod for 4 doses or 2 mg/kg qod for 7 doses
Amphotericin B (deoxycholate)	IV	0.5–1 mg/kg qod or qd (total: up to ~20 mg/kg)
Oral alternatives		
Ketoconazole	PO	600 mg/d for 28 days[e]
Itraconazole	PO	200 mg bid for 28 days[e]
Dapsone	PO	100 mg bid for 6 weeks[e]
MUCOSAL LEISHMANIASIS		
First-line		
Pentavalent antimony[b]	IV, IM	20 mg Sb^V/kg qd for 28 days
Alternatives		
Amphotericin B (deoxycholate)	IV	1 mg/kg qod or qd (total: usually ~20–40 mg/kg)
Pentamidine isethionate	IV, IM	2–4 mg/kg qod or thrice weekly for ≥15 doses

[a] See text for additional details. To maximize effectiveness and minimize toxicity, the listed regimens should be individualized according to the particularities of the case.

[b] The Centers for Disease Control and Prevention (CDC) provides the pentavalent antimonial (Sb^V) compound sodium stibogluconate (Pentostam; Glaxo Wellcome, PLC, United Kingdom; 100 mg Sb^V/mL) to U.S.-licensed physicians through the CDC Drug Service (404-639-3670). The other widely used pentavalent antimonial compound, meglumine antimonate (Glucantime; Rhône Poulenc, France; 85 mg Sb^V/mL), is available primarily in Spanish- and French-speaking areas of the world.

[c] The lipid formulations of amphotericin B include liposomal amphotericin B, amphotericin B lipid complex, and amphotericin B cholesteryl sulfate. The U.S. Food and Drug Administration recently approved the following regimen of liposomal amphotericin B for immunocompetent patients: 3 mg/kg qd on days 1–5, 14, and 21, for a total of 21 mg/kg; for immunosuppressed patients, the approved regimen is 4 mg/kg qd on days 1–5, 10, 17, 24, 31, and 38, for a total of 40 mg/kg. Alternative regimens that have been proposed for immunocompetent patients include treatment on days 1–5 and 10 with 3–4 mg/kg qd for cases from Europe or Brazil, with 3 mg/kg qd for cases from Africa, and with 2–3 mg/kg qd for cases from India.

[d] Not commercially available as of this writing.

[e] Adult dosage.

ease include pancytopenia—anemia, leukopenia (neutropenia, marked eosinopenia, relative lymphocytosis and monocytosis), and thrombocytopenia—as well as hypergammaglobulinemia (chiefly involving IgG, from polyclonal B cell activation) and hypoalbuminemia. Causes of anemia can include bone-marrow infiltration, hypersplenism, autoimmune hemolysis, and bleeding.

Some patients develop post–kala-azar dermal leishmaniasis. This syndrome is manifested by skin lesions (including macules, papules, nodules, and patches) that typically are most prominent on the face. These lesions can develop during therapy or within a few months thereafter (e.g., in East Africa) or can develop years later (e.g., in India); relapse of visceral infection can occur. Persons with persistent skin lesions can serve as reservoir hosts of infection.

Viscerotropic leishmaniasis caused by *L. tropica*, which typically is dermotropic, was recognized among U.S. soldiers who participated in Operation Desert Storm in the Persian Gulf. The affected persons had light parasite burdens and nonspecific manifestations of visceral infection (e.g., fatigue, fever, and gastrointestinal symptoms).

DIAGNOSIS   Although molecular techniques are under investigation, parasitologic diagnosis of visceral leishmaniasis has traditionally been accomplished by demonstration of the parasite on stained slides or in cultures of a tissue aspirate or a biopsy specimen (e.g., of spleen, liver, bone marrow, or lymph node). The diagnostic yield is highest for splenic aspiration (specifically, as high as 98% vs. <90% for other specimens), but this procedure can cause hemorrhage.

Patients with florid kala-azar commonly have relatively heavy parasite burdens, develop high titers of antibody to *Leishmania* (diagnostically useful but not protective), and have undetectable *Leishmania*-specific cell-mediated immunity (with leishmanin skin-test reactivity as well as lymphocyte proliferation and IFN-γ responses to leishmanial antigens typically noted only after recovery). In contrast, viscerotropic leishmaniasis can be difficult to diagnose because of a light parasite burden and a minimal antibody response. A promising noninvasive serologic method for diagnosing kala-azar uses nitrocellulose paper strips impregnated with K39, a recombinant leishmanial polypeptide; this technique is being field-tested.

The differential diagnosis of visceral leishmaniasis includes other tropical infectious diseases that cause fever or organomegaly (e.g., typhoid fever, miliary tuberculosis, brucellosis, malaria, tropical splenomegaly syndrome, and schistosomiasis) as well as diseases such as leukemia and lymphoma. Post–kala-azar dermal leishmaniasis should be differentiated from syphilis, yaws, and leprosy.

℞ TREATMENT   Because persons who have kala-azar generally die if not appropriately treated, highly effective therapy is essential, as is close monitoring for bleeding and intercurrent infectious conditions such as pneumonia and diarrhea. Outside of India, treatment with a pentavalent antimonial compound still is common (Table 215-2). The use of an alternative parenteral agent (Table 215-2) should be considered even for first-line therapy if unresponsiveness to Sb^V therapy is prevalent, as it is in India, or if nonantimonial therapy would be advantageous for other reasons (e.g., toxicity profile or duration of therapy).

A major advance has been the advent of lipid formulations of amphotericin B, in which various lipids have replaced deoxycholate. These formulations, which passively target amphotericin to macrophage-rich organs, are more costly than conventional amphotericin B but are associated with less nephrotoxicity and can be given in shorter courses. Other parenteral alternatives that have merit in some settings include the aminoglycoside paromomycin (the chemical equivalent of aminosidine; not commercially available as of this writing), which has been used as monotherapy (in India) or as an adjunct to Sb^V, and pentamidine. The oral agent miltefosine is being evaluated in clinical trials and preliminarily appears to be highly effective and acceptably tolerated.

Typically, patients feel better and become afebrile during the first week of treatment. Abnormal laboratory findings and splenomegaly may take weeks or months to resolve. The best indicator of permanent cure is freedom from clinical relapse during at least 6 months of follow-up. Repeat tissue sampling is indicated if the patient's status is in question. The persistence of some parasites is not necessarily a poor prognostic indicator, whereas the apparent absence of parasites does not ensure that the patient will not have a relapse.

VISCERAL LEISHMANIASIS IN PERSONS INFECTED WITH HIV   Visceral leishmaniasis has become an important opportunistic infection among persons infected with HIV-1 in geographic areas in which both infections are endemic. To date, most dual infections have been reported from southern Europe, where *L. infantum* (of the *L. donovani* complex) is endemic. In patients infected with HIV, even relatively avirulent *Leishmania* strains can disseminate to the viscera. Clinical leishmaniasis in coinfected patients can represent newly acquired or reactivated infection; most coinfected patients with clinically evident leishmaniasis have fewer than 200 CD4+ lymphocytes per microliter. Recent data suggest that leishmaniasis is a cofactor in the pathogenesis of HIV infection; the lipophosphoglycan (a major surface molecule) of *L. donovani* induces transcription of HIV in CD4+ cells.

A diagnosis of visceral leishmaniasis should be considered for patients infected with HIV who have ever been in leishmaniasis-endemic areas and who have manifestations such as unexplained fever, organomegaly, anemia, or pancytopenia. Coinfected patients can develop unusual manifestations of visceral leishmaniasis, in part because of atypical localization of the parasite (e.g., in the gastrointestinal tract).

The diagnostic sensitivity of classic serologic methods is lower in coinfected than in immunocompetent patients (~50% vs. >90%). However, parasitologic diagnosis by noninvasive means is easier in coinfected patients. Parasites are more commonly found in the circulating blood monocytes of these patients; the sensitivities are ~50% for a Giemsa-stained peripheral-blood smear and ~70% for culture of a buffy-coat preparation. Invasive methods of parasitologic diagnosis (e.g., microscopic examination or culture of a bone marrow aspirate) typically are highly sensitive, especially for previously untreated patients, who commonly have heavy parasite burdens.

Coinfected patients may initially respond well to standard antileishmanial therapy, albeit with more drug toxicity than is experienced by most immunocompetent persons. However, coinfected patients commonly have a chronic or relapsing course, seemingly irrespective of the drug regimens used for induction and suppression therapy.

CUTANEOUS LEISHMANIASIS

Cutaneous leishmaniasis has traditionally been classified as New World (American) or Old World disease. Local names for New World disease include *chiclero ulcer*, *pian bois* (bush yaws), and *uta*; those for Old World disease include *oriental sore*, *bouton d'orient*, *Aleppo evil*, and *Baghdad boil*. More than 90% of the world's cases of cutaneous leishmaniasis occur in Afghanistan, Algeria, Iran, Iraq, Saudi Arabia, Syria, Brazil, and Peru. In the Americas, the leishmaniasis-endemic area extends from southern Texas to northern Argentina; the etiologic agents typically are those of the *L. mexicana* complex and the *Viannia* subgenus (Table 215-1) but also include *L. major*–like organisms and *L. chagasi*. Old World cutaneous leishmaniasis is caused by *L. tropica*, *L. major*, and *L. aethiopica* as well as by *L. infantum* and *L. donovani*.

CLINICAL MANIFESTATIONS   The incubation period for clinically evident disease typically ranges from weeks to months. The first manifestation is usually a papule at the site of the sandfly bite but can be regional lymphadenopathy (sometimes bubonic) in *L. (V.) braziliensis* infection. Most skin lesions evolve from papular to nodular to ulcerative, with a central depression (which can be several centimeters in diameter) surrounded by a raised indurated border (Fig. 215-2). Some lesions persist as nodules or plaques. Multiple primary lesions, satellite lesions, regional adenopathy, sporotrichoid subcuta-

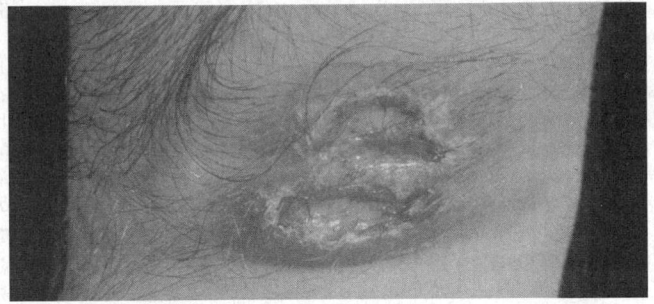

FIGURE 215-2 Ulcerative skin lesions with raised outer borders on the arm of a patient with New World (American) cutaneous leishmaniasis acquired in Costa Rica. *(Photograph courtesy of Dr. A. Wright.)*

neous nodules, lesion pain or pruritus, and secondary bacterial infection are variably present. The infecting species, the location of the lesion, and the host's immune response are among the determinants of the clinical manifestations and chronicity of untreated lesions. For example, in the New World, lesions caused by *L. mexicana* tend to be smaller and less chronic than those caused by *L. (V.) braziliensis*; in the Old World, *L. major* tends to cause "wet" exudative lesions that are less chronic than the "dry" lesions with central crusting that are caused by *L. tropica*. The spontaneous resolution of lesions does not preclude reactivation or reinfection.

The polyparasitic and oligoparasitic ends of the spectrum of cutaneous leishmaniasis are respectively represented by the rare syndromes of diffuse cutaneous leishmaniasis (DCL) and leishmaniasis recidivans, both of which are notoriously difficult to treat. DCL, caused by *L. aethiopica* (Old World) or by the *L. mexicana* complex (New World), develops in the context of *Leishmania*-specific anergy and is manifested by chronic, disseminated, nonulcerative skin lesions; on histopathologic examination of specimens from these lesions, abundant parasites but few lymphocytes are noted. Leishmaniasis recidivans, a hyperergic variant with scarce parasites, is usually caused by *L. tropica* and manifested by a chronic solitary lesion on the cheek that expands slowly despite central healing.

DIAGNOSIS Dermal scrapings of debrided ulcerative lesions are useful for histologic examination, aspirates of skin lesions and lymph nodes for in vitro culture, and biopsy specimens for both examination and culture. Although examination of histologic sections of biopsy specimens can help exclude other diagnoses, amastigotes appear larger and are more easily recognizable on Giemsa-stained thin smears (e.g., smears of dermal scrapings, touch preparations of biopsy specimens). As lesions age, amastigotes become scarcer, and parasitologic confirmation becomes more difficult.

Serologic testing is an insensitive means for diagnosing cutaneous leishmaniasis; antibody titers usually are at most minimally elevated except in patients who have DCL. In contrast, leishmanin skin-test reactivity usually develops during active infection in persons who have simple cutaneous or recidivans leishmaniasis but not in those who have DCL.

Cutaneous leishmaniasis is frequently confused with tropical, traumatic, and venous-stasis ulcers; foreign-body reactions; superinfected insect bites; myiasis; impetigo; fungal infections (e.g., sporotrichosis); mycobacterial infections; and other diseases (e.g., sarcoidosis, neoplasms). DCL and leishmaniasis recidivans should be differentiated from lepromatous leprosy and lupus vulgaris, respectively.

℞ **TREATMENT** Decisions about whether and how to treat cutaneous leishmaniasis should take into account whether mucosal dissemination is possible (as it is in the Americas with some organisms in the *Viannia* subgenus; Table 215-1) as well as the location (e.g., on the face), number, size, evolution, and chronicity of the cutaneous lesions. When optimal effectiveness is important, intravenous or intramuscular Sb^V therapy is recommended (Table 215-2). In studies in Colombia (predominantly with the *Viannia* subgenus), relatively short courses of treatment with pentamidine (Table 215-2) were effective (cure rate, 96%) and quite well tolerated. Thus pentamidine may be a good parenteral alternative to Sb^V. The clinical response to antileishmanial therapy begins with lessening induration; healing often continues after the end of therapy. Relapse typically is manifested by clinical reactivation at the margin of the lesion.

Although many oral agents have been touted for treatment of leishmaniasis, even those that are the most effective typically are moderately active at best and are effective only against some *Leishmania* species or strains. The oral agent miltefosine is being evaluated. In the New World, ketoconazole has some activity against *L. mexicana* and *L. (V.) panamensis* and may be more active than itraconazole (at least against the *Viannia* subgenus), which is better tolerated (Table 215-2). Dapsone has looked promising in India but not in Colombia. Adjunctive immunotherapy remains highly experimental but may be useful in DCL. Local or topical therapy can be considered for some cases of infection in which there is no risk of mucosal dissemination (e.g., for relatively benign lesions caused by *L. mexicana* or *L. major*). Examples of local approaches include the application of an ointment containing paromomycin and methylbenzethonium chloride (not licensed in the United States), the intralesional administration of Sb^V, heat therapy, and cryotherapy.

MUCOSAL LEISHMANIASIS

Leishmanial infection of the naso-oropharyngeal mucosa is a relatively rare but potentially disfiguring metastatic complication of cutaneous leishmaniasis. Mucosal disease develops despite antileishmanial cell-mediated immunity and most commonly is caused by organisms of the *Viannia* subgenus, typically *L. (V.) braziliensis* but also *L. (V.) panamensis* and *L. (V.) guyanensis*. Although mucosal disease usually becomes clinically evident within several years after the healing of the original cutaneous lesions, cutaneous and mucosal lesions can coexist or appear decades apart. Typically, the original cutaneous lesions of patients who develop mucosal disease were not treated or were suboptimally treated.

Mucosal involvement generally is manifested first by persistent unusual nasal symptoms (e.g., epistaxis), with erythema and edema of the nasal mucosa, and then by progressive, ulcerative, naso-oropharyngeal destruction. Supportive laboratory data (e.g., a positive serologic test) are useful, but the scarcity of amastigotes makes parasitologic confirmation difficult. The differential diagnosis includes sarcoidosis, neoplasms, midline granuloma, rhinoscleroma, paracoccidioidomycosis, histoplasmosis, leprosy, syphilis, and tertiary yaws.

Treatment with a pentavalent antimonial compound is moderately effective for mild mucosal disease, whereas advanced disease may not respond to such treatment or may relapse repeatedly (Table 215-2). Amphotericin B (deoxycholate) is the best alternative drug currently available. Patients who develop signs of respiratory compromise during therapy may benefit from the concomitant administration of glucocorticoids.

BIBLIOGRAPHY

ALVAR J et al: *Leishmania* and human immunodeficiency virus coinfection: The first 10 years. Clin Microbiol Rev 10:298, 1997

BERMAN JD: Human leishmaniasis: Clinical, diagnostic, and chemotherapeutic developments in the last 10 years. Clin Infect Dis 24:684, 1997

———: Editorial response: U.S. Food and Drug Administration approval of AmBisome (liposomal amphotericin B) for treatment of visceral leishmaniasis. Clin Infect Dis 28:49, 1999

BERNIER R et al: The lipophosphoglycan of *Leishmania donovani* up-regulates HIV-1 transcription in T cells through the nuclear factor-κB elements. J Immunol 160:2881, 1998

HERWALDT BL: Leishmaniasis. Lancet 354:1191, 1999

———, BERMAN JD: Recommendations for treating leishmaniasis with sodium stibogluconate (Pentostam) and review of pertinent clinical studies. Am J Trop Med Hyg 46:296, 1992

JHA TK et al: Miltefosine, an oral agent, for the treatment of Indian visceral leishmaniasis. N Engl J Med 341:1795, 1999

KENNEY RT et al: Splenic cytokine responses in Indian kala-azar before and after treatment. J Infect Dis 177:815, 1998

LAGUNA F et al: Treatment of visceral leishmaniasis in HIV-infected patients: A randomized trial comparing meglumine antimonate with amphotericin B. AIDS 13:1063, 1999

MAGILL AJ et al: Visceral infection caused by *Leishmania tropica* in veterans of Operation Desert Storm. N Engl J Med 328:1383, 1993

MEYERHOFF A: U.S. Food and Drug Administration approval of AmBisome (liposomal amphotericin B) for treatment of visceral leishmaniasis. Clin Infect Dis 28:42, 1999

REED SG: Diagnosis of leishmaniasis. Clin Dermatol 14:471, 1996

SUNDAR S et al: Rapid accurate field diagnosis of Indian visceral leishmaniasis. Lancet 351:563, 1998

WEIGLE K, SARAVIA NG: Natural history, clinical evolution, and the host-parasite interaction in New World cutaneous leishmaniasis. Clin Dermatol 14:433, 1996

WORLD HEALTH ORGANIZATION: Control of the leishmaniases. Technical Report Series 793. Geneva, World Health Organization, 1990

216 *Louis V. Kirchhoff*

TRYPANOSOMIASIS

CHAGAS' DISEASE

DEFINITION Chagas' disease, or American trypanosomiasis, is a zoonosis caused by the protozoan parasite *Trypanosoma cruzi*. Acute Chagas' disease is usually a mild febrile illness that results from initial infection with the organism. After spontaneous resolution of the acute illness, most infected persons remain for life in the indeterminate phase of chronic Chagas' disease, which is characterized by subpatent parasitemia, easily detectable antibodies to *T. cruzi*, and an absence of symptoms. In a minority of chronically infected patients, cardiac and gastrointestinal lesions develop that can result in serious morbidity and even death.

LIFE CYCLE AND TRANSMISSION *T. cruzi* is transmitted among its mammalian hosts by hematophagous triatomine insects, often called reduviid bugs. The insects become infected by sucking blood from animals or humans who have circulating parasites. Ingested organisms multiply in the gut of the triatomines, and infective forms are discharged with the feces at the time of subsequent blood meals. Transmission to a second vertebrate host occurs when breaks in the skin, mucous membranes, or conjunctivae become contaminated with bug feces that contain infective parasites. *T. cruzi* also can be transmitted by the transfusion of blood donated by infected persons, from mother to fetus, and in laboratory accidents.

PATHOLOGY An indurated inflammatory lesion called a *chagoma* often appears at the site of the parasite's entry. Local histologic changes include the presence of parasites within leukocytes and cells of subcutaneous tissues and the development of interstitial edema, lymphocytic infiltration, and reactive hyperplasia of adjacent lymph nodes. After dissemination of the organisms through the lymphatics and the bloodstream, muscles (including the myocardium) may become heavily parasitized. The characteristic pseudocysts present in sections of infected tissues are intracellular aggregates of multiplying parasites.

The pathogenesis of chronic Chagas' disease is poorly understood. The heart is the organ most commonly affected, and changes include biventricular enlargement, thinning of the ventricular walls, apical aneurysms, and mural thrombi. Widespread lymphocytic infiltration, diffuse interstitial fibrosis, and atrophy of myocardial cells are often demonstrated, but parasites are rarely seen in myocardial tissue. Conduction-system involvement often affects the right branch and the left anterior branch of the bundle of His. In chronic Chagas' disease of the gastrointestinal tract (megadisease), the esophagus and colon may exhibit varying degrees of dilatation. On microscopic examination, focal inflammatory lesions with lymphocytic infiltration are seen,

and the number of neurons in the myenteric plexus may be markedly reduced.

EPIDEMIOLOGY *T. cruzi* is found only in the Americas. Wild and domestic mammals harboring *T. cruzi* and infected triatomines are found in spotty distributions from the southern United States to southern Argentina. Humans become involved in the cycle of transmission when infected vectors take up residence in the primitive wood, adobe, and stone houses common in much of Latin America. Thus, human *T. cruzi* infection is a health problem primarily among the poor in rural areas of Central and South America. Most new *T. cruzi* infections in rural settings occur in children, but the incidence is unknown because most cases go undiagnosed. Thousands of individuals also become infected every year through blood transfusions in urban areas. Several dozen patients with HIV and chronic *T. cruzi* infections who underwent acute recrudescence of the latter have been described. These patients generally presented with *T. cruzi* brain abscesses, a manifestation of the illness that does not occur in immunocompetent persons. Currently, it is estimated that 16 to 18 million people, more than a third of whom live in Brazil, are chronically infected with *T. cruzi*. Chronic Chagas' disease is a major cause of morbidity and mortality in many Latin American countries, including Mexico, since many chronically infected persons eventually develop symptomatic cardiac lesions or gastrointestinal disease.

In recent years, the rate of *T. cruzi* transmission has been decreasing in several endemic countries as a result of successful vector and blood-bank control programs. A major program in the "southern cone" nations of South America (Uruguay, Paraguay, Bolivia, Brazil, Chile, and Argentina), begun in 1991, has provided the framework for much of the progress achieved. If current trends continue, transmission will be essentially eliminated in much of the endemic range by the year 2003.

Acute Chagas' disease is rare in the United States. Five cases of autochthonous transmission and four instances of transmission by blood transfusion have been reported. Moreover, in the last 26 years, seven laboratory-acquired infections and nine imported cases of acute Chagas' disease were reported to the Centers for Disease Control and Prevention (CDC). In contrast, the prevalence of chronic *T. cruzi* infections in the United States has increased considerably in recent years. Since the mid-1970s, enormous numbers of Latin Americans have emigrated to the United States. In one study conducted in Washington, D.C., 5% of Salvadoran and Nicaraguan immigrants were found to have chronic *T. cruzi* infections. Estimates based on the latter study and on studies done in several United States blood banks put the total number of infected immigrants now living in the United States at more than 50,000. The presence of these carriers of *T. cruzi* creates a substantial risk of transmission by blood transfusion, as is evidenced by the four transfusion-associated cases just cited.

CLINICAL COURSE The first signs of acute Chagas' disease develop at least 1 week after invasion by the parasites. When the organisms enter through a break in the skin, an indurated area of erythema and swelling (the chagoma), accompanied by local lymphadenopathy, may appear. Romaña's sign—the classic finding in acute Chagas' disease, which consists of unilateral painless edema of the palpebrae and periocular tissues—can result when the conjunctiva is the portal of entry. These initial local signs are followed by malaise, fever, anorexia, and edema of the face and lower extremities. A morbilliform rash may also appear. Generalized lymphadenopathy and hepatosplenomegaly may develop. Severe myocarditis develops rarely; most deaths in acute Chagas' disease are due to heart failure. Neurologic signs are not common, but meningoencephalitis has been reported. The acute symptoms resolve spontaneously in virtually all patients, who then enter the asymptomatic or indeterminate phase of chronic *T. cruzi* infection.

Symptomatic chronic Chagas' disease becomes apparent years or even decades after the initial infection. The heart is commonly involved, and symptoms are caused by rhythm disturbances, cardiomyopathy, and thromboembolism. Right bundle-branch block is the most common electrocardiographic abnormality, but other types of atrioventricular block, premature ventricular contractions, and tachy-

and bradyarrhythmias occur frequently. Cardiomyopathy often results in right-sided or biventricular heart failure. Embolization of mural thrombi to the brain or other areas may take place. Patients with mega-esophagus suffer from dysphagia, odynophagia, chest pain, and regurgitation. Aspiration can occur, especially during sleep, and repeated episodes of aspiration pneumonitis are common. Weight loss, cachexia, and pulmonary infection can result in death. Patients with megacolon are plagued by abdominal pain and chronic constipation, and advanced megacolon can cause obstruction, volvulus, septicemia, and death.

DIAGNOSIS The diagnosis of acute Chagas' disease requires the detection of parasites. Microscopic examination of fresh anticoagulated blood or of the buffy coat is the simplest way to see the motile organisms. Parasites also can be seen in Giemsa-stained thin and thick blood smears. When repeated attempts to visualize the organisms are unsuccessful, mouse inoculation, culture of blood in specialized media, or xenodiagnosis can be performed. In the last technique, uninfected triatomine insects are allowed to feed on the patient's blood. When done properly, all of these methods yield positive results in a high proportion of patients with acute Chagas' disease and in at least half of those with chronic infections. Since early treatment of acute Chagas' disease is extremely important, however, the decision to initiate therapy for *T. cruzi* infection despite negative wet preparations and smears must be made on clinical and epidemiologic grounds before the results of these indirect methods become available. Serologic testing is of limited usefulness in diagnosing acute Chagas' disease.

The diagnosis of chronic Chagas' disease is made by the detection of antibodies that bind to *T. cruzi* antigens. Demonstration of the parasite is not of primary importance. Several highly sensitive serologic tests for antibodies to *T. cruzi* are used widely in Latin America, including complement-fixation and immunofluorescence tests and enzyme-linked immunosorbent assays (ELISAs). However, a persistent problem with these conventional assays is the occurrence of false-positive reactions, typically with sera from patients who have other parasitic infections or autoimmune diseases. For this reason, it is generally recommended that positivity in one assay be confirmed by two other tests and that well-characterized positive and negative comparison sera be included in each run. A highly sensitive and specific method for detecting antibodies to *T. cruzi* [approved by the Clinical Laboratory Improvement Amendment (CLIA) and available in the author's laboratory] employs immunoprecipitation of radiolabeled *T. cruzi* antigens and electrophoresis. Serodiagnostic assays that employ recombinant *T. cruzi* proteins as target antigens are being developed, as are tests based on the amplification of *T. cruzi* DNA sequences by polymerase chain reaction. However, these tests are not yet available for general use.

℞ **TREATMENT** Therapy for Chagas' disease is unsatisfactory. Nifurtimox is the only drug active against *T. cruzi* that is available in the United States. In acute Chagas' disease, nifurtimox markedly reduces the duration of symptoms and parasitemia and decreases the mortality rate. Nevertheless, its efficacy at eradicating parasites is low. Limited studies have shown that only ~70% of acute infections are cured parasitologically by a full course of treatment. Despite its limitations, nifurtimox treatment should be initiated as early as possible in acute Chagas' disease. Moreover, when laboratory accidents occur in which it appears likely that *T. cruzi* infection could become established, nifurtimox therapy should be initiated without waiting for clinical or parasitologic indications of infection.

Common adverse effects of nifurtimox include abdominal pain, anorexia, nausea, vomiting, and weight loss. Neurologic reactions to the drug may include restlessness, disorientation, insomnia, twitching, paresthesia, polyneuritis, and seizures. These symptoms usually disappear when the dosage is reduced or treatment is discontinued. The recommended daily dosage is 8 to 10 mg/kg for adults, 12.5 to 15 mg/kg for adolescents, and 15 to 20 mg/kg for children 1 to 10 years of age. The drug should be given orally in four divided doses each day, and therapy should be continued for 90 to 120 days. Nifurtimox is

available from the Drug Service of the CDC in Atlanta, Georgia (telephone number, 770-639-3670).

Benznidazole is a second agent used to treat Chagas' disease. Its efficacy is similar to that of nifurtimox, and its adverse effects include peripheral neuropathy, rash, and granulocytopenia. The recommended oral dosage is 5 mg/kg per day for 60 days. Benznidazole is used widely in Latin America.

The question of whether patients in the indeterminate or chronic symptomatic phases of Chagas' disease should be treated with nifurtimox or benznidazole has been debated for years. Studies of *T. cruzi*–infected laboratory animals and humans suggest that elimination of the parasites reduces the appearance or progression of cardiac pathology. In view of these findings, an international panel of experts has recommended that all patients infected with *T. cruzi* be treated with one drug or the other, regardless of their clinical status or the duration of infection.

The usefulness of allopurinol, fluconazole, and itraconazole for the treatment of acute Chagas' disease has been studied extensively in laboratory animals and to a lesser extent in humans. None of these drugs has exhibited a level of anti–*T. cruzi* activity that warrants its use in patients. Studies in mice have shown that recombinant interferon γ decreases the duration and severity of acute *T. cruzi* infection; however, its usefulness in persons with acute Chagas' disease has not been evaluated systematically.

Patients who develop cardiac and/or gastrointestinal disease in association with *T. cruzi* infection should be referred to appropriate subspecialists for further evaluation and treatment. Cardiac transplantation is an option for patients with end-stage chagasic cardiopathies. Postoperative prophylaxis with nifurtimox or benznidazole should be considered because without it the immunosuppression required after surgery has been shown to result in reactivation of *T. cruzi* infection, often with serious consequences or even death.

PREVENTION Since drug therapy is unsatisfactory and vaccines are not available, the control of *T. cruzi* transmission in endemic countries must depend on reduction of domiciliary vector populations by spraying of insecticides, improvement of housing, and education. In addition, in endemic areas, programs for the screening of donated blood for *T. cruzi* need to be expanded and improved to reduce rates of transmission by transfusion. Tourists traveling in endemic areas should avoid sleeping in dilapidated houses outside urban areas. Mosquito nets and insect repellent provide additional protection.

In the United States, the question of how best to avoid transmission of *T. cruzi* by blood transfusion is not easily resolved. Since no assay for *T. cruzi* infection has received clearance from the Food and Drug Administration (FDA) for use in blood banks, serologic screening is not yet an option. The FDA currently mandates the use of a questionnaire for identifying and deferring donors at high risk for *T. cruzi* infection. This approach may be effective and not reduce the blood supply intolerably, but it is important to bear in mind that approaches based solely on questionnaires have not been entirely successful at eliminating transfusion-associated transmission of other infectious agents.

In view of the possibly serious consequences of chronic *T. cruzi* infection, it would be prudent for all immigrants from endemic regions to be tested for evidence of infection. Identification of infected persons is also important because the implantation of pacemakers benefits some patients who develop ominous rhythm disturbances. The possibility of congenital transmission is yet another justification for screening.

Laboratory personnel should wear gloves and eye protection when working with *T. cruzi* and infected vectors.

SLEEPING SICKNESS

DEFINITION Sleeping sickness, or human African trypanosomiasis (HAT), is caused by flagellated protozoan parasites that belong to the *T. brucei* complex and are transmitted to humans by tsetse flies. In untreated patients, the trypanosomes first cause a febrile illness that is followed months or years later by progressive neurologic impairment and death.

THE PARASITES AND THEIR TRANSMISSION The East African (*rhodesiense*) and the West African (*gambiense*) forms of sleeping sickness are caused, respectively, by two trypanosome subspecies: *T. brucei rhodesiense* and *T. brucei gambiense*. These subspecies are morphologically indistinguishable but cause illnesses that are epidemiologically and clinically distinct. The parasites are transmitted by blood-sucking tsetse flies of the genus *Glossina*. The insects acquire the infection when they ingest blood from infected mammalian hosts. After many cycles of multiplication in the midgut of the vector, the parasites migrate to the salivary glands. Their transmission takes place when they are inoculated during a subsequent blood meal. The injected trypanosomes multiply in the blood and other extracellular spaces and evade immune destruction in mammalian hosts for long periods by undergoing antigenic variation, in which the antigenic structure of their surface coat of glycoproteins changes periodically.

PATHOGENESIS AND PATHOLOGY A self-limited inflammatory lesion (trypanosomal chancre) may appear a week or so after the bite of an infected tsetse fly. A systemic febrile illness then evolves as the parasites are disseminated through the lymphatics and bloodstream. Systemic HAT without central nervous system (CNS) involvement is generally referred to as *stage I disease*. In this stage, widespread lymphadenopathy and splenomegaly reflect marked lymphocytic and histiocytic proliferation and invasion of morular cells, which are plasmacytes that may be involved in the production of IgM. Endarteritis, with perivascular infiltration of both parasites and lymphocytes, may develop in lymph nodes and spleen. Myocarditis develops frequently in patients with stage I disease and is especially common in *T. b. rhodesiense* infections.

Hematologic manifestations that accompany stage I HAT include moderate leukocytosis, thrombocytopenia, and anemia. High levels of immunoglobulins, consisting primarily of polyclonal IgM, are a constant feature, and heterophile antibodies, antibodies to DNA, and rheumatoid factor are often detected. High levels of antigen-antibody complexes may play a role in the tissue damage and increased vascular permeability that facilitate dissemination of the parasites.

Stage II disease involves invasion of the CNS. The presence of trypanosomes in perivascular areas is accompanied by intense infiltration of mononuclear cells. Abnormalities in cerebrospinal fluid (CSF) include increased pressure, elevated total protein concentration, and pleocytosis. In addition, trypanosomes are frequently found in CSF.

EPIDEMIOLOGY The trypanosomes that cause sleeping sickness are found only in Africa. Approximately 50 million persons are at risk of acquiring HAT, and tens of thousands of new cases occur every year. Precise data are not available because health statistics are often incomplete in the developing countries where HAT is endemic. Sleeping sickness has undergone a resurgence in recent years, with major epidemics in the Sudan, Ivory Coast, Chad, the Central African Republic, and several other endemic countries.

Humans are the only reservoir of *T. b. gambiense*, which occurs in widely distributed foci in tropical rain forests of Central and West Africa. Gambiense trypanosomiasis is primarily a problem in rural populations; tourists rarely become infected. Trypanotolerant antelope species in savanna and woodland areas of Central and East Africa are the principal reservoir of *T. b. rhodesiense*. Cattle also can become infected but generally succumb to the parasite. Since risk results for the most part from contact with tsetse flies that feed on wild animals, humans acquire *T. b. rhodesiense* infection only incidentally, usually while working in areas where infected game and vectors are present. In addition, occasional cases occur among visitors to game parks in East Africa. During the past 22 years, 21 cases of imported HAT have

been reported to the CDC, most of which were caused by *T. b. rhodesiense*.

CLINICAL COURSE A painful trypanosomal chancre appears in some patients at the site of inoculation of the parasite. Hematogenous and lymphatic dissemination (stage I disease) is marked by the onset of fever. Typically, bouts of high temperatures lasting several days are separated by afebrile periods. Lymphadenopathy is prominent in *T. b. gambiense* trypanosomiasis. The nodes are discrete, movable, rubbery, and nontender. Cervical nodes are often visible, and enlargement of the nodes of the posterior cervical triangle, or Winterbottom's sign, is a classic finding. Pruritus and maculopapular rashes are common. Inconstant findings include malaise, headache, arthralgias, weight loss, edema, hepatosplenomegaly, and tachycardia.

CNS invasion (stage II disease) is characterized by the insidious development of protean neurologic manifestations that are accompanied by progressive abnormalities in the CSF. A picture of progressive indifference and daytime somnolence develops (hence the designation "sleeping sickness"), sometimes alternating with restlessness and insomnia at night. A listless gaze accompanies a loss of spontaneity, and speech may become halting and indistinct. Extrapyramidal signs may include choreiform movements, tremors, and fasciculations. Ataxia is frequent, and the patient may appear to have Parkinson's disease, with a shuffling gait, hypertonia, and tremors. In the final phase, progressive neurologic impairment ends in coma and death.

The most striking difference between the West African and East African trypanosomiases is that the latter illness tends to follow a more acute course. Typically, in tourists, systemic signs of infection, such as fever, malaise, and headache, appear before the end of the trip or shortly after the return home. Persistent tachycardia unrelated to fever is common early in the course of *T. b. rhodesiense* trypanosomiasis, and death may result from arrhythmias and congestive heart failure before CNS disease develops. In general, untreated *T. b. rhodesiense* trypanosomiasis leads to death in a matter of weeks to months, often without a clear distinction between the hemolymphatic and CNS stages.

DIAGNOSIS A definitive diagnosis of HAT requires detection of the parasite. If a chancre is present, fluid should be expressed and examined directly by light microscopy for the highly motile trypanosomes. The fluid also should be fixed and stained with Giemsa. Material obtained by needle aspiration of lymph nodes early in the course of the illness should be examined similarly. Examination of wet preparations and Giemsa-stained thin and thick films of serial blood samples is also useful. If parasites are not seen in blood, efforts should be made to concentrate the organisms; the simplest method involves the use of quantitative buffy coat analysis tubes (QBC, Becton-Dickinson, Franklin Lakes, NJ). In these tubes, which are coated with acridine orange, the parasites are separated from blood cells by centrifugation and are easily seen under light microscopy because of the stain. The buffy coat from 10 to 15 mL of anticoagulated blood or the pellet obtained by centrifugation of the eluate from 25 to 50 mL of blood passed through a DEAE-cellulose column also can be examined. Trypanosomes may be seen in material aspirated from the bone marrow; the aspirate can be inoculated into liquid culture medium, as can blood, buffy coat, lymph node aspirates, and CSF. Finally, *T. b. rhodesiense* infection can be detected by inoculation of these specimens into mice or rats, which results in patent parasitemias in a week or two. Although this method is highly sensitive for the detection of *T. b. rhodesiense*, it does not detect *T. b. gambiense* because of host specificity.

It is essential to examine CSF from all patients in whom HAT is suspected. An increase in the CSF cell count is the first abnormality to be detected; increases in opening pressure and in levels of total protein and IgM develop later. Trypanosomes may be seen in the sediment of centrifuged CSF. Any CSF abnormality in a patient in whom trypanosomes have been found at other sites must be viewed as pathognomonic for CNS involvement and thus must prompt specific treatment for CNS disease.

A number of serologic assays are available to aid in the diagnosis of HAT, but their variable sensitivity and specificity mandate that de-

℞ **TREATMENT** The drugs traditionally used for treatment of HAT are suramin, pentamidine, and organic arsenicals. An addition to this list is eflornithine (difluoromethylornithine), which was approved by the FDA in November 1990 for the treatment of West African trypanosomiasis. In the United States these drugs can be obtained from the CDC. Therapy for HAT must be individualized on the basis of the infecting organism (*T. b. gambiense* or *T. b. rhodesiense*), the presence or absence of CNS disease, adverse reactions, and (occasionally) drug resistance. The choices of drugs for the treatment of HAT are summarized in Table 216-1.

Suramin is highly effective against stage I disease. However, it can cause serious adverse effects and must be administered under the close supervision of a physician. A 100- to 200-mg intravenous test dose should be administered to detect hypersensitivity. The dosage for adults is 1 g intravenously on days 1, 3, 7, 14, and 21. The regimen for children is 20 mg/kg (maximum, 1 g) intravenously on days 1, 3, 7, 14, and 21. The drug is given by slow intravenous infusion of a freshly prepared 10% aqueous solution. Approximately 1 patient in 20,000 has an immediate, severe, and potentially fatal reaction to the drug, developing nausea, vomiting, shock, and seizures. Less severe reactions include fever, photophobia, pruritus, arthralgias, and skin eruptions. Renal damage is the most common important adverse effect of suramin. Transient proteinuria often appears during treatment. A urinalysis should be done before each dose, and treatment should be discontinued if proteinuria increases or if casts and red cells appear in the sediment. Suramin should not be given to patients with renal insufficiency.

Eflornithine is highly effective for treatment of both stages of West African trypanosomiasis. In the trials on which the FDA based its approval, this agent cured more than 90% of 600 patients with stage II disease. The recommended treatment schedule is 400 mg/kg per day intravenously in four divided doses for 2 weeks. Adverse reactions include diarrhea, anemia, thrombocytopenia, seizures, and hearing loss. The high dosage and duration of therapy required are disadvantages that make widespread use of eflornithine difficult.

Pentamidine is the alternative drug for patients with stage I HAT, although some *T. b. rhodesiense* infections are unresponsive to this agent. The dose for both adults and children is 4 mg/kg per day intramuscularly or intravenously for 10 days. Frequent, immediate adverse reactions include nausea, vomiting, tachycardia, and hypotension. These reactions are usually transient and do not warrant cessation of therapy. Other adverse reactions include nephrotoxicity, abnormal liver function tests, neutropenia, rashes, hypoglycemia, and sterile abscesses.

The arsenical melarsoprol is the drug of choice for the treatment of East African trypanosomiasis with CNS involvement. Melarsoprol cures both stages of the disease and therefore is also indicated for the treatment of stage I disease in patients who fail to respond to or cannot tolerate suramin and/or pentamidine. However, because of its relatively high toxicity, melarsoprol is never the first choice for the treatment of stage I disease. The drug should be given to adults in three courses of 3 days each. The dosage is 2 to 3.6 mg/kg per day intravenously in three divided doses for 3 days followed 1 week later by 3.6 mg/kg per day, also in three divided doses and for 3 days. The latter course is repeated 10 to 21 days later. In debilitated patients, suramin is administered for 2 to 4 days before therapy with melarsoprol is initiated. An 18-mg initial dose of the latter drug, followed by progressive increases to the standard dose, has been recommended. For children, a total of 18 to 25 mg/kg should be given over 1 month. A starting dose of 0.36 mg/kg intravenously should be increased gradually to a maximum of 3.6 mg/kg at 1- to 5-day intervals, for a total of 9 or 10 doses.

Melarsoprol is highly toxic and should be administered with great care. The incidence of reactive encephalopathy has been reported to be as high as 18% in some series. Clinical manifestations of reactive encephalopathy include high fever, headache, tremor, impaired speech, seizures, and even coma and death. Treatment with melarsoprol should be discontinued at the first sign of encephalopathy but may be restarted cautiously at lower doses a few days after signs have resolved. Extravasation of the drug results in intense local reactions. Vomiting, abdominal pain, nephrotoxicity, and myocardial damage can occur.

The treatment of patients with stage II East African disease who cannot tolerate melarsoprol is problematic. The combination of the arsenical tryparsamide and suramin is one possible approach, but its efficacy is limited because suramin does not penetrate the CNS well and tryparsamide is much less effective against *T. b. rhodesiense* than it is against *T. b. gambiense*. The schedule for tryparsamide therapy is 30 mg/kg (maximum, 2 g) in a single intravenous dose every 5 days for a total of 12 doses; that for suramin treatment is 10 mg/kg intravenously every 5 days, also for a total of 12 injections. Tryparsamide can cause encephalopathy, fever, vomiting, abdominal pain, rash, tinnitus, and a variety of ocular symptoms. Alternatively, eflornithine can be administered as outlined above to patients who cannot tolerate melarsoprol, but, as noted, its effectiveness against *T. b. rhodesiense* is variable.

PREVENTION HAT poses complex public-health and epizootic problems in Africa. Considerable progress has been made in some areas through control programs that focus on eradication of vectors and drug treatment of infected humans; however, there is no consensus on the best approach to solving the overall problem, and major epidemics continue to occur. Individuals can reduce their risk of acquiring trypanosomiasis by avoiding areas known to harbor infected insects, by wearing protective clothing, and by using insect repellent. Chemoprophylaxis is not recommended, and no vaccine is available to prevent transmission of the parasites.

BIBLIOGRAPHY

CHAGAS' DISEASE

BOCCHI EA et al: Higher incidence of malignant neoplasms after heart transplantation for treatment of chronic Chagas' heart disease. J Heart Lung Transplant 17:399, 1998

GOMES ML et al: Chagas' disease diagnosis: Comparative analysis of parasitologic, molecular, and serologic methods. Am J Trop Med Hyg 60:205, 1999

GUZMAN BRACHO C et al: Risk of transmission of *Trypanosoma cruzi* by blood transfusion in Mexico [Spanish]. Pan Am J Public Health 4:94, 1998

KIRCHHOFF LV: American trypanosomiasis (Chagas' disease): A persistent problem in Latin America now affects the United States. N Engl J Med 329:639, 1993

——: American trypanosomiasis (Chagas' disease). Gastroenterol Clin North Am 25:517, 1996

—— et al: Increased specificity of serodiagnosis of Chagas' disease by detection of antibody to the 72- and 90-kilodalton glycoproteins of *Trypanosoma cruzi*. J Infect Dis 155:561, 1987

LEIBY DA et al: Seroepidemiology of *Trypanosoma cruzi*, etiologic agent of Chagas' disease, in U.S. blood donors. J Infect Dis 176:1047, 1997

OCHS DE et al: Postmortem diagnosis of autochthonous acute chagasic myocarditis by PCR amplification of a species-specific DNA sequence of *Trypanosoma cruzi*. Am J Trop Med Hyg 54:526, 1996

PARADA H et al: Cardiac involvement is a constant finding in acute Chagas' disease: A clinical, parasitological and histopathological study. Int J Cardiol 60:49, 1997

Table 216-1 Treatment of Human African Trypanosomiases[a]

Causative Organism	Clinical Stage	
	I (Normal CSF)	II (Abnormal CSF)
T. brucei gambiense (West African)	Suramin or eflornithine Alternative: Pentamidine	Eflornithine Alternative: Tryparsamide plus suramin
T. brucei rhodesiense (East African)	Suramin Alternative: Pentamidine	Melarsoprol

[a] For doses and duration, see text.

SARTORI AM et al: Follow-up of 18 patients with human immunodeficiency virus infection and chronic Chagas' disease, with reactivation of Chagas' disease causing cardiac disease in three patients. Clin Infect Dis 26:177, 1998

SCHMUNIS GA et al: Interruption of Chagas' disease transmission through vector elimination. Lancet 348:1171, 1996

SLEEPING SICKNESS

DONELSON JE et al: Multiple mechanisms of immune evasion by African trypanosomes. Mol Biochem Parasitol 91:51, 1998

Drugs for parasitic infections. Med Lett Drugs Ther 40:1, 1998

EKWANZALA M et al: In the heart of darkness: Sleeping sickness in Zaire. Lancet 348: 1427, 1996

HUNTER CA, KENNEDY PGE: Immunopathology in central nervous system human African trypanosomiasis. J Neuroimmunol 36:91, 1992

JORDAN AM: *Trypanosomiasis Control and African Rural Development*. London, Longman, 1986

PEPIN J, MILORD F: The treatment of African trypanosomiasis. Adv Parasitol 33:1, 1994

STERNBERG JM: Immunobiology of African trypanosomiasis. Chem Immunol 70:186, 1998

TRUC P et al: Parasitological diagnosis of human African trypanosomiasis: A comparison of the QBC® and miniature anion-exchange centrifugation techniques. Trans R Soc Trop Med Hyg 92:288, 1998

217 Lloyd H. Kasper

TOXOPLASMA INFECTION

DEFINITION Toxoplasmosis is the disease caused by infection with the obligate intracellular parasite *Toxoplasma gondii*. Acute infection acquired after birth may be asymptomatic but frequently results in the chronic persistence of cysts within the tissues of the host. Both acute and chronic toxoplasmosis are conditions in which the parasite is responsible for the development of clinically evident disease, including lymphadenopathy, encephalitis, myocarditis, and pneumonitis. Congenital toxoplasmosis is an infection of newborns that results from the transplacental passage of parasites from an infected mother to the fetus. These infants usually are asymptomatic at birth but later manifest a wide range of signs and symptoms, including chorioretinitis, strabismus, epilepsy, and psychomotor retardation.

ETIOLOGY *T. gondii* is an intracellular coccidian that infects both birds and mammals. There are two distinct stages in the life cycle of *T. gondii*: the nonfeline and feline stages. In the nonfeline stage, tissue cysts that contain bradyzoites or sporulated oocysts are ingested by an intermediate host (e.g., a human, mouse, sheep, or pig). The cyst is rapidly digested by the acidic-pH gastric secretions. Bradyzoites or sporozoites are released, enter the small-intestinal epithelium, and transform into rapidly dividing tachyzoites. The tachyzoites can infect and replicate in all mammalian cells except red blood cells. Once attached to the host cell, the parasite penetrates the cell and forms a parasitophorous vacuole within which it divides. Parasite replication continues until the number of parasites within the cell approaches a critical mass and the cell ruptures, releasing parasites that infect adjoining cells.

As a result of this process, an infected organ soon shows evidence of cytopathology. Most tachyzoites are eliminated by means of the host's humoral and cell-mediated immune responses. Tissue cysts containing many bradyzoites develop 7 to 10 days after the systemic tachyzoite infection. These tissue cysts occur in a variety of host organs but persist principally within the central nervous system (CNS) and muscle. The development of this chronic stage completes the nonfeline portion of the life cycle. Active infection in the immunocompromised host is most likely due to the spontaneous release of encysted parasites that undergo rapid transformation into tachyzoites within the CNS.

The principal stage in the life cycle of the parasite takes place in the cat (the definitive host) and its prey. The parasite's sexual phase is defined by the formation of oocysts within the feline host. This enteroepithelial cycle begins with the ingestion of the bradyzoite tissue cysts and culminates after several intermediate stages in the production of gametes. Gamete fusion produces a zygote, which envelops itself in a rigid wall and is secreted in the feces as an unsporulated oocyst. After 2 to 3 days of exposure to air at ambient temperature, the noninfectious oocyst sporulates to produce eight sporozoite progeny. The sporulated oocyst can be ingested by an intermediate host, such as a person emptying a cat's litter box, a pig rummaging in a barnyard, or perhaps a mouse. It is in the intermediate host that the parasite completes its life cycle.

EPIDEMIOLOGY *T. gondii* infects a wide range of mammals and birds. Its seroprevalence depends on the locale and the age of the population. Generally, hot arid climatic conditions are associated with a low prevalence of infection. In the United States and most European countries, the prevalence of seroconversion increases with age and exposure. For example, in the United States, 5 to 30% of individuals 10 to 19 years old and 10 to 67% of those over the age of 50 years show serologic evidence of exposure; seroprevalence increases by approximately 1% per year. In Central America, France, Turkey, and Brazil, the seroprevalence is higher.

TRANSMISSION **Oral Transmission** The principal source of human *Toxoplasma* infection remains uncertain. Transmission usually takes place by the oral route and can be attributable to ingestion of either sporulated oocysts from contaminated soil or bradyzoites from undercooked meat. During acute feline infection, a cat may excrete as many as 100 million parasites per day. These very stable sporozoite-containing oocysts are highly infectious and may remain viable for many years in the soil. Humans infected during a well-documented outbreak of oocyst-transmitted infection develop stage-specific antibodies to the oocyst/sporozoite.

Children and adults also can acquire infection from tissue cysts containing bradyzoites. The ingestion of a single cyst is all that is required for human infection. Undercooking or insufficient freezing of meat is an important source of infection in the developed world. In the United States, 10 to 20% of lamb products and 25 to 35% of pork products show evidence of cysts that contain bradyzoites. The incidence in beef is much lower—perhaps as low as 1%. Direct ingestion of bradyzoite cysts in these various meat products leads to acute infection.

Transmission via Blood or Organs In addition to oral transmission, direct transmission of the parasite by blood or organ products during transplantation takes place at a low rate. Viable parasites can be cultured from refrigerated anticoagulated blood, which may be a source of infection in individuals receiving blood transfusions. *T. gondii* infection also has been reported in kidney and heart transplant recipients who were uninfected before transplantation.

Transplacental Transmission About one-third of all women who acquire infection with *T. gondii* during pregnancy transmit the parasite to the fetus; the remainder give birth to normal, uninfected babies. Of the various factors that influence fetal outcome, gestational age at the time of infection is the most critical (see below). Few data support a role for recrudescent maternal infection as the source of congenital disease. Thus, women who are seropositive before pregnancy usually are protected against acute infection and do not give birth to congenitally infected neonates.

The following general guidelines can be used to evaluate congenital infection. There is essentially no risk if the mother becomes infected ≥6 months before conception. If infection is acquired <6 months before conception, the likelihood of transplacental infection increases as the interval between infection and conception decreases. In pregnancy, if the mother becomes infected during the first trimester, the incidence of transplacental infection is lowest (about 15%), but the disease in the neonate is most severe. If maternal infection occurs during the third trimester, the incidence of transplacental infection is greatest (65%), but the infant is usually asymptomatic at birth. Infected infants who are normal at birth may have a higher incidence of learning disabilities and chronic neurologic sequelae than uninfected children.

Only a small proportion (20%) of women infected with *T. gondii* develop clinical signs of infection. Often the diagnosis is first appreciated when routine postconception serologic tests show evidence of specific antibody.

PATHOGENESIS Upon the host's ingestion of either tissue cysts containing bradyzoites or oocysts containing sporozoites, the parasites are released from the cysts by a digestive process. Bradyzoites are resistant to the effect of pepsin and invade the host's gastrointestinal tract. Within enterocytes, the parasites undergo morphologic transformation, giving rise to invasive tachyzoites. These tachyzoites induce a parasite-specific secretory IgA response. From the gastrointestinal tract, parasites are disseminated to a variety of organs, particularly lymphatic tissue, skeletal muscle, myocardium, retina, placenta, and the CNS. At these sites, the parasite infects host cells, replicates, and invades the adjoining cells. In this fashion, the hallmarks of the infection develop: cell death and focal necrosis surrounded by an acute inflammatory response.

In the normal immune host, both the humoral and the cellular immune responses control infection; parasite virulence and tissue tropism may be strain specific. Tachyzoites are sequestered by a variety of immune mechanisms, including induction of parasiticidal antibody, activation of macrophages with radical intermediates, production of interferon γ (IFN-γ), and stimulation of cytotoxic T lymphocytes of the CD8+ phenotype. These antigen-specific lymphocytes are capable of killing both extracellular parasites and target cells infected with parasites. As tachyzoites are cleared from the acutely infected host, tissue cysts containing bradyzoites begin to appear, usually within the CNS and the retina. In the immunocompromised or fetal host, the immune factors necessary to control the spread of tachyzoite infection are lacking. This altered immune state allows the persistence of tachyzoites and gives rise to the progressive focal destruction that results in organ failure (i.e., necrotizing encephalitis, pneumonia, and myocarditis).

Persistence of infection with cysts containing bradyzoites is common in the immunocompetent host. This lifelong infection usually remains subclinical. Although bradyzoites are in a slow metabolic phase, cysts do degenerate and rupture within the CNS. This degenerative process, with the development of new bradyzoite-containing cysts, is the most probable source of recrudescent infection in immunocompromised individuals and the most likely stimulus for the persistence of antibody titers in the immunocompetent host.

PATHOLOGY Cell death and focal necrosis due to replicating tachyzoites induce an intense mononuclear inflammatory response in any tissue or cell type infected. Tachyzoites rarely can be visualized by routine histopathologic staining of these inflammatory lesions. However, immunofluorescence staining with parasitic antigen-specific antibodies can reveal either the organism itself or evidence of antigen. In contrast to this inflammatory process caused by tachyzoites, bradyzoite-containing cysts cause inflammation only at the early stages of development, and even this inflammation may be a response to the presence of tachyzoite antigens. Once the cysts reach maturity, the inflammatory process can no longer be detected, and the cysts remain immunologically quiescent within the brain matrix until they rupture.

Lymph Nodes During acute infection, lymph node biopsy demonstrates characteristic findings, including follicular hyperplasia and irregular clusters of tissue macrophages with eosinophilic cytoplasm. Granulomas rarely are evident in these specimens. Although tachyzoites are not usually visible, they can be sought either by subinoculation of infected tissue into mice, with resultant disease, or by the polymerase chain reaction (PCR). PCR amplification of DNA fragments representing either p30 (SAG-1) or p22 (SAG-2) surface antigen or B1 antigen is an effective and sensitive assay for establishing infection of lymph node tissue by tachyzoites.

Eyes In the eye, infiltrates of monocytes, lymphocytes, and plasma cells may produce uni- or multifocal lesions. Granulomatous lesions and chorioretinitis can be observed in the posterior chamber following acute necrotizing retinitis. Other ocular complications of infection include iridocyclitis, cataracts, and glaucoma.

Central Nervous System During CNS involvement, both focal and diffuse meningoencephalitis can be documented, with evidence of necrosis and microglial nodules. Necrotizing encephalitis in patients without AIDS is characterized by small diffuse lesions with perivascular cuffing in contiguous areas. In the AIDS population, polymorphonuclear leukocytes may be present in addition to monocytes, lymphocytes, and plasma cells. Cysts containing bradyzoites frequently are found contiguous with the necrotic tissue border.

Lungs Among patients with AIDS who die of toxoplasmosis, 40 to 70% have involvement of the heart and lung. Interstitial pneumonitis can develop in the neonate and the immunocompromised patient. Thickened and edematous alveolar septa infiltrated with mononuclear and plasma cells are apparent. This inflammation may extend to the endothelial walls. Tachyzoites and bradyzoite-containing cysts have been observed within the alveolar membrane. Superimposed bronchopneumonia can be caused by other microbial agents.

Heart Cysts and aggregates of parasites in cardiac muscle tissue are evident in patients with AIDS who die of toxoplasmosis. Focal necrosis surrounded by inflammatory cells is associated with hyaline necrosis and disrupted myocardial cells. Pericarditis is associated with toxoplasmosis in some patients.

Other Sites Pathologic changes during disseminated infection are similar to those described for the lymph nodes, eyes, and CNS. In patients with AIDS, the skeletal muscle, pancreas, stomach, and kidneys can be involved, with necrosis, invasion by inflammatory cells, and (rarely) the presence of tachyzoites detectable by routine staining. Large necrotic lesions may cause direct tissue destruction. In addition, secondary effects from acute infection of these various organs, including pancreatitis, myositis, and glomerulonephritis, have been reported.

HOST IMMUNE RESPONSE Acute *Toxoplasma* infection evokes a cascade of protective immune responses in the normal host. *Toxoplasma* enters the host at the gut mucosal level and evokes a mucosal immune response that includes the production of antigen-specific secretory IgA. Titers of serum IgA antibody directed at p30 (SAG-1) have been shown to be a useful marker of congenital and acute toxoplasmosis. Milk-whey IgA from acutely infected mothers contains a high titer of antibody to *T. gondii* and can block infection of enterocytes in vitro. In mice, IgA intestinal secretions directed at the parasite are abundant and are associated with the induction of mucosal T cells.

Within the host, *T. gondii* rapidly induces detectable levels of both IgM and IgG serum antibodies. Monoclonal gammopathy of the IgG class can occur in congenitally infected infants. IgM levels may be increased in newborns with congenital infection. The polyclonal IgG antibodies evoked by infection are parasiticidal in vitro in the presence of serum complement and are the basis for the Sabin-Feldman dye test. However, cell-mediated immunity is the major protective response evoked by the parasite during host infection. Macrophages are activated following phagocytosis of antibody-opsonized parasites. This activation can lead to death of the parasite by either an oxygen-dependent or an oxygen-independent process. If the parasite is not phagocytosed and enters the macrophage by active penetration, it continues to replicate, and this replication may represent the mechanism for transport and dissemination to distant organs. *Toxoplasma* stimulates a robust interleukin (IL) 12 response by human dendritic cells. The CD4+ and CD8+ T cell responses are antigen-specific and further stimulate the production of a variety of important lymphokines that expand the T cell and natural killer cell repertoire. *T. gondii* is a potent inducer of a T$_{\rm H}$1 phenotype, with IL-12 and IFN-γ playing an essential role in the control of the parasites' growth in the host. Regulation of the inflammatory response is at least partially under the control of a T$_{\rm H}$2 response that includes the production of IL-4 and IL-10 in seropositive individuals. Both asymptomatic patients and those with active infection may show a depression in the ratio of CD4+ to CD8+ lymphocytes. This shift may be correlated with a disease syndrome but is not necessarily correlated with disease outcome. Human T cell clones of both the CD4+ and the CD8+ phenotypes are cytolytic against parasite-infected macrophages. These T cell clones produce cytokines that are "microbistatic." IL-18, IL-7, and IL-15 upregulate the production of IFN-γ and may be important during acute and chronic infection. The effect of IFN-γ may be paradoxical, with stimulation of a host downregulatory response as well.

Although in patients with AIDS *T. gondii* infection is believed to be recrudescent, determination of antibody titers is not helpful in establishing reactivation. Because of the severe depletion in CD4+ T cells, quite frequently there is no observed increase in antibody titer during exacerbation of infection. T cells from AIDS patients with reactivation of toxoplasmosis fail to secrete both IFN-γ and IL-2. This alteration in the production of these critical immune cytokines contributes to the persistence of infection. *Toxoplasma* infection frequently develops late in the course of AIDS, when the loss of T cell–dependent protective mechanisms, particularly CD8+ T cells, becomes most pronounced.

CLINICAL MANIFESTATIONS   In persons whose immune systems are intact, acute toxoplasmosis is usually asymptomatic and self-limited. This condition can go unrecognized in 80 to 90% of adults and children with acquired infection. The asymptomatic nature of this infection makes diagnosis difficult in mothers infected during pregnancy. In contrast, the wide range of clinical manifestations in congenitally infected children includes severe neurologic complications such as hydrocephalus, microcephaly, mental retardation, and chorioretinitis. If prenatal infection is severe, multiorgan failure and subsequent intrauterine fetal death can occur. In children and adults, chronic infection can persist throughout life, with little consequence to the immunocompetent host.

Toxoplasmosis in the Immunocompetent Person   The most common manifestation of acute toxoplasmosis is cervical lymphadenopathy. The nodes may be single or multiple, are usually nontender, are discrete, and vary in firmness. Lymphadenopathy also may be found in suboccipital, supraclavicular, inguinal, and mediastinal areas. Generalized lymphadenopathy occurs in 20 to 30% of symptomatic patients. Between 20 and 40% of patients with lymphadenopathy also have headache, malaise, fatigue, and fever [usually with a temperature of <40°C (<104°F)]. A smaller proportion of symptomatic individuals have myalgia, sore throat, abdominal pain, maculopapular rash, meningoencephalitis, and confusion. Rare complications associated with infection in the normal immune host include pneumonia, myocarditis, encephalopathy, pericarditis, and polymyositis. Symptoms associated with acute infection usually resolve within several weeks, although the lymphadenopathy may persist for some months. In a recent epidemic, toxoplasmosis was diagnosed correctly in only 3 of the 25 patients who consulted physicians. If toxoplasmosis is considered in the differential diagnosis, routine laboratory and serologic screening should be performed before node biopsy.

The results of routine laboratory studies are usually unremarkable except for minimal lymphocytosis, an elevated sedimentation rate, and a nominal increase in liver aminotransferases. Evaluation of cerebrospinal fluid (CSF) in cases with evidence of encephalopathy or meningoencephalitis shows an elevation of intracranial pressure, mononuclear pleocytosis (10 to 50 cells/mL), a slight increase in protein concentration, and (occasionally) an increase in the gamma globulin level. PCR amplification of the *Toxoplasma* DNA target sequence in the CSF may be beneficial. The CSF of chronically infected individuals is normal.

Ocular Infection   Infection with *T. gondii* is estimated to cause 35% of all cases of chorioretinitis in the United States and Europe. Most ocular involvement is believed to be due to congenital infection, with a very low incidence following acquired infection. Between 1 and 3% of all patients with AIDS develop debilitating chorioretinitis due to *T. gondii*. A variety of ocular manifestations are documented, including blurred vision, scotoma, photophobia, and eye pain. Macular

involvement occurs with loss of central vision, and nystagmus is secondary to poor fixation. Involvement of the extraocular muscles may lead to disorders of convergence and to strabismus. Ophthalmologic examination should be undertaken in newborns with suspected congenital infection. As the inflammation resolves, vision improves, but episodic flare-ups of chorioretinitis, which progressively destroy retinal tissue and lead to glaucoma, are common.

The ophthalmologic examination reveals yellow-white, cotton-like patches with indistinct margins of hyperemia. As the lesions age, white plaques with distinct borders and black spots within the retinal pigment become more apparent. Lesions usually are located near the posterior pole of the retina; they may be single but are more commonly multiple. Congenital lesions may be unilateral or bilateral and show evidence of massive chorioretinal degeneration with extensive fibrosis. Surrounding these areas of involvement are a normal retina and vasculature. In patients with AIDS, retinal lesions are often large, with diffuse retinal necrosis, and include both free tachyzoites and cysts containing bradyzoites. Toxoplasmic chorioretinitis may be a prodrome to the development of encephalitis.

Infection of the Immunocompromised Person   Patients with AIDS and those receiving immunosuppressive therapy for lymphoproliferative disorders are at greatest risk for developing acute toxoplasmosis. This predilection may be due either to reactivation of latent infection or to acquisition of parasites from exogenous sources such as blood or transplanted organs. In individuals with AIDS, more than 95% of cases of *Toxoplasma* encephalitis are believed to be due to recrudescent infection. In most of these cases, encephalitis develops when the CD4+ cell count falls below 100/μL. In the immunocompromised individual, the disease may be rapidly fatal if untreated. Thus accurate diagnosis and initiation of appropriate therapy are necessary to prevent fulminant infection.

Toxoplasmosis is a principal opportunistic infection of the CNS in persons with AIDS. Although geographic origin may be related to frequency of infection, it has no correlation with the severity of disease in the immunocompromised host. Individuals with AIDS who are seropositive for *T. gondii* are at a very high risk for developing encephalitis. In the United States, about one-third of the 15 to 40% of adult patients with AIDS who are latently infected with the parasite develop *Toxoplasma* encephalitis.

The signs and symptoms of acute toxoplasmosis in the immunocompromised patient are principally within the CNS. More than 50% of patients with clinical manifestations have intracerebral involvement. Clinical findings at the time of presentation range from nonfocal to focal dysfunction. These findings include encephalopathy, meningoencephalitis, and mass lesions. Patients may present with altered mental status (75%), fever (10 to 72%), seizures (33%), headaches (56%), and focal neurologic findings (60%), including motor deficits, cranial nerve palsies, movement disorders, dysmetria, visual-field loss, and aphasia. Patients who present with evidence of diffuse cortical dysfunction develop evidence of focal neurologic disease as the infection progresses. This altered condition is due not only to the necrotizing encephalitis caused by direct invasion of the parasite but also to secondary effects, including vasculitis, edema, and hemorrhage. The onset of infection can range from an insidious process over several weeks to an acute confusional state with fulminant focal deficits, including hemiparesis, hemiplegia, visual-field defects, localized headache, and focal seizures.

Although lesions can occur anywhere within the CNS, the areas most involved appear to be the brainstem, basal ganglia, pituitary gland, and corticomedullary junction. Brainstem involvement gives rise to a variety of neurologic dysfunctions, including cranial nerve palsy, dysmetria, and ataxia. With basal ganglionic infection, patients may develop hydrocephalus, choreiform movements, and choreoathetosis. Because *Toxoplasma* usually causes encephalitis, meningeal involvement is uncommon, and thus CSF findings may be unremarkable or may include a modest increase in cell count and in protein—but not glucose—concentration.

Cerebral toxoplasmosis needs to be differentiated from other opportunistic infections or tumors within the CNS of those afflicted with AIDS. The differential diagnosis includes herpes simplex encephalitis, cryptococcal meningitis, progressive multifocal leukoencephalopathy, and primary CNS lymphoma. Involvement of the pituitary gland can give rise to panhypopituitarism and hyponatremia from inappropriate secretion of vasopressin (antidiuretic hormone). AIDS-dementia complex may present as cognitive impairment, attention loss, and altered memory. Brain biopsy in those patients who have been treated for *Toxoplasma* encephalitis but who continue to exhibit neurologic dysfunction often fails to identify organisms.

Autopsies of patients infected with *Toxoplasma* have demonstrated the involvement of multiple organs, including the lungs, gastrointestinal tract, pancreas, skin, eyes, heart, and liver. *Toxoplasma* pneumonia can occur and can be confused with *Pneumocystis carinii* infection. Respiratory involvement usually presents as dyspnea, fever, and a nonproductive cough and may rapidly progress to acute respiratory failure with hemoptysis, metabolic acidosis, hypotension, and (occasionally) disseminated intravascular coagulation. Histopathologic studies demonstrate necrosis and a mixed cellular infiltrate. The presence of organisms is a helpful diagnostic indicator, but organisms can also be found in healthy tissue. Infection of the heart is usually asymptomatic but can be associated with cardiac tamponade or biventricular failure. Infections of the gastrointestinal tract and the liver have been documented.

A presumptive clinical diagnosis of toxoplasmic encephalitis in patients with AIDS is based on clinical presentation, history of exposure as evidenced by positive serology, and radiologic evaluation. When these criteria are used, the predictive value is as high as 80%. More than 97% of patients with AIDS and toxoplasmosis have IgG antibody to the parasite in their sera. IgM serum antibody is usually not demonstrable. Intrathecal antibody to *T. gondii* may be present. Neuroradiologic evaluation should include double-dose contrast computed tomography (CT) of the head. By this test, single and frequently multiple contrast-enhancing lesions (<2 cm) may be identified. Magnetic resonance imaging (MRI) usually demonstrates multiple lesions and provides a more sensitive evaluation of the efficacy of therapy than does CT. Patients with primary CNS lymphoma are four times more likely than patients with *Toxoplasma* encephalitis to have solitary lesions on an MRI scan. A therapeutic trial of anti-*Toxoplasma* medications is frequently used to assess the diagnosis. Treatment of presumptive *Toxoplasma* encephalitis with pyrimethamine/clindamycin results in quantifiable clinical improvement in more than 50% of patients by day 3. By day 7, more than 90% of treated patients show evidence of improvement. In contrast, if patients fail to respond or have lymphoma, clinical signs and symptoms worsen by day 7. Patients in this category require brain biopsy with or without a change in therapy. This procedure can now be performed by a stereotactic CT-guided method that reduces the potential for complications. Brain biopsy for *T. gondii* identifies organisms in 50 to 75% of cases. Some studies indicate that PCR amplification of target genes significantly increases the sensitivity of detection of parasites.

Congenital Toxoplasmosis Between 400 and 4000 infants born each year in the United States are affected by congenital toxoplasmosis. Infection of the placenta leads to hematogenous infection of the fetus. As has already been stated, the proportion of fetuses that become infected increases but the clinical severity of the infection declines as gestation proceeds. Persistence of the parasite can ultimately result in reactivation and further damage decades later. Factors associated with relatively severe disabilities include delayed diagnosis and initiation of therapy, neonatal hypoxia and hypoglycemia, profound visual impairment, uncorrected hydrocephalus, and increased intracranial pressure. If treated appropriately, upwards of 70% of children have normal developmental, neurologic, and ophthalmologic findings at follow-up evaluations. Treatment for 1 year with pyrimethamine and sulfonamide is tolerated with minimal toxicity (see below).

DIAGNOSIS **Tissue and Body Fluids** The diagnosis of acute toxoplasmosis can be made by isolation of the parasite from blood or other body fluids after subinoculation of the sample into the peritoneal cavity of mice. Mice should be tested for organisms in the peritoneal fluid 6 to 10 days after inoculation. If no parasites are found in the mouse's peritoneal fluid, its anti-*Toxoplasma* serum titer can be evaluated 4 to 6 weeks after inoculation. Isolation of *T. gondii* from the patient's body fluids reflects acute infection, whereas isolation from biopsied tissue is an indication only of the presence of tissue cysts and should not be misinterpreted as acute toxoplasmosis. Persistent parasitemia in patients with latent, asymptomatic infection is rare. Histologic examination of lymph nodes may suggest the characteristic changes described above. Demonstration of tachyzoites in lymph nodes establishes the diagnosis of acute toxoplasmosis. Like subinoculation into mice, histologic demonstration of cysts containing bradyzoites confirms prior infection with *T. gondii* but is nondiagnostic for acute infection.

Serology The procedures just described have great diagnostic value but are limited by difficulties encountered either in the growth of parasites in vivo or in the identification of tachyzoites by histochemical methods. Serologic testing has become the routine method of diagnosis. A wide range of serologic tests that can be used to measure antibody to *T. gondii* are available commercially.

Diagnosis of acute infection with *T. gondii* can be established by detection of the simultaneous presence of IgG and IgM antibody to *Toxoplasma* in serum. The presence of circulating IgA favors the diagnosis of an acute infection. The Sabin-Feldman dye test, the indirect fluorescent antibody test, and the enzyme-linked immunosorbent assay (ELISA) all satisfactorily measure circulating IgG antibody to *Toxoplasma*. Positive IgG titers (>1:10) can be detected as early as 2 to 3 weeks after infection. These titers usually peak at 6 to 8 weeks and decline slowly to a new baseline level that persists for life. It is necessary to measure the serum IgM titer in concert with the IgG titer to better establish the time of infection. The methods currently available for this determination are the double-sandwich IgM-ELISA and the IgM-immunosorbent assay (IgM-ISAGA). Both of these assays are specific and sensitive, and their use precludes the false-positive results associated with rheumatoid factor and antinuclear antibody. The double-sandwich IgA-ELISA is more sensitive than the IgM-ELISA for detecting congenital infection in the fetus and newborn.

The Immunocompetent Adult or Child For the patient who presents with lymphadenopathy only, a positive IgM titer is an indication of acute infection—and an indication for therapy, if that is clinically warranted (see "Treatment" below). The serum IgM titer should be determined again in 3 weeks. An elevation in the IgG titer without an increase in the IgM titer suggests that infection is present but that it is not acute. If there is a borderline increase in either IgG or IgM, the titers should be assessed again in 3 to 4 weeks.

Ocular Toxoplasmosis Because of the congenital nature of ocular toxoplasmosis, the serum antibody titer may not correlate with the presence of active lesions in the fundus. In general, a positive IgG titer (measured in undiluted serum if necessary) in conjunction with typical lesions establishes the diagnosis. If lesions are atypical and the titer is in the low-positive range, the diagnosis is presumptive. The parasitic antigen-specific polyclonal IgG assay as well as the parasitic antigen-specific PCR may facilitate the diagnosis.

The Immunocompromised Host As discussed above, in patients with AIDS, the presence of IgG and radiologic findings consistent with toxoplasmosis are grounds for a presumptive diagnosis. Attempts to evaluate rising IgG titers or to determine whether IgM is present are not productive. Serologic evidence of infection virtually always precedes the development of *Toxoplasma* encephalitis. It is therefore important to determine the *Toxoplasma* antibody status of all patients infected with HIV. Antibody titers may range from negative to 1:1024 in patients with AIDS and *Toxoplasma* encephalitis. Fewer than 3% of patients have no demonstrable antibody to *Toxoplasma* at the time of diagnosis. Determination of the intrathecal antibody titer may be useful in identifying prior infection. PCR amplification of genetic material of the parasite found in the CSF may prove diagnostically beneficial in the future.

Patients with toxoplasmic encephalitis have focal or multifocal abnormalities demonstrable by CT or MRI. These findings are not pathognomonic of *Toxoplasma* infection since 40% of CNS lymphomas are multifocal and 50% are ring-enhancing. Lesions on MRI scan are multiple and are located in both hemispheres, with the basal ganglia and corticomedullary junction most commonly involved. For both MRI and CT scans, the rate of false-negative results is approximately 10%. The finding of a single lesion on an MRI scan increases the suspicion of primary lymphoma and strengthens the argument for the performance of a brain biopsy.

Now used in some centers, SPECT (single-photon emission CT) has been touted as a definitive means of detecting or ruling out *Toxoplasma* infection when a CNS lesion is suspected. In the future, SPECT may well be widely used for this purpose.

As in other conditions, the radiologic response may lag behind the clinical response. Resolution of lesions may take from 3 weeks to 6 months. Some patients show clinical improvement despite worsening radiographic findings.

A presumptive diagnosis of *Toxoplasma* encephalitis should prompt the immediate initiation of therapy. After 3 weeks, repeat radiologic studies should detect improvement. If glucocorticoids have been administered, radiologic studies should be repeated at the time of discontinuation to determine whether an exacerbation of disease has occurred. If the patient's clinical condition becomes worse, performance of a biopsy must be strongly considered.

Congenital Infection   The issue of concern when a pregnant woman has evidence of recent *T. gondii* infection is obviously whether the fetus is infected. PCR of the amniotic fluid to detect the B1 gene of the parasite has replaced fetal blood sampling. Serologic diagnosis is based on the persistence of IgG antibody or a positive IgM titer after the first week of life (a time frame that excludes placental leak). The IgG determination should be repeated every 2 months. An increase in IgM beyond the first week of life is indicative of acute infection. However, up to 25% of infected newborns may be seronegative and have normal routine physical examinations. Thus assessment of the eye and the brain, with ophthalmologic testing, CSF evaluation, and radiologic studies, is important in establishing the diagnosis.

TREATMENT   Current therapeutic protocols are directed at folate metabolism, protein synthesis, or nucleic acid synthesis of the parasite. Pyrimethamine and trimethoprim inhibit the enzyme dihydrofolate reductase. Inhibitors of protein synthesis, including clindamycin, chlortetracycline, and azithromycin, affect growth of the parasite. Inhibitors of purine synthesis, such as arprinocid, may prove to be important. Atovaquone, which blocks pyrimidine salvage, has demonstrated activity against both *T. gondii* and *P. carinii*.

Immunologically competent adults and older children who have only lymphadenopathy do not require specific therapy unless they have persistent and severe symptoms. Patients with ocular toxoplasmosis should be treated for 1 month with pyrimethamine plus either sulfadiazine or clindamycin. Prenatal antibiotic therapy can reduce the number of infants severely affected by *Toxoplasma* infection.

Congenital Infection   Congenitally infected neonates are treated with daily oral pyrimethamine (0.5 to 1 mg/kg) and sulfadiazine (100 mg/kg) for 1 year. In addition, therapy with spiramycin (100 mg/kg per day) plus prednisone (1 mg/kg per day) has been shown to be efficacious for congenital infection.

Infection in Immunocompromised Patients   Patients with AIDS should be treated for acute toxoplasmosis; in the immunocompromised patient, toxoplasmosis is rapidly fatal if untreated. The main-

stay of treatment for *Toxoplasma* encephalitis in immunocompromised patients is a combination regimen. Administered together for 4 to 6 weeks or until radiologic improvement is documented, pyrimethamine (a 200-mg loading dose followed by 50 to 75 mg/d) and sulfadiazine (4 to 6 g/d in four divided doses) block folic acid metabolism and reduce the parasite burden. Leucovorin (calcium folinate, 10 to 15 mg/d) is given as an adjunct to prevent the bone marrow toxicity associated with pyrimethamine. Both pyrimethamine and sulfadiazine cross the blood-brain barrier. A prominent consequence of dual therapy is the high incidence of associated toxicity (40%). Rash may develop during the first 3 weeks in up to 20% of patients but does not preclude the use of this combination. Other complications include hematologic effects, crystalluria, hematuria, radiolucent renal stones, and nephrotoxicity. During therapy, serum levels of these drugs may be erratic, but such fluctuations have not been correlated with these complications.

Pyrimethamine and sulfadiazine are active only against the tachyzoite stage of the parasite. Thus, after immunocompromised patients complete the initial 4- to 6-week course, they must receive lifelong suppressive therapy with pyrimethamine (25 to 50 mg/d) and sulfadiazine (2 to 4 g/d). If sulfadiazine cannot be tolerated, a combination of pyrimethamine (75 mg/d) plus clindamycin (450 mg tid) can be used. It is possible that pyrimethamine (50 to 75 mg/d) is sufficient for chronic suppressive therapy.

Alternative Regimens   Alternative therapies have been established because of the toxicity associated with the long-term antimicrobial therapy necessary for many individuals infected with *T. gondii*. Dapsone (diaminodiphenyl sulfone), with its longer serum half-life and decreased toxicity, is an effective alternative to sulfadiazine. Spiramycin, which has been used in Europe to treat pregnant women, reduces transplacental transmission. However, spiramycin has been ineffective as primary prophylaxis in patients with AIDS. Clindamycin is well absorbed from the gastrointestinal tract, and serum levels peak 1 to 2 h after administration. The combination of oral pyrimethamine (25 to 75 mg/d) plus intravenous clindamycin (1200 to 4800 mg/d) is effective for patients with AIDS who have *Toxoplasma* encephalitis. Toxic effects of clindamycin include nausea, vomiting, neutropenia, rash, and pseudomembranous colitis. Other macrolides that have been evaluated include roxithromycin, clarithromycin, and azithromycin. Evidence suggests that the macrolides are not beneficial by themselves, but a combination of pyrimethamine and clarithromycin appears to be effective. Atovaquone (750 mg tid or qid) is an optional agent for the treatment of individuals who are intolerant of other agents. Glucocorticoids can be used to treat intracerebral edema, but their benefit has not yet been established. It is difficult to assess the benefit of glucocorticoids when they are administered in conjunction with anti-*Toxoplasma* medication. Anticonvulsants are sometimes necessary for the treatment of seizures, but attention should be given to the potential interaction between sulfadiazine and phenytoin. A regimen of trimethoprim-sulfamethoxazole or dapsone plus pyrimethamine with leucovorin may prevent the development of *Toxoplasma* encephalitis in individuals infected with HIV who are seropositive for *T. gondii* after their CD4+ T lymphocyte count falls to 100/μL.

PREVENTION   The chances of primary infection with *Toxoplasma* can be reduced by not eating undercooked meat and by avoiding oocyst-contaminated material (i.e., a cat's litter box). Meat should be heated to 60°C or frozen to kill cysts. Hands should be washed thoroughly after work in the garden, and all fruits and vegetables should be washed. Blood intended for transfusion into *Toxoplasma*-seronegative immunocompromised individuals should be screened for antibody to *T. gondii*. Although such serologic screening is not routinely performed, seronegative women should be screened for evidence of infection several times during pregnancy if they are exposed to environmental conditions that put them at risk for infection with *T. gondii*. HIV-positive individuals should adhere closely to these preventive measures.

FICHERA ME, ROOS DS: A plastid organelle as a drug target in apicomplexa parasites. Nature 390:407, 1997

FOULON W et al: Treatment of toxoplasmosis during pregnancy. Am J Obstet Gynecol 180:410, 1999

HOWE D, SIBLEY LD: *T. gondii* comprises three clonal lineages: Correlation of genotype with human disease. J Infect Dis 172:1561, 1995

MCLEOD R et al: Immunogenetics in pathogenesis of and protection against toxoplasmosis. Curr Top Microbiol Immunol 219:95, 1996

METS MB et al: Eye manifestations of congenital toxoplasmosis. Am J Ophthalmol 123:1, 1997

PODZAMCZER D et al: Intermittent trimethoprim-sulfamethoxazole compared with dapsone-pyrimethamine for the simultaneous primary prophylaxis of *Pneumocystis* pneumonia and toxoplasmosis in patients infected with HIV. Ann Intern Med 122:755, 1995

REMINGTON JS et al: Toxoplasmosis, in *Infectious Diseases of the Fetus and Newborn Infant*, 4th ed, JS Remington, JO Klein (eds). Philadelphia, Saunders, 1994

ROBERTS F et al: Evidence for the shikimato pathway in apicomplexa parasites. Nature 393:801, 1998

SEGUIN R, KASPER LH: Sensitized lymphocytes and CD40 ligation augment IL-12 production by human dendritic cells in response to *T. gondii*. J Infect Dis 179:467, 1999

VILLENA I et al: Pyrimethamine-sulfadoxine treatment of congenital toxoplasmosis. Scand J Infect Dis 30:295, 1998

218 *Peter F. Weller*

PROTOZOAL INTESTINAL INFECTIONS AND TRICHOMONIASIS

PROTOZOAL INFECTIONS

GIARDIASIS *Giardia lamblia* is a cosmopolitan protozoal parasite that inhabits the small intestines of humans and other mammals. Giardiasis is one of the most common parasitic diseases worldwide and causes both endemic and epidemic intestinal disease and diarrhea.

Life Cycle and Epidemiology Infection follows the ingestion of the environmentally hardy cysts, which excyst in the small intestine, releasing trophozoites that multiply by binary fission, occasionally to enormous numbers. *Giardia* remains a pathogen of the proximal small bowel and does not disseminate hematogenously. Trophozoites remain free in the lumen or attach to the mucosal epithelium by means of a ventral sucking disk. As a trophozoite encounters altered conditions, it forms a morphologically distinct cyst, which is the stage of the parasite usually found in the feces. Trophozoites may be present and even predominate in loose or watery stools, but it is the resistant cyst that survives outside the body and is responsible for transmission. Cysts do not tolerate heating, desiccation, or continued exposure to feces but do remain viable for months in cold fresh water. The number of cysts excreted varies widely but can approach 10^7 per gram of stool.

Giardia infections are common in both developed and developing countries. Ingestion of as few as 10 cysts is sufficient to cause infection in humans. Because cysts are infectious when excreted or shortly thereafter, person-to-person transmission occurs where fecal hygiene is poor. Giardiasis, as a symptomatic or an asymptomatic infection, is especially prevalent in day-care centers; person-to-person spread also takes place in other institutional settings with poor fecal hygiene and during homosexual contact. If food is contaminated with *Giardia* cysts after cooking or preparation, food-borne transmission can occur. Waterborne transmission accounts for episodic infections (e.g., in campers and other travelers) and for massive epidemics in metropolitan areas. Surface water, ranging from mountain streams to large municipal res-

ervoirs, can become contaminated with fecally derived *Giardia* cysts; outmoded water systems are subject to cross-contamination from leaking sewer lines. The efficacy of water as a means of transmission is enhanced by the small infectious inoculum of *Giardia*, the prolonged survival of cysts in cold water, and the resistance of cysts to killing by routine chlorination methods that are adequate for controlling bacteria. Viable cysts can be eradicated from water by either boiling or filtration. In the United States, *Giardia* is a common agent identified in waterborne epidemics of gastroenteritis; it is also common in developing countries.

The importance of animal reservoirs as sources of infection for humans is unclear. *Giardia* parasites morphologically similar to those in humans are found in a large number of mammals, including beavers from reservoirs implicated in epidemics, dogs, cats, and ruminants. Although the high degree of isolate heterogeneity noted in humans is consistent with infections originating from different animal sources, animals have not been directly established as sources of human infection.

Giardiasis, like cryptosporidiosis, creates a significant economic burden because of the costs incurred in the installation of water filtration systems required to prevent waterborne epidemics, in the management of epidemics that involve large communities, and in the evaluation and treatment of endemic infections.

Pathophysiology The reasons that some, but not all, infected patients develop clinical manifestations and the mechanisms by which *Giardia* causes alterations in small-bowel function are largely unknown. Although trophozoites adhere to the epithelium, they do not cause invasive or locally destructive alterations. The lactose intolerance and significant malabsorption that develop in a minority of infected adults and children are clinical signs of the loss of brush border enzyme activities. In most infections the morphology of the bowel is unaltered, but in a few cases—usually in chronically infected, symptomatic patients—the histopathologic findings (including flattened villi) and the clinical manifestations resemble those of tropical sprue and gluten-sensitive enteropathy. The pathogenesis of diarrhea in giardiasis is not known.

The natural history of *Giardia* infection varies markedly. Infections may be aborted, transient, recurrent, or chronic. Parasite as well as host factors may be important in determining the course of infection and disease. Both cellular and humoral responses develop in human infections, but their precise roles in the control of infection and/or disease are unknown. Because patients with hypogammaglobulinemia commonly suffer from prolonged, severe infections that are poorly responsive to treatment, humoral immune responses appear to be important. The greater susceptibility of the young than of the old and of newly exposed persons than of chronically exposed populations also suggests that at least partial protective immunity may develop. Although no strains of the parasite that are clearly nonpathogenic have been identified, *Giardia* isolates vary biochemically and biologically. The marked biochemical differences among some isolates may help account for the different courses of infection in experimentally infected humans and animals. The surface of trophozoites is covered by a family of related cysteine-rich proteins that undergo surface antigenic variation and may contribute to prolonged and/or repeated infections.

Clinical Manifestations Disease manifestations of giardiasis range from asymptomatic carriage to fulminant diarrhea and malabsorption. Most infected persons are asymptomatic, but in epidemics the proportion of symptomatic cases may be higher. Symptoms may develop suddenly or gradually. In persons with acute giardiasis, symptoms develop after an incubation period that lasts at least 5 to 6 days and usually 1 to 3 weeks. Prominent early symptoms include diarrhea, abdominal pain, bloating, belching, flatus, nausea, and vomiting. Although diarrhea is common, upper intestinal manifestations such as nausea, vomiting, bloating, and abdominal pain may predominate. The duration of acute giardiasis is usually in excess of 1 week, although diarrhea often subsides. Individuals with chronic giardiasis may present with or without having experienced an antecedent acute symptomatic episode. Diarrhea is not necessarily prominent, but increased flatus, loose stools, sulfurous burping, and (in some instances) weight loss occur. Symptoms may be continual or episodic and can persist for years. Some persons who have relatively mild symptoms for long periods recognize the extent of their discomfort only in retrospect. Fever, the presence of blood and/or mucus in the stools, and other signs and symptoms of colitis are uncommon and suggest a different diagnosis or a concomitant illness. Symptoms tend to be intermittent yet recurring and gradually debilitating, in contrast with the acute disabling symptoms associated with many enteric bacterial infections. Because of the less severe illness and the propensity for chronic infections, patients may seek medical advice late in the course of the illness; however, disease can be severe, resulting in malabsorption, weight loss, growth retardation, dehydration, and (in rare cases) death. A number of extraintestinal manifestations have been described, such as urticaria, anterior uveitis, and arthritis; whether these are caused by giardiasis or concomitant processes is unclear.

Giardiasis can be life-threatening in patients with hypogammaglobulinemia and is typically difficult to treat and eradicate. *Giardia* infections can complicate other preexisting intestinal diseases, such as cystic fibrosis. Although *Giardia* can cause enteric illness in patients with AIDS, neither the course of infection nor the response to treatment differs for patients with and without AIDS.

Diagnosis Giardiasis is diagnosed by the detection of parasite antigen in the feces or by the identification of cysts in the feces or of trophozoites in the feces or small intestines. Cysts are oval, measure 8 to 12 μm $\times$ 7 to 10 μm, and characteristically contain four nuclei. Trophozoites are pear-shaped, dorsally convex, flattened parasites with two nuclei and four pairs of flagella. The diagnosis is sometimes difficult to establish. Direct examination of fresh or properly preserved stools as well as concentration methods should be used. Because cyst excretion is variable and may be undetectable at times, repeated examination of stool, sampling of duodenal fluid, and biopsy of the small intestine may be required to detect the parasite. Tests for parasitic antigen in stool are at least as sensitive and specific as good microscopic examinations and are easier to perform. All of these methods occasionally yield false-negative results.

℞ TREATMENT Cure rates with metronidazole (250 mg tid for 5 days) are usually >80%; those with furazolidone (100 mg qid for 7 to 10 days) are somewhat lower. The latter agent is frequently used to treat children because it is available as a palatable elixir that is not bitter. Quinacrine, the first effective drug for the treatment of giardiasis, is available from a limited number of pharmacies. Albendazole (400 mg/d for 5 days) may be effective.

Patients in whom initial treatment fails can be re-treated with a longer course. Almost all patients respond to therapy and are cured, although some with chronic giardiasis experience delayed resolution of symptoms after eradication of *Giardia*. Those who remain infected after repeated treatments should be evaluated for reinfection through family members, close personal contacts, and environmental sources as well as for hypogammaglobulinemia. In cases refractory to multiple treatment courses, prolonged therapy with metronidazole (750 mg tid for 21 days) has been successful. Tinidazole, not available in the United States, is considered more effective than metronidazole or quinacrine. When children attending day-care centers infect an entire family, treatment of all infected family members, including asymptomatic carriers, may be required to prevent reinfection. Paromomycin, an oral aminoglycoside that is not well absorbed, can be given to symptomatic pregnant women, although the experience accumulated thus far is not a sufficient basis on which to judge how often this agent either eradicates infection or ameliorates symptoms.

Prevention Although *Giardia* is extremely infectious, disease can be prevented by the exclusive consumption of noncontaminated food and water. Cooking food adequately and boiling or filtering potentially contaminated water prevent infection.

CRYPTOSPORIDIOSIS The coccidian parasite *Cryptosporidium* is now known to cause diarrheal disease in immunocompetent human hosts and to be especially common among persons with AIDS or other forms of immunodeficiency.

Life Cycle and Epidemiology Cryptosporidiosis is acquired by the consumption of oocysts (50% infectious dose: ~132 oocysts in nonimmune individuals), which excyst to liberate sporozoites that in turn enter and infect intestinal epithelial cells. The parasite's further development involves both asexual and sexual cycles, which produce forms capable of infecting other epithelial cells and of generating oocysts that are passed in the feces. *Cryptosporidium* spp. infect a number of animals and can spread from infected animals to humans. Since oocysts are immediately infectious when passed in feces, person-to-person transmission takes place in day-care centers and among household contacts and medical providers. Waterborne transmission accounts for infections in travelers and for common-source epidemics. Oocysts are quite hardy and resist killing by routine chlorination. Both drinking water and recreational water (e.g., pools, waterslides) have been increasingly recognized as sources of infection.

Pathophysiology Although intestinal epithelial cells harbor the parasite in an intracellular vacuole, the means by which secretory diarrhea is elicited remain uncertain. No characteristic pathologic changes are found by biopsy. The distribution of infection can be spotty within the principal site of infection, the small bowel. Cryptosporidia are found in some patients in the pharynx, stomach, and large bowel and at times in the respiratory tract. Especially in patients with AIDS, involvement of the biliary tract can cause papillary stenosis, sclerosing cholangitis, or cholecystitis.

Clinical Manifestations Asymptomatic infections can occur in both immunocompetent and immunocompromised hosts. In immunocompetent persons, symptoms develop after an incubation period of about a week and consist principally of watery nonbloody diarrhea, at times in conjunction with abdominal pain, nausea, anorexia, fever, and/or weight loss. In these hosts, the illness usually subsides after 1 to 2 weeks, whereas in immunocompromised hosts, especially those with AIDS, diarrhea can be chronic, persistent, and remarkably profuse, causing clinically significant fluid and electrolyte depletion. Stool volumes may range from 1 to 25 L/d. Weight loss, wasting, and abdominal pain may be severe. Biliary tract involvement can manifest as midepigastric or right upper quadrant pain.

Diagnosis Evaluation usually starts with fecal examination for small oocysts, which are 4 to 5 μm in diameter and are smaller than the fecal stages of most other parasites. Detection is enhanced by evaluation of stools (obtained on multiple days) by several techniques, including modified acid-fast and direct immunofluorescent stains and enzyme immunoassays. Cryptosporidia also can be identified by light and electron microscopy at the apical surfaces of intestinal epithelium from biopsy specimens of the small bowel and, less frequently, the large bowel.

℞ TREATMENT To date, no chemotherapeutic agents effective against *Cryptosporidium* have been identified, although paromomycin (500 to 750 mg qid) may be partially effective for some patients infected with HIV. Improvement in immune status with antiretroviral therapy can lead to amelioration of cryptosporidiosis. Otherwise, treatment includes supportive care with replacement of fluids and electrolytes and administration of antidiarrheal agents. Biliary tract obstruction may require papillotomy or T-tube placement. Prevention requires minimizing exposure to infectious oocysts in human or animal feces. Use of submicron water filters may minimize acquisition of infection from drinking water.

ISOSPORIASIS The coccidian parasite *Isospora belli* causes human intestinal disease. Infection is acquired by the consumption of oocysts, after which the parasite invades intestinal epithelial cells and undergoes both sexual and asexual cycles of development. Oocysts excreted in stool are not immediately infectious but must undergo further maturation. Although *I. belli* infects many animals, little is known about the epidemiology or prevalence of this parasite in humans. It appears to be most common in tropical and subtropical countries. Acute infections can begin abruptly with fever, abdominal pain, and watery nonbloody diarrhea and can last for weeks or months. In patients who have AIDS or are immunocompromised for other reasons, infections often are not self-limited but rather resemble cryptosporidiosis, with chronic, profuse watery diarrhea. Eosinophilia, which is not found in other enteric protozoan infections, may be detectable. The diagnosis is usually made by detection of the large (~25-μm) oocysts in stool by modified acid-fast staining. Oocyst excretion may be low-level and intermittent; if repeated stool examinations are unrevealing, sampling of duodenal contents by aspiration or small-bowel biopsy (often with electron-microscopic examination) may be necessary.

In contrast to cryptosporidiosis, isosporiasis responds to chemotherapy. Trimethoprim-sulfamethoxazole (160/800 mg qid for 10 days and then bid for 3 weeks) has been effective; for patients intolerant of sulfonamides, pyrimethamine (50 to 75 mg/d) can be used. Relapses can occur in persons with AIDS and necessitate maintenance therapy with trimethoprim-sulfamethoxazole (160/800 mg three times a week) or combined sulfadoxine (500 mg) and pyrimethamine (25 mg) once weekly.

CYCLOSPORIASIS Coccidian parasites of the genus *Cyclospora* have been identified as the causative organisms in diarrheal illness formerly ascribed to blue-green algal or *Cyanobacteria*-like forms. This parasite is globally distributed: illness due to *Cyclospora cayetanensis* has been reported in the United States, Asia, Africa, Latin America, and Europe. The epidemiology of this parasite has not yet been fully defined, but waterborne transmission and especially transmission in imported raspberries have been recognized. The full spectrum of illness attributable to *Cyclospora* has not been delineated. Some patients may harbor the infection without symptoms, but many with cyclosporiasis have diarrhea, flulike symptoms, and flatulence and burping. The illness can be self-limited, can wax and wane, or (in many cases) can involve prolonged diarrhea, anorexia, and upper gastrointestinal symptoms, with sustained fatigue and weight loss in some instances. Diarrheal illness may persist for longer than a month. *Cyclospora* can cause enteric illness in patients infected with HIV, albeit at an unknown frequency.

The parasite is detectable in epithelial cells of small-bowel biopsy samples and elicits secretory diarrhea by an unknown means. The absence of fecal blood and leukocytes indicates that disease due to *Cyclospora* is not caused by destruction of the small-bowel mucosa. The diagnosis can be made by detection of spherical 8- to 10-μm oocysts in the stool, although routine stool O and P examinations are not sufficient. Specific fecal examinations must be requested to detect the oocysts, which are variably acid-fast and are fluorescent when viewed with ultraviolet light microscopy. Cyclosporiasis should be considered in the differential diagnosis of prolonged diarrhea, with or without a history of travel by the patient to other countries.

Cyclosporiasis is effectively treated with trimethoprim-sulfamethoxazole (160/800 mg bid for 7 days). Patients infected with HIV, however, may experience relapses after such treatment and thus may require longer-term suppressive maintenance therapy.

MICROSPORIDIOSIS Microsporidia are obligate intracellular spore-forming protozoa that infect many animals and cause disease in humans, especially as opportunistic pathogens in AIDS. Microsporidia are members of a distinct phylum, Microspora, which contains dozens of genera and hundreds of species. The various microsporidia are differentiated by their developmental life cycles, by ultrastructural features, and by molecular taxonomy based on ribosomal RNA. The complex life cycles of the organisms result in the production of infectious spores. Currently, six genera of microsporidia—*Encephalitozoon*, *Pleistophora*, *Nosema*, *Vittaforma*, *Trachipleistophora*, and *Enterocytozoon*—are recognized as causes of human disease; a seventh genus—*Microsporidium*, which includes organisms of uncertain taxonomic status—also causes disease in humans. Though some microsporidia are probably prevalent causes of self-limited or asymptomatic infections in immunocompetent patients, little is known of how microsporidiosis is acquired.

Microsporidiosis is most common among patients with AIDS, less common among patients with other types of immunocompromise, and rare among immunocompetent hosts. In patients with AIDS, intestinal infections with *Enterocytozoon bieneusi* and *Encephalitozoon* (formerly *Septata*) *intestinalis* are increasingly recognized to contribute to chronic diarrhea and wasting; these infections are found in 10 to 40% of patients with chronic diarrhea. Both organisms have been found in the biliary tracts of patients with cholecystitis. *E. intestinalis* may also disseminate to cause fever, diarrhea, sinusitis, cholangitis, and bronchiolitis. In patients with AIDS, *E. hellem* has caused superficial keratoconjunctivitis as well as sinusitis, respiratory tract disease, and disseminated infection. Myositis due to *Pleistophora* has been documented. *Nosema*, *Vittaforma*, and *Microsporidium* have caused stromal keratitis associated with trauma in immunocompetent patients.

Microsporidia are small gram-positive organisms with mature spores measuring 0.5 to 2 μm $\times$ 1 to 4 μm. Diagnosis of microsporidial infections in tissue often requires electron microscopy, although intracellular spores can be visualized by light microscopy with hematoxylin and eosin, Giemsa, or tissue Gram's stains. For the diagnosis of intestinal microsporidiosis, modified trichrome or chromotrope 2R-based staining and Uvitex 2B or calcofluor fluorescent staining reveal spores in smears of feces or duodenal aspirates. Definitive therapies for microsporidial infections remain to be established. For superficial keratoconjunctivitis due to *E. hellem*, topical therapy with fumagillin suspension has shown promise (Chap. 211). For enteric infections with *E. bieneusi* and *E. intestinalis* in HIV-infected patients, therapy with albendazole may be efficacious (Chap. 211).

OTHER INTESTINAL PROTOZOA **Balantidiasis** *Balantidium coli* is a large ciliated protozoal parasite that can produce a spectrum of large-intestinal disease analogous to amebiasis. The parasite is widely distributed in the world. Since it infects pigs, cases in humans are more common where pigs are raised; in Muslim countries, rodents may be important carriers. Infective cysts can be transmitted from person to person and through water, but many cases are due to the ingestion of cysts derived from porcine feces in association with slaughtering, with use of pig feces for fertilizer, or with contamination of water supplies by pig feces.

Ingested cysts liberate trophozoites, which reside and replicate in the large bowel. Many patients remain asymptomatic, but some have persisting intermittent diarrhea, and a few develop more fulminant dysentery. In symptomatic individuals, the pathology in the bowel—both gross and microscopic—is similar to that seen in amebiasis, with varying degrees of mucosal invasion, focal necrosis, and ulceration. Balantidiasis, unlike amebiasis, does not spread hematogenously to other organs. The diagnosis is usually made by detection of the trophozoite stage in stool or sampled colonic tissue. Tetracycline (500 mg qid for 10 days) is an effective therapeutic agent.

***Blastocystis hominis* Infection** *B. hominis*, long considered a nonpathogenic yeast, is believed by some to be a protozoan capable of causing intestinal disease, although its taxonomy and inherent pathogenicity remain uncertain. Some patients who pass *B. hominis* in their stools are asymptomatic, whereas others have diarrhea and associated intestinal symptoms. Diligent evaluation reveals other potential bacterial, viral, or protozoal causes of diarrhea in some but not all patients with symptoms. Because the pathogenicity of *B. hominis* is uncertain and because therapy for *Blastocystis* infection is neither specific nor uniformly effective, patients with prominent intestinal symptoms should be fully evaluated for other infectious causes of diarrhea. If diarrheal symptoms associated with *Blastocystis* are prominent, either metronidazole (750 mg tid for 10 days) or iodoquinol (650 mg tid for 20 days) can be used.

***Dientamoeba fragilis* Infection**   *D. fragilis* is unique among intestinal protozoa in that it has a trophozoite stage but not a cyst stage. How trophozoites survive to transmit infection is not known, but the unusually high prevalence of *D. fragilis* infection among persons with pinworm infection raises the possibility that eggs or larvae of *Enterobius* facilitate the transmission of *D. fragilis*. When symptoms develop in patients with *D. fragilis* infection, they are generally mild and include intermittent diarrhea, abdominal pain, and anorexia. The diagnosis is made by the detection of trophozoites in stool; the lability of these forms accounts for the greater yield when fecal samples are preserved immediately after collection. Since fecal excretion rates vary, examination of several samples obtained on alternate days increases the rate of detection. Iodoquinol (650 mg tid for 20 days), paromomycin (25 to 30 mg/kg per day in three doses for 7 days), or tetracycline (500 mg qid for 10 days) is appropriate for treatment.

Sarcosporidiosis   Various *Sarcocystis* spp. of coccidian parasites are widely distributed agents of infection in numerous animals. These parasites have an obligatory cycle of development involving two hosts. Sexual reproduction occurs in the intestine, with sporocysts passed in the feces; asexual multiplication leads to the development of muscle cysts. Humans can develop intestinal infections—albeit apparently infrequently—by ingesting muscle-stage cysts in undercooked pork or beef. While the full spectrum of the intestinal disease is not defined, a diarrheal illness can ensue, and sporocysts are found in the stool. Alternatively, ingestion of fecally derived sporocysts can lead to the development of cysts in striated or cardiac muscle. Some patients experience muscle pain and swelling, but the frequency and nature of symptoms elicited by muscle involvement are not clear, and these cysts, measuring 100 to 325 μm, also have been found incidentally in muscle specimens. Muscle-stage infections are not followed by further spread in humans. No specific therapy exists for either intestinal or muscle-stage *Sarcocystis* infections in humans.

TRICHOMONIASIS

Various species of trichomonads can be found in the mouth (in association with periodontitis) and occasionally in the gastrointestinal tract. *Trichomonas vaginalis*—one of the most prevalent protozoal parasites in the United States—is a pathogen of the genitourinary tract and a major cause of symptomatic vaginitis.

Life Cycle and Epidemiology   *T. vaginalis* is a pear-shaped, actively motile organism that measures about 10 by 7 μm, replicates by binary fission, and inhabits the lower genital tract of females and the urethra and prostate of males. In the United States, it accounts for about 3 million infections per year in women. While the organism can survive for a few hours in moist environments and could be acquired by direct contact, person-to-person venereal transmission accounts for virtually all cases of trichomoniasis. Its prevalence is greatest among persons with multiple sexual partners and among those with other sexually transmitted diseases.

Clinical Manifestations   Most men infected with *T. vaginalis* are asymptomatic, although some develop urethritis and a few have epididymitis or prostatitis. In contrast, infection in women, which has an incubation period of 5 to 28 days, is usually symptomatic and manifests with malodorous vaginal discharge (often yellow), vulvar erythema and itching, dysuria or urinary frequency (in 30 to 50% of pa-

tients), and dyspareunia. These manifestations, however, do not clearly distinguish trichomoniasis from other types of infectious vaginitis.

Diagnosis   Detection of motile trichomonads by microscopy of wet mounts of vaginal or prostatic secretions has been the conventional means of diagnosis. Although such microscopy provides an immediate diagnosis, its sensitivity for the detection of *T. vaginalis* is only ~50 to 60% in routine evaluations of vaginal secretions. Direct immunofluorescent antibody staining is more sensitive (70 to 90%) than wet-mount examinations. *T. vaginalis* can be recovered from the urethra of both males and females and is detectable in males after prostatic massage. Culture of the parasite is the most sensitive means of detection; however, the facilities for culture are not generally available, and detection of the organism takes 3 to 7 days.

℞ TREATMENT   Metronidazole is the mainstay of treatment and may be given either as a single 2-g dose or as 250 mg tid for 7 days. All sexual partners must be treated concurrently to prevent reinfection, especially from asymptomatic males. Alternatives to metronidazole for treatment during pregnancy are not readily available, although use of 100-mg clotrimazole vaginal suppositories nightly for 2 weeks may cure some infections in pregnant women. Reinfection often accounts for apparent treatment failures, but strains of *T. vaginalis* exhibiting high-level resistance to metronidazole have been encountered. Treatment of these resistant infections with higher oral doses, parenteral doses, or concurrent oral and vaginal doses of metronidazole has been successful.

BIBLIOGRAPHY

CHAPPELL CL et al: Infectivity of *Cryptosporidium parvum* in heathy adults with pre-existing anti–*C. parvum* serum immunoglobulin G. Am J Trop Med Hyg 60:157, 1999

EBERHARD ML et al: Laboratory diagnosis of *Cyclospora* infections. Arch Pathol Lab Med 121:792, 1997

EBRAHIMZADEH A, BOTTONE EJ: Persistent diarrhea caused by *Isospora belli*: Therapeutic response to pyrimethamine and sulfadiazine. Diagn Microbiol Infect Dis 26:87, 1996

FLEMING CA et al: A foodborne outbreak of *Cyclospora cayetanensis* at a wedding: Clinical features and risk factors for illness. Arch Intern Med 158:1121, 1998

GRIFFITHS JK: Human cryptosporidiosis: Epidemiology, transmission, clinical disease, treatment, and diagnosis. Adv Parasitol 40:37, 1998

HERWALDT BL, BEACH MJ: The return of *Cyclospora* in 1997: Another outbreak of cyclosporiasis in North America associated with imported raspberries. Cyclospora Working Group. Ann Intern Med 130:210, 1999

HORIKI N et al: Epidemiologic survey of *Blastocystis hominis* infection in Japan. Am J Trop Med Hyg 56:370, 1997

HOXIE NJ et al: Cryptosporidiosis-associated mortality following a massive waterborne outbreak in Milwaukee, Wisconsin. Am J Public Health 87:2032, 1997

KOTLER DP, ORENSTEIN JM: Clinical syndromes associated with microsporidiosis. Adv Parasitol 40:321, 1998

KRAMER MH et al: First reported outbreak in the United States of cryptosporidiosis associated with a recreational lake. Clin Infect Dis 26:27, 1998

LENGERICH EJ et al: Severe giardiasis in the United States. Clin Infect Dis 18:760, 1994

MANABE YC et al: Cryptosporidiosis in patients with AIDS: Correlates of disease and survival. Clin Infect Dis 27:536, 1998

MANK TG et al: Sensitivity of microscopy versus enzyme immunoassay in the laboratory diagnosis of giardiasis. Eur J Clin Microbiol Infect Dis 16:615, 1997

MOLINA JM et al: Albendazole for treatment and prophylaxis of microsporidiosis due to *Encephalitozoon intestinalis* in patients with AIDS: A randomized double-blind controlled trial. J Infect Dis 177:1373, 1998

OBERHUBER G et al: Giardiasis: A histologic analysis of 567 cases. Scand J Gastroenterol 32:48, 1997

ORTEGA YR et al: *Cyclospora cayetanensis*. Adv Parasitol 40:399, 1998

PETRIN D et al: Clinical and microbiological aspects of *Trichomonas vaginalis*. Clin Microbiol Rev 11:300, 1998

STEINER TS et al: Protozoal agents: What are the dangers for the public water supply? Annu Rev Med 48:329, 1997

219

Leo X. Liu, Peter F. Weller

TRICHINELLA AND OTHER TISSUE NEMATODES

Nematodes are elongated, symmetric roundworms. Parasitic nematodes of medical significance may be broadly classified as intestinal or tissue nematodes, but such a classification system is imprecise. This chapter covers trichinellosis, visceral and ocular larva migrans, cutaneous larva migrans, cerebral angiostrongyliasis, and gnathostomiasis. All are zoonotic infections caused by incidental exposure to infectious nematodes. The clinical symptoms of these infections are due largely to invasive larval stages that (except in the case of *Trichinella*) do not reach maturity in humans.

TRICHINELLOSIS Trichinellosis develops after the ingestion of meat containing cysts of *Trichinella*—for example, pork or other meat from a carnivore. While most infections are mild and asymptomatic, heavy infections can cause severe enteritis, periorbital edema, myositis, and (infrequently) death.

Life Cycle and Epidemiology Five species of *Trichinella* are now recognized as causes of infection in humans. Two species are distributed worldwide: *T. spiralis*, which is found in a great variety of carnivorous and omnivorous animals, and *T. pseudospiralis*, which is found in mammals and birds. *T. nativa* is present in Arctic regions and infects bears; *T. nelsoni* is found in equatorial Africa, where it is common among felid predators and scavengers such as hyenas and bush pigs; and *T. bitovi* is found in temperate areas of Europe and western Asia among carnivores but not among domestic swine.

After the consumption of trichinous meat by the host, encysted larvae are liberated by digestive acid and pepsin (Fig. 219-1). The larvae invade the small-bowel mucosa and mature rapidly into adult worms. After about 1 week, female worms release newborn larvae that migrate via the circulation to striated muscle. The larvae of all species except *T. pseudospiralis* then encyst by inducing a radical transformation in the muscle cell architecture. Although host immune responses may help to expel adult worms, they have little effect on muscle-dwelling larvae.

Human trichinellosis is most often caused by the ingestion of infected pork products and thus can occur in almost any location where the meat of domestic or wild swine is eaten. Human trichinellosis also may be acquired from the meat of other animals, including dogs (in parts of Asia and Africa), horses (in Italy and France), and bears and walruses (in northern regions). Although cattle (being herbivores) are not natural hosts of *Trichinella*, beef has been implicated in outbreaks when contaminated or adulterated with trichinous pork. Laws that prohibit the feeding of uncooked garbage to pigs have greatly reduced the transmission of trichinellosis in the United States. About 40 cases of trichinellosis are reported annually in this country, but most mild cases probably remain undiagnosed. Recent U.S. outbreaks have been attributable to undercooked ethnic pork dishes, homemade and commercial sausage, wild boar meat, and walrus meat.

Pathogenesis and Clinical Features Clinical symptoms of trichinellosis arise from the successive phases of parasite enteric invasion, larval migration, and muscle encystment (Fig. 219-1). Most light infections (those with <10 larvae per gram of muscle) are asymptomatic, whereas heavy infections (which can involve >50 larvae per gram of muscle) can be life-threatening. Invasion of the gut by large numbers of parasites occasionally provokes diarrhea during the first week after infection. Abdominal pain, constipation, nausea, or vomiting also may be prominent. The prolonged and fulminant diarrhea

noted with Arctic trichinellosis probably reflects a response to repeated infection.

Symptoms due to larval migration and muscle invasion begin to appear in the second week after infection. The migrating *Trichinella* larvae provoke a marked local and systemic hypersensitivity reaction, with fever and hypereosinophilia. Periorbital and facial edema is common, as are hemorrhages in the subconjunctivae, retina, and nail beds ("splinter" hemorrhages). A maculopapular rash, headache, cough, dyspnea, or dysphagia sometimes develops. Myocarditis with tachyarrhythmias or heart failure—and, less commonly, encephalitis or pneumonitis—may develop and accounts for most deaths of patients with trichinellosis.

Upon onset of larval encystment in muscle 2 to 3 weeks after infection, symptoms of myositis with myalgias, muscle edema, and weakness develop, usually overlapping with the inflammatory reactions to migrating larvae. The most commonly involved muscle groups include the extraocular muscles; the biceps; and the muscles of the jaw, neck, lower back, and diaphragm. Peaking about 3 weeks after infection, symptoms subside only gradually during a prolonged convalescence.

Laboratory Findings and Diagnosis Blood eosinophilia develops in >90% of patients with symptomatic trichinellosis and may peak at a level of >50% between 2 and 4 weeks after infection. Serum levels of IgE and muscle enzymes, including creatine phosphokinase, lactate dehydrogenase, and aspartate aminotransferase, are elevated in most symptomatic patients. Patients should be questioned thoroughly

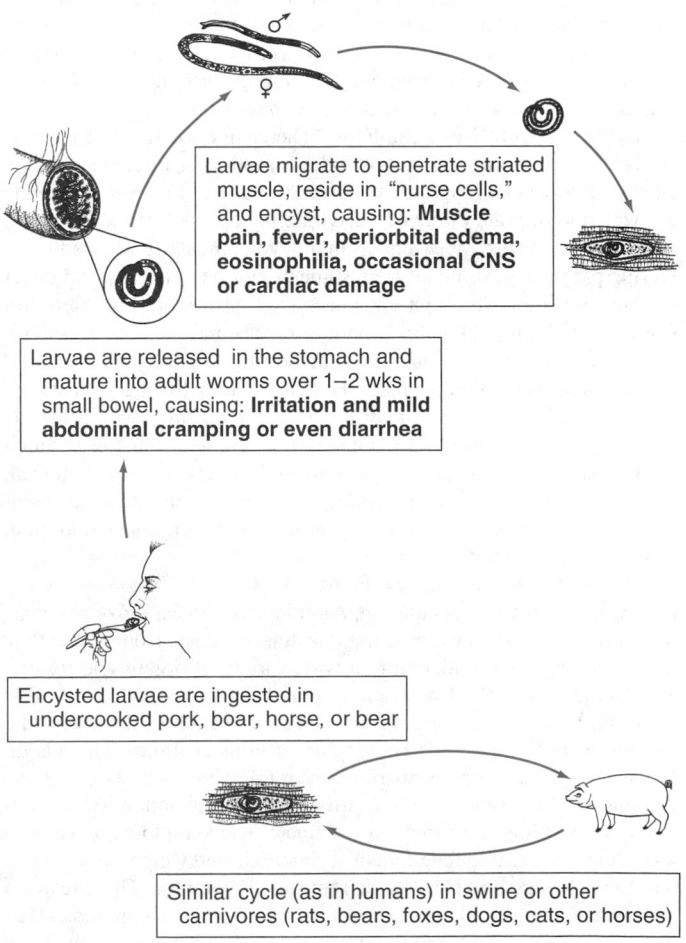

Larvae migrate to penetrate striated muscle, reside in "nurse cells," and encyst, causing: **Muscle pain, fever, periorbital edema, eosinophilia, occasional CNS or cardiac damage**

Larvae are released in the stomach and mature into adult worms over 1–2 wks in small bowel, causing: **Irritation and mild abdominal cramping or even diarrhea**

Encysted larvae are ingested in undercooked pork, boar, horse, or bear

Similar cycle (as in humans) in swine or other carnivores (rats, bears, foxes, dogs, cats, or horses)

FIGURE 219-1 Life cycle of *Trichinella. (From Bruschi and Murrell, with permission.)*

about their consumption of pork or wild-animal meat and about illness in other individuals who ate the same meat. A presumptive clinical diagnosis can be based on fevers, eosinophilia, periorbital edema, and myalgias after a suspect meal. A rise in the titer of parasite-specific antibody, which usually does not occur until after the third week of infection, confirms the diagnosis. Alternatively, a definitive diagnosis requires surgical biopsy of at least 1 g of involved muscle; the yields are highest near tendon insertions. The fresh muscle tissue should be compressed between glass slides and examined microscopically, because larvae may be overlooked by examination of routine histopathologic sections alone.

℞ TREATMENT Current anthelmintic drugs are ineffective against *Trichinella* larvae in muscle. Fortunately, most lightly infected patients recover uneventfully with bed rest, antipyretics, and analgesics. Glucocorticoids like prednisone (1 mg/kg daily for 5 days) are beneficial for severe myositis and myocarditis. Mebendazole and albendazole, like thiabendazole, appear to be active against enteric stages of the parasite, but their efficacy against encysted larvae has not been conclusively demonstrated.

Prevention Larvae may be killed by cooking pork until it is no longer pink or by freezing it at $-15°C$ for 3 weeks. However, Arctic *T. nativa* larvae in walrus or bear meat are relatively resistant and may remain viable despite freezing.

VISCERAL AND OCULAR LARVA MIGRANS Visceral larva migrans is a syndrome caused by nematodes that are normally parasitic for nonhuman host species. In humans, the nematode larvae do not typically develop into adult worms but instead migrate through host tissues and elicit eosinophilic inflammation. The most common form of visceral larva migrans is toxocariasis due to larvae of the canine ascarid *Toxocara canis* or, less commonly, the feline ascarid *T. cati*. Rare cases with eosinophilic meningoencephalitis have been caused by the raccoon ascarid *Baylisascaris procyonis*.

Life Cycle and Epidemiology The canine roundworm *T. canis* is distributed among dogs worldwide. Ingestion of infective eggs by dogs is followed by liberation of *Toxocara* larvae, which penetrate the gut wall and migrate intravascularly into the canine liver, muscle, and other tissues, where most remain in a developmentally arrested state. During pregnancy, some larvae resume migration in bitches and infect puppies prenatally (through transplacental transmission) or after birth (through suckling). Thus, in lactating bitches and puppies, larvae return to the intestinal tract and develop into adult worms, which produce eggs that are released in the feces. Humans acquire toxocariasis mainly by eating soil contaminated by puppy feces containing infective *T. canis* eggs. Visceral larva migrans is most common among children who habitually eat dirt, but most toxocaral infections are subclinical. Reported rates of *Toxocara* seropositivity range from 2% in an unselected American population to >20% among kindergarten children in the United States and England.

Pathogenesis and Clinical Features Clinical disease most commonly afflicts preschool children. After humans ingest *Toxocara* eggs, the larvae hatch and penetrate the intestinal mucosa, from which they are carried by the circulation to a wide variety of organs and tissues. The larvae invade the liver, lungs, central nervous system, and other sites, releasing toxic products and provoking intense local eosinophilic granulomatous responses. The degree of clinical illness depends on larval number and tissue distribution, reinfection, and host immune responses. Most light infections are asymptomatic and may be manifest only by blood eosinophilia. Characteristic symptoms of visceral larva migrans include fever, malaise, anorexia and weight loss, cough, wheezing, and rashes. Hepatosplenomegaly is common. These features are often accompanied by extraordinary peripheral eosinophilia, which may approach 90%. Uncommonly, seizures or behavioral disorders develop. The rare deaths in this disease are due to severe neurologic, pneumonic, or myocardial involvement.

Diagnosis In addition to prominent eosinophilia, leukocytosis and hypergammaglobulinemia are usually evident. Transient pulmonary infiltrates are apparent on chest x-rays of about half of patients with symptoms of pneumonitis. The clinical diagnosis can be confirmed by an enzyme-linked immunosorbent assay for toxocaral antibodies. Stool examination, while important in the evaluation of unexplained eosinophilia, is worthless for toxocariasis, since the larvae do not develop into egg-producing adults in humans.

The ocular form of the larva migrans syndrome occurs when *Toxocara* larvae invade the eye. An eosinophilic granulomatous mass, most commonly in the posterior pole of the retina, develops around the entrapped larva. The retinal lesion can mimic retinoblastoma in appearance, and mistaken diagnosis of the latter condition can lead to unnecessary enucleation. The spectrum of eye involvement also includes endophthalmitis, uveitis, and chorioretinitis. Unilateral visual disturbances, strabismus, and eye pain are the most common presenting symptoms. In contrast to visceral larva migrans, ocular toxocariasis usually develops in older children or young adults with no history of pica; these patients seldom have eosinophilia or visceral manifestations.

℞ TREATMENT The vast majority of *Toxocara* infections are self-limited and resolve without specific therapy. In patients with severe myocardial, central nervous system, or pulmonary involvement, glucocorticoids may be employed to reduce inflammatory complications. Available anthelmintic drugs, including diethylcarbamazine, mebendazole, and albendazole, have not been shown conclusively to alter the course of larva migrans. Control measures include prohibiting dog excreta in public parks and playgrounds, deworming dogs, and preventing pica in children. Treatment of ocular disease is unsatisfactory, and the role of glucocorticoids or anthelmintic drugs in management is controversial.

CUTANEOUS LARVA MIGRANS Cutaneous larva migrans ("creeping eruption") is a serpiginous skin eruption caused by burrowing larvae of animal hookworms, usually the dog and cat hookworm *Ancylostoma braziliense*. The larvae hatch from eggs passed in dog and cat feces and mature in the soil. Humans become infected after skin contact with soil in areas frequented by dogs and cats, such as areas underneath house porches or scrub vegetation. Cutaneous larva migrans is especially prevalent among children and in regions with warm humid climates, including the southeastern United States.

After larvae penetrate the skin, erythematous lesions form along the tortuous tracts of their migration through the dermal-epidermal junction; the larvae advance several centimeters in a day. The intensely pruritic lesions may occur anywhere on the body and can be numerous if the patient has lain on the ground. Vesicles and bullae may form later. The animal hookworm larvae do not mature in humans and, without treatment, will die out after several weeks, with resolution of skin lesions. The diagnosis is made readily on clinical grounds, and a skin biopsy only rarely yields diagnostic parasite material. Symptoms can be alleviated by thiabendazole administered orally (25 mg/kg bid) or topically (10% aqueous or petroleum jelly suspension) for 2 to 5 days, by ivermectin (a single dose of 150 to 200 μg/kg), or by albendazole (200 mg bid for 2 days).

***ANGIOSTRONGYLUS CANTONENSIS* INFECTION** *A. cantonensis*, the rat lungworm, is the most common cause of human eosinophilic meningitis.

Life Cycle and Epidemiology This infection occurs principally in Southeast Asia and the Pacific Basin. *A. cantonensis* larvae produced by adult worms in the rat lung migrate to the gastrointestinal tract and are expelled with the feces. They develop into infective larvae in land snails and slugs. Humans acquire the infection by ingesting raw infected mollusks; vegetables contaminated by mollusk slime; or crabs, freshwater shrimp, and certain marine fish that have themselves eaten infected mollusks. The larvae then migrate to the brain.

Pathogenesis and Clinical Features The parasites eventually die in the central nervous system, but not before initiating pathologic consequences that, in heavy infections, can result in permanent neurologic sequelae or death. Migrating larvae cause proteolytic damage and marked local eosinophilic inflammation and hemorrhage, with subsequent necrosis and granuloma formation around dying worms. Clinical symptoms develop between 2 and 35 days after the ingestion of larvae. Patients usually present with an insidious or abrupt excruciating frontal, occipital, or bitemporal headache. Neck stiffness, nausea and vomiting, and paresthesias are also common. Fever, cranial and extraocular nerve palsies, seizures, paralysis, and lethargy are uncommon.

Laboratory Findings Examination of the cerebrospinal fluid is mandatory in suspected cases and usually reveals an elevated opening pressure, a white blood cell count of 150 to 2000/μL, and an eosinophilic pleocytosis of >20%. The protein concentration is usually elevated and the glucose level normal. The motile larvae of *A. cantonensis* are only rarely seen in the cerebrospinal fluid. Peripheral-blood eosinophilia may be mild. The diagnosis is generally based on the clinical presentation of eosinophilic meningitis together with a compatible epidemiologic history.

℞ **TREATMENT** Specific chemotherapy is not of benefit in angiostrongyliasis; larvicidal agents may actually exacerbate inflammatory brain lesions. Management consists of supportive measures, including the administration of analgesics, sedatives, and—in severe cases—glucocorticoids. In most patients, cerebral angiostrongyliasis has a self-limited course, and recovery is complete. The infection may be prevented by adequately cooking snails, crabs, and prawns and inspecting vegetables for mollusk infestation. Other parasitic causes of eosinophilic meningitis in endemic areas may include gnathostomiasis, paragonimiasis, schistosomiasis, and neurocysticercosis.

GNATHOSTOMIASIS Infection of human tissues with larvae of *Gnathostoma spinigerum* can cause eosinophilic meningoencephalitis, migratory cutaneous swellings, or invasive masses of the eye and visceral organs.

Life Cycle and Epidemiology Human gnathostomiasis occurs in many countries and is notably endemic in Southeast Asia and parts of China and Japan. In nature, the mature adult worms parasitize the gastrointestinal tract of dogs and cats. First-stage larvae hatch from eggs passed into water and are ingested by *Cyclops* species (water fleas). Infective third-stage larvae develop in the flesh of many animal species (including fish, frogs, eels, snakes, chickens, and ducks) that have eaten either infected *Cyclops* or another infected second intermediate host. Humans typically acquire the infection by eating raw or undercooked fish or poultry. The raw fish dishes of *somfak* in Thailand and *sashimi* in Japan account for most cases of human gnathostomiasis. Some cases in Thailand result from the local practice of applying frog or snake flesh as a poultice.

Pathogenesis and Clinical Features Clinical symptoms are due to the aberrant migration of a single larva into cutaneous, visceral, neural, or ocular tissues. After invasion, larval migration may cause local inflammation, with pain, cough, or hematuria accompanied by fever and eosinophilia. Painful, itchy, migratory swellings may develop in the skin, particularly in the distal extremities or periorbital area. Cutaneous swellings usually last about a week but often recur intermittently over many years. Larval invasion of the eye can provoke a sight-threatening inflammatory response. Finally, invasion of the central nervous system results in eosinophilic meningitis with myeloencephalitis, a serious complication due to ascending larval migration along a large nerve track. Patients characteristically present with agonizing radicular pain and paresthesias in the trunk or a limb, which are followed shortly by paraplegia. Cerebral involvement, with focal hemorrhages and tissue destruction, is often fatal.

Diagnosis and Treatment Cutaneous migratory swellings with marked peripheral eosinophilia, supported by an appropriate geographic and dietary history, generally constitute an adequate basis for a clinical diagnosis of gnathostomiasis. However, patients may present with ocular or cerebrospinal involvement without antecedent cutaneous swellings. In the latter case, eosinophilic pleocytosis is demonstrable (usually along with hemorrhagic or xanthochromic cerebrospinal fluid), but worms are almost never recovered from the cerebrospinal fluid. Surgical removal of the parasite from subcutaneous or ocular tissue, though rarely feasible, is both diagnostic and therapeutic. Albendazole (400 to 800 mg daily for 21 days) may be helpful. At present, cerebrospinal involvement is managed with supportive measures and generally with a course of glucocorticoids. Gnathostomiasis can be prevented by adequate cooking of fish and poultry in endemic areas.

BIBLIOGRAPHY

BALDISSEROTTO M et al: Ultrasound findings in children with toxocariasis: Report on 18 cases. Pediatr Radiol 29:316, 1999

BRUSCHI F, MURRELL KD: Trichinellosis, in *Tropical Infectious Diseases: Principles, Pathogens and Practice,* RL Guerrant et al (eds). Philadelphia, Churchill Livingstone, 1999, pp 917–926

DIAZ CAMACHO SP et al: Clinical manifestations and immunodiagnosis of gnathostomiasis in Culiacan, Mexico. Am J Trop Med Hyg 59:908, 1998

HOTEZ PJ: Visceral and ocular larva migrans. Semin Neurol 13:175, 1993

JELINEK T et al: Cutaneous larva migrans in travelers: Synopsis of histories, symptoms, and treatment of 98 patients. Clin Infect Dis 19:1062, 1994

JONGWUTIWES S et al: First outbreak of human trichinellosis caused by *Trichinella pseudospiralis.* Clin Infect Dis 26:111, 1998

KAPEL CM et al: Freeze tolerance, morphology, and RAPD-PCR identification of *Trichinella nativa* in naturally infected Arctic foxes. J Parasitol 85:144, 1999

LUCCHINA LC et al: Dermatology and the recently returned traveler: Infectious diseases with dermatologic manifestations. Int J Dermatol 36:167, 1997

MOORHEAD A et al: Trichinellosis in the United States, 1991–1996: Declining but not gone. Am J Trop Med Hyg 60:66, 1999

WELLER PF, LIU LX: Eosinophilic meningitis. Semin Neurol 13:161, 1993

220 *Peter F. Weller, Thomas B. Nutman*

INTESTINAL NEMATODES

More than a billion people worldwide are infected with one or more species of intestinal nematodes. Table 220-1 summarizes biologic and clinical features of infections due to the major intestinal parasitic nematodes. These parasites are most common in regions with poor fecal sanitation, particularly in developing countries in the tropics and subtropics but also in the United States. Although nematode infections are not usually fatal, they contribute to malnutrition and diminished work capacity. Humans may on occasion be infected with nematode parasites that ordinarily infect animals; these zoonotic infections include trichostrongyliasis, anisakiasis, capillariasis, and abdominal angiostrongyliasis.

Intestinal nematodes are roundworms; they range in length from 1 mm to many centimeters when mature (Table 220-1). Their life cycles are complex and highly varied; some species, including *Strongyloides stercoralis* and *Enterobius vermicularis*, can be transmitted directly from person to person, while others, such as *Ascaris lumbricoides*, *Necator americanus*, and *Ancylostoma duodenale*, require a soil phase for development. Because most helminth parasites do not self-replicate, the acquisition of a heavy burden of adult worms requires repeated exposure to the parasite in its infectious stage, whether larva or egg. Hence, clinical disease, as opposed to asymptomatic infection, generally develops only with prolonged residence in an endemic area. In persons with marginal nutrition, intestinal helminth infections may impair growth and development. Eosinophilia and elevated serum IgE levels are features of many helminthic infections and, when unexplained, should always prompt a search for occult helminthiasis. Significant protective immunity to intestinal nematodes appears not to develop in humans, although mechanisms of parasite im-

Table 220-1 Major Human Intestinal Parasitic Nematodes

Feature	Parasitic Nematode				
	Ascaris lumbricoides (Roundworm)	*Necator americanus, Ancylostoma duodenale* (Hookworm)	*Strongyloides stercoralis*	*Trichuris trichiura* (Whipworm)	*Enterobius vermicularis* (Pinworm)
Global prevalence in humans (millions)	1273	1277	50	902	300
Endemic areas	Worldwide	Hot, humid regions	Hot, humid regions	Worldwide	Worldwide
Infective stage	Egg	Filariform larva	Filariform larva	Egg	Egg
Route of infection	Oral	Percutaneous	Percutaneous or auto-infection	Oral	Oral
Gastrointestinal location of worms	Jejunal lumen	Jejunal mucosa	Small-bowel mucosa	Cecum, colonic mucosa	Cecum, appendix
Adult worm size	15–40 cm	7–12 mm	2 mm	30–50 mm	8–13 mm (female)
Pulmonary passage of larvae	Yes	Yes	Yes	No	No
Incubation period[a] (days)	60–75	40–100	17–28	70–90	35–45
Longevity	1 y	*N. americanus*: 2–5 y *A. duodenale*: 6–8 y	Decades (owing to autoinfection)	5 y	2 months
Fecundity (eggs/day/worm)	240,000	*N. americanus*: 4000–10,000 *A. duodenale*: 10,000–25,000	5000–10,000	3000–7000	2000
Principal symptoms	Rarely gastrointestinal or biliary obstruction	Iron-deficiency anemia in heavy infection	Gastrointestinal symptoms; malabsorption or sepsis in hyperinfection	Gastrointestinal symptoms, anemia	Perianal pruritus
Diagnostic stage	Eggs in stool	Eggs in fresh stool, larvae in old stool	Larvae in stool or duodenal aspirate; sputum in hyperinfection	Eggs in stool	Eggs from perianal skin on cellulose acetate tape
Treatment	Mebendazole Albendazole Pyrantel pamoate Piperazine citrate	Mebendazole Pyrantel pamoate Albendazole	1. Ivermectin 2. Albendazole 3. Thiabendazole	Mebendazole Albendazole	Mebendazole Pyrantel pamoate Albendazole

[a] Time from infection to egg production by mature female worm.

mune evasion and host immune responses to these infections have not been elucidated in detail.

ASCARIASIS *A. lumbricoides* is the largest intestinal nematode parasite of humans, reaching up to 40 cm in length. Most infected individuals have low worm burdens and are asymptomatic. Clinical disease arises from larval migration in the lungs or effects of the adult worms in the intestines.

Life Cycle Adult worms live in the lumen of the small intestine. Mature female *Ascaris* worms are extraordinarily fecund, each producing up to 240,000 eggs a day, which pass with the feces. Ascarid eggs, which are remarkably resistant to environmental stresses, become infective after several weeks of maturation in the soil and can remain infective for years. After infective eggs are swallowed, larvae hatched in the intestine invade the mucosa, migrate through the circulation to the lungs, break into the alveoli, ascend the bronchial tree, and return via swallowing to the small intestine, where they develop into adult worms. Between 2 and 3 months elapse between initial infection and egg production. The adult worms live for ~1 to 2 years.

Epidemiology *Ascaris* is widely distributed in tropical and subtropical regions as well as in other humid areas, including the rural southeastern United States. Transmission typically occurs through fecally contaminated soil and is due either to a lack of sanitary facilities or to the use of human manure ("night soil") as fertilizer. With their propensity for hand-to-mouth fecal carriage, younger children in impoverished rural areas are most affected. Infection outside endemic areas, though uncommon, can occur from eggs borne on transported vegetables.

Clinical Features During the lung phase of larval migration, about 9 to 12 days after egg ingestion, patients may develop an irritating nonproductive cough and burning substernal discomfort that is aggravated by coughing or deep inspiration. Dyspnea and blood-tinged

sputum are less common. Fever is usually reported, with temperatures sometimes exceeding 38.5°C (101.3°F). Eosinophilia develops during this symptomatic phase and subsides slowly over weeks. Chest x-rays may reveal evidence of eosinophilic pneumonitis (Löffler's syndrome), with round or oval infiltrates a few millimeters to several centimeters in size. These infiltrates may be transient and intermittent, clearing after several weeks. Where there is seasonal transmission of the parasite, seasonal pneumonitis with eosinophilia may develop in previously infected and sensitized hosts.

In established infections, adult worms in the small intestine usually cause no symptoms. In heavy infections, particularly in children, a large bolus of entangled worms can cause pain and small-bowel obstruction, sometimes complicated by perforation, intussusception, or volvulus. Single worms may cause disease when they migrate into aberrant sites. A large worm can enter and occlude the biliary tree, causing biliary colic, cholecystitis, cholangitis, pancreatitis, or (rarely) intrahepatic abscesses. Migration of an adult worm up the esophagus can provoke coughing and oral expulsion of the worm. In highly endemic areas, intestinal and biliary ascariasis can rival acute appendicitis and gallstones as causes of surgical acute abdomen.

Laboratory Findings Most cases of ascariasis can be diagnosed by the microscopic detection of characteristic mamillated *Ascaris* eggs (65 by 45 μm) in fecal samples. Occasionally, patients present after passing an adult worm—identifiable by its large size and smooth cream-colored surface—in the stool or through the mouth or nose. During the early transpulmonary migratory phase, when eosinophilic pneumonitis occurs, larvae can be found in sputum or gastric aspirates before diagnostic eggs appear in the stool. The eosinophilia that is prominent during this early stage usually decreases to minimal levels in established infection. The large adult worms may be visualized, occasionally serendipitously, on contrast studies of the gastrointestinal tract. A plain abdominal film may reveal masses of worms in gas-filled loops of bowel in patients with intestinal obstruction. Pancreatico-biliary worms can be detected by ultrasound and endoscopic retrograde cholangiopancreatography; the latter method also has been used to extract biliary *Ascaris* worms.

Rx **TREATMENT** Ascariasis should always be treated to prevent potentially serious complications. Mebendazole or albendazole (which is considered an investigational drug by the Food and Drug Administration for this indication) is effective. These benzimidazoles are contraindicated in pregnancy and in heavy infections, in which they may provoke ectopic migration. Pyrantel pamoate and piperazine citrate are safe in pregnancy. Mild diarrhea and abdominal pain are uncommon side effects of these agents. Partial intestinal obstruction should be managed with nasogastric suction, intravenous fluid administration, and instillation of piperazine through the nasogastric tube, but complete obstruction and its severe complications require immediate surgical intervention.

HOOKWORM One-fourth of the world's population is infected with one of the two hookworm species (*A. duodenale* and *N. americanus*). Most infected individuals are asymptomatic. Hookworm disease develops from a combination of factors—a heavy worm burden, a prolonged duration of infection, and an inadequate iron intake—and results in iron-deficiency anemia and, on occasion, hypoproteinemia.

Life Cycle Adult hookworms, which are about 1 cm long, use buccal teeth (*Ancylostoma*) or cutting plates (*Necator*) to attach to the small-bowel mucosa and suck blood (0.2 mL/d per *Ancylostoma* adult) and interstitial fluid. The adult hookworms produce thousands of eggs daily. The eggs are deposited with feces in soil, where rhabditiform larvae hatch and develop over a 1-week period into infectious filariform larvae. Infective larvae penetrate the skin and reach the lungs by way of the bloodstream. There they invade alveoli and ascend the airways before being swallowed and reaching the small intestine. The prepatent period from skin invasion to appearance of eggs in the feces is about 6 to 8 weeks, but it may be longer with *A. duodenale*. Larvae of *A. duodenale*, if swallowed, can survive and develop directly in the intestinal mucosa. Adult hookworms may survive over a decade but usually live about 6 to 8 years for *A. duodenale* and 2 to 5 years for *N. americanus*.

Epidemiology *A. duodenale* is prevalent in southern Europe, North Africa, and northern Asia, and *N. americanus* is the predominant species in the western hemisphere and equatorial Africa. The two species overlap in many tropical regions, particularly Southeast Asia. In most areas, older children have the greatest incidence and intensity of hookworm infection. In rural areas where fields are fertilized with night soil, older working adults also may be heavily affected.

Clinical Features Most hookworm infections are asymptomatic. Infective larvae may provoke pruritic maculopapular dermatitis ("ground itch") at the site of skin penetration as well as serpiginous tracts of subcutaneous migration (similar to cutaneous larva migrans) in previously sensitized hosts. Larvae migrating through the lungs occasionally cause mild transient pneumonitis, but this condition develops less frequently in hookworm infection than in ascariasis. In the early intestinal phase, infected persons may develop epigastric pain (often with postprandial accentuation), inflammatory diarrhea, or other abdominal symptoms accompanied by eosinophilia. The major consequence of chronic hookworm infection is iron deficiency. Symptoms are minimal if iron intake is adequate, but marginally nourished individuals develop symptoms of progressive iron-deficiency anemia and hypoproteinemia, including weakness, shortness of breath, and skin depigmentation.

Laboratory Findings The diagnosis is established by the finding of characteristic 40- by 60-μm oval hookworm eggs in the feces. Stool-concentration procedures may be required to detect light infections. Eggs of the two species are indistinguishable. In a stool sample that is not fresh, the eggs may have hatched to release rhabditiform larvae, which need to be differentiated from those of *S. stercoralis*.

Hypochromic microcytic anemia, occasionally with eosinophilia or hypoalbuminemia, is characteristic of hookworm disease.

Rx **TREATMENT** Hookworm infection can be eradicated with several safe and highly effective anthelmintic drugs, including mebendazole, albendazole, and pyrantel pamoate (Chap. 212). Mild iron-deficiency anemia often can be treated with oral iron alone. Severe hookworm disease with protein loss and malabsorption necessitates nutritional support and oral iron replacement along with deworming.

Ancylostoma caninum This parasite, the canine hookworm, has been identified as a cause of human eosinophilic enteritis, especially in northeastern Australia. In this zoonotic infection, adult hookworms attach to the small intestine (where they may be visualized by endoscopy) and elicit abdominal pain and intense local eosinophilia. Treatment with mebendazole (100 mg twice daily for 3 days) is effective.

STRONGYLOIDIASIS *S. stercoralis* is distinguished by its ability, unusual among helminths, to replicate in the human host. This capacity permits ongoing cycles of autoinfection as infective larvae are internally produced. Strongyloidiasis can thus persist for decades without further exposure of the host to exogenous infective larvae. In immunocompromised hosts, large numbers of invasive *Strongyloides* larvae can disseminate widely and can be fatal.

Life Cycle In addition to a parasitic cycle of development, *Strongyloides* can undergo a free-living cycle of development in the soil. This adaptability facilitates the parasite's survival in the absence of mammalian hosts. Rhabditiform larvae passed in feces can transform into infectious filariform larvae either directly or after a free-living phase of development. Humans acquire strongyloidiasis when filariform larvae in fecally contaminated soil penetrate the skin or mucous membranes. The larvae then travel through the bloodstream to the lungs, where they break into the alveolar spaces, ascend the bronchial tree, are swallowed, and thereby reach the small intestine. There the larvae mature into adult worms that penetrate the mucosa of the proximal small bowel. The minute (2-mm-long) parasitic adult female worms reproduce by parthenogenesis; parasitic adult males do not exist. Eggs hatch locally in the intestinal mucosa, releasing rhabditiform larvae that migrate to the lumen and pass with the feces into soil. Alternatively, rhabditiform larvae in the bowel can develop directly into filariform larvae that penetrate the colonic wall or perianal skin and enter the circulation to repeat the migration that establishes ongoing internal reinfection. This autoinfection cycle allows strongyloidiasis to persist for decades after the host has left an endemic area.

Epidemiology *S. stercoralis* is spottily distributed in tropical areas and other hot, humid regions and is particularly common in Southeast Asia, sub-Saharan Africa, and Brazil. In the United States, the parasite is endemic in parts of the South and is found in residents of mental institutions who practice poor hygiene and in immigrants and military veterans who have lived in endemic areas abroad.

Clinical Features In uncomplicated strongyloidiasis, many patients are asymptomatic or have mild cutaneous and/or abdominal symptoms. Recurrent urticaria, often involving the buttocks and wrists, is the most common cutaneous manifestation. Migrating larvae can elicit a pathognomonic serpiginous eruption, *larva currens* ("running larva")—a pruritic, raised, erythematous lesion that advances as rapidly as 10 cm/h along the course of larval migration. Adult parasites burrow into the duodenojejunal mucosa and can cause abdominal (usually midepigastric) pain, which resembles peptic ulcer pain except that it is aggravated by food ingestion. Nausea, diarrhea, gastrointestinal bleeding, mild chronic colitis, and weight loss can occur. Small-bowel obstruction may develop with early, heavy infection. Pulmonary symptoms are rare in uncomplicated strongyloidiasis. Eosinophilia is common, with levels fluctuating over time.

The ongoing autoinfection cycle of strongyloidiasis is normally contained by unknown factors of the host's immune system. Abrogation of host immunity, especially with glucocorticoid therapy and much less commonly with other immunosuppressive medications, leads to hyperinfection, with the generation of large numbers of filariform larvae. Colitis, enteritis, or malabsorption may develop. In disseminated strongyloidiasis, larvae may invade not only gastrointestinal tissues and the lungs but also the central nervous system, peritoneum, liver, and kidney. Moreover, bacteremia may develop because of the entry of enteric flora through disrupted mucosal barriers. Gram-negative sepsis, pneumonia, or meningitis may complicate or dominate the clinical course. Eosinophilia is often absent in severely infected patients. Disseminated strongyloidiasis, particularly in patients with unsuspected infection who are given glucocorticoids, can be fatal. Strongyloidiasis is a frequent complication of infection with human T cell lymphotropic virus type I, but disseminated strongyloidiasis is not common among patients infected with HIV.

Diagnosis   In uncomplicated strongyloidiasis, the finding of rhabditiform larvae in feces is diagnostic. The eggs are almost never detectable because they hatch in the intestine. Rhabditiform larvae are 200 to 250 μm long, with a short buccal cavity that distinguishes them from hookworm rhabditiform larvae. Single stool examinations detect only about one-third of uncomplicated infections, in which few larvae are passed. Serial examinations and the use of the agar plate detection method improve the sensitivity of stool diagnosis. In uncomplicated— but not hyperinfection—strongyloidiasis, stool examinations may be repeatedly negative. If stool examinations are negative, *Strongyloides* can be assayed by sampling of the duodenojejunal contents by aspiration or biopsy. An enzyme-linked immunosorbent assay for antibodies to excretory-secretory or somatic antigens of *Strongyloides* is a sensitive method of diagnosing uncomplicated infections. In disseminated strongyloidiasis, filariform larvae (550 μm long) should be sought in stool as well as in samples obtained from sites of potential larval migration, including sputum, bronchoalveolar lavage fluid, or surgical drainage fluid.

℞   **TREATMENT**   Even in the asymptomatic state, strongyloidiasis must be treated because of the potential for fatal hyperinfection. Ivermectin (200 μg/kg daily for 1 or 2 days) is more effective and better tolerated than thiabendazole (25 mg/kg bid for 2 days), whose common adverse effects include nausea, vomiting, diarrhea, dizziness, and neuropsychiatric disturbances. Because thiabendazole is not uniformly effective, stool examinations, eosinophil counts, and monitoring of clinical symptoms should be continued after treatment. For disseminated strongyloidiasis, treatment should be extended for at least 5 to 7 days or until the parasites are eradicated.

Strongyloides fülleborni   This unusual species, which has been encountered in Africa and Papua New Guinea, is thought to be transmitted from person to person and through maternal milk. *S. fülleborni* releases membranous sacs filled with eggs into the stool. Most commonly affected are infants and young children, who present with abdominal distention, respiratory distress, vomiting, or diarrhea.

TRICHURIASIS   Most infections with the whipworm *Trichuris trichiura* are asymptomatic, but heavy infections may cause gastrointestinal symptoms. Like the other soil-transmitted helminths, whipworm is distributed globally in the tropics and subtropics and is most common among poor children.

Life Cycle   A broad posterior section and a thin anterior portion give *Trichuris* its characteristic whiplike shape. The adult worms reside in the colon and cecum, the anterior portions threaded into the superficial mucosa. Thousands of eggs laid daily by adult female worms pass with the feces and mature in the soil. After ingestion, infective eggs hatch in the duodenum, releasing larvae that mature before migrating to the large bowel. The entire cycle takes about 3 months, and adult worms may live for several years.

Clinical Features   Tissue reactions to whipworms are mild. Most infected individuals have no symptoms or eosinophilia. Heavy infec-

tions may result in abdominal pain, anorexia, and bloody or mucoid diarrhea resembling inflammatory bowel disease. Rectal prolapse can result from massive infections in children, who often suffer from malnourishment and other diarrheal illnesses. Moderately heavy whipworm burdens also contribute to growth retardation.

Diagnosis and Treatment   The characteristic 50- by 20-μm lemon-shaped whipworm eggs are readily detected on stool examination. Adult worms, which are 3 to 5 cm long, occasionally can be seen on proctoscopy. Mebendazole or albendazole is safe and effective for treatment (Chap. 212).

ENTEROBIASIS (PINWORM)   *E. vermicularis* is more common in temperate countries than in the tropics. More than 40 million Americans, particularly schoolchildren, are estimated to be infected with pinworms.

Life Cycle and Epidemiology   *Enterobius* adult worms are about 1 cm long and dwell in the bowel lumen. The gravid female worm migrates nocturnally out into the perianal region and releases up to 10,000 immature eggs. The eggs become infective within hours and are transmitted by hand-to-mouth passage. The larvae hatch and mature entirely within the intestine. This life cycle takes about 1 month, and adult worms survive for about 2 months. Self-infection results from perianal scratching and transport of infective eggs on the hands or under the nails to the mouth. Owing to the ease of person-to-person spread, pinworm infections are common among family members and institutionalized populations.

Clinical Features   Most pinworm infections are asymptomatic. Perianal pruritus is the cardinal symptom. The itching is often worse at night owing to the nocturnal migration of the female worms, and it may lead to excoriation and bacterial superinfection. Heavy infections have been claimed to cause abdominal pain and weight loss. On rare occasions, pinworms invade the female genital tract, causing vulvovaginitis and pelvic or peritoneal granulomas. Eosinophilia or elevated levels of serum IgE are rare.

Diagnosis   Since pinworm eggs are not usually released in the bowel, the diagnosis cannot be made by looking for eggs in the feces. Instead, eggs deposited in the perianal region are detected by the application of clear cellulose acetate tape to the perianal region in the morning. After the tape is transferred to a microscope slide, low-power examination will reveal the characteristic pinworm eggs, which are oval, measure 55 by 25 μm, and are flattened along one side.

℞   **TREATMENT**   All affected individuals should be given a dose of mebendazole or pyrantel pamoate, with treatment repeated after 10 to 14 days (Chap. 212). Treatment of household members is also advocated to eliminate asymptomatic reservoirs of potential reinfection.

TRICHOSTRONGYLIASIS   *Trichostrongylus* species that are normally parasites of herbivorous animals occasionally infect humans, particularly in Asia and Africa. This parasite has been termed *pseudo hookworm* because of similarities to the hookworms in life cycle and egg morphology. Humans acquire the infection by accidentally ingesting *Trichostrongylus* larvae on contaminated leafy vegetables. The larvae do not migrate in humans but mature directly into adult worms in the small bowel. These worms ingest far less blood than hookworms; most infected people are asymptomatic, but heavy infections may give rise to mild anemia and eosinophilia. *Trichostrongylus* eggs encountered on stool examination resemble those of hookworms but are larger (85 by 115 μm). Appropriate treatment consists of mebendazole or albendazole (Chap. 212).

ANISAKIASIS   Anisakiasis is a gastrointestinal infection caused by the accidental ingestion in uncooked saltwater fish of nematode larvae belonging to the family Anisakidae. The incidence of anisakiasis in the United States has increased as a result of the growing popularity of raw fish dishes. Most cases occur in Japan, the Netherlands, and Chile, where raw fish—sushi, pickled green herring, and seviche, respectively—are national culinary staples. Anisakid nematodes parasitize large sea mammals such as whales, dolphins, and seals. As part of a complex parasitic life cycle involving marine food chains, infectious larvae migrate to the musculature of a variety of fish. Both *Anisakis simplex* and *Pseudoterranova decipiens* have been implicated in human anisakiasis, but an identical gastric syndrome may be caused by the red larvae of eustrongylid parasites of fish-eating birds.

When humans consume infected raw fish, live larvae may be coughed up within 48 h. Alternatively, larvae may immediately penetrate the mucosa of the stomach. Within hours, violent upper abdominal pain accompanied by nausea and occasionally vomiting ensues, mimicking an acute abdomen. The diagnosis can be established by direct visualization on upper endoscopy, outlining of the worm by contrast radiographic studies, or histopathologic examination of extracted tissue. In experienced hands, the first technique is preferable because extraction of the burrowing larvae by endoscopic technique is curative. In addition, larvae may pass to the small bowel, where they penetrate the mucosa and provoke a vigorous eosinophilic granulomatous response. Symptoms may appear 1 or 2 weeks after the infective meal, with intermittent abdominal pain, diarrhea, nausea, and fever resembling the manifestations of Crohn's disease. The diagnosis may be suggested by barium studies and confirmed by curative surgical resection of a granuloma in which the worm is embedded. Anisakid eggs are not found in the stool, since the larvae do not mature in humans. Anisakid larvae in saltwater fish are killed by cooking to 60°C, freezing at −20°C for 3 days, or commercial blast freezing, but not usually by salting, marinating, or cold smoking. No medical treatment is available; if possible, surgical or endoscopic removal should be undertaken.

CAPILLARIASIS Intestinal capillariasis is caused by ingestion of raw fish infected with *Capillaria philippinensis*. Subsequent autoinfection can lead to a severe wasting syndrome. The disease occurs in the Philippines and Thailand and, on occasion, elsewhere in Asia. The natural cycle of *C. philippinensis* involves fish from fresh and brackish water. When humans eat infected raw fish, the larvae mature in the intestine into adult worms, which produce invasive larvae that cause intestinal inflammation and villus loss. Capillariasis has an insidious onset with nonspecific abdominal pain and watery diarrhea. If untreated, progressive autoinfection can lead to protein-losing enteropathy and severe malabsorption and ultimately to death from cachexia, cardiac failure, or superinfection. The diagnosis is established by identification of the characteristic peanut-shaped (20- by 40-μm) eggs on stool examination. Severely ill patients require hospitalization and supportive therapy in addition to prolonged anthelmintic treatment with mebendazole or albendazole (Chap. 212).

ABDOMINAL ANGIOSTRONGYLIASIS Abdominal angiostrongyliasis is found in Latin America and Africa. The zoonotic parasite *Angiostrongylus costaricensis* causes eosinophilic ileocolitis after the ingestion of contaminated vegetation. *A. costaricensis* normally parasitizes the cotton rat and other rodents, with slugs and snails serving as intermediate hosts. Humans become infected by accidentally ingesting infective larvae in mollusk slime deposited on fruits and vegetables; children are at highest risk. The larvae penetrate the gut wall and migrate to the mesenteric artery, where they develop into adult worms. Eggs deposited in the gut wall provoke an intense eosinophilic granulomatous reaction, and adult worms may cause mesenteric arteritis, thrombosis, or frank bowel infarction. Symptoms may mimic those of appendicitis, including abdominal pain and tenderness, fever, vomiting, and a palpable mass in the right iliac fossa. Leukocytosis and eosinophilia are prominent. A barium enema may reveal ileocecal filling defects, but a definitive diagnosis is usually made surgically with partial bowel resection. Pathologic study reveals a thickened bowel wall with eosinophilic granulomas surrounding the *Angiostrongylus* eggs. In nonsurgical cases, the diagnosis rests solely on clinical grounds because larvae and eggs cannot be detected in the stool. Medical therapy for abdominal angiostrongyliasis (thiabendazole; Chap. 212) is of uncertain efficacy. Careful observation and surgical resection for severe symptoms are the mainstays of treatment.

BIBLIOGRAPHY

BECKINGHAM IJ et al: Management of hepatobiliary and pancreatic *Ascaris* infestation in adults after failed medical treatment. Br J Surg 85:907, 1998

CHAN M-S:The global burden of intestinal nematode infections—fifty years on. Parasitol Today 13:438, 1997

CROESE J et al: Human enteric infection with canine hookworms. Ann Intern Med 120: 369, 1994

CROSS JH: Intestinal capillariasis. Clin Microbiol Rev 5:120, 1992

DUARTE Z et al: Abdominal angiostrongyliasis in Nicaragua: A clinico-pathological study on a series of 12 case reports. Ann Parasitol Hum Comp 66:259, 1991

GENTA RM et al: Strongyloidiasis in US veterans of the Vietnam and other wars. JAMA 258:49, 1987

GOTUZZO E et al: *Strongyloides stercoralis* hyperinfection associated with human T cell lymphotropic virus type-1 infection in Peru. Am J Trop Med Hyg 60:146, 1999

GYORKOS TW et al: Intestinal parasite infection in the Kampuchean refugee population 6 years after resettlement in Canada. J Infect Dis 166:413, 1992

HAQUE AK et al: Pathogenesis of human strongyloidiasis: Autopsy and quantitative parasitological analysis. Mod Pathol 7:276, 1994

HOTEZ PJ, PRITCHARD DI: Hookworm infection. Sci Am 272:68, 1995

OCHOA B: Surgical complications of ascariasis. World J Surg 15:222, 1991

REEDER MM: The radiological and ultrasound evaluation of ascariasis of the gastrointestinal, biliary, and respiratory tracts. Semin Roentgenol 33:57, 1998

SCHANTZ PM: The dangers of eating raw fish (editorial). N Engl J Med 320:1143, 1989

TAKABE K et al: Anisakidosis: A cause of intestinal obstruction from eating sushi. Am J Gastroenterol 93:1172, 1998

UPARANUKRAW P et al: Fluctuations of larval excretion in *Strongyloides stercoralis* infection. Am J Trop Med Hyg 60:967, 1999

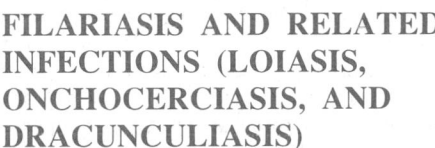

221

Thomas B. Nutman, Peter F. Weller

FILARIASIS AND RELATED INFECTIONS (LOIASIS, ONCHOCERCIASIS, AND DRACUNCULIASIS)

Filarial worms are nematodes that dwell in the subcutaneous tissues and the lymphatics. Eight filarial species infect humans (Table 221-1); of these, four—*Wuchereria bancrofti, Brugia malayi, Onchocerca volvulus,* and *Loa loa*—are responsible for most serious filarial infections. Filarial parasites, which infect an estimated 170 million persons worldwide, are transmitted by specific species of mosquitoes or other arthropods and have a complex life cycle including infective larval stages carried by insects and adult worms that reside in either lymphatic or subcutaneous tissues of humans. The offspring of adults are microfilariae, which, depending on their species, are 200 to 250 μm long and 5 to 7 μm wide, may or may not be enveloped in a loose sheath, and either circulate in the blood or migrate through the skin (Table 221-1). To complete the life cycle, microfilariae are ingested by the arthropod vector and develop over 1 to 2 weeks into new infective larvae. Adult worms live for many years, whereas microfilariae survive from 3 to 36 months.

Usually, infection is established only with repeated and prolonged exposures to infective larvae. Since the clinical manifestations of filarial diseases develop relatively slowly, these infections should be considered chronic diseases with possible long-term debilitating effects. In terms of the nature, severity, and timing of clinical manifestations, patients with filariasis who are native to endemic areas and undergo lifelong exposure may differ significantly from those who are travelers or who have recently moved to these areas. Characteristically, the disease is more acute and intense in newly exposed individuals than in natives of endemic areas.

LYMPHATIC FILARIASIS

Lymphatic filariasis is caused by *W. bancrofti, B. malayi,* or *B. timori.* The threadlike adult parasites reside in lymphatic channels or

Table 221-1 Characteristics of the Filariae

Organism	Periodicity	Distribution	Vector	Location of Adult	Microfilarial Location	Sheath
Wuchereria bancrofti	Nocturnal	Cosmopolitan areas worldwide, including South America and Africa	*Culex* (mosquitoes)	Lymphatic tissue	Blood	+
		Mainly India	*Anopheles* (mosquitoes)			
		China, Indonesia	*Aedes* (mosquitoes)			
	Subperiodic	Eastern Pacific	*Aedes* (mosquitoes)	Lymphatic tissue	Blood	+
Brugia malayi	Nocturnal	Southeast Asia, Indonesia, India	*Mansonia, Anopheles* (mosquitoes)	Lymphatic tissue	Blood	+
	Subperiodic	Indonesia, Southeast Asia	*Coquillettidia, Mansonia* (mosquitoes)	Lymphatic tissue	Blood	+
B. timori	Nocturnal	Indonesia	*Anopheles* (mosquitoes)	Lymphatic tissue	Blood	+
Loa loa	Diurnal	West and Central Africa	*Chrysops* (deerflies)	Subcutaneous tissue	Blood	+
Onchocerca volvulus	None	South and Central America, Africa	*Simulium* (blackflies)	Subcutaneous tissue	Skin, eye	−
Mansonella ozzardi	None	South and Central America Caribbean	*Culicoides* (midges) *Simulium* (blackflies)	Undetermined site	Blood	−
M. perstans	None	South and Central America, Africa	*Culicoides* (midges)	Body cavities, mesentery, perirenal tissue	Blood	−
M. streptocerca	None	West and Central Africa	*Culicoides* (midges)	Subcutaneous tissue	Skin	−

lymph nodes, where they may remain viable for more than two decades.

EPIDEMIOLOGY *W. bancrofti*, the most widely distributed human filarial parasite, affects an estimated 115 million people and is found throughout the tropics and subtropics, including Asia and the Pacific Islands, Africa, areas of South America, and the Caribbean basin. Humans are the only definitive host for the parasite. Generally, the subperiodic form is found only in the Pacific Islands; elsewhere, *W. bancrofti* is nocturnally periodic. (Nocturnally periodic forms of microfilariae are scarce in peripheral blood by day and increase at night, whereas subperiodic forms are present in peripheral blood at all times and reach maximal levels in the afternoon.) Natural vectors for *W. bancrofti* are *Culex fatigans* mosquitoes in urban settings and anopheline or aedean mosquitoes in rural areas.

Brugian filariasis due to *B. malayi* occurs primarily in China, India, Indonesia, Korea, Japan, Malaysia, and the Philippines. *B. malayi* also has two forms distinguished by the periodicity of microfilaremia. The more common nocturnal form is transmitted in areas of coastal rice fields, while the subperiodic form is found in forests. *B. malayi* naturally infects cats as well as humans. *B. timori* exists only on islands of the Indonesian archipelago.

PATHOLOGY The principal pathologic changes result from inflammatory damage to the lymphatics, which is caused by adult worms and not by microfilariae. Adult worms live in afferent lymphatics or sinuses of lymph nodes and cause lymphatic dilatation and thickening of the vessel walls. The infiltration of plasma cells, eosinophils, and macrophages in and around the infected vessels, along with endothelial and connective tissue proliferation, leads to tortuosity of the lymphatics and damaged or incompetent lymph valves. Lymphedema and chronic-stasis changes with hard or brawny edema develop in the overlying skin. These consequences of filariasis are due both to direct effects of the worms and to the immune response of the host to the parasite. These immune responses are believed to cause the granulomatous and proliferative processes that precede total lymphatic obstruction. It is thought that the vessel remains patent as long as the worm remains viable and that death of the worm leads to enhanced granulomatous reaction and fibrosis. Lymphatic obstruction results, and, despite collateralization of the lymphatics, lymphatic function is compromised.

CLINICAL FEATURES The most common presentations of the lymphatic filariases are asymptomatic (or subclinical) microfilaremia, hydrocele, acute adenolymphangitis (ADL), and chronic lymphatic disease. In areas where *W. bancrofti* or *B. malayi* is endemic,

the overwhelming majority of infected individuals have few overt clinical manifestations of filarial infection despite large numbers of circulating microfilariae in the peripheral blood. Although they may be clinically asymptomatic, virtually all persons with *W. bancrofti* or *B. malayi* microfilaremia have some degree of subclinical disease that includes microscopic hematuria and/or proteinuria, dilated (and tortuous) lymphatics (visualized by imaging), and—in men—scrotal lymphangiectasia (detectable by ultrasound). Despite these findings, the majority of individuals appear to remain clinically asymptomatic for years; relatively few progress to the acute and chronic stages of infection.

ADL is characterized by high fever, lymphatic inflammation (lymphangitis and lymphadenitis), and transient local edema. The lymphangitis is retrograde, extending peripherally from the lymph node draining the area where the adult parasites reside. Regional lymph nodes are often enlarged, and the entire lymphatic channel can become indurated and inflamed. Concomitant local thrombophlebitis can occur as well. In brugian filariasis, a single local abscess may form along the involved lymphatic tract and subsequently rupture to the surface. The lymphadenitis and lymphangitis involve both the upper and lower extremities in both bancroftian and brugian filariasis, but involvement of the genital lymphatics occurs almost exclusively with *W. bancrofti* infection. This genital involvement can be manifested by funiculitis, epididymitis, scrotal pain, and tenderness. In endemic areas, another type of acute disease—dermatolymphangioadenitis (DLA)—is recognized as a syndrome that includes high fever, chills, myalgias, and headache. Edematous inflammatory plaques clearly demarcated from normal skin are seen. Vesicles, ulcers, and hyperpigmentation may also be noted. There is often a history of trauma, burns, radiation, insect bites, punctiform lesions, or chemical injury. Entry lesions, especially in the interdigital area, are common. DLA is often diagnosed as cellulitis.

If lymphatic damage progresses, transient lymphedema can develop into *lymphatic obstruction* and the permanent changes associated with elephantiasis. Brawny edema follows early pitting edema, and thickening of the subcutaneous tissues and hyperkeratosis occur. Fissuring of the skin develops, as do hyperplastic changes. Superinfection of these poorly vascularized tissues becomes a problem. In bancroftian filariasis, in which genital involvement is common, hydroceles may develop; in advanced stages, this condition may evolve into scrotal lymphedema and scrotal elephantiasis. Furthermore, if there is obstruction of the retroperitoneal lymphatics, the increased renal lymphatic pressure leads to rupture of the renal lymphatics and the development of chyluria, which is usually intermittent and most prominent in the morning.

The clinical manifestations of filarial infections in travelers or transmigrants who have recently entered an endemic region are distinctive. Given a sufficient number of bites by infected vectors, usually over a 3- to 6-month period, recently exposed patients can develop acute lymphatic or scrotal inflammation with or without urticaria and localized angioedema. Lymphadenitis of epitrochlear, axillary, femoral, or inguinal lymph nodes is often followed by retrogradely evolving lymphangitis. Acute attacks are short-lived and, in contrast to filarial fevers in patients native to endemic areas, are usually not accompanied by fever. With prolonged exposure to infected mosquitoes, these attacks, if untreated, become more severe and lead to permanent lymphatic inflammation and obstruction.

DIAGNOSIS A definitive diagnosis can be made only by detection of the parasites and hence can be difficult. Adult worms localized in lymphatic vessels or nodes are largely inaccessible. Microfilariae can be found in blood, in hydrocele fluid, or (occasionally) in other body fluids. Such fluids can be examined microscopically, either directly or—for greater sensitivity—after concentration of the parasites by the passage of fluid through a polycarbonate cylindrical pore filter (pore size, 3 μm) or by the centrifugation of fluid fixed in 2% formalin (Knott's concentration technique). The timing of blood collection is critical and should be based on the periodicity of the microfilariae in the endemic region involved. Many infected individuals do not have microfilaremia, and definitive diagnosis in such cases can be difficult. Assays for circulating antigens of *W. bancrofti* permit the diagnosis of microfilaremic and cryptic (amicrofilaremic) infection. Two tests are commercially available: one is an enzyme-linked immunosorbent assay (ELISA) and the other a rapid-format immunochromatographic card test. Both assays have sensitivities that range from 96 to 100% and specificities that approach 100%. There are currently no tests for circulating antigens in brugian filariasis.

Polymerase chain reaction (PCR)–based assays for DNA of *W. bancrofti* and *B. malayi* in blood have been developed. A number of studies indicate that this diagnostic method is of equivalent or greater sensitivity compared with parasitologic methods, detecting patent infection in almost all infected subjects.

In cases of suspected lymphatic filariasis, examination of the scrotum or the female breast using high-frequency ultrasound in conjunction with Doppler techniques may result in the identification of motile adult worms within dilated lymphatics. Worms may be visualized in the lymphatics of the spermatic cord in up to 80% of infected men. Live adult worms have a distinctive pattern of movement within the lymphatic vessels (termed the *filaria dance sign*).

Radionuclide lymphoscintigraphic imaging of the limbs reliably demonstrates widespread lymphatic abnormalities in both asymptomatic microfilaremic persons and those with clinical manifestations of lymphatic pathology. While of potential utility in the delineation of anatomic changes associated with infection, lymphoscintigraphy is unlikely to assume primacy in the diagnostic evaluation of individuals with suspected infection; it is principally a research tool, and the radionuclide-protein conjugates are not commercially available or approved by the U.S. Food and Drug Administration (FDA).

Eosinophilia and elevated serum concentrations of IgE and antifilarial antibody support the diagnosis of lymphatic filariasis. There is, however, extensive cross-reactivity between filarial antigens and antigens of other helminths, including the common intestinal roundworms; thus, interpretations of serologic findings can be difficult. In addition, residents of endemic areas can become sensitized to filarial antigens through exposure to infected mosquitoes without having patent filarial infections.

In acute episodes, lymphatic filariasis must be distinguished from thrombophlebitis, infection, and trauma. Retrogradely evolving lymphangitis is a characteristic feature that helps distinguish filarial lymphangitis from typically ascending bacterial lymphangitis. Chronic filarial lymphedema must be distinguished from the lymphedema of malignancy, postoperative scarring, trauma, chronic edematous states, and congenital lymphatic system abnormalities.

℞ **TREATMENT** With new definitions of clinical syndromes in lymphatic filariasis and new tools to assess clinical status (e.g., ultrasound, lymphoscintigraphy, circulating filarial antigen assays), approaches to treatment based on infection status can be considered. Diethylcarbamazine (DEC, 6 mg/kg daily for 12 days), which has both macro- and microfilaricidal properties, remains the treatment of choice for the individual with active lymphatic filariasis (microfilaremia, antigen positivity, or adult worms on ultrasound), although albendazole (400 mg twice daily for 21 days) has demonstrated macrofilaricidal efficacy.

As has already been mentioned, a growing body of evidence indicates that, although they may be asymptomatic, virtually all persons with *W. bancrofti* or *B. malayi* microfilaremia have some degree of subclinical disease (hematuria, proteinuria, abnormalities on lymphoscintigraphy). Thus, early treatment of asymptomatic persons is recommended to prevent further lymphatic damage. For ADL, supportive treatment (including the administration of antipyretics and analgesics) is recommended, as is antibiotic therapy if secondary bacterial infection is likely. Similarly, because lymphatic disease is associated with the presence of adult worms, treatment with DEC is recommended for microfilaria-negative adult-worm carriers.

In persons with chronic manifestations of lymphatic filariasis, treatment regimens that emphasize hygiene, prevention of secondary bacterial infections, and physiotherapy have gained wide acceptance for morbidity control. These regimens are similar to those recommended for lymphedema of most nonfilarial causes and known by a variety of names, including *complex decongestive physiotherapy* and *complex lymphedema therapy*. Hydroceles can be drained repeatedly or managed surgically. In patients with chronic manifestations of lymphatic filariasis, drug treatment should be reserved for cases with evidence of active infection.

The recommended course of DEC treatment (12 days; total dose, 72 mg/kg) has remained standard for many years; however, data indicate that single-dose DEC treatment with 6 mg/kg may be equally efficacious. The 12-day course provides more rapid short-term microfilarial suppression. Regimens that utilize single-dose DEC or ivermectin or combinations of single doses of albendazole and either DEC or ivermectin have all been demonstrated to have a sustained microfilaricidal effect.

Side effects of DEC treatment include fever, chills, arthralgias, headaches, nausea, and vomiting. Both the development and the severity of these reactions are directly related to the number of microfilariae circulating in the bloodstream and may represent an acute hypersensitivity reaction to the antigens being released by dead and dying parasites.

PREVENTION AND CONTROL Avoidance of mosquito bites is usually not feasible for residents of endemic areas, but visitors should make use of insect repellent and mosquito nets. DEC can kill developing forms of filarial parasites and has been shown to be useful as a prophylactic agent in humans.

Community-based intervention is the current approach to elimination of lymphatic filariasis as a public health problem. The underlying tenet of this approach is that mass annual distribution of antimicrofilarial chemotherapy (albendazole with either DEC or ivermectin) will profoundly suppress microfilaremia. If the suppression is sustained, then transmission can be interrupted. As an added benefit, these combinations have secondary effects on gastrointestinal helminths. An alternative approach to the control of lymphatic filariasis is the use of salt fortified with DEC. Community use of DEC-fortified salt dramatically reduces microfilarial density with no apparent adverse reactions. Community education and clinical care for persons already suffering from the chronic sequelae of lymphatic filariasis are important components of filariasis control and elimination programs.

TROPICAL PULMONARY EOSINOPHILIA

Tropical pulmonary eosinophilia (TPE) is a distinct syndrome that develops in some individuals infected with lymphatic filarial species. This syndrome affects males and females at a ratio of 4:1, often during the third decade of life. The majority of cases have been reported from India, Pakistan, Sri Lanka, Brazil, and Southeast Asia.

CLINICAL FEATURES The main features include a history of residence in filarial endemic regions, paroxysmal cough and wheezing that are usually nocturnal (and probably related to the nocturnal periodicity of microfilariae), weight loss, low-grade fever, adenopathy, and pronounced blood eosinophilia (>3000 eosinophils/μL). Chest x-rays may be normal but generally show increased bronchovascular markings; diffuse miliary lesions or mottled opacities may be present in the middle and lower lung fields. Tests of pulmonary function show restrictive abnormalities in most cases and obstructive defects in half. Total serum IgE levels (10,000 to 100,000 ng/mL) and antifilarial antibody titers are characteristically elevated.

PATHOLOGY In TPE there is rapid clearance of microfilariae and parasite antigens from the bloodstream by the lungs, and the clinical symptoms result from allergic and inflammatory reactions elicited by the cleared parasites. In some subjects, trapping of microfilariae in other reticuloendothelial organs can cause hepatomegaly, splenomegaly, or lymphadenopathy. A prominent, eosinophil-enriched, intra-alveolar infiltrate is often reported. In the absence of successful treatment, interstitial fibrosis can lead to progressive pulmonary damage.

DIFFERENTIAL DIAGNOSIS TPE must be distinguished from asthma, Löffler's syndrome, allergic bronchopulmonary aspergillosis, allergic granulomatosis with angiitis (Churg-Strauss syndrome), the systemic vasculitides (most notably periarteritis nodosa and Wegener's granulomatosis), chronic eosinophilic pneumonia, and the idiopathic hypereosinophilic syndrome. In addition to a geographic history of filarial exposure, useful features for distinguishing TPE include wheezing that is solely nocturnal, very high levels of antifilarial antibodies, and a rapid initial response to treatment with DEC.

℞ **TREATMENT** DEC is used at a dosage of 4 to 6 mg/kg of body weight per day for 14 days. Symptoms usually resolve within 3 to 7 days after the initiation of therapy. Relapse, which occurs in ~12 to 25% of cases (sometimes after an interval of years), requires re-treatment.

ONCHOCERCIASIS

Onchocerciasis ("river blindness") is caused by the filarial nematode *O. volvulus*, which infects an estimated 13 million individuals. The majority of individuals infected with *O. volvulus* live in the equatorial region of Africa extending from the Atlantic coast to the Red Sea. About 70,000 persons are infected in Guatemala and Mexico, with smaller foci in Venezuela, Colombia, Brazil, Ecuador, Yemen, and Saudi Arabia. Onchocerciasis is the second leading cause of infectious blindness worldwide.

ETIOLOGY AND EPIDEMIOLOGY Infection in humans begins with the deposition of infective larvae on the skin by the bite of an infected blackfly. The larvae develop into adults, which are typically found in subcutaneous nodules. About 7 months to 3 years after infection, the gravid female releases microfilariae that migrate out of the nodule and throughout the tissues, concentrating in the dermis. Infection is transmitted to other persons when a female fly ingests microfilariae from the host's skin and these microfilariae then develop into infective larvae. Adult *O. volvulus* females and males are about 40 to 60 cm and 3 to 6 cm in length, respectively. The life span of adults can be as long as 18 years, with an average of ~9 years. Because the blackfly vector breeds along free-flowing rivers and streams (particularly in rapids) and generally restricts its flight to an area within several kilometers of these breeding sites, both biting and disease transmission are most intense in these locations.

PATHOLOGY Onchocerciasis affects primarily the skin, eyes, and lymph nodes. In contrast to that in lymphatic filariasis, the damage in onchocerciasis is elicited by microfilariae and not by adults. In the skin, there are mild but chronic inflammatory changes that can result in loss of elastic fibers, atrophy, and fibrosis. The subcutaneous nodules, or onchocercomata, consist primarily of fibrous tissues surrounding the adult worm, often with a peripheral ring of inflammatory cells. In the eye, neovascularization and corneal scarring lead to corneal opacities and blindness. Inflammation in the anterior and posterior chambers frequently results in anterior uveitis, chorioretinitis, and optic atrophy. Although punctate opacities are due to an inflammatory reaction surrounding dead or dying microfilariae, the pathogenesis of most manifestations of onchocerciasis is still unclear.

CLINICAL FEATURES **Skin** Pruritus and rash are the most frequent manifestations of onchocerciasis. The pruritus can be incapacitating; the rash is typically a papular eruption that is generalized rather than localized to a particular region of the body. Long-term infection results in exaggerated and premature wrinkling of the skin, loss of elastic fibers, and epidermal atrophy that can lead to loose, redundant skin and hypo- or hyperpigmentation. Localized eczematoid dermatitis can cause hyperkeratosis, scaling, and pigmentary changes. Such lesions are often seen in the lower extremities but can be distributed more extensively.

Onchocercomata These subcutaneous nodules, which can be palpable and/or visible, contain the adult worm. In African patients, they are common over the coccyx and sacrum, the trochanter of the femur, the lateral anterior crest, and other bony prominences; in Latin American patients, they tend to develop preferentially in the upper part of the body, particularly on the head, neck, and shoulders. Nodules vary in size and characteristically are firm and not tender. It has been estimated that, for every palpable nodule, there are four deeper nonpalpable ones.

Ocular Tissue Visual impairment is the most serious complication of onchocerciasis and usually affects only those persons with moderate or heavy infections. Lesions may develop in all parts of the eye. The most common early finding is conjunctivitis with photophobia. In the cornea, punctate keratitis—consisting of acute inflammatory reactions surrounding dying microfilariae manifested as "snowflake" opacities—is frequent in younger patients and resolves without apparent complications. Sclerosing keratitis occurs in 1 to 5% of infected persons and is the leading cause of onchocercal blindness in Africa. Anterior uveitis and iridocyclitis develop in ~5% of infected persons in Africa. In Latin America, complications of the anterior uveal tract (pupillary deformity) may cause secondary glaucoma. Characteristic chorioretinal lesions develop as a result of atrophy and hyperpigmentation of the retinal pigment epithelium. Constriction of the visual field and frank optic atrophy may occur.

Lymph Nodes Mild to moderate lymphadenopathy is frequent, particularly in the inguinal and femoral areas, where the enlarged nodes may hang down in response to gravity ("hanging groin"), sometimes predisposing to inguinal and femoral hernias.

Systemic Manifestations Some heavily infected individuals develop cachexia with loss of adipose tissue and muscle mass. Among adults who become blind, there is a three- to fourfold increase in the mortality rate.

DIAGNOSIS Definitive diagnosis depends on the detection of an adult worm in an excised nodule or, more commonly, of microfilariae in a skin snip. Skin snips are obtained with a corneal-scleral punch, which collects a blood-free skin biopsy sample extending to just below the epidermis, or by lifting of the skin with the tip of a needle and excision of a small (1- to 3-mm) piece with a sterile scalpel blade. The biopsy tissue is incubated in tissue culture medium or in saline on a glass slide or flat-bottomed microtiter plate. After incubation for 2 to 4 h (or occasionally overnight in light infections), microfilariae emergent from the skin can be visualized by low-power microscopy.

Eosinophilia and elevated serum IgE levels are common but, because they occur in many parasitic infections, are not diagnostic in themselves. Assays to detect specific antibodies to *Onchocerca* and PCR to detect onchocercal DNA in skin snips are now in use in specialized laboratories and are highly sensitive and specific.

The *Mazzotti test* is a provocative technique that can be used in cases where the diagnosis of onchocerciasis is still in doubt (i.e., when skin snips and ocular examination reveal no microfilariae). A small dose of DEC (0.5 to 1.0 mg/kg) is given orally; the development or exacerbation of pruritus or rash within hours is highly suggestive of onchocerciasis.

℞ **TREATMENT** The main goals of therapy are to prevent the development of irreversible lesions and to alleviate symptoms. Surgical excision is recommended when nodules are located on the head (because of the proximity of microfilaria-producing adult worms to the eye), but chemotherapy is the mainstay of management. Ivermectin, a semisynthetic macrocyclic lactone active against microfilariae, is the first-line agent for the treatment of onchocerciasis. It is given orally in a single dose of 150 μg/kg, either yearly or semiannually. After treatment, most individuals have few or no reactions. Pruritus, cutaneous edema, and/or maculopapular rash occurs in ~1 to 10% of treated individuals. In areas of Africa coendemic for *O. volvulus* and *L. loa*, however, ivermectin is contraindicated (as it is for pregnant or breastfeeding women) because of severe posttreatment encephalopathy seen in patients, especially children, who are heavily microfilaremic for *L. loa* (>2000 to 5000 microfilariae per milliliter). Although ivermectin treatment results in a marked drop in microfilarial density, its effect can be short-lived (<6 months in some cases). Thus, it is occasionally necessary to give ivermectin more frequently for persistent symptoms. No currently available agent kills adult *O. volvulus*.

PREVENTION Vector control has been beneficial in highly endemic areas in which breeding sites are vulnerable to insecticide spraying, but most areas endemic for onchocerciasis are not suited to this type of control. Community-based administration of ivermectin every 6 to 12 months is now being used to interrupt transmission in endemic areas. This measure, in conjunction with vector control, has already helped reduce the prevalence of disease in endemic foci in Africa and Latin America. No drug has proven useful for prophylaxis of *O. volvulus* infection.

LOIASIS

ETIOLOGY AND EPIDEMIOLOGY Loiasis is caused by *L. loa* (the African eye worm), which is present in the rain forests of West and Central Africa. Adult parasites (females, 50 to 70 mm long and 0.5 mm wide; males, 25 to 35 mm long and 0.25 mm wide) live in subcutaneous tissues; microfilariae circulate in the blood with a diurnal periodicity that peaks between 12:00 noon and 2:00 P.M.

CLINICAL FEATURES Manifestations of loiasis in natives of endemic areas may differ from those in temporary residents or visitors. Among the indigenous population, loiasis is often an asymptomatic infection with microfilaremia. Infection may be recognized only after subconjunctival migration of an adult worm or may be manifested by episodic Calabar swellings, evanescent localized areas of angioedema and erythema developing on the extremities and less frequently at other sites. Nephropathy, encephalopathy, and cardiomyopathy are rare. In patients who are not residents of endemic areas, allergic symptoms predominate, episodes of Calabar swelling tend to be more frequent and debilitating, microfilaremia is rare, and eosinophilia and increased levels of antifilarial antibodies are characteristic.

PATHOLOGY The pathogenesis of the manifestations of loiasis is poorly understood. Calabar swellings are thought to result from a hypersensitivity reaction to the adult worm.

DIAGNOSIS Definitive diagnosis of loiasis requires the detection of microfilariae in the peripheral blood or the isolation of the adult worm from the eye or from a subcutaneous biopsy specimen from a site of swelling developing after treatment. PCR-based assays for the detection of *L. loa* DNA in blood are now available in specialized laboratories and are highly sensitive and specific. In practice, the diagnosis must often be based on a characteristic history and clinical presentation, blood eosinophilia, and elevated levels of antifilarial antibodies, particularly in travelers to an endemic region, who are usually amicrofilaremic. Other clinical findings in the latter individuals include hypergammaglobulinemia, elevated levels of serum IgE, and elevated leukocyte and eosinophil counts.

℞ **TREATMENT** DEC (8 to 10 mg/kg per day for 21 days) is effective against both the adult and the microfilarial forms of *L. loa*, but multiple courses are frequently necessary before the disease resolves completely. In cases of heavy microfilaremia, allergic or other inflammatory reactions can take place during treatment, including central nervous system involvement with coma and encephalitis. Heavy infections can be treated initially with apheresis to remove the microfilariae and with glucocorticoids (40 to 60 mg of prednisone per day) followed by doses of DEC (0.5 mg/kg per day). If antifilarial treatment has no adverse effects, the prednisone dose can be rapidly tapered and the dose of DEC gradually increased to 8 to 10 mg/kg per day.

Albendazole and ivermectin (although not approved by the FDA) have been shown to be effective in reducing microfilarial loads. DEC (300 mg weekly) is an effective prophylactic regimen for loiasis.

STREPTOCERCIASIS

Mansonella streptocerca, found mainly in the tropical forest belt of Africa from Ghana to Zaire, is transmitted by biting midges. The major clinical manifestations involve the skin and include pruritus, papular rashes, and pigmentation changes. Many infected individuals have inguinal adenopathy, although most are asymptomatic. The diagnosis is made by detection of the characteristic microfilariae in skin snips. DEC (6 mg/kg per day in divided doses for 14 to 21 days) is effective in killing both microfilariae and adult worms. As in onchocerciasis, treatment is sometimes accompanied by urticaria, arthralgias, myalgias, headaches, and abdominal discomfort. Ivermectin at a single dose of 150 μg/kg leads to sustained suppression of microfilariae in the skin and is likely to assume primacy in the treatment of streptocerciasis.

MANSONELLA PERSTANS INFECTION

Mansonella perstans, distributed across the center of Africa and in northeastern South America, is transmitted by midges. Adult worms reside in serous cavities—pericardial, pleural, and peritoneal—as well as in the mesentery and the perirenal and retroperitoneal tissues. Microfilariae circulate in the blood without periodicity. The clinical and pathologic features of the infection are poorly defined. Most patients appear to be asymptomatic, but manifestations may include transient angioedema and pruritus of the arms, face, or other parts of the body (analogous to the Calabar swellings of loiasis); fever; headache; arthralgias; and right upper quadrant pain. Occasionally, pericarditis and hepatitis occur. The diagnosis is based on the demonstration of microfilariae in blood or serosal effusions. Perstans filariasis is often associated with peripheral blood eosinophilia and antifilarial antibody elevations. Although DEC (8 to 10 mg/kg per day for 21 days) is the standard therapeutic agent, there is little evidence that it is effective. Cure is indicated by the disappearance of symptoms and eosinophilia; multiple courses of therapy are usually required. Both mebendazole (100 mg twice daily for 30 days) and albendazole (400 mg twice daily for 10 days) have been reported to be effective.

MANSONELLA OZZARDI INFECTION

The distribution of *Mansonella ozzardi* is restricted to Central and South America and certain Caribbean islands. Adult worms are rarely recovered from humans. Microfilariae circulate in the blood without periodicity. Although this organism has often been considered non-pathogenic, headache, articular pain, fever, pulmonary symptoms, adenopathy, hepatomegaly, pruritus, and eosinophilia have been ascribed to *M. ozzardi* infection. Diagnosis is made by the detection of microfilariae in peripheral blood. Ivermectin (a single dose of 6 mg) has been shown to be effective in treating this infection.

DRACUNCULIASIS (GUINEA WORM INFECTION)

ETIOLOGY AND EPIDEMIOLOGY   Dracunculiasis, caused by *Dracunculus medinensis*, is a parasitic infection whose incidence has declined dramatically because of global eradication efforts. Current estimates suggest that there are only 78,000 cases worldwide, the majority in Sudan. Humans acquire this infection when they ingest water containing infective larvae derived from *Cyclops*, a crustacean that is the intermediate host. Larvae penetrate the stomach or intestinal wall, mate, and mature. The adult male probably dies; the female *Dracunculus* develops over a year and migrates to subcutaneous tissues, usually in the lower extremity. As the thin female *Dracunculus*, ranging in length from 300 cm to 1 m, approaches the skin, a blister forms that, over days, breaks down and forms an ulcer. When the blister opens, large numbers of motile, rhabditiform larvae can be released into stagnant water; ingestion by *Cyclops* completes the life cycle.

CLINICAL FEATURES   Few or no clinical manifestations of dracunculiasis are evident until just before the blister forms, when there is an onset of fever and generalized allergic symptoms, including periorbital edema, wheezing, and urticaria. The emergence of the worm is associated with local pain and swelling. When the blister ruptures (usually as a result of immersion in water), the adult worm releases larva-rich fluid, and this release is associated with a relief of symptoms. The shallow ulcer surrounding the emerging adult worm heals over weeks to months. Such ulcers, however, can become secondarily infected, the result being cellulitis, local inflammation, abscess formation, or (uncommonly) tetanus. Occasionally, the adult worm does not emerge but becomes encapsulated and calcified.

DIAGNOSIS   The diagnosis is based on the findings developing with the emergence of the adult worm, as described above.

℞ **TREATMENT**   Gradual extraction of the worm by winding of a few centimeters on a stick each day remains the common and effective practice. Worms may be excised surgically. The administration of thiabendazole (25 mg/kg twice daily for 3 days) or metronidazole (250 mg three times daily for 10 days) may relieve symptoms but has no proven activity against the worm.

PREVENTION   Prevention, which remains the only real control measure, depends on the provision of safe drinking water.

ZOONOTIC FILARIAL INFECTIONS

Dirofilariae that affect primarily dogs, cats, and raccoons and *Brugia* parasites that affect small mammals occasionally infect humans incidentally. Because humans are an abnormal host, the parasites never develop fully. Pulmonary dirofilarial infection caused by the canine heartworm *Dirofilaria immitis* generally presents in humans as a solitary pulmonary nodule. Chest pain, hemoptysis, and cough are uncommon. Infections with *D. repens* (from dogs) or *D. tenuis* (from raccoons) can cause local subcutaneous nodules in humans. Zoonotic *Brugia* infection can produce isolated lymph node enlargement. Eosinophilia levels and antifilarial antibody titers are not commonly el-

evated. Excisional biopsy is both diagnostic and curative; these infections usually do not respond to chemotherapy.

BIBLIOGRAPHY

ADDISS DA, DREYER G: Treatment of lymphatic filariasis, in *Lymphatic Filariasis*, TB Nutman (ed). London, Imperial College Press, 1999, pp 151–199

BURNHAM GJ: Onchocerciasis. Lancet 351:1341, 1998

DREYER G et al: Acute attacks in the extremities of persons living in an area endemic for bancroftian filariasis: Differentiation of two syndromes. Trans R Soc Trop Med Hyg 93:413, 1999

FREEDMAN DO et al: Lymphoscintigraphic analysis of lymphatic abnormalities in symptomatic and asymptomatic human filariasis. J Infect Dis 170:927, 1994

GARDON J et al: Serious reactions after mass treatment of onchocerciasis with ivermectin in an area endemic for *Loa loa* infection. Lancet 350:18, 1997

HOPKINS DR: Perspectives from the dracunculiasis eradication programme. Bull World Health Organ 76(Suppl 2):38, 1998

KLION AD et al: Loiasis in endemic and non-endemic populations: Immunologically mediated differences in clinical presentation. J Infect Dis 163:1318, 1991

MCCARTHY JS: Diagnosis of lymphatic filarial infections, in *Lymphatic Filariasis*, TB Nutman (ed). London, Imperial College Press, 1999, pp 127–149

NOROES J et al: Occurrence of living adult *Wuchereria bancrofti* in the scrotal area of men with microfilaraemia. Trans R Soc Trop Med Hyg 90:55, 1996

ORIHEL TC, EBERHARD ML: Zoonotic filariasis. Clin Microbiol Rev 11:366, 1998

OTTESEN EA et al: The role of albendazole in programmes to eliminate lymphatic filariasis. Parasitol Today 15:382, 1999

WHO EXPERT COMMITTEE ON ONCHOCERCIASIS: Onchocerciasis and its control: Fourth report. Technical Report Series No. 852, Geneva, WHO, 1995

| 222 | *Adel A.F. Mahmoud* |

SCHISTOSOMIASIS AND OTHER TREMATODE INFECTIONS

Trematodes, or flatworms, are a group of morphologically and biologically heterogeneous parasitic helminths that belong to the phylum Platyhelminthes. Human infection with trematodes occurs in many geographic areas and can cause considerable morbidity and mortality. For clinical purposes, the significant trematode infections of humans may be divided according to the tissues invaded by adult flukes: blood, biliary tree, intestines, and lungs (Table 222-1).

Trematodes share some common morphologic features, including macroscopic size (from 1 cm to several cm); dorsoventral, flattened, bilaterally symmetric bodies (adult worms); and the prominence of two suckers. Except for the schistosomes, all trematodes that parasitize humans are hermaphroditic. The life cycle of trematodes involves a definitive host (mammalian/human), in which adult worms initiate sexual reproduction, and an intermediate host (snails, fish, etc.), in which asexual multiplication of the larval forms occurs. More than one intermediate host may be necessary for some species of trematodes. Human infection is initiated either by direct penetration of intact skin or by ingestion. Upon maturation within the human host, adult flukes initiate sexual reproduction that results in egg production. Helminth ova leave the definitive host in excreta or sputum and, upon reaching suitable environmental conditions, they hatch, releasing free-living miracidia that must find a specific snail intermediate host. After asexual reproduction, cercariae are released from infected snails; these organisms either infect humans (schistosomes) or must find another intermediate host to allow encystment into metacercariae.

The host-parasite relationship in trematode infections is a product of the biologic features of these organisms: they are multicellular, undergo several developmental changes within the host, and usually result in chronic infections. In general, the distribution of worm infections in human populations is overdispersed; i.e., it follows a negative binomial mathematical relationship in which most infected individuals harbor low worm burdens while a small percentage are heavily infected. It is the heavily infected minority who are particularly prone to disease sequelae and who represent an epidemiologically significant

Table 222-1 Major Human Trematode Infections

Trematode	Transmission	Endemic Area(s)
BLOOD FLUKES		
Shistosoma mansoni	Skin penetration by cercariae	Africa, South America, Middle East
S. japonicum	Skin penetration by cercariae	China, Philippines, Indonesia
S. intercalatum	Skin penetration by cercariae	West Africa
S. mekongi	Skin penetration by cercariae	Southeast Asia
S. haematobium	Skin penetration by cercariae	Africa, Middle East
BILIARY (HEPATIC) FLUKES		
Clonorchis sinensis	Ingestion of metacercariae in freshwater fish	Far East
Opisthorchis viverrini	Ingestion of metacercariae in freshwater fish	Far East, Thailand
O. felineus	Ingestion of metacercariae in freshwater fish	Far East, Europe
Fasciola hepatica	Ingestion of metacercariae on aquatic plants or in water	Worldwide
F. gigantica	Ingestion of metacercariae on aquatic plants or in water	Sporadic, Africa
INTESTINAL FLUKES		
Fasciolopsis buski	Ingestion of metacercariae on aquatic plants	Southeast Asia
Heterophyes heterophyes	Ingestion of metacercariae in freshwater or brackish-water fish	Far East, North Africa
LUNG FLUKES		
Paragonimus westermani	Ingestion of metacercariae in crayfish or crabs	Global except North America and Europe

reservoir of infection in endemic areas. It is important to appreciate that worms do not multiply within the definitive host and that they have a relatively long life span, ranging from a few months to a few years. Morbidity and mortality due to trematode infections reflect a multifactorial process that results from the tipping of a delicate balance based on the intensity of infection and the host reactions that initiate and modulate pathologic outcome. The genetics of the parasite and the human host contribute to the outcome of infection and disease. Furthermore, infections with trematodes that migrate through or reside in host tissues are associated with a moderate to high degree of peripheral blood eosinophilia; this association is of significance in protective and immunopathologic sequelae and is a useful clinical indicator of infection.

_____ *Approach to the Patient* _____

The approach to individuals with suspected trematode infection begins with the question: Where have you been? Details of geographic history, exposure to freshwater bodies, and indulgence in local eating habits without ensuring safety of food and drink are all essential elements in the history. The workup plan must include a detailed physical examination and tests appropriate for the suspected infection. Diagnosis is based either on detection of the relevant stage of the parasite in excreta, sputum, or (rarely) tissue samples or on sensitive and specific serologic tests. Consultation with physicians familiar with these infections or with the U.S. Centers for Disease Control and Prevention (CDC) is helpful in guiding diagnosis and selecting therapy.

BLOOD FLUKES: SCHISTOSOMIASIS

Human schistosomiasis is caused by five species of this parasitic trematode belonging to the subclass Digenea: the intestinal species *Schistosoma mansoni*, *S. japonicum*, *S. mekongi*, and *S. intercalatum* and the urinary species *S. haematobium*. Infection may cause considerable morbidity in the intestines, liver, and urinary tract, and a proportion of affected individuals die. Other schistosome species (e.g., avian species) may invade human skin but then die in subcutaneous tissue, producing only self-limiting cutaneous manifestations.

Information on the prevalence and geographic distribution of human schistosomiasis is inexact. The five species are estimated to infect 200 to 300 million people in South America, the Caribbean, Africa, the Middle East, and Southeast Asia. The total population living under conditions favoring transmission approximates double or triple that number—a fact reflecting the public health significance of schistosomiasis.

ETIOLOGY Human infection is initiated by penetration of intact skin with infective cercariae. These organisms are released from infected snails in freshwater bodies; they measure ~2 mm in length and possess an anterior and a ventral sucker that attaches to the skin surface and facilitates penetration. Once in the subcutaneous tissue, the organism transforms into the next stage: the schistosomula. This transformation involves morphologic, membrane, and immunologic changes, prominent among which is the transformation of the cercarial outer membrane from a trilaminar to a heptalaminar structure that is then maintained throughout the life span of the worms in humans. The transformation to a heptalaminar structure is thought to be the schistosome's main adaptive mechanism for survival in humans. Schistosomula begin their migration within 2 to 4 days via venous or lymphatic vessels, reaching the lungs and finally the liver parenchyma. Sexually mature worms descend in pairs into the venous system at specific anatomic locations: intestinal veins (*S. mansoni*, *S. japonicum*, *S. mekongi*, and *S. intercalatum*) and vesical veins (*S. haematobium*). Adult gravid females then travel against venous blood flow to small tributaries, where they deposit their ova intravascularly. Schistosome ova have specific morphologic features that can be used to differentiate species. Aided by enzymatic secretions through minipores in eggshells, ova move through the venous wall, traversing host tissues to reach the lumen of the intestinal or urinary tract, and are voided with stools or urine. Approximately 50% of ova, however, fail in their attempt to be transported to the outside environment and are either retained in host tissues locally (intestines or urinary tract) or carried by venous blood flow to the liver and other organs. Schistosome ova that reach freshwater bodies hatch, releasing free-living miracidia that seek the snail intermediate host to undergo several asexual multiplication cycles. Finally, infective cercariae are shed from snails.

Adult schistosome worms measure ~1 to 2 cm in length. The male is slightly shorter, with a flattened body; its edges curve anteriorly to form the gynecophoral canal, in which mature adult females are usually held. The females are longer, slender, and rounded in cross-section. The precise nature of biochemical and reproductive exchanges between the two sexes is unknown, as are the regulatory mechanisms for pairing. Adult schistosomes parasitize specific sites in the host venous system. What guides adult intestinal schistosomes to branches of the superior or inferior mesenteric veins or adult *S. haematobium* worms to the vesical plexus is unknown. In addition, the evasion mechanisms by which adult worms inhibit the coagulation cascade and the effector arms of the host immune responses are not fully understood.

A systematic examination of schistosomal molecular phylogeny as well as gene structure and organization has begun. Analysis of the sequence of nuclear ribosome and internal transcribed spacer 2 and mitochondrial 16 sRNA indicates that human schistosomes may be divided into three monophyletic groups: the *S. haematobium* group, including *S. haematobium* and *S. intercalatum*; the *S. mansoni* group, including *S. mansoni* and *S. rodhaini*; and a group containing the two Asian schistosomes, *S. japonicum* and *S. mekongi*. These molecular groupings coincide with results of previous attempts to use morphologic or nucleic acid data to produce a taxonomic framework. In other studies, the schistosome genome was determined to be made up of 16 chromosomes; sexual differentiation is related to the presence of ZW chromosomes in females and ZZ chromosomes in males.

EPIDEMIOLOGY   The distribution of schistosome infection and related disease syndromes in human populations is dependent on both parasite and host factors. In endemic areas, the rate of yearly onset of new infection, or incidence, is low. Prevalence, on the other hand, starts to be appreciable by the age of 3 to 4 years and builds to a maximum that varies by endemic region (up to 100%) in the 15- to 20-year age group. Prevalence then stabilizes or decreases slightly in older age groups (>40 years). Intensity of infection (as measured by fecal or urinary egg counts, which correlate with adult worm burdens in most circumstances) follows the increase in prevalence up to the age of 15 to 20 years and then declines markedly in older age groups. This decline may reflect acquisition of resistance, or it may be due to changes in water contact patterns, since older people are exposed less. Furthermore, the unique distribution of schistosomes in human populations, which fits a negative binomial pattern (see above), may be due to heterogeneity of worm populations, with some more invasive than others; alternatively, it may be due to differences in the genetic susceptibility of host populations.

Disease due to schistosomiasis is the outcome of parasitologic, host, and additional infectious, nutritional, and environmental factors. Most of the disease syndromes relate to the presence of one or more of the parasite stages in the human host. The distribution of disease manifestations in the populations of endemic areas correlates with the intensity and duration of infection as well as with the age and genetic susceptibility of the host. Overall, disease manifestations are clinically relevant in only a small proportion of persons infected with any of the intestinal schistosomes. In contrast, urinary schistosomiasis manifests clinically in most infected individuals.

Patients with both HIV infection and schistosomiasis have been found to excrete far fewer eggs in their stools than those infected with *S. mansoni* alone. The two groups have responded equally to treatment with praziquantel.

PATHOGENESIS AND IMMUNITY   During the invasive stage, cercaria-associated dermatitis reflects dermal and subdermal inflammatory responses—both humoral and cell-mediated. As the parasites approach sexual maturity and the commencement of oviposition, acute schistosomiasis or Katayama fever (a serum sickness–like illness; see "Clinical Features," below) may occur. The associated antigen excess results in the formation of soluble immune complexes, which may be deposited in several tissues, initiating the sequence of pathologic events. In chronic schistosomiasis, most disease manifestations are due to eggs retained in host tissue. The granulomatous response around these ova is cell-mediated and is regulated both positively and negatively by a cascade of cytokine, cellular, and humoral responses. Granuloma formation begins with recruitment of a host of inflammatory cells in response to antigens secreted by the living organism within the ova. Cells recruited initially include phagocytes, antigen-specific T cells, and eosinophils. Fibroblasts, giant cells, and B lymphocytes predominate later. Once activated, T cells produce cytokines [such as tumor necrosis factor α (TNF-α), interleukin (IL) 2, IL-4, and IL-5, which in turn activate endothelial cells] and produce specific chemokines such as monocyte chemotactic protein 1 (MCP-1). The result is recruitment of the cellular elements that organize in the form of granulomas around parasite eggs. These lesions reach a size many times that of the eggs, thus inducing organomegaly and obstruction. Immunomodulation or downregulation of host responses to schistosome eggs plays a significant role in limiting the extent of the granulomatous lesions—and consequently disease—in chronically infected experimental animals or humans. The underlying mechanisms involve another cascade of regulatory cytokines (IL-10, IL-12) and idiotypic antibodies. Subsequent to the granulomatous response, fibrosis sets in, resulting in more permanent disease sequelae. Because schistosomiasis is a chronic infection, the accumulation of antigen-antibody complexes results in deposits in renal glomeruli and may cause significant kidney disease.

The better-studied pathologic sequelae in schistosomiasis are those observed in liver disease. Ova that are carried by portal blood embolize to the liver. Because of their size (~150 × 60 μm in the case of *S. mansoni*), they lodge at presinusoidal sites, where granulomas are formed. The granulomas contribute to the liver enlargement observed in infected individuals. Schistosomal hepatomegaly is also associated with certain class I and class II HLA markers; its genetic basis appears to be multigenic. Presinusoidal portal blockage causes several hemodynamic changes, including portal hypertension and associated development of portosystemic collaterals at the esophagogastric junction and other sites. Esophageal varices are most likely to break and cause repeated episodes of hematemesis. Because changes in liver hemodynamics in schistosomiasis are slow, compensatory arterialization of blood flow through the liver is established. While this compensatory mechanism may be associated with certain metabolic side effects, the retention of hepatocyte perfusion may permit the maintenance of normal liver function for several years.

After granuloma formation, the second most significant pathologic change in the liver relates to the onset of fibrosis. It is characteristically periportal (Symmers' clay-pipe stem fibrosis) but may be diffuse. Fibrosis, when diffuse, may be seen in areas of egg deposition and granuloma formation, but it is also seen in distant locations such as portal tracts. Schistosomiasis alone results in pure fibrotic lesions in the liver; cirrhosis occurs when other nutritional or infectious agents (e.g., hepatitis B or C virus) are involved. In recent years, it has been recognized that deposition of fibrotic tissue in the extracellular matrix results from the interaction of T lymphocytes with cells of the fibroblast series; several cytokines, such as IL-2, IL-4, IL-1, and transforming growth factor β (TGF-β), are known to stimulate fibrogenesis. The process may be dependent on the genetic constitution of the host. Furthermore, regulatory cytokines that can suppress fibrogenesis, such as interferon γ (IFN-γ) or IL-12, may play a role in modulating the response.

While the above description focuses on granuloma formation and fibrosis of the liver, similar processes occur in urinary schistosomiasis. Granuloma formation at the lower end of the ureters obstructs urinary flow, with subsequent development of hydroureter and hydronephrosis. Similar lesions in the urinary bladder cause the protrusion of papillomatous structures into its cavity; these may ulcerate and/or bleed. The chronic stage of infection is associated with scarring and deposition of calcium in the bladder wall.

Immunomodulation is an essential mechanism in shaping the clinical and pathologic outcome of schistosomiasis. While most detailed immunologic analyses have been performed in experimental animals, enough evidence exists from studies in humans to delineate the suppression of T cell responses in association with active infections and a regulatory role for IL-10.

Studies on immunity to schistosomiasis, whether innate or acquired, have expanded our knowledge of the components of these responses and the target antigens. The concept of innate immunity is illustrated by the inability of avian schistosomes, which cause swimmers' itch, to reach maturity in humans. The critical question, however, is whether humans acquire immunity to schistosomes. Epidemiologic evidence suggests the onset of acquired immunity during the course of infection in young adults. Curative treatment of infection divides populations in endemic areas into those who acquire reinfection rapidly (susceptible) and those who follow a protracted course (resistant). This difference may be explained by differences in transmission, immunologic response, or genetic susceptibility. The mechanism of acquired immunity involves antibodies, complement, and several effector cells, particularly eosinophils. Furthermore, the intensity of schistosome infection has been correlated with a region in chromosome 5. In other studies, several protective schistosome antigens have been identified as vaccine candidates.

CLINICAL FEATURES   In general, disease manifestations of schistosomiasis occur in three stages, which vary not only by species but also by intensity of infection and other host factors, such as age and genetics. During the phase of cercarial invasion, a form of dermatitis may be observed. This so-called swimmers' itch occurs most often with *S. mansoni* and *S. japonicum* infections, manifesting 2 or

3 days after invasion as an itchy maculopapular rash on the affected areas of the skin. The condition is particularly severe when humans are exposed to avian schistosomes. This form of cercarial dermatitis is seen around the freshwater lakes in the northern United States, particularly in the spring. Cercarial dermatitis is a self-limiting clinical entity. During worm maturation and at the beginning of oviposition (i.e., 4 to 8 weeks after skin invasion), acute schistosomiasis or Katayama fever—a serum sickness–like syndrome with fever, generalized lymphadenopathy, and hepatosplenomegaly—may develop. Individuals suffering from acute schistosomiasis show a high degree of peripheral blood eosinophilia. Parasite-specific antibodies may be detected before schistosome eggs are identified in excreta. Acute schistosomiasis has become an important clinical entity worldwide because of increased travel to endemic areas. Travelers are exposed to the parasite while swimming or wading in freshwater bodies and upon their return present with the acute manifestations of the disease. The course of acute schistosomiasis is generally benign, but deaths are occasionally reported in association with heavy exposure to schistosomes.

The main clinical manifestations of chronic schistosomiasis are species-dependent. Intestinal species (*S. mansoni*, *S. japonicum*, *S. mekongi*, and *S. intercalatum*) cause intestinal and hepatosplenic disease as well as several manifestations associated with portal hypertension. During the intestinal phase, which may begin a few months after infection and may last for years, symptomatic patients characteristically have colicky abdominal pain and bloody diarrhea. Patients may also report fatigue and an inability to perform daily routine functions and may show evidence of growth retardation. The severity of intestinal schistosomiasis is often related to the intensity of the worm burden. The disease runs a chronic course but rarely progresses to a functional level (e.g., malabsorption) or to anatomic lesions of the gut. The exception is colonic polyposis, which has been seen in some endemic areas, such as Egypt.

The hepatosplenic phase of disease manifests early (during the first year of infection, particularly in children) with enlargement of the liver due to parasite-induced granulomatous lesions. Hepatomegaly is seen in ~15 to 20% of infected individuals when whole communities in endemic areas are studied. It correlates roughly with the intensity of infection, occurs more often in children than in adults, and may be related to specific HLA haplotypes. In subsequent phases of infection, presinusoidal blockage of blood flow leads to portal hypertension and splenomegaly. Moreover, portal hypertension may lead to varices at the lower end of the esophagus and at other sites. Patients with schistosomal liver disease may have right-upper-quadrant "dragging" pain during the hepatomegaly phase, and this pain may move to the left upper quadrant as splenomegaly progresses. Bleeding from esophageal varices may, however, be the first clinical manifestation of this phase. Patients may experience repeated bleeding but seem to tolerate its impact, since an adequate total hepatic blood flow permits normal liver function for a considerable period in schistosomal hepatomegaly. In late-stage disease, typical fibrotic changes occur along with liver function deterioration and the onset of ascites, hypoalbuminemia, and defects in coagulation. Intercurrent viral infections of the liver or nutritional deficiencies may well accelerate or exacerbate the deterioration of hepatic function.

The extent and severity of intestinal and hepatic disease in schistosomiasis mansoni and japonica have been well described. While it was originally thought that *S. japonicum* might induce more severe disease manifestations because the adult worms can produce ten times more eggs than *S. mansoni*, subsequent field studies have not supported this claim. Clinical observations of individuals infected with *S. mekongi* or *S. intercalatum* have been less detailed, partly because of the far more limited geographic distribution of these organisms.

The clinical manifestations of *S. haematobium* infection occur relatively early and involve a relatively high percentage of individuals. Up to 80% of children infected with *S. haematobium* have dysuria, frequency, and hematuria, which may be terminal. Urine examination reveals blood and albumin as well as an unusually high frequency of bacterial urinary tract infection. These manifestations correlate with

intense infection, the presence of urinary bladder granulomas, and subsequent ulceration. Along with the local effects of granuloma formation in the urinary bladder, obstruction of the lower end of the ureters results in hydroureter and hydronephrosis, which can be seen in 25 to 50% of infected children. As infection progresses, bladder granulomas undergo fibrosis; the result is the presence of typical sandy patches visible on cystoscopy. In many endemic areas, an association between squamous cell carcinoma of the bladder and *S. haematobium* infection has been observed. Such malignancy is detected in a younger age group than transitional cell carcinoma. In fact, *S. haematobium* has now been classified as a human carcinogen.

Significant disease may occur in other organs during chronic schistosomiasis. Most important is disease in the lungs and central nervous system; other locations, such as the skin and the genital organs, are far less frequently affected. In pulmonary schistosomiasis, embolized eggs lodge in small arterioles, producing acute necrotizing arteriolitis and granuloma formation. During *S. mansoni* and *S. japonicum* infection, schistosome eggs reach the lungs after the development of portosystemic collateral circulation; in *S. haematobium* infection, ova may reach the lungs directly via connections between the vesical and systemic circulation. After the development of arteriolitis and granuloma formation, fibrous tissue deposition is detected and leads to endarteritis obliterans, pulmonary hypertension, and cor pulmonale. This clinical entity is an uncommon presentation during chronic schistosomiasis. The most frequent symptoms are cough, fever, and dyspnea; ascites and hemoptysis are less frequently encountered. Cor pulmonale may be diagnosed radiologically on the basis of prominent right side of the heart and dilation of the pulmonary artery. Frank evidence of right-sided heart failure may be seen in late cases.

Central nervous system schistosomiasis is important but less frequent than pulmonary schistosomiasis. It characteristically occurs as cerebral disease due to *S. japonicum* infection. Migratory worms deposit eggs in the brain and induce a granulomatous response. The frequency of this manifestation among infected individuals in some endemic areas (e.g., the Philippines) is calculated at 2 to 4%. Jacksonian epilepsy due to *S. japonicum* infection is the second most common cause of epilepsy in these areas. *S. mansoni* and *S. haematobium* infections have been associated with transverse myelitis. This syndrome is thought to be due to eggs traveling to the venous plexus around the spinal cord. In schistosomiasis mansoni, transverse myelitis is usually seen in the chronic stage after the development of portal hypertension and portosystemic shunts, which allow ova to travel to the spinal cord veins. This proposed sequence of events has been challenged because of a few reports of transverse myelitis occurring early in the course of *S. mansoni* infection. More information is needed to confirm these observations. During schistosomiasis haematobia, ova may travel through communication between vesical and systemic veins, resulting in spinal cord disease that may be detected at any stage of infection. Pathologic study of lesions in schistosomal transverse myelitis may reveal eggs along with necrotic or granulomatous lesions. Patients usually present with acute or rapidly progressing lower-leg weakness accompanied by sphincter dysfunction.

DIAGNOSIS Physicians in areas not endemic for schistosomiasis face considerable diagnostic challenges. In the most common clinical presentation, a returning traveler exhibits symptoms and signs of any of the acute syndromes of schistosomiasis—namely, cercarial dermatitis or Katayama fever. Central to correct diagnosis is a thorough inquiry into travel history and exposure to freshwater bodies, whether slow or fast running. Differential diagnosis of fever in returned travelers includes a spectrum of infections whose etiologies are viral (e.g., Dengue fever), bacterial (e.g., enteric fever, leptospirosis), rickettsial, or protozoal (e.g., malaria). In cases of Katayama fever, prompt diagnosis is essential and is based on clinical presentation, high-level peripheral blood eosinophilia, and a positive serologic assay for schistosomal antibodies. Two tests are available at the CDC: the Falcon assay screening test/enzyme-linked immunosorbent assay (FAST-

ELISA) and the confirmatory enzyme-linked immunoelectrotransfer blot (EITB). Both tests are highly sensitive and ~96% specific. In some instances, examination of stool or urine for ova may yield positive results.

Individuals with established infection are diagnosed by a combination of geographic history, characteristic clinical presentation, and presence of schistosome ova in excreta. The diagnosis may also be established with the serologic assays mentioned above or with those that detect circulating schistosome antigens. These assays can be applied either to blood or to other body fluids (e.g., cerebrospinal fluid). For stool examination, the Kato thick smear or any other concentration method generally identifies all but the most lightly infected individuals. Urine may be examined by microscopy of sediment or by filtration of a known volume through Nuclepore filters. Kato thick smear and Nuclepore filtration provide quantitative data on the intensity of infection, which is of value in assessing the degree of tissue damage and in monitoring the effect of chemotherapy. Finally, schistosome infection may be diagnosed by examination of tissue samples, typically rectal biopsies; other biopsy procedures (e.g., liver biopsy) are not needed, except in special circumstances.

Differential diagnosis of schistosomal hepatomegaly must include viral hepatitis of all etiologies, miliary tuberculosis, malaria, visceral leishmaniasis, ethanol abuse, and causes of hepatic and portal vein obstruction. Of patients with these conditions, only a few may present with organomegaly and relatively intact liver function. The differential diagnosis of hematuria in *S. haematobium* infection includes bacterial cystitis, tuberculosis, urinary stones, and malignancy.

℞ **TREATMENT**   Treatment of schistosomiasis depends on the stage of infection and the clinical presentation. Other than topical dermatologic applications for relief of itching, no specific treatment is indicated for cercarial dermatitis caused by avian schistosomes. Therapy for acute schistosomiasis or Katayama fever needs to be adjusted appropriately for each case. While antischistosomal chemotherapy is indicated, it does not address immediate pathologic changes. In severe acute schistosomiasis, management in an acute-care setting is necessary, with supportive measures and consideration of glucocorticoid treatment. Once the acute critical phase is over, specific chemotherapy is indicated. For all individuals with infection established by either the demonstration of schistosome eggs or positive serology, treatment to eradicate the parasite should be administered. The drug of choice is praziquantel, which—depending on the infecting species (Table 222-2)—is administered orally as 40 or 60 mg/kg in two or three doses over a single day. Praziquantel treatment results in parasitologic cure in ~85% of cases and reduces egg counts by >90%. Few side effects

Table 222-2   Drug Therapy for Human Trematode Infections

Infection	Drug of Choice	Adult Dose and Duration
BLOOD FLUKES		
S. mansoni, S. intercalatum, S. haematobium	Praziquantel	20 mg/kg, 2 doses in 1 day
S. japonicum, S. mekongi	Praziquantel	20 mg/kg, 3 doses in 1 day
BILIARY FLUKES		
C. sinensis, O. viverrini, O. felineus	Praziquantel	25 mg/kg, 3 doses in 1 day
F. hepatica, F. gigantica	Triclabendazole	10 mg/kg once
INTESTINAL FLUKES		
F. buski, H. heterophyes	Praziquantel	25 mg/kg, 3 doses in 1 day
LUNG FLUKES		
P. westermani	Praziquantel	25 mg/kg, 3 doses per day for 2 days

have been encountered, and those that do develop usually do not interfere with completion of treatment. Other antischistosomal chemotherapeutic agents are currently considered only as alternatives when praziquantel is unavailable. The effect of antischistosomal treatment on disease manifestations varies by stage. Early hepatomegaly and bladder lesions are known to resolve following chemotherapy, but the late established manifestations, such as fibrosis, do not change. Additional management modalities are needed for individuals with other manifestations, such as hepatocellular failure or recurrent hematemesis. The use of these interventions is guided by general medical and surgical principles.

PREVENTION AND CONTROL   Since transmission of schistosomiasis is dependent on human behavior, it is theoretically possible to devise an effective preventive strategy. The geographic distribution of infections in endemic regions of the world is not clearly demarcated. It is therefore prudent for travelers to avoid contact with all freshwater bodies, irrespective of the speed of water flow or unsubstantiated claims of safety. Some topical agents, when applied to the skin, may conceivably inhibit cercarial penetration, but none of these agents is currently available. If exposure occurs, a follow-up visit with a health care provider is strongly recommended. Prevention of infection in inhabitants of endemic areas is a significant challenge. People of these regions use freshwater bodies for sanitary, domestic, recreational, and agricultural purposes. In the absence of adequate alternatives, several control measures have been used, including application of molluscicides, provision of sanitary water and means for sewage disposal, chemotherapy, and health education. Current recommendations to countries endemic for schistosomiasis emphasize the use of multiple approaches. Particularly with the advent of a single-oral-dose, safe, and effective antischistosomal agent, chemotherapy has been most successful in reducing the intensity of infection and reversing disease. The duration of this positive impact depends on transmission dynamics in a specific endemic region. The ultimate goal of research on prevention and control is the development of a vaccine. Although there are a few promising leads, this goal is probably not within reach during the next decade or so.

LIVER (BILIARY) FLUKES

Several species of biliary fluke infecting humans are particularly common in Southeast Asia and Russia. Other species are transmitted in Europe, Africa, and the Americas. On the basis of their migratory pathway in humans, these infections may be divided into the *Clonorchis* and *Fasciola* groups.

CLONORCHIASIS AND OPISTHORCHIASIS   Infection with *C. sinensis*, the Chinese or oriental fluke, is endemic among fish-eating mammals in Southeast Asia. Humans are an incidental host; the prevalence of human infection is highest in China, Vietnam, and Korea. Infection with *Opisthorchis viverrini* and *O. felineus* is zoonotic in cats and dogs. Transmission to humans occurs occasionally, particularly in Thailand (*O. viverrini*) and in Southeast Asia and eastern Europe (*O. felineus*). Data on the exact geographic distribution of these infectious agents in human populations are rudimentary.

Infection with any of these three species is established by ingestion of raw or inadequately cooked freshwater fish harboring metacercariae. These organisms excyst in the duodenum, releasing larvae that travel through the ampulla of Vater and mature into adult worms in the bile canaliculi. Mature flukes are flat and elongated, measuring 1 to 2 cm in length. The hermaphroditic worms reproduce by releasing small operculated eggs, which pass with bile into the intestines and are voided with stools. The life cycle is completed in the environment in specific freshwater snails (the first intermediate host) and encystment of metacercariae in freshwater fish.

Except for late sequelae, the exact clinical syndromes caused by clonorchiasis and opisthorchiasis are not well defined. Since most infected individuals harbor a low worm burden, many are asymptomatic. Moderate to heavy infection may be associated with vague right-upper-quadrant pain. In contrast, chronic or repeated infection is associated with manifestations such as cholangitis, cholangiohepatitis, and biliary obstruction. Cholangiocarcinoma is epidemiologically related to *C. sinensis* infection in China and to *O. viverrini* infection in northeastern Thailand. This association has resulted in the classification of these infectious agents as human carcinogens.

FASCIOLIASIS Infections with *F. hepatica* and *F. gigantica* are worldwide zoonoses that are particularly endemic in sheep-raising countries. Human cases have been reported in South America, Europe, Africa, Australia, and the Far East. Recent estimates indicate a worldwide prevalence of 17 million cases. High endemicity has been reported in certain areas of Peru and Bolivia. In most endemic areas the predominant species is *F. hepatica*, but in Asia and Africa a varying degree of overlap with *F. gigantica* has been observed.

Humans acquire fascioliasis by ingestion of metacercariae attached to certain aquatic plants, such as watercress. Infection may also be acquired by consumption of contaminated water or ingestion of food items washed with such water. Acquisition of human infection through consumption of freshly prepared raw liver containing immature flukes has been reported. Infection is initiated when metacercariae excyst, penetrate the gut wall, and travel through the peritoneal cavity to invade the liver capsule. Adult worms finally reach the bile ducts, where they produce large operculated eggs, which are voided in the bile and through the gastrointestinal tract to the outside environment. The flukes' life cycle is completed in specific snails (the first intermediate host) and encystment on aquatic plants.

The clinical features of fascioliasis relate to the intensity of infection, but even more to the stage of infection. Acute disease develops during the parasites' migration (1 to 2 weeks after infection) and includes fever, right-upper-quadrant pain, hepatomegaly, and eosinophilia. Computed tomography of the liver may show migratory tracks. Symptoms and signs usually subside as the parasites reach their final habitat. In individuals with chronic infection, bile duct obstruction and biliary cirrhosis are infrequently demonstrated. No relation to hepatic malignancy has been ascribed to fascioliasis.

DIAGNOSIS The diagnosis of infection with any of the biliary flukes depends on a high degree of suspicion, the elicitation of an appropriate geographic history, and stool examination for the characteristically shaped parasite ova. Additional evidence may be obtained by documenting peripheral blood eosinophilia or imaging the liver. Serologic testing is helpful, particularly in lightly infected individuals.

℞ **TREATMENT** Drug therapy (praziquantel or triclabendazole) is summarized in Table 222-2. Patients with anatomic lesions in the biliary tract or malignancy are managed according to general medical guidelines.

INTESTINAL FLUKES

Two species of intestinal flukes cause human infection in defined geographic areas worldwide. The large *Fasciolopsis buski* (adults measure 2 by 7 cm) is endemic in Southeast Asia, while the smaller *Heterophyes heterophyes* is found in the Nile Delta of Egypt and in the Far East. Infection is initiated by ingestion of metacercariae attached to aquatic plants (*F. buski*) or encysted in freshwater or brackish-water fish (*H. heterophyes*). Flukes mature in human intestines, and eggs are passed with stools. Most individuals infected with intestinal flukes are asymptomatic. In heavy *F. buski* infection, diarrhea, abdominal pain, and malabsorption may be encountered. Heavy infection with *H. heterophyes* may be associated with abdominal pain and mucous diarrhea. The diagnosis is established by detection of the characteristically shaped ova in stool samples. The drug of choice for treatment is praziquantel (Table 222-2).

LUNG FLUKES

Infection with the lung fluke *Paragonimus westermani* and related species (e.g., *P. africanus*) is endemic in many parts of the world, excluding North America and Europe. Endemicity is particularly noticeable in West Africa, Central and South America, and Asia. In nature, the reservoir hosts of *P. westermani* are wild and domestic felines. In Africa, *P. africanus* has been found in other species, such as dogs. Adult lung flukes, which are 7 to 12 mm in length, are found encapsulated in the lungs of infected persons. In rare circumstances, flukes are found encysted in the central nervous system (cerebral paragonimiasis) or abdominal cavity. Humans acquire lung fluke infection by ingesting infective metacercariae encysted in the muscles and viscera of crayfish and freshwater crabs. In endemic areas, these crustaceans are consumed either raw or pickled. Once the organisms reach the duodenum, they excyst, penetrate the gut wall, and travel through the peritoneal cavity, diaphragm, and pleural space to reach the lungs. Mature flukes are found in the bronchioles surrounded by cystic lesions. Parasite eggs are either expectorated with sputum or swallowed and passed to the outside environment with feces. The life cycle is completed in snails and freshwater crustacea.

When maturing flukes lodge in lung tissues, they cause hemorrhage and necrosis, resulting in cyst formation. The adjacent lung parenchyma shows evidence of inflammatory infiltration, predominantly by eosinophils. Cysts usually measure 1 to 2 cm in diameter and may contain 1 or 2 worms each. With the onset of oviposition, cysts usually rupture in adjacent bronchioles—an event allowing ova to exit from the human host. Older cysts develop thickened walls, which may undergo calcification. During the active phase of paragonimiasis, lung tissues surrounding parasite cysts may contain evidence of pneumonia, bronchitis, bronchiectasis, and fibrosis.

Pulmonary paragonimiasis is particularly symptomatic in persons with moderate to heavy infection. Productive cough with brownish sputum or frank hemoptysis associated with peripheral blood eosinophilia is usually the presenting feature. Chest examination may reveal signs of pleurisy. In chronic cases, bronchitis or bronchiectasis may predominate, but these conditions rarely proceed to lung abscess. Imaging of the lungs demonstrates characteristic features, including patchy densities, cavities, pleural effusion, and ring shadows. Cerebral paragonimiasis presents as either space-occupying lesions or epilepsy. Pulmonary paragonimiasis is diagnosed by the detection of parasite ova in sputum and/or stools. Serology is of considerable help in egg-negative cases and in cerebral paragonimiasis. The drug of choice for treatment is praziquantel (Table 222-2). Other medical or surgical management may be needed for pulmonary or cerebral lesions.

CONTROL AND PREVENTION OF TISSUE FLUKES

For residents of nonendemic areas who are visiting an endemic region, the only effective preventive measure is to avoid ingestion of local plants, fish, or crustaceans; if their ingestion is necessary, they should be washed or cooked thoroughly. Instruction on water and food preparation and consumption should be included in physicians' advice to travelers (Chap. 123). Interruption of transmission among residents of endemic areas depends on avoiding ingestion of the infective stage of the helminths and appropriate disposal of feces and sputum to prevent the hatching of eggs in the environment. These two approaches rely greatly on socioeconomic development and health education. In countries where economic progress has resulted in financial and social improvements, transmission has decreased. The third approach to control in endemic communities entails selective use of chemotherapy for individuals posing the highest risk of transmission—i.e., those with heavy infections. The availability of praziquantel—a broad-spectrum, safe, and effective antihelminthic agent—provides a means for reducing the reservoirs of infection in human populations. However, the existence of most of these helminths as zoonoses in several animal species complicates control efforts.

BIBLIOGRAPHY

Drugs for parasitic infections. Med Lett Drugs Ther 40:1, 1998

GUYATT H et al: Assessing the public health importance of *Schistosoma mansoni* in different endemic areas: Attributable fraction estimates as an approach. Am J Trop Med Hyg 53:660, 1995

LIU LX, HARINASUTA KT: Liver and intestinal flukes. Gastroenterol Clin North Am 25: 627, 1996

MAHMOUD AAFM (ed): Parasitic lung diseases, in *Lung Biology in Health and Disease*, vol 101, C Lenfaut (ex ed). New York, Marcel Dekker, 1997, pp 1–235

————: Schistosomiasis from the bench to the field, in *Tropical Medicine: Science and Practice*, G Pasvol and S Hoffman (eds). London, Imperial College Press, 2000

MAS-COMA MS et al: Epidemiology of human fascioliasis: A review and proposed new classification. Bull World Health Organ 77:340, 1999

MONTENEGRO SML et al: Cytokine production in acute versus chronic human schistosomiasis: The cross-regulatory role of interferon γ and interleukin-10 in the responses of peripheral blood mononuclear cells and splenocytes to parasite antigens. J Infect Dis 179:1502, 1999

SUBRAMANIAN AK et al: Long-term suppression of adult bladder morbidity and severe hydronephrosis following selective population chemotherapy for *Schistosoma haematobium*. Am J Trop Med Hyg 61:476, 1999

TSANG VCW, WILKINS PP: Immunodiagnosis of schistosomiasis. Immunol Invest 26: 175, 1997

VISSER LG et al: Outbreak of acute schistosomiasis among travelers returning from Mali, West Africa. Clin Infect Dis 20:280, 1995

223   *A. Clinton White, Jr., Peter F. Weller*

CESTODES

Cestodes, or tapeworms, are segmented worms. The adults reside in the gastrointestinal tract, but the larvae can be found in almost any organ. Human tapeworm infections can be divided into two major clinical groups. In one group, humans are the definitive hosts, and the adult tapeworms live in the gastrointestinal tract (*Taenia saginata*, *Diphyllobothrium*, *Hymenolepis*, and *Dipylidium caninum*). In the other, humans are intermediate hosts, and larval-stage parasites are present in the tissues. Diseases in this category include echinococcosis, sparganosis, and coenurosis. For *T. solium*, the human may be either the definitive or the intermediate host.

The ribbon-shaped tapeworm attaches to the intestinal mucosa by means of sucking cups or grooves located on the head (scolex). Behind the scolex is a short, narrow neck from which proglottids (segments) form. As each proglottid matures, it is displaced further back from the neck by the formation of new, less mature segments. The progressively elongating chain of attached proglottids, called the *strobila*, constitutes the bulk of the tapeworm. The length varies among species. In some, the tapeworm may consist of more than 1000 proglottids and may be several meters long. As each proglottid becomes gravid, eggs are released. Since eggs of the different *Taenia* species are morphologically identical, differences in the morphology of the scolex or proglottids provide the basis for diagnostic identification to the species level. Most human tapeworms require at least one intermediate host for complete larval development. After ingestion by an intermediate host, an egg releases the larval oncosphere, which penetrates the intestinal mucosa. The oncosphere migrates to tissues and develops into an encysted form known as a *cysticercus* (single scolex), a *coenurus* (multiple scolices), or a *hydatid* (cyst with daughter cysts, each containing several protoscolices). Ingestion by the definitive host of tissues containing a cyst enables a scolex to develop into a tapeworm.

TAENIASIS SAGINATA   The beef tapeworm *T. saginata* occurs in all countries where raw or undercooked beef is eaten. It is most prevalent in sub-Saharan African and Middle Eastern countries.

Etiology and Pathogenesis   Humans are the only definitive host for the adult stage of *T. saginata*. This tapeworm, which can reach 8 m in length, inhabits the upper jejunum and has a scolex with four prominent suckers and 1000 to 2000 proglottids. Each gravid segment has 15 to 30 uterine branches (in contrast to 8 to 12 for *T. solium*). The eggs are indistinguishable from those of *T. solium*; each measures 30 to 40 μm and has a thick brown striated shell containing the embryo. Eggs deposited on vegetation can live for months to years until they are ingested by cattle or other herbivores. The embryo released after ingestion invades the intestinal wall and is carried to striated muscle, where it transforms into a cysticercus. When ingested in raw or undercooked beef, this form can infect humans. After the cysticercus is ingested, it takes about 2 months for an adult worm to develop.

Clinical Manifestations   Patients become aware of the infection most commonly by noting passage of proglottids in their feces. The proglottids are often motile, and patients may experience perianal discomfort when proglottids are discharged. Mild abdominal pain or discomfort, nausea, change in appetite, weakness, and weight loss can occur with *T. saginata* infection.

Diagnosis   The diagnosis is made by the detection of eggs or proglottids in the stool. Eggs may also be present in the perianal area; thus, if proglottids or eggs are not found in the stool, the perianal region should be examined with use of a cellophane-tape swab (as in pinworm infection). Distinguishing *T. saginata* from *T. solium* requires examination of mature proglottids or the scolex. Serologic tests are not helpful diagnostically. Eosinophilia and elevated levels of serum IgE may be detected.

℞ TREATMENT   A single dose of praziquantel (5 to 10 mg/kg) is highly effective.

Prevention   The major method of preventing infection is the adequate cooking of beef; exposure to temperatures as low as 56°C for 5 min will destroy cysticerci. Refrigeration or salting for long periods or freezing at −10°C for 9 days also kills cysticerci in beef. General preventive measures include inspection of beef and proper disposal of human feces.

TAENIASIS SOLIUM AND CYSTICERCOSIS   The pork tapeworm *T. solium* can cause two distinct forms of infection. The form that develops depends on whether humans are infected with adult tapeworms in the intestine or with larval forms in the tissues (cysticercosis). Humans are the only definitive hosts for *T. solium*; pigs are the usual intermediate hosts, although dogs, cats, and sheep may harbor the larval forms. *T. solium* exists worldwide but is most prevalent in Latin America, Africa, South and Southeast Asia, and eastern Europe. Cysticercosis occurs in industrialized nations largely as a result of the immigration of infected persons from endemic areas.

Etiology and Pathogenesis   The adult tapeworm generally resides in the upper jejunum. Its globular scolex attaches by both sucking disks and two rows of hooklets. Often only one adult worm is present, but that worm may live for years. The tapeworm, usually about 3 m in length, may have as many as 1000 proglottids, each of which produces up to 50,000 eggs. Groups of three to five proglottids are generally released and excreted into the feces, and the eggs in these proglottids are infective for both humans and animals. The eggs may survive in the environment for several months. After ingestion by the intermediate host, eggs embryonate, penetrate the intestinal wall, and are carried to many tissues, with a predilection for striated muscle of the neck, tongue, and trunk. Within 60 to 90 days, the encysted larval stage develops. These cysticerci can survive for long periods. Humans acquire infections that lead to intestinal tapeworms by ingesting undercooked pork containing cysticerci. Infections that cause human cysticercosis follow the ingestion of *T. solium* eggs, usually from fecally contaminated food. Autoinfection may occur if an individual with an egg-producing tapeworm ingests eggs derived from his or her own feces.

Clinical Manifestations   Intestinal infections with *T. solium* may be asymptomatic. Epigastric discomfort, nausea, a sensation of hunger, weight loss, and diarrhea are infrequent. Fecal passage of proglottids may be noted by patients.

In cysticercosis, the clinical manifestations are entirely different.

Cysticerci can be found anywhere in the body, most commonly in the brain and the skeletal muscle. The clinical presentation of cysticercosis depends on the number and location of cysticerci as well as the extent of associated inflammatory responses or scarring. Neurologic manifestations are the most common. When inflammation surrounds cysticerci in the brain parenchyma, seizures are frequent. These seizures may be generalized, focal, or Jacksonian. Hydrocephalus results from obstruction of cerebrospinal fluid (CSF) flow by cysticerci and accompanying inflammation or by CSF outflow obstruction from arachnoiditis. Signs of increased intracranial pressure, including headache, nausea, vomiting, changes in vision, dizziness, ataxia, or confusion, are often evident. Patients with hydrocephalus may develop papilledema or display altered mental status. When cysticerci develop at the base of the brain or in the subarachnoid space, they cause chronic meningitis or arachnoiditis, communicating hydrocephalus, or strokes.

Diagnosis The diagnosis of intestinal *T. solium* infection is made by the detection of eggs or proglottids, as described for *T. saginata*. In cysticercosis, diagnosis can be difficult. A consensus conference has proposed absolute, major, minor, and epidemiologic criteria for diagnosis (Table 223-1). Diagnostic certainty is possible only with definite demonstration of the parasite (absolute criteria). This task can be accomplished by histologic observation of the parasite in excised tissue, by funduscopic visualization of the parasite in the eye (in the anterior chamber, vitreous, or subretinal spaces), or by neuroimaging studies demonstrating cystic lesions containing a scolex. In most cases, diagnostic certainty is not possible. Instead, a clinical diagnosis is made on the basis of a combination of clinical presentation, radiographic studies, serologic tests, and exposure history.

Neuroimaging findings suggestive of neurocysticercosis constitute the primary major diagnostic criterion. These findings include cystic lesions with or without enhancement (e.g., ring enhancement), one or more calcifications (which may also have associated enhancement), or focal enhancing lesions. Cysticerci in the brain parenchyma are usually 5 to 10 mm in diameter and rounded. Cystic lesions in the subarachnoid space or fissures may enlarge up to 5 cm in diameter and may be lobulated. For cysticerci within the subarachnoid space or ventricles, the walls may be very thin and the cyst fluid is often isodense with CSF. Thus, obstructive hydrocephalus or enhancement of the basilar meninges may be the only finding on computed tomography (CT) in neurocysticercosis. Cysticerci in the ventricles or subarachnoid space are usually visible to an experienced neuroradiologist on magnetic resonance imaging (MRI) or with intraventricular contrast injection. CT is more sensitive than MRI in identifying calcified lesions, whereas MRI is better for identifying cystic lesions and enhancement. Typical

cigar-shaped calcifications in muscle are a second major diagnostic criterion.

The third major diagnostic criterion is detection of specific antibodies to cysticerci. While most tests employing unfractionated antigen have high rates of false-positive and -negative results, this problem can be overcome by using the more specific immunoblot assay. An immunoblot assay using lentil-lectin purified glycoproteins has >99% specificity and is highly sensitive. However, patients with single intracranial lesions or with calcifications may be seronegative. With this assay, serum samples provide greater diagnostic sensitivity than CSF. However, CSF may be useful when only unfractionated antigens are used.

Minor diagnostic criteria include the presence of subcutaneous nodules, punctate soft tissue or intracranial calcifications, clinical manifestations suggestive of neurocysticercosis (such as seizures, hydrocephalus, or altered mental status), or disappearance of lesions in conjunction with anticysticercal drug therapy. Epidemiologic criteria include current or prior residence in an endemic area, frequent travel to an endemic area, or exposure to a tapeworm carrier or household member infected with *T. solium*. Diagnosis is confirmed in patients with a combination of either two major criteria or one major criterion with two minor criteria and one epidemiologic criterion. The fulfillment of one major criterion and two other criteria or of three minor criteria with epidemiologic exposure supports a probable diagnosis. While the CSF is usually abnormal in neurocysticercosis, CSF abnormalities are not pathognomonic. Patients may have CSF pleocytosis with a predominance of lymphocytes, neutrophils, or eosinophils. The protein level in CSF may be elevated; the glucose concentration is usually normal but may be depressed.

TREATMENT Intestinal *T. solium* infection is treated with a single dose of praziquantel (5 to 10 mg/kg). However, praziquantel can evoke an inflammatory response in the central nervous system if concomitant cryptic cysticercosis is present.

The management of neurocysticercosis focuses primarily on symptomatic treatment of seizures or hydrocephalus. Seizures can usually be controlled with anticonvulsants. If parenchymal lesions resolve without development of calcifications and patients remain free of seizures, anticonvulsant therapy can usually be discontinued after 2 years. Four placebo-controlled trials failed to identify any clinical advantage of antiparasitic drugs for parenchymal neurocysticercosis. However, trends toward faster resolution of neuroradiologic abnormalities were observed. Thus, some authorities favor use of antiparasitic drugs, including praziquantel (50 to 60 mg/kg daily in three divided doses for 15 days or 100 mg/kg in three doses given over a single day) or albendazole (15 mg/kg per day for 8 to 28 days). Both agents may exacerbate the inflammatory response around the dying parasite, exacerbating seizures or hydrocephalus. Thus, patients receiving these drugs should be carefully monitored. High-dose glucocorticoids can be used during treatment or if symptoms worsen. Since glucocorticoids induce first-pass metabolism of praziquantel and may decrease its antiparasitic effect, cimetidine should be coadministered to inhibit praziquantel metabolism.

For patients with hydrocephalus, the emergent reduction of intracranial pressure is the mainstay of therapy. In the case of obstructive hydrocephalus, this task requires either a diverting procedure, such as ventriculoperitoneal shunting, or removal of the cysticerci by craniotomy or via ventriculoscopy. Historically, shunts have usually failed. However, low failure rates have been attained with treatment with antiparasitic drugs or chronic glucocorticoids or with use of flow-sensitive shunts. In patients with subarachnoid cysts, glucocorticoids are needed to reduce arachnoiditis and accompanying vasculitis. Patients may benefit from prolonged courses of antiparasitic drugs and shunting for hydrocephalus. In patients with elevated intracranial pressure due to multiple inflamed lesions, glucocorticoids are the mainstay of therapy, and antiparasitic drugs should be avoided until the elevated pressure resolves. For ocular and spinal medullary lesions, drug-induced

Table 223-1 Proposed Diagnostic Criteria for Human Cysticercosis, 1996

1. Absolute criteria
   a. Demonstration of cysticerci by histologic or microscopic examination of biopsy material
   b. Visualization of the parasite in the eye by funduscopy
   c. Neuroradiologic demonstration of cystic lesions containing a scolex
2. Major criteria
   a. Neuroradiologic lesions suggestive of neurocysticercosis
   b. Demonstration of antibodies to cysticerci in serum by immunoblot or in cerebrospinal fluid by immunoblot or ELISA
   c. Identification of characteristic "cigar-shaped" calcifications on soft tissue x-rays
3. Minor criteria
   a. Presence of subcutaneous nodules suggestive of cysticerci
   b. Punctate calcifications on radiographic studies
   c. Clinical manifestations suggestive of neurocysticercosis
   d. Disappearance of intracranial lesions during treatment with anticysticercal drugs
4. Epidemiologic criteria
   a. Residence in a cysticercosis-endemic area
   b. Frequent travel to a cysticercosis-endemic area
   c. Household contact with an individual infected with *Taenia solium*

NOTE: ELISA, enzyme-linked immunosorbent assay.
SOURCE: Modified from Del Brutto et al.

inflammation may cause irreversible damage. Most patients should be managed surgically, although case reports have described cures with medical therapy.

Prevention   Measures for the prevention of intestinal *T. solium* infection consist of the application to pork of precautions similar to those described above for beef with regard to *T. saginata* infection. The prevention of cysticercosis involves minimizing the opportunities for ingestion of fecally derived eggs by means of good personal hygiene, effective fecal disposal, and treatment and prevention of human intestinal infections.

ECHINOCOCCOSIS   Echinococcosis is an infection of humans caused by the larval stage of *Echinococcus granulosus*, *E. multilocularis*, or *E. vogeli*. *E. granulosus*, which produces unilocular cystic lesions, is prevalent in areas where livestock is raised in association with dogs. This tapeworm species is found in Australia, Argentina, Chile, Africa, eastern Europe, the Middle East, New Zealand, and the Mediterranean region, particularly Lebanon and Greece. *E. multilocularis*, which causes multilocular alveolar lesions that are locally invasive, is found in Alpine, sub-Arctic, or Arctic regions, including Canada, the United States, and central and northern Europe and Asia. *E. vogeli* causes polycystic hydatid disease and is found only in Central and South America. Like other cestodes, echinococcal species have both intermediate and definitive hosts. The definitive hosts are dogs that pass eggs in their feces. Cysts develop in the intermediate hosts—sheep, cattle, humans, goats, camels, and horses for *E. granulosus* and mice and other rodents for *E. multilocularis*—after the ingestion of eggs. When a dog ingests beef or lamb containing cysts, the life cycle is completed.

Etiology   The small (5 mm long) adult *E. granulosus* worm, which lives for 5 to 20 months in the jejunum of dogs, has only three proglottids—one immature, one mature, and one gravid. The gravid segment splits to release eggs that are morphologically similar to *Taenia* eggs and are extremely hardy. After humans ingest the eggs, embryos escape from the eggs, penetrate the intestinal mucosa, enter the portal circulation, and are carried to various organs, most commonly the liver and lungs. Larvae develop into fluid-filled unilocular hydatid cysts that consist of an external membrane and an inner germinal layer. Daughter cysts develop from the inner aspect of the germinal layer, as do germinating cystic structures called *brood capsules*. New larvae, called *protoscolices*, develop in large numbers within the brood capsule. The cysts expand slowly over a period of years.

The life cycle of *E. multilocularis* is similar except that small rodents serve as the intermediate hosts. The cyst of *E. multilocularis*, however, is quite different in that the larval form remains in the proliferative phase, the hydatid cyst is always multilocular, and vesicles progressively invade the host tissue by peripheral extension of processes from the germinal layer.

Clinical Manifestations   Slowly enlarging echinococcal cysts generally remain asymptomatic until their expanding size or their space-occupying effect in an involved organ elicits symptoms. The liver and the lungs are the most common sites of these cysts. Since a period of years elapses before cysts enlarge sufficiently to cause symptoms, they may be discovered incidentally on a routine x-ray or ultrasound study.

Patients with hepatic echinococcosis who are symptomatic most often present with abdominal pain or a palpable mass in the right upper quadrant. Compression of a bile duct or leakage of cyst fluid into the biliary tree may mimic recurrent cholelithiasis, and biliary obstruction can result in jaundice. Rupture of or episodic leakage from a hydatid cyst may produce fever, pruritus, urticaria, eosinophilia, or anaphylaxis. Pulmonary hydatid cysts may rupture into the bronchial tree or peritoneal cavity and produce cough, chest pain, or hemoptysis. Rupture of hydatid cysts may lead to multifocal dissemination of protoscolices, which can form additional cysts. Rupture can occur spontaneously or at surgery. Other presentations are due to the involvement

of bone (invasion of the medullary cavity with slow bone erosion producing pathologic fractures), the central nervous system (space-occupying lesions), and the heart (conduction defects, pericarditis).

The cysts of *E. multilocularis* characteristically present as a slowly growing hepatic tumor, with progressive destruction of the liver and extension into vital structures. Patients commonly complain of upper quadrant and epigastric pain, and obstructive jaundice may be apparent. A minority of patients experience the metastasis of lesions to the lung and brain.

Diagnosis   Radiographic and related imaging studies are important in detecting and evaluating echinococcal cysts. Plain films will define pulmonary cysts—usually as rounded irregular masses of uniform density—but may miss cysts in other organs unless there is cyst wall calcification (as occurs in the liver). MRI, CT, and ultrasound reveal well-defined cysts with thick or thin walls. When older cysts contain a layer of hydatid sand that is rich in accumulated scolices, these imaging methods may detect this fluid layer of different density. However, the most pathognomonic finding, if demonstrable, is that of daughter cysts within the larger cyst. This finding, like eggshell or mural calcification on CT, is indicative of *E. granulosus* infection and helps to distinguish the cyst from carcinomas, bacterial or amebic liver abscesses, or hemangiomas. CT of alveolar hydatid cysts reveals indistinct solid masses with central necrosis and plaquelike calcifications.

A specific diagnosis can be made by the examination of aspirated fluids for scoliceal hooklets, but diagnostic aspiration is not usually recommended because of the risk of fluid leakage resulting in either dissemination of infection or anaphylactic reactions. Serodiagnostic assays can be useful, although a negative test does not exclude the diagnosis of echinococcosis. Cysts in the liver elicit positive antibody responses in ~90% of cases, whereas up to 50% of individuals with cysts in the lungs are seronegative. Detection of antibody to specific echinococcal antigens by immunoblotting has the highest degree of specificity.

℞ **TREATMENT**   Therapy for echinococcosis is based on considerations of the size, location, and manifestations of cysts and the overall health of the patient. Surgery has traditionally been the principal definitive method of treatment; *E. granulosus* cysts are excised, or tissue containing *E. multilocularis* cysts is resected. Risks at surgery from leakage of fluid include anaphylaxis and dissemination of infectious scolices. The latter complication has been minimized by the instillation of scolicidal solutions such as hypertonic saline or ethanol, which may cause hypernatremia, intoxication, or sclerosing cholangitis. Albendazole, which is active against *Echinococcus*, should be administered adjunctively, beginning before resection and continuing for several weeks for *E. granulosus* and for up to 2 years for *E. multilocularis*. Percutaneous *a*spiration, *i*nfusion of scolicidal agents, and *r*easpiration (PAIR) can be used instead of surgery in many cases of cystic echinococcosis. PAIR is contraindicated for superficially located cysts (because of the risk of rupture), for cysts with multiple thick internal septal divisions (honeycombing pattern), and for cysts communicating with the biliary tree. Therapy with albendazole (15 mg/kg daily in two divided doses) should be initiated at least 4 days before the procedure and continued for at least 4 weeks afterward. Ultrasound- or CT-guided aspiration allows confirmation of the diagnosis by demonstration of protoscolices in the aspirate. Either alcohol or hypertonic saline should then be infused. Daughter cysts within the primary cyst may need to be punctured separately. In experienced hands, this approach yields rates of cure and relapse equivalent to those following surgery, with less perioperative morbidity and shorter hospitalization. Medical therapy with albendazole alone for 12 weeks to 6 months results in cure in ~30% of cases and improvement in another 50%. Many of the failures are subsequently treated successfully with PAIR or additional courses of medical therapy. Response to treatment is best assessed by serial imaging studies with attention to cyst size and consistency.

Prevention   In endemic areas, echinococcosis can be prevented by administering praziquantel to infected dogs, by denying dogs access to infected animals, or by vaccinating sheep. Limitation of the number of stray dogs is helpful in reducing the prevalence of infection among humans.

HYMENOLEPIASIS NANA Infection with *Hymenolepis nana*, the dwarf tapeworm, is the most common of all the cestode infections. *H. nana* is endemic in both temperate and tropical regions of the world. Infection is spread by fecal/oral contamination and is common among institutionalized children.

Etiology and Pathogenesis *H. nana* is the only cestode of humans that does not require an intermediate host. Both the larval and adult phases take place in the human. The adult, the smallest tapeworm parasitizing humans, is about 2 cm long and dwells in the proximal ileum. Proglottids, which are quite small and are rarely seen in the stool, release spherical eggs 30 to 44 μm in diameter, each of which contains an oncosphere with six hooklets. The eggs are immediately infective and are unable to survive in the external environment for more than 10 days. *H. nana* can also be acquired by the ingestion of infected insects (especially larval meal-worms and larval fleas). When the egg is ingested by a new host, the oncosphere is freed and penetrates the intestinal villi, becoming a cysticercoid larva. Larvae migrate back into the intestinal lumen, attach to the mucosa, and mature over 10 to 12 days into adult worms. Eggs may also hatch before passing into the stool, causing internal autoinfection with increasing numbers of intestinal worms. Although the life span of adult *H. nana* is only about 4 to 10 weeks, the autoinfection cycle perpetuates the infection.

Clinical Manifestations *H. nana* infection, even with many intestinal worms, is usually asymptomatic. When infection is intense, anorexia, abdominal pain, and diarrhea develop.

Diagnosis Infection is diagnosed by the finding of eggs in the stool.

℞ **TREATMENT** Praziquantel (25 mg/kg once) is the treatment of choice, since it acts against both the adult worms and the cysticercoids in the intestinal villi.

Prevention Good personal hygiene and improved sanitation can eradicate the disease. Epidemics have been controlled by mass chemotherapy coupled with improved hygiene.

HYMENOLEPIASIS DIMINUTA *Hymenolepis diminuta*, a cestode of rodents, occasionally infects small children, who ingest the adult worm in uncooked cereal foods contaminated by fleas and other insects in which larvae develop. Infection is usually asymptomatic and is diagnosed by the detection of eggs in the stool. Treatment with praziquantel results in cure in most cases.

DIPHYLLOBOTHRIASIS *Diphyllobothrium latum* and other *Diphyllobothrium* species are found in the lakes, rivers, and deltas of the northern hemisphere, Central Africa, and Chile.

Etiology and Pathogenesis The adult worm, the longest tapeworm (up to 25 m), attaches to the ileal and occasionally to the jejunal mucosa by its suckers, which are located on its elongated scolex. The adult worm has 3000 to 4000 proglottids, which release approximately 1 million eggs daily into the feces. If an egg reaches water, it hatches and releases a free-swimming embryo that can be eaten by small freshwater crustaceans (*Cyclops* or *Diaptomus* species). After an infected crustacean containing a developed procercoid is swallowed by a fish, the larva migrates into the fish's flesh and grows into a plerocercoid, or sparganum larva. Humans acquire the infection by ingesting infected raw fish. Within 3 to 5 weeks, the tapeworm matures into an adult in the human intestine.

Clinical Manifestations Most *D. latum* infections are asymptomatic, although manifestations may include transient abdominal discomfort, diarrhea, vomiting, weakness, and weight loss. Occasionally, infection can cause acute abdominal pain and intestinal obstruction; in rare cases cholangitis or cholecystitis may be produced by migrating proglottids. Because the tapeworm absorbs large quantities of vitamin B_{12} and interferes with ileal B_{12} absorption, vitamin B_{12} deficiency can develop. Up to 2% of infected patients, especially the elderly, have megaloblastic anemia resembling pernicious anemia and may exhibit neurologic sequelae of B_{12} deficiency.

Diagnosis The diagnosis is made readily by the detection of the characteristic eggs in the stool. The eggs possess a single shell with an operculum at one end and a knob at the other. Mild to moderate eosinophilia may be detected.

℞ **TREATMENT** Praziquantel (5 to 10 mg/kg once) is highly effective. Parenteral vitamin B_{12} should be given if B_{12} deficiency is manifest.

Prevention Infection can be prevented by heating fish to 54°C for 5 min or by freezing it at -18°C for 24 h. Placing fish in brine with a high salt concentration for long periods kills the eggs.

DIPYLIDIASIS *Dipylidium caninum*, a common tapeworm of dogs and cats, may accidentally infect humans. Dogs, cats, and occasionally humans become infected by ingesting fleas harboring cysticercoids. Children are more likely to become infected than adults. Most infections are asymptomatic, but abdominal pain, diarrhea, anal pruritus, urticaria, eosinophilia, or passage of segments in the stool may occur. The diagnosis is made by the detection of proglottids in the stool. As in *D. latum* infection, therapy consists of praziquantel. Prevention requires anthelmintic treatment and flea control for pet dogs or cats.

SPARGANOSIS Humans can be infected by the sparganum, or plerocercoid larva, of a diphyllobothrid tapeworm of the genus *Spirometra*. Infection can be acquired by the consumption of water containing infected *Cyclops*; by the ingestion of infected snakes, birds, or mammals; or by the application of infected flesh as poultices. The worm migrates slowly in tissues, and infection commonly presents as a subcutaneous swelling. Periorbital tissues can be involved, and ocular sparganosis may destroy the eye. Surgical excision is used to treat localized sparganosis.

COENUROSIS This rare infection of humans by the larval stage (coenurus) of the dog tapeworm *Taenia multiceps* or *T. serialis* results in a space-occupying cystic lesion. As in cysticercosis, involvement of the central nervous system and subcutaneous tissue is most common. Both definitive diagnosis and treatment require surgical excision of the lesion. Chemotherapeutic agents generally are not effective.

BIBLIOGRAPHY

AMMANN RW, ECKERT J: Cestodes: *Echinococcus*. Gastroenterol Clin North Am 25:655, 1996

BOTERO D et al: Taeniasis and cysticercosis. Infect Dis Clin North Am 7:683, 1993

DEL BRUTTO OH et al: Proposal for diagnostic criteria for human cysticercosis and neurocysticercosis. J Neurol Sci 142:1, 1996

FLISSER A: Taeniasis and cysticercosis due to *Taenia solium*. Prog Clin Parasitol 4:77, 1994

FRANCHI C et al: Long-term evaluation of patients with hydatidosis treated with benzimidazole carbamates. Clin Infect Dis 29:304, 1999

GIL-GRANDE LA et al: Randomised controlled trial of efficacy of albendazole in intraabdominal hydatid disease. Lancet 342:1269, 1993

KAMMERER WS, SCHANTZ PM: Echinococcal disease. Infect Dis Clin North Am 7:605, 1993

KHUROO MS et al: Percutaneous drainage compared with surgery for hepatic hydatid cysts. N Engl J Med 337:881, 1997

PAWLOWSKI Z, SCHANTZ P (eds): Advances in clinical management of cystic echinococcosis. Acta Trop 64:1; 67:1, 1997

SALINAS R, PRASAD K: Drugs in neurocysticercosis (tapeworm infection of the brain), in *The Cochrane Library*, issue 4. Oxford, Update Software, 1998

SCHAEFER JW, KHAN MY: Echinococcosis (hydatid disease): Lessons from experience with 59 patients. Rev Infect Dis 13:243, 1991

SCHANTZ PM, KRAMER HJ: Larval cestode infections: Cysticercosis and echinococcosis. Curr Opin Infect Dis 8:342, 1995

SCHARF D: Neurocysticercosis: Two hundred thirty eight cases from a California hospital. Arch Neurol 46:77, 1989

WHITE AC JR: Neurocysticercosis: A major cause of neurologic disease worldwide. Clin Infect Dis 24:101, 1997

———: Neurocysticercosis: Updates on epidemiology, pathogenesis, diagnosis and management. Annu Rev Med 51:187, 2000

——— et al: *Taenia solium* cysticercosis: Host-parasite interactions and the immune response. Chem Immunol 66:209, 1997

WORLD HEALTH ORGANIZATION INFORMAL WORKING GROUP ON ECHINOCOCCOSIS: Guidelines for treatment of cystic and alveolar echinococcosis in humans. Bull World Health Organ 74:231, 1996

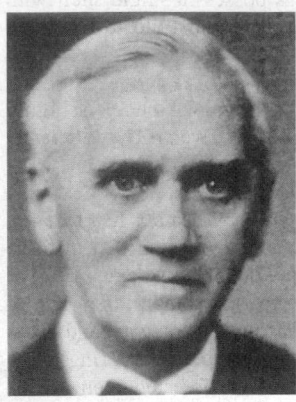

Alexander Fleming was born on August 6, 1881, the youngest child of Hugh and Grace Fleming in Lochfield, Scotland. After attending local schools, he moved to London to join his two brothers, Tom and John, and attended Regent Street Polytechnic for two years. At age 16 he became a shipping clerk, but with the good fortune of a legacy of 250 British pounds from an uncle, he decided to enroll in medical school at St. Mary's in London. Fleming was a brilliant student, capturing virtually every academic prize. More important, when he graduated in 1906 he joined the laboratory of Almroth Wright, his future mentor. During World War I, Fleming and Wright moved to Boulogne, France, where they tended the wounds of injured soldiers. At the end of the war, Fleming returned to St. Mary's to become assistant director of the Inoculation Department. Although Fleming was a skilled laboratory worker, his laboratory was not very neat, as he stacked old culture plates on his bench until there was no more room. In 1928 he was growing various strains of staphylococcus and prepared some culture plates just before leaving for 2 weeks of vacation. On his return he saw one plate that was contaminated with a mold and observed that no bacteria were growing around the mold. In 1929 he published a paper entitled "On the Antibacterial Actions of Cultures of a Penicillium."

In the 1930s, Fleming used penicillin primarily to prepare pure strains of bacteria for vaccines. He no doubt felt that enhanced natural immunity with vaccines, rather than chemotherapy, would be the future treatment of bacterial infections in humans. Moreover, he observed that staphylococci developed rapid immunity to penicillin in culture and that penicillin was unstable; in the impure state, large quantities would be necessary to treat humans. In fact, had it not been for the work of Florey and Chain on penicillin at Oxford, the drug might have remained of interest only to bacteriologists and not to physicians caring for patients.

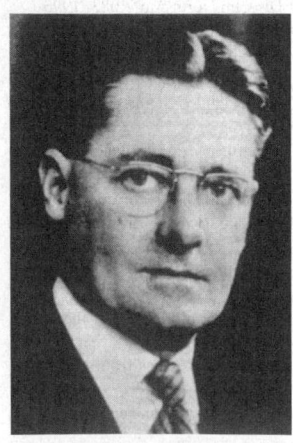

Howard Florey was born in Adelaide, Australia, on September 24, 1898, the only son of Joseph and Bertha Florey. He attended Saint Peter's Collegiate School in Adelaide and then attended medical school at the University of Adelaide. After graduation, Florey studied at Oxford University in England on a Rhodes scholarship. He spent a year abroad in the United States as a Rockefeller Fellow and then completed his Ph.D. at Cambridge in 1927 under the direction of the internationally renowned biochemist, Frederick G. Hopkins. In 1932 Florey was appointed Chair in Pathology at the University of Sheffield; and then in 1936 he became director of Oxford's Sir William Dunn School of Pathology. It was there that Florey began his long association with Ernst Chain. With a mutual interest in antibacterial chemicals produced by microbes, Florey and Chain began to study the crude form of penicillin, which could be obtained from the culture medium in which the mold, *Penicillium notatum*, had been grown. In 1940 Florey and his co-workers published a paper, "Penicillin as a Chemotherapeutic Agent," which showed that mice infected with fatal doses of staphylococci or clostridia (gangrene) uniformly survived when treated with penicillin. Moreover, in contrast to earlier attempts to develop chemotherapeutic agents, penicillin demonstrated no evidence of toxicity.

The initial stumbling block for its use in humans was that it took hundreds of gallons of culture media to yield enough penicillin to treat a single individual. This problem was overcome in Florey's laboratory, and in 1941 infections in 10 humans were treated with penicillin and the results reported in a paper entitled "Further Observations of Penicillin." Great Britain was in the throes of World War II and could not provide adequate funding to produce enough penicillin for widespread use. Florey went to the United States and convinced the American Office of Scientific Research, along with industry, to fund the effort. This led to the widespread use of penicillin to treat the casualties during the Normandy invasion.

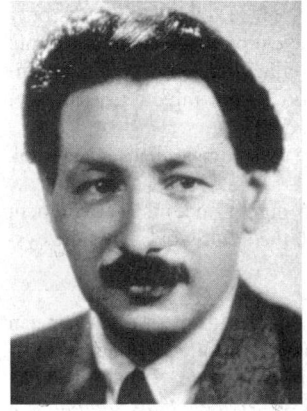

Ernst Chain was born in Berlin, Germany, on June 19, 1906, the son of Michael, an immigrant from White Russia, and Margarete, his German wife. Both Russian and German were spoken at home, where music was important and Ernst became an accomplished pianist. He attended the Luisen *Gymnasium* (German high school) and then the Friedrich Wilhelm University. Ernst earned his degree in 1930 in chemistry and physiology. After graduation he worked first at the Kaiser-Wilhelm Institute and then the Charité Hospital in Berlin in biochemical research. With the rise of Nazism and being a Jew, Chain left Germany and worked with Sir Frederick G. Hopkins at Cambridge from 1933 to 1935. He then went as a lecturer in clinical pathology to Sir William Dunn School of Pathology at Oxford where he met Howard Florey. In 1939 they began to work on penicillin together with some funding from the Rockefeller Institute. Chain focused on the fundamental chemical properties and structure of penicillin. Eventually penicillin was identified by x-ray analysis of the crystals as a beta-lactam in 1945. In 1948 he moved to Rome and with Beecham researchers, Chain discovered a process for producing 6-aminopenicillanic acid from which all known penicillins could be produced by a simple reaction. This observation led to the production of an oral penicillin. In 1961 he returned to Britain to Imperial College, University of London, as Chair of Biochemistry where he facilitated the movement of discoveries from the laboratory to pilot studies and then to production.

REFERENCES

1. Aaseng N: *The Disease Fighters*. Minneapolis, Lerner Publications, 1987
2. Magill FN (ed): *Nobel Prize Winners: Physiology or Medicine*, vol 2. Pasadena, Salem Press, 1993
3. Schrier RW: *A Salute to Nobel Laureates in Physiology and Medicine*, Proceedings of the Association of American Physicians 108(1): Jan 1996
4. Sourkes TL: *Nobel Prize Winners in Medicine and Physiology 1901–1965*. London, Abelard-Schuman, 1967

Robert W. Schrier, MD

Section 1
DIAGNOSIS

224

Eugene Braunwald

APPROACH TO THE PATIENT WITH HEART DISEASE

The symptoms caused by heart disease result most commonly from myocardial ischemia, from disturbance of the contraction and/or relaxation of the myocardium, from obstruction to blood flow, or from an abnormal cardiac rhythm or rate. Ischemia is manifest most frequently as chest discomfort, while reduction of the pumping ability of the heart commonly leads to weakness and fatigability or, when severe, produces cyanosis, hypotension, syncope, and elevated intravascular pressure behind a failing ventricle. The latter results in abnormal fluid accumulation, which in turn leads to dyspnea, orthopnea, and systemic or pulmonary edema. Obstruction to blood flow, as in valvular stenosis, can cause symptoms resembling those resulting from congestive heart failure. Cardiac arrhythmias often develop suddenly, and the resulting signs and symptoms—palpitation, dyspnea, hypotension, presyncope and syncope—generally occur abruptly and may disappear as rapidly as they develop. Ischemic heart disease, by far the most common form of heart disease in adults, may present with chest discomfort but also as heart failure, tachyarrhythmia, and sudden cardiac death.

Myocardial or coronary function that may be adequate at rest may be inadequate during exertion. Thus a history of chest discomfort and/or dyspnea that appears only during activity is characteristic of heart disease, while the opposite pattern, i.e., the appearance of these symptoms at rest and their remission during exertion, is rarely observed in patients with organic heart disease.

Many patients with cardiocirculatory disease also may be asymptomatic, both at rest and during exertion, but may present an abnormal physical finding, such as a heart murmur, elevated arterial pressure, or an abnormality of the electrocardiogram (ECG) or of the cardiac silhouette on the chest roentgenogram. Patients may exhibit asymptomatic ischemia on an exercise stress test. In some asymptomatic patients the first clinical event may be catastrophic—sudden cardiac death, acute myocardial infarction, or stroke.

Diseases of the heart and circulation are so common and the laity is so well acquainted with the major symptoms resulting from these disorders that patients, and occasionally physicians, erroneously attribute many noncardiac complaints to cardiovascular disease. The combination of the widespread fear of heart disease with the deep-seated emotional connotations concerning this organ's function results in the frequent development of symptoms that mimic those of organic disease in persons with normal cardiovascular systems. The unraveling of symptoms and signs due to organic heart disease from those not directly related is an important and challenging task in such patients.

Patients in whom heart disease has been confirmed, especially those who have experienced a major cardiovascular event such as a myocardial infarction or a serious arrhythmia, are often frightened and anxious about hospital discharge and resuming normal activity, including sexual relations. Attention to these matters is vital in the care of cardiac patients.

Dyspnea, one of the cardinal manifestations of heart failure, is not limited to patients with heart disease but is also observed in conditions as diverse as pulmonary disease, marked obesity, and anxiety (Chap.

32). Similarly, chest discomfort may result from a variety of causes other than myocardial ischemia (Chap. 13). Whether heart disease is responsible for these symptoms can frequently be determined by carrying out a careful clinical examination. Noninvasive testing using electrocardiography at rest and during exercise (Chap. 226), echocardiography (Chap. 227), roentgenography, and myocardial imaging usually provides important additional information to permit the correct interpretation of symptoms; more specialized invasive examinations (catheterization and angiography; Chap. 228) are occasionally necessary.

DIAGNOSIS As outlined by the New York Heart Association, the elements of a complete cardiac diagnosis include consideration of the following:

1. *The underlying etiology.* Is the disease congenital, infectious, hypertensive, or ischemic in origin?
2. *The anatomic abnormalities.* Which chambers are involved? Are they hypertrophied, dilated, or both? Which valves are affected? Are they regurgitant and/or stenotic? Is there pericardial involvement? Has there been a myocardial infarction?
3. *The physiologic disturbances.* Is an arrhythmia present? Is there evidence of congestive heart failure or of myocardial ischemia?

One example may serve to illustrate the importance of establishing a complete diagnosis. The identification of myocardial ischemia as the etiology of a patient's exertional chest discomfort is of great clinical importance. However, the simple recognition of ischemia is insufficient to formulate a therapeutic strategy or prognosis until the underlying anatomic abnormalities responsible for the myocardial ischemia, e.g., coronary atherosclerosis or aortic stenosis, are identified and a judgment made as to whether other physiologic disturbances that cause an imbalance between myocardial oxygen supply and demand, such as severe anemia, thyrotoxicosis, or supraventricular tachycardia, play a contributory role.

The fourth element of the diagnosis involves an assessment of *functional disability*. How strenuous is the physical activity required to elicit symptoms? The functional classification provided by the New York Heart Association has been found to be useful (Table 224-1).

The establishment of a correct and complete cardiac diagnosis often commences with the history and physical examination (Chap. 225). Indeed the clinical examination remains the basis for the diagnosis of a wide variety of disorders (Table 224-2). The clinical examination may then be supplemented by four types of laboratory tests: (1) ECG (Chap. 226); (2) chest roentgenogram; (3) noninvasive graphic examinations [echocardiogram, radionuclide and imaging techniques] (Chap. 227); and occasionally (4) specialized invasive examinations, i.e., cardiac catheterization, angiocardiography, and coronary angiography (Chap. 228).

In the diagnostic process, the results obtained from each of these several modalities should be analyzed independently of one another as well as together. Only in this way can one avoid overlooking a subtle, though important, finding. For example, an ECG should be obtained in every patient suspected of heart disease. It may provide the critical clue in establishing the correct diagnosis, e.g., the finding of a mild atrioventricular conduction disturbance in a patient with unexplained syncope, even when all other methods of examination reveal no abnormal findings, can be the clue that advanced heart block and asystole might be the cause and can dictate electrophysiologic

Table 224-1   New York Heart Association Functional Classification

Class I	Class III
No limitation of physical activity	Marked limitation of physical activity
No symptoms with ordinary exertion	Less than ordinary activity causes symptoms
Class II	Asymptomatic at rest
Slight limitation of physical activity	Class IV
Ordinary activity causes symptoms	Inability to carry out any physical activity without discomfort
	Symptoms at rest

SOURCE: Modified from The Criteria Committee of the New York Heart Association.

testing. On the other hand, when combined intelligently with the results of other methods of examination, the ECG may provide essential confirmatory data. Thus, the knowledge that a patient has an apical diastolic rumbling murmur may direct particular attention to the P waves, and the recognition of electrocardiographic left atrial enlargement supports the suggestion that the murmur is caused by mitral stenosis. The diagnosis can then be confirmed by echocardiography, a technique that can also determine the severity of the obstruction and its effects on pulmonary artery pressure and on right and left ventricular function.

Family History   In eliciting the history of a patient with known or suspected cardiovascular disease, particular attention should be directed to the family history. Familial clustering is common in many forms of heart disease. Mendelian transmission of single-gene defects may occur, as in hypertrophic cardiomyopathy (Chap. 238), the Marfan syndrome (Chap. 351), and sudden death associated with a prolonged QT syndrome (Chap. 230). Essential hypertension or coronary atherosclerosis are often polygenic disorders. While familial transmission may be less obvious than in the single-gene disorders, it is also helpful in assessing risk and prognosis. Familial clustering of cardiovascular diseases may occur not only on a genetic basis but also may be related to familial dietary or behavior patterns, such as excessive ingestion of salt or calories or cigarette smoking.

Assessment of Functional Impairment   When an attempt is made to determine the severity of functional impairment in a patient with heart disease, it is helpful to ascertain with as much precision as possible the level of activity and the rate at which it is performed before symptoms develop. Thus, breathlessness that occurs after running up two long flights of stairs denotes far less functional impairment than similar symptoms occurring after taking a few steps on the level. Also, the degree of customary physical activity at work and during recreation should be considered. The development of two-flight dyspnea in a marathon runner may be far more significant than the development of one-flight dyspnea in a previously sedentary person. Similarly, the history must include a detailed consideration of the patient's therapeutic regimen. For example, the persistence or development of edema, breathlessness, and other manifestations of heart failure in a patient whose diet is rigidly restricted in sodium content and who is receiving optimal doses of diuretics is far more grave than are similar manifestations in the absence of these measures. In an effort to determine the rate of progression of symptoms, and thereby of the severity

Table 224-2   Conditions in Which Clinical Examination Is an Important Determinant of Diagnosis: Confirmation by Echocardiography Is Often Useful

Mitral valve prolapse	Tricuspid regurgitation
Congestive heart failure	Aortic stenosis
Cardiac tamponade	Acute pulmonary hypertension
Hypertension	Chronic pulmonary hypertension
Mitral stenosis	High-output states
Chronic mitral regurgitation	Atrial septal defect
Chronic aortic regurgitation	Anginal syndrome

of the underlying illness, it may be useful to ascertain what, if any, specific tasks the patient could carry out 1 year earlier that he or she cannot carry out at present.

Electrocardiogram   (See also Chap. 226)   Although an ECG should be recorded in every patient with known or suspected heart disease, with the exception of the identification of arrhythmias and of acute myocardial infarction, it rarely permits establishment of a specific diagnosis. In the absence of other abnormal findings, electrocardiographic changes must not be overinterpreted. The range of normal electrocardiographic findings is wide, and the tracing can be affected significantly by many noncardiac factors, such as age, body habitus, and serum electrolyte concentrations.

Natural History   The natural history of cardiovascular disease must be appreciated. Cardiovascular disorders often present acutely, as in a previously asymptomatic patient with extensive coronary atherosclerosis who develops an acute myocardial infarction or the previously asymptomatic patient with hypertrophic cardiomyopathy whose first clinical manifestation is syncope or even sudden death. However, in both instances, the alert physician may recognize the patient at risk of these complications long before they occur and can often take measures to prevent their occurrence. For example, the patient with acute myocardial infarction may well have had risk factors for atherosclerosis for many years. Had these been recognized, their elimination or reduction might have delayed or even prevented the infarction. Similarly, the patient with hypertrophic cardiomyopathy may have had a heart murmur for years, and a positive family history might have led to an echocardiographic examination and the recognition of the condition and appropriate therapy long before the acute manifestations.

PITFALLS IN CARDIOVASCULAR MEDICINE   Increasing subspecialization in internal medicine and the perfection of advanced diagnostic techniques in cardiology can lead to several undesirable consequences. Examples include:

1. Failure by the *noncardiologist* to recognize important cardiac manifestations of systemic illnesses. Examples of the latter are (a) stroke (atrial fibrillation, mitral stenosis); (b) skeletal muscular dystrophies (associated with cardiomyopathy); (c) hemochromatosis (associated with myocardial infiltration and restrictive cardiomyopathy); (d) congenital deafness (associated with prolonged QT interval and serious cardiac arrhythmias); (e) Raynaud's disease (associated with primary pulmonary hypertension and coronary vasospasm); (f) connective tissue disorders, e.g., the Marfan syndrome, (aortic dilatation and aneurysm, prolapsed mitral valve); (g) hyperthyroidism (heart failure, atrial fibrillation); (h) hypothyroidism (pericardial effusion, coronary artery disease); (i) rheumatoid arthritis (pericarditis, aortic valve disease); (j) scleroderma (cor pulmonale, myocardial fibrosis, pericarditis); (k) systemic lupus erythematosus (valvulitis, myocarditis, pericarditis); and (l) sarcoidosis (arrhythmias, cardiomyopathy). In patients with these and other systemic disorders a cardiovascular examination should be carried out to identify and estimate the severity of cardiovascular involvement.

2. Failure by the cardiologist to recognize underlying systemic disorders, such as those listed above, in patients with a cardiac disorder. Patients with heart disease should be assessed for the frequent *noncardiac* manifestations of systemic disorders with cardiovascular manifestations. For example, Lyme disease should be considered in patients with unexplained fluctuating atrioventricular block. A cardiovascular abnormality may provide the clue critical to the recognition of some systemic disorders. For instance, unexplained atrial fibrillation may provide the first clue to the diagnosis of thyrotoxicosis.

3. Overreliance on and overutilization of laboratory tests, particularly invasive techniques for the examination of the cardiovascular system. Cardiac catheterization and coronary arteriography (Chap. 228) provide precise diagnostic information under many circumstances. For example, they aid in establishing a specific anatomic diagnosis, which, in turn, may be critical to developing a therapeutic plan in patients with known or suspected ischemic heart disease. Although a great deal of attention has been lavished on these expensive

examinations, it should be recognized that they serve to *supplement*, not *supplant*, a careful examination carried out by clinical and noninvasive techniques. A coronary arteriogram should not be carried out in lieu of a careful history in patients with chest pain suspected of having ischemic heart disease. Although coronary arteriography may establish whether the coronary arteries are obstructed, the results often do not provide a definite answer to the question of whether a patient's complaint of chest pain is attributable to coronary arteriosclerosis. Catheterization of the left side of the heart is all too frequently employed to assess patients with valvular heart disease when echocardiographic examination would actually provide more useful information.

Despite the enormous value of these invasive tests in certain circumstances, they entail some small risk to the patient, involve discomfort and substantial cost, and place a strain on existing medical facilities. Therefore, they should be carried out only if, after clinical examination and assessment by noninvasive tests, the results of the invasive examination can be expected to modify the patient's management.

℞ **TREATMENT** After a complete diagnosis has been established, a number of therapeutic options are usually available. Several examples may be used to demonstrate some of the principles of cardiovascular therapeutics:

1. In the absence of evidence of heart disease, a clear, definitive statement to that effect should be made and the patient should *not* be asked to return at intervals for repeated examinations. If there is no evidence for disease, such continued attention may lead to the patient developing inappropriate anxiety and fixation on the heart.

2. If there is no evidence of cardiovascular disease but the patient has one or more risk factors for the development of ischemic heart disease (Chap. 242), a plan for their reduction should be developed and the patient should be retested at intervals to assess that he or she is complying and that these risk factors are in fact being reduced.

3. Asymptomatic or mildly symptomatic patients with valvular heart disease that is anatomically severe should be evaluated periodically, every 6 to 12 months, by clinical and noninvasive examinations. Early signs of deterioration of ventricular function can be detected in this manner and in appropriate patients may signify the need for surgical treatment before the development of disabling symptoms, irreversible myocardial damage, and excessive risk of surgical treatment (Chap. 236).

4. It is critical to establish clear criteria for deciding on the form of treatment (medical, percutaneous coronary intervention, or surgical revascularization) in patients with ischemic heart disease (Chap. 244). Mechanical revascularization, i.e., the latter two modalities, represents a major therapeutic advance in the treatment of this most common form of heart disease in developed nations, but these techniques are probably being employed too frequently in the United States; the mere presence of angina pectoris and/or the demonstration of critical coronary arterial narrowing at angiography should not reflexly evoke a decision to treat the patient surgically or by percutaneous coronary intervention. Instead, coronary revascularization should be limited to those patients with ischemic heart disease who have not responded adequately to medical treatment (e.g., intractable angina) or in whom the procedure has been shown to improve the natural history (e.g., threevessel coronary artery disease with left ventricular dysfunction.)

BIBLIOGRAPHY

BRAUNWALD E, ZIPES D, LIBBY P (eds): *Heart Disease*, 6th ed. Philadelphia, Saunders, 2001

CONSTANT J: *Bedside Cardiology*, 4th ed. Boston, Little, Brown, 1993

THE CRITERIA COMMITTEE OF THE NEW YORK HEART ASSOCIATION: *Nomenclature and Criteria for Diagnosis*, 9th ed. Boston, Little, Brown, 1994

HURST JW: *Cardiovascular Diagnosis: The Initial Examination*. St. Louis, Mosby, 1993

MARRIOTT HJL: *Bedside Cardiac Diagnosis*. Philadelphia, Lippincott, 1993

O'ROURKE RA et al: The history, physical examination, and cardiac auscultation, in *Hurst's The Heart*, 9th ed, RW Alexander et al (eds). New York, McGraw-Hill, 1998, pp 229–342

VANDEN BELT J: The history, in *Classic Teachings in Clinical Cardiology: A Tribute to W. Proctor Harvey*, M Chizner (ed). Cedar Grove, NJ, Laennec, 1996, pp 41–54

---

225 *Robert A. O'Rourke, Eugene Braunwald*

PHYSICAL EXAMINATION OF THE CARDIOVASCULAR SYSTEM

A meticulous physical examination is an often inadequately utilized low-cost method for assessing the cardiovascular system and frequently provides important information for the appropriate selection of additional tests. First, the general physical appearance should be evaluated. The patient may appear tired because of a chronic low cardiac output; the respiratory rate may be rapid in cases of pulmonary venous congestion. Central cyanosis, often associated with clubbing of the fingers and toes, indicates right-to-left cardiac or extracardiac shunting or inadequate oxygenation of blood by the lungs. Cyanosis in the distal extremities, cool skin, and increased sweating result from vasoconstriction in patients with severe heart failure (Chap. 36). Noncardiovascular details can be equally important. For example, infective endocarditis is the likely diagnosis in patients with petechiae, Osler's nodes, and Janeway lesions (Chap. 126).

The blood pressure should be taken in both arms and with the patient supine and upright; the heart rate should be timed for 30 s. Orthostatic hypotension and tachycardia may indicate a reduced blood volume, while resting tachycardia may be due to heart failure.

Careful examination of the optic fundi is essential (Chap. 246), and the retinal vessels may show evidence of systemic hypertension, arteriosclerosis, or embolism. The latter may result from atherosclerosis in larger arteries (e.g., the carotid) or may represent a complication of valvular heart disease (e.g., endocarditis).

Palpation of the peripheral arterial pulses in the upper and lower extremities is necessary to define the adequacy of systemic blood flow and to detect the presence of occlusive arterial lesions. It is also important to examine both legs for evidence of edema, varicose veins, or thrombophlebitis (Chap. 248). The cardiovascular examination includes careful evaluation of both the carotid arterial and the jugular venous pulses, as well as deliberate precordial palpation and attentive cardiac auscultation.

ARTERIAL PRESSURE PULSE The normal central aortic pulse wave is characterized by a fairly rapid rise to a somewhat rounded peak (Fig. 225-1). The anacrotic shoulder, present on the ascending limb, occurs at the time of peak rate of aortic flow just before maximum pressure is reached. The less steep descending limb is interrupted by a sharp downward deflection, coincident with aortic valve closure, called the *incisura*. As the pulse wave is transmitted peripherally, the initial upstroke becomes steeper, the anacrotic shoulder becomes less apparent, and the incisura is replaced by the smoother dicrotic notch. Accordingly, palpation of a peripheral arterial pulse (e.g., the radial pulse) frequently gives less information than examination of a more central pulse (e.g., the carotid pulse) regarding alterations in left ventricular ejection or aortic valve function. However, certain findings, such as the bisferiens pulse of aortic regurgitation or pulsus alternans, are more evident in peripheral arteries (Fig. 225-2). The carotid pulse is best examined with the sternocleidomastoid muscle relaxed and with the head rotated slightly toward the examiner. In palpating the brachial arterial pulse, the examiner can support the subject's relaxed elbow with the right arm while compressing the brachial pulse with the thumb. The usual technique is to compress the artery

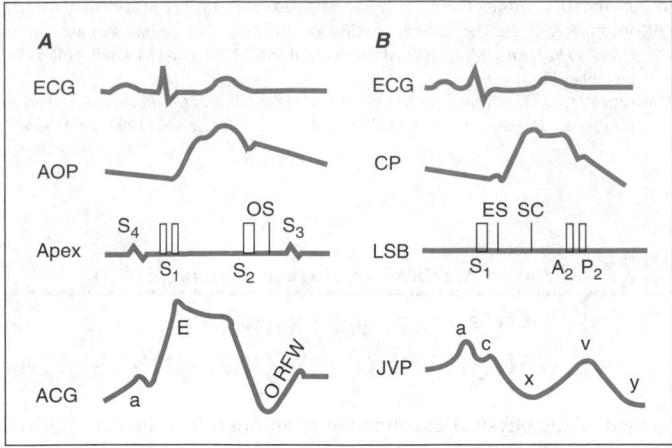

FIGURE 225-1 *A.* Schematic representation of electrocardiogram, aortic pressure pulse (AOP), phonocardiogram recorded at the apex, and apex cardiogram (ACG). On the phonocardiogram, S_1, S_2, S_3, and S_4 represent the first through fourth heart sounds; OS represents the opening snap of the mitral valve, which occurs coincident with the O point of the apex cardiogram. S_3 occurs coincident with the termination of the rapid-filling wave (RFW) of the ACG, while S_4 occurs coincident with the *a* wave of the ACG. *B.* Simultaneous recording of electrocardiogram, indirect carotid pulse (CP), phonocardiogram along the left sternal border (LSB), and indirect jugular venous pulse (JVP). ES, ejection sound; SC, systolic click.

with the thumb or forefinger until the maximum pulse is sensed. Varying degrees of pressure should then be applied while concentrating on the separate phases of the pulse wave. This method, known as *trisection*, is useful for assessing the sharpness of the upstroke, systolic peak, and diastolic slope of the arterial pulse. In most normal persons, a dicrotic wave is not palpable.

A small weak pulse, *pulsus parvus*, is common in conditions with a diminished left ventricular stroke volume, a narrow pulse pressure, and increased peripheral vascular resistance (Fig. 225-2). A *hypokinetic* pulse may be due to hypovolemia, to left ventricular failure, to restrictive pericardial disease, or to mitral valve stenosis. In aortic valve stenosis, the delayed systolic peak, *pulsus tardus*, results from obstruction to left ventricular ejection. In contrast, a large, bounding (*hyperkinetic*) pulse is usually associated with an increased left ventricular stroke volume, a wide pulse pressure, and a decrease in peripheral vascular resistance. This pattern occurs characteristically in

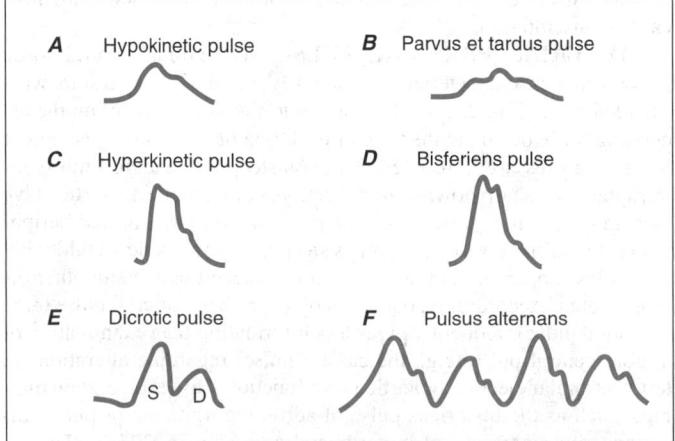

FIGURE 225-2 Schematic representation of arterial pulse waveforms that occur with alterations in cardiac hemodynamics, which may result from normal physiologic responses or may be due to cardiac disease. S, systole; D, diastole. [*Modified from RA O'Rourke, in Hurst's The Heart, 9th ed, RW Alexander et al (eds). New York, McGraw-Hill, 1990, with permission.*]

patients with an elevated stroke volume, as in complete heart block; with hyperkinetic circulation due to anxiety, anemia, exercise, or fever; or with a rapid runoff of blood from the arterial system (as caused by a patent ductus arteriosus or peripheral arteriovenous fistula). Patients with mitral regurgitation or a ventricular septal defect may also have a bounding pulse, since vigorous left ventricular ejection produces a rapid upstroke in the arterial pulse, even though the duration of systole and the forward stroke volume may be reduced. In aortic regurgitation, the rapidly rising, bounding arterial pulse results from an increased left ventricular stroke volume and an increased rate of ventricular ejection.

The *bisferiens pulse*, which has two systolic peaks, is characteristic of aortic regurgitation (with or without accompanying stenosis) and of hypertrophic cardiomyopathy (Chap. 238). In the latter condition, the pulse wave upstroke rises rapidly and forcefully, producing the first systolic peak ("percussion wave"). A brief decline in pressure follows because of the sudden midsystolic decrease in the rate of left ventricular ejection, when severe obstruction often develops. This pressure trough is followed by a smaller and more slowly rising positive pulse wave ("tidal wave") produced by continued ventricular ejection and by reflected waves from the periphery. The *dicrotic pulse* has two palpable waves, one in systole and one in diastole. It usually denotes a very low stroke volume, particularly in patients with dilated cardiomyopathy.

Pulsus alternans is a pattern in which there is regular alteration of the pressure pulse amplitude, despite a regular rhythm (Fig. 225-2). It is due to alternating left ventricular contractile force, usually indicates severe impairment of left ventricular function, and commonly occurs in patients who also have a loud third heart sound. Pulsus alternans may also occur during or following paroxysmal tachycardia or for several beats following a premature beat in patients without heart disease. In *pulsus bigeminus*, there is also a regular alteration of pressure pulse amplitude, but it is caused by a premature ventricular contraction that follows each regular beat. In *pulsus paradoxus*, the decrease in systolic arterial pressure that normally accompanies the reduction in arterial pulse amplitude during inspiration is accentuated. In patients with pericardial tamponade (Chap. 239), airway obstruction, or superior vena cava obstruction, the decrease in systolic arterial pressure frequently exceeds the normal decrease of 10 mmHg and the peripheral pulse may disappear completely during inspiration.

Simultaneous palpation of the radial and femoral arterial pulses, which normally are virtually coincident, is important to rule out aortic coarctation, in which the latter pulse is weakened and delayed (Chap. 234).

JUGULAR VENOUS PULSE (JVP) The two main objectives of the examination of the neck veins are inspection of their waveform and estimation of the central venous pressure (CVP). In most patients, the right internal jugular vein is best for both purposes. Usually, the pulsation of the internal jugular vein is greatest when the trunk is inclined by less than 30°. In patients with elevated venous pressure, it may be necessary to elevate the trunk further, sometimes to as much as 90°. When the neck muscles are relaxed, shining a beam of light tangentially across the skin overlying the vein exposes the pulsations of the internal jugular vein. Simultaneous palpation of the left carotid artery aids the examiner in deciding which pulsations are venous and in relating the venous pulsations to their timing in the cardiac cycle.

The normal JVP reflects phasic pressure changes in the right atrium and consists of two or sometimes three positive waves and two negative troughs (Fig. 225-1). The positive presystolic *a* wave is produced by venous distention due to right atrial contraction and is the dominant wave in the JVP, particularly during inspiration. Large *a* waves indicate that the right atrium is contracting against an increased resistance (Fig. 225-3), such as occurs with tricuspid stenosis or more commonly with increased resistance to right ventricular filling (pulmonary hypertension or pulmonic stenosis). Large *a* waves also occur during arrhythmias whenever the right atrium contracts while the tricuspid valve is closed by right ventricular systole. Such "cannon" *a* waves may occur regularly (as during junctional rhythm) or irregularly (as in

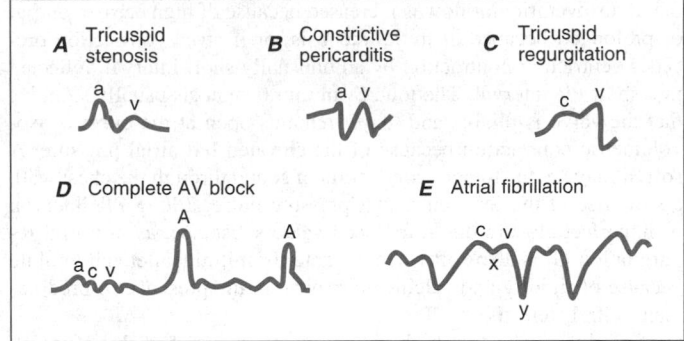

| A Tricuspid stenosis | B Constrictive pericarditis | C Tricuspid regurgitation |

FIGURE 225-3 Abnormal jugular venous pulse waveforms commonly present in patients with cardiac disease and/or arrhythmias. See text. [*Modified from RA O'Rourke, in Hurst's The Heart, 9th ed, RW Alexander et al (eds). New York, McGraw-Hill, 1990, with permission.*]

atrioventricular dissociation with ventricular tachycardia or complete heart block). The *a* wave is absent in patients with atrial fibrillation, and there is an increased delay between the *a* wave and the carotid arterial pulse in patients with first-degree atrioventricular block.

The *c* wave, often observed in the JVP, is a positive wave produced by the bulging of the tricuspid valve into the right atrium during right ventricular isovolumetric systole and by the impact of the carotid artery adjacent to the jugular vein. The *x* descent is due both to atrial relaxation and to the downward displacement of the tricuspid valve during ventricular systole. The *x* descent wave during systole is often accentuated in patients with constrictive pericarditis (Fig. 225-3), but the nadir of this wave is reduced with right ventricular dilation and is often reversed in tricuspid regurgitation. The positive, late systolic *v* wave results from the increasing volume of blood in the right atrium during ventricular systole when the tricuspid valve is closed. Tricuspid regurgitation causes the *v* wave to be more prominent; when tricuspid regurgitation becomes severe, the combination of a prominent *v* wave and obliteration of the *x* descent results in a single large positive systolic wave. After the *v* wave peaks, the right atrial pressure falls because of the decreased bulging of the tricuspid valve into the right atrium as right ventricular pressure declines and the tricuspid valve opens (Fig. 225-3).

This negative descending limb—the *y* descent of the JVP—is produced mainly by the opening of the tricuspid valve and the subsequent rapid inflow of blood into the right ventricle. A rapid, deep *y* descent in early diastole occurs with severe tricuspid regurgitation. A venous pulse characterized by a sharp *y* descent, a deep *y* trough, and a rapid ascent to the baseline is seen in patients with constrictive pericarditis or with severe right-sided heart failure and a high venous pressure. A slow *y* descent in the JVP suggests an obstruction to right ventricular filling, as occurs with tricuspid stenosis or right atrial myxoma.

The right internal jugular is the best vein to use for accurate estimation of the CVP. The sternal angle is used as the reference point, because the center of the right atrium lies approximately 5 cm below the sternal angle in the average patient, regardless of body position. The patient is examined at the optimal degree of trunk elevation for visualization of venous pulsations. The vertical distance between the top of the oscillating venous column and the level of the sternal angle is determined; generally it is less than 3 cm (3 cm + 5 cm = 8 cm blood). The most common cause of a high venous pressure is an elevated right ventricular diastolic pressure. In patients suspected of having right ventricular failure who have a normal CVP at rest, the abdominojugular reflux test may be helpful. The palm of the examiner's hand is placed over the abdomen, and firm pressure is applied for 10 s or more. In normal persons, this maneuver does not alter the jugular venous pressure significantly, but when right heart function is impaired, the upper level of venous pulsation usually increases. A positive abdominojugular test is best defined as an increase in JVP during 10 s of firm midabdominal compression followed by a rapid

drop in pressure of 4 cm blood on release of the compression. The most common cause of a positive test is right-sided heart failure secondary to elevated left heart filling pressures. Also, abdominal compression may elicit the JVP pattern typical of tricuspid regurgitation when the resting pulse wave is normal. *Kussmaul's sign*—an increase rather than the normal decrease in the CVP during inspiration—is most often caused by severe right-sided heart failure; it is a frequent finding in patients with constrictive pericarditis or right ventricular infarction.

PRECORDIAL PALPATION The location, amplitude, duration, and direction of the cardiac impulse usually can be best appreciated with the fingertips. The normal left ventricular apex impulse is located at or medial to the left midclavicular line in the fourth or fifth intercostal space and is a tapping, early systolic outward thrust localized to a point usually less than 2.5 cm in diameter. It is due primarily to recoil of the heart as blood is ejected and should be evaluated with the patient supine and in the left lateral position. Left ventricular hypertrophy results in exaggeration of the amplitude, duration, and often size of the normal left ventricular thrust. The impulse may be displaced laterally and downward into the sixth or seventh interspace, particularly in patients with a left ventricular volume load such as occurs in cases of aortic regurgitation or dilated cardiomyopathy.

Additional abnormal features that are detectable at the left ventricular apex include marked presystolic distention of the left ventricle, which is often accompanied by a fourth heart sound in patients with an excessive left ventricular pressure load or myocardial ischemia/infarction, and a prominent early diastolic rapid-filling wave, which is often accompanied by a third heart sound in patients with left ventricular failure or mitral valve regurgitation (Fig. 225-1). A double systolic apical impulse is often palpable in patients with hypertrophic cardiomyopathy.

Right ventricular hypertrophy often results in a sustained systolic lift at the lower left parasternal area, which starts in early systole and is synchronous with the left ventricular apical impulse.

Abnormal precordial pulsations occur during systole in patients with left ventricular dyssynergy due to ischemic heart disease or to diffuse myocardial disease from some other cause. These pulsations often occur in patients with a recent myocardial infarction and may be present in some patients only during episodes of angina. They are most commonly felt in the left midprecordium one or two interspaces above and/or 1 to 2 cm medial to the left ventricular apex. A systolic bulge occurring in the region of the apex is difficult to distinguish from the impulse of left ventricular hypertrophy.

A left parasternal lift is frequently present in patients with severe mitral regurgitation. This pulsation occurs distinctly later than the left ventricular apical impulse, is synchronous with the *v* wave in the left atrial pressure curve, and is due to anterior displacement of the right ventricle by an enlarged, expanding left atrium. A similar impulse occurs to the right of the sternum in some patients with severe tricuspid regurgitation and a giant right atrium. Pulsation of the right sternoclavicular joint may indicate a right-sided aortic arch or aneurysmal dilation of the ascending aorta. Pulmonary artery pulsation is often visible and palpable in the second left intercostal space. While it may be normal in children or thin young adults, this pulsation usually denotes pulmonary hypertension, increased pulmonary blood flow, or poststenotic pulmonary artery dilation.

Thrills are palpable, low-frequency vibrations associated with heart murmurs. The systolic murmur of mitral regurgitation may be palpated at the cardiac apex. When the palm of the hand is placed over the precordium, the thrill of aortic stenosis crosses the palm toward the right side of the neck, while the thrill of pulmonic stenosis radiates more often to the left side of the neck. The thrill due to a ventricular septal defect is usually located in the third and fourth intercostal spaces near the left sternal border.

Percussion should be performed in each patient to identify normal or abnormal position of the heart, stomach, and liver. However, in patients with a normal cardiac situs, percussion adds little to careful inspection and palpation in the recognition of cardiac enlargement.

CARDIAC AUSCULTATION

To obtain the most information from cardiac auscultation, the observer should keep in mind several principles: (1) Auscultation should be performed in a quiet room to avoid the distracting noises of normal activity. (2) For optimal auscultation, attention must be focused on the phase of the cardiac cycle during which the auscultatory event is expected to occur. (3) The timing of a heart sound or murmur can be determined accurately from its relation to other observable events in the cardiac cycle—the carotid arterial pulse, the apical impulse, or the JVP. (4) To define the significance of a cardiac sound or murmur, it is often necessary to observe alterations in its timing or intensity during various physiologic and/or pharmacologic interventions (Table 225-1).

HEART SOUNDS   The major components of heart sounds are vibrations associated with the abrupt acceleration or deceleration of blood in the cardiovascular system. Studies using simultaneous echocardiographic-phonocardiographic recordings indicate that the first and second heart sounds are produced primarily by the closure of the atrioventricular (AV) and semilunar valves and the events that accompany these closures. The intensity of the *first heart sound* (S_1) is influenced by (1) the position of the mitral leaflets at the onset of ventricular systole; (2) the rate of rise of the left ventricular pressure pulse; (3) the presence or absence of structural disease of the mitral valve; and (4) the amount of tissue, air, or fluid between the heart and the stethoscope. S_1 is louder if diastole is shortened because of tachycar-

Table 225-1   Effects of Physiologic and Pharmacologic Interventions on the Intensity of Heart Murmurs and Sounds

Respiration   Systolic murmurs due to TR or pulmonic blood flow through a normal or stenotic valve and diastolic murmurs of TS or PR generally increase with inspiration, as do right-sided S_3 and S_4. Left-sided murmurs and sounds usually are louder during expiration.

Valsalva maneuver   Most murmurs decrease in length and intensity. Two exceptions are the systolic murmur of HCM, which usually becomes much louder, and that of MVP, which becomes longer and often louder. Following release of the Valsalva maneuver, right-sided murmurs tend to return to control intensity earlier than left-sided murmurs.

After VPB or AF   Murmurs originating at normal or stenotic semilunar valves increase in the cardiac cycle following a VPB or in the cycle after a long cycle length in AF. By contrast, systolic murmurs due to AV valve regurgitation either do not change, diminish (papillary muscle dysfunction), or become shorter (MVP).

Positional changes   With *standing*, most murmurs diminish, two exceptions being the murmur of HCM, which becomes louder, and that of MVP, which lengthens and often is intensified. With *squatting*, most murmurs become louder, but those of HCM and MVP usually soften and may disappear. Passive leg raising usually produces the same results.

Exercise   Murmurs due to blood flow across normal or obstructed valves (e.g., PS, MS) become louder with both isotonic and submaximal isometric (handgrip) exercise. Murmurs of MR, VSD, and AR also increase with handgrip exercise. However, the murmur of HCM often decreases with near maximum handgrip exercise. Left-sided S_4 and S_3 are often accentuated by exercise, particularly when due to ischemic heart disease.

Pharmacologic interventions   During the initial relative hypotension following amyl nitrite inhalation, murmurs of MR, VSD, and AR decrease, while murmurs of aortic stenosis or sclerosis increase. During the later tachycardia phase, murmurs of MS and right-sided lesions also increase. The response in MVP often is biphasic (first softer and then louder than control). The arterial constrictor phenylephrine tends to produce the opposite effects.

Transient arterial occlusion   Transient external compression of both arms by bilateral cuff inflation to 20 mmHg over peak systolic pressure augments the murmurs of MR, VSD, and AR, but not murmurs due to other causes.

NOTE: TR, tricuspid regurgitation; TS, tricuspid stenosis; PR, pulmonic regurgitation; HCM, hypertrophic cardiomyopathy; MVP, mitral valve prolapse; PS, pulmonic stenosis; MS, mitral stenosis; MR, mitral regurgitation; VSD, ventricular septal defect; AR, aortic regurgitation; VPB, ventricular premature beat; and AF, atrial fibrillation.

dia, if atrioventricular flow is increased because of high cardiac output or prolonged because of mitral stenosis, or if atrial contraction precedes ventricular contraction by an unusually short interval, reflected in a short PR interval. The loud S_1 in mitral stenosis usually signifies that the valve is pliable and that it remains open at the onset of isovolumetric contraction because of the elevated left atrial pressure. A soft S_1 may be due to poor conduction of sound through the chest wall, a slow rise of the left ventricular pressure pulse, a long PR interval, or imperfect closure due to reduced valve substance, as in mitral regurgitation. S_1 is also soft when the anterior mitral leaflet is immobile because of rigidity and calcification, even in the presence of predominant mitral stenosis.

Splitting of the two high-pitched components of S_1 by 10 to 30 ms is a normal phenomenon (Fig. 225-1). The first component of S_1 is attributed to mitral valve closure, and the second to tricuspid valve closure. Widening of the S_1 is due most often to complete right bundle branch block and the resulting delay in onset of the right ventricular pressure pulse. Reversed splitting of the S_1, in which the mitral component follows the tricuspid component, may be present in patients with severe mitral stenosis, left atrial myxoma, and left bundle branch block.

Splitting of the *second heart sound* (S_2) into audibly distinct aortic (A_2) and pulmonic (P_2) components occurs normally during inspiration, when the augmented inflow into the right ventricle increases its stroke volume and ejection period and thus delays closure of the pulmonic valve. P_2 is coincident with the incisura of the pulmonary artery pressure curve, which is separated from the right ventricular pressure tracing by an interval termed the "hangout time." The absolute value of this interval reflects the resistance to pulmonary blood flow and the impedance characteristics of the pulmonary vascular bed. This interval is prolonged, and physiologic splitting of S_2 is accentuated, in conditions associated with right ventricular volume overload and a distensible pulmonary vascular bed. However, in patients with an increase in pulmonary vascular resistance, the hangout time is markedly reduced, and narrow splitting of S_2 is present. Splitting that persists with expiration (heard best at the pulmonic area or left sternal border) is usually abnormal when the patient is in the upright position. Such splitting may be due to many causes: delayed activation of the right ventricle (right bundle branch block); left ventricular ectopic beats; a left ventricular pacemaker; prolongation of right ventricular contraction with an increased right ventricular pressure load (pulmonary embolism or pulmonic stenosis); or delayed pulmonic valve closure because of right ventricular volume overload associated with right ventricular failure or diminished impedance of the pulmonary vascular bed and a prolonged hangout time (atrial septal defect).

In pulmonary hypertension, P_2 is loud, and splitting of the second heart sound may be diminished, normal, or accentuated, depending on the cause of the pulmonary hypertension, the pulmonary vascular resistance, and the presence or absence of right ventricular decompensation. Early aortic valve closure, occurring with mitral regurgitation or a ventricular septal defect, may also produce splitting that persists during expiration. It may also occur with constrictive pericarditis. In patients with an atrial septal defect, the proportion of right atrial filling contributed by the left atrium and the venae cavae varies reciprocally during the respiratory cycle, so that right atrial inflow remains relatively constant. Therefore, the volume and duration of right ventricular ejection are not significantly increased by inspiration, and there is little inspiratory exaggeration of the splitting of S_2. This phenomenon, termed *fixed splitting* of the second heart sound, is of considerable diagnostic value.

A delay in aortic valve closure causing P_2 to precede A_2 results in so-called reversed (paradoxic) splitting of S_2. Splitting is then maximal in expiration and decreases during inspiration with the normal delay of pulmonic valve closure. The most common causes of reversed splitting of S_2 are left bundle branch block and delayed excitation of the left ventricle from a right ventricular ectopic beat. Mechanical prolongation of left ventricular systole, resulting in reversed splitting of S_2, may also be caused by severe aortic outflow obstruction, a large aorta-to-pulmonary artery shunt, systolic hypertension, and ischemic heart disease or cardiomyopathy with left ventricular failure. P₂ is normally softer than A₂ in the second left intercostal space; a P₂ that is greater than A₂ in this area suggests pulmonary hypertension, except in patients with atrial septal defect.

The *third heart sound* (S₃) is a low-pitched sound produced in the ventricle 0.14 to 0.16 s after A₂, at the termination of rapid filling. This sound is frequent in normal children and in patients with high cardiac output. However, in patients over 40 years old, an S₃ usually indicates impairment of ventricular function, AV valve regurgitation, or other conditions that increase the rate or volume of ventricular filling. The left-sided S₃ is best heard with the bell piece of the stethoscope at the left ventricular apex during expiration and with the patient in the left lateral position. The right-sided S₃ is best heard at the left sternal border or just beneath the xiphoid and is usually louder with inspiration. Often it is accompanied by the systolic murmur of functional tricuspid regurgitation. Third heart sounds often disappear with treatment of heart failure.

An S₃ that is earlier (0.10 to 0.12 s after A₂) and higher-pitched than normal (a pericardial knock) often occurs in patients with constrictive pericarditis (Chap. 239); its presence depends on the restrictive effect of the adherent pericardium, which halts diastolic filling abruptly.

The *opening snap* (OS) is a brief, high-pitched, early diastolic sound, which is usually due to stenosis of an AV valve, most often the mitral valve. It is generally heard best at the lower left sternal border and radiates well to the base of the heart. The A₂-OS interval is inversely related to the height of the mean left atrial pressure and ranges from 0.04 to 0.12 s. In the second intercostal space, an OS is often confused with P₂. However, careful auscultation will reveal both components of S₂, followed by the OS. The OS of tricuspid stenosis occurs later in diastole than the mitral OS and is often overlooked in patients with more prominent mitral valve disease.

The *fourth heart sound* (S₄) is a low-pitched, presystolic sound produced in the ventricle during ventricular filling; it is associated with an effective atrial contraction and is best heard with the bell piece of the stethoscope. The sound is absent in patients with atrial fibrillation. The S₄ occurs when diminished ventricular compliance increases the resistance to ventricular filling, and it is frequently present in patients with systemic hypertension, aortic stenosis, hypertrophic cardiomyopathy, ischemic heart disease, and acute mitral regurgitation. Most patients with an acute myocardial infarction and sinus rhythm have an audible S₄. The fourth heart sound is frequently accompanied by visible and palpable presystolic distention of the left ventricle. It is loudest at the left ventricular apex when the patient is in the left lateral position and is accentuated by mild isotonic or isometric exercise in the supine position. The right-sided S₄ is present in patients with right ventricular hypertrophy secondary to either pulmonic stenosis or pulmonary hypertension and frequently accompanies a prominent presystolic *a* wave in the JVP.

An S₄ frequently accompanies delayed AV conduction even in the absence of clinically detectable heart disease. The incidence of an audible S₄ increases with increasing age. Whether an audible S₄ in adults without other evidence of cardiac disease is abnormal remains controversial.

The *ejection sound* is a sharp, high-pitched event occurring in early systole and closely following the first heart sound. Ejection sounds occur in the presence of semilunar valve stenosis and in conditions associated with dilation of the aorta or pulmonary artery. The aortic ejection sound is usually heard best at the left ventricular apex and the second right intercostal space; the pulmonary ejection sound is loudest at the upper left sternal border. The latter, unlike most other right-sided acoustical events, is heard better during expiration.

Nonejection or *midsystolic clicks*, occurring with or without a late systolic murmur, often denote prolapse of one or both leaflets of the mitral valve (Chap. 236). They also may be caused by tricuspid valve prolapse. They probably result from chordae tendineae that are functionally unequal in length on either or both AV valves and are heard best along the lower left sternal border and at the left ventricular apex. Systolic clicks may be single or multiple, and they may occur at any time in systole but are usually later than the systolic ejection sound.

HEART MURMURS (See also Chap. 34) Cardiac murmurs result from vibrations set up in the bloodstream and the surrounding heart and great vessels as a result of turbulent blood flow, the formation of eddies, and cavitation (bubble formation as a result of sudden decrease in pressure).

The intensity (loudness) of murmurs may be graded from I to VI. A grade I murmur is so faint that it can be heard only with special effort; a grade IV murmur is commonly accompanied by a thrill; and a grade VI murmur is audible with the stethoscope removed from contact with the chest. The configuration of a murmur may be crescendo, decrescendo, crescendo-decrescendo (diamond-shaped), or plateau. The precise time of onset and time of cessation of a murmur depend on the instant in the cardiac cycle at which an adequate pressure difference between two chambers arises and disappears (Fig. 225-4).

The location on the chest wall where the murmur is best heard and the areas to which it radiates can aid in identifying the cardiac structure from which the murmur originates. For example, the murmur of aortic valve stenosis is usually loudest in the second right intercostal space and radiates to the carotid arteries. By contrast, the murmur of mitral regurgitation is most often loudest at the cardiac apex. It may radiate to the left sternal border and base of the heart when the posterior mitral leaflet is predominantly involved or to the axilla and back when the anterior leaflet is more severely affected. In the latter case, the regurgitant blood is directed toward the posterior left atrial wall.

It is often difficult to classify a cardiac murmur with certainty on the basis of its timing, configuration, location, radiation, pitch, or intensity. However, by noting changes in the characteristics of the murmur during maneuvers that alter cardiac hemodynamics, the auscultator can often identify its correct origin and significance (Table 225-1).

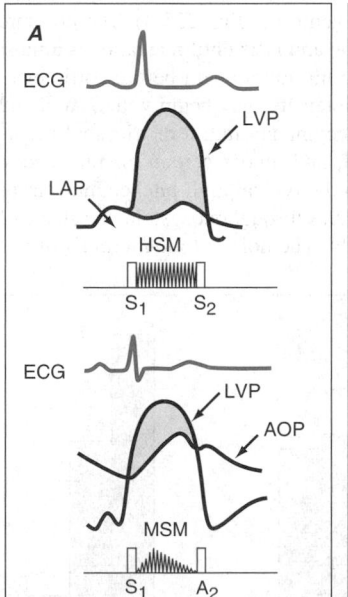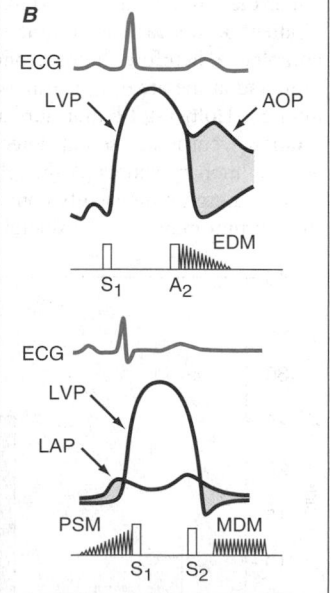

FIGURE 225-4 *A.* Schematic representation of ECG, aortic pressure (AOP), left ventricular pressure (LVP), and left atrial pressure (LAP). The shaded areas indicate a transvalvular pressure difference during systole. HSM, holosystolic murmur; MSM, midsystolic murmur. *B.* Graphic representation of ECG, aortic pressure (AOP), left ventricular pressure (LVP) and left atrial pressure (LAP) with shaded areas indicating transvalvular diastolic pressure difference. EDM, early diastolic murmur; PSM, presystolic murmur; MDM, middiastolic murmur.

Accentuation of a murmur during inspiration (a maneuver that augments systemic venous return) implies that it originates on the right side of the circulation; expiratory exaggeration has less significance. Prolonged expiratory pressure against a closed glottis (i.e., the Valsalva maneuver) reduces the intensity of most murmurs by diminishing both right and left ventricular filling (i.e., ventricular preload). The systolic murmur associated with *hypertrophic cardiomyopathy* and the late systolic murmur due to *mitral valve prolapse* are exceptions and may be paradoxically accentuated during the Valsalva maneuver. Murmurs due to flow across a normal or obstructed semilunar valve increase in intensity in the cycle following a premature ventricular beat or a long RR interval in atrial fibrillation. In contrast, murmurs due to AV valve regurgitation or a ventricular septal defect do not change appreciably during the beat following a prolonged diastole. Standing, which decreases left ventricular volume, accentuates the murmur of hypertrophic cardiomyopathy and occasionally the murmur due to mitral valve prolapse. Squatting, which increases both venous return and systemic arterial resistance and thus ventricular afterload, increases most murmurs, except those due to hypertrophic cardiomyopathy and mitral regurgitation due to a prolapsed mitral valve, which often decrease. Sustained handgrip exercise, which increases systemic arterial pressure and heart rate, often accentuates the murmurs of mitral regurgitation, aortic regurgitation, and mitral stenosis but usually diminishes those due to aortic stenosis or hypertrophic cardiomyopathy. Pharmacologic interventions include inhalation of amyl nitrite, which reduces systemic arterial pressure and increases blood flow, thereby increasing the intensity of murmurs due to valvular stenosis while diminishing those due to aortic or mitral regurgitation (Table 225-1). Transient external arterial occlusion by the inflation of bilateral arm cuffs to 20 mmHg (2.66 kPa) above systolic blood pressure for 5 s usually intensifies murmurs due to left-sided regurgitant lesions; this method is applicable to almost all patients and does not require administration of any drug.

Systolic Murmurs   *Holosystolic (pansystolic) murmurs* are generated when there is flow between two chambers that have widely different pressures throughout systole, such as the left ventricle and either the left atrium or the right ventricle (Fig. 225-4). The pressure gradient occurs early in contraction and lasts until relaxation is almost complete. Therefore, holosystolic murmurs begin before aortic ejection, and at the area of maximal intensity they begin with S_1 and end after S_2. Holosystolic murmurs accompany mitral or tricuspid regurgitation, ventricular septal defect, and, under certain circumstances, aortopulmonary shunts. Although the typical high-pitched murmur of mitral regurgitation usually continues throughout systole, the shape of the murmur may vary considerably. The holosystolic murmurs of mi-

tral regurgitation and ventricular septal defect are augmented by transient exercise and are diminished by lowering the left ventricular systolic pressure by inhalation of amyl nitrite. The murmur of tricuspid regurgitation associated with pulmonary hypertension is holosystolic and frequently increases during inspiration. Not all patients with mitral or tricuspid regurgitation or ventricular septal defect have holosystolic murmurs (Chap. 236). Often, a mild valvular regurgitant jet, detected by color flow Doppler techniques, is not associated with an audible murmur despite optimal auscultation. Such regurgitant jets usually do not indicate clinical heart disease. Trivial mitral regurgitation can be detected by Doppler in up to 45% of normal individuals; tricuspid regurgitation in up to 70%; and pulmonic regurgitation in up to 88%. Normal aortic regurgitation is encountered much less frequently, and its incidence increases with advancing age (Fig. 225-5).

Midsystolic murmurs, also called *systolic ejection murmurs*, which are often crescendo-decrescendo in shape, occur when blood is ejected across the aortic or pulmonic outflow tracts (Fig. 225-4). The murmur starts shortly after S_1, when the ventricular pressure becomes high enough to open the semilunar valve. As the velocity of ejection increases, the murmur gets louder; as ejection declines, it diminishes. The murmur ends before the ventricular pressure falls enough to permit closure of the aortic or pulmonic leaflets. When the semilunar valves are normal, an increased flow rate (as occurs in states of elevated cardiac output), ejection into a dilated vessel beyond the valve, or increased transmission of sound through a thin chest wall may be responsible for this murmur. Most benign, functional murmurs are midsystolic and originate from the pulmonary outflow tract. Valvular or subvalvular obstruction of either ventricle may also cause such a midsystolic murmur, the intensity being related to the flow rate.

The murmur of aortic stenosis is the prototype of the left-sided midsystolic murmur. The location and radiation of this murmur are influenced by the direction of the high-velocity jet within the aortic root. In *valvular aortic stenosis*, the murmur is usually maximal in the second right intercostal space, with radiation into the neck. In *supravalvular aortic stenosis*, the murmur is occasionally loudest even higher, with disproportionate radiation into the right carotid artery. In hypertrophic cardiomyopathy, the midsystolic murmur originates in the left ventricular cavity and is usually maximal at the lower left sternal edge and apex, with relatively little radiation to the carotids. When the aortic valve is immobile (calcified), the aortic closure sound (A_2) may be soft and inaudible so that the length and configuration of the murmur are difficult to determine. Midsystolic murmurs also occur in patients with mitral regurgitation or, less frequently, tricuspid regurgitation resulting from papillary muscle dysfunction. Such murmurs due to mitral regurgitation are often confused with those originating in the aorta, particularly in elderly patients.

The patient's age and the area of maximal intensity aid in determining the significance of midsystolic murmurs. Thus, in a young adult with a thin chest and a high velocity of blood flow, a faint or moderate midsystolic murmur heard only in the pulmonic area is usually without clinical significance, while a somewhat louder murmur in the aortic area may indicate congenital aortic stenosis. In elderly patients, pulmonic flow murmurs are rare, while aortic systolic murmurs are common and may be due to aortic dilation, to a significant degree of valvular aortic stenosis, or to nonstenotic thickening of the aortic valve leaflets. Midsystolic aortic and pulmonic murmurs are intensified after amyl nitrite inhalation and during the cardiac cycle following a premature ventricular beat, while those due to mitral regurgitation are unchanged or softer. Aortic systolic murmurs are diminished by interventions that increase aortic impedance, such as transient arterial occlu-

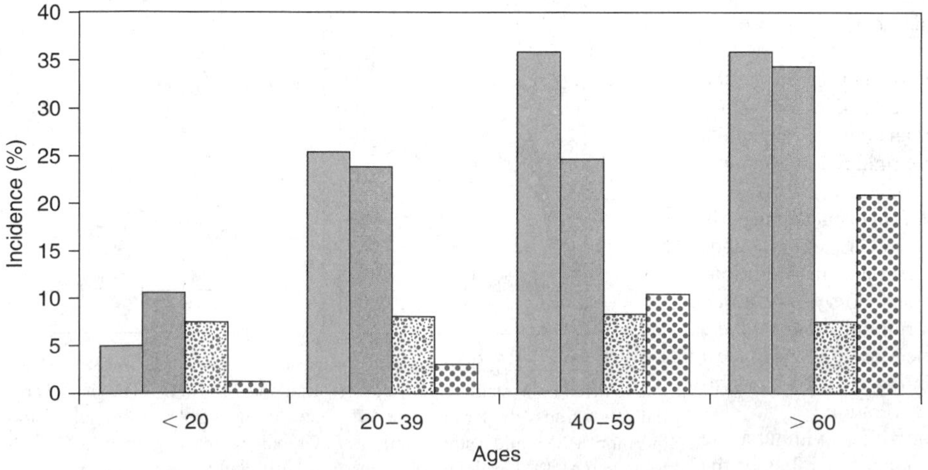

FIGURE 225-5   Percent incidence of mitral (shaded blue), tricuspid (shaded gray), pulmonic (stippled blue), and aortic (blue dots) regurgitation by Doppler echocardiography in clinically normal subjects at various ages. (*Modified from Choong et al.*)

sion. Echocardiography or cardiac catheterization may be necessary to separate a prominent and exaggerated functional murmur from one due to congenital or acquired semilunar valve stenosis.

Early systolic murmurs begin with the first heart sound and end in midsystole. In *large ventricular septal defects with pulmonary hypertension*, the shunting at the end of systole may be small or absent, resulting in an early systolic murmur. A similar murmur may occur with very *small muscular ventricular septal defects*, the shunt being interrupted in late systole. An early systolic murmur is a feature of *tricuspid regurgitation occurring in the absence of pulmonary hypertension*. This lesion is common in narcotics abusers with infective endocarditis, in whom a tall regurgitant right atrial *v* wave reaches the level of the normal right ventricular pressure in late systole, confining the murmur to early systole. Patients with acute mitral regurgitation into a noncompliant left atrium and a large *v* wave often have a loud early systolic murmur that diminishes as the pressure gradient between the left ventricle and left atrium decreases in late systole (Chap. 236).

Late systolic murmurs are faint or moderately loud, high-pitched apical murmurs that start well after ejection and do not mask either heart sound. They are probably related to papillary muscle dysfunction caused by infarction or ischemia of these muscles or to their distortion by left ventricular dilation. They may appear only during angina but are common in patients with myocardial infarction or diffuse myocardial disease. Late systolic murmurs following midsystolic clicks are due to late systolic mitral regurgitation caused by prolapse of the mitral valve into the left atrium (Chap. 236).

Diastolic Murmurs *Early diastolic murmurs* (Fig. 225-4) begin with or shortly after S_2, as soon as the corresponding ventricular pressure falls enough below that in the aorta or pulmonary artery. The high-pitched murmurs of aortic regurgitation or of pulmonic regurgitation due to pulmonary hypertension are generally decrescendo, since there is a progressive decline in the volume or rate of regurgitation during diastole. Faint, high-pitched murmurs of aortic regurgitation are difficult to hear unless they are specifically sought by applying firm pressure with the diaphragm over the left midsternal border while the patient sits leaning forward and holds a breath in full expiration. The diastolic murmur of aortic regurgitation is enhanced by an acute elevation of the arterial pressure, such as occurs with handgrip exercise; it diminishes with a decrease in arterial pressure, as with amyl nitrite inhalation. The diastolic murmur of congenital pulmonic regurgitation without pulmonary hypertension is low- to medium-pitched. The onset of this murmur is delayed because the regurgitant flow is minimal at the onset of pulmonic valve closure when the reverse pressure gradient responsible for the regurgitation is negligible.

Middiastolic murmurs usually arise from the mitral or tricuspid valves (Fig. 225-4), occur during early ventricular filling, and are due to disproportion between valve orifice size and flow rate. Such murmurs may be quite loud (grade III), despite only slight AV valve stenosis, when there is normal or increased blood flow. Conversely, the murmurs may be soft or even absent despite severe obstruction if the cardiac output is markedly reduced. When stenosis is marked, the diastolic murmur is prolonged, and the duration of the murmur is more reliable than its intensity as an index of the severity of valve obstruction.

The low-pitched, middiastolic murmur of mitral stenosis characteristically follows the OS. It should be specifically sought by placing the bell of the stethoscope at the site of the left ventricular impulse, which is best localized with the patient on the left side. Frequently, the murmur of mitral stenosis is present only at the left ventricular apex, and it may be increased in intensity by mild supine exercise or by inhalation of amyl nitrite. In tricuspid stenosis, the middiastolic murmur is localized to a relatively limited area along the left sternal edge and may be louder during inspiration.

Middiastolic murmurs may be generated across the mitral valve in cases of mitral regurgitation, patent ductus arteriosus, or ventricular septal defect, and across the tricuspid valve in cases of tricuspid regurgitation or atrial septal defect. These murmurs are related to the torrential flow across an AV valve, usually follow an S_3, and tend to

occur with large left-to-right shunts or severe AV valve regurgitation. A soft middiastolic murmur may sometimes be heard in patients with acute rheumatic fever (Carey-Coombs murmur). It has been attributed to inflammation of the mitral valve cusps or excessive left atrial blood flow as a consequence of mitral regurgitation.

In acute, severe aortic regurgitation, the left ventricular diastolic pressure may exceed the left atrial pressure, resulting in a middiastolic murmur due to "diastolic mitral regurgitation." In severe, chronic aortic regurgitation, a murmur is frequently present that may be either middiastolic or presystolic (Austin-Flint murmur). This murmur appears to originate at the anterior mitral valve leaflet when blood enters the left ventricle simultaneously from both the aortic root and the left atrium.

Presystolic murmurs begin during the period of ventricular filling that follows atrial contraction and therefore occur in sinus rhythm. They are usually due to AV valve stenosis and have the same quality as the middiastolic filling rumble, but they are usually crescendo, reaching peak intensity at the time of a loud S_1. The presystolic murmur corresponds to the AV valve gradient, which may be minimal until the moment of right or left atrial contraction. It is the presystolic murmur that is most characteristic of tricuspid stenosis and sinus rhythm. A right or left *atrial myxoma* may occasionally cause either middiastolic or presystolic murmurs that resemble the murmurs of mitral or tricuspid stenosis.

Continuous Murmurs These begin in systole, peak near S_2, and continue into all or part of diastole. These murmurs result from continuous flow due to a communication between high- and low-pressure areas that persists through the end of systole and the beginning of diastole. A *patent ductus arteriosus* causes a continuous murmur as long as the pressure in the pulmonary artery is much below that in the aorta. The murmur is intensified by elevation of the systemic arterial pressure and is reduced by amyl nitrite inhalation. When pulmonary hypertension is present, the diastolic portion may disappear, leaving the murmur confined to systole. A continuous murmur is uncommon in cases of aortopulmonary septal defect, which usually is associated with severe pulmonary hypertension. Surgically produced connections and the subclavian–pulmonary artery anastomosis result in murmurs similar to that of a patent ductus.

Continuous murmurs may result from congenital or acquired *systemic arteriovenous fistula*, *coronary arteriovenous fistula*, anomalous origin of the left coronary artery from the pulmonary artery, and communications between the *sinus of Valsalva and the right side of the heart*. Continuous murmurs may also occur in patients with a small atrial septal defect with a high left atrial pressure. Murmurs associated with *pulmonary arteriovenous fistulas* may be continuous but are usually only systolic. Continuous murmurs may also be due to disturbances of flow pattern in constricted systemic (e.g., renal) or pulmonary arteries when marked pressure differences between the two sides of the narrow segment persist; a continuous murmur in the back may be present in *coarctation of the aorta*; *pulmonary embolism* may cause continuous murmurs in partially occluded vessels.

In nonconstricted arteries, continuous murmurs may be due to rapid flow through a tortuous bed. Such murmurs typically occur within the bronchial arterial collateral circulation in cyanotic patients with severe pulmonary outflow obstruction. The "mammary souffle," an innocent murmur heard over the breasts during late pregnancy and in the early postpartum period, may be systolic or continuous. The innocent cervical venous hum is a continuous murmur usually audible over the medial aspect of the right supraclavicular fossa with the patient upright. The hum is usually louder during diastole and can be abolished instantaneously by digital compression of the ipsilateral internal jugular vein. Transmission of a loud venous hum to the area below the clavicles may result in a mistaken diagnosis of patent ductus arteriosus.

Pericardial Friction Rub These adventitious sounds may have presystolic, systolic, and early diastolic scratchy components, may be confused with a murmur or extracardiac sound when heard only in systole. It is best appreciated with the patient upright and leaning forward and may be accentuated during inspiration.

The evaluation of the patient with a heart murmur may vary greatly depending on many of the considerations discussed above. These include the intensity of the cardiac murmur, its timing in the cardiac cycle, its location and radiation, and its response to various physiologic maneuvers. Also of importance are the presence or absence of cardiac and noncardiac symptoms and whether other cardiac or noncardiac physical findings suggest that the cardiac murmur is clinically significant. The skill and confidence of the cardiac auscultator, the relative costs of various diagnostic approaches, and the accuracy and reliability of additional tests in the laboratory where they are performed are also important factors. One systematic approach to the patient with a heart murmur is depicted in Fig. 34-3. This algorithm is particularly applicable to children and adults under age 40.

BIBLIOGRAPHY

BRAUNWALD E: The clinical examination, in *Primary Cardiology*, L Goldman, E Braunwald (eds). Philadelphia, Saunders, 1998, pp 27–43

———: Physical examination of the heart and circulation, in *Heart Disease*, 6th ed, E Braunwald et al (eds). Philadelphia, Saunders, 2001

CHOONG CY et al: Prevalence of valvular regurgitation by Doppler echocardiography in patients with structurally normal hearts by 2-dimensional echocardiography. Am Heart J 117:636, 1989

CLEMENT DL, COHN JN: Salvaging the history, physical examination and doctor-patient relationship in a technological cardiology environment. J Am Coll Cardiol 33:892, 1999

CRAWFORD MH: *Examination of the Heart, Part 2: Inspection and Palpation of Venous and Arterial Pulses*. Chicago, American Heart Association, 1990

EILEN SD et al: Accuracy of precordial palpation for detecting increased left ventricular volume. Ann Intern Med 99:628, 1983

EWY GA: The abdominojugular test: Technique and hemodynamic correlates. Ann Intern Med 109:456, 1988

LEMBO NJ et al: Bedside diagnosis of systolic murmurs. N Engl J Med 318:1572, 1988

O'ROURKE RA: Approach to a patient with a heart murmur, in *Primary Cardiology*, L Goldman, E Braunwald (eds). Philadelphia, Saunders, 1998, pp 155–173

PERLOFF JK (ed): *Physical Examination of the Heart and Circulation*, 2d ed. Philadelphia, Saunders, 1990

SHAVER JA: Cardiac auscultation: A cost-effective diagnostic skill. Curr Probl Cardiol 20(7):441, 1995

YOSHIDA K et al: Color Doppler evaluation of valvular regurgitation in normals. Circulation 78:840, 1988

226   *Ary L. Goldberger*

ELECTROCARDIOGRAPHY

The electrocardiogram (ECG or EKG) is a graphic recording of electric potentials generated by the heart. The signals are detected by means of metal electrodes attached to the extremities and chest wall and are then amplified and recorded by the electrocardiograph. ECG *leads* actually display the instantaneous *differences* in potential between these electrodes.

The clinical utility of the ECG derives from its immediate availability as a noninvasive, inexpensive, and highly versatile test. In addition to its use in detecting arrhythmias, conduction disturbances, and myocardial ischemia, electrocardiography may reveal other findings related to life-threatening metabolic disturbances (e.g., hyperkalemia) or increased susceptibility to sudden cardiac death (e.g., QT prolongation syndromes). The advent of coronary thrombolysis or angioplasty in the early therapy of acute myocardial infarction (Chap. 243) has refocused particular attention on the sensitivity and specificity of ECG signs of myocardial ischemia.

ELECTROPHYSIOLOGY   (See also Chaps. 229 and 230)

Depolarization of the heart is the initiating event for cardiac contraction. The electric currents that spread through the heart are produced by three components: cardiac pacemaker cells, specialized conduction tissue, and the heart muscle itself. The ECG, however, records only the depolarization (stimulation) and repolarization (recovery) potentials generated by the atrial and ventricular myocardium. Under resting conditions, myocardial cells are *polarized*; that is, they carry an electric charge on their surface due to transmembrane ion concentration differences. The charge measured across atrial and ventricular cell membranes is about 90 mV, with the inside negative relative to the outside. When these cells are stimulated above a critical threshold potential, they rapidly depolarize and transiently reverse their membrane polarity. This depolarization process spreads in a wavelike manner through the atria and ventricles. The return of myocardial fibers to their original resting state occurs during repolarization.

The depolarization stimulus for the normal heartbeat originates in the sinoatrial (SA) *node* (Fig. 226-1) or *sinus node*, a collection of *pacemaker* cells. These cells fire spontaneously; that is, they exhibit *automaticity*. The first phase of cardiac electrical activation is the spread of the depolarization wave through the right and left atria, followed by atrial contraction. Next, the impulse stimulates pacemaker and specialized conduction tissues in the atrioventricular (AV) nodal and His-bundle areas; together, these two regions constitute the AV junction. The bundle of His bifurcates into two main branches, the right and left bundles, which rapidly transmit depolarization wavefronts to the right and left ventricular myocardium by way of Purkinje fibers. The main left bundle bifurcates into two primary subdivisions, a left anterior fascicle and a left posterior fascicle. The depolarization wavefronts then spread through the ventricular wall, from endocardium to epicardium, triggering ventricular contraction.

Since the cardiac depolarization and repolarization waves have direction and magnitude, they can be represented by vectors. *Vectorcardiograms* that measure and display these instantaneous potentials are no longer used much in clinical practice. However, the general principles of vector analysis remain fundamental to understanding the genesis of normal and pathologic ECG waveforms. Vector analysis illustrates a central concept of electrocardiography—that the ECG records the complex spatial and temporal summation of electrical potentials from multiple myocardial fibers conducted to the surface of the body. This principle accounts for inherent limitations in both ECG *sensitivity* (activity from certain cardiac regions may be canceled out or may be too weak to be recorded) and *specificity* (the same vectorial sum can result from either a selective gain or a loss of forces in opposite directions).

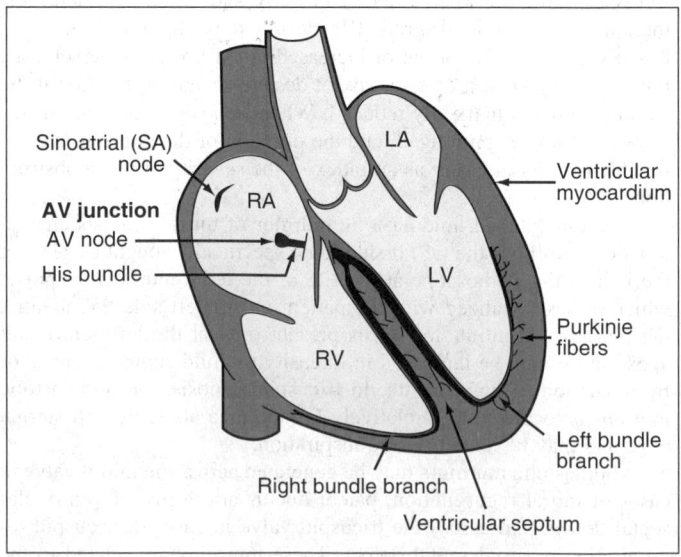

FIGURE 226-1 Schematic of the cardiac conduction system.

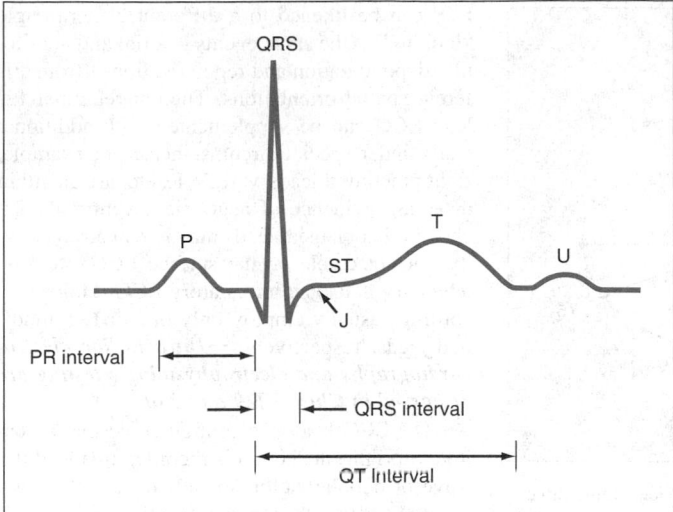

FIGURE 226-2 Basic ECG waveforms and intervals. Not shown is the R-R interval, the time between consecutive QRS complexes.

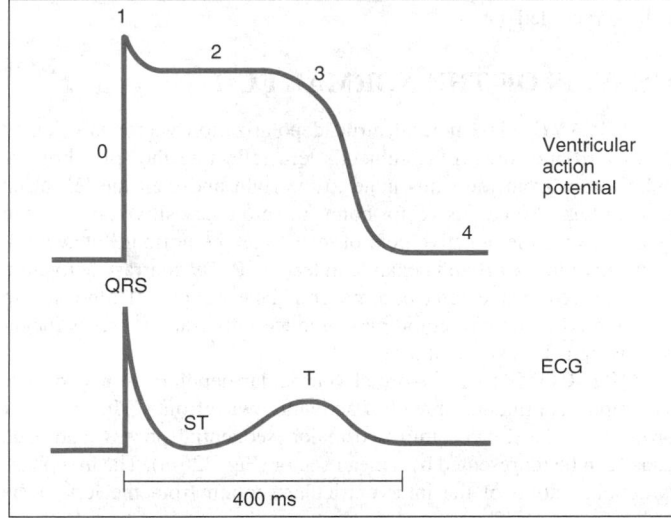

FIGURE 226-3 The QRS-T cycle corresponds to different phases of the ventricular action potential as described in Chap. 229.

ECG WAVEFORMS AND INTERVALS The ECG waveforms are labeled alphabetically, beginning with the P wave, which represents atrial depolarization (Fig. 226-2). The QRS complex represents ventricular depolarization, and the ST-T-U complex (ST segment, T wave, and U wave) represents ventricular repolarization. The J point is the junction between the end of the QRS complex and the beginning of the ST segment. Atrial repolarization is usually too low in amplitude to be detected, but it may become apparent in such conditions as acute pericarditis or atrial infarction.

The QRS-T waveforms of the surface (extracellular) ECG correspond in a general way with the different phases of simultaneously obtained ventricular *action potentials*, the intracellular recordings from single myocardial fibers (Fig. 226-3) (Chap. 229). The rapid upstroke (phase 0) of the action potential corresponds to the onset of QRS. The plateau (phase 2) corresponds to the

isoelectric ST segment, and active repolarization (phase 3) to the inscription of the T wave. Factors that decrease the slope of phase 0 by impairing the influx of Na^+ (e.g., drugs such as quinidine or procainamide, or hyperkalemia) tend to increase QRS duration. Conditions that prolong phase 2 (amiodarone, hypocalcemia) increase the QT interval. In contrast, shortening of ventricular repolarization (phase 2), as by digitalis or hypercalcemia, abbreviates the ST segment.

The electrocardiogram is ordinarily recorded on special graph paper which is divided into 1-mm² gridlike boxes (Fig. 226-4). Since the ECG paper speed is generally 25 mm/s, the smallest (1 mm) horizontal divisions correspond to 0.04 s (40 ms), with heavier lines at intervals of 0.20 s (200 ms). Vertically, the ECG graph measures the amplitude of a given wave or deflection (1 mV = 10 mm with standard calibration; the voltage criteria for hypertrophy mentioned below are given in millimeters). There are four major ECG intervals: R-R, PR, QRS, and QT (Fig. 226-2). The heart rate (beats per minute) can be readily computed from the interbeat (R-R) interval by dividing the number of large (0.20 s) time units between consecutive R waves into 300 or the number of small (0.04 s) units into 1500. The PR interval measures the time (normally 120 to 200 ms) between atrial and ventricular depolarization, which includes the physiologic delay imposed by stimulation of cells in the AV junction area. The QRS interval (normally 100 ms or less) reflects the duration of ventricular depolarization. The QT interval includes both ventricular depolarization and repolarization times and varies inversely with the heart rate. A rate-related ("corrected") QT interval, QT_c, can be calculated as $QT/\sqrt{R\text{-}R}$ and normally is ≤ 0.44 s.

The QRS complex is subdivided into specific deflections or waves. If the initial QRS deflection in a given lead is negative, it is termed a *Q wave*; the first positive deflection is termed an *R wave*. A negative deflection after an R wave is an *S wave*. Subsequent positive or negative waves are labeled R′ and S′, respectively. Lowercase letters (qrs) are used for waves of relatively small amplitude. An entirely negative QRS complex is termed a *QS wave*.

ECG LEADS The 12 conventional ECG leads record the difference in potential between electrodes placed on the surface of the body. These leads are divided into two groups: six extremity (limb) leads and six chest (precordial) leads. The extremity leads record potentials transmitted onto the *frontal plane* (Fig. 226-5A), and the chest leads record potentials transmitted onto the *horizontal plane* (Fig. 226-5B). The six extremity leads are further subdivided into three *bipolar* leads (I, II, and III) and three *unipolar* leads (aVR, aVL, and aVF). Each bipolar lead measures the difference in potential between electrodes at two extremities: lead I = left arm−right arm voltages, lead II = left leg−right arm, and lead III = left leg−left arm. The unipolar

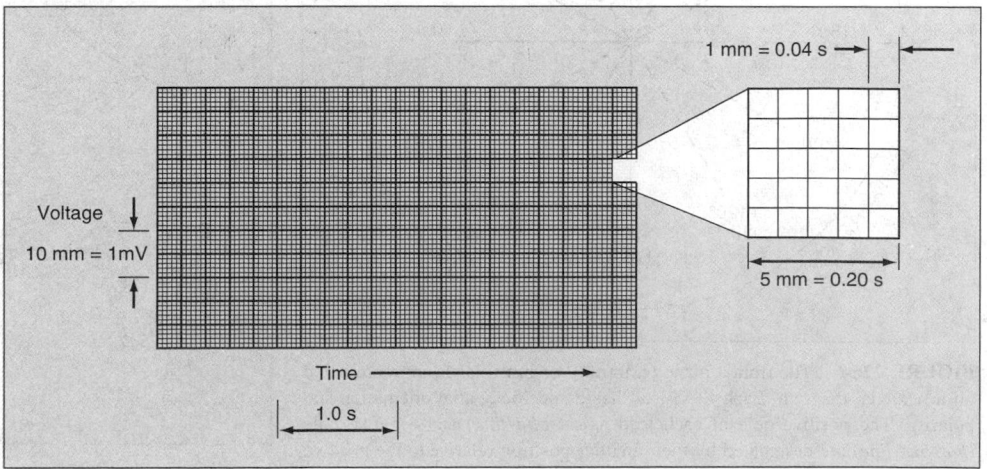

FIGURE 226-4 The ECG graph paper records the time (interval) between cardiac electrical events along the horizontal axis and their amplitude (voltage) along the vertical axis.

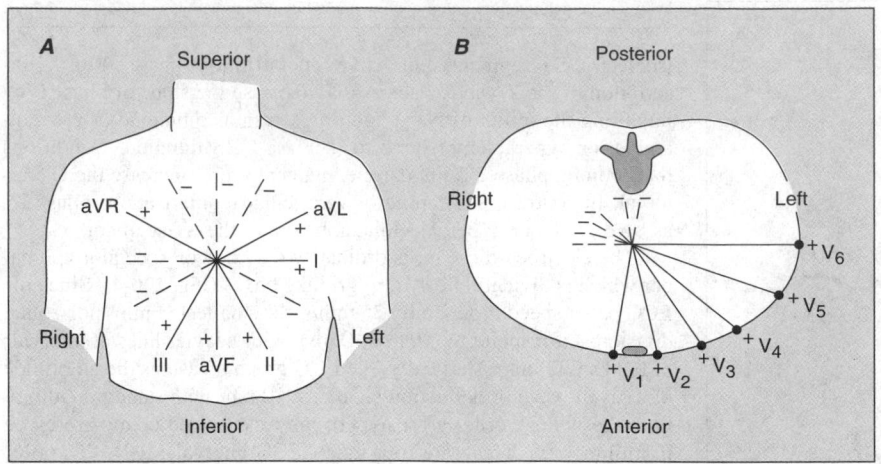

FIGURE 226-5 The six frontal plane (*A*) and six horizontal plane (*B*) leads provide a three-dimensional representation of cardiac electrical activity.

leads measure the voltage (V) at one locus relative to an electrode (called the *central terminal* or *indifferent electrode*) that has approximately zero potential. Thus, aVR = right arm, aVL = left arm, and aVF = left leg (foot). The lowercase *a* indicates that these unipolar potentials are electrically augmented by 50 percent. The right leg electrode functions as a ground. The spatial orientation and polarity of the six frontal plane leads is represented on the hexaxial diagram (Fig. 226-6).

The six chest leads (Fig. 226-7) are unipolar recordings obtained by electrodes in the following positions: lead V_1, fourth intercostal space, just to the right of the sternum; lead V_2, fourth intercostal space, just to the left of the sternum; lead V_3, midway between V_2 and V_4; lead V_4, midclavicular line, fifth intercostal space; lead V_5, anterior axillary line, same level as V_4; and lead V_6, midaxillary line, same level as V_4 and V_5.

Together, the frontal and horizontal plane electrodes provide a three-dimensional representation of cardiac electrical activity. Each

lead can be likened to a different camera angle "looking" at the same events—atrial and ventricular depolarization and repolarization—from different spatial orientations. The conventional 12-lead ECG can be supplemented with additional leads under special circumstances. For example, right precordial leads V_3R, V_4R, etc. are useful in detecting evidence of acute right ventricular ischemia. Esophageal leads may reveal atrial activity not detectable on the surface ECG. Bedside telemetry units and ambulatory ECG (Holter) recordings usually employ only one or two modified leads, respectively. →*Intracardiac electrocardiography and electrophysiologic testing are discussed in Chaps. 229 and 230.*

The ECG leads are configured so that a positive (upright) deflection is recorded in a lead if a wave of depolarization spreads toward the positive pole of that lead, and a negative deflection if the wave spreads toward the negative pole. If the mean orientation of the depolarization vector is at right angles to a given lead axis, a biphasic (equally positive and negative) deflection will be recorded.

GENESIS OF THE NORMAL ECG

P WAVE The normal atrial depolarization vector is oriented downward and toward the subject's left, reflecting the spread of depolarization from the sinus node to the right and then the left atrial myocardium. Since this vector points toward the positive pole of lead II and toward the negative pole of lead aVR, the normal P wave will be positive in lead II and negative in lead aVR. By contrast, activation of the atria from an ectopic pacemaker in the lower part of either atrium or in the AV junction region may produce retrograde P waves (negative in lead II, positive in lead aVR).

QRS COMPLEX Normal ventricular depolarization proceeds as a rapid, continuous spread of activation wavefronts. This complex process can be divided into two major, sequential phases, and each phase can be represented by a mean vector (Fig. 226-8). The first phase is depolarization of the interventricular septum from the left to the right (vector 1). The second results from the simultaneous depolarization of the main mass of the right and left ventricles; it is normally dominated by the more massive left ventricle, so that vector 2 points leftward and posteriorly. Therefore, a right precordial lead (V_1) will record this biphasic depolarization process with a small positive deflection (septal r wave) followed by a larger negative deflection (S

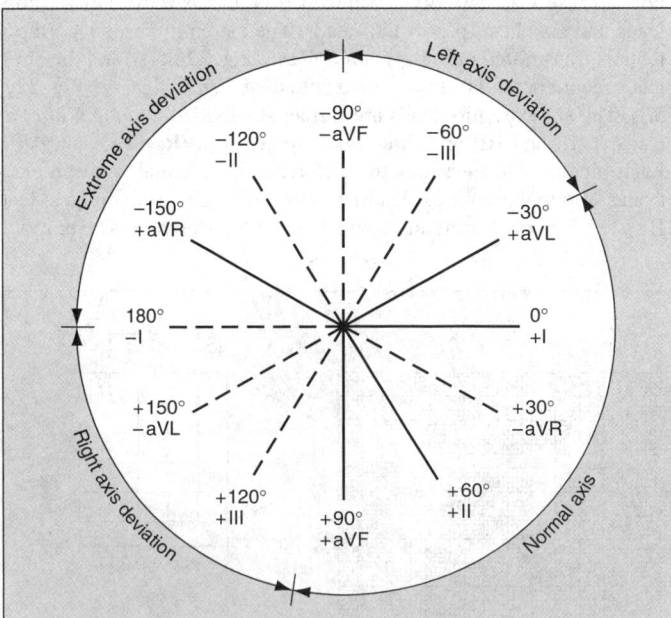

FIGURE 226-6 The frontal plane (extremity or limb) leads are represented on a hexaxial diagram. Each ECG lead has a specific spatial orientation and polarity. The positive pole of each lead axis (*solid line*) and negative pole (*hatched line*) are designated by their angular position relative to the positive pole of lead I (0°). The mean electrical axis of the QRS complex is measured with respect to this display.

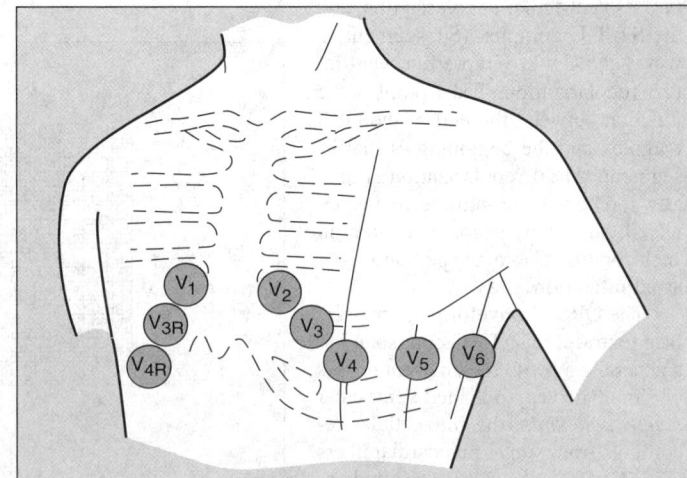

FIGURE 226-7 The horizontal plane (chest or precordial) leads are obtained with electrodes in the locations shown.

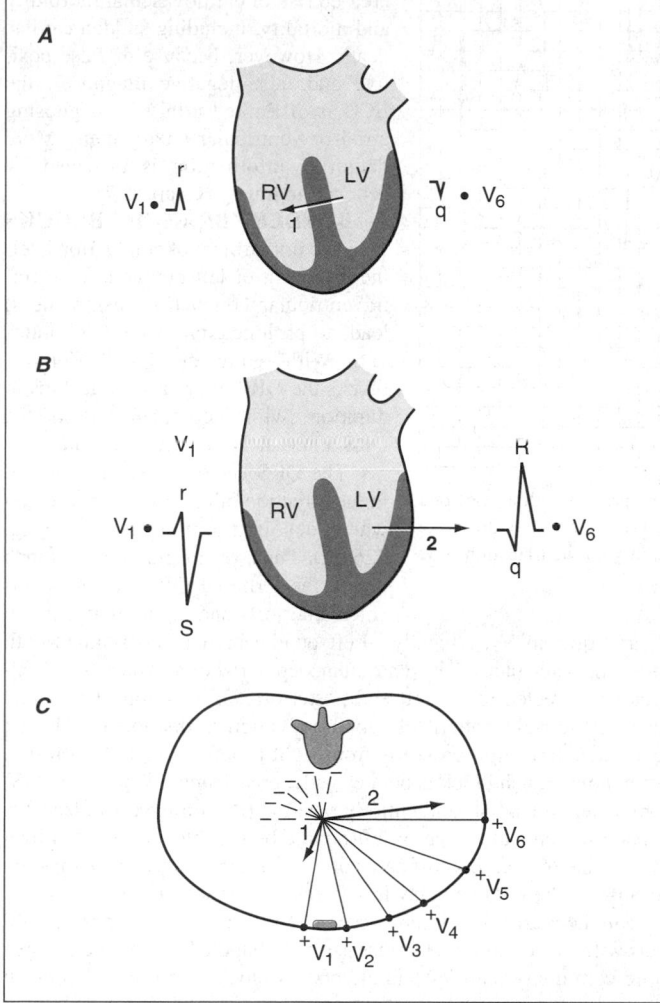

FIGURE 226-8 Ventricular depolarization can be divided into two major phases, each represented by a vector. *A.* The first phase (*arrow 1*) denotes depolarization of the ventricular septum, beginning on the left side and spreading to the right. This process is represented by a small "septal" r wave in lead V_1 and a small septal q wave in lead V_6. *B.* Simultaneous depolarization of the left and right ventricles (LV and RV) constitutes the second phase. Vector 2 is oriented to the left and posteriorly, reflecting the electrical predominance of the LV. *C.* Vectors (*arrows*) representing these two phases are shown in reference to the horizontal plane leads. (*After Goldberger, 1999.*)

wave). A left precordial lead, e.g., V_6, will record the same sequence with a small negative deflection (septal q wave) followed by a relatively tall positive deflection (R wave). Intermediate leads show a relative increase in R-wave amplitude (normal R-wave progression) and a decrease in S-wave amplitude progressing across the chest from the right to left. The precordial lead where the R and S waves are of approximately equal amplitude is referred to as the *transition zone* (usually V_3 or V_4) (Fig. 226-9).

The QRS pattern in the extremity leads may vary considerably from one normal subject to another depending on the *electrical axis* of the QRS, which describes the mean orientation of the QRS vector with reference to the six frontal plane leads. Normally, the QRS axis ranges from $-30°$ to $+100°$ (Fig. 226-6). An axis more negative than $-30°$ is referred to as *left axis deviation*, while an axis more positive than $+100°$ is referred to as *right axis deviation*. Left axis deviation may occur as a normal variant but is more commonly associated with left ventricular hypertrophy, a block in the anterior fascicle of the left bundle system (left anterior fascicular block or hemiblock), or inferior myocardial infarction. Right axis deviation also may occur as a normal variant (particularly in children and young adults), as a spurious find-

ing due to reversal of the left and right arm electrodes, or in conditions such as right ventricular overload (acute or chronic), infarction of the lateral wall of the left ventricle, dextrocardia, left pneumothorax, or left posterior fascicular block.

T WAVE AND U WAVE Normally, the mean T-wave vector is oriented roughly concordant with the mean QRS vector. Since depolarization and repolarization are electrically opposite processes, this normal QRS–T-wave vector concordance indicates that repolarization must normally proceed in the reverse direction from depolarization (i.e., from ventricular epicardium to endocardium). The normal U wave is a small, rounded deflection (≤ 1 mm) that follows the T wave and usually has the same polarity as the T wave. An abnormal increase in U-wave amplitude is most commonly due to drugs (e.g., quinidine, procainamide, disopyramide) or hypokalemia. Very prominent U waves are a marker of increased susceptibility to the *torsades de pointes* type of ventricular tachycardia (Chap. 230). Inversion of the U wave in the precordial leads is abnormal and may be a subtle sign of ischemia.

MAJOR ECG ABNORMALITIES

CARDIAC ENLARGEMENT AND HYPERTROPHY
Right atrial overload (acute or chronic) may lead to an increase in P-wave amplitude (≥ 2.5 mm) (Fig. 226-10). Left atrial overload typically produces a biphasic P wave in V_1 with a broad negative component or a broad (≥ 120 ms), often notched P wave in one or more limb leads (Fig. 226-10). This pattern also may occur with left atrial conduction delays in the absence of actual atrial enlargement, leading to the more general designation of *left atrial abnormality*.

Right ventricular hypertrophy due to a pressure load (as from pulmonic valve stenosis or pulmonary artery hypertension) is characterized by a relatively tall R wave in lead V_1 ($R \geq S$ wave), usually with right axis deviation (Fig. 226-11); alternatively, there may be a qR pattern in V_1 or V_3R. ST depression and T-wave inversion in the right to midprecordial leads are also often present. This so-called ventricular strain pattern is attributed to repolarization abnormalities in hypertrophied muscle. Right ventricular hypertrophy due to ostium secundum–type atrial septal defects, with the accompanying right ventricular volume overload, is commonly associated with an incomplete or complete right bundle branch block pattern with a rightward QRS axis.

Acute cor pulmonale due to pulmonary embolism (Chap. 261) for example, may be associated with a normal ECG or a variety of abnormalities. Sinus tachycardia is the most common arrhythmia, although other tachyarrhythmias, such as atrial fibrillation or flutter, may occur. The QRS axis may shift to the right, sometimes in concert with the so-called $S_1Q_3T_3$ pattern (prominence of the S wave in lead I, Q wave in lead III, with T-wave inversion in lead III). Acute right ventricular dilation also may be associated with poor R-wave progression and T-wave inversions in V_1 to V_4 (right ventricular "strain") simulating acute anterior infarction. A right ventricular conduction disturbance may appear.

Chronic cor pulmonale due to obstructive lung disease (Chap. 237) usually does not produce the classic ECG patterns of right ventricular hypertrophy noted above. Instead of tall right precordial R waves, chronic lung disease more typically is associated with small R waves in right to midprecordial leads (poor R-wave progression) due in part to downward displacement of the diaphragm and the heart. Low-voltage complexes are commonly present, owing to hyperaeration of the lungs.

A number of different voltage criteria for *left ventricular hypertrophy* (Fig. 226-11) have been proposed on the basis of the presence of tall left precordial R waves and deep right precordial S waves [e.g., $SV_1 + (RV_5$ or $RV_6) \geq 35$ mm; or $(RV_5$ or $RV_6) \geq 25$ mm]. Repolarization abnormalities (ST depression with T-wave inversions) also may appear (left ventricular "strain" pattern) in leads with prominent

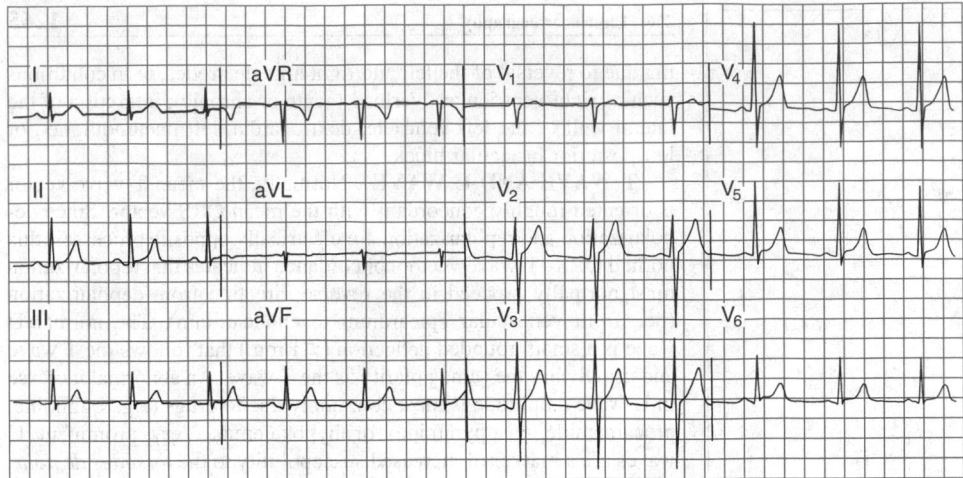

FIGURE 226-9 Normal electrocardiogram from a healthy subject. Sinus rhythm is present with a heart rate of 75 beats per minute. PR interval is 0.16 s; QRS interval (duration) is 0.08 s; QT interval is 0.36 s; the mean QRS axis is about +70°. The precordial leads show normal R-wave progression with the transition zone (R wave = S wave) in lead V_3.

R waves. However, prominent precordial voltages may occur as a normal variant, especially in athletic or thin-chested individuals. Left ventricular hypertrophy may increase limb lead voltage (e.g., RaVL ≥ 11 to 13 mm, RaVF ≥ 20 mm; $R_1 + S_{III} ≥ 25$ mm) with or without increased precordial voltage. The presence of left atrial abnormality increases the likelihood of underlying left ventricular hypertrophy in cases with borderline voltage criteria. Left ventricular hypertrophy often progresses to incomplete or complete left bundle branch block. The sensitivity of conventional voltage criteria for left ventricular hypertrophy is decreased in obese persons and in women. ECG evidence for left ventricular hypertrophy is a major noninvasive marker of in-

creased risk of cardiovascular morbidity and mortality, including sudden cardiac death. However, because of false-positive and false-negative diagnoses, the ECG is of limited utility in diagnosing atrial or ventricular enlargement. More definitive information is provided by echocardiography (Chap. 227).

BUNDLE BRANCH BLOCKS
Intrinsic impairment of conduction in either the right or left bundle system (intraventricular conduction disturbances) leads to prolongation of the QRS interval. With complete bundle branch blocks the QRS interval is ≥ 120 ms in duration; with incomplete blocks the QRS interval is between 100 and 120 ms. The QRS vector is usually oriented in the direction of the myocardial region where depolarization is delayed (Fig. 226-12). Thus, with right bundle branch block, the terminal QRS vector is oriented anteriorly and to the right (rSR′ in V_1 and qRS in V_6, typically). Left bundle branch block alters both early and later phases of ventricular depolarization. The major QRS vector is directed to the left and posteriorly. In addition, the normal early left-to-right pattern of septal activation is disrupted such that septal depolarization proceeds from right to left as well. As a result, left bundle branch block generates wide, predominantly negative (QS) complexes in lead V_1 and entirely positive (R) complexes in lead V_6. A pattern identical to that of left bundle branch block, preceded by a sharp spike, is seen in most cases of electronic right ventricular pacing because of the relative delay in left ventricular activation.

Bundle branch block may occur in a variety of conditions. In subjects without structural heart disease, right bundle branch block is seen more commonly than left bundle branch block. Right bundle branch block also occurs with heart disease, both congenital (e.g., atrial septal defect) and acquired (e.g., valvular, ischemic). Left bundle branch block is often a marker of one of four underlying conditions: ischemic heart disease, long-standing hypertension, severe aortic valve disease, and cardiomyopathy. Bundle branch blocks may be chronic or intermittent. A bundle branch block may be rate-related; for example, often it occurs when the heart rate exceeds some critical value.

Bundle branch blocks and depolarization abnormalities secondary to artificial pacemakers not only affect ventricular depolarization (QRS) but are also characteristically associated with *secondary repolarization* (ST-T) abnormalities. With bundle branch blocks, the T-wave is typically opposite in polarity to the last deflection of the QRS (Fig. 226-12). This discordance of the QRS–T-wave vectors is caused by the altered sequence of repolarization that occurs secondary to altered depolarization. In contrast, *primary repolarization* abnormalities are independent of QRS changes and are related instead to actual alterations in the electrical properties of the myocardial fibers themselves (for example, in the resting membrane potential or action potential duration), not just to changes in the sequence of repolarization. Ischemia, electrolyte imbalance, and drugs such as digitalis all cause such primary ST–T-wave changes. Primary and secondary T-wave changes may coexist. For example, T-wave inversions in the right precordial leads with left bundle branch block or in the left precordial leads with right bundle branch block may be important markers of underlying ischemia or other abnormalities.

Partial blocks ("hemiblocks") in the left bundle system (left anterior or posterior fascicular blocks) generally do not prolong the QRS duration substantially but instead are associated with shifts in the frontal plane QRS axis (leftward or rightward, respectively). More complex combinations of fascicular and bundle branch blocks may occur involving the left and right bundle system. Examples of *bifascicular block* include right bundle branch block and left posterior fascicular

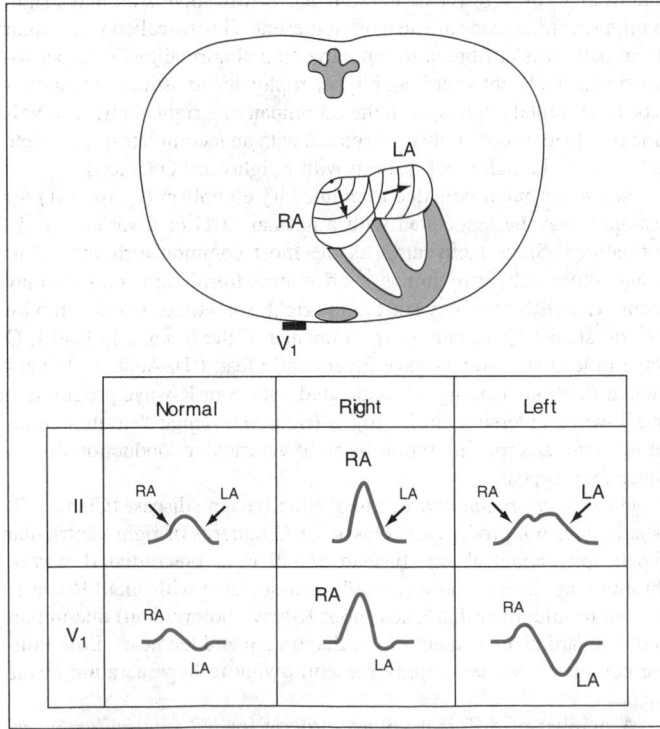

FIGURE 226-10 Right atrial (RA) overload may cause tall, peaked P waves in the limb or precordial leads. Left atrial (LA) abnormality may cause broad, often notched P waves in the limb leads and a biphasic P wave in lead V_1 with a prominent negative component representing delayed depolarization of the LA. *(After MK Park, WG Guntheroth: How to Read Pediatric ECGs, 2d ed. St. Louis, Mosby–Year Book, 1987.)*

block, right bundle branch block with left anterior fascicular block, and complete left bundle branch block. Chronic bifascicular block in an asymptomatic individual is associated with a relatively low risk of progression to high-degree AV heart block. In contrast, new bifascicular block with acute anterior myocardial infarction carries a much greater risk of complete heart block. Alternation of right and left bundle branch block is a sign of *trifascicular disease*. However, the presence of a prolonged PR interval and bifascicular block does not necessarily indicate trifascicular involvement, since this combination may arise with AV node disease and bifascicular block. Intraventricular conduction delays also can be caused by extrinsic (toxic) factors that slow ventricular conduction, particularly hyperkalemia or drugs (type 1 antiarrhythmic agents, tricyclic antidepressants, phenothiazines).

Prolongation of QRS duration does not necessarily indicate a conduction delay but may be due to *preexcitation* of the ventricles via a bypass tract, as in the Wolff-Parkinson-White (WPW) syndrome (Chap. 230) and related variants. The diagnostic triad of WPW consists of a wide QRS complex associated with a relatively short PR interval and slurring of the initial part of the QRS (delta wave), the latter effect due to aberrant activation of ventricular myocardium. The presence of a bypass tract predisposes to reentrant supraventricular tachyarrhythmias (Chap. 230).

MYOCARDIAL ISCHEMIA AND INFARCTION (See also Chap. 243)   The ECG is a cornerstone in the diagnosis of acute and chronic ischemic heart disease. The findings depend on several key factors: the nature of the process [reversible (i.e., ischemia) versus irreversible (i.e., infarction)], the duration (acute versus chronic), extent (transmural versus subendocardial), and localization (anterior versus inferoposterior), as well as the presence of other underlying abnormalities (ventricular hypertrophy, conduction defects).

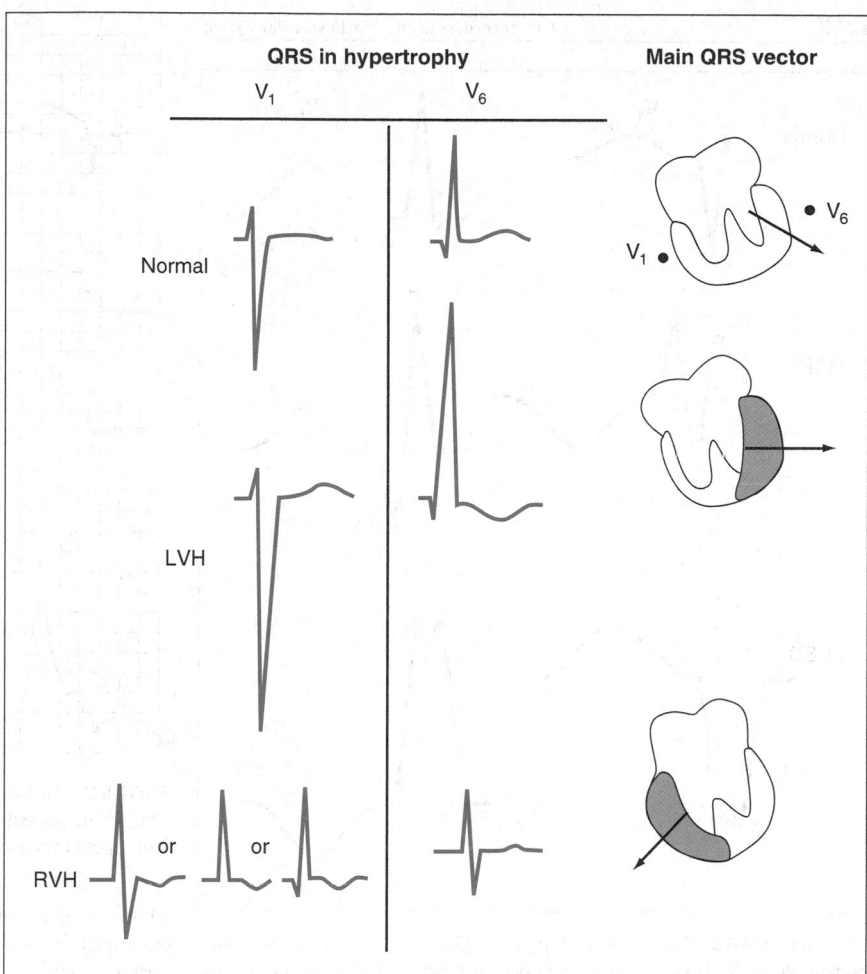

FIGURE 226-11   Left ventricular hypertrophy (LVH) increases the amplitude of electrical forces directed to the left and posteriorly. In addition, repolarization abnormalities may cause ST-segment depression and T-wave inversion in leads with a prominent R wave ("strain" pattern). Right ventricular hypertrophy (RVH) may shift the QRS vector to the right; this effect usually is associated with an R, RS, or qR complex in lead V_1. T-wave inversions may be present in right precordial leads ("strain" pattern).

Ischemia exerts complex time-dependent effects on the electrical properties of myocardial cells. Severe, acute ischemia lowers the resting membrane potential and shortens the duration of the action potential. Such changes cause a voltage gradient between normal and ischemic zones. As a consequence, current flows between these regions. These so-called currents of injury are represented on the surface ECG by deviation of the ST segment (Fig. 226-13). When the acute ischemia is *transmural*, the ST vector is usually shifted in the direction of the outer (epicardial) layers, producing ST elevations and sometimes, in the earliest stages of ischemia, tall, positive so-called hyperacute T waves over the ischemic zone. With ischemia confined primarily to the *subendocardium*, the ST vector typically shifts toward the subendocardium and ventricular cavity, so that overlying (e.g., anterior precordial) leads show ST-segment depression (with ST elevation in lead aVR). Multiple factors affect the amplitude of acute ischemic ST deviations. Profound ST elevation or depression in multiple leads usually indicates very severe ischemia. From a clinical viewpoint, the division of acute myocardial infarction into ST segment elevation and non-ST elevation (NSTEMI) types is useful since the efficacy of acute reperfusion therapy is limited to the former group (Chap. 243).

The ECG leads are more helpful in localizing regions of ST elevation than non-ST elevation ischemia. For example, acute transmural anterior wall ischemia is reflected by ST elevations or increased T-wave positivity (Fig. 226-14) in one or more of the precordial leads (V_1 to V_6) and leads I and aVL. Anteroseptal ischemia produces these changes in leads V_1 to V_3, apical or lateral ischemia in leads V_4 to V_6. Transmural inferior wall ischemia produces changes in leads II, III, and aVF. Posterior wall ischemia may be indirectly recognized by *reciprocal* ST depressions in leads V_1 to V_3. Prominent reciprocal ST depressions in these leads also occur with certain inferior wall infarcts, particularly those with posterior or lateral wall extension. Right ventricular ischemia usually produces ST elevations in right-sided chest leads (Fig. 226-7). When ischemic ST elevations occur as the earliest sign of acute infarction, they are typically followed within a period ranging from hours to days by evolving T-wave inversions and often by Q waves occurring in the same lead distribution. (T-wave inversions due to evolving or chronic ischemia correlate with prolongation of repolarization and are often associated with QT lengthening.) Reversible transmural ischemia, for example, due to coronary vasospasm (Prinzmetal's variant angina), may cause transient ST-segment elevations without development of Q waves. Depending on the severity and duration of such ischemia, the ST elevations may either resolve completely in minutes or be followed by T-wave inversions that persist for hours or even days. Patients with ischemic chest pain who present with deep T-wave inversions in multiple precordial leads (e.g., V_1 to V_4) with or without cardiac enzyme elevations typically have severe obstruction in the left anterior descending coronary artery system (Fig. 226-15). In contrast, patients whose baseline ECG already shows abnormal T-wave inversions may develop T-wave normalization (pseudonormalization) during episodes of acute transmural ischemia.

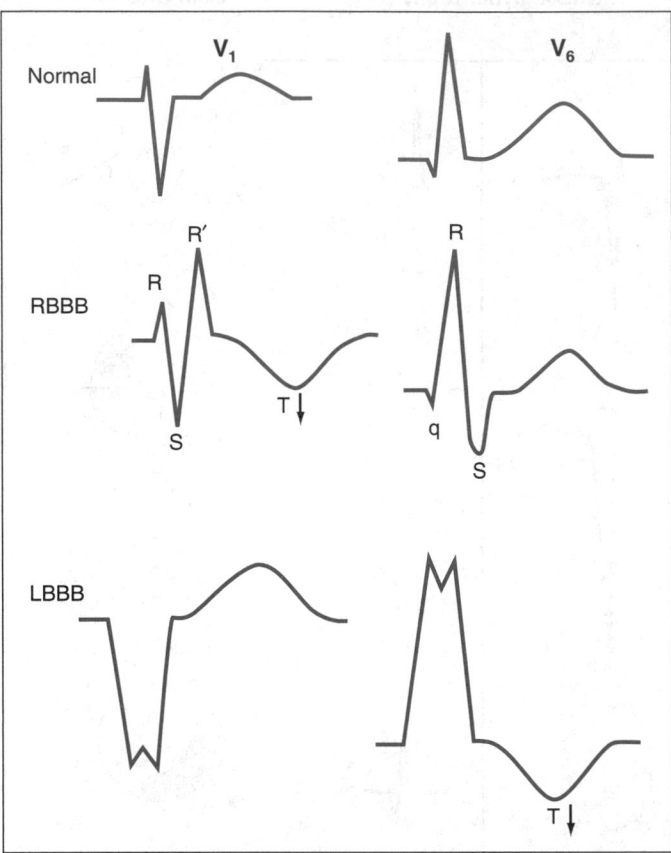

FIGURE 226-12   Comparison of typical QRS-T patterns in right bundle branch block (RBBB) and left bundle branch block (LBBB) with the normal pattern in leads V_1 and V_6. Note the secondary T-wave inversions (*arrows*) in leads with an rSR′ complex with RBBB and in leads with a wide R wave with LBBB.

With infarction, depolarization (QRS) changes often accompany repolarization (ST-T) abnormalities. Necrosis of sufficient myocardial tissue may lead to decreased R-wave amplitude or frank abnormal Q waves in the anterior or inferior leads (Fig. 226-16). Previously, abnormal Q waves were considered to be markers of transmural myocardial infarction, while subendocardial infarcts were thought not to produce Q waves. However, careful ECG-pathology correlative studies have indicated that transmural infarcts may occur without Q waves and that subendocardial (nontransmural) infarcts may sometimes be associated with Q waves. Therefore, infarcts are more appropriately classified as "Q-wave" or "non-Q-wave." The major acute ECG

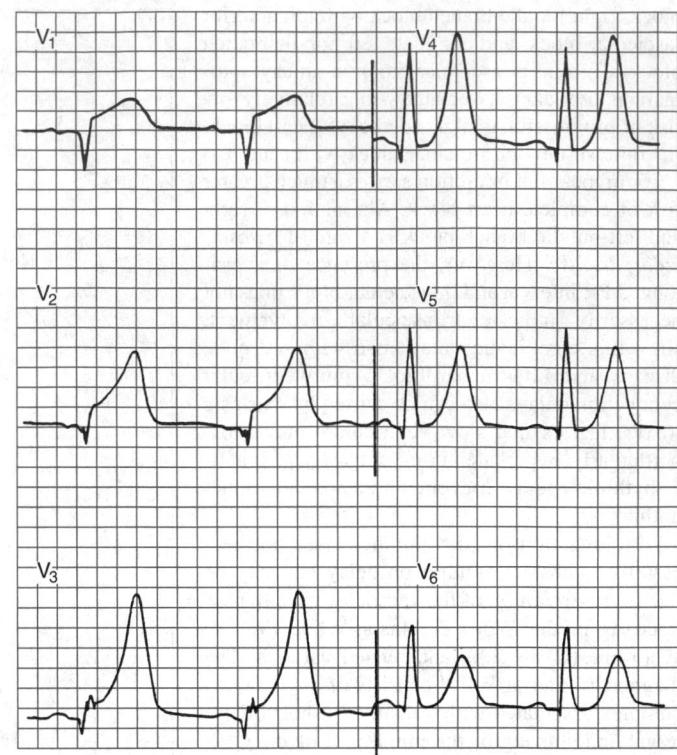

FIGURE 226-14   Hyperacute phase of anteroseptal myocardial infarction (MI). Note the tall positive T waves (V_2 to V_3) along with ST-segment elevations and Q waves (V_1 to V_3).

changes in syndromes of ischemic heart disease are schematically summarized in Fig. 226-17. Loss of depolarization forces due to posterior or lateral infarction may cause reciprocal increases in R-wave amplitude in leads V_1 and V_2 without diagnostic Q waves in any of the conventional leads. Atrial infarction may be associated with PR-segment deviations due to an atrial current of injury, changes in P-wave morphology, or atrial arrhythmias. In the weeks and months following infarction, these ECG changes may persist or begin to resolve. Complete normalization of the ECG following Q-wave infarction is uncommon but may occur, particularly with smaller infarcts. In contrast, ST-segment elevations that persist for several weeks or more after a Q-wave infarct usually correlate with a severe underlying wall motion disorder (akinetic or dyskinetic zone), although not necessarily a frank ventricular aneurysm.

ECG changes due to ischemia may occur spontaneously or may be provoked by various exercise protocols (stress electrocardiography) (Chap. 244). In patients with severe ischemic heart disease, exercise testing is most likely to elicit signs of subendocardial ischemia (horizontal or downsloping ST depression in multiple leads). ST-segment elevation during exercise is most often observed after a Q-wave infarct. This repolarization change does not necessarily indicate active ischemia but correlates strongly with the presence of an underlying ventricular wall motion abnormality. However, in patients *without* prior infarction, transient ST-segment elevation with exercise is a reliable sign of transmural ischemia.

The ECG has important limitations in both sensitivity and specificity in the diagnosis of ischemic heart disease. Although a single normal ECG does not exclude ischemia or even acute infarc-

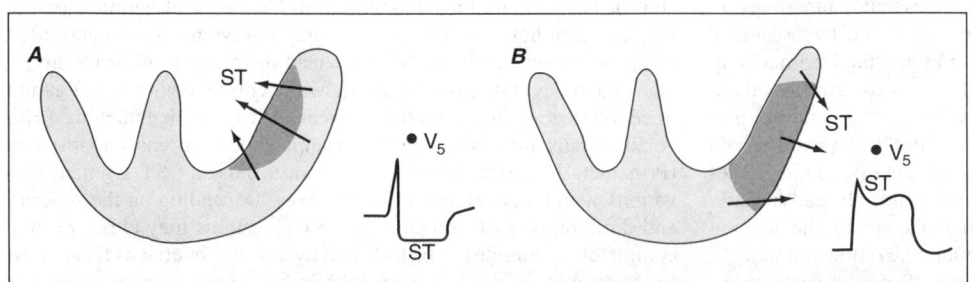

FIGURE 226-13   Acute ischemia causes a current of injury. With predominant subendocardial ischemia (*A*), the resultant ST vector will be directed toward the inner layer of the affected ventricle and the ventricular cavity. Overlying leads therefore will record ST depression. With ischemia involving the outer ventricular layer (*B*) (transmural or epicardial injury), the ST vector will be directed outward. Overlying leads will record ST elevation.

tion, a normal ECG *throughout* the course of an acute infarct is distinctly uncommon. Prolonged chest pain without diagnostic ECG changes, therefore, should always prompt a careful search for other noncoronary causes of chest pain (Chap. 13). Furthermore, the diagnostic changes of acute or evolving ischemia are often masked by the presence of left bundle branch block, electronic ventricular pacemaker patterns, and WPW preexcitation. On the other hand, clinicians may overdiagnose ischemia or infarction based on the presence of ST-segment elevations or depressions, T-wave inversions, tall positive T waves, or Q waves *not* related to ischemic heart disease (pseudoinfarct patterns). For example, ST-segment elevations simulating ischemia may occur with acute pericarditis (Fig. 226-18) or myocarditis, or as a normal variant ("early repolarization" pattern). Similarly, tall, positive T waves do not invariably represent hyperacute ischemic changes but also may be caused by normal variants, hyperkalemia, cerebrovascular injury, and left ventricular volume overload due to mitral or aortic regurgitation, among other causes. ST-segment elevations and tall, positive T waves are common findings in leads V_1 and V_2 in left bundle branch block or left ventricular hypertrophy in the absence of ischemia. The differential diagnosis of Q waves (Table 226-1) includes physiologic or positional variants, ventricular hypertrophy, acute or chronic noncoronary myocardial injury, hypertrophic cardiomyopathy, and ventricular conduction disorders. Digitalis, ventricular hypertrophy, hypokalemia, and a variety of other factors may cause ST-segment depression mimicking subendocardial ischemia. Prominent T-wave inversion may occur with ventricular hypertrophy, cardiomyopathy, myocarditis, and cerebrovascular injury (particularly intracranial bleeds; Fig. 226-19), among many other conditions.

METABOLIC FACTORS AND DRUG EFFECTS A variety of metabolic and pharmacologic agents alter the ECG and, in par-

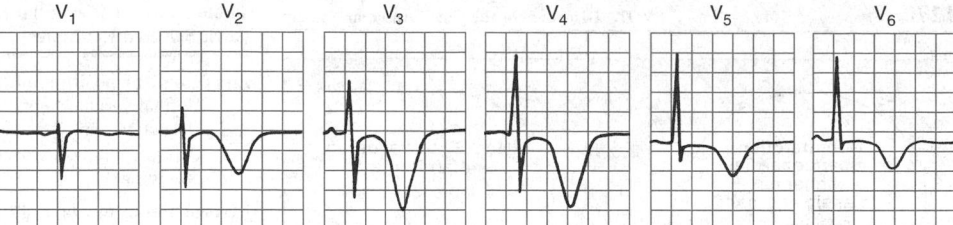

FIGURE 226-15 Severe anterior wall ischemia (with or without infarction) may cause prominent T-wave inversions in the precordial leads. This pattern is usually associated with a high-grade stenosis of the left anterior descending coronary artery.

ticular, cause changes in repolarization (ST-T-U) and sometimes QRS prolongation. Certain life-threatening electrolyte disturbances may be diagnosed initially and monitored from the ECG. *Hyperkalemia* produces a sequence of changes usually beginning with narrowing and peaking (tenting) of the T waves. Further elevation of extracellular K^+ leads to AV conduction disturbances, diminution in P-wave amplitude, and widening of the QRS interval. Severe hyperkalemia eventually causes cardiac arrest with a slow sinusoidal type of mechanism ("sine-wave" pattern) followed by asystole. *Hypokalemia* (Fig. 226-19) prolongs ventricular repolarization, often with prominent U waves. Prolongation of the QT interval (Fig. 226-19) is also seen with drugs that increase the duration of the ventricular action potential—type 1A antiarrhythmic agents and related drugs (e.g., quinidine, disopyramide, procainamide, tricyclic antidepressants, phenothiazines) and type III agents (amiodarone, sotalol). Marked QT prolongation, sometimes with deep, wide T-wave inversions, may occur with intracranial bleeds, particularly subarachnoid hemorrhage ("CVA T-wave" pattern) (Fig. 226-19). Systemic *hypothermia* (Fig. 226-19) also prolongs repolarization, usually with a distinctive convex elevation of the J point (Osborn wave). *Hypocalcemia* typically prolongs the QT interval (ST portion), while *hypercalcemia* shortens it (Fig. 226-20). Digitalis glycosides also shorten the QT interval, often with a characteristic "scooping" of the ST–T-wave complex (*digitalis effect*).

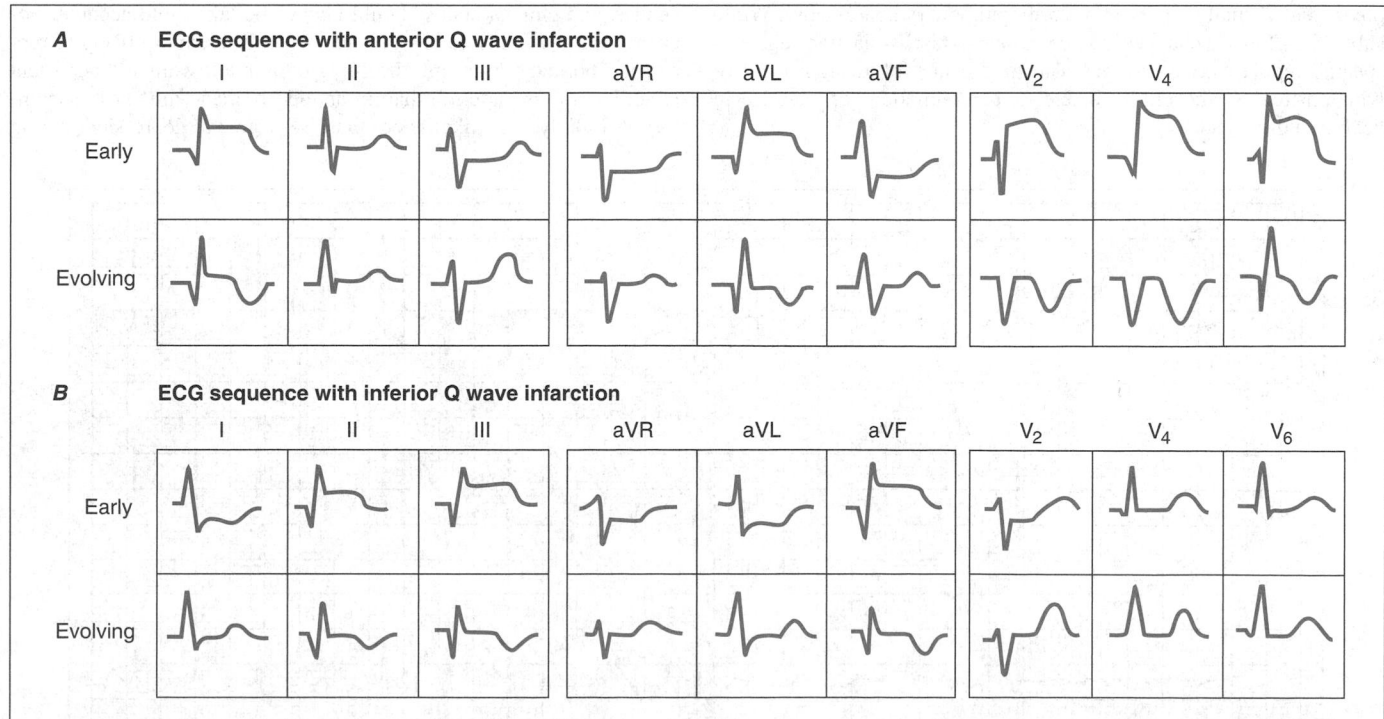

FIGURE 226-16 Sequence of depolarization and repolarization changes with (*A*) acute anterior and (*B*) acute inferior wall Q-wave infarctions. With anterior infarcts, ST elevation in leads I, aVL, and the precordial leads may be accompanied by reciprocal ST depressions in leads II, III, and aVF. Conversely, acute inferior (or posterior) infarcts may be associated with reciprocal ST depressions in leads V_1 to V_3. (*After Goldberger, 1999.*)

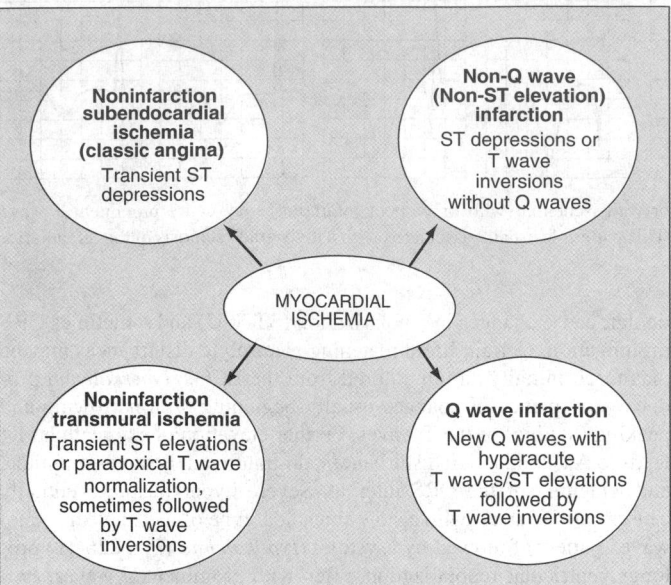

FIGURE 226-17 Variability of ECG patterns with acute myocardial ischemia. The ECG also may be normal or nonspecifically abnormal. Furthermore, these categorizations are not mutually exclusive. For example, a non-ST elevation infarct may evolve into a Q-wave infarct; ST elevations may be followed by a non-Q-wave infarct; or ST depressions and T-wave inversions may be followed by a Q-wave infarct. *(After Goldberger, 1991.)*

Many other factors are associated with ECG changes, particularly alterations in ventricular repolarization. T-wave flattening, minimal T-wave inversions or slight ST-segment depression ("nonspecific ST–T-wave changes") may occur with a variety of electrolyte and acid-base disturbances, a variety of infectious processes, central nervous system disorders, endocrine abnormalities, many drugs, ischemia, hypoxia, and virtually any type of cardiopulmonary abnormality. While subtle ST–T-wave changes may be markers of ischemia, transient nonspecific repolarization changes also may occur following a meal or with postural (orthostatic) change, hyperventilation, or exercise in healthy individuals.

Table 226-1 Differential Diagnosis of Q Waves (with Selected Examples)

Physiologic or positional factors
1. Normal variant "septal" q waves
2. Normal variant Q waves in V_1 to V_2, aVL, III, and aVF
3. Left pneumothorax or dextrocardia: loss of lateral R-wave progression

Myocardial injury or infiltration
1. Acute processes: myocardial ischemia or infarction, myocarditis, hyperkalemia
2. Chronic processes: myocardial infarction, idiopathic cardiomyopathy, myocarditis, amyloid, tumor, sarcoid, scleroderma, Chagas' disease, echinococcus cyst

Ventricular hypertrophy/enlargement
1. Left ventricular (poor R-wave progression[a])
2. Right ventricular (reversed R-wave progression[b] or poor R-wave progression, particularly with chronic obstructive lung disease)
3. Hypertrophic cardiomyopathy (may simulate anterior, inferior, posterior, or lateral infarcts)

Conduction abnormalities
1. Left bundle branch block (poor R-wave progression[b])
2. Wolff-Parkinson-White patterns

---

[a] Small or absent R waves in the right to midprecordial leads.
[b] Progressive decrease in R-wave amplitude from V_1 to the mid- or lateral precordial leads.
SOURCE: After Goldberger, 1991.

ELECTRICAL ALTERNANS Electrical alternans—a beat-to-beat alternation in one or more components of the ECG signal—is a common type of nonlinear cardiovascular response to a variety of perturbations. For example, total electrical alternans (P-QRS-T) with sinus tachycardia is a relatively specific sign of pericardial effusion, often with cardiac tamponade. The mechanism relates to a periodic swinging motion of the heart in the effusion at a frequency exactly one-half the heart rate. ST-T alternans is a sign of electrical instability and may precede ventricular fibrillation.

CLINICAL INTERPRETATION OF THE ECG Accurate analysis of ECGs requires thoroughness and care. The patient's age, gender, and clinical status should always be taken into account. For example, T-wave inversions in leads V_1 to V_3 are more likely to represent a normal variant in a healthy young adult woman ("persistent juvenile T-wave pattern") than in an elderly man with chest discomfort. Similarly, the likelihood that ST-segment depression during

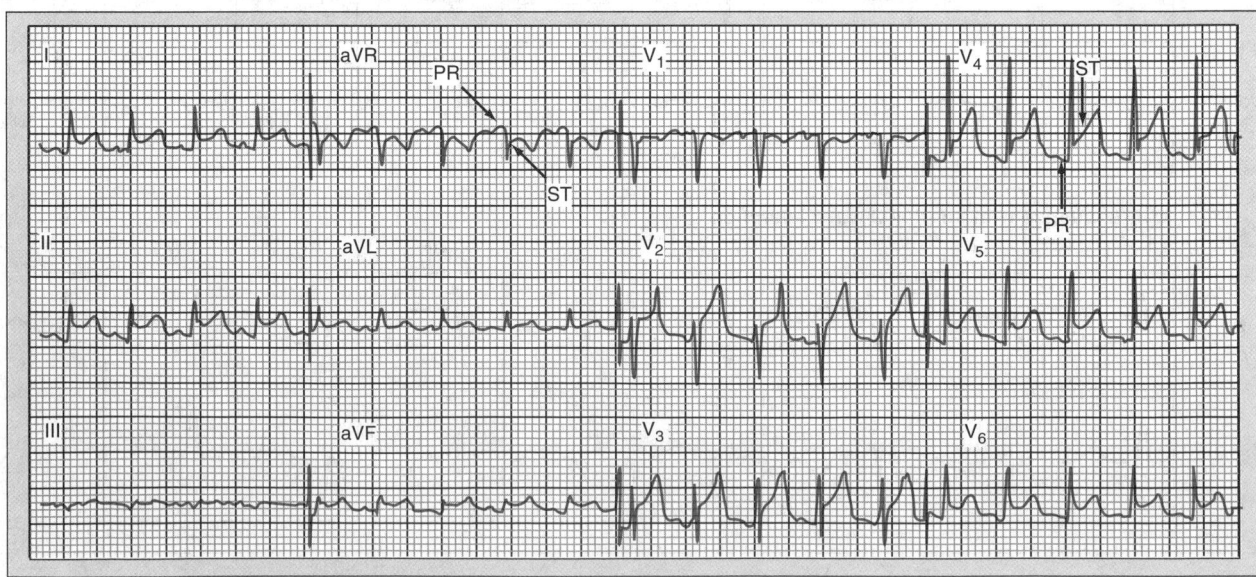

FIGURE 226-18 Acute pericarditis often produces diffuse ST-segment elevations (in this case in leads I, II, aVF, and V_2 to V_6) due to a ventricular current of injury. Note also the characteristic PR-segment deviation (opposite in polarity to the ST segment) due to a concomitant atrial injury current.

exercise testing represents ischemia depends partly on the prior probability of coronary artery disease.

Many mistakes in ECG interpretation are errors of omission. Therefore, a systematic approach is desirable. The following 14 points should be analyzed carefully in every ECG: (1) standardization (calibration) and technical features (including lead placement and artifacts); (2) heart rate; (3) rhythm; (4) PR interval; (5) QRS interval; (6) QT interval; (7) P waves; (8) QRS voltages; (9) mean QRS electrical axis; (10) precordial R-wave progression; (11) abnormal Q waves; (12) ST segments; (13) T waves; (14) U waves.

Only after analyzing all these points should the interpretation be formulated. Where appropriate, important clinical correlates or inferences should be mentioned. For example, prolonged ventricular repolarization with prominent U waves should suggest hypokalemia or drug toxicity (e.g., due to quinidine or procainamide) (Fig. 226-19). The combination of left atrial abnormality (enlargement) and signs of right ventricular hypertrophy suggests mitral stenosis. Low voltage with sinus tachycardia raises the possibility of pericardial tamponade or chronic obstructive lung disease. Sinus tachycardia with QRS and QT (U) prolongation suggests tricyclic antidepressant overdose (Fig. 226-19). Comparison with previous ECGs is essential. →*The diagnosis and management of specific cardiac arrhythmias and conduction disturbances are discussed in Chaps. 229 and 230.*

COMPUTERIZED ELECTROCARDIOGRAPHY   Computerized ECG systems are increasingly used. Digital systems provide for convenient storage and immediate retrieval of thousands of ECG records. In recent years, computer programs for ECG analysis have become more reliable. However, despite these advances, computer interpretation of ECGs has important limitations. Incomplete or inaccurate readings are most likely with arrhythmias and complex abnormalities. Therefore, computerized interpretation (including measurements of basic ECG intervals) should not be accepted without careful physician review.

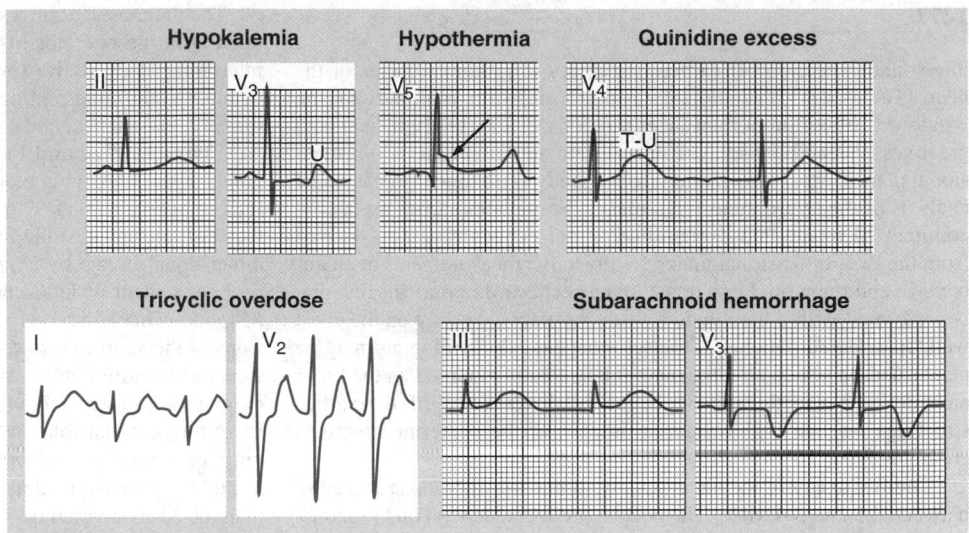

FIGURE 226-19   A variety of metabolic derangements, drug effects, and other factors may prolong ventricular repolarization with QT prolongation or prominent U waves. Repolarization prolongation, particularly if due to hypokalemia or pharmacologic agents, indicates increased susceptibility to torsades de pointes type ventricular tachycardia. Hypothermia is associated with a distinctive convex "hump" at the J point (Osborn wave, *arrow*). Note QRS and QT prolongation along with sinus tachycardia in the case of tricyclic antidepressant overdose.

BIBLIOGRAPHY

BRADY WJ et al: Electrocardiographic manifestations: Patterns that confound the EKG diagnosis of acute myocardial infarction—left bundle branch block, ventricular paced rhythm, and left ventricular hypertrophy. J Emerg Med 18:71, 2000

GOLDBERGER AL: *Myocardial Infarction: Electrocardiographic Differential Diagnosis*, 4th ed. St. Louis, Mosby–Year Book, 1991

GOLDBERGER AL: *Clinical Electrocardiography: A Simplified Approach*, 6th ed. St. Louis, Mosby, 1999

MIRVIS DM: *Electrocardiography: A Physiologic Approach.* St. Louis, Mosby–Year Book, 1993

MIRVIS DM, GOLDBERGER AL: Electrocardiography, in *Heart Disease: A Textbook of Cardiovascular Medicine*, 6th ed, E Braunwald, DP Zipes, P Libby (eds). Philadelphia, Saunders, 2001

227

Rick A. Nishimura, Raymond J. Gibbons, A. Jamil Tajik

NONINVASIVE CARDIAC IMAGING: ECHOCARDIOGRAPHY AND NUCLEAR CARDIOLOGY

Cardiovascular imaging has significantly enhanced the practice of cardiology over the past few decades. Two-dimensional echocardiography is able to visualize the heart directly in real time using ultrasound, providing instantaneous assessment of the myocardium, valves, pericardium, and great vessels. Doppler echocardiography measures the velocity of moving red blood cells and has become a noninvasive alternative to cardiac catheterization for assessment of hemodynamics. Transesophageal echocardiography has provided a new window for high-resolution imaging of posterior structures of the heart, particularly the left atrium, mitral valve, and aorta. Nuclear cardiology uses isotopes to assess myocardial perfusion and function and has contributed greatly to the evaluation of patients with ischemic heart disease. This chapter provides an overview of the basic concepts of both echocardiography and nuclear cardiology and the clinical indications for each procedure.

ECHOCARDIOGRAPHY

TWO-DIMENSIONAL ECHOCARDIOGRAPHY   Basic Principles   Two-dimensional echocardiography uses the principle of

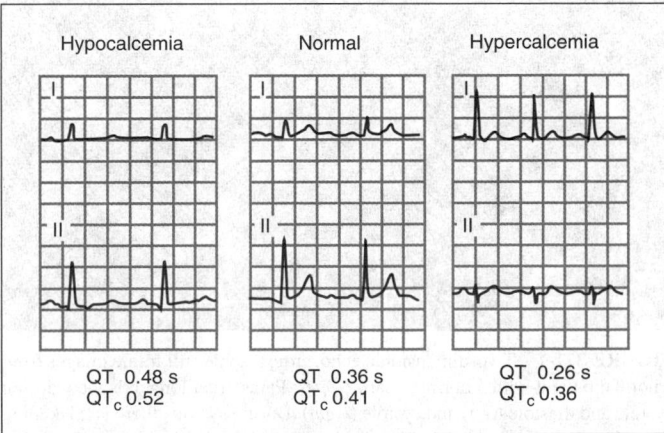

FIGURE 226-20   Prolongation of the Q-T interval (ST-segment portion) is typical of hypocalcemia. Hypercalcemia may cause abbreviation of the ST segment and shortening of the QT interval.

ultrasound reflection off cardiac structures to produce images of the heart (Table 227-1). The imaging is performed from multiple acoustic windows with different transducer rotations so that the entire heart and great vessels can be displayed in real time and in various two-dimensional planes. Most information from a study is obtained from a visual analysis of the two-dimensional images. Some laboratories use a concomitant M-mode study (one-dimensional echocardiogram) derived from the two-dimensional image for objective measurements of chamber size and function. For a transthoracic echocardiogram, the imaging is performed with a hand-held transducer placed directly on the chest wall. In selected patients, a transesophageal echocardiogram may be performed, in which an ultrasound transducer is mounted on the tip of an endoscope placed in the esophagus and directed towards the cardiac structures, so that high-resolution images of the posterior structures are obtained.

The frequency of the ultrasound used in clinical practice is usually between 2.5 and 5.0 MHz. The images produced depend on the acoustic reflection of the ultrasound off the various structures. Ultrasound passes readily through liquid, such as blood or pericardial fluid, and these are displayed as black on the two-dimensional image. When ultrasound is reflected off more solid structures, such as the myocardium and valves, there is a gray scale display. Structures such as calcium produce intense acoustic reflection and are displayed as bright white on the two-dimensional image. In a standard echocardiographic examination, the images are obtained from parasternal, apical, subcostal, and suprasternal windows. Multiple transducer rotations and angulations from each window are used to ensure that all parts of the cardiac structures are imaged. Most echocardiographic studies are recorded on videotape for off-line analysis, but direct digital acquisition units are enhancing the ability for storage and retrieval of images.

Current echocardiographic machines are portable, which allows them to be wheeled directly to the patient's bedside. Thus, a major advantage of echocardiography over other imaging modalities is the ability to obtain instantaneous images of the cardiac structures for immediate interpretation, even in emergency or trauma units or in critical care settings.

A limitation of a two-dimensional echocardiogram performed via a transthoracic approach is the inability to obtain high-quality images in all patients, especially those with a thick chest wall or severe lung disease. Ultrasound waves are poorly transmitted through lung parenchyma. In patients with inadequate transthoracic echocardiographic images, transesophageal echocardiography can be performed.

Table 227-1 Clinical Uses of Echocardiography

Two-Dimensional Echocardiography	**Stress Echocardiography**
Cardiac chambers	Two-dimensional
Chamber size	Myocardial ischemia
Left ventricular	Viable myocardium
Hypertrophy	Doppler
Regional wall motion abnormalities	Valve disease
Valve	**Transesophageal Echocardiography**
Morphology and motion	Inadequate transthoracic images
Pericardium	Aortic disease
Effusion	Infective endocarditis
Tamponade	Source of embolism
Masses	Valve prosthesis
Great vessels	Intraoperative
Doppler Echocardiography	
Valve stenosis	
Gradient	
Valve area	
Valve regurgitation	
Semiquantitation	
Intracardiac pressures	
Volumetric flow	
Diastolic filling	
Intracardiac shunts	

The diagnostic accuracy of an echocardiogram is highly dependent upon both the operator of the echocardiographic equipment and the interpreter of the study. There are many important technical aspects to obtaining and interpreting the two-dimensional images, requiring training, experience, and expertise.

Chamber Size and Function   Two-dimensional echocardiography is an ideal imaging modality for assessing left ventricular size and function (Fig. 227-1). A qualitative assessment of the cavity size of the ventricle and systolic function can be made directly from the two-dimensional image by experienced observers (Fig. 227-2). Quantitative assessment of left ventricular size and function can be made by M-mode echocardiography (measuring systolic and diastolic dimensions of the short axis of the left ventricle) or quantitative two-dimensional echocardiography. With quantitative two-dimensional echocardiography, endocardial outlines of the left ventricular cavity are traced in systole and diastole and the left ventricular cavity areas are then fitted to computer models of the left ventricle to obtain systolic and diastolic volumes, making it more cumbersome and less reproducible than the M-mode method. However, the M-mode method can be used only in patients with symmetrically contracting ventricles, as the M-mode samples only the septum and free wall at the mid-ventricle level. The presence or absence of regional wall motion abnormalities can be visually assessed by examining endocardial motion as well as wall thickening. M-mode and two-dimensional echocardiography are useful in the diagnosis of left ventricular hypertrophy, seen as an increase in wall thickness. Other chamber sizes are assessed by visual analysis, including the left atrium and right-sided chambers. There is no method for quantitative analysis of right ventricular size and function by two-dimensional echocardiography, due to the complex geometry of the right ventricle.

Valve Abnormalities (See also Chap. 236)   Valve morphology and motion can be visualized by two-dimensional echocardiography (Figs. 227-1 and 227-2). Leaflet thickness and mobility, valve calcification, and the appearance of subvalvular and supravalvular struc-

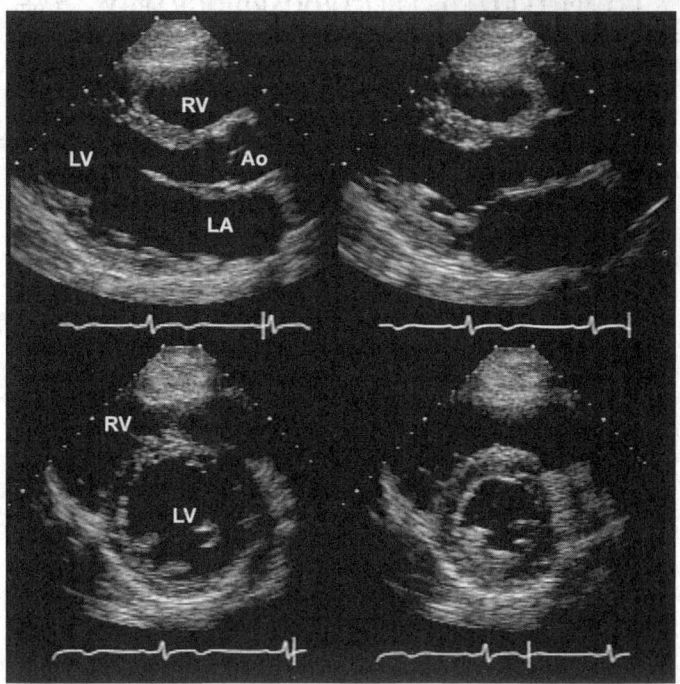

FIGURE 227-1   Two-dimensional echocardiographic still frame images from a normal patient with a normal heart. *Upper*: Parasternal long axis view during systole and diastole (*left*) and systole (*right*). During systole, there is thickening of the myocardium and reduction in the size of the left ventricle (LV). The valve leaflets are thin and open widely. *Lower*: Parasternal short axis view during diastole (*left*) and systole (*right*) demonstrating a decrease in the left ventricular cavity size during systole as well as an increase in wall thickening. LA, left atrium; RV, right ventricle; Ao, aorta.

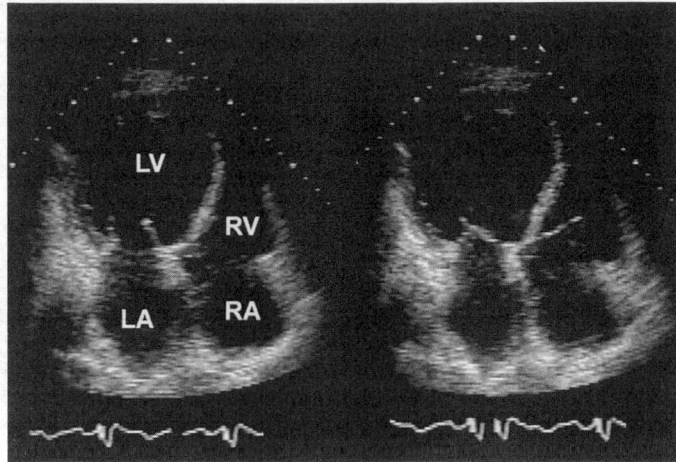

FIGURE 227-2 Apical four-chamber view from a patient with a dilated cardiomyopathy. The left ventricle (LV) is dilated, and there is little change in the LV cavity size from diastole (*left*) to systole (*right*). RV, right ventricle; LA, left atrium.

tures can be assessed. Valve stenosis is reliably diagnosed by the thickening and decreased mobility of the valve. Two-dimensional echocardiography is the "gold standard" for the diagnosis of mitral stenosis, which produces typical tethering and diastolic doming. The severity of the stenosis can be obtained from a direct planimeter measurement of the mitral valve orifice from the short axis view. The presence and etiology of stenosis of the semilunar valves can be made by two-dimensional echocardiography (**Plate I-1**). Estimating the severity of the stenosis by two-dimensional echocardiography alone is less reliable and requires Doppler echocardiography. The diagnosis of valvular regurgitation must be made by Doppler echocardiography, but two-dimensional echocardiography is valuable for determining the etiology of the regurgitation. Annular dilatation, prolapse, flail leaflets, vegetation, and rheumatic involvement can be diagnosed and the left ventricular response to volume overload can be assessed by two-dimensional echocardiography.

Pericardial Disease (See also Chap. 239) Two-dimensional echocardiography is the imaging modality of choice for the detection of pericardial effusion, which is easily visualized as a black echolucent ovoid structure surrounding the heart. In the hemodynamically unstable patient with pericardial tamponade, typical echo findings of right ventricular collapse, right atrial collapse, and a dilated inferior vena cava are seen (see Fig. 239-1). In patients with subclinical tamponade, these two-dimensional echocardiographic features may not be present, but the diagnosis of elevated pericardial pressure can be made by Doppler findings of variations of inflow velocities with respiration (see Figs. 239-2 and 239-4). Echocardiographically guided pericardiocentesis has now become a standard of care. A two-dimensional echocardiogram can directly visualize the location of the pericardial fluid in relationship to the entry point, and this technique has led to a low complication rate. Increased thickness of the pericardium is difficult to assess by two-dimensional echocardiography. Subtle clues to pericardial constriction can be seen on two-dimensional echocardiography from enhanced ventricular interaction, but Doppler imaging is required for confirmation of this diagnosis.

Intracardiac Masses (See also Chap. 240) Intracardiac masses can be visualized on two-dimensional echocardiography, provided that image quality is adequate. Solid masses appear as echo-dense structures, which can be located inside the cardiac chambers or infiltrating into the myocardium or pericardium (see Fig. 240-1). Although an echocardiographic examination cannot provide pathologic confirmation of the etiology of a mass, there are several instances in which the diagnosis of the mass can be suspected from its appearance, mobility, and the concomitant abnormalities seen. *Left ventricular thrombus* appears as an echo-dense structure, usually in the apical region associated with regional wall motion abnormalities. The appearance and mobility of the thrombus are predictive of embolic events. *Atrial myxoma* can be diagnosed by the appearance of a well-circumscribed mobile mass with attachments to the atrial septum. Prominent benign structures, such as *lipomatous infiltration of the atrial septum* and a *calcified mitral annulus*, may appear as cardiac masses. The high-resolution images provided by transesophageal echocardiography may be required for further delineation of myocardial masses.

Aortic Disease (See also Chap. 247) Two-dimensional echocardiography can provide information on diseases of the aorta. The proximal ascending aorta, the arch, and the distal descending aorta can usually be visualized via the transthoracic approach. For patients in whom a dilated aorta is well visualized, two-dimensional echocardiography can be used for serial follow-up. Aortic dissection can be diagnosed when an intimal flap is visualized on a transthoracic echocardiogram. However, the definitive diagnosis of an aortic dissection usually requires a transesophageal echocardiogram (**Plate I-2**).

DOPPLER ECHOCARDIOGRAPHY **Basic Principles** Doppler echocardiography uses ultrasound reflecting off moving red blood cells to measure the velocity of blood flow across valves, within cardiac chambers, and through the great vessels. Normal and abnormal blood flow patterns can be assessed noninvasively. Color flow Doppler imaging (**Plates I-1 and I-2**) displays the blood velocities in real time superimposed upon a two-dimensional echocardiographic image. The different colors indicate the direction of blood flow (blue towards and red away from the transducer), with green color superimposed when there is turbulent flow. Thus regurgitant lesions and shunts may be assessed by color flow Doppler. Pulsed-wave Doppler measures the blood flow velocity in a specific location on the two-dimensional echocardiographic image and displays the velocities in a spectral pattern using time as the *x*-axis. Continuous-wave Doppler echocardiography can measure high velocities of blood flow directed along the line of the Doppler beam, such as occur in the presence of valve stenosis, valve regurgitation, or intracardiac shunts. These high velocities can be used to determine intracardiac pressure gradients by a modified Bernoulli equation:

$$\text{Pressure change} = 4 \times (\text{velocity})^2$$

In this equation, the contribution from viscous friction and flow acceleration to the change in pressure is assumed to be negligible. The derived pressure gradient can be used to determine intracardiac pressures and stenosis severity.

Valve Gradients (See also Chap. 236) In the presence of valvular stenosis, there is an increase in the velocity of blood flow across the stenotic valve. A continuous-wave Doppler beam can be placed into this jet of blood, and the measured velocity used to determine an instantaneous gradient across the valve by applying the modified Bernoulli equation. Integration of this velocity over time provides an accurate measurement of the mean gradient across the valve. If the Doppler beam is directed parallel to the jet, the Doppler-derived valve gradient is accurate and reproducible and correlates with that obtained from cardiac catheterization. Since the valve gradient is dependent upon transvalvular flow, a valve area should be derived noninvasively. An accurate assessment of the mean gradient and valve area can be obtained in most patients, provided that the Doppler beam is parallel to the stenotic jet. The Doppler examination is highly operator-dependent, especially in patients with aortic stenosis. If the Doppler beam is not parallel to the stenotic jet, there may be a significant underestimation of the valve gradient. In patients with mitral stenosis, it is technically easier to align the Doppler beam with the stenotic jet; thus the mean transmitral gradient is usually accurate and reproducible. A Doppler-derived transmitral gradient may be more reliable than that obtained by conventional cardiac catheterization, given the inherent errors that may occur with a pulmonary artery wedge pressure measurement.

Valvular Regurgitation (See also Chap. 236) Valvular regurgitation is diagnosed by Doppler echocardiography when there is an abnormal retrograde flow across the valve. Color flow imaging is the Doppler method used most frequently to detect valve regurgitation by visualization of a high-velocity turbulent jet in the chamber proximal to the regurgitant valve. The sensitivity of Doppler echocardiography for the detection of regurgitant lesions is high, and even trivial or mild regurgitation in the absence of clinical auscultatory evidence of a regurgitant murmur may be detected. The size and extent of the color flow jet into the receiving cardiac chamber provide a qualitative estimate of the severity of regurgitation, but there are many limitations to using color jet size alone. Indirect clues for the severity of valvular regurgitation are available from other Doppler interrogation sites (e.g., intensity of a continuous-wave signal, volume of forward flow across a regurgitant valve). Methods for quantitation of regurgitation severity are now available, such as the measurement of the proximal isovelocity surface area, and these may be employed for determining effective orifice area and regurgitant volumes. As with other quantitative Doppler measurements, these methods are operator-dependent, and reliable data require an experienced high-volume laboratory.

Intracardiac Pressures These can be calculated from the peak continuous-wave Doppler signal of a regurgitant lesion. The Bernoulli equation is applied to the peak velocity to obtain the pressure gradient between two cardiac chambers. This is commonly applied to a tricuspid regurgitant jet, from which the systolic pressure gradient between the right atrium and right ventricle can be calculated. Adding an assumed right atrial pressure to this gradient will give a derived right ventricular systolic pressure. Change in pressure over time during isovolumic contraction can be derived from a mitral regurgitation signal. This measurement provides an index of systolic contractility.

Cardiac Output Volume flow rates can be reliably measured noninvasively from Doppler echocardiography. Using the hydrodynamic principle of flow through a rigid tube, the volume of flow can be calculated from the area of an orifice through which blood flows multiplied by the time of the velocity. The most accurate site for this measurement is through the left ventricular outflow tract. The product of the outflow area and velocity provides a beat-to-beat measurement of stroke volume, which, when multiplied by heart rate, provides a measurement of cardiac output.

Diastolic filling (See also Chap. 231) Doppler echocardiography allows noninvasive evaluation of ventricular diastolic filling. The transmitral velocity curves reflect the relative pressure gradients between the left atrium and left ventricle throughout the diastolic filling period. They are influenced by the rate of ventricular relaxation, the driving force across the valve, and the compliance of the left ventricle. There is a progression of diastolic dysfunction in disease states, which can be assessed by Doppler flow velocity curves (Fig. 227-3). In the early phase of diastolic dysfunction there is primarily an abnormality of relaxation, with decreased early transmitral flow and a compensatory increase in flow during atrial contraction. As disease progresses, there is a higher left atrial pressure and reduced compliance of the left ventricle, resulting in a higher early transmitral velocity and shortening of the deceleration of flow in early diastole, termed *restriction to filling*. These transmitral flow curves can be used to estimate ventricular filling pressures and to determine prognosis in certain disease entities. The addition of Doppler interrogation of pulmonary venous flow as well as right-sided chamber flow provides further information concerning the diastolic properties.

Congenital Heart Disease (See also Chap. 234) Doppler echocardiography has been useful in the evaluation of patients with congenital heart disease. Congenital stenotic or regurgitant valve lesions can be assessed. The detection and semiquantitation of intracardiac shunts is possible by Doppler echocardiography. Patency of surgical shunts and conduits can be determined.

STRESS ECHOCARDIOGRAPHY (See also Chap. 244) Two-dimensional and Doppler echocardiography are usually per-

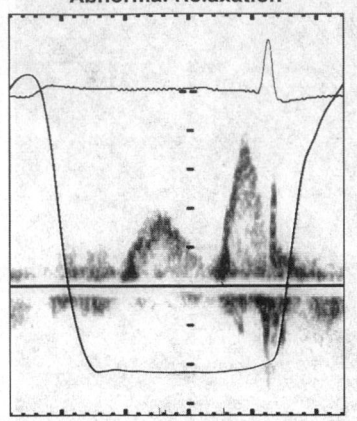
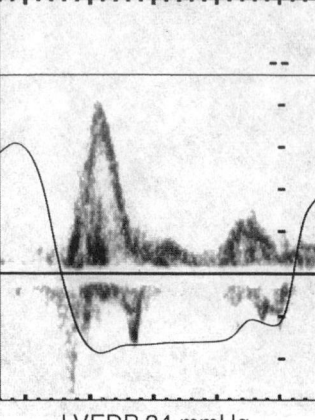

Abnormal Relaxation   **Restriction**

LVEDP 6 mmHg   LVEDP 34 mmHg

FIGURE 227-3 High-fidelity left ventricular pressure curve superimposed upon a mitral inflow velocity curve obtained by Doppler echocardiography. The ratio of early and late diastolic flows is termed an *E:A ratio. Left*: In early stages of diastolic dysfunction, there is an abnormality of relaxation. There is a decrease in the early diastolic filling and an increase with filling at atrial contraction, resulting in a low E:A ratio of 0.5, with deceleration time (DT) of 280 ms. In this instance, the left ventricular end-diastolic pressure (LVEDP) is low at 6 mmHg. *Right*: As diastolic dysfunction progresses, there is a restriction to filling, in which there is a high early diastolic velocity and low velocity at atrial contraction resulting in a high E:A ratio of 3.0, with DT of 120 ms. In this instance, the LVEDP is markedly elevated to 34 mmHg. The DT reflects the rate of decline of the early velocity and is a measure of the effective operative compliance of the left ventricle. (See text for explanation.)

formed in the resting state. Further information can be obtained by reimaging during either exercise or pharmacologic stress. The primary indications for stress echocardiography are to confirm the suspicion of coronary artery disease and estimate its severity. Doppler stress testing provides additional information for the patient with valvular heart disease.

The response of the myocardium to ischemia consists of a cascade of events. A decrease in systolic contraction of the ischemic area, termed a *regional wall motion abnormality*, occurs before symptoms or electrocardiographic changes. During a stress echocardiogram, two-dimensional echocardiographic images at rest and during stress are digitized and displayed in a side-by-side format so that induced regional wall motion abnormalities may be detected. Changes in overall systolic function as well as end-systolic volume are also assessed. New regional wall motion abnormalities, a decline in ejection fraction, and an increase in end-systolic volume with stress are all indicators of myocardial ischemia (Fig. 227-4).

Stress testing is usually done with exercise protocols using either upright treadmill or bicycle exercise. The echocardiographic imaging is done at baseline and then immediately after exercise. In patients who are not able to exercise, pharmacologic testing can be performed by infusing dobutamine, which increases myocardial oxygen demand. Dobutamine echocardiography has also been used to assess myocardial viability in patients with poor systolic function and concomitant coronary artery disease. In this type of study, dobutamine is given at a low dose of 5 to 10 μg/kg per minute. In the presence of viable myocardium, an increase in the systolic contraction of the myocardium is evident.

There are limitations to stress echocardiography. It is important that the images be obtained as soon as possible after exercise is stopped since regional wall motion abnormalities may dissipate rapidly with time. Optimal image quality is essential for proper interpretation, and this depends on not only patient habitus but also the ability of the sonographer to obtain the image. Interpretation of the images is highly operator-dependent, and thus this technique requires an experienced echocardiographer.

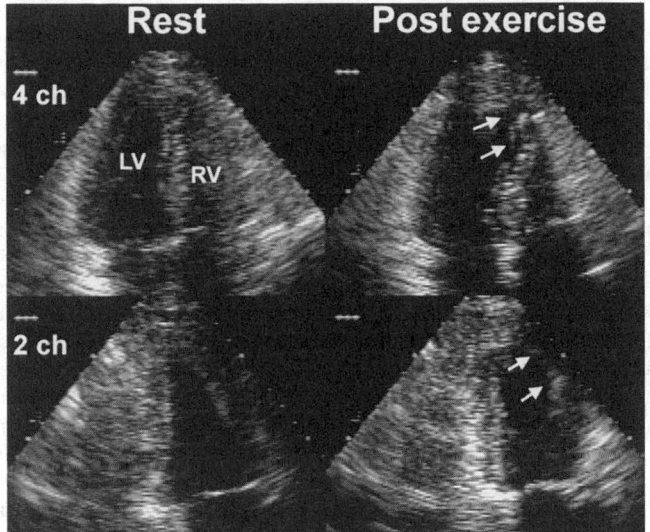

FIGURE 227-4 Stress echocardiographic images in a patient with known coronary artery disease. *Left*: The systolic views from a patient in the resting state is shown. The upper frame is taken from a four-chamber view and the lower frame is taken from a two-chamber view. *Right*: The systolic views are shown immediately after exercise. The arrows point to the appearance of a regional wall motion abnormality in the anterior and apical segments. LV, left ventricle; RV, right ventricle. *(From Oh JK et al, with permission.)*

Doppler echocardiography can be used at rest and during exercise in patients with valvular heart disease to determine the hemodynamic response to stress. Gradients across stenotic valves can be measured at rest and immediately after exercise, which provides information previously obtained by right heart catheterization during exercise. Pulmonary pressures can be obtained from the tricuspid regurgitation velocities at rest and during exercise.

TRANSESOPHAGEAL ECHOCARDIOGRAPHY This technique has provided a new window on the heart. Because of the close proximity of the esophagus to the heart, high-resolution images of posterior structures are consistently obtained. Transesophageal echocardiography should be performed when further information is required after comprehensive two-dimensional and Doppler transthoracic echocardiograms. Diseases of the aorta, such as aortic dissection, can be readily diagnosed and quantitated by transesophageal echocardiography (**Plate I-2**; Chap. 247). Defining the source of embolism is a common indication for transesophageal echocardiography, as abnormalities such as atrial thrombi, patent foramen ovale, and aortic debris can be detected. Other masses, particularly those in the atria, can be visualized. The presence of vegetations for the diagnosis of infective endocarditis and its complications can be assessed by transesophageal echocardiography (Chap. 126). The evaluation of suspected abnormalities of a mitral prosthesis is an indication for transesophageal echocardiography, as the posterior imaging window will avoid the problems of acoustic reflection caused by the prosthetic valve seen with transthoracic echocardiography. Transesophageal echocardiography can be used during cardiac surgery to guide various operations, such as mitral valve repair and septal myectomy. When limited information is obtained from a transthoracic echocardiogram due to poor imaging windows, transesophageal echocardiography can be useful.

ADVANCES IN ECHOCARDIOGRAPHY There are several areas of technological advances in the field of echocardiography. Digital conversion of images allows zoom functions and endless loop playback and facilitates storage and retrieval. Harmonic imaging is a technologic advance that may significantly improve image quality, particularly in patients with poor acoustic windows. Echo contrast agents containing microbubbles cause reflection of ultrasound waves and produce bright echo-dense images. Newer contrast agents have been developed that traverse the pulmonary circulation, entering the left-sided chambers from an intravenous injection. Two-dimensional echocardiographic imaging during the appearance of echo contrast in the left ventricle enhances definition of the endocardial border. The appearance of contrast directly in the myocardium may be useful for examining myocardial blood flow. Three-dimensional reconstruction of ultrasound images is an exciting new area of investigation that will add further to the utility of echocardiography.

NUCLEAR CARDIOLOGY

BASIC PRINCIPLES OF NUCLEAR CARDIOLOGY All nuclear cardiology studies depend upon the injection into the patient of an isotope that emits photons, generally gamma rays generated during radioactive decay when the nucleus of an isotope changes from one energy level to a lower one. Radionuclide imaging uses a special camera that images these photons. A common problem with all nuclear studies is that photons are emitted in all directions from the point of origin, and scattering, attenuation, and absorption of the photons can occur. The higher the energy of the isotope, the less chance for scatter or absorption.

The two most commonly used isotopes are technetium 99m (^{99m}Tc) and thallium 201 (^{201}Tl). Technetium is used in both myocardial perfusion studies and radionuclide angiography and is formed on site from molybdenum 99 (^{99}Mo). The parent compound has a half-life of 66 h and thus is easily transported. ^{99m}Tc, which is a metastable compound, is constantly formed from ^{99}Mo in the on-site generator. During the decay of ^{99m}Tc to ^{99}Tc, photons are emitted with a characteristic 140-keV photopeak and a half-life of 6 h. ^{201}Tl, on the other hand, needs to be generated in a cyclotron facility and transported as a finished product, with a half-life of 73 h. The thallium isotope decay process is more complex than that of technetium, with most photons in the 80-keV range. Due to its higher energy and shorter half-life, technetium is a more desirable imaging agent.

ASSESSMENT OF VENTRICULAR FUNCTION Equilibrium radionuclide angiography, also known as *multiple-gated blood pool imaging*, is useful for the noninvasive assessment of ventricular function. It involves the imaging of ^{99m}Tc-labeled albumin or red cells that are uniformly distributed throughout the blood volume. Resting images of the blood pool of isotopes within the cardiac chambers are obtained by electrocardiographic gating through multiple cycles, so that sufficient counts can be detected to obtain an image. This requires that the heart rate be reasonably constant without significant arrhythmia. Resting images are usually obtained in the anterior, lateral, and left anterior oblique views. Each image lasts approximately 2 to 4 min.

Ejection fraction is determined by a count-based program from equilibrium radionuclide angiography; this does not require any assumptions regarding the geometry of the ventricle. It provides an accurate, reproducible method for assessment of left ventricular function. Regional wall motion analysis can be done by visual qualitative assessment, although there are programs for quantitative analysis. Left ventricular volume can also be assessed by a count-based method, using a regression equation. Other clinical variables that can be obtained include size and function of the right ventricle, size of atrial chambers and great vessels, and diastolic filling parameters. The severity of valvular regurgitant lesions can be assessed by measurement of a regurgitant fraction, which compares right ventricular stroke volume with left ventricular stroke volume.

First-pass radionuclide angiography is an alternative method for the noninvasive assessment of ventricular function. In contrast to equilibrium radionuclide angiography, first-pass radionuclide angiography involves the recording of the movement of a bolus of radionuclide during its "first pass" through the central circulation. This does not require labeling of red blood cells. ^{99m}Tc is utilized because of its low cost and short half-life. During this testing, the passage of the radioisotope through the right atrium, right ventricle, pulmonary circulation, left atrium, left ventricle, and aorta is recorded with a high count (usually multicrystal) camera. The high count rates allow temporal definition of the passage of the bolus. The change in counts of a sample placed over a ventricle reflects its function. One major advantage of first-pass angiography is the short acquisition time required, as an injected bolus will complete its passage within 30 s. In contrast to equilibrium radionuclide angiography, the right and left sides of the heart can be scanned separately. The disadvantage of first-pass radionuclide angiography compared to equilibrium testing is its poorer resolution of ventricular wall motion. It is also inaccurate in instances where the injected bolus becomes delayed in its transit, such as with severe tricuspid regurgitation or pulmonary hypertension.

Ejection fraction and regional wall motion may also be assessed using gating of single-photon emission computed tomographic (SPECT) myocardial perfusion images using technetium-labeled perfusion agents (see below).

ASSESSMENT OF MYOCARDIAL PERFUSION Myocardial perfusion imaging by nuclear techniques is now widely applied for the evaluation of ischemic heart disease. Injection of radioisotopes at rest and during stress is performed to produce images of myocardial regional uptake proportional to regional blood flow. With maximal exercise, myocardial blood flow is increased up to fivefold above the resting condition. In the presence of a fixed coronary stenosis, there is an inability to increase myocardial perfusion in the territory supplied by the stenosis, creating a flow differential and inhomogeneous distribution of the isotope (see Fig. 244-2). In patients who are unable to exercise, pharmacologic agents are used to increase blood flow and create similar inhomogeneities. The preferred pharmacologic agents are adenosine or dipyridamole, which increase blood flow to a similar degree as exercise. In patients with bronchospastic lung disease, which is a contraindication to the use of adenosine or dipyridamole, dobutamine may be used as an alternative, although it does not increase blood flow to the same extent.

^{201}Tl is a potassium analogue and is avidly taken up by viable myocardial cells. The degree of uptake is related directly to the coronary blood flow. An initial injection is usually performed at peak exercise, and hypoperfused myocardium will have less thallium uptake than a region of normal perfusion (see Fig. 244-2). Over the next several hours, a complex process occurs that is known as "redistribution." There is a continuous input of thallium into the myocardium from a large reservoir of thallium in the blood pool. At the same time, thallium continuously washes out of portions of the myocardium at a rate that is dependent on local myocardial perfusion. The final result is that a region of ischemia that initially appears as an area of reduced uptake becomes apparently normal over time; this redistribution is seen on delayed imaging. In regions of fibrosis (infarction), there will be no redistribution on delayed imaging. A "reinjection" of an additional small amount of thallium before acquisition of the delayed images enhances the detection of ischemia. The presence of redistribution in areas of hypokinesia has been associated with recovery of left ventricular function after revascularization.

Other findings on thallium imaging may be of considerable clinical importance. Increased lung uptake of thallium may be seen immediately after stress and assessed either quantitatively or qualitatively. This finding reflects increased pulmonary capillary wedge pressure during stress. It occurs in the presence of severe coronary artery disease and/or left ventricular dysfunction. It provides important adverse prognostic information that is incremental to other clinical, stress, and coronary angiographic variables. Thallium images may also show evidence of transient poststress left ventricular dilatation. This finding is also associated with severe coronary artery disease and/or left ventricular dysfunction as well as with an adverse prognosis.

^{99m}Tc-labeled compounds have a higher photon energy and shorter half-life than ^{201}Tl, permitting the injection of larger doses. As a result, these compounds generally provide higher quality scans with fewer artifacts. Three technetium-labeled agents have been approved for general use: teboroxime, tetrofosmin, and sestamibi. The latter is the best

studied of these agents and is currently used most frequently. Like thallium, sestamibi distributes to the myocardium in relation to blood flow, and its uptake requires a viable myocardial cell and an intact cell membrane. It is transported through the cytoplasm and bound to the mitochondria in a nearly irreversible fashion. Compared to thallium, there is far less redistribution. As a result, the agent must generally be injected twice—once at rest and once during stress.

Myocardial Perfusion Imaging Protocols (Plate I-1) The use of ^{201}Tl usually involves one of three protocols. The first protocol (stress-redistribution-delayed imaging) involves stress imaging, followed by redistribution imaging 3 or 4 h later (see Fig. 244-2). If fixed defects are present, delayed imaging is performed at a later time (usually 24 h) to detect additional redistribution. The second protocol (stress-redistribution-reinjection) also involves stress images and redistribution images 3 or 4 h later. In those patients with fixed defects on redistribution imaging, reinjection of a small amount of thallium is then performed. Repeat imaging is performed approximately 30 min later to identify a difference in myocardial uptake consistent with ischemia. In the third protocol (stress-reinjection-delayed imaging) patients are reinjected with a small amount of thallium before performing delayed imaging at 3 or 4 h. In those patients who have fixed defects on these reinjection images, more delayed imaging is then performed (usually at 24 h) in order to detect redistribution of both the initial stress dose as well as the reinjection dose. All three protocols therefore involve the use of stress images and delayed images in all patients, with a third set of images in a small subset of patients in order to improve the detection of thallium redistribution.

Stress imaging with sestamibi may utilize a 2-day protocol with different days for the injections of sestamibi at rest and during stress. Either the stress image or the rest image may be performed first. The protocol may also be carried out in one day. When the rest study is performed first a low dose is used, followed by a stress study using a larger injected dose. Alternatively, the order of these two studies may be reversed.

COMPARISON OF THALLIUM AND SESTAMIBI Both ^{201}Tl and ^{99m}Tc sestamibi provide clinically useful myocardial perfusion images in the majority of patients. The choice between the two is often dictated by local experience and economics. However, in selected patients, there may be factors that suggest a clear advantage for one or the other. The relative advantages of both agents are listed in Table 227-2.

NUCLEAR CARDIOLOGY IN CLINICAL DECISION MAKING Stress-myocardial-perfusion imaging with either ^{201}Tl or ^{99m}Tc sestamibi plays a pivotal role in both the diagnosis and risk stratification of patients with established or suspected coronary artery disease.

For the diagnosis of coronary artery disease, stress-myocardial-perfusion imaging is an appropriate initial test (as opposed to a treadmill exercise electrocardiogram) in patients with left bundle branch

Table 227-2   Relative Advantages of Thallium-201 and Technetium-99m Sestamibi

Thallium
  Lower radiopharmaceutical cost
  Greater experience, including long-term prognostic value
  Measurement of increased pulmonary uptake
  Detection of resting ischemia (hibernating myocardium)
Sestamibi
  Better image quality (particularly in obese patients or female patients with breast attenuation)
  Ventricular function assessment (first-pass or gated SPECT)
  Shorter imaging times (lower cost)
  Shorter imaging protocols (patient/scheduling convenience)
  Acute imaging in myocardial infarction (myocardium at risk) and unstable angina (chest pain triage)
  Superior quantification, particularly of resting perfusion defect (infarct size)

NOTE: SPECT, single-positron emission computed tomography.

block, an electronically paced ventricular rhythm, >1 mm of ST segment depression at rest, or prior coronary artery revascularization, or in patients who are unable to exercise to a level high enough to give meaningful results. Stress-myocardial-perfusion imaging is also performed as a second test to clarify the significance of an equivocal treadmill exercise electrocardiogram.

For risk stratification, stress perfusion imaging can identify the extent, severity, and location of ischemia. These findings are often pivotal in defining the need for coronary angiography and coronary revascularization. Normal stress-myocardial-perfusion scans are highly predictive of both the absence of significant coronary artery disease and a low risk of cardiac death (less than 1% per year); coronary angiography is usually not required. Patients with markedly abnormal myocardial perfusion scans (large stress-induced defects, multiple stress-induced defects of moderate size, large fixed defect with left ventricular dilatation or increased ^{201}Tl lung uptake) are at high risk (>3 percent annual mortality rate). In such patients, coronary angiography and possible revascularization are appropriate.

POSITRON EMISSION TOMOGRAPHY (PET) The underlying physics of PET scanning is quite different from that involved in the standard radionuclide techniques described above. The annihilation of the positron leads to the simultaneous emission of two very high energy (511 keV) photons in opposite directions. These can then be imaged by a series of detectors placed in a ring around the patient. The very high energy of the photons results in far less scatter and attenuation than with conventional nuclear cardiology techniques. The sophistication of the required equipment and the associated expense have generally limited the availability of this technique. PET cameras are considerably more expensive than conventional nuclear cardiology cameras. The radiopharmaceuticals involved require a cyclotron for production and generally have half-lives that are so short that transportation beyond the immediate local region is not feasible.

Positron emitters can be employed to study both myocardial blood flow and myocardial metabolism. Nitrogen-13 ammonia, oxygen-15 water, and rubidium-82 have all been employed to assess myocardial blood flow. They permit measurement of absolute regional blood flows, in contrast to the relative blood flows that are assessed with ^{201}Tl or ^{99m}Tc sestamibi. This advantage has been utilized for research purposes but has not yet been exploited clinically. Myocardial metabolism is most often assessed using fluorine-18 deoxyglucose. This agent permits the detection and quantification of exogenous glucose utilization in areas of hypoperfused myocardium.

The clinical application of PET scanning that has been most well studied is the assessment of myocardial viability. The pattern of enhanced fluorodeoxyglucose uptake in regions of decreased perfusion (termed *glucose/blood flow "mismatch"*) indicates the presence of ischemic myocardium that has preferentially shifted its metabolic substrate towards glucose rather than fatty acid or lactate. This pattern identifies regions of ischemic or hibernating myocardium that are likely to improve in function after revascularization (Chap. 244).

Careful studies have consistently shown the ability of PET to identify ischemic or hibernating myocardium in 10 to 20% of regions that would be classified as fibrotic (infarcted) by ^{201}Tl or ^{99m}Tc sestamibi. For that reason, this technique is generally regarded as the "gold standard" for the assessment of myocardial viability. However, because of its greater cost, national clinical practice guidelines have suggested that its usage be restricted to the specific situations where it is most beneficial.

Within the past few years, specially modified conventional gamma cameras have been employed to image fluorodeoxyglucose in an attempt to avoid the expense related to cameras dedicated to PET. The limited evidence available suggests that this approach is inferior to standard PET.

BIBLIOGRAPHY

BELLER GA: Perfusion imaging: 50th Anniversary Historical Article. J Am Coll Cardiol 34:49, 1999

FLEISCHMANN KE et al: Exercise echocardiography or exercise SPECT imaging? A meta-analysis of diagnostic test performance. JAMA 180(10):913, 1998

GIBBONS RJ: Role of nuclear cardiology for determining management of patients with stable coronary artery disease. J Nucl Cardiol 1 (Suppl):S118–130, 1994

——— et al: Long-term outcome of patients with intermediate-risk exercise electrocardiograms who do not have myocardial perfusion defects on radionuclide imaging. Circulation (in press).

——— et al: Infarct size measured by SPECT imaging with technetium-99m sestamibi—a measure of the efficacy of therapy in acute myocardial infarction. Circulation (in press).

NISHIMURA RA, TAJIK AJ: Evaluation of diastolic filling of the left ventricle in health and disease: Doppler echocardiography is the clinicians' Rosetta stone. J Am Coll Cardiol 30(1):8, 1997

OH JK et al: *The Echo Manual*, 2d ed. Lippincott-Williams & Wilkins, Philadelphia 1999

RITCHIE JL et al: ACC/AHA guidelines for clinical use of radionuclide imaging: A report of the ACC/AHA task force on practice guidelines. J Am Coll Cardiol 25:521, 1995

228 *Donald S. Baim, William Grossman*

DIAGNOSTIC CARDIAC CATHETERIZATION AND ANGIOGRAPHY

Despite progressive improvements in noninvasive techniques, cardiac catheterization remains a key clinical tool for assessing the anatomy and physiology of the heart and its associated vasculature. It involves the insertion of small (diameter, 2 to 3 mm), hollow plastic tubes or catheters into a peripheral artery or vein under local anesthesia, and passage of their tips into the heart for pressure measurement or for the injection of a liquid radiographic contrast agent. The findings characterize the extent and severity of cardiac disease and thereby help in deciding on the most appropriate plan for medical, surgical, or catheter-based treatment. While most patients with coronary artery disease (CAD) or valvular disease can be managed using only clinical and noninvasive test data, more than 1.5 million cardiac catheterization and angiographic procedures are performed each year for diagnostic or interventional purposes, or both. This chapter focuses on the uses of cardiac catheterization as a diagnostic tool. →*For further discussion of catheter-based interventions, see Chap. 245.*

INDICATIONS, CONTRAINDICATIONS, AND COMPLICATIONS **Indications** Given the expense and small, but real, risks of cardiac catheterization, it is not performed routinely whenever cardiac disease is diagnosed or suspected. Instead, cardiac catheterization is recommended only when there is a need to confirm the presence of a clinically suspected condition, define its anatomic and physiologic severity, and determine whether important associated conditions are present. This need most commonly arises when a patient is experiencing limiting or escalating symptoms of cardiac dysfunction (Chap. 232) or myocardial ischemia (Chap. 244) or when objective measures (such as exercise testing or echocardiography) suggest that the patient has a high risk of progressing to rapid functional deterioration, myocardial infarction, or other adverse events. Under these circumstances, catheterization is often a prelude to treatment by cardiac surgery or a catheter-based intervention. In the past, cardiac catheterization was considered mandatory in *all* patients being considered for cardiac surgery. Today, many patients with congenital or valvular heart disease can undergo surgical correction based solely on clinical and noninvasive test data; however, cardiac catheterization and coronary arteriography remain the only techniques that can define coronary anatomy with sufficient precision to support decisions regarding coronary surgery or catheter-based interventions in patients with CAD. In patients with other forms of heart disease (e.g., dilated cardiomyopathy, valvular heart disease), cardiac catheterization can provide hemody-

Table 228-1   Relative Contraindications to Cardiac Catheterization and Angiography

Uncontrolled ventricular irritability: increased risk of ventricular tachycardia and fibrillation during catheterization if ventricular irritability is uncontrolled

Uncorrected hypokalemia or digitalis toxicity

Uncorrected hypertension: predisposes to myocardial ischemia and/or heart failure during angiography

Intercurrent febrile illness

Decompensated heart failure: especially acute pulmonary edema, unless catheterization can be done with patient sitting up

Anticoagulated state: prothrombin time >18 s

Severe allergy to radiographic contrast agent

Severe renal insufficiency and/or anuria: unless dialysis is planned to remove fluid and radiographic contrast load

namic characterization essential for the design of an appropriate medical regimen as well as for an assessment of prognosis.

Contraindications   When there is a clinical "need to know," there are very few absolute contraindications in a patient who understands and accepts the associated risks. Some relative contraindications to cardiac catheterization, however, are listed in Table 228-1. Most center on factors that increase the risk of the procedure above the baseline mortality risk of roughly 1 in 1000 for clinically stable patients. This risk is increased more than tenfold in patients with severe symptoms, certain types of coronary anatomy, valve disease, left ventricular dysfunction, or severe noncardiac disease, as outlined in Table 228-2.

Complications   Beyond the mortality risk, cardiac catheterization carries a 1 in 1000 risk of stroke or myocardial infarction. Other problems, such as transient tachy- or bradyarrhythmias or bruising or bleeding at the catheter insertion site, occur in fewer than 1% of patients and respond to drug therapy, countershock, or vascular surgical repair, without long-term sequelae. Although serious, problems such as cardiac perforation or arterial dissection are very rare in the modern era of cardiac catheterization.

Some patients, however, are intolerant of the iodinated contrast agents used for angiography, which may produce transient deterioration in renal function (particularly in patients with baseline renal dysfunction or proteinuria who are not adequately prehydrated) or *allergic reactions* ranging from urticaria to frank anaphylaxis in sensitive patients. These allergic reactions can be suppressed by pretreatment with glucocorticoids (prednisone, 20 to 40 mg every 6 h), conventional antihistamines (e.g., diphenhydramine, 25 mg every 6 h), and H_2 antagonists (cimetidine, 300 mg every 6 h), starting 18 to 24 h prior to

Table 228-2   Patient Characteristics Associated with Increased Mortality from Cardiac Catheterization

Age: Infants (<1 month old) and the elderly (>80 years old) are at increased risk of death during cardiac catheterization. Elderly women appear to be at higher risk than elderly men.

Functional class: Mortality in class IV patients is more than 10 times greater than in class I–II patients.

Severity of coronary obstruction: Mortality for patients with left main coronary artery disease is more than 10 times greater than in patients with one- or two-vessel disease.

Valvular heart disease: Especially when severe and combined with coronary disease, is associated with a higher risk of death at cardiac catheterization than coronary artery disease alone.

Left ventricular dysfunction: Mortality in patients with a left ventricular ejection fraction <30% is more than 10 times greater than in patients with an ejection fraction ≥50%.

Severe noncardiac disease: Patients with renal insufficiency, insulin-requiring diabetes, advanced cerebrovascular and/or peripheral vascular disease, or severe pulmonary insufficiency have an increased incidence of death and other major complications from cardiac catheterization.

the procedure. Despite these precautions, occasional individuals still develop anaphylactic reactions during radiographic contrast angiography, and intravenous epinephrine must be at hand to treat such instances. Alternatively, one of the newer nonionic contrast agents may be used with less risk of a severe allergic reaction. Unlike the original high-osmolar agents, the newer low-osmolar contrast agents (including true nonionic contrast agents and the ionic dimer ioxaglate) have a lesser myocardial depressant effect and produce fewer side effects (hypotension, nausea, bradycardia, or a sensation of marked warmth following injection) than earlier high-osmolar agents. They are, however, somewhat more expensive than traditional high-osmolar ionic agents, so that many catheterization laboratories reserve their use for patients who are at higher risk for contrast-related problems.

TECHNIQUES

Cardiac catheterization is performed with the patient in the fasting state and awake but sedated. Although cardiac catheterization used to be performed exclusively as an inpatient procedure, current practice is to perform most elective procedures on an outpatient basis, with the patient discharged 4 to 6 h after the procedure is completed. Typical preprocedure sedatives include diazepam (Valium, 5 to 10 mg orally) or midazolam (Versed, 1 mg intravenously). It is also customary to give the antihistamine diphenhydramine (Benadryl, 25 to 50 mg orally) before the procedure in the hope of suppressing minor allergic reactions to iodinated contrast. Since cardiac catheterization is a sterile procedure, prophylactic antibiotics are not necessary. To minimize the risks of bleeding at the local catheter insertion site, patients who have been anticoagulated chronically with warfarin should have this agent discontinued at least 48 h prior to the procedure, so that the INR falls below 2.

Most (>95%) cardiac catheterizations are performed by the percutaneous femoral technique, in which a needle puncture is performed in the femoral artery (for left heart catheterization) and the femoral vein (for right heart catheterization). A flexible guidewire is inserted through this needle, allowing placement of a vascular access sheath through which the desired catheters can be advanced. This percutaneous technique has been modified for other sites, including the brachial and even the radial artery. The brachial or radial approach has an advantage in the patient with peripheral vascular disease involving the abdominal aorta and iliac or femoral arteries or in whom immediate postprocedure ambulation is desired, but it involves some limitations in the range of devices that can be used if the diagnostic procedure evolves into a catheter-based intervention. With these alternatives, the original cut-down, or Sones, technique of cardiac catheterization by direct exposure of the brachial artery and vein in the antecubital fossa is rarely used.

Cardiac catheterization may include a variety of different measurements of pressure and flow (hemodynamics) as well as a variety of different contrast injections recorded as x-ray movies (angiography). The exact types of testing performed in any given procedure depend on the nature of the clinical problem being evaluated. In patients with CAD, the procedure may include only left ventriculography and coronary angiography, while in patients with valvular heart disease, full left and right heart hemodynamic studies may be performed.

RIGHT HEART CATHETERIZATION   Measurement of the pressures in the right side of the heart was once a routine part of each cardiac catheterization, but it is now used in fewer than 25% of procedures because it adds little to the evaluation of the patient with CAD. It is still useful, however, when significant left and/or right ventricular dysfunction, valve disease, myopericardial disease, or intracardiac shunting is suspected. The right heart catheterization procedure is similar to the placement of a Swan-Ganz catheter at the bedside in the intensive care unit, except that it is performed under fluoroscopic guidance. A balloon flotation catheter is advanced from a suitable vein (femoral, brachial, subclavian, or internal jugular) into the superior vena cava, where blood is sampled for oximetry. The

Pressures (mmHg)	
Systemic arterial	
Peak systolic/end-diastolic	100–140/60–90
Mean	70–105
Left ventricle	
Peak systolic/end-diastolic	100–140/3–12
Left atrium (or pulmonary capillary wedge)	
Mean	2–10
a wave	3–15
v wave	3–15
Pulmonary artery	
Peak systolic/end-diastolic	15–30/4–12
Mean	9–18
Right ventricle	
Peak systolic/end-diastolic	15–30/2–8
Right atrium	
Mean	2–8
a wave	2–10
v wave	2–10
Resistances [(dyn·s)/cm^5]	
Systemic vascular resistance	700–1600
Pulmonary vascular resistance	20–130
Cardiac index [(L/min)/m^2]	2.6–4.2
Oxygen consumption index [(L/min)/m^2]	110–150
Arteriovenous oxygen difference (mL/L)	30–50

catheter is then positioned in the right atrium, where pressure is measured. The balloon is inflated with air (or carbon dioxide, if intracardiac shunting is supected) and advanced sequentially into the right ventricle, pulmonary artery, and pulmonary artery wedge position. Pressure is recorded at each of these locations, with normal values for pressures measured during cardiac catheterization summarized in Table 228-3. After the pulmonary wedge pressure (which approximates left atrial pressure) is recorded, the balloon is deflated so that pulmonary artery pressure can be monitored and blood samples obtained for oximetry. Comparison of oxygen saturations in the superior and inferior vena cava, the chambers of the right heart, and pulmonary artery permits assessment of the presence of a left-to-right shunt at the atrial, ventricular, or pulmonary artery level, which will be manifested as an increase ("step-up") in oxygen saturation of blood as it traverses these vessels and chambers.

Measurement of Cardiac Output   Measurements of the pulmonary artery and aortic oxygen content and oxygen consumption allow calculation of the cardiac output by the Fick principle, which states that

$$Q \text{ (L/min)} = \frac{O_2 \text{ consumption (mL/min)}}{\text{arteriovenous } O_2 \text{ difference (mL/L)}}$$

In order to compare individuals of different body weights and sizes, O_2 consumption and cardiac output (Q) are commonly divided by body surface area. Normal values for O_2 consumption and cardiac output are given in Table 228-3. What is calculated by dividing O_2 consumption by the arteriovenous O_2 difference across the lungs (estimated pulmonary venous − pulmonary arterial O_2 content) is actually the pulmonary blood flow (Q_p). In patients with left-to-right shunt at the atrial, ventricular, or pulmonary artery levels, pulmonary blood flow will exceed systemic blood flow. In such cases, systemic blood flow (Q_s) is calculated by dividing O_2 consumption by the systemic arteriovenous O_2 difference. The latter is calculated as the systemic arterial blood O_2 content minus the mixed venous blood O_2 content as estimated using blood from the chamber immediately proximal to the level of the shunt. The Fick method is most dependable when the cardiac output is low and the arteriovenous oxygen difference is large.

Another approach to the measurement of cardiac output during right heart catheterization is the thermodilution technique, in which a thermistor is mounted on the tip of a balloon flotation catheter and positioned in the pulmonary artery. Cold dextrose solution or saline is injected via a proximal port on the catheter into the vena cava or right atrium, and the change in temperature monitored at the thermistor is integrated electronically. This integral is inversely proportional to the volume flow rate past the thermistor, and if the temperatures of the injectate and pulmonary artery blood are measured, cardiac output (actually, pulmonary blood flow) can be calculated. In contrast to the Fick method, the indicator-dilution method is least reliable when the cardiac output is low.

LEFT HEART CATHETERIZATION   Whether performed using the femoral, brachial, or radial approach, the left heart catheter is advanced under fluoroscopic guidance into the central aorta, where pressure is measured and recorded. Next, the catheter is advanced in retrograde fashion across the aortic valve into the left ventricle, where pressure is measured. If a right heart catheter is in place, this is an appropriate time for simultaneous measurement and recording of left heart, right heart, and peripheral arterial pressures together with a determination of cardiac output by either thermodilution or the Fick principle. These measures allow assessment of possible pressure gradients across the mitral and aortic valves, and catheter pullback on the right side permits assessment of possible gradients across the pulmonic and tricuspid valves. Simultaneous measurement of pressures and cardiac output provides the data for calculation of systemic and pulmonary vascular resistances. The resistance to blood flow through the systemic vascular bed is

$$SVR = 80(MAP - RA)/SBF$$

where *SVR* is systemic vascular resistance [(dyn·s)/cm^5], *MAP* and *RA* are mean aortic and right atrial pressures (mmHg), 80 is a constant for converting to metric units, and *SBF* is systemic blood flow (L/min). Resistance to blood flow through the pulmonary vascular bed is

$$PVR = 80(PA - PCW \text{ or } LA)/PBF$$

where *PVR* is pulmonary vascular resistance [(dyn·s)/cm^5]; *PA*, *PCW*, and *LA* are pulmonary artery, pulmonary capillary wedge, and left atrial mean pressures, respectively (mmHg); and *PBF* is pulmonary blood flow (L/min). Normal values for pulmonary and systemic vascular resistances are given in Table 228-3.

When valvular stenosis is present, the measurements of the upstream and downstream pressures and flow allow calculation of the valve orifice using the Gorlin formula.

$$A = flow/K\sqrt{\Delta P}$$

where *A* is the valve orifice area (cm^2), *flow* is the blood flow (mL/s) across the stenotic valve; ΔP is the mean pressure gradient (mmHg) during the period of blood flow; and *K* is a constant (44.3 for the aortic valve and 37.7 for the mitral valve).

As seen in Fig. 228-1, normal left ventricular and aortic pressures are essentially equal during systole, while normal left atrial (pulmonary capillary wedge) and left ventricular pressures are equal during diastole in the normal heart. The presence of a systolic pressure gradient between the left ventricle and aorta indicates obstruction at the level of the aortic valve (e.g., calcific *aortic stenosis*) or at subaortic level (e.g., *hypertrophic obstructive cardiomyopathy*). Similarly, the presence of a diastolic pressure gradient between the left atrium (or pulmonary capillary wedge pressure) and the left ventricle generally indicates *mitral stenosis*, although it may also be seen in rare conditions such as cor triatriatum and left atrial myxoma. An example of a large diastolic pressure gradient in a patient with mitral stenosis is seen in Fig. 228-2. As seen in Fig. 228-3, patients with significant mitral regurgitation may have a prominent *v* wave in the pulmonary capillary wedge pressure, which often increases substantially during modest exercise. Severe *aortic regurgitation* produces a widening of

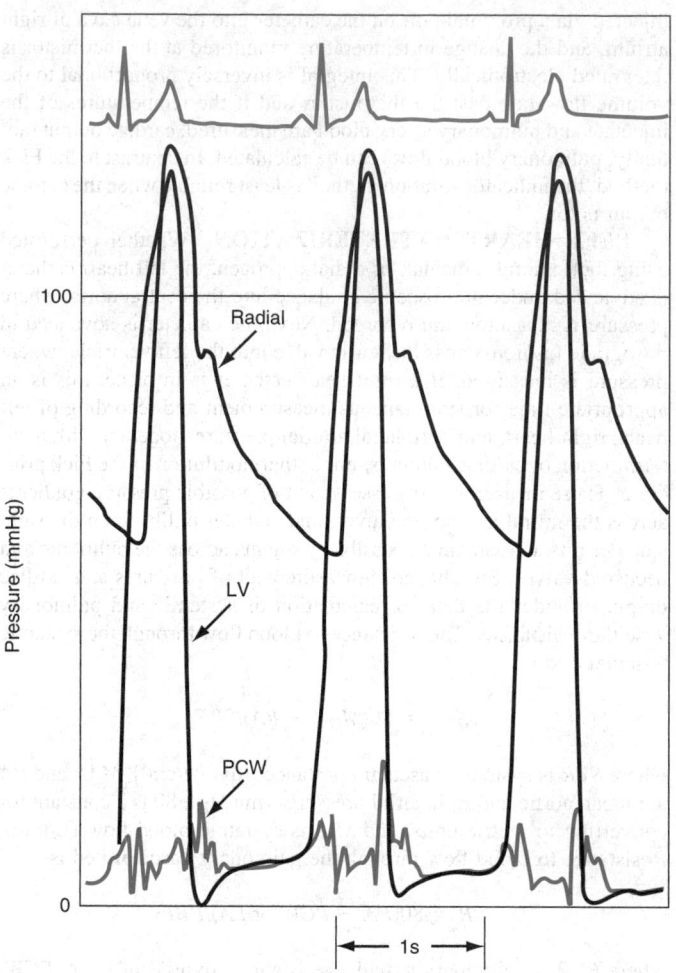

FIGURE 228-1 Left ventricular (LV), radial artery, and pulmonary capillary wedge (PCW) pressures in a patient with normal cardiovascular function. Note the absence of a pressure gradient between the LV and radial artery in systole and between the LV and PCW in diastole.

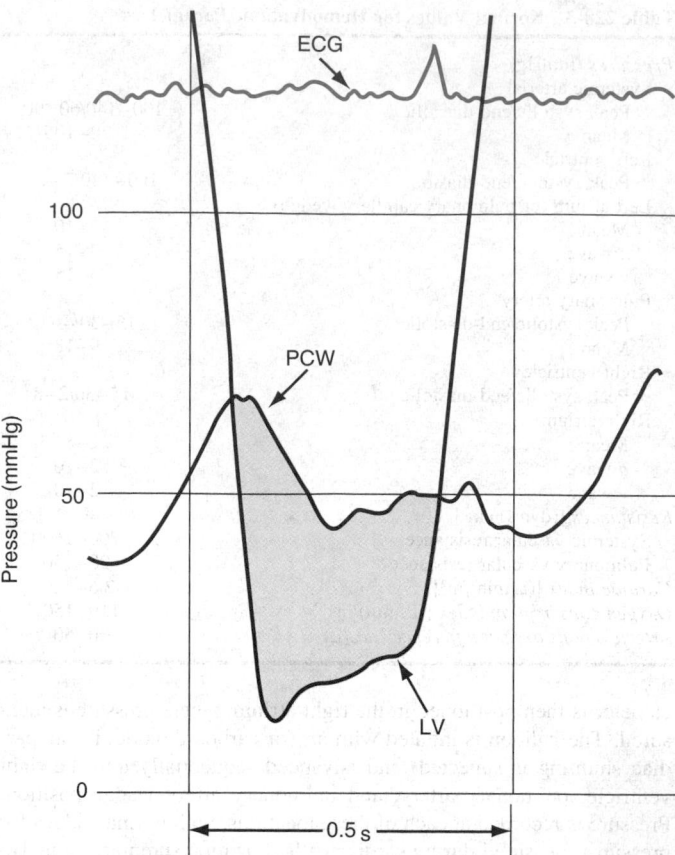

FIGURE 228-2 Pulmonary capillary wedge (PCW) and left ventricular (LV) pressure tracings in a 40-year-old woman with mitral stenosis. This patient also had systemic hypertension and significant elevation of her LV diastolic pressure. *[From BA Carabello, W Grossman, in Grossman's Cardiac Catheterization, Angiography, and Intervention, 6th ed, DS Baim, W Grossman (eds). Baltimore, Lippincott Williams & Wilkins, 2000.]*

the aortic pulse pressure, with equilibration of aortic and left ventricular pressures in diastole (Fig. 228-4). Right-sided pressures exhibit a characteristic deformity in the presence of valvular heart disease affecting the tricuspid or pulmonic valves. In patients with severe *tricuspid regurgitation*, the right atrial pressure resembles the right ventricular pressure closely in appearance. Mean right atrial pressure and right ventricular end-diastolic pressure are both elevated in tricuspid regurgitation. In *tricuspid stenosis*, there is a pressure gradient between the right atrium and ventricle during diastole.

Abnormalities in pressure waveforms may also be suggestive of conditions such as *cardiac tamponade* or *pericardial constriction* (Chap. 239). In both conditions there is equalization of left and right ventricular diastolic pressures. However, in constrictive pericarditis, nearly all ventricular filling occurs shortly after mitral and tricuspid valve opening; after this period of rapid filling, ventricular volumes cannot increase further owing to the constricting pericardium. This abnormality produces an abrupt early ventricular diastolic pressure rise with a mid- and late-ventricular pressure plateau, giving the so-called square root sign (Fig. 228-5). In contrast, in tamponade there is equalization of diastolic pressures with a gradual increase throughout diastole.

Congestive heart failure due to myocardial contractile dysfunction is associated with characteristic alterations in the ventricular pressure waveforms seen at cardiac catheterization. Neither the rise nor the decline in isovolumic pressure is as steep as in the normal heart. The reduced slopes of pressure rise and decline are associated with an

abbreviated ejection period, giving the left ventricular pressure tracing a triangular appearance (Fig. 228-6). Also, the pressure decline does not continue to zero, so the minimal left ventricular pressure may be elevated. This hemodynamic finding correlates with an increased ventricular end-systolic volume, which is a sign of depressed contractile function of the left ventricular myocardium.

CARDIAC ANGIOGRAPHY

LEFT VENTRICULOGRAPHY   Following the measurement of cardiac pressures, the angiographic portion of the cardiac catheterization usually begins with left ventriculography—the injection of radiographic contrast material directly into the left ventricular cavity. A power injector is used to inject 30 to 45 mL of radiographic contrast material into the left ventricular chamber at a rate of 10 to 12 mL/s. The resulting radiographic images are recorded, and the left ventricular silhouette is defined at end-diastole and end-systole. This permits calculation of the left ventricular chamber volumes and ejection fraction, as well as qualitative assessment of regional wall motion abnormalities. The normal left ventricle ejects 50 to 80% of its end-diastolic volume with each beat; i.e., its *ejection fraction* is 0.50 to 0.80. In adults, normal values for left ventricular volumes are, for end-diastolic volume, 72 ± 15 mL/m^2 (mean $\pm$ standard deviation) and, for end-systolic volume, 20 ± 8 mL/m^2. Regional abnormalities of wall motion are illustrated in Fig. 228-7 and include diminished inward motion of a myocardial segment (*hypokinesis*), absence of inward movement of a myocardial segment (*akinesis*), and paradoxical systolic expansion of a regional myocardial segment (*dyskinesis*).

Left ventriculography is usually performed in the right anterior oblique projection, which allows assessment of the mitral and aortic valves. Mitral regurgitation is easily visualized as the leakage of radiographic contrast material back into the left atrium during left ventricular systole. Its severity can be estimated qualitatively using a grading system of 1+ (mild; radiographic contrast material clears with each beat and never opacifies the entire left atrium) to 4+ (severe; opacification of the entire left atrium occurs within one beat, and contrast material can be seen refluxing into the pulmonary veins).

Left ventriculography performed in the *left* anterior oblique projection permits detection of abnormal communications, such as a ventricular septal defect (Chap. 234). In the most common form of hypertrophic cardiomyopathy (idiopathic hypertrophic subaortic stenosis; Chap. 238), left ventriculography in this projection shows anterior motion of the anterior leaflet of the mitral valve during systole and bulging of the interventricular septum into the left ventricular cavity, especially in the subaortic region. Mural thrombi within the left ventricular chamber may be well visualized during left ventriculography; they occur most commonly in the left ventricular apex.

AORTOGRAPHY Rapid injection of radiographic contrast material into the ascending aorta allows detection of abnormalities that involve the aorta and aortic valve. When suspected clinically, aortography permits detection and qualitative assessment of the severity of abnormalities such as aortic regurgitation, which is graded using a 1+ to 4+ scale, as for mitral regurgitation. Abnormal communications between the aorta and right side of the heart, such as a patent ductus arteriosus or ruptured aneurysm of a sinus of Valsalva, may be visualized. Aortography can permit identification of aortic aneurysm and of aortic dissection (Chap. 247) by visualizing an intimal flap within the aortic lumen.

CORONARY ANGIOGRAPHY This common procedure involves the selective injection of a radiographic contrast agent into the coronary arteries. Placement of the catheter tip into the right and left coronary arteries is carried out under fluoroscopic guidance, and contrast agent is injected by hand during recording of the radiographic image. Each coronary artery is usually viewed in several projections to permit assessment of the severity of stenosis and to minimize the overlap of adjacent vessels. In addition to the detection of coronary artery stenoses, coronary angiography is useful for the detection of congenital abnormalities of the coronary circulation, coronary arteriovenous fistulas, and patency of coronary artery bypass grafts. Examples of normal and abnormal coronary anatomy are shown in Figs. 228-8 and 228-9. The location, severity, and morphology of the stenotic lesions can be analyzed in great detail, and the resulting information is essential to planning either bypass surgery or catheter-based intervention (Fig. 228-10). This is usually done by visual estimation of percent diameter stenosis of each lesion relative to the "uninvolved" adjacent reference segment, with stenosis > 50% taken as being hemodynamically significant (interfering with maximal increases in perfusion of the subserved myocardial territory during stress).

POSTPROCEDURE CARE The average cardiac catheterization procedure takes between 30 and 45 min. Intravenous heparin (2000 to 3000 IU) may or may not be given at the time of catheter insertion. At the completion of the procedure, heparin may be reversed

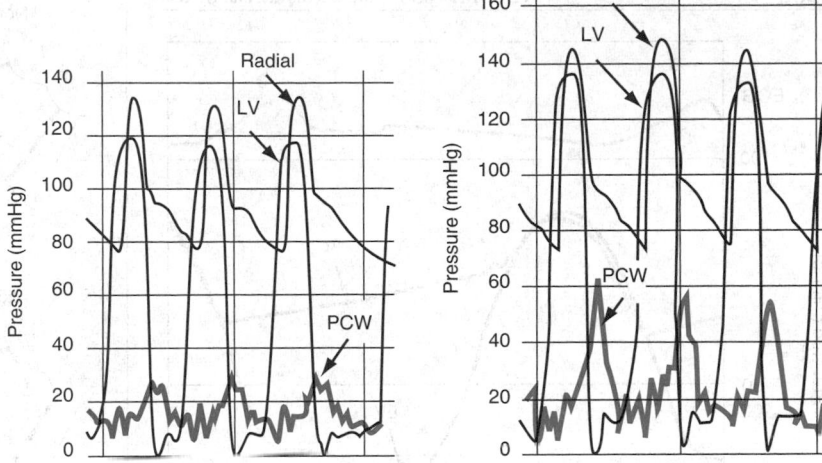

FIGURE 228-3 Hemodynamic findings at rest and during exercise in a patient with mitral regurgitation. Left ventricular (LV), pulmonary capillary wedge (PCW), and radial artery pressure tracings are shown before (*left*) and during (*right*) the sixth minute of supine bicycle exercise. PCW mean pressure and *v* wave increase substantially with exercise. [*From BH Lorell, W Grossman, in Grossman's Cardiac Catheterization, Angiography, and Intervention, 6th ed, DS Baim, W Grossman (eds). Baltimore, Lippincott Williams & Wilkins, 2000.*]

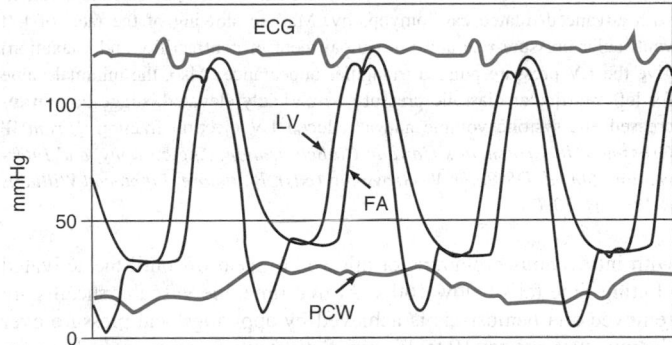

FIGURE 228-4 Severe aortic regurgitation. There is equilibration between the left ventricular (LV) and aortic or femoral artery (FA) pressures in diastole. Also, LV diastolic pressure exceeds pulmonary capillary wedge (PCW) pressure early in diastole, indicating premature closure of the mitral valve (a characteristic feature of severe aortic regurgitation). [*From W Grossman, in Grossman's Cardiac Catheterization, Angiography, and Intervention, 6th ed, DS Baim, W Grossman (eds). Baltimore, Lippincott Williams & Wilkins, 2000.*]

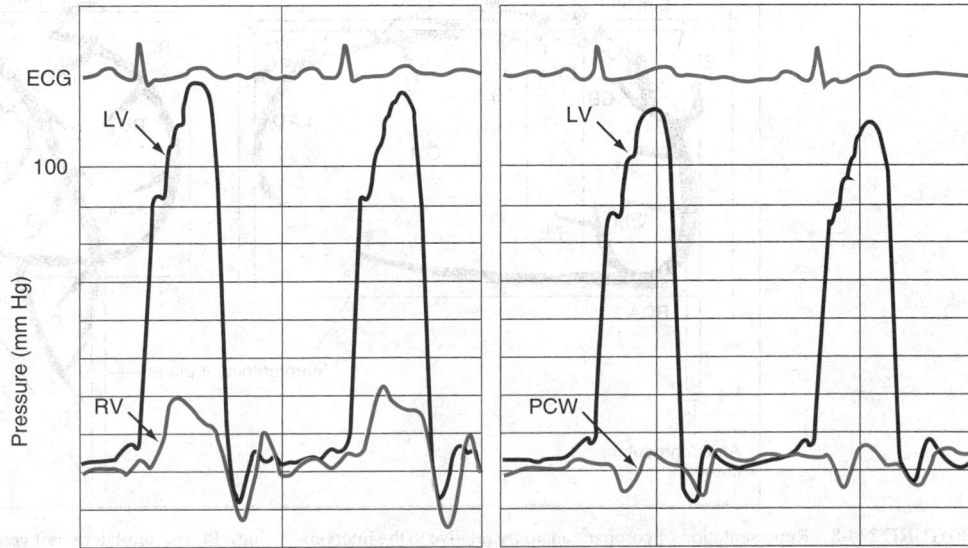

FIGURE 228-5 Left ventricular (LV), right ventricular (RV), and pulmonary capillary wedge (PCW) pressure tracings in a patient with severe constrictive pericarditis. Note the diastolic dip and plateau ("square root sign") pattern for left and right ventricular diastolic pressures (*left*). The wedge pressure (*right*) shows early systolic and early diastolic dips.

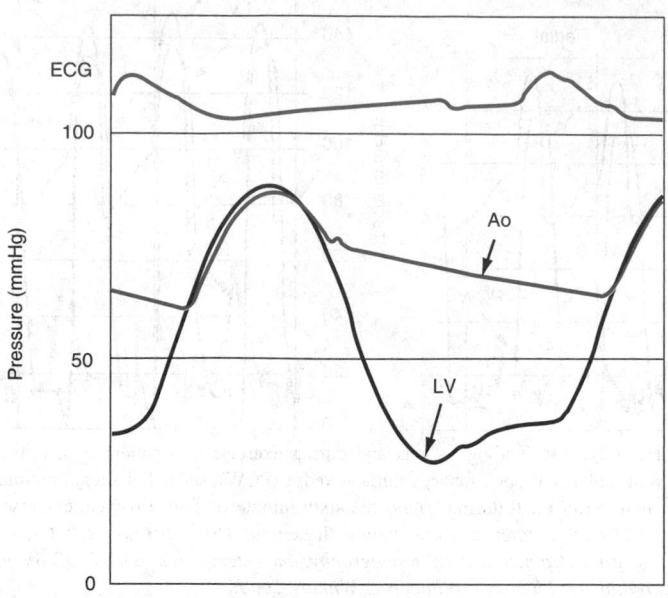

FIGURE 228-6   Left ventricular (LV) and aortic (Ao) pressures in a patient with advanced dilated cardiomyopathy. Marked slowing of the rates of left ventricular pressure rise and fall (impairment of contractility and relaxation) give the LV pressure pulse a triangular appearance. Also, the minimal value for left ventricular diastolic pressure is markedly elevated, suggesting an increased end-systolic volume and a reduced LV ejection fraction. *[From W Grossman, in Grossman's Cardiac Catheterization, Angiography, and Intervention, 6th ed, DS Baim, W Grossman (eds). Baltimore, Lippincott Williams & Wilkins, 2000.]*

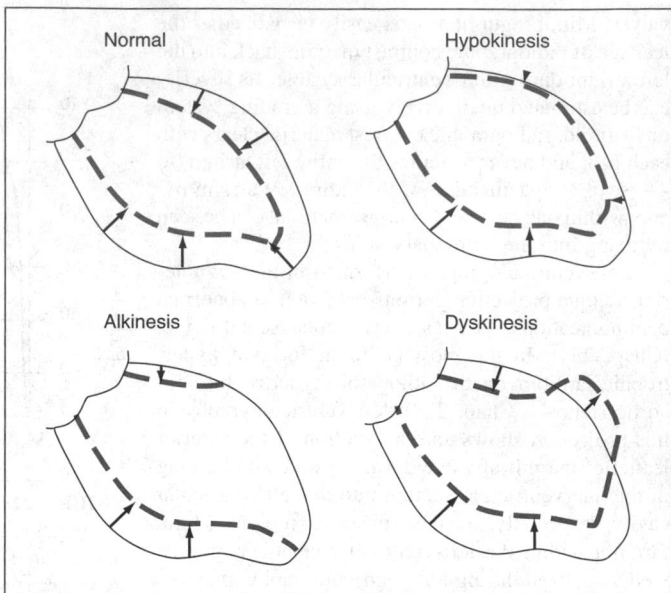

FIGURE 228-7   Diagrammatic representation of end-diastolic (*solid line*) and end-systolic (*dashed line*) silhouettes of left ventricular cineangiograms in various forms of localized wall motion disorder in patients with coronary heart disease. Normal wall motion is symmetric; a patient with *hypokinesis* exhibits reduced contraction, seen here over the anterior and apical surfaces; a patient with *akinesis* exhibits absent wall motion, seen here over the anteroapical surface; a patient with *dyskinesis* exhibits paradoxic bulging of a small portion of the anterior wall with systole.

with intravenous protamine or allowed to wear off until the activated clotting time falls below 160 s. At that time, the vascular sheaths are removed and hemostasis is achieved by applying local pressure over the puncture site for 10 to 15 min. Patients then remain at bed rest for

4 to 6 h before ambulating and being discharged to home. A variety of devices for sealing the arterial puncture site can allow a shorter period of bed rest and earlier ambulation. Patients with suitable anatomy may return at a later date for either catheter-based intervention or bypass surgery, although it is now common practice to perform a catheter-based intervention during the same procedure as the diagnostic cardiac catheterization, if appropriate.

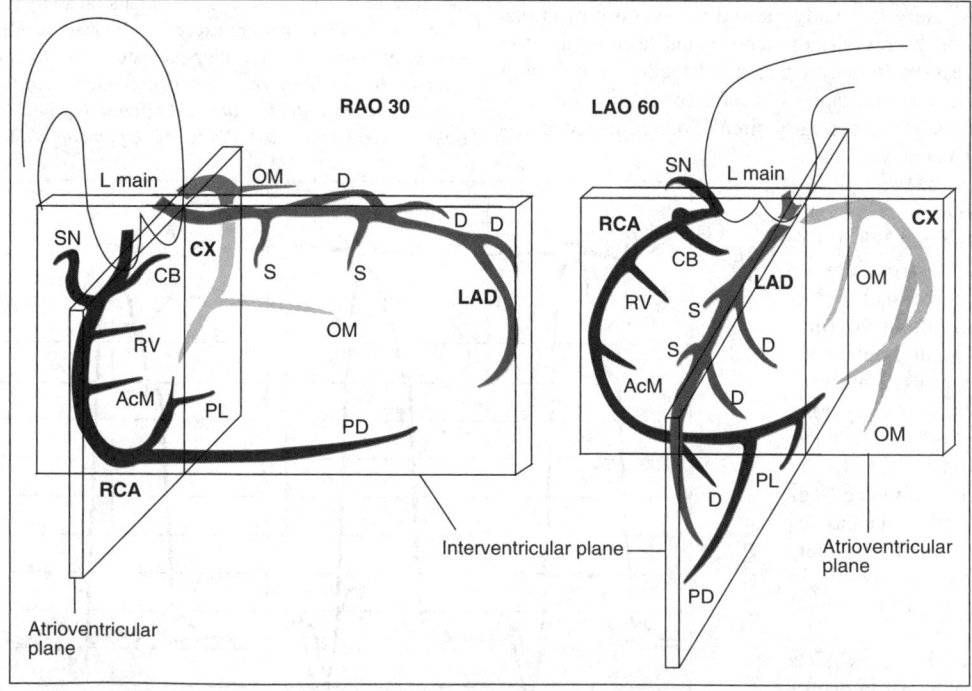

FIGURE 228-8   Representation of coronary anatomy relative to the interventricular and atrioventricular valve planes. Coronary branches are indicated as L Main (left main), LAD (left anterior descending), D (diagonal), S (septal), CX (circumflex), OM (obtuse marginal), RCA (right coronary artery), CB (conus branch), SN (sinus node), AcM (acute marginal), PD (posterior descend-

ing), PL (posterolateral left ventricular). RAO, right anterior oblique, LAO, left anterior oblique. *[From DS Baim, W Grossman, in Grossman's Cardiac Catheterization, Angiography, and Intervention, 6th ed, DS Baim, W Grossman (eds). Baltimore, Lippincott Williams & Wilkins, 2000.]*

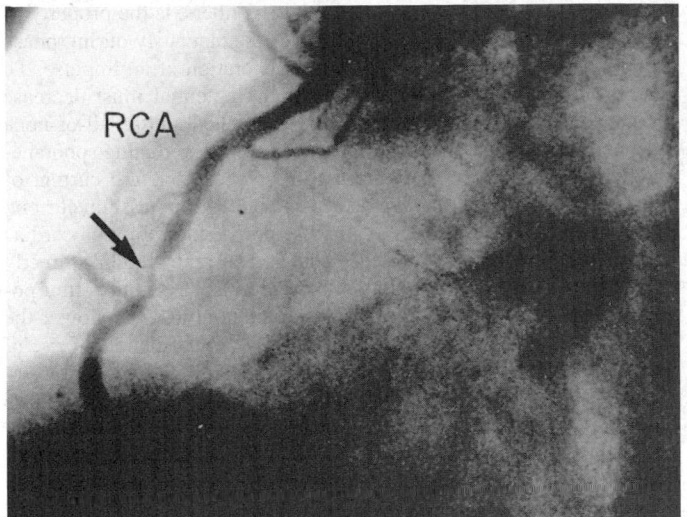

FIGURE 228-9　Coronary angiogram showing a right coronary artery (RCA) with a severe (95%) stenosis at its midpoint (*arrow*).

BIBLIOGRAPHY

BAIM DS, GROSSMAN W (eds): *Grossman's Cardiac Catheterization, Angiography, and Intervention,* 6th ed. Baltimore, Lippincott Williams & Wilkins, 2000

DAVIDSON CJ et al: Cardiac catheterization, in *Heart Disease,* 6th ed, E Braunwald (ed). Philadelphia, Saunders, 2001

JOHNSON LW, KRONE R: Cardiac catheterization 1991: A report of the Registry of the Society for Cardiac Angiography and Interventions (SCA&I). Cathet Cardiovasc Diagn 28:219, 1993

KERN MJ et al: Interpretation of cardiac pathophysiology from pressure waveform anal-

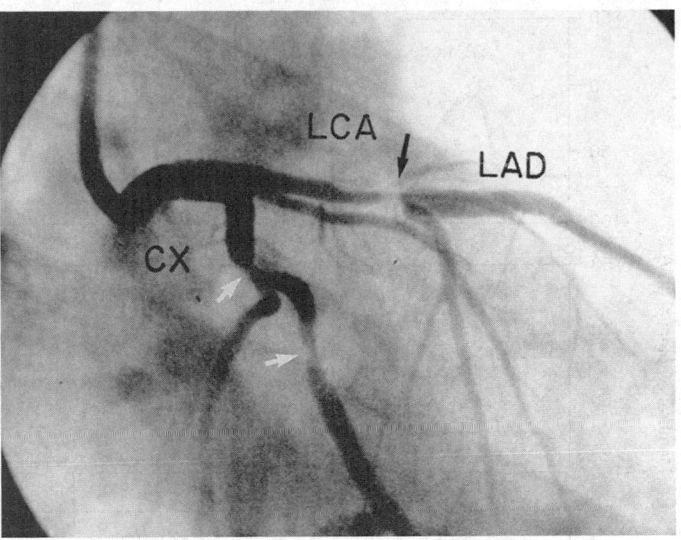

FIGURE 228-10　Coronary angiogram of a left coronary artery (LCA) with a tight stenosis in the proximal left anterior descending (LAD) artery (*black arrow*) immediately prior to the origin of a large septal branch. The circumflex artery (CX) has two moderately severe stenoses (*white arrows*).

ysis: Simultaneous left and right ventricular pressure measurements. Cathet Cardiovasc Diagn 28:51, 1993

SCANLON PJ et al: AHA/ACC guidelines or coronary angiography—executive summary and recommendations. Circulation 99:2345, 1999

Section 2
DISORDERS OF RHYTHM

229

Mark E. Josephson, Peter Zimetbaum

THE BRADYARRHYTHMIAS: DISORDERS OF SINUS NODE FUNCTION AND AV CONDUCTION DISTURBANCES

ANATOMY OF THE CONDUCTING SYSTEM　Under normal conditions, the pacemaker function of the heart resides in the sinoatrial (SA) node, which lies at the junction of the right atrium and superior vena cava. The SA node is approximately 1.5 cm long and 2 to 3 mm wide and is supplied by the sinus node artery, which arises from either the right coronary artery (60%) or the left circumflex coronary artery (40%). Once the impulse exits the sinus node and perinodal tissue, it traverses the atrium until it reaches the atrioventricular (AV) node. The blood supply of the AV node is derived from the posterior descending coronary artery (90%). The AV node lies at the base of the interatrial septum just above the tricuspid annulus and anterior to the coronary sinus. The electrophysiologic properties of the AV node result in slow conduction, which is responsible for the normal delay in AV conduction, i.e., the PR interval.

The bundle of His emerges from the AV node, enters the fibrous skeleton of the heart, and courses anteriorly across the membranous interventricular septum. It has a dual blood supply from the AV nodal artery and a branch of the anterior descending coronary artery. The branching (distal) portion of the bundle of His gives rise to a broad sheet of fibers that course over the left side of the interventricular septum to form the left bundle branch and a narrow cable-like structure on the right side that forms the right bundle branch. The arborization of both the right and left bundle branches gives rise to the distal His-Purkinje system, which ultimately extends throughout the endocardium of the right and left ventricles.

The SA node, atrium, and AV node are significantly influenced by autonomic tone. Vagal influences depress automaticity of the SA node, depress conduction, and prolong refractoriness in the tissue surrounding the SA node; inhomogeneously decrease atrial refractoriness and slow atrial conduction; and prolong AV nodal conduction and refractoriness. Sympathetic influences exert the opposite effect.

ELECTROPHYSIOLOGIC PRINCIPLES

In the resting state, the interior of most cardiac cells, with the exception of the SA and AV nodes, is approximately −80 to −90 mV, negative with respect to a reference extracellular electrode. The resting membrane potential is determined primarily by the concentration gradient of potassium across the cell membrane. Activation of cardiac cells results from movement of ions across the cell membrane, causing a transient depolarization known as the *action potential*. The ionic species responsible for the action potential varies among the cardiac tissues, and the configuration of the action potential is therefore unique to each tissue (Fig. 229-1).

The action potential of the His-Purkinje system and ventricular myocardium has five phases (Fig. 229-2). The rapid depolarizing current (phase 0) is mainly determined by an influx of sodium into my-

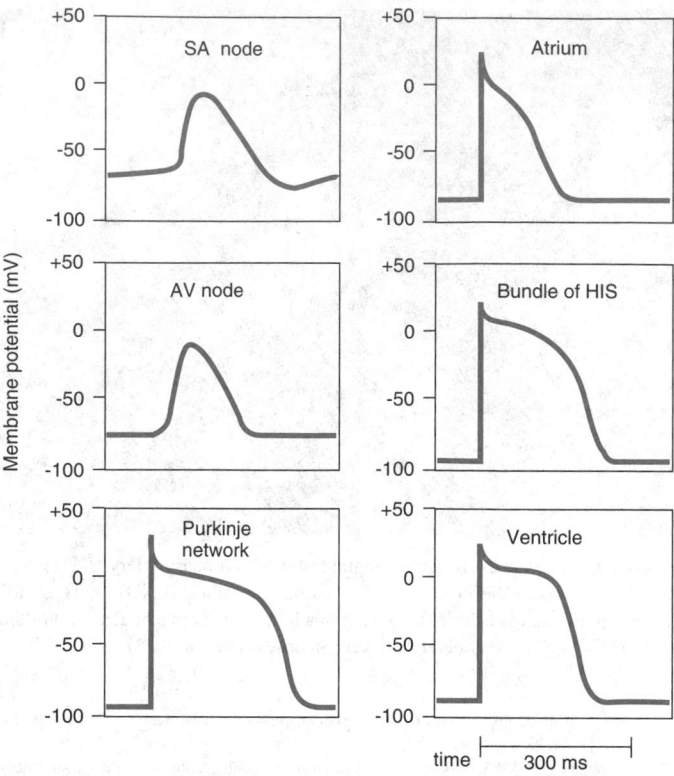

FIGURE 229-1   Action potential configurations in different regions of the mammalian heart. *(From AM Katz, Physiology of the Heart, 2e, New York, Raven, 1992, with permission.)*

ocardial cells followed by a secondary (slower) influx of calcium, which produces a slow inward current. The repolarization phases of the action potential (phases 1 to 3) are primarily related to outward flux of potassium. The resting membrane potential is phase 4.

The bradyarrhythmias result from abnormalities either of impulse formation, i.e., automaticity, or of conduction. *Automaticity,* which is normally observed in the sinus node, the specialized fibers of the His-

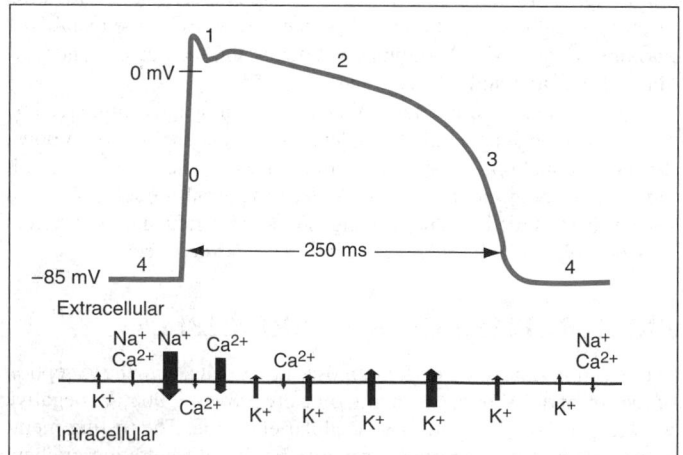

FIGURE 229-2   Schematic representation of the action potential in normal ventricle depicting the direction, strength, and period of flow of the ionic currents underlying the action potential. The arrow's direction and size indicate whether current is inward- or outward-directed and the approximate current strength of the ion identified at the arrow's base. The horizontal position of the arrow corresponds to the same moment in the time course of action potential (see text). The five phases of the action potential are indicated by the numerals placed along the waveform. *(From Ten Eick et al, Prog Cardiovasc Dis 24(2): 157, 1981, with permission.)*

Purkinje system, and some specialized atrial fibers, is the property of a cardiac cell that causes it to depolarize spontaneously during phase 4 of the action potential, leading to the generation of an impulse. To exhibit automaticity, the resting membrane potential must decrease spontaneously until threshold potential is reached and an all-or-none regenerative response occurs. The ionic currents producing spontaneous diastolic depolarization appear to involve the inward current of either sodium or calcium and a decreasing outward potassium current. The velocity of *conduction,* i.e., impulse propagation through cardiac tissues, depends on the magnitude of inward current, which is directly related to the rate of rise and amplitude of phase 0 of the action potential. The more positive the threshold potential and the slower the rate of depolarization toward threshold, the slower is the rate of rise of phase 0 of the action potential and the slower is the conduction velocity. Disease states or drugs may result in lower rates of rise of phase 0 at any given membrane potential. Passive membrane properties (e.g., intracellular resistance and intercellular coupling) can also affect impulse propagation. Propagation is more rapid parallel to fiber orientation than transverse to it, a property termed *anisotropic conduction.*

Refractoriness is a property of cardiac cells that defines the period of recovery that cells require after being discharged before they can be reexcited by a stimulus. The *absolute refractory period* is defined by that portion of the action potential during which no stimulus, regardless of its strength, can evoke another response. The *effective refractory period* is that part of the action potential during which a stimulus can evoke only a local, nonpropagated response. The *relative refractory period* extends from the end of the effective refractory period to the time that the tissue is fully recovered. During this time, a stimulus of greater than threshold strength is required to evoke a response, which is propagated more slowly than normal. In the normal His-Purkinje system or ventricular myocytes, excitability is recovered following completion of the action potential, and evoked responses have characteristics similar to the spontaneous normal response. In the AV node, recovery of excitability occurs well after completion of the action potential.

INTRACARDIAC RECORDINGS OF THE SPECIALIZED CONDUCTING SYSTEM   Electrode catheters allow the recording of activation of portions of the specialized conducting system, including the bundle of His. To obtain a recording from the bundle of His, the electrode catheter is positioned across the tricuspid valve (Fig. 229-3). The interval from local atrial depolarization in the His bundle recording to the onset of depolarization of the His bundle deflection is called the *AH interval* (normal = 60 to 125 ms) and represents an indirect method of assessing AV nodal conduction time. The interval from the beginning of the His bundle deflection to the earliest onset of ventricular activation, as measured from any of multiple-surface electrocardiogram (ECG) leads or the intracardiac ventricular electrogram, is called the *HV interval* (normal = 35 to 55 ms) and represents conduction time through the His-Purkinje system. Electrode catheters can be positioned in the area of the sinus node to record high right atrial activity. Left atrial activity may be recorded directly via a catheter placed across a patent foramen ovale or indirectly using a catheter inserted into the coronary sinus. The atrial activation sequence may be "mapped," and sites of intra- and interatrial conduction abnormalities may be ascertained.

SINUS NODE DYSFUNCTION

The SA node is normally the dominant cardiac pacemaker because its intrinsic discharge rate is the highest of all potential cardiac pacemakers. Its responsiveness to alterations in autonomic nervous system tone is responsible for the normal acceleration of heart rate during exercise and the slowing that occurs during rest and sleep. Increases in sinus rate normally result from an increase in sympathetic tone acting via β-adrenergic receptors and/or a decrease in parasympathetic tone acting via muscarinic receptors. Slowing of the heart rate is normally due to opposite alterations. In adults, the normal sinus rate under basal conditions is 60 to 100 beats per minute. *Sinus bradycardia* is said to exist when the sinus rate is less than 60 beats per minute, and *sinus*

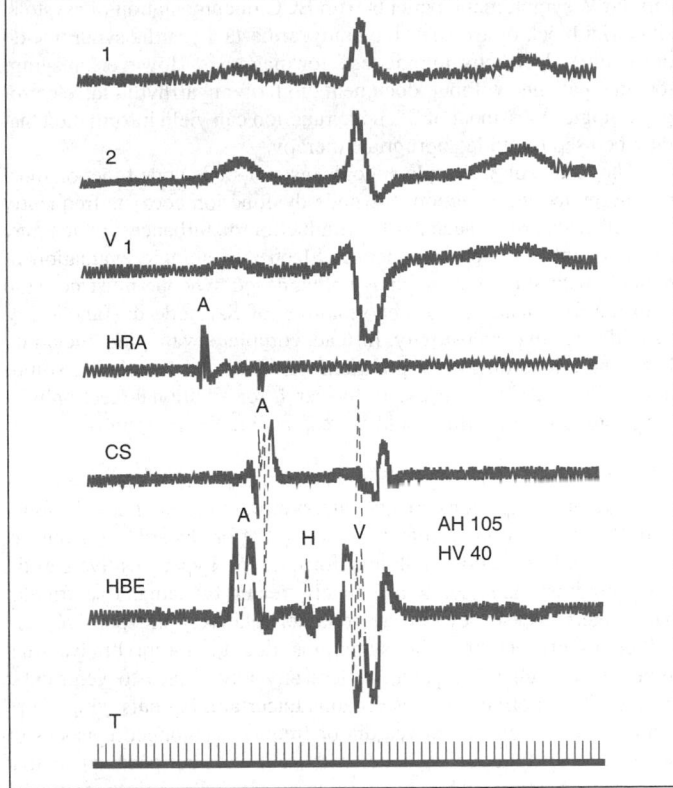

FIGURE 229-3 Normal intracardiac recording. Surface ECG leads I, II, and V₁ are displayed with intracardiac ECGs from the high right atrium (HRA), left atrium from the coronary sinus (CS), and AV junction to obtain a His bundle electrogram (HBE). T, time lines; A, atrial activation; H, His bundle activation; V, ventricular activation. Atrial activation begins in the HRA and spreads inferiorly to the low atrial septum, as recorded in the HBE, and the left atrium, as recorded in the CS. The AH and HV intervals represent AV nodal and His-Purkinje conduction times, respectively. Vertical lines = 0.10 s. *(From ME Josephson, SF Seides, Clinical Cardiac Electrophysiology: Techniques and Interpretations. Philadelphia, Lea & Febiger, 1979, with permission.)*

tachycardia when it exceeds 100 beats per minute. However, there is wide variation among individuals, and rates less than 60 beats per minute do not necessarily indicate pathologic states. For example, trained athletes often exhibit resting rates under 50 beats per minute due to increases in vagal tone. Normal elderly individuals may also show marked sinus bradycardia at rest.

ETIOLOGY SA node dysfunction is most often found in the elderly as an isolated phenomenon. Although interruption of the blood supply to the SA node may produce dysfunction, the correlation between obstruction of the sinus node artery and clinical evidence of SA node dysfunction is poor. Specific disease states associated with SA node dysfunction include senile amyloidosis and other conditions associated with infiltration of the atrial myocardium. Sinus bradycardia is associated with hypothyroidism, advanced liver disease, hypothermia, typhoid fever, and brucellosis; it occurs during episodes of hypervagotonia (vasovagal syncope), severe hypoxia, hypercapnia, acidemia, and acute hypertension. However, most cases of SA node dysfunction are due to idiopathic degeneration or are secondary to pharmacologic agents.

MANIFESTATIONS Although marked (≤50 beats per minute) sinus bradycardia may cause fatigue and other symptoms due to inadequate cardiac output, more commonly sinus node dysfunction is manifest as paroxysmal dizziness, presyncope, or syncope.

These symptoms usually result from abrupt, prolonged sinus pauses caused by failure of sinus impulse formation (sinus arrest) or block of conduction of sinus impulses to the surrounding atrial tissue (sinus exit block). In either case, the ECG manifestation is a prolonged period (>3 s) of atrial asystole. In some patients, SA node dysfunction is accompanied by abnormalities in AV conduction. In addition to the absence of atrial activity, lower pacemakers fail to emerge during the sinus pauses, resulting in periods of ventricular asystole and syncope. Occasionally, SA node dysfunction is manifested by an inadequate acceleration in sinus rate in response to a stress such as exercise or fever. In some patients, SA node dysfunction may become manifest only in the presence of certain cardioactive drugs: cardiac glycosides, β-adrenergic blocking drugs, calcium channel blockers, amiodarone, and other antiarrhythmic agents. These agents, which do not usually cause sinus node dysfunction in normal people, may unmask evidence of sinus node dysfunction in susceptible individuals.

The *sick sinus syndrome* refers to a combination of symptoms (dizziness, confusion, fatigue, syncope, and congestive heart failure) caused by SA node dysfunction and manifested by marked sinus bradycardia, sinoatrial block, or sinus arrest. Because these symptoms are nonspecific, and because ECG manifestations of sinus node dysfunction are often intermittent, it may be difficult to prove that such symptoms are actually caused by SA node dysfunction.

Atrial tachyarrhythmias such as atrial fibrillation, atrial flutter, or atrial tachycardia may be accompanied by SA node dysfunction. The *bradycardia-tachycardia syndrome* refers to paroxysmal atrial arrhythmia that upon termination is followed by prolonged sinus pauses (Fig. 229-4) or in which there are alternating periods of tachyarrhythmia and bradyarrhythmia. Syncope or presyncope may result from failure of the sinus node to recover function following suppression of automaticity by atrial tachyarrhythmia.

DIAGNOSIS *First-degree sinoatrial exit block* denotes a prolonged conduction time from the SA node to the surrounding atrial tissue. It cannot be recognized on a standard (surface) ECG but requires invasive intracardiac recordings, which can detect this condition indirectly, by measuring the sinus response to atrial premature beats, or directly, by recording SA node electrograms. *Second-degree sinoatrial exit block* denotes the intermittent failure of conduction of sinus impulses to the surrounding atrial tissue; it is manifested as the intermittent absence of P waves (Fig. 229-5). *Third-degree*, or *complete, sinoatrial block* is characterized by a lack of atrial activity or by the presence of an ectopic subsidiary atrial pacemaker. On the standard ECG it cannot be distinguished from sinus arrest, but direct intracardiac recordings of SA node activity permit this distinction. The *bradycardia-tachycardia syndrome* is manifested on the standard ECG as tachyarrhythmias (Fig. 229-4). Most often these are atrial flutter or fibrillation, although any tachycardia during which the atria are activated may cause overdrive suppression of the sinus node resulting in clinical appearance of this syndrome.

The most important step in the diagnosis is to correlate symptoms with ECG evidence of SA node dysfunction. While ambulatory ECG (Holter) monitoring remains a mainstay in evaluating sinus node function, most episodes of syncope are paroxysmal and unpredictable. Sin-

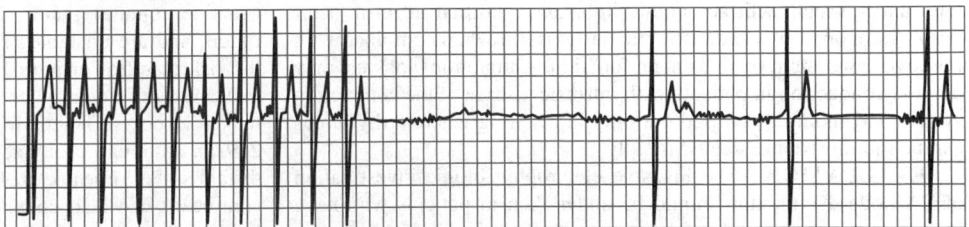

FIGURE 229-4 Tachycardia-bradycardia syndrome. Rhythm strip of ECG lead II showing spontaneous cessation of supraventricular tachycardia followed by a 6-s pause prior to resumption of sinus activity. The patient was asymptomatic during supraventricular tachycardia, but the sinus pause caused severe light-headedness.

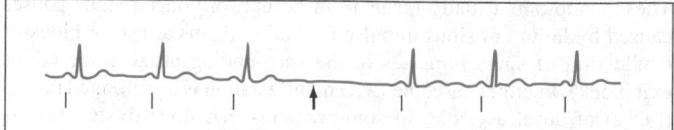

FIGURE 229-5   Second-degree sinoatrial exit block. Surface ECG denoting abrupt absence of P wave during sinus rhythm. Prior to the pause, the sinus rate is regular. The interval of the pause is exactly twice the basal sinus cycle length. The arrow marks the appropriate location for the absent P wave. SA exit block can be 2:1 as above or longer, as shown in Fig. 229-6.

gle and even multiple 24-h Holter monitor recordings may fail to include a symptomatic episode.

Caution must be taken in interpreting the Holter monitor results. For instance, a pause during sleep is often a normal finding associated with heightened vagal tone. This should not be interpreted as sinus node dysfunction requiring pacemaker implantation.

Continuous-loop event records represent a more specific diagnostic tool. These devices may be worn for prolonged periods of time and allow close correlation between electrocardiographic findings and symptoms. They do require the patient's ability to activate the monitor at the time of symptoms. More recently, an implantable event recorder, which can be interrogated like a pacemaker, has been developed for patients with rare events.

The response to carotid sinus pressure and pharmacologic autonomic "denervation" of the heart may be helpful. Carotid sinus pressure can be particularly useful in patients in whom paroxysmal dizziness or syncope is compatible with the hypersensitive carotid sinus syndrome (Chap. 21). In such patients, the response can be dramatic, and sinus pauses in excess of 5 s may occur. Although pauses in excess of 3 s are considered abnormal, in elderly patients such pauses are common and do not necessarily signify a diagnostic response. This is a major limitation of the use of carotid sinus pressure as a diagnostic test in the elderly. The other noninvasive test of SA node function involves the use of pharmacologic agents to manipulate the autonomic nervous system and assess the balance of parasympathetic and sympathetic activity on the sinus node. Physiologic or pharmacologic maneuvers that are vagomimetic (Valsalva maneuver or phenylephrine-induced hypertension), vagolytic (atropine), sympathomimetic (isoproterenol or hypotension by nitroprusside), or sympatholytic (β-adrenergic blocking agents) can be utilized, singly and in combination. These studies are designed to test the response of the sinus node to autonomic stimulation and inhibition and thereby characterize the status of autonomic regulation of the sinus node. Abnormalities of the autonomic control of sinus function are particularly common in patients in whom asymptomatic sinus bradycardia is documented.

Intrinsic Heart Rate   This is a manifestation of the primary activity of the SA node, and its determination requires chemical autonomic blockade of the heart with a combination of atropine and a beta blocker. Normal values of intrinsic heart rate (in beats per minute) are calculated by the formula $118.1 - (0.57 \times \text{age})$. The use of autonomic blockade can separate patients with asymptomatic sinus bradycardia into a group with primary sinus node dysfunction (slow intrinsic heart rate) and a group with autonomic imbalance (normal intrinsic heart rate). Autonomic blockade is particularly useful when combined with invasive assessment of sinus node function. Autonomic blockade may depress conduction in patients with intrinsic disease of the conduction system and should be carried out only in a setting where arrhythmias can be monitored and treated rapidly.

EVALUATION   The invasive electrophysiologic investigation of SA node dysfunction should be undertaken in patients who have had symptoms compatible with SA node dysfunction and in whom no documentation of the arrhythmia responsible for these symptoms has been obtained by prolonged Holter monitoring. Asymptomatic patients with sinus bradycardia need *not* be tested, since no therapy is indicated.

Similarly, symptomatic patients with ECG documentation of asystole, sinoatrial block or arrest, or the bradycardia-tachycardia syndrome do not require electrophysiologic tests for diagnosis. However, in symptomatic patients without documentation of an arrhythmia, electrophysiologic assessment of SA node function can yield information that may be used to guide appropriate therapy.

The results of electrophysiologic tests of sinus node function must be interpreted with caution. SA node dysfunction coexists frequently with other disorders such as AV conduction disturbances, which may cause symptoms such as syncope. Electrophysiologic evaluation of patients with symptoms such as undiagnosed syncope must not stop with the demonstration of abnormalities of SA node dysfunction or carotid sinus hypersensitivity. Instead, complete evaluation, including His bundle recordings and programmed atrial and ventricular stimulation (Chap. 230), is necessary to search for additional electrophysiologic abnormalities that could be responsible for symptoms.

TREATMENT   Permanent pacemakers (p. 1290) are the mainstay of therapy for patients with symptomatic SA node dysfunction. Patients with intermittent paroxysms of bradycardia or sinus arrest and with the cardioinhibitory form of the hypersensitive carotid sinus syndrome are usually adequately treated by demand ventricular pacemakers. These devices are reliable, relatively inexpensive, and suffice to prevent episodic symptoms due to abrupt bradycardia. Whether dual-chamber pacing offers any advantages to ventricular pacing in such circumstances remains uncertain. Patients with symptomatic chronic sinus bradycardia or frequent prolonged episodes of sinus node dysfunction do better with dual-chamber pacemakers that preserve the normal AV activation sequence. Although theoretically an atrial demand pacemaker should be adequate for patients with SA node dysfunction, the frequent accompaniment of dysfunction in other portions of the cardiac conduction system usually mandates placement of a pacemaker capable of ventricular pacing. Recent studies suggest that AV sequential pacing may also be useful in preventing atrial fibrillation, an important component of the bradycardia-tachycardia syndrome.

AV CONDUCTION DISTURBANCES

The specialized cardiac conducting system normally ensures synchronous conduction of each sinus impulse from the atria to the ventricles. Abnormalities of conduction of the sinus impulse to the ventricles may portend the development of heart block, which can ultimately lead to syncope or cardiac arrest. In order to evaluate the clinical significance of conduction abnormalities, the physician must assess (1) the site of conduction disturbance, (2) the risk of progression to complete block, and (3) the probability that a subsidiary escape rhythm arising distal to the site of block will be electrophysiologically and hemodynamically stable. This latter point is perhaps the most important, since the rate and stability of the escape pacemaker determine what symptoms result from heart block. The escape pacemaker following AV nodal block is usually in the His bundle, which generally has a stable rate of 40 to 60 beats per minute and is associated with a QRS complex of normal duration (in the absence of a preexisting intraventricular conduction defect). This contrasts with escape rhythms arising in the distal His-Purkinje system, which have lower intrinsic rates (25 to 45 beats per minute), manifest wide QRS complexes with prolonged duration, and are unstable. Thus, the most important issue is to assess the risk of infra- or intra-His block (which always mandates a pacemaker) or AV nodal block in which the frequency of the escape pacemaker is not sufficient to meet hemodynamic requirements (Table 229-1). Although prolonged QRS complexes are invariable when the distal His-Purkinje pacemakers form the escape mechanism, wide QRS complexes can also coexist with AV nodal block and a His bundle rhythm. Therefore, QRS morphology alone may not be adequate to identify the site of block.

ETIOLOGY   The AV node is supplied by the parasympathetic and sympathetic nervous systems and is sensitive to variations in au-

1. Atrial activation times: Measurement of intraatrial conduction times. Prolonged activation times may be associated with atrial flutter or fibrillation.
2. Measurement of AH and HV intervals: Prolongation of AH interval (>125 ms) or prolongation of the HV interval (>55 ms) may help localize the site of delay.
3. Incremental atrial pacing: To determine the cycle length at which block occurs in the AV node and/or His-Purkinje system. Block below the His bundle at rates of <150 beats per minute portends the development of infra-His block.

tonomic tone. Chronic slowing of AV nodal conduction may be seen in highly trained athletes who have hypervagotonia at rest. A variety of diseases and drugs can also influence AV nodal conduction. These include acute processes such as myocardial infarction (particularly inferior), coronary spasm (usually of the right coronary artery), digitalis intoxication, excesses of beta and/or calcium blockers, acute infections such as viral myocarditis, acute rheumatic fever, infectious mononucleosis, and miscellaneous disorders such as Lyme disease, sarcoidosis, amyloidosis, and neoplasms, particularly cardiac mesotheliomas. AV nodal block may also be congenital.

Two degenerative diseases are commonly responsible for damage to the specialized conducting system and produce AV block usually associated with bundle branch block (Chap. 226). In *Lev's disease*, there is calcification and sclerosis of the fibrous cardiac skeleton, which frequently involves the aortic and mitral valves, the central fibrous body, and the summit of the ventricular septum. *Lenegre's disease* appears to be a primary sclerodegenerative disease within the conducting system itself with no involvement of the myocardium or the fibrous skeleton of the heart. These two diseases are probably the most common causes of isolated chronic heart block in adults. Hypertension and aortic and/or mitral stenosis are specific disorders that either accelerate the degeneration of the conducting system or have a direct effect by calcification and fibrosis involving the conducting system.

First-degree AV block, more properly termed *prolonged AV conduction*, is classically characterized by a PR interval >0.20 s, but use of this value may be misleading in terms of clinical significance. Since the PR interval is determined by atrial, AV nodal, and His-Purkinje activation, delay in any one or more of these structures can contribute to a prolonged PR interval. In the presence of a QRS complex of normal duration, a PR interval >0.24 s almost invariably is due to a delay within the AV node. If the QRS is prolonged, delays may be present at any of the levels mentioned above. Delay within the His-Purkinje system is always accompanied by a prolonged QRS duration but can occur with a relatively normal PR interval (Fig. 229-6). However, as indicated below, it is only with intracardiac recordings that the exact site of delay can be determined.

Second-degree heart block (intermittent AV block) is present when some atrial impulses fail to conduct to the ventricles. Mobitz type I second-degree AV block (AV Wenckebach block) is characterized by progressive PR interval prolongation prior to block of an atrial impulse (Fig. 229-7A). The pause that follows is less than fully compensatory (i.e., is less than two normal sinus intervals), and the PR interval of the first conducted impulse is shorter than the last conducted atrial impulse prior to the blocked P wave. Usually the difference between the longest and shortest PR intervals exceeds 100 ms. This type of block is almost always localized to the AV node and associated with a normal QRS duration, although bundle branch block may be present. It is seen most often as a transient abnormality with inferior wall infarction or with drug intoxication, particularly digitalis, beta blockers, and occasionally calcium channel antagonists. This type of block can also be observed in normal individuals with heightened vagal tone. Although Mobitz type I block can progress to complete heart block, this is uncommon, except in the setting of acute inferior wall myocardial infarction. Even when it does, however, the heart block is usually well tolerated because the escape pacemaker usually arises in the

proximal His bundle and provides a stable rhythm. As a result, the presence of Mobitz type I second-degree AV block rarely mandates aggressive therapy. Therapeutic decisions depend on the ventricular response and the symptoms of the patient. If the ventricular rate is adequate and the patient is asymptomatic, observation is sufficient.

In Mobitz type II second-degree AV block, conduction fails suddenly and unexpectedly without a preceding change in PR intervals (Fig. 229-7B). It is generally due to disease of the His-Purkinje system and is most often associated with a prolonged QRS duration. When Mobitz type II block occurs with a normal QRS duration, an intra-His site of block should be expected (Fig. 229-7C). It is important to recognize this type of block because it has a high incidence of progression to complete heart block with an unstable, slow, lower escape pacemaker. Therefore, pacemaker implantation is necessary in this condition. Mobitz type II block may occur in the setting of anteroseptal infarction or in the primary or secondary sclerodegenerative or calcific disorders of the fibrous skeleton of the heart. In so-called high-degree AV block there are periods of two or more consecutively blocked P waves, but intermittent conduction can be demonstrated. Block is usually in the His-Purkinje system, but simultaneous block in the AV node may also be present. Regardless of the site of origin of the escape rhythm, if it is slow and the patient is symptomatic, a cardiac pacemaker is mandatory.

Third-degree AV block is present when no atrial impulse propagates to the ventricles. If the QRS complex of the escape rhythm is of normal duration, occurs at a rate of 40 to 55 beats per minute, and increases with atropine or exercise, AV nodal block is probable. Congenital complete AV block is usually localized to the AV node. If the block is within the His bundle, the escape pacemaker is usually less responsive to these perturbations. If the escape rhythm of the QRS is wide and associated with rates ≤40 beats per minute, block is usually localized in, or distal to, the His bundle and mandates a pacemaker, since the escape rhythm in this setting is unreliable (Fig. 229-8). Some patients with infra-His bundle block are capable of retrograde conduction. In such patients, a "pacemaker syndrome" (see below) may develop if a simple ventricular pacemaker is used. Dual-chamber pacemakers eliminate this potential problem.

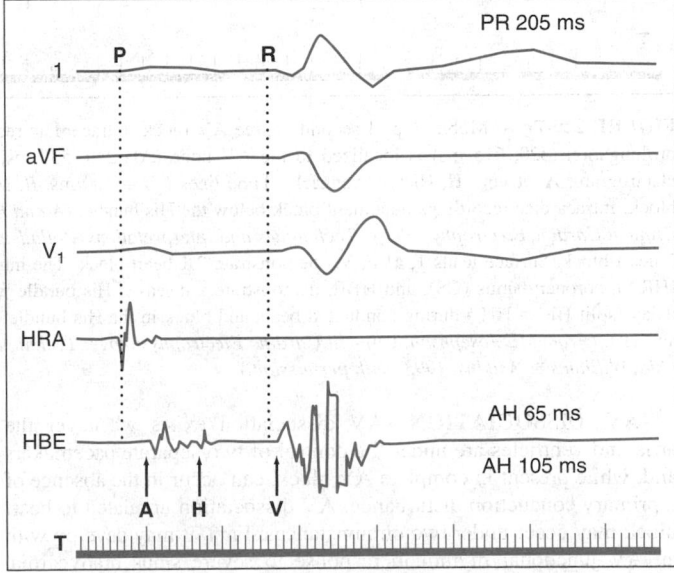

FIGURE 229-6 Example of marked His-Purkinje system disease with a relatively normal PR interval. Surface leads I, aVF, and V_1 are shown with electrograms from the high right atrium (HRA), His bundle electrogram (HBE), and time lines (T). The QRS shows right bundle branch block and left anterior hemiblock; the PR interval is minimally elevated at 205 ms, but the HV interval exceeds 100 ms. Such a prolonged HV interval mandates a pacemaker.

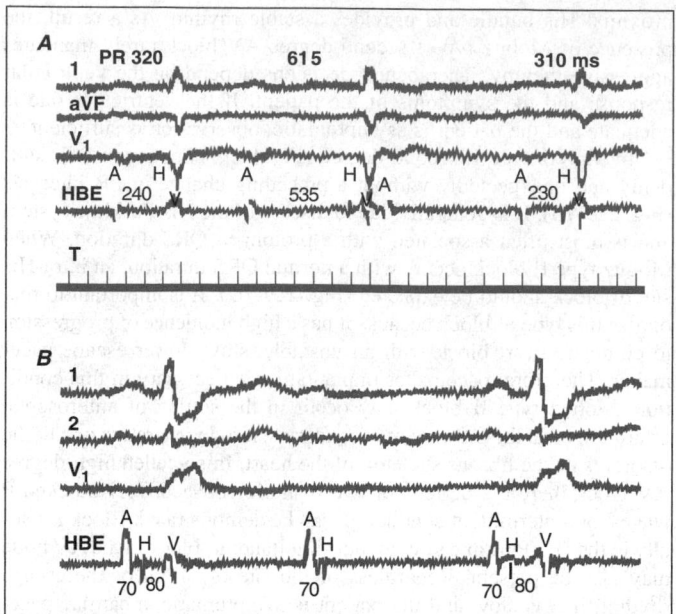

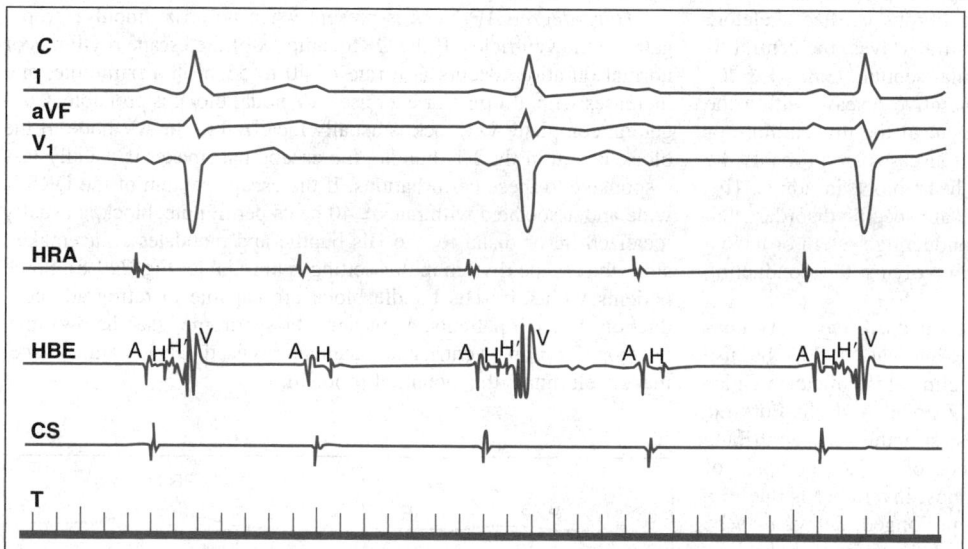

FIGURE 229-7 *A.* Mobitz type I second-degree AV block. Intracardiac recordings demonstrate that the PR prolongation (320, 615 ms) is localized to the AV node (AH 240, 535 ms, respectively). HBE, His bundle electrogram; A, atrium; H, His; V, ventricle. Time lines (T) = 100 ms. *B.* Mobitz type II second-degree AV block. Intracardiac recordings document block below the His bundle. *(A and B from ME Josephson, SF Seides, Clinical Cardiac Electrophysiology: Techniques and Interpretations. Philadelphia, Lea & Febiger, 1979.) C.* 2: 1 heart block. Surface leads 1, aVF, V$_1$, demonstrate 2:1 heart block. The intracardiac leads, high right atrium (HRA), coronary sinus (CS), and HBE, demonstrate a diseased His bundle with marked intra-His conduction delay (split-His = HH′) during conducted beats and block in the His bundle every other beat (i.e., between H and H′). *(From ME Josephson, Clinical Cardiac Electrophysiology: Techniques and Interpretations. Philadelphia, Williams & Wilkins, 1993, with permission.)*

escape rhythm is slow and results in symptoms. Second, AV dissociation can be caused by an enhanced lower (junctional or ventricular) pacemaker that competes with normal sinus rhythm and frequently exceeds it. This has been called *interference AV dissociation* because the rapid lower pacemaker results in bombardment of the AV node in a retrograde fashion, rendering it refractory to the normal sinus impulses. Thus failure of antegrade conduction is a physiologic response in this circumstance. Interference dissociation commonly occurs during ventricular tachycardia, accelerated junctional or ventricular rhythms seen with digitalis intoxication, myocardial ischemia and/or infarction, or local irritation following cardiac surgery. The accelerated rhythm should be treated with either antiarrhythmic drugs (Chap. 230), removal of an offending drug, or correction of the metabolic abnormality or ischemia.

INTRACARDIAC ELECTROCARDIOGRAPHIC RE-CORDINGS IN DIAGNOSIS AND MANAGEMENT The main therapeutic decision in patients with AV conduction disturbance is whether or not a permanent pacemaker is required, and a number of circumstances exist in which His bundle electrocardiography can be a useful diagnostic tool upon which to base this decision. It is unquestionable that patients with *symptomatic* second- or third-degree AV block should be paced, and therefore, these patients do not require electrophysiologic study. However, intracardiac ECG recordings can be useful in at least the following four groups of patients:

1. *Patients with syncope and bundle branch or bifascicular block without documentation of AV block.* In such patients, the demonstration of marked infra-His bundle conduction disturbances, i.e., a prolonged HV interval (>100 ms), may usually be taken as an indication of the need for the insertion of the permanent pacemaker. Complete electrophysiologic evaluation, including atrial and ventricular programmed stimulation, is indicated to help identify other possible cardiac etiologies for the syncope. Since the incidence of significant advanced AV block is low in *asymptomatic* patients who have bifascicular block, electrophysiologic evaluation or permanent pacemakers are not cost-effective. In this group, observation appears most reasonable.

2. *Patients with 2:1 AV conduction.* Intracardiac recordings are necessary to ascertain the site of the conduction disturbance because the typical ECG features of Mobitz type I or Mobitz type II block cannot be discerned during a 2:1 pattern of AV conduction on the surface ECG. Intracardiac recordings may demonstrate that AV nodal block, intra-His bundle block, infra-His bundle block, or combinations of block may be responsible (Figs. 229-7 and 229-8). A surface ECG finding that suggests an infra-His bundle lesion is the presence of alternating bundle branch block associated with changing PR intervals. Intracardiac recordings in such patients confirm that the block is almost always in the His-Purkinje system. Increasing block with exercise or following atropine suggests intra- or infra-His block (Table 229-2). The finding of infra- or intra-His bundle block in patients with asymptomatic second-degree AV block mandates pacemaker therapy because of the high likelihood of the development of symptomatic high-grade AV block and syncope.

3. *Patients with Wenckebach block in the presence of bundle branch block.* This situation, particularly when the maximal change in PR interval is ≤ 50 ms, can suggest intra- or infra-His Wenckebach

AV DISSOCIATION AV dissociation exists whenever the atria and ventricles are under the control of two separate pacemakers and, while present in complete AV block, can occur in the absence of a primary conduction disturbance. AV dissociation unrelated to heart block may occur under two circumstances: First, it may develop with an AV junctional rhythm in response to severe sinus bradycardia. When the sinus rate and the escape rate are similar and the P waves occur just before, in, or following the QRS complex, *isorhythmic AV dissociation* is said to be present. Treatment usually consists of removal of the offending cause of sinus bradycardia (i.e., discontinuation of digitalis, beta blockers, or calcium antagonists), accelerating the sinus node by vagolytic agents, or insertion of a pacemaker if the

block, in which case a pacemaker is mandated. Intracardiac recordings are necessary to make this diagnosis.

4. *Asymptomatic patients with third-degree AV block*. In such patients, electrophysiologic studies may be useful in assessing the stability of the junctional pacemaker. Pacing is indicated when the His bundle escape pacemaker is shown to be unstable by an inadequate response to exercise, atropine, or isoproterenol or by a prolonged junctional recovery time following ventricular pacing.

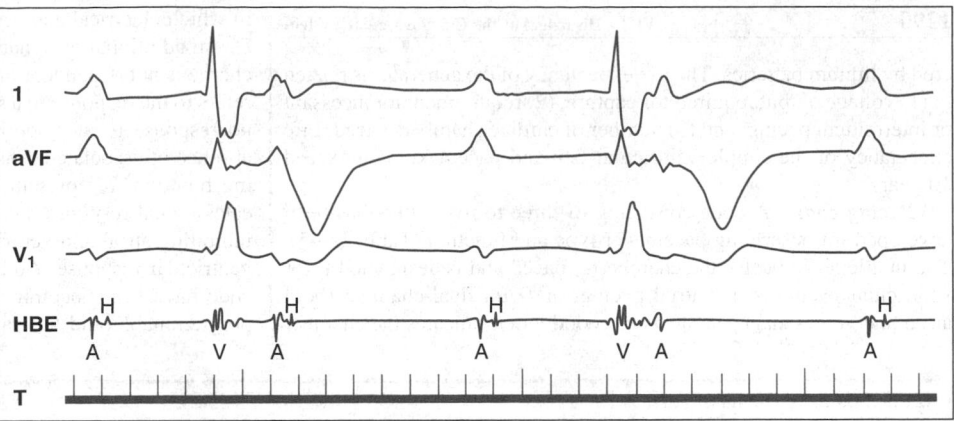

FIGURE 229-8 Third-degree AV block. The figure shows surface leads 1, aVF, V₁, and an intracardiac His bundle recording (HBE). Complete heart block is evident on the surface leads. The intracardiac recording demonstrates an absence of QRS deflection (V) after a His bundle (H) spike. This indicates block below the His bundle. Note that following the second QRS complex (V), there is an atrial (A) deflection indicating retrograde conduction. Retrograde conduction is often present when block is in the His-Purkinje system but is virtually never present when block is in the AV node. *(From ME Josephson, Clinical Cardiac Electrophysiology: Techniques and interpretations, Philadelphia, Williams & Wilkins, 1993.)*

GENETIC CONSIDERATIONS

A number of congenital and familial syndromes involving the cardiac conduction system have been described. An example of a congenital condition that is transmitted but not genetic is congenital complete heart block associated with material systemic lupus erythematosus. This disorder is associated with maternal IgG autoantibodies to several ribonucleoproteins that are transplacentally transmitted to the fetus and damage the fetal AV node. The fetal conduction disease is generally clinically evident by the second trimester and is associated with significant fetal mortality and neonatal requirement of cardiac pacing.

The embryonic development of the cardiac septa and conduction system occur together, and clinical disorders have been described, including the Holt-Oram syndrome, an autosomal dominant disorder including upper limb dysplasia and atrial septal defect, often with conduction disturbances in the AV node. Studies of families with a high incidence of congenital heart disease, including ostium secundum atrial septal defect and conduction disorders in the AV node, have identified the gene NKX2-5 on chromosome 5q35 as important in the regulation of septation and in the development and function of the AV node. A familial syndrome of progressive complete heart block has also long been recognized. The gene for this disorder has been mapped to a region on chromosome 19q13. Familial disorders of SA node function have also been described, but specific details of abnormal genetic sites are not available. ∎

TREATMENT **Pharmacologic Therapy** Pharmacologic therapy is usually reserved for acute situations. Atropine (0.5 to 2.0 mg intravenously) and isoproterenol (1 to 4 μg/min intravenously) are useful in increasing heart rate and decreasing symptoms in patients with sinus bradycardia or AV block localized to the AV node. They have an insignificant effect on lower pacemakers. In patients with neurovascular syncope, beta blockers and disopyramide have been suggested as methods to depress left ventricular function and decrease mechanoreceptor-related reflexes. Mineralocorticoids, ephedrine, and theophylline have also been reported to be of benefit to occasional patients. Unfortunately, no controlled study has shown that any of these pharmacologic modalities works in a predictable fashion in all patients. Further work on delineating different mechanisms in different patient groups may allow us to apply pharmacologic agents more appropriately. Long-term therapy of bradyarrhythmias is best accomplished by pacemakers.

Pacemakers External energy sources can be used to stimulate the heart when disorders in impulse formation and/or transmission lead to symptomatic bradyarrhythmias. Pacer stimuli can be applied to the atria and/or ventricles. Indications for pacemaker insertion are listed in the guidelines summarized on p. 1290.

Temporary pacing This is usually instituted to provide immediate stabilization prior to permanent pacemaker placement or to provide pacemaker support when a bradycardia is precipitated by what is presumed to be a transient event such as ischemia or drug toxicity. Temporary pacing is usually achieved by the transvenous insertion of an electrode catheter with the catheter positioned in the right ventricular apex and attached to an external generator. This procedure is associated with a small risk of cardiac perforation, infection at the insertion site, and thromboembolism; the risk of the latter two complications increases markedly if the pacing wire is left in place for more than 48 h. The development of an entirely external transthoracic cardiac pacing system may preclude the need for transvenous pacing in selected patients. However, occasional failure of ventricular capture and significant discomfort related to the large current required for effective transthoracic ventricular stimulation preclude the uniform use of this approach.

Permanent pacing This mode of pacing is instituted for persistent or intermittent symptomatic bradycardia not related to a self-limiting precipitating factor or for documented infranodal second- or third-degree AV block. Permanent pacing leads are usually inserted transvenously through the subclavian or cephalic vein with the leads positioned in the right atrial appendage for atrial pacing and the right ventricular apex for ventricular pacing. The leads are then attached to the pulse generator, which is inserted into a subcutaneous pocket below the clavicle. Epicardial lead placement is used when (1) transvenous access cannot be obtained; (2) the chest is already open, i.e., in the course of a cardiac operation; and (3) adequate endocardial lead placement cannot be achieved. Most pacemaker generators are pow-

Table 229-2 Site of 2:1 Atrioventricular Block

Characteristic	Observation—Site of Block
1. QRS width	BBB—anywhere
	Normal QRS—in AV node or His bundle
2. PR interval of conducted P wave	>0.30 s—in AV node
	≤0.16 s—in HPS or His bundle[a]
3. Atropine or exercise	Improve conduction—in AV node
	Worsen conduction—in HPS or His bundle[a]
4. CSP	Worsen conduction—in AV node
	Improve conduction—in HPS or His bundle[a]
5. Retrograde conduction	Present—in HPS or His bundle[a]
	Absent—may be anywhere

[a] Use of a pacemaker is indicated.

NOTE: BBB, bundle branch block; HPS, His-Purkinje system; CSP, carotid sinus pressure.

ered by lithium batteries. The life expectancy of the generator is related to (1) voltage output required for capture, (2) requirement for incessant or intermittent pacing, and (3) number of cardiac chambers paced. Life expectancy of the simple ventricular demand pacemaker can exceed 10 years.

Pacing code   A code consisting of three to five letters has been developed for describing pacemaker type and function (Table 229-3). The first letter indicates the chamber(s) paced and is designated *V* for ventricular pacing, *A* for atrial pacing, or *D* for dual-chamber (both atrial and ventricular) pacing. The second letter indicates the chamber

in which electrical activity is sensed and is also indicated by *A*, *V*, or *D*. An additional designation, *O*, has been used when pacemaker discharge is not dependent on a sensed electrical activity. The third letter refers to the response to a sensed electric signal. The letter *O* represents no response to an underlying electric signal, usually related to the absence of associated sensing function; *I* represents inhibition of pacing function; *T* represents triggering of pacing function; and *D* indicates a dual response, i.e., spontaneous atrial and ventricular activity inhibiting atrial and ventricular pacing and atrial activity triggering a ventricular response. Additional fourth and fifth letters of the pacing code have been recommended to indicate whether the pacemaker is programmable and has rate modulation (fourth) and whether special

---

Guidelines for Permanent Pacing*

Acquired AV Block in Adults

Class I
1. Complete heart block, permanent or intermittent, at any anatomic level, associated with any anatomic level, associated with any one of the following complications:
   a. Symptomatic bradycardia. In the presence of complete heart block, symptoms must be presumed to be due to the heart block unless proved to be otherwise.
   b. Congestive heart failure.
   c. Ectopic rhythms and other medical conditions that require drugs that suppress the automaticity of escape pacemakers and result in symptomatic bradycardia.
   d. Documented periods of asystole ≥ 3.0 s or any escape rate < 40 beats per minute in symptom-free patients.
   e. Confusional states that clear with temporary pacing.
   f. Post-AV junction ablation, myotonic dystrophy.
2. Second-degree AV block, permanent or intermittent, regardless of the type or the site of block, with symptomatic bradycardia.
3. Atrial fibrillation, atrial flutter, or rare cases of supraventricular tachycardia with complete heart block or advanced AV block, bradycardia, and any of the conditions described under a. The bradycardia must be related to digitalis or drugs known to impair AV conduction.

Class II
1. Asymptomatic complete heart block, permanent or intermittent, at any anatomic site, with ventricular rates of 40 beats per minute or faster.
2. Asymptomatic type II second-degree AV block, permanent or intermittent.
3. Asymptomatic type I second-degree AV block at infra-His or intra-His levels.

Class III
1. First-degree AV block.
2. Asymptomatic type I second-degree AV block at the supra-His (AV node) level.

After Myocardial Infarction

Class I
1. Persistent advanced second-degree AV block or complete heart block after acute myocardial infarction with block in the His-Purkinje system (bilateral bundle branch block).
2. Transient advanced AV block and associated bundle branch block.

Class II
1. Persistent advanced block at the AV node.

Class III
1. Transient AV conduction disturbances in the absence of intraventricular conduction defects.
2. Transient AV block in the presence of isolated left anterior hemiblock.
3. Acquired left anterior hemiblock in the absence of AV block.
4. Persistent first-degree AV block in the presence of bundle branch block not demonstrated previously.

Bifascicular and Trifascicular Block

Class I
1. Bifascicular block with intermittent complete heart block associated with symptomatic bradycardia.

2. Bifascicular or trifascicular block with intermittent type II second-degree AV block without symptoms attributable to the heart block.

Class II
1. Bifascicular or trifascicular block with syncope that is not proved to be due to complete heart block, but other possible causes for syncope are not identifiable.
2. Markedly prolonged HV (>100 ms).
3. Pacing-induced infra-His block.

Class III
1. Fascicular block without AV block or symptoms.
2. Fascicular block with first-degree AV block without symptoms.

Sinus Node Dysfunction

Class I
1. Sinus node dysfunction with documented symptomatic bradycardia. In some patients this will occur as a consequence of long-term (essential) drug therapy of a type and dose for which there are no acceptable alternatives.

Class II
1. Sinus node dysfunction, occurring spontaneously or as a result of necessary drug therapy, with heart rates < 40 beats per minute when a clear association between significant symptoms consistent with bradycardia and the actual presence of bradycardia has not been documented.

Class III
1. Sinus node dysfunction in asymptomatic patients, including those in whom substantial sinus bradycardia (heart rate < 40 beats per minute) is a consequence of long-term drug treatment.
2. Sinus node dysfunction in patients in whom symptoms suggestive of bradycardia are clearly documented not to be associated with a slow heart rate.

Hypersensitive Carotid Sinus and Neurovascular Syndromes

Class I
1. Recurrent syncope associated with clear, spontaneous events provoked by carotid sinus stimulation; minimal carotid sinus pressure induces asystole of >3 s duration in the absence of any medication that depresses the sinus node or AV conduction.

Class II
1. Recurrent syncope without clear, provocative events and with a hypersensitive cardioinhibitory response.
2. Syncope with associated bradycardia reproduced by a head-up tilt with or without isoproterenol or other forms of provocative maneuvers and in which a temporary pacemaker and a second provocative test can establish the likely benefits of a permanent pacemaker.

Class III
1. A hyperactive cardioinhibitory response to carotid sinus stimulation in the absence of symptoms.
2. Vague symptoms, such as dizziness, light-headedness, or both, with a hyperactive cardioinhibitory response to carotid sinus stimulation.
3. Recurrent syncope, light-headedness, or dizziness in the absence of a cardioinhibitory response.

---

* Class I: agreement that permanent pacemaker should be implanted. Class II: divergence of opinion regarding need for implantation. Class III: agreement that pacemaker is unnecessary.

SOURCE: Guidelines for The Implantation of Cardiac Pacemakers and Antiarrhythmic Devices. Am Coll Cardiol/Am Heart Assoc.

antitachycardia functions are available (i.e., antitachycardia pacing, *T*, and delivery of high- or low-energy shocks). In the fourth category, *M* represents multiprogrammability and *R* represents rate response ("physiologic") pacing. It follows from the described code that the standard VVIR (ventricular demand pacemaker) paces the ventricle, senses the ventricle, is inhibited by sensed spontaneous ventricular activity, and has rate modulation, while the DDDR pulse generator is capable of sensing and pacing both the atria and ventricles and has a dual response to the sensed atrial and ventricular activity as described above (Fig. 229-9). Both pacemakers have rate modulation (*R*). "Physiologic" pacemakers use sensors (muscular activity, respiratory rate, temperature, O_2 saturation, QT interval, etc.) as methods to allow the pacemaker to increase the heart rate in response to physiologic demands, i.e., exercise. These pacemakers are essential when chronotropic incompetence is present and an increase in heart rate is required to enhance physiologic performance. Studies have shown that such "physiologic" pacemakers improve exercise tolerance and relieve symptoms to a greater degree than fixed-rate pacemakers.

Selection of the appropriate pacemaker and pacing mode depends on the clinical condition and the type of bradyarrhythmia being treated. The two most common pacing mode selections are DDD and VVI. DDD provides AV sequential pacing, which is ideally suited for the relatively young and active patient who has intact sinus node function or intermittent dysfunction and high-grade persistent or intermittent AV block. The DDD mode will allow for physiologic atrial sensed and ventricular paced rates and improve exercise tolerance. AV synchrony and dual-chamber pacing may also be desirable in patients with borderline hemodynamic reserve who are dependent on atrial contribution to cardiac output and in those patients who develop the pacemaker syndrome (see below) in response to ventricular demand pacing.

Rate-responsive DDD (i.e., DDDR) pacing is indicated when chronotropic incompetence is present in a patient who requires AV synchrony. The DDD pacing mode is contraindicated in chronic atrial fibrillation or flutter, because rapid and irregular ventricular pacing will occur to the upper rate limit. In some cases this will produce a more rapid ventricular rate than the patient's own rate in the absence of a pacemaker. DDD pacemakers must either automatically switch (i.e., mode-switching function) or be reprogrammed to the VVI mode. Almost all such pacemakers are now combined with some form of rate responsiveness so that when the device functions in the VVI mode, it also will respond to physiologic demands (VVIR).

Chronotropic insufficiency (i.e., the inability of the sinus rate to accelerate) is a contraindication for a DDD pacemaker, since such a pacemaker will act as a "fixed-rate" pacemaker at the programmed lower rate. In these situations, a rate-adaptive or "physiologic" pacemaker is indicated (VVIR or DDDR). In patients with impaired sinus node function or chronic atrial fibrillation, a sensor-driven, rate-adaptive pacemaker must be implanted. As mentioned earlier, these pacemakers automatically adjust ventricular pacing rates to a sensed indicator of exertion. The DDD pacing mode may also be contraindicated in patients with intermittent or persistent ventriculoatrial conduction, who may develop pacemaker-mediated tachycardia (see below).

Programmability of pacemakers This allows for modification of

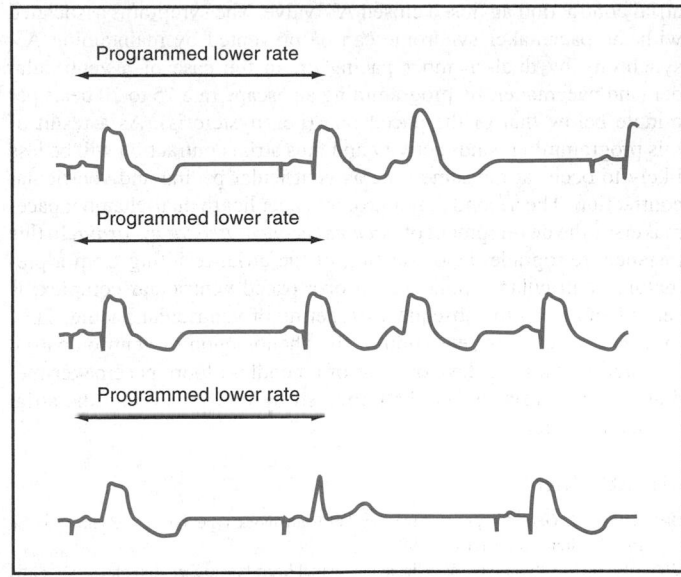

FIGURE 229-9 Normally functioning DDD pacemaker. All three panels show a lead II rhythm strip at 50 mm/s. The programmed lower rate is approximately 55 beats per minute. (*Top*) AV sequential pacing with a paced AV interval of 160 ms is shown for the first two complexes. A VPC occurs and is sensed, resetting the cycle. (*Middle*) The first beat is AV paced, but spontaneous sinus P waves and APC trigger a ventricular paced complex with a sensed P to QRS of 120 ms. (*Bottom*) After the first AV paced complex, a paced atrial complex conducts to the ventricle with a PR of 120 ms, inhibiting the ventricular pacemaker.

pacing function after implantation and for adaptation to changes in clinical needs. Pacemaker programming is accomplished by activation of the programming head positioned over the implanted pulse generator after making the desired changes in programmable parameters (Table 229-3). A radio frequency system is routinely used to communicate the program to the pacemaker. A high degree of sophistication is required to recognize the presence and causes of pacemaker malfunction and their treatment.

Complications Adverse effects of permanent pacing are usually associated with failure or malfunction of the pacing system. These problems are usually secondary to over- or undersensing, output failure, and/or lead fracture or displacement. Two other problems may occur. The *pacemaker syndrome* consists of fatigue, dizziness, syncope, and distressing pulsations in the neck and chest and can be associated with adverse hemodynamic effects. The pathophysiologic contributors to the pacemaker syndrome include (1) loss of atrial contribution to ventricular systole; (2) vasodepressor reflex initiated by cannon *a* waves, which are caused by atrial contractions against a closed tricuspid valve and observed in the jugular venous pulse (Chap. 225); and (3) systemic and pulmonary venous regurgitation due to

Table 229-3 The NASPE/BPEG Generic Pacemaker Code

	I	II	III	IV	V
Position Category	**Chamber(s) Paced**	**Chamber(s) Sensed**	**Response to Sensing**	**Programmability, Rate Modulation**	**Antitachyarrhythmia Function(s)**
	O, None	O, None	O, None	O, None	O, None
	A, Atrium	A, Atrium	T, Triggered	P, Simple programmable	P, pacing (antitachyarrhythmia)
	V, Ventricle	V, Ventricle	I, Inhibited	M, Multiprogrammable	S, Shock
	D, Dual (A + V)	D, Dual (A + V)	D, Dual (T + I)	C, Communicating	D, Dual (P + S)
				R, Rate modulation	
Manufacturer's designation	S, single (A or V)	S, (A or V)			

SOURCE: From DP Zipes, in E Braunwald (ed): *Heart Disease: A Textbook of Cardiovascular Medicine*, 5th ed. Philadelphia, Saunders, 1997.

atrial contraction against a closed AV valve. The symptoms associated with the pacemaker syndrome can be prevented by maintaining AV synchrony by dual-chamber pacing or, in the case of a ventricular demand pacemaker, by programming an escape rate 15 to 20 beats per minute below that of the paced rate (i.e., hysteresis). As a result of this programming, sinus activity and thus atrial contraction will be less likely to occur at the same time as ventricular pacing and ventricular contraction. The second major problem peculiar to dual-chamber pacemakers is the development of *pacemaker-mediated tachycardia*. In this instance, retrograde depolarization of the atria, resulting from a premature ventricular depolarization or a paced ventricular complex, is sensed and leads to subsequent triggering of ventricular pacing. This, in turn, can result in repetition of the phenomenon of ventriculoatrial conduction with the development of an endless-loop, pacemaker-mediated tachycardia. It may be corrected by reprogramming the atrial refractory period.

BIBLIOGRAPHY

BRINK P et al: Gene for progressive familial heart block type 1 maps to chromosome 19q13. Circulation 91:1633, 1995

BUYON J et al: Autoimmune associated congenital heart block: Demographics, mortality, morbidity and recurrence rates obtained from a national neonatal lupus registry. J Am Coll Cardiol 31:1685, 1998

DREIFUS LS et al: Guidelines for implantation of cardiac pacemakers and antiarrhythmic devices: A report of the American College of Cardiology/American Heart Association Task Force on Assessment of Diagnostic and Therapeutic Cardiovascular Procedures (Committee on Pacemaker Implantation). J Am Coll Cardiol 18:1, 1991

ELLENBOGEN KA et al: New insights into pacemaker syndrome gained from hemodynamic, humoral and vascular responses during ventriculo-atrial pacing. Am J Cardiol 65(1):53, 1990

GROH SS, ZIPES DP: Cardiac pacemakers, in *Heart Disease: A Textbook of Cardiovascular Medicine*, 6th ed, E Braunwald et al (eds). Philadelphia, Saunders, 2001

HUANG SK et al: Carotid sinus hypersensitivity in patients with unexplained syncope: Clinical, electrophysiologic and long-term follow-up observations. Am Heart J 116:989, 1988

JOSEPHSON ME: *Clinical Electrophysiology*, 2d ed. Philadelphia, Lea and Febiger, 1993, chaps 4, 5, 6, 13

MENDES LA, DAVIDOFF R: Cardiogenic seizure with bradyarrhythmia: Documentation of the mechanism during asytole. Am Heart J 125:1786, 1993

MICHAËLSON M, JANZON A: Isolated congenital complete atrioventricular block in adult life. A prospective study. Circulation 92:442, 1995

SCHOTT J et al: Congenital heart disease caused by mutations in the transcription factor NKX2-5. Science, in press

SRA JS et al: Comparison of cardiac pacing with drug therapy in the treatment of neurocardiogenic (vasovagal) syncope with bradycardia or asystole. N Engl J Med 328:1085, 1993

WALLER BF et al: Anatomy, histology and pathology of the cardiac conduction system: Part II. Clin Cardiol 16:347, 1993

230   *Mark E. Josephson, Peter Zimetbaum*

THE TACHYARRHYTHMIAS

AF atrial fibrillation	PSVT paroxysmal supraventricular tachycardias
APCs atrial premature complexes	
AV atrioventricular	SVT supraventricular tachycardia
CAST cardiac arrhythmia suppression trial	VA ventriculoatrial
	VF ventricular fibrillation
ECG electrocardiogram	VPCs ventricular premature complexes
ICD implantable cardioverter/defibrillator	
	VT ventricular tachycardia
LQTS long QT syndrome	WPW Wolff-Parkinson-White
MAT multifocal atrial tachycardia	

MECHANISMS OF TACHYARRHYTHMIAS

Tachyarrhythmias may be divided into disorders of impulse propagation and disorders of impulse formation.

REENTRY   Disorders of impulse propagation (reentry) are generally considered to be the most common mechanism of sustained paroxysmal tachyarrhythmia. The requirements for initiating reentry include (1) electrophysiologic inhomogeneity (i.e., differences in conduction and/or refractoriness) in two or more regions of the heart connected with each other to form a potentially closed loop; (2) unidirectional block in one pathway; (3) slow conduction over an alternative pathway, allowing time for the initially blocked pathway to recover excitability; and (4) reexcitation of the initially blocked pathway to complete a loop of activation (Fig. 230-1). Repetitive circulation of the impulse over this loop can produce a sustained tachyarrhythmia. While anatomic obstacles may underlie reentry and provide an inexcitable center around which the impulse can circulate, they are not essential. Reentrant arrhythmias can be reproducibly initiated and terminated by premature complexes and rapid stimulation. The response of these arrhythmias to stimulation can help distinguish them from arrhythmias caused by triggered activity.

ENHANCED AUTOMATICITY   Disorders of impulse formation can be subdivided into tachyarrhythmias caused by enhanced automaticity and those caused by triggered activity. In addition to the sinus node, automatic pacemaker activity can be observed in specialized atrial fibers, fibers of the atrioventricular (AV) junction, and Purkinje fibers (Chap. 229). Myocardial cells do not normally possess pacemaker activity. Enhancement of normal automaticity in latent pacemaker fibers or the development of abnormal automaticity due to partial depolarization of the resting membrane occurs as a consequence of a variety of pathophysiologic states, which include (1) increased endogenous or exogenous catecholamines, (2) electrolyte disturbances (e.g., hyperkalemia), (3) hypoxia or ischemia, (4) mechanical effects (e.g., stretch), and (5) drugs (e.g., digitalis). Tachycardia caused by automaticity cannot be started or stopped by pacing.

TRIGGERED ACTIVITY   Rhythms due to triggered activity are events that do not occur spontaneously but require a change in cardiac electrical frequency as a trigger. Triggered activity may be caused by early afterdepolarizations, which occur during phases 2 and 3 of the action potential, or delayed afterdepolarizations, which occur following completion of phase 3 of the action potential (Fig. 229-2). Triggered activity has been observed in atrial, ventricular, and His-Purkinje tissue under conditions such as increased local catecholamine concentration, hyperkalemia, hypercalcemia, and digitalis intoxication (delayed afterdepolarizations) or during bradycardia, hypokalemia, or

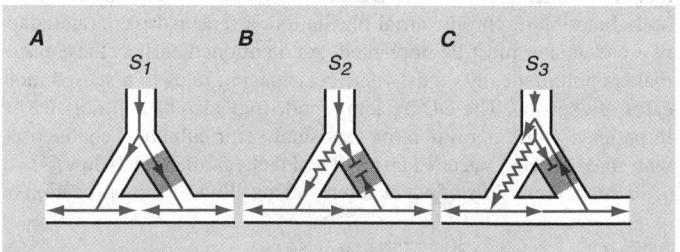

FIGURE 230-1   Schema of reentry. Y branching of the Purkinje system to ventricular muscle is shown in panels *A* through *C*. The right limb (*gray area*) of the Purkinje system has a longer refractory period than the left. *A*. During a slow stimulated rate (S_1), conduction proceeds normally over both Purkinje fibers, resulting in collision in the ventricular muscle. *B*. An early premature stimulus (S_2) results in block in the Purkinje fiber on the right and slow conduction down the left. The impulse conducts through the ventricle and attempts to reenter the initial site of block but fails because this site has not fully recovered excitability. *C*. An earlier stimulus (S_3) again results in block on the left. The resulting slower propagation down the left fiber provides enough time for the initial site of block to recur and allows the impulse to conduct through it to produce a reentrant circuit.

other situations prolonging action potential duration (early afterdepolarizations). All of these conditions produce an accumulation of intracellular calcium. With increasing amplitude of the afterdepolarizations, threshold can be reached and repetitive activity produced. The exact role of triggered activity in spontaneous clinical arrhythmias is unknown, but tachyarrhythmias associated with digitalis intoxication, accelerated idioventricular rhythm in acute infarction and/or reperfusion, and exercise-induced ventricular tachycardia (VT) are believed to be caused by triggered activity due to delayed afterdepolarizations. *Torsade de pointes* ("twisting of the points"; polymorphic VT associated with long QT intervals) may be caused by triggered activity due to early afterdepolarizations, although reentry may also be operative.

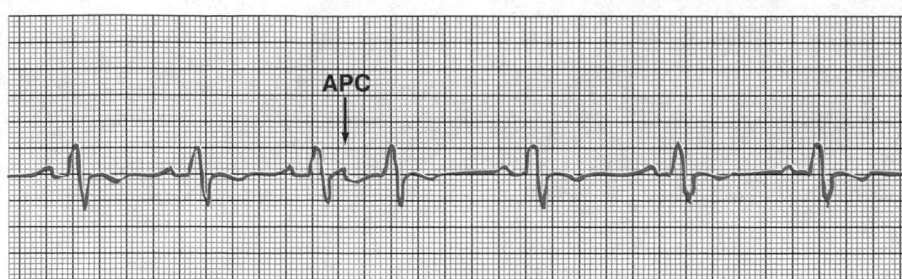

FIGURE 230-2 ECG lead II. Sinus rhythm with one atrial premature complex (*arrow*). Note the difference in P-wave configuration between sinus and the premature atrial complexes. In addition, note that the PR interval of the premature complex is prolonged, due to slowed conduction of the premature impulse through the AV conduction system.

The use of electrophysiologic studies, i.e., intracardiac recordings and programmed stimulation, has greatly expanded the understanding of the mechanisms of tachyarrhythmias. In addition to helping diagnose arrhythmias, these techniques may be of value in determining the most appropriate types of therapy because they allow the physician to observe the hemodynamic and symptomatic consequences of the arrhythmia in the presence or absence of therapy. Electrophysiologic studies of tachycardias require the positioning of multiple electrode catheters at critical areas within the heart. These electrodes must be capable of both stimulating and recording from multiple sites in the atria and/or ventricles.

PREMATURE COMPLEXES

ATRIAL PREMATURE COMPLEXES (APC) APCs can be found on 24-h Holter monitoring in over 60% of normal adults. APCs are usually asymptomatic and benign, although at times they may be associated with palpitations. In susceptible patients, they can initiate paroxysmal supraventricular tachycardias. APCs may originate from any location in either atrium, and they are recognized on the electrocardiogram (ECG) as early P waves with a morphology that differs from the sinus P wave (Fig. 230-2). While APCs usually conduct to the ventricles when they occur late in the cardiac cycle, early APCs may reach the AV conduction system while it is still in its relative refractory period, resulting in a conduction delay manifested by prolonged PR interval following the premature P wave (Fig. 230-2). Very early APCs may even block in the AV node if this structure is encountered during its effective refractory period. APCs, whether conducted or not, are usually followed by a pause before a return to sinus activity. Most commonly, an APC enters and resets the sinus node, so the sum of the pre- and postextrasystolic PP intervals is less than the sum of two sinus PP intervals (Fig. 230-2). In this case, the pause is said to be less than fully compensatory. The QRS complex following most APCs is normal, although early APCs may be followed by aberrantly conducted QRS complexes due to the premature complex falling within the relative refractory period of the His-Purkinje system.

Since most APCs are asymptomatic, treatment is not required. When they cause palpitations or trigger paroxysmal supraventricular tachycardias (see below), treatment may be useful. Factors that precipitate APCs, such as alcohol, tobacco, or adrenergic stimulants, should be identified and eliminated; in their absence, mild sedation or the use of a beta blocker may be tried.

AV JUNCTIONAL COMPLEXES The site of origin of these complexes is thought to be in the bundle of His, since the normal AV node in vivo possesses no automaticity. AV junctional complexes are less common than either atrial or ventricular premature complexes and are more often associated with cardiac disease or digitalis intoxication. Junctional premature impulses can conduct both antegradely to the ventricles and retrogradely to the atrium and, on rare occasions, may fail to conduct in either direction. Premature AV junctional complexes can be recognized by normal-appearing QRS complexes that are not preceded by a P wave. Retrograde P waves (inverted in leads II, III, and aVF) may be observed after the QRS complex.

While often asymptomatic, junctional premature complexes may be associated with palpitations and cause cannon *a* waves, which may result in distressing pulsations in the neck. When symptomatic, they should be treated like APCs.

VENTRICULAR PREMATURE COMPLEXES (VPCs) These are among the most common arrhythmias and occur in patients with and without heart disease. Of adult males, ≥60% will exhibit VPCs during a 24-h Holter monitoring. In patients without heart disease, VPCs have not been shown to be associated with any increased incidence in mortality or morbidity. VPCs may occur in up to 80% of patients with previous myocardial infarction, and in this setting, if frequent (>10 per hour) and/or complex (occurring in couplets), they have been associated with increased mortality. However, cardiac mortality in such patients usually occurs in association with significantly impaired ventricular function. While frequent and complex ventricular ectopy is an independent risk factor, it is not as strong a risk factor as is impaired ventricular function. Moreover, even though ventricular tachycardia and/or fibrillation may be the basis for the sudden death in these patients, this does not a priori establish a cause-and-effect relation between spontaneous ectopy and life-threatening ventricular tachycardia or fibrillation. Very early cycle (R-on-T) VPCs have been stated by some to increase the risk of sudden death. Although this has been observed during acute ischemia and in the setting of QT prolongation, frequently, VT or fibrillation is precipitated by VPCs that occur after the T wave of the prior beat.

VPCs are recognized by wide (usually >0.14 s), bizarre QRS complexes that are not preceded by P waves (Fig. 230-3*A*). They may bear a relatively fixed relationship to the preceding sinus complex (i.e., fixed coupled VPCs). When fixed coupling is not present and the interval between VPCs has a common denominator, *ventricular parasystole* is said to be present (Fig. 230-4). Under these circumstances, the VPCs are a manifestation of abnormal automaticity of a protected ventricular focus. Because this focus is not penetrated by sinus impulses, it is not reset by them, and the interectopic intervals remain relatively fixed (≤120 ms variation of mean RR cycle length).

VPCs may occur singly; in patterns of bigeminy, in which every sinus beat is followed by a VPC; in trigeminy, in which two sinus beats are followed by a VPC; in quadrigeminy, etc. Two successive VPCs are termed *pairs* or *couplets*, while three or more consecutive VPCs are termed *ventricular tachycardia* when the rate exceeds 100 beats per minute (Fig. 230-3*B*). VPCs may have similar morphologies (monomorphic, or uniform) or different morphologies (polymorphic, or multiformed).

Most commonly, VPCs are not conducted retrogradely to the atrium to reset the sinoatrial node. Thus they produce a fully compensatory pause; i.e., the interval between conducted sinus beats that

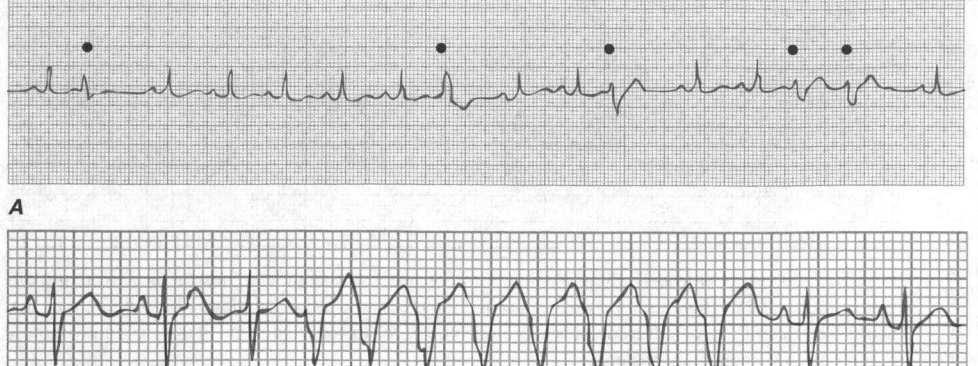

A

B

FIGURE 230-3 *A*. Single ventricular ectopy. During sinus rhythm, five premature ventricular complexes (filled circles) occur. Note that the QRS configuration is bizarre and different from that during sinus rhythm. The premature ventricular complexes are not preceded by P waves. The QRS widths of the premature complexes are 120–160 ms and multiple morphologies are present. The pause following the premature complexes is fully compensatory, the sinus beat after the premature complex occurring on time. *B*. Nonsustained ventricular tachycardia (VT). Following two sinus beats, an atrial premature contraction with long PR interval initiates an 8-beat run of wide complex tachycardia. Atrial activity can be seen following the fourth and seventh beats. The greater number of QRS complexes compared with P waves confirms the diagnosis of VT.

bracket the VPC equals two basic RR intervals. Ventricular impulses may also manifest retrograde conduction to the atrium and cause inverted P waves in leads II, III, and aVF. This retrograde atrial activation can reset the sinus node, and the pause that results may therefore be less than compensatory. In many instances, the VPC will not be associated with retrograde ventriculoatrial (VA) conduction but may block retrogradely in the AV node. This renders the AV node refractory to the subsequent sinus beat and causes slowed conduction (i.e., prolonged PR interval) or block of the next sinus P wave. This prolonged PR interval is said to be a manifestation of concealed retrograde conduction of the ventricular impulse into the AV node. A VPC that does not produce any manifestation of retrograde concealed conduction and fails to influence the oncoming sinus impulse is termed an *interpolated VPC*.

VPCs can cause palpitations or neck pulsations secondary to either the occurrence of cannon *a* waves or the increased force of contraction due to postextrasystolic potentiation of ventricular contractility. Pa-

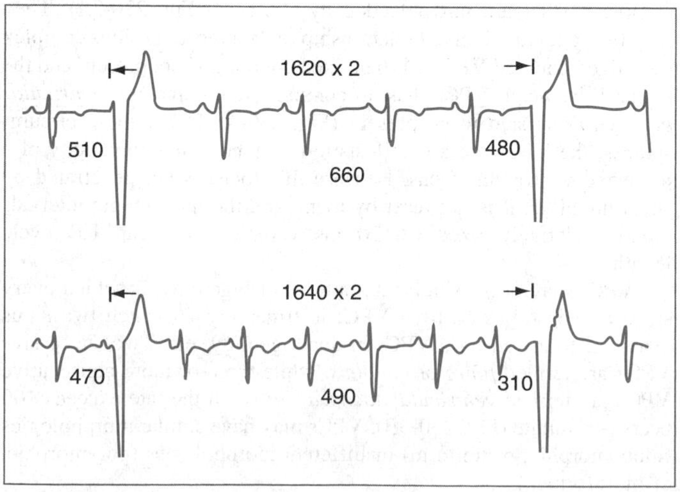

FIGURE 230-4 Ventricular parasystole. At varying sinus cycle lengths during exercise, interectopic intervals remain constant at 1620 to 1640 ms. However, the coupling intervals between sinus and ectopic complexes vary between 510 and 310 ms.

tients with frequent VPCs or bigeminy may rarely develop syncope or lightheadedness because the VPCs do not result in an adequate stroke volume and the cardiac output is reduced by the "halving" of the heart rate.

℞ TREATMENT In the absence of cardiac disease, isolated asymptomatic VPCs, regardless of configuration and frequency, need no treatment. When arrhythmias are symptomatic, the symptoms should first be addressed by either allaying the patient's anxiety or, if this is not successful, reducing the frequency of the VPCs with antiarrhythmic agents. β-Adrenergic blockers may be successful in managing VPCs that occur primarily in the daytime or under stressful situations and in specific settings such as mitral valve prolapse and thyrotoxicosis. While other antiarrhythmic agents may be tried should this be unsuccessful, their risk may outweigh any benefits. In patients with cardiac disease, frequent VPCs are associated with an increased risk of sudden and nonsudden cardiac death, and many physicians have attempted to eliminate or reduce the frequency of these VPCs in an attempt to reduce this risk. However, the cause-and-effect relationship of the VPCs to fatal events has never been established. The ability of pharmacologic antiarrhythmic therapy guided by continuous ECG monitoring to reduce the risk of sudden death in postmyocardial infarction patients with frequent (≥ 6 per minute) VPCs was tested by the Cardiac Arrhythmia Suppression Trial (CAST). This study compared mortality in patients whose ectopy was suppressed by one of three agents (encainide, flecainide, or moricizine) and then randomized to treat with either the "effective" drug or placebo. After a mean follow-up of 2 years, the study was discontinued because both the sudden death and overall mortality rate were significantly increased in patients receiving antiarrhythmic agents. This study has shown that in patients having the characteristics of the study population, abolition of ventricular ectopy by pharmacologic therapy cannot be used as a marker to define reduction of the risk of sudden death after myocardial infarction and, in fact, may increase mortality. Recent studies have evaluated the use of electrophysiologic testing and implantable cardioverter/defibrillator (ICD) placement in the management of patients at high risk for sudden death (i.e., those with left ventricular ejection fractions <40% and nonsustained VT). These studies have found that induction of a sustained ventricular arrhythmia through programmed electrical stimulation selects a group of these patients whose prognosis is improved with implantation of a defibrillator. These studies have found no correlation between the rate, morphology, or duration of nonsustained episodes of VT and the likelihood of having a sustained ventricular arrhythmia.

Antiarrhythmic agents can also produce the lethal arrhythmias that they are given to prevent (proarrhythmic effects). Thus therapy directed toward VPCs in the setting of chronic cardiac disease may result in an inappropriate and costly use of agents without proven efficacy and with potential side effects in many patients. The high incidence of side effects and the frequent exacerbation of arrhythmias caused by all antiarrhythmic drugs make it mandatory to monitor patients being treated with such agents.

In acute myocardial infarction, the greatest incidence of primary ventricular fibrillation occurs within the first 24 h (Chap. 243). Temporary prophylactic antiarrhythmic therapy with lidocaine or procainamide was formerly recommended for all patients with acute infarction, regardless of the presence or degree of spontaneous ectopy.

However, failure to improve overall survival and drug toxicity have led most physicians to recommend prophylactic antiarrhythmic therapy only to young patients with complicated infarctions, where a favorable risk-benefit ratio may be obtained. Other studies have shown that intravenous beta blockers may also reduce the incidence of primary ventricular fibrillation.

TACHYCARDIAS

Tachycardias refer to arrhythmias with three or more complexes at rates exceeding 100 beats per minute; they occur more often in structurally diseased than in normal hearts. Those paroxysmal tachycardias that are initiated by APCs or VPCs are considered to be due to reentry, except some of the digitalis-induced tachyarrhythmias, which are probably due to triggered activity (see below).

If the patient is hemodynamically stable, an attempt should be made to determine the mechanism and origin of the tachycardia, since this will usually lead to an appropriate therapeutic decision. Information to be obtained from the ECG includes (1) the presence, frequency, morphology, and regularity of P waves and QRS complexes; (2) the relationship between atrial and ventricular activity; (3) a comparison of the QRS morphology during sinus rhythm and during the tachycardia; and (4) the response to carotid sinus massage or other vagal maneuvers. It is useful first to compare a 12-lead ECG during the tachycardia with one recorded during sinus rhythm. One can also utilize the electrodes situated at the end of a flexible pacing catheter inserted into the esophagus behind the left atrium to record atrial activity.

Observation of the jugular venous pulse can provide clues to the presence of atrial activity and its relationship to ventricular ectopy. Intermittent cannon *a* waves suggest AV dissociation, while persistent cannon *a* waves suggest 1:1 VA conduction. Flutter waves may be seen or no atrial activity may be apparent, as in the presence of atrial flutter and fibrillation, respectively. The arterial pulse may also manifest AV dissociation or atrial fibrillation by demonstrating variations in amplitude. A first heart sound of variable intensity during a regular rhythm also suggests AV dissociation or atrial fibrillation (AF).

Carotid sinus pressure should only be applied while the patient is electrocardiographically monitored with resuscitative equipment available to manage the rare episode of asystole and/or ventricular fibrillation associated with this procedure. Carotid sinus massage should not be performed in patients with carotid arterial bruits. The patient should be positioned flat with the neck extended. Massage of one carotid bulb at a time should be performed by applying firm pressure just underneath the angle of the jaw for up to 5 s. Alternative vagomimetic maneuvers include the Valsalva maneuver, immersion of the face in cold water, and administration of 5 to 10 mg edrophonium.

SINUS TACHYCARDIA In the adult, sinus tachycardia is said to be present when the heart rate exceeds 100 beats per minute (bpm): sinus tachycardia rarely exceeds 200 bpm and is not a primary arrhythmia; instead, it represents a physiologic response to a variety of stresses, such as fever, volume depletion, anxiety, exercise, thyrotoxicosis, hypoxemia, hypotension, or congestive heart failure. Sinus tachycardia has a gradual onset and offset. The ECG demonstrates P waves with sinus contour preceding each QRS complex. Carotid sinus pressure usually produces modest slowing with a gradual return to the previous rate upon cessation. This contrasts with the response of paroxysmal supraventricular tachycardias, which may slow slightly and terminate abruptly.

℞ **TREATMENT** Sinus tachycardia should not be treated as a primary arrhythmia, since it is almost always a physiologic response to a demand placed on the heart. As such, the therapy should be directed to the primary disorder. This may involve institution of digitalis and/or diuretics for heart failure and oxygen for hypoxemia, treatment of thyrotoxicosis, volume repletion, aspirin for fever, or tranquilizers for emotional upset.

ATRIAL FIBRILLATION AF is a common arrhythmia that may occur in paroxysmal and persistent forms. It may be seen in normal subjects, particularly during emotional stress or following surgery, exercise, acute alcoholic intoxication, or a prominent surge of vagal tone (i.e., vasovagal response). It may also occur in patients with heart or lung disease who develop acute hypoxia, hypercapnia, or metabolic or hemodynamic derangements. Persistent AF usually occurs in patients with cardiovascular disease, most commonly rheumatic heart disease, nonrheumatic mitral valve disease, hypertensive cardiovascular disease, chronic lung disease, atrial septal defect, and a variety of miscellaneous cardiac abnormalities. AF may be the presenting finding in thyrotoxicosis. So-called lone AF, which occurs in patients without underlying heart disease, often represents the tachycardia phase of the tachycardia-bradycardia syndrome.

The morbidity associated with AF is related to (1) excessive ventricular rate, which in turn may lead to hypotension, pulmonary congestion, or angina pectoris in susceptible individuals; (2) the pause following cessation of AF, which can cause syncope; (3) systemic embolization, which occurs most commonly in patients with rheumatic heart disease (Table 230-1); (4) loss of the contribution of atrial contraction to cardiac output, which may cause fatigue; and (5) anxiety secondary to palpitations. In patients with severe cardiac dysfunction, particularly those with hypertrophied, noncompliant ventricles, the combination of the loss of the atrial contribution to ventricular filling and the abbreviated filling period due to the rapid ventricular rate in AF can produce marked hemodynamic instability, resulting in hypotension, syncope, or heart failure. In patients with mitral stenosis, in whom ventricular filling time is critical, development of AF with a rapid ventricular rate may precipitate pulmonary edema (Chap. 236). AF may also cause a cardiomyopathy related to persistent rapid rates (so-called tachycardia-induced cardiomyopathy).

AF is characterized by disorganized atrial activity without discrete P waves on the surface ECG (Fig. 230-5A). Atrial activation is manifested by an undulating baseline or by more sharply inscribed atrial deflections of varying amplitude and frequency ranging from 350 to 600 beats per minute. The ventricular response is irregularly irregular. This results from the large number of atrial impulses that penetrate the AV node, making it partially refractory to subsequent impulses. This effect of nonconducted atrial impulses to influence the response to subsequent atrial impulses is termed *concealed conduction*. As a result, the ventricular response is relatively slow, considering the actual atrial rate. AF may convert to atrial flutter, especially in response to antiarrhythmic drugs like quinidine or flecainide. If AF converts to atrial flutter, which has a slower atrial rate, the effect of concealed conduction may be diminished, and a paradoxic increase in the ventricular response may occur. The main factor determining the rate of the ventricular response is the functional refractory period of the AV node or the most rapid paced rate at which 1:1 conduction through the AV node can be observed.

If, in the presence of AF, the ventricular rhythm becomes regular and slow (e.g., 30 to 60 bpm), complete heart block is suggested, and if the ventricular rhythm is regular and rapid (e.g., ≥100 bpm), a tachycardia arising in the AV junction or ventricle should be suspected. Digitalis intoxication is a common cause of both phenomena.

Table 230-1 Factors Associated with High Risk of Stroke in Patients with Atrial Fibrillation

1. Age >65
2. Hypertension
3. Rheumatic heart disease
4. Prior stroke or TIA
5. Diabetes mellitus
6. Congestive heart failure
7. Left atrial dimension >5 cm

NOTE: TIA, transient ischemic attack.

V₁

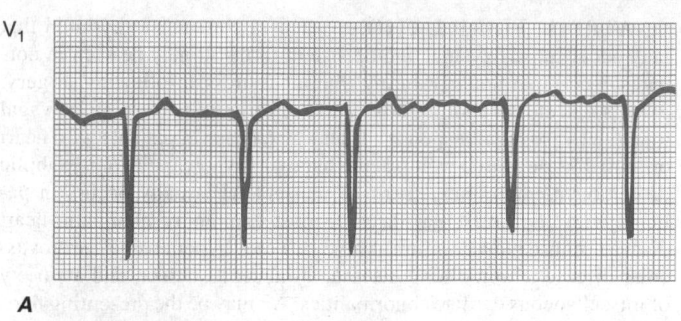

A

II

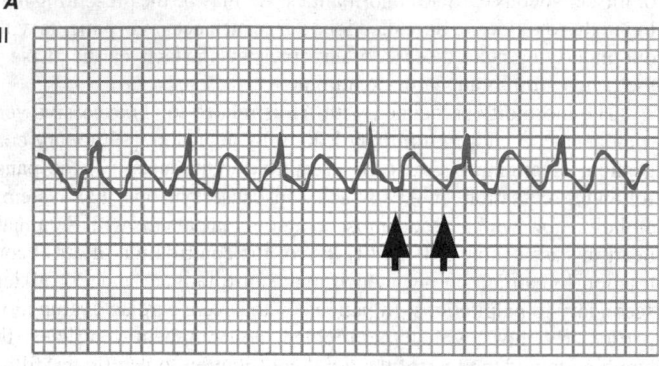

B

FIGURE 230-5   Atrial fibrillation and atrial flutter. *A.* Lead V₁ demonstrating an irregular ventricular rhythm associated with poorly defined irregular atrial activity consistent with atrial fibrillation. *B.* Lead II demonstrates atrial flutter, identified by the regular "sawtooth-like" activity (*arrows*) at an atrial rate of 300 bpm with 2:1 ventricular response.

Patients with AF exhibit a loss of *a* waves in the jugular venous pulse and variable pulse pressures in the carotid arterial pulse. The first heart sound usually varies in intensity. On echocardiography, the left atrium is frequently enlarged, and in patients in whom the left atrial diameter exceeds 4.5 cm, it may be difficult to convert AF to sinus rhythm and/or maintain the latter, despite therapy.

℞ **TREATMENT**   In acute AF, a precipitating factor such as fever, pneumonia, alcoholic intoxication, thyrotoxicosis, pulmonary emboli, congestive heart failure, or pericarditis should be sought. When such a factor is present, therapy should be directed toward the primary abnormality. If the patient's clinical status is severely compromised, electrical cardioversion is the treatment of choice. In the absence of severe cardiovascular compromise, slowing of ventricular rate becomes the initial therapeutic goal. This may be most rapidly accomplished with β-adrenergic blockers and/or calcium channel antagonists. Both prolong the refractory period of the AV node and slow conduction within it. When catecholamine levels or sympathetic nervous system tone is likely to be elevated, beta blockers may be favored. Digitalis preparations are less effective, take longer to act, and are associated with more toxicity. Conversion to sinus rhythm may then be attempted. Prior to cardioversion, precautions must be taken to reduce the risk of systemic embolization. Patients should be anticoagulated to an INR of at least 1.8 for the prior 3 consecutive weeks or have had AF for <48 h. Alternatively, for those patients with AF for >48 h who are not anticoagulated, a transesophageal echocardiogram can exclude the presence of left atrial thrombus and allow safe cardioversion. Following cardioversion, anticoagulation must be maintained for at least 4 weeks until atrial mechanical function returns to normal.

Antiarrhythmic medications in either oral or intravenous form may be employed but are only modestly effective in restoring sinus rhythm. When antiarrhythmic agents such as the quinidine-like drugs (type 1A) or the flecainide-like agents (type 1C) are used (Table 230-2), it is important to increase AV node refractoriness prior to administering such drugs because their vagolytic effect and/or their ability to convert

Table 230-2   Classification of Antiarrhythmic Drugs

Class I	Drugs that reduce maximal velocity of phase of depolarization (V_max) due to block of inward Na⁺ current in tissue with fast response action potentials A ↓ V_max at all heart rates and ↑ action potential duration, e.g., quinidine, procainamide, disopyramide B Little effect at slow rates on V_max in normal tissue; ↓ V_max in partially depolarized cells with fast response action potentials Effects increased at faster rates No change or ↓ in action potential duration, e.g., lidocaine, phenytoin, tocainide, mexiletine C ↓ V_max at normal rates in normal tissue Minimal effect on action potential duration, e.g., flecainide, propafenone, moricizine
Class II	Antisympathetic agents, e.g., propranolol and other β-adrenergic blockers: ↓ SA nodal automaticity, ↑ AV nodal refractoriness, and ↓ AV nodal conduction velocity
Class III	Agents that prolong action potential duration in tissue with fast-response action potentials, e.g., bretylium, amiodarone, sotalol
Class IV	Calcium (slow) channel blocking agents: ↓ conduction velocity and ↑ refractoriness in tissue with slow-response action potentials, e.g., verapamil, diltiazem

Drugs that cannot be classified by this schema:
Digitalis
Adenosine

NOTE: SA, sinoatrial; AV, atrioventricular.

AF to atrial flutter may reduce the concealed conduction in the AV node and lead to an excessively rapid ventricular response. β-Adrenergic blockers are especially useful in this regard.

Direct-current electrical cardioversion is a highly effective method to restore sinus rhythm, either as a primary method of therapy or following the failure of antiarrhythmic medications. Electrical cardioversion is accomplished through the delivery of at least 200 W · s of energy between electrodes placed to the right of the sternum and the cardiac apex or to the left of the scapula. If external cardioversion is unsuccessful, internal cardioversion with energy delivered between two catheters inside the heart or one inside and a patch outside the heart may prove effective.

It is unlikely that patients with chronic AF will convert to and remain in sinus rhythm in the presence of long-standing rheumatic heart disease and/or when the atria are markedly enlarged. It is also unlikely for patients with recurrent, paroxysmal lone AF to be converted to and maintained in sinus rhythm.

The goal of therapy in patients in whom AF cannot be converted to sinus rhythm is control of the ventricular response. This can usually be accomplished by digitalis, beta blockers, or calcium channel blockers singly or in combination. In occasional patients, the ventricular response cannot be controlled by pharmacologic therapy alone. In such patients, the creation of complete heart block by radiofrequency catheter ablation of the AV junction followed by permanent pacemaker implantation is appropriate. Surgical or direct-current catheter ablation of the AV junction is rarely required to achieve AV block.

If sinus rhythm is restored electrically or pharmacologically, quinidine or related agents as well as the class IC agents (e.g., flecainide), sotalol, or amiodarone may be used to prevent recurrence. In patients in whom cardioversion is unsuccessful or in whom AF has recurred or is likely to recur despite antiarrhythmic therapy, it is probably wisest to allow the patient to remain in AF and to control the ventricular response with calcium antagonists, β-adrenergic blockers, or digitalis glycosides. Since such patients are always at risk of systemic embolization, particularly in the presence of organic heart disease, chronic anticoagulation must be considered (Table 230-3). Chronic anticoagulation is particularly important in the elderly, where the attributable

Age, years	Risk Factors[a]	Recommendations
<65	Absent	Aspirin
	Present	Warfarin [target INR 2.5 (range 2.0–3.0)]
65–75	Absent	Aspirin or warfarin
	Present	Warfarin [target INR 2.5 (range 2.0–3.0)]
>75	All patients	Warfarin [target INR 2.5 (range 2.0–3.0)]

[a] Risk factors are prior transient ischemic attack, systemic embolus or stroke, hypertension, poor left ventricular function, rheumatic mitral valve disease, prosthetic heart valve.
SOURCE: From A Laupacis et al: Chest 114:579S, 1998.

risk of AF for stroke approaches 30%. Several studies have now demonstrated conclusively that the incidence of embolization in patients with AF not associated with valvular heart disease is reduced by chronic anticoagulation with warfarin-like agents. Aspirin also may be effective for this purpose in patients who are not at high risk for stroke. Although anticoagulation may be associated with hemorrhagic complications, the risk is largely associated with INRs above the recommended range of 1.8 to 3.0. Recommendations for the selection of antiarrhythmic medications to prevent the recurrence of AF are shown in Fig. 230-6.

Ablation therapy for cure of AF is an active area of investigation. This therapy is particularly attractive for the small subset of patients who have a focal atrial tachycardia that degenerates into AF. These automatic foci are often located in the pulmonary veins, and a targeted ablation in these areas may be curative. While ablation of these foci is possible, the procedure can result in pulmonary vein stenosis, pulmonary hypertension, and stroke. Further technologic advances are necessary before this procedure can be more widely and safely performed. A more morbid approach involves making multiple lesions in the right and left atria (MAZE procedure) to compartmentalize the electrical conductance of these chambers and disallow the propagation of fibrillatory waves. The morbidity, mortality, and success rate of such catheter-based procedures renders them experimental at this time.

ATRIAL FLUTTER This arrhythmia occurs most often in patients with organic heart disease. Flutter may be paroxysmal, in which

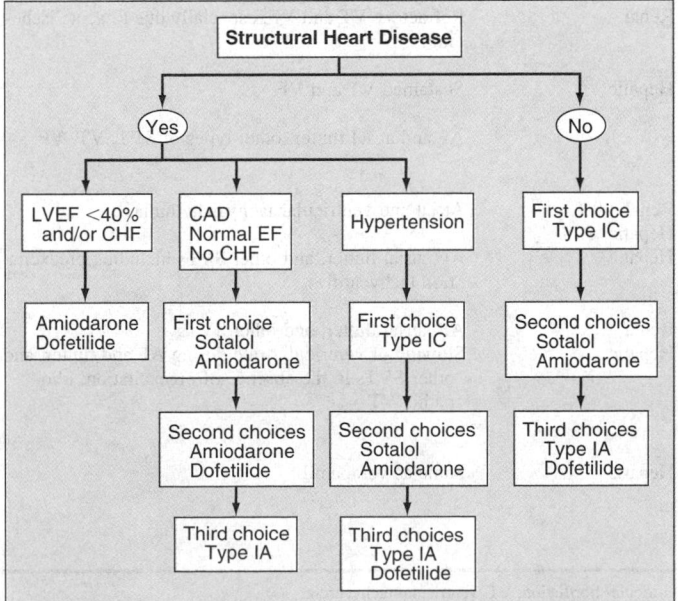

FIGURE 230-6 Recommendations for the selection of antiarrhythmic medications to prevent the recurrence of atrial fibrillation. See Tables 230-2 and 230-4 for definition of types IA and IC drugs. An atrioventricular nodal blocking agent (i.e., beta blocker, calcium channel blocker, or digoxin) should be added to all type IC and IA agents as well as to dofetilide. LVEF, left ventricular ejection fraction; CHF, congestive heart failure; CAD, coronary artery disease; EF, ejection fraction.

case there is usually a precipitating factor, such as pericarditis or acute respiratory failure, or it may be persistent. Atrial flutter (as well as AF) is very common during the first week following open-heart surgery. Atrial flutter is usually less long-lived than is AF, although on occasion it may persist for months to years. Most commonly, if it lasts for more than a week, atrial flutter will convert to AF. Systemic embolization is less common in atrial flutter than in AF.

Atrial flutter is characterized by an atrial rate between 250 and 350 bpm. Typically, the ventricular rate is half the atrial rate, i.e., approximately 150 bpm. If the atrial rate is slowed to <220 beats per minute by antiarrhythmic agents such as quinidine, which also possess vagolytic properties, the ventricular rate may rise suddenly because of the development of 1:1 AV conduction. Classically, flutter waves are seen as regular sawtooth-like atrial activity, most prominent in the inferior leads (Fig. 230-5D). When the ventricular response is regular and not a simple fraction of the atrial rate, complete AV block is present, which may be a manifestation of digitalis toxicity. Activation mapping suggests that atrial flutter is a form of atrial reentry localized to the right atrium.

TREATMENT The most effective treatment of atrial flutter is direct-current cardioversion, which can be accomplished at low energy (25 to 50 W · s) under mild sedation. Higher energies (100 to 200 W · s) are often used because they are less likely to cause AF, which not infrequently occurs following lower energy delivery. Although atrial flutter is associated with a slightly lower risk of embolization than AF, the same precautions should be followed in regard to anticoagulation as are used with AF. In patients who develop atrial flutter following open-heart surgery or recurrent flutter in the setting of acute myocardial infarction, particularly if they are being treated with digitalis, atrial pacing (using temporary pacing wires implanted at the time of operation or a pacing lead inserted into the atrium pervenously) at rates of 115 to 130% of the atrial flutter rate can usually convert the atrial flutter to sinus rhythm. Atrial pacing may also result in the conversion of atrial flutter to AF, which allows for easier control of the ventricular response. If immediate conversion of atrial flutter is not mandated by the patient's clinical status, the ventricular response should first be slowed by blocking the AV node with a beta blocker, calcium antagonist, or digitalis. Digitalis is the least effective and occasionally converts atrial flutter into AF. Once AV nodal conduction is slowed with any of these drugs, an attempt to convert flutter to sinus rhythm using a class I (A or C) agent or amiodarone should be made. Increasing doses of the drug selected are administered until the rhythm converts or side effects occur. Ibutilide is a new antiarrhythmic agent that is administered intravenously and appears to be particularly effective for conversion of atrial flutter to sinus rhythm.

Quinidine, other Class IA drugs, flecainide, propafenone, sotalol, and amiodarone (Table 230-4) may be useful in preventing recurrences of atrial flutter. Radiofrequency ablation is a highly effective treatment for patients with the most typical forms of atrial flutter, which are due to reentry around the tricuspid valve in a counterclockwise or clockwise fashion. The coronary sinus and inferior vena cava cause the wavefront of activation to pass between them and the tricuspid valve. Ablation of the narrowed isthmus using radiofrequency energy can cure flutter in >85% of cases.

PAROXYSMAL SUPRAVENTRICULAR TACHYCARDIAS (PSVT) In most cases, functional differences in conduction and refractoriness in the AV node or the presence of an AV bypass tract provide the substrate for the development of PSVT (previously termed *paroxysmal atrial tachycardia*). Electrophysiologic studies have demonstrated that reentry is responsible for the vast majority of cases of PSVT (Fig. 230-7). Reentry has been localized to the sinus node, atrium, AV node, or a macroreentrant circuit involving conduction in the antegrade direction through the AV node and retrograde through an AV bypass tract. Such a bypass tract may also conduct

Table 230-4 Drugs Used to Treat Cardiac Tachyarrhythmias

Drug	Mode of Administration	$t_{1/2}$ (oral), h	Route of Metabolism	Clinical Effects and/or Indications for Use
Digoxin	IV, 0.25–1.5 mg Oral, 0.75–1.5 mg loading dose over 12–24 h Maintenance, 0.23–0.50 mg/kg	36	Renal	Slowing of ventricular rate during AF, flutter, and other atrial tachycardias in the absence of preexcitation; slowing, termination, and/or prevention of SVT due to AV nodal reentry and AV reentry utilizing bypass tracts; may terminate or prevent intra-atrial reentrant tachycardias; ineffective in prevention of automatic atrial tachycardias
Adenosine	IV bolus, 6–12 mg	<10s		Acute termination of regular reentrant SVT involving the AV node
Quinidine (class IA)	Oral, 200–400 mg q6h	8–9	Hepatic, 80% Renal, 20%	Atrial and ventricular tachyarrhythmias; all types of SVT; control of ventricular rate in patients with preexcitation and AF and flutter
Procainamide (class IA)	IV, 40–50 mg/min to total of 10–20 mg/kg. Oral, 500–1000 mg q6h (sustained-release forms)	3–5	Hepatic, 50% Renal, 50%	Same as quinidine
Disopyramide (class IA)	Oral, 100–300 mg q6h	8–9	Hepatic, 50% Renal, 50%	Same as quinidine
Lidocaine (class IB)	IV, 20–50 mg/min to total of 5 mg/kg loading dose, followed by 1–4 mg/kg	1–2	Hepatic	VT and VF, especially during acute ischemia and myocardial infarction
Phenytoin (class IB)	IV, 20 mg/kg to total dose of 1000 mg Oral, 1000-mg loading dose over 24 h Maintenance, 100–400 mg/d	18–36	Hepatic	Tachyarrhythmias induced by digitalis; occasionally effective for ventricular tachyarrhythmias not induced by digitalis alone or in combination with other antiarrhythmic agents; polymorphic VT associated with increased QT interval
Mexiletine (class IB)	Oral, 100–300 mg q6–8h	9–12	Hepatic	Ventricular tachyarrhythmias; secondary agent in combination with other class 1 medication
Flecainide (class IC)	Oral, begin at 50–100 mg bid, increase by ≤50 mg in 4-day intervals to a maximum of mg daily	7–23	Hepatic, 75% Renal, 25%	Supraventricular tachyarrhythmias including atrial fibrillation and flutter; also ventricular arrhythmias refractory to other medications or radiofrequency ablation
Propafenone (class IC)	Oral, 150–300 mg q8h	5–8	Hepatic	Same as flecainide
Moricizine (class IC)	Oral, 200–400 mg q8h	2–6	Hepatic	Same as flecainide
Beta blockers (class II) e.g., metoprolol	IV, load with 5–10 mg q5min for 3 doses, then 3 mg q6h Oral, 25–100 mg bid	3–4	Hepatic	Slowing of ventricular rate during AF, atrial flutter, and other atrial tachyarrhythmias in the absence of preexcitation; SVT due to AV nodal reentry; reentry utilizing bypass tracts; arrhythmias (e.g., VT) induced by exercise or occurring in the presence of hyperthyroidism; polymorphic VT associated with congenital long QT syndrome
Bretylium (class III)	IV, 1–2 mg/kg per min to total load, 5–10 mg/kg Maintenance, 0.5–2 mg/kg	8–14	Renal	Refractory VT and VF, especially due to acute ischemia
Amiodarone (class III)	IV, 5–10 mg/kg load over 20 min, then 1 g/24 h		Hepatic	Sustained VT and VF
	Oral, load 800–1600 mg/d for 1 week, then 400–600 mg/d for 3 weeks, then 200–400 mg/d thereafter	13–103		AF and atrial flutter, other types of SVT, VT, VF
Sotalol (class III)	Oral, 80–320 mg q12h	10–20	Renal, 90% Hepatic, 10%	Atrial and ventricular tachyarrhythmias
Ibutilide (class III)	IV, <60 kg: 0.01 mg/kg over 10 min IV, ≥60 kg: 1 mg over 10 min, repeat after 10 min if no effect	2–6	Hepatic	AF, atrial flutter, and other SVTs including preexcitation tachycardias
Dofetilide	125–250 mg PO bid	8–12	Renal	AF, atrial flutter, and other SVTs
Calcium channel blockers (class IV) e.g., verapamil	IV, 2.5–10 mg over 1–2 min to total of 0.15 mg/kg Oral, 240–480 qd	6–24	Hepatic	Slowing of ventricular rate during AF and flutter, and other SVTs in the absence of preexcitation; idiopathic VT
Diltiazem	IV, load with 0.25 mg/kg over 2 min; if needed, repeat after 15 min with 0.35 mg over 2 min Maintenance, 10–15 mg/h		Hepatic	Same as verapamil

NOTE: AF, atrial fibrillation; AV, atrioventricular; SVT, supraventricular tachycardia; VF, ventricular fibrillation; VT, ventricular tachycardia.

antegradely, in which case the Wolff-Parkinson-White (WPW) syndrome is said to be present. When the bypass tract manifests only retrograde conduction, it is termed a *concealed bypass tract* (Fig. 230-7B). In these cases, the QRS complex during sinus rhythm is normal. In the absence of the WPW syndrome, reentry through the AV node or through a concealed bypass tract makes up more than 90% of all PSVTs.

AV NODAL REENTRANT TACHYCARDIA There is no age or disease predisposition for the development of AV nodal reentrant tachycardia, the most common cause of supraventricular tachy-

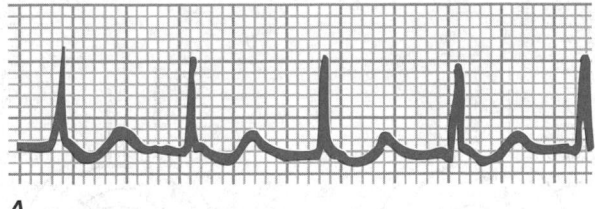

A

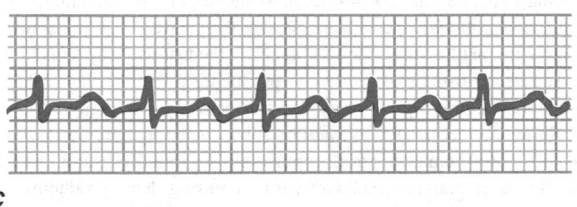

B

C

FIGURE 230-7 Examples of reentrant supraventricular tachycardia (SVT). *A.* AV nodal reentry. No P waves are visible. *B.* AV reentry using a concealed bypass tract. Inverted retrograde P waves are superimposed on the T wave. *C.* Intraatrial reentry. Inverted P waves follow the T waves and precede the QRS complex.

cardia. It is, however, more commonly observed in women. It usually presents as a regular narrow QRS complex tachycardia at rates of 120 to 250 bpm. APCs that initiate the arrhythmia are almost always associated with a prolonged PR interval. Retrograde P waves may be absent, buried in the QRS complex, or appear as distortions at the terminal parts of the QRS complex (Fig. 230-7*A*).

AV nodal reentrant PSVT (Fig. 230-8) can be reproducibly initiated and terminated by appropriately timed atrial premature stimuli. The onset of the tachycardia is almost always associated with prolongation of the PR interval due to marked AV nodal conduction delay (prolonged AH interval) following the APC that is critical for the genesis of the arrhythmia. The sudden prolongation of the AH interval is consistent with the concept of dual AV nodal pathways: a *fast pathway*, which exhibits rapid conduction and a long refractory period, and a *slow pathway*, which has a short refractory period but conducts slowly. During sinus rhythm, only conduction over the fast pathway is manifest, resulting in a normal PR interval (Fig. 230-8). Atrial extrastimuli at a critical coupling interval are blocked in the fast pathway because of its longer refractory period and are conducted slowly through the slow pathway. If conduction down the slow pathway is slow enough to allow the previously refractory fast pathway time to recover excitability, a single atrial (echo) reentrant beat or sustained tachycardia ensues. A critical balance between conduction velocity and refractoriness within the node is required to sustain AV nodal reentry. Retrograde atrial and antegrade ventricular activation occur simultaneously, explaining why P waves may not be apparent on the surface ECG.

Clinical Features AV nodal reentry may produce palpitations, syncope, and heart failure depending on the rate and duration of the arrhythmia and the presence and severity of any underlying heart disease. Hypotension and syncope may occur because of the sudden loss of the atrial contribution to ventricular filling; this can also lead to a marked increase in atrial pressure, acute pulmonary edema, and a reduction in ventricular filling. Simultaneous atrial and ventricular contraction produces cannon *a* waves with each heartbeat.

℞ TREATMENT In patients without hypotension, vagal maneuvers, particularly carotid sinus massage, can terminate the arrhythmia in 80% of cases. If hypotension is present, raising the blood pressure by the cautious use of intravenous phenylephrine in 0.1-mg increments may terminate the arrhythmia alone or in combination with carotid sinus pressure. If these maneuvers are unsuccessful, verapamil (2.5 to 10 mg intravenously) or adenosine (6 to 12 mg intravenously) is the agent of choice. We prefer to use adenosine because of its extremely short half-life, lessening the consequences of any side effects. Beta blockers may also be used to slow or terminate the tachycardia but are agents of second choice. Digitalis glycosides have a slower onset of action and should *not* be used for acute therapy. When these drugs fail to terminate the tachycardia, or when the tachycardia is recurrent, atrial or ventricular pacing via a temporary pacemaker inserted pervenously may be used to terminate the arrhythmia. However, if severe ischemia and/or hypotension is caused by the tachycardia, dc cardioversion should be considered.

AV nodal reentry can usually be prevented by the use of drugs that act primarily on the antegrade slow pathway (such as digitalis, beta blockers, or calcium channel antagonists) or on the fast pathway (class IA or IC; Table 230-4). We favor initial therapy with beta blockers, calcium channel antagonists, or digoxin because the risk-benefit ratio associated with treatment with these agents is more favorable than that of IA or IC agents. Drugs most likely to avert recurrences prevent induction of the arrhythmias by programmed stimulation. This technique utilizes temporary pacemaker catheters connected to a physiologic stimulator capable of variable rate pacing and stimulation with one or more precisely timed premature impulses. In symptomatic patients who require chronic therapy, radiofrequency catheter modification of the AV node should be considered. This technique can cure AV nodal reentry in >90% of cases and has been proven to be safe, although a 1 to 2% risk of AV block requiring a permanent pacemaker exists.

AV REENTRANT TACHYCARDIA PSVT due to AV reentry incorporates a concealed AV bypass tract as part of the tachycardia circuit. Thus the impulse passes antegradely from the atria through the AV node and His-Purkinje system to the ventricles and then retrogradely through the (concealed) bypass tract back to the atrium. Patients with this disorder manifest the same type of PSVT as do patients with the WPW syndrome (see below), but the bypass tract cannot conduct in an antegrade direction during sinus rhythm or other atrial tachyarrhythmias.

AV reentrant tachycardia can be initiated and terminated by either APCs or VPCs. Initiation of PSVT by a VPC is virtually diagnostic of AV reentry. Alternation of the QRS complexes occurs in approximately one-third of such tachycardias. Since atrial activation must follow ventricular activation during AV reentry, the P wave usually occurs after the QRS complex (Fig. 230-7*B*).

Atrial activation mapping is of major value in evaluating the origin of these tachycardias. Most concealed bypass tracts are left-sided. Thus, during PSVT or during ventricular pacing, the earliest activation sequence is recorded in the left atrium, usually via a catheter in the coronary sinus. This eccentric atrial activation is quite distinct from the normal retrograde activation sequence in which the earliest activation of the atria is in the area of the AV junction. The ability of a ventricular stimulus to conduct to the atrium at a time when the bundle

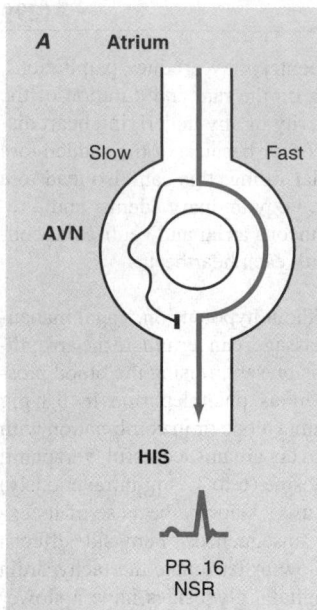 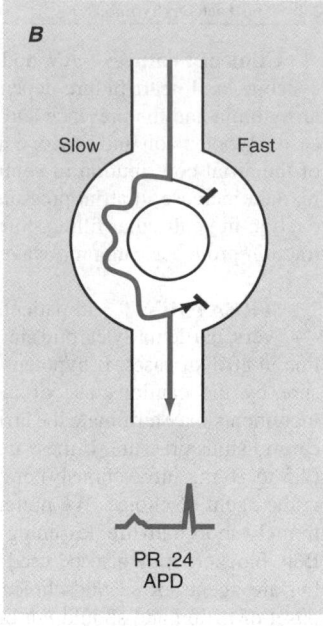 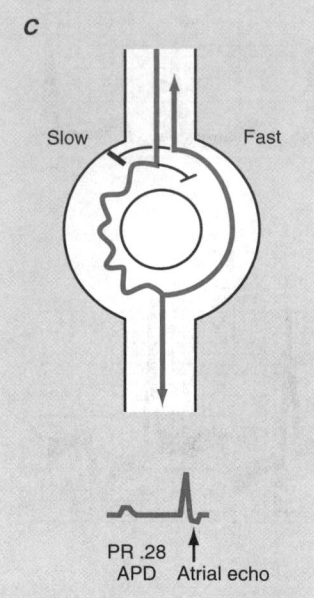 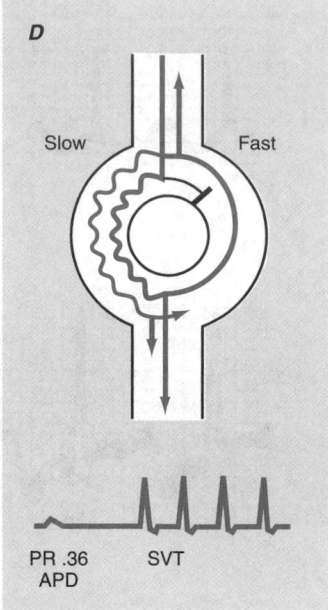

FIGURE 230-8 Mechanism of AV nodal reentry: The atrium, AV node (AVN), and His bundle are shown schematically. The AV node is longitudinally dissociated into two pathways, slow and fast, with different functional properties (see text). In each panel of this diagram, blue lines denote excitation in the AV node, which is manifest on the surface electrocardiogram, while black lines denote conduction, which is concealed and not apparent on the surface electrocardiogram. *A.* During sinus rhythm (NSR) the impulse from the atrium conducts down both pathways. However, only conduction over the fast pathway is manifest on the surface ECG, producing a normal PR interval of 0.16 s. *B.* An atrial premature depolarization (APD) blocks in the fast pathway. The impulse conducts over the slow pathway to the His bundle and ventricles, producing a PR interval of 0.24 s. Because the impulse is premature, conduction over the slow pathway occurs more slowly than it would during sinus rhythm. *C.* A more premature atrial impulse blocks in the fast pathway, conducting with increased delay in the slow pathway, producing a PR interval of 0.28 s. The impulse conducts retrogradely up the fast pathway producing a single atrial echo. Sustained reentry is prevented by subsequent block in the slow pathway. *D.* A still more premature atrial impulse blocks initially in the fast pathway, conducting over the slow pathway with increasing delay producing a PR interval of 0.36 s. Retrograde conduction occurs over the fast pathway and reentry occurs, producing a sustained tachycardia (SVT). *(After ME Josephson: Clinical Cardiac Electrophysiology, 2d ed. Phildelphia, Lea & Febiger, 1993.)*

of His is refractory and the termination of the tachycardia by a ventricular stimulus that does not reach the atrium are diagnostic of retrograde conduction over a concealed bypass tract.

℞ **TREATMENT** This is similar to the treatment for AV nodal reentry tachycardia. Although pharmacologic agents may be used, patients who require chronic therapy should be considered candidates for radiofrequency catheter ablation of the bypass tract. This requires detailed electrophysiologic study to exclude other arrhythmias that may be responsible for patients' symptoms and to determine the location of the bypass tract(s). The efficacy of this procedure exceeds 90%, with minimal risks. In the remaining small number of patients failing catheter ablation, surgical ablation or pharmacologic therapy can be used.

SINUS NODE REENTRY AND OTHER ATRIAL TACHYCARDIAS Reentry in the region of the sinus node or within the atria is invariably initiated by APCs. These arrhythmias are less common than AV nodal or AV reentry and are more often associated with underlying cardiac disease. During sinus node reentry, the P-wave morphology is identical to that occurring in sinus rhythm, but the PR interval is prolonged. This is in contrast to sinus tachycardia, in which the PR interval tends to shorten. With intraatrial reentry, the P-wave configuration differs from that during sinus rhythm, and the PR interval is prolonged (Fig. 230-7C).

℞ **TREATMENT** Sinus node and atrial reentrant arrhythmias are managed like other reentrant PSVTs, except that catheter ablation is less successful because multiple foci may be present.

NONREENTRANT ATRIAL TACHYCARDIAS These may be a manifestation of digitalis intoxication or may be associated with severe pulmonary or cardiac disease, with hypokalemia, or with the administration of theophylline or adrenergic drugs. Multifocal atrial tachycardia (MAT) (Fig. 230-9) is particularly common following theophylline administration. By definition, MAT requires three or more consecutive P waves of different morphologies at rates greater than 100 beats per minute. MAT usually has an irregular ventricular rate because of varying AV conduction. There is a high incidence of atrial fibrillation (50 to 70%) in patients with MAT. Treatment should be directed at the underlying disorder. The digitalis-induced arrhythmias are caused by triggered activity. In such atrial tachycardias with AV block secondary to digitalis intoxication, the atrial rate rarely exceeds 180 bpm, and typically 2:1 block is present. Atrial arrhythmias

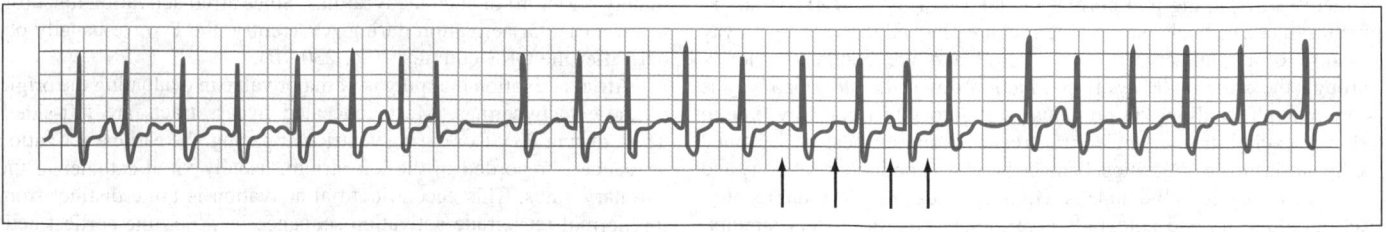

FIGURE 230-9 Multifocal atrial tachycardia. A lead I rhythm strip demonstrates a multifocal atrial tachycardia defined by ≥3 consecutive P waves of variable morphology and rate >100 bpm (*arrows*).

precipitated by digitalis can usually be treated by withdrawal of the drug.

Automatic atrial tachycardias not caused by digitalis are difficult to terminate, and in such cases the main goal of therapy should be to control the ventricular response, either by drugs that affect the AV node, such as digitalis, beta blockers, or calcium channel antagonists, or by ablation techniques. Catheter ablation and surgery have been employed to eradicate the arrhythmia's focus or create heart block for rate control.

PREEXCITATION (WPW) SYN-DROME The most frequently encountered type of ventricular preexcitation is that associated with AV bypass tracts. These connections are composed of strands of atrial-like muscle which may occur almost anywhere around the AV rings. The term *Wolff-Parkinson-White syndrome* is applied to patients with both preexcitation on the ECG and paroxysmal tachycardias. AV bypass tracts can be associated with certain congenital abnormalities, the most important of which is Ebstein's anomaly.

AV bypass tracts that conduct in an antegrade direction produce a typical ECG pattern of a short PR interval (<0.12 s), a slurred upstroke of the QRS complex (delta wave), and a wide QRS complex. This pattern results from a fusion of activation of the ventricles over both the bypass tract and the AV nodal His-Purkinje system (Fig. 230-10). The relative contribution of activation over each system determines the amount of preexcitation.

During PSVT in WPW, the impulse is usually conducted antegradely over the normal AV system and retrogradely through the bypass tract. The characteristics are identical to those described on p. 1299. Rarely (approximately 5%), tachycardias occurring in patients with WPW will exhibit a reverse pattern with antegrade conduction through the bypass tract and retrograde conduction through the normal AV system. This produces a tachycardia with a wide QRS complex in which the ventricles are totally activated by the bypass tract. Atrial flutter and AF also occur commonly in patients with WPW syndrome. Since the bypass tract does not have the same decremental conducting properties as the AV node, the ventricular responses during atrial flutter or fibrillation may be unusually rapid and may cause ventricular fibrillation (VF).

The goals of electrophysiologic evaluation in patients suspected of having the WPW syndrome are (1) to confirm the diagnosis, (2) to localize the bypass tract and determine how many bypass tracts are present, (3) to demonstrate the role of the bypass tract in the genesis of the arrhythmias, (4) to determine the potential for the development of possibly life-threatening rates during atrial flutter or fibrillation, and (5) to evaluate therapeutic options.

℞ **TREATMENT** Pharmacologic therapy is aimed at altering the electrophysiologic properties (i.e., refractoriness or conduction velocity) of one or more components of the reentrant circuit. This is most often accomplished by agents such as beta blockers or calcium channel blockers that slow conduction and increase refractoriness of the AV node or by agents such as quinidine or flecainide that slow conduction and increase refractoriness primarily in the bypass tract. Some drugs may affect multiple sites (Fig. 230-11).

Acute management of episodes of PSVT in patients with WPW syndrome is similar to that of PSVT in patients with concealed bypass tracts.

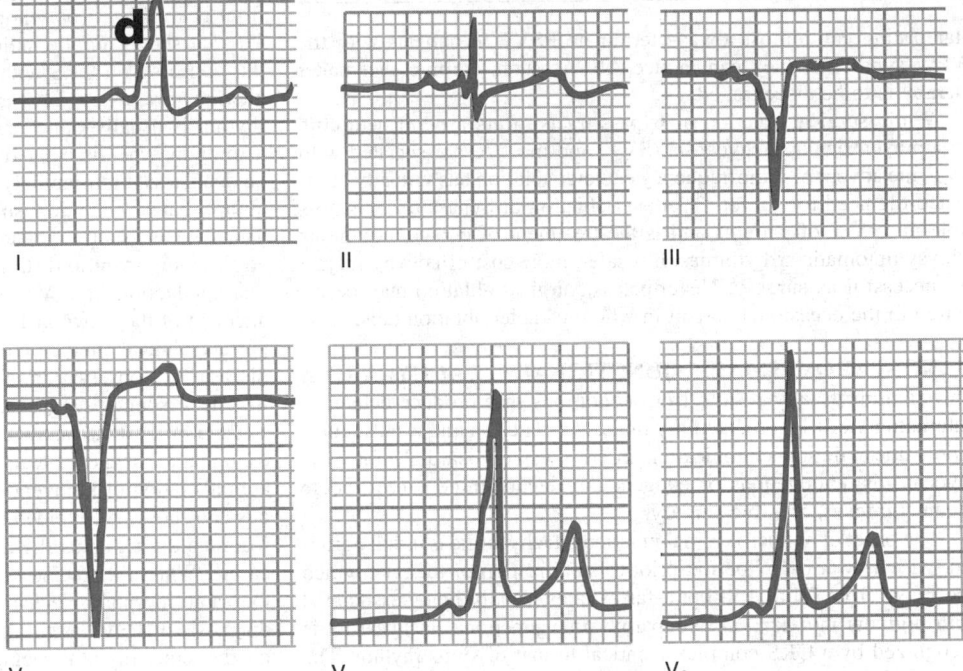

FIGURE 230-10 ECG in Wolff-Parkinson-White syndrome. There is a short PR interval (0.11 s), a wide QRS complex (0.12 s), and slurring on the upstroke of the QRS produced by early ventricular activation over the bypass tract (delta wave, d in lead I). The negative delta waves in V_1 are diagnostic of a right-sided bypass tract. Note the Q wave (negative delta wave) in lead III, mimicking myocardial infarction.

In patients with the WPW syndrome and AF, dc cardioversion should be carried out if there is a life-threatening, rapid ventricular response. In non-life–threatening situations, lidocaine (3 to 5 mg/kg) or procainamide (15 mg/kg) administered intravenously over 15 to 20 min will usually slow the ventricular response. More recently, ibutilide has become available as an alternative therapy for preexcitation tachycardia. Caution should be employed when using digitalis or intravenous verapamil in patients with the WPW syndrome and AF, since these drugs can shorten the refractory period of the accessory pathway and can increase the ventricular rate, thereby placing the patient at increased risk for VF. Chronic oral therapy with verapamil is not associated with this risk. In addition to these drugs, beta-blocking agents are of no utility in controlling the ventricular response during AF when conduction proceeds over the bypass tract. Although atrial or ventric-

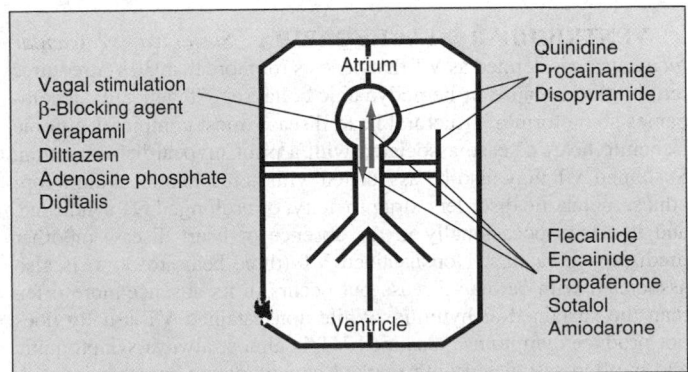

FIGURE 230-11 Site of action of antiarrhythmic agents in the Wolff-Parkinson-White syndrome. The atrium, ventricle, antegrade conduction through the AV node (↓), retrograde conduction through the AV node (↑), and the bypass tract are shown. Drugs on the left affect antegrade AV nodal conduction. Type IA drugs on the upper right affect retrograde conduction over the node and antegrade conduction over the bypass tract. Drugs on the lower right affect conduction in both directions in the AV node and the bypass tract.

ular pacing can almost always terminate PSVT in patients with the WPW syndrome, they can induce AF. As such, chronic pacemaker therapy is to be discouraged.

While surgical ablation of bypass tracts offers a permanent cure of supraventricular tachycardia (SVT) and most AFs associated with SVT, the advent of radiofrequency catheter ablation has virtually eliminated the need for surgery. Catheter ablation of bypass tracts is possible in >90% of patients and is the treatment of choice in patients with symptomatic arrhythmias. It is safer, more cost-effective, and just as successful as surgery. Nevertheless, surgical ablation may be required in the occasional patient in whom catheter ablation fails.

NONPAROXYSMAL   JUNCTIONAL   TACHYCARDIA
This rhythm usually results from conditions that produce enhanced automaticity or triggered activity in the AV junction and is most commonly due to digitalis intoxication, inferior wall myocardial infarction, myocarditis, endogenous or exogenous catecholamine excess, acute rheumatic fever, or valve surgery.

The onset of nonparoxysmal junctional tachycardia is usually gradual, with a "warm-up" period prior to stabilization of the rate, which can range from 70 to 150 bpm, faster rates usually being associated with digitalis intoxication. Nonparoxysmal junctional tachycardia is recognized by a QRS complex identical to that of sinus rhythm. The rate can be influenced by autonomic tone and can be increased by catecholamines, vagolytic agents, or exercise and slowed somewhat by carotid sinus pressure. When this rhythm is due to digitalis intoxication, it usually is associated with AV block and/or dissociation. Soon after cardiac surgery, retrograde conduction is more likely to be present because of the heightened sympathetic state.

℞ **TREATMENT**   This is directed toward elimination of the underlying etiologic factors. Since digitalis is the most common cause of this rhythm, discontinuation of this drug is indicated. If the rhythm is associated with other serious manifestations of digitalis intoxication, such as ventricular or atrial irritability, active intervention with lidocaine or a beta blocker may be useful, and in some instances, use of digitalis antibodies (Fab fragments) should be considered. Cardioversion of this rhythm should not be attempted, particularly in the setting of digitalis intoxication. When AV conduction is intact, atrial pacing can capture and override the junctional focus and provide the AV synchrony necessary to maximize cardiac output. Nonparoxysmal junctional tachycardia is usually not a chronic, recurrent problem, and attention to the acute precipitating events can often resolve the tachycardia.

VENTRICULAR   TACHYCARDIA   *Sustained ventricular tachycardia* is defined as VT that persists for more than 30 s or requires termination because of hemodynamic collapse. VT generally accompanies some form of structural heart disease, most commonly chronic ischemic heart disease associated with a prior myocardial infarction. Sustained VT may also be associated with nonischemic cardiomyopathies, metabolic disorders, drug toxicity, or prolonged QT syndrome, and it occurs occasionally in the absence of heart disease or other predisposing factors. Nonsustained VT (three beats to 30 s) is also associated with cardiac disease but occurs in its absence more often than the sustained arrhythmia. While nonsustained VT usually does not produce symptoms, sustained VT is almost always symptomatic and is often associated with marked hemodynamic compromise and/or the development of myocardial ischemia. A fixed anatomic substrate, not acute ischemia, is responsible for most recurrent episodes of sustained uniform VT. Acute ischemia appears to have little role in the genesis of sustained uniform VT associated with chronic infarction but may play a role in the degeneration of stable VT into VF or initiation of polymorphic VT. Most episodes of VF begin with VT.

The ECG diagnosis of VT is suggested by a wide-complex QRS tachycardia at a rate exceeding 100 bpm. The QRS configuration during any episode of VT may be uniform (monomorphic), or it may vary from beat to beat (polymorphic). *Bidirectional tachycardia* refers to VT that shows an alternation in QRS amplitude and axis. Typically this appears as a QRS with a right bundle branch block pattern with alternating superior (leftward) and inferior axes (rightward). While the rhythm is usually quite regular, slight irregularity may exist. Atrial activity may be dissociated from ventricular activity, or the atria may be depolarized retrogradely. The onset of the tachycardia is generally abrupt, but in nonparoxysmal tachycardias it can be gradual. Paroxysmal VT is usually initiated by a VPC.

It is important to distinguish SVT with aberration of intraventricular conduction from VT because the clinical implications and management of these two arrhythmias are totally different. The most important clinical predictor of VT is the presence of structural heart disease. The observation of intermittent cannon *a* waves and varying first heart sounds suggests AV dissociation and is diagnostic of VT. In a majority of cases, the diagnosis can and should be made by close examination of the 12-lead ECG. Pharmacologic maneuvers, such as administration of intravenous verapamil or adenosine, can be hazardous and should be avoided. It is always useful to have a 12-lead ECG recorded during sinus rhythm for comparison with that during tachycardia. When the tracing obtained during sinus rhythm demonstrates the same morphologic features as those during the tachycardia, the diagnosis of PSVT with aberration is favored. An infarction pattern on the sinus rhythm tracing suggests the potential presence of the anatomic substrate necessary for VT. Characteristics of the 12-lead ECG during the tachycardia that suggest a ventricular origin for the arrhythmia are (1) a QRS complex >0.14 s in the absence of antiarrhythmic therapy, (2) AV dissociation (with or without fusion or captured beats) or variable retrograde conduction (Fig. 230-12), (3) a superior QRS axis in the presence of a right bundle branch block pattern, (4) concordance of the QRS pattern in all precordial leads (i.e., all positive or all negative deflections), and (5) other QRS patterns (morphology) with prolonged duration that are inconsistent with typical right or left bundle branch block patterns. (See Table 230-5 for a detailed synopsis of ECG criteria that favor the diagnosis of VT over SVT for wide complex tachycardia.) A wide, complex, bizarre tachycardia that is very irregular suggests AF with conduction over an AV bypass tract. Similarly, a QRS complex in excess of 0.20 s is uncommon during VT in the absence of drug therapy and is more common with preexcitation. Intravenous verapamil will stop most recalcitrant SVTs involving the AV junction, but it is rarely effective for VT. Because of this property, verapamil has been utilized to attempt to differentiate SVT with aberrant conduction from VT. However, this is extremely hazardous, since intravenous verapamil can precipitate cardiac arrest in patients with VT.

It has been possible to replicate sustained uniform VT in more than 95% of patients with this arrhythmia using programmed electrical stimulation. In most patients the tachycardia is initiated with ventricular premature stimuli. A sustained monomorphic VT with a morphology identical to that of the spontaneous arrhythmia is the rule. The clinical significance of polymorphic VT initiated by programmed stimulation is not clear, since more aggressive stimulation (i.e., the use of three or four extrastimuli) can induce polymorphic VT and even VF in some normal subjects and in patients who have never had a clinical arrhythmia.

Sustained uniform VT can be terminated by programmed stimulation or rapid pacing in at least 75% of patients; the remainder require cardioversion. The ability to reproducibly initiate and terminate a sustained, uniform VT permits assessment of pharmacologic and electrical therapy of these arrhythmias.

The reproducible termination of VT by programmed stimulation permits evaluation of the effectiveness of antitachycardia pacemakers for long-term therapy of paroxysmal episodes of arrhythmia. Unfortunately, rapid pacing, the most effective form of therapy, can accelerate the tachycardia and/or produce VF. Therefore, antitachycardia pacing is a viable form of therapy only when the pacing device includes backup defibrillation capabilities.

Clinical Features Symptoms resulting from VT depend on the ventricular rate, duration of the tachycardia, and presence and extent of underlying cardiac disease. When the tachycardia is rapid and associated with severe myocardial dysfunction and cerebrovascular disease, hypotension and syncope are common. However, the presence of hemodynamic stability does not preclude a diagnosis of VT. The rate, loss of the atrial contribution to ventricular filling, and abnormal sequence of ventricular activation are important factors producing a decreased cardiac output during VT.

The *prognosis* of VT depends on the underlying disease state. If sustained VT develops within the first 6 weeks following acute myocardial infarction, the prognosis is poor, with a 75% mortality rate at 1 year. Patients with nonsustained VT following myocardial infarction have a threefold greater risk of death

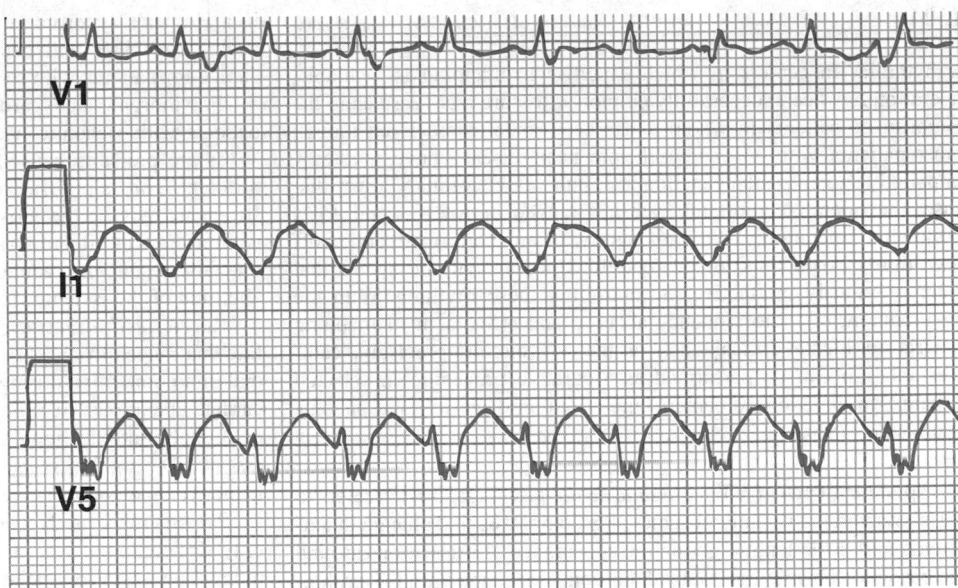

FIGURE 230-12 Ventricular tachycardia with AV dissociation. P waves are dissociated from the underlying wide complex rhythm (best seen on lead V₁).

than a comparable group of patients without this arrhythmia. However, a cause-and-effect relationship between the nonsustained tachycardia and subsequent sudden death has not been established. Patients without heart disease who have uniform VT have a good prognosis and an extremely low risk of sudden death.

[Rx] **TREATMENT** The risk-benefit ratio of treating each specific type of VT should be considered before beginning therapy. This is important because antiarrhythmic agents can produce or exacerbate the very arrhythmias that they are given to prevent. In general, patients with VT but without organic heart disease have a benign course; such patients with asymptomatic, nonsustained VT need not be treated because their prognosis will not be affected. An exception is the patient with congenital long QT syndrome. Such patients have recurrent polymorphic VT and a high mortality from sudden death if untreated. Patients with sustained VT in the absence of heart disease usually require therapy because the arrhythmia causes symptoms. These tachycardias may respond to beta blockers; verapamil; class IA, IC, or III agents; or amiodarone. In patients with VT and organic heart disease, if marked hemodynamic compromise is present or if there is evidence of ischemia, congestive heart failure, or central nervous system hypoperfusion, the rhythm should be promptly terminated by dc cardioversion (see below). If the patient with organic heart disease tolerates the VT well, pharmacologic therapy may be tried. Procainamide is probably the most effective agent for acute therapy. It may or may not terminate the tachycardia but almost always slows the rate. In stable patients in whom these drugs do not terminate the arrhythmia, a pacing catheter can be inserted pervenously into the right ventricular apex, and the tachycardia can be terminated by overdrive pacing.

Programmed stimulation is probably the most effective way to select the appropriate antiarrhythmic agent to prevent recurrent, sustained VT. After demonstrating that the tachycardia can be initiated reproducibly in the absence of antiarrhythmic agents, drugs can be studied serially, and the drug that prevents initiation of the tachycardia can be selected; long-term (>2 years) successful prevention of the arrhythmia can then be expected in 80% of patients if a complete stimulation protocol is used following drug administration. Failure to perform a complete protocol will lead to recurrences, which are often blamed on the lack of utility of programmed stimulation as a method of evaluating drug efficacy. Drug levels demonstrated to be successful in the laboratory need to be maintained chronically. Unfortunately, prevention of inducible VT is expected in only 50% of cases. Use of Holter monitor for guided therapy, although advocated by some, is of less value.

Antitachycardia pacing has been used as a means to terminate tachycardias that have been reproducibly terminated by pacing in the electrophysiology laboratory. Automatic antitachycardia pacing devices are not used alone because pacing during VT may accelerate tachycardia, converting a stable arrhythmia into an unstable one and resulting in severe hemodynamic compromise. However, devices combining antitachycardia pacing with an ICD (see below) afford a "backup" means of terminating unstable arrhythmias.

The advent of endocardial catheter and intraoperative mapping led to the development of surgical techniques for the management of VT. Activation mapping permits localization of the site of origin of the

Table 230-5 Wide Complex Tachycardia

ECG CRITERIA THAT FAVOR VENTRICULAR TACHYCARDIA

1. AV dissociation
2. QRS width: >0.14 s with RBBB configuration
             >0.16 s with LBBB configuration
3. QRS axis: Left axis deviation with RBBB morphology
             Extreme left axis deviation (northwest axis) with LBBB morphology
4. Concordance of QRS in precordial leads
5. Morphologic patterns of the QRS complex
       RBBB: Mono- or biphasic complex in V₁
             RS (*only with left axis deviation*) or QS in V₆

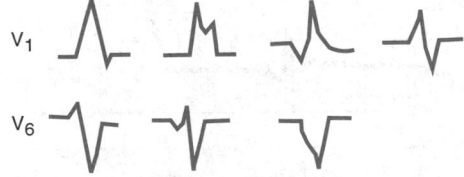

    LBBB: Broad R wave in V₁ or V₂ ≥0.04 s
             Onset of QRS to nadir of S wave in V₁ or V₂ of ≥0.07 s
             Notched downslope of S wave in V₁ or V₂
             Q wave in V₆

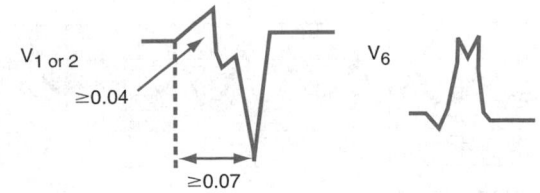

NOTE: AV, atrioventricular; BBB, bundle branch block.

arrhythmia. In centers in which expertise in mapping is available, operation has been successfully employed to cure tachycardias in the majority of patients in whom it has been undertaken. Even though most patients with VT and ischemic heart disease have markedly impaired left ventricular function and multivessel coronary artery disease, the operative mortality rate has ranged between 8 and 15%. Following operation, >90% of survivors are controlled either off (two-thirds of patients) or on (one-third) antiarrhythmic agents that were previously ineffective in controlling these rhythms. With the development of radiofrequency ablation and refinement of mapping criteria to locate critical sites of the VT circuit, precisely, catheter ablation can be performed as a curative procedure in selected patients. In experienced centers cure of VT in these *selected* patients approaches 75%.

Specific Types of VT   *Torsade de pointes* (Fig. 230-13) refers to VT characterized by polymorphic QRS complexes that change in amplitude and cycle length, giving the appearance of oscillations around the baseline. This rhythm is, by definition, associated with QT prolongation. The latter may result from electrolyte disturbances (particularly hypokalemia and hypomagnesemia), use of a variety of antiarrhythmic drugs (especially quinidine), phenothiazines and tricyclic antidepressants, liquid protein diets, intracranial events, and bradyarrhythmias, particularly third-degree AV block. It also may occur as a congenital anomaly that most often presents with torsade de pointes (syncope or sudden death) at a young age.

The electrocardiographic hallmark is polymorphic VT preceded by marked QT prolongation, often in excess of 0.60 s. These patients often have multiple episodes of nonsustained polymorphic VT associated with recurrent syncope, but they also may develop VF and sudden cardiac death.

Therapy should be directed at removing the precipitating factors, i.e., correcting metabolic abnormalities and removing drugs that have induced the prolonged QT interval. In the setting of drug-induced torsade de pointes, atrial or ventricular overdrive pacing and the administration of magnesium have also been useful in terminating and preventing the arrhythmia. For patients with the congenital prolonged QT interval syndrome, β-adrenergic blocking agents have been the mainstay of therapy; agents that shorten the QT interval may also be useful (e.g., phenytoin). Cervicothoracic sympathectomy has been proposed as a form of therapy for congenital prolonged QT syndrome, but it is not often effective as the sole therapy. Pacing in combination with beta blockers and sympathectomy has been used by some investigators when beta blockers fail, but it is not uniformly successful and results

in a Horner's syndrome. More recently, ICDs with dual chambered pacing capability and beta blockers have become the treatment of choice for patients with recurrent episodes despite beta blockers.

Polymorphic tachycardias associated with normal QT intervals in patients with ischemic heart disease that are initiated by "R-on-T" VPCs are probably caused by reentry, and their treatment is totally different. This is not true torsade de pointes. In such cases, class I or III agents may be the most effective form of therapy and should be administered in full antiarrhythmic doses. However, these arrhythmias may also result from acute, severe ischemia and will only respond to abolition of the ischemia, usually by revascularization.

Accelerated idioventricular rhythm, also termed *slow VT*, with a rate that ranges from 60 to 120 bpm, usually occurs in acute myocardial infarction, often during reperfusion. It may also be seen following cardiac operations; in patients with cardiomyopathy, rheumatic fever, or digitalis intoxication; and in patients with no evidence of heart disease. The rhythm is usually transient and rarely causes significant hemodynamic compromise or symptoms.

Treatment is rarely necessary and should usually be considered only if symptoms arise due to impaired hemodynamics, most commonly due to AV dissociation. In most cases, atropine can accelerate the sinus rate to overdrive the ventricular rhythm.

VENTRICULAR FLUTTER AND VENTRICULAR FIBRILLATION (Fig. 230-14; See also Chap. 39)   These arrhythmias occur most often in patients with ischemic heart disease. They also occur following administration of antiarrhythmic drugs, particularly those that induce prolonged QT intervals and torsade de pointes (see above), in patients with severe hypoxia or ischemia, and in those with WPW who develop AF with an extremely rapid ventricular response (p. 1299). Electrical accidents frequently cause cardiac arrest due to the development of VF. The onset of these arrhythmias is rapidly followed by loss of consciousness and, if untreated, death. Episodes of cardiac arrest recorded during Holter monitoring reveal that approximately three-fourths of the sudden deaths are due to VT or VF.

In patients with nonischemic VF, the onset usually begins with a short run of rapid VT, which is initiated by a relatively late coupled VPC. In patients with acute myocardial infarction or ischemia, however, VF is usually precipitated by a single early ventricular complex beat falling on the T wave (the vulnerable period), which produces a rapid VT that degenerates into VF (Fig. 230-14).

The clinical setting in which VF occurs is important. Most patients who have primary VF within the first 48 h of the onset of acute infarction have a good long-term prognosis, with a very low rate of recurrence or sudden cardiac death. Their short-term mortality may, however, be slightly increased. In contrast, patients who experience VF unassociated with the development of acute myocardial infarction

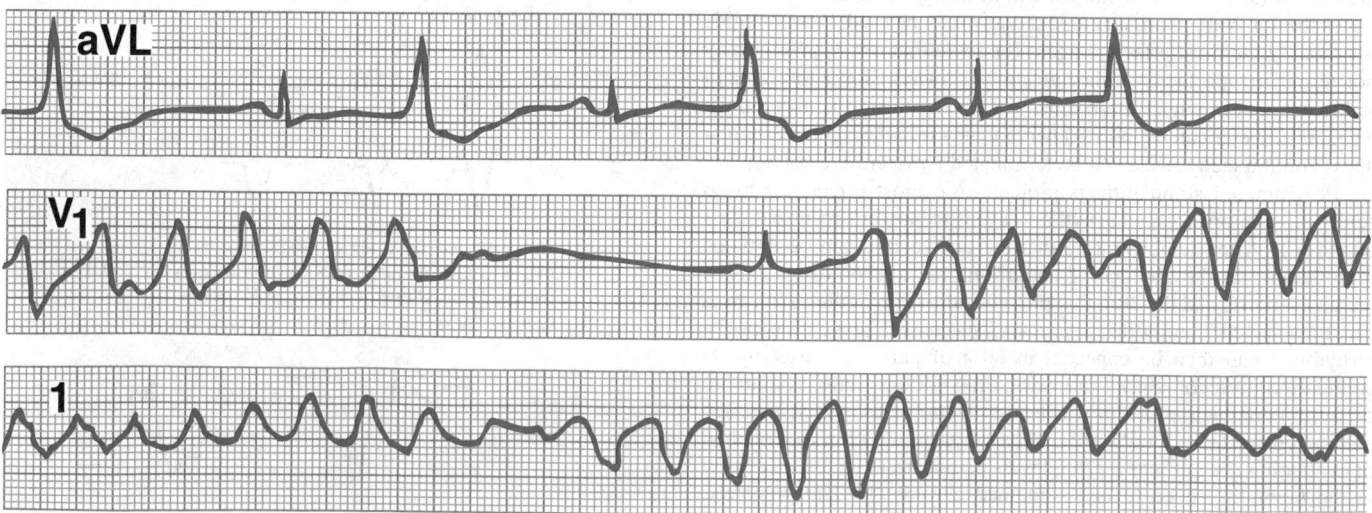

FIGURE 230-13   Rhythm strips of patients with drug (disopyramide)-induced torsade de pointes. The polymorphic ventricular tachycardia is associated with very long QT intervals.

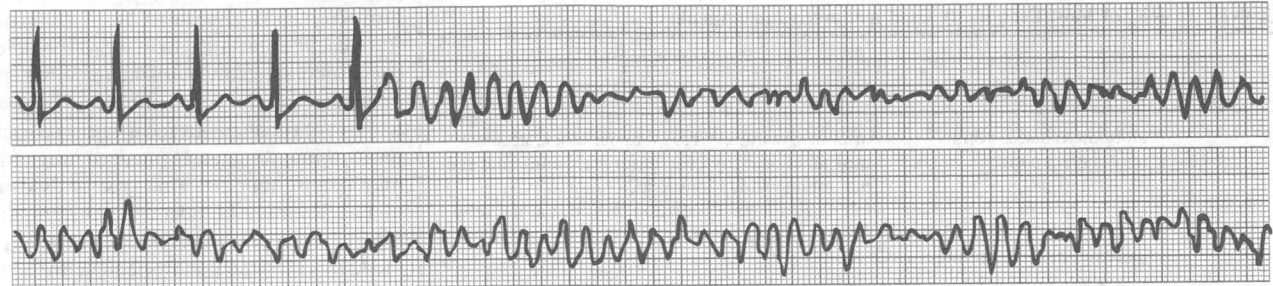

FIGURE 230-14 Ventricular fibrillation. In a patient with coronary disease, ventricular fibrillation is initiated by an early ventricular premature complex that produces a rapid polymorphic ventricular tachycardia which rapidly degenerates to ventricular fibrillation (note the undulating baseline with indistinguishable systole and diastole).

have a recurrence rate of 20 to 30% in the year following the event (Chap. 39).

Ventricular flutter usually appears as a sine wave with a rate between 150 and 300 bpm. These oscillations make it impossible to assign a specific morphology to the arrhythmia and in some cases to distinguish it from rapid VT. VF is recognized by grossly irregular undulations of varying amplitudes, contours, and rates (Fig. 230-14). Electrophysiologic studies have demonstrated that regardless of the apparent gross irregularity on the surface ECG, VF usually starts out with a rapid repetitive sequence of VT that ultimately breaks down into multiple wavelets of reentry.

Electrophysiologic studies have been useful in patients who have been resuscitated from cardiac arrest. In approximately 70% of patients with prior infarction, programmed stimulation can reproducibly initiate a sustained VT. Ablation may be possible in some of these patients, particularly if the VT can be slowed so that it can be mapped. Several recent secondary prevention trials have demonstrated superior survival (3 years) in patients treated with ICDs versus amiodarone (Table 230-6). However, in patients with ejection fractions >35% or <20%, survival was comparable. Further subgroup analysis is necessary to identify those patients most likely to be benefited by ICDs.

GENETIC CONSIDERATIONS Many advances have been made in the identification of genes responsible for syndromes associated with ventricular tachycardias and sudden cardiac death. Four specific examples include the congenital long QT syndrome (LQTS), hypertrophic obstructive cardiomyopathy (Chap. 238), arrhythmogenic right ventricular dysplasia, and the Brugada syndrome. The latter is a recently described disorder characterized by the electrocardiographic profile of a pseudo bundle branch block pattern with ST elevation and terminal T-wave inversion in leads V_1-V_3 (Fig. 230-15). The clinical presentation is VF in patients with structurally normal hearts. A mutation in the cardiac sodium channel, SCN 5A, is believed to be responsible. While the same gene is responsible for the LQTS, the mutation is different in the two syndromes. ■

TREATMENT

Pharmacologic Antiarrhythmic Therapy Prior to initiation of pharmacologic antiarrhythmic therapy, potential aggravating factors such as transient metabolic abnormalities, congestive heart failure, or acute ischemia must be corrected; in some cases this may suffice to control arrhythmias. In addition, the potential role of drugs as a cause or exacerbating factor in the development of the arrhythmia must be

Table 230-6 Trials of ICD Therapy vs. Antiarrythmic Drugs (AAD): VT/VF Patients

	AVID			CIDS	CASH
Protocol	ICD vs. empiric amiodarone or sotolol (mainly amiodarone)			ICD vs. empiric amiodarone	ICD vs. empiric amiodarone, metoprolol, and propafenone[a]
Sample size	$n = 1016$ AAD = 509 ICD = 507			$n = 659$ Amiodarone = 331 ICD = 328	$n = 346$ Amiodarone = 92 Metoprolol = 97 Propafenone* = 58 ICD = 99
Patient inclusion criteria	Survivors of VF VT with syncope VT with EF ≤ 40%			Survivors of VF VT with syncope VT with EF ≤ 35% and cycle length ≤ 400 ms	Survivors of VF (no EF requirement)
Mortality in "drug" or "control" arm	17.7% 1 year	25.3% 2 years	35.9% 3 years	30% 3 years	19.6% 2 years
Mortality in ICD arm	10.7% 1 year	18.4% 2 years	24.6% 3 years	25% 3 years	12.1% 2 years
Reduction in mortality with ICD	39% 1 year	27% 2 years	31% 3 years	20% 3 years	37% 2 years

[a] Following an interim analysis in March, 1992, enrollment in propafenone arm was discontinued because mortality was increased significantly over mortality in the ICD arm.
NOTE: EF, ejection fraction; ICD, implanted cardioverter/defibrillator; VF, ventricular fibrillation; VT, ventricular tachycardia.
SOURCES: AVID Investigators: N Engl J Med 337(22):1576, 1997; K Kuck, S Connolly: ACC NewsOnline, 1998.

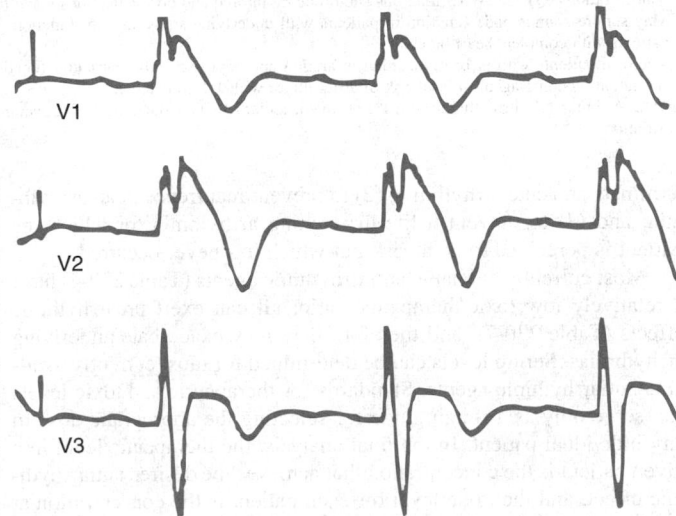

FIGURE 230-15 Brugada syndrome. Note ST elevation with terminal T wave inversion in leads V_1-V_3 mimicking right bundle branch block.

considered. It must be recognized that we do not have a good understanding of the effects of antiarrhythmic agents on the spontaneous onset of tachyarrhythmias. In some cases, they may facilitate the onset.

Antiarrhythmic drugs are used in three principal situations: (1) to

Table 230-7   Toxicity of Most Frequently Used Antiarrhythmic Agents

Drug	Nonarrhythmic Toxicity	Proarrhythmic Toxicity			
		TDP[a]	A Flutter 1:1	VT/VF	Bradycardia
Digoxin	Anorexia, nausea, vomiting, visual changes	Atrial tachycardia, VT, AV nodal block, accelerated junctional rhythms, atrial and ventricular premature depolarizations; acceleration of ventricular rate during atrial fibrillation or flutter in the presence of preexcitation			
Quinidine[b]	Anorexia, nausea, vomiting, diarrhea, cinchonism, tinnitus, hearing and visual changes, thrombocytopenia, hemolytic anemia, rash, potentiation of digoxin levels	2%	++	++	+
Procainamide[b]	Lupus erythematosus–like syndrome, anorexia, nausea	2%	+	++	+
Disopyramide[b]	Anticholinergic actions: dry mouth, urinary retention, visual disturbances (avoid in narrow-angle glaucoma) constipation, congestive heart failure	2%	+	++	+
Lidocaine	Dizziness, confusion, delirium, seizures, coma; side effects potentiated by liver and heart failure	—	—	—	+[b]
Mexiletine	Ataxia, tremor, gait disturbances, rash, vomiting	—	—	—	—
Flecainide	Dizziness, nausea	Rare	+++	++	++
Propafenone[c]	Taste disturbance, bronchospasm	Rare	+++	++	++
Amiodarone	Pulmonary infiltrates and fibrosis, hepatitis, hypo- and hyperthyroidism, photosensitivity, peripheral neuropathy, tremor	Rare	+++	+++	+++
Sotalol	Bronchospasm	+++	+	+	+++

[a] TDP (torsade de pointes) occurs most often in the setting of slow heart rates, QT prolongation, and hypokalemia or hypomagnesemia and at the time of conversion from atrial fibrillation to sinus rhythm. QT prolongation and torsade de pointes are not dose-related phemonema. QRS prolongation is a dose-related phenomena and will occur at toxic concentrations. QT and WRS intervals should be monitored and dose reductions made for interval prolongations.

[b] May suppress sinus node function in patients with underlying sinus node dysfunction. May suppress escape foci in patients with complete heart block.

[c] Avoid in patients with prior myocardial infarction and depressed left ventricular function. Use in combination with AV nodal blocking agent to limit risk of atrial flutter with 1:1 conduction.

NOTE: A flutter 1:1, atrial flutter with 1:1 atrioventricular (AV) conduction; VT/VF, ventricular tachycardia/ventricular fibrillation.

terminate an acute arrhythmia; (2) to prevent recurrence of an arrhythmia; and (3) to prevent a life-threatening arrhythmia for which the patient is perceived to be at risk but which has never occurred.

Most currently available antiarrhythmic agents (Table 230-4) have a relatively low toxic/therapeutic ratio; all can exert proarrhythmic effects (Table 230-7), and therefore they may exacerbate underlying arrhythmias. Serum levels can be determined for most currently available antiarrhythmic agents. Standards for therapeutic and toxic levels can serve only as a rough guide for selecting the appropriate dose in any individual patient. In the final analysis, the therapeutic level in a given patient is the concentration that achieves the desired antiarrhythmic effect, and the toxic level for each patient is the concentration at which undesirable side effects occur. Since many adverse effects are directly related to drug concentrations, the lowest serum level that achieves an effective antiarrhythmic response should be chosen.

In order to determine the therapeutic level for a patient, one must have a standard to judge drug efficacy. For a patient with an incessant arrhythmia, antiarrhythmic drugs may be administered empirically until the arrhythmia is suppressed. If a reproducible precipitating factor such as exercise can be identified, serial drug testing during such a provocative maneuver may be performed. Unfortunately, most arrhythmias are sporadic and occur unpredictably without identifiable precipitating factors. In these cases, if one waits to observe spontaneous recurrences on each antiarrhythmic drug, assessment of drug efficacy may require months. This type of assessment of efficacy may be adequate for arrhythmias that are not life-threatening. However, this mode of assessment is inadequate for arrhythmias that compromise hemodynamic stability, result in syncope, or cause cardiac arrest. In such cases, two methods for determination of arrhythmic drug efficacy have been utilized. The first, which consists of continuous ECG monitoring in the control state and then in the presence of antiarrhythmic drugs, has been used in order to determine the effect that each drug has on spontaneous atrial or ventricular ectopy. This method presupposes that the mechanism responsible for sustained arrhythmias is the same as that causing isolated premature depolarizations (which may or may not be true) and that therefore eradication of isolated ectopy will correlate with prevention of sustained arrhythmias. This method has a number of limitations. First, patients frequently show marked degrees of spontaneous variation in frequency of ectopy, which may mimic antiarrhythmic drug effects. Second, 25 to 30% of patients with sustained ventricular arrhythmias such as VT or VF demonstrate only rare spontaneous ectopy. Finally, many patients demonstrate a dissociation between the effects of antiarrhythmic agents on spontaneous ectopy and the effects of the same agent on sustained arrhythmias.

An alternative method to assess drug efficacy is programmed stimulation. Numerous studies have demonstrated that most clinically occurring supraventricular and ventricular tachyarrhythmias may be reproducibly initiated and terminated safely using this technique. Studies are performed initially in a baseline state in the absence of antiarrhythmic drugs. If the patient's clinical arrhythmia can be reproducibly initiated, then the ability of individual antiarrhythmic drugs to prevent reinduction of the arrhythmia can be assessed either after the drug is administered intravenously or after several days of oral loading in order to achieve a steady-state serum concentration. Use of this method assumes that (1) the induced and spontaneous arrhythmias are identical, and (2) prevention of induction of arrhythmias will correlate with prevention of recurrent spontaneous tachycardias on the same drug regimen. This technique has been validated in patients with a variety of reentrant PSVTs, VT, and VF. The technique is safe when carefully performed, the potential complications being those of any intravascular catheterization. Appropriate interpretation of the results of programmed stimulation is critically dependent on correlating the patient's spontaneous arrhythmias with those induced in the laboratory, with regard to rate and morphology, in order to be certain that the arrhythmia induced in the laboratory represents the same arrhythmia that occurred spontaneously and caused symptoms.

Classification of Antiarrhythmic Drugs   A number of classifications of antiarrhythmic drugs have been proposed; the most frequently used is a modification of one proposed by Vaughan-Williams (Table 230-2). This classification is based in part on the ability of antiarrhythmic drugs to modify the cardiac cellular (1) excitatory cur-

(phase 4 depolarization). These effects of the drugs on isolated cardiac cells are thought to account for some of the antiarrhythmic properties of the drugs. Thus depression of excitatory currents by class I and class IV antiarrhythmics results in slowing of conduction velocity and may interrupt arrhythmias by blocking conduction in areas of marginal excitability, where conduction velocity is already slow. Class III antiarrhythmics allegedly exert their action by increasing refractoriness through prolongation of the action potential duration. However, this classification has a number of limitations. The electrophysiologic effects of these drugs in vivo may differ from their effects on isolated cells. Also, the effects of heart rate and fiber geometry are not considered. Not all drugs (e.g., adenosine) fit into the classifications. Finally, some drugs (e.g., amiodarone) exhibit properties consistent with multiple classes. The uses, actions, and toxic actions of currently available antiarrhythmic drugs are summarized in Tables 230-4 and 230-7.

Electrical Therapy of Tachyarrhythmias • *Pacemakers*

Cardiac pacing can be used to terminate and in selected cases prevent recurrent supraventricular and ventricular arrhythmias. Because many tachyarrhythmias appear to be due to a reentrant mechanism with the impulse traveling in a circuit, a properly timed paced impulse can penetrate and prematurely depolarize part of the circuit, rendering it refractory to the next circulating wavefront and thereby interrupting the circus movement. Pacing therapy for arrhythmias is generally reserved for patients whose arrhythmias are refractory to drug therapy and who remain hemodynamically stable during the tachycardia. All forms of pacing therapy require repeated demonstration of their effectiveness and reliability in terminating the arrhythmias during electrophysiologic testing prior to implantation of the pacing device.

The type of pacing device and modality selected for arrhythmia termination depends on (1) the rate of the tachycardia (rates >160 bpm are rarely terminated by a single premature stimulus), (2) the type of arrhythmia (atrial flutter and VT are rarely terminated by single extrastimuli), and (3) concomitant drug therapy.

Because many tachycardias cannot be terminated by single premature stimuli, pacemakers have been developed that allow for multiple extrastimuli (burst pacing) to be introduced. In the current era, antitachycardia pacing is almost exclusively for ventricular arrhythmias because of the success of radiofrequency ablative therapy for supraventricular arrhythmias.

Cardiac pacing has also been used to prevent ventricular tachyarrhythmias. Polymorphic VT associated with a long QT interval and bradycardia (torsade de pointes, p. 1304) is most likely to respond. Pacing the atrium and/or ventricle at rates between 90 and 120 bpm appears to increase the homogeneity of electrical recovery and markedly reduces the propensity for a recurrence of arrhythmias.

Pacemakers may be self-contained or energized by an external radiofrequency source. The self-contained pacemaker may function automatically [i.e., it incorporates an arrhythmia recognition program (circuit)], or it may be activated by an external magnet. The major advantage of a fully automatic system is that there is no need for the patient to recognize the arrhythmia in order for termination to occur. The advantages of the externally activated system (rarely used today) include (1) the decreased risk of unnecessary treatment because of faulty sensing, and (2) the opportunity to initiate monitoring at the time of attempted termination of arrhythmia. This type of monitoring is frequently helpful if pacing techniques are employed to terminate VT, given the risk of acceleration of the arrhythmia by pacing.

The limitations of pacing therapy are primarily related to (1) the changes in the characteristics of the arrhythmia over time such that programmed pacing parameters no longer terminate the tachycardia, (2) the risk of acceleration of the tachycardia with the development of AF when stimulating the atrium and the development of rapid VT and VF when stimulating the ventricles, and (3) inappropriate recognition of supraventricular tachyarrhythmias as ventricular tachycardias, leading to delivery of therapy unnecessarily, which can initiate VT or VF. Future pacing generators that can perform cardioversion and defibril-

lation will increase the applicability of pacing therapy for the treatment of arrhythmias (see below).

Cardioversion and defibrillation Electrical cardioversion and defibrillation remain the most reliable methods for terminating arrhythmias. By depolarizing all or at least a large portion of excitable myocardium in a near homogeneous fashion, the electrical shock can interrupt reentrant arrhythmias. External cardioversion is routinely performed by placing two paddles 12 cm in diameter in firm contact with the chest wall, with one paddle usually located to the right of the sternum at the level of the second rib and the other in the left anterior axillary line in the fifth intercostal space. If the patient is conscious, a short-acting barbiturate to act as an anesthetic or an amnesic drug such as diazepam or medazolam should be administered to prevent patient discomfort. A person skilled in maintaining an airway should be present.

Energy is delivered synchronously with the QRS complex for all arrhythmias except ventricular flutter and VF, since asynchronous shocks can produce VF. The amount of energy used will vary with the type of tachycardia being treated. With the exception of AF, SVTs can frequently be terminated with energy levels in the range of 25 to 50 W · s, while AF usually requires ≥100 W · s for termination. For terminating VT, energy levels ≥100 W · s should probably be employed. While energies as low as 25 W · s may be used successfully, they also have a higher incidence of producing VF or AF. At least 200 W · s of energy should be used for initial attempts at terminating VF. If the initial shock fails, all repeated attempts at defibrillation should be with the maximum energy that the defibrillator is capable of delivering (320 to 400 W · s).

Indications for cardioversion depend on the clinical setting and the patient's general condition. Any tachycardia (except sinus tachycardia) that produces hypotension, myocardial ischemia, or heart failure warrants consideration of prompt termination using external cardioversion. Arrhythmias that fail to terminate with pharmacologic therapy may also be terminated by electrical cardioversion. Transient bradycardias and supraventricular and ventricular irritability following cardioversion are common and usually do not warrant antiarrhythmic intervention.

Implanted cardioverter/defibrillator ICD devices have been developed that will promptly recognize and terminate life-threatening ventricular arrhythmias. These devices can deliver <1 to 40 W · s, the amount of which can be programmed. Current devices have antitachycardia pacing capabilities such that VT can be sensed and terminated without resorting to a painful shock. In such devices, high-energy shocks are reserved for hypotensive VT, acceleration of VT, or failure to terminate VT after a programmed duration (Fig. 230-16). ICDs now can be implanted transvenously, and some are small enough to be implanted in a manner similar to pacemakers. Clinical trials testing the function of these devices in patients with drug-refractory ventricular arrhythmias have demonstrated survival from sudden death at 1 year ranging between 92 and 100%. Currently, ICDs should be considered for patients with VT that is not hemodynamically tolerated. As mentioned earlier, recent randomized trials suggest that ICDs confer improved mortality over amiodarone in patients with hemodynamically untolerated VT and a cardiac arrest not due to reversible causes (Table 230-6). Finally, they are indicated for patients with depressed left ventricular function, prior myocardial infarction, nonsustained and sustained VT at electrophysiologic study (Table 230-8). Guidelines for their use are given in Table 230-9.

The most frequent problem with the ICD has been its inappropriate discharge in the absence of sustained ventricular arrhythmias. Additional potential problems include an increase in defibrillation threshold and decrease in tachycardia rates below the rate cut-off of the device in response to many antiarrhythmic drugs. Permanently implanted ventricular pacemakers may interfere with the device's ability to sense VF. This can be avoided by using committed bipolar pacing systems that are better able to sense local ventricular activity. Diagnostic fea-

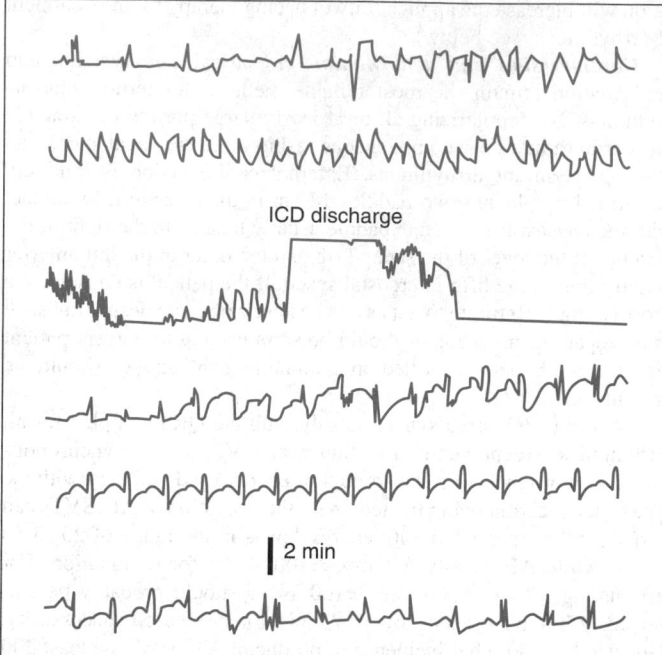

FIGURE 230-16 Normally functioning implantable defibrillators. A continuous Holter monitoring tracing is shown. On the top strip, a rapid polymorphic tachycardia is initiated which beats more uniformly. The automatic implantable cardioverter/defibrillator (ICD) senses the rhythm and delivers a shock which restores sinus rhythm.

tures of newer, all-in-one devices are able to identify the probable cause of an ICD discharge (e.g., AF, SVT, fractured lead) and to adjust pharmacologic therapy or reprogram the device to avoid such inappropriate shocks. These newer devices have the capability to take a "second look" prior to shock delivery and thus may abort delivery for self-terminating arrhythmias. In addition, the range of candidates suitable for implantation will be expanded because the newer devices have the capability of shock therapy for patients whose arrhythmias do not cause loss of consciousness.

Table 230-9   ACC/AHA Guidelines for ICD Implantation

CLASS 1[a]

1. Cardiac arrest due to VF or VT not due to a transient or reversible cause.
2. Spontaneous sustained VT.
3. Syncope of undetermined origin with clinically relevant, hemodynamically significant sustained VT or VF induced at EP study when drug therapy is ineffective, not tolerated, or not preferred.
4. Nonsustained VT with coronary disease, prior MI, LV dysfunction, and inducible VF or sustained VT at EP study that is not suppressible by a class I antiarrhythmic drug.

CLASS 2[b]

1. Cardiac arrest presumed to be due to VF when EP testing is precluded by other medical conditions.
2. Severe symptoms attributable to sustained ventricular tachyarrhythmias while awaiting cardiac transplantation.
3. Familial or inherited conditions with a high risk for life-threatening ventricular tachyarrhythmias such as long QT syndrome or hypertrophic cardiomyopathy.
4. Nonsustained VT with coronary artery disease, prior MI, and LV dysfunction, and inducible sustained VT or VF at EP study.
5. Recurrent syncope of undetermined etiology in the presence of ventricular dysfunction and inducible ventricular arrhythmias at EP study, when other causes of syncope have been excluded.

CLASS 3[c]

1. Syncope of undetermined cause in a patient without inducible ventricular tachyarrhythmias
2. Incessant VT or VF
3. VF or VT resulting from arrhythmias amenable to surgical or catheter ablation; for example, atrial arrhythmias associated with the Wolff-Parkinson-White syndrome, right ventricular outflow tract VT, idiopathic LV tachycardia, or fascicular VT.
4. Ventricular tachyarrhythmias due to a transient or reversible disorder.

[a] Evidence and/or agreement that procedure is indicated.
[b] Divergence in evidence opinion that procedure is indicated.
[c] Evidence/agreement that procedure is not indicated or is harmful.
NOTE: EP, electrophysiology; LV, left ventricular; MI, myocardial infarction; VF, ventricular fibrillation, VT, ventricular tachycardia.
SOURCE: Adapted from American College of Cardiology/American Heart Association: J Am Coll Cardiol 31:1175, 1998.

Newer generations of ICDs are smaller and frequently allow placement of a second lead in the right atria. This lead senses atrial activity and provides enhanced discrimination of atrial from ventricular electrical activity. This enhanced discrimination of SVT from VT prevents inappropriate shocks for SVT that may be misinterpreted as VT and allows the device to switch from a dual-chamber to a single-chamber device should an SVT-like AF develop. These dual-chamber devices also allow AV sequential pacing. Finally, ICDs are now available that have defibrillation coils in the right atrium as well as right ventricle. These devices are suited for patients with infrequent but highly symptomatic atrial fibrillation. Patients with these atrial defibrillators can activate the device themselves and terminate their atrial fibrillation without going to the hospital.

Ablative Therapy for Arrhythmias
Catheter-based mapping techniques have provided a nonoperative approach to the identification and cure of a variety of arrhythmias. In fact, catheter ablation techniques are now the procedures of choice for symptomatic patients with (1) concealed or manifest (WPW) bypass tracts, (2) AV nodal reentrant SVT, (3) typical atrial flutter, and (4) poorly controlled ventricular responses to atrial arrhythmias, most commonly AF. Successful ablation of bypass tracts and modifications of the AV node by radiofrequency energy are extremely successful and

Table 230-8   ICD Therapy for Primary Prevention of Sudden Cardiac Death

	MADIT	MUSTT
Protocol	ICD vs. conventional (AAD, primarily empiric amiodarone)	EP-guided Rx (AAD or ICD) vs. control

Sample size	n = 196
	    Conventional = 101
	    ICD = 95
		n = 704
		    EP-guided Rx = 351
		    Control = 353

Patient inclusion	S/P MI, EF ≤ 35% NSVT, inducible sustained VT not suppressible by procainamide	CAD, EF ≤ 40%, NSVT, inducible sustained VT
Total mortality	Conventional = 39% ICD = 16% (27 months)	Control = 48% EP-guided Rx = 42% AAD = 55% ICD = 24% (60 months)
Reduction in mortality by ICD	54%	55% (vs. control or AAD)
SCD or cardiac arrest	Conventional = 13% ICD = 3.2%	Control = 32% EP-guided Rx = 25% AAD = 37% ICD = 9%
Reduction in SCD or cardiac arrest by ICD	62.5%	75% (vs. control or AAD)

NOTE: AAD, antiarrhythmic drug; CAD, coronary artery disease; EF, ejection fraction; EP, electrophysiology; ICD, implantable cardioverter/defibrillator; MADIT, multicenter automatic defibrillator trial; MUSTT, multicenter unsustained tachycardia trial; NSVT, nonsustained ventricular tachycardia; RX, therapy; SCD, sudden cardiac death; S/P MI, status post-myocardial infarction; VT, ventricular tachycardia.
SOURCE: From Buxton; Moss.

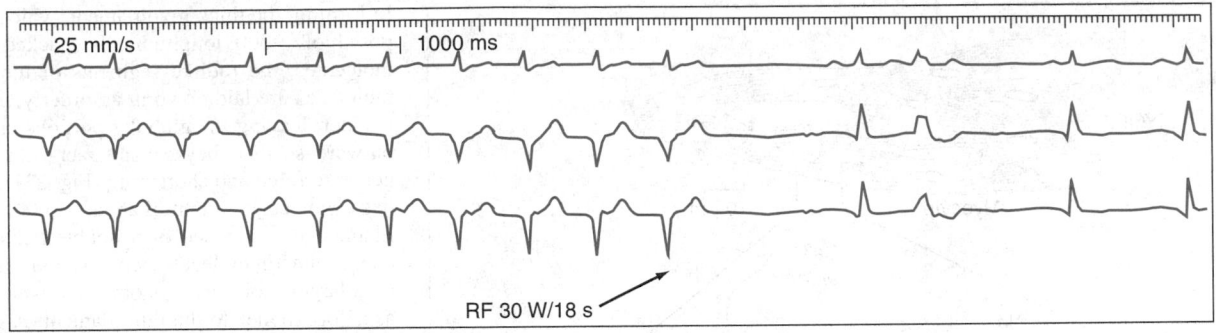

FIGURE 230-17 Radiofrequency ablation of idiopathic ventricular tachycardia in a patient with prior infarction. Leads I, II, and III are shown. Ventricular tachycardia with a right bundle branch block and left axis deviation is shown in a patient with a prior inferior wall infarction. Radiofrequency applied to the site of origin terminates the tachycardia.

cost effective and are the procedure of choice for patients with recurrent episodes. The creation of AV block with implantation of a pacemaker is the method of choice in managing patients with AF and poorly controlled ventricular response. Idiopathic VTs (Fig. 230-17) and some VTs that are associated with coronary artery disease are also amenable to ablation, but the result is less successful than for ablation of SVTs.

Surgical therapy is now relegated to cases of sustained VT associated with coronary artery disease when operative intervention is needed for coronary bypass surgery and/or aneurysmectomy or VT associated with specific structural abnormalities (e.g., idiopathic left ventricle aneurysm, s/p surgery for tetralogy of Fallot). It also may be undertaken for the unusual instances of failed catheter ablation for SVTs associated with bypass tracts.

BIBLIOGRAPHY

BRUGADA R et al: Identification of a genetic locus for familial atrial fibrillation. N Engl J Med 336:905, 1997

BUXTON AE et al: A randomized study of the prevention of sudden death in patients with coronary artery disease. N Engl J Med 341:1882, 1999

GILLIS AM: Pacing to prevent atrial fibrillation. Cardiol Clin 18:25, 2000

GREGORATAS G: ACC/AHA Guidelines for Implantation of Cardiac Pacemakers and Antiarrhythmia Devices: A report of the American College of Cardiology/American Heart Association Task Force on Practice Guidelines (Committee on Pacemaker Implantation). J Am Coll Cardiol 31:1175, 1998

HOLMES DR JR et al: The effect of medical and surgical treatment on subsequent sudden cardiac death in patients with coronary artery disease. A report from the Coronary Artery Surgery Study. Circulation 73:1254, 1986

HUANG DT et al: Hybrid pharmacologic and ablative therapy: A novel and effective approach for the management of atrial fibrillation. J Cardiovasc Electrophysiol 9:462, 1998

KIRCHOFF CJHJ, JOSEPHSON ME: In *Role of Anisotopy in Clinical Arrhythmias*, PM Spooner, RW Joyner, J Jalife (eds): New York, Futura, 1998, pp 135–157

LEVY S: Classification system of atrial fibrillation. Curr Opin Cardiol 15:54, 2000

MOSS AJ et al: Improved survival with an implanted defibrillator in patients with coronary disease at high risk for ventricular arrhythmia. N Engl J Med 335:1933, 1996

OLGIN JE, MILES W: Ablation of atrial tachycardia, in I Singer, S Barold, AJ Camm (eds): Pharmacologic Therapy in the 21st Century. New York, Futura, 1998, pp 197–217

PRIORI SG: Genetic and molecular basis of cardiac arrhythmias: Impact on clinical management. Circulation 99:518, 1995

ROY D et al: Amiodarone to prevent recurrence of atrial fibrillation. Canadian trial of Atrial Fibrillation Investigators. N Engl J Med 342:913, 2000

WYSE DG: Pharmacologic therapy in patients with ventricular tachyarrhythmias. Cardiol Clin 11:65, 1993

ZIPES DP: Specific arrhythmias: Diagnosis and treatment, in *Heart Disease: A Textbook of Cardiovascular Medicine,* 6th ed, E Braunwald (ed). Philadelphia, Saunders, 2001

Section 3

DISORDERS OF THE HEART

231

Eugene Braunwald

NORMAL AND ABNORMAL MYOCARDIAL FUNCTION

CELLULAR BASIS OF CARDIAC CONTRACTION

THE CARDIAC ULTRASTRUCTURE About three-fourths of the ventricular *myocardium* is composed of individual striated muscle cells (myocytes), normally 17 to 25 μm in diameter and 60 to 140 μm in length (Fig. 231-1*A*). Each fiber contains multiple, rodlike cross-banded strands (myofibrils) that run the length of the fiber and are, in turn, composed of serially repeating structures, the sarcomeres. The cytoplasm between the myofibrils contains other cell constituents (Fig. 231-1*B*), such as the single centrally located nucleus, numerous mitochondria, and intracellular membrane system, the sarcoplasmic reticulum.

The *sarcomere*, the structural and functional unit of contraction, is delimited by two adjacent dark lines, the Z lines (Fig. 231-1*C*). The distance between Z lines varies with the degree of contraction or stretch of the muscle and ranges between 1.6 and 2.2 μm. Within the confines of the sarcomere are alternating light and dark bands, giving the myocardial fibers their striated appearance under the light microscope. At the center of the sarcomere is a dark band of constant length (1.5 μm), the A band, which is flanked by two lighter bands, the I bands, which are of variable length. The sarcomere of heart muscle, like that of skeletal muscle, is made up of two sets of interdigitating myofilaments (Fig. 232-1*D*). Thicker filaments, composed principally of the protein myosin, traverse the A band. They are about 10 nm (100 Å) in diameter, with tapered ends, and measure 1.5 to 1.6 μm in length. Thinner filaments, composed primarily of actin, course from the Z line through the I band into the A band. They are approximately 5 nm (50 Å) in diameter and 1.0 μm in length. Thus there is overlapping of thick and thin filaments only within the A band, while the I band contains only thin filaments (Fig. 232-1*C*). On electron-micro-

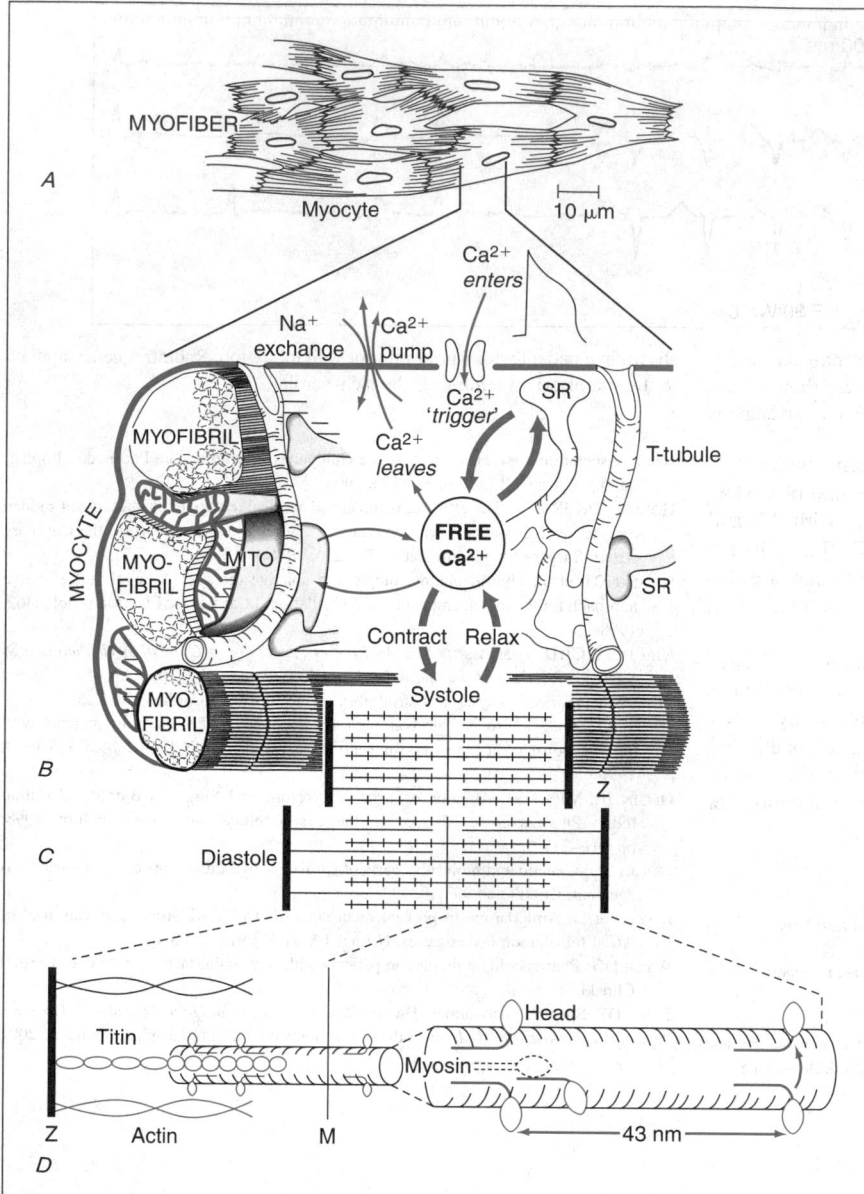

In forming the thick myofilament, which is composed of ~300 longitudinally stacked myosin molecules, the rodlike segments of the myosin molecules are laid down in an orderly, polarized manner, leaving the globular portions projecting outward so that they can interact with actin to generate force and shortening (Fig. 231-2). *Actin* has a molecular weight of about 47,000. The thin filament is composed of a double helix of two chains of actin molecules wound about each other on a larger molecule, tropomyosin, which serves as a "backbone" to the thin filament. A group of these regulatory proteins, troponins C, I, and T, are spaced at regular intervals on this filament (Fig. 231-3). In contrast to myosin, actin has no intrinsic enzymatic activity, but it has the ability to combine reversibly with myosin in the presence of ATP and Ca^{2+}. The latter activates the myosin ATPase, which in turn breaks down ATP, the energy source for contraction. In relaxed muscle this interaction is inhibited by tropomyosin. *Titin* (Fig. 231-1D) is a large, flexible, myofibrillar protein that connects myosin to the Z line. Its stretching is believed to contribute to the elasticity of the heart.

During activation of the myocyte, Ca^{2+} becomes attached to troponin C, which results in a conformational change in the regulatory protein tropomyosin, which in turn exposes the actin cross-bridge interaction sites. Repetitive interaction between myosin heads and actin filaments is termed *cross-bridge cycling*, which results in sliding of the actin along the myosin filaments, ultimately causing muscle shortening and/or the development of tension. The splitting of ATP, which is synthesized in the mitochondria, then dissociates the myosin cross-bridge from the actin. In the presence of ATP (Fig. 231-2), linkages between actin and myosin filaments are made and broken cyclically as long as sufficient Ca^{2+} is present; these linkages cease when $[Ca^{2+}]$ falls below a critical level, and the troponin-tropomyosin complex once more prevents interactions between the myosin cross-bridges and the actin filaments. Intracytoplasmic Ca^{2+} is a principal mediator of the inotropic state of the heart; the fundamental action of most positive inotropic drugs, including the digitalis glycosides, β-adrenergic agonists, and phosphodiesterase inhibitors, is to raise the $[Ca^{2+}]$ in the vicinity of the myofilaments. Cyclic AMP enhances the phosphorylation of troponin I, a protein that accelerates cardiac relaxation.

FIGURE 231-1 *A.* Microscopic evidence of heart muscle. *B.* Cardiac contraction and relaxation result from changing concentrations of Ca^{2+} ions in the myocardial cytosol. Ca^{2+} ions are shown schematically as entering via the calcium channel, which opens in response to the wave of depolarization that travels along the sarcolemma. These Ca^{2+} ions "trigger" the release of more calcium from the sarcoplasmic reticulum (SR) and thereby initiate a contraction-relaxation cycle. Eventually, the small amount of calcium that has entered the cell leaves, predominantly by a Na^+-Ca^{2+} exchanger with a lesser role for the sarcolemmal calcium pump. *C.* The varying actin-myosin overlap is shown for systole and diastole. *D.* The myosin heads, attached to the thick filaments, interact with the thin actin filaments. *(Reprinted with permission. Copyright 1997 LH Opie.)*

scopic examination, bridges may be seen to extend between the thick and thin filaments within the A band.

THE CONTRACTILE PROCESS The sliding model for muscle rests on the fundamental observation that the thick and thin filaments are constant in overall length during both contraction and relaxation. With activation, the actin filaments are propelled further into the A band. In the process, the A band remains constant in length, whereas the I band shortens and the Z lines move toward one another.

The *myosin* molecule is a complex, asymmetric fibrous protein with a molecular weight of about 500,000; it has a rodlike portion that is about 150 nm (1500 Å) in length with a globular portion at its end (Fig. 231-1D). This globular portion of the myosin is the site of ATPase activity and also forms the bridges between the myosin and actin.

The *sarcoplasmic reticulum* (SR) (Fig. 231-1B) is a complex network of anastomosing intracellular channels that invests the myofibrils. It is less profuse in cardiac than in skeletal muscle. Its longitudinally disposed membrane-lined tubules are closely applied to the surfaces of individual sarcomeres but have no direct continuity with the outside of the cell. However, closely related to the SR, both structurally and functionally, are the transverse tubules, or T system, formed by tubelike invaginations of the sarcolemma that extend into the myocardial fiber along the Z lines, i.e., the ends of the sarcomeres.

CARDIAC ACTIVATION At rest, the cardiac cell is polarized, i.e., the interior has a negative charge relative to the outside of the cell, with a transmembrane potential of −80 to −100 mV (Chap. 229). The sarcolemma, which in the resting state is largely impermeable to Na^+, has a Na^+- and K^+-stimulating pump energized by ATP that extrudes Na$^+$ from the cell; the pump plays a critical role in establishing this resting potential. Thus, on the inside of the cell [K$^+$] is relatively high and [Na$^+$] is far lower, while in the extracellular milieu [Na$^+$] is high and [K$^+$] is low. At the same time, in the resting state, the extracellular [Ca^{2+}] greatly exceeds the free intracellular [Ca^{2+}].

During the plateau of the action potential (phase 2) there is a slow inward current through L-type Ca^{2+} channels in the sarcolemma (Fig. 231-4). The absolute quantity of Ca^{2+} that crosses the surface membrane is relatively small and itself appears to be incapable of bringing about full activation of the contractile apparatus. The depolarizing current not only extends across the surface of the cell but penetrates deeply into the cell by way of the ramifying T system; this Ca^{2+} current triggers the release of much larger quantities of Ca^{2+} from the SR, a process termed *Ca^{2+}-induced Ca^{2+} release*.

The Ca^{2+} released from the SR then diffuses toward the sarcomere and, as already described, combines with troponin C. By repressing this inhibitor of contraction, Ca^{2+} activates the myofilaments to shorten. During repolarization the activity of the Ca^{2+} pump in the SR reaccumulates Ca^{2+} against a concentration gradient, and the Ca^{2+} is stored by its attachment to a protein *calsequestrin*. This is an energy-requiring process that lowers the [Ca^{2+}] in the vicinity of the myofibrils to a level that inhibits the actin-myosin interaction responsible for contraction and in this manner leads to relaxation. Also, there is an exchange of Ca^{2+} for Na$^+$ at the sarcolemma, reducing the cytoplasmic [Ca^{2+}]. Thus, the combination of the cell membrane, transverse tubules, and SR, with their ability to transmit the action potential, to release, and then to reaccumulate Ca^{2+}, appears to play a fundamental role in the rhythmic contraction and relaxation of heart muscle.

The ATP formed from substrate oxidation is the principal source of energy for almost all of the mechanical work of contraction performed by the myocardial cell. The high-energy phosphate stores in ATP are in equilibrium with those in the form of creatine phosphate. The activity of myosin ATPase determines the rate of forming and breaking of the actin-myosin cross-bridges and ultimately the velocity of muscle contraction.

THE ROLE OF MUSCLE LENGTH In all striated muscle, including cardiac muscle, the force of contraction depends on initial muscle length. The sarcomere length associated with the most forceful contraction is approximately 2.2 μm. At this length the two sets of myofilaments of the sarcomere are configured so as to provide the greatest area for their interaction. The length of the sarcomere also regulates the extent of activation of the contractile system, i.e., its sensitivity to Ca^{2+}. According to this concept, termed *length-dependent activation*, at the optimal sarcomere length of 2.2 μm, the myofilament sensitivity to Ca^{2+} is maximal.

The relation between the initial length of the muscle fibers and the developed force is of prime importance for the function of heart muscle. This forms the basis of the Frank-Starling relation (Starling's law of the heart), which states that, within limits, the force of ventricular contraction is a function of the end-diastolic length of the cardiac muscle, which in turn is closely related to the ventricular end-diastolic volume.

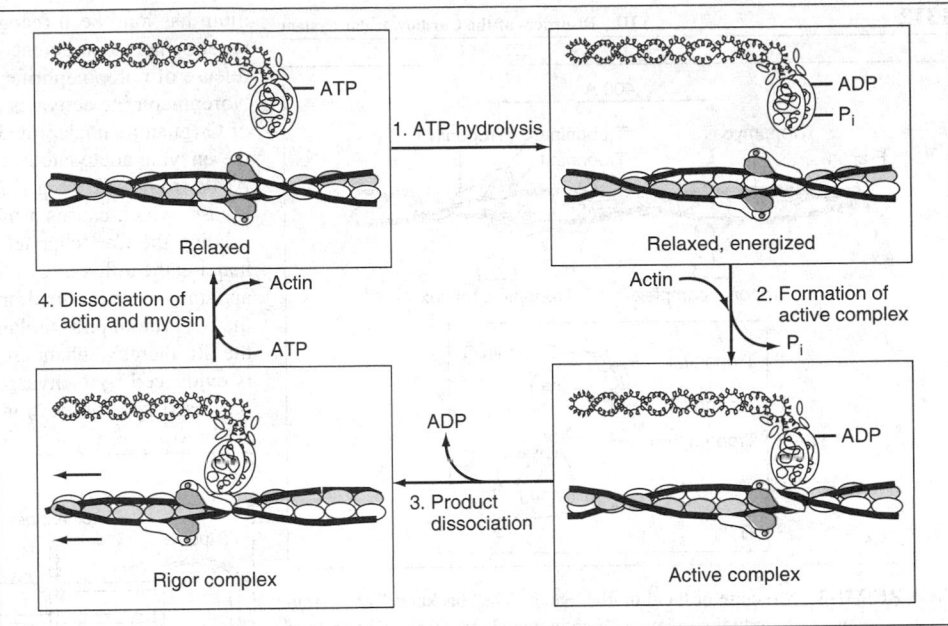

FIGURE 231-2 Reaction mechanism of actomyosin ATPase, simplified to show four steps. In relaxed muscle (*upper left*), ATP bound to the myosin cross-bridge dissociates the thick and thin filaments. *Step 1:* Hydrolysis of myosin-bound ATP by the ATPase site on the myosin head transfers the chemical energy of the nucleotide to the activated cross-bridge (*upper right*). When cytosolic Ca^{2+} concentration is low, as in relaxed muscle, the reaction cannot proceed because tropomyosin and the troponin complex on the thin filament do not allow the active sites on actin to interact with the cross-bridges. Therefore, even though the cross-bridges are energized, they cannot interact with actin. *Step 2:* When Ca^{2+} binding to troponin C has exposed active sites on the thin filament, actin interacts with the myosin cross-bridges to form an active complex (lower right) in which the energy derived from ATP is retained in the actin-bound cross-bridge, whose orientation has not yet shifted. *Step 3:* The muscle contracts when ADP dissociates from the cross-bridge; this step leads to the formation of the low-energy rigor complex (lower left), in which the chemical energy derived from ATP hydrolysis has been expended to perform mechanical work (the "rowing" motion of the cross-bridge). *Step 4:* The muscle returns to its resting state, and the cycle ends when a new molecule of ATP binds to the rigor complex and dissociates the cross-bridge from the thin filament. This cycle continues until calcium is dissociated from troponin C in the thin filament, which causes the contractile proteins to return to the resting state with the cross-bridge in the energized state. [*From AM Katz, in WS Colucci (ed): Heart Failure: Cardiac Function and Dysfunction, in Atlas of Heart Diseases, 2d ed, E Braunwald (series ed). Philadelphia, Current Medicine, 1999.*]

MYOCARDIAL MECHANICS

THE FORCE-VELOCITY CURVE The mechanical activity of striated muscle, skeletal and cardiac, may be expressed externally in two ways: by shortening and by the development of tension. In both forms of striated muscle the velocity of shortening is inversely related to the tension development, an expression of the so-called force-velocity relation (Fig. 231-5). Expressed simply, the greater the load the muscle is called upon to lift, the lower the velocity (and extent) of shortening, and vice versa. Skeletal muscle fibers have a single, essentially fixed, force-velocity curve; i.e., at any given muscle length, the inverse relation between force and velocity is fixed. The contractile activity of skeletal muscle is controlled by varying the frequency of nerve impulses stimulating the muscle, and thereby the number of contractions of each fiber per unit of time, as well as by the number of muscle fibers, i.e., motor units, that contact, while the contractile properties of each individual fiber remain constant. Although the muscle's resting length also influences the characteristics of contraction, this variable remains essentially fixed in vivo because of the muscles' skeletal attachments. In contrast to skeletal muscle, the number of myocardial cells and within them the myofibrils and sarcomeres that become activated during each contraction is constant. However, the contractile activity of the myocardium is readily altered under physiologic conditions by changes in resting fiber length and by changes

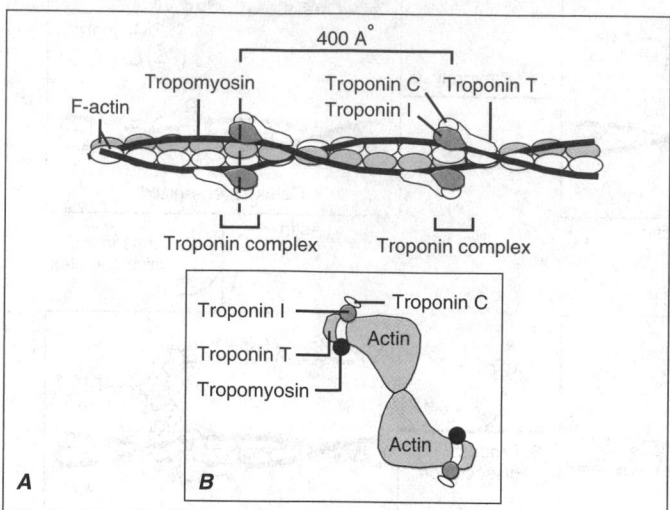

FIGURE 231-3 Structure of the thin filament. *A*. The "backbone" of the thin filament, seen in a longitudinal view, is F-actin, which contains two strands of actin monomers (light blue and white). Troponin complexes, made up of one molecule each of troponin C, troponin I, and troponin T, are distributed at approximately 40-nm (400-Å) intervals along the thin filament. Elongated tropomyosin molecules (solid line in the grooves between the two actin strands). *B*. A cross-section of the thin filament at the level where the troponin complexes are located shows probable relationships between actin, tropomyosin, and the three components of the troponin complex. The strength of the bond linking troponin I and actin varies, depending on whether Ca²⁺ is bound to troponin C. [*Adapted from AM Katz, in WS Colucci (ed): Heart Failure: Cardiac Function and Dysfunction, in Atlas of Heart Diseases, 2d ed, E Braunwald (series ed). Philadelphia, Current Medicine, 1999, with permission of the publisher.*]

in the inotropic state, i.e., the contractility, both of which shift the myocardial force-velocity curve. Many neurohumoral influences affect contractility, but the most important influence is the adrenergic nervous system operating via its neurotransmitter, norepinephrine.

VENTRICULAR EJECTION AND FILLING

Analysis of the heart as a pump has classically centered on the relation between the end-diastolic volume of the ventricle (which is related to the length of the muscle fibers) and its stroke volume (the Frank-Starling relation). The end-diastolic or "filling" pressure of the ventricle is sometimes used as a surrogate for the end-diastolic volume. In the heart-lung preparation the stroke volume varies directly with the diastolic fiber length (preload) and inversely with the arterial resistance (afterload), and as the heart fails it delivers a progressively smaller stroke volume from a normal or even elevated end-diastolic volume. The relation between the ventricular end-diastolic pressure and the stroke work of the ventricle (the ventricular function curve) provides a useful definition of the level of *myocardial contractility* (also termed the contractile, or inotropic, state of the ventricle). An increase in ventricular contractility is accompanied by a shift of the ventricular function curve upward and to the left [greater stroke work at any level of ventricular end-diastolic pressure (or volume), or lower end-diastolic pressure at any level of stroke work], while depression of contractility is characterized by a shift downward and to the right (Fig. 231-6).

During the adrenergic stimulation of the myocardium that accompanies exercise, relatively little change in ventricular end-diastolic volume occurs, while cardiac output, aortic flow velocity, stroke work, and the rate of ventricular pressure development are all augmented, reflecting an increase in myocardial contractility.

The important influence of the adrenergic neurotransmitter, norepinephrine (Chap. 72), on the mechanical properties of the myocar-

dium has long been recognized. Direct stimulation of the cardiac adrenergic nerves augments ventricular function as a consequence of the release of norepinephrine from adrenergic nerve endings in the heart. Norepinephrine activates myocardial β receptors and through a series of G (guanine nucleotide binding) protein mediated changes activates the enzyme adenylate cyclase, which leads to the formation of cyclic AMP from ATP (Fig. 231-7). The latter, in turn, activates protein kinase, which causes a more rapid, forceful contraction by phosphorylating the Ca²⁺ channel in the myocardial sarcolemma, thereby enhancing the influx of Ca²⁺ into the myocyte. Ca²⁺ acts on the contractile apparatus, as described on p. 1311. Cyclic AMP also phosphorylates the SR protein phospholamban, which increases the uptake of Ca²⁺ by the SR, thereby enhancing the rate of relaxation. Adrenergic activation is evidenced by tachycardia, a reduction in cardiac dimensions, and increased rates of ejection and filling.

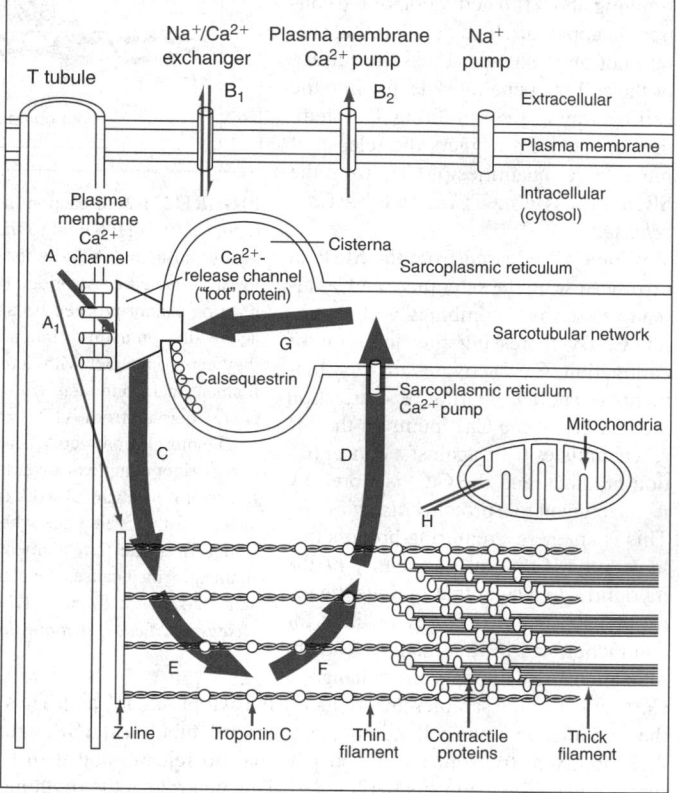

FIGURE 231-4 The Ca²⁺ fluxes and key structures involved in cardiac excitation-contraction coupling. The *arrows* denote the direction of Ca²⁺ fluxes. The thickness of each arrow indicates the magnitude of the calcium flux. Two Ca²⁺ cycles regulate excitation-contraction coupling and relaxation. The larger cycle is entirely intracellular and involves Ca²⁺ fluxes into and out of the sarcoplasmic reticulum, and Ca²⁺ binding to and release from troponin C. The smaller extracellular Ca²⁺ cycle occurs when this cation moves into and out of the cell. The action potential opens plasma membrane Ca²⁺ channels to allow passive entry of Ca²⁺ into the cell from the extracellular fluid (*arrow A*). Only a small portion of the Ca²⁺ that enters the cell directly activates the contractile proteins (*arrow A₁*). The extracellular cycle is completed when Ca²⁺ is actively transported back out to the extracellular fluid by way of two plasma membrane fluxes mediated by the sodium-calcium exchanger (*arrow B₁*) and the plasma membrane calcium pump (*arrow B₂*). In the intracellular Ca²⁺ cycle, passive Ca²⁺ release occurs through channels in the cisternae (*arrow C*) and initiates contraction, and active Ca²⁺ uptake by the Ca²⁺ pump of the sarcotubular network (*arrow D*) relaxes the heart. Diffusion of Ca²⁺ within the sarcoplasmic reticulum (*arrow G*) returns this activator cation to the cisternae, where it is stored in a complex with calsequestrin and other calcium-binding proteins. Ca²⁺ released from the sarcoplasmic reticulum initiates systole when it binds to troponin C (*arrow E*). Lowering of cytosolic [Ca²⁺] by the SR cause this ion to dissociate from troponin (*arrow F*) and relaxes the heart. Ca²⁺ may also move between mitochondria and cytoplasm (H). (*Adapted from Katz, with permission.*)

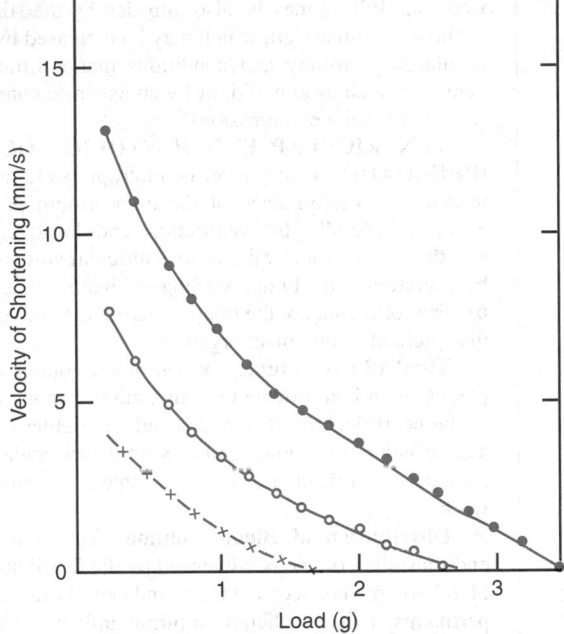

FIGURE 231-5 Effects of the addition of norepinephrine (NE) and the development of heart failure on the force-velocity relation of the cat papillary muscle. NE induces an increase in the velocity of shortening at any load, in the maximum force and isometric contraction (Po), and in the maximum velocity of zero load shortening (V_{max}). Heart failure has the opposite effect. *Key:* o, control; -x-x, failure. *(Modified from E Braunwald in Heart Disease, 4th ed. Philadelphia, Saunders, 1992.)*

ASSESSMENT OF CARDIAC FUNCTION

Several techniques are available for defining impaired cardiac function in patients. With the patient at rest, and at a normal or elevated ventricular end-diastolic pressure, the cardiac output and stroke volume may be depressed in the presence of heart failure, but not uncommonly these variables are within normal limits. A more sensitive index is the ejection fraction, i.e., the ratio of stroke volume to end-diastolic volume (normal value 67 ± 8%), which may be estimated by radiocontrast or radionuclide angiography or echocardiography, and it is frequently depressed in systolic heart failure even when the stroke volume itself is normal. Alternatively, the detection of abnormally elevated ventricular end-diastolic volumes (normal value 70 ± 20 mL/m²) in the presence of a normal stroke volume signifies impairment of left ventricular systolic function. A limitation of cardiac output, ejection fraction, and ventricular volume in the assessment of cardiac function is that these variables are influenced strongly by ventricular loading conditions. Thus, a depressed ejection fraction and lowered cardiac output may be observed in patients with normal ventricular function but reduced preload, as occurs in hypovolemia, or with increased afterload, as occurs in acutely elevated arterial pressure.

The end-systolic left ventricular pressure-volume relationship is a particularly useful index of ventricular performance since it is independent of both preload and afterload (Fig. 231-8). At any level of myocardial contractility, left ventricular end-systolic volume varies inversely with end-systolic pressure; as contractility declines, end-systolic volume (at any level of end-systolic pressure) rises. Noninvasive techniques, particularly echocardiography and radionuclide angiography (Chap. 227), are of great value in the clinical assessment of myocardial function. They provide measurements of end-systolic volume (or end-systolic dimension) that can be related to systolic arterial pressure. In addition, they provide convenient measurements of ejection fraction and systolic shortening rate and allow measurement of ventricular filling (see below).

Exercise A useful technique for evaluating ventricular performance involves the measurement of the circulatory changes occurring during exercise. Thus, left ventricular performance may be estimated

accurately by measuring the left ventricular end-diastolic pressure, cardiac output, and total-body O_2 consumption at rest and during exercise. In persons with normal cardiac function, the cardiac output rises by more than 500 mL/min for each 100-mL increase in O_2 consumption per minute. The left ventricular end-diastolic pressure at rest is less than 12 mmHg and changes little during exercise, while cardiac output, and to a lesser extent stroke volume, rise, the latter especially when exercise is carried out in the upright position. The failing left ventricle, on the other hand, is characterized by an elevation of end-diastolic pressure during exercise to above 12 mmHg, accompanied by either no change or a fall in stroke volume and a subnormal increase in cardiac output related to the increase in minute O_2 consumption. The overall performance of the cardiopulmonary system in delivering oxygen to the metabolizing tissue can also be estimated by measuring the maximal O_2 consumption achieved during escalating treadmill exercise ($\dot{V}_{maxO_2}$). Normal values exceed 20 mL/min per kilogram, while values under 10 mL/min per kilogram represent severe impairment of function, usually seen in patients with severe heart failure and a poor prognosis.

The potential value of stressing the left ventricle in assessing its performance is emphasized by the fact that the normal range of left ventricular end-diastolic pressure, cardiac index, and ventricular stroke work in the resting state are wide, with values that frequently overlap those seen in patients with ventricular dysfunction.

DIASTOLIC FUNCTION (Fig. 231-9) This important variable is best assessed by continuously measuring the flow velocity across the mitral valve using Doppler echocardiography. Normally, the velocity of inflow is more rapid in early diastole than during atrial systole; with impaired relaxation the rate of early diastolic filling declines, while the rate of presystolic filling rises. With severe impairment of filling the pattern is "pseudo-normalized" and early ventricular filling becomes more rapid as left atrial pressure upstream to the stiff left ventricle rises.

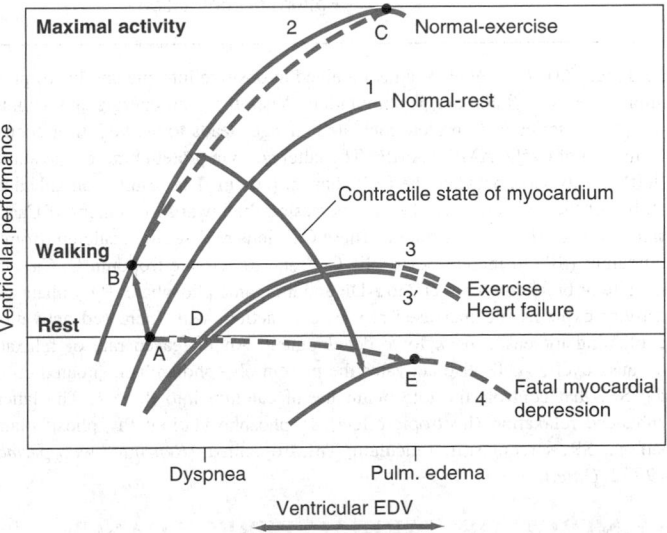

FIGURE 231-6 Diagram showing the interrelations among influences on ventricular end-diastolic volume (EDV) through stretching of the myocardium and the contractile state of the myocardium. Levels of ventricular EDV associated with filling pressures that result in dyspnea and pulmonary edema are shown on the abscissa. Levels of ventricular performance required when the subject is at rest, while walking, and during maximal activity are designated on the ordinate. The broken lines are the descending limbs of the ventricular-performance curves, which are rarely seen during life but which show the level of ventricular performance if end-diastolic volume could be elevated to very high levels. For further explanation see text. *(Modified from E Braunwald et al: Mechanisms of Contraction of the Normal and Failing Heart. Boston, Little, Brown, 1976.)*

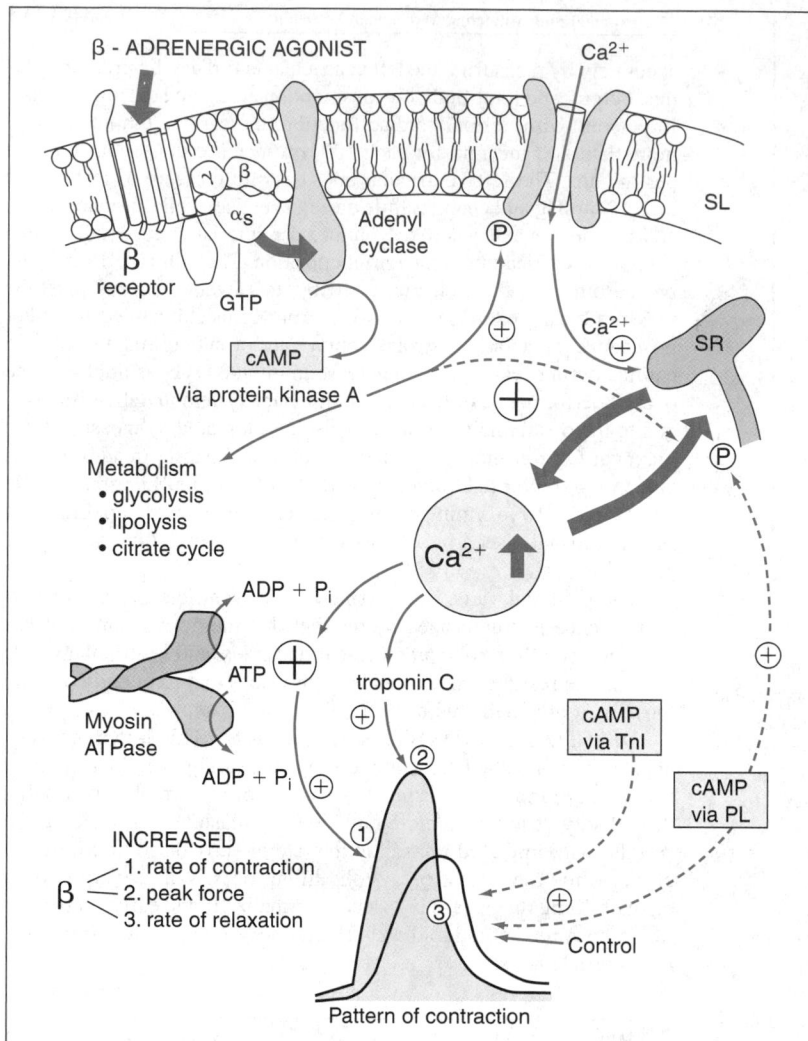

FIGURE 231-7 Signal systems involved in positive intropic and lusitropic (enhanced relaxation) effects of β-adrenergic stimulation. When the β-adrenergic agonist interacts with the β receptor, a series of G protein-mediated changes leads to activation of adenylate cyclase and formation of cyclic AMP (cAMP). The latter acts via protein kinase A to stimulate metabolism (left) and to phosphorylate the Ca^{2+} channel protein. The result is an enhanced opening probability of the Ca^{2+} channel, thereby increasing the inward movement of Ca^{2+} ions through the sarcolemma (SL) of the T tubule. These Ca^{2+} ions release more calcium from the sarcoplasmic reticulum (SR) to increase cytosolic Ca^{2+} and to activate troponin C. Ca^{2+} ions also increase the rate of breakdown of ATP to ADP and inorganic phosphate (P_i). Enhanced myosin ATPase activity explains the increased rate of contraction, with increased activation of troponin C explaining increased peak force development. An increased rate of relaxation is explained because cyclic AMP also activates the protein phospholamban, situated on the membrane of the SR, that controls the rate of uptake of calcium into the SR. The latter effect explains enhanced relaxation (lusitropic effect). P, phosphorylation; PL, phospholamban; SL, sarcolemma; SR, sarcoplasmic reticulum; TnI, troponin I. *(Reprinted with permission. Copyright 1997 L Opie.)*

CONTROL OF CARDIAC PERFORMANCE AND OUTPUT

The extent of shortening of heart muscle and, therefore, the stroke volume of the intact ventricle are determined by three influences: (1) the length of the muscle at the onset of contraction, i.e., the preload; (2) the inotropic state of the muscle, i.e., the position of its force-velocity-length relation and its end-diastolic–shortening–relation; and (3) the tension that the muscle is called upon to develop during contraction, i.e., the afterload. Within wide limits, heart rate determines the cardiac output at any stroke volume as long as the other three influences remain constant. Ventricular filling is influenced by the extent and speed of myocardial relaxation, which in turn is determined by the rate of uptake of Ca^{2+} by the SR; the latter may be reduced by

ischemia. Filling may be also impeded by the stiffness of the ventricular wall, which may be increased by ventricular hypertrophy and conditions that infiltrate the ventricle, such as amyloid, or by an extrinsic constraint (e.g., pericardial compression).

VENTRICULAR END-DIASTOLIC VOLUME (PRELOAD) At any level of inotropic state and afterload, the performance of the myocardium is influenced profoundly by ventricular end-diastolic fiber length and therefore by diastolic ventricular volume, i.e., by operation of the Frank-Starling mechanism (Fig. 231-6). The following are the major determinants of ventricular preload in the intact organism:

Total Blood Volume When blood volume is depleted, as in hemorrhage or dehydration, venous return to the heart declines (Chap. 38) and ventricular end-diastolic volume (preload) falls, as does ventricular performance, as reflected in stroke volume and ventricular work.

Distribution of Blood Volume The ventricular end-diastolic volume is influenced by the distribution of blood volume between the intra- and extrathoracic compartments. This distribution in turn is influenced by the following:

1. *Body position.* Gravitational forces pool blood in dependent portions of the body; upright posture augments extrathoracic at the expense of intrathoracic blood volume and reduces ventricular work.

2. *Intrathoracic pressure.* Normally, mean intrathoracic pressure is negative, which increases thoracic blood volume and ventricular end-diastolic volume and enhances the return of blood to the heart, particularly during inspiration, when this pressure becomes more negative. Elevation of intrathoracic pressure, as occurs during the Valsalva maneuver or prolonged bouts of coughing or with positive-pressure ventilation, has the opposite effect. It impedes venous return, diminishes intrathoracic blood volume, and reduces stroke volume and ventricular work.

3. *Intrapericardial pressure.* When this pressure is elevated, as in pericardial tamponade (Chap. 239), there is interference with cardiac filling, and the resultant reduction in ventricular diastolic volume reduces stroke volume and ventricular work.

4. *Venous tone.* The venous system is not a simple system of passive conduits between the systemic capillary bed and the right atrium. Instead, the smooth muscle in the walls of the venules and veins responds to a variety of neural and humoral stimuli. Venoconstriction occurs during muscular exercise, deep respiration, fright, or marked hypovolemic shock, reducing extrathoracic and augmenting intrathoracic and intraventricular blood volumes and ventricular performance.

5. *The pumping action of skeletal muscle.* During muscular exercise the contracting skeletal muscles squeeze blood out of the venous bed and, with the aid of the venous valves, displace it centrally, thereby increasing intrathoracic blood volume, ventricular end-diastolic volume, and ventricular work.

Atrial Contraction Vigorous, appropriately timed atrial contraction augments ventricular filling and end-diastolic volume. The atrial contribution to ventricular filling, the so-called atrial kick, is of particular importance in patients with concentric ventricular hypertrophy. In such patients, the loss of atrial systole (as occurs with the development of atrial fibrillation) reduces ventricular end-diastolic pressure and volume, ultimately lowering myocardial performance. The atrial contribution to ventricular filling may also be reduced by atrioventricular dissociation, prolongation or abbreviation of the P-R interval, and depression of atrial contractility.

INOTROPIC STATE (MYOCARDIAL CONTRACTILITY) A number of factors determine the level of ventricular performance at any given ventricular end-diastolic volume, i.e., the position of the ventricular function curve (Fig. 231-6) as well as the position of the left ventricular pressure-volume plane (Fig. 231-8). These influences may be considered to operate by modifying myocardial force-velocity relations. In the final analysis, most of these influences act by altering the [Ca^{2+}] in the vicinity of the myofilaments, which in turn trigger cross-bridge cycling (p. 1293).

Adrenergic Nerve Activity (See also Chap. 72) The quantity of norepinephrine released by adrenergic nerve endings in the heart is determined by the adrenergic nerve impulse traffic; alterations in the frequency of these nerve impulses modify the quantity of norepinephrine released and acting on the β-adrenergic receptors in the myocardium. This mechanism is the most important one that acutely modifies myocardial contractility under physiologic conditions.

Circulating Catecholamines (See also Chap. 72) When it is stimulated by adrenergic nerve impulse, the adrenal medulla releases catecholamines, which, when they reach the heart, augment both heart rate and myocardial contractility.

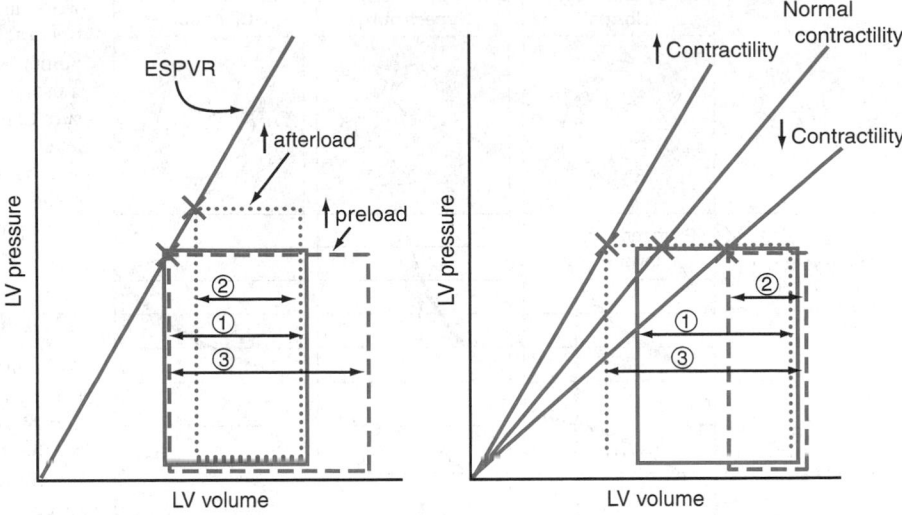

FIGURE 231-8 The responses of the left ventricle to increased afterload, increased preload, and increased and reduced contractility are shown in the pressure-volume plane. ESPVR, end-systolic pressure-volume relation; E_{ES}, the slope of the end-systolic pressure-volume relation. *Left.* Effects of increases in preload and afterload on the pressure-volume loop. Since there has been no change in contractility, ESPVR is unchanged. With an increase in afterload, stroke volume falls (1 → 2); with an increase in preload, stroke volume rises (1 → 3). *Right.* With increased myocardial contractility, the normal ESPVR moves to the left of the normal line (lower end-systolic volume at any end-systolic pressure) and stroke volume rises (1 → 3). With reduced myocardial contractility, the ESPVR moves to the right; end-systolic volume is increased and stroke volume falls (1 → 2).

The Force-Frequency Relation The position of the myocardial force-velocity curve is also influenced by the rate and rhythm of cardiac contraction; e.g., ventricular extrasystoles result in postextrasystolic potentiation, presumably by increasing the quantity of Ca^{2+} that enters the cardiac cell. The contractility of the normal (but not the failing) heart is augmented by an increase in frequency of contraction.

Exogenously Administered Inotropic Agents Isoproterenol, dopamine, dobutamine, and other sympathomimetic agents, cardiac glycosides, Ca^{2+}, amrinone, milrinone, and other phosphodiesterase inhibitors all improve the myocardial force-velocity relation and therefore may be used to stimulate ventricular performance.

Physiologic Depressants Included among these are severe myocardial hypoxia, ischemia, and acidosis. Acting either singly or in combination, these influences depress the myocardial force-velocity curve and left ventricular work at any given ventricular end-diastolic volume.

Pharmacologic Depressants These include many antiarrhythmic drugs such as procainamide and disopyramide; calcium antagonists such as verapamil; beta blockers; and large doses of barbiturates, alcohol, and general anesthetics as well as many other drugs.

Loss of Myocytes When a sufficiently large portion of ventricular myocardium becomes nonfunctional or necrotic, as occurs transiently during ischemia (Chap. 244) and permanently in myocardial infarction (Chap. 243), total ventricular performance at any given level of end-diastolic volume becomes depressed. Programmed cell death (apoptosis) can also cause loss of myocytes and, when sufficiently widespread, can impair ventricular function and cause heart failure.

Intrinsic Myocardial Depression Although the fundamental mechanisms responsible for depression of myocardial contractility in most cases of chronic congestive heart failure secondary to prolonged ventricular overload or cardiomyopathy remain to be elucidated (p. 1316), it is now apparent that in this condition the inotropic state of individual surviving myocytes is depressed, and as a consequence the ventricular performance at any ventricular preload and afterload is lowered.

VENTRICULAR AFTERLOAD The stroke volume is ultimately a function of the extent of ventricular fiber shortening. In the intact heart, as in isolated cardiac muscle, the velocity and extent of shortening of ventricular muscle fibers at any level of preload and myocardial contractility are inversely related to the afterload, i.e., the load that opposes shortening. In the intact heart the afterload may be defined as the tension or stress developed in the ventricular wall during ejection. Therefore, the afterload is determined by the aortic pressure as well as the volume and thickness of the ventricular cavity. Laplace's law indicates that the tension of the myocardial fiber is a function of the product of the intracavitary ventricular pressure and ventricular radius divided by the wall thickness. Therefore, at any given level of aortic pressure, the afterload faced by a dilated left ventricle of normal thickness is higher than that encountered by a normal-sized ventricle. Conversely, at the same aortic pressure and ventricular diastolic volume, the afterload of a thick-walled ventricle is lower than of a thin-walled chamber. The aortic pressure, in turn, is determined by the peripheral vascular resistance, the physical characteristics of the arterial tree, and the volume of blood it contains at the onset of ejection.

The critical role played by the ventricular afterload in cardiovascular regulation is shown in Fig. 231-10. As already noted, increases in both preload and contractility increase myocardial fiber shortening, while increases in afterload reduce it. The extent of myocardial fiber shortening and left ventricular size are the determinants of stroke volume. Arterial pressure, in turn, is related to the product of cardiac output and systemic vascular resistance, while afterload is a function of left ventricular volume, wall thickness, and arterial pressure. An increase in arterial pressure induced by vasoconstriction, for example, augments afterload, which opposes myocardial fiber shortening, reducing stroke volume. This in turn tends to limit the increase in pressure.

When myocardial contractility becomes impaired and the ventricle dilates, afterload rises and becomes increasingly important in determining cardiac output. Increases in afterload may result from neural and humoral stimuli that occur in response to a fall in cardiac output. This increased afterload may reduce cardiac output further while myocardial oxygen requirements are increased. This can cause a vicious cycle. Treatment with vasodilators has the opposite effect; by reducing afterload, cardiac output rises (Chap. 232).

Under normal circumstances, the various influences acting on cardiac performance enumerated above interact in a complex fashion to maintain cardiac output at a level appropriate to the requirements of the metabolizing tissues, and interference with any one of these mechanisms may not influence the cardiac output. For example, a moderate reduction of blood volume *or* the loss of the atrial contribution to

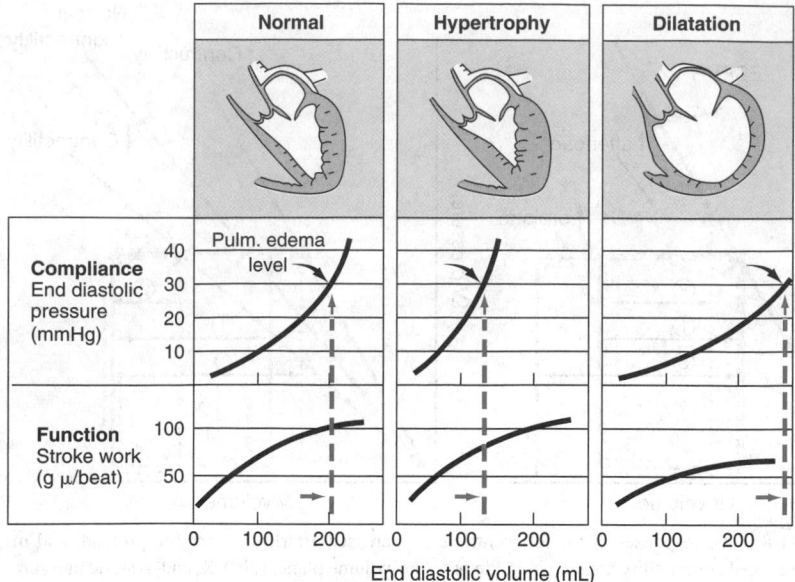

	Normal	Hypertrophy	Dilatation

FIGURE 231-9 Relationship between left ventricular end-diastolic volume and (1) end-diastolic pressure (*top*), describing the *compliance* of the left ventricle, i.e., its *diastolic* properties; and (2) left ventricular stroke work (*bottom*), describing the ventricle's *systolic* function curve. The normal left ventricle (*left*) reaches an end-diastolic pressure of 30 mmHg (pulmonary edema level) when its end-diastolic volume is elevated to 200 mL. The concentrically hypertrophied left ventricle (*center*) exhibits normal systolic function since the relation between left ventricular end-diastolic volume and stroke work is unchanged, but there is "diastolic failure" in that end-diastolic pressure reaches pulmonary edema level (i.e., 30 mmHg) at a lower level than normal (i.e., 130 mL). The dilated ventricle (*right*) exhibits "systolic failure" in that the maximal stroke work and the stroke volume at any level of end-diastolic volume are depressed. The left ventricle displays increased diastolic compliance, i.e., distensibility, with a higher than normal end-diastolic volume (280 mL) required to reach the pulmonary edema level. (*Reprinted with permission from R Gorlin, Prim Cardiol 6:84, 1980.*)

ventricular contraction can ordinarily be sustained without a reduction in the cardiac output at rest. Other factors, such as increases in the frequency of adrenergic nerve impulses to the heart and in heart rate, will, in a normal individual, serve as compensatory mechanisms, augment contractility, and sustain cardiac output.

EXERCISE The hemodynamic changes that occur normally during exercise in the upright position are complex (Fig. 231-6). Hyperventilation, the pumping action of the exercising muscles, and the venoconstriction during exercise all augment venous return and hence ventricular filling and preload. Simultaneously, the increase in the adrenergic nerve impulse traffic to the myocardium, the increased concentration of circulating catecholamines, and the tachycardia that occur during exercise combine to augment the contractile state of the myocardium (Fig. 231-6, curves 1 and 2) and lead to an elevation of stroke

work and stroke volume, without change or even a reduction of end-diastolic pressure and volume (Fig. 231-6, points A and B). Vasodilatation occurs in the exercising muscles, thus tending to limit the increase in arterial pressure that would otherwise occur as cardiac output rises to levels as high as five times basal during maximal exercise. This vasodilatation ultimately allows the achievement of a greatly elevated cardiac output during exercise, at an arterial pressure only moderately higher than in the resting state.

THE FAILING HEART

Although heart failure may be readily described as a clinical syndrome, characterized by well-known symptoms and physical signs (Chap. 232), a precise physiologic or biochemical definition is far more difficult. However, from the clinical point of view, heart failure may be considered to be the condition in which *an abnormality of cardiac function is responsible for the inability of the heart to pump blood at a rate commensurate with the requirements of the metabolizing tissues and/or allows it to do so only from an abnormally elevated ventricular diastolic volume.* Abnormalities during systole and/or diastole may be present in heart failure (Fig. 231-9). In so-called *systolic heart failure* (p. 1320), an impairment of myocardial contractility causes weakened systolic contraction, which leads, ultimately, to a reduction in stroke volume and cardiac output, inadequate ventricular emptying, cardiac dilatation, and often elevation of ventricular diastolic pressure. Idiopathic dilated cardiomyopathy (Chap. 238) is the prototype of systolic heart failure. In *diastolic heart failure* (p. 1320), the principal abnormality is impaired relaxation and filling of the ventricle, which leads to an elevation of ventricular diastolic pressure at any given diastolic volume (Fig. 231-9). Failure of relaxation can be functional and transient, as during ischemia, which reduced the ATP required for the SR pump to lower cytoplasmic Ca^{2+}. Chronically impaired ventricular filling can be caused by a stiffened, thickened ventricle. Typical conditions in which diastolic failure occurs are restrictive cardiomyopathy secondary to infiltrative conditions, such as amyloidosis or hemochromatosis, as well as hypertrophic cardiomyopathy (Chap. 238). The concentric hypertrophy associated with chronic hypertension can also impair ventricular filling but rarely causes overt heart failure. In many patients with cardiac hypertrophy and dilatation, systolic and diastolic failure coexist; the left ventricle both empties and fills abnormally. There may be cardiac dilatation, but the ventricle's pressure-volume relation is shifted, raising the ventricular diastolic pressure at any given volume.

Although a defect in myocardial contraction is characteristic of systolic heart failure, many conditions may cause such a defect. These include a primary abnormality in the heart muscle, as occurs in cardiomyopathy, or an abnormality secondary to a chronic excessive work load as in hypertension or valvular heart disease. In ischemic heart disease, systolic heart failure results from a loss in the quantity of normally contracting cells (secondary to myocardial necrosis and apoptosis) and/or from transient loss of function in reversibly ischemic (hibernating) myocardium (Chap. 244).

Heart failure should be distinguished from conditions that resemble it, such as (1) states of circulatory insufficiency in which myocardial function is not primarily impaired, such as cardiac tamponade or hemorrhagic shock; (2) conditions in which there is circulatory congestion because of abnormal salt and water retention but in which there is no serious disturbance of the heart's function, such as acute glomerulonephritis; and

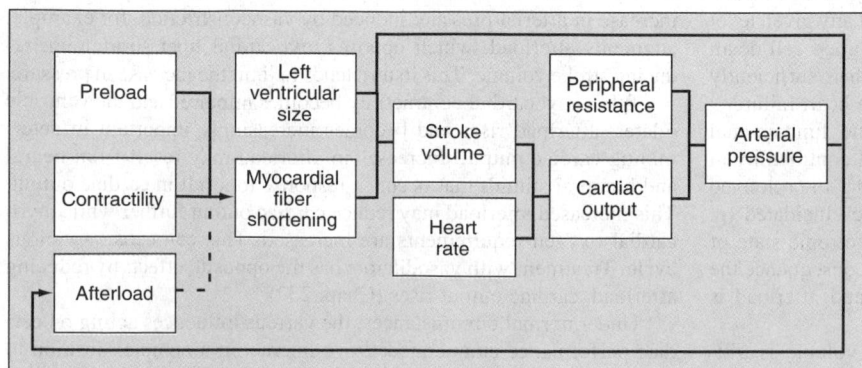

FIGURE 231-10 Scheme of interactions among various components that regulate cardiac activity. Solid lines indicate an augmenting effect; broken line represents an inhibiting effect. (*From E Braunwald, N Engl J Med 290:1124–1129, 1420–1425, 1974.*)

(3) conditions in which a normal myocardium is suddenly presented with a load that exceeds its capacity, such as accelerated hypertension or rupture of a valve cusp secondary to infective endocarditis.

ADAPTIVE MECHANISMS A number of mechanisms aid the heart faced with an increased hemodynamic burden (such as pressure or volume overload) or that has sustained loss of myocardium or contractility. These mechanisms include the following:

1. The *Frank-Starling mechanism* operating through an increase in preload (p. 1314). As outlined above, an increase in the end-diastolic volume of the ventricle is associated with stretching of the sarcomeres, which increases the interaction between actin and myosin filaments and their sensitivity to Ca^{2+}. Ventricular dilatation may become maladaptive when it becomes excessive, as may occur in severe aortic or mitral regurgitation; this increases wall stress through the operation of LaPlace's law and reduces shortening.

2. *Increased afterload*, as occurs in aortic stenosis and hypertension, also augments wall tension, leading to concentric hypertrophy, which in turn restores elevated ventricular wall stress to normal. However, ventricular hypertrophy impairs ventricular filling, and if the hypertrophy is insufficient to restore wall stress to normal, the ventricle dilates and this increases wall stress further, leading to a vicious circle.

3. *Redistribution of a subnormal cardiac output* away from the skin, skeletal muscle, and kidneys with maintenance of blood flow to the brain and the heart.

4. *Neurohumoral adjustments*, which tend to maintain arterial pressure and are discussed in Chap. 72. Like the other adaptive mechanisms, when neurohumoral adjustments are severe and chronic they impair cardiac function (see below).

BIOCHEMICAL ABNORMALITIES IN HEART FAILURE There is no unifying theory providing a biochemical basis for heart failure. However, a number of abnormalities have been described.

Reduction in Cardiac Efficiency The common forms of low-output systolic heart failure, secondary to coronary atherosclerosis, hypertension, cardiomyopathy, and certain valvular and congenital lesions, are characterized by an absolute or a relative reduction in the external work delivered by the heart, while myocardial oxygen consumption remains normal or nearly so. Therefore, the external efficiency, i.e., the ratio of external work performed to energy consumed, is often depressed.

Alterations in Energy Metabolism When heart failure occurs in the presence of acute or chronic ischemia, it can be attributed to reduced myocardial energy supplies. Severe ventricular hypertrophy and/or dilatation of any etiology can also cause relative ischemia, especially in the subendocardium, and this can impair both ventricular contraction and filling. In some forms of experimental and clinical heart failure without ischemia, myocardial energy stores in the form of creatine phosphate are decreased, as is the activity of the enzyme creatin kinase required for the shuttling of high-energy phosphate between creatine phosphate and adenosine diphosphate, suggesting that reductions in myocardial energy reserves may play a role.

Alterations in Regulatory Proteins Changes in the cardiac regulatory proteins frequently occur in chronic heart failure. These include a reduction of myosin ATPase activity, which may be caused by an alteration in the expression of troponin T and/or of myosin light chain kinase 2, alterations that could be responsible for lowering the rate of interaction between myosin and actin myofilaments, leading to systolic heart failure.

Abnormalities of Excitation-Contraction Coupling Substantial evidence supports the view that in many forms of heart failure the delivery of Ca^{2+} to the contractile sites is reduced, thereby impairing cardiac performance (Table 231-1). However, the molecular basis of this abnormality—indeed of the subcellular structures involved, i.e., the sarcolemma, T tubules, and/or SR—has yet to be defined. There is, however, evidence for a reduction in the activity of the Ca^{2+} release channel in the SR and of messenger RNAs of the proteins regulating Ca^{2+} movements. These include the sarcolemmal Ca^{2+} channels, the Ca^{2+} release channels, and the Ca^{2+} uptake pump, which play critical roles in the movement of Ca^{2+} between the SR and the cytoplasm.

Table 231-1 Calcium Homeostasis in Failing Human Myocardium

Intracellular Calcium Concentration	Calcium-Handling Proteins (mRNA Levels)
Basal (diastolic) ↑	Voltage-dependent Ca^{2+} channels ↓
Peak (systolic) ↓	Na^+/Ca^{2+} exchanger ↑
Rate of fall ↓	SR Ca^{2+}-ATPase ↓
	Phospholamban ↓
	Phospholamban/SR Ca^{2+} ATPase ↑
	Ca^{2+} release channel ↓
	Calsequestrin ↔

SOURCE: From DB Sawyer, WS Colucci, in WS Colucci (ed): *Heart Failure: Cardiac Function and Dysfunction*, in *Atlas of Heart Diseases*, 2d ed, E Braunwald (series ed). Philadelphia, Current Medicine, 1999.

Impaired expression of the genes encoding these proteins can impair both myocardial contraction and relaxation and thereby contribute to the development of heart failure.

NEUROHUMORAL AND CYTOKINE ADJUSTMENTS A reduction in cardiac performance evokes a series of neurohumoral adjustments, which, at different times, may be adaptive and maladaptive. Although they are useful because they maintain arterial perfusion pressure in the face of a sudden reduction of cardiac output, these neurohumoral adjustments increase the hemodynamic burden and oxygen requirements of the failing ventricle (Fig. 231-11).

The Adrenergic Nervous System In patients with heart failure the levels of circulating norepinephrine may be markedly elevated, reflecting the increased activity of the adrenergic nervous system; indeed the prognosis in patients with heart failure varies inversely with the concentration of plasma norepinephrine. This increased activity of the adrenergic neurons supports ventricular contractility in *acute* heart failure. Heart failure is intensified when large doses of β-adrenergic blocking agents are administered acutely, providing evidence for the protective action of adrenergic nervous activation. However, the *chronic* adrenergic stimulation that occurs in heart failure may increase afterload by raising vascular resistance, cause cardiac arrhythmias, and may damage myocytes further, perhaps by causing Ca^{2+} overload.

The density of adrenergic receptors, their coupling to G proteins,

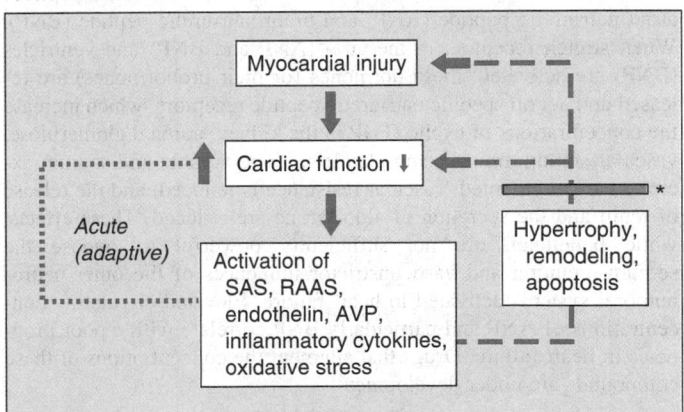

FIGURE 231-11 Interplay between cardiac function and neurohumoral and cytokine systems. Myocardial injury, of many etiologies, can depress cardiac function, which in turn causes activation of the sympathoadrenal system (SAS) and the renin-angiotensin-aldosterone system (RAAS) and the elaboration of endothelin, arginine vasopressin (AVP), and cytokines such as tumor necrosis factor (TNF) α. In acute heart failure (*left*), these are adaptive and tend to maintain arterial pressure and cardiac function. In chronic heart failure (*right*), they cause maladaptive hypertrophic remodeling and apoptosis, which cause further myocardial injury and impairment of cardiac function. The horizontal line on the right (*) shows that chronic maladaptive influences can be inhibited by angiotensin converting enzyme inhibitors, β-adrenergic blockers, angiotensin type I receptor blockers, aldosterone antagonists, and endothelin type A blockers.

and the concentration of cardiac norepinephrine stores are all reduced in chronic, severe heart failure. These changes are accompanied by a reduction in the activity of adenylate cyclase, which may lower the intracellular concentration of cyclic AMP. The latter in turn reduces the activation of protein kinase, the phosphorylation of Ca^{2+} channels, transarcolemmal Ca^{2+} entry, as well as the phosphorylation of phospholamban, a protein in the SR, which reduces the reuptake of Ca^{2+} by the latter (Fig. 231-7). Changes in the G proteins, which couple the β receptor to the catalytic adenylate cyclase (which is responsible for the production of cyclic AMP), may also occur in heart failure, with increased activity of the inhibitory subunit.

The Renin-Angiotensin-Aldosterone System When cardiac output declines, the renin-angiotensin-aldosterone system (Chap. 331) is activated. Concentrations of both circulating angiotensin II and aldosterone are increased, the former contributing to excess vasoconstriction and the latter to the retention of salt and water and perhaps to cardiac fibrosis. The local (tissue) renin-angiotensin system is also activated in heart failure. Patients with heart failure are usually improved by blocking this system with angiotensin-converting enzyme inhibitors, angiotensin II receptor blockers, and aldosterone antagonists (Chap. 232).

Endothelin The concentration of circulatory endothelin, a polypeptide that is a very powerful vasoconstrictor, is increased in heart failure. A number of studies have shown that blockade of endothelin receptors improves left ventricular function in patients and experimental animals with heart failure.

Tumor Necrosis Factor α The overexpression of a number of cytokines also appears to play a prominent role in the pathogenesis of heart failure. It has now been well established that patients exhibit elevated levels of tumor necrosis factor (TNF) α, both in the circulation and in cardiac muscle; the pathophysiologic significance of this finding is just unfolding. Transgenic mice with overexpressed cardiac TNF-α have systolic dysfunction, myocarditis, ventricular dilatation, heart failure, and shortened survival. The infusion of TNF-α impairs ventricular function, and this can be reversed with a TNF-α antagonist.

Vasodilator Peptides A number of vasodilator peptides are released by the dilated heart. Best known are the natriuretic peptides atrial natriuretic peptide (ANP) and brain natriuretic peptide (BNP). When stretch receptors in the atria (ANP and BNP) and ventricles (BNP) are activated, these hormones (or their prohormones) are released and act on specific natriuretic peptide receptors, which increase the concentrations of cyclic GMP in the kidney, adrenal glomerulose, vascular smooth muscle, and platelets. Urine volume and sodium excretion are augmented, vascular resistance is reduced, and the release of renin and the secretion of aldosterone are reduced. These effects, while beneficial, are not sufficiently powerful to oppose the sodium-retaining and vasoconstrictor influences of the other neurohumoral systems activated in heart failure. Elevated circulating concentrations of ANP and particularly BNP correlate with a poor prognosis in heart failure. Drugs that augment the concentrations of these compounds are under development.

Figure 231-11 illustrates current concepts of neurohumoral-cytokine activation in heart failure. The activation of the adrenergic nervous system and the renin-angiotensin-aldosterone system and the enhanced elaboration of endothelin and arginine vasopressin appear to be adaptive in *acute*, severe heart failure. However, they all appear to exert a maladaptive response in chronic heart failure. Inflammatory cytokines and oxidative stress are emerging as potent noxious stimuli as well. Together they result in a vicious circle, causing myocyte hypertrophy, remodeling, and cell death, the latter often due to myocardial apoptosis, all resulting in further impairment of cardiac function and myocardial injury. Effective agents that interfere with the adverse effects of these stimuli on cardiac function, such as endothelin receptor blockers and TNF-α antagonists, are becoming available, and these neurohumoral and cytokine blockers appear capable of interrupting the vicious circle.

HEART FAILURE—A DISTURBANCE OF THE MYOCARDIAL PUMP In the final analysis, in systolic heart failure the basic problem is depression of the myocardial force-velocity relationship and of the length–active tension curve, reflecting reductions in the contractile state of the myocardium (Fig. 231-6, curves 1 to 3, Fig. 231-8, right). In diastolic failure there is upward displacement of the diastolic pressure–volume relation (Fig. 231-9). In many instances, cardiac output and external ventricular performance at rest are within normal limits but are maintained at these levels only by an increased end-diastolic fiber length and an elevated ventricular end-diastolic volume, i.e., through the operation of the Frank-Starling mechanism (Fig. 231-6, points A to D). The elevation of left ventricular preload is associated with increases in the pulmonary capillary pressure, contributing to the dyspnea experienced by patients with heart failure, while elevation of right ventricular preload raises systemic venous pressure and contributes to the development of edema. The improvement of contractility that normally accompanies augmented adrenergic activity during exercise is attenuated or even prevented by norepinephrine depletion and downregulation of myocardial β receptors, which occur in severe heart failure (Fig. 231-6, curves 3 and 3').

The factors that augment ventricular filling during exercise in the normal individual push the failing myocardium along its flattened length–active tension curve, and although the left ventricle may perform somewhat better at this higher diastolic volume, this occurs only as a consequence of an inordinate elevation of ventricular end-diastolic volume and pressure and, therefore, of the pulmonary capillary pressure. The latter intensifies dyspnea and therefore plays an important role in limiting the intensity of exercise that the patient can perform. Left ventricular failure becomes fatal when the myocardial length–active tension curve is depressed (Fig. 231-6, curve 4) to the point at which cardiac performance fails to satisfy the requirements of the peripheral tissues even at rest, and/or the left ventricular end-diastolic and pulmonary capillary pressures are elevated to levels that result in pulmonary edema (Fig. 231-6, point E).

BIBLIOGRAPHY

ANVERSA P et al: Myocyte death in heart failure. Curr Opin Cardiol 11:245, 1996

ARAI M et al: Sarcoplasmic reticulum gene expression in cardiac hypertrophy and heart failure. Circ Res 74:555, 1994

COLUCCI WS (ed): *Heart Failure: Cardiac Function and Dysfunction*, in *Atlas of Heart Diseases*, 2d ed, E Braunwald (series ed). Philadelphia, Current Medicine, 1999

———, BRAUNWALD E: Pathophysiology of heart failure, in *Heart Disease*, 6th ed, E Braunwald (ed). Philadelphia, Saunders, 2001

HEIN S et al: Altered expression of titin and contractile proteins in failing human myocardium. J Mol Cell Biol 26:1291, 1994

KATZ AM: *Heart Failure*, New York, Raven, 2000, pp 381

LITTLE WC, BRAUNWALD E: Assessment of cardiac function, in *Heart Disease*, 6th ed, E Braunwald (ed). Philadelphia, Saunders, 2001

OPIE LH: Mechanisms of cardiac contraction and relaxation, in *Heart Disease*, 6th ed, E Braunwald (ed). Philadelphia, Saunders, 2001

SCHWARTZ K, MERCADIER J-J: Molecular and cellular biology of heart failure. Curr Opin Cardiol 11:227, 1996

SOLARO RJ et al: Regulatory proteins and diastolic relaxation, in *Diastolic Relaxation of the Heart*, BH Lorell, W Grossman (eds). Boston, Kluwer Academic, 1994, pp 43–53

WOLFF MR et al: Rate of tension development in cardiac muscle varies with level of activator calcium. Circ Res 76:154, 1995

232   *Eugene Braunwald*

HEART FAILURE

Heart failure (HF) is the pathophysiologic state in which an abnormality of *cardiac* function is responsible for the failure of the heart to pump blood at a rate commensurate with the requirements of the metabolizing tissues *and/or* allows it to do so only from an abnormally elevated diastolic volume. HF is frequently, but not always, caused by a defect in myocardial contraction, and then the term *myocardial failure* is appropriate. The latter may result from a primary abnormality in heart muscle, as occurs in the cardiomyopathies, in viral myocarditis (Chap. 238), and with excessive programmed cell death (apoptosis). HF also results commonly from coronary atherosclerosis, which interferes with cardiac contraction by causing myocardial infarction and ischemia. HF may also occur in valvular and/or congenital heart disease in which the heart muscle is damaged by the long-standing excessive hemodynamic burden imposed by the valvular abnormality or cardiac malformation.

In other patients with HF, however, a similar clinical syndrome is present but without any detectable abnormality of *myocardial* function. In some of these patients the normal heart is suddenly presented with a mechanical load that exceeds its capacity, such as an acute hypertensive crisis, rupture of an aortic valve cusp, or massive pulmonary embolism. HF in the presence of normal myocardial function also occurs in chronic conditions in which there is impaired filling of the ventricles due to a mechanical abnormality such as tricuspid and/or mitral stenosis, constrictive pericarditis without myocardial involvement, endocardial fibrosis, and some forms of hypertrophic cardiomyopathy. In many patients with HF, particularly those with valvular or congenital heart disease, there is a combination of impaired myocardial function and hemodynamic overload.

Heart failure should be distinguished from (1) conditions in which there is circulatory congestion secondary to abnormal salt and water retention but in which there is no disturbance of cardiac function per se, as occurs in renal failure; and (2) noncardiac causes of inadequate cardiac output, such as hypovolemic shock (Chap. 38).

The ventricles respond to a chronically increased hemodynamic burden with the development of hypertrophy (Fig. 232-1). When the ventricle is called on to deliver an elevated cardiac output for prolonged periods, as in valvular regurgitation, it develops *eccentric hypertrophy*, i.e., cavity dilatation, with an increase in muscle mass so that the ratio between wall thickness and ventricular cavity size remains relatively constant early in the process. With chronic pressure overload, as in valvular aortic stenosis or untreated hypertension, *concentric ventricular hypertrophy* develops; in this condition the ratio between wall thickness and ventricular cavity size increases. In both eccentric and concentric hypertrophy, a stable hyperfunctioning state may exist for many years, but myocardial function may ultimately deteriorate, leading to HF. Often at this time, the ventricle dilates and the ratio between wall thickness and cavity size declines, leading to increased stress on each unit of myocardium, further dilatation, and a vicious circle.

Heart failure represents a major public health problem in industrialized nations. It appears to be the only common cardiovascular condition that is increasing in prevalence and incidence. In the United States, HF is responsible for almost 1 million hospital admissions and 40,000 deaths annually. Since HF is more common in the elderly, its prevalence is likely to continue to increase as the population ages.

CAUSES OF HEART FAILURE

In evaluating patients with HF, it is important to identify not only the *underlying* but also the *precipitating cause*. The cardiac abnormality produced by a congenital or acquired lesion such as valvular aortic stenosis may exist for many years and cause no clinical disability. Frequently, however, clinical manifestations of HF are precipitated for the first time in the course of some acute disturbance that places an additional load on a myocardium that is chronically excessively burdened (see below). Such a heart may be compensated but have little additional reserve, and the additional load imposed by a precipitating cause results in further deterioration of cardiac function. Identification of such precipitating causes is of critical importance because their

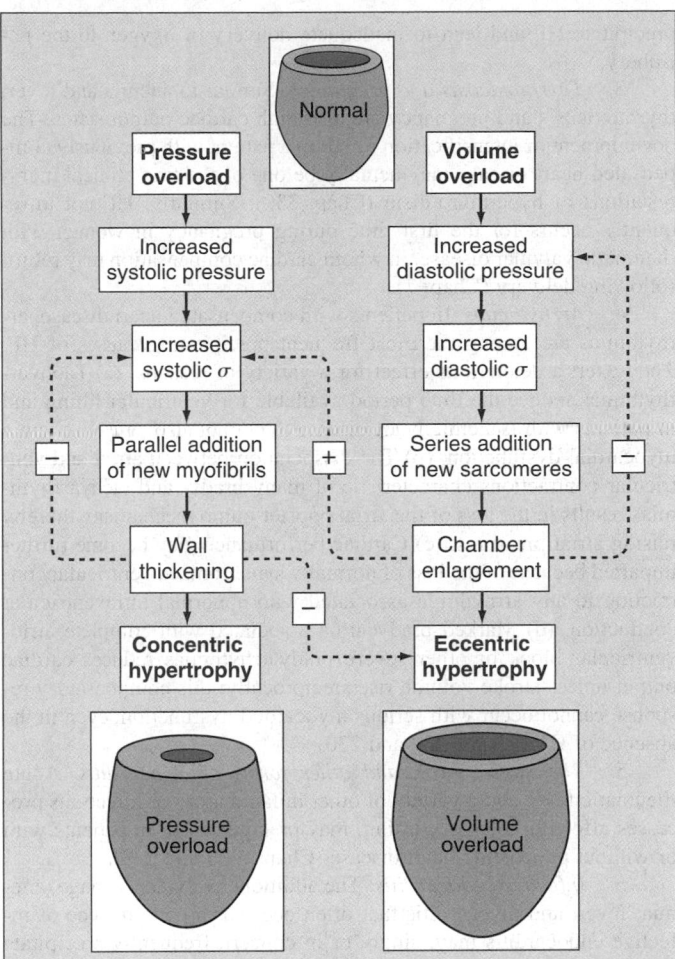

FIGURE 232-1 Patterns of ventricular hypertrophy. Specific patterns of ventricular remodeling occur in response to the imposed augmentation in work load. A pattern of hypertrophic growth characterized as concentric, in which increased mass is out of proportion to chamber volume, is particularly effective in reducing systolic wall stress (σ) under conditions of heightened pressure load. In contrast, in volume overload conditions, in which the major stimulus is diastolic loading, a predominant finding is a great increase in the cavity size or volume. Although there can be extensive increases in mass, the relationship between mass and volume is either preserved or, in severe cases, reduced. The fundamental response is generated by cellular hypertrophy. However, the configuration of the new contractile tissue is specific and offsets the mechanical stimulus. [*Modified from W Grossman et al in NR Alpert (ed): Perspectives in Cardiovascular Research. Myocardial Hypertrophy and Failure, vol 7. New York, Raven Press, 1993, with permission.*]

prompt alleviation may be lifesaving. In the absence of underlying heart disease, these acute disturbances do not by themselves lead to HF.

PRECIPITATING CAUSES

1. *Infection.* Patients with pulmonary vascular congestion due to left ventricular failure are more susceptible to pulmonary infection than are normal persons; any infection may precipitate HF. The resulting fever, tachycardia, and hypoxemia and the increased metabolic demands may place a further burden on an overloaded, but compensated, myocardium of a patient with chronic heart disease.

2. *Anemia.* In the presence of anemia, the oxygen needs of the metabolizing tissues can be met only by an increase in the cardiac output (Chap. 61). Although such an increase in cardiac output can be sustained by a normal heart, a diseased, overloaded, but otherwise compensated heart may be unable to augment sufficiently the volume of blood that it delivers to the periphery. In this manner, the combination of anemia and previously compensated heart disease can

precipitate HF and lead to inadequate delivery of oxygen to the periphery.

3. *Thyrotoxicosis and pregnancy.* Similar to anemia and fever, thyrotoxicosis and pregnancy are also high cardiac output states. The development or intensification of HF in a patient with previously compensated heart disease may actually be one of the first clinical manifestations of hyperthyroidism (Chap. 330). Similarly, HF not infrequently occurs for the first time during pregnancy in women with rheumatic valvular disease, in whom cardiac compensation may return following delivery (Chap. 7).

4. *Arrhythmias.* In patients with compensated heart disease, arrhythmias are among the most frequent precipitating causes of HF. They exert a deleterious effect for a variety of reasons: (a) Tachyarrhythmias reduce the time period available for ventricular filling and in patients with ischemic heart disease they may also cause ischemic myocardial dysfunction. (b) The dissociation between atrial and ventricular contractions characteristic of many brady- and tachyarrhythmias results in the loss of the atrial booster pump mechanism, thereby raising atrial pressures. (c) Cardiac performance may become further impaired because of the loss of normally synchronized ventricular contraction in any arrhythmia associated with abnormal intraventricular conduction. (d) Marked bradycardia associated with complete atrioventricular block or other severe bradyarrhythmias reduces cardiac output unless stroke volume rises reciprocally; this compensatory response cannot occur with serious myocardial dysfunction, even in the absence of HF (Chaps. 229 and 230).

5. *Rheumatic, viral, and other forms of myocarditis.* Acute rheumatic fever and a variety of other inflammatory or infectious processes affecting the myocardium may precipitate HF in patients with or without preexisting heart disease (Chaps. 235 and 238).

6. *Infective endocarditis.* The additional valvular damage, anemia, fever, and myocarditis that often occur as a consequence of infective endocarditis may, singly or in concert, frequently precipitate HF (Chap. 126).

7. *Physical, dietary, fluid, environmental, and emotional excesses.* The sudden augmentation of sodium intake as with a large meal, the inappropriate discontinuation of pharmaceuticals to treat HF, blood transfusions, physical overexertion, excessive environmental heat or humidity, and emotional crises all may precipitate HF in patients with heart disease who were previously compensated.

8. *Systemic hypertension.* Rapid elevation of arterial pressure, as may occur in some instances of hypertension of renal origin or upon discontinuation of antihypertensive medication in patients with essential hypertension, may result in cardiac decompensation (Chap. 246).

9. *Myocardial infarction.* In patients with chronic but compensated ischemic heart disease, a fresh infarct, sometimes otherwise silent clinically, may further impair ventricular function and precipitate HF (Chap. 243).

10. *Pulmonary embolism.* Physically inactive patients with low cardiac output are at increased risk of developing thrombi in the veins of the lower extremities or the pelvis. Pulmonary emboli may result in further elevation of pulmonary arterial pressure, which in turn may produce or intensify ventricular failure. In the presence of pulmonary vascular congestion, such emboli also may cause pulmonary infarction (Chap. 261).

A systematic search for these precipitating causes should be made in every patient with the new development or recent intensification of HF. If properly recognized, the precipitating cause of HF usually can be treated more effectively than the underlying cause. Therefore, the prognosis in patients with HF in whom a precipitating cause can be identified, treated, and eliminated is more favorable than in patients in whom the underlying disease process has progressed to the point of producing HF without a precipitating cause.

FORMS OF HEART FAILURE

HF may be described as *systolic* or *diastolic*, *high-output* or *low-output*, *acute* or *chronic*, *right-sided* or *left-sided*, and *forward* or *backward*. These descriptors are often useful in a clinical setting, particularly early in the patient's course, but late in the course of chronic HF the differences between them often become blurred.

SYSTOLIC VERSUS DIASTOLIC FAILURE   The distinction between these two forms of HF, described in Fig. 231-9, relates to whether the principal abnormality is the inability of the ventricle to contract normally and expel sufficient blood (systolic failure) or to relax and/or fill normally (diastolic failure). The major clinical manifestations of systolic failure relate to an inadequate cardiac output with weakness, fatigue, reduced exercise tolerance, and other symptoms of hypoperfusion, while in diastolic HF the manifestations relate principally to the elevation of filling pressures. Many patients, particularly those who have both ventricular hypertrophy *and* dilatation, exhibit abnormalities both of contraction and relaxation coexist.

Diastolic HF may be caused by increased resistance to ventricular inflow and reduced ventricular diastolic capacity (constrictive pericarditis and restrictive, hypertensive, and hypertrophic cardiomyopathy), impaired ventricular relaxation (acute myocardial ischemia), and myocardial fibrosis and infiltration (restrictive cardiomyopathy).

HIGH-OUTPUT VERSUS LOW-OUTPUT HEART FAILURE   It is useful to classify patients with HF into those with a low cardiac output, i.e., *low-output HF*, and those with an elevated cardiac output, i.e., *high-output HF*. The former occurs secondary to ischemic heart disease, hypertension, dilated cardiomyopathy, and valvular and pericardial disease, while the latter is seen in patients with HF and hyperthyroidism, anemia, pregnancy, arteriovenous fistulas, beriberi, and Paget's disease. In clinical practice, however, low-output and high-output HF cannot always be readily distinguished. The normal range of cardiac output is wide [2.2 to 3.5 $(L/min)/m^2$]; in many patients with so-called low-output HF, the cardiac output may actually be just within the normal range at rest (although lower than it had been previously), but it fails to rise normally during exertion. On the other hand, in patients with so-called high-output HF, the output may not exceed the upper limits of normal (although it would have been elevated had it been measured before HF supervened); rather, it may have fallen to within normal limits. Regardless of the *absolute* level of the cardiac output, however, cardiac failure may be said to be present when the characteristic clinical manifestations described below are accompanied by a depression of the curve relating ventricular end-diastolic volume to cardiac performance (see Fig. 231-6).

An integral physiologic component of *systolic* HF is the delivery of an inadequate quantity of oxygen required by the metabolizing tissues. In the absence of peripheral shunting of blood, this is reflected in an abnormal widening of the normal arterial–mixed venous oxygen difference (35 to 50 mL/L in the basal state). In mild cases, such an abnormality may not be present at rest but becomes evident only during exertion or other hypermetabolic states. In patients with high cardiac output states, such as those associated with arteriovenous fistula or thyrotoxicosis, the arterial–mixed venous oxygen difference is normal or low. The mixed venous oxygen saturation is raised by the admixture of blood that has been diverted away from the metabolizing tissues, and it may be presumed that even in these patients the delivery of oxygen to the latter is reduced despite the normal or even elevated mixed venous oxygen saturation. When HF occurs in such patients, the arterial–mixed venous oxygen difference, regardless of the absolute value, still exceeds the level that existed prior to the development of HF. Therefore, the cardiac output, though normal or even elevated, is lower than before HF supervened.

In most forms of high-output HF, the heart is called on to pump abnormally large quantities of blood in order to deliver the oxygen required by the metabolizing tissues. The hemodynamic burden placed on the myocardium by the increased flow load resembles that produced by chronic aortic regurgitation. In addition, thyrotoxicosis and beriberi may also impair myocardial metabolism directly, while very severe anemia may interfere with myocardial function by producing myocardial anoxia, especially in the subendocardium and in the presence of underlying obstructive coronary artery disease.

ACUTE VERSUS CHRONIC HEART FAILURE The prototype of *acute HF* is the sudden development of a large myocardial infarction or rupture of a cardiac valve in a patient who previously was entirely well. *Chronic HF* is typically observed in patients with dilated cardiomyopathy or multivalvular heart disease that develops or progresses slowly. Acute HF is usually predominantly systolic, and the sudden reduction in cardiac output often results in systemic hypotension without peripheral edema. In contrast, in chronic HF, arterial pressure is ordinarily well maintained until very late in the course, but there is often accumulation of edema.

RIGHT-SIDED VERSUS LEFT-SIDED HEART FAILURE Many of the clinical manifestations of HF result from the accumulation of excess fluid behind either one or both ventricles (Chaps. 32 and 37). This fluid usually localizes upstream to (behind) the ventricle that is initially affected. For example, patients in whom the left ventricle is hemodynamically overloaded (e.g., aortic stenosis) or weakened (e.g., postmyocardial infarction) develop dyspnea and orthopnea as a result of pulmonary congestion, a condition referred to as *left-sided HF*. In contrast, when the underlying abnormality affects the right ventricle primarily (e.g., congenital valvular pulmonic stenosis or pulmonary hypertension secondary to pulmonary thromboembolism), symptoms resulting from pulmonary congestion are uncommon, and edema, congestive hepatomegaly, and systemic venous distention, i.e., clinical manifestations of *right-sided HF*, are more prominent. When HF has existed for months or years, such localization of excess fluid behind the failing ventricle may no longer exist. For example, patients with long-standing aortic valve disease or systemic hypertension may develop ankle edema, congestive hepatomegaly, and systemic venous distention late in the course of their disease, even though the abnormal hemodynamic burden initially was placed on the left ventricle. This occurs in part because of the secondary pulmonary hypertension and resultant right-sided HF but also because of the retention of salt and water characteristic of HF (Chap. 37). The muscle bundles composing both ventricles are continuous, and both ventricles share a common wall, the interventricular septum. Also, biochemical changes that occur in HF and that may be involved in the impairment of myocardial function (Chap. 231), such as norepinephrine depletion and alterations in the activity of myosin ATPase, occur in the myocardium of *both* ventricles, regardless of the specific chamber on which the abnormal hemodynamic burden is placed initially.

BACKWARD VERSUS FORWARD HEART FAILURE For many years a controversy has revolved around the question of the mechanism of the clinical manifestations resulting from HF. The concept of *backward HF* contends that in HF, one or the other ventricle fails to discharge its contents or fails to fill normally. As a consequence, the pressures in the atrium and venous system behind the failing ventricle rise, and retention of sodium and water occurs as a consequence of the elevation of systemic venous and capillary pressures and the resultant transudation of fluid into the interstitial space (Chap. 37). In contrast, the proponents of the *forward HF* hypothesis maintain that the clinical manifestations of HF result directly from an inadequate discharge of blood into the arterial system. According to this concept, salt and water retention is a consequence of diminished renal perfusion and excessive proximal tubular sodium reabsorption and of excessive distal tubular reabsorption through activation of the renin-angiotensin-aldosterone (RAA) system.

A rigid distinction between *backward* and *forward* HF (like a rigid distinction between right and left HF) is artificial, since both mechanisms appear to operate to varying extents in most patients with HF. However, the rate of onset of HF often influences the clinical manifestations. For example, when a large portion of the left ventricle is suddenly destroyed, as in myocardial infarction, although stroke vol-

ume and blood pressure are suddenly reduced (both manifestations of forward failure), the patient may succumb to acute pulmonary edema, a manifestation of backward failure. If the patient survives the acute insult, clinical manifestations resulting from a chronically depressed cardiac output, including the abnormal retention of fluid within the systemic vascular bed, may develop. Similarly, in the case of massive pulmonary embolism, the right ventricle may dilate and the systemic venous pressure may rise to high levels (backward failure), or the patient may develop shock secondary to low cardiac output (forward failure), but this low-output state may have to be maintained for some days before sodium and water retention sufficient to produce peripheral edema occurs.

REDISTRIBUTION OF CARDIAC OUTPUT In HF, systemic blood flow is redistributed so that the delivery of oxygen to vital organs, such as the brain and myocardium, is maintained at normal or near-normal levels, while flow to less critical areas, such as the cutaneous and muscular beds and the viscera, is reduced. This redistribution serves as an important compensatory mechanism when cardiac output is reduced. It is most marked when a patient with HF exercises, but as HF advances, redistribution occurs even in the basal state. Vasoconstriction mediated by the adrenergic nervous system is largely responsible for redistribution, which in turn may be responsible for many of the clinical manifestations of HF, such as fluid accumulation (reduction of renal blood flow), low-grade fever (reduction of cutaneous flow), and fatigue (reduction of muscle flow).

SALT AND WATER RETENTION (See also Chap. 37) When the volume of blood pumped by the left ventricle into the systemic vascular bed is reduced, a complex sequence of adjustments occurs that ultimately results in the abnormal accumulation of fluid. On the one hand, many of the troubling clinical manifestations of HF are secondary to this excessive retention of fluid; on the other, this abnormal fluid accumulation and the expansion of blood volume that accompanies it also constitute an important compensatory mechanism that tends to maintain cardiac output and therefore perfusion of the vital organs. Except in the terminal stages of HF, the ventricle operates on an ascending, albeit depressed and flattened, function curve (Fig. 231-6, p. 1313), and the augmented ventricular end-diastolic volume and pressure characteristic of HF must be regarded as helping to maintain the reduced cardiac output, despite causing pulmonary and/or systemic venous congestion.

Congestive HF is also characterized by a complex series of neurohumoral adjustments. The activation of the adrenergic nervous system is discussed on p. 1315; there is also activation of the RAA system and increased release of antidiuretic hormone and endothelin. These influences elevate systemic vascular resistance and enhance sodium and water retention and potassium excretion. These actions are, to a minor extent, opposed by the release of atrial and brain natriuretic peptide, which also occurs in congestive HF. Patients with severe HF may exhibit a reduced capacity to excrete a water load, which may result in dilutional hyponatremia. In the presence of HF, effective filling of the systemic arterial bed is reduced, a condition that initiates the renal and hormonal changes mentioned above (Fig. 37-2).

The elevation of systemic venous pressure and the alterations of renal and adrenal function characteristic of HF vary in their relative importance in the production of edema in different patients. The RAA axis is activated most intensely by acute HF, and its activity tends to decline as HF becomes chronic. In patients with tricuspid valve disease or constrictive pericarditis, the elevated venous pressure and the transudation of fluid from systemic capillaries appear to play the dominant role in edema formation. On the other hand, severe edema may be present in patients with ischemic or hypertensive heart disease, in whom systemic venous pressure is within normal limits or is only minimally elevated. In such patients, the retention of salt and water is probably due primarily to a redistribution of cardiac output and a concomitant reduction in renal perfusion, as well as activation of the RAA axis. Regardless of the mechanisms involved in fluid retention, untreated patients with chronic congestive HF have elevations of total blood volume, interstitial fluid volume, and body sodium. These abnormalities diminish after clinical compensation has been achieved by effective treatment, especially with diuretics.

CLINICAL MANIFESTATIONS OF HEART FAILURE

DYSPNEA Respiratory distress that occurs as the result of increased effort in breathing is the most common symptom of HF (Chap. 32). In early HF, dyspnea is observed only during activity, when it may simply represent an aggravation of the breathlessness that occurs normally under these circumstances. As HF advances, however, dyspnea appears with progressively less strenuous activity and ultimately is present even when the patient is at rest. The principal difference between exertional dyspnea in normal persons and in patients with HF is the degree of activity necessary to induce this symptom. Cardiac dyspnea is observed most frequently in patients with elevations of pulmonary venous and capillary pressures. Such patients usually have engorged pulmonary vessels and interstitial pulmonary edema, which may be evident on radiologic examination. This interstitial pulmonary edema reduces the compliance of the lungs and thereby increases the work of the respiratory muscles required to inflate the lungs. The activation of receptors in the lungs results in the rapid, shallow breathing characteristic of cardiac dyspnea. The oxygen cost of breathing is increased by the excessive work of the respiratory muscles. This is coupled with the diminished delivery of oxygen to these muscles, which occurs as a consequence of the reduced cardiac output and which may contribute to fatigue of the respiratory muscles and the sensation of shortness of breath.

Orthopnea Dyspnea in the recumbent position is usually a later manifestation of HF than exertional dyspnea. Orthopnea occurs because of the redistribution of fluid from the abdomen and lower extremities into the chest during recumbency causing an increase in the pulmonary capillary hydrostatic pressure, as well as elevation of the diaphragm accompanying supine posture. Patients with orthopnea must elevate their heads on several pillows at night and frequently awaken short of breath or coughing (the so-called nocturnal cough) if their heads slip off the pillows. The sensation of breathlessness is usually relieved by sitting upright, since this position reduces venous return and pulmonary capillary pressure, and many patients report that they find relief from sitting in front of an open window. In advanced HF, orthopnea may become so severe that patients cannot lie down at all and must spend the entire night in a sitting position. On the other hand, in other patients with long-standing, severe left ventricular failure, symptoms of pulmonary congestion may actually diminish with time as the function of the right ventricle becomes impaired.

Paroxysmal (Nocturnal) Dyspnea This term refers to attacks of severe shortness of breath and coughing that generally occur at night, usually awaken the patient from sleep, and may be quite frightening. Though simple orthopnea may be relieved by sitting upright at the side of the bed with legs dependent, in the patient with paroxysmal nocturnal dyspnea, coughing and wheezing often persist even in this position. Paradoxical nocturnal dyspnea may be caused in part by the depression of the respiratory center during sleep, which may reduce ventilation sufficiently to lower arterial oxygen tension, particularly in patients with interstitial lung edema and reduced pulmonary compliance. Also, ventricular function may be further impaired at night because of reduced adrenergic stimulation of myocardial function. *Cardiac asthma* is closely related to paroxysmal nocturnal dyspnea and nocturnal cough and is characterized by wheezing secondary to bronchospasm—most prominent at night. *Acute pulmonary edema* (Chap. 32) is a severe form of cardiac asthma due to marked elevation of

pulmonary capillary pressure leading to alveolar edema, associated with extreme shortness of breath, rales over the lung fields, and the transudation and expectoration of blood-tinged fluid. If not treated promptly, acute pulmonary edema may be fatal.

CHEYNE-STOKES RESPIRATION Also known as *periodic respiration* or *cyclic respiration*, Cheyne-Stokes respiration is characterized by diminished sensitivity of the respiratory center to arterial P_{CO_2}. There is an apneic phase, during which the arterial P_{O_2} falls and the arterial P_{CO_2} rises. These changes in the arterial blood stimulate the depressed respiratory center, resulting in hyperventilation and hypocapnia, followed in turn by recurrence of apnea. Cheyne-Stokes respiration occurs most often in patients with cerebral atherosclerosis and other cerebral lesions, but the prolongation of the circulation time from the lung to the brain that occurs in HF, particularly in patients with hypertension and coronary artery disease and associated cerebral vascular disease, also appears to precipitate this form of breathing.

FATIGUE AND WEAKNESS These nonspecific but common symptoms of HF are related to the reduction of perfusion of skeletal muscle. Exercise capacity is reduced by the limited ability of the failing heart to increase its output and deliver oxygen to the exercising muscle.

ABDOMINAL SYMPTOMS Anorexia and nausea associated with abdominal pain and fullness are frequent complaints and may be related to the congested liver and portal venous system.

CEREBRAL SYMPTOMS In severe HF, particularly in elderly patients with accompanying cerebral arteriosclerosis, reduced cerebral perfusion, and arterial hypoxemia, there may be alterations in the mental state characterized by confusion, difficulty in concentration, impairment of memory, headache, insomnia, and anxiety. *Nocturia* is common in HF and may contribute to insomnia.

PHYSICAL FINDINGS (See Chap. 225) In moderate HF, the patient is in no distress at rest except that he or she may be uncomfortable when lying flat for more than a few minutes. In more severe HF, the pulse pressure may be diminished, reflecting a reduction in stroke volume, and the diastolic arterial pressure may be elevated as a consequence of generalized vasoconstriction. In acute HF, severe hypotension may be present. There may be cyanosis of the lips and nail beds (Chap. 36) and sinus tachycardia, and the patient may insist on sitting upright. *Systemic venous pressure* is often abnormally elevated in HF, and this may be reflected in distention of the jugular veins. In the early stages of HF, the venous pressure may be normal at rest but may become abnormally elevated during and immediately after exertion as well as with sustained pressure on the abdomen (positive abdominojugular reflux).

Third and fourth heart sounds are often audible but are not specific for HF, and *pulsus alternans*, i.e., a regular rhythm in which there is alternation of strong and weak cardiac contractions and therefore alternation in the strength of the peripheral pulses, may be present. Pulsus alternans, a sign of severe HF, may be detected by sphygmomanometry and in more severe instances by palpation; it frequently follows an extrasystole and is observed most commonly in patients with cardiomyopathy or hypertensive or ischemic heart disease.

Pulmonary Rales Moist, inspiratory, crepitant rales and dullness to percussion over the lung bases are common in patients with HF and elevated pulmonary venous and capillary pressures. In patients with pulmonary edema, rales may be heard widely over both lung fields; they are frequently coarse and sibilant and may be accompanied by expiratory wheezing. Rales may, however, be caused by many conditions other than left ventricular failure. Some patients with long-standing HF have no rales because of increased lymphatic drainage of alveolar fluid.

Cardiac Edema (See Chap. 37) This is usually symmetric and dependent, occurring in the legs, particularly in the pretibial region and ankles in ambulatory patients, in whom it is most prominent in the evening. Cardiac edema occurs in the sacral region of patients who are bed-ridden. Pitting edema of the arms and face occurs rarely and then only late in the course of HF.

Hydrothorax and Ascites Pleural effusion in congestive HF results from the elevation of pleural capillary pressure and transudation of fluid into the pleural cavities. Since the pleural veins drain into *both* the systemic and pulmonary veins, hydrothorax occurs most commonly with marked elevation of pressure in both venous systems but also may be seen with marked elevation of pressure in either venous bed. It is more frequent in the right pleural cavity than in the left. *Ascites* also occurs as a consequence of transudation and results from increased pressure in the hepatic veins and the veins draining the peritoneum (Chap. 46). Marked ascites occurs most frequently in patients with tricuspid valve disease and constrictive pericarditis.

Congestive Hepatomegaly An enlarged, tender, pulsating liver also accompanies systemic venous hypertension and is observed not only in the same conditions in which ascites occurs but also in milder forms of HF from any cause. With prolonged, severe hepatomegaly, as in patients with tricuspid valve disease or chronic constrictive pericarditis, enlargement of the spleen, i.e., congestive splenomegaly, may also occur.

Jaundice This is a late finding in HF and is associated with elevations of both the direct- and indirect-reacting bilirubin; it results from impairment of hepatic function secondary to hepatic congestion and the hepatocellular hypoxia associated with central lobular atrophy. Hepatic enzymes are frequently elevated. If hepatic congestion occurs acutely, the jaundice may be severe and the enzymes strikingly elevated.

Cardiac Cachexia With severe chronic HF there may be serious weight loss and cachexia because of (1) elevation of circulating concentrations of tumor necrosis factor; (2) elevation of the metabolic rate, which results in part from the extra work performed by the respiratory muscles, the increased oxygen needs of the hypertrophied heart, and/or the discomfort associated with severe HF; (3) anorexia, nausea, and vomiting due to central causes, to digitalis intoxication, or to congestive hepatomegaly and abdominal fullness; (4) impairment of intestinal absorption due to congestion of the intestinal veins; and (5) rarely, due to protein-losing enteropathy in patients with particularly severe failure of the right side of the heart.

Other Manifestations With reduction of blood flow, the extremities may be cold, pale, and diaphoretic. Urine flow is depressed, and the urine contains albumin and has a high specific gravity and a low concentration of sodium. In addition, prerenal azotemia may be present. In patients with long-standing severe HF, impotence and depression are common.

ROENTGENOGRAPHIC AND ECHOCARDIOGRAPHIC FINDINGS In addition to the enlargement of the particular chambers characteristic of the lesion responsible for HF, distention of pulmonary veins and redistribution to the apices is common in patients with HF and elevated pulmonary vascular pressures. Also, pleural effusions may be evident and associated with interlobar effusions.

DIFFERENTIAL DIAGNOSIS The diagnosis of congestive HF may be established by observing some combination of the clinical manifestations of HF described above, together with the findings characteristic of one of the etiologic forms of heart disease. Table 232-1 shows the Framingham criteria, which are useful in the diagnosis of HF. Since chronic HF is often associated with cardiac enlargement, the diagnosis should be questioned, but is by no means excluded, when all chambers are normal in size. Two-dimensional echocardiography (Chap. 227) is particularly useful in assessing the dimensions of each cardiac chamber. HF is sometimes difficult to distinguish from pulmonary disease, and the differential diagnosis is discussed in Chap. 32. Pulmonary embolism also presents many of the manifestations of HF, but hemoptysis, pleuritic chest pain, a right ventricular lift, and the characteristic mismatch between ventilation and perfusion on lung scan should point to this diagnosis (Chap. 261).

Ankle edema may be due to varicose veins, cyclic edema, or grav-

Table 232-1 Framingham Criteria for Diagnosis of Congestive Heart Failure[a]

MAJOR CRITERIA

Paroxysmal nocturnal dyspnea
Neck vein distention
Rales
Cardiomegaly
Acute pulmonary edema
S_3 gallop
Increased venous pressure (>16 cmH$_2$O)
Positive hepatojugular reflux

MINOR CRITERIA

Extremity edema
Night cough
Dyspnea on exertion
Hepatomegaly
Pleural effusion
Vital capacity reduced by one-third from normal
Tachycardia (≥120 bpm)

MAJOR OR MINOR

Weight loss ≥4.5 kg over 5 days' treatment

[a] To establish a clinical diagnosis of congestive heart failure by these criteria, at least one major and two minor criteria are required.
SOURCE: KKL Ho et al, Circulation 88:107, 1993.

itational effects (Chap. 37), but in these patients there is no jugular venous hypertension at rest or with pressure over the abdomen. Edema secondary to renal disease can usually be recognized by appropriate renal function tests and urinalysis and is rarely associated with elevation of venous pressure. Enlargement of the liver and ascites occur in patients with hepatic cirrhosis and also may be distinguished from HF by normal jugular venous pressure and absence of a positive abdominojugular reflux.

TREATMENT (See Practice Guidelines) The treatment of HF may be divided into four components: (1) removal of the precipitating cause, (2) correction of the underlying cause, (3) prevention of deterioration of cardiac function, and (4) control of the congestive HF state. The first two components are discussed in other chapters together with each specific disease entity or complication. Examples of removal of precipitating causes are the treatment of pneumococcal pneumonia or the restoration of sinus rhythm in a patient with atrial fibrillation. In many instances, surgical treatment will correct or at least alleviate the underlying cause of HF. The third component of the treatment of HF, i.e., the prevention of deterioration of cardiac function, involves the administration of angiotensin-converting enzyme (ACE) inhibitors and β-adrenergic blockers as well as reduction of cardiac work load. Control of the congestive heart failure state requires reduction of the excessive retention of salt and water as well as enhancement of myocardial contractility. The vigor with which each of these measures is pursued in any individual patient should depend on the severity of HF and the tempo of the disease. Following effective treatment, recurrence of the clinical manifestations of HF can often be prevented by continuing those measures that were originally effective.

While a simple rule for the treatment of all patients with HF cannot be formulated because of its varied etiologies, hemodynamic features, clinical manifestations, and severity of HF, insofar as the treatment of chronic congestive failure is concerned, the administration of an ACE inhibitor retards the development of HF and should be begun early in patients with left ventricular systolic dysfunction (ejection fraction < 0.40), even if they are asymptomatic. Then, as symptoms develop, simple measures such as moderate restriction of activity and sodium intake and oral diuretics should be tried. β-adrenergic receptor blockers and digitalis glycosides are given for patients with systolic HF. If

---

Practice Guidelines for Heart Failure

I. Evaluation
  A. Assess functional status by NY Heart Association classification
  B. Assess fluid status to determine need for diuretics
  C. Assess left ventricular (LV) ejection fraction to distinguish between systolic, diastolic, or combined HF (echocardiography or radionuclide angiography)
  D. Assess invasive hemodynamics in patients unresponsive to treatment and/or transplant candidates

II. Prevention
  A. Control coronary risk factors (Chap. 241)
  B. Institute reperfusion strategies in acute myocardial infarction (Chap. 242)
  C. Prescribe ACE inhibition and/or beta blockade in patients with LV dysfunction without HF

III. General therapeutic measures
  A. Restrict salt intake to <3 g qd
  B. Recommend regular, moderate exercise
  C. Avoid antiarrhythmic agents for asymptomatic arrhythmias
  D. Avoid nonsteroidal anti-inflammatory agents
  E. Provide influenzal and pneumococcal immunization

IV. Diuretics
  A. Administer diuretics for all pts with HF with fluid accumulation to achieve normal jugular venous pressure and relief of edema
  B. Weigh daily to select/adjust dose
  C. Treat diuretic resistance
    1. IV administration
    2. Use ≥2 diuretics in combination (e.g. furosemide and metolazone)
  D. Administer short-term dopamine to enhance renal blood flow

V. ACE inhibitors
  A. Administer to all patients with LV systolic failure and LV dysfunction without heart failure
  B. Contraindications:
    1. High-output angioedema or anuric renal failure
    2. Pregnancy
    3. Hypotension
    4. Creatinine > 265 μmol/L (3 mg/dL)
    5. Serum K > 5.5 mmol/L
    6. Bilateral renal artery stenosis.

VI. β-Adrenergic blockers
  A. Administer to all NYHA class II or III pts with systolic HF, often together with ACE inhibitors and diuretics
  B. Contraindications
    1. Bronchospastic disease
    2. Symptomatic bradycardia or advanced heart block
    3. Instability

VII. Digitalis
  A. Use in pts with LV systolic HF along with diuretics, ACE inhibitors, beta blocker; especially useful in pts with atrial fibrillation

VIII. Other measures
  A. Consider hydralazine-iosorbide combination in patients intolerant of ACE inhibition
  B. Use angiotensin-receptor blocker in pts who develop angioedema or cough with ACE inhibitor
  C. Consider spironolactone in patients with class IV symptoms
  D. Do *not* use calcium antagonists for treatment of heart failure and avoid them for treatment of angina or hypertension in pts with heart failure

IX. Antiarrhythmic therapy
  A. Antiarrhythmic drugs (Chap. 230) are not recommended for pts with asymptomatic or nonsustained ventricular arrhythmias
  B. Class I antiarrhythmics should be avoided except in acute life-threatening arrhythmias
  C. Class III antiarrhythmics, especially amiodarone, may be used to treat atrial arrhythmias but not for the prevention of sudden death.

SOURCE: Modified from Packer and Cohn.

---

these measures are insufficient, the next step is more rigorous restriction of salt intake and higher doses and multiple diuretics. If HF persists, hospitalization with rigid salt restriction, bed rest, intravenous vasodilators, and positive inotropic agents are tried. Assisted circulation and cardiac transplantation (Chap. 233) are considered for patients with severe, intractable HF and a poor prognosis.

Prevention of Deterioration of Myocardial Infarction   Chronic activation of the RAA axis and of the sympathetic nervous systems in HF result in a maladaptive response and cause further deterioration of cardiac function and/or potentially fatal arrhythmias (Chap. 231). Drugs that block these two systems have been found to be useful in the management of HF (Tables 232-2 and 232-3).

Angiotensin-converting enzyme inhibitors   In many patients with HF, the left ventricular afterload is increased as a consequence of the several neural and humoral influences that act to constrict the peripheral vascular bed. In addition to the vasoconstriction, the ventricular end-diastolic and -systolic volumes rise in systolic HF. As a consequence of the operation of Laplace's law, which relates myocardial wall tension to the product of intraventricular pressure and radius (both of which may become elevated in HF), the aortic impedance, i.e., the force that opposes left ventricular ejection, or the ventricular afterload, rises, which reduces stroke volume (Fig. 231-10, p. 1316). In many patients with systolic HF, a modest reduction of systemic vascular resistance and afterload elevates the stroke volume and reduces the elevated ventricular filling pressure of the failing ventricle.

The pharmacologic reduction of impedance to left ventricular ejection with an ACE inhibitor represents an important component of the management of HF. This approach may be particularly helpful in (but is by no means limited to) patients with systolic HF due to myocardial infarction (Chap. 243), and in patients with valvular regurgitation (Chap. 236). ACE inhibition should not be used in hypotensive patients. In patients with both acute and chronic systolic HF who are treated with ACE inhibitors, cardiac output rises, the pulmonary wedge pressure falls, the signs and symptoms of HF are relieved, and a new steady state is achieved in which cardiac output is higher and afterload lower with no or only mild reduction of arterial pressure. The administration of ACE inhibitors has been shown to prevent or retard the development of HF in patients with left ventricular dysfunction without HF, to reduce symptoms, enhance exercise performance, and to reduce long-term mortality when they are begun in such patients shortly after acute myocardial infarction. These beneficial effects are related only in part to the salutary hemodynamic effects, i.e., the reduction of preload and afterload. Their major effect appears to be on inhibition of local (tissue) renin-angiotensin systems.

Lisinopril in doses of 20 mg qd or enalapril 10 mg bid have been shown to be useful in the management of heart failure.

Angiotensin Receptor Blockers   In patients who cannot tolerate ACE inhibitors (because of cough, angioneurotic edema, leukopenia),

Table 232-2   Overview of Angiotensin-Converting Enzyme Inhibitors in Heart Failure

	Odds Ratio	95% Confidence Interval
Total mortality	0.77	0.67–0.88
Mortality or hospitalization	0.65	0.57–0.74
Progressive heart failure	0.69	0.58–0.83
Sudden death	0.91	0.73–1.12
Fatal myocardial infarction	0.82	0.60–1.11
Total mortality		
Class 1	0.75	0.46–1.23
Class 2	0.83	0.68–1.01
Class 3	0.76	0.60–0.96
Class 4	0.55	0.36–0.84
EF >0.25	0.98	0.78–1.23
EF ≤0.25	0.69	0.57–0.85

NOTE: EF, ejection fraction
SOURCE: From Garg and Yusuf. Copyright 1995, American Medical Association.

Table 232-3 Clinical Trials in Heart Failure

	Beta Blockade		Aldosterone Antagonist
Trial name	CIBIS II	MERIT-HF	RALES
Drug	Bisoprolol (B1 selective)	Metoprolol (B1 selective)	Spironolactone
Age (avg, years)	61	64	65
CAD%	50	65	54
Male %	80	77	73
NYHA II %		41	
III %	83	55	71
IV	17	4	29
ACE I %	90	90	95
LVEF %	28	28	<35%
Placebo Annual mortality, %	13	10	22
Mortality reduction			
All cause	34	34	30
Sudden death	42	41	29
Pump failure death	26	49	36
Hospital admissions for HF	32		35

an angiotensin II receptor blocker (type AT1) antagonist (e.g., losartan 50 mg qid) may be used instead.

Aldosterone Antagonist The activation of the RAA axis in HF increases not only circulating and tissue angiotensin II but also aldosterone. The latter, in addition to causing sodium retention and worsening edema (Chaps. 331 and 37), causes sympathetic activation, myocardial, vascular, and perivascular fibrosis and reduces arterial compliance. In one large multicenter trial in patients with advanced heart failure and reduced ejection fraction (RALES), spironolactone, 25 mg/d reduced total mortality, as well as sudden death and death from pump failure (Table 232-3). Since spironolactone is also a useful diuretic (see below), its widespread use in systolic heart failure should be considered.

β-adrenoceptor blockers While the abrupt administration of large doses of β-adrenergic receptor blockers can intensify HF, the administration of gradually escalating doses of metoprolol, carvedilol, and bisoprolol have been reported to improve the symptoms of HF, and to reduce all-cause death, cardiovascular death, sudden death, and pump failure death (Table 232-3). In patients with moderately severe HF (classes II and III), the administration of 12.5 mg metoprolol CR/XL qd, increasing over 4 weeks to a target dose of 200 mg qid, has been shown to be beneficial. β-Adrenoceptor blockers are not indicated in HF patients who are unstable, in New York Heart Association Class IV, in HF patients shortly after acute myocardial infarction, or in those with HF and normal ejection fraction, i.e., with diastolic HF.

Reduction of Cardiac Work Load This consists of reducing physical activity, instituting emotional rest, and reducing afterload (see above). Modest restriction of physical activity in mild cases and rest in bed or in a chair in severe failure are useful. In acute, severe failure, meals should be small in quantity, but more frequent, and every effort should be made to diminish the patient's anxiety; sometimes drugs such as diazepam (2 to 5 mg tid) for several days are useful. Physical and emotional rest tends to lower arterial pressure and reduce the load on the myocardium by diminishing the requirements for cardiac output.

Reduced physical exertion should be continued for several days after the patient's condition has stabilized. The hazards of phlebothrombosis and pulmonary embolism which occur with bed rest may be reduced with anticoagulants, leg exercises, and elastic stockings. *Absolute* bed rest is rarely required or advisable, and the patient should ordinarily be encouraged to sit in a chair. Heavy sedation should be avoided. In ambulatory patients with chronic, moderately severe HF, additional periods of rest on weekends frequently allow continuation of gainful employment. Following recovery from HF, the patient's activities should be assessed, and often, professional, community, and/or family responsibilities should be curtailed. Intermittent rest during the day (e.g., a scheduled 1-h nap or rest following lunch) and the avoidance of strenuous exertion are often helpful. Regular, nonexhausting exercise such as walking or riding a stationary-bicycle ergometer as tolerated should be employed once the patient has become compensated. Weight reduction by restriction of caloric intake in obese patients with HF also diminishes cardiac work load and is an essential component of the therapeutic program.

Control of Excessive Fluid Many of the clinical manifestations of HF result from expansion of the extracellular fluid volume. A negative sodium balance can be achieved by reducing the dietary intake and increasing the urinary excretion of this ion with the aid of diuretics. Rarely, in severe HF, mechanical removal of extracellular fluid by means of thoracentesis and paracentesis may be necessary.

Diet In patients with mild HF, symptomatic improvement may result simply from reducing the sodium intake, particularly if accompanied by periods of physical rest. The normal diet contains approximately 6 to 10 g sodium chloride; this intake can be reduced by half simply by excluding salt-rich foods and salt added at the table. Reduction of the ordinary dietary intake to approximately one-fourth of normal may be achieved if, in addition, all salt is omitted from cooking. In patients with severe HF who have fluid accumulation despite diuretic therapy (see below), the dietary intake of sodium chloride should be reduced to between 500 and 1000 mg, and in order to achieve this, milk, cheese, bread, cereals, canned vegetables and soups, some salted cuts of meat, and some fresh vegetables (including spinach, celery, and beets) must be eliminated. A variety of fresh fruit, green vegetables, specially processed breads and milk, and salt substitutes are permissible. Late in the course of HF, dilutional hyponatremia may develop in patients who are unable to excrete a water load, sometimes because of excessive secretion of antidiuretic hormone. In such cases, water intake as well as sodium intake must be restricted.

Calories should be restricted in obese patients with HF. In patients with severe HF and cardiac cachexia, on the other hand, an attempt must be made to maintain nutritional intake and to avoid caloric and vitamin deficiencies; nutritional supplements may be in order.

Diuretics Diuretics should be given to relieve fluid accumulation and thus reduce or prevent edema and jugular venous distention. A variety of diuretic agents are available (Table 246-6, p. 1422), and almost all are effective in patients with mild HF. However, in the more severe forms of HF, the selection of diuretics is more difficult, and abnormalities in serum electrolytes must be taken into account. Overtreatment must be avoided, since the resultant hypovolemia may reduce cardiac output, interfere with renal function, and produce profound weakness and lethargy.

THIAZIDE DIURETICS These agents are used widely and are useful by themselves in patients with mild HF and in combination with other diuretics in those with severe HF. In patients with chronic mild or moderate HF, the continued administration of a thiazide diuretic abolishes or diminishes the need for rigid dietary sodium restriction, although salty foods and table salt still should be avoided. Thiazide diuretics reduce the reabsorption of sodium and chloride in the first half of the distal convoluted tubule and a portion of the cortical ascending limb of the loop of Henle, and water follows the unreabsorbed salt. Thiazides fail to increase free water clearance and in some instances reduce it. This may result in the excretion of a hypertonic urine and may contribute to dilutional hyponatremia. As a consequence of increased delivery of sodium to the distal nephron, sodium-potassium ion exchange is enhanced, and kaliuresis results. In contrast to the loop diuretics, which enhance calcium excretion, the thiazides have the opposite effect.

Thiazide diuretics are effective and useful in the treatment of HF as long as the glomerular filtration rate exceeds approximately 50% of normal. Chlorothiazide is administered in doses of up to 500 mg every 6 h. Many derivatives of this compound are available but differ principally in dosage and duration of action. Chlorthalidone (25 to 50 mg/d) is especially useful since it may be administered once daily.

Potassium depletion and metabolic alkalosis (the latter due to increased H^+ secretion as a substitute for the depleted intracellular stores of potassium) are the chief adverse metabolic effects following prolonged administration of the thiazides, of metolazone, and of the loop diuretics. Hypokalemia may seriously enhance the dangers of digitalis intoxication (see below), and induce fatigue and lethargy; these may be prevented by oral supplementation with potassium chloride or preferably by the addition of a potassium-retaining diuretic, such as a spironolactone or triamterene. Other side effects of thiazides include reduction of the excretion of uric acid, which may lead to hyperuricemia, and impaired glucose tolerance, which rarely may precipitate hyperosmolar coma in poorly regulated diabetic patients. Skin rashes, thrombocytopenia, and granulocytopenia have also been reported.

METOLAZONE   This quinethazone derivative has a site of action and potency similar to those of the thiazides but has been reported to be effective in the presence of moderate renal failure. The usual dose is 5 to 10 mg/d. Metolazone may be added to thiazide and loop diuretics in severe HF.

FUROSEMIDE, BUMETANIDE, ETHACRYNIC ACID, PIRETANIDE, AND TORSEMIDE   These "loop" diuretics are similar physiologically but differ chemically from one another. These drugs reversibly inhibit the reabsorption of sodium, potassium, and chloride in the thick ascending limb of Henle's loop, apparently by blocking a cotransport system in the luminal membrane. They may induce renal cortical vasodilatation and can produce rates of urine formation that may be as high as one-fourth of the glomerular filtration rate. Metabolic alkalosis may be caused by a large increase in the urinary excretion of chloride, hydrogen, and potassium ions. Hypokalemia, hyperuricemia, and hyperglycemia are observed occasionally, as with thiazide diuretics. The reabsorption of free water is decreased. All five of these drugs are readily absorbed orally, are excreted in the bile and urine, and are usually effective both intravenously and by mouth. Weakness, nausea, and dizziness may complicate the administration of all loop diuretics; ethacrynic acid has been associated with transient or even permanent deafness as well as with skin rash and granulocytopenia.

These powerful diuretics are useful in all forms of HF, particularly in patients with otherwise refractory HF and pulmonary edema. They have been shown to be effective in patients with hypoalbuminemia, hyponatremia, hypochloremia, hypokalemia, and with reductions in the glomerular filtration rate and to produce a diuresis in patients in whom thiazide diuretics and aldosterone antagonists, alone and in combination, are ineffective. In patients with refractory HF, the action of loop diuretics may be potentiated by intravenous administration and by the addition of other diuretics, i.e., thiazides, metozalone, osmotic diuretics, and the potassium-sparing diuretics—spironolactone, triamterene, and amiloride.

ALDOSTERONE ANTAGONISTS   These agents act on the cortical collecting ducts, are relatively weak, and therefore are rarely indicated as sole agents. However, their potassium-sparing properties make them particularly useful in conjunction with the more potent kaliuretic agents, i.e., the loop diuretics, thiazides, and metozalone. The potassium-sparing agents fall into two classes.

The spironolactones resemble aldosterone structurally and act by competitive inhibition of aldosterone, thereby blocking the exchange between sodium and both potassium and hydrogen in the distal tubules and collecting ducts. These agents produce a sodium diuresis, and in contrast to the thiazides, ethacrynic acid, and furosemide, they result in potassium retention. Although secondary hyperaldosteronism exists in some patients with congestive HF, the spironolactones are effective even in patients in whom the serum aldosterone concentration is within normal limits.

Spironolactone may be administered in doses of 25 mg daily to 50 mg three to four times daily by mouth. The maximal effect of this regimen is not observed for approximately 4 days. Spironolactones are most effective when administered in combination with loop and/or thiazide diuretics. The opposing action of these drugs on urine and serum potassium makes possible a sodium diuresis without either hyper- or hypokalemia when spironolactone and one of these other agents are administered in combination. Also, since spironolactone, triamterene, and amiloride act on the distal tubule, they are particularly effective when used in combination with one of these other diuretics that act more proximally. Spironolactone, triamterene, and amiloride should not be administered alone to patients with hyperkalemia, renal failure, or hyponatremia. Reported complications of Aldactone A include nausea, epigastric distress, mental confusion, drowsiness, gynecomastia, and erythematous eruptions.

As mentioned above, a lower dose of spironolactone (25 mg/d), which exerts little if any diuretic effect, has been shown to prolong life in patients with advanced HF (Table 232-3).

Triamterene and *amiloride* exert renal effects similar to those of the spironolactones; i.e., they block sodium reabsorption and secondarily inhibit potassium secretion in the distal tubules. However, their action does not depend on the presence of aldosterone. The effective dose of triamterene is 100 mg once or twice daily, and that of amiloride is 5 mg daily. Side effects include nausea, vomiting, diarrhea, headache, granulocytopenia, eosinophilia, and skin rash. Both triamterene and the chemically unrelated diuretic amiloride resemble Aldactone A in that their diuretic potency is not great, but they are effective in preventing the hypokalemia characteristic of loop diuretics and thiazides. A number of diuretic preparations contain a combination of a thiazide and either triamterene or amiloride in a single capsule. They may be useful in patients who develop hypokalemia with a thiazide but should not be used in patients with impaired renal function and/or hyperkalemia.

When *choosing a diuretic*, orally administered loop diuretics or thiazides are the agents of choice in the treatment of chronic cardiac edema of mild to moderate degree in patients without hyperglycemia, hyperuricemia, or hypokalemia. Spironolactones, triamterene, and amiloride are not potent diuretics when used alone, but they potentiate the thiazide and loop diuretics. Loop diuretics, given alone or with spironolactone or triamterene, are the agents of choice in patients with severe HF refractory to other diuretics. In very severe HF, the combination of a loop diuretic, a thiazide, and a potassium-sparing diuretic is required.

Vasodilators   Direct vasodilators may be useful in patients with severe, acute HF who demonstrate systemic vasoconstriction despite ACE inhibitor therapy. The ideal vasodilator for the treatment of *acute* HF should have a rapid onset and brief duration of action when administered by intravenous infusion; sodium nitroprusside (0.1 to 3.0 μg/kg per minute) qualifies as such a drug, but its use requires careful monitoring of the arterial pressure and, if possible, of the pulmonary artery wedge pressure. The combination of hydralazine (up to 300 mg qd orally) and isosorbide diuretics (up to 160 mg qd orally) may be useful for chronic oral administration.

Enhancement of Myocardial Contractility • Digitalis   The improvement of myocardial contractility by means of cardiac glycosides is useful in the control of HF. *Digoxin*, which has a half-life of 1.6 days, is filtered in the glomeruli and secreted by the renal tubules. Significant reductions of the glomerular filtration rate reduce the elimination of digoxin and, therefore, may prolong digoxin's effect, allowing it to accumulate to toxic levels. In patients with normal renal function, a plateau concentration in the blood and tissue is reached after 5 days of daily maintenance treatment without a loading dose (see Fig. 70-2).

MECHANISM OF ACTION   The most important effect of digitalis on cardiac muscle is to shift its force-velocity relation upward (Fig. 231-5, p. 1313). Cardiac glycosides inhibit the monovalent cation transport enzyme–coupled Na^+,K^+-ATPase and increase intracellular sodium content; this, in turn, increases intracellular Ca^{2+} through a

Na$^+$-Ca^{2+} exchange carrier mechanism. The increased myocardial uptake of Ca^{2+} augments Ca^{2+} released to the myofilaments during excitation and, therefore, invokes a positive inotropic response.

Cardiac glycosides also produce alterations in the electrical properties of both the contractile cells and the specialized automatic cells, leading to increased automaticity and ectopic impulse activity. They also prolong the effective *refractory period* of the atrioventricular node and thereby slow ventricular rate in atrial flutter and fibrillation.

USE IN HEART FAILURE Digitalis is particularly effective in patients with systolic HF complicated by atrial flutter and fibrillation and a rapid ventricular rate, who benefit from both slowing of the ventricular rate and the positive inotropic effect. Although digitalis does not improve survival in patients with systolic HF and sinus rhythm, it reduces the need for hospitalization. By stimulating myocardial contractility moderately, digitalis improves ventricular emptying; i.e., it increases cardiac output, augments the ejection fraction, promotes diuresis, and reduces the elevated diastolic pressure and volume and the end-systolic volume of the failing ventricle. This action reduces symptoms resulting from pulmonary vascular congestion and elevated systemic venous pressure. Digitalis is of little or no value in patients with HF, sinus rhythm, and the following conditions: hypertrophic cardiomyopathy, myocarditis, mitral stenosis, chronic constrictive pericarditis, and any form of diastolic HF.

The maintenance dose of digoxin is 0.25 mg qd for most adults; in the elderly and others with mild impairment of renal function, it is 0.125 mg qd. Loading doses, four times the maintenance dose, may be administered in acute systolic failure.

DIGITALIS INTOXICATION This is a serious and potentially fatal complication. Advanced age, acute myocardial infarction or ischemia, hypoxemia, magnesium depletion, renal insufficiency, hypercalcemia, electrical cardioversion, and hypothyroidism all may reduce tolerance to digitalis. The most common precipitating cause of digitalis intoxication, however, is depletion of potassium stores, which often occurs in patients with HF as a result of diuretic therapy and secondary hyperaldosteronism.

Anorexia, nausea, and vomiting are among the earliest signs of digitalis intoxication. The most frequent disturbances of cardiac rhythm are ventricular premature beats, bigeminy, ventricular tachycardia, and, rarely, ventricular fibrillation. Atrioventricular block of varying degrees of severity may occur. Nonparoxysmal atrial tachycardia with variable atrioventricular block is characteristic of digitalis intoxication. Chronic digitalis intoxication may be insidious in onset and characterized by exacerbations of HF, weight loss, cachexia, neuralgias, gynecomastia, yellow vision, and delirium.

The administration of quinidine, verapamil, amiodarone, and propafenone to patients receiving digoxin raises the serum concentration of the latter by reducing both the renal and nonrenal elimination of digoxin and by reducing its volume of distribution. These drugs increase the propensity to digitalis intoxication, and the dose of digitalis should be reduced by half in patients receiving these drugs.

TREATMENT OF DIGITALIS INTOXICATION When tachyarrhythmias result from digitalis intoxication, withdrawal of the drug and treatment with β-adrenoceptor blocker or lidocaine are indicated. If hypokalemia is present, potassium should be administered cautiously and by the oral route. Fab fragments of purified, intact digitalis antibodies are a potentially lifesaving approach to the treatment of severe intoxication.

Sympathomimetic amines (See also Chap. 72) Two sympathomimetic amines that act largely on β-adrenergic receptors—dopamine and dobutamine—improve myocardial contractility (Table 72-1) and are effective in the management of HF; they must be administered by constant intravenous infusion for up to 1 week and are useful in patients with intractable, severe HF, particularly those with a reversible component, such as exists in patients who have undergone cardiac surgery, in patients with acute myocardial infarction and shock or pulmonary edema, and in patients with refractory HF as a "bridge" to transplantation. While these sympathomimetic amines improve the hemodynamics and symptoms in these conditions, it is not clear that they

improve survival. Their administration should be accompanied by careful and continuous monitoring of the electrocardiogram, arterial pressure, and, if possible, pulmonary artery wedge pressure.

Dopamine is a naturally occurring immediate precursor of norepinephrine and has a combination of actions that makes it particularly useful in the treatment of a variety of hypotensive states of HF. At very low doses, i.e., 1 to 2 (μg/kg)/min, it dilates renal and mesenteric blood vessels through stimulation of specific dopaminergic receptors, thereby augmenting renal and mesenteric blood flow and sodium excretion. In the range of 2 to 10 (μg/kg)/min, dopamine stimulates myocardial β_1 receptors but induces relatively little tachycardia, while at higher doses it also stimulates α-adrenergic receptors and elevates arterial pressure.

Dobutamine is a synthetic catecholamine that acts on β_1, β_2, and α receptors. It exerts a potent inotropic action, has only a modest cardioaccelerating effect, and lowers peripheral vascular resistance, but since it simultaneously raises cardiac output, it may not lower systemic arterial pressure in patients with severe HF. Dobutamine, given in continuous infusions of 2.5 to 10 (μg/kg)/min, is useful in the treatment of acute HF without hypotension.

A major problem with sympathomimetics is the loss of responsiveness, apparently due to "downregulation" of adrenergic receptors, which becomes evident within 8 h of continuous administration. This problem may be managed by intermittent therapy.

Phosphodiesterase inhibitors These bipyridines, amrinone and milrinone, are noncatecholamine, nonglycoside agents that exert both positive inotropic and vasodilator actions by inhibiting a specific phosphodiesterase. They are suitable for intravenous use only; by simultaneously stimulating cardiac contractility and dilating the systemic vascular bed they reverse the major hemodynamic abnormalities associated with intractable HF. Amrinone and milrinone may be administered for the same conditions in which sympathomimetics are useful and may be employed together with dopamine or dobutamine.

Other Measures • *Anticoagulants* Patients with severe HF are at increased risk of pulmonary emboli secondary to venous thrombosis and of systemic emboli secondary to intracardiac thrombi and should be treated with warfarin. Patients with HF and atrial fibrillation, previous venous thrombosis, and pulmonary or systemic emboli are at especially high risk and should receive heparin followed by warfarin.

Diastolic heart failure The major goal in the treatment of this condition is to eliminate or reduce the causes of diastolic dysfunction, such as ventricular hypertrophy, fibrosis, or ischemia. The second is to reduce pulmonary and/or systemic venous congestion, a major consequence of diastolic dysfunction.

Management of arrhythmias (See also Chap. 230) Premature ventricular contractions and episodes of asymptomatic ventricular tachycardia are common in advanced HF. Sudden death, presumably due to ventricular fibrillation, is responsible for about one-half of all deaths in this condition. (The remainder are due to failure of the cardiac pump.) The management of arrhythmias should commence with correction of electrolyte and acid-base disturbances (Chaps. 49 and 50), especially diuretic-induced hypokalemia, as well as digitalis intoxication (see above). Treatment with class I antiarrhythmics such as quinidine, procainamide, or flecainide (Chap. 230) is fraught with danger because these drugs are proarrhythmic in patients with HF. Amiodarone, a class III antiarrhythmic, on the other hand, is well tolerated and is the drug of choice for patients with heart failure and atrial fibrillation. Patients who have been resuscitated from sudden death, those with syncope or presyncope due to ventricular arrhythmias, and those with asymptomatic ventricular tachyarrhythmias in whom ventricular tachycardia can be induced during electrophysiologic testing should be considered for the implantable automatic defibrillator. This may prevent recurrence of the arrhythmia and sudden death; back-up pacing may prevent sudden death due to bradyarrhythmias.

Refractory heart failure When the response to ordinary treatment is inadequate, HF is considered to be refractory. Before assuming that this condition simply reflects advanced, terminal, myocardial depression, careful consideration must be given to several possibilities: (1) an underlying and overlooked cause of the heart disease that may be amenable to specific surgical or medical therapy, such as infective endocarditis, hypertension, thyrotoxicosis, or silent aortic or mitral stenosis; (2) one or a combination of the precipitating causes of HF, such as pulmonary or urinary tract infection, recurrent pulmonary emboli, arterial hypoxemia, anemia, or arrhythmia; and (3) complications of overly vigorous therapy, such as digitalis intoxication, hypovolemia, or electrolyte imbalance. Recognition and proper treatment of the aforementioned complications are likely to restore responsiveness to therapy.

Hyponatremia is a manifestation of advanced refractory HF. It may be a complication of overaggressive diuresis leading to reduced glomerular filtration rate and decreased delivery of NaCl to the diluting sites in the distal tubule. Hyponatremia may also result from nonosmotic stimuli for the continued secretion of antidiuretic hormone. Therapy involves improvement of the cardiovascular status, if possible (sometimes requiring the administration of a sympathomimetic amine), as well as temporary cessation of diuretic therapy and restriction of oral water intake. Hypertonic saline is very rarely indicated because total-body sodium is usually elevated, not depressed, in HF.

The combination of the intravenously administered vasodilator sodium nitroprusside, a phosphodiesterase inhibitor (amrinone or milrinone), together with a sympathomimetic amine (dopamine or dobutamine) often results in additive effects, raising cardiac output and lowering filling pressure.

In hospitalized patients with refractory HF, therapy guided by hemodynamic measurements provided by a balloon flotation (Swan-Ganz) catheter may be helpful. The goal of manipulating diuretics, vasodilators, and inotropic agents is to achieve a pulmonary capillary wedge pressure of 15 to 18 mmHg, a right atrial pressure of 5 to 8 mmHg, a cardiac index > 2.2 (L/min)/m^2, and a systemic vascular resistance of 800 to 1200 dyne · s/cm^5. Once these values are achieved, an attempt should be made to convert the patient from intravenous to oral vasodilator therapy.

Assisted circulation/cardiac transplantation   When patients with HF become unresponsive to a combination of all the aforementioned therapeutic measures, are in New York Heart Association class IV, and are deemed unlikely to survive 1 year, they should be considered for temporary assisted circulation and/or cardiac transplantation (see Chap. 233).

Treatment of Acute Pulmonary Edema   Pulmonary edema secondary to left ventricular failure or mitral stenosis is described in Chap. 32. It is life-threatening and must be considered a medical emergency. As is the case for the more chronic forms of HF, in the treatment of pulmonary edema, attention must be directed to identifying and removing any precipitating causes of decompensation, such as an arrhythmia or infection. However, because of the acute nature of the problem, a number of additional nonspecific measures are necessary. If it does not delay treatment unduly, recording pulmonary vascular pressures through a Swan-Ganz catheter and intraarterial pressure directly is advisable. The first six measures listed below are ordinarily applied simultaneously or nearly so.

1. Morphine is administered intravenously repetitively, as needed, in doses from 2 to 5 mg. This drug reduces anxiety, reduces adrenergic vasoconstrictor stimuli to the arteriolar and venous beds, and thereby helps to break a vicious cycle. Naloxone should be available in case respiratory depression occurs.

2. Because the alveolar edema interferes with O_2 diffusion resulting in arterial hypoxemia, 100% O_2 should be administered, preferably under positive pressure. The latter increases intraalveolar pressure, reduces transudation of fluid from the alveolar capillaries, and impedes venous return to the thorax, reducing pulmonary capillary pressure.

3. The patient should be maintained in the sitting position, with the legs dangling along the side of the bed, if possible, which tends to reduce venous return.

4. Intravenous loop diuretics, such as furosemide or ethacrynic acid (40 to 100 mg) or bumetanide (1 mg), will, by rapidly establishing a diuresis, reduce circulating blood volume and thereby hasten the relief of pulmonary edema. In addition, when given intravenously, furosemide also exerts a venodilator action, reduces venous return, and thereby improves pulmonary edema even before the diuresis commences.

5. Afterload reduction is achieved with intravenous sodium nitroprusside at 20 to 30 μg/min in patients whose systolic arterial pressures exceed 100 mmHg.

6. Inotropic support should be provided by dopamine or dobutamine as described on p. 1327. Patients with systolic HF who are not receiving digitalis should receive 0.75 to 1.0 mg digoxin intravenously over 15 min.

7. Sometimes, aminophylline (theophylline ethylenediamine), 240 to 480 mg intravenously, is effective in diminishing bronchoconstriction, increasing renal blood flow and sodium excretion, and augmenting myocardial contractility.

8. If the above-mentioned measures are not sufficient, rotating tourniquets should be applied to the extremities.

After these emergency measures have been instituted and the precipitating factors treated, the diagnosis of the underlying cardiac disorder responsible for the pulmonary edema must be established, if it is not already known. After stabilization of the patient's condition, a long-range strategy for prevention of future episodes of pulmonary edema must be established, and this may require surgical treatment.

PROGNOSIS

The prognosis in patients with HF depends primarily on the nature of the underlying heart disease and on the presence or absence of a precipitating factor that can be treated. When one of the latter can be identified and removed, the outlook for immediate survival is far better than if HF occurs without any obvious precipitating cause. In the latter situation, survival usually ranges between 6 months and 4 years depending on the severity (Fig. 232-2). The long-term prognosis is more favorable when the underlying forms of heart disease, e.g., valvular heart disease, can be treated effectively. The prognosis can be estimated by observing the response to treatment. When clinical improvement occurs with only modest dietary sodium restriction and small doses of diuretics, the outlook is far better than if, in addition to these measures, intensive diuretic therapy and vasodilators are necessary. Other factors that have been shown to be associated with a poor prog-

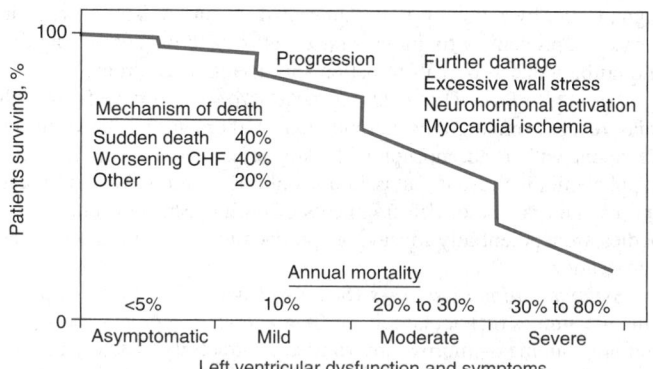

FIGURE 232-2   The natural history of congestive heart failure (CHF). Once left ventricular systolic dysfunction is present, it usually progresses, albeit not predictably. As left ventricular dysfunction progresses and symptoms increase, mortality rate increases and the process becomes inexorable. Myocyte loss and fibrosis become irreversible. An effective preventive measure must be introduced before onset or early in the course of progressive left ventricular dysfunction. *(From Massie and Shah, with permission.)*

nosis include a severely depressed ejection fraction (<25%), a reduced maximal O_2 uptake [<10 (mL/kg)/min], the inability to walk on the level and at a normal pace for more than 3 min, reduced (<133 mEq/L) serum sodium concentration, reduced (<3 mEq/L) serum potassium concentration, elevated circulating atrial and brain natriuretic peptide and norepinephrine concentrations, as well as frequent ventricular extrasystoles. A large fraction of patients with HF die suddenly, presumably of ventricular fibrillation. Unfortunately, there is no evidence that this complication can be prevented by the administration of antiarrhythmic agents. See guideline material.

BIBLIOGRAPHY

BRISTOW M et al: Clinical management of heart failure, in *Heart Disease*, 6th ed, E Braunwald (ed). Philadelphia, Saunders, 2001

BRISTOW MR: Beta adrenergic receptor blockade in chronic heart failure. Circulation 101: 558, 2000

CIBIS II INVESTIGATORS AND COMMITTEES: The Cardiac Insufficiency Bisoprolol Study II (CIBIS II): A randomised trial. Lancet 353:9–13, 1999

COLUCCI WS, BRAUNWALD E (eds): *Heart Failure: Cardiac Function and Dysfunction*, in *Atlas of Heart Diseases*, 2d ed, E Braunwald (series ed). Philadelphia, Current Medicine, 1999

COLUCCI WS et al: Clinical aspects of heart failure, in *Heart Disease*, 6th ed, E Braunwald (ed). Philadelphia, Saunders, 2001

FRANCIS GS et al: Neurohumoral activation in preclinical heart failure. Remodeling and the potential for intervention. Circulation 87 (Suppl 5):IV90, 1993

GARG R, YUSUF S: Overview of randomized trials of angiotensin-converting enzyme inhibitors on mortality and morbidity in patients with heart failure. Collaborative Group on ACE Inhibitor Trials. JAMA 274:462, 1995

GHEORGHIADE M et al: Current medical therapy for advanced heart failure. Heart Lung 29:16, 2000

KUBO SH, COHN JN: Long-term treatment of the ambulatory patient with heart failure, in *Cardiovascular Therapeutics*, TW Smith (ed). Philadelphia, Saunders, 1996, pp 210–231

MASSIE BM, SHAH NH: The heart failure epidemic: Magnitude of the problem and potential mitigating approaches. Curr Opin Cardiol 11:221, 1996

MERIT-HF STUDY GROUP: Effect of metoprolol CR/XL in chronic heart failure: Metoprolol CR/XL Randomised Intervention Trial in Congestive Heart Failure (MERIT-HF). Lancet 353:2001, 1999

PACKER M, COHN JN (eds): Consensus recommendations for the management of chronic heart failure. Am J Cardiol 83:1a-38a, 1999

PITT B et al: The effect of spironolactone on morbidity and mortality in patients with severe heart failure. N Engl J Med 341:709, 1999

WILCOX CS: Diuretics, in *The Kidney*, 6th ed, BM Brenner (ed). Philadelphia, Saunders, 2000, pp 2219–2252

sume a functional life after transplantation. It is estimated that only 2000 potential donors in the United States, for a pool of at least 20,000 candidates based on current guidelines, become available yearly. Attempts to increase donor awareness in both physicians and the public are being made. Optimal candidates for this procedure are those who would be expected to return to a functional life if their hearts were replaced (Table 233-1). This requires a mentally vigorous, medically compliant person who has not suffered extensive other end-stage organ damage from cardiac failure, does not have other systemic disease such as severe diabetes mellitus or collagen vascular disease, or is not positive for HIV. Long-standing pulmonary hypertension or recurrent pulmonary emboli and infarction may result in irreversible pulmonary hypertension leading to intraoperative death. Several heart transplant centers have initiated cardiac transplantation for newborns with left ventricular hypoplasia, but long-term survival experience is still very limited.

Timing of the recommendation to undergo cardiac transplantation can be difficult and requires assessment of the patient's current disability, stability of course, and likelihood of surviving the next 6 to 12 months. Generally, left ventricular ejection fractions under 15 to 20% and presence of serious ventricular arrhythmias indicate a 1-year survival rate of 50% or less. Estimating prognosis remains very challenging. A maximal oxygen uptake during exercise (maximal $\dot{V}_{O_2}$) of <10 mL O_2 per kilogram per minute usually indicates poor likelihood of survival for 1 year and has been a criterion for transplant candidacy in some programs. Maximal $\dot{V}_{O_2}$ values between 10 and 14 mL O_2 per kilogram per minute are in a borderline range, with values >14 usually predicting good 1- to 2-year survival. The increasing acceptance of cardiac transplantation as a treatment modality for heart failure without a corresponding increase in donor availability has led to prolonged waiting times of as much as 2 years or more. This longer waiting time has led to more rigorous medical care of the patient awaiting transplant with meticulous monitoring of electrolytes, fluid status, and overall well-being. Aggressive therapy for congestive heart failure with high-dose angiotensin-converting enzyme inhibitors and beta blockers and meticulous monitoring of serum electrolytes and renal function have led to stabilization and many times some improvement in the functional status of patients awaiting a donor. This has led to as many as 30 to 40% of listed patients being placed "on hold" based on their improved status. Whether these patients can maintain their improved

233 *John S. Schroeder*

CARDIAC TRANSPLANTATION

Orthotopic allograft cadaver cardiac transplantation as a treatment for end-stage cardiac disease achieved its thirty-third anniversary on December 7, 2000. On that day in 1967 Dr. Christiaan Barnard accomplished the first successful cardiac transplant in a human, quickly followed by Dr. Norman Shumway and Dr. Richard Lower at Stanford University. After an initial early wave of enthusiasm, the problems of immunosuppression slowed application of the procedure until the introduction of cyclosporine in 1980. A subsequent worldwide expansion of cardiac transplantation has resulted in approximately 2500 cardiac transplants per year, with further increases limited only by the donor supply. Current 1- and 5-year survival rates of 85 and 70% indicate that cardiac transplantation is the therapy of choice in patients with end-stage heart disease who are unlikely to survive the next 6 to 12 months.

INDICATIONS AND SELECTION OF CANDIDATES
The limited donor supply and relatively high cost of cardiac transplantation have restricted it to patients most likely to survive and re-

Table 233-1   Indications and Contraindications for Cardiac Transplantation

Indications
1. End-stage heart disease that limits prognosis for survival over 2 years or severely limits daily quality of life despite optimal medical and other surgical therapy
2. No secondary exclusion criteria
3. Suitable psychosocial profile and social support system
4. Suitable physiologic/chronologic age

Exclusion Criteria
1. Active infectious process
2. Recent pulmonary infarction
3. Insulin-requiring diabetes with evidence of end-organ damage
4. Irreversible pulmonary hypertension [pulmonary vascular resistance (PVR) poorly responsive to nitroprusside with PVR > 2 or pulmonary systolic pressure > 50 mmHg at peak dose or at mean arterial pressure of 65–70 mmHg]
5. Presence of circulating cytotoxic antibodies
6. Presence of active peptic ulcer disease
7. Active or recent malignancy
8. Presence of severe chronic obstructive pulmonary disease or chronic bronchitis
9. Substance or alcohol abuse
10. Presence of peripheral or cerebrovascular disease
11. Other systemic diseases that would jeopardize rehabilitation posttransplant

state or will subsequently deteriorate remains to be seen. Recurrent hospitalizations may be required. Patients may become dopamine/dobutamine-dependent to maintain adequate cardiac output. This dependency on an inotropic agent plus the need for a balloon flotation catheter for hemodynamic monitoring moves the patient to the highest priority (1a) for a donor heart.

In addition to these pharmacologic bridges to transplantation, mechanical bridges are occasionally used where pharmacologic therapy is no longer effective. Three approaches are currently used. The first is intraaortic balloon pumping, which can increase cardiac output by 15 to 20%. The second is a left ventricular assist device (LVAD), which empties blood via a tube placed in the apex of the left ventricle and pumps it with an electrically driven "bellows-type" mechanism into the abdominal aorta. This approach is highly effective and has been used for several months with successful subsequent transplantation. Limitations include right ventricular failure and/or high pulmonary vascular resistance, since the LVAD does not "unload" the right ventricle. Blood clotting in the device remains a problem, in addition to the obvious problems of infection. Finally, total mechanical heart replacement is also applied in some transplant centers. This complete replacement circumvents the problem of right ventricular failure but is limited by the greater complexity of the device, which can lead to clotting and systemic emboli. Patients who underwent mechanical assistance *and* received a donor heart have 1-year survival statistics similar to those who went directly to transplantation.

Tissue cross-matching between donor and recipient has generally not been done because of difficulty in obtaining good matches and lack of correlation between match and outcome. Size, ABO matching, negative lymphocyte cross-match, and avoidance of a transplantation from a cytomegalovirus (CMV)-positive donor to a CMV-negative recipient are more important.

OPERATIVE PROCEDURE The surgeon removes the diseased heart but leaves the posterior wall of the right atrium in place and the superior and inferior venae cavae intact. The posterior wall of the left atrium is also left in situ with pulmonary veins intact. The donor heart is then removed in toto with the posterior wall of the right and left atria incised, which allows suturing of left atrial donor rim to recipient rim and right atrial donor rim to recipient rim, with anastomosis of the aorta and pulmonary artery.

IMMUNOSUPPRESSION AND REJECTION Controlling rejection while avoiding the adverse side effects of immunosuppressive agents is pivotal to successful transplantation. Rejection is characterized by perivascular infiltration of killer T lymphocytes, which migrate into the myocardium and cause cellular necrosis if not checked. Since early rejection can be silent, it is important to detect it before necrosis occurs. Immunologic monitoring of activated T lymphocytes in peripheral blood offers clues to the timing of a rejection process but has not been sufficiently reliable to dictate antirejection therapy. Therefore, repeated percutaneous transvenous right ventricular endomyocardial biopsies via the right internal jugular vein are required for histologic determination of the state of immunosuppression and rejection.

One widely used scheme for grading the stages of rejection is as follows: cannot rule out rejection, mild early rejection, moderate rejection, and severe rejection. Serial biopsies are taken every 1 to 2 weeks early after transplantation, with gradually widening intervals depending on the patient's course and rejection history. Prolongation of isovolumic relaxation time measured by echocardiography may also provide early clues to rejection.

Immunosuppressive therapy regimens vary but usually include triple therapy with cyclosporine, azathioprine, and prednisone. The immunosuppressive agent tacrolimus, as either "rescue therapy" for graft rejection unresponsive to cyclosporine or as initial immunosuppressive therapy, is increasingly popular. Another immunosuppressive agent, mycophenolate mofetil, has been introduced initially as a substitute

for azathioprine, and in one trial appeared to be superior in reducing transplant coronary atherosclerosis and mortality. Prophylactic courses of monoclonal antibody OKT3 or antithymocyte globulin may also be given early after transplantation. Careful monitoring of the adverse side effects of these agents is extremely important because they include nephrotoxicity, bone marrow suppression, and opportunistic infections. For discussion of immunosuppressive drugs, see Chap. 272.

EARLY COURSE AND COMPLICATIONS It is rare for a cardiac transplant patient to have a completely uncomplicated postoperative course. In the immediate postoperative period, right-sided heart failure due to pulmonary vascular disease is most life-threatening. During the 2 to 3 weeks after transplantation, the patient is hospitalized with meticulous monitoring for evidence of rejection and infections, repeated percutaneous transvenous endomyocardial biopsies, and adjustment of immunosuppressive drugs. During the ensuing 4 to 6 weeks, infectious complications, including bacterial, viral, and protozoan infections, are common. A successful transplant program requires a highly aggressive and sophisticated approach to diagnosis and therapy of infections in the immunocompromised host. CMV infection involving multiple organs is common and accelerates graft rejection as well. Prophylaxis with ganciclovir can dramatically reduce severe CMV infections and graft rejection, leading to less morbidity and improved survival. Depending on the degree of cardiac cachexia preoperatively, the patient is usually functional at 1 week and discharged from the hospital at 2 to 3 weeks if no major complication occurs.

The average first-year cost ranges from $100,000 to $150,000, depending on the need for repeated hospitalization and cardiac biopsies, and is occasionally much higher. Yearly costs for immunosuppressive agents range from $10,000 to $30,000, in addition to the expense of medical surveillance for rejection or complications.

PHYSIOLOGY AND FUNCTION Since the allografted heart remains denervated, cardiac function differs from that of the innervated heart during both rest and exercise. The electrocardiogram of a recipient shows two P waves; the P wave of the recipient's heart reflects the residual sinus node and posterior walls of the remaining native atria but is dissociated from the QRS, since the depolarization impulse does not cross the suture line. Although it does not control donor heart rate, the recipient's sinus node remains innervated and under the influence of the autonomic nervous system. The donor sinus node controls the rate of the transplanted heart. The donor heart's P wave has a regular PR interval, reflecting conduction to the ventricles. Since the controlling sinus node is denervated, it maintains a heart rate of 100 to 110 beats per minute, and rate increase depends on alterations in chronotropic agents perfusing the sinus node. Partial reinnervation may occur in some patients late after transplantation. This is manifested primarily by the occurrence of angina-like symptoms in patients who have developed accelerated graft atherosclerosis (see below).

Ventricular function in response to isometric and isotonic exercise has been studied extensively. The early response to exercise is more dependent on the Frank-Starling mechanism and change in ventricular volume and filling pressure. As exercise proceeds and catecholamines are released with their positive inotropic and chronotropic effects, cardiac output begins to rise. The cardiac transplant recipient can achieve approximately 70% of the maximal cardiac output expected for his or her age, easily sufficient for the stresses of everyday life.

LATE COURSE AND COMPLICATIONS Although the rejection process partially subsides, lifelong administration of immunosuppressive drugs, albeit at lower doses, is still required and remains a hazard. Infectious complications and unsuspected rejection continue to occur, requiring ongoing surveillance and monitoring. Routine cardiac biopsies are performed at 3-month intervals to monitor for unsuspected early rejection. Acute rejection or infection predominates in the first year after transplantation. Chronic rejection (i.e., accelerated coronary vascular disease) becomes the most important cause of death after the first year. The process is a fibrointimal hyperplasia that can go undetected by coronary arteriography at first and then cause diffuse atherosclerotic changes. Risk factors for its development may include repeated rejection episodes and elevated lipid levels. CMV infections have also been associated with higher frequency of this disease. Immunocytochemistry on endomyocardial biopsies in cardiac transplant recipients has shown a high incidence of arterial endothelial cell activation, as reflected by the presence of intercellular adhesion molecule 1 and histocompatibility antigen HLA-DR during the first 3 months after transplantation. The presence of these markers has been associated with a high risk of the subsequent development of graft coronary artery atherosclerosis, with death or the need for a second transplant. Thus, activation of the arterial/arteriolar endothelium predicts development of coronary artery disease in and the subsequent failure of the transplanted heart.

Angina is rare, and patients may present with sudden death or silent myocardial infarction. This diffuse accelerated vascular process affects both proximal and distal coronary vessels so that standard approaches, such as angioplasty or coronary artery bypass grafting, are not generally useful but occasionally are successful.

Uncontrolled trials with anticoagulation, aspirin, and improved immunosuppression with cyclosporine have done little to lower this frequency; 40 to 50% of patients show arteriographic evidence of coronary vascular disease 5 years after transplantation. Retransplantation has been employed for some patients with severe graft atherosclerosis, but it is limited by the scarcity of donors and poorer survival expectations after the second transplant. Diltiazem has been reported to reduce the severity and occurrence of this accelerated vascular process when started at the time of transplantation. Calcium channel blockers are the agents of choice for cyclosporine-induced hypertension, a common complication in the posttransplant patient. Pravastatin and simvastatin have been reported not only to lower lipid levels but also to reduce graft vessel coronary artery disease and improve survival. Administration of one of these drugs is advisable for all heart transplant recipients. A comparative trial of azathioprine versus mycophenolate mofetil reported less graft disease and cardiovascular mortality in the latter group.

In addition to the well-known hazards of long-term glucocorticoid usage, the immunosuppressed patient is at increased risk for neoplasia. An unusual form of lymphoma can occur frequently in extranodal locations, which is linked to prior Epstein-Barr viral infection. This lymphoma can be polyclonal or monoclonal, is associated with excessive immunosuppression, and may respond to simply lowering doses of cyclosporine and administration of acyclovir rather than requiring more aggressive chemo- or radiotherapy. Many cases regress fully and do not recur.

HEART-LUNG TRANSPLANTATION

Patients with congenital heart disease with Eisenmenger's complex (Chap. 234) or primary pulmonary hypertension (Chap. 260) are now considered for heart-lung transplantation. The surgical technique is similar to that for heart transplantation, except that the pulmonary venous attachments to the left atrium are left intact, and a tracheal anastomosis is required. The postoperative period is more complex, since the lungs may be rejected separately from the heart, requiring repeated endobronchoscopic biopsies when rejection is suspected. The immunosuppressive regimen is similar to that for heart transplants, except that glucocorticoids are avoided in the first 1 to 2 weeks to allow healing of the tracheal anastamosis. Long-term survival has in the past been limited by obliterative bronchiolitis due to chronic unrecognized rejection; survival rates have been approximately 60% at 1 year and 50% at 2 years but appear to be improving. Heart-lung transplants have also been applied to primary pulmonary hypertension, but more recent experience with single-lung transplants for these patients has been satisfactory, thus utilizing scarce donors more effectively. Single-lung transplants are also being applied increasingly for patients with advanced emphysema. Double-lung transplants for pa-tients with cystic fibrosis have also become the operation of choice for this group. →*For further discussion, see Chap. 267.*

BIBLIOGRAPHY

BENIAMINOVITZ A et al: Prevention of rejection in cardiac transplantation by blockade of the interleukin-2 receptor with a monoclonal antibody. N Engl J Med 342:613, 2000

HOSENPUD JD et al: The Registry of the International Society for Heart and Lung Transplantation: Fifteenth official Report—1998. Transplantation 17:656, 1999

HUNT SA: Current status of cardiac transplantation. JAMA 280:1692, 1998

KAPADIA SR et al: Intravascular ultrasound imaging after cardiac transplantation: Advantage of multi-vessel imaging. J Heart Lung Trans 19:167, 2000

KOBASHIGAWA JA: Mycophenolate mofetil in cardiac transplantation. Curr Opin Cardiol 13:117, 1998

LABARRERE CA et al: Endothelial activation and development of coronary artery disease in transplanted human hearts. JAMA 278:1169, 1997

ROBBINS R, REITZ B: Therapy of heart failure: Heart-lung transplantation, in E Braunwald, D Zipes, P Libby (eds): *Heart Disease*, 6th ed. Philadelphia, Saunders, 2001

WENKE K et al: Simvastatin reduces graft vessel disease and mortality after heart transplantation: A four year randomized trial. Circulation 96:1398, 1997

---

234   *William F. Friedman, John S. Child*

CONGENITAL HEART DISEASE IN THE ADULT

Congenital heart disease complicates approximately 1% of all live births. It occurs in about 4% of offspring of women with congenital heart disease. Substantial numbers of affected infants reach adulthood because of successful medical and/or surgical management, or because the alteration caused in cardiovascular physiology is well tolerated.

ETIOLOGY AND PREVENTION   Congenital cardiovascular malformations are generally the result of aberrant embryonic development of a normal structure, or failure of such a structure to progress beyond an early stage of embryonic or fetal development. Malformations are due to complex multifactorial genetic and environmental causes. Recognized chromosomal aberrations and mutations of single genes account for <10% of all cardiac malformations (Table 234-1).

The presence of a cardiac malformation as one component of the multiple system involvement in Down's, Turner's, and the trisomy 13-15(D1) and 17-18 (E) syndromes may be anticipated in occasional pregnancies by detection of abnormal chromosomes in fetal cells obtained from amniotic fluid or chorionic villus biopsy. Identification in such cells of the enzyme disorders characteristic of Hurler's syndrome, homocystinuria, or type II glycogen storage disease may also allow one to predict cardiac disease.

PATHOPHYSIOLOGY   The anatomic and physiologic changes in the heart and circulation due to any specific congenital cardiocirculatory lesion are not static but rather progress from prenatal life to adulthood. Thus, malformations that are benign or escape detection in childhood may become clinically significant in the adult. For example, the functionally normal, congenitally bicuspid aortic valve may thicken and calcify with time, resulting in significant aortic stenosis; or the well-tolerated left-to-right shunt of an atrial septal defect may not result in cardiac decompensation, with or without pulmonary hypertension, until the fourth or fifth decade.

Pulmonary Hypertension   This is a common companion of many congenital cardiac lesions, and the status of the pulmonary vascular bed is often the principal determinant of the clinical manifestations, the course, and the feasibility of surgical repair. Increases in pulmonary arterial pressure result from elevation of pulmonary blood flow and/or resistance, the latter due sometimes to an increase in vascular tone but usually the result of obstructive, obliterative structural

Table 234-1 Syndromes with Associated Cardiovascular Involvement

Syndrome (Genetic Locus)	Major Cardiovascular Manifestations	Major Noncardiac Abnormalities
HERITABLE AND POSSIBLY HERITABLE		
Ellis–van Creveld	Single atrium or atrial septal defect	Chondrodystrophic dwarfism, nail dysplasia, polydactyly
TAR (thrombocytopenia-absent radius)	Atrial septal defect, tetralogy of Fallot	Radial aplasia or hypoplasia, thrombocytopenia
Holt-Oram (12q21–q3)	Atrial septal defect (other defects common)	Skeletal upper limb defect, hypoplasia of clavicles
Kartagener	Dextrocardia	Situs inversus, sinusitis, bronchiectasis
Laurence-Moon-Biedl-Bardet	Variable defects	Retinal pigmentation, obesity, polydactyly
Noonan (12q24)	Pulmonic valve dysplasia, cardiomyopathy (usually hypertrophic)	Webbed neck, pectus excavatum, cryptorchidism
Tuberous sclerosis (type 1—4q); type 2—16p)	Rhabdomyoma, cardiomyopathy	Phakomatosis, bone lesions, hamartomatous skin lesions
Multiple lentigines (LEOPARD) syndrome	Pulmonic stenosis	Basal cell nevi, broad facies, rib anomalies, deafness
Rubenstein-Taybi (16p13.3)	Patent ductus arteriosus (others)	Broad thumbs and toes, hypoplastic maxilla, slanted palpebral fissures
Familial deafness	Arrhythmias, sudden death	Sensorineural deafness
Weber-Osler-Rendu (9q33)	Arteriovenous fistulas (lung, liver, mucous membranes)	Multiple telangiectasias
Apert (10q26)	Ventricular septal defect	Craniosynostosis, midfacial hypoplasia, syndactyly
Crouzon (10q26, 4p16.3)	Patent ductus arteriosus, aortic coarctation	Ptosis with shallow orbits, craniosynostosis, maxillary hypoplasia
Hypertrophic cardiomyopathy (locus heterogeneity, 14q11.2–12, 1q32, 15q22, 11p11.2, etc.)	Asymmetric septal hypertrophy	Family history of sudden death
Incontinentia pigmenti	Patent ductus arteriosus	Irregular pigmented skin lesions, patchy alopecia, hypodontia
Alagille (arteriohepatic dysplasia) (20p12)	Peripheral pulmonic stenosis, pulmonic stenosis	Biliary hypoplasia, vertebral anomalies, prominent forehead, deep-set eyes
Catch-22 (DiGeorge) (22q11)	Interrupted aortic arch, tetralogy of Fallot, truncus arteriosus	Thymic hypoplasia or aplasia, parathyroid aplasia or hypoplasia, abnormal facies
Shprintzen (velocardiofacial) (22q11.2)	Ventricular septal defect, tetralogy of Fallot, right aortic arch	Cleft palate, prominent nose, slender hands, learning disability
Williams (7q11.23)	Supravalvular aortic stenosis, peripheral pulmonic stenosis	Mental deficiency, elfin facies, loquacious personality, hoarse voice
Long QT (Jervell and Lange-Nielsen, Romano-Ward) (11p15.5, 7q35, 3p21, 21q22)	Long QT interval, ventricular arrhythmias	Family history of sudden death, congenital deafness (not in Romano-Ward)
Friedreich's ataxia (9q)	Cardiomyopathy and conduction defects	Ataxia, speech defect, degeneration of spinal cord dorsal columns
Muscular dystrophy	Cardiomyopathy	Pseudohypertrophy of calf muscles, weakness of trunk and proximal limb muscles
Cystic fibrosis (7q)	Cor pulmonale	Pancreatic insufficiency, malabsorption, chronic lung disease
Sickle cell anemia	Cardiomyopathy, mitral regurgitation	Hemoglobin SS
Conradi-Hunermann	Ventricular septal defect, patent ductus arteriosus	Asymmetrical limb shortness, early punctate mineralization, large skin pores
Cockayne	Accelerated atherosclerosis	Cachectic dwarfism, retinal pigment abnormalities, photosensitivity dermatitis
Progeria	Accelerated atherosclerosis	Premature aging, alopecia, atrophy of subcutaneous fat, skeletal hypoplasia
CONNECTIVE TISSUE DISORDERS		
Cutis laxa	Peripheral pulmonic stenosis	Generalized disruption of elastic fibers, diminished skin resilience, hernias
Ehlers-Danlos (2q31)	Arterial dilatation and rupture, mitral regurgitation	Hyperextensible joints, hyperelastic and friable
Marfan (15q21.1)	Aortic dilatation, aortic and mitral incompetence	Gracile habitus, arachnodactyly with hyperextensibility, lens subluxation
Osteogenesis imperfecta (4.17)	Aortic incompetence	Fragile bones, blue sclerae
Pseudoxanthoma elasticum	Peripheral and coronary arterial disease	Degeneration of elastic fibers in skin, retinal angioid streaks
INBORN ERRORS OF METABOLISM		
Pompe disease	Glycogen storage disease of heart	Acid maltase deficiency, muscular weakness
Homocystinuria	Aortic and pulmonary arterial dilatation, intravascular thrombosis	Cystathionine synthetase deficiency, lens subluxation, osteoporosis
Mucopolysaccharidoses: Hurler; Hunter	Multivalvular and coronary and great artery disease, cardiomyopathy	Hurler: Deficiency of α-L-iduronidase, corneal clouding, coarse features, growth and mental retardation
		Hunter: Deficiency of L-iduranosulfate sulfatase, coarse facies, clear cornea, growth and mental retardation

(continued)

Table 234-1—*(continued)*

Syndrome (Genetic Locus)	Major Cardiovascular Manifestations	Major Noncardiac Abnormalities
Morquio; Scheie; Maroteaux-Lamy	Aortic regurgitation	Morquio: Deficiency of *N*-acetylhexosamine sulfate sulfatase, cloudy cornea, severe bone changes involving vertebrae and epiphyses Scheie: Deficiency of α-L-iduronidase, cloudy cornea, normal intelligence, peculiar facies Maroteaux-Lamy: Deficiency of arylsulfatase B, cloudy cornea, osseous changes
CHROMOSOMAL ABNORMALITIES		
Trisomy 21 (Down syndrome)	Endocardial cushion defect, atrial or ventricular septal defect, tetralogy of Fallot	Hypotonia, hyperextensible joints, mongoloid facies, mental retardation
Trisomy 13 (D)	Ventricular septal defect, RV patent ductus arteriosus, double-outlet RV	Single midline intracerebral ventricle with midfacial defects, polydactyly, nail changes, mental retardation
Trisomy 18 (E)	Congenital polyvalvular dysplasia, ventricular septal defect, patent ductus	Clenched hand, short sternum, low arch dermal ridge pattern on fingertips, mental retardation
Cri du chat (short-arm deletion-5)	Ventricular septal defect	Cat cry, microcephaly, antimongoloid slant of palpebral fissures, mental retardation
XO (Turner)	Coarctation of aorta, bicuspid aortic valve, aortic dilatation	Short female, broad chest, lymphedema, webbed neck
XXXY and XXXXX	Patent ductus arteriosus	XXXY: Hypogenitalism, mental retardation, radial-ulnar synostosis XXXXX: Small hands, incurving of fifth fingers, mental retardation
SPORADIC DISORDERS		
VATER association	Ventricular septal defect	Vertebral anomalies, anal atresia, tracheo-esophageal fistula, radial and renal anomalies
CHARGE association	Tetralogy of Fallot (other defects common)	Colobomas, choanal atresia, mental and growth deficiency, genital and ear anomalies
Cornelia de Lange	Ventricular septal defect	Micromelia, synophrys, mental and growth deficiency
TERATOGENIC DISORDERS		
Rubella	Patent ductus arteriosus, pulmonic valvular and/or arterial stenosis, atrial septal defect	Cataracts, deafness, microcephaly
Alcohol	Ventricular septal defect (other defects)	Microcephaly, growth and mental deficiency, short palpebral fissures, smooth philtrum, thin upper lip
Dilantin	Pulmonic stenosis, aortic stenosis, coarctation, patent ductus arteriosus	Hypertelorism, growth and mental deficiency, short phalanges, bowed upper lip
Thalidomide	Variable	Phocomelia
Lithium	Ebstein's anomaly, tricuspid atresia	None

SOURCE: Modified from WF Friedman.

changes within the pulmonary vascular bed. Because pulmonary vascular obstructive disease can be the determining factor in assessing the advisability of operation, it is important to quantitate and compare pulmonary to systemic flows and resistances in patients with severe pulmonary hypertension. The causes of pulmonary vascular obstructive disease are unknown, although increased pulmonary blood flow, increased pulmonary arterial blood pressure, elevated pulmonary venous pressure, erythrocytosis, systemic hypoxemia, acidosis, and the bronchial circulation have been implicated. The designation *Eisenmenger syndrome* is applied to patients with a large communication between the two circulations at the aortopulmonary, ventricular, or atrial levels and bidirectional or predominantly right-to-left shunts because of high-resistance and obstructive pulmonary hypertension. No specific treatment has proved beneficial for obstructive pulmonary vascular disease, although both single lung transplantation with intracardiac defect repair, and total heart-lung transplantation show promise (Chaps. 233 and 267).

Erythrocytosis The chronic hypoxemia in cyanotic congenital heart disease results in *erythrocytosis* due to increased erythropoietin production (Chap. 36). The commonly used term *polycythemia* is a misnomer because white cell counts are normal and platelet counts are normal to decreased. Cyanotic patients with erythrocytosis may have compensated or decompensated hematocrits. Compensated erythrocytosis with iron-replete equilibrium hematocrits rarely results in symptoms of hyperviscosity at hematocrits <65% and occasionally

not even with hematocrits ≥70%. Therapeutic phlebotomy is rarely required in compensated erythrocytosis. In contrast, patients with decompensated erythrocytosis fail to establish equilibrium with unstable, rising hematocrits and recurrent hyperviscosity symptoms. Therapeutic phlebotomy, a two-edged sword, allows temporary relief of symptoms but begets instability of the hematocrit and compounds the problem by iron depletion. Iron-deficiency symptoms are usually indistinguishable from those of hyperviscosity; progressive symptoms after recurrent phlebotomy are usually due to iron depletion with hypochromic microcytosis. Iron depletion results in a larger number of smaller (microcytic) hypochromic red cells that are less capable of carrying oxygen and less deformable in the microcirculation. Because these microcytes are less deformable in the microcirculation and there are more of them relative to the plasma volume, the viscosity is greater than for an equivalent hematocrit with fewer, larger, iron-replete, deformable cells. As such, iron-depleted erythrocytosis results in increasing symptoms due to decreased oxygen delivery to the tissues.

Hemostasis is abnormal in cyanotic congenital heart disease, due in part to the increased blood volume and engorged capillaries, abnormalities in platelet function and sensitivity to aspirin or nonsteroidal anti-inflammatory agents, and abnormalities of the extrinsic and intrinsic coagulation system. Oral contraceptives are contraindicated for cyanotic women because of the enhanced risk of vascular thrombosis.

The risk of stroke is greatest in children younger than 4 years with cyanotic heart disease and iron deficiency, often with dehydration as an aggravating cause. In contrast, adults with cyanotic congenital heart disease do not appear to be at increased risk for stroke, unless there are excessive injudicious phlebotomies, inappropriate use of aspirin or anticoagulants, or the presence of atrial arrhythmias or infective endocarditis.

Symptoms of hyperviscosity can be produced in any cyanotic patient with erythrocytosis if dehydration causes a reduction of plasma volume. Phlebotomy, when required for symptoms of hyperviscosity not due to dehydration or iron deficiency, is a simple outpatient removal of 500 mL of blood over 45 min with isovolumetric replacement with isotonic saline (5% dextrose if congestive heart failure exists). Acute phlebotomy without volume replacement is contraindicated. Iron repletion in decompensated iron-depleted erythrocytosis ameliorates iron-deficiency symptoms but must be done gradually to avoid a sudden excessive rise in hematocrit and resultant hyperviscosity.

Pregnancy The physiologic alterations during normal gestation (Chap. 7) can create symptoms and physical findings that may be attributed erroneously to heart disease. Dyspnea due to the hormonal influence of progesterone and elevation of the diaphragm in association with peripheral edema and fatigability may be attributed inappropriately to heart failure. The jugular venous pulsations normally become more apparent after the twentieth week. Elevation of the diaphragm can cause basal rales (which disappear with deep breathing). Both ventricles are more easily palpated due to the normal increase in ventricular volumes and elevation of the diaphragm. Third heart sounds, already relatively frequent in normal nongravid young women, increase in frequency and intensity with pregnancy because of increased heart rate and volume of flow across the mitral and tricuspid valves. Midsystolic murmurs across the pulmonary outflow tract and supraclavicular systolic murmurs are caused by increased cardiac output. Venous hums and mammary souffles are usual during pregnancy.

These normal circulatory changes may impinge upon the woman's cardiac reserve. The mother is most at risk if she has a cardiovascular lesion associated with pulmonary vascular disease and pulmonary hypertension (e.g., Eisenmenger's physiology or mitral stenosis) or left ventricular (LV) outflow tract obstruction (e.g., aortic stenosis) but also risks death with any malformation that may cause heart failure or a hemodynamically important arrhythmia (Table 234-2). The fetus is most at risk in the presence of maternal cyanosis, heart failure, or pulmonary hypertension. Women with aortic coarctation or Marfan's syndrome are at risk for aortic dissection. Patients with cyanotic heart disease, pulmonary hypertension, or Marfan's syndrome should not become pregnant; those with correctable lesions should be counseled about the risks of pregnancy with an uncorrected malformation versus repair and later pregnancy. The effect of pregnancy in postoperative patients depends on the outcome of the repair including the presence and severity of residua, sequelae, or complications. Contraception is an important topic with such patients. Tubal ligation should be considered in those in whom pregnancy is strictly contraindicated.

INFECTIVE ENDOCARDITIS (See also Chap. 126) Routine antimicrobial prophylaxis is recommended for most patients with congenital heart disease whether operated on or not. Antibiotic prophylaxis is not uniformly effective. Nonetheless, it is recommended for all dental procedures, gastrointestinal and genitourinary surgery, and diagnostic procedures such as proctosigmoidoscopy and cystoscopy. The clinical and bacteriologic profile of infective endocarditis in patients with congenital heart disease has changed with the advent of intracardiac surgery and of prosthetic devices. Two major predisposing causes of infective endocarditis are a susceptible cardiovascular substrate and a source of bacteremia. Prophylaxis includes both chemotherapeutic (antimicrobial) and nonchemotherapeutic (hygienic) measures. Meticulous dental and skin care is required.

EXERCISE Advice on athletics and exercise is governed by the nature of the exercise and by the type and severity of the congenital cardiovascular lesion. Patients with lesions characterized by LV outflow tract obstruction, if more than mild to moderate, or pulmonary vascular disease, risk syncope or even sudden death. In Fallot's tetralogy, isotonic exercise–induced decrease in systemic vascular resistance relative to the right ventricular (RV) outflow obstruction augments the right-to-left shunt, increases hypoxemia, and causes an increase in subjective breathlessness due to the response of the respiratory center to the changes in blood gases and pH.

INSURABILITY AND EMPLOYABILITY Most patients with congenital heart disease must pay significantly more than standard life insurance rates, assuming their anomaly places them in a category that companies have determined is eligible for insurance. A paucity of actuarial survival data beyond adolescence for persons with most congenital cardiac lesions that have undergone operative repair has made it difficult to convince insurance companies to offer reasonable cost insurance even to individual patients whose long-term prognosis is quite good.

Employment is affected by the patient's physical capacity relative to the type of job sought. Job discrimination exists, often because the employer is reluctant to accept health insurance responsibilities. Eligibility for some occupations is governed by public safety regulations, e.g., airline pilots, bus drivers.

SPECIFIC CARDIAC DEFECTS

Table 234-3 provides a classification of cardiac anomalies that recognizes the general categories of clinical presentation, functional consequences, and site of origin of congenital defects.

Categorizing the defect(s) in an individual patient requires an answer to a number of basic questions. Is the patient acyanotic or cyanotic? Is pulmonary arterial blood flow increased or not? Does the malformation originate in the left or right side of the heart? Which is the dominant ventricle? Is pulmonary hypertension present or not? With the above information as a foundation, the use of more refined diagnostic techniques such as transthoracic (precordial) and transesophageal echocardiography and Doppler imaging, magnetic resonance imaging, and/or hemodynamic study and angiocardiography leads to a precise anatomic and functional assessment.

ACYANOTIC CONGENITAL HEART DISEASE WITH A LEFT-TO-RIGHT SHUNT

ATRIAL SEPTAL DEFECT This common cardiac anomaly in adults occurs more frequently in females. The *sinus venosus* type occurs high in the atrial septum near the entry of the superior vena cava and is associated frequently with anomalous connection of pul-

Table 234-2   Tolerance of Pregnancy by Patients with Various Congenital Cardiac Malformations

Well Tolerated	Intermediate Effect	Poorly Tolerated
NYHA class I	NYHA class II–III	NYHA class IV
Left-right shunts without PHTN	Repaired transposition of the great arteries	Right-left shunt, unrepaired cyanotic heart disease
Aortic or mitral valvular regurgitation (mild-moderate)	Fontan repairs	PHTN and/or pulmonary vascular disease (e.g., Eisenmenger's, "primary PHTN")
Pulmonic or tricuspid regurgitation (if low pressure, even severe)	Aortic or mitral stenosis (moderate)	Aortic or mitral stenosis (severe)
Pulmonic stenosis (mild-moderate)	Ebstein's anomaly	Pulmonic stenosis (severe)
Well-repaired tetralogy of Fallot		Marfan's or aortic coarctation

NOTE: NYHA, New York Heart Association; PHTN, pulmonary hypertension.

monary veins from the right lung to the junction of the superior vena cava and right atrium (RA). *Ostium primum* anomalies are a form of atrioventricular septal defect that lie immediately adjacent to the atrioventricular valves, either of which may be deformed and incompetent. Ostium primum defects occur commonly in patients with Down's syndrome, although the more complex atrioventricular septal defects with a common atrioventricular valve and a posterior defect of the basal portion of the interventricular septum are more characteristic of this chromosomal defect. The most common atrial septal defect involves the fossa ovalis, is midseptal in location, and is of the *ostium secundum* type. This type of defect should not be confused with a *patent foramen ovale*. Anatomic obliteration of the foramen ovale ordinarily follows its functional closure soon after birth, but residual "probe patency" is a normal variant; atrial septal defect denotes a true deficiency of the atrial septum and implies functional and anatomic patency.

The magnitude of the left-to-right shunt through an atrial septal defect depends on the defect size, the diastolic properties of both ventricles, and the relative impedance in the pulmonary and systemic circulations. The left-to-right shunt causes diastolic over-loading of the RV and increased pulmonary blood flow.

Patients with atrial septal defect are usually asymptomatic in early life, although there may be some physical underdevelopment and an increased tendency for respiratory infections; cardiorespiratory symptoms occur in many older patients. Beyond the fourth decade, a significant number of patients develop atrial arrhythmias, pulmonary arterial hypertension, bidirectional and then right-to-left shunting of blood, and cardiac failure. Patients exposed to the chronic environmental hypoxia of high altitude tend to develop pulmonary hypertension at younger ages. In some older patients, left-to-right shunting across the defect increases as progressive systemic hypertension and/or coronary artery disease result in reduced compliance of the LV.

Physical Examination Examination usually reveals a prominent RV cardiac impulse and palpable pulmonary artery pulsation. The first heart sound is normal or split, with accentuation of the tricuspid valve closure sound. Increased flow across the pulmonic valve is responsible for a midsystolic pulmonary ejection murmur. The second heart sound is widely split and is relatively fixed in relation to respiration. A mid-diastolic rumbling murmur, loudest at the fourth intercostal space and

Table 234-3 Classification of Congenital Heart Disease

ACYANOTIC WITH LEFT-TO-RIGHT SHUNT

I. Atrial level shunt
   A. Atrial septal defect
      1. Ostium primum
      2. Ostium secundum
      3. Sinus venosus
   B. Atrial septal defect with mitral stenosis (Lutembacher's syndrome)
   C. Partial anomalous pulmonary venous connection
II. Ventricular level shunt
   A. Ventricular septal defect
      1. Inlet septum
      2. Muscular septum
      3. Perimembranous septum
      4. Infundibular septum
   B. Ventricular septal defect with aortic regurgitation
   C. Ventricular septal defect with left ventricular to right atrial shunt

III. Aortic root to right heart shunt
   A. Ruptured sinus of Valsalva aneurysm
   B. Coronary arteriovenous fistula
   C. Anomalous origin of the left coronary artery from the pulmonary trunk
IV. Aortopulmonary level shunt
   A. Aortopulmonary window
   B. Patent ductus arteriosus
V. Multiple level shunts
   A. Complete common atrioventricular canal
   B. Ventricular septal defect with atrial septal defect
   C. Ventricular septal defect with patent ductus arteriosus

ACYANOTIC WITHOUT A SHUNT

I. Left heart malformations
   A. Congenital obstruction to left atrial inflow
      1. Pulmonary vein stenosis
      2. Mitral stenosis
      3. Cor triatriatum
   B. Mitral regurgitation
      1. Atrioventricular septal (endocardial cushion)
      2. Congenitally corrected transposition of the great arteries
      3. Anomalous origin of the left coronary artery from the pulmonary trunk
      4. Miscellaneous (double-orifice mitral valve, congenital perforations, accessory commissures with anomalous chordal insertion, congenitally short or absent chordae, cleft posterior leaflet, parachute mitral valve, etc.)
   C. Primary dilated endocardial fibroelastosis

   D. Aortic stenosis
      1. Discrete subvalvular
      2. Valvular
      3. Supravalvular
   E. Aortic valve regurgitation
   F. Coarctation of the aorta
II. Right heart malformations
   A. Acyanotic Ebstein's anomaly of the tricuspid valve
   B. Pulmonic stenosis
      1. Subinfundibular
      2. Infundibular
      3. Valvular
      4. Supravalvular (stenosis of pulmonary artery and its branches)
   C. Congenital pulmonary valve regurgitation
   D. Idiopathic dilatation of the pulmonary trunk

CYANOTIC

I. Increased pulmonary blood flow
   A. Complete transposition of the great arteries
   B. Double-outlet right ventricle of the Taussig-Bing type
   C. Truncus arteriosus
   D. Total anomalous pulmonary venous connection
   E. Single ventricle without pulmonic stenosis
   F. Common atrium
   G. Tetralogy of Fallot with pulmonary atresia and increased collateral arterial flow
   H. Tricuspid atresia with large ventricular septal defect and no pulmonic stenosis
   I. Hypoplastic left heart (aortic atresia, mitral atresia)

II. Normal or decreased pulmonary blood flow
   A. Tricuspid atresia
   B. Ebstein's anomaly with right-to-left atrial shunt
   C. Pulmonary atresia with intact ventricular septum
   D. Pulmonic stenosis or atresia with ventricular septal defect (tetralogy of Fallot)
   E. Pulmonic stenosis with right-to-left atrial shunt
   F. Complete transposition of the great arteries with pulmonic stenosis
   G. Double-outlet right ventricle with pulmonic stenosis
   H. Single ventricle with pulmonic stenosis
   I. Pulmonary arteriovenous fistula
   J. Vena caval to left atrial communication

OTHER

I. Congenitally corrected transposition of the great arteries

II. The cardiac malpositions
III. Congenital complete heart block

SOURCE: Modified from JK Perloff, *The Clinical Recognition of Congenital Heart Disease,* Philadelphia, Saunders, 1991.

along the left sternal border, reflects increased flow across the tricuspid valve. In patients with ostium primum defects, an apical thrill and holosystolic murmur indicate associated mitral or tricuspid incompetence or a ventricular septal defect.

The physical findings are altered when an increase in the pulmonary vascular resistance results in diminution of the left-to-right shunt. Both the pulmonary and tricuspid murmurs decrease in intensity, the pulmonic component of the second heart sound and a systolic ejection sound are accentuated, the two components of the second heart sound may fuse, and a diastolic murmur of pulmonic regurgitation appears. Cyanosis and clubbing accompany the development of a right-to-left shunt.

In adults with an atrial septal defect and atrial fibrillation, the physical findings may be confused with the findings of mitral stenosis with pulmonary hypertension because the tricuspid flow murmur and widely split second heart sound may be mistakenly thought to represent the diastolic murmur of mitral stenosis and the mitral "opening snap," respectively.

Electrocardiogram   In patients with an ostium secundum defect, the electrocardiogram (ECG) usually shows right axis deviation and an rSr' pattern in the right precordial leads representing delayed posterobasal activation of the ventricular septum and enlargement of the RV outflow tract. An ectopic atrial pacemaker or first-degree heart block occurs occasionally in patients with defects of the sinus venosus type. In patients with an ostium primum defect, the RV conduction defect is characteristically accompanied by left axis deviation and by superior orientation and counterclockwise rotation of the QRS loop in the frontal plane. Varying degrees of RV and RA hypertrophy may occur with each type of defect, depending on the height of the pulmonary artery pressure. *Chest roentgenograms* reveal enlargement of the RA and RV, dilatation of the pulmonary artery and its branches, and increased pulmonary vascular marking.

Echocardiogram   This test shows pulmonary arterial and RV dilatation, and anterior systolic (paradoxical) or flat interventricular septal motion if a significant RV volume overload is present. The defect may be visualized directly from subcostal, right parasternal, or apical echocardiographic windows. In most institutions, two-dimensional echocardiography, supplemented by conventional or color Doppler flow examination, has supplanted cardiac catheterization as the confirmatory test for atrial septal defect. Transesophageal echocardiography is indicated if the transthoracic echocardiogram is ambiguous, which is often the case with sinus venosus defects. Cardiac catheterization is then performed if inconsistencies exist in the clinical data, if significant pulmonary hypertension or associated malformations are suspected, or if coronary artery disease is a possibility.

℞ **TREATMENT**   Operative repair, ideally in children age 3 to 6 years, should be advised for all patients with uncomplicated atrial septal defects in whom there is significant left-to-right shunting, i.e., with pulmonary-to-systemic flow ratios exceeding ~2.0:1.0. Excellent results may be anticipated, at low risk, even in patients older than 40 years in the absence of pulmonary hypertension. The defect is closed, usually with a patch of pericardium or of prosthetic material, with the patient on cardiopulmonary bypass. In patients with ostium primum defects, cleft, deformed, and incompetent valves often require repair. Intraoperative transesophageal echocardiography is used to monitor the surgical results of mitral valve repair. Operation should not be carried out in patients with small defects and trivial left-to-right shunts, or in those with severe pulmonary vascular disease without a significant left-to-right shunt.

Patients with atrial septal defect of the sinus venosus or ostium secundum types rarely die before the fifth decade. During the fifth and sixth decades the incidence of progressive symptoms, often leading to severe disability, increases substantially. Medical management should include prompt treatment of respiratory tract infections, antiarrhythmic medications for atrial fibrillation or supraventricular tachycardia, and the usual measures for hypertension, coronary disease, or heart failure (Chap. 232), if these complications occur. The risk of infective endocarditis is quite low unless the defect is complicated by valvular regurgitation or has recently been repaired with a patch (Chap. 126).

VENTRICULAR SEPTAL DEFECT   Defects of the ventricular septum are common as isolated defects and as one component of a combination of anomalies. The opening is usually single and situated in the membranous portion of the septum. The functional disturbance is dependent primarily on its size and on the status of the pulmonary vascular bed, rather than on the location of the defect. Only small or moderate-size defects are usually seen initially in adulthood as most patients with isolated large defects come to medical and, often, surgical attention very early in life.

A wide spectrum exists in the natural history of ventricular septal defect, ranging from spontaneous closure to congestive cardiac failure and death in early infancy. Within this spectrum is the possible development of pulmonary vascular obstruction, RV outflow tract obstruction, aortic regurgitation, and infective endocarditis. Spontaneous closure is more common in patients born with a small ventricular septal defect and occurs in early childhood in most patients.

Patients with large ventricular septal defects and pulmonary hypertension are those at greatest risk for developing pulmonary vascular obstruction. Thus, large defects should be corrected surgically early in life when pulmonary vascular disease is still reversible or not yet developed. In patients with severe pulmonary vascular obstruction (Eisenmenger syndrome), symptoms in adult life consist of exertional dyspnea, chest pain, syncope, and hemoptysis. The right-to-left shunt leads to cyanosis, clubbing, and erythrocytosis. In all patients, the degree to which pulmonary vascular resistance is elevated before operation is a critical factor determining prognosis. If the pulmonary vascular resistance is one-third or less of the systemic value, progression of pulmonary vascular disease after operation is unusual. However, if a moderate to severe increase in pulmonary vascular resistance exists preoperatively, either no change or a progression of pulmonary vascular disease is common postoperatively.

RV outflow tract obstruction develops in ~5 to 10% of patients who present in infancy with a moderate to large left-to-right shunt. With time, as subvalvular RV outflow tract obstruction progresses, the findings in these patients begin to resemble more closely those of the cyanotic tetralogy of Fallot.

In ~5% of patients, incompetence of the aortic valve results from insufficient cusp tissue or prolapse of the cusp through the interventricular defect; the aortic regurgitation then complicates and usually dominates the clinical course.

Two-dimensional *echocardiography* with conventional or color Doppler examination can usually define the number and location of defects in the ventricular septum and detect associated anomalies. Hemodynamic and angiographic study may be employed to assess the status of the pulmonary vascular bed and clarify details of the altered anatomy.

℞ **TREATMENT**   Surgery is not recommended for patients with normal pulmonary arterial pressures with small shunts (pulmonary-to-systemic flow ratios of less than 1.5 to 2.0:1.0). Operative correction is indicated when there is a moderate to large left-to-right shunt with a pulmonary-to-systemic flow ratio >1.5:1.0 or 2.0:1.0, in the absence of prohibitively high levels of pulmonary vascular resistance.

PATENT DUCTUS ARTERIOSUS   The ductus arteriosus is a vessel leading from the bifurcation of the pulmonary artery to the aorta just distal to the left subclavian artery. Normally, the vascular channel is open in the fetus but closes immediately after birth. The flow across the ductus is determined by the pressure and resistance relationships between the systemic and pulmonary circulations and by the cross-sectional area and length of the ductus. In most adults with this anomaly, pulmonary pressures are normal and a gradient and shunt from aorta to pulmonary artery persist throughout the cardiac cycle, resulting in a characteristic thrill and a continuous "machinery" murmur with a late systolic accentuation at the upper left sternal edge. In adults who were born with a large left-to-right shunt through the ductus arteriosus, pulmonary vascular obstruction (Eisenmenger syndrome) with pulmonary hypertension, right-to-left shunting, and cyanosis have usually developed. Severe pulmonary vascular disease results in reversal of flow through the ductus, unoxygenated blood is shunted to the descending aorta, and the toes, but not the fingers, become cyanotic and clubbed, a finding termed *differential cyanosis*. The leading causes of death in adults with patent ductus are cardiac failure and infective endocarditis; occasionally severe pulmonary vascular obstruction may cause aneurysmal dilatation, calcification, and rupture of the ductus.

℞ **TREATMENT** In the absence of severe pulmonary vascular disease and predominant left-to-right shunting of blood, the patent ductus should be surgically ligated or divided. Transcatheter closure is experimental, using coils, buttons, plugs, and umbrellas. Thoracoscopic surgical approaches are considered experimental. Operation should be deferred for several months in patients treated successfully for infective endocarditis, because the ductus may remain somewhat edematous and friable.

AORTIC ROOT TO RIGHT HEART SHUNTS

The three most common causes of aortic root to right heart shunts are congenital aneurysm of an aortic sinus of Valsalva with fistula, coronary arteriovenous fistula, and anomalous origin of the left coronary artery from the pulmonary trunk. *Aneurysm of an aortic sinus of Valsalva* consists of a separation or lack of fusion between the media of the aorta and the annulus fibrosis of the aortic valve. Rupture usually occurs in the third or fourth decade of life; most often the aorticocardiac fistula is between the right coronary cusp and the RV, but occasionally, when the noncoronary cusp is involved, the fistula drains into the RA. Abrupt rupture causes chest pain, bounding pulses, a continuous murmur accentuated in diastole, and volume overload of the heart. Diagnosis is confirmed by two-dimensional and Doppler echocardiographic studies; cardiac catheterization quantitates the left-to-right shunt, and thoracic aortography visualizes the fistula. Medical management is directed at cardiac failure, arrhythmias, or endocarditis. At operation, the aneurysm is closed and amputated, and the aortic wall is reunited with the heart, either by direct suture or with a prosthesis.

Coronary arteriovenous fistula, an unusual anomaly, consists of a communication between a coronary artery and another cardiac chamber, usually the coronary sinus, RA, or RV. The shunt is usually of small magnitude, and myocardial blood flow is not usually compromised. Potential complications include infective endocarditis, thrombus formation with occlusion or distal embolization, rupture of an aneurysmal fistula, and rarely, pulmonary hypertension and congestive failure. A loud, superficial, continuous murmur at the lower or midsternal border usually prompts a further evaluation of asymptomatic patients. Doppler echocardiography demonstrates the site of drainage; if the site of origin is proximal, it may be detectable by two-dimensional echocardiography. Retrograde thoracic aortography or coronary arteriography permits identification of the size and anatomic features of the fistulous tract, which may be closed by suture or transcatheter obliteration.

The third anomaly causing a shunt from the aortic root to the right heart is *anomalous origin of the left coronary artery from the pulmonary artery*. Myocardial infarction and fibrosis commonly lead to death within the first year, though up to 20% of patients survive to adolescence and beyond without surgical correction. The diagnosis is supported by the ECG findings of an anterolateral myocardial infarction. Operative management of adults consists of coronary artery bypass with an internal mammary artery graft or saphenous vein–coronary artery graft.

ACYANOTIC CONGENITAL HEART DISEASE WITHOUT A SHUNT

CONGENITAL AORTIC STENOSIS Malformations that cause obstruction to LV outflow include congenital valvular aortic stenosis, discrete subaortic stenosis, supravalvular aortic stenosis, and hypertrophic obstructive cardiomyopathy (Chap. 238).

Valvular Aortic Stenosis This malformation occurs three to four times more often in males than in females. The congenital bicuspid aortic valve, which is not necessarily stenotic, is one of the most common congenital malformations of the heart, although it may go undetected in early life. Because bicuspid valves may become stenotic

with time or be the site of infective endocarditis, the lesion may be difficult to distinguish in adults from acquired rheumatic or degenerative calcific aortic stenosis.

The dynamics of blood flow associated with a congenitally deformed, rigid aortic valve commonly lead to thickening of the cusps and, in later life, to calcification. Hemodynamically significant obstruction causes concentric hypertrophy of the LV wall and dilatation of the ascending aorta.→*The clinical manifestations and hemodynamic abnormalities are discussed in Chap. 236.*

℞ **TREATMENT** The medical management of congenital valvular aortic stenosis includes prophylaxis against infective endocarditis and, in patients with diminished cardiac reserve, the administration of digitalis and diuretics and sodium restriction while awaiting operation. If severe aortic stenosis is present, strenuous physical activity should be avoided even when the patient is asymptomatic, and participation in competitive sports should probably be restricted in patients with milder degrees of obstruction. Aortic valve replacement is indicated in adults with critical obstruction, i.e., with an aortic valve area <0.5 cm^2/m^2, with symptoms secondary to LV dysfunction or myocardial ischemia, or with hemodynamic evidence of LV dysfunction. In asymptomatic children or adolescents or young adults with critical aortic stenosis without valvular calcification or these features, aortic balloon valvuloplasty is often useful (Chap. 245). If surgery is contraindicated in older patients because of a complicating medical problem such as malignancy or renal or hepatic failure, balloon valvuloplasty may provide short-term improvement. It may serve as a bridge to aortic valve replacement in patients with severe heart failure.

Subaortic Stenosis The most common form of subaortic stenosis is the *idiopathic hypertrophic* variety, also termed *hypertrophic cardiomyopathy*, which is present at birth in about one-third of the patients and is discussed in Chap. 238. In contrast, both clinically and physiologically, the *discrete* form of subaortic stenosis resembles valvular aortic stenosis. The lesion usually consists of a membranous diaphragm or fibrous ring encircling the LV outflow tract just beneath the base of the aortic valve. Echocardiography demonstrates the subaortic obstruction; Doppler studies show turbulence proximal to the aortic valve and also detect and quantitate the pressure gradient and severity of aortic regurgitation. Treatment consists of excision of the membrane or fibrous ridge.

Supravalvular Aortic Stenosis This anomaly consists of a localized or diffuse narrowing of the ascending aorta originating just above the level of the coronary arteries at the superior margin of the sinuses of Valsalva. In contrast to other forms of aortic stenosis, the coronary arteries are subjected to elevated systolic pressures from the LV, are often dilated and tortuous, and are susceptible to premature atherosclerosis. New information indicates that a genetic defect for the anomaly is located in the same chromosomal subunit as elastin on chromosome 7.

COARCTATION OF THE AORTA Narrowing or constriction of the lumen of the aorta may occur anywhere along its length but is most common distal to the origin of the left subclavian artery near the insertion of the ligamentum arteriosum. Coarctation occurs in ~7% of patients with congenital heart disease, is twice as common in males as in females, and is most frequent in patients with gonadal dysgenesis. Clinical manifestations depend on the site and extent of obstruction and the presence of associated cardiac anomalies, most commonly a bicuspid aortic valve. Aneurysmal arterial dilatation of the circle of Willis produces a high risk of sudden rupture and death.

Most children and young adults with isolated, discrete coarctation are asymptomatic. Headache, epistaxis, cold extremities, and claudication with exercise may occur, and attention is usually directed to the cardiovascular system when a heart murmur or hypertension in the upper extremities and absence, marked diminution, or delayed pulsations in the femoral arteries are detected on physical examination.

Enlarged and pulsatile collateral vessels may be palpated in the intercostal spaces anteriorly, in the axillae, or posteriorly in the interscapular area. The upper extremities and thorax may be more developed than the lower extremities. A midsystolic murmur over the anterior part of the chest, back, and spinous processes may become continuous if the lumen is narrowed sufficiently to result in a high-velocity jet across the lesion throughout the cardiac cycle. Additional systolic and continuous murmurs over the lateral thoracic wall may reflect increased flow through dilated and tortuous collateral vessels. The ECG usually reveals LV hypertrophy. Roentgenograms may show a dilated left subclavian artery high on the left mediastinal border and a dilated ascending aorta. Indentation of the aorta at the site of coarctation and pre- and poststenotic dilatation (the "3" sign) along the left paramediastinal shadow are almost pathognomonic. Notching of the ribs, an important radiographic sign, is due to erosion by dilated collateral vessels. Two-dimensional echocardiography from para- or suprasternal windows identifies the site and length of coarctation, while Doppler studies record and quantitate the pressure gradient. Transesophageal echocardiography and magnetic resonance imaging or digital angiography allow visualization of the length and severity of the obstruction and the associated collateral arteries. In adults, cardiac catheterization is indicated primarily to evaluate the coronary arteries.

The chief hazards result from severe hypertension and include the development of cerebral aneurysms and hemorrhage, rupture of the aorta, premature coronary arteriosclerosis, LV failure, and infective endocarditis.

℞ **TREATMENT**   Treatment is usually surgical; resection and end-to-end anastomosis or subclavian flap angioplasty are used commonly, although it may be necessary to use a tubular graft, patch, or bypass conduit if the narrowed segment is long. Systemic hypertension postoperatively, in the absence of residual coarctation, appears to be related to the duration of preoperative hypertension. Percutaneous balloon dilatation is controversial in native unoperated aortic coarctation but commonly successful for postsurgical recoarctation, often with deployment of a stent.

PULMONARY STENOSIS WITH INTACT VENTRICULAR SEPTUM   Obstruction to RV outflow may be localized to the supravalvular, valvular, or subvalvular levels or occur at a combination of these sites. Multiple sites of narrowing of the peripheral pulmonary arteries are a feature of *rubella embryopathy* and may occur with both the familial and sporadic forms of supravalvular aortic stenosis. Valvular pulmonic stenosis is the most common form of isolated RV obstruction.

The severity of the obstructing lesion, rather than the site of narrowing, is the most important determinant of the clinical course. In the presence of a normal cardiac output, a peak systolic transvalvular pressure gradient between 50 and 80 mmHg is considered to be moderate stenosis; levels below and above that range are classified as mild and severe, respectively. Patients with mild pulmonic stenosis are generally asymptomatic and demonstrate little or no progression in the severity of obstruction with age. In patients with more significant stenosis, the severity may increase with time. Symptoms vary with the degree of obstruction. Fatigue, dyspnea, RV failure, and syncope may limit the activity of older patients, in whom moderate or severe obstruction may prevent an augmentation of cardiac output with exercise. In patients with severe obstruction, the systolic pressure in the RV may exceed that in the LV, since the ventricular septum is intact. RV ejection is prolonged with moderate or severe stenosis, and the sound of pulmonary valve closure is delayed and soft. RV hypertrophy reduces the compliance of that chamber, and a forceful RA contraction is necessary to augment RV filling. A fourth heart sound, prominent *a* waves in the jugular venous pulse, and, occasionally, presystolic pulsations of the liver reflect vigorous atrial contraction. The clinical diagnosis is supported by a right parasternal lift and harsh systolic

ejection murmur and thrill at the upper left sternal border, typically preceded by a systolic ejection sound, if the obstruction is valvular. The holosystolic decrescendo murmur of tricuspid regurgitation may accompany severe pulmonic stenosis, especially in the presence of congestive heart failure. Cyanosis usually reflects right-to-left shunting through a patent foramen ovale or atrial septal defect. In patients with supravalvular or peripheral pulmonary arterial stenosis, the murmur is systolic or continuous and is best heard over the area of narrowing, with radiation to the peripheral lung fields.

The ECG may be helpful in assessing the degree of RV obstruction. In mild cases, the ECG is often normal, whereas moderate and severe stenoses are associated with right axis deviation and RV hypertrophy. A ventricular strain pattern, as well as high-amplitude P waves in leads II and V_1, indicating RA enlargement, is associated with severe stenosis. The chest roentgenogram with mild or moderate pulmonic stenosis often shows a heart of normal size and normal vascularity of the lungs. In the presence of valvular stenosis, poststenotic dilatation of the main and left pulmonary arteries may be evident. With severe obstruction and resultant RV failure, RA and RV enlargement are generally evident. The pulmonary vascularity may be reduced with severe stenosis, RV failure, and/or a right-to-left shunt at the atrial level. Two-dimensional echocardiography visualizes pulmonary valve morphology; the outflow tract pressure gradient can be estimated by Doppler ultrasonography.

℞ **TREATMENT**   The cardiac catheter technique of balloon valvuloplasty (Chap. 228) is usually effective. Direct surgical relief of moderate and severe obstruction may be accomplished at a low risk. Multiple stenoses of the peripheral pulmonary arteries are usually inoperable, but narrowing of a single branch or at the bifurcation of the main pulmonary trunk may be corrected.

CYANOTIC CONGENITAL HEART DISEASE WITH INCREASED PULMONARY BLOOD FLOW

COMPLETE TRANSPOSITION OF THE GREAT ARTERIES   In this condition the aorta arises from the RV to the right of and anterior to the pulmonary artery, which emerges from the LV (Fig. 234-1, *left panel*). This results in two separate and parallel circulations, and some communication between them must exist after birth to sustain life. Most patients have an interatrial communication, two-thirds have a patent ductus arteriosus, and about one-third have

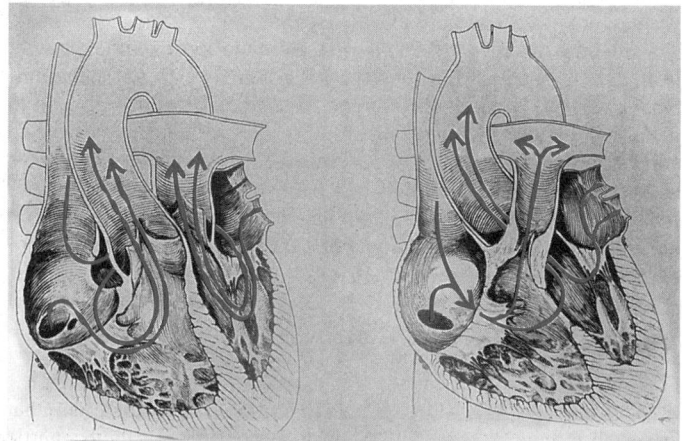

FIGURE 234-1   Complete transposition of the great arteries is depicted in the left panel. The aorta arises from the RV and the pulmonary artery from the LV. The only mixing between the two circulations occurs across a patent foramen ovale. In the right panel, the tetralogy of Fallot cartoon illustrates the two most important anatomic findings, a large ventricular septal defect and RV outflow tract obstruction. A right-to-left shunt is shown across the ventricular septum.

an associated ventricular septal defect. Transposition is more common in males and accounts for ~10% of cyanotic heart disease.

The course is determined by the degree of tissue hypoxia, the ability of each ventricle to sustain an increased work load in the presence of reduced coronary arterial oxygenation, the nature of the associated cardiovascular anomalies, and the status of the pulmonary vascular bed. Pulmonary vascular obstruction develops by 1 to 2 years of age in patients with an associated large ventricular septal defect or large patent ductus arteriosus in the absence of obstruction to LV outflow.

℞ **TREATMENT** The balloon or blade catheter or surgical creation or enlargement of an interatrial communication in the neonate is the simplest procedure for providing increased intracardiac mixing of systemic and pulmonary venous blood. Systemic–pulmonary artery anastomosis may be indicated in the patient with severe obstruction to LV outflow and diminished pulmonary blood flow. Intracardiac repair may be accomplished by rearranging the venous returns (intraatrial switch, i.e., Mustard or Senning operation) so that the systemic venous blood is directed to the mitral valve and thence to the LV and pulmonary artery, while the pulmonary venous blood is diverted through the tricuspid valve and RV to the aorta. The late survival after these repairs is good, but late sudden death is the most worrisome feature. Preferably, this malformation is corrected in infancy by transposing both coronary arteries to the posterior artery and transecting, contraposing, and anastomosing the aorta and pulmonary arteries (arterial switch operation). For those patients with a ventricular septal defect in whom it is necessary to bypass a severely obstructed LV outflow tract, corrective operation employs an intracardiac ventricular baffle and extracardiac prosthetic conduit to replace the pulmonary artery (Rastelli procedure).

SINGLE VENTRICLE This is a family of complex lesions with both atrioventricular valves or a common atrioventricular valve opening to a single ventricular chamber. Associated anomalies include abnormal great artery positional relationships, pulmonic valvular or subvalvular stenosis, and subaortic stenosis.

Survival to adulthood depends on a relatively normal pulmonary blood flow and good ventricular function. Modifications of the Fontan approach are generally applied to these patients with creation of a pathway(s) from the systemic veins to the pulmonary arteries.

CYANOTIC CONGENITAL HEART DISEASE WITH DECREASED PULMONARY BLOOD FLOW

TRICUSPID ATRESIA This malformation is characterized by atresia of the tricuspid valve, an interatrial communication, and, frequently, hypoplasia of the RV and pulmonary artery. The clinical picture is usually dominated by severe cyanosis due to obligatory admixture of systemic and pulmonary venous blood in the LV. The ECG characteristically shows RA enlargement, left axis deviation, and LV hypertrophy.

Atrial septostomy and palliative operations to increase pulmonary blood flow, often by anastomosis of a systemic artery or vein to a pulmonary artery, may allow survival to the second or third decade. A Fontan atriopulmonary connection may then allow functional correction in those patients with normal or low pulmonary arterial resistance pressure and good LV function.

EBSTEIN'S ANOMALY Characterized by a downward displacement of the tricuspid valve into the RV, due to anomalous attachment of the tricuspid leaflets, the Ebstein tricuspid valve tissue is dysplastic and results in tricuspid regurgitation. The abnormally situated tricuspid orifice produces an "atrialized" portion of the RV lying between the atrioventricular ring and the origin of the valve, which is continuous with the RA chamber. Often the RV is hypoplastic. Although the clinical manifestations are variable, some patients come to initial attention because of progressive cyanosis from right-to-left atrial shunting, or symptoms due to tricuspid regurgitation and RV

dysfunction, or paroxysmal atrial tachyarrhythmias. Diagnostic findings by two-dimensional echocardiography include the abnormal positional relation between the tricuspid and mitral valves with apical displacement of the septal tricuspid leaflet. Tricuspid regurgitation is quantitated by Doppler examination. Surgical approaches include prosthetic replacement of the tricuspid valve when the leaflets are tethered or repair of the native valve.

TETRALOGY OF FALLOT The four components of the tetralogy of Fallot are ventricular septal defect, obstruction to RV outflow, aortic override (straddle) of the ventricular septal defect, and RV hypertrophy (Fig. 234-1, right panel).

The severity of RV outflow obstruction determines the clinical presentation. The severity of hypoplasia of the RV outflow tract varies from mild to complete (pulmonary atresia). Pulmonary valve stenosis and supravalvular and peripheral pulmonary arterial obstruction may coexist; rarely there is unilateral absence of a pulmonary artery (usually the left). A right-sided aortic arch and descending aorta occur in ~25% of patients with tetralogy.

The relationship between the resistance to blood flow from the ventricles into the aorta and into the pulmonary vessels plays a major role in determining the hemodynamic and clinical picture. Thus, the severity of obstruction to RV outflow is of fundamental significance. When the obstruction is severe, the pulmonary blood flow is reduced markedly, and a large volume of desaturated systemic venous blood is shunted from right to left across the ventricular septal defect. Severe cyanosis and erythrocytosis occur, and symptoms and sequelae of systemic hypoxemia are prominent. In many infants and children the obstruction is mild but progressive.

The ECG ordinarily shows RV and, less often, RA hypertrophy. Radiologic examination characteristically reveals a normal-sized, boot-shaped heart (*coeur en sabot*) with prominence of the RV and a concavity in the region of the pulmonary conus. The pulmonary vascular markings are typically diminished, and the aortic arch and knob may be on the right side. Two-dimensional echocardiography from the parasternal or subcostal windows demonstrates the malalignment of the ventricular septal defect and the subpulmonary stenosis. Selective angiocardiography with RV injection provides architectural details of the RV outflow tract, pulmonary valve and annulus, and caliber of the main branches of the pulmonary artery; coronary arteriography identifies the anatomy and course of the coronary arteries.

℞ **TREATMENT** Factors that may complicate the treatment of patients with tetralogy of Fallot include infective endocarditis, paradoxic embolism, excessive erythrocytosis, coagulation defects, and cerebral infarction or abscess. Corrective operation is advisable at some point for almost all patients with this anomaly. Successful correction avoids progressive infundibular obstruction, delayed growth, and complications due to hypoxemia and excessive erythrocytosis. The size of the pulmonary arteries rather than the age or size of the infant or child is the most important determinant in establishing candidacy for primary repair. Pronounced hypoplasia of the pulmonary arteries is a relative contraindication for an early corrective surgical procedure. When this problem is present, a palliative operation, such as creation of a systemic arterial–pulmonary arterial shunt, is carried out and is usually followed by complete correction, which can be carried out at a lower risk later in childhood.

OTHER FORMS OF CONGENITAL HEART DISEASES

CONGENITALLY CORRECTED TRANSPOSITION The two fundamental anatomic abnormalities in this malformation are transposition of the ascending aorta and pulmonary trunk and inversion of the ventricles. This arrangement results in desaturated systemic venous blood passing from the RA through the mitral valve to the LV and into the pulmonary trunk, whereas arterialized pulmonary venous blood flows from the left atrium (LA) through the tricuspid valve to the RV and into the aorta. Thus, the circulation is corrected functionally. The clinical presentation, course, and prognosis of patients with congenitally corrected transposition vary depending on the nature and severity of any complicating intracardiac anomalies. Ebstein-type anomalies of the left-side tricuspid atrioventricular valve, ventricular septal defect, obstruction to outflow from the venous ventricle, and congenital heart block are often associated with corrected transposition. The diagnosis of the malformation and associated lesions can often be established by two-dimensional echocardiography and Doppler examination.

MALPOSITIONS OF THE HEART   Positional anomalies refer to conditions in which the cardiac apex is in the right side of the chest (dextrocardia), or at the midline (mesocardia), or in which there is a normal location of the heart in the left side of the chest but abnormal position of the viscera (isolated levocardia). Knowledge of the position of the abdominal organs and of the branching pattern of the main stem bronchi is important in categorizing these malpositions. When dextrocardia occurs without situs inversus, when the visceral situs is indeterminate, or if isolated levocardia is present, associated, often complex, multiple cardiac anomalies are usually present. In contrast, mirror-image dextrocardia is usually observed with complete situs inversus, which occurs most frequently in individuals whose hearts are otherwise normal.

SURGICALLY MODIFIED CONGENITAL HEART DISEASE

Because of the enormous strides in cardiovascular surgical techniques that have occurred in the past 20 years, a large number of long-term survivors of corrective operations in infancy and childhood have reached adulthood. These patients are often challenging because of the diversity of anatomic, hemodynamic, and electrophysiologic residua and sequelae of cardiac operations.

The proper care of the survivor of operation for congenital heart disease requires that the clinician understand the details of the malformation before operation; pay meticulous attention to the details of the operative procedure; and recognize the postoperative residua (conditions left totally or partially uncorrected), the sequelae (conditions caused by surgery), and the complications that may have resulted from the operation. With the exception of ligation and division of an uncomplicated patent ductus arteriosus, almost every other surgical repair of an anomaly leaves behind or causes some abnormality of the heart and circulation that may range from trivial to serious. Intraoperative transesophageal echocardiography assists in detecting unsuspected lesions, in monitoring the repair, and in verifying a satisfactory result or directing further repair. Thus, even with results that are considered clinically to be good to excellent, continued long-term postoperative follow-up is advisable.

Table 234-4 lists the categories of common late postoperative problems. Cardiac operations importantly involving the atria, such as closure of atrial septal defect, repair of total or partial anomalous pulmonary venous return, or venous switch corrections of complete transposition of the great arteries (the Mustard or Senning operations), may be followed years later by sinus node or atrioventricular node dysfunction or by atrial arrhythmias. Intraventricular surgery may also result in electrophysiologic consequences, including complete heart block necessitating pacemaker insertion to avoid sudden death. In ad-

Table 234-4   Potential Late Postoperative Problems

Residual shunts	Arrhythmias and conduction defects
Residual ventricular outflow obstruction	Myocardial dysfunction
	Prosthetic valve malfunction
Residual valvular anomalies	Prosthetic conduit obstruction
Systemic arterial hypertension	Infective endocarditis
Pulmonary vascular obstruction	

dition, valvular problems may arise late after initial cardiac operation. An example is the progressive stenosis of an initially nonobstructive bicuspid aortic valve in the patient who underwent aortic coarctation repair. Such aortic valves may also be the site of infective endocarditis. After repair of the ostium primum atrial septal defect, the cleft mitral valve may become progressively incompetent. Tricuspid regurgitation may also be progressive in the postoperative patient with tetralogy of Fallot if RV outflow tract obstruction was not relieved adequately at initial surgery. In many patients with surgically modified congenital heart disease, inadequate relief of an obstructive lesion, or a residual regurgitant lesion, or a residual shunt will cause or hasten the onset of clinical signs and symptoms of myocardial dysfunction. Despite a good hemodynamic repair, many patients with a subaortic RV develop RV decompensation and signs of "left heart failure." In many patients, particularly those who were cyanotic for many years before operation, a preexisting compromise in ventricular performance is due to the original underlying malformation.

A final category of postoperative problems involves the use of prosthetic valves, patches, or conduits in the operative repair. The special risks include infective endocarditis, thrombus formation, and premature degeneration and calcification of the prosthetic materials. There are many patients in whom extracardiac conduits are required to correct the circulation functionally and often to carry blood to the lungs from the RA or RV. These conduits may develop intraluminal obstruction, and, if they include a prosthetic valve, it may show progressive calcification and thickening.

BIBLIOGRAPHY

BRICKNER ME et al: Congenital heart disease in adults. N Engl J Med 342:256, 334, 2000

BURN J et al: Recurrence risks in offspring of adults with major heart defects: Results from first cohort of British collaborative study. Lancet 351:311, 1998

CHILD JS (section editor): Congenital heart disease. Curr Treatment Options Cardiovasc Med 1:301-379, 1999

CONNELLY MS et al: Canadian consensus conference on adult congenital heart disease 1996. Can J Cardiol 14:395, 1998

FRIEDMAN WF: Congenital heart disease in infancy and childhood, in *Heart Disease*, 6th ed, E Braunwald et al (eds). Philadelphia, Saunders, 2001

GATZOULIS MA et al: Atrial arrhythmia after surgical closure of atrial septal defects in adults. N Engl J Med 340:839, 1999

LIP GYH et al: Percutaneous balloon valvuloplasty for congenital pulmonary valve stenosis in adults. Clin Cardiol 22:733, 1999

MORRIS CD et al: Thirty-year incidence of infective endocarditis after surgery for congenital heart defect. JAMA 279:599, 1998

NIWA K et al: Eisenmenger syndrome in adults: Ventricular septal defect, truncus arteriosus, univentricular heart. J Am Coll Cardiol 34:223, 1999

SAIDI AS et al: Outcome of pregnancy following intervention for coarctation of the aorta. Am J Cardiol 82:786, 1998

235   *Edward L. Kaplan*

RHEUMATIC FEVER

In many parts of the world, especially in industrialized countries, acute rheumatic fever is less common than it was during the early and mid-years of the twentieth century. In the late 1940s, patients with rheumatic fever and rheumatic heart disease accounted for more than half of schoolchildren recognized to have cardiovascular problems in the United States. During the Second World War, there were more than 20,000 cases of acute rheumatic fever in U.S. Navy personnel alone. The incidence of rheumatic fever has declined remarkably in the industrialized countries of the world, where the disease has become rare. However, in many developing countries, which account for almost two-thirds of the world's population, streptococcal infections, rheumatic fever, and rheumatic heart disease remain a very significant public health problem. The magnitude of the problem in these countries today is similar to that in North America 50 years ago.

The decreased incidence of acute rheumatic fever and the low prevalence of rheumatic heart disease in industrialized countries have led many physicians and public health authorities to the incorrect conclusion that these conditions are no longer a problem. However, starting in the 1980s, unexpected scattered outbreaks of acute rheumatic fever among both adults and children in North America have confirmed the capacity for this potentially serious illness to reappear and pose significant public health problems. Neither antimicrobial agents nor other public health measures have been totally effective in the control of rheumatic fever in the industrialized or industrializing world.

EPIDEMIOLOGY The epidemiology of acute rheumatic fever is identical to that of group A streptococcal upper respiratory tract infections (Chap. 140). As is the case for streptococcal sore throat, acute rheumatic fever most often occurs in children; the peak age-related incidence is between 5 and 15 years. Most initial attacks in adults take place at the end of the second and beginning of the third decades of life. Rarely, initial attacks occur as late as the fourth decade and recurrent attacks have been documented as late as the fifth decade.

Epidemiologic risk factors classically associated with individual attacks and especially with outbreaks of acute rheumatic fever include lower standards of living, especially crowding; the disease has been more common among socially and economically disadvantaged populations. However, the outbreaks in the United States in the late 1980s and early 1990s cannot be explained entirely by these factors. The large Utah outbreak of more than 500 cases during 13 years has affected primarily middle class patients with ready access to medical care. Therefore, one can conclude that the organism itself as well as the degree of host/herd immunity to the prevalent serotypes in an affected community are equally important risk factors.

Studies have shown that approximately 3% of individuals with untreated group A streptococcal pharyngitis will develop rheumatic fever. The epidemiology of rheumatic fever is also influenced by the serotypes of group A streptococci present in a population. The concept of "rheumatogenecity" of specific strains is largely based upon epidemiologic evidence associating certain serotypes with rheumatic fever (e.g., serotypes 1, 3, 5, 6, 18, etc.). Mucoid isolates are frequently associated with virulence and with rheumatic fever.

PATHOGENESIS More than half a century ago the pioneering studies of Lancefield differentiated beta-hemolytic streptococci into serologic groups. This ultimately led to the association of infection by the group A organism of the pharynx and tonsils (not of the skin) and the subsequent development of acute rheumatic fever. However, the mechanism(s) responsible for the development of rheumatic fever after an infection remains incompletely defined. Historically, approaches to understanding the pathogenesis of rheumatic fever have been grouped into three major categories: (1) direct infection by the group A streptococcus; (2) a toxic effect of streptococcal extracellular products on the host tissues; and (3) an abnormal or dysfunctional immune response to one or more as yet unidentified somatic or extracellular antigens produced by all (or perhaps only by some) group A streptococci.

There is insufficient evidence to support direct infection of the heart as the inciting event. Additionally, while toxins such as streptolysin O and others have been postulated to have a pathogenetic role, there is relatively little convincing evidence of this at the present time. Major efforts have focused on an abnormal immune response by the human host to one or more group A streptococcal antigens.

The hypothesis of "antigenic mimicry" between human and group A streptococcal antigens has been studied extensively and has concentrated on two interactions. The first is the similarity between the group-specific carbohydrate of the group A streptococcus and the glycoprotein of heart valves; the second involves the molecular similarity among the streptococcal cell membrane, streptococcal M protein sarcolemma, and other moieties of the human myocardial cell.

The possibility of a predisposing genetic influence in some individuals is one of the most tantalizing of the incompletely understood factors that might contribute to susceptibility to rheumatic fever. The precise genetic factors influencing the attack rate have never been adequately defined. Observations have been described that support the concept that this nonsuppurative sequel to a group A streptococcal upper respiratory tract infection results from an abnormal immune response by the human host. Thus, differences in immune responses to streptococcal antigens have been reported. Further, new data suggest that a unique surface marker on non-T lymphocytes in patients with rheumatic fever and rheumatic heart disease may prove helpful in defining which individuals are susceptible to developing rheumatic fever after a streptococcal infection because of abnormal immune responses.

DIAGNOSIS There is no specific laboratory test that can establish a diagnosis of rheumatic fever. The diagnosis, therefore, is a clinical one but requires supporting evidence from the clinical microbiology and clinical immunology laboratories. Because of the variety of signs and symptoms associated with the rheumatic fever syndrome, in 1944 Jones first proposed criteria to assist the clinician in standardizing the diagnosis of rheumatic fever. The most recent modification of the *Jones criteria* (Updated Jones Criteria) was published in 1992 by a Special Writing Group of the American Heart Association (Table 235-1).

There are five criteria termed *major* because they are most commonly found in patients with rheumatic fever: carditis, migratory polyarthritis, Sydenham's chorea, subcutaneous nodules, and erythema marginatum.

The *carditis* of acute rheumatic fever is a pancarditis involving the pericardium, myocardium, and endocardium. In most published series, between 40 and 60% of patients with acute rheumatic fever have evidence of carditis, which is characterized by one or more of the following: sinus tachycardia, the murmur of mitral regurgitation, an S_3 gallop, a pericardial friction rub, and cardiomegaly. The introduction of echocardiography has assisted in the identification of subtle abnormalities of the mitral valve, and these may be present in an additional 20% of patients who do not have an audible heart murmur. A prolonged PR interval and evidence of heart failure may be present as well, but these are nonspecific and may be found in a number of other diseases.

Healing of the rheumatic valvulitis may cause fibrous thickening and adhesion, resulting in the most serious complication of rheumatic fever, i.e., valvular stenosis and/or regurgitation (Chap. 236). The mitral valve is involved most frequently, followed by the aortic valve. However, isolated aortic valve disease as a consequence of acute rheumatic fever is quite rare. In patients with aortic valve disease due to rheumatic fever, the mitral valve is almost always simultaneously affected. Even minor degrees of rheumatic valvular involvement can lead to susceptibilities to infective endocarditis (Chap. 126). Although rheumatic pericarditis can cause a serous effusion, fibrin deposits, and even pericardial calcification, it does not lead to constrictive pericarditis.

A *migratory polyarthritis* is present in as many as 75% of cases, most often affecting the ankles, wrists, knees, and elbows over a period of days. It usually does not affect the small joints of the hands or feet

Table 235-1 The Jones Criteria for Rheumatic Fever, Updated 1992

Major Criteria	Minor Criteria
Carditis	Clinical
Migratory polyarthritis	Fever
Sydenham's chorea	Arthralgia
Subcutaneous nodules	Laboratory
Erythema marginatum	Elevated acute phase reactants
	Prolonged PR interval

plus

Supporting evidence of a recent group A streptococcal infection (e.g., positive throat culture or rapid antigen detection test; and/ or elevated or increasing streptococcal antibody test)

SOURCE: Modified from the Special Writing Group of the American Heart Association.

and seldom involves the hip joints. Since salicylates and other anti-inflammatory drugs usually cause prompt resolution of joint symptoms, it is important that the clinician *not* prescribe these medications until it is determined whether the arthritis is migratory. The arthritis of acute rheumatic fever is extremely painful. Pain can be controlled with codeine or similar analgesics until the diagnosis is established. The difference between arthralgia (subjective joint pain) and arthritis (joint pain and swelling) must be understood. Too often, arthralgia is used (incorrectly) as a major criterion.

Sydenham's chorea occurs in fewer than 10% of patients with rheumatic fever. The latent period between the onset of the initiating streptococcal infection and the onset of Sydenham's chorea may be as long as several months. While differing from the other manifestations, this central nervous system disorder is a part of the rheumatic fever complex and should be managed as such. Many patients who appear to have only chorea may present several decades later with evidence of typical rheumatic valvular disease. There is no definitive laboratory test for establishing a diagnosis of Sydenham's chorea, and the diagnosis is one of exclusion. Patients with Sydenham's chorea should be given secondary prophylaxis for prevention of recurrent attacks, even if they do not appear to have rheumatic heart disease.

Subcutaneous nodules and *erythema marginatum* are rare major manifestations, usually present in fewer than 10% of cases. Subcutaneous nodules are found over extensor surfaces of joints, are seen most often in patients with long-standing rheumatic heart disease, and are extremely rare in patients experiencing an initial attack. Erythema marginatum is an uncommon manifestation. It is an evanescent macular eruption with rounded borders—usually concentrated on the trunk.

The *minor criteria* (Table 235-1) are nonspecific and may be present in many clinical conditions.

To fulfill the Jones criteria, either two major criteria, or one major criterion and two minor criteria, *plus* evidence of an antecedent streptococcal infection are required. The latter may be provided by recovery of the organism on culture or by evidence of an immune response to one of the commonly measured group A streptococcal antibodies (e.g., anti-streptolysin O, anti-deoxyribonuclease B, anti-hyaluronidase). Since the accurate diagnosis of rheumatic fever has future medical and financial implications, the clinician is obligated to evaluate any patient completely until the suspected diagnosis is either established or excluded.

Both the clinical microbiology and the clinical immunology laboratories have important roles in confirming the diagnosis of rheumatic fever. An attempt should be made to recover the organism from a throat culture, although group A streptococci can be recovered from the upper respiratory tract of only 25 to 40% of patients at the time the diagnosis is made. If a rapid antigen detection test is used but is negative, a confirmatory throat culture must be performed. It is helpful to obtain two or three cultures from the throat at the time the diagnosis is suspected but before initiating antibiotic therapy in order to confirm the presence of the organism.

At least 80% of patients with acute rheumatic fever have an elevated anti-streptolysin O titer at presentation. If one employs two additional streptococcal antibody tests such as the anti-DNAse B or anti-hyaluronidase test, the percentage of patients who show evidence of a preceding group A streptococcal infection will rise to more than 95%. While an initially elevated titer is convincing, being able to demonstrate a rise in titer from the acute to the convalescent phase is a more reliable means of documenting the recent infection. If three antibody tests are done and there is no evidence of a preceding infection, the diagnosis must be seriously reconsidered.

℞ **TREATMENT**　　There are two necessary therapeutic approaches to patients with acute rheumatic fever: anti-streptococcal antibiotic therapy and therapy for the clinical manifestations of the disease. At the time of diagnosis, *all* patients with acute rheumatic fever should be treated as if they have a group A streptococcal infection, whether or not the organism is recovered by culture. In addition to the relatively large percentage of such patients who may have a negative throat culture at the time of diagnosis, others may have only a few organisms present in the throat. Conventional antibiotic treatment should be started immediately: a complete 10-day course in adults of either oral penicillin V (500 mg twice daily), or erythromycin (250 mg four times daily) for those with penicillin allergy. Many choose intramuscular benzathine penicillin G (a single intramuscular injection of 1.2 million units) for the treatment of the presumed streptococcal infection; this will also serve as the first dose of secondary prophylaxis for the prevention of recolonization of the upper respiratory tract in the future. Intramuscular benzathine penicillin G has been reported to result in a transient elevation of the erythrocyte sedimentation rate, which can prove confusing in the acute phase of the disease.

Following the initial anti-streptococcal therapy, secondary prophylaxis should be initiated to prevent subsequent colonization of the upper respiratory tract with group A streptococci. Recommendations of the American Heart Association and of the World Health Organization are for intramuscular injection of 1.2 million units of benzathine penicillin G every 4 weeks or for oral penicillin V (250 mg twice daily) or oral sulfadiazine (1.0 g daily). Recent studies have shown that in those individuals who are at high risk for recurrence of rheumatic fever, intramuscular benzathine penicillin G given every 3 weeks is more effective in reducing the risk of recurrence. Since it is known that the risk of recurrence of rheumatic fever is highest during the first 5 years after the attack, secondary prophylaxis is always given for at least this period. After that the decision to continue or discontinue secondary prophylaxis is dependent upon whether the patient has documented rheumatic heart disease and whether the patient is at high risk of exposure to streptococci (e.g., students, school teachers, medical and military personnel, etc.). Many believe that those with documented recurrences and/or documented rheumatic valvular heart disease should receive secondary prophylaxis for life. The duration of prophylaxis is often individualized for specific patients.

Medical therapy for the manifestations of rheumatic fever depends on the clinical status of the patient. For adult patients with the arthritis of rheumatic fever, salicylates in doses escalating to 2 g four times daily are very effective and will result in marked clinical improvement, often within 12 h. When this prompt relief does not occur, one should reexamine the original diagnosis. Salicylates may be given for 4 to 6 weeks and gradually tapered so as to prevent a rebound. The erythrocyte sedimentation rate is one method for determining the rate of taper for salicylates. Usually this requires at least 2 weeks. There are no conclusive data to support using nonsteroidal anti-inflammatory drugs for acute rheumatic fever. There is no indication for the use of steroids (usually prednisone) solely for the treatment of the arthritis of rheumatic fever.

Most experienced physicians believe that there is a role for steroids in patients with severe carditis accompanied by congestive heart failure. However, neither salicylates nor glucocorticoids influence the future development of valvular heart disease. In adults, prednisone can be started in doses as high as 30 mg four times daily in especially severe cases, and, as the patient improves, salicylates can be added during the tapering of the steroid dose; this may require 4 to 6 weeks.

In the presence of congestive heart failure, conventional medical measures (Chap. 232) are indicated. In the past, patients with acute rheumatic fever were kept at complete bed rest for months. This is inappropriate unless there is a specific reason such as persistent active carditis or severe heart failure. Patients with arthritis will begin to feel better very soon after anti-inflammatory therapy with salicylates is begun. They may be released from bed rest but should not resume full activity until signs of inflammatory process have abated and the acute-phase reactants have returned to normal.

BIBLIOGRAPHY

COMMITTEE ON RHEUMATIC FEVER, ENDOCARDITIS AND KAWASAKI DISEASE OF THE COUNCIL ON CARDIOVASCULAR DISEASE IN THE YOUNG OF THE AMERICAN HEART ASSOCIATION: Treatment of acute streptococcal pharyngitis and prevention of rheumatic fever: A statement for health professionals. Pediatrics 96:758, 1995

DAJANI A: Rheumatic fever, in *Heart Disease*, 6th ed, E Braunwald et al (eds). Philadelphia, Saunders, 2001

KAPLAN EL: Global assessment of rheumatic fever and rheumatic heart disease at the close of the century. The influences and dynamics of population and pathogens: A failure to realize prevention? (The T. Duckett Jones Memorial Lecture.) Circulation 88:1964, 1993

KAPLAN EL: The group A streptococcal upper respiratory tract carrier state: An enigma. J Pediatr 97:337, 1980

KIM EJ: Index of suspicion. Diagnosis: acute rheumatic fever (ARF). Pediatr Rev 21:21, 26, 2000

NARULA J et al (eds): Rheumatic fever, in *American Registry of Pathology*. Washington, DC, 1999

SPECIAL WRITING GROUP OF THE COMMITTEE ON RHEUMATIC FEVER, ENDOCARDITIS AND KAWASAKI DISEASE OF THE COUNCIL ON CARDIOVASCULAR DISEASE IN THE YOUNG OF THE AMERICAN HEART ASSOCIATION: Guidelines for the diagnosis of rheumatic fever. Jones criteria, 1992 Update. JAMA 268:2069, 1992

STEVENS DL, KAPLAN EL (eds): *Streptococcal Infections: Clinical Aspects, Microbiology, and Molecular Pathogenesis*. New York, Oxford Univ Press, 2000

VEASY GL et al: Persistence of acute rheumatic fever in the intermountain area of the United States. J Pediatr 24:9, 1994

236   *Eugene Braunwald*

VALVULAR HEART DISEASE

AF	atrial fibrillation	MVP	mitral valve prolapse
AR	aortic regurgitation	MVR	mitral valve replacement
AS	aortic stenosis	OS	opening snap
AVR	aortic valve replacement	PA	pulmonary arterial
CO	cardiac output	PAP	pulmonary arterial pressure
EF	ejection fraction	PR	pulmonary regurgitation
LA	left atrium	RA	right atrial
LV	left ventricle	RV	right ventricle
MR	mitral regurgitation	TR	tricuspid regurgitation
MS	mitral stenosis	TS	tricuspid stenosis

The role of physical examination in the evaluation of patients with valvular disease is also considered in Chap. 225; of electrocardiography in Chap. 226; of echocardiography in Chap. 227; and of cardiac catheterization and angiography in Chap. 228.

MITRAL STENOSIS

ETIOLOGY AND PATHOLOGY   Two-thirds of all patients with mitral stenosis (MS) are female. MS is generally rheumatic in origin; very rarely, it is congenital. Pure or predominant MS occurs in approximately 40% of all patients with rheumatic heart disease. In others, lesser degrees of MS may accompany mitral regurgitation (MR) and aortic valve lesions. With reductions in the incidence of acute rheumatic fever, particularly in temperate climates and developed nations, the incidence of MS is declining. In rheumatic stenosis the valve leaflets are diffusely thickened by fibrous tissue and/or calcific deposits. The mitral commissures fuse, the chordae tendineae fuse and shorten, the valvular cusps become rigid, and these changes, in turn, lead to narrowing at the apex of the funnel-shaped (fish-mouth) valve. Although the initial insult to the mitral valve is rheumatic, the later changes may be a nonspecific process resulting from trauma to the valve caused by altered flow patterns due to the initial deformity. Calcification of the stenotic mitral valve immobilizes the leaflets and narrows the orifice further. Thrombus formation and arterial embolization may arise from the calcific valve itself, but more frequently arise from the dilated left atrium (LA) in patients with atrial fibrillation (AF).

PATHOPHYSIOLOGY   In normal adults the mitral valve orifice is 4 to 6 cm². In the presence of significant obstruction, i.e., when the orifice is less than approximately 2 cm², blood can flow from the LA to the left ventricle (LV) only if propelled by an abnormally elevated left atrioventricular pressure gradient (see Fig. 228-2), the hemodynamic hallmark of MS. When the mitral valve opening is reduced to 1 cm², a LA pressure of approximately 25 mmHg is required to maintain a normal cardiac output (CO). The elevated pulmonary venous and pulmonary arterial (PA) wedge pressures reduce pulmonary compliance, contributing to exertional dyspnea. The first bouts of dyspnea are usually precipitated by clinical events that increase the rate of blood flow across the mitral orifice, resulting in further elevation of the LA pressure (see below). To assess the severity of obstruction, both the transvalvular pressure gradient and the flow rate must be measured (Chap. 228). The latter depends not only on the CO but on the heart rate as well. An increase in heart rate shortens diastole proportionately more than systole and diminishes the time available for flow across the mitral valve. Therefore, at any given level of CO, tachycardia augments the transvalvular gradient and elevates further the LA pressure. (Similar considerations apply to the tricuspid valve.)

The LV diastolic pressure is normal in isolated MS; coexisting aortic valve disease, systemic hypertension, MR, ischemic heart disease, and perhaps the residua of damage produced by rheumatic myocarditis are sometimes responsible for elevations that reflect impaired LV function and/or reduced LV compliance. LV dysfunction, as reflected in reduced LV ejection fraction (EF), occurs in about one-fourth of patients with severe, chronic MS and may be a consequence of prolonged reduction of preload and/or extension of scarring from the valve into the adjacent myocardium. In pure MS and sinus rhythm, the elevated LA and PA wedge pressures exhibit a prominent atrial contraction (*a* wave) and a gradual pressure decline after mitral valve opening (*y* descent) (see Fig. 228-4). In severe MS and whenever the pulmonary vascular resistance is significantly increased, the pulmonary arterial pressure (PAP) is elevated even when the patient is at rest, and in extreme cases it may approach the systemic arterial pressure. Further elevations of LA, PA wedge, and PAP occur during exercise. When the PA systolic pressure exceeds approximately 50 mmHg in patients with MS, or for that matter with any lesion affecting the left side of the heart, the increased right ventricle (RV) afterload impedes the emptying of this chamber, and the RV end-diastolic pressure and volume usually rise.

Cardiac Output   The hemodynamic response to mitral obstruction ranges from a normal CO and a high left atrioventricular pressure gradient to a markedly reduced CO and low transvalvular pressure gradient. In most patients with moderate MS, the CO is normal or almost so at rest but rises subnormally during exertion. In patients with severe MS, particularly those in whom the pulmonary vascular resistance is strikingly elevated, the CO is subnormal at rest and may fail to rise or may even decline during activity.

Pulmonary Hypertension   The clinical and hemodynamic features of MS are influenced importantly by the level of the PAP. Pulmonary hypertension results from (1) passive backward transmission of the elevated LA pressure; (2) pulmonary arteriolar constriction, which presumably is triggered by LA and pulmonary venous hypertension (reactive pulmonary hypertension); (3) interstitial edema in the walls of the small pulmonary vessels; and (4) organic obliterative changes in the pulmonary vascular bed. Severe pulmonary hypertension results in tricuspid regurgitation (TR) and pulmonary incompetence as well as right-sided heart failure. The changes in the pulmonary vascular bed also may be considered to exert a protective effect; the elevated precapillary resistance reduces the likelihood of symptoms of pulmonary congestion by reducing the surge of blood into the pulmonary capillary bed during activity. However, this protection occurs at the expense of a reduced, fixed CO.

SYMPTOMS   In temperate climates the latent period between the initial attack of rheumatic carditis (in the increasingly rare circumstances in which a history of one can be elicited) and the development of symptoms due to MS is generally about two decades; most patients begin to experience disability in the fourth decade. Studies carried out before the development of mitral valvotomy revealed that once a patient with MS became seriously symptomatic, the disease progressed continuously to death within 2 to 5 years. In economically deprived areas, in tropical and subtropical climates, particularly on the Indian subcontinent, in Central America, and in the Middle East, MS tends to progress more rapidly and frequently causes serious symptoms in patients less than the age of 20 years. In contrast, slowly progressive MS in the elderly is being recognized with increasing frequency in the United States and western Europe.

When valvular obstruction is mild, the physical signs of MS may be present without symptoms. However, even in patients whose mitral orifices are large enough to accommodate a normal blood flow with only mild elevations of LA pressure, marked elevations of this pressure leading to dyspnea and cough may be precipitated by severe exertion, excitement, fever, severe anemia, paroxysmal tachycardia, sexual intercourse, pregnancy, and thyrotoxicosis. As MS progresses, lesser stresses precipitate dyspnea, and the patient becomes limited in daily activities. The redistribution of blood from the dependent portions of the body to the lungs, which occurs when the recumbent position is assumed, leads to orthopnea and paroxysmal nocturnal dyspnea. *Pulmonary edema* develops when there is a sudden surge in flow across a markedly narrowed mitral orifice. When moderately severe MS has existed for several years, *atrial arrhythmias*—premature contractions, paroxysmal tachycardia, flutter, and AF—occur with increasing frequency. The rapid ventricular rate associated with untreated or inadequately treated AF is frequently responsible for acute exacerbations of dyspnea. The development of permanent AF often marks a turning point in the patient's course and is generally associated with acceleration of the rate at which symptoms progress.

Hemoptysis (Chap. 33) results from rupture of pulmonary-bronchial venous connections secondary to pulmonary venous hypertension. It occurs most frequently in patients who have elevated LA pressures without markedly elevated pulmonary vascular resistances and is almost never fatal.

As the severity of MS progresses and the pulmonary vascular resistance rises or when tricuspid stenosis (TS) or TR develop, symptoms secondary to pulmonary congestion sometimes diminish, and the episodes of acute pulmonary edema and hemoptysis may become reduced in frequency and severity. The elevation of pulmonary vascular resistance further increases RV systolic pressure, leading to RV failure, fatigue, abdominal discomfort due to hepatic congestion, and edema.

Recurrent pulmonary emboli (Chap. 261), sometimes with infarction, are an important cause of morbidity and mortality late in the course of MS. *Pulmonary infections*, i.e., bronchitis, bronchopneumonia, and lobar pneumonia, commonly complicate untreated MS. *Infective endocarditis* (Chap. 126) is rare in pure MS but is not uncommon in patients with combined MS and MR. *Chest pain* occurs in about 10% of patients with severe MS; it may be due to pulmonary hypertension or myocardial ischemia secondary to accompanying coronary atherosclerosis.

Pulmonary Changes   In addition to the aforementioned changes in the pulmonary vascular bed, fibrous thickening of the walls of the alveoli and pulmonary capillaries occurs commonly in MS. The vital capacity, total lung capacity, maximal breathing capacity, and oxygen uptake per unit of ventilation are reduced (Chap. 250), and the latter fails to rise normally during exertion. Pulmonary compliance falls further as pulmonary capillary pressure rises during exercise. In some patients, airway resistance is abnormally increased. These alterations in pulmonary mechanics contribute to an increase in the work of breathing and dyspnea. The diffusing capacity may be reduced, particularly during exertion, as a result of structural changes in the diffusing surface and reduction of the pulmonary capillary blood volume. These changes in the lungs are due, in part, to increased transudation of fluid from the pulmonary capillaries into the interstitial and alveolar spaces. However, the increased capacity of the pulmonary lymphatic system to drain excess fluid retards the development of alveolar edema.

Thrombi and Emboli   *Thrombi* may form in the left atria, particularly in the enlarged atrial appendages of patients with MS. If they *embolize*, they do so most commonly to the brain, kidneys, spleen, and extremities. Embolization occurs much more frequently in patients with AF or other unstable atrial arrhythmias, in older patients, and in those with a reduced cardiac output. However, systemic embolization may be the presenting complaint in otherwise asymptomatic patients with mild MS. At operation, thrombi are not found more frequently in the LA of patients with a past history of embolization than in those without this complication, indicating that usually the freshly formed clots are the ones that dislodge. Patients who have had one or more systemic emboli have an increased predilection for further embolic episodes. Rarely, a large pedunculated thrombus or a free-floating clot may suddenly obstruct the stenotic mitral orifice. Such "ball valve" thrombi produce syncope, angina, and changing auscultatory signs with alterations in position, findings that resemble those produced by an LA myxoma (Chap. 240).

PHYSICAL FINDINGS   (See also Chap. 225)   **Inspection and Palpation**   In patients with severe MS, there may be a malar flush with pinched and blue facies. In patients with sinus rhythm and severe pulmonary hypertension or associated TS, the jugular venous pulse reveals prominent *a* waves due to vigorous right atrial systole. In patients with AF, the jugular pulse reveals only a single expansion during systole (*c-v* wave). The systemic arterial pressure is usually normal or slightly low. A RV tap along the left sternal border signifies an enlarged RV. A diastolic thrill is frequently present at the cardiac apex, particularly with the patient in the left lateral recumbent position.

Auscultation   The first heart sound (S_1) is generally accentuated and snapping, and since the mitral valve does not close until the LV pressure reaches the level of the elevated LA pressure, this sound is often slightly delayed, causing a prolonged Q-S_1 interval on the phonocardiogram. The pulmonary component of the second heart sound (P_2) is often accentuated, and the two components of the second heart sound (S_2) are closely split. A pulmonary systolic ejection click may be heard in patients with severe pulmonary hypertension. The opening snap (OS) of the mitral valve is most readily audible in expiration at, or just medial to, the cardiac apex but also may be easily heard along the left sternal edge or at the base of the heart. This sound generally follows the sound of aortic valve closure (A_2) by 0.05 to 0.12 s; that is, it follows P_2. Since the OS occurs when the LV pressure falls below the LA pressure, the time interval between A_2 and OS varies inversely with the severity of the MS. The intensities of the OS and S_1 correlate with the mobility of the anterior mitral leaflet.

The OS is followed by a low-pitched, rumbling, diastolic murmur, heard best at the apex with the patient in the left lateral recumbent position (see Fig. 225-4). It is accentuated by mild exercise (e.g., a few rapid sit-ups) carried out just before auscultation. In general, the duration of this murmur correlates with the severity of the stenosis. In patients with sinus rhythm, the murmur often reappears or becomes reaccentuated during atrial systole, as atrial contraction reelevates the rate of blood flow across the narrowed orifice. Soft (grade I or II/VI) systolic murmurs are commonly heard at the apex or along the left sternal border in patients with pure MS and do not necessarily signify the presence of MR. Hepatomegaly, ankle edema, ascites, and pleural effusion, particularly in the right pleural cavity, may occur in patients with MS and RV failure.

Associated Lesions   With severe pulmonary hypertension, a pansystolic murmur produced by functional TR may be audible along the left sternal border. Characteristically, this murmur is accentuated by inspiration and diminishes during forced expiration (Carvallo's sign) or during performance of the Valsalva maneuver; it should not be confused with the apical pansystolic murmur of MR.

The recognition of associated MR is of considerable clinical importance in patients with MS. A presystolic murmur and an accentuated S_1 speak against the presence of serious associated MR, but when the S_1 and/or the OS are soft or absent in a patient with mitral valve disease who also has an apical systolic murmur, it is likely that significant MR and/or serious calcification of the deformed mitral valve leaflets are present. A third heart sound (S_3) at the apex often signifies that the MR is serious; this sound is generally duller, is lower pitched, and follows the OS. Occasionally, in patients with pure MS, physical signs may falsely suggest MR. A RV S_3 and an enlarged RV that forms the cardiac apex may give the erroneous impression of LV enlargement. The rumbling diastolic murmur of MS become less prominent or may even disappear and be replaced by the systolic murmur of functional TR, which is mistaken for MR. When CO is markedly reduced in a patient with MS, the typical auscultatory findings, including the diastolic rumbling murmur, may not be detectable (silent MS), but they may reappear as compensation is restored. Associated TS also tends to obscure many of the physical signs of MS.

The Graham Steell murmur of pulmonary regurgitation (PR), a high-pitched, diastolic, decrescendo blowing murmur along the left sternal border, results from dilatation of the pulmonary valve ring and occurs in patients with mitral valve disease and severe pulmonary hypertension. This murmur may be indistinguishable from the more common murmur produced by aortic regurgitation (AR), except that it is rarely audible at the second right intercostal space and may disappear after successful surgical treatment of the MS.

LABORATORY EXAMINATION **Electrocardiogram** In MS and sinus rhythm, the P wave usually suggests LA enlargement (see Fig. 226-10). It may become tall and peaked in lead II and upright in lead V_1 when severe pulmonary hypertension or TS complicates MS and right atrial (RA) enlargement occurs. The QRS complex is usually normal. However, with severe pulmonary hypertension, right axis deviation and RV hypertrophy are often present.

Roentgenogram The earliest changes are straightening of the left border of the cardiac silhouette, prominence of the main pulmonary arteries, dilatation of the upper lobe pulmonary veins, and backward displacement of the esophagus by an enlarged LA. In severe MS, however, all chambers and vessels upstream to the narrowed valve are prominent, including both atria, pulmonary arteries and veins, RV, and superior vena cava. Kerley B lines are fine, dense, opaque, horizontal lines that are most prominent in the lower and midlung fields and that result from distention of interlobular septa and lymphatics with edema when the resting mean LA pressure exceeds approximately 20 mmHg.

Echocardiogram (See also Chap. 227) This is the most sensitive and specific noninvasive method for diagnosing MS. Transthoracic two-dimensional color flow Doppler echocardiographic imaging and Doppler ultrasound provide critical information, including an estimate of the transvalvular gradient and of mitral orifice size, the presence and severity of accompanying MR, the extent of restriction of valve leaflets, their thickness, and the degree of distortion of the subvalvular apparatus, and the anatomic suitability for balloon mitral valvotomy. In addition, echocardiography provides an assessment of the size of the cardiac chambers, an estimation of the PAP, and an indication of the presence and severity of associated TR and PR. Transesophageal echocardiography provides superior images and should be employed when transthoracic imaging is inadequate for guiding therapy.

DIFFERENTIAL DIAGNOSIS Significant MR may also be associated with a prominent diastolic murmur at the apex, but this murmur commences slightly later in patients with MR than in patients with MS, and there is often clear-cut evidence of LV enlargement. An apical pansystolic murmur of at least grade III/VI intensity as well as an S_3 should arouse the suspicion of significant associated MR. Similarly, the apical middiastolic murmur associated with AR (Austin Flint murmur) may be mistaken for MS. TS, which occurs rarely in the absence of MS, may mask many of the clinical features of MS. Echocardiography is particularly useful in detecting MS in patients who have or are suspected of having other valve lesions and in defining the severity of the various lesions.

Primary pulmonary hypertension (Chap. 260) results in a number of the clinical and laboratory features of MS. It occurs most frequently in young women. However, the OS and diastolic rumbling murmur are absent, and the pulmonary artery wedge and LA pressures are normal, as is the size of the LA on echocardiography. *Atrial septal defect* (Chap. 234) also may be mistaken for MS; in both conditions

there is often clinical, electrocardiographic, and roentgenographic evidence of RV enlargement and accentuation of the pulmonary vascularity. The widely split S_2 of atrial septal defect may be confused with the mitral OS, and the diastolic flow murmur across the tricuspid valve may be mistaken for the mitral diastolic murmur. However, the absence of LA enlargement and of Kerley B lines and the demonstration of fixed splitting of S_2 favor atrial septal defect over MS.

Left atrial myxoma (Chap. 240) may obstruct LA emptying, causing dyspnea, a diastolic murmur, and hemodynamic changes resembling those of MS. However, patients with an LA myxoma often have features suggestive of a systemic disease, such as weight loss, fever, anemia, systemic emboli, and elevated erythrocyte sedimentation rate and serum IgG concentration. Usually an OS is not audible, and the auscultatory findings may change markedly with body position. The diagnosis can be established by the demonstration of a characteristic echo-producing mass in the LA with two-dimensional echocardiography.

CARDIAC CATHETERIZATION AND ANGIOCARDIOGRAPHY Left heart catheterization is useful for clarifying the picture when there is a discrepancy between clinical and echocardiographic findings (see Fig. 228-2). It is helpful in assessing associated lesions such as aortic stenosis (AS) and AR. Catheterization and coronary arteriography are not usually necessary to aid in the decision about surgery in younger patients with typical findings of severe obstruction on clinical examination and echocardiography. In males over 45 years of age, females over 55 years of age, and younger patients with coronary risk factors, especially those with positive noninvasive stress tests for myocardial ischemia, coronary angiography is usually advisable preoperatively to detect patients with critical coronary obstructions that should be bypassed at the time of operation. Catheterization and LV angiography are also indicated in most patients who have undergone balloon mitral valvotomy or previous mitral valve operations and who have redeveloped serious symptoms.

℞ TREATMENT In the asymptomatic adolescent with mitral valve disease, penicillin prophylaxis of β-hemolytic streptococcal infections (Chap. 235) and prophylaxis for infective endocarditis (Chap. 126) are important. In symptomatic patients, some improvement usually occurs with restriction of sodium intake and maintenance doses of oral diuretics. Digitalis glycosides do not alter the hemodynamics and usually do not benefit patients with pure MS and sinus rhythm but are necessary for slowing the ventricular rate of patients with AF. Small doses of beta blockers (e.g., atenolol 25 to 50 mg/d) may be added when cardiac glycosides fail to control ventricular rate in such patients. Anticoagulants should be administered for at least 1 year to patients with MS who have suffered systemic and/or pulmonary embolization and permanently to those with AF.

If AF is of relatively recent origin in a patient whose MS is not severe enough to warrant balloon mitral valvotomy or surgical valvotomy, reversion to sinus rhythm pharmacologically or by means of electrical countershock is indicated. Usually this reversion should be undertaken after the patient has had 3 weeks of anticoagulant treatment. Conversion to sinus rhythm is rarely helpful in patients with severe MS, particularly those in whom the LA is especially enlarged or in whom AF has been present for more than 1 year, since sinus rhythm is rarely sustained.

Mitral valvotomy Unless there is a specific contraindication, mitral valvotomy is indicated in the symptomatic patient with isolated MS whose effective orifice is less than approximately 1.0 cm²/m² body surface area, or <1.6 cm² in normal-sized adults. Mitral valvotomy can be carried out by two techniques: percutaneous balloon mitral valvotomy and surgical valvotomy. In balloon mitral valvotomy (Figs. 236-1 and 236-2), a catheter is directed into the LA after transseptal puncture and a balloon (Inoue balloon) is directed across the valve and inflated in the valvular orifice. This has become the procedure of choice for patients with uncomplicated MS.

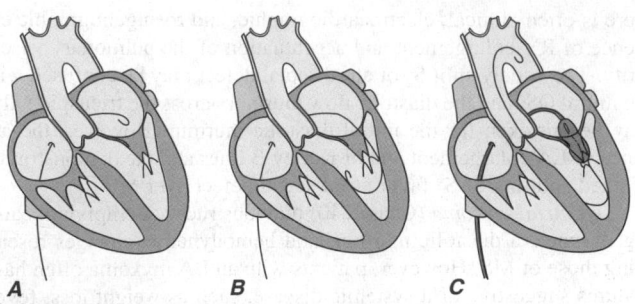

FIGURE 236-1 Technique of double balloon mitral valvuloplasty. *A.* The position of the guidewire in the left atrium after left atrial puncture using the Brockenbrough needle. *B.* The position of the guidewire as it is advanced into the left ventricle across the stenotic mitral valve. C. Partial inflation of a balloon catheter across the stenotic mitral valve. *[From JP Srebro, TA Ports, Catheter-balloon valvuloplasty, in K Chatterjee et al (eds): Cardiology: An Illustrated Text. Philadelphia, Lippincott, 1991.]*

An "open" valvotomy with cardiopulmonary bypass is usually preferable to closed valvotomy. In addition to opening the valve commissures, it is important to loosen any subvalvular fusion of papillary muscles and chordae tendineae and to remove large deposits of calcium, thereby improving valvular function, as well as to remove atrial thrombi.

Valvotomy, whichever technique is used, usually results in striking symptomatic and hemodynamic improvement and prolongs survival. In uncomplicated cases, the mortality rate is <2%. However, there is no evidence that the procedure improves the prognosis of patients with slight or no functional impairment unless they develop severe pulmonary hypertension on exertion. Therefore, unless recurrent systemic embolization has occurred, valvotomy is *not* recommended for patients who are entirely asymptomatic, regardless of hemodynamic findings. When there is little symptomatic improvement after valvotomy, it is likely that the procedure was ineffective, that it induced MR, or that associated valvular or myocardial disease was present. The recurrence of symptoms several years after what appeared to be a satisfactory initial result is usually due to an inadequate valvotomy, but progression of other valvular lesions, mitral restenosis, or some combination of these conditions also may be responsible. About half of all patients undergoing mitral valvotomy require reoperation by 10 years. In the pregnant patient with MS, valvotomy should be carried out if pulmonary congestion occurs despite intensive medical treatment.

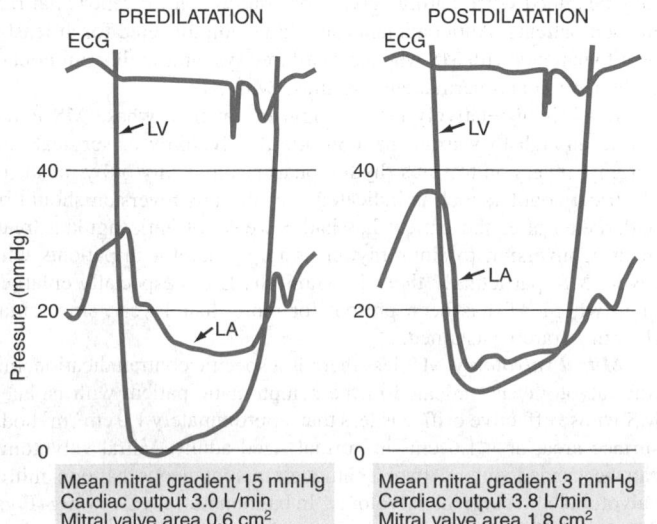

FIGURE 236-2 Simultaneous left atrial (LA) and left ventricular (LV) pressure before and after balloon mitral valvuloplasty in a patient with severe mitral stenosis. *[From Braunwald (Courtesy of Raymond G. McKay, MD).]*

Table 236-1   Mortality Rates After Valve Replacement and Repair

Operative Category	Number	Operative Mortality (%)
AVR (isolated)	26,317	4.3
MVR (isolated)	13,936	6.4
Multiple valve replacement	3,840	9.6
AVR + CAB	22,713	8.0
MVR + CAB	8,788	15.3
Multiple valve replacement + CAB	1,424	18.8
AVR + any valve repair	938	7.4
MVR + any valve repair	1,266	12.5
Aortic valve repair	597	5.9
Mitral valve repair	4,167	3.0
Tricuspid valve repair	144	13.9

NOTE: AVR, aortic valve replacement; CAB, coronary artery bypass; MVR, mitral valve replacement.
SOURCE: Modified from WRE Jamieson et al.

In patients with MS and significant associated MR, those in whom the valve has been severely distorted by previous transcatheter or operative manipulation, or those in whom the surgeon does not find it possible to improve valve function significantly, mitral valve replacement (MVR) may have to be carried out. Since the operative mortality rate of isolated MVR is still approximately 6% (Table 236-1), and since there are long-term complications of valve replacement, patients in whom preoperative evaluation suggests the possibility that MVR may be required should be operated on only if they have critical MS, i.e., an orifice <0.6 cm²/m² body surface area and are in New York Heart Association class III, i.e., symptomatic with ordinary activity, despite optimal medical therapy. The overall 10-year survival of surgical survivors is approximately 70%. Long-term prognosis is worse in older patients and those with marked disability and striking depression of the cardiac index preoperatively.

MITRAL REGURGITATION

ETIOLOGY   Chronic rheumatic heart disease is the cause of severe MR in about one-third of cases. In contrast to MS, rheumatic MR occurs more frequently in males. The rheumatic process produces rigidity, deformity, and retraction of the valve cusps and commissural fusion, as well as shortening, contraction, and fusion of the chordae tendineae. Mitral valve prolapse (MVP), an important cause of MR, is considered in the next section. MR also may occur as a congenital anomaly (Chap. 234), most commonly as a defect of the endocardial cushions (atrioventricular cushion defects). MR may occur with fibrosis of a papillary muscle in patients with healed myocardial infarction as well as in patients with infarction involving the base of a papillary muscle. Transient MR also may occur during periods of ischemia involving a papillary muscle or the adjacent myocardium and may accompany bouts of angina pectoris. MR may occur with marked LV enlargement of any cause in which dilatation of the mitral annulus and lateral displacement of the papillary muscles interfere with coaptation of the valve leaflets. In hypertrophic cardiomyopathy, the anterior leaflet of the mitral valve is displaced anteriorly during systole, leading to regurgitation (Chap. 238). Calcification of the mitral annulus of unknown cause, presumably degenerative, which occurs most commonly in elderly women, also can be responsible for significant MR. Acute MR may occur secondary to infective endocarditis involving the valve or chordae tendineae, in acute myocardial infarction with rupture of a papillary muscle or one of its heads, as a consequence of trauma, or after chordal rupture.

Regardless of cause, severe MR is often progressive, since enlargement of the LA places tension on the posterior mitral leaflet, pulling it away from the mitral orifice and thereby aggravating the valvular dysfunction. Similarly, the dilatation of the LV increases the regurgitation, which in turn enlarges the LA and LV further, causing chordal rupture and resulting in a vicious circle; hence the aphorism, "mitral regurgitation begets mitral regurgitation."

PATHOPHYSIOLOGY The resistance to LV emptying is reduced in patients with MR. As a consequence, the LV is decompressed into the LA during ejection, and with the reduction in LV size there is a rapid decline in LV tension. The initial compensation to acute MR is more complete LV emptying. However, LV volume increases progressively as the severity of the regurgitation increases and as LV function deteriorates. This increase in LV volume is often accompanied by a depressed forward CO. The regurgitant volume varies directly with the LV systolic pressure and the size of the regurgitant orifice; the latter, in turn, is influenced profoundly by the extent of LV dilatation.

The v wave in the LA pressure pulse is usually prominent (see Fig. 228-3). During early diastole, as the distended LA empties, there is a particularly rapid y descent (as long as there is no associated MS). In chronic MR, there is often an increase in LV compliance, so that LV volume rises with little elevation in LV diastolic pressure. The effective (forward) CO is usually reduced in seriously symptomatic patients. A brief, early diastolic atrioventricular pressure gradient may occur in patients with pure MR as a result of the very rapid flow of blood across a normal-sized mitral orifice.

The prompt appearance of contrast material in the LA after its injection into the LV signifies the presence of MR. The regurgitant volume can be measured by determining the difference between the total LV stroke volume, estimated angiocardiographically, and the effective forward stroke volume determined by the Fick method (Chap. 228). In severe cases, as much as 50% of the total LV stroke volume regurgitates with each beat. Qualitative, but clinically useful, estimates of the severity of regurgitation may be made by observation on cineangiograms of the degree of LA opacification after the injection of contrast material into the LV. Color flow Doppler imaging is most commonly used for this purpose (see below).

The compliance, i.e., the pressure-volume relationship, of the LA and pulmonary venous bed affects the clinical picture. Patients with acute MR usually have *normal or reduced compliance*, little enlargement of the LA, but marked elevation of the LA pressure, particularly of the v wave. Pulmonary edema is common. Patients with a *marked increase in LA compliance* are at the opposite end of the spectrum, having long-standing, severe MR, marked enlargement of the LA, and normal or only slightly elevated LA and PA pressures. These patients usually complain of severe fatigue and exhaustion secondary to a low CO, while symptoms resulting from pulmonary congestion are less prominent; AF is almost invariably present. Most common are patients whose clinical and hemodynamic features are between those in the two aforementioned groups, with variable degrees of enlargement of the LA and with significant elevation of the LA pressure. Symptoms are secondary to a combination of reduced forward CO and pulmonary congestion.

SYMPTOMS Fatigue, exertional dyspnea, and orthopnea are the most prominent complaints in patients with chronic, severe MR. Systemic embolism occurs less frequently than in MS. Right-sided heart failure, with painful hepatic congestion, ankle edema, distended neck veins, ascites, and TR, occurs in patients with MR who have associated pulmonary vascular disease and marked pulmonary hypertension. In patients with acute, severe MR, LV failure with acute pulmonary edema is common.

PHYSICAL FINDINGS The arterial pressure is usually normal, and in patients with severe MR the arterial pulse may show a sharp upstroke. The jugular venous pulse shows abnormally prominent *a* waves in patients with sinus rhythm and marked pulmonary hypertension and prominent *v* waves in those with accompanying severe TR. A systolic thrill is often palpable at the cardiac apex, the LV is hyperdynamic with a brisk systolic impulse and a palpable rapid-filling wave, and the apex beat is often displaced laterally. An RV tap and the shock of pulmonary valve closure may be palpable in patients with marked pulmonary hypertension.

Auscultation The S_1 is generally absent, soft, or buried in the systolic murmur; indeed, an accentuated mitral closure sound is useful in excluding severe MR. In patients with severe MR, the aortic valve

may close prematurely, resulting in wide splitting of the S_2. An OS indicates associated MS but does not exclude predominant regurgitation. A low-pitched S_3 occurring 0.12 to 0.17 s after the aortic valve closure sound, i.e., at the completion of the rapid-filling phase of the LV, is believed to be caused by the sudden tensing of the papillary muscles, chordae tendineae, and valve leaflets and is an important auscultatory feature of severe MR. The absence of an S_3 indicates that if MR exists, it may not be severe. The S_3 may be followed by a short, rumbling, diastolic murmur, even in the absence of MS. A fourth heart sound (S_4) is often audible in patients with acute, severe MR of recent onset who are in sinus rhythm. A presystolic murmur is not ordinarily heard with isolated MR but is present in patients with sinus rhythm and associated MS.

A systolic murmur of at least grade III/VI intensity, is the most characteristic auscultatory finding in severe MR. It is usually holosystolic (see Fig. 225-4), but it may be decrescendo and cease in late systole in patients with acute, severe MR when the tall v wave in the LA pressure pulse reduces the late systolic LV-LA (reverse) pressure gradient. In MR due to papillary muscle dysfunction or MVP, the systolic murmur commences in midsystole (see below). The systolic murmur is usually most prominent at the apex and radiates into the axilla. However, in patients with ruptured chordae tendineae or primary involvement of the posterior mitral leaflet, the regurgitant jet strikes the LA wall adjacent to the aortic root. In this situation, the systolic murmur is transmitted to the base of the heart and therefore may be confused with the murmur of AS. In patients with ruptured chordae tendineae the systolic murmur may have a cooing or "sea gull" quality, while a flail leaflet may cause a murmur with a musical quality. The systolic murmur of MR is intensified by isometric strain but is reduced during the Valsalva maneuver.

LABORATORY EXAMINATION **Electrocardiogram** In patients with sinus rhythm there is evidence of LA enlargement, but RA enlargement also may be present when pulmonary hypertension is severe. Chronic, severe MR is generally associated with AF. In many patients there is no clear-cut electrocardiographic evidence of enlargement of either ventricle. In others the signs of LV hypertrophy are present.

Roentgenogram The LA and LV are the dominant chambers; in chronic cases, the former may be massively enlarged and forms the right border of the cardiac silhouette. Pulmonary venous congestion, interstitial edema, and Kerley B lines are sometimes noted. Marked calcification of the mitral leaflets occurs commonly in patients with long-standing combined MR and MS. Calcification of the mitral annulus may be visualized.

Echocardiogram Color flow Doppler imaging is the most accurate noninvasive technique for the detection and estimation of MR. Two-dimensional echocardiography is useful for assessing LV function from end systolic and end-diastolic volumes and EF. The LA is usually enlarged and/or exhibits increased pulsations; the LV may be hyperdynamic. Findings that help to determine the etiology of MR can often be identified by two-dimensional echocardiography. Transesophageal imaging provides greater detail than transthoracic imaging. With ruptured chordae tendineae or a flail leaflet, coarse, errative motion of the involved leaflets may be noted. Vegetations associated with infective endocarditis, incomplete coaptation of the anterior and posterior mitral leaflets, and annular calcification, as well as MR secondary to LV dilatation, aneurysm, or dyskinesis may be recognized. The echocardiogram in patients with MVP is described in the next section.

℞ **TREATMENT** **Medical** The nonsurgical management of patients with severe MR begins with restricting those physical activities that regularly produce dyspnea and excessive fatigue, reducing sodium intake, and enhancing sodium excretion with the appropriate use of diuretics (Chap. 232). Vasodilators and digitalis glycosides increase the forward output of the failing LV. Intravenous nitroprusside or nitroglycerin to reduce afterload and thereby the volume of regurgitant flow are useful in stabilizing patients with acute and/or severe MR. Angiotensin-converting enzyme inhibitors are useful in the treatment of chronic MR. The same considerations as in patients with MS apply to the reversion of AF to sinus rhythm. In the late stages of heart failure anticoagulants and leg binders are used to diminish the likelihood of venous thrombi and pulmonary emboli.

Surgical   In the selection of patients with severe MR for surgical treatment, the chronic, often slowly progressive nature of the condition must be balanced against the immediate and long-term risks associated with valve reconstruction or replacement. Patients with MR who are asymptomatic or who are limited only during strenuous exertion are not considered to be candidates for surgical treatment, since their condition may remain stable for many years. By contrast, unless there are contraindications, surgical treatment should be offered to patients with severe MR whose limitations do not allow full time employment or the performance of normal household activities despite optimal medical management. Surgical treatment of severe MR is indicated even for asymptomatic patients or those with mild symptoms when LV dysfunction is progressive, with LV ejection fraction declining below 60% and/or end-systolic cavity dimension on echocardiography rising above 50 mm. In patients with impaired LV function, the risk of surgery rises sharply, the recovery of LV performance is incomplete, and the long-term survival is reduced (Fig. 236-3). However, conservative management has little to offer these patients, so operative treatment may be indicated even at an advanced stage of the disease; and occasionally, the clinical and hemodynamic improvement that follows surgical treatment of patients with advanced disease is dramatic. Though most patients who survive surgery appear to be greatly improved, some degree of myocardial dysfunction may persist.

When surgical treatment is contemplated, left-sided heart catheterization and angiocardiography may be helpful in confirming the presence of severe MR in patients in whom there is a discrepancy between the clinical picture and the echocardiographic findings; these procedures may also aid in detecting and assessing the severity of associated valve lesions. Importantly, coronary arteriography identifies patients who require concomitant coronary revascularization.

Surgical treatment of MR, especially that caused by valves that are markedly deformed, with shrunken, calcified leaflets secondary to rheumatic fever, requires MVR with a prosthesis. However, in an increasing fraction of patients, particularly those with severe annular dilatation, flail leaflets, MVP, ruptured chordae, or infective endocarditis, reconstruction of the mitral valve apparatus (mitral valvuloplasty) and/or mitral annuloplasty with an annuloplasty ring may be successful. Valve reconstruction should be carried out whenever feasible since the operative risk is about half (~3%) of that associated with MVR (Table 236-1). Also, reconstruction spares the patient the long-term adverse consequences of valve replacement (i.e., thromboembolic and hemorrhagic complications in the case of mechanical

prostheses and late valve failure necessitating repeat valve replacement in the case of bioprostheses). In addition, by preserving the integrity of the papillary muscles and subvalvular apparatus, mitral valvuloplasty maintains LV function.

MITRAL VALVE PROLAPSE

MVP, also variously termed the *systolic click-murmur syndrome, Barlow's syndrome, floppy-valve syndrome,* and *billowing mitral leaflet syndrome,* is a relatively common, but highly variable, clinical syndrome resulting from diverse pathogenic mechanisms of the mitral valve apparatus. Among these are excessive or redundant mitral leaflet tissue, which is commonly involved with myxomatous degeneration and greatly increased concentration of acid mucopolysaccharide. It is a frequent finding in patients with heritable disorders of connective tissue, including the Marfan syndrome (Chap. 351), osteogenesis imperfecta, and the Ehler-Danlos syndrome. In most patients with MVP, however, myxomatous degeneration is confined to the mitral (or less commonly the tricuspid or aortic) valves without other clinical or pathologic manifestations of disease; the posterior leaflet is usually more affected than the anterior, and the mitral valve annulus is often greatly dilated. In many patients, elongated redundant chordae tendineae cause or contribute to the regurgitation.

In most patients with MVP, the cause is unknown, but in some it appears to be a genetically determined collagen tissue disorder. A reduction in the production of type III collagen has been incriminated, and electron microscopy has revealed fragmentation of collagen fibrils. MVP may be associated with thoracic skeletal deformities similar to but not as severe as those in the Marfan syndrome, including a high arched palate and alterations of the chest and thoracic spine, including the so-called straight back syndrome. MVP also may occur as a sequel of acute rheumatic fever, in ischemic heart disease, and in cardiomyopathies, as well as in 20% of patients with ostium secundum atrial septal defect.

MVP may lead to excessive stress on the papillary muscles, which in turn leads to dysfunction and ischemia of the papillary muscles and subjacent ventricular myocardium; rupture of chordae tendineae and progressive annular dilatation and calcification also contribute to valvular regurgitation, which then places more stress on the diseased mitral valve apparatus, thereby creating a vicious cycle. The electrocardiographic changes (see below) and ventricular arrhythmias appear to result from regional ventricular dysfunction related to increased stress placed on the papillary muscles.

CLINICAL FEATURES   MVP is more common in females. It affects individuals in a wide age range but most commonly between the ages of 14 and 30 years. The clinical course is often benign. MVP may also be observed in older (>50 years) patients, often males, and in them MR is more often severe and requires surgical treatment. There is an increased familial incidence for some patients, suggesting an autosomal dominant form of inheritance. MVP encompasses a broad spectrum of severities in patients, ranging from only a systolic click and murmur and mild prolapse of the posterior leaflet of the mitral valve to severe MR due to chordal rupture and massive prolapse of both leaflets. In many patients, this condition progresses over years or decades.

Most patients are asymptomatic and remain so for their entire lives. However, MVP is now the most common cause of isolated severe MR requiring surgical treatment in North America. Arrhythmias, most commonly ventricular premature contractions and paroxysmal supraventricular and ventricular tachycardia, have been reported and may cause palpitations, light-headedness, and syncope. Sudden death has been noted but is a very rare complication. Many patients have chest pain that is difficult to evaluate. It is often substernal, prolonged, poorly related to exertion, and rarely resembles typical angina pectoris. Transient cerebral ischemic attacks secondary to emboli from the mitral valve due to endothelial disruption have been reported. Infective endocarditis may occur in patients with MR associated with MVP.

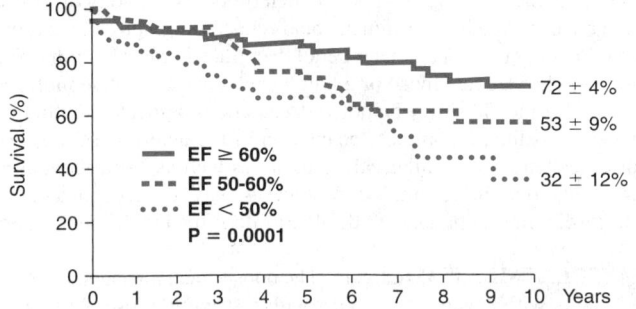

FIGURE 236-3   Late survival rates of patients surviving surgical correction of MR according to preoperative echocardiographic ejection fraction (EF). *(From M Enriquez-Sarano et al: Echocardiographic prediction of survival after surgical correction of organic mitral regurgitation. Circulation 90:833, 1994, with permission.)*

Auscultation The most important finding is the mid- or late (nonejection) systolic click, which occurs 0.14 s or more after the S_1 and is thought to be generated by the sudden tensing of slack, elongated chordae tendineae or by the prolapsing mitral leaflet when it reaches its maximum excursion. Systolic clicks may be multiple and may be followed by a high-pitched, late systolic crescendo-decrescendo murmur, which occasionally is "whooping" or "honking," and is heard best at the apex. The click and murmur occur earlier with standing, during the strain of the Valsalva maneuver, and any intervention that decreases LV volume, exaggerating the propensity of mitral leaflet prolapse. Conversely, squatting and isometric exercise, which increase LV volume, diminish mitral prolapse, and the click-murmur complex is delayed and may even disappear. Some patients have a midsystolic click without the murmur; others have the murmur without a click. Still others have both sounds at different times.

LABORATORY EXAMINATION The *electrocardiogram* most commonly is normal but may show biphasic or inverted T waves in leads II, III, and aVF, and occasionally supraventricular or ventricular premature contractions. *Two-dimensional echocardiography* is particularly effective in identifying the abnormal position and prolapse of the mitral valve leaflets; a useful echocardiographic definition of MVP is systolic displacement (in the parasternal view) of the mitral valve leaflets by at least 2 mm into the LA superior to the plane of the mitral annulus. Thickening of the mitral valve leaflets identifies a subgroup of patients at higher risk of infective endocarditis and the development of severe MR. Prolapse of the tricuspid and/or aortic valve may be found. *Color-imaging* and *Doppler studies* are helpful in revealing and evaluating accompanying MR. *Angiocardiography* generally shows prolapse of the posterior and sometimes of both mitral valve leaflets.

TREATMENT The management of patients with MVP consists of reassurance of the asymptomatic patient without severe MR or arrhythmias and the prevention of infective endocarditis with antibiotic prophylaxis in patients with a systolic murmur and/or thickening of mitral valve leaflets on endocardiography. Beta blockers have been found to relieve chest pain. If symptomatic tachyarrhythmias have occurred, antiarrhythmic agents as dictated by electrophysiologic studies should be administered. If the patient is symptomatic from severe MR, mitral valve repair (or rarely, replacement) is indicated. Antiplatelet aggregation agents such as aspirin should be given to patients with transient ischemic attacks, and if these are not effective, anticoagulants should be used.

AORTIC STENOSIS

AS occurs in about one-fourth of all patients with chronic valvular heart disease; approximately 80% of adult patients with symptomatic valvular AS are male.

ETIOLOGY AS in adults may be congenital in origin, it may be secondary to rheumatic inflammation of the aortic valve, or it may be due to degenerative calcification of the aortic cusps of unknown cause. The *congenitally affected valve* may already be stenotic at birth (Chap. 234) and may become progressively more fibrotic, calcified, and stenotic. In other cases the valve may be congenitally deformed, usually bicuspid, without serious narrowing of the aortic orifice during childhood; its abnormal architecture makes its leaflets susceptible to otherwise ordinary hemodynamic stresses, which ultimately lead to valvular thickening, calcification, increased rigidity, and narrowing of the aortic orifice.

Rheumatic endocarditis of the aortic leaflets produces commissural fusion, sometimes resulting in a bicuspid valve. This condition in turn, makes the leaflets more susceptible to trauma and ultimately leads to fibrosis, calcification, and further narrowing. By the time the obstruction to LV outflow causes serious clinical disability, the valve is usually a rigid calcified mass, and careful examination may make it difficult or even impossible to determine the etiology of the underlying process. Rheumatic AS is almost always associated with rheumatic

involvement of the mitral valve. A rheumatic etiology is favored by a history of active rheumatic fever and by associated severe AR.

Age-related degenerative calcific AS (also known as senile or sclerocalcific AS) is now the most common cause of AS in adults in North America and Western Europe. About 30% of persons >65 years exhibit aortic valve sclerosis, many of whom have a systolic murmur of AS but without obstruction, while an additional 2% exhibit frank stenosis.

OTHER FORMS OF OBSTRUCTION TO LEFT VENTRICULAR OUTFLOW Besides valvular AS, three other lesions may be responsible for obstruction to LV outflow.

1. *Hypertrophic cardiomyopathy* (Chap. 238). This condition is characterized by marked hypertrophy of the LV and involves in particular the interventricular septum; it may cause subaortic obstruction.
2. *Discrete congenital subvalvular AS* (Chap. 234). This congenital anomaly is produced by either a membranous diaphragm or a fibrous ridge just below the aortic valve.
3. *Supravalvular AS* (Chap. 234). This uncommon congenital anomaly is produced by narrowing of the ascending aorta or by a fibrous diaphragm with a small opening just above the aortic valve.

PATHOPHYSIOLOGY The obstruction to LV outflow produces a systolic pressure gradient between the LV and aorta. When severe obstruction is suddenly produced experimentally, the LV responds by dilatation and reduction of stroke volume. However, in patients the obstruction may be present at birth and/or increases gradually over the course of many years, and LV output is maintained by the presence of concentric LV hypertrophy. This serves as a useful compensatory mechanism because it reduces toward normal the systolic stress developed by the myocardium. A large transaortic valvular pressure gradient may exist for many years without a reduction of CO or LV dilatation; ultimately, however, these changes occur.

A peak systolic pressure gradient >50 mmHg in the face of a normal cardiac output or an effective aortic orifice less than approximately 0.5 cm^2/m^2 body surface area, i.e., less than approximately one-third of the normal orifice, is generally considered to represent critical obstruction to LV outflow. The elevated LV end-diastolic pressure observed in many patients with severe AS signifies the presence of LV dilatation and/or diminished compliance of the hypertrophied LV wall. A large *a* wave in the LA pressure pulse is usually present. Loss of an appropriately timed, vigorous atrial contraction, as occurs in AF or atrioventricular dissociation, may result in a rapid aggravation of symptoms. Although the CO at rest is within normal limits in most patients with severe AS, it usually fails to rise normally during exercise. Late in the course the CO and LV–aortic pressure gradient decline, and the mean LA, PA, and RV pressures rise.

The hypertrophied LV muscle mass elevates myocardial oxygen requirements. In addition, even in the absence of obstructive coronary artery disease, there may be interference with coronary blood flow, because the pressure compressing the coronary arteries exceeds the coronary perfusion pressure, often causing ischemia, especially in the subendocardium and during tachycardia both in the presence and in the absence of coronary arterial narrowing.

A significant fraction of patients with rheumatic AS has associated mitral valve disease. AS intensifies the severity of accompanying MR by increasing the pressure driving blood from the LV to the LA.

SYMPTOMS AS is rarely of hemodynamic or clinical importance until the valve orifice has narrowed to approximately 0.5 cm^2/m^2 body surface area in adults. Even critical AS may exist for many years without producing any symptoms because of the ability of the hypertrophied LV to generate the elevated intraventricular pressures required for a normal stroke volume.

Most patients with pure or predominant AS have gradually increasing obstruction for years but do not become symptomatic until the sixth to eighth decades. Exertional dyspnea, angina pectoris, and syncope are the three cardinal symptoms. Often there is a history of insidious progression of fatigue and dyspnea associated with gradual curtailment of activities. *Dyspnea* results primarily from elevation of the pulmonary capillary pressure caused by elevations of LA and LV diastolic pressures secondary to reduced compliance and/or LV dilatation. *Angina pectoris* usually develops somewhat later and reflects an imbalance between the augmented myocardial oxygen requirements and reduced oxygen availability; the former results from the increased myocardial mass and intraventricular pressure, while the latter may result from accompanying coronary artery disease, which is not uncommon in patients with AS, as well as from compression of the coronary vessels by the hypertrophied myocardium. Therefore, angina may occur in severe AS even without obstructive epicardial coronary artery disease. *Exertional syncope* may result from a decline in arterial pressure caused by vasodilatation in the exercising muscles and inadequate vasoconstriction in nonexercising muscles in the face of a fixed CO or from a sudden fall in CO produced by an arrhythmia.

Since the CO at rest is usually well maintained until late in the course, marked fatigability, weakness, peripheral cyanosis, and other clinical manifestations of a low CO are usually not prominent until this stage is reached. Orthopnea, paroxysmal nocturnal dyspnea, and pulmonary edema, i.e., symptoms of LV failure, also occur only in the advanced stages of the disease. Severe pulmonary hypertension leading to RV failure and systemic venous hypertension, hepatomegaly, AF, and TR are usually late findings in patients with isolated, severe AS.

When AS and MS coexist, the reduction of cardiac output induced by MS lowers the pressure gradient across the aortic valve and thereby masks many of the clinical findings produced by AS. Left heart catheterization is helpful in defining the relative importance of each valvular abnormality.

PHYSICAL FINDINGS The rhythm is generally regular until very late in the course; at other times, AF should suggest the possibility of associated mitral valve disease. The systemic arterial pressure is usually within normal limits. In the late stages, however, when stroke volume declines, the systolic pressure may fall and the pulse pressure narrow. Systemic hypertension is unusual in patients with marked AS, and a basal systolic arterial pressure >200 mmHg essentially excludes severe narrowing of this valve. The peripheral arterial pulse, as palpated in the carotid or brachial arteries, rises slowly to a delayed sustained peak (pulsus parvus et tardus) (see Fig. 225-2*B*). In the elderly, the stiffening of the arterial wall may mask this important physical sign. A palpable double systolic arterial pulse, the so-called bisferiens pulse, excludes pure or predominant AS and signifies dominant AR. In the late stages of AS, when the pulse pressure is reduced, the pulse amplitude may be so small that the anacrotic nature of the pulse and the delay in its upstroke may become difficult to appreciate. In many patients the *a* wave in the jugular venous pulse is accentuated. This results from the diminished distensibility of the RV cavity caused by the bulging, hypertrophied interventricular septum.

The LV impulse is usually active and displaced laterally, reflecting the presence of LV hypertrophy. A double apical impulse may be recognized, particularly with the patient in the left lateral recumbent position. A systolic thrill is generally present at the base of the heart, in the jugular notch, and along the carotid arteries. In patients who do not have marked pulmonary emphysema, a thick chest wall, thoracic deformity, or heart failure, the absence of a systolic thrill suggests that the AS is relatively mild.

Auscultation An early systolic ejection sound, actually the OS of the aortic valve, is frequently audible in children and adolescents with congenital noncalcific valvular AS. This sound usually disappears when the valve becomes calcified and rigid. As AS increases in severity, LV systole may become prolonged so that the aortic valve closure sound no longer precedes the pulmonic valve closure sound, and the two components may become synchronous, or aortic valve closure may even follow pulmonic valve closure, causing paradoxic

splitting of the S_2 (Chap. 225). The sound of aortic valve closure can be heard most frequently in patients with AS who have pliable valves, and calcification diminishes the intensity of this sound. Frequently, an S_4 is audible at the apex and reflects the presence of LV hypertrophy and an elevated LV end-diastolic pressure; an S_3 generally occurs when the LV dilates.

The murmur of AS is characteristically an ejection (mid) systolic murmur that commences shortly after the S_1, increases in intensity to reach a peak toward the middle of ejection, and ends just before aortic valve closure (see Fig. 225-4). It is characteristically low-pitched, rough, and rasping in character, loudest at the base of the heart, most commonly in the second right intercostal space. It is transmitted upward along the carotid arteries. Occasionally, it is transmitted downward and to the apex where it may be confused with the systolic murmur of MR; the latter, however, is usually holosystolic. In almost all patients with severe obstruction, the murmur is at least grade III/VI. In patients with mild degrees of obstruction or in those with severe stenosis with heart failure in whom the stroke volume and therefore the transvalvular flow rate are reduced, the murmur may be relatively soft and brief.

LABORATORY EXAMINATION **Electrocardiogram** The main finding in most patients with severe AS is LV hypertrophy (see Fig. 226-10). In advanced cases, ST-segment depression and T-wave inversion (LV "strain") in standard leads I and aVL and in the left precordial leads are evident. However, there is no close correlation between the electrocardiogram and the hemodynamic severity of obstruction, and the absence of electrocardiographic signs of LV hypertrophy does not exclude severe obstruction. The presence of LA enlargement should suggest the possibility of associated mitral valve disease.

Roentgenogram The chest roentgenogram may show no or little overall cardiac enlargement for many years, since the development of concentric LV hypertrophy is the initial response to obstruction to LV outflow. Hypertrophy without dilatation may produce some rounding of the cardiac apex in the frontal projection and slight backward displacement in the lateral view; critical AS is often associated with post-stenotic dilatation of the ascending aorta. Aortic calcification is usually readily apparent on fluoroscopic examination or by echocardiography; *the absence of valvular calcification in an adult suggests that severe valvular AS is not present*. In later stages of the disease as the LV dilates, there is increasing roentgenographic evidence of LV enlargement; pulmonary congestion; and enlargement of the LA, PA, and right side of the heart.

Echocardiogram The key findings are LV hypertrophy and, in patients with valvular calcification (i.e., most adult patients with symptomatic AS), multiple, bright, thick, echoes from within the aortic root. Eccentricity of the aortic valve cusps is characteristic of congenitally bicuspid valves (**Plate I-3**). Transesophageal imaging displays the obstructed orifice extremely well. LV dilatation and reduced systolic shortening reflect impairment of LV function. The transaortic valvular gradient can be estimated by Doppler echocardiography. Echocardiography is particularly useful for identifying valvular abnormalities such as MS and AR, which sometimes accompany AS, and for differentiating valvular AS from obstructive hypertrophic cardiomyopathy.

Catheterization Catheterization of the left side of the heart and coronary arteriography should generally be carried out in patients suspected of having severe AS who are being considered for operative treatment. These investigations are especially indicated in the following:

1. Patients with clinical signs of AS and symptoms of myocardial ischemia, in whom associated coronary artery disease is suspected. An effort should be made to determine whether AS or coronary atherosclerosis is primarily responsible for the symptoms, and coronary arteriography should be carried out in an effort to identify patients who require coronary bypass grafting at the time of aortic valve surgery.

2. Patients with multivalvular disease, in whom the role played by each valvular deformity should be defined to aid in the planning of definitive operative treatment.

3. Young, asymptomatic patients with noncalcific congenital AS, to define the severity of obstruction to LV outflow, since operation [which does not usually require aortic valve replacement (AVR)] or balloon valvotomy may be indicated for them if severe AS is present, even in the absence of symptoms. Balloon valvotomy may follow left heart catheterization immediately.

4. Patients in whom it is suspected that the obstruction to LV outflow may not be at the aortic valve but rather in the sub- or supravalvular regions.

NATURAL HISTORY Death in patients with severe AS occurs most commonly in the seventh and eighth decades. Based on data obtained at postmortem examination in patients not treated surgically, the average time to death after the onset of various symptoms was as follows: angina pectoris, 3 years; syncope, 3 years; dyspnea, 2 years; and congestive heart failure, 1.5 to 2 years. Moreover, in >80% of patients who died with AS, symptoms had existed for <4 years. Congestive heart failure was considered to be the cause of death in one-half to two-thirds of patients. Among adults dying with valvular AS, sudden death, which presumably results from an arrhythmia, occurred in 10 to 20% and at an average age of 60 years. However, most sudden deaths occur in patients who had previously been symptomatic.

℞ **TREATMENT** All patients with moderate or severe AS require careful periodic follow-up. In patients with severe AS, strenuous physical activity should be avoided even in the asymptomatic stage. Digitalis glycosides, sodium restriction, and the cautious administration of diuretics are indicated in the treatment of congestive heart failure, but care must be taken to avoid volume depletion since this may cause a marked reduction of CO. While nitroglycerin is helpful in relieving angina pectoris, vasodilator therapy for heart failure is usually of little value and may, in fact, be harmful.

Surgical Treatment The most critical decision in the management of AS concerns the advisability of surgical treatment which, in most adults with calcific AS and critical obstruction (aortic orifice <0.5 cm²/m² body surface area), consists of AVR. In most instances, it is prudent to postpone operation in patients with severe calcific AS who are asymptomatic (unless they exhibit LV dysfunction), since their future course is difficult to predict and they may continue to do well for many years. However, they should be followed carefully by clinical examination for the development of symptoms and by serial echocardiograms for evidence of deteriorating LV function. Operation is generally indicated in patients with severe AS who are asymptomatic, irrespective of their LV function, as well as those who exhibit LV dysfunction, even if they are asymptomatic. In patients without heart failure, the operative risk of AVR is approximately 4% (Table 236-1).

When angina pectoris, syncope, or LV decompensation develops in adults with severe valvular AS, the outlook, despite medical treatment, is very poor and can be improved significantly by AVR. The operative risk is considerably lower than the risk of nonoperative treatment; moreover, the symptomatic improvement in some survivors of operation has been remarkable. Regression of LV hypertrophy may occur after relief of obstruction.

Operation should, if possible, be carried out before frank LV failure develops; at this late stage, the operative risk is high (15 to 20%), and evidence of myocardial disease may persist even when the operation is technically successful. Furthermore, long-term postoperative survival also correlates inversely with preoperative LV dysfunction. Nonetheless, in view of the very poor prognosis of such patients when they are treated medically, there is usually little choice but to advise surgical treatment. In patients in whom severe AS and coronary artery disease coexist, relief of the AS and revascularization of the myocardium by means of aortocoronary bypass grafting may result in striking clinical and hemodynamic improvement.

Because many patients with calcific AS are elderly, particular attention must be directed to the adequacy of hepatic, renal, and pulmonary function before AVR is recommended. The mortality rate depends to a substantial extent on the patient's preoperative clinical and hemodynamic state. The 10-year survival rate of patients with AVR is approximately 60%. Approximately 30% of bioprosthetic valves evidence primary valve failure in 10 years, requiring re-replacement, and an approximately equal percentage of patients with mechanical prostheses develop significant hemorrhagic complications as a consequence of treatment with anticoagulants.

Percutaneous Balloon Aortic Valvuloplasty This procedure is preferable to operation in children and young adults with congenital, noncalcific AS. It is not commonly used in elderly patients with severe calcific AS because of a high restenosis rate. Nonetheless, this procedure has been used successfully in patients who are too ill or frail to undergo operation, in patients with life-threatening AS and advanced extracardiac disease, and as a "bridge to operation" in patients with severe LV dysfunction.

AORTIC REGURGITATION

ETIOLOGY AR may be caused by primary valve disease or by primary aortic root disease.

Primary Valve Disease Approximately three-fourths of patients with pure or predominant valvular AR are males; females predominate among patients with AR who have associated mitral valve disease. In approximately two-thirds of patients with AR the disease is rheumatic in origin, resulting in thickening, deformity, and shortening of the individual aortic valve cusps, changes that prevent their proper opening during systole and closure during diastole. A rheumatic origin is less common in patients with isolated AR. Acute AR may result from infective endocarditis, which can develop on a valve previously affected by rheumatic disease, a congenitally deformed valve, or, rarely, a normal aortic valve, and perforate or erode one or more of the leaflets. Patients with congenital membranous subaortic stenosis often develop thickening of the aortic valve leaflets, which makes the valves particularly susceptible to endocarditis. AR also may occur in patients with congenital bicuspid aortic valves. Prolapse of an aortic cusp, resulting in progressive chronic AR, occurs in approximately 15% of patients with ventricular septal defect (Chap. 234). Congenital fenestrations of the aortic valve occasionally produce mild AR. Although traumatic rupture of the aortic valve is an uncommon cause of acute AR, it does represent the most frequent serious lesion in patients surviving nonpenetrating cardiac injuries. The coexistence of hemodynamically significant AS with AR usually excludes all the rarer forms of AR because it occurs almost exclusively in patients whose AR is rheumatic or congenital in origin. In patients with AR due to primary valvular disease, dilatation of the aortic annulus may occur secondarily and intensify the regurgitation.

Primary Aortic Root Disease AR, both acute and chronic, also may be due entirely to marked aortic dilatation, i.e., aortic root disease, without primary involvement of the valve leaflets; widening of the aortic annulus and separation of the aortic leaflets are responsible for the AR (Chap. 247). Cystic medial necrosis of the ascending aorta, which may or may not be associated with other manifestations of the Marfan syndrome, idiopathic dilatation of the aorta, osteogenesis imperfecta, and severe hypertension all may widen the aortic annulus and lead to progressive AR. Occasionally, AR is caused by retrograde dissection of the aorta involving the aortic annulus. Syphilis and ankylosing rheumatoid spondylitis may be associated with cellular infiltration and scarring of the media of the thoracic aorta, leading to aortic dilatation, aneurysm formation, and severe regurgitation. In syphilis of the aorta, the involvement of the intima may narrow the coronary ostia, which in turn may be responsible for myocardial ischemia.

PATHOPHYSIOLOGY The total stroke volume ejected by the LV (i.e., the sum of the effective forward stroke volume and the volume of blood that regurgitates back into the LV) is increased in patients with AR. In patients with wide-open (free) AR, the volume of regurgitant flow may equal the effective forward stroke volume. In contrast to MR, in which a fraction of the LV stroke volume is delivered into the low-pressure LA, in AR the entire LV stroke volume is ejected into a high-pressure zone, the aorta. An increase in the LV end-diastolic volume (increased preload) constitutes the major hemodynamic compensation for AR. The dilatation of the LV allows this chamber to eject a larger stroke volume without requiring any increase in the relative shortening of each myofibril. Therefore, severe AR may occur with a normal effective forward stroke volume and a normal left ventricular/ejection fraction (EF) [total (forward plus regurgitant) stroke volume/end-diastolic volume], together with an elevated LV end-diastolic pressure and volume. However, through the operation of Laplace's law (which holds that myocardial wall tension is the product of intracavitary pressure and LV radius), LV dilatation increases the LV systolic tension required to develop any given level of systolic pressure. As LV function deteriorates, the end-diastolic volume rises and the forward stroke volume and EF decline. Deterioration of LV function often precedes the development of symptoms. Considerable thickening of the LV wall also occurs with chronic AR, and at autopsy the hearts of these patients may be among the largest encountered, sometimes weighing >1000 g.

The reverse pressure gradient from aorta to LV, which is responsible for the AR flow, falls progressively during diastole (see Fig. 228-4), accounting for the decrescendo nature of the diastolic murmur. Equilibration between aortic and LV pressures may occur toward the end of diastole in patients with severe AR, particularly when the heart rate is slow, and the LV end-diastolic pressure may be elevated, occasionally to extremely high levels (>40 mmHg). Rarely, in acute, severe AR, the LV pressure exceeds the LA pressure toward the end of diastole, and this reversed pressure gradient closes the mitral valve prematurely or causes diastolic MR.

In patients with severe AR, the effective forward CO usually is normal or only slightly reduced at rest, but often it fails to rise normally during exertion. Early signs of LV dysfunction include reduction in the EF, determined by echocardiography or radionuclide angiography. In advanced stages there may be considerable elevation of the LA, PA wedge, PA, and RV pressures and lowering of the forward CO at rest.

Myocardial ischemia may occur in patients with AR because myocardial oxygen requirements are elevated by both LV dilatation and elevated LV systolic tension. However, the major portion of coronary blood flow occurs during diastole, when arterial pressure is subnormal, thereby reducing coronary perfusion pressure. This combination of increased oxygen demand and reduced supply may cause myocardial ischemia, particularly of the subendocardium.

HISTORY   A family history may frequently be elicited from patients with AR associated with the Marfan syndrome. A history compatible with infective endocarditis may sometimes be elicited from patients with rheumatic or congenital involvement of the aortic valve, and the infection often precipitates or seriously aggravates preexisting symptoms. Ankylosing spondylitis is usually self-evident.

Chronic, severe AR may have a long latent period, and patients may remain relatively asymptomatic for as long as 10 to 15 years. However, uncomfortable awareness of the heartbeat, especially on lying down, may be an early complaint. Sinus tachycardia during exertion or with emotion or premature ventricular contractions may produce particularly uncomfortable palpitations, as well as head pounding. These complaints may persist for many years before the development of exertional dyspnea, usually the first symptom of diminished cardiac reserve. The dyspnea is followed by orthopnea, paroxysmal nocturnal dyspnea, and excessive diaphoresis. Chest pain occurs frequently, even in younger patients, and it is not necessary to invoke the presence of coronary artery disease to explain this symptom in patients with severe AR. Anginal pain may develop at rest as well as during exertion. Nocturnal angina may be a particularly troublesome symptom, and it may be accompanied by marked diaphoresis. The anginal episodes can be prolonged and often do not respond satisfac-

torily to sublingual nitroglycerin. Systemic fluid accumulation, including congestive hepatomegaly and ankle edema may develop late in the course of the disease.

In patients with acute, severe AR, as may occur in infective endocarditis or trauma, the LV cannot dilate sufficiently to maintain stroke volume, and LV diastolic pressure rises rapidly with associated elevations of LA and PA wedge pressures. Pulmonary edema and/or cardiogenic shock may develop rapidly.

PHYSICAL FINDINGS   In severe AR, the jarring of the entire body and the bobbing motion of the head with each systole can be appreciated, and the abrupt distention and collapse of the larger arteries are easily visible. The examination should be directed toward the detection of conditions predisposing to AR, such as the Marfan syndrome, rheumatoid spondylitis, and ventricular septal defect.

Arterial Pulse   A rapidly rising "water-hammer" pulse, which collapses suddenly as arterial pressure falls rapidly during late systole and diastole (Corrigan's pulse), and capillary pulsations, an alternate flushing and paling of the skin at the root of the nail while pressure is applied to the tip of the nail (Quincke's pulse), are characteristic of free AR. A booming, "pistol-shot" sound can be heard over the femoral arteries (Traube's sign), and a to-and-fro murmur (Duroziez's sign) is audible if the femoral artery is lightly compressed with a stethoscope.

The arterial pulse pressure is widened, with an elevation of the systolic pressure, sometimes to as high as 300 mmHg, and a depression of the diastolic pressure. The measurement of arterial diastolic pressure with a sphygmomanometer may be complicated by the fact that systolic sounds are frequently heard with the cuff completely deflated. However, the level of cuff pressure at the time of muffling of the Korotkoff sounds generally corresponds fairly closely to the true intraarterial diastolic pressure. The severity of AR does not always correlate directly with the arterial pulse pressure, and severe regurgitation may exist in patients with arterial pressures in the range of 140/60 mmHg. As the disease progresses and the LV end-diastolic pressure rises markedly, the arterial diastolic pressure may actually rise also, since the aortic diastolic pressure cannot fall below the LV end-diastolic pressure.

Palpation   The LV impulse is heaving and displaced laterally and inferiorly. The systolic expansion and diastolic retraction of the apex are prominent and contrast with the sustained systolic thrust characteristic of severe AS. A diastolic thrill is often palpable along the left sternal border, and a prominent systolic thrill may be palpable in the jugular notch and transmitted upward along the carotid arteries. This thrill and the accompanying systolic murmur are due to the markedly increased blood flow across the aortic orifice and do not necessarily signify the coexistence of AS. In many patients with pure AR or with combined AS and AR, the carotid arterial pulse is bisferiens, i.e., with two systolic waves separated by a trough.

Auscultation   In patients with severe AR, the aortic valve closure sound is usually absent. An S₃ and systolic ejection sound are frequently audible, and occasionally, an S₄ also may be heard. The murmur of AR is typically a high-pitched, blowing, decrescendo diastolic murmur, heard best in the third intercostal space along the left sternal border (see Fig. 225-4). In patients with mild AR, this murmur is brief, but as the severity increases, generally becomes louder and longer, indeed holodiastolic. When the murmur is soft, it can be heard best with the diaphragm of the stethoscope and with the patient sitting up, leaning forward, and with the breath held in forced expiration. In patients in whom the AR is caused by primary valvular disease, the diastolic murmur is usually louder along the left than the right sternal border. However, when the murmur is heard best along the right sternal border, it suggests that the AR is caused by aneurysmal dilatation of the aortic root. "Cooing" or musical diastolic murmurs suggest eversion of an aortic cusp vibrating in the regurgitant stream. Unless it is trivial in magnitude, the AR is usually accompanied by peripheral signs such as a widened pulse pressure or a collapsing pulse. By contrast, with the Graham Steell murmur of pulmonary regurgitation, which may be confused with the diastolic murmur of AR, there usually is clinical evidence of severe pulmonary hypertension, including a loud and palpable pulmonary component of the S_2.

A midsystolic ejection murmur is frequently audible in AR. It is generally heard best at the base of the heart and is transmitted along the carotid vessels. This murmur may be quite loud without signifying aortic obstruction; it is often higher pitched, shorter, and less rasping in quality than the ejection systolic murmur heard in patients with predominant AS. A third murmur frequently heard in patients with severe AR is the Austin Flint murmur, a soft, low-pitched, rumbling middiastolic bruit. It is probably produced by the displacement of the anterior leaflet of the mitral valve by the AR stream but does not appear to be associated with hemodynamically significant mitral obstruction. Both the Austin Flint murmur and the rumbling diastolic murmur of MS are loudest at the apex, but the murmur of MS is usually accompanied by a loud S_1 and immediately follows the OS of the mitral valve, whereas the Austin Flint murmur is often shorter in duration than the murmur of MS; in patients with sinus rhythm the latter exhibits presystolic accentuation. The auscultatory features of AR are intensified by isometric exercise such as strenuous handgrip, which augments systemic resistance, and reduced by inhalation of amyl nitrite. A blowing holosystolic murmur at the apex, which is transmitted to the axilla, also may be heard in patients with AR who have marked LV dilatation and functional MR.

In acute, severe AR, the elevation of LV end-diastolic pressure may lead to early closure of the mitral valve, an associated middiastolic sound, a soft or absent S_1, a pulse pressure that is not particularly wide, and a soft, short diastolic murmur.

LABORATORY EXAMINATION **Electrocardiogram** In patients with mild AR, there may be no electrocardiographic abnormalities, but with severe, chronic AR, the electrocardiographic signs of LV hypertrophy become manifest (Chap. 226). In addition, these patients frequently exhibit ST-segment depression and T-wave inversion in leads I, aVL, V_5, and V_6 ("LV strain"). Left axis deviation and/or QRS prolongation denote diffuse myocardial disease, generally associated with patchy fibrosis, and usually signify a poor prognosis.

Roentgenogram In severe chronic AR, the apex is displaced downward and to the left in the frontal projection, and frequently the cardiac shadow extends below the left diaphragm. LV enlargement also may be apparent in the left anterior oblique and lateral projections, in which the LV is displaced posteriorly and encroaches on the spine. In patients in whom primary valvular disease is responsible for the AR, the ascending aorta and aortic knob may be moderately dilated. When AR is caused by primary disease of the aortic wall, aneurysmal dilatation of the aorta may be noted, and the aorta may fill the retrosternal space in the lateral view.

Echocardiogram Increased systolic excursion of the posterior left ventricular wall is evident; the extent and velocity of wall motion are normal or even supernormal, until myocardial contractility declines. A rapid, high-frequency fluttering of the anterior mitral leaflet produced by the impact of the regurgitant jet is a characteristic finding. The echocardiogram is also useful in determining the cause of AR, by detecting dilatation of the aortic annulus (**Plate I-3**). Thickening and failure of coaptation of the leaflets also may be noted. Color flow Doppler echocardiographic imaging is very sensitive in the detection of AR, and Doppler echocardiography is helpful in assessing its severity. Serial two-dimensional echocardiography is valuable in evaluating LV performance and in detecting progressive myocardial dysfunction.

Cardiac Catheterization and Angiography In addition to providing an accurate confirmation of the magnitude of regurgitation and the status of LV function, the condition of the coronary arterial bed may be evaluated preoperatively.

℞ **TREATMENT** Although operation constitutes the principal treatment of AR and should be carried out before the development of heart failure, the latter usually responds briefly to treatment with digitalis glycosides, salt restriction, diuretics, and vasodilators, espe-

cially ACE inhibitors. Digitalis also may be indicated in patients with severe regurgitation and dilated left ventricles without frank LV failure. Cardiac arrhythmias and infections are poorly tolerated in patients with free AR and must be treated promptly and vigorously. Although nitroglycerin and long-acting nitrates are not as helpful in relieving anginal pain as in patients with ischemic heart disease, they are worth a trial. Long-acting nifedipine has been found to delay the need for operation. Patients with syphilitic aortitis should receive a full course of penicillin therapy (Chap. 172).

Surgical Treatment In deciding on the advisability and proper timing of surgical treatment, two points should be kept in mind: (1) patients with chronic AR usually do not become symptomatic until after the development of myocardial dysfunction, and (2) surgical treatment often does not restore normal LV function. Therefore, in patients with severe AR, careful clinical follow-up and noninvasive testing with echocardiography at approximately 6-month intervals are necessary if operation is to be undertaken at the optimal time, i.e., *after* the onset of LV dysfunction but *prior* to the development of severe symptoms. Operation can be deferred as long as the patient both remains asymptomatic and retains normal LV function. In general, operation should be carried out even in asymptomatic patients with progressive LV dysfunction and an LVEF <55% or a LV end-systolic volume >55 mL/m². (The latter has been referred to as the "55/55 rule.")

AVR with a suitable mechanical or tissue prosthesis is generally necessary in patients with rheumatic AR and in many patients with other forms of regurgitation. Rarely, when a leaflet has been perforated during an episode of infective endocarditis or torn from its attachments to the aortic annulus, surgical repair may be possible. When AR is due to aneurysmal dilatation of the annulus and ascending aorta rather than to primary valvular involvement, it may be possible to reduce the regurgitation by narrowing the annulus or by excising a portion of the aortic root without replacing the valve. More frequently, however, regurgitation can be eliminated only by replacing the aortic valve, excising the dilated or aneurysmal ascending aorta responsible for the regurgitation, and replacing the latter with a graft. This formidable procedure entails a higher risk than isolated AVR.

As in patients with other valvular abnormalities, both the operative risk and the late mortality are largely dependent on the stage of the disease and on myocardial function at the time of operation. The overall operative mortality for isolated AVR is 4.3% (Table 236-1). However, patients with marked cardiac enlargement and prolonged LV dysfunction experience an operative mortality rate of approximately 10% and a late mortality rate of approximately 5% per year due to LV failure despite a technically satisfactory operation. Nonetheless, because of the very poor prognosis with medical management, even patients with LV failure should be considered for operation.

ACUTE AORTIC REGURGITATION Infective endocarditis, aortic dissection, and trauma are the most common causes of severe, acute AR. Since the LV has not had time to dilate in this condition, stroke volume declines and ventricular diastolic pressure rises markedly; the arterial pulse pressure is often not markedly widened, and the physical signs characteristic of severe chronic AR may be absent. Premature closure of the mitral valve is common and can be recognized by echocardiography. The S_1 is soft or absent; the aortic diastolic murmur is characteristically brief. Patients present with pulmonary congestion and edema, as well as hypotension secondary to a low cardiac output. Acute, severe AR requires prompt surgical treatment, which may be lifesaving.

TRICUSPID STENOSIS

TS, a relatively uncommon valvular lesion in North America and western Europe, is more common in tropical and subtropical climates, especially on the Indian subcontinent, and in Latin America. It is generally rheumatic in origin and is more common in women than in men. It does not occur as an isolated lesion but is usually associated with MS. Hemodynamically significant TS occurs in 5 to 10% of patients with severe MS; rheumatic TS is commonly associated with some degree of TR.

PATHOPHYSIOLOGY A diastolic pressure gradient between the RA and RV can be recorded with a double-lumen cardiac catheter. It is augmented when the transvalvular blood flow increases during inspiration and declines during expiration. A mean diastolic pressure gradient >4 mmHg is usually sufficient to elevate the mean RA pressure to levels that result in systemic venous congestion and, unless sodium intake has been restricted and diuretics administered, it is associated with ascites and edema, sometimes severe. In patients with sinus rhythm, the RA *a* wave may be extremely tall and may even approach the level of the RV systolic pressure. The resting CO is usually depressed and fails to rise during exercise. The low CO is responsible for the normal or only slightly elevated LA, PA, and RV systolic pressures despite the presence of MS.

SYMPTOMS Since the development of MS generally precedes that of TS, many patients initially have symptoms of pulmonary congestion. Amelioration of these symptoms should raise the possibility that TS may be developing. Characteristically, patients complain of relatively little dyspnea for the degree of hepatomegaly, ascites, and edema that they have. Fatigue secondary to a low cardiac output and discomfort due to refractory edema, ascites, and marked hepatomegaly are common in patients with TS and/or TR. In some patients, TS may be suspected for the first time when symptoms of RV failure persist after an adequate mitral valvulotomy.

PHYSICAL FINDINGS Since TS usually occurs in the presence of other obvious valvular disease, the diagnosis may be missed unless it is specifically considered and searched for. Severe TS is associated with marked hepatic congestion, often resulting in cirrhosis, jaundice, serious malnutrition, anasarca, and ascites. Congestive hepatomegaly and, in cases of severe tricuspid valve disease, splenomegaly are present. The jugular veins are distended, and in patients with sinus rhythm there may be giant *a* waves. The *v* waves are less conspicuous, and since tricuspid obstruction impedes RA emptying during diastole, there is a slow *y* descent. In patients with sinus rhythm there may be prominent presystolic pulsations of the enlarged liver as well.

On auscultation, the pulmonic valve closure sound is not accentuated, and occasionally, an OS of the tricuspid valve may be heard approximately 0.06 s after pulmonic valve closure. The diastolic murmur of TS has many of the qualities of the diastolic murmur of MS, and since TS almost always occurs in the presence of MS, the less common valvular lesion may be missed. However, the tricuspid murmur is generally heard best along the left lower sternal margin and over the xiphoid process and is most prominent during presystole in patients with sinus rhythm. The diastolic murmur is reduced in amplitude as the stethoscope is inched laterally, only to intensify or reappear as the mitral murmur at the apex. The murmur of TS is augmented during inspiration, and it is reduced during expiration and particularly during the strain of Valsalva maneuver, when tricuspid blood flow is reduced. This finding is often most easily elicited when the patient is in the erect position.

LABORATORY EXAMINATION The electrocardiographic features of RA enlargement (Chap. 226) include tall, peaked P waves in lead II, as well as prominent, upright P waves in lead V_1. The *absence* of electrocardiographic evidence of renovascular hypertension (RVH) in a patient with right-sided heart failure who is believed to have MS should suggest associated tricuspid valve disease. The chest roentgenogram in patients with combined TS and MS show particular prominence of the RA and superior vena cava without much enlargement of the PA and with less evidence of pulmonary vascular congestion than occurs in patients with isolated MS. On echocardiographic

examination, the tricuspid valve is usually thickened; the transvalvular gradient can be estimated by Doppler echocardiography.

℞ **TREATMENT** Patients with TS generally exhibit marked systemic venous congestion; intensive salt restriction and diuretic therapy are required during the preoperative period. Such a preparatory period may diminish hepatic congestion and thereby improve hepatic function sufficiently so that the risks of operation are diminished. Surgical relief of the TS should be carried out, preferably at the time of mitral valvotomy, in patients with moderate or severe TS who have mean diastolic pressure gradients exceeding approximately 4 mmHg and tricuspid orifices less than 1.5 to 2.0 cm². TS is almost always accompanied by significant TR. Open-heart repair may permit substantial improvement of tricuspid valve function. If this cannot be accomplished, the tricuspid valve may have to be replaced with a prosthesis, preferably a large bioprosthetic valve.

TRICUSPID REGURGITATION

Most commonly, TR is functional and secondary to marked dilatation of the RV and the tricuspid annulus. Functional TR may complicate RV enlargement of any cause, including inferior wall infarcts that involve the RV, and it is commonly seen in the late stages of heart failure due to rheumatic or congenital heart disease with severe pulmonary hypertension, as well as in ischemic heart disease, cardiomyopathy, and cor pulmonale. It is in part reversible if pulmonary hypertension is relieved. Rheumatic fever may produce organic TR, often associated with TS. Infarction of RV papillary muscles, tricuspid valve prolapse, carcinoid heart disease, endomyocardial fibrosis, infective endocarditis, and trauma all may produce TR. Less commonly, TR results from congenitally deformed tricuspid valves, and it occurs with defects of the atrioventricular canal as well as with Ebstein's malformation of the tricuspid valve (Chap. 234).

As is the case for TS, the clinical features of TR result primarily from systemic venous congestion and reduction of CO. With the onset of TR in patients with pulmonary hypertension, symptoms of pulmonary congestion diminish, but the clinical manifestations of right-sided heart failure become intensified. The neck veins are distended with prominent *v* waves; and marked hepatomegaly, ascites, pleural effusions, edema, systolic pulsations of the liver, and positive hepatojugular reflux are common. A prominent RV pulsation along the left parasternal region and a blowing holosystolic murmur along the lower left sternal margin, which may be intensified during inspiration and reduced during expiration or the strain of the Valsalva maneuver, are characteristic findings; AF is usually present.

The electrocardiogram usually shows changes characteristic of the lesion responsible for the enlargement of the RV that leads to TR. Roentgenographic examination usually reveals enlargement of both the RA and RV. Echocardiography may be helpful by demonstrating RV dilatation and prolapsing or flail tricuspid leaflets; the diagnosis of TR can be made by color flow Doppler echocardiography, and the severity estimated by Doppler examination. The latter is also useful in estimating PA pressure.

In patients with severe TR, the CO is usually markedly reduced, and the RA pressure pulse may exhibit no *x* descent during early systole but a prominent *c-v* wave with a rapid *y* descent. The mean RA and the RV end-diastolic pressures are often elevated.

℞ **TREATMENT** Isolated TR, in the absence of pulmonary hypertension, such as that occurring as a consequence of infective endocarditis or trauma, is usually well tolerated and does not require operation. Indeed, even total excision of an infected tricuspid valve is often well tolerated if the PA pressure is normal. Treatment of the underlying cause of heart failure usually reduces the severity of functional TR. In patients with mitral valve disease and TR secondary to pulmonary hypertension and massive RV enlargement, effective surgical correction of the mitral valvular abnormality results in lowering of the PA pressures and gradual reduction or disappearance of the TR without direct treatment of the tricuspid valve. However, recovery may be much more rapid in patients with severe secondary TR if, at the time of mitral valve surgery, tricuspid annuloplasty (generally with the insertion of a plastic ring), open tricuspid valve repair, or, in the rare instance of severe organic tricuspid valve disease, tricuspid valve replacement is performed. Surgical treatment of the TR also should be carried out in patients with severe regurgitation secondary to deformity of the tricuspid valve due to rheumatic fever, particularly those *without* severe pulmonary hypertension.

PULMONIC VALVE DISEASE

The pulmonic valve is affected by rheumatic fever far less frequently than are the other valves, and it is uncommonly the seat of infective endocarditis. The most common *acquired* abnormality affecting the pulmonic valve is regurgitation secondary to dilatation of the pulmonic valve ring as a consequence of severe pulmonary hypertension. This produces the Graham Steell murmur, a high-pitched, decrescendo, diastolic blowing murmur along the left sternal border, which is difficult to differentiate from the far more common murmur produced by AR. It is usually of little hemodynamic significance; indeed, surgical removal or destruction of the pulmonic valve by infective endocarditis does not produce heart failure unless serious pulmonary hypertension is also present. The *carcinoid syndrome* may cause pulmonic stenosis and/or regurgitation. →*Congenital pulmonic stenosis is discussed in Chap. 234.*

VALVE REPLACEMENT

The results of replacement of any valve are dependent primarily on (1) the patient's myocardial function and general medical condition at the time of operation, (2) the technical abilities of the operative team and the quality of the postoperative care, and (3) the durability, hemodynamic characteristics, and thrombogenicity of the prosthesis. Increased operative mortality is associated with the higher levels of preoperative functional disability and pulmonary hypertension. Late complications of replacement of any valve, which are declining in incidence, include paravalvular leakage, thromboemboli, bleeding due to anticoagulants, mechanical dysfunction of the prosthesis, and infective endocarditis.

The considerations involved in the choice between a bioprosthetic (tissue) and artificial mechanical valve are similar in the mitral and aortic positions and in the treatment of stenotic, regurgitant, or mixed lesions. All patients who have undergone replacement of any valve with a mechanical prosthesis must be maintained permanently on anticoagulants, but this treatment imposes a hazard of hemorrhage. The primary advantage of bioprostheses over mechanical prostheses is the reduction of thromboembolic complications; and except for patients with chronic AF, few such instances have been associated with their use. The major disadvantage of bioprosthetic valves is their mechanical deterioration, the incidence of which is inversely proportional with age. This results in the need to replace the prosthesis in 30% of patients by 10 years and in 50% by 15 years. Bioprostheses are ordinarily not used in younger patients (<35 years) because of accelerated deterioration but are particularly useful in the elderly (>70 years), in whom there is more concern about chronic anticoagulation than about long-term (>15 years) valve durability. These valves are also indicated in women who expect to become pregnant, as well as others in whom anticoagulation may be contraindicated. Alternative bioprostheses are homograft (allograft) aortic valves obtained from cadavers and cryopreserved, pericardial autografts as well as pulmonary autograft transplanted into the aortic position. In patients without contraindications to anticoagulants, particularly those under 65 years, a mechanical prosthesis may be preferable. Many surgeons now select the St. Jude prosthesis, a double-disk tilting prosthesis, for replacement of both aortic and mitral valves because of somewhat more favorable hemodynamic characteristics and a suggestion of lower thrombogenicity.

BIBLIOGRAPHY

BONOW RO et al: ACC/AHA Guidelines for the management of patients with valvular heart disease. J Am Coll Cardiol 32:1486, 1998

BRAUNWALD E: Valvular heart disease, in *Heart Disease*, 6th ed, E Braunwald, D Zipes, P Libby (eds). Philadelphia, Saunders, 2001

BYRNE JG et al: Repair versus replacement of mitral valve for treating severe ischemic mitral regurgitation. Coron Artery Dis 11:31, 2000

CANNEGIETER SC et al: Oral anticoagulant treatment in patients with mechanical heart valves: How to reduce the risk of thromboembolic and bleeding complications. J Intern Med 245:369, 1999

CARABELLO BA, CRAWFORD FA: Valvular heart disease. N Engl J Med 337:32, 1997

HA JW et al: Tricuspid stenosis and regurgitation: Doppler and color flow echocardiography and cardiac catheterization findings. Clin Cardiol 23:51, 2000

JAMIESON WRE et al: Risk stratification for cardiac valve replacement. National Cardiac Surgery Database. Ann Thorac Surg 67:943, 1999

KIRKLIN JW, BARRATT-BOYES BG: Part III. Acquired valvular heart disease, in *Cardiac Surgery*, 2d ed, JW Kirklin, DG Barratt-Boyes (eds). New York, Wiley, 1993, p 425

KVIDAL P et al: Observed and relative survival after aortic valve replacement. J Am Coll Cardiol 35:747, 2000

OTTO CM (ed): *Valvular Heart Disease*. Philadelphia, Saunders, 1999, 468 pp

RAHIMTOOLA S (ed): *Valvular Heart Disease*, in *Atlas of Heart Diseases*, vol 11, E Braunwald (series ed). Philadelphia, Current Medicine, 1996

SENTHILNATHAN V et al: Heart valves: Which is the best choice? Cardiovasc Surg 7:393, 1999

VON SEGESSER LK et al: Less invasive aortic valve surgery: Rationale and technique. Eur J Cardiothorac Surg 15:781, 1999

237 Eugene Braunwald

COR PULMONALE

DEFINITIONS *Cor pulmonale* is defined as enlargement of the right ventricle (RV) secondary to abnormalities of the lungs, thorax, pulmonary ventilation, or circulation. It sometimes leads to RV failure, with an elevation of transmural RV end-diastolic pressure. Cor pulmonale and RV failure may be acute, as in pulmonary thromboembolism; or chronic, as in stable, severe chronic obstructive lung disease (COLD); or "acute on chronic," as in COLD with a superimposed infection and intensification of hypoxia. Approximately 20% of hospital admissions for heart failure are caused by RV failure associated with cor pulmonale. More than half of the patients with COLD have cor pulmonale, and this condition constitutes between 5 and 10% of all adult heart diseases in the United States. Cor pulmonale constitutes a higher percentage of all forms of heart disease in countries where the incidence of COLD is higher, such as the United Kingdom, and in areas such as Mexico City where air pollution is severe.

NORMAL FUNCTION OF THE PULMONARY CIRCULATION

The pulmonary circulation is interposed between the right and left ventricles for the purpose of gas exchange, the filtering out of particles, and the chemical modification of the blood, such as the conversion of angiotensin I to angiotensin II. Normally, flow through the pulmonary vascular bed depends not only on the pumping action of the RV but also on respiratory movements and on the filling and contraction of the left ventricle. Respiratory motion facilitates pulmonary blood flow by enhancing venous return into the thorax on inhalation; the positive pressure of exhalation then aids in propelling blood into the systemic vascular bed.

The stroke volume of the RV, as of the left, is regulated by its preload, contractility, and afterload (Chap. 231). Since the RV is a

Table 237-1   Cor Pulmonale

Mechanisms	Responses	Characteristics
PULMONARY VASCULAR DISEASES		
Emboli, large or multiple	Fall in cardiac output due to acute obstruction	Acute cor pulmonale Right ventricular distention Shock
Emboli, small; vasculitis; widespread lung damage (ARDS)	Pulmonary hypertension due to widespread hypoxia and microvascular obstruction	Subacute cor pulmonale Right ventricular distention Breathlessness and fever
Emboli, medium and recurrent; primary pulmonary hypertension; diet or drug vasopathy	Pulmonary hypertension due to vascular obstruction Low or normal cardiac output	Chronic cor pulmonale Right heart hypertrophy Breathlessness
RESPIRATORY DISEASES		
Obstructive Chronic bronchitis and emphysema; chronic asthma	Pulmonary hypertension due to hypoxia, vascular stretching, and loss of vessels Heart beat impeded externally by lung hyperinflation Normal or high output	Chronic cor pulmonale "Blue bloater" or "Pink puffer" (see Chap. 258)
Restrictive 1. Intrinsic: interstitial fibrosis, lung resection	Hypertension due to hypoxia, vascular distortion and loss Normal or low output	Chronic cor pulmonale Breathlessness Hyperventilation
2. Extrinsic: obesity, myxedema, muscle weakness, kyphoscoliosis, upper airway obstruction, diminished respiratory drive, high altitude	Hypertension due to alveolar hypoxia Normal or high output	Chronic cor pulmonale Peripheral edema Hypoventilation

NOTE: ARDS, acute respiratory distress syndrome.

relatively thin, compliant reservoir, acute changes in venous return (e.g., an increase with inhalation and decline with exhalation) can occur with little change in transmural RV pressure. However, the ability of the RV to increase its systolic pressure is limited. Normally, the RV afterload, which is closely related to the pulmonary artery pressure, is low. The pulmonary artery pressure normally rises slightly when blood is displaced into the chest at the start of exercise; on assuming recumbency; or with cold, anxiety, or pain. A driving pressure of only about 5 cmH$_2$O between the pulmonary artery (15 cmH$_2$O) and the left atrium (10 cmH$_2$O) normally propels the entire cardiac output of approximately 5 L/min at rest through the lungs, and only a modest increase in pressure is necessary to drive a flow of up to 25 L/min through the pulmonary capillary bed during maximal exercise.

The resistance of the pulmonary circulation (R), i.e., the pulmonary vascular resistance (Chap. 228), is calculated as the intravascular driving pressure (DP), i.e., pulmonary artery pressure minus pulmonary venous or left atrial pressure, divided by the pulmonary blood flow rate ($\dot{Q}$). The caliber of a distensible vessel depends on its transmural pressure. Calculated R increases when vessels collapse, narrow, or lengthen, or when the viscosity of the blood increases.

$$ R = \frac{Kl\mu}{r^4} $$

where K = constant; l = length; r = radius; and μ = viscosity. Calculated R decreases with increasing pulmonary blood flow because pulmonary vessels are distended and collapsed vessels are recruited.

PATHOPHYSIOLOGY   The severity of RV enlargement in cor pulmonale is a function of the increase in afterload. When the pulmonary vascular resistance is elevated and relatively fixed, as in pulmonary vascular or severe parenchymal lung disease, an elevation in cardiac output as occurs with physical exertion can elevate pulmonary artery pressure markedly. RV afterload may be augmented when the lungs are hyperinflated, as in COLD, due to the compression of the

alveolar capillaries and the lengthening of the pulmonary vessels. RV afterload can also increase when lung volume is reduced following extensive pulmonary resection, as well as in restrictive lung diseases in which pulmonary vessels are compressed and distorted. RV afterload rises with hypoxic pulmonary vasoconstriction caused by hypoxia or acidosis, which are important causes of pulmonary hypertension. Hypoxic vasoconstriction in regions of the lung affected by disease distributes blood flow to normally ventilated regions. Hypoxic vasoconstriction results from alveolar, rather than intravascular, hypoxia and is exaggerated by hypercapnia, probably because of the associated acidosis. When the hematocrit becomes markedly elevated with chronic hypoxemia (secondary polycythemia), the increase in blood viscosity can also aggravate the pulmonary hypertension. Chronic hypoxic pulmonary vasoconstriction may cause pulmonary vascular disease with endothelial swelling and medial hypertrophy (see below).

The elevation of RV afterload responsible for cor pulmonale is caused principally by pulmonary vascular or parenchymal disease. The principal syndromes and their pathophysiologic mechanisms are summarized in Table 237-1.

PULMONARY VASCULAR DISEASES

In these conditions the RV afterload is elevated as a consequence of restriction to pulmonary blood flow. In cor pulmonale secondary to pulmonary vascular disease, pulmonary hypertension is usually more severe than in pulmonary parenchymal disease. Chronic cor pulmonale secondary to pulmonary vascular disease may result from repeated pulmonary emboli, pulmonary vasculitis, pulmonary vasoconstriction secondary to high altitude, congenital heart disease with left-to-right shunting (e.g., atrial or ventricular septal defect, patent ductus arteriosus; Chap. 234), as well as pulmonary venoocclusive disease. When the cause of elevated pulmonary vascular resistance responsible for cor pulmonale cannot be defined, the condition is referred to as *primary pulmonary hypertension* (Chap. 260).

COR PULMONALE DUE TO PULMONARY EMBOLI   This condition is associated with two distinct syndromes.

Acute Cor Pulmonale   It has been estimated that in the United States about 50,000 people die each year from pulmonary thromboembolism (Chap. 261). Probably half die within the first hour from acute right heart failure due to massive or multiple emboli. A sudden, large embolic burden causes a low-output state resulting from the RV's inability to generate the pressure necessary to drive blood through the acutely compromised pulmonary vascular bed. Depression of cardiac output can also occur with a moderate-sized embolism if the pulmonary circulation has been critically compromised by previous pulmonary vascular or parenchymal disease. The RV begins to fail when systolic pressure is forced to double acutely, i.e., to exceed approximately 50 mmHg. Acute RV failure secondary to pulmonary embolism is suggested by the history of the sudden onset of severe dyspnea and cardiovascular collapse in a patient with, or predisposed to, venous thrombosis.

Clinical manifestations   Acute RV failure causes pallor, sweating, hypotension, and a rapid pulse of small amplitude. The neck veins are distended and often exhibit prominent *v* waves secondary to tricuspid regurgitation. The liver may be pulsatile, distended, and tender. A systolic murmur of tricuspid regurgitation along the left sternal border may be accompanied by a presystolic (S₄) gallop sound. Arterial blood gas frequently shows reduced Pa_{O_2} due to ventilation/perfusion mismatching and a low Pa_{CO_2} due to hyperventilation.

℞ **TREATMENT** If the cardiac output remains adequate to sustain the patient during the critical first 2 or 3 h, endogenous thrombolysis usually results in fragmentation of the clot and the pulmonary artery pressure returns to normal rapidly. Although it has been shown that treatment with thrombolytic agents lyses clots more rapidly than does heparin (Chap. 261), this therapy is probably indicated only when cardiac output is critically reduced and the RV fails. In acute cor pulmonale [and in RV failure due to acute RV infarction (Chap. 243)], an increase in RV preload can be achieved by a cautious expansion of blood volume, which helps to maintain cardiac output. When hypoxic pulmonary vasoconstriction contributes to pulmonary hypertension, inhalation of 100% O_2 reduces RV afterload.

Chronic Cor Pulmonale Secondary to Pulmonary Vascular Disease In contrast to acute, massive thromboembolism, when the elevation in pulmonary vascular resistance and the RV hypertrophy develop gradually, higher pulmonary vascular pressures, sometimes even approaching systemic arterial levels, may be generated. Chronic cor pulmonale can be caused by recurrent, medium-sized emboli that fail to lyse, but organize, resulting in chronic thromboembolic pulmonary hypertension. Particles from intravenous drug abuse, parasites, or tumor tissue that embolizes into the pulmonary vascular bed may also cause persistent pulmonary hypertension. Chronic cor pulmonale can also be caused by *primary pulmonary hypertension* (Chap. 260) or any chronic widespread vasculitis, such as occurs in association with collagen vascular disorders and that may affect the pulmonary vascular bed, particularly the CREST syndrome (Chap. 313).

Clinical Manifestations Dyspnea and tachypnea are characteristic features of pulmonary hypertension secondary to pulmonary vascular disease. They may be distressing during mild exertion or even at rest and are *not* relieved by sitting upright. An unproductive cough is another frequent complaint. Anterior chest pain, due to acute dilation of the root of the pulmonary artery or RV ischemia, can occur. The elevation in systemic venous pressure can cause hepatomegaly and ankle edema.

Occasionally there is cyanosis due to arterial hypoxemia and low cardiac output. A RV heave may be palpable along the left sternal border or in the epigastrium, and a high-pitched pulmonary ejection click may be audible to the left of the upper sternum. The second (pulmonary) component of the second heart sound is intensified and may be palpable; fixed narrow splitting of the second heart sound and a right ventricular protodiastolic gallop (S₃) that may increase during inspiration can be present. A systolic murmur of tricuspid regurgitation, which is augmented by inspiration, is often audible; occasionally, a diastolic murmur of pulmonary regurgitation is also heard. Prominent *a* (and sometimes also *v*) waves in the jugular venous pulse are evident. The onset of RV failure is reflected by an increase of venous pressure, the development of larger *v* waves associated with increasing tricuspid regurgitation, a positive hepatojugular reflux, and a gallop rhythm with both third and fourth heart sounds. These physical findings of RV failure can disappear rapidly when pulmonary artery pressure is reduced by relief of hypoxemia.

Hypocapnia due to alveolar hyperventilation is an important feature of chronic pulmonary hypertension secondary to pulmonary vascular disease. Usually there are no abnormalities on spirometry, but the ratio of dead space to tidal volume may be high, particularly when large-vessel obstruction is present. The diffusing capacity of the lung is reduced when the pulmonary vascular disease is associated with a capillary vasculitis and/or loss of capillary blood volume. Typically,

exertion causes a marked fall in Pa_{O_2}. The assessment of exercise capacity may be a useful way of following changes in the severity of pulmonary vascular disease in patients with chronic cor pulmonale, because exercise ability is limited by cardiac output and the latter, in turn, by the severity of the pulmonary vascular obstruction.

Laboratory Examination On *radiologic examination* the pulmonary trunk and hilar vessels are enlarged, as is the descending right pulmonary artery. Ventilation and perfusion lung scans and systemic venography showing deep vein thrombosis in the lower extremities are helpful in confirming the diagnosis of embolic pulmonary vascular disease. In the presence of severe pulmonary hypertension, the *electrocardiogram* (ECG) shows P pulmonale, right axis deviation, and RV hypertrophy (Chap. 226).

Echocardiography allows measurement of the thickness of the RV wall and may show enlargement of the RV cavity in relation to the left. The interventricular septum may be displaced leftward and may move paradoxically during the cardiac cycle. Pulmonary artery and RV systolic pressure can be estimated from measurement of the peak tricuspid regurgitant flow and pulmonic regurgitant flow with Doppler echocardiography.

Magnetic resonance imaging is useful for measuring RV mass, wall thickness, cavity volume, and ejection fraction.

Failure of the RV ejection fraction (measured by radionuclide ventriculography) to increase on exercise is a good indicator of pulmonary hypertension and/or intrinsic RV dysfunction. *Myocardial perfusion scintigraphy* with thallium 201 or sestamibi is also useful in diagnosing cor pulmonale, since the hypertrophied RV is visualized by these radionuclides. (Normally the RV is not imaged by these radionuclides because of the much greater uptake by the left ventricle.)

Cardiac catheterization provides precise measurement of pulmonary vascular pressures, calculation of pulmonary vascular resistance, and their responses to oxygen and vasodilators. Catheterization is sometimes helpful in patients with cor pulmonale to exclude congenital and left heart diseases, and it allows pulmonary angiography to be carried out to confirm the nature of the pulmonary vascular obstruction. Measurements of pulmonary vascular pressure and flow during exercise may reveal abnormal pressure increments of pulmonary artery systolic and diastolic and RV diastolic pressures and an inadequate responses of cardiac output.

Lung biopsy can be useful in demonstrating vasculitis in some types of pulmonary vascular disease such as the collagen vascular diseases, rheumatoid arthritis, and Wegener's granulomatosis.

PARENCHYMAL PULMONARY DISEASES

The pathogenesis of cor pulmonale in patients with chronic parenchymal pulmonary disease is shown in Fig. 237-1. Cor pulmonale may be caused by both obstructive and restrictive lung diseases, more frequently the former. In these conditions there are usually only modest elevations of pulmonary artery pressure. The development of cor pulmonale confers a poor prognosis on patients with respiratory disease, not because RV failure cannot be treated, but because it reflects the seriousness of the underlying pulmonary disease.

CHRONIC OBSTRUCTIVE LUNG DISEASE (See also Chap. 258) This is the most common cause of chronic cor pulmonale. The enlargement of the RV is attributed to the mild-to-moderate pulmonary hypertension that is common in severe obstructive bronchitis and emphysema. Pulmonary artery systolic pressure is typically in the range of 50 to 60 mmHg, far below the systemic levels that may occur in patients with congenital heart disease and in those with primary pulmonary hypertension. Patients with cor pulmonale due to COLD usually have an advanced form of the disease with $FEV_1 <$ 1.0 L and $Pa_{O_2} <$ 60 mmHg (Chap. 250). RV failure secondary to COLD often occurs when there is "acute-on-chronic" respiratory failure with intensification of hypoxemia.

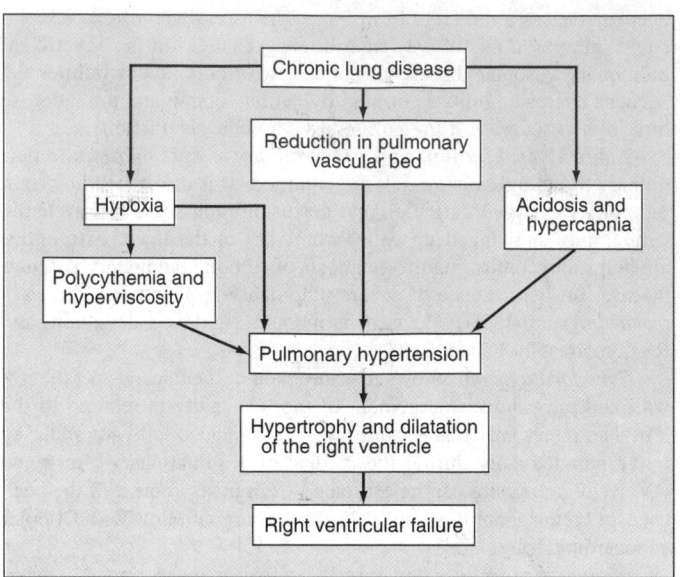

```
          ┌─────────────────────────┐
          │  Chronic lung disease   │
          └─────────────────────────┘
          ┌─────────────────────────┐
          │ Reduction in pulmonary  │
          │     vascular bed        │
          └─────────────────────────┘
 ┌──────────┐                    ┌──────────────┐
 │ Hypoxia  │                    │ Acidosis and │
 └──────────┘                    │ hypercapnia  │
                                 └──────────────┘
 ┌───────────────┐
 │ Polycythemia  │
 │and hyperviscosity│
 └───────────────┘
          ┌─────────────────────────┐
          │ Pulmonary hypertension  │
          └─────────────────────────┘
          ┌─────────────────────────┐
          │ Hypertrophy and dilatation │
          │   of the right ventricle  │
          └─────────────────────────┘
          ┌─────────────────────────┐
          │ Right ventricular failure │
          └─────────────────────────┘
```

FIGURE 237-1 Pathogenesis of cor pulmonale. *[Reproduced with permission from WR Summer, in LJ Rubin (ed): Pulmonary Heart Disease. Boston, Martinus Nijhoff, 1984, p 285.]*

Pulmonary hypertension in COLD is caused by one or more of the following:

1. Pulmonary vasoconstriction secondary to alveolar hypoxia, acidemia, and hypercapnia. When these vasoconstrictor stimuli persist, medial thickening of the smaller muscular arteries develops by the mechanical effects of the high lung volume on the pulmonary vessels.
2. The loss of small vessels in the vascular bed in regions of emphysema and lung destruction.
3. The increased cardiac output and blood viscosity caused by polycythemia secondary to hypoxia.

Of these causes, hypoxia is the most important. Pulmonary artery pressure rises further on exercise and often falls acutely on inspiration of 100% O_2. Cardiac output tends to be high in the absence of heart failure if hypoxia and hypercapnia are present. Because of the importance of hypoxic pulmonary vasoconstriction in causing pulmonary hypertension, the hypoventilating "blue bloater" with alveolar hypoxia and hypercapnia more frequently suffers from pulmonary hypertension and consequent cor pulmonale than does the emphysematous "pink puffer" without alveolar hypoxia. Ischemic left ventricular dysfunction is a frequent accompaniment since patients with cor pulmonale secondary to COLD usually have a history of heavy cigarette smoking, a major risk factor for ischemic heart disease. The elevation of pulmonary artery pressure may be secondary, in part, to the increase in left atrial pressure resulting from left heart dysfunction. Almost half of all patients who die with cor pulmonale due to COLD also have left ventricular hypertrophy on postmortem examination.

Right ventricular failure often complicates cor pulmonale when patients with COLD develop ventilatory failure and/or a superimposed acute respiratory infection with hypoxia and hypercapnia, and worsening of pulmonary hypertension. Both supraventricular and ventricular arrhythmias may occur. The liver is engorged, tender, and displaced downward by the low diaphragm; a hepatojugular reflux may be present.

An exacerbation of airway obstruction elevates intrathoracic pressure, which impedes venous return, raises jugular venous pressure, and may cause peripheral edema. The venous hypertension due to airflow obstruction declines, sometimes very rapidly, with relief of the obstruction.

Pathology The RV hypertrophies progressively in COLD. The main pulmonary arteries are enlarged, and the muscular pulmonary arteries show prominent longitudinal muscle, fibrosis, and elastic changes that continue into the arterioles, where the media becomes muscularized. The small vessels and capillaries are distorted or disappear in regions of lung hyperinflation.

Clinical Manifestations A history of a productive cough and dyspnea, perhaps with wheezing, is frequently elicited. Breathlessness limits the patient's ability in the minor stresses of daily living. Frequently there is a history of emergency hospital admissions because of respiratory infection, sometimes necessitating mechanical ventilation. In breathing oxygen, there may be increasing somnolence or other symptoms of hypercapnia such as recurring headaches, confusion, and even vomiting which, when combined with blurred optic discs (also due to cerebral vasodilation), constitutes the "pseudo tumor cerebri" syndrome. Hypoxia due to hypoventilation is usually worse at night.

Physical findings Often there is nicotine staining of the fingers, a tell-tale sign reflecting many years of heavy cigarette smoking. The skin may be warm and the arterial pulse bounding in the high cardiac output state induced by hypoxia and hypercapnia. The distention of the chest due to the airflow obstruction and the presence of rhonchi and wheezes secondary to chronic bronchitis usually make cardiac auscultation difficult. A right-sided protodiastolic gallop sound (S_3) and a systolic murmur of tricuspid regurgitant may be audible. Signs of right heart failure are, as discussed above, difficult to separate from those due to severe airflow obstruction. Peripheral edema may worsen with elevation of systemic venous pressure when atrial fibrillation occurs or when pulmonary infection supervenes. A positive hepatojugular reflux suports the diagnosis of RV failure.

Laboratory Examination *Pulmonary function studies* show marked airflow obstruction with hypoxemia and hypercapnia. Exercise is limited by ventilatory rather than cardiac dysfunction until RV failure develops. The *chest roentgenogram* reveals hyperinflation, which makes the degree of right heart enlargement difficult to assess. The central pulmonary arteries are large, but at the periphery the vessels are narrowed and disappear, particularly in regions of the lungs that are markedly emphysematous. The ECG is relatively insensitive in demonstrating right heart enlargement because the enlarged lungs are poor electrical conductors and the inspiratory position of the chest is associated with a vertically positioned heart. Arrhythmias, particularly atrial fibrillation and multifocal atrial tachycardia, are common.

Echocardiographic imaging is often difficult because of the air in the distended lungs but usually reveals an increased cross-section of the right ventricular cavity, abnormal thickening of the RV wall, and pulmonary hypertension. Myocardial perfusion scintigraphy shows an abnormally high ratio of right-to-left ventricular uptake.

Right heart catheterization can be carried out at the bedside with a balloon-tipped, flow-directed, multilumen catheter fitted with thermocouples for measuring cardiac output by thermodilution (Chap. 228). The pulmonary artery wedge pressure is usually normal at rest in patients with uncomplicated cor pulmonale. Cardiac catheterization may be useful in assessing the severity of the pulmonary hypertension and its response to respiring oxygen.

℞ TREATMENT First, medical management of the acute and/or chronic lung disease must be optimal (Chaps. 258 and 265). Acute respiratory infection, often the precipitant of RV failure, must be treated promptly and vigorously. Alveolar hypoxia at rest and during exertion and sleep should be corrected by improving alveolar ventilation through relieving the airflow obstruction and by judiciously increasing the inspired O_2 concentration. Long-term O_2 therapy is helpful in patients with severe COLD and reduces pulmonary artery pressure and pulmonary vascular resistance. When the lung disease improves and pulmonary vasoconstriction secondary to the alveolar hypoxia and hypercapnia are corrected, tachypnea and the signs attributed to right heart failure are relieved. Bronchodilators and antibiotics lessen airflow obstruction, and diuretics relieve the edema. Loop diuretics must be used with care since they may cause a metabolic alkalosis and thereby blunt the respiratory drive. Digitalis should be used cautiously in the presence of overt RV failure, and small phlebotomies should be considered when the hematocrit exceeds 55 to 60%. Inhalation of nitric oxide and infusion of prostacyclin are undergoing evaluation as agents to reduce pulmonary hypertension.

The prognosis in cor pulmonale depends on that of the underlying pulmonary disease.

RESTRICTIVE LUNG DISEASES (See also Chap. 259) Cor pulmonale in a variety of restrictive disorders of the lung is often associated with obliteration of the pulmonary vascular bed by lung destruction and fibrosis. Treatment of the underlying disorder and management of RV failure, as described above, are indicated.

DISORDERS OF VENTILATION A variety of disorders of the neuromuscular apparatus, diaphragm, and chest wall cause pulmonary hypertension and cor pulmonale secondary to chronic hypoxia and/or compression of pulmonary vessels. Disorders of ventilatory control, including the sleep apnea syndrome, and upper airways obstruction may be responsible for chronic hypoxia, secondary pulmonary hypertension, cor pulmonale, and eventual RV failure. Management consists of treating the underlying disorder, as discussed in Chaps. 263 and 264; the inhalation of oxygen; and the management of RV failure with diuretics and digoxin.

CHRONIC MOUNTAIN SICKNESS (MONGE'S DISEASE) Residents at high altitudes with chronic hypoxia and secondary polycythemia may develop pulmonary hypertension and cor pulmonale. Psychiatric symptoms—confusion and loss of mental acuity—are common features. Descent to a lower altitude and/or cautious phlebotomy result in lowering of pulmonary artery pressure and relief of symptoms.

BIBLIOGRAPHY

HARALDSSON A et al: Comparison of inhaled nitric oxide and inhaled aerosolized prostacyclin in the evaluation of heart transplant candidates with elevated pulmonary vascular resistance. Chest 114:780, 1998

INCALZI RA et al: Electrocardiographic signs of cor pulmonale: A negative prognostic finding in chronic obstructive pulmonary disease. Circulation 99:1600, 1999

JAIN D, ZARET BJ: Assessment of right ventricular function. Role of nuclear imaging techniques. Cardiol Clin 10:23, 1992

LOH E: Cor pulmonale, in *Cardiopulmonary Diseases and Cardiac Tumors*, S Goldhaber (ed), in *Atlas of Heart Diseases*, vol 3, E Braunwald (series ed). Philadelphia, Current Medicine, 1995, pp 1.1–1.24

MACNEE W: Pathophysiology of cor pulmonale in chronic obstructive pulmonary disease. Am J Respir Crit Care Med 150:833, 1994

RAPAPORT E: Cor pulmonale, in *Textbooks of Respiratory Medicine*, JF Murray, JA Nadel (eds). Philadelphia, Saunders, 2000

RICH S: Cor pulmonale, in *Heart Disease*, 6th ed, E Braunwald (ed). Philadelphia, Saunders, 2001

TUTAR E et al: Echocardiographic evaluation of left ventricular diastolic function in chronic cor pulmonale. Am J Cardiol 83:1414, 1999

VIZZA CD et al: Right and left ventricular dysfunction in patients with severe pulmonary disease. Chest 113:576, 1998

WEITZENBLUM E et al: Benefit from long-term O₂ therapy in chronic obstructive pulmonary disease patients. Respiration 59(Suppl I):14, 1992

——— et al: Pulmonary hemodynamics in patients with chronic obstructive pulmonary disease before and during an episode of peripheral edema. Chest 105:1377, 1994

238

Joshua Wynne, Eugene Braunwald

THE CARDIOMYOPATHIES AND MYOCARDITIDES

The cardiomyopathies are diseases that involve the myocardium directly and are not the result of hypertension or congenital, valvular, coronary, arterial, or pericardial abnormalities.* When the cardiomyopathies are classified on an etiologic basis, two fundamental forms are recognized: (1) a primary type, consisting of heart muscle disease of unknown cause; and (2) a secondary type, consisting of myocardial disease of known cause or associated with a disease involving other organ systems (Table 238-1). (In the World Health Organization classification, *specific cardiomyopathy* is used to describe heart muscle diseases associated with certain systemic or cardiac disorders; examples include hypertensive and metabolic cardiomyopathy.) In many cases, however, it is not possible to arrive at a specific etiologic diagnosis, and thus it is often more desirable to classify the cardiomyopathies on the basis of differences in their pathophysiology and clinical presentation (Tables 238-2 and 238-3).

DILATED CARDIOMYOPATHY

Left and/or right ventricular systolic pump function is impaired, leading to progressive cardiac enlargement, a process called *remodeling*, and often, but not invariably, producing symptoms of congestive heart failure. There is, however, no close correlation between the degree of contractile dysfunction and the severity of symptoms. Mural thrombi may be present, particularly in the left ventricular apex. Histologic examination reveals extensive areas of interstitial and perivascular fibrosis. Myocyte necrosis and cellular infiltration may be present but are not prominent.

Although no cause is apparent in many cases, dilated cardiomyopathy is probably the end result of myocardial damage produced by a variety of toxic, metabolic, or infectious agents. Dilated cardiomyopathy may be the late sequel of acute viral myocarditis, possibly mediated through an immunologic mechanism. Most commonly a disease of middle-aged men and more common in African Americans than in whites, it may occur in any patient population. The prevalence of this condition appears to be increasing. A reversible form of dilated cardiomyopathy may be found with alcohol abuse, pregnancy, selenium deficiency, hypophosphatemia, hypocalcemia, thyroid disease, cocaine use, and chronic uncontrolled tachycardia. Approximately 20% of patients have familial forms of the disease, with mutations of genes encoding myocardial structure proteins as well as transcription factors that control the expression of other myocyte genes. The disease is genetically heterogeneous; autosomal dominant, autosomal recessive, and X-linked transmission have been documented.

Right ventricular dysplasia is a unique cardiomyopathy marked by progressive replacement of the right ventricular wall with adipose tissue. Often associated with ventricular arrhythmias, the clinical course is variable, but sudden death is a constant threat. Catheter ablation of putative arrhythmia sites and insertion of an implantable cardioverter-defibrillator are often employed.

CLINICAL MANIFESTATIONS Symptoms of left- and right-sided congestive failure (Chap. 232), manifested by exertional

---

*Diffuse myocardial fibrosis secondary to multiple myocardial scars produced by extensive coronary arterial narrowing and occlusion can impair left ventricular function and is frequently referred to as *ischemic cardiomyopathy*. This is a colloquial use of the term, however, and should be avoided; the term *cardiomyopathy* should be restricted to a condition *primarily* involving heart muscle. In so-called ischemic cardiomyopathy the *primary* involvement is of the coronary vessels.

Table 238-1   Etiologic Classification of Cardiomyopathies

PRIMARY MYOCARDIAL INVOLVEMENT

Idiopathic (D,R,H)
Familial (D,R,H)
Eosinophilic endomyocardial disease (R)
Endomyocardial fibrosis (R)

SECONDARY MYOCARDIAL INVOLVEMENT

Infective (D)	Connective tissue disorders (D)
Viral myocarditis	Systemic lupus erythematosus
Bacterial myocarditis	Polyarteritis nodosa
Fungal myocarditis	Rheumatoid arthritis
Protozoal myocarditis	Progressive systemic sclerosis
Metazoal myocarditis	Dermatomyositis
Spirochetal	Infiltrations and granulomas (R,D)
Rickettsial	Amyloidosis
Metabolic (D)	Sarcoidosis
Familial storage disease (D,R)	Malignancy
Glycogen storage disease	Neuromuscular (D)
Mucopolysaccharidoses	Muscular dystrophy
Hemochromatosis	Myotonic dystrophy
Fabry's disease	Friedreich's ataxia (H,D)
Deficiency (D)	Sensitivity and toxic reactions (D)
Electrolytes	Alcohol
Nutritional	Radiation
	Drugs
	Peripartum heart disease (D)

NOTE: The principal clinical manifestation(s) of each etiologic grouping is denoted by D (dilated), R (restrictive), or H (hypertrophic) cardiomyopathy.
SOURCE: Adapted from the WHO/ISFC task force report on the definition and classification of cardiomyopathies, 1980.

dyspnea, fatigue, orthopnea, paroxysmal nocturnal dyspnea, peripheral edema, and palpitations, develop gradually in most patients. Some patients have left ventricular dilatation for months or even years before becoming symptomatic. Others develop symptoms after recovery from a viral infection. Although vague chest pain may be present, typical angina pectoris is unusual and suggests the presence of concomitant ischemic heart disease. Systemic embolism, stroke, and syncope may occur.

PHYSICAL EXAMINATION   Variable degrees of cardiac enlargement and findings of congestive heart failure are noted. In patients with advanced disease, the pulse pressure is narrow and the jugular venous pressure is elevated. Third and fourth heart sounds are common, and mitral or tricuspid regurgitation may occur.

LABORATORY EXAMINATIONS   The chest roentgenogram demonstrates enlargement of the cardiac silhouette due to left ventricular enlargement, although generalized cardiomegaly is often seen. The lung fields may demonstrate evidence of pulmonary venous hypertension and interstitial or alveolar edema. The electrocardiogram often shows sinus tachycardia or atrial fibrillation, ventricular arrhythmias, left atrial abnormality, diffuse nonspecific ST-T wave abnormalities, and sometimes intraventricular conduction defects and low voltage. Echocardiography and radionuclide ventriculography show left ventricular dilatation, with normal or minimally thickened or thinned walls, and systolic dysfunction (reduced ejection fraction).

Cardiac catheterization and coronary angiography are usually performed to exclude ischemic heart disease, although hemodynamic monitoring may occasionally be helpful in the management of the

Table 238-2   Clinical Classification of Cardiomyopathies

1. Dilated: Left and/or right ventricular enlargement, impaired systolic function, congestive heart failure, arrhythmias, emboli
2. Restrictive: Endomyocardial scarring or myocardial infiltration resulting in restriction to left and/or right ventricular filling
3. Hypertrophic: Disproportionate left ventricular hypertrophy, typically involving septum more than free wall, with or without an intraventricular systolic pressure gradient; usually of a nondilated left ventricular cavity

acutely decompensated patient. The left ventricular end-diastolic, left atrial, and pulmonary capillary wedge pressures are usually elevated; when failure of the right side of the heart supervenes, the right ventricular end-diastolic, right atrial, and central venous pressures also rise. Angiography reveals a dilated, diffusely hypokinetic left ventricle, often with some degree of mitral regurgitation; the coronary arteries are normal, thereby excluding so-called ischemic cardiomyopathy. Transvenous endomyocardial biopsy is usually not necessary in idiopathic or familial dilated cardiomyopathy, in which it reveals nonspecific findings of myocyte hypertrophy and fibrosis. However, it may be helpful in the recognition of secondary cardiomyopathies such as myocardial infiltration with amyloid and of acute myocarditis.

℞ TREATMENT   Most patients pursue an inexorably downhill course, and the majority, particularly those over 55 years of age, die within 3 years of the onset of symptoms. African Americans are more likely to suffer progressive heart failure and death than Caucasians. Spontaneous improvement or stabilization occurs in about a quarter of patients. Death is due to either congestive heart failure or ventricular tachy- or bradyarrhythmia; sudden death is a constant threat. Systemic embolization is a concern, and patients with heart failure secondary to cardiomyopathy should be considered for chronic anticoagulation. Standard therapy of heart failure with salt restriction, angiotensin-converting enzyme (ACE) inhibitors, diuretics, and digitalis produces symptomatic improvement (Chap. 232). An angiotensin II receptor blocker may be substituted in ACE-intolerant patients. Most ambulatory patients profit as well from the addition of a β-adrenergic blocker. Some patients with dilated cardiomyopathy who have biopsy evidence of myocardial inflammation have been treated with immunosuppressive therapy, but long-term evidence of efficacy is lacking. Alcohol should be avoided because of its cardiac toxic effects. Antiarrhythmic agents are best avoided for fear of proarrhythmic and other side effects, unless they are needed to treat symptomatic or serious arrhythmias. Insertion of an implantable cardioverter-defibrillator is useful in patients with malignant arrhythmias. In patients with advanced disease who are refractory to medical therapy, cardiac transplantation should be considered (Chap. 233).

ALCOHOLIC CARDIOMYOPATHY   Individuals who consume large quantities of alcohol over many years may develop a clinical picture identical to idiopathic dilated cardiomyopathy; indeed, alcoholic cardiomyopathy is the major form of secondary dilated cardiomyopathy in the western world. Ceasing alcohol consumption before severe heart failure has developed may halt the progression or even reverse the course of this disease, unlike the idiopathic variety, which is marked by progressive deterioration. Alcoholic patients with advanced heart failure have a poor prognosis, particularly if they continue to drink; fewer than one-quarter survive 3 years. The key to the treatment of alcoholic cardiomyopathy is total and permanent abstinence.

A second presentation of alcoholic cardiotoxicity may be found in individuals without overt heart failure and consists of recurrent supraventricular or ventricular tachyarrhythmias. Termed the *holiday heart syndrome*, it typically appears after a drinking binge; atrial fibrillation is seen most frequently, followed by atrial flutter and ventricular premature depolarizations. Other patients develop left ventricular hypertrophy, perhaps related to concomitant systemic hypertension; they may present with symptoms of pulmonary congestion due to abnormal diastolic stiffness (diminished compliance) of the left ventricle (Chap. 231).

PERIPARTUM CARDIOMYOPATHY (See Chap. 7)   Cardiac dilatation and congestive heart failure of unexplained cause may develop during the last trimester of pregnancy or within 6 months after delivery; most women develop symptoms in the month before or immediately after delivery. The cause of this disorder is unknown, but in some patients endomyocardial biopsy has shown evidence of a myocarditis. Necropsy shows cardiac enlargement, often with mural thrombi, along with histologic evidence of myocardial degeneration and fibrosis. The patient who develops peripartum cardiomyopathy typically is multiparous, African American, and over the age of 30, although the disease may be found in a wide spectrum of patients. The symptoms, signs, and treatment are similar to those in patients with idiopathic dilated cardiomyopathy. The mortality rate is quite variable but may be as high as 25 to 50%. The prognosis in these patients appears to be closely related to whether the heart size returns to normal after the first episode of congestive heart failure. If it does, subsequent pregnancies may sometimes be well tolerated; if the heart remains enlarged, however, further pregnancies frequently produce increasing myocardial damage, ultimately leading to refractory congestive heart failure and death. Those who recover should be encouraged to avoid further pregnancies, particularly if cardiomegaly persists.

NEUROMUSCULAR DISEASE (See also Chap. 381) Cardiac involvement is common in many of the muscular dystrophies. In *Duchenne's progressive muscular dystrophy*, mutations in a gene that encodes a cardiac structural protein called *dystrophin* lead to myocyte death. Myocardial involvement is most frequently indicated by a distinctive and unique electrocardiographic pattern consisting of tall R waves in right precordial leads with an R/S ratio greater than 1.0, often associated with deep Q waves in the limb and lateral precordial leads. These electrocardiographic abnormalities appear to result from selective transmural necrosis of the posterobasal left ventricle and associated papillary muscle. A variety of supraventricular and ventricular arrhythmias are frequently found. Rapidly progressive congestive heart failure may develop despite extended periods of apparent circulatory stability during which the only detectable abnormalities are in the electrocardiogram. *Myotonic dystrophy* is characterized by a variety of electrocardiographic abnormalities, especially disorders of impulse formation and conduction, but other overt clinical evidence of heart disease is uncommon. Because of these abnormalities, syncope and sudden death are major hazards; in appropriate patients, insertion of a permanent pacemaker may be effective. In *limb-girdle dystrophy* and *fascioscapulohumeral dystrophy*, cardiac involvement is uncommon and seldom severe, although arrhythmias and conduction disturbances may be seen on occasion. Involvement of the heart is very common in *Friedreich's ataxia* (manifested by abnormal electrocardiographic or echocardiographic findings), with as many as half the patients developing cardiac symptoms. The electrocardiogram most commonly demonstrates ST-segment and T-wave abnormalities. The echocardiogram may demonstrate left ventricular hypertrophy, with either symmetric or asymmetric hypertrophy of the left ventricular septum compared with the free wall. Although morphologically similar to some cases of hypertrophic cardiomyopathy, cellular disarray is lacking.

DRUGS A variety of pharmacologic agents may damage the myocardium acutely, producing a pattern of inflammation (myocarditis), or they may lead to chronic damage of the type seen with idiopathic dilated cardiomyopathy (Chap. 71). Certain drugs produce only electrocardiographic abnormalities, while others may precipitate fulminant congestive heart failure and death.

The anthracycline derivatives, particularly *doxorubicin* (Adriamycin), are powerful antineoplastic agents that, when given in high doses (more than 550 mg/m² for doxorubicin), may produce fatal heart failure. The incidence of heart failure is related not only to the dose of the drug but also to the presence or absence of several risk factors

Table 238-3   Laboratory Evaluation of the Cardiomyopathies

	Dilated	Restrictive	Hypertrophic
Chest roentgenogram	Moderate to marked cardiac silhouette enlargement Pulmonary venous hypertension	Mild cardiac silhouette enlargement	Mild to moderate cardiac silhouette enlargement
Electrocardiogram	ST-segment and T-wave abnormalities	Low voltage, conduction defects	ST-segment and T-wave abnormalities Left ventricular hypertrophy Abnormal Q waves
Echocardiogram	Left ventricular dilatation and dysfunction	Increased left ventricular wall thickness Normal or mildly reduced systolic function	Asymmetric septal hypertrophy (ASH) Systolic anterior motion (SAM) of the mitral valve
Radionuclide studies	Left ventricular dilatation and dysfunction (RVG)	Normal or mildly reduced systolic function (RVG)	Vigorous systolic function (RVG) Perfusion defect (^{201}Tl)
Cardiac catheterization	Left ventricular dilatation and dysfunction Elevated left- and often right-sided filling pressures Diminished cardiac output	Normal or mildly reduced systolic function Elevated left- and right-sided filling pressures	Vigorous systolic function Dynamic left ventricular outflow obstruction Elevated left- and right-sided filling pressures

NOTE: RVG, radionuclide ventriculogram; ^{201}Tl, thallium 201.

(cardiac irradiation, age >70 years, underlying heart disease, hypertension, treatment with cyclophosphamide); at any dose, patients with these risk factors have an eight- to tenfold greater frequency of developing heart failure than do patients lacking them. Radionuclide ventriculography and echocardiography, usually combined with exercise stress, may document preclinical deterioration of left ventricular function and allow appropriate dose adjustments; by so monitoring left ventricular function, it is often possible to continue doxorubicin even in patients at high risk for developing heart failure. Efforts to modify the dose schedule by giving the drug more slowly, along with the selective use of potentially cardioprotective agents such as the iron-chelator dexrazoxone, have further reduced the risk of cardiotoxicity. Some patients with congestive heart failure, even those with severe depression of left ventricular function, have demonstrated recovery of cardiac function with aggressive management with ACE inhibitors and diuretics. In others, late asymptomatic contractile dysfunction is common, even in those without initial cardiotoxicity. Children may demonstrate reduced myocardial hypertrophy and mass over time, presumably due to doxorubicin's inhibition of myocardial cell growth.

High-dose *cyclophosphamide* may produce congestive heart failure acutely or within 2 weeks of administration; a characteristic histopathologic feature is myocardial edema and hemorrhagic necrosis. Rarely, patients treated with *5-fluorouracil* will develop chest pain and electrocardiographic changes of myocardial ischemia or infarction. Electrocardiographic changes and arrhythmias may result from treatment with tricyclic antidepressants, the phenothiazines, emetine, lithium, and various aerosol propellants. *Cocaine abuse* is associated with a variety of life-threatening cardiac complications, including sudden death, myocarditis, dilated cardiomyopathy, and acute myocardial infarction (resulting from coronary spasm and/or thrombosis with or without underlying coronary artery stenosis). Nitrates and calcium channel blockers have been used to treat cocaine-induced cardiotoxicities; β-adrenergic blockers should be avoided.

HYPERTROPHIC CARDIOMYOPATHY

Hypertrophic cardiomyopathy (HCM) is characterized by left ventricular hypertrophy, typically of a nondilated chamber, without obvious cause such as hypertension or aortic stenosis. It is found in about 1 in 500 of the general population. Two features of HCM have attracted the greatest attention: (1) heterogeneous left ventricular hypertrophy, often with preferential hypertrophy of the interventricular septum resulting in asymmetric septal hypertrophy; and (2) a dynamic left ventricular outflow tract pressure gradient, related to a narrowing of the subaortic area as a consequence of the midsystolic apposition of the anterior mitral valve leaflet against the hypertrophied septum, i.e., systolic anterior motion (SAM) of the mitral valve. Initial studies of this disease emphasized the dynamic "obstructive" features, and it has been termed *idiopathic hypertrophic subaortic stenosis* and *hypertrophic obstructive cardiomyopathy*. It has become clear, however, that only about one-quarter of patients with HCM demonstrate an outflow tract pressure gradient. The ubiquitous pathophysiologic abnormality is not systolic but rather *diastolic* dysfunction (Chap. 231), characterized by increased stiffness of the hypertrophied muscle. This results in elevated diastolic filling pressures and is present despite a hyperdynamic left ventricle.

The pattern of hypertrophy is distinctive in HCM and differs from that seen in secondary hypertrophy (as in hypertension). Most patients have striking regional variations in the extent of hypertrophy in different portions of the left ventricle, and the majority demonstrate a ventricular septum whose thickness is disproportionately increased when compared with the free wall. Other patients may demonstrate disproportionate involvement of the apex or left ventricular free wall; 10% or more of patients have concentric involvement of the ventricle. A bizarre and disorganized arrangement of cardiac muscle cells in the septum occurs, with disorganization of the myofibrillar architecture, along with a variable degree of myocardial fibrosis and thickening of the small intramural coronary arteries. In some children, systolic compression of an intramyocardial segment of a coronary artery may lead to ischemia and death.

GENETIC CONSIDERATIONS   About half of all patients with HCM have a positive family history compatible with autosomal-dominant transmission, and more than 100 different mutations have been identified. About 40% of these are associated with mutations of the cardiac β-myosin heavy chain gene on chromosome 14, with certain mutations associated with more malignant prognoses. About 15% have a mutation of the cardiac troponin T gene on chromosome 1, 20% a mutation of myosin-binding protein C (chromosome 11), and about 5% a mutation of the α-tropomyosin gene. The remainder of familial cases are due to mutations of other genes such as the gene for troponin I. Echocardiographic studies have confirmed that about one-third of the first-degree relatives of patients with familial HCM have evidence of the disease, although in many of these patients the extent of hypertrophy is mild, no outflow tract pressure gradient is present, and symptoms are not prominent. Since the hypertrophic characteristics may not be apparent in childhood and often appear first in adolescence, a single normal echocardiogram in a child does not exclude the presence of the disease. Many sporadic cases of HCM probably represent spontaneous mutations. ■

HEMODYNAMICS   In contrast to the obstruction produced by a fixed narrowed orifice, such as valvular aortic stenosis, the pressure gradient in HCM, when present, is dynamic and may change between examinations and even from beat to beat. Obstruction appears to result from further narrowing of an already small left ventricular outflow tract by SAM of the mitral valve against the hypertrophied septum. While SAM is occasionally found in a variety of conditions besides HCM, it is *always* found when obstruction is present in HCM. Three basic mechanisms are involved in the production and intensification of the dynamic pressure gradient: (1) increased left ventricular contractility, (2) decreased ventricular volume (preload), and (3) decreased aortic impedance and pressure (afterload). Interventions that increase myocardial contractility, such as exercise, sympathomimetic amines, and digitalis glycosides, and those that reduce ventricular volume, such as the Valsalva maneuver, sudden standing, nitroglycerin, amyl nitrite, or tachycardia, may all cause an increase in the gradient and the mur-

mur. Conversely, elevation of arterial pressure by phenylephrine, squatting, sustained handgrip, augmentation of venous return by passive leg raising, and expansion of the blood volume all increase ventricular volume and ameliorate the gradient and murmur.

CLINICAL FEATURES   The clinical course of HCM is highly variable. Many patients are asymptomatic or mildly symptomatic and may be relatives of patients with known disease. Unfortunately, the first clinical manifestation of the disease may be sudden death, frequently occurring in children and young adults, often during or after physical exertion. In symptomatic patients, the most common complaint is dyspnea, largely due to increased stiffness of the left ventricular walls, which impairs ventricular filling and leads to elevated left ventricular diastolic and left atrial pressures. Other symptoms include angina pectoris, fatigue, syncope, and near-syncope ("graying-out spells"). Symptoms are not closely related to the presence or severity of an outflow pressure gradient. Most patients with gradients demonstrate a double or triple apical precordial impulse, a rapidly rising carotid arterial pulse, and a fourth heart sound. The hallmark of obstructive HCM is a systolic murmur, which is typically harsh, diamond-shaped, and usually begins well after the first heart sound, since ejection is unimpeded early in systole. The murmur is best heard at the lower left sternal border as well as at the apex, where it is often more holosystolic and blowing in quality, no doubt due to the mitral regurgitation that usually accompanies obstructive HCM.

LABORATORY EVALUATION   The *electrocardiogram* commonly shows left ventricular hypertrophy and widespread, deep, broad Q waves that suggest an old myocardial infarction. Many patients demonstrate arrhythmias, both atrial (supraventricular tachycardia or atrial fibrillation) and ventricular (ventricular tachycardia), during ambulatory (Holter) monitoring. *Chest roentgenography* may be normal, although a mild to moderate increase in the cardiac silhouette is common. The mainstay of the diagnosis of HCM is the *echocardiogram*, which demonstrates left ventricular hypertrophy, often with the septum 1.3 or more times the thickness of the high posterior left ventricular free wall. The septum may demonstrate an unusual "ground-glass" appearance, probably related to its abnormal cellular architecture and myocardial fibrosis. SAM of the mitral valve is found in patients with pressure gradients. The left ventricular cavity typically is small in HCM, with vigorous posterior wall motion but reduced septal excursion. A rare form of HCM, characterized by apical hypertrophy, is often associated with giant negative T waves on the electrocardiogram and a "spade-shaped" left ventricular cavity on angiography; it usually has a benign clinical course. *Radionuclide scintigraphy* with thallium 201 frequently reveals evidence of myocardial perfusion defects even in asymptomatic patients.

Although cardiac catheterization is not required to diagnose HCM, the two typical *hemodynamic* features are an elevated left ventricular diastolic pressure due to diminished left ventricular compliance and, when obstruction is present, a systolic pressure gradient between the body of the left ventricle and the subaortic region. When a gradient is not present, it can be induced in some patients by provocative maneuvers such as infusion of isoproterenol, inhalation of amyl nitrite, or the Valsalva maneuver.

TREATMENT   Since sudden death often occurs during or just after physical exertion, competitive sports and probably strenuous activity should be proscribed. Dehydration should be avoided, and diuretics should be used with caution. β-Adrenergic blockers are often used and ameliorate angina pectoris and syncope in one-third to one-half of patients. Resting intraventricular pressure gradients are usually unchanged, although these drugs may limit the increase in the gradient that occurs during exercise. It is not known whether β-adrenergic blockers offer any protection against sudden death. Amiodarone appears to be effective in reducing the frequency of supraventricular as well as life-threatening ventricular arrhythmias, and anecdotal data suggest that it may reduce the risk of sudden death. Verapamil and diltiazem may reduce the stiffness of the ventricle, reduce the elevated diastolic pressures, increase exercise tolerance, and, in some instances, reduce the severity of outflow tract pressure gradients, although adverse side effects occur in about one-quarter of patients. Nifedipine should be avoided. The combination of beta blockers and calcium antagonists should be used with caution. Disopyramide has been used in some patients to reduce left ventricular contractility and the outflow pressure gradient.

If atrial fibrillation occurs, a strenuous effort should be made to restore and then maintain sinus rhythm. Dual-chamber permanent pacing with a short PR interval has been reported to improve symptoms and reduce the outflow gradient in some patients with severe symptoms, presumably by altering the pattern of ventricular depolarization and contraction. Infarction of the interventricular septum induced by ethanol injections into the septal artery has also been reported to reduce obstruction. The insertion of an implantable cardioverter defibrillator should be considered in patients surviving cardiac arrest and those with high-risk ventricular tachyarrhythmias (Chap. 230). A surgical myotomy/myectomy of the hypertrophied septum may result in lasting symptomatic improvement in about three-quarters of severely symptomatic patients with large pressure gradients who are unresponsive to medical management. The effect of any of these therapies on the natural history is not clear. Digitalis, diuretics, nitrates, vasodilators, and β-adrenergic agonists are best avoided if possible, particularly in patients with known left ventricular outflow tract pressure gradients. Even social alcohol ingestion may produce sufficient vasodilatation to exacerbate an outflow pressure gradient.

First-degree relatives of patients with HCM should be screened by echocardiography.

PROGNOSIS The natural history of HCM is variable, although many patients never exhibit any clinical manifestations. Others demonstrate an improvement of symptoms with time. Atrial fibrillation is common late in the course of the disease; its onset may lead to an increase in symptoms, due to loss of the atrial contribution to filling of the thickened ventricle. Infective endocarditis occurs in fewer than 10% of patients, and endocarditis prophylaxis is indicated, particularly in patients with resting obstruction and mitral regurgitation. Progression of HCM to left ventricular dilatation and dysfunction without an outflow pressure gradient has been reported but is unusual; in about 5 to 10% of patients, however, some degree of left ventricular systolic impairment, wall thinning, and chamber enlargement occurs over time. The major cause of mortality in HCM is sudden death, which may occur in asymptomatic patients or interrupt an otherwise stable course in symptomatic ones. Predictors of sudden death include age less than 30 years, ventricular tachycardia on ambulatory monitoring, marked ventricular hypertrophy, syncope (especially in children), genetic mutations associated with an increased risk, and a family history of sudden death. There is no correlation between the risk of sudden death and the severity of symptoms or the presence or severity of an outflow tract pressure gradient.

RESTRICTIVE CARDIOMYOPATHY

The hallmark of the restrictive cardiomyopathies is abnormal diastolic function (Chap. 231); the ventricular walls are excessively rigid and impede ventricular filling. Myocardial fibrosis, hypertrophy, or infiltration due to a variety of causes is usually responsible. The infiltrative diseases, which represent important causes for secondary restrictive cardiomyopathy, may also show some impairment of systolic function. Myocardial involvement with *amyloid* is a common cause of secondary restrictive cardiomyopathy, although restriction is also seen in hemochromatosis, glycogen deposition, endomyocardial fibrosis, sarcoidosis, Fabry's disease, the eosinophilias, and scleroderma; in the transplanted heart and following mediastinal radiation; and in neoplastic infiltration and myocardial fibrosis of diverse causes. In many of these conditions, particularly those with substantial concomitant endocardial involvement, partial obliteration of the ventricular cavity by fibrous tissue and thrombus contributes to the abnormally increased

resistance to ventricular filling. Thromboembolic complications ensue in about a third of patients.

The inability of the ventricle to fill limits cardiac output and raises filling pressure. Therefore, exercise intolerance and dyspnea are usually the most prominent symptoms. As a result of persistently elevated venous pressure, these patients commonly have dependent edema, ascites, and an enlarged, tender, and often pulsatile liver. The jugular venous pressure is elevated and does not fall normally, or it may rise with inspiration (Kussmaul's sign). The heart sounds may be distant, and third and fourth heart sounds are common. In contrast to constrictive pericarditis, which the restrictive cardiomyopathies resemble in many respects, the apex impulse is usually easily palpable, and mitral regurgitation is more common. The electrocardiogram often shows low-voltage, nonspecific ST-T-wave changes and various arrhythmias. Pericardial calcification on x-ray, which would suggest constrictive pericarditis, is absent. Echocardiography typically reveals symmetrically thickened left ventricular walls and normal or slightly reduced ventricular volumes and systolic function. Doppler recordings demonstrate accentuated early diastolic filling. Cardiac catheterization shows a decreased cardiac output, elevation of the right and left ventricular end-diastolic pressures, and a dip-and-plateau configuration of the diastolic portion of the ventricular pressure pulse resembling that seen in constrictive pericarditis.

Differentiation from constrictive pericarditis may be challenging (Chap. 239). This distinction is of importance because the latter condition is potentially curable by operation. Helpful in the differentiation of these two diseases are right ventricular transvenous endomyocardial biopsy (by revealing myocardial infiltration or fibrosis in restrictive cardiomyopathy) and computed tomography or magnetic resonance imaging (by demonstrating a thickened pericardium in constrictive pericarditis). Treatment is usually disappointing, except for hemochromatosis (where desferoxamine has been helpful in reducing myocardial iron content). Chronic anticoagulation is often recommended to reduce the risk of embolization from the heart.

ENDOMYOCARDIAL FIBROSIS This is a progressive disease of unknown cause that occurs most commonly in children and young adults residing in tropical and subtropical Africa, particularly Uganda and Nigeria. Endomyocardial fibrosis is a frequent cause of heart failure in Africa, accounting for up to one-quarter of deaths due to heart disease. The condition is characterized by fibrous endocardial lesions of the inflow portion of the right or left ventricle (or both) and often involves the atrioventricular valves, producing valvular regurgitation. The apex of the ventricles may be obliterated by a mass of thrombus and fibrous tissue. In some ways this disease resembles eosinophilic endomyocardial disease (see below), although they occur in quite different geographic areas and age groups and generally are felt to be different diseases.

The clinical picture depends on which ventricle and atrioventricular valve show predominant involvement; left-sided involvement results in symptoms of pulmonary congestion, while predominant right-sided disease presents features of a restrictive cardiomyopathy. Medical treatment is often disappointing, and surgical excision of the fibrotic endocardium and replacement of the involved atrioventricular valve have led to substantial symptomatic improvement in some patients.

EOSINOPHILIC ENDOMYOCARDIAL DISEASE Also called *Loeffler's endocarditis* and *fibroplastic endocarditis*, this disease appears to be a subcategory of the hypereosinophilic syndrome in which the heart is predominantly involved, with cardiac damage the apparent result of the toxic effects of eosinophilic proteins. Typically, the endocardium of either or both ventricles thickens markedly, with involvement of the underlying myocardium. Large mural thrombi may develop in either ventricle, thereby compromising the size of the ventricular cavity and serving as a source of pulmonary and systemic emboli. Hepatosplenomegaly and localized eosinophilic infiltration of other organs are usually present. Management usually includes diuretics, afterload-reducing agents, and anticoagulation. The use of glucocorticoids and cytotoxic drugs (hydroxyurea in particular) appears to have improved survival substantially. Surgical treatment, as for endomyocardial fibrosis, may be helpful in selected patients.

DIFFERENTIAL DIAGNOSIS   Involvement of the heart is the most frequent cause of death in *primary amyloidosis* (Chap. 319), while clinically significant cardiac involvement is uncommon in the secondary form. Focal deposits of amyloid in elderly patients (*senile cardiac amyloidosis*) are common and usually clinically insignificant. Aspiration of abdominal fat or biopsy of the rectal mucosa, gingiva, liver, kidney, or myocardium permits the diagnosis to be made before death in over three-quarters of cases. The heart is firm, rubbery, and noncompliant, and four clinical presentations (alone or in combination) are seen: (1) diastolic dysfunction (restrictive cardiomyopathy), (2) systolic dysfunction, (3) arrhythmias and conduction disturbances, and (4) orthostatic hypotension. The two-dimensional echocardiogram may be helpful in making the diagnosis of amyloidosis and may show a thickened myocardial wall with a distinctive "speckled" appearance. Chemotherapy, often with alkylating agents, appears to have improved survival in specific cases, but the overall prognosis is poor.

Hemochromatosis (Chap. 345) is often the result of multiple transfusions or a hemoglobinopathy; the familial (autosomal recessive) form should be suspected if cardiomyopathy occurs in the setting of diabetes mellitus, hepatic cirrhosis, and increased skin pigmentation. The diagnosis may be confirmed by endomyocardial biopsy. Phlebotomy may be of some benefit if employed early in the course of the disease. Continuous subcutaneous administration of deferoxamine may reduce body iron stores and result in clinical improvement.

Myocardial *sarcoidosis* (Chap. 318) is generally associated with other manifestations of systemic disease and may cause restrictive as well as congestive features, since cardiac infiltration by sarcoid granulomas results not only in increased stiffness of the myocardium but also in diminished systolic contractile function. A variety of arrhythmias, including high-grade atrioventricular block, have been noted. A common cardiac manifestation of systemic sarcoidosis is right heart overload due to pulmonary artery hypertension as a result of parenchymal pulmonary involvement. The *carcinoid syndrome* results in endocardial fibrosis and stenosis and/or regurgitation of the tricuspid and/or pulmonary valve (Chap. 236); morphologically similar lesions have been seen with the use of the anorexic agents fenfluramine and phentermine.

MYOCARDITIDES

Myocarditis, i.e., cardiac inflammation, is most commonly the result of an infectious process. Myocarditis may also result from a hypersensitivity to drugs or may be caused by radiation, chemicals, or physical agents. In an unknown number of cases, acute myocarditis progresses to chronic dilated cardiomyopathy. While almost every infectious agent is capable of producing myocarditis (Table 238-1), clinically significant acute myocarditis in the United States is caused most commonly by viruses, especially coxsackievirus B. The clinical manifestations range from an asymptomatic state, with the presence of myocarditis inferred only by the finding of transient electrocardiographic ST-T-wave abnormalities, to a fulminant condition with arrhythmias, heart failure, and death. In some patients, myocarditis simulates acute myocardial infarction, with chest pain, electrocardiographic changes, and elevated serum levels of myocardial enzymes.

The physical examination is often normal, although more severe cases may show a muffled first heart sound, along with a third heart sound and a murmur of mitral regurgitation. A pericardial friction rub may be audible in patients with associated pericarditis.

Though viral myocarditis is most often self-limited and without sequelae, severe involvement may recur, and it is likely that acute viral myocarditis occasionally progresses to a chronic form and to dilated cardiomyopathy. Patients with viral myocarditis often give a history of a preceding upper respiratory febrile illness or a flulike syndrome, and viral nasopharyngitis or tonsillitis may be evident clinically. The isolation of virus from the stool, pharyngeal washings, or other body fluids and changes in specific antibody titers are helpful clinically. Endomyocardial biopsy, carried out early in the illness, may show round-cell infiltration and necrosis of adjacent myocytes.

Experimental studies suggest that exercise may be deleterious in patients with viral myocarditis, and strenuous activity should be proscribed until the electrocardiogram has returned to normal. Patients who develop congestive heart failure respond to the usual measures (ACE inhibitors, diuretics, and salt restriction), but they appear to be unusually sensitive to digitalis. Arrhythmias are common and are occasionally difficult to manage. Deaths attributed to heart failure, tachyarrhythmias, and heart block have been reported, and it seems prudent to monitor the electrocardiogram of patients with arrhythmias, especially during the acute illness.

HIV MYOCARDITIS   (See also Chap. 309)   Many HIV-infected patients have subclinical cardiac involvement, including pericardial effusion, right-sided chamber enlargement, and neoplastic involvement. Overt clinical involvement is seen in 10% of HIV patients, and the most common finding is left ventricular dysfunction that in some cases appears to be due to infiltration of the myocardium by the virus itself. In other patients, the heart is affected by any of the various opportunistic infections common in AIDS, such as toxoplasmosis, as well as by cardiac metastases in Kaposi's sarcoma. The clinical manifestations of cardiac involvement may be incorrectly attributed to concurrent noncardiac problems such as pneumonia. This is unfortunate, since the dilated cardiomyopathy of HIV infection may respond at least transiently to standard therapy with digitalis, diuretics, and ACE inhibitors.

BACTERIAL MYOCARDITIS   Bacterial involvement of the heart is uncommon, but when it does occur, it is usually as a complication of bacterial endocarditis (typically due to *Staphylococcus aureus* and enterococci). Myocardial abscess formation may involve the valve rings and interventricular septum. *Diphtheritic myocarditis* develops in over one-quarter of the patients with diphtheria, is one of the most serious complications, and is the most common cause of death (Chap. 141). Cardiac damage is due to the liberation of a toxin that inhibits protein synthesis and leads to a dilated, flabby, hypocontractile heart; the conducting system is frequently involved as well. Cardiomegaly and severe congestive heart failure typically appear after the first week of illness. Prompt therapy with antitoxin is crucial; antibiotic therapy is also indicated but is of less urgency.

CHAGAS' DISEASE   Chagas' disease, caused by the protozoan *Trypanosoma cruzi* and transmitted by an insect vector (Chap. 216), produces an extensive myocarditis that typically becomes evident years after the initial infection. It is one of the most common causes of heart disease encountered in Central and South America; in rural endemic areas 20 to 75% of the population may be affected. An increasing number of cases are found in the United States as patients migrate from endemic areas. Although only about 1% of infected individuals have an acute illness, which may include acute myocarditis, upwards of one-third develop chronic myocardial damage many years later. The chronic form is characterized by dilatation of several cardiac chambers, fibrosis and thinning of the ventricular wall, aneurysm formation (especially at the left ventricular apex), and mural thrombi. Chronic progressive heart failure is the rule and is associated with poor survival. The electrocardiogram is abnormal in most patients with cardiac involvement and typically shows right bundle branch block and left anterior hemiblock, which may progress to complete atrioventricular block. The *echocardiogram* may reveal a unique pattern of hypokinesis of the posterior left ventricular wall and relatively preserved septal motion. Ventricular arrhythmias are common and are seen especially during and after exertion; oral amiodarone appears to be particularly effective in treating ventricular tachyarrhythmias. The cause of death is either intractable congestive heart failure or an arrhythmia, with a minority of patients dying from embolic phenomena.

TREATMENT Therapy is directed toward amelioration of the congestive heart failure and arrhythmias; progressive conduction system disease and heart block may require implantation of a pacemaker. Anticoagulation (if feasible) may reduce the risk of thromboembolism. Medical therapy is often unsatisfactory or unavailable (especially in poor rural areas), however, and a more promising tactic in endemic areas has been the institution of public health measures, particularly the use of insecticides to eliminate the vector.

GIANT CELL MYOCARDITIS This rare myocarditis of unknown cause is characterized by the presence of multinucleated giant cells in the myocardium. It usually causes rapidly fatal congestive heart failure and arrhythmia in young to middle-aged adults. At necropsy, the distinctive features include cardiac enlargement, ventricular thrombi, grossly visible serpiginous areas of myocardial necrosis in both ventricles, and microscopic evidence of giant cells within an extensive inflammatory infiltrate. The cause of giant cell myocarditis remains obscure, although it occurs in association with thymoma, systemic lupus erythematosus, and thyrotoxicosis. While treatment with immunosuppressive therapy may help in some patients, cardiac transplantation is the treatment of choice.

LYME CARDITIS (See also Chap. 176) Lyme disease is caused by a tick-borne spirochete and is most common in the Northeast, upper Midwest, and Pacific Coastal regions of the United States during the summer months. About 10% of patients develop symptomatic cardiac involvement during the acute phase of the disease. Atrioventricular nodal conduction abnormalities are the most common manifestations of involvement, and may lead to syncope. Concomitant myopericarditis is not uncommon, and mild asymptomatic left ventricular dysfunction may occur. Intravenous ceftriaxone or penicillin is used in all but the mildest forms of Lyme carditis, in which case oral amoxicillin or doxycycline is employed. Hospitalization with electrocardiographic monitoring is indicated in patients with second- or third-degree atrioventricular block. A temporary pacemaker may be needed for symptomatic heart block; the utility of glucocorticoids in reversing heart block is uncertain, but they are usually employed. Long-term cardiac manifestations of Lyme disease are uncommon.

BIBLIOGRAPHY

BORGGREFE M, BREITHARDT G: Is the implantable defibrillator indicated in patients with hypertrophic cardiomyopathy and aborted sudden death? J Am Coll Cardiol 31: 1086, 1998

BRODSKY GL et al: Lamin A/C gene mutation associated with dilated cardiomyopathy with variable skeletal muscle involvement. Circulation 101:473, 2000

BROWN CS, BERTOLET BD: Peripartum cardiomyopathy: A comprehensive review. Am J Obstet Gynecol 178:409, 1998

DEC GW, FUSTER V: Medical progress: Idiopathic dilated cardiomyopathy. N Engl J Med 331:1564, 1994

DOEVENDANS PA: Hypertrophic cardiomyopathy: Do we have the algorithm for life and death? Circulation 10:1224, 2000

FAUCHIER L et al: Comparison of long-term outcome of alcoholic and idiopathic dilated cardiomyopathy. Eur Heart J 21:306, 2000

FRUSTACI A et al: Giant cell myocarditis responding to immunosuppressive therapy. Chest 117:905, 2000

GARG A et al: The ineffectiveness of immunosuppressive therapy in lymphocytic myocarditis: An overview. Ann Intern Med 129:317, 1998

HAGAR JM, RAHIMTOOLA SH: Chagas' heart disease. Curr Probl Cardiol 20:827, 1995

KUSHWAHA SS et al: Restrictive cardiomyopathy. N Engl J Med 336:267, 1997

KYLE RA: Amyloidosis. Circulation 91:1269, 1995

LEIDEN JM: The genetics of dilated cardiomyopathy—emerging clues to the puzzle. N Engl J Med 337:1080, 1997

MACHADO CR et al: Cardiac autonomic denervation in congestive heart failure: Comparison of Chagas' heart disease with other dilated cardiomyopathy. Hum Pathol 31:3, 2000

MARON BJ et al: Impact of laboratory molecular diagnosis on contemporary diagnostic criteria for genetically transmitted cardiovascular diseases: Hypertrophic cardiomyopathy, long-QT syndrome, and Marfan syndrome. Circulation 98:1460, 1998

MASON JW et al: A clinical trial of immunosuppressive therapy for myocarditis. N Engl J Med 333:269, 1995

NIIMURA H et al: Mutations in the gene for cardiac myosin-binding protein C and late-onset familial hypertrophic cardiomyopathy. N Engl J Med 338:1248, 1998

RICHARDSON P et al: Report of the 1995 World Health Organization/International Society and Federation of Cardiology Task Force on the Definition and Classification of Cardiomyopathies. Circulation 93:841, 1996

ROBIOLIO PA et al: Carcinoid heart disease. Correlation of high serotonin levels with valvular abnormalities detected by cardiac catheterization and echocardiography. Circulation 92:790, 1995

SANGHA O et al: Lack of cardiac manifestations among patients with previously treated Lyme disease. Ann Intern Med 128:346, 1998

SINGAL PK, ILISKOVIC N: Doxorubicin-induced cardiomyopathy. N Engl J Med 339:900, 1998

SORAJJA P et al: Pacing in hypertrophic cardiomyopathy. Cardiol Clin 18:67, 2000

THANIGARAJ S, PEREZ JE: Apical hypertrophic cardiomyopathy: Echocardiographic diagnosis with the use of intravenous contrast image enhancement. J Am Soc Echocardiogr 13:146, 2000

WYNNE J, BRAUNWALD E: The cardiomyopathies and myocarditides, in *Heart Disease*, 6th ed, E. Braunwald (ed). Philadelphia, Saunders, 2001

239 *Eugene Braunwald*

PERICARDIAL DISEASE

NORMAL FUNCTIONS OF THE PERICARDIUM The visceral pericardium is a serous membrane that is separated by a small quantity (15 to 50 mL) of fluid, an ultrafiltrate of plasma, from a fibrous sac, the parietal pericardium. The pericardium normally prevents sudden dilatation of the cardiac chambers during exercise and with hypervolemia. As the result of the development of a negative intrapericardial pressure during ejection, the pericardial sac facilitates atrial filling during ventricular systole. The pericardium also restricts the anatomic position of the heart, minimizes friction between the heart and surrounding structures, prevents displacement of the heart and kinking of the great vessels, and probably retards the spread of infections from the lungs and pleural cavities to the heart. Notwithstanding the foregoing, total absence of the pericardium does not produce obvious clinical disease. In partial left pericardial defects the main pulmonary artery and left atrium may bulge through the defect; very rarely, herniation and subsequent strangulation of the left atrium may cause sudden death.

ACUTE PERICARDITIS

Acute pericarditis, by far the most common pathologic process involving the pericardium, may be classified both clinically and etiologically (Table 239-1). Pain, a pericardial friction rub, electrocardiographic changes, and pericardial effusion with cardiac tamponade and paradoxic pulse are cardinal manifestations of many forms of acute pericarditis and will be considered prior to a discussion of the most common forms of the disorder.

Chest pain is an important but not invariable symptom in various forms of acute pericarditis (Chap. 13); it is usually present in the acute infectious types and in many of the forms presumed to be related to hypersensitivity or autoimmunity. Pain is often absent in a slowly developing tuberculous, postirradiation, neoplastic, or uremic pericarditis. The pain of pericarditis is often severe. It is characteristically retrosternal and left precordial, referred to the back and the left trapezius ridge. Often the pain is pleuritic consequent to accompanying pleural inflammation, i.e., sharp and aggravated by inspiration, coughing, and changes in body position, but sometimes it is a steady, constricting pain that radiates into either arm or both arms and resembles that of myocardial ischemia; therefore, confusion with myocardial infarction is common. Characteristically, however, pericardial pain may be relieved by sitting up and leaning forward and is intensified by lying supine. The differentiation of acute myocardial infarction from acute pericarditis becomes perplexing when, with acute pericarditis, the serum creatine kinase level rises, presumably because of concomitant involvement of the epicardium. However, these enzyme

Table 239-1   Classification of Pericarditis

CLINICAL CLASSIFICATION

I. Acute pericarditis (<6 weeks)
  A. Fibrinous
  B. Effusive (serous or sanguineous)
II. Subacute pericarditis (6 weeks to 6 months)
  A. Effusive-constrictive
  B. Constrictive
III. Chronic pericarditis (<6 months)
  A. Constrictive
  B. Effusive
  C. Adhesive (nonconstrictive)

ETIOLOGIC CLASSIFICATION

I. Infectious pericarditis
  A. Viral (coxsackievirus A and B, echovirus, mumps, adenovirus, hepatitis, HIV)
  B. Pyogenic (pneumococcus, streptococcus, staphylococcus, *Neisseria, Legionella*)
  C. Tuberculous
  D. Fungal (histoplasmosis, coccidioidomycosis, *Candida,* blastomycosis)
  E. Other infections (syphilitic, protozoal, parasitic)
II. Noninfectious pericarditis
  A. Acute myocardial infarction
  B. Uremia
  C. Neoplasia
    1. Primary tumors (benign or malignant, mesothelioma)
    2. Tumors metastatic to pericardium (lung and breast cancer, lymphoma, leukemia)
  D. Myxedema
  E. Cholesterol
  F. Chylopericardium
  G. Trauma
    1. Penetrating chest wall
    2. Nonpenetrating
  H. Aortic dissection (with leakage into pericardial sac)
  I. Postirradiation
  J. Familial Mediterranean fever
  K. Familial pericarditis
    1. Mulibrey nanism[a]
  L. Acute idiopathic
  M. Whipple's Disease
  N. Sarcoidosis
III. Pericarditis presumably related to hypersensitivity or autoimmunity
  A. Rheumatic fever
  B. Collagen vascular disease (SLE, rheumatoid arthritis, ankylosing spondylitis, scleroderma, acute rheumatic fever, Wegener's granulomatosis)
  C. Drug-induced (e.g., procainamide, hydralazine, phenytoin, isoniazide, minoxidil, anticoagulants, methysergide)
  D. Postcardiac injury
    1. Postmyocardial infarction (Dressler's syndrome)
    2. Postpericardiotomy
    3. Posttraumatic

[a] An autosomal recessive syndrome, characterized by growth failure, muscle hypotonia, hepatomegaly, ocular changes, enlarged cerebral ventricles, mental retardation, and chronic constrictive pericarditis.

elevations, if they occur, are quite modest, given the extensive electrocardiographic ST-segment elevation in pericarditis.

The *pericardial friction rub* is the most important physical sign of acute pericarditis; it may have up to three components per cardiac cycle and is high-pitched, scratching, and grating, as described in Chap. 225; it can sometimes be elicited only when firm pressure with the diaphragm of the stethoscope is applied to the chest wall at the left lower sternal border. It is heard most frequently during expiration with the patient in the sitting position. The rub is often inconstant and the loud to-and-fro leathery sound may disappear within a few hours, possibly to reappear the following day.

The *electrocardiogram* (ECG) in acute pericarditis without massive effusion usually displays changes secondary to acute subepicar-

dial inflammation (see Fig. 226-18, p. 1270). There is widespread elevation of the ST segments, often with upward concavity, involving two or three standard limb leads and V_2 to V_6, with reciprocal depressions only in aVR and sometimes V_1. Usually there are no significant changes in QRS complexes, except for some reduction in voltage in patients with large pericardial effusions. After several days, the ST segments return to normal, and only then do the T waves become inverted. In contrast, in acute myocardial infarction, reciprocal depression of ST segments is usually more prominent; QRS changes occur, particularly the development of Q waves, as well as notching and loss of R-wave amplitude; and T-wave inversions usually occur within hours *before* the ST segments have become isoelectric. Sequential ECGs are useful in distinguishing acute pericarditis from acute myocardial infarction. In the latter, elevated ST segments return to normal within hours. Early repolarization is a normal variant and may also cause widespread ST-segment elevation, most prominent in left precordial leads. However, in this condition the T waves are usually tall and the ST/T ratio is under 0.25, but this ratio is higher in acute pericarditis. Depression of the PR segment (below the TP segment) is also common and reflects atrial involvement. With large pericardial effusions, the QRS voltage is reduced; atrial premature beats and atrial fibrillation are sometimes noted.

PERICARDIAL EFFUSION   In acute pericarditis, pericardial effusion is usually associated with pain and/or the above-mentioned ECG changes characteristic of pericarditis and an enlargement of the cardiac silhouette. Pericardial effusion is especially important clinically when it develops within a relatively short time, since it may lead to cardiac tamponade (see below). Differentiation from cardiac enlargement may be difficult on physical examination, but heart sounds tend to become faint with pericardial effusion; the friction rub may disappear, and the apex impulse may vanish, but sometimes it remains palpable, albeit medial to the left border of cardiac dullness. The base of the left lung may be compressed by pericardial fluid, producing Ewart's sign, a patch of dullness beneath the angle of the left scapula. The chest roentgenogram may show a "water bottle" configuration of the cardiac silhouette but may also be normal or almost so. Lucent pericardial fat lines may be seen deep within the cardiopericardial silhouette. Fluoroscopic examination may show the ventricular pulsations to be diminished. Pericardial effusion is common after cardiac surgery and myocardial infarction.

Diagnosis   *Echocardiography* is the most effective diagnostic laboratory technique available, since it is sensitive, specific, simple, noninvasive, may be performed at the bedside, and can identify accompanying cardiac tamponade (see below). The presence of pericardial fluid is recorded by two-dimensional transthoracic echocardiography as a relatively echo-free space between the posterior pericardium and left ventricular epicardium in patients with small effusions and as a space between the anterior right ventricle and the parietal pericardium just beneath the anterior chest wall in those with larger effusions. In the latter the heart may swing freely within the pericardial sac; when severe, the extent of this motion alternates and may be associated with electrical alternans. Echocardiography allows localization and estimation of the quantity of pericardial fluid. The diagnosis of pericardial fluid or thickening may be confirmed by computed tomography (CT) or magnetic resonance imaging (MRI); these techniques may be superior to echocardiography in detecting loculated pericardial effusions and pericardial thickening.

Pericardiocentesis   When pericardial fluid is removed for diagnostic and/or therapeutic purposes, a needle attached to a properly grounded ECG lead is inserted into the pericardial space, usually through a subxiphoid approach, and, if possible, using echocardiographic control. Intrapericardial pressure should be measured before fluid is withdrawn. Pericardial effusion nearly always has the physical characteristics of an exudate. Bloody fluid is commonly due to tuberculosis or tumor but may also be found in the effusion of rheumatic fever, post-cardiac injury, and post-myocardial infarction (especially following the administration of anticoagulant), and in uremic pericarditis. Transudative pericardial effusions may occur in heart failure.

CARDIAC TAMPONADE The accumulation of fluid in the pericardium in an amount sufficient to cause serious obstruction to the inflow of blood to the ventricles results in cardiac tamponade. This complication may be fatal if it is not recognized and treated promptly. The three most common causes of tamponade are neoplastic disease, idiopathic pericarditis, and uremia. Tamponade may also result from bleeding into the pericardial space either following cardiac operations and trauma (including cardiac perforation during diagnostic procedures) or from tuberculosis and hemopericardium. The latter may occur when a patient with any form of acute pericarditis is treated with anticoagulants.

The three principal features of tamponade are elevation of intracardiac pressures, limitation of ventricular filling, and reduction of cardiac output. The quantity of fluid necessary to produce this critical state may be as small as 200 mL when the fluid develops rapidly or more than 2000 mL in slowly developing effusions when the pericardium has had the opportunity to stretch and adapt to an increasing volume. The volume of fluid required to produce tamponade also varies directly with the thickness of the ventricular myocardium and inversely with the thickness of the parietal pericardium.

Table 239-2 lists the features that distinguish cardiac tamponade from constrictive pericarditis. The classic findings of falling arterial pressure, rising venous pressure, and faint heart sounds usually occur only with severe, acute tamponade, as occurs with cardiac trauma or rupture. Tamponade may also develop more slowly, and under these circumstances the clinical manifestations may resemble those of heart failure, including dyspnea, orthopnea, hepatic engorgement, and jugular venous hypertension. A high index of suspicion for cardiac tamponade is required, since, in many instances, no obvious cause for pericardial disease is apparent. Tamponade should be considered in any patient with hypotension and elevation of jugular venous pressure with a prominent x descent; in contrast to constrictive pericarditis, in which the y descent is prominent (Chap. 225), in cardiac tamponade it is diminutive or absent. A positive Kussmaul sign (see below) is rare in cardiac tamponade, as is a pericardial knock. Their presence suggests that an organizing process and epicardial constriction are present in addition to effusion. A widening of the area of flatness to percussion across the anterior aspect of the chest wall, a paradoxical pulse (see below), hypotension, relatively clear lung fields, diminished pulsations of the cardiac silhouette on fluoroscopy, enlargement of the cardiac silhouette (especially in subacute or chronic tamponade), reduction in amplitude of the QRS complexes, and *electrical alternans* of the P, QRS, and T waves should raise the suspicion of cardiac tamponade.

Paradoxical Pulse This important clue to the presence of cardiac tamponade consists of *a greater than normal (10 mmHg) inspiratory decline in systolic arterial pressure*. When severe, it may be detected by palpating weakness or disappearance of the arterial pulse during inspiration, but usually sphygmomanometric measurement of systolic pressure during slow respiration is required.

Table 239-2 Features That Distinguish Cardiac Tamponade from Constrictive Pericarditis and Similar Clinical Disorders

Characteristic	Tamponade	Constrictive Pericarditis	Restrictive Cardiomyopathy	RVMI[a]
Clinical				
Pulsus paradoxus	Common	Usually absent	Rare	Rare
Jugular veins				
Prominent y descent	Absent	Usually present	Rare	Rare
Prominent x descent	Present	Usually present	Present	Rare
Kussmaul's sign	Absent	Present	Absent	Absent
Third heart sound	Absent	Absent	Rare	May be present
Pericardial knock	Absent	Often present	Absent	Absent
Electrocardiogram				
Low ECG voltage	May be present	May be present	May be present	Absent
Electrical alternans	May be present	Absent	Absent	Absent
Echocardiography				
Thickened pericardium	Absent	Present	Absent	Absent
Pericardial calcification	Absent	Often present	Absent	Absent
Pericardial effusion	Present	Absent	Absent	Absent
RV size	Usually small	Usually normal	Usually normal	Enlarged
Myocardial thickness	Normal	Normal	Usually increased	Normal
Right atrial collapse and RVDC	Present	Absent	Absent	Absent
Increased early filling, ↑ mitral flow velocity	Absent	Present	Present	May be present
Exaggerated respiratory variation in flow velocity	Present	Present	Absent	Absent
CT/MRI				
Thickened/calcific pericardium	Absent	Present	Absent	Absent
Cardiac catheterization				
Equalization of diastolic procedures	Usually present	Usually present	Usually absent	Absent or present
Cardiac biopsy helpful?	No	No	Sometimes	No

[a] RV, right ventricle; RVMI, right ventricular myocardial infarction; RVDC, right ventricular diastolic collapse; ECG, electrocardiograph.
SOURCE: From GM Brockington et al, Cardiol Clin 8:645, 1990.

Since both ventricles share a tight incompressible covering, i.e., the pericardial sac, the inspiratory enlargement of the right ventricle in cardiac tamponade compresses and reduces left ventricular volume; leftward bulging of the interventricular septum further reduces the left ventricular cavity as the right ventricle enlarges during inspiration. Thus in cardiac tamponade the normal inspiratory augmentation of right ventricular volume causes an exaggerated reciprocal reduction in left ventricular volume. Also, respiratory distress increases the fluctuations in intrathoracic pressure, which exaggerates the mechanism just described. Right ventricular infarction (Chap. 243) may resemble cardiac tamponade with hypotension, elevated jugular venous pressure, an absent y descent in the jugular venous pulse, and occasionally pulsus paradoxus. The differences between these two conditions are shown in Table 239-2.

Paradoxical pulse occurs not only in cardiac tamponade but also in approximately one-third of patients with constrictive pericarditis. Paradoxical pulse is not pathognomonic of pericardial disease because it may be observed in some cases of hypovolemic shock, acute and chronic obstructive airways disease, and pulmonary embolus.

Low-pressure tamponade refers to mild tamponade in which the intrapericardial pressure is increased from its slightly subatmospheric levels to +5 to +10 mmHg; in some instances hypovolemia coexists. As a consequence, the central venous pressure is normal or only slightly elevated, while arterial pressure is unaffected and there is no paradoxical pulse. The patients are asymptomatic or complain of mild weakness and dyspnea. The diagnosis is aided by echocardiography, and both hemodynamic and clinical manifestations improve following pericardiocentesis.

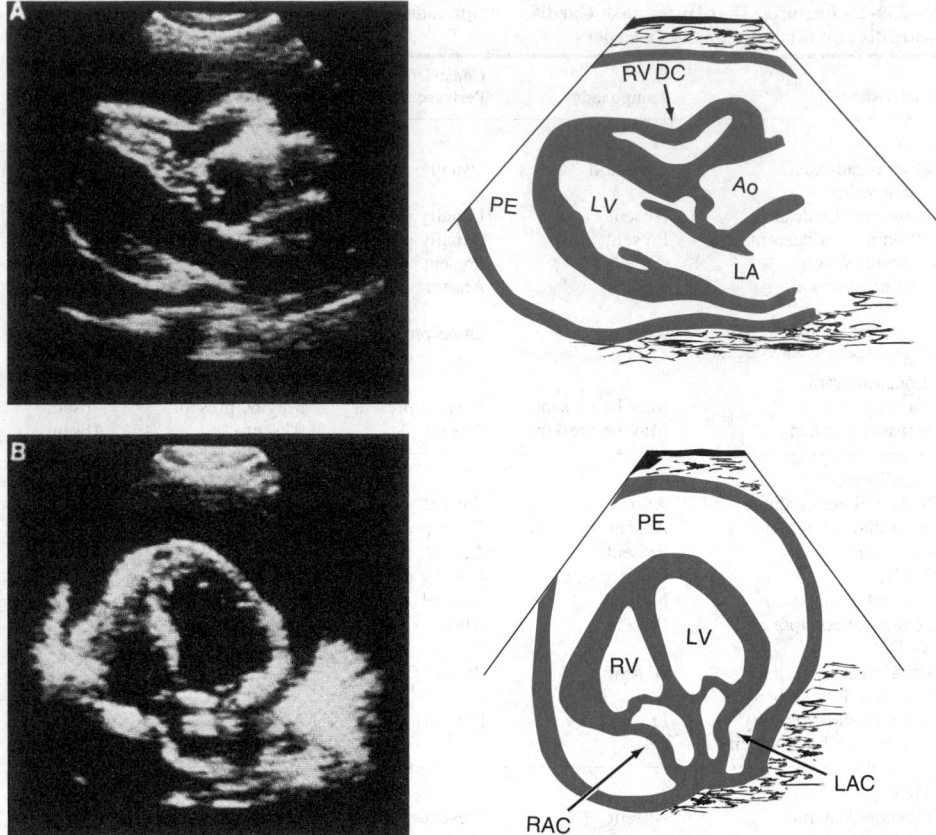

FIGURE 239-1 Parasternal long-axis (*A*) and apical four-chamber (*B*) images from a patient with cardiac tamponade, demonstrating the presence of right ventricular diastolic collapse and right atrial collapse. In this patient, even the left atrium is seen to collapse because of tamponade. LV, left ventricle; LA, left atrium; Ao, aorta; PE, pericardial effusion; RVDC, right ventricular diastolic collapse; RAC, right atrial collapse; LAC, left atrial collapse. (*From Cujer et al.*)

sion is carried out, an attempt should be made to remove as much fluid as possible. Surgical drainage through a limited thoracotomy may be required in recurrent tamponade and/or when it is necessary to obtain tissue for diagnosis.

VIRAL OR IDIOPATHIC FORM OF ACUTE PERICARDITIS In some cases of this common disorder, an A or B coxsackievirus or the virus of influenza, echovirus, mumps, herpes simplex, chickenpox, adenovirus, or Epstein-Barr has been isolated from pericardial fluid and/or appropriate elevations in viral antibody titers have been noted. In many instances, acute pericarditis occurs in association with illnesses of known viral origin and, presumably, are caused by the same agent. Commonly, there is an antecedent infection of the respiratory tract, but in many patients such an association is not evident and viral isolation and serologic studies are negative. Most frequently, a viral causation cannot be established; the term *acute idiopathic pericarditis* is then appropriate. Acute pericarditis is a common complication in patients infected with AIDS (Chap. 309). It may be caused by HIV itself; by opportunistic infections, such as cytomegalovirus and tuberculosis; or by associated neoplasms, such as lymphoma or Kaposi's sarcoma.

Acute pericarditis occurs at all ages

Diagnosis Since immediate treatment of cardiac tamponade may be lifesaving, prompt measures to establish the diagnosis by echocardiography should be undertaken (Fig 239-1). When pericardial effusion causes tamponade, during inspiration right ventricular diameter increases while left ventricular diameter and mitral valve opening decrease. Often the right ventricular cavity is reduced in diameter, and there is late diastolic inward motion (collapse) of the right ventricular free wall and of the right atrium. Doppler ultrasound shows exaggerated pulmonic (and tricuspid) flow during inspiration, with reciprocal changes in aortic (and mitral) flow (Fig 239-2).

If measured, the pericardial pressure is elevated and equal to the right atrial pressure. There is "equalization" of pressures, i.e., the pulmonary artery wedge is equal, or close, to right atrial, right ventricular, and pulmonary artery diastolic pressures. The "square root" sign in the ventricular pressure pulses and the prominent *y* descent in atrial and jugular venous pressure are characteristic of constrictive pericarditis (see below) and are rarely present in tamponade.

℞ **TREATMENT** Patients with acute pericarditis should be observed frequently for the development of an effusion; if a large effusion is present, the patient should be hospitalized and watched closely for signs of tamponade. In the presence of an effusion, arterial and venous pressures and heart rate should be monitored or followed carefully and serial echocardiograms obtained. If manifestations of tamponade appear, pericardiocentesis must be carried out at once, since relief of the intrapericardial pressure may be lifesaving. It is helpful, though not essential, to carry this out in the catheterization laboratory with hemodynamic and fluoroscopic monitoring. A small catheter advanced over the needle inserted into the pericardial cavity may be left in place to allow draining of the pericardial space if fluid reaccumulates. When a *diagnostic* pericardiocentesis of a large effu-

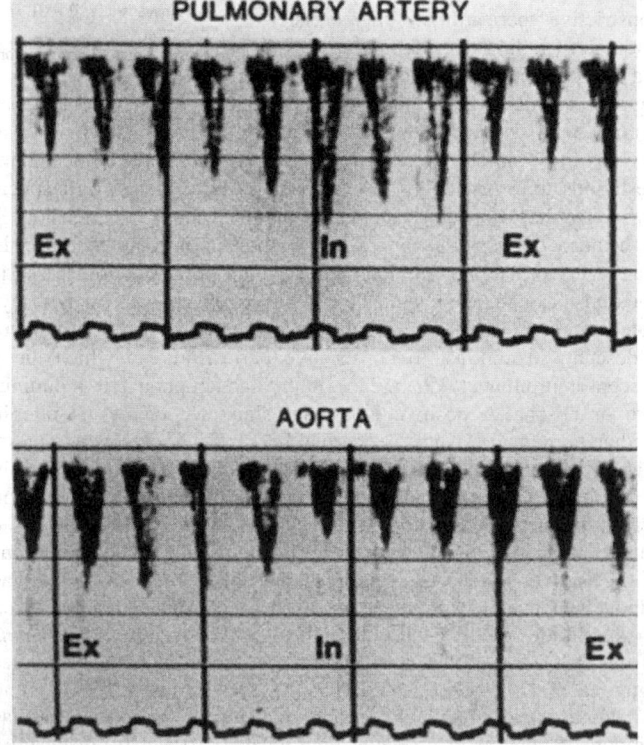

FIGURE 239-2 Pulmonary artery and aortic blood flow velocity recordings in cardiac tamponade. There is a marked increase in the pulmonary flow velocity during inspiration. Simultaneously, there is a marked decrease in aortic flow velocity. In, inspiration; Ex, expiration. (*From Cujer et al.*)

but is more frequent in young adults. Regardless of the specific cause, the clinical manifestations are similar. Acute pericarditis is often associated with pleural effusions and pneumonitis. The almost simultaneous development of fever and precordial pain, often 10 to 12 days after a presumed viral illness, constitutes an important feature in the differentiation of acute pericarditis from myocardial infarction, in which pain precedes fever. The constitutional symptoms are usually mild to moderate, but occasionally the initial symptoms are stormy, the temperature rising to 40°C. A pericardial friction rub is often audible. The disease ordinarily runs its course in a few days to 4 weeks, but one or more recurrences occur in about one-fourth of patients. Although accumulation of some pericardial fluid is common, tamponade is unusual, and constrictive pericarditis is a possible complication. The ST-segment alterations in the ECG usually disappear after 1 or more weeks, but the abnormal T waves may persist for several years and be a source of confusion in persons without a clear history of pericarditis. Pleuritis and pneumonitis frequently accompany pericarditis. Granulocytosis followed by lymphocytosis is common.

℞ **TREATMENT** There is no specific therapy, but bed rest and anti-inflammatory treatment with aspirin, if necessary up to 900 mg qid, may be given. If this is ineffective, one of the nonsteroidal anti-inflammatory agents, such as indomethacin (25 to 75 mg qid) or a glucocorticoid (e.g., prednisone, 40 to 80 mg daily) usually suppresses the clinical manifestations of the acute illness and may be useful in patients in whom the purulent and tuberculous forms of pericarditis have been excluded. Anticoagulants should be avoided. After the patient has been asymptomatic and afebrile for about a week, the dose of the anti-inflammatory agent is gradually tapered. When recurrences are multiple, frequent, disabling, and continue beyond 2 years, pericardiectomy may be effective in terminating the illness.

POST-CARDIAC INJURY SYNDROME Acute pericarditis may appear under a variety of circumstances that have one common feature: previous injury to the myocardium, with blood in the pericardial cavity. The syndrome may develop after a cardiac operation (postpericardiotomy syndrome); after cardiac trauma (Chap. 240), e.g., a stab wound, contusions after a nonpenetrating blow to the chest; or after perforation of the heart with a catheter. Rarely, it follows myocardial infarction.

The clinical picture of the post-cardiac injury syndrome mimics acute viral or acute idiopathic pericarditis. The principal symptom is the pain of acute pericarditis, which usually develops 1 to 4 weeks following the cardiac injury but sometimes appears only after an interval of months. Recurrences of pericarditis are common and may occur up to 2 years or more after the injury. Fever with temperature up to 40°C, pericarditis, pleuritis, and pneumonitis are the outstanding features, and the bout of illness usually subsides in 1 or 2 weeks. The pericarditis may be of the fibrinous variety, or it may be a pericardial effusion, which is often serosanguineous, and may be accompanied by arthralgias, but rarely causes tamponade. Leukocytosis, an increased sedimentation rate, and electrocardiographic changes typical of acute pericarditis also may occur.

The mechanisms responsible for this syndrome have not been identified, but they are probably the result of a hypersensitivity reaction in which the antigen originates from injured myocardial tissue and/or pericardium; the suggested designation of *post-cardiac injury syndrome* for this group of disorders implies that they may have a common pathogenetic mechanism. Circulating autoantibodies to myocardium occur frequently, but their precise role has not been defined. Viral infection may also play an etiologic role, since antiviral antibodies are often elevated in patients who develop this syndrome following cardiac surgery.

Often no treatment is necessary aside from aspirin and analgesics. The management of pericardial effusion and tamponade has already been discussed. When the illness is followed by a series of disabling recurrences, therapy with a nonsteroidal anti-inflammatory agent or a glucocorticoid is usually effective.

Differential Diagnosis Since there is no specific test for *acute idiopathic pericarditis*, the diagnosis is one of exclusion. Consequently, all other disorders that may be associated with acute fibrinous pericarditis must be considered. A common diagnostic error is mistaking acute viral or idiopathic pericarditis for acute myocardial infarction and vice versa. When it is associated with *acute myocardial infarction*, acute fibrinous pericarditis may be confused with acute viral or idiopathic pericarditis; this complication of infarction, described in Chap. 243, is characterized by fever, pain, and a friction rub in the first 4 days following the development of the infarct (to be distinguished from the pericarditis in Dressler's syndrome, which is a form of post-cardiac injury pericarditis and which occurs a week or two following myocardial infarction). ECG abnormalities (such as the appearance of Q waves, brief ST-segment elevations with reciprocal changes, and earlier T-wave changes in myocardial infarction) and the extent of the elevations of myocardial enzymes are helpful in differentiating pericarditis from acute myocardial infarction.

Pericarditis secondary to post-cardiac injury is differentiated from acute idiopathic pericarditis chiefly by timing. If it occurs within a few weeks of a myocardial infarction or a chest blow, it may be justified to conclude that the two are probably related. If the infarct has been silent or the chest blow forgotten, the relationship to the pericarditis may not be recognized.

It is important to distinguish *pericarditis due to collagen vascular disease* from acute idiopathic pericarditis. Most important in the differential diagnosis is the pericarditis due to systemic lupus erythematosus (SLE; Chap. 311) or drug-induced (procainamide or hydralazine) lupus. In these conditions, pain is often present; sometimes in SLE the pericarditis appears as an asymptomatic effusion, and rarely, tamponade develops. When pericarditis occurs in the absence of any obvious underlying disorder, the diagnosis may be made on discovery of lupus erythematosus cells or a rise in the titer of antinuclear antibodies. Acute pericarditis may complicate the viral, pyogenic, mycobacterial, and fungal infections that occur in AIDS. Acute pericarditis is an occasional complication of *rheumatoid arthritis*, *scleroderma*, and *polyarteritis nodosa*, and other evidence of these diseases is usually obvious. Asymptomatic pericardial effusion is also frequent in these disorders. It is important to question every patient with acute pericarditis about the ingestion of procainamide, hydralazine, isoniazid, cromolyn, and minoxidil, since these drugs can cause this syndrome.

The pericarditis of *acute rheumatic fever* is generally associated with evidence of severe pancarditis and with cardiac murmurs (Chap. 235). *Pyogenic (purulent) pericarditis* is usually secondary to cardiothoracic operations, immunosuppressive therapy, rupture of the esophagus into the pericardial sac, or rupture of a ring abscess in a patient with infective endocarditis and with septicemia complicating aseptic pericarditis. It is accompanied by fever, chills, septicemia, and evidence of infection elsewhere. *Tuberculous pericarditis* (Chap. 169) may present as an acute pericarditis associated with fever, weight loss, and other clinical manifestations of active systemic tuberculosis; the diagnosis may be aided by a positive tuberculin test and evidence of pulmonary or mediastinal tuberculosis. Tubercle bacilli can be cultured from the pericardial space only infrequently, and a biopsy of the pericardium with bacteriologic and histologic examination may be required. Alternatively, tuberculous pericarditis may present as a chronic asymptomatic effusion, as subacute effusive-constrictive pericarditis, or as frank chronic constrictive pericarditis (see below).

Uremic pericarditis (Chap. 270) occurs in up to one-third of patients with chronic uremia and is seen most frequently in patients undergoing chronic hemodialysis. It may be fibrinous and is generally associated with an effusion that may be sanguineous. A friction rub is common, but pain is usually absent. Treatment with an anti-inflammatory agent and intensification of hemodialysis is usually adequate. Occasionally, tamponade occurs and pericardiocentesis is required. When uremic pericarditis is recurrent, persistent, or very troubling, pericardiectomy may be necessary. Pericarditis due to *neoplastic diseases* results from extension or invasion of metastatic tumors (most commonly carcinoma of the lung and breast, malignant melanoma, lymphoma, and leukemia) to the pericardium; pain, atrial arrhythmias, and tamponade are complications that occur occasionally. *Mediastinal irradiation* for neoplasm may cause acute pericarditis and/or chronic constrictive pericarditis after eradication of the tumor. Unusual causes of acute pericarditis include syphilis, fungal infection (histoplasmosis, blastomycosis, aspergillosis, and candidiasis), and parasitic infestation (amebiasis, toxoplasmosis, echinococcosis, trichinosis).

CHRONIC PERICARDIAL EFFUSIONS   Chronic pericardial effusions are sometimes encountered in patients without an antecedent history of acute pericarditis. They may cause few symptoms per se, and their presence may be detected by finding an enlarged cardiac silhouette on chest roentgenogram.

Tuberculosis   This is a common cause of chronic pericardial effusion, although less so in the United States than in other parts of the world (Chap. 169). The clinical picture is that of a chronic, systemic illness in a patient with pericardial effusion. It is important to consider this condition in a middle-aged or elderly person with fever and enlargement of the cardiac silhouette of undetermined origin, with or without elevation of venous pressure. Weight loss, fever, and fatigability are sometimes observed. Inasmuch as treatment is quite effective, overlooking a tuberculous pericardial effusion may have serious consequences. A chest roentgenogram for pulmonary tuberculosis should be obtained, and a search for tuberculosis in other organs carried out; tuberculin skin tests should be performed and repeated after several weeks. If the etiology of chronic pericardial effusion remains obscure, a pericardial biopsy, preferably by a limited thoracotomy, should be performed. If definitive evidence is then still lacking but the specimen shows caseation necrosis, antituberculous chemotherapy is indicated. If the biopsy specimen shows a thickened pericardium, pericardiectomy should be carried out in order to prevent the development of constriction.

Other Causes of Chronic Pericardial Effusion   *Myxedema* may be responsible for a pericardial effusion that is sometimes massive but rarely, if ever, causes cardiac tamponade. The cardiac silhouette is markedly enlarged, and an echocardiogram is necessary to distinguish cardiomegaly from pericardial effusion. The diagnosis of myxedema is frequently overlooked. It is important, therefore, to carry out appropriate tests for thyroid function (Chap. 330) as well as echocardiography in patients with an enlarged cardiac outline of undetermined origin. *Cholesterol pericardial disease* is sometimes associated with myxedema. It is characterized by large pericardial effusions with a high cholesterol content, which may induce an inflammatory response and constrictive pericarditis.

Neoplasms, SLE, rheumatoid arthritis, mycotic infections, radiation therapy, pyogenic infections, severe chronic anemia, and chylopericardium may also cause chronic pericardial effusion and should be considered and specifically looked for in such patients.

Aspiration and analysis of the pericardial fluid are often helpful in diagnosis. In infections the organism can often be identified by smear or culture. Grossly sanguineous pericardial fluid results most commonly from a neoplasm, tuberculosis, uremia, or slow leakage from an aortic aneurysm.

CHRONIC CONSTRICTIVE PERICARDITIS

This disorder results when the healing of an acute fibrinous or serofibrinous pericarditis or a chronic pericardial effusion is followed by obliteration of the pericardial cavity with the formation of granulation tissue. The latter gradually contracts and forms a firm scar, encasing the heart and interfering with filling of the ventricles. In some reports, a high percentage of cases has been of tuberculous origin. In North America, tuberculosis is now an infrequent cause. Chronic constrictive pericarditis may also follow purulent infection, trauma, cardiac oper-

ation of any type, mediastinal irradiation, histoplasmosis, neoplastic disease (especially breast cancer, lung cancer, and lymphoma), acute viral or idiopathic pericarditis, rheumatoid arthritis, SLE, and chronic renal failure with uremia treated by chronic dialysis. In many patients the cause of the pericardial disease is undetermined, and in them an asymptomatic or forgotten bout of viral pericarditis, acute or idiopathic, may have been the inciting event. The heart may also be constricted and compressed by malignant tumors or organized blood clot in the pericardial cavity.

The basic physiologic abnormality in symptomatic patients with chronic constrictive pericarditis, as in those with cardiac tamponade, is the inability of the ventricles to fill because of the limitations imposed by the rigid, thickened pericardium or the tense pericardial fluid. In constrictive pericarditis, ventricular filling is unimpeded during early diastole but is reduced abruptly when the elastic limit of the pericardium is reached, while in cardiac tamponade, ventricular filling is impeded throughout diastole. In chronic constrictive pericarditis, ventricular end-diastolic and stroke volumes are reduced and the end-diastolic pressures in both ventricles and the mean pressures in the atria, pulmonic veins, and systemic veins are all elevated to similar levels, i.e., within 5 mmHg. The fibrotic process may extend into the myocardium and cause myocardial scarring, and venous congestion may then be due to the combined effects of the myocardial and pericardial lesions. Despite these hemodynamic changes, myocardial function may be normal or only slightly impaired.

In constrictive pericarditis, the central venous and right and left atrial pressure pulses display an M-shaped contour, with prominent *x* and *y* descents; the *y* descent, which is absent or diminished in cardiac tamponade, is the most prominent deflection in constrictive pericarditis and is interrupted by a rapid rise in pressure during early diastole, when ventricular filling is impeded by the constricting pericardium. These characteristic changes are transmitted to the jugular veins, where they may be recognized by inspection. In constrictive pericarditis, the ventricular pressure pulses in both ventricles exhibit characteristic "square root" signs during diastole (Fig. 239-3). These hemodynamic changes, although characteristic, are not pathognomonic of constrictive pericarditis but may also be observed in cardiomyopathies characterized by restriction of ventricular filling (Chap. 238).

CLINICAL AND LABORATORY FINDINGS (Table 239-2) Weakness, fatigue, weight gain, increased abdominal girth, abdominal discomfort, and edema are common. The patient often appears to be

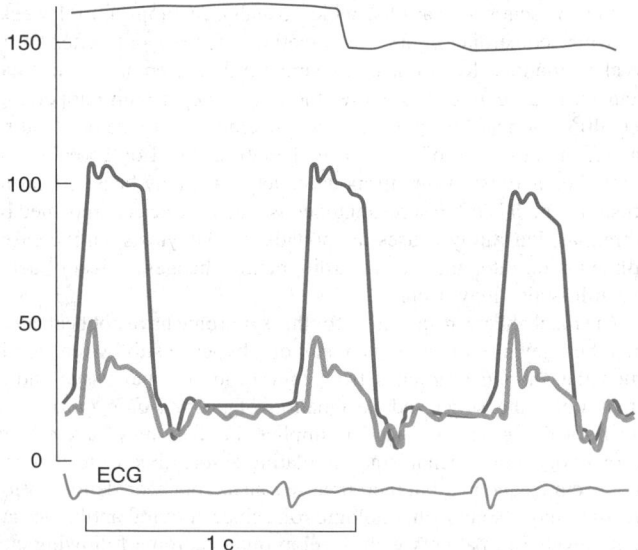

FIGURE 239-3   Left (LV) and right ventricular (RV) pressure recording from a patient with constrictive pericarditis showing the characteristic dip and plateau ("square root" sign) in both ventricular pressure pulses. End-diastolic pressures are equal in the two ventricles. *[Modified from BH Lorell, W Grossman, in W Grossman (ed): Cardiac Catheterization and Angiography. Philadelphia, Lea & Febiger, 1986, p 430.]*

chronically ill with decreased skeletal muscle mass and a protuberant abdomen. Exertional dyspnea is common, and orthopnea may occur, although it is usually not severe. Acute left ventricular failure (acute pulmonary edema) is very uncommon. The cervical veins are distended and may remain so even after intensive diuretic treatment, and venous pressure may fail to decline during inspiration (Kussmaul's sign). The latter is frequent in chronic pericarditis but may also occur in tricuspid stenosis, right ventricular infarction, and restrictive cardiomyopathy. The pulse pressure is normal or reduced. In about one-third of the cases a paradoxical pulse can be detected. Congestive hepatomegaly is pronounced and may impair hepatic function; ascites is common and is usually more prominent than dependent edema. In about half of patients the heart is normal in size; if it is enlarged, the enlargement is rarely extreme. The apical pulse is reduced in intensity, retracts in systole, and moves outward in diastole. The heart sounds may be distant; an early third heart sound, i.e., a pericardial knock, occurring 0.09 to 0.12 s after aortic valve closure that coincides with a sudden deceleration in ventricular filling, is often conspicuous, and murmurs are usually absent. Because of the high sustained venous pressure, congestive splenomegaly may make the spleen palpable. In the absence of infective endocarditis or tricuspid valve disease, splenomegaly in a patient with congestive heart failure should arouse suspicion of constrictive pericarditis. Protein-losing gastroenteropathy, due to impaired lymphatic drainage from the small intestine, and marked proteinuria or hypoalbuminemia may complicate chronic constrictive pericarditis.

The *ECG* frequently displays low voltage of the QRS complex and diffuse flattening or inversion of the T waves. P mitrale may be present in patients with sinus rhythm; atrial fibrillation is present in about one-third of patients. The *chest roentgenogram* shows a normal or slightly enlarged heart, sometimes with pericardial calcification.

Inasmuch as the usual physical signs of cardiac disease (murmurs, cardiac enlargement) may be inconspicuous or absent in chronic constrictive pericarditis, hepatic enlargement and dysfunction associated with intractable ascites may lead to a mistaken diagnosis of cirrhosis of the liver. This error can be avoided if the neck veins are inspected carefully in patients with ascites and hepatomegaly. *Given a clinical picture resembling hepatic cirrhosis, but with the added feature of distended neck veins, careful search for calcification of the pericardium by chest roentgenography and CT or MRI should be carried out and may disclose this curable or remediable form of heart disease.*

The echocardiogram typically shows pericardial thickening, atrial enlargement, dilatation of the inferior vena cava and hepatic veins, and a sharp halt in ventricular filling in early diastole, with normal ventricular systolic function; there is a distinctive pattern of transvalvular flow velocity on Doppler echocardiography. There is an exaggerated reduction in blood flow velocity in the pulmonary veins and across the mitral valve during inspiration, with the opposite occurring during expiration. Diastolic flow velocity in the vena cavae into the right atrium and across the tricuspid valve increases in an exaggerated manner during inspiration and declines during expiration (Fig. 239-4). However, echocardiography cannot definitively exclude the diagnosis. MRI and CT scanning, especially the latter (Fig. 239-5), are more accurate than echocardiography in establishing or excluding the presence of a thickened pericardium. Pericardial thickening and even pericardial calcification, however, are not synonymous with constrictive pericarditis since they may occur without seriously impairing ventricular filling.

DIFFERENTIAL DIAGNOSIS Like cor pulmonale (Chap. 237), chronic constrictive pericarditis may be associated with severe systemic venous hypertension but little pulmonary congestion; the heart usually is not enlarged, and a paradoxical pulse may be present. However, in cor pulmonale advanced parenchymal pulmonary disease is usually obvious and venous pressure *falls* during inspiration, i.e., Kussmaul's sign is negative. *Tricuspid stenosis* (Chap. 236) may also simulate chronic constrictive pericarditis; congestive hepatomegaly, splenomegaly, ascites, and venous distention may be equally prominent, and the manifestations of left-sided heart failure may be incon-

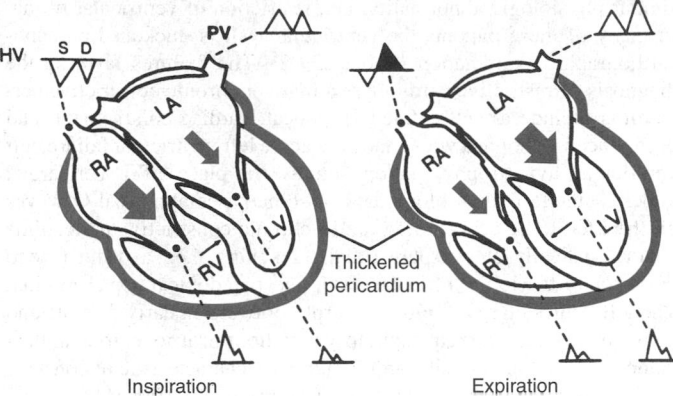

FIGURE 239-4   Schematic of respiratory variation in transvalvular and central venous flow velocities in constrictive pericarditis. With inspiration, the driving pressure gradient from the pulmonary capillaries to the left cardiac chambers decreases, resulting in a decrease in mitral and diastolic pulmonary venous (PV) flow velocity. The decreased left ventricular filling results in ventricular septal shift to the left (small arrow), allowing augmented flow to the right-sided chambers, shown as increased tricuspid inflow and diastolic hepatic venous (HV) flow velocity (downward deflection = increased flow to the right atrium) because the cardiac volume is relatively fixed as a result of the thickened shell of pericardium. The opposite changes occur during expiration. D, diastole; LA, left atrium; LV, left ventricle; RA, right atrium; RV, right ventricle; S, systole. *(From Oh et al.)*

spicuous. However, in tricuspid stenosis, a characteristic murmur as well as mitral stenosis are usually present. In tricuspid stenosis, a paradoxical pulse and a steep, deep *y* descent in the jugular venous pulse do not occur, serving to differentiate it from chronic constrictive pericarditis.

Because constrictive pericarditis can be corrected surgically, it is important, though often difficult, to distinguish chronic constrictive pericarditis from restrictive cardiomyopathy (Chap. 238), which has a

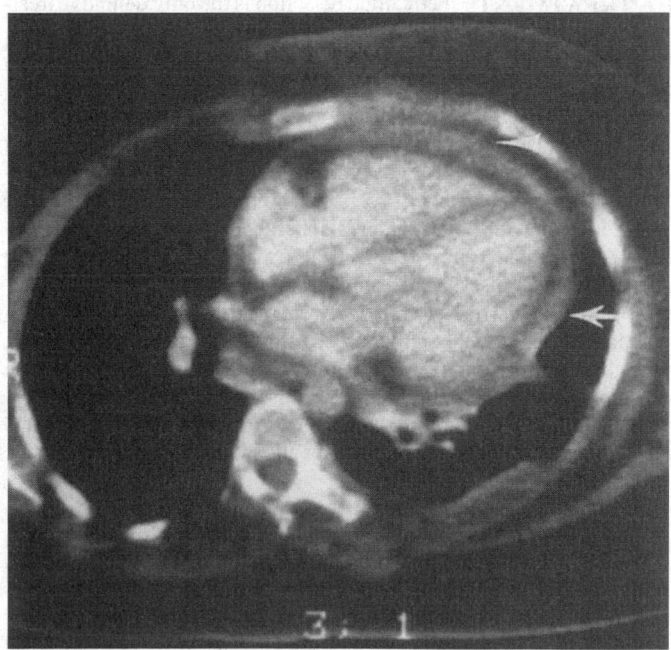

FIGURE 239-5   Computed tomographic scan showing thickened pericardium encases the right (arrowhead) and left ventricles (arrow), producing constriction. The cause of the constriction was thought to be an inflammatory process. *[From W Stanford, in LP Elliott (ed): The Fundamentals of Cardiac Imaging in Infants, Children and Adults. Philadelphia, Lippincott, 1991, p 418, with permission.]*

similar physiologic abnormality, i.e., restriction of ventricular filling. In many of these patients the ventricular wall is thickened on echocardiographic examination (Table 239-2). The features favoring the diagnosis of restrictive cardiomyopathy over chronic constrictive pericarditis include a well-defined apex beat, cardiac enlargement, and pronounced orthopnea with attacks of acute left ventricular failure, left ventricular hypertrophy, gallop sounds (in place of a pericardial knock), bundle branch block, and in some cases abnormal Q waves on the ECG. The echocardiogram in chronic constrictive pericarditis characteristically shows pericardial thickening, i.e., a distinct echo posterior to the left ventricular wall, and paradoxical septal motion. The left ventricular wall moves sharply outward in early diastole and then remains flat. Marked respiratory variations in atrioventricular flow velocities on Doppler echocardiography are characteristic of constrictive pericarditis but not restrictive cardiomyopathy (Fig. 239-4). The definitive diagnosis of restrictive cardiomyopathy, when it is due to an infiltrative disease such as amyloidosis, can often be established by endomyocardial biopsy. CT scanning and MRI are very useful in distinguishing between restrictive cardiomyopathy and chronic constrictive pericarditis. In the former, the ventricular walls are hypertrophied, while in the latter the pericardium is thickened and sometimes calcified.

When a patient has progressive, disabling, and unresponsive congestive failure and displays any of the features of constrictive heart disease, the most careful and detailed clinical and laboratory studies must be carried out in order to detect or exclude constrictive pericarditis, since the latter is usually curable.

Occult Constrictive Disease   Patients with this condition may have unexplained fatigue, dyspnea, and chest pain. No overt manifestations of pericardial disease are present, but following the rapid intravenous infusion of 1 L of saline solution, diastolic equilibration of intracardiac atrial and ventricular pressures found in overt constrictive pericarditis occur. Although symptomatic improvement may follow pericardiectomy, this procedure should not be carried out in asymptomatic persons.

TREATMENT   Pericardial resection is the only definitive treatment of constrictive pericarditis, but dietary sodium restriction and diuretics are useful during preoperative preparation. The benefits derived from cardiac decortication are often striking, and the improvement, though slight at first, usually is progressive over a period of months. The risk of this operation depends on the extent of penetration of the myocardium by the calcific process, by the severity of myocardial atrophy, by the extent of secondary impairment of hepatic and/or renal function, and by the patient's general condition. Operative mortality is in the range of 3 to 10%; the patients with the most severe and/or advanced disease are at highest risk. Therefore, surgical treatment should be carried out relatively early in the course.

Many cases of constrictive pericarditis are of tuberculous origin. Antituberculous therapy during the phase of effusion may prevent the development of constriction, and such therapy should be carried out before and after operation if a tuberculous origin can be diagnosed, is suspected, or cannot be excluded in a patient with chronic constrictive pericarditis (Chap. 169).

Subacute Effusive-Constrictive Pericarditis   This form of pericardial disease is characterized by the combination of a tense effusion in the pericardial space and constriction of the heart by thickened pericardium. It shares a number of features both with chronic pericardial effusion (p. 1366) producing cardiac compression and with pericardial constriction. It may be caused by tuberculosis, multiple attacks of acute idiopathic pericarditis, radiation, traumatic pericarditis, uremia, and scleroderma. The heart is generally enlarged, and a paradoxical pulse and a prominent x descent (without a prominent y descent) are present in the atrial and jugular venous pressure pulses. Following pericardiocentesis, the physiologic findings may change from those of cardiac

tamponade to those of pericardial constriction, with a "square root" sign in the ventricular pressure pulse and a prominent y descent in the atrial and jugular venous pressure pulses. Furthermore, the intrapericardial pressure and the central venous pressure may decline, but not to normal. In many patients the condition progresses to the chronic constrictive form of the disease. Wide excision of both the visceral and parietal pericardium is usually effective.

OTHER DISORDERS OF THE PERICARDIUM

Pericardial cysts appear as rounded or lobulated deformities of the cardiac silhouette, most commonly at the right cardiophrenic angle. They do not cause symptoms, and their major clinical significance lies in the possibility of confusion with a tumor, ventricular aneurysm, or massive cardiomegaly. *Tumors* involving the pericardium are most commonly secondary to malignant neoplasms originating in or invading the mediastinum, including carcinoma of the bronchus and breast, lymphoma, and melanoma. The most common *primary* malignant tumor is the mesothelioma. The usual clinical picture of malignant pericardial tumor is an insidiously developing, often bloody, pericardial effusion. Surgical exploration is required to establish a definitive diagnosis and to carry out definitive or, more commonly, palliative treatment.

BIBLIOGRAPHY

CUJER B et al: Echocardiography in pericardial diseases, in *Marcus' Cardiac Imaging: A Companion to Braunwald's Heart Disease*, 2d ed, DJ Skorton et al (eds). Philadelphia, Saunders, 1996, pp 404–419

FOWLER NO: Constrictive pericarditis: Its history and current status. Clin Cardiol 18:341, 1995

HEIDENREICH PA et al: Pericardial effusions in AIDS: Incidence and survival. Circulation 92:3229, 1995

HOIT BD, SHAW D: The paradoxical pulse in tamponade, mechanisms and echocardiographic correlates. Echocardiography 11:477, 1994

KHAN AH: The postcardiac injury syndromes. Clin Cardiol 15:67, 1992

LING LH et al: Calcific constrictive pericarditis: Is it still with us? Ann Intern Med 132:444, 2000

OH JK et al: Diagnostic role of Doppler echocardiography in constrictive pericarditis. J Am Coll Cardiol 23:154, 1994

SAGRISTA SAULEDA J et al: Purulent pericarditis: Review of a 20-year experience in a general hospital. J Am Coll Cardiol 22:1661, 1993

SHABETAI R: Treatment of pericardial disease, in *Cardiovascular Therapeutics: A Companion to Braunwald's Heart Disease*, TW Smith (ed). Philadelphia, Saunders, 1996, pp 742–750

SPODICK D: Pericardial diseases, in *Heart Disease*, 6th ed, E Braunwald, D Zipes, P Libby (eds): Philadelphia, Saunders, 2001

TSANG TS et al: Outcomes of primary and secondary treatment of pericardial effusion in patients with malignancy. Mayo Clin Proc 75:248, 2000

VAITKUS PT, KUSSMAUL WG: Treatment of malignant pericardial effusion. JAMA 272:59, 1994

ZAYAS R et al: Incidence of specific etiology and role of methods for specific etiologic diagnosis of primary acute pericarditis. Am J Cardiol 75:378, 1995

240   *Wilson S. Colucci, Daniel T. Price*

CARDIAC TUMORS, CARDIAC MANIFESTATIONS OF SYSTEMIC DISEASES, AND TRAUMATIC CARDIAC INJURY

TUMORS OF THE HEART

PRIMARY TUMORS   Primary tumors of the heart are rare. Approximately three-quarters are histologically benign, and the remainder, which in almost all cases are sarcomas, are malignant (Table 240-1). Because all cardiac tumors have the potential for causing life-

Table 240-1   Relative Incidence of Primary Tumors of the Heart

Type	Number	Percent
Benign	199	58.0
Myxoma	114	33.2
Rhabdomyoma	20	5.8
Fibroma	20	5.8
Hemangioma	17	5.0
Atrioventricular nodal	10	2.9
Granular cell	4	1.2
Lipoma	2	0.6
Paraganglioma	2	0.6
Myocytic hamartoma	2	0.6
Histiocytoid cardiomyopathy	2	0.6
Inflammatory psuedotumor	2	0.6
Other benign tumors	4	1.2
Malignant	144	42.0
Sarcoma	137	39.9
Lymphoma	7	2.1

SOURCE: Modified from A Burke; R Virmani: *Atlas of Tumor Pathology. Tumors of the Heart and Great Vessels.* Washington, DC, Armed Forces Institute of Pathology 1996, p 231.

threatening complications, and many are now curable by surgery, it is important that the diagnosis be made whenever possible.

Clinical Presentation   Cardiac tumors may present with a wide array of cardiac and noncardiac manifestations. The location and the size of the tumor are the major determinants of the specific signs and symptoms, many of which are present in more common forms of heart disease, such as chest pain, syncope, heart failure, murmurs, arrhythmias, conduction disturbances, and pericardial effusion with or without tamponade.

Myxoma   Myxomas are the most common type of primary cardiac tumor in all age groups, accounting for one-third to one-half of all cases at postmortem and for about three-quarters of the tumors treated surgically. They occur at all ages, most commonly in the third through sixth decades. There is a female predilection. Although most myxomas are sporadic, some are familial with autosomal dominant transmission or are part of a syndrome that involves a complex of abnormalities including lentigines or pigmented nevi, primary nodular adrenal cortical disease with or without Cushing's syndrome, myxomatous mammary fibroadenomas, testicular tumors, and/or pituitary adenomas with gigantism or acromegaly. Certain constellations of findings have been referred to as the *NAME* syndrome (nevi, atrial myxoma, myxoid neurofibroma, and ephelides) or the *LAMB* syndrome (lentigines, atrial myxoma, and blue nevi). Approximately 7% of cardiac myxomas are familial or part of the syndrome myxoma with the complex of abnormalities described above.

Pathologically, myxomas are gelatinous structures consisting of myxoma cells imbedded in a stroma rich in glycosaminoglycans. Most are pedunculated on a fibrovascular stalk and average 4 to 8 cm in diameter. The majority are solitary and located in the atria, particularly the left, where they arise from the interatrial septum in the vicinity of the fossa ovalis. In contrast to sporadic tumors, familial or syndrome myxoma tumors tend to occur in younger individuals, be multiple or ventricular in location, and have more postoperative recurrences, probably reflecting their multicentric nature.

Myxomas commonly present with obstructive, embolic, or constitutional signs and symptoms. The most common clinical presentation mimics that of mitral valve disease, either stenosis due to tumor prolapse into the mitral orifice or regurgitation due to tumor-induced valvular trauma. Ventricular myxomas may cause outflow obstruction similar to that caused by subaortic or subpulmonic stenosis. The symptoms and signs of myxoma may be of sudden onset or positional in nature, reflecting changes in tumor position due to gravity. An auscultatory finding, termed a "tumor plop," is a characteristic low-pitched sound that may be audible during early or middiastole and is thought to result from the tumor abruptly stopping as it strikes the ventricular wall. Myxomas may also present with peripheral or pulmonary emboli, or constitutional signs and symptoms including fever, weight loss, cachexia, malaise, arthralgia, rash, clubbing, Raynaud's phenomenon, hypergammaglobulinemia, anemia, polycythemia, leukocytosis, elevated erythrocyte sedimentation rate, thrombocytopenia, or thrombocytosis. Not surprisingly, myxomas are frequently misdiagnosed as endocarditis, collagen vascular disease, or noncardiac tumor.

Two-dimensional transthoracic or transesophageal echocardiography is useful in the diagnosis of cardiac myxoma and allows determination of the site of tumor attachment and tumor size, which are important considerations in the planning of surgical excision (Fig. 240-1). Computed tomography and particularly magnetic resonance imaging may provide important information regarding size, shape, composition, and surface characteristics of the tumor. Because myxomas may be familial, echocardiographic screening of first-degree relatives is appropriate, particularly if the patient is young and has multiple tumors or evidence of syndrome myxoma. Although cardiac catheterization and angiography have previously been performed routinely before surgery, catheterization of the chamber from which the tumor arisees is attended by the risk of tumor emboli. Catheterization is no longer considered mandatory when adequate noninvasive information is available and other cardiac diseases (e.g., coronary artery disease) are not considered likely.

TREATMENT   Surgical excision utilizing cardiopulmonary bypass is indicated and is generally curative. Myxomas recur in approximately 12 to 22% of familial cases and in about 1 to 2% of sporadic cases. Tumor recurrence is most likely due to multifocal lesions in the former and inadequate resection in the latter.

Other Benign Tumors   Cardiac *lipomas*, although relatively common, are usually incidental findings at postmortem examination. However, they may grow as large as 15 cm and may present with symptoms due to mechanical interference with cardiac function, arrhythmias, or conduction disturbances, or as an abnormality of the cardiac silhouette on chest x-ray. *Papillary fibroelastomas*, similarly, are relatively common findings on cardiac valves or the adjacent endothelium at postmortem, but seldom result in clinical symptoms. Occasionally, these growths may cause mechanical interference with valve function. *Rhabdomyomas* and *fibromas*, the most frequent tu-

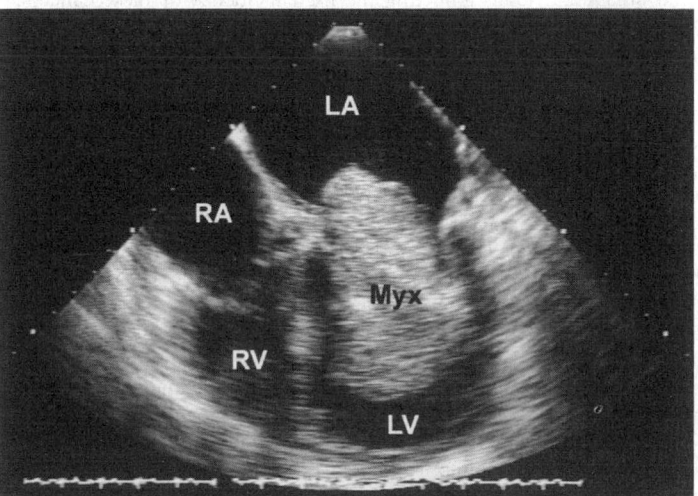

FIGURE 240-1   Transthoracic echocardiogram during diastole demonstrating a large myocardial mass, which is an atrial myxoma (Myx) that prolapses into the left ventricle (LV). RA, right atrium; RV, right ventricle. *(Courtesy of Dr. Rick Nishimura.)*

mors in infants and children, most commonly occur in the ventricles and therefore produce signs and symptoms by mechanical obstruction that may mimic valvular stenosis, congestive heart failure, restrictive or hypertrophic cardiomyopathy, and pericardial constriction. Rhabdomyomas are probably hamartomatous growths; are multiple in 90% of cases; and may be associated with tuberous sclerosis, adenoma sebaceum, and benign kidney tumors in approximately 30% of patients. Calcification of a cardiac tumor strongly suggests that it is a fibroma, although myxomas and sarcomas also may be calcified. *Hemangiomas* and *mesotheliomas* are generally small tumors, most often intramyocardial in location, and may cause atrioventricular conduction disturbances and even sudden death as a result of their propensity for location in the region of the AV node. Other benign tumors arising from the heart include *teratoma, chemodectoma, neurilemoma, granular cell myoblastoma,* and *bronchogenic cysts.*

Sarcoma   Almost all primary cardiac malignancies are sarcomas, which may be of several histologic types. In general, these tumors are characterized by a rapidly downhill course leading to the patient's death in weeks to months from the time of presentation as a result of hemodynamic compromise, local invasion, or distant metastases. Sarcomas commonly involve the right side of the heart, and because of their rapid growth, invasion of the pericardial space and obstruction of the cardiac chambers or venae cavae are common. Sarcomas can also occur on the left side of the heart and may be mistaken for myxomas.

℞ **TREATMENT**   At the time of presentation these tumors have often spread too extensively for surgical excision. Although scattered reports exist of palliation with surgery, radiotherapy, and/or chemotherapy, the overall experience with cardiac sarcomas is poor. The one exception appears to be cardiac lymphosarcomas, which may respond to a combination of chemo- and radiotherapy.

TUMORS METASTATIC TO THE HEART   Tumors metastatic to the heart are many times more common than primary tumors; and as the life expectancy of patients with various forms of malignant neoplasms is extended by more effective therapy, the frequency of cardiac metastases will also increase. Although cardiac metastases occur in 1 to 20% of all tumor types, the relative incidence is especially high in malignant melanoma and, to a somewhat lesser extent, in leukemia and lymphoma. In absolute numbers, the most common primary originating sites of cardiac metastases are carcinoma of the breast and lung, reflecting the high incidence of these cancers. Cardiac metastases almost always occur in the setting of widespread primary disease, and most often either primary or metastatic disease exists elsewhere in the thoracic cavity. Nevertheless, a cardiac metastasis may occasionally be the initial presentation of a tumor elsewhere in the body.

Cardiac metastases reach the heart from the blood stream, the lymphatics, or by direct invasion. They generally are small, firm nodules. Diffuse infiltration may also occur, especially with sarcomas or hematologic neoplasms. The pericardium is most often involved, followed by myocardial involvement of any chamber, and, rarely, by involvement of the endocardium or cardiac valves.

Cardiac metastases result in clinical manifestations only about 10% of the time and rarely are the cause of death. In most instances the metastases are not the cause of the presenting clinical features but occur in the setting of a previously recognized malignant neoplasm. Although cardiac metastases may present with a large number of nonspecific signs and symptoms, the most common are dyspnea, signs of acute pericarditis, cardiac tamponade, a rapid increase in the cardiac silhouette on chest x-ray, new onset of ectopic tachyarrhythmia or AV block, and congestive heart failure. As with primary cardiac tumors, the clinical presentation is more closely related to the location and size of the tumor rather than histologic type. Many of these signs and symptoms also occur with myocarditis, pericarditis, or cardiomyopathy resulting from radiotherapy or chemotherapy.

Electrocardiographic findings are nonspecific. On chest roentgenography the cardiac silhouette is most often normal but may reveal a pericardial effusion or bizarre contour. Echocardiography is useful for the diagnosis of pericardial effusion and the visualization of larger metastases. Computed tomography, magnetic resonance imaging, and radionuclide imaging with gallium or thallium may provide useful anatomic information. Angiography may delineate discrete lesions, and pericardiocentesis can allow a specific cytologic diagnosis.

℞ **TREATMENT**   Because most patients with cardiac metastases have widespread disease, therapy generally consists of treatment of the primary tumor. Symptomatic malignant effusions are treated by removal of fluid by pericardiocentesis, with or without concomitant instillation of a sclerosing agent (e.g., tetracycline), or placement of a pericardial window for drainage to the pleural space to palliate symptoms and delay or prevent reaccumulation of the effusion.

CARDIAC EFFECTS OF CANCER THERAPY   →*See Chap. 238.*

CARDIOVASCULAR MANIFESTATIONS OF SYSTEMIC DISEASES

DIABETES MELLITUS (See also Chap. 333)   There is an increased incidence of large vessel atherosclerosis and myocardial infarction in patients with both insulin- and non-insulin-dependent diabetes mellitus. Coronary artery disease is the most common cause of death in adults with diabetes mellitus. Diabetes mellitus is an independent risk factor for coronary artery disease (Chap. 241), and the incidence of coronary artery disease is related to the duration of diabetes. In patients with diabetes mellitus, myocardial infarctions are not only more frequent but also tend to be larger in size and more likely to result in complications such as heart failure, shock, and death. Patients with diabetes mellitus are more likely to have an abnormal or absent pain response to myocardial ischemia, probably as a result of generalized autonomic nervous system dysfunction. Ambulatory electrocardiographic monitoring has shown that up to 90% of episodes of ischemia are silent in diabetic patients with coronary artery disease; the presentation of ischemia may be exertional or episodic dyspnea, flash pulmonary edema, arrhythmias, heart block, or syncope. Since coronary artery disease is more common in in patients with diabetes mellitus and often is not associated with typical anginal symptoms, the threshold for the diagnosis should be low, particularly when the duration of disease is long and concomitant risk factors for coronary artery disease (e.g., hypertension, smoking, hyperlipidemia) are present.

Patients with diabetes mellitus may also have myocardial dysfunction characteristic of a restrictive cardiomyopathy in the absence of large-vessel (epicardial) coronary artery disease, with abnormal relaxation of the myocardium, and evidenced clinically by elevated left ventricular filling pressures. Histologically, these patients have interstitial fibrosis with increased amounts of collagen, glycoprotein, triglycerides, and cholesterol in the myocardial interstitium; and in some cases intimal thickening, hyaline deposition, and inflammatory changes have been observed in small intramural arteries. Patients with diabetes mellitus have an increased risk of developing clinical heart failure, even after correction for the presence of coronary artery disease, hypertension, and obesity, and it is likely that diabetic cardiomyopathy contributes to excessive cardiovascular morbidity and mortality in these patients. There is some evidence that insulin therapy results in an amelioration of the myocardial dysfunction.

MALNUTRITION AND VITAMIN DEFICIENCY MALNUTRITION (See also Chap. 74)   In patients whose intake of protein, calories, or both is severely deficient, the heart may become thin, pale, and flabby with myofibrillar atrophy and interstitial edema. The systolic pressure and cardiac output are low, and the pulse pressure is

factors, including reduced serum oncotic pressure and myocardial dysfunction. Such profound states of malnutrition, termed *marasmus* in the case of caloric deficiency and *kwashiorkor* in the case of relative protein deficiency, are most common in underdeveloped countries. However, significant nutritional heart disease may also occur in developed nations, particularly in patients with chronic diseases such as AIDS, in patients with anorexia nervosa, and in patients with severe cardiac failure in whom gastrointestinal hypoperfusion and venous congestion may lead to anorexia and malabsorption. Open-heart surgery poses increased risk in malnourished patients, and they may benefit from preoperative hyperalimentation.

Thiamine Deficiency (Beriberi) (See also Chap. 75)   In many cases, malnutrition is accompanied by thiamine deficiency, although this hypovitaminosis may also occur in the presence of an adequate protein and caloric intake, particularly in the Far East, where polished rice deficient in thiamine may be a major dietary component. In western nations, the widespread use of thiamine-enriched flour limits the presence of deficiency primarily to alcoholics and food faddists. The measurement of the thiamine-pyrophosphate effect (TPPE) can biochemically quantitate thiamine stores. An elevated TPPE, indicative of thiamine deficiency, has been found in 20 to 90% of patients with chronic heart failure. The deficiency appears to result from both reduced dietary intake and a diuretic-induced increase in the urinary excretion of thiamine. The acute administration of thiamine to these patients increases the left ventricular ejection fraction and the excretion of salt and water.

Clinically, there is usually evidence of generalized malnutrition, peripheral neuropathy, glossitis, and anemia. The characteristic cardiovascular syndrome is heart failure with increased cardiac output, tachycardia, and often elevated filling pressures in the left and right sides of the heart. The major cause of the high-output state is vasomotor depression, the precise mechanism of which is not understood but which leads to a reduced systemic vascular resistance. The cardiac examination reveals a wide pulse pressure, tachycardia, a third heart sound, and, frequently, an apical systolic murmur. The electrocardiogram may show decreased voltage, a prolonged QT interval, and T-wave abnormalities. The chest x-ray generally shows a large heart with signs of congestive heart failure. The response to thiamine is often dramatic, with an increase in systemic vascular resistance, decrease in cardiac output, clearing of pulmonary congestion, and a reduction in heart size often occurring in 12 to 48 h. Although the response to digitalis and diuretics may be poor before thiamine therapy, these agents may be important *after* thiamine is given, since the left ventricle may not be capable of dealing with the increased workload presented by the return of vascular tone.

Vitamin B₆, B₁₂, and Folate Deficiency (See also Chap. 241) These vitamin cofactors in the metabolism of homocysteine probably contribute to the majority of cases of hyperhomocysteinemia in the general population. Hyperhomocysteinemia is associated with increased risk of atherosclerosis. Supplementation of these vitamins has reduced the incidence of hyperhomocysteinemia in the United States. The clinical benefit of normalizing elevated homocysteine levels, however, remains unproven.

OBESITY (See also Chap. 77)   Severe obesity, particularly when it occurs in an upper-body distribution, is associated with an increase in cardiovascular morbidity and mortality. Although obesity itself is not considered a disease, there is clearly an increased prevalence of hypertension, glucose intolerance, and atherosclerotic coronary artery disease in obese patients. In addition, these patients have a distinct abnormality of the cardiovascular system characterized by increases in total and central blood volumes, cardiac output, and left ventricular filling pressure. The elevated cardiac output appears to be required to support the metabolic needs of the excessive adipose tissue. Left ventricular filling pressure is often at the upper limits of normal and rises excessively with exercise. As a result of chronic volume overload, eccentric cardiac hypertrophy with cardiac dilatation and abnormal ventricular function may develop. Pathologically, there are

left and, in some cases, right ventricular hypertrophy and generalized cardiac dilatation, which is not due simply to fatty infiltration of the myocardium. Although these patients may develop pulmonary congestion, peripheral edema, and exercise intolerance, the recognition of these findings may be difficult in massively obese patients.

Weight reduction is the most effective therapy and results in reduction in blood volume and in the return of cardiac output toward normal. However, rapid weight reduction may be dangerous, as cardiac arrhythmias and sudden death due to electrolyte imbalance have been described. Digitalis, sodium restriction, and diuretics may also be useful. This form of heart disease should be distinguished from the Pickwickian syndrome (Chap. 263), which may share several of the cardiovascular features of heart disease secondary to severe obesity but, in addition, frequently has components of central apnea, hypoxemia, pulmonary hypertension, and cor pulmonale.

THYROID DISEASE (See also Chap. 330)   Thyroid hormone exerts a major influence on the cardiovascular system by a number of direct and indirect mechanisms, and not surprisingly, cardiovascular effects are prominent in both hypo- and hyperthyroidism. Thyroid hormone causes increases in total-body metabolism and oxygen consumption that indirectly place an increased workload on the heart. In addition, although the exact mechanism has not been defined, thyroid hormone exerts direct inotropic, chronotropic, and dromotropic effects that are similar to those seen with adrenergic stimulation (e.g., tachycardia, increased cardiac output). Thyroid hormone increases the synthesis of myosin and of Na⁺,K⁺-ATPase, as well as the density of myocardial beta-adrenergic receptors.

Hyperthyroidism   Cardiovascular presentations of hyperthyroidism include palpitations, systolic hypertension, fatigue, or, in patients with underlying heart disease, angina or heart failure. Sinus tachycardia is found in about 40% of patients and atrial fibrillation in about 15%. Other findings include a hyperdynamic precordium, a widened pulse pressure, an increase in the intensity of the first heart sound and the pulmonic component of the second heart sound, and a third heart sound. An increased incidence of mitral valve prolapse has been associated with hyperthyroidism, and in some cases there may be a midsystolic murmur heard best at the left sternal border with or without a systolic ejection click. A *Means-Lerman scratch* is a systolic scratchy sound, heard at the left second intercostal space during expiration; it is thought to result from the rubbing of the hyperdynamic pericardium against the pleura. Elderly patients with hyperthyroidism, so-called apathetic hyperthyroidism, may present with only the cardiovascular manifestations of thyrotoxicosis, such as atrial fibrillation, which may be resistant to therapy until the hyperthyroidism is controlled. Angina pectoris and congestive heart failure are unusual unless there is coexistent underlying heart disease, and in many cases symptoms resolve with treatment of the hyperthyroidism.

Hypothyroidism   Cardiac manifestations of hypothyroidism include a reduction in cardiac output, stroke volume, heart rate, blood pressure, and pulse pressure. In about one-third of patients there is a pericardial effusion which only rarely results in tamponade. Increased capillary permeability results in pleural and pericardial effusions. Other clinical signs include cardiomegaly, bradycardia, weak arterial pulses, and distant heart sounds. Although the signs and symptoms of myxedema may suggest the diagnosis of congestive heart failure, in the absence of other cardiac disease, myocardial failure is uncommon. The electrocardiogram generally shows sinus bradycardia and low voltage and may show prolongation of the QT interval, decreased P-wave voltage, prolonged AV conduction time, intraventricular conduction disturbances, and nonspecific ST-T wave abnormalities. Chest x-ray may show cardiomegaly, often with a "water bottle" configuration, pleural effusions, and, in some cases, evidence of congestive heart failure. Pathologically, the heart is pale, dilated, and flabby, often with myofibrillar swelling, loss of striations, and interstitial fibrosis.

Patients with hypothyroidism frequently have elevations of cholesterol and triglycerides and severe atherosclerotic coronary artery disease. Before treatment with thyroid hormone, patients with hypothyroidism frequently do not have angina pectoris, presumably because of the low metabolic demands made by their condition. However, angina and myocardial infarction may be precipitated during initiation of thyroid hormone replacement, especially in elderly patients with underlying heart disease. Therefore, replacement should be done with care, starting with low doses that are increased gradually.

MALIGNANT CARCINOID (See also Chap. 93)   These tumors elaborate a variety of vasoactive amines (e.g., serotonin), kinins, indoles, and other substances believed to be responsible for the diarrhea, flushing, and labile blood pressure in these patients. The cardiac lesions due to gastrointestinal carcinoids are almost exclusively in the right side of the heart and occur only when there are hepatic metastases, suggesting that the substance responsible for the cardiac lesions is inactivated by passage through the liver and lungs. Similar lesions occur in the left side of the heart when there exists a right-to-left shunt or the tumor is located in the lungs. These lesions are fibrous plaques on the endothelium of the cardiac chambers, valves, and great vessels. These plaques, which result in distortion of the cardiac valves, consist of smooth-muscle cells embedded in a stroma of acid mucopolysaccharide and collagen and presumably result from healing of endothelial injury. The clinical syndrome is most often that of tricuspid regurgitation, pulmonic stenosis, or both. In some cases a high-output state may occur, presumably as a result of a decrease in systemic vascular resistance due to a vasoactive substance released by the tumor. Progression of the cardiac lesions does not appear to be affected by treatment with serotonin antagonists, and in some severely symptomatic patients valve replacement is indicated. Coronary artery spasm, presumably due to a circulating vasoactive substance, may occur in patients with carcinoid syndrome.

PHEOCHROMOCYTOMA (See also Chap. 332)   In addition to causing labile or sustained hypertension, the high circulating levels of catecholamines may also cause direct myocardial injury. Focal myocardial necrosis and inflammatory cell infiltration are present in about 50% of patients who die with pheochromocytoma and may contribute to clinically significant left ventricular failure and pulmonary edema. Left ventricular function and congestive heart failure may resolve after removal of the tumor. In addition, hypertension results in left ventricular hypertrophy.

RHEUMATOID ARTHRITIS AND THE COLLAGEN VASCULAR DISEASES   Rheumatoid Arthritis   (See also Chap. 312)   There may be inflammation of any or all parts of the heart in patients with rheumatoid arthritis. Pericarditis is the most common cause of clinically apparent disease and may be found by echocardiography in 10 to 50% of all patients with rheumatoid arthritis, particularly those with subcutaneous nodules. However, only a small fraction of these patients have clinical evidence of pericarditis, which usually follows a benign course but occasionally may progress to cardiac tamponade or constrictive pericarditis. The pericardial fluid is generally an exudate, with decreased concentrations of complement and glucose and elevated cholesterol. Coronary arteritis with intimal inflammation and edema is present in about 20% of cases but only rarely results in angina pectoris or myocardial infarction. The cardiac valves, most often the mitral and aortic, may be involved by inflammation and granuloma formation that in some cases may cause clinically significant regurgitation due to valve deformity. Myocarditis rarely results in cardiac dysfunction.

Treatment is directed at the underlying rheumatoid arthritis and may include glucocorticoids. Pericardiectomy is usually required in cases of tamponade or persistent effusion.

Seronegative Arthropathies   The seronegative arthropathies (Chaps. 315 and 324), ankylosing spondylitis, Reiter's syndrome, psoriatic arthritis, and the arthritides associated with ulcerative colitis and regional enteritis may be accompanied by a pancarditis and proximal aortitis; the latter may result in aortic regurgitation and may extend into the anterior mitral valve ring and/or AV node. Conduction disturbances are common, occurring in up to one-third of patients; they are more common in patients with aortic valve disease and appear to be associated with the presence of the HLA-B27 antigen. Both aortic regurgitation and AV block are more common in patients with peripheral joint involvement and long-standing disease; treatment with aortic valve replacement and permanent pacemaker placement may be required. Up to one-fifth of patients with peripheral joint involvement and disease for more than 30 years have significant aortic regurgitation. Occasionally, aortic regurgitation precedes the onset of arthritis, and, therefore, the diagnosis of a seronegative arthritis should be considered in young males with isolated aortic regurgitation.

Systemic Lupus Erythematosus (SLE) (See also Chap. 311)   Pericarditis is common, occurring in about two-thirds of patients, and generally pursues a benign course, although rarely tamponade or constriction may result. The characteristic *endocardial lesions* of SLE, described by Libman and Sacks, consist of wartlike lesions most often located at the angles of the AV valves or on the ventricular surface of the mitral valve. Hemodynamically important valvular regurgitation is rare. Patients with the antiphospholipid syndrome have a higher incidence of cardiovascular abnormalities, including valvular disease (particularly regurgitant lesions), a variety of thrombotic disorders (venous and arterial thrombosis, thrombocytopenia, premature stroke), myocardial infarction, pulmonary hypertension, and cardiomyopathy. Myocarditis generally parallels the activity of the disease, and although common histologically, seldom results in clinical heart failure unless associated with hypertension. Although arteritis of large coronary arteries may rarely result in myocardial ischemia, there is also an increased frequency of coronary atherosclerosis that may be related to hypertension or glucocorticoid therapy.

TRAUMATIC HEART DISEASE

Cardiac damage may be due to either penetrating or nonpenetrating injuries. The most frequent cause of a *nonpenetrating injury* is the impact of the chest against the steering wheel of an automobile. The absence of external signs of thoracic trauma does not exclude serious injury of the heart. Although the commonest injury is myocardial contusion, any structure of the heart may be affected by the trauma.

Myocardial contusions are often not immediately recognized in trauma patients due to focus on more obvious injuries. Myocardial contusion may cause arrhythmias, bundle branch block, or electrocardiographic abnormalities resembling those of infarction or pericarditis, and so it is important to bear trauma in mind as a cause of otherwise unexplained electrocardiographic changes. Serum creatine kinase (CK) MB isoenzyme levels are increased in about 20% of patients, but false-positive elevations of MB may occur in the presence of massive injuries associated with large increases in total CK. Cardiac troponin levels may have a greater diagnostic value than CK-MB. Echocardiography can detect abnormal wall motion and the presence of pericardial effusion, in addition to aiding in diagnosis of other forms of cardiac trauma. Myocardial contusion may produce positive radionuclide scans and regional impairment of ventricular function, as occurs in myocardial infarction (Chap. 243). Pericardial effusion may occur weeks or even months after the accident. In these cases, the pericardial effusion is a manifestation of the postcardiac injury syndrome, which resembles the postpericardiotomy syndrome (Chap. 239).

Rupture of the heart valves or the supporting structures leads to acute valvular incompetence. The presence of a loud heart murmur followed by the development of rapidly progressive heart failure after trauma heralds this diagnosis, which can be made by either transthoracic or transesophageal echocardiography.

The most serious consequence of nonpenetrating injury is myocardial rupture, leading to tamponade or intracardiac shunting. Although it is generally immediately fatal, up to 40 percent of patients with cardiac rupture have been reported to survive long enough to reach a specialized trauma center. Hemopericardium may also follow tearing of a pericardial vessel or coronary artery.

Rupture of the aorta is a common consequence of nonpenetrating chest trauma. Indeed, rupture of the aorta at the isthmus or just above the aortic valve is the most common vascular deceleration injury. The clinical presentation is similar to that in aortic dissection (Chap. 247). The arterial pressure and pulse amplitude may be increased in the upper extremities and decreased in the lower extremities, and on chest roentgenogram there may be widening of the mediastinum. Occasionally, aortic rupture is limited by the aortic adventitia and results in a silent false aneurysm that may be discovered months or years after the injury.

Penetrating injuries of the heart, produced by bullets or stab wounds, usually result in immediate or very rapid death because of hemopericardium or massive hemorrhage. However, up to half of such patients may survive if they are resuscitated and/or survive long enough to reach a specialized trauma center. Perforation complicating the placement of an intravenous intracardiac catheter or pacemaker lead is another common cause of penetrating injuries to the heart and great vessels.

When great vessel rupture is due to a penetrating injury, there is usually a hemothorax and, less often, a hemopericardium. Hematoma formation may compress major vessels, and arteriovenous fistulae may form, sometimes resulting in high-output congestive heart failure.

Patients who suffer penetrating injuries of the heart should be carefully examined several weeks after the event to rule out a ventricular septal defect or mitral regurgitation that may have gone undetected at the time of emergency surgery. Sometimes the patient survives the acute incident and presents with a cardiac murmur and congestive heart failure. A left-to-right shunt due to traumatic ventricular septal defect, aortopulmonary artery fistula, or coronary arteriovenous fistula may be suspected and confirmed by cardiac catheterization and angiocardiography.

℞ **TREATMENT** The treatment of an uncomplicated myocardial contusion, with or without myocardial infarction, is similar to that for a myocardial infarction, except that anticoagulation is contraindicated, and should include monitoring for the development of complications such as arrhythmia and cardiac rupture (Chap. 243). Acute myocardial failure resulting from the rupture of a valve usually re-

quires operative correction. Immediate thoracotomy should be carried out for most cases of penetrating injury or if there is evidence of cardiac tamponade and/or shock regardless of the type of trauma. Pericardiocentesis may be helpful in patients with tamponade, but usually only as holding maneuver on the way to the operating room. Pericardial hemorrhage often leads to constriction, which must be treated by decortication.

BIBLIOGRAPHY

COLUCCI WS et al: Primary tumors of the heart, in *Heart Disease*, 6th ed, E Braunwald et al (eds). Philadelphia, Saunders, 2001

DUFLOU J et al: Sudden cardiac death as a result of heart disease in morbid obesity. Am Heart J 130:306, 1996

HOFFMAN : Rheumatic diseases and the heart, in *Heart Disease*, 6th ed, E Braunwald et al (eds). Philadelphia, Saunders, 2001

KLEIN I: Thyroid hormone and the cardiovascular system. Am J Med 88:631, 1990

KLUKE MH, MAYER RJ: Carcinoid tumors. N Engl J Med 340:858, 1999

MATTOX : Traumatic heart disease, in *Heart Disease*, 6th ed, E Braunwald et al (eds). Philadelphia, Saunders, 2001

MCALLISTER HA Jr et al: Tumors of the heart and pericardium. Curr Probl Cardiol 24: 57, 1999

NATAN DM: Long-term complications of diabetes mellitus. N Engl J Med 328:1676, 1993

O'NEILL TW et al: The heart in ankylosing spondylitis. Ann Rheum Dis 51:705, 1992

PRETRE R, CHILCOTT M: Blunt trauma to the heart and great vessels. N Engl J Med. 336: 626, 1997

REYMAN K: Cardiac myxomas. N Engl J Med 333:1610, 1995

RHEE PM et al: Penetrating cardiac injuries: a population-based study. J Trauma 45:366, 1998

ROBERTS WC: A unique heart disease associated with a unique cancer: carcinoid heart disease. Am J Cardiol 80:251, 1997

———, HIGH ST: The heart in systemic lupus erythematosus. Curr Probl Cardiol 24:1, 1999

SHIMON I et al: Improved left ventricular function after thiamine supplementation in patients with congestive heart failure receiving long-term furosemide therapy. Am J Med 98:485, 1995

SOWERS JR: Diabetes mellitus and cardiovascular disease in women. Arch Intern Med 158:617, 1998

WELCH GN, LOSCALZO J: Homocysteine and atherothrombosis. N Engl J Med 338:1042, 1998

Section 4
VASCULAR DISEASE

241 *Peter Libby*

THE PATHOGENESIS OF ATHEROSCLEROSIS

HDL	high-density lipoproteins	PAI	plasminogen-activator inhibitor
ICAM	intercellular adhesion molecule	PDGF	platelet-derived growth factors
IFN	interferon	TGF	transforming growth factor
IL	interleukin	TNF	tumor necrosis factor
LDL	low-density lipoprotein	VCAM	vascular cell adhesion molecule
Lp(a)	lipoprotein		

Atherosclerosis is the leading cause of death and disability in the developed world. Despite our familiarity with this disease, some of its fundamental characteristics remain poorly recognized and understood. Although many generalized or systemic risk factors predispose to its development, atherosclerosis affects various regions of the circulation preferentially and yields distinct clinical manifestations depending on the particular circulatory bed affected. Atherosclerosis of the coronary

arteries commonly causes myocardial infarction (Chap. 243) and angina pectoris (Chap. 244). Atherosclerosis of the arteries supplying the central nervous system frequently provokes strokes and transient cerebral ischemia (Chap. 361). In the peripheral circulation, atherosclerosis causes intermittent claudication and gangrene and can jeopardize limb viability (Chap. 248). Involvement of the splanchnic circulation can cause mesenteric ischemia. Atherosclerosis can affect the kidneys either directly (e.g., renal artery stenosis) or as a frequent site of atheroembolic disease (Chap. 278).

Even within a given arterial bed, atherosclerosis tends to occur focally, typically in certain predisposed regions. In the coronary circulation, for example, the proximal left anterior descending coronary artery exhibits a particular predilection for developing atherosclerotic occlusive disease. Likewise, atherosclerosis preferentially affects the proximal portions of the renal arteries and, in the extracranial circulation to the brain, the carotid bifurcation. Indeed, atherosclerotic lesions often form at branching points of arteries, regions of disturbed blood flow. Not all manifestations of atherosclerosis result from stenotic, occlusive disease. Ectasia and development of aneurysmal disease, for example, frequently occur in the aorta (Chap. 247). The mechanisms that underlie this discontinuous anatomic distribution of atherosclerosis remain uncertain.

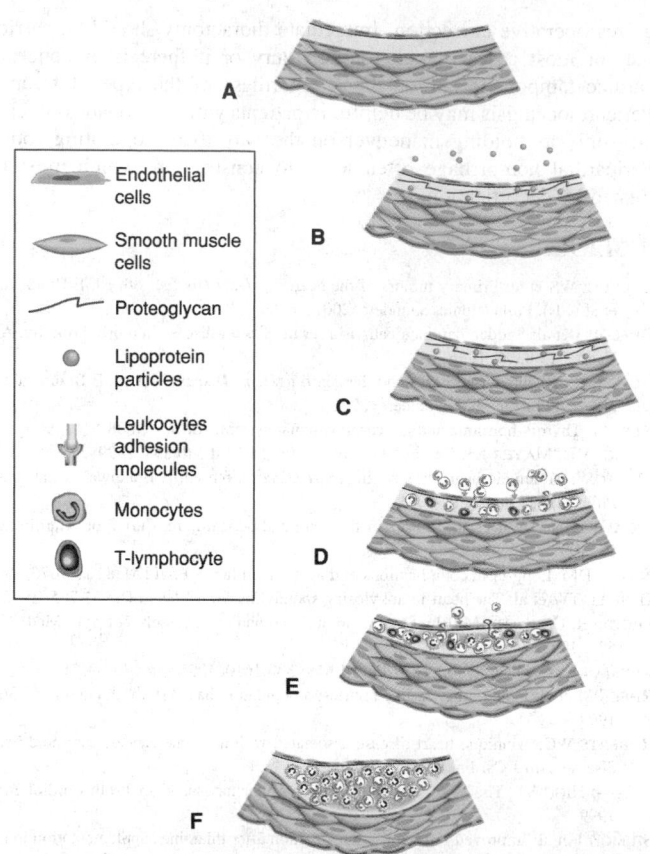

Endothelial cells

Smooth muscle cells

Proteoglycan

Lipoprotein particles

Leukocytes adhesion molecules

Monocytes

T-lymphocyte

FIGURE 241-1 *A*. The normal artery. The normal artery consists of three layers. The intima, lined by a monolayer of endothelial cells in contact with the blood, contains resident smooth-muscle cells embedded in extracellular matrix. The internal elastic lamina forms the border of the intima with the underlying tunica media. The media contains layers of smooth-muscle cells

Atherosclerosis manifests itself focally not only in space, as just described, but in time as well. Atherogenesis in humans typically occurs over a period of many years, usually many decades. Growth of atherosclerotic plaques probably does not occur in a smooth linear fashion, but rather discontinuously, with periods of relative quiescence punctuated by periods of rapid evolution. After a generally prolonged "silent" period, atherosclerosis may become clinically manifest. The clinical expressions of atherosclerosis may be chronic, as in the development of stable, effort-induced angina pectoris or of predictable and reproducible intermittent claudication. Alternatively, a much more dramatic acute clinical event, such as myocardial infarction, a cerebrovascular accident, or sudden cardiac death, may first herald the presence of atherosclerosis. Other individuals may never experience clinical manifestations of arterial disease despite the presence of widespread atherosclerosis demonstrated post mortem.

INITIATION OF ATHEROSCLEROSIS   Lipoprotein Accumulation and Modification • *Fatty streak formation*   An integrated view of experimental results in animals and study of human atherosclerosis suggests that the "fatty streak" represents the initial lesion of atherosclerosis (Fig. 241-1). The formation of these early lesions of atherosclerosis most often seems to arise from focal increases in the content of lipoproteins within regions of the intima (Fig. 241-1*B*). This accumulation of lipoprotein particles may not result simply from an increased permeability, or "leakiness," of the overlying endothelium. Rather, these lipoproteins may collect in the intima of arteries because they bind to constituents of the extracellular matrix, increasing the residence time of the lipid-rich particles within the arterial wall. Lipoproteins that accumulate in the extracellular space of the intima of arteries often associate with proteoglycan molecules of

FIGURE 241-1—*(continued)*

invested with a collagen- and elastin-rich extracellular matrix. Elastic arteries such as the aorta contain concentric lamellae of smooth-muscle cells sandwiched between dense bands of elastin. Muscular arteries have a looser organization of smooth-muscle cells dispersed within the matrix. The external elastic lamina forms the border of the media with the adventitia. The adventitia contains nerves and some mast cells and is the origin of the vasa vasorum, which supply blood to the outer two-thirds of the tunica media.

B. Accumulation of lipoprotein particles. Lipoprotein particles can accumulate in the intima of arteries, particularly when the ambient concentration is increased by hypercholesterolemic states. The lipoprotein particles often associate with constituents of the extracellular matrix, notably proteoglycans. Sequestration within the intima separates lipoproteins from some plasma antioxidants and can favor oxidative modification. Such modified lipoprotein particles may trigger a local inflammatory response responsible for signaling subsequent steps in lesion formation.

C. Adhesion of leukocytes. In hypercholesterolemia, adhesion of mononuclear leukocytes to the luminal endothelial occurs early. The augmented expression of various adhesion molecules for leukocytes probably triggers this first step in the recruitment of white blood cells to the site of a nascent arterial lesion.

D. Penetration of leukocytes. Once adherent, some white blood cells will migrate into the intima. The directed migration of leukocytes probably depends on chemoattractant factors including modified lipoprotein particles themselves and chemoattractant cytokines such as the chemokine macrophage chemoattractant protein 1 produced by vascular wall cells in response to modified lipoproteins.

E. Accumulation of leukocytes. Leukocytes resident in the evolving fatty streak can divide and exhibit augmented expression of receptors for modified lipoproteins (scavenger receptors). These mononuclear phagocytes imbibe lipids and transform into foam cells whose cytoplasm is filled with lipid droplets.

F. Formation of the fibrous cap and lipid core. As the fatty streak evolves into a more complicated atherosclerotic lesion, smooth-muscle cells accumulate within the expanding intima and the amount of extracellular matrix increases. The fibrous cap, formed of extracellular matrix elaborated by the smooth-muscle cells in the intima, characteristically overlies a lipid core filled with macrophages. In addition to dividing, these cells in the lipid core can die, releasing their lipid contents into the extracellular space.

the arterial extracellular matrix. At sites of lesion formation, the balance of different matrix constituents may vary in important ways. Of the three major classes of proteoglycans, for example, a relative excess of heparan sulfate molecules in relation to keratan sulfate or chondritin sulfate may promote the retention of lipoprotein particles by binding them and slowing their egress from nascent lesions.

Lipoprotein particles in the extracellular space of the intima, particularly those bound to matrix macromolecules, may undergo chemical modifications. Accumulating evidence supports a pathogenic role for such modifications of lipoproteins in atherogenesis. Two types of such alterations in lipoproteins bear particular interest in the context of understanding how risk factors actually promote atherogenesis: oxidation and nonenzymatic glycation.

Lipoprotein oxidation   Lipoproteins sequestered from plasma antioxidants in the extracellular space of the intima may be particularly susceptible to oxidative modification. Oxidatively modified low-density lipoprotein (LDL), rather than being a defined homogenous entity, actually comprises a variable and incompletely defined mixture. Both the lipid and protein moieties of these particles can participate in oxidative modification. Modifications of the lipids may include formation of hydroperoxides, lysophospholipids, oxysterols, and aldehydic breakdown products of fatty acids. Recently recognized phospholipid oxidation products include palmitoyl-oxovaleroyl-glycero-phosphoryl choline (POVPC), palmitoyl-glutaroyl-glycerophosphoryl choline (PGPC), and epoxyisoprostane E_2-glycero-phosphocholine (PEIPC). Modifications of the apoprotein moieties may include breaks in the peptide backbone as well as derivatization of certain amino acid residues. The side chain amino group of lysine may condense with components of the oxidized lipids (4-hydroxynonenol, or malondialdehyde). A more recently recognized modification may result from local hypochlorous acid production by inflammatory cells within the plaque, giving rise to chlorinated species such as chlorotyrosyl moieties. Ongoing work is characterizing specific chemical constituents of oxidized lipoproteins responsible for various biologic effects. Examples include oxovaleryl-phosphoryl choline. Considerable evidence supports the presence of such chemical entities in atherosclerotic lesions.

Nonenzymatic glycation In diabetic patients with sustained hyperglycemia, nonenzymatic glycation of apolipoproteins and other arterial proteins likely occurs that may likewise alter their function and propensity to accelerate atherogenesis. A good deal of experimental work suggests that both oxidatively modified and glycated lipoproteins or their constituents can contribute to many of the subsequent cellular events of lesion development.

Leukocyte Recruitment After the accumulation of extracellular lipid, recruitment of leukocytes occurs as a second step in formation of the fatty streak (Fig. 241-1C). The white blood cell types typically found in the evolving atheroma include primarily cells of the mononuclear lineage: monocytes and lymphocytes. A number of adhesion molecules or receptors for leukocytes expressed on the surface of the arterial endothelial cell likely participate in the recruitment of leukocytes to the nascent fatty streak. Adhesion molecules of particular interest include vascular cell adhesion molecule (VCAM) 1 and intercellular adhesion molecule (ICAM) 1 (members of the immunoglobulin gene superfamily) and P-selectin (a member of a distinct family of leukocyte receptors known as selectins). Lysophosphatidylcholine, a constituent of oxidatively modified LDL, can augment expression of VCAM-1. This example illustrates how the accumulation of lipoproteins in the arterial intima may link mechanistically with leukocyte recruitment and subsequent events in lesion formation.

Laminar shear forces, such as those encountered in most regions of normal arteries, can also suppress the expression of leukocyte adhesion molecules such as VCAM-1. Sites of predilection for forming atherosclerotic lesions (e.g., branch points) often have disturbed laminar flow. Ordered laminar shear of normal blood flow augments the production of nitric oxide by endothelial cells. This molecule, in addition to its vasodilator properties, can act at the low levels constitutively produced by arterial endothelium as a local anti-inflammatory autacoid, for example, limiting local VCAM-1 expression. These examples indicate how hemodynamic forces may influence the cellular events that underlie atherosclerotic lesion initiation and illustrate a potential explanation for the focal distribution of atherosclerotic lesions at certain sites predetermined by altered flow patterns.

Once adherent to the surface of the arterial endothelial cell via interaction with a receptor such as VCAM-1, the monocytes and lymphocytes penetrate the endothelial layer and take up residence in the intima (Fig. 241-1D). In addition to products of modified lipoproteins, cytokines (a class of protein mediators of inflammation) can regulate the expression of adhesion molecules involved in leukocyte recruitment. For example, the cytokines interleukin (IL) 1 or tumor necrosis factor (TNF) α induce or augment the expression of VCAM-1 and ICAM-1 on endothelial cells. Because modified lipoproteins can induce cytokine release from vascular wall cells, this pathway may provide an additional link between accumulation and modification of lipoproteins and leukocyte recruitment. The directed migration of leukocytes into the arterial wall may also result from the actions of modified lipoprotein. For example, oxidized LDL may promote the chemotaxis of leukocytes. Also, oxidatively modified lipoproteins can elicit the production by vascular wall cells of chemoattractant cytokines such as monocyte chemoattractant protein 1.

Foam-cell formation Once resident within the intima, the mononuclear phagocytes differentiate into macrophages and transform into lipid-laden foam cells. Transformation of mononuclear phagocytes into foam cells requires the uptake of lipoprotein particles by receptor-mediated endocytosis. One might suppose that the well-known recognized receptor for LDL mediates this lipid uptake. Patients or animals lacking effective LDL receptors due to genetic alterations (e.g., familial hypercholesterolemia), however, have abundant arterial lesions and extraarterial xanthomata rich in macrophage-derived foam-cells. Also, the exogenous cholesterol suppresses expression of the LDL receptor, such that under hypercholesterolemic conditions the level of this cell-surface receptor for LDL decreases. Candidates for alternative receptors that can mediate lipid-loading of foam cells include a growing number of macrophage "scavenger" receptors, which preferentially endocytose modified lipoproteins, and other receptors for oxidized LDL or β-VLDL (very low density lipoprotein), a type of lipoprotein commonly encountered in certain hypercholesterolemic states (Chap. 344). By imbibing lipids from the extracellular space, the mononuclear phagocytes bearing such scavenger receptors may remove lipoproteins from the developing lesion. Some lipid-loaded macrophages may leave the artery wall, functioning to clear lipid from the artery. Lipid accumulation, and hence propensity to form atheroma, ensues if the amount of lipid entering the artery wall exceeds that exported by mononuclear phagocytes or other pathways. Macrophages may thus play a vital role in the dynamic economy of lipid accumulation in the arterial wall during atherogenesis. Some lipid-laden foam cells within the expanding intimal lesion perish. Some of the death of foam cells may result from a program of cell death known as *apoptosis*. This death of mononuclear phagocytes results in formation of the lipid-rich center of more complicated atherosclerotic plaques, often called the *necrotic core* of the lesion.

Macrophages taking up modified lipoproteins, much like intrinsic vascular wall cells, may elaborate cytokines and growth factors that can further signal some of the cellular events in lesion complication. A number of growth factors or cytokines elaborated by mononuclear phagocytes can stimulate smooth-muscle cell proliferation and production of extracellular matrix, which accumulates in atherosclerotic plaques. IL-1 and TNF-α are examples of cytokines that can induce local production of growth factors such as forms of platelet-derived growth factor, fibroblast growth factor, and others that may play a role in plaque evolution and complication. Other cytokines, notably interferon (IFN) γ derived from activated T cells within lesions, can inhibit smooth-muscle proliferation and synthesis of interstitial forms of collagen. These examples illustrate how atherogenesis likely depends on a complex balance between mediators that can promote lesion formation and other pathways that can mitigate the atherogenic process.

Factors That Modulate Inhibition of Atheroma Elaboration of small molecules by activated mononuclear phagocytes and vascular wall cells in the evolving lesion may also modulate atherogenesis. Notably, reactive oxygen species can modulate growth of smooth-muscle cells, activate inflammatory gene expression via the nuclear factor kappa B (NFκB) transcriptional control system, and annihilate NO radicals, decreasing the effect of this endogenous vasodilator. However, the macrophage in the lesion may be activated to express the inducible form of the enzyme that can synthesize NO, known as inducible NO synthase. This high-capacity form of the enzyme can produce relatively large, potentially cytotoxic amounts of NO radicals. While at low concentrations of ·NO produced by the constitutive NO synthase in endothelial cells, this radical may produce beneficial effects; when overproduced by activated phagocytes, it may prove deleterious.

Export by phagocytes may constitute one response to local lipid overload in the evolving lesion. Another mechanism, reverse cholesterol transport mediated by high-density lipoproteins (HDL), may provide an independent pathway for lipid removal from atheroma. Multiple observational studies have established a tight inverse relationship between the level of HDL cholesterol and the risk for coronary events. Increased HDL may explain why premenopausal women have less atherosclerosis than age-matched men. In various in vitro models, HDL can mediate net cholesterol removal from lipid-laden macrophages. This process likely involves a family of scavenger receptors (the "B" family), highly expressed by steroidogenic tissues and by cells within atheroma as well. Such "reverse cholesterol transport" may also pertain during human atherogenesis and help to explain HDL's protective effect on lesion formation.

Although clear evidence supports lipoprotein disorders as predisposing factors for atheroma formation, other etiologies may contribute to or modulate atherogenesis (Table 242-1). For example, hypertension constitutes an independent risk factor for coronary events. Male gender and the postmenopausal state also augment the risk of developing coronary artery disease. Premenopausal women have increased HDL levels compared to age-matched men. However, a favorable lipoprotein pattern only partially accounts for the protection against atherosclerosis conferred by the premenopausal state. Thus, as yet poorly understood direct effects of estrogens on the arterial wall may account for some of this benefit. Studies in progress are investigating possible mechanisms of estrogen's possible "vasculoprotective" effect and the role of estrogen replacement therapy as an antiatherogenic strategy in postmenopausal women.

Diabetes mellitus accelerates atherogenesis. In addition to the well-known microvascular complications of diabetes (Chap. 333), macrovascular disease such as atherosclerosis causes a great deal of excess mortality in the diabetic populations. Diabetes-associated dyslipidemias strongly promote atherogenesis. In particular, the constellation of insulin resistance, high triglycerides, and low HDL, often in association with central adiposity and hypertension frequent in type 2 diabetic patients, seems to accelerate atherogenesis potently. As noted above, hyperglycemia may promote the nonenzymatic glycation of LDL. LDL modified in this manner, like oxidatively modified LDL, may signal many of the initial events in atherogenesis. Other lipoproteins such as triglyceride-rich particles or lipoprotein (a) [Lp(a)] may also prove particularly atherogenic.

Lp(a) (often pronounced "lipoprotein little a" to distinguish it from apolipoprotein AI and others found in HDL) provides a potential link between hemostasis and blood lipids. The Lp(a) particle consists of an apoprotein (a) molecule bound by a sulfhydryl link to the apolipoprotein B moiety of a LDL particle. Apoprotein (a) has homology with plasminogen and may inhibit fibrinolysis by competing with plasminogen. Other risk factors for atherosclerosis related to blood clotting include elevated levels of fibrinogen or of the inhibitor of fibrinolysis, plasminogen-activator inhibitor (PAI) 1. Another nonlipid risk factor for coronary events, elevated levels of *homocysteine*, may act by promoting thrombosis, although the pathophysiology of this association is uncertain at present.

The relationship between *tobacco use* and atherosclerosis also remains poorly understood (Chap. 390). The rapid reduction in risk for cardiac events after cessation of cigarette smoking implies that tobacco may promote thrombosis or some other determinant of plaque stability as well as evolution of the atherosclerotic lesion itself. For example, tobacco smokers have elevated fibrinogen levels, a variable associated with increased atherosclerosis and acute cardiovascular events.

In other situations, antecedent inflammatory states may predispose towards atherosclerosis. For example, *Kawasaki disease* in childhood may promote development of vascular lesions in the arteries of adults (Chap. 317). Infectious agents continue to be proposed as instigators or potentiators of atherogenesis. Both viral and microbial pathogens have been invoked in this context (e.g., Herpesviridiae, including cytomegalovirus, or *Chlamydia*). In some patients, immune or autoimmune reactions may contribute to atherogenesis. In the particular example of the accelerated form of coronary arteriopathy that plagues heart transplant recipients, immunologic factors may contribute importantly to the pathogenesis. The roles of the immune response and of infectious diseases in usual atherosclerosis remain speculative.

Known genetic defects in lipoprotein metabolism account for only a fraction of the familial risk for coronary artery disease. Thus, other as yet undefined genetic factors must contribute to coronary risk. Mechanisms of disease susceptibility involving the arterial wall might account for some of the genetic predisposition to atherosclerosis unexplained by lipoprotein disorders. Application of molecular genetic techniques should help identify new polymorphisms linked to coronary risk and may eventually shed light on new pathophysiologic mechanisms. For example, some data suggest a link between certain alleles of the genes encoding angiotensin-converting enzyme or PAI-1 with increased risk of myocardial infarction. Large studies currently in progress should clarify these and other potential markers of genetic susceptibility to atherosclerosis.

ATHEROMA EVOLUTION AND COMPLICATION   Involvement of Arterial Smooth-Muscle Cells   Although the fatty streak commonly precedes the development of a more advanced atherosclerotic plaque, not all fatty streaks progress to yield atheroma. Fatty streaks occur in populations not prone to develop late lesions (e.g., indigenous Africans). These findings raise several questions. Why do some fatty streaks progress to fibrous lesions but not others? By what mechanisms do fatty streaks evolve into more complex lesions? While accumulation of lipid-laden macrophages is the hallmark of the fatty streaks, accumulation of fibrous tissue typifies the more advanced atherosclerotic lesion. The smooth-muscle cell synthesizes the bulk of the extracellular matrix of the complex atherosclerotic lesion. Hence, arrival of smooth-muscle cells and their elaboration of extracellular matrix probably provides a critical transition, yielding a fibrofatty lesion in place of a simple accumulation of macrophage-derived foam cells.

Recent research has provided insight into the mechanisms that may trigger migration and proliferation of smooth-muscle cells into and within the evolving intimal lesion and signal the accumulation of extracellular matrix. Cytokines and growth factors elicited by modified lipoproteins or other agents from both vascular wall cells and infiltrating leukocytes can modulate functions of the smooth-muscle cell. For example, platelet-derived growth factors (PDGF) elaborated by activated endothelial cells can stimulate the migration of smooth-muscle cells. In this manner, smooth-muscle cells resident in the tunica media may migrate into the intima. Various growth factors produced locally can stimulate the proliferation of both resident smooth-muscle cells in the intima and those that have migrated from the media. Transforming growth factor (TGF) β, among other mediators, potently stimulates interstitial collagen production by smooth-muscle cells. These mediators may arise not only from neighboring vascular cells or leukocytes (a "paracrine" pathway) but in some instances from the same cell that responds to the factor (an "autocrine" pathway). Together, these alterations in smooth-muscle cells, signaled by these mediators acting at short distances, can hasten transformation of the fatty streak into a more fibrous smooth-muscle cell and extracellular matrix–rich lesion.

In addition to locally produced mediators, atherogenic risk factor signals related to blood coagulation and thrombosis likely contribute to atheroma evolution and complication. Current evidence suggests that fatty streak formation begins without frank denuding endothelial injury or desquamation. In advanced fatty streaks, however, microscopic breaches in endothelial integrity may occur. Microthrombi rich in platelets can form at such sites of limited endothelial denudation, due to exposure of the highly thrombogenic extracellular matrix of underlying basement membrane. Activated platelets release numerous factors that can promote the fibrotic response. In addition to PDGF and TGF-β, low-molecular-weight mediators such as serotonin can also alter smooth-muscle function. Most of these microthrombi probably resolve without clinical manifestation by a process of local fibrinolysis, resorption, and endothelial repair.

As atherosclerotic lesions advance, abundant plexi of microvessels develop in connection with the artery's vasa vasorum. These newly developing microvascular networks may contribute to lesion complication in several ways. These blood vessels provide an abundant surface area for leukocyte trafficking and may serve as the portal of entry and exit of white blood cells from the established atheroma. The plaques' microvessels may also furnish foci for intraplaque hemorrhage. Like the neovessels in the diabetic retina, microvessels of the plaque may be friable and prone to rupture and produce focal hemorrhage. Such a vascular leak leads to thrombosis in situ and thrombin

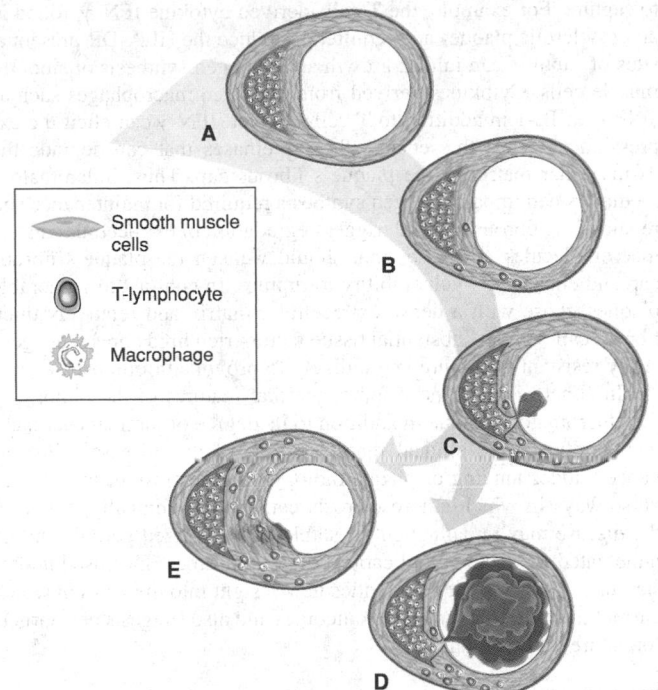

FIGURE 241-2 Plaque rupture, thrombosis, and healing. *A.* Arterial remodeling during atherogenesis. During the initial part of the life history of an atheroma, growth is often outward, preserving the caliber of lumen. This phenomenon of "compensatory enlargement" accounts in part for the tendency of coronary arteriography to underestimate the degree of atherosclerosis.

B. Focal inflammation characterizes unstable atherosclerotic plaques. Foci of inflammation often occur in atheroma. Analysis of lesions that have ruptured and caused fatal myocardial infarction characteristically show a prominent infiltration of macrophages and T lymphocytes. Both the leukocytes and the intrinsic vascular cells around points of plaque rupture show markers of inflammatory activation.

C. Rupture of the plaque's fibrous cap causes thrombosis. Physical disruption of the atherosclerotic plaque commonly causes arterial thrombosis by allowing blood coagulant factors to contact thrombogenic collagen found in the

generation from prothrombin. In addition to its role in blood coagulation, thrombin can modulate many aspects of vascular cell function including stimulation of proliferation and cytokine release from smooth-muscle cells and production of growth factors such as PDGF from endothelial cells. Atherosclerotic plaques often contain fibrin and hemosiderin, indicating episodes of intraplaque hemorrhage as an element in plaque complication.

As they advance, atherosclerotic plaques also accumulate calcium. Proteins specialized in binding of calcium usually associated with bone also occur in atherosclerotic lesions. For example, osteocalcin, osteopontin, and bone morphogenetic proteins localize in atherosclerotic plaques. In fact, complication of the atherosclerotic plaque recapitulates many aspects of bone formation.

Traditionally, atherosclerosis research has focused much attention on proliferation of smooth-muscle cells, yet these cells actually replicate rather slowly in complicated atherosclerotic lesions. Estimates of the rate of smooth-muscle cell division at a given time point in such lesions show replicative rate below 1%. Such observations do not exclude bursts of proliferative activity at certain junctures in the history of an atheroma, perhaps in association with local thrombin generation due to microvascular hemorrhage or formation of a microthrombus at a site of localized endothelial denudation, as discussed above. On the other hand, cell death has been recognized as a component of atherogenesis since the time of Virchow in the mid-nineteenth century. Indeed, complex atheroma often have a primarily fibrous character lacking the hypercellular appearance of less advanced lesions and actually exhibiting a paucity of smooth-muscle cells. This relative lack

FIGURE 241-2—*(continued)*
arterial extracellular matrix and tissue factor produced by macrophage-derived foam cells in the lipid core of lesions. In this manner, sites of plaque rupture form the nidus for thrombi. The normal artery wall possesses several fibrinolytic or antithrombotic mechanisms that tend to resist thrombosis and lyse clots that begin to form in situ. Such antithrombotic or thrombolytic molecules include thrombomodulin, tissue and urokinase-type plasminogen activators, heparan sulfate proteoglycans, prostacyclin, and nitric oxide. When the clot overwhelms the endogenous fibrinolytic mechanisms, it may propagate and lead to arterial occlusion (*E*). In some cases, the thrombus may lyse or organize into a mural thrombus without occluding the vessel. Such instances may be clinically silent. The subsequent thrombin-induced fibrosis and healing causes a fibroproliferative response that can lead to a more fibrous lesion, one that can produce an eccentric plaque that causes a hemodynamically significant stenosis (*D*).

D. Healing of a mural thrombus leads to lesion fibrosis and progression and luminal narrowing. Local thrombin activation can stimulate smooth-muscle proliferation. Proteins released from platelets including platelet-derived growth factors and transforming growth factor β may also augment collagen production by smooth-muscle cells and modulate their growth. In this way, a nonocclusive mural thrombus, even if clinically silent or causing unstable angina rather than infarction, can provoke a healing response that can promote lesion fibrosis and luminal encroachment. Such a sequence of events may convert a "vulnerable" atheroma with a thin fibrous cap prone to rupture into a more "stable" fibrous plaque with a reinforced cap. Angioplasty of unstable coronary lesions may "stabilize" the lesions by a similar mechanism, producing a wound followed by healing.

E. Plaque rupture with a propagated, occlusive thrombus can cause acute myocardial infarction. When a stable, occlusive thrombus forms in a coronary artery, the consequences depend on the degree of existing collateral vessels. In a patient with chronic multivessel, occlusive coronary artery disease, collateral channels have usually formed. In such circumstances, even a total arterial occlusion may not lead to myocardial infarction, or may produce an unexpectedly modest or a non-Q-wave infarct because of collateral flow. In the patient with less advanced disease and without substantial stenotic lesions to provide a stimulus to collateral vessel formation, sudden plaque rupture and arterial occlusion commonly produce Q wave infarction. These are the types of patients who may present with myocardial infarction or sudden death as a first manifestation of coronary atherosclerosis.

of smooth-muscle cells in advanced atheroma may result from the ultimate predominance of cytostatic mediators such as TGF-β or IFN-γ, which can inhibit smooth-muscle cell proliferation. Also, smooth-muscle cells as well as macrophages in advanced atherosclerotic lesions can undergo programmed cell death, or apoptosis. Some of the same cytokines that activate atherogenic functions of vascular wall cells can also trigger the program of apoptosis in these cells.

Thus, during the evolution of the atherosclerotic plaque, a complex balance between entry and egress of lipoproteins and leukocytes, cell proliferation and cell death, extracellular matrix production and remodeling, as well as calcification and neovascularization contribute to lesion formation. Multiple and often competing signals trigger these various cellular events. Increasingly, we appreciate links between atherogenic risk factors and the altered behavior of intrinsic vascular wall cells and infiltrating leukocytes that underlie the complex pathogenesis of these lesions.

CLINICAL SYNDROMES OF ATHEROSCLEROSIS

Atherosclerotic lesions occur ubiquitously in western societies. Most atheroma produce no symptoms, and many never cause clinical manifestations. Numerous patients with diffuse atherosclerosis may succumb to unrelated illnesses without ever having experienced a clinically significant manifestation of atherosclerosis. What accounts for this variability in the clinical expression of atherosclerotic disease?

Arterial remodeling during atheroma formation (Fig. 241-2*A*) represents a frequently overlooked but clinically important feature of lesion evolution. During the initial phases of atheroma development, the plaque usually grows outward, in an abluminal direction. Vessels affected by atherogenesis tend to increase in diameter, a phenomenon known as *compensatory enlargement*, a type of vascular remodeling. The growing atheroma does not encroach upon the arterial lumen until the burden of atherosclerotic plaque exceeds approximately 40% of the area encompassed by the internal elastic lamina. Thus, during much of its life history, an atheroma will not cause stenosis that can limit blood flow.

Flow-limiting stenoses commonly form later in the history of the plaque. Many such plaques manifest themselves by stable syndromes such as demand-induced angina pectoris or intermittent claudication in the extremities. In the coronary and other circulations, even occlusion due to atheroma does not invariably lead to infarction. The hypoxic stimulus of repeated bouts of ischemia characteristically induces formation of collateral vessels in the myocardium, mitigating the consequences of an acute occlusion of an epicardial coronary artery. On the other hand, we now appreciate that many lesions that cause acute or unstable atherosclerotic syndromes, particularly in the coronary circulation, may arise from atherosclerotic plaques that do not produce a flow-limiting stenosis. Such lesions may produce only minimal luminal irregularities on traditional angiograms and often do not meet the traditional criteria for "significance" by arteriography. Instability of such nonocclusive stenoses may explain the frequency of myocardial infarction as an initial manifestation of coronary artery disease (in about a third of cases) in patients who report no prior history of angina pectoris, a syndrome usually caused by flow-limiting stenoses.

Pathologic studies afford considerable insight into the microanatomic substrate underlying "instability" of plaques that are not critically stenotic. A superficial erosion of the endothelium or a frank plaque rupture or fissure usually produces the thrombus that causes episodes of unstable angina pectoris or the occlusive and relatively persistent thrombus that causes acute myocardial infarction (Fig. 241-2C). In the case of carotid atheroma, a deeper ulceration that provides a nidus for formation of platelet thrombi may underlie the unstable syndromes that cause transient ischemic attacks.

Rupture of the plaque's fibrous cap (Fig. 241-2C) permits contact of coagulation factors in the blood with highly thrombogenic tissue factor expressed by macrophage foam cells in the plaque's lipid-rich core. If the ensuing thrombus is nonocclusive or transient, the episode of plaque disruption may not cause symptoms or may result in ischemic symptoms such as rest angina. Occlusive thrombi that endure will often cause acute myocardial infarction, particularly in the absence of a well-developed collateral circulation supplying the affected territory. Repetitive episodes of plaque disruption and healing provide one likely mechanism of transition of the fatty streak to a more complex fibrous lesion (Fig. 241-2D). The healing process in arteries, as in skin wounds, involves the laying down of new extracellular matrix and fibrosis.

Not all atheroma exhibit the same propensity to rupture. Studies of the pathology of culprit lesions that have caused acute myocardial infarction reveal several characteristic features. Plaques that have proven vulnerable tend to have thin fibrous caps, relatively large lipid cores, and a high content of macrophages. Morphometric studies of such culprit lesions show that macrophages and T lymphocytes predominate at the site of plaque rupture. On the other hand, sites of plaque rupture contain relatively few smooth-muscle cells. The cells that concentrate at sites of plaque rupture bear markers of inflammatory activation. The presence of the transplantation, or histocompatibility, antigen HLA-DR provides one convenient gauge of the degree of inflammation in cells in atheroma. Resting cells in normal arteries seldom express this transplantation antigen. However, macrophages and smooth-muscle cells at sites of human coronary artery plaque disruption do bear this inducible cell-surface marker. Therefore, the presence of HLA-DR-positive macrophages and T cells indicates an ongoing inflammatory response at sites of plaque rupture.

Inflammatory mediators may actually regulate processes that govern the integrity of the plaque's fibrous cap and hence its propensity to rupture. For example, the T cell–derived cytokine IFN-γ, found in atherosclerotic plaques and required to induce the HLA-DR present at sites of rupture, can inhibit growth and collagen synthesis of smooth-muscle cells. Cytokines derived from activated macrophages such as TNF-α or IL-1 in addition to T cell–derived IFN-γ can elicit the expression of genes that encode the proteinases that can degrade the extracellular matrix of the plaque's fibrous cap. Thus, inflammatory mediators can impair collagen synthesis required for maintenance and repair of the fibrous cap and trigger degradation of extracellular matrix macromolecules, processes that should weaken the plaque's fibrous cap and enhance its vulnerability to rupture. In contrast to vulnerable plaques, those with a dense extracellular matrix and relatively thick fibrous cap without substantial tissue factor–rich lipid cores seem generally resistant to rupture and unlikely to provoke thrombosis.

In conclusion, we now appreciate that features of the biology of the atheromatous plaque in addition to its degree of luminal encroachment influence the clinical manifestations of this disease. This enhanced understanding of plaque biology provides insight into the diverse ways in which atherosclerosis can present clinically, and why the disease may remain silent or stable for prolonged periods and be punctuated by acute complications at certain times. Increased understanding of atherogenesis provides new insight into the ways in which current therapies may improve outcomes and also suggests new targets for future intervention.

BIBLIOGRAPHY

DAVIES MJ: The composition of coronary-artery plaques. N Engl J Med 336:1312, 1997

FUSTER V et al: Pathogenesis of coronary disease: The biologic role of risk factors. J Am Coll Cardiol 27:964, 1996

LIBBY P: The molecular bases of the acute coronary syndromes. Circulation 91:2844, 1995

LIBBY P: The vascular biology of atherosclerosis, in *Heart Disease*, 6th ed., E Braunwald, D Zipes, P Libby (eds). Philadelphia, Saunders, 2001

ROSS R: Atherosclerosis—an inflammatory disease. N Engl J Med 340:115, 1999

WITZUM JL, BERLINER JA: Oxidized phospholipids and isoprostanes in atherosclerosis. Curr Opin Lipidol 9:441, 1998

| 242 | *Peter Libby* |

PREVENTION AND TREATMENT OF ATHEROSCLEROSIS

Atherosclerosis remains the major cause of death and premature disability in developed societies. Moreover, current predictions estimate that by the year 2020 cardiovascular diseases, notably atherosclerosis, will become the leading global cause of total disease burden, defined as the years subtracted from healthy life by disability or premature death. Substantial success has been achieved in recent years in reducing morbidity and mortality due to acute coronary events. However, the opportunity for treating the underlying disease process, atherosclerosis, and preventing its acute complications presents an enormous challenge and opportunity at the same time.

THE CONCEPT OF ATHEROSCLEROTIC RISK FACTORS

During the first half of the twentieth century, animal experiments and clinical observation linked certain variables, such as hypercholesterolemia, to the risk of atherosclerotic events. The systematic study of risk factors in humans, however, began approximately mid-century. The prospective, community-based Framingham Heart Study provided rigorous support for the concept that hypercholesterolemia, hypertension, and other factors correlated with cardiovascular risk. Similar observational studies performed in the United States and abroad provided independent support for the concept of "risk factors" for cardiovascular disease. Numerous studies, including the Seven Countries Study per-

Modifiable risk factors	Unmodifiable risk factors
By life-style	Age
Smoking	Male gender
Obesity	Genetics
Physical inactivity	
By pharmacotherapy and or life-style	
Lipid disorders	
Hypertension	
Insulin resistance	

formed by Keys and colleagues, suggested a link between dietary habits and cardiovascular risk based upon population studies.

From a practical viewpoint, it is useful to group the cardiovascular risk factors that have emerged from such studies into two categories: (1) those modifiable by lifestyle and/or pharmacotherapy, and (2) those that are essentially unmodifiable (Table 242-1). The weight of evidence supporting various risk factor differs. For example, hypercholesterolemia and hypertension indubitably predict coronary risk, but other so-called nontraditional risk factors, such as levels of homocysteine, lipoprotein (a) [Lp(a)], or infection, remain controversial. It is worth distinguishing further between factors that actually participate in the pathogenesis of atherosclerosis and those that may merely serve as markers of risk without themselves playing a primary role in pathogenesis. The sections below will consider some of these risk factors and approaches to their modification.

LIPID DISORDERS (See also Chap. 344) Abnormalities in plasma lipoproteins and derangements in lipid metabolism rank as the most firmly established and best understood risk factors for atherosclerosis. Descriptions of the lipoprotein classes, and a detailed explication of lipoprotein metabolism are given in Chap. 344. The mechanisms by which lipoproteins may influence atherogenesis are considered in Chap. 241. Therefore this section will focus on preventive aspects of treatment of lipid disorders.

Current national guidelines recommend cholesterol screening in all adults. The screen should include a fasting lipid profile [total cholesterol, triglycerides, low-density lipoprotein (LDL) cholesterol and high-density lipoprotein (HDL) cholesterol]. Dietary measures, including specific consultation by practitioners with training in nutrition, should be offered to all patients with hyperlipidemia as defined by the National Cholesterol Education Project Adult Treatment Panel II (Table 242-2). A "normal" total cholesterol level should not falsely reassure individuals with additional risk factors for coronary heart disease or when the HDL level is below 1 mmol/L (40 mg/dL). Many patients with established atherosclerosis fall into this category. Such individuals should receive particular encouragement to adopt life-style measures such as diet and exercise aimed at increasing their HDL levels.

The addition of drug therapy to dietary and other nonpharmacologic measures to reduce the risk of atherosclerotic events in asymptomatic patients without manifest vascular disease remains unsettled. In asymptomatic patients with heterozygous familial hypercholesterolemia, LDL lowering by pharmacologic measures reduces atherosclerosis in both men and women. The West of Scotland Study established that lipid lowering with the HMG-CoA inhibitor pravastatin can effectively reduce cardiac events and total mortality in a cohort of patients with hypercholesterolemia but without prior myocardial infarction (Table 242-3). The recent AFCAPS/TexCAPS Study showed that treatment with lovastatin similarly reduced coronary events in patients without previous myocardial infarction but with "average" total and LDL cholesterol levels and somewhat decreased HDL levels.

Although the role of drug therapy in primary prevention of the manifestations of atherosclerosis remains incompletely defined, abundant evidence establishes the benefit of drug therapy in patients with hypercholesterolemia and established coronary artery disease (Table 242-3). A number of well-designed and -executed large-scale clinical trials have now shown that treatment with statins reduces recurrent myocardial infarction, reduces strokes, and lessens the need for revascularization or hospitalization for unstable angina pectoris. These studies have enrolled patients in numerous countries on at least three continents and encompass individuals with clearly elevated levels of cholesterol and those with "average" total and LDL cholesterol levels.

Lipid-lowering therapies do not appear to exert their beneficial effect on cardiovascular events by causing a marked "regression" of obstructive coronary lesions. Angiographically monitored studies of lipid lowering have shown at best a modest reduction in coronary artery stenoses over the duration of study. Yet these same studies consistently show substantial decreases in coronary events. These results suggest that the mechanism of benefit of lipid lowering does not require a substantial reduction in the fixed stenoses. Rather, the benefit may derive from "stabilization" of atherosclerotic lesions without decreased stenosis. Such stabilization of atherosclerotic lesions and the attendant decrease in coronary events may result from the egress of lipids or by favorably influencing aspects of the biology of atherogenesis discussed in Chap. 241. In addition, as sizeable lesions may protrude abluminally rather than into the lumen, shrinkage of such plaques might not be apparent on angiograms.

The benefit of LDL lowering by HMG-CoA reductase inhibitor (statin) therapy on cardiovascular events seems to require 6 to 24 months of treatment. Improvement of vasomotor responses to endothelial-dependent vasodilators occurs much more rapidly, requiring 6 months or less. Thus, HMG-CoA reductase inhibitors may act by two or more mechanisms on the arteries of hypercholesterolemic individuals. The relatively rapid improvement in endothelial-dependent vasomotion may reflect enhanced production or reduced destruction of the endogenous vasodilator nitric oxide at the level of the arterial endothelium. Reduction in the thrombotic complications of atherosclerosis, such as myocardial infarction or unstable angina, probably requires more prolonged treatment to effect removal of lipid from deeper within the atheroma, yielding improvements in the biology underlying plaque destabilization described in Chap. 241.

Our current understanding of the mechanism by which elevated LDL levels promote atherogenesis relates to oxidative modification of these particles within the artery wall, promoting formation of macrophage-derived foam cells and providing a stimulus for inflammation (Chap. 241). These concepts have given rise to considerable interest in the possibility that antioxidants, either dietary or pharmacologic, might reduce atherogenesis. Considerable experimental evidence supports this notion. In addition, many observational studies show a correlation of antioxidant consumption and reduced cardiovascular risk. Rigorous, controlled clinical trial evidence, however, has not yet proven the effectiveness of antioxidant therapy, whether dietary or with supplements of vitamins or drugs, for prevention or treatment of

Table 242-2 Treatment Decisions Based on LDL Cholesterol Level

Patient Category	Initiation Level, mmol/L (mg/dL)		LDL Goal, mmol/L (mg/dL)	
	Dietary Therapy	Drug Treatment	Dietary Therapy	Drug Treatment
Without CHD and with fewer than two risk factors	≥4.1(160)	≥4.9(190)	<4.1(160)	<4.1(160)
Without CHD and with two or more risk factors	≥3.4(130)	≥4.1(160)	<3.4(130)	<3.4(130)
With CHD	>2.6(100)	≥3.4(130)	≤2.6(100)	≤2.6(100)

NOTE: LDL, low-density lipoprotein; CHD, coronary heart disease.
SOURCE: From the guidelines issued by the National Cholesterol Education Project Adult Treatment Panel II: JAMA 269:3025, 1993.

Table 242-3 Selected Clinical Trials of Statin Therapy for Prevention of Coronary or CHD Events

Trial	Previous MI	Lipids	Before lipid lowering, mmol/L (mg/dL)	Decrease in cholesterol, mmol/L(mg/dL)	CHD event reduction, %
WOSCOPS	−	Total cholesterol	7.0(272)	0.52(20)	31
		LDL	5.0(192)	0.67(26)	
AFCAPS/TexCAPS	−	Total cholesterol	5.7(220)	0.47(18)	36
		LDL	4.0(156)	0.65(25)	
4S	+	Total cholesterol	6.7(261)	0.65(25)	34
		LDL	4.9(188)	0.91(35)	
CARE	+	Total cholesterol	5.4(209)	0.52(20)	24
		LDL	3.6(139)	0.72(28)	
LIPID	+	Total cholesterol	5.7(219)	0.47(18)	24
		LDL	3.9(150)	0.65(25)	

NOTE: MI, myocardial infarction; CHD, coronary heart disease; LDL, low-density lipoprotein.
SOURCES: WOSCOPS: J Shepherd et al: West of Scotland Coronary Prevention Study Group. N Engl J Med 333:1301, 1995. AFCAPS/TexCAPS: JR Downs et al: Air Force/Texas Coronary Atherosclerosis Prevention Study. JAMA 279:1615, 1998. 4S: Anonymous: The Scandinavian Simvastin Survival Study. Lancet 344:1383, 1994. CARE: FM Sacks et al: Cholesterol and Recurrent Events Trial (CARE) Investigators. N Engl J Med 335:1001, 1996. LIPID: Anonymous: The Long-Term Intervention with Pravastatin in Ischemic Disease (LIPID) Study Group. N Engl J Med 339:1349, 1998.

atherosclerosis. Indeed, controlled trials with β-carotene have demonstrated no reduction in cardiovascular events. For these reasons, as its efficacy remains speculative, it is premature to consider antioxidant administration as a replacement for established therapies. Furthermore, general use of such treatments, particularly in lower risk individuals, should await the results of rigorous prospective studies designed to define the doses, appropriate patient groups, and evaluate the possibility of adverse or unwanted effects of antioxidants.

HYPERTENSION (See also Chap. 246) The preponderance of epidemiologic data supports a relationship between hypertension and atherosclerotic risk. Clinical trial evidence available since the 1970s established that pharmacologic treatment of hypertension can reduce the risk of stroke and heart failure. However, clinical trial evidence demonstrating reduced risk of coronary events due to antihypertensive therapy has lagged. At present, the combined weight of the evidence supports a reduction in coronary risk by antihypertensive therapy. Some of the difficulty in demonstrating this benefit may derive from the potentially adverse effects of certain classes of antihypertensive drugs on the lipid profile, notably, thiazide diuretics and beta-blocking agents. Indeed, studies of patients with previous myocardial infarction or reduced left ventricular function have shown that treatment with angiotensin-converting enzyme (ACE) inhibitors can reduce the risk of coronary events, an unanticipated outcome. Therefore "lipid-neutral" antihypertensive agents such as ACE inhibitors or α_1-adrenergic blocking agents merit consideration in patients with other risk factors for coronary artery disease or with established atherosclerosis.

DIABETES MELLITUS AND INSULIN RESISTANCE (See also Chap. 333) Most patients with diabetes mellitus die of atherosclerosis and its complications. Secular trends towards aging of the population and increased girth will make type 2 (noninsulin-dependent) diabetes mellitus an increasing public health problem in the coming years. The criteria for diagnosis of diabetes have recently undergone revision. Currently, a fasting plasma glucose level of 6.9 mmol/L (125 mg/dL) establishes the diagnosis of diabetes. In the intermediate range, plasma glucose levels between 6.1 and 6.9 mmol/L (110 and 125 mg/dL) indicate impaired fasting glucose. Thus, fasting glucose >6.1 mmol/L (110 mg/dL) indicates abnormal glucose tolerance. These definitions based on fasting plasma glucose alone obviate the need for performing glucose tolerance tests.

A major feature of elevated cardiovascular risk in patients with type 2 diabetes probably relates to the abnormal lipoprotein profile associated with insulin resistance known as *diabetic dyslipidemia*. While diabetic patients may often have LDL cholesterol levels near average, the LDL particles tend to be smaller and denser and thus more atherogenic (Chap. 344). Other features of diabetic dyslipidemia include low HDL and elevated triglycerides. Establishing that strict glycemic control reduces the risk of macrovascular complications of di-

abetes has proven much more elusive than the established beneficial effects on microvascular complications such as retinopathy or renal disease. In the absence of clear-cut evidence that tight glycemic control reduces coronary risk in diabetic patients, attention to other aspects of risk in this patient population assumes even greater importance. In this regard, recent clinical trials have demonstrated unequivocal benefit of HMG-CoA reductase inhibitor therapy in diabetic patients, including those with "average" LDL cholesterol levels. Having diabetes places patients in the same risk category as those with established atherosclerotic disease. Therefore, recent guidelines promulgated by the American Diabetes Association recommend an aggressive approach to lipid lowering in the diabetic population, as supported by recent clinical trials. These guidelines establish a target LDL cholesterol level of 2.6 mmol/L (100 mg/dL) for the patient with diabetes.

MALE GENDER/POSTMENOPAUSAL STATE Decades of observational studies have verified excess coronary risk in males compared with premenopausal females. After menopause, however, coronary risk accelerates in women. At least part of the apparent protection against coronary heart disease in premenopausal women derives from their relatively higher HDL levels compared with those of men. After menopause, HDL values fall in concert with increased coronary risk. Estrogen therapy lowers LDL cholesterol and raises HDL cholesterol, changes that should decrease coronary risk. A multitude of observational studies has suggested that estrogen-replacement therapy (ERT) reduces coronary risk. Substantial experimental data support the biologic plausibility of a beneficial effect of estrogen in reducing atherosclerotic events, but a number of potential confounding factors render clinical trials necessary to establish the cardiovascular benefits of ERT. In men, high-dose estrogen treatment caused excess mortality, probably due to increased thromboembolic complications.

The recently reported Heart and Estrogen/Progestin Replacement Study (HERS) has highlighted the need for clinical trial evidence to substantiate the observational and experimental data regarding estrogen's beneficial effects on the vasculature and lipid profile. In this trial, postmenopausal female survivors of acute myocardial infarction were randomized to an estrogen/progestin combination or to placebo. This study showed no overall reduction in recurrent coronary events in the active treatment arm. Indeed, early in the 5-year course of this trial, there was a trend toward an actual increase in vascular events in the treated women. As in the previous Coronary Drug Project trial, the excess events may have resulted from an increase in thromboembolism. HERS does not definitively exclude a potential benefit of other combinations of estrogens with progestins or a benefit of estrogens alone in patients lacking a uterus. A more prolonged follow-up might have disclosed an accrual of benefit in the treatment group, as the excess events appeared in the first years of the trial in the treated group. Moreover, drugs of the selective estrogen receptor modulator class might dissociate the increased risk of breast and/or uterine cancer from cardiovascular benefit. This possibility will likewise require randomized clinical trial evidence evaluating coronary events to validate widespread application. The current quandary surrounding ERT as a means of reducing cardiovascular risk highlights the need for redoubled attention to known modifiable risk factors in women. In the recent clinical trials with HMG-CoA reductase inhibitors, women, when included, have derived benefits at least commensurate with those seen in men. Data from HERS itself showed that application of lipid-lowering therapy to female survivors of myocardial infarction lagged far behind guidelines. Choices regarding ERT in postmenopausal women remain complex. Physicians should work together with women to provide information and help weigh the risks and benefits of ERT, taking personal preferences into account.

DYSREGULATED COAGULATION OR FIBRINOLYSIS

Thrombosis ultimately causes the gravest complications of atherosclerosis. The propensity to form thrombi and/or to lyse clots once they form could clearly influence the manifestations of atherosclerosis. Thrombosis provoked by atheroma rupture and subsequent healing may promote plaque growth, as described in Chap. 241. Certain individual characteristics can influence thrombosis or fibrinolysis and have received attention as potential coronary risk factors. For example, fibrinogen levels correlate with coronary risk and provide information regarding coronary risk independent of the lipoprotein profile. Elevated fibrinogen levels might promote a thrombotic diathesis. Alternatively, fibrinogen, an acute-phase reactant, may serve as a marker of inflammation rather than directly participating in the pathogenesis of coronary events.

The stability of an arterial thrombus depends on the balance between fibrinolytic factors, such as plasmin, and inhibitors of the fibrinolytic system, such as plasminogen activator inhibitor (PAI) 1. Certain genotypes of the PAI-1 gene appear to correlate with increased coronary risk. Yet, overall, the levels of tissue plasminogen activator and PAI-1 in plasma have not proven to add information beyond the lipid profile to assessment of cardiovascular risk. Likewise, the role of Lp(a) (Chap. 344) as a modulator of fibrinolysis remains controversial. Apo Lp(a) has high homology to plasminogen but lacks the enzymatic activity of this fibrinolytic molecule. Thus, Lp(a) might antagonize fibrinolysis, serving as a type of "dominant negative" competitor of plasminogen. However, in vivo evidence for this mechanism, and, indeed, the independent contribution of Lp(a), is clouded by difficulties in standardizing the assays and the highly polymorphic nature of this protein in humans.

HOMOCYSTEINE

A large body of literature suggests a relationship between hyperhomocysteinemia and coronary events. Several mutations in the enzymes involved in homocysteine accumulation correlate with thrombosis and, in some studies, coronary risk. Although thrombosis and atherosclerosis seem intimately linked, direct evidence of an atherogenic effect of hyperhomocysteinemia in humans remains weak. The role of hyperhomocysteinemia in atherosclerotic complications, however, has important practical implications. The plasma level of homocysteine can vary with diet. Nutritional supplementation with folic acid can lower homocysteine levels in many individuals. A substantial portion of the elderly population in the United States has only a marginal sufficiency of folate intake. A fortification of the American diet with folic acid, aimed at reduction of neural tube defects, is lowering homocysteine levels in the population at large. Recommending a diet rich in folate or consumption of multivitamin supplements containing folic acid should be considered in individuals with atherosclerosis out of proportion to traditional or established risk factors and with elevated levels of homocysteine. The possibility that folate treatment might mask pernicious anemia should be considered when advising such supplementation. No clinical trial evidence currently establishes a reduction in coronary events in patients with hyperhomocysteinemia treated with folate.

INFECTION/INFLAMMATION

Recent years have witnessed a resurgence of interest in the possibility that infections may cause or contribute to atherosclerosis. A spate of recent publications has furnished evidence in support for a role of *Chlamydia pneumoniae*, cytomegalovirus, or other infectious agents in atherosclerosis and restenosis following coronary intervention. Some microorganisms exist in human atherosclerotic plaques. However, seroepidemiologic evidence for an association between infection with various agents and atherosclerosis remains inconclusive. Several ongoing large trials of antibiotic treatment in survivors of myocardial infarction may provide support for an etiologic or contributory role of microbial infection in recurrent coronary events. Even if positive, however, such clinical trials would neither inculpate any particular microorganisms nor even prove that a benefit derived from the antimicrobial action of the agent employed.

Although direct infection may not cause atherosclerosis, the infectious agents and the host defenses against these invaders might potentiate atherogenesis, acting as inflammatory stimuli. Just as inflammation may mediate some of the altered arterial biology in response to hyperlipoproteinemia, so might infectious agents incite an inflammatory response that could promote atherosclerosis and its complications. Thus, microbial pathogens might act in concert with traditional risk factors to accelerate atherogenesis or cause complication or aggravation of existing atheroma.

In this regard, evidence is accumulating that markers of inflammation correlate with coronary risk. For example, elevated plasma levels of C-reactive protein (CRP) can prospectively predict risk of myocardial infarction and correlate with outcome of patients with acute coronary syndromes. As in the case of fibrinogen, elevated levels of the acute-phase reactant CRP may merely reflect ongoing inflammation rather than a direct etiologic role for CRP in coronary artery disease. It remains uncertain whether elevations in acute-phase reactants such as fibrinogen or CRP serve as a marker for the overall atherosclerotic burden, and hence of coronary events. Alternatively, the elevation in acute-phase reactants could reflect extravascular inflammation that could potentiate atherosclerosis or its complications. In all likelihood, both factors contribute to elevation of inflammatory markers in patients at risk for coronary events. These observations raise the possibility that anti-inflammatory therapies might reduce atherosclerotic events. Indeed, lipid-lowering therapy may reduce coronary events in part by reducing the inflammatory aspects of the pathogenesis of atherosclerosis.

LIFE-STYLE MODIFICATION

The prevention of atherosclerosis presents a long-term challenge to all health care professionals and for public health policy. Both individual practitioners and organizations providing health care should strive to help patients optimize their risk factor profile long before atherosclerotic disease might become manifest. The care plan for all patients seen by internists should include measures to assess and minimize cardiovascular risk. Physicians must counsel patients regarding the health risks of tobacco use and provide guidance regarding smoking cessation. Likewise, physicians should advise all patients about prudent dietary and exercise habits for maintaining ideal body weight. The recent National Institutes of Health Consensus Panel on Physical Activity and Cardiovascular Health established a goal of accumulating at least 30 min of moderate-intensity physical activity on a daily basis. Obesity, particularly the male pattern of centripetal or visceral fat accumulation, can promote an atherogenic dyslipidemia characterized by elevated triglycerides, a low HDL level, and glucose intolerance. Physicians should encourage their patients to take responsibility for behavior related to modifiable risk factors for development of premature atherosclerotic disease. Conscientious counseling and patient education may forestall the need for pharmacologic measures intended to reduce coronary risk.

ISSUES IN RISK ASSESSMENT

A growing panel of markers of coronary risk presents a perplexing array to the practitioner. Such markers include size fractionation of LDL particles, measurement of concentrations of homocysteine, Lp(a), fibrinogen, CRP, and PAI-1, among others. In general, such specialized tests add little to the information available from a careful history and physical examination and measurement of a plasma lipoprotein profile and fasting blood sugar. Evaluation of such specialized markers might be considered in individuals without evident risk factors other than premature vascular disease or a worrisome family history. A similar confusion surrounds the use of specialized radiographic estimations of coronary artery calcification. Information is accumulating that the amount of calcium determined by such techniques as electron beam computed tomography correlates with coronary risk. However, the utility of using such estimates of coronary artery calcium content as a guide to therapy remains unproven, particularly in asymptomatic individuals. Inappropriate use of such imaging modalities might promote excessive inva-

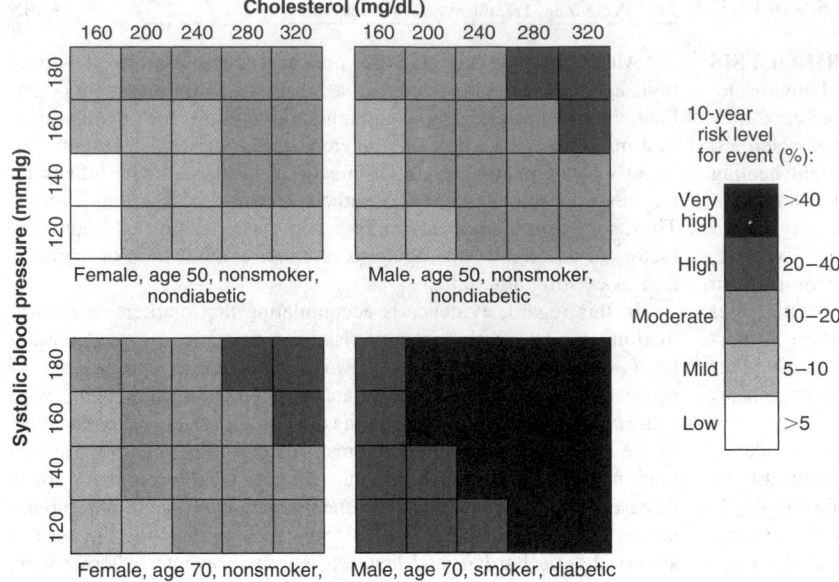

Cholesterol (mg/dL)

FIGURE 242-1 *The multi-factorial nature of coronary risk*: examples from the European Treatment Guidelines. Shown are four matrices derived from the guidelines currently used in Europe to stratify individuals for treatment. Each matrix shows differing levels of systolic blood pressure (columns) and increasing levels of serum cholesterol (rows). The 10-year risk levels for a coronary heart disease event are plotted according to the scale shown on the far right. The darkness of the color indicates higher risk. These examples illustrate the differences between a female (top left matrix) versus a male (top right matrix), both age 50 and nonsmokers. The bottom pair of matrices illustrate the risk ascribed to individuals both age 70, one with three additional risk factors (male gender, tobacco use, and diabetes mellitus, lower right) versus a nonsmoking, nondiabetic female (lower left). *(From D Wood et al: Prevention of coronary heart disease in clinical practice. Summary of recommendations of the Second Joint Task Force of European and other Societies on Coronary Prevention. Hypertension 16:1407, 1998.)*

sive diagnostic and therapeutic procedures. Widespread application of such modalities for screening should await proof that clinical benefit derives from their application.

THE CONCEPT OF GLOBAL RISK

Adoption of hygienic life-style changes to ameliorate coronary risk entails little expense or possibility of adverse effects. In contrast, pharmacotherapy can prove costly. Although lipid-lowering drugs such as the HMG-CoA reductase inhibitors have proven exceedingly well tolerated in clinical trials, the use of these or other lipid-lowering agents could produce adverse reactions in some individuals. The decision to initiate drug treatment for reduction of risk of atherosclerotic events requires careful consideration, particularly in the setting of "primary prevention" or in patients without known atherosclerotic disease. In this regard, it is prudent to consider not only the LDL cholesterol but also the individual patient's global cardiovascular risk. For example, an individual with an average LDL but a low HDL, hypertension, and a family history of premature coronary artery disease might warrant initiation of drug therapy more than an individual with the same LDL level in the absence of the other risk factors. Rather than considering plasma lipoprotein values in isolation, current European guidelines reserve drug treatment for individuals with a calculated absolute coronary heart disease risk of greater than 20% over 10 years. The calculation of coronary risk includes taking gender, smoking history, and systolic blood pressure into account, in addition to plasma cholesterol levels. This policy illustrates how estimations of global risk may be applied to optimize decisions regarding initiation of drug therapy to prevent atherosclerotic events (Fig. 242-1).

THE CHALLENGE OF IMPLEMENTATION: CHANGING PHYSICIAN AND PATIENT BEHAVIOR Enormous strides have been made in the prevention and treatment of atherosclerosis. Despite declining age-adjusted rates of coronary death, cardio-

vascular mortality is on the rise due to the aging of the population overall. There is a powerful global trend toward increased atherosclerotic disease. Enormous challenges remain regarding translation of the current evidence base into practice. The obstacles to implementation of current evidence-based prevention and treatment of atherosclerosis include economics, education, physician awareness, and patient adherence to recommended regimens. Future goals in the field of treatment of atherosclerosis should include application of the current knowledge regarding risk factor management and, when appropriate, drug therapy.

BIBLIOGRAPHY

ANONYMOUS: Management of dyslipidemia in adults with diabetes. Diabetes Care 22 (Suppl 1):S56, 1999

BROWN BG et al: Lipid lowering and plaque regression: New insights into prevention of plaque disruption and clinical events in coronary disease. Circulation 87:1781, 1993

GAZIANO JM, MANSON JE, RIDKER PM: Primary and secondary prevention of coronary heart disease, in *Heart Disease*, 6th ed., E Braunwald, D Zipes, P Libby (eds). Philadelphia, Saunders, 2001

GOTTO AM Jr.: Lipid-lowering therapy for the primary prevention of coronary heart disease. J Am Coll Cardiol 33:2078, 1999

LIBBY P et al: Roles of infectious agents in atherosclerosis and restenosis: An assessment of the evidence and need for future research. Circulation 96:4095, 1997

MURRAY CH, LOPEZ AD: Alternative projections of mortality and disability by cause 1990–2020: Global Burden of Disease Study. Lancet 349:1498, 1997

PETITTI DB: Hormone replacement therapy and heart disease prevention: Experimentation trumps observation. JAMA 280:650, 1998

RIDKER P, LIBBY P: Nontraditional coronary risk factors and vascular biology: The frontiers of preventive cardiology. J Invest Med 46:338, 1998

243

Elliott M. Antman, Eugene Braunwald

ACUTE MYOCARDIAL INFARCTION

ACE angiotensin-converting enzyme	LMWHs low-molecular-weight
AIVR accelerated idioventricular	heparin preparations
rhythm	LV left ventricular
AMI acute myocardial infarction	MI myocardial infarction
APSAC anisoylated plasminogen	MR mitral regurgitation
streptokinase activator complex	NSTEMI non-ST elevation MI
AV atrioventricular	PCI percutaneous coronary
CHF congestive heart failure	intervention
CK creatine phosphokinase	rPA reteplase
cTnI cardiac-specific troponin I	RV right ventricular
cTnT cardiac-specific troponin T	tPA tissue plasminogen activator
ECG electrocardiogram	UFH unfractionated heparin

Acute myocardial infarction (AMI) is one of the most common diagnoses in hospitalized patients in industrialized countries. In the United States, approximately 1.1 million AMIs occur each year. The mortality rate with AMI is approximately 30%, with more than half of these deaths occurring before the stricken individual reaches the hospital. Although the mortality rate after admission for AMI has declined by about 30% over the last two decades, approximately 1 of every 25 patients who survives the initial hospitalization dies in the first year after AMI. Survival is markedly reduced in elderly patients (over age 75), whose mortality rate is 20% at 1 month and 30% at 1 year after AMI.

AMI generally occurs when coronary blood flow decreases abruptly after a thrombotic occlusion of a coronary artery previously narrowed by atherosclerosis. Slowly developing, high-grade coronary artery stenoses usually do not precipitate AMI because of the development of a rich collateral network over time. Instead, AMI occurs when a coronary artery thrombus develops rapidly at a site of vascular injury. This injury is produced or facilitated by factors such as cigarette smoking, hypertension, and lipid accumulation. In most cases, infarction occurs when an atherosclerotic plaque fissures, ruptures, or ulcerates and when conditions (local or systemic) favor thrombogenesis, so that a mural thrombus forms at the site of rupture and leads to coronary artery occlusion. Histologic studies indicate that the coronary plaques prone to rupture are those with a rich lipid core and a thin fibrous cap (Chap. 241). After an initial platelet monolayer forms at the site of the ruptured plaque, various agonists (collagen, ADP, epinephrine, serotonin) promote platelet activation. After agonist stimulation of platelets, there is production and release of thromboxane A_2 (a potent local vasoconstrictor), further platelet activation, and potential resistance to thrombolysis.

In addition to the generation of thromboxane A_2, activation of platelets by agonists promotes a conformational change in the glycoprotein IIb/IIIa receptor (Chap. 116). Once converted to its functional state, this receptor develops a high affinity for amino acid sequences on soluble adhesive proteins (i.e., integrins) such as von Willebrand factor (vWF) and fibrinogen. Since vWF and fibrinogen are multivalent molecules, they can bind to two different platelets simultaneously, resulting in platelet cross-linking and aggregation.

The coagulation cascade is activated on exposure of tissue factor in damaged endothelial cells at the site of the ruptured plaque. Factors VII and X are activated, ultimately leading to the conversion of prothrombin to thrombin, which then converts fibrinogen to fibrin (Chap. 117). Fluid-phase and clot-bound thrombin participate in an autoamplification reaction that leads to further activation of the coagulation cascade. The culprit coronary artery eventually becomes occluded by a thrombus containing platelet aggregates and fibrin strands.

In rare cases, AMI may be due to coronary artery occlusion caused by coronary emboli, congenital abnormalities, coronary spasm, and a wide variety of systemic—particularly inflammatory—diseases. The amount of myocardial damage caused by coronary occlusion depends on (1) the territory supplied by the affected vessel, (2) whether or not the vessel becomes totally occluded, (3) the duration of coronary occlusion, (4) the quantity of blood supplied by collateral vessels to the affected tissue, (5) the demand for oxygen of the myocardium whose blood supply has been suddenly limited, (6) native factors that can produce early spontaneous lysis of the occlusive thrombus, and (7) the adequacy of myocardial perfusion in the infarct zone when flow is restored in the occluded epicardial coronary artery.

Patients at increased risk of developing AMI include those with multiple coronary risk factors (Chap. 241) and those with unstable angina or Prinzmetal's variant angina (Chap. 244). Less common underlying medical conditions predisposing patients to AMI include hypercoagulability, collagen vascular disease, cocaine abuse, and intracardiac thrombi or masses that can produce coronary emboli.

CLINICAL PRESENTATION

In up to one-half of cases, a precipitating factor appears to be present before AMI, such as vigorous physical exercise, emotional stress, or a medical or surgical illness. Although AMI may commence at any time of the day or night, circadian variations have been reported such that clusters are seen in the morning within a few hours of awakening. The increased frequency early in the day may be due to a combination of an increase in sympathetic tone and an increased tendency to thrombosis between 6:00 A.M. and 12 noon.

Pain is the most common presenting complaint in patients with AMI. In some instances, it may be severe enough to be described as the worst pain the patient has ever felt. The pain is deep and visceral; adjectives commonly used to describe it are *heavy, squeezing,* and *crushing,* although occasionally it is described as stabbing or burning (Chap. 13). It is similar in character to the discomfort of angina pectoris but usually is more severe and lasts longer. Typically the pain involves the central portion of the chest and/or the epigastrium, and on occasion it radiates to the arms. Less common sites of radiation include the abdomen, back, lower jaw, and neck. The frequent location of the pain beneath the xiphoid and patients' denial that they may be suffering a heart attack are chiefly responsible for the common mistaken impression of indigestion. The pain of AMI may radiate as high as the occipital area but not below the umbilicus. It is often accompanied by weakness, sweating, nausea, vomiting, anxiety, and a sense of impending doom. The pain may commence when the patient is at rest. When the pain begins during a period of exertion, it does not usually subside with cessation of activity, in contrast to angina pectoris.

Although pain is the most common presenting complaint, it is by no means always present. The proportion of painless AMIs is greater in patients with diabetes mellitus, and it increases with age. In the elderly, AMI may present as sudden-onset breathlessness, which may progress to pulmonary edema. Other less common presentations, with or without pain, include sudden loss of consciousness, a confusional state, a sensation of profound weakness, the appearance of an arrhythmia, evidence of peripheral embolism, or merely an unexplained drop in arterial pressure. The pain of AMI can simulate pain from acute pericarditis (Chap. 239), pulmonary embolism (Chap. 261), acute aortic dissection (Chap. 247), costochondritis, and gastrointestinal disorders. These conditions should therefore be considered in the differential diagnosis.

PHYSICAL FINDINGS Most patients are anxious and restless, attempting unsuccessfully to relieve the pain by moving about in bed, altering their position, and stretching. Pallor associated with perspiration and coolness of the extremities occurs commonly. The combination of substernal chest pain persisting for >30 min and diaphoresis strongly suggests AMI. Although many patients have a normal pulse rate and blood pressure within the first hour of AMI, about one-fourth of patients with anterior infarction have manifestations of sympathetic nervous system hyperactivity (tachycardia and/or hypertension), and up to one-half with inferior infarction show evidence of parasympathetic hyperactivity (bradycardia and/or hypotension).

The precordium is usually quiet, and the apical impulse may be difficult to palpate. In patients with anterior wall infarction, an abnormal systolic pulsation caused by dyskinetic bulging of infarcted myocardium may develop in the periapical area within the first days of the illness and then may resolve. Other physical signs of ventricular dysfunction that may be present include, in order of decreasing incidence, fourth (S_4) and third (S_3) heart sounds, decreased intensity of heart sounds, and, in more severe cases, paradoxical splitting of the second heart sound (Chap. 225). A transient apical systolic murmur due to dysfunction of the mitral valve apparatus may be midsystolic or late systolic in timing. A pericardial friction rub is heard in many patients with transmural AMI at some time in the course of the disease, if they are examined frequently. The carotid pulse is often decreased in volume, reflecting reduced stroke volume. Jugular venous distention with clear lung fields should raise suspicion of right ventricular infarction. Temperature elevations up to 38°C may be observed during the first week after AMI; however, a temperature exceeding 38°C should prompt a search for other causes. The arterial pressure is variable; in most patients with transmural infarction, systolic pressure declines by approximately 10 to 15 mmHg from the preinfarction state.

LABORATORY FINDINGS

Myocardial infarction (MI) progresses through the following temporal stages: (1) acute (first few hours to 7 days), (2) healing (7 to 28 days), and (3) healed (29 days and beyond). When evaluating the results of diagnostic tests for AMI, the temporal phase of the infarction process must be considered. The laboratory tests of value in confirming the diagnosis may be divided into 4 groups: (1) electrocardiogram (ECG), (2) serum cardiac markers, (3) cardiac imaging, and (4) nonspecific indexes of tissue necrosis and inflammation.

ELECTROCARDIOGRAM The electrocardiographic manifestations of AMI are described in Chap. 226. During the initial stage of the acute phase of MI, total occlusion of the infarct artery produces ST-segment elevation. Most patients initially presenting with ST-segment elevation evolve Q waves on the ECG and are ultimately diagnosed as having sustained a Q-wave MI. A small proportion may sustain only a non-Q-wave MI. When the obstructing thrombus is not totally occlusive, obstruction is transient, or if a rich collateral network is present, no ST-segment elevation is seen. Such patients are initially considered to be experiencing either unstable anigna or a non-ST-segment elevation MI (NSTEMI). Among patients presenting without ST-segment elevation, if a serum cardiac marker is detected and no Q wave develops, the diagnosis of non-Q-wave MI is ultimately made. A minority of patients who present initially without ST-segment elevation may develop a Q-wave MI. Previously it was believed that transmural MI is present if the ECG demonstrates Q waves or loss of R waves, and nontransmural MI may be present if the ECG shows only transient ST-segment and T-wave changes. However, electrocardiographic-pathologic correlations are far from perfect; and therefore a more rational nomenclature for designating electrocardiographic infarction is now commonly in use, with the terms Q-wave and non-Q-wave MI replacing the terms transmural and nontransmural MI, respectively.

The presentations that comprise the spectrum ranging from unstable angina through non-Q-wave MI to Q-wave MI are called the *acute coronary syndromes* (Fig. 243-1). This classification scheme provides a conceptual framework for interpreting the diagnostic and prognostic information gleaned from serum cardiac marker measurements as well as for planning antithrombotic therapy.

SERUM CARDIAC MARKERS Certain proteins, called *serum cardiac markers*, are released into the blood in large quantities

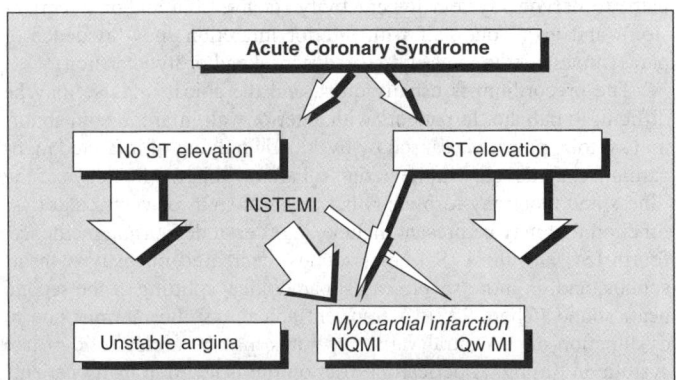

FIGURE 243-1 Acute coronary syndromes. Patients with ischemic discomfort may present with or without ST-segment elevation on the ECG. Of patients with ST-segment elevation, most (*large arrow*) ultimately develop a Q-wave AMI (QwMI), while a few (*small arrow*) develop a non-Q-wave AMI (NQMI). Patients who do not present without ST-segment elevation are suffering from either unstable angina or a non-ST segment elevation MI (NSTEMI) (*large arrows*), a distinction that is ultimately made on the presence or absence of a serum cardiac marker such as CKMB or a cardiac troponin detected in the blood. Most patients presenting with NSTEMI ultimately develop a NQMI on the ECG; a few may develop a QwMI. The spectrum of clinical presentations ranging from unstable angina through NQMI and QwMI are referred to as the actue coronary syndromes. *[Adapted from EM Antman, E Braunwald: Acute myocardial infarction, in Heart Disease, A Textbook of Cardiovascular Medicine, 5th ed, E Braunwald (ed). Philadelphia, Saunders, 1997.]*

from necrotic heart muscle after AMI. The rate of liberation of specific proteins differs depending on their intracellular location and molecular weight, and the local blood and lymphatic flow. The temporal pattern of protein release is of diagnostic importance, but contemporary urgent reperfusion strategies necessitate making a decision (based largely on a combination of clinical and ECG findings) before the results of blood tests have returned from the central laboratory. Rapid whole-blood bedside assays for serum cardiac markers are now available and may facilitate management decisions, particularly in patients with nondiagnostic ECGs.

Creatine phosphokinase (CK) rises within 4 to 8 h and generally returns to normal by 48 to 72 h. An important drawback of total CK measurement is its lack of specificity for AMI, as CK may be elevated with skeletal muscle trauma. A two- to threefold elevation of total CK may follow an intramuscular injection, for example. This ambiguity may lead to the erroneous diagnosis of AMI in a patient who has been given an intramuscular injection of a narcotic for chest pain of noncardiac origin. Other potential sources of total CK elevation are (1) skeletal muscular diseases, including muscular dystrophy, myopathies, and polymyositis; (2) electrical cardioversion; (3) hypothyroidism; (4) stroke; (5) surgery; and (6) skeletal muscle damage secondary to trauma, convulsions, and prolonged immobilization.

The MB isoenzyme of CK has the advantage over total CK that it is not present in significant concentrations in extracardiac tissue and therefore is considerably more specific. However, cardiac surgery, myocarditis, and electrical cardioversion often result in elevated serum levels of the MB isoenzyme. A ratio (relative index) of CKMB mass: CK activity ≥ 2.5 suggests but is not diagnostic of a myocardial rather than a skeletal muscle source for the CKMB elevation. This ratio is less useful when levels of total CK are high owing to skeletal muscle injury or when the total CK level is within the normal range but CKMB is elevated.

Rather than attempting to make the diagnosis of AMI on the basis of a single measurement of CK and CKMB, clinicians should evaluate a series of measurements obtained over the first 24 h. Skeletal muscle release of CKMB typically produces a "plateau" pattern, whereas AMI produces a CKMB elevation that peaks approximately 20 h after the onset of coronary occlusion. When released into the circulation, the myocardial form of CKMB (CKMB2) is acted on by the enzyme carboxypeptidase, which cleaves a lysine residue from the carboxyl terminus to produce an isoform (CKMB1) with a different electrophoretic mobility. A CKMB2:CKMB1 ratio of >1.5 is highly sensitive for the diagnosis of AMI, particularly 4 to 6 h after the onset of coronary occlusion.

Cardiac-specific troponin T (cTnT) and *cardiac-specific troponin I (cTnI)* have amino acid sequences different from those of the skeletal muscle forms of these proteins. These differences have permitted the development of quantitative assays for cTnT and cTnI with highly specific monoclonal antibodies. Since cTnT and cTnI are not normally detectable in the blood of healthy individuals but may increase after AMI to levels over 20 times higher than the cutoff value (usually set only slightly above the noise level of the assay), the measurement of cTnT or cTnI is of considerable diagnostic usefulness, and they are now the preferred biochemical markers for MI. The cardiac troponins are particularly valuable when there is clinical suspicion of either skeletal muscle injury or a small MI that may be below the detection limit for CK and CKMB measurements. Levels of cTnI may remain elevated for 7 to 10 days after AMI, and cTnT levels may remain elevated for up to 10 to 14 days. Thus, measurement of cTnT or cTnI has replaced measurement of lactate dehydrogenase (LDH) and its isoenzymes in patients with suspected MI who come to medical attention more than 24 to 48 h after the onset of symptoms.

Myoglobin is released into the blood within only a few hours of the onset of AMI. Although myoglobin is one of the first serum cardiac markers that rises above the normal range after AMI, it lacks cardiac specificity, and it is rapidly excreted in the urine, so that blood levels return to the normal range within 24 h of the onset of infarction.

Many hospitals are using cTnT or cTnI rather than CKMB as the routine serum cardiac marker for diagnosis of AMI, although any of these analytes remains clinically acceptable. It is not cost-effective to measure both a cardiac-specific troponin and CKMB at all time points in every patient. However, in view of the prolonged elevation of cardiac-specific troponins (>1 week), episodes of recurrent ischemic discomfort and suspected recurrent MI are more readily diagnosed with a serum cardiac marker that remains elevated in the blood more briefly, such as CKMB or myoglobin.

While it has long been recognized that the total quantity of protein released correlates with the size of the infarct, the peak protein concentration correlates only weakly with infarct size. Recanalization of a coronary artery occlusion (either spontaneously or by mechanical or pharmacologic means) in the early hours of AMI causes earlier and higher peaking (at about 8 to 12 h after reperfusion) of serum cardiac markers.

Characteristic rises occur in serum cardiac markers in virtually all patients with clinically proven MI. CK and CKMB levels generally do not rise in unstable angina. However, approximately one-third of patients who are considered to have unstable angina on the basis of a lack of CK or CKMB elevation have elevations of cTnT or cTnI, probably indicating the presence of microinfarction. The finding of an elevated cardiac-specific troponin level, even in the presence of normal CK and CKMB values, is indicative of an adverse prognosis, and such patients should be considered to have sustained MI and managed as described below.

For the purposes of confirming the diagnosis of MI, serum cardiac markers should be measured on admission, 6 to 9 h after admission, and 12 to 24 h after admission if the diagnosis remains uncertain.

The *nonspecific reaction* to myocardial injury is associated with polymorphonuclear leukocytosis, which appears within a few hours after the onset of pain, persists for 3 to 7 days, and often reaches levels of 12,000 to 15,000 leukocytes per microliter. The erythrocyte sedimentation rate rises more slowly than the white blood cell count, peaking during the first week and sometimes remaining elevated for 1 or 2 weeks.

CARDIAC IMAGING *Two-dimensional echocardiography* (Chap. 227) is the most frequently employed imaging modality in patients with AMI. Abnormalities of wall motion are almost universally present. Even when no ST-segment elevation is seen, echocardiographically detectable wall motion abnormalities may be observed. Although AMI cannot be distinguished from an old myocardial scar or from acute severe ischemia by echocardiography, the ease and safety of the procedure make its use appealing as a screening tool. In the emergency department setting, early detection of the presence or absence of wall motion abnormalities by echocardiography can aid in management decisions, such as whether the patient should receive reperfusion therapy [e.g., thrombolysis or a percutaneous coronary intervention (PCI)]. Echocardiographic estimation of left ventricular (LV) function is useful prognostically; detection of reduced function serves as an indication for therapy with an angiotensin-converting enzyme inhibitor (see "Angiotensin-Converting Enzyme Inhibitors," below). Echocardiography may also identify the presence of right ventricular (RV) infarction, ventricular aneurysm, pericardial effusion, and LV thrombus. In addition, Doppler echocardiography is useful in the detection and quantitation of a ventricular septal defect and mitral regurgitation, two serious complications of AMI (see below).

Several radionuclide imaging techniques are available for evaluating patients with suspected AMI. However, these imaging modalities are used less often than echocardiography because they are more cumbersome and they lack sensitivity and specificity in many clinical circumstances. Myocardial perfusion imaging with ^{201}Tl or ^{99m}Tc-sestamibi, which are distributed in proportion to myocardial blood flow and concentrated by viable myocardium (Chap. 244) reveal a defect ("cold spot") in most patients during the first few hours after development of a transmural infarct. However, although perfusion scanning is extremely sensitive, it cannot distinguish acute infarcts from chronic scars and thus is not specific for the diagnosis of *acute* MI. Radionuclide ventriculography, carried out with ^{99m}Tc-labeled red blood cells, frequently demonstrates wall motion disorders and reduction in the ventricular ejection fraction in patients with AMI. While of value in assessing the hemodynamic consequences of infarction and in aiding in the diagnosis of RV infarction when the RV ejection fraction is depressed, this technique is also quite nonspecific, as many cardiac abnormalities other than MI alter the radionuclide ventriculogram.

MANAGEMENT

PREHOSPITAL CARE The prognosis in AMI is largely related to the occurrence of two general classes of complications: (1) electrical complications (arrhythmias) and (2) mechanical problems ("pump failure"). Most out-of-hospital deaths from AMI are due to the sudden development of ventricular fibrillation. The vast majority of deaths due to ventricular fibrillation occur within the first 24 h of the onset of symptoms, and, of these, over half occur in the first hour. Therefore, the major elements of prehospital care of patients with suspected AMI include (1) recognition of symptoms by the patient and prompt seeking of medical attention; (2) rapid deployment of an emergency medical team capable of performing resuscitative maneuvers, including defibrillation; and (3) expeditious transportation of the patient to a hospital facility that is continuously staffed by physicians and nurses skilled in managing arrhythmias, providing advanced cardiac life support, and (4) expeditious implementation of reperfusion therapy. The biggest delay usually occurs not during transportation to the hospital but rather between the onset of pain and the patient's decision to call for help. This delay can best be reduced by education of the public by health care professionals concerning the significance of chest pain and the importance of seeking early medical attention. Increasingly, monitoring and treatment are carried out by trained personnel in the ambulance, further shortening the time between the onset of the infarction and appropriate treatment.

INITIAL MANAGEMENT IN THE EMERGENCY DEPARTMENT In the emergency department, the goals for the management of patients with suspected AMI include control of cardiac pain, rapid identification of patients who are candidates for urgent reperfusion therapy, triage of lower-risk patients to the appropriate location in the hospital, and avoidance of inappropriate discharge of patients with AMI. Many aspects of the treatment of AMI are initiated in the emergency department and then continued during the in-hospital phase of management.

Aspirin is now considered an essential element in the management of patients with suspected AMI and is effective across the entire spectrum of acute coronary syndromes (Fig. 243-2 and 243-3). Rapid inhibition of cyclooxygenase in platelets followed by a reduction of thromboxane A_2 levels is achieved by buccal absorption of a chewed 160 to 325 mg tablet in the emergency department. This measure should be followed by daily oral administration of aspirin in a dose of 160 to 325 mg.

Since patients with AMI may develop hypoxemia secondary to ventilation-perfusion abnormalities from LV failure and intrinsic pulmonary disease, it has been a common practice to routinely administer *supplemental oxygen*. In patients whose arterial oxygen saturation is normal as estimated by pulse oximetry or measured by an arterial blood gas specimen, supplemental oxygen is of limited if any clinical benefit and therefore is not cost effective. However, when hypoxemia is present, oxygen should be administered by nasal prongs or face mask (2 to 4 L/min) for the first 6 to 12 h after infarction; the patient should then be reassessed to determine if there is a continued need for such treatment.

CONTROL OF PAIN *Morphine* is a very effective analgesic for the pain associated with AMI. However, it may reduce sympathetically mediated arteriolar and venous constriction, and the resulting venous pooling may reduce cardiac output and arterial pressure. This complication does not contraindicate the use of morphine. Hypotension associated with venous pooling usually responds promptly to elevation of the legs, but in some patients volume expansion with intra-

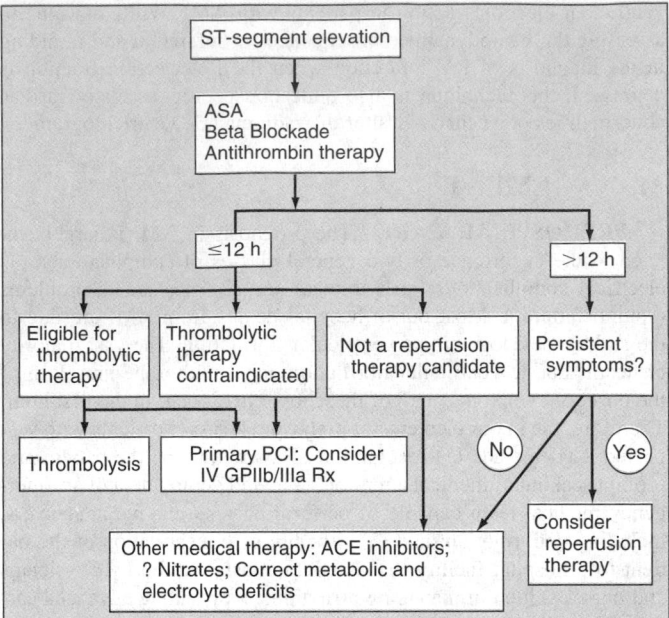

FIGURE 243-2 Management strategy for patients suspected of having an ST-segment elevation. AMI patients should receive aspirin (ASA), beta blockers (in the absence of contraindications), and an antithrombin (particularly if a relatively fibrin-specific thrombolytic agent is used). Adjunctive antithrombin therapy is probably not required for patients receiving streptokinase. Patients treated within 12 h who are eligible for thrombolytic therapy should expeditiously receive such treatment or be considered for primary percutaneous transluminal coronary angioplasty (PCI). Immediate, primary PCI is also to be considered when lytic therapy is contraindicated. An intravenous glycoprotein IIb/IIIa (GPIIb/IIIa) inhibitor may be helpful for reducing thrombotic complications during primary PCI. *[Modified from EM Antman: Overview of medical therapy, in RM Califf (ed): Acute Myocardial Infarction and Other Acute Ischemic Syndromes, in E Braunwald (Series ed): Atlas of Heart Diseases, vol. 8. Philadelphia, Current Medicine 1996.]*

venous saline is required. The patient may experience diaphoresis and nausea, but these events usually pass and are replaced by a feeling of well-being associated with the relief of pain. Morphine also has a vagotonic effect and may cause bradycardia or advanced degrees of heart block, particularly in patients with posteroinferior infarction. These side effects usually respond to atropine (0.5 mg intravenously). Morphine is routinely administered by repetitive (every 5 min) intravenous injection of small doses (2 to 4 mg) rather than by the subcutaneous administration of a larger quantity, because absorption may be unpredictable by the latter route.

Before morphine is administered, sublingual *nitroglycerin* can be given safely to most patients with AMI. Up to three 0.4-mg doses should be administered at about 5-min intervals. In addition to diminishing or abolishing chest discomfort, nitroglycerin, once considered contraindicated in the setting of AMI, may be capable of both decreasing myocardial oxygen demand (by lowering preload) and increasing myocardial oxygen supply (by dilating infarct-related coronary vessels or collateral vessels). In patients whose initially favorable response to sublingual nitroglycerin is followed by the return of chest pain, particularly if accompanied by other evidence of ongoing ischemia such as further ST-segment or T-wave shifts, the use of intravenous nitroglycerin should be considered. Therapy with nitrates should be avoided in patients who present with low systolic arterial pressure (<100 mmHg) or in whom there is clinical suspicion of right ventricular infarction (inferior infarction on electrocardiogram, elevated jugular venous pressure, clear lungs, and hypotension). Nitrates should not be administered to patients who have taken the phosphodiasterase 5 inhibitor sildenafil for erectile dysfunction within the preceding 24 h

since it may potentiate the hypotensive effects of nitrates. An idiosyncratic reaction to nitrates, consisting of sudden marked hypotension, sometimes occurs but can usually be reversed promptly by the rapid administration of intravenous atropine.

Intravenous *beta blockers* are also useful in the control of the pain of AMI. These drugs control pain effectively in some patients, presumably by diminishing myocardial oxygen demand and hence ischemia. More important, there is evidence that intravenous beta blockers reduce in-hospital mortality, particularly in high-risk patients (see "β-Adrenoceptor Blockers," below). A commonly employed regimen is metoprolol, 5 mg every 2 to 5 min for a total of three doses, provided the patient has a heart rate >60 beats per minute (bpm), systolic pressure >100 mmHg, a PR interval <0.24 s, and rales that are no higher than 10 cm up from the diaphragm. Fifteen minutes after the last intravenous dose, an oral regimen is initiated of 50 mg every 6 h for 48 h followed by 100 mg every 12 h.

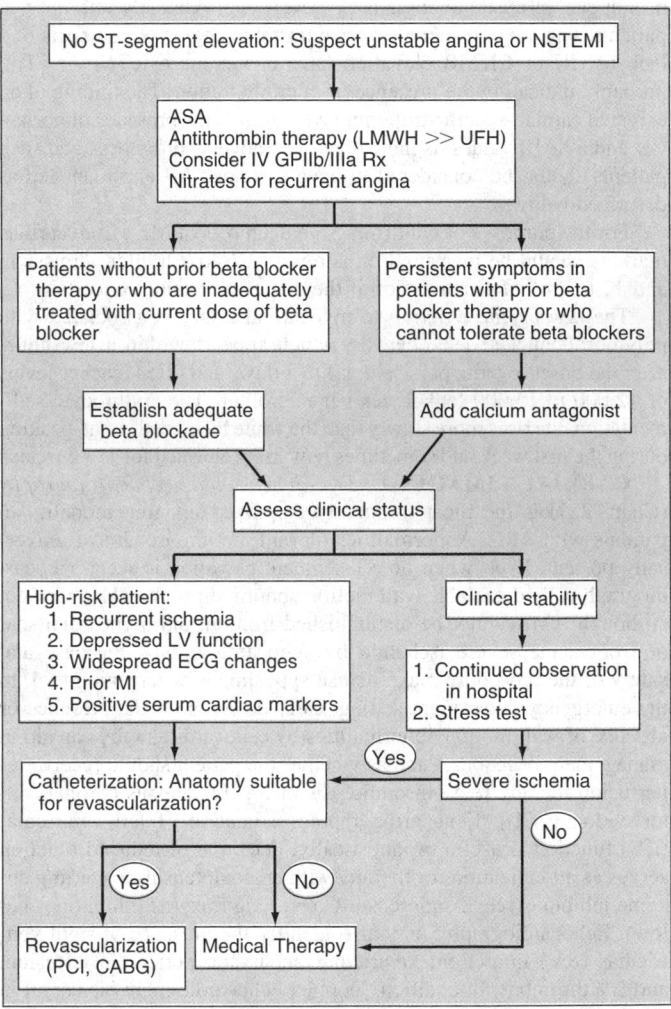

FIGURE 243-3 Management strategy for patients with unstable angina and AMI without ST-segment elevation. These patients should be treated with an antithrombin and aspirin. Nitrates should be administered for recurrent episodes of angina. The risk of death and cardiac ischemic events may be reduced in high risk patients if an intravenous GPIIb/IIIa inhibitor is administered. Adequate beta blockade should be established; when that is not possible or contraindications exist, a calcium antagonist can be considered. Patients at high risk should be triaged to cardiac catheterization with plans for revascularization if clinically suitable, while patients who are clinically stable can be treated more conservatively with continued observation in the hospital and consideration of a stress test to screen for any provocable myocardial ischemia. CABG, coronary artery bypass grafting; LV, left ventricular. *[Modified from EM Antman: Overview of medical therapy, in RM Califf (ed): Acute Myocardial Infarction and Other Acute Ischemic Syndromes, in E Braunwald (Series ed): Atlas of Heart Diseases, vol. 8. Philadelphia, Current Medicine 1996.]*

Unlike beta blockers, calcium antagonists are of little value in the acute setting, and there is evidence that short-acting dihydropyridines may be associated with an increased mortality risk.

MANAGEMENT STRATEGIES (Figs. 243-2 and 243-3) The primary tool for screening patients and making triage decisions is the initial 12-lead ECG. When ST-segment elevation in at least two contiguous leads of at least 2 mm in V1-V3 and 1 mm in other leads is present, a patient should be considered a candidate for *reperfusion therapy* (Fig. 243-2). If no contraindications are present (see "Contraindications and Complications," under "Thombolysis," below), thrombolytic therapy should ideally be initiated within 30 min. The process of selecting patients for thrombolysis versus primary PCI (angioplasty, or stenting) (Chap. 245) is discussed below. In the absence of ST-segment elevation, thrombolysis is not helpful, and evidence exists suggesting that it may be harmful. Pharmacotherapy for patients presenting without ST-segment elevation (Fig. 243-3) typically includes measures to control cardiac pain (as discussed above), aspirin, antithrombin therapy (preferably with low-molecular-weight heparin), and infusion of nitroglycerin as needed to control recurrent ischemia. For high-risk patients an intravenous infusion of a glycoprotein IIb/IIIa inhibitor should be considered. Further management recommendations for patients without ST-segment elevation are outlined in Fig. 243-3.

LIMITATION OF INFARCT SIZE The quantity of myocardium that becomes necrotic as a consequence of a coronary artery occlusion is determined by factors other than just the site of occlusion. While the central zone of the infarct contains necrotic tissue that is irretrievably lost, the fate of the surrounding ischemic myocardium may be improved by timely restoration of coronary perfusion, reduction of myocardial oxygen demands, prevention of the accumulation of noxious metabolites, and blunting of the impact of mediators of reperfusion injury (e.g., calcium overload and oxygen-derived free radicals). Up to one-third of patients with AMI may achieve *spontaneous* reperfusion of the infarct-related coronary artery within 24 h and experience improved healing of infarcted tissue. Reperfusion either pharmacologically (by thrombolysis) or mechanically (by angioplasty and/or stenting) accelerates the process of opening the occluded infarct-related artery in those patients in whom spontaneous thrombolysis ultimately would have occurred and also greatly increases the number of patients in whom restoration of flow in the infarct-related artery is accomplished. Timely restoration of flow in the epicardial infarct-related artery combined with improved perfusion of the downstream zone of infarcted myocardium results in a limitation of infarct size. Protection of the ischemic myocardium by the maintenance of an optimal balance between myocardial oxygen supply and demand through pain control, treatment of congestive heart failure, and minimization of tachycardia and hypertension extends the "window" of time for the salvage of myocardium by reperfusion strategies.

Glucocorticoids and nonsteroidal anti-inflammatory agents, with the exception of aspirin, should be avoided in the setting of AMI. They can impair infarct healing and increase the risk of myocardial rupture, and their use may result in a larger infarct scar. In addition, they can increase coronary vascular resistance, thereby potentially reducing flow to ischemic myocardium.

THROMBOLYSIS The thrombolytic agents tissue plasminogen activator (tPA), streptokinase, anisoylated plasminogen streptokinase activator complex (APSAC) and reteplase (rPA) have been approved by the Food and Drug Administration for intravenous use in the setting of AMI. These drugs all act by promoting the conversion of plasminogen to plasmin, which subsequently lyses fibrin thrombi. Although considerable emphasis was first placed on a distinction between more fibrin-specific agents, such as tPA, and non-fibrin-specific agents, such as streptokinase, it is now recognized that these differences are only relative, as some degree of systemic fibrinolysis occurs with tPA. The principal goal of thrombolysis is prompt restoration of coronary arterial patency.

When assessed angiographically, flow in the culprit coronary artery is described by a simple qualitative scale called the TIMI grading

system: grade 0 indicates complete occlusion of the infarct-related artery; grade 1 indicates some penetration of the contrast material beyond the point of obstruction but without perfusion of the distal coronary bed; grade 2 indicates perfusion of the entire infarct vessel into the distal bed but with flow that is delayed compared with that of a normal artery; and grade 3 indicates full perfusion of the infarct vessel with normal flow. Early reports frequently lumped TIMI grades 2 and 3 under the general category of *patency*, but it is now recognized that grade 3 flow is the goal of reperfusion therapy, because full perfusion of the infarct-related coronary artery yields far better results in terms of infarct size, maintenance of LV function, and reduction of both short- and long-term mortality rates. Relatively new methods of angiographic assessment of the efficacy of thrombolysis include counting the number of frames required on the cine film for dye to flow from the origin of the infarct-related artery to a landmark in the distal vascular bed (TIMI frame count) and determining the rate of entry and exit of contrast dye from the microvasculature in the myocardial infarct zone (TIMI Myocardial Perfusion Grade).

Thrombolytic therapy can reduce the relative risk of in-hospital death by up to 50% when administered within the first hour of the onset of symptoms of AMI, and much of this benefit is maintained for at least 10 years. Appropriately used thrombolytic therapy appears to reduce infarct size, limit LV dysfunction, and reduce the incidence of serious complications such as septal rupture, cardiogenic shock, and malignant ventricular arrhythmias. Since myocardium can be salvaged only before it has been irreversibly injured, the timing of reperfusion therapy, by thrombolysis or a catheter-based approach, is of extreme importance in achieving maximum benefit. While the upper time limit depends on specific factors in individual patients, it is clear that "every minute counts" and that patients treated within 1 to 3 h of the onset of symptoms generally benefit most. Although reduction of the mortality rate is more modest, the therapy remains of benefit for many patients seen 3 to 6 h after the onset of infarction, and some benefit appears to be possible up to 12 h, especially if chest discomfort is still present and ST segments remain elevated in ECG leads that do not yet demonstrate new Q waves. In addition to the possibility of early treatment, clinical factors that favor proceeding with thrombolytic therapy include anterior wall injury, hemodynamically complicated infarction, and widespread ECG evidence of myocardial jeopardy. Although patients (younger than 65 years) achieve a greater relative reduction in the mortality rate than elderly patients, the higher *absolute* mortality rate (15 to 25%) in elderly patients results in similar absolute reductions in the mortality rates for both age groups.

Intriguing data are accumulating to indicate that improved ventricular function and reduced mortality may also be achieved by *late coronary reperfusion*. The benefits of late reperfusion cannot be attributed to a reduction of infarct size but appear to result from improvement of tissue healing in the infarct zone with prevention of infarct expansion, enhancement of collateral flow, improvement of myocardial contractile performance, and reduction in the tendency to electrical instability. In addition, *hibernating myocardium* (i.e., poorly contractile myocardium in a zone that is supplied by a stenotic infarct-related coronary artery with slow antegrade perfusion, Chap. 244) may show improved contraction after angioplasty to increase coronary blood flow.

tPA is more effective than streptokinase at restoring full perfusion—i.e., TIMI grade 3 coronary flow—and has a small edge in improving survival as well. The current recommended regimen of tPA consists of a 15-mg bolus followed by 50 mg intravenously over the first 30 min, followed by 35 mg over the next 60 min. Streptokinase is administered as 1.5 million units (MU) intravenously over 1 h. Reteplase is administered in a double bolus regimen consisting of a 10-MU bolus given over 2 to 3 min followed by a second 10-MU bolus 30 min later.

Promising new pharmacologic regimens for reperfusion combine an intravenous glycoprotein IIb/IIIa inhibitor with a reduced dose of a thrombolytic agent. Such combination reperfusion regimens appear to facilitate the rate and extent of thrombolysis by inhibiting platelet aggregation, weakening the clot structure, and allowing penetration of the thrombolytic agent deeper into the clot.

Contraindications and Complications   Clear contraindications to the use of thrombolytic agents include a history of cerebrovascular hemorrhage at any time, a nonhemorrhagic stroke or other cerebrovascular event within the past year, marked hypertension (a reliably determined systolic arterial pressure >180 mmHg and/or a diastolic pressure >110 mmHg) at any time during the acute presentation, suspicion of aortic dissection, and active internal bleeding (excluding menses). While advanced age is associated with an increase in hemorrhagic complications, the benefit of thrombolytic therapy in the elderly appears to justify its use if no other contraindications are present and the amount of myocardium in jeopardy appears to be substantial.

Relative contraindications to thrombolytic therapy, which require careful assessment of the risk:benefit ratio, include current use of anticoagulants (international normalized ratio ≥2), a recent (<2 weeks) invasive or surgical procedure or prolonged (>10 min) cardiopulmonary resuscitation, known bleeding diasthesis, pregnancy, a hemorrhagic ophthalmic condition (e.g., hemorrhagic diabetic retinopathy), active peptic ulcer disease, and a history of severe hypertension that is currently adequately controlled. Because of the risk of an allergic reaction, patients should not receive streptokinase if that agent had been received within the preceding 5 days to 2 years.

Allergic reactions to streptokinase occur in approximately 2% of patients who receive it. While a minor degree of hypotension occurs in 4 to 10% of patients given this agent, marked hypotension occurs, although rarely, in association with severe allergic reactions.

Hemorrhage is the most frequent and potentially the most serious complication. Because bleeding episodes that require transfusion are more common when patients require invasive procedures, unnecessary venous or arterial interventions should be avoided in patients receiving thrombolytic agents. Hemorrhagic stroke is the most serious complication and occurs in approximately 0.5 to 0.9% of patients being treated with these agents. This rate increases with advancing age, with patients older than 70 years experiencing roughly twice the rate of intracranial hemorrhage as those younger than 65 years. Large-scale intervention trials have suggested that the rate of intracranial hemorrhage with tPA or rPA is slightly higher than that with streptokinase.

Routine angiography after thrombolysis with the intent of performing a PCI on underlying coronary artery stenoses in the culprit vessel is not recommended. Higher rates of abrupt closure of the infarct-related coronary artery with a need for urgent coronary artery bypass surgery as well as a trend toward an increase in mortality rate have been noted with this approach. Instead, after thrombolytic therapy, cardiac catheterization and coronary angiography should be carried out if there is evidence of either (1) failure of reperfusion (persistent chest pain and ST-segment elevation beyond 90 min) in which case a *rescue PCI* should be considered, or (2) coronary artery reocclusion (reelevation of ST segments and/or recurrent chest pain) or the development of recurrent ischemia (such as recurrent angina in the early hospital course or a positive exercise stress test before discharge), in which case an *elective PCI* should be considered. Coronary artery bypass surgery should be reserved for patients whose coronary anatomy is unsuited to angioplasty but in whom revascularization appears to be advisable because of extensive jeopardized myocardium or recurrent ischemia.

Primary Percutaneous Coronary Intervention (See also Chap. 245)   PCI, usually angioplasty and/or stenting without preceding thrombolysis, is also effective in restoring perfusion in AMI when carried out on an emergency basis in the first few hours of MI. It has the advantage of being applicable to patients who have contraindications to thrombolytic therapy but otherwise are considered appropriate candidates for reperfusion. It appears to be more effective than thrombolysis in opening occluded coronary arteries and, *when performed by experienced operators in dedicated medical centers*, is associated with better short-term and long-term clinical outcomes. It remains to be determined whether the advantages of primary PCI reported from organized research efforts can be replicated in routine clinical practice. However, PCI is expensive in terms of personnel and facilities, and its applicability is seriously limited by its availability, around the clock, in only a minority of hospitals.

HOSPITAL PHASE MANAGEMENT

CORONARY CARE UNITS   These units are routinely equipped with a system that permits continuous monitoring of the cardiac rhythm of each patient and hemodynamic monitoring in selected patients. Defibrillators, respirators, noninvasive transthoracic pacemakers, and facilities for introducing pacing catheters and flow-directed balloon-tipped catheters are also usually available. Equally important is the organization of a highly trained team of nurses who can recognize arrhythmias; adjust the dosage of antiarrhythmic, vasoactive, and anticoagulant drugs; and perform cardiac resuscitation, including electroshock, when necessary.

Patients should be admitted to a coronary care unit early in their illness when it is expected that they will derive benefit from the sophisticated and expensive care provided. The availability of electrocardiographic monitoring and trained personnel outside the coronary care unit has made it possible to admit lower-risk patients (e.g., those not hemodynamically compromised and without active arrhythmias) to "intermediate care units."

The duration of stay in the coronary care unit is dictated by the ongoing need for intensive care. If AMI has been ruled out (ideally within 8 to 12 h) and symptoms are controlled with oral therapy, patients may be transferred out of the coronary care unit. Also, patients who have a confirmed AMI but who are considered to be at low risk (no prior infarction and no persistent chest discomfort, congestive heart failure, hypotension, or cardiac arrhythmias) may be safely transferred out of the coronary care unit in 24 to 36 h.

Activity   Factors that increase the work of the heart during the initial hours of infarction may increase the size of the infarct. Therefore, patients with AMI should be kept at bed rest for the first 12 h. However, in the absence of complications, patients should be encouraged, under supervision, to resume an upright posture by dangling their feet over the side of the bed and sitting in a chair within the first 24 h. This practice is both psychologically beneficial and usually results in a reduction in the pulmonary capillary wedge pressure. In the absence of hypotension and other complications, by the second or third day patients typically are ambulating in their room with increasing duration and frequency, and they may shower or stand at the sink to bathe. By day 3 or 4 after infarction, patients should be increasing their ambulation progressively to a goal of 600 ft at least three times a day.

Diet   Because of the risk of emesis and aspiration soon after MI, patients should receive either nothing or only clear liquids by mouth for the first 4 to 12 h. The typical coronary care unit diet should provide ≤30% of total calories as fat and have a cholesterol content of ≤300 mg/d. Complex carbohydrates should make up 50 to 55% of total calories. Portions should not be unusually large, and the menu should be enriched with foods that are high in potassium, magnesium, and fiber but low in sodium. Diabetes mellitus and hypertriglyceridemia are managed by restriction of concentrated sweets in the diet.

Bowels   Bed rest and the effect of the narcotics used for the relief of pain often lead to constipation. A bedside commode rather than a bedpan, a diet rich in bulk, and the routine use of a stool softener such as dioctyl sodium sulfosuccinate (200 mg/d) are recommended. If the patient remains constipated despite these measures, a laxative can be prescribed. Contrary to prior belief, it is safe to perform a gentle rectal examination on patients with AMI.

Sedation   Many patients require sedation during hospitalization to withstand the period of enforced inactivity with tranquillity. Diazepam (5 mg), oxazepam (15 to 30 mg), or lorazepam (0.5 to 2 mg), given three or four times daily, is usually effective. An additional dose of any of the above medications may be given at night to ensure adequate sleep. Attention to this problem is especially important during the first few days in the coronary care unit, where the atmosphere of 24-h vigilance may interfere with the patient's sleep. However, sedation is no substitute for reassuring, quiet surroundings. Many drugs used in the coronary care unit, such as atropine, H_2 blockers, and narcotics, can produce delirium, particularly in the elderly. This effect should not be confused with agitation, and it is wise to conduct a thorough review of the patient's medications before arbitrarily prescribing additional doses of anxiolytics.

PHARMACOTHERAPY

ANTITHROMBOTIC AGENTS The use of antiplatelet and antithrombin therapy during the initial phase of AMI is based on extensive laboratory and clinical evidence that thrombosis plays an important role in the pathogenesis of this condition. The primary goal of treatment with antiplatelet and antithrombin agents is to establish and maintain patency of the infarct-related artery. A secondary goal is to reduce the patient's tendency to thrombosis and thus the likelihood of mural thrombus formation or deep venous thrombosis, either of which could result in pulmonary embolization. The degree to which antiplatelet and antithrombin therapy achieves these goals partly determines how effectively it reduces the risk of mortality from AMI.

As noted previously (see "Initial Management in the Emergency Department," above), aspirin is the standard antiplatelet agent for patients with AMI. The most compelling evidence for the benefits of antiplatelet therapy (mainly with aspirin) in AMI is found in the comprehensive overview by the Antiplatelet Trialists' Collaboration. Data from nearly 20,000 patients with AMI enrolled in nine randomized trials were pooled and revealed a reduction in the mortality rate from 11.7% in control patients to 9.3% in patients receiving antiplatelet agents. This difference corresponds to the prevention of 24 deaths for every 1000 patients treated. Similarly, 2 strokes and 12 recurrent infarctions are prevented for every 1000 patients treated with antiplatelet therapy.

The glycoprotein IIb/IIIa receptor is the focus of intense investigation by basic and clinical scientists (Chap. 116). Because platelet-rich thrombi are more resistant to thrombolytic agents than platelet-poor thrombi and because platelet aggregates appear to play a role in reocclusion after initially successful thrombolysis, glycoprotein IIb/IIIa inhibition may facilitate thrombolysis and reduce the rate of reocclusion of reperfused vessels. Compounds have been developed that block the glycoprotein IIb/IIIa receptor. These drugs appear useful for preventing thrombotic complications in patients with AMI undergoing PCI and reduce the rate of the composite endpoint of death and recurrent AMI in the medical management of patients without ST-segment elevation at presentation.

The standard antithrombin agent used in clinical practice is unfractionated heparin (UFH). Despite numerous clinical trials, the precise role of heparin in patients treated with thrombolytic agents remains uncertain. The available data fail to show any convincing benefit of UFH with respect to either coronary arterial patency or mortality rate when UFH is added to a regimen of aspirin and a non-fibrin-specific thrombolytic agent such as streptokinase. Although not conclusively proven, it appears that the immediate administration of intravenous UFH, in addition to a regimen of aspirin and tPA, helps to facilitate thrombolysis and to establish and maintain patency of the infarct-related artery. This effect is achieved at the cost of a small increased risk of bleeding. Most clinicians who use tPA also administer a bolus and infusion of UFH, which should be administered as a bolus of 60 U/kg followed by a maintenance infusion of 12 U/kg per hour. The activated partial thromboplastin time during maintenance therapy should be 1.5 to 2 times the control value.

An alternative to UFH for anticoagulation of patients with AMI that is being used with increased frequency are the low-molecular-weight heparin preparations (LMWHs), which are formed by enzymatic or chemical depolymerization to produce saccharide chains of

varying length but with a mean molecular weight of about 5000 Da. The LMWHs have several advantages over UFH including an increased anti-factor Xa:IIa ratio, decreased sensitivity to platelet factor IV, a more stable reliable anticoagulant effect, and enhanced bioavailability, thereby permitting administration via the subcutaneous route. Because of the stable anticoagulant effect when LMWHs are used, routine monitoring of hematologic tests such as the activated partial thromboplastin time (aPTT) is not required. Although the LMWHs share many pharmacologic similarities, they also vary in a number of important features; and therefore these agents should be considered individually rather than as members of an interchangeable class of compounds. Of the LMWHs, nadroparin and dalteparin have been found to be similar to UFH in therapeutic effectiveness, while enoxaparin (1 mg/kg subcutaneously every 12 h) appears to be superior to UFH for reducing the mortality rate and cardiac ischemic events in patients with AMI who do not present with ST-segment elevation. Direct comparisons among the LMWHs have not been carried out.

Patients with an anterior location of the infarction, severe LV dysfunction, congestive heart failure, a history of embolism, two-dimensional echocardiographic evidence of mural thorombus, or atrial fibrillation are at increased risk of systemic or pulmonary thromboembolism. Such individuals should receive full therapeutic levels of antithrombin therapy (UFH or LMWHs) while hospitalized, followed by at least 3 months of warfarin therapy.

BETA-ADRENOCEPTOR BLOCKERS The benefits of beta blockers in patients with AMI can be divided into those that occur immediately when the drug is given acutely and those that accrue over the long term when the drug is given for secondary prevention after an index infarction. Acute intravenous beta blockade improves the myocardial oxygen supply-demand relationship, decreases pain, reduces infarct size, and decreases the incidence of serious ventricular arrhythmias. An overview of the data from 27,000 patients enrolled in nine randomized trials in the prethrombolytic era indicates that intravenous followed by oral beta blockade is associated with a 15% relative reduction in mortality, nonfatal reinfarction, and nonfatal cardiac arrest. In patients who undergo thrombolysis soon after the onset of chest pain, no incremental reduction in mortality rate is seen with beta blockers, but recurrent ischemia and reinfarction are reduced.

Beta blocker therapy after AMI thus is useful for most patients except those in whom it is specifically contraindicated (patients with heart failure or severely compromised LV function, heart block, orthostatic hypotension, or a history of asthma) and perhaps those whose excellent long-term prognosis (defined as an expected mortality rate of <1% per year) markedly diminishes any potential benefit (patients younger than 55 years with normal ventricular function, no complex ventricular ectopy, and no angina).

Although the data supporting the use of beta blockers in patients with AMI who do not present with ST-segment elevation are limited, the available evidence suggests that even among such patients, the use of beta blockers decreases the rates of cardiovascular mortality and reinfarction, and increases the probability of long-term survival.

ANGIOTENSIN CONVERTING ENZYME INHIBITORS Angiotensin-converting enzyme (ACE) inhibitors reduce the mortality rate after AMI, and the mortality benefits are additive to those achieved with aspirin and beta blockers. The maximum benefit is seen in high-risk patients (those who are elderly or have an anterior infarction, a prior infarction, and/or globally depressed LV function), but evidence suggests that a short-term benefit occurs when ACE inhibitors are prescribed unselectively to all hemodynamically stable patients with AMI (i.e., those with a systolic pressure >100 mmHg). The mechanism involves a reduction in ventricular remodeling after infarction (see "Ventricular Dysfunction," below) with a subsequent reduction in the risk of congestive heart failure (CHF). The rate of recurrent infarction also may be lower in patients treated chronically with ACE inhibitors after infarction.

ACE inhibitors should be prescribed within 24 h to all patients with AMI and overt CHF as well as to hemodynamically stable patients with ST-segment elevation or left bundle branch block. There is little evidence to support the immediate use of ACE inhibitors in patients with AMI who present without ST-segment changes or only with ST-segment depression without CHF. Before hospital discharge, LV function should be assessed with an imaging study. ACE inhibitors should be continued indefinitely in patients who have clinically evident CHF, in patients whom an imaging study shows a reduction in global LV function or a large regional wall motion abnormality, or in those who are hypertensive.

OTHER AGENTS   Although the actual impact on the mortality rate is slight (three to four lives saved per 1000 patients treated), *nitrates* (intravenous or oral) may be useful in the relief of pain associated with AMI. Favorable effects on the ischemic process and ventricular remodeling (see below) have led many physicians to routinely use intravenous nitroglycerin (5 to 10 μg/min initial dose and up to 200 μg/min as long as hemodynamic stability is maintained) for the first 24 to 48 h after the onset of infarction.

Results of multiple trials of different calcium antagonists have failed to establish a role for these agents in the treatment of most patients with AMI, in contrast to the more consistent data that exist for other drugs (e.g., beta blockers, aspirin, thrombolytic agents). The routine use of calcium antagonists cannot be recommended.

A metabolic supportive measure that has shown promise in several small-scale trials of patients with AMI is the administration of a solution of glucose-insulin-potassium (GIK). A GIK infusion lowers the concentration of plasma free fatty acids and improves ventricular performance. Strict control of blood glucose in diabetic patients with AMI has been shown to reduce the mortality rate. It remains to be determined whether infusions of GIK should be administered to all patients with AMI.

Intracellular *magnesium* levels are frequently reduced in patients with AMI, but this deficit is not adequately reflected in serum measurements, as magnesium is predominantly an intracellular ion and <1% of its total body stores is intravascular. Whether giving routine empirical supplemental infusions of magnesium to high-risk patients with AMI is beneficial remains an open question. At present, serum magnesium should be measured in all patients on admission, and any demonstrated deficits should be corrected to minimize the risk of arrhythmias. There does not appear to be any benefit in the routine use of magnesium when it is administered relatively late (after more than 6 h) or to patients with an uncomplicated AMI who have a low mortality risk. Its role in high-risk patients is under investigation.

COMPLICATIONS AND THEIR TREATMENT

VENTRICULAR DYSFUNCTION   After AMI, the LV undergoes a series of changes in shape, size, and thickness in both the infarcted and noninfarcted segments. This process is referred to as *ventricular remodeling* and generally precedes the development of clinically evident CHF in the months to years after infarction. Soon after AMI, the LV begins to dilate. Acutely, this results from expansion of the infarct (i.e., slippage of muscle bundles, disruption of normal myocardial cells, and tissue loss within the necrotic zone, resulting in disproportionate thinning and elongation of the infarct zone). Later, lengthening of the noninfarcted segments occurs as well. The overall chamber enlargement that occurs is related to the size and location of the infarct, with greater dilation following infarction of the apex of the LV and causing more marked hemodynamic impairment, more frequent heart failure, and a poorer prognosis. Progressive dilation and its clinical consequences may be ameliorated by therapy with ACE inhibitors and other vasodilators (e.g., nitrates). Thus, in patients with an ejection fraction <40%, regardless of whether or not heart failure is present, ACE inhibitors should be prescribed.

HEMODYNAMIC ASSESSMENT   Pump failure is now the primary cause of in-hospital death from AMI. The extent of ischemic

necrosis correlates well with the degree of pump failure and with mortality, both early (within 10 days of infarction) and later. The most common clinical signs are pulmonary rales and S_3 and S_4 gallop rhythms. Pulmonary congestion is also frequently seen on the chest roentgenogram. Elevated LV filling pressure and elevated pulmonary artery pressure are the characteristic hemodynamic findings, but these findings may result from a reduction of ventricular compliance (diastolic failure) and/or a reduction of stroke volume with secondary cardiac dilation (systolic failure) (Chap. 231).

A classification originally proposed by Killip divides patients into four groups: class I, no signs of pulmonary or venous congestion; class II, moderate heart failure as evidenced by rales at the lung bases, S_3 gallop, tachypnea, or signs of failure of the right side of the heart, including venous and hepatic congestion; class III, severe heart failure, pulmonary edema; and class IV, shock with systolic pressure <90 mmHg and evidence of peripheral vasoconstriction, peripheral cyanosis, mental confusion, and oliguria. When this classification was established in 1967, the expected hospital mortality rate of patients in these classes was as follows: class I, 0 to 5%; class II, 10 to 20%; class III, 35 to 45%; and class IV, 85 to 95%. With advances in management, the mortality rate in each class has fallen, perhaps by as much as one-third to one-half.

Hemodynamic evidence of abnormal LV function appears when contraction is seriously impaired in 20 to 25% of the LV. Infarction of ≥40% of the LV usually results in cardiogenic shock (see below). Positioning of a balloon flotation catheter in the pulmonary artery permits monitoring of LV filling pressure; this technique is useful in patients who exhibit hypotension and/or clinical evidence of CHF. Cardiac output can also be determined with a pulmonary artery catheter. With the addition of intraarterial pressure monitoring, systemic vascular resistance can be calculated as a guide to adjusting vasopressor and vasodilator therapy. Some patients with AMI have markedly elevated LV filling pressures (>22 mmHg) and normal cardiac indexes [>2.6 and >3.6 L/(min/m²)], while others have relatively low LV filling pressures (<15 mmHg) and reduced cardiac indexes. The former patients usually benefit from diuresis, while the latter may respond to volume expansion by means of intravenous administration of colloid-containing solutions.

Hypovolemia   Hypovolemia is an easily corrected condition that may contribute to the hypotension and vascular collapse associated with AMI in some patients. It may be secondary to previous diuretic use, to reduced fluid intake during the early stages of the illness, and/or to vomiting associated with pain or medications. Consequently, hypovolemia should be identified and corrected in patients with AMI and hypotension before more vigorous forms of therapy are begun. Central venous pressure reflects RV rather than LV filling pressure and is an inadequate guide for adjustment of blood volume, since LV function is almost always affected much more adversely than RV function in patients with AMI. The optimal LV filling or pulmonary artery wedge pressure may vary considerably among patients. Each patient's ideal level (generally ~20 mmHg) is reached by cautious fluid administration during careful monitoring of oxygenation and cardiac output. Eventually, the cardiac output level plateaus, and further increases in LV filling pressure only increase congestive symptoms and decrease systemic oxygenation without raising arterial pressure.

TREATMENT   The management of CHF in association with AMI is similar to that of acute heart failure secondary to other forms of heart disease (avoidance of hypoxemia, diuresis, afterload reduction, inotropic support) (Chap. 232), except that the benefits of digitalis administration to patients with AMI are unimpressive. By contrast, diuretic agents are extremely effective, as they diminish pulmonary congestion in the presence of systolic and/or diastolic heart failure. Left ventricular filling pressure falls and orthopnea and dyspnea improve after the intravenous administration of furosemide or other loop diuretics. These drugs should be used with caution, however, as they can result in a massive diuresis with associated decreases in plasma volume, cardiac output, systemic blood pressure, and hence coronary perfusion. Nitrates in various forms may be used to decrease preload and congestive symptoms. Oral isosorbide dinitrate, topical nitroglycerin ointment, or intravenous nitroglycerin all have the advantage over a diuretic of lowering preload through venodilation without decreasing the total plasma volume. In addition, nitrates may improve ventricular compliance if ischemia is present, as ischemia causes an elevation of LV filling pressure. The patient with pulmonary edema is treated as described in Chap. 232, but vasodilators must be used with caution to prevent serious hypotension. As noted earlier, ACE inhibitors are an ideal class of drugs for management of ventricular dysfunction after AMI, especially for the long term.

CARDIOGENIC SHOCK In recent years, efforts to reduce infarct size and prompt treatment of ongoing ischemia and other complications of MI appear to have reduced the incidence of cardiogenic shock from 20% to about 7%. Only 10% of patients with this condition present with it on admission, while 90% develop it during hospitalization. Typically, patients who develop cardiogenic shock have severe multivessel coronary artery disease with evidence of "piecemeal" necrosis extending outward from the original infarct zone (Fig. 243-4).

Cardiogenic shock should be considered to be a form of severe LV failure. This syndrome is characterized by marked hypotension with systolic arterial pressure of <80 mmHg and a markedly reduced cardiac index [<1.8 L/(min/m^2)] in the face of an elevated LV filling (pulmonary capillary wedge) pressure (>18 mmHg). Hypotension alone is not a basis for the diagnosis of cardiogenic shock, because many patients who make an uneventful recovery have serious hypotension (systolic pressure of <80 mmHg) for several hours. Such patients often have low LV filling pressures, and their hypotension usually resolves with the administration of intravenous fluids. In contrast to hypovolemic hypotension, cardiogenic shock is generally associated

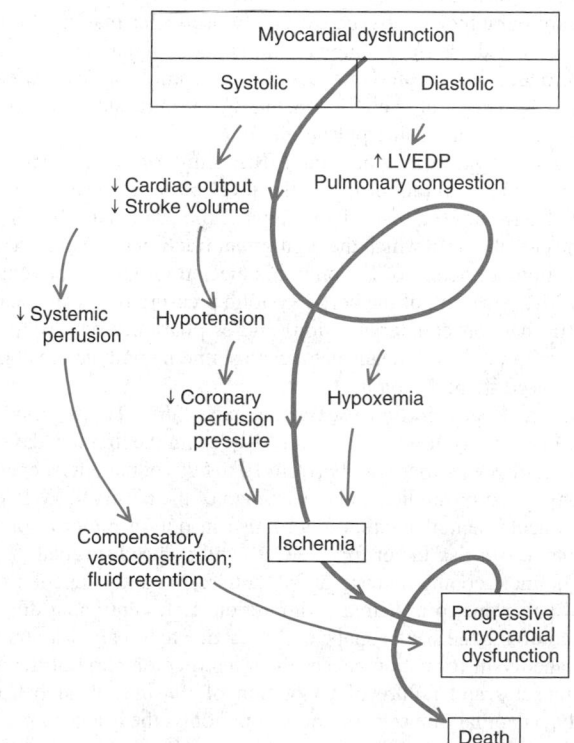

FIGURE 243-4 Pathophysiology of cardiogenic shock: Systolic and diastolic myocardial dysfunction occurs after MI, resulting in pulmonary congestion and a reduction in cardiac output. Systemic and coronary hypoperfusion occur, resulting in progressive ischemia. Although a number of compensatory mechanisms are activated in an attempt to support the circulation, these compensatory mechanisms may become maladaptive and produce a worsening of hemodynamics. A vicious circle of progressive myocardial dysfunction occurs that ultimately results in death if it is not interrupted. LVEDP, left ventricular end-diastolic pressure. *(From Hollenberg et al.)*

with a mortality rate of >70%; however, recent efforts to restore perfusion by coronary angioplasty or surgical revascularization suggest that this high mortality rate can be lowered by as much as one-half.

Risk factors for the in-hospital development of shock include advanced age, a depressed LV ejection fraction on admission, a large infarct, previous MI, and a history of diabetes mellitus. Patients with several of these risk factors should be considered for cardiac catheterization and mechanical reperfusion (by PCI or surgery) before the development of shock.

Pathophysiology of Severe Power Failure A marked reduction in the quantity of contracting myocardium is the cause of cardiogenic shock in AMI. The initial insult reduces arterial pressure, and the reduction in coronary perfusion pressure and myocardial blood flow initiates a vicious cycle that impairs myocardial function further and may increase the size of the infarct (Fig. 243-4). Arrhythmias and metabolic acidosis also contribute to this deterioration, because they are the result of inadequate perfusion. This positive feedback loop accounts for the high mortality rate associated with the shock syndrome.

TREATMENT The physiology and ominous prognosis of cardiogenic shock dictate that all patients with this condition should, if possible, have continuous monitoring of arterial pressure and of LV filling pressure (as reflected in the pulmonary capillary wedge pressure measured with a pulmonary artery balloon catheter) as well as frequent determinations of cardiac output. When pulmonary edema coexists, endotracheal intubation may be necessary to ensure oxygenation. The relief of pain is important, as some vasodepressor reflex activity may be a response to severe pain. However, narcotics should be used cautiously, in view of their propensity to lower arterial pressure. The primary objective of treatment is to maintain coronary perfusion by raising the arterial blood pressure with vasopressors (see below), intraaortic balloon counterpulsation, and manipulation of blood volume to a level that ensures an optimum LV filling pressure (~20 mmHg). The latter may require either infusion of crystalloid or diuresis.

Vasopressors Various intravenous drugs may be used to augment arterial pressure and cardiac output in patients with cardiogenic shock. All have important disadvantages or problems, and none has been shown to change the outcome in patients with established shock. *Isoproterenol* is a sympathomimetic amine that is now rarely used in the treatment of shock due to MI. Although this agent increases contractility, it also produces peripheral vasodilation and increases the heart rate. The resulting increase in myocardial oxygen consumption and reduction of coronary perfusion pressure may extend the area of ischemic injury. *Norepinephrine* (Chap. 72) is a potent α-adrenergic agonist with powerful vasoconstrictor properties that also possesses β-adrenergic activity and therefore enhances contractility. Because the increase in afterload and contractility associated with its use causes a marked increase in myocardial oxygen consumption, norepinephrine should be reserved for patients in desperate situations or for those with cardiogenic shock and reduced systemic vascular resistance. It should be started at a dosage of 2 to 4 μg/min. If pressure cannot be maintained with a dosage of 15 μg/min, it is unlikely that a further increase will be beneficial.

Dopamine (Chap. 72) is useful in many patients with severe power failure. At low doses (2 to 10 μg/kg per min), the drug has positive chronotropic and inotropic effects as a consequence of β receptor stimulation. At higher doses, a vasoconstrictor effect results from α receptor stimulation. At lower doses ($\leq$2 μg/kg per min), dopamine also has the unique effect of dilating the renal and splanchnic vascular beds, and it apparently has little effect on myocardial oxygen consumption. Intravenous dopamine is started at an infusion rate of 2 to 5 μg/kg per min, and the dosage is increased every 2 to 5 min up to a maximum of 20 to 50 μg/kg per min. Systolic arterial blood pressure should be maintained at ~90 mmHg. *Dobutamine* is a synthetic sympathomimetic amine with positive inotropic action and minimal positive chronotropic or peripheral vasoconstrictive activity in the usual dosage range of 2.5 to 10 μg/kg per min. It should not be used when a vaso-constrictor effect is required. However, in patients with less profound degrees of hypotension, dobutamine may be an extremely useful agent, particularly if positive chronotropy is to be avoided.

Amrinone and *milrinone* are positive inotropic agents without cat-echolamine structure or activity that inhibit phosphodiesterase. These drugs resemble dobutamine in pharmacologic activity, although they have a more potent vasodilating action. For amrinone, an initial load-ing dose of 0.75 mg/kg is given over 2 to 3 min. If effective, it is followed by an infusion of 5 to 10 μg/kg per min. If necessary, the dose may then be increased up to 15 μg/kg per min for short periods. Milrinone is given as a loading dose of 50 μg/kg over 10 min followed by a maintenance infusion of 0.375 to 0.75 μg/kg per min.

Aortic Counterpulsation In cardiogenic shock, mechanical as-sistance with an intraaortic balloon pumping (IABP) system capable of augmenting both diastolic pressure and cardiac output may be help-ful. A sausage-shaped balloon at the end of a catheter is introduced percutaneously into the aorta via the femoral artery, and the balloon is automatically inflated during early diastole, thereby augmenting cor-onary blood flow. The balloon collapses in early systole, thereby re-ducing the afterload against which LV ejection takes place. Improve-ment in hemodynamic status has been achieved with balloon pumping in a large number of patients. In the absence of early revascularization, however, long-term survival after this mode of therapy in patients with cardiogenic shock is still disappointing. Intraaortic balloon pumping may best be reserved for patients whose condition merits mechanical (surgical or angioplastic) intervention (e.g., patients with continuing ischemia, ventricular septal rupture, or mitral regurgitation) and in whom a successful result is likely to reverse the cardiogenic shock. This technique is contraindicated if aortic regurgitation is present or aortic dissection is suspected.

Therapy for the shock syndrome secondary to MI, while improving gradually as a result of meticulous attention to the details outlined above, continues to be disappointing overall because a large fraction of patients with the syndrome have large areas of infarcted myocar-dium with severe, diffuse coronary atherosclerosis. The SHOCK trial was a randomized study comparing emergency revascularization (PCI or coronary artery bypass grafting) with initial medical stabilization and delayed revascularization as clinically indicated for patients with cardiogenic shock. Although the 30-day mortality rates in the two groups did not differ significantly, the 6-month and 1-year mortality rates in the emergency revascularization group were significantly lower than the corresponding rates in the stabilization and delayed revascularization group. Patients younger than 75 years showed par-ticular benefit from emergency revascularization. However, few pa-tients developing cardiogenic shock have prompt access to these ex-pensive techniques. It is hoped that the widespread and early application of thrombolytic therapy will reduce the amount of myo-cardium that becomes necrotic and thereby reduce the incidence of this syndrome.

RIGHT VENTRICULAR INFARCTION Approximately one-third of patients with inferoposterior infarction demonstrate at least a minor degree of RV necrosis. An occasional patient with inferopos-terior LV infarction also has extensive RV infarction, and rare patients present with infarction limited primarily to the RV. Clinically signif-icant RV infarction causes signs of severe RV failure [jugular venous distention, Kussmaul's sign (Chap. 225), hepatomegaly] with or with-out hypotension. ST-segment elevations of right-sided precordial ECG leads, particularly lead V_4R, are frequently present in the first 24 h in patients with RV infarction. Two-dimensional echocardiography is helpful in determining the degree of RV dysfunction. Catheterization of the right side of the heart often reveals a distinctive hemodynamic pattern resembling cardiac tamponade or constrictive pericarditis (steep right atrial "y" descent and an early diastolic dip and plateau in

right ventricular waveforms) (Chap. 239). Therapy consists of volume expansion to maintain adequate RV preload and efforts to improve LV performance with attendant reduction in pulmonary capillary wedge and pulmonary arterial pressures.

MECHANICAL CAUSES OF HEART FAILURE Free Wall Rupture Myocardial rupture is a dramatic complication of AMI that is most likely to occur during the first week after the onset of symptoms; its frequency increases with the age of the patient. First infarction, a history of hypertension, no history of angina pectoris, and a relatively large Q-wave infarct are associated with a higher incidence of cardiac rupture. The clinical presentation typically is a sudden loss of pulse, blood pressure and consciousness while the ECG continues to show sinus rhythm (apparent electromechanical dissociation or pulseless electrical activity). The myocardium continues to contract, but forward flow is not maintained as blood escapes into the pericar-dium. Cardiac tamponade (Chap. 239) ensues, and closed-chest mas-sage is ineffective. This condition is almost universally fatal, although dramatic cases of urgent pericardiotensis followed by successful sur-gical repair have been reported.

Ventricular Septal Defect The pathogenesis of perforation of the ventricular septum is similar to that of free wall rupture, but the chance of successful therapy is greater. Patients with ventricular septal rupture present with sudden, severe LV failure in association with the appearance of a pansystolic murmur, often accompanied by a para-sternal thrill. It is often impossible to differentiate this condition from rupture of a papillary muscle with resulting mitral regurgitation (MR), and the presence in both conditions of a tall "v" wave in the pulmonary capillary wedge pressure further complicates the differentiation. The diagnosis of ventricular septal defect can be established by the dem-onstration of a left-to-right shunt (i.e., an oxygen step-up at the level of the RV) by means of limited cardiac catheterization performed at the bedside with a flow-directed balloon catheter. Color flow Doppler echocardiography can also be extremely useful for making this diag-nosis at the bedside. A prolonged period of hemodynamic compromise may produce end-organ damage and other complications that can be avoided by early intervention, including nitroprusside infusion and intraaortic balloon counterpulsation.

The pathophysiology of acute MR is similar to that of acute ven-tricular septal perforation in that the level of aortic systolic pressure partly determines the regurgitant volume, the principal difference be-ing the chamber into which the regurgitant fraction is ejected. In septal perforation, a fraction of LV output is ejected into the right ventricle. As in MR, lowering of the aortic systolic pressure by mechanical (in-traaortic balloon counterpulsation) and/or pharmacologic (nitroglyc-erin or nitroprusside) means can decrease the hemodynamic compro-mise caused by perforation.

Mitral Regurgitation (See also Chap. 236)   The reported inci-dence of apical systolic murmurs of MR during the first few days after the onset of AMI varies widely (from 10 to 50% of patients) depending on the population studied and the acumen of the observers. While MR causes acute hemodynamic compromise in only a minority of these patients, it is a risk factor for late CHF and reduced survival.

The most common cause of MR after AMI is dysfunction of the mitral valve due to ischemia or infarction. Left ventricular dilatation or alteration in the size or shape of the LV due to impaired contractility or to aneurysm formation causes disordered contraction of the papil-lary muscles and failure of coaptation of the mitral valve leaflets. Rarely, a papillary muscle, or, more commonly, the head of a papillary muscle, may rupture. Then, LV function deteriorates dramatically, with superimposition of severe MR. The major element in the differ-ential diagnosis is perforation of the ventricular septum as discussed above. Surgical repair or replacement of the mitral valve may lead to dramatic improvement in patients in whom acute heart failure re-sults primarily from severe MR due to papillary muscle rupture or dysfunction and in whom global ventricular function is relatively good.

If aortic systolic pressure is lowered in patients with MR, a greater fraction of the LV output will be ejected antegrade, thus lessening the regurgitant fraction. To this end, both intraaortic balloon counterpulsation (IABC), which lowers the aortic systolic pressure mechanically, and the infusion of nitroglycerin or sodium nitroprusside, which reduce systemic vascular resistance, have been used with success in the interim management of patients with severe MR in the presence of AMI. Ideally, definitive operative treatment should be postponed until pulmonary congestion has cleared and the infarct has had time to heal. However, if the patient's hemodynamic and/or clinical condition does not improve or stabilize, surgical treatment should be undertaken, even in the acute stage.

ARRHYTHMIAS (See also Chaps. 229 and 230) The incidence of arrhythmias after AMI is higher in patients seen early after the onset of symptoms. The mechanisms responsible for infarction-related arrhythmias include autonomic nervous system imbalance, electrolyte disturbances, ischemia, and slowed conduction in zones of ischemic myocardium. An arrhythmia can usually be managed successfully if trained personnel and appropriate equipment are available when it develops. Since most deaths from arrhythmia occur during the first few hours after infarction, the effectiveness of treatment relates directly to the speed with which patients come under medical observation. The prompt management of arrhythmias constitutes a significant advance in the treatment of myocardial infarction.

Ventricular Premature Beats Infrequent, sporadic ventricular premature depolarizations occur in almost all patients with AMI and do not require therapy. Whereas in the past, frequent, multifocal, or early diastolic ventricular extrasystoles (so-called warning arrhythmias) were routinely treated with antiarrhythmic drugs to reduce the risk of development of ventricular tachycardia and ventricular fibrillation, pharmacologic therapy is now reserved for patients with sustained ventricular arrhythmias. Prophylactic antiarrhythmic therapy (either intravenous lidocaine early or oral agents later) is contraindicated for ventricular premature beats in the absence of clinically important ventricular tachyarrhythmias, as such therapy may actually increase the mortality rate. β-Adrenoceptor blocking agents are effective in abolishing ventricular ectopic activity in patients with AMI and in the prevention of ventricular fibrillation. As described above (see "β-Adrenoceptor Blockers"), they should be used routinely in patients without contraindications. In addition, hypokalemia and hypomagnesemia are risk factors for ventricular fibrillation in patients with AMI; the serum potassium concentration should be adjusted to approximately 4.5 mmol/L and magnesium to about 2.0 mmol/L.

Ventricular Tachycardia and Fibrillation Within the first 24 h of AMI, ventricular tachycardia and fibrillation can occur without prior warning arrhythmias. The occurrence of ventricular fibrillation can be reduced by prophylactic administration of intravenous lidocaine. However, prophylactic use of lidocaine has not been shown to reduce overall mortality from AMI. In fact, in addition to causing possible noncardiac complications, lidocaine may predispose to an excess risk of bradycardia and asystole. For these reasons, and with earlier treatment of active ischemia, more frequent use of beta-blocking agents, and the nearly universal success of electrical cardioversion or defibrillation, routine prophylactic antiarrhythmic drug therapy is no longer recommended. It should be reserved for patients who cannot reach a hospital or for those treated in hospitals that lack the constant presence in the coronary care unit of a physician or nurse trained in the recognition and treatment of ventricular fibrillation.

Sustained ventricular tachycardia that is well tolerated hemodynamically should be treated with an intravenous regimen of lidocaine (bolus of 1.0 to 1.5 mg/kg; infusion of 20 to 50 μg/kg per min), procainamide (bolus of 15 mg/kg over 20 to 30 min; infusion of 1 to 4 mg/min), or amiodarone (bolus of 75 to 150 mg over 10 to 15 min followed by infusion of 1.0 mg/min for 6 h and then 0.5 mg/min); if it does not stop promptly, electroversion should be used (Chap. 230). An unsynchronized discharge of 200 to 300 J (defibrillation) is used immediately in patients with ventricular fibrillation or when ventricular tachycardia causes hemodynamic deterioration. Ventricular tachycardia or fibrillation that is refractory to electroshock may be more responsive after the patient is treated with epinephrine (1 mg intra-venously or 10 mL of a 1:10,000 solution via the intracardiac route), bretylium (a 5 mg/kg bolus), or amiodarone (a 75 to 150 mg bolus).

Ventricular arrhythmias, including the unusual form of ventricular tachycardia known as *torsade de pointes* (Chap. 230), may occur in patients with AMI as a consequence of other concurrent problems (such as hypoxia, hypokalemia, or other electrolyte disturbances) or of the toxic effects of an agent being administered to the patient (such as digoxin or quinidine). A search for such secondary causes should always be undertaken.

Although the in-hospital mortality rate is increased, the long-term survival is good in patients who survive to hospital discharge after *primary* ventricular fibrillation, i.e., ventricular fibrillation that is a primary response to acute ischemia and is not associated with predisposing factors such as CHF, shock, bundle branch block, or ventricular aneurysm. This result is in sharp contrast to the poor prognosis for patients who develop ventricular fibrillation *secondary* to severe pump failure. For patients who develop ventricular tachycardia or ventricular fibrillation late in their hospital course (i.e., after the first 48 h), the mortality rate is increased both in-hospital and during long-term follow-up. Such patients should be considered for electrophysiologic study (Chap. 230).

Accelerated Idioventricular Rhythm Accelerated idioventricular rhythm (AIVR, "slow ventricular tachycardia"), a ventricular rhythm with a rate of 60 to 100 beats per minute, occurs in 25% of patients with AMI. It often occurs transiently during thrombolytic therapy at the time of reperfusion. The rate of AIVR is usually similar to that of the sinus rhythm that precedes and follows it, and this similarity of rate plus the relatively minor hemodynamic effects make this rhythm more difficult to detect except by electrocardiographic monitoring. For the most part, AIVR is benign and does not presage the development of classic ventricular tachycardia. Most episodes of AIVR do not require treatment if the patient is monitored carefully, as degeneration into a more serious arrhythmia is rare, and, if it occurs, AIVR can generally be readily treated with a drug that increases the sinus rate (atropine).

Supraventricular Arrhythmias Sinus tachycardia is the most common supraventricular arrhythmia. If it occurs secondary to another cause (such as anemia, fever, heart failure, or a metabolic derangement), the primary problem should be treated first. However, if it appears to be due to sympathetic overstimulation, for example, as part of a hyperdynamic state, then treatment with a beta blocker is indicated. Other common arrhythmias in this group are atrial flutter and atrial fibrillation, which are often secondary to LV failure. Digoxin is usually the treatment of choice for supraventricular arrhythmias if heart failure is present. If heart failure is absent, beta blockers, verapamil, or diltiazem are suitable alternatives for controlling the ventricular rate, as they may also help to control ischemia. If the abnormal rhythm persists for >2 h with a ventricular rate in excess of 120 beats per minute, or if tachycardia induces heart failure, shock, or ischemia (as manifested by recurrent pain or ECG changes), a synchronized electroshock (100 to 200 J) should be used.

Accelerated junctional rhythms have diverse causes but may occur in patients with inferoposterior infarction. Digitalis excess must be ruled out. In some patients with severely compromised LV function, the loss of appropriately timed atrial systole results in a marked decrease in cardiac output. Right atrial or coronary sinus pacing is indicated in such instances.

Sinus Bradycardia Treatment of sinus bradycardia is indicated if hemodynamic compromise results from the slow heart rate. Atropine is the most useful drug for increasing heart rate and should be given intravenously in doses of 0.5 mg initially. If the rate remains below 50 to 60 bpm, additional doses of 0.2 mg, up to a total of 2.0 mg, may be given. Persistent bradycardia (<40 bpm) despite atropine may be treated with electrical pacing. Isoproterenol should be avoided.

Atrioventricular and Intraventricular Conduction Disturbances (See also Chap. 229) Both the in-hospital mortality rate and the post-discharge mortality rate of patients who have complete atrioventricular (AV) block in association with anterior infarction are markedly higher than those of patients who develop AV block with inferior infarction. This difference is related to the fact that heart block in inferior infarction is commonly a result of increased vagal tone and/or the release of adenosine and therefore is transient. In anterior wall infarction, heart block is usually related to ischemic malfunction of the conduction system, which commonly is associated with extensive myocardial necrosis.

Temporary electrical pacing provides an effective means of increasing the heart rate of patients with bradycardia due to AV block. However, acceleration of the heart rate may have only a limited impact on prognosis in patients with anterior wall infarction and complete heart block in whom the large size of the infarct is the major factor determining outcome. It should be carried out if it improves hemodynamics, however. Pacing does appear to be beneficial in patients with inferoposterior infarction who have complete heart block associated with heart failure, hypotension, marked bradycardia, or significant ventricular ectopic activity. A subgroup of these patients, those with RV infarction, often respond poorly to ventricular pacing because of the loss of the atrial contribution to ventricular filling. In such patients, dual-chamber AV sequential pacing may be required.

External noninvasive pacing electrodes should be positioned in a "demand" mode for patients with sinus bradycardia (rate <50 bpm) that is unresponsive to drug therapy, Mobitz II second-degree AV block, third-degree heart block, or bilateral bundle branch block (e.g., right bundle branch block plus left anterior fascicular block). Retrospective studies suggest that permanent pacing may reduce the long-term risk of sudden death due to bradyarrhythmias in the rare patient who develops combined persistent bifascicular and transient third-degree heart block during the acute phase of MI.

OTHER COMPLICATIONS   Recurrent Chest Discomfort Recurrent angina develops in ~25% of patients hospitalized for AMI. This percentage is even higher in patients who undergo successful thrombolysis. Since recurrent or persistent ischemia often heralds extension of the original infarct or reinfarction in a new myocardial zone and is associated with a doubling of risk after AMI, patients with these symptoms should be considered for repeat thrombolysis or referred for prompt coronary arteriography and mechanical revascularization. Repeat administration of a thrombolytic agent is an alternative to early mechanical revascularization.

Pericarditis (See also Chap. 239)   Pericardial friction rubs and/or pericardial pain are frequently encountered in patients with transmural AMI. This complication can usually be managed with aspirin (650 mg qid). It is important to diagnose the chest pain of pericarditis accurately, since failure to recognize it may lead to the erroneous diagnosis of recurrent ischemic pain and/or infarct extension, with resulting inappropriate use of anticoagulants, nitrates, beta blockers, or coronary arteriography. When it occurs, complaints of pain radiating to either trapezius muscle is helpful since such a pattern of discomfort is typical of pericarditis but rarely occurs with ischemic discomfort. Anticoagulants potentially could cause tamponade in the presence of acute pericarditis (as manifested by either pain or persistent rub) and therefore should not be used unless there is a compelling indication.

Thromboembolism Clinically apparent thromboembolism complicates AMI in ~10% of cases, but embolic lesions are found in 20% of patients in necropsy series, suggesting that thromboembolism is often clinically silent. Thromboembolism is considered to be at least an important contributing cause of death in 25% of patients with AMI who die after admission to the hospital. Arterial emboli originate from LV mural thrombi, while most pulmonary emboli arise in the leg veins.

Thromboembolism typically occurs in association with large infarcts (especially anterior), CHF, and a LV thrombus detected by echocardiography. The incidence of arterial embolism from a clot originating in the ventricle at the site of an infarction is small but real. Two-dimensional echocardiography reveals LV thrombi in about one-third of patients with anterior wall infarction but in few patients with inferior or posterior infarction. Arterial embolism often presents as a major complication, such as hemiparesis when the cerebral circulation is involved or hypertension if the renal circulation is compromised. When a thrombus has been clearly demonstrated by echocardiographic or other techniques or when a large area of regional wall motion abnormality is seen even in the absence of a detectable mural thrombus, systemic anticoagulation should be undertaken (in the absence of contraindications), as the incidence of embolic complications appears to be markedly lowered by such therapy. The appropriate duration of therapy is unknown, but 3 to 6 months is probably prudent.

Left Ventricular Aneurysm The term *ventricular aneurysm* is usually used to describe *dyskinesis* or local expansile paradoxical wall motion. Normally functioning myocardial fibers must shorten more if stroke volume and cardiac output are to be maintained in patients with ventricular aneurysm; if they cannot, overall ventricular function is impaired. True aneurysms are composed of scar tissue and neither predispose to nor are associated with cardiac rupture.

The complications of LV aneurysm do not usually occur for weeks to months after AMI; they include CHF, arterial embolism, and ventricular arrhythmias. Apical aneurysms are the most common and the most easily detected by clinical examination. The physical finding of greatest value is a double, diffuse, or displaced apical impulse. Ventricular aneurysms are readily detected by two-dimensional echocardiography, which may also reveal a mural thrombus in an aneurysm.

Rarely, myocardial rupture may be contained by a local area of pericardium, along with organizing thrombus and hematoma. Over time, this *pseudoaneurysm* enlarges, maintaining communication with the LV cavity through a narrow neck. Because a pseudoaneurysm often ruptures spontaneously, it should be surgically repaired if recognized.

POSTINFARCTION RISK STRATIFICATION AND MANAGEMENT

Many clinical factors have been identified that are associated with an increase in cardiovascular risk after initial recovery from AMI. Some of the most important factors include persistent ischemia (spontaneous or provoked), depressed LV ejection fraction (<40%), rales above the lung bases on physical examination or congestion on chest radiograph, and symptomatic ventricular arrhythmias. Other features associated with increased risk include a history of previous myocardial infarction, age over 70 years, diabetes, prolonged sinus tachycardia, hypotension, ST-segment changes at rest without angina ("silent ischemia"), an abnormal signal-averaged ECG, nonpatency of the infarct-related coronary artery (if angiography is undertaken), and persistent advanced heart block or a new intraventricular conduction abnormality on the ECG. Therapy must be individualized on the basis of the relative importance of the risk(s) present.

The goal of preventing reinfarction and death after recovery from AMI has led to strategies to evaluate risk after infarction. Early after AMI, this evaluation generally involves the use of noninvasive testing. In stable patients, submaximal exercise stress testing may be carried out before hospital discharge to detect residual ischemia and ventricular ectopy and to provide the patient with a guideline for exercise in the early recovery period. Alternatively, or in addition, a maximal (symptom-limited) exercise stress test may be carried out 4 to 6 weeks after infarction. Evaluation of LV function at rest and during exercise is usually warranted as well. Recognition of a depressed LV ejection fraction by echocardiography or radionuclide ventriculography identifies patients who should receive ACE inhibitors (see "Angiotensin-Converting Enzyme Inhibitors," above). Patients in whom angina is induced at relatively low workloads, those who have a large reversible defect on perfusion imaging or a depressed ejection fraction, those with demonstrable ischemia, and those in whom exercise provokes symptomatic ventricular arrhythmias should be considered at high risk for recurrent MI or death from arrhythmia; and cardiac catheterization with coronary angiography and/or invasive electrophysiologic evaluation is advised.

Exercise tests also aid in formulating an individualized exercise prescription, which can be much more vigorous in patients who tolerate exercise without any of the above-mentioned adverse signs. Additionally, predischarge stress testing may provide an important psychological benefit, building the patient's confidence by demonstrating a reasonable exercise tolerance. Furthermore, particularly when no arrhythmias or signs of ischemia are identified, the patient benefits by the physician's reassurance that objective evidence suggests no immediate jeopardy.

In many hospitals a cardiac rehabilitation program with progressive exercise is initiated in the hospital and continued after discharge. Ideally, such programs should include an educational component that informs patients about their disease and its risk factors.

The usual duration of hospitalization for an uncomplicated AMI is about 5 days. The remainder of the convalescent phase may be accomplished at home. During the first 2 weeks, the patient should be encouraged to increase activity by walking about the house and outdoors in good weather. Normal sexual activity may be resumed during this period. After 2 weeks, the physician must regulate the patient's activity on the basis of exercise tolerance. Most patients will be able to return to work within 2 to 4 weeks.

SECONDARY PREVENTION OF INFARCTION

Various secondary preventive measures are at least partly responsible for the improvement in the long-term mortality and morbidity rates after AMI. Long-term treatment with an antiplatelet agent (usually aspirin) after AMI is associated with a 25% reduction in the risk of recurrent infarction, stroke, or cardiovascular mortality (36 fewer events for every 1000 patients treated). In addition, in patients taking aspirin chronically, AMIs tend to be smaller and are more likely to be non-Q-wave in nature. An alternative antiplatelet agent that may be used for secondary prevention in patients intolerant of aspirin is the ADP receptor antagonist clopidogrel (75 mg orally daily). ACE inhibitors should be used indefinitely by patients with clinically evident heart failure, a moderate decrease in global ejection fraction, or a large regional wall motion abnormality to prevent late ventricular remodeling and recurrent ischemic events.

The chronic routine use of oral β-adrenoceptor blockers for at least 2 years after AMI is supported by well-conducted, placebo-controlled trials that have convincingly demonstrated reductions in the rates of total mortality, sudden death, and, in some instances, reinfarction. In contrast, calcium antagonists are not recommended for routine secondary prevention.

Evidence suggests that warfarin lowers the risk of late mortality and the incidence of reinfarction after AMI. Since studies comparing aspirin and warfarin therapy separately or in combination have not yet been completed, most physicians prescribe aspirin routinely for all patients without contraindications and add warfarin for patients at increased risk of embolism (see "Thromboembolism," above).

Finally, risk factors for *atherosclerosis* (Chap. 241) should be discussed with the patient, and, when possible, favorably modified. In particular, efforts should be made to ensure the cessation of smoking and the control of hypertension and hyperlipidemia (the target low-density lipoprotein level is <100 mg/dL). In addition, regular physical exercise and reduction of emotional stress should be encouraged. The benefits of hormone replacement therapy in postmenopausal women recovering from MI remain controversial. The initiation of a combination of estrogen plus progestin is associated with an increased risk of cardiovascular events within the first year but may reduce events in later years (HERS Trial). Thus, hormone replacement therapy prevention of coronary events should not be given *de novo* to postmenopausal women after AMI. Postmenopausal women already taking estrogen plus progestin at the time of AMI may continue that therapy.

BIBLIOGRAPHY

AMERICAN HEART ASSOCIATION: *Heart and Stroke Facts: 2000 Statistical Supplement.* Dallas, American Heart Association, 2000

ANTMAN EM, BRAUNWALD E: Acute myocardial infarction, in *Heart Disease*, 6th ed, E Braunwald, Zipes DP, Libby P (eds). Philadelphia, Saunders, 2001

——— et al: Abciximab facilitates the rate and extent of thrombolysis: Results of the Thrombolysis in Myocardial Infarction (TIMI) 14 trial. Circulation 99:2720, 1999

——— et al: Assessment of the treatment effect of enoxaparin for unstable angina/non-Q-wave myocardial infarction: TIMI 11B-ESSENCE meta-analysis. Circulation 100: 1602, 1999

BARRON HV et al: Use of reperfusion therapy for acute myocardial infarction in the United States: Data from the National Registry of Myocardial Infarction 2. Circulation 97: 1150, 1998

CAIRNS JA et al: Antithrombotic agents in coronary artery disease. Chest 114:611S, 1998

FALK E et al: Coronary plaque disruption. Circulation 92:657, 1995

FIBRINOLYTIC THERAPY TRIALISTS (FTT) COLLABORATIVE GROUP: Indications for fibrinolytic therapy in suspected acute myocardial infarction: Collaborative overview of early mortality and major morbidity results from all randomised trials of more than 1000 patients. Lancet 343:311, 1994

FUTTERMAN LG, LEMBERG L: Update on management of acute myocardial infarction: Facilitated percutaneous coronary intervention. Am J Crit Care 9:70, 2000

GOLDMAN LE, EISENBERG MJ: Identification and management of patients with failed thrombolysis after acute myocardial infarction. Ann Intern Med 132:556, 2000

GOTTLIEB SS et al: Effect of beta-blockade on mortality among high-risk and low-risk patients after myocardial infarction. N Engl J Med 339:489, 1998

HOCHMAN JS et al: Early revascularization in acute myocardial infarction complicated by cardiogenic shock. N Engl J Med 341:625, 1999

HOLLENBERG SM et al: Cardiogenic shock. Ann Intern Med 131:47, 1999

KINCH JW, RYAN TJ: Right ventricular infarction. N Engl J Med 330:1211, 1994

MICHAELS AD, GOLDSCHLAGER N: Risk stratification after acute myocardial infarction in the reperfusion era. Prog Cardiovasc Dis 42:273, 2000

NATIONAL HEART ATTACK ALERT PROGRAM COORDINATING COMMITTEE—60 MINUTES TO TREATMENT WORKING GROUP: Emergency department: Rapid identification and treatment of patients with acute myocardial infarction. Ann Emerg Med 23:311, 1994

PFEFFER JM et al: Angiotensin-converting enzyme inhibition and ventricular remodeling after myocardial infarction. Annu Rev Physiol 57:805, 1995

RYAN TJ et al: 1999 Update: ACC/AHA guidelines for the management of patients with acute myocardial infarction. A report of the American College of Cardiology/American Heart Association Task Force on Practice Guidelines (Committee on Management of Acute Myocardial Infarction). J Am Coll Cardiol 34:890, 1999

SCARBOROUGH RM et al: Platelet glycoprotein IIb/IIIa antagonists: What are the relevant issues concerning their pharmacology and clinical use? Circulation 100:437, 1999

THE GUSTO INVESTIGATORS: An international randomized trial comparing four thrombolytic strategies for acute myocardial infarction. N Engl J Med 329:673, 1993

TIEFEBRUNN AJ et al: Clinical experience with primary percutaneous transluminal coronary angioplasty compared with alteplase (recombinant tissue-type plasminogen activator) in patients with acute myocardial infarction: A report from the Second National Registry of Myocardial Infarction (NRMI-2). J Am Coll Cardiol 31:1240, 1998

TOPOL EJ: Acute myocardial infarction: Thrombolysis. Heart 83:122, 2000

YUSUF S et al: Beta blockade during and after myocardial infarction: An overview of the randomized trials. Prog Cardiovasc Dis 27:335, 1985

ZIMMERMAN J et al: Diagnostic marker cooperative study for the diagnosis of myocardial infarction. Circulation 99:1671, 1999

244

Andrew P. Selwyn, Eugene Braunwald

ISCHEMIC HEART DISEASE

ETIOLOGY AND PATHOPHYSIOLOGY

Ischemia refers to a lack of oxygen due to inadequate perfusion, which results from an imbalance between oxygen supply and demand. The most common cause of myocardial ischemia is atherosclerotic disease of epicardial coronary arteries. Ischemic heart disease (IHD) is the most common, serious, chronic, life-threatening illness in the United States, where more than 11 million persons have IHD. This condition causes more deaths and disability and incurs greater economic costs than any other illness in the developed world.

By reducing the lumen of the coronary arteries, atherosclerosis reduces myocardial perfusion in the basal state or limits appropriate increases in perfusion when the demand for flow is augmented, as occurs during exertion or excitement. Coronary blood flow can also be limited by spasm, arterial thrombi, and, rarely, coronary emboli as well as by ostial narrowing due to luetic aortitis. Congenital abnormalities, such as anomalous origin of the left anterior descending coronary artery from the pulmonary artery, may cause myocardial ischemia and infarction in infancy, but this cause is very rare in adults. Myocardial ischemia can also occur if myocardial oxygen demands are markedly increased, as in severe ventricular hypertrophy due to aortic stenosis. The latter can present with angina that is indistinguishable from that caused by coronary atherosclerosis. A reduction in the oxygen-carrying capacity of the blood, as in extremely severe anemia or in the presence of carboxyhemoglobin, is a rare cause of myocardial ischemia. Not infrequently, two or more causes of ischemia will coexist, such as an increase in oxygen demand due to left ventricular hypertrophy and a reduction in oxygen supply secondary to coronary atherosclerosis and anemia. Often such a combination leads to clinical manifestations of ischemia.

Although the large epicardial coronary arteries are capable of constriction and relaxation, in healthy persons they serve largely as conduits and are referred to as *conductance vessels*, while the intramyocardial arterioles normally exhibit striking changes in tone and are therefore referred to as *resistance vessels*. Abnormal constriction or failure of normal dilation of the coronary resistance vessels can also cause ischemia. When it causes angina this condition is referred to as *microvascular angina*.

The normal coronary circulation is dominated and controlled by the heart's requirements for oxygen. This need is met by the ability of the coronary vascular bed to vary its resistance (and therefore blood flow) considerably while the myocardium extracts a high and relatively fixed percentage of oxygen. Normally, intramyocardial resistance vessels demonstrate an immense capacity for dilation. For example, the changing oxygen needs with exercise and emotional stress affect coronary vascular resistance and in this manner regulate the supply of oxygen and substrate to the myocardium (*metabolic regulation*). The coronary resistance vessels also adapt to physiologic alterations in blood pressure in order to maintain coronary blood flow at levels appropriate to myocardial needs (*autoregulation*).

CORONARY ATHEROSCLEROSIS (See also Chap. 241) Epicardial coronary arteries are a major site of atherosclerotic disease. The major risk factors for atherosclerosis [high plasma low-density lipoprotein (LDL), low plasma high-density lipoprotein (HDL), cigarette smoking, hypertension, and diabetes mellitus] are thought to disturb the normal functions of the vascular endothelium. These functions include local control of vascular tone, maintenance of an anticoagulant surface, and defense against inflammatory cells. The loss of these defenses leads to inappropriate constriction, luminal clot formation, and abnormal interactions with blood monocytes and platelets. The latter leads to subintimal collections of fat, cells, and debris (i.e., atherosclerotic plaques), which develop at irregular rates in different segments of the epicardial coronary tree and lead eventually to segmental reductions in cross-sectional area (stenosis). The relationship between pulsatile flow and luminal stenosis is complex, but experiments have shown that when a stenosis reduces the cross-sectional area by approximately 75%, a full range of increases in flow to meet increased myocardial demand is not possible. When the luminal area is reduced by more than approximately 80%, blood flow at rest may be reduced, and further minor decreases in the stenotic orifice can reduce coronary flow dramatically and cause myocardial ischemia.

Segmental atherosclerotic narrowing of epicardial coronary arteries is caused most commonly by the formation of a plaque, which is subject to fissuring, hemorrhage, and thrombosis. Any of these events can temporarily worsen the obstruction, reduce coronary blood flow, and cause clinical manifestations of myocardial ischemia, as described below. The location of the obstruction will influence the quantity of myocardium rendered ischemic and thus determine the severity of the clinical manifestations. Severe coronary narrowing and myocardial ischemia are frequently accompanied by the development of collateral vessels, especially when the narrowing develops gradually. When well developed, such vessels can, by themselves, provide sufficient blood flow to sustain the viability of the myocardium at rest but not during conditions of increased demand.

Once stenosis of a proximal epicardial artery has reduced the cross-sectional area by more than approximately 70%, the distal resistance vessels (when they function normally) dilate to reduce vascular resistance and maintain coronary blood flow. A pressure gradient develops across the proximal stenosis, and poststenotic pressure falls. When the resistance vessels are maximally dilated, myocardial blood flow becomes dependent on the pressure in the coronary artery distal to the obstruction. In these circumstances ischemia in the region perfused by the stenotic artery can be precipitated by increases in myocardial oxygen demands caused by physical activity, emotional stress, and/or tachycardia. Changes in the caliber of the stenosed coronary artery due to physiologic vasomotion, loss of endothelial control of dilation, pathologic spasm, or small platelet plugs can all upset the critical balance between oxygen supply and demand and thus precipitate myocardial ischemia.

EFFECTS OF ISCHEMIA The inadequate perfusion induced by coronary atherosclerosis may cause transient disturbances of the mechanical, biochemical, and electrical functions of the myocardium. The abrupt development of severe ischemia, as occurs with total or subtotal occlusion, is associated with almost instantaneous failure of normal muscle contraction and relaxation. The relatively poor perfusion of the subendocardium causes more intense ischemia of this portion of the wall. Ischemia of large portions of the ventricle will cause transient left ventricular failure, and if the papillary muscles are involved, mitral regurgitation can complicate this event. When ischemia is transient, it may be associated with angina pectoris; when it is prolonged, it can lead to myocardial necrosis and scarring with or without the clinical picture of acute myocardial infarction (Chap. 243). Coronary atherosclerosis is a focal process that usually causes nonuniform ischemia. Regional disturbances of ventricular contractility cause segmental akinesis or, in severe cases, bulging (dyskinesia), which can greatly reduce myocardial pump function.

Underlying these mechanical disturbances are a wide range of abnormalities in cell metabolism, function, and structure. When oxygenated, the normal myocardium metabolizes fatty acids and glucose to carbon dioxide and water. With severe oxygen deprivation, fatty acids cannot be oxidized, and glucose is broken down to lactate; intracellular pH is reduced, as are the myocardial stores of high-energy phosphates, ATP, and creatine phosphate. Impaired cell membrane function leads to potassium leakage and the uptake of sodium by myocytes. The severity and duration of the imbalance between myocardial oxygen supply and demand will determine whether the damage is reversible (0 to 20 min for total occlusion) or whether it is permanent, with subsequent myocardial necrosis (>20 min).

Ischemia also causes characteristic changes in the electrocardiogram (ECG) such as repolarization abnormalities, as evidenced by inversion of the T wave and, when more severe, by displacement of the ST segment (Chap. 226). Transient ST-segment depression often reflects subendocardial ischemia, while transient ST-segment elevation is thought to be caused by more severe transmural ischemia. Another important consequence of myocardial ischemia is electrical instability, which may lead to ventricular tachycardia or ventricular fibrillation (Chap. 230). Most patients who die suddenly from IHD do so as a result of ischemia-induced malignant ventricular tachyarrhythmias (Chap. 39).

ASYMPTOMATIC VERSUS SYMPTOMATIC ISCHEMIC HEART DISEASE (IHD) Postmortem studies on accident victims and military casualties in western countries have shown that coronary atherosclerosis often begins to develop prior to age 20 and is widespread even among adults who were asymptomatic during life.

When all age groups are considered, IHD is the most common cause of death not only in men but also in women (Chap. 6). Exercise stress tests in asymptomatic persons may show evidence of silent myocardial ischemia, i.e., exercise-induced ECG changes not accompanied by angina; coronary angiographic studies of such persons may reveal obstructive [coronary artery disease (CAD) (Chap. 228)]. Postmortem examination of patients with obstructive CAD without a history of any clinical manifestations of myocardial ischemia often shows macroscopic scars secondary to myocardial infarction in regions supplied by diseased coronary arteries. According to population studies, approximately 25% of patients who survive acute myocardial infarction may not reach medical attention, and these patients carry the same adverse prognosis as those who present with the classic clinical syndrome (Chap. 243). Sudden death may be unheralded and is a common presenting manifestation of IHD (Chap. 39). Patients can also present with cardiomegaly and heart failure secondary to ischemic damage of the left ventricular myocardium that may have caused no symptoms prior to the development of heart failure; this condition is referred to as *ischemic cardiomyopathy*. In contrast to the asymptomatic phase of IHD, the symptomatic phase is characterized by chest discomfort due to either angina pectoris or acute myocardial infarction (Chap. 243). Having entered the symptomatic phase, the patient may exhibit a stable or progressive course, revert to the asymptomatic stage, or suddenly die.

STABLE ANGINA PECTORIS

This episodic clinical syndrome is due to transient myocardial ischemia. Various diseases that cause myocardial ischemia as well as the numerous forms of discomfort with which it may be confused are discussed in Chap. 13. Males constitute approximately 70% of all patients with angina pectoris and an even greater fraction of those younger than 50 years of age.

HISTORY The typical patient with angina is a 50- to 60-year-old man or 65- to 75-year-old woman who seeks medical help for chest discomfort, usually described as heaviness, pressure, squeezing, smothering, or choking and only rarely as frank pain. When the patient is asked to localize the sensation, he or she will typically press on the sternum, sometimes with a clenched fist, to indicate a squeezing, central, substernal discomfort. This symptom is usually crescendo-decrescendo in nature and lasts 1 to 5 min. Angina can radiate to the left shoulder and to both arms and especially to the ulnar surfaces of the forearm and hand. It can also arise in or radiate to the back, neck, jaw, teeth, and epigastrium.

Although episodes of angina are typically caused by exertion (e.g., exercise, hurrying, or sexual activity) or emotion (e.g., stress, anger, fright, or frustration) and are relieved by rest, they may also occur at rest (see "Unstable Angina Pectoris," p. 1408) and at night while the patient is recumbent (angina decubitus). The patient may be awakened at night distressed by typical chest discomfort and dyspnea. Nocturnal angina may be due to episodic tachycardia or activities such as micturition. It can also be due to the expansion of the intrathoracic blood volume that occurs with recumbency, which causes an increase in cardiac size and myocardial oxygen demand that lead to ischemia and transient left ventricular failure.

The threshold for the development of angina pectoris varies from person to person and may vary by time of day and emotional state. Many patients report a fixed threshold for angina, which occurs predictably at a certain level of activity. In these patients coronary stenosis and myocardial oxygen supply are fixed and ischemia is precipitated by an increase in myocardial oxygen demand. In other patients the threshold for angina may vary considerably within any given day and from day to day. In such patients variations in oxygen supply, most likely due to changes in coronary vascular tone, may play an important role. A patient may report symptoms upon minor exertion in the morning (a short walk or shaving) yet by midday may be capable of much greater effort without symptoms. Angina may also be precipitated by unfamiliar tasks, a heavy meal, or exposure to cold.

Sharp, fleeting chest pain or prolonged, dull aches localized to the left submammary area are rarely due to myocardial ischemia. However, angina pectoris may be atypical in location and may not be strictly related to provoking factors. In addition, this symptom may exacerbate and remit over days, weeks, or months. Its occurrence can be seasonal, being more frequent in the winter in temperate climates. Anginal "equivalents" are symptoms of myocardial ischemia other than angina. These include dyspnea, fatigue, and faintness and are more common in the elderly.

Systematic questioning of the patient with suspected IHD is important to uncover a positive family history of premature IHD (under the age of 45 years in first-degree male relatives and under 55 in female relatives), diabetes, hyperlipidemia, hypertension, cigarette smoking, and other risk factors for coronary atherosclerosis. The history of typical angina pectoris establishes the diagnosis of IHD until proven otherwise. In patients with atypical angina (Chap. 13), coexistence of advanced age, male sex, the postmenopausal state, and risk factors for atherosclerosis (Chap. 241) increase the likelihood of important coronary disease.

PHYSICAL EXAMINATION The physical examination is often normal in the patient with stable angina. Rarely, the general examination reveals signs of risk factors associated with coronary atherosclerosis such as xanthelasma, xanthomas (Chap. 241), or diabetic skin lesions. There may also be signs of anemia, thyroid disease, and nicotine stains on the fingertips from cigarette smoking. Palpation can reveal thickened or absent peripheral arteries, signs of cardiac enlargement, and abnormal contraction of the cardiac impulse (left ventricular akinesia or dyskinesia). Examination of the fundi may reveal increased light reflexes and arteriovenous nicking as evidence of hypertension (Table 35-2), while auscultation can uncover arterial bruits, a third and/or fourth heart sound, and, if acute ischemia or previous infarction has impaired papillary muscle function, an apical systolic murmur due to mitral regurgitation. These auscultatory signs are best appreciated with the patient in the left decubitus position. Aortic stenosis, aortic regurgitation (Chap. 236), pulmonary hypertension (Chap. 260), and hypertrophic cardiomyopathy (Chap. 238) must be excluded, since these disorders may cause angina in the absence of coronary atherosclerosis. Examination during an anginal attack is useful, since ischemia can cause transient left ventricular failure with the appearance of a third and/or fourth heart sound, a dyskinetic cardiac apex, mitral regurgitation, and even pulmonary edema.

LABORATORY EXAMINATION Although the diagnosis of IHD can be made with confidence from the clinical examination, a number of simple laboratory tests can be helpful. The urine should be examined for evidence of diabetes mellitus and renal disease, since both of these conditions accelerate atherosclerosis. Similarly, examination of the blood should include measurements of lipids (cholesterol—total, low density, high density—and triglycerides), glucose, creatinine, hematocrit, and, if indicated based on the physical examination, thyroid function. A chest x-ray is important, since it may show the consequences of IHD, i.e., cardiac enlargement, ventricular aneurysm, or signs of heart failure. These signs can support the diagnosis of IHD and are important in assessing the degree of cardiac damage and the effects of treatment for heart failure.

Electrocardiogram A 12-lead ECG recorded at rest is normal in about half the patients with typical angina pectoris, but there may be signs of an old myocardial infarction (Chap. 226). Although repolarization abnormalities, i.e., T-wave and ST-segment changes and intraventricular conduction disturbances at rest, are suggestive of IHD, they are nonspecific, since they can also occur in pericardial, myocardial, and valvular heart disease or transiently with anxiety, changes in posture, drugs, or esophageal disease. Typical ST-segment and T-wave changes that accompany episodes of angina pectoris and disappear thereafter are more specific. The most characteristic changes include displacement of the ST segment that is similar in every way to that induced during a stress test (see below). The ST segment is usually depressed during angina but may be elevated—sometimes strikingly so—in Prinzmetal's angina.

Stress Testing The most widely used test both for the diagnosis of IHD and establishing the prognosis involves recording the 12-lead ECG before, during, and after exercise on a treadmill or using a bicycle ergometer. The test consists of a standardized incremental increase in external workload while the patient's ECG, symptoms, and arm blood pressure are monitored. Performance is usually symptom-limited, and the test is discontinued upon evidence of chest discomfort, severe shortness of breath, dizziness, fatigue, ST-segment depression of >0.2 mV (2 mm), a fall in systolic blood pressure exceeding 10 mmHg, or the development of a ventricular tachyarrhythmia. This test seeks to discover any limitation in exercise performance and establish the relationship between chest discomfort and the typical ECG signs of myocardial ischemia. The ischemic ST-segment response is generally defined as flat depression of the ST segment of more than 0.1 mV below the baseline (i.e., the PR segment) and lasting longer than 0.08 s (Fig. 244-1). Upsloping or junctional ST-segment changes are not considered characteristic of ischemia and do not constitute a positive test. Although T-wave abnormalities, conduction disturbances, and ventricular arrhythmias that develop during exercise should be noted, they are also not diagnostic. Negative exercise tests in which the target heart rate (85% of maximal heart rate for age and sex) is not achieved are considered to be nondiagnostic. When applying and interpreting ECG stress testing, one must first consider the probability that CAD exists in the patient or population under study (i.e., pretest probability). Overall, false-positive or -negative results can occur in one-third of cases. However, a positive result on exercise indicates that the likelihood of CAD is 98% in males over 50 years of age with a history of typical angina pectoris who develop chest discomfort during the test. The likelihood decreases progressively and significantly if the patient has atypical or no chest pain by history and/or during the test. The incidence of false-positive tests is significantly increased in asymptomatic men under the age of 40 or in premenopausal women with no risk factors for premature atherosclerosis. It is also increased in patients taking cardioactive drugs, such as digitalis and quinidine, or in those with intraventricular conduction disturbances, resting abnormalities of the ST segment and T wave, myocardial hypertrophy, or abnormal serum potassium levels. Obstructive disease limited to the circumflex coronary artery may result in a false-negative stress test since the posterior portion of the heart which this vessel supplies is not well represented on the surface 12-lead ECG. Since the overall

sensitivity of exercise stress electrocardiography is only about 75%, a negative result does not exclude CAD, although it makes the likelihood of three-vessel or left main CAD extremely unlikely.

The physician should be present throughout the exercise test, and it is important to measure total duration of exercise, the times to the onset of ischemic ST-segment change and chest discomfort, the external work performed (generally expressed as a stage of exercise), and the internal cardiac work performed; the last is represented by the heart rate–blood pressure product. The depth of the ST-segment depression and the time needed for recovery of these ECG changes are also important. Because the risks of exercise testing are small but real— estimated at one fatality and two nonfatal complications per 10,000 tests—equipment for resuscitation should be available. Modified (heart rate–limited rather than symptom-limited) exercise tests can be performed safely in patients as early as 6 days after myocardial infarction. Contraindications to exercise stress testing include acute myocardial infarction (<4–5 days), rest angina <48 h, unstable rhythm, severe aortic stenosis, acute myocarditis, uncontrolled heart failure, and active infective endocarditis.

The normal response to graded exercise includes a progressive increase in heart rate and blood pressure. Failure of the blood pressure to increase or an actual decrease in blood pressure with signs of ischemia during the test is an important adverse prognostic sign, since it may reflect ischemia-induced global left ventricular dysfunction. The development of angina and/or severe (>0.2 mV) ST-segment depression at a low workload, i.e., before completion of stage II of the Bruce protocol, and ST-segment depression that persists for more than 5 min after the termination of exercise increases the specificity of the test and suggests severe ischemic heart disease and a high risk of future adverse events.

When the resting ECG is abnormal (e.g., Wolff-Parkinson-White syndrome, >1 mm of resting ST-segment depression, left bundle branch block, paced ventricular rhythm), information gained from an exercise test can be enhanced by stress myocardial perfusion imaging after the intravenous administration of a radioisotope such as thallium 201 or technetium 99m sestamibi during exercise (or a pharmacologic stress) (Chap. 227); the imaging is carried out both immediately after cessation of exercise to detect reversible ischemia and 4 h later to confirm reversible ischemia and regions of infarction (Fig. 244-2).

An important fraction of patients who need noninvasive stress testing to identify myocardial ischemia and increased risk of coronary events cannot exercise because of peripheral vascular or musculoskeletal disease, exertional dyspnea, or deconditioning. In these circumstances intravenous dipyridamole or adenosine can be used in place of exercise. The development of a transient perfusion defect with a tracer such as radioactive thallium or technetium 99m sestamibi is used to detect myocardial ischemia. Ambulatory monitoring of the ECG can assess myocardial ischemia as episodes of ST-segment depression. These techniques are sensitive and capable of identifying patients with ischemia who are at increased risk of coronary events.

Two-dimensional echocardiography of the left ventricle can assess both global and regional wall motion abnormalities due to myocardial infarction or persistent ischemia (Chap. 227). Stress (exercise or dobutamine) echocardiography may cause the emergence of regions of akinesis or dyskinesis not present at rest. Stress echocardiography, like stress myocardial perfusion imaging, is more sensitive than exercise electrocardiography in the diagnosis of IHD. The relative advantages of stress echocardiography and stress radionuclide perfusion imaging in the diagnosis of IHD are shown in Table 244-1.

Echocardiography or radionuclide angiography should be carried out to assess left ventricular function in patients with chronic stable angina and in patients with a history of a prior myocardial infarction, pathologic Q waves, or clinical evidence of heart failure.

Coronary Arteriography (See also Chap. 228) This diagnostic method outlines the coronary anatomy and can be used to detect important evidence of coronary atherosclerosis or to exclude this condition. By this means, one can assess the severity of obstructive lesions and, when coronary arteriography is combined with left ventricular

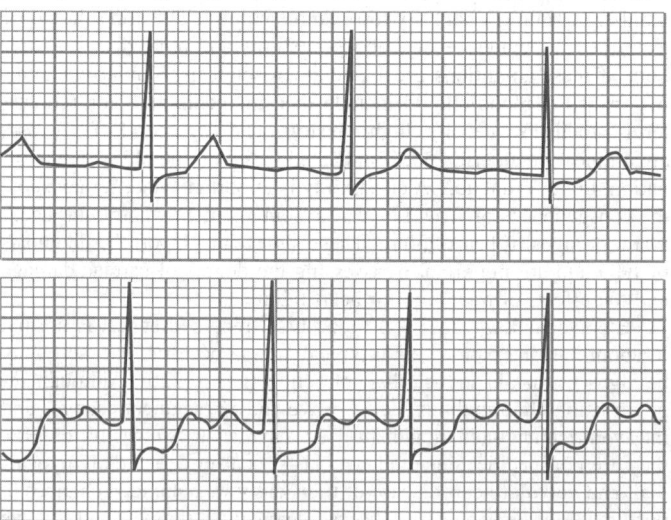

FIGURE 244-1 Lead V_4 at rest (*top*) and after $4\frac{1}{2}$ min of exercise (*bottom*). There is 3 mm (0.3 mV) of horizontal ST-segment depression, indicating a positive test for ischemia. [*Modified from BR Chaitman, in E Braunwald et al (eds): Heart Disease, 6th ed, Philadelphia, Saunders, 2001.*]

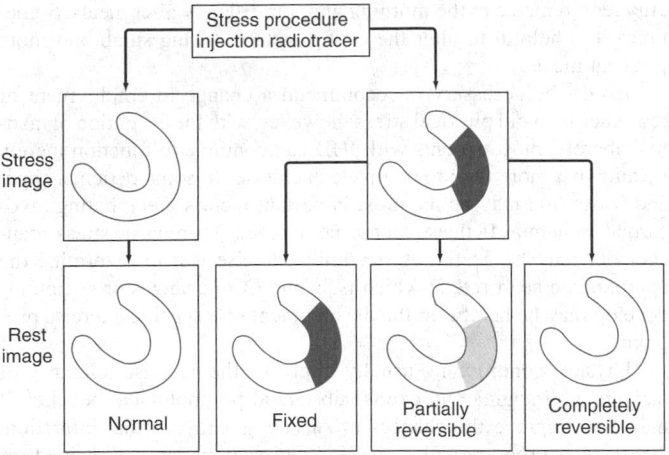

FIGURE 244-2 Interpretation of stress (exercise) and rest myocardial perfusion images. A normal image will show homogeneous accumulation of radiotracer on the exercise and rest (or delayed) image. An area with decreased uptake of the radiotracer (which appears as a darker area on a perfusion image) is referred to as a *defect*. A patient with a fixed perfusion defect will have an abnormal exercise image and an identical rest or delayed redistribution image (scarring). A partially reversible perfusion defect appears as an abnormal exercise image and an improved but still abnormal rest image (ischemia and scarring). A reversible perfusion defect appears as an abnormal exercise image and a normal rest or delayed image (ischemia). *[From FJ Wackers, in GA Beller (ed), Chronic Ischemic Heart Disease, in E Braunwald (series ed), Atlas of Heart Diseases, Philadelphia, Current Medicine, 1994.]*

angiocardiography, can evaluate both global and regional function of the left ventricle.

Indications Coronary arteriography is indicated in (1) patients with chronic stable angina pectoris who are severely symptomatic despite medical therapy and who are being considered for revascularization, i.e., a percutaneous coronary intervention (PCI) or coronary artery bypass grafting (CABG); (2) patients with troublesome symptoms that present diagnostic difficulties in whom there is need to confirm or rule out the diagnosis of IHD; (3) patients with known or possible angina pectoris who have survived sudden cardiac death; and (4) patients judged to be at high risk of sustaining coronary events based on signs of severe ischemia on noninvasive testing, regardless of the presence or severity of symptoms (see below).

Examples of other clinical situations include:

1. Patients with chest discomfort suggestive of angina pectoris but a negative or nondiagnostic stress test who require a definitive diagnosis for guiding medical management, alleviating psychological stress, career or family planning, or insurance purposes.
2. Patients who have been admitted repeatedly to the hospital for suspected acute myocardial infarction but in whom this diagnosis has not been established and in whom the presence or absence of CAD should be determined.
3. Patients with careers that involve the safety of others (e.g., airline pilots) who have questionable symptoms, suspicious or positive noninvasive tests, and in whom there are reasonable doubts about the state of the coronary arteries.
4. Patients with aortic stenosis or hypertrophic cardiomyopathy and angina in whom the chest pain could be due to IHD.
5. Male patients aged 45 and females aged 55 years of age or older who are to undergo a cardiac operation, such as valve replacement or repair and who may or may not have clinical evidence of myocardial ischemia.
6. Patients who are at high risk after myocardial infarction because of the recurrence of angina or the presence of heart failure, frequent ventricular premature contractions, or signs of ischemia in the stress test.
7. Patients with angina pectoris, regardless of severity, in whom noninvasive testing indicates a high risk of coronary events.

8. Patients in whom coronary spasm or another nonatherosclerotic cause of myocardial ischemia (e.g., coronary artery anomaly, Kawasaki's disease) is suspected.

PROGNOSIS

The principal prognostic indicators in patients with IHD are the functional state of the left ventricle, the location and severity of coronary artery narrowing, and the severity or activity of myocardial ischemia. Angina pectoris of recent onset, unstable angina, angina that is unresponsive or poorly responsive to medical therapy or is accompanied by symptoms of congestive heart failure all indicate an increased risk for adverse coronary events. The same is true for the physical signs of heart failure, episodes of pulmonary edema, transient third heart sounds, or mitral regurgitation or for echocardiographic (or roentgenographic) evidence of cardiac enlargement. An abnormal resting ECG or positive evidence of myocardial ischemia during a stress test also indicates increased risk. Most importantly, the following signs during noninvasive testing indicate a high risk for coronary events: a strongly positive exercise test showing onset of myocardial ischemia at low workloads [≥0.1 mV ST-segment depression before completion of stage II (Bruce protocol) of the exercise test; ≥0.2 mV ST depression in any stage; ST depression for >5 min following the cessation of exercise; a decline in systolic pressure >10 mmHg during exercise; the development of ventricular tachyarrhythmias during exercise]; the development of large or multiple perfusion defects or increased lung uptake during stress radioisotope perfusion imaging; and a decrease in left ventricular ejection fraction during exercise on radionuclide ventriculography or during stress echocardiography. Conversely, patients who can complete stage III of the Bruce exercise protocol and have a normal stress perfusion scan or negative stress echocardiographic evaluation are at very low risk of future coronary events.

On cardiac catheterization, elevations in left ventricular end-diastolic pressure and ventricular volume and a reduced ejection fraction are the most important signs of left ventricular dysfunction and are associated with a poor prognosis. Patients with chest discomfort but normal left ventricular function and normal coronary arteries have an excellent prognosis. In patients with normal left ventricular function and mild angina but with critical stenoses (≥70% luminal diameter) of one, two, or three epicardial coronary arteries, the 5-year mortality rates are approximately 2, 8, and 11 percent, respectively. Obstructive lesions of the left anterior descending coronary artery proximal to the origin of the first septal artery are associated with a greater risk than are lesions of the right or left circumflex coronary artery, since the former vessel usually perfuses a greater quantity of myocardium. Stenosis (>50% luminal diameter) of the left main coronary artery is

Table 244-1 Comparative Advantages of Stress Echocardiography and Stress Radionuclide Perfusion Imaging in Diagnosis of CAD

Advantages of stress echocardiography
  1. Higher specificity
  2. Versatility—more extensive evaluation of cardiac anatomy and function
  3. Greater convenience/efficacy/availability
  4. Lower cost

Advantages of stress perfusion imaging
  1. Higher technical success rate
  2. Higher sensitivity—especially for single vessel coronary disease involving the left circumflex
  3. Better accuracy in evaluating possible ischemia when multiple resting LV wall motion abnormalities are present
  4. More extensive published data base—especially in evaluation of prognosis

SOURCE: ACC/AHA/ACP-ASIM Guidelines for the Management of Patients with Chronic Stable Angina: A report of the American College of Cardiology/American Heart Association Task Force on Practice Guidelines (Committee on Management of Patients with Chronic Stable Angina). J Am Coll Cardiol 33:2092, 1999.

associated with a mortality rate of about 15% per year. The segmental atherosclerotic plaques in epicardial arteries go through phases of inflammatory cellular activity, degeneration, endothelial instability, abnormal vasomotion, platelet aggregation, and fissuring or hemorrhage. These factors can temporarily worsen the stenosis and cause abnormal reactivity of the vessel wall, thus exacerbating the manifestations of ischemia. The recent onset of symptoms, the appearance of severe ischemia during stress testing, and unstable angina pectoris (p. 1508) all reflect episodes of rapid progression in coronary lesions.

With any degree of obstructive CAD, mortality is greatly increased when left ventricular function is impaired; conversely, at any level of left ventricular function, the prognosis is influenced importantly by the quantity of myocardium perfused by the critically obstructed vessels. Therefore, it is useful to collect all the evidence substantiating past myocardial damage (ECG and ventriculographic evidence of myocardial infarction), residual left ventricular function (ejection fraction and wall motion), and risk of future damage from coronary events (extent of coronary disease and severity of ischemia defined by noninvasive stress testing). The larger the amount of established myocardial necrosis, the less the heart is able to withstand additional damage and the poorer the prognosis. All the above signs of past damage plus the risk of future damage should be considered indicators of risk.

TREATMENT Each patient must be evaluated individually with respect to his or her expectations and goals, control of symptoms, and prevention of adverse clinical outcomes such as myocardial infarction and premature death. The degree of disability as well as the physical and emotional stress that precipitate angina must be carefully recorded in order to set treatment goals. Each management plan should consist of the following: (1) explanation and reassurance, (2) identification and treatment of aggravating conditions, (3) adaptation of activity, (4) treatment of risk factors that will decrease the occurrence of adverse coronary outcomes, (5) drug therapy for angina, and (6) consideration of mechanical revascularization.

Explanation and Reassurance Patients with IHD need to understand their condition as best they can and to realize that a long and useful life is possible even though they suffer from angina pectoris or have experienced and recovered from an acute myocardial infarction. Offering case histories of persons in public life who have lived with coronary disease as well as results of national studies showing improved outcomes can be of great value when encouraging patients to resume or maintain activity and return to their occupation. A planned program of rehabilitation can encourage patients to lose weight, improve exercise tolerance, and control risk factors with more confidence.

Identification and Treatment of Aggravating Conditions A number of conditions may either increase oxygen demand or decrease oxygen supply to the myocardium and may precipitate or exacerbate angina. Aortic valve disease and hypertrophic cardiomyopathy may cause angina and should be excluded or treated. Obesity, hypertension, and hyperthyroidism may be managed successfully in order to reduce the frequency of anginal attacks. Decreased myocardial oxygen supply may be due to reduced oxygenation of the blood (e.g., in pulmonary disease or, when carboxyhemoglobin is present, due to cigarette or cigar smoking) or decreased oxygen-carrying capacity (e.g., in anemia). Correction of these abnormalities, if present, may reduce or even eliminate angina pectoris.

Adaptation of Activity Therapy of angina due to episodes of myocardial ischemia consists of eliminating the discrepancy between the demand of the heart muscle for oxygen and the ability of the coronary circulation to meet this demand. Most patients can be made to understand this fundamental concept and utilize it in the rational programming of activity. Many tasks that ordinarily evoke angina may be accomplished without symptoms simply by reducing the speed at which they are performed. Patients must appreciate the diurnal variation in their tolerance of certain activities and should reduce their energy requirements in the morning and immediately after meals. Sometimes it is helpful to alter the eating pattern, taking small and more frequent meals.

It may be necessary to recommend a change in employment or residence to avoid physical stress; however, with the exception of manual laborers, most patients with IHD can continue to function merely by allowing more time to complete each task. In some patients, anger and frustration may be the most important factors precipitating myocardial ischemia. If these cannot be avoided, training in stress management may be useful. A treadmill exercise test to determine the approximate heart rate at which ischemic ECG changes or symptoms develop may be helpful in the development of a specific exercise program.

Physical conditioning usually improves the exercise tolerance of patients with angina and exerts substantial psychological benefits. It may also improve the chances of surviving a myocardial infarction. An exercise program within the limits of each patient's threshold for the development of angina pectoris should be encouraged.

Treatment of Risk Factors Although the treatment of risk factors was developed for the primary prevention of coronary atherosclerosis, there is growing evidence that it can reduce the occurrence of angina, myocardial infarction, and death both in subjects without proven IHD as well as in those with a history of chronic angina or an acute coronary syndrome. A *family history* of premature IHD is an important indicator of increased risk and should trigger a search for treatable risk factors such as hyperlipidemia, hypertension, and diabetes. *Obesity* impairs the treatment of other risk factors and increases the risk of adverse coronary events. In addition, obesity is often accompanied by two other risk factors—hypertension and hyperlipidemia. The treatment of obesity and these accompanying risk factors is an important component of any management plan.

Cigarette smoking accelerates coronary atherosclerosis in both sexes and at all ages and increases the risk of myocardial infarction and death. By increasing myocardial oxygen needs and reducing oxygen supply it aggravates angina. Smoking cessation studies have demonstrated important benefits with a significant decline in the occurrence of these adverse outcomes. The physician's message must be clear and strong and supported by programs that achieve and monitor abstinence (Chap. 390). *Hypertension* (Chaps. 35 and 246) is associated with increased risk of adverse clinical events from coronary atherosclerosis as well as stroke. In addition, the left ventricular hypertrophy that results from sustained hypertension aggravates ischemia. There is evidence that long-term, effective treatment of hypertension can decrease the occurrence of adverse coronary events. *Diabetes mellitus* (Chap. 333) accelerates coronary and peripheral atherosclerosis and is frequently associated with dyslipidemias and increases in the risk of angina, myocardial infarction, and sudden coronary death. Strict control of the dyslipidemia that is frequently found in diabetic patients is essential, as described below.

Treatment of dyslipidemia The adverse interactions between the atherogenic lipids (LDL, triglycerides, and lipid remnants) play a critical role in the development of atherosclerosis and the ischemic syndromes. The treatment of dyslipidemia is central when aiming for long-term relief from angina, reduced need for revascularization, and reduction in myocardial infarction and death. Epidemiology, angiographic trials, and controlled trails have shown that (1) men over 45 years and women over 55 years with two risk factors (family history of premature IHD, cigarette smoking, hypertension, diabetes mellitus) or evidence of atherosclerotic disease should have a total cholesterol $\leq$ 5.17 mmol/L ($\leq$200 mg/dL), LDL $\leq$ 2.58 mmol/L ($\leq$100 mg/dL), and HDL $\geq$ 1.03 mmol/L ($\leq$40 mg/dL); and (2) diabetic patients any age need to achieve the same goals as the likelihood of adverse coronary events is so high. The controlled trials have shown equal benefit for women, the elderly, and even smokers. The control of lipids can be achieved by the combination of a diet low in saturated fatty acids, exercise, and weight loss. Frequently, HMG CoA reductase inhibitors (statins) are required and can lower LDL cholesterol (25 to 60%), raise HDL cholesterol (5 to 9%), and lower triglycerides (5 to 45%). Niacin and fibrates can be used to raise HDL cholesterol and lower triglycerides (Chaps. 242 and 341).

Risk reduction in women with IHD The incidence of clinical IHD in premenopausal women is very low. However, following the menopause, the atherogenic risk factors increase (e.g., increased LDL, reduced HDL) and the rate of clinical coronary events accelerates to the levels observed in men. Women have not given up cigarette smoking as effectively as have men. Diabetes mellitus, which is more common in women, greatly increases the occurrence of clinical IHD and amplifies the deleterious effects of hypertension, hyperlipidemia, and smoking. Cardiac catheterization and coronary revascularization are often applied more sparingly in women and at a later, and more severe, stage of the disease than in men. These factors likely explain the modest increase in complications. Although many of the clinical trials to date have not represented women adequately, the evidence is that when cholesterol lowering, beta blockers after myocardial infarction, and CABG are applied in the appropriate patient groups, women enjoy the same benefits of improved outcome as do men.

Drug Therapy The commonly used drugs for angina pectoris are summarized in Table 244-2.

Nitrates This valuable class of drugs in the management of angina pectoris acts by causing systemic venodilation, thereby reducing myocardial wall tension and oxygen requirements, as well as by dilating the epicardial coronary vessels and increasing blood flow in collateral vessels. The absorption of these agents is most rapid and complete through the mucous membranes. For this reason, nitroglycerin is administered sublingually in tablets of 0.4 or 0.6 mg. Patients with angina should be instructed to take the medication both to relieve angina and also in anticipation of stress (exercise or emotional) that is likely to induce an episode. The value of this prophylactic use of the drug cannot be overemphasized.

Headache and a pulsating feeling in the head are the most common side effects of nitroglycerin and fortunately only rarely become disturbing at the doses usually required to relieve or prevent angina. Nitroglycerin deteriorates with exposure to air, moisture, and sunlight, so that if the drug neither relieves discomfort or headache nor produces a slight sensation of burning at the sublingual site of absorption, the preparation may be inactive and a fresh supply should be obtained. If relief is not achieved after the first dose of nitroglycerin, a second or third dose may be given at 5-min intervals. If discomfort continues despite treatment, the patient should consult a physician or report promptly to a hospital emergency room for evaluation of possible unstable angina or acute myocardial infarction (Chap. 243).

A diary of angina and nitroglycerin use may be valuable for detecting changes in the frequency or severity of discomfort that may signify the development of unstable angina pectoris and/or herald an impending myocardial infarction.

None of the long-acting nitrates is as effective as sublingual nitroglycerin for the acute relief of angina. These preparations can be swallowed, chewed, or administered as a patch or paste by the transdermal route. They can provide effective plasma levels for up to 24 h, but the therapeutic response is highly variable. Different preparations and/or administration during the daytime should be tried only to prevent discomfort in the individual patient while avoiding side effects such as

Table 244-2   Drugs Commonly Used for Angina Pectoris

Drug	Usual Dose	Side Effects	Contraindications
NITRATES			
Sublingual NTG	0.3–0.6 mg	Flushing, headache	Intolerance of side effects
Isosorbide dinitrate SR			
Oral	10–60 mg q8h	Flushing, headache, tolerance after 24 h	As above, worsening ischemia on withdrawal
Sublingual	2.5–10 mgq4–6h		
Transdermal NTG patch	0.4–1.2 mg/h for 12–14 h	Flushing, headache, tolerance after 24 h	As above, worsening ischemia on withdrawal
Isosorbide-5-monitrate			
Oral	20–30 mg bid	Flushing, headache, tolerance after 24 h	As above, worsening ischemia on withdrawal
Oral SR	60–240 mg once daily		
BETA BLOCKERS			
Propranolol	20–80 mg qid	Depression, constipation, impotence, bronchospasm, heart failure, bradycardia	Asthma, AV conduction block, heart failure
Metoprolol	25–200 mg bid	As above	As above
Atenolol	50–150 mg once daily	As above	As above
CALCIUM CHANNEL BLOCKING DRUGS			
Nifedipine XL	30–90 mg daily	Hypotension, flushing, edema, worsening angina	Hypotension, intolerance of side effects
Diltiazem SR	60–120 mg bid	Constipation, AV conduction block, worsening heart failure	AV conduction block, impaired LV function, bradycardia
Verapamil SR	180–240 mg daily	Constipation, AV conduction block, worsening heart failure	AV conduction delay, impaired LV function, bradycardia
Amlodipine	5–10 mg daily	Edema	Intolerance of side effects

NOTE: NTG, nitroglycerin; SR, slow release; XL, slow release preparation.

headache and dizziness. Individual dose titration is important in order to prevent side effects. Useful preparations include isosorbide dinitrate (10 to 60 mg PO bid or tid), nitroglycerin ointment (0.5 to 2.0 in. qid), or sustained-release transdermal patches (5 to 25 mg/d). The nitrates likely bind to guanylate cyclase in vascular smooth muscle cells, oxidize sulfhydryl groups, and are converted to *S*-nitrosothiols. This leads to an increase in cyclic guanosine monophosphate which causes relaxation of vascular smooth muscle. Tolerance with loss of efficacy develops with 12 to 24 h of continuous exposure to all of the long-acting nitrates due to depletion of sulfhydryl groups and to counter-regulatory alterations in intravascular fluid balance with fluid retention. In order to minimize the effects of tolerance, the minimum effective dose should be used and a minimum of 8 h each day kept free of the drug so as to restore any useful response(s).

Beta blockers (See also Chap. 72) These drugs represent an important component of the pharmacologic treatment of angina pectoris. They reduce myocardial oxygen demand by inhibiting the increases in heart rate and myocardial contractility caused by adrenergic activation. Beta blockade reduces these variables most strikingly during exercise while causing only small reductions in heart rate, cardiac output, and arterial pressure at rest. Long-acting beta-blocking drugs (atenolol, 50 to 100 mg/d, and nadolol, 40 to 80 mg/d) offer the advantage of once-a-day dosage (Tables 72-1 and 244-2). The therapeutic aims include relief of angina and ischemia. These drugs can also reduce mortality and reinfarction when given to patients after myocardial infarction. Relative contraindications to the use of beta blockers include asthma and reversible airway obstruction in patients with chronic lung disease, atrioventricular conduction disturbances, severe bradycardia, Raynaud's phenomenon, and a history of depression. Side effects include fatigue, impotence, cold extremities, intermittent claudication, bradycardia (sometimes severe), impaired atrioventricular conduction, left ventricular failure, bronchial asthma, and intensification of the hypoglycemia produced by oral hypoglycemic agents and insulin. Reducing the dose or even discontinuation of the drug may be necessary if these side effects develop and persist.

Calcium antagonists   Slow-release nifedipine (30 to 90 mg once daily), verapamil (80 to 120 mg tid), diltiazem (30 to 90 mg qid), amlodipine (2.5 to 10 mg daily), and other calcium antagonists are coronary vasodilators that produce variable and dose-dependent reductions in myocardial oxygen demand, contractility, and arterial pressure. These combined pharmacologic effects are advantageous and make these agents effective in the treatment of angina pectoris. They are indicated when beta blockers are contraindicated, poorly tolerated, or ineffective. Verapamil and diltiazem may produce symptomatic disturbances in cardiac conduction and bradyarrhythmias, exert negative inotropic actions, and are more likely to worsen left ventricular failure, particularly when used in patients with left ventricular dysfunction. Although useful effects are usually achieved when calcium antagonists are combined with beta blockers and nitrates, careful individual titration of dose is essential with these potent combinations. Variant (Prinzmetal's) angina responds particularly well to calcium antagonists, supplemented when necessary by nitrates. Nifedipine as well as other calcium antagonists are now formulated as long-acting preparations including diltiazem (60 to 120 mg twice daily) and verapamil (180 to 240 mg once daily).

Verapamil should not ordinarily be combined with beta blockers because of the combined effects on heart rate and contractility. Diltiazem can be combined with beta blockers with caution and only in patients with normal ventricular function and no conduction disturbances. Nifedipine or amlodipine and the beta blockers have complementary actions on coronary blood supply and myocardial oxygen demands. While the former decreases blood pressure and dilates coronary arteries, the latter slows heart rate and decreases contractility. Nifedipine and the other second-generation dihydropyridine calcium antagonists (nicardipine, isradipine, amlodipine, and felodipine) are potent vasodilators and useful in the simultaneous treatment of angina and hypertension. Short-acting dihydropyridines should be avoided because of the risk of precipitating infarction, particularly in the absence of beta blockers.

Choice between beta blockers and calcium antagonists for initial therapy   Since beta blockers have been shown to improve life expectancy following myocardial infarction (p. 1393), they may be preferable in patients with chronic IHD. However, calcium antagonists are indicated in patients with the following: (1) angina and a history of asthma or chronic obstructive pulmonary disease; (2) sick-sinus syndrome or significant atrioventricular conduction disturbances; (3) Prinzmetal's angina; (4) symptomatic peripheral vascular disease; and (5) adverse reactions to beta blockers—depression, sexual disturbances, fatigue. Many patients with angina do well with a combination of a beta blocker and dihydropyridine calcium antagonist.

Antiplatelet drugs   Aspirin is an irreversible inhibitor of platelet cyclooxygenase activity and thereby interferes with platelet activation. Chronic administration of 100 to 325 mg orally per day has been shown to reduce coronary events in asymptomatic adult men, patients with asymptomatic ischemia after myocardial infarction, patients with chronic stable angina, and patients with or who have survived unstable angina and myocardial infarction. Administration of this drug should be considered in all patients with IHD in the absence of side effects such as gastrointestinal bleeding, allergy, or dyspepsia. Clopidogrel is an oral agent that blocks ADP receptor–mediated platelet aggregation. It provides the same benefits as aspirin, if not better, particularly if aspirin causes the side effects listed above.

In summary, a regimen of exercise, smoking cessation, treatment of hypertension and dyslipidemia, aspirin, and beta blockers after infarction are medical interventions that reduce angina, the need for revascularization, myocardial infarction and coronary death.

Treatment af angina and heart failure   Transient left ventricular failure with angina can be controlled by the use of nitrates. For patients with established congestive heart failure the increased left ventricular wall tension raises myocardial oxygen demand. Treatment of conges-tive heart failure with angiotensin-converting enzyme inhibitors, diuretics, and digitalis (Chap. 232) will decrease heart size, wall tension, and myocardial oxygen demands, which, in turn, will help to control angina and ischemia. Nocturnal angina can often be relieved by the treatment of heart failure; however, there is no proven benefit when these drugs are used in patients with angina, a normal heart size, and no evidence of heart failure. Nitrates are particularly useful and can simultaneously improve the disturbed hemodynamics of congestive heart failure by vasodilatation, thereby reducing preload, and relieve angina by preventing or reversing myocardial ischemia. There is some evidence that amlodipine is a calcium antagonist that is well tolerated by patients with left ventricular dysfunction and a valuable agent in the treatment of angina in patients with heart failure. The combination of congestive heart failure and angina in patients with IHD usually indicates a poor prognosis and warrants serious consideration of cardiac catheterization and mechanical revascularization.

CORONARY REVASCULARIZATION

While the basic management of patients with CAD, which is a lifelong condition, is medical, as described above, many patients are improved by coronary revascularization procedures, as described below. These interventions should be employed in conjunction with but do not replace the continuing need to modify risk factors.

PERCUTANEOUS CORONARY INTERVENTION (See also Chap. 245) PCI, most commonly percutaneous transluminal coronary angioplasty (PTCA) or stenting, is a widely used method to achieve revascularization of the myocardium in patients with symptomatic IHD and suitable stenoses of epicardial coronary arteries. Whereas patients with stenosis of the left main coronary artery and those with three-vessel CAD (especially with associated impaired left ventricular function) who require revascularization are best treated with CABG, PCI is widely employed in patients with symptoms and evidence of ischemia due to stenoses of one or two vessels, and even selected patients with three-vessel disease, and may offer many advantages over surgery.

Indications and Patient Selection   The most common clinical indication for PCI is angina pectoris, stable or unstable, accompanied by evidence of ischemia in an exercise test. PCI is more effective than medical therapy for the relief of angina. The value of this procedure in reducing the occurrence of coronary death and myocardial infarction has not been established, and therefore it is not generally indicated in asymptomatic or mildly symptomatic patients. PCI can be used to treat stenoses in native coronary arteries as well as in bypass grafts in patients who have recurrent angina following coronary artery surgery. This is an important indication when the technical difficulties and the increased mortality that accompanies reoperation are considered. PCI has also been carried out in patients with recent total occlusion (within 3 months) of a coronary artery and severe angina; in this group the primary success rate is slightly decreased.

Risks   When coronary stenoses are discrete and symmetric, two and three vessels can be dilated in sequence. However, case selection is essential in order to avoid a prohibitive risk of complications. Advanced age, stenoses with thrombus, left ventricular dysfunction, stenosis of an artery perfusing a large segment of myocardium without collaterals, long eccentric or irregular stenoses, and calcified plaques all increase the likelihood of complications but are not absolute contraindications, while left main coronary artery stenosis *is* generally regarded as an absolute contraindication. The major complications are usually due to dissection or thrombosis with vessel occlusion, uncontrolled ischemia, and ventricular failure. Oral aspirin and intravenous heparin are always given to reduce coronary thrombus formation. In unstable angina and when intracoronary thrombus is seen, the use of specific platelet glycoprotein receptor antagonists further reduce thrombotic complications and increase success. In experienced hands, the overall mortality rate should be less than 0.5%, the need for emergency coronary surgery less than 1%, and the occurrence of clinical myocardial infarction less than 2%. Minor complications occur in 5 to 10% of patients and include occlusion of a branch of a coronary artery, myocardial infarction with release of CK-MB into the circulation, and complications of arterial catheterization.

Efficacy Primary success, i.e., adequate dilation (an increase in luminal diameter to a residual diameter obstruction <50%) with relief of angina, is achieved in approximately 95% of cases. Recurrent stenosis of the dilated vessels occurs in 30 to 45% of cases within 6 months of PTCA, and angina will recur within 6 to 12 months in 25% of cases. This recurrence of symptoms and restenosis is more common in patients with diabetes mellitus, unstable angina, incomplete dilation of the stenosis, dilation of the left anterior descending coronary artery, and stenoses containing thrombi. Dilation of arteries that are totally occluded and of stenotic or occluded vein grafts also exhibits a high incidence of restenosis. It is usual clinical practice to administer aspirin for months after the procedure. Although aspirin and the antiplatelet drug Clopidogrel may help prevent acute coronary thrombosis during and shortly following PCI, there are no controlled clinical trials that have demonstrated that these medications or any other can clearly reduce the incidence of restenosis. Successful deployment of a metal stent lowers the restenosis rate to 10 to 30% at 6 months but initially requires vigorous antiplatelet therapy (aspirin and Clopidogrel). There is early evidence that local radiation can further reduce restenosis.

If patients do not develop restenosis or angina within the first year after angioplasty, the prognosis for maintaining improvement over the subsequent 4 years is excellent. If restenosis occurs, PTCA can be repeated with the same success and risk, but the likelihood of restenosis increases with the third or subsequent attempt.

Successful PCI produces effective relief of angina in over 95% of cases and has been shown to be more effective than medical therapy for up to 2 years. Between 30 and 50% of patients with symptomatic IHD who require revascularization can be treated by PCI and need not undergo CABG. Successful PCI is less invasive and expensive than CABG, usually requires only 1 to 2 days in the hospital, and permits considerable savings in the initial cost of care. Successful PCI also allows earlier return to work and the resumption of an active life. However, this economic benefit is reduced over time because of the greater need for follow-up and for repeat procedures.

CORONARY ARTERY BYPASS GRAFTING In CABG, a section of a vein (usually the saphenous) is used to form a connection between the aorta and the coronary artery distal to the obstructive lesion. Alternatively, anastomosis of one or both of the internal mammary arteries or a radial artery to the coronary artery distal to the obstructive lesion may be employed and is now preferred whenever possible.

Although some indications for coronary artery bypass surgery are controversial, certain areas of agreement exist:

1. The operation is relatively safe, with mortality rates less than 1% in patients without serious comorbid disease and normal left ventricular function, when the procedure is performed by an experienced surgical team.
2. Intraoperative and postoperative mortality increase with the degree of ventricular dysfunction, comorbidities, age above 80 years, and surgical inexperience. The effectiveness and risk of CABG vary widely depending on case selection and the skill and experience of the surgical team.
3. Occlusion of vein grafts is observed in 10 to 20% during the first postoperative year and in approximately 2% per year during 5- to 7-year follow-up and 4% per year thereafter. Long-term patency rates are considerably higher for internal mammary and radial artery implantations; in patients with left anterior descending coronary artery obstruction, survival is better when coronary bypass involves the internal mammary artery rather than a saphenous vein. Graft patency and outcomes are improved by meticulous treatment of risk factors, particularly dyslipidemia.
4. Angina is abolished or greatly reduced in approximately 90% of

patients following complete revascularization. Although this is usually associated with graft patency and restoration of blood flow, the pain may also have been alleviated as a result of infarction of the ischemic segment or a placebo effect. Within 3 years, angina recurs in about one-fourth of patients but is rarely severe.

5. CABG does not appear to reduce the incidence of myocardial infarction in patients with chronic IHD; perioperative myocardial infarction occurs in 5 to 10% of cases, but in most instances these infarcts are small and have little effect on left ventricular function.
6. Mortality is reduced by operation in patients with stenosis of the left main coronary artery as well as in patients with three- or two-vessel disease with significant obstruction of the proximal left anterior descending coronary artery. The survival benefit is greater in patients with abnormal left ventricular function (ejection fraction <50%). Mortality *may* also be reduced in the following patients: (1) with one- or two-vessel CAD without significant proximal left anterior descending artery CAD but with high-risk criteria on noninvasive testing; (2) with obstructive CAD who have survived sudden cardiac death or sustained ventricular tachycardia; (3) who have undergone previous CABG and who have multiple saphenous vein graft stenoses, especially of a graft supplying the left anterior descending coronary artery; and (4) with prior PCI recurrent stenosis, and high-risk criteria on noninvasive testing.

Indications for CABG are usually based on the severity of symptoms, coronary anatomy, and ventricular function. The ideal candidate is male, less than 75 years of age, has no other complicating disease, has troublesome or disabling symptoms that are not adequately controlled by medical therapy or does not tolerate medical therapy and wishes to lead a more active life, and has severe stenoses of several epicardial coronary arteries with objective evidence of myocardial ischemia as a cause of the chest discomfort. Great symptomatic benefit can be anticipated in such patients.

Congestive heart failure and/or left ventricular dysfunction (ejection fraction <40%), advanced age (>75 years), reoperation, urgent need for surgery, and the presence of diabetes are all associated with higher perioperative mortality.

Left ventricular dysfunction can be due to noncontractile segments that are viable (hibernating myocardium). These can be detected by using radionuclide scans of myocardial perfusion and metabolism, positron emission tomography, or delayed scanning with thallium-201 or by return of contractile function provoked by low-dose dobutamine. Revascularization can return function and improve survival.

The Choice Between PCI and CABG (See Table 244-3) A number of randomized trials have compared PTCA and CABG in patients with multivessel CAD who were suitable technically for both procedures. The redevelopment of angina requiring repeat coronary angiography and repeat revascularization due to restenosis was higher in the PTCA group. However, the occurrence of death or myocardial infarction has been found to be similar between both groups for up to 5 years. In patients with diabetes plus disease of two or more coronary arteries, bypass surgery results in significantly better outcomes and survival and should be the technique of choice. In addition, the recurrence of angina and stenosis and the need for additional revascularization was much higher in the angioplasty group (about 50%) than in the surgery group (about 10%). Based on these trials and observational studies, we now recommend that patients with an unacceptable level of angina despite optimal medical management should be considered for revascularization. Patients with single- or two-vessel disease with normal or slightly depressed global left ventricular function and anatomically suitable lesions are ordinarily advised initially to undergo PCI (Chap. 245). Patients with two- or three-vessel disease and impaired global left ventricular function (left ventricular ejection fraction <45%) or diabetes mellitus or those with left main disease or other

Table 244-3 Comparison of Revascularization Procedures in Multivessel Disease

Procedure	Advantages	Disadvantages
Percutaneous coronary intervention (PCI)	Less invasive Shorter hospital stay Lower initial cost Easily repeated Effective in relieving symptoms	Restenosis High incidence of incomplete revascularization Unknown effect on outcomes in patients with severe left ventricular dysfunction Limited to specific anatomic subsets Poor outcome in diabetics with 2 or 3 vessel coronary disease
Coronary artery bypass grafting (CABG)	Effective in relieving symptoms Improved survival in certain subsets Ability to achieve complete revascularization	Cost Increased risk of a repeat procedure due to late graft closure Morbidity and mortality of major surgery

SOURCE: Modified from DP Faxon, in GA Beller (ed), *Chronic Ischemic Heart Disease,* in E Braunwald (series ed), *Atlas of Heart Diseases,* Philadelphia, Current Medicine, 1994.

lesions unsuitable for catheter-based procedures should be considered for CABG as the initial method of revascularization (Table 244-3).

UNSTABLE ANGINA PECTORIS

The following three patient groups may be said to have unstable angina pectoris: (1) patients with new onset (<2 months) angina that is severe and/or frequent (≥3 episodes per day); (2) patients with accelerating angina, i.e., those with chronic stable angina who develop angina that is distinctly more frequent, severe, prolonged, or precipitated by less exertion than previously; (3) those with angina at rest. Five mechanisms for unstable angina have been described: (1) a nonocclusive thrombus—often a platelet plug—overlying a fissured atherosclerotic plaque; (2) dynamic obstruction—either spasm of an epicardial coronary artery, as in Prinzmetal's variant angina (see below), or abnormal vasoconstriction of the coronary microcirculation, as in microvascular angina; (3) severe, organic luminal narrowing, as in restenosis following a PCI; (4) arterial inflammation leading to thrombosis; and (5) increase in myocardial oxygen demands caused by conditions such as tachycardia, fever, and thyrotoxicosis in the presence of fixed, severe coronary obstruction. More than one of these may be operative.

When unstable angina is accompanied by objective ECG evidence of transient myocardial ischemia (ST-segment changes and/or T-wave inversions during episodes of chest pain), it is associated with critical stenoses in one or more major epicardial coronary arteries in about 85% of cases.

R**TREATMENT** The management of unstable angina is outlined in Fig. 244-3. The patient is admitted to the hospital, placed at rest, sedated, and reassured. In all instances, concomitant conditions that can intensify ischemia, such as tachycardia, hypertension, diabetes mellitus, cardiomegaly, heart failure, arrhythmias, thyrotoxicosis, and any acute febrile illness, should be sought and vigorously treated. Acute myocardial infarction should be ruled out by means of serial ECGs and measurements of plasma cardiac enzyme activity.

Continuous ECG monitoring should be carried out. Since thrombus formation frequently complicates this condition, intravenous heparin should be given for 3 to 5 days to maintain the partial thrombo-

plastin time at 2 to 2.5 times control, together with or followed by oral aspirin at a dose of 325 mg/d. Alternatively, low-molecular-weight heparin (e.g., enoxaparin, 1 mg/kg subcutaneously b.i.d.) may be used. High-risk unstable angina patients, i.e., those with rest pain, and ST-segment deviations and/or release of a marker of myocardial injury (such as troponin I or T) should also receive an intravenous infusion of a platelet GpIIb/IIIa inhibitor. A beta blocker should be administered and a calcium antagonist added if ischemia persists despite the aforementioned therapy, but with caution and an awareness of the possible side effects discussed above. Dosages of these agents should be raised rapidly, but the patient must be observed carefully to avoid bradycardia, heart failure, and hypotension. Nitroglycerin should be given by the sublingual route as needed for symptoms. Intravenous nitroglycerin is quite effective, especially in patients with episodes of ischemia that are particularly severe or prolonged. It is begun at a dosage of 10 μg/min and is raised in 5 μg/min increments to a level at which chest pain is abolished but systolic arterial pressure is maintained or reduced only slightly and other side effects are avoided. After initial stabilization, either an early invasive strategy (coronary angiography and revascularization) or early conservative strategy (continued medical therapy) can be pursued (Fig. 244-3).

The majority of patients (approximately 80%) improve with rest and medical treatment over a 48-h period. If angina at rest and/or ECG evidence of ischemia persist despite 24 to 48 h of the comprehensive treatment described above, then cardiac catheterization and coronary arteriography should be performed in patients with no obvious contraindications for revascularization. If the anatomy is suitable, PCI can be performed. If the coronary anatomy is not suitable for PCI, CABG should be considered to relieve symptoms and myocardial ischemia and as a means of preventing myocardial damage. The factors that influence the choice between catheter-based and surgical revascularization are similar to those in chronic stable angina.

In the early conservative strategy, if the patient's symptoms and signs are controlled on medical therapy, a diagnostic exercise ECG or perfusion scan or, if exercise is not possible, a pharmacologic stress test (p. 1402) should be carried out near the time of hospital discharge. If there is evidence of severe myocardial ischemia and/or evidence of a high risk of coronary events (p. 1402), consideration should be given to catheterization and, depending on the findings, revascularization. Following discharge, patients with unstable angina should be managed similar to chronic angina patients (p. 1404). Severe obstructive CAD is often present in patients with unstable angina who respond to medical therapy. Many patients in whom the unstable state is controlled are left with severe chronic stable angina and ultimately require mechanical revascularization.

PRINZMETAL'S VARIANT ANGINA This relatively uncommon form of unstable angina is characterized by recurrent, prolonged attacks of severe ischemia, caused by episodic focal spasm of an epicardial coronary artery. Approximately three-fourths of patients with Prinzmetal's angina exhibit a mild or moderately severe fixed obstruction (with a luminal diameter 50 to 70% of normal) within 1 cm of the site of spasm. Patients with this condition are often smokers and are younger than patients with unstable angina secondary to coronary atherosclerosis. Ischemic pain usually occurs at rest, sometimes awakens the patient from sleep, and is characterized by multilead ST-segment elevation. The diagnosis may be confirmed by detecting transient spasm occurring spontaneously or following a provocative stimulus (intracoronary acetylcholine, hyperventilation) on coronary arteriography. While long-term survival is excellent, complications include episodes of disabling pain, myocardial infarction, serious ventricular arrhythmias, atrioventricular block, and, rarely, sudden death.

R**TREATMENT** Management of the acute attack consists of multiple doses of sublingual nitroglycerin, an intravenous infusion of nitroglycerin, and short-acting nifedipine (10 to 30 mg); hypotension should be avoided. In chronic management, long-acting nitrates and calcium antagonists are useful. Beta blockers are of little value, while prazosin, a selective alpha-adrenoceptor blocker, may be useful. Occasionally, mechanical revascularization is helpful in patients with accompanying severe discrete obstructive lesions.

ASYMPTOMATIC (SILENT) ISCHEMIA

Obstructive CAD, acute myocardial infarction, and transient myocardial ischemia are frequently asymptomatic. During continuous ambulatory ECG monitoring, the majority of ambulatory patients with typical chronic stable angina are found to have objective evidence of myocardial ischemia (ST-segment depression) during episodes of chest discomfort while they are active outside the hospital, but many of these patients also appear to have more frequent episodes of asymptomatic ischemia. In addition, there is a large (but as yet unknown) number of totally asymptomatic people with severe coronary atherosclerosis who exhibit ST-segment changes during activity. Some of these patients exhibit higher thresholds to electrically induced pain, others show higher endorphin levels, and still others may be diabetic patients with autonomic dysfunction.

Evidence of frequent episodes of ischemia (symptomatic and asymptomatic) during daily life appears to indicate an increased likelihood of adverse coronary events such as death and myocardial infarction. The widespread use of exercise ECG during routine examinations has also defined some of these heretofore unrecognized patients with asymptomatic CAD. Longitudinal studies have demonstrated an increased incidence of coronary events (sudden death, myocardial infarction, and angina) in asymptomatic patients with positive exercise tests. In addition, patients with asymptomatic ischemia after suffering a myocardial infarction are at greater risk for a second coronary event.

℞ TREATMENT The management of patients with asymptomatic ischemia must be individualized. Thus, the physician should consider the following: (1) the degree of positivity of the stress test, particularly the stage of exercise at which ECG signs of ischemia appear, the magnitude and number of the perfusion defect(s) on thallium scintigraphy, and the change in left ventricular ejection fraction which occurs on radionuclide ventriculography or echocardiography during ischemia and/or during exercise; (2) the ECG leads showing a positive response, with changes in the anterior precordial leads indicating a less favorable prognosis than changes in the inferior leads; and (3) the patient's age, occupation, and general medical condition. Most would agree that an asymptomatic 45-year-old commercial airline pilot with 0.4-mV ST-segment depression in leads V_1 to V_4 during mild exercise should undergo coronary arteriography, whereas the asymptomatic, sedentary 75-year-old retiree with 0.1-mV ST-segment depression in leads II and III during maximal activity need not. However, there is no consensus about the appropriate procedure in the large majority of patients for whom the situation is less extreme. Patients with evidence of severe ischemia on noninvasive testing (as outlined

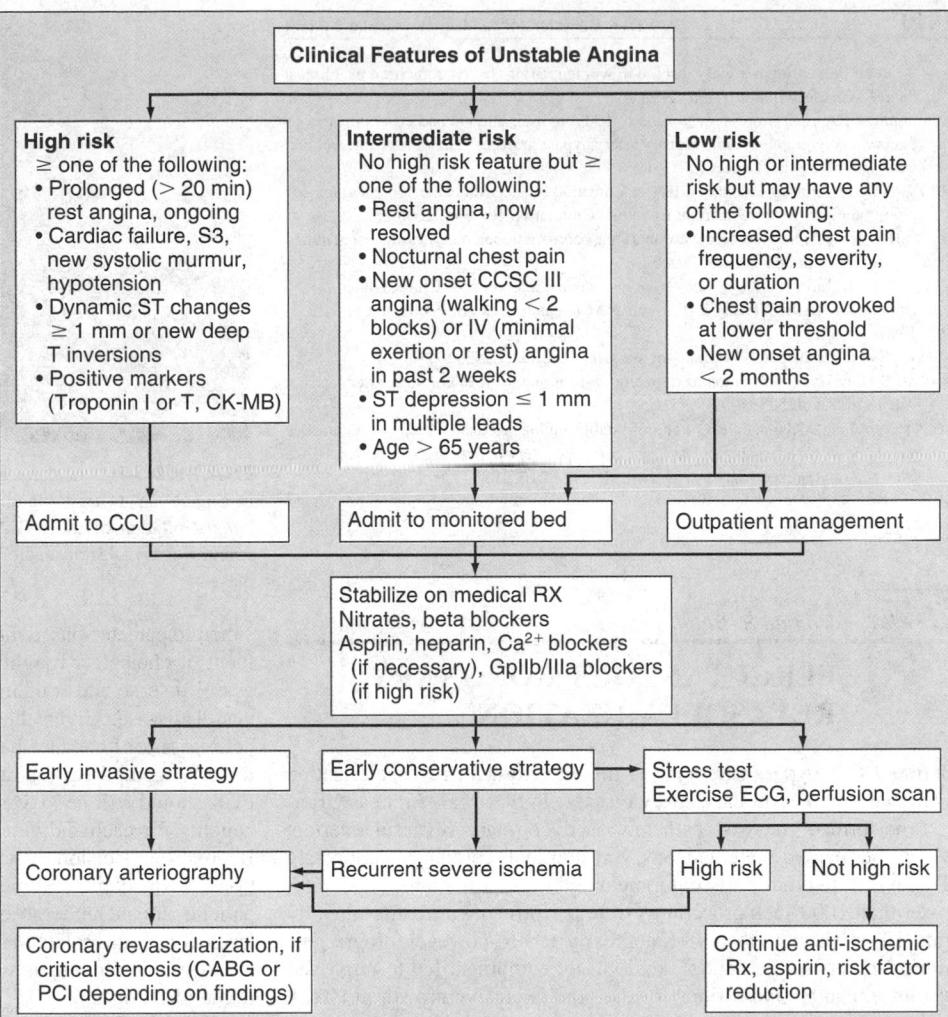

FIGURE 244-3 Management algorithm for unstable angina. CCSC, Canadian Cardiovascular Society classification; CCU, coronary care unit; CABG, coronary artery bypass grafting; PCI, percutaneous coronary intervention. *(Modified from Braunwald et al.)*

earlier) should undergo coronary arteriography. Asymptomatic patients with silent ischemia, three-vessel CAD, and impaired left ventricular function may be considered appropriate candidates for CABG.

The treatment of risk factors, particularly lipid lowering as described above, as well as the use of aspirin and beta blockers have been shown to reduce events and improve outcomes in asymptomatic as well as symptomatic patients with ischemia and proven CAD. While the incidence of asymptomatic ischemia can be reduced by treatment with beta blockers, calcium channel antagonists, and long-acting nitrates, it is not clear whether this is necessary or desirable in patients who have not suffered a myocardial infarction. However, there is evidence that beta-adrenoceptor blockade begun 7 to 35 days after acute myocardial infarction improves survival (Chap. 243).

BIBLIOGRAPHY

BRAUNWALD E et al: Diagnosing and managing unstable angina. Circulation 90:613, 1994

CAIRNS JA et al: Antithrombotic agents in coronary artery disease. Chest 114:61S, 1998

CREAGER MA et al: Results of the CAPTURE trial. Clopidogrel versus aspirin in patients at risk of ischemic events. Vasc Med 3:257, 1998

FARMER JA et al: Aggressive lipid therapy in the statin era. Prog Cardiovasc Dis 41:71, 1998

FAVOLARO RG et al: Landmarks in the development of coronary artery bypass surgery. Circulation 98:466, 1998

GERSH BJ et al: Chronic ischemic heart disease, in *Heart Disease*, 6th ed, E Braunwald et al (eds). Philadelphia, Saunders, 2001

GOTTO AM Jr et al: Risk factor modification: Rationale for management of dyslipidemia. Am J Med 104:6S, 1998

———— et al: Preventing coronary disease in women: Brief observations from the clinical data. J Women's Health 7:195, 1998

HENDERSON RA et al: Long-term results of RITA-1 trial, clinical and cost comparisons of coronary angioplasty and coronary artery bypass grafting. Randomized intervention treatment of angina. Lancet 352:1419, 1998

HE ZX et al: Severity of coronary artery calcification by electron beam computed tomography predicts silent myocardial ischemia. Circulation 101:244, 2000

HEUSCH G et al: Alpha-adrenergic coronary vasoconstriction and myocardial ischemia in humans. Circulation 101:689, 2000

KING SB et al: Balloon angioplasty versus new device intervention: Clinical outcomes. A comparison of the NHLBI PTCA and NACI registries. J Am Coll Cardiol 31:558, 1998

MAYER S et al: Prinzmetal's variant angina. Clin Cardiol 21:243, 1998

NAKAO S et al: Hyperventilation as a specific test for diagnosis of coronary artery spasm. Am J Cardiol 80:545, 1997

SOLOMON AJ et al: Management of chronic stable angina: Medical therapy, percutaneous transluminal coronary angioplasty, and coronary artery bypass graft surgery. Lessons from the randomized trials. Ann Intern Med 128:216, 1998

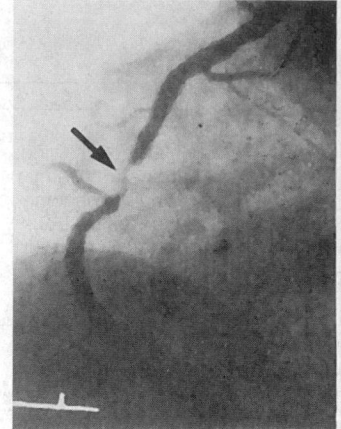
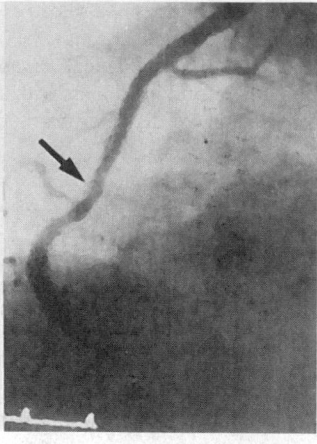

FIGURE 245-1   Focal discrete stenosis of the mid-right coronary angioplasty in a patient with unstable angina, shown before (*left panel*) and after (*right panel*) inflation of the PTCA balloon catheter. The lesion is typical of the straightforward lesion anatomy treated by early (pre-1985) coronary angioplasty.

245   *Donald S. Baim*

PERCUTANEOUS CORONARY REVASCULARIZATION

Before 1977, bypass surgery was the only form of revascularization available to treat coronary artery disease. In that year, Andreas Gruntzig performed the first catheter-based coronary revascularization, which he named percutaneous transluminal coronary angioplasty (PTCA). With crude early equipment and limited anatomic capability, fewer than 1000 such procedures were performed worldwide annually until 1981. Through the 1980s and early 1990s, however, progressive improvements in the balloon angioplasty equipment led to improved results, expanded indications for use, and explosive growth in PTCA to the point that in the United States, the annual number of procedures (~300,000) roughly matched the number of surgical bypass operations. This growth has been sustained during the late 1990s with the introduction of a number of newer devices (including stents and atherectomy devices) that further improved the acute success and safety as well as the long-term durability of what is now known more broadly as percutaneous coronary revascularization (PCR) or intervention (PCI). The current annual number of PCRs (~600,000) is thus now greater than the number of coronary bypass operations (~400,000). The dominant role that catheter-based intervention has assumed in the treatment of coronary artery disease has led to definition of the field known as *interventional cardiology*, which now has its own fellowship requirements and Board certification of additional qualifications based on training (a specialized interventional cardiology fellowship beyond basic cardiology training), ongoing experience (75 procedures per year), and a written examination.

All catheter-based coronary interventions are derivatives of diagnostic cardiac catheterization (Chap. 228), in which catheters are introduced into the arterial circulation by needle puncture, advanced into the heart under fluoroscopic guidance, and used for pressure measurements or injections of radio-opaque liquid contrast agents. Interventional procedures differ in that the catheter placed into the ostium of the narrowed coronary artery has a slightly larger diameter, and its lumen is used to convey a flexible, steerable guidewire (diameter <0.5 mm) down the coronary artery lumen, through the narrowing, and into the vessel beyond. This guidewire then serves as the rail over which angioplasty balloons or other therapeutic devices are run to enlarge the narrowed segment of coronary artery (Fig. 245-1). Because PCR is performed with local anesthesia and requires only a short (1- to 2-day) hospitalization, its use in suitable patients can greatly decrease expense and recovery time compared to those associated with coronary bypass surgery. Not all types of coronary narrowing are well

suited to catheter-based intervention, but such intervention is the treatment of choice for roughly 70% of patients with symptomatic single vessel disease and roughly 20% of patients with symptomatic three-vessel disease. Given these anatomic restrictions and the small but definite risk of catheter-based intervention (elective mortality rate 0.4 to 1.0%, compared to a rate of 1 to 3% for elective surgical bypass), PCR should still be viewed as an invasive procedure whose risks and benefits for each individual patient need to be weighed before use. Beyond the decision of which patients should undergo revascularization (versus continued medical management), the selection of which patients should undergo catheter-based rather than surgical revascularization requires detailed understanding of both clinical and coronary angiographic factors, as well as the applicability of various interventional techniques.

INDICATIONS   The main indication for PCR remains the presence of one or more coronary stenoses that are approachable by catheter-based techniques and are thought to be responsible for a clinical syndrome that warrants revascularization. Moreover, the risks and benefits of revascularization by PCR should compare favorably with those of surgery. In patients with significant narrowing of a single coronary artery, the main benefit of revascularization lies in relief of anginal symptoms rather than in increasing their already good prognosis with medical therapy. By contrast, for the patient with significant left main stenosis or multivessel disease, revascularization may both relieve angina *and* improve long-term survival. Most patients with multivessel coronary disease, however, currently undergo surgical rather than catheter-based revascularization, particularly when one or more vessels supplying significant areas of viable myocardium are not well-suited to PCR (owing to chronic total occlusion or other unfavorable anatomic features). In patients for whom either PCR or bypass surgery is a possible treatment for multivessel coronary artery disease, a number of randomized trials have suggested that the two procedures have equivalent in-hospital and 3- to 5-year mortality rates, but that more patients undergoing PCR (40 to 50% versus 7 to 10% surgical patients) will require a second revascularization procedure (generally a repeat PCR to treat restenosis) by 5 years to maintain an equivalent level of symptom relief. One exception may be diabetic patients with multivessel coronary artery disease, for whom some studies have suggested better survival with surgical treatment than with PCR.

The clinical indications for PCR cover the spectrum from patients with unstable angina or acute infarction to patients with silent ischemia, as summarized in the 1999 guidelines. For most patients, PCR is used to treat anatomically approachable lesions that are responsible for the clinical syndrome of *moderately severe, chronic, stable angina*, which persists despite medical antianginal therapy (Chap. 244). Approximately 15% of current patients undergoing PCR, however, have only mild anginal symptoms despite suitable coronary anatomy but have objective evidence of ischemia on noninvasive testing (i.e., an abnormal exercise test). At the other extreme, many patients have more pressing indications for revascularization, including unstable angina or even acute myocardial infarction (with or without prior thrombolytic therapy). An aggressive approach to the treatment of unstable angina involving initial stabilization with beta blockers, nitrates, heparin, and antiplatelet agents (aspirin and frequently a platelet glycoprotein IIb/IIIa receptor blocker), followed by diagnostic catheterization and same-procedure PCR of the underlying blockage, offers the patient a more rapid return to work, fewer readmissions and late revascularizations, and potentially a reduction in late events compared to prolonged initial trials of medical therapy before proceeding with invasive evaluation and treatment.

In the early 1980s the introduction of intravenous fibrinolytic agents to reopen the occluded infarct-related vessel was a major advance in the treatment of acute myocardial infarction (Chap. 243). It seemed reasonable that PCR might further improve the results of thrombolytic therapy by treating the underlying atherosclerotic stenosis, opening those arteries that failed to reperfuse with a thrombolytic alone and preventing the 10 to 20% incidence of in-hospital reocclusion that occurs after even successful thrombolysis. Randomized trials, however, showed that none of the routine PCR strategies tested after thrombolytic administration improved the outcome more than a "watchful waiting" strategy in which PCR was reserved for patients with spontaneous or exercise-induced ischemia. In contrast, there is evidence that *primary* or direct angioplasty (used instead of thrombolytic therapy) can reduce the in-hospital mortality rate (from roughly 7 to 4%) when performed promptly by a skilled operator (Fig. 245-2). Another advantage of PCR is that it can be performed even in the approximately 30% of patients with acute myocardial infarction with contraindications to thrombolytic therapy.

As the clinical indications for PCR have broadened, so have its anatomic capabilities. PCR thus is no longer restricted to proximal, discrete, subtotal, concentric, noncalcified lesions, as was the case initially. Calcified, complex, or diffuse disease lesions respond well to coronary stent placement, sometimes after pretreatment with rotational atherectomy. Even totally occluded coronary arteries (particularly ones that have been occluded for less than 6 months) can be crossed and dilated effectively, although the success rate remains somewhat lower than for subtotal lesions (60% versus 90% for subtotal stenotic lesions). In addition to lesions in the native coronary tree, obstructions in saphenous vein (Fig. 245-3) or internal mammary artery bypass grafts also can be dilated successfully to treat postbypass angina. If multiple lesions are responsible for the clinical syndrome, they generally can be dilated during a single procedure.

RESULTS The success rate for PCR exceeds 95% for dilating a target lesion so that its residual diameter stenosis is <50% (<30% when a stent has been used), without producing an associated complication. About half of the failures result from inability to cross the target lesion with the guidewire or balloon catheter, particularly when that target lesion is a chronic total occlusion. With balloon dilatation alone, some local dissection is present in virtually all successful procedures. Before the introduction of stent technology (see below), more extensive dissection (particularly in association with local thrombus formation or vasospasm) led to abrupt closure of the dilated segment soon after withdrawal of the balloon catheter, and necessitated emergency bypass surgery in approximately 3% of angioplasty attempts. However, such dissections are now routinely treated by stent placement, reducing the incidence of emergency bypass surgery to <1%. Other than dissection, the main hazards of PCR concern spasm, thrombosis, and perforation.

Coronary spasm is controlled by the routine use of vasodilators (nitrates and calcium channel antagonists), whereas thrombosis is con-

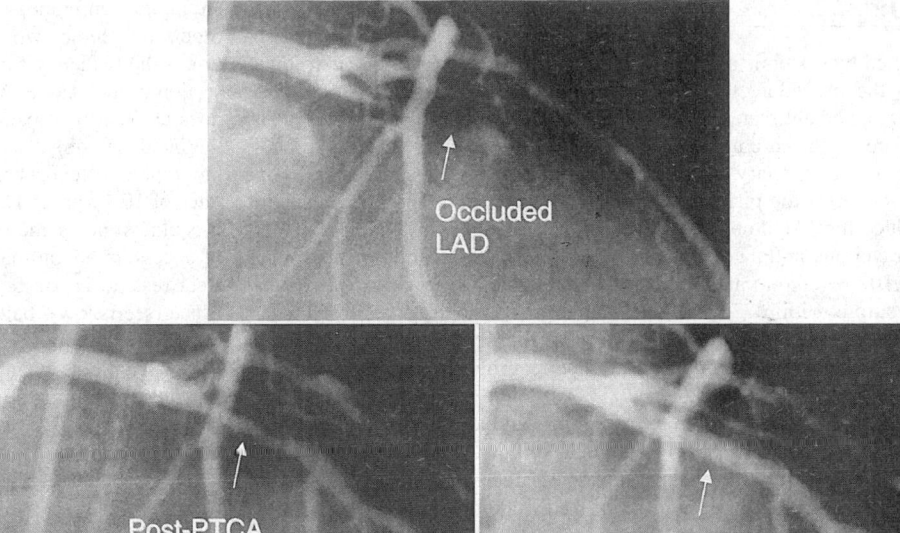

FIGURE 245-2 Left coronary angiogram in a patient with acute anterior myocardial infarction and cardiogenic shock shows occlusion of the proximal left anterior descending coronary artery (*top panel, arrow*) with only faint filling beyond the obstructing thrombus. After initial PTCA (*lower left panel*), there is restored antegrade flow with residual stenosis. After stent placement (*lower right panel*), there is no residual stenosis and brisk flow. This improvement was associated with reversal of shock hemodynamics, including normalization of severe lactic acidosis.

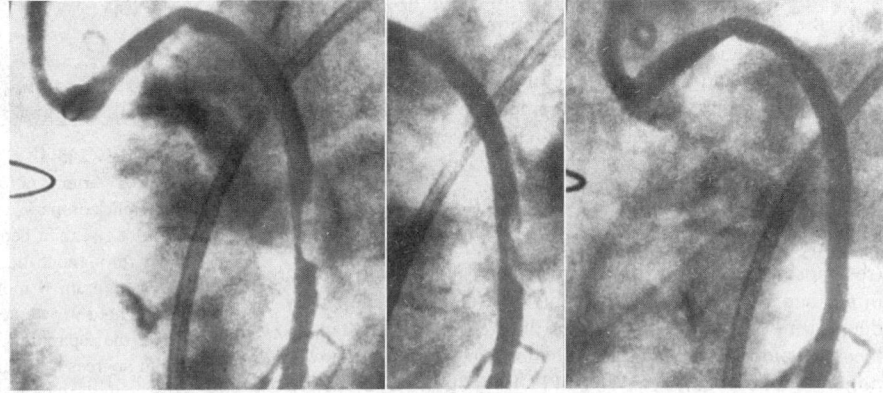

FIGURE 245-3 Stent placement in a diseased saphenous vein graft. *Left*: Severe eccentric stenosis in an 8-year-old saphenous vein graft to the left anterior descending coronary artery. *Middle*: After balloon angioplasty, the lumen remains stenotic due to elastic recoil of the vessel wall and disruption (dissection) of the plaque. *Right*: After placement of a coronary stent, both recoil and dissection have been overcome, providing a large smooth lumen.

trolled by systemic anticoagulation (heparin, 7000 to 10,000 units during the procedure to maintain an activated clotting time of 250 to 300 s), and antiplatelet therapy (aspirin, 325 mg/d starting at least 24 h before PCR and continued for at least 3 to 6 months after the procedure). If a coronary stent has been placed, aspirin is supplemented by a blocker of the platelet ADP receptor (ticlopidine or clopidogrel) to reduce the likelihood of stent thrombosis (see below). Newer potent intravenous antiplatelet agents (blockers of the platelet glycoprotein IIb/IIIa receptors) may reduce further the incidence of ischemic complications within 72 h of PCR, and are used prophylactically in what are perceived to be high-risk interventions or provisionally in interventions that have left behind an imperfect mechanical result (e.g., an unstented distal dissection).

Perforation of a coronary artery was an extremely rare complication of conventional balloon angioplasty but may occur in up to 1% of patients undergoing more aggressive atherectomy procedures (see below). Even small perforations of the distal vessel by the angioplasty guidewire may lead to significant hemopericardium requiring urgent pericardiocentesis in the setting of intense anticoagulant and antiplatelet therapy. Finally, catheter-based interventions are subject to all of the complications of diagnostic catheterization, including adverse reactions to iodinated contrast agents and groin hematoma. By and large, however, catheter-based coronary revascularization has reached the point of being a safe and effective alternative to surgical revascularization.

FOLLOW-UP   After successful PCR of all "culprit" lesions, marked improvement or complete resolution of the presenting ischemic syndrome should be evident. In approximately 20% of patients, however, evidence of recurrent ischemia develops within 6 months, due to restenosis of the dilated segment. This restenosis appears to result from excessive local fibrointimal proliferation and vessel constriction, occurring in response to the local injury that is part of enlarging the stenotic lumen. When recurrent ischemia develops more than 6 months after PCR, it usually reflects progression of disease at another site, rather than restenosis. Whether due to restenosis or disease progression, most post-PCR problems can be treated by repeat PCR, so that only about 10% of patients require bypass surgery during the 5 years after a successful procedure. When a patient has provided evidence of severe obstructive coronary atherosclerosis requiring revascularization, either by bypass surgery or PCR, the opportunity to implement an aggressive program to reduce atherosclerotic risk factors and thereby slow the pace of development of new lesions should not be overlooked (Chap. 244).

NONBALLOON TECHNIQUES   Conventional balloon angioplasty (PTCA) was the only catheter-based coronary revascularization technique that was widely available before 1990. Although it offered anatomic versatility and acceptable short- and long-term results, the difficulty of using this technique for certain anatomic lesion types (e.g., calcified eccentric, ostial, thrombus-containing, or bifurcation lesions) and the persistence of problems such as abrupt closure and restenosis fostered the development of a number of newer, nonballoon techniques that include stent placement and atherectomy. These treatments moved from clinical investigation to routine clinical practice during the early 1990s and now account for 70 to 80% of percutaneous coronary interventions. Used appropriately, these new techniques have improved the success, safety, and long-term results (restenosis rate) in most lesion types. Most of these procedures cost more than PTCA, but much of this cost can be recouped by the reduction in long-term expenses for the treatment of restenosis. Given these developments, stand-alone balloon angioplasty is now used in a minority of procedures (20% of all PCRs), although adjunctive balloon angioplasty is still routinely used to pre- or postdilate, before or after a newer interventional device.

STENTS   Stents are metallic scaffolds that are inserted into a diseased vessel segment in their collapsed form and are then expanded (by balloon expansion, or by self-expansion after removal of a con-

straining membrane) to establish a normal-appearing vessel lumen. Stents overcome two of the principal limitations of balloon dilatation—the tendency for elastic recoil of the vessel wall and local dissection of the plaque. As such, stents provide a larger acute lumen than does conventional balloon angioplasty, which allows them to reduce the incidence of subsequent restenosis by roughly one-third (e.g., angiographic restenosis rates of 20% versus 33%, and clinical restenosis rates of 10% versus 16 to 20%). When in-stent restenosis does occur, it is almost never the result of stent crush but rather the consequence of excessive neointimal hyperplasia within the stent (Fig. 245-4). In-stent restenosis can be treated by atherectomy to remove the excess tissue (see below), balloon dilatation, and then local delivery of β or γ radiation to suppress neointimal regrowth.

Two balloon-expandable stent designs were approved by the Food and Drug Administration (FDA) in the early 1990s—a wire coil design for use in stabilizing actual or threatened abrupt closure and a slotted tube design for elective treatment of native coronary lesions. After their release, the efficacy of the slotted tube design was demonstrated in a variety of other circumstances, including restenotic lesions and saphenous vein grafts (Fig. 245-3). In the late 1990s, a number of second generation stent designs were developed that offer easier delivery to tortuous or distal lesions as well as a wider variety of sizes and lengths. The approval of these devices has allowed them to completely replace the first generation devices in clinical practice (Fig. 245-5). Still further refinements in stent coverings (to seal aneurysms or perforations) and coatings (to suppress stent thrombosis and in-stent proliferation) are in progress.

Early experience suggested that metallic stents were prone to thrombotic occlusion, either acute (<24 h) or subacute (1 to 14 days with a peak at 6 days), and that an aggressive anticoagulation regimen (aspirin, dipyridamole, and warfarin) was needed to prevent such thrombosis. This aggressive anticoagulant regimen reduced the incidence of stent thrombosis to ~3% but led to longer hospitalization and an increased incidence of local vascular complications at the femoral arterial entry site. Subsequent data suggested that many of these thrombotic complications were the result of incomplete stent expansion and that more attention to full initial deployment would allow the same stents to be used with only antiplatelet drugs (aspirin plus the platelet ADP-receptor blockers, ticlopidine or clopidogrel) with more

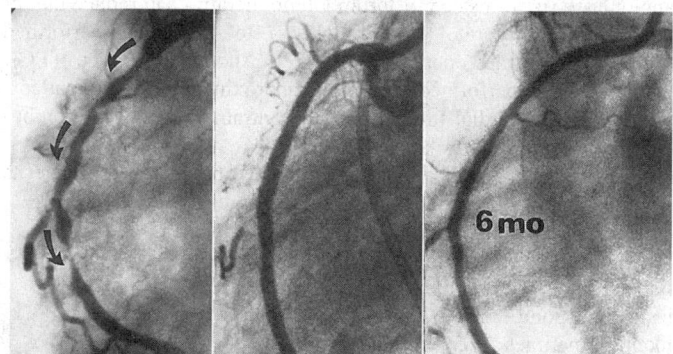

FIGURE 245-4   Short- and long-term results in a long lesion in the right coronary artery. *Left*: A long (~50 mm) area of disease (*arrows*) is present in the right coronary artery. *Right center*: Contrast injection after placement of two long second generation stents (25 and 35 mm long) shows excellent patency throughout the proximal- and mid-portions of the vessel. *Right*: Follow-up angiogram 6 months after stent placement shows mild lumen reduction throughout the stented segment due to neointimal hyperplasia within the stent (note the separation between the stent shadows and the contrast-filled lumen. Mild degrees of proliferative narrowing are benign and common within stents (particularly long stents such as this one). Had the degree of lumen reduction been greater and associated with recurrent symptoms or an abnormal exercise test, however, re-intervention would have been performed with a debulking technique (e.g., rotational atherectomy) followed by balloon angioplasty, and possibly local radiation delivery (brachytherapy) to inhibit excessive tissue regrowth.

acceptable thrombosis and vascular complication rates (each <1%). This rapid evolution in devices, concomitant medications, and indications has led to the dominance of stent placement in catheter-based coronary revascularization, with placement of one or more stents in 70 to 80% of all procedures.

Atherectomy Whereas both balloon angioplasty and stent placement enlarge the coronary lumen by displacing plaque, atherectomy catheters enlarge the lumen by removing plaque mass from the treated lesion. Directional atherectomy achieves this result by use of a special catheter with a windowed steel cylinder at its tip. Inflation of a low-pressure positioning balloon on the back of the cylinder presses plaque into the window, where it is cut and trapped by a spinning cup-shaped cutter. This device was the first (1990) approved nonballoon technology to reach clinical practice, and it is still the treatment of choice for noncalcified lesions at the origin of the left anterior descending artery or at major coronary bifurcations (Fig. 245-6). Although its efficacy over conventional balloon angioplasty has been demonstrated, the ease and result of stent placement are much greater for most other lesion types. Rotational atherectomy uses burrs of various sizes (diameter 1.25 to 2.50 mm) that are coated on their leading half with small diamond chips. The burr is spun at 140,000 to 160,000 rpm as it is advanced through a coronary lesion over a leading guidewire. As the burr is advanced, the diamond chips grind through the obstructing plaque, and pulverize it into small (5 to 25 μm) particles, which pass through the distal coronary microcirculation. This device has emerged as an effective treatment for long (>20 mm), calcified, ostial lesions or in-stent restenotic lesions, frequently followed by balloon dilation or stent placement. *Extraction* atherectomy uses a combination of distal cutting blades rotating at low speed and continuous vacuum aspiration to remove coronary obstructions. The device has limited cutting efficiency, and its use is now confined to softer lesions (e.g., atherosclerotic saphenous vein grafts) or thrombotic lesions. Newer aspiration devices based on the Bernoulli principle appear better able to remove clot and cause less vessel disruption.

Although it is not mechanical, laser light [at wavelengths from the ultraviolet (308 mm) to the midinfrared (2000 μm)] can be delivered to obstructing coronary plaques through bundles of small optical fibers housed in flexible catheters whose outer diameter is between 1.2 and 2.0 mm. When these catheters are pulsed with laser energy as they are advanced through a coronary obstruction over a guidewire, they can ablate noncalcified coronary plaque by a combination of photoacoustic (blast), thermal, and photochemical effects. Although lasers have been used to treat ostial as well as diffuse coronary lesions, acceptance of the technique has been limited by the expense of the device and the fact that these lesions can be treated by other techniques, such as rotational atherectomy.

SUMMARY With the development of new techniques such as stent placement and atherectomy, new drug regimens, and a preponderance of "evidence-based" practices, over the last 20 years catheter-based revascularization (PCR) has developed from a procedural curiosity to one of the mainstays of coronary revascularization. As short- and long-term results have improved and the number of procedures has continued to grow, the pace of development, if anything, has intensified.

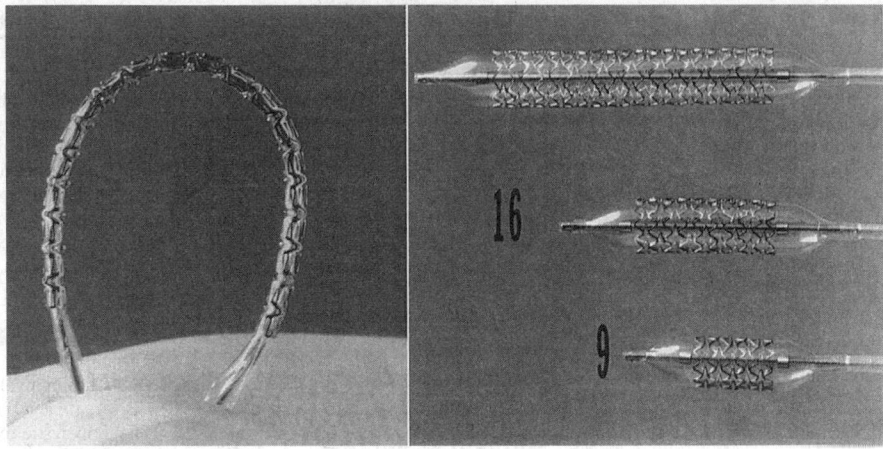

FIGURE 245-5 Second generation stent. *Left*: The flexibility typical of second generation stents is shown in bending the collapsed stent on its delivery balloon. *Right*: The same stent design is shown in its balloon-expanded configuration, in some of the available lengths [32 mm (top), 16 mm, and 9 mm]. The availability of a variety of second generation stents since 1997 has helped make stent placement a part of more than 70% of all PCRs.

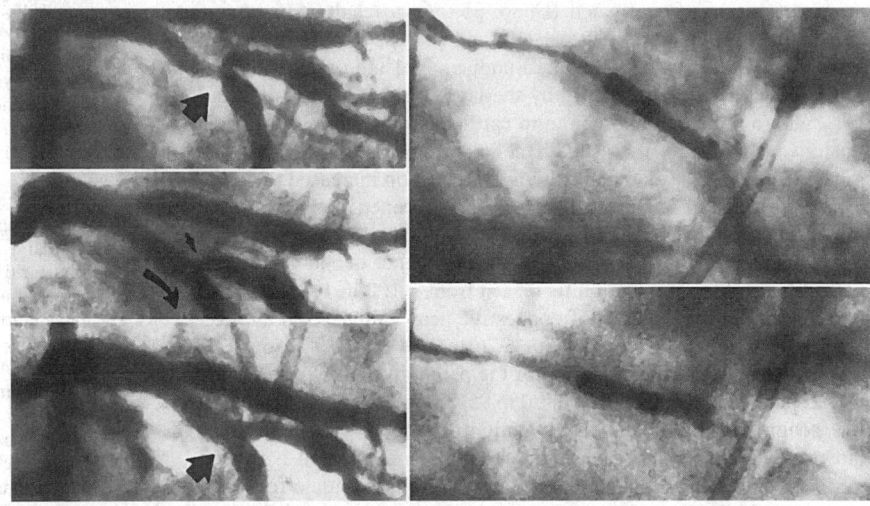

FIGURE 245-6 Treatment of a bifurcation lesion in the circumflex coronary artery. *Upper left*: Stenosis (*arrow*) involves both the main circumflex and a large marginal branch. *Upper right*: Directional atherectomy as performed in the main circumflex. *Middle left*: Interim result after atherectomy in the main circumflex shows resolution of stenosis in that vessel (*curved arrow*) but persistent stenosis in the marginal branch (*small arrow*). *Lower right*: Additional atherectomy cuts are made in the marginal branch. *Lower left*: The final result (*arrow*) shows no residual stenosis in either the main circumflex or the marginal branch.

BIBLIOGRAPHY

BAIM DS: Coronary angioplasty, in *Cardiac Catheterization, Angiography and Intervention*, 6th ed, D Baim, W Grossman (eds). Baltimore, Lippincott, Williams & Wilkins, 2000

CARROZZA JP et al: Coronary intervention: Angioplasty, stents, and atherectomy, in *Evidence Based Cardiology*, S Yusuf et al (eds). London, BMJ Books, 1998

DETRE KM et al: Coronary revascularization in diabetic patients—a comparison of the randomized and observational components of the Bypass Angioplasty Revascularization Investigation (BARI). Circulation 99:633, 1999

FISCHMAN DL et al: A randomized comparison of coronary stent placement and balloon angioplasty in the treatment of coronary artery disease. N Engl J Med 331:496, 1994

GIBBONS RJ et al: ACC/AHA/ACP-ASIM guidelines for the management of patients with chronic stable angina—executive summary and recommendations. Circulation 99: 2829, 1999

HIRSHFELD JW et al: Recommendations for the assessment and maintenance of proficiency in coronary interventional procedures. J Am Coll Cardiol 31:722, 1998

KONG DF et al: Outcomes of therapeutic agents that block the platelet glycoprotein IIb/IIIa integrin in ischemic heart disease. Circulation 98:2829, 1998

KUNTZ RE, BAIM DS: Defining coronary restenosis: Newer clinical and angiographic
    paradigms. Circulation 88:1310, 1993
LEON MB et al: A randomized trial comparing three anti-thrombotic drug regimens fol-
    lowing coronary-artery stenting. N Engl J Med 339:1665, 1998
POPMA J: Interventional cardiology, in *Heart Disease*, 6th ed, E Braunwald, D Zipes, P
    Libby (eds). Philadelphia, Saunders, 2001
WEAVER WD et al: Comparison of primary coronary angioplasty and intravenous throm-
    bolytic therapy for acute myocardial infarction—a quantitative review. JAMA 278:
    2093, 1997

246 *Gordon H. Williams*

HYPERTENSIVE VASCULAR DISEASE

An elevated arterial pressure is probably the most important public
health problem in developed countries. It is common, asymptomatic,
readily detectable, usually easily treatable, and often leads to lethal
complications if left untreated (Chap. 35). As a result of extensive
educational programs in the late 1960s and 1970s by both private and
government agencies, the number of undiagnosed and/or untreated patients was reduced significantly by the late 1980s to a level of about
25%, with a concomitant decline in cardiovascular mortality. Unfortunately, by the mid-1990s, this beneficial trend began to wane. The
number of undiagnosed patients with hypertension increased to nearly
33%, the decline in cardiovascular mortality flattened, and the number
of individuals with chronic diseases with untreated or poorly treated
hypertension increased. For example, the prevalence of end-stage renal
disease per million population increased from <100 in 1982 to >250
in 1995, and the prevalence of congestive heart failure from ages 55
to 75 more than doubled between 1976 to 1980 and 1988 to 1991.
Thus, although our understanding of the pathophysiology of elevated
arterial pressure has increased, in 90 to 95% of cases the etiology (and
thus potentially the means of prevention or cure) is still largely unknown. As a consequence, in most cases the hypertension is treated
nonspecifically, resulting in a large number of minor side effects and
a relatively high (50 to 60%) noncompliance rate.

PREVALENCE The prevalence of hypertension depends on
both the racial composition of the population studied and the criteria
used to define the condition. In a white suburban population like that
in the Framingham Study, nearly one-fifth of individuals have blood
pressures >160/95, while almost one-half have pressures >140/90.
An even higher prevalence has been documented in the nonwhite population. In females the prevalence is closely related to age, with a
substantial increase occurring after age 50. This increase is presumably
related to the hormonal changes of menopause, although the mechanism is unclear. Thus, the ratio of hypertension frequency in women
versus men increases from 0.6 to 0.7 at age 30 to 1.1 to 1.2 at age 65.

The prevalence of various forms of secondary hypertension depends on the nature of the population studied and on how extensive
the evaluation is. There are no available data to define the frequency
of secondary hypertension in the general population, although in middle-aged males it has been reported to be 6%. On the other hand, in
referral centers where patients undergo an extensive evaluation, it has
been reported to be as high as 35%. The various forms of hypertension
are outlined in Table 246-1, and their relative frequencies are given in
Table 246-2.

ESSENTIAL HYPERTENSION

Patients with arterial hypertension and no definable cause are said to
have *primary*, *essential*, or *idiopathic hypertension*. Undoubtedly, the
primary difficulty in uncovering the mechanism(s) responsible for the
hypertension in these patients is attributable to the variety of systems

Table 246-1 Classification of Arterial Hypertension

SYSTOLIC HYPERTENSION WITH WIDE PULSE PRESSURE

I. Decreased compliance of aorta (arteriosclerosis)
II. Increased stroke volume
   A. Aortic regurgitation
   B. Thyrotoxicosis
   C. Hyperkinetic heart syndrome
   D. Fever
   E. Arteriovenous fistula
   F. Patent ductus arteriosus

**SYSTOLIC AND DIASTOLIC HYPERTENSION (INCREASED PERIPHERAL
VASCULAR RESISTANCE)**

I. Renal
   A. Chronic pyelonephritis
   B. Acute and chronic glomerulonephritis
   C. Polycystic renal disease
   D. Renovascular stenosis or renal infarction
   E. Most other severe renal diseases (arteriolar nephrosclerosis, diabetic
      nephropathy, etc.)
   F. Renin-producing tumors
II. Endocrine
   A. Oral contraceptives
   B. Adrenocortical hyperfunction
      1. Cushing's disease and syndrome
      2. Primary hyperaldosteronism
      3. Congenital or hereditary adrenogenital syndromes
         (17α-hydroxylase and 11β-hydroxylase defects)
   C. Pheochromocytoma
   D. Myxedema
   E. Acromegaly
III. Neurogenic
   A. Psychogenic
   B. Diencephalic syndrome
   C. Familial dysautonomia (Riley-Day)
   D. Polyneuritis (acute porphyria, lead poisoning)
   E. Increased intracranial pressure (acute)
   F. Spinal cord section (acute)
IV. Miscellaneous
   A. Coarctation of aorta
   B. Increased intravascular volume (excessive transfusion, polycythemia
      vera)
   C. Polyarteritis nodosa
   D. Hypercalcemia
   E. Medications, e.g., glucocorticoids, cyclosporine
V. Unknown etiology
   A. Essential hypertension (>90% of all cases of hypertension)
   B. Toxemia of pregnancy
   C. Acute intermittent porphyria

**Table 246-2 Prevalence of Various Forms of Hypertension in the
General Population and in Specialized Referral Clinics[a]**

Diagnosis	General Population, %	Specialty Clinic, %
Essential hypertension	92–94	65–85
Renal hypertension:		
Parenchymal	2–3	4–5
Renovascular	1–2	4–16
Endocrine hypertension:		
Primary aldosteronism	0.3	0.5–12
Cushing's syndrome	<0.1	0.2
Pheochromocytoma	<0.1	0.2
Oral contraceptive–induced	0.5–1	1–2
Miscellaneous	0.2	1

[a] Estimates based on a number of reports in the literature.

that are involved in the regulation of arterial pressure—peripheral and/
or central adrenergic, renal, hormonal, and vascular—and to the complexity of the interrelations of these systems. Several abnormalities
have been described in patients with essential hypertension, often with
a claim that one or more of them are primarily responsible for the
hypertension. While it is still uncertain whether these individual ab-

normalities are primary or secondary, varying expressions of a single disease process or reflective of separate disease entities, the accumulating data increasingly support the latter hypothesis. Therefore, just as pneumonia is caused by a variety of infectious agents, even though the clinical picture observed may be similar, so essential hypertension likely has a number of distinct causes. Thus, the distinction between primary and secondary hypertension has become blurred, and the approach to both the diagnosis and therapy of hypertensive patients has been modified. For example, when a group of patients with essential hypertension is separated into a distinct subset (e.g., low-renin essential hypertension), the patients have not been reclassified as having a form of secondary hypertension but rather remain in the essential hypertensive group. In this chapter, individuals in whom a specific structural organ or gene defect is responsible for hypertension are defined as having a *secondary* form of hypertension. In contrast, individuals in whom generalized or functional abnormalities may be the cause of hypertension, even if the abnormalities are discrete, are defined as having *essential* hypertension.

§ GENETIC CONSIDERATIONS   Genetic factors have long been assumed to be important in the genesis of hypertension. Data supporting this view can be found in animal studies as well as in population studies in humans. One approach has been to assess the correlation of blood pressure in families (familial aggregation). From these studies, the minimum size of the genetic factor can be expressed by a correlation coefficient of approximately 0.2. However, the variation in the size of the genetic factor in different studies reemphasizes the probably heterogeneous nature of the essential hypertensive population. In addition, most studies support the concept that the inheritance is probably multifactorial or that a number of different genetic defects each have an elevated blood pressure as one of their phenotypic expressions. Finally, both monogenic defects (e.g., glucocorticoid-remediable aldosteronism and Liddle's syndrome) and susceptibility genes (e.g., the angiotensinogen and α adducin genes) have now been reported which have as one of their consequences an increased arterial pressure (see below and Chap. 331). Yet, as can be seen in Table 246-3, most studies of likely genes have failed to document linkage

Table 246-3 Genesis Hypothesized to be Involved in Essential Hypertension

Gene	Intermediate Phenotype Used	Association	Linkage
11β Hydroxylase/aldosterone synthase	Urine 18 OH cortisol	Not done	Positive
β Subunit epithelial sodium channel	None	Not done	Positive
Angiotensinogen	Severe, early-onset hypertension	Positive	Positive
Angiotensin-converting enzyme	None	Negative[a]	Negative
Renin	None	Negative	Negative
Angiotensin II AT1 receptor	None	Negative	Negative
Glucocorticoid receptor	Increased plasma cortisol	Positive	Not done
Renal kallikrein	None	Negative	Not done
Endothelin 1	None	Negative	Not done
Insulin receptor	None	Positive	Not done
Human SA locus	None	Positive	Negative
α Adducin	None	Positive	Not done
Endothelial cell adducin	None	Positive	Not done
Endothelial cell NO synthase	None	Positive	Not done
Apoliproprotein C III	None	Positive	Not done
Lipoprotein lipase	None	Positive	Not done

[a] One positive study.
NOTE: OH, hydroxy; NO, nitric oxide.
SOURCE: From GH Williams, NDL Fisher, in E Braunwald (ed): *The Genetics of Human Hypertension in Heart Disease, Update 5.* Philadelphia, Saunders, 1995.

or consistent association with hypertension. However, uncertainty exists as to the validity of these negative conclusions. A positive relationship between hypertension and a gene could be obscured by the high probability of a false-negative result because of the heterogeneity of the hypertensive population. Thus, intermediate phenotypes in the hypertensive population need to be identified to differentiate patients into more homogeneous subgroups; the role of a specific candidate gene can then be more readily assessed. Such an approach is illustrated in Table 246-4. ∎

ENVIRONMENT   A number of environmental factors have been implicated in the development of hypertension, including salt intake, obesity, occupation, alcohol intake, family size, and crowding. These factors have all been assumed to be important in the increase in blood pressure with age in more affluent societies, in contrast to the decline in blood pressure with age in less affluent groups.

SALT SENSITIVITY   The environmental factor that has received the greatest attention is salt intake. Even this factor illustrates the heterogeneous nature of the essential hypertensive population, in that the blood pressure in only approximately 60% of hypertensives is particularly responsive to the level of sodium intake. The cause of this special sensitivity to salt varies, with primary aldosteronism, bilateral renal artery stenosis, renal parenchymal disease, and low-renin essential hypertension accounting for about half the patients. In the remainder, the pathophysiology is still uncertain, but postulated contributing factors include chloride intake, calcium intake, a generalized cellular membrane defect, insulin resistance, and "nonmodulation" (see below).

ROLE OF RENIN   Renin is an enzyme secreted by the juxtaglomerular cell of the kidney and linked with aldosterone in a negative feedback loop (Chap. 331). While a variety of factors can modify its rate of secretion, the primary determinant is the volume status of the individual, particularly as related to changes in dietary sodium intake. The end product of the action of renin on its substrate is the generation of the peptide angiotensin II. The response of target tissues to this peptide is uniquely determined by the prior dietary electrolyte intake. For example, sodium intake normally modulates adrenal and renal vascular responses to angiotensin II. With sodium restriction, adrenal responses are enhanced and the renal vascular responses reduced. Sodium loading has the opposite effect. The range of plasma renin activities observed in hypertensive subjects is broader than in normotensive individuals. In consequence, some hypertensive patients have been defined as having *low-renin* and others as having *high-renin* essential hypertension.

Low-Renin Essential Hypertension   Approximately 20% of patients who by all other criteria have essential hypertension have suppressed plasma renin activity. This situation is more common in individuals of African descent than in white patients. Though these patients are not hypokalemic, they have been reported to have expanded extracellular fluid volumes, and it has been suggested but not proved that they have sodium retention and renin suppression due to excessive production of an unidentified mineralocorticoid. On the other hand, some, but not all, studies have suggested that the adrenal cortex of some of these patients has an increased sensitivity to angi-

Table 246-4 Role of Intermediate Phenotypes in Genetic Analysis

Gene	Phenotype Intermediate	Distant
Converting enzyme ⎫ Angiotensinogen ⎬	Angiotensin II effect on kidney	Increases BP Increases BP
Aldo synthase	Increases 18 OH cortisol	Increases BP
Kallikrein	Decreases urine kallikrein	Increases BP
Na⁺/H⁺ exchanger	Increases Na/Li CTT	Increases BP

NOTE: BP, blood pressure; OH, hydroxy; CTT, countertransport.
SOURCE: From GH Williams, NDL Fisher, in E Braunwald (ed): *The Genetics of Human Hypertension in Heart Disease, Update 5.* Philadelphia, Saunders, 1995.

otensin II as the underlying mechanism. Not only does this hypothesis potentially explain their low plasma renin activity, it also suggests the cause of their hypertension. On a diet with a normal or high sodium content, aldosterone production will not be suppressed normally, leading to a mild degree of hyperaldosteronism with its resulting increased sodium retention, volume expansion, and increase in blood pressure. Since this altered sensitivity has been reported even in patients with normal-renin hypertension, it is likely that patients with low-renin hypertension are not a distinct subset but rather form part of a continuum of patients with essential hypertension.

Nonmodulating Essential Hypertension   Another subset of hypertensive patients has an adrenal defect opposite to that observed in some low-renin patients—a reduced adrenal response to sodium restriction. In these individuals, sodium intake does not modulate either adrenal or renal vascular responses to angiotensin II. Hypertensives in this subset have been termed *nonmodulators* because of the absence of the sodium-mediated modulation of target tissue responses to angiotensin II. These individuals make up 25 to 30% of the hypertensive population, have plasma renin activity levels that are normal to high if measured when the patient is on a low-salt diet, and have hypertension that is salt-sensitive because of a defect in the kidney's ability to excrete sodium appropriately. They also are more insulin-resistant than ohter hypertensive patients, and the pathophysiologic characteristics can be corrected by the administration of a converting-enzyme inhibitor. Furthermore, the nonmodulation characteristic appears to be genetically determined (associated with a certain allele of the angiotensinogen gene). Thus, nonmodulators are probably the most completely characterized intermediate phenotype in the hypertensive population.

High-Renin Essential Hypertension   Approximately 15% of patients with essential hypertension have plasma renin activity levels above the normal range. It has been suggested that plasma renin plays an important role in the pathogenesis of the elevated arterial pressure in these patients. However, most studies have found that saralasin (a substance that, like losartan, acts as a competitive antagonist of angiotensin II) significantly reduces blood pressure in fewer than half of these patients. This finding has led some investigators to postulate that the elevated renin levels and blood pressure may both be secondary to an increase in adrenergic system activity. It has been proposed that, in patients with angiotensin-dependent high-renin hypertension whose arterial pressures are lowered by an angiotensin II antagonist, the mechanism responsible for the increase in renin and, therefore, for the hypertension is the nonmodulating defect.

SODIUM ION VERSUS CHLORIDE OR CALCIUM   Most studies assessing the role of salt in the hypertensive process have assumed that it is the sodium ion that is important. However, some investigators have suggested that the chloride ion may be equally important. This suggestion is based on the observation that feeding chloride-free sodium salts to salt-sensitive hypertensive animals fails to increase arterial pressure. Calcium has also been implicated in the pathogenesis of some forms of essential hypertension. A low-calcium intake has been associated with an increase in blood pressure in epidemiologic studies; an increase in leukocyte cytosolic calcium levels has been reported in some hypertensives. Finally, calcium entry blockers are effective antihypertensive agents. Several studies have reported a potential link between the salt-sensitive forms of hypertension and calcium. It has been postulated that salt loading in combination with a defect in the kidney's ability to excrete salt may lead to a secondary increase in circulating natriuretic factors. One of these factors, the so-called digitalis-like natriuretic factor, inhibits ouabain-sensitive Na^+, K^+-ATPase and thereby leads to intracellular calcium accumulation and a hyperreactive vascular smooth muscle.

CELL MEMBRANE DEFECT   Another postulated explanation for salt-sensitive hypertension is a generalized cell membrane defect. This hypothesis derives most of its data from studies on circulating blood elements, particularly red blood cells, in which abnormalities in the transport of sodium across the cell membrane have

been documented. Since both increases and decreases in the activity of different transport systems have been reported, it is likely that some abnormalities are primary and some are secondary. It has been assumed that this abnormality in sodium transport reflects an undefined alteration in the cell membrane and that this defect occurs in many, perhaps all, cells of the body, particularly the vascular smooth-muscle cells. The defect leads to an abnormal accumulation of calcium in vascular smooth muscle, resulting in a heightened vascular responsiveness to vasoconstrictor agents. This defect has been proposed to be present in 35 to 50% of essential hypertensive persons on the basis of studies using red cells. Other studies suggest that the abnormality in red cell sodium transport is not fixed but can be modified by environmental factors.

The common final pathway in all these hypotheses is an increase in cytosolic calcium resulting in increased vascular reactivity. However, as described above, several mechanisms might produce this calcium accumulation.

INSULIN RESISTANCE   Insulin resistance and/or hyperinsulinemia have been suggested as being responsible for the increased arterial pressure in some patients with hypertension. While it is clear that a substantial fraction of the hypertensive population has insulin resistance and hyperinsulinemia, it is less certain that this is more than an association. Insulin resistance is common in patients with non-insulin-dependent diabetes mellitus (NIDDM) or obesity. Both obesity and NIDDM are more common in hypertensive than in normotensive subjects. However, several studies have found that hyperinsulinemia and insulin resistance are present even in lean hypertensive patients without NIDDM, suggesting that this relationship is more than a coincidence. As noted earlier, these individuals seem to be concentrated in the nonmodulation phenotype.

Hyperinsulinemia can increase arterial pressure by one or more of four mechanisms. An underlying assumption in each case is that some, but not all, of the target tissues of insulin are resistant to its effects. Specifically, tissues involved in glucose homeostasis are resistant (thereby producing the hyperinsulinemia), while tissues involved in the hypertensive process are not. First, hyperinsulinemia produces renal sodium retention (at least acutely) and increases sympathetic activity. Either or both of these effects could lead to an increase in arterial pressure. Another mechanism is vascular smooth-muscle hypertrophy secondary to the mitogenic action of insulin. Third, insulin also modifies ion transport across the cell membrane, thereby potentially increasing the cytosolic calcium levels of insulin-sensitive vascular or renal tissues. This mechanism would increase arterial pressure for reasons similar to those described above for the membrane-defect hypothesis. Finally, insulin resistance may be a marker for another pathologic process, e.g., nonmodulation, which could be the primary mechanism increasing blood pressure. It is important to point out, however, that the role of insulin in controlling arterial pressure is only vaguely understood, and, therefore, its potential as a pathogenic factor in hypertension remains unclear.

Few of the features of hypertension discussed above remain constant in a given patient. Some may be a reflection of the current metabolic and hormonal status of the patient rather than a permanent feature of the disease process. For example, at one point a patient might have insulin resistance secondary to obesity, which could lead to sodium retention, intravascular volume expansion, and renin suppression. This patient would be labeled as having "low-renin essential hypertension." If the patient lost weight, however, the salt-retaining tendency would be reversed. If the blood pressure did not normalize, the patient might then have "normal or high-renin essential hypertension." Thus, the features reviewed above should not be considered mutually exclusive or permanent characteristics in a given patient with hypertension.

FACTORS THAT MODIFY THE COURSE OF ESSENTIAL HYPERTENSION   Age, race, sex, smoking, alcohol intake, serum cholesterol, glucose intolerance, and weight may all alter the prognosis of this disease. The younger the patient when hypertension is first noted, the greater is the reduction in life expectancy if the hypertension is left untreated. In the United States, urban blacks have

Black race
Youth
Male sex
Persistent diastolic pressure >115 mmHg
Smoking
Diabetes mellitus
Hypercholesterolemia
Obesity
Excess alcohol intake
Evidence of end organ damage
  1. Cardiac
     a. Cardiac enlargement
     b. Electrocardiographic signs of ischemia or left ventricular strain
     c. Myocardial infarction
     d. Congestive heart failure
  2. Eyes
     a. Retinal exudates and hemorrhages
     b. Papilledema
  3. Renal: impaired renal function
  4. Nervous system: cerebrovascular accident

about twice the prevalence of hypertension as whites and more than four times the hypertension-induced morbidity rate. At all ages and in both white and nonwhite populations, females with hypertension fare better than males up to the age of 65, and the prevalence of hypertension in premenopausal females is substantially less than that in age-matched males or postmenopausal women. Yet, compared with their normotensive counterparts, females with hypertension run the same relative risk of a morbid cardiovascular event as males do. Accelerated atherosclerosis is an invariable companion of hypertension. Thus, it is not surprising that independent risk factors associated with the development of atherosclerosis, such as an elevated serum cholesterol, glucose intolerance, and/or cigarette smoking, significantly enhance the effect of hypertension on mortality rate regardless of age, sex, or race (Chap. 241). There also is no question that a positive correlation exists between obesity and arterial pressure. A gain in weight is associated with an increased frequency of hypertension in persons with normal blood pressure, and weight loss in obese persons with hypertension lowers their arterial pressure and, if they are being treated for hypertension, the intensity of therapy required to keep them normotensive. Whether these changes are mediated by changes in insulin resistance is unknown.

NATURAL HISTORY Because essential hypertension is a heterogeneous disorder, variables other than the arterial pressure modify its course. Thus, the probability of developing a morbid cardiovascular event with a given arterial pressure may vary as much as 20-fold depending on whether associated risk factors are present (Table 246-5). Although exceptions have been reported, most untreated adults with hypertension will develop further increases in arterial pressure with time. Furthermore, it has been demonstrated from both actuarial data and experience in the era prior to effective therapy that untreated hypertension is associated with a shortening of life by 10 to 20 years, usually related to an acceleration of the atherosclerotic process, with the rate of acceleration in part related to the severity of the hypertension. Even individuals who have relatively mild disease—i.e., without evidence of end organ damage—that is left untreated for 7 to 10 years have a high risk of developing significant complications. Nearly 30% will exhibit atherosclerotic complications, and more than 50% will have end organ damage related to the hypertension itself, such as cardiomegaly, congestive heart failure, retinopathy, a cerebrovascular accident, and/or renal insufficiency. Thus, even in its mild forms, hypertension is a progressive and lethal disease if left untreated.

SECONDARY HYPERTENSION

As noted earlier, in only a small minority of patients with elevated arterial pressure can a specific cause be identified. Yet these patients should not be ignored for at least two reasons: (1) correction of the cause may cure their hypertension, and (2) these secondary forms of the disease may provide insight into the etiology of essential hypertension. Nearly all the secondary forms of hypertension are related to an alteration in hormone secretion and/or renal function and are discussed in detail in other chapters.

RENAL HYPERTENSION (See also Chap. 278) Hypertension produced by renal disease is the result of either (1) a derangement in the renal handling of sodium and fluids leading to volume expansion or (2) an alteration in renal secretion of vasoactive materials resulting in a systemic or local change in arteriolar tone. The main subdivisions of renal hypertension are renovascular hypertension, including preeclampsia and eclampsia, and renal parenchymal hypertension. A simple explanation for *renal vascular hypertension* is that decreased perfusion of renal tissue due to stenosis of a main or branch renal artery activates the renin-angiotensin system, described in Chap. 331. Circulating angiotensin II elevates arterial pressure by directly causing vasoconstriction, by stimulating aldosterone secretion with resulting sodium retention, and/or by stimulating the adrenergic nervous system. In practice, only about one-half of patients with renovascular hypertension have an absolute elevation in renin activity in peripheral plasma, although when renin measurements are referenced against an index of sodium balance, a much higher fraction have inappropriately high values.

Activation of the renin-angiotensin system has also been offered as an explanation for the hypertension in both acute and chronic *renal parenchymal disease*. In this formulation, the only difference between renovascular and renal parenchymal hypertension is that the decreased perfusion of renal tissue in the latter case results from inflammatory and fibrotic changes involving multiple small intrarenal vessels. There are enough differences between the two conditions, however, to suggest that other mechanisms are active in renal parenchymal disease. Specifically, (1) peripheral plasma renin activity is elevated far less frequently in renal parenchymal than in renovascular hypertension; (2) cardiac output is said to be normal in renal parenchymal hypertension (unless uremia and anemia are present) but slightly elevated in renovascular hypertension; (3) circulatory responses to tilting and to the Valsalva maneuver are exaggerated in the latter condition; and (4) blood volume tends to be high in patients with severe renal parenchymal disease and low in patients with severe unilateral renovascular hypertension. Alternative explanations for the hypertension in renal parenchymal disease include the possibilities that the damaged kidneys (1) produce an unidentified vasopressor substance other than renin, (2) fail to produce a necessary humoral vasodilator substance (perhaps prostaglandin or bradykinin), (3) fail to inactivate circulating vasopressor substances, and/or (4) are ineffective in disposing of sodium. In the last case, the retained sodium would be responsible for the hypertension as outlined earlier. Although all these explanations, including participation of the renin-angiotensin system, probably have some validity in individual patients, the hypothesis involving sodium retention is particularly attractive. It is supported by the observation that those patients with chronic pyelonephritis or polycystic renal disease who are salt wasters do not develop hypertension and by the observation that removal of salt and water by dialysis or diuretics is effective in controlling arterial pressure in most patients with renal parenchymal disease.

A rare form of renal hypertension results from the excess secretion of renin by juxtaglomerular cell tumors or nephroblastomas. The initial presentation is similar to that of hyperaldosteronism, with hypertension, hypokalemia, and overproduction of aldosterone. However, in contrast to primary aldosteronism, peripheral renin activity is *elevated instead of subnormal*. This disease can be distinguished from other forms of secondary aldosteronism by the presence of normal renal function and unilateral increases in renal vein renin concentration without a renal artery lesion.

ENDOCRINE HYPERTENSION   **Adrenal Hypertension** Hypertension is a feature of a variety of adrenal cortical abnormalities. In *primary aldosteronism* (Chap. 331), there is a clear relationship between the aldosterone-induced sodium retention and the hypertension. Normal individuals given aldosterone develop hypertension only if they also ingest sodium. Since aldosterone causes sodium retention by stimulating renal tubular exchange of sodium for potassium, hypokalemia is a prominent feature in most patients with primary aldosteronism, and, therefore, the measurement of serum potassium provides a simple screening test. The effect of sodium retention and volume expansion in chronically suppressing plasma renin activity is critical for the definitive diagnosis. In most clinical situations, plasma renin activity and plasma or urinary aldosterone levels parallel each other, but in patients with primary aldosteronism, aldosterone levels are high and relatively fixed because of autonomous aldosterone secretion, whereas plasma renin activity levels are suppressed and respond sluggishly to sodium depletion. Primary aldosteronism may be secondary to either a tumor or bilateral adrenal hyperplasia. It is important to distinguish between these two conditions preoperatively, since the hypertension in the latter case is usually not modified by operation.

The sodium-retaining effect of large amounts of glucocorticoids (perhaps resulting in part from saturation of the 11β-hydroxysteroid hydrogenase enzyme system in the kidney by the increased concentration of cortisol) also offers an explanation for the hypertension in severe cases of Cushing's syndrome (Chap. 331). Moreover, increased production of mineralocorticoids has also been documented in some patients with Cushing's syndrome. However, the hypertension in many cases of Cushing's syndrome does not seem volume-dependent, leading investigators to speculate that it may be secondary to glucocorticoid-induced production of renin substrate (angiotensin-mediated hypertension). In the forms of the adrenogenital syndrome due to C-11 or C-17 hydroxylase deficiency (Chap. 331), deoxycorticosterone accounts for the sodium retention and the resulting hypertension, which is accompanied by suppression of plasma renin activity.

In patients with pheochromocytoma (Chap. 332), increased secretion of epinephrine and norepinephrine by a tumor (most often located in the adrenal medulla) causes excessive stimulation of adrenergic receptors, which results in peripheral vasoconstriction and cardiac stimulation. This diagnosis is confirmed by demonstrating increased urinary excretion of epinephrine and norepinephrine and/or their metabolites.

Acromegaly (See also Chap. 328)   Hypertension, coronary atherosclerosis, and cardiac hypertrophy are frequent complications of this condition.

Hypercalcemia (See also Chap. 340)   The hypertension that occurs in up to one-third of patients with hyperparathyroidism ordinarily can be attributed to renal parenchymal damage due to nephrolithiasis and nephrocalcinosis. However, increased calcium levels can also have a direct vasoconstrictive effect. In some cases, the hypertension disappears when the hypercalcemia is corrected. Thus, paradoxically, the increased serum calcium level in hyperparathyroidism raises blood pressure, while epidemiologic studies suggest that a high calcium intake lowers blood pressure. To further confuse the issue, calcium entry–blocking agents are effective antihypertensive agents. Additional studies are needed to resolve these seemingly conflicting observations.

Oral Contraceptives   Several years ago, a common cause of endocrine hypertension was the use of estrogen-containing oral contraceptives. However, several studies have since suggested that this is no longer true, probably owing to the lower estrogen content of modern oral contraceptives. In patients receiving these agents who do become hypertensive, the mechanism is likely to be activation of the renin-angiotensin-aldosterone system. Thus, both volume (aldosterone) and vasoconstrictor (angiotensin II) factors are important. The estrogen component of oral contraceptive agents stimulates the hepatic synthesis of the renin substrate angiotensinogen, which in turn favors the increased production of angiotensin II and secondary aldosteronism. Some women taking oral contraceptives have increased plasma concentrations of angiotensin II and aldosterone with some increase in

arterial pressure. However, only a small number actually have an increase in arterial pressure to a level >140/90, and, in about half of these, the hypertension will remit within 6 months of stopping the drug.

Why some women taking oral contraceptives develop hypertension and others do not is unclear but may be related to (1) increased vascular sensitivity to angiotensin II, (2) the presence of mild renal disease, (3) familial factors (over one-half have a positive family history for hypertension), (4) age (hypertension is significantly more prevalent in women over age 35), (5) the estrogen content of the contraceptive, and/or (6) obesity. Indeed some investigators have suggested that the oral contraceptives are simply unmasking women with essential hypertension.

COARCTATION OF THE AORTA (See also Chap. 234) The hypertension associated with coarctation may be caused by the constriction itself or perhaps by the changes in the renal circulation, which result in an unusual form of renal arterial hypertension. The diagnosis of coarctation is usually evident from physical examination and routine x-ray findings.

EFFECTS OF HYPERTENSION

Patients with hypertension die prematurely; the most common cause of death is heart disease, with stroke and renal failure also frequent, particularly in patients with significant retinopathy.

EFFECTS ON THE HEART   Cardiac compensation for the excessive workload imposed by increased systemic pressure is at first sustained by concentric left ventricular hypertrophy, characterized by an increase in wall thickness. Ultimately, the function of this chamber deteriorates, the cavity dilates, and the symptoms and signs of heart failure appear (Chap. 231). Angina pectoris may also occur because of the combination of accelerated coronary arterial disease and increased myocardial oxygen requirements as a consequence of the increased myocardial mass (Chap. 244). On physical examination, the heart is enlarged and has a prominent left ventricular impulse. The sound of aortic closure is accentuated, and there may be a faint murmur of aortic regurgitation. Presystolic (atrial, fourth) heart sounds appear frequently in hypertensive heart disease, and a protodiastolic (ventricular, third) heart sound or summation gallop rhythm may be present. Electrocardiographic changes of left ventricular hypertrophy (Chap. 226) may occur, but the electrocardiogram substantially underestimates the frequency of cardiac hypertrophy compared with that observed with the echocardiogram. Evidence of ischemia or infarction may be observed late in the disease. Most deaths due to hypertension result from myocardial infarction or congestive heart failure. Recent data suggest that some of the myocardial damage may be mediated by aldosterone in the presence of a normal/high salt intake rather than just the increased blood pressure or an increase in angiotensin II levels per se.

NEUROLOGIC EFFECTS   The neurologic effects of longstanding hypertension may be divided into retinal and central nervous system changes. Because the retina is the only tissue in which the arteries and arterioles can be examined directly, repeated ophthalmoscopic examination provides the opportunity to observe the progress of the vascular effects of hypertension (Table 35-2). The Keith-Wagener-Barker classification of the *retinal changes* in hypertension has provided a simple and excellent means for serial evaluation of hypertensive patients. Increasing severity of hypertension is associated with focal spasm and progressive general narrowing of the arterioles, as well as the appearance of hemorrhages, exudates, and papilledema. These retinal lesions often produce scotomata, blurred vision, and even blindness, especially when there is papilledema or hemorrhages of the macular area. Hypertensive lesions may develop acutely and, if therapy results in significant reduction of blood pressure, may show rapid resolution. Rarely, these lesions resolve without therapy. In contrast, retinal arteriolosclerosis results from endothelial and muscular proliferation, and it accurately reflects similar changes in other organs. Sclerotic changes do not develop as rapidly as hypertensive lesions, nor do they regress appreciably with therapy. As a consequence of increased wall thickness and rigidity, sclerotic arterioles distort and compress the veins where the two vessel types cross in their common fibrous sheath, and the reflected light streak from the arterioles is changed by the increased opacity of the vessel wall.

Central nervous system dysfunction also occurs frequently in patients with hypertension. Occipital headaches, most often occurring in the morning, are among the most prominent early symptoms of hypertension. Dizziness, light-headedness, vertigo, tinnitus, and dimmed vision or syncope may also be observed, but the more serious manifestations are due to vascular occlusion, hemorrhage, or encephalopathy (Chap. 361). The pathogeneses of the former two disorders are quite different. *Cerebral infarction* is secondary to the increased atherosclerosis observed in hypertensive patients, whereas *cerebral hemorrhage* is the result of both the elevated arterial pressure and the development of cerebral vascular microaneurysms (Charcot-Bouchard aneurysms). Only age and arterial pressure are known to influence the development of the microaneurysms. Thus, it is not surprising that arterial pressure shows a better association with cerebral hemorrhage than with either cerebral or myocardial infarction.

Hypertensive encephalopathy consists of the following symptom complex: severe hypertension, disordered consciousness, increased intracranial pressure, retinopathy with papilledema, and seizures. The pathogenesis is uncertain but is probably not related to arteriolar spasm or cerebral edema. Focal neurologic signs are infrequent and, if present, suggest that infarction, hemorrhage, or transient ischemic attacks are more likely diagnoses. Although some investigators have suggested that prompt lowering of arterial pressure in these patients may adversely affect cerebral blood flow, most studies indicate that this is not the case.

EFFECTS ON THE KIDNEY (See also Chap. 278) Arteriosclerotic lesions of the afferent and efferent arterioles and the glomerular capillary tufts are the most common renal vascular lesions in hypertension and result in a decreased glomerular filtration rate and tubular dysfunction. Proteinuria and microscopic hematuria occur because of glomerular lesions, and approximately 10% of the deaths caused by hypertension result from renal failure. Blood loss in hypertension occurs not only from renal lesions; epistaxis, hemoptysis, and metrorrhagia also occur frequently in these patients.

Approach to the Patient

The detailed initial evaluation of the hypertensive patient is outlined in Chap. 35. It includes the critical elements of the history, physical examination, and basic laboratory investigation that aid in arriving at appropriate diagnostic and therapeutic decisions (Table 35-2).

DIAGNOSIS OF SECONDARY HYPERTENSION Certain clues from the history, physical examination, and basic laboratory studies may suggest an unusual cause for the hypertension and dictate the need for special studies. For example, the abrupt onset of severe hypertension and/or the onset of hypertension of any severity in a patient under the age of 25 or over the age of 50 should lead to laboratory tests to exclude renovascular hypertension and pheochromocytoma. A history of headaches, palpitations, anxiety attacks, unusual sweating, hyperglycemia, and weight loss should also lead to tests to exclude pheochromocytoma. The presence of an abdominal bruit should lead to a workup for renovascular hypertension, and the finding on physical examination of bilateral upper abdominal masses consistent with polycystic renal disease should lead to the performance of an abdominal ultrasound examination or intravenous pyelogram (IVP). An elevated creatinine or blood urea nitrogen level, associated with proteinuria and hematuria, should prompt a detailed workup for renal insufficiency (Chap. 268). Special studies for secondary hypertension are also indicated if there is therapeutic failure with the initial drug program. The specific diagnostic measures depend on the most likely causes of secondary hypertension.

Pheochromocytoma (See also Chap. 332) The easiest and best screening procedure for pheochromocytoma is the measurement of catecholamines and their metabolites in a 24-h urine sample collected while the patient is hypertensive. Measurement of plasma catecholamine levels may also be useful. These tests may be indicated even in patients who do not have episodic hypertension, since over half the patients with pheochromocytoma have fixed hypertension. Provocative tests are seldom, if ever, indicated, although occasionally a suppressive test may be useful.

Cushing's Syndrome (See also Chap. 331) A 24-h urine test for cortisol and creatinine or the administration of 1 mg of dexamethasone at bedtime, followed by the measurement of plasma cortisol at 7 to 10 A.M., is the best test to screen for the presence of Cushing's syndrome. A urine cortisol level of <2750 nmol (100 μg) or suppression of the plasma cortisol level to <140 nmol/L (5 μg/dL) effectively rules out Cushing's syndrome.

Renovascular Hypertension (See also Chap. 278) Over the past decades the standard approach to screen for renovascular hypertension has progressed from the rapid-sequence IVP to one of three noninvasive techniques: the captopril-enhanced radionuclide renal scan (the preferred choice), a duplex Doppler flow study, or magnetic resonance (MRI) angiography. However, perhaps the most sensitive and specific screening test, the spiral computed tomography (CT) scan, which gives a three-dimensional view, unfortunately also requires giving an intravenous contrast agent.

The definitive test for surgically correctable renal disease is the combination of a renal angiogram and renal vein renin determinations. The renal arteriogram both establishes the presence of a renal arterial lesion and aids in the determination of whether the lesion is due to atherosclerosis or to one of the fibrous or fibromuscular dysplasias. It does not, however, prove that the lesion is responsible for the hypertension, nor does it permit prediction of the chances of surgical cure. It must be noted that (1) renal artery stenosis is a frequent finding by angiography and at postmortem in normotensive individuals, and (2) essential hypertension is a common condition and may occur in combination with renal arterial stenosis that is not responsible for the hypertension. Bilateral renal vein catheterization for measurement of plasma renin activity is therefore used to assess the functional significance of any lesion noted on arteriography. When one kidney is ischemic and the other is normal, all the renin released comes from the involved kidney. In the most straightforward situation, the ischemic kidney has a significantly higher venous plasma renin activity than the normal kidney, by a factor of 1.5 or more. Moreover, the renal venous blood draining the uninvolved kidney exhibits levels similar to those in the inferior vena cava below the entrance of the renal veins.

Significant benefit from operative correction may be anticipated in at least 80% of patients with the findings described above if care is taken to prepare the patient properly before renal vein blood sampling, i.e., by discontinuing renin-suppressing drugs, such as beta blockers, for at least 10 days; restricting the patient to a low-sodium intake for 4 days; and/or giving a converting-enzyme inhibitor for 24 h. When obstructing lesions in the *branches* of the renal arteries are demonstrated by arteriography, an attempt to obtain blood samples from the main *branches* of the renal vein should be made in an effort to identify a localized intrarenal arterial lesion responsible for the hypertension.

Primary Aldosteronism (See also Chap. 331) These patients usually exhibit hypokalemia. Diuretic therapy often complicates the picture when the hypokalemia is first observed and needs to be assessed. Given the presence of hypokalemia, the relation between plasma renin activity and the aldosterone level becomes the key to the diagnosis of primary aldosteronism. The aldosterone concentration or excretion rate is high and plasma renin activity is low in primary aldosteronism, and these levels are relatively unaffected by changes in sodium balance. Thus, the aldosterone:renin ratio is high. A critical part of the evaluation after primary aldosteronism has been established is to determine whether disease is unilateral or bilateral, because surgical removal of the lesion usually reduces arterial pressure only in patients with unilateral disease.

Plasma Renin Activity Measurements   Some studies have suggested that the plasma renin level should be measured in most hypertensive patients and related to a 24-h urine sodium excretion rate to assess whether high, low, or normal renin levels are present. It has been proposed that this information may be important for both therapeutic and prognostic reasons. However, as noted earlier, it is unclear, on the basis of the available data and treatment programs, that these random measurements are really useful except in patients with findings suggestive of renal vascular disease or mineralocorticoid excess in whom lateralizing renal vein renin levels or suppressed peripheral renin levels may be of diagnostic and/or therapeutic significance.

TREATMENT   Indications for Therapy   Virtually every patient with a diastolic arterial pressure that persistently exceeds 90 mmHg, or any patient over 65 years of age with a systolic arterial pressure >160 mmHg, is a candidate for diagnostic studies and for subsequent treatment. Furthermore, at any given level of blood pressure elevation, the ultimate risk of developing hypertensive vascular complications is greater in men than in women, in younger than in older persons, and in diabetic than nondiabetic patients. It may be argued, then, that it is hard to justify producing the uncomfortable side effects of therapy in, for example, an asymptomatic woman over 70 years of age with a diastolic pressure of 90 mmHg. On the other hand, it is easy to justify side effects in a man of 30 with a diastolic pressure exceeding 110 mmHg because such a person may be expected to receive the greatest benefit from therapy. Fortunately, the choice of treatment is such that a satisfactory program to control arterial pressure with minimal side effects can be developed for most patients, particularly as more studies assessing the impact of specific therapeutic agents on the patient's quality of life are reported.

A reasonable guideline would be that all patients with a diastolic pressure repeatedly >90 mmHg or systolic pressure >140 mmHg should be treated unless specific contraindications exist. Patients with isolated *systolic* hypertension (levels >160 mmHg with diastolic pressure <89 mmHg) should also be treated if they are over age 65. It is uncertain that individuals under age 65 who have isolated systolic hypertension will benefit from therapy until the results of a well-controlled, prospective study are completed. Patients with labile hypertension or isolated systolic hypertension who are not treated should have regular follow-up examinations at 6-month intervals because of the frequent development of progressive and/or sustained hypertension. Finally, if coronary artery disease or associated cardiovascular risks are present, then treatment of a patient with a lower blood pressure may be warranted. For example, patients with angina pectoris or diabetes mellitus with diastolic blood pressures between 85 and 90 mmHg may be candidates for antihypertensive therapy.

What should the blood pressure goal be? Previously it was assumed that 140/90 mmHg was the desired level. This still seems reasonable for nondiabetic patients since the Hypertension Optimal Treatment (HOT) study did not detect a significant difference in cardiovascular risk between patients with treatment goal diastolic blood pressures of 90 and 80 mmHg. However, in patients with diabetes this is not the case. In the UK Prospective Diabetes Study (UKPDS), individuals with a blood pressure of 144/82 mmHg had a substantially lower risk compared to those with a blood pressure of 154/87 mmHg. The HOT study investigators documented a similar finding in their diabetic subset. Thus, it seems reasonable to target a blood pressure in the normal range for diabetic patients, i.e., 130/85 mmHg. While not definitively proven, it seems prudent to use the same goal in all young and middle-aged patients depending on what other cardiovascular risk factors are present. For elderly individuals, a goal of 140/90 mmHg is appropriate, although definitive data for lowering systolic blood pressure below 160 mmHg is still lacking. Importantly, how aggressive one should be in achieving these blood pres-

sure goals depends on the number and severity of other risk factors present.

The identification of an operable form of secondary hypertension does not automatically mean that surgical treatment is indicated. The decision depends on the age and general health of the patient, the natural history of the lesion, and the response of the arterial pressure to drug therapy. In patients with renovascular hypertension, the feasibility of renal angioplasty, the advantages of surgical repair versus nephrectomy, and the degree of overall renal functional impairment must be considered. Age and general health are important in patients with renovascular hypertension due to arteriosclerosis, because there is no evidence that repair of the stenosis increases life expectancy in the elderly patient with other evidence of vascular disease. Knowledge of the natural history of the disease is especially important when making a decision in the case of a young patient with renal artery stenosis due to fibrous dysplasia. If the arteriographic appearance suggests that the stenosis is due to intimal or subadventitial fibroplasia, the lesion may be expected to progress, and operation or angioplasty is required. Medial fibroplasia, on the other hand, often remains stable, and operation or angioplasty may not be necessary if pressure can be controlled by drug therapy.

The decision regarding operation should also be considered carefully in patients with primary aldosteronism when neither abdominal CT nor bilateral adrenal venous sampling for aldosterone demonstrates a tumor, because such patients may prove to have multinodular hyperplasia. In that case, bilateral adrenalectomy would be required to eliminate the aldosterone excess, and, even then, hypertension would usually persist. If hypokalemia can be controlled by an aldosterone receptor antagonist, e.g., spironolactone, or other drug therapy and arterial pressure lowered with antihypertensive agents, then it is reasonable to withhold operative treatment.

GENERAL MEASURES   Nondrug therapeutic intervention is probably indicated in all patients with sustained hypertension and probably in most with labile hypertension. The general measures employed include (1) relief of stress, (2) dietary management, (3) regular aerobic exercise, (4) weight reduction (if needed), and (5) control of other risk factors contributing to the development of arteriosclerosis. Relief of emotional and environmental stress is one of the reasons for the improvement in hypertension that occurs when a patient is hospitalized. Though it is usually impossible to extricate the hypertensive patient from all internal and external stresses, he or she should be advised to avoid unnecessary tensions. In rare instances, it may be appropriate to recommend a change of job or of life-style. It has been suggested that relaxation techniques may also lower arterial pressure. However, it is uncertain that these techniques alone have much long-term effect.

Dietary management has three aspects:

1.   Because of the documented efficacy of sodium restriction and volume contraction in lowering blood pressure, patients previously were instructed to curtail sodium intake drastically. Some investigators have suggested that this is not necessary. They base their conclusion on two observations: (1) In many patients the blood pressure is not sensitive to the level of sodium intake, and (2) diuretics provide another method of decreasing body sodium stores in individuals whose blood pressure is sodium-sensitive. However, meta-analyses of previous diet studies have documented a 5-mmHg reduction in systolic pressure and a 2.6-mmHg reduction in diastolic pressure when sodium intake is reduced by approximately 75 meq/d. In addition, several reports have documented that, while mild sodium restriction has little if any direct action on blood pressure, it significantly potentiates the efficacy of nearly all antihypertensive agents. Thus, by making it possible to control blood pressure with lower doses of drugs, sodium restriction leads to a reduction in side effects. In addition, it is quite clear that in some hypertensive patients, as noted above, the level of sodium intake does influence the blood pressure. Thus, since there is no apparent risk to mild sodium restriction, the most practical approach now is to advise mild dietary sodium restriction (up to 5 g NaCl per

day), which can be achieved by eliminating all additions of salt to food that is prepared normally. Some studies have also reported a lowering of arterial pressure related to an *increase* in potassium and/or calcium intake. For example, in one meta-analysis, dietary potassium supplements of 50 to 120 meq/d reduced blood pressure by about the same amount as salt restriction (by 6 mmHg systolic and 3.4 mmHg diastolic). While the advisability of these forms of dietary alteration is still controversial, the fact that a moderately high calcium intake (1.5 g elemental calcium daily) probably also reduces the extent of age-related osteoporosis, combined with the results of the potassium supplementation studies, indicate that they are probably useful adjuncts. A particularly useful approach is the DASH (Dietary Approaches to Stop Hypertension) diet, which uses natural foods that are high in potassium and low in saturated and total fat. This diet significantly lowered blood pressure in borderline and stage 1 hypertensive subjects (see Table 35-1 for definitions).

2. Caloric restriction should be urged for patients who are over weight. Some obese patients will show a significant reduction in blood pressure simply as a consequence of weight loss. In the Trial of Antihypertensive Interventions and Management (TAIM) study, weight reduction (average 4.4 kg over 6 months) lowered blood pressure by 2.5 mmHg.

3. A restriction in the intake of cholesterol and saturated fats is recommended, as this diet modification may diminish the incidence of arteriosclerotic complications. Reducing alcohol intake to <15 mL daily is also beneficial. Regular exercise is indicated within the limits of the patient's cardiovascular status. Not only is exercise helpful in controlling weight, but there is also evidence that physical conditioning itself may lower arterial pressure. Isotonic exercises (jogging, swimming) are better than isometric exercises (weight lifting) since the latter, if anything, raises arterial pressure. The dietary management outlined above is aimed at the control of other risk factors. Probably the most significant additional step that could be taken in this area would be to convince the smoker to give up cigarettes.

DRUG THERAPY FOR HYPERTENSION
(Table 246-6)

To make rational use of antihypertensive drugs, the sites and mechanisms of their action must be understood. In general, there are six classes of drugs: diuretics, antiadrenergic agents, vasodilators, calcium entry blockers, angiotensin-converting enzyme (ACE) inhibitors, and angiotensin receptor antagonists.

DIURETICS (See also Chap. 232) The thiazides are the most frequently used and most extensively investigated members of this group, and their early effect is certainly related to sodium diuresis and volume depletion. A reduction in peripheral vascular resistance has also been reported by some workers to be important in the long term. Traditionally, thiazide diuretics have formed the cornerstone of most therapeutic programs designed to lower arterial pressure, and they are usually effective within 3 to 4 days. Furthermore, they have been shown to reduce mortality and morbidity in long-term trials. However, in recent years there has been increasing resistance to their routine use, primarily because of their adverse metabolic effects, which include hypokalemia due to renal potassium loss, hyperuricemia due to uric acid retention, carbohydrate intolerance, and hyperlipidemia. These effects are minimized if the dose is kept below the equivalent of 25 mg/d of hydrochlorothiazide. The more potent loop-acting diuretics furosemide and bumetanide have also been shown to be antihypertensive but have been used less extensively for this indication, primarily because of their shorter duration of action. Spironolactone causes renal sodium loss by blocking the effect of mineralocorticoids, and, therefore, it may be more effective in patients whose mineralocorticoid levels are excessive, such as patients with primary or secondary aldosteronism. However, a clinical trial in heart failure using low doses of spironolactone achieved a 30% reduction in mortality, suggesting that an aldosterone receptor antagonist may be beneficial even when aldosterone levels are relatively normal. Although they do not compete directly with aldosterone, triamterene and amiloride act at the same site as spironolactone to impede sodium reabsorption. They are effective in the same situations as an aldosterone receptor antagonist, except that triamterene has little intrinsic antihypertensive effect. Their major disadvantage is that they can produce hyperkalemia, particularly in patients with impaired renal function. Any of these three potassium-sparing diuretics can also be given along with thiazide diuretics to minimize renal potassium loss.

ANTIADRENERGIC AGENTS (See also Chap. 72) These drugs act at one or more sites—centrally on the vasomotor center, in peripheral neurons, where they modify catecholamine release, or in target tissues, where they block adrenergic receptor sites. Drugs that appear to have predominant *central actions* are *clonidine, methyldopa, guanabenz,* and *guanfacine.* These drugs and their metabolites are predominantly α-receptor agonists. Stimulation of α_2 receptors in the vasomotor centers of the brain *reduces* sympathetic outflow, thereby reducing arterial pressure. Usually a fall in cardiac output and heart rate also occurs, more commonly with clonidine and guanabenz, but the baroreceptor reflex is intact. Thus, postural symptoms are absent. However, rebound hypertension may occur rarely when these drugs, particularly clonidine and guanabenz, are stopped. This effect is probably secondary to an increase in norepinephrine release, which is inhibited by these agents owing their agonist effect on presynaptic α receptors. They are usually not used as first-line therapy.

Another class of antiadrenergic agents consists of the *ganglionic blocking drugs,* which are used infrequently now. Because of their side effects, ganglionic blocking agents are now usually reserved for the rapid lowering of arterial pressure by parenteral administration of the short-acting agent *trimethaphan* in patients with severe hypertension.

Various drugs act at *postganglionic adrenergic nerve endings,* but they are rarely used now because of their side effects. *Guanethidine* and its shorter-acting analogue guanadrel block the release of norepinephrine from adrenergic nerve endings. They usually reduce cardiac output and lower systolic more than diastolic blood pressure. They also produce a greater postural effect than the other drugs that act at the nerve endings, and orthostatic hypotension is a frequent side effect.

The last group of drugs affecting the adrenergic system are those that block the *peripheral adrenergic receptors,* α, β, or both (Chap. 72).

α-Adrenergic Receptor Blockers These agents also usually are not used as first-line therapy. *Phentolamine* and *phenoxybenzamine* block the action of norepinephrine at α-adrenergic receptor sites. These two compounds block both presynaptic (α_2) and postsynaptic (α_1) α receptors, and the former action accounts for the tolerance that develops. *Prazosin* is more effective because it selectively blocks only *postsynaptic α receptors,* i.e., α_1 receptors. Thus, presynaptic α activity remains, suppressing norepinephrine release, and tolerance occurs only infrequently. Accordingly, prazosin produces less tachycardia but more postural hypotension than direct-acting vasodilators, such as hydralazine, and rarely can produce substantial hypotension following the first dose. Its use has decreased with a report of its association with an increase in cardiovascular events.

β-Adrenergic Receptor Blockers (See also Chap. 244) A number of effective *β-adrenergic receptor blocking agents* are available that block sympathetic effects on the heart and should be most effective in reducing cardiac output and in lowering arterial pressure when there is increased cardiac sympathetic nerve activity. These agents *are* often used as first-line therapy. In addition, they block the adrenergic nerve–mediated release of renin from the renal juxtaglomerular cells. This action may be an important component of their blood pressure–lowering action. β-Adrenergic blockers are particularly useful when employed in conjunction with vascular smooth-muscle relaxants, which tend to evoke a reflex increase in heart rate, and with diuretics, the administration of which often results in an elevation of circulating renin activity. In practice, beta blockers appear to be effective even when there is no evidence of increased sympathetic tone, with about

Table 246-6   Drugs Used in Treatment of Hypertension—Listed According to Site of Action

Site of Action	Drug	Dosage	Indications	Contraindications/Cautions	Frequent or Peculiar Side Effects
DIURETICS					
Renal tubule	Thiazides: e.g., hydro-chlorothiazide	Depends on specific drug Oral: 12.5–25 mg daily	Mild hypertension; as adjunct in treatment of moderate to severe hypertension	Diabetes mellitus, hyperuricemia, primary aldosteronism	Potassium depletion, hyperglycemia, hyperuricemia, hypercholesterolemia, dermatitis, purpura, depression, hypercalcemia
	Loop-acting: e.g., furosemide	Oral: 20–80 mg 2 or 3 times a day	Mild hypertension; as adjunct in severe or malignant hypertension, particularly with renal failure	Hyperuricemia, primary aldosteronism	Potassium depletion, hyperuricemia, hyperglycemia, hypocalcemia, blood dyscrasias, rash, nausea, vomiting, diarrhea
	Potassium-sparing: Spironolactone	Oral: 25 mg 2 to 4 times daily	Hypertension due to hypermineralocorticoidism; as adjunct to thiazide therapy	Renal failure	Hyperkalemia, diarrhea, gynecomastia menstrual irregularities
	Triamterene	Oral: 25–100 mg daily	}		} Hyperkalemia, nausea, vomiting, leg cramps, nephrolithiasis, GI disturbances
	Amiloride	Oral: 5–10 mg daily	}		
ANTIADRENERGIC AGENTS					
Central	Clonidine	Oral: 0.05–0.6 mg twice daily	Mild to moderate hypertension, renal disease with hypertension		Postural hypotension, drowsiness, dry mouth, rebound hypertension after abrupt withdrawal, insomnia
	Guanabenz	Oral: 4–16 mg twice daily			
	Guanfacine	Oral: 1–3 mg daily			
	Methyldopa (also acts by blocking sympathetic nerves)	Oral: 250–1000 mg twice daily IV: 250–1000 mg every 4–6 h (tolerance may develop)	Mild to moderate hypertension (oral), malignant hypertension (IV)	Pheochromocytoma, active hepatic disease (IV), during MAO inhibitor administration	Postural hypotension, sedation, fatigue, diarrhea, impaired ejaculation, fever, gynecomastia, lactation, positive Coombs' tests (occasionally associated with hemolysis), chronic hepatitis, acute ulcerative colitis, lupus-like syndrome
Autonomic ganglia	Trimethaphan	IV: 1–6 mg/min	Severe or malignant hypertension	Severe coronary artery disease, cerebrovascular insufficiency, diabetes mellitus (on hypoglycemic therapy), glaucoma, prostatism	Postural hypotension, visual symptoms, dry mouth, constipation, urinary retention, impotence
Nerve endings	Guanethidine	Oral: 10–150 mg daily	Moderate to severe hypertension	Pheochromocytoma, severe coronary artery disease, cerebrovascular insufficiency, during MAO inhibitor administration	Postural hypotension, bradycardia, dry mouth, diarrhea, impaired ejaculation, fluid retention, asthma
	Guanadrel	Oral: 5–50 mg twice daily			
α Receptors	Phentolamine	IV: 1–5 mg bolus	Suspected or proved pheochromocytoma	Severe coronary artery disease	Tachycardia, weakness, dizziness, flushing
	Phenoxybenza-mine	Oral: 10–50 mg once or twice daily (tolerance may develop)	Proved pheochromocytoma		Postural hypotension, tachycardia, miosis, nasal congestion, dry mouth
	Prazosin	Oral: 1–10 mg twice daily	Mild to moderate hypertension	Use with caution in the elderly	Sudden syncope, headache, sedation, dizziness, tachycardia, anticholinergic effect, fluid retention
	Terazosin	Oral: 1–20 mg daily			
	Doxazosin	Oral: 1–16 mg daily			
β Receptors	Propranolol	Oral: 10–120 mg 2 to 4 times daily	Mild to moderate hypertension (especially with evidence of hyperdynamic circulation); as adjunct to hydralazine therapy	Congestive heart failure, asthma, diabetes mellitus (on hypoglycemic therapy), during MAO inhibitor administration, COPD, sick sinus syndrome, 2d or 3d degree heart block	Dizziness, depression, bronchospasm, nausea, vomiting, diarrhea, constipation, heart failure, fatigue, Raynaud's phenomenon, hallucinations, hypertriglyceridemia, hypercholesterolemia, psoriasis; sudden withdrawal may precipitate angina or myocardial injury in patients with heart disease
	Metoprolol	Oral: 25–150 mg twice daily			
	Nadolol	Oral: 20–120 mg daily			
	Atenolol	Oral: 25–100 mg daily			
	Timolol	Oral: 5–15 mg twice daily			
	Betaxolol	Oral: 10–20 mg daily			

(continued)

Table 246-6—*(continued)*

Site of Action	Drug	Dosage	Indications	Contraindications/Cautions	Frequent or Peculiar Side Effects
	Carteolol	Oral: 2.5–10 mg daily			
	Pindolol	Oral: 5–30 mg twice daily			Less resting bradycardia than other beta blockers
	Acebutolol	Oral: 200–600 mg twice daily			
α/β Receptors	Labetalol	Oral: 100–600 mg twice daily IV: 2 mg/min			Similar to beta blockers with more postural effects
	Carvediol	Oral: 12.5–50 mg daily or in divided doses			
VASODILATORS					
Vascular smooth muscle	Hydralazine	Oral: 10–75 mg 4 times daily IV or IM: 10–50 mg every 6 h (tolerance may develop)	As adjunct in treatment of moderate to severe hypertension (oral), malignant hypertension (IV or IM), renal disease with hypertension	Lupus erythematosus, severe coronary artery disease	Headache, tachycardia, angina pectoris, anorexia, nausea, vomiting, diarrhea, lupuslike syndrome, rash, fluid retention
	Minoxidil	Oral: 2.5–40 mg twice daily	Severe hypertension	Severe coronary artery disease	Tachycardia, aggravates angina, marked fluid retention, hair growth on face and body, coarsening of facial features, possible pericardial effusions
	Diazoxide	IV: 1–3 mg/kg up to 150 mg rapidly	Severe or malignant hypertension	Diabetes mellitus, hyperuricemia, congestive heart failure	Hyperglycemia, hyperuricemia, sodium retention
	Nitroprusside	IV: 0.5–8 (μg/kg)/min	Malignant hypertension		Apprehension, weakness, diaphoresis, nausea, vomiting, muscle twitching, cyanide toxicity
ANGIOTENSIN-CONVERTING ENZYME INHIBITORS					
Converting enzyme	Captopril	Oral: 12.5–75 mg twice daily	Mild to severe hypertension, renal artery stenosis	Renal failure (reduction of dose), bilateral renal artery stenosis, pregnancy	Leukopenia, pancytopenia, hypotension, cough, angioedema, urticarial rash, fever, loss of taste, acute renal failure in bilateral renal artery stenosis, hyperkalemia
	Benazepril	Oral: 5–40 mg daily			Same as captopril, but little evidence for leukopenia, but perhaps increased frequency of cough and angioedema. All can be given once daily, but side effects are reduced if one-half dose is given twice daily. Fosinopril is excreted more in bile than the others.
	Enalapril	Oral: 2.5–40 mg daily			
	Enalaprilat	IV: 0.625–1.25 mg over 5 min every 6–8 h			
	Fosinopril	Oral: 10–40 mg daily			
	Lisinopril	Oral: 5–40 mg daily			
	Quinapril	Oral: 5–80 mg daily			
	Ramipril	Oral: 1.25–20 mg daily			
	Trandolapril	Oral: 1–4 mg daily			
ANGIOTENSIN RECEPTOR ANTAGONISTS					
	Losartan	Oral: 25–50 mg once or twice daily	Mild to severe hypertension, renal artery stenosis	Pregnancy, bilateral renal artery stenosis	Hypotension, acute renal failure in bilateral renal artery stenosis, hyperkalemia
	Valsartan	Oral: 80–320 mg			
	Irbesartan	Oral: 150–300 mg daily			

(continued)

Site of Action	Drug	Dosage	Indications	Contraindications/Cautions	Frequent or Peculiar Side Effects
CALCIUM CHANNEL ANTAGONISTS					
Vascular smooth muscle	Dihydropyridines: Nifedipine XL	Oral: 30–90 mg daily	Mild to moderate hypertension	Heart failure, 2d or 3d degree heart block	Tachycardia, flushing, gastrointestinal disturbances, hyperkalemia, edema, headache
	Amlodipine	Oral: 2.5–10 mg daily			
	Felodipine XL	Oral: 5–10 mg daily			
	Isradipine	Oral: 2.5–10 mg daily			
	Nicardipine	Oral: 20–40 mg 3 times daily			
	Benzothiazepines: Diltiazem	Oral: 30–90 mg 4 times daily or as CD form 180–300 mg daily	Mild to moderate hypertension	Heart failure, 2d or 3d degree heart block	Same as amlodipine, except no tachycardia or edema, but can cause heart block, constipation, and liver dysfunction
	Phenylalkylamine: Verapamil	Oral: 30–120 mg 4 times daily or as SR form 120–480 mg daily	Mild to moderate hypertension	Heart failure, 2d or 3d degree heart block	

NOTE: MAO, monoamine oxidase; COPD, chronic obstructive pulmonary disease; XL, CD, SR are long-acting or sustained-release formulations.

one-half or more of all hypertensive patients showing a fall in pressure. Furthermore, like diuretics, they have been shown to reduce morbidity and mortality in long-term clinical trials. However, these agents can precipitate congestive heart failure and asthma in susceptible individuals, and they must be used with caution in diabetic patients receiving hypoglycemic therapy because they inhibit the usual sympathetic responses to hypoglycemia. Cardioselective beta-blocking agents (so-called beta$_1$ blockers, e.g., metoprolol, atenolol) have been developed and may be superior to nonselective beta blockers such as propranolol and timolol in patients with bronchospasm. Nadolol, a nonselective beta blocker, unlike other drugs of this class, is excreted unchanged in the urine and has a half-life of 14 to 20 h; only one dose a day is required. Atenolol also usually needs to be given only once a day. Pindolol and acebutolol are nonselective beta blockers that have partial agonist activity and, therefore, produce less bradycardia. Labetalol exerts both α- and β-adrenergic blocking actions. It is usually not used as first-line therapy as there is no mortality study in which it has been tested. Thus, it lowers arterial pressure not only by the same complex actions as do beta blockers but also directly by reducing systemic vascular resistance. Usually it has a more rapid onset of action but produces more postural symptoms and chronic sexual dysfunction than the other beta blockers.

VASODILATORS These agents are usually not used for initial therapy. *Hydralazine* is the most versatile of the drugs that cause direct relaxation of vascular smooth muscle; it is effective both orally and parenterally and acts mainly on arterial resistance rather than on venous capacitance vessels, as evidenced by lack of postural effects. Unfortunately, the effect of hydralazine on peripheral resistance is partly negated by a reflex increase in sympathetic discharge that raises heart rate and cardiac output. This response limits the usefulness of hydralazine, especially in patients with severe coronary artery disease. However, the efficacy of hydralazine can be increased if it is given in conjunction with a beta blocker or a drug such as methyldopa or clonidine, all of which block reflex sympathetic stimulation of the heart. A serious side effect of doses of hydralazine exceeding 300 mg/d has been the production of a lupus erythematosus–like syndrome.

Minoxidil is even more potent than hydralazine but unfortunately produces significant hypertrichosis and fluid retention and, therefore, is mainly limited to patients with severe hypertension and renal insufficiency.

Diazoxide, a thiazide derivative, is restricted in its application to acute situations. It is not a diuretic; in fact, it causes sodium retention. However, like other thiazides, it reduces carbohydrate tolerance. It must be given rapidly intravenously to guarantee an effect. It begins to act immediately to lower blood pressure, and its effects may last for several hours. *Nitroprusside* given intravenously also acts as a direct vasodilator, with onset and offset of actions that are almost immediate. *Nitroglycerin* is a third direct-acting vasodilator useful as an intravenous agent. These latter three drugs are useful only for the treatment of hypertensive emergencies (Table 246-7).

Table 246-7 Therapeutic Agents Used to Treat Malignant Hypertension

Drug	Route	Starting Dose	Onset	Peak	Duration	Oral Preparation Available
			Time Course of Action			
IMMEDIATE ONSET						
Nitroprusside	Continuous IV	0.25 μg/kg/min	<1 min	1–2 min	2–5 min	No
Nitroglycerin	Continuous IV	5 μg/min	1–5 min	2–6 min	3–10 min	No
Diazoxide	IV bolus	50 mg q 5–10 min up to 600 mg	1–5 min	2–4 min	4–12 h	No
Fenoldopan	Continuous IV	0.1–0.3 μg/kg per min	<5 min	5–10 min	30 min	No
Esmolol	Continuous IV	250–500 μg/min × 1 min; then 50–100 μg/kg per min × 4 min	1–2 min	2–3 min	10–20 min	No
DELAYED ONSET						
Enalaprilat	IV	1.25 mg q 6 h	10–15 min	3–4 h	6–24 h	Yes
Hydralazine	IV, IM	5–10 mg q 20 min × 3	10–20 min	20–40 min	4–12 h	Yes
Labetalol	IV	20–80 mg q 10 min up to 300 mg	5 min	20–30 min	3–6 h	Yes
Nicardipine	IV	5–15 mg/h	5–10 min	20–40 min	1–4 h	Yes

ACE INHIBITORS Drugs from several of the categories discussed above have been shown to possess an additional action resulting in inhibition of renin secretion. These include clonidine, reserpine, methyldopa, and beta blockers. A second group of drugs inhibit the enzyme converting angiotensin I into angiotensin II—ACE. These agents are an increasingly popular choice for initial therapy. They are useful because they not only inhibit the generation of a potent vasoconstrictor (angiotensin II) but also may retard the degradation of a potent vasodilator (bradykinin), alter prostaglandin production (an effect most notable with captopril), and can modify the activity of the adrenergic nervous system. They are especially useful in renal or renovascular hypertension and in diabetic patients, as well as in accelerated and malignant hypertension. However, in patients with bilateral renal artery stenosis, rapid deterioration of renal function may occur. They are also as effective in mild, uncomplicated hypertension as beta blockers and thiazides—and have fewer side effects, particularly ones that adversely affect the patient's quality of life.

These drugs should be used with caution when the renin system is activated (e.g., by severe heart failure, prior diuretic therapy, or substantial salt restriction) to avoid profound hypotension. Usually, diuretics are stopped 2 to 3 days before administration of an ACE inhibitor is begun and are added back later if needed.

ANGIOTENSIN RECEPTOR ANTAGONISTS These drugs have effects similar to those of ACE inhibitors. However, instead of blocking the production of angiotensin II, they competitively inhibit its binding to the angiotensin II AT$_1$ receptor subtype. Their utility and tolerability are similar to those of the ACE inhibitors, but they do not cause cough or angioedema.

CALCIUM CHANNEL ANTAGONISTS There are three subclasses of calcium channel antagonists: the phenylalkylamine derivatives (e.g., verapamil), the benzothiazepines (e.g., diltiazem), and the dihydropyridines (e.g., amlodipine). To date, there is only one therapeutic agent in each of the first two classes but a number of agents in the third class. All three subclasses modify calcium entry into cells by interacting with specific binding sites on the α_1 subunit of the L-type voltage-dependent calcium channel. Thus, since there are other calcium channels (e.g., the T and N types), the actions of these drugs only partially modify total calcium transport into cells. The relative specificity of each agent stems from the fact that each class has a unique binding site on the α_1 subunit, and these sites are variably expressed in different tissues. Thus, while agents from all three subclasses cause vasodilation, usually only dihydropyridines produce reflex tachycardia. Diltiazem and verapamil can both slow atrioventricular conduction—a feature not observed with the dihydropyridines. While calcium channel antagonists are also useful in angina pectoris (Chap. 244), because of their negative inotropic actions, they should be used with caution in hypertensive patients with heart failure. Considerable controversy has surrounded the use of calcium channel antagonists in the treatment of hypertension. In part the controversy was secondary to the inadequacy of the data and the confusion between the use of short-acting agents (e.g., nifedipine) and long-acting agents. Several facts have helped partially to resolve this controversy. First has been the general recognition that despite its previously frequent use as an antihypertensive agent, short-acting nifedipine rarely, if ever, should be used to treat hypertension, since it has been reported to increase the incidence of acute coronary events. Second, the results of the SYST-EUR (Systolic Hypertension in Europe) trial documented that a long-acting calcium channel antagonist reduced mortality to an extent equivalent to that previously reported for diuretics and beta blockers. Thus, long-acting calcium channel antagonists are often used as first-line therapy.

APPROACH TO DRUG THERAPY The aim of drug therapy is to use the agents just described, alone or in combination, to return arterial pressure to normal levels with minimal side effects. Ideally, one would choose a therapeutic program that specifically corrects the underlying defect resulting in the elevated blood pressure—for example, treatment with spironolactone for patients with primary aldosteronism. As our knowledge of the mechanisms underlying the hypertension in individual patients increases, more specific drug programs will become available. Such programs presumably will result in normalization of blood pressure with fewer side effects. In the absence of this information, an empirical approach is used, which takes into consideration efficacy, safety, impact on the quality of life, compliance, ease of administration, and cost. When used in combination, drugs are chosen for their different sites of action. However, except for those patients with severe hypertension (average diastolic blood pressure >130 mmHg), in whom intensive therapy with several agents simultaneously is usually required, most patients are treated *initially* with a single agent.

Since many effective antihypertensive agents are available, a number of useful therapeutic regimens have been developed. There are two major authoritative groups who have treatment guidelines when the patient's condition does not require a specific approach: World Health Organization–International Society of Hypertension (WHO-ISH) (Figs. 246-1 and 246-2) and the Sixth U.S. Joint National Committee (JNC) on Prevention, Detection, Evaluation, and Treatment of High Blood Pressure (JNC VI). In the absence of specific therapy, their approaches are similar in most respects, relying heavily on the results of randomized clinical trials (Table 246-8), except for which drugs should be used to initiate therapy. JNC VI recommends starting with diuretics and/or beta blockers because they are the ones where mortality trials have demonstrated a positive effect of treatment. The WHO-ISH guidelines recommends initiating therapy with any of six classes of agents (Table 246-9). The different recommendations, in part, reflect the fact that the WHO-ISH committee reviewed more recent data from mortality clinical trials that, in one case, documented a reduction in morbidity and mortality with a long-acting calcium

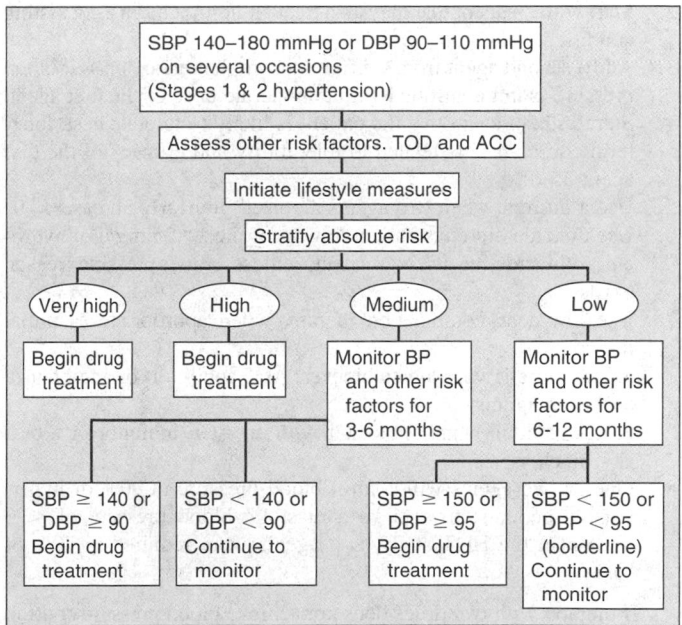

FIGURE 246-1 Initiation of treatment in patients with hypertension. See Table 246-9 for listing of classes of agents to use initially. In the initial evaluation the patients are stratified for cardiovascular risk using three categories: level of blood pressure (stages 1 to 3 varying from low to high risk); the presence of risk factors—smoking, obesity, male gender, etc.—which vary from 0 factors (low risk) to three or more factors (high risk equivalent to having diabetes mellitus), target organ damage (TOD), or diabetes (both high risk if present regardless of other risk factors); and clinical cardiovascular or renal disease (very high risk if present regardless of other risk factors). SBP, systolic blood pressure; DBP, diastolic blood pressure; TOD, target organ damage (previous WHO stage 2 hypertension); ACC, associated clinical conditions including clinical cardiovascular disease and renal disease (previous WHO stage 3 hypertension). (*Adapted with permission from 1999 WHO.*)

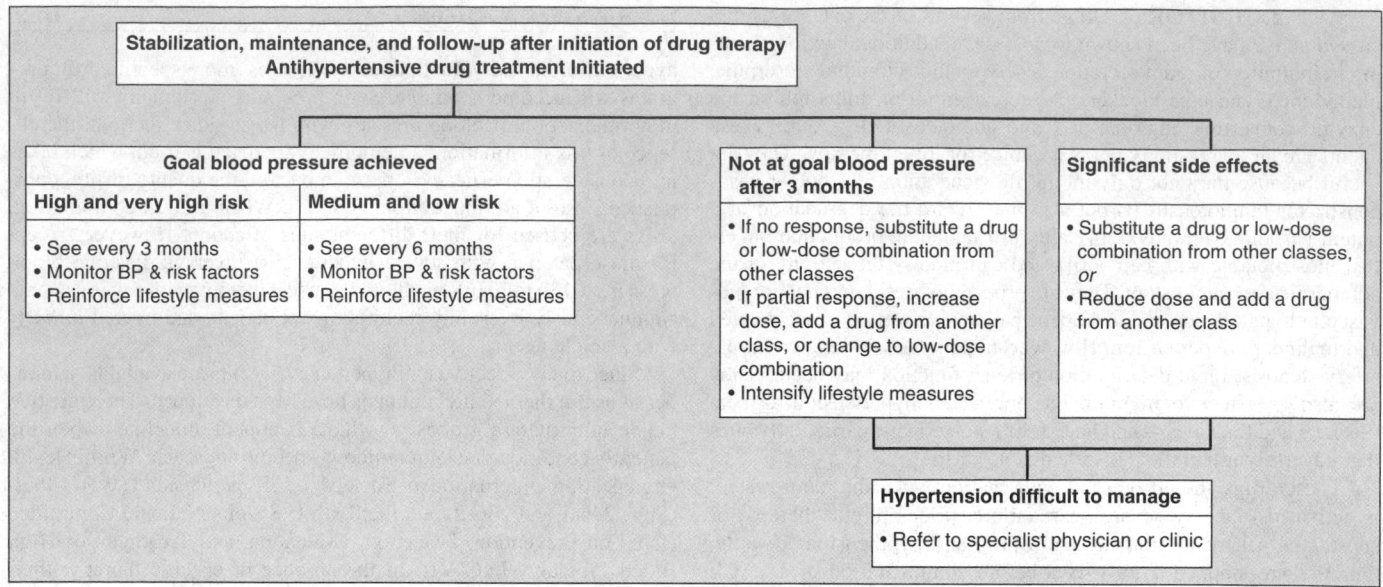

FIGURE 246-2 Approach to the hypertensive patient after initiating anti-hypertensive drug treatment. See Fig. 246-1 for initial steps and definition of risk and Table 246-9 for initial choice of agents. *(Adapted with permission from 1999 WHO.)*

channel antagonist versus placebo that was similar to previous reports for diuretics and beta blockers and, in another case, reported that ACE inhibitors were as effective as beta blockers and diuretics in reducing mortality (Table 246-8).

There are several critical caveats common to both approaches:

1. Start with a low dose of an agent and, if blood pressure is not controlled, increase only moderately.
2. Start with an agent that may also treat and/or not harm a coexisting condition.
3. Add a second agent from a different, complementary class if blood pressure is not controlled with a moderate dose of the first agent.
4. Start with an agent that the patient is likely to tolerate best; long-term compliance is related to tolerability and efficacy of the first agent used.
5. Use a diuretic when two agents are used, in nearly all cases.
6. Use thiazide diuretics only at low doses, i.e., ≤25 mg/d of hydrochlorothiazide or its equivalent, unless some pressing reason exists.
7. Use low-dose combination therapy when appropriate as initial therapy:
   a. A diuretic with a beta blocker, ACE inhibitor, or angiotensin II antagonist;
   b. A calcium channel blocker with an ACE inhibitor or a beta blocker
8. One or two agents will control blood pressure in 90% of hypertensive patients; to achieve a diastolic blood pressure of <90 mmHg in the HOT study, two agents were required in 70% of cases.

If therapy with two drugs does not achieve blood pressure control, the primary agent should be increased to full dose, e.g., 100 mg of captopril or atenolol, 20 mg of enalapril, or 360 mg of diltiazem. If the blood pressure is still not controlled, then a detailed search for a secondary cause of hypertension, as outlined above, is indicated. If none is found, then a dietary assessment will often reveal a high sodium intake. With reduction in salt intake to 5 g/d or less, blood pressure is often controlled. If the blood pressure is still not controlled, then the primary agent should be switched, maintaining the thiazide. Caution should be used if an ACE inhibitor was not the original agent, as administration of such an agent to a patient who is already taking a diuretic occasionally may lead to profound hypotension. If none of these changes produces better control of arterial pressure, then the combination of a calcium channel antagonist and an ACE inhibitor, or

triple therapy, usually with a diuretic, ACE inhibitor, and hydralazine, may be effective.

If the blood pressure is controlled, then a stepwise reduction in the dose and/or withdrawal of some of the agents should be carried out to determine the minimal therapeutic program that will maintain the blood pressure at 140/90 mmHg or less. Whether triple or quadruple drug therapy is warranted to lower blood pressure further is uncertain.

Fewer than 5% of patients will still be hypertensive at this point. For these, one first should consider the reasons for therapeutic failure, as shown in Table 246-10. If none can be identified, then one of the other agents, such as one of the vasodilators listed in Table 246-6 (e.g., hydralazine) or an antiadrenergic agent (e.g., prazosin or clonidine), should be added. If blood pressure is controlled, previous drugs are withdrawn sequentially to determine the minimal therapeutic program that will maintain a normal blood pressure.

While the recommendations outlined above are satisfactory for a large majority of patients, it is important to use a flexible approach, because individual patients may respond differently to individual drugs and drug combinations. For those patients requiring multiple drugs, once the appropriate combination has been found, the use of a single formulation with the appropriate combination of drugs may simplify the regimen and thereby increase compliance. Every effort should be made to reduce the number of times each day the patients must interrupt their schedules for the medication. Pharmacologic treatment of essential hypertension is usually lifelong, and since most patients are asymptomatic, compliance with a complex regimen may be a serious problem, particularly if the therapeutic regimen has a negative impact on the quality of the patient's life. Finally, it is uncertain what level of arterial pressure should be accepted as representing adequate control. It is clear that reducing diastolic blood pressure to <90 mmHg is appropriate and reduces morbidity and/or mortality.

Five groups of patients with hypertension require special consideration because of associated conditions. These groups are considered in the following sections.

RENAL DISEASE Reduction of arterial pressure in hypertensive patients with impaired renal function is often accompanied initially by an increase in serum creatinine. This change does not represent further structural renal damage and should not deter the physician from continuing the therapy, since achievement of blood pressure control may eventually reduce the value toward normal. However, if serum creatinine increases in a patient treated with a converting-enzyme inhibitor, care needs to be exercised, because these patients may have bilateral renal artery disease. Their renal function will continue to de-

Table 246-8   Randomized Clinical Trials in Hypertension

Trial Reference	Patient Number and Characteristics	Trial Arms	Endpoints	Results	Conclusion
SYST-EUR, Staessen et al, 1997	4695, >60 years old 2 years' follow-up	Nitrendipine/enalapril or HTZ Placebo	Primary: Death, all cardiovascular events, strokes	Active treatment reduced total stroke rate 42% ($p = .003$); nonfatal stroke decreased 44% ($p = .007$). All fatal and nonfatal cardiac endpoints declined 26% ($p = .03$). Cardiovascular mortality decreased 27% ($p = .07$).	Among elderly patients with isolated systolic hypertension, nitrendipine reduced cardiovascular complications; treatment of 1000 patients for 5 years with this regimen may prevent 29 strokes and/or 53 major cardiovascular endpoints
SYST-EUR, Tuomilehto et al, 1999	4695 (diabetic = 492) >60 years old 2 years' follow-up	Nitrendipine/enalapril or HTZ Placebo	Primary: Death, all cardiovascular events, strokes	In diabetics total mortality reduced 55%; mortality from cardiovascular disease by 76%; all cardiovascular events combined by 69%; nonfatal stroke by 73% Reductions in mortality and all cardiovascular events were significantly larger among diabetic than nondiabetic patients ($p = .04$ to $.01$).	Calcium channel antagonist significantly reduces cardiovascular morbidity and mortality in elder hypertensive patients; the effect is greater in diabetic than nondiabetic subjects
CAPPP Trial, Hansson et al, 1999	10,985, age 25–66, diastolic BP $\geq$ 100 mmHg 2–3 years' follow-up	Captopril Diuretics/beta blocker	Primary: Composite of fatal and nonfatal myocardial infarction, stroke, and other cardiovascular deaths	Primary endpoint relative risk 1.05, $p = .52$; Cardiovascular mortality was lower with captopril, relative risk 0.77, $p = .092$ Fatal and nonfatal stroke was more common with captopril, relative risk 1.25, $p = .044$	Captopril and conventional treatment did not differ in preventing cardiovascular morbidity and mortality
HOT Study, Hansson et al, 1998	18,790, 50–80 years with diastolic BP 100–115 mmHg 3–4 years' follow-up	Felodipine plus four other agents to reduce diastolic BP to 90 mmHg or 85 mmHg or 80 mmHg	Major cardiovascular events	Lowest cardiovascular mortality occurred at 86.5 mmHg; further reduction below these BPs was safe but no further reduction in risk; in patients with diabetes, a 51% reduction in cardiovascular events in target group = 80 mmHg compared with target group = 90 mmHg (p for trend = .006)	Intensive lowering of BP was associated with a low rate of cardiovascular events down to a diastolic BP of 82.6 mmHg
DASH Trial, Appel et al, 1997	459 with diastolic blood pressure 80–95 mmHg; 8 wks. Sodium intake and body weight were maintained constant.	Diet rich in fruits and vegetables Diet rich in fruits, vegetables, and low-fat dairy products Control (average U.S. diet)	Blood pressure.	Combination diet reduced systolic and diastolic BP by 5.5 and 3.0 mmHg more than the control diet ($p < .001$); the fruit and vegetable diet had an intermediate effect	A diet rich in fruits, vegetables, and low-fat dairy food can substantially lower BP
Messerli et al, 1998	Meta-analysis of efficacy of beta blockers vs. Diuretics as first-line therapy for elderly patients (60 years) with hypertension Approximate mean of 5 years' follow-up	Diuretics, 8 trials Beta blockers, 2 trials	Cerebrovascular events, coronary heart disease, stroke mortality, cardiovascular mortality, all-cause mortality	Diuretics significantly reduced cerebrovascular events odds ratio (0.61), coronary heart disease odds ratio (0.74), stroke mortality odds ratio (0.67), cardiovascular mortality odds ratio (0.75), and all-cause mortality odds ratio (0.86); beta blockers significantly reduced only cerebrovascular events odds ratio (0.74)	In elderly patients with hypertension, first-line diuretics reduced morbidity and mortality better than beta blockers

NOTE: HTZ, hydrochlorothiazine; BP, blood pressure.

Table 246-9 Guidelines for Selecting Drug Treatment of Hypertension

Class of Drug	Compelling Indications	Possible Indications	Compelling Contraindications	Possible Contraindications
Diuretics	Heart failure Elderly patients Systolic hypertension	Diabetes	Gout	Dyslipidemia Sexually active males
β-Blockers	Angina After myocardial infarct Tachyarrhythmias	Heart failure Pregnancy Diabetes	Asthma and COPD Heart block[a]	Dyslipidemia Athletes and physically active patients Peripheral vascular disease
ACE inhibitors	Heart failure Left ventricular dysfunction After myocardial infarct Diabetic nephropathy		Pregnancy Hyperkalaemia Bilateral renal artery stenosis	
Calcium antagonists	Angina Elderly patients Systolic hypertension	Peripheral vascular disease	Heart block[b]	Congestive heart failure[c]
α-Blockers	Prostatic hypertrophy	Glucose intolerance Dyslipidaemia		Orthostatic hypotension
Angiotensin II antagonists	ACE inhibitor cough	Heart failure	Pregnancy Bilateral renal artery stenosis Hyperkalaemia	

[a] Grade 2 or 3 atrioventricular block.
[b] Grade 2 or 3 atrioventricular block with verapamil or diltiazem.
[c] Verapamil or diltiazem.

NOTE: COPD, chronic obstructive pulmonary disease; ACE, angiotensin-converting enzyme.
SOURCE: Adapted with permission from 1999 WHO.

teriorate as long as the converting-enzyme inhibitor is given. Thus, converting-enzyme inhibitors should be used cautiously in patients with impaired renal function, and renal function should be assessed frequently (every 4 to 5 days) for the first 3 weeks. While converting-enzyme inhibitors are contraindicated in patients with bilateral renal artery stenosis, these are the drugs of choice in patients with unilateral renal artery stenosis and a normally functioning contralateral kidney and probably also in patients with chronic renal failure with or without diabetes mellitus.

CORONARY ARTERY DISEASE In these patients, who also may be taking cardiac glycosides, thiazides should be used judiciously, and a reduction in serum potassium levels should be watched for and, if found, should be corrected rapidly. Beta blockers should be withdrawn carefully, if at all, in these patients. Finally, calcium channel antagonists and converting-enzyme inhibitors may be useful in these patients because they minimize a number of potential adverse reactions that accompany the use of other therapeutic agents, particularly nonspecific vasodilators.

DIABETES MELLITUS The diabetic patient with hypertension is particularly challenging to treat because many of the agents used to lower blood pressure can affect glucose metabolism adversely. Converting-enzyme inhibitors may be particularly useful in these individuals. They have no known adverse effects on glucose or lipid metabolism and minimize the development of diabetic nephropathy by reducing renal vascular resistance and renal perfusion pressure—the primary factor underlying renal deterioration in these patients.

PREGNANCY The patient who is pregnant and hypertensive or who develops hypertension during pregnancy (pregnancy-induced hy-

Table 246-10 Reasons for Poor Therapeutic Response in Patients with Hypertension

Inadequate patient compliance
Volume expansion
  Caused by excessive sodium intake
  Caused by nondiuretic antihypertensive agent
  Caused by renal damage
Excessive weight gain
Inadequate doses
Drug antagonism
Cold remedies
Sympathomimetics
Oral contraceptives (estrogens)
Adrenal steroids
Secondary forms of hypertension

pertension, preeclampsia, eclampsia) is particularly difficult to treat. Because it is uncertain whether autoregulation of uterine blood flow occurs, lowering blood pressure in the pregnant hypertensive patient may result in reduced placental and fetal perfusion. Thus, a conservative approach to lowering blood pressure is usually indicated. In the second and third trimesters, antihypertensive agents are often not indicated unless the diastolic pressure exceeds 95 mmHg. In general, severe salt restriction and/or diuretics are not used because of the associated increase in fetal wastage. Beta blockers need to be used cautiously for similar reasons. Methyldopa and hydralazine, and to a lesser extent calcium channel antagonists, are the antihypertensive agents used most often, because they have no known adverse effects on the fetus. Little is known about the safety of other antihypertensive agents in pregnancy, except that nitroprusside and converting-enzyme inhibitors may cause adverse effects on the fetus and are contraindicated.

ELDERLY PATIENTS Hypertensive patients who are over age 65, and particularly those over age 75, offer substantial challenges to the physician. Several studies have reported that healthy elderly patients, whether male or female, who are treated with relatively modest doses of antihypertensive agents show a substantial reduction in strokes and stroke-related deaths. This is true whether the patient has systolic and diastolic hypertension or isolated systolic hypertension. What is not clear from these studies is how broadly the results can be extrapolated, since the studies were performed in healthy elderly patients, while many such patients have other diseases. Thus, in the elderly hypertensive patient, individualization of therapy still seems warranted.

Probably fewer than one-third of hypertensive patients in the United States are being treated effectively. Only a small number of these failures are related to drug unresponsiveness. Most are related to (1) failure to detect hypertension, (2) failure to institute effective treatment of an asymptomatic hypertensive patient, and (3) failure of the asymptomatic hypertensive patient to adhere to therapy. To help with the latter problem, patients must be educated to continue treatment once an effective regimen has been identified. Side effects and inconveniences of treatment must be minimized or counteracted in order to obtain the patient's continued cooperation.

MALIGNANT HYPERTENSION

In addition to marked blood pressure elevation in association with papilledema and retinal hemorrhages and exudates, the full-blown picture of malignant hypertension may include manifestations of hypertensive encephalopathy, such as severe headache, vomiting, visual disturbances (including transient blindness), transient paralyses, convulsions, stupor, and coma. These manifestations have been attributed to spasm of cerebral vessels and to cerebral edema. In some patients who have died, multiple small thrombi have been found in the cerebral vessels. Cardiac decompensation and rapidly declining renal function are other critical features of malignant hypertension. Oliguria may, in fact, be the presenting feature. The vascular lesion characteristic of malignant hypertension is fibrinoid necrosis of the walls of small arteries and arterioles, and this development can be reversed by effective antihypertensive therapy.

The pathogenesis of malignant hypertension is unknown. However, at least two independent processes—dilation of cerebral arteries and generalized arteriolar fibrinoid necrosis—contribute to the associated signs and symptoms. The cerebral arteries dilate because the normal autoregulation of cerebral blood flow decompensates as a result of the markedly elevated arterial pressure. Cerebral blood flow therefore is excessive, producing the encephalopathy associated with malignant hypertension. Many patients also show evidence of a microangiopathic hemolytic anemia; this secondary phenomenon could contribute to the deterioration of renal function. Most patients also have elevated levels of peripheral plasma renin activity and increased aldosterone production, and these effects may be involved in causing vascular damage.

Perhaps fewer than 1% of hypertensive patients develop the malignant phase, which can occur in the course of both essential and secondary hypertension. Rarely, it is the first recognized manifestation of the blood pressure problem, and it is unusual for it to occur in patients under treatment. The average age at diagnosis is 40, and men are affected more often than women. Prior to the availability of effective therapy, the life expectancy after diagnosis of malignant hypertension was less than 2 years, with most deaths being due to renal failure, cerebral hemorrhage, or congestive heart failure. With the advent of effective antihypertensive therapy, at least half the patients survive for more than 5 years.

℞ **TREATMENT** Malignant hypertension is a medical emergency that requires immediate therapy. However, it needs to be distinguished from severe hypertension, since overly aggressive therapy in malignant hypertension could result in a potentially hazardous reduction in myocardial and cerebral perfusion. The initial aims of therapy should be (1) correction of medical complications and (2) reduction of diastolic pressure by one-third, but not to a level <95 mmHg. The drugs available for treatment of malignant hypertension can be divided into two groups on the basis of time of onset of action (Table 246-7). Those in the first group act within a few minutes but are not satisfactory for long-term management. If the patient is having convulsions, and if arterial pressure must be reduced rapidly, then one from the immediate-acting group should be used.

The first three agents in this group require continuous infusion and close monitoring. *Nitroprusside* is given by continuous intravenous infusion at a dose of 0.25 to 8.0 μg/kg per min. It is probably the agent of choice in this condition, since it dilates both arterioles and veins. It has the advantage over the ganglionic blockers of not being associated with the development of tachyphylaxis and can be used for days with few side effects. The dosage must be controlled with an infusion pump. *Nitroglycerin* affects veins more than arterioles and is given by continuous infusion at a rate of 5 to 100 μg/min. It is particularly useful in the treatment of hypertension following coronary bypass surgery, myocardial infarction, left ventricular failure, or unstable angina pectoris. *Diazoxide* is the easiest agent to administer, for no individual titration of dosage is required. However, it is probably less effective than the other agents. It primarily affects arteriolar and not venous tone. A dose of 50 to 100 mg is given rapidly intravenously, and the antihypertensive effect appears in 1 to 5 min. The same dose can be repeated in 5 to 10 min, if necessary, or when the pressure begins to rise, usually after several hours. The total dose should not exceed 600 mg/d. In an occasional patient, pressure may drop below normal levels after diazoxide administration. This drug should not be

used in patients in whom aortic dissection or myocardial infarction is suspected. Because it can increase the force of myocardial contraction, often a beta blocker is given concomitantly. *Enalaprilat*, an intravenous form of the ACE inhibitor *enalapril*, has also proven effective, particularly in individuals with left heart failure. Finally, intravenous *labetalol* may be particularly useful in patients with a myocardial infarct or angina because it prevents an increase in heart rate. However, it may be ineffective in patients previously treated with beta blockers and is contraindicated in patients with heart failure, asthma, bradycardia, or heart block. It may also serve as an alternative therapy in patients with eclampsia who are unresponsive to hydralazine.

Patients given any of these agents also should receive other medications effective for long-term control. Those in the second group in Table 246-7 require 30 min or more to produce their full effect, but they have the advantage of being satisfactory for subsequent oral administration and for long-term management of the patient's hypertension. If such a delay in the achievement of the full effect is acceptable, intravenous *hydralazine* is effective in many patients within 10 min; an effective protocol involves giving 10-mg doses intravenously every 10 to 15 min until the desired effect has been obtained or until a total of 50 mg has been administered. The total amount required for response may then be repeated intramuscularly or intravenously every 6 h. Hydralazine should be used with caution in patients with significant coronary artery disease and should be avoided in patients manifesting myocardial ischemia or aortic dissection. It is effective in preeclampsia. *Esmolol*, a beta blocker with an onset of action of 1 to 2 min, is particularly useful in aortic dissection and for perioperative hypertensive crisis. Its major disadvantage is that it can have a negative inotropic effect. Its use in individuals with congestive heart failure, obstructive lung disease, or asthma is problematic.

Furosemide is an important adjunct to the therapy just discussed. Given either orally or intravenously, it serves to maintain sodium diuresis in the face of a falling arterial pressure and thus will speed recovery from encephalopathy and congestive heart failure as well as maintain the sensitivity to the primary antihypertensive drug. Digitalis (Chap. 232) may also be indicated if there is evidence of cardiac decompensation.

In patients with malignant hypertension in whom the existence of pheochromocytoma is suspected, urine should be collected for measurement of the products of catecholamine metabolism, and drugs that might release additional catecholamines, such as methyldopa, reserpine, and guanethidine, must be avoided. The parenteral drug of choice in these patients is phentolamine, administered with care to avoid a precipitous reduction in arterial pressure.

There is hope even for patients who fail to respond sufficiently to any of the forms of therapy and who show progressive deterioration in renal function. In some, a period of peritoneal dialysis or hemodialysis to deplete extracellular fluid has resulted in better blood pressure control and eventual improvement in renal function. In other patients with refractory hypertension and renal failure who do not respond to volume depletion or hypotensive therapy, including minoxidil administration—particularly those with marked elevation of plasma renin activity—bilateral nephrectomy has resulted in amelioration of hypertension; subsequently, these patients have been maintained on chronic dialysis or have received renal homografts. However, bilateral nephrectomy should be avoided where possible because (1) the loss of renal erythropoietin will contribute to the associated anemia, (2) vitamin D metabolism may be adversely affected, and (3) all residual renal function will be lost.

BIBLIOGRAPHY

APPEL LJ et al: A clinical trial of the effects of dietary patterns on blood pressure. DASH Collaborative Research Group N Engl J Med 336:1117, 1997

CONLIN PH, WILLIAMS GH: Use of calcium blockers in hypertension. Adv Intern Med, 43:533, 1998

DAHLOF B et al: Morbidity and mortality in the Swedish Trial in Old Patients with Hypertension (STOP-Hypertension). Lancet 338:1281, 1991

DE WARDENER HE: Salt reduction and cardiovascular risk: The anatomy of a myth. J Hum Hypertens 13:1, 1999

DOMINICZAK AF et al: Genes and hypertension: From gene mapping in experimental models to vascular gene transfer strategies. Hypertension 35:164, 2000

GRIFFITH LE et al: The influence of dietary and nondietary calcium supplementation on blood pressure. Am J Hypertens 12:84, 1999

HANSSON L et al: Effects of intensive blood-pressure lowering and low-dose aspirin in patients with hypertension: Principal results of the Hypertension Optimal Treatment (HOT) randomized trial. Lancet 351:1755, 1998

——— et al: Effect of angiotensin-converting-enzyme inhibition compared with conventional therapy of cardiovascular morbidity and mortality in hypertension: The Captopril Prevention Project (CAPPP) randomized trial. Lancet 353:611, 1999

HIRSCHL MM: Guidelines for the drug treatment of hypertensive crises. Drugs 50:991, 1995

JAFFE LS, SEELY EW: The heterogeneity of the blood pressure response to hormonal contraceptives. Curr Opin Endo Diab 2:257, 1995

JULIUS S et al: Overweight and hypertension: A 2-way street? Hypertension 35:807, 2000

KAPLAN N: Systemic hypertension: Mechanisms and diagnosis, in *Heart Disease*, 6th ed, E Braunwald et al (eds). Philadelphia, WB Saunders, 2001

LAKSHMAN MR et al: Diuretics and beta-blockers do not have adverse effects at 1 year on plasma lipid and lipoprotein profiles in men with hypertension. Arch Intern Med 159:551, 1999

MESSERLI FG, GRODZICKI T: Antihypertensive therapy in the elderly: Evidence-based guidelines and reality. Arch Intern Med 159:1621, 1999

——— et al: Are beta-blockers efficacious as first line therapy for hypertension in the elderly? A systematic review. JAMA 279:1903, 1998

MORTENSEN RM, WILLIAMS GH: Aldosterone action (physiology), in *Endocrinology*, 4th ed, LJ DeGroot et al (eds). Philadelphia, Saunders, 2000

PRISANT LM, MOSER M: Hypertension in the elderly: Can we improve results of therapy? Arch Intern Med 160:283, 2000

PUSCHETT JB: Diuretics and the therapy of hypertension. Am J Med Sci 319:1, 2000

Sixth Report of the Joint National Committee on Prevention, Detection, Evaluation, and Treatment of High Blood Pressure. Arch Intern Med 157:2413, 1997

STAESSEN JA et al: Randomized double-blind comparison of placebo and active treatment for older patients with isolated systolic hypertension. The Systolic Hypertension in Europe (SYST-EUR) trial investigators. Lancet 350:757, 1997

WARNOCK DG: Low renin hypertension in the next milennium. Semin Nephrol 20:40, 2000

WILLIAMS GH: Quality of life considerations in therapeutic decision-making: Antihypertensive therapy as a model, in *Aging, Health and Healing*, M Bergener et al (eds). New York, Springer, 1995, p 257

1999 World Health Organization–International Society of Hypertension Guidelines for the Management of Hypertension. J Hypertens 17:151, 1999

247

Victor J. Dzau, Mark A. Creager

DISEASES OF THE AORTA

The aorta is the conduit through which the blood ejected from the left ventricle is delivered to the systemic arterial bed. In adults, its diameter is approximately 3 cm at the origin, 2.5 cm in the descending portion in the thorax, and 1.8 to 2 cm in the abdomen. The aortic wall consists of a thin intima composed of endothelium, subendothelial connective tissue, and an internal elastic lamina; a thick tunica media composed of smooth-muscle cells and extracellular matrix; and an adventitia composed primarily of connective tissue enclosing the vasa vasorum and nervi vascularis. In addition to its conduit function, the viscoelastic and compliant properties of the aorta also subserve a buffering function. The aorta is distended during systole to enable a portion of the stroke volume to be stored, and it recoils during diastole so that blood continues to flow to the periphery. Because of its continuous exposure to high pulsatile pressure and shear stress, the aorta is particularly prone to injury and disease resulting from mechanical trauma (Table 247-1). The aorta is also more prone to rupture than any other vessel, especially with the development of aneurysmal dilatation, since its

Table 247-1   Diseases of the Aorta: Etiology and Associated Factors

Aortic aneurysm	Aortic occlusion
Atherosclerosis	Atherosclerosis
Cystic medial necrosis	Thromboembolism
Tuberculosis	**Aortitis**
Syphilitic infection	Syphilitic aortitis
Mycotic infection	Rheumatic aortitis
Rheumatic aortitis	Takayasu's arteritis
Trauma	Giant cell arteritis
Aortic dissection	
Cystic medial necrosis	
Systemic hypertension	
Atherosclerosis	
Takayasu's arteritis	
Giant cell arteritis	

wall tension, as governed by Laplace's law (i.e., proportional to the product of pressure and radius), would be increased.

AORTIC ANEURYSM

An *aneurysm* is defined as a pathologic dilatation of a segment of a blood vessel. A *true aneurysm* involves all three layers of the vessel wall and is distinguished from a *pseudoaneurysm*, in which the intimal and medial layers are disrupted and the dilatation is lined by adventitia only and sometimes by perivascular clot. Aneurysms also may be classified accordingly to their gross appearance. A *fusiform aneurysm* affects the entire circumference of a segment of the vessel, resulting in a diffusely dilated lesion. In contrast, a *saccular aneurysm* involves only a portion of the circumference, resulting in an outpouching of the vessel wall. Aortic aneurysms are also classified according to location, i.e., abdominal versus thoracic. Aneurysms of the descending thoracic aorta are usually contiguous with infradiaphragmatic aneurysms and are referred to as *thoracoabdominal aortic aneurysms*.

ETIOLOGY   The most common pathologic condition associated with aortic aneurysm is *atherosclerosis*. It is controversial whether atherosclerosis itself actually causes aortic aneurysms or whether atherosclerosis develops as a secondary event in the dilated aorta. Causality is implied by studies that have shown that many patients with aortic aneurysms have coexisting risk factors for atherosclerosis (Chap. 241), particularly cigarette smoking, as well as atherosclerosis in other blood vessels. Seventy-five percent of atherosclerotic aneurysms are located in the distal abdominal aorta, below the renal arteries.

Cystic medial necrosis is the term used to describe the degeneration of collagen and elastic fibers in the tunica media of the aorta, as well as the loss of medial cells that are replaced by multiple clefts of mucoid material. Cystic medial necrosis characteristically affects the proximal aorta, results in circumferential weakness and dilatation, and leads to development of fusiform aneurysms involving the ascending aorta and the sinuses of Valsalva. This condition is particularly prevalent in patients with Marfan syndrome and Ehrlers-Danlos syndrome type IV (Chap. 351) but also occurs in pregnant women, in patients with hypertension, and in those with valvular heart disease. Sometimes it appears as an isolated condition in patients without any other apparent disease. Familial clusterings of aortic aneurysms occur in 20% of patients, suggesting a hereditary basis of the disease. A mutation of the gene encoding type III procollagen has been implicated. *Syphilis* (Chap. 172) is a relatively uncommon cause of aortic aneurysm. Syphilitic periaortitis and mesoaortitis damage elastic fibers, resulting in thickening and weakening of the aortic wall. Approximately 90% of syphilitic aneurysms are located in the ascending aorta or aortic arch. *Tuberculous aneurysms* (Chap. 169) typically affect the thoracic aorta and result from direct extension of infection from hilar lymph nodes or contiguous abscesses or from bacterial seeding. Loss of aortic wall elasticity results from granulomatous destruction of the medial layer. A *mycotic aneurysm* is a rare condition that develops as a result of staphylococcal, streptococcal, or salmonella infections of the aorta,

usually at an atherosclerotic plaque. These aneurysms are usually saccular. Blood cultures are often positive and reveal the nature of the
infecting agent.

Vasculitides associated with aortic aneurysm include Takayasu's
arteritis and giant cell arteritis, which may cause aneurysms of the
aortic arch and descending thoracic aorta. Spondyloarthropathies such
as ankylosing spondylitis, rheumatoid arthritis, psoriatic arthritis, relapsing polychondritis, Behçet's syndrome, and Reiter's syndrome are
associated with dilatation of the ascending aorta. *Traumatic aneurysms*
may develop after penetrating or non-penetrating chest trauma and
most commonly affect the descending thoracic aorta just beyond the
site of insertion of the ligamentum arteriosum. *Congenital aortic aneurysms* may be primary or associated with anomalies such as a bicuspid aortic valve or aortic coarctation.

THORACIC AORTIC ANEURYSMS The clinical manifestations and natural history of thoracic aortic aneurysms depend on their
location. Cystic medial necrosis is the most common cause of ascending aortic aneurysms, whereas atherosclerosis is the condition most
frequently associated with aneurysms of the aortic arch and descending
thoracic aorta. The average growth rate of thoracic aneurysms is 0.1
to 0.4 cm per year. The risk of rupture is related to the size of the
aneurysm and the presence of symptoms; it increases substantially for
ascending aortic aneurysms >6 cm and descending thoracic aneurysms >7 cm. Most thoracic aortic aneurysms are asymptomatic.
However, compression or erosion of adjacent tissue by aneurysms may
cause symptoms such as chest pain, shortness of breath, cough, hoarseness, or dysphagia. Aneurysmal dilatation of the ascending aorta may
cause congestive heart failure as a consequence of aortic regurgitation;
and compression of the superior vena cava may produce congestion
of the head, neck, and upper extremities.

A chest x-ray may be the first test to suggest the diagnosis of a
thoracic aortic aneurysm. Findings include widening of the mediastinal
shadow and displacement or compression of the trachea or left mainstem bronchus. Two-dimensional echocardiography, and particularly
transesophageal echocardiography, can be used to assess the proximal
ascending aorta and descending thoracic aorta. Both contrast-
enhanced computed tomography (CT) and magnetic resonance imaging (MRI) are sensitive and specific tests for assessment of aneurysms
of the thoracic aorta. In asymptomatic patients whose aneurysms are
too small to justify surgery, noninvasive testing with either contrast-
enhanced CT or MRI should be performed at least every 6 to 12
months to monitor expansion. Contrast aortography is frequently required preoperatively to assess the length of the aneurysm and involvement of branch vessels.

Patients with thoracic aortic aneurysms, and particularly patients
with Marfan syndrome who have evidence of aortic root dilatation,
should receive long-term beta-blocker therapy. Additional medical
therapy should be given, as necessary, to control hypertension. Operative repair with placement of a prosthetic graft is indicated in patients with symptomatic thoracic aortic aneurysms and in those in
whom the aortic diameter is >6 cm. In patients with Marfan syndrome,
thoracic aortic aneurysms >5 cm should be considered for surgery.

ABDOMINAL AORTIC ANEURYSMS Abdominal aortic
aneurysms occur more frequently in males than in females, and the
incidence increases with age. Abdominal aortic aneurysms may affect
1 to 2% of men older than 50 years. At least 90% of all abdominal
aortic aneurysms are affected by atherosclerosis, and most of these
aneurysms are below the level of the renal arteries. Prognosis is related
to both the size of the aneurysm and the severity of coexisting coronary
artery and cerebrovascular disease. The risk of rupture increases with
the size of the aneurysm. The 5-year risk of rupture for aneurysms <5
cm is 1 to 2%, whereas it is 20 to 40% for aneurysms >5 cm in
diameter. The formation of mural thrombi within the aneurysm may
predispose to peripheral embolization.

An abdominal aortic aneurysm commonly produces no symptoms.
It is usually detected on routine examination as a palpable, pulsatile,
and nontender mass, or it is an incidental finding during an abdominal
x-ray or ultrasound performed for other reasons. However, as abdom-

inal aortic aneurysms expand, they may become painful. Some patients
complain of strong pulsations in the abdomen; others experience pain
in the chest, lower back, or scrotum. Aneurysmal pain is usually a
harbinger of rupture and represents a medical emergency. More often,
acute rupture occurs without any prior warning, and this complication
is always life-threatening. Rarely, there is leakage of the aneurysm
with severe pain and tenderness. Acute pain and hypotension occur
with rupture of the aneurysm, which requires emergency operation.

Abdominal radiography may demonstrate the calcified outline of
the aneurysm. However, about 25% of aneurysms are not calcified and
cannot be visualized by plain x-ray. An abdominal ultrasound can
delineate the transverse and longitudinal dimensions of an abdominal
aortic aneurysm and may detect mural thrombus. Abdominal ultrasound in useful for serial documentation of aneurysm size and can be
used to screen patients at risk for developing aortic aneurysm, such as
those with affected siblings, peripheral atherosclerosis, or peripheral
artery aneurysms. CT with contrast and MRI are accurate, noninvasive
tests to determine the location and size of abdominal aortic aneurysms.
Contrast aortography is used commonly for the evaluation of patients
with aneurysms before surgery; but the procedure carries a small risk
of complications, such as bleeding, allergic reactions, and atheroembolism. This technique is useful in documenting the length of the aneurysm, especially its upper and lower limits, and the extent of associated atherosclerotic vascular disease. However, since the presence of
mural clots may reduce the luminal size, aortography may underestimate the diameter of an aneurysm.

TREATMENT Operative repair of the aneurysm and insertion
of a prosthetic graft is indicated for abdominal aortic aneurysms
of any size that are expanding rapidly or are associated with symptoms.
For asymptomatic aneurysms, operation is indicated if the diameter is
>5 cm. Operation may be recommended in patients with aneurysm
diameters of 4 to 5 cm, except for patients with exceptionally high
operative risk. However, in a recent randomized trial of patients with
abdominal aortic aneurysms <5.5 cm, there was no difference in the
6-year mortality rate between those followed with ultrasound surveillance and those undergoing elective aneurysm repair. Thus, serial noninvasive follow-up of smaller aneurysms (<5 cm) is an alternative to
immediate surgery. Percutaneous placement of endovascular stent
grafts (Fig. 247-1) for treatment of infrarenal abdominal aortic aneurysms is currently available for selected patients, and initial reports
have been favorable.

In surgical candidates, careful preoperative cardiac and general
medical evaluations (followed by appropriate therapy of complicating
conditions) are essential. Preexisting coronary artery disease, congestive heart failure, pulmonary disease, diabetes, and advanced age add
to the risk of surgery. Perioperative management should include the
placement of a Swan-Ganz catheter and arterial line to monitor and
optimize left ventricular filling pressure, cardiac output, and arterial
pressure, especially during clamping and unclamping of the aorta, as
well as during the immediate postoperative period. With careful preoperative cardiac evaluation and postoperative care the operative mortality rate approximates 1 to 2%. After acute rupture, the mortality rate
of emergent operation generally exceeds 50%.

AORTIC DISSECTION

Aortic dissection is caused by a circumferential or, less frequently,
transverse tear of the intima. It often occurs along the right lateral wall
of the ascending aorta where the hydraulic shear stress is high. Another
common site is the descending thoracic aorta just below the ligamentum arteriosum. The initiating event is either a primary intimal tear
with secondary dissection into the media or a medial hemorrhage that
dissects into and disrupts the intima. The pulsatile aortic flow then
dissects along the elastic lamellar plates of the aorta and creates a false
lumen. The dissection usually propagates distally down the descending

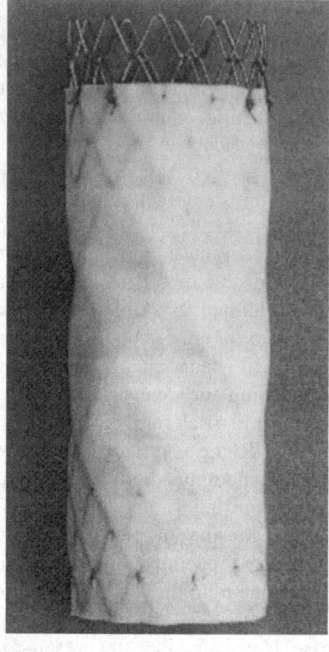
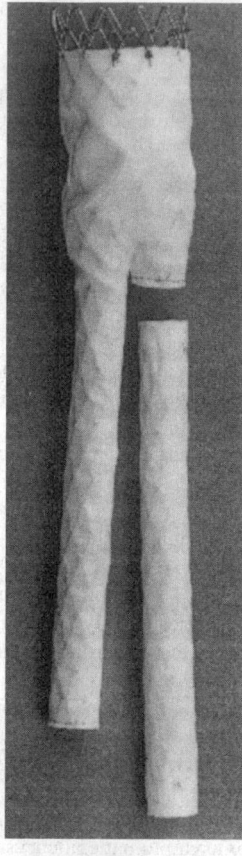

FIGURE 247-1 Example of stent grafts used for the endoluminal treatment of infrarenal aortic aneurysms. The left panel shows a straight stent graft that is inserted into the abdominal aorta. The right panel shows a bifurcated graft with two components that are inserted separately and then joined. *(From Blum et al., with permission.)*

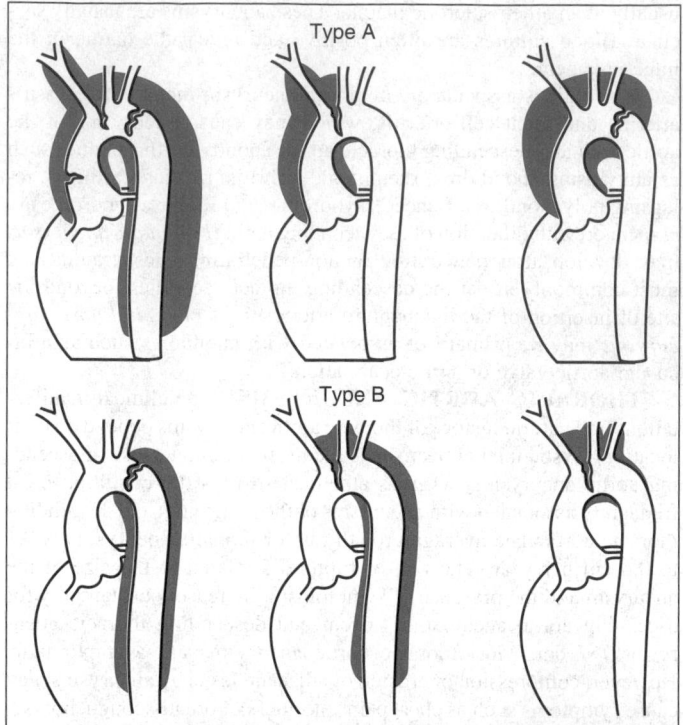

FIGURE 247-2 Classification of aortic dissections. Stanford classification: Type A dissections (*top panels*) involve the ascending aorta independent of site of tear and distal extension; type B dissections (*bottom panels*) involve transverse and/or descending aorta without involvement of the ascending aorta. DeBakey classification: Type I dissection involves ascending to descending aorta (*top left*); type II dissection is limited to ascending or transverse aorta, without descending aorta (*top center + top right*); type III dissection involves descending aorta only (*bottom left*). [*From DC Miller, in RM Doroghazi, EE Slater (eds): Aortic Dissection. New York, McGraw-Hill, 1983, with permission.*]

aorta and into its major branches, but it also may propagate proximally. In some cases, a secondary distal intimal disruption occurs, resulting in the reentry of blood from the false to the true lumen.

There are at least two important pathologic and radiologic variants: intramural hematoma without an intimal flap and penetrating ulcer. The clinical picture and therapeutic management of intramural hematoma are similar to those for classic aortic dissection. By contrast, penetrating ulcers are usually localized and are not associated with extensive propagation. They are primarily found in the distal portion of the descending thoracic aorta and are associated with extensive atherosclerotic disease. The ulcer can erode beyond the intimal border, leading to medial hematoma, and may progress to false aneurysm formation or rupture.

DeBakey and coworkers initially classified aortic dissections as type I, in which an intimal tear occurs in the ascending aorta but which involves the descending aorta as well; type II, in which the dissection is limited to the ascending aorta; and type III, in which the intimal tear is located in the descending area with distal propagation of the dissection (Fig. 247-2). Another classification (Stanford) is that of type A, in which the dissection involves the ascending aorta (proximal dissection), and type B, in which it is limited to the descending aorta (distal dissection). From a management standpoint, classification into type A or B is more practical and useful, since DeBakey types I and II are managed in a similar manner.

The factors that predispose to aortic dissection include systemic hypertension, a coexisting condition in 70% of patients, and cystic medial necrosis. Aortic dissection is the major cause of morbidity and mortality in patients with Marfan syndrome (Chap. 351) and similarly may affect patients with Ehlers-Danlos syndrome. The incidence is also increased in patients with inflammatory aortitis (i.e., Takayasu's arteritis, giant cell arteritis), congenital aortic valve anomalies (e.g., bicuspid valve), in those with coarctation of the aorta, and in otherwise normal women during the third trimester of pregnancy.

CLINICAL MANIFESTATIONS The peak incidence is in the sixth and seventh decades. Men are more affected than women by a ratio of 2:1. The presentations of aortic dissection and its variants are the consequences of intimal tear, dissecting hematoma, occlusion of involved arteries, and compression of adjacent tissues. Acute aortic dissection presents with the sudden onset of pain (Chap. 13), which is often described as very severe and tearing and is associated with diaphoresis. The pain may be localized to the front or back of the chest, often the interscapular region, and typically migrates with propagation of the dissection. Other symptoms include syncope, dyspnea, and weakness. Physical findings may include hypertension or hypotension, loss of pulses, aortic regurgitation, pulmonary edema, and neurologic findings due to carotid artery obstruction (hemiplegia, hemianesthesia) or spinal cord ischemia (paraplegia). Bowel ischemia, hematuria, and myocardial ischemia have all been observed. These clinical manifestations reflect complications resulting from the dissection occluding the major arteries. Furthermore, clinical manifestations may result from the compression of adjacent structures (e.g., superior cervical ganglia, superior vena cava, bronchus, esophagus) by the expanding dissection causing aneursymal dilatation, and include Horner's syndrome, superior vena caval syndrome, hoarseness, dysphagia, and airway compromise. Hemopericardium and cardiac tamponade may complicate a type A lesion with retrograde dissection. Acute aortic regurgitation is an important and common (>50%) complication of proximal dissection. It is the outcome of either a circumferential tear that widens the aortic root or a disruption of the annulus by dissecting hematoma that tears a leaflet(s) or displaces it below the line of closure. Signs of aortic regurgitation include bounding pulses, a wide pulse pressure, a diastolic murmur often radiating along the right sternal border, and evidence of congestive heart failure. The clinical manifestation depends on the severity of the regurgitation.

In dissections involving the ascending aorta, the chest x-ray often reveals a widened superior mediastinum. A pleural effusion (usually left-sided) also may be present. This effusion is typically serosanguinous and not indicative of rupture unless accompanied by hypotension and falling hematocrit. In dissections of the descending thoracic aorta, a widened mediastinum also may be observed on chest x-ray. In addition, the descending aorta may appear to be wider than the ascending portion. An electrocardiogram that shows no evidence of ischemia is helpful in distinguishing aortic dissection from myocardial infarction. Rarely, the dissection involves the right or left coronary ostium and causes acute myocardial infarction. The diagnosis of aortic dissection can be established by aortography or by the use of noninvasive techniques such as echocardiography, CT, or MRI. Aortography may be used to document the diagnosis; identify the entry point, the intimal flap, and the false and true lumina; and to establish the extent of dissection into the major arteries. Coronary angiography may be performed concomitantly in high-risk patients in the evaluation and preparation for surgery. The sensitivity of aortography is 70% for visualizing an intimal flap, 56% for the site of intimal tear, and 87% for false lumen. It is unable to recognize intramural hemorrhage. Transthoracic echocardiography can be performed simply and rapidly and has an overall sensitivity of 60 to 85%. For diagnosing proximal ascending aortic dissections, its sensitivity exceeds 80%; it is less useful for detecting dissection of the arch and descending thoracic aorta. Transesophageal echocardiography (Fig. 247-3) requires greater skill and patient cooperation but is very accurate in identifying dissections of the ascending and descending thoracic aorta, but not the arch, achieving 98% sensitivity and approximately 90% specificity. CT and MRI are both highly accurate in identifying the intimal flap and the extent of the dissection; each has a sensitivity and specificity exceeding 90%. They are useful in recognizing intramural hemorrhage and penetrating ulcers. MRI also can detect blood flow, which may be useful in characterizing antegrade versus retrograde dissection. These noninvasive tests are now becoming the diagnostic procedures of choice. Their relative utility depends on the availability and expertise in individual institutions as well as on the hemodynamic stability of the patient, with CT and MRI obviously less suitable for more unstable patients.

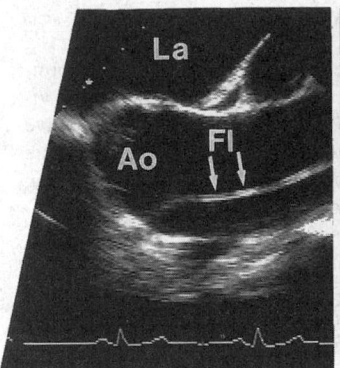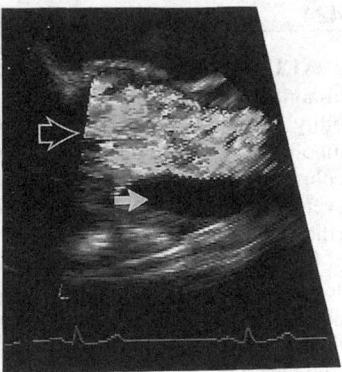

FIGURE 247-3 Aortic dissection. *Left.* Transesophageal echocardiogram of the ascending aorta demonstrating a freely mobile flap within the lumen of the vessel. Ao, aorta; La, left atrium; Fl, flap. *Right.* When color Doppler was superimposed on the image, the true lumen (*open arrow*) was easily separated from the false lumen (*solid arrow*).

℞ **TREATMENT** Medical therapy should be initiated as soon as the diagnosis is considered. The patient should be admitted to an intensive care unit for monitoring hemodynamics and urine output. Unless hypotension is present, therapy should be aimed at reducing cardiac contractility and systemic arterial pressure, and thereby shear stress. For acute dissection, unless contraindicated, β-adrenergic blockers should be administered parenterally, using intravenous propranolol, metoprolol, or the short-acting esmolol to achieve a heart rate of approximately 60 beats per minute. This should be accompanied by sodium nitroprusside infusion to lower systolic blood pressure to 120 mmHg or less. Labetalol (Chap. 246), a drug with both β- and α-adrenergic blocking properties, also has been used as a parenteral agent in the acute therapy of dissection.

The calcium channel antagonists, verapamil and diltiazem, may be used intravenously if nitroprusside or labetalol cannot be employed. Experience with calcium antagonists is limited. Direct vasodilators, such as diazoxide and hydralazine, are contraindicated because these agents can increase hydraulic shear and may propagate dissection.

Emergent or urgent surgical correction is the preferred treatment for ascending aortic dissections (type A) and complicated type B dissections including those characterized by propagation, compromise of major aortic branches, impending rupture, or continued pain. Surgery involves excision of the intimal flap, obliteration of the false lumen, and placement of an interposition graft. A composite valve-graft conduit is used if the aortic valve is disrupted. The overall in-hospital mortality rate after surgical treatment of patients with aortic dissection is reported to be 15 to 20%. The major causes of perioperative mortality and morbidity include myocardial infarction, paraplegia, renal failure, tamponade, hemorrhage, and sepsis. Recent reports of the use of endoluminal stent grafts in selected patients with type B dissection have been encouraging. Other transcatheter techniques, such as fenestration of the intimal flaps and stenting of narrowed branch vessels to increase flow to compromised organs, are also under investigation. For uncomplicated and stable distal dissection (type B), medical therapy is the preferred treatment. The in-hospital mortality rate of medically treated patients with type B dissection is 15 to 20%. Long-term therapy for patients with aortic dissection (with or without surgery) consists of the control of hypertension and reduction of cardiac contractility with the use of beta blockers plus other antihypertensive agents such as angiotensin-converting enzyme inhibitor or calcium antagonist. Patients with chronic type B dissection should be followed on an outpatient basis every 6 to 12 months by contrast-enhanced CT or MRI to detect propagation. Patients with Marfan syndrome are at high risk for postdissection complications. The long-term prognosis for patients with treated dissections is generally good with careful follow-up; the 10-year survival rate is approximately 60%.

AORTIC OCCLUSION

CHRONIC ATHEROSCLEROTIC OCCLUSIVE DISEASE
Atherosclerosis may affect the thoracic and abdominal aorta, but occlusive aortic disease caused by atherosclerosis usually is confined to the distal abdominal aorta below the renal arteries. Frequently the disease extends to the iliac arteries (Chap. 248). Claudication characteristically involves the lower back, buttocks, and thighs and may be associated with impotence in males (Leriche syndrome). The severity of the symptoms depends on the adequacy of collaterals. With sufficient collateral blood flow, a complete occlusion of the abdominal aorta may occur without the development of ischemic symptoms. The physical findings include absence of femoral and other distal pulses bilaterally and the detection of an audible bruit over the abdomen (usually at or below the umbilicus) and the common femoral arteries. Atrophic skin, loss of hair, and coolness of the lower extremities are usually observed. In advanced ischemia, rubor on dependency and pallor on elevation can be seen.

The diagnosis is usually established by the physical examination and noninvasive testing, including leg pressure measurements, Doppler velocity analysis, and pulse volume recordings. The anatomy may be defined by abdominal aortography before revascularization. Operative treatment is indicated in patients with debilitating symptoms and/or with the development of leg ischemia.

ACUTE OCCLUSION Acute occlusion in the distal abdominal aorta represents a medical emergency because it threatens the viability of the lower extremities. It usually results from an occlusive embolus that almost always originates from the heart. Rarely, acute occlusion may occur as the result of in situ thrombosis in a preexisting severely narrowed segment of the aorta or plaque rupture and hemorrhage into such an area.

The clinical picture is one of acute ischemia of the lower extremities. Severe rest pain, coolness, and pallor of the lower extremities and the absence of distal pulses bilaterally are the usual manifestations. Diagnosis should be established rapidly by aortography. Emergency thrombectomy or revascularization is indicated.

AORTITIS

Aortitis frequently affects the ascending aorta and may result in aneurysmal dilatation and aortic regurgitation; it occasionally obstructs branch vessels of the aorta.

SYPHILITIC AORTITIS This late manifestation of luetic infection (Chap. 172) usually affects the proximal ascending aorta, particularly the aortic root, resulting in aortic dilatation and aneurysm formation. Syphilitic aortitis may occasionally involve the aortic arch or the descending aorta. The aneurysms may be saccular or fusiform and are usually asymptomatic, but compression of and erosion into adjacent structures may result in symptoms; rupture also may occur.

The initial lesion is an obliterative endarteritis of the vasa vasorum, especially in the adventitia. This is an inflammatory response to the invasion of the adventitia by the spirochetes. Destruction of the aortic media occurs as the spirochetes spread into this layer, usually via the lymphatics accompanying the vasa vasorum. Destruction of collagen and elastic tissues leads to dilation of the aorta, scar formation, and calcification. These changes account for the characteristic radiographic appearance of a calcified ascending aortic aneurysm.

The disease typically presents as an incidental radiographic finding 15 to 30 years after initial infection. Symptoms may result from aortic regurgitation, narrowing of coronary ostia due to syphilitic aortitis, compression of adjacent structures (e.g., esophagus), or rupture. Diagnosis is established by a positive serologic test, i.e., rapid plasmin reagin (RPR) or fluorescent treponemal antibody. Treatment includes penicillin and surgical excision and repair.

RHEUMATIC AORTITIS Rheumatoid arthritis (Chap. 312), ankylosing spondylitis (Chap. 315), psoriatic arthritis (Chap. 324), Reiter's syndrome (Chap. 315), Behçet's syndrome (Chap. 316), relapsing polychondritis, and inflammatory bowel disorders may all be associated with aortitis involving the ascending aorta. The inflammatory lesions usually involve the ascending aorta and may extend to the sinuses of Valsalva, the mitral valve leaflets, and adjacent myocardium. The clinical manifestations are aneurysm, aortic regurgitation, and involvement of the cardiac conduction system.

TAKAYASU'S ARTERITIS Inflammatory diseases of the aortic arch resulting in obstruction of the aorta and its major arteries characterize this major group of diseases. Takayasu's arteritis is also termed *pulseless disease* because of the frequent occlusion of the large arteries originating from the aorta. It also may involve the descending thoracic and abdominal aorta and occlude large branches such as the renal arteries. Aortic aneurysms may also occur. The pathology is a panarteritis, characterized by mononuclear cells and occasionally giant cells, with marked intimal hyperplasia, medial and adventitial thickening, and, in chronic form, fibrotic occlusion. The disease is most prevalent in young females of Asian descent. During the acute stage, fever, malaise, weight loss, and other systemic symptoms may be evident. An elevation of the erythrocyte sedimentation rate is common. The chronic stages of the disease present with symptoms related to large artery occlusion, such as upper extremity claudication, cerebral ischemia, and syncope. The chronic disease is intermittently active. Since the process is progressive and there is no definitive therapy, the

prognosis is usually poor. Glucocorticoids and immunosuppressive agents have been reported to be effective in some patients during the acute phase. Occasionally, anticoagulation prevents thrombosis and complete occlusion of a large artery. Surgical bypass of a critically stenotic artery may be necessary.

GIANT CELL ARTERITIS (See also Chap. 317) This vasculitis occurs in older individuals and affects women more often than men. Primarily large and medium-sized arteries are affected. The pathology is that of focal granulomatous lesions involving the entire arterial wall. It may be associated with polymyalgia rheumatica. Obstruction of medium-sized arteries (e.g., temporal and ophthalmic arteries) and of major branches of the aorta and the development of aortitis and aortic regurgitation are some of the complications of the disease. High-dose glucocorticoid therapy may be effective when given early.

BIBLIOGRAPHY

BLANCHARD JF et al: Risk factors for abdominal aortic aneurysm: results of a case-control study. Am J Epidem 151:575, 2000

BLUM U et al: Endoluminal stent-grafts for infrarenal abdominal aortic aneurysms. N Engl J Med 336:13, 1997

CREAGER MA et al: Aneurysmal disease of the aorta and its branches, in *Vascular Medicine*, J Loscalzo et al (eds). Boston, Little, Brown, 1996, pp 907–925

DAKE MD et al: Endovascular stent-graft placement for the treatment of acute aortic dissection. N Engl J Med 340:1546, 1999

HAGAN PG et al: The International Registry of Acute Aortic Dissection (IRAD): New insights into an old disease. JAMA 283:897, 2000

HASHIMOTO H: Takayasu's arteritis and giant cell (temporal or cranial) arteritis. Intern Med 39:4, 2000

ISSELBACHER EM et al: Diseases of the aorta, in *Heart Disease*, 6th ed, E Braunwald (ed). Philadelphia, Saunders, 2001

NIENABER CA et al: Nonsurgical reconstruction of thoracic aortic dissection by stent-graft placement. N Engl J Med 340:1539, 1999

O'GARA PT, DESANCTIS RN: Aortic dissection in vascular medicine. J Loscalzo et al (eds). Boston, Little, Brown, 1996, pp 927–950

PALOMBI M et al: Endovascular treatment of a ruptured thoracic aortic aneurysm. Eur J Vasc Endovasc Surg 19:101, 2000

THE UK SMALL ANEURYSM TRIAL PARTICIPANTS: Mortality results from randomised controlled trial of early elective surgery or ultrasonographic surveillance for small abdominal aortic aneurysms. Lancet 352:1649, 1998

248 VASCULAR DISEASES OF THE EXTREMITIES

Mark A. Creager, Victor J. Dzau

ARTERIAL DISORDERS

PERIPHERAL ARTERIAL DISEASE Atherosclerosis (arteriosclerosis obliterans) is the leading cause of occlusive arterial disease of the extremities in patients over 40 years old; the highest incidence occurs in the sixth and seventh decades of life. As in patients with atherosclerosis of the coronary and cerebral vasculature, there is an increased prevalence of peripheral atherosclerotic disease in individuals with diabetes mellitus, hypercholesterolemia, hypertension, or hyperhomocysteinemia and in cigarette smokers.

Pathology (See also Chap. 241) Segmental lesions causing stenosis or occlusion are usually localized in large and medium-sized vessels. The pathology of the lesions includes atherosclerotic plaques with calcium deposition, thinning of the media, patchy destruction of muscle and elastic fibers, fragmentation of the internal elastic lamina, and thrombi composed of platelets and fibrin. The primary sites of involvement are the abdominal aorta and iliac arteries (30% of symptomatic patients), the femoral and popliteal arteries (80 to 90% of patients), and the more distal vessels, including the tibial and peroneal arteries (40 to 50% of patients). Atherosclerotic lesions occur preferentially at arterial branch points, sites of increased turbulence, altered shear stress, and intimal injury. Involvement of the distal vasculature is most common in elderly individuals and patients with diabetes mellitus.

Clinical Evaluation The most common *symptom* is intermittent claudication, which is defined as a pain, ache, cramp, numbness, or a sense of fatigue in the muscles; it occurs during exercise and is relieved by rest. The site of claudication is distal to the location of the occlusive lesion. For example, buttock, hip, and thigh discomfort occurs in patients with aortoiliac disease (Leriche syndrome), whereas calf claudication develops in patients with femoral-popliteal disease. Symptoms are far more common in the lower than in the upper extremities because of the higher incidence of obstructive lesions in the former region. In patients with severe arterial occlusive disease, critical limb ischemia may develop. Patients will complain of rest pain or a feeling of cold or numbness in the foot and toes. Frequently, these symptoms occur at night when the legs are horizontal and improve when the legs are in a dependent position. With severe ischemia, rest pain may be persistent.

Important *physical findings* of peripheral arterial disease include decreased or absent pulses distal to the obstruction, the presence of bruits over the narrowed artery, and muscle atrophy. With more severe disease, hair loss, thickened nails, smooth and shiny skin, reduced skin temperature, and pallor or cyanosis are frequent physical signs. In addition, ulcers or gangrene may occur. Elevation of the legs and repeated flexing of the calf muscles produce pallor of the soles of the feet, whereas rubor, secondary to reactive hyperemia, may develop when the legs are dependent. The time required for rubor to develop or for the veins in the foot to fill when the patient's legs are transferred from an elevated to a dependent position is related to the severity of the ischemia and the presence of collateral vessels. Patients with severe ischemia may develop peripheral edema because they keep their legs in a dependent position much of the time. Ischemic neuritis can result in numbness and hyporeflexia.

Noninvasive Testing The history and physical examination are usually sufficient to establish the diagnosis of peripheral arterial disease. An objective assessment of the severity of disease is obtained by noninvasive techniques. These include digital pulse volume recordings, Doppler flow velocity waveform analysis, duplex ultrasonography (which combines B-mode imaging and pulse-wave Doppler examination), segmental pressure measurements, transcutaneous oximetry, stress testing (usually using a treadmill), and tests of reactive hyperemia. In the presence of significant peripheral arterial disease, the volume displacement in the leg is decreased with each pulse, and the Doppler velocity contour becomes progressively flatter. Duplex ultrasonography is often useful in detecting stenotic lesions in native arteries and bypass grafts.

Arterial pressure can be recorded noninvasively along the legs by serial placement of sphygmomanometric cuffs and use of a Doppler device to auscultate or record blood flow. Normally, systolic blood pressure in the legs and arms is similar. Indeed, ankle pressure may be slightly higher than arm pressure due to pulse-wave reflection. In the presence of hemodynamically significant stenoses, the systolic blood pressure in the leg is decreased. Thus, if one were to obtain a ratio of the ankle and brachial artery pressures, it would be ≥ 1.0 in normal individuals and < 1.0 in patients with peripheral arterial disease. A ratio of < 0.5 is consistent with severe ischemia.

Treadmill testing allows the physician to assess functional limitations objectively. Decline of the ankle-brachial systolic pressure ratio immediately after exercise may provide further support for the diagnosis of peripheral arterial disease in patients with equivocal symptoms and findings on examination. Exercise testing also allows simultaneous evaluation for the presence of coronary artery disease.

Contrast angiography should not be used for routine diagnostic testing but is performed prior to potential revascularization. It is useful in defining the anatomy to assist operative planning and is also indicated if nonsurgical interventions are being considered, such as percutaneous transluminal angioplasty (PTA) or thrombolysis. Recent studies have suggested that magnetic resonance angiography has diagnostic accuracy comparable to that of contrast angiography.

Prognosis The natural history of patients with peripheral arterial disease is influenced primarily by the extent of coexisting coronary artery and cerebral vascular disease. Studies using coronary angiography have estimated that approximately one-half of patients with symptomatic peripheral arterial disease also have significant coronary artery disease. Life-table analysis has indicated that patients with claudication have a 70% 5-year and a 50% 10-year survival rate. Most deaths are either sudden or secondary to myocardial infarction. The likelihood of symptomatic progression of peripheral arterial disease appears less than the chance of succumbing to coronary artery disease. Approximately 75% of nondiabetic patients who present with mild to moderate claudication remain symptomatically stable or improve. Deterioration is likely to occur in the remainder, with approximately 5% of the group ultimately undergoing amputation. The prognosis is worse in patients who continue to smoke cigarettes or who have diabetes mellitus.

TREATMENT Therapeutic options include supportive measures, pharmacologic treatment, nonoperative interventions, and surgery. Supportive measures include meticulous care of the feet, which should be kept clean and protected against excessive drying with moisturizing creams. Well-fitting and protective shoes are advised to reduce trauma. Sandals and shoes made of synthetic materials that do not "breathe" should be avoided. Elastic support hose should be avoided, as they reduce blood flow to the skin. In patients with ischemia at rest, shock blocks under the head of the bed together with a canopy over the feet may improve perfusion pressure and ameliorate some of the rest pain.

Treatment of associated factors that contribute to the development of atherosclerosis should be initiated. The importance of discontinuing cigarette smoking cannot be overemphasized. The physician must assume a major role in this life-style modification. It is important to control blood pressure in hypertensive patients but to avoid hypotensive levels. Treatment of hypercholesterolemia is advocated, although reduction in cholesterol levels has not been shown unequivocally to reverse peripheral atherosclerotic lesions. However, it has been shown to prevent or to slow progression of the disease and to improve survival in patients with coronary atherosclerosis. Patients with claudication should also be encouraged to exercise regularly and at progressively more strenuous levels. Supervised exercise training programs may improve muscle efficiency and prolong walking distance. Patients also should be advised to walk for 30 to 45 min daily, stopping at the onset of claudication and resting until the symptoms resolve before resuming ambulation.

Pharmacologic Management This form of treatment of patients with peripheral arterial disease has not been as successful as the medical treatment of coronary artery disease (Chap. 244). In particular, vasodilators as a class have not proved to be beneficial. During exercise, peripheral vasodilation occurs distal to sites of significant arterial stenoses. As a result, perfusion pressure falls, often to levels less than that generated in the interstitial tissue by the exercising muscle. Drugs such as α-adrenergic blocking agents, calcium channel antagonists, papaverine, and other vasodilators have not been shown to be effective in patients with peripheral arterial disease. Pentoxifylline, a substituted xanthine derivative, has been reported to decrease blood viscosity and to increase red cell flexibility, thereby increasing blood flow to the microcirculation and enhancing tissue oxygenation. Several placebo-controlled studies have reported that pentoxifylline increased the duration of exercise in patients with claudication, but its efficacy has not been confirmed in all clinical trials. Cilostazol, a phosphodiesterase inhibitor with vasodilator and antiplatelet properties, has been reported to increase claudication distance and recently received an indication for treatment of peripheral arterial disease by the U.S. Food and Drug Administration. Other drugs are being studied that potentially may improve claudication, such as L-arginine, which is the precursor of the endothelium-dependent vasodilator, nitric oxide, and vasodilator prostaglandins. Several studies have suggested that long-term parenteral administration of vasodilator prostaglandins decreases pain and facilitates healing of ulcers in patients with severe limb ischemia. Clinical trials with angiogenic growth factors such as vascular endothelial growth factor (VEGF) and basic fibroblast growth factor (bFGF) are proceeding. A preliminary report suggested that intramuscular gene transfer of DNA encoding VEGF may promote collateral blood vessel growth in patients with critical limb ischemia.

Platelet inhibitors, particularly aspirin, reduce the risk of adverse cardiovascular events in patients with peripheral atherosclerosis. Clopidogril, a drug that inhibits platelet aggregation via its effect on ADP-dependent platelet-fibrinogen binding, appears to be more effective than aspirin in reducing cardiovascular morbidity and mortality in patients with peripheral arterial disease. The anticoagulants heparin and warfarin have not been shown to be effective in patients with chronic peripheral arterial disease but may be useful in acute arterial obstruction secondary to thrombosis or systemic embolism. Similarly, thrombolytic intervention using drugs such as streptokinase, urokinase, or recombinant tissue plasminogen activator (tPA) may have a role in the treatment of acute thrombotic arterial occlusion but is not effective in patients with chronic arterial occlusion secondary to atherosclerosis.

Revascularization Revascularization procedures, including nonoperative as well as operative interventions, are usually reserved for patients with progressive, severe, or disabling symptoms and ischemia at rest, as well as for individuals who must be symptom-free because of their occupation. Angiography should be performed mainly in patients who are being considered for a revascularization procedure. Nonoperative interventions include PTA, stent placement, and atherectomy (Chap. 245). PTA of the iliac artery is associated with a higher success rate than PTA of the femoral and popliteal arteries. Approximately 90 to 95% of iliac PTAs are initially successful, and the 3-year patency rate is in excess of 75%. Patency rates may be higher if a stent is placed in the iliac artery. The initial success rate for femoral-popliteal PTA is approximately 80%, with a 60% 3-year patency rate. Patency rates are influenced by the severity of pretreatment stenoses; the prognosis of total occlusive lesions is worse than that of nonocclusive stenotic lesions.

Several operative procedures are available for treating patients with aortoiliac and femoral-popliteal artery disease. The preferred operative procedure depends on the location and extent of the obstruction(s) and general medical condition of the patient. Operative procedures for aortoiliac disease include aortobifemoral bypass, axillofemoral bypass, femoral-femoral bypass, and aortoiliac endarterectomy. The most frequently used procedure is the aortobifemoral bypass using knitted Dacron grafts. Immediate graft patency approaches 99%, and 5- and 10-year graft patency in survivors is in excess of 90 and 80%, respectively. Operative complications include myocardial infarction and stroke, infection of the graft, peripheral embolization, and sexual dysfunction from interruption of autonomic nerves in the pelvis. Operative mortality ranges from 1 to 3%, mostly due to ischemic heart disease.

Operative therapy for femoral-popliteal artery disease includes in situ and reverse autogenous saphenous vein bypass grafts, placement of polytetrafluoroethylene (PTFE) or other synthetic grafts, and thromboendarterectomy. Operative mortality ranges from 1 to 3%. The long-term patency rate depends on the type of graft used, the location of the distal anastomosis, and the patency of runoff vessels beyond the anastomosis. Patency rates of femoral-popliteal saphenous vein bypass grafts at 1 year approach 90% and at 5 years, 70 to 80%. Five-year patency rates of infrapopliteal saphenous vein bypass grafts are 60 to 70%. In contrast, 5-year patency rates of infrapopliteal PTFE grafts are less than 30%. Lumbar sympathectomy alone or as an adjunct to aortofemoral reconstruction has fallen into disfavor.

Preoperative cardiac risk assessment may identify individuals especially likely to experience an adverse cardiac event during the perioperative period. Patients with angina, prior myocardial infarction, ventricular ectopy, heart failure, or diabetes are among those at increased risk. Noninvasive tests, such as treadmill testing (if feasible), dipyridamole thallium or sestamibi scintigraphy, dobutamine echocardiography, and ambulatory ischemia monitoring permit further stratification of patient risk (Chap. 245). Patients with abnormal test results require close supervision and adjunctive management with antianginal medications. It is not known whether coronary angiography and coronary arterial revascularization reduce overall perioperative mortality in high-risk patients undergoing peripheral vascular surgery, but cardiac catheterization should be considered in patients suspected of having left main or three-vessel coronary artery disease.

FIBROMUSCULAR DYSPLASIA This is a hyperplastic disorder affecting medium-sized and small arteries. It occurs predominantly in females and usually involves renal and carotid arteries but can affect extremity vessels such as the iliac and subclavian arteries. The histologic classification includes intimal, medial, and periadventitial dysplasia. Medial dysplasia is the most common type and is characterized by hyperplasia of the media with or without fibrosis of the elastic membrane. It is identified angiographically by a "string of beads" appearance caused by thickened fibromuscular ridges contiguous with thin, less involved portions of the arterial wall. When limb vessels are involved, clinical manifestations are similar to those for atherosclerosis, including claudication and rest pain. PTA and surgical reconstruction have been beneficial in patients with debilitating symptoms or threatened limbs.

THROMBOANGIITIS OBLITERANS Thromboangiitis obliterans (Buerger's disease) is an inflammatory occlusive vascular disorder involving small and medium-sized arteries and veins in the distal upper and lower extremities. Cerebral, visceral, and coronary vessels may also be affected. This disorder develops most frequently in men under age 40. The prevalence is higher in Asians and individuals of eastern European descent. While the cause of thromboangiitis obliterans is not known, there is a definite relationship to cigarette smoking in patients with this disorder.

In the initial stages of thromboangiitis obliterans, polymorphonuclear leukocytes infiltrate the walls of the small and medium-sized arteries and veins. The internal elastic lamina is preserved, and thrombus may develop in the vascular lumen. As the disease progresses, mononuclear cells, fibroblasts, and giant cells replace the neutrophils. Later stages are characterized by perivascular fibrosis and recanalization.

The clinical features of thromboangiitis obliterans often include a triad of claudication of the affected extremity, Raynaud's phenomenon (p. 1438), and migratory superficial vein thrombophlebitis. Claudication is usually confined to the calves and feet or the forearms and hands, because this disorder primarily affects distal vessels. In the presence of severe digital ischemia, trophic nail changes, painful ulcerations, and gangrene may develop at the tips of the fingers. The physical examination shows normal brachial and popliteal pulses but reduced or absent radial, ulnar, and/or tibial pulses. Arteriography is helpful in making the diagnosis. Smooth, tapering segmental lesions in the distal vessels are characteristic, as are collateral vessels at sites of vascular occlusion. Proximal atherosclerotic disease is usually absent. The diagnosis can be confirmed by excisional biopsy and pathologic examination of an involved vessel.

There is no specific treatment except abstention from tobacco. The prognosis is worse in individuals who continue to smoke, but results are discouraging even in those who do stop smoking. Arterial bypass of the larger vessels may be used in selected instances, as well as local debridement, depending on the symptoms and severity of ischemia. Antibiotics may be useful; anticoagulants and glucocorticoids are not helpful. If these measures fail, amputation may be required.

VASCULITIS Other vasculitides may affect the arteries supplying the upper and lower extremities. →*Takayasu's arteritis and giant cell (temporal) arteritis are discussed in Chap. 317.*

ACUTE ARTERIAL OCCLUSION This results in the sudden cessation of blood flow to an extremity. The severity of ischemia and the viability of the extremity depend on the location and extent of the occlusion and the presence and subsequent development of collateral blood vessels. There are two principal causes of acute arterial occlusion: embolism and thrombus in situ.

The most common sources of arterial emboli are the heart, aorta, and large arteries. Cardiac disorders that cause thromboembolism include atrial fibrillation, both chronic and paroxysmal; acute myocardial infarction; ventricular aneurysm; cardiomyopathy; infectious and marantic endocarditis; prosthetic heart valves; and atrial myxoma. Emboli to the distal vessels may also originate from proximal sites of atherosclerosis and aneurysms of the aorta and large vessels. Less frequently, an arterial occlusion results paradoxically from a venous thrombus that has entered the systemic circulation via a patent foramen ovale or other septal defect. Arterial emboli tend to lodge at vessel bifurcations because the vessel caliber decreases at these sites; in the lower extremities, emboli lodge most frequently in the femoral artery, followed by the iliac artery, aorta, and popliteal and tibioperoneal arteries.

Acute arterial thrombosis in situ occurs most frequently in atherosclerotic vessels at the site of a stenosis or aneurysm and in arterial bypass grafts. Trauma to an artery may also result in the formation of an acute arterial thrombus. Arterial occlusion may complicate arterial punctures and placement of catheters. Less frequent causes include the thoracic outlet compression syndrome, which causes subclavian artery occlusion, and entrapment of the popliteal artery by abnormal placement of the medial head of the gastrocnemius muscle. Polycythemia and hypercoagulable disorders (Chaps. 110 and 118) are also associated with acute arterial thrombosis.

Clinical Features The symptoms of an acute arterial occlusion depend on the location, duration, and severity of the obstruction. Often, severe pain, paresthesia, numbness, and coldness develop in the involved extremity within 1 h. Paralysis may occur with severe and persistent ischemia. Physical findings include loss of pulses distal to the occlusion, cyanosis or pallor, mottling, decreased skin temperature, muscle stiffening, loss of sensation, weakness, and/or absent deep tendon reflexes. If acute arterial occlusion occurs in the presence of an adequate collateral circulation, as is often the case in acute graft occlusion, the symptoms and findings may be less impressive. In this situation, the patient complains about an abrupt decrease in the distance walked before claudication occurs or of modest pain and paresthesia. Pallor and coolness are evident, but sensory and motor functions are generally preserved. The diagnosis of acute arterial occlusion is usually apparent from the clinical presentation. Arteriography is useful for confirming the diagnosis and demonstrating the location and extent of occlusion.

Ɍx **TREATMENT** Once the diagnosis is made, the patient should be anticoagulated with intravenous heparin to prevent propagation of the clot. In cases of severe ischemia of recent onset, and particularly when limb viability is jeopardized, immediate intervention to ensure reperfusion is indicated. Surgical thromboembolectomy or arterial bypass procedures are used to restore blood flow to the ischemic extremity promptly, particularly when a large proximal vessel is occluded.

Intraarterial thrombolytic therapy is effective when acute arterial occlusion is caused by a thrombus in an atherosclerotic vessel or arterial bypass graft. Thrombolytic therapy may also be indicated when the patient's overall condition contraindicates surgical intervention or when smaller distal vessels are occluded, thus preventing surgical access. One approach for administering intraarterial urokinase is to give 240,000 IU/h for 4 h, followed by 120,000 IU/h for a maximum of 48 h. Intraarterial recombinant tPA may be administered at infusion rates of 1 mg/h or 0.05 mg/kg per hour. Meticulous observation for hemorrhagic complications is required during intraarterial thrombolytic therapy.

If the limb is not in jeopardy, a more conservative approach that includes observation and administration of anticoagulants may be taken. Anticoagulation prevents recurrent embolism and reduces the likelihood of thrombus propagation. It can be initiated with intravenous heparin and followed by oral warfarin. Recommended dosages are the same as those used for deep vein thrombosis (see below). Emboli resulting from infectious endocarditis, the presence of prosthetic heart valves, or atrial myxoma often require surgical intervention to remove the cause.

ATHEROEMBOLISM Atheroembolism constitutes a subset of acute arterial occlusion. In this condition, multiple small deposits of fibrin, platelet, and cholesterol debris embolize from proximal atherosclerotic lesions or aneurysmal sites. Atheroembolism may occur after intraarterial procedures. Since the emboli tend to lodge in the small vessels of the muscle and skin and may not occlude the large vessels, distal pulses usually remain palpable. Patients complain of acute pain and tenderness at the site of embolization. Digital vascular occlusion may result in ischemia and the "blue toe" syndrome; digital necrosis and gangrene may develop. Localized areas of tenderness, pallor, and livedo reticularis (see below) occur at sites of emboli. Skin or muscle biopsy may demonstrate cholesterol crystals.

Ischemia resulting from atheroemboli is notoriously difficult to treat. Usually neither surgical revascularization procedures nor thrombolytic therapy is helpful because of the multiplicity, composition, and distal location of the emboli. Some evidence suggests that platelet inhibitors prevent atheroembolism. Surgical intervention to remove or bypass the atherosclerotic vessel or aneurysm that causes the recurrent atheroemboli may be necessary.

THORACIC OUTLET COMPRESSION SYNDROME This is a symptom complex resulting from compression of the neurovascular bundle (artery, vein, or nerves) at the thoracic outlet as it courses through the neck and shoulder. Cervical ribs, abnormalities of the scalenus anticus muscle, proximity of the clavicle to the first rib, or abnormal insertion of the pectoralis minor muscle may compress the subclavian artery and brachial plexus as these structures pass from the thorax to the arm. Patients may develop shoulder and arm pain, weakness, paresthesia, claudication, Raynaud's phenomenon, and even ischemic tissue loss and gangrene. Examination is often normal unless provocative maneuvers are performed. Occasionally, distal pulses are decreased or absent and digital cyanosis and ischemia may be evident. Tenderness may be present in the supraclavicular fossa. Abducting the affected arm by 90° and externally rotating the shoulder may precipitate symptoms. Several additional maneuvers are used to confirm the diagnosis of vascular compression and to suggest the location of the abnormality. These include the scalene maneuver (extension of the neck and rotation of the head to the side of the symptoms), the costoclavicular maneuver (posterior rotation of shoulders), and the hyperabduction maneuver (raising the arm 180°), which may cause subclavian bruits and loss of pulses in the arm. A chest x-ray will indicate the presence of cervical ribs. The electromyogram will be abnormal if the brachial plexus is involved.

Ɍx **TREATMENT** Most patients can be managed conservatively. They should be advised to avoid the positions that cause symptoms. Many patients benefit from shoulder girdle exercises. Surgical procedures such as removal of the first rib or resection of the scalenus anticus muscle are necessary occasionally for relief of symptoms or treatment of ischemia.

ARTERIOVENOUS FISTULA Abnormal communications between an artery and a vein, bypassing the capillary bed, may be congenital or acquired. Congenital arteriovenous fistulas are the result of persistent embryonic vessels that fail to differentiate into arteries and veins; they may be associated with birthmarks, can be located in almost any organ of the body, and frequently occur in the extremities. Acquired arteriovenous fistulas are either created to provide vascular access for hemodialysis or occur as a result of a penetrating injury such as a gunshot or knife wound or as complications of arterial catheterization or surgical dissection. An infrequent cause of arteriovenous fistula is rupture of an arterial aneurysm into a vein.

The clinical features depend on the location and size of the fistula. Frequently, a pulsatile mass is palpable, and a thrill and bruit lasting throughout systole and diastole are present over the fistula. With long-standing fistulas, clinical manifestations of chronic venous insufficiency, including peripheral edema, large, tortuous varicose veins, and stasis pigmentation become apparent because of the high venous pressure. Evidence of ischemia may occur in the distal portion of the extremity. Skin temperature is higher over the arteriovenous fistula. Large arteriovenous fistulas may result in an increased cardiac output with consequent cardiomegaly and high-output heart failure (Chap. 232).

Diagnosis The diagnosis is often evident from the physical examination. Compression of a large arteriovenous fistula may cause reflex slowing of the heart rate (Nicoladoni-Branham sign). Arteriography can confirm the diagnosis and is useful in demonstrating the site and size of the arteriovenous fistula.

℞ **TREATMENT** Management of arteriovenous fistulas may involve surgery, radiotherapy, or embolization. Congenital arteriovenous fistulas are often difficult to treat because the communications may be numerous and extensive, and new ones frequently develop after ligation of the most obvious ones. Many of these lesions are best treated conservatively using elastic support hose to reduce the consequences of venous hypertension. Occasionally, embolization with autologous material, such as fat or muscle, or with hemostatic agents, such as gelatin sponges or silicon spheres, is used to obliterate the fistula. Acquired arteriovenous fistulas are usually amenable to surgical treatment that involves division or excision of the fistula. Occasionally, autogenous or synthetic grafting is necessary to reestablish continuity of the artery and vein.

RAYNAUD'S PHENOMENON Raynaud's phenomenon is characterized by episodic digital ischemia, manifested clinically by the sequential development of digital blanching, cyanosis, and rubor of the fingers or toes following cold exposure and subsequent rewarming. Emotional stress may also precipitate Raynaud's phenomenon. The color changes are usually well demarcated and are confined to the fingers or toes. Typically, one or more digits will appear white when the patient is exposed to a cold environment or touches a cold object. The blanching, or pallor, represents the ischemic phase of the phenomenon and results from vasospasm of digital arteries. During the ischemic phase, capillaries and venules dilate, and cyanosis results from the deoxygenated blood that is present in these vessels. A sensation of cold or numbness or paresthesia of the digits often accompanies the phases of pallor and cyanosis.

With rewarming, the digital vasospasm resolves, and blood flow into the dilated arterioles and capillaries increases dramatically. This "reactive hyperemia" imparts a bright red color to the digits. In addition to rubor and warmth, patients often experience a throbbing, painful sensation during the hyperemic phase. Although the triphasic color response is typical of Raynaud's phenomenon, some patients may develop only pallor and cyanosis; others may experience only cyanosis.

Pathophysiology Raynaud originally proposed that cold-induced episodic digital ischemia was secondary to exaggerated reflex sympathetic vasoconstriction. This theory is supported by the fact that α-adrenergic blocking drugs as well as sympathectomy decrease the frequency and severity of Raynaud's phenomenon in some patients. An alternative hypothesis is that the digital vascular responsiveness to cold or to normal sympathetic stimuli is enhanced. It is also possible that normal reflex sympathetic vasoconstriction is superimposed on local digital vascular disease or that there is enhanced adrenergic neuroeffector activity.

Raynaud's phenomenon is broadly separated into two categories: the idiopathic variety, termed *Raynaud's disease*, and the secondary variety, which is associated with other disease states or known causes of vasospasm (Table 248-1).

Table 248-1 Classification of Raynaud's Phenomenon

Primary or idiopathic Raynaud's phenomenon: Raynaud's disease
Secondary Raynaud's phenomenon
  Collagen vascular diseases: scleroderma, systemic lupus erythematosus, rheumatoid arthritis, dermatomyositis, polymyositis
  Arterial occlusive diseases: atherosclerosis of the extremities, thromboangiitis obliterans, acute arterial occlusion, thoracic outlet syndrome
  Pulmonary hypertension
  Neurologic disorders: intervertebral disk disease, syringomyelia, spinal cord tumors, stroke, poliomyelitis, carpal tunnel syndrome
  Blood dyscrasias: cold agglutinins, cryoglobulinemia, cryofibrinogenemia, myeloproliferative disorders, Waldenström's macroglobulinemia
  Trauma: vibration injury, hammer hand syndrome, electric shock, cold injury, typing, piano playing
  Drugs: ergot derivatives, methysergide, β-adrenergic receptor blockers, bleomycin, vinblastine, cisplatin

Raynaud's Disease This appellation is applied when the secondary causes of Raynaud's phenomenon have been excluded. Over 50% of patients with Raynaud's phenomenon have Raynaud's disease. Women are affected about five times more often than men, and the age of presentation is usually between 20 and 40 years. The fingers are involved more frequently than the toes. Initial episodes may involve only one or two fingertips, but subsequent attacks may involve the entire finger and may include all the fingers. The toes are affected in 40% of patients. Although vasospasm of the toes usually occurs in patients with symptoms in the fingers, it may happen alone. Rarely, the earlobes and the tip of the nose are involved. Raynaud's phenomenon occurs frequently in patients who also have migraine headaches or variant angina. These associations suggest that there may be a common predisposing cause for the vasospasm.

Results of physical examination often are entirely normal; the radial, ulnar, and pedal pulses are normal. The fingers and toes may be cool between attacks and may perspire excessively. Thickening and tightening of the digital subcutaneous tissue (*sclerodactyly*) develop in 10% of patients. Angiography of the digits for diagnostic purposes is not indicated.

In general, patients with Raynaud's disease appear to have the milder forms of Raynaud's phenomenon. Fewer than 1% of these patients lose a part of a digit. After the diagnosis is made, the disease improves spontaneously in approximately 15% of patients and progresses in about 30%.

Secondary Causes of Raynaud's Phenomenon Raynaud's phenomenon occurs in 80 to 90% of patients with systemic sclerosis (scleroderma) and is the presenting symptom in 30% (Chap. 313). It may be the only symptom of scleroderma for many years. Abnormalities of the digital vessels may contribute to the development of Raynaud's phenomenon in this disorder. Ischemic fingertip ulcers may develop and progress to gangrene and autoamputation. About 20% of patients with systemic lupus erythematosus (SLE) have Raynaud's phenomenon (Chap. 311). Occasionally, persistent digital ischemia develops and may result in ulcers or gangrene. In most severe cases, the small vessels are occluded by a proliferative endarteritis. Raynaud's phenomenon occurs in about 30% of patients with dermatomyositis or polymyositis (Chap. 382). It frequently develops in patients with rheumatoid arthritis and may be related to the intimal proliferation that occurs in the digital arteries.

Atherosclerosis of the extremities is a frequent cause of Raynaud's phenomenon in men over age 50. Thromboangiitis obliterans is an uncommon cause of Raynaud's phenomenon but should be considered in young men, particularly in those who are cigarette smokers. The development of cold-induced pallor in these disorders may be confined to one or two digits of the involved extremity. Occasionally, Raynaud's phenomenon may follow acute occlusion of large and medium-sized arteries by a thrombus or embolus. Embolization of atheroembolic debris may cause digital ischemia. The latter situation often involves one or two digits and should not be confused with Raynaud's phenomenon. In patients with the thoracic outlet syndrome, Raynaud's phenomenon may result from diminished intravascular pressure, stimulation of sympathetic fibers in the brachial plexus, or a combination of both. Raynaud's phenomenon occurs in patients with primary pulmonary hypertension (Chap. 260); this is more than coincidental and may reflect a neurohumoral abnormality that affects both the pulmonary and digital circulations.

A variety of blood dyscrasias may be associated with Raynaud's phenomenon. Cold-induced precipitation of plasma proteins, hyperviscosity, and aggregation of red cells and platelets may occur in patients with cold agglutinins, cryoglobulinemia, or cryofibrinogenemia. Hyperviscosity syndromes that accompany myeloproliferative disorders and Waldenström's macroglobulinemia should also be considered in the initial evaluation of patients with Raynaud's phenomenon.

Raynaud's phenomenon occurs often in patients whose vocations require the use of vibrating hand tools, such as chain saws or jackhammers. The frequency of Raynaud's phenomenon also seems to be increased in pianists and typists. Electric shock injury to the hands or frostbite may lead to the later development of Raynaud's phenomenon.

Several drugs have been causally implicated in Raynaud's phenomenon. These include ergot preparations, methysergide, β-adrenergic receptor antagonists, and the chemotherapeutic agents bleomycin, vinblastine, and cisplatin.

℞ **TREATMENT** Most patients with Raynaud's phenomenon experience only mild and infrequent episodes. These patients need reassurance and should be instructed to dress warmly and avoid unnecessary cold exposure. In addition to gloves and mittens, patients should protect the trunk, head, and feet with warm clothing to prevent cold-induced reflex vasoconstriction. Tobacco use is contraindicated.

Drug treatment should be reserved for the severe cases. The calcium channel antagonists, especially nifedipine and diltiazem, decrease the frequency and severity of Raynaud's phenomenon. Adrenergic blocking agents, such as reserpine, have been shown to increase nutritional blood flow to the fingers. Some, but not all, patients achieve satisfactory results with long-term reserpine therapy. Moreover, systemic use of this drug is limited by side effects of hypotension, nasal stuffiness, lethargy, and depression. The postsynaptic α_1-adrenergic antagonist prazosin has been used with favorable responses. Doxazosin and terazosin may also be effective. Other sympatholytic agents, such as methyldopa, guanethidine, and phenoxybenzamine, may be useful in some patients. Surgical sympathectomy is helpful in some patients who are unresponsive to medical therapy, but benefit is often transient.

ACROCYANOSIS In this condition, there is arterial vasoconstriction and secondary dilation of the capillaries and venules with resulting persistent cyanosis of the hands and, less frequently, the feet. Cyanosis may be intensified by exposure to a cold environment. Women are affected much more frequently than men, and the age of onset is usually less than 30 years. Generally, patients are asymptomatic but seek medical attention because of the discoloration. Examination reveals normal pulses, peripheral cyanosis, and moist palms. Trophic skin changes and ulcerations do *not* occur. The disorder can be distinguished from Raynaud's phenomenon because it is persistent and not episodic, the discoloration extends proximally from the digits, and blanching does not occur. Ischemia secondary to arterial occlusive disease can usually be excluded by the presence of normal pulses. Central cyanosis and decreased arterial oxygen saturation are not present. Patients should be reassured and advised to dress warmly and avoid cold exposure. Pharmacologic intervention is not indicated.

LIVEDO RETICULARIS In this condition, localized areas of the extremities develop a mottled or netlike appearance of reddish to blue discoloration. The mottled appearance may be more prominent following cold exposure. The idiopathic form of this disorder occurs equally in men and women, and the most common age of onset is in the third decade. Patients with the idiopathic form are usually asymptomatic and seek attention for cosmetic reasons. Livedo reticularis can also occur following atheroembolism (see above). Rarely, skin ulcerations develop. Patients should be reassured and advised to avoid cold environments. No drug treatment is indicated.

PERNIO (CHILBLAINS) This is a vasculitic disorder associated with exposure to cold; acute forms have been described. Raised erythematous lesions develop on the lower part of the legs and feet in cold weather. These are associated with pruritus and a burning sensation, and they may blister and ulcerate. Pathologic examination demonstrates angiitis characterized by intimal proliferation and perivascular infiltration of mononuclear and polymorphonuclear leukocytes. Giant cells may be present in the subcutaneous tissue. Patients should avoid exposure to cold, and ulcers should be kept clean and protected with sterile dressings. Sympatholytic drugs may be effective in some patients.

ERYTHROMELALGIA (ERYTHERMALGIA) This disorder is characterized by burning pain and erythema of the extremities. The feet are involved more frequently than the hands, and males are affected more frequently than females. Erythromelalgia may occur at any age but is most common in middle age. It may be primary or secondary to myeloproliferative disorders such as polycythemia vera and essential thrombocytosis, or it may occur as an adverse effect of drugs such as nifedipine or bromocriptine. Patients complain of burning in the extremities that is precipitated by exposure to a warm environment and aggravated by a dependent position. The symptoms are relieved by exposing the affected area to cool air or water or by elevation. Erythromelalgia can be distinguished from ischemia secondary to peripheral arterial disorders and peripheral neuropathy because the peripheral pulses are present and the neurologic examination is normal. There is no specific treatment; aspirin may produce relief in patients with erythromelalgia secondary to myeloproliferative disease. Treatment of associated disorders in secondary erythromelalgia may be helpful.

FROSTBITE In this condition, tissue damage results from severe environmental cold exposure or from direct contact with a very cold object. Tissue injury results from both freezing and vasoconstriction. Frostbite usually affects the distal aspects of the extremities or exposed parts of the face, such as the ears, nose, chin, and cheeks. Superficial frostbite involves the skin and subcutaneous tissue. Patients experience pain or paresthesia, and the skin appears white and waxy. After rewarming, there is cyanosis and erythema, wheal- and-flare formation, edema, and superficial blisters. Deep frostbite involves muscle, nerves, and deeper blood vessels. It may result in edema of the hand or foot, vesicles and bullae, tissue necrosis, and gangrene.

Initial treatment is rewarming, performed in an environment where reexposure to freezing conditions will not occur. Rewarming is accomplished by immersion of the affected part in a water bath at temperatures of 40 to 44°C (104 to 111°F). Massage, application of ice water, and extreme heat are contraindicated. The injured area should be cleansed with soap or antiseptic and sterile dressings applied. Analgesics are often required during rewarming. Antibiotics are used if there is evidence of infection. The efficacy of sympathetic blocking drugs is not established. Following recovery, the affected extremity may exhibit increased sensitivity to cold.

VENOUS DISORDERS

Veins in the extremities can be broadly classified as either superficial or deep. In the lower extremity, the superficial venous system includes the greater and lesser saphenous veins and their tributaries. The deep veins of the leg accompany the major arteries. Perforating veins connect the superficial and deep systems at multiple locations. Bicuspid valves are present throughout the venous system to direct the flow of venous blood centrally.

VENOUS THROMBOSIS The presence of thrombus within a superficial or deep vein and the accompanying inflammatory response in the vessel wall is termed *venous thrombosis* or *thrombophlebitis*. Initially, the thrombus is composed principally of platelets and fibrin. Red cells become interspersed with fibrin, and the thrombus tends to propagate in the direction of blood flow. The inflammatory response in the vessel wall may be minimal or characterized by granulocyte infiltration, loss of endothelium, and edema.

The factors that predispose to venous thrombosis were initially described by Virchow in 1856 and include stasis, vascular damage, and hypercoagulability. Accordingly, a variety of clinical situations are associated with increased risk of venous thrombosis (Table 248-2). Venous thrombosis may occur in more than 50% of patients having orthopedic surgical procedures, particularly those involving the hip or knee, and in 10 to 40% of patients who undergo abdominal or thoracic operations. The prevalence of venous thrombosis is particularly high in patients with cancer of the pancreas, lungs, genitourinary tract, stomach, and breast. Approximately 10 to 20% of patients with idiopathic deep vein thrombosis have or develop clinically overt cancer; there is no consensus on whether these individuals should be subjected to intensive diagnostic workup to search for occult malignancy. Risk of thrombosis is increased following trauma, such as fractures of the spine, pelvis, femur, and tibia. Immobilization, regardless of the underlying disease, is a major predisposing cause of venous thrombosis. This fact may account for the relatively high incidence in patients with acute myocardial infarction or congestive heart failure. The incidence of venous thrombosis is increased during pregnancy, particularly in the third trimester and in the first month postpartum, and in individuals who use oral contraceptives or receive postmenopausal hormone replacement therapy. A variety of clinical disorders that produce systemic hypercoagulability, including resistance to activated protein C (factor V Leiden); antithrombin III, protein C, and protein S deficiencies; antiphospholipid syndrome; SLE; myeloproliferative diseases; dysfibrinogenemia; and disseminated intravascular coagulation, are associated with venous thrombosis. Venulitis occurring in thromboangiitis obliterans, Behçet's disease, and homocysteinuria may also cause venous thrombosis.

DEEP VENOUS THROMBOSIS   The most important consequences of this disorder are pulmonary embolism (Chap. 261) and the syndrome of chronic venous insufficiency. Deep venous thrombosis of the iliac, femoral, or popliteal veins is suggested by unilateral leg swelling, warmth, and erythema. Tenderness may be present along the course of the involved veins, and a cord may be palpable. There may be increased tissue turgor, distention of superficial veins, and the appearance of prominent venous collaterals. In some patients, deoxygenated hemoglobin in stagnant veins imparts a cyanotic hue to the limb, a condition called *phlegmasia cerulea dolens*. In markedly edematous legs, the interstitial tissue pressure may exceed the capillary perfusion pressure, causing pallor, a condition designated *phlegmasia alba dolens*.

The diagnosis of deep venous thrombosis of the calf is often difficult to make at the bedside. This is so because only one of multiple veins may be involved, allowing adequate venous return through the remaining patent vessels. The most common complaint is calf pain.

Examination may reveal posterior calf tenderness, warmth, increased tissue turgor or modest swelling, and, rarely, a cord. Increased resistance or pain during dorsiflexion of the foot (Homans' sign) is an unreliable diagnostic sign.

Deep venous thrombosis occurs less frequently in the upper extremity than in the lower extremity, but the incidence is increasing because of greater utilization of indwelling central venous catheters. The clinical features and complications are similar to those described for the leg.

Diagnosis   The noninvasive test used most often to diagnose deep venous thrombosis is duplex venous ultrasonography (B-mode, i.e., two-dimensional, imaging, and pulse-wave Doppler interrogation). By imaging the deep veins, thrombus can be detected either by direct visualization or by inference when the vein does not collapse on compressive maneuvers. The Doppler ultrasound measures the velocity of blood flow in veins. This velocity is normally affected by respiration and by manual compression of the foot or calf. Flow abnormalities occur when deep venous obstruction is present. The positive predictive value of duplex venous ultrasonography approaches 95% for proximal deep vein thrombosis. In the calf, because calf veins are more difficult to visualize than proximal veins, the sensitivity of this technique is only 50 to 75%, although its specificity is 95%.

Impedance plethysmography measures changes in venous capacitance during physiologic maneuvers. Venous obstruction blunts the normal changes in venous capacitance that occur following inflation and deflation of a thigh cuff. The predictive value of this test for detecting occlusive thrombi in proximal veins is approximately 90%. However, it is much less sensitive for diagnosing deep venous thrombosis of the calves.

Magnetic resonance imaging (MRI) is another noninvasive means to detect deep vein thrombosis. Its diagnostic accuracy for assessing proximal deep vein thrombosis is similar to that of duplex ultrasonography. It is useful in patients with suspected thrombosis of the superior and inferior venae cavae or pelvic veins.

Deep venous thrombosis can also be diagnosed by venography. Contrast medium is injected into a superficial vein of the foot and directed to the deep system by the application of tourniquets. The presence of a filling defect or absence of filling of the deep veins is required to make the diagnosis.

Deep vein thrombosis must be differentiated from a variety of disorders that cause unilateral leg pain or swelling, including muscle rupture, trauma, or hemorrhage; a ruptured popliteal cyst; and lymphedema. It may be difficult to distinguish swelling caused by the postphlebitic syndrome from that due to acute recurrent deep venous thrombosis. Leg pain may also result from nerve compression, arthritis, tendinitis, fractures, and arterial occlusive disorders. A careful history and physical examination can usually determine the cause of these symptoms.

Table 248-2   Conditions Associated with an Increased Risk for Development of Venous Thrombosis

Surgery
  Orthopedic, thoracic, abdominal, and genitourinary procedures
Neoplasms
  Pancreas, lung, ovary, testes, urinary tract, breast, stomach
Trauma
  Fractures of spine, pelvis, femur, or tibia; spinal cord injuries
Immobilization
  Acute myocardial infarction, congestive heart failure, stroke, postoperative convalescence
Pregnancy
Estrogen use (for replacement or contraception)
Hypercoagulable states
  Resistance to activated protein C; deficiencies of antithrombin III, protein C, or protein S; antiphospholipid antibodies; myeloproliferative diseases; dysfibrinogenemia; disseminated intravascular coagulation
Venulitis
  Thromboangiitis obliterans, Behçet's disease, homocysteinuria
Previous deep vein thrombosis

℞ **TREATMENT   Anticoagulants** (See also Chap. 261)   Prevention of pulmonary embolism is the most important reason for treating patients with deep vein thrombosis, since in the early stages the thrombus may be loose and poorly adherent to the vessel wall. Patients should be placed in bed, and the affected extremity should be elevated above the level of the heart until the edema and tenderness subside. Anticoagulants prevent thrombus propagation and allow the endogenous lytic system to operate. Initial therapy should include either unfractionated heparin or low-molecular-weight heparin. Unfractionated heparin should be administered intravenously as an initial bolus of 7500 to 10,000 IU, followed by a continuous infusion of 1000 to 1500 IU/h. The rate of the heparin infusion should be adjusted so that the activated partial thromboplastin time (aPTT) is approximately twice the control value. Subcutaneous injection of heparin has been used as an alternative form of therapy. In fewer than 5% of patients, heparin therapy may cause thrombocytopenia. Infrequently, these patients develop arterial thrombosis and ischemia. Low-molecular-weight (4000 to 6000 Da) heparins are reported to be as effective as or better than conventional, unfractionated heparin in preventing extension or recurrence of venous thrombosis. Depending on the specific preparation, low-molecular-weight heparin is administered subcutaneously, in fixed doses, once or twice daily; for example, the dose of enoxaparin is 1 mg/kg subcutaneously bid. The incidence of thrombocytopenia is less with low-molecular-weight heparin than with conventional preparations. Hirudin, a direct thrombin inhibitor, may be used as initial anticoagulant therapy for patients in whom heparin is contraindicated because of heparin-induced thrombocytopenia. Warfarin is administered during the first week of treatment with heparin and may be started as early as the first day of heparin treatment if the aPTT is therapeutic. It is important to overlap heparin treatment with oral anticoagulant therapy for at least 4 to 5 days because the full anticoagulant effect of warfarin is delayed. The dose of warfarin should be adjusted to maintain the prothrombin time at an international normalized ratio (INR) of 2.0 to 3.0.

Anticoagulant treatment is indicated for patients with proximal deep vein thrombosis, since pulmonary embolism may occur in approximately 50% of untreated individuals. The use of anticoagulants for isolated deep vein thrombosis of the calf is controversial. However, approximately 20 to 30% of calf thrombi propagate to the thigh, thereby increasing the risk of pulmonary embolism. The overall incidence of pulmonary embolism in patients presenting initially with deep calf vein thrombosis is 5 to 20%. Also, isolated calf vein thrombosis has been identified as a cause of embolic stroke via a patent foramen ovale. Therefore, patients with calf vein thrombosis should either receive anticoagulants or be followed with serial noninvasive tests to determine whether proximal propagation has occurred. Anticoagulant treatment should be continued for at least 3 to 6 months for patients with acute idiopathic deep vein thrombosis and for those with a temporary risk factor for venous thrombosis to decrease the chance of recurrence. The duration of treatment is indefinite for patients with recurrent deep vein thrombosis and for those in whom associated causes, such as malignancy or hypercoagulability, have not been eliminated. If treatment with anticoagulants is contraindicated because of a bleeding diathesis or risk of hemorrhage, protection from pulmonary embolism can be achieved by mechanically interrupting the flow of blood through the inferior vena cava. Inferior vena cava plication generally has been replaced by percutaneous insertion of a filter.

Thrombolytics Thrombolytic drugs such as streptokinase, urokinase, and tPA may also be used, but there is no evidence that thrombolytic therapy is more effective than anticoagulants in preventing pulmonary embolism. However, early administration of thrombolytic drugs may accelerate clot lysis, preserve venous valves, and decrease the potential for developing postphlebitic syndrome.

Prophylaxis Prophylaxis should be considered in clinical situations where the risk of deep vein thrombosis is high. Low-dose unfractionated heparin (5000 units 2 h prior to surgery and then 5000 units every 8 to 12 h postoperatively), warfarin, and external pneumatic compression are all useful. Low-dose heparin reduces the risk of deep vein thrombosis associated with thoracic and abdominal surgery and with prolonged bed rest. Low-molecular-weight heparins have been shown to prevent deep vein thrombosis in patients undergoing general or orthopedic surgery and in acutely ill medical patients. They are said to be more effective than conventional heparin and to cause an equal or lower incidence of bleeding. Danaparoid, a low-molecular-weight heparinoid, may be used for prophylaxis in patients undergoing hip surgery. Warfarin in a dose that yields a prothrombin time equivalent to an INR of 2.0 to 3.0 is effective in preventing deep vein thrombosis associated with bone fractures and orthopedic surgery. Warfarin is started the night before surgery and continued throughout the convalescent period. External pneumatic compression devices applied to the legs are used to prevent deep vein thrombosis when even low doses of heparin or warfarin might cause serious bleeding, as during neurosurgery or transurethral resection of the prostate.

SUPERFICIAL VEIN THROMBOSIS Thrombosis of the greater or lesser saphenous veins or their tributaries—i.e., superficial vein thrombosis—does not result in pulmonary embolism. It is asso-

ciated with intravenous catheters and infusions, occurs in varicose veins, and may develop in association with deep vein thrombosis. Migrating superficial vein thrombosis is often a marker for a carcinoma and may also occur in patients with vasculitides, such as thromboangiitis obliterans. The clinical features of superficial vein thrombosis are easily distinguished from those of deep vein thrombosis. Patients complain of pain localized to the site of the thrombus. Examination reveals a reddened, warm, and tender cord extending along a superficial vein. The surrounding area may be red and edematous.

℞ **TREATMENT** Treatment is primarily supportive. Initially, patients can be placed at bed rest with leg elevation and application of warm compresses. Nonsteroidal antiinflammatory drugs may provide analgesia but may also obscure clinical evidence of thrombus propagation. If a thrombosis of the greater saphenous vein develops in the thigh and extends toward the saphenofemoral vein junction, it is reasonable to consider anticoagulant therapy to prevent extension of the thrombus into the deep system and a possible pulmonary embolism.

VARICOSE VEINS Varicose veins are dilated, tortuous superficial veins that result from defective structure and function of the valves of the saphenous veins, from intrinsic weakness of the vein wall, from high intraluminal pressure, or, rarely, from arteriovenous fistulas. Varicose veins can be categorized as primary or secondary. Primary varicose veins originate in the superficial system and occur two to three times as frequently in women as in men. Approximately half of patients have a family history of varicose veins. Secondary varicose veins result from deep venous insufficiency and incompetent perforating veins or from deep venous occlusion causing enlargement of superficial veins that are serving as collaterals.

Patients with venous varicosities are often concerned about the cosmetic appearance of their legs. Symptoms consist of a dull ache or pressure sensation in the legs after prolonged standing; it is relieved with leg elevation. The legs feel heavy, and mild ankle edema develops occasionally. Extensive venous varicosities may cause skin ulcerations near the ankle. Superficial venous thrombosis may be a recurring problem, and, rarely, a varicosity ruptures and bleeds. Visual inspection of the legs in the dependent position usually confirms the presence of varicose veins.

Varicose veins can usually be treated with conservative measures. Symptoms often decrease when the legs are elevated periodically, when prolonged standing is avoided, and when elastic support hose are worn. External compression stockings provide a counterbalance to the hydrostatic pressure in the veins. Small symptomatic varicose veins can be treated with sclerotherapy, in which a sclerosing solution is injected into the involved varicose vein and a compression bandage is applied. Surgical therapy usually involves extensive ligation and stripping of the greater and lesser saphenous veins and should be reserved for patients who are very symptomatic, suffer recurrent superficial vein thrombosis, and/or develop skin ulceration. Surgical therapy may also be indicated for cosmetic reasons.

CHRONIC VENOUS INSUFFICIENCY Chronic venous insufficiency may result from deep vein thrombosis and/or valvular incompetence. Following deep vein thrombosis, the delicate valve leaflets become thickened and contracted so that they cannot prevent retrograde flow of blood; the vein becomes rigid and thick-walled. Although most veins recanalize after an episode of thrombosis, the large proximal veins may remain occluded. Secondary incompetence develops in distal valves because high pressures distend the vein and separate the leaflets. Primary deep venous valvular dysfunction may also occur without previous thrombosis. Patients with venous insufficiency often complain of a dull ache in the leg that worsens with prolonged standing and resolves with leg elevation. Examination demonstrates increased leg circumference, edema, and superficial varicose veins. Erythema, dermatitis, and hyperpigmentation develop along the distal aspect of the leg, and skin ulceration may occur near the medial and lateral malleoli. Cellulitis may be a recurring problem. Patients should be advised to avoid prolonged standing or sitting; frequent leg elevation is helpful. Graduated compression stockings should be worn during the day. These efforts should be intensified if skin ulcers develop. Ulcers should be treated with applications of wet to dry dressings and, occasionally, dilute topical antibiotic solutions. Commercially available dressings comprising antiseptic solutions and compressive bandages may be applied and should be changed weekly until healing occurs. Recurrent ulceration and severe edema may be treated by surgical interruption of incompetent communicating veins. Rarely, surgical valvuloplasty and bypass of venous occlusions are employed.

LYMPHATIC DISORDERS

Lymphatic capillaries are blind-ended tubes formed by a single layer of endothelial cells. The absent or widely fenestrated basement membrane of lymphatic capillaries allows access to interstitial proteins and particles. Lymphatic capillaries merge to form larger vessels which contain smooth muscle and are capable of vasomotion. Small and medium-sized lymphatic vessels empty into progressively larger channels, most of which drain into the thoracic duct. The lymphatic circulation is involved in the absorption of interstitial fluid and in the response to infection.

LYMPHEDEMA　Lymphedema may be categorized as primary or secondary (Table 248-3). The prevalence of primary lymphedema is approximately 1 per 10,000 individuals. Primary lymphedema may be secondary to agenesis, hypoplasia, or obstruction of the lymphatic vessels. It may be associated with Turner syndrome, Klinefelter syndrome, Noonan syndrome, the yellow nail syndrome, the intestinal lymphangiectasia syndrome, and lymphangiomyomatosis. Women are affected more frequently than men. There are three clinical subtypes: congenital lymphedema, which appears shortly after birth; lymphedema praecox, which has its onset at the time of puberty; and lymphedema tarda, which usually begins after age 35. Familial forms of congenital lymphedema (Milroy's disease) and lymphedema praecox (Meige's disease) may be inherited in an autosomal dominant manner with variable penetrance; autosomal or sex-linked recessive forms are less common.

Secondary lymphedema is an acquired condition resulting from damage to or obstruction of previously normal lymphatic channels (Table 248-3). Recurrent episodes of bacterial lymphangitis, usually caused by streptococci, are a very common cause of lymphedema. The most common cause of secondary lymphedema worldwide is filariasis (Chap. 221). Tumors, such as prostate cancer and lymphoma, can also obstruct lymphatic vessels. Both surgery and radiation therapy for breast carcinoma may cause lymphedema of the upper extremity. Less common causes include tuberculosis, contact dermatitis, lymphogranuloma venereum, rheumatoid arthritis, pregnancy, and self-induced or factitious lymphedema following application of tourniquets.

Lymphedema is generally a painless condition, but patients may

experience a chronic dull, heavy sensation in the leg, and most often they are concerned about the appearance of the leg. Lymphedema of the lower extremity, initially involving the foot, gradually progresses up the leg so that the entire limb becomes edematous. In the early stages, the edema is soft and pits easily with pressure. In the chronic stages, the limb has a woody texture, and the tissues become indurated and fibrotic. At this point the edema may no longer be pitting. The limb loses its normal contour, and the toes appear square. Lymphedema should be distinguished from other disorders that cause unilateral leg swelling, such as deep vein thrombosis and chronic venous insufficiency. In the latter condition, the edema is softer, and there is often evidence of a stasis dermatitis, hyperpigmentation, and superficial venous varicosities.

The evaluation of patients with lymphedema should include diagnostic studies to clarify the cause. Abdominal and pelvic ultrasound and computed tomography can be used to detect obstructing lesions such as neoplasms. MRI may reveal edema in the epifascial compartment and identify lymph nodes and enlarged lymphatic channels. Lymphoscintigraphy and lymphangiography are rarely indicated, but either can be used to confirm the diagnosis or to differentiate primary from secondary lymphedema. Lymphoscintigraphy involves the injection of radioactively labeled technetium-containing colloid into the distal subcutaneous tissue of the affected extremity. In lymphangiography, contrast material is injected into a distal lymphatic vessel that has been isolated and cannulated. In primary lymphedema, lymphatic channels are absent, hypoplastic, or ectatic. In secondary lymphedema, lymphatic channels are usually dilated, and it may be possible to determine the level of obstruction.

Rₓ **TREATMENT**　Patients with lymphedema of the lower extremities must be instructed to take meticulous care of their feet to prevent recurrent lymphangitis. Skin hygiene is important, and emollients can be used to prevent drying. Prophylactic antibiotics are often helpful, and fungal infection should be treated aggressively. Patients should be encouraged to participate in physical activity; frequent leg elevation can reduce the amount of edema. Physical therapy, including massage to facilitate lymphatic drainage, may be helpful. Patients can be fitted with graduated compression hose to reduce the amount of lymphedema that develops with upright posture. Occasionally, intermittent pneumatic compression devices can be applied at home to facilitate reduction of the edema. Diuretics are contraindicated and may cause depletion of intravascular volume and metabolic abnormalities. Recently, microsurgical lymphatico-venous anastomotic procedures have been performed to rechannel lymph flow from obstructed lymphatic vessels into the venous system.

Table 248-3　Causes of Lymphedema

Primary
  Congenital (includes Milroy's disease)
  Lymphedema praecox (includes Meige's disease)
  Lymphedema tarda
Secondary
  Recurrent lymphangitis
  Filariasis
  Tuberculosis
  Neoplasm
  Surgery
  Radiation therapy

BIBLIOGRAPHY

AQEL MB, OLIN JW: Thromboangiitis obliterans (Buerger's disease). Vasc Med 2:61, 1997

BAUMGARTNER I et al: Constitutive expression of VEGF165 after intramuscular gene transfer promotes collateral vessel development in patients with critical limb ischemia. Circulation 97:1114, 1998

DAWSON DL et al: Cilostazol has beneficial effects in treatment of intermittent claudication. Circulation 98:678, 1998

DORMANDY JA, RUTHERFORD RB: Management of peripheral arterial disease (PAD). J Vasc Surg 31:51, 2000

DE CATERINA R: Endothelial dysfunctions: Common denominators in vascular disease. Curr Opin Lipid 11:9, 2000

GOULD MK et al: Low-molecular-weight heparins compared with unfractionated heparin for treatment of acute venous thrombosis. Ann Intern Med 130:789, 1999

KEARON C et al: A comparison of three months of anticoagulation with extended anticoagulation for a first episode of idiopathic venous thromobembolism. N Engl J Med 340:901, 1999

LOSCALZO J et al:*Vascular Medicine*, 2d ed. Boston, Little, Brown, 1996

SZUBA A, ROCKSON SG: Lymphedema: Classification, diagnosis and therapy. Vasc Med 3:145, 1998

THE COLUMBUS INVESTIGATORS: Low-molecular-weight heparin in the treatment of patients with venous thromboembolism. N Engl J Med 337:657, 1997

WORKING PARTY ON THROMBOLYSIS IN THE MANAGEMENT OF LIMB ISCHEMIA: Thrombolysis in the management of lower limb peripheral arterial occlusion—a consensus document. Am J Cardiol 81:207, 1998

APPENDICES

A

LABORATORY VALUES OF CLINICAL IMPORTANCE

INTRODUCTORY COMMENTS

All laboratory appendices should be interpreted with caution since normal values differ widely among clinical laboratories. The values given in this Appendix are meant primarily for use with this text. In preparing the Appendix, the editors have taken into account the fact that the system of international units (SI, système international d'unités) is now used in most countries and in most medical and scientific journals.[1] However, clinical laboratories in many countries continue to report values in traditional units. Therefore, both systems are used in the Appendix. Values in SI units appear first and traditional units appear in parentheses after the SI units. The dual system is also used in the text except for (1) those instances in which the numbers remain the same but only the terminology is changed (mmol/L for meq/L or IU/L for mIU/mL), when only the SI units are given; and (2) most pressure measurements (e.g., blood and cerebrospinal fluid pressures), when the traditional units (mmHg, mmH2O) are used. In all other instances in the text the SI unit is followed by the traditional unit in parentheses. The SI base units, SI derived units, other units of measure referred to in Appendix A, and SI prefixes are listed in Tables A-1 to A-3. Conversions from one system to another can be made as follows:

$$mmol/L = \frac{mg/dL \times 10}{\text{atomic weight}}$$

$$mg/dL = \frac{mmol/L \times \text{atomic weight}}{10}$$

TABLE A-1 RADIATION-DERIVED UNITS

Quantity	Old Unit	SI Unit	Name for SI Unit (and Abbreviation)	Conversion
Activity	curie (Ci)	Disintegrations per second (dps)	becquerel (Bq)	1 Ci = 3.7 × 10^{10} Bq 1 mCi = 37 mBq 1 μCi = 0.037 MBq or 37 GBq 1 Bq = 2.703 × 10^{-11} Ci
Absorbed dose	rad	joule per kilogram (J/kg)	gray (Gy)	1 Gy = 100 rad 1 rad = 0.01 Gy 1 mrad = 10^{-3} cGy
Exposure	roentgen (R)	coulomb per kilogram (C/kg)	—	1 C/kg = 3876 R 1 R = 2.58 × 10^{-4} C/kg 1 mR = 258 pC/kg
Dose equivalent	rem	joule per kilogram (J/kg)	sievert (Sv)	1 Sv = 100 rem 1 rem = 0.01 Sv 1 mrem = 10 μSv

[1]Young DS: Implementation of SI units for clinical laboratory data. Ann Intern Med 106:114, 1987

TABLE A-2 BODY FLUIDS AND OTHER MASS DATA

	Reference Range	
	SI Units	Conventional Units
Ascitic fluid: See Chap. 46		
Body fluid, total volume (lean) of body weight	50% (in obese) to 70%	
Intracellular	0.3–0.4 of body weight	
Extracellular	0.2–0.3 of body weight	
Blood		
Total volume		
Males	69 mL per kg body weight	
Females	65 mL per kg body weight	
Plasma volume		
Males	39 mL per kg body weight	
Females	40 mL per kg body weight	
Red blood cell volume		
Males	30 mL per kg body weight	1.15–1.21 L/m² of body surface area
Females	25 mL per kg body weight	0.95–1.00 L/m² of body surface area

TABLE A-3 CEREBROSPINAL FLUID[a]

Constituent	Reference Range	
	SI Units	Conventional Units
Osmolarity	292–297 mmol/kg water	292–297 mOsm/L
Electrolytes		
Sodium	137–145 mmol/L	137–145 meq/L
Potassium	2.7–3.9 mmol/L	2.7–3.9 meq/L
Calcium	1.0–1.5 mmol/L	2.1–3.0 meq/L
Magnesium	1.0–1.2 mmol/L	2.0–2.5 meq/L
Chloride	116–122 mmol/L	116–122 meq/L
CO_2 content	20–24 mmol/L	20–24 meq/L
P_{CO_2}	6–7 kPa	45–49 mmHg
pH	7.31–7.34	
Glucose	2.2–3.9 mmol/L	40–70 mg/dL
Lactate	1–2 mmol/L	10–20 mg/dL
Total protein	0.2–0.5 g/L	20–50 mg/dL
Albumin	0.066–0.442 g/L	6.6–44.2 mg/dL
IgG	0.009–0.057 g/L	0.9–5.7 mg/dL
IgG index[b]	0.29–0.59	
Oligoclonal bands (OGB)	<2 bands not present in matched serum sample	
Ammonia	15–47 μmol/L	25–80 μg/dL
Creatinine	44–168 μmol/L	0.5–1.9 mg/dL
Myelin basic protein	<4 μg/L	
CSF pressure		50–180 mmH2O
CSF volume (adult)	~150 mL	
Leukocytes		
Total	<5 per μL	
Differential:		
Lymphocytes	60–70%	
Monocytes	30–50%	
Neutrophils	None	

[a] Since cerebrospinal fluid concentrations are equilibrium values, measurements of the same parameters in blood plasma obtained at the same time are recommended. However, there is a time lag in attainment of equilibrium, and cerebrospinal levels of plasma constituents that can fluctuate rapidly (such as plasma glucose) may not achieve stable values until after a significant lag phase.

[b] $\text{IgG index} = \dfrac{\text{CSF IgG(mg/dL)} \times \text{serum albumin(g/dL)}}{\text{Serum IgG(g/dL)} \times \text{CSF albumin(mg/dL)}}$

TABLE A-4 CHEMICAL CONSTITUENTS OF BLOOD

Constituent	Specimen	Reference Range SI Units	Conventional Units
Acetoacetate	P	$<100\ \mu$mol/L	<1 mg/dL
Albumin	S	35–55 g/L	3.5–5.5 g/dL
Aldolase		0–100 nkat/L	0–6 U/L
Alpha$_1$ antitrypsin	S	0.8–2.1 g/L	85–213 mg/dL
Alpha fetoprotein (adult)	S	$<30\ \mu$g/L	<30 ng/mL
Aminotransferases	S		
Aspartate (AST, SGOT)		0–0.58 μkat/L	0–35 U/L
Alanine (ALT, SGPT)		0–0.58 μkat/L	0–35 U/L
Ammonia, as NH_3	P	6–47 μmol/L	10–80 μg/dL
Amylase	S	0.8–3.2 μkat/L	60–180 U/L
Angiotensin-converting enzyme (ACE)		<670 nkat/L	<40 U/L
Anticonvulsant drug levels: see Table 360-8			
Arterial blood gases			
[$HCO_3{}^-$]		21–28 mmol/L	21–30 meq/L
P_{CO_2}		4.7–5.9 kPa	35–45 mmHg
pH		7.38–7.44	
P_{O_2}		11–13 kPa	80–100 mmHg
β-Hydroxybutyrate	P	$<300\ \mu$mol/L	<3 mg/dL
Bilirubin, total	S (Malloy-Evelyn)	5.1–17 μmol/L	0.3–1.0 mg/dL
Direct	S	1.7–5.1 μmol/L	0.1–0.3 mg/dL
Indirect	S	3.4–12 μmol/L	0.2–0.7 mg/dL
Calcium, ionized		1.1–1.4 mmol/L	4.5–5.6 mg/dL
Calcium	P	2.2–2.6 mmol/L	9–10.5 mg/dL
Carbon dioxide content	P (sea level)	21–30 mmol/L	21–30 meq/L
Carbon dioxide tension (P_{CO_2})	Arterial blood (sea level)	4.7–5.9 kPa	35–45 mmHg
Carbon monoxide content	Blood	Symptoms with 20% saturation of hemoglobin	
Chloride	S (as Cl^-)	98–106 mmol/L	98–106 meq/L
Cholesterol: see Table A-9			
Complement	S		
C3		0.55–1.20 g/L	55–120 mg/dL
C4		0.20–0.50 g/L	20–50 mg/dL
Coproporphyrins (types I and III)	U	150–460 μmol/d	100–300 μg/d
Creatine kinase	S (total)		
Females		0.17–1.17 μkat/L	10–70 U/L
Males		0.42–1.50 μkat/L	25–90 U/L
Creatine kinase-MB		0–7 μg/L	
Creatinine	S	$<133\ \mu$mol/L	<1.5 mg/dL
Erythropoietin	S	5–36 U/L	
Fatty acids, free (nonesterified)	P	180 mg/L	<18 mg/dL
Ferritin	S		
Women		10–200 μg/L	10–200 ng/mL
Men		15–400 μg/L	15–400 ng/mL
Fibrinogen: See "Hematologic Evaluations: Platelets and Coagulation Parameters"			
Fibrinogen split products: See "Hematologic Evaluations: Platelets and Coagulation Parameters"			
Glucose (fasting)	P		
Normal		4.2–6.4 mmol/L	75–115 mg/dL
Diabetes mellitus		>7.8 mmol/L	>140 mg/dL
Glucose, 2 h postprandial	P		
Normal		<7.8 mmol/L	<140 mg/dL
Impaired glucose tolerance		7.8–11.1 mmol/L	140–200 mg/dL
Diabetes mellitus		>11.1 mmol/L	>200 mg/dL
Hemoglobin	B (sea level)		
Male		140–180 g/L	14–18 g/dL
Female		120–160 g/L	12–16 g/dL
Hemoglobin A_{1c} Up to 6% of total hemoglobin			
Iron	S	9–27 μmol/L	50–150 μg/dL
Iron-binding capacity	S	45–66 μmol/L	250–370 μg/dL
Saturation		0.2–0.45	20–45%
Lactate dehydrogenase	S	1.7–3.2 μkat/L	100–190 U/L
Lactate dehydrogenase isoenzymes	S (agarose)		
Fraction 1 (of total)		0.14–0.25	14–26%
Fraction 2		0.29–0.39	29–39%
Fraction 3		0.20–0.25	20–26%
Fraction 4		0.08–0.16	8–16%
Fraction 5		0.06–0.16	6–16%

(continued)

Constituent	Specimen	Reference Range	
		SI Units	**Conventional Units**
Lactate	P, venous	0.6–1.7 mmol/L	5–15 mg/dL
Lipase	S	0–2.66 μkat/L	0–160 U/L
Lipids: see Table A-9			
Lipids, triglyceride: S see "Triglycerides"			
Lipoprotein: see Table A-9			
Lipoprotein (a)	S	0–300 mg/L	0–3 mg/dL
Magnesium	S	0.8–1.2 mmol/L	1.8–3 mg/dL
Myoglobin	S		
Male		19–92 μg/L	
Female		12–76 μg/L	
Osmolality	P	285–295 mmol/kg serum water	285–295 mosmol/kg serum water
Oxygen content	B, arterial (sea level)		17–21 vol%
	B, venous arm (sea level)		10 to 16 vol%
Oxygen percent saturation (sea level)	B, arterial	0.97 mol/mol	97%
	B, venous, arm	0.60–0.85 mol/mol	60–85%
Oxygen tension (P_{O_2})	Blood	11–13 kPa	80–100 mmHg
pH	B	7.38–7.44	
Phosphatase, acid	S	0.90 nkat/L	0–5.5 U/L
Phosphatase, alkaline	S	0.5–2.0 nkat/L	30–120 U/L
Phosphorus, inorganic	S	1.0–1.4 mmol/L	3–4.5 mg/dL
Porphobilinogen	U	None	None
Potassium	S	3.5–5.0 mmol/L	3.5–5.0 meq/L
Prostate-specific antigen (PSA)	S		
Female		<0.5 μg/L	<0.5 ng/mL
Male: <40 years		0.0–2.0 μg/L	0.0–2.0 ng/mL
≥40 years		0.0–4.0 μg/L	0.0–4.0 ng/mL
PSA, free, in males 45–75 years, with PSA values between 4 and 20 μg/mL	S	>0.25 associated with benign prostatic hyperplasia	>25% associated with benign prostatic hyperplasia
Protein, total	S	55–80 g/L	5.5–8.0 g/dL
Protein fractions	S		
Albumin		35–55 g/L	3.5–5.5 g/dL (50–60%)
Globulin		20–35 g/L	2.0–3.5 g/dL (40–50%)
Alpha$_1$		2–4 g/L	0.2–0.4 g/dL (4.2–7.2%)
Alpha$_2$		5–9 g/L	0.5–0.9 g/dL (6.8–12%)
Beta		6–11 g/L	0.6–1.1 g/dL (9.3–15%)
Gamma		7–17 g/L	0.7–1.7 g/dL (13–23%)
Pyruvate	P, venous	60–170 μmol/L	0.5–1.5 mg/dL
Sodium	S	136–145 mmol/L	136–145 meq/L
Transferrin	S	2.3–3.9 g/L	230–390 mg/dL
Triglycerides	S	<1.8 mmol/L	<160 mg/dL
Troponin I	S	0–0.4 μg/L	0–0.4 ng/mL
Troponin T	S	0–0.1 μg/L	0–0.1 ng/mL
Urea nitrogen	S	3.6–7.1 mmol/L	10–20 mg/dL
Uric acid:	S		
Men		150–480 μmol/L	2.5–8.0 mg/dL
Women		90–360 μmol/L	1.5–6.0 mg/dL
Urobilinogen	U	1.7–5.9 μmol/d	1–3.5 mg/d

NOTE: B, blood; P, plasma; S, serum; U, urine.

Drug	Therapeutic Range		Toxic Level	
	Conventional Units	SI Units	Conventional Units	SI Units
Acetaminophen	10–30 μg/mL	66–199 μmol/L	>200 μg/mL	>1324 μmol/L
Amikacin				
Peak	25–35 μg/mL	43–60 μmol/L	>35 μg/mL	>60 μmol/L
Trough	4–8 μg/mL	6.8–13.7 μmol/L	>10 μg/mL	>17 μmol/L
Amitriptyline	120–250 ng/mL	433–903 nmol/L	>500 ng/mL	>1805 nmol/L
Amphetamine	20–30 ng/mL	148–222 nmol/L	>200 ng/mL	>1480 nmol/L
Barbiturates, most short-acting			>20 mg/L	>88 μmol/L
Bromide			>1250 μg/mL	>15.6 mmol/L
Carbamazepine	6–12 μg/mL	26–51 μmol/L	>15 μg/mL	>63 μmol/L
Chlordiazepoxide	700–1000 ng/mL	2.34–3.34 μmol/L	>5000 ng/mL	>16.7 μmol/L
Clonazepam	15–60 ng/mL	48–190 nmol/L	>80 ng/mL	>254 nmol/L
Clozapine	200–350 ng/mL	0.6–1 μmol/L		
Cocaine	100–500 ng/mL	330–1650 nmol/L	>1000 ng/mL	>3300 nmol/L
Desipramine	75–300 ng/mL	281–1125 nmol/L	>400 ng/mL	>1500 nmol/L
Diazepam	100–1000 ng/mL	0.35–351 μmol/L	>5000 ng/mL	>17.55 μmol/L
Digoxin	0.8–2.0 ng/mL	1.0–2.6 nmol/L	>2.5 ng/mL	>3.2 umol/L
Doxepin	30–150 ng/mL	107–537 nmol/L	>500 ng/mL	>1790 nmol/L
Ethanol			>300 mg/dL	>65 mmol/L
Behavioral changes	>20 mg/dL	>4.3 mmol/L		
Legal intoxication	>80 mg/dL	>17 mmol/L		
Ethosuximide	40–100 μg/mL	283–708 μmol/L	>150 μg/mL	>1062 μmol/L
Flecainide	0.2–1.0 μg/mL	0.5–2.4 μmol/L	>1.0 μg/mL	>2.4 μmol/L
Gentamicin				
Peak	8–10 μg/mL	16.7–20.9 μmol/L	>10 μg/mL	>21 μmol/L
Trough	<2–4 μg/mL	<4.2–8.4 μmol/L	>4 μg/mL	>8.4 μmol/L
Imipramine	125–250 ng/mL	446–893 nmol/L	>500 ng/mL	>1784 nmol/L
Lidocaine	1.5–6.0 μg/mL	6.4–26 μmol/L		
CNS or cardiovascular depression			6–8 μg/mL	26–34.2 μmol/L
Seizures, obtundation, decreased cardiac output			>8 μg/mL	>34.2 μmol/L
Lithium	0.6–1.2 meq/L	0.6–1.2 nmol/L	>2 meq/L	>2 mmol/L
Methadone	100–400 ng/mL	0.32–1.29 μmol/L	>2000 ng/mL	>6.46 μmol/L
Methotrexate	Variable	Variable		
Low-dose (1–2 weeks)			>9.1 ng/mL	>20 nmol/L
High-dose (48 h)			>227 ng/mL	>0.5 μmol/L
Morphine	10–80 ng/mL	35–280 μmol/L	>200 ng/mL	>700 nmol/L
Nitroprusside (as thiocyanate)	6–29 μg/mL	103–499 μmol/L		
Nortriptyline	50–170 ng/mL	190–646 nmol/L	>500 ng/mL	>1.9 μmol/L
Phenobarbital	10–40 μg/mL	43–170 μmol/L		
Slowness, ataxia, nystagmus			35–80 μg/mL	151–345 μmol/L
Coma with reflexes			65–117 μg/mL	280–504 μmol/L
Coma without reflexes			>100 μg/mL	>430 μmol/L
Phenytoin	10–20 μg/mL	40–79 μmol/L	>20 μg/mL	>79 μmol/L
Procainamide	4–10 μg/mL	17–42 μmol/L	>10–12 μg/mL	>42–51 μmol/L
Quinidine	2–5 μg/mL	6–15 μmol/L	>6 μg/mL	>18 μmol/L
Salicylates	150–300 μg/mL	1086–2172 μmol/L	>300 μg/mL	>2172 μmol/L
Theophylline	8–20 μg/mL	44–111 μmol/L	>20 μg/mL	>110 μmol/L
Thiocyanate				
After nitroprusside infusion	6–29 μg/mL	103–499 μmol/L		
Nonsmoker	1–4 μg/mL	17–69 μmol/L	>120 μg/mL	>2064 μmol/L
Smoker	3–12 μg/mL	52–206 μmol/L		
Tobramycin				
Peak	8–10 μg/mL	17–21 μmol/L	>10 μg/mL	>21 μmol/L
Trough	<4 μg/mL	<9 μmol/L	>4 μg/mL	>9 μmol/L
Valproic acid	50–150 μg/mL	347–1040 μmol/L	>150 μg/mL	>1040 μmol/L
Vancomycin				
Peak	18–26 μg/mL	12–18 μmol/L		
Trough	5–10 μg/mL	3–7 μmol/L	>80–100 μg/mL	>55–69 μmol/L

TABLE A-6 CIRCULATORY FUNCTION TESTS

Test	Results: Reference Range SI Units (Range)	Conventional Units (Range)
Arteriovenous oxygen difference	30–50 mL/L	30–50 mL/L
Cardiac output (Fick)	2.5–3.6 L/m² of body surface area per min	2.5–3.6 L/m² of body surface area per min
Contractility indexes		
Max. left ventricular dp/dt	220 kPa/s (176–250 kPa/s)	1650 mmHg/s (1320–1880 mmHg/s)
(dp/dt)/DP when DP = 5.3 kPa (40 mmHg)(DP, diastolic pressure)	(37.6 ± 12.2)/s	(37.6 ± 12.2)/s
Mean normalized systolic ejection rate (angiography)	3.32 ± 0.84 end-diastolic volumes per second	3.32 ± 0.84 end-diastolic volumes per second
Mean velocity of circumferential fiber shortening (angiography)	1.66 ± 0.42 circumferences per second	1.66 ± 0.42 circumferences per second
Ejection fraction: stroke volume/end-diastolic volume (SV/EDV)	0.67 (0.55–0.78)	0.67 (0.55–0.78)
End-diastolic volume	75 mL/m² (60–88 mL/m²)	75 mL/m² (60–88 mL/m²)
End-systolic volume	25 mL/m² (20–33 mL/m²)	25 mL/m² (20–33 mL/m²)
Left ventricular work		
Stroke work index	30–110 (g·m)/m²	30–110 (g·m)/m²
Left ventricular minute work index	1.8–6.6 [(kg·m)/m²]/min	1.8–6.6 [(kg·m)/m²]/min
Oxygen consumption index	110–150 mL	110–150 mL

Test	Results: Reference Range SI Units (Range)	Conventional Units (Range)
Maximum oxygen uptake	35 mL/min (20–60 mL/min)	35 mL/min (20–60 mL/min)
Pulmonary vascular resistance	2–12 (kPa·s)/L	20–120 (dyn·s)/cm⁵
Systemic vascular resistance	77–150 (kPa·s)/L	770–1500 (dyn·s)/cm⁵

TABLE A-7 NORMAL VALUES OF DOPPLER ECHOCARDIOGRAPHIC MEASUREMENTS IN ADULTS

	Range	Mean
RVD (cm)	0.9 to 2.6	1.7
LVID (cm)	3.5 to 5.7	4.7
Posterior LV wall thickness (cm)	0.6 to 1.1	0.9
IVS wall thickness (cm)	0.6 to 1.1	0.9
Left atrial dimension (cm)	1.9 to 4.0	2.9
Aortic root dimension (cm)	2.0 to 3.7	2.7
Aortic cusps separation (cm)	1.5 to 2.6	1.9
Percentage of fractional shortening	34 to 44%	36%
Mitral flow (m/s)	0.6 to 1.3	0.9
Tricuspid flow (m/s)	0.3 to 0.7	0.5
Pulmonary artery (m/s)	0.6 to 0.9	0.75
Aorta (m/s)	1.0 to 1.7	1.35

NOTE: RVD, right ventricular dimension; LVID, left ventricular internal dimension; LV, left ventricle; IVS, interventricular septum.
SOURCE: From H Feigenbaum, *Echocardiography*, 5th ed, Philadelphia. Lea & Febiger, 1994

TABLE A-8 GASTROINTESTINAL TESTS. SEE ALSO "STOOL ANALYSIS"

Test	Results SI Units	Conventional Units
Absorption tests		
D-Xylose: after overnight fast, 25 g xylose given in oral aqueous solution		
Urine, collected for following 5 h	33–53 mmol (or >20% of ingested dose)	5–8 g (or >20% of ingested dose)
Serum, 1 h after dose	1.7–2.7 mmol/L	25–40 mg/dL
Vitamin A: a fasting blood specimen is obtained and 200,000 units of vitamin A in oil is given orally	Serum level should rise to twice fasting level in 3–5 h	Serum level should rise to fasting level in 3–5 h
Bentiromide test (pancreatic function): 500 mg bentiromide (chymex) orally; *p*-aminobenzoic acid (PABA) measured		
Plasma		>3.6 (±1.1) µg/mL at 90 min
Urine	>50% recovered in 6 h	>50% recovered in 6 h
Gastric juice		
Volume		
24 h	2–3 L	2–3 L
Nocturnal	600–700 mL	600–700 mL
Basal, fasting	30–70 mL/h	30–70 mL/h
Reaction		
pH	1.6–1.8	1.6–1.8
Titratable acidity of fasting juice	4–9 µmol/s	15–35 meq/h
Acid output		
Basal		
Females (mean ± 1 SD)	0.6 ± 0.5 µmol/s	2.0 ± 1.8 meq/h
Males (mean ± 1 SD)	0.8 ± 0.6 µmol/s	3.0 ± 2.0 meq/h
Maximal (after SC histamine acid phosphate, 0.004 mg/kg body weight, and preceded by 50 mg promethazine, or after betazole, 1.7 mg/kg body weight, or pentagastrin, 6 µg/kg body weight)		
Females (mean ± 1 SD)	4.4 ± 1.4 µmol/s	16 ± 5 meq/h
Males (mean ± 1 SD)	6.4 ± 1.4 µmol/s	23 ± 5 meq/h
Basal acid output/maximal acid output ratio	≤0.6	≤0.6
Gastrin, serum	40–200 µg/L	40–200 pg/mL
Secretin test (pancreatic exocrine function): 1 unit/kg body weight, IV		
Volume (pancreatic juice) in 80 min	>2.0 mL/kg	>2.0 mL/kg
Bicarbonate concentration	>80 mmol/L	>80 meq/L
Bicarbonate output in 30 min	>10 mmol	>10 meq

Substance	Specimen	Reference Range SI Units	Reference Range Conventional Units	Substance	Specimen	Reference Range SI Units	Reference Range Conventional Units
Adrenocorticotropin (ACTH), 8 A.M.	P	1.3–16.7 pmol/L	6.0–76.0 pg/mL	Growth hormone, after 100 g oral glucose		<2 μg/L	<2 ng/mL
Aldosterone, 8 A.M., (patient supine, 100 mmol/L Na and 60–100 mmol/L K intake)	P	<220 pmol/L	<8 ng/dL	Hemoglobin A$_{1c}$	WB	0.038–0.064	3.8–6.4%
				17-Hydroxycorticosteroids	U	5.5–28 μmol/d	2–10 mg/d
Aldosterone	U	14–53 nmol/d	5–19 μg/d	5-Hydroxyindoleacetic acid (5-HIAA)	U	≤31.4 μmol/d	≤6 mg/d
Androstenedione	P			17-Hydroxyprogesterone	P		
Women		3.5–7.0 nmol/L	1–2 ng/mL	Women			
Men		3.0–5.0 nmol/L	0.8–1.3 ng/mL	Follicular phase		0.6–3 nmol/L	0.2–1.0 μg/L
Angiotensin II, 8 A.M.	P	10–30 nmol/L	10–30 pg/mL	Luteal phase		1.5–10.6 nmol/L	0.5–3.5 μg/L
Arginine vasopressin (AVP), random fluid intake	P	1.4–5.6 pmol/L	1.5–6.0 ng/L	Men		0.2–9.0 nmol/L	0.06–3.0 μg/L
				Insulin, fasting	S, P	43–186 pmol/L	6–26 μU/mL
Calciferols (vitamin D)	P			Insulin-like growth factor (somatomedin C, IGF-1/ SM C)	S		
1,25-dihydroxyvitamin D [1,25(OH)$_2$D]		40–160 pmol/L	16–65 pg/mL	16–24 years		182–780 μg/L	182–780 ng/mL
25-hydroxyvitamin D [25(OH)D]		20–200 nmol/L	8–80 ng/mL	25–39 years		114–492 μg/L	114–492 ng/mL
				40–54 years		90–360 μg/L	90–360 ng/mL
Calcitonin	P			>54 years		71–290 μg/L	71–290 ng/mL
Women		≤8 ng/L	≤8 pg/mL	17-Ketosteroids	U		
Men		≤4 ng/L	≤4 pg/mL	Women		20–59 μmol/d	6–17 mg/d
Catecholamines				Men		20–69 μmol/d	6–20 mg/d
Epinephrine	U	<275 nmol/d	<50 μg/d	Oxytocin			
Free	U	<590 nmol/d	<100 μg/d	Random		1–4 pmol/L	1.25–5 ng/L
Metanephrine	U	<7 μmol/d	<1.3 mg/d	Ovulatory peak in women		4–8 pmol/L	5–10 ng/L
Norepinephrine	U	89–473 nmol/d	15–80 μg/d	Parathyroid hormone	S	10–60 ng/L	10–60 pg/mL
Vanillylmandelic acid (VMA)	U	<40 μmol/d	<8 mg/d	Parathyroid hormone–related protein	P	<1.3 pmol/L	<1.3 pmol/L
Chorionic gonadotropin, β subunit (β-hCG), men and nonpregnant women	P	<3 IU/L	<3 mIU/mL	Progesterone	P		
				Women, luteal, peak		6–60 nmol/L	2–20 ng/mL
Cortisol				Men, prepubertal girls, preovulatory women, postmenopausal women		<6 nmol/L	<2 ng/mL
Free	U	25–140 nmol/d	10–50 μg/d				
8 A.M.	P	140–690 nmol/L	5–25 μg/dL				
4 P.M.	P	80–330 nmol/L	3–12 μg/dL	Prolactin	S	2–15 μg/L	2–15 ng/mL
Dehydroepiandrosterone (DHEA)	P	7–31 nmol/L	2–9 ng/dL	Radioactive iodine uptake, 24 h (range varies in different areas due to variations in iodine intake)			5–30%
11-Deoxycortisol (compound S)	P	<30 nmol/L	<1 μg/dL				
DHEA sulfate	P	1.3–6.8 μmol/L	500–2500 μg/dL	Renin (adult, normal-Na diet)	P		
Estradiol	P			Supine		0.08–0.83 ng/(L·s)	0.3–3.0 ng/(mL·h)
Women (higher at ovulation)		70–220 pmol/L	20–60 pg/mL	Upright		0.28–2.5 ng/(L·s)	1.0–9.0 ng/(mL·h)
Men		<180 pmol/L	<50 pg/mL	Resin triiodothyronine (T$_3$)		0.25–0.35	25–35%
Gastrin	S	40–200 ng/L	40–200 pg/mL	Reverse T$_3$ (rT$_3$)	P	0.15–0.61 nmol/L	10–40 ng/dL
Glucagon	P	50–100 ng/L	50–100 pg/mL	Semen analysis: see Chap. 335			
Gonadotropins				T$_3$	P	1.1–2.9 nmol/L	70–190 ng/dL
Follicle-stimulating hormone (FSH)	P			Testosterone	P		
Women				Women		<3.5 nmol/L	<1 ng/mL
Mature, premenopausal, except at ovulation		1.4–9.6 IU/L	1.4–9.6 mIU/mL	Men		10–35 nmol/L	3–10 ng/mL
				Prepubertal boys and girls		0.17–0.7 nmol/L	0.05–0.2 ng/mL
Ovulatory surge		2.3–21 IU/L	2.3–21 mIU/mL	Thyroglobulin	S	0–60 μg/L	0–60 ng/mL
Postmenopausal		34–96 IU/L	34–96 mIU/mL	Thyroid stimulating hormone (TSH)		0.4–5.0 mU/L	0.4–5.0 μU/mL
Men		0.9–15 IU/L	0.9–15 mIU/mL	Thyroxine (T$_4$)	SR	64–154 nmol/L	5–12 μg/dL
Luteinizing hormone (LH)	P						
Children, prepubertal		1.0–5.9 IU/L	1.0–5.9 mIU/mL				
Women							
Mature, premenopausal, except at ovulation		0.8–26 IU/L	0.8–26 mIU/mL				
Ovulatory surge		25–57 IU/L	25–57 mIU/mL				
Postmenopausal		40–104 IU/L	40–104 mIU/mL				
Men		1.3–13 IU/L	1.3–13 mIU/mL				

NOTE: P, plasma; S, serum; SR; serum radioimmunoassay; U, urine; WB, whole blood.

TABLE A-10   CLASSIFICATION OF TOTAL CHOLESTEROL, LDL-CHOLESTEROL, AND HDL-CHOLESTEROL VALUES

	Total Plasma Cholesterol		LDL-Cholesterol		HDL-Cholesterol	
	SI, mmol/L	C, mg/dL	SI, mmol/L	C, mg/dL	SI, mmol/L	C, mg/dL
Desirable	<5.2	<200	<3.36	<130	>1.55	>60
Borderline	5.20–6.18	200–239	3.36–4.11	130–159	0.9–1.55	35–60
Undesirable	≥6.21	≥240	≥4.14	≥160	<0.9	<35

NOTE: LDL, low-density lipoprotein; HDL, high-density lipoprotein; SI, SI units; C, conventional units
SOURCE: Modified from the report of the Expert Panel on Detection, Evaluation, and Treatment of High Blood Cholesterol in Adults: Second Report of the National Cholesterol Education Program (NCEP) expert panel on detection, evaluation, and treatment of high blood cholesterol (Adult Treatment Panel II). Circulation 89:1329, 1994.

TABLE A-11   VITAMINS AND TRACE MINERALS

		Reference Range	
	Specimen	SI Units	Conventional Units
Carotenoids	S	0.9–5.6 μmol/L	50–300 μg/dL
Ceruloplasmin	S	270–370 mg/L	27–37 ng/dL
Copper	S	11–22 μmol/L	70–140 μg/dL
Folic acid	RC	340–1020 nmol/L cells	150–450 ng/mL cells
Folic acid	S	7–36 nmol/L cells	3–16 ng/mL cells
Lead	S	<1 μmol/L	<20 μg/dL
Vitamin A	S	0.7–3.5 μmol/L	20–100 μg/dL
Vitamin B_1 (thiamine)	S	0–75 nmol/L	0–2 μg/dL
Vitamin B_2 (riboflavin)	S	106–638 nmol/L	4–24 μg/dL
Vitamin B_6	P	20–121 nmol/L	5–30 ng/ml
Vitamin B_{12}	S	148–443 pmol/L	200–600 pg/mL
Vitamin C (ascorbic acid)	S	23–57 μmol/L	0.4–1.0 mg/dL
Vitamin D_3, 1,25-dihydroxy	S	60–108 pmol/L	25–45 pg/mL
Vitamin D_3, 25-hydroxy	P		
Summer		37.4–200 nmol/L	15–80 ng/mL
Winter		34.9–105 nmol/L	14–42 ng/mL
Vitamin E	S	12–42 μmol/L	5–18 μg/mL
Zinc	S	11.5–18.5 μmol/L	75–120 μg/dL

NOTE: P, plasma; RC, red cells; S, serum.

TABLE A-12   PULMONARY FUNCTION TESTS

See Table A-19: Summary of Values Useful in Pulmonary Physiology

TABLE A-13   RENAL FUNCTION TESTS

	Reference Range	
	SI Units	Conventional Units
Clearances (corrected to 1.72 m² body surface area):		
Measures of glomerular filtration rate:		
Inulin clearance (Cl)		
Males (mean ± 1 SD)	2.1 ± 0.4 mL/s	124 ± 25.8 mL/min
Females (mean ± 1 SD)	2.0 ± 0.2 mL/s	119 ± 12.8 mL/min
Endogenous creatinine clearance	1.5–2.2 mL/s	91–130 mL/min
Urea	1.0–1.7 mL/s	60–100 mL/min
Measures of effective renal plasma flow and tubular function:		
p-Aminohippuric acid clearance (Cl_{PAH}):		
Males (mean ± 1 SD)	10.9 ± 2.7 mL/s	654 ± 163 mL/min
Females (mean ± 1 SD)	9.9 ± 1.7 mL/s	594 ± 102 mL/min
Concentration and dilution test:		
Specific gravity of urine:		
After 12-h fluid restriction	≥1.025	≥1.025
After 12-h deliberate water intake	≤1.003	≤1.003
Protein excretion, urine	<0.15 g/d	<150 mg/d
Males	0–0.06 g/d	0–60 mg/d
Females	0–0.09 g/d	0–90 mg/d
Specific gravity, maximal range	1.002–1.028	1.002–1.028
Tubular reabsorption, phosphorus	0.79–0.94 of filtered load	79–94% of filtered load

TABLE A-14   HEMATOLOGIC EVALUATIONS. SEE ALSO "CHEMICAL CONSTITUENTS OF BLOOD"

	Reference Range			Reference Range	
	SI Units	Conventional Units		SI Units	Conventional Units
Bone marrow: see Table A-6			Platelets and coagulation parameters:		
Carboxyhemoglobin			Alpha$_2$ antiplasmin		70–130%
Nonsmoker	0–0.023	0–2.3%	Antithrombin III		80–120%
Smoker	0.021–0.042	2.1–4.2%	Bleeding time (Simplate)	<7 min	<7 min
Erythrocyte			Euglobulin lysis time	>2 h	>2 h
Count	4.15–4.90 × 10^{12}/L	4.15–4.90 × 10^6/mm^3	Factor II		60–100%
			Factor V		60–100%
Distribution width	0.13–0.15	13–15%	Factor VII		60–100%
Glucose-6-phosphate dehydrogenase	0.78 ± 0.13 MU/mol Hb	12.1 ± 2 IU/g Hb	Factor IX		60–100%
			Factor X		60–100%
Life span			Factor XI		60–100%
Normal survival	120 days	120 days	Factor XII		60–100%
Chromium-labeled, half-life ($t_{1/2}$)	28 days	28 days	Factor XIII		60–100%
Mean corpuscular hemoglobin (MCH)	28–33 pg/cell	28–33 pg/cell	Fibrinogen	2–4 g/L	200–400 mg/dL
			Plasminogen		2.4–4.4 CTA U/mL
Mean corpuscular hemoglobin concentration (MCHC)	320–360 g/L	32–36 g/dL	Protein C (antigenic assay)		58–148%
			Protein S (antigenic assay)		58–148%
Mean corpuscular volume (MCV)	86–98 fl	86–98 μm^3	Partial thromboplastin time (activated PTT) comparable to control		
Ham's test (acid serum)	Negative	Negative	Prothrombin time (quick one-stage) control ± 1 s		
Haptoglobin (serum)	0.5–2.2 g/L	50–220 mg/dL			
Hematocrit			Platelets	130–400 × 10^9/L	130,000–400,000/mm^3
Males	0.42–0.52	42–52%			
Females	0.37–0.48	37–48%	Thrombin time control ± 3 s		
Hemoglobin			von Willebrand's antigen		60–150%
Plasma	0.01–0.05 g/L	1–5 mg/dL	Protoporphyrin, free erythrocyte (FEP)	0.28–0.64 μmol/L of red blood cells	16–36 μg/dL of red blood cells
Whole blood					
Males	8.1–11.2 mmol/L	13–18 g/dL			
Females	7.4–9.9 mmol/L	12–16 g/dL	Red cells: see "Erythrocytes"		
Hemoglobin A$_2$ (HbA$_2$)	0.015–0.035	1.5–3.5%	Schilling test, orally administered vitamin B$_{12}$ excreted		7–40%
Hemoglobin, fetal (HbF)	<0.02	<2%	in urine		
Leukocytes			Sedimentation rate		
Alkaline phosphatase (LAP)	0.2–1.6 μkat/L	13–100 μ/L	Westergren, <50 years of age		
			Males		0–15 mm/h
Count	4.3–10.8 × 10^9/L	4.3–10.8 × 10^3/mm^3	Females		0–20 mm/h
			Westergren, >50 years of age		
Differential			Males		0–20 mm/h
Neutrophils	0.45–0.74	45–74%	Females		0–30 mm/h
Bands	0–0.04	0–4%	Sucrose hemolysis	Negative	Negative
Lymphocytes	0.16–0.45	16–45%	Viscosity		
Monocytes	0.04–0.10	4–10%	Plasma	1.7–2.1	1.7–2.1
Eosinophils	0–0.07	0–7%	Serum	1.4–1.8	1.4–1.8
Basophils	0–0.02	0–2%	White blood cells: see "Leukocytes"		
T cells: see Chap. 309					
Methemoglobin: <2 mg/L (<2 μg/mL)					
Osmotic fragility					
Slight hemolysis		0.45–0.39%			
Complete hemolysis	0.33–0.30%				

TABLE A-15   DIFFERENTIAL NUCLEATED CELL COUNTS OF BONE MARROW

	Normal, Mean %[a]	Range, %[b]		Normal, Mean %[a]	Range, %[b]
Myeloid	56.7		Erythroid	25.6	
Neutrophilic series	53.6		Pronormoblasts	0.6	0.2–1.3
Myeloblast	0.9	0.2–1.5	Basophilic normoblasts	1.4	0.5–2.4
Promyelocyte	3.3	2.1–4.1	Polychromatophilic normoblasts	21.6	17.9–29.2
Myelocyte	12.7	8.2–15.7			
Metamyelocyte	15.9	9.6–24.6	Orthochromatic normoblasts	2.0	0.4–4.6
Band	12.4	9.5–15.3	Megakaryocytes	<0.1	
Segmented			Lymphoreticular	17.8	
Eosinophilic series	3.1	1.2–5.3	Lymphocytes	16.2	11.1–23.2
Basophilic series	<0.1	0–0.2	Plasma cells	2.3	0.4–3.9
			Reticulum cells	0.3	0–0.9

[a] From MM Wintrobe et al, *Clinical Hematology,* 8th ed. Philadelphia, Lea & Febiger, 1981.
[b] Range observed in 12 healthy men.

	Specimen	Reference Range	
		SI Units	**Conventional Units**
α_2 Antitrypsin (adult)	S	0.76–1.89 g/L	76–189 mg/dL
Antiglomerular basement membrane antibodies	S		
Qualitative		Negative	Negative
Quantitative		<5 kU/L	<5 U/mL
Antineutrophil cytoplasmic autoantibodies, cytoplasmic (C-ANCA)	S		
Qualitative		Negative	Negative
Quantitative (antibodies to proteinase 3)		<2.8 kU/L	<2.8 U/mL
Antineutrophil cytoplasmic autoantibodies, perinuclear (P-ANCA)	S		
Qualitative		Negative	Negative
Quantitative (antibodies to myeloperoxidase)		<1.4 kU/L	<1.4 U/mL
Autoantibodies			
Antiadrenal antibody	S	NA	Negative at 1:10 dilution
Anti-double stranded (native) DNA	S	NA	Negative at 1:10 dilution
Antigranulocyte antibody	S	NA	Negative
Anti-Jo-1 antibody	S	NA	Negative
Anti-La antibody	S	NA	Negative
Antimitochondrial antibody	S	NA	Negative
Antinuclear antibody	S	NA	Negative at 1:40 dilution
Antiparietal cell antibody	S	NA	Negative at 1:20 dilution
Anti-Ro antibody	S	NA	Negative
Anti-RNP antibody	S	NA	Negative
Anti-Scl-70 antibody	S	NA	Negative
Anti-Smith antibody	S	NA	Negative
Anti-smooth-muscle antibody	S	NA	Negative at 1:20 dilution
Antithyroglobulin antibody	S	NA	Negative
Antithyroid antibody	S	<0.3 kIU/L	<0.3 IU/mL
Bence Jones protein	S	NA	None detected
Qualitative	U	NA	None detected in a 50-fold concentration
Quantitative	U		
Kappa		<0.03 g/L	<2.5 mg/dL
Lambda		<0.05 g/L	<5.0 mg/dL
C1 esterase-inhibitor protein	S		
Antigenic		0.12–0.25 g/L	12.4–24.5 mg/dL
Functional		Present	Present
Complement			
C3 (adult)	S	0.86–1.84 g/L	86–184 mg/dL
C4 (adult)	S	0.20–0.58 g/L	20–58 mg/dL
Total complement (adult)	S	63–145 kU/L	63–145 U/mL
Factor B	S	0.17–0.42 g/L	17–42 mg/dL
Cryoproteins	S	NA	None detected
CSF	CSF		
Agarose electrophoresis		NA	No banding seen in an 80-fold concentration
Quantitation of albumin (adult)		0.11–0.51 g/L	11.0–50.9 mg/dL
Quantitation of IgG (adult)		0.0–0.08 g/L	0.0–8.0 mg/dL
Immunoglobulins	S		
IgA		0.9–3.2 g/L	90–325 mg/dL
IgD		0–0.08 g/L	0–8 mg/dL
IgE		<0.00025 g/L	<0.025 mg/dL
IgG		8.0–15.0 g/L	800–1500 mg/dL
IgM		0.45–1.5 g/L	45–150 mg/dL
Rheumatoid factor	S, JF	<30 kIU/L	<30 IU/mL
Serum protein electrophoresis	S	NA	Normal pattern
T cells: see Chap. 309			
Viscosity	S	1.4–1.8 relative viscosity units, as compared with water	1.4–1.8 relative viscosity units, as compared with water

NOTE: CSF, cerebrospinal fluid; JF, joint fluid; S, serum; U, urine; NA, not applicable.   SOURCE: Adapted from A Kratz, KB Lewandrowski: N Engl J Med 339:1063, 1998.

TABLE A-17 STOOL ANALYSIS

	Reference Range	
	SI Units	Conventional Units
Bulk		
Wet weight	<197.5 (115 ± 41)g/d	<197.5 (115 ± 41) g/d
Dry weight	<66.4 (34 ± 15) g/d	<66.4 (34 ± 15) g/d
α_1 Antitrypsin	0.98 (±0.17) mg/g dry weight	0.98 (±0.17) mg/g dry weight
Coproporphyrin	600–1500 nmol/d	400–1000 μg/d
Fat (on diet containing at least 50 g fat), measured on a ≥ 3-day collection		
Fat		
Percent of dry weight	<0.30	<30.4%
Coefficient of fat absorption	>0.95	>95%
Fatty acid		
Free	0.01–0.10	1–10% of dry matter
Combined as soap	0.005–0.12	0.5–12% of dry matter
Nitrogen	<1.7 (1.4 ± 0.2) g/d	<1.7 (1.4 ± 0.2) g/d
Protein content	Minimal	Minimal
Urobilinogen	68–470 μmol/d	40–280 mg/d
Water	~0.65	~65%

TABLE A-18 URINE ANALYSIS

	Reference Range	
	SI Units	Conventional Units
Acidity, titratable	20–40 mmol/d	20–40 meq/d
Ammonia	30–50 mmol/d	30–50 meq/d
Amylase		4–400 U/L
Amylase/creatinine clearance ratio [(Cl_{am}/Cl_{cr}) × 100]	1–5	1–5
Calcium (10 meq/d or 200-mg/d dietary calcium)	<7.5 mmol/d	<300 mg/d
Creatine, as creatinine		
Women	<760 μmol/d	<100 mg/d
Men	<380 μmol/d	<50 mg/d
Creatinine	8.8–14 mmol/d	1.0–1.6 g/d
Glucose, true (oxidase method)	0.3–1.7 mmol/d	50–300 mg/d
5-Hydroxyindoleacetic acid (5-HIAA)	10–47 μmol/d	2–9 mg/d
Protein	<0.15 g/d	<150 mg/d
Potassium (varies with intake)	25–100 mmol/d	25–100 meq/d
Sodium (varies with intake)	100–260 mmol/d	100–260 meq/d

TABLE A-19 SUMMARY OF VALUES USEFUL IN PULMONARY PHYSIOLOGY

	Symbol	Typical Values	
		Man Aged 40, 75 kg, 175 cm Tall	Woman Aged 40, 60 kg, 160 cm Tall
PULMONARY MECHANICS			
Spirometry—volume-time curves			
Forced vital capacity	FVC	4.8 L	3.3 L
Forced expiratory volume in 1 s	FEV_1	3.8 L	2.8 L
FEV_1/FVC	FEV_1%	76%	77%
Maximal midexpiratory flow	MMF (FEF 25–27)	4.8 L/s	3.6 L/s
Maximal expiratory flow rate	MEFR (FEF 200–1200)	9.4 L/s	6.1 L/s
Spirometry—flow-volume curves			
Maximal expiratory flow at 50% of expired vital capacity	V_{max} 50 (FEF 50%)	6.1 L/s	4.6 L/s
Maximal expiratory flow at 75% of expired vital capacity	V_{max} 75 (FEF 75%)	3.1 L/s	2.5 L/s
Resistance to airflow:			
Pulmonary resistance	RL (R_L)	<3.0 (cmH$_2$O/s)/L	
Airway resistance	Raw	<2.5 (cmH$_2$O/s)/L	
Specific conductance	SGaw	>0.13 cmH$_2$O/s	
Pulmonary compliance			
Static recoil pressure at total lung capacity	Pst TLC	25 ± 5 cmH$_2$O	
Compliance of lungs (static)	CL	0.2 L cmH$_2$O	
Compliance of lungs and thorax	C(L + T)	0.1 L cmH$_2$O	
Dynamic compliance of 20 breaths per minute	C dyn 20	0.25 ± 0.05 L/cmH$_2$O	
Maximal static respiratory pressures:			
Maximal inspiratory pressure	MIP	>90 cmH$_2$O	>50 cmH$_2$O
Maximal expiratory pressure	MEP	>150 cmH$_2$O	>120 cmH$_2$O
LUNG VOLUMES			
Total lung capacity	TLC	6.4 L	4.9 L
Functional residual capacity	FRC	2.2 L	2.6 L
Residual volume	RV	1.5 L	1.2 L
Inspiratory capacity	IC	4.8 L	3.7 L
Expiratory reserve volume	ERV	3.2 L	2.3 L
Vital capacity	VC	1.7 L	1.4 L
GAS EXCHANGE (SEA LEVEL)			
Arterial O$_2$ tension	Pa$_{O_2}$	12.7 ± 0.7 kPa (95 ± 5 mmHg)	
Arterial CO$_2$ tension	Pa$_{CO_2}$	5.3 ± 0.3 kPa (40 ± 2 mmHg)	
Arterial O$_2$ saturation	Sa$_{O_2}$	0.97 ± 0.02 (97 ± 2%)	
Arterial blood pH	pH	7.40 ± 0.02	
Arterial bicarbonate	HCO$_3^-$	24 + 2 meq/L	
Base excess	BE	0 ± 2 meq/L	
Diffusing capacity for carbon monoxide (single breath)	DL$_{CO}$	0.42 mLCO/s/mmHg (25 mL CO/min/mmHg)	
Dead space volume	V$_D$	2 ml/kg body wt	
Physiologic dead space; dead space-tidal volume ratio	V$_D$/V$_T$		
Rest		≤35% V$_T$	
Exercise		≤20% V$_T$	
Alveolar-arterial difference for O$_2$	P(A − a)$_{O_2}$	≤2.7 kPa ≤20 kPa (≤20 mmHg)	

INSTRUCTIONS FOR COLLECTION AND TRANSPORT OF SPECIMENS FOR CULTURE

It is absolutely essential that the microbiology laboratory be informed of the site of origin of the sample to be cultured and of the infections that are suspected. This information determines the selection of culture media and the length of culture time.

Type of Culture (Synonyms)	Specimen	Minimum Volume	Container	Other Considerations
BLOOD				
Blood, routine (blood culture for aerobes, anaerobes, and yeasts)	Whole blood	10 mL in each of 2 bottles for adults and children; 5 mL, if possible, in each of 2 bottles for infants; less for neonates	See below.[a]	See below.[b]
Blood for fungi/*Mycobacterium* spp.	Whole blood	10 mL in each of 2 bottles, as for routine blood cultures, or in Isolator tube requested from laboratory	Same as for routine blood culture	Specify "hold for extended incubation," since fungal agents may require 4 weeks or more to grow.
Blood, Isolator (lysis centrifugation)	Whole blood	10 mL	Isolator tubes	Use mainly for isolation of fungi, *Mycobacterium,* or other fastidious aerobes and for elimination of antibiotics from cultured blood in which organisms are concentrated by centrifugation.
RESPIRATORY TRACT				
Nose	Swab from nares	1 swab	Sterile culturette or similar transport system containing holding medium	Swabs made of calcium alginate may be used.
Throat	Swab of posterior pharynx, ulcerations, or areas of suspected purulence	1 swab	Sterile culturette or similar swab specimen collection system containing holding medium	See below.[c]
Sputum	Fresh sputum (not saliva)	2 mL	Commercially available sputum collection system or similar sterile container with screw cap	*Cause for rejection:* Care must be taken to ensure that the specimen is sputum and not saliva. Examination of Gram's stain, with number of epithelial cells and PMNs noted, can be an important part of the evaluation process. Induced sputum specimens should not be rejected.
Bronchial aspirates	Transtracheal aspirate, bronchoscopy specimen, or bronchial aspirate	1 mL of aspirate or brush in transport medium	Sterile aspirate or bronchoscopy tube, bronchoscopy brush in a separate sterile container	Special precautions may be required, depending on diagnostic considerations (e.g., *Pneumocystis*).
STOOL				
Stool for routine culture; stool for *Salmonella, Shigella,* and *Campylobacter*	Rectal swab or (preferably) fresh, randomly collected stool	1 g of stool or 2 rectal swabs	Plastic-coated cardboard cup or plastic cup with tight-fitting lid. Other leak-proof containers are also acceptable.	If *Vibrio* spp. are suspected, the laboratory must be notified, and appropriate collection/transport methods should be used.
Stool for *Yersinia, E. coli* O157	Fresh, randomly collected stool	1 g	Plastic-coated cardboard cup or plastic cup with tight-fitting lid	*Limitations:* Procedure requires enrichment techniques.
Stool for *Aeromonas* and *Plesiomonas*	Fresh, randomly collected stool	1 g	Plastic-coated cardboard cup or plastic cup with tight-fitting lid	*Limitations:* Stool should not be cultured for these organisms unless also cultured for other enteric pathogens.
UROGENITAL TRACT				
Urine	Clean-voided urine specimen or urine collected by catheter	0.5 mL	Sterile, leak-proof container with screw cap or special urine transfer tube	See below.[d]
Urogenital secretions	Vaginal or urethral secretions, cervical swabs, uterine fluid, prostatic fluid, etc.	1 swab or 0.5 mL of fluid	Transwab containing Amies transport medium or similar system containing holding medium for *Neisseria gonorrhoeae;* modified Todd-Hewitt broth for group B *Streptococcus* surveillance cultures	Vaginal swab samples for "routine culture" should be discouraged whenever possible unless a particular pathogen is suspected. For detection of multiple organisms (e.g., group B *Streptococcus, Trichomonas, Chlamydia,* or *Candida* spp.), 1 swab per test should be obtained.

(continued)

Cerebrospinal fluid (lumbar puncture)	Spinal fluid	1 mL for routine cultures; ≥5 mL for *Mycobacterium*	Sterile tube with tight-fitting cap	Do not refrigerate; transfer to laboratory as soon as possible.
Body fluids	Aseptically aspirated body fluids	1 mL for routine cultures	Sterile tube with tight-fitting cap. Specimen may be left in syringe used for collection if the syringe is capped before transport.	For some body fluids (e.g., peritoneal lavage samples), increased volumes are helpful for isolation of small numbers of bacteria.
Biopsy and aspirated materials	Tissue removed at surgery, bone, anticoagulated bone marrow, biopsy samples, or other specimens from normally sterile areas	1 mL of fluid or a 1-g piece of tissue	Sterile "culturette"-type swab or similar transport system containing holding medium. Sterile bottle or jar should be used for tissue specimens.	Accurate identification of specimen and source is critical. Enough tissue should be collected for both microbiologic and histopathologic evaluations.
Wounds	Purulent material or abscess contents obtained from wound or abscess without contamination by normal microflora	2 swabs or 0.5 mL of aspirated pus	Culturette swab or similar transport system or sterile tube with tight-fitting screw cap. For simultaneous anaerobic cultures, send specimen in anaerobic transport device or closed syringe.	*Collection:* Abscess contents or other fluids should be collected in a syringe (see above) when possible to provide an adequate sample volume and an anaerobic environment.

SPECIAL RECOMMENDATIONS

Fungi	Specimen types listed above may be used. When urine or sputum is cultured for fungi, a first morning specimen is usually preferred.	1 mL or as specified above for individual listing of specimens. Large volumes may be useful for urinary fungi.	Sterile, leak-proof container with tight-fitting cap	*Collection:* Specimen should be transported to microbiology laboratory within 1 h of collection. Contamination with normal flora from skin, rectum, vaginal tract, or other body surfaces should be avoided.
Mycobacterium (acid-fast bacilli)	Sputum, tissue, urine, body fluids	10 mL of fluid or small piece of tissue. Swabs should not be used.	Sterile container with tight-fitting cap	Detection of *Mycobacterium* spp. is improved by use of concentration techniques. Smears and cultures of pleural, peritoneal, and pericardial fluids often have low yields. Multiple cultures from the same patient are encouraged. Culturing in liquid media shortens the time to detection.
Legionella	Pleural fluid, lung biopsy, bronchoalveolar lavage fluid, bronchial/transbronchial biopsy. Rapid transport to laboratory is critical.	1 mL of fluid; any size tissue sample, although a 0.5-g sample should be obtained when possible	—	—
Anaerobic organisms	Aspirated specimens from abscesses or body fluids	1 mL of aspirated fluid or 2 swabs	An appropriate anaerobic transport device is required.[e]	Specimens cultured for obligate anaerobes should be cultured for facultative bacteria as well.
Viruses[f]	Respiratory secretions, wash aspirates from respiratory tract, nasal swabs, blood samples (including buffy coats), vaginal and rectal swabs, swab specimens from suspicious skin lesions, stool samples (in some cases)	1 mL of fluid, 1 swab, or 1 g of stool in each appropriate transport medium	Fluid or stool samples in sterile containers or swab samples in viral culturette devices (kept on ice but not frozen) are generally suitable. Plasma samples and buffy coats in sterile collection tubes should be kept at 4 to 8°C. If specimens are to be shipped or kept for a long time, freezing at −80°C is usually adequate.	Most samples for culture are transported in holding medium containing antibiotics to prevent bacterial overgrowth and viral inactivation. Many specimens should be kept cool but not frozen, provided they are transported promptly to the laboratory. Procedures and transport media vary with the agent to be cultured and the duration of transport.

[a] For samples from adults and children, two bottles (smaller for pediatric samples) should be used: one with dextrose phosphate, tryptic soy, or another appropriate broth and the other with thioglycollate or another broth containing reducing agents appropriate for isolation of obligate anaerobes. For special situations (e.g., suspected fungal infection, culture-negative endocarditis, or mycobacteremia), different blood collection systems may be used (Isolator systems; see table).

[b] *Collection:* An appropriate disinfecting technique should be used on both the bottle septum and the patient. Do not allow air bubbles to get into anaerobic broth bottles. *Special considerations:* There is no more important clinical microbiology test than the detection of blood-borne pathogens. The rapid identification of bacterial and fungal agents is a major determinant of patients' survival. Bacteria may be present in blood either continuously (as in endocarditis, overwhelming sepsis, and the early stages of salmonellosis and brucellosis) or intermittently (as in most other bacterial infections, in which bacteria are shed into the blood on a sporadic basis). Most blood culture systems employ two separate bottles containing broth medium: one that is vented in the laboratory for the growth of facultative and aerobic organisms and a second that is maintained under anaerobic conditions. In cases of suspected continuous bacteremia/fungemia, two or three samples should be drawn before the start of therapy, with additional sets obtained if fastidious organisms are thought to be involved. For intermittent bacteremia, two or three samples should be obtained at least 1 h apart during the first 24 h.

[c] Normal microflora includes alpha-hemolytic streptococci, saprophytic *Neisseria* spp., diphtheroids, and *Staphylococcus* spp. Aerobic culture of the throat ("routine") includes screening for and identification of beta-hemolytic *Streptococcus* spp. and other potentially pathogenic organisms. Although considered components of the normal microflora, organisms such as *Staphylococcus aureus*, *Haemophilus influenzae*, and *Streptococcus pneumoniae* will be identified by most laboratories, if requested. When *Neisseria gonorrhoeae* or *Corynebacterium diphtheriae* is suspected, a special culture request is recommended.

[d] (1) Clean-voided specimens, midvoid specimens, and Foley or indwelling catheter specimens that yield ≥50,000 organisms/mL and from which no more than three species are isolated should have organisms identified. (2) Straight-catheterized, bladder-tap, and similar urine specimens should undergo a complete workup (identification and susceptibility testing) for all potentially pathogenic organisms, regardless of colony count. (3) Certain clinical problems (e.g., acute dysuria in women) may warrant identification and susceptibility testing of isolates present at concentrations of <50,000 organisms/mL.

[e] Aspirated specimens in capped syringes or other transport devices designed to limit oxygen exposure are suitable for the cultivation of obligate anaerobes. A variety of commercially available transport devices may be used. Contamination of specimens with normal microflora from the skin, rectum, vaginal vault, or another body site should be avoided. Collection containers for aerobic culture (such as dry swabs) and inappropriate specimens (such as refrigerated samples; expectorated sputum; stool; gastric aspirates; and vaginal, throat, nose, and rectal swabs) should be rejected as unsuitable.

[f] Laboratories generally use diverse methods to detect viral agents, and the specific requirements for each specimen should be checked before a sample is sent.

INDEX

Bold number indicates the start of the main discussion of the topic; numbers with "f" and "t" refer to figure and table pages; italic roman numerals refer to the Color Atlas plates.

ISBN 0-07-118319-1

90000

9 780071 183192

BRAUNWALD/I.E.
SETCODE

ISBN 0-07-118320-5

90000

9 780071 183208

BRAUNWALD/I.E.
VOL. 1

ISBN 0-07-913686-9

90000

9 780079 136862

BRAUNWALD/U.S.
SETCODE

ISBN 0-07-007273-6

90000

9 780070 072732

BRAUNWALD/U.S.
VOL. 1

TOPICAL CONTENTS